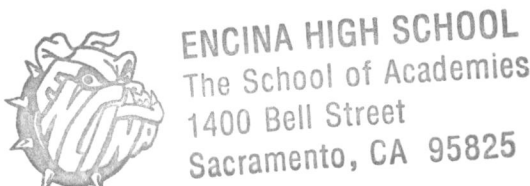

PDR MEDICAL DICTIONARY

SECOND EDITION

PDR®

Medical Dictionary

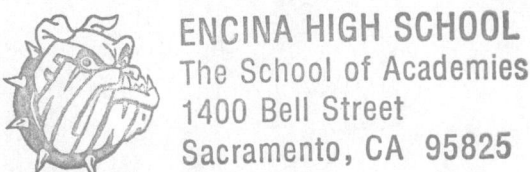

ENCINA HIGH SCHOOL
The School of Academies
1400 Bell Street
Sacramento, CA 95825

PDR MEDICAL DICTIONARY

SECOND EDITION

PDR®
Medical Dictionary

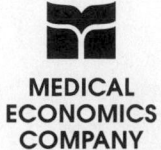

MEDICAL
ECONOMICS
COMPANY

Senior Managing Editor: Maureen Barlow Pugh
Managing Editor: Barbara Werner
New Terms Editor: Thomas W. Filardo, MD
Copy Editors: Peter W. Binns, Linda G. Francis, Raymond Lukens, Bonnie Montgomery
Chief On-Line Editor: Barbara L. Ferretti
On-Line Editors: Kathryn J. Cadle, Dana Workman
Proofreaders: Peter W. Binns; David A. Bloom, MD; Alfred J. Bollet, MD; Ted Burk; Regina Lavette Davis; John A. Day, Jr., MD, FCCP; Richard Diamanti; John H. Dirckx, MD; Thomas W. Filardo, MD; Linda G. Francis; John M. Last, MD, FRACP, FRCPC; Raymond Lukens; Kate Mason, CMT; Joan Sarchese
Database Programmers: Dave Marcus, Lexi-Comp Inc., Hudson, OH
Art Director: Jonathan Dimes
Illustrations: Neil O. Hardy
Additional artwork by: Mary Anna Barratt-Dimes, Kathryn Born, Rob Duckwall, Timothy Hengst, Mikki Senkarik, Michael Schenk, Larry Ward
Graphic preparation assistance: Susan Caldwell, Jennifer Clements, Thomas Dolan, Christina Nihira
Design: Dan Pfisterer

Database design by Lexi-Comp Inc., Hudson, OH
Printed in the United States of America by World Color, Inc.

Library of Congress Cataloging-in-Publication Data

Stedman, Thomas Lathrop, 1853-1938.
    Stedman's medical dictionary.—27th ed.
      p.; cm.
    ISBN 0-683-40007-X (regular)—ISBN 0-683-40008-8 (deluxe)
    1. Medicine—Dictionaries. I. Title: Medical dictionary. II. Title.
    [DNLM: 1. Medicine—Dictionary—English. W 13 S812m 1999]
  R121 .S8 1999
  610'.3—dc21

                                 99-056094

00 01 02 03 04 05
1 2 3 4 5

CONTENTS

With its combination of PDR's unparalleled database of pharmaceutical names and an exhaustive lexicon of medical terminology, the *PDR" Medical Dictionary* is a truly unique professional resource. Now in a completely revised and updated 2nd edition, it includes not only the very latest brand and generic drugs, but also the newest nomenclature in such rapidly changing fields as biotechnology, biochemistry, genetics, embryology, radiology, and neurology. Here in one convenient volume, you'll find all the basic information you need to keep pace with the explosive changes taking place throughout all the health sciences.

New in This Edition

This edition of the *PDR Medical Dictionary* has been critically reviewed and revised by consultants representing 44 medical specialties. Revisions of genetics, bacteriology, gross anatomy, and laboratory medicine were especially extensive. Veterinary medicine terms were revised to focus on that terminology relevant to human medicine.

New Terms Editor   Thomas Filardo, MD creates the position of New Terms Editor with this edition. As a generalist, he has taken a holistic view of the dictionary and has suggested to the specialty consultants new terms for inclusion. He has also adjudicated submissions from the consultants, with a view toward achieving a more consistent, complete, and correct reference.

New Specialties   We have added consultants in oncology, pediatrics, pulmonology, and emergency medicine, reflecting the increasing importance of these specialties.

Terminologia Anatomica   For many years, the Federative Committee on Anatomical Terminology has been working on changing the official anatomy nomenclature from *Nomina Anatomica* [NA] to *Terminologia Anatomica* [TA]. The committee's official TA Latin and English anatomical terms have been approved by the International Federation of Associations of Anatomists.

At the printing of this edition, the committee had completed the new terminology for Gross Anatomy and Neuroanatomy, but was still at work on Embryology, Cytology, and Histology. This edition, therefore, reflects the TA terminology for Gross Anatomy and Neuroanatomy but retains the NA nomenclature for Embryology, Cytology, and Histology. Please note that we have by no means deleted the Gross Anatomy and Neuroanatomy *Nomina Anatomica* Latin terms from the dictionary; they are simply not designated as NA anymore.

As we did in the 1st edition, we list anatomical definitions where readers are most likely to look—at the English translations of the Latin terms.

Genus Finder   To find the binomial designation and definition of an organism (except viruses) in the dictionary, you must look under the genus name. Yet in much of the medical literature, the genus component of a binomial is abbreviated even at first reference, and the genus is never identified. Readers who do not know the genus name will have trouble finding the definition in a dictionary.

Our new *Genus Finder* solves this problem. All binomial names in the dictionary are cross-referenced by the species name. For example, to identify *P. falciparum,* look in the *Genus Finder* under "falciparum" and find *Plasmodium*. Then take your search to the pages of the dictionary under *Plasmodium,* where you will find the entry and its definition.

Because virus nomenclature does not abbreviate the genus name, viruses are not included in *Genus Finder.*

Anatomy Tables   In the first appendix of this dictionary, you will find three large anatomy tables. Taken with revisions from Dr. Keith Moore's *Clinically Oriented Anatomy, 4th Edition,* these tables list all the arteries, nerves, and muscles of the body, along with relevant information, and reflect the *Terminologia Anatomica* nomenclature.

The Art Program   Our goal for the art program was to use images and tables that would expand and clarify the meanings of the dictionary terms. To that end, our consultants and editors, under the direction of Art Director Jonathan Dimes, have reviewed every submitted image for clarity, scientific accuracy, and currency. The result is more than 1,050 color illustrations, photographs, and tables.

In this edition are three insert sections totaling 64 pages of full color anatomy and diagnostic medicine images. The quick-reference, 32-page anatomical atlas near the center of the book showcases art from *adam.com,* the award-winning medical education software company. A complete index containing each structure precedes these richly labeled illustrations.

We are also proud to present over 400 illustrations created by renowned medical artist Neil O. Hardy. Mr. Hardy's exceptional 50-year career has been highlighted by numerous honors, including the Association of Medical Illustrators' Lifetime Achievement Award.

Within the A to Z section there are over 700 illustrations, many with multiple images to help the reader better understand a topic. A symbol beside an entry—a white letter "I" in a solid blue square (🔲)—indicates that the entry is illustrated, either on that page or in the inserts.

Readers can easily locate any image using the Illustration Index on page xix in the front section of the book. Simply look up the term in the Illustration Index to find the page number of the illustration.

Continuing Features

Yes, we have added new features to make the *PDR Medical Dictionary* more accessible, informative, and comprehensive, but we've left others unchanged because they have served our readers well and distinguish us from other medical dictionaries.

High Profile Terms   "High profile" terms are concepts that so profoundly affect the practice of medicine that they warrant more than the standard dictionary definition. John Dirckx, MD, Etymology consultant and internist, wrote the high profile terms for this edition. With the help of our consultants, Dr. Dirckx identified 130 such terms, 51 of which he expanded and extensively revised from the previous edition. All others are new with this edition. These terms appear in the A to Z section of the book, highlighted between two blue horizontal rules.

Word Finder   We have continued our practice of publishing a long list of multiple-term entries in the front of the book. The purpose of this list is to identify where in the dictionary a multiple-term entry is defined—the main challenge in a dictionary organized, as this one is, in main entry/subentry format. All of the definitions involving "cochlear," for example, do not appear at "cochlear"; instead, they appear as subentries of these other, organizing entries:

> aqueduct; area; canal; canaliculus; duct; implant; joint; labyrinth; nerve; nucleus; part; prosthesis; recess; root; window.

For more information about using *Word Finder*, see page WF 1, the section immediately preceding the A- Z section.

Easy-to-Find Subentries   We continue our practice of putting each subentry on a new line to help readers quickly find the information they need.

Cross-References in Blue   Many entries do not have definitions; they are synonyms that point readers to the main term where the definition appears. We have printed all these synonyms in blue, signaling readers to look up the word in blue to find the definition.

Building Blocks   Approximately 1,200 Greek and Latin word parts account for about 90 percent of medical language, so learning these word parts helps one understand the vocabulary. We've marked these suffixes, prefixes, and combining forms with the universal symbol for recycling △ in the margins of the A to Z section, and we've listed them on page 2007.

Precision Thumb Tabs   On every page is a green thumb tab with the first two letters of the last word on that page. We call this a strategic thumb index because it enables readers to know exactly where they are in the alphabet whenever they open the book. This is another feature that helps readers find what they want quickly.

Working Dictionary   This is a working dictionary, a record of a living language, and words are formed, spelled, pronounced, and defined as they are actually used. Every dictionary contains words that by philological standards are misformed, misspelled, mispronounced, or misused. A dictionary may suggest standards, but it cannot enforce them. The *PDR Medical Dictionary*, therefore, serves as a guide for those who wish to speak and write more precisely and to coin new terms more accurately.

Acknowledgments

Editing a volume such as this is much larger than any one person. A team of consultants, editors, artists, proofreaders, and database experts are responsible for this book. We at *Physicians' Desk Reference* are grateful, first and foremost, to the consultants in the medical specialties for writing and revising the more than 100,000 entries in this dictionary.

We are especially grateful to Dr. Dirckx and Dr. Filardo who, in addition to their contracted work, provided expert assistance on everything from questions of usage and spelling to the value of an illustration.

Special thanks are due Managing Editor, Barbara Werner, and Chief Online Editor, Barbara Ferretti, for bringing their skill, diligence, dedication, and good humor to the multitudinous tasks they performed for this edition.

Also indispensable in the development of any truly useful reference work is another large group—the thousands of users whose comments, suggestions, additions, and corrections guide the evolution of the work. We welcome your suggestions for further improvements. Please feel free to call us toll-free at 1-800-922-0937 or fax us at 201-722-2680.

R. Donald Allison, PhD **Biochemistry**
Associate Scientist, Department of Biochemistry and Molecular Biology, University of Florida College of Medicine, Gainesville, FL

Douglas R. Bacon, MD, MA **Biography and Eponyms**
Associate Professor and Vice Chairman for Education, Department of Anesthesiology, State University of New York at Buffalo; Chief of Anesthesiology Service, Buffalo VA Medical Center, Buffalo, NY

John Bennett, MD **Mycology**
Head, Clinical Mycology Section, Laboratory of Clinical Investigation, National Institute of Allergy and Infectious Diseases, Bethesda, MD

David A. Bloom, MD **Urology and Urologic Surgery**
Chief, Pediatric Urology, Professor of Surgery, The University of Michigan & Mott Children's Hospital, Ann Arbor, MI

Alfred Jay Bollet, MD **Internal Medicine**
Clinical Professor of Medicine, Yale University School of Medicine, New Haven, CT

David G. Bostwick, MD **Pathology**
Consultant and Professor of Pathology and Urology, Mayo Clinic and Mayo Medical School, Rochester, MN

Michael J. Burridge, BVM&S, MPVM, PhD **Veterinary Medicine**
Professor, Department of Pathobiology, College of Veterinary Medicine, University of Florida, Gainesville, FL

Philip M. Buttaravoli, MD, FACEP **Emergency Medicine**
Medical Director, Emergency Department, Palm Beach Gardens Medical Center, Palm Beach Gardens, FL

Patricia Charache, MD **Bacteriology**
Professor of Pathology, Medicine, and Oncology, Departments of Pathology and Medicine, Johns Hopkins Medical Institutions, Baltimore, MD

Barbara A. Conley, MD **Oncology**
Senior Investigator, Clinical Investigations Branch, Cancer Therapy Evaluation Program, National Cancer Institute, Rockville, MD

Arthur F. Dalley II, PhD **Gross Anatomy**
Professor of Cell Biology, Director of Gross Anatomy, Department of Cell Biology, Vanderbilt University School of Medicine, Nashville, TN; President, American Association of Clinical Anatomists

John A. Day, Jr., MD, FCCP **Pulmonary Disease**
Assistant Professor of Medicine, University of Massachusetts Medical School, Attending Physician, Division of Pulmonary and Critical Care, St. Vincent Hospital and University of Massachusetts Memorial Health Care, Worcester, MA

John H. Dirckx, MD **Etymologies and High Profile Terms**
Director, University of Dayton Health Center, Dayton, OH

Thomas W. Filardo, M.D. **New Terms Editor**
Physician-Consultant, Evendale, OH

Clair A. Francomano, MD **Genetics**
Clinical Director, National Human Genome Research Institute, National Institutes of Health, Bethesda, MD

Paul J. Friedman, MD   **Radiology**
Professor of Radiology and Chief of Thoracic Radiology, School of Medicine, University of California, San Diego, CA

Lynne S. Garcia, MS, MT(ASCP), CLS(NCA), F(AAM)   **Tropical Medicine/Parasitology**
Department of Pathology and Laboratory Medicine, UCLA Medical Center, Los Angeles, CA

Steven I. Gutman, MD, MBA Pathology, Hematology, and Laboratory Medicine/Stains and Procedures
Director, Division of Clinical Laboratory Devices, Division of Clinical Laboratory Devices, Food and Drug Administration, Rockville, MD

Duane E. Haines, PhD   **Neuroanatomy**
Professor of Anatomy, Chairman, Department of Anatomy, The University of Mississippi Medical Center, Jackson, MS

David E. Hall, MD   **Pediatrics**
Clinical Associate Professor of Pediatrics, Emory University School of Medicine, Childrens Healthcare of Atlanta at Scottish Rite, Atlanta, GA

Iain Kalfas, MD   **Neurosurgery**
Department of Neurosurgery, Cleveland Clinic Foundation, Cleveland, OH

John B. Kerrison, MD   **Ophthalmology**
Assistant Chief of Service, Wilmer Eye Institute, Johns Hopkins Hospital, Baltimore, MD

John M. Last, MD, FRACP, FRCPC   **Medical Statistics and Epidemiology**
Professor Emeritus, Department of Epidemiology and Community Medicine, University of Ottawa, Ottawa, Ontario, Canada

Stanley S. Lefkowitz, PhD   **Immunology and Virology**
Professor, Department of Microbiology and Immunology, Texas Tech University Health Sciences Center, Lubbock, TX

David N. Menton, PhD   **Histology**
Associate Professor of Anatomy, Washington University School of Medicine, St. Louis, MO

Edward D. Miller, MD   **Anesthesiology**
The Frances Watt Baker, M.D., and Lenox D. Baker, Jr., M.D., Dean of the Medical Faculty, Chief Executive Officer, Johns Hopkins Medicine, Johns Hopkins School of Medicine, Baltimore, MD

John B. Mulliken, MD   **Plastic and Reconstructive Surgery**
Associate Professor of Surgery, Harvard Medical School; Director, Craniofacial Centre, Children's Hospital, Boston, MA

Martin L. Nusynowitz, MD   **Nuclear Medicine**
Professor, Radiology, Internal Medicine, and Pathology, University of Texas Medical Branch at Galveston, Galveston, TX

J. Patrick O'Leary, MD   **General Surgery**
The Isidore Cohn, Jr., Professor and Chairman of Surgery, Louisiana State University Medical School, New Orleans, LA

Sharon T. Phelan, MD   **Obstetrics and Gynecology**
Associate Professor, Department of Obstetrics and Gynecology, University of Alabama at Birmingham, Birmingham, AL

Ronald B. Ponn, MD   **Thoracic Surgery**
Assistant Clinical Professor and Associate Section Chief of Cardiothoracic Surgery, Yale University School of Medicine and Yale-New Haven Hospital, New Haven, CT

Richard Prayson, MD   **Neuropathology**
Department of Anatomic Pathology, The Cleveland Clinic Foundation, Cleveland, OH

Arthur Raines, PhD   **Pharmacology and Toxicology**
Professor Emeritus of Pharmacology and Neurology, Department of Pharmacology, Georgetown University
Medical Center, Washington, DC

George S. Schuster, DDS, MS, PhD   **Dentistry**
Ione and Arthur Merritt Professor, Chairman, Department of Oral Biology and Maxillofacial Pathology,
Medical College of Georgia, School of Dentistry, Augusta, GA

Sheldon M. Schuster, PhD   **Biotechnology**
Professor, Biochemistry and Molecular Biology, Program Director, Biotechnology Program, University of
Florida, Gainesville, FL

James B. Snow, Jr., M.D., FACS   **Otorhinolaryngology**
Former Director, National Institute on Deafness and Other Communication Disorders, National Institutes of
Health, Bethesda, MD; Professor Emeritus of Otorhinolaryngology, University of Pennsylvania School of
Medicine, Philadelphia, PA

David H. Spodick MD, DSc   **Cardiology**
Professor of Medicine, University of Massachusetts Medical School; Lecturer in Medicine, Tufts University
School of Medicine; Lecturer in Medicine, Boston University School of Medicine; Director of Clinical
Cardiology and Director of Cardiovascular Fellowship Training, St. Vincent Hospital, Worcester, MA

Kathleen K. Sulik, PhD   **Embryology**
Professor, Department of Cell Biology and Anatomy, University of North Carolina, Chapel Hill, NC

Asa J. Wilbourn, MD   **Neurology**
Director, EMG Laboratory, The Cleveland Clinic Foundation, Clinical Professor of Neurology, Case-Western
Reserve University School of Medicine, Cleveland, OH

Colin Wood, MD   **Dermatology**
Professor Emeritus of Pathology, University of Maryland School of Medicine, Baltimore, MD

Douglas D. Woodruff, MD   **Psychiatry/Psychology**
Private Practice, Baltimore, MD

David B. Young, PhD   **Physiology**
Professor, Physiology and Biophysics, University of Mississippi Medical Center, Jackson, MS

Joseph D. Zuckerman, MD   **Orthopaedics**
Walter A. L. Thompson Professor of Orthopaedic Surgery, New York University School of Medicine;
Chairman, NYU-Hospital for Joint Diseases, Department of Orthopaedic Surgery, New York, NY

Janine Denis Cook, PhD, Department of Medical and Research Technology, University of Maryland School of Medicine. Contributing Editor, Laboratory Reference Range Values appendix

Show-Hong Duh, PhD, DABCC, Department of Pathology, University of Maryland School of Medicine. Contributing Editor, Laboratory Reference Range Values appendix

Doris L. Lefkowitz, PhD, Associate Professor, Department of Biological Sciences, Texas Tech University, Lubbock, TX. Contributing Editor, Immunology

John B. Imboden, MD, Associate Professor of Psychiatry, Johns Hopkins University School of Medicine, Baltimore, MD. Contributing Editor, Psychiatry

Nicola Ho, MD, Fellow, Medical Genetics Branch, National Human Genome Research Institute, National Institutes of Health, Bethesda, MD. Contributing Editor, Genetics

Ivan Damjanov, MD, PhD, Professor, Department of Pathology, The University of Kansas School of Medicine, Kansas City, KS. Contributing Editor, Pathology

Linda A. Smith, PhD, CLS(NCA), Associate Professor and Graduate Program Director, Department of Clinical Laboratory Science, University of Texas Health Science Center, San Antonio, TX. Contributing Editor, Blood Groups appendix

Artwork in this edition of *Stedman's Medical Dictionary* was created or adapted by the following individuals (see Illustration Sources for sources of adaptations):

All artwork in the anatomy insert, **imagery © 1999 adam.com™.** All rights reserved.

Mary Anna Barratt-Dimes, Parkton, MD. 23, 41, 93, 101, 159, 169, 215, 308, 352, 377, 438, 442, 456, 492, 577, 659, 441, 802 (hemoglobin), 808, 817, 825, 831, 833, 878, 879, 881, 895, 951, 970, 1092, 1226, 1329, 1420, 1504, 1519, 1530, 1564, 1584, 1767, 1860, 1862, 1864, 1900 (tympanogram), 1933 (vasopressin), 1952, 1979

Kathryn Born, Arlington, TX. 1460 (prostate examination)

Michael Budowick, Munich, Germany. 128

Susan Caldwell, Pikesville, MD, created all tables in the A–Z section of this book.

Robert Demarest, Hawthorne, NJ. 1273

Duckwall Productions, Baltimore, MD. 830, 1282

Neil O. Hardy. Westport, CT. 2, 5, 10, 22, 53, 54, 55, 60, 70, 79, 80, 84, 97, 120, 145, 135, 138, 158, 164, 170, 180, 182, 189, 190, 201, 206, 209, 210, 211, 212, 223, 233, 247, 253, 259 (burns), 264, 266, 270, 274, 277, 279, 281, 293, 296, 298, 302, 207, 331, 353, 354, 355 (systemic circulation), 358, 366, 374, 382, 383, 385, 399, 413, 415, 437, 446, 463, 464, 465, 475, 481, 494, 500, 524, 525, 532, 535, 540, 543, 544, 545, 548, 560, 562 (abdominal retractor), 574, 576, 580, 581, 600, 608, 609, 617, 620, 636, 658, 670, 673, 678, 681, 684, 686, 689, 695, 696, 697, 702, 710, 711, 712, 724, 728, 732, 734, 743, 749, 752, 761, 766, 774, 777, 779, 783, 797, 802 (hemodialysis), 805, 806, 813, 839, 852, 858, 864, 874, 884, 887, 900, 903, 904, 905, 906, 915, 918, 925, 934, 937, 944, 949, 952, 968, 975, 980, 984, 999, 1018, 1028, 1032, 1035, 1040, 1051, 1061 (Heimlich maneuver), 1069 (massage), 1070, 1074, 1090, 1091, 1121 (mitosis), 1127, 1132, 1134, 1184, 1160, 1176 (myopia), 1181, 1183, 1184, 1190, 1194, 1195, 1202, 1209, 1210, 1221, 1245, 1246, 1247, 1249, 1257 (olfaction), 1271, 1272 (male and female organs), 1281 (ossicle), 1285, 1287, 1291, 1298, 1300, 1302, 1303, 1306, 1333, 1345, 1346, 1351, 1358, 1359, 1389, 1391, 1394, 1395, 1403, 1412, 1416, 1423, 1438, 1441, 1449, 1460 (prostate), 1484, 1486, 1492, 1497, 1540, 1554, 1555, 1558, 1559, 1562, 1563, 1599, 1629, 1635, 1644, 1646, 1647, 1649, 1650, 1656, 1666, 1671, 1674, 1676, 1677, 1679, 1681, 1695, 1696, 1698, 1701, 1738, 1740, 1744, 1778, 1783, 1784, 1785, 1788, 1794, 1799, 1832, 1841, 1845 (tooth), 1847, 1852 (trachea), 1853, 1855, 1857, 1863, 1871, 1897, 1900 (monozygotic twins), 1904, 1911, 1919, 1926, 1927, 1931, 1933 (vasectomy), 1936, 1945, 1951, 1953, 1957, 1968, 1974, 1980, 1991, B8 (bronchoscopy), B9 (laparoscopy), B11, B14, B15

Timothy Hengst, Thousand Oaks, CA. 63

Siri Mills, Munich, Germany. 791, 1341, 1882, 1886

Michael Schenk, Jackson, MS. 6, 87, 271, 286, 486, 676, 812, 896, 1200, 1385, 1574

Mikki Senkarik, San Antonio, TX. 78, 150, 184, 187, 282, 381, 531, 562 (ECG placement), 682, 865, 1061 (Leopold maneuver), 1068 (nonbreathing mask), 1297, 1710, 1956, 2002, B1, B2, B3, B8 (esophagoduodenoscope), B9 (thoracoscopy), B10 (colonoscope)

Larry Ward, Salt Lake City, UT. 628, 763, 790, 1068 (oxygen mask), 1069 (rectal mass), 1262, 1485, 1708, 1844

Courtesy of Acuson Computed Sonography Corporation. Mountain View, CA. 1905, B11

Courtesy of Advanced Technology Laboratory. Bothell, WA. B11 (obstetrical sonography)

From Agur AMR and Lee M. *Grant's Atlas of Anatomy* (9th ed.). Baltimore: Williams & Wilkins, 1991. 385

Courtesy of American Academy of Dermatology. Schamburg, IL. C8 (bulla, macule, nodule, papule, patch, plaque, pustule, tumor, vesicle wheal), C9 (cherry angioma, crust, ecchymosis, erosion, fissure, keloid, scale, telangiectasia, ulcer)

Courtesy of American Cancer Society, Inc. Atlanta, GA. C12 (malignant melanoma)

Courtesy of American Society of Clinical Pathologists Journal. Chicago, IL. C16 (Giardia lamblia)

Courtesy of American Society of Microbiology. Washington, DC. 808

Adapted from *Application Manual: Cytokines/Chemokine Manual*, PharMingen Corporation. San Diego, CA. 1998. 453, 454

From Ballenger JJ & Snow JB. *Otorhinolaryngology: Head and Neck Surgery* (15th ed.). Baltimore: Williams & Wilkins, 1996. 218, 250, 532

Courtesy of Baschat A, MD. Center for Advanced Fetal Care, University of Maryland School of Medicine. Baltimore, MD. C11 (Doppler flow, fetal heart)

From Bear MF, Connors BW, Paradiso MA. *Neuroscience: Exploring the Brain*. Baltimore: Williams & Wilkins, 1996. 830

Courtesy of Bennett J, PhD. National Institutes of Health. Bethesda, MD. 233, C1 (methenamine silver stain), C7 (Aspergillus hyphae, histoplasmosis, mycetoma), C15 (normal brain MRI)

From Bickley LS, MD. *Bates' Guide to Physical Examination and History Taking* (7th ed.). Philadelphia: Lippincott Williams & Wilkins, 1999. C8 (vitiligo), C15 (Down syndrome, clubbing, cyanosis, jaundice, facial nerve palsy, Babinski response, Brushfield spots)

From Brant WE & Helms CA. *Fundamentals of Diagnostic Radiology* (2nd ed.). Baltimore: Williams & Wilkins, 1999. 250, 430, 520, 584, 671, 681, 711, 842, 1623, 1639, B11 (ovarian carcinoma, cleft lip), B13 (mesothelioma), B14 (bronchiectasis, breast cancer mammogram, normal mammogram, mammography, CT liver scan)

Adapted from Braunwald E, Fauci AS, Isselbacher KJ, Kasper DL, Hauser SL, Longo DL, Jameson JL. *Harrison's Principles of Medicine* [book on CD-ROM] (14th Ed). New York: McGraw-Hill Companies, 1998. 38, 290, 5841683

Courtesy of Brinkley W, PhD. Baylor College of Medicine, Houston, TX. 320

Courtesy of Bristow RE, MD. Johns Hopkins School of Medicine. Baltimore, MD. B9 (laparoscopic biopsy, normal pelvis)

Burtis CA, Ashwood ER, Aldrich JE. *Tietz Fundamentals of Clinical Chemistry* (4th ed.). Philadelphia: WB Saunders Company, 1996. 847, 859, 1056

Courtesy of Caughman WF, DDS, Fazier KB, DDS, Haywood VB, DMD. Carbamide peroxide whitening of nonvital single discolored teeth: case reports. *Quintessance International*, 30: 155–161, 1999. B7 (bleached maxillary teeth)

Courtesy of Cavallucci D, CDA, EFDA, RDH. Harcum College, Bryn Mawr, PA. 674

Adapted from Chaffee EE, RN, MN & Greisheimer, MD, PhD. *Basic Physiology and Anatomy* (3rd ed.). Philadelphia: JB Lippincott Company, 1974. 120, 189, 274, 307, 353, 409, 463, 545, 617, 697, 724, 962, 968, 1028, 1141, 1210, 1438, 1649, 1695, 1761, 1785, 1853

Courtesy of Chai T, MD, & Sklar G, MD. University of Maryland School of Medicine. Baltimore, MD. B9 (bladder tumor through scope, catheter in ureters)

Courtesy of College of American Pathologists, Chicago, IL. C16 (granular cast, uric acid, hyaline crystals)

Adapted from Collier L & Mahy BWJ. *Topley & Wilson's Microbiology and Microbial Infections* (9th ed.) Vol. 1. London: Arnold Publications, 1998. 1261

From Daffner RH. *Clinical Radiology: The Essentials* (2nd ed.). Baltimore: Williams & Wilkins, 1998. 1470, B11 (previa placenta), B12 (radiography), B13 (P. carinii pneumonia, pulmonary edema), B14 (brain hematoma, lung carcinoma), B15 (brain MRI–multiple sclerosis, herniated nucleus pulposus), C13 (nodular metastasis), C14 (breast carcinoma, colon carcinoma, prostatic carcinoma, Ewing tumor)

From Damjanov I, MD. *Histopathology: A Color Atlas and Textbook*. Baltimore: Williams & Wilkins, 1996. C13 (actinic keratosis, squamous cell carcinoma, Bowen disease, glioblastoma, liposarcoma, lymphoma, nodular melanoma, neuroblastoma, retinoblastoma, teratoma, pituitary adenoma, Wilms tumor)

From Danzi JT, Landma S. *Case Atlas of Gastroenterology*. Baltimore: Williams & Wilkins, 1995. B8 (Barrett esophagus, gastric polyp)

Adapted from Danforth N, MD & Scott JR, MD. *Danforth's Obstetrics and Gynecology* (8th ed.). Philadelphia: Lippincott Williams & Wilkins, 1999. 1329

From Davis RL, MD, Robertson DM, MD, MSC, FRCDC. *Textbook of Neuropathology* (3rd ed.). Baltimore: Williams & Wilkins, 1997. 219

Courtesy of Day JA, MD. University of Massachusetts School of Medicine, Boston, MA. B12 (ARDS, lobar collapse), B13 (interstitial lung disease)

Courtesy of Dirckx JH, MD. University of Dayton Health Center, Dayton, OH. 1021, 1777

Courtesy of Dura Pharmaceuticals, San Diego, CA. B9 (intraoperative cholangiography)

Fadem B & Simring S. *High-Yield Psychiatry*. Baltimore: Lippincott Williams & Wilkins, 1998. Tables–anxiety, antianxiety agents, anti-depressants, antimanic agents, antipsychotic medications, development of a normal child, mental disorders, mood disorders, sleeping

From Feinsilver SH & Fein A. *Textbook of Bronchoscopy*. Baltimore: Williams & Wilkins, 1995. B8 (bronchus, carina, trachea, vocal folds)

From Fuller J, RN, PhD & Schaller-Ayers J, RNC, MNSc, PhD. *A Nursing Approach* (2nd ed.), 1994. 628, 636, 763, 790, 1069, 1139, 1485, 1744, 1844, 1857

Adapted from Garcia LS & Bruckner DA. *Diagnostic Medical Parasitology* (3rd ed.). Washington DC: ASM Press, 1997. 394

From Gartner LP & Hiatt JL. *Color Atlas of Histology* (2nd ed.). Baltimore: Williams & Wilkins, 1994. 390, 1594, C2 (basophil, eosinophil, monocyte, neutrophil)

Courtesy of General Electric Medical Systems. Milwaukee, WI. B15 (magnetic resonance imaging, torn knee meniscus), B16 (nuclear lung scan, positron emission tomography)

From Georgiade NG, Riefkohl R, Levine LS. Georgiade, GS. *Plastic, Maxillofacial and Reconstructive Surgery* (3rd ed.) Baltimore: Williams & Wilkins, 1996. 684

From Goodheart HP, MD. *A Photoguide of Common Skin Disorders: Diagnosis and Management*. Baltimore: Lippincott Williams & Wilkins: 1999. C4 (folliculitis, Henöch-Schonlein purpura), C5 (molluscum contagiosum), C8 (Acanthosis nigrans, pilomatricoma cyst, dermatomyositis), C9 (excoriation, lichenification), C11 (drug eruption, erythema multiforme, erythema nodosum, Stevens-Johnson syndrome), C12 (neurofibromatosis), C15 (exophthalmia, myxedema)

From Halstead CL, Blozis GG, Drinnan AJ, Gier RE. *Physical Evaluation of Dental Patient*. St. Louis: CV Mosby Company, 1982. 1845

Courtesy of Hawke M, MD. Toronto, Canada. B5 (cholesteatoma, normal tympanic membrane, tympanosclerosis)

Courtesy of Haywood VB, DMD. School of Dentistry, Medical College of Georgia, Augusta, GA. B7 (vital bleaching)

Courtesy of Haywood VB, DMD. Extended bleaching of tetracycline-stained teeth: a case report. *Contemporary Esthetics and Restorative Practice*. Jamesburg, NJ: Dental Learning Systems Co., Inc. 1 (1): 14-17, 1997. B7 (tetracycline-stained teeth)

Courtesy of Hoag Memorial Presbyterian Hospital. Newport Beach, CA. B16 (bone scan)

Adapted from Kapikian AZ. *Journal of the American Medical Association*. Chicago, IL: American Medical Association., 1993. Vol. 269:627. 1967

From Kini SR. *Color Atlas of Differential Diagnosis in Exfoliative and Aspiration Cytopathology*. Baltimore: Williams & Wilkins, 1998. 1257, C13 (ependymomas)

From Koneman EW, Allen SD, Janda WM, Schreckenberger PC, Winn WC, Jr. *Color Atlas and Textbook of Diagnostic Microbiology* (4th & 5th eds.). Philadelphia: Lippincott, 1992 & 1997. C1 (methenamine silver stain, *Chlamydia*, *Clostridium tetani*, *Escherichia coli*, hematoxylin and eosin stain, benign pancreatic acinar tissue, Periodic acid-Schiff stain, Papanicolaou stain, *Streptococcus pneumoniae*, Warthin-Starry stain), C4 (pseudomonas), C5 (influenza A virus), C6 (A. lumbricoides egg, malarial parasites, pinworm ova), C7 (*Candida albicans*, *Alternaria* (*Penicillium*), *Isospora belli*, microsporum gypseum)

From Kuby J. *Immunology*. (3rd ed.). New York: WH Freeman Company, 1997. 38, 171, 873, 881, 882, 883

Courtesy of Last JM, MD. University of Ottawa, Ontario, Canada. 1063

From Lee RG, Foerster J, Lukens J, Paraskevas F, Greer JP, Rodgers GM. *Wintrobe's Clinical Hematology* (10th ed.) Vol.1. Baltimore: Williams & Wilkins, 1998. C2 (neutrophilic myelocyte), C3 (reticulocyte)

Courtesy of Life Art. The Life Art Professional Collection–Surgery Collection. 326, 1082, 1121

Adapted from Male D, Roitt I, Brostoff J. *Immunology: An Illustrated Outline*. (5th ed.). London: CV Mosby Company, 1998. 392, 1067, 1125

Adapted from Martin FN. *Introduction to Audiology* (5th ed.). Englewood Cliffs, NJ: Prentice Hall, 1994. 1900

From McArdle WD, Katch FL, & Katch VL. *Essentials of Exercise Physiology*. Philadelphia: Lea & Febiger, 1994. 1915

From McClatchey K. *Clinical Laboratory Medicine*. Baltimore: Williams & Wilkins, 1994. 449, C2 (erythroblasts), C3 (Heinz body), C4 (E.M. bacterial cell, gonococci), C5 (Burkitt lymphoma), C16 (bone marrow aspirate, waxy cast, cystine crystals, calcium oxalate crystals, red blood cells, white blood cells, whole chromosome probe)

Courtesy of McKenzie SB, Clare N, Burns C, Larson L, Metz J. *Textbook of Hematology* (2nd ed.). Baltimore: Williams & Wilkins, 1996. 347, 1414, 1816, C1 (Wright-Giemsa stain), C2 (megakaryoblast, promyelocyte), C3 (aplastic, blood, hemolytic, microcytic, sickle cell anemias; anisocytosis, basophilic stippling, macrocytosis, microcytosis, poikilocytosis, reticulocytes, spherocytosis)

Copyright from Mediclip: The Complete Medical Image Source. Clinical Images OB/GYN. 1920

Adapted from Melnick JL, Adelberg EA, Brooks GF, Jawetz E, Morse SA, Butel JS. *Jawetz Melnick and Adelberg's Medical Microbiology* (21st ed.). New York, NY: McGraw Hill, 1998. 316, 815, 1965

From Mims C, Playfair J, Roitt I, Wakelin D, R Williams. *Medical Microbiology* (2nd ed.). London: CV Mosby Company, 1998. 1971

From Ming SC & Goldman H. *Pathology of the Gastrointestinal Tract* (2nd ed.). Baltimore: Williams & Wilkins, 1998. C12 (benign stomach tumor, malignant stromal tumor, ulcerative carcinoma)

Courtesy of Mission Hospital Regional Medical Center. Mission Viego, CA. B8 (gastritis, esophageal varices), B10 (colon polypectomy), B11 (sonogram)

From Moore KL, PhD, FRSM, FIAC & Dalley AF II, PhD. *Clinically Oriented Anatomy* (4th ed.). Baltimore: Lippincott Williams & Wilkins, 1999. Tabular material: arteries, muscle, nerve and vein tables for use in the appendices

Adapted from *Morbidity and Mortality Weekly Report Series*. Atlanta: Centers for Disease Control and Prevention, 1991. Vol 40 RR03. 1500

From Naeim F. *Pathology of Bone Marrow* (2nd ed.). Baltimore: Williams & Wilkins, 1998. C1 (Prussia blue stain)

From Neville BW, Damm DD, White DK. *Color Atlas of Clinical Oral Pathology* (2nd ed.). Baltimore: Williams & Wilkins, 1998. 39, 691, C10 (ameloblastoma, aphthous ulcerations, cancer of tongue, *Candida albicans*, cheilitis, Behcet disease, herpangina, herpes stomatitis, leukoplakia, oral hairy leukoplakia, commissural lip pits, mucocele, Fordyce granules, stomatitis)

Courtesy of Newport Diagnostic Center, Newport Beach, CA. B16 (Alzheimer's and normal brain PET scans)

Courtesy of Olympus America, Inc., Melville, NY. B9 (thoracoscopy), B10 (colonoscope)

Courtesy of Orange Coast College, Costa Mesa, CA. 595

Courtesy of Peroukta R, MD. Cockeysville, MD. B14 (arthroscopy, ACL graft, normal meniscus, meniscal tear)

Courtesy of Philips Medical Systems. Shelton, CT. B14 (computed tomography)

From Pillitteri A, PhD, RN, PNP. *Maternal & Child Health Nursing: Care of the Childbearing & Childrearing Family* (3rd ed.). Philadelphia: Lippincott Williams & Wilkins, 1998. 78, 282, 464, 878, 879, 1061, 2002

Courtesy of Potter, B, DDS. School of Dentistry, Medical College of Georgia, Augusta, GA. B6 (cephalometric radiograph, radiograph, endosteal implant, mixed dentation, radiolucent, recurrent decay, root canal, unerupted third molar)

From Rassner G. translated by WHC Burgdorf. *Atlas of Dermatology* (3rd ed.). Philadelphia: Lea & Febiger, 1994. 18, 259, 552, 566, 815, 1036, 1216, 1317, 1339, 1604, 1931, C4 (impetigo), C6 (elephantiasis), C8 (Peutz–Jeghers syndrome), C9 (hemangioma), C11 (allergic contact dermatitis, dermatitis herpetiformis, polymorphic light eruption, photodermatitis, radiodermatitis), C12 (angiosarcoma, Bowen disease, actinic keratosis, lentigo maligna melanoma, pyogenic granuloma, seborrheic keratoses), C15 (Paget disease)

From Roche Lexikon Medizin (3rd ed.). Munich, Germany: Urban & Schwarzenberg, 1993. 3, 8, 16, 25, 26, 39, 82, 98, 128, 133, 135, 151, 159, 183, 286, 251, 300, 337, 351, 355, 420, 442, 514, 567, 568, 590, 591, 608, 676, 698, 699, 731, 769, 791, 806, 833, 881, 894, 957, 962, 968, 1038, 1054, 1060, 1080, 1169, 1175, 1185, 1207, 1216, 1269, 1281, 1341, 1358, 1368, 1371, 1388, 1408, 1421, 1424, 1472, 1480, 1489, 1530, 1561, 1567, 1603, 1611, 1648, 1672, 1677, 1808, 1852, 1882, 1886, 1990, 1997, 2003) B4 (blepharitis, coloboma iridis, hyphema, retinal tear), B8 (laryngeal carcinoma), B10 (ulcerative colitis, diverticulosis), B15 (meningioma), B16 (thyroid uptake, liver scan) C2 (blood cells, lymphocytes), C3 (pernicious anemia erythrocytes), C4 (staphylococci, streptococci, mycobacterium tuberculosis), C5 (AIDS virus, herpes zoster, hepatitis B), C9 (rosacea), C12 (neurofibromatosis, keratoacanthoma), C16 (ferning of cervical mucus)

Adapted from Rosdahl Bunker C, RN, BSN, MA. *Textbook of Basic Nursing* (7th ed.). Philadelphia: Lippincott Williams & Wilkins, 1999. 63, 904

Courtesy of Ross MH. *Histology: A Text and Atlas* (3rd ed.). Baltimore: Williams & Wilkins, 1995. 311, 939, 1208

From Sanders CV, Nesbitt LT, Jr. *The Skin and Infection: A Color Atlas and Text*. Baltimore: Williams & Wilkins, 1995. 1185, C4 (Lyme disease, erysipelas, lepromatous leprosy, staphylococci, streptococci), C5 (erythema infectiosum, hepatitis B, hepatitis C, genital herpes, infectious mononucleosis, hemorrhagic varicella, plantar wart), C6 (cutaneous larva migrans, pediculosis capitis, pediculosis pubis, scabies), C7 (cryptococcus, tinea capitis, tinea pedis, tinea versicolor), C10 (Strawberry tongue), C12 (Kaposi sarcoma)

Courtesy of Scheie Eye Institute. Philadelphia, PA. B4 (glaucomatus, papilledema, normal retina, retinal detachment, diabetic retinopathy, hypertensive retinopathy)

Courtesy of Schuster GS, DDS, PhD. School of Dentistry, Medical College of Georgia, Augusta, GA. B6 (dental chart).

From Seshan SV, D'Agati V, Appel GA, Churg, J. *Renal Disease: Classification and Atlas of Tubulo-interstitial and Vascular Diseases*. Baltimore: Williams & Wilkins, 1998. 162, 514

Courtesy of Sheen, G, DDS, MS. School of Dentistry, Medical College of Georgia, Augusta, GA. B7 (restoration replacement, veneer hypoplasty, resin veneer diastema, resin-bonded bridge, porcelain crowns).

Adapted from Skarin AT, Dorfman DM: Non-Hodgkin's lymphoma: current classification and management. *CA: A Cancer Journal for Clinicians*. Baltimore: Williams & Wilkins. 1997. Vol. 47 No 6. 1046

Courtesy of Skin Cancer Foundation. New York, NY. C12 (basal cell carcinoma, squamous cell carcinoma)

From Smeltzer SC & Bare BG. *Brunner & Suddarth's Textbook of Medical Surgical-Nursing* (8th ed.). Philadelphia: JB Lippincott Company, 1996. 150, 187, 247, 377, 381, 531, 562, 682, 865, 1297, 1298, 1430, 1485, 1600, 1666, 1710, 1864, 1956, B8 (fiberoptic bronchoscopy, esophagoduodenoscope), B9 (laparoscopy, thoracoscopy), B10 (colonoscopy), B11 (sonography), B14 (x-ray), B15 (MRI imaging)

Stites DP, Terr AI, Parslow TG. *Basic and Clinical Medical Immunology* (8th ed.). New York, NY: McGraw Hill, 1994. 880

Adapted from Suddarth Smith, D. *Lippincott's Manual of Nursing Practice* (5th ed.). Philadelphia: JB Lippincott Company, 1991. 465, 608, 1346, 1708, 1788

From Sun T. *Parasitic Disorders* (2nd ed.). Baltimore: Williams & Wilkins, 1998. 447, 597, 539, C6 (acanthamoeba, elephantiasis, *Giardia lamblia*, taenia eggs, trichomonas hominis)

From Sun T, Tenenbaum MJ, Greenspan J. *Journal of Infectious Disease*. Chicago, IL: University of Chicago Press, 1993. Vol 238; 248. C6 (*Babesia* organism)

Courtesy of Temple University Hospital. Philadelphia, PA. B8 (bronchoscopy)

Courtesy of Underwood L, MD & Underwood RD, MD. Mission Viejo, CA. C4 (syphilis), C9 (petechia)

Courtesy of Wang F, MD. Orange, CA. B16 (ventilation and perfusion scans)

Courtesy of Welch Allyn, Inc. Skaneateles Falls, NY. B4 (eye exam, ophthalmoscope), B5 (exostosis, foreign body, otomycosis, otitis externa, otitis media, otoscope, otoscopy, perforation), C11 (allergic rhinitis, nasal polyps)

From Wilcox RB. *High-Yield Biochemistry*. Baltimore: Lippincott Williams & Wilkins, 1999. 443, 1527, 1860

From Willis MC. *Medical Terminology: The Language of Health Care*. Baltimore: Williams & Wilkins, 1996. 987, 1411, 1569

From Yochum TR & Rowe LJ. *Essentials of Skeletal Radiology* (2nd ed.). Baltimore: Williams & Wilkins, 1996. 632, 1176

Courtesy of Zucker-Franklin D, PhD. New York University Medical Center, New York, NY. C2 (monocyte), C3 (reticulocyte)

ILLUSTRATION INDEX

The Illustration and Tables Indices provide a quick way to find any image in this book. The page number listed next to each term indicates where readers can find an illustration for that term.

Terms followed by the letter "A" and a page number indicate that the image can be found in the first color insert, the 32-page anatomy atlas. Terms accompanied by the letter "B" and a page number indicate that the image can be found in the second insert, diagnostic imagery and anatomical positions. Terms listed with the letter "C" and a page number show the image can be found in the third insert, the diseases and ailments section.

To find the definition of the illustrated term, simply look up the word in bold. Readers can identify whether a term in the A-Z section is illustrated—either at the term itself or in the inserts —if the term is accompanied by this symbol: (▣)

HIGH PROFILE TERMS IN THIS EDITION

activator, tissue plasminogen
AIDS
angioplasty, percutaneous transluminal coronary
antibody, monoclonal
antigen, prostate-specific
antileukotriene
antioxidant
apnea, obstructive sleep
apoptosis
asthma, bronchial
atherosclerosis
carcinoma
carcinoma, breast
carcinoma, prostate
care, end-of-life
care, managed
Chlamydia pneumoniae
ciguatera
CLIA
cloning
cocaine
colposcopy
complex, histocompatibility
cytogenetics
cytokine
dehydroepiandrosterone (DHEA)
depression, major
diabetes mellitus
diabetes, gestational
Diagnostic and Statistical Manual of Mental Disorders

diet, low fat
directive, advance
disease, Alzheimer
disease, cat-scratch
disease, Creutzfeldt-Jakob
disease, gastroesophageal reflux
disease, Lyme
ehrlichiosis
encephalopathy, bovine spongiform
excision, loop
fasciitis, necrotizing
fever, rheumatic
fingerprinting, DNA
flunitrazepam
fluoroquinolone
folic acid
Framingham Heart Study
gene, BRCA1, BRCA2
gene, tumor suppressor
Ginkgo biloba
Helicobacter pylori
hepatitis
herpesvirus 8
HMO
homocysteine
hospitalist
Human Genome Project
γ-hydroxybutyrate
hypertension
immunotherapy
infarction, myocardial
inhibitor, α-glucosidase
inhibitor, HMG CoA reductase

inhibitor, protease
insulin, lispro
interferon
knife, gamma
laparoscopy
leptin
leukoplakia, hairy
lipoprotein
lipoprotein (a)
load, viral
mammography
medicine, alternative
melatonin
meningitis, meningococcal
mouse, knockout
nephropathy, diabetic
neuropathy, diabetic
nicotine
nitric oxide
nurse practitioner
obesity
oncogene
osteoporosis
parvovirus B19
pill, morning after
prion
probe
psychopharmacology
radiation, background
radical, free
raloxifene
reaction, polymerase chain
resistance, drug
resistance, insulin
retinopathy, diabetic
retrovirus

risks, radiation
schizophrenia
smallpox
stroke
suicide, physician-assisted
syndrome, fragile X
syndrome, premenstrual
syndrome, shaken baby
syndrome, sudden infant death
system, Bethesda
system, cytochrome P-450
tamoxifen citrate
telomerase
Terminologia Anatomica
test, stress
testing, genetic
therapy, gene
therapy, estrogen replacement
therapy, thrombolytic
tobacco
tomography, positron emission
trabeculoplasty, laser
trial, clinical
tuberculosis
ultrasonography, Doppler
universal precautions
virus, Ebola
virus, human papilloma
wellness
workaholic
wort, St. John's

Main Entry-Subentry Format

Stedman's Medical Dictionary differs in organization from general English dictionaries. The two primary kinds of entries in *Stedman's* are main entries and subentries. A main entry is the single-word noun under which multiple-word subentries are grouped. Main entries appear in bold and flush with the margin. Pronunciations in parentheses follow the main entries. Subentries are grouped alphabetically under their governing main entry. For example:

main entry → **groove** (groov). A narrow elongated depression or furrow on any surface. SEE ALSO sulcus

subentry →   **alveolobuccal g.,** the upper and lower half of the buccal vestibule. . . .

To locate a subentry term, the reader must refer to the main entry:

To find	Look under
myocardial infarction	infarction
hemorrhagic fever	fever
Q fever	
carcinoid tumor	
giant cell tumor of bone	tumor
Wilms tumor	

    Verbs, adjectives, adverbs, combining forms, prefixes, abbreviations, and symbols follow the general rules of indexing and thus are located as main entries.

    Compound words that usually are written closed up as one word or hyphenated are located as main entries rather than as subentries under the portion of the term that would otherwise represent the main entry. For example, "aftercontraction" is located in the A's rather than under contraction; "self-hypnosis" is located in the S's rather than under hypnosis.

    Multiple-word chemical and drug terms generally are located at the first word of a term, unless the term includes a general noun that would be considered a kind or type. For example:

To find	Look under
adrenergic blocking agent (a type of agent)	agent
Agent Orange (a specific compound)	Agent Orange
bile acid (a type of acid)	acid
acid red (a stain that is neither an acid nor red)	acid red
ribonucleic acid (a molecule rather than an acid)	ribonucleic acid

Tips on Finding Multiple-Word Terms

- Look in the *Word Finder* on page WF1, immediately preceding the A–Z section

- For Genus species, look in the *Genus Finder*, on page GF1, immediately preceding the *Word Finder*.

- Look at the alphabetical location of the specific words making up the term

- Look under another main entry that is similar to the term you are looking for

- Look at cross-references

To find	Look under
a surgical procedure	operation
	technique
	method
a disease	syndrome
	disease

ALPHABETIZATION

Main Entries

Main entries are alphabetized letter by letter as spelled, rather than word by word as in a telephone directory:

blood	cross
blood bank	crossbreed
bloodletting	cross-cylinder
blood purple	crossing-over of genes
bloodstream	cross-matching
blood vessel	crossway

Prepositional phrases, especially Latin expressions, are considered in alphabetization:

To find	**Look under**
ante cibum	the A's
in vitro	the I's

Spelled-out Greek letters and configurational forms also are considered in alphabetization:

To find	**Look under**
α-naphthylurea	the N's
alpha-blocker	the A's
L-dopa	the D's
levodopa	the L's

Capitalized words (proper nouns) precede lowercase words (common nouns):

Streptococcus	appears before streptococcus
Down	appears before down

Exceptions

For alphabetization, *Stedman's* disregards the following: prepositions, conjunctions, articles, apostrophes of possessive terms, spaces, punctuation, Greek letters (e.g., α, β, γ), numbers, configurational characters, (e.g., D-, +, −), and italicized forms (e.g., *p-, N-, cis-*), whether as prefixes or as interior components in compound chemical terms.

Subentries

Subentries are alphabetized letter by letter following the same rules given above for main entries but with some additional significant differences.

In subentry terms (as well as throughout definitions of both main entries and subentries), the governing main entry is represented by its initial letter if it is singular; by addition of an apostrophe and "s" if it is a regular plural; or by a spelled-out form if it is an irregular plural of a plural Latin word. For example:

crest	**gyrus**
gluteal c.	angular g.
c. of greater tubercle	gyri breves insulae
inguinal c.	central gyri
c.'s of nail bed	g. dentales
nasal c.	hort gyri of insula
c. of neck rib	gyri temporalis transversi

Regardless of its form, the main entry word is disregarded in alphabetization of subentries, as are prepositions, conjunctions, articles, and possessive forms.

Spelling

For alphabetizing letter by letter, spelling disregards spaces, punctuation, Greek letters, numbers, configurational characters, and italicized forms.

Alternative spellings, especially those of prefixed combining forms, are given as main entries with cross-references to the various spellings:

curet. SEE curette.

hem-, hema-. Blood. SEE ALSO hemat-, hemato-, hemo-. [G. *haima*]

kyto- SEE cyto-.

Alternative spellings that have been superseded are also given as main entries with cross-references to the currently used spellings:

oari-, oario- Obsolete term for an ovary. SEE oo-, oophor-, ovario-.
[G. *ōarion*, a small egg, dim. of *ōon*, egg].

pleio- rarely used alternative spelling for pleo-.

Differences in British and American spellings, particularly those at or near the beginning of a word, are handled by prefix main entries cross-referenced from the British spelling to the American spellings:

ae- For words so beginning and not found here, SEE UNDER e-.
oe- For words so beginning and not found here, SEE e-.

British spellings within compound words may change the alphabetical location of some entries:

	British	**American**
ae* for e	aetiology	etiology
	faeces	feces
oe for e	coeliac	celiac
	oedema	edema
	diarrhoea	diarrhea
our for or	tumour	tumor
re for er	fibre	fiber

Surnames, used as biographical main entry cross-references to associated eponymic terms, are also alphabetized by their most commonly used spellings. Users should keep in mind spelling variations such as "a/ae," "o/oe," "u/ue," and "Mac/Mc." For names beginning with prefixes, such as "Van," "van der," "von," "de," which may be used with or without the prefix, cross-reference main entries direct the user to the proper location. Regardless of the form of a surname (e.g., "Crohn," "Bence Jones," "d'Herelle," "von Willebrand," "Loeffler" or "Löffler"), the name is alphabetized letter by letter as spelled.

ORGANIZATION OF ENTRIES AND CROSS-REFERENCES

The definition is given at only one location for two or more synonymous terms. Entries for the other synonymous terms are cross-referenced to the term where the definition is to be found. This system is also used for obsolete or outmoded terms, for spelling variations, or when there is a definite preference dictated by its us-

---

* "Ae" in the combining form "aero-" is accepted spelling in both usages, as in "aerosol," "anaerobe," and other words derived from the G. *aer*, air. "Aeroplane"/"airplane" is a well-known exception.

age. The practice of placing a definition at only one location primarily serves to focus all of the information concerning a term at a single place, rather than strictly as an indicator of preference. It also keeps the size of *Stedman's* manageable by avoiding duplication of definitions.

Main Entries

Defined main entries usually are constructed as follows: (1) boldface entry word followed by its abbreviation or symbol (if any) in parentheses, (2) pronunciation in parentheses, (3) the definition proper, and (4) the derivation in brackets.

> **electrocardiogram (ECG, EKG)** (ē-lek-trō-kar′dē -ō-gram). Graphic record of the heart's integrated action currents obtained with the electrocardiograph. [electro- + G. *kardia*, heart, + *gramma*, a drawing]

If the main entry is used in its own definition, it is abbreviated to its first letter or to its accepted abbreviation, e.g., "b." for "bone," "DNA" for "deoxyribonucleic acid," "Hb" for "hemoglobin."

Boldface numbers followed by a period distinguish multiple definitions, but their numerical sequence does not necessarily indicate importance or preference:

> **mesocardia** (mez′ō-kar′d ē-ă). **1.** Atypical position of the heart in a central position in the chest, as in early embryonic life. **2.** Plural of mesocardium. [meso- + G. *kardia*, heart]

Synonyms follow the final definition of a term and are preceded by "SYN." A lightface number in parentheses following a synonym indicates the particular definition of that term with which the boldface entry word is synonymous. If an entry or main entry is followed by a synonym and no other definition (the synonym will appear in blue), readers must refer to the synonym to find the definition.

> **nephropathy** (ne-frop′ă-thē). Any disease of the kidney. SYN nephrosis (1); [nephro- +G. *pathos*, suffering]

> **analgesic n.** SYN analgesic *nephritis*.

Systematic names of defined trivial or generic chemical and drug terms appear at the beginning of the definition, along with the molecular formula:

> **acetone** (as′e-tōn). CH_3COCH_3; a colorless, volatile, inflammable liquid; extremely small amounts are . . . SYN dimethyl ketone.

> **aspirin** (as′pi-rin). $C_6H_4(OCOCH_3)COOH$; a widely used analgesic, antipyretic, and anti-inflammatory agent; also used as an antiplatelet agent. SYN acetylsalicylic acid.

Subentries

Defined subentries are organized much like main entries, as described above. Pronunciation and derivation are provided when the principal words making up the subentry term are not provided as main entries in the vocabulary, as in the following example:

> **folie**
> **f. à deux** (ă-du), identical or similar mental disorders, such as a paranoid fixation, usually affecting two members of the same family living together. SYN shared psychotic disorder. [Fr. two]

In the definition, the main entry word, whenever used, is abbreviated to its first letter or to its accepted abbreviation as a space-saving device, e.g., "b." for "bone," "DNA" for "deoxyribonucleic acid," "Hb" for "hemoglobin."

Boldface numbers in parentheses distinguish multiple definitions, but their numerical sequence does not necessarily indicate importance or preference:

> **age**
>> **developmental a., (1)** a. estimated by anatomic development since implantation; SYN fetal a. **(2) (DA),** a. of an individual estimated from the degree of anatomic, physiologic, mental, and emotional maturation.

Cross-References

Cross-references may be main entries or subentries or may be part of a main entry or subentry definition. They may direct the user to a defined entry or to an entry where additional or related information can be found. *Stedman's* uses the following types of cross-references:

Synonym A word that has the same meaning as the entry. When a synonym occurs at a term without a definition, it appears in blue after "SYN." For example:

> **boil** (boyl). SYN furuncle. [A.S. *byl*, a swelling]

When the relevant synonym is a multiple-word term located as a subentry, the governing main entry word under which it will be found is italicized, as in the following example:

> **candle-power** (kan′dl-pow′er). SYN luminous *intensity.*

When the synonym cross-reference is from one subentry to another subentry under the same main entry, the main entry word is abbreviated, as in the following example:

> **calculus**
>> **arthritic c.** gouty *tophus.*
>> **biliary c.** gallstone.
>> **dendritic c.** staghorn c.
>> **nephritic c.** obsolete term for renal c.

SEE
Refers the reader to a term with a meaning similar to the entry.

SEE ALSO
Refers the reader to a term with further information about the entry.

Cf. *(L. confer, compare)* **and q.v.** *(L. quod vide, which see)*
Refers the reader to comparative or related information, but with a less direct relationship than a SEE ALSO reference.

Obsolete term for
The term is no longer widely used. Refers the reader to the term in current use.

Eponyms

Eponyms are terms that are named after people and places. A brief biography appears at a person's name, along with a cross-reference to the eponym.

> **Hoffman,** Johann, German neurologist, 1857–1919. SEE H. muscular *atrophy, phenomenon, reflex, sign*; Werdnig-H. *disease,* Werdnig-H. muscular *atrophy.*
>
> **Sylvius,** (DuBois, de le Boë). Le Böe, Franciscus (François), Dutch physician, anatomist, and physiologist, 1614–1672. SEE sylvian *angle,* sylvian *aqueduct,* sylvian *fissure,* sylvian *line,* sylvian *point,* sylvian *valve,* sylvian *ventricle*; *fossa* of S.; *vallecula* sylvii.
>
> **Wilms,** Max, German surgeon, 1867–1918. SEE W. tumor.

Reflecting the trend in current publications, this edition of *Stedman's* has dropped the possessive form for eponymous terms.

Abbreviations and Symbols

Abbreviations and symbols, as well as acronyms and other contractions, are included in the vocabulary if they are accepted usage as opposed to ad hoc creations. They are located as main entries, generally as cross-references to the spelled-out terms where they are cited parenthetically in boldface immediately after the boldface entry word(s):

Cyt Symbol for cytosine

cytosine (Cyt) (si′to-sen). 4-Amino-2(1H)-pyrimidinone; a. . . .

PET Abbreviation for positron emission *tomography*
tomography
  positron emission t. (PET), tomographic imaging of local. . . .

stat. Abbreviation for L. *statim*, at once, immediately.
statim (stat.) (sta′tim) [L.]. At once; immediately.

Some abbreviations and symbols are self-explanatory or are more appropriately defined at their entries than at a contrived entry for the spelled-out terms:

b.i.d. Abbreviation for L. *bis in die,* twice a day.

FUO Abbreviation for fever of unknown origin.

PUVA Acronym for oral administration of *p*soralen and subsequent exposure to long wavelength ultraviolet light (*uv-a*); used to treat psoriasis.

QCO_2 Symbol for the microliters STPD of CO_2 given off per milligram of tissue per hour.

Abbreviations may appear with or without periods. Some nomenclature conventions have eliminated the period from certain types of abbreviations. General use of periods with most abbreviations is progressively declining, but in some instances periods are retained to avoid confusion.

PRONUNCIATION

Conventions

Phonetic spelling for pronunciation appears in parentheses immediately after the boldface entry word(s). Pronunciations follow main entries except where redundant because the phonetic spelling is the same as the spelling of the boldface entry word(s). Pronunciations are not given for subentries except words in Latin, where a prime (′) indicates the stressed syllable.

The phonetic system used is a basic one and has only a few conventions:

- Two diacritical marks are used; the macron (ˉ) for long vowels; and the breve (˘) for short vowels.

- Principal stressed syllables are followed by a prime (′); monosyllables do not have a stress mark.

- Other syllables are separated by dots.

The following pronunciation key provides examples and consonant sounds encountered in the phonetic system. No attempt has been made to accommodate the slurred sounds common in speech or regional variations in speech sounds. Note that a vowel with a breve (˘) is used for the indefinite vowel sound of the schwa (ə). Native pronunciation of foreign words is approximated as closely as possible.

Pronunciation Key

Vowels

ā	day, care, guage		f	fit
a	mat, damage		g	got
ă	about, para		h	hit
ah	father		j	jade
aw	fall, cause, raw		k	kept
ē	be, equal, ear		ks	tax
ě	taken, genesis		kw	quit
e	term, learn		l	law
ī	pie		m	me
ĭ	pit, sieve, build		n	no
ō	note, for, so		ng	ring
o	not, oncology, ought		p	pan
oo	food		r	rot
ow	cow, out		s	so, miss
oy	troy, void		sh	should
ū	unit, curable		t	ten
ŭ	cut		th	thin, with
			v	very

Consonants

b	bad		w	we
ch	child		y	yes
d	dog		z	zero
dh	this, smooth		zh	azure, measure

In some words the initial sound is not that of the initial letter(s), or the initial letter(s) is not sounded or has a different sound, as in the following examples:

aerobe (ar'ob)	phthalein (thal'e-in)
eimuria (ime're-a)	pneumonia (nu-mo'ne-a)
gnathic (nath'ik)	psychology (si-kol'o-je)
knuckle (nuk-l)	ptosis (to'sis)
oedipism (ed'i-pizm)	xanthoma (zan-tho'ma)

MEDICAL ETYMOLOGY

Organization

The origin or etymology of a boldface entry term is given in square brackets [ ] at the end of the entry. Of necessity, derivations are brief and as simple as possible to facilitate memory and promote association with similar derivatives. The information provided has three basic components: (1) the abbreviation of the language to which the original word(s) belongs; (2) in italics, the original word(s) from which the term is derived; and (3) the English translation of the word(s). For Greek and Latin verbs, the first-person singular present form, rather than the infinitive, is used for more ready recognition of the root word; however, the English translation is given in the infinitive:

> **diphtheria** (dif-thēr′ē-ă). A specific infectious disease. . . . SYN diphtheritis. [G. *diphthera*, leather]

> **graph** (graf). **1.** A line or tracing. . . . [G. *graphō*, to write].

> **union** (ūn′yŭn)]. **1.** The joining or amalgamation. . . . [L. *unus*, one]

When the boldface entry term has the same or approximately the same meaning and/or spelling as the word(s) from which it is derived, the redundant material is not included in the derivation, as in the following examples:

> **idea** (ī-dē′ă). Any mental image or concept. [G. semblance]

> **locus,** pl. **loci** (lō′kŭs, lō′sī). **1.** A place; usually, a. . . . [L.]

Derivations frequently include additional components, especially when a derivation involves compound words or more than one word from one or more languages. A Greek or Latin verb may be hyphenated to indicate that the second part of the word exists as a simple verb with the same or approximately the same meaning, qualified by the addition of an adjectival or adverbial prefix; if the simple verb undergoes a change when forming part of a compound verb, that change is also shown:

> **apocrine** (ap′ō-krin). Denoting a mechanism of glandular secretion in which the apical portion of secretory cells is shed and incorporated into the secretion. SEE ALSO a. *gland*. [G. *apo-krinō*, to separate]

> **component** (kom-pō′nent). An element forming a part of the whole. [L. *com-pono*, pp. *-positus*, to place together]

When words originating from more than one language are part of a derivation, the language of each word and the word's English translation are given; when the words are from the same language, the language is indicated only for the first word:

> **apicectomy** (ap-i-sek′tō-mē). **1.** Opening and exenteration of air cells. . . . [L. *apex*, summit or tip, + G. *ektomē*, excision]

> **gonarthrotomy** (gon-ar-throt′ō-mē). Incision into the knee joint. [G. *gony*, knee, + *arthron*, joint, + *tomē*, incision]

Prefixes and Suffixes

Combining forms used as prefixes or within compound words are listed in the vocabulary as boldface main entries with their own bracketed derivations and full definitions. They are preceded by the recycle symbol (△). When combining forms appear in bracketed derivations of other boldface entry terms that follow alphabetically in the vocabulary, their language of origin and English translation are not given:

△ **neur-, neuri-, neuro-.** Nerve, nerve tissue, the nervous system. [G. *neuron*]

neuralgia (nū-ral′jē-ă). Pain of a severe, throbbing, or stabbing character in the course or distribution of a nerve. SYN neurodynia. [neur- + G. *algos*, pain]

Combining forms used as suffixes and terminations are also listed in the vocabulary as boldface main entries with their own bracketed derivations and full definitions. When used in bracketed derivations of other boldface entry items, the language of origin is indicated (only if different from the preceding word), and the English translation is given:

△ **-osis,** pl. **-oses**. Suffix, properly added only to words formed from G. roots, meaning a process, condition, or state, usually abnormal or diseased. It denotes. . . . [G.]

halitosis (hal-i-tō′sis). A foul odor from the mouth. SYN fetor oris, ozostomia, stomatodysodia. [L. *halitus*, breath, + G. *-osis*, condition]

ABBREVIATIONS AND SYMBOLS USED IN THE DICTIONARY

The abbreviations and symbols below are used in the derivations and definitions of entries in the dictionary. They should be distinguished from the abbreviations and symbols given as entries in the vocabulary or accompanying the spelled-out entry words that they represent, as discussed above.

acc.	accusative	EC	Enzyme Commission
adj.	adjective	e.g.	L. exempli gratia, for example
Am.Ind.	American Indian		
Ar.	Arabic	Eng.	English
A.S.	Anglo-Saxon	etym.	etymology
Br.	British	fem.	feminine
c., ca	L. circa, about	Fr.	French
cf.	L. confer, compare	fr.	from
Ch.	Chinese	fut.	future
char.	character	G.	Greek
C.I.	Colour Index	Gael.	Gaelic
D.	Dutch	gen.	genitive
dial.	dialect	Ger.	German
dim.	diminutive	Hind.	Hindu

Ice.	Icelandic	O.H.G.	Old High German
i.e.	L. id est, that is	O.N.	Old Norse
Ind.	Indian	p.	participle
It.	Italian	Pers.	Persian
Jap.	Japanese	Pg.	Portuguese
L.	Latin	pl.	plural
L.L.	Late Latin	pp.	past participle
masc.	masculine	priv.	privative, negative
M.E.	Middle English	pr.p.	present participle
Med.L., Mediev. L.	Medieval Latin	q.v.	L. quod vide, which see
Mod.L.	Modern Latin	Sansk.	Sanskrit
myth.	mythological	Sc.	Scandinavian
N.A.	*Nomina Anatomica*	sing.	singular
neut.	neuter	Sp.	Spanish
N.G.	New Guinea	Sw.	Swedish
ntr.	neuter	T.A.	*Terminologia Anatomica*
obs.	obsolete	thr.	through
O.E.	Old English	U.S.	United States
O.Fr.	Old French	W.Af.	West African

In biographical data, * denotes year of birth when year of death is not given, and † denotes year of death when year of birth is not given.

GUIDE TO PHARMACEUTICAL NAMES

Whether you need to check a spelling, locate brand-name drugs containing a particular generic ingredient, or identify a product's manufacturer, this convenient compilation of brand and generic drug names will provide the answer you seek. The section is organized alphabetically, with brand and generic entries integrated throughout. Brand names are shown in upper and lower case, followed in parentheses by the manufacturer. Generic names are shown underlined and in upper case. Below each generic name you'll find a list of brands containing the ingredient. Additional information on any of the listed brands and their manufacturers can be found in *Physicians' Desk Reference*.

A

ABACAVIR SULFATE
  Ziagen Oral Solution (GLAXO WELLCOME)
  Ziagen Tablets (GLAXO WELLCOME)
ABBO-CODE INDEX (ABBOTT)
ABBOKINASE (ABBOTT)
ABBOKINASE OPEN-CATH (ABBOTT)

ABCIXIMAB
  ReoPro Vials (LILLY)
ABELCET INJECTION (LIPOSOME)
ABSCENTS DEODORIZING POWDER
  (GORDON)

ACARBOSE
  Precose Tablets (BAYER)
ACCOLATE TABLETS (ASTRAZENECA)
ACCUPRIL TABLETS (PARKE-DAVIS)
ACCUTANE CAPSULES (ROCHE LABS)
ACCUZYME DEBRIDING OINTMENT
  (HEALTHPOINT)

ACEBUTOLOL HYDROCHLORIDE
  Acebutolol Hydrochloride Capsules (MYLAN)
  Acebutolol Hydrochloride Capsules (WATSON)
  Sectral Capsules (WYETH-AYERST)
ACEBUTOLOL HYDROCHLORIDE
  CAPSULES (MYLAN)
ACEBUTOLOL HYDROCHLORIDE
  CAPSULES (WATSON)
ACEBUTOLOL HYDROCHLORIDE
  CAPSULES (ESI LEDERLE)
ACEL-IMUNE (LEDERLE LABS)
ACEON TABLETS (2 MG, 4 MG, 8 MG)
  (SOLVAY)
ACES ANTIOXIDANT SOFT GELS (CARLSON)

ACETAMINOPHEN
  Acetaminophen Oral Solution (Cherry)
    (ROXANE)
  Acetaminophen Oral Solution USP
    (PHARMACEUTICAL ASSOCIATES)
  Acetaminophen Tablets (ROXANE)
  Acetaminophen and Codeine Phosphate Oral
    Solution USP
    (PHARMACEUTICAL ASSOCIATES)
  Acetaminophen and Codeine Phosphate Oral
    Solution and Tablets (ROXANE)
  Acetaminophen and Codeine Phosphate
    Tablets, USP CIII (WATSON)
  Alumadrine Tablets (FLEMING)
  Anabar Caplets (LUNSCO)
  Anolor 300 Capsules (BLANSETT)
  Aspirin Free Excedrin Caplets (BRISTOL-MYERS)
  Aspirin Free Excedrin Geltabs (BRISTOL-MYERS)
  Axocet Capsules (SAVAGE)

  Benadryl Allergy/Cold Tablets
    (WARNER-LAMBERT)
  Benadryl Allergy/Sinus Headache Caplets &
    Gelcaps (WARNER-LAMBERT)
  Bupap Tablets (ECR)
  Butalbital, Acetaminophen and Caffeine
    Tablets USP (MALLINCKRODT)
  Butalbital, Caffeine, and Acetaminophen
    Tablets, USP (WATSON)
  Capital and Codeine Oral Suspension
    (CARNRICK)
  Children's Tylenol Allergy-D Liquid and
    Chewable Tablets (MCNEIL CONSUMER)
  Children's Tylenol Cold Liquid and Chewable
    Tablets (MCNEIL CONSUMER)
  Children's Tylenol Cold Plus Cough
    Suspension Liquid and Chewable Tablets
    (MCNEIL CONSUMER)
  Children's Tylenol Flu Suspension Liquid
    (MCNEIL CONSUMER)
  Children's Tylenol Sinus Liquid and Chewable
    Tablets (MCNEIL CONSUMER)
  Children's Tylenol Soft-Chew Chewable
    Tablets, Elixir, and Suspension Liquid
    (MCNEIL CONSUMER)
  Darvocet-N 100 Tablets (LILLY)
  Darvocet-N 50 Tablets (LILLY)
  Endocet Tablets, USP CII (ENDO GENERICS)
  Esgic Capsules (FOREST)
  Esgic Tablets (FOREST)
  Esgic-Plus Tablets (FOREST)
  Excedrin Extra-Strength Caplets
    (BRISTOL-MYERS)
  Excedrin Extra-Strength Geltabs
    (BRISTOL-MYERS)
  Excedrin Extra-Strength Tablets
    (BRISTOL-MYERS)
  Excedrin Migraine Caplets (BRISTOL-MYERS)
  Excedrin Migraine Tablets (BRISTOL-MYERS)
  Excedrin P.M. Caplets (BRISTOL-MYERS)
  Excedrin P.M. Geltabs (BRISTOL-MYERS)
  Excedrin P.M. Tablets (BRISTOL-MYERS)
  Fiorpap Tablets (GENEVA)
  Hycomine Compound Tablets (ENDO LABS)
  Hydrocet Capsules (CARNRICK)
  Hydrocodone Bitartrate and APAP Tablets,
    USP CIII (WATSON)
  Hydrocodone Bitartrate and Acetaminophen
    Capsules (MALLINCKRODT)
  Hydrocodone Bitartrate and Acetaminophen
    Elixir (MALLINCKRODT)
  Hydrocodone Bitartrate and Acetaminophen
    Elixir (PHARMACEUTICAL ASSOCIATES)
  Hydrocodone Bitartrate and Acetaminophen
    Tablets, USP (MALLINCKRODT)
  Hydrocodone Bitartrate/Acetaminophen Tablets,
    USP CIII (ENDO GENERICS)

  Infants' Tylenol Cold Decongestant and Fever
    Reducer Concentrated Drops
    (MCNEIL CONSUMER)
  Infants' Tylenol Cold Decongestant and Fever
    Reducer Concentrated Drops Plus Cough
    (MCNEIL CONSUMER)
  Infants' Tylenol Concentrated Drops
    (MCNEIL CONSUMER)
  Junior Strength Tylenol Coated Caplets and
    Soft-Chew Chewable Tablets
    (MCNEIL CONSUMER)
  Lorcet 10/650 Tablets (FOREST)
  Lorcet Plus Tablets (FOREST)
  Lorcet-HD Capsules (FOREST)
  Lortab 10/500 Tablets (UCB)
  Lortab 2.5/500 Tablets (UCB)
  Lortab 5/500 Tablets (UCB)
  Lortab 7.5/500 Tablets (UCB)
  Lortab Elixir (UCB)
  Medigesic Capsules (U.S. PHARMACEUTICAL)
  Midrin Capsules (CARNRICK)
  Norco Tablets CIII (WATSON)
  Norel Plus Capsules (U.S. PHARMACEUTICAL)
  Oxycodone and Acetaminophen Capsules, USP
    (MALLINCKRODT)
  Oxycodone and Acetaminophen Capsules, USP
    CII (WATSON)
  Oxycodone and Acetaminophen Tablets, USP
    (MALLINCKRODT)
  Oxycodone and Acetaminophen Tablets, USP
    CII (WATSON)
  Pacaps Capsules (LUNSCO)
  Percocet Tablets (ENDO LABS)
  Phenaphen with Codeine Capsules (ROBINS)
  Phrenilin Forte Capsules (CARNRICK)
  Phrenilin Tablets (CARNRICK)
  Propoxyphene Hydrochloride and
    Acetaminophen Tablets (MYLAN)
  Propoxyphene Hydrochloride and
    Acetaminophen Tablets, USP CIV (WATSON)
  Propoxyphene Napsylate and Acetaminophen
    Tablets (MYLAN)
  Protid Tablets (LUNSCO)
  Roxilox Capsules (ROXANE)
  Sedapap Tablets 50 mg/650 mg (MERZ)
  Sinulin Tablets (CARNRICK)
  Sinutab Sinus Allergy MS Caplets and Tablets
    (WARNER-LAMBERT)
  Sinutab Sinus MS Without Drowsiness Caplets
    and Tablets (WARNER-LAMBERT)
  Sudafed Cold & Cough Liquid Caps
    (WARNER-LAMBERT)
  Sudafed Cold & Sinus Liquid Caps
    (WARNER-LAMBERT)
  Sudafed Severe Cold Formula MS Caplets and
    Tablets (WARNER-LAMBERT)
  Sudafed Sinus MS Caplets and Tablets
    (WARNER-LAMBERT)

UNDERLINE DENOTES GENERIC NAME

Talacen Caplets (SANOFI)

Tylenol Allergy Sinus NightTime, Maximum Strength Caplets (MCNEIL CONSUMER)

Tylenol Allergy Sinus, Maximum Strength Caplets, Gelcaps, and Geltabs (MCNEIL CONSUMER)

Tylenol Arthritis Extended Relief Caplets (MCNEIL CONSUMER)

Tylenol Cold Complete Formula, Multi-Symptom Tablets and Caplets (MCNEIL CONSUMER)

Tylenol Cold Non-Drowsy, Multi-Symptom Caplets and Gelcaps (MCNEIL CONSUMER)

Tylenol Cold Severe Congestion Non-Drowsy, Multi-Symptom Caplets (MCNEIL CONSUMER)

Tylenol Extra Strength Adult Liquid Pain Reliever (MCNEIL CONSUMER)

Tylenol Extra Strength Gelcaps, Geltabs, Caplets, and Tablets (MCNEIL CONSUMER)

Tylenol Flu NightTime, Maximum Strength Gelcaps (MCNEIL CONSUMER)

Tylenol Flu NightTime, Maximum Strength Liquid (MCNEIL CONSUMER)

Tylenol Flu NightTime, Maximum Strength Powder (MCNEIL CONSUMER)

Tylenol Flu Non-Drowsy, Maximum Strength Gelcaps (MCNEIL CONSUMER)

Tylenol PM Pain Reliever/Sleep Aid, Extra Strength Caplets, Geltabs, and Gelcaps (MCNEIL CONSUMER)

Tylenol Regular Strength Caplets and Tablets (MCNEIL CONSUMER)

Tylenol Severe Allergy Caplets (MCNEIL CONSUMER)

Tylenol Sinus NightTime, Maximum Strength Caplets (MCNEIL CONSUMER)

Tylenol Sinus Non-Drowsy, Maximum Strength Geltabs, Gelcaps, Caplets, and Tablets (MCNEIL CONSUMER)

Tylenol Sore Throat, Maximum Strength Adult Liquid (MCNEIL CONSUMER)

Tylenol with Codeine Elixir (ORTHO-MCNEIL)

Tylenol with Codeine Tablets (ORTHO-MCNEIL)

Tylox Capsules (ORTHO-MCNEIL)

ViTelle Lurline PMS Tablets (FIELDING)

Vicodin ES Tablets (KNOLL LABS)

Vicodin HP Tablets (KNOLL LABS)

Vicodin Tablets (KNOLL LABS)

VitaMinophen (MAYOR)

Vitamist Intra-Oral Spray Dietary Supplements (MAYOR)

Wygesic Tablets (WYETH-AYERST)

Zebutal Capsules (HORIZON)

Zydone Tablets (ENDO LABS)

ACETAMINOPHEN ORAL SOLUTION USP (PHARMACEUTICAL ASSOCIATES)

ACETAMINOPHEN ORAL SOLUTION (CHERRY) (ROXANE)

ACETAMINOPHEN TABLETS (ROXANE)

ACETAMINOPHEN AND CODEINE PHOSPHATE ORAL SOLUTION USP (PHARMACEUTICAL ASSOCIATES)

ACETAMINOPHEN AND CODEINE PHOSPHATE ORAL SOLUTION AND TABLETS (ROXANE)

ACETAMINOPHEN AND CODEINE PHOSPHATE TABLETS, USP CIII (WATSON)

ACETAMINOPHEN TABLETS 325 MG (PADDOCK)

ACETAZOLAMIDE SODIUM FOR INJECTION, USP (BEDFORD)

ACETIC ACID

Aci-Jel Therapeutic Vaginal Jelly (ORTHO-MCNEIL)

Otic Domeboro Solution (BAYER)

VoSoL HC Otic Solution (WALLACE)

0.25% ACETIC ACID IRRIGATION, USP (AQUALITE) (ABBOTT)

ACETOHYDROXAMIC ACID

Lithostat Tablets (MISSION)

ACETYLCYSTEINE

Acetylcysteine Solution (ROXANE)

Acetylcysteine Solution USP, Mucosil (DEY)

ACETYLCYSTEINE SOLUTION (ROXANE)

ACETYLCYSTEINE SOLUTION USP, MUCOSIL (DEY)

ACETYLCYSTEINE SOLUTION, USP (BEDFORD)

ACHROMYCIN V CAPSULES (LEDERLE LABS)

ACI-JEL THERAPEUTIC VAGINAL JELLY (ORTHO-MCNEIL)

ACITRETIN

Soriatane Capsules (ROCHE LABS)

ACLOVATE CREAM (GLAXO WELLCOME)

ACLOVATE OINTMENT (GLAXO WELLCOME)

ACNE MASK (NEUTROGENA)

ACRIVASTINE

Semprex-D Capsules (MEDEVA)

A.C.S. CLOSURE SYSTEM NEEDLES AND SUTURES (ALCON)

HP ACTHAR GEL (RHONE-POULENC RORER)

ACTHIB (PASTEUR MERIEUX CONNAUGHT)

ACTHREL FOR INJECTION (FERRING)

ACTICAL TABLETS (USANA)

ACTICIN CREAM (BERTEK)

ACTIDOSE WITH SORBITOL SUSPENSION (PADDOCK)

ACTIDOSE-AQUA SUSPENSION (PADDOCK)

ACTIFED COLD & ALLERGY TABLETS (WARNER-LAMBERT)

ACTIGALL CAPSULES (NOVARTIS)

ACTIMMUNE (INTERMUNE)

ACTIQ (ABBOTT)

ACTIS VENOUS FLOW CONTROLLER (VIVUS)

ACTIVASE I.V. (GENENTECH)

ACTONEL TABLETS (PROCTER & GAMBLE PHARMACEUTICALS)

ACTOS TABLETS (TAKEDA)

ACULAR OPHTHALMIC SOLUTION (ALLERGAN)

ACULAR PF OPHTHALMIC SOLUTION (ALLERGAN)

ACYCLOVIR

Acyclovir Capsules and Tablets (MYLAN)

Acyclovir Capsules and Tablets, Caps 200 mg, Tabs 400 mg, 800 mg (NOVOPHARM)

Zovirax Capsules (GLAXO WELLCOME)

Zovirax Ointment 5% (GLAXO WELLCOME)

Zovirax Suspension (GLAXO WELLCOME)

Zovirax Tablets (GLAXO WELLCOME)

ACYCLOVIR CAPSULES (ESI LEDERLE)

ACYCLOVIR CAPSULES & TABLETS (APOTHECON)

ACYCLOVIR CAPSULES AND TABLETS (MYLAN)

ACYCLOVIR CAPSULES AND TABLETS, CAPS 200 MG, TABS 400 MG, 800 MG (NOVOPHARM)

ACYCLOVIR INJECTION (ESI LEDERLE)

ACYCLOVIR SODIUM

Zovirax for Injection (GLAXO WELLCOME)

ACYCLOVIR SODIUM FOR INJECTION (BEDFORD)

ACYCLOVIR SODIUM FOR INJECTION (APOTHECON)

ACYCLOVIR TABLETS (ESI LEDERLE)

ACYCLOVIR TABLETS AND CAPSULES (SCHEIN)

ADAGEN INJECTION (ENZON)

ADALAT CAPSULES (BAYER)

ADALAT CC TABLETS (BAYER)

ADAPALENE

Differin Gel (GALDERMA)

Differin Solution (GALDERMA)

ADDERALL TABLETS (SHIRE RICHWOOD)

ADEKS MULTIVITAMIN SUPPLEMENT (SCANDIPHARM)

ADEKS PEDIATRIC DROPS (SCANDIPHARM)

ADENOCARD INJECTION (FUJISAWA)

ADENOSCAN (FUJISAWA)

ADENOSINE

Adenocard Injection (FUJISAWA)

Adenoscan (FUJISAWA)

ADIPEX-P CAPSULES (GATE)

ADIPEX-P TABLETS (GATE)

ADRENALIN CHLORIDE SOLUTION (MONARCH)

ADRENOCORTICOTROPIC HORMONE

HP Acthar Gel (RHONE-POULENC RORER)

ADRIAMYCIN PFS/RDF INJECTION (PHARMACIA & UPJOHN)

ADRUCIL INJECTION (PHARMACIA & UPJOHN)

ADSORBONAC (ALCON P.R.)

ADVANCE, EXTEND, RENEW (MAYOR)

AEROBID INHALER SYSTEM (FOREST)

AEROBID-M INHALER SYSTEM (FOREST)

AEROCHAMBER AND AEROCHAMBER WITH MASK (FOREST)

AEROLATE LIQUID (FLEMING)

AEROLATE JR. T.D. CAPSULES (FLEMING)

AEROLATE SR. T.D. CAPSULES (FLEMING)

AEROLATE III T.D. CAPSULES (FLEMING)

AGENERASE CAPSULES (GLAXO WELLCOME)

AGENERASE ORAL SOLUTION (GLAXO WELLCOME)

AGGRASTAT INJECTION (MERCK)

AGGRASTAT INJECTION PREMIXED (MERCK)

AGRYLIN CAPSULES (ROBERTS)

AH-CHEW CHEWABLE TABLETS (WE)

AH-CHEW D CHEWABLE TABLETS (WE)

AIRET INHALATION SOLUTION (MEDEVA)

AKINETON INJECTION (KNOLL LABS)

AKINETON TABLETS (KNOLL LABS)

AKNE-MYCIN OINTMENT (HEALTHPOINT)

ALATROFLOXACIN MESYLATE

Trovan I.V. (PFIZER)

ALBALON OPHTHALMIC SOLUTION (ALLERGAN)

ALBAMYCIN CAPSULES (PHARMACIA & UPJOHN)

ALBENDAZOLE

Albenza Tablets (SMITHKLINE BEECHAM)

ALBENZA TABLETS (SMITHKLINE BEECHAM)

ALBUMARC 5% SOLUTION (AMERICAN RED CROSS)

ALBUMARC 25% SOLUTION (AMERICAN RED CROSS)

ALBUMIN (HUMAN)

Albumarc 25% Solution (AMERICAN RED CROSS)

Albumarc 5% Solution (AMERICAN RED CROSS)

Albumin (Human) 25% (IMMUNO)

Albumin (Human) 5% (IMMUNO)

Albuminar-25, U.S.P. (CENTEON)

Albuminar-5, U.S.P. (CENTEON)

Albutein 25% Solution (ALPHA)

Albutein 5% Solution (ALPHA)

Buminate 25% Solution, USP (BAXTER HEALTHCARE)

UNDERLINE DENOTES GENERIC NAME

Buminate 5% Solution, USP
  (BAXTER HEALTHCARE)
Human Albumin Grifols 20% Solution
  (GRIFOLS)
Plasbumin-20 (BAYER BIOLOGICAL)
Plasbumin-25 (BAYER BIOLOGICAL)
Plasbumin-5 (BAYER BIOLOGICAL)
ALBUMIN (HUMAN) 5% (IMMUNO)
ALBUMIN (HUMAN) 25% (IMMUNO)
ALBUMINAR-5, U.S.P. (CENTEON)
ALBUMINAR-25, U.S.P. (CENTEON)
ALBUTEIN 5% SOLUTION (ALPHA)
ALBUTEIN 25% SOLUTION (ALPHA)

ALBUTEROL

Albuterol Inhalation Aerosol (DEY)
Albuterol Tablets (MYLAN)
Proventil Inhalation Aerosol (SCHERING)
Ventolin Inhalation Aerosol and Refill
  (GLAXO WELLCOME)
ALBUTEROL INHALATION AEROSOL (DEY)
ALBUTEROL INHALATION AEROSOL
  (APOTHECON)

ALBUTEROL SULFATE

Airet Inhalation Solution (MEDEVA)
Albuterol Sulfate Inhalation Solutions (DEY)
Albuterol Sulfate Tablets (LEDERLE STANDARD)
Albuterol Tablets (GENEVA)
Albuterol Tablets, 2mg, 4mg (NOVOPHARM)
Combivent Inhalation Aerosol
  (BOEHRINGER INGELHEIM)
Proventil HFA Inhalation Aerosol (SCHERING)
Proventil Inhalation Solution 0.083%
  (SCHERING)
Proventil Repetabs Tablets (SCHERING)
Proventil Solution for Inhalation 0.5%
  (SCHERING)
Proventil Syrup (SCHERING)
Proventil Tablets (SCHERING)
Ventolin Inhalation Solution
  (GLAXO WELLCOME)
Ventolin Nebules Inhalation Solution
  (GLAXO WELLCOME)
Ventolin Rotacaps for Inhalation
  (GLAXO WELLCOME)
Ventolin Syrup (GLAXO WELLCOME)
Volmax Extended-Release Tablets (MURO)
ALBUTEROL SULFATE INHALATION
  SOLUTIONS (DEY)
ALBUTEROL SULFATE TABLETS
  (LEDERLE STANDARD)
ALBUTEROL TABLETS (MYLAN)
ALBUTEROL TABLETS (GENEVA)
ALBUTEROL TABLETS, 2MG, 4MG
  (NOVOPHARM)
ALCAINE (ALCON P.R.)

ALCLOMETASONE DIPROPIONATE

Aclovate Cream (GLAXO WELLCOME)
Aclovate Ointment (GLAXO WELLCOME)
5% ALCOHOL & 5% DEXTROSE
  INJECTION (ABBOTT)
ALCON SURGICAL SYSTEM
  (IRRIGATION/ASPIRATION KITS;
  PHACOEMULSIFICATION KITS) (ALCON)
ALDACTAZIDE TABLETS (SEARLE)
ALDACTONE TABLETS (SEARLE)
ALDARA CREAM, 5% (3M)

ALDESLEUKIN

Proleukin for Injection (CHIRON)
ALDOCLOR TABLETS (MERCK)
ALDOMET TABLETS (MERCK)
ALDOMET ESTER HCL INJECTION
  (MERCK)
ALDORIL TABLETS (MERCK)

ALENDRONATE SODIUM

Fosamax Tablets (MERCK)
ALESSE-21 TABLETS (WYETH-AYERST)
ALESSE-28 TABLETS (WYETH-AYERST)
ALFENTA INJECTION (TAYLOR)
ALFENTANIL HCL INJECTION (BAXTER)

ALFENTANIL HYDROCHLORIDE

Alfenta Injection (TAYLOR)
Alfentanil HCl Injection (BAXTER)
ALFERON N INJECTION (INTERFERON)
ALGINATE STYPTIC GAUZE (PEDINOL)

ALITRETINOIN

Panretin Gel (LIGAND)
ALKA-AID (ANTACID) (VITALINE)
ALKERAN FOR INJECTION
  (GLAXO WELLCOME)
ALKERAN TABLETS (GLAXO WELLCOME)
ALLEGRA CAPSULES
  (HOECHST MARION ROUSSEL)
ALLEGRA-D EXTENDED-RELEASE
  TABLETS (HOECHST MARION ROUSSEL)
ALL-FLEX ARCING SPRING DIAPHRAGM
  (SEE ORTHO DIAPHRAGM KITS)
  (ORTHO-MCNEIL)

ALLOPURINOL

Allopurinol Tablets (PAR)
Allopurinol Tablets (MYLAN)
Zyloprim Tablets (FARO)

ALLOPURINOL SODIUM

Aloprim for Injection (NABI)
ALLOPURINOL TABLETS (PAR)
ALLOPURINOL TABLETS (MYLAN)
ALMORA TABLETS (FOREST)
ALOE GRANDE CREME & LOTION
  (GORDON)
ALOMIDE OPHTHALMIC SOLUTION
  (ALCON)
ALOPRIM FOR INJECTION (NABI)
ALORA TRANSDERMAL SYSTEM
  (PROCTER & GAMBLE PHARMACEUTICALS)
ALPHA KERI MOISTURE RICH
  CLEANSING BAR (BRISTOL-MYERS)
ALPHA KERI MOISTURE RICH SHOWER
  AND BATH OIL (BRISTOL-MYERS)

ALPHA1-PROTEINASE INHIBITOR (HUMAN)

Prolastin (BAYER BIOLOGICAL)
ALPHAGAN OPHTHALMIC SOLUTION
  (ALLERGAN)
ALPHANATE SOLVENT
  DETERGENT/HEAT TREATED (ALPHA)
ALPHANINE SD SOLVENT DETERGENT
  TREATED/VIRUS FILTERED (ALPHA)

ALPRAZOLAM

Alprazolam Tablets (PAR)
Alprazolam Tablets (MYLAN)
Alprazolam Tablets (GENEVA)
Alprazolam Tablets (LEDERLE STANDARD)
Alprazolam Tablets, USP CIV (WATSON)
Xanax Tablets (PHARMACIA & UPJOHN)
ALPRAZOLAM TABLETS (PAR)
ALPRAZOLAM TABLETS (MYLAN)
ALPRAZOLAM TABLETS (GENEVA)
ALPRAZOLAM TABLETS
  (LEDERLE STANDARD)
ALPRAZOLAM TABLETS, USP CIV
  (WATSON)

ALPROSTADIL

Caverject Sterile Powder
  (PHARMACIA & UPJOHN)
Edex for Injection (SCHWARZ)
MUSE Urethral Suppository (VIVUS)
Prostin VR Pediatric Sterile Solution
  (PHARMACIA & UPJOHN)

ALPROSTADIL INJECTION, USP (BEDFORD)
ALTACE CAPSULES (MONARCH)

ALTEPLASE, RECOMBINANT

Activase I.V. (GENENTECH)
ALTERRA (ST. JOHN'S WORT)
  (UPSHER-SMITH)

ALTRETAMINE

Hexalen Capsules (U.S. BIOSCIENCE)
ALU-CAP CAPSULES (3M)
ALUMADRINE TABLETS (FLEMING)

ALUMINUM ACETATE

Otic Domeboro Solution (BAYER)

ALUMINUM CHLORIDE

Drysol Solution (PERSON & COVEY)
Xerac AC Solution (PERSON & COVEY)

ALUMINUM HYDROXIDE

Alu-Cap Capsules (3M)
Alu-Tab Tablets (3M)
Aluminum Hydroxide Gel Concentrate
  (PHARMACEUTICAL ASSOCIATES)
Aluminum Hydroxide Gel USP
  (PHARMACEUTICAL ASSOCIATES)
Amphojel Suspension (WYETH-AYERST)
Amphojel Tablets (WYETH-AYERST)
Fast-Acting Mylanta Liquid Antacid
  (J&J – MERCK)
Maalox Magnesia and Alumina Oral
  Suspension (NOVARTIS CONSUMER)
Maximum Strength Fast-Acting Mylanta Liquid
  (J&J – MERCK)
Maximum Strength Maalox Antacid/Anti-Gas
  Liquid (NOVARTIS CONSUMER)
ALUMINUM HYDROXIDE GEL USP
  (PHARMACEUTICAL ASSOCIATES)
ALUMINUM HYDROXIDE GEL
  CONCENTRATE
  (PHARMACEUTICAL ASSOCIATES)
ALUMINUM PASTE (PADDOCK)
ALUPENT INHALATION AEROSOL
  (BOEHRINGER INGELHEIM)
ALUPENT INHALATION SOLUTION
  (BOEHRINGER INGELHEIM)
ALUPENT SYRUP (BOEHRINGER INGELHEIM)
ALUPENT TABLETS (BOEHRINGER INGELHEIM)
ALU-TAB TABLETS (3M)

AMANTADINE HYDROCHLORIDE

Amantadine Hydrochloride Syrup USP
  (PHARMACEUTICAL ASSOCIATES)
Amantadine Hydrochloride Syrup, USP
  (ENDO GENERICS)
Symmetrel Syrup (ENDO LABS)
Symmetrel Tablets (ENDO LABS)
AMANTADINE HYDROCHLORIDE SYRUP
  USP (PHARMACEUTICAL ASSOCIATES)
AMANTADINE HYDROCHLORIDE SYRUP,
  USP (ENDO GENERICS)
AMARYL TABLETS
  (HOECHST MARION ROUSSEL)
AMBENYL COUGH SYRUP (FOREST)
AMBENYL D SYRUP (FOREST)
AMBIEN TABLETS (SEARLE)
AMBISOME FOR INJECTION (FUJISAWA)

AMCINONIDE

Cyclocort Topical Cream 0.1% (FUJISAWA)
Cyclocort Topical Lotion 0.1% (FUJISAWA)
Cyclocort Topical Ointment 0.1% (FUJISAWA)
AMEN TABLETS (CARNRICK)
AMERGE TABLETS (GLAXO WELLCOME)
AMERICAINE ANESTHETIC LUBRICANT
  (MEDEVA)
AMERICAINE OTIC TOPICAL
  ANESTHETIC EAR DROPS (MEDEVA)

UNDERLINE DENOTES GENERIC NAME

AMICAR SYRUP, TABLETS, AND INJECTION (IMMUNEX)
AMIDATE (ETOMIDATE INJECTION) AMPUL, ABBOJECT (ABBOTT)

AMIFOSTINE

Ethyol for Injection (ALZA)

AMIKACIN SULFATE

Amikacin Sulfate Injection, USP (ELKINS-SINN)
AMIKACIN SULFATE INJECTION, USP (BEDFORD)
AMIKACIN SULFATE INJECTION, USP (ELKINS-SINN)
AMIKIN INJECTION (APOTHECON)
AMILORIDE HCL AND HCTZ TABLETS, USP (WATSON)
AMILORIDE HCL TABLETS (PAR)

AMILORIDE HYDROCHLORIDE

Amiloride HCl Tablets (PAR)
Amiloride HCl and HCTZ Tablets, USP (WATSON)
Amiloride Hydrochloride and Hydrochlorothiazide Tablets (MYLAN)
Amiloride Hydrochloride and Hydrochlorothiazide Tablets, USP (ENDO GENERICS)
Midamor Tablets (MERCK)
Moduretic Tablets (MERCK)
AMILORIDE HYDROCHLORIDE AND HYDROCHLOROTHIAZIDE TABLETS (MYLAN)
AMILORIDE HYDROCHLORIDE AND HYDROCHLOROTHIAZIDE TABLETS, USP (ENDO GENERICS)

AMINO ACID PREPARATIONS

C + Zinc (MAYOR)
CardioCare (MAYOR)
GinkgoMist (MAYOR)
HeartBar (COOKE)
L-Carnitine USP 500mg Chewable Wafers, 250mg Tablets, 500mg Caplets, and 500mg Capsules (VITALINE)
Marlyn Formula 50 Capsules (MARLYN)
NephrAmine Injection (R&D)
Revitalizer (MAYOR)
Vitamist Intra-Oral Spray Dietary Supplements (MAYOR)

AMINOBENZOATE POTASSIUM

Potaba Capsules (GLENWOOD)
Potaba Powder (GLENWOOD)
Potaba Tablets (GLENWOOD)

AMINOCAPROIC ACID

Amicar Syrup, Tablets, and Injection (IMMUNEX)
Aminocaproic Acid Injection (ELKINS-SINN)
AMINOCAPROIC ACID INJECTION (ELKINS-SINN)
AMINO-CERV CREME (MILEX)

AMINOHIPPURATE SODIUM

Aminohippurate Sodium 'PAH' Injection (MERCK)
AMINOHIPPURATE SODIUM 'PAH' INJECTION (MERCK)

AMINOPHYLLINE

Aminophylline Oral Solution (ROXANE)
AMINOPHYLLINE 250 MG, 10 ML, AMPUL & VIAL (ABBOTT)
AMINOPHYLLINE 500 MG, 20 ML, AMPUL & VIAL (ABBOTT)
AMINOPHYLLINE ORAL SOLUTION (ROXANE)

AMINOSALICYLIC ACID

Paser Granules (JACOBUS)

AMINOSYN 3.5% M (ABBOTT)
AMINOSYN 5% (ABBOTT)
AMINOSYN 7% (ABBOTT)
AMINOSYN 7% TPN KIT (ABBOTT)
AMINOSYN 7% WITH ELECTROLYTES (ABBOTT)
AMINOSYN 7% WITH ELECTROLYTES TPN KIT (ABBOTT)
AMINOSYN 8.5% (ABBOTT)
AMINOSYN 8.5% TPN KIT (ABBOTT)
AMINOSYN 8.5% WITH ELECTROLYTES (ABBOTT)
AMINOSYN 10% (ABBOTT)
AMINOSYN 10% TPN KIT (ABBOTT)
AMINOSYN-HBC 7% (ABBOTT)
AMINOSYN II 7% (ABBOTT)
AMINOSYN II 8.5% (ABBOTT)
AMINOSYN II 10% (ABBOTT)
AMINOSYN II IN DEXTROSE, NUTRIMIX DUAL CHAMBER (ABBOTT)
AMINOSYN-PF 7% AND 10% (ABBOTT)
AMINOSYN WITH DEXTROSE, NUTRIMIX DUAL CHAMBER (ABBOTT)
AMIODARONE HCL TABLETS (PAR)

AMIODARONE HYDROCHLORIDE

Amiodarone HCl Tablets (PAR)
Amiodarone Tablets, 200 mg (NOVOPHARM)
Cordarone Intravenous (WYETH-AYERST)
Cordarone Tablets (WYETH-AYERST)
Pacerone Tablets (UPSHER-SMITH)
AMIODARONE TABLETS, 200 MG (NOVOPHARM)
AMITRIPTYLINE HCL TABLETS (GENEVA)

AMITRIPTYLINE HYDROCHLORIDE

Amitriptyline HCl Tablets (GENEVA)
Amitriptyline Hydrochloride Tablets (MYLAN)
Chlordiazepoxide and Amitriptyline Hydrochloride Tablets (MYLAN)
Elavil Injection (ASTRAZENECA)
Elavil Tablets (ASTRAZENECA)
Etrafon 2-10 Tablets (2-10) (SCHERING)
Etrafon Tablets (2-25) (SCHERING)
Etrafon-Forte Tablets (4-25) (SCHERING)
Limbitrol DS Tablets (ICN)
Limbitrol Tablets (ICN)
Perphenazine and Amitriptyline Hydrochloride Tablets (MYLAN)
Perphenazine/Amitriptyline HCl Tablets (GENEVA)
Perphenazine/Amitriptyline Hydrochloride Tablets, USP (WATSON)
Triavil Tablets (LOTUS)
AMITRIPTYLINE HYDROCHLORIDE TABLETS (MYLAN)

AMLEXANOX

Aphthasol Oral Paste (BLOCK)

AMLODIPINE BESYLATE

Lotrel Capsules (NOVARTIS)
Norvasc Tablets (PFIZER)
AMMONIUM CHLORIDE (ABBOTT)

AMMONIUM LACTATE

Lac-Hydrin 12% Cream (WESTWOOD-SQUIBB)
Lac-Hydrin 12% Lotion (WESTWOOD-SQUIBB)

AMOXAPINE

Amoxapine Tablets (GENEVA)
Amoxapine Tablets, USP (WATSON)
AMOXAPINE TABLETS (GENEVA)
AMOXAPINE TABLETS, USP (WATSON)

AMOXICILLIN

Amoxicillin Capsules (PAR)
Amoxicillin Oral Suspension (PAR)
PREVPAC (TAP)
AMOXICILLIN CAPSULES (PAR)

AMOXICILLIN CAPSULES AND ORAL SUSPENSION (SEE TRIMOX) (APOTHECON)
AMOXICILLIN CAPSULES USP AND ORAL SUSPENSION, CAPS 250 MG, 500 MG, O.S. 125 MG/5 ML, 250 MG/5 ML (NOVOPHARM)
AMOXICILLIN ORAL SUSPENSION (PAR)
AMOXICILLIN TABLETS (CHEWABLE), 125 MG, 250 MG (NOVOPHARM)
AMOXICILLIN TABLETS, USP (CHEWABLE) (APOTHECON)

AMOXICILLIN TRIHYDRATE

Amoxicillin Capsules USP and Oral Suspension, Caps 250 mg, 500 mg, O.S. 125 mg/5 mL, 250 mg/5 mL (NOVOPHARM)
Amoxicillin Tablets (Chewable), 125 mg, 250 mg (NOVOPHARM)
Amoxil Capsules, Tablets and Chewable Tablets (SMITHKLINE BEECHAM)
Amoxil Pediatric Drops, Powder for Oral Suspension (SMITHKLINE BEECHAM)
Augmentin Powder for Oral Suspension and Chewable Tablets (SMITHKLINE BEECHAM)
Augmentin Tablets (SMITHKLINE BEECHAM)
AMOXIL CAPSULES, TABLETS AND CHEWABLE TABLETS (SMITHKLINE BEECHAM)
AMOXIL PEDIATRIC DROPS, POWDER FOR ORAL SUSPENSION (SMITHKLINE BEECHAM)

AMPHETAMINE ASPARTATE

Adderall Tablets (SHIRE RICHWOOD)

AMPHETAMINE SULFATE

Adderall Tablets (SHIRE RICHWOOD)
AMPHOCIN INJECTION (PHARMACIA & UPJOHN)
AMPHOJEL SUSPENSION (WYETH-AYERST)
AMPHOJEL TABLETS (WYETH-AYERST)

AMPHOTERICIN B

Abelcet Injection (LIPOSOME)
AmBisome for Injection (FUJISAWA)

AMPICILLIN

Ampicillin Capsules (PAR)
Ampicillin Oral Suspension (PAR)
AMPICILLIN CAPSULES (PAR)
AMPICILLIN CAPSULES AND ORAL SUSPENSION (SEE PRINCIPEN) (APOTHECON)
AMPICILLIN FOR INJECTION USP AND IN ADD-VANTAGE VIALS (APOTHECON)
AMPICILLIN ORAL SUSPENSION (PAR)

AMPICILLIN SODIUM

Unasyn for Injection (PFIZER)

AMPRENAVIR

Agenerase Capsules (GLAXO WELLCOME)
Agenerase Oral Solution (GLAXO WELLCOME)

AMYLASE

Arco-Lase Plus Tablets (ARCO)
Arco-Lase Tablets (ARCO)
Donnazyme Tablets (ROBINS)
Ku-Zyme Capsules (SCHWARZ)
Ku-Zyme HP Capsules (SCHWARZ)
Kutrase Capsules (SCHWARZ)
AMYTAL SODIUM VIALS (LILLY)
ANABAR CAPLETS (LUNSCO)
ANADROL-50 TABLETS (UNIMED)
ANAFRANIL CAPSULES (NOVARTIS)

ANAGRELIDE HYDROCHLORIDE

Agrylin Capsules (ROBERTS)
ANA-KIT ANAPHYLAXIS EMERGENCY TREATMENT KIT (BAYER ALLERGY)
ANALPRAM HC LOTION 2.5% (FERNDALE)

UNDERLINE DENOTES GENERIC NAME

ANALPRAM-HC RECTAL CREAM 1% AND 2.5% (FERNDALE)
ANAMINE SYRUP (MERZ)
ANAMINE T. D. CAPSULES (MERZ)
ANAPLEX DM COUGH SYRUP (ECR)
ANAPLEX HD COUGH SYRUP (ECR)
ANAPROX TABLETS (ROCHE LABS)
ANAPROX DS TABLETS (ROCHE LABS)

ANASTROZOLE
Arimidex Tablets (ASTRAZENECA)
ANATUSS DM SYRUP (MERZ)
ANATUSS LA TABLETS (MERZ)
ANATUSS SYRUP (MERZ)
ANATUSS TABLETS (MERZ)
ANCEF FOR INJECTION (SMITHKLINE BEECHAM)
ANCOBON CAPSULES (ICN)
ANDRODERM TRANSDERMAL SYSTEM CIII (WATSON)
ANDROID CAPSULES, 10 MG (ICN)
ANECTINE INJECTION (GLAXO WELLCOME)
ANESTACON JELLY (POLYMEDICA)

ANISTREPLASE
Eminase (ROBERTS)
ANOLOR 300 CAPSULES (BLANSETT)
ANSAID TABLETS (PHARMACIA & UPJOHN)
ANTABUSE TABLETS (WYETH-AYERST)
ANTHRA-DERM OINTMENT 1%, 1/2%, 1/4%, 1/10% (DERMIK)

ANTHRALIN
Dritho-Scalp 0.25%, 0.5% Cream (DERMIK)
Drithocreme 0.1%, 0.25%, 0.5%, 1.0% (HP) Cream (DERMIK)
Micanol 1% Cream (BIOGLAN)

ANTI-THYMOCYTE GLOBULIN
Thymoglobulin for Injection (SANGSTAT)
ANTICOAGULANT CITRATE PHOSPHATE DEXTROSE SOLUTION, USP (ABBOTT)

ANTIHEMOPHILIC FACTOR (HUMAN)
Alphanate Solvent Detergent/Heat Treated (ALPHA)
Hemofil M (BAXTER HEALTHCARE)
Humate-P Concentrate (CENTEON)
Koate-DVI (BAYER BIOLOGICAL)
Koate-HP (BAYER BIOLOGICAL)
Monarc-M (AMERICAN RED CROSS)
Monoclate-P Concentrate (CENTEON)

ANTIHEMOPHILIC FACTOR (PORCINE)
Hyate:C (SPEYWOOD)

ANTIHEMOPHILIC FACTOR (RECOMBINANT)
BeneFix for Injection (GENETICS)
Helixate Concentrate (CENTEON)
Kogenate (BAYER BIOLOGICAL)
NovoSeven (NOVO NORDISK)
Recombinate (BAXTER HEALTHCARE)

ANTI-INHIBITOR COAGULANT COMPLEX
Autoplex T (NABI)
Feiba VH Immuno (IMMUNO)
ANTILIRIUM INJECTABLE (FOREST)
ANTI-OXIDANT (MAYOR)
ANTIOXIDANT FORMULA (ADVANCED) (VITALINE)

ANTIPYRINE
Auralgan Otic Solution (WYETH-AYERST)
Tympagesic Ear Drops (SAVAGE)

ANTITHROMBIN III
Thrombate III (BAYER BIOLOGICAL)
ANTIVENIN (BLACK WIDOW SPIDER ANTIVENIN) (MERCK)

ANTIVENIN (MICRURUS FULVIUS) (WYETH-AYERST)

ANTIVENIN (MICRURUS FULVIUS)
Antivenin (Micrurus fulvius) (WYETH-AYERST)
ANTIVERT, ANTIVERT/25, & ANTIVERT/50 TABLETS (PFIZER)
ANTURANE CAPSULES (NOVARTIS)
ANTURANE TABLETS (NOVARTIS)
ANUSOL HC-1 OINTMENT (WARNER-LAMBERT)
ANUSOL HEMORRHOIDAL OINTMENT (WARNER-LAMBERT)
ANUSOL HEMORRHOIDAL SUPPOSITORIES (WARNER-LAMBERT)
ANUSOL-HC CREAM 2.5% (MONARCH)
ANUSOL-HC SUPPOSITORIES (MONARCH)
ANZEMET INJECTION (HOECHST MARION ROUSSEL)
ANZEMET TABLETS (HOECHST MARION ROUSSEL)
A-OK OPHTHALMIC KNIVES (ALCON)
APAP & CODEINE TABLETS, #2, #3 AND #4 (DURAMED)
APHRODYNE CAPLETS (STAR)
APHTHASOL ORAL PASTE (BLOCK)
A.P.L. (WYETH-AYERST)
APLIGRAF (NOVARTIS)
APLISOL INJECTION (PARKEDALE)
APRESAZIDE CAPSULES (NOVARTIS)
APRESOLINE HYDROCHLORIDE TABLETS (NOVARTIS)

APROTININ
Trasylol Injection (BAYER)
AQUABASE (PADDOCK)
AQUAMEPHYTON INJECTION (MERCK)
AQUANIL LOTION (PERSON & COVEY)
AQUANIL HC LOTION (PERSON & COVEY)
AQUAPHOR GAUZE (BEIERSDORF)
AQUAPHOR HEALING OINTMENT (BEIERSDORF)
AQUAPHOR ORIGINAL OINTMENT (BEIERSDORF)
AQUASOL A PARENTERAL (ASTRAZENECA LP)
AQUASOL E (ASTRAZENECA LP)
AQUATENSEN TABLETS (WALLACE)
ARALEN HYDROCHLORIDE INJECTION (SANOFI)
ARALEN TABLETS (SANOFI)
ARAMINE INJECTION (MERCK)
ARAVA TABLETS (HOECHST MARION ROUSSEL)
ARCO-CEE TABLETS (ARCO)
ARCO-LASE TABLETS (ARCO)
ARCO-LASE PLUS TABLETS (ARCO)
ARCORET TABLETS (ARCO)
ARCORET W/IRON TABLETS (ARCO)
ARCOTINIC LIQUID (ARCO)
ARCOTINIC TABLETS (ARCO)

ARDEPARIN SODIUM
Normiflo Injection (WYETH-AYERST)
Normiflo Injection in Tubex (WYETH-AYERST)
ARDUAN FOR INJECTION (ORGANON)
AREDIA FOR INJECTION (NOVARTIS)
ARICEPT TABLETS (EISAI)
ARICEPT TABLETS (PFIZER)
ARIMIDEX TABLETS (ASTRAZENECA)
ARISTOCORT A 0.025% CREAM (FUJISAWA)
ARISTOCORT A 0.1% CREAM (FUJISAWA)
ARISTOCORT A 0.5% CREAM (FUJISAWA)
ARISTOCORT A 0.1% OINTMENT (FUJISAWA)
ARISTOCORT SUSPENSION (FORTE PARENTERAL) (FUJISAWA)
ARISTOCORT SUSPENSION (INTRALESIONAL) (FUJISAWA)

ARISTOSPAN SUSPENSION (INTRA-ARTICULAR) (FUJISAWA)
ARISTOSPAN SUSPENSION (INTRALESIONAL) (FUJISAWA)
ARMOUR THYROID TABLETS (FOREST)
AROMATIC CASCARA FLUIDEXTRACT (ROXANE)
AROMATIC CASCARA FLUIDEXTRACT USP (PHARMACEUTICAL ASSOCIATES)
ARTANE ELIXIR (LEDERLE LABS)
ARTANE TABLETS (LEDERLE LABS)
ARTHRIFLEX (MAYOR)
ARTHROPAN LIQUID (PURDUE FREDERICK)
ARTHROTEC TABLETS (SEARLE)
ASACOL DELAYED-RELEASE TABLETS (PROCTER & GAMBLE PHARMACEUTICALS)
ARTHRITIS PAIN ASCRIPTIN (NOVARTIS CONSUMER)
ENTERIC ASCRIPTIN (NOVARTIS CONSUMER)
MAXIMUM STRENGTH ASCRIPTIN (NOVARTIS CONSUMER)
REGULAR STRENGTH ASCRIPTIN (NOVARTIS CONSUMER)

ASPARAGINASE
Elspar for Injection (MERCK)

ASPIRIN
Butalbital, Aspirin, Caffeine, and Codeine Phosphate Capsules, USP (ENDO GENERICS)
Butalbital, Aspirin, Caffeine, and Codeine Phosphate Capsules, USP CIII (WATSON)
Carisoprodol and Aspirin Tablets (PAR)
Darvon Compound-65 Pulvules (LILLY)
Easprin Tablets (LOTUS)
Ecotrin Enteric Coated Aspirin Low, Regular and Maximum Strength Tablets (SMITHKLINE BEECHAM CONSUMER)
Endodan Tablets, USP CII (ENDO GENERICS)
Equagesic Tablets (WYETH-AYERST)
Excedrin Extra-Strength Caplets (BRISTOL-MYERS)
Excedrin Extra-Strength Geltabs (BRISTOL-MYERS)
Excedrin Extra-Strength Tablets (BRISTOL-MYERS)
Excedrin Migraine Caplets (BRISTOL-MYERS)
Excedrin Migraine Tablets (BRISTOL-MYERS)
Fiortal Capsules (GENEVA)
Fiortal w/Codeine Capsules (GENEVA)
Halfprin Tablets (KRAMER)
Methocarbamol and Aspirin Tablets (PAR)
Norgesic Forte Tablets (3M)
Norgesic Tablets (3M)
Orphenadrine Citrate, Aspirin and Caffeine Tablets (MYLAN)
Orphengesic Forte Tablets (PAR)
Orphengesic Tablets (PAR)
Oxycodone and Aspirin Tablets, USP CII (WATSON)
Percodan Tablets (ENDO LABS)
Percodan-Demi Tablets (ENDO LABS)
Propoxyphene Hydrochloride, Aspirin and Caffeine Capsules (MYLAN)
Robaxisal Tablets (ROBINS)
Roxiprin Tablets (ROXANE)
Soma Compound Tablets (WALLACE)
Soma Compound w/Codeine Tablets (WALLACE)
Synalgos-DC Capsules (WYETH-AYERST)
Talwin Compound Caplets (SANOFI)
ASPIRIN SUPPOSITORIES 300 MG, 600 MG (PADDOCK)
ASPIRIN TABLETS, ENTERIC-COATED 325 MG (PADDOCK)
ASTELIN NASAL SPRAY (WALLACE)

UNDERLINE DENOTES GENERIC NAME

ASTRAMORPH/PF INJECTION, USP (PRESERVATIVE-FREE) (ASTRAZENECA LP)
ATACAND TABLETS (ASTRAZENECA LP)
ATAMET TABLETS (ATHENA)
ATAPRYL TABLETS (ATHENA)
ATARAX TABLETS & SYRUP (PFIZER)

ATENOLOL

Atenolol Tablets (MYLAN)
Atenolol Tablets (GENEVA)
Atenolol Tablets (LEDERLE STANDARD)
Atenolol Tablets, 50 mg, 100 mg (NOVOPHARM)
Atenolol and Chlorthalidone Tablets (MYLAN)
Tenoretic Tablets (ASTRAZENECA)
Tenormin Tablets and I.V. Injection (ASTRAZENECA)

ATENOLOL AND /ATENOLOL WITH CHLORTHALIDONE TABLETS (SCHEIN)
ATENOLOL AND CHLOROTHALIDONE TABLETS (APOTHECON)
ATENOLOL TABLETS (MYLAN)
ATENOLOL TABLETS (GENEVA)
ATENOLOL TABLETS (LEDERLE STANDARD)
ATENOLOL AND CHLORTHALIDONE TABLETS (MYLAN)
ATENOLOL TABLETS, 50 MG, 100 MG (NOVOPHARM)
ATGAM STERILE SOLUTION (PHARMACIA & UPJOHN)
ATIVAN INJECTION (BAXTER)
ATIVAN INJECTION (WYETH-AYERST)
ATIVAN TABLETS (WYETH-AYERST)
ATIVAN IN TUBEX (WYETH-AYERST)

ATORVASTATIN CALCIUM

Lipitor Tablets (PFIZER)
Lipitor Tablets (PARKE-DAVIS)

ATOVAQUONE

Mepron Suspension (GLAXO WELLCOME)

ATRACURIUM BESYLATE

Atracurium Besylate Injection (BAXTER)
Tracrium Injection (GLAXO WELLCOME)

ATRACURIUM BESYLATE INJECTION (BAXTER)
ATRACURIUM BESYLATE INJECTION (BEDFORD)
ATRACURIUM BESYLATE INJECTION (ESI LEDERLE)
ATROHIST PEDIATRIC CAPSULES (MEDEVA)
ATROHIST PEDIATRIC SUSPENSION DYE-FREE (MEDEVA)
ATROHIST PLUS TABLETS (MEDEVA)
ATROMID-S CAPSULES (WYETH-AYERST)
ATROPINE 0.05 MG/ML, 5 ML, ABBOJECT SYRINGE (ABBOTT)
ATROPINE 0.1 MG/ML, 5 ML, 10 ML, ABBOJECT SYRINGE (ABBOTT)

ATROPINE SULFATE

Arco-Lase Plus Tablets (ARCO)
Atrohist Plus Tablets (MEDEVA)
Atropine Sulfate Injection (ELKINS-SINN)
Atropine Sulfate Injection, USP (BAXTER)
Diphenoxylate Hydrochloride & Atropine Sulfate Oral Solution (ROXANE)
Diphenoxylate Hydrochloride and Atropine Sulfate Tablets (MYLAN)
Diphenoxylate Hydrochloride and Atropine Sulfate Tablets, USP (MALLINCKRODT)
Donnatal Capsules (ROBINS)
Donnatal Elixir (ROBINS)
Donnatal Extentabs (ROBINS)
Donnatal Tablets (ROBINS)
Enlon-Plus Injection (BAXTER)
Lomotil Liquid (SEARLE)
Lomotil Tablets (SEARLE)
Lonox Tablets (GENEVA)
Motofen Tablets (CARNRICK)
Prosed/DS Tablets (STAR)
Urised Tablets (POLYMEDICA)

ATROPINE SULFATE INJECTION (ELKINS-SINN)
ATROPINE SULFATE INJECTION, USP (BAXTER)
ATROPINE SULFATE VIALS (LILLY)
ATROVENT INHALATION AEROSOL (BOEHRINGER INGELHEIM)
ATROVENT INHALATION SOLUTION (BOEHRINGER INGELHEIM)
ATROVENT NASAL SPRAY 0.03% (BOEHRINGER INGELHEIM)
ATROVENT NASAL SPRAY 0.06% (BOEHRINGER INGELHEIM)
A/T/S TOPICAL GEL (MEDICIS)
A/T/S TOPICAL SOLUTION (MEDICIS)
ATTENUVAX (MERCK)
AUGMENTIN POWDER FOR ORAL SUSPENSION AND CHEWABLE TABLETS (SMITHKLINE BEECHAM)
AUGMENTIN TABLETS (SMITHKLINE BEECHAM)
AURALGAN OTIC SOLUTION (WYETH-AYERST)

AUROTHIOGLUCOSE

Solganal Injectable Suspension (SCHERING)

AUTOPLEX T (NABI)
AVALIDE TABLETS (BRISTOL-MYERS SQUIBB)
AVANDIA TABLETS (SMITHKLINE BEECHAM)
AVAPRO TABLETS (SANOFI)
AVAPRO TABLETS (BRISTOL-MYERS SQUIBB)
AVC CREAM (MONARCH)
AVC SUPPOSITORIES (MONARCH)
AVENTYL HCL LIQUID (LILLY)
AVENTYL PULVULES (LILLY)
AVITA CREAM (BERTEK)
AVITA GEL (BERTEK)
AVONEX (BIOGEN)
AXID PULVULES (LILLY)
AXOCET CAPSULES (SAVAGE)
AYGESTIN TABLETS (ESI LEDERLE)
AZACTAM FOR INJECTION (DURA)
AZACTAM FOR INJECTION (BRISTOL-MYERS SQUIBB)

AZATADINE MALEATE

Rynatan Tablets (WALLACE)
Trinalin Repetabs Tablets (KEY)

AZATHIOPRINE

Imuran Injection (FARO)
Imuran Tablets (FARO)

AZATHIOPRINE SODIUM FOR INJECTION, USP (BEDFORD)

AZELAIC ACID

Azelex Cream (ALLERGAN)

AZELASTINE HYDROCHLORIDE

Astelin Nasal Spray (WALLACE)

AZELEX CREAM (ALLERGAN)

AZITHROMYCIN DIHYDRATE

Zithromax Capsules, 250 mg (PFIZER)
Zithromax Tablets, 250 mg (PFIZER)
Zithromax Tablets, 600 mg (PFIZER)
Zithromax for IV Infusion (PFIZER)
Zithromax for Oral Suspension, 1 g (PFIZER)
Zithromax for Oral Suspension, 300 mg, 600 mg, 900 mg, 1200 mg (PFIZER)

AZMACORT INHALATION AEROSOL (RHONE-POULENC RORER)
AZOPT OPHTHALMIC SUSPENSION (ALCON)

AZTREONAM

Azactam for Injection (DURA)

AZULFIDINE EN-TABS TABLETS (PHARMACIA & UPJOHN)
AZULFIDINE TABLETS (PHARMACIA & UPJOHN)

B

B & O SUPPRETTES NO. 15A & NO. 16A (POLYMEDICA)
B-COMPLEX '50' REGULAR AND CONTROLLED TIME RELEASE (VITALINE)
B-COMPLEX '100' REGULAR AND CONTROLLED TIME RELEASE (VITALINE)
B12 (MAYOR)

BACAMPICILLIN HYDROCHLORIDE

Spectrobid Tablets (PFIZER)

BACITRACIN

Sterile Bacitracin USP for Injection (PADDOCK)

BACITRACIN STERILE POWDER, USP (PHARMACIA & UPJOHN)
STERILE BACITRACIN USP FOR INJECTION (PADDOCK)
BACITRACIN USP MICRONIZED POWDER (PADDOCK)

BACITRACIN ZINC

Betadine Brand First Aid Antibiotics & Moisturizer Ointment (PURDUE FREDERICK)
Betadine Brand Plus First Aid Antibiotics & Pain Reliever Ointment (PURDUE FREDERICK)
Cortisporin Ointment (MONARCH)
Cortisporin Ophthalmic Ointment Sterile (MONARCH)
Neosporin + Pain Relief Maximum Strength Ointment (WARNER-LAMBERT)
Neosporin Ophthalmic Ointment Sterile (MONARCH)
Neosporin Original Ointment (WARNER-LAMBERT)
Polysporin Ointment (WARNER-LAMBERT)
Polysporin Powder (WARNER-LAMBERT)

BACLOFEN

Baclofen Tablets, USP (WATSON)

BACLOFEN TABLETS, USP (SCHEIN)
BACLOFEN TABLETS, USP (WATSON)
BACTRIM I.V. INFUSION (ROCHE LABS)
BACTRIM PEDIATRIC SUSPENSION (ROCHE LABS)
BACTRIM TABLETS (ROCHE LABS)
BACTRIM DS TABLETS (ROCHE LABS)
BACTROBAN CREAM (SMITHKLINE BEECHAM)
BACTROBAN NASAL (SMITHKLINE BEECHAM)
BACTROBAN OINTMENT (SMITHKLINE BEECHAM)
BALANCED SALT SOLUTION (ABBOTT)
BALNETAR (WESTWOOD-SQUIBB)

BALSAM PERU

Granulex Aerosol (BERTEK)

BANALG HOSPITAL STRENGTH ARTHRITIC PAIN RELIEVER (FOREST)
BANALG LINIMENT (FOREST)
BANCAP HC CAPSULES (FOREST)
BARBIDONNA TABLETS (WALLACE)
BAR-TEST (GLENWOOD)

BASILIXIMAB

Simulect for Injection (NOVARTIS)

BAYCOL TABLETS (BAYER)

UNDERLINE DENOTES GENERIC NAME

BAYGAM (BAYER BIOLOGICAL)
BAYHEP B (BAYER BIOLOGICAL)
BAYRAB (BAYER BIOLOGICAL)
BAYRHO-D FULL DOSE (BAYER BIOLOGICAL)
BAYRHO-D MINI-DOSE (BAYER BIOLOGICAL)
BAYTET (BAYER BIOLOGICAL)

BCG, LIVE (INTRAVESICAL)

TheraCys (PASTEUR MERIEUX CONNAUGHT)
Tice BCG, BCG Live (ORGANON)
BEBULIN VH IMMUNO (IMMUNO)

BECAPLERMIN

Regranex Gel (ORTHO-MCNEIL)

BECLOMETHASONE DIPROPIONATE

Beclovent Inhalation Aerosol and Refill
(GLAXO WELLCOME)
Beconase Inhalation Aerosol
(GLAXO WELLCOME)
Vancenase AQ Double Strength Nasal Spray
0.084% (SCHERING)
Vancenase AQ Nasal Spray 0.042%
(SCHERING)
Vancenase Nasal Inhaler (SCHERING)
Vancenase PocketHaler Nasal Inhaler
(SCHERING)
Vanceril Double Strength Inhalation Aerosol
(SCHERING)
Vanceril Inhalation Aerosol (SCHERING)

BECLOMETHASONE DIPROPIONATE
MONOHYDRATE

Beconase AQ Nasal Spray (GLAXO WELLCOME)
**BECLOVENT INHALATION AEROSOL AND
REFILL** (GLAXO WELLCOME)
BECONASE INHALATION AEROSOL
(GLAXO WELLCOME)
BECONASE AQ NASAL SPRAY
(GLAXO WELLCOME)
BEELITH TABLETS (BEACH)
BEEPEN-VK TABLETS (SMITHKLINE BEECHAM)

BELLADONNA ALKALOIDS

B & O Supprettes No. 15A & No. 16A
(POLYMEDICA)
Respa-A.R.M. Tablets (RESPA)
**BELLADONNA AND OPIUM
SUPPOSITORIES 16.2 MG/30 MG AND
16.2 MG/60 MG CII** (PADDOCK)
BELLERGAL-S TABLETS (NOVARTIS)
BENADRYL ALLERGY CHEWABLES
(WARNER-LAMBERT)
**BENADRYL ALLERGY KAPSEAL
CAPSULES** (WARNER-LAMBERT)
BENADRYL ALLERGY LIQUID
(WARNER-LAMBERT)
**BENADRYL ALLERGY ULTRATAB
TABLETS** (WARNER-LAMBERT)
BENADRYL ALLERGY/COLD TABLETS
(WARNER-LAMBERT)
**BENADRYL ALLERGY/CONGESTION
LIQUID** (WARNER-LAMBERT)
**BENADRYL ALLERGY/CONGESTION
TABLETS** (WARNER-LAMBERT)
**BENADRYL ALLERGY/SINUS HEADACHE
CAPLETS & GELCAPS** (WARNER-LAMBERT)
BENADRYL DYE-FREE ALLERGY LIQUID
(WARNER-LAMBERT)
**BENADRYL DYE-FREE ALLERGY LIQUI-
GELS** (WARNER-LAMBERT)
**BENADRYL ITCH RELIEF STICK EXTRA
STRENGTH** (WARNER-LAMBERT)
**BENADRYL ITCH STOPPING CREAM
ORIGINAL AND EXTRA STRENGTH**
(WARNER-LAMBERT)
**BENADRYL ITCH STOPPING GEL
ORIGINAL AND EXTRA STRENGTH**
(WARNER-LAMBERT)

**BENADRYL ITCH STOPPING SPRAY
ORIGINAL AND EXTRA STRENGTH**
(WARNER-LAMBERT)
BENADRYL PARENTERAL (PARKE-DAVIS)

BENAZEPRIL HYDROCHLORIDE

Lotrel Capsules (NOVARTIS)

BENDROFLUMETHIAZIDE

Corzide 40/5 Tablets (BRISTOL-MYERS SQUIBB)
Corzide 80/5 Tablets (BRISTOL-MYERS SQUIBB)
BENEFIX FOR INJECTION (GENETICS)
BENEMID TABLETS (MERCK)
BENOQUIN CREAM 20% (ICN)
BENOXYL-5 LOTION (STIEFEL)
BENOXYL-10 LOTION (STIEFEL)
BENSULFOID CREAM (ECR)
**BENTYL CAPSULES, TABLETS,
INJECTABLE, SYRUP**
(HOECHST MARION ROUSSEL)
BENYLIN ADULT FORMULA
(WARNER-LAMBERT)
BENYLIN EXPECTORANT (WARNER-LAMBERT)
BENYLIN MULTI-SYMPTOM
(WARNER-LAMBERT)
BENYLIN PEDIATRIC (WARNER-LAMBERT)
BENZAC AC 2 1/2, 5 & 10 GEL (GALDERMA)
BENZAC AC WASH 2 1/2, 5 & 10
(GALDERMA)
5 BENZAGEL ACNE GEL (DERMIK)
10 BENZAGEL ACNE GEL (DERMIK)

BENZALKONIUM CHLORIDE

Ony-Clear Solution (PEDINOL)
BENZAMYCIN TOPICAL GEL (DERMIK)

BENZOCAINE

Americaine Anesthetic Lubricant (MEDEVA)
Americaine Otic Topical Anesthetic Ear Drops
(MEDEVA)
Auralgan Otic Solution (WYETH-AYERST)
Cetacaine Topical Anesthetic (CETYLITE)
Hurricaine Topical Anesthetic Aerosol Spray,
2 oz. Wild Cherry (BEUTLICH)
Hurricaine Topical Anesthetic Gel: 1 oz. Wild
Cherry, Fresh Mint, Pina Colada,
Watermelon, 1/6 oz. Wild Cherry,
Watermelon (BEUTLICH)
Hurricaine Topical Anesthetic Liquid: 1 oz.
Wild Cherry and Pina Colada .25 ml Dry
Handle Swab Wild Cherry, 1/6 oz. Wild
Cherry (BEUTLICH)
Hurricaine Topical Anesthetic Spray Extension
Tubes (200) (BEUTLICH)
Hurricaine Topical Anesthetic Spray Kit
(BEUTLICH)
Tympagesic Ear Drops (SAVAGE)

BENZOIC ACID

Prosed/DS Tablets (STAR)
Urised Tablets (POLYMEDICA)
BENZOIN COMPOUND TINCTURE USP
(PADDOCK)

BENZONATATE

Tessalon Perles (FOREST)

BENZOYL PEROXIDE

10 Benzagel Acne Gel (DERMIK)
5 Benzagel Acne Gel (DERMIK)
Benzac AC 2 1/2, 5 & 10 Gel (GALDERMA)
Benzac AC Wash 2 1/2, 5 & 10 (GALDERMA)
Benzamycin Topical Gel (DERMIK)
Brevoxyl-4 Cleansing Lotion (STIEFEL)
Brevoxyl-4 Creamy Wash (STIEFEL)
Brevoxyl-4 Gel (STIEFEL)
Brevoxyl-8 Cleansing Lotion (STIEFEL)
Brevoxyl-8 Creamy Wash (STIEFEL)
Brevoxyl-8 Gel (STIEFEL)
PanOxyl 10 Acne Gel (STIEFEL)

PanOxyl 5 Acne Gel (STIEFEL)
PanOxyl AQ 10 Acne Gel (STIEFEL)
PanOxyl AQ 2 1/2 Acne Gel (STIEFEL)
PanOxyl AQ 5 Acne Gel (STIEFEL)
Triaz Cleanser (MEDICIS)
Triaz Gel (MEDICIS)
Vanoxide-HC Acne Lotion (DERMIK)

BENZTROPINE MESYLATE

Benztropine Mesylate Tablets (PAR)
Cogentin Injection (MERCK)
Cogentin Tablets (MERCK)
BENZTROPINE MESYLATE TABLETS (PAR)

BEPRIDIL HYDROCHLORIDE

Vascor Tablets (ORTHO-MCNEIL)

BERACTANT

Survanta Intratracheal Suspension (ROSS)
BEROCCA TABLETS (ROCHE LABS)
BEROCCA PLUS TABLETS (ROCHE LABS)

BETA CAROTENE

ACES Antioxidant Soft Gels (CARLSON)
Eucerin Q10 Anti-Wrinkle Sensitive Skin
Creme (BEIERSDORF)
BETADINE AEROSOL SPRAY
(PURDUE FREDERICK)
BETADINE ANTISEPTIC GAUZE PAD
(PURDUE FREDERICK)
**BETADINE BRAND FIRST AID
ANTIBIOTICS & MOISTURIZER
OINTMENT** (PURDUE FREDERICK)
**BETADINE BRAND PLUS FIRST AID
ANTIBIOTICS & PAIN RELIEVER
OINTMENT** (PURDUE FREDERICK)
BETADINE MEDICATED DOUCHE
(PURDUE FREDERICK)
**BETADINE MEDICATED DISPOSABLE
DOUCHE** (PURDUE FREDERICK)
**BETADINE PRE-MIXED MEDICATED
DISPOSABLE DOUCHE** (PURDUE FREDERICK)
BETADINE MEDICATED DOUCHE KIT
(PURDUE FREDERICK)
BETADINE MOUTHWASH/GARGLE
(PURDUE FREDERICK)
BETADINE OINTMENT (PURDUE FREDERICK)
**BETADINE PERINEAL WASH
CONCENTRATE KIT** (PURDUE FREDERICK)
BETADINE PREPSTICK APPLICATOR
(PURDUE FREDERICK)
BETADINE SHAMPOO (PURDUE FREDERICK)
BETADINE SKIN CLEANSER
(PURDUE FREDERICK)
BETADINE SOLUTION (PURDUE FREDERICK)
BETADINE SOLUTION SWAB AID
(PURDUE FREDERICK)
BETADINE SOLUTION SWABSTICKS
(PURDUE FREDERICK)
BETADINE SURGICAL SCRUB
(PURDUE FREDERICK)
BETADINE SURGI-PREP SPONGE-BRUSH
(PURDUE FREDERICK)
**BETADINE VISCOUS FORMULA
ANTISEPTIC GAUZE PAD**
(PURDUE FREDERICK)
**BETAGAN OPHTHALMIC SOLUTION
WITH C CAP COMPLIANCE CAP Q.D.
AND B.I.D.** (ALLERGAN)

BETAINE

SAMe Plus (NUTRACEUTICS)

BETAMETHASONE ACETATE

Celestone Soluspan Injectable Suspension
(SCHERING)

BETAMETHASONE DIPROPIONATE

Diprolene AF Cream 0.05% (SCHERING)
Diprolene Gel 0.05% (SCHERING)

UNDERLINE DENOTES GENERIC NAME

Diprolene Lotion 0.05% (SCHERING)
Diprolene Ointment 0.05% (SCHERING)
Lotrisone Cream (SCHERING)

BETAMETHASONE SODIUM PHOSPHATE

Celestone Soluspan Injectable Suspension
(SCHERING)

BETAPACE TABLETS (BERLEX)

BETASEPT SURGICAL SCRUB
(PURDUE FREDERICK)

BETASERON FOR SC INJECTION (BERLEX)

BETAXOLOL HYDROCHLORIDE

Betoptic S Ophthalmic Suspension (ALCON)
Kerlone Tablets (SEARLE)

BETAZYME (BETAINE HCL) (VITALINE)

BETHANECHOL CHLORIDE

Urecholine Injection (MERCK)
Urecholine Tablets (MERCK)

BETOPTIC S OPHTHALMIC SUSPENSION
(ALCON)

BETULINE LINIMENT (FERNDALE)

BEVITAMEL TABLETS (WESTLAKE)

BIAVAX II (MERCK)

**BIAXIN (CLARITHROMYCIN) (SEE
ABBOTT LABORATORIES)** (ROSS)

BIAXIN FILMTAB TABLETS (ABBOTT)

BIAXIN FOR ORAL SUSPENSION (ABBOTT)

BICALUTAMIDE

Casodex Tablets (ASTRAZENECA)

BICILLIN C-R 900/300 INJECTION
(WYETH-AYERST)

BICILLIN C-R 900/300 IN TUBEX
(WYETH-AYERST)

BICILLIN C-R INJECTION (WYETH-AYERST)

BICILLIN C-R IN TUBEX (WYETH-AYERST)

BICILLIN L-A INJECTION (WYETH-AYERST)

BICILLIN L-A IN TUBEX (WYETH-AYERST)

BICITRA (ALZA)

BICNU
(BRISTOL-MYERSSQUIBBONCOLOGY/IMMUNOLOGY)

BILBERRY

VitaSight (MAYOR)
Vitamist Intra-Oral Spray Dietary Supplements
(MAYOR)

BILTRICIDE TABLETS (BAYER)

BIO ST. JOHN'S CAPSULES (PHARMANEX)

BIOBRANE TEMPORARY BURN DRESSING
(BERTEK)

BIOFLAVONOIDS

Peridin-C Tablets (BEUTLICH)

**BIOGINKGO 27/7 EXTRA STRENGTH
TABLETS** (PHARMANEX)

BIOHIST LA TABLETS (WAKEFIELD)

BION TEARS LUBRICANT EYE DROPS
(ALCON)

BIOTIN

Biotin Capsules (MERICON)
Mega-B Tablets (ARCO)
Megadose Tablets (ARCO)

BIOTIN CAPSULES (MERICON)

BIOTIN FORTE 3MG (VITALINE)

BIOTIN FORTE 5MG (VITALINE)

BIPERIDEN HYDROCHLORIDE

Akineton Injection (KNOLL LABS)
Akineton Tablets (KNOLL LABS)

BISACODYL

Dulcolax Suppositories (NOVARTIS CONSUMER)
Dulcolax Tablets (NOVARTIS CONSUMER)
Evac-Q-Kwik (SAVAGE)
Fleet Bisacodyl Laxatives (FLEET)
Fleet Prep Kits (FLEET)

BISACODYL SUPPOSITORIES 10 MG
(PADDOCK)

BISACODYL TABLETS 5 MG (PADDOCK)

BISACODYL UNISERTS SUPPOSITORIES
(UPSHER-SMITH)

BISMUTH SUBSALICYLATE

Pepto-Bismol Maximum Strength Liquid
(PROCTER & GAMBLE)
Pepto-Bismol Original Liquid, Original and
Cherry Tablets and Easy-To-Swallow
Caplets (PROCTER & GAMBLE)

BISOPROLOL FUMARATE

Zebeta Tablets (LEDERLE LABS)
Ziac Tablets (LEDERLE LABS)

BITOLTEROL MESYLATE

Tornalate Metered Dose Inhaler (DURA)
Tornalate Solution for Inhalation, 0.2% (DURA)

BLACK WIDOW SPIDER ANTIVENIN
(EQUINE)

Antivenin (Black Widow Spider Antivenin)
(MERCK)

BLENOXANE
(BRISTOL-MYERSSQUIBBONCOLOGY/IMMUNOLOGY)

BLEOMYCIN SULFATE

Blenoxane
(BRISTOL-MYERSSQUIBBONCOLOGY/IMMUNOLOGY)

BLEPH-10 OPHTHALMIC OINTMENT
(ALLERGAN)

BLEPH-10 OPHTHALMIC SOLUTION
(ALLERGAN)

BLEPHAMIDE OPHTHALMIC OINTMENT
(ALLERGAN)

BLEPHAMIDE OPHTHALMIC SUSPENSION
(ALLERGAN)

BLOCADREN TABLETS (MERCK)

BLUE-GREEN SEA SPRAY (MAYOR)

BONA-BACILLUS CAPSULES (WESTLAKE)

BONINE CHEWABLE TABLETS
(PFIZER CONSUMER)

BONTRIL PDM TABLETS (CARNRICK)

BONTRIL SLOW-RELEASE CAPSULES
(CARNRICK)

BORON 6MG (VITALINE)

BOROPAK (GLENWOOD)

**BOTOX PURIFIED NEUROTOXIN
COMPLEX** (ALLERGAN)

BOTULINUM TOXIN TYPE A

Botox Purified Neurotoxin Complex
(ALLERGAN)

BRASIVOL BASE (STIEFEL)

BRASIVOL FINE (STIEFEL)

BRASIVOL MEDIUM (STIEFEL)

BRASIVOL ROUGH (STIEFEL)

BREEZEE MIST FOOT POWDER (PEDINOL)

BREONESIN CAPSULES (SANOFI)

BRETHAIRE INHALER (NOVARTIS)

BRETHINE AMPULS (NOVARTIS)

BRETHINE TABLETS (NOVARTIS)

**BRETYLIUM TOSYLATE IN 5%
DEXTROSE INJECTION (50 MG/ML)**
(ABBOTT)

BREVIBLOC INJECTION (BAXTER)

BREVICON (WATSON)

BREVICON-21 TABLETS (SEARLE)

BREVICON-28 TABLETS (SEARLE)

BREVITAL SODIUM FOR INJECTION, USP
(JONES)

BREVOXYL-4 CLEANSING LOTION
(STIEFEL)

BREVOXYL-8 CLEANSING LOTION
(STIEFEL)

BREVOXYL-4 CREAMY WASH (STIEFEL)

BREVOXYL-8 CREAMY WASH (STIEFEL)

BREVOXYL-4 GEL (STIEFEL)

BREVOXYL-8 GEL (STIEFEL)

BRIMONIDINE TARTRATE

Alphagan Ophthalmic Solution (ALLERGAN)

BRINZOLAMIDE

Azopt Ophthalmic Suspension (ALCON)

BROMELAIN 500MG (VITALINE)

**BROMFED CAPSULES (EXTENDED-
RELEASE)** (MURO)

**BROMFED-PD CAPSULES (EXTENDED-
RELEASE)** (MURO)

BROMI-LOTION (GORDON)

BROMI-TALC (GORDON)

BROMI-TALC PLUS (GORDON)

BROMOCRIPTINE MESYLATE

Bromocriptine Mesylate Capsules (GENEVA)
Bromocriptine Mesylate Tablets (GENEVA)

BROMOCRIPTINE MESYLATE CAPSULES
(GENEVA)

BROMOCRIPTINE MESYLATE TABLETS
(GENEVA)

BROMPHENIRAMINE MALEATE

Anaplex DM Cough Syrup (ECR)
Bromfed Capsules (Extended-Release) (MURO)
Bromfed-PD Capsules (Extended-Release)
(MURO)
Dallergy-JR Capsules (LASER)
Dimetane-DX Cough Syrup (ROBINS)
Lodrane Allergy Capsules (ECR)
Lodrane LD Capsules (ECR)
Lodrane Liquid (ECR)
Poly-Histine CS Syrup (SANOFI)
Poly-Histine DM Syrup (SANOFI)
Respahist Capsules (RESPA)
Ultrabrom Capsules (WE)
Ultrabrom PD Capsules (WE)

BRONCHOLATE SYRUP (SANOFI)

**BSS AND BSS PLUS IRRIGATION
SOLUTION ADMINISTRATION SET**
(ALCON)

**BSS IRRIGATION SOLUTION (15 ML, 30
ML, 250 ML, 500 ML)** (ALCON)

**BSS PLUS IRRIGATION SOLUTION (250
ML, 500 ML)** (ALCON)

BUCET CAPSULES (FOREST)

BUDESONIDE

Pulmicort Turbuhaler Inhalation Powder
(ASTRAZENECA LP)
Rhinocort Nasal Inhaler (ASTRAZENECA LP)

BUFFERIN (BRISTOL-MYERS)

ARTHRITIS STRENGTH BUFFERIN
(BRISTOL-MYERS)

EXTRA STRENGTH BUFFERIN
(BRISTOL-MYERS)

**BUFFERIN LOW DOSE (81 MG) ADULT
REGIMEN** (BRISTOL-MYERS)

BUMETANIDE

Bumetanide Injection, USP (BAXTER)
Bumetanide Tablets (MYLAN)

BUMETANIDE INJECTION, USP (BAXTER)

BUMETANIDE INJECTION, USP (BEDFORD)

BUMETANIDE TABLETS (MYLAN)

BUMEX INJECTION (ROCHE LABS)

BUMEX TABLETS (ROCHE LABS)

BUMINATE 5% SOLUTION, USP
(BAXTER HEALTHCARE)

BUMINATE 25% SOLUTION, USP
(BAXTER HEALTHCARE)

BUPAP TABLETS (ECR)

BUPIVACAINE HYDROCHLORIDE

Sensorcaine Injection (ASTRAZENECA LP)
Sensorcaine with Epinephrine Injection
(ASTRAZENECA LP)
Sensorcaine-MPF Injection (ASTRAZENECA LP)

Sensorcaine-MPF Spinal Injection
(ASTRAZENECA LP)

Sensorcaine-MPF with Epinephrine Injection
(ASTRAZENECA LP)

**BUPIVACAINE HYDROCHLORIDE
INJECTION, USP, 0.25%, 0.5%, 0.75%,
AMPUL, ABBOJECT SYRINGE** (ABBOTT)

BUPRENEX INJECTABLE
(RECKITT & COLMAN)

BUPRENORPHINE HYDROCHLORIDE

Buprenex Injectable (RECKITT & COLMAN)

BUPROPION HYDROCHLORIDE

Wellbutrin SR Sustained-Release Tablets
(GLAXO WELLCOME)

Wellbutrin Tablets (GLAXO WELLCOME)

Zyban Sustained-Release Tablets
(GLAXO WELLCOME)

BUROW'S SOLUTION

Pedi-Boro Soak Paks (PEDINOL)

BUSPAR TABLETS (BRISTOL-MYERS SQUIBB)

BUSPIRONE HYDROCHLORIDE

BuSpar Tablets (BRISTOL-MYERS SQUIBB)

BUSPIRONE TABLETS, USP (APOTHECON)

BUSULFAN

Myleran Tablets (GLAXO WELLCOME)

BUTABARBITAL

Pyridium Plus Tablets (WARNER CHILCOTT)

BUTALBITAL

Anolor 300 Capsules (BLANSETT)

Axocet Capsules (SAVAGE)

Bupap Tablets (ECR)

Butalbital, Acetaminophen and Caffeine
Tablets USP (MALLINCKRODT)

Butalbital, Aspirin, Caffeine, and Codeine
Phosphate Capsules, USP (ENDO GENERICS)

Butalbital, Aspirin, Caffeine, and Codeine
Phosphate Capsules, USP CIII (WATSON)

Butalbital, Caffeine, and Acetaminophen
Tablets, USP (WATSON)

Esgic Capsules (FOREST)

Esgic Tablets (FOREST)

Esgic-Plus Tablets (FOREST)

Fiorpap Tablets (GENEVA)

Fiortal Capsules (GENEVA)

Fiortal w/Codeine Capsules (GENEVA)

Medigesic Capsules (U.S. PHARMACEUTICAL)

Pacaps Capsules (LUNSCO)

Phrenilin Forte Capsules (CARNRICK)

Phrenilin Tablets (CARNRICK)

Sedapap Tablets 50 mg/650 mg (MERZ)

Zebutal Capsules (HORIZON)

**BUTALBITAL, ASPIRIN, CAFFEINE, AND
CODEINE PHOSPHATE CAPSULES, USP
CIII** (WATSON)

**BUTALBITAL, CAFFEINE, AND
ACETAMINOPHEN TABLETS, USP**
(WATSON)

**BUTALBITAL, ASPIRIN, CAFFEINE, AND
CODEINE PHOSPHATE CAPSULES, USP**
(ENDO GENERICS)

**BUTALBITAL, ACETAMINOPHEN AND
CAFFEINE TABLETS USP** (MALLINCKRODT)

BUTENAFINE HYDROCHLORIDE

Mentax Cream (BERTEK)

BUTESIN PICRATE OINTMENT (ABBOTT)

BUTIBEL ELIXIR & TABLETS (WALLACE)

BUTISOL SODIUM ELIXIR (WALLACE)

BUTISOL SODIUM TABLETS (WALLACE)

BUTORPHANOL TARTRATE

Butorphanol Tartrate Injection, USP (BAXTER)

Stadol NS Nasal Spray
(BRISTOL-MYERS SQUIBB)

**BUTORPHANOL TARTRATE INJECTION,
USP** (BAXTER)

**BUTORPHANOL TARTRATE INJECTION,
USP** (BEDFORD)

BUTYL AMINOBENZOATE

Cetacaine Topical Anesthetic (CETYLITE)

C

C + ZINC (MAYOR)

CABERGOLINE

Dostinex Tablets (PHARMACIA & UPJOHN)

CAFERGOT SUPPOSITORIES (NOVARTIS)

CAFFEINE

Anolor 300 Capsules (BLANSETT)

Aspirin Free Excedrin Caplets (BRISTOL-MYERS)

Aspirin Free Excedrin Geltabs (BRISTOL-MYERS)

Butalbital, Aspirin, Caffeine, and Codeine
Phosphate Capsules, USP (ENDO GENERICS)

Butalbital, Aspirin, Caffeine, and Codeine
Phosphate Capsules, USP CIII (WATSON)

Butalbital, Caffeine, and Acetaminophen
Tablets, USP (WATSON)

Darvon Compound-65 Pulvules (LILLY)

Ercaf Tablets (GENEVA)

Esgic Capsules (FOREST)

Esgic Tablets (FOREST)

Esgic-Plus Tablets (FOREST)

Excedrin Extra-Strength Caplets
(BRISTOL-MYERS)

Excedrin Extra-Strength Geltabs
(BRISTOL-MYERS)

Excedrin Extra-Strength Tablets
(BRISTOL-MYERS)

Excedrin Migraine Caplets (BRISTOL-MYERS)

Excedrin Migraine Tablets (BRISTOL-MYERS)

Fiorpap Tablets (GENEVA)

Fiortal Capsules (GENEVA)

Fiortal w/Codeine Capsules (GENEVA)

Hycomine Compound Tablets (ENDO LABS)

Medigesic Capsules (U.S. PHARMACEUTICAL)

Norgesic Forte Tablets (3M)

Norgesic Tablets (3M)

Orphenadrine Citrate, Aspirin and Caffeine
Tablets (MYLAN)

Orphengesic Forte Tablets (PAR)

Orphengesic Tablets (PAR)

Pacaps Capsules (LUNSCO)

Propoxyphene Hydrochloride, Aspirin and
Caffeine Capsules (MYLAN)

Synalgos-DC Capsules (WYETH-AYERST)

Wigraine Tablets (ORGANON)

Zebutal Capsules (HORIZON)

**CAFFEINE AND SODIUM BENZOATE
INJECTION, USP** (BEDFORD)

CAFFEINE ANHYDROUS

Butalbital, Acetaminophen and Caffeine
Tablets USP (MALLINCKRODT)

CALADRYL CLEAR LOTION
(WARNER-LAMBERT)

CALADRYL CREAM FOR KIDS
(WARNER-LAMBERT)

CALADRYL LOTION (WARNER-LAMBERT)

CALAMINE

Caladryl Cream For Kids (WARNER-LAMBERT)

Caladryl Lotion (WARNER-LAMBERT)

CALAN TABLETS (SEARLE)

CALAN SR CAPLETS (SEARLE)

**CAL-CARB FORTE (500MG ELEMENTAL
CALCIUM)** (VITALINE)

CALCET TABLETS (MISSION)

CALCET PLUS TABLETS (MISSION)

CALCIBIND ORAL POWDER (MISSION)

CALCI-CHEW TABLETS (R&D)

CALCIFEDIOL

Calderol Capsules (ORGANON)

CALCIFEROL DROPS (SCHWARZ)

CALCIFEROL IN OIL INJECTION
(SCHWARZ)

CALCIJEX INJECTION (ABBOTT)

**CALCILO XD LOW-CALCIUM/VITAMIN D-
FREE INFANT FORMULA WITH IRON**
(ROSS)

CALCIMAR INJECTION, SYNTHETIC
(RHONE-POULENC RORER)

CALCI-MIX CAPSULES (R&D)

CALCIPOTRIENE

Dovonex Cream 0.005% (WESTWOOD-SQUIBB)

Dovonex Ointment 0.005% (WESTWOOD-SQUIBB)

Dovonex Scalp Solution 0.005%
(WESTWOOD-SQUIBB)

CALCITONIN-SALMON

Calcimar Injection, Synthetic
(RHONE-POULENC RORER)

Calcitonin-Salmon Injection, Synthetic
(ASTRAZENECA LP)

Miacalcin Injection (NOVARTIS)

Miacalcin Nasal Spray (NOVARTIS)

**CALCITONIN-SALMON INJECTION,
SYNTHETIC** (ASTRAZENECA LP)

CALCITRIOL

Calcijex Injection (ABBOTT)

Rocaltrol Capsules (ROCHE LABS)

Rocaltrol Oral Solution (ROCHE LABS)

CALCIUM

Calcet Plus Tablets (MISSION)

Calcet Tablets (MISSION)

Fosfree Tablets (MISSION)

Mission Prenatal F.A. Tablets (MISSION)

Mission Prenatal H.P. Tablets (MISSION)

Mission Prenatal Tablets (MISSION)

Osteo-CalMag (MAYOR)

Vitamist Intra-Oral Spray Dietary Supplements
(MAYOR)

CALCIUM ACETATE

PhosLo Tablets (BRAINTREE)

**CALCIUM ACETATE 0.5 MEQ/ML
INJECTION** (ABBOTT)

CALCIUM CARBONATE

Calci-Chew Tablets (R&D)

Calci-Mix Capsules (R&D)

Calcium Carbonate Tablets & Oral Suspension
(ROXANE)

Children's Mylanta Upset Stomach Relief
Liquid (J&J – MERCK)

Children's Mylanta Upset Stomach Relief
Tablets (J&J – MERCK)

Fast-Acting Mylanta Antacid Tablets
(J&J – MERCK)

Florical Capsules and Tablets (MERICON)

Maximum Strength Fast-Acting Mylanta
Antacid Tablets (J&J – MERCK)

Monocal Tablets (MERICON)

Mylanta Supreme Liquid (J&J – MERCK)

Nephro-Calci Tablets (R&D)

Osteomax (NUTRACEUTICS)

Quick Dissolve Maalox Antacid Tablets,
Maximum Strength (NOVARTIS CONSUMER)

Quick Dissolve Maalox Antacid Tablets,
Regular Strength (NOVARTIS CONSUMER)

ViTelle Nesentials Tablets (formerly Gerimed)
(FIELDING)
**CALCIUM CARBONATE TABLETS &
ORAL SUSPENSION** (ROXANE)
CALCIUM CARBONATE, USP (LILLY)
**CALCIUM CHLORIDE 10%, (1.4 MEQ/ML)
ABBOJECT** (ABBOTT)

CALCIUM CITRATE

ActiCal Tablets (USANA)
Chelated Mineral Tablets (USANA)
Citracal Caplets + D (MISSION)
Citracal Liquitabs (MISSION)
Citracal Tablets (MISSION)
CALCIUM CITRATE 250MG (VITALINE)
**CALCIUM DISODIUM VERSENATE
INJECTION** (3M)
**CALCIUM GLUCEPTATE INJECTION
AMPUL & ABBOJECT (0.9 MEQ/ML)**
(ABBOTT)

CALCIUM GLUCONATE

Calcium Gluconate Tablets (ROXANE)
CALCIUM GLUCONATE TABLETS (ROXANE)

CALCIUM PANTOTHENATE

Mega-B Tablets (ARCO)

CALCIUM PHOSPHATE, DIBASIC

ViTelle Nesentials Tablets (formerly Gerimed)
(FIELDING)
CALDEROL CAPSULES (ORGANON)

CALFACTANT

Infasurf Intratracheal Suspension (FOREST)
CALICYLIC CREME (GORDON)
CALM COLON CAPSULES (SAMRA)
CAL-MAG ASPARTATE (VITALINE)
CALPHOSAN INJECTION (GLENWOOD)

CAMELLIA SINENSIS

Tegreen 97 Capsules (PHARMANEX)

CAMPHOR

Panalgesic Gold Topical Liquid (ECR)
CAMPTOSAR INJECTION
(PHARMACIA & UPJOHN)

CANDESARTAN CILEXETIL

Atacand Tablets (ASTRAZENECA LP)
CANTIL TABLETS (HOECHST MARION ROUSSEL)
CAPASTAT SULFATE INJECTION (DURA)

CAPECITABINE

Xeloda Tablets (ROCHE LABS)
**CAPITAL AND CODEINE ORAL
SUSPENSION** (CARNRICK)
CAPITROL SHAMPOO (WESTWOOD-SQUIBB)

CAPREOMYCIN SULFATE

Capastat Sulfate Injection (DURA)
CAPSAICIN CREAM 0.025% (FERNDALE)
CAPSAICIN-HP CREAM 0.075% (FERNDALE)

CAPTOPRIL

Captopril Tablets (PAR)
Captopril Tablets (MYLAN)
Captopril Tablets, 12.5 mg, 25 mg, 50 mg,
100 mg (NOVOPHARM)
Captopril Tablets, USP (WATSON)
Captopril Tablets, USP (ENDO GENERICS)
Captopril and Hydrochlorothiazide Tablets
(MYLAN)
Captopril and Hydrochlorothiazide Tablets,
USP (ENDO GENERICS)
**CAPTOPRIL AND
HYDROCHLOROTHIAZIDE TABLETS,
USP** (ENDO GENERICS)
CAPTOPRIL TABLETS (PAR)
CAPTOPRIL TABLETS (MYLAN)
CAPTOPRIL TABLETS (ESI LEDERLE)

**CAPTOPRIL AND
HYDROCHLOROTHIAZIDE TABLETS**
(MYLAN)
**CAPTOPRIL TABLETS, 12.5 MG, 25 MG,
50 MG, 100 MG** (NOVOPHARM)
CAPTOPRIL TABLETS, USP (WATSON)
CAPTOPRIL TABLETS, USP (APOTHECON)
CAPTOPRIL TABLETS, USP (ENDO GENERICS)
**CAPTOPRIL/HYDROCHLOROTHIAZIDE
TABLETS, USP** (APOTHECON)
CARAFATE SUSPENSION
(HOECHST MARION ROUSSEL)
CARAFATE TABLETS
(HOECHST MARION ROUSSEL)

CARBAMAZEPINE

Carbatrol Capsules (SHIRE RICHWOOD)
Tegretol Chewable Tablets (NOVARTIS)
Tegretol Suspension (NOVARTIS)
Tegretol Tablets (NOVARTIS)
Tegretol-XR Tablets (NOVARTIS)

CARBAMIDE PEROXIDE

Murine Ear Wax Removal System/Murine Ear
Drops (ROSS)
CARBATROL CAPSULES (SHIRE RICHWOOD)

CARBENICILLIN INDANYL SODIUM

Geocillin Tablets (PFIZER)

CARBETAPENTANE TANNATE

Rynatuss Pediatric Suspension (WALLACE)
Rynatuss Tablets (WALLACE)
Tussi-12 Suspension (WALLACE)
CARBEX TABLETS (ENDO LABS)

CARBIDOPA

Atamet Tablets (ATHENA)
Carbidopa and Levodopa Tablets, USP
(ENDO GENERICS)
Sinemet CR Tablets (DUPONT)
Sinemet Tablets (DUPONT)
**CARBIDOPA AND LEVODOPA TABLETS,
USP** (ENDO GENERICS)

CARBINOXAMINE MALEATE

Rondec Oral Drops (DJ PHARMA)
Rondec Syrup (DJ PHARMA)
Rondec Tablet (DJ PHARMA)
Rondec-DM Oral Drops (DJ PHARMA)
Rondec-DM Syrup (DJ PHARMA)
Rondec-TR Tablet (DJ PHARMA)
CARBISET (GLENWOOD)

CARBOPLATIN

Paraplatin for Injection
(BRISTOL-MYERSSQUIBBONCOLOGY/IMMUNOLOGY)
CARDENE CAPSULES (ROCHE LABS)
CARDENE I.V. (WYETH-AYERST)
CARDENE SR CAPSULES (ROCHE LABS)
CARDIOCARE (MAYOR)
CARDIOQUIN TABLETS (PURDUE FREDERICK)
CARDIOTROPIN (NUTRACEUTICS)
CARDIZEM CD CAPSULES
(HOECHST MARION ROUSSEL)
CARDIZEM INJECTABLE
(HOECHST MARION ROUSSEL)
CARDIZEM LYO-JECT SYRINGE
(HOECHST MARION ROUSSEL)
CARDIZEM MONOVIAL
(HOECHST MARION ROUSSEL)
CARDIZEM SR CAPSULES
(HOECHST MARION ROUSSEL)
CARDIZEM TABLETS
(HOECHST MARION ROUSSEL)
CARDURA TABLETS (PFIZER)

CARISOPRODOL

Carisoprodol Tablets (GENEVA)
Carisoprodol Tablets (WATSON)

Carisoprodol and Aspirin Tablets (PAR)
Soma Compound Tablets (WALLACE)
Soma Compound w/Codeine Tablets
(WALLACE)
Soma Tablets (WALLACE)
CARISOPRODOL AND ASPIRIN TABLETS
(PAR)
CARISOPRODOL TABLETS (GENEVA)
CARISOPRODOL TABLETS (WATSON)
CARISOPRODOL TABLETS, USP (SCHEIN)

CARMUSTINE (BCNU)

BiCNU
(BRISTOL-MYERSSQUIBBONCOLOGY/IMMUNOLOGY)
Gliadel Wafer (RHONE-POULENC RORER)
CARNITOR INJECTION (SIGMA-TAU)
CARNITOR TABLETS AND SOLUTION
(SIGMA-TAU)

CARTEOLOL HYDROCHLORIDE

Cartrol Filmtab Tablets (ABBOTT)
CARTROL FILMTAB TABLETS (ABBOTT)

CARVEDILOL

Coreg Tablets (SMITHKLINE BEECHAM)

CASANTHRANOL

Docusate Sodium with Casanthranol
(PHARMACEUTICAL ASSOCIATES)
Peri-Colace Capsules and Syrup (ROBERTS)

CASCARA SAGRADA

Aromatic Cascara Fluidextract (ROXANE)
Aromatic Cascara Fluidextract USP
(PHARMACEUTICAL ASSOCIATES)
Milk of Magnesia Cascara Suspension
(PHARMACEUTICAL ASSOCIATES)
Milk of Magnesia-Cascara Suspension
Concentrated (ROXANE)
CASODEX TABLETS (ASTRAZENECA)
CASTELLANI PAINT MODIFIED (PEDINOL)

CASTOR OIL

Granulex Aerosol (BERTEK)
Hydrisinol Creme (PEDINOL)
Hydrisinol Lotion (PEDINOL)
CASTOR OIL USP (PADDOCK)
CATAFLAM TABLETS (NOVARTIS)
**CATALYTIC FORMULA (PROTEOLYTIC
ENZYMES)** (VITALINE)
CATAPRES TABLETS (BOEHRINGER INGELHEIM)
CATAPRES-TTS (BOEHRINGER INGELHEIM)
CAVERJECT STERILE POWDER
(PHARMACIA & UPJOHN)

CAYANNE

Ex. O (MAYOR)
Vitamist Intra-Oral Spray Dietary Supplements
(MAYOR)
C-B TIME CAPSULES (ARCO)
C-B TIME LIQUID (ARCO)
C-B TIME 500 TABLETS (ARCO)
CEBOCAP CAPSULES (FOREST)
CECLOR CD TABLETS (DURA)
CECLOR PULVULES (LILLY)
CECLOR SUSPENSION (LILLY)
CECON SOLUTION (ABBOTT)
CEDAX CAPSULES (SCHERING)
CEDAX ORAL SUSPENSION (SCHERING)
CEENU CAPSULES
(BRISTOL-MYERSSQUIBBONCOLOGY/IMMUNOLOGY)

CEFACLOR

Ceclor CD Tablets (DURA)
Ceclor Pulvules (LILLY)
Ceclor Suspension (LILLY)
Cefaclor Capsules and Powders for Oral
Suspension (MYLAN)
Cefaclor Capsules, 250 mg, 500 mg
(NOVOPHARM)

CEFACLOR CAPSULES AND POWDERS FOR ORAL SUSPENSION (MYLAN)
CEFACLOR CAPSULES, 250 MG, 500 MG (NOVOPHARM)
CEFACLOR CAPSULES, USP (APOTHECON)
CEFACLOR FOR ORAL SUSPENSION, USP (APOTHECON)

CEFADROXIL

Duricef Capsules (BRISTOL-MYERS SQUIBB)
Duricef Oral Suspensions (BRISTOL-MYERS SQUIBB)
Duricef Tablets (BRISTOL-MYERS SQUIBB)
CEFADROXIL CAPSULES, USP (APOTHECON)

CEFAMANDOLE NAFATE

Mandol Vials (LILLY)
CEFAZOLIN FOR INJECTION USP (APOTHECON)

CEFAZOLIN SODIUM

Ancef for Injection (SMITHKLINE BEECHAM)
Kefzol Vials, ADD-Vantage (LILLY)

CEFDINIR

Omnicef Capsules (PARKE-DAVIS)
Omnicef for Oral Suspension (PARKE-DAVIS)

CEFEPIME HYDROCHLORIDE

Maxipime for Injection (DURA)

CEFIXIME

Suprax Tablets (LEDERLE LABS)
Suprax for Oral Suspension (LEDERLE LABS)
CEFIZOX FOR INTRAMUSCULAR OR INTRAVENOUS USE (FUJISAWA)
CEFIZOX FOR INTRAMUSCULAR OR INTRAVENOUS USE PHARMACY BULK PACKAGE (FUJISAWA)
CEFIZOX FOR INTRAVENOUS INFUSION (FUJISAWA)
CEFIZOX FOR INTRAVENOUS USE IN GALAXY PLASTIC CONTAINER (FUJISAWA)
CEFOBID INTRAVENOUS/INTRAMUSCULAR (PFIZER)
CEFOBID PHARMACY BULK PACKAGE - NOT FOR DIRECT INFUSION (PFIZER)
CEFOL FILMTAB TABLETS (ABBOTT)

CEFOPERAZONE SODIUM

Cefobid Intravenous/Intramuscular (PFIZER)
Cefobid Pharmacy Bulk Package - Not for Direct Infusion (PFIZER)
CEFOTAN FOR INJECTION (ASTRAZENECA)
CEFOTAN INJECTION (ASTRAZENECA)

CEFOTAXIME SODIUM

Claforan (HOECHST MARION ROUSSEL)

CEFOTETAN DISODIUM

Cefotan Injection (ASTRAZENECA)
Cefotan for Injection (ASTRAZENECA)

CEFOXITIN SODIUM

Mefoxin Premixed Intravenous Solution (MERCK)
Mefoxin for Injection (MERCK)

CEFPODOXIME PROXETIL

Vantin Tablets and Oral Suspension (PHARMACIA & UPJOHN)

CEFPROZIL

Cefzil Tablets (BRISTOL-MYERS SQUIBB)
Cefzil for Oral Suspension (BRISTOL-MYERS SQUIBB)

CEFTAZIDIME

Ceptaz (GLAXO WELLCOME)
Fortaz (GLAXO WELLCOME)
Tazicef for Injection (SMITHKLINE BEECHAM)
Tazidime Vials, Faspak & ADD-Vantage (LILLY)

CEFTIBUTEN DIHYDRATE

Cedax Capsules (SCHERING)
Cedax Oral Suspension (SCHERING)
CEFTIN FOR ORAL SUSPENSION (GLAXO WELLCOME)
CEFTIN TABLETS (GLAXO WELLCOME)

CEFTIZOXIME SODIUM

Cefizox for Intramuscular or Intravenous Use (FUJISAWA)
Cefizox for Intramuscular or Intravenous Use Pharmacy Bulk Package (FUJISAWA)
Cefizox for Intravenous Infusion (FUJISAWA)
Cefizox for Intravenous Use in Galaxy Plastic Container (FUJISAWA)

CEFTRIAXONE SODIUM

Rocephin Injectable Vials, ADD-Vantage, Galaxy, Bulk (ROCHE LABS)

CEFUROXIME

Zinacef (GLAXO WELLCOME)

CEFUROXIME AXETIL

Ceftin Tablets (GLAXO WELLCOME)
Ceftin for Oral Suspension (GLAXO WELLCOME)

CEFUROXIME SODIUM

Kefurox Vials, ADD-Vantage (LILLY)
CEFZIL FOR ORAL SUSPENSION (BRISTOL-MYERS SQUIBB)
CEFZIL TABLETS (BRISTOL-MYERS SQUIBB)
CELEBREX CAPSULES (PFIZER)
CELEBREX CAPSULES (SEARLE)

CELECOXIB

Celebrex Capsules (PFIZER)
Celebrex Capsules (SEARLE)
CELESTONE PHOSPHATE INJECTION (SCHERING)
CELESTONE SOLUSPAN INJECTABLE SUSPENSION (SCHERING)
CELESTONE SYRUP (SCHERING)
CELESTONE TABLETS (SCHERING)
CELEXA TABLETS (FOREST)
CELLCEPT CAPSULES (ROCHE LABS)
CELLCEPT INTRAVENOUS (ROCHE LABS)
CELLCEPT ORAL SUSPENSION (ROCHE LABS)
CELLCEPT TABLETS (ROCHE LABS)

CELLULASE

Arco-Lase Plus Tablets (ARCO)
Arco-Lase Tablets (ARCO)
Ku-Zyme Capsules (SCHWARZ)
Kutrase Capsules (SCHWARZ)

CELLULOSE

Unifiber (NICHE)

CELLULOSE SODIUM PHOSPHATE

Calcibind Oral Powder (MISSION)
CELLUVISC LUBRICANT EYE DROPS (ALLERGAN)
CELONTIN KAPSEALS (PARKE-DAVIS)
CENESTIN TABLETS (DURAMED)
CENOLATE AMPULES (500 MG/ML) (ABBOTT)
CEO-TWO EVACUANT SUPPOSITORY (BEUTLICH)

CEPHALEXIN

Cephalexin Capsules USP and Oral Suspension, Caps 250 mg, 500 mg, O.S. 125 mg/mL, 250 mg/mL (NOVOPHARM)
Cephalexin Capsules and Powders for Oral Suspension (MYLAN)
Cephalexin Capsules, USP (LEDERLE STANDARD)
Keflex Oral Suspension (DISTA)
Keflex Pulvules (DISTA)
CEPHALEXIN CAPSULES (ESI LEDERLE)
CEPHALEXIN CAPSULES, USP (LEDERLE STANDARD)
CEPHALEXIN CAPSULES AND FOR ORAL SUSPENSION USP (APOTHECON)
CEPHALEXIN CAPSULES AND POWDERS FOR ORAL SUSPENSION (MYLAN)
CEPHALEXIN CAPSULES USP AND ORAL SUSPENSION, CAPS 250 MG, 500 MG, O.S. 125 MG/ML, 250 MG/ML (NOVOPHARM)

CEPHALEXIN HYDROCHLORIDE

Keftab Tablets (DJ PHARMA)
CEPHALEXIN ORAL SUSPENSION (ESI LEDERLE)
CEPHULAC SOLUTION (HOECHST MARION ROUSSEL)
CEPTAZ (GLAXO WELLCOME)
CEREBYX INJECTION (PARKE-DAVIS)
CEREZYME FOR INJECTION (GENZYME)

CERIVASTATIN SODIUM

Baycol Tablets (BAYER)
CEROSE-DM (WYETH-AYERST)
CERTIVA INJECTION (NORTH AMERICAN VACCINE)
CERUBIDINE FOR INJECTION (BEDFORD)
CERUMENEX EARDROPS (PURDUE FREDERICK)
CERVIDIL VAGINAL INSERT (FOREST)
CETACAINE TOPICAL ANESTHETIC (CETYLITE)
CETAMIDE OINTMENT (ALCON)
CETAPHIL GENTLE CLEANSING BAR (GALDERMA)
CETAPHIL ANTIBACTERIAL GENTLE CLEANSING BAR (GALDERMA)
CETAPHIL GENTLE SKIN CLEANSER (GALDERMA)
CETAPHIL OILY SKIN CLEANSER (GALDERMA)
CETAPHIL MOISTURIZING CREAM (GALDERMA)
CETAPHIL MOISTURIZING LOTION (GALDERMA)
CETAPRED OINTMENT (ALCON)

CETIRIZINE HYDROCHLORIDE

Zyrtec Syrup (PFIZER)
Zyrtec Tablets (PFIZER)

CETYL ALCOHOL

Exosurf Neonatal for Intratracheal Suspension (GLAXO WELLCOME)
CETYLCIDE G STERILANT (CETYLITE)
CETYLCIDE II GERMICIDAL CONCENTRATE (CETYLITE)
CETYLITE AIRFRESH DEODORIZER (CETYLITE)
CETYLITE SKIN SCREEN PROTECTIVE SKIN LOTION (CETYLITE)

CHARCOAL, ACTIVATED

Actidose with Sorbitol Suspension (PADDOCK)
Actidose-Aqua Suspension (PADDOCK)
Charcoal Plus DS Enteric Coated Tablets (KRAMER)
CHARCOAL PLUS DS ENTERIC COATED TABLETS (KRAMER)
CHELATED MINERAL TABLETS (USANA)
CHEMET CAPSULES (SANOFI)
CHIBROXIN STERILE OPHTHALMIC SOLUTION (MERCK)
CHIROCAINE INJECTION (PURDUE PHARMA)
CHLOR-3 (FLEMING)

CHLORAL HYDRATE
  Chloral Hydrate Syrup USP
    (PHARMACEUTICAL ASSOCIATES)
CHLORAL HYDRATE SYRUP USP
  (PHARMACEUTICAL ASSOCIATES)
CHLORAMBUCIL
  Leukeran Tablets (GLAXO WELLCOME)
CHLORDIAZEPOXIDE
  Chlordiazepoxide and Amitriptyline
    Hydrochloride Tablets (MYLAN)
  Limbitrol DS Tablets (ICN)
  Limbitrol Tablets (ICN)
**CHLORDIAZEPOXIDE AND
  AMITRIPTYLINE HYDROCHLORIDE
  TABLETS** (MYLAN)
CHLORDIAZEPOXIDE HYDROCHLORIDE
  Chlordiazepoxide Hydrochloride Capsules CIV
    (WATSON)
  Librium Capsules (ICN)
  Librium for Injection (ICN)
**CHLORDIAZEPOXIDE HYDROCHLORIDE
  CAPSULES CIV** (WATSON)
CHLORESIUM OINTMENT (RYSTAN)
CHLORESIUM SOLUTION (RYSTAN)
CHLORESIUM TABLETS (RYSTAN)
CHLORESIUM TOOTHPASTE (RYSTAN)
CHLORHEXIDINE GLUCONATE
  Betasept Surgical Scrub (PURDUE FREDERICK)
  Hibiclens Antimicrobial Skin Cleanser
    (ASTRAZENECA)
  Hibistat Germicidal Hand Rinse
    (ASTRAZENECA)
  Hibistat Towelette (ASTRAZENECA)
  Periogard Oral Rinse (COLGATE ORAL)
CHLOROETHANE
  Gebauer's Ethyl Chloride (GEBAUER)
CHLOROMYCETIN OTIC (MONARCH)
CHLOROPHYLLIN COPPER COMPLEX
SODIUM
  Chloresium Ointment (RYSTAN)
  Chloresium Solution (RYSTAN)
  Derifil Tablets (RYSTAN)
  Panafil Ointment (HEALTHPOINT)
CHLOROPROCAINE HYDROCHLORIDE
  Nesacaine Injection (ASTRAZENECA LP)
  Nesacaine-MPF Injection (ASTRAZENECA LP)
**CHLOROPROCAINE HYDROCHLORIDE
  INJECTION, USP** (BEDFORD)
CHLOROPTIC OPHTHALMIC OINTMENT
  (ALLERGAN)
CHLOROPTIC OPHTHALMIC SOLUTION
  (ALLERGAN)
CHLOROQUINE HYDROCHLORIDE
  Aralen Hydrochloride Injection (SANOFI)
CHLOROQUINE PHOSPHATE
  Aralen Tablets (SANOFI)
CHLOROTHIAZIDE
  Aldoclor Tablets (MERCK)
  Chlorothiazide Tablets (MYLAN)
  Diuril Oral Suspension (MERCK)
  Diuril Tablets (MERCK)
CHLOROTHIAZIDE SODIUM
  Diuril Sodium Intravenous (MERCK)
CHLOROTHIAZIDE TABLETS (MYLAN)
CHLOROXYLENOL
  Cortane-B Ear Drops (BLANSETT)
  Cortane-B Otic Vials (BLANSETT)
  Cortic Ear Drops (EVERETT)
  Gordochom Solution (GORDON)
  Zoto-HC Ear Drops (HORIZON)

CHLORPHENIRAMINE
  Nalex-A Liquid (BLANSETT)
CHLORPHENIRAMINE MALEATE
  Ah-Chew Chewable Tablets (WE)
  Alumadrine Tablets (FLEMING)
  Ana-Kit Anaphylaxis Emergency Treatment Kit
    (BAYER ALLERGY)
  Anaplex HD Cough Syrup (ECR)
  Atrohist Pediatric Capsules (MEDEVA)
  Atrohist Plus Tablets (MEDEVA)
  Biohist LA Tablets (WAKEFIELD)
  Children's Tylenol Cold Liquid and Chewable
    Tablets (MCNEIL CONSUMER)
  Children's Tylenol Cold Plus Cough
    Suspension Liquid and Chewable Tablets
    (MCNEIL CONSUMER)
  Children's Tylenol Flu Suspension Liquid
    (MCNEIL CONSUMER)
  D.A. Chewable Tablets (DJ PHARMA)
  D.A. II Tablets (DJ PHARMA)
  Dallergy Caplets, Syrup, Tablets (LASER)
  Donatussin Drops (LASER)
  Donatussin Syrup (LASER)
  Dura-Vent/DA Tablets (DJ PHARMA)
  Endal-HD (FOREST)
  Extendryl Chewable Tablets (FLEMING)
  Extendryl Sr. & Jr. Capsules (FLEMING)
  Extendryl Syrup (FLEMING)
  Histussin HC Syrup (SANOFI)
  Hycomine Compound Tablets (ENDO LABS)
  Kronofed-A Kronocaps (FERNDALE)
  Kronofed-A-Jr. Kronocaps (FERNDALE)
  Mescolor Tablets (HORIZON)
  Nalex-A Tablets (BLANSETT)
  Nolamine Timed-Release Tablets (CARNRICK)
  Norel DM Liquid (U.S. PHARMACEUTICAL)
  Norel Plus Capsules (U.S. PHARMACEUTICAL)
  Omnihist L.A. Tablets (WE)
  Ornade Spansule Capsules
    (SMITHKLINE BEECHAM)
  Pediacof Syrup (SANOFI)
  Propade Extended-Release Capsules
    (MALLINCKRODT)
  Protid Tablets (LUNSCO)
  Respa-A.R.M. Tablets (RESPA)
  Sinulin Tablets (CARNRICK)
  Sinutab Sinus Allergy MS Caplets and Tablets
    (WARNER-LAMBERT)
  Sudafed Cold & Allergy Tablets
    (WARNER-LAMBERT)
  Tussend Syrup (MONARCH)
  Tussend Tablets (MONARCH)
  Tylenol Allergy Sinus, Maximum Strength
    Caplets, Gelcaps, and Geltabs
    (MCNEIL CONSUMER)
  Tylenol Cold Complete Formula, Multi-
    Symptom Tablets and Caplets
    (MCNEIL CONSUMER)
CHLORPHENIRAMINE POLISTIREX
  Tussionex Pennkinetic Extended-Release
    Suspension (MEDEVA)
CHLORPHENIRAMINE TANNATE
  Atrohist Pediatric Suspension Dye-Free
    (MEDEVA)
  Rynatan-P Pediatric Suspension (WALLACE)
  Rynatan-S Pediatric Suspension (WALLACE)
  Rynatuss Pediatric Suspension (WALLACE)
  Rynatuss Tablets (WALLACE)
  Tanafed Suspension (HORIZON)
  Tussi-12 Suspension (WALLACE)
CHLORPROMAZINE
  Thorazine Suppositories (SMITHKLINE BEECHAM)
CHLORPROMAZINE HCL TABLETS
  (GENEVA)

CHLORPROMAZINE HYDROCHLORIDE
  Chlorpromazine HCl Tablets (GENEVA)
  Chlorpromazine Hydrochloride Injection
    (ELKINS-SINN)
  Chlorpromazine Hydrochloride Intensol
    (ROXANE)
  Thorazine Ampuls (SMITHKLINE BEECHAM)
  Thorazine Concentrate (SMITHKLINE BEECHAM)
  Thorazine Multi-dose Vials
    (SMITHKLINE BEECHAM)
  Thorazine Spansule Capsules
    (SMITHKLINE BEECHAM)
  Thorazine Syrup (SMITHKLINE BEECHAM)
  Thorazine Tablets (SMITHKLINE BEECHAM)
**CHLORPROMAZINE HYDROCHLORIDE
  INJECTION** (ELKINS-SINN)
**CHLORPROMAZINE HYDROCHLORIDE
  INTENSOL** (ROXANE)
CHLORPROPAMIDE
  Chlorpropamide Tablets (MYLAN)
  Diabinese Tablets (PFIZER)
CHLORPROPAMIDE TABLETS (MYLAN)
CHLORTHALIDONE
  Atenolol and Chlorthalidone Tablets (MYLAN)
  Chlorthalidone Tablets (MYLAN)
  Clorpres Tablets (BERTEK)
  Combipres Tablets (BOEHRINGER INGELHEIM)
  Hygroton Tablets (RHONE-POULENC RORER)
  Tenoretic Tablets (ASTRAZENECA)
  Thalitone Tablets (MONARCH)
CHLORTHALIDONE TABLETS (MYLAN)
CHLOR-TRIMETON INJECTION (SCHERING)
CHLORZOXAZONE
  Chlorzoxazone Tablets, USP (WATSON)
  Parafon Forte DSC Caplets (ORTHO-MCNEIL)
CHLORZOXAZONE TABLETS, USP
  (WATSON)
**CHOLEDYL SA EXTENDED-RELEASE
  TABLETS** (WARNER CHILCOTT)
CHOLERA VACCINE (WYETH-AYERST)
CHOLERA VACCINE
  Cholera Vaccine (WYETH-AYERST)
CHOLESTIN CAPSULES (PHARMANEX)
CHOLESTYRAMINE
  Cholestyramine Oral Solution, Regular and
    Light, Reg 4g/9g, Light 4g/5g (NOVOPHARM)
  Prevalite Powder (UPSHER-SMITH)
**CHOLESTYRAMINE FOR ORAL
  SUSPENSION LIGHT, USP** (APOTHECON)
**CHOLESTYRAMINE FOR ORAL
  SUSPENSION, USP** (APOTHECON)
**CHOLESTYRAMINE ORAL SOLUTION,
  REGULAR AND LIGHT, REG 4G/9G,
  LIGHT 4G/5G** (NOVOPHARM)
CHOLINE BITARTRATE
  Mega-B Tablets (ARCO)
  Megadose Tablets (ARCO)
CHOLINE MAGNESIUM TRISALICYLATE
  Trilisate Liquid (PURDUE FREDERICK)
  Trilisate Tablets (PURDUE FREDERICK)
CHOLOXIN (KNOLL LABS)
CHONDROITIN SULFATE
  ArthriFlex (MAYOR)
  Vitamist Intra-Oral Spray Dietary Supplements
    (MAYOR)
CHONDRO-PRO ARTHRITIS FORMULA
  (MDR FITNESS)
CHORIONIC GONADOTROPIN
  A.P.L. (WYETH-AYERST)
  Novarel for Injection (FERRING)
  Pregnyl for Injection (ORGANON)
  Profasi for Injection (SERONO)

CHROMAGEN CAPSULES (SAVAGE)
CHROMAGEN FA CAPSULES (SAVAGE)
CHROMAGEN FORTE CAPSULES (SAVAGE)
CHROMAGEN OB CAPSULES (SAVAGE)

CHROMIUM

Slender-Mist (MAYOR)
Vitamist Intra-Oral Spray Dietary Supplements
(MAYOR)
CHROMIUM 10 ML (4 MCG/ML) (ABBOTT)
CHROMIUM GTF 1MG (VITALINE)

CHROMIUM PICOLINATE

Chelated Mineral Tablets (USANA)
CHROMIUM PICOLINATE 1.6 MG
(MERICON)
**CHROMIUM PICOLINATE 200 AND
500MCG** (VITALINE)
CHRONULAC SOLUTION
(HOECHST MARION ROUSSEL)
**CHYMODIACTIN (CHYMOPAPAIN FOR
INJECTION)** (KNOLL LABS)

CICLOPIROX OLAMINE

Loprox Cream (MEDICIS)
Loprox Lotion (MEDICIS)

CIDOFOVIR

Vistide Injection (GILEAD)

CILASTATIN

Primaxin I.M. (MERCK)
Primaxin I.V. (MERCK)

CILOSTAZOL

Pletal Tablets (OTSUKA AMERICA)
Pletal Tablets (PHARMACIA & UPJOHN)
CILOXAN OPHTHALMIC OINTMENT
(ALCON)
CILOXAN OPHTHALMIC SOLUTION
(ALCON)

CIMETIDINE

Cimetidine Tablets (MYLAN)
Cimetidine Tablets (GENEVA)
Cimetidine Tablets (LEDERLE STANDARD)
Cimetidine Tablets, 200 mg (NOVOPHARM)
Cimetidine Tablets, 300 mg (NOVOPHARM)
Cimetidine Tablets, 400 mg (NOVOPHARM)
Cimetidine Tablets, 800 mg (NOVOPHARM)
Cimetidine Tablets, USP (ENDO GENERICS)
Tagamet Tablets (SMITHKLINE BEECHAM)
CIMETIDINE HCL ORAL SOLUTION
(ROXANE)

CIMETIDINE HYDROCHLORIDE

Cimetidine HCl Oral Solution (ROXANE)
Cimetidine Hydrochloride Injection
(ENDO GENERICS)
Cimetidine Hydrochloride Oral Solution
(ENDO GENERICS)
Cimetidine Hydrochloride Oral Solution
(PHARMACEUTICAL ASSOCIATES)
Tagamet Injection (SMITHKLINE BEECHAM)
Tagamet Liquid (SMITHKLINE BEECHAM)
**CIMETIDINE HYDROCHLORIDE
INJECTION** (ENDO GENERICS)
**CIMETIDINE HYDROCHLORIDE ORAL
SOLUTION** (ENDO GENERICS)
**CIMETIDINE HYDROCHLORIDE ORAL
SOLUTION** (PHARMACEUTICAL ASSOCIATES)
CIMETIDINE TABLETS (MYLAN)
CIMETIDINE TABLETS (GENEVA)
CIMETIDINE TABLETS (LEDERLE STANDARD)
CIMETIDINE TABLETS, USP
(ENDO GENERICS)
CIMETIDINE TABLETS, 200 MG
(NOVOPHARM)
CIMETIDINE TABLETS, 300 MG
(NOVOPHARM)

CIMETIDINE TABLETS, 400 MG
(NOVOPHARM)
CIMETIDINE TABLETS, 800 MG
(NOVOPHARM)
CINOBAC CAPSULES, 250MG, 500MG
(OCLASSEN)
CIPRO HC OTIC SUSPENSION (ALCON)
CIPRO I.V. (BAYER)
CIPRO I.V. PHARMACY BULK PACKAGE
(BAYER)
CIPRO ORAL SUSPENSION (BAYER)
CIPRO TABLETS (BAYER)

CIPROFLOXACIN

Cipro I.V. (BAYER)
Cipro I.V. Pharmacy Bulk Package (BAYER)
Cipro Oral Suspension (BAYER)

CIPROFLOXACIN HYDROCHLORIDE

Ciloxan Ophthalmic Ointment (ALCON)
Ciloxan Ophthalmic Solution (ALCON)
Cipro HC Otic Suspension (ALCON)
Cipro Tablets (BAYER)

CISAPRIDE

Propulsid Suspension (JANSSEN)
Propulsid Tablets (JANSSEN)

CISATRACURIUM BESYLATE

Nimbex Injection (GLAXO WELLCOME)

CISPLATIN

Platinol-AQ Injection
(BRISTOL-MYERSSQUIBBONCOLOGY/IMMUNOLOGY)

CITALOPRAM HYDROBROMIDE

Celexa Tablets (FOREST)
CITANEST SOLUTIONS (ASTRAZENECA LP)
CITRACAL LIQUITABS (MISSION)
CITRACAL TABLETS (MISSION)
CITRACAL CAPLETS + D (MISSION)
CITRADERM FACIAL COMPLEX CREAM
(PEDINOL)

CITRIC ACID

Bicitra (ALZA)
Polycitra Syrup and Polycitra-LC Syrup (ALZA)
Polycitra-K Crystals (ALZA)
Polycitra-K Oral Solution (ALZA)
Potassium Citrate and Citric Acid Oral
Solution USP
(PHARMACEUTICAL ASSOCIATES)
Renacidin Irrigation (GUARDIAN)
Sodium Citrate and Citric Acid Oral Solution
USP (PHARMACEUTICAL ASSOCIATES)
CITROLITH TABLETS (BEACH)

CLADRIBINE

Leustatin Injection (ORTHO BIOTECH)
CLAFORAN (HOECHST MARION ROUSSEL)

CLARITHROMYCIN

Biaxin Filmtab Tablets (ABBOTT)
Biaxin for Oral Suspension (ABBOTT)
PREVPAC (TAP)
CLARITIN REDITABS (SCHERING)
CLARITIN SYRUP (SCHERING)
CLARITIN TABLETS (SCHERING)
**CLARITIN-D 12 HOUR EXTENDED
RELEASE TABLETS** (SCHERING)
**CLARITIN-D 24 HOUR EXTENDED
RELEASE TABLETS** (SCHERING)

CLAVULANATE POTASSIUM

Augmentin Powder for Oral Suspension and
Chewable Tablets (SMITHKLINE BEECHAM)
Augmentin Tablets (SMITHKLINE BEECHAM)
Timentin for Injection (SMITHKLINE BEECHAM)
**CLEAR EYES ACR
ASTRINGENT/LUBRICANT EYE
REDNESS RELIEVER DROPS** (ROSS)

CLEAR EYES CLR SOOTHING DROPS
(ROSS)
**CLEAR EYES LUBRICANT EYE REDNESS
RELIEVER DROPS** (ROSS)

CLEMASTINE FUMARATE

Clemastine Fumarate Syrup (GENEVA)
Clemastine Fumarate Tablets (GENEVA)
CLEMASTINE FUMARATE SYRUP (GENEVA)
CLEMASTINE FUMARATE TABLETS
(GENEVA)
CLEOCIN HCL CAPSULES
(PHARMACIA & UPJOHN)
**CLEOCIN PEDIATRIC FLAVORED
GRANULES** (PHARMACIA & UPJOHN)
**CLEOCIN PHOSPHATE STERILE
SOLUTION** (PHARMACIA & UPJOHN)
CLEOCIN T TOPICAL GEL
(PHARMACIA & UPJOHN)
CLEOCIN T TOPICAL LOTION
(PHARMACIA & UPJOHN)
CLEOCIN T TOPICAL SOLUTION
(PHARMACIA & UPJOHN)
CLEOCIN VAGINAL CREAM
(PHARMACIA & UPJOHN)
CLIMARA TRANSDERMAL SYSTEM
(BERLEX)
CLINDA-DERM SOLUTION (PADDOCK)
CLINDAMYCIN HCL CAPSULES, USP
(SCHEIN)

CLINDAMYCIN HYDROCHLORIDE

Cleocin HCl Capsules (PHARMACIA & UPJOHN)

CLINDAMYCIN PHOSPHATE

Cleocin Phosphate Sterile Solution
(PHARMACIA & UPJOHN)
Cleocin T Topical Gel (PHARMACIA & UPJOHN)
Cleocin T Topical Lotion
(PHARMACIA & UPJOHN)
Cleocin T Topical Solution
(PHARMACIA & UPJOHN)
Cleocin Vaginal Cream (PHARMACIA & UPJOHN)
Clindets Pledgets (STIEFEL)
CLINDETS PLEDGETS (STIEFEL)
CLINORIL TABLETS (MERCK)

CLOBETASOL PROPIONATE

Cormax Cream (OCLASSEN)
Cormax Ointment (OCLASSEN)
Cormax Scalp Application (OCLASSEN)
Embeline E Cream (HEALTHPOINT)
Temovate Cream (GLAXO WELLCOME)
Temovate E Emollient (GLAXO WELLCOME)
Temovate Gel (GLAXO WELLCOME)
Temovate Ointment (GLAXO WELLCOME)
Temovate Scalp Application
(GLAXO WELLCOME)

CLOCORTOLONE PIVALATE

Cloderm Cream (HEALTHPOINT)
CLODERM CREAM (HEALTHPOINT)

CLOFIBRATE

Atromid-S Capsules (WYETH-AYERST)
Clofibrate Capsules USP, 500 mg
(NOVOPHARM)
CLOFIBRATE CAPSULES USP, 500 MG
(NOVOPHARM)
CLOMID TABLETS
(HOECHST MARION ROUSSEL)

CLOMIPHENE CITRATE

Clomid Tablets (HOECHST MARION ROUSSEL)
Clomiphene Citrate Tablets (WATSON)
Serophene Tablets (SERONO)
CLOMIPHENE CITRATE TABLETS
(WATSON)
CLOMIPHENE TABLETS (PAR)

UNDERLINE DENOTES GENERIC NAME

CLOMIPRAMINE CAPSULES, 25 MG, 50 MG, 75 MG (NOVOPHARM)
CLOMIPRAMINE HCL CAPSULES (GENEVA)

CLOMIPRAMINE HYDROCHLORIDE

Clomipramine Capsules, 25 mg, 50 mg, 75 mg (NOVOPHARM)
Clomipramine HCl Capsules (GENEVA)
Clomipramine Hydrochloride Capsules (MYLAN)
Clomipramine Hydrochloride Capsules (WATSON)
CLOMIPRAMINE HYDROCHLORIDE CAPSULES (MYLAN)
CLOMIPRAMINE HYDROCHLORIDE CAPSULES (WATSON)

CLONAZEPAM

Clonazepam CIV Tablets, 0.5 mg, 1 mg, 2 mg (NOVOPHARM)
Clonazepam Tablets (PAR)
Clonazepam Tablets (MYLAN)
Clonazepam Tablets, USP CIV (WATSON)
Klonopin Tablets (ROCHE LABS)
CLONAZEPAM CIV TABLETS, 0.5 MG, 1 MG, 2 MG (NOVOPHARM)
CLONAZEPAM TABLETS (PAR)
CLONAZEPAM TABLETS (MYLAN)
CLONAZEPAM TABLETS, USP CIV (WATSON)

CLONIDINE

Catapres-TTS (BOEHRINGER INGELHEIM)
CLONIDINE HCL TABLETS (LEDERLE STANDARD)

CLONIDINE HYDROCHLORIDE

Catapres Tablets (BOEHRINGER INGELHEIM)
Clonidine HCl Tablets (LEDERLE STANDARD)
Clonidine Hydrochloride Tablets (MYLAN)
Clorpres Tablets (BERTEK)
Combipres Tablets (BOEHRINGER INGELHEIM)
Duraclon Injection (ROXANE)
CLONIDINE HYDROCHLORIDE TABLETS (MYLAN)

CLOPIDOGREL BISULFATE

Plavix Tablets (SANOFI)
Plavix Tablets (BRISTOL-MYERS SQUIBB)

CLORAZEPATE DIPOTASSIUM

Clorazepate Dipotassium Tablets (MYLAN)
Clorazepate Dipotassium Tablets CIV (WATSON)
Tranxene T-TAB Tablets (ABBOTT)
Tranxene-SD Half Strength Tablets (ABBOTT)
Tranxene-SD Tablets (ABBOTT)
CLORAZEPATE DIPOTASSIUM TABLETS (MYLAN)
CLORAZEPATE DIPOTASSIUM TABLETS CIV (WATSON)
CLORAZEPATE TABLETS CIV, 3.75 MG, 7.5MG, 15 MG (NOVOPHARM)
CLORPACTIN WCS-90 (GUARDIAN)
CLORPRES TABLETS (BERTEK)

CLOTRIMAZOLE

Fungoid Solution (PEDINOL)
Lotrimin Cream 1% (SCHERING)
Lotrimin Lotion 1% (SCHERING)
Lotrimin Topical Solution 1% (SCHERING)
Lotrisone Cream (SCHERING)
Mycelex Troche (ALZA)
Mycelex-G 500 mg Vaginal Tablets (BAYER)

CLOZAPINE

Clozapine Tablets (MYLAN)
Clozaril Tablets (NOVARTIS)
CLOZAPINE TABLETS (MYLAN)
CLOZARIL TABLETS (NOVARTIS)

COAL TAR

DHS Tar Gel Shampoo (PERSON & COVEY)
DHS Tar Shampoo (PERSON & COVEY)
Zetar Emulsion (DERMIK)

COCAINE HYDROCHLORIDE

Cocaine Hydrochloride Topical Solution (ROXANE)
Cocaine Hydrochloride Topical Solution (ASTRAZENECA LP)
COCAINE HYDROCHLORIDE TOPICAL SOLUTION (ROXANE)
COCAINE HYDROCHLORIDE TOPICAL SOLUTION (ASTRAZENECA LP)

CODEINE PHOSPHATE

Acetaminophen and Codeine Phosphate Oral Solution USP (PHARMACEUTICAL ASSOCIATES)
Acetaminophen and Codeine Phosphate Oral Solution and Tablets (ROXANE)
Acetaminophen and Codeine Phosphate Tablets, USP CIII (WATSON)
Butalbital, Aspirin, Caffeine, and Codeine Phosphate Capsules, USP (ENDO GENERICS)
Butalbital, Aspirin, Caffeine, and Codeine Phosphate Capsules, USP CIII (WATSON)
Capital and Codeine Oral Suspension (CARNRICK)
Codeine Phosphate Oral Solution (ROXANE)
Codeine Phosphate in Tubex (WYETH-AYERST)
Codimal PH Syrup (SCHWARZ)
Fiortal w/Codeine Capsules (GENEVA)
Guaifenesin Syrup with Codeine (PHARMACEUTICAL ASSOCIATES)
Nucofed Capsules (MONARCH)
Nucofed Pediatric Expectorant Syrup (MONARCH)
Pediacof Syrup (SANOFI)
Phenaphen with Codeine Capsules (ROBINS)
Phenergan VC with Codeine Syrup (WYETH-AYERST)
Phenergan with Codeine Syrup (WYETH-AYERST)
Poly-Histine CS Syrup (SANOFI)
Promethazine Hydrochloride and Codeine Phosphate Syrup (PHARMACEUTICAL ASSOCIATES)
Robitussin A-C Syrup (ROBINS)
Robitussin-DAC Syrup (ROBINS)
Soma Compound w/Codeine Tablets (WALLACE)
Tussi-Organidin NR Liquid (WALLACE)
Tussi-Organidin-S NR Liquid (WALLACE)
Tylenol with Codeine Elixir (ORTHO-MCNEIL)
Tylenol with Codeine Tablets (ORTHO-MCNEIL)
CODEINE PHOSPHATE IN TUBEX (WYETH-AYERST)
CODEINE PHOSPHATE INJECTION (WYETH-AYERST)
CODEINE PHOSPHATE ORAL SOLUTION (ROXANE)

CODEINE SULFATE

Codeine Sulfate Tablets (ROXANE)
CODEINE SULFATE TABLETS (ROXANE)
CODEINE SULFATE TABLETS (KNOLL LABS)
CODICLEAR DH SYRUP (SCHWARZ)
CODIMAL DH SYRUP (SCHWARZ)
CODIMAL DM SYRUP (SCHWARZ)
CODIMAL PH SYRUP (SCHWARZ)

COENZYME Q-10

CardioCare (MAYOR)
Coenzyme Q10 200mg, 100mg & 60mg Chewable Wafers, 200mg, 60mg and 25mg Tablets, and 60mg Softgels (VITALINE)

Eucerin Q10 Anti-Wrinkle Sensitive Skin Creme (BEIERSDORF)
Q-Bid (NUTRACEUTICS)
Vitamist Intra-Oral Spray Dietary Supplements (MAYOR)
COENZYME Q10 200MG, 100MG & 60MG CHEWABLE WAFERS, 200MG, 60MG AND 25MG TABLETS, AND 60MG SOFTGELS (VITALINE)
COENZYME Q-10 CHEWABLE TABLETS (WESTLAKE)
CO-GEL TABLETS (ARCO)
COGENTIN INJECTION (MERCK)
COGENTIN TABLETS (MERCK)
CO-GESIC TABLETS (SCHWARZ)
COGNEX CAPSULES (PARKE-DAVIS)
COLACE CAPSULES, SYRUP, LIQUID (ROBERTS)
COLACE GLYCERIN SUPPOSITORIES (ROBERTS)
COLACE MICROENEMA (ROBERTS)
COLBENEMID TABLETS (MERCK)

COLCHICINE

ColBENEMID Tablets (MERCK)
COLCHICINE INJECTION, USP (BEDFORD)
COLCHICINE TABLETS (ABBOTT)
COLCHICINE TABLETS, USP (SCHEIN)
COLESTID TABLETS (PHARMACIA & UPJOHN)
COLESTID/FLAVORED COLESTID FOR ORAL SUSPENSION (PHARMACIA & UPJOHN)

COLESTIPOL HYDROCHLORIDE

Colestid Tablets (PHARMACIA & UPJOHN)
Colestid/Flavored Colestid for Oral Suspension (PHARMACIA & UPJOHN)

COLFOSCERIL PALMITATE

Exosurf Neonatal for Intratracheal Suspension (GLAXO WELLCOME)

COLISTIMETHATE SODIUM

Coly-Mycin M Parenteral (MONARCH)

COLISTIN SULFATE

Cortisporin-TC Otic Suspension (MONARCH)
COLISTIN SULFATE USP POWDER (PADDOCK)

COLLAGENASE

Collagenase Santyl Ointment (KNOLL LABS)
COLLAGENASE SANTYL OINTMENT (KNOLL LABS)
COLLOIDAL MINERALS (MAYOR)
COLY-MYCIN M PARENTERAL (MONARCH)
COLYTE FOR ORAL SOLUTION (SCHWARZ)
COLYTE - FLAVORED FOR ORAL SOLUTION (SCHWARZ)
COLYTE WITH FLAVOR PACKS FOR ORAL SOLUTION (SCHWARZ)
COMBIPATCH TRANSDERMAL SYSTEM (RHONE-POULENC RORER)
COMBIPRES TABLETS (BOEHRINGER INGELHEIM)
COMBIVENT INHALATION AEROSOL (BOEHRINGER INGELHEIM)
COMBIVIR TABLETS (GLAXO WELLCOME)
COMPAZINE MULTI-DOSE VIALS (SMITHKLINE BEECHAM)
COMPAZINE SPANSULE CAPSULES (SMITHKLINE BEECHAM)
COMPAZINE SUPPOSITORIES (SMITHKLINE BEECHAM)
COMPAZINE SYRUP (SMITHKLINE BEECHAM)
COMPAZINE TABLETS (SMITHKLINE BEECHAM)
COMPAZINE VIALS (SMITHKLINE BEECHAM)
COMPETE (MISSION)
COMTREX ACUTE HEAD COLD & SINUS RELIEF (BRISTOL-MYERS)

UNDERLINE DENOTES GENERIC NAME

COMTREX ALLERGY-SINUS TREATMENT, MAXIMUM STRENGTH (BRISTOL-MYERS)
COMTREX DEEP CHEST COLD & CONGESTION RELIEF NON-DROWSY (BRISTOL-MYERS)
COMTREX MAXIMUM STRENGTH MULTI-SYMPTOM COLD & FLU RELIEF (BRISTOL-MYERS)
COMTREX MAXIMUM STRENGTH MULTI-SYMPTOM DAY/NIGHT (BRISTOL-MYERS)
COMTREX MAXIMUM STRENGTH MULTI-SYMPTOM NON-DROWSY (BRISTOL-MYERS)
COMVAX (MERCK)
CONDYLOX GEL (OCLASSEN)
CONDYLOX TOPICAL SOLUTION (OCLASSEN)
COPAXONE FOR INJECTION (TEVA MARION)

COPPER

Chelated Mineral Tablets (USANA)
ParaGard T 380A Intrauterine Copper Contraceptive (ORTHO-MCNEIL)
COPPER 10 ML (0.4 MG/ML) (ABBOTT)
COQUINONE CAPSULES (USANA)
CORDARONE INTRAVENOUS (WYETH-AYERST)
CORDARONE TABLETS (WYETH-AYERST)
CORDARONE TABLETS, 200 MG (WYETH-AYERST)
CORDRAN LOTION (OCLASSEN)
CORDRAN OINTMENT 0.025%, 30G, 60G (OCLASSEN)
CORDRAN OINTMENT 0.05%, 15G, 30G, 60G (OCLASSEN)
CORDRAN SP CREAM 0.025%, 30G, 60G (OCLASSEN)
CORDRAN SP CREAM 0.05%, 15G, 30G, 60G (OCLASSEN)
CORDRAN TAPE (OCLASSEN)

CORDYCEPS SINENSIS

CordyMax Cs-4 Capsules (PHARMANEX)
CORDYMAX CS-4 CAPSULES (PHARMANEX)
COREG TABLETS (SMITHKLINE BEECHAM)
CORLOPAM INJECTION (NEUREX)
CORMAX CREAM (OCLASSEN)
CORMAX OINTMENT (OCLASSEN)
CORMAX SCALP APPLICATION (OCLASSEN)
CORTANE-B EAR DROPS (BLANSETT)
CORTANE-B OTIC AQUEOUS (BLANSETT)
CORTANE-B OTIC LOTION (BLANSETT)
CORTANE-B OTIC PLAIN (BLANSETT)
CORTANE-B OTIC VIALS (BLANSETT)
CORT-DOME HIGH POTENCY SUPPOSITORIES (BAYER)
CORTEF ORAL SUSPENSION (PHARMACIA & UPJOHN)
CORTEF TABLETS (PHARMACIA & UPJOHN)
CORTENEMA (SOLVAY)
CORTIC EAR DROPS (EVERETT)
CORTICAINE CREAM (UCB)

CORTICORELIN OVINE TRIFLUTATE

Acthrel for Injection (FERRING)
CORTIFOAM (SCHWARZ)

CORTISONE ACETATE

Cortone Acetate Injectable Suspension (MERCK)
Cortone Acetate Tablets (MERCK)
CORTISONE ACETATE TABLETS, USP (PHARMACIA & UPJOHN)
CORTISPORIN CREAM (MONARCH)
CORTISPORIN OINTMENT (MONARCH)
CORTISPORIN OPHTHALMIC OINTMENT STERILE (MONARCH)
CORTISPORIN OPHTHALMIC SUSPENSION STERILE (MONARCH)

CORTISPORIN OTIC SOLUTION STERILE (MONARCH)
CORTISPORIN OTIC SUSPENSION STERILE (MONARCH)
CORTISPORIN-TC OTIC SUSPENSION (MONARCH)
CORTONE ACETATE INJECTABLE SUSPENSION (MERCK)
CORTONE ACETATE TABLETS (MERCK)
CORTROSYN FOR INJECTION (ORGANON)
CORVERT INJECTION (PHARMACIA & UPJOHN)
CORZIDE (SEE BRISTOL-MYERS SQUIBB COMPANY) (APOTHECON)
CORZIDE 40/5 TABLETS (BRISTOL-MYERS SQUIBB)
CORZIDE 80/5 TABLETS (BRISTOL-MYERS SQUIBB)
COSAMIN DS CAPSULES (NUTRAMAX)
COSMEGEN FOR INJECTION (MERCK)
COSOPT STERILE OPHTHALMIC SOLUTION (MERCK)

COSYNTROPIN

Cortrosyn for Injection (ORGANON)
COTAZYM CAPSULES (ORGANON)
COTAZYM-S CAPSULES (ORGANON)
COUMADIN FOR INJECTION (DUPONT)
COUMADIN TABLETS (DUPONT)
COVERA-HS TABLETS (SEARLE)
COVERLET (BEIERSDORF)
COVERLET EYE OCCLUSOR (BEIERSDORF)
COVERLET O.R. (BEIERSDORF)
COVER-ROLL (BEIERSDORF)
COVER-STRIP (BEIERSDORF)
COZAAR TABLETS (MERCK)

CREATINE PHOSPHATE

Cardiotropin (NUTRACEUTICS)
CREON 5 CAPSULES (SOLVAY)
CREON 10 CAPSULES (SOLVAY)
CREON 20 CAPSULES (SOLVAY)
CRINONE 4% GEL (SERONO)
CRINONE 8% GEL (SERONO)
CRIXIVAN CAPSULES (MERCK)

CROMOLYN SODIUM

Cromolyn Sodium Inhalation Solution USP (DEY)
Gastrocrom Oral Concentrate (MEDEVA)
Intal Inhaler (RHONE-POULENC RORER)
Intal Nebulizer Solution (RHONE-POULENC RORER)
Opticrom Ophthalmic Solution (ALLERGAN)
CROMOLYN SODIUM INHALATION SOLUTION USP (DEY)
PRESCRIPTION STRENGTH CRUEX CREAM (NOVARTIS CONSUMER)
CRUEX SPRAY POWDER (NOVARTIS CONSUMER)
PRESCRIPTION STRENGTH CRUEX SPRAY POWDER (NOVARTIS CONSUMER)
CRUEX SQUEEZE POWDER (NOVARTIS CONSUMER)
CUPRIMINE CAPSULES (MERCK)
CUTINOVA LINE - ADVANCED WOUND CARE (BEIERSDORF)
CUTIVATE CREAM (GLAXO WELLCOME)
CUTIVATE OINTMENT (GLAXO WELLCOME)
CV CO-FACTORS (VITALINE)
CYANOCOBALAMIN (VIT. B12) INJECTION (ELKINS-SINN)
CYANOJECT-10 (MERZ)
CYANOJECT-30 (MERZ)
CYCLINEX-1 AMINO ACID-MODIFIED MEDICAL FOOD WITH IRON (ROSS)
CYCLINEX-2 AMINO ACID-MODIFIED MEDICAL FOOD (ROSS)

CYCLOBENZAPRINE HCL TABLETS (GENEVA)

CYCLOBENZAPRINE HYDROCHLORIDE

Cyclobenzaprine HCl Tablets (GENEVA)
Cyclobenzaprine Hydrochloride Tablets (MYLAN)
Cyclobenzaprine Hydrochloride Tablets, USP (WATSON)
Cyclobenzaprine Hydrochloride Tablets, USP (ENDO GENERICS)
Flexeril Tablets (MERCK)
CYCLOBENZAPRINE HYDROCHLORIDE TABLETS (MYLAN)
CYCLOBENZAPRINE HYDROCHLORIDE TABLETS, USP (WATSON)
CYCLOBENZAPRINE HYDROCHLORIDE TABLETS, USP (ENDO GENERICS)
CYCLOBENZAPRINE HCL TABLETS, USP (SCHEIN)
CYCLOCORT TOPICAL CREAM 0.1% (FUJISAWA)
CYCLOCORT TOPICAL LOTION 0.1% (FUJISAWA)
CYCLOCORT TOPICAL OINTMENT 0.1% (FUJISAWA)
CYCLOGYL OPHTHALMIC SOLUTION (ALCON)
CYCLOMYDRIL OPHTHALMIC SOLUTION (ALCON)

CYCLOPHOSPHAMIDE

Cytoxan Tablets (BRISTOL-MYERSSQUIBBONCOLOGY/IMMUNOLOGY)
Cytoxan for Injection (BRISTOL-MYERSSQUIBBONCOLOGY/IMMUNOLOGY)

CYCLOSERINE

Seromycin Capsules (DURA)

CYCLOSPORINE

Neoral Oral Solution for Microemulsion (NOVARTIS)
Neoral Soft Gelatin Capsules for Microemulsion (NOVARTIS)
Sandimmune I.V. Ampuls for Infusion (NOVARTIS)
Sandimmune Oral Solution (NOVARTIS)
Sandimmune Soft Gelatin Capsules (NOVARTIS)
SangCya Oral Solution (SANGSTAT)
CYCRIN TABLETS (ESI LEDERLE)
CYKLOKAPRON AMPOULE (PHARMACIA & UPJOHN)
CYLERT (PEMOLINE) (SEE ABBOTT LABORATORIES) (ROSS)
CYLERT TABLETS (ABBOTT)
CYLERT CHEWABLE TABLETS (ABBOTT)

CYPROHEPTADINE HYDROCHLORIDE

Periactin Syrup (MERCK)
Periactin Tablets (MERCK)
CYSTAGON CAPSULES (MYLAN)

CYSTAMINE BITARTRATE

Cystagon Capsules (MYLAN)
CYSTEINE HYDROCHLORIDE INJECTION (ABBOTT)
CYSTITOMES & CANNULAS (ALCON)
CYSTOSPAZ TABLETS (POLYMEDICA)
CYSTOSPAZ-M CAPSULES (POLYMEDICA)

CYTARABINE

Cytosar-U Sterile Powder (PHARMACIA & UPJOHN)
CYTARABINE FOR INJECTION, USP (BEDFORD)

CYTARABINE LIPOSOME

DepoCyt Injection (CHIRON)
CYTOGAM INTRAVENOUS (MEDIMMUNE)

UNDERLINE DENOTES GENERIC NAME

CYTOMEGALOVIRUS IMMUNE GLOBULIN
  CytoGam Intravenous (MEDIMMUNE)
CYTOMEL TABLETS (JONES)
CYTOSAR-U STERILE POWDER
  (PHARMACIA & UPJOHN)
CYTOTEC TABLETS (SEARLE)
CYTOVENE CAPSULES (ROCHE LABS)
CYTOVENE-IV (ROCHE LABS)
CYTOXAN FOR INJECTION
  (BRISTOL-MYERSSQUIBBONCOLOGY/IMMUNOLOGY)
CYTOXAN TABLETS
  (BRISTOL-MYERSSQUIBBONCOLOGY/IMMUNOLOGY)

D

D.A. CHEWABLE TABLETS (DJ PHARMA)
D.A. II TABLETS (DJ PHARMA)

DACARBAZINE
  DTIC-Dome (BAYER)

DACLIZUMAB
  Zenapax for Injection (ROCHE LABS)

DACTINOMYCIN
  Cosmegen for Injection (MERCK)
DALLERGY CAPLETS, SYRUP, TABLETS
  (LASER)
DALLERGY-JR CAPSULES (LASER)
DALMANE CAPSULES (ICN)

DALTEPARIN SODIUM
  Fragmin Injection (PHARMACIA & UPJOHN)

DANAPAROID SODIUM
  Orgaran Injection (ORGANON)

DANAZOL
  Danocrine Capsules (SANOFI)
DANOCRINE CAPSULES (SANOFI)
DANTRIUM CAPSULES
  (PROCTER & GAMBLE PHARMACEUTICALS)
DANTRIUM INTRAVENOUS
  (PROCTER & GAMBLE PHARMACEUTICALS)

DANTROLENE SODIUM
  Dantrium Capsules
    (PROCTER & GAMBLE PHARMACEUTICALS)
  Dantrium Intravenous
    (PROCTER & GAMBLE PHARMACEUTICALS)

DAPSONE
  Dapsone Tablets USP (JACOBUS)
DAPSONE TABLETS USP (JACOBUS)
DARANIDE TABLETS (MERCK)
DARAPRIM TABLETS (GLAXO WELLCOME)
DARVOCET-N 50 TABLETS (LILLY)
DARVOCET-N 100 TABLETS (LILLY)
DARVON COMPOUND-65 PULVULES (LILLY)
DARVON PULVULES (LILLY)
DARVON-N TABLETS (LILLY)

DAUNORUBICIN CITRATE LIPOSOME
  DaunoXome Injection (GILEAD)

DAUNORUBICIN HYDROCHLORIDE
  Cerubidine for Injection (BEDFORD)
**DAUNORUBICIN HYDROCHLORIDE
  INJECTION** (BEDFORD)
DAUNOXOME INJECTION (GILEAD)
DAYALETS FILMTAB (ABBOTT)
DAYALETS PLUS IRON FILMTAB (ABBOTT)
DAYPRO CAPLETS (SEARLE)
DDAVP INJECTION 4 MCG/ML
  (RHONE-POULENC RORER)

DDAVP NASAL SPRAY
  (RHONE-POULENC RORER)
DDAVP RHINAL TUBE
  (RHONE-POULENC RORER)
DDAVP TABLETS (RHONE-POULENC RORER)
DEBROX DROPS
  (SMITHKLINE BEECHAM CONSUMER)
DECADRON ELIXIR (MERCK)
DECADRON TABLETS (MERCK)
DECADRON PHOSPHATE INJECTION
  (MERCK)
**DECADRON PHOSPHATE STERILE
  OPHTHALMIC OINTMENT** (MERCK)
**DECADRON PHOSPHATE STERILE
  OPHTHALMIC SOLUTION** (MERCK)
DECADRON-LA STERILE SUSPENSION
  (MERCK)
DECA-DURABOLIN INJECTION (ORGANON)
DECAJECT-5 (MERZ)
DECAJECT-L.A. (MERZ)
DECLOMYCIN TABLETS (LEDERLE LABS)
DECONSAL II TABLETS (MEDEVA)
DECUBITENE OXYGENATED OIL
  (FERNDALE)
DEFEN-L.A. TABLETS (HORIZON)

DEFEROXAMINE MESYLATE
  Desferal Vials (NOVARTIS)
DEHYDRATED ALCOHOL INJECTION, USP
  (ABBOTT)

DEHYDROEPIANDROSTERONE (DHEA)
  DHEA (MAYOR)
  Vitamist Intra-Oral Spray Dietary Supplements
    (MAYOR)
DELATESTRYL INJECTION (BTG)

DELAVIRDINE MESYLATE
  Rescriptor Tablets (PHARMACIA & UPJOHN)
DELTASONE TABLETS (PHARMACIA & UPJOHN)
DEMADEX TABLETS AND INJECTION
  (ROCHE LABS)

DEMECARIUM BROMIDE
  Humorsol Sterile Ophthalmic Solution (MERCK)

DEMECLOCYCLINE HYDROCHLORIDE
  Declomycin Tablets (LEDERLE LABS)
DEMEROL SYRUP (SANOFI)
DEMEROL TABLETS (SANOFI)
DEMSER CAPSULES (MERCK)
DEMULEN 1/35-21 TABLETS (SEARLE)
DEMULEN 1/35-28 TABLETS (SEARLE)
DEMULEN 1/50-21 TABLETS (SEARLE)
DEMULEN 1/50-28 TABLETS (SEARLE)
DENAVIR CREAM
  (SMITHKLINE BEECHAM CONSUMER)

DENILEUKIN DIFTITOX
  Ontak Vials (LIGAND)
DEPACON INJECTION (ABBOTT)
DEPAKENE CAPSULES (ABBOTT)
DEPAKENE SYRUP (ABBOTT)
DEPAKOTE SPRINKLE CAPSULES (ABBOTT)
DEPAKOTE TABLETS (ABBOTT)
DEPEN TITRATABLE TABLETS (WALLACE)
DEPOCYT INJECTION (CHIRON)
DEPO-ESTRADIOL STERILE SOLUTION
  (PHARMACIA & UPJOHN)
DEPOJECT-40 (MERZ)
DEPOJECT-80 (MERZ)
**DEPO-MEDROL STERILE AQUEOUS
  SUSPENSION** (PHARMACIA & UPJOHN)
**DEPO-MEDROL STERILE AQUEOUS
  SUSPENSION AND SINGLE-DOSE VIAL**
  (PHARMACIA & UPJOHN)
**DEPONIT TRANSDERMAL DELIVERY
  SYSTEM** (SCHWARZ)

**DEPO-PROVERA CONTRACEPTIVE
  INJECTION** (PHARMACIA & UPJOHN)
**DEPO-PROVERA STERILE AQUEOUS
  SUSPENSION** (PHARMACIA & UPJOHN)
DEPO-TESTADIOL STERILE SOLUTION
  (PHARMACIA & UPJOHN)
**DEPO-TESTOSTERONE STERILE
  SOLUTION** (PHARMACIA & UPJOHN)
DERIFIL TABLETS (RYSTAN)
DERMABASE (PADDOCK)
DERMAMIST SPRAY (FERNDALE)
DERMA-SMOOTHE/FS TOPICAL OIL (HILL)
DERMATOP EMOLLIENT CREAM
  (ORTHO DERMATOLOGICAL)
DERMATOP OINTMENT
  (ORTHO DERMATOLOGICAL)
**PRESCRIPTION STRENGTH DESENEX
  CREAM** (NOVARTIS CONSUMER)
**DESENEX FOOT AND SNEAKER SHAKE
  POWDER** (NOVARTIS CONSUMER)
**DESENEX FOOT AND SNEAKER SPRAY
  POWDER** (NOVARTIS CONSUMER)
DESENEX OINTMENT (NOVARTIS CONSUMER)
DESENEX SHAKE POWDER
  (NOVARTIS CONSUMER)
**PRESCRIPTION STRENGTH DESENEX
  SPRAY LIQUID** (NOVARTIS CONSUMER)
DESENEX SPRAY POWDER
  (NOVARTIS CONSUMER)
**PRESCRIPTION STRENGTH DESENEX
  SPRAY POWDER** (NOVARTIS CONSUMER)
DESFERAL VIALS (NOVARTIS)

DESFLURANE
  Suprane Liquid for Inhalation (BAXTER)
DESIPRAMINE HCL TABLETS (GENEVA)

DESIPRAMINE HYDROCHLORIDE
  Desipramine HCl Tablets (GENEVA)
  Desipramine Hydrochloride Tablets (WATSON)
  Norpramin Tablets (HOECHST MARION ROUSSEL)
**DESIPRAMINE HYDROCHLORIDE
  TABLETS** (WATSON)

DESMOPRESSIN ACETATE
  DDAVP Injection 4 mcg/mL
    (RHONE-POULENC RORER)
  DDAVP Nasal Spray (RHONE-POULENC RORER)
  DDAVP Rhinal Tube (RHONE-POULENC RORER)
  DDAVP Tablets (RHONE-POULENC RORER)
  Desmopressin Acetate Injection (FERRING)
  Desmopressin Acetate Rhinal Tube (FERRING)
  Stimate Nasal Spray (CENTEON)
DESMOPRESSIN ACETATE INJECTION
  (FERRING)
DESMOPRESSIN ACETATE RHINAL TUBE
  (FERRING)
DESOGEN TABLETS (ORGANON)

DESOGESTREL
  Desogen Tablets (ORGANON)
  Mircette Tablets (ORGANON)
  Ortho-Cept 21 Tablets (ORTHO-MCNEIL)
  Ortho-Cept 28 Tablets (ORTHO-MCNEIL)

DESONIDE
  DesOwen Cream (GALDERMA)
  DesOwen Lotion (GALDERMA)
  DesOwen Ointment (GALDERMA)
  Tridesilon Cream (BAYER)
  Tridesilon Ointment (BAYER)
DESOWEN CREAM (GALDERMA)
DESOWEN LOTION (GALDERMA)
DESOWEN OINTMENT (GALDERMA)

DESOXIMETASONE
  Topicort Cream (MEDICIS)
  Topicort Gel (MEDICIS)
  Topicort LP Cream (MEDICIS)

UNDERLINE DENOTES GENERIC NAME

Topicort Ointment (MEDICIS)
DESOXYN GRADUMET TABLETS (ABBOTT)
DESOXYN TABLETS (ABBOTT)
DESQUAM-E 2.5 EMOLLIENT GEL
(WESTWOOD-SQUIBB)
DESQUAM-E 5 EMOLLIENT GEL
(WESTWOOD-SQUIBB)
DESQUAM-E 10 EMOLLIENT GEL
(WESTWOOD-SQUIBB)
DESQUAM-X 10 BAR (WESTWOOD-SQUIBB)
DESQUAM-X 5 GEL (WESTWOOD-SQUIBB)
DESQUAM-X 10 GEL (WESTWOOD-SQUIBB)
DESQUAM-X 5 WASH (WESTWOOD-SQUIBB)
DESQUAM-X 10 WASH (WESTWOOD-SQUIBB)
DESYREL DIVIDOSE TABLETS (APOTHECON)
DETACHOL ADHESIVE REMOVER
(FERNDALE)
DETROL TABLETS (PHARMACIA & UPJOHN)

DEXAMETHASONE

Decadron Elixir (MERCK)
Decadron Tablets (MERCK)
Dexamethasone Intensol (ROXANE)
Dexamethasone Tablets (PAR)
Dexamethasone Tablets and Oral Solution
(ROXANE)
TobraDex Ophthalmic Ointment (ALCON)
TobraDex Ophthalmic Suspension (ALCON)

DEXAMETHASONE ACETATE

Decadron-LA Sterile Suspension (MERCK)
DEXAMETHASONE ACETATE USP
MICRONIZED POWDER (PADDOCK)
DEXAMETHASONE INTENSOL (ROXANE)

DEXAMETHASONE SODIUM PHOSPHATE

Decadron Phosphate Injection (MERCK)
Decadron Phosphate Sterile Ophthalmic
Ointment (MERCK)
Decadron Phosphate Sterile Ophthalmic
Solution (MERCK)
Dexamethasone Sodium Phosphate Injection
(ELKINS-SINN)
NeoDecadron Sterile Ophthalmic Ointment
(MERCK)
NeoDecadron Sterile Ophthalmic Solution
(MERCK)
DEXAMETHASONE SODIUM PHOSPHATE
INJECTION (ELKINS-SINN)
DEXAMETHASONE SODIUM PHOSPHATE
USP POWDER (PADDOCK)
DEXAMETHASONE TABLETS (PAR)
DEXAMETHASONE TABLETS AND ORAL
SOLUTION (ROXANE)
DEXEDRINE SPANSULE CAPSULES
(SMITHKLINE BEECHAM)
DEXEDRINE TABLETS (SMITHKLINE BEECHAM)

DEXRAZOXANE

Zinecard for Injection (PHARMACIA & UPJOHN)

DEXTRAN 70

Bion Tears Lubricant Eye Drops (ALCON)
Tears Naturale Free Lubricant Eye Drops
(ALCON)
Tears Naturale II Lubricant Eye Drops
(ALCON)
6% DEXTRAN 70 W/V & 5% DEXTROSE
INJECTION (ABBOTT)
6% DEXTRAN 70 W/V & 0.9% SODIUM
CHLORIDE INJECTION (ABBOTT)

DEXTROAMPHETAMINE SACCHARATE

Adderall Tablets (SHIRE RICHWOOD)

DEXTROAMPHETAMINE SULFATE

Adderall Tablets (SHIRE RICHWOOD)
Dexedrine Spansule Capsules
(SMITHKLINE BEECHAM)
Dexedrine Tablets (SMITHKLINE BEECHAM)

DextroStat Tablets (SHIRE RICHWOOD)

DEXTROMETHORPHAN HYDROBROMIDE

Anaplex DM Cough Syrup (ECR)
Anatuss DM Syrup (MERZ)
Benylin Adult Formula (WARNER-LAMBERT)
Benylin Expectorant (WARNER-LAMBERT)
Benylin Multi-Symptom (WARNER-LAMBERT)
Benylin Pediatric (WARNER-LAMBERT)
Children's Sudafed Cough & Cold Liquid
(WARNER-LAMBERT)
Children's Tylenol Cold Plus Cough
Suspension Liquid and Chewable Tablets
(MCNEIL CONSUMER)
Children's Tylenol Flu Suspension Liquid
(MCNEIL CONSUMER)
Codimal DM Syrup (SCHWARZ)
Diabe-Tuss DM Syrup (PADDOCK)
Dimetane-DX Cough Syrup (ROBINS)
Donatussin Syrup (LASER)
Duratuss DM Elixir (UCB)
Fenesin DM Tablets (DJ PHARMA)
Guaifenesin Syrup and Dextromethorphan
(PHARMACEUTICAL ASSOCIATES)
Infants' Tylenol Cold Decongestant and Fever
Reducer Concentrated Drops Plus Cough
(MCNEIL CONSUMER)
Muco-fen 800 DM Tablets (WAKEFIELD)
Muco-fen DM Tablets (WAKEFIELD)
Norel DM Liquid (U.S. PHARMACEUTICAL)
Phenergan with Dextromethorphan Syrup
(WYETH-AYERST)
Poly-Histine DM Syrup (SANOFI)
Profen II DM Liquid (WAKEFIELD)
Profen II DM Tablets (WAKEFIELD)
Protuss-DM Tablets (HORIZON)
Respa-DM Tablets (RESPA)
Rondec-DM Oral Drops (DJ PHARMA)
Rondec-DM Syrup (DJ PHARMA)
Safe Tussin 30 Liquid (KRAMER)
Sudafed Cold & Cough Liquid Caps
(WARNER-LAMBERT)
Sudafed Severe Cold Formula MS Caplets and
Tablets (WARNER-LAMBERT)
Syn-Rx DM Tablets 14 Day Treatment
Regimen (MEDEVA)
Trikof-D Tablets (RESPA)
Tussafed-EX Syrup (EVERETT)
Tussafed-LA Caplets (EVERETT)
Tussi-Organidin DM NR Liquid (WALLACE)
Tussi-Organidin DM-S NR Liquid (WALLACE)
Tylenol Cold Complete Formula, Multi-
Symptom Tablets and Caplets
(MCNEIL CONSUMER)
Tylenol Cold Non-Drowsy, Multi-Symptom
Caplets and Gelcaps (MCNEIL CONSUMER)
Tylenol Cold Severe Congestion Non-Drowsy,
Multi-Symptom Caplets (MCNEIL CONSUMER)
Tylenol Flu NightTime, Maximum Strength
Liquid (MCNEIL CONSUMER)
Tylenol Flu Non-Drowsy, Maximum Strength
Gelcaps (MCNEIL CONSUMER)

DEXTROSE

Glutose 15, Glutose 45 (Oral Glucose Gel)
(PADDOCK)
ViTelle Nestrex Tablets (FIELDING)
Xylocaine-MPF 1.5% Solution with Dextrose
7.5% (ASTRAZENECA LP)
Xylocaine-MPF 5% with Glucose 7.5%
(ASTRAZENECA LP)
2.5% DEXTROSE & 1/2 STR LACTATED
RINGER'S INJECTION (ABBOTT)
2.5% DEXTROSE & 0.45% SODIUM
CHLORIDE INJECTION, USP (ABBOTT)
5% DEXTROSE & LACTATED RINGER'S
INJECTION (ABBOTT)

5% DEXTROSE & 0.15% POT CHL
INJECTION (20 MEQ) (ABBOTT)
5% DEXTROSE & 0.224% POT CHL
INJECTION (30 MEQ) (ABBOTT)
5% DEXTROSE & 0.3% POT CHL
INJECTION (40 MEQ) (ABBOTT)
5% DEXTROSE & RINGER'S INJECTION
(ABBOTT)
5% DEXTROSE & 0.225% SODIUM
CHLORIDE WITH 0.075% POTASSIUM
CHLORIDE INJECTION (10 MEQ)
(ABBOTT)
5% DEXTROSE & 0.225% SODIUM
CHLORIDE WITH 0.15% POTASSIUM
CHLORIDE INJECTION (20 MEQ)
(ABBOTT)
5% DEXTROSE & 0.225% SODIUM
CHLORIDE WITH 0.224% POTASSIUM
CHLORIDE INJECTION (30 MEQ)
(ABBOTT)
5% DEXTROSE & 0.225% SODIUM
CHLORIDE WITH 0.3% POTASSIUM
CHLORIDE INJECTION (40 MEQ)
(ABBOTT)
5% DEXTROSE & 0.3% SODIUM
CHLORIDE WITH 0.075% POTASSIUM
CHLORIDE INJECTION (10 MEQ)
(ABBOTT)
5% DEXTROSE & 0.3% SODIUM
CHLORIDE WITH 0.15% POTASSIUM
CHLORIDE INJECTION (20 MEQ)
(ABBOTT)
5% DEXTROSE & 0.3% SODIUM
CHLORIDE WITH 0.224% POTASSIUM
CHLORIDE INJECTION (30 MEQ)
(ABBOTT)
5% DEXTROSE & 0.45% SODIUM
CHLORIDE WITH 0.075% POTASSIUM
CHLORIDE INJECTION (10 MEQ)
(ABBOTT)
5% DEXTROSE & 0.45% SODIUM
CHLORIDE WITH 0.15% POTASSIUM
CHLORIDE INJECTION (20 MEQ)
(ABBOTT)
5% DEXTROSE & 0.45% SODIUM
CHLORIDE WITH 0.224% POTASSIUM
CHLORIDE INJECTION (30 MEQ)
(ABBOTT)
5% DEXTROSE & 0.45% SODIUM
CHLORIDE WITH 0.3% POTASSIUM
CHLORIDE INJECTION (40 MEQ)
(ABBOTT)
5% DEXTROSE & 0.225% SODIUM
CHLORIDE INJECTION, USP (ABBOTT)
5% DEXTROSE & 0.3% SODIUM
CHLORIDE INJECTION, USP (ABBOTT)
5% DEXTROSE & 0.45% SODIUM
CHLORIDE INJECTION, USP (ABBOTT)
5% DEXTROSE & 0.9% SODIUM
CHLORIDE INJECTION, USP (ABBOTT)
10% DEXTROSE & 0.9% SODIUM
CHLORIDE INJECTION, USP (ABBOTT)
2.5% DEXTROSE INJECTION, USP (ABBOTT)
5% DEXTROSE INJECTION, USP (ABBOTT)
5% DEXTROSE INJECTION, USP (ADD-
VANTAGE) (ABBOTT)
5% DEXTROSE INJECTION, USP
(PARTIAL FILL) (ABBOTT)
10% DEXTROSE INJECTION, USP (ABBOTT)
20% DEXTROSE INJECTION, USP (ABBOTT)
30% DEXTROSE INJECTION, USP (ABBOTT)
40% DEXTROSE INJECTION, USP (ABBOTT)
50% DEXTROSE INJECTION, USP (ABBOTT)
60% DEXTROSE INJECTION, USP (ABBOTT)
70% DEXTROSE INJECTION, USP (ABBOTT)
DEXTROSTAT TABLETS (SHIRE RICHWOOD)

UNDERLINE DENOTES GENERIC NAME

D-FEDA II TABLETS (WE)
DHCPLUS CAPSULES (PURDUE FREDERICK)
D.H.E. 45 INJECTION (NOVARTIS)
DHEA (MAYOR)
DHS SHAMPOO (PERSON & COVEY)
DHS CLEAR SHAMPOO (PERSON & COVEY)
DHS SAL SHAMPOO (PERSON & COVEY)
DHS TAR SHAMPOO (PERSON & COVEY)
DHS TAR GEL SHAMPOO (PERSON & COVEY)
DHS ZINC SHAMPOO (PERSON & COVEY)
DIABETA TABLETS
   (HOECHST MARION ROUSSEL)
DIABE-TUSS DM SYRUP (PADDOCK)
DIABINESE TABLETS (PFIZER)
DIAMOX INTRAVENOUS (LEDERLE LABS)
**DIAMOX SEQUELS (SUSTAINED
   RELEASE)** (LEDERLE LABS)
DIAMOX TABLETS (LEDERLE LABS)
DIASTAT RECTAL DELIVERY SYSTEM
   (ELAN)

DIAZEPAM

   Diastat Rectal Delivery System (ELAN)
   Diazepam Injection (ELKINS-SINN)
   Diazepam Injection, USP (BAXTER)
   Diazepam Intensol (ROXANE)
   Diazepam Oral Solution (ROXANE)
   Diazepam Tablets (MYLAN)
   Diazepam Tablets (LEDERLE STANDARD)
   Valium Injectable (ROCHE LABS)
   Valium Tablets (ROCHE PRODUCTS)
DIAZEPAM INJECTION (ELKINS-SINN)
DIAZEPAM INJECTION, USP (BAXTER)
DIAZEPAM INTENSOL (ROXANE)
DIAZEPAM ORAL SOLUTION (ROXANE)
DIAZEPAM TABLETS (MYLAN)
DIAZEPAM TABLETS (LEDERLE STANDARD)

DIAZOXIDE

   Hyperstat I.V. Injection (SCHERING)
DIBENZYLINE CAPSULES
   (SMITHKLINE BEECHAM)

DICHLORALPHENAZONE

   Midrin Capsules (CARNRICK)

DICHLORPHENAMIDE

   Daranide Tablets (MERCK)
**DICLOFENAC NA TABLETS, 50 MG, 75
MG** (NOVOPHARM)

DICLOFENAC POTASSIUM

   Cataflam Tablets (NOVARTIS)
   Diclofenac Potassium Immediate Release
     Tablets (GENEVA)
   Diclofenac Potassium Tablets (MYLAN)
   Diclofenac Potassium Tablets (WATSON)
**DICLOFENAC POTASSIUM IMMEDIATE
RELEASE TABLETS** (GENEVA)
DICLOFENAC POTASSIUM TABLETS
   (MYLAN)
DICLOFENAC POTASSIUM TABLETS
   (WATSON)

DICLOFENAC SODIUM

   Arthrotec Tablets (SEARLE)
   Diclofenac Na Tablets, 50 mg, 75 mg
     (NOVOPHARM)
   Diclofenac Sodium Delayed-Release Tablets
     (GENEVA)
   Diclofenac Sodium Ophthalmic Drops
     (GENEVA)
   Diclofenac Sodium Tablets (ROXANE)
   Voltaren Tablets (NOVARTIS)
   Voltaren-XR Tablets (NOVARTIS)
**DICLOFENAC SODIUM DELAYED-
RELEASE TABLETS** (GENEVA)
**DICLOFENAC SODIUM OPHTHALMIC
DROPS** (GENEVA)

DICLOFENAC SODIUM TABLETS (ROXANE)
DICLOXACILLIN SODIUM CAPSULES
   (APOTHECON)
**DICLOXACILLIN SODIUM CAPSULES AND
ORAL SUSPENSION USP (SEE
DYNAPEN)** (APOTHECON)
DICUMAROL TABLETS (ABBOTT)

DICYCLOMINE HYDROCHLORIDE

   Dicyclomine Hydrochloride Capsules (WATSON)
   Dicyclomine Hydrochloride Capsules, USP
     (ENDO GENERICS)
   Dicyclomine Hydrochloride Tablets (WATSON)
   Dicyclomine Hydrochloride Tablets, USP
     (ENDO GENERICS)
**DICYCLOMINE HYDROCHLORIDE
CAPSULES** (WATSON)
**DICYCLOMINE HYDROCHLORIDE
CAPSULES, USP** (ENDO GENERICS)
**DICYCLOMINE HYDROCHLORIDE
TABLETS** (WATSON)
**DICYCLOMINE HYDROCHLORIDE
TABLETS, USP** (ENDO GENERICS)

DIDANOSINE

   Videx Chewable Tablets
     (BRISTOL-MYERSSQUIBBONCOLOGY/IMMUNOLOGY)
   Videx Pediatric Powder for Oral Solution
     (BRISTOL-MYERSSQUIBBONCOLOGY/IMMUNOLOGY)
   Videx Powder for Oral Solution
     (BRISTOL-MYERSSQUIBBONCOLOGY/IMMUNOLOGY)
DIDREX TABLETS (PHARMACIA & UPJOHN)
DIDRONEL I.V. INFUSION (MGI)
DIDRONEL TABLETS
   (PROCTER & GAMBLE PHARMACEUTICALS)

DIENESTROL

   Ortho Dienestrol Cream (ORTHO-MCNEIL)

DIETHYLPROPION HYDROCHLORIDE

   Diethylpropion Hydrochloride Extended
     Release Tablets CIV (WATSON)
   Diethylpropion Hydrochloride Tablets CIV
     (WATSON)
**DIETHYLPROPION HYDROCHLORIDE
TABLETS CIV** (WATSON)
**DIETHYLPROPION HYDROCHLORIDE
EXTENDED RELEASE TABLETS CIV**
   (WATSON)

DIFENOXIN HYDROCHLORIDE

   Motofen Tablets (CARNRICK)
DIFFERIN GEL (GALDERMA)
DIFFERIN SOLUTION (GALDERMA)

DIFLORASONE DIACETATE

   Maxiflor Cream (ALLERGAN)
   Maxiflor Ointment (ALLERGAN)
   Psorcon Cream 0.05% (DERMIK)
   Psorcon E Cream (DERMIK)
   Psorcon E Ointment (DERMIK)
   Psorcon Ointment 0.05% (DERMIK)
**DIFLUCAN TABLETS, INJECTION, AND
ORAL SUSPENSION** (PFIZER)

DIFLUNISAL

   Diflunisal Tablets, USP (ENDO GENERICS)
   Dolobid Tablets (MERCK)
DIFLUNISAL TABLETS, USP (ENDO GENERICS)
DIGESTIVE ENZYMES (VITALINE)
DIGIBIND (GLAXO WELLCOME)

DIGOXIN

   Digoxin Elixir (ROXANE)
   Digoxin Injection (ELKINS-SINN)
   Digoxin in Tubex (WYETH-AYERST)
   Lanoxicaps (GLAXO WELLCOME)
   Lanoxin Elixir Pediatric (GLAXO WELLCOME)
   Lanoxin Injection (GLAXO WELLCOME)
   Lanoxin Injection Pediatric (GLAXO WELLCOME)

   Lanoxin Tablets (GLAXO WELLCOME)
DIGOXIN ELIXIR (ROXANE)

DIGOXIN IMMUNE FAB (OVINE)

   Digibind (GLAXO WELLCOME)
DIGOXIN IN TUBEX (WYETH-AYERST)
DIGOXIN INJECTION (ELKINS-SINN)
DIGOXIN INJECTION (WYETH-AYERST)

DIHYDROCODEINE BITARTRATE

   Synalgos-DC Capsules (WYETH-AYERST)

DIHYDROERGOTAMINE MESYLATE

   D.H.E. 45 Injection (NOVARTIS)
   Migranal Nasal Spray (NOVARTIS)
DILACOR XR CAPSULES (WATSON)
DILANTIN INFATABS (PARKE-DAVIS)
DILANTIN KAPSEALS (PARKE-DAVIS)
DILANTIN-125 SUSPENSION (PARKE-DAVIS)
DILATRATE-SR CAPSULES (SCHWARZ)
DILAUDID AMPULES (KNOLL LABS)
DILAUDID COUGH SYRUP (KNOLL LABS)
DILAUDID INJECTION (KNOLL LABS)
**DILAUDID MULTIPLE DOSE VIALS
(STERILE SOLUTION)** (KNOLL LABS)
DILAUDID ORAL LIQUID (KNOLL LABS)
DILAUDID POWDER (KNOLL LABS)
DILAUDID RECTAL SUPPOSITORIES
   (KNOLL LABS)
DILAUDID TABLETS 2 MG AND 4 MG
   (KNOLL LABS)
DILAUDID TABLETS - 8 MG (KNOLL LABS)
DILAUDID-HP INJECTION (KNOLL LABS)
**DILAUDID-HP LYOPHILIZED POWDER
250MG** (KNOLL LABS)
DILOR ELIXIR (SAVAGE)
DILOR INJECTION (SAVAGE)
DILOR-200 TABLETS (SAVAGE)
DILOR-400 TABLETS (SAVAGE)
DILOR-G LIQUID (SAVAGE)
DILOR-G TABLETS (SAVAGE)
**DILTIAZEM EXTENDED RELEASE
CAPSULES** (WATSON)

DILTIAZEM HYDROCHLORIDE

   Cardizem CD Capsules
     (HOECHST MARION ROUSSEL)
   Cardizem Injectable
     (HOECHST MARION ROUSSEL)
   Cardizem Lyo-Ject Syringe
     (HOECHST MARION ROUSSEL)
   Cardizem Monovial
     (HOECHST MARION ROUSSEL)
   Dilacor XR Capsules (WATSON)
   Diltiazem Extended Release Capsules
     (WATSON)
   Diltiazem Hydrochloride Extended-release
     Capsules (once-a-day) (MYLAN)
   Diltiazem Hydrochloride Extended-release
     Capsules (twice-a-day) (MYLAN)
   Diltiazem Hydrochloride Injection (BAXTER)
   Diltiazem Hydrochloride Tablets (MYLAN)
   Diltiazem Hydrochloride Tablets (WATSON)
   Diltiazem Hydrochloride Tablets
     (LEDERLE STANDARD)
   Tiazac Capsules (FOREST)
**DILTIAZEM HYDROCHLORIDE
EXTENDED-RELEASE CAPSULES
(ONCE-A-DAY)** (MYLAN)
**DILTIAZEM HYDROCHLORIDE
EXTENDED-RELEASE CAPSULES
(TWICE-A-DAY)** (MYLAN)
**DILTIAZEM HYDROCHLORIDE
INJECTION** (BAXTER)
**DILTIAZEM HYDROCHLORIDE
INJECTION** (BEDFORD)
DILTIAZEM HYDROCHLORIDE TABLETS
   (MYLAN)

UNDERLINE DENOTES GENERIC NAME

DILTIAZEM HYDROCHLORIDE TABLETS
(WATSON)
DILTIAZEM HYDROCHLORIDE TABLETS
(LEDERLE STANDARD)
DILUENT (FLAVORED) FOR ORAL USE
(ROXANE)

DIMENHYDRINATE

Dimenhydrinate in Tubex (WYETH-AYERST)
VitaMotion-S (MAYOR)
Vitamist Intra-Oral Spray Dietary Supplements
(MAYOR)
DIMENHYDRINATE IN TUBEX
(WYETH-AYERST)
DIMENHYDRINATE INJECTION
(WYETH-AYERST)
DIMETANE-DX COUGH SYRUP (ROBINS)

DIMETHICONE

Eucerin Plus Alpha Hydroxy Creme
(BEIERSDORF)
Eucerin Tri-Lipid Replenishing Lotion
(BEIERSDORF)

DINOPROSTONE

Cervidil Vaginal Insert (FOREST)
Prepidil Gel (PHARMACIA & UPJOHN)
Prostin E2 Suppositories
(PHARMACIA & UPJOHN)
DIOVAN CAPSULES (NOVARTIS)
DIOVAN HCT TABLETS (NOVARTIS)

DIOXYBENZONE

Solaquin Forte 4% Cream (ICN)
Solaquin Forte 4% Gel (ICN)
DIPENTUM CAPSULES (PHARMACIA & UPJOHN)

DIPHENHYDRAMINE CITRATE

Excedrin P.M. Caplets (BRISTOL-MYERS)
Excedrin P.M. Geltabs (BRISTOL-MYERS)
Excedrin P.M. Tablets (BRISTOL-MYERS)
DIPHENHYDRAMINE HCL INJECTION
(WYETH-AYERST)

DIPHENHYDRAMINE HYDROCHLORIDE

Benadryl Allergy Chewables
(WARNER-LAMBERT)
Benadryl Allergy Kapseal Capsules
(WARNER-LAMBERT)
Benadryl Allergy Liquid (WARNER-LAMBERT)
Benadryl Allergy Ultratab Tablets
(WARNER-LAMBERT)
Benadryl Allergy/Cold Tablets
(WARNER-LAMBERT)
Benadryl Allergy/Congestion Liquid
(WARNER-LAMBERT)
Benadryl Allergy/Congestion Tablets
(WARNER-LAMBERT)
Benadryl Allergy/Sinus Headache Caplets &
Gelcaps (WARNER-LAMBERT)
Benadryl Dye-Free Allergy Liqui-gels
(WARNER-LAMBERT)
Benadryl Dye-Free Allergy Liquid
(WARNER-LAMBERT)
Benadryl Itch Relief Stick Extra Strength
(WARNER-LAMBERT)
Benadryl Itch Stopping Cream Original and
Extra Strength (WARNER-LAMBERT)
Benadryl Itch Stopping Gel Original and Extra
Strength (WARNER-LAMBERT)
Benadryl Itch Stopping Spray Original and
Extra Strength (WARNER-LAMBERT)
Benadryl Parenteral (PARKE-DAVIS)
Children's Tylenol Allergy-D Liquid and
Chewable Tablets (MCNEIL CONSUMER)
Diphenhydramine Hydrochloride Elixir USP
(PHARMACEUTICAL ASSOCIATES)
Diphenhydramine Hydrochloride Injection
(ELKINS-SINN)

Diphenhydramine Hydrochloride in Tubex
(WYETH-AYERST)
Dytuss (LUNSCO)
Maximum Strength Unisom SleepGels
(PFIZER CONSUMER)
Simply Sleep Caplets (MCNEIL CONSUMER)
Tylenol Allergy Sinus NightTime, Maximum
Strength Caplets (MCNEIL CONSUMER)
Tylenol Flu NightTime, Maximum Strength
Gelcaps (MCNEIL CONSUMER)
Tylenol Flu NightTime, Maximum Strength
Powder (MCNEIL CONSUMER)
Tylenol PM Pain Reliever/Sleep Aid, Extra
Strength Caplets, Geltabs, and Gelcaps
(MCNEIL CONSUMER)
Tylenol Severe Allergy Caplets
(MCNEIL CONSUMER)
**DIPHENHYDRAMINE HYDROCHLORIDE
ELIXIR USP** (PHARMACEUTICAL ASSOCIATES)
**DIPHENHYDRAMINE HYDROCHLORIDE
IN TUBEX** (WYETH-AYERST)
**DIPHENHYDRAMINE HYDROCHLORIDE
INJECTION** (ELKINS-SINN)

DIPHENOXYLATE HYDROCHLORIDE

Diphenoxylate Hydrochloride & Atropine
Sulfate Oral Solution (ROXANE)
Diphenoxylate Hydrochloride and Atropine
Sulfate Tablets (MYLAN)
Diphenoxylate Hydrochloride and Atropine
Sulfate Tablets, USP (MALLINCKRODT)
Lomotil Liquid (SEARLE)
Lomotil Tablets (SEARLE)
Lonox Tablets (GENEVA)
**DIPHENOXYLATE HYDROCHLORIDE &
ATROPINE SULFATE ORAL SOLUTION**
(ROXANE)
**DIPHENOXYLATE HYDROCHLORIDE AND
ATROPINE SULFATE TABLETS** (MYLAN)
**DIPHENOXYLATE HYDROCHLORIDE AND
ATROPINE SULFATE TABLETS, USP**
(MALLINCKRODT)
**DIPHTHERIA & TETANUS TOXOIDS
ADSORBED PUROGENATED**
(LEDERLE LABS)
**DIPHTHERIA & TETANUS TOXOIDS
ADSORBED USP (FOR PEDIATRIC USE)
(DT)** (PASTEUR MERIEUX CONNAUGHT)

DIPHTHERIA & TETANUS TOXOIDS
ADSORBED, (FOR PEDIATRIC USE)

Diphtheria & Tetanus Toxoids Adsorbed
Purogenated (LEDERLE LABS)

DIPHTHERIA & TETANUS TOXOIDS AND
ACELLULAR PERTUSSIS VACCINE
ADSORBED

Acel-Imune (LEDERLE LABS)
Certiva Injection (NORTH AMERICAN VACCINE)
Infanrix (SMITHKLINE BEECHAM)
Tripedia (PASTEUR MERIEUX CONNAUGHT)

DIPHTHERIA & TETANUS TOXOIDS AND
PERTUSSIS VACCINE ADSORBED

Diphtheria and Tetanus Toxoids and Pertussis
Vaccine Adsorbed USP (For Pediatric Use)
(PASTEUR MERIEUX CONNAUGHT)

DIPHTHERIA & TETANUS TOXOIDS AND
PERTUSSIS WITH HAEMOPHILUS B
CONJUGATE VACCINE

Tetramune (LEDERLE LABS)
**DIPHTHERIA AND TETANUS TOXOIDS
AND PERTUSSIS VACCINE ADSORBED
USP (FOR PEDIATRIC USE)**
(PASTEUR MERIEUX CONNAUGHT)

DIPOTASSIUM PHOSPHATE

Uro-KP-Neutral Tablets (STAR)

DIPRIVAN INJECTABLE EMULSION
(ASTRAZENECA)
DIPROLENE AF CREAM 0.05% (SCHERING)
DIPROLENE GEL 0.05% (SCHERING)
DIPROLENE LOTION 0.05% (SCHERING)
DIPROLENE OINTMENT 0.05% (SCHERING)
DIPROSONE CREAM 0.05% (SCHERING)
DIPROSONE LOTION 0.05% (SCHERING)
DIPROSONE OINTMENT 0.05% (SCHERING)
DIPROSONE TOPICAL AEROSOL 0.1%
(SCHERING)

DIPYRIDAMOLE

Dipyridamole Injection (ELKINS-SINN)
Dipyridamole Tablets (LEDERLE STANDARD)
Persantine Tablets (BOEHRINGER INGELHEIM)
DIPYRIDAMOLE INJECTION (BEDFORD)
DIPYRIDAMOLE INJECTION (ELKINS-SINN)
DIPYRIDAMOLE TABLETS
(LEDERLE STANDARD)

DIRITHROMYCIN

Dynabac Tablets (SANOFI)
DISALCID CAPSULES (3M)
DISALCID TABLETS (3M)
DISOBROM TABLETS (GENEVA)

DISODIUM PHOSPHATE

Uro-KP-Neutral Tablets (STAR)

DISOPYRAMIDE PHOSPHATE

Norpace CR Capsules (SEARLE)
Norpace Capsules (SEARLE)
**DISOPYRAMIDE PHOSPHATE CAPSULES,
USP** (SCHEIN)

DISULFIRAM

Antabuse Tablets (WYETH-AYERST)
DITROPAN TABLETS AND SYRUP (ALZA)
**DITROPAN XL EXTENDED RELEASE
TABLETS** (ALZA)
DIUCARDIN TABLETS (WYETH-AYERST)
DIURIL ORAL SUSPENSION (MERCK)
DIURIL TABLETS (MERCK)
DIURIL SODIUM INTRAVENOUS (MERCK)
DIUTENSEN-R TABLETS (WALLACE)

DIVALPROEX SODIUM

Depakote Sprinkle Capsules (ABBOTT)
Depakote Tablets (ABBOTT)
**DML FACIAL MOISTURIZER WITH
SUNSCREEN** (PERSON & COVEY)
DML-FORTE CREAM (PERSON & COVEY)
DML-LOTION (PERSON & COVEY)
DOAN'S EXTRA STRENGTH ANALGESIC
(NOVARTIS CONSUMER)
EXTRA STRENGTH DOAN'S P.M.
(NOVARTIS CONSUMER)
**DOAN'S REGULAR STRENGTH
ANALGESIC** (NOVARTIS CONSUMER)

DOBUTAMINE

Dobutamine Injection, USP (ASTRAZENECA LP)

DOBUTAMINE HYDROCHLORIDE

Dobutamine Hydrochloride Injection (BAXTER)
Dobutrex Solution Vials (LILLY)
**DOBUTAMINE HYDROCHLORIDE
INJECTION** (BAXTER)
**DOBUTAMINE HYDROCHLORIDE
INJECTION** (ELKINS-SINN)
DOBUTAMINE INJECTION, USP (BEDFORD)
DOBUTAMINE INJECTION, USP
(ASTRAZENECA LP)
DOBUTREX SOLUTION VIALS (LILLY)

DOCETAXEL

Taxotere for Injection Concentrate
(RHONE-POULENC RORER)

DOCOSAHEXAENOIC ACID (DHA)
SuperEPA Softgels (ADVANCED NUTRITIONAL)

DOCUSATE SODIUM
Colace Capsules, Syrup, Liquid (ROBERTS)
Colace Microenema (ROBERTS)
Docusate Sodium Liquid
(PHARMACEUTICAL ASSOCIATES)
Docusate Sodium Syrup (ROXANE)
Docusate Sodium Syrup USP
(PHARMACEUTICAL ASSOCIATES)
Docusate Sodium with Casanthranol
(PHARMACEUTICAL ASSOCIATES)
Peri-Colace Capsules and Syrup (ROBERTS)
Senokot-S Tablets (PURDUE FREDERICK)
DOCUSATE SODIUM CAPSULES 100 MG, 250 MG (PADDOCK)
DOCUSATE SODIUM CAPSULES W/CASANTHRANOL 100 MG/30 MG (PADDOCK)
DOCUSATE SODIUM LIQUID (PHARMACEUTICAL ASSOCIATES)
DOCUSATE SODIUM SYRUP (ROXANE)
DOCUSATE SODIUM SYRUP USP (PHARMACEUTICAL ASSOCIATES)
DOCUSATE SODIUM WITH CASANTHRANOL (PHARMACEUTICAL ASSOCIATES)

DOLASETRON MESYLATE
Anzemet Injection (HOECHST MARION ROUSSEL)
Anzemet Tablets (HOECHST MARION ROUSSEL)
DOLOBID TABLETS (MERCK)
DOLOPHINE HYDROCHLORIDE TABLETS AND INJECTION (ROXANE)
DOME-PASTE BANDAGE (UNNA'S BOOT) (BAYER)
DONATUSSIN DROPS (LASER)
DONATUSSIN SYRUP (LASER)
DONATUSSIN DC SYRUP (LASER)

DONEPEZIL HYDROCHLORIDE
Aricept Tablets (EISAI)
Aricept Tablets (PFIZER)

DONG QUAI
ArthriFlex (MAYOR)
Vitamist Intra-Oral Spray Dietary Supplements (MAYOR)
DONNAGEL LIQUID (WYETH-AYERST)
DONNATAL CAPSULES (ROBINS)
DONNATAL ELIXIR (ROBINS)
DONNATAL EXTENTABS (ROBINS)
DONNATAL TABLETS (ROBINS)
DONNAZYME TABLETS (ROBINS)

DOPAMINE HYDROCHLORIDE
Dopamine Hydrochloride Injection (ELKINS-SINN)
DOPAMINE HYDROCHLORIDE IN 5% DEXTROSE INJECTION (800, 1600, 3200 MCG/ML) (ABBOTT)
DOPAMINE HYDROCHLORIDE INJECTION (ELKINS-SINN)
DOPRAM INJECTABLE (ROBINS)
DORAL TABLETS (WALLACE)

DORNASE ALFA
Pulmozyme Inhalation Solution (GENENTECH)
DORYX COATED PELLET FILLED CAPSULES (WARNER CHILCOTT)

DORZOLAMIDE HYDROCHLORIDE
Cosopt Sterile Ophthalmic Solution (MERCK)
Trusopt Sterile Ophthalmic Solution (MERCK)
DOSTINEX TABLETS (PHARMACIA & UPJOHN)
DOVONEX CREAM 0.005% (WESTWOOD-SQUIBB)
DOVONEX OINTMENT 0.005% (WESTWOOD-SQUIBB)

DOVONEX SCALP SOLUTION 0.005% (WESTWOOD-SQUIBB)

DOXACURIUM CHLORIDE
Nuromax Injection (GLAXO WELLCOME)

DOXAPRAM HYDROCHLORIDE
Dopram Injectable (ROBINS)

DOXAZOSIN MESYLATE
Cardura Tablets (PFIZER)
DOXEPIN HCL CAPSULES (PAR)

DOXEPIN HYDROCHLORIDE
Doxepin HCl Capsules (PAR)
Doxepin Hydrochloride Capsules (MYLAN)
Doxepin Hydrochloride Capsules, USP (WATSON)
Sinequan Capsules (PFIZER)
Sinequan Oral Concentrate (PFIZER)
Zonalon Cream (BIOGLAN)
DOXEPIN HYDROCHLORIDE CAPSULES (MYLAN)
DOXEPIN HYDROCHLORIDE CAPSULES, USP (WATSON)
DOXIL INJECTION (ALZA)

DOXORUBICIN HYDROCHLORIDE
Adriamycin PFS/RDF Injection (PHARMACIA & UPJOHN)
Doxil Injection (ALZA)
Rubex for Injection (BRISTOL-MYERSSQUIBBONCOLOGY/IMMUNOLOGY)
DOXORUBICIN HYDROCHLORIDE FOR INJECTION, USP (BEDFORD)
DOXORUBICIN HYDROCHLORIDE INJECTION, USP (BEDFORD)

DOXYCYCLINE CALCIUM
Vibramycin Calcium Oral Suspension Syrup (PFIZER)

DOXYCYCLINE HYCLATE
Doryx Coated Pellet Filled Capsules (WARNER CHILCOTT)
Doxycycline Hyclate Capsules and Tablets (MYLAN)
Periostat Capsules (COLLAGENEX)
Vibra-Tabs Film Coated Tablets (PFIZER)
Vibramycin Hyclate Capsules (PFIZER)
Vibramycin Hyclate Intravenous (PFIZER)
DOXYCYCLINE HYCLATE CAPSULES AND TABLETS (MYLAN)

DOXYCYCLINE MONOHYDRATE
Monodox Capsules (OCLASSEN)
Vibramycin Monohydrate for Oral Suspension (PFIZER)

DOXYLAMINE SUCCINATE
Tylenol Flu NightTime, Maximum Strength Liquid (MCNEIL CONSUMER)
Tylenol Sinus NightTime, Maximum Strength Caplets (MCNEIL CONSUMER)
Unisom SleepTabs (PFIZER CONSUMER)
DR'S. CREAM (GEBAUER)
DRISDOL 50,000 UNIT CAPSULES (SANOFI)
DRISDOL IN PROPYLENE GLYCOL (SANOFI)
DRITHOCREME 0.1%, 0.25%, 0.5%, 1.0% (HP) CREAM (DERMIK)
DRITHO-SCALP 0.25%, 0.5% CREAM (DERMIK)

DRONABINOL
Marinol Capsules (ROXANE)
Marinol Capsules (UNIMED)

DROPERIDOL
Fentanyl Citrate and Droperidol Injection (ASTRAZENECA LP)

DROXIA CAPSULES (BRISTOL-MYERSSQUIBBONCOLOGY/IMMUNOLOGY)
DRYSOL SOLUTION (PERSON & COVEY)
DTIC-DOME (BAYER)
DULCOLAX SUPPOSITORIES (NOVARTIS CONSUMER)
DULCOLAX TABLETS (NOVARTIS CONSUMER)
DUOVISC VISCOELASTIC SYSTEM (ALCON)
DUPHALAC SOLUTION (SOLVAY)
DURACID (FIELDING)
DURACLON INJECTION (ROXANE)
DURADRIN CAPSULES (DURAMED)
DURAGESIC TRANSDERMAL SYSTEM (JANSSEN)
DURAMORPH INJECTION (BAXTER)
DURAMORPH INJECTION (ELKINS-SINN)
DURANEST INJECTIONS (ASTRAZENECA LP)
DURATEARS NATURALE LUBRICANT EYE OINTMENT (ALCON)
DURATUSS DM ELIXIR (UCB)
DURATUSS G TABLETS (UCB)
DURATUSS HD ELIXIR (UCB)
DURATUSS TABLETS (UCB)
DURA-VENT TABLETS (DJ PHARMA)
DURA-VENT/DA TABLETS (DJ PHARMA)
DURICEF CAPSULES (BRISTOL-MYERS SQUIBB)
DURICEF ORAL SUSPENSIONS (BRISTOL-MYERS SQUIBB)
DURICEF TABLETS (BRISTOL-MYERS SQUIBB)
DYAZIDE CAPSULES (SMITHKLINE BEECHAM)
DYLIX ELIXIR (LUNSCO)
DYNABAC TABLETS (SANOFI)
DYNACIN CAPSULES (MEDICIS)
DYNACIRC CAPSULES (NOVARTIS)
DYNACIRC CR TABLETS (NOVARTIS)
DYNAPEN (DICLOXACILLIN SODIUM) ORAL SUSPENSION (APOTHECON)

DYPHYLLINE
Dilor Elixir (SAVAGE)
Dilor Injection (SAVAGE)
Dilor-200 Tablets (SAVAGE)
Dilor-400 Tablets (SAVAGE)
Dilor-G Liquid (SAVAGE)
Dilor-G Tablets (SAVAGE)
Dylix Elixir (LUNSCO)
Lufyllin Elixir (WALLACE)
Lufyllin Tablets (WALLACE)
Lufyllin-400 Tablets (WALLACE)
Lufyllin-GG Elixir (WALLACE)
Lufyllin-GG Tablets (WALLACE)
DYRENIUM CAPSULES (SMITHKLINE BEECHAM)
DYTUSS (LUNSCO)

E

E + SELENIUM (MAYOR)
E-PHEROL (D-ALPHA TOCOPHEROL) 400 I.U. (VITALINE)
EASPRIN TABLETS (LOTUS)
ECHINACEA + G (MAYOR)
ECHINACEA 125MG/GOLDENSEAL 125MG (VITALINE)

ECHINACEA ANGUSTIFOLIA
Echinacea + G (MAYOR)
Vitamist Intra-Oral Spray Dietary Supplements (MAYOR)
EC-NAPROSYN DELAYED-RELEASE TABLETS (ROCHE LABS)

UNDERLINE DENOTES GENERIC NAME

ECONAZOLE NITRATE
　Spectazole Cream (ORTHO DERMATOLOGICAL)
ECONOPRED (ALCON P.R.)
ECONOPRED PLUS (ALCON P.R.)
**ECONOPRED PLUS OPHTHALMIC
　SUSPENSION** (ALCON)
**ECOTRIN ENTERIC COATED ASPIRIN
　LOW, REGULAR AND MAXIMUM
　STRENGTH TABLETS**
　(SMITHKLINE BEECHAM CONSUMER)
EDECRIN TABLETS (MERCK)
EDECRIN SODIUM INTRAVENOUS (MERCK)

EDETATE CALCIUM DISODIUM
　Calcium Disodium Versenate Injection (3M)
EDEX FOR INJECTION (SCHWARZ)

EDROPHONIUM CHLORIDE
　Enlon Injection (BAXTER)
　Enlon-Plus Injection (BAXTER)
　Reversol Injection (ORGANON)
　Tensilon Injectable (ICN)
E.E.S. 200 LIQUID (ABBOTT)
E.E.S. 400 FILMTAB TABLETS (ABBOTT)
E.E.S. 400 LIQUID (ABBOTT)
E.E.S. GRANULES (ABBOTT)

EFAVIRENZ
　Sustiva Capsules (DUPONT)
EFFEXOR TABLETS (WYETH-AYERST)
EFFEXOR TABLETS, 25 MG (WYETH-AYERST)
EFFEXOR TABLETS, 37.5 MG
　(WYETH-AYERST)
EFFEXOR TABLETS, 50 MG (WYETH-AYERST)
EFFEXOR TABLETS, 75 MG (WYETH-AYERST)
EFFEXOR TABLETS, 100 MG
　(WYETH-AYERST)
EFFEXOR XR CAPSULES (WYETH-AYERST)
EFFEXOR XR CAPSULES, 150 MG
　(WYETH-AYERST)
EFFEXOR XR CAPSULES, 37.5 MG
　(WYETH-AYERST)
EFFEXOR XR CAPSULES, 75 MG
　(WYETH-AYERST)
EFUDEX CREAM (ICN)
EFUDEX TOPICAL SOLUTIONS (ICN)
E-GEMS SOFT GELS (CARLSON)

EICOSAPENTAENOIC ACID (EPA)
　SuperEPA Softgels (ADVANCED NUTRITIONAL)
8-MOP CAPSULES (ICN)
ELA-MAX CREAM (FERNDALE)
ELA-MAX 5 CREAM (FERNDALE)
ELASTOMULL (BEIERSDORF)
ELASTOPLAST (BEIERSDORF)
ELAVIL INJECTION (ASTRAZENECA)
ELAVIL TABLETS (ASTRAZENECA)
ELDEPRYL CAPSULES (SOMERSET)
ELDERCAPS (MERZ)
ELDERTONIC (MERZ)
ELDOPAQUE 2% CREAM (ICN)
ELDOPAQUE FORTE 4% CREAM (ICN)
ELDOQUIN 2% CREAM (ICN)
ELDOQUIN FORTE 4% CREAM (ICN)

ELECTROLYTE SOLUTION
　Kaolectrolyte (BRECKENRIDGE)
　Pedialyte Oral Electrolyte Maintenance
　　Solution (ROSS)
　Rehydralyte Oral Electrolyte Rehydration
　　Solution (ROSS)
ELIMITE CREAM (ALLERGAN)
ELIXOPHYLLIN ELIXIR (FOREST)
ELIXOPHYLLIN-GG ORAL SOLUTION
　(FOREST)
ELIXOPHYLLIN-KI ELIXIR (FOREST)
ELMIRON CAPSULES (ALZA)
ELOCON CREAM 0.1% (SCHERING)
ELOCON LOTION 0.1% (SCHERING)

ELOCON OINTMENT 0.1% (SCHERING)
ELSPAR FOR INJECTION (MERCK)
EMADINE OPHTHALMIC SOLUTION
　(ALCON)
EMBELINE E CREAM (HEALTHPOINT)
EMCYT CAPSULES (PHARMACIA & UPJOHN)
EMGEL 2% TOPICAL GEL
　(GLAXO WELLCOME)
EMINASE (ROBERTS)
EMLA CREAM (ASTRAZENECA LP)
EMLA ANESTHETIC DISC (ASTRAZENECA LP)
EMOLLIA-CREME & LOTION (GORDON)
EMPTY EVACUATED CONTAINER (ABBOTT)
**EMULSOIL (SELF-EMULSIFYING CASTOR
　OIL)** (PADDOCK)
E-MYCIN DELAYED-RELEASE TABLETS
　(KNOLL LABS)

ENALAPRIL MALEATE
　Lexxel Tablets (ASTRAZENECA LP)
　Vaseretic Tablets (MERCK)
　Vasotec Tablets (MERCK)

ENALAPRILAT
　Vasotec I.V. Injection (MERCK)
ENBREL FOR INJECTION (IMMUNEX)
ENBREL FOR INJECTION (WYETH-AYERST)
ENDAFED CAPSULES (FOREST)
ENDAL EXPECTORANT (FOREST)
ENDAL TABLETS (FOREST)
ENDAL-HD (FOREST)
ENDAL-HD PLUS (FOREST)
ENDOCET TABLETS, USP CII
　(ENDO GENERICS)
ENDODAN TABLETS, USP CII
　(ENDO GENERICS)
**ENDRATE SOLUTION, AMPULES (150
　MG/ML)** (ABBOTT)
ENDURON TABLETS (ABBOTT)
ENDURONYL FORTE TABLETS (ABBOTT)
ENDURONYL TABLETS (ABBOTT)
ENFAMIL NATALINS RX TABLETS
　(MEAD JOHNSON)

ENFLURANE
　Ethrane Liquid for Inhalation (BAXTER)
ENGERIX-B (SMITHKLINE BEECHAM)
ENGYSTOL TABLETS (HEEL)
ENLON INJECTION (BAXTER)
ENLON-PLUS INJECTION (BAXTER)

ENOXACIN
　Penetrex Tablets (RHONE-POULENC RORER)

ENOXAPARIN SODIUM
　Lovenox Injection (RHONE-POULENC RORER)
ENTEX CAPSULES (DURA)
ENTEX LA TABLETS (DURA)
ENTEX LIQUID (DURA)
ENTEX PSE TABLETS (DURA)
**ENUCLENE CLEANING/LUBRICATING
　SOLUTION FOR ARTIFICIAL EYES**
　(ALCON)
ENVIRO-STRESS (VITALINE)
ENZONE CREAM (FOREST)

EPHEDRINE HYDROCHLORIDE
　Broncholate Syrup (SANOFI)
　Kie Syrup (LASER)

EPHEDRINE SULFATE
　Marax Tablets & DF Syrup (PFIZER)
EPHEDRINE SULFATE INJECTION, USP
　(BEDFORD)
**EPHEDRINE SULFATE, INJECTION (50
　MG/ML)** (ABBOTT)

EPHEDRINE TANNATE
　Rynatuss Pediatric Suspension (WALLACE)
　Rynatuss Tablets (WALLACE)

EPIFOAM (SCHWARZ)
**EPIFRIN STERILE OPHTHALMIC
　SOLUTION** (ALLERGAN)
EPILYT LOTION (STIEFEL)
EPINAL OPHTHALMIC SOLUTION (ALCON)

EPINEPHRINE
　EpiPen Auto-Injector (DEY)
　EpiPen Jr. Auto-Injector (DEY)
　Epinephrine Injection (ELKINS-SINN)
　Epinephrine in Tubex (WYETH-AYERST)
　Lidocaine Hydrochloride & Epinephrine
　　Injection (ELKINS-SINN)
　Sensorcaine with Epinephrine Injection
　　(ASTRAZENECA LP)
　Xylocaine with Epinephrine Injection
　　(ASTRAZENECA LP)
EPINEPHRINE 1:10,000, 10 ML., ABBOJECT
　(ABBOTT)

EPINEPHRINE BITARTRATE
　Sensorcaine-MPF with Epinephrine Injection
　　(ASTRAZENECA LP)

EPINEPHRINE HYDROCHLORIDE
　Ana-Kit Anaphylaxis Emergency Treatment Kit
　　(BAYER ALLERGY)
EPINEPHRINE IN TUBEX (WYETH-AYERST)
EPINEPHRINE INJECTION (ELKINS-SINN)
EPINEPHRINE INJECTION (1:1000)
　(WYETH-AYERST)
EPIPEN AUTO-INJECTOR (DEY)
EPIPEN JR. AUTO-INJECTOR (DEY)
EPIPEN TRAINER (DEY)
EPIVIR ORAL SOLUTION (GLAXO WELLCOME)
EPIVIR TABLETS (GLAXO WELLCOME)
EPIVIR-HBV ORAL SOLUTION
　(GLAXO WELLCOME)
EPIVIR-HBV TABLETS (GLAXO WELLCOME)

EPOETIN ALFA
　Epogen for Injection (AMGEN)
　Procrit for Injection (ORTHO BIOTECH)
EPOGEN FOR INJECTION (AMGEN)

EPOPROSTENOL SODIUM
　Flolan for Injection (GLAXO WELLCOME)

EPTIFIBATIDE
　Integrilin Injection (COR)
　Integrilin Injection (KEY)
EQUAGESIC TABLETS (WYETH-AYERST)
EQUANIL TABLETS (WYETH-AYERST)
ERCAF TABLETS (GENEVA)
ERGAMISOL TABLETS (JANSSEN)

ERGOCALCIFEROL
　Calciferol Drops (SCHWARZ)
　Calciferol in Oil Injection (SCHWARZ)
ERGOMAR TABLETS (LOTUS)

ERGOTAMINE TARTRATE
　Ercaf Tablets (GENEVA)
　Ergomar Tablets (LOTUS)
　Wigraine Tablets (ORGANON)
ERGOTRATE MALEATE (BEDFORD)
ERYC DELAYED-RELEASE CAPSULES
　(WARNER CHILCOTT)
ERYCETTE TOPICAL SOLUTION
　(ORTHO DERMATOLOGICAL)
ERYDERM TOPICAL SOLUTION (ABBOTT)
ERYGEL TOPICAL GEL (ALLERGAN)
ERYMAX TOPICAL SOLUTION (ALLERGAN)
ERYPED 200 & ERYPED 400 (ABBOTT)
ERYPED DROPS (ABBOTT)
ERYPED CHEWABLE TABLETS (ABBOTT)
ERY-TAB TABLETS (ABBOTT)
ERYTHRA-DERM SOLUTION (PADDOCK)
ERYTHROCIN ADD-VANTAGE KITS
　(ABBOTT)

UNDERLINE DENOTES GENERIC NAME

ERYTHROCIN LACTOBIONATE-I.V.
(ABBOTT)
ERYTHROCIN PIGGYBACK (ABBOTT)
**ERYTHROCIN STEARATE FILMTAB
TABLETS** (ABBOTT)

ERYTHROMYCIN

A/T/S Topical Gel (MEDICIS)
A/T/S Topical Solution (MEDICIS)
Akne-Mycin Ointment (HEALTHPOINT)
Benzamycin Topical Gel (DERMIK)
Emgel 2% Topical Gel (GLAXO WELLCOME)
Ery-Tab Tablets (ABBOTT)
Eryc Delayed-Release Capsules
(WARNER CHILCOTT)
Erycette Topical Solution
(ORTHO DERMATOLOGICAL)
Erygel Topical Gel (ALLERGAN)
Erymax Topical Solution (ALLERGAN)
Erythromycin Base Filmtab Tablets (ABBOTT)
Erythromycin Delayed-Release Capsules, USP
(ABBOTT)
Ilotycin Ophthalmic Ointment (DISTA)
PCE Dispertab Tablets (ABBOTT)
Theramycin Z Topical Solution (BIOGLAN)
**ERYTHROMYCIN BASE FILMTAB
TABLETS** (ABBOTT)
**ERYTHROMYCIN DELAYED-RELEASE
CAPSULES, USP** (ABBOTT)

ERYTHROMYCIN ETHYLSUCCINATE

E.E.S. 200 Liquid (ABBOTT)
E.E.S. 400 Filmtab Tablets (ABBOTT)
E.E.S. 400 Liquid (ABBOTT)
E.E.S. Granules (ABBOTT)
EryPed 200 & EryPed 400 (ABBOTT)
EryPed Chewable Tablets (ABBOTT)
EryPed Drops (ABBOTT)
Erythromycin Ethylsuccinate Tablets (MYLAN)
Erythromycin Ethylsuccinate/ Sulfisoxazole
Acetyl Oral Suspension
(LEDERLE STANDARD)
Pediazole Suspension (ROSS)
**ERYTHROMYCIN ETHYLSUCCINATE
TABLETS** (MYLAN)
**ERYTHROMYCIN ETHYLSUCCINATE/
SULFISOXAZOLE ACETYL ORAL
SUSPENSION** (LEDERLE STANDARD)

ERYTHROMYCIN LACTOBIONATE

Sterile Erythromycin Lactobionate for Injection
(LEDERLE STANDARD)
**STERILE ERYTHROMYCIN
LACTOBIONATE FOR INJECTION**
(LEDERLE STANDARD)

ERYTHROMYCIN STEARATE

Erythrocin Stearate Filmtab Tablets (ABBOTT)
Erythromycin Stearate Tablets (MYLAN)
ERYTHROMYCIN STEARATE TABLETS
(MYLAN)
ERYTHROMYCIN USP POWDER (PADDOCK)
ESGIC CAPSULES (FOREST)
ESGIC TABLETS (FOREST)
ESGIC-PLUS TABLETS (FOREST)
ESIDRIX TABLETS (NOVARTIS)
ESKALITH CAPSULES (SMITHKLINE BEECHAM)
**ESKALITH CR CONTROLLED RELEASE
TABLETS** (SMITHKLINE BEECHAM)

ESMOLOL HYDROCHLORIDE

Brevibloc Injection (BAXTER)
ESTAR GEL (WESTWOOD-SQUIBB)

ESTAZOLAM

Estazolam Tablets CIV (WATSON)
ProSom Tablets (ABBOTT)
ESTAZOLAM TABLETS CIV (WATSON)
ESTINYL TABLETS (SCHERING)

**ESTRACE CREAM (SEE BRISTOL-MYERS
SQUIBB COMPANY)** (APOTHECON)
ESTRACE VAGINAL CREAM
(BRISTOL-MYERS SQUIBB)
ESTRADERM TRANSDERMAL SYSTEM
(NOVARTIS)

ESTRADIOL

Alora Transdermal System
(PROCTER & GAMBLE PHARMACEUTICALS)
Climara Transdermal System (BERLEX)
CombiPatch Transdermal System
(RHONE-POULENC RORER)
Estrace Vaginal Cream
(BRISTOL-MYERS SQUIBB)
Estradiol Tablets (MYLAN)
Estradiol Tablets, USP (WATSON)
Estring Vaginal Ring (PHARMACIA & UPJOHN)
Gynodiol Tablets (FIELDING)
Vivelle Transdermal System (NOVARTIS)
Vivelle-Dot Transdermal System (NOVARTIS)
ESTRADIOL TABLETS (MYLAN)
ESTRADIOL TABLETS (DURAMED)
ESTRADIOL TABLETS (ESI LEDERLE)
ESTRADIOL TABLETS, USP (APOTHECON)
ESTRADIOL TABLETS, USP (WATSON)

ESTRAMUSTINE PHOSPHATE SODIUM

Emcyt Capsules (PHARMACIA & UPJOHN)
ESTRATAB TABLETS (0.3, 0.625, 2.5 MG)
(SOLVAY)
ESTRATEST TABLETS (SOLVAY)
ESTRATEST H.S. TABLETS (SOLVAY)
ESTRING VAGINAL RING
(PHARMACIA & UPJOHN)

ESTROGENS, CONJUGATED, SYNTHETIC A

Cenestin Tablets (DURAMED)

ESTROGENS, CONJUGATED

Premarin Intravenous (WYETH-AYERST)
Premarin Tablets (WYETH-AYERST)
Premarin Vaginal Cream (WYETH-AYERST)
Premphase Tablets (WYETH-AYERST)
Prempro Tablets (WYETH-AYERST)

ESTROGENS, ESTERIFIED

Estratab Tablets (0.3, 0.625, 2.5 mg) (SOLVAY)
Estratest H.S. Tablets (SOLVAY)
Estratest Tablets (SOLVAY)
Menest Tablets (MONARCH)

ESTROPIPATE

Estropipate Tablets, USP (WATSON)
Ogen Tablets (PHARMACIA & UPJOHN)
Ortho-Est Tablets (WOMEN FIRST)
ESTROPIPATE TABLETS, USP (WATSON)
ESTROSTEP 21 TABLETS (PARKE-DAVIS)
ESTROSTEP FE TABLETS (PARKE-DAVIS)

ETANERCEPT

Enbrel for Injection (IMMUNEX)
Enbrel for Injection (WYETH-AYERST)

ETHACRYNATE SODIUM

Edecrin Sodium Intravenous (MERCK)

ETHACRYNIC ACID

Edecrin Tablets (MERCK)

ETHAMBUTOL HYDROCHLORIDE

Myambutol Tablets (DURA)
Myambutol Tablets (LEDERLE LABS)
ETHAMOLIN INJECTION, 5% (CYPROS)

ETHANOLAMINE OLEATE

Ethamolin Injection, 5% (CYPROS)

ETHCHLORVYNOL

Placidyl Capsules (ABBOTT)

ETHINYL ESTRADIOL

Alesse-21 Tablets (WYETH-AYERST)

Alesse-28 Tablets (WYETH-AYERST)
Brevicon-21 Tablets (SEARLE)
Brevicon-28 Tablets (SEARLE)
Demulen 1/35-21 Tablets (SEARLE)
Demulen 1/35-28 Tablets (SEARLE)
Demulen 1/50-21 Tablets (SEARLE)
Demulen 1/50-28 Tablets (SEARLE)
Desogen Tablets (ORGANON)
Estinyl Tablets (SCHERING)
Estrostep 21 Tablets (PARKE-DAVIS)
Estrostep Fe Tablets (PARKE-DAVIS)
Ethynodiol Diacetate and Ethinyl Estradiol
Tablets, USP (ZOVIA) (WATSON)
Levlen 21 Tablets (BERLEX)
Levlen 28 Tablets (BERLEX)
Levlite 21 Tablets (BERLEX)
Levlite 28 Tablets (BERLEX)
Levora Tablets (WATSON)
Lo/Ovral Tablets (WYETH-AYERST)
Lo/Ovral-28 Tablets (WYETH-AYERST)
Loestrin 21 Tablets (PARKE-DAVIS)
Loestrin Fe Tablets (PARKE-DAVIS)
Mircette Tablets (ORGANON)
Modicon 21 Tablets (ORTHO-MCNEIL)
Modicon 28 Tablets (ORTHO-MCNEIL)
Necon 0.5/35 Tablets (WATSON)
Necon 1/35 Tablets (WATSON)
Necon 10/11 Tablets (WATSON)
Nordette-21 Tablets (WYETH-AYERST)
Nordette-28 Tablets (WYETH-AYERST)
Norethindrone and Ethinyl Estradiol Tablets,
USP (NECON) (WATSON)
Norinyl 1 + 35-21 Tablets (SEARLE)
Norinyl 1 + 35-28 Tablets (SEARLE)
Ortho Tri-Cyclen 21 Tablets (ORTHO-MCNEIL)
Ortho Tri-Cyclen 28 Tablets (ORTHO-MCNEIL)
Ortho-Cept 21 Tablets (ORTHO-MCNEIL)
Ortho-Cept 28 Tablets (ORTHO-MCNEIL)
Ortho-Cyclen 21 Tablets (ORTHO-MCNEIL)
Ortho-Cyclen 28 Tablets (ORTHO-MCNEIL)
Ortho-Novum 1/35 21 Tablets (ORTHO-MCNEIL)
Ortho-Novum 1/35 28 Tablets (ORTHO-MCNEIL)
Ortho-Novum 10/11 21 Tablets
(ORTHO-MCNEIL)
Ortho-Novum 10/11 28 Tablets
(ORTHO-MCNEIL)
Ortho-Novum 7/7/7 21 Tablets (ORTHO-MCNEIL)
Ortho-Novum 7/7/7 28 Tablets (ORTHO-MCNEIL)
Ovcon 35 Tablets (BRISTOL-MYERS SQUIBB)
Ovcon 50 Tablets (BRISTOL-MYERS SQUIBB)
Ovral Tablets (WYETH-AYERST)
Ovral-28 Tablets (WYETH-AYERST)
Preven Emergency Contraceptive Kit
(GYNETICS)
Tri-Levlen 21 Tablets (BERLEX)
Tri-Levlen 28 Tablets (BERLEX)
Tri-Norinyl 21 Tablets (SEARLE)
Tri-Norinyl 28 Tablets (SEARLE)
Triphasil-21 Tablets (WYETH-AYERST)
Triphasil-28 Tablets (WYETH-AYERST)
Trivora Tablets (WATSON)
Zovia 1/35E Tablets (WATSON)
Zovia 1/50E Tablets (WATSON)

ETHIODIZED OIL

Ethiodol Injection (SAVAGE)
ETHIODOL INJECTION (SAVAGE)

ETHIONAMIDE

Trecator-SC Tablets (WYETH-AYERST)
ETHMOZINE TABLETS (ROBERTS)

ETHOSUXIMIDE

Zarontin Capsules (PARKE-DAVIS)
Zarontin Syrup (PARKE-DAVIS)
ETHRANE LIQUID FOR INHALATION
(BAXTER)

ETHYNODIOL DIACETATE
 Demulen 1/35-21 Tablets (SEARLE)
 Demulen 1/35-28 Tablets (SEARLE)
 Demulen 1/50-21 Tablets (SEARLE)
 Demulen 1/50-28 Tablets (SEARLE)
 Ethynodiol Diacetate and Ethinyl Estradiol
  Tablets, USP (ZOVIA) (WATSON)
 Zovia 1/35E Tablets (WATSON)
 Zovia 1/50E Tablets (WATSON)
**ETHYNODIOL DIACETATE AND ETHINYL
 ESTRADIOL TABLETS, USP (ZOVIA)**
 (WATSON)
ETHYOL FOR INJECTION (ALZA)

ETIDOCAINE HYDROCHLORIDE
 Duranest Injections (ASTRAZENECA LP)

ETIDRONATE DISODIUM
 Didronel I.V. Infusion (MGI)
 Didronel Tablets
  (PROCTER & GAMBLE PHARMACEUTICALS)

ETODOLAC
 Etodolac Capsules (WATSON)
 Etodolac Capsules (ENDO GENERICS)
 Etodolac Capsules and Tablets (MYLAN)
 Etodolac Tablets (PAR)
 Etodolac Tablets (WATSON)
 Etodolac Tablets (ENDO GENERICS)
 Etodolac Tablets, 400 mg, 500 mg
  (NOVOPHARM)
 Lodine Capsules (WYETH-AYERST)
 Lodine Tablets (WYETH-AYERST)
 Lodine XL Extended-Release Tablets
  (WYETH-AYERST)
ETODOLAC CAPSULES (WATSON)
ETODOLAC CAPSULES (ESI LEDERLE)
ETODOLAC CAPSULES (ENDO GENERICS)
ETODOLAC CAPSULES AND TABLETS
 (MYLAN)
ETODOLAC TABLETS (PAR)
ETODOLAC TABLETS (WATSON)
ETODOLAC TABLETS (ESI LEDERLE)
ETODOLAC TABLETS (ENDO GENERICS)
ETODOLAC TABLETS, 400 MG, 500 MG
 (NOVOPHARM)
ETOMIDATE INJECTION (BEDFORD)
ETOPOPHOS FOR INJECTION
 (BRISTOL-MYERSSQUIBBONCOLOGY/IMMUNOLOGY)

ETOPOSIDE
 VePesid Capsules
  (BRISTOL-MYERSSQUIBBONCOLOGY/IMMUNOLOGY)
 VePesid for Injection
  (BRISTOL-MYERSSQUIBBONCOLOGY/IMMUNOLOGY)
ETOPOSIDE INJECTION (BEDFORD)

ETOPOSIDE PHOSPHATE
 Etopophos for Injection
  (BRISTOL-MYERSSQUIBBONCOLOGY/IMMUNOLOGY)
ETRAFON 2-10 TABLETS (2-10) (SCHERING)
ETRAFON TABLETS (2-25) (SCHERING)
ETRAFON-FORTE TABLETS (4-25)
 (SCHERING)

EUCALYPTOL
 Cool Mint Listerine (WARNER-LAMBERT)
 FreshBurst Listerine (WARNER-LAMBERT)
 Listerine Antiseptic (WARNER-LAMBERT)
**EUCERIN GENTLE HYDRATING
 CLEANSER** (BEIERSDORF)
**EUCERIN ORIGINAL MOISTURIZING
 CREME** (BEIERSDORF)
**EUCERIN ORIGINAL MOISTURIZING
 LOTION** (BEIERSDORF)
**EUCERIN PROTECTIVE MOISTURE
 LOTION SPF 25** (BEIERSDORF)
**EUCERIN TRI-LIPID REPLENISHING
 LOTION** (BEIERSDORF)

**EUCERIN PLUS ALPHA HYDROXY
 CREME** (BEIERSDORF)
**EUCERIN PLUS ALPHA HYDROXY
 LOTION** (BEIERSDORF)
**EUCERIN PLUS RENEWAL ALPHA
 HYDROXY SPF 15** (BEIERSDORF)
**EUCERIN Q10 ANTI-WRINKLE SENSITIVE
 SKIN CREME** (BEIERSDORF)
EUDAL SR TABLETS (FOREST)
EULEXIN CAPSULES (SCHERING)
EUPHORBIUM NASAL SPRAY (HEEL)
EURAX CREAM (WESTWOOD-SQUIBB)
EURAX LOTION (WESTWOOD-SQUIBB)
EVAC-Q-KWIK (SAVAGE)
EVISTA TABLETS (LILLY)
EX. O (MAYOR)
ASPIRIN FREE EXCEDRIN CAPLETS
 (BRISTOL-MYERS)
ASPIRIN FREE EXCEDRIN GELTABS
 (BRISTOL-MYERS)
EXCEDRIN EXTRA-STRENGTH CAPLETS
 (BRISTOL-MYERS)
EXCEDRIN EXTRA-STRENGTH GELTABS
 (BRISTOL-MYERS)
EXCEDRIN EXTRA-STRENGTH TABLETS
 (BRISTOL-MYERS)
EXCEDRIN MIGRAINE CAPLETS
 (BRISTOL-MYERS)
EXCEDRIN MIGRAINE GELTABS
 (BRISTOL-MYERS)
EXCEDRIN MIGRAINE TABLETS
 (BRISTOL-MYERS)
EXCEDRIN P.M. CAPLETS (BRISTOL-MYERS)
EXCEDRIN P.M. GELTABS (BRISTOL-MYERS)
EXCEDRIN P.M. TABLETS (BRISTOL-MYERS)
EXELDERM CREAM 1.0%
 (WESTWOOD-SQUIBB)
EXELDERM SOLUTION 1.0%
 (WESTWOOD-SQUIBB)
EXGEST LA TABLETS (CARNRICK)
**EX LAX REGULAR STRENGTH LAXATIVE
 PILLS** (NOVARTIS CONSUMER)
EX LAX GENTLE STRENGTH CAPLETS
 (NOVARTIS CONSUMER)
**EX LAX MAXIMUM STRENGTH
 LAXATIVE PILLS** (NOVARTIS CONSUMER)
**EX LAX REGULAR STRENGTH
 CHOCOLATED LAXATIVE PIECES**
 (NOVARTIS CONSUMER)
EX LAX STOOL SOFTENER CAPLETS
 (NOVARTIS CONSUMER)
**EXOSURF NEONATAL FOR
 INTRATRACHEAL SUSPENSION**
 (GLAXO WELLCOME)
EXSEL LOTION/SHAMPOO (ALLERGAN)
EXTENDRYL CHEWABLE TABLETS
 (FLEMING)
EXTENDRYL SR. & JR. CAPSULES
 (FLEMING)
EXTENDRYL SYRUP (FLEMING)
EYE PAK SURGICAL DRAPES (ALCON)
**EYE STREAM EYE IRRIGATING
 SOLUTION** (ALCON)
E-Z SPACER (WE)
E-Z SPACER AND MASK (WE)
E-Z SPACER MASK (WE)

F

FACTOR VIII (AHF, AHG)
 Alphanate Solvent Detergent/Heat Treated
  (ALPHA)

FACTOR IX (HUMAN)
 AlphaNine SD Solvent Detergent Treated/Virus
  Filtered (ALPHA)
 Mononine Concentrate (CENTEON)

FACTOR IX COMPLEX
 Bebulin VH Immuno (IMMUNO)
 Konyne 80 (BAYER BIOLOGICAL)
 Profilnine SD Solvent Detergent Treated
  (ALPHA)
 Proplex T (BAXTER HEALTHCARE)
FACTREL (WYETH-AYERST)

FAMCICLOVIR
 Famvir Tablets (SMITHKLINE BEECHAM)

FAMOTIDINE
 Pepcid AC Tablets (J&J – MERCK)
 Pepcid Injection (MERCK)
 Pepcid Injection Premixed (MERCK)
 Pepcid RPD Orally Disintegrating Tablets
  (MERCK)
 Pepcid Tablets (MERCK)
 Pepcid for Oral Suspension (MERCK)
FAMVIR TABLETS (SMITHKLINE BEECHAM)
FANSIDAR TABLETS (ROCHE LABS)
FARESTON TABLETS (SCHERING)
FASTIN CAPSULES (SMITHKLINE BEECHAM)
FATTIBASE (PADDOCK)
FEIBA VH IMMUNO (IMMUNO)

FELBAMATE
 Felbatol Oral Suspension (WALLACE)
 Felbatol Tablets (WALLACE)
FELBATOL ORAL SUSPENSION (WALLACE)
FELBATOL TABLETS (WALLACE)
FELDENE CAPSULES (PFIZER)

FELODIPINE
 Lexxel Tablets (ASTRAZENECA LP)
 Plendil Extended-Release Tablets
  (ASTRAZENECA LP)
FEMARA TABLETS (NOVARTIS)
FENESIN TABLETS (DJ PHARMA)
FENESIN DM TABLETS (DJ PHARMA)

FENOFIBRATE
 Tricor Capsules, Micronized (ABBOTT)

FENOLDOPAM MESYLATE
 Corlopam Injection (NEUREX)

FENOPROFEN CALCIUM
 Fenoprofen Calcium Tablets (MYLAN)
 Fenoprofen Calcium Tablets
  (LEDERLE STANDARD)
 Nalfon Capsules (DISTA)
FENOPROFEN CALCIUM TABLETS (MYLAN)
FENOPROFEN CALCIUM TABLETS
 (LEDERLE STANDARD)

FENTANYL
 Duragesic Transdermal System (JANSSEN)

FENTANYL CITRATE
 Actiq (ABBOTT)
 Fentanyl Citrate Injection (Preservative-Free)
  (ELKINS-SINN)
 Fentanyl Citrate Injection, USP (BAXTER)
 Fentanyl Citrate and Droperidol Injection
  (ASTRAZENECA LP)
**FENTANYL CITRATE AND DROPERIDOL
 INJECTION** (ASTRAZENECA LP)
**FENTANYL CITRATE INJECTION
 (PRESERVATIVE-FREE)** (ELKINS-SINN)
FENTANYL CITRATE INJECTION, USP
 (BAXTER)
FENTANYL INJECTION, AMPUL, VIAL
 (ABBOTT)

UNDERLINE DENOTES GENERIC NAME

FENTANYL ORALET (ORAL TRANSMUCOSAL FENTANYL CITRATE) CII (ABBOTT)
FEOSOL CAPLETS
(SMITHKLINE BEECHAM CONSUMER)
FEOSOL ELIXIR
(SMITHKLINE BEECHAM CONSUMER)
FEOSOL TABLETS
(SMITHKLINE BEECHAM CONSUMER)
FEOSTAT DROPS (FOREST)
FEOSTAT SUSPENSION (FOREST)
FEOSTAT TABLETS (FOREST)
FERATAB TABLETS (UPSHER-SMITH)
FERO-FOLIC-500 FILMTAB TABLETS
(ABBOTT)
FERO-GRAD-500 FILMTAB TABLETS
(ABBOTT)
FERRLECIT INJECTION (SCHEIN)

FERROUS FUMARATE

Chromagen Capsules (SAVAGE)
Chromagen FA Capsules (SAVAGE)
Chromagen Forte Capsules (SAVAGE)
Estrostep Fe Tablets (PARKE-DAVIS)
Fetrin Capsules (LUNSCO)
Fumatinic Capsules (LASER)
Hemocyte Plus Tabules (U.S. PHARMACEUTICAL)
Hemocyte Tablets (U.S. PHARMACEUTICAL)
Hemocyte-F Tablets (U.S. PHARMACEUTICAL)
Loestrin Fe Tablets (PARKE-DAVIS)
Nephro-Fer Rx Tablets (R&D)
Nephro-Fer Tablets (R&D)
Nephro-Vite + Fe Tablets (R&D)
Trinsicon Capsules (UCB)
Vi-Daylin/F Multivitamin + Iron Chewable
Tablets With Fluoride (ROSS)

FERROUS GLUCONATE

Megadose Tablets (ARCO)
FERROUS GLUCONATE TABLETS
(UPSHER-SMITH)
FERROUS GLUCONATE TABLETS 324 MG
(PADDOCK)

FERROUS SULFATE

Feosol Elixir (SMITHKLINE BEECHAM CONSUMER)
Feosol Tablets
(SMITHKLINE BEECHAM CONSUMER)
Fero-Folic-500 Filmtab Tablets (ABBOTT)
Ferrous Sulfate Liquid
(PHARMACEUTICAL ASSOCIATES)
Iberet-Folic-500 Filmtab Tablets (ABBOTT)
Vi-Daylin/F ADC Vitamins + Iron Drops
With Fluoride (ROSS)
Vi-Daylin/F Multivitamin + Iron Drops With
Fluoride (ROSS)
ViTelle Irospan Capsules (FIELDING)
ViTelle Irospan Tablets (FIELDING)
FERROUS SULFATE LIQUID
(PHARMACEUTICAL ASSOCIATES)
FERROUS SULFATE TABLETS 324 MG
(PADDOCK)
FERTINEX FOR INJECTION (SERONO)
FETRIN CAPSULES (LUNSCO)

FEXOFENADINE HYDROCHLORIDE

Allegra Capsules (HOECHST MARION ROUSSEL)
Allegra-D Extended-Release Tablets
(HOECHST MARION ROUSSEL)

FILGRASTIM

Neupogen for Injection (AMGEN)

FINASTERIDE

Propecia Tablets (MERCK)
Proscar Tablets (MERCK)
FIORICET TABLETS (NOVARTIS)
FIORICET WITH CODEINE CAPSULES
(NOVARTIS)

FIORINAL CAPSULES (NOVARTIS)
FIORINAL WITH CODEINE CAPSULES
(NOVARTIS)
FIORPAP TABLETS (GENEVA)
FIORTAL CAPSULES (GENEVA)
FIORTAL W/CODEINE CAPSULES (GENEVA)
FLAGYL 375 CAPSULES (SEARLE)
FLAGYL ER TABLETS (SEARLE)
FLAGYL I.V. (SCS)
FLAGYL I.V. RTU (SCS)
FLAGYL TABLETS (SEARLE)
FLAREX OPHTHALMIC SUSPENSION
(ALCON)
**FLAVONEX FLAVORED ENERGY
SUPPLEMENT** (ROSS)

FLAVOXATE HYDROCHLORIDE

Urispas Tablets (ALZA)

FLAXSEED OIL

Blue-Green Sea Spray (MAYOR)
Vitamist Intra-Oral Spray Dietary Supplements
(MAYOR)

FLECAINIDE ACETATE

Tambocor Tablets (3M)
FLEET BISACODYL LAXATIVES (FLEET)
FLEET ENEMA (FLEET)
FLEET ENEMA FOR CHILDREN (FLEET)
FLEET GLYCERIN LAXATIVES (FLEET)
FLEET MINERAL OIL ENEMA (FLEET)
FLEET PHOSPHO-SODA (FLEET)
FLEET PREP KITS (FLEET)
**FLEXDERM HYDROGEL WOUND
DRESSING** (BERTEK)
FLEXERIL TABLETS (MERCK)
FLEXOJECT (MERZ)
FLEXZAN WOUND DRESSING (BERTEK)
FLOLAN FOR INJECTION
(GLAXO WELLCOME)
FLOMAX CAPSULES (BOEHRINGER INGELHEIM)
FLONASE NASAL SPRAY (GLAXO WELLCOME)
FLORICAL CAPSULES AND TABLETS
(MERICON)
FLORINEF TABLETS (APOTHECON)
FLORVITE DROPS .25MG (EVERETT)
FLORVITE + IRON DROPS .25 + .5 MG
(EVERETT)
FLORVITE TABLETS 0.5 + 1 MG (EVERETT)
FLORVITE + IRON TABLETS .5 + 1 MG
(EVERETT)
**FLOVENT 44 MCG INHALATION
AEROSOL** (GLAXO WELLCOME)
**FLOVENT 110 MCG INHALATION
AEROSOL** (GLAXO WELLCOME)
**FLOVENT 220 MCG INHALATION
AEROSOL** (GLAXO WELLCOME)
FLOVENT ROTADISK 50 MCG
(GLAXO WELLCOME)
FLOVENT ROTADISK 100 MCG
(GLAXO WELLCOME)
FLOVENT ROTADISK 250 MCG
(GLAXO WELLCOME)
FLOXIN I.V. (ORTHO-MCNEIL)
FLOXIN OTIC SOLUTION (DAIICHI)
FLOXIN TABLETS (ORTHO-MCNEIL)

FLOXURIDINE

Sterile FUDR (ROCHE LABS)

FLUCONAZOLE

Diflucan Tablets, Injection, and Oral
Suspension (PFIZER)

FLUCYTOSINE

Ancobon Capsules (ICN)
FLUDARA FOR INJECTION (BERLEX)

FLUDARABINE PHOSPHATE

Fludara for Injection (BERLEX)

FLUMADINE SYRUP (FOREST)
FLUMADINE TABLETS (FOREST)

FLUMAZENIL

Romazicon Injection (ROCHE LABS)

FLUNISOLIDE

Aerobid Inhaler System (FOREST)
Aerobid-M Inhaler System (FOREST)
Nasalide Nasal Spray (DURA)
Nasarel Nasal Solution 0.025% (DURA)

FLUOCINOLONE ACETONIDE

Derma-Smoothe/FS Topical Oil (HILL)
FS Shampoo (HILL)
Fluonid Topical Solution (ALLERGAN)
Synalar Cream (MEDICIS)
Synalar Ointment (MEDICIS)
Synalar Topical Solution (MEDICIS)
Synemol Cream (MEDICIS)

FLUOCINONIDE

Lidex Cream (MEDICIS)
Lidex Gel (MEDICIS)
Lidex Ointment (MEDICIS)
Lidex Topical Solution (MEDICIS)
Lidex-E Cream (MEDICIS)
FLUOGEN INJECTION (PARKEDALE)
FLUONID TOPICAL SOLUTION (ALLERGAN)
FLUORESCITE INJECTION (ALCON)
FLUORI-METHANE (GEBAUER)
FLUOROPLEX TOPICAL CREAM
(ALLERGAN)
FLUOROPLEX TOPICAL SOLUTION
(ALLERGAN)

FLUOROURACIL

Efudex Cream (ICN)
Efudex Topical Solutions (ICN)
Fluoroplex Topical Cream (ALLERGAN)
Fluoroplex Topical Solution (ALLERGAN)
FLUOROURACIL INJECTION (ICN)
FLUOTHANE (WYETH-AYERST)

FLUOXETINE HYDROCHLORIDE

Prozac Pulvules & Liquid, Oral Solution
(DISTA)
**FLUPHENAZINE DECANOATE INJECTION,
USP** (BEDFORD)
FLUPHENAZINE HCL TABLETS (PAR)
FLUPHENAZINE HCL TABLETS (GENEVA)

FLUPHENAZINE HYDROCHLORIDE

Fluphenazine HCl Tablets (PAR)
Fluphenazine HCl Tablets (GENEVA)
Fluphenazine Hydrochloride Elixir USP
(PHARMACEUTICAL ASSOCIATES)
Fluphenazine Hydrochloride Oral Solution USP
(Concentrate) (PHARMACEUTICAL ASSOCIATES)
Fluphenazine Hydrochloride Tablets (MYLAN)
**FLUPHENAZINE HYDROCHLORIDE
ELIXIR USP** (PHARMACEUTICAL ASSOCIATES)
**FLUPHENAZINE HYDROCHLORIDE ORAL
SOLUTION USP (CONCENTRATE)**
(PHARMACEUTICAL ASSOCIATES)
**FLUPHENAZINE HYDROCHLORIDE
TABLETS** (MYLAN)

FLURANDRENOLIDE

Cordran Lotion (OCLASSEN)
Cordran Tape (OCLASSEN)
FLURAZEPAM HCL CAPSULES (PAR)

FLURAZEPAM HYDROCHLORIDE

Flurazepam HCl Capsules (PAR)
Flurazepam Hydrochloride Capsules (MYLAN)
**FLURAZEPAM HYDROCHLORIDE
CAPSULES** (MYLAN)

FLURBIPROFEN

Flurbiprofen Tablets (MYLAN)

UNDERLINE DENOTES GENERIC NAME

Flurbiprofen Tablets (GENEVA)
Flurbiprofen Tablets, 50 mg, 100 mg
(NOVOPHARM)
FLURBIPROFEN TABLETS (MYLAN)
FLURBIPROFEN TABLETS (GENEVA)
**FLURBIPROFEN TABLETS, 50 MG, 100
MG** (NOVOPHARM)

FLUTAMIDE

Eulexin Capsules (SCHERING)

FLUTICASONE PROPIONATE

Cutivate Cream (GLAXO WELLCOME)
Cutivate Ointment (GLAXO WELLCOME)
Flonase Nasal Spray (GLAXO WELLCOME)
Flovent 110 mcg Inhalation Aerosol
(GLAXO WELLCOME)
Flovent 220 mcg Inhalation Aerosol
(GLAXO WELLCOME)
Flovent 44 mcg Inhalation Aerosol
(GLAXO WELLCOME)
Flovent Rotadisk 100 mcg (GLAXO WELLCOME)
Flovent Rotadisk 250 mcg (GLAXO WELLCOME)
Flovent Rotadisk 50 mcg (GLAXO WELLCOME)
FLUTTER (SCANDIPHARM)

FLUVASTATIN SODIUM

Lescol Capsules (NOVARTIS)
FLUVIRIN (MEDEVA)

FLUVOXAMINE MALEATE

Luvox Tablets (25, 50, 100 mg) (SOLVAY)
FLUZONE (PASTEUR MERIEUX CONNAUGHT)
FML FORTE OPHTHALMIC SUSPENSION
(ALLERGAN)
FML OPHTHALMIC SUSPENSION
(ALLERGAN)
FML S.O.P. OPHTHALMIC OINTMENT
(ALLERGAN)
FML-S OPHTHALMIC SUSPENSION
(ALLERGAN)
FOLACIN (MAYOR)
**FOLGARD (FOLIC ACID, VITAMIN B-6,
VITAMIN B-12 COMBINATION)**
(UPSHER-SMITH)

FOLIC ACID

Bevitamel Tablets (WESTLAKE)
Cefol Filmtab Tablets (ABBOTT)
Chromagen FA Capsules (SAVAGE)
Chromagen Forte Capsules (SAVAGE)
Fero-Folic-500 Filmtab Tablets (ABBOTT)
Folacin (MAYOR)
Folic Acid Injection (LEDERLE STANDARD)
Hemocyte-F Elixir (U.S. PHARMACEUTICAL)
Hemocyte-F Tablets (U.S. PHARMACEUTICAL)
Iberet-Folic-500 Filmtab Tablets (ABBOTT)
Mega-B Tablets (ARCO)
Megadose Tablets (ARCO)
Mission Prenatal F.A. Tablets (MISSION)
Mission Prenatal H.P. Tablets (MISSION)
Mission Prenatal Tablets (MISSION)
Nephro-Fer Rx Tablets (R&D)
Nephro-Vite + Fe Tablets (R&D)
Nephro-Vite Rx Tablets (R&D)
Nephro-Vite Tablets (R&D)
Niferex-150 Forte Capsules (SCHWARZ)
Nu-Iron Plus Elixir (MERZ)
Trinsicon Capsules (UCB)
VitaZac (MAYOR)
Vitafol Caplets (EVERETT)
Vitamist Intra-Oral Spray Dietary Supplements
(MAYOR)
FOLIC ACID INJECTION
(LEDERLE STANDARD)
FOLIC ACID INJECTION, USP (BEDFORD)
FOLIC ACID TABLETS, USP (SCHEIN)
FOLIC ACID/B12 POWDER (VITALINE)
FOLLISTIM FOR INJECTION (ORGANON)

FOLLITROPIN ALFA

Gonal-F for Injection (SERONO)

FOLLITROPIN BETA

Follistim for Injection (ORGANON)
FORANE LIQUID FOR INHALATION
(BAXTER)
FORMA-RAY (GORDON)
FORMADON (GORDON)

FORMALDEHYDE

Formalyde-10 Spray (PEDINOL)
Lazerformalyde Solution (PEDINOL)
FORMALYDE-10 SPRAY (PEDINOL)
FORTAZ (GLAXO WELLCOME)
FORTOVASE CAPSULES (ROCHE LABS)
FOSAMAX TABLETS (MERCK)

FOSCARNET SODIUM

Foscavir Injection (ASTRAZENECA LP)
FOSCAVIR INJECTION (ASTRAZENECA LP)

FOSFOMYCIN TROMETHAMINE

Monurol Sachet (FOREST)
FOSFREE TABLETS (MISSION)

FOSINOPRIL SODIUM

Monopril Tablets (BRISTOL-MYERS SQUIBB)

FOSPHENYTOIN SODIUM

Cerebyx Injection (PARKE-DAVIS)
FOSTEX 10% BENZOYL PEROXIDE BAR
(BRISTOL-MYERS)
**FOSTEX 10% BENZOYL PEROXIDE
(VANISH) GEL** (BRISTOL-MYERS)
FOSTEX 10% BENZOYL PEROXIDE WASH
(BRISTOL-MYERS)
FOSTEX MEDICATED CLEANSING BAR
(BRISTOL-MYERS)
**FOSTEX MEDICATED CLEANSING
CREAM** (BRISTOL-MYERS)
FOSTRIL (WESTWOOD-SQUIBB)
FOTOTAR CREAM (ICN)
**4-WAY FAST ACTING NASAL SPRAY -
REGULAR & MENTHOLATED
FORMULAS** (BRISTOL-MYERS)
4-WAY LONG LASTING NASAL SPRAY
(BRISTOL-MYERS)
**4-WAY NASAL MOISTURIZING SALINE
MIST** (BRISTOL-MYERS)
FRAGMIN INJECTION (CENTOCOR)
FRAGMIN INJECTION (PHARMACIA & UPJOHN)
FREE FORM AMINO ACID COMPLEX
(VITALINE)
FS SHAMPOO (HILL)
STERILE FUDR (ROCHE LABS)
FULVICIN P/G TABLETS (SCHERING)
FULVICIN P/G 165 & 330 TABLETS
(SCHERING)
FULVICIN-U/F TABLETS (SCHERING)
FUMATINIC CAPSULES (LASER)
**FUNGIZONE CREAM, LOTION AND
OINTMENT** (APOTHECON)
FUNGIZONE FOR TISSUE CULTURE
(APOTHECON)
FUNGIZONE INTRAVENOUS (APOTHECON)
FUNGOID SOLUTION (PEDINOL)
FUNGOID TINCTURE (PEDINOL)
**FUNGOID TINCTURE TOPICAL
ANTIFUNGAL TREATMENT KIT**
(PEDINOL)
FURACIN SOLUBLE DRESSING (ROBERTS)
FURACIN TOPICAL CREAM (ROBERTS)
FURADANTIN ORAL SUSPENSION (DURA)
FURADANTIN ORAL SUSPENSION
(PROCTER & GAMBLE PHARMACEUTICALS)

FURAZOLIDONE

Furoxone Liquid (ROBERTS)
Furoxone Tablets (ROBERTS)

FUROSEMIDE

Furosemide Injection (Preservative-Free)
(ELKINS-SINN)
Furosemide Injection, USP (BAXTER)
Furosemide Tablets (MYLAN)
Furosemide Tablets (GENEVA)
Furosemide Tablets & Oral Solution (ROXANE)
Furosemide Tablets, USP (WATSON)
**FUROSEMIDE INJECTION
(PRESERVATIVE-FREE)** (ELKINS-SINN)
FUROSEMIDE INJECTION, USP (BAXTER)
FUROSEMIDE TABLETS (MYLAN)
FUROSEMIDE TABLETS (GENEVA)
FUROSEMIDE TABLETS (LEDERLE STANDARD)
**FUROSEMIDE TABLETS & ORAL
SOLUTION** (ROXANE)
FUROSEMIDE TABLETS, USP (WATSON)
FUROXONE LIQUID (ROBERTS)
FUROXONE TABLETS (ROBERTS)

G

GABAPENTIN

Neurontin Capsules (PARKE-DAVIS)
GABITRIL FILMTAB TABLETS (ABBOTT)
GALIUM-HEEL LIQUID (HEEL)
**GAMIMUNE N, 5% SOLVENT/DETERGENT
TREATED** (BAYER BIOLOGICAL)
**GAMIMUNE N, 10%
SOLVENT/DETERGENT TREATED**
(BAYER BIOLOGICAL)
GAMMAGARD S/D (BAXTER HEALTHCARE)
GAMMAR-P I.V. (CENTEON)

GANCICLOVIR

Cytovene Capsules (ROCHE LABS)

GANCICLOVIR SODIUM

Cytovene-IV (ROCHE LABS)
GANTANOL TABLETS (ROCHE LABS)
GANTRISIN PEDIATRIC SUSPENSION
(ROCHE LABS)
GARAMYCIN CREAM 0.1% (SCHERING)
GARAMYCIN INJECTABLE (SCHERING)
GARAMYCIN OINTMENT 0.1% (SCHERING)
**GARAMYCIN OPHTHALMIC OINTMENT
STERILE** (SCHERING)
**GARAMYCIN OPHTHALMIC SOLUTION
STERILE** (SCHERING)

GARLIC EXTRACT

Echinacea + G (MAYOR)
Vitamist Intra-Oral Spray Dietary Supplements
(MAYOR)
GARLIC FORTE 3 (VITALINE)
GASTROCROM ORAL CONCENTRATE
(MEDEVA)
**GAS-X EXTRA STRENGTH ANTIGAS
LIQUIDS** (NOVARTIS CONSUMER)
**GAS-X EXTRA STRENGTH ANTIGAS
SOFTGELS** (NOVARTIS CONSUMER)
**GAS-X EXTRA STRENGTH ANTIGAS
CHEWABLE TABLETS**
(NOVARTIS CONSUMER)
**GAS-X REGULAR STRENGTH ANTIGAS
CHEWABLE TABLETS**
(NOVARTIS CONSUMER)
**GAVISCON REGULAR STRENGTH
ANTACID TABLETS**
(SMITHKLINE BEECHAM CONSUMER)
**GAVISCON EXTRA STRENGTH ANTACID
TABLETS** (SMITHKLINE BEECHAM CONSUMER)

UNDERLINE DENOTES GENERIC NAME

GAVISCON REGULAR STRENGTH LIQUID
ANTACID (SMITHKLINE BEECHAM CONSUMER)
GAVISCON EXTRA STRENGTH LIQUID
ANTACID (SMITHKLINE BEECHAM CONSUMER)
GEBAUER'S ETHYL CHLORIDE (GEBAUER)

GELATIN
Gelfilm Sterile Film (PHARMACIA & UPJOHN)
Gelfilm Sterile Ophthalmic Film
(PHARMACIA & UPJOHN)
Gelfoam Sterile Powder
(PHARMACIA & UPJOHN)

GELATIN SPONGE
Gelfoam Dental Packs (PHARMACIA & UPJOHN)
Gelfoam Sterile Compressed Sponge
(PHARMACIA & UPJOHN)
Gelfoam Sterile Sponge (PHARMACIA & UPJOHN)
GELFILM STERILE FILM
(PHARMACIA & UPJOHN)
GELFILM STERILE OPHTHALMIC FILM
(PHARMACIA & UPJOHN)
GELFOAM DENTAL PACKS
(PHARMACIA & UPJOHN)
GELFOAM STERILE POWDER
(PHARMACIA & UPJOHN)
GELFOAM STERILE SPONGE
(PHARMACIA & UPJOHN)
GELFOAM STERILE COMPRESSED
SPONGE (PHARMACIA & UPJOHN)
GELOCAST (BEIERSDORF)

GEMCITABINE HYDROCHLORIDE
Gemzar for Injection (LILLY)

GEMFIBROZIL
Gemfibrozil Tablets (MYLAN)
Lopid Tablets (PARKE-DAVIS)
GEMFIBROZIL TABLETS (MYLAN)
GEMZAR FOR INJECTION (LILLY)
GENOPTIC OPHTHALMIC OINTMENT
(ALLERGAN)
GENOPTIC OPHTHALMIC SOLUTION
(ALLERGAN)
GENOTROPIN LYOPHILIZED POWDER
(PHARMACIA & UPJOHN)
GENTAMICIN PREMIX ADD-VANTAGE
PRODUCTS (ABBOTT)

GENTAMICIN SULFATE
Garamycin Cream 0.1% (SCHERING)
Garamycin Injectable (SCHERING)
Garamycin Ointment 0.1% (SCHERING)
Garamycin Ophthalmic Ointment Sterile
(SCHERING)
Garamycin Ophthalmic Solution Sterile
(SCHERING)
Gentamicin Sulfate Injection (ELKINS-SINN)
GENTAMICIN SULFATE IN 0.9% SODIUM
CHLORIDE INJECTION (0.8, 0.9, 1.0, 1.2,
1.4 MG/ML) (ABBOTT)
GENTAMICIN SULFATE INJECTION
(ELKINS-SINN)
GENTAMICIN SULFATE USP POWDER
(PADDOCK)
GEOCILLIN TABLETS (PFIZER)
GEREF FOR INJECTION (SERONO)
GFS-2000 CAPSULES (WESTLAKE)

GINGER
VitaMotion-S (MAYOR)
Vitamist Intra-Oral Spray Dietary Supplements
(MAYOR)

GINKGO BILOBA
BioGinkgo 27/7 Extra Strength Tablets
(PHARMANEX)
GinkgoMist (MAYOR)
VitaSight (MAYOR)
VitaZac (MAYOR)

Vitamist Intra-Oral Spray Dietary Supplements
(MAYOR)
GINKGO BILOBA EXTRACT 60 MG
(MERICON)
GINKGO BILOBA PLUS (VITALINE)
GINKGOMIST (MAYOR)

GLATIRAMER ACETATE
Copaxone for Injection (TEVA MARION)
GLAUCON (ALCON P.R.)
GLIADEL WAFER (RHONE-POULENC RORER)

GLIMEPIRIDE
Amaryl Tablets (HOECHST MARION ROUSSEL)

GLIPIZIDE
Glipizide Tablets (MYLAN)
Glipizide Tablets (GENEVA)
Glipizide Tablets, USP (WATSON)
Glipizide Tablets, USP (ENDO GENERICS)
Glucotrol Tablets (PFIZER)
Glucotrol XL Extended Release Tablets
(PFIZER)
GLIPIZIDE TABLETS (MYLAN)
GLIPIZIDE TABLETS (GENEVA)
GLIPIZIDE TABLETS, USP (ENDO GENERICS)
GLIPIZIDE TABLETS, USP (WATSON)

GLOBULIN, IMMUNE (HUMAN)
BayGam (BAYER BIOLOGICAL)
BayRho-D Full Dose (BAYER BIOLOGICAL)
BayRho-D Mini-Dose (BAYER BIOLOGICAL)
Gamimune N, 10% Solvent/Detergent Treated
(BAYER BIOLOGICAL)
Gamimune N, 5% Solvent/Detergent Treated
(BAYER BIOLOGICAL)
Gammagard S/D (BAXTER HEALTHCARE)
Gammar-P I.V. (CENTEON)
Iveegam (IMMUNO)
MICRhoGAM (ORTHO-CLINICAL)
Panglobulin (AMERICAN RED CROSS)
Polygam S/D (AMERICAN RED CROSS)
RhoGAM (ORTHO-CLINICAL)
Sandoglobulin I.V. (NOVARTIS)
Venoglobulin-S 10% Solution Solvent
Detergent Treated (ALPHA)
Venoglobulin-S 5% Solution Solvent Detergent
Treated (ALPHA)
GLOFIL-125 INJECTION (CYPROS)
GLUCAGEN (GLUCAGON (RDNA ORIGIN)
FOR INJECTION) DIAGNOSTIC KIT
(BEDFORD)

GLUCAGON
Glucagon for Injection Vials and Emergency
Kit (LILLY)
GLUCAGON FOR INJECTION VIALS AND
EMERGENCY KIT (LILLY)

GLUCONO-DELTA-LACTONE
Renacidin Irrigation (GUARDIAN)
GLUCOPHAGE TABLETS
(BRISTOL-MYERS SQUIBB)

GLUCOSAMINE HYDROCHLORIDE
Cosamin DS Capsules (NUTRAMAX)

GLUCOSAMINE SULFATE
ArthriFlex (MAYOR)
Vitamist Intra-Oral Spray Dietary Supplements
(MAYOR)
GLUCOSAMINE SULFATE 500 MG
(MERICON)
GLUCOSAMINE SULFATE 500MG WITH
CHONDROITIN SULFATE 200MG
(VITALINE)
GLUCOTROL TABLETS (PFIZER)
GLUCOTROL XL EXTENDED RELEASE
TABLETS (PFIZER)
GLUTANAC CAPSULES (WESTLAKE)

GLUTAREX-1 AMINO ACID-MODIFIED
MEDICAL FOOD WITH IRON (ROSS)
GLUTAREX-2 AMINO ACID-MODIFIED
MEDICAL FOOD (ROSS)
GLUTOL (PADDOCK)
GLUTOSE 15, GLUTOSE 45 (ORAL
GLUCOSE GEL) (PADDOCK)

GLYBURIDE
DiaBeta Tablets (HOECHST MARION ROUSSEL)
Glyburide Micronized Tablets, USP, 1.5 mg,
3.0 mg, 6.0 mg (NOVOPHARM)
Glyburide Tablets (MYLAN)
Glyburide Tablets USP, 1.25 mg, 2.5 mg, 5
mg (NOVOPHARM)
Glynase PresTab Tablets
(PHARMACIA & UPJOHN)
Micronase Tablets (PHARMACIA & UPJOHN)
GLYBURIDE MICRONIZED TABLETS, USP,
1.5 MG, 3.0 MG, 6.0 MG (NOVOPHARM)
GLYBURIDE TABLETS (MYLAN)
GLYBURIDE TABLETS USP, 1.25 MG, 2.5
MG, 5 MG (NOVOPHARM)

GLYCERIN
Aci-Jel Therapeutic Vaginal Jelly
(ORTHO-MCNEIL)
Auralgan Otic Solution (WYETH-AYERST)
Eucerin Q10 Anti-Wrinkle Sensitive Skin
Creme (BEIERSDORF)
Fleet Glycerin Laxatives (FLEET)
1.5% GLYCINE IRRIGATION, USP (FLEX
& AQUALITE) (ABBOTT)
1.5% GLYCINE IRRIGATION/AQUALITE
(ABBOTT)

GLYCOPYRROLATE
Robinul Forte Tablets (HORIZON)
Robinul Injectable (BAXTER)
Robinul Injectable (ROBINS)
Robinul Tablets (HORIZON)
GLYNASE PRESTAB TABLETS
(PHARMACIA & UPJOHN)
GLY-OXIDE LIQUID
(SMITHKLINE BEECHAM CONSUMER)
GLYSET TABLETS (PHARMACIA & UPJOHN)
GLYTUSS TABS (MERZ)

GOLD SODIUM THIOMALATE
Myochrysine Injection (MERCK)

GOLDENSEAL
Echinacea + G (MAYOR)
Vitamist Intra-Oral Spray Dietary Supplements
(MAYOR)
GOLYTELY AND PINEAPPLE FLAVOR
GOLYTELY FOR ORAL SOLUTION
(BRAINTREE)

GONADORELIN HYDROCHLORIDE
Factrel (WYETH-AYERST)
GONAL-F FOR INJECTION (SERONO)
GONIOSCOPIC PRISM SOLUTION (ALCON)
GORDOCHOM SOLUTION (GORDON)
GORDOFILM (GORDON)
GORDOGESIC CREME (GORDON)
GORDON'S NO. 5 SPRAY FOOT POWDER
(GORDON)
GORDON'S UREA 22% (GORDON)
GORDON'S UREA 40% (GORDON)
GORDON'S VITE A CREME & LOTION
(GORDON)
GORDON'S VITE E CREME (GORDON)
GORMEL CREME & LOTION (GORDON)

GOSERELIN ACETATE
Zoladex (ASTRAZENECA)
Zoladex 3-month (ASTRAZENECA)

UNDERLINE DENOTES GENERIC NAME

GRAFTSKIN
Apligraf (NOVARTIS)

GRAMICIDIN
Neosporin Ophthalmic Solution Sterile
(MONARCH)

GRANISETRON HYDROCHLORIDE
Kytril Injection (SMITHKLINE BEECHAM)
Kytril Tablets (SMITHKLINE BEECHAM)
GRANULEX AEROSOL (BERTEK)

GRAPE SEED
Pine Bark and Grape Seed (MAYOR)
Vitamist Intra-Oral Spray Dietary Supplements
(MAYOR)
GREEN SOAP TINCTURE USP (PADDOCK)

GREPAFLOXACIN HYDROCHLORIDE
Raxar Tablets (GLAXO WELLCOME)
**GRIFULVIN V TABLETS MICROSIZE AND
ORAL SUSPENSION MICROSIZE**
(ORTHO DERMATOLOGICAL)
GRIPP-HEEL TABLETS (HEEL)
GRISACTIN CAPSULES (WYETH-AYERST)
GRISACTIN TABLETS (WYETH-AYERST)
GRISEOFULVIN (ESI LEDERLE)

GRISEOFULVIN
Fulvicin P/G 165 & 330 Tablets (SCHERING)
Fulvicin P/G Tablets (SCHERING)
Grifulvin V Tablets Microsize and Oral
Suspension Microsize
(ORTHO DERMATOLOGICAL)
Gris-PEG Tablets (ALLERGAN)
Grisactin Capsules (WYETH-AYERST)
Grisactin Tablets (WYETH-AYERST)
GRISEOFULVIN ULTRA (ESI LEDERLE)
GRIS-PEG TABLETS (ALLERGAN)
GUAIFED CAPSULES (MURO)
GUAIFED-PD CAPSULES (MURO)

GUAIFENESIN
Anatuss DM Syrup (MERZ)
Anatuss LA Tablets (MERZ)
Benylin Expectorant (WARNER-LAMBERT)
Benylin Multi-Symptom (WARNER-LAMBERT)
Broncholate Syrup (SANOFI)
Codiclear DH Syrup (SCHWARZ)
D-Feda II Tablets (WE)
Deconsal II Tablets (MEDEVA)
Defen-L.A. Tablets (HORIZON)
Dilaudid Cough Syrup (KNOLL LABS)
Dilor-G Liquid (SAVAGE)
Dilor-G Tablets (SAVAGE)
Donatussin DC Syrup (LASER)
Donatussin Drops (LASER)
Donatussin Syrup (LASER)
Dura-Vent Tablets (DJ PHARMA)
Duratuss DM Elixir (UCB)
Duratuss G Tablets (UCB)
Duratuss HD Elixir (UCB)
Duratuss Tablets (UCB)
Entex Capsules (DURA)
Entex LA Tablets (DURA)
Entex Liquid (DURA)
Entex PSE Tablets (DURA)
Exgest LA Tablets (CARNRICK)
Fenesin DM Tablets (DJ PHARMA)
Fenesin Tablets (DJ PHARMA)
Guai-Vent/PSE Tablets (DJ PHARMA)
Guaifed Capsules (MURO)
Guaifed-PD Capsules (MURO)
Guaifenesin Syrup (ROXANE)
Guaifenesin Syrup USP
(PHARMACEUTICAL ASSOCIATES)
Guaifenesin Syrup and Dextromethorphan
(PHARMACEUTICAL ASSOCIATES)

Guaifenesin Syrup with Codeine
(PHARMACEUTICAL ASSOCIATES)
Humibid L.A. Tablets (MEDEVA)
Hycotuss Expectorant Syrup (ENDO LABS)
Hydrocodone Bitartrate and Guaifenesin
Expectorant (PHARMACEUTICAL ASSOCIATES)
Lufyllin-GG Elixir (WALLACE)
Lufyllin-GG Tablets (WALLACE)
Muco-fen 1200 Tablets (WAKEFIELD)
Muco-fen 800 DM Tablets (WAKEFIELD)
Muco-fen 800 Tablets (WAKEFIELD)
Muco-fen DM Tablets (WAKEFIELD)
Muco-fen LA Tablets (WAKEFIELD)
Nasatab LA Tablets (ECR)
Nucofed Pediatric Expectorant Syrup
(MONARCH)
Organidin NR Liquid (WALLACE)
Organidin NR Tablets (WALLACE)
Pneumomist Tablets (ECR)
Pneumotussin HC Cough Syrup (ECR)
Pneumotussin Tablets (ECR)
Profen II DM Liquid (WAKEFIELD)
Profen II DM Tablets (WAKEFIELD)
Profen II Tablets (WAKEFIELD)
Profen LA Tablets (WAKEFIELD)
Protuss-DM Tablets (HORIZON)
Respa-1st Tablets (RESPA)
Respa-DM Tablets (RESPA)
Respa-GF Tablets (RESPA)
Respaire-SR Capsules 60, 120 (LASER)
Robitussin A-C Syrup (ROBINS)
Robitussin-DAC Syrup (ROBINS)
Safe Tussin 30 Liquid (KRAMER)
Sinutab Non-Drying Liquid Caps
(WARNER-LAMBERT)
Sinuvent Tablets (WE)
Slo-Phyllin GG Capsules
(RHONE-POULENC RORER)
Slo-Phyllin GG Syrup (RHONE-POULENC RORER)
Sudafed Cold & Cough Liquid Caps
(WARNER-LAMBERT)
Sudafed Non-Drying Sinus Liquid Caps
(WARNER-LAMBERT)
Syn-Rx DM Tablets 14 Day Treatment
Regimen (MEDEVA)
Syn-Rx Tablets 14 Day Treatment Regimen
(MEDEVA)
Triaminic Expectorant DH
(NOVARTIS CONSUMER)
Trikof-D Tablets (RESPA)
Tussafed-EX Syrup (EVERETT)
Tussafed-HC Syrup (EVERETT)
Tussafed-LA Caplets (EVERETT)
Tussend Expectorant Liquid (MONARCH)
Tussi-Organidin DM NR Liquid (WALLACE)
Tussi-Organidin DM-S NR Liquid (WALLACE)
Tussi-Organidin NR Liquid (WALLACE)
Tussi-Organidin-S NR Liquid (WALLACE)
Tylenol Cold Severe Congestion Non-Drowsy,
Multi-Symptom Caplets (MCNEIL CONSUMER)
Vicodin Tuss Expectorant (KNOLL LABS)
Zephrex LA Tablets (SANOFI)
Zephrex Tablets (SANOFI)
GUAIFENESIN AC (ESI LEDERLE)
GUAIFENESIN DAC (ESI LEDERLE)
GUAIFENESIN SYRUP (ROXANE)
GUAIFENESIN SYRUP USP
(PHARMACEUTICAL ASSOCIATES)
GUAIFENESIN SYRUP WITH CODEINE
(PHARMACEUTICAL ASSOCIATES)
**GUAIFENESIN SYRUP AND
DEXTROMETHORPHAN**
(PHARMACEUTICAL ASSOCIATES)
**GUAIMAX-D EXTENDED-RELEASE
TABLETS** (SCHWARZ)
GUAI-VENT/PSE TABLETS (DJ PHARMA)

GUANABENZ ACETATE
Guanabenz Acetate Tablets, USP (WATSON)
Wytensin Tablets (WYETH-AYERST)
GUANABENZ ACETATE TABLETS, USP
(WATSON)

GUANADREL SULFATE
Hylorel Tablets (MEDEVA)

GUANFACINE HYDROCHLORIDE
Guanfacine Hydrochloride Tablets, USP
(WATSON)
Guanfacine Tablets (PAR)
Guanfacine Tablets (MYLAN)
Tenex Tablets (ROBINS)
**GUANFACINE HYDROCHLORIDE
TABLETS** (ESI LEDERLE)
**GUANFACINE HYDROCHLORIDE
TABLETS, USP** (WATSON)
GUANFACINE TABLETS (PAR)
GUANFACINE TABLETS (MYLAN)
GUANIDINE HYDROCHLORIDE TABLETS
(KEY)
GYNODIOL TABLETS (FIELDING)

H

HABITROL TRANSDERMAL SYSTEM
(NOVARTIS CONSUMER)

HAEMOPHILUS B CONJUGATE VACCINE
ActHIB (PASTEUR MERIEUX CONNAUGHT)
Comvax (MERCK)
HibTITER (LEDERLE LABS)
Liquid PedvaxHIB (MERCK)
OmniHIB (SMITHKLINE BEECHAM)
ProHIBiT (PASTEUR MERIEUX CONNAUGHT)
HALCION TABLETS (PHARMACIA & UPJOHN)
HALDOL DECANOATE 50 INJECTION
(ORTHO-MCNEIL)
HALDOL DECANOATE 100 INJECTION
(ORTHO-MCNEIL)
**HALDOL INJECTION, TABLETS AND
CONCENTRATE** (ORTHO-MCNEIL)
HALFPRIN TABLETS (KRAMER)

HALOBETASOL PROPIONATE
Ultravate Cream 0.05% (WESTWOOD-SQUIBB)
Ultravate Ointment 0.05% (WESTWOOD-SQUIBB)
HALOG CREAM 0.1% (WESTWOOD-SQUIBB)
HALOG OINTMENT 0.1% (WESTWOOD-SQUIBB)
HALOG SOLUTION 0.1% (WESTWOOD-SQUIBB)
HALOG-E CREAM 0.1% (WESTWOOD-SQUIBB)

HALOPERIDOL
Haldol Injection, Tablets and Concentrate
(ORTHO-MCNEIL)
Haloperidol Oral Solution USP (Concentrate)
(PHARMACEUTICAL ASSOCIATES)
Haloperidol Tablets (MYLAN)
Haloperidol Tablets (GENEVA)

HALOPERIDOL DECANOATE
Haldol Decanoate 100 Injection
(ORTHO-MCNEIL)
Haldol Decanoate 50 Injection (ORTHO-MCNEIL)
HALOPERIDOL DECANOATE INJECTION
(BEDFORD)
**HALOPERIDOL ORAL SOLUTION USP
(CONCENTRATE)**
(PHARMACEUTICAL ASSOCIATES)
HALOPERIDOL TABLETS (MYLAN)
HALOPERIDOL TABLETS (GENEVA)

UNDERLINE DENOTES GENERIC NAME

HALOTHANE

Fluothane (WYETH-AYERST)

HAVRIX (SMITHKLINE BEECHAM)

HEAD & SHOULDERS DANDRUFF SHAMPOO (PROCTER & GAMBLE)

HEAD & SHOULDERS DANDRUFF SHAMPOO DRY SCALP (PROCTER & GAMBLE)

HEAD & SHOULDERS INTENSIVE TREATMENT DANDRUFF AND SEBORRHEIC DERMATITIS SHAMPOO (PROCTER & GAMBLE)

HEARTBAR (COOKE)

HELIXATE CONCENTRATE (CENTEON)

HEMABATE STERILE SOLUTION (SALES RESTRICTED TO HOSPITALS ONLY) (PHARMACIA & UPJOHN)

HEMIN

Panhematin for Injection (ABBOTT)

HEMOCYTE TABLETS (U.S. PHARMACEUTICAL)

HEMOCYTE PLUS TABULES (U.S. PHARMACEUTICAL)

HEMOCYTE-F ELIXIR (U.S. PHARMACEUTICAL)

HEMOCYTE-F TABLETS (U.S. PHARMACEUTICAL)

HEMOFIL M (BAXTER HEALTHCARE)

HEMORRHOIDAL-HC UNISERTS SUPPOSITORIES (HEMRIL-HC) (UPSHER-SMITH)

HEPARIN FLUSH KITS (WYETH-AYERST)

HEPARIN FLUSH KITS IN TUBEX (WYETH-AYERST)

HEPARIN FLUSH 2 ML KITS (WYETH-AYERST)

HEPARIN LOCK FLUSH SOLUTION (WYETH-AYERST)

HEPARIN LOCK FLUSH SOLUTION IN TUBEX (WYETH-AYERST)

HEPARIN SODIUM

Hep-Lock (Heparin Lock Flush Solution) (ELKINS-SINN)

Hep-Lock (Preservative-Free Heparin Lock Flush Solution) (ELKINS-SINN)

Heparin Flush Kits in Tubex (WYETH-AYERST)

Heparin Lock Flush Solution (WYETH-AYERST)

Heparin Lock Flush Solution in Tubex (WYETH-AYERST)

Heparin Sodium Injection (ELKINS-SINN)

Heparin Sodium Injection (WYETH-AYERST)

Heparin Sodium Vials (LILLY)

Heparin Sodium in Tubex (WYETH-AYERST)

HEPARIN SODIUM IN 0.45% SODIUM CHLORIDE INJECTION (50 & 100 UNITS/ML) (ABBOTT)

HEPARIN SODIUM IN 5% DEXTROSE INJECTION (50 & 100 UNITS/ML) (ABBOTT)

HEPARIN SODIUM INJECTION (ELKINS-SINN)

HEPARIN SODIUM INJECTION (WYETH-AYERST)

HEPARIN SODIUM INJECTION, USP, STERILE SOLUTION (PHARMACIA & UPJOHN)

HEPARIN SODIUM IN TUBEX (WYETH-AYERST)

HEPARIN SODIUM VIALS (LILLY)

HEPATITIS A VACCINE, INACTIVATED

Havrix (SMITHKLINE BEECHAM)

Vaqta (MERCK)

HEPATITIS B IMMUNE GLOBULIN (HUMAN)

BayHep B (BAYER BIOLOGICAL)

Nabi-HB (NABI)

HEPATITIS B VACCINE, RECOMBINANT

Comvax (MERCK)

Engerix-B (SMITHKLINE BEECHAM)

Recombivax HB (MERCK)

HEP-FORTE CAPSULES (MARLYN)

HEP-LOCK (HEPARIN LOCK FLUSH SOLUTION) (ELKINS-SINN)

HEP-LOCK (PRESERVATIVE-FREE HEPARIN LOCK FLUSH SOLUTION) (ELKINS-SINN)

HERBAL ANTIOXIDANT FORMULA WITH PYCNOGENOL (VITALINE)

HERBALS, MULTIPLE

Calm Colon Capsules (SAMRA)

Vitamist Intra-Oral Spray Dietary Supplements (MAYOR)

HERCEPTIN I.V. (GENENTECH)

HESPERIDIN COMPLEX

Peridin-C Tablets (BEUTLICH)

HESPERIDIN METHYL CHALCONE

Peridin-C Tablets (BEUTLICH)

HETASTARCH

6% Hetastarch in 0.9% Sodium Chloride Injection (BAXTER)

6% HETASTARCH IN 0.9% SODIUM CHLORIDE INJECTION (BAXTER)

HEXACHLOROPHENE

pHisoHex Cleanser (SANOFI)

HEXALEN CAPSULES (U.S. BIOSCIENCE)

HEXAVITAMIN TABLETS (UPSHER-SMITH)

HIBICLENS ANTIMICROBIAL SKIN CLEANSER (ASTRAZENECA)

HIBICLENS PACKETTES (ASTRAZENECA)

HIBICLENS SPONGE/BRUSH WITH NAIL CLEANER (ASTRAZENECA)

HIBISTAT GERMICIDAL HAND RINSE (ASTRAZENECA)

HIBISTAT TOWELETTE (ASTRAZENECA)

HIBTITER (LEDERLE LABS)

HIPREX (HOECHST MARION ROUSSEL)

HISTOPLASMIN, DILUTED (MONARCH)

HISTUSSIN D LIQUID (SANOFI)

HISTUSSIN HC SYRUP (SANOFI)

HIVID TABLETS (ROCHE LABS)

HMS OPHTHALMIC SUSPENSION (ALLERGAN)

HOMATROPINE METHYLBROMIDE

Hycodan Syrup (ENDO LABS)

Hycodan Tablets (ENDO LABS)

HOMEOPATHIC FORMULATIONS

CoQuinone Capsules (USANA)

Mega Antioxidant Tablets (USANA)

Proflavanol Tablets (USANA)

Traumeel Injection Solution (HEEL)

Vertigoheel Liquid in Oral Vials (HEEL)

Vertigoheel Oral Drops (HEEL)

Vertigoheel Tablets (HEEL)

HOMINEX-1 AMINO ACID-MODIFIED MEDICAL FOOD WITH IRON (ROSS)

HOMINEX-2 AMINO ACID-MODIFIED MEDICAL FOOD (ROSS)

HOMOSALATE

Solbar AVO Lotion SPF 32 (PERSON & COVEY)

HUMALOG (LILLY)

HUMAN ALBUMIN GRIFOLS 20% SOLUTION (GRIFOLS)

HUMAN INSULIN DELIVERY SYSTEMS (DURABLE, DISPOSABLE) (NOVO NORDISK)

HUMATE-P CONCENTRATE (CENTEON)

HUMATIN (MONARCH)

HUMATROPE VIALS AND CARTRIDGES (LILLY)

HUMEGON FOR INJECTION (ORGANON)

HUMIBID L.A. TABLETS (MEDEVA)

HUMORSOL STERILE OPHTHALMIC SOLUTION (MERCK)

HUMULIN 50/50, 100 UNITS (LILLY)

HUMULIN 70/30, 100 UNITS (LILLY)

HUMULIN 70/30 PEN (LILLY)

HUMULIN L, 100 UNITS (LILLY)

HUMULIN N, 100 UNITS (LILLY)

HUMULIN R REGULAR (U-500) (LILLY)

HUMULIN R, 100 UNITS (LILLY)

HUMULIN U, 100 UNITS (LILLY)

HUMULIN 70/30 CARTRIDGE (LILLY)

HUMULIN N NPH CARTRIDGE (LILLY)

HUMULIN N NPH PEN (LILLY)

HUMULIN R REGULAR CARTRIDGE (LILLY)

HURRICAINE TOPICAL ANESTHETIC AEROSOL SPRAY, 2 OZ. WILD CHERRY (BEUTLICH)

HURRICAINE TOPICAL ANESTHETIC GEL: 1 OZ. WILD CHERRY, FRESH MINT, PINA COLADA, WATERMELON, 1/6 OZ. WILD CHERRY, WATERMELON (BEUTLICH)

HURRICAINE TOPICAL ANESTHETIC LIQUID: 1 OZ. WILD CHERRY AND PINA COLADA .25 ML DRY HANDLE SWAB WILD CHERRY, 1/6 OZ. WILD CHERRY (BEUTLICH)

HURRICAINE TOPICAL ANESTHETIC SPRAY EXTENSION TUBES (200) (BEUTLICH)

HURRICAINE TOPICAL ANESTHETIC SPRAY KIT (BEUTLICH)

HYALGAN SOLUTION (SANOFI)

HYALURONIDASE

Wydase, Lyophilized (WYETH-AYERST)

HYATE:C (SPEYWOOD)

HYCAMTIN FOR INJECTION (SMITHKLINE BEECHAM)

HYCODAN SYRUP (ENDO LABS)

HYCODAN TABLETS (ENDO LABS)

HYCOMINE COMPOUND TABLETS (ENDO LABS)

HYCOMINE SYRUP (ENDO LABS)

HYCOMINE PEDIATRIC SYRUP (ENDO LABS)

HYCOTUSS EXPECTORANT SYRUP (ENDO LABS)

HYDERGINE LIQUID (NOVARTIS)

HYDERGINE LC LIQUID CAPSULES (NOVARTIS)

HYDERGINE ORAL TABLETS (NOVARTIS)

HYDRALAZINE HCL TABLETS (PAR)

HYDRALAZINE HCL TABLETS (LEDERLE STANDARD)

HYDRALAZINE HYDROCHLORIDE

Hydra-Zide Capsules (PAR)

Hydralazine HCl Tablets (PAR)

Hydralazine HCl Tablets (LEDERLE STANDARD)

HYDRA-ZIDE CAPSULES (PAR)

HYDREA CAPSULES (BRISTOL-MYERSSQUIBBONCOLOGY/IMMUNOLOGY)

HYDRISALIC GEL (PEDINOL)

HYDRISINOL CREME (PEDINOL)

HYDRISINOL LOTION (PEDINOL)

HYDROCET CAPSULES (CARNRICK)

HYDROCHLOROTHIAZIDE

Aldactazide Tablets (SEARLE)

Aldoril Tablets (MERCK)

Amiloride HCl and HCTZ Tablets, USP (WATSON)

Amiloride Hydrochloride and Hydrochlorothiazide Tablets (MYLAN)

Amiloride Hydrochloride and Hydrochlorothiazide Tablets, USP (ENDO GENERICS)

Avalide Tablets (BRISTOL-MYERS SQUIBB)
Captopril and Hydrochlorothiazide Tablets
  (MYLAN)
Captopril and Hydrochlorothiazide Tablets,
  USP (ENDO GENERICS)
Diovan HCT Tablets (NOVARTIS)
Dyazide Capsules (SMITHKLINE BEECHAM)
Hydra-Zide Capsules (PAR)
HydroDIURIL Tablets (MERCK)
Hydrochlorothiazide Oral Solution (ROXANE)
Hydrochlorothiazide Tablets
  (LEDERLE STANDARD)
Hyzaar 100-25 Tablets (MERCK)
Hyzaar 50-12.5 Tablets (MERCK)
Inderide LA Long-Acting Capsules
  (WYETH-AYERST)
Inderide Tablets (WYETH-AYERST)
Maxzide Tablets (BERTEK)
Maxzide-25 mg Tablets (BERTEK)
Methyldopa & Hydrochlorothiazide Tablets
  (LEDERLE STANDARD)
Methyldopa and Hydrochlorothiazide Tablets
  (MYLAN)
Methyldopa/Hydrochlorothiazide Tablets, USP
  (ENDO GENERICS)
Microzide Capsules (WATSON)
Moduretic Tablets (MERCK)
Prinzide Tablets (MERCK)
Propranolol Hydrochloride and
  Hydrochlorothiazide Tablets (MYLAN)
Spironolactone and Hydrochlorothiazide Tablets
  (MYLAN)
Timolide Tablets (MERCK)
Triamterene and Hydrochlorothiazide Capsules
  and Tablets (MYLAN)
Triamterene and Hydrochlorothiazide Tablets,
  USP (WATSON)
Triamterene/HCTZ (Dyazide) 37.5mg/25mg
  Capsules (GENEVA)
Triamterene/HCTZ (Maxzide) 75mg/50mg
  Tablets (GENEVA)
Triamterene/HCTZ (mini-Maxzide)
  37.5mg/25mg Tablets (GENEVA)
Triamterene/HCTZ 50mg/25mg Capsules
  (GENEVA)
Uniretic Tablets (SCHWARZ)
Vaseretic Tablets (MERCK)
Zestoretic Tablets (ASTRAZENECA)
Ziac Tablets (LEDERLE LABS)
**HYDROCHLOROTHIAZIDE ORAL
SOLUTION** (ROXANE)
HYDROCHLOROTHIAZIDE TABLETS
(LEDERLE STANDARD)

HYDROCODONE BITARTRATE

Anaplex HD Cough Syrup (ECR)
Codiclear DH Syrup (SCHWARZ)
Codimal DH Syrup (SCHWARZ)
Donatussin DC Syrup (LASER)
Duratuss HD Elixir (UCB)
Endal-HD (FOREST)
Histussin D Liquid (SANOFI)
Histussin HC Syrup (SANOFI)
Hycodan Syrup (ENDO LABS)
Hycodan Tablets (ENDO LABS)
Hycomine Compound Tablets (ENDO LABS)
Hycomine Pediatric Syrup (ENDO LABS)
Hycomine Syrup (ENDO LABS)
Hycotuss Expectorant Syrup (ENDO LABS)
Hydrocet Capsules (CARNRICK)
Hydrocodone Bitartrate and APAP Tablets,
  USP CIII (WATSON)
Hydrocodone Bitartrate and Acetaminophen
  Capsules (MALLINCKRODT)
Hydrocodone Bitartrate and Acetaminophen
  Elixir (MALLINCKRODT)

Hydrocodone Bitartrate and Acetaminophen
  Elixir (PHARMACEUTICAL ASSOCIATES)
Hydrocodone Bitartrate and Acetaminophen
  Tablets, USP (MALLINCKRODT)
Hydrocodone Bitartrate and Guaifenesin
  Expectorant (PHARMACEUTICAL ASSOCIATES)
Hydrocodone Bitartrate/Acetaminophen Tablets,
  USP CIII (ENDO GENERICS)
Lorcet 10/650 Tablets (FOREST)
Lorcet Plus Tablets (FOREST)
Lorcet-HD Capsules (FOREST)
Lortab 10/500 Tablets (UCB)
Lortab 2.5/500 Tablets (UCB)
Lortab 5/500 Tablets (UCB)
Lortab 7.5/500 Tablets (UCB)
Lortab Elixir (UCB)
Nalex DH Liquid (BLANSETT)
Norco Tablets CIII (WATSON)
Pneumotussin HC Cough Syrup (ECR)
Pneumotussin Tablets (ECR)
Protuss Liquid (HORIZON)
Protuss-D Liquid (HORIZON)
Triaminic Expectorant DH
  (NOVARTIS CONSUMER)
Tussafed-HC Syrup (EVERETT)
Tussend Expectorant Liquid (MONARCH)
Tussend Syrup (MONARCH)
Tussend Tablets (MONARCH)
Vicodin ES Tablets (KNOLL LABS)
Vicodin HP Tablets (KNOLL LABS)
Vicodin Tablets (KNOLL LABS)
Vicodin Tuss Expectorant (KNOLL LABS)
Vicoprofen Tablets (KNOLL LABS)
Zydone Tablets (ENDO LABS)
**HYDROCODONE BITARTRATE AND
ACETAMINOPHEN CAPSULES**
(MALLINCKRODT)
**HYDROCODONE BITARTRATE AND
ACETAMINOPHEN ELIXIR**
(MALLINCKRODT)
**HYDROCODONE BITARTRATE AND
ACETAMINOPHEN ELIXIR**
(PHARMACEUTICAL ASSOCIATES)
**HYDROCODONE BITARTRATE AND
ACETAMINOPHEN TABLETS**
(ESI LEDERLE)
**HYDROCODONE BITARTRATE AND
ACETAMINOPHEN TABLETS, USP**
(MALLINCKRODT)
**HYDROCODONE BITARTRATE AND APAP
TABLETS, USP CIII** (WATSON)
**HYDROCODONE BITARTRATE AND
GUAIFENESIN EXPECTORANT**
(PHARMACEUTICAL ASSOCIATES)
**HYDROCODONE
BITARTRATE/ACETAMINOPHEN
TABLETS, USP CIII** (ENDO GENERICS)

HYDROCODONE POLISTIREX

Tussionex Pennkinetic Extended-Release
  Suspension (MEDEVA)
**HYDROCOL HYDROCOLLOID WOUND
DRESSING** (BERTEK)
A-HYDROCORT (ABBOTT)

HYDROCORTISONE

Anusol-HC Cream 2.5% (MONARCH)
Aquanil HC Lotion (PERSON & COVEY)
Cipro HC Otic Suspension (ALCON)
Cortane-B Ear Drops (BLANSETT)
Cortane-B Otic Vials (BLANSETT)
Cortenema (SOLVAY)
Cortic Ear Drops (EVERETT)
Cortisporin Ointment (MONARCH)
Cortisporin Ophthalmic Ointment Sterile
  (MONARCH)

Cortisporin Ophthalmic Suspension Sterile
  (MONARCH)
Cortisporin Otic Solution Sterile (MONARCH)
Cortisporin Otic Suspension Sterile (MONARCH)
Hydrocortone Tablets (MERCK)
Hytone Cream 2 1/2% (DERMIK)
Hytone Lotion 2 1/2% (DERMIK)
Hytone Ointment 2 1/2% (DERMIK)
LactiCare-HC Lotion, 1% (STIEFEL)
LactiCare-HC Lotion, 2 1/2% (STIEFEL)
Lazersporin-C Solution (PEDINOL)
Nutracort Lotion (HEALTHPOINT)
Pediotic Suspension Sterile (MONARCH)
Penecort Cream (ALLERGAN)
Penecort Topical Solution (ALLERGAN)
ProctoCream-HC 2.5% (SCHWARZ)
Proctocort Cream (MONARCH)
Vanoxide-HC Acne Lotion (DERMIK)
VoSoL HC Otic Solution (WALLACE)
Vytone Cream 1% (DERMIK)
Zoto-HC Ear Drops (HORIZON)

HYDROCORTISONE ACETATE

Analpram HC Lotion 2.5% (FERNDALE)
Analpram-HC Rectal Cream 1% and 2.5%
  (FERNDALE)
Anusol HC-1 Ointment (WARNER-LAMBERT)
Anusol-HC Suppositories (MONARCH)
Cortifoam (SCHWARZ)
Cortisporin Cream (MONARCH)
Cortisporin-TC Otic Suspension (MONARCH)
Epifoam (SCHWARZ)
Hydrocortone Acetate Injectable Suspension
  (MERCK)
Pramosone Cream (FERNDALE)
Pramosone Lotion (FERNDALE)
Pramosone Ointment (FERNDALE)
ProctoFoam-HC (SCHWARZ)
Proctocort Suppositories (MONARCH)
Terra-Cortil Ophthalmic Suspension (PFIZER)

HYDROCORTISONE BUTYRATE

Locoid Cream (FERNDALE)
Locoid Lipocream Cream (FERNDALE)
Locoid Ointment (FERNDALE)
Locoid Topical Solution (FERNDALE)
HYDROCORTISONE CREAM 1% (MERICON)
HYDROCORTISONE LOTION 1% (MERICON)

HYDROCORTISONE PROBUTATE

Pandel Cream (SAVAGE)

HYDROCORTISONE SODIUM PHOSPHATE

Hydrocortone Phosphate Injection, Sterile
  (MERCK)
**HYDROCORTISONE USP MICRONIZED
POWDER** (PADDOCK)
**HYDROCORTISONE VALERATE CREAM
AND OINTMENT** (APOTHECON)
**HYDROCORTISONE ACETATE USP
MICRONIZED POWDER** (PADDOCK)
**HYDROCORTISONE ACETATE
SUPPOSITORIES 25 MG** (PADDOCK)
HYDROCORTONE TABLETS (MERCK)
**HYDROCORTONE ACETATE INJECTABLE
SUSPENSION** (MERCK)
**HYDROCORTONE PHOSPHATE
INJECTION, STERILE** (MERCK)
HYDROCREAM BASE (PADDOCK)
HYDRODIURIL TABLETS (MERCK)

HYDROFLUMETHIAZIDE

Diucardin Tablets (WYETH-AYERST)
HYDROMORPHONE HCL INJECTION
(WYETH-AYERST)
HYDROMORPHONE HCL INJECTION
(ASTRAZENECA LP)
**HYDROMORPHONE HCL USP NON-
STERILE POWDER CII** (PADDOCK)

HYDROMORPHONE HCL SUPPOSITORIES 3 MG CII (PADDOCK)

HYDROMORPHONE HYDROCHLORIDE

Dilaudid Ampules (KNOLL LABS)
Dilaudid Cough Syrup (KNOLL LABS)
Dilaudid Injection (KNOLL LABS)
Dilaudid Multiple Dose Vials (Sterile Solution) (KNOLL LABS)
Dilaudid Oral Liquid (KNOLL LABS)
Dilaudid Powder (KNOLL LABS)
Dilaudid Rectal Suppositories (KNOLL LABS)
Dilaudid Tablets - 8 mg (KNOLL LABS)
Dilaudid Tablets 2 mg and 4 mg (KNOLL LABS)
Dilaudid-HP Injection (KNOLL LABS)
Dilaudid-HP Lyophilized Powder 250mg (KNOLL LABS)
Hydromorphone HCl Injection (ASTRAZENECA LP)
Hydromorphone Hydrochloride Injection (ELKINS-SINN)
Hydromorphone Hydrochloride Tablets and Oral Solution (ROXANE)
Hydromorphone Hydrochloride Tablets, USP (MALLINCKRODT)
Hydromorphone Hydrochloride Tablets, USP CII (ENDO GENERICS)
Hydromorphone Hydrochloride in Tubex (WYETH-AYERST)

HYDROMORPHONE HYDROCHLORIDE IN TUBEX (WYETH-AYERST)

HYDROMORPHONE HYDROCHLORIDE INJECTION (ELKINS-SINN)

HYDROMORPHONE HYDROCHLORIDE TABLETS AND ORAL SOLUTION (ROXANE)

HYDROMORPHONE HYDROCHLORIDE TABLETS, USP (MALLINCKRODT)

HYDROMORPHONE HYDROCHLORIDE TABLETS, USP CII (ENDO GENERICS)

HYDROQUINONE

Eldopaque Forte 4% Cream (ICN)
Eldoquin Forte 4% Cream (ICN)
Lustra Cream (MEDICIS)
Lustra-AF Cream (MEDICIS)
Melanex Topical Solution (NEUTROGENA)
Solaquin Forte 4% Cream (ICN)
Solaquin Forte 4% Gel (ICN)

HYDROXYCHLOROQUINE SULFATE

Hydroxychloroquine Sulfate Tablets (MYLAN)
Hydroxychloroquine Sulfate Tablets (GENEVA)
Hydroxychloroquine Sulfate Tablets, USP (WATSON)
Plaquenil Tablets (SANOFI)

HYDROXYCHLOROQUINE SULFATE TABLETS (MYLAN)

HYDROXYCHLOROQUINE SULFATE TABLETS (GENEVA)

HYDROXYCHLOROQUINE SULFATE TABLETS, USP (WATSON)

HYDROXYPROPYL CELLULOSE

Lacrisert Sterile Ophthalmic Insert (MERCK)

HYDROXYPROPYL METHYLCELLULOSE

Bion Tears Lubricant Eye Drops (ALCON)
Tears Naturale Free Lubricant Eye Drops (ALCON)
Tears Naturale II Lubricant Eye Drops (ALCON)

HYDROXYUREA

Droxia Capsules (BRISTOL-MYERSSQUIBBONCOLOGY/IMMUNOLOGY)
Hydrea Capsules (BRISTOL-MYERSSQUIBBONCOLOGY/IMMUNOLOGY)
Hydroxyurea Capsules (PAR)

HYDROXYUREA CAPSULES (PAR)

HYDROXYZINE HCL INJECTION, ABBOJECTS, AMPULS, VIALS, SYRINGES (ABBOTT)

HYDROXYZINE HYDROCHLORIDE

Atarax Tablets & Syrup (PFIZER)
Hydroxyzine Hydrochloride Injection (ELKINS-SINN)
Hydroxyzine Hydrochloride Tablets, USP (WATSON)
Marax Tablets & DF Syrup (PFIZER)
Vistaril Intramuscular Solution (PFIZER)

HYDROXYZINE HYDROCHLORIDE INJECTION (ELKINS-SINN)

HYDROXYZINE HYDROCHLORIDE TABLETS, USP (WATSON)

HYDROXYZINE PAMOATE

Hydroxyzine Pamoate Capsules (WATSON)
Vistaril Capsules (PFIZER)
Vistaril Oral Suspension (PFIZER)

HYDROXYZINE PAMOATE CAPSULES (WATSON)

HYGROTON TABLETS (RHONE-POULENC RORER)

HYLAN G-F 20

Synvisc (WYETH-AYERST)

HYLOREL TABLETS (MEDEVA)

HYOSCYAMINE

Cystospaz Tablets (POLYMEDICA)
Urised Tablets (POLYMEDICA)

HYOSCYAMINE HYDROBROMIDE

Pyridium Plus Tablets (WARNER CHILCOTT)

HYOSCYAMINE SULFATE

Arco-Lase Plus Tablets (ARCO)
Atrohist Plus Tablets (MEDEVA)
Cystospaz-M Capsules (POLYMEDICA)
Donnatal Capsules (ROBINS)
Donnatal Elixir (ROBINS)
Donnatal Extentabs (ROBINS)
Donnatal Tablets (ROBINS)
Kutrase Capsules (SCHWARZ)
Levbid Extended-Release Tablets (SCHWARZ)
Levsin Drops (SCHWARZ)
Levsin Elixir (SCHWARZ)
Levsin Injection (SCHWARZ)
Levsin Tablets (SCHWARZ)
Levsin/SL Tablets (SCHWARZ)
Levsinex Timecaps (SCHWARZ)
Prosed/DS Tablets (STAR)

HYPERICUM

Bio St. John's Capsules (PHARMANEX)
VitaZac (MAYOR)
Vitamist Intra-Oral Spray Dietary Supplements (MAYOR)

HYPERSTAT I.V. INJECTION (SCHERING)

HYTAKEROL CAPSULES (SANOFI)

HYTONE CREAM 2 1/2% (DERMIK)

HYTONE LOTION 2 1/2% (DERMIK)

HYTONE OINTMENT 2 1/2% (DERMIK)

HYTRIN CAPSULES (ABBOTT)

HYZAAR 50-12.5 TABLETS (MERCK)

HYZAAR 100-25 TABLETS (MERCK)

I

IBERET-FOLIC-500 FILMTAB TABLETS (ABBOTT)

IBU TABLETS (PAR)

IBUPROFEN

Children's Motrin Chewable Tablets (MCNEIL CONSUMER)
Children's Motrin Oral Suspension (MCNEIL CONSUMER)
IBU Tablets (PAR)
Ibuprofen Suspension (PAR)
Ibuprofen Tablets (PAR)
Ibuprofen Tablets (MYLAN)
Infants' Motrin Concentrated Drops (MCNEIL CONSUMER)
Junior Strength Motrin Caplets (MCNEIL CONSUMER)
Junior Strength Motrin Chewable Tablets (MCNEIL CONSUMER)
Motrin Cold & Flu Caplets (MCNEIL CONSUMER)
Motrin IB Pain Reliever Tablets, Caplets, and Gelcaps (MCNEIL CONSUMER)
Motrin Sinus Headache Caplets (MCNEIL CONSUMER)
Motrin Suspension, Oral Drops, Chewable Tablets, and Caplets (MCNEIL CONSUMER)
Vicoprofen Tablets (KNOLL LABS)

IBUPROFEN SUSPENSION (PAR)

IBUPROFEN TABLETS (PAR)

IBUPROFEN TABLETS (MYLAN)

IBUTILIDE FUMARATE

Corvert Injection (PHARMACIA & UPJOHN)

IDAMYCIN INJECTION (PHARMACIA & UPJOHN)

IDAMYCIN PFS INJECTION (PHARMACIA & UPJOHN)

IDARUBICIN HYDROCHLORIDE

Idamycin PFS Injection (PHARMACIA & UPJOHN)

IFEX FOR INJECTION (BRISTOL-MYERSSQUIBBONCOLOGY/IMMUNOLOGY)

IFOSFAMIDE

Ifex for Injection (BRISTOL-MYERSSQUIBBONCOLOGY/IMMUNOLOGY)

I-KNIFE OPHTHALMIC KNIFE (ALCON)

ILETIN II, LENTE (PORK), 100 UNITS (LILLY)

ILETIN II, NPH (PORK), 100 UNITS (LILLY)

ILETIN II, REGULAR (PORK), 100 UNITS (LILLY)

ILOTYCIN OPHTHALMIC OINTMENT (DISTA)

IMDUR TABLETS (KEY)

IMIGLUCERASE

Cerezyme for Injection (GENZYME)

IMIPENEM

Primaxin I.M. (MERCK)
Primaxin I.V. (MERCK)

IMIPRAMINE HCL TABLETS (PAR)

IMIPRAMINE HCL TABLETS (GENEVA)

IMIPRAMINE HYDROCHLORIDE

Imipramine HCl Tablets (PAR)
Imipramine HCl Tablets (GENEVA)

IMIQUIMOD

Aldara Cream, 5% (3M)

IMITREX INJECTION (GLAXO WELLCOME)

IMITREX NASAL SPRAY (GLAXO WELLCOME)

IMITREX TABLETS (GLAXO WELLCOME)

IMMUNOCAL (IMMUNOTEC)

IMODIUM CAPSULES (MCNEIL CONSUMER)

IMODIUM A-D CAPLETS AND LIQUID (MCNEIL CONSUMER)

IMODIUM ADVANCED CHEWABLE TABLETS (MCNEIL CONSUMER)

UNDERLINE DENOTES GENERIC NAME

IMOGAM RABIES - HT
(PASTEUR MERIEUX CONNAUGHT)
IMOVAX RABIES I.D. VACCINE
(PASTEUR MERIEUX CONNAUGHT)
IMOVAX RABIES VACCINE
(PASTEUR MERIEUX CONNAUGHT)
IMURAN INJECTION (FARO)
IMURAN TABLETS (FARO)

INDAPAMIDE

Indapamide Tablets (PAR)
Indapamide Tablets (MYLAN)
Indapamide Tablets, USP (WATSON)
Lozol Tablets (RHONE-POULENC RORER)
INDAPAMIDE TABLETS (PAR)
INDAPAMIDE TABLETS (MYLAN)
INDAPAMIDE TABLETS, USP (WATSON)
INDERAL INJECTABLE (WYETH-AYERST)
INDERAL LA LONG-ACTING CAPSULES
(WYETH-AYERST)
INDERAL TABLETS (WYETH-AYERST)
INDERIDE LA LONG-ACTING CAPSULES
(WYETH-AYERST)
INDERIDE TABLETS (WYETH-AYERST)

INDINAVIR SULFATE

Crixivan Capsules (MERCK)
INDOCIN CAPSULES (MERCK)
INDOCIN I.V. (MERCK)
INDOCIN ORAL SUSPENSION (MERCK)
INDOCIN SUPPOSITORIES (MERCK)
INDOCIN SR CAPSULES (MERCK)

INDOMETHACIN

Indocin Capsules (MERCK)
Indocin Oral Suspension (MERCK)
Indocin SR Capsules (MERCK)
Indocin Suppositories (MERCK)
Indomethacin Capsules (MYLAN)
Indomethacin Capsules, 25 mg, 50 mg
(NOVOPHARM)
Indomethacin Extended-Release Capsules, USP
(ENDO GENERICS)
INDOMETHACIN CAPSULES (MYLAN)
INDOMETHACIN CAPSULES
(LEDERLE STANDARD)
**INDOMETHACIN CAPSULES, 25 MG, 50
MG** (NOVOPHARM)
**INDOMETHACIN EXTENDED-RELEASE
CAPSULES, USP** (ENDO GENERICS)

INDOMETHACIN SODIUM TRIHYDRATE

Indocin I.V. (MERCK)
INFANRIX (SMITHKLINE BEECHAM)
INFASURF INTRATRACHEAL SUSPENSION
(FOREST)
INFED INJECTION (SCHEIN)
INFERGEN (AMGEN)

INFLIXIMAB

Remicade for IV Injection (CENTOCOR)

INFLUENZA VIRUS VACCINE

Fluogen Injection (PARKEDALE)
Fluvirin (MEDEVA)
Fluzone (PASTEUR MERIEUX CONNAUGHT)
Influenza Virus Vaccine, Trivalent, Types A
& B, FluShield, 1999-2000 Formula
(WYETH-AYERST)
Influenza Virus Vaccine, Trivalent, Types A
& B, FluShield, 1999-2000 Formula, in
Tubex (WYETH-AYERST)
**INFLUENZA VIRUS VACCINE,
TRIVALENT, TYPES A & B,
FLUSHIELD, 1999-2000 FORMULA**
(WYETH-AYERST)

**INFLUENZA VIRUS VACCINE,
TRIVALENT, TYPES A & B,
FLUSHIELD, 1999-2000 FORMULA, IN
TUBEX** (WYETH-AYERST)
**INFUMORPH 200 AND INFUMORPH 500
STERILE SOLUTIONS** (ELKINS-SINN)

INOSITOL

Amino-Cerv Creme (MILEX)
Mega-B Tablets (ARCO)
Megadose Tablets (ARCO)
INSPIREASE DRUG DELIVERY SYSTEM
(SCHERING)
INSTA-GLUCOSE (ICN)

INSULIN LISPRO, HUMAN

Humalog (LILLY)

INSULIN, HUMAN NPH

Humulin N NPH Cartridge (LILLY)
Humulin N NPH Pen (LILLY)
Humulin N, 100 Units (LILLY)
Novolin N Human Insulin 10 ml Vials
(NOVO NORDISK)
Novolin N PenFill 1.5 ml Cartridges
(NOVO NORDISK)
Novolin N Prefilled Syringe Disposable Insulin
Delivery System (NOVO NORDISK)

INSULIN, HUMAN REGULAR

Humulin R Regular (U-500) (LILLY)
Humulin R Regular Cartridge (LILLY)
Humulin R, 100 Units (LILLY)
NovoPen 1.5 Insulin Delivery Device
(NOVO NORDISK)
Novolin R Human Insulin 10 ml Vials
(NOVO NORDISK)
Novolin R PenFill 1.5 ml Cartridges
(NOVO NORDISK)
Novolin R Prefilled Syringe Disposable Insulin
Delivery System (NOVO NORDISK)
Velosulin BR Human Insulin 10 ml Vials
(NOVO NORDISK)

INSULIN, HUMAN REGULAR AND HUMAN
NPH MIXTURE

Humulin 50/50, 100 Units (LILLY)
Humulin 70/30 Cartridge (LILLY)
Humulin 70/30 Pen (LILLY)
Humulin 70/30, 100 Units (LILLY)
Novolin 70/30 Human Insulin 10 ml Vials
(NOVO NORDISK)
Novolin 70/30 PenFill 1.5 ml Cartridges
(NOVO NORDISK)
Novolin 70/30 Prefilled Disposable Insulin
Delivery System (NOVO NORDISK)

INSULIN, HUMAN, ZINC SUSPENSION

Humulin L, 100 Units (LILLY)
Humulin U, 100 Units (LILLY)
Novolin L Human Insulin 10 ml Vials
(NOVO NORDISK)

INSULIN, NPH

Iletin II, NPH (Pork), 100 Units (LILLY)
Purified Pork NPH Isophane Insulin
(NOVO NORDISK)

INSULIN, REGULAR

Iletin II, Regular (Pork), 100 Units (LILLY)
Purified Pork Regular Insulin (NOVO NORDISK)

INSULIN, ZINC SUSPENSION

Iletin II, Lente (Pork), 100 Units (LILLY)
Purified Pork Lente Insulin (NOVO NORDISK)
INTAL INHALER (RHONE-POULENC RORER)
INTAL NEBULIZER SOLUTION
(RHONE-POULENC RORER)
INTEGRILIN INJECTION (COR)
INTEGRILIN INJECTION (KEY)

INTERFERON ALFA-2A, RECOMBINANT

Roferon-A Injection (ROCHE LABS)

INTERFERON ALFA-2B, RECOMBINANT

Intron A for Injection (SCHERING)
Rebetron Combination Therapy (SCHERING)

INTERFERON ALFACON-1

Infergen (AMGEN)

INTERFERON ALFA-N3 (HUMAN
LEUKOCYTE DERIVED)

Alferon N Injection (INTERFERON)

INTERFERON BETA-1A

Avonex (BIOGEN)

INTERFERON BETA-1B

Betaseron for SC Injection (BERLEX)

INTERFERON GAMMA-1B

Actimmune (INTERMUNE)
INTRAOCULAR LENSES (ALCON)

INTRINSIC FACTOR CONCENTRATE

Trinsicon Capsules (UCB)
INTRON A FOR INJECTION (SCHERING)

INULIN

Inulin and Sodium Chloride Injection (CYPROS)
**INULIN AND SODIUM CHLORIDE
INJECTION** (CYPROS)
INVERSINE TABLETS (MERCK)
INVIRASE CAPSULES (ROCHE LABS)

IODOQUINOL

Vytone Cream 1% (DERMIK)
Yodoxin Tablets (GLENWOOD)
IONAMIN CAPSULES (MEDEVA)
IOPIDINE OPHTHALMIC SOLUTION
(ALCON)
IPECAC SYRUP USP (PADDOCK)
IPOL (PASTEUR MERIEUX CONNAUGHT)

IPRATROPIUM BROMIDE

Atrovent Inhalation Aerosol
(BOEHRINGER INGELHEIM)
Atrovent Inhalation Solution
(BOEHRINGER INGELHEIM)
Atrovent Nasal Spray 0.03%
(BOEHRINGER INGELHEIM)
Atrovent Nasal Spray 0.06%
(BOEHRINGER INGELHEIM)
Combivent Inhalation Aerosol
(BOEHRINGER INGELHEIM)
Ipratropium Bromide Inhalation Solution (DEY)
**IPRATROPIUM BROMIDE INHALATION
SOLUTION** (DEY)

IPRIFLAVONE

Osteo I.P. (NUTRACEUTICS)

IRBESARTAN

Avalide Tablets (BRISTOL-MYERS SQUIBB)
Avapro Tablets (SANOFI)
Avapro Tablets (BRISTOL-MYERS SQUIBB)

IRINOTECAN HYDROCHLORIDE

Camptosar Injection (PHARMACIA & UPJOHN)
IROMIN-G TABLETS (MISSION)

IRON

Calcet Plus Tablets (MISSION)
Feosol Caplets
(SMITHKLINE BEECHAM CONSUMER)
Fero-Grad-500 Filmtab Tablets (ABBOTT)
Fosfree Tablets (MISSION)
Iromin-G Tablets (MISSION)
Mission Prenatal F.A. Tablets (MISSION)
Mission Prenatal H.P. Tablets (MISSION)
Mission Prenatal Tablets (MISSION)

IRON DEXTRAN

INFeD Injection (SCHEIN)

UNDERLINE DENOTES GENERIC NAME

ISMELIN TABLETS (NOVARTIS)
ISMO TABLETS (WYETH-AYERST)
ISMOTIC ISOSORBIDE SOLUTION (ALCON)

ISOETHARINE
 Isoetharine Inhalation Solution (ROXANE)
ISOETHARINE INHALATION SOLUTION
 (ROXANE)

ISOFLURANE
 Forane Liquid for Inhalation (BAXTER)
ISOFLURANE, USP (APOTHECON)

ISOMETHEPTENE MUCATE
 Midrin Capsules (CARNRICK)

ISONIAZID
 Rifamate Capsules (HOECHST MARION ROUSSEL)
 Rifater (HOECHST MARION ROUSSEL)
ISONIAZID TABLETS 300 MG (PADDOCK)

ISOPROPYL MYRISTATE
 Eucerin Original Moisturizing Lotion
 (BEIERSDORF)
ISOPROTERENOL HCL 1:5,000 5 ML,
 UNIVERSAL ADD SYRINGE (ABBOTT)
ISOPROTERENOL HCL 1:5,000 10 ML,
 UNIVERSAL ADD SYRINGE (ABBOTT)
ISOPROTERENOL HCL 1:50,000, 10 ML,
 ABBOJECT (ABBOTT)

ISOPROTERENOL HYDROCHLORIDE
 Isoproterenol Hydrochloride Injection
 (ELKINS-SINN)
ISOPROTERENOL HYDROCHLORIDE
 INJECTION (ELKINS-SINN)
ISOPTIN SR TABLETS (KNOLL LABS)
ISOPTO ATROPINE (ALCON P.R.)
ISOPTO CARBACHOL (ALCON P.R.)
ISOPTO CARPINE (ALCON P.R.)
ISOPTO CETAPRED (ALCON P.R.)
ISOPTO HOMATROPINE (ALCON P.R.)
ISOPTO HYOSCINE (ALCON P.R.)
ISORDIL SUBLINGUAL TABLETS, 2.5 MG
 (WYETH-AYERST)
ISORDIL SUBLINGUAL TABLETS, 5 MG
 (WYETH-AYERST)
ISORDIL 5 TITRADOSE TABLETS, 5 MG
 (WYETH-AYERST)
ISORDIL 20 TITRADOSE TABLETS, 20 MG
 (WYETH-AYERST)
ISORDIL 30 TITRADOSE TABLETS, 30 MG
 (WYETH-AYERST)
ISORDIL SUBLINGUAL TABLETS
 (WYETH-AYERST)
ISORDIL TITRADOSE TABLETS
 (WYETH-AYERST)

ISOSORBIDE DINITRATE
 Dilatrate-SR Capsules (SCHWARZ)
 Isordil Sublingual Tablets (WYETH-AYERST)
 Isordil Titradose Tablets (WYETH-AYERST)
 Isosorbide Dinitrate Tablets (PAR)
 Isosorbide Dinitrate Tablets (GENEVA)
 Sorbitrate Chewable Tablets (ASTRAZENECA)
 Sorbitrate Oral Tablets (ASTRAZENECA)
ISOSORBIDE DINITRATE TABLETS (PAR)
ISOSORBIDE DINITRATE TABLETS
 (GENEVA)

ISOSORBIDE MONONITRATE
 Imdur Tablets (KEY)
 Ismo Tablets (WYETH-AYERST)
 Monoket Tablets (SCHWARZ)
ISOTRATE ER TABLETS (APOTHECON)

ISOTRETINOIN
 Accutane Capsules (ROCHE LABS)
ISOXSUPRINE HCL TABLETS (GENEVA)

ISOXSUPRINE HYDROCHLORIDE
 Isoxsuprine HCl Tablets (GENEVA)
I-SPEAR SURGICAL EYE SPONGE (ALCON)

ITRACONAZOLE
 Sporanox Capsules (JANSSEN)
 Sporanox Injection (JANSSEN)
 Sporanox Injection (ORTHO BIOTECH)
 Sporanox Oral Solution (JANSSEN)
 Sporanox Oral Solution (ORTHO BIOTECH)
I-VALEX-1 AMINO ACID-MODIFIED
 MEDICAL FOOD WITH IRON (ROSS)
I-VALEX-2 AMINO ACID-MODIFIED
 MEDICAL FOOD (ROSS)
IVEEGAM (IMMUNO)

IVERMECTIN
 Stromectol Tablets (MERCK)

J

JAPANESE ENCEPHALITIS VACCINE
INACTIVATED
 JE-Vax (PASTEUR MERIEUX CONNAUGHT)
JE-VAX (PASTEUR MERIEUX CONNAUGHT)

K

K-MAG ASPARTATE (POTASSIUM &
 MAGNESIUM) (VITALINE)
KABIKINASE LYOPHILIZED POWDER
 (PHARMACIA & UPJOHN)
KADIAN CAPSULES (FAULDING)
KANTREX CAPSULES (APOTHECON)
KANTREX INJECTION (APOTHECON)
KANTREX PEDIATRIC INJECTION
 (APOTHECON)
KAOLECTROLYTE (BRECKENRIDGE)

KAOLIN
 Kaolin-Pectin Suspension (ROXANE)
KAOLIN-PECTIN SUSPENSION (ROXANE)

KAVA-KAVA
 VitaZac (MAYOR)
 Vitamist Intra-Oral Spray Dietary Supplements
 (MAYOR)
KAY CIEL ORAL SOLUTION (FOREST)
KAY CIEL POWDER PACKETS (FOREST)
KAYEXALATE POWDER (SANOFI)
K-DUR MICROBURST RELEASE SYSTEM
 ER TABLETS (KEY)
KEFLEX ORAL SUSPENSION (DISTA)
KEFLEX PULVULES (DISTA)
KEFTAB TABLETS (DJ PHARMA)
KEFUROX VIALS, ADD-VANTAGE (LILLY)
KEFZOL VIALS, ADD-VANTAGE (LILLY)
KENAJECT-40 (MERZ)
KENALOG CREAM, LOTION, AND
 OINTMENT (APOTHECON)
KENALOG IN ORABASE (APOTHECON)
KENALOG SPRAY AEROSOL (APOTHECON)
KENALOG-10 AND KENALOG-40
 SUSPENSION (APOTHECON)
KERI ANTI-BACTERIAL HAND LOTION
 (BRISTOL-MYERS)
KERI CREAM (BRISTOL-MYERS)

KERI CORT-10 CREAM (BRISTOL-MYERS)
KERI LOTION - ORIGINAL FORMULA,
 SENSITIVE SKIN FRAGRANCE - FREE,
 AND SILKY SMOOTH (BRISTOL-MYERS)
KERLONE TABLETS (SEARLE)
KETALAR (MONARCH)
KETAMINE HYDROCHLORIDE
 INJECTION, USP (BEDFORD)

KETOCONAZOLE
 Ketoconazole Tablets, 200 mg (NOVOPHARM)
 Nizoral 2% Cream (MCNEIL CONSUMER)
 Nizoral 2% Shampoo (MCNEIL CONSUMER)
 Nizoral A-D Shampoo (MCNEIL CONSUMER)
 Nizoral Tablets (JANSSEN)
KETOCONAZOLE TABLETS, 200 MG
 (NOVOPHARM)
KETONEX-1 AMINO ACID-MODIFIED
 MEDICAL FOOD WITH IRON (ROSS)
KETONEX-2 AMINO ACID-MODIFIED
 MEDICAL FOOD (ROSS)

KETOPROFEN
 Ketoprofen Capsules (MYLAN)
 Ketoprofen Capsules (LEDERLE STANDARD)
 Orudis Capsules (WYETH-AYERST)
 Oruvail Capsules (WYETH-AYERST)
KETOPROFEN CAPSULES (MYLAN)
KETOPROFEN CAPSULES
 (LEDERLE STANDARD)
KETOPROFEN EXTENDED RELEASE
 CAPSULES (SCHEIN)
KETOPROFEN SR CAPSULES (ESI LEDERLE)

KETOROLAC TROMETHAMINE
 Acular Ophthalmic Solution (ALLERGAN)
 Acular PF Ophthalmic Solution (ALLERGAN)
 Ketorolac Tromethamine Tablets (MYLAN)
 Toradol IM Injection, IV Injection
 (ROCHE LABS)
 Toradol Tablets (ROCHE LABS)
KETOROLAC TROMETHAMINE
 INJECTION USP (BEDFORD)
KETOROLAC TROMETHAMINE TABLETS
 (MYLAN)
KIE SYRUP (LASER)
KIONEX POWDER (PADDOCK)
KLARON LOTION 10% (DERMIK)
KLONOPIN TABLETS (ROCHE LABS)
K-LOR POWDER PACKETS (ABBOTT)
KLOR-CON/EF TABLETS (UPSHER-SMITH)
KLOR-CON 8/KLOR-CON 10 TABLETS
 (UPSHER-SMITH)
KLOR-CON POWDER (UPSHER-SMITH)
KLOR-CON/25 POWDER (UPSHER-SMITH)
KLORVESS 10% LIQUID (NOVARTIS)
KLORVESS EFFERVESCENT GRANULES
 (NOVARTIS)
KLOTRIX TABLETS (APOTHECON)
K-LYTE EFFERVESCENT TABLETS
 (APOTHECON)
K-LYTE DS EFFERVESCENT TABLETS
 (APOTHECON)
K-LYTE/CL TABLETS (APOTHECON)
K-LYTE/CL 50 EFFERVESCENT TABLETS
 (APOTHECON)
KOATE-DVI (BAYER BIOLOGICAL)
KOATE-HP (BAYER BIOLOGICAL)
KOGENATE (BAYER BIOLOGICAL)
KONYNE 80 (BAYER BIOLOGICAL)
K-PHOS M.F. TABLETS (BEACH)
K-PHOS NEUTRAL TABLETS (BEACH)
K-PHOS NO. 2 TABLETS (BEACH)
K-PHOS ORIGINAL (SODIUM FREE)
 TABLETS (BEACH)
KRISTALOSE FOR ORAL SOLUTION
 (BERTEK)
KRONOFED-A KRONOCAPS (FERNDALE)

UNDERLINE DENOTES GENERIC NAME

KRONOFED-A-JR. KRONOCAPS (FERNDALE)
K-TAB FILMTAB TABLETS (ABBOTT)
KUDROX SUSPENSION (SCHWARZ)
KUTAPRESSIN INJECTION (SCHWARZ)
KUTRASE CAPSULES (SCHWARZ)
KU-ZYME CAPSULES (SCHWARZ)
KU-ZYME HP CAPSULES (SCHWARZ)
KYTRIL INJECTION (SMITHKLINE BEECHAM)
KYTRIL TABLETS (SMITHKLINE BEECHAM)

L

LABETALOL HCL TABLETS (WATSON)
LABETALOL HCL TABLETS, USP (APOTHECON)
LABETALOL HYDROCHLORIDE
  Labetalol HCl Tablets (WATSON)
  Normodyne Injection (SCHERING)
  Normodyne Tablets (SCHERING)
  Trandate Injection (FARO)
  Trandate Tablets (FARO)
LABETALOL HYDROCHLORIDE INJECTION, USP (BEDFORD)
LAC-HYDRIN 12% CREAM (WESTWOOD-SQUIBB)
LAC-HYDRIN 12% LOTION (WESTWOOD-SQUIBB)
LAC-HYDRIN FIVE LOTION (WESTWOOD-SQUIBB)
LACRISERT STERILE OPHTHALMIC INSERT (MERCK)
LACTAID ORIGINAL STRENGTH CAPLETS (MCNEIL CONSUMER)
LACTAID EXTRA STRENGTH CAPLETS (MCNEIL CONSUMER)
LACTAID ULTRA CAPLETS AND CHEWABLE TABLETS (MCNEIL CONSUMER)
LACTAID DROPS (MCNEIL CONSUMER)
LACTASE (BETA-D-GALACTOSIDASE)
  Lactaid Drops (MCNEIL CONSUMER)
  Lactaid Extra Strength Caplets (MCNEIL CONSUMER)
  Lactaid Original Strength Caplets (MCNEIL CONSUMER)
  Lactaid Ultra Caplets and Chewable Tablets (MCNEIL CONSUMER)
LACTATED RINGER'S INJECTION, USP (ABBOTT)
LACTATED RINGERS FOR IRRIGATION (FLEX) (ABBOTT)
LACTIC ACID
  Lactinol Lotion (PEDINOL)
  Lactinol-E Creme (PEDINOL)
LACTICARE LOTION (STIEFEL)
LACTICARE-HC LOTION, 1% (STIEFEL)
LACTICARE-HC LOTION, 2 1/2% (STIEFEL)
LACTINOL LOTION (PEDINOL)
LACTINOL-E CREME (PEDINOL)
LACTOCAL-F TABLETS (LASER)
LACTRASE CAPSULES (SCHWARZ)
LACTULOSE
  Duphalac Solution (SOLVAY)
  Kristalose for Oral Solution (BERTEK)
  Lactulose Solution (MYLAN)
  Lactulose Solution (ROXANE)
  Lactulose Solution USP (PHARMACEUTICAL ASSOCIATES)
LACTULOSE SOLUTION (MYLAN)
LACTULOSE SOLUTION (ROXANE)

LACTULOSE SOLUTION USP (PHARMACEUTICAL ASSOCIATES)
LADYMATE (MAYOR)
LAMICTAL TABLETS (GLAXO WELLCOME)
LAMICTAL CHEWABLE DISPERSIBLE TABLETS (GLAXO WELLCOME)
LAMISIL SOLUTION, 1% (NOVARTIS)
LAMISIL TABLETS (NOVARTIS)
LAMIVUDINE
  Combivir Tablets (GLAXO WELLCOME)
  Epivir Oral Solution (GLAXO WELLCOME)
  Epivir Tablets (GLAXO WELLCOME)
  Epivir-HBV Oral Solution (GLAXO WELLCOME)
  Epivir-HBV Tablets (GLAXO WELLCOME)
LAMOTRIGINE
  Lamictal Chewable Dispersible Tablets (GLAXO WELLCOME)
  Lamictal Tablets (GLAXO WELLCOME)
LAMPRENE CAPSULES (NOVARTIS)
LANOXICAPS (GLAXO WELLCOME)
LANOXIN ELIXIR PEDIATRIC (GLAXO WELLCOME)
LANOXIN INJECTION (GLAXO WELLCOME)
LANOXIN INJECTION PEDIATRIC (GLAXO WELLCOME)
LANOXIN TABLETS (GLAXO WELLCOME)
LANSOPRAZOLE
  PREVPAC (TAP)
  Prevacid Delayed-Release Capsules (TAP)
LARIAM TABLETS (ROCHE LABS)
LARODOPA TABLETS (ROCHE LABS)
LASIX TABLETS (HOECHST MARION ROUSSEL)
LAZERCREME (PEDINOL)
LAZERFORMALYDE SOLUTION (PEDINOL)
LAZERSPORIN-C SOLUTION (PEDINOL)
L-CARNITINE CAPSULES (R&D)
L-CARNITINE USP 500MG CHEWABLE WAFERS, 250MG TABLETS, 500MG CAPLETS, AND 500MG CAPSULES (VITALINE)
L-CYSTINE
  Amino-Cerv Creme (MILEX)
LECITHIN
  PhosChol 900 Softgels (AMERICAN LECITHIN)
  PhosChol Concentrate (AMERICAN LECITHIN)
LEFLUNOMIDE
  Arava Tablets (HOECHST MARION ROUSSEL)
LEPIRUDIN
  Refludan (HOECHST MARION ROUSSEL)
LESCOL CAPSULES (NOVARTIS)
LEUCOVORIN CALCIUM
  Leucovorin Calcium Tablets (ROXANE)
  Leucovorin Calcium Tablets (IMMUNEX)
  Leucovorin Calcium for Injection (IMMUNEX)
  Leucovorin Calcium for Injection (Preservative-Free) (ELKINS-SINN)
LEUCOVORIN CALCIUM FOR INJECTION (BEDFORD)
LEUCOVORIN CALCIUM FOR INJECTION (IMMUNEX)
LEUCOVORIN CALCIUM FOR INJECTION (PRESERVATIVE-FREE) (ELKINS-SINN)
LEUCOVORIN CALCIUM TABLETS (ROXANE)
LEUCOVORIN CALCIUM TABLETS (IMMUNEX)
LEUKERAN TABLETS (GLAXO WELLCOME)
LEUKINE (IMMUNEX)
LEUPROLIDE ACETATE
  Lupron Depot 3.75 mg (TAP)
  Lupron Depot 7.5 mg (TAP)
  Lupron Depot–3 Month 11.25 mg (TAP)

  Lupron Depot–3 Month 22.5 mg (TAP)
  Lupron Depot–4 Month 30 mg (TAP)
  Lupron Depot-PED 7.5 mg, 11.25 mg and 15 mg (TAP)
  Lupron Injection (TAP)
  Lupron Injection Pediatric (TAP)
LEUPROLIDE ACETATE INJECTION (BEDFORD)
LEUSTATIN INJECTION (ORTHO BIOTECH)
LEVALBUTEROL HYDROCHLORIDE
  Xopenex Inhalation Solution (SEPRACOR)
LEVAMISOLE HYDROCHLORIDE
  Ergamisol Tablets (JANSSEN)
LEVAQUIN INJECTION (ORTHO-MCNEIL)
LEVAQUIN TABLETS (ORTHO-MCNEIL)
LEVATOL TABLETS (SCHWARZ)
LEVBID EXTENDED-RELEASE TABLETS (SCHWARZ)
LEVLEN 21 TABLETS (BERLEX)
LEVLEN 28 TABLETS (BERLEX)
LEVLITE 21 TABLETS (BERLEX)
LEVLITE 28 TABLETS (BERLEX)
LEVOBUPIVACAINE HYDROCHLORIDE
  Chirocaine Injection (PURDUE PHARMA)
LEVOCARNITINE
  Cardiotropin (NUTRACEUTICS)
  Carnitor Injection (SIGMA-TAU)
  Carnitor Tablets and Solution (SIGMA-TAU)
  L-Carnitine Capsules (R&D)
  L-Carnitine USP 500mg Chewable Wafers, 250mg Tablets, 500mg Caplets, and 500mg Capsules (VITALINE)
  Slender-Mist (MAYOR)
  Vitamist Intra-Oral Spray Dietary Supplements (MAYOR)
LEVODOPA
  Atamet Tablets (ATHENA)
  Carbidopa and Levodopa Tablets, USP (ENDO GENERICS)
  Sinemet CR Tablets (DUPONT)
  Sinemet Tablets (DUPONT)
LEVO-DROMORAN INJECTABLE (ICN)
LEVO-DROMORAN TABLETS (ICN)
LEVOFLOXACIN
  Levaquin Injection (ORTHO-MCNEIL)
  Levaquin Tablets (ORTHO-MCNEIL)
LEVOMETHADYL ACETATE HYDROCHLORIDE
  Orlaam Oral Solution (ROXANE)
LEVONORGESTREL
  Alesse-21 Tablets (WYETH-AYERST)
  Alesse-28 Tablets (WYETH-AYERST)
  Levlen 21 Tablets (BERLEX)
  Levlen 28 Tablets (BERLEX)
  Levlite 21 Tablets (BERLEX)
  Levlite 28 Tablets (BERLEX)
  Levora Tablets (WATSON)
  Nordette-21 Tablets (WYETH-AYERST)
  Nordette-28 Tablets (WYETH-AYERST)
  Norplant System (WYETH-AYERST)
  Plan B Tablets (WOMEN'S CAPITAL)
  Preven Emergency Contraceptive Kit (GYNETICS)
  Tri-Levlen 21 Tablets (BERLEX)
  Tri-Levlen 28 Tablets (BERLEX)
  Triphasil-21 Tablets (WYETH-AYERST)
  Triphasil-28 Tablets (WYETH-AYERST)
  Trivora Tablets (WATSON)
LEVORA (LEVONORGESTREL AND ETHINYL ESTRADIOL TABLETS USP) (SCS)
LEVORA TABLETS (WATSON)

UNDERLINE DENOTES GENERIC NAME

LEVORPHANOL TARTRATE
Levo-Dromoran Injectable (ICN)
Levo-Dromoran Tablets (ICN)
Levorphanol Tartrate Tablets (ROXANE)
LEVORPHANOL TARTRATE TABLETS
(ROXANE)
LEVOTHROID TABLETS (FOREST)

LEVOTHYROXINE SODIUM
Levothroid Tablets (FOREST)
Levoxyl Tablets (JONES)
Synthroid Injection (KNOLL)
Synthroid Tablets (KNOLL)
**LEVOTHYROXINE SODIUM FOR
INJECTION** (BEDFORD)
LEVOTHYROXINE SODIUM TABLETS
(ESI LEDERLE)
LEVOXYL TABLETS (JONES)
LEVSIN DROPS (SCHWARZ)
LEVSIN ELIXIR (SCHWARZ)
LEVSIN INJECTION (SCHWARZ)
LEVSIN TABLETS (SCHWARZ)
LEVSIN/SL TABLETS (SCHWARZ)
LEVSINEX TIMECAPS (SCHWARZ)
LEXXEL TABLETS (ASTRAZENECA LP)
**L-GLUTAMINE WITH CHOLINE AND
INOSITOL** (VITALINE)

L-HISTIDINE
NephrAmine Injection (R&D)
LIBRAX CAPSULES (ICN)
LIBRIUM CAPSULES (ICN)
LIBRIUM FOR INJECTION (ICN)
LIDEX CREAM (MEDICIS)
LIDEX GEL (MEDICIS)
LIDEX OINTMENT (MEDICIS)
LIDEX TOPICAL SOLUTION (MEDICIS)
LIDEX-E CREAM (MEDICIS)
LIDOCAINE VISCOUS 2% (ROXANE)

LIDOCAINE
ELA-Max 5 Cream (FERNDALE)
ELA-Max Cream (FERNDALE)
EMLA Anesthetic Disc (ASTRAZENECA LP)
EMLA Cream (ASTRAZENECA LP)
Lidocaine Viscous 2% (ROXANE)
Lidoderm Patch (ENDO LABS)
Xylocaine 10% Oral Spray (ASTRAZENECA LP)
Xylocaine 5% Ointment (ASTRAZENECA LP)
**LIDOCAINE HCL INJECTION, 0.2% IN 5%
DEXTROSE** (ABBOTT)
**LIDOCAINE HCL INJECTION, 0.4% IN 5%
DEXTROSE** (ABBOTT)
**LIDOCAINE HCL INJECTION, 0.8% IN 5%
DEXTROSE** (ABBOTT)
LIDOCAINE HCL INJECTION, USP (BAXTER)
**LIDOCAINE HCL INJECTION, USP, 1%, 5
ML, ABBOJECT** (ABBOTT)
**LIDOCAINE HCL INJECTION, USP, 1%, 5
ML, STERILE PACK ABBOJECT** (ABBOTT)
**LIDOCAINE HCL INJECTION, USP, 2%, 5
ML, ABBOJECT** (ABBOTT)
**LIDOCAINE HCL INJECTION, USP, 2%, 5
ML, STERILE PACK ABBOJECT** (ABBOTT)
**LIDOCAINE HCL INJECTION, USP, 5%
WITH 7.5% DEXTROSE** (ABBOTT)
**LIDOCAINE HCL INJECTION, USP, 20%, 5
ML, 1 GRAM-PINTOP, U.A.S.** (ABBOTT)
**LIDOCAINE HCL INJECTION, USP, 20%,
10 ML, 2 GRAM-PINTOP, U.A.S.** (ABBOTT)
LIDOCAINE HCL TOPICAL SOLUTION
(ROXANE)

LIDOCAINE HYDROCHLORIDE
Anestacon Jelly (POLYMEDICA)
Lidocaine HCl Injection, USP (BAXTER)
Lidocaine HCl Topical Solution (ROXANE)

Lidocaine Hydrochloride & Epinephrine
Injection (ELKINS-SINN)
Lidocaine Hydrochloride Injection
(ELKINS-SINN)
Lidocaine Hydrochloride Injection
(Preservative-Free) (ELKINS-SINN)
Xylocaine 2% Jelly (ASTRAZENECA LP)
Xylocaine 2% Viscous Solution
(ASTRAZENECA LP)
Xylocaine 4% Topical Solution
(ASTRAZENECA LP)
Xylocaine Injection (ASTRAZENECA LP)
Xylocaine Injection for Ventricular
Arrhythmias (ASTRAZENECA LP)
Xylocaine with Epinephrine Injection
(ASTRAZENECA LP)
Xylocaine-MPF 1.5% Solution with Dextrose
7.5% (ASTRAZENECA LP)
Xylocaine-MPF 4% Sterile Solution
(ASTRAZENECA LP)
Xylocaine-MPF 5% with Glucose 7.5%
(ASTRAZENECA LP)
**LIDOCAINE HYDROCHLORIDE
INJECTION** (ELKINS-SINN)
**LIDOCAINE HYDROCHLORIDE
INJECTION (PRESERVATIVE-FREE)**
(ELKINS-SINN)
**LIDOCAINE HYDROCHLORIDE &
EPINEPHRINE INJECTION** (ELKINS-SINN)
LIDODERM PATCH (ENDO LABS)
LIGHTPLAST PRO (BEIERSDORF)
LIMBITROL TABLETS (ICN)
LIMBITROL DS TABLETS (ICN)
LINCOCIN CAPSULES (PHARMACIA & UPJOHN)
LINCOCIN STERILE SOLUTION
(PHARMACIA & UPJOHN)

LINDANE
Lindane Lotion USP 1% (ALPHARMA)
Lindane Shampoo USP 1% (ALPHARMA)
LINDANE LOTION USP 1% (ALPHARMA)
LINDANE SHAMPOO USP 1% (ALPHARMA)
LIORESAL TABLETS (NOVARTIS)

LIOTHYRONINE SODIUM
Cytomel Tablets (JONES)
Triostat Injection (JONES)

LIOTRIX
Thyrolar Tablets (FOREST)

LIPASE
Arco-Lase Plus Tablets (ARCO)
Arco-Lase Tablets (ARCO)
Donnazyme Tablets (ROBINS)
Ku-Zyme Capsules (SCHWARZ)
Ku-Zyme HP Capsules (SCHWARZ)
Kutrase Capsules (SCHWARZ)
LIPITOR TABLETS (PFIZER)
LIPITOR TABLETS (PARKE-DAVIS)
LIPOSYN II 10% AND 20% (ABBOTT)
LIQUADERM-A (PADDOCK)
LIQUA-GEL (PADDOCK)
LIQUI-DOSS (FERNDALE)

LISINOPRIL
Prinivil Tablets (MERCK)
Prinzide Tablets (MERCK)
Zestoretic Tablets (ASTRAZENECA)
Zestril Tablets (ASTRAZENECA)
LISTERINE ANTISEPTIC (WARNER-LAMBERT)
COOL MINT LISTERINE (WARNER-LAMBERT)
FRESHBURST LISTERINE (WARNER-LAMBERT)
**LISTERMINT ALCOHOL-FREE
MOUTHWASH** (WARNER-LAMBERT)

LITHIUM CARBONATE
Eskalith CR Controlled Release Tablets
(SMITHKLINE BEECHAM)

Eskalith Capsules (SMITHKLINE BEECHAM)
Lithium Carbonate Capsules & Tablets
(ROXANE)
Lithobid Slow-Release Tablets (SOLVAY)
**LITHIUM CARBONATE CAPSULES &
TABLETS** (ROXANE)

LITHIUM CITRATE
Lithium Citrate Syrup (ROXANE)
LITHIUM CITRATE SYRUP (ROXANE)
LITHOBID SLOW-RELEASE TABLETS
(SOLVAY)
LITHOSTAT TABLETS (MISSION)

LIVER PREPARATIONS
Hep-Forte Capsules (MARLYN)
Trinsicon Capsules (UCB)
L-LYSINE HCL 1000MG (VITALINE)
**10% LMD W/V AND 5% DEXTROSE
INJECTION** (ABBOTT)
**10% LMD W/V AND 0.9% SODIUM
CHLORIDE INJECTION** (ABBOTT)
LOCOID CREAM (FERNDALE)
LOCOID LIPOCREAM CREAM (FERNDALE)
LOCOID OINTMENT (FERNDALE)
LOCOID TOPICAL SOLUTION (FERNDALE)
LODINE CAPSULES (WYETH-AYERST)
LODINE CAPSULES, 300 MG (WYETH-AYERST)
LODINE TABLETS (WYETH-AYERST)
LODINE TABLETS, 200 MG (WYETH-AYERST)
LODINE TABLETS, 400 MG (WYETH-AYERST)
**LODINE XL EXTENDED-RELEASE
TABLETS** (WYETH-AYERST)
LODRANE ALLERGY CAPSULES (ECR)
LODRANE LD CAPSULES (ECR)
LODRANE LIQUID (ECR)
LOESTRIN 21 TABLETS (PARKE-DAVIS)
LOESTRIN FE TABLETS (PARKE-DAVIS)

LOMEFLOXACIN HYDROCHLORIDE
Maxaquin Tablets (UNIMED)
LOMOTIL LIQUID (SEARLE)
LOMOTIL TABLETS (SEARLE)

LOMUSTINE (CCNU)
CeeNU Capsules
(BRISTOL-MYERSSQUIBBONCOLOGY/IMMUNOLOGY)
LONOX TABLETS (GENEVA)
LO/OVRAL TABLETS (WYETH-AYERST)
LO/OVRAL-28 TABLETS (WYETH-AYERST)
LOPERAMIDE HCL CAPSULES (GENEVA)

LOPERAMIDE HYDROCHLORIDE
Imodium A-D Caplets and Liquid
(MCNEIL CONSUMER)
Imodium Advanced Chewable Tablets
(MCNEIL CONSUMER)
Imodium Capsules (MCNEIL CONSUMER)
Loperamide HCl Capsules (GENEVA)
Loperamide Hydrochloride Capsules (MYLAN)
Loperamide Hydrochloride Capsules USP, 2
mg (NOVOPHARM)
Loperamide Hydrochloride Oral Solution
(ROXANE)
**LOPERAMIDE HYDROCHLORIDE
CAPSULES** (MYLAN)
**LOPERAMIDE HYDROCHLORIDE
CAPSULES USP, 2 MG** (NOVOPHARM)
**LOPERAMIDE HYDROCHLORIDE ORAL
SOLUTION** (ROXANE)
LOPID TABLETS (PARKE-DAVIS)
LOPRESSOR TABLETS (NOVARTIS)
LOPRESSOR HCT TABLETS (NOVARTIS)
LOPROX CREAM (MEDICIS)
LOPROX LOTION (MEDICIS)
LORABID SUSPENSION AND PULVULES
(LILLY)

LORACARBEF
Lorabid Suspension and Pulvules (LILLY)

LORATADINE
Claritin Reditabs (SCHERING)
Claritin Syrup (SCHERING)
Claritin Tablets (SCHERING)
Claritin-D 12 Hour Extended Release Tablets (SCHERING)
Claritin-D 24 Hour Extended Release Tablets (SCHERING)

LORAZEPAM
Ativan Injection (BAXTER)
Ativan Injection (WYETH-AYERST)
Ativan Tablets (WYETH-AYERST)
Ativan in Tubex (WYETH-AYERST)
Lorazepam Intensol (ROXANE)
Lorazepam Tablets (MYLAN)
Lorazepam Tablets (GENEVA)
Lorazepam Tablets, USP CIV (WATSON)
LORAZEPAM CARTRIDGE (ESI LEDERLE)
LORAZEPAM INTENSOL (ROXANE)
LORAZEPAM TABLETS (MYLAN)
LORAZEPAM TABLETS (GENEVA)
LORAZEPAM TABLETS (ESI LEDERLE)
LORAZEPAM TABLETS, USP CIV (WATSON)
LORCET 10/650 TABLETS (FOREST)
LORCET PLUS TABLETS (FOREST)
LORCET-HD CAPSULES (FOREST)
LORTAB 2.5/500 TABLETS (UCB)
LORTAB 5/500 TABLETS (UCB)
LORTAB 7.5/500 TABLETS (UCB)
LORTAB 10/500 TABLETS (UCB)
LORTAB ELIXIR (UCB)

LOSARTAN POTASSIUM
Cozaar Tablets (MERCK)
Hyzaar 100-25 Tablets (MERCK)
Hyzaar 50-12.5 Tablets (MERCK)
LOTENSIN TABLETS (NOVARTIS)
LOTENSIN HCT TABLETS (NOVARTIS)
LOTREL CAPSULES (NOVARTIS)
LOTRIMIN CREAM 1% (SCHERING)
LOTRIMIN LOTION 1% (SCHERING)
LOTRIMIN TOPICAL SOLUTION 1% (SCHERING)
LOTRISONE CREAM (SCHERING)

LOVASTATIN
Mevacor Tablets (MERCK)
LOVENOX INJECTION (RHONE-POULENC RORER)
LOWILA CAKE (WESTWOOD-SQUIBB)
LOW-OGESTREL (NORGESTREL AND ETHINYL ESTRADIOL TABLETS, USP) (WATSON)
LOXAPINE CAPSULES, USP (WATSON)

LOXAPINE HYDROCHLORIDE
Loxapine Capsules, USP (WATSON)
Loxitane C Oral Concentrate (WATSON)
Loxitane IM (WATSON)

LOXAPINE SUCCINATE
Loxitane Capsules (WATSON)
LOXITANE CAPSULES (WATSON)
LOXITANE C ORAL CONCENTRATE (WATSON)
LOXITANE IM (WATSON)
LOZOL TABLETS (RHONE-POULENC RORER)
LTA II KIT (ABBOTT)
LTA KIT, PREATTACHED (ABBOTT)
LTA PEDIATRIC KIT (ABBOTT)
LUBRIDERM DAILY UV LOTION WITH SUNSCREEN (WARNER-LAMBERT)
LUDIOMIL TABLETS (NOVARTIS)
LUFYLLIN ELIXIR (WALLACE)
LUFYLLIN TABLETS (WALLACE)

LUFYLLIN-400 TABLETS (WALLACE)
LUFYLLIN-EPG TABLETS (WALLACE)
LUFYLLIN-GG ELIXIR (WALLACE)
LUFYLLIN-GG TABLETS (WALLACE)
LUPRON DEPOT 3.75 MG (TAP)
LUPRON DEPOT 7.5 MG (TAP)
LUPRON DEPOT–3 MONTH 11.25 MG (TAP)
LUPRON DEPOT–3 MONTH 22.5 MG (TAP)
LUPRON DEPOT–4 MONTH 30 MG (TAP)
LUPRON DEPOT-PED 7.5 MG, 11.25 MG AND 15 MG (TAP)
LUPRON INJECTION (TAP)
LUPRON INJECTION PEDIATRIC (TAP)
LURIDE DROPS 50 ML (COLGATE ORAL)
LURIDE LOZI-TABS TABLETS (COLGATE ORAL)
LUSTRA CREAM (MEDICIS)
LUSTRA-AF CREAM (MEDICIS)

LUTEIN
VitaSight (MAYOR)
Vitamist Intra-Oral Spray Dietary Supplements (MAYOR)
LUVOX TABLETS (25, 50, 100 MG) (SOLVAY)

LYME DISEASE VACCINE (RECOMBINANT OSPA)
LYMErix (SMITHKLINE BEECHAM)
LYMERIX (SMITHKLINE BEECHAM)
LYMPHOMYOSOT LIQUID (HEEL)
LYMPHOMYOSOT TABLETS (HEEL)
LYSODREN TABLETS (BRISTOL-MYERSSQUIBBONCOLOGY/IMMUNOLOGY)

M

MAXIMUM STRENGTH MAALOX ANTACID/ANTI-GAS LIQUID (NOVARTIS CONSUMER)
MAALOX ANTI-GAS TABLETS, REGULAR STRENGTH AND EXTRA STRENGTH (NOVARTIS CONSUMER)
MAALOX MAGNESIA AND ALUMINA ORAL SUSPENSION (NOVARTIS CONSUMER)
QUICK DISSOLVE MAALOX ANTACID TABLETS, MAXIMUM STRENGTH (NOVARTIS CONSUMER)
QUICK DISSOLVE MAALOX ANTACID TABLETS, REGULAR STRENGTH (NOVARTIS CONSUMER)
MACROBID CAPSULES (PROCTER & GAMBLE PHARMACEUTICALS)
MACRODANTIN CAPSULES (PROCTER & GAMBLE PHARMACEUTICALS)

MAFENIDE ACETATE
Sulfamylon Cream (BERTEK)
Sulfamylon Topical Solution (BERTEK)
MAG-CARB CAPSULES (R&D)

MAGNESIUM
ActiCal Tablets (USANA)
Chelated Mineral Tablets (USANA)
Osteo-CalMag (MAYOR)
Vitamist Intra-Oral Spray Dietary Supplements (MAYOR)

MAGNESIUM CARBONATE
Mag-Carb Capsules (R&D)
Renacidin Irrigation (GUARDIAN)

MAGNESIUM CHLORIDE
Chlor-3 (FLEMING)
Slow-Mag Tablets (ROBERTS)

MAGNESIUM CITRATE
Evac-Q-Kwik (SAVAGE)
Fleet Prep Kits (FLEET)

MAGNESIUM GLUCONATE
Magonate Natal Liquid (FLEMING)
Magonate Tablets and Liquid (FLEMING)

MAGNESIUM HYDROXIDE
Fast-Acting Mylanta Antacid Tablets (J&J – MERCK)
Fast-Acting Mylanta Liquid Antacid (J&J – MERCK)
Maalox Magnesia and Alumina Oral Suspension (NOVARTIS CONSUMER)
Maximum Strength Fast-Acting Mylanta Antacid Tablets (J&J – MERCK)
Maximum Strength Fast-Acting Mylanta Liquid (J&J – MERCK)
Maximum Strength Maalox Antacid/Anti-Gas Liquid (NOVARTIS CONSUMER)
Milk of Magnesia & Milk of Magnesia-Concentrated Flavored (ROXANE)
Milk of Magnesia Cascara Suspension (PHARMACEUTICAL ASSOCIATES)
Milk of Magnesia Concentrate (PHARMACEUTICAL ASSOCIATES)
Milk of Magnesia USP (PHARMACEUTICAL ASSOCIATES)
Milk of Magnesia-Cascara Suspension Concentrated (ROXANE)
Mylanta Supreme Liquid (J&J – MERCK)

MAGNESIUM LACTATE
MagTab SR Caplets (NICHE)

MAGNESIUM OXIDE
Beelith Tablets (BEACH)
Mag-Ox 400 Tablets (BLAINE)
Uro-Mag Capsules (BLAINE)

MAGNESIUM SALICYLATE
Magsal Tablets (U.S. PHARMACEUTICAL)
MAGNESIUM SULFATE 12.5%, 8 ML, PINTOP (ABBOTT)
MAGNESIUM SULFATE 50% W/V AMPOULES, VIALS & ABBOJECT (ABBOTT)
MAGONATE NATAL LIQUID (FLEMING)
MAGONATE TABLETS AND LIQUID (FLEMING)
MAG-OX 400 TABLETS (BLAINE)
MAGSAL TABLETS (U.S. PHARMACEUTICAL)
MAGTAB SR CAPLETS (NICHE)

MALATHION
Ovide Lotion (MEDICIS)
MALTSUPEX POWDER, LIQUID, TABLETS (WALLACE)
MANDELAMINE TABLETS (WARNER CHILCOTT)
MANDOL VIALS (LILLY)

MANGANESE
Chelated Mineral Tablets (USANA)
MANGANESE 10 ML (1 MG/ML) (ABBOTT)
MANGANESE 15MG (VITALINE)

MANGANESE ASCORBATE
Cosamin DS Capsules (NUTRAMAX)
5% MANNITOL INJECTION, USP (ABBOTT)
10% MANNITOL INJECTION, USP (ABBOTT)
15% MANNITOL INJECTION, USP (ABBOTT)
20% MANNITOL INJECTION, USP (ABBOTT)
25% MANNITOL INJECTION, USP (ABBOTT)
MANTADIL CREAM (MONARCH)
MAOLATE TABLETS (PHARMACIA & UPJOHN)

MAPROTILINE HYDROCHLORIDE
Maprotiline Hydrochloride Tablets (MYLAN)

Maprotiline Hydrochloride Tablets, USP
(WATSON)
**MAPROTILINE HYDROCHLORIDE
TABLETS** (MYLAN)
**MAPROTILINE HYDROCHLORIDE
TABLETS, USP** (WATSON)
MARAX TABLETS & DF SYRUP (PFIZER)
MARBLEN SUSPENSION (FLEMING)
MARINE LIPID CONCENTRATE 1200MG
(VITALINE)
MARINOL CAPSULES (ROXANE)
MARINOL CAPSULES (UNIMED)
MARLYN FORMULA 50 CAPSULES
(MARLYN)
**MASSENGILL DOUCHES, TOWELETTES
AND CLEANSING WASH**
(SMITHKLINE BEECHAM CONSUMER)
MASTISOL LIQUID ADHESIVE (FERNDALE)
MATERNA TABLETS (LEDERLE LABS)
MATULANE CAPSULES (SIGMA-TAU)
MAVIK TABLETS (KNOLL)
MAXAIR AUTOHALER (3M)
MAXAIR INHALER (3M)
MAXALT TABLETS (MERCK)
**MAXALT-MLT ORALLY DISINTEGRATING
TABLETS** (MERCK)
MAXAQUIN TABLETS (UNIMED)
MAXIDEX OINTMENT (ALCON)
MAXIDEX SUSPENSION (ALCON P.R.)
MAXIFLOR CREAM (ALLERGAN)
MAXIFLOR OINTMENT (ALLERGAN)
**MAXIMUM FORMULA RED, BLUE AND
GREEN (MULTIVITAMIN-
MULTIMINERAL)** (VITALINE)
MAXIPIME FOR INJECTION (DURA)
MAXIPIME FOR INJECTION
(BRISTOL-MYERS SQUIBB)
MAXITROL OINTMENT (ALCON)
MAXITROL SUSPENSION (ALCON P.R.)
**MAXIVATE CREAM, LOTION &
OINTMENT 0.05%** (WESTWOOD-SQUIBB)
MAXZIDE TABLETS (BERTEK)
MAXZIDE-25 MG TABLETS (BERTEK)
MAY-VITA ELIXIR (MERZ)
**MDR FITNESS TABS FOR MEN AND
WOMEN** (MDR FITNESS)

MEASLES & RUBELLA VIRUS VACCINE
LIVE
M-R-VAX II (MERCK)

MEASLES VIRUS VACCINE LIVE
Attenuvax (MERCK)

MEASLES, MUMPS & RUBELLA VIRUS
VACCINE LIVE
M-M-R II (MERCK)
MEBARAL TABLETS (SANOFI)

MEBENDAZOLE
Vermox Chewable Tablets (MCNEIL CONSUMER)

MECAMYLAMINE HYDROCHLORIDE
Inversine Tablets (MERCK)

MECHLORETHAMINE HYDROCHLORIDE
Mustargen for Injection (MERCK)
MECHOLYL OINTMENT (GORDON)
MECLIZINE HCL TABLETS (PAR)
MECLIZINE HCL TABLETS (GENEVA)

MECLIZINE HYDROCHLORIDE
Antivert, Antivert/25, & Antivert/50 Tablets
(PFIZER)
Bonine Chewable Tablets (PFIZER CONSUMER)
Meclizine HCl Tablets (PAR)
Meclizine HCl Tablets (GENEVA)
Meclizine Hydrochloride Tablets (WATSON)
MECLIZINE HYDROCHLORIDE TABLETS
(WATSON)

MECLOFENAMATE SODIUM
Meclofenamate Sodium Capsules (MYLAN)
MECLOFENAMATE SODIUM CAPSULES
(MYLAN)
MEDIGESIC CAPSULES
(U.S. PHARMACEUTICAL)
MEDIPLAST (BEIERSDORF)
MEDIPLEX ULTRA TABULES
(U.S. PHARMACEUTICAL)
MEDROL TABLETS (PHARMACIA & UPJOHN)
MEDROL TABLETS AND DOSEPAK
(PHARMACIA & UPJOHN)

MEDROXYPROGESTERONE ACETATE
Amen Tablets (CARNRICK)
Cycrin Tablets (ESI LEDERLE)
Depo-Provera Contraceptive Injection
(PHARMACIA & UPJOHN)
Depo-Provera Sterile Aqueous Suspension
(PHARMACIA & UPJOHN)
Premphase Tablets (WYETH-AYERST)
Prempro Tablets (WYETH-AYERST)
Provera Tablets (PHARMACIA & UPJOHN)

MEFENAMIC ACID
Ponstel Kapseals (PARKE-DAVIS)

MEFLOQUINE HYDROCHLORIDE
Lariam Tablets (ROCHE LABS)
MEFOXIN FOR INJECTION (MERCK)
**MEFOXIN PREMIXED INTRAVENOUS
SOLUTION** (MERCK)
MEGA ANTIOXIDANT TABLETS (USANA)
MEGA-B TABLETS (ARCO)
MEGA-B WITH C (ARCO)
MEGACE ORAL SUSPENSION
(BRISTOL-MYERSSQUIBBONCOLOGY/IMMUNOLOGY)
MEGACE TABLETS
(BRISTOL-MYERSSQUIBBONCOLOGY/IMMUNOLOGY)
MEGADOSE TABLETS (ARCO)

MEGESTROL ACETATE
Megace Oral Suspension
(BRISTOL-MYERSSQUIBBONCOLOGY/IMMUNOLOGY)
Megace Tablets
(BRISTOL-MYERSSQUIBBONCOLOGY/IMMUNOLOGY)
Megestrol Acetate Tablets (PAR)
Megestrol Acetate Tablets (ROXANE)
MEGESTROL ACETATE TABLETS (PAR)
MEGESTROL ACETATE TABLETS (ROXANE)
MELANEX TOPICAL SOLUTION
(NEUTROGENA)
MELATONIN (MAYOR)

MELATONIN
Bevitamel Tablets (WESTLAKE)
Melatonin (MAYOR)
Vitamist Intra-Oral Spray Dietary Supplements
(MAYOR)
**MELATONIN FORTE 3MG WITH KAVA
KAVA** (VITALINE)
MELLARIL CONCENTRATE (NOVARTIS)
MELLARIL TABLETS (NOVARTIS)
MELLARIL-S ORAL SUSPENSION
(NOVARTIS)

MELPHALAN
Alkeran Tablets (GLAXO WELLCOME)

MELPHALAN HYDROCHLORIDE
Alkeran for Injection (GLAXO WELLCOME)
MENEST TABLETS (MONARCH)

MENINGOCOCCAL POLYSACCHARIDE
VACCINE
Menomune-A/C/Y/W-135
(PASTEUR MERIEUX CONNAUGHT)
MENOMUNE-A/C/Y/W-135
(PASTEUR MERIEUX CONNAUGHT)

MENOTROPINS
Humegon for Injection (ORGANON)
Pergonal for Injection (SERONO)
Repronex for Intramuscular Injection (FERRING)
MENTAX CREAM (BERTEK)

MENTHOL
Cool Mint Listerine (WARNER-LAMBERT)
FreshBurst Listerine (WARNER-LAMBERT)
Listerine Antiseptic (WARNER-LAMBERT)
Panalgesic Gold Cream (ECR)
Panalgesic Gold Topical Liquid (ECR)
Thera-Gesic Creme (MISSION)
MEPERGAN FORTIS CAPSULES
(WYETH-AYERST)
MEPERGAN INJECTION (WYETH-AYERST)
MEPERGAN IN TUBEX (WYETH-AYERST)
MEPERIDINE HCL INJECTION
(WYETH-AYERST)
**MEPERIDINE HCL INJECTION (10 MG/ML,
PCA VIALS)** (ABBOTT)

MEPERIDINE HYDROCHLORIDE
Demerol Syrup (SANOFI)
Demerol Tablets (SANOFI)
Mepergan Injection (WYETH-AYERST)
Mepergan in Tubex (WYETH-AYERST)
Meperidine Hydrochloride Injection
(ELKINS-SINN)
Meperidine Hydrochloride Injection, USP
(ASTRAZENECA LP)
Meperidine Hydrochloride Injection, USP -
Dosette (BAXTER)
Meperidine Hydrochloride Injection, USP -
Tubex (BAXTER)
Meperidine Hydrochloride Syrup (ROXANE)
Meperidine Hydrochloride Tablets (ROXANE)
Meperidine Hydrochloride Tablets, USP CII
(WATSON)
Meperidine Hydrochloride in Tubex
(WYETH-AYERST)
**MEPERIDINE HYDROCHLORIDE IN
TUBEX** (WYETH-AYERST)
**MEPERIDINE HYDROCHLORIDE
INJECTION** (ELKINS-SINN)
**MEPERIDINE HYDROCHLORIDE
INJECTION, USP - DOSETTE** (BAXTER)
**MEPERIDINE HYDROCHLORIDE
INJECTION, USP - TUBEX** (BAXTER)
**MEPERIDINE HYDROCHLORIDE
INJECTION, USP** (ASTRAZENECA LP)
MEPERIDINE HYDROCHLORIDE SYRUP
(ROXANE)
MEPERIDINE HYDROCHLORIDE TABLETS
(ROXANE)
**MEPERIDINE HYDROCHLORIDE
TABLETS, USP CII** (WATSON)

MEPHOBARBITAL
Mebaral Tablets (SANOFI)
MEPHYTON TABLETS (MERCK)

MEPIVACAINE HYDROCHLORIDE
Polocaine Injection, USP (ASTRAZENECA LP)
Polocaine-MPF Injection, USP
(ASTRAZENECA LP)

MEPROBAMATE
Equagesic Tablets (WYETH-AYERST)
Equanil Tablets (WYETH-AYERST)
Meprobamate Tablets CIV (WATSON)
Miltown Tablets (WALLACE)
MEPROBAMATE TABLETS CIV (WATSON)
MEPRON SUSPENSION (GLAXO WELLCOME)

MERCAPTOPURINE
Purinethol Tablets (GLAXO WELLCOME)
MERIDIA CAPSULES (KNOLL)

MEROPENEM
Merrem I.V. (ASTRAZENECA)
MERREM I.V. (ASTRAZENECA)
MERUVAX II (MERCK)

MESALAMINE
Asacol Delayed-Release Tablets
(PROCTER & GAMBLE PHARMACEUTICALS)
Pentasa Capsules (ROBERTS)
Rowasa Rectal Suspension Enema 4.0
grams/unit (60 mL) (SOLVAY)
**MESALAMINE (5-AMINOSALICYLIC ACID)
POWDER** (PADDOCK)
MESANTOIN TABLETS (NOVARTIS)
MESCOLOR TABLETS (HORIZON)

MESNA
Mesnex Injection
(BRISTOL-MYERSSQUIBBONCOLOGY/IMMUNOLOGY)
MESNEX INJECTION
(BRISTOL-MYERSSQUIBBONCOLOGY/IMMUNOLOGY)

MESORIDAZINE BESYLATE
Serentil Ampuls (BOEHRINGER INGELHEIM)
Serentil Concentrate (BOEHRINGER INGELHEIM)
Serentil Tablets (BOEHRINGER INGELHEIM)
MESTINON SYRUP (ICN)
MESTINON TABLETS (ICN)
MESTINON TIMESPAN TABLETS (ICN)

MESTRANOL
Necon 1/50 Tablets (WATSON)
Norethindrone and Mestranol Tablets, USP
(NECON) (WATSON)
Norinyl 1 + 50-21 Tablets (SEARLE)
Norinyl 1 + 50-28 Tablets (SEARLE)
Ortho-Novum 1/50 28 Tablets (ORTHO-MCNEIL)
**METAMUCIL ORIGINAL TEXTURE
POWDER, ORANGE FLAVOR**
(PROCTER & GAMBLE)
**METAMUCIL ORIGINAL TEXTURE
POWDER, REGULAR FLAVOR**
(PROCTER & GAMBLE)
**METAMUCIL SMOOTH TEXTURE
POWDER, ORANGE FLAVOR**
(PROCTER & GAMBLE)
**METAMUCIL SMOOTH TEXTURE
POWDER, SUGAR-FREE, ORANGE
FLAVOR** (PROCTER & GAMBLE)
**METAMUCIL SMOOTH TEXTURE
POWDER, SUGAR-FREE, REGULAR
FLAVOR** (PROCTER & GAMBLE)
**METAMUCIL WAFERS, APPLE CRISP AND
CINNAMON SPICE FLAVORS**
(PROCTER & GAMBLE)

METAPROTERENOL SULFATE
Alupent Inhalation Aerosol
(BOEHRINGER INGELHEIM)
Alupent Inhalation Solution
(BOEHRINGER INGELHEIM)
Alupent Syrup (BOEHRINGER INGELHEIM)
Alupent Tablets (BOEHRINGER INGELHEIM)
Metaproterenol Sulfate Inhalation Solution
(ROXANE)
Metaproterenol Sulfate Inhalation Solution USP
(DEY)
**METAPROTERENOL SULFATE
INHALATION SOLUTION** (ROXANE)
**METAPROTERENOL SULFATE
INHALATION SOLUTION USP** (DEY)

METARAMINOL BITARTRATE
Aramine Injection (MERCK)
**METASTRON (SEE UNDER MEDI-PHYSICS,
INC., AMERSHAM HEALTHCARE)**
(ASTRAZENECA)

METAXALONE
Skelaxin Tablets (CARNRICK)

METFORMIN HYDROCHLORIDE
Glucophage Tablets (BRISTOL-MYERS SQUIBB)
METHADONE HCL POWDER (ROXANE)

METHADONE HYDROCHLORIDE
Dolophine Hydrochloride Tablets and Injection
(ROXANE)
Methadone HCl Powder (ROXANE)
Methadone Hydrochloride Diskets (Dispersible
Tablets) (ROXANE)
Methadone Hydrochloride Oral Concentrate
(ROXANE)
Methadone Hydrochloride Oral Solution &
Tablets (ROXANE)
Methadose Dispersible Tablets (MALLINCKRODT)
Methadose Oral Concentrate (MALLINCKRODT)
Methadose Oral Tablets (MALLINCKRODT)
**METHADONE HYDROCHLORIDE DISKETS
(DISPERSIBLE TABLETS)** (ROXANE)
**METHADONE HYDROCHLORIDE ORAL
CONCENTRATE** (ROXANE)
**METHADONE HYDROCHLORIDE ORAL
SOLUTION & TABLETS** (ROXANE)
METHADOSE ORAL CONCENTRATE
(MALLINCKRODT)
METHADOSE DISPERSIBLE TABLETS
(MALLINCKRODT)
METHADOSE ORAL TABLETS
(MALLINCKRODT)
METHAGUAL (GORDON)

METHAMPHETAMINE HYDROCHLORIDE
Desoxyn Gradumet Tablets (ABBOTT)
A-METHAPRED (ABBOTT)

METHAZOLAMIDE
Methazolamide Tablets (GENEVA)
Methazolamide Tablets (LEDERLE STANDARD)
METHAZOLAMIDE TABLETS (GENEVA)
METHAZOLAMIDE TABLETS
(LEDERLE STANDARD)

METHENAMINE
Prosed/DS Tablets (STAR)
Urised Tablets (POLYMEDICA)
METHENAMINE, FOR TIMED BURNING
(LILLY)

METHENAMINE HIPPURATE
Urex Tablets (3M)

METHENAMINE MANDELATE
Mandelamine Tablets (WARNER CHILCOTT)
Uroqid-Acid No. 2 Tablets (BEACH)
METHERGINE INJECTION (NOVARTIS)
METHERGINE TABLETS (NOVARTIS)

METHIMAZOLE
Tapazole Tablets (JONES)

METHIONINE
Amino-Cerv Creme (MILEX)

METHOCARBAMOL
Methocarbamol Tablets (GENEVA)
Methocarbamol Tablets (WATSON)
Methocarbamol Tablets (LEDERLE STANDARD)
Methocarbamol and Aspirin Tablets (PAR)
Robaxin Injectable (ROBINS)
Robaxin Tablets (ROBINS)
Robaxin-750 Tablets (ROBINS)
Robaxisal Tablets (ROBINS)
**METHOCARBAMOL AND ASPIRIN
TABLETS** (PAR)
METHOCARBAMOL TABLETS (GENEVA)
METHOCARBAMOL TABLETS (WATSON)
METHOCARBAMOL TABLETS
(LEDERLE STANDARD)
METHOCARBAMOL TABLETS, USP (SCHEIN)

METHOHEXITAL SODIUM
Brevital Sodium for Injection, USP (JONES)
METHOTREXATE INJECTION, USP
(BEDFORD)

METHOTREXATE SODIUM
Methotrexate Sodium Tablets, Injection, for
Injection and LPF Injection (IMMUNEX)
Methotrexate Tablets (MYLAN)
Methotrexate Tablets (ROXANE)
Rheumatrex Dose Pack (LEDERLE LABS)
METHOTREXATE SODIUM TABLETS
(ESI LEDERLE)
**METHOTREXATE SODIUM TABLETS,
INJECTION, FOR INJECTION AND LPF
INJECTION** (IMMUNEX)
METHOTREXATE TABLETS (MYLAN)
METHOTREXATE TABLETS (ROXANE)
METHOTREXATE TABLETS (LEDERLE LABS)

METHOXAMINE HYDROCHLORIDE
Vasoxyl Injection (GLAXO WELLCOME)

METHOXSALEN
8-MOP Capsules (ICN)
Oxsoralen Lotion 1% (ICN)
Oxsoralen-Ultra Capsules (ICN)

METHSCOPOLAMINE NITRATE
Ah-Chew Chewable Tablets (WE)
D.A. Chewable Tablets (DJ PHARMA)
D.A. II Tablets (DJ PHARMA)
Dallergy Caplets, Syrup, Tablets (LASER)
Dura-Vent/DA Tablets (DJ PHARMA)
Extendryl Chewable Tablets (FLEMING)
Extendryl Sr. & Jr. Capsules (FLEMING)
Extendryl Syrup (FLEMING)
Mescolor Tablets (HORIZON)
Omnihist L.A. Tablets (WE)

METHSUXIMIDE
Celontin Kapseals (PARKE-DAVIS)

METHYCLOTHIAZIDE
Aquatensen Tablets (WALLACE)
Diutensen-R Tablets (WALLACE)
Enduron Tablets (ABBOTT)
Methyclothiazide Tablets (MYLAN)
METHYCLOTHIAZIDE TABLETS (MYLAN)

METHYL SALICYLATE
Cool Mint Listerine (WARNER-LAMBERT)
FreshBurst Listerine (WARNER-LAMBERT)
Listerine Antiseptic (WARNER-LAMBERT)
Panalgesic Gold Cream (ECR)
Panalgesic Gold Topical Liquid (ECR)
Thera-Gesic Creme (MISSION)

METHYLDOPA
Aldoclor Tablets (MERCK)
Aldomet Tablets (MERCK)
Aldoril Tablets (MERCK)
Methyldopa & Hydrochlorothiazide Tablets
(LEDERLE STANDARD)
Methyldopa Tablets (MYLAN)
Methyldopa Tablets (LEDERLE STANDARD)
Methyldopa Tablets, USP (ENDO GENERICS)
Methyldopa and Hydrochlorothiazide Tablets
(MYLAN)
Methyldopa/Hydrochlorothiazide Tablets, USP
(ENDO GENERICS)
**METHYLDOPA &
HYDROCHLOROTHIAZIDE TABLETS**
(LEDERLE STANDARD)
METHYLDOPA TABLETS (MYLAN)
METHYLDOPA TABLETS
(LEDERLE STANDARD)
**METHYLDOPA AND
HYDROCHLOROTHIAZIDE TABLETS**
(MYLAN)

UNDERLINE DENOTES GENERIC NAME

METHYLDOPA TABLETS, USP
(ENDO GENERICS)
METHYLDOPA/HYDROCHLOROTHIAZIDE TABLETS, USP (ENDO GENERICS)
METHYLDOPATE HYDROCHLORIDE
　Aldomet Ester HCl Injection (MERCK)
METHYLENE BLUE
　Prosed/DS Tablets (STAR)
　Urised Tablets (POLYMEDICA)
　Urolene Blue Tablets (STAR)
METHYLIN TABLETS (MALLINCKRODT)
METHYLPHENIDATE HCL TABLETS
(GENEVA)
**METHYLPHENIDATE HCL TABLETS, USP
C II** (SCHEIN)
METHYLPHENIDATE HYDROCHLORIDE
　Methylin Tablets (MALLINCKRODT)
　Methylphenidate HCL Tablets (GENEVA)
　Methylphenidate Sustained Release Tablets
　　(GENEVA)
　Ritalin Hydrochloride Tablets (NOVARTIS)
　Ritalin-SR Tablets (NOVARTIS)
**METHYLPHENIDATE HYDROCHLORIDE
EXTENDED-RELEASE TABLETS, USP**
(APOTHECON)
**METHYLPHENIDATE HYDROCHLORIDE
TABLETS, USP** (APOTHECON)
**METHYLPHENIDATE SUSTAINED
RELEASE TABLETS** (GENEVA)
METHYLPREDNISOLONE
　Medrol Tablets (PHARMACIA & UPJOHN)
　Methylprednisolone Tablets (PAR)
　Methylprednisolone Tablets (WATSON)
METHYLPREDNISOLONE ACETATE
　Depo-Medrol Sterile Aqueous Suspension
　　(PHARMACIA & UPJOHN)
METHYLPREDNISOLONE SODIUM
SUCCINATE
　Solu-Medrol Sterile Powder
　　(PHARMACIA & UPJOHN)
METHYLPREDNISOLONE TABLETS (PAR)
METHYLPREDNISOLONE TABLETS
(WATSON)
METHYLPREDNISOLONE TABLETS
(DURAMED)
METHYLTESTOSTERONE
　Android Capsules, 10 mg (ICN)
　Estratest H.S. Tablets (SOLVAY)
　Estratest Tablets (SOLVAY)
　Testred Capsules, 10 mg (ICN)
　Virilon Capsules (STAR)
METICORTEN TABLETS (SCHERING)
**METIMYD OPHTHALMIC
OINTMENT–STERILE** (SCHERING)
**METIMYD OPHTHALMIC
SUSPENSION–STERILE** (SCHERING)
METOCLOPRAMIDE
　Metoclopramide Injection, USP (BAXTER)
　Metoclopramide Intensol (ROXANE)
　Metoclopramide Oral Solution (ROXANE)
METOCLOPRAMIDE HYDROCHLORIDE
　Metoclopramide Hydrochloride Tablets
　　(WATSON)
　Metoclopramide Oral Solution USP
　　(PHARMACEUTICAL ASSOCIATES)
　Reglan Injectable (ROBINS)
　Reglan Syrup (ROBINS)
　Reglan Tablets (ROBINS)
**METOCLOPRAMIDE HYDROCHLORIDE
TABLETS** (WATSON)
METOCLOPRAMIDE INJECTION, USP
(BAXTER)

METOCLOPRAMIDE INTENSOL (ROXANE)
METOCLOPRAMIDE ORAL SOLUTION
(ROXANE)
**METOCLOPRAMIDE ORAL SOLUTION
USP** (PHARMACEUTICAL ASSOCIATES)
METOCLOPRAMIDE TABLETS (ESI LEDERLE)
METOLAZONE
　Mykrox Tablets (MEDEVA)
　Zaroxolyn Tablets (MEDEVA)
METOPIRONE CAPSULES (NOVARTIS)
METOPROLOL INJECTABLE (GENEVA)
METOPROLOL SUCCINATE
　Toprol-XL Tablets (ASTRAZENECA LP)
METOPROLOL TARTRATE
　Metoprolol Injectable (GENEVA)
　Metoprolol Tartrate Tablets (MYLAN)
　Metoprolol Tartrate Tablets (GENEVA)
　Metoprolol Tartrate Tablets, 50 mg, 100 mg
　　(NOVOPHARM)
　Metoprolol Tartrate Tablets, USP (WATSON)
METOPROLOL TARTRATE TABLETS
(MYLAN)
METOPROLOL TARTRATE TABLETS
(GENEVA)
METOPROLOL TARTRATE TABLETS, USP
(APOTHECON)
**METOPROLOL TARTRATE TABLETS, 50
MG, 100 MG** (NOVOPHARM)
METOPROLOL TARTRATE TABLETS, USP
(WATSON)
METRIC 21 TABLETS (FIELDING)
METROCREAM (GALDERMA)
METROGEL (GALDERMA)
METROGEL-VAGINAL GEL (3M)
METROLOTION (GALDERMA)
METRONIDAZOLE
　Flagyl 375 Capsules (SEARLE)
　Flagyl ER Tablets (SEARLE)
　Flagyl I.V. RTU (SCS)
　MetroCream (GALDERMA)
　MetroGel (GALDERMA)
　MetroGel-Vaginal Gel (3M)
　MetroLotion (GALDERMA)
　Noritate Cream (DERMIK)
METRONIDAZOLE HYDROCHLORIDE
　Flagyl I.V. (SCS)
**METRONIDAZOLE INJECTION, USP (5
MG/ML)** (ABBOTT)
METYROSINE
　Demser Capsules (MERCK)
MEVACOR TABLETS (MERCK)
**MEXILETINE CAPSULES, 150 MG, 200 MG,
250 MG** (NOVOPHARM)
MEXILETINE HCL CAPSULES (GENEVA)
MEXILETINE HYDROCHLORIDE
　Mexiletine Capsules, 150 mg, 200 mg, 250
　　mg (NOVOPHARM)
　Mexiletine HCl Capsules (GENEVA)
　Mexiletine Hydrochloride Capsules (ROXANE)
　Mexiletine Hydrochloride Capsules, USP
　　(WATSON)
　Mexitil Capsules (BOEHRINGER INGELHEIM)
**MEXILETINE HYDROCHLORIDE
CAPSULES** (ROXANE)
**MEXILETINE HYDROCHLORIDE
CAPSULES, USP** (WATSON)
MEXITIL CAPSULES (BOEHRINGER INGELHEIM)
**MEZLIN FOR INTRAVENOUS OR
INTRAMUSCULAR USE** (BAYER)
MEZLIN PHARMACY BULK PACKAGE
(BAYER)

MEZLOCILLIN SODIUM
　Mezlin Pharmacy Bulk Package (BAYER)
　Mezlin for Intravenous or Intramuscular Use
　　(BAYER)
MIACALCIN INJECTION (NOVARTIS)
MIACALCIN NASAL SPRAY (NOVARTIS)
MICANOL 1% CREAM (BIOGLAN)
MICARDIS TABLETS (BOEHRINGER INGELHEIM)
MICONAZOLE NITRATE
　Monistat-Derm Cream
　　(ORTHO DERMATOLOGICAL)
MICRAININ TABLETS (WALLACE)
MICRHOGAM (ORTHO-CLINICAL)
MICRONASE TABLETS
(PHARMACIA & UPJOHN)
MICRONOR TABLETS (ORTHO-MCNEIL)
MICROSPONGE SURGICAL EYE SPONGE
(ALCON)
MICROZIDE CAPSULES (WATSON)
MIDAMOR TABLETS (MERCK)
MIDAZOLAM HYDROCHLORIDE
　Versed Injection (ROCHE LABS)
　Versed Syrup (ROCHE LABS)
MIDODRINE HYDROCHLORIDE
　ProAmatine Tablets (ROBERTS)
MIDRIN CAPSULES (CARNRICK)
MIGLITOL
　Glyset Tablets (PHARMACIA & UPJOHN)
MIGRANAL NASAL SPRAY (NOVARTIS)
MILK OF MAGNESIA USP
(PHARMACEUTICAL ASSOCIATES)
**MILK OF MAGNESIA & MILK OF
MAGNESIA-CONCENTRATED
FLAVORED** (ROXANE)
MILK OF MAGNESIA CONCENTRATE
(PHARMACEUTICAL ASSOCIATES)
**MILK OF MAGNESIA CASCARA
SUSPENSION** (PHARMACEUTICAL ASSOCIATES)
MILK OF MAGNESIA USP (PADDOCK)
**MILK OF MAGNESIA-CASCARA
SUSPENSION CONCENTRATED** (ROXANE)
MILKINOL (SCHWARZ)
MILRINONE LACTATE
　Primacor Injection (SANOFI)
MILTOWN TABLETS (WALLACE)
MINERAL OIL (PHARMACEUTICAL ASSOCIATES)
MINERAL OIL
　Anusol Hemorrhoidal Ointment
　　(WARNER-LAMBERT)
　Aquaphor Healing Ointment (BEIERSDORF)
　Aquaphor Original Ointment (BEIERSDORF)
　Eucerin Original Moisturizing Creme
　　(BEIERSDORF)
　Eucerin Original Moisturizing Lotion
　　(BEIERSDORF)
　Eucerin Plus Alpha Hydroxy Creme
　　(BEIERSDORF)
　Eucerin Plus Alpha Hydroxy Lotion
　　(BEIERSDORF)
　Fleet Mineral Oil Enema (FLEET)
　Mineral Oil (PHARMACEUTICAL ASSOCIATES)
　Mineral Oil Topical Light (ROXANE)
MINERAL OIL TOPICAL LIGHT (ROXANE)
MINERAL SUPPLEMENTS
　Colloidal Minerals (MAYOR)
　Vitamist Intra-Oral Spray Dietary Supplements
　　(MAYOR)
MINIPRESS CAPSULES (PFIZER)
**MINITRAN TRANSDERMAL DELIVERY
SYSTEM** (3M)
MINIT-RUB ANALGESIC OINTMENT
(BRISTOL-MYERS)
MINIZIDE CAPSULES (PFIZER)

UNDERLINE DENOTES GENERIC NAME

MINOCIN INTRAVENOUS (LEDERLE LABS)
MINOCIN ORAL SUSPENSION
(LEDERLE LABS)
MINOCIN PELLET-FILLED CAPSULES
(LEDERLE LABS)
MINOCYCLINE HCL CAPSULES
(ESI LEDERLE)
MINOCYCLINE HCL CAPSULES, USP
(SCHEIN)

MINOCYCLINE HYDROCHLORIDE

Dynacin Capsules (MEDICIS)
Minocin Intravenous (LEDERLE LABS)
Minocin Oral Suspension (LEDERLE LABS)
Minocin Pellet-Filled Capsules (LEDERLE LABS)
Vectrin Capsules (WARNER CHILCOTT)

MINOXIDIL

Minoxidil Tablets (PAR)
MINOXIDIL TABLETS (PAR)
MINTEZOL SUSPENSION (MERCK)
MINTEZOL CHEWABLE TABLETS (MERCK)
MIOSTAT INTRAOCULAR MIOTIC
SOLUTION (ALCON)
MIRADON TABLETS (SCHERING)
MIRALAX POWDER FOR ORAL
SOLUTION (BRAINTREE)
MIRAPEX TABLETS (PHARMACIA & UPJOHN)
MIRCETTE TABLETS (ORGANON)

MIRTAZAPINE

Remeron Tablets (ORGANON)

MISOPROSTOL

Arthrotec Tablets (SEARLE)
Cytotec Tablets (SEARLE)
MISSION PRENATAL TABLETS (MISSION)
MISSION PRENATAL F.A. TABLETS
(MISSION)
MISSION PRENATAL H.P. TABLETS
(MISSION)
MITHRACIN FOR INTRAVENOUS USE
(BAYER)

MITOMYCIN (MITOMYCIN-C)

Mitomycin for Injection, USP (SUPERGEN)
Mutamycin for Injection
(BRISTOL-MYERSSQUIBBONCOLOGY/IMMUNOLOGY)
MITOMYCIN FOR INJECTION, USP
(BEDFORD)
MITOMYCIN FOR INJECTION, USP
(SUPERGEN)

MITOTANE

Lysodren Tablets
(BRISTOL-MYERSSQUIBBONCOLOGY/IMMUNOLOGY)

MITOXANTRONE HYDROCHLORIDE

Novantrone for Injection (IMMUNEX)
MITROLAN TABLETS (ROBINS)
MIVACRON INJECTION (GLAXO WELLCOME)

MIVACURIUM CHLORIDE

Mivacron Injection (GLAXO WELLCOME)
M-M-R II (MERCK)
MOBAN ORAL CONCENTRATE (ENDO LABS)
MOBAN TABLETS (ENDO LABS)

MODAFINIL

Provigil Tablets (CEPHALON)
MODERIL TABLETS (PFIZER)
MODICON 21 TABLETS (ORTHO-MCNEIL)
MODICON 28 TABLETS (ORTHO-MCNEIL)
MODURETIC TABLETS (MERCK)

MOEXIPRIL HYDROCHLORIDE

Uniretic Tablets (SCHWARZ)
Univasc Tablets (SCHWARZ)
MOISTUREL CREAM (WESTWOOD-SQUIBB)
MOISTUREL LOTION (WESTWOOD-SQUIBB)

MOISTUREL SENSITIVE SKIN CLEANSER
(WESTWOOD-SQUIBB)

MOLINDONE HYDROCHLORIDE

Moban Oral Concentrate (ENDO LABS)
Moban Tablets (ENDO LABS)

MOMETASONE FUROATE

Elocon Cream 0.1% (SCHERING)
Elocon Lotion 0.1% (SCHERING)
Elocon Ointment 0.1% (SCHERING)

MOMETASONE FUROATE MONOHYDRATE

Nasonex Nasal Spray (SCHERING)
MONARC-M (AMERICAN RED CROSS)

MONASCUS PURPUREUS WENT

Cholestin Capsules (PHARMANEX)
MONISTAT-DERM CREAM
(ORTHO DERMATOLOGICAL)

MONOBENZONE

Benoquin Cream 20% (ICN)
MONOCAL TABLETS (MERICON)
MONOCLATE-P CONCENTRATE (CENTEON)
MONODOX CAPSULES (OCLASSEN)

MONOFLUOROPHOSPHATE

Monocal Tablets (MERICON)
MONO-GESIC TABLETS (SCHWARZ)
MONOKET TABLETS (SCHWARZ)
MONONINE CONCENTRATE (CENTEON)
MONOPRIL TABLETS (BRISTOL-MYERS SQUIBB)
MONO-VACC TEST (O.T.)
(PASTEUR MERIEUX CONNAUGHT)

MONTELUKAST SODIUM

Singulair Chewable Tablets (MERCK)
Singulair Tablets (MERCK)
MONUROL SACHET (FOREST)

MORICIZINE HYDROCHLORIDE

Ethmozine Tablets (ROBERTS)

MORPHINE SULFATE

Astramorph/PF Injection, USP (Preservative-
Free) (ASTRAZENECA LP)
Duramorph Injection (BAXTER)
Duramorph Injection (ELKINS-SINN)
Infumorph 200 and Infumorph 500 Sterile
Solutions (ELKINS-SINN)
Kadian Capsules (FAULDING)
MS Contin Tablets (PURDUE FREDERICK)
MSIR Oral Capsules (PURDUE FREDERICK)
MSIR Oral Solution (PURDUE FREDERICK)
MSIR Oral Solution Concentrate
(PURDUE FREDERICK)
MSIR Oral Tablets (PURDUE FREDERICK)
Morphine Sulfate (Immediate Release)
Concentrated Oral Solution
(ASTRAZENECA LP)
Morphine Sulfate Extended-Release Tablets CII
(ENDO GENERICS)
Morphine Sulfate Immediate Release Oral
Solution (ASTRAZENECA LP)
Morphine Sulfate Injection (ELKINS-SINN)
Morphine Sulfate Injection, USP - Dosette
(BAXTER)
Morphine Sulfate Injection, USP - Tubex
(BAXTER)
Morphine Sulfate Injection, USP for
Intravenous Infusion (ASTRAZENECA LP)
Morphine Sulfate Injection, USP for
Intravenous Injection (ASTRAZENECA LP)
Morphine Sulfate Injection, USP for
Intravenous Use After Dilution
(ASTRAZENECA LP)
Morphine Sulfate Oral Solution & Tablets
(ROXANE)
Morphine Sulfate in Tubex (WYETH-AYERST)
Oramorph SR Tablets (ROXANE)

RMS Suppositories CII (UPSHER-SMITH)
Roxanol 100 Concentrated Oral Solution
(ROXANE)
Roxanol Concentrated Oral Solution (ROXANE)
Roxanol-T Oral Solution (ROXANE)
MORPHINE SULFATE EXTENDED-
RELEASE TABLETS CII (ENDO GENERICS)
MORPHINE SULFATE (IMMEDIATE
RELEASE) CONCENTRATED ORAL
SOLUTION (ASTRAZENECA LP)
MORPHINE SULFATE IMMEDIATE
RELEASE ORAL SOLUTION
(ASTRAZENECA LP)
MORPHINE SULFATE IN TUBEX
(WYETH-AYERST)
MORPHINE SULFATE INJECTION
(ELKINS-SINN)
MORPHINE SULFATE INJECTION
(WYETH-AYERST)
MORPHINE SULFATE INJECTION, USP
FOR INTRAVENOUS INFUSION
(ASTRAZENECA LP)
MORPHINE SULFATE INJECTION, USP
FOR INTRAVENOUS INJECTION
(ASTRAZENECA LP)
MORPHINE SULFATE INJECTION, USP -
DOSETTE (BAXTER)
MORPHINE SULFATE INJECTION, USP -
TUBEX (BAXTER)
MORPHINE SULFATE INJECTION, USP (1
& 5 MG/ML, PCA VIALS) (ABBOTT)
MORPHINE SULFATE INJECTION, USP
FOR INTRAVENOUS USE AFTER
DILUTION (ASTRAZENECA LP)
MORPHINE SULFATE ORAL SOLUTION &
TABLETS (ROXANE)
MORPHINE SULFATE USP POWDER CII
(PADDOCK)
MORPHINE SULFATE SUPPOSITORIES 5
MG, 10 MG, 20 MG, 30 MG CII
(PADDOCK)
MORPHINE SULFATE VIALS & SOLUBLE
TABLETS (LILLY)
MOTOFEN TABLETS (CARNRICK)
CHILDREN'S MOTRIN CHEWABLE
TABLETS (MCNEIL CONSUMER)
CHILDREN'S MOTRIN ORAL SUSPENSION
(MCNEIL CONSUMER)
MOTRIN SUSPENSION, ORAL DROPS,
CHEWABLE TABLETS, AND CAPLETS
(MCNEIL CONSUMER)
MOTRIN COLD & FLU CAPLETS
(MCNEIL CONSUMER)
MOTRIN IB PAIN RELIEVER TABLETS,
CAPLETS, AND GELCAPS
(MCNEIL CONSUMER)
INFANTS' MOTRIN CONCENTRATED
DROPS (MCNEIL CONSUMER)
JUNIOR STRENGTH MOTRIN CAPLETS
(MCNEIL CONSUMER)
JUNIOR STRENGTH MOTRIN CHEWABLE
TABLETS (MCNEIL CONSUMER)
MOTRIN SINUS HEADACHE CAPLETS
(MCNEIL CONSUMER)
MOTRIN TABLETS (PHARMACIA & UPJOHN)
M-R-VAX II (MERCK)
MS CONTIN TABLETS (PURDUE FREDERICK)
MSIR ORAL CAPSULES (PURDUE FREDERICK)
MSIR ORAL SOLUTION (PURDUE FREDERICK)
MSIR ORAL SOLUTION CONCENTRATE
(PURDUE FREDERICK)
MSIR ORAL TABLETS (PURDUE FREDERICK)
MSTA MUMPS SKIN TEST ANTIGEN
(PASTEUR MERIEUX CONNAUGHT)
MUCO-FEN 800 DM TABLETS (WAKEFIELD)
MUCO-FEN 800 TABLETS (WAKEFIELD)

UNDERLINE DENOTES GENERIC NAME

MUCO-FEN 1200 TABLETS (WAKEFIELD)
MUCO-FEN DM TABLETS (WAKEFIELD)
MUCO-FEN LA TABLETS (WAKEFIELD)
MUCOMYST-10 AND MUCOMYST-20
　(APOTHECON)
MULTIMINERAL PLUS ADVANCED
　FORMULA (VITALINE)
MULTIPLE
　ADULT/CHILDREN'S/PRENATAL
　FORMULAS (MAYOR)

MUMPS SKIN TEST ANTIGEN

　MSTA Mumps Skin Test Antigen
　　(PASTEUR MERIEUX CONNAUGHT)

MUMPS VIRUS VACCINE, LIVE

　Mumpsvax (MERCK)
MUMPSVAX (MERCK)

MUPIROCIN

　Bactroban Ointment (SMITHKLINE BEECHAM)

MUPIROCIN CALCIUM

　Bactroban Cream (SMITHKLINE BEECHAM)
　Bactroban Nasal (SMITHKLINE BEECHAM)
MURINE EAR WAX REMOVAL
　SYSTEM/MURINE EAR DROPS (ROSS)
MURINE TEARS LUBRICANT EYE DROPS
　(ROSS)
MURINE TEARS PLUS LUBRICANT
　REDNESS RELIEVER EYE DROPS (ROSS)

MUROMONAB-CD3

　Orthoclone OKT3 Sterile Solution
　　(ORTHO BIOTECH)
MUSE URETHRAL SUPPOSITORY (VIVUS)
MUSTARGEN FOR INJECTION (MERCK)
MUTAMYCIN FOR INJECTION
　(BRISTOL-MYERSSQUIBBONCOLOGY/IMMUNOLOGY)
M.V.I. PEDIATRIC FOR INFUSION
　(ASTRAZENECA LP)
M.V.I.-12 MULTI-VITAMIN INFUSION
　(ASTRAZENECA LP)
MYAMBUTOL TABLETS (DURA)
MYAMBUTOL TABLETS (LEDERLE LABS)
MYCELEX TROCHE (BAYER)
MYCELEX TWIN PACK (BAYER)
MYCELEX-G 500 MG VAGINAL TABLETS
　(BAYER)
MYCOBUTIN CAPSULES
　(PHARMACIA & UPJOHN)
MYCOLOG-II CREAM AND OINTMENT
　(APOTHECON)

MYCOPHENOLATE MOFETIL

　CellCept Capsules (ROCHE LABS)
　CellCept Oral Suspension (ROCHE LABS)
　CellCept Tablets (ROCHE LABS)

MYCOPHENOLATE MOFETIL
HYDROCHLORIDE

　CellCept Intravenous (ROCHE LABS)
MYCOSTATIN CREAM (WESTWOOD-SQUIBB)
MYCOSTATIN ORAL SUSPENSION
　(APOTHECON)
MYCOSTATIN ORAL TABLETS (NYSTATIN
　TABLETS USP) (APOTHECON)
MYCOSTATIN PASTILLES
　(BRISTOL-MYERSSQUIBBONCOLOGY/IMMUNOLOGY)
MYCOSTATIN TOPICAL POWDER
　(WESTWOOD-SQUIBB)
MYDFRIN 2.5% (ALCON P.R.)
MYDRIACYL (ALCON P.R.)
MYKROX TABLETS (MEDEVA)
CHILDREN'S MYLANTA UPSET STOMACH
　RELIEF LIQUID (J&J – MERCK)
CHILDREN'S MYLANTA UPSET STOMACH
　RELIEF TABLETS (J&J – MERCK)
MYLANTA DOUBLE STRENGTH TABLETS
　(J&J – MERCK)

FAST-ACTING MYLANTA ANTACID
　TABLETS (J&J – MERCK)
MAXIMUM STRENGTH FAST-ACTING
　MYLANTA ANTACID TABLETS
　(J&J – MERCK)
FAST-ACTING MYLANTA LIQUID
　ANTACID (J&J – MERCK)
MAXIMUM STRENGTH FAST-ACTING
　MYLANTA LIQUID (J&J – MERCK)
MYLANTA GAS RELIEF GELCAPS
　(J&J – MERCK)
MYLANTA GAS RELIEF TABLETS
　(J&J – MERCK)
MAXIMUM STRENGTH MYLANTA GAS
　RELIEF TABLETS (J&J – MERCK)
MYLANTA GELCAPS ANTACID
　(J&J – MERCK)
MYLANTA SUPREME LIQUID (J&J – MERCK)
MYLANTA TABLETS (J&J – MERCK)
MYLERAN TABLETS (GLAXO WELLCOME)
MYLICON INFANTS' DROPS (J&J – MERCK)
MYOCHRYSINE INJECTION (MERCK)
MYOFLEX ANALGESIC CREAM
　(NOVARTIS CONSUMER)
MYSOLINE SUSPENSION (ELAN)
MYSOLINE TABLETS (ELAN)
MYTELASE CHLORIDE CAPLETS (SANOFI)
MYTREX CREAM (SAVAGE)
MYTREX OINTMENT (SAVAGE)

N

NABI-HB (NABI)

NABUMETONE

　Relafen Tablets (SMITHKLINE BEECHAM)
N-ACETYLCYSTEINE 500MG (VITALINE)

NADOLOL

　Corzide 40/5 Tablets (BRISTOL-MYERS SQUIBB)
　Corzide 80/5 Tablets (BRISTOL-MYERS SQUIBB)
　Nadolol Tablets (MYLAN)
NADOLOL TABLETS (MYLAN)
NADOLOL TABLETS, USP (APOTHECON)

NAFARELIN ACETATE

　Synarel Nasal Solution for Central Precocious
　　Puberty (SEARLE)
　Synarel Nasal Solution for Endometriosis
　　(SEARLE)
NAFCILLIN FOR INJECTION USP AND IN
　ADD-VANTAGE VIALS (APOTHECON)

NAFTIFINE HYDROCHLORIDE

　Naftin Cream (ALLERGAN)
　Naftin Gel (ALLERGAN)
NAFTIN CREAM (ALLERGAN)
NAFTIN GEL (ALLERGAN)
NAIL SCRUB WITH BRUSH (PEDINOL)

NALBUPHINE HYDROCHLORIDE

　Nalbuphine Hydrochloride Injection
　　(ASTRAZENECA LP)
　Nubain Injection (ENDO LABS)
NALBUPHINE HYDROCHLORIDE
　INJECTION (ABBOTT)
NALBUPHINE HYDROCHLORIDE
　INJECTION (ASTRAZENECA LP)
NALDECON SYRUP, TABLETS, PEDIATRIC
　DROPS, PEDIATRIC SYRUP AND LIQUI-
　GELS (APOTHECON)
NALEX A LIQUID (BLANSETT)
NALEX EXPECTORANT (BLANSETT)

NALEX DH LIQUID (BLANSETT)
NALEX-A LIQUID (BLANSETT)
NALEX-A TABLETS (BLANSETT)
NALFON CAPSULES (DISTA)

NALIDIXIC ACID

　NegGram Caplets (SANOFI)
　NegGram Suspension (SANOFI)

NALMEFENE HYDROCHLORIDE

　Revex Injection (BAXTER)
NALOXONE HCL INJECTION, USP (BAXTER)

NALOXONE HYDROCHLORIDE

　Naloxone HCl Injection, USP (BAXTER)
　Naloxone Hydrochloride Injection (ELKINS-SINN)
　Narcan Injection (ENDO LABS)
　Pentazocine and Naloxone HCl Tablets, USP
　　CIV (WATSON)
　Talwin Nx Tablets (SANOFI)
NALOXONE HYDROCHLORIDE
　INJECTION (ELKINS-SINN)

NALTREXONE HYDROCHLORIDE

　ReVia Tablets (DUPONT)

NANDROLONE DECANOATE

　Deca-Durabolin Injection (ORGANON)

NAPHAZOLINE HYDROCHLORIDE

　Naphcon-A Ophthalmic Solution (ALCON)
NAPHCON (ALCON P.R.)
NAPHCON-A OPHTHALMIC SOLUTION
　(ALCON)
NAPRELAN TABLETS (CARNRICK)
NAPROSYN SUSPENSION (ROCHE LABS)
NAPROSYN TABLETS (ROCHE LABS)

NAPROXEN

　EC-Naprosyn Delayed-Release Tablets
　　(ROCHE LABS)
　Naprosyn Suspension (ROCHE LABS)
　Naprosyn Tablets (ROCHE LABS)
　Naproxen Oral Suspension (ROXANE)
　Naproxen Tablets (MYLAN)
　Naproxen Tablets (GENEVA)
　Naproxen Tablets (WATSON)
　Naproxen Tablets (LEDERLE STANDARD)
　Naproxen Tablets, 250 mg (NOVOPHARM)
　Naprosyn Tablets, 375 mg (NOVOPHARM)
　Naproxen Tablets, 500 mg (NOVOPHARM)
NAPROXEN ORAL SUSPENSION (ROXANE)

NAPROXEN SODIUM

　Anaprox DS Tablets (ROCHE LABS)
　Anaprox Tablets (ROCHE LABS)
　Naprelan Tablets (CARNRICK)
　Naproxen Sodium Tablets (MYLAN)
　Naproxen Sodium Tablets (GENEVA)
　Naproxen Sodium Tablets (WATSON)
　Naproxen Sodium Tablets, 275 mg, 550 mg
　　(NOVOPHARM)
NAPROXEN SODIUM TABLETS (WATSON)
NAPROXEN SODIUM TABLETS, 275 MG,
　550 MG (NOVOPHARM)
NAPROXEN TABLETS (MYLAN)
NAPROXEN TABLETS (GENEVA)
NAPROXEN TABLETS (WATSON)
NAPROXEN TABLETS (LEDERLE STANDARD)
NAPROXEN SODIUM TABLETS (MYLAN)
NAPROXEN SODIUM TABLETS (GENEVA)
NAPROXEN TABLETS, 250 MG (NOVOPHARM)
NAPROXEN TABLETS, 375 MG (NOVOPHARM)
NAPROXEN TABLETS, 500 MG (NOVOPHARM)
NAPROXEN TABLETS, USP (SCHEIN)
NAQUA TABLETS (SCHERING)

NARATRIPTAN HYDROCHLORIDE

　Amerge Tablets (GLAXO WELLCOME)
NARCAN INJECTION (ENDO LABS)
NARDIL TABLETS (PARKE-DAVIS)

UNDERLINE DENOTES GENERIC NAME

NAROPIN INJECTION (ASTRAZENECA LP)
NASACORT AQ NASAL SPRAY
(RHONE-POULENC RORER)
NASACORT NASAL INHALER
(RHONE-POULENC RORER)
NASALIDE NASAL SPRAY (DURA)
NASAREL NASAL SOLUTION 0.025%
(DURA)
NASATAB LA TABLETS (ECR)
NASCOBAL GEL (SCHWARZ)
NASONEX NASAL SPRAY (SCHERING)
NATACYN OPHTHALMIC SUSPENSION
(ALCON)
NATAFORT TABLETS (WARNER CHILCOTT)
NATURETIN-5 TABLETS (APOTHECON)
NAVANE CAPSULES (PFIZER)
NAVANE CONCENTRATE (PFIZER)
NAVANE INTRAMUSCULAR (PFIZER)
NAVELBINE INJECTION (GLAXO WELLCOME)
NEBCIN VIALS, HYPORETS & ADD-
VANTAGE (LILLY)
NECON 0.5/35 TABLETS (WATSON)
NECON 1/35 TABLETS (WATSON)
NECON 1/50 TABLETS (WATSON)
NECON 10/11 TABLETS (WATSON)

NEDOCROMIL SODIUM

Tilade Inhaler (RHONE-POULENC RORER)

NEFAZODONE HYDROCHLORIDE

Serzone Tablets (BRISTOL-MYERS SQUIBB)
NEGGRAM CAPLETS (SANOFI)
NEGGRAM SUSPENSION (SANOFI)

NELFINAVIR MESYLATE

Viracept Oral Powder (AGOURON)
Viracept Tablets (AGOURON)
NEMBUTAL ELIXIR (ABBOTT)
NEMBUTAL SODIUM CAPSULES (ABBOTT)
NEMBUTAL SODIUM SOLUTION (ABBOTT)
NEMBUTAL SODIUM SUPPOSITORIES
(ABBOTT)
NEO-CALGLUCON SYRUP (NOVARTIS)
NEODECADRON STERILE OPHTHALMIC
OINTMENT (MERCK)
NEODECADRON STERILE OPHTHALMIC
SOLUTION (MERCK)

NEOMYCIN

Neosporin + Pain Relief Maximum Strength
Cream (WARNER-LAMBERT)
Neosporin + Pain Relief Maximum Strength
Ointment (WARNER-LAMBERT)
Neosporin Original Ointment
(WARNER-LAMBERT)

NEOMYCIN SULFATE

Cortisporin Cream (MONARCH)
Cortisporin Ointment (MONARCH)
Cortisporin Ophthalmic Ointment Sterile
(MONARCH)
Cortisporin Ophthalmic Suspension Sterile
(MONARCH)
Cortisporin Otic Solution Sterile (MONARCH)
Cortisporin Otic Suspension Sterile (MONARCH)
Cortisporin-TC Otic Suspension (MONARCH)
Lazersporin-C Solution (PEDINOL)
NeoDecadron Sterile Ophthalmic Ointment
(MERCK)
NeoDecadron Sterile Ophthalmic Solution
(MERCK)
Neosporin G.U. Irrigant Sterile (MONARCH)
Neosporin Ophthalmic Ointment Sterile
(MONARCH)
Neosporin Ophthalmic Solution Sterile
(MONARCH)
Pediotic Suspension Sterile (MONARCH)
NEOMYCIN SULFATE USP MICRONIZED
POWDER (PADDOCK)

NEORAL SOFT GELATIN CAPSULES FOR
MICROEMULSION (NOVARTIS)
NEORAL ORAL SOLUTION FOR
MICROEMULSION (NOVARTIS)
NEOSAR INJECTION (PHARMACIA & UPJOHN)
NEOSPORIN + PAIN RELIEF MAXIMUM
STRENGTH CREAM (WARNER-LAMBERT)
NEOSPORIN + PAIN RELIEF MAXIMUM
STRENGTH OINTMENT (WARNER-LAMBERT)
NEOSPORIN G.U. IRRIGANT STERILE
(MONARCH)
NEOSPORIN OPHTHALMIC OINTMENT
STERILE (MONARCH)
NEOSPORIN OPHTHALMIC SOLUTION
STERILE (MONARCH)
NEOSPORIN ORIGINAL OINTMENT
(WARNER-LAMBERT)

NEOSTIGMINE BROMIDE

Prostigmin Tablets (ICN)

NEOSTIGMINE METHYLSULFATE

Neostigmine Methylsulfate Injection
(ELKINS-SINN)
Neostigmine Methylsulfate Injection, USP
(BAXTER)
Prostigmin Injectable (ICN)
NEOSTIGMINE METHYLSULFATE
INJECTION (ELKINS-SINN)
NEOSTIGMINE METHYLSULFATE
INJECTION, USP (BAXTER)
NEO-SYNEPHRINE OPHTHALMIC
SOLUTION (SANOFI)
NEPHRAMINE INJECTION (R&D)
NEPHRO-CALCI TABLETS (R&D)
NEPHROCAPS (FLEMING)
NEPHRO-FER TABLETS (R&D)
NEPHRO-FER RX TABLETS (R&D)
NEPHRO-VITE TABLETS (R&D)
NEPHRO-VITE + FE TABLETS (R&D)
NEPHRO-VITE RX TABLETS (R&D)
NEPTAZANE TABLETS (LEDERLE LABS)
NESACAINE INJECTION (ASTRAZENECA LP)
NESACAINE-MPF INJECTION
(ASTRAZENECA LP)
NESTABS CBF TABLETS (FIELDING)
NESTABS FA (FIELDING)

NETILMICIN SULFATE

Netromycin Injection 100 mg/ml (SCHERING)
NETROMYCIN INJECTION 100 MG/ML
(SCHERING)
NEUMEGA FOR INJECTION (GENETICS)
NEUPOGEN FOR INJECTION (AMGEN)
NEURONTIN CAPSULES (PARKE-DAVIS)
NEUT ABBO-VIAL & PINTOP (ABBOTT)
NEUTREXIN FOR INJECTION
(U.S. BIOSCIENCE)
NEUTROGENA ANTISEPTIC (NEUTROGENA)
NEUTROGENA CLEANSING BAR FOR
ACNE-PRONE SKIN (NEUTROGENA)
NEUTROGENA CLEANSING BAR FOR
DRY SKIN (NEUTROGENA)
NEUTROGENA CLEANSING BAR FOR
DRY SKIN FRAGRANCE-FREE
(NEUTROGENA)
NEUTROGENA CLEANSING BAR FOR
OILY SKIN (NEUTROGENA)
NEUTROGENA CLEANSING BAR
ORIGINAL FORMULA (NEUTROGENA)
NEUTROGENA CLEANSING BAR
ORIGINAL FORMULA FRAGRANCE-
FREE (NEUTROGENA)
NEUTROGENA CLEANSING WASH
(NEUTROGENA)
NEUTROGENA COSMETICS (NEUTROGENA)
NEUTROGENA EXTRA GENTLE
CLEANSER (NEUTROGENA)

NEUTROGENA EXTRA GENTLE
CLEANSING BAR (NEUTROGENA)
NEUTROGENA HEALTHY SKIN ANTI-
WRINKLE CREAM WITH STABILIZED
RETINOL (NEUTROGENA)
NEUTROGENA HEALTHY SKIN FACE
LOTION WITH SPF 15 (NEUTROGENA)
NEUTROGENA LIP MOISTURIZER
(NEUTROGENA)
LIQUID NEUTROGENA (NEUTROGENA)
LIQUID NEUTROGENA, FRAGRANCE
FREE (NEUTROGENA)
NEUTROGENA MOISTURE (NEUTROGENA)
NEUTROGENA MOISTURE SPF 15
UNTINTED (NEUTROGENA)
NEUTROGENA MOISTURE SPF 15 WITH
SHEER TINT (NEUTROGENA)
NEUTROGENA NON-DRYING CLEANSER
(NEUTROGENA)
NEUTROGENA NORWEGIAN FORMULA
EMULSION (NEUTROGENA)
NEUTROGENA NORWEGIAN FORMULA
HAND CREAM (NEUTROGENA)
NEUTROGENA RAINBATH (NEUTROGENA)
NEUTROGENA SENSITIVE SKIN
SUNBLOCK SPF 17 (NEUTROGENA)
NEUTROGENA SHAMPOO (NEUTROGENA)
NEUTROGENA SUNBLOCK SPF 15
(NEUTROGENA)
NEUTROGENA SUNBLOCK SPF 30
(NEUTROGENA)
NEUTROGENA T/DERM TAR EMOLLIENT
(NEUTROGENA)
NEUTROGENA VEHICLE/N (NEUTROGENA)
NEUTROGENA VEHICLE/N MILD
(NEUTROGENA)

NEVIRAPINE

Viramune Oral Suspension (ROXANE)
Viramune Tablets (ROXANE)

NIACIN

GinkgoMist (MAYOR)
Niacor Tablets (UPSHER-SMITH)
Niaspan Extended-Release Tablets (KOS)
Slo-Niacin Tablets (UPSHER-SMITH)
Vitamist Intra-Oral Spray Dietary Supplements
(MAYOR)
NIACIN TABLETS USP (APOTHECON)

NIACINAMIDE

Mega-B Tablets (ARCO)
NIACOR TABLETS (UPSHER-SMITH)
NIASPAN EXTENDED-RELEASE TABLETS
(KOS)

NICARDIPINE

Nicardipine Capsules (PAR)
NICARDIPINE CAPSULES (PAR)

NICARDIPINE HYDROCHLORIDE

Cardene I.V. (WYETH-AYERST)
Nicardipine Hydrochloride Capsules (MYLAN)
NICARDIPINE HYDROCHLORIDE
CAPSULES (MYLAN)
NICODERM CQ PATCH
(SMITHKLINE BEECHAM CONSUMER)
NICORETTE GUM
(SMITHKLINE BEECHAM CONSUMER)

NICOTINE

Habitrol Transdermal System
(NOVARTIS CONSUMER)
Nicoderm CQ Patch
(SMITHKLINE BEECHAM CONSUMER)
Nicotine Patch (PAR)
Nicotrol Inhaler (MCNEIL CONSUMER)
Nicotrol Nasal Spray (MCNEIL CONSUMER)
Nicotrol Patch (MCNEIL CONSUMER)

UNDERLINE DENOTES GENERIC NAME

NICOTINE PATCH (PAR)

NICOTINE POLACRILEX

Nicorette Gum
(SMITHKLINE BEECHAM CONSUMER)

NICOTINE TRANSDERMAL SYSTEM, USP
(SCHEIN)

NICOTINEX ELIXIR (FLEMING)

NICOTROL INHALER (MCNEIL CONSUMER)

NICOTROL NASAL SPRAY
(MCNEIL CONSUMER)

NICOTROL PATCH (MCNEIL CONSUMER)

NIFEDIPINE

Adalat CC Tablets (BAYER)
Adalat Capsules (BAYER)
Nifedipine Capsules, 10 mg (NOVOPHARM)
Procardia Capsules (PFIZER)
Procardia XL Extended Release Tablets
(PFIZER)

NIFEDIPINE CAPSULES, 10 MG
(NOVOPHARM)

NIFEREX ELIXIR (SCHWARZ)

NIFEREX TABLETS (SCHWARZ)

NIFEREX-150 CAPSULES (SCHWARZ)

NIFEREX-150 FORTE CAPSULES (SCHWARZ)

NIFEREX-PN TABLETS (SCHWARZ)

NIFEREX-PN FORTE TABLETS (SCHWARZ)

NILANDRON TABLETS
(HOECHST MARION ROUSSEL)

NILUTAMIDE

Nilandron Tablets (HOECHST MARION ROUSSEL)

NIMBEX INJECTION (GLAXO WELLCOME)

NIMODIPINE

Nimotop Capsules (BAYER)

NIMOTOP CAPSULES (BAYER)

NIPENT FOR INJECTION (SUPERGEN)

NISOLDIPINE

Sular Tablets (ASTRAZENECA)

NITE-CAL CALCIUM (MDR FITNESS)

NITRAZINE PAPER (APOTHECON)

NITRO-BID IV (HOECHST MARION ROUSSEL)

NITRO-BID OINTMENT
(HOECHST MARION ROUSSEL)

NITRODISC (ROBERTS)

**NITRO-DUR TRANSDERMAL INFUSION
SYSTEM** (KEY)

NITROFURANTOIN

Furadantin Oral Suspension (DURA)
Macrodantin Capsules
(PROCTER & GAMBLE PHARMACEUTICALS)
Nitrofurantoin Capsules (MYLAN)

NITROFURANTOIN CAPSULES (MYLAN)

NITROFURANTOIN MONOHYDRATE

Macrobid Capsules
(PROCTER & GAMBLE PHARMACEUTICALS)

NITROGARD TABLETS (FOREST)

NITROGLYCERIN

Deponit Transdermal Delivery System
(SCHWARZ)
Minitran Transdermal Delivery System (3M)
Nitro-Dur Transdermal Infusion System (KEY)
Nitroglycerin Transdermal System (MYLAN)
Nitrol Ointment (SAVAGE)
Nitrolingual Spray (RHONE-POULENC RORER)
Nitrostat Tablets (PARKE-DAVIS)

**NITROGLYCERIN TRANSDERMAL
SYSTEM** (MYLAN)

NITROL OINTMENT (SAVAGE)

NITROLINGUAL SPRAY
(RHONE-POULENC RORER)

NITROPRESS (ABBOTT)

NITROSTAT TABLETS (PARKE-DAVIS)

NIX CREME RINSE (WARNER-LAMBERT)

NIZATIDINE

Axid Pulvules (LILLY)

NIZORAL 2% CREAM (MCNEIL CONSUMER)

NIZORAL 2% SHAMPOO (MCNEIL CONSUMER)

NIZORAL A-D SHAMPOO (MCNEIL CONSUMER)

NIZORAL TABLETS (JANSSEN)

NO DOZ MAXIMUM STRENGTH
(BRISTOL-MYERS)

NOLAHIST TABLETS (CARNRICK)

NOLAMINE TIMED-RELEASE TABLETS
(CARNRICK)

NOLVADEX TABLETS (ASTRAZENECA)

NORCO TABLETS CIII (WATSON)

NORCURON FOR INJECTION (ORGANON)

NORDETTE-21 TABLETS (WYETH-AYERST)

NORDETTE-28 TABLETS (WYETH-AYERST)

NORDITROPIN FOR INJECTION
(NOVO NORDISK)

NOREL DM LIQUID (U.S. PHARMACEUTICAL)

NOREL PLUS CAPSULES
(U.S. PHARMACEUTICAL)

NORETHINDRONE

Brevicon-21 Tablets (SEARLE)
Brevicon-28 Tablets (SEARLE)
Micronor Tablets (ORTHO-MCNEIL)
Modicon 21 Tablets (ORTHO-MCNEIL)
Modicon 28 Tablets (ORTHO-MCNEIL)
Necon 0.5/35 Tablets (WATSON)
Necon 1/35 Tablets (WATSON)
Necon 1/50 Tablets (WATSON)
Necon 10/11 Tablets (WATSON)
Nor-QD Tablets (WATSON)
Norethindrone and Ethinyl Estradiol Tablets,
USP (NECON) (WATSON)
Norethindrone and Mestranol Tablets, USP
(NECON) (WATSON)
Norinyl 1 + 35-21 Tablets (SEARLE)
Norinyl 1 + 35-28 Tablets (SEARLE)
Norinyl 1 + 50-21 Tablets (SEARLE)
Norinyl 1 + 50-28 Tablets (SEARLE)
Ortho-Novum 1/35 21 Tablets (ORTHO-MCNEIL)
Ortho-Novum 1/35 28 Tablets (ORTHO-MCNEIL)
Ortho-Novum 1/50 28 Tablets (ORTHO-MCNEIL)
Ortho-Novum 10/11 21 Tablets
(ORTHO-MCNEIL)
Ortho-Novum 10/11 28 Tablets
(ORTHO-MCNEIL)
Ortho-Novum 7/7/7 21 Tablets (ORTHO-MCNEIL)
Ortho-Novum 7/7/7 28 Tablets (ORTHO-MCNEIL)
Ovcon 35 Tablets (BRISTOL-MYERS SQUIBB)
Ovcon 50 Tablets (BRISTOL-MYERS SQUIBB)
Tri-Norinyl 21 Tablets (SEARLE)
Tri-Norinyl 28 Tablets (SEARLE)

NORETHINDRONE ACETATE

Aygestin Tablets (ESI LEDERLE)
CombiPatch Transdermal System
(RHONE-POULENC RORER)
Estrostep 21 Tablets (PARKE-DAVIS)
Estrostep Fe Tablets (PARKE-DAVIS)
Loestrin 21 Tablets (PARKE-DAVIS)
Loestrin Fe Tablets (PARKE-DAVIS)

**NORETHINDRONE AND ETHINYL
ESTRADIOL TABLETS, USP (NECON)**
(WATSON)

**NORETHINDRONE AND MESTRANOL
TABLETS, USP (NECON)** (WATSON)

NORFLEX EXTENDED-RELEASE TABLETS
(3M)

NORFLEX INJECTION (3M)

NORFLOXACIN

Chibroxin Sterile Ophthalmic Solution (MERCK)
Noroxin Tablets (MERCK)
Noroxin Tablets (ROBERTS)

NORGESIC TABLETS (3M)

NORGESIC FORTE TABLETS (3M)

NORGESTIMATE

Ortho Tri-Cyclen 21 Tablets (ORTHO-MCNEIL)
Ortho Tri-Cyclen 28 Tablets (ORTHO-MCNEIL)
Ortho-Cyclen 21 Tablets (ORTHO-MCNEIL)
Ortho-Cyclen 28 Tablets (ORTHO-MCNEIL)

NORGESTREL

Lo/Ovral Tablets (WYETH-AYERST)
Lo/Ovral-28 Tablets (WYETH-AYERST)
Ovral Tablets (WYETH-AYERST)
Ovral-28 Tablets (WYETH-AYERST)
Ovrette Tablets (WYETH-AYERST)

NORINYL 1 + 35-21 TABLETS (SEARLE)

NORINYL 1 + 35-28 TABLETS (SEARLE)

NORINYL 1 + 50-21 TABLETS (SEARLE)

NORINYL 1 + 50-28 TABLETS (SEARLE)

NORINYL TABLETS (WATSON)

NORITATE CREAM (DERMIK)

NORMIFLO INJECTION (WYETH-AYERST)

NORMIFLO INJECTION IN TUBEX
(WYETH-AYERST)

NORMODYNE INJECTION (SCHERING)

NORMODYNE TABLETS (SCHERING)

**NORMOSOL-M & 5% DEXTROSE
INJECTION** (ABBOTT)

NORMOSOL-R (ABBOTT)

**NORMOSOL-R & 5% DEXTROSE
INJECTION** (ABBOTT)

NORMOSOL-R PH 7.4 (ABBOTT)

NOROXIN TABLETS (MERCK)

NOROXIN TABLETS (ROBERTS)

NORPACE CAPSULES (SEARLE)

NORPACE CR CAPSULES (SEARLE)

NORPLANT SYSTEM (WYETH-AYERST)

NORPRAMIN TABLETS
(HOECHST MARION ROUSSEL)

NOR-QD TABLETS (WATSON)

NORTRIPTYLINE HCL CAPSULES (GENEVA)

NORTRIPTYLINE HCL CAPSULES, USP
(SCHEIN)

NORTRIPTYLINE HYDROCHLORIDE

Nortriptyline HCl Capsules (GENEVA)
Nortriptyline Hydrochloride Capsules (MYLAN)

**NORTRIPTYLINE HYDROCHLORIDE
CAPSULES** (MYLAN)

NORVASC TABLETS (PFIZER)

NORVIR CAPSULES (ABBOTT)

NORVIR ORAL SOLUTION (ABBOTT)

NOVACET LOTION (MEDICIS)

NOVAFED A CAPSULES
(HOECHST MARION ROUSSEL)

NOVANTRONE FOR INJECTION (IMMUNEX)

NOVAREL FOR INJECTION (FERRING)

NOVOFINE 30 DISPOSABLE NEEDLE
(NOVO NORDISK)

**NOVOLIN 70/30 HUMAN INSULIN 10 ML
VIALS** (NOVO NORDISK)

**NOVOLIN 70/30 PENFILL 1.5 ML
CARTRIDGES** (NOVO NORDISK)

**NOVOLIN 70/30 PREFILLED DISPOSABLE
INSULIN DELIVERY SYSTEM**
(NOVO NORDISK)

**NOVOLIN 70/30 PENFILL 3 ML
CARTRIDGES** (NOVO NORDISK)

**NOVOLIN L HUMAN INSULIN 10 ML
VIALS** (NOVO NORDISK)

**NOVOLIN N HUMAN INSULIN 10 ML
VIALS** (NOVO NORDISK)

**NOVOLIN N PENFILL 1.5 ML
CARTRIDGES** (NOVO NORDISK)

NOVOLIN N PENFILL 3 ML CARTRIDGES
(NOVO NORDISK)

**NOVOLIN N PREFILLED SYRINGE
DISPOSABLE INSULIN DELIVERY
SYSTEM** (NOVO NORDISK)

UNDERLINE DENOTES GENERIC NAME

NOVOLIN R HUMAN INSULIN 10 ML VIALS (NOVO NORDISK)
NOVOLIN R PENFILL 3 ML CARTRIDGES (NOVO NORDISK)
NOVOLIN R PENFILL 1.5 ML CARTRIDGES (NOVO NORDISK)
NOVOLIN R PREFILLED SYRINGE DISPOSABLE INSULIN DELIVERY SYSTEM (NOVO NORDISK)
NOVOPEN 1.5 INSULIN DELIVERY DEVICE (NOVO NORDISK)
NOVOPEN 3 INSULIN DELIVERY DEVICE (NOVO NORDISK)
NOVOSEVEN (NOVO NORDISK)
NUBAIN INJECTION (ENDO LABS)
NUCOFED CAPSULES (MONARCH)
NUCOFED CAPSULES AND SYRUP CIII (MONARCH)
NUCOFED EXPECTORANT SYRUP CIII (MONARCH)
NUCOFED PEDIATRIC EXPECTORANT SYRUP CV (MONARCH)
NUCOFED PEDIATRIC EXPECTORANT SYRUP (MONARCH)
NU-IRON 150 CAPSULES (MERZ)
NU-IRON ELIXIR (MERZ)
NU-IRON PLUS ELIXIR (MERZ)
NU-IRON V TABLETS (MERZ)
NULYTELY, CHERRY FLAVOR NULYTELY AND LEMON-LIME FLAVOR NULYTELY FOR ORAL SOLUTION (BRAINTREE)
NUMORPHAN INJECTION (ENDO LABS)
NUMORPHAN SUPPOSITORIES (ENDO LABS)
NUPERCAINAL HC 1% (NOVARTIS CONSUMER)
NUPERCAINAL HEMORRHOIDAL AND ANESTHETIC OINTMENT (NOVARTIS CONSUMER)
NUPERCAINAL SUPPOSITORIES (NOVARTIS CONSUMER)
NUPRIN (BRISTOL-MYERS)
NUPRIN BACKACHE (BRISTOL-MYERS)
NUROMAX INJECTION (GLAXO WELLCOME)
NUTRACORT LOTION (HEALTHPOINT)
NUTR-E-SOL LIQUID (ADVANCED NUTRITIONAL)
NUTRISION CAPSULES (WESTLAKE)
NUTRISURE OTC TABLETS (WESTLAKE)
NUTROPIN AQ INJECTION (GENENTECH)
NUTROPIN FOR INJECTION (GENENTECH)
NYDRAZID INJECTION (APOTHECON)
NYSTATIN
  Mycostatin Pastilles (BRISTOL-MYERSSQUIBBONCOLOGY/IMMUNOLOGY)
  Mytrex Cream (SAVAGE)
  Mytrex Ointment (SAVAGE)
  Nystatin Oral Suspension, Powder (LEDERLE STANDARD)
  Nystop Topical Powder USP (PADDOCK)
  Paddock Nystatin USP for Extemporaneous Preparation of Oral Suspension (PADDOCK)
  Pedi-Dri Topical Powder (PEDINOL)
NYSTATIN ORAL SUSPENSION, POWDER (LEDERLE STANDARD)
PADDOCK NYSTATIN USP FOR EXTEMPORANEOUS PREPARATION OF ORAL SUSPENSION (PADDOCK)
NYSTOP TOPICAL POWDER USP (PADDOCK)

O

OBEGYN (FLEMING)

OCEAN (NASAL MIST) (FLEMING)
OCEANS-12 (FLEMING)

OCTOCRYLENE
  Solbar PF Cream SPF 50 (PABA Free) (PERSON & COVEY)
  Solbar PF Liquid SPF 30 (PERSON & COVEY)

OCTREOTIDE ACETATE
  Sandostatin LAR Depot (NOVARTIS)

OCTYL METHOXYCINNAMATE
  Eucerin Plus Renewal Alpha Hydroxy SPF 15 (BEIERSDORF)
  Eucerin Protective Moisture Lotion SPF 25 (BEIERSDORF)
  Lubriderm Daily UV Lotion with Sunscreen (WARNER-LAMBERT)
  Solbar AVO Lotion SPF 32 (PERSON & COVEY)
  Solbar PF Cream SPF 50 (PABA Free) (PERSON & COVEY)
  Solbar PF Liquid SPF 30 (PERSON & COVEY)

OCTYL SALICYLATE
  Eucerin Plus Renewal Alpha Hydroxy SPF 15 (BEIERSDORF)
  Eucerin Protective Moisture Lotion SPF 25 (BEIERSDORF)
  Lubriderm Daily UV Lotion with Sunscreen (WARNER-LAMBERT)
OCUCEL LINT-FREE SURGICAL PRODUCTS (ALCON)
OCUFEN OPHTHALMIC SOLUTION (ALLERGAN)
OCUFLOX OPHTHALMIC SOLUTION (ALLERGAN)

OFLOXACIN
  Floxin I.V. (ORTHO-MCNEIL)
  Floxin Otic Solution (DAIICHI)
  Floxin Tablets (ORTHO-MCNEIL)
  Ocuflox Ophthalmic Solution (ALLERGAN)
OGEN TABLETS (PHARMACIA & UPJOHN)
OIL OF OLAY COMPLETE UV PROTECTIVE MOISTURE CREAM SPF 15 - REGULAR AND FRAGRANCE FREE (PROCTER & GAMBLE)
OIL OF OLAY COMPLETE UV PROTECTIVE MOISTURE LOTION SPF 15 - REGULAR AND FRAGRANCE FREE (PROCTER & GAMBLE)
OILATUM-AD SOAP FREE CLEANSER (STIEFEL)
OILATUM CLEANSING BAR (SCENTED) (STIEFEL)
OILATUM CLEANSING BAR (UNSCENTED) (STIEFEL)
OIL-FREE ACNE WASH (NEUTROGENA)

OLANZAPINE
  Zyprexa Tablets (LILLY)

OLOPATADINE HYDROCHLORIDE
  Patanol Ophthalmic Solution (ALCON)

OLSALAZINE SODIUM
  Dipentum Capsules (PHARMACIA & UPJOHN)

OMEPRAZOLE
  Prilosec Delayed-Release Capsules (ASTRAZENECA LP)
OMNICEF CAPSULES (PARKE-DAVIS)
OMNICEF FOR ORAL SUSPENSION (PARKE-DAVIS)
OMNIHIB (SMITHKLINE BEECHAM)
OMNIHIST L.A. TABLETS (WE)
ONCASPAR (RHONE-POULENC RORER)
ONCOVIN SOLUTION VIALS (LILLY)

ONDANSETRON
  Zofran ODT Orally Disintegrating Tablets (GLAXO WELLCOME)

ONDANSETRON HYDROCHLORIDE
  Zofran Injection (GLAXO WELLCOME)
  Zofran Injection Premixed (GLAXO WELLCOME)
  Zofran Oral Solution (GLAXO WELLCOME)
  Zofran Tablets (GLAXO WELLCOME)
ONTAK VIALS (LIGAND)
ON-THE-SPOT ACNE TREATMENT (NEUTROGENA)
ONY-CLEAR SOLUTION (PEDINOL)
OPHTHETIC OPHTHALMIC SOLUTION (ALLERGAN)
OPIUM & BELLADONNA RECTAL SUPPOSITORIES (WYETH-AYERST)

OPIUM ALKALOIDS
  B & O Supprettes No. 15A & No. 16A (POLYMEDICA)
OPIUM TINCTURE, USP (LILLY)

OPRELVEKIN
  Neumega for Injection (GENETICS)
OPTEMP STERILE DISPOSABLE CAUTERY (ALCON)
OPTICROM OPHTHALMIC SOLUTION (ALLERGAN)
OPTILETS-500 FILMTAB (ABBOTT)
OPTILETS-M-500 FILMTAB (ABBOTT)
OPTIMINE TABLETS (SCHERING)
ORAMORPH SR TABLETS (ROXANE)
ORAP TABLETS (GATE)
ORA-PLUS (PADDOCK)
ORA-SWEET (PADDOCK)
ORA-SWEET SF (PADDOCK)
ORETON METHYL BUCCAL TABLETS (SCHERING)
ORETON METHYL TABLETS (SCHERING)
ORGANIDIN NR LIQUID (WALLACE)
ORGANIDIN NR TABLETS (WALLACE)
ORGARAN INJECTION (ORGANON)
ORINASE TABLETS (PHARMACIA & UPJOHN)
ORLAAM ORAL SOLUTION (ROXANE)

ORLISTAT
  Xenical Capsules (ROCHE LABS)
ORNADE SPANSULE CAPSULES (SMITHKLINE BEECHAM)

ORPHENADRINE CITRATE
  Norflex Extended-Release Tablets (3M)
  Norflex Injection (3M)
  Norgesic Forte Tablets (3M)
  Norgesic Tablets (3M)
  Orphenadrine Citrate Extended-release Tablets (MYLAN)
  Orphenadrine Citrate, Aspirin and Caffeine Tablets (MYLAN)
  Orphengesic Forte Tablets (PAR)
  Orphengesic Tablets (PAR)
ORPHENADRINE CITRATE ER TABLETS (SCHEIN)
ORPHENADRINE CITRATE EXTENDED-RELEASE TABLETS (MYLAN)
ORPHENADRINE CITRATE, ASPIRIN AND CAFFEINE TABLETS (MYLAN)
ORPHENGESIC TABLETS (PAR)
ORPHENGESIC FORTE TABLETS (PAR)
ORTHO COIL SPRING DIAPHRAGM (SEE ORTHO DIAPHRAGM KITS) (ORTHO-MCNEIL)
ORTHO DIAPHRAGM KITS – ALL-FLEX ARCING SPRING; ORTHO COIL SPRING (ORTHO-MCNEIL)
ORTHO DIENESTROL CREAM (ORTHO-MCNEIL)

ORTHO TRI-CYCLEN 21 TABLETS
(ORTHO-MCNEIL)
ORTHO TRI-CYCLEN 28 TABLETS
(ORTHO-MCNEIL)
ORTHO-CEPT 21 TABLETS (ORTHO-MCNEIL)
ORTHO-CEPT 28 TABLETS (ORTHO-MCNEIL)
ORTHOCLONE OKT3 STERILE SOLUTION
(ORTHO BIOTECH)
ORTHO-CYCLEN 21 TABLETS
(ORTHO-MCNEIL)
ORTHO-CYCLEN 28 TABLETS
(ORTHO-MCNEIL)
ORTHO-EST TABLETS (WOMEN FIRST)
ORTHO-NOVUM 1/35 21 TABLETS
(ORTHO-MCNEIL)
ORTHO-NOVUM 1/35 28 TABLETS
(ORTHO-MCNEIL)
ORTHO-NOVUM 1/50 28 TABLETS
(ORTHO-MCNEIL)
ORTHO-NOVUM 7/7/7 21 TABLETS
(ORTHO-MCNEIL)
ORTHO-NOVUM 7/7/7 28 TABLETS
(ORTHO-MCNEIL)
ORTHO-NOVUM 10/11 21 TABLETS
(ORTHO-MCNEIL)
ORTHO-NOVUM 10/11 28 TABLETS
(ORTHO-MCNEIL)
ORUDIS CAPSULES (WYETH-AYERST)
ORUDIS CAPSULES, 75 MG (WYETH-AYERST)
ORUVAIL CAPSULES (WYETH-AYERST)
**OS-CAL 250 + D, 500, 500 + D, AND 500
CHEWABLE TABLETS**
(SMITHKLINE BEECHAM CONSUMER)
OSMOGLYN ORAL OSMOTIC AGENT
(ALCON)
OSTEO I.P. (NUTRACEUTICS)
OSTEO-CALMAG (MAYOR)
OSTEOMAX (NUTRACEUTICS)
OSTIDERM (PEDINOL)
OSTIDERM ROLL-ON (PEDINOL)
OTIC DOMEBORO SOLUTION (BAYER)
OTOBIOTIC OTIC SOLUTION (SCHERING)
OTRIVIN NASAL DROPS
(NOVARTIS CONSUMER)
OTRIVIN PEDIATRIC NASAL DROPS
(NOVARTIS CONSUMER)
OTRIVIN NASAL SPRAY
(NOVARTIS CONSUMER)
**OVCON (SEE BRISTOL-MYERS SQUIBB
COMPANY)** (APOTHECON)
OVCON 35 TABLETS (BRISTOL-MYERS SQUIBB)
OVCON 50 TABLETS (BRISTOL-MYERS SQUIBB)
OVIDE LOTION (MEDICIS)
OVRAL TABLETS (WYETH-AYERST)
OVRAL-28 TABLETS (WYETH-AYERST)
OVRETTE TABLETS (WYETH-AYERST)
OX-ABSORB (VITALINE)
**OXACILLIN CAPSULES USP AND FOR
ORAL SOLUTION** (APOTHECON)
**OXACILLIN FOR INJECTION USP AND IN
ADD-VANTAGE VIALS** (APOTHECON)
OXANDRIN TABLETS (BTG)

OXANDROLONE
  Oxandrin Tablets (BTG)

OXAPROZIN
  Daypro Caplets (SEARLE)

OXAZEPAM
  Oxazepam Capsules (GENEVA)
OXAZEPAM CAPSULES (GENEVA)
OXAZEPAM CAPSULES (ESI LEDERLE)

OXICONAZOLE NITRATE
  Oxistat Cream (GLAXO WELLCOME)
  Oxistat Lotion (GLAXO WELLCOME)
OXISTAT CREAM (GLAXO WELLCOME)

OXISTAT LOTION (GLAXO WELLCOME)
OXSORALEN LOTION 1% (ICN)
OXSORALEN-ULTRA CAPSULES (ICN)

OXTRIPHYLLINE
  Choledyl SA Extended-Release Tablets
  (WARNER CHILCOTT)

OXYBENZONE
  Eucerin Plus Renewal Alpha Hydroxy SPF 15
  (BEIERSDORF)
  Lubriderm Daily UV Lotion with Sunscreen
  (WARNER-LAMBERT)
  Solaquin Forte 4% Cream (ICN)
  Solbar AVO Lotion SPF 32 (PERSON & COVEY)
  Solbar PF Cream SPF 50 (PABA Free)
  (PERSON & COVEY)
  Solbar PF Liquid SPF 30 (PERSON & COVEY)

OXYBUTYNIN CHLORIDE
  Ditropan Tablets and Syrup (ALZA)
  Ditropan XL Extended Release Tablets (ALZA)
  Oxybutynin Chloride Syrup USP
  (PHARMACEUTICAL ASSOCIATES)
  Oxybutynin Chloride Tablets (WATSON)
OXYBUTYNIN CHLORIDE SYRUP USP
(PHARMACEUTICAL ASSOCIATES)
OXYBUTYNIN CHLORIDE TABLETS
(WATSON)
**OXYCODONE AND ACETAMINOPHEN
CAPSULES, USP CII** (WATSON)
**OXYCODONE AND ACETAMINOPHEN
CAPSULES, USP** (MALLINCKRODT)
**OXYCODONE AND ACETAMINOPHEN
TABLETS, USP CII** (WATSON)
**OXYCODONE AND ACETAMINOPHEN
TABLETS, USP** (MALLINCKRODT)
OXYCODONE & APAP CAPSULES
(DURAMED)
**OXYCODONE AND ASPIRIN TABLETS,
USP CII** (WATSON)

OXYCODONE HYDROCHLORIDE
  Endocet Tablets, USP CII (ENDO GENERICS)
  Endodan Tablets, USP CII (ENDO GENERICS)
  OxyContin Tablets (PURDUE PHARMA)
  OxyFast Oral Concentrate Solution
  (PURDUE PHARMA)
  OxyIR Capsules (PURDUE PHARMA)
  Oxycodone Hydrochloride Tablets, USP CII
  (WATSON)
  Oxycodone and Acetaminophen Capsules, USP
  (MALLINCKRODT)
  Oxycodone and Acetaminophen Capsules, USP
  CII (WATSON)
  Oxycodone and Acetaminophen Tablets, USP
  (MALLINCKRODT)
  Oxycodone and Acetaminophen Tablets, USP
  CII (WATSON)
  Oxycodone and Aspirin Tablets, USP CII
  (WATSON)
  Percocet Tablets (ENDO LABS)
  Percodan Tablets (ENDO LABS)
  Percodan-Demi Tablets (ENDO LABS)
  Percolone Tablets (ENDO LABS)
  Roxicodone Tablets, Oral Solution & Intensol
  (ROXANE)
  Roxilox Capsules (ROXANE)
  Roxiprin Tablets (ROXANE)
  Tylox Capsules (ORTHO-MCNEIL)
**OXYCODONE HYDROCHLORIDE
TABLETS, USP CII** (WATSON)

OXYCODONE TEREPHTHALATE
  Endodan Tablets, USP CII (ENDO GENERICS)
  Percodan Tablets (ENDO LABS)
  Percodan-Demi Tablets (ENDO LABS)
  Roxiprin Tablets (ROXANE)
OXYCONTIN TABLETS (PURDUE PHARMA)

**OXYFAST ORAL CONCENTRATE
SOLUTION** (PURDUE PHARMA)
OXYIR CAPSULES (PURDUE PHARMA)

OXYMETHOLONE
  Anadrol-50 Tablets (UNIMED)

OXYMORPHONE HYDROCHLORIDE
  Numorphan Injection (ENDO LABS)
  Numorphan Suppositories (ENDO LABS)

OXYQUINOLINE SULFATE
  Aci-Jel Therapeutic Vaginal Jelly
  (ORTHO-MCNEIL)

OXYTETRACYCLINE
  Terramycin Intramuscular Solution (PFIZER)

OXYTETRACYCLINE HYDROCHLORIDE
  Terra-Cortril Ophthalmic Suspension (PFIZER)
  Terramycin with Polymyxin B Sulfate
  Ophthalmic Ointment (PFIZER)
  Urobiotic-250 Capsules (PFIZER)

P

PACAPS CAPSULES (LUNSCO)
PACERONE TABLETS (UPSHER-SMITH)

PACLITAXEL
  Taxol Injection
  (BRISTOL-MYERSSQUIBBONCOLOGY/IMMUNOLOGY)

PADIMATE O (OCTYL DIMETHYL PABA)
  Solaquin Forte 4% Cream (ICN)
  Solaquin Forte 4% Gel (ICN)

PALIVIZUMAB
  Synagis Intramuscular (MEDIMMUNE)
PALS INTERNAL DEODORANT (GLENWOOD)

PAMABROM
  ViTelle Lurline PMS Tablets (FIELDING)
PAMELOR CAPSULES (NOVARTIS)

PAMIDRONATE DISODIUM
  Aredia for Injection (NOVARTIS)
PANAFIL OINTMENT (HEALTHPOINT)
PANALGESIC GOLD CREAM (ECR)
PANALGESIC GOLD TOPICAL LIQUID
(ECR)
PANCREASE CAPSULES (ORTHO-MCNEIL)
PANCREASE MT CAPSULES (ORTHO-MCNEIL)

PANCREATIN
  Donnazyme Tablets (ROBINS)
PANCREATIN 4X 600MG (VITALINE)
PANCREATIN 8X 900MG (VITALINE)

PANCRELIPASE
  Cotazym Capsules (ORGANON)
  Cotazym-S Capsules (ORGANON)
  Creon 10 Capsules (SOLVAY)
  Creon 20 Capsules (SOLVAY)
  Creon 5 Capsules (SOLVAY)
  Ku-Zyme HP Capsules (SCHWARZ)
  Pancrease Capsules (ORTHO-MCNEIL)
  Pancrease MT Capsules (ORTHO-MCNEIL)
  Ultrase Capsules (SCANDIPHARM)
  Ultrase MT Capsules (SCANDIPHARM)
  Viokase Powder (AXCAN)
  Viokase Tablets (AXCAN)
  Zymase Capsules (ORGANON)
**PANCREZYME 4X (VEGETARIAN
PANCREATIN)** (VITALINE)

UNDERLINE DENOTES GENERIC NAME

PANCURONIUM BROMIDE
Pancuronium Bromide Injection (BAXTER)
Pancuronium Bromide Injection (ELKINS-SINN)
Pavulon Injection (ORGANON)
PANCURONIUM BROMIDE INJECTION (BAXTER)
PANCURONIUM BROMIDE INJECTION (ELKINS-SINN)
PANDEL CREAM (SAVAGE)
PANGLOBULIN (AMERICAN RED CROSS)
PANHEMATIN FOR INJECTION (ABBOTT)
PANMYCIN CAPSULES (PHARMACIA & UPJOHN)
PANOXYL 5 ACNE GEL (STIEFEL)
PANOXYL 10 ACNE GEL (STIEFEL)
PANOXYL AQ 2 1/2 ACNE GEL (STIEFEL)
PANOXYL AQ 5 ACNE GEL (STIEFEL)
PANOXYL AQ 10 ACNE GEL (STIEFEL)
PANOXYL BAR 5 (STIEFEL)
PANOXYL BAR 10 (STIEFEL)
PANRETIN GEL (LIGAND)
PANTETHINE CAPSULES (WESTLAKE)
PANTOTHENIC ACID 500MG (VITALINE)
PAPAIN
Accuzyme Debriding Ointment (HEALTHPOINT)
Panafil Ointment (HEALTHPOINT)
PAPAVERINE HYDROCHLORIDE INJECTION, USP (BEDFORD)
PARA-AMINOBENZOIC ACID
Mega-B Tablets (ARCO)
PARAFON FORTE DSC CAPLETS (ORTHO-MCNEIL)
PARAGARD T 380A INTRAUTERINE COPPER CONTRACEPTIVE (ORTHO-MCNEIL)
PARAPLATIN FOR INJECTION (BRISTOL-MYERSSQUIBBONCOLOGY/IMMUNOLOGY)
PARCODE PRODUCT LIST (PARKE-DAVIS)
PARICALCITOL
Zemplar Injection (ABBOTT)
PARLODEL CAPSULES (NOVARTIS)
PARLODEL SNAPTABS (NOVARTIS)
PARNATE TABLETS (SMITHKLINE BEECHAM)
PAROXETINE HYDROCHLORIDE
Paxil Oral Suspension (SMITHKLINE BEECHAM)
Paxil Tablets (SMITHKLINE BEECHAM)
PASER GRANULES (JACOBUS)
PATANOL OPHTHALMIC SOLUTION (ALCON)
PAVULON INJECTION (ORGANON)
PAXIL ORAL SUSPENSION (SMITHKLINE BEECHAM)
PAXIL TABLETS (SMITHKLINE BEECHAM)
PAXIPAM TABLETS (SCHERING)
PAZO HEMORRHOID OINTMENT (BRISTOL-MYERS)
PBZ TABLETS (NOVARTIS)
PBZ-SR TABLETS (NOVARTIS)
PCE DISPERTAB TABLETS (ABBOTT)
PECTIN
Kaolin-Pectin Suspension (ROXANE)
PEDAMETH CAPSULES (FOREST)
PEDAMETH LIQUID (FOREST)
PEDIACOF SYRUP (SANOFI)
PEDIAFLOR DROPS (ROSS)
PEDIALYTE ORAL ELECTROLYTE MAINTENANCE SOLUTION (ROSS)
PEDIAPRED ORAL SOLUTION (MEDEVA)
PEDIASURE COMPLETE LIQUID NUTRITION (ROSS)
PEDIAZOLE SUSPENSION (ROSS)
PEDI-BORO SOAK PAKS (PEDINOL)
PEDI-DRI TOPICAL POWDER (PEDINOL)
PEDIOTIC SUSPENSION STERILE (MONARCH)

PEDI-PRO FOOT POWDER (PEDINOL)
LIQUID PEDVAXHIB (MERCK)
PEGADEMASE BOVINE
Adagen Injection (ENZON)
PEGASPARGASE
Oncaspar (RHONE-POULENC RORER)
PEMOLINE
Cylert Chewable Tablets (ABBOTT)
Cylert Tablets (ABBOTT)
PENBUTOLOL SULFATE
Levatol Tablets (SCHWARZ)
PENCICLOVIR
Denavir Cream (SMITHKLINE BEECHAM CONSUMER)
PENECORT CREAM (ALLERGAN)
PENECORT TOPICAL SOLUTION (ALLERGAN)
PENETREX TABLETS (RHONE-POULENC RORER)
PENICILLAMINE
Cuprimine Capsules (MERCK)
Depen Titratable Tablets (WALLACE)
PENICILLIN G BENZATHINE
Bicillin C-R 900/300 Injection (WYETH-AYERST)
Bicillin C-R 900/300 in Tubex (WYETH-AYERST)
Bicillin C-R Injection (WYETH-AYERST)
Bicillin C-R in Tubex (WYETH-AYERST)
Bicillin L-A Injection (WYETH-AYERST)
Bicillin L-A in Tubex (WYETH-AYERST)
PENICILLIN G POTASSIUM
Pfizerpen for Injection (PFIZER)
PENICILLIN G PROCAINE
Bicillin C-R 900/300 Injection (WYETH-AYERST)
Bicillin C-R 900/300 in Tubex (WYETH-AYERST)
Bicillin C-R Injection (WYETH-AYERST)
Bicillin C-R in Tubex (WYETH-AYERST)
Wycillin Injection (WYETH-AYERST)
Wycillin in Tubex (WYETH-AYERST)
PENICILLIN V POTASSIUM
Penicillin V Potassium Suspension (PAR)
Penicillin V Potassium Tablets (PAR)
PENICILLIN V POTASSIUM SUSPENSION (PAR)
PENICILLIN V POTASSIUM TABLETS (PAR)
PENTASA CAPSULES (ROBERTS)
PENTAZOCINE AND NALOXONE HCL TABLETS, USP CIV (WATSON)
PENTAZOCINE HYDROCHLORIDE
Pentazocine and Naloxone HCl Tablets, USP CIV (WATSON)
Talacen Caplets (SANOFI)
Talwin Compound Caplets (SANOFI)
Talwin Nx Tablets (SANOFI)
PENTOBARBITAL SODIUM
Nembutal Sodium Capsules (ABBOTT)
Nembutal Sodium Solution (ABBOTT)
Nembutal Sodium Suppositories (ABBOTT)
Pentobarbital Sodium in Tubex (WYETH-AYERST)
PENTOBARBITAL SODIUM IN TUBEX (WYETH-AYERST)
PENTOBARBITAL SODIUM INJECTION (WYETH-AYERST)
PENTOSAN POLYSULFATE SODIUM
Elmiron Capsules (ALZA)
PENTOSTATIN
Nipent for Injection (SUPERGEN)

PENTOTHAL (THIOPENTAL SODIUM FOR INJECTION) (ABBOTT)
PENTOTHAL KIT (ABBOTT)
PENTOTHAL RTM SYRINGE (ABBOTT)
PENTOXIFYLLINE
Pentoxifylline Extended-release Tablets (MYLAN)
Pentoxil Tablets (UPSHER-SMITH)
Trental Tablets (HOECHST MARION ROUSSEL)
PENTOXIFYLLINE ER TABLETS (ESI LEDERLE)
PENTOXIFYLLINE EXTENDED-RELEASE TABLETS (MYLAN)
PENTOXIL TABLETS (UPSHER-SMITH)
PEPCID AC TABLETS (J&J – MERCK)
PEPCID INJECTION (MERCK)
PEPCID INJECTION PREMIXED (MERCK)
PEPCID FOR ORAL SUSPENSION (MERCK)
PEPCID RPD ORALLY DISINTEGRATING TABLETS (MERCK)
PEPCID TABLETS (MERCK)
PEPPERMINT
Ex. O (MAYOR)
Vitamist Intra-Oral Spray Dietary Supplements (MAYOR)
PEPTO-BISMOL MAXIMUM STRENGTH LIQUID (PROCTER & GAMBLE)
PEPTO-BISMOL ORIGINAL LIQUID, ORIGINAL AND CHERRY TABLETS AND EASY-TO-SWALLOW CAPLETS (PROCTER & GAMBLE)
PERCOCET TABLETS (ENDO LABS)
PERCODAN TABLETS (ENDO LABS)
PERCODAN-DEMI TABLETS (ENDO LABS)
PERCOLONE TABLETS (ENDO LABS)
PERDIEM FIBER THERAPY (NOVARTIS CONSUMER)
PERDIEM OVERNIGHT RELIEF (NOVARTIS CONSUMER)
PERGOLIDE MESYLATE
Permax Tablets (ATHENA)
PERGONAL FOR INJECTION (SERONO)
PERIACTIN SYRUP (MERCK)
PERIACTIN TABLETS (MERCK)
PERI-COLACE CAPSULES AND SYRUP (ROBERTS)
PERIDIN-C TABLETS (BEUTLICH)
PERINDOPRIL ERBUMINE
Aceon Tablets (2 mg, 4 mg, 8 mg) (SOLVAY)
PERIOGARD ORAL RINSE (COLGATE ORAL)
PERIOSTAT CAPSULES (COLLAGENEX)
PERMAX TABLETS (ATHENA)
PERMETHRIN
Acticin Cream (BERTEK)
Elimite Cream (ALLERGAN)
Nix Creme Rinse (WARNER-LAMBERT)
PERMITIL ORAL CONCENTRATE (SCHERING)
PERMITIL TABLETS (SCHERING)
PERNOX SCRUB CLEANSER (WESTWOOD-SQUIBB)
PERPHENAZINE
Etrafon 2-10 Tablets (2-10) (SCHERING)
Etrafon Tablets (2-25) (SCHERING)
Etrafon-Forte Tablets (4-25) (SCHERING)
Perphenazine Tablets (GENEVA)
Perphenazine and Amitriptyline Hydrochloride Tablets (MYLAN)
Perphenazine/Amitriptyline HCl Tablets (GENEVA)
Perphenazine/Amitriptyline Hydrochloride Tablets, USP (WATSON)
Triavil Tablets (LOTUS)

UNDERLINE DENOTES GENERIC NAME

Trilafon Concentrate (SCHERING)
Trilafon Injection (SCHERING)
Trilafon Tablets (SCHERING)
**PERPHENAZINE AND AMITRIPTYLINE
HYDROCHLORIDE TABLETS** (MYLAN)
PERPHENAZINE TABLETS (GENEVA)
**PERPHENAZINE/AMITRIPTYLINE HCL
TABLETS** (GENEVA)
**PERPHENAZINE/AMITRIPTYLINE
HYDROCHLORIDE TABLETS, USP**
(WATSON)
PERSANTINE TABLETS
(BOEHRINGER INGELHEIM)

PETROLATUM

Aquaphor Healing Ointment (BEIERSDORF)
Aquaphor Original Ointment (BEIERSDORF)
Eucerin Original Moisturizing Creme
(BEIERSDORF)

PETROLATUM, WHITE

Prophyllin CCC Topical, Emollient Ointment
(RYSTAN)
PFIZERPEN FOR INJECTION (PFIZER)
PHENAPHEN WITH CODEINE CAPSULES
(ROBINS)

PHENAZOPYRIDINE HYDROCHLORIDE

Prodium Tablets (BRECKENRIDGE)
Pyridium Plus Tablets (WARNER CHILCOTT)
Pyridium Tablets (WARNER CHILCOTT)
Urobiotic-250 Capsules (PFIZER)

PHENDIMETRAZINE TARTRATE

Bontril PDM Tablets (CARNRICK)
Bontril Slow-Release Capsules (CARNRICK)
Prelu-2 (ROXANE)

PHENELZINE SULFATE

Nardil Tablets (PARKE-DAVIS)
PHENERGAN INJECTION (WYETH-AYERST)
PHENERGAN SUPPOSITORIES
(WYETH-AYERST)
PHENERGAN SYRUP FORTIS
(WYETH-AYERST)
PHENERGAN SYRUP PLAIN (WYETH-AYERST)
PHENERGAN TABLETS (WYETH-AYERST)
PHENERGAN TABLETS, 25 MG
(WYETH-AYERST)
PHENERGAN IN TUBEX (WYETH-AYERST)
PHENERGAN VC SYRUP (WYETH-AYERST)
PHENERGAN VC WITH CODEINE SYRUP
(WYETH-AYERST)
PHENERGAN WITH CODEINE SYRUP
(WYETH-AYERST)
**PHENERGAN WITH
DEXTROMETHORPHAN SYRUP**
(WYETH-AYERST)
**PHENEX-1 AMINO ACID-MODIFIED
MEDICAL FOOD WITH IRON** (ROSS)
**PHENEX-2 AMINO ACID-MODIFIED
MEDICAL FOOD** (ROSS)

PHENINDAMINE TARTRATE

Nolahist Tablets (CARNRICK)
Nolamine Timed-Release Tablets (CARNRICK)

PHENIRAMINE MALEATE

Naphcon-A Ophthalmic Solution (ALCON)
Poly-Histine Elixir (SANOFI)
Poly-Histine-D Capsules (SANOFI)
Poly-Histine-D Elixir (SANOFI)
Poly-Histine-D Ped Caps (SANOFI)
Triaminic Expectorant DH
(NOVARTIS CONSUMER)
Triaminic Rx Pediatric Oral Solution
(NOVARTIS CONSUMER)

PHENOBARBITAL

Arco-Lase Plus Tablets (ARCO)

Donnatal Capsules (ROBINS)
Donnatal Elixir (ROBINS)
Donnatal Extentabs (ROBINS)
Donnatal Tablets (ROBINS)
Phenobarbital Elixir
(PHARMACEUTICAL ASSOCIATES)
PHENOBARBITAL ELIXIR
(PHARMACEUTICAL ASSOCIATES)

PHENOBARBITAL SODIUM

Phenobarbital Sodium Injection (ELKINS-SINN)
Phenobarbital Sodium in Tubex
(WYETH-AYERST)
PHENOBARBITAL SODIUM IN TUBEX
(WYETH-AYERST)
PHENOBARBITAL SODIUM INJECTION
(ELKINS-SINN)
PHENOBARBITAL SODIUM INJECTION
(WYETH-AYERST)
PHENOBARBITAL, USP (LILLY)
PHENOJECT-50 (MERZ)

PHENOL

Sore Throat Spray
(PHARMACEUTICAL ASSOCIATES)

PHENOXYBENZAMINE HYDROCHLORIDE

Dibenzyline Capsules (SMITHKLINE BEECHAM)

PHENTERMINE HYDROCHLORIDE

Adipex-P Capsules (GATE)
Adipex-P Tablets (GATE)
Fastin Capsules (SMITHKLINE BEECHAM)

PHENTERMINE RESIN

Ionamin Capsules (MEDEVA)
**PHENTOLAMINE MESYLATE FOR
INJECTION, USP** (BEDFORD)

PHENYL SALICYLATE

Prosed/DS Tablets (STAR)
Urised Tablets (POLYMEDICA)

PHENYLALANINE

Pro Endorphin (NUTRACEUTICS)

PHENYLEPHRINE HYDROCHLORIDE

Ah-Chew Chewable Tablets (WE)
Ah-Chew D Chewable Tablets (WE)
Anaplex HD Cough Syrup (ECR)
Atrohist Plus Tablets (MEDEVA)
Codimal DH Syrup (SCHWARZ)
Codimal DM Syrup (SCHWARZ)
Codimal PH Syrup (SCHWARZ)
D.A. Chewable Tablets (DJ PHARMA)
D.A. II Tablets (DJ PHARMA)
Dallergy Caplets, Syrup, Tablets (LASER)
Donatussin DC Syrup (LASER)
Donatussin Drops (LASER)
Donatussin Syrup (LASER)
Dura-Vent/DA Tablets (DJ PHARMA)
Endal-HD (FOREST)
Entex Capsules (DURA)
Entex Liquid (DURA)
Extendryl Chewable Tablets (FLEMING)
Extendryl Sr. & Jr. Capsules (FLEMING)
Extendryl Syrup (FLEMING)
Histussin HC Syrup (SANOFI)
Hycomine Compound Tablets (ENDO LABS)
Nalex DH Liquid (BLANSETT)
Nalex-A Liquid (BLANSETT)
Nalex-A Tablets (BLANSETT)
Neo-Synephrine Ophthalmic Solution (SANOFI)
Norel DM Liquid (U.S. PHARMACEUTICAL)
Omnihist L.A. Tablets (WE)
Pediacof Syrup (SANOFI)
Phenergan VC Syrup (WYETH-AYERST)
Phenergan VC with Codeine Syrup
(WYETH-AYERST)

Phenylephrine Hydrochloride Injection
(ELKINS-SINN)
Phenylephrine Hydrochloride Injection, USP
(BAXTER)
Protid Tablets (LUNSCO)
Respa-A.R.M. Tablets (RESPA)
Tussafed-EX Syrup (EVERETT)
Tussafed-HC Syrup (EVERETT)
Tympagesic Ear Drops (SAVAGE)
**PHENYLEPHRINE HYDROCHLORIDE
INJECTION** (ELKINS-SINN)
**PHENYLEPHRINE HYDROCHLORIDE
INJECTION, USP** (BAXTER)

PHENYLEPHRINE TANNATE

Atrohist Pediatric Suspension Dye-Free
(MEDEVA)
Rynatan-P Pediatric Suspension (WALLACE)
Rynatan-S Pediatric Suspension (WALLACE)
Rynatuss Pediatric Suspension (WALLACE)
Rynatuss Tablets (WALLACE)
Tussi-12 Suspension (WALLACE)

PHENYLPROPANOLAMINE
HYDROCHLORIDE

Alumadrine Tablets (FLEMING)
Atrohist Plus Tablets (MEDEVA)
Dura-Vent Tablets (DJ PHARMA)
Entex Capsules (DURA)
Entex LA Tablets (DURA)
Entex Liquid (DURA)
Exgest LA Tablets (CARNRICK)
Hycomine Pediatric Syrup (ENDO LABS)
Hycomine Syrup (ENDO LABS)
Nolamine Timed-Release Tablets (CARNRICK)
Norel Plus Capsules (U.S. PHARMACEUTICAL)
Ornade Spansule Capsules
(SMITHKLINE BEECHAM)
Poly-Histine CS Syrup (SANOFI)
Poly-Histine DM Syrup (SANOFI)
Poly-Histine-D Capsules (SANOFI)
Poly-Histine-D Elixir (SANOFI)
Poly-Histine-D Ped Caps (SANOFI)
Profen II DM Liquid (WAKEFIELD)
Profen II DM Tablets (WAKEFIELD)
Profen II Tablets (WAKEFIELD)
Profen LA Tablets (WAKEFIELD)
Propade Extended-Release Capsules
(MALLINCKRODT)
Propagest Tablets (CARNRICK)
Respa-A.R.M. Tablets (RESPA)
Sinulin Tablets (CARNRICK)
Sinuvent Tablets (WE)
Triaminic Expectorant DH
(NOVARTIS CONSUMER)
Triaminic Rx Pediatric Oral Solution
(NOVARTIS CONSUMER)
Trikof-D Tablets (RESPA)

PHENYLTOLOXAMINE

Nalex-A Liquid (BLANSETT)

PHENYLTOLOXAMINE CITRATE

Anabar Caplets (LUNSCO)
Kutrase Capsules (SCHWARZ)
Nalex-A Tablets (BLANSETT)
Poly-Histine Elixir (SANOFI)
Poly-Histine-D Capsules (SANOFI)
Poly-Histine-D Elixir (SANOFI)
Poly-Histine-D Ped Caps (SANOFI)

PHENYLTOLOXAMINE DIHYDROGEN
CITRATE

Magsal Tablets (U.S. PHARMACEUTICAL)
Norel Plus Capsules (U.S. PHARMACEUTICAL)

PHENYTOIN

Dilantin Infatabs (PARKE-DAVIS)
Dilantin-125 Suspension (PARKE-DAVIS)

UNDERLINE DENOTES GENERIC NAME

PHENYTOIN SODIUM
Dilantin Kapseals (PARKE-DAVIS)
Extended Phenytoin Sodium Capsules (MYLAN)
Phenytoin Sodium Injection (ELKINS-SINN)
**EXTENDED PHENYTOIN SODIUM
CAPSULES** (MYLAN)
PHENYTOIN SODIUM INJECTION
(ELKINS-SINN)
PHISOHEX CLEANSER (SANOFI)
PHOSCHOL CONCENTRATE
(AMERICAN LECITHIN)
PHOSCHOL GOLD (AMERICAN LECITHIN)
PHOSCHOL 900 SOFTGELS
(AMERICAN LECITHIN)
PHOSLO TABLETS (BRAINTREE)

PHOSPHATIDYLCHOLINE
PhosChol 900 Softgels (AMERICAN LECITHIN)
PhosChol Concentrate (AMERICAN LECITHIN)
PHOSPHATIDYL-SERINE CAPSULES
(WESTLAKE)
**PHOSPHOLINE IODIDE FOR
OPHTHALMIC SOLUTION** (WYETH-AYERST)
PHOTOFRIN FOR INJECTION (SANOFI)
PHRENILIN FORTE CAPSULES (CARNRICK)
PHRENILIN TABLETS (CARNRICK)
PHYSIOSOL IRRIGATION (AQUALITE)
(ABBOTT)

PILOCARPINE HYDROCHLORIDE
Salagen Tablets (MGI)
PILOPINE HS GEL (ALCON)
PIMA SYRUP (FLEMING)

PIMOZIDE
Orap Tablets (GATE)

PINDOLOL
Pindolol Tablets (MYLAN)
Pindolol Tablets (GENEVA)
Pindolol Tablets, 10 mg (NOVOPHARM)
Pindolol Tablets, 5 mg (NOVOPHARM)
Pindolol Tablets, USP (WATSON)
PINDOLOL TABLETS (MYLAN)
PINDOLOL TABLETS (GENEVA)
PINDOLOL TABLETS, 5 MG (NOVOPHARM)
PINDOLOL TABLETS, 10 MG (NOVOPHARM)
PINDOLOL TABLETS, USP (WATSON)

PINE BARK
Pine Bark and Grape Seed (MAYOR)
Vitamist Intra-Oral Spray Dietary Supplements
(MAYOR)
PINE BARK AND GRAPE SEED (MAYOR)

PIOGLITAZONE HYDROCHLORIDE
Actos Tablets (TAKEDA)

PIPECURONIUM BROMIDE
Arduan for Injection (ORGANON)

PIPERACILLIN SODIUM
Pipracil (LEDERLE LABS)
Zosyn (LEDERLE LABS)
Zosyn Pharmacy Bulk Package (LEDERLE LABS)
Zosyn in Galaxy Containers (LEDERLE LABS)
PIPRACIL (LEDERLE LABS)

PIRBUTEROL ACETATE
Maxair Autohaler (3M)
Maxair Inhaler (3M)

PIROXICAM
Feldene Capsules (PFIZER)
Piroxicam Capsules (MYLAN)
Piroxicam Capsules, 10 mg, 20 mg
(NOVOPHARM)
Piroxicam Capsules, USP (WATSON)
PIROXICAM CAPSULES (MYLAN)
PIROXICAM CAPSULES USP (SCS)

PIROXICAM CAPSULES, 10 MG, 20 MG
(NOVOPHARM)
PIROXICAM CAPSULES, USP (WATSON)
PITOCIN (MONARCH)
PITRESSIN (MONARCH)
PLACIDYL CAPSULES (ABBOTT)
PLAN B TABLETS (WOMEN'S CAPITAL)
PLAQUENIL TABLETS (SANOFI)
PLASBUMIN-5 (BAYER BIOLOGICAL)
PLASBUMIN-20 (BAYER BIOLOGICAL)
PLASBUMIN-25 (BAYER BIOLOGICAL)

PLASMA FRACTIONS, HUMAN
BayRab (BAYER BIOLOGICAL)
BayRho-D Full Dose (BAYER BIOLOGICAL)
BayRho-D Mini-Dose (BAYER BIOLOGICAL)

PLASMA PROTEIN FRACTION (HUMAN)
Plasmanate (BAYER BIOLOGICAL)
PLASMANATE (BAYER BIOLOGICAL)
PLATINOL-AQ INJECTION
(BRISTOL-MYERSSQUIBBONCOLOGY/IMMUNOLOGY)
PLAVIX TABLETS (SANOFI)
PLAVIX TABLETS (BRISTOL-MYERS SQUIBB)
PLEGISOL (ABBOTT)
PLENDIL EXTENDED-RELEASE TABLETS
(ASTRAZENECA LP)
PLETAL TABLETS (OTSUKA AMERICA)
PLETAL TABLETS (PHARMACIA & UPJOHN)

PLICAMYCIN
Mithracin for Intravenous Use (BAYER)
PMS (MAYOR)

PNEUMOCOCCAL VACCINE, POLYVALENT
Pneumovax 23 (MERCK)
Pnu-Imune 23 (LEDERLE LABS)
PNEUMOMIST TABLETS (ECR)
PNEUMOTUSSIN HC COUGH SYRUP (ECR)
PNEUMOTUSSIN TABLETS (ECR)
PNEUMOVAX 23 (MERCK)
PNS UNNA BOOT (PEDINOL)
PNU-IMUNE 23 (LEDERLE LABS)
PODOCON-25 LIQUID (PADDOCK)

PODOFILOX
Condylox Gel (OCLASSEN)
Condylox Topical Solution (OCLASSEN)

PODOPHYLLIN
Podocon-25 Liquid (PADDOCK)
POLARAMINE EXPECTORANT (SCHERING)
POLARAMINE SYRUP (SCHERING)
POLARAMINE TABLETS (SCHERING)
POLARMINE REPETABS TABLETS
(SCHERING)

POLIOVIRUS VACCINE INACTIVATED
Ipol (PASTEUR MERIEUX CONNAUGHT)
POLOCAINE INJECTION, USP
(ASTRAZENECA LP)
POLOCAINE-MPF INJECTION, USP
(ASTRAZENECA LP)
POLYBASE (PADDOCK)
**POLYCITRA SYRUP AND POLYCITRA-LC
SYRUP** (ALZA)
POLYCITRA-K CRYSTALS (ALZA)
POLYCITRA-K ORAL SOLUTION (ALZA)

POLYETHYLENE GLYCOL
Colyte - Flavored for Oral Solution (SCHWARZ)
Colyte for Oral Solution (SCHWARZ)
Colyte with Flavor Packs for Oral Solution
(SCHWARZ)
GoLYTELY and Pineapple Flavor GoLYTELY
for Oral Solution (BRAINTREE)
MiraLax Powder for Oral Solution
(BRAINTREE)

NuLYTELY, Cherry Flavor NuLYTELY and
Lemon-Lime Flavor NuLYTELY for Oral
Solution (BRAINTREE)
POLYGAM S/D (AMERICAN RED CROSS)
POLY-HISTINE CS SYRUP (SANOFI)
POLY-HISTINE DM SYRUP (SANOFI)
POLY-HISTINE ELIXIR (SANOFI)
POLY-HISTINE-D CAPSULES (SANOFI)
POLY-HISTINE-D ELIXIR (SANOFI)
POLY-HISTINE-D PED CAPS (SANOFI)
POLYMYXIN B SULFATE (BEDFORD)

POLYMYXIN B SULFATE
Betadine Brand First Aid Antibiotics &
Moisturizer Ointment (PURDUE FREDERICK)
Betadine Brand Plus First Aid Antibiotics &
Pain Reliever Ointment (PURDUE FREDERICK)
Cortisporin Cream (MONARCH)
Cortisporin Ointment (MONARCH)
Cortisporin Ophthalmic Ointment Sterile
(MONARCH)
Cortisporin Ophthalmic Suspension Sterile
(MONARCH)
Cortisporin Otic Solution Sterile (MONARCH)
Cortisporin Otic Suspension Sterile (MONARCH)
Lazersporin-C Solution (PEDINOL)
Neosporin + Pain Relief Maximum Strength
Cream (WARNER-LAMBERT)
Neosporin + Pain Relief Maximum Strength
Ointment (WARNER-LAMBERT)
Neosporin G.U. Irrigant Sterile (MONARCH)
Neosporin Ophthalmic Ointment Sterile
(MONARCH)
Neosporin Ophthalmic Solution Sterile
(MONARCH)
Neosporin Original Ointment
(WARNER-LAMBERT)
Pediotic Suspension Sterile (MONARCH)
Polysporin Ointment (WARNER-LAMBERT)
Polysporin Powder (WARNER-LAMBERT)
Polytrim Ophthalmic Solution (ALLERGAN)
Terramycin with Polymyxin B Sulfate
Ophthalmic Ointment (PFIZER)
POLYMYXIN B SULFATE USP POWDER
(PADDOCK)
POLY-PRED OPHTHALMIC SUSPENSION
(ALLERGAN)

POLYSACCHARIDE IRON COMPLEX
Hemocyte-F Elixir (U.S. PHARMACEUTICAL)
Niferex Elixir (SCHWARZ)
Niferex Tablets (SCHWARZ)
Niferex-150 Capsules (SCHWARZ)
Niferex-150 Forte Capsules (SCHWARZ)
Nu-Iron 150 Capsules (MERZ)
Nu-Iron Elixir (MERZ)
Nu-Iron Plus Elixir (MERZ)
Nu-Iron V Tablets (MERZ)
POLYSPORIN OINTMENT (WARNER-LAMBERT)
**POLYSPORIN OPHTHALMIC OINTMENT
STERILE** (MONARCH)
POLYSPORIN POWDER (WARNER-LAMBERT)
POLYTAR SHAMPOO (STIEFEL)
POLYTAR SOAP (STIEFEL)

POLYTHIAZIDE
Minizide Capsules (PFIZER)
Renese Tablets (PFIZER)
POLYTRIM OPHTHALMIC SOLUTION
(ALLERGAN)
PONSTEL KAPSEALS (PARKE-DAVIS)

PORFIMER SODIUM
Photofrin for Injection (SANOFI)
POST-OPERATIVE KITS (ALCON)
POTABA CAPSULES (GLENWOOD)
POTABA POWDER (GLENWOOD)
POTABA TABLETS (GLENWOOD)

UNDERLINE DENOTES GENERIC NAME

POTASSIUM ACETATE 40 MEQ VIAL,
PINTOP & FLIPTOP (ABBOTT)

POTASSIUM ACID PHOSPHATE

K-Phos M.F. Tablets (BEACH)
K-Phos No. 2 Tablets (BEACH)
K-Phos Original (Sodium Free) Tablets
(BEACH)

POTASSIUM BICARBONATE

Klor-Con/EF Tablets (UPSHER-SMITH)

POTASSIUM BITARTRATE

Ceo-Two Evacuant Suppository (BEUTLICH)

POTASSIUM CHLORIDE

Chlor-3 (FLEMING)
Colyte - Flavored for Oral Solution (SCHWARZ)
Colyte for Oral Solution (SCHWARZ)
Colyte with Flavor Packs for Oral Solution
(SCHWARZ)
GoLYTELY and Pineapple Flavor GoLYTELY
for Oral Solution (BRAINTREE)
K-Dur Microburst Release System ER Tablets
(KEY)
K-Lor Powder Packets (ABBOTT)
K-Tab Filmtab Tablets (ABBOTT)
Klor-Con 8/Klor-Con 10 Tablets
(UPSHER-SMITH)
Klor-Con Powder (UPSHER-SMITH)
Klor-Con/25 Powder (UPSHER-SMITH)
NuLYTELY, Cherry Flavor NuLYTELY and
Lemon-Lime Flavor NuLYTELY for Oral
Solution (BRAINTREE)
Potassium Chloride Oral Solution (ROXANE)
Potassium Chloride Oral Solution USP 10%
(PHARMACEUTICAL ASSOCIATES)
Potassium Chloride Oral Solution USP 20%
(PHARMACEUTICAL ASSOCIATES)
Rum-K (FLEMING)

POTASSIUM CHLORIDE EXTENDED-
RELEASE CAPSULES, USP (ESI LEDERLE)

POTASSIUM CHLORIDE INJECTION
AMPOULES & VIALS, PINTOP &
UNIVERSAL ADDITIVE SYRINGE
(ABBOTT)

POTASSIUM CHLORIDE ORAL SOLUTION
(ROXANE)

POTASSIUM CHLORIDE ORAL SOLUTION
USP 10% (PHARMACEUTICAL ASSOCIATES)

POTASSIUM CHLORIDE ORAL SOLUTION
USP 20% (PHARMACEUTICAL ASSOCIATES)

POTASSIUM CITRATE

Citrolith Tablets (BEACH)
Evac-Q-Kwik (SAVAGE)
Polycitra Syrup and Polycitra-LC Syrup (ALZA)
Polycitra-K Crystals (ALZA)
Polycitra-K Oral Solution (ALZA)
Potassium Citrate and Citric Acid Oral
Solution USP
(PHARMACEUTICAL ASSOCIATES)
Urocit-K Tablets (MISSION)

POTASSIUM CITRATE AND CITRIC ACID
ORAL SOLUTION USP
(PHARMACEUTICAL ASSOCIATES)

POTASSIUM CL EXTENDED RELEASE
TABLETS (APOTHECON)

POTASSIUM GUAIACOLSULFONATE

Protuss Liquid (HORIZON)
Protuss-D Liquid (HORIZON)

POTASSIUM IODIDE

Chelated Mineral Tablets (USANA)
Kie Syrup (LASER)
Pediacof Syrup (SANOFI)
Pima Syrup (FLEMING)
Potassium Iodide Oral Solution (ROXANE)
SSKI Solution (UPSHER-SMITH)

POTASSIUM IODIDE ORAL SOLUTION
(ROXANE)

POTASSIUM PHOSPHATE

K-Phos Neutral Tablets (BEACH)

POTASSIUM PHOSPHATE 15 MM VIAL &
FLIPTOP (ABBOTT)

POTASSIUM PHOSPHATE 45 MM VIAL
(ABBOTT)

POVIDONE IODINE

Betadine Medicated Douche
(PURDUE FREDERICK)
Betadine Ointment (PURDUE FREDERICK)
Betadine PrepStick Applicator
(PURDUE FREDERICK)
Betadine Skin Cleanser (PURDUE FREDERICK)
Betadine Solution (PURDUE FREDERICK)
Betadine Surgical Scrub (PURDUE FREDERICK)

PRALIDOXIME CHLORIDE

Protopam Chloride for Injection
(WYETH-AYERST)

PRAMIPEXOLE DIHYDROCHLORIDE

Mirapex Tablets (PHARMACIA & UPJOHN)

PRAMOSONE CREAM (FERNDALE)

PRAMOSONE LOTION (FERNDALE)

PRAMOSONE OINTMENT (FERNDALE)

PRAMOXINE HYDROCHLORIDE

Analpram HC Lotion 2.5% (FERNDALE)
Analpram-HC Rectal Cream 1% and 2.5%
(FERNDALE)
Anusol Hemorrhoidal Ointment
(WARNER-LAMBERT)
Betadine Brand Plus First Aid Antibiotics &
Pain Reliever Ointment (PURDUE FREDERICK)
Caladryl Clear Lotion (WARNER-LAMBERT)
Caladryl Cream For Kids (WARNER-LAMBERT)
Caladryl Lotion (WARNER-LAMBERT)
Cortane-B Ear Drops (BLANSETT)
Cortane-B Otic Vials (BLANSETT)
Cortic Ear Drops (EVERETT)
Epifoam (SCHWARZ)
Neosporin + Pain Relief Maximum Strength
Cream (WARNER-LAMBERT)
Neosporin + Pain Relief Maximum Strength
Ointment (WARNER-LAMBERT)
Pramosone Cream (FERNDALE)
Pramosone Lotion (FERNDALE)
Pramosone Ointment (FERNDALE)
Prax Lotion (FERNDALE)
ProctoFoam-HC (SCHWARZ)
Zoto-HC Ear Drops (HORIZON)

PRANDIN TABLETS (0.5, 1, AND 2 MG)
(NOVO NORDISK)

PRAVACHOL TABLETS
(BRISTOL-MYERS SQUIBB)

PRAVASTATIN SODIUM

Pravachol Tablets (BRISTOL-MYERS SQUIBB)

PRAX LOTION (FERNDALE)

PRAZIQUANTEL

Biltricide Tablets (BAYER)

PRAZOSIN HCL CAPSULES
(LEDERLE STANDARD)

PRAZOSIN HYDROCHLORIDE

Minipress Capsules (PFIZER)
Minizide Capsules (PFIZER)
Prazosin HCl Capsules (LEDERLE STANDARD)
Prazosin Hydrochloride Capsules (MYLAN)

PRAZOSIN HYDROCHLORIDE CAPSULES
(MYLAN)

PRECARE PRENATAL MULTI-
VITAMIN/MINERAL (UCB)

PRECOSE TABLETS (BAYER)

PRED FORTE OPHTHALMIC SUSPENSION
(ALLERGAN)

PRED-G OPHTHALMIC OINTMENT
(ALLERGAN)

PRED-G OPHTHALMIC SUSPENSION
(ALLERGAN)

PRED MILD OPHTHALMIC SUSPENSION
(ALLERGAN)

PREDNICARBATE

Dermatop Emollient Cream
(ORTHO DERMATOLOGICAL)
Dermatop Ointment (ORTHO DERMATOLOGICAL)

PREDNISOLONE

Prednisolone Syrup (MYLAN)
Prednisolone Syrup, USP (WE)
Prelone Syrup (MURO)

PREDNISOLONE ACETATE

Blephamide Ophthalmic Ointment (ALLERGAN)
Blephamide Ophthalmic Suspension
(ALLERGAN)

PREDNISOLONE SODIUM PHOSPHATE

Pediapred Oral Solution (MEDEVA)

PREDNISOLONE SYRUP (MYLAN)

PREDNISOLONE SYRUP, USP (WE)

PREDNISONE

Prednisone Intensol (ROXANE)
Prednisone Oral Solution (ROXANE)
Prednisone Tablets (ROXANE)
Prednisone Tablets (WATSON)
Sterapred 5 mg 12 Day Unipak (MERZ)
Sterapred 5 mg Unipak (MERZ)
Sterapred DS 12 Day Unipak (MERZ)
Sterapred DS Unipak (MERZ)

PREDNISONE INTENSOL (ROXANE)

PREDNISONE ORAL SOLUTION (ROXANE)

PREDNISONE TABLETS (ROXANE)

PREDNISONE TABLETS (WATSON)

PREDNISONE TABLETS, USP (SCHEIN)

PREGNYL FOR INJECTION (ORGANON)

PRELONE SYRUP (MURO)

PRELU-2 (ROXANE)

PREMARIN INTRAVENOUS (WYETH-AYERST)

PREMARIN TABLETS (WYETH-AYERST)

PREMARIN VAGINAL CREAM
(WYETH-AYERST)

PREMPHASE TABLETS (WYETH-AYERST)

PREMPRO TABLETS (WYETH-AYERST)

PRENATAL PLUS TABLETS (ESI LEDERLE)

PRENATE ULTRA TABLETS (SANOFI)

PREPIDIL GEL (PHARMACIA & UPJOHN)

PRESUN SENSITIVE SUNBLOCK 28
(WESTWOOD-SQUIBB)

PRESUN ULTRA CREAM 15
(WESTWOOD-SQUIBB)

PRESUN ULTRA CREAM 30
(WESTWOOD-SQUIBB)

PRESUN ULTRA GEL 15 (WESTWOOD-SQUIBB)

PRESUN ULTRA GEL 30 (WESTWOOD-SQUIBB)

PRESUN ULTRA SPRAY 27
(WESTWOOD-SQUIBB)

PREVACID DELAYED-RELEASE CAPSULES
(TAP)

PREVALITE POWDER (UPSHER-SMITH)

PREVEN EMERGENCY CONTRACEPTIVE
KIT (GYNETICS)

PREVIDENT 5000 PLUS DENTAL CREAM
(COLGATE ORAL)

PREVPAC (TAP)

PRIFTIN TABLETS (HOECHST MARION ROUSSEL)

PRILOCAINE

EMLA Anesthetic Disc (ASTRAZENECA LP)
EMLA Cream (ASTRAZENECA LP)

UNDERLINE DENOTES GENERIC NAME

PRILOSEC DELAYED-RELEASE CAPSULES
(ASTRAZENECA LP)
PRIMACOR INJECTION (SANOFI)
PRIMAQUINE PHOSPHATE TABLETS
(SANOFI)
PRIMAXIN I.M. (MERCK)
PRIMAXIN I.V. (MERCK)
PRIMIDONE
Mysoline Suspension (ELAN)
Mysoline Tablets (ELAN)
**PRINCIPEN CAPSULES, FOR ORAL
SUSPENSION, AND PEDIATRIC DROPS**
(APOTHECON)
PRINIVIL TABLETS (MERCK)
PRINZIDE TABLETS (MERCK)
PRISCOLINE HYDROCHLORIDE AMPULS
(NOVARTIS)
PRO ENDORPHIN (NUTRACEUTICS)
PRO-BANTHINE TABLETS (ROBERTS)
PROAMATINE TABLETS (ROBERTS)
PROBENECID
Benemid Tablets (MERCK)
ColBENEMID Tablets (MERCK)
Probenecid Tablets (MYLAN)
**PROBENECID AND PROBENECID WITH
COLCHICINE TABLETS, USP** (SCHEIN)
PROBENECID TABLETS (MYLAN)
PROCAINAMIDE HYDROCHLORIDE
Procainamide Hydrochloride Injection
(ELKINS-SINN)
Procanbid Extended-Release Tablets (MONARCH)
**PROCAINAMIDE HYDROCHLORIDE
INJECTION** (ELKINS-SINN)
**PROCAINAMIDE HYDROCHLORIDE
INJECTION, USP** (ABBOTT)
**PROCAINE HYDROCHLORIDE INJECTION
1% & 2% VIAL** (ABBOTT)
**PROCANBID EXTENDED-RELEASE
TABLETS** (MONARCH)
PROCARBAZINE HYDROCHLORIDE
Matulane Capsules (SIGMA-TAU)
PROCARDIA CAPSULES (PFIZER)
**PROCARDIA XL EXTENDED RELEASE
TABLETS** (PFIZER)
PROCEDURE PACKS (ALCON)
PROCHLORPERAZINE
Compazine Multi-dose Vials
(SMITHKLINE BEECHAM)
Compazine Spansule Capsules
(SMITHKLINE BEECHAM)
Compazine Suppositories
(SMITHKLINE BEECHAM)
Compazine Syrup (SMITHKLINE BEECHAM)
Compazine Tablets (SMITHKLINE BEECHAM)
Compazine Vials (SMITHKLINE BEECHAM)
Prochlorperazine Tablets (PAR)
PROCHLORPERAZINE EDISYLATE
Prochlorperazine Edisylate Injection
(ELKINS-SINN)
**PROCHLORPERAZINE EDISYLATE
INJECTION** (ELKINS-SINN)
PROCHLORPERAZINE MALEATE
Prochlorperazine Maleate Tablets (MYLAN)
**PROCHLORPERAZINE MALEATE
TABLETS** (MYLAN)
PROCHLORPERAZINE TABLETS (PAR)
PROCRIT FOR INJECTION (ORTHO BIOTECH)
PROCTOCORT CREAM (MONARCH)
PROCTOCORT CREAM & SUPPOSITORIES
(MONARCH)
PROCTOCORT SUPPOSITORIES (MONARCH)
PROCTOCREAM-HC 2.5% (SCHWARZ)
PROCTOFOAM-HC (SCHWARZ)

PROCTOFOAM-NS (NON-STEROID)
(SCHWARZ)
PRODERM (BERTEK)
PRODIUM TABLETS (BRECKENRIDGE)
PROFASI FOR INJECTION (SERONO)
PROFEN II DM LIQUID (WAKEFIELD)
PROFEN II DM TABLETS (WAKEFIELD)
PROFEN II TABLETS (WAKEFIELD)
PROFEN LA TABLETS (WAKEFIELD)
PROFENAL OPHTHALMIC SOLUTION
(ALCON)
**PROFILNINE SD SOLVENT DETERGENT
TREATED** (ALPHA)
PROFLAVANOL TABLETS (USANA)
**PROGESTASERT INTRAUTERINE
PROGESTERONE CONTRACEPTIVE
SYSTEM** (ALZA)
PROGESTERONE
Crinone 4% Gel (SERONO)
Crinone 8% Gel (SERONO)
Prometrium Capsules (100 mg) (SOLVAY)
**PROGESTERONE USP MICRONIZED
POWDER** (PADDOCK)
**PROGESTERONE USP WETTABLE
MICROCRYSTALLINE POWDER**
(PADDOCK)
PROGRAF (FUJISAWA)
PROHIBIT (PASTEUR MERIEUX CONNAUGHT)
PROLASTIN (BAYER BIOLOGICAL)
PROLEUKIN FOR INJECTION (CHIRON)
PROLEX DH LIQUID (BLANSETT)
PROLEX DM LIQUID (BLANSETT)
PROLIXIN DECANOATE INJECTION
(APOTHECON)
PROLIXIN ELIXIR (APOTHECON)
PROLIXIN ENANTHATE INJECTION
(APOTHECON)
PROLIXIN INJECTION (APOTHECON)
PROLIXIN ORAL CONCENTRATE
(APOTHECON)
PROLIXIN TABLETS (APOTHECON)
PROLOPRIM TABLETS (MONARCH)
PROMETHAZINE HCL SYRUP PLAIN
(ESI LEDERLE)
PROMETHAZINE HCL TABLETS
(ESI LEDERLE)
**PROMETHAZINE HCL AND CODEINE
PHOSPHATE SYRUP** (ESI LEDERLE)
**PROMETHAZINE HCL AND
DEXTROMETHORPHAN
HYDROBROMIDE SYRUP** (ESI LEDERLE)
**PROMETHAZINE HCL AND
PHENYLEPHRINE HCL SYRUP**
(ESI LEDERLE)
**PROMETHAZINE HCL, PHENYLEPHRINE
HCL AND CODEINE PHOSPHATE
SYRUP** (ESI LEDERLE)
PROMETHAZINE HCL TABLETS (GENEVA)
PROMETHAZINE HYDROCHLORIDE
Mepergan Injection (WYETH-AYERST)
Mepergan in Tubex (WYETH-AYERST)
Phenergan Injection (WYETH-AYERST)
Phenergan Suppositories (WYETH-AYERST)
Phenergan Syrup Fortis (WYETH-AYERST)
Phenergan Syrup Plain (WYETH-AYERST)
Phenergan Tablets (WYETH-AYERST)
Phenergan VC Syrup (WYETH-AYERST)
Phenergan VC with Codeine Syrup
(WYETH-AYERST)
Phenergan in Tubex (WYETH-AYERST)
Phenergan with Codeine Syrup
(WYETH-AYERST)
Phenergan with Dextromethorphan Syrup
(WYETH-AYERST)
Promethazine HCl Tablets (GENEVA)

Promethazine Hydrochloride Injection
(ELKINS-SINN)
Promethazine Hydrochloride and Codeine
Phosphate Syrup
(PHARMACEUTICAL ASSOCIATES)
**PROMETHAZINE HYDROCHLORIDE AND
CODEINE PHOSPHATE SYRUP**
(PHARMACEUTICAL ASSOCIATES)
**PROMETHAZINE HYDROCHLORIDE
INJECTION** (ELKINS-SINN)
PROMETRIUM CAPSULES (100 MG)
(SOLVAY)
**PRONESTYL CAPSULES, TABLETS AND
INJECTION** (APOTHECON)
PRONESTYL-SR TABLETS (APOTHECON)
**PROPADE EXTENDED-RELEASE
CAPSULES** (MALLINCKRODT)
PROPAFENONE HYDROCHLORIDE
Rythmol Tablets – 150mg, 225mg, 300mg
(KNOLL LABS)
PROPAGEST TABLETS (CARNRICK)
**PROPANOLOL HCL LONG-ACTING
CAPSULES** (ESI LEDERLE)
PROPANTHELINE BROMIDE
Propantheline Bromide Tablets (ROXANE)
PROPANTHELINE BROMIDE TABLETS
(ROXANE)
PROPECIA TABLETS (MERCK)
**PRO-PHREE PROTEIN-FREE ENERGY
MODULE WITH IRON, VITAMINS &
MINERALS** (ROSS)
**PROPHYLLIN CCC TOPICAL, EMOLLIENT
OINTMENT** (RYSTAN)
**PROPHYLLIN CCC WET DRESSING
POWDER** (RYSTAN)
**PROPIMEX-1 AMINO ACID-MODIFIED
MEDICAL FOOD WITH IRON** (ROSS)
**PROPIMEX-2 AMINO ACID-MODIFIED
MEDICAL FOOD** (ROSS)
**PROPINE OPHTHALMIC SOLUTION WITH
C CAP COMPLIANCE CAP B.I.D.**
(ALLERGAN)
PROPLEX T (BAXTER HEALTHCARE)
PROPOFOL
Diprivan Injectable Emulsion (ASTRAZENECA)
Propofol Injectable Emulsion 1% (BAXTER)
PROPOFOL INJECTABLE EMULSION 1%
(BAXTER)
**PROPOXYPHENE HYDROCHLORIDE
CAPSULES** (MYLAN)
PROPOXYPHENE HYDROCHLORIDE
Darvon Compound-65 Pulvules (LILLY)
Darvon Pulvules (LILLY)
Propoxyphene Hydrochloride Capsules (MYLAN)
Propoxyphene Hydrochloride and
Acetaminophen Tablets (MYLAN)
Propoxyphene Hydrochloride and
Acetaminophen Tablets, USP CIV (WATSON)
Propoxyphene Hydrochloride, Aspirin and
Caffeine Capsules (MYLAN)
Wygesic Tablets (WYETH-AYERST)
**PROPOXYPHENE HYDROCHLORIDE AND
ACETAMINOPHEN TABLETS, USP CIV**
(WATSON)
**PROPOXYPHENE HYDROCHLORIDE,
ASPIRIN AND CAFFEINE CAPSULES**
(MYLAN)
**PROPOXYPHENE HYDROCHLORIDE AND
ACETAMINOPHEN TABLETS** (MYLAN)
PROPOXYPHENE NAPSYLATE
Darvocet-N 100 Tablets (LILLY)
Darvocet-N 50 Tablets (LILLY)
Darvon-N Tablets (LILLY)

UNDERLINE DENOTES GENERIC NAME

Propoxyphene Napsylate and Acetaminophen Tablets (MYLAN)
PROPOXYPHENE NAPSYLATE AND ACETAMINOPHEN TABLETS (MYLAN)
PROPRANOLOL HCL INTENSOL (ROXANE)

PROPRANOLOL HYDROCHLORIDE

Inderal Injectable (WYETH-AYERST)
Inderal LA Long-Acting Capsules (WYETH-AYERST)
Inderal Tablets (WYETH-AYERST)
Inderide LA Long-Acting Capsules (WYETH-AYERST)
Inderide Tablets (WYETH-AYERST)
Propranolol HCl Intensol (ROXANE)
Propranolol Hydrochloride Oral Solution (ROXANE)
Propranolol Hydrochloride Tablets (MYLAN)
Propranolol Hydrochloride Tablets, USP (WATSON)
Propranolol Hydrochloride and Hydrochlorothiazide Tablets (MYLAN)
PROPRANOLOL HYDROCHLORIDE ORAL SOLUTION (ROXANE)
PROPRANOLOL HYDROCHLORIDE TABLETS (MYLAN)
PROPRANOLOL HYDROCHLORIDE AND HYDROCHLOROTHIAZIDE TABLETS (MYLAN)
PROPRANOLOL HYDROCHLORIDE TABLETS, USP (WATSON)
PROPULSID SUSPENSION (JANSSEN)
PROPULSID TABLETS (JANSSEN)

PROPYLTHIOURACIL

Propylthiouracil Tablets (LEDERLE STANDARD)
PROPYLTHIOURACIL TABLETS (LEDERLE STANDARD)
PRO-Q SKIN PROTECTANT (FERNDALE)
PROSCAR TABLETS (MERCK)
PROSED/DS TABLETS (STAR)
PROS-FORTE (VITALINE)
PROSHIELD CORNEAL COLLAGEN SHIELD (ALCON)
PROSOM TABLETS (ABBOTT)
PROSTIGMIN INJECTABLE (ICN)
PROSTIGMIN TABLETS (ICN)
PROSTIN E2 SUPPOSITORIES (PHARMACIA & UPJOHN)
PROSTIN VR PEDIATRIC STERILE SOLUTION (PHARMACIA & UPJOHN)

PROTAMINE SULFATE

Protamine Sulfate Injection (Preservative-Free) (ELKINS-SINN)
Protamine Sulfate Vials (LILLY)
PROTAMINE SULFATE INJECTION (PRESERVATIVE-FREE) (ELKINS-SINN)
PROTAMINE SULFATE VIALS (LILLY)

PROTEASE

Arco-Lase Plus Tablets (ARCO)
Arco-Lase Tablets (ARCO)
Donnazyme Tablets (ROBINS)
Ku-Zyme Capsules (SCHWARZ)
Ku-Zyme HP Capsules (SCHWARZ)
Kutrase Capsules (SCHWARZ)
PROTEOLYTIC FORMULA (PROTEOLYTIC ENZYMES) (VITALINE)
PROTEXIN ORAL BREATH SPRAY (CETYLITE)
PROTEXIN ORAL RINSE CONCENTRATE (CETYLITE)
PROTID TABLETS (LUNSCO)

PROTIRELIN

Thyrel TRH (FERRING)
PROTOPAM CHLORIDE FOR INJECTION (WYETH-AYERST)

PROTRIPTYLINE HYDROCHLORIDE

Vivactil Tablets (MERCK)
PROTROPIN FOR INJECTION (GENENTECH)
PROTUSS LIQUID (HORIZON)
PROTUSS-D LIQUID (HORIZON)
PROTUSS-DM TABLETS (HORIZON)
PROVENTIL INHALATION AEROSOL (SCHERING)
PROVENTIL HFA INHALATION AEROSOL (SCHERING)
PROVENTIL INHALATION SOLUTION 0.083% (SCHERING)
PROVENTIL REPETABS TABLETS (SCHERING)
PROVENTIL SOLUTION FOR INHALATION 0.5% (SCHERING)
PROVENTIL SYRUP (SCHERING)
PROVENTIL TABLETS (SCHERING)
PROVERA TABLETS (PHARMACIA & UPJOHN)
PROVIGIL TABLETS (CEPHALON)
PROVIMIN PROTEIN-VITAMIN-MINERAL FORMULA COMPONENT WITH IRON (ROSS)
PROVISC OPHTHALMIC VISCOSURGICAL DEVICE (ALCON)
PROVOL (PYGEUM AFRICANUM) (UPSHER-SMITH)
PROZAC PULVULES & LIQUID, ORAL SOLUTION (DISTA)
PROZAC SCORED TABLETS (LILLY)
PSEUDOEPHEDRINE HCL TABLETS (GENEVA)

PSEUDOEPHEDRINE HYDROCHLORIDE

Actifed Cold & Allergy Tablets (WARNER-LAMBERT)
Allegra-D Extended-Release Tablets (HOECHST MARION ROUSSEL)
Anaplex DM Cough Syrup (ECR)
Anatuss DM Syrup (MERZ)
Anatuss LA Tablets (MERZ)
Atrohist Pediatric Capsules (MEDEVA)
Benadryl Allergy/Cold Tablets (WARNER-LAMBERT)
Benadryl Allergy/Congestion Liquid (WARNER-LAMBERT)
Benadryl Allergy/Congestion Tablets (WARNER-LAMBERT)
Benadryl Allergy/Sinus Headache Caplets & Gelcaps (WARNER-LAMBERT)
Benylin Multi-Symptom (WARNER-LAMBERT)
Biohist LA Tablets (WAKEFIELD)
Bromfed Capsules (Extended-Release) (MURO)
Bromfed-PD Capsules (Extended-Release) (MURO)
Children's Sudafed Cough & Cold Liquid (WARNER-LAMBERT)
Children's Sudafed Nasal Decongestant Chewables (WARNER-LAMBERT)
Children's Sudafed Nasal Decongestant Liquid (WARNER-LAMBERT)
Children's Tylenol Allergy-D Liquid and Chewable Tablets (MCNEIL CONSUMER)
Children's Tylenol Cold Liquid and Chewable Tablets (MCNEIL CONSUMER)
Children's Tylenol Cold Plus Cough Suspension Liquid and Chewable Tablets (MCNEIL CONSUMER)
Children's Tylenol Flu Suspension Liquid (MCNEIL CONSUMER)
Children's Tylenol Sinus Liquid and Chewable Tablets (MCNEIL CONSUMER)
D-Feda II Tablets (WE)
Dallergy-JR Capsules (LASER)
Deconsal II Tablets (MEDEVA)
Defen-L.A. Tablets (HORIZON)
Dimetane-DX Cough Syrup (ROBINS)

Duratuss HD Elixir (UCB)
Duratuss Tablets (UCB)
Entex PSE Tablets (DURA)
Guai-Vent/PSE Tablets (DJ PHARMA)
Guaifed Capsules (MURO)
Guaifed-PD Capsules (MURO)
Histussin D Liquid (SANOFI)
Infants' Tylenol Cold Decongestant and Fever Reducer Concentrated Drops (MCNEIL CONSUMER)
Infants' Tylenol Cold Decongestant and Fever Reducer Concentrated Drops Plus Cough (MCNEIL CONSUMER)
Kronofed-A Kronocaps (FERNDALE)
Kronofed-A-Jr. Kronocaps (FERNDALE)
Lodrane LD Capsules (ECR)
Lodrane Liquid (ECR)
Mescolor Tablets (HORIZON)
Motrin Cold & Flu Caplets (MCNEIL CONSUMER)
Motrin Sinus Headache Caplets (MCNEIL CONSUMER)
Nasatab LA Tablets (ECR)
Nucofed Capsules (MONARCH)
Nucofed Pediatric Expectorant Syrup (MONARCH)
Protuss-D Liquid (HORIZON)
Protuss-DM Tablets (HORIZON)
Pseudoephedrine HCl Tablets (GENEVA)
Pseudoephedrine Hydrochloride Syrup USP (PHARMACEUTICAL ASSOCIATES)
Pseudoephedrine Hydrochloride Tablets (ROXANE)
Respa-1st Tablets (RESPA)
Respahist Capsules (RESPA)
Respaire-SR Capsules 60, 120 (LASER)
Robitussin-DAC Syrup (ROBINS)
Rondec Oral Drops (DJ PHARMA)
Rondec Syrup (DJ PHARMA)
Rondec Tablet (DJ PHARMA)
Rondec-DM Oral Drops (DJ PHARMA)
Rondec-DM Syrup (DJ PHARMA)
Rondec-TR Tablet (DJ PHARMA)
Semprex-D Capsules (MEDEVA)
Sinutab Non-Drying Liquid Caps (WARNER-LAMBERT)
Sinutab Sinus Allergy MS Caplets and Tablets (WARNER-LAMBERT)
Sinutab Sinus MS Without Drowsiness Caplets and Tablets (WARNER-LAMBERT)
Sudafed 12 Hour Tablets (WARNER-LAMBERT)
Sudafed 24 Hour Tablets (WARNER-LAMBERT)
Sudafed Cold & Allergy Tablets (WARNER-LAMBERT)
Sudafed Cold & Cough Liquid Caps (WARNER-LAMBERT)
Sudafed Cold & Sinus Liquid Caps (WARNER-LAMBERT)
Sudafed Nasal Decongestant 30 mg Tablets (WARNER-LAMBERT)
Sudafed Non-Drying Sinus Liquid Caps (WARNER-LAMBERT)
Sudafed Severe Cold Formula MS Caplets and Tablets (WARNER-LAMBERT)
Sudafed Sinus MS Caplets and Tablets (WARNER-LAMBERT)
Syn-Rx DM Tablets 14 Day Treatment Regimen (MEDEVA)
Syn-Rx Tablets 14 Day Treatment Regimen (MEDEVA)
Tussafed-LA Caplets (EVERETT)
Tussend Expectorant Liquid (MONARCH)
Tussend Syrup (MONARCH)
Tussend Tablets (MONARCH)
Tylenol Allergy Sinus NightTime, Maximum Strength Caplets (MCNEIL CONSUMER)

UNDERLINE DENOTES GENERIC NAME

Tylenol Allergy Sinus, Maximum Strength
Caplets, Gelcaps, and Geltabs
(MCNEIL CONSUMER)
Tylenol Cold Complete Formula, Multi-
Symptom Tablets and Caplets
(MCNEIL CONSUMER)
Tylenol Cold Non-Drowsy, Multi-Symptom
Caplets and Gelcaps (MCNEIL CONSUMER)
Tylenol Cold Severe Congestion Non-Drowsy,
Multi-Symptom Caplets (MCNEIL CONSUMER)
Tylenol Flu NightTime, Maximum Strength
Gelcaps (MCNEIL CONSUMER)
Tylenol Flu NightTime, Maximum Strength
Liquid (MCNEIL CONSUMER)
Tylenol Flu NightTime, Maximum Strength
Powder (MCNEIL CONSUMER)
Tylenol Flu Non-Drowsy, Maximum Strength
Gelcaps (MCNEIL CONSUMER)
Tylenol Sinus NightTime, Maximum Strength
Caplets (MCNEIL CONSUMER)
Tylenol Sinus Non-Drowsy, Maximum
Strength Geltabs, Gelcaps, Caplets, and
Tablets (MCNEIL CONSUMER)
Ultrabrom Capsules (WE)
Ultrabrom PD Capsules (WE)
Zephrex LA Tablets (SANOFI)
Zephrex Tablets (SANOFI)
**PSEUDOEPHEDRINE HYDROCHLORIDE
SYRUP USP** (PHARMACEUTICAL ASSOCIATES)
**PSEUDOEPHEDRINE HYDROCHLORIDE
TABLETS** (ROXANE)

PSEUDOEPHEDRINE SULFATE

Claritin-D 12 Hour Extended Release Tablets
(SCHERING)
Claritin-D 24 Hour Extended Release Tablets
(SCHERING)
Rynatan Tablets (WALLACE)
Trinalin Repetabs Tablets (KEY)

PSEUDOEPHEDRINE TANNATE

Tanafed Suspension (HORIZON)
PSORCON CREAM 0.05% (DERMIK)
PSORCON E CREAM (DERMIK)
PSORCON E OINTMENT (DERMIK)
PSORCON OINTMENT 0.05% (DERMIK)

PSYLLIUM PREPARATIONS

Metamucil Original Texture Powder, Orange
Flavor (PROCTER & GAMBLE)
Metamucil Original Texture Powder, Regular
Flavor (PROCTER & GAMBLE)
Metamucil Smooth Texture Powder, Orange
Flavor (PROCTER & GAMBLE)
Metamucil Smooth Texture Powder, Sugar-
Free, Orange Flavor (PROCTER & GAMBLE)
Metamucil Smooth Texture Powder, Sugar-
Free, Regular Flavor (PROCTER & GAMBLE)
Metamucil Wafers, Apple Crisp and Cinnamon
Spice Flavors (PROCTER & GAMBLE)
Perdiem Fiber Therapy (NOVARTIS CONSUMER)
Perdiem Overnight Relief
(NOVARTIS CONSUMER)
**PTG, ALCON APPLANATION
PNEUMATONOGRAPH** (ALCON)
**PULMICORT TURBUHALER INHALATION
POWDER** (ASTRAZENECA LP)
PULMOZYME INHALATION SOLUTION
(GENENTECH)
PURGE (FLEMING)
PURIFIED PORK LENTE INSULIN
(NOVO NORDISK)
PURIFIED PORK NPH ISOPHANE INSULIN
(NOVO NORDISK)
PURIFIED PORK REGULAR INSULIN
(NOVO NORDISK)
PURINETHOL TABLETS (GLAXO WELLCOME)

PYRAZINAMIDE

Pyrazinamide Tablets (LEDERLE LABS)
Pyrazinamide Tablets (LEDERLE STANDARD)
Rifater (HOECHST MARION ROUSSEL)
PYRAZINAMIDE TABLETS (LEDERLE LABS)
PYRAZINAMIDE TABLETS
(LEDERLE STANDARD)
PYRIDIUM TABLETS (WARNER CHILCOTT)
PYRIDIUM PLUS TABLETS
(WARNER CHILCOTT)

PYRIDOSTIGMINE BROMIDE

Mestinon Syrup (ICN)
Mestinon Tablets (ICN)
Mestinon Timespan Tablets (ICN)
Regonol Injection (ORGANON)

PYRILAMINE MALEATE

Codimal DH Syrup (SCHWARZ)
Codimal DM Syrup (SCHWARZ)
Codimal PH Syrup (SCHWARZ)
Poly-Histine Elixir (SANOFI)
Poly-Histine-D Capsules (SANOFI)
Poly-Histine-D Elixir (SANOFI)
Poly-Histine-D Ped Caps (SANOFI)
Triaminic Expectorant DH
(NOVARTIS CONSUMER)
Triaminic Rx Pediatric Oral Solution
(NOVARTIS CONSUMER)

PYRILAMINE TANNATE

Atrohist Pediatric Suspension Dye-Free
(MEDEVA)
Rynatan-P Pediatric Suspension (WALLACE)
Rynatan-S Pediatric Suspension (WALLACE)

PYRIMETHAMINE

Daraprim Tablets (GLAXO WELLCOME)

PYRITHIONE ZINC

DHS Zinc Shampoo (PERSON & COVEY)
Head & Shoulders Dandruff Shampoo
(PROCTER & GAMBLE)
Head & Shoulders Dandruff Shampoo Dry
Scalp (PROCTER & GAMBLE)
PYROGALLIC ACID OINTMENT (GORDON)

Q

Q-BID (NUTRACEUTICS)
**QUELICIN (SUCCINYLCHOLINE
CHLORIDE INJECTION) AMPUL &
VIAL, PINTOP** (ABBOTT)
QUESTRAN FOR ORAL SUSPENSION
(APOTHECON)
**QUESTRAN LIGHT FOR ORAL
SUSPENSION** (APOTHECON)

QUETIAPINE FUMARATE

Seroquel Tablets (ASTRAZENECA)
QUIBRON CAPSULES (MONARCH)
QUIBRON-T/SR ACCUDOSE TABLETS
(MONARCH)
QUINAGLUTE DURA-TABS TABLETS
(BERLEX)

QUINAPRIL HYDROCHLORIDE

Accupril Tablets (PARKE-DAVIS)
QUINIDEX EXTENTABS (ROBINS)

QUINIDINE GLUCONATE

Quinaglute Dura-Tabs Tablets (BERLEX)
Quinidine Gluconate Injection, USP (LILLY)
**QUINIDINE GLUCONATE ER TABLETS,
USP** (SCHEIN)

QUINIDINE GLUCONATE INJECTION, USP
(LILLY)

QUINIDINE POLYGALACTURONATE

Cardioquin Tablets (PURDUE FREDERICK)

QUINIDINE SULFATE

Quinidex Extentabs (ROBINS)
Quinidine Sulfate Tablets (LEDERLE STANDARD)
QUINIDINE SULFATE E-R (ESI LEDERLE)
QUINIDINE SULFATE TABLETS
(LEDERLE STANDARD)

QUININE SULFATE

Quinine Sulfate Capsules, USP (WATSON)
Quinine Sulfate Tablets, USP (WATSON)
QUININE SULFATE CAPSULES, USP
(WATSON)
QUININE SULFATE TABLETS, USP
(WATSON)

R

RABIES IMMUNE GLOBULIN (HUMAN)

BayRab (BAYER BIOLOGICAL)
Imogam Rabies - HT
(PASTEUR MERIEUX CONNAUGHT)

RABIES VACCINE

Imovax Rabies I.D. Vaccine
(PASTEUR MERIEUX CONNAUGHT)
Imovax Rabies Vaccine
(PASTEUR MERIEUX CONNAUGHT)
Rabies Vaccine Adsorbed
(SMITHKLINE BEECHAM)
Rabies Vaccine RabAvert (CHIRON)
RABIES VACCINE ADSORBED
(SMITHKLINE BEECHAM)
RABIES VACCINE RABAVERT (CHIRON)

RALOXIFENE HYDROCHLORIDE

Evista Tablets (LILLY)

RAMIPRIL

Altace Capsules (MONARCH)

RANITIDINE BISMUTH CITRATE

Tritec Tablets (GLAXO WELLCOME)
RANITIDINE HCL CAPSULES (GENEVA)
RANITIDINE HCL TABLETS (GENEVA)
**RANITIDINE HCL TABLETS, 150 MG, 300
MG** (NOVOPHARM)

RANITIDINE HYDROCHLORIDE

Ranitidine HCl Capsules (GENEVA)
Ranitidine HCl Tablets (GENEVA)
Ranitidine HCl Tablets, 150 mg, 300 mg
(NOVOPHARM)
Ranitidine Tablets (PAR)
Ranitidine Tablets (MYLAN)
Ranitidine Tablets (WATSON)
Zantac 150 EFFERdose Granules
(GLAXO WELLCOME)
Zantac 150 EFFERdose Tablets
(GLAXO WELLCOME)
Zantac 150 GELdose Capsules
(GLAXO WELLCOME)
Zantac 150 Tablets (GLAXO WELLCOME)
Zantac 300 GELdose Capsules
(GLAXO WELLCOME)
Zantac 300 Tablets (GLAXO WELLCOME)
Zantac 75 (WARNER-LAMBERT)
Zantac Injection (GLAXO WELLCOME)
Zantac Injection Premixed (GLAXO WELLCOME)
Zantac Syrup (GLAXO WELLCOME)

UNDERLINE DENOTES GENERIC NAME

RANITIDINE TABLETS (PAR)
RANITIDINE TABLETS (MYLAN)
RANITIDINE TABLETS (WATSON)
RANITIDINE TABLETS (APOTHECON)
RAUZIDE TABLETS (APOTHECON)
RAXAR TABLETS (GLAXO WELLCOME)
RCF ROSS CARBOHYDRATE FREE SOY
   FORMULA BASE WITH IRON (ROSS)
REBETRON COMBINATION THERAPY
   (SCHERING)
RECOMBINATE (BAXTER HEALTHCARE)
RECOMBIVAX HB (MERCK)
REDIPAK (RESPIRATORY THERAPY
   UNIT) PRODUCTS: (WYETH-AYERST)
REDIPAK UNIT DOSE MEDICATIONS
   (WYETH-AYERST)
REDIPAK UNIT DOSE MEDICATIONS
   (STRIP PACK AND/OR INDIVIDUALLY
   WRAPPED) PRODUCTS: (WYETH-AYERST)
REDOX (NUTRACEUTICS)
REFLUDAN (HOECHST MARION ROUSSEL)
REFRESH PLUS LUBRICANT EYE DROPS
   (ALLERGAN)
REFRESH P.M. LUBRICANT EYE
   OINTMENT (ALLERGAN)
REFRESH TEARS LUBRICANT EYE
   DROPS (ALLERGAN)
REGLAN INJECTABLE (ROBINS)
REGLAN SYRUP (ROBINS)
REGLAN TABLETS (ROBINS)
REGONOL INJECTION (ORGANON)
REGRANEX GEL (ORTHO-MCNEIL)
REHYDRALYTE ORAL ELECTROLYTE
   REHYDRATION SOLUTION (ROSS)
RELAFEN TABLETS (SMITHKLINE BEECHAM)
RE-LEAF (MAYOR)
RELEASE ANTIADHESIVE (CETYLITE)
REMERON TABLETS (ORGANON)
REMICADE FOR IV INJECTION (CENTOCOR)

REMIFENTANIL HYDROCHLORIDE

   Ultiva for Injection (GLAXO WELLCOME)
RENACIDIN IRRIGATION (GUARDIAN)
RENAGEL CAPSULES (GENZYME)
RENAL MULTIVITAMIN FORMULA
   (VITALINE)
RENAL MULTIVITAMIN FORMULA PLUS
   IRON (VITALINE)
RENAL MULTIVITAMIN FORMULA WITH
   ZINC (VITALINE)
RENESE TABLETS (PFIZER)
RENOVA CREAM (ORTHO DERMATOLOGICAL)
REOPRO VIALS (LILLY)
REOPRO VIALS (CENTOCOR)

REPAGLINIDE

   Prandin Tablets (0.5, 1, and 2 mg)
   (NOVO NORDISK)
REPAN-CF TABLETS (EVERETT)
REPAN TABLETS (EVERETT)
REPRONEX FOR INTRAMUSCULAR
   INJECTION (FERRING)
REQUIP TABLETS (SMITHKLINE BEECHAM)

RESCINNAMINE

   Moderil Tablets (PFIZER)
RESCRIPTOR TABLETS
   (PHARMACIA & UPJOHN)

RESERPINE

   Diutensen-R Tablets (WALLACE)

RESORCINOL

   Bensulfoid Cream (ECR)
RESPA-1ST TABLETS (RESPA)
RESPA-A.R.M. TABLETS (RESPA)
RESPA-DM TABLETS (RESPA)
RESPA-GF TABLETS (RESPA)
RESPAHIST CAPSULES (RESPA)

RESPAIRE-SR CAPSULES 60, 120 (LASER)
RESTORIL CAPSULES (NOVARTIS)
RESVERATROL FORTE (GRAPE SEED
   AND GRAPE SKIN EXTRACTS) (VITALINE)
RETAVASE VIALS (CENTOCOR)

RETEPLASE

   Retavase Vials (CENTOCOR)
RETIN-A CREAM/GEL/LIQUID
   (ORTHO DERMATOLOGICAL)
RETIN-A MICRO MICROSPHERE, 0.1%
   (ORTHO DERMATOLOGICAL)
RETINOIC ACID USP POWDER (TRANS)
   (PADDOCK)
RETROVIR CAPSULES (GLAXO WELLCOME)
RETROVIR IV INFUSION (GLAXO WELLCOME)
RETROVIR SYRUP (GLAXO WELLCOME)
RETROVIR TABLETS (GLAXO WELLCOME)
REVERSOL INJECTION (ORGANON)
REVEX INJECTION (BAXTER)
REVIA TABLETS (DUPONT)
REVITALIZER (MAYOR)
REZULIN TABLETS (PARKE-DAVIS)
R-GENE 10 INJECTION
   (PHARMACIA & UPJOHN)
RHEUMATREX DOSE PACK (LEDERLE LABS)
RHINOCORT NASAL INHALER
   (ASTRAZENECA LP)

RHO (D) IMMUNE GLOBULIN (HUMAN)

   BayRho-D Full Dose (BAYER BIOLOGICAL)
   BayRho-D Mini-Dose (BAYER BIOLOGICAL)
   MICRhoGAM (ORTHO-CLINICAL)
   RhoGAM (ORTHO-CLINICAL)
   WinRho SDF (NABI)
RHOGAM (ORTHO-CLINICAL)

RIBAVIRIN

   Rebetron Combination Therapy (SCHERING)
   Virazole (ICN)

RICINOLEIC ACID

   Aci-Jel Therapeutic Vaginal Jelly
   (ORTHO-MCNEIL)

RIFABUTIN

   Mycobutin Capsules (PHARMACIA & UPJOHN)
RIFADIN CAPSULES
   (HOECHST MARION ROUSSEL)
RIFADIN IV (HOECHST MARION ROUSSEL)
RIFAMATE CAPSULES
   (HOECHST MARION ROUSSEL)

RIFAMPIN

   Rifadin Capsules (HOECHST MARION ROUSSEL)
   Rifadin IV (HOECHST MARION ROUSSEL)
   Rifamate Capsules (HOECHST MARION ROUSSEL)
   Rifater (HOECHST MARION ROUSSEL)

RIFAPENTINE

   Priftin Tablets (HOECHST MARION ROUSSEL)
RIFATER (HOECHST MARION ROUSSEL)
RILUTEK TABLETS (RHONE-POULENC RORER)

RILUZOLE

   Rilutek Tablets (RHONE-POULENC RORER)
RIMACTANE CAPSULES (GENEVA)
RIMACTANE CAPSULES (NOVARTIS)

RIMANTADINE HYDROCHLORIDE

   Flumadine Syrup (FOREST)
   Flumadine Tablets (FOREST)
RINGER'S INJECTION, USP (ABBOTT)
RINGER'S IRRIGATION, USP (AQUALITE)
   (ABBOTT)

RISEDRONATE SODIUM

   Actonel Tablets
   (PROCTER & GAMBLE PHARMACEUTICALS)
RISPERDAL ORAL SOLUTION (JANSSEN)
RISPERDAL TABLETS (JANSSEN)

RISPERIDONE

   Risperdal Oral Solution (JANSSEN)
   Risperdal Tablets (JANSSEN)
RITALIN HYDROCHLORIDE TABLETS
   (NOVARTIS)
RITALIN-SR TABLETS (NOVARTIS)

RITONAVIR

   Norvir Capsules (ABBOTT)
   Norvir Oral Solution (ABBOTT)
RITUXAN FOR INFUSION (IDEC)
RITUXAN I.V. (GENENTECH)

RITUXIMAB

   Rituxan I.V. (GENENTECH)
   Rituxan for Infusion (IDEC)

RIZATRIPTAN BENZOATE

   Maxalt Tablets (MERCK)
   Maxalt-MLT Orally Disintegrating Tablets
   (MERCK)
RMS SUPPOSITORIES CII (UPSHER-SMITH)
ROBAXIN INJECTABLE (ROBINS)
ROBAXIN TABLETS (ROBINS)
ROBAXIN-750 TABLETS (ROBINS)
ROBAXISAL TABLETS (ROBINS)
ROBINUL FORTE TABLETS (HORIZON)
ROBINUL INJECTABLE (BAXTER)
ROBINUL INJECTABLE (ROBINS)
ROBINUL TABLETS (HORIZON)
ROBITUSSIN A-C SYRUP (ROBINS)
ROBITUSSIN-DAC SYRUP (ROBINS)
ROCALTROL CAPSULES (ROCHE LABS)
ROCALTROL ORAL SOLUTION
   (ROCHE LABS)
ROCEPHIN INJECTABLE VIALS, ADD-
   VANTAGE, GALAXY, BULK (ROCHE LABS)

ROCURONIUM BROMIDE

   Zemuron Injection (ORGANON)

ROFECOXIB

   Vioxx Oral Suspension (MERCK)
   Vioxx Tablets (MERCK)
ROFERON-A INJECTION (ROCHE LABS)
ROMAZICON INJECTION (ROCHE LABS)
RONDEC ORAL DROPS (DJ PHARMA)
RONDEC SYRUP (DJ PHARMA)
RONDEC TABLET (DJ PHARMA)
RONDEC-DM ORAL DROPS (DJ PHARMA)
RONDEC-DM SYRUP (DJ PHARMA)
RONDEC-TR TABLET (DJ PHARMA)

ROPINIROLE HYDROCHLORIDE

   Requip Tablets (SMITHKLINE BEECHAM)

ROPIVACAINE HYDROCHLORIDE

   Naropin Injection (ASTRAZENECA LP)

ROSIGLITAZONE MALEATE

   Avandia Tablets (SMITHKLINE BEECHAM)
ROSS METABOLIC FORMULA SYSTEM
   (ROSS)
ROTASHIELD FOR ORAL
   ADMINISTRATION (WYETH-AYERST)

ROTAVIRUS VACCINE, LIVE, ORAL,
TETRAVALENT

   RotaShield for Oral Administration
   (WYETH-AYERST)
ROWASA RECTAL SUSPENSION ENEMA
   4.0 GRAMS/UNIT (60 ML) (SOLVAY)
ROWASA SUPPOSITORY (500 MG) (SOLVAY)
ROXANOL 100 CONCENTRATED ORAL
   SOLUTION (ROXANE)
ROXANOL CONCENTRATED ORAL
   SOLUTION (ROXANE)
ROXANOL-T ORAL SOLUTION (ROXANE)
ROXICODONE TABLETS, ORAL
   SOLUTION & INTENSOL (ROXANE)
ROXILOX CAPSULES (ROXANE)

UNDERLINE DENOTES GENERIC NAME

ROXIPRIN TABLETS (ROXANE)
RUBELLA & MUMPS VIRUS VACCINE LIVE
  Biavax II (MERCK)
RUBELLA VIRUS VACCINE LIVE
  Meruvax II (MERCK)
RUBEX FOR INJECTION
  (BRISTOL-MYERSSQUIBBONCOLOGY/IMMUNOLOGY)
RUM-K (FLEMING)
RVPAQUE CREAM (ICN)
RYNA LIQUID (WALLACE)
RYNA-C LIQUID (WALLACE)
RYNATAN TABLETS (WALLACE)
RYNATAN-P PEDIATRIC SUSPENSION
  (WALLACE)
RYNATAN-S PEDIATRIC SUSPENSION
  (WALLACE)
RYNATUSS TABLETS (WALLACE)
RYNATUSS PEDIATRIC SUSPENSION
  (WALLACE)
**RYTHMOL TABLETS – 150MG, 225MG,
300MG** (KNOLL LABS)

S

S-ADENOSYLMETHIONINE
  SAMe Plus (NUTRACEUTICS)
SAFE TUSSIN 30 LIQUID (KRAMER)
SAIZEN FOR INJECTION (SERONO)
SAL-ACID PLASTERS (PEDINOL)
SALACTIC FILM (PEDINOL)
SALAGEN TABLETS (MGI)
SALFLEX TABLETS (CARNRICK)
SALICYLAMIDE
  Anabar Caplets (LUNSCO)
SALICYLIC ACID
  DHS Sal Shampoo (PERSON & COVEY)
  Hydrisalic Gel (PEDINOL)
  Sal-Acid Plasters (PEDINOL)
  Sal-Plant Gel (PEDINOL)
  Salactic Film (PEDINOL)
SALICYLIC ACID & SULFUR SOAP
  (STIEFEL)
SALICYLIC ACID CLEANSING BAR
  (STIEFEL)
**SALINE SOLUTION (SEE SODIUM
CHLORIDE INJECTION)** (WYETH-AYERST)
SALIVA SUBSTITUTE (ROXANE)
SALIVART (GEBAUER)
SALMETEROL XINAFOATE
  Serevent Diskus (GLAXO WELLCOME)
  Serevent Inhalation Aerosol
    (GLAXO WELLCOME)
SAL-PLANT GEL (PEDINOL)
SALSALATE
  Disalcid Capsules (3M)
  Disalcid Tablets (3M)
  Salflex Tablets (CARNRICK)
SALUTENSIN TABLETS (ROBERTS)
SALUTENSIN-DEMI TABLETS (ROBERTS)
SAME PLUS (NUTRACEUTICS)
**SANDIMMUNE I.V. AMPULS FOR
INFUSION** (NOVARTIS)
SANDIMMUNE ORAL SOLUTION (NOVARTIS)
SANDIMMUNE SOFT GELATIN CAPSULES
  (NOVARTIS)
SANDOGLOBULIN I.V. (NOVARTIS)
SANDOSTATIN INJECTION (NOVARTIS)
SANDOSTATIN LAR DEPOT (NOVARTIS)

SANGCYA ORAL SOLUTION (SANGSTAT)
SANOREX TABLETS (NOVARTIS)
SANSERT TABLETS (NOVARTIS)
SAQUINAVIR
  Fortovase Capsules (ROCHE LABS)
SAQUINAVIR MESYLATE
  Invirase Capsules (ROCHE LABS)
SARAPIN (HIGH CHEMICAL)
SARGRAMOSTIM
  Leukine (IMMUNEX)
SARNA LOTION (STIEFEL)
SARRACENIACEAE
  Sarapin (HIGH CHEMICAL)
SASTID SOAP (STIEFEL)
SBR-LIPOCREAM (FERNDALE)
SCANDICAL (SCANDIPHARM)
SCANDISHAKE (SCANDIPHARM)
SCANDISHAKE–LACTOSE FREE
  (SCANDIPHARM)
**SCANDISHAKE–SWEETENED WITH
ASPARTAME** (SCANDIPHARM)
SCLEROMATE INJECTION (GLENWOOD)
SCOPOLAMINE
  Transderm Scop Transdermal Therapeutic
    System (NOVARTIS CONSUMER)
SCOPOLAMINE HYDROBROMIDE
  Atrohist Plus Tablets (MEDEVA)
  Donnatal Capsules (ROBINS)
  Donnatal Elixir (ROBINS)
  Donnatal Extentabs (ROBINS)
  Donnatal Tablets (ROBINS)
SEBIZON LOTION (SCHERING)
SEBULEX DANDRUFF SHAMPOO
  (WESTWOOD-SQUIBB)
**SEBULEX DANDRUFF SHAMPOO WITH
CONDITIONERS** (WESTWOOD-SQUIBB)
SEBULON SHAMPOO (WESTWOOD-SQUIBB)
SEBUTONE TAR SHAMPOO
  (WESTWOOD-SQUIBB)
SECONAL SODIUM (LILLY)
SECTRAL CAPSULES (WYETH-AYERST)
SECTRAL CAPSULES, 200 MG
  (WYETH-AYERST)
SEDAPAP TABLETS 50 MG/650 MG (MERZ)
SELEGILINE HCL CAPSULES (WATSON)
SELEGILINE HCL TABLETS (WATSON)
SELEGILINE HCL TABLETS (ESI LEDERLE)
SELEGILINE HCL TABLETS, 5 MG
  (NOVOPHARM)
SELEGILINE HYDROCHLORIDE
  Ataptryl Tablets (ATHENA)
  Carbex Tablets (ENDO LABS)
  Eldepryl Capsules (SOMERSET)
  Selegiline HCl Capsules (WATSON)
  Selegiline HCl Tablets (WATSON)
  Selegiline HCl Tablets, 5 mg (NOVOPHARM)
  Selegiline Hydrochloride Tablets, USP
    (ENDO GENERICS)
**SELEGILINE HYDROCHLORIDE TABLETS,
USP** (APOTHECON)
**SELEGILINE HYDROCHLORIDE TABLETS,
USP** (ENDO GENERICS)
SELENIUM
  ACES Antioxidant Soft Gels (CARLSON)
  Chelated Mineral Tablets (USANA)
  E + Selenium (MAYOR)
  Revitalizer (MAYOR)
  Vitamist Intra-Oral Spray Dietary Supplements
    (MAYOR)
SELENIUM 200MCG (VITALINE)
SELENIUM SULFIDE
  Exsel Lotion/Shampoo (ALLERGAN)

  Head & Shoulders Intensive Treatment
    Dandruff and Seborrheic Dermatitis
    Shampoo (PROCTER & GAMBLE)
  Selsun Blue Dandruff Shampoo (ROSS)
  Selsun Rx 2.5% Lotion, USP (ROSS)
SELSUN BLUE DANDRUFF SHAMPOO
  (ROSS)
SELSUN RX 2.5% LOTION, USP (ROSS)
SEMPREX-D CAPSULES (MEDEVA)
SENNA
  Perdiem Overnight Relief
    (NOVARTIS CONSUMER)
  Senokot Children's Syrup (PURDUE FREDERICK)
  Senokot Granules (PURDUE FREDERICK)
  Senokot Tablets (PURDUE FREDERICK)
  Senokot-S Tablets (PURDUE FREDERICK)
  SenokotXTRA Tablets (PURDUE FREDERICK)
  X-Prep Liquid (PURDUE FREDERICK)
SENOKOT GRANULES (PURDUE FREDERICK)
SENOKOT SYRUP (PURDUE FREDERICK)
SENOKOT CHILDREN'S SYRUP
  (PURDUE FREDERICK)
SENOKOT TABLETS (PURDUE FREDERICK)
SENOKOT-S TABLETS (PURDUE FREDERICK)
SENOKOTXTRA TABLETS
  (PURDUE FREDERICK)
SENSORCAINE INJECTION (ASTRAZENECA LP)
**SENSORCAINE WITH EPINEPHRINE
INJECTION** (ASTRAZENECA LP)
SENSORCAINE-MPF INJECTION
  (ASTRAZENECA LP)
SENSORCAINE-MPF SPINAL INJECTION
  (ASTRAZENECA LP)
**SENSORCAINE-MPF WITH EPINEPHRINE
INJECTION** (ASTRAZENECA LP)
SEPTRA I.V. INFUSION (MONARCH)
SEPTRA SUSPENSION (MONARCH)
SEPTRA GRAPE SUSPENSION (MONARCH)
SEPTRA TABLETS (MONARCH)
SEPTRA DS TABLETS (MONARCH)
SER-AP-ES TABLETS (NOVARTIS)
SERENTIL AMPULS (BOEHRINGER INGELHEIM)
SERENTIL CONCENTRATE
  (BOEHRINGER INGELHEIM)
SERENTIL TABLETS (BOEHRINGER INGELHEIM)
SEREVENT DISKUS (GLAXO WELLCOME)
SEREVENT INHALATION AEROSOL
  (GLAXO WELLCOME)
SERMORELIN ACETATE
  Geref for Injection (SERONO)
SEROMYCIN CAPSULES (DURA)
SEROPHENE TABLETS (SERONO)
SEROQUEL TABLETS (ASTRAZENECA)
SEROSTIM FOR INJECTION (SERONO)
SERTRALINE HYDROCHLORIDE
  Zoloft Tablets (PFIZER)
SERZONE TABLETS (BRISTOL-MYERS SQUIBB)
SEVELAMER HYDROCHLORIDE
  Renagel Capsules (GENZYME)
SFC LOTION (STIEFEL)
SHARPER FOCUS (VITALINE)
SHEPARD'S CREAM LOTION (DERMIK)
SHEPARD'S SKIN CREAM (DERMIK)
SIBUTRAMINE HYDROCHLORIDE
MONOHYDRATE
  Meridia Capsules (KNOLL)
SILDENAFIL CITRATE
  Viagra Tablets (PFIZER)
SILVADENE CREAM 1% (MONARCH)
**SILVER NITRATE SOLUTIONS 10%, 25%,
50%** (GORDON)
SILVER SULFADIAZINE
  SSD AF Cream (PAR)

UNDERLINE DENOTES GENERIC NAME

SSD Cream (PAR)
Silvadene Cream 1% (MONARCH)
Silver Sulfadiazine Cream (WATSON)
SILVER SULFADIAZINE CREAM (WATSON)

SIMETHICONE

Fast-Acting Mylanta Liquid Antacid
  (J&J – MERCK)
Imodium Advanced Chewable Tablets
  (MCNEIL CONSUMER)
Maximum Strength Fast-Acting Mylanta Liquid
  (J&J – MERCK)
Maximum Strength Maalox Antacid/Anti-Gas
  Liquid (NOVARTIS CONSUMER)
Maximum Strength Mylanta Gas Relief
  Tablets (J&J – MERCK)
Mylanta Gas Relief Gelcaps (J&J – MERCK)
Mylanta Gas Relief Tablets (J&J – MERCK)
Mylicon Infants' Drops (J&J – MERCK)
**SIMILAC PM 60/40 LOW-IRON INFANT
  FORMULA** (ROSS)
SIMPLY SLEEP CAPLETS
  (MCNEIL CONSUMER)
SIMULECT FOR INJECTION (NOVARTIS)

SIMVASTATIN

Zocor Tablets (MERCK)
SINEMET TABLETS (DUPONT)
SINEMET CR TABLETS (DUPONT)
SINEQUAN CAPSULES (PFIZER)
SINEQUAN ORAL CONCENTRATE (PFIZER)
SINGLET TABLETS
  (SMITHKLINE BEECHAM CONSUMER)
SINGULAIR TABLETS (MERCK)
SINGULAIR CHEWABLE TABLETS (MERCK)
SINULIN TABLETS (CARNRICK)
**SINUTAB SINUS ALLERGY MS CAPLETS
  AND TABLETS** (WARNER-LAMBERT)
**SINUTAB SINUS MS WITHOUT
  DROWSINESS CAPLETS AND TABLETS**
  (WARNER-LAMBERT)
SINUTAB NON-DRYING LIQUID CAPS
  (WARNER-LAMBERT)
SINUVENT TABLETS (WE)
SKELAXIN TABLETS (CARNRICK)
SKELID TABLETS (SANOFI)
SLENDER-MIST (MAYOR)
SLO-BID GYROCAPS (RHONE-POULENC RORER)
SLO-NIACIN TABLETS (UPSHER-SMITH)
SLO-PHYLLIN 80 SYRUP
  (RHONE-POULENC RORER)
SLO-PHYLLIN GG CAPSULES
  (RHONE-POULENC RORER)
SLO-PHYLLIN GG SYRUP
  (RHONE-POULENC RORER)
SLO-PHYLLIN TABLETS
  (RHONE-POULENC RORER)
SLOW-K EXTENDED-RELEASE TABLETS
  (NOVARTIS)
SLOW-MAG TABLETS (ROBERTS)
SMOKE-LESS (MAYOR)
**SODIUM ACETATE 40 MEQ, 100 MEQ
  AND 200 MEQ VIALS** (ABBOTT)

SODIUM ACID PHOSPHATE

K-Phos M.F. Tablets (BEACH)
K-Phos No. 2 Tablets (BEACH)
Uroqid-Acid No. 2 Tablets (BEACH)

SODIUM BICARBONATE

Ceo-Two Evacuant Suppository (BEUTLICH)
Colyte - Flavored for Oral Solution (SCHWARZ)
Colyte for Oral Solution (SCHWARZ)
Colyte with Flavor Packs for Oral Solution
  (SCHWARZ)
GoLYTELY and Pineapple Flavor GoLYTELY
  for Oral Solution (BRAINTREE)

NuLYTELY, Cherry Flavor NuLYTELY and
  Lemon-Lime Flavor NuLYTELY for Oral
  Solution (BRAINTREE)
**4.2% SODIUM BICARBONATE INJECTION,
  10 MEQ IN 10 ML ABBOJECT
  (NEONATAL)** (ABBOTT)
**5% SODIUM BICARBONATE INJECTION,
  USP** (ABBOTT)
**7.5% SODIUM BICARBONATE INJECTION,
  44.6 MEQ IN 50 ML AMPUL OR
  ABBOJECT** (ABBOTT)
**8.4% SODIUM BICARBONATE INJECTION,
  10 MEQ IN 10 ML ABBOJECT
  (PEDIATRIC)** (ABBOTT)
**8.4% SODIUM BICARBONATE INJECTION,
  50 MEQ IN 50 ML ABBOJECT OR
  FLIPTOP VIAL** (ABBOTT)
SODIUM BICARBONATE TABLETS (LILLY)

SODIUM CHLORIDE

6% Hetastarch in 0.9% Sodium Chloride
  Injection (BAXTER)
Chlor-3 (FLEMING)
Colyte - Flavored for Oral Solution (SCHWARZ)
Colyte for Oral Solution (SCHWARZ)
Colyte with Flavor Packs for Oral Solution
  (SCHWARZ)
GoLYTELY and Pineapple Flavor GoLYTELY
  for Oral Solution (BRAINTREE)
Inulin and Sodium Chloride Injection (CYPROS)
NuLYTELY, Cherry Flavor NuLYTELY and
  Lemon-Lime Flavor NuLYTELY for Oral
  Solution (BRAINTREE)
Sodium Chloride Inhalation Solution (ROXANE)
Sodium Chloride Inhalation Solutions USP
  (DEY)
Sodium Chloride Injection (Preservative-Free)
  (ELKINS-SINN)
Sodium Chloride Injection, Bacteriostatic
  (ELKINS-SINN)
Sodium Chloride, Bacteriostatic in Tubex
  (WYETH-AYERST)
SODIUM CHLORIDE 0.9% (WYETH-AYERST)
5% SODIUM CHLORIDE (ABBOTT)
**SODIUM CHLORIDE INHALATION
  SOLUTION** (ROXANE)
**SODIUM CHLORIDE INHALATION
  SOLUTIONS USP** (DEY)
**0.45% SODIUM CHLORIDE INJECTION,
  USP** (ABBOTT)
0.9% SODIUM CHLORIDE INJECTION
  (ABBOTT)
**0.9% SODIUM CHLORIDE INJECTION,
  USP (ADD-VANTAGE)** (ABBOTT)
**0.9% SODIUM CHLORIDE INJECTION,
  USP (PARTIAL FILL)** (ABBOTT)
**SODIUM CHLORIDE INJECTION,
  BACTERIOSTATIC** (ELKINS-SINN)
**SODIUM CHLORIDE INJECTION,
  BACTERIOSTATIC** (WYETH-AYERST)
**SODIUM CHLORIDE INJECTION
  (PRESERVATIVE-FREE)** (ELKINS-SINN)
**0.45% SODIUM CHLORIDE IRRIGATION,
  USP (AQUALITE)** (ABBOTT)
**0.9% SODIUM CHLORIDE IRRIGATION,
  USP (FLEX AND AQUALITE)** (ABBOTT)
SODIUM CHLORIDE SOLUTION, 0.9%
  (WYETH-AYERST)
**SODIUM CHLORIDE, BACTERIOSTATIC
  IN TUBEX** (WYETH-AYERST)
SODIUM CHLORIDE, USP (LILLY)

SODIUM CHONDROITIN SULFATE

Cosamin DS Capsules (NUTRAMAX)

SODIUM CITRATE

Bicitra (ALZA)
Citrolith Tablets (BEACH)

Polycitra Syrup and Polycitra-LC Syrup (ALZA)
Sodium Citrate and Citric Acid Oral Solution
  USP (PHARMACEUTICAL ASSOCIATES)
**SODIUM CITRATE AND CITRIC ACID
  ORAL SOLUTION USP**
  (PHARMACEUTICAL ASSOCIATES)

SODIUM FERRIC GLUCONATE

Ferrlecit Injection (SCHEIN)

SODIUM FLUORIDE

Florical Capsules and Tablets (MERICON)
Listermint Alcohol-Free Mouthwash
  (WARNER-LAMBERT)
Luride Drops 50 ml (COLGATE ORAL)
Luride Lozi-Tabs Tablets (COLGATE ORAL)
Pediaflor Drops (ROSS)
PreviDent 5000 Plus Dental Cream
  (COLGATE ORAL)
Vi-Daylin/F ADC Vitamins + Iron Drops
  With Fluoride (ROSS)
Vi-Daylin/F ADC Vitamins Drops With
  Fluoride (ROSS)
Vi-Daylin/F Multivitamin + Iron Chewable
  Tablets With Fluoride (ROSS)
Vi-Daylin/F Multivitamin + Iron Drops With
  Fluoride (ROSS)
Vi-Daylin/F Multivitamin Chewable Tablets
  With Fluoride (ROSS)
Vi-Daylin/F Multivitamin Drops With Fluoride
  (ROSS)

SODIUM HYALURONATE

Hyalgan Solution (SANOFI)
SODIUM HYDROXIDE 10% (GORDON)

SODIUM IOTHALAMATE

Glofil-125 Injection (CYPROS)

SODIUM LACTATE

Eucerin Plus Alpha Hydroxy Creme
  (BEIERSDORF)
Eucerin Plus Alpha Hydroxy Lotion
  (BEIERSDORF)
**SODIUM LACTATE INJECTION, USP, 1/6
  MOLAR** (ABBOTT)

SODIUM NITROPRUSSIDE

Sodium Nitroprusside Injection (BAXTER)
SODIUM NITROPRUSSIDE INJECTION
  (BAXTER)

SODIUM OXYCHLOROSENE

Clorpactin WCS-90 (GUARDIAN)

SODIUM PHOSPHATE

Fleet Enema (FLEET)
Fleet Enema for Children (FLEET)
Fleet Phospho-Soda (FLEET)
Fleet Prep Kits (FLEET)
K-Phos Neutral Tablets (BEACH)
Uro-KP-Neutral Tablets (STAR)
SODIUM PHOSPHATE 45 MMOL (ABBOTT)

SODIUM POLYSTYRENE SULFONATE

Kayexalate Powder (SANOFI)
Kionex Powder (PADDOCK)

SODIUM PROPIONATE

Amino-Cerv Creme (MILEX)
**SODIUM SULAMYD OPHTHALMIC
  OINTMENT 10%-STERILE** (SCHERING)
**SODIUM SULAMYD OPHTHALMIC
  SOLUTION 10%-STERILE** (SCHERING)
**SODIUM SULAMYD OPHTHALMIC
  SOLUTION 30% STERILE** (SCHERING)

SODIUM SULFACETAMIDE

Novacet Lotion (MEDICIS)
Sulfacet-R Lotion (DERMIK)
Sulfacet-R Tint Free Lotion (DERMIK)

SODIUM SULFATE

Colyte - Flavored for Oral Solution (SCHWARZ)
Colyte for Oral Solution (SCHWARZ)
Colyte with Flavor Packs for Oral Solution (SCHWARZ)
GoLYTELY and Pineapple Flavor GoLYTELY for Oral Solution (BRAINTREE)

SODIUM TETRADECYL SULFATE

Sotradecol Injection (ELKINS-SINN)
SOFGUARD FLEXIBLE EYE SHIELD (ALCON)
SOLAQUIN 2% CREAM (ICN)
SOLAQUIN FORTE 4% CREAM (ICN)
SOLAQUIN FORTE 4% GEL (ICN)
SOLBAR AVO LOTION SPF 32 (PERSON & COVEY)
SOLBAR PF CREAM SPF 50 (PABA FREE) (PERSON & COVEY)
SOLBAR PF LIQUID SPF 30 (PERSON & COVEY)
SOLGANAL INJECTABLE SUSPENSION (SCHERING)
SOLU-CORTEF STERILE POWDER (PHARMACIA & UPJOHN)
SOLU-MEDROL STERILE POWDER (PHARMACIA & UPJOHN)
SOMA TABLETS (WALLACE)
SOMA COMPOUND TABLETS (WALLACE)
SOMA COMPOUND W/CODEINE TABLETS (WALLACE)

SOMATREM

Protropin for Injection (GENENTECH)

SOMATROPIN

Genotropin Lyophilized Powder (PHARMACIA & UPJOHN)
Humatrope Vials and Cartridges (LILLY)
Norditropin for Injection (NOVO NORDISK)
Nutropin AQ Injection (GENENTECH)
Nutropin for Injection (GENENTECH)
Saizen for Injection (SERONO)
Serostim for Injection (SERONO)
SONATA CAPSULES (WYETH-AYERST)
SORBIDON HYDRATE (GORDON)

SORBITOL

Actidose with Sorbitol Suspension (PADDOCK)
Sorbitol Solution USP (PHARMACEUTICAL ASSOCIATES)
SORBITOL SOLUTION (UPSHER-SMITH)
SORBITOL SOLUTION USP (PHARMACEUTICAL ASSOCIATES)
SORBITOL SOLUTION USP 70% (PADDOCK)
SORBITOL-MANNITOL IRRIGATION (FLEX & AQUALITE) (ABBOTT)
SORBITRATE CHEWABLE TABLETS (ASTRAZENECA)
SORBITRATE ORAL TABLETS (ASTRAZENECA)
SORBSAN WOUND DRESSING (BERTEK)
SORE THROAT SPRAY (PHARMACEUTICAL ASSOCIATES)
SORIATANE CAPSULES (ROCHE LABS)

SOTALOL HYDROCHLORIDE

Betapace Tablets (BERLEX)
SOTRADECOL INJECTION (ELKINS-SINN)
SPANTUSS LIQUID (ARCO)
SPANTUSS TABLETS (ARCO)

SPARFLOXACIN

Zagam Tablets (BERTEK)
SPEC-T SORE THROAT ANESTHETIC LOZENGES (APOTHECON)
SPECTAZOLE CREAM (ORTHO DERMATOLOGICAL)
SPECTROBID TABLETS (PFIZER)

SPIRONOLACTONE

Aldactazide Tablets (SEARLE)
Aldactone Tablets (SEARLE)
Spironolactone Tablets (MYLAN)
Spironolactone Tablets (GENEVA)
Spironolactone and Hydrochlorothiazide Tablets (MYLAN)
SPIRONOLACTONE TABLETS (MYLAN)
SPIRONOLACTONE TABLETS (GENEVA)
SPIRONOLACTONE AND HYDROCHLOROTHIAZIDE TABLETS (MYLAN)

SPIRULINA

Blue-Green Sea Spray (MAYOR)
Vitamist Intra-Oral Spray Dietary Supplements (MAYOR)
SPORANOX CAPSULES (JANSSEN)
SPORANOX CAPSULES (ORTHO BIOTECH)
SPORANOX INJECTION (JANSSEN)
SPORANOX INJECTION (ORTHO BIOTECH)
SPORANOX ORAL SOLUTION (JANSSEN)
SPORANOX ORAL SOLUTION (ORTHO BIOTECH)
SQUIBB COD LIVER OIL (ROBERTS)
SQUIBB MINERAL OIL (ROBERTS)
SSD CREAM (PAR)
SSD AF CREAM (PAR)
SSKI SOLUTION (UPSHER-SMITH)
ST. JOHN'S WORT 300MG (VITALINE)
ST. JOHN'S WORT 150 MG (MERICON)
STADOL (SEE BRISTOL-MYERS SQUIBB COMPANY) (APOTHECON)
STADOL NS NASAL SPRAY (BRISTOL-MYERS SQUIBB)

STANOZOLOL

Winstrol Tablets (SANOFI)

STARCH

Anusol Hemorrhoidal Suppositories (WARNER-LAMBERT)

STAVUDINE

Zerit Capsules (BRISTOL-MYERSSQUIBBONCOLOGY/IMMUNOLOGY)
Zerit for Oral Solution (BRISTOL-MYERSSQUIBBONCOLOGY/IMMUNOLOGY)
STELAZINE CONCENTRATE (SMITHKLINE BEECHAM)
STELAZINE MULTI-DOSE VIALS (SMITHKLINE BEECHAM)
STELAZINE TABLETS (SMITHKLINE BEECHAM)
STERAPRED 5 MG UNIPAK (MERZ)
STERAPRED 5 MG 12 DAY UNIPAK (MERZ)
STERAPRED DS UNIPAK (MERZ)
STERAPRED DS 12 DAY UNIPAK (MERZ)
STERILE WATER FOR INHALATION USP (DEY)
STERI-UNITS SINGLE DOSE SURGICAL DROPS (ALCON)
STILPHOSTROL AMPULES (BAYER)
STIMATE NASAL SPRAY (CENTEON)
STIMULEAN (VITALINE)
STREPTASE FOR INFUSION (ASTRAZENECA LP)

STREPTOKINASE

Streptase for Infusion (ASTRAZENECA LP)

STREPTOMYCIN SULFATE

Streptomycin Sulfate Injection (PFIZER)
STREPTOMYCIN SULFATE INJECTION (PFIZER)

STREPTOZOCIN

Zanosar Sterile Powder (PHARMACIA & UPJOHN)
STRESS (MAYOR)
STRESS DEFENSE TABS (MDR FITNESS)
STRESS-600 TABLETS (UPSHER-SMITH)

STRESS-600 WITH ZINC TABLETS (UPSHER-SMITH)
STROMECTOL TABLETS (MERCK)
STROVITE FORTE CAPLETS (EVERETT)
STROVITE FORTE SYRUP (EVERETT)
STROVITE PLUS CAPLETS (EVERETT)
STROVITE TABLETS (EVERETT)

SUCCIMER

Chemet Capsules (SANOFI)

SUCCINYLCHOLINE CHLORIDE

Anectine Injection (GLAXO WELLCOME)
Succinylcholine Chloride Injection (ORGANON)
SUCCINYLCHOLINE CHLORIDE INJECTION (ORGANON)

SUCRALFATE

Carafate Suspension (HOECHST MARION ROUSSEL)
Carafate Tablets (HOECHST MARION ROUSSEL)
Sucralfate Tablets (WATSON)
SUCRALFATE TABLETS (WATSON)
SUDAFED 12 HOUR TABLETS (WARNER-LAMBERT)
SUDAFED 24 HOUR TABLETS (WARNER-LAMBERT)
CHILDREN'S SUDAFED COUGH & COLD LIQUID (WARNER-LAMBERT)
CHILDREN'S SUDAFED NASAL DECONGESTANT CHEWABLES (WARNER-LAMBERT)
CHILDREN'S SUDAFED NASAL DECONGESTANT LIQUID (WARNER-LAMBERT)
SUDAFED COLD & ALLERGY TABLETS (WARNER-LAMBERT)
SUDAFED COLD & COUGH LIQUID CAPS (WARNER-LAMBERT)
SUDAFED COLD & SINUS LIQUID CAPS (WARNER-LAMBERT)
SUDAFED NASAL DECONGESTANT 30 MG TABLETS (WARNER-LAMBERT)
SUDAFED NON-DRYING SINUS LIQUID CAPS (WARNER-LAMBERT)
SUDAFED SEVERE COLD FORMULA MS CAPLETS AND TABLETS (WARNER-LAMBERT)
SUDAFED SINUS MS CAPLETS AND TABLETS (WARNER-LAMBERT)
SUFENTA INJECTION (TAYLOR)

SUFENTANIL CITRATE

Sufenta Injection (TAYLOR)
Sufentanil Citrate Injection (ELKINS-SINN)
Sufentanil Citrate Injection, USP (BAXTER)
SUFENTANIL CITRATE INJECTION (ELKINS-SINN)
SUFENTANIL CITRATE INJECTION, USP (BAXTER)
SULAMYD OPHTHALMIC OINTMENT STERILE (SCHERING)
SULAMYD OPHTHALMIC SOLUTION STERILE (SCHERING)
SULAR TABLETS (ASTRAZENECA)

SULBACTAM SODIUM

Unasyn for Injection (PFIZER)

SULFABENZAMIDE

Sultrin Triple Sulfa Cream (ORTHO-MCNEIL)

SULFACETAMIDE

Sultrin Triple Sulfa Cream (ORTHO-MCNEIL)

SULFACETAMIDE SODIUM

Blephamide Ophthalmic Ointment (ALLERGAN)
Blephamide Ophthalmic Suspension (ALLERGAN)
Klaron Lotion 10% (DERMIK)

Sulamyd Ophthalmic Ointment Sterile
(SCHERING)
Sulamyd Ophthalmic Solution Sterile
(SCHERING)
SULFACET-R LOTION (DERMIK)
SULFACET-R TINT FREE LOTION (DERMIK)
SULFAMETH/TRIMETHOPRIM SS & D/S TABLETS, USP (SCHEIN)

SULFAMETHIZOLE
Urobiotic-250 Capsules (PFIZER)

SULFAMETHOXAZOLE
Bactrim DS Tablets (ROCHE LABS)
Bactrim I.V. Infusion (ROCHE LABS)
Bactrim Pediatric Suspension (ROCHE LABS)
Bactrim Tablets (ROCHE LABS)
Septra DS Tablets (MONARCH)
Septra Grape Suspension (MONARCH)
Septra I.V. Infusion (MONARCH)
Septra Suspension (MONARCH)
Septra Tablets (MONARCH)
Sulfamethoxazole & Trimethoprim Concentrate
for Injection (ELKINS-SINN)
Sulfamethoxazole & Trimethoprim Tablets
(LEDERLE STANDARD)
SULFAMETHOXAZOLE & TRIMETHOPRIM CONCENTRATE FOR INJECTION (ELKINS-SINN)
SULFAMETHOXAZOLE & TRIMETHOPRIM TABLETS (LEDERLE STANDARD)
SULFAMETHOXAZOLE AND TRIMETHOPRIM TABLETS (ESI LEDERLE)
SULFAMYLON CREAM (BERTEK)
SULFAMYLON TOPICAL SOLUTION (BERTEK)

SULFANILAMIDE
AVC Cream (MONARCH)
AVC Suppositories (MONARCH)

SULFASALAZINE
Azulfidine EN-tabs Tablets
(PHARMACIA & UPJOHN)
Sulfasalazine Tablets (WATSON)
SULFASALAZINE TABLETS (WATSON)

SULFATHIAZOLE
Sultrin Triple Sulfa Cream (ORTHO-MCNEIL)

SULFISOXAZOLE ACETYL
Erythromycin Ethylsuccinate/ Sulfisoxazole
Acetyl Oral Suspension
(LEDERLE STANDARD)
Pediazole Suspension (ROSS)
SULFOXYL LOTION REGULAR (STIEFEL)
SULFOXYL LOTION STRONG (STIEFEL)

SULFUR
Bensulfoid Cream (ECR)
Novacet Lotion (MEDICIS)
Sulfacet-R Lotion (DERMIK)
Sulfacet-R Tint Free Lotion (DERMIK)
SULFUR SOAP (STIEFEL)

SULINDAC
Clinoril Tablets (MERCK)
Sulindac Tablets (MYLAN)
Sulindac Tablets (GENEVA)
Sulindac Tablets (LEDERLE STANDARD)
Sulindac Tablets, USP (ENDO GENERICS)
SULINDAC TABLETS (MYLAN)
SULINDAC TABLETS (GENEVA)
SULINDAC TABLETS (LEDERLE STANDARD)
SULINDAC TABLETS, USP (SCHEIN)
SULINDAC TABLETS, USP (ENDO GENERICS)
SULTRIN TRIPLE SULFA CREAM (ORTHO-MCNEIL)

SUMATRIPTAN
Imitrex Nasal Spray (GLAXO WELLCOME)

SUMATRIPTAN SUCCINATE
Imitrex Injection (GLAXO WELLCOME)
Imitrex Tablets (GLAXO WELLCOME)
SUMYCIN TABLETS, CAPSULES AND SYRUP (APOTHECON)
SUNBLOCK STICK SPF25 (NEUTROGENA)
SUNKIST CHILDREN'S CHEWABLE MULTIVITAMINS - COMPLETE (NOVARTIS CONSUMER)
SUNKIST CHILDREN'S CHEWABLE MULTIVITAMINS - PLUS EXTRA C (NOVARTIS CONSUMER)
SUNKIST VITAMIN C - CHEWABLE (NOVARTIS CONSUMER)
SUNKIST VITAMIN C ROLLS (NOVARTIS CONSUMER)
SUNLESS TANNING LOTION – BODY (NEUTROGENA)
SUNLESS TANNING LOTION – FACE (NEUTROGENA)
SUPEREPA SOFTGELS (ADVANCED NUTRITIONAL)
SUPEROXIDE DISMUTASE (VITALINE)
SUPPRELIN INJECTION (ROBERTS)
SUPRANE LIQUID FOR INHALATION (BAXTER)
SUPRAX FOR ORAL SUSPENSION (LEDERLE LABS)
SUPRAX TABLETS (LEDERLE LABS)
SURBEX 750 WITH ZINC FILMTAB (ABBOTT)
SURBEX WITH C FILMTAB (ABBOTT)
SURBEX-T FILMTAB (ABBOTT)
SURMONTIL CAPSULES (WYETH-AYERST)
SURVANTA INTRATRACHEAL SUSPENSION (ROSS)
SUSPENDOL-S (PADDOCK)
SUSTIVA CAPSULES (DUPONT)
SYLLACT POWDER (WALLACE)
SYMBIOTROPIN (NUTRACEUTICS)
SYMMETREL SYRUP (ENDO LABS)
SYMMETREL TABLETS (ENDO LABS)
SYNAGIS INTRAMUSCULAR (MEDIMMUNE)
SYNALAR CREAM (MEDICIS)
SYNALAR OINTMENT (MEDICIS)
SYNALAR TOPICAL SOLUTION (MEDICIS)
SYNALGOS-DC CAPSULES (WYETH-AYERST)
SYNAREL NASAL SOLUTION FOR CENTRAL PRECOCIOUS PUBERTY (SEARLE)
SYNAREL NASAL SOLUTION FOR ENDOMETRIOSIS (SEARLE)
SYNEMOL CREAM (MEDICIS)
SYN-RX TABLETS 14 DAY TREATMENT REGIMEN (MEDEVA)
SYN-RX DM TABLETS 14 DAY TREATMENT REGIMEN (MEDEVA)
SYNTHROID INJECTION (KNOLL)
SYNTHROID TABLETS (KNOLL)
SYNTOCINON INJECTION (NOVARTIS)
SYNVISC (WYETH-AYERST)
SYPRINE CAPSULES (MERCK)

T

T/GEL EXTRA STRENGTH THERAPEUTIC SHAMPOO (4% NEUTAR) (NEUTROGENA)
T/GEL THERAPEUTIC CONDITIONER (NEUTROGENA)
T/GEL THERAPEUTIC SHAMPOO (2% NEUTAR) (NEUTROGENA)
MAXIMUM STRENGTH T/SAL THERAPEUTIC SHAMPOO (3% SALICYLIC ACID) (NEUTROGENA)

TACRINE HYDROCHLORIDE
Cognex Capsules (PARKE-DAVIS)

TACROLIMUS
Prograf (FUJISAWA)
TAGAMET HB 200 TABLETS (SMITHKLINE BEECHAM CONSUMER)
TAGAMET INJECTION (SMITHKLINE BEECHAM)
TAGAMET LIQUID (SMITHKLINE BEECHAM)
TAGAMET TABLETS (SMITHKLINE BEECHAM)
TALACEN CAPLETS (SANOFI)
TALWIN COMPOUND CAPLETS (SANOFI)
TALWIN NX TABLETS (SANOFI)
TAMBOCOR TABLETS (3M)

TAMOXIFEN CITRATE
Nolvadex Tablets (ASTRAZENECA)

TAMSULOSIN HYDROCHLORIDE
Flomax Capsules (BOEHRINGER INGELHEIM)
TANAFED SUSPENSION (HORIZON)
TAO CAPSULES (PFIZER)
TAPAZOLE TABLETS (JONES)
TARKA TABLETS (KNOLL)
TASMAR TABLETS (ROCHE LABS)
TAVIST ALLERGY 12 HOUR RELIEF ANTIHISTAMINE (FORMERLY TAVIST-1) (NOVARTIS CONSUMER)
TAVIST D 12 HOUR RELIEF ANTIHISTAMINE/NASAL DECONGESTANT (NOVARTIS CONSUMER)
TAVIST SINUS PAIN RELIEVER/NASAL DECONGESTANT (NOVARTIS CONSUMER)
TAVIST SYRUP (NOVARTIS)
TAVIST TABLETS (NOVARTIS)
TAXOL INJECTION (BRISTOL-MYERSSQUIBBONCOLOGY/IMMUNOLOGY)
TAXOTERE FOR INJECTION CONCENTRATE (RHONE-POULENC RORER)

TAZAROTENE
Tazorac Gel (ALLERGAN)
TAZICEF FOR INJECTION (SMITHKLINE BEECHAM)
TAZIDIME VIALS, FASPAK & ADD-VANTAGE (LILLY)

TAZOBACTAM SODIUM
Zosyn (LEDERLE LABS)
Zosyn Pharmacy Bulk Package (LEDERLE LABS)
Zosyn in Galaxy Containers (LEDERLE LABS)
TAZORAC GEL (ALLERGAN)
TE ANATOXAL BERNA (BERNA)
TEARS NATURALE FREE LUBRICANT EYE DROPS (ALCON)
TEARS NATURALE II LUBRICANT EYE DROPS (ALCON)
TECZEM TABLETS (HOECHST MARION ROUSSEL)
TEGREEN 97 CAPSULES (PHARMANEX)
TEGRETOL CHEWABLE TABLETS (NOVARTIS)
TEGRETOL SUSPENSION (NOVARTIS)
TEGRETOL TABLETS (NOVARTIS)
TEGRETOL-XR TABLETS (NOVARTIS)

TELMISARTAN
Micardis Tablets (BOEHRINGER INGELHEIM)

TEMAZEPAM
Temazepam Capsules (PAR)
Temazepam Capsules (MYLAN)

Temazepam Capsules (GENEVA)
TEMAZEPAM CAPSULES (PAR)
TEMAZEPAM CAPSULES (MYLAN)
TEMAZEPAM CAPSULES (GENEVA)
TEMOVATE CREAM (GLAXO WELLCOME)
TEMOVATE E EMOLLIENT
(GLAXO WELLCOME)
TEMOVATE GEL (GLAXO WELLCOME)
TEMOVATE OINTMENT (GLAXO WELLCOME)
TEMOVATE SCALP APPLICATION
(GLAXO WELLCOME)
**TEMPRA 1 ASPIRIN FREE INFANT
DROPS, TEMPRA 2 ASPIRIN FREE
TODDLER SYRUP** (BRISTOL-MYERS)
**TEMPRA QUICKLETS ASPIRIN FREE
JUNIOR AND CHILDREN'S STRENGTHS**
(BRISTOL-MYERS)
TENEX TABLETS (ROBINS)

TENIPOSIDE

Vumon for Injection
(BRISTOL-MYERSSQUIBBONCOLOGY/IMMUNOLOGY)
TENORETIC TABLETS (ASTRAZENECA)
**TENORMIN TABLETS AND I.V.
INJECTION** (ASTRAZENECA)
TENSILON INJECTABLE (ICN)
TENUATE TABLETS/DOSPAN
(HOECHST MARION ROUSSEL)
TERAZOL 3 VAGINAL CREAM
(ORTHO-MCNEIL)
TERAZOL 3 VAGINAL SUPPOSITORIES
(ORTHO-MCNEIL)
TERAZOL 7 VAGINAL CREAM
(ORTHO-MCNEIL)

TERAZOSIN HYDROCHLORIDE

Hytrin Capsules (ABBOTT)

TERBINAFINE HYDROCHLORIDE

Lamisil Tablets (NOVARTIS)

TERBUTALINE SULFATE

Brethine Ampuls (NOVARTIS)
Brethine Tablets (NOVARTIS)

TERCONAZOLE

Terazol 3 Vaginal Cream (ORTHO-MCNEIL)
Terazol 3 Vaginal Suppositories
(ORTHO-MCNEIL)
Terazol 7 Vaginal Cream (ORTHO-MCNEIL)
**TERRA-CORTRIL OPHTHALMIC
SUSPENSION** (PFIZER)
**TERRAMYCIN INTRAMUSCULAR
SOLUTION** (PFIZER)
**TERRAMYCIN WITH POLYMYXIN B
SULFATE OPHTHALMIC OINTMENT**
(PFIZER)
TESLAC TABLETS
(BRISTOL-MYERSSQUIBBONCOLOGY/IMMUNOLOGY)
TESSALON PERLES (FOREST)
TESTODERM TRANSDERMAL SYSTEMS
(ALZA)

TESTOLACTONE

Teslac Tablets
(BRISTOL-MYERSSQUIBBONCOLOGY/IMMUNOLOGY)

TESTOSTERONE

Androderm Transdermal System CIII (WATSON)
Testoderm Transdermal Systems (ALZA)

TESTOSTERONE CYPIONATE

Virilon IM Injection (STAR)

TESTOSTERONE ENANTHATE

Delatestryl Injection (BTG)
**TESTOSTERONE USP MICRONIZED NON-
STERILE POWDER CIII** (PADDOCK)
**TESTOSTERONE PROPIONATE USP
MICRONIZED NON-STERILE POWDER
CIII** (PADDOCK)

TESTRED CAPSULES, 10 MG (ICN)
TESTURIA (WYETH-AYERST)

TETANUS & DIPHTHERIA TOXOIDS
ADSORBED

Tetanus & Diphtheria Toxoids Adsorbed
Purogenated (LEDERLE LABS)
Tetanus and Diphtheria Toxoids Adsorbed For
Adult Use (PASTEUR MERIEUX CONNAUGHT)
**TETANUS & DIPHTHERIA TOXOIDS
ADSORBED PUROGENATED**
(LEDERLE LABS)
**TETANUS AND DIPHTHERIA TOXOIDS
ADSORBED FOR ADULT USE**
(PASTEUR MERIEUX CONNAUGHT)

TETANUS IMMUNE GLOBULIN (HUMAN)

BayTet (BAYER BIOLOGICAL)
**TETANUS TOXOID ADSORBED
PUROGENATED** (LEDERLE LABS)
TETANUS TOXOID ADSORBED USP
(PASTEUR MERIEUX CONNAUGHT)
TETANUS TOXOID USP
(PASTEUR MERIEUX CONNAUGHT)

TETANUS TOXOID, ADSORBED

TE Anatoxal Berna (BERNA)
Tetanus Toxoid Adsorbed Purogenated
(LEDERLE LABS)

TETRACAINE HYDROCHLORIDE

Cetacaine Topical Anesthetic (CETYLITE)
TETRACYCLINE HCL CAPSULES
(LEDERLE STANDARD)

TETRACYCLINE HYDROCHLORIDE

Achromycin V Capsules (LEDERLE LABS)
Tetracycline HCl Capsules
(LEDERLE STANDARD)
Tetracycline Hydrochloride Capsules (MYLAN)
**TETRACYCLINE HYDROCHLORIDE
CAPSULES** (MYLAN)
TETRACYCLINE OINTMENT 3%
(LEDERLE STANDARD)
TETRAMUNE (LEDERLE LABS)

THALIDOMIDE

Thalomid Capsules (CELGENE)
THALITONE TABLETS (MONARCH)
THALOMID CAPSULES (CELGENE)
THAM SOLUTION (ABBOTT)
THEO-24 EXTENDED RELEASE CAPSULES
(UCB)
THEOCHRON TABLETS (FOREST)
**THEO-DUR EXTENDED-RELEASE
TABLETS** (KEY)
THEOLAIR TABLETS (3M)

THEOPHYLLINE

Aerolate III T.D. Capsules (FLEMING)
Aerolate Jr. T.D. Capsules (FLEMING)
Aerolate Liquid (FLEMING)
Aerolate Sr. T.D. Capsules (FLEMING)
Marax Tablets & DF Syrup (PFIZER)
Slo-Phyllin 80 Syrup (RHONE-POULENC RORER)
Slo-Phyllin GG Capsules
(RHONE-POULENC RORER)
Slo-Phyllin GG Syrup (RHONE-POULENC RORER)
Slo-Phyllin Tablets (RHONE-POULENC RORER)
Slo-bid Gyrocaps (RHONE-POULENC RORER)
Theo-24 Extended Release Capsules (UCB)
Theo-Dur Extended-Release Tablets (KEY)
Theo-X Extended-Release Tablets (CARNRICK)
Theolair Tablets (3M)
Theophylline Oral Solution (ROXANE)
Uni-Dur Extended-Release Tablets (KEY)
Uniphyl 400 mg and 600 mg Tablets
(PURDUE FREDERICK)

**THEOPHYLLINE IN 5% DEXTROSE
INJECTION (0.4, 0.8, 1.6, 2, 3.2, 4
MG/ML)** (ABBOTT)
THEOPHYLLINE ORAL SOLUTION
(ROXANE)
THEO-X EXTENDED-RELEASE TABLETS
(CARNRICK)
THERACYS (PASTEUR MERIEUX CONNAUGHT)
**THERAFLU FLU AND COLD HOT LIQUID
MEDICINE** (NOVARTIS CONSUMER)
**THERAFLU FLU, COLD & COUGH
LEMON FLAVORED HOT LIQUID
MEDICINE** (NOVARTIS CONSUMER)
**THERAFLU MAXIMUM STRENGTH
NIGHTTIME FLU, COLD & COUGH
LEMON FLAVORED HOT LIQUID
MEDICINE** (NOVARTIS CONSUMER)
**THERAFLU MAXIMUM STRENGTH NO
DROWSINESS FLU, COLD & COUGH
LEMON FLAVORED HOT LIQUID
MEDICINE** (NOVARTIS CONSUMER)
**THERAFLU MAXIMUM STRENGTH SORE
THROAT & COLD APPLE CINNAMON
FLAVORED HOT LIQUID MEDICINE**
(NOVARTIS CONSUMER)
**THERAFLU MAXIMUM STRENGTH SORE
THROAT & COUGH CHERRY
FLAVORED HOT LIQUID MEDICINE**
(NOVARTIS CONSUMER)
**THERAFLU MAXIMUM STRENGTH NON-
DROWSY FLU, COLD & COUGH
CAPLETS** (NOVARTIS CONSUMER)
**THERAFLU MAXIMUM STRENGTH
NIGHTTIME FLU, COLD & COUGH
CAPLETS** (NOVARTIS CONSUMER)
THERA-GESIC CREME (MISSION)
THERAGRAN HEMATINIC (APOTHECON)
**THERAGRAN, HIGH POTENCY
MULTIVITAMINS** (BRISTOL-MYERS)
**THERAGRAN, HIGH POTENCY
MULTIVITAMIN LIQUID WITH
MINERALS** (BRISTOL-MYERS)
**THERAGRAN STRESS FORMULA HIGH
POTENCY MULTIVITAMINS WITH
MINERALS AND VITAMIN C & E**
(BRISTOL-MYERS)
**THERAGRAN-M, HIGH POTENCY
MULTIVITAMINS** (BRISTOL-MYERS)
THERAMYCIN Z TOPICAL SOLUTION
(BIOGLAN)
**THERAPEUTIC B COMPLEX WITH
VITAMIN C CAPSULES** (UPSHER-SMITH)
THERAPEUTIC MINERAL ICE
(BRISTOL-MYERS)
**THERAPEUTIC MINERAL ICE EXERCISE
FORMULA** (BRISTOL-MYERS)
THERAPEUTIC MULTIVITAMIN TABLETS
(UPSHER-SMITH)
**THERAPEUTIC MULTIVITAMIN WITH
MINERALS TABLETS** (UPSHER-SMITH)

THIABENDAZOLE

Mintezol Chewable Tablets (MERCK)
Mintezol Suspension (MERCK)

THIAMINE HYDROCHLORIDE

Thiamine Hydrochloride Injection (ELKINS-SINN)
THIAMINE HYDROCHLORIDE INJECTION
(ELKINS-SINN)

THIAMINE MONONITRATE

Mega-B Tablets (ARCO)

THIOGUANINE

Thioguanine Tablets, Tabloid Brand
(GLAXO WELLCOME)
**THIOGUANINE TABLETS, TABLOID
BRAND** (GLAXO WELLCOME)

UNDERLINE DENOTES GENERIC NAME

THIOLA TABLETS (MISSION)

THIOPENTAL SODIUM

Thiopental Sodium for Injection, USP
(BAXTER)

THIOPENTAL SODIUM FOR INJECTION, USP (BAXTER)

THIOPLEX FOR INJECTION (IMMUNEX)

THIORIDAZINE HCL INTENSOL (ROXANE)

THIORIDAZINE HCL TABLETS (GENEVA)

THIORIDAZINE HYDROCHLORIDE

Thioridazine HCl Intensol (ROXANE)
Thioridazine HCl Tablets (GENEVA)
Thioridazine Hydrochloride Tablets (MYLAN)

THIORIDAZINE HYDROCHLORIDE TABLETS (MYLAN)

THIOTEPA

Thioplex for Injection (IMMUNEX)

THIOTHIXENE

Navane Capsules (PFIZER)
Thiothixene Capsules (MYLAN)
Thiothixene Capsules (GENEVA)

THIOTHIXENE CAPSULES (MYLAN)

THIOTHIXENE CAPSULES (GENEVA)

THIOTHIXENE HYDROCHLORIDE

Navane Concentrate (PFIZER)
Navane Intramuscular (PFIZER)

THONZONIUM BROMIDE

Cortisporin-TC Otic Suspension (MONARCH)

THORAZINE AMPULS (SMITHKLINE BEECHAM)

THORAZINE CONCENTRATE (SMITHKLINE BEECHAM)

THORAZINE MULTI-DOSE VIALS (SMITHKLINE BEECHAM)

THORAZINE SPANSULE CAPSULES (SMITHKLINE BEECHAM)

THORAZINE SUPPOSITORIES (SMITHKLINE BEECHAM)

THORAZINE SYRUP (SMITHKLINE BEECHAM)

THORAZINE TABLETS (SMITHKLINE BEECHAM)

THROMBATE III (BAYER BIOLOGICAL)

THROMBIN

Thrombin-JMI (JONES)

THROMBIN-JMI (JONES)

THYMOGLOBULIN FOR INJECTION (SANGSTAT)

THYMOL

Cool Mint Listerine (WARNER-LAMBERT)
FreshBurst Listerine (WARNER-LAMBERT)
Listerine Antiseptic (WARNER-LAMBERT)

THYMUS 200 (VITALINE)

THYREL TRH (FERRING)

THYROGEN FOR INJECTION (GENZYME)

THYROID

Armour Thyroid Tablets (FOREST)

THYROLAR TABLETS (FOREST)

THYROTROPIN ALFA

Thyrogen for Injection (GENZYME)

TIAGABINE HYDROCHLORIDE

Gabitril Filmtab Tablets (ABBOTT)

TIAMATE TABLETS (HOECHST MARION ROUSSEL)

TIAZAC CAPSULES (FOREST)

TICAR FOR INJECTION (SMITHKLINE BEECHAM)

TICARCILLIN DISODIUM

Ticar for Injection (SMITHKLINE BEECHAM)
Timentin for Injection (SMITHKLINE BEECHAM)

TICE BCG, BCG LIVE (ORGANON)

TICLID TABLETS (ROCHE LABS)

TICLOPIDINE HCL TABLETS (PAR)

TICLOPIDINE HYDROCHLORIDE

Ticlid Tablets (ROCHE LABS)

TIGAN CAPSULES (ROBERTS)

TIGAN INJECTABLE (ROBERTS)

TIGAN SUPPOSITORIES (ROBERTS)

TILADE INHALER (RHONE-POULENC RORER)

TILUDRONATE DISODIUM

Skelid Tablets (SANOFI)

TIMENTIN FOR INJECTION (SMITHKLINE BEECHAM)

TIMOLIDE TABLETS (MERCK)

TIMOLOL MALEATE

Blocadren Tablets (MERCK)
Cosopt Sterile Ophthalmic Solution (MERCK)
Timolide Tablets (MERCK)
Timolol Maleate Tablets (MYLAN)
Timolol Maleate Tablets, USP (ENDO GENERICS)
Timoptic Sterile Ophthalmic Solution (MERCK)
Timoptic in Ocudose (MERCK)
Timoptic-XE Sterile Ophthalmic Gel Forming Solution (MERCK)

TIMOLOL MALEATE TABLETS (MYLAN)

TIMOLOL MALEATE TABLETS, USP (ENDO GENERICS)

TIMOPTIC IN OCUDOSE (MERCK)

TIMOPTIC STERILE OPHTHALMIC SOLUTION (MERCK)

TIMOPTIC-XE STERILE OPHTHALMIC GEL FORMING SOLUTION (MERCK)

TIN-BEN DISPENSER (FERNDALE)

TIN-CO-BEN DISPENSER (FERNDALE)

TINE TEST PPD (LEDERLE LABS)

TIOPRONIN

Thiola Tablets (MISSION)

TIROFIBAN HYDROCHLORIDE

Aggrastat Injection (MERCK)
Aggrastat Injection Premixed (MERCK)

TI-SCREEN SUNSCREENS, SUNBLOCK, SPORTSGEL, AND LIP PROTECTANT (PEDINOL)

TITANIUM DIOXIDE

Eucerin Protective Moisture Lotion SPF 25 (BEIERSDORF)

TIZANIDINE HYDROCHLORIDE

Zanaflex Tablets (ATHENA)

TOBI SOLUTION FOR INHALATION (PATHOGENESIS)

TOBRADEX OPHTHALMIC OINTMENT (ALCON)

TOBRADEX OPHTHALMIC SUSPENSION (ALCON)

TOBRAMYCIN

TOBI Solution for Inhalation (PATHOGENESIS)
TobraDex Ophthalmic Ointment (ALCON)
TobraDex Ophthalmic Suspension (ALCON)

TOBRAMYCIN SULFATE

Nebcin Vials, Hyporets & ADD-Vantage (LILLY)
Tobramycin Sulfate Injection (LEDERLE STANDARD)

TOBRAMYCIN SULFATE INJECTION (LEDERLE STANDARD)

TOBRAMYCIN SULFATE INJECTION USP (APOTHECON)

TOCAINIDE HYDROCHLORIDE

Tonocard Tablets (ASTRAZENECA LP)

TOFRANIL TABLETS (NOVARTIS)

TOFRANIL-PM CAPSULES (NOVARTIS)

TOLAZAMIDE

Tolazamide Tablets (MYLAN)

TOLAZAMIDE TABLETS (MYLAN)

TOLBUTAMIDE

Tolbutamide Tablets (MYLAN)

TOLBUTAMIDE TABLETS (MYLAN)

TOLCAPONE

Tasmar Tablets (ROCHE LABS)

TOLECTIN 200 TABLETS (ORTHO-MCNEIL)

TOLECTIN 600 TABLETS (ORTHO-MCNEIL)

TOLECTIN DS CAPSULES (ORTHO-MCNEIL)

TOLINASE TABLETS (PHARMACIA & UPJOHN)

TOLMETIN SODIUM

Tolectin 200 Tablets (ORTHO-MCNEIL)
Tolectin 600 Tablets (ORTHO-MCNEIL)
Tolectin DS Capsules (ORTHO-MCNEIL)
Tolmetin Sodium Capsules USP, 400 mg (NOVOPHARM)
Tolmetin Sodium Capsules and Tablets (MYLAN)

TOLMETIN SODIUM CAPSULES AND TABLETS (MYLAN)

TOLMETIN SODIUM CAPSULES USP, 400 MG (NOVOPHARM)

TOLTERODINE TARTRATE

Detrol Tablets (PHARMACIA & UPJOHN)

TONOCARD TABLETS (ASTRAZENECA LP)

TOPAMAX SPRINKLE CAPSULES (ORTHO-MCNEIL)

TOPAMAX TABLETS (ORTHO-MCNEIL)

TOPICLUDE OCCLUSIVE DRESSING (FERNDALE)

TOPICORT CREAM (MEDICIS)

TOPICORT GEL (MEDICIS)

TOPICORT OINTMENT (MEDICIS)

TOPICORT LP CREAM (MEDICIS)

TOPIRAMATE

Topamax Sprinkle Capsules (ORTHO-MCNEIL)
Topamax Tablets (ORTHO-MCNEIL)

TOPOTECAN HYDROCHLORIDE

Hycamtin for Injection (SMITHKLINE BEECHAM)

TOPROL-XL TABLETS (ASTRAZENECA LP)

TORADOL IM INJECTION, IV INJECTION (ROCHE LABS)

TORADOL TABLETS (ROCHE LABS)

TOREMIFENE CITRATE

Fareston Tablets (SCHERING)

TORNALATE METERED DOSE INHALER (DURA)

TORNALATE SOLUTION FOR INHALATION, 0.2% (DURA)

TORSEMIDE

Demadex Tablets and Injection (ROCHE LABS)

TOTAL FORMULA 1, 2 AND 3 (MULTIVITAMIN-MULTIMINERAL) (VITALINE)

TOTAL-E SOFTGELS (WESTLAKE)

TOTEPHAN CREME (PEDINOL)

T-PHYL TABLETS (PURDUE FREDERICK)

TPN ELECTROLYTES (ABBOTT)

TRACRIUM INJECTION (GLAXO WELLCOME)

TRAMADOL HYDROCHLORIDE

Ultram Tablets (ORTHO-MCNEIL)

TRANDATE INJECTION (FARO)

TRANDATE TABLETS (FARO)

TRANDOLAPRIL

Mavik Tablets (KNOLL)
Tarka Tablets (KNOLL)

TRANSDERM SCOP TRANSDERMAL THERAPEUTIC SYSTEM (NOVARTIS CONSUMER)

TRANSDERM-NITRO (NOVARTIS)

TRANXENE T-TAB TABLETS (ABBOTT)

UNDERLINE DENOTES GENERIC NAME

**TRANXENE-SD HALF STRENGTH
TABLETS** (ABBOTT)
TRANXENE-SD TABLETS (ABBOTT)

TRANYLCYPROMINE SULFATE

Parnate Tablets (SMITHKLINE BEECHAM)

TRASTUZUMAB

Herceptin I.V. (GENENTECH)
TRASYLOL INJECTION (BAYER)
TRAUMEEL GEL (HEEL)
TRAUMEEL INJECTION SOLUTION (HEEL)
TRAUMEEL OINTMENT (HEEL)
TRAUMEEL ORAL DROPS (HEEL)
TRAUMEEL ORAL LIQUID IN VIALS
(HEEL)
TRAUMEEL TABLETS (HEEL)
TRAZODONE HCL TABLETS (GENEVA)

TRAZODONE HYDROCHLORIDE

Trazodone HCl Tablets (GENEVA)
**TRAZODONE HYDROCHLORIDE
TABLETS, USP** (APOTHECON)
TRAZODONE TABLETS, USP (SCHEIN)
TRECATOR-SC TABLETS (WYETH-AYERST)
TRENTAL TABLETS
(HOECHST MARION ROUSSEL)

TRETINOIN

Avita Cream (BERTEK)
Avita Gel (BERTEK)
Renova Cream (ORTHO DERMATOLOGICAL)
Retin-A Cream/Gel/Liquid
(ORTHO DERMATOLOGICAL)
Retin-A Micro Microsphere, 0.1%
(ORTHO DERMATOLOGICAL)
Tretinoin Cream (GENEVA)
Vesanoid Capsules (ROCHE LABS)
TRETINOIN CREAM (GENEVA)
TRI-CHLOR (GORDON)
TRIAD CAPSULES (FOREST)

TRIAMCINOLONE ACETONIDE

Aristocort A 0.025% Cream (FUJISAWA)
Aristocort A 0.1% Cream (FUJISAWA)
Aristocort A 0.1% Ointment (FUJISAWA)
Aristocort A 0.5% Cream (FUJISAWA)
Azmacort Inhalation Aerosol
(RHONE-POULENC RORER)
Mytrex Cream (SAVAGE)
Mytrex Ointment (SAVAGE)
Nasacort AQ Nasal Spray
(RHONE-POULENC RORER)
Nasacort Nasal Inhaler
(RHONE-POULENC RORER)
**TRIAMCINOLONE ACETONIDE USP
MICRONIZED POWDER** (PADDOCK)

TRIAMCINOLONE DIACETATE

Aristocort Suspension (Forte Parenteral)
(FUJISAWA)
Aristocort Suspension (Intralesional) (FUJISAWA)

TRIAMCINOLONE HEXACETONIDE

Aristospan Suspension (Intra-articular)
(FUJISAWA)
Aristospan Suspension (Intralesional)
(FUJISAWA)
**TRIAMINIC AM COUGH &
DECONGESTANT** (NOVARTIS CONSUMER)
TRIAMINIC AM DECONGESTANT
(NOVARTIS CONSUMER)
TRIAMINIC DM COUGH RELIEF
(NOVARTIS CONSUMER)
TRIAMINIC EXPECTORANT
(NOVARTIS CONSUMER)
TRIAMINIC EXPECTORANT DH
(NOVARTIS CONSUMER)

**TRIAMINIC INFANT ORAL
DECONGESTANT DROPS**
(NOVARTIS CONSUMER)
TRIAMINIC NIGHT TIME
(NOVARTIS CONSUMER)
**TRIAMINIC RX PEDIATRIC ORAL
SOLUTION** (NOVARTIS CONSUMER)
TRIAMINIC SEVERE COLD & FEVER
(NOVARTIS CONSUMER)
TRIAMINIC SORE THROAT
(NOVARTIS CONSUMER)
TRIAMINIC SYRUP COLD & ALLERGY
(NOVARTIS CONSUMER)
**TRIAMINIC TRIAMINICOL COLD &
COUGH** (NOVARTIS CONSUMER)

TRIAMTERENE

Dyazide Capsules (SMITHKLINE BEECHAM)
Dyrenium Capsules (SMITHKLINE BEECHAM)
Maxzide Tablets (BERTEK)
Maxzide-25 mg Tablets (BERTEK)
Triamterene and Hydrochlorothiazide Capsules
and Tablets (MYLAN)
Triamterene and Hydrochlorothiazide Tablets,
USP (WATSON)
Triamterene/HCTZ (Dyazide) 37.5mg/25mg
Capsules (GENEVA)
Triamterene/HCTZ (Maxzide) 75mg/50mg
Tablets (GENEVA)
Triamterene/HCTZ (mini-Maxzide)
37.5mg/25mg Tablets (GENEVA)
Triamterene/HCTZ 50mg/25mg Capsules
(GENEVA)
**TRIAMTERENE AND
HYDROCHLOROTHIAZIDE CAPSULES
AND TABLETS** (MYLAN)
**TRIAMTERENE AND
HYDROCHLOROTHIAZIDE TABLETS,
USP** (WATSON)
**TRIAMTERENE/HCTZ 50MG/25MG
CAPSULES** (GENEVA)
TRIAMTERENE/HCTZ CAPSULES (DURAMED)
**TRIAMTERENE/HCTZ (DYAZIDE)
37.5MG/25MG CAPSULES** (GENEVA)
**TRIAMTERENE/HCTZ (MINI-MAXZIDE)
37.5MG/25MG TABLETS** (GENEVA)
**TRIAMTERENE/HCTZ (MAXZIDE)
75MG/50MG TABLETS** (GENEVA)
TRIAVIL TABLETS (LOTUS)
TRIAZ CLEANSER (MEDICIS)
TRIAZ GEL (MEDICIS)

TRIAZOLAM

Halcion Tablets (PHARMACIA & UPJOHN)
Triazolam Tablets (PAR)
Triazolam Tablets (ROXANE)
TRIAZOLAM TABLETS (PAR)
TRIAZOLAM TABLETS (ROXANE)
**TRICHOTINE POWDER, VAGINAL
DOUCHE** (SCHWARZ)
TRICITRATES ORAL SOLUTION
(PHARMACEUTICAL ASSOCIATES)

TRICLOSAN

Cetaphil Antibacterial Gentle Cleansing Bar
(GALDERMA)
TRICOR CAPSULES, MICRONIZED (ABBOTT)
TRIDESILON CREAM (BAYER)
TRIDESILON OINTMENT (BAYER)
TRIDIONE DULCET TABLETS (ABBOTT)

TRIENTINE HYDROCHLORIDE

Syprine Capsules (MERCK)

TRIETHANOLAMINE POLYPEPTIDE OLEATE-
CONDENSATE

Cerumenex Eardrops (PURDUE FREDERICK)
TRIFLUOPERAZINE HCL TABLETS
(GENEVA)

TRIFLUOPERAZINE HYDROCHLORIDE

Stelazine Concentrate (SMITHKLINE BEECHAM)
Stelazine Multi-dose Vials
(SMITHKLINE BEECHAM)
Stelazine Tablets (SMITHKLINE BEECHAM)
Trifluoperazine HCl Tablets (GENEVA)
Trifluoperazine Hydrochloride Tablets (MYLAN)
**TRIFLUOPERAZINE HYDROCHLORIDE
TABLETS** (MYLAN)

TRIFLURIDINE

Viroptic Ophthalmic Solution, 1% Sterile
(MONARCH)
TRIHEXYPHENIDYL HCL TABLETS, USP
(WATSON)
TRIHEXYPHENIDYL HCL TABLETS, USP
(SCHEIN)

TRIHEXYPHENIDYL HYDROCHLORIDE

Artane Elixir (LEDERLE LABS)
Artane Tablets (LEDERLE LABS)
Trihexyphenidyl HCl Tablets, USP (WATSON)
Trihexyphenidyl Hydrochloride Elixir USP
(PHARMACEUTICAL ASSOCIATES)
**TRIHEXYPHENIDYL HYDROCHLORIDE
ELIXIR USP** (PHARMACEUTICAL ASSOCIATES)
TRIHIBIT (SEE ACTHIB AND TRIPEDIA)
(PASTEUR MERIEUX CONNAUGHT)
TRIKOF-D TABLETS (RESPA)
TRILAFON CONCENTRATE (SCHERING)
TRILAFON INJECTION (SCHERING)
TRILAFON TABLETS (SCHERING)
TRI-LEVLEN 21 TABLETS (BERLEX)
TRI-LEVLEN 28 TABLETS (BERLEX)
TRILISATE LIQUID (PURDUE FREDERICK)
TRILISATE TABLETS (PURDUE FREDERICK)
**TRIMETHOBENZAMIDE HCL
SUPPOSITORIES 100 MG, 200 MG**
(PADDOCK)

TRIMETHOBENZAMIDE HYDROCHLORIDE

Tigan Capsules (ROBERTS)
Tigan Injectable (ROBERTS)
Tigan Suppositories (ROBERTS)

TRIMETHOPRIM

Bactrim DS Tablets (ROCHE LABS)
Bactrim I.V. Infusion (ROCHE LABS)
Bactrim Pediatric Suspension (ROCHE LABS)
Bactrim Tablets (ROCHE LABS)
Septra DS Tablets (MONARCH)
Septra Grape Suspension (MONARCH)
Septra I.V. Infusion (MONARCH)
Septra Suspension (MONARCH)
Septra Tablets (MONARCH)
Sulfamethoxazole & Trimethoprim Concentrate
for Injection (ELKINS-SINN)
Sulfamethoxazole & Trimethoprim Tablets
(LEDERLE STANDARD)

TRIMETHOPRIM SULFATE

Polytrim Ophthalmic Solution (ALLERGAN)

TRIMETREXATE GLUCURONATE

Neutrexin for Injection (U.S. BIOSCIENCE)

TRIMIPRAMINE MALEATE

Surmontil Capsules (WYETH-AYERST)
**TRIMOX CAPSULES, FOR ORAL
SUSPENSION AND CHEWABLE
TABLETS** (APOTHECON)
TRIMPEX TABLETS (ROCHE LABS)
TRINALIN REPETABS TABLETS (KEY)
**TRI-NORINYL (NORETHINDRONE AND
ESTRADIOL) TABLETS** (WATSON)
TRI-NORINYL 21 TABLETS (SEARLE)
TRI-NORINYL 28 TABLETS (SEARLE)
TRINSICON CAPSULES (UCB)
TRIOSTAT INJECTION (JONES)
TRIPEDIA (PASTEUR MERIEUX CONNAUGHT)

UNDERLINE DENOTES GENERIC NAME

TRIPHASIL-21 TABLETS (WYETH-AYERST)
TRIPHASIL-28 TABLETS (WYETH-AYERST)
TRIPROLIDINE HYDROCHLORIDE
   Actifed Cold & Allergy Tablets
    (WARNER-LAMBERT)
TRISTOJECT (MERZ)
TRITEC TABLETS (GLAXO WELLCOME)
TRIVORA TABLETS (WATSON)
TROBICIN STERILE POWDER
   (PHARMACIA & UPJOHN)
TROGLITAZONE
   Rezulin Tablets (PARKE-DAVIS)
TROLEANDOMYCIN
   Tao Capsules (PFIZER)
TRONOLANE ANESTHETIC CREAM FOR HEMORRHOIDS (ROSS)
TRONOLANE HEMORRHOIDAL SUPPOSITORIES (ROSS)
TRONOTHANE HYDROCHLORIDE CREAM
   (ABBOTT)
TROVAFLOXACIN MESYLATE
   Trovan Tablets (PFIZER)
TROVAN I.V. (PFIZER)
TROVAN TABLETS (PFIZER)
TRUSOPT STERILE OPHTHALMIC SOLUTION (MERCK)
TRYPSIN
   Granulex Aerosol (BERTEK)
T-STAT 2.0% TOPICAL SOLUTION AND PADS (WESTWOOD-SQUIBB)
TUBERCULIN, OLD
   Mono-Vacc Test (O.T.)
    (PASTEUR MERIEUX CONNAUGHT)
   Tuberculin, Old, Tine Test (LEDERLE LABS)
TUBERCULIN, PURIFIED PROTEIN DERIVATIVE, DILUTED
   Aplisol Injection (PARKEDALE)
TUBERCULIN, PURIFIED PROTEIN DERIVATIVE, MULTIPLE PUNCTURE DEVICE
   Tine Test PPD (LEDERLE LABS)
TUBERCULIN, PURIFIED PROTEIN DERIVATIVE FOR MANTOUX TEST
   Tubersol (PASTEUR MERIEUX CONNAUGHT)
TUBERCULIN, OLD, TINE TEST
   (LEDERLE LABS)
TUBERSOL (PASTEUR MERIEUX CONNAUGHT)
TUBEX CLOSED INJECTION SYSTEM PRODUCTS (WYETH-AYERST)
TUBEX INJECTOR (WYETH-AYERST)
TUBOCURARINE CHLORIDE INJECTION USP (APOTHECON)
TUBOCURARINE CHLORIDE INJECTION, USP (ABBOTT)
TUCKS MEDICATED PADS
   (WARNER-LAMBERT)
TUCKS TAKE ALONGS TOWELETTES
   (WARNER-LAMBERT)
TUINAL PULVULES (LILLY)
TUMS REGULAR, TUMS EX, AND TUMS ULTRA ANTACID/CALCIUM SUPPLEMENT TABLETS
   (SMITHKLINE BEECHAM CONSUMER)
TUSSAFED DROPS (EVERETT)
TUSSAFED SYRUP (EVERETT)
TUSSAFED-EX SYRUP (EVERETT)
TUSSAFED-HC SYRUP (EVERETT)
TUSSAFED-LA CAPLETS (EVERETT)
TUSSEND TABLETS OR SYRUP CIII
   (MONARCH)
TUSSEND EXPECTORANT SYRUP CIII
   (MONARCH)

TUSSEND EXPECTORANT LIQUID
   (MONARCH)
TUSSEND SYRUP (MONARCH)
TUSSEND TABLETS (MONARCH)
TUSSI-12 SUSPENSION (WALLACE)
TUSSIONEX PENNKINETIC EXTENDED-RELEASE SUSPENSION (MEDEVA)
TUSSI-ORGANIDIN NR LIQUID (WALLACE)
TUSSI-ORGANIDIN DM NR LIQUID
   (WALLACE)
TUSSI-ORGANIDIN DM-S NR LIQUID
   (WALLACE)
TUSSI-ORGANIDIN-S NR LIQUID (WALLACE)
TYLENOL EXTRA STRENGTH ADULT LIQUID PAIN RELIEVER
   (MCNEIL CONSUMER)
TYLENOL ALLERGY SINUS, MAXIMUM STRENGTH CAPLETS, GELCAPS, AND GELTABS (MCNEIL CONSUMER)
TYLENOL ALLERGY SINUS NIGHTTIME, MAXIMUM STRENGTH CAPLETS
   (MCNEIL CONSUMER)
TYLENOL ARTHRITIS EXTENDED RELIEF CAPLETS (MCNEIL CONSUMER)
CHILDREN'S TYLENOL ALLERGY-D LIQUID AND CHEWABLE TABLETS
   (MCNEIL CONSUMER)
CHILDREN'S TYLENOL COLD LIQUID AND CHEWABLE TABLETS
   (MCNEIL CONSUMER)
CHILDREN'S TYLENOL COLD PLUS COUGH SUSPENSION LIQUID AND CHEWABLE TABLETS (MCNEIL CONSUMER)
CHILDREN'S TYLENOL FLU SUSPENSION LIQUID (MCNEIL CONSUMER)
CHILDREN'S TYLENOL SINUS LIQUID AND CHEWABLE TABLETS
   (MCNEIL CONSUMER)
CHILDREN'S TYLENOL SOFT-CHEW CHEWABLE TABLETS, ELIXIR, AND SUSPENSION LIQUID (MCNEIL CONSUMER)
TYLENOL COLD COMPLETE FORMULA, MULTI-SYMPTOM TABLETS AND CAPLETS (MCNEIL CONSUMER)
TYLENOL COLD NON-DROWSY, MULTI-SYMPTOM CAPLETS AND GELCAPS
   (MCNEIL CONSUMER)
TYLENOL COLD SEVERE CONGESTION NON-DROWSY, MULTI-SYMPTOM CAPLETS (MCNEIL CONSUMER)
TYLENOL EXTRA STRENGTH GELCAPS, GELTABS, CAPLETS, AND TABLETS
   (MCNEIL CONSUMER)
TYLENOL FLU NIGHTTIME, MAXIMUM STRENGTH GELCAPS (MCNEIL CONSUMER)
TYLENOL FLU NIGHTTIME, MAXIMUM STRENGTH LIQUID (MCNEIL CONSUMER)
TYLENOL FLU NIGHTTIME, MAXIMUM STRENGTH POWDER (MCNEIL CONSUMER)
TYLENOL FLU NON-DROWSY, MAXIMUM STRENGTH GELCAPS (MCNEIL CONSUMER)
INFANTS' TYLENOL COLD DECONGESTANT AND FEVER REDUCER CONCENTRATED DROPS
   (MCNEIL CONSUMER)
INFANTS' TYLENOL COLD DECONGESTANT AND FEVER REDUCER CONCENTRATED DROPS PLUS COUGH (MCNEIL CONSUMER)
INFANTS' TYLENOL CONCENTRATED DROPS (MCNEIL CONSUMER)
JUNIOR STRENGTH TYLENOL COATED CAPLETS AND SOFT-CHEW CHEWABLE TABLETS (MCNEIL CONSUMER)

TYLENOL PM PAIN RELIEVER/SLEEP AID, EXTRA STRENGTH CAPLETS, GELTABS, AND GELCAPS
   (MCNEIL CONSUMER)
TYLENOL REGULAR STRENGTH CAPLETS AND TABLETS
   (MCNEIL CONSUMER)
TYLENOL SEVERE ALLERGY CAPLETS
   (MCNEIL CONSUMER)
TYLENOL SINUS NIGHTTIME, MAXIMUM STRENGTH CAPLETS (MCNEIL CONSUMER)
TYLENOL SINUS NON-DROWSY, MAXIMUM STRENGTH GELTABS, GELCAPS, CAPLETS, AND TABLETS
   (MCNEIL CONSUMER)
TYLENOL SORE THROAT, MAXIMUM STRENGTH ADULT LIQUID
   (MCNEIL CONSUMER)
TYLENOL WITH CODEINE ELIXIR
   (ORTHO-MCNEIL)
TYLENOL WITH CODEINE TABLETS
   (ORTHO-MCNEIL)
TYLOX CAPSULES (ORTHO-MCNEIL)
TYLOXAPOL
   Exosurf Neonatal for Intratracheal Suspension
   (GLAXO WELLCOME)
TYMPAGESIC EAR DROPS (SAVAGE)
TYPHIM VI (PASTEUR MERIEUX CONNAUGHT)
TYPHOID VACCINE (WYETH-AYERST)
TYPHOID VACCINE
   Typhoid Vaccine (WYETH-AYERST)
TYPHOID VACCINE LIVE ORAL TY21A
   Vivotif Berna (BERNA)
TYPHOID VI POLYSACCHARIDE VACCINE
   Typhim Vi (PASTEUR MERIEUX CONNAUGHT)
TYREX-2 AMINO ACID-MODIFIED MEDICAL FOOD (ROSS)
TYROMEX-1 AMINO ACID-MODIFIED MEDICAL FOOD WITH IRON (ROSS)

U

ULTANE (SEVOFLURANE) (ABBOTT)
ULTIVA FOR INJECTION (GLAXO WELLCOME)
ULTRA G.I. CAPSULES (WESTLAKE)
ULTRABROM CAPSULES (WE)
ULTRABROM PD CAPSULES (WE)
ULTRA-CAROTENOIDS CAPSULES
   (WESTLAKE)
ULTRA-LIPOIC FORTE CAPSULES
   (WESTLAKE)
ULTRAM TABLETS (ORTHO-MCNEIL)
ULTRASE CAPSULES (SCANDIPHARM)
ULTRASE MT CAPSULES (SCANDIPHARM)
ULTRASONIC CLEANER (CETYLITE)
ULTRAVATE CREAM 0.05%
   (WESTWOOD-SQUIBB)
ULTRAVATE OINTMENT 0.05%
   (WESTWOOD-SQUIBB)
UNASYN FOR INJECTION (PFIZER)
UNDECYLENIC ACID
   Gordochom Solution (GORDON)
UNI-DUR EXTENDED-RELEASE TABLETS
   (KEY)
UNIFIBER (NICHE)
UNIPHYL 400 MG AND 600 MG TABLETS
   (PURDUE FREDERICK)
UNIQUE E VITAMIN E CAPSULES (GRACE)

UNDERLINE DENOTES GENERIC NAME

UNIRETIC TABLETS (SCHWARZ)
MAXIMUM STRENGTH UNISOM
  SLEEPGELS (PFIZER CONSUMER)
UNISOM SLEEPTABS (PFIZER CONSUMER)
UNIVASC TABLETS (SCHWARZ)

UREA
  Accuzyme Debriding Ointment (HEALTHPOINT)
  Amino-Cerv Creme (MILEX)
  Eucerin Plus Alpha Hydroxy Creme
    (BEIERSDORF)
  Eucerin Plus Alpha Hydroxy Lotion
    (BEIERSDORF)
  Panafil Ointment (HEALTHPOINT)
UREACIN-10 LOTION (PEDINOL)
UREACIN-20 CREME (PEDINOL)
UREAPHIL (ABBOTT)
URECHOLINE INJECTION (MERCK)
URECHOLINE TABLETS (MERCK)
UREX TABLETS (3M)
URISED TABLETS (POLYMEDICA)
URISPAS TABLETS (ALZA)
UROBIOTIC-250 CAPSULES (PFIZER)
UROCIT-K TABLETS (MISSION)

UROFOLLITROPIN
  Fertinex for Injection (SERONO)

UROKINASE
  Abbokinase (ABBOTT)
  Abbokinase Open-Cath (ABBOTT)
URO-KP-NEUTRAL TABLETS (STAR)
UROLENE BLUE TABLETS (STAR)
UROLOGIC G IRRIGATION (AQUALITE)
  (ABBOTT)
URO-MAG CAPSULES (BLAINE)
URO-PRO CAPSULES (WESTLAKE)
UROQID-ACID NO. 2 TABLETS (BEACH)
URSO TABLETS (SCHWARZ)
URSO TABLETS 250 MG (AXCAN)

URSODIOL
  Urso Tablets (SCHWARZ)
  Urso Tablets 250 mg (AXCAN)

V

VALACYCLOVIR HYDROCHLORIDE
  Valtrex Caplets (GLAXO WELLCOME)
VALISONE CREAM, 0.1% (SCHERING)
VALISONE LOTION 0.1% (SCHERING)
VALISONE OINTMENT 0.1% (SCHERING)
VALISONE REDUCED STRENGTH CREAM
  .01% (SCHERING)
VALIUM INJECTABLE (ROCHE LABS)
VALIUM TABLETS (ROCHE PRODUCTS)

VALPROATE SODIUM
  Depacon Injection (ABBOTT)

VALPROIC ACID
  Depakene Capsules (ABBOTT)
  Depakene Syrup (ABBOTT)
  Valproic Acid Syrup (WATSON)
VALPROIC ACID SYRUP (WATSON)

VALRUBICIN
  Valstar Sterile Solution for Intravesical
    Instillation (MEDEVA)

VALSARTAN
  Diovan Capsules (NOVARTIS)
  Diovan HCT Tablets (NOVARTIS)
VALSTAR STERILE SOLUTION FOR
  INTRAVESICAL INSTILLATION (MEDEVA)

VALTREX CAPLETS (GLAXO WELLCOME)
VANCENASE AQ NASAL SPRAY 0.042%
  (SCHERING)
VANCENASE AQ DOUBLE STRENGTH
  NASAL SPRAY 0.084% (SCHERING)
VANCENASE NASAL INHALER (SCHERING)
VANCENASE POCKETHALER NASAL
  INHALER (SCHERING)
VANCERIL INHALATION AEROSOL
  (SCHERING)
VANCERIL DOUBLE STRENGTH
  INHALATION AEROSOL (SCHERING)
VANCOCIN HCL CAPSULES & PULVULES
  (LILLY)
VANCOCIN HCL ORAL SOLUTION (LILLY)
VANCOCIN HCL, VIALS & ADD-VANTAGE
  (LILLY)
VANCOMYCIN HCL INJECTION
  (ESI LEDERLE)
VANCOMYCIN HCL INJECTION
  (LEDERLE STANDARD)

VANCOMYCIN HYDROCHLORIDE
  Vancocin HCl Capsules & Pulvules (LILLY)
  Vancocin HCl Oral Solution (LILLY)
  Vancocin HCl, Vials & ADD-Vantage (LILLY)
  Vancomycin HCl Injection
    (LEDERLE STANDARD)
VANOXIDE ACNE LOTION (DERMIK)
VANOXIDE-HC ACNE LOTION (DERMIK)
VANTIN TABLETS AND ORAL
  SUSPENSION (PHARMACIA & UPJOHN)
VAQTA (MERCK)

VARICELLA VIRUS VACCINE LIVE
  Varivax (MERCK)
VARIVAX (MERCK)
VARNAL CAVITY VARNISH (CETYLITE)
VASCOR TABLETS (ORTHO-MCNEIL)
VASCOR TABLETS (SEE ORTHO-MCNEIL
  PHARMACEUTICAL) (WALLACE)
VASERETIC TABLETS (MERCK)
VASODILAN TABLETS (APOTHECON)
VASOTEC I.V. INJECTION (MERCK)
VASOTEC TABLETS (MERCK)
VASOXYL INJECTION (GLAXO WELLCOME)
VECTRIN CAPSULES (WARNER CHILCOTT)

VECURONIUM BROMIDE
  Norcuron for Injection (ORGANON)
VEETIDS TABLETS AND FOR ORAL
  SUSPENSION (APOTHECON)
VELBAN VIALS (LILLY)
VELOSEF CAPSULES AND FOR ORAL
  SUSPENSION (APOTHECON)
VELOSULIN BR HUMAN INSULIN 10 ML
  VIALS (NOVO NORDISK)

VENLAFAXINE HYDROCHLORIDE
  Effexor Tablets (WYETH-AYERST)
  Effexor XR Capsules (WYETH-AYERST)
VENOGLOBULIN-S 5% SOLUTION
  SOLVENT DETERGENT TREATED
  (ALPHA)
VENOGLOBULIN-S 10% SOLUTION
  SOLVENT DETERGENT TREATED
  (ALPHA)
VENTOLIN INHALATION AEROSOL AND
  REFILL (GLAXO WELLCOME)
VENTOLIN INHALATION SOLUTION
  (GLAXO WELLCOME)
VENTOLIN NEBULES INHALATION
  SOLUTION (GLAXO WELLCOME)
VENTOLIN ROTACAPS FOR INHALATION
  (GLAXO WELLCOME)
VENTOLIN SYRUP (GLAXO WELLCOME)
VEPESID CAPSULES
  (BRISTOL-MYERSSQUIBBONCOLOGY/IMMUNOLOGY)

VEPESID FOR INJECTION
  (BRISTOL-MYERSSQUIBBONCOLOGY/IMMUNOLOGY)
VERAPAMIL HCL EXTENDED RELEASE
  TABLETS (DURAMED)
VERAPAMIL HCL SR PELLET-FILLED
  CAPS (SCHEIN)
VERAPAMIL HCL TABLETS (GENEVA)

VERAPAMIL HYDROCHLORIDE
  Calan SR Caplets (SEARLE)
  Calan Tablets (SEARLE)
  Covera-HS Tablets (SEARLE)
  Isoptin SR Tablets (KNOLL LABS)
  Tarka Tablets (KNOLL)
  Verapamil HCl Tablets (GENEVA)
  Verapamil Hydrochloride Extended-release
    Capsules and Tablets (MYLAN)
  Verapamil Hydrochloride Tablets (MYLAN)
  Verapamil Hydrochloride Tablets, USP
    (WATSON)
  Verelan Capsules (SCHWARZ)
  Verelan PM Capsules (SCHWARZ)
VERAPAMIL HYDROCHLORIDE TABLETS
  (MYLAN)
VERAPAMIL HYDROCHLORIDE
  EXTENDED-RELEASE CAPSULES AND
  TABLETS (MYLAN)
VERAPAMIL HYDROCHLORIDE TABLETS,
  USP (WATSON)
VERELAN CAPSULES (SCHWARZ)
VERELAN PM CAPSULES (SCHWARZ)
VERMOX CHEWABLE TABLETS
  (MCNEIL CONSUMER)
VERSED INJECTION (ROCHE LABS)
VERSED SYRUP (ROCHE LABS)
VERTIGOHEEL LIQUID IN ORAL VIALS
  (HEEL)
VERTIGOHEEL ORAL DROPS (HEEL)
VERTIGOHEEL TABLETS (HEEL)
VESANOID CAPSULES (ROCHE LABS)
VESPRIN INJECTION (APOTHECON)
VEXOL OPHTHALMIC SUSPENSION
  (ALCON)
VIAGRA TABLETS (PFIZER)
VIBRAMYCIN CALCIUM ORAL
  SUSPENSION SYRUP (PFIZER)
VIBRAMYCIN HYCLATE CAPSULES
  (PFIZER)
VIBRAMYCIN HYCLATE INTRAVENOUS
  (PFIZER)
VIBRAMYCIN MONOHYDRATE FOR
  ORAL SUSPENSION (PFIZER)
VIBRA-TABS FILM COATED TABLETS
  (PFIZER)
VICKS 44 COUGH RELIEF
  (PROCTER & GAMBLE)
VICKS 44D COUGH & HEAD
  CONGESTION RELIEF (PROCTER & GAMBLE)
VICKS 44E COUGH & CHEST
  CONGESTION RELIEF (PROCTER & GAMBLE)
PEDIATRIC VICKS 44E COUGH & CHEST
  CONGESTION RELIEF (PROCTER & GAMBLE)
VICKS 44M COUGH, COLD & FLU
  RELIEF (PROCTER & GAMBLE)
PEDIATRIC VICKS 44M COUGH & COLD
  RELIEF (PROCTER & GAMBLE)
VICKS CHLORASEPTIC SORE THROAT
  LOZENGES (PROCTER & GAMBLE)
VICKS CHLORASEPTIC SORE THROAT
  SPRAY (PROCTER & GAMBLE)
VICKS COUGH DROPS, MENTHOL &
  CHERRY FLAVORS (PROCTER & GAMBLE)
VICKS DAYQUIL MULTI-SYMPTOM
  COLD/FLU RELIEF LIQUID &
  LIQUICAPS (PROCTER & GAMBLE)

VICKS DAYQUIL SINUS PRESSURE & PAIN RELIEF WITH IBUPROFEN (PROCTER & GAMBLE)
CHILDREN'S VICKS NYQUIL COLD/COUGH RELIEF (PROCTER & GAMBLE)
VICKS NYQUIL LIQUICAPS (PROCTER & GAMBLE)
VICKS NYQUIL LIQUID (PROCTER & GAMBLE)
VICKS SINEX 12 HOUR NASAL SPRAY AND ULTRA FINE MIST FOR SINUS RELIEF (PROCTER & GAMBLE)
VICKS SINEX NASAL SPRAY AND ULTRA FINE MIST FOR SINUS RELIEF (PROCTER & GAMBLE)
VICKS VAPOR INHALER (PROCTER & GAMBLE)
VICKS VAPORUB CREAM (PROCTER & GAMBLE)
VICKS VAPORUB OINTMENT (PROCTER & GAMBLE)
VICKS VAPOSTEAM (PROCTER & GAMBLE)
VICODIN TABLETS (KNOLL LABS)
VICODIN ES TABLETS (KNOLL LABS)
VICODIN HP TABLETS (KNOLL LABS)
VICODIN TUSS EXPECTORANT (KNOLL LABS)
VICON-C CAPSULES (UCB)
VICON FORTE CAPSULES (UCB)
VICON PLUS CAPSULES (UCB)
VICOPROFEN TABLETS (KNOLL LABS)
VI-DAYLIN ADC VITAMINS DROPS (ROSS)
VI-DAYLIN ADC VITAMINS + IRON DROPS (ROSS)
VI-DAYLIN MULTIVITAMIN CHEWABLE TABLETS (ROSS)
VI-DAYLIN MULTIVITAMIN + IRON CHEWABLE TABLETS (ROSS)
VI-DAYLIN MULTIVITAMIN DROPS (ROSS)
VI-DAYLIN MULTIVITAMIN + IRON DROPS (ROSS)
VI-DAYLIN MULTIVITAMIN LIQUID (ROSS)
VI-DAYLIN MULTIVITAMIN + IRON LIQUID (ROSS)
VI-DAYLIN/F ADC VITAMINS DROPS WITH FLUORIDE (ROSS)
VI-DAYLIN/F ADC VITAMINS + IRON DROPS WITH FLUORIDE (ROSS)
VI-DAYLIN/F MULTIVITAMIN CHEWABLE TABLETS WITH FLUORIDE (ROSS)
VI-DAYLIN/F MULTIVITAMIN + IRON CHEWABLE TABLETS WITH FLUORIDE (ROSS)
VI-DAYLIN/F MULTIVITAMIN DROPS WITH FLUORIDE (ROSS)
VI-DAYLIN/F MULTIVITAMIN + IRON DROPS WITH FLUORIDE (ROSS)
VIDEX POWDER FOR ORAL SOLUTION (BRISTOL-MYERSSQUIBBONCOLOGY/IMMUNOLOGY)
VIDEX PEDIATRIC POWDER FOR ORAL SOLUTION (BRISTOL-MYERSSQUIBBONCOLOGY/IMMUNOLOGY)
VIDEX CHEWABLE TABLETS (BRISTOL-MYERSSQUIBBONCOLOGY/IMMUNOLOGY)

VINBLASTINE SULFATE
  Velban Vials (LILLY)
VINBLASTINE SULFATE FOR INJECTION, USP (BEDFORD)
VINCASAR INJECTION (PHARMACIA & UPJOHN)

VINCRISTINE SULFATE
  Oncovin Solution Vials (LILLY)

VINORELBINE TARTRATE
  Navelbine Injection (GLAXO WELLCOME)
VIOKASE (PADDOCK)

VIOKASE POWDER (AXCAN)
VIOKASE TABLETS (AXCAN)
VIOXX ORAL SUSPENSION (MERCK)
VIOXX TABLETS (MERCK)
VIQUIN FORTE CREAM (ICN)
VIRACEPT ORAL POWDER (AGOURON)
VIRACEPT TABLETS (AGOURON)
VIRAMUNE ORAL SUSPENSION (ROXANE)
VIRAMUNE TABLETS (ROXANE)
VIRAZOLE (ICN)
VIRILON CAPSULES (STAR)
VIRILON IM INJECTION (STAR)
VIROPTIC OPHTHALMIC SOLUTION, 1% STERILE (MONARCH)
VISCOAT OPHTHALMIC VISCOSURGICAL DEVICE (ALCON)
VISKEN TABLETS (NOVARTIS)
VISTARIL CAPSULES (PFIZER)
VISTARIL INTRAMUSCULAR SOLUTION (PFIZER)
VISTARIL ORAL SUSPENSION (PFIZER)
VISTIDE INJECTION (GILEAD)
VITA-RAY CREME (GORDON)
VITA-CALCIUM (CALCIUM AND VITAMIN D) (VITALINE)
VITADYE LOTION (ICN)
VITAFOL CAPLETS (EVERETT)
VITAFOL SYRUP (EVERETT)
VITAFOL-PN CAPLETS (EVERETT)
VITA-MAG (MAGNESIUM) (VITALINE)
VITAMIN A 10,000 I.U. (VITALINE)

VITAMIN A
  ACES Antioxidant Soft Gels (CARLSON)
  Aquasol A Parenteral (ASTRAZENECA LP)
  LazerCreme (PEDINOL)
  Megadose Tablets (ARCO)
  Revitalizer (MAYOR)
  Vi-Daylin ADC Vitamins + Iron Drops (ROSS)
  Vi-Daylin ADC Vitamins Drops (ROSS)
  Vi-Daylin/F ADC Vitamins + Iron Drops With Fluoride (ROSS)
  Vi-Daylin/F ADC Vitamins Drops With Fluoride (ROSS)
  Vitamist Intra-Oral Spray Dietary Supplements (MAYOR)

VITAMIN B1
  Mega-B Tablets (ARCO)

VITAMIN B2
  Mega-B Tablets (ARCO)

VITAMIN B6
  Beelith Tablets (BEACH)
  Folacin (MAYOR)
  Marlyn Formula 50 Capsules (MARLYN)
  Mega-B Tablets (ARCO)
  ViTelle Lurline PMS Tablets (FIELDING)
  ViTelle Nestrex Tablets (FIELDING)
  VitaMotion-S (MAYOR)
  Vitamist Intra-Oral Spray Dietary Supplements (MAYOR)

VITAMIN B12
  B12 (MAYOR)
  Bevitamel Tablets (WESTLAKE)
  Chromagen Capsules (SAVAGE)
  Chromagen FA Capsules (SAVAGE)
  Chromagen Forte Capsules (SAVAGE)
  Cyanocobalamin (Vit. B12) Injection (ELKINS-SINN)
  Fetrin Capsules (LUNSCO)
  Folacin (MAYOR)
  Fumatinic Capsules (LASER)
  GinkgoMist (MAYOR)
  Hemocyte-F Elixir (U.S. PHARMACEUTICAL)
  Mega-B Tablets (ARCO)
  Nascobal Gel (SCHWARZ)

  Niferex-150 Forte Capsules (SCHWARZ)
  Nu-Iron Plus Elixir (MERZ)
  Trinsicon Capsules (UCB)
  VitaZac (MAYOR)
  Vitamist Intra-Oral Spray Dietary Supplements (MAYOR)

VITAMIN B COMPLEX
  Mega-B Tablets (ARCO)
  Pine Bark and Grape Seed (MAYOR)
  Revitalizer (MAYOR)
  Slender-Mist (MAYOR)
  Stress (MAYOR)
  VitaMinophen (MAYOR)
  Vitamist Intra-Oral Spray Dietary Supplements (MAYOR)

VITAMIN B COMPLEX WITH VITAMIN C
  Cefol Filmtab Tablets (ABBOTT)
  Hemocyte Plus Tabules (U.S. PHARMACEUTICAL)
  Iberet-Folic-500 Filmtab Tablets (ABBOTT)
  Megadose Tablets (ARCO)
  Nephro-Vite + Fe Tablets (R&D)
  Nephro-Vite Rx Tablets (R&D)
  Nephro-Vite Tablets (R&D)
  ViTelle Nesentials Tablets (formerly Gerimed) (FIELDING)
VITAMIN B-6 CONTROLLED TIME RELEASE 200MG (VITALINE)
VITAMIN B-12 2500MCG SUBLINGUAL TABLETS (VITALINE)

VITAMIN C
  ACES Antioxidant Soft Gels (CARLSON)
  C + Zinc (MAYOR)
  CardioCare (MAYOR)
  Chromagen Capsules (SAVAGE)
  Chromagen FA Capsules (SAVAGE)
  Chromagen Forte Capsules (SAVAGE)
  CitraDerm Facial Complex Cream (PEDINOL)
  Fero-Folic-500 Filmtab Tablets (ABBOTT)
  Fero-Grad-500 Filmtab Tablets (ABBOTT)
  Fetrin Capsules (LUNSCO)
  Fumatinic Capsules (LASER)
  Peridin-C Tablets (BEUTLICH)
  Proflavanol Tablets (USANA)
  Trinsicon Capsules (UCB)
  Vi-Daylin ADC Vitamins + Iron Drops (ROSS)
  Vi-Daylin ADC Vitamins Drops (ROSS)
  Vi-Daylin/F ADC Vitamins + Iron Drops With Fluoride (ROSS)
  Vi-Daylin/F ADC Vitamins Drops With Fluoride (ROSS)
  ViTelle Irospan Capsules (FIELDING)
  ViTelle Irospan Tablets (FIELDING)
  Vitamist Intra-Oral Spray Dietary Supplements (MAYOR)
VITAMIN C 1000MG CONTROLLED TIME RELEASE (VITALINE)
VITAMIN C 1000MG WITH CITRUS BIOFLAVONOIDS (VITALINE)
VITAMIN C BUFFERED POWDER (VITALINE)

VITAMIN D
  ActiCal Tablets (USANA)
  Citracal Caplets + D (MISSION)
  Megadose Tablets (ARCO)
  Osteo-CalMag (MAYOR)
  Vi-Daylin ADC Vitamins + Iron Drops (ROSS)
  Vi-Daylin ADC Vitamins Drops (ROSS)
  Vi-Daylin/F ADC Vitamins + Iron Drops With Fluoride (ROSS)
  Vi-Daylin/F ADC Vitamins Drops With Fluoride (ROSS)
  Vitamist Intra-Oral Spray Dietary Supplements (MAYOR)
VITAMIN D, USP (SANOFI)
VITAMIN D3 400 I.U. (VITALINE)

UNDERLINE DENOTES GENERIC NAME

VITAMIN E

ACES Antioxidant Soft Gels (CARLSON)
Blue-Green Sea Spray (MAYOR)
C + Zinc (MAYOR)
CardioCare (MAYOR)
Cefol Filmtab Tablets (ABBOTT)
E + Selenium (MAYOR)
E-Gems Soft Gels (CARLSON)
Eucerin Q10 Anti-Wrinkle Sensitive Skin
 Creme (BEIERSDORF)
Lactinol-E Creme (PEDINOL)
LazerCreme (PEDINOL)
Megadose Tablets (ARCO)
Nutr-E-Sol Liquid (ADVANCED NUTRITIONAL)
Revitalizer (MAYOR)
Unique E Vitamin E Capsules (GRACE)
Vitamist Intra-Oral Spray Dietary Supplements
 (MAYOR)
VITAMIN E 400 I.U. SOFTGELS (VITALINE)

VITAMIN K1

AquaMEPHYTON Injection (MERCK)
Mephyton Tablets (MERCK)
VITAMINOPHEN (MAYOR)
VITAMINS (SANOFI)

VITAMINS, MULTIPLE

Anti-Oxidant (MAYOR)
Calcet Plus Tablets (MISSION)
HeartBar (COOKE)
M.V.I. Pediatric for Infusion (ASTRAZENECA LP)
M.V.I.-12 Multi-Vitamin Infusion
 (ASTRAZENECA LP)
Materna Tablets (LEDERLE LABS)
Mega Antioxidant Tablets (USANA)
Nephro-Vite Rx Tablets (R&D)
Nephro-Vite Tablets (R&D)
Nephrocaps (FLEMING)
Vi-Daylin Multivitamin Chewable Tablets
 (ROSS)
Vi-Daylin Multivitamin Drops (ROSS)
Vi-Daylin Multivitamin Liquid (ROSS)
Vi-Daylin/F Multivitamin + Iron Chewable
 Tablets With Fluoride (ROSS)
Vi-Daylin/F Multivitamin + Iron Drops With
 Fluoride (ROSS)
Vi-Daylin/F Multivitamin Chewable Tablets
 With Fluoride (ROSS)
Vi-Daylin/F Multivitamin Drops With Fluoride
 (ROSS)
ViTelle Nesentials Tablets (formerly Gerimed)
 (FIELDING)
Vitamist Intra-Oral Spray Dietary Supplements
 (MAYOR)

VITAMINS, PRENATAL

Chromagen OB Capsules (SAVAGE)
Enfamil Natalins Rx Tablets (MEAD JOHNSON)
Lactocal-F Tablets (LASER)
Mission Prenatal F.A. Tablets (MISSION)
Mission Prenatal H.P. Tablets (MISSION)
Mission Prenatal Tablets (MISSION)
Niferex-PN Forte Tablets (SCHWARZ)
Niferex-PN Tablets (SCHWARZ)
Obegyn (FLEMING)
Precare Prenatal Multi-Vitamin/Mineral (UCB)
Prenate Ultra Tablets (SANOFI)
ViTelle Nestabs OTC Tablets (FIELDING)

VITAMINS WITH FLUORIDE

Vi-Daylin/F ADC Vitamins + Iron Drops
 With Fluoride (ROSS)
Vi-Daylin/F ADC Vitamins Drops With
 Fluoride (ROSS)
Vi-Daylin/F Multivitamin + Iron Chewable
 Tablets With Fluoride (ROSS)
Vi-Daylin/F Multivitamin + Iron Drops With
 Fluoride (ROSS)

Vi-Daylin/F Multivitamin Chewable Tablets
 With Fluoride (ROSS)
Vi-Daylin/F Multivitamin Drops With Fluoride
 (ROSS)

VITAMINS WITH IRON

Calcet Plus Tablets (MISSION)
Fosfree Tablets (MISSION)
Hemocyte Plus Tabules (U.S. PHARMACEUTICAL)
Iberet-Folic-500 Filmtab Tablets (ABBOTT)
Iromin-G Tablets (MISSION)
Materna Tablets (LEDERLE LABS)
Mission Prenatal F.A. Tablets (MISSION)
Mission Prenatal H.P. Tablets (MISSION)
Mission Prenatal Tablets (MISSION)
NataFort Tablets (WARNER CHILCOTT)
Nephro-Vite + Fe Tablets (R&D)
Trinsicon Capsules (UCB)
Vi-Daylin ADC Vitamins + Iron Drops (ROSS)
Vi-Daylin Multivitamin + Iron Chewable
 Tablets (ROSS)
Vi-Daylin Multivitamin + Iron Drops (ROSS)
Vi-Daylin Multivitamin + Iron Liquid (ROSS)
Vi-Daylin/F ADC Vitamins + Iron Drops
 With Fluoride (ROSS)
Vi-Daylin/F Multivitamin + Iron Chewable
 Tablets With Fluoride (ROSS)
Vi-Daylin/F Multivitamin + Iron Drops With
 Fluoride (ROSS)

VITAMINS WITH MINERALS

ArthriFlex (MAYOR)
Eldercaps (MERZ)
Eldertonic (MERZ)
Fosfree Tablets (MISSION)
Hemocyte Plus Tabules (U.S. PHARMACEUTICAL)
Hep-Forte Capsules (MARLYN)
Immunocal (IMMUNOTEC)
Iromin-G Tablets (MISSION)
M.V.I. Pediatric for Infusion (ASTRAZENECA LP)
MDR Fitness Tabs for Men and Women
 (MDR FITNESS)
Materna Tablets (LEDERLE LABS)
May-Vita Elixir (MERZ)
Mediplex Ultra Tabules (U.S. PHARMACEUTICAL)
Megadose Tablets (ARCO)
Multiple Adult/Children's/Prenatal Formulas
 (MAYOR)
Nestabs CBF Tablets (FIELDING)
Niferex-PN Forte Tablets (SCHWARZ)
Niferex-PN Tablets (SCHWARZ)
Nu-Iron V Tablets (MERZ)
Osteomax (NUTRACEUTICS)
Precare Prenatal Multi-Vitamin/Mineral (UCB)
Prenate Ultra Tablets (SANOFI)
Strovite Forte Caplets (EVERETT)
Strovite Forte Syrup (EVERETT)
ViTelle Nesentials Tablets (formerly Gerimed)
 (FIELDING)
Vicon Forte Capsules (UCB)
VitaSight (MAYOR)
Vitafol Caplets (EVERETT)
Vitafol Syrup (EVERETT)
Vitafol-PN Caplets (EVERETT)
Vitamist Intra-Oral Spray Dietary Supplements
 (MAYOR)
**VITAMIST INTRA-ORAL SPRAY DIETARY
SUPPLEMENTS** (MAYOR)
VITAMOTION-S (MAYOR)
VITASIGHT (MAYOR)
VITAZAC (MAYOR)
VITELLE IROSPAN CAPSULES (FIELDING)
VITELLE IROSPAN TABLETS (FIELDING)
VITELLE LURLINE PMS TABLETS
 (FIELDING)
**VITELLE NESENTIALS TABLETS
(FORMERLY GERIMED)** (FIELDING)

VITELLE NESTABS OTC TABLETS
 (FIELDING)
VITELLE NESTREX TABLETS (FIELDING)
VIVACTIL TABLETS (MERCK)
VIVELLE TRANSDERMAL SYSTEM
 (NOVARTIS)
VIVELLE-DOT TRANSDERMAL SYSTEM
 (NOVARTIS)
VIVOTIF BERNA (BERNA)
VI-ZAC CAPSULES (UCB)
VOLMAX EXTENDED-RELEASE TABLETS
 (MURO)
VOLTAREN TABLETS (NOVARTIS)
VOLTAREN-XR TABLETS (NOVARTIS)
VOSOL HC OTIC SOLUTION (WALLACE)
VUMON FOR INJECTION
 (BRISTOL-MYERSSQUIBBONCOLOGY/IMMUNOLOGY)
VYTONE CREAM 1% (DERMIK)

W

WARFARIN SODIUM

Coumadin Tablets (DUPONT)
Coumadin for Injection (DUPONT)
**WATER FOR INJECTION
BACTERIOSTATIC 30 ML FLIPTOP**
 (ABBOTT)
**WATER FOR INJECTION,
BACTERIOSTATIC** (ELKINS-SINN)
**WATER FOR INJECTION, STERILE, USP,
AMPS, VIAL** (ABBOTT)
**WATER FOR IRRIGATION, STERILE, USP
(FLEX AND AQUALITE)** (ABBOTT)
**WATER FOR RESPIRATORY THERAPY,
STERILE (FLEX)** (ABBOTT)

WATER, BACTERIOSTATIC

Water For Injection, Bacteriostatic
 (ELKINS-SINN)

WATER, STERILE

Sterile Water for Inhalation USP (DEY)
WELLBUTRIN TABLETS (GLAXO WELLCOME)
**WELLBUTRIN SR SUSTAINED-RELEASE
TABLETS** (GLAXO WELLCOME)
WESTCORT CREAM 0.2%
 (WESTWOOD-SQUIBB)
WESTCORT OINTMENT 0.2%
 (WESTWOOD-SQUIBB)
WIGRAINE TABLETS (ORGANON)
WINRHO SDF (NABI)
WINSTROL TABLETS (SANOFI)

WITCH HAZEL

Tucks Medicated Pads (WARNER-LAMBERT)
Tucks Take Alongs Towelettes
 (WARNER-LAMBERT)
WONDER ICE (PEDINOL)
WYAMINE SULFATE INJECTION
 (WYETH-AYERST)
WYCILLIN INJECTION (WYETH-AYERST)
WYCILLIN IN TUBEX (WYETH-AYERST)
WYDASE, LYOPHILIZED (WYETH-AYERST)
WYDASE, STABILIZED SOLUTION
 (WYETH-AYERST)
WYGESIC TABLETS (WYETH-AYERST)
WYTENSIN TABLETS (WYETH-AYERST)

UNDERLINE DENOTES GENERIC NAME

X

X-PREP KIT 1 (PURDUE FREDERICK)
X-PREP KIT 2 (PURDUE FREDERICK)
XANAX TABLETS (PHARMACIA & UPJOHN)
XELODA TABLETS (ROCHE LABS)
XENICAL CAPSULES (ROCHE LABS)
XERAC AC SOLUTION (PERSON & COVEY)
XOPENEX INHALATION SOLUTION
   (SEPRACOR)
X-PREP LIQUID (PURDUE FREDERICK)
XYLOCAINE INJECTION (ASTRAZENECA LP)
XYLOCAINE INJECTION FOR
   VENTRICULAR ARRHYTHMIAS
   (ASTRAZENECA LP)
XYLOCAINE 2% JELLY (ASTRAZENECA LP)
XYLOCAINE 2.5% OINTMENT
   (ASTRAZENECA LP)
XYLOCAINE 5% OINTMENT
   (ASTRAZENECA LP)
XYLOCAINE 10% ORAL SPRAY
   (ASTRAZENECA LP)
XYLOCAINE 4% TOPICAL SOLUTION
   (ASTRAZENECA LP)
XYLOCAINE 2% VISCOUS SOLUTION
   (ASTRAZENECA LP)
XYLOCAINE WITH EPINEPHRINE
   INJECTION (ASTRAZENECA LP)
XYLOCAINE-MPF 1.5% SOLUTION WITH
   DEXTROSE 7.5% (ASTRAZENECA LP)
XYLOCAINE-MPF 4% STERILE SOLUTION
   (ASTRAZENECA LP)
XYLOCAINE-MPF 5% WITH GLUCOSE
   7.5% (ASTRAZENECA LP)

Y

YELLOW FEVER VACCINE
   YF-Vax (PASTEUR MERIEUX CONNAUGHT)
YF-VAX (PASTEUR MERIEUX CONNAUGHT)
YOCON TABLETS (GLENWOOD)
YODOXIN TABLETS (GLENWOOD)

YOHIMBINE HYDROCHLORIDE
   Aphrodyne Caplets (STAR)
   Yohimbine Hydrochloride Tablets (WATSON)
YOHIMBINE HYDROCHLORIDE TABLETS
   (WATSON)

Z

ZAFIRLUKAST
   Accolate Tablets (ASTRAZENECA)
ZAGAM TABLETS (BERTEK)

ZALCITABINE
   Hivid Tablets (ROCHE LABS)

ZALEPLON
   Sonata Capsules (WYETH-AYERST)
ZANAFLEX TABLETS (ATHENA)

ZANOSAR STERILE POWDER
   (PHARMACIA & UPJOHN)
ZANTAC 150 EFFERDOSE GRANULES
   (GLAXO WELLCOME)
ZANTAC 150 EFFERDOSE TABLETS
   (GLAXO WELLCOME)
ZANTAC 150 GELDOSE CAPSULES
   (GLAXO WELLCOME)
ZANTAC 300 GELDOSE CAPSULES
   (GLAXO WELLCOME)
ZANTAC 150 TABLETS (GLAXO WELLCOME)
ZANTAC 300 TABLETS (GLAXO WELLCOME)
ZANTAC INJECTION (GLAXO WELLCOME)
ZANTAC INJECTION PREMIXED
   (GLAXO WELLCOME)
ZANTAC SYRUP (GLAXO WELLCOME)
ZANTAC 75 (WARNER-LAMBERT)
ZARONTIN CAPSULES (PARKE-DAVIS)
ZARONTIN SYRUP (PARKE-DAVIS)
ZAROSEN DESENSITIZER (CETYLITE)
ZAROXOLYN TABLETS (MEDEVA)
ZBT BABY POWDER (GLENWOOD)
ZEASORB POWDER (STIEFEL)
ZEASORB-AF LOTION/POWDER (STIEFEL)
ZEASORB-AF POWDER (STIEFEL)
ZEBETA TABLETS (LEDERLE LABS)
ZEBUTAL CAPSULES (HORIZON)
ZEEL OINTMENT (HEEL)
ZEEL TABLETS (HEEL)
ZEMPLAR INJECTION (ABBOTT)
ZEMURON INJECTION (ORGANON)
ZENAPAX FOR INJECTION (ROCHE LABS)
ZEPHIRAN CHLORIDE AQUEOUS
   SOLUTION (SANOFI)
ZEPHREX TABLETS (SANOFI)
ZEPHREX LA TABLETS (SANOFI)
ZERIT CAPSULES
   (BRISTOL-MYERSSQUIBBONCOLOGY/IMMUNOLOGY)
ZERIT FOR ORAL SOLUTION
   (BRISTOL-MYERSSQUIBBONCOLOGY/IMMUNOLOGY)
ZESTORETIC TABLETS (ASTRAZENECA)
ZESTRIL TABLETS (ASTRAZENECA)
ZETAR EMULSION (DERMIK)
ZETAR SHAMPOO (DERMIK)
ZIAC TABLETS (LEDERLE LABS)
ZIAGEN ORAL SOLUTION
   (GLAXO WELLCOME)
ZIAGEN TABLETS (GLAXO WELLCOME)

ZIDOVUDINE
   Combivir Tablets (GLAXO WELLCOME)
   Retrovir Capsules (GLAXO WELLCOME)
   Retrovir IV Infusion (GLAXO WELLCOME)
   Retrovir Syrup (GLAXO WELLCOME)
   Retrovir Tablets (GLAXO WELLCOME)

ZILEUTON
   Zyflo Filmtab Tablets (ABBOTT)
ZINACEF (GLAXO WELLCOME)

ZINC
   C + Zinc (MAYOR)
   Calcet Plus Tablets (MISSION)
   Mission Prenatal F.A. Tablets (MISSION)
   Vitamist Intra-Oral Spray Dietary Supplements
      (MAYOR)
ZINC 10 ML (1 MG/1 ML) (ABBOTT)

ZINC ACETATE
   Benadryl Itch Relief Stick Extra Strength
      (WARNER-LAMBERT)
   Benadryl Itch Stopping Cream Original and
      Extra Strength (WARNER-LAMBERT)
   Benadryl Itch Stopping Spray Original and
      Extra Strength (WARNER-LAMBERT)
   Caladryl Clear Lotion (WARNER-LAMBERT)

ZINC CITRATE
   Chelated Mineral Tablets (USANA)

ZINC GLUCONATE
   Megadose Tablets (ARCO)
ZINC GLUCONATE LOZENGES (MERICON)

ZINC OXIDE
   Anusol Hemorrhoidal Ointment
      (WARNER-LAMBERT)
   Eucerin Protective Moisture Lotion SPF 25
      (BEIERSDORF)
ZINC OXIDE OINTMENT (MERICON)

ZINC SULFATE
   Hemocyte Plus Tabules (U.S. PHARMACEUTICAL)
ZINC SULFATE CAPSULES (UPSHER-SMITH)
ZINC SULFATE TABS & CAPS (MERICON)
ZINC-220 (50MG ELEMENTAL ZINC)
   (VITALINE)
ZINCATE CAPSULES 220 MG (PADDOCK)
ZINCFRIN (ALCON P.R.)
ZINECARD FOR INJECTION
   (PHARMACIA & UPJOHN)
ZITHROMAX CAPSULES, 250 MG (PFIZER)
ZITHROMAX FOR IV INFUSION (PFIZER)
ZITHROMAX FOR ORAL SUSPENSION, 1
   G (PFIZER)
ZITHROMAX FOR ORAL SUSPENSION, 300
   MG, 600 MG, 900 MG, 1200 MG (PFIZER)
ZITHROMAX TABLETS, 250 MG (PFIZER)
ZITHROMAX TABLETS, 600 MG (PFIZER)
ZITHROMAX Z-PAK (PFIZER)
ZNP BAR (STIEFEL)
ZOCOR TABLETS (MERCK)
ZOFRAN INJECTION (GLAXO WELLCOME)
ZOFRAN INJECTION PREMIXED
   (GLAXO WELLCOME)
ZOFRAN ODT ORALLY DISINTEGRATING
   TABLETS (GLAXO WELLCOME)
ZOFRAN ORAL SOLUTION
   (GLAXO WELLCOME)
ZOFRAN TABLETS (GLAXO WELLCOME)
ZOLADEX (ASTRAZENECA)
ZOLADEX 3-MONTH (ASTRAZENECA)

ZOLMITRIPTAN
   Zomig Tablets (ASTRAZENECA)
ZOLOFT TABLETS (PFIZER)

ZOLPIDEM TARTRATE
   Ambien Tablets (SEARLE)
ZOMIG TABLETS (ASTRAZENECA)
ZONALON CREAM (BIOGLAN)
ZONE A FORTE LOTION (FOREST)
ZONE A LOTION 1% (FOREST)
ZORPRIN TABLETS (PAR)
ZOSYN (LEDERLE LABS)
ZOSYN IN GALAXY CONTAINERS
   (LEDERLE LABS)
ZOSYN PHARMACY BULK PACKAGE
   (LEDERLE LABS)
ZOTO-HC EAR DROPS (HORIZON)
ZOVIA 1/35E TABLETS (WATSON)
ZOVIA 1/50E TABLETS (WATSON)
ZOVIRAX CAPSULES (GLAXO WELLCOME)
ZOVIRAX FOR INJECTION
   (GLAXO WELLCOME)
ZOVIRAX OINTMENT 5% (GLAXO WELLCOME)
ZOVIRAX SUSPENSION (GLAXO WELLCOME)
ZOVIRAX TABLETS (GLAXO WELLCOME)
ZYBAN SUSTAINED-RELEASE TABLETS
   (GLAXO WELLCOME)
ZYDONE TABLETS (ENDO LABS)
ZYFLO FILMTAB TABLETS (ABBOTT)
ZYLOPRIM TABLETS (FARO)
ZYMASE CAPSULES (ORGANON)
ZYPREXA TABLETS (LILLY)
ZYRTEC SYRUP (PFIZER)
ZYRTEC TABLETS (PFIZER)

UNDERLINE DENOTES GENERIC NAME

The following pages (GF1-GF5) contain a list of genus species terms from the A to Z vocabulary. These terms are arranged alphabetically by species name. Use *Genus Finder* when you want to find the definition for a genus species but don't know the genus name. For example, if you want to find the definition for "B. abortus," look under "abortus" in the *Genus Finder,* and you will find "Brucella." Then look up "Brucella" in the A to Z vocabulary to find the definition for "Brucella abortus." *Genus Finder* can also serve as a handy reference if you just need the spelling of a genus species.

Genus Finder

A

abortus: Brucella
abscessus: Mycobacterium
aceti: Turbatrix
acidophilum: Thermoplasma
acidophilus: Lactobacillus
acidovorans: Pseudomonas
acnes: Corynebacterium;
 Propionibacterium
aconitus: Anopheles
actinoides: Thysanosoma
actinomycetemcomitans:
 Actinobacillus; Haemophilus
aegypti: Aedes
aegyptius: Haemophilus
aerofaciens: Eubacterium
aerogenes: Enterobacter;
 Pasteurella; Peptococcus
aeruginosa: Pseudomonas
aethiopica: Leishmania
aethiopicum: Plasmodium
africae: Rickettsia
africana: Actinomadura;
 Taenia
afzelii: Borrelia
agalactiae: Streptococcus
ajacis: Delphinium
akamushi: Leptotrombidium;
 Trombicula
akari: Rickettsia
albicans: Candida
albimanus: Anopheles
albitarsus: Anopheles
albopictus: Aedes;
 Dermacentor
album: Veratrum
albus: Streptomyces
alcalescens subsp.
 alcalescens: Veillonella
alcalescens subsp. dispar:
 Veillonella
alcalesens: Veillonella
alcalifaciens: Providencia
alfreddugesi: Trombicula
alginolyticus: Vibrio
amalonatica: Citrobacter;
 Levinea
ambiguus: Passalurus
americana: Cochliomyia
americanum: Amblyomma
amycolatum:
 Corynebacterium

anaerobius:
 Peptostreptococcus
anatipestifer: Moraxella
anatolicum: Hyalomma
anatolicum anatolicum:
 Hyalomma
andersoni: Dermacentor
anginosus: Streptococcus
anitrata: Lingelsheimia
annua: Artemisia
annularis: Anopheles
annulipes: Anopheles
anomalus: Hoplopsyllus
anserina: Borrelia
anseris: Amidostomum
anthracis: Bacillus
anthropophaga: Cordylobia
aphrophilus: Haemophilus
apiospermum: Monosporium;
 Scedosporium
apiostomum:
 Oesophagostomum
aquasalis: Anopheles
aquatile: Flavobacterium
arabiensis: Anopheles
argentipes: Phlebotomus
armata: Taenia
armillatus: Armillifer;
 Porocephalus
asaccharolytica:
 Porphyromonas
asaccharolyticus:
 Peptostreptococcus
asini: Strongylus
asteroides: Nocardia
atlanticus: Aedes
atypica: Veillonella
audouinii: Microsporum
aureus: Staphylococcus
austeni: Culicoides
australiensis: Bipolaris
australis: Rickettsia
avium: Mycobacterium;
 Trypanosoma
avium-intracellulare
 complex: Mycobacterium
axanthum: Acholeplasma
axei: Trichostrongylus
aztecus: Anopheles

B

bacilliformis: Bartonella
bacteriovorus: Bdellovibrio

balabacensis: Anopheles
balatus: Acarus
bancrofti: Wuchereria
barbirostris: Anopheles
bellator: Anopheles
belli: Isospora
berghei: Plasmodium
bieneusi: Enterocytozoon
bifermentans: Clostridium
bifidum: Bifidobacterium
bigemina: Isospora
biloba: Ginkgo
bisonis: Cooperia
bivia: Prevotella
bivius: Bacteroides
botulinum: Clostridium
bovih'ominis: Sarcocystis
bovis: Actinomyces;
 Cysticercus;
 Mycobacterium;
 Streptococcus
boydii: Allescheria;
 Pseudallescheria; Shigella
bozemanii: Legionella
brasiliensis: Nocardia;
 Paracoccidioides
brazilianum: Plasmodium
braziliense: Ancylostoma
braziliensis: Leishmania
braziliensis braziliensis:
 Leishmania
braziliensis guyanensis:
 Leishmania
braziliensis panamensis:
 Leishmania
breve: Flavobacterium;
 Gymnodinium
brevicaeca: Heterophyes
brevicaudum:
 Oesophagostomum
brevis: Bacillus; Lactobacillus
bronchialis: Cyathostoma
bronchiseptica: Bordetella
brucei: Trypanosoma
brucei brucei: Trypanosoma
brucei gambiense:
 Trypanosoma
brucei rhodesiense:
 Trypanosoma
brumpti: Oesophagostomum
brunnipes: Anopheles
buccale: Mycoplasma

buccalis: Amoeba;
 Entamoeba; Leptotrichia;
 Trichomonas
buchneri: Lactobacillus
bulgaricus: Lactobacillus
burgdorferi: Borrelia
burgdorferi sensu lato:
 Borrelia
burgdorferi sensu stricto:
 Borrelia
burnetii: Coxiella; Rickettsia
buski: Fasciolopsis
bütschlii: Iodamoeba
butyricum: Clostridium
butzleri: Arcobacter

C

caballus: Aedes
cadaveris: Clostridium
caesar: Lucilia
cajennense: Amblyomma
calcitrans: Stomoxys
calcoaceticus: Acinetobacter
californiensis: Thelazia
callipaeda: Thelazia
campestris: Anopheles
canicularis: Anthomyia
canimorsus: Capnocytophaga
caninum: Ancylostoma;
 Dipylidium
canis: Brucella; Ehrlichia;
 Isospora; Microsporum;
 Rickettsia; Toxocara
canis, var. distortum:
 Microsporum
canium: Neospora
cantonensis: Angiostrongylus
capillaris: Muellerius
capillatus: Solenopotes
capillosus: Bacteroides
capitatus: Blastoschizomyces
capricola: Trichostrongylus
capsulatum: Histoplasma
carateum: Treponema
carinii: Pneumocystis
carnis: Clostridium
carrionii: Cladosporium
casei: Lactobacillus; Philopia;
 Piophila
catanella: Gonyaulax
catarrhalis: Branhamella;
 Moraxella; Neisseria
catenaformis: Lactobacillus

cati: Notoedres
caucasica: Borrelia
caudatus: Bodo
caviae: Neisseria; Nocardia
cayetanensis: Cyclospora
cellulosae: Cysticercus
cepacia: Burkholderia;
  Pseudomonas
cerebralis: Coenurus
cereus: Bacillus
cervi: Setaria
ceylanicum: Ancylostoma
ceylonica: Haemadipsa
chaffeensis: Ehrlichia
chattoni: Entamoeba
chauvoei: Clostridium
chelonae: Mycobacterium
chelonae subsp. abscessus:
  Mycobacterium
cheopis: Pulex
chinensis: Phlebotomus
cholerae: Vibrio
cinaedi: Helicobacter
cinnabarina: Haemaphysalis
circulans: Bacillus
cladosporioides:
  Cladosporium
clavatus: Aspergillus
cloacae: Enterobacter
cochlearium: Clostridium
coli: Amoeba; Balantidium;
  Campylobacter; Entamoeba;
  Escherichia
colubriformis:
  Trichostrongylus
columbianum:
  Oesophagostomum
combesi: Eubacterium
concentricum: Trichophyton
concinna: Haemaphysalis
concisus: Campylobacter
conglomeratus: Micrococcus
congolense: Trypanosoma
congolensis: Dermatophilus
conjunctivae: Dirofilaria
conorii: Rickettsia
constellatus: Peptococcus;
  Streptococcus
contortum: Eubacterium
cookei: Ixodes
cordatum: Diphyllobothrium
cordatus: Bothriocephalus
coriaceus: Ornithodoros
corneum: Nosema
coronata: Entomophthora
corrodens: Bacteroides;
  Eikenella
corticale: Cryptostroma
corymbosa: Rivea
costaricensis:
  Angiostrongylus;
  Morerastrongylus
crassicollis: Taenia
crispatum: Eubacterium
crispatus: Lactobacillus
crocidurae: Borrelia

crucians: Anopheles
cruzi: Anopheles;
  Schizotrypanum;
  Trypanosoma
culicifacies: Anopheles
culicis: Agamomermis
cuniculi: Encephalitozoon;
  Treponema
curcas: Jatropha
curticei: Cooperia
curvatus: Lactobacillus
cyaniventris: Dermatobia
cynomolgi: Plasmodium

D

dammini: Ixodes
damnosum: Simulium
darlingi: Anopheles
dassonvillei: Nocardiopsis
davtiani: Teladorsagia
delbrueckii: Lactobacillus
deliensis: Trombicula
demarquayi: Mansonella
demerariensis: Taenia
deminutus: Ternidens
dendriticum:
  Diphyllobothrium
denitrificans: Listeria
dentalis: Amoeba
dentata: Taenia
dentatum: Oesophagostomum
dentatus: Stephanurus
denticola: Prevotella;
  Treponema
dentium: Bifidobacterium
dentocariosa: Rothia
dentrificans: Jonesia
dermatitidis: Blastomyces
destruens: Hyphomyces
difficile: Clostridium
diminuta: Hymenolepis;
  Pseudomonas
dimorphon: Trypanosoma
diphtheriae: Corynebacterium
disiens: Bacteroides;
  Prevotella
dispar: Entamoeba
distasonis: Bacteroides
divergens: Babesia
diversus: Citrobacter; Levinea
doloresi: Gnathostoma
donovani: Leishmania
donovani archibaldi:
  Leishmania
donovani chagasi: Leishmania
donovani donovani:
  Leishmania
donovani infantum:
  Leishmania
dorsalis: Aedes
ducreyi: Haemophilus
dumoffii: Legionella
duodenale: Ancylostoma
durans: Streptococcus
duttonii: Borrelia

E

echidninus: Laelaps
edentatus: Strongylus
elegans: Cunninghamella
enterica subsp. choleraesuis:
  Salmonella
enterica subsp. enteritidis:
  Salmonella
enterica subsp. paratyphi A:
  Salmonella
enterica subsp. paratyphi B:
  Salmonella
enterica subsp. typhi:
  Salmonella
enterica subsp.
  typhimurium: Salmonella
enterocolitica: Yersinia
epidermidis: Staphylococcus
equi: Corynebacterium;
  Ehrilichia; Ehrlichia;
  Rhodococcus
equina: Setaria; Taenia
equinum: Trichophyton;
  Trypanosoma
equinus: Strongylus
equiperdum: Trypanosoma
equorum: Ascaris; Parascaris
erraticus: Ornithodoros
escomelis: Trypanosoma
esculenta: Gyromitra; Helvella
evansi: Trypanosoma
evolutus: Peptostreptococcus

F

faecalis: Enterococcus;
  Streptococcus
faecium: Enterococcus
falciparum: Plasmodium
fallax: Clostridium
farcinica: Nocardia
fasciatus: Pulex
faucium: Mycoplasma
feeleii: Legionella
felineus: Opisthorchis
felis: Isospora
fennelliae: Helicobacter
fermentans: Mycoplasma
fermentum: Lactobacillus
ferrugineum: Microsporum
fetus: Campylobacter; Vibrio
fetus subsp. jejuni:
  Campylobacter
fieldingi: Cooperia
filamentosum: Eubacterium
flava: Neisseria
flavescens: Neisseria
flavirostris: Anopheles
flaviscutellata: Lutzomyia
flaviscutellatus: Phlebotomus
flavus: Aspergillus
flexneri: Shigella

dysenteriae: Amoeba;
  Shigella

fluorescens: Pseudomonas
fluvialis: Vibrio
fluviatilis: Anopheles
foetidus: Peptostreptococcus
foetus: Trichomonas
folliculorum: Acarus;
  Demodex
fortuitum: Mycobacterium
fragilis: Bacteroides;
  Dientamoeba
frederiksenii: Yersinia
freeborni: Anopheles
freudenreichii:
  Propionibacterium
freundii: Citrobacter;
  Escherichia
fulvum: Microsporum
fumigatus: Aspergillus
funestus: Anopheles
furcosus: Bacteroides
furens: Culicoides
furfur: Malassezia
furnissii: Vibrio
furunculosa: Leishmania
fusiformis: Sarcocystis

G

gallinacea: Echidnophaga
gallinae: Acarus;
  Dermanyssus; Microsporum
gallinarum: Trichomonas
gambiae: Anopheles
gambiense: Trypanosoma
garinii: Borrelia
genitalis: Treponema
genitalium: Mycoplasma
georgianum:
  Oesophagostomum
gibsonii: Nocardia;
  Streptomyces
gigantica: Fasciola
gingivalis: Entamoeba
glabrata: Candida
glandulifera: Jatropha
glucuronolyticum:
  Corynebacterium
gondii: Toxoplasma
gonorrhoeae: Neisseria
gormanii: Legionella
gracilis: Euglena
granularum: Acholeplasma;
  Mycoplasma
granulomatis:
  Calymmatobacterium
granulosis: Noguchia
granulosus: Echinococcus
grayi: Listeria
gypseum: Microsporum

H

haematobium: Schistosoma
haemolysans: Neisseria
haemolyticum:
  Arcanobacterium;

Clostridium;
Corynebacterium
haemolyticus: Haemophilus;
Staphylococcus
hartmanni: Entamoeba
hawaiiensis: Bipolaris
hebraeum: Amblyomma
heilmannii: Helicobacter
hellum: Encephalitozoon
hemipterus: Cimex
hemolyticus: Bacillus
henselae: Bartonella
heparinolytica: Prevotella
hepatica: Capillaria; Fasciola
hermsi: Ornithodoros
hermsii: Borrelia
heterophyes: Heterophyes
hians: Diphyllobothrium
hinshawii: Arizona
hinzii: Bordetella
hirudinaceus:
Macracanthorhynchus
hispanica: Borrelia
hispidum: Gnathostoma
histolytica: Amoeba;
Entamoeba
histolyticum: Clostridium
histolyticus: Bacillus
hofmannii: Corynebacterium
hollisae: Vibrio
holmesii: Bordetella
hominis: Blastocystis;
Cardiobacterium;
Dermatobia;
Gastrodiscoides;
Gastrodiscus; Mycoplasma;
Octomitus; Sarcocystis;
Staphylococcus; Taenia;
Trichomonas; Trypanosoma
hominivorax: Cochliomyia
honei: Rickettsia
hordei: Acarus
houghtoni: Diphyllobothrium
hydatigena: Taenia
hydrophila: Aeromonas
hyodysenteriae: Treponema
hyointestinalis:
Campylobacter

I

ignotum: Trypanosoma
illustris: Lucilia
ilocanum: Echinostoma
immitis: Dirofilaria
inconstans: Proteus
indologenes: Kingella
inflatum: Scedosporium
influenzae: Haemophilus
infundibulum: Choanotaenia
innominatum: Clostridium
inornata: Culiseta
insidiosa: Erysipelothrix
insidiosum: Pythium
intercalatum: Schistosoma

intermedia: Prevotella;
Yersinia
intermedius: Lutzomyia;
Peptostreptococcus;
Streptococcus
interrogans: Leptospira
intestinale: Encephalitozoon
intestinalis: Giardia; Lamblia
intracellulare:
Mycobacterium
invicta: Solenopsis
irritans: Pulex; Siphona
israelii: Actinomyces

J

japonica: Rickettsia; Scopolia
japonicum: Schistosoma
jeanselmei: Exophiala
jeikeium: Corynebacterium
jejuni: Campylobacter
jensenii: Lactobacillus;
Propionibacterium
jeyporiensis: Anopheles

K

kansasii: Mycobacterium
karwari: Anopheles
katsuradai: Heterophyes
kellicotti: Paragonimus
kingae: Kingella; Moraxella
knowlesi: Plasmodium
kochi: Plasmodium
koseri: Citrobacter
kristensenii: Yersinia
kweiyangensis: Anopheles

L

labranchiae: Anopheles
lactis: Streptococcus
lacunata: Moraxella
lahorensis: Ornithodoros
laidlawii: Acholeplasma;
Mycoplasma
lamblia: Giardia
lanceolata: Hymenolepis
lari: Campylobacter
laryngeus:
Mammomonogamus
latina: Actinomadura
latum: Diphyllobothrium
latus: Bothriocephalus;
Dibothriocephalus
latyschewii: Borrelia
leachi: Haemaphysalis
lectularia: Acanthia
lectularius: Cimex
lentum: Eubacterium
leonina: Toxascaris
leprae: Mycobacterium
lesteri: Anopheles
leucocelaenus: Aedes
leucosphyrus: Anopheles
lewisi: Trypanosoma

lignieresii: Actinobacillus
lilacinus: Paecilomyces
limosum: Eubacterium
lindemanni: Sarcocystis
linguloides: Diphyllobothrium
loboi: Loboa
longbeachae: Legionella
longior: Tyroglyphus
longipalpis: Lutzomyia;
Phlebotomus
longispicularis:
Trichostrongylus
longispiculata: Nematodirella
lova: Dracunculus
lumbricoides: Ascaris
lupi: Spirocerca
lurida: Nocardia
luteola: Auchmeromyia
luteus: Micrococcus

M

macrorchis: Prosthogonimus
mactans: Latrodectus
maculatum: Amblyomma
maculatus: Anopheles
maculipennis: Anopheles
madagascariensis:
Inermicapsifer; Taenia
madurae: Nocardia
magnus: Peptostreptococcus
major: Leishmania;
Phlebotomus
majus: Habronema
malariae: Plasmodium
malayanum: Echinostoma
malayensis: Schistosoma
malayi: Brugia; Wuchereria
malaysiensis: Angiostrongylus
mallei: Burkholderia;
Pseudomonas
malonatica: Levinea
maltophilia: Pseudomonas;
Stenotrophomonas;
Xanthomonas
mangiferae: Nattrassia
mansoni: Bothriocephalus;
Diphyllobothrium;
Oxyspirura; Schistosoma;
Spirometra
mansonoides:
Bothriocephalus;
Diphyllobothrium;
Spirometra
marcescens: Serratia
marginatum: Hyalomma
marginatus: Dermacentor
marianum: Mycobacterium
marinum: Mycobacterium
marshalli: Marshallagia
matruchotii: Corynebacterium
mattheei: Schistosoma
maydis: Ustilago
mazzottii: Borrelia
medinensis: Dracunculus
mediterranei: Nocardia

megastoma: Habronema
megaterium: Bacillus
megninii: Trichophyton
mekongi: Schistosoma
melanimon: Aedes
melaninogenica: Prevotella
melaninogenicus: Bacteroides
melanura: Culiseta
melitensis: Brucella
melophagium: Trypanosoma
meningisepticum:
Flavobacterium
meningitidis: Neisseria
mentagrophytes:
Trichophyton
mesenteroides: Leuconostoc
messeae: Anopheles
metel: Datura
metschnikovii: Vibrio
mexicana: Leishmania
mexicana amazonensis:
Leishmania
mexicana garnhami:
Leishmania
mexicana mexicana:
Leishmania
mexicana pifanoi: Leishmania
mexicana venezuelensis:
Leishmania
micdadei: Legionella
micros: Peptostreptococcus
microstoma: Habronema
microti: Babesia;
Mycobacterium
miescheriana: Sarcocystis
milleri: Streptococcus
milnei: Culicoides
mimicus: Vibrio
minima: Taenia
minimus: Anopheles
minus: Spirillum
minutissimum:
Corynebacterium
minutum: Eubacterium
mirabilis: Proteus
mitchellae: Aedes
mitis: Streptococcus
mobilis: Klebsiella
moniliforme: Eubacterium
moniliformis: Streptobacillus
monocytogenes: Listeria
morbillorum: Gemella;
Peptostreptococcus;
Streptococcus
morganii: Morganella; Proteus
morsitans: Glossina
mortiferum: Fusobacterium
moshkovskii: Entamoeba
moubata complex:
Ornithodoros
mucosum: Treponema
multiceps: Multiceps
multiformis: Haverhillia
multilocularis: Echinococcus
multipapillosa: Parafilaria

multocida: Pasteurella
muscae: Habronema
muscaria: Amanita
mutans: Streptococcus
mystax: Toxocara

N

naeslundii: Actinomyces
nana: Hymenolepis
nana, var. fraterna:
  Hymenolepis
nanum: Microsporum
neavei: Simulium
necrophorum: Fusobacterium
neoformans: Cryptococcus
nidulans: Aspergillus
niger: Aspergillus;
  Peptococcus
nigrescens: Mermis
nigrificans: Clostridium;
  Desulfotomaculum
nigripalpus: Culex
nigromaculis: Aedes
nihonkaiense:
  Diphyllobothrium
nilotica: Limnatis
nipponicum: Gnathostoma
nodosus: Bacteroides;
  Dichelobacter
noguchi: Phlebotomus
nonliquefaciens: Moraxella
nova: Nocardia
novyi: Clostridium
nucleatum: Fusobacterium

O

obermeieri: Spirochaeta
occidentalis: Dermacentor
ochraceum: Simulium
oculi: Dracunculus
odontolyticus: Actinomyces
oedematiens: Clostridium
oncophora: Cooperia
orale: Mycoplasma
oralis: Bacteroides; Prevotella
orbiculare: Pityrosporum
orcini: Diphyllobothrium
orientalis: Nocardia;
  Phlebotomus
orientalis subsp. lurida:
  Amycolatopsis
oris: Bacteroides; Prevotella
osloensis: Moraxella
otitidiscaviarum: Nocardia
ovale: Pityrosporum;
  Plasmodium
ovalis: Malassezia
ovatum: Loxotrema
ovis: Taenia;
  Tetratrichomonas;
  Trichomonas
oxytoca: Klebsiella
ozaenae: Klebsiella
ozzardi: Mansonella

P

pachydermatis: Malassezia
pacificum: Diphyllobothrium
pacificus: Ixodes
paleopneumoniae:
  Peptostreptococcus
pallidipes: Glossina
pallidum: Treponema
palpalis: Glossina
papatasii: Phlebotomus
pappilipes: Ornithodoros
parabotulinum: Clostridium
parahaemolyticus:
  Haemophilus; Vibrio
parainfluenzae: Haemophilus
parapertussis: Bordetella
parapsilosis: Candida
paraputrificum: Clostridium
paratropicalis: Haemophilus
paratuberculosis:
  Mycobacterium
parkeri: Borrelia;
  Ornithodoros
parva var. crescens:
  Emmonsia
parva var. parva: Emmonsia
parvula: Veillonella
parvula subsp. atypica:
  Veillonella
parvula subsp. parvula:
  Veillonella
parvula subsp. rodentium:
  Veillonella
parvulus: Peptostreptococcus
parvum: Chrysosporium;
  Corynebacterium;
  Cryptosporidium;
  Eubacterium
pectinata: Cooperia
pelliertieri: Actinomadura
penetrans: Pulex; Sarcopsylla;
  Tunga
perfoliata: Anoplocephala
perfringens: Clostridium
perniciosus: Phlebotomus
persarum: Dracunculus
persica: Borrelia
persicolor: Microsporum
perstans: Mansonella
persulcatus: Ixodes
pertenue: Treponema
pertussis: Bordetella
peruensis: Lutzomyia
peruviana: Leishmania
pestis: Pasteurella; Yersinia
phagocytophila: Ehrlichia
phalloides: Amanita
pharyngis: Mycoplasma
phenylpyruvica: Moraxella
philippina: Taenia
philippinensis: Capillaria
phlebotomum: Bunostomum
phlei: Mycobacterium

phosphoreum:
  Photobacterium
physalis: Physalia
pifanoi: Leishmania
pilulifera: Euphorbia
pipiens: Culex
piscicida: Flavobacterium;
  Pseudomonas
pisiformis: Taenia
plagarumbelli:
  Peptostreptococcus
plantarum: Lactobacillus
plebeius: Vaginulus
plicatilis: Spirochaeta
pneumoniae: Chlamydia;
  Klebsiella; Mycoplasma;
  Streptococcus
pneumoniae subsp. ozaenae:
  Klebsiella
pneumophila: Legionella
pneumosintes: Bacteroides
poeciloides: Eubacterium
polecki: Entamoeba
polymyxa: Bacillus
polynesiensis: Aedes
praeacuta: Tissierella
praeacutus: Bacteroides
procyonis: Baylisascaris
productus: Peptostreptococcus
prolificans: Scedosporium
prolixus: Rhodnius
propionica: Arachnia
propionicus:
  Propionibacterium
proteus: Amoeba
prowazekii: Rickettsia
prunifolium: Viburnum
pseudoalcaligenes:
  Pseudomonas
pseudodiphtheriticum:
  Corynebacterium
pseudomallei: Burkholderia;
  Pseudomonas
pseudopunctipennis:
  Anopheles
pseudospiralis.: Trichinella
pseudotortuosum:
  Eubacterium
pseudotuberculosis:
  Pasteurella; Yersinia
psittaci: Chlamydia; Rickettsia
pteronyssinus:
  Dermatophagoides
pulchrum: Gongylonema
pumilis: Bacillus
punctata: Cooperia
punjatensis: Ceratophyllus
purpureus: Rhinoestrus
putredinis: Bacteroides
putrefaciens: Alteromonas;
  Pseudomonas
putrescentiae: Tyrophagus
putridus: Peptostreptococcus
pylori: Campylobacter;
  Helicobacter
pyogenes: Streptococcus

pyogenes albus:
  Staphylococcus
pyogenes aureus:
  Staphylococcus
pyriformis: Tetrahymena

Q

quadrilobata: Taenia
quadrimaculatus: Anopheles
quadrispinulatum:
  Oesophagostomum
quadrumanus: Chiropsalmus
quartum: Eubacterium
quinquecirrha: Chrysaora
quinquefasciatus: Culex
quintana: Bartonella
quintum: Eubacterium

R

radiatum: Oesophagostomum
radiatus: Strongylus
ramosum: Clostridium
rangeli: Trypanosoma
ratellina: Grisonella
rathouisi: Fasciolopsis
reconditum: Dipetalonema
rectale: Eubacterium
recurrentis: Borrelia
redikorzevi: Ixodes
reflexus: Argas
regina: Phormia
renale: Dioctophyma
restuans: Culex
reticulatus: Dermacentor
rettgeri: Proteus; Providencia
rhinaria: Linguatula
rhinoscleromatis: Klebsiella
rhizoglypticus hyacinthi:
  Acarus
rhodesiense: Trypanosoma
rhusiopathiae: Erysipelothrix
richteri: Solenopsis
ricinus: Ixodes
rickettsii: Rickettsia
ringeri: Paragonimus
risticii: Ehrlichia
rivolta: Isospora
rodentium: Veillonella
romeroi: Pyrenochaeta
rosati: Neotestudina
rosea: Vinca
rubrocoerulea var. praecox:
  Ipomoea
rubrum: Trichophyton
rudis: Ornithodoros
rugglesi: Simulium

S

saginata: Taenia
sagitta: Dipus
sakazakii: Enterobacter
salinarius: Culex
salivarium: Mycoplasma

salivarius: Lactobacillus; Streptococcus
salmincola: Nanophyetus; Troglotrema
saltans: Bodo
sanguineus: Rhipicephalus
sanguis: Streptococcus
sapiens: Homo
saprophyticus: Staphylococcus
sardinae: Eimeria
savigni: Ornithodoros
scabei: Acarus
scabiei: Sarcoptes
scapularis: Ixodes
schneideri: Elaeophora
schoenleinii: Trichophyton
scoticum: Diphyllobothrium
scrofulaceum: Mycobacterium
seeberi: Rhinosporidium
segnis: Haemophilus
sennetsu: Ehrlichia; Rickettsia
seoi: Gymnophalloides
septicum: Clostridium
septique: Vibrion
sergenti: Phlebotomus
serialis: Coenurus; Multiceps
sericata: Lucilia; Phaenicia
serotina: Prunus
serrata: Linguatula
serraticeps: Pulex
sexalatus: Physocephalus
shigelloides: Plesiomonas
siamense: Gnathostoma
sibirica: Rickettsia
sicca: Neisseria
simiae: Trypanosoma
simii: Trichophyton
simulans: Staphylococcus
sinensis: Clonorchis; Opisthorchis
sinuatum: Entoloma
slovaca: Rickettsia
smegmatis: Mycobacterium
solium: Taenia
sollicitans: Aedes
somaliensis: Streptomyces
sonnei: Shigella
sordellii: Clostridium
spatulata: Cooperia
sphaericus: Bacillus
sphenoides: Clostridium
spicifera: Bipolaris
spiniger: Heterodoxus
spinigera: Haemaphysalis

spinigerum: Gnathostoma
spinipalpis: Ixodes
spiralis: Acuaria; Trichinella
splanchnicus: Bacteroides
sporogenes: Clostridium
sputorum: Campylobacter; Vibrio
stegomyiae: Myxococcidium
stephanostomum: Oesophagostomum
stephensi: Anopheles
stilesi: Stephanofilaria
stramonium: Datura
streptocerca: Dipetalonema; Mansonella
striatum: Corynebacterium
strongylina: Ascarops
stuartii: Providencia
studeri: Bertiella
stutzeri: Pseudomonas
subflava: Neisseria
subtilis: Bacillus
suihominis: Sarcocystis
suis: Balantidium; Brucella; Isospora; Trichomonas; Trichuris; Trypanosoma
sundaicus: Anopheles
superpictus: Anopheles

T

taeniaeformis: Hydatigera; Taenia
taeniorhynchus: Aedes
talaje: Alectorobius
talajé: Ornithodoros
tarsalis: Culex
tenax: Trichomonas
tenella: Sarcocystis
tenue: Eubacterium
tenuis: Trichostrongylus
terreus: Aspergillus
tertium: Clostridium
tetani: Clostridium
tetraptera: Aspiculuris
theileri: Trypanosoma
thermosaccharolyticum: Clostridium
thetaiotamicron: Bacteroides
tholozani: Ornithodoros
thuringiensis: Bacillus
tonsurans: Trichophyton
tortuosum: Eubacterium
toruloidea: Hendersonula

trachomatis: Chlamydia
transvalensis: Nocardia
triatomae: Trypanosoma
trichiura: Trichuris
trichodectis: Cryptocystis
trichodes: Lactobacillus
trigonocephalum: Bunostomum
triseriatus: Aedes
tritici: Pyemotes
trivittatus: Aedes
tropica: Leishmania
tropicalis: Candida
tropica major: Leishmania
tropica mexicana: Leishmania
tsutsugamushi: Orientia; Rickettsia
tubaeforme: Ancylostoma
tuberculosis: Mycobacterium
tucumana: Mansonella
tularensis: Francisella; Pasteurella
turicata: Ornithodoros
turicatae: Borrelia
typhi: Rickettsia; Salmonella
typhosa: Salmonella

U

ugandense: Trypanosoma
ulcerans: Mycobacterium
urealyticum: Ureaplasma
urens: Jatropha
ureolyticus: Bacteroides
urinarius: Bodo

V

vaccae: Mycobacterium
vaginalis: Gardnerella; Trichomonas
vanbreuseghemi: Microsporum
variabilis: Dermacentor
varians: Micrococcus
variegatum: Amblyomma; Hyalomma
variegatus: Aedes
vasiformis: Saksenaea
venezuelensis: Borrelia; Ornithodoros
ventricosus: Haemodipsus; Pediculoides; Strongylus

ventriculi: Sarcina
venulosum: Oesophagostomum
verrucarum: Phlebotomus
verrucosum: Trichophyton
verrucosus: Ornithodoros
versicolor: Ipomoea
vesicularis: Pseudomonas
vexans: Aedes
violaceum: Cardiobacterium; Chromobacterium; Trichophyton
virginiana: Prunus
viridans: Streptococcus
viride: Veratrum
viridis: Euglena
viscosus: Actinomyces
vitrinus: Trichostrongylus
vitulorum: Neoascaris
vivax: Plasmodium; Trypanosoma
viverrini: Opisthorchis
vivipara: Probstymayria
vogeli: Echinococcus
volutans: Spirillum
volvulus: Onchocerca
vulgaris: Proteus; Strongylus
vulnificus: Vibrio
vulpis: Crenosoma; Trichuris

W

wadsworthii: Legionella
watsoni: Cladorchis
welchii: Clostridium
werneckii: Cladosporium; Exophiala
westermani: Paragonimus
whippelii: Tropheryma
winthemi: Margaropus

X

xenopi: Mycobacterium
xerosis: Corynebacterium
(Xylohypha) bantianum: Cladosporium

Z

zeae: Ustilago
zoohelcum: Weeksella

Genus Finder

The following pages (WF1-WF122) contain a list of multiword (or subentry) terms from the A to Z vocabulary. These terms are arranged alphabetically by their first word(s). Use *Word Finder* when you want to find the definition for a subentry, but don't know the main, governing word. For example, if you want to find the definition for "Aaron sign," look under "Aaron" in the *Word Finder* and you will find "sign." Then look up "sign" in the A to Z vocabulary to find the definition for "Aaron sign." *Word Finder* can also serve as a handy reference if you just need the spelling of a term.

A

α′: hemolysis

α: fetoprotein; granules; helix; hemolysin; thalassemia; thalassemia intermedia

A: bands; bile; cells; chain; disks; fibers; wave

A1: segment of anterior cerebral artery

A2: segment of anterior cerebral artery

α₁-: antitrypsin; lipoprotein

A₂: thalassemia

A-: DNA; strabismus

α-: keto acid dehydrogenase

aaa: disease

Aagenaes: syndrome

Aaron: sign

Aarskog-Scott: syndrome

abacterial thrombotic: endocarditis

Abadie: sign of tabes dorsalis

abapical: pole

abarticular: gout

Abbe: flap

Abbé: condenser

Abbott: artery; stain for spores; tube

ABC: leads

A.B.C.: process

abdominal: angina; aorta; apoplexy; aura; ballottement; canal; cavity; dropsy; fibromatosis; fissure; fistula; guarding; hernia; hysterectomy; hysteropexy; hysterotomy; lymph nodes; migraine; myomectomy; nephrectomy; ostium of uterine tube; pad; part of aorta; part of esophagus; part of pectoralis major (muscle); part of peripheral autonomic plexuses and ganglia; part of thoracic duct; part of ureter; pool; pregnancy; pressure; pulse; reflexes; regions; respiration; ring; sac; salpingectomy; salpingo-oophorectomy;

salpingotomy; section; testis; typhoid; zones

abdominal aortic (nervous): plexus

abdominal external oblique: muscle

abdominal internal oblique: muscle

abdominal muscle deficiency: syndrome

abdominocardiac: reflex

abdominojugular: reflux

abdominopelvic: cavity

abdominopelvic splanchnic: nerves

abdominoperineal: resection

abdominothoracic: arch

abdominovaginal: hysterectomy

abducens: eminence; nerve; nucleus

abducent: nerve [CN VI]

abductor: muscle; muscle of great toe; muscle of little finger; muscle of little toe

abductor digiti minimi: muscle of foot; muscle of hand

abductor hallucis: muscle

abductor pollicis brevis: muscle

abductor pollicis longus: muscle

abductor spasmodic: dysphonia

Abegg: rule

Abell-Kendall: method

Abelson murine leukemia: virus

Abernethy: fascia

aberrant: artery; bundles; complex; ducts; ductules; ganglion; goiter; hemoglobin; regeneration

aberrant bile: ducts

aberrant obturator: artery

aberrant ventricular: conduction

abnormal: cleavage of cardiac valve; correspondence; occlusion

abnormal ST: segment

ABO: antigens; factors

ABO hemolytic: disease of the newborn

aborted: systole

aborted ectopic: pregnancy

abortion: rate

abortive: neurofibromatosis; transduction

abortus: bacillus

abraded: wound

Abrahams: sign

Abrams heart: reflex

abrasive: strip

abscopal: effect

absence: seizure

absent: state

absolute: agraphia; alcohol; dehydration; glaucoma; hemianopia; humidity; hydration; hyperopia; leukocytosis; oils; pressure; scale; scotoma; system of units; temperature; threshold; unit; viscosity; zero

absolute cell: increase

absolute intensity threshold: acuity

absolute refractory: period

absolute terminal innervation: ratio

absorbable gelatin: film; sponge

absorbable surgical: suture

absorbancy: index

absorbed: dose

absorbent: cotton; points; system; vessels

absorption: band; cell; chromatography; coefficient; collapse; fever; lines; spectrum

absorptive: cells of intestine

abstinence: symptoms; syndrome

abstract: intelligence; thinking

a-c: interval

Acanthamoeba: medium

acanthocytosis with: chorea

acapnial: alkalosis

acarine: dermatosis

accelerated: conduction; eruption; hypertension; reaction; rejection

accelerator: factor; fibers; globulin; nerves

acceptor: RNA; site

acceptor splicing: site

access: opening

accessory: adrenal; atrium; auricles; branch of middle meningeal artery; breast; canal; cartilage; cell; chromosome; flocculus; gland; ligaments; lymph nodes; molecules; nerve [CN XI]; nipple; nuclei of optic tract; organs; organs of the eye; pancreas; placenta; portion of spinal accessory nerve; process of lumbar vertebra; root of tooth; sign; spleen; structures; symptom; thyroid; tragus; tubercle

accessory cephalic: vein

accessory cuneate: nucleus

accessory flexor: muscle of foot

accessory hemiazygos: vein

accessory lacrimal: glands

accessory meningeal: artery; branch; branch of middle meningeal artery

accessory nasal: cartilages

accessory nerve: lymph nodes; trunk

accessory obturator: artery

accessory olivary: nuclei

accessory pancreatic: duct

accessory parotid: gland

accessory phrenic: nerves

accessory plantar: ligaments

accessory quadrate: cartilage

accessory saphenous: vein

accessory suprarenal: glands

accessory thyroid: gland

accessory vertebral: vein

accessory visual: apparatus; structures

accessory volar: ligaments

accident: neurosis

accidental: abortion; host; hypothermia; image; murmur; myiasis; parasite; symptom

acclimating: fever

accolé: forms

accommodation: phosphene; reflex

accommodative: asthenopia; convergence; insufficiency; strabismus

accommodative convergence-accommodation: ratio

accompanying: vein; vein of hypoglossal nerve

accoucheur: hand

accretion: lines

accretionary: growth

accumulation: analysis; disease

acentric: chromosome; fragment

acephalgic: migraine

acetabular: artery; branch; fossa; labrum; lip; margin; notch

acetate replacement: factor

acetic: fermentation; solution

acetone: body; chloroform; compound; fixative; test

acetone-insoluble: antigen

aceto-orcein: stain

acetosoluble: albumin

acetyl: value

acetyl-activating: enzyme

Achard: syndrome

Achard-Thiers: syndrome

Achenbach: syndrome

achievement: age; motive; quotient; test

Achilles: bursa; reflex; tendon

achlorhydric: anemia

acholuric: jaundice

achondroplastic: dwarfism

achrestic: anemia

achromatic: apparatus; lens; objective; threshold; vision

acid: agglutination; alcohol; carboxypeptidase; cell; deoxyribonuclease; dextran; dextrin; dyspepsia; fuchsin; gland; indigestion; intoxication; maltase; oxide; phosphatase; radical; reaction; rigor; salt; seromucoid; stain; sulfate; tartrate; tide; wave

α_1**-acid:** glycoprotein

acid-ash: diet

acid-base: balance; equilibrium

acid etch cemented: splint

acid-etched: restoration

acidic: amino acid; dyes

acidified serum: test

acidophil: adenoma; cell; granule

acidophilic: leukocyte

acidophilus: milk

acid perfusion: test

acid phosphatase: test for semen

acid reflux: test

acinar: carcinoma; cell

acinar cell: tumor

acinic cell: adenocarcinoma; carcinoma

acinotubular: gland

acinous: cell; gland

ackee: poisoning

acne: keloid

acorn-tipped: catheter

Acosta: disease

acoustic: agraphia; aphasia; area; cell; crest; enhancement; impedance; lemniscus; lens; meatus; nerve; neurilemoma; neurinoma; neuroma; papilla; pressure; radiation; reflex; schwannoma; shadow; spots; striae; teeth; tetanus; tolerance; tubercle; tumor; vesicle

acoustical: surround

acousticofacial: ganglion

acousticopalpebral: reflex

acoustic reference: level

acoustic stimulation: test

acquired: agammaglobulinemia; character; cuticle; drives; hyperlipoproteinemia; hypogammaglobulinemia; ichthyosis; immunity; leukoderma; leukopathia; megacolon; methemoglobinemia; nevus; pellicle; reflex; sensitivity; toxoplasmosis in adults; trichoepithelioma

acquired centric: relation

acquired eccentric: relation

acquired epileptic: aphasia

acquired hemolytic: anemia; icterus

acquired immunodeficiency: syndrome

acquired tufted: angioma

acral lentiginous: melanoma

Acrel: ganglion

acrid: poison

acridine: dyes

acrocentric: chromosome

acrodynic: erythema

acrofacial: dysostosis; syndrome

acromegalic: gigantism

acromelic: dwarfism

acromesomelic: dwarfism

acromial: anastomosis of the thoracoacromial artery; angle; artery; branch of suprascapular artery; branch of thoracoacromial artery; end of clavicle; extremity of clavicle; facet of clavicle; part of deltoid (muscle); plexus; process; reflex

acromial arterial: network

acromial articular: facies of clavicle; surface of clavicle

acromioclavicular: disk; joint; ligament

acromion: presentation

acromiothoracic: artery

acroparesthesia: syndrome

acrosomal: cap; granule; vesicle

acrylic: resin

acrylic resin: base; tooth; tray

ACTH-producing: adenoma

ACTH stimulation: test

actin: filament

actinic: cheilitis; conjunctivitis; dermatitis; granuloma; keratitis; keratosis; porokeratosis; prurigo; ray; reticuloid

actinide: elements

actinium: emanation

actinomycotic: appendicitis

action: current; potential; tremor

activated: acetaldehyde; amino acid; atom; carboxylic acid; charcoal; choline; fatty acid; glucose; hydrogen; macrophage; resin; sludge; state

activated clotting: time

activated partial thromboplastin: time

activated sludge: method

activation: analysis

active: acetate; aldehyde; anaphylaxis; carbon dioxide; caries; center; congestion; electrode; formaldehyde; formate; formyl; glycoaldehyde; hyperemia; immunity; immunization; inflammation; labor; methionine; methyl; movement; mutant; placebo; principle; prophylaxis; psychoanalysis; pyruvate; repressor; site; splint; succinate; sulfate; transport; treatment; vasoconstriction; vasodilation

active length-tension: curve

activities of daily living: scale

activity: coefficient

actual: cautery

acupuncture: anesthesia

acute: abdomen; abscess; alcoholism; angle; appendicitis; ataxia; chalazion; cholecystitis; chorea; delirium; glaucoma; glomerulonephritis; goiter; histoplasmosis; inflammation; malaria; mania; nephritis; nephrosis; pyelonephritis; rejection; rhinitis; rickets; schizophrenia; trypanosomiasis; urticaria

acute adrenocortical: insufficiency

acute African sleeping: sickness

acute anterior: poliomyelitis

acute ascending: paralysis

acute bacterial: endocarditis

acute brachial: radiculitis

acute bulbar: poliomyelitis

acute catarrhal: conjunctivitis

acute cellular: rejection

acute compression: triad

acute contagious: conjunctivitis

acute crescentic: glomerulonephritis

acute cutaneous: leishmaniasis

acute decubitus: ulcer

acute disseminated: encephalomyelitis

acute epidemic: conjunctivitis; leukoencephalitis

acute febrile neutrophilic: dermatosis

acute fibrinous: pericarditis

acute follicular: conjunctivitis

acute fulminating: meningococcemia

acute fulminating meningococcal: septicemia

acute hallucinatory: paranoia

acute hemorrhagic: conjunctivitis; encephalitis; glomerulonephritis; leukoencephalitis; pancreatitis

acute idiopathic: polyneuritis

acute inclusion body: encephalitis

acute infectious nonbacterial: gastroenteritis

acute inflammatory: polyneuropathy

acute inflammatory demyelinating: polyradiculoneuropathy

acute intermittent: porphyria

acute interstitial: nephritis; pneumonia; pneumonitis

acute invasive: aspergillosis

acute isolated: myocarditis

acute lobar: nephrosis

acute massive liver: necrosis

acute motor axonal: neuropathy

acute multifocal placoid pigment: epitheliopathy

acute necrotizing: encephalitis; myelitis

acute necrotizing hemorrhagic: encephalomyelitis; leukoencephalitis

acute necrotizing ulcerative: gingivitis

acute organic brain: syndrome

acute parenchymatous: hepatitis

acute phase: protein; reactants; reaction; response

acute poststreptococcal: glomerulonephritis

acute primary hemorrhagic: meningoencephalitis

acute promyelocytic: leukemia

acute pulmonary: alveolitis

acute radiation: syndrome

acute recurrent: rhabdomyolysis

acute reflex bone: atrophy

acute respiratory distress: syndrome

acute retinal: necrosis

acute rheumatic: arthritis

acute scalp: cellulitis

acute schizophrenic: episode

acute sensory motor axonal: neuropathy

acute situational: reaction

acute splenic: tumor

acute stress: reaction

acute transverse: myelitis

acute vascular: purpura

acute viral: conjunctivitis

acute yellow: atrophy of the liver

acyclic: compound

acyl-activating: enzyme

acyl carrier: protein

acylmercaptan: bond

Adair-Koshland-Némethy-Filmer: model

adamantine: membrane

Adams-Stokes: disease; syncope; syndrome

adansonian: classification

adaptation: diseases; syndrome of Selye

adaptive: behavior; enzyme; hypertrophy

adaptive behavior: scales

adaptor: hypothesis

addictive: drug

Addis: count; test

Addison: anemia; disease

Addison-Biermer: disease

Addison clinical: planes

addisonian: anemia; crisis; syndrome

addition: compound; mutation

addition-deletion: mutation

additive: effect; model

addressin: ligands

adductor: canal; compartment of thigh; hiatus; muscle; muscle of great toe; muscle of thumb; reflex; tubercle of femur

adductor brevis: muscle

adductor hallucis: muscle

adductor longus: muscle

adductor magnus: muscle

adductor minimus: muscle

adductor pollicis: muscle

adductor spasmodic: dysphonia

Aden: fever; ulcer

adeno-associated: virus

adenoid: facies; tissue; tumor

adenoidal-pharyngeal-conjunctival: virus

adenoid cystic: carcinoma

adenomatoid: tumor

adenomatoid odontogenic: tumor

adenomatous: goiter; hyperplasia; polyp; polyposis coli

adenosatellite: virus

adenosquamous: carcinoma

adequal: cleavage

adequate: stimulus

adherence: syndrome

adherent: leukoma; pericardium; placenta

adhering: junctions

adhesion: dyspepsia; molecules; phenomenon; test

adhesive: arachnoiditis; atelectasis; bandage; capsulitis; inflammation; otitis; pericarditis; peritonitis; phlebitis; pleurisy; tape; vaginitis

adhesive absorbent: dressing

Adie: pupil; syndrome

adipokinetic: hormone

adipose: capsule; cell; degeneration; folds of the pleura; fossae; infiltration; tissue; tumor

adiposogenital: degeneration; dystrophy; syndrome

adjacent: angle

adjustable: articulator

adjustable axis: face-bow

adjustable occlusal: pivot

adjustment: disorders

adjuvant: chemotherapy; vaccine

Adler: test

adlerian: psychoanalysis; psychology

admaxillary: gland

adnexal: adenoma; carcinoma

adolescent: albuminuria; crisis; medicine

adolescent round: back

adoptive: immunity; immunotherapy

ADP: ribosylation

adrenal: androgen; apoplexy; body; capsule; cortex; crisis; gland; hermaphroditism; hypertension; leukodystrophy; rest; virilism

adrenal androgen-stimulating: hormone

adrenal cortex: injection

adrenal cortical: carcinoma; syndrome

adrenaline: reversal

adrenal virilizing: syndrome

adrenal weight: factor

α-adrenergic: receptors

β-adrenergic: receptors

adrenergic: amine; blockade; fibers; neurotransmitter; receptors

β-adrenergic blocking: agent

α-adrenergic blocking: agent

adrenergic blocking: agent

adrenergic neuronal blocking: agent

β-adrenergic receptor blocking: agent

α-adrenoceptor: antagonist

adrenocortical: adenoma; hormones; insufficiency

adrenocorticotropic: hormone; peptide

adrenocorticotropic releasing: factor

adrenogenital: syndrome

adrenomedullary: hormones

adrenomimetic: amine

β-adrenoreceptor: antagonist

adrenotropic: hormone

Adson: forceps; maneuver; test

adsorption: chromatography; theory of narcosis

adult: hypophosphatasia; medulloepithelioma; rickets; tuberculosis

adult foveomacular retinal: dystrophy

adult lactase: deficiency

adult-onset: diabetes

adult pseudohypertrophic muscular: dystrophy

adult respiratory distress: syndrome

adult T-cell: leukemia; lymphoma

advance: directive

advanced multiple-beam equalization: radiography

advancement: flap

adventitial: cell; neuritis

adventitious: albuminuria; bursa; cyst

adventitious breath: sounds

adverse: reaction

adversive: movement

adynamic: ileus

A-E: amputation

Aeby: plane

aerial: mycelium; sickness

aerobic: dehydrogenase; respiration

aerodynamic: theory

aerogenic: tuberculosis

aerosol: generator

aerospace: medicine

aestivoautumnal: fever

AFA: fixative

affect: displacement; hunger; memory; spasms

affective: disorders; personality; psychosis; tone

afferent: fibers; lymphatic; nerve; vessel

afferent glomerular: arteriole

afferent loop: syndrome

affinity: antibody; chromatography; column

afibrillar: cementum

AFORMED: phenomenon

African: histoplasmosis; trypanosomiasis

African endomyocardial: fibrosis

African furuncular: myiasis

African hemorrhagic: fever

African horse sickness: virus

African sleeping: sickness

African tick: fever

African tick-bite: fever

afterloading: radiation; screw

afunctional: occlusion

A/G: ratio

Ag-AS: stain

agene: process

age-related macular: degeneration

age-specific: rate

agglutinating: antibody

agglutination: test

agglutinative: thrombus

aggregate: anaphylaxis; glands

aggregated lymphatic: follicles of small intestine; follicles of vermiform appendix; nodules

aggregated lymphoid: nodules; nodules of small intestine

aggressive: angiomyxoma; instinct

aggressive infantile: fibromatosis

agitated: depression

aglossia-adactylia: syndrome

agminate: glands

agnogenic myeloid: metaplasia

agonal: clot; infection; leukocytosis; rhythm; thrombus

agranular: cortex; leukocyte

agranular endoplasmic: reticulum

agranulocytic: angina

AH: interval

AH conduction: time

Ahumada-Del Castillo: syndrome

Aicardi: syndrome

AIDS: dementia

AIDS dementia: complex

AIDS-related: complex; virus

air: bladder; bronchogram; cells; cells of auditory tube; conduction; dose; embolism; pollution; sac; sickness; splint; syringe; thermometer; tube; vesicles

air-bone: gap

airborne: infection

airbrasive: technique

air-conditioner: lung

air contrast: enema

air contrast barium: enema

air-gap: radiography; technique

airplane: splint

airport: malaria

air-slaked: lime

airspace-filling: pattern

airway: pattern; resistance

airway pressure release: ventilation

Airy: disk

A-K: amputation

Akabane: virus

akamushi: disease

Åkerlund: deformity

akinetic: mutism; seizure

ala central: lobule

alactic oxygen: debt

Alagille: syndrome

Åland Island: albinism

Alanson: amputation

alar: artery of nose; chest; folds of intrapatellar synovial fold; lamina of neural tube; ligaments; part of nasalis muscle; plate of neural tube; process; spine

alarm: reaction

alaryngeal: speech

Albarran: glands; test

Albarran y Dominguez: tubules

albedo: retinae

Albers-Schönberg: disease

Albert: disease; stain; suture

Albini: nodules

albino: rats

Albinus: muscle

Albrecht: bone

Albright: disease; syndrome

Albright hereditary: osteodystrophy

albumin-globulin: ratio

albuminized: iron

albuminocytologic: dissociation

albuminoid: degeneration

albuminous: cell; gland; swelling

albuminuric: retinitis

Alcock: canal

alcohol: addiction; diuresis

alcohol amnestic: syndrome

alcohol-glycerin: fixative

alcoholic: cardiomyopathy; cirrhosis; deterioration; extract; fermentation; hyalin; myocardiopathy; pneumonia; polyneuropathy; psychoses; tincture

alcoholic hyaline: bodies

alcoholic withdrawal: tremor

alcohol withdrawal: delirium

aldehyde: fuchsin; reaction

Alder: anomaly; bodies

aldol: condensation

aldosterone: antagonist

Aldrich: syndrome

alecithal: ovum

Aleppo: boil

aleukemic: leukemia; myelosis

Aleutian mink disease: virus

Alexander: disease; hearing impairment; law

alexin: unit

Alezzandrini: syndrome

algid: malaria; stage

algid pernicious: fever

algoid: cell

Alice in Wonderland: syndrome

alicyclic: compounds

alignment: curve; mark

alimentary: apparatus; canal; diabetes; glycosuria; hyperinsulinism; lipemia; osteopathy; pentosuria; system; tract

alimentary tract: smear

aliphatic: compound

alisphenoid: cartilage

alizarin: indicator

alkali: metal; reserve; therapy

alkali denaturation: test

alkali earth: metal

alkaline: earths; phosphatase; reaction; RNase; tide; toluidine blue O; water; wave

alkaline-ash: diet

alkaline earth: elements

alkaline milk: drip

alkaline reflux: gastritis

alkylating: agent

allantoenteric: diverticulum

allantoic: bladder; cyst; diverticulum; fluid; sac; stalk; vesicle

allantoid: membrane

allantoidoangiopagous: twins

allelic: exclusion; gene

Allen: test

Allen-Doisy: test; unit

Allen-Masters: syndrome

allergenic: extract

allergic: angiitis; conjunctivitis; coryza; eczema; extract; granulomatosis; inflammation; purpura; reaction; rhinitis

allergic bronchopulmonary: aspergillosis

allergic contact: dermatitis

allergic granulomatous: angiitis

Allgrove: syndrome

allied: reflexes

alligator: forceps; skin

Allis: forceps

all or none: law

allogeneic: antigen; graft; inhibition

allograft: rejection

allomeric: function

allopathic: keratoplasty

allosteric: enzyme; site

allotypic: determinants; marker

alloxan: diabetes

Almeida: disease

Almén: test for blood

Alpers: disease

Alpha: tests

alpha: alcoholism; angle; blocking; cells of anterior lobe of hypophysis; cells of pancreas; error; fibers; granule; particle; radiation; ray; rhythm; substance; units; wave

alpha-: oxidation

alpha methyl: dopa

Alpine: scurvy

Alport: syndrome

Alström: syndrome

ALT:AST: ratio

Altemeier: operation

alterative: inflammation

altercursive: intubation

alternate: hemianesthesia

alternate binaural loudness balance: test

alternate cover: test

alternate day: strabismus

alternating: current; hemiplegia; mydriasis; pulse; strabismus; tremor

alternating light: test

alternative: hypothesis; inheritance; medicine; splicing; tremor

altitude: chamber; disease; erythremia; sickness

altitudinal: hemianopia

Altmann: fixative; granule; theory

Altmann anilin-acid fuchsin: stain

Altmann-Gersh: method

Alu: sequences

alu: family

alu-equivalent: family

alum: whey

aluminum: penicillin

alveolar: abscess; adenocarcinoma; air; angle; arch of mandible; arch of maxilla; atrophy; body; bone; border; canals of maxilla; cell; crest; duct; foramina of maxilla; gas; gingiva; gland; index; macrophage; mucosa; osteitis; part of mandible; pattern; periosteum; point; pores; process of maxilla; ridge; sac; septum; ventilation; yokes

alveolar-arterial oxygen: difference

alveolar cell: carcinoma

alveolar dead: space

alveolar duct: emphysema

alveolar gas: equation

alveolar hydatid: cyst

alveolar soft part: sarcoma

alveolar supporting: bone

alveolobuccal: groove; sulcus

alveolocapillary: block; membrane

alveolodental: canals; ligament; membrane

alveololabial: groove; sulcus

alveololingual: groove; sulcus

alveolonasal: line

Alzheimer: dementia; disease; sclerosis

Alzheimer type I: astrocyte

Alzheimer type II: astrocyte

Am: antigens

amacrine: cell

Amadori: rearrangement

amalgam: carrier; matrix; strip; tattoo

amaranth: solution

amaurotic: mydriasis; nystagmus; pupil

amaurotic cat: eye

amber: codon; mutant; mutation; suppressor

Amberg lateral sinus: line

ambient: cistern

ambiguous: genitalia

ambiguous atrioventricular: connections
ambiguous external: genitalia
ambiguus: nucleus
amblyogenic: period
amboceptor: unit
Amboyna: button
Ambu: bag
ambulant: edema; erysipelas; plague
ambulatory: anesthesia; automatism; schizophrenia; surgery; typhoid
amebic: abscess; colitis; dysentery; granuloma; vaginitis
ameboid: cell; movement
amelanotic: melanoma
ameloblastic: fibroma; fibrosarcoma; layer; odontoma; sarcoma
ameloblastic adenomatoid: tumor
ameloblastomatous: craniopharyngioma
amelodental: junction
amenorrhea-galactorrhea: syndrome
American: leishmaniasis; tarantula; trypanosomiasis
American Law Institute: rule
American Sign: Language
Ames: assay; test
amide: oximes
amino: sugars
amino-: terminal
amino acid: activation; analysis; reagent
amino acid activating: enzyme
4-aminobutyrate: pathway
p-aminohippurate: clearance
δ-aminolevulinate dehydratase: porphyria
Ammon: fissure; horn; prominence
ammonia: assimilation; detoxication; fixation; rash
ammoniacal: urine
ammoniated: mercuric chloride; mercury; tincture
amnemonic: agraphia
amnestic: aphasia; syndrome
amniocardiac: vesicle
amnioembryonic: junction
amniogenic: cells
amnion: ring
amnionic: adhesions; amputation; band; cavity; corpuscle; duct; ectoderm; fluid; fold; raphe; sac
amnionic fluid: embolism; index; syndrome
amorphous: fraction of adrenal cortex;

hydroxyapatite; phosphorus; silicon
amorphous insulin zinc: suspension
amorphous selenium: plate
AMPA: receptor
Ampère: postulate
amphibolic: fistula
amphiprotic: solvent
amphophil: granule
amphoric: rale; resonance; respiration; voice
amphoric voice: sound
amphoteric: electrolyte; element; reaction
amphotropic: virus
amplifier: host
amplitude of: accommodation; convergence
ampullar: abortion; pregnancy
ampullary: aneurysm; crest; crest (of semicircular ducts); crura of semicircular ducts; cupula; folds of uterine tube; groove; sulcus; type of renal pelvis
ampullary membranous: limbs of semicircular ducts
amputating: ulcer
amputation: knife; neuroma
Amsel: criteria
Amsler: chart; grid; test
Amsterdam: syndrome
Amussat: valve; valvula
amygdaloclaustral: area
amygdaloid: body; complex; fossa; nucleus; tubercle
amygdalopiriform transition: area
amylaceous: corpuscle
amylase-creatinine clearance: ratio
amylic: fermentation
amylogenic: body
amyloid: angiopathy; bodies of the prostate; degeneration; kidney; nephrosis; protein; tumor
amyotrophic lateral: sclerosis
AN: interval
anabiotic: cell
anabolic: steroid
anaclitic: depression; psychotherapy
anacrotic: limb; pulse
anaerobic: cellulitis; dehydrogenase; pneumonia; respiration
anagen: effluvium
anal: atresia; canal; cleft; columns; crypts; cushions; ducts; erotism; fascia; fissure; fistula; gland; membrane; orifice; pecten; phase; pit; plate; reflex;

region; sinuses; triangle; valves; verge
analeptic: enema
analgesic: cuirass; nephritis; nephropathy
anal skin: tag
anal transitional: zone
analytic: chemistry; psychiatry; study; therapy
analytical: psychology; sensitivity; specificity
analyzing: rod
anamnestic: reaction; response
anaphase: lag
anaphylactic: antibody; intoxication; reaction; shock
anaphylactoid: crisis; purpura; shock
anaplastic: astrocytoma; carcinoma; cell; oligodendroglioma
anaplastic large cell: lymphoma
anaplerotic: reaction
anarthritic rheumatoid: disease
anastomosing: fibers; vessel
anastomotic: branch; branch of middle meningeal artery with lacrimal artery; stricture; ulcer; veins; vessel
anatomic: airway; pathology; position; rigidity; sphincter; tooth; tubercle; wart
anatomical: age; conjugate; crown; element; neck of humerus; root
anatomical internal: os of uterus
anatomic dead: space
anatrophic: nephrotomy
anchor: splint
anchorage: dependence
anchoring: fibrils; villus
ancillary: ports
anconal: fossa
anconeus: muscle
ancylostoma: dermatitis
Andernach: ossicles
Anders: disease
Andersch: ganglion; nerve
Andersen: disease
Anderson: splint
Anderson-Collip: test
Anderson and Goldberger: test
Andes: virus
Andral: decubitus
androgen: unit
androgen binding: protein
androgenic: alopecia; hormone; zone
androgen insensitivity: syndrome

androgen resistance: syndromes
android: obesity; pelvis
anechoic: chamber
Anel: method
anemic: anoxia; halo; hypoxia; infarct; murmur
anergic: leishmaniasis
aneroid: manometer
anesthesia: machine; record
anesthetic: circuit; depth; ether; gas; index; leprosy; shock; vapor
anestrous: ovulation
aneurysm: needle
aneurysmal: bruit; cough; murmur; sac; varix
aneurysmal bone: cyst
angel: wing
Angelman: syndrome
Angelucci: syndrome
Anger: camera
anginose: scarlatina
angioblastic: cells; cyst
angiodysgenetic: myelomalacia
angiofollicular mediastinal lymph node: hyperplasia
angiogenesis: factor
angiography: catheter
angioid: streaks
angioimmunoblastic: lymphadenopathy with dysproteinemia
angiolithic: degeneration; sarcoma
angiolymphoid: hyperplasia with eosinophilia
angioneurotic: edema
angioosteohypertrophy: syndrome
angiopathic: neurasthenia
angiopathic hemolytic: anemia
angioplasty: balloon
angiotensin: receptor
angiotensin-converting: enzyme
angiotensin-converting enzyme: inhibitors
angiotensin receptor: blockers
Angle: classification of malocclusion
angle: recession
angle of: convergence
angle-closure: glaucoma
Ångström: law; scale; unit
angular: acceleration; aldehyde; aperture; artery; cheilitis; conjunctivitis; convolution; curvature; gyrus; incisure; methyl; notch; spine; stomatitis; vein
anhepatic: jaundice
anhepatogenous: jaundice

Word Finder

anhidrotic ectodermal: dysplasia

anhydrous: alcohol; chloral; lanolin

anicteric: hepatitis; leptospirosis

anicteric virus: hepatitis

aniline: fuchsin

animal: charcoal; dextran; force; graft; magnetism; model; pole; psychology; soap; starch; toxin; viruses; wax

animal protein: factor

anion: gap

anion-exchange: resin

anionic: detergents

anionic neutrophil-activating: peptide

anisometropic: amblyopia

anisotropic: disks; lipid

Anitschkow: cell; myocyte

ankle: bone; clonus; jerk; joint; reflex; region

ankle-foot: orthosis

ankyloglossia superior: syndrome

ankylosed: tooth

ankylosing: hyperostosis; spondylitis

annealing: lamp; tray

annectent: gyrus

annihilation: radiation

annulate: lamellae

annuloaortic: ectasia

annuloplasty: ring

annulospiral: ending; organ

anococcygeal: body; ligament; nerve

anocutaneous: line

anodal: current

anodal closure: contraction

anodal opening: contraction

anode: rays

anogenital: band; raphe

anomalous: complex; conduction; trichromatism; uterus; viscosity

anomalous atrioventricular: excitation

anomalous mitral: arcade

anomalous pulmonary venous: connections, total or partial

anomalous retinal: correspondence

anomeric: carbon

anomic: aphasia

anonymous: veins

anorectal: angle; flexure; junction; lymph nodes; spasm; syndrome

anorectoperineal: muscles

anosognosic: epilepsy; seizures

anospinal: center

anovular: menstruation

anovular ovarian: follicle

anovulational: menstruation

anovulatory: cycle

anoxemia: test

anoxic: anoxia

ANP: receptors

ANP clearance: receptors

Anrep: effect; phenomenon

anserine: bursa; bursitis

ansiform: lobule

ansoparamedian: fissure

antagonistic: muscles; reflexes

antalgic: gait

antebrachial: fascia

antebrachial flexor: retinaculum

antecedent: sign

antecubital: space

antegonial: notch

antegrade: block; cardioplegia; conduction; cystography; pyelography; urography

antemortem: clot; thrombus

antenatal: diagnosis

anterior: aphasia; arch of atlas; asynclitism; belly of digastric muscle; border; border of body of pancreas; border of eyelids; border of fibula; border of lung; border of pancreas; border of radius; border of testis; border of tibia; border of ulna; branch; branch of the renal artery; canaliculus of chorda tympani; cells; centriole; chamber of eyeball; choroiditis; column; column of medulla oblongata; commissure; commissure of the larynx; compartment of arm; compartment of forearm; compartment of leg; compartment of thigh; component of force; crus of stapes; curvature; cusp of left atrioventricular valve; cusp of mitral valve; cusp of right atrioventricular valve; cusp of tricuspid valve; divisions of (trunks of) brachial plexus; embryotoxon; epithelium of cornea; extremity of caudate nucleus; extremity of spleen; fascicle of palatopharyngeus (muscle); fasciculus proprius; fontanelle; fovea; funiculus; guide; horn; layer of rectus sheath; layer of thoracolumbar fascia; ligament of fibular head;

ligament of Helmholtz; ligament of malleus; limb of internal capsule; limb of stapes; lip of external os of uterus; lip of uterine os; lobe of hypophysis; margin; mediastinoscopy; mediastinotomy; mediastinum; megalophthalmos; naris; neuropore; notch of auricle; notch of cerebellum; notch of ear; nuclei of thalamus; nucleus; nucleus; nucleus of trapezoid body; occlusion; part; part of anterior commissure of brain; part of diaphragmatic surface of liver; part of fornix of vagina; part of pons; part of tongue; pillar of fauces; pillar of fornix; pituitary; pole of eyeball; pole of lens; portion of left medial segment IV of liver; process of malleus; pyramid; rami of cervical nerves; rami of lumbar nerves; rami of sacral nerves; rami of thoracic nerves; ramus of lateral sulcus of cerebrum; ramus of spinal nerve; recess; recess of tympanic membrane; region of arm; region of elbow; region of forearm; region of knee; region of leg; region of neck; region of thigh; region of wrist; rhinoscopy; rhizotomy; root of spinal nerve; scleritis; sclerotomy; segment; sinuses; staphyloma; surface; surface of arm; surface of cornea; surface of elbow; surface of eyelids; surface of forearm; surface of iris; surface of kidney; surface of leg; surface of lens; surface of lower limb; surface of maxilla; surface of patella; surface of petrous part of temporal bone; surface of prostate; surface of radius; surface of suprarenal gland; surface of thigh; surface of ulna; surface of uterus; symblepharon; synechia; thoracotomy; tooth; triangle of neck; tubercle of atlas; tubercle of cervical vertebrae; tubercle of thalamus; urethra; urethritis; uveitis; vein of septum pellucidum; vitrectomy; wall of middle ear; wall of

stomach; wall of tympanic cavity; wall of vagina

anterior abdominal cutaneous: branch of intercostal nerve

anterior acoustic: stria

anterior ampullary: nerve

anterior amygdaloid: area

anterior antebrachial: nerve; region

anterior apprehension: test

anterior articular: surface of dens

anterior atlanto-occipital: membrane

anterior auricular: branches of superficial temporal artery; groove; muscle; nerves; vein

anterior axillary: fold; line; lymph nodes

anterior basal: branch; branch of superior basal vein (of right and left inferior pulmonary veins); vein

anterior basal (bronchopulmonary): segment [S VIII]

anterior basal segmental: artery

anterior brachial: region

anterior (bronchopulmonary): segment [S III]

anterior cardiac: veins

anterior carpal: region

anterior cecal: artery

anterior central: convolution; gyrus

anterior cerebellar: notch

anterior cerebral: artery; veins

anterior cervical: lymph nodes; region

anterior cervical intertransversarii: muscles

anterior cervical intertransverse: muscles

anterior chamber: trabecula

anterior chamber cleavage: syndrome

anterior choroidal: artery

anterior ciliary: arteries; veins

anterior circumflex humeral: artery; vein

anterior clear: space

anterior clinoid: process

anterior communicating: artery

anterior condyloid: canal of occipital bone; foramen

anterior conjunctival: artery

anterior corneal: dystrophy

anterior coronary periarterial: plexus

anterior corticospinal: tract
anterior costotransverse: ligament
anterior cranial: base; fossa
anterior cruciate: ligament
anterior crural: nerve; region
anterior cubital: region
anterior cutaneous: branches of femoral nerve; branches of intercostal nerves; branch of iliohypogastric nerve; nerves of abdomen
anterior deep cervical: lymph nodes
anterior elastic: layer
anterior ethmoidal: artery; cells; nerve
anterior ethmoidal air: cells
anterior external arcuate: fibers
anterior facial: height; vein
anterior femoral cutaneous: nerves
anterior focal: point
anterior gastric: branches of anterior vagal trunk
anterior glandular: branch of superior thyroid artery
anterior gray: column; commissure
anterior ground: bundle
anterior horn: cell
anterior humeral circumflex: artery
anterior hypothalamic: area; nucleus; region
anterior inferior cerebellar: artery
anterior inferior iliac: spine
anterior inferior renal: segment
anterior inferior segmental: artery of kidney
anterior intercondylar: area of tibia
anterior intercostal: arteries; branches of internal thoracic artery; veins
anterior intermediate: groove; sulcus
anterior interosseous: artery; nerve
anterior interpositus: nucleus
anterior interventricular: artery; branch of left coronary artery; groove; sulcus
anterior intestinal: portal
anterior intraoccipital: joint; synchondrosis
anterior jugular: lymph nodes; vein
anterior junction: line
anterior knee: region
anterior labial: arteries; branches of deep external

pudendal artery; commissure; nerves; veins
anterior lacrimal: crest
anterior lateral malleolar: artery
anterior lateral nasal: branches of anterior ethmoidal artery
anterior/lateral/posterior glandular: branches of superior thyroid artery
anterior and lateral thoracic: regions
anterior limiting: lamina; layer of cornea; ring
anterior lingual: gland
anterior longitudinal: ligament
anterior lunate: lobule
anterior medial malleolar: artery
anterior median: fissure of medulla oblongata; fissure of spinal cord; line
anterior mediastinal: arteries; lymph nodes
anterior medullary: velum
anterior meningeal: artery; branch (of anterior ethmoidal artery)
anterior meniscofemoral: ligament
anterior myocardial: infarction
anterior nasal: spine; spine of maxilla
anterior ocular: segment
anterior olfactory: nucleus
anterior palatine: arch; foramen
anterior palpebral: margin
anterior paracentral: gyrus
anterior parietal: artery
anterior parolfactory: sulcus
anterior pectoral cutaneous: branch of intercostal nerves
anterior pelvic: exenteration
anterior perforated: substance
anterior perforating: arteries
anterior periventricular: nucleus
anterior peroneal: artery
anterior piriform: gyrus
anterior pituitary: gonadotropin
anterior pituitary-like: hormone
anterior pontomesencephalic: vein
(anterior and posterior) radicular: arteries
(anterior and posterior) superior pancreaticoduodenal: artery

(anterior and posterior) vestibular: veins
anterior primary: division
anterior pyramidal: fasciculus; tract
anterior quadrigeminal: body
anterior raphespinal: tract
anterior rectus: muscle of head
anterior sacrococcygeal: ligament
anterior sacroiliac: ligaments
anterior sacrosciatic: ligament
anterior scalene: muscle
anterior scrotal: branch of deep external pudendal artery; nerves; veins
anterior segmental: artery
anterior semicircular: canals
anterior septal: branches of anterior ethmoidal artery
anterior serratus: muscle
anterior spinal: artery
anterior spinocerebellar: tract
anterior spinothalamic: tract
anterior sternoclavicular: ligament
anterior superficial cervical: lymph nodes
anterior superior alveolar: arteries; branches of infraorbital nerve; nerves
anterior superior dental: arteries
anterior superior iliac: spine
anterior superior renal: segment
anterior superior segmental: artery of kidney
anterior supraclavicular: nerve
anterior talar articular: surface of calcaneus
anterior talofibular: ligament
anterior talotibial: ligament
anterior tarsal tendinous: sheaths
anterior tegmental: decussation
anterior temporal: artery; branch
anterior thalamic: radiation; tubercle
anterior tibial: artery; bursa; lymph node; muscle; nerve; node; veins
anterior tibial compartment: syndrome
anterior tibial recurrent: artery
anterior tibiofibular: ligament
anterior tibiotalar: ligament; part of deltoid ligament; part

of medial ligament of ankle joint
anterior transverse temporal: gyrus
anterior trigeminothalamic: tract
anterior tympanic: artery
anterior urethral: valve
anterior vertebral: vein
anterior vestibular: artery
anterior white: commissure
anterodorsal: nucleus of thalamus
anterofacial: dysplasia
anterograde: amnesia; block; conduction; memory
anteroinferior: surface of pancreas
anteroinferior myocardial: infarction
anterolateral: column of spinal cord; cordotomy; fontanelle; groove; sulcus; surface of arytenoid cartilage; surface of (shaft of) humerus; system; tract; tractotomy
anterolateral central: arteries
anterolateral myocardial: infarction
anterolateral striate: arteries
anterolateral thalamostriate: arteries
anteromedial: nucleus; nucleus of thalamus; surface of shaft of humerus
anteromedial central: arteries; branches
anteromedial frontal: branch of callosomarginal artery
anteromedial intermuscular: septum
anteromedial thalamostriate: arteries
anteromedian: groove
anteroposterior: diameter of the pelvic inlet; projection
anteroseptal myocardial: infarction
anterosuperior: surface of body of pancreas
anteroventral: nucleus of thalamus
anthracotic: tuberculosis
anthrax: septicemia; toxin
anthropoid: pelvis
anthroponotic cutaneous: leishmaniasis
antialopecia: factor
antianemic: factor; principle
antiangiogenesis: factor
antianxiety: agent
anti–basement membrane: antibody; glomerulonephritis; nephritis
antiberiberi: factor; vitamin

antibiotic: enterocolitis; sensitivity
antibiotic sensitivity: test
anti–black-tongue: factor
antibody: excess
antibody-combining: site
antibody deficiency: disease; syndrome
antibody-dependent cell-mediated: cytotoxicity
anticardiolipin: antibodies
anticoagulant: therapy
anticoding: strand
anticomplementary: factor; serum
anti-D: immunoglobulin
antidermatitis: factor
antidiuretic: hormone
antidyskinetic: agent
antiepithelial: serum
antifoaming: agents
anti-G: suit
antigen: excess; interferon; peptides; unit
antigen-antibody: complex; reaction
antigen-binding: site
antigenic: competition; complex; determinant; drift; shift
antigen-presenting: cells
antigen-responsive: cell
antigen-sensitive: cell
antiglobulin: test
antigravity: muscles
antihemophilic: factor A; factor B; globulin; globulin A; globulin B; plasma
antihemorrhagic: factor; vitamin
antihuman: globulin
antihuman globulin: test
antiidiotype: antibody; autoantibody
anti–kidney serum: nephritis
antilymphocyte: globulin; serum
anti-MAG: antibody
antimicrobial: spectrum
anti-Monson: curve
anti-müllerian: hormone
antineuritic: factor; vitamin
antineutrophil cytoplasmic: antibodies; antibody
antinuclear: antibody; factor
antiparallel: strand
antipellagra: factor
antipernicious anemia: factor
antiphospholipid: antibodies
antipodal: cone
anti-Pr cold: autoagglutinin
antipsychotic: agent
antirabies: serum
antirachitic: vitamins
antireflection: coating
antireticular cytotoxic: serum

antiscorbutic: vitamin
antisense: DNA; RNA; strand; therapy
antiseptic: dressing
antiserum: anaphylaxis
antisocial: personality
antisocial personality: disorder
antisterility: factor; vitamin
antitermination: protein
antithrombin: test
antithyroglobulin: antibody
antitoxic: serum
antitoxin: rash; unit
antitragicus: muscle
antitragohelicine: fissure
antitrypsin: deficiency
α_1-antitrypsin: deficiency
α_1-antitrypsin deficiency: panniculitis
antitryptic: index
antitumor: enzyme; protein
antivenene: unit
antiviral: immunity; protein
Anton: syndrome
Antoni type A: neurilemoma
Antoni type B: neurilemoma
antral: follicle; lavage; pouch; sphincter
Antyllus: method
anular: band; cartilage; cataract; ligament; ligament of radius; ligament of stapes; ligaments of trachea; lipid; pancreas; part of fibrous digital sheath of digits of hand and foot; placenta; plexus; pulley; scleritis; scotoma; sphincter; staphyloma; stricture; synechia; syphilid
anvil: sound
anxiety: disorders; dream; hysteria; neurosis; reaction; syndrome
anxiety tension: state
anxious: delirium
aortic: aneurysm; arch; arches; area (of auscultation); atresia; bifurcation; bodies; bulb; coarctation; dissection; dwarfism; facies; foramen; glomera; hiatus; impression of left lung; incompetence; insufficiency; isthmus; knob; knuckle; murmur; nerve; nipple; notch; opening; orifice; ostium; reflex; regurgitation; sac; sinus; spindle; stenosis; sulcus; valve; vestibule; window
aortic arch: syndrome
aortic body: tumor
aortic lymphatic: plexus
aortico-left ventricular: tunnel

aorticopulmonary: window
aorticorenal: ganglia
aortic-pulmonic: window
aortic septal: defect
aortic sinus: aneurysm
aortoannular: ectasia
aortocoronary: bypass
aortoiliac: bypass
aortoiliac occlusive: disease
aortopulmonary: septum; window
aortorenal: bypass
AP: projection
APACHE: score
apallic: state; syndrome
apathetic: thyrotoxicosis
apatite: calculus
A-pattern: esotropia; exotropia; strabismus
A-P-C: virus
APC: compound
ape: fissure; hand
aperiodic: biopolymer
aperiosteal: amputation
Apert: hirsutism; syndrome
aperture: diaphragm
apex: beat; impulse; pneumonia
apex anterior: angulation
apex posterior: angulation
Apgar: score
aphakic: eye; glaucoma
aphonic: pectoriloquy
aphthous: stomatitis
apical: abscess; angle; area; branch of inferior lobar branch of right pulmonary artery; branch of right superior pulmonary vein; cap; complex; dendrite; foramen of tooth; gland; granuloma; infarction; infection; ligament of dens; periodontitis; process; space; vein
apical-aortic: conduit
apical axillary: lymph nodes
apical (bronchopulmonary): segment [S I]
apical dental: foramen
apical ectodermal: ridge
apical lordotic: projection
apical periodontal: abscess; cyst
apical segmental: artery; artery of superior lobar artery of right lung
apicoposterior: artery; branch of left superior pulmonary vein; vein
apicoposterior (bronchopulmonary): segment [SI + SII]
aplanatic: lens
aplastic: anemia; lymph
apnea-hypopnea: index

apneic: oxygenation; pause
apneustic: breathing
apochromatic: lens; objective
apocrine: adenoma; carcinoma; chromhidrosis; gland; hidrocystoma; metaplasia; miliaria
apocrine sweat: glands
apolar: bond; cell; interaction
aponeurogenic: ptosis
aponeurotic: fibroma; reflex
apophysary: point
apophysial: fracture
apoplectic: cyst; retinitis
apothecaries: weight
apparent: leukonychia; viscosity
appendiceal: abscess
appendicular: artery; colic; lymph nodes; muscle; skeleton; vein
apperceptive: mass
appetite: juice
appetitive: behavior
applanation: tonometer
apple jelly: nodules
applied: anatomy; anthropology; chemistry
appliqué: forms
apposition: suture
appositional: growth
approach-approach: conflict
approach-avoidance: conflict
approximal: surface of tooth
approximation: suture
Apt: test
aptitude: test
APUD: cells
apyretic: typhoid
aquagenic: pruritus
aqueduct: veil
aqueductal: intubation
aqueous: chambers; flare; humor; phase; solution; vaccine; vein
aqueous influx: phenomenon
aquo-: ion
arachnoid: cyst; foramen; granulations; membrane; trabecula; villi
arachnoidal: granulations
arachnoidea: mater cranialis; mater encephali
Aran-Duchenne: disease
Arantius: ligament; nodule; ventricle
arborescent: cataract
arborization: block
arc: perimeter
arc-flash: conjunctivitis
arch: bar; form; length; wire
archaic-paralogical: thinking
arched: crest
archenteric: canal
arch length: deficiency
arch-loop-whorl: system

arciform: arteries; veins of kidney

arcon: articulator

arcuate: arteries of kidney; artery (of foot) (inconstant); crest; crest of arytenoid cartilage; eminence; fasciculus; fibers; fibers of cerebrum; line; line of ilium; line of rectus sheath; nucleus; nucleus of thalamus; scotoma; uterus; veins of kidney; zone

arcuate popliteal: ligament

arcuate pubic: ligament

ardent: fever; spirits

areolar: choroiditis; choroidopathy; glands; tissue; tubercles

areolar venous: plexus

argentaffin: cells; granules

Argentinean hemorrhagic: fever

Argentine hemorrhagic fever: virus

arginine: oxytocin; vasopressin; vasotocin

argininosuccinic: aciduria

arginosuccinate lyase: deficiency

argon: laser

Argyll Robertson: pupil

argyrophilic: cells; fibers

Arias-Stella: effect; phenomenon; reaction

aristotelian: method

Aristotle: anomaly

arithmetic: mean

Arlt: operation; sinus

arm: bone; phenomenon

Armanni-Ebstein: change; kidney

armed: macrophage; rostellum

Armitage-Doll: model

armor: heart

armored: heart

Army Alpha: tests

Army Beta: tests

Army General Classification: Test

Arndt: law

Arndt-Gottron: syndrome

Arneth: classification; count; formula; index; stages

Arnold: bodies; bundle; canal; ganglion; nerve; tract

Arnold-Chiari: deformity; malformation; syndrome

aromatase: inhibitors

aromatic: bitters; castor oil; compound; series; water

aromatic ammonia: spirit

arousal: function; reaction

arrector: muscle of hair

arrector pili: muscles

arrest: signal

arrest of active phase: dystocia

arrest of descent: dystocia

arrested: tuberculosis

arrested dental: caries

Arrhenius: doctrine; equation; law

Arrhenius-Madsen: theory

arrow: poison

arrow point: tracing

Arruga: forceps

arsenic: pigmentation

arsenical: keratosis; polyneuropathy

arseniureted: hydrogen

arterial: arcades; arches of colon; arches of ileum; arches of jejunum; arch of lower eyelid; arch of upper eyelid; blood; bulb; canal; capillary; circle of cerebrum; cone; duct; flap; forceps; grooves; hyperemia; hypotension; ligament; line; murmur; nephrosclerosis; plexus; sclerosis; segments of kidney; spider; tension; transfusion; vein; wave

arterial switch: operation

arterial thoracic outlet: syndrome

arteriocapillary: sclerosis

arteriococcygeal: gland

arteriolar: nephrosclerosis; network; sclerosis

arteriolosclerotic: kidney

arteriolovenular: anastomosis; bridge

arteriosclerotic: aneurysm; gangrene; kidney; retinopathy

arteriovenous: anastomosis; aneurysm; fistula; nicking; shunt

arteriovenous carbon dioxide: difference

arteriovenous oxygen: difference

arthritic: atrophy; calculus

arthritic general: pseudoparalysis

arthrodial: articulation; cartilage; joint

Arthus: phenomenon; reaction

articular: branches; capsule; cartilage; cavity; chondrocalcinosis; circumference of head of radius; circumference of head of ulna; corpuscles; crepitus; crescent; crest; disk; disk of acromioclavicular joint; disk of distal radioulnar joint; disk of sternoclavicular joint; disk of

temporomandibular joint; eminence of temporal bone; facet; facet of head of fibula; facet of head of rib; facet of lateral malleolus; facet of medial malleolus; facet of radial head; facet of tubercle of rib; fossa of temporal bone; fracture; gout; labrum; lamella; leprosy; lip; margin; meniscus; muscle; muscle of elbow; muscle of knee; nerve; network; pit of head of radius; process; rheumatism; sensibility; surface; surface of acromion; surface of arytenoid cartilage; surface of mandibular fossa of temporal bone; surface on calcaneus for cuboid bone; surface of patella; tubercle of temporal bone

articularis cubiti: muscle

articularis genus: muscle

articular vascular: circle; network; network of elbow; network of knee; plexus

articulated: skeleton

articulating: paper

articulation: disorders

artificial: anatomy; ankylosis; crown; dentition; eye; fever; heart; insemination; intelligence; kidney; melanin; pacemaker; pneumothorax; pupil; radioactivity; respiration; selection; sphincter; stone; tears; ventilation

artificial active: immunity

artificial Carlsbad: salt

artificial Kissingen: salt

artificial membrane: rupture

artificial passive: immunity

artificial Vichy: salt

artistic: anatomy

arycorniculate: synchondrosis

aryepiglottic: fold; muscle; part of oblique arytenoid muscle

arylated: alkyl

arylsulfatase A: deficiency

arylsulfatase B: deficiency

arytenoepiglottidean: fold

arytenoid: cartilage; dislocation; glands; subluxation; swelling

arytenoidal articular: surface of cricoid

asbestos: bodies; corn; liner; wart

ascending: aorta; artery; branch; branch of the inferior mesenteric artery;

branch of superficial cervical artery; cholangitis; colon; current; degeneration; myelitis; neuritis; paralysis; part of aorta; part of duodenum; part of trapezius (muscle); process; pyelonephritis; ramus of lateral sulcus of cerebrum

ascending cervical: artery

ascending frontal: convolution; gyrus

ascending lumbar: vein

ascending palatine: artery

ascending parietal: convolution; gyrus

ascending pharyngeal: artery; plexus

ascertainment: bias

Ascher: syndrome

Ascher aqueous influx: phenomenon

Aschheim-Zondek: test

Aschner: phenomenon; reflex

Aschner-Dagnini: reflex

Aschoff: bodies; cell; nodules

Ascoli: reaction; test

ascorbate-cyanide: test

Aselli: gland; pancreas

aseptic: fever; necrosis; surgery

asexual: dwarfism; generation; reproduction

Ashby: method

ashen: tuber; tubercle; wing

Asherman: syndrome

ash-leaf: macule

Ashman: phenomenon

ashy: dermatosis

asialoglycoprotein: receptor

Asian: influenza

Asiatic: cholera; schistosomiasis

asiderotic: anemia

Askanazy: cell

Ask-Upmark: kidney

Asperger: disorder

aspermatogenic: sterility

aspheric: lens

asphyxiating thoracic: chondrodystrophy; dysplasia; dystrophy

aspirating: needle

aspiration: biopsy; pneumonia

asplenia: syndrome

Assam: fever

assassin: bug

assertive: conditioning; training

Assézat: triangle

assident: sign; symptom

assimilation: pelvis; sacrum

assist-control: ventilation

assisted: circulation; respiration; ventilation

assisted cephalic: delivery

assisted reproductive: technology

assistive: movement

Assmann tuberculous: infiltrate

associated: antagonist; movements

association: areas; constant; cortex; fibers; mechanism; neurosis; system; test; time; tract

associative: aphasia; reaction; strength

assortative: mating

astacoid: rash

astatic: seizure

asteroid: body; hyalosis

asthenic: personality

asthenic personality: disorder

asthma: crystals

asthmatic: bronchitis

asthmatoid: wheeze

astigmatic: dial; lens

Astler-Coller: classification

astral: fibers

astroglia: cell

Astwood: test

asymmetric: chondrodystrophy; disulfide

asymmetric fetal growth: restriction

asymmetric motor: neuropathy

asymptomatic: neurosyphilis

asynchronous pulse: generator

A/T: cloning

atactic: abasia; agraphia

atavistic: epiphysis

ataxia telangiectasia: syndrome

ataxic: aphasia; breathing; dysarthria; gait; paramyotonia; paraplegia

atelectatic: rale

ateliotic: dwarfism

atheromatous: degeneration; embolism; plaque

atherosclerotic: aneurysm

athlete's: foot; heart

athletic: heart

atlantic: part of vertebral artery

atlantoaxial: joint

atlanto-occipital: articulation; joint; membrane

atmospheric: pressure

atomic: core; heat; number; theory; volume; weight

atomic absorption: spectrophotometry

atomic mass: unit

atomistic: psychology

atonic: bladder; dyspepsia; ectropion; entropion; epiphora; seizure; ulcer

atopic: allergy; asthma; cataract; dermatitis; eczema; keratoconjunctivitis; reagin

ATP: citrate (*pro*-3*S*)-lyase; cobalamin adenoxyltransferase

atrabiliary: capsule

atraumatic: needle; suture

atresic: teratosis

atretic: corpus luteum

atretic ovarian: follicle

atrial: appendage; arteries; auricle; auricula; bigeminy; branches; capture; complex; diastole; dissociation; echo; extrasystole; fibrillation; flutter; gallop; kick; myxoma; septostomy; sound; standstill; systole; tachycardia

atrial anastomotic: branch of circumflex branch of left coronary artery

atrial capture: beat

atrial chaotic: tachycardia

atrial fusion: beat

atrial natriuretic: factor; peptide

atrial septal: defect

atrial synchronous pulse: generator

atrial transport: function

atrial triggered pulse: generator

atrial ventricular canal: defect

atrial-well: technique

atriosystolic: murmur

atrioventricular: band; block; bundle; canal; conduction; connections; dissociation; extrasystole; gradient; groove; interval; node; septum; sulcus; valves

atrioventricular canal: cushions

atrioventricular junctional: bigeminy; rhythm; tachycardia

atrioventricular nodal: branch

atrophic: arthritis; excavation; gastritis; glossitis; heterochromia; inflammation; kidney; pharyngitis; rhinitis; thrombosis; vaginitis

atropine: test

attached: craniotomy; gingiva

attached cranial: section

attachment: apparatus

attack: rate

attending: physician; staff; surgeon

attention: span

attention deficit: disorder

attention deficit hyperactivity: disorder

attenuated: tuberculosis; vaccine; virus

attenuation: compensation

attitudinal: reflexes

attraction: sphere

attributable: risk

atypical: achromatopsia; fibroxanthoma; gingivitis; lipoma; measles; mycobacteria; pneumonia; pseudocholinesterase

atypical absence: seizure

atypical antipsychotic: agent

atypical endometrial: hyperplasia

atypical facial: neuralgia

atypical glandular: cells of undetermined significance

atypical melanocytic: hyperplasia

atypical squamous: cells of undetermined significance

atypical trigeminal: neuralgia

atypical verrucous: endocarditis

Au: antigen

Aub-DuBois: table

Aubert: phenomenon

audiogenic: seizure

auditory: agnosia; alternans; aphasia; area; aura; canal; capsule; cortex; fatigue; feedback; field; ganglion; hairs; hallucination; hyperesthesia; lemniscus; localization; nerve; neuropathy; nucleus; organ; ossicles; pathway; pits; placodes; process; prosthesis; reflex; striae; strings; teeth; threshold; tract; tube; vesicle

auditory brainstem: response

auditory oculogyric: reflex

auditory receptor: cells

Auenbrugger: sign

Auer: bodies; rods

Auerbach: ganglia; plexus

Aufrecht: sign

Auger: electron

augmentation: mammaplasty

augmented: lead

augmented histamine: test

augmentor: fibers; nerves

Aujeszky disease: virus

aural: myiasis; vertigo

auramine O fluorescent: stain

auricular: appendage; appendectomy; appendix; arc; branch of occipital artery; branch of posterior auricular artery; branch of vagus nerve; canaliculus; cartilage; complex;

extrasystole; fissure; ganglion; index; ligaments; muscles; notch; point; reflex; standstill; surface of ilium; surface of sacrum; systole; tachycardia; triangle; tubercle; veins

auricularis anterior: muscle

auricularis posterior: muscle

auricularis superior: muscle

auriculoinfraorbital: plane

auriculopalpebral: reflex

auriculopressor: reflex

auriculotemporal: nerve

auriculotemporal nerve: syndrome

auriculoventricular: groove; interval

auropalpebral: reflex

Aus: antigen

ausculatory: triangle

auscultatory: alternans; gap; percussion; sound

Auspitz: sign

aussage: test

Austin Flint: murmur; phenomenon

Australia: antigen

Australian bat: Lyssavirus

Australian Q: fever

Australian tick: typhus

Australian X: disease; encephalitis

Australian X disease: virus

autacoid: substance

authoritarian: personality

authority: figure

autistic: disorder; parasite

autochthonous: ideas; malaria; parasite

autocrine: hypothesis

autoerythrocyte: sensitization

autoerythrocyte sensitization: syndrome

autogeneic: graft

autogenous: control; keratoplasty; union; vaccine

autohemolysis: test

autoimmune: disease; thyroiditis

autoimmune hemolytic: anemia

autoimmune neonatal: thrombocytopenia

autokinetic: effect

autologous: graft; protein

autolytic: enzyme

automated differential leukocyte: counter

automated lamellar: keratectomy

automatic: audiometer; audiometry; beat; condenser; contraction; epilepsy; plugger

automatic auditory brainstem: response
automatic gain: control
automotor: seizure
autonomic: division of nervous system; epilepsy; ganglia; imbalance; nerve; part; part of peripheral nervous system; plexuses; seizure
autonomic motor: neuron
autonomic nerve: fibers
autonomic nervous: system
autonomic neurogenic: bladder
autonomic (visceral motor): nuclei
autonomous: psychotherapy
autoparenchymatous: metaplasia
autophagic: vacuole
autoplastic: graft
autopolymer: resin
autoscopic: phenomenon
autoserum: therapy
autosomal: gene
autumn: fever
auxanographic: method
auxetic: growth
auxiliary: abutment
auxotrophic: mutant; strains
AV: difference; interval; junction
A-V: valves
available arch: length
avalanche: conduction
avascular: necrosis
Avellis: syndrome
average flow: rate
average pulse: magnitude
aversion: therapy
aversive: behavior; conditioning; control; stimulus; training
avian: sarcoma
avian encephalomyelitis: virus
avian influenza: virus
avian lymphomatosis: virus
avian neurolymphomatosis: virus
avian pneumoencephalitis: virus
avian viral arthritis: virus
aviation: medicine
aviator's: disease
avidity: antibody
AV junctional: rhythm; tachycardia
Avogadro: constant; hypothesis; law; number; postulate
avoidance: conditioning; training
avoidance-avoidance: conflict

avoidant: disorder of adolescence; disorder of childhood; personality
avoidant personality: disorder
A-V strabismus: syndrome
avulsed: wound
avulsion: fracture
axial: ametropia; aneurysm; angle; cataract; current; filament; hyperopia; illumination; muscle; myopia; neuritis; plane; plate; point; projection; section; skeleton; surfaces; view; walls of the pulp chambers
axial pattern: flap
axilla: thermometer
axillary: anesthesia; arch; artery; cavity; fascia; fold; fossa; glands; hairs; line; lymph nodes; nerve; plexus; region; sheath; space; thermometer; thoracotomy; triangle; vein
axillary arch: muscle
axillary lymphatic: plexus
axillary sweat: glands
axiolabiolingual: plane
axiomesiodistal: plane
axis: corpuscle; cylinder; deviation; ligament of malleus; shift; traction
axis-traction: forceps
axoaxonic: synapse
axodendritic: synapse
axon: degeneration; hillock; reflex; terminals
axonal: degeneration; polyneuropathy; process
axonal terminal: boutons
axon loss: polyneuropathy
axoplasmic: transport
axosomatic: synapse
Ayala: index; quotient
Ayerza: disease; syndrome
Ayre: brush
azin: dyes
azo: dyes; itch
azocarmine: dyes
Azorean: disease
azotemic: retinitis
azotobacter: nuclease
Aztec: ear
azure: lunula of nails
azurophil: granule
azygoesophageal: recess
azygos: artery of vagina; fissure; lobe of right lung; vein

B

β_1-: lipoprotein
β_2-: microglobulin

β: corynebacteriophage; hemolysin; hemolysis; phage; thalassemia
β_{1C}: globulin
B: bile; cell; chain; fibers; lymphocyte; virus; wave
B19: virus
B_T: factor
B-: DNA
β-: microglobulin
β-δ: thalassemia
Babbitt: metal
Babcock: tube
Babès: nodes
Babinski: phenomenon; reflex; sign; syndrome
baby: tooth
baby bottle: syndrome
Baccelli: sign
Bachman: test
Bachmann: bundle
Bachman-Pettit: test
bacillary: angiomatosis; dysentery; layer
Bacillus anthracis: toxin
bacillus Calmette-Guérin: vaccine
back: cross; mutation; pressure; tooth
back-action: plugger
backboard: splint
back of foot: reflex
background: level; radiation
back table: procedure
back vertex: power
backward: curvature
backward heart: failure
backwash: ileitis
Bacon: anoscope
bacterial: allergy; antagonism; capsule; cast; cystitis; encephalitis; endarteritis; endocarditis; growth; hemolysin; interference; peliosis; pericarditis; photosynthesis; plaque; pneumonia; toxin; translocation; vaginosis; vegetations; virus
bacterial food: poisoning
bacteriocin: factors
bacteriocinogenic: plasmids
bacteriogenic: agglutination
bacteriolytic: serum
bacteriophage: immunity; plaque; resistance; typing
bacteriostatic: agent
bacteriotropic: substance
Baehr-Lohlein: lesion
Baelz: disease
Baer: law; vesicle
Baermann: concentration
Baeyer: theory
bag of: waters
bag: ventilation
Baggenstoss: change

Bagolini: test
Baillarger: bands; lines
Bailliart: ophthalmodynamometer
Bainbridge: reflex
baked: tongue
Baker: cyst
baker: eczema; itch
Baker acid: hematein
Baker pyridine: extraction
baking: soda
Balamuth aqueous egg yolk infusion: medium
balance: theory
balanced: anesthesia; articulation; bite; diet; occlusion; polymorphism; translocation
balancing: contact; side
balancing occlusal: surface
balancing side: condyle
balanic: hypospadias
balanitic: epispadias
balantidial: dysentery
Balbani: ring
bald: tongue
Baldy: operation
Balint: syndrome
Balkan: beam; frame; nephropathy; splint
Ball: operation
ball: thrombus; valve; variance
Ballance: sign
ballerina-foot: pattern
balloon: atrioseptostomy; catheter; cell; septostomy; sickness
balloon cell: nevus
balloon counter: pulsation
ballooning: degeneration
balloon-tip: catheter
ballpoint pen: technique
ball and socket: abutment; joint
ball-valve: thrombus
ball valve: action
Baló: disease
Baltic myoclonus: disease
Bamberger: albuminuria; disease; sign
Bamberger-Marie: disease; syndrome
Bamberger-Pins-Ewart: sign
bamboo: hair; spine
banana: sign
bancroftian: filariasis
band: cell; centrifugation; neutrophil
bandage contact: lens
bandbox: resonance
Bandl: ring
bandpass: filter
band-shaped: keratopathy
Bang: disease
Bankart: lesion
Bannister: disease

Word Finder

Bannwarth: syndrome
Banti: disease; syndrome
bar: clasp
Bárány: sign
Bárány caloric: test
Barbados: leg
barbed: broach
barber: itch
barber pilonidal: sinus
bar clasp: arm
Barclay-Baron: disease
bar clip: attachments
Barcoo: rot; vomit
Barcroft-Warburg: apparatus; technique
Bardet-Biedl: syndrome
Bardinet: ligament
bare: area of liver; area of stomach
bare lymphocyte: syndrome
barium: enema
bar joint: denture
Barkan: membrane; operation
Barkman: reflex
Barkow: ligaments
Barlow: disease; maneuver; syndrome; test
Barmah Forest: virus
Barnes: curve; zone
barometric: pressure
baroreceptor: nerve
Barraquer: disease; method
Barr chromatin: body
Barré: sign
barrel: chest; distortion
barrel-shaped: thorax
Barrett: epithelium; esophagus; metaplasia; syndrome
barrier: contraceptive
bar-sleeve: attachments
Bart: syndrome
Barth: hernia; syndrome
Bartholin: abscess; anus; cyst; cystectomy; duct; gland
Barton: bandage; forceps; fracture
Bartonella: anemia
Bartter: syndrome
Baruch: law
baryta: water
basal: age; anesthesia; body; bone; cell; cistern; corpuscle; crest of cochlear duct; diet; encephalocele; ganglia; gland; granule; lamina; lamina of choroid; lamina of ciliary body; lamina of cochlear duct; lamina of neural tube; lamina of semicircular duct; layer; layer of choroid; layer of ciliary body; membrane of semicircular duct; metabolism; nuclei; nucleus of Ganser; part; part of left

and right inferior pulmonary arteries; part of occipital bone; plate of neural tube; ridge; rod; seat; sphincter; striations; substantia; surface; tuberculosis; vein; vein of Rosenthal
basal body: temperature
basal cell: adenoma; carcinoma; epithelioma; hyperplasia; layer; nevus; papilloma
basal cell nevus: syndrome
basal joint: reflex
basal laminar: drusen
basal linear: drusen
basal metabolic: rate
basaloid: carcinoma; cell
basal seat: area
basal skull: fracture
basal squamous cell: carcinoma
basal tentorial: branch of internal carotid artery
Basan: syndrome
base: composition; deficit; excess; hospital; increase at low levels; line; material; metal; pair; plate; projection; units; view
baseball: finger
Basedow: disease; goiter; pseudoparaplegia
baseline: tonus; variability of fetal heart rate
baseline fetal heart: rate
basement: lamina; membrane
baseplate: wax
basibregmatic: axis
basic: amino acid; diet; dyes; esotropia; exotropia; fuchsin; oxide; personality; proteins; reaction; salt; stain
basic electrical: rhythm
basic fuchsin-methylene blue: stain
basic personality: type
basicranial: axis; flexure
basifacial: axis
basilar: angle; apophysis; artery; bone; cartilage; cell; crest of cochlear duct; fibrocartilage; impression; index; invagination; lamina; leptomeningitis; membrane of cochlear duct; meningitis; migraine; papilla; part of occipital bone; part of pons; parts; process; process of occipital bone; prognathism; sinus; sulcus; vertebra
basilar pontine: sulcus
basilar venous: plexus
basilic: vein
basinasal: line
basioccipital: bone

basipharyngeal: canal
basisphenoid: bone
basivertebral: veins
basket: cell; nucleus
basolateral amygdaloid: nucleus
basomedial amygdaloid: nucleus
basophil: adenoma; cell of anterior lobe of hypophysis; granule; substance
basophilic: degeneration; leukemia; leukocyte; leukocytosis; leukopenia; substance
basosquamous: carcinoma
Bassen-Kornzweig: syndrome
Bassini: herniorrhaphy; operation
Bassler: sign
Bassora: gum
Bastedo: sign
bat: ear
batch: analyzer; culture
bath: itch; pruritus
bathing trunk: nevus
Batista: procedure
Batson: plexus
Batten: disease
Batten-Mayou: disease
battered child: syndrome
battered spouse: syndrome
Battey: bacillus
Battista: operation
Battle: sign
battle: fatigue
battledore: placenta
Baudelocque: diameter; operation
Baudelocque uterine: circle
Bauer: syndrome
Bauer chromic acid leucofuchsin: stain
Bauer-Kirby: test
Bauhin: gland; valve
Baumé: scale
Baumès: symptom
Baumgarten: glands; veins
bauxite: pneumoconiosis
Bayes: theorem
Bayesian: hypothesis
Bayley: Scales of Infant Development
bayonet: apposition; forceps; hair
Bayou: virus
Bazett: formula
Bazex: syndrome
Bazin: disease
B6 bronchus: sign
B cell: co-receptor; receptors
B cell differentiating: factor
B cell differentiation/growth: factors
B cell stimulatory: factor 2
BCG: vaccine

B-E: amputation
Bea: antigens
beaded: hair
beak: sign
beaked: pelvis
beaker: cell
Beale: cell
bearing-down: pain
beat-to-beat: variability of fetal heart rate
Beau: lines
Bechterew: band; disease; nucleus; sign
Bechterew-Mendel: reflex
Beck: method; triad
Becker: antigen; disease; nevus; stain for spirochetes
Becker muscular: dystrophy
Becker-type tardive muscular: dystrophy
Beckmann: apparatus
Beckwith-Wiedemann: syndrome
Béclard: anastomosis; hernia; triangle
Becquerel: rays
bed: rest; sore
Bednar: aphthae; tumor
bedside: radiography
bee: toxin
beechwood: sugar
Beer: knife; law
beer: heart
Beer-Lambert: law
beet: sugar
beet-: tongue
Beevor: sign
Begg light wire differential force: technique
Béguez César: disease
behavior: chain; disorder; modification; reflex; therapy
behavioral: epidemic; genetics; health; manifestation; medicine; pathogen; psychology
behavioral observation: audiometry
behavioristic: psychology
Behçet: disease; syndrome
behind-the-ear: hearing aid
Behr: disease; syndrome
Behring: law
BEI: test
Békésy: audiometer; audiometry
Belgian Congo: anemia
Bell: law; muscle; palsy; phenomenon; spasm
bell: sound; stage
belladonna: extract; tincture
bell clapper: deformity
Bellini: ducts; ligament
Bell-Magendie: law
bellmetal: resonance
bellows: murmur

Bell respiratory: nerve
bell-shaped: crown
Belsey: fundoplication; procedure
Belsey Mark: operation
belt: test
Bence Jones: albumin; cylinders; myeloma; proteins; proteinuria; reaction
bench: testing
Bender gestalt: test
Bender Visual Motor Gestalt: test
bending: fracture
Benedek: reflex
Benedict: solution; test for glucose
Benedict-Hopkins-Cole: reagent
Benedict-Roth: apparatus; calorimeter
Benedikt: syndrome
benign: albuminuria; cementoblastoma; dyskeratosis; fructosuria; glycosuria; hypertension; lymphadenosis; lymphocytoma cutis; lymphoma of the rectum; mesothelioma; mesothelioma of genital tract; myoclonus of infancy; nephrosclerosis; stupor; tumor
benign bone: aneurysm
benign childhood: epilepsy with centrotemporal spikes
benign coital: cephalalgia
benign congenital: hypotonia
benign dry: pleurisy
benign essential: tremor
benign exertional: headache
benign familial: chorea; icterus
benign familial chronic: pemphigus
benign giant lymph node: hyperplasia
benign infantile: myoclonus
benign inoculation: lymphoreticulosis; reticulosis
benign juvenile: melanoma
benign lymphoepithelial: lesion
benign migratory: glossitis
benign monoclonal: gammopathy
benign mucosal: pemphigoid
benign myalgic: encephalomyelitis
benign neonatal: convulsions
benign paroxysmal: peritonitis; torticollis of infancy

benign paroxysmal positional: vertigo
benign positional: vertigo
benign prostatic: hyperplasia; hypertrophy
benign rheumatoid: nodules
benign tertian: fever; malaria
Bennett: angle; fracture; movement
Bennhold Congo red: stain
Bensley specific: granules
bentiromide: test
bentonite flocculation: test
benzene: nucleus; ring
benzidine: test
benzoinated: lard
benzyl: penicillin
Beradinelli: syndrome
Bérard: aneurysm
Berardinelli: syndrome
Béraud: valve
Berg: stain
Berger: cells; disease; rhythm; space
Berger focal: glomerulonephritis
Bergman: sign
Bergmann: cords; fibers
Bergmeister: papilla
beriberi: heart
Berkefeld: filter
Berlin: edema
berloque: dermatitis
Bernard: canal; duct; puncture
Bernard-Cannon: homeostasis
Bernard-Horner: syndrome
Bernard-Sergent: syndrome
Bernard-Soulier: disease; syndrome
Bernays: sponge
Bernhardt: disease; formula
Bernhardt-Roth: syndrome
Bernheim: syndrome
Bernoulli: distribution; effect; law; principle; theorem
Bernstein: test
Berry: ligaments
berry: aneurysm; cell
Berson: test
Berthelot: reaction
Berthollet: law
Bertin: bones; columns; ligament; ossicles
beryllium: granuloma
Besnier: prurigo
Besnier-Boeck-Schaumann: disease; syndrome
Best: disease
best: frequency
Best carmine: stain
Beta: tests
beta: alcoholism; angle; cell of anterior lobe of hypophysis; cell of pancreas; error; fibers; granule;

particle; radiation; ray; rhythm; wave
beta-: oxidation
beta-oxidation-condensation: theory
betel: cancer
Bethesda: classification; system; unit
Betke-Kleihauer: test
Bettendorff: test
betula: oil
Betz: cells
Beuren: syndrome
Bevan-Lewis: cells
bevelled: anastomosis
Bezold: abscess; ganglion
Bezold-Jarisch: reflex
BH: interval
Bi: antigen
Bial: test
Bianchi: nodule
biauricular: axis
biaxial: joint
bi bi: reaction
bicameral: abscess
bicanalicular: sphincter
BICAP: cautery
biceps: muscle of arm; muscle of thigh; reflex
biceps brachii: muscle
biceps femoris: muscle; reflex
Bichat: canal; fat-pad; fissure; fossa; ligament; membrane; protuberance; tunic
bicipital: aponeurosis; fascia; groove; rib; ridges; tuberosity
bicipitoradial: bursa
Bickel: ring
biclonal: gammopathy; peak
biconcave: lens
bicondylar: articulation; joint
biconvex: lens
bicornate: uterus
bicoudate: catheter
bicuspid: tooth; valve
bidirectional: replication
bidirectional ventricular: tachycardia
bidiscoidal: placenta
Biebl: loop
Biederman: sign
Bielschowsky: disease; sign; stain
Biemond: syndrome
Bier: amputation; hyperemia; method
Biermer: anemia; disease
Biernacki: sign
Biesiadecki: fossa
bifid: epiglottis; penis; rib; thumb; tongue; uterus; uvula
bifidus: factor
bifocal: lens; spectacles
biforate: uterus
bifoveal: fixation

bifurcate: ligament
bifurcated: ligament
bifurcation: lymph nodes
big: ACTH
Bigelow: ligament; septum
bigeminal: bodies; pregnancy; pulse; rhythm
bilaminar: blastoderm
bilateral: hermaphroditism; left-sidedness; pleurisy; synchrony
bilateral medial orbital: ecchymoses
Bile: antigen
bile: capillary; cyst; duct; gastritis; papilla; peritonitis; pigments; salts; thrombus
bile: acids; alcohol
bile acid tolerance: test
bi-leaflet: valve
bile esculin: test
bile pigment: hemoglobin
bile salt: agar
bile solubility: test
bilharzial: appendicitis; dysentery; granuloma
biliaropancreatic: ampulla
biliary: atresia; calculus; canaliculus; cirrhosis; colic; duct; ductules; dyskinesia; fistula; glands; steatorrhea; xanthomatosis
bilious: headache; pneumonia; typhoid of Griesinger; vomit
bilious remittent: fever; malaria
bilirubin: encephalopathy
Bill: maneuver
Billings: method
billowing mitral valve: syndrome
Billroth: cords; operation I; operation II; venae cavernosae
Billroth I: anastomosis
Billroth II: anastomosis
bilocular: joint; stomach
bilocular femoral: hernia
bimalleolar: fracture
bimanual: palpation; percussion; version
bimaxillary: protrusion
bimaxillary dentoalveolar: protrusion
bimaxillary protrusive: occlusion
binangle: chisel
binary: combination; complex; digit; fission; nomenclature; process
binasal: hemianopia
binaural: stethoscope
binaural alternate loudness balance: test
binding: constant; energy
Binet: age; scale; test

Binet-Simon: scale
Bing: reflex
Bingham: flow; model; plastic
binocular: fixation; heterochromia; loupe; microscope; ophthalmoscope; parallax; rivalry; vision
binomial: distribution
Binswanger: disease; encephalopathy
biochemical: genetics; metastasis; modulation; pharmacology; profile
biochemical oxygen: demand
bioelectric: potential
biogenetic: law
biogenic: amines
biologic: assay; chemistry; control; evolution; half-life; hemolysis; immunotherapy; psychiatry; time; valve
biological: coefficient; sampling; vector
biological standard: unit
biologic response: modifier
biomedical: engineering; model
biometrical: school
Biondi-Heidenhain: stain
biophysical: profile
biopsy: needle
biopsychosocial: model
biorbital: angle
Biot: breathing; respiration; sign
Biot breathing: sign
biotic: community; factors; potential
biotinidase: deficiency
biparietal: diameter
bipartite: uterus; vagina
bipedicle: flap
bipennate: muscle
biphasic: insulin; response
biplane: angiography
bipolar: cautery; cell; disorder; lead; neuron; psychosis; taxis; version
Birbeck: granule
Birch-Hirschfeld: stain
Bird: sign
bird: face; unit
bird-breeder's: disease; lung
birdseed: agar
bird shot: retinochoroiditis
bird's nest: filter
birth: canal; control; defect; fracture; palsy; rate; trauma; weight
birthing: center
Bischof: myelotomy
biscuit: bite
bisferious: pulse
Bishop: score; sphygmoscope
Biskra: boil; button

bismuth: line
bite: analysis; fork; gauge; plane; rim
bitemporal: hemianopia
bitewing: film; radiograph
bithermal caloric: test
biting: louse; pressure; strength
Bitot: spots
bitter: orange peel; orange peel, dried; orange peel, fresh; orange peel oil; peptides; principles; tonic; water
bitter almond: oil
Bittner: agent; virus
Bittner milk: factor
Bittorf: reaction
biundulant: meningoencephalitis
biuret: reaction; reagent; test
bivalent: antibody; chromosome
bivalent gas gangrene: antitoxin
bivalve: speculum
biventer: lobule
biventral: lobule
Bixler type: hypertelorism
Bizzozero: corpuscle
Bizzozero red: cells
Bjerrum: scotoma; screen; sign
Björk-Shiley: valve
Björnstad: syndrome
B-K: amputation
BK: virus
Black: classification; formula
black: box; cataract; death; eye; fever; heel; lead; line; lung; measles; mustard; piedra; plague; sickness; spore; tarantula; tongue; urine; vomit
Black Creek Canal: virus
black currant: rash
black-dot: ringworm
black hairy: tongue
black imported fire: ant
blackwater: fever
bladder: calculus; compliance; ear; reflex; schistosomiasis; stone
blade: bone
Blagden: law
Blainville: ears
Blalock: shunt
Blalock-Hanlon: operation
Blalock-Taussig: operation; shunt
bland: diet; embolism; infarct
Blandin: gland
blanket: suture
Blasius: duct
blast: cell; crisis; injury

blastodermic: disk; layers; vesicle
blastomycetic: dermatitis
blastoporic: canal
Blatin: syndrome
bleached: wax
bleaching: powder
blear: eye
bleary: eye
bleeding: polyp; time
blending: inheritance
blighted: ovum
blind: boil; enema; fistula; foramen of frontal bone; foramen of the tongue; gut; headache; passage; spot; study; test
blinding: disease; glare
blind loop: syndrome
blind nasotracheal: intubation
blink: reflex; response
blister: agent
blistering: collodion
blistering distal: dactylitis
Bloch: reaction
Bloch-Sulzberger: disease; syndrome
block: anesthesia; vertebrae
block design: test
blocked: aerogastria; reading frame
blocking: activity; agent; antibody
Blocq: disease
Blom-Singer: valve
blood: agar; albumin; blister; calculus; capillary; cast; cell; circulation; clot; corpuscle; count; crisis; crystals; cyst; disk; dyscrasia; gases; group; island; islet; lymph; mole; motes; pH; plasma; plastid; plate; poisoning; pressure; serum; spots; substitute; sugar; tumor; type; vessel
blood-air: barrier
blood-aqueous: barrier
blood-brain: barrier
blood-cerebrospinal fluid: barrier
blood gas: analysis
blood group: agglutinins; agglutinogens; antibodies; antigen; antiserums; substance; systems
blood group-specific: substances A and B
bloodless: amputation; decerebration; operation; phlebotomy
blood plasma: fractions
blood pool: imaging
blood-testis: barrier
blood-thymus: barrier
blood urea: nitrogen

blood-vascular: system
blood volume: nomogram
Bloom: syndrome
Blount: disease
Blount-Barber: disease
blowout: pipette
blow-out: fracture
blubber: finger
blue: atrophy; baby; cataract; dextran; disease; edema; fever; line; nevus; ointment; pus; sclera; spot; vision
blueberry muffin: baby
blue cone: monochromatism
blue diaper: syndrome
blue dome: cyst
blue dot: sign
blue-green: algae; bacteria; bacterium
blue pus: bacillus
blue rubber-bleb: nevi
blue toe: syndrome
bluetongue: virus
Blumberg: sign
Blumenau: nucleus
Blumenbach: clivus
Blumer: shelf
blunt duct: adenosis
blunted: affect
blunt-end: ligation
blunt-ended: DNA
boat: conformation; form
boat-shaped: abdomen
Bochdalek: foramen; ganglion; gap; muscle; valve
Bock: ganglion; nerve
Bockhart: impetigo
Bodansky: unit
Bödecker: index
Bodian copper-PROTARGOL: stain
body: cavity; image; language; mechanics; plethysmograph; schema; stalk
body dysmorphic: disorder
body mass: index
body righting: reflexes
body-weight: ratio
Boeck: disease; sarcoid
Boeck and Drbohlav Locke-egg-serum: medium
Boehmer: hematoxylin
Boerhaave: syndrome
Bogros: space
Bogros serous: membrane
Bohn: nodules
Bohr: atom; effect; equation; magneton; theory
boiling: point
Boley: gauge
Bolivian hemorrhagic: fever
Bolivian hemorrhagic fever: virus
Boll: cells
Bollinger: granules
Bolognini: symptom

bolster: finger
bolus: dressing
bomb: calorimeter
Bombay: phenomenon; trait
bone: abscess; ache; age; block; canaliculus; cell; charcoal; chips; conduction; corpuscle; cyst; density; flap; forceps; graft; infarct; island; marrow; matrix; phosphate; plate; resorption; salt; sclerosis; sensibility; tissue; wax
bone block: fusion
bone Gla: protein
bone marrow: dose; embolism; transplantation
Bonhoeffer: sign
Bonnet: capsule
Bonnet-Dechaume-Blanc: syndrome
Bonney: test
Bonnier: syndrome
Bonwill: triangle
bony: ampullae of semicircular canals; ankylosis; crepitus; heart; labyrinth; limbs of semicircular canals; palate; part of external acoustic meatus; part of nasal septum; part of pharyngotympanic (auditory) tube; part of skeletal system
bony nasal: septum
bony semicircular: canals
Böök: syndrome
booster: dose; response
BOR: syndrome
Bordeaux: mixture
border: cells; molding; movements; seal
borderline: case; hypertension; leprosy; personality
borderline ovarian: tumor
borderline personality: disorder
border tissue: movements
Bordet and Gengou: reaction
Bordet-Gengou: bacillus; phenomenon
Bordet-Gengou potato blood: agar
Börjeson-Forssman-Lehmann: syndrome
Born: method of wax plate reconstruction
Borna disease: virus
Bornholm: disease
Bornholm disease: virus
Borrel blue: stain
Borst-Jadassohn type intraepidermal: epithelioma
bosch: yaws
Bosin: disease

Boston: exanthema; opium
Botallo: duct; foramen; ligament
bothropic: antitoxin
Bothrops: antitoxin
botryoid: sarcoma
botryoid odontogenic: cyst
Böttcher: canal; cells; crystals; ganglion; space
botulinum: antitoxin
botulinus: toxin
botulism: antitoxin
Bouchard: disease
Bouchut: tube
Bouffardi white: mycetoma
Bouillaud: disease
Bouin: fixative
bound: water
boundary: lamina
bouquet: fever
Bourgery: ligament
Bourneville: disease
Bourneville-Pringle: disease
boutonneuse: fever
boutonnière: deformity
bovine: antitoxin; brucellosis; colloid; ketosis; rhinoviruses
bovine leukemia: virus
bovine leukosis: virus
bovine papular stomatitis: virus
bovine serum: albumin
bovine spongiform: encephalopathy
bovine virus diarrhea: virus
bow-: leg
Bowditch: effect; law
bowel: bypass; movement; sounds
bowel bypass: syndrome
Bowen: disease
Bowenoid: cells
bowenoid: papulosis
Bowen precancerous: dermatosis
Bowie: stain
Bowles type: stethoscope
Bowman: capsule; disks; gland; layer; membrane; muscle; probe; space; theory
Bowman-Birk: inhibitor
box: jelly
boxer's: ear; fracture
boxing: wax
Boyd communicating perforation: veins
Boyden: meal; sphincter
Boyer: bursa; cyst
Boyle: law
Bozeman: operation; position
Bozeman-Fritsch: catheter
Bozzolo: sign
BP: fistula
Braasch: bulb; catheter
brachial: anesthesia; artery; fascia; gland; lymph nodes;

muscle; neuritis; plexitis; plexus; veins
brachial autonomic: plexus
brachial birth: palsy
brachialis: muscle
brachial plexus: injury; neuropathy
brachiocephalic: arteritis; lymph nodes
brachiocephalic (arterial): trunk
brachioradial: muscle; reflex
brachioradialis: muscle
Bracht: maneuver
Bracht-Wächter: lesion
brachypellic: pelvis
Bradbury-Eggleston: syndrome
Bradford: frame
bradykinetic: analysis
bradykinin-potentiating: peptide
bradytachycardia: syndrome
Brailsford-Morquio: disease
Brain: reflex
brain: attack; box; cicatrix; concussion; congestion; contusion; death; edema; laceration; lipid; mantle; murmur; potential; sand; stem; sugar; swelling; wave
brain-heart infusion: agar
brainstem: glioma; hemorrhage
brainstem auditory evoked: potential
brainstem evoked: response
brain wave: complex; cycle
branch: migration
branched: calculus
branched chain: ketoaciduria; ketonuria
brancher deficiency: glycogenosis
brancher glycogen storage: disease
branchial: apparatus; arches; cartilages; clefts; cyst; fissure; fistula; groove; mesoderm; pouches
branchial cleft: cyst
branchial efferent: column
branching: enzyme; factor; type of renal pelvis
branchiomeric: muscles
branchiomotor: nuclei
branchiootorenal: dysplasia; syndrome
Brandt-Andrews: maneuver
brandy: nose
Branham: sign
branny: desquamation; tetter
Brasdor: method
brass founder's: ague; fever
brassy: body; cough
BRAT: diet

Braun: anastomosis
Braune: canal; muscle; valve
brawny: arm; edema; scleritis
Braxton Hicks: contraction; sign; version
Brazelton Neonatal Behavioral Assessment: Scale
Brazil: wax
Brazilian: blastomycosis; pemphigus
Brazilian hemorrhagic: fever
Brazilian purpuric: fever
Brazilian spotted: fever
BRCA1: gene
BRCA2: gene
BrDu-: banding
bread: pill
bread-and-butter: pericardium
break: shock
breakbone: fever
breakoff: phenomenon
breast: bone; pang; pump
breath: analysis; sounds; test
breath-holding: test
breathing: bag; reserve
Breda: disease
breech: delivery; extraction; presentation
bregmatic: fontanelle
bregmatolambdoid: arc
bregmocardiac: reflex
Brenner: tumor
Breschet: bones; canals; hiatus; sinus; vein
Brescia-Cimino: fistula
Breslow: thickness
Breus: mole
Brewer: infarcts
brewers': yeast
brickdust: deposit
Bricker: operation
brickmaker's: anemia
bridge: corpuscle
bridging hepatic: necrosis
bridle: stricture; suture
brief: psychotherapy
Brigg: test
Bright: disease
brightness difference: threshold
Brill: disease
Brill-Symmers: disease
Brill-Zinsser: disease
Brimacombe: fragment
Brinell hardness: number
Briquet: ataxia; disease; syndrome
Brissaud: disease; infantilism; reflex
Brissaud-Marie: syndrome
bristle: cell
British: gum
British thermal: unit
brittle: bones; diabetes

broad: fascia; ligament of the uterus; spectrum
Broadbent: law; sign
broad beta: disease
broadest: muscle of back
broad-spectrum: antibiotic
Broca: angles; aphasia; area; center; field; fissure; formula; pouch
Broca basilar: angle
Broca diagonal: band
Broca facial: angle
Broca parolfactory: area
Broca visual: plane
Brock: operation; syndrome
Brockenbrough: sign
Brocq: disease
Brödel bloodless: line
Brodie: abscess; bursa; disease; fluid; knee; ligament
Brodmann: areas
Broesike: fossa
bromide: acne
bromine: water
bromphenol: test
Brompton: cocktail
bromsulphalein: test
bronchial: adenoma; arteries; arteriography; asthma; atresia; branches of thoracic aorta; breathing; bud; calculus; fremitus; glands; mucosa; pneumonia; polyp; respiration; stenosis; tubes; veins; voice
bronchial breath: sounds
bronchial mucous gland: adenoma
bronchic: cells
bronchiolar: adenocarcinoma; carcinoma
bronchiolar exocrine: cell
bronchioloalveolar: adenocarcinoma
bronchiolo-alveolar: carcinoma
bronchitic: asthma
bronchoalveolar: carcinoma; fluid; lavage
broncho-aortic: constriction
bronchobiliary: fistula
bronchocavitary: fistula
bronchoesophageal: fistula; muscle
bronchoesophageus: muscle
bronchogenic: carcinoma; cyst
bronchomediastinal (lymphatic): trunk
bronchopleural: fistula
bronchopleural-cutaneous: fistula
bronchopulmonary: dysplasia; lymph nodes;

segment; sequestration; spirochetosis
bronchoscopic: brush; smear
bronchovesicular: respiration
bronchovesicular breath: sounds
bronchus-associated lymphoid: tissue
Brönsted: acid; base; theory
bronze: diabetes
bronze baby: syndrome
bronzed: diabetes; disease; skin
brood: capsules; cell
Brooke: ileostomy; tumor
brother: complex
Broviac: catheter
brow: presentation
Brown: syndrome
brown: atrophy; edema; fat; induration of the lung; layer; lung; pellicle; striae; tumor
brown adipose: tissue
Brown-Adson: forceps
Brown-Brenn: stain
brownian: motion; movement
brownian-Zsigmondy: movement
Browning: vein
Brown-Séquard: paralysis; syndrome
Bruce: protocol
brucella strain 19: vaccine
Bruch: glands; membrane
Bruck: disease
Brücke: muscle; tunic
Brücke-Bartley: phenomenon
Brudzinski: sign
Brug: filariasis
Brugsch: syndrome
Brumpt white: mycetoma
Brunn: membrane; nest; reaction
Brunner: glands
Bruns: ataxia; nystagmus
Brunschwig: operation
brush: biopsy; border; burn; catheter
brush burn: abrasion
Brushfield: spots
Brushfield-Wyatt: disease
brush heap: structure
Bruton: agammaglobulinemia
Bryant: traction; triangle
BSP: test
bubble gum: dermatitis
bubbling: rale
bubonic: plague
buccal: angles; artery; branches of facial nerve; caries; cavity; curve; digestion; embrasure; fat-pad; flange; gingiva; glands; lymph node; nerve; occlusion; pit; region; root

of tooth; smear; surface; tablet; vestibule
buccinator: crest; muscle; nerve; node
buccocervical: ridge
buccogingival: ridge
buccolingual: diameter; dimension; relation
bucconasal: membrane
bucconeural: duct
bucco-occlusal: angle
buccopharyngeal: fascia; membrane; part of superior pharyngeal constrictor
Büchner: extract; funnel
Buchwald: atrophy
Buck: extension; fascia; traction
buck: tooth
bucket-handle: incision; tear
buckled: aorta
buckled innominate: artery
buckthorn: polyneuropathy
Bucky: diaphragm
bud: fission; stage
Budd: syndrome
Budd-Chiari: syndrome
Budde: process
buddeized: milk
Budge: center
Budin obstetrical: joint
Buerger: disease
buffalo: hump; neck; type
buffer: capacity; index; pair; value; value of the blood
buffered crystalline: penicillin G
buffy: coat
buffy coat: concentration
bulbar: apoplexy; conjunctiva; myelitis; palsy; paralysis; pulse; ridge; septum
bulbar corticonuclear: fibers
bulbocavernosus: muscle; reflex
bulboid: corpuscles
bulbomimic: reflex
bulboreticulospinal: tract
bulbosacral: system
bulbospongiosus: muscle
bulbourethral: gland
bulbous: bougie
bulboventricular: loop; ridge
bulging eye: disease
bulk: modulus
bulky: disease; lymphadenopathy
bull: neck
bulldog: forceps; head
bullet: bubo; forceps
bullous: edema; edema vesicae; emphysema; impetigo of newborn; keratopathy; myringitis; pemphigoid; syphilid

bullous congenital ichthyosiform: erythroderma
bull's-eye: maculopathy
Bumke: pupil
bundle: bone
bundle-branch: block
Bunnell: suture
Bunsen-Roscoe: law
Bunsen solubility: coefficient
Bunyamwera: fever; virus
bunyavirus: encephalitis
buoyant: density
bur: drill
Burchard-Liebermann: reaction
Burdach: column; fasciculus; nucleus; tract
Burdwan: fever
Burger: triangle
Bürger-Grütz: disease; syndrome
Burgundy: pitch
buried: flap; penis; suture
Burkitt: lymphoma
Burlew: disk; wheel
burner: syndrome
Burnett: syndrome
burning: tongue
burning drops: sign
burning foot: syndrome
burning mouth: syndrome
burning tongue: syndrome
burning vulva: syndrome
Burn and Rand: theory
Burns: ligament; space
Burns falciform: process
burnt: alum
Burow: solution; triangle; vein
burr: cell
burrowing: hairs
bursal: abscess; cyst; synovitis
Burton: line
Buruli: ulcer
Bury: disease
Busacca: nodules
Buschke: disease
Buschke-Löwenstein: tumor
Buschke-Ollendorf: syndrome
bush: yaws
Busquet: disease
butanol-extractable: iodine
butanol-extractable iodine: test
butter: stools
butterfly: eruption; fragment; lung; patch; pattern; rash; vertebra
button: suture
buttonhole: iridectomy; stenosis
buttress: plate
buyo cheek: cancer
Buzzard: maneuver
Bwamba: fever; virus
By: antigen

Byars: flap
Byler: disease
by-product: material
bystander: lysis
Byzantine arch: palate

C

C: bile; cell; chain; factors; fibers; gene; terminus; value; wave
C1: esterase
CA: virus
CA-125: antigen
CA-15-3: antigen
CA-19-9: antigen
CAAT: box
cabbage: goiter
Cabot-Locke: murmur
Cabot ring: bodies
cacao: butter
cachectic: diarrhea; edema; endocarditis; fever; pallor
cadaveric: rigidity; spasm
caddis: worm
caeruleun: nucleus
caerulospinal: tract
cafe: coronary
café au lait: spots
Caffey: disease; syndrome
Caffey-Kempe: syndrome
Caffey-Silverman: syndrome
Cagot: ear
Cain: complex
caisson: disease; sickness
Cajal: cell
Cajal astrocyte: stain
cake: alum; kidney
caked: breast
Calabar: swelling
calabash: curare
calcaneal: anastomosis; apophysitis; arteries; bone; branches; gait; petechiae; process of cuboid; region; sulcus; tendon; tuber; tubercle; tuberosity
calcaneal arterial: network
calcaneal articular: surface of talus
calcaneocuboid: joint; ligament
calcaneofibular: ligament
calcaneonavicular: ligament
calcaneotibial: ligament
calcareous: conjunctivitis; corpuscles; degeneration; infiltration; metastasis; pancreatitis
calcarine: artery; branch of medial occipital artery; fasciculus; fissure; spur; sulcus
calcic: water
calcific: bursitis; pancreatitis
calcification: lines of Retzius

calcific nodular aortic: stenosis
calcified: cartilage
calcifying epithelial odontogenic: tumor
calcifying and keratinizing odontogenic: cyst
calcifying odontogenic: cyst
calcined: magnesia
calcinuric: diabetes
calcitonin gene-related: peptide
calcium: antagonist; gout; pump; rigor; sign; tungstate
calcium channel: blocker
calcium channel-blocking: agent
calcium pyrophosphate deposition: disease
calculated mean: organism
calculated serum: osmolality
Caldani: ligament
Caldwell: projection; view
Caldwell-Luc: operation
Caldwell-Moloy: classification
calf: bone; pump
calibration: curve; interval
caliceal: diverticulum
caliciform: cell
California: encephalitis; virus
California psychological inventory: test
caliper: micrometer
Calkins: sign
Callahan: method
Callander: amputation
Call-Exner: bodies
Callison: fluid
callosal: convolution; gyrus; sulcus
callosomarginal: artery; fissure; sulcus
Calmette: test
Calmette-Guérin: bacillus; vaccine
calomel: electrode
Calori: bursa
caloric: nystagmus; test; value
calorigenic: action
Calot: triangle
calvarial: hook
Calvé-Perthes: disease
calyciform: ending
cambium: layer
CAMP: factor; test
camp: fever; hospital
Campbell: ligament; sound
Camper: chiasm; fascia; ligament; line; plane
camphorated: menthol; phenol
cAMP receptor: protein
camptomelic: dwarfism; syndrome

Canada: balsam; snakeroot; turpentine
canalicular: adenoma; ducts; sphincter
Canavan: disease; sclerosis
Canavan-van Bogaert-Bertrand: disease
cancellous: bone; tissue
cancer: bodies; family
cancer antigen 125: test
cane: sugar
canicola: fever
canine: adenovirus 1; amebiasis; carcinoma 1; eminence; fossa; leishmaniasis; prominence; spasm; tooth
canine distemper: virus
canities: poliosis
canker: sores
Cannizzaro: reaction
Cannon: theory
Cannon: point; ring
cannon: wave
cannon: sound
cannonball: pulse
Cannon-Bard: theory
Cantelli: sign
cantering: rhythm
canthal: hypertelorism
cantharidal: collodion
cantharis: camphor
canthomeatal: plane
cantilever: beam; bridge
Cantor: tube
caoutchouc: pelvis
cap: splint; stage
capeline: bandage
Capgras: phenomenon; syndrome
Capillaria: granuloma
capillary: angioma; arteriole; attraction; bed; circulation; drainage; fracture; fragility; hemangioma; hemangioma of infancy; lake; lamina of choroid; loop; nevus; pulse; vein; vessel
capillary fragility: test
capillary permeability: factor
capillary resistance: test
capillary zone: electrophoresis
Capim: viruses
capital: operation
capitate: bone
capitular: joint
Caplan: nodules; syndrome
capon: unit
capon-comb: unit
capped: uterus
capping: proteins
Capps: reflex
capsular: advancement; antigen; branches of intrarenal arteries; branches of renal artery; cataract;

**cirrhosis of liver; ligament; space
capsular flap: pyeloplasty
capsular precipitation: reaction
capsule: cell; forceps
capsulolenticular: cataract
capture-recapture: method
Capuron: points
caput: epididymis
car: sickness
Carabelli: tubercle
Caraparu: virus
carbacrylamine: resins
carbamino: compound
carbamylcholine: chloride
carbohydrate: loading; metabolism
carbohydrate-induced: hyperlipemia
carbohydrate utilization: test
carbol: fuchsin
carbol-fuchsin: paint
carbol-thionin: stain
carbon: autotrophy
carbonated: water
carbonate dehydratase: inhibitor
carbon dioxide: acidosis; content; cycle; electrode; elimination
carbon dioxide combining: power
carbon dioxide-free: water
carbon disulfide: poisoning
carbonic: anhydrase
carbonic acid: gas
carbonic anhydrase: inhibitor
carbonic anhydrase II deficiency: syndrome
carbon monoxide: hemoglobin; poisoning
carbonmonoxy: myoglobin
carboxy: terminal
carboxylic acid: ester
carboxymethyl: cellulose
carcinoembryonic: antigen
carcinoid: flush; syndrome; tumor
carcinomatous: encephalomyelopathy; implants; myelopathy; myopathy; neuromyopathy; pericarditis
Carden: amputation
cardiac: accident; albuminuria; alternation; aneurysm; antrum; arrest; arrhythmia; asthma; catheter; cirrhosis; competence; contractility; cycle; decompression; diuretic; dropsy; dyspnea; dysrhythmia; edema; failure; ganglia; gating; gland; glands; glands of esophagus;

Word Finder

glands of stomach; glycosides; heterotaxia; histiocyte; hormone; impression of diaphragmatic surface of liver; impression on lung; impulse; incompetence; index; infarction; insufficiency; jelly; liver; lung; mapping; massage; monitor; murmur; muscle; neurosis; notch; notch of left lung; opening; orifice; output; part of stomach; polyp; prominence; reserve; segment; shock; skeleton; souffle; sound; standstill; syncope; tamponade; telemetry; tube; veins

cardiac depressor: reflex
cardiac fibrous: skeleton
cardiac lymphatic: ring
cardiac muscle: tissue; wrap
cardiac (nervous): plexus
cardiac valve: prosthesis
cardiac valvular: incompetence
cardial: notch; orifice; part of stomach
cardinal: ligament; points; symptom; veins
cardinal ocular: movements
cardioarterial: interval
cardiodiaphragmatic: angle
cardioesophageal: junction; relaxation
cardiofacial: syndrome
cardiogenic: plate; shock
cardiohepatic: angle; triangle
cardioid: condenser
cardiophrenic: angle
cardioplegic: arrest
cardiopulmonary: arrest; bypass; murmur; resuscitation; transplantation
cardiopulmonary splanchnic: nerves
cardiorespiratory: murmur
cardiothoracic: ratio
cardiotoxic: myolysis
cardiovascular: radiology; syphilis; system
Carey Coombs: murmur
carinal: lymph nodes
carinate: abdomen
Carlen: tube
Carman: sign
Carmody-Batson: operation
carnassial: tooth
carnauba: wax
carneous: degeneration; mole
Carnett: sign
Carney: complex
carnitine: deficiency
Carnoy: fixative
Caroli: disease; syndrome

β-carotene-cleavage: enzyme
caroticoclinoid: ligament
caroticotympanic: arteries (of internal carotid artery); canaliculi; nerves
carotid: arteries; body; branch of glossopharyngeal nerve (CN IX); bruit; bulb; canal; duct; endarterectomy; foramen; ganglion; groove; pulse; sheath; shudder; sinus; sulcus; triangle; tubercle; wall of middle ear; wall of tympanic cavity
carotid body: tumor
carotid-cavernous: fistula
carotid sinus: branch; nerve; reflex; syncope; syndrome; test
carp: mouth
carpal: arches; artery; bones; canal; groove; joints; tunnel
carpal articular: surface of radius
carpal tendinous: sheaths
carpal tunnel: syndrome
Carpenter: syndrome
Carpentier-Edwards: valve
carpometacarpal: joints; joint of thumb; ligaments (dorsal and palmar)
carpopedal: spasm
Carrel: treatment
Carrel-Lindbergh: pump
carrier: cell; electrophoresis; screening; state; strain
Carrington: disease
Carrión: disease
Carr-Price: reaction; test
Carr-Purcell: experiment
carrying: angle; capacity
Carter black: mycetoma
cartesian: nomogram
cartilage: bone; capsule; cell; knife; lacuna; matrix; space
cartilage-hair: hypoplasia
cartilaginous: articulation; joint; neurocranium; part of external acoustic meatus; part of nasal septum; part of pharyngotympanic (auditory) tube; part of skeletal system; septum; tissue; viscerocranium
Carus: circle; curve
Carvallo: sign
Casal: necklace
cascade: stomach
case: management
case control: study
case fatality: rate; ratio
caseous: abscess; degeneration; necrosis; osteitis; pneumonia; tubercle
Casoni: antigen
Casoni intradermal: test

Casoni skin: test
Casselberry: position
Casser: fontanelle
Casser perforated: muscle
cassette: mutagenesis
cassia: cinnamon
Castellani: bronchitis; paint
Castellani-Low: sign
Castile: soap
casting: flask; ring; wax
Castle intrinsic: factor
Castleman: disease
castration: anxiety; cells; complex
cat: unit
catabolite: repression
catabolite gene: activator
catabolite (gene) activator: protein
catacrotic: pulse
catadicrotic: pulse
catalatic: reaction
catalytic: antibody; center
catamenial: pneumothorax
cataract: lens; needle; spoon
cataract-oligophrenia: syndrome
catarrhal: asthma; fever; gastritis; inflammation; ophthalmia
catastrophe: theory
catastrophic: reaction
catatonic: dementia; excitement; pupil; rigidity; schizophrenia; stupor
catatropic: image
cat-bite: disease; fever
catchment: area
catechol: estrogen
categorical: trait
caterpillar: cell; dermatitis; rash
caterpillar-hair: ophthalmia
catgut: suture
catheter: embolus; fever; gauge; guide
catheter coiling: sign
cathodal closure: contraction
cathodal duration: tetanus
cathodal opening: clonus; contraction
cathode: rays
cathode ray: oscilloscope; tube
cation-anion: difference
cation-exchange: resin
cationic: detergents
catscratch: disease; fever
cat's cry: syndrome
cat's-eye: pupil; syndrome
Cattell Infant Intelligence: Scale
Catu: virus
cauda: epididymis
cauda equina: syndrome

caudal: anesthesia; canal; flexure; ligament; neuropore; retinaculum; sheath; vertebrae
caudal neurosecretory: system
caudal pancreatic: artery
caudal pharyngeal: complex
caudal pontine reticular: nucleus
caudal transtentorial: herniation
caudal transverse: fissure
caudate: branches of left branch of portal vein; lobe; nucleus; process
caudolenticular gray: bridges
cauliflower: ear
causal: additivity; independence; treatment
caustic: alkali; potash; soda
cautery: conization; knife
caval: fold; opening of diaphragm; valve
cavalry: bone
cave: sickness
cavernous: angioma; arteries; bodies of anal canal; body of clitoris; body of penis; branch of cavernous part of internal carotid artery; groove; hemangioma; lymphangiectasis; nerves of clitoris; nerves of penis; part of internal carotid artery; plexus of clitoris; plexus of penis; rale; resonance; respiration; rhonchus; sinus; space; spaces of corpora cavernosa; spaces of corporus spongiosum; tissue; transformation of portal vein; veins of penis; voice
cavernous nervous: plexus
cavernous sinus: branch of internal carotid artery; syndrome
cavernous (vascular): plexus of conchae
cavernous voice: sound
caviar: lesion
cavity: liner; margin; preparation; wall
cavity line: angle
cavity preparation: base; form
cavopulmonary: anastomosis; shunt
cavosurface: angle; bevel
Cazenave: vitiligo
CB: lead
C-banding: stain
C carbohydrate: antigen
CD4/CD8: count
CDE: antigens
cDNA: clone; library

ceasmic: teratosis

cecal: arteries; folds; foramen of frontal bone; foramen of the tongue; hernia; recess; volvulus

Cecil: urethroplasty

cecocentral: scotoma

Ceelen-Gellerstedt: syndrome

Celestin: tube

celiac: artery; axis; branches of posterior vagal trunk; branches of vagus nerve; disease; ganglia; lymph nodes; plexus; rickets; sprue; syndrome

celiac (arterial): trunk

celiac (lymphatic): plexus

celiac (nervous): plexus

celiacoduodenal: part of suspensory muscle (ligament) of duodenum

celiac plexus: reflex

celiotomy: incision

cell: body; bridges; center; culture; cycle; determination; fusion; hybridization; inclusions; line; marker; matrix; membrane; nest; organelle; plate; sap; strain; transformation; wall

cell adhesion: molecule

cell-bound: antibody

cell-mediated: immunity; reaction

cell surface: marker

cellular: biology; biophysics; cartilage; embolism; immunodeficiency with abnormal immunoglobulin synthesis; infiltration; mosaicism; pathology; polyp; spill; tenacity; tumor

cellular blue: nevus

cellular immune: theory

cellular immunity deficiency: syndrome

cellulitic: phlegmasia

celluloid: strip

cellulose tape: technique

cell wall–defective: bacteria

CELO: virus

celomic: bay

celomic metaplasia: theory of endometriosis

Celsius: scale

Celsus: kerion; vitiligo

cement: base; corpuscle; disease; line

cemental: caries

cementing: substance

cementodentinal: junction

cementoenamel: junction

cementoossifying: fibroma

cementum: hyperplasia

centigrade: scale

centimeter-gram-second: system; unit

central: amputation; apnea; apparatus; artery; artery of retina; bearing; body; bone; bone of ankle; bradycardia; callus; canal; canals of cochlea; canal of spinal cord; canal of the vitreous; cataract; chromatolysis; complex; deafness; dogma; ganglioneuroma; gyri; illumination; implantation; incisor; inhibition; lacteal; lobule; lobule of cerebellum; necrosis; neuritis; nucleus; osteitis; paralysis; part of lateral ventricle; pit; placenta previa; pneumonia; scotoma; spindle; sulcus; sulcus of insula; tendon of diaphragm; tendon of perineum; veins of liver; vein of suprarenal gland; vision

central amygdaloid: nucleus

central angiospastic: retinitis; retinopathy

central areolar choroidal: atrophy; dystrophy; sclerosis

central axillary: lymph nodes

central-bearing: device; point

central-bearing tracing: device

central cloudy corneal: dystrophy of François

central cord: syndrome

central core: disease

central crystalline corneal: dystrophy of Snyder

Central European tick-borne: fever

Central European tick-borne encephalitis: virus

central excitatory: state

central fibrous: body

central gray: substance

centralization: phenomenon

central lateral: nucleus of thalamus

central and lateral intermediate: substances

central limit: theorem

central mesenteric: lymph nodes

central nervous: system

central ossifying: fibroma

central palmar: space

central pontine: myelinolysis

central retinal: artery; fovea; vein

central serous: choroidopathy; retinopathy

central sulcal: artery

central superior mesenteric: lymph nodes

central tegmental: fasciculus; tract

central terminal: electrode

central thalamic: radiation

central transactional: core

central type: neurofibromatosis

central venous: catheter; pressure

centrencephalic: epilepsy

centriacinar: emphysema

centric: contact; fusion; occlusion; position

centric jaw: relation

centrifugal: casting; current; nerve

centrifugal fast: analyzer

centrilobular: emphysema

centripetal: current; nerve

centroacinar: cell

centrofacial: lentiginosis

centrolecithal: egg; ovum

centromedian: nucleus

centromere banding: stain

centromeric: index

centronuclear: myopathy

cephalic: angle; curve; flexure; index; pole; presentation; replacement; tetanus; triangle; vein; vein of forearm; version

cephalic arterial: rami

cephalocaudal: axis

cephalomedullary: angle

cephalometric: analysis; radiograph; tracing

cephalo-oculocutaneous: telangiectasia

cephalo-orbital: index

cephalopalpebral: reflex

cephalopelvic: disproportion

cephalorrhachidian: index

cephalotrigeminal: angiomatosis

ceramide lactoside: lipidosis

ceramo-metal: casting

ceratocricoid: ligament; muscle

ceratoglossus: muscle

ceratopharyngeal: part of middle constrictor muscle of pharynx; part of middle pharyngeal constrictor (muscle) of pharynx

cercopithecrine: herpesvirus

cerebellar: arteries; astrocytoma; ataxia; atrophy; cortex; cyst; falx; fissures; fossa; frenulum; gait; nuclei; pyramid; rigidity; speech; sulci; syndrome; tentorium; tonsil; veins

cerebellohypothalamic: fibers

cerebellomedullary: cistern

cerebellomedullary malformation: syndrome

cerebelloolivary: fibers

cerebellopontile: angle

cerebellopontine: angle; cisternography; recess

cerebellopontine angle: syndrome; tumor

cerebellorubral: tract

cerebellospinal: fibers

cerebellothalamic: tract

cerebral: angiography; anthrax; aqueduct; arteries; arteriography; calculus; cladosporiosis; compression; cortex; death; decompression; decortication; diataxia; dominance; dysplasia; edema; falx; fissures; flexure; gigantism; gyri; hemisphere; hemorrhage; hernia; index; lacuna; layer of retina; lipidosis; lobes; localization; malaria; palsy; part of arachnoid; part of dura mater; part of internal carotid artery; peduncle; porosis; rheumatism; sinuses; sphingolipidosis; sulci; surface; tetanus; thrombosis; trigone; tuberculosis; veins; ventricles; vesicle; vomiting

cerebral amyloid: angiopathy

cerebral arterial: circle

cerebrohepatorenal: syndrome

cerebroretinal: angiomatosis

cerebroside: lipidosis; lipoidosis

cerebrospinal: axis; fever; fluid; index; meningitis; nematodiasis; pressure; system

cerebrospinal fluid: otorrhea; rhinorrhea

cerebrotendinous: xanthomatosis

cerebrovascular: accident; disease

Cerenkov: radiation

ceroid: lipofuscinosis

certified: milk

certified pasteurized: milk

certified reference: material

certified registered: nurse anesthetist

cerulean: cataract

ceruminous: glands

cervical: amputation; anchorage; anesthesia; auricle; branch of facial nerve; canal; cap; diverticulum; duct; dysplasia; enlargement; enlargement of spinal cord; fibrositis; flexure; glands;

Word Finder

glands of uterus; hydrocele;
hygroma; hyperesthesia;
ligament of uterus; line;
loop; lordosis; margin;
margin of tooth; myelogram;
myositis; myospasm; nerves
[C1–C8]; nystagmus;
orthosis; part of esophagus;
part of internal carotid
artery; part of spinal cord;
part of thoracic duct; part of
vertebral artery; patagium;
pleura; plexus; pregnancy;
rib; segments of spinal cord
[C1–C8]; sinus; smear;
spondylosis; triangle; vein;
vertebrae [C1–C7]; vesicle;
zone; zone of tooth
cervical aortic: knuckle
cervical compression:
   syndrome
cervical disk: syndrome
cervical fusion: syndrome
cervical iliocostal: muscle
cervical interspinal: muscle
cervical interspinales:
   muscles
cervical intraepithelial:
   neoplasia
cervical longissimus: muscle
cervical rib: syndrome
cervical rib and band:
   syndrome
cervical rotator: muscles
cervical splanchnic: nerves
cervical tension: syndrome
cervicoaxillary: canal
cervicolumbar: phenomenon
cervicooculoacoustic:
   syndrome
cervicothoracic: ganglion;
   orthosis; transition
cervicovaginal: artery
cesarean: hysterectomy;
   operation; section
Cestan-Chenais: syndrome
C1 esterase: inhibitor
Ceylon: cinnamon; moss
CF: antibody; lead; test
C group: viruses
Chaddock: reflex; sign
Chadwick: sign
Chagas: disease
Chagas-Cruz: disease
chagasic: myocardiopathy
Chagres: virus
chain: ganglia; reaction; reflex
α **chain:** disease
chain-compensated:
   spirometer
chair: form
chalice: cell
challenge: diet
chalybeate: water
Chamberlain: line; procedure
Chamberlen: forceps

Champy: fixative
Chance: fracture
chancriform: pyoderma;
   syndrome
chancroidal: bubo
chandelier: sign
Chandler: syndrome
change: blindness
Chantemesse: reaction
chaos: theory
chaotic: heart; rhythm
character: analysis; disorder;
   neurosis
characteristic: curve;
   emission; frequency;
   radiation
characterizing: group
Charcot: arteries; disease;
   gait; joint; syndrome; triad;
   vertigo
Charcot-Böttcher:
   crystalloids
Charcot-Bouchard: aneurysm
Charcot intermittent: fever
Charcot-Leyden: crystals
Charcot-Marie-Tooth:
   disease
Charcot-Neumann: crystals
Charcot-Robin: crystals
Charcot-Weiss-Baker:
   syndrome
Chargaff: rule
CHARGE: association;
   syndrome
charge: nurse
charge transfer: complex;
   system
Charles: law
Charlouis: disease
Charnley hip: arthroplasty
Charrière: scale
Charters: method
Chassaignac: space; tubercle
Chauffard: syndrome
Chaussier: areola; line; sign
Chayes: method
Cheadle: disease
Cheatle: slit
check: ligaments of eyeball,
   medial and lateral; ligaments
   of medial and lateral rectus
   muscles; ligaments of
   odontoid
Chédiak-Higashi: disease;
   syndrome
Chédiak-Steinbrinck-
   Higashi: anomaly;
   syndrome
cheek: bone; muscle; tooth
cheese: maggot
cheese worker's: lung
cheesy: abscess; pus
chemical: antidote; attraction;
   burn; cautery; ceptor;
   complexity; conjunctivitis;
   depilatory; dermatitis;

diabetes; energy; equation;
evolution; formula; kinetics;
knife; modification; peeling;
peritonitis; pneumonia;
potential; pregnancy;
prophylaxis; ray; repair;
sampling; senses; shift;
solution; sympathectomy;
taxonomy; thyroidectomy
chemically cured: resin
chemical shift: artifact
chemiosmotic: theory
chemotherapeutic: index
Cheney: syndrome
cherry: angioma
cherry-red: spot
cherry-red spot myoclonus:
   syndrome
cherubic: facies
chest: index; leads; radiology;
   wall
Chevalier-Jackson: dilator
chevron: incision
chewing: cycle; force
Cheyne-Stokes: psychosis;
   respiration
chi: sequence; structure
Chian: turpentine
Chiari: disease; net; syndrome
Chiari-Budd: syndrome
Chiari-Frommel: syndrome
Chiari II: syndrome
chiasma: syndrome
chiasmatic: cistern; groove;
   sulcus
Chicago: disease
chicken: breast
chicken embryo lethal
   orphan: virus
chicken fat: clot
chickenpox: immunoglobulin;
   virus
chickenpox immune: globulin
   (human)
Chick-Martin: test
chiclero: ulcer
chief: agglutinin; artery of
   thumb; cell; cell of corpus
   pineale; cell of parathyroid
   gland; cell of stomach;
   complaint
Chievitz: layer; organ
chikungunya: virus
Chilaiditi: syndrome
chilblain: lupus; lupus
   erythematosus
CHILD: syndrome
child: abuse; psychiatry;
   psychology
childbearing: age
childbed: fever
childhood: epilepsy with
   occipital paroxysms;
   hypophosphatasia;
   schizophrenia; tuberculosis
childhood absence: epilepsy

childhood muscular:
   dystrophy
childhood type: tuberculosis
Chilean: saltpeter
chimeric: antibodies; molecule
chimney sweep's: cancer
chimpanzee coryza: agent
chin: cap; jerk; muscle; reflex
Chinese: cinnamon; ginger;
   wax
Chinese restaurant:
   syndrome
chip: syringe
chiral: crystal
chi-square: distribution; test
chloride: shift
chlorinated: lime; paraffin
chlorine: acne; water
chlorohemin: crystals
chloropercha: method
chlorophyll: unit
chloroprocaine: penicillin O
chlorotic: anemia
chlorotriazine: dyes
choanal: atresia; polyp
chocolate: agar; cyst
Chodzko: reflex
choked: disk
cholangiolitic: hepatitis
cholangitic: abscess
cholecystoduodenal: fistula
choledoch: duct
choledochal: cyst; sphincter
choledochoduodenal: junction
cholera: agar; bacillus; toxin;
   vaccine
choleraic: diarrhea
cholera-red: reaction
choleric: jaundice
cholestatic: hepatitis; jaundice
cholestatic hepatosis: icterus
   gravidarum
cholesterinized: antigen
cholesterol: cleft; embolism;
   granuloma
cholesterol ester storage:
   disease
cholesterol ester transport:
   proteins
cholesteryl ester storage:
   disease
cholestyramine: resin
cholinergic: agent; blockade;
   fibers; neurotransmitter;
   receptors; urticaria
cholinesterase: inhibitor
chondrification: center
chondrin: ball
chondrodystrophic: dwarfism
chondroectodermal: dysplasia
chondroglossus: muscle
chondroid: syringoma; tissue
chondromyxoid: fibroma
chondropharyngeal: part of
   middle constrictor muscle of
   pharynx; part of middle

pharyngeal constrictor (muscle) of pharynx
chondroxiphoid: ligament
Chopart: amputation; joint
chorda: saliva
choreic: movement
chorioallantoic: graft; membrane; placenta
chorioamnionic: placenta
choriocapillary: layer
chorionic: ectoderm; gonadotropin; plate; sac; villi
chorionic gonadotropic: hormone
chorionic gonadotropin: unit
chorionic growth: hormone-prolactin
chorionic villus: biopsy
choroid: blood vessels; branches; enlargement; fissure; glomus; line; membrane; plexus; plexus of fourth ventricle; plexus of lateral ventricle; plexus of third ventricle; skein; vein; veins of eye
choroidal: fissure; neovascularization; ring
choroidal vascular: atrophy
choroplethic: map
Chotzen: syndrome
Chr^a: antigens
Christchurch: chromosome
Christensen-Krabbe: disease
Christian: disease; syndrome
Christison: formula
Christmas: disease; factor
chromaffin: body; cell; reaction; system; tissue; tumor
chromate: stain for lead
chromatic: aberration; apparatus; audition; fiber; granule; spectrum; vision
chromatin: body; network; nucleolus; particles
chromatography: paper
chrome: alum; ulcer
chrome alum hematoxylin-phloxine: stain
chrome-cobalt: alloys
chromic: catgut
chromic phosphate P 32 colloidal: suspension
chromidial: apparatus; net; substance
chromophil: granule; substance
chromophobe: adenoma; cells of anterior lobe of hypophysis; granules
chromosomal: deletion; gap; region; RNA; syndrome; trait

chromosomal instability: syndromes
chromosome: aberration; band; map; mapping; mosaicism; pair; satellite
chronic: abscess; alcoholism; anaphylaxis; appendicitis; ataxia; bronchitis; cholecystitis; conjunctivitis; eczema; glaucoma; glomerulonephritis; hepatitis; histoplasmosis; inflammation; malaria; nephritis; pancreatitis; pleurisy; pneumonia; pyelonephritis; rejection; rheumatism; rhinitis; shock; soroche; tamponade; trypanosomiasis; ulcer; urticaria; vertigo
chronic absorptive: arthritis
chronic acholuric: jaundice
chronic actinic: keratopathy
chronic active: hepatitis; inflammation
chronic active liver: disease
chronic adrenocortical: insufficiency
chronic African sleeping: sickness
chronic allograft: rejection
chronic anterior: poliomyelitis
chronic atrophic: polychondritis; thyroiditis; vulvitis
chronic bacillary: diarrhea
chronic bullous: dermatosis of childhood
chronic cicatrizing: enteritis
chronic constrictive: pericarditis
chronic cutaneous: leishmaniasis
chronic cystic: mastitis
chronic desquamative: gingivitis
chronic diffuse sclerosing: osteomyelitis
chronic discoid: lupus erythematosus
chronic endemic: fluorosis
chronic eosinophilic: pneumonia
chronic familial: icterus; jaundice; polyneuritis
chronic fibrosing: alveolitis; pancreatitis
chronic fibrous: thyroiditis
chronic focal sclerosing: osteomyelitis
chronic follicular: conjunctivitis
chronic granulocytic: leukemia

chronic granulomatous: disease
chronic hemorrhagic villous: synovitis
chronic hypertensive: disease
chronic hypertrophic: vulvitis
chronic hyperventilation: syndrome
chronic idiopathic: jaundice; xanthomatosis
chronic inflammatory demyelinating: polyneuropathy
chronic interstitial: hepatitis; salpingitis
chronic lymphadenoid: thyroiditis
chronic lymphocytic: lymphoma; thyroiditis
chronic mediastinal: histoplasmosis
chronic mountain: sickness
chronic myelocytic: leukemia
chronic myelogenous: leukemia
chronic myeloid: leukemia
chronic necrotizing: aspergillosis
chronic nonleukemic: myelosis
chronic obstructive pulmonary: disease
chronic persistent: hepatitis
chronic persisting: hepatitis
chronic posterior: laryngitis
chronic progressive: chorea
chronic progressive external: ophthalmoplegia
chronic progressive syphilitic: meningoencephalitis
chronic relapsing: pancreatitis
chronic subglottic: laryngitis
chronic ulcerative: proctitis
chronologic: age
Churg-Strauss: syndrome
Chvostek: sign
chyle: cistern; corpuscle; cyst; fistula; peritonitis; vessel
chyliform: ascites
chylomicron retention: disease
chylous: arthritis; ascites; hydrothorax; urine
chymotropic: pigment
α-chymotrypsin-induced: glaucoma
Ciaccio: glands; stain
Cianca: syndrome
cicatricial: alopecia; conjunctivitis; ectropion; entropion; horn
cicatrization: atelectasis
cigarette: drain
cigarette-paper: scars

ciliary: blepharitis; body; border of iris; canals; cartilage; crown; disk; dyskinesis; folds; ganglion; glands; ligament; margin of iris; movement; muscle; part of retina; poliosis; process; ring; staphyloma; wreath; zone; zonule
ciliary ganglionic: plexus
ciliated: epithelium
ciliospinal: center; reflex
cinchona: bark
cinematic: amputation
cineplastic: amputation
cingular: branch of callosomarginal artery
cingulate: convolution; gyrus; herniation; sulcus
cingulum: rest
circadian: rhythm
Circe: effect
circinate: retinitis; retinopathy
circle absorption: anesthesia
circular: amputation; bandage; dichroism; fibers; folds of small intestine; layer of detrusor (muscle) of urinary bladder; layer of muscle coat of small intestine; layer of muscular coat; layers of muscular tunics; layer of tympanic membrane; reaction; sinus; sulcus of insula; sulcus of Reil
circulation: time
circulatory: arrest; collapse; system
circumalveolar: fixation
circumanal: glands
circumduction: gait
circumferential: cartilage; clasp; fibrocartilage; implantation; lamella; wiring
circumferential clasp: arm
circumferential pontine: branches of pontine arteries
circumflex: branch of left coronary artery; branch of posterior tibial artery; nerve; veins
circumflex femoral: arteries
circumflex fibular: artery; branch (of posterior tibial artery)
circumflex humeral: arteries
circumflex iliac: arteries
circumflex peroneal: branch of posterior tibial artery
circumflex scapular: artery; vein
circummandibular: fixation
circumscribed: craniomalacia; myxedema; peritonitis; pyocephalus

circumscribed posterior: keratoconus

circumsporozoite: protein

circumvallate: papillae

circumventricular: organs

circumzygomatic: fixation; wiring

circus: movement; rhythm

cirsoid: aneurysm; varix

cis: configuration

cis: phase

13-*cis*-: retinoic acid

cis-acting: locus; protein

cisternal: puncture

cis/trans: test

citrate: intoxication

citrate-cleavage: enzyme

citrated: calcium carbimide

citric acid: cycle

citrovorum: factor

Civatte: bodies; disease

Civinini: canal; ligament; process

CL: lead

Clado: anastomosis; band; ligament; point

Clagett: procedure for empyema

Claisen: condensation

clamp: forceps

clamshell: incision; thoracotomy

clang: association

Clapton: line

Clara: cell

Clark: electrode; level

Clarke: cells; column; nucleus

Clarke-Hadfield: syndrome

Clark weight: rule

clasp: arm; bar; guideline

clasping: reflex

clasp-knife: effect; rigidity; spasticity

class: switching

class I: antigens; molecule

classic: hemophilia; migraine

classical: conditioning; genetics

classical cesarean: section

classic cervical rib: syndrome

classic choroidal: neovascularization

classifiable: character

class II: antigens; molecule

class III: antigens

clastic: anatomy

clathrate: crystal

Clauberg: test; unit

Claude: syndrome

Claudius: cells; fossa

claustral: layer

clavate: papillae

clavicular: branch of thoracoacromial artery; facet; head of pectoralis major muscle; notch of

sternum; part of deltoid (muscle); part of pectoralis major (muscle); percussion

clavicular articular: facet of acromion

clavipectoral: fascia; triangle

claw: foot; hand

Claybrook: sign

clay shoveler's: fracture

clean intermittent bladder: catheterization

cleansing: cream

clear: cell; layer of epidermis

clear cell: acanthoma; adenocarcinoma; carcinoma; carcinoma of kidney; carcinoma of salivary glands; hidradenoma

clearing: factors; medium

clear liquid: diet

cleavage: cavity; cell; division; lines; product; site; spindle

cleaved: cell

cleft: hand; lip; nose; palate; spine; tongue

cleidocranial: dysostosis; dysplasia

Cleland: nomenclature; reagent

clenched fist: sign

clerical: spectacles

Clevenger: fissure

click: syndrome

clicking: rale; tinnitus

client-centered: therapy

climacteric: syndrome

climatic: bubo; keratopathy

climatic droplike: keratopathy

climbing: fibers

clinical: anatomy; burden; chemistry; crown; depression; diagnosis; epidemiology; eruption; fitness; genetics; indicator; lethal; medicine; nurse specialist; path; pathology; pharmacologist; pharmacology; pharmacy; psychology; recording; root of tooth; sensitivity; spectrometry; spectroscopy; thermometer; trial

clinical end: point

clinical practice: guidelines

clinoid: process

clip: forceps

clipped: speech

clitoral: recession

clivus: branches of cerebral part of internal carotid artery

cloacal: exstrophy; membrane; plate; theory

cloacogenic: carcinoma

clomiphene: test

clonal: aging; expansion

clonal deletion: theory

clonal selection: theory

clonic: convulsion; seizure

clonidine growth hormone stimulation: test

cloning: vector

clonogenic: assay; cell

Cloquet: canal; hernia; septum; space

close: bite

closed: anesthesia; bite; circle; comedo; dislocation; drainage; fracture; hospital; laparoscopy; reading frame; reduction of fractures; surgery; system

closed-angle: glaucoma

closed chain: compound

closed chest: massage

closed circuit: method

closed head: injury

closed loop: obstruction

closed skull: fracture

closing: contraction; membranes; snap; volume

clostridial: myonecrosis

Clostridium perfringens: enterotoxin

Clostridium perfringens **alpha:** toxin

Clostridium perfringens **beta:** toxin

Clostridium perfringens **epsilon:** toxin

Clostridium perfringens **iota:** toxin

closure: principle

clot retraction: time

clotting: factor; time

clouding of: consciousness

Cloudman: melanoma

cloudy: swelling; urine

cloverleaf: model; skull

cloverleaf skull: syndrome

club: foot; hair; hand; moss

clubbed: digit; fingers; penis

clue: cell

cluster: analysis; headache; sample

cluster of differentiation (CD): antigen

Clutton: joints

CO₂: narcosis

coagulation: factor; necrosis; time; vitamin

coal tar: naphtha

coal worker's: pneumoconiosis

coaptation: splint; suture

coarctate: retina

coarse: dispersion; tremor

coated: pit; tongue; vesicle

Coats: disease

Cobb: method; syndrome

cobbler's: suture

cobra: hemotoxin; toxin

cobra venom: cofactor; factor

cocarde: reaction

coccidioidal: granuloma

coccidioidin: test

coccygeal: body; bone; cornu; dimple; fistula; foveola; ganglion; gland; horn; joint; ligament; muscle; nerve [Co]; part of spinal cord; plexus; segment of spinal cord [Co]; sinus; vertebrae [Co1–Co4]; whorl

coccygeus: muscle

Cochin China: diarrhea

cochlear: aqueduct; area; branch of labyrinthine artery; branch of vestibulocochlear artery; canal; canaliculus; cupula; drill-out; duct; dysplasia; ganglion; implant; joint; labyrinth; nerve; nuclei; part of vestibulocochlear nerve; potential; prosthesis; recess; root of VIII nerve; window

cochlear hair: cells

cochleariform: process

cochleo-orbicular: reflex

cochleopalpebral: reflex

cochleopupillary: reflex

cochleostapedial: reflex

Cochrane: collaboration

Cockayne: disease; syndrome

Cockett communicating perforating: veins

cockscomb: ulcer

coconut: sound

codeine: phosphate; sulfate

codfish: vertebrae

coding: sequence; strand

Codman: triangle; tumor

codominant: allele; gene; inheritance; trait

Coe: virus

coelomic: metaplasia

coenzyme: factor

coffee-ground: vomit

Coffey: suspension

Coffin-Lowry: syndrome

Coffin-Siris: syndrome

Cogan: dystrophy; syndrome

Cogan-Reese: syndrome

cognitive: development; dissonance; psychology; therapy

cognitive dissonance: theory

cognitive laterality: quotient

cogwheel: phenomenon; respiration; rigidity

cogwheel ocular: movements

cohesive: gold

Cohnheim: area; field

cohort: study

coil: gland

coiled: artery of the uterus

coin: lesion of lungs; test

coincidental: evolution
cointegrate: structure
coital: headache
Coiter: muscle
cold: abscess; agglutination; agglutinin; allergy; antibody; autoagglutinin; autoantibody; cautery; chain; cream; erythema; gangrene; hemolysin; light; nodule; pack; snare; sore; stage; ulcer; urticaria; virus
cold agglutinin: syndrome
cold bend: test
cold-blooded: animal
cold cure: resin
cold hemagglutinin: disease
cold knife: conization
cold pressor: test
cold-reactive: antibody
cold-rigor: point
cold-sensitive: enzyme; mutant
Cole-Cecil: murmur
colic: arteries; branch of ileocolic artery; impression on liver; impression of spleen; intussusception; lymph nodes; sphincter; surface of spleen; teniae; veins
coliform: bacilli
collagen: disease; fiber; fibrils; helix; implantation; injection
collagenous: colitis; pneumoconiosis
collapse: therapy
collapsing: pulse
collar: bone; incision
collar-button: abscess
collared: flagellate
collar-stud: chalazion
collateral: artery; branches of posterior intercostal arteries 3–11; branch of intercostal nerves; circulation; eminence; fissure; hyperemia; inheritance; ligament; sulcus; trigone; vessel
collateral digital: artery
collective: unconscious
Colles: fascia; fracture; ligament; space
Collet-Sicard: syndrome
collicular: artery
Collier: sign; tract
collier: lung
Collier tucked lid: sign
colliquative: albuminuria; degeneration; diarrhea; necrosis; sweat
Collis: gastroplasty
Collis-Belsey: fundoplication; procedure
collision: tumor

Collis-Nissen: fundoplication
collodion: baby
colloid: acne; adenoma; bath; bodies; cancer; carcinoma; corpuscle; cyst; degeneration; goiter; system; theory of narcosis
colloidal: dispersion; gel; metal; silicon dioxide; silver iodide; solution
colloidal gold: reaction; test
colloidal radioactive: gold
colobomatous: microphthalmia
colocutaneous: fistula
coloileal: fistula
colon: bacillus
colon cutoff: sign
colonic: diverticula; fistula; smear
colony-forming: unit
colony-stimulating: factors
color: aberration; agnosia; blindness; constancy; hearing; radical; scotoma; sense; spectrum; taste
Colorado tick: fever
Colorado tick fever: virus
color-contrast: microscope
colored: vision
colorimetric: titration
colorimetric caries susceptibility: test
colostomy: bag
colostrum: corpuscle
colovaginal: fistula
colovesical: fistula
Columbia Mental Maturity: Scale
Columbia S. K.: virus
column: cells; chromatography
columnar: epithelium; layer
coma: aberration; cast; scale; vigil
combat: exhaustion; neurosis
comb-growth: test
combination: beat; chemotherapy; restoration
combination oral: contraceptive
combined: glaucoma; immunodeficiency; methods; pregnancy; sclerosis; version
combined fat- and carbohydrate-induced: hyperlipemia
combined immunodeficiency: syndrome
combined system: disease
combining: weight
comblike: septum
combustion: equivalent
Comby: sign
comet: sign
comet tail: sign

comfort: zone
comitant: artery of median nerve; strabismus
comma: bacillus; bundle of Schultze; tract of Schultze
command: hallucination
commando: operation; procedure
commemorative: sign
commensal: parasite
comminuted: fracture
comminuted skull: fracture
commissural: cell; cheilitis; fibers; myelotomy
commisural: pits
common: antigen; baldness; crus of semicircular ducts; migraine; opsonin; salt; wart
common basal: vein
common bile: duct
common cardinal: veins
common carotid: artery; plexus
common carotid nervous: plexus
common cochlear: artery
common cold: virus
common facial: vein
common fibular: nerve
common flexor: sheath (of hand)
common hepatic: artery; duct
common iliac: artery; lymph nodes; vein
common interosseous: artery
common membranous: limb of membranous semicircular ducts; limb of semicircular ducts
common modiolar: vein
common palmar digital: artery; nerves
common peroneal: nerve
common peroneal tendon: sheath
common plantar digital: artery; nerves
common tendinous: ring of extraocular muscles
common variable: immunodeficiency
communicable: disease
communicating: artery; branch; branch of anterior interosseous nerve with ulnar nerve; branch of chorda tympani to lingual nerve; branch of chorda tympani with lingual nerve; branches of auriculotemporal nerve with facial nerve; branches of lingual nerve with hypoglossal nerve; branches of spinal nerves; branches of sympathetic trunk; branch of

facial nerve with glossopharyngeal nerve; branch of facial nerve with tympanic plexus; branch of fibular artery; branch of glossopharyngeal nerve with auricular branch of vagus nerve; branch of intermediate nerve with tympanic plexus; branch of internal laryngeal nerve with recurrent laryngeal nerve; branch of lacrimal nerve with zygomatic nerve; branch of median nerve with ulnar nerve; branch of nasociliary nerve with ciliary ganglion; branch of otic ganglion to auriculotemporal nerve; branch of otic ganglion to chorda tympani; branch of otic ganglion with chorda tympani; branch of otic ganglion with medial pterygoid nerve; branch of otic ganglion with meningeal branch of mandibular nerve; branch of peroneal artery; branch of radial nerve with ulnar nerve; branch of superficial radial nerve with ulnar nerve; branch of superior laryngeal nerve with recurrent laryngeal nerve; branch of tympanic plexus with auricular branch of vagus nerve; hematoma; hydrocele; hydrocephalus; junction; rami of sympathetic trunk
community: dentistry; medicine; nurse; psychiatry; psychology
community-acquired: pneumonia
community health: nurse
compact: bone; substance
companion: artery to sciatic nerve; lymph nodes of accessory nerve; vein; veins
comparative: anatomy; medicine; pathology; physiology; psychology
comparator: microscope
compartment: syndrome
compensated: acidosis; alkalosis; glaucoma
compensated metabolic: alkalosis
compensated respiratory: acidosis; alkalosis
compensating: curve; emphysema; ocular
compensation: neurosis

compensatory: circulation; hypertrophy; hypertrophy of the heart; pause; polycythemia
competing: risk
competitive: antagonist; inhibition
competitive binding: assay
competitor: DNA
complement: factor I; fixation; system; unit
complemental: air
complementarity determining: regions
complementary: air; colors; DNA; hypertrophy; medicine; role; strand; structures
complement binding: assay
complement chemotactic: factor
complement-fixation: reaction; test
complement-fixing: antibody
complete: abortion; achromatopsia; antibody; antigen; ascertainment; blood count; carcinogen; cataract; cleavage; denture; disinfectant; fistula; hemianopia; hernia; iridoplegia; mastoidectomy; medium; metamorphosis; tetanus; transduction
complete androgen insensitivity: syndrome
complete atrioventricular: dissociation
complete AV: block
complete denture: impression
completely in the canal: hearing aid
complete posterior laryngeal: cleft
complex: fracture; joint; locus; odontoma; sound
complex endometrial: hyperplasia
complex febrile: convulsion
complex learning: processes
complex motor: seizure
complex partial: seizure
complex pleural: effusion
complex precipitated: epilepsy
complicated: cataract; migraine
component: management
composite: flap; graft; joint; resin
composite dental: cement
compound: aneurysm; articulation; caries; character; cyst; dislocation; eye; fracture; gland; heterozygote; joint; lens;

lipids; microscope; nevus; odontoma; pregnancy; presentation; protein; restoration
compound action: potential
compound granule: cell
compound hyperopic: astigmatism
compound myopic: astigmatism
compound skull: fracture
comprehensive medical: care
compressed: sponge; tablet; yeast
compressible cavernous: bodies
compression: anesthesia; cyanosis; molding; neuropathy; paralysis; plate; plating; retinopathy; syndrome; thrombosis
compressive: myelopathy; nystagmus; strength
compressor urethra: muscle
Compton: effect; scatter
compulsive: idea; neurosis; personality
computed: perimetry; radiography; tomography
computer: model; simulation
computerized axial: tomography
Concato: disease
concave: lens; mirror
concavoconcave: lens
concavoconvex: lens
concealed: conduction; hemorrhage; hernia; penis
concentrated human red blood: corpuscle
concentration: gradient
concentric: fibroma; hypertrophy; lamella
concept: formation
concerted: evolution; model
conchal: cartilage; crest; crest of body of maxilla; crest of palatine bone
conchoidal: bodies
concomitant: immunity; strabismus; symptom
concordance: rate
concordant: alternans; alternation
concordant atrioventricular: connections
concordant changes: electrocardiogram
concrete: oils; operations; seborrhea; thinking
concurrent: disinfection; validity
concussion: cataract; myelitis
condensation: compound
condensed: milk
condensing: enzyme; osteitis

conditional: probability
conditional-lethal: mutant
conditionally lethal: mutant
conditioned: avitaminosis; hemolysis; insomnia; reflex; response; stimulus
conditioning: therapy
conduct: disorder
conducting: airway; system of heart
conduction: analgesia; anesthesia; aphasia; block
conductive: hearing impairment; heat
condylar: articulation; axis; canal; fossa; guidance; guide; joint; process of mandible
condylar emissary: vein
condylar guidance: inclination
condylar hinge: position
condyle: cord; path
condyloid: canal; process
cone: cell of retina; degeneration; disks; dystrophy; fiber; granule; vision
cone-rod retinal: dystrophy
confidence: interval
confluent: articulation; smallpox
confluent and reticulate: papillomatosis
confocal: microscope
conformational: map
confrontation: method
confusion: colors
congelation: urticaria
congenic: strain
congenital: afibrinogenemia; amputation; anemia; aplasia of thymus; baldness; bronchiectasis; cataract; choreoathetosis; conus; dysphagocytosis; elephantiasis; epulis of newborn; fibrosis of the extraocular muscles; glaucoma; hydrocele; hydrocephalus; hypophosphatasia; hypothyroidism; lymphedema; megacolon; methemoglobinemia; myxedema; nevus; nystagmus; pancytopenia; paramyotonia; pneumonia; stridor; syphilis; torticollis; toxoplasmosis; valve
congenital adrenal: hyperplasia
congenital aplastic: anemia
congenital atonic: pseudoparalysis
congenital cerebellar: atrophy

congenital cerebral: aneurysm
congenital diaphragmatic: hernia
congenital dyserythropoietic: anemia
congenital dysplastic: angiectasia; angiomatosis
congenital ectodermal: defect; dysplasia
congenital erythropoietic: porphyria
congenital facial: diplegia
congenital generalized: fibromatosis
congenital heart: block
congenital hemolytic: anemia; icterus; jaundice
congenital hereditary endothelial: dystrophy
congenital hip: dysplasia
congenital hypoplastic: anemia
congenital ichthyosiform: erythroderma
congenital lobar: emphysema
congenital microvillus: atrophy
congenital nonregenerative: anemia
congenital pulmonary arteriovenous: fistula
congenital pyloric: stenosis
congenital rubella: syndrome
congenital sebaceous: hyperplasia
congenital selective glucose and galactose: malabsorption
congenital spastic: paraplegia
congenital sutural: alopecia
congenital total: lipodystrophy
congenital virilizing adrenal: hyperplasia
congestive: cardiomyopathy; cirrhosis; splenomegaly
congestive heart: failure
Congolian red: fever
congophilic: angiopathy
Congo red: paper
congruent: points
congruous: hemianopia
conic: papillae
conical: catheter; cornea; lobules of epididymis; papillae
conjoined: anastomosis; tendon; twins
conjoined asymmetrical: twins
conjoined equal: twins
conjoined symmetrical: twins
conjoined unequal: twins
conjoint: tendon; therapy
conjugal: cancer

conjugate: acid; axis; deviation of the eyes; diameter of pelvic inlet; diameter of pelvic outlet; division; foci; foramen; gaze; movement of eyes; nystagmus; point

conjugate acid-base: pair

conjugated: antigen; bilirubin; compound; estrogen; hapten; protein

conjugated double: bonds

conjugative: plasmid

conjunctival: arteries; cul-de-sac; fornix; glands; layer of bulb; layer of eyelids; reflex; ring; sac; varix; veins

Conn: syndrome

connecting: cartilage; stalk; tubule

connective: tissue; tumor

connective-tissue: disease

connective tissue: cell; group

connector: bar

Connell: suture

conoid: ligament; process; tubercle (of clavicle)

Conradi: disease; line

Conradi-Hünermann: disease; syndrome

consecutive: amputation; aneurysm; angiitis; esotropia

consensual: reaction; validation

consensual light: reflex

conservative: replication; treatment

consistency: principle

consolidation: chemotherapy

consonating: rale

constancy: phenomenon

constant: coupling; region

constant field: equation

constant infusion: pump

constitutional: cause; formula; hirsutism; psychology; reaction; symptom; thrombopathy; ulcer

constitutional hepatic: dysfunction

constitutive: enzyme; heterochromatin

constriction: hyperemia; ring

constrictive: bronchiolitis; endocarditis; pericarditis

construct: validity

constructional: agraphia; apraxia

consulting: staff

consumption: coagulopathy

contact: allergy; area; catalysis; ceptor; cheilitis; dermatitis; hypersensitivity; hysteroscope; illumination; inhibition; lens; point; surface of tooth

contagious: disease; ecthyma

contagious ecthyma (pustular dermatitis): virus of sheep

contagious pustular: dermatitis

contagious pustular stomatitis: virus

contained disk: herniation

content: analysis; validity

contig: map

contingency: table

continued: fever

continuous: arrhythmia; beam; capillary; clasp; culture; eruption; murmur; phase; spectrum; suture; tremor; variable; variation

continuous ambulatory peritoneal: dialysis

continuous bar: retainer

continuous epidural: anesthesia

continuous flow: analyzer

continuous interleaved: sampling

continuous loop: wiring

continuous otoacoustic: emission

continuous passive: motion

continuous positive airway: pressure

continuous positive pressure: ventilation

continuous random: variable

continuous spinal: anesthesia

continuous wave: laser

contour: lines of Owen

contraceptive: device; sponge

contracted: foot; kidney; pelvis

contractile: stricture; vacuole

contraction: band

contraction band: necrosis

contraction stress: test

contractual: psychiatry; psychotherapy

contractural: diathesis

contracture: deformity

contralateral: hemiplegia; reflex; sign

contralateral routing of: signals

contrast: agent; bath; echocardiography; enema; enhancement; material; medium; sensitivity; stain

contrast sensitivity: testing

contrasuppressor: cells

contrecoup: injury of brain

control: animal; experiment; gene; group; syringe

controlled: respiration; substance; ventilation

controlled mechanical: ventilation

control release: suture

convalescent: carrier; serum

convective: heat

convenience: form

conventional: animal; signs; thoracoplasty; tomography

convergence: excess; insufficiency; nucleus of Perlia

convergence-retraction: nystagmus

convergent: evolution; squint; strabismus

converging: meniscus

conversion: disorder; electron; hysteria; neurosis; reaction

conversion hysteria: neurosis

conversive: heat

convex: lens; mirror

convexoconcave: lens

convexoconvex: lens

convoluted: bone; gland; part of kidney lobule; tubule of kidney

convoluted seminiferous: tubule

convulsant: threshold

convulsive: seizure; state; therapy; tic

cooing: murmur

Cooke: speculum

cooled-knife: method

Cooley: anemia

Coolidge: tube

coolie: itch

Coombs: murmur; serum; test

Cooper: fascia; hernia; herniotome; ligaments

cooperative: enzyme

cooperativity: model

Cooper-Rand artificial: larynx

coordinate covalent: bond

Cope: clamp

copia: elements

copolymer: resin

copper: cataract; colic; nose; protein

copper phosphate: cement

copper sulfate: method

Coppet: law

copra: itch

coracoacromial: arch; ligament

coracobrachial: bursa; muscle

coracobrachialis: muscle

coracoclavicular: ligament

coracohumeral: ligament

coracoid: process; tuberosity

coral: calculus

coralliform: cataract

cord: blood; hydrocele

cordate: pelvis

cordiform: uterus

cordy: pulse

core: particle; pneumonia

Cori: cycle; disease; ester

corkscrew: vessels

corn: ergot; sugar

corneal: astigmatism; corpuscles; decompensation; dystrophy; ectasia; facet; graft; layer of epidermis; lens; limbus; margin; pannus; reflex; space; spot; staphyloma; transplantation; trepanation; vertex

corneal endothelial: polymorphism

Cornelia de Lange: syndrome

corneocyte: envelope

corneoscleral: junction; part of trabecular tissue of sclera

Corner: tampon

Corner-Allen: test; unit

corniculate: cartilage; tubercle

corniculopharyngeal: ligament

cornified: layer of nail

cornmeal: agar

cornoid: lamella

cornual: pregnancy

coronal: epispadias; hypospadias; plane; pulp; section; suture

coronary: angiography; arteriosclerosis; arteritis; artery; atherectomy; cataract; endarterectomy; failure; groove; insufficiency; ligament of knee; ligament of liver; node; occlusion; plexus; sinus; steal; sulcus; tendon; thrombosis; valve; vein

coronary artery: aneurysm; bypass

coronary care: unit

coronary nodal: rhythm

coronary ostial: stenosis

coronary perfusion: pressure

coronary-prone: behavior

coronary sinus: rhythm

coronoid: fossa of humerus; process; process of the mandible; process of the ulna

corpora lutea: cyst

corpus: epididymis

corpuscular: lymph; radiation

corpus luteum: hematoma

corpus luteum deficiency: syndrome

corpus luteum hormone: unit

corralin: yellow

corrected: dextrocardia; transposition of the great vessels

corrective emotional: experience

correlation: coefficient

correlational: method

correlative: differentiation

Correra: line
Corrigan: disease; pulse; sign
corrosion: preparation
corrosive: sublimate; ulcer
corrugator: muscle
corrugator cutis: muscle of anus
corrugator supercilii: muscle
Corti: arch; canal; cells; ganglion; membrane; organ; pillars; rods; tunnel
Corti auditory: teeth
cortical: apraxia; arches of kidney; arteries; audiometry; blindness; bone; cataract; convexity; deafness; dysgenesis; dysplasia; epilepsy; hormones; implantation; lobules of kidney; osteitis; part; part of middle cerebral artery; sensibility; substance
cortical amygdaloid: nucleus
cortical radiate: arteries
corticobasal: degeneration
corticobulbar: fibers; tract
corticomesencephalic: fibers
corticonuclear: fibers
corticopontine: fibers; tract
corticoreticular: fibers
corticorubral: fibers
corticospinal: fibers; tract
corticosteroid-binding: globulin; protein
corticosteroid-induced: glaucoma
corticothalamic: fibers
corticotropic: hormone
corticotropin-releasing: factor; hormone
Corvisart: facies
corymbose: syphilid
coryneform: bacteria
cosmetic: dermatitis; surgery
cosmic: rays
costal: angle; arch; cartilage; chondritis; facets; fringe; groove; line of pleural reflection; margin; notches; part of diaphragm; part of parietal pleura; pit of transverse process; pleura; pleurisy; process; respiration; surface; surface of lung; surface of scapula; tuberosity
costal arch: reflex
Costen: syndrome
costimulatory: molecule
costoaxillary: vein
costocervical: artery
costocervical (arterial): trunk
costochondral: joints; junctions; syndrome
costoclavicular: ligament; line; syndrome

costocolic: ligament
costodiaphragmatic: recess
costomediastinal: recess; sinus
costopectoral: reflex
costophrenic: angle; sulcus
costophrenic septal: lines
costotransverse: foramen; joint; ligament
costovertebral: angle; joints
costoxiphoid: angle; ligament
cot: death
Cotard: syndrome
Cotte: operation
Cotton: effect
cotton-dust: asthma
cotton-fiber: embolism
cotton-mill: fever
cotton-root: bark
cotton-wool: patches; spots
Cotunnius: aqueduct; canal; liquid; space
cotyledonary: placenta
cotyloid: cavity; joint; ligament; notch
couching: needle
cough: fracture; reflex
Coumel: tachycardia
Councilman: body
counseling: psychology
count: density
counter: transference
counter-: shock
countercurrent: distribution; mechanism
counting: chamber
coup: injury of brain
coupled: beats; pulse; rhythm
coupling: defect; factors; interval; phase
Cournand: dip
Courvoisier: gallbladder; law; sign
Couvelaire: uterus
covalent: modification
cove: plane
cover: glass; test
covert: sensitization
cover-uncover: test
cow: face; kidney
Cowden: disease
Cowdry type A inclusion: bodies
Cowdry type B inclusion: bodies
CO$_2$-withdrawal seizure: test
cowl: muscle
Cowling: rule
cow milk: anemia
Cowper: cyst; gland; ligament
cowpox: virus
coxal: bone
coxitic: scoliosis
coxsackie: encephalitis; virus
CR: lead
crab: hand; yaws

Crabtree: effect
crack: cocaine
cracked: heel
cracked-pot: resonance; sound
crackling: jaw; rale
cradle: cap
Crafoord: clamp
Cramer wire: splint
Crampton: line; muscle; test
Crandall: syndrome
cranial: arachnoid mater; arteritis; base; bones; capacity; cavity; dura mater; flexure; fontanelles; index; nerves; neuropore; part of parasympathetic part of autonomic division of nervous system; root of accessory nerve; sinuses; sutures; synchondroses; vault; vertebra
(cranial) extradural: space
cranial pia: mater
cranial synovial: joints
craniocardiac: reflex
craniocarpotarsal: dysplasia; dystrophy
craniocervical: part of peripheral autonomic plexuses and ganglia
craniodiaphysial: dysplasia
craniofacial: angle; appliance; axis; dysostosis; fixation; surgery
craniofacial dysjunction: fracture
craniofacial suspension: wiring
craniometaphysial: dysplasia
craniometric: points
craniopharyngeal: canal; duct
craniosacral: division of autonomic nervous system
craniosacral nervous: system
craniospinal sensory: ganglia
crater: arc
cravat: bandage
C-reactive: protein
cream of: tartar
crease: wound
creatine kinase: isoenzymes
creatinine: clearance; coefficient
creative: thinking
Credé: maneuvers; methods
creep: recovery
creeping: eruption; myiasis; thrombosis; ulcer
cremaster: muscle
cremasteric: artery; fascia; reflex
creola: bodies
crepitant: rale
crescendo: angina; murmur; sleep
crescent: cell; sign

crescentic: lobules of the cerebellum
CREST: syndrome
Cresylecht violet: stain
Creutzfeldt-Jakob: disease
crevicular: epithelium; fluid
crib: death
cribriform: area of the renal papilla; fascia; foramina; hymen; plate of ethmoid bone
cribrous: lamina
Crichton-Browne: sign
cricoarytenoid: articulation; joint; ligament
cricoarytenoid articular: capsule
cricoesophageal: tendon
cricoid: cartilage
cricoid split: operation
cricopharyngeal: achalasia; ligament; myotomy; part of inferior constrictor (muscle) of pharynx
cricopharyngeus: muscle
cricosantorinian: ligament
cricothyroid: artery; articulation; branch of superior thyroid artery; joint; membrane; muscle
cricothyroid articular: capsule
cricotracheal: ligament; membrane
cricovocal: membrane
cri-du-chat: syndrome
Crigler-Najjar: disease; syndrome
Crile: clamp
Crimean: fever
Crimean-Congo hemorrhagic: fever
Crimean-Congo hemorrhagic fever: virus
criminal: abortion; anthropology; hygiene; insanity; irresponsibility; psychology
crisis: intervention
crisscross: heart
criterion-related: validity
critical: angle; illumination; limit; organ; pathway; period; pH; point; pressure; rate; temperature
critical care: unit
critical flicker fusion: frequency
critical illness: polyneuropathy
critical micelle: concentration
crocodile: tears
crocodile tears: syndrome
Crocq: disease
Crohn: disease
Cronkhite-Canada: syndrome

Crooke: granules
Crooke hyaline: change; degeneration
Crookes: glass
Crookes-Hittorf: tube
Crosby: capsule
cross: agglutination; birth; circulation; flap; hybridization; infection; mating; section; tolerance
cross-: reaction
crossbite: tooth
cross-cultural: psychiatry
cross-cut: bur
crossed: anesthesia; aphasia; cylinders; diplopia; embolism; eyes; fixation; hemianesthesia; hemianopia; hemiplegia; immunoelectrophoresis; jerk; laterality; paralysis; reflex; reflex of pelvis
crossed adductor: jerk; reflex
crossed extension: reflex
crossed knee: jerk; reflex
crossed pyramidal: tract
crossed renal: ectopia
crossed spino-adductor: reflex
crossed testicular: ectopia
cross-level: bias
cross-linked: polymer; resin
cross-over: study
cross-reacting: agglutinin; antibody; material
cross-sectional: echocardiography; method; study
cross-table lateral: projection
crotalaria: poisoning
Crotalus: antitoxin; toxin
croup-associated: virus
croupous: bronchitis; laryngitis; lymph; membrane
Crouzon: disease; syndrome
crowding: phenomenon
Crowe-Davis mouth: gag
Crow-Fukase: syndrome
crowing: inspiration
crown: cavity; flask; glass; pulp; tubercle
crown-heel: length
crown-rump: length
crucial: bandage; ligament
cruciate: anastomosis; eminence; ligament of the atlas; ligament of leg; ligaments of knee; muscle
cruciform: eminence; ligament of atlas; loops; part of fibrous digital sheath; part of fibrous sheath; pulley
crude: calcium sulfide; death rate; drug; urine

crural: arch; fascia; fossa; hernia; ring; septum; sheath; triangle
crural interosseous: nerve
crush: kidney; syndrome
crusted: ringworm; scabies; tetter
crutch: palsy; paralysis
Cruveilhier: disease; fascia; fossa; joint; ligaments; plexus
Cruveilhier-Baumgarten: disease; murmur; sign; syndrome
Cruz: trypanosomiasis
cry: reflex
crypt: abscesses
cryptogenic: cirrhosis; epilepsy; infection; pyemia; septicemia
cryptogenic fibrosing: alveolitis
cryptophthalmus: syndrome
cryptorchid: testis
crystal: rash; structure
crystalline: capsule; cataract; digitalin; interface; lens
crystalline insulin zinc: suspension
crystallized: trypsin
crystal violet: vaccine
Csillag: disease
"C" sliding: osteotomy
CT: number; pelvimetry; unit
Cuban: itch
cube: pessary
cubic: centimeter; niter
cubital: anastomosis; bone; fossa; joint; lymph nodes; nerve
cubital tunnel: syndrome
cuboid: bone
cuboidal: carcinoma; epithelium
cuboidal articular: surface of calcaneus
cuboideonavicular: joint; ligaments
cuboidodigital: reflex
cued: speech
cuirass: respirator; ventilator
cul-de-sac: smear
Cullen: sign
Culp: pyeloplasty
cultivated: yeast
cultural: anthropology; shock
culture: medium
Culver: root
Cummer: classification; guideline
Cumulative: Index Medicus
cumulative: action; dose; effect
cumulative trauma: disorders
cuneate: fasciculus; funiculus; nucleus; tubercle

cuneiform: bone; cartilage; cataract; lobe; nucleus; part of vomer; tubercle
cuneocerebellar: fibers; tract
cuneocuboid: joint; ligaments
cuneocuboid interosseous: ligament
cuneometatarsal: joints
cuneometatarsal interosseous: ligaments
cuneonavicular: articulation; joint; ligaments
cuneospinal: fibers
cup biopsy: forceps
Cupid's: bow
cupping: glass
cupular: cecum of the cochlear duct; part of epitympanic recess
cupular blind: sac
cupuliform: cataract
curative: dose
curb: tenotomy
curd: soap
curdy: pus
curlicue: ureter
Curling: ulcer
currant jelly: clot; stool; thrombus
current of: injury
Curschmann: spirals
curvature: aberration; hyperopia; myopia
Cushing: basophilism; disease; disease of the omentum; effect; phenomenon; response; suture; syndrome; syndrome medicamentosus
Cushing pituitary: basophilism
cusp: angle; height
cuspal: interference
cuspid: tooth
cuspless: tooth
cutaneomeningospinal: angiomatosis
cutaneomucouveal: syndrome
cutaneous: absorption; albinism; ancylostomiasis; anthrax; apoplexy; blastomycosis; branch of anterior branch of obturator nerve; branch of mixed nerve; branch of obturator nerve; diphtheria; emphysema; gangrene; glands; hemorrhoids; horn; larva migrans; layer of tympanic membrane; leishmaniasis; lupus erythematosus; meningioma; muscle; nerve; pseudolymphoma; reflex; schistosomiasis japonica; test; tuberculosis;

ureterostomy; vasculitis; vein
cutaneous cervical: nerve
cutaneous focal: mucinosis
cutaneous graft versus host: reaction
cutaneous leishmaniasis: granuloma
cutaneous loop: ureterostomy
cutaneous pupil: reflex
cutaneous tuberculin: test
cuticular: drusen
cutireaction: test
cutis: plate
cutting: edge; forceps; needle; teeth
cuttlefish: disk
cuvette: oximeter
Cuvier: ducts; veins
cyanide: poisoning
cyanide-nitroprusside: test
cyanobacteriumlike: bodies
cyanogenic: glycoside
cyanose: tardive
cyanotic: asphyxia; atrophy; atrophy of the liver; induration
cycle length: alternans
cycle-specific: agent
cyclic: adenylic acid; albuminuria; compound; esotropia; guanosine 3′,5′-monophosphate; neutropenia; nucleotide; peptide; phosphate; phosphoric acid; strabismus; uridine 3′,5′-monophosphate; vomiting
cyclopian: eye
cyclothymic: disorder; personality
cyclothymic personality: disorder
cylinder: retinoscopy
cylindrical: bronchiectasis; epithelium; joint; lens
cylindroid: aneurysm
cylindromatous: carcinoma
Cyon: nerve
cysteine: hydrolases
cystic: acne; artery; bronchiectasis; carcinoma; diathesis; disease of the breast; disease of renal medulla; duct; fibrosis; goiter; hygroma; hyperplasia; hyperplasia of the breast; kidney; lung; lymphangiectasis; lymph node; mole; node; polyp; veins
cystic adenomatoid: malformation
cystic duct: cholangiography
cysticercus: disease
cystic gall: duct

cystic medial: necrosis
cystic papillomatous: craniopharyngioma
cystine: bridge; calculus
cystine storage: disease
cystinotic: leukocyte
cystoduodenal: ligament
cystohepatic: triangle
cystoid: maculopathy
cystoid macular: edema
cystoscopic: urography
cythemolytic: icterus
cytochrome: system
cytochrome P-450: system
cytocrine: secretion
cytogenetic: map
cytogenic: reproduction
cytoid: bodies
cytokeratin: filaments
cytologic: examination; screening; smear; specimen
cytologic filter: preparation
cytomegalic: cells
cytomegalic inclusion: disease
cytomegalovirus: disease
cytopathic: effect
cytopathogenic: virus
cytophagic histiocytic: panniculitis
cytophil: group
cytophilic: antibody
cytoplasmic: bridges; inheritance; matrix
cytoplasmic inclusion: bodies
cytoreductive: therapy
cytostatic: chemotherapy
cytotonic: enterotoxin
cytotoxic: cell; chemotherapy; reaction
cytotrophoblastic: cells; shell
cytotropic: antibody
cytotropic antibody: test
Czapek-Dox: medium
Czapek solution: agar
Czerny: suture
Czerny-Lembert: suture

D

D: antigen; cell; enzyme; loop; wave
D-: 3-hydroxybutyric acid dehydrogenase; proline reductase
Daae: disease
Da Fano: stain
daily: dose
Dakin: fluid; solution
Dakin-Carrel: treatment
Dale: reaction
Dale-Feldberg: law
Dalen-Fuchs: nodules
Dalrymple: sign
Dalton: law
Dalton-Henry: law
Dam: unit

Damus-Kaye-Stancel: procedure
Damus-Stancel-Kaye: anastomosis
Dana: operation
Dance: sign
dancing: chorea
Dandy: operation
dandy: fever
Dandy-Walker: syndrome
Dane: particles; stain
Danforth: sign
Danielssen: disease
Danielssen-Boeck: disease
Danubian endemic familial: nephropathy
Danysz: phenomenon
DAPI: stain
DA pregnancy: test
dapsone: neuropathy
d'Arcet: metal
Darier: disease; sign
dark: adaptation; cells; reaction
dark-adapted: eye
dark-field: condenser; illumination; microscope
dark-ground: illumination
Darling: disease
d'Arsonval: current; galvanometer
dartoic: tissue
dartos: fascia; muscle
darwinian: ear; evolution; reflex; theory; tubercle
date: boil; fever
datum: plane
Datura: poisoning
Daubenton: angle; line; plane
daughter: cell; colony; cyst; isotope; star
Davidoff: cells
Davidson: syringe
Daviel: operation; spoon
Davies: disease
Davis: graft
Davis battery model of: transduction
Davis interlocking: sound
dawn: phenomenon
Dawson: encephalitis
Day: test
day: blindness; hospital; residue; sight
dazzling: glare
D-dimer: test
dead: fingers; nerve; pulp; space; tooth; tracts
dead arm: syndrome
dead-end: host
dead fetus: syndrome
dead-in-bed: syndrome
deadly: agaric; nightshade
deamidizing: enzymes
deaminating: enzymes
Dean fluorosis: index

death: instinct; rate; trance
Deaver: incision; method
DeBakey: classification; forceps
de Bordeau: theory
debrancher: deficiency
debranching: enzymes; factors
debranching deficiency limit: dextrinosis
Debré: phenomenon
Debré-Sémélaigne: syndrome
debulking: operation
decapacitation: factor
decarboxylated: dopa
decay: constant; theory
decentered: lens
decerebrate: rigidity; state
decidual: cast; cell; endometritis; fissure; reaction
deciduate: placenta
deciduous: dentition; membrane; skin; tooth
decision: analysis
declamping: phenomenon; shock
de Clerambault: syndrome
decomposition of: movement
decompression: chamber; disease; operations; sickness
decorticate: rigidity; state
decoy: cell
decremental: conduction
decubital: gangrene
decubitus: film; radiograph; ulcer
de-emetinized: ipecacuanha
deep: artery of arm; artery of clitoris; artery of penis; artery of thigh; artery of tongue; bite; branch; branch of the lateral plantar nerve; branch of the medial circumflex femoral artery; branch of the medial plantar artery; branch of radial nerve; branch of the superior gluteal artery; branch of the transverse cervical artery; branch of the ulnar nerve; cell; cortex; fascia; fascia of arm; fascia of forearm; fascia of leg; fascia of neck; fascia of penis; fascia of thigh; head of flexor pollicis brevis; lamina; layer; layer of levator palpebrae superioris; layer of temporal fascia; muscles of back; part of anterior compartment of forearm; part of external anal sphincter; part of flexor retinaculum; part of masseter (muscle); part of palpebral part of orbicularis

oculi (muscle); part of parotid gland; part of posterior (flexor) compartment of leg; percussion; reflex; scleritis; sensibility; veins of clitoris; veins of penis; vein of thigh
deep abdominal: reflexes
deep anterior cervical: lymph nodes
deep auricular: artery
deep brachial: artery
deep cardiac: plexus
deep cerebral: veins
(deep) cervical: fascia
deep cervical: artery; vein
deep circumflex iliac: artery; vein
deep crural: arch
deep dorsal: vein of clitoris; vein of penis
deep dorsal sacrococcygeal: ligament
deep epigastric: artery; vein
deep facial: vein
deep femoral: vein
deep fibular: nerve
deep flexor: muscle of fingers
deep gray: layer of superior colliculus
deep hypothermic: arrest
deep infrapatellar: bursa
deep inguinal: lymph nodes; ring
deep lateral cervical: lymph nodes
deep lingual: artery; vein
deep lymph: vessel
deep middle cerebral: vein
deep palmar: branch of ulnar artery
deep palmar (arterial): arch
deep palmar venous: arch
deep parotid: lymph nodes
deep perineal: fascia; pouch; space
deep peroneal: nerve
deep petrosal: nerve
deep plantar: artery; branch of dorsalis pedis artery
deep posterior sacrococcygeal: ligament
deep punctate: keratitis
deep temporal: artery; nerves; veins
deep tendon: reflex
deep transitional: gyrus
deep transverse: muscle of perineum
deep transverse metacarpal: ligament
deep transverse metatarsal: ligament
deep transverse perineal: muscle

deep white: layer of superior colliculus; layer [TA] of superior colliculus
deer-fly: disease; fever
Deetjen: bodies
def caries: index
defective: bacteriophage; organism; phage; probacteriophage; prophage; virus
defective interfering: particle
defense: mechanism; reflex
defensive: circle; medicine
deferent: canal; duct
deferential: artery
deferential (nervous): plexus
deferred: shock
defervescent: stage
deficiency: anemia; disease; mutant; symptom
definitive: callus; host; lysosomes; method; prosthesis
deflective occlusal: contact
degenerative: arthritis; chorea; index; inflammation; myopia
degenerative joint: disease
degloving: injury
deglutition: apnea; pneumonia; reflex; syncope
Degos: acanthoma; disease; syndrome
degree of: kindred
Dehio: test
dehydrated: alcohol
dehydration: fever
dehydrocholate: test
deionized: water
deiterospinal: tract
Deiters: cells; nucleus
Deiters terminal: frames
déjà vu: phenomenon
Dejerine: disease; reflex; sign
Dejerine hand: phenomenon
Dejerine-Klumpke: palsy; syndrome
Dejerine-Roussy: syndrome
Dejerine-Sottas: disease
Delafield: hematoxylin
de Lange: syndrome
delayed: allergy; coma after hypoxia; conduction; dentition; eruption; flap; graft; hypersensitivity; puberty; reaction; reflex; sensation; suture
delayed reaction: experiment
Delbet: sign
Del Castillo: syndrome
deletion: mutation
Delhi: sore
delimiting: keratotomy
delphian: node
delta: agent; alcoholism; antigen; bilirubin; cell of anterior lobe of hypophysis;

cell of pancreas; fibers; granule; hepatitis; rhythm; virus; wave
deltoid: branch; crest; eminence; impression; ligament; muscle; region; tubercle (of spine of scapula); tuberosity (of humerus)
deltoideopectoral: triangle; trigone
deltopectoral: flap; triangle
delusional: disorder
demand: pacemaker
demand pulse: generator
demarcation: current; line of retina; potential
Demarquay: sign
dematiaceous: fungi
demigauntlet: bandage
demilune: body
demodectic: acariasis; blepharitis; mange
Demoivre: formula
demonstration: ophthalmoscope
De Morgan: spots
de Morsier: syndrome
de Musset: sign
demyelinated: myelitis
demyelinating: disease; encephalopathy; polyneuropathy
denaturation: temperature of DNA
denatured: alcohol; protein
dendriform: keratitis
dendritic: calculus; cataract; cell; depolarization; process; spines; thorns
dendritic corneal: ulcer
dengue: fever; virus
dengue hemorrhagic: fever
dengue shock: syndrome
Denis Browne: pouch; splint
Denman spontaneous: evolution
Dennie: line
Dennie-Morgan: fold
Denonvilliers: aponeurosis; ligament
dense: bodies
dense-deposit: disease
density: gradient
density gradient: centrifugation
dental: abscess; anatomy; anesthesia; ankylosis; apparatus; arch; articulation; biomechanics; biophysics; branches; bulb; calculus; canals; caps; caries; cast; cement; cord; crest; crypt; curing; cuticle; drill; dysfunction; engineering; fistula; floss; follicle;

forceps; formula; furnace; geriatrics; germ; granuloma; groove; hygienist; impaction; implants; index; jurisprudence; lamina; ledge; lever; lymph; material; neck; nerve; orthopedics; osteoma; papilla; pathology; plaque; polyp; process; prophylaxis; prosthesis; prosthetics; pulp; pump; rami; ridge; sac; sealant; senescence; shelf; surgeon; syringe; tubercle; tubules; ulcer; wedge
dentary: center
dentate: fascia; fissure; fracture; gyrus; ligament of spinal cord; line; nucleus of cerebellum; suture
dentatorubral: fibers
dentatorubral cerebellar: atrophy with polymyoclonus
dentatothalamic: fibers; tract
denticulate: hymen; ligament
dentigerous: cyst
dentin: bridge; dysplasia; globule
dentinal: canals; fibers; fluid; papilla; pulp; sheath; tubules
dentinocemental: junction
dentinoenamel: junction
dentoalveolar: joint
dentogingival: lamina
denture: base; border; brush; characterization; edge; esthetics; flange; flask; foundation; hyperplasia; packing; prognosis; retention; space; stability
denture basal: surface
denture-bearing: area
denture foundation: area; surface
denture impression: surface
denture occlusal: surface
denture polished: surface
denture sore: mouth
denture-supporting: area; structures
Denucé: ligament
denumerable: character
Denver: classification; shunt
Denver Developmental Screening: Test
Denys-Drash: syndrome
Denys-Leclef: phenomenon
deodorized: opium
deoxy: sugar
dependent: beat; drainage; edema; personality; variable
dependent personality: disorder
depersonalization: disorder; syndrome
de Pezzer: catheter
depletion: response

depletional: hyponatremia
depolarizing: block; relaxant
depot: injection; reaction; therapy
depressed: fracture
depressed skull: fracture
depressive: neurosis; psychosis; reaction; stupor; syndrome
depressor: fibers; muscle of epiglottis; muscle of eyebrow; muscle of lower lip; muscle of septum; nerve of Ludwig; reflex
depressor anguli oris: muscle
depressor labii inferioris: muscle
depressor septi nasi: muscle
depressor supercilii: muscle
deprivation: amblyopia; dwarfism
depth: compensation; dose; perception; psychology; recording
de Quervain: disease; fracture; tenosynovitis; thyroiditis
derby hat: fracture
Dercum: disease
derivative: chromosome
derived: protein
dermal: bone; graft; leishmanoid; papillae; ridges; sinus; system; tuberculosis
dermal duct: tumor
dermal-fat: graft
dermatan: sulfate
dermatitis-arthritis-tenosynovitis: syndrome
dermatitis-causing: caterpillar
dermatogenic: torticollis
dermatologic: paste
dermatomal: distribution
dermatomic: area
dermatopathic: lymphadenitis; lymphadenopathy
dermoepidermal: interface
dermoid: cyst; cyst of ovary; tumor
dermolytic bullous: dermatosis
dermotuberculin: reaction
De Sanctis-Cacchione: syndrome
Desault: bandage
Descartes: law
Descemet: membrane
descending: aorta; artery of knee; branch; branch of anterior segmental artery of left and right lungs; branch of hypoglossal nerve; branch of lateral circumflex femoral artery; branch of medial

circumflex femoral artery; branch of occipital artery; branch of posterior segmental artery of left and right lungs; branch of superficial cervical artery; colon; current; degeneration; neuritis; nucleus of the trigeminus; part of aorta; part of duodenum; part of facial canal; part of iliofemoral ligament; part of trapezius (muscle); tract of trigeminal nerve

descending anterior: branch
descending genicular: artery
descending palatine: artery
descending posterior: branch
descending scapular: artery
Deschamps: needle
descriptive: anatomy; myology; psychiatry; statistics
DES (diethylstilbestrol): daughter
desensitizing: paste
desert: fever; sore
desiccated: liver; pituitary
design: denture
Desmarres: dacryoliths; retractor
desmoid: tumor
desmoplastic: fibroma; medulloblastoma; trichoepithelioma
desmoplastic cerebral: astrocytoma
desmoplastic malignant: melanoma
desmoplastic small cell: tumor
desmoteric: medicine
desoxy: sugar
despeciated: antitoxin
D'Éspine: sign
desquamative: pneumonia
desquamative inflammatory: vaginitis
desquamative interstitial: pneumonia
destructive: distillation
detachable: balloon
detached: craniotomy; retina
detached cranial: section
detector: coil
determinant: group
determinate: cleavage
detrusor: areflexia; compliance; hyperreflexia; instability; muscle; pressure; stability
detrusor sphincter: dyssynergia
Deutschländer: disease

developmental: age; anatomy; anomaly; disability; grooves; lines; psychology
developmental hip: dysplasia
Deventer: pelvis
deviational: nystagmus
Devic: disease
devil: grip
Devine: exclusion
devitalized: tooth
Devonshire: colic
dew: itch; point
Dewar: flask
de Wecker: scissors
dexamethasone suppression: test
df caries: index
Dharmendra: antigen
d'Herelle: phenomenon
dhobie mark: dermatitis
D.I.: particle
Di: antigen
diabetic: acidosis; amyotrophy; arthropathy; cataract; coma; dermopathy; diet; fetopathy; gangrene; gingivitis; glomerulosclerosis; lipemia; myelopathy; nephropathy; neuropathy; polyneuropathy; polyradiculopathy; puncture; retinitis; retinopathy
diabetic neuropathic: cachexia
diabetic thoracic: radiculopathy
diabetogenic: factor
diachronic: study
diagnosis-related: group
diagnostic: anesthesia; audiometry; cast; radiology; sensitivity; specificity; ultrasound
diagnostic diphtheria: toxin
diagonal: band; conjugate; section
diagonal conjugate: diameter
diagonalis: stria
dial: manometer
dialysis: dementia; shunt
dialysis disequilibrium: syndrome
dialysis encephalopathy: syndrome
diamond: disk; fuchsin; skin
Diamond-Blackfan: anemia; syndrome
diamond cutting: instruments
diamond-shaped: murmur
Diamond TYM: medium
Diana: complex
diaper: dermatitis; rash
diaphragm: pessary
diaphragmatic: constriction of esophagus; flutter; hernia; ligament of the

mesonephros; pacemaker; part of parietal pleura; peritonitis; pleura; pleurisy; surface
diaphragmatic myocardial: infarction
diaphysial: center; dysplasia
diarthrodial: cartilage; joint
diastasis: cordis
diastatic skull: fracture
diastolic: afterpotential; murmur; pressure; shock; thrill
diastrophic: dwarfism; dysplasia
diathermic: therapy
diatomaceous: earth
diazo: reaction; reagent; stain for argentaffin granules
diazonium: salts
dibasic: acid; amino acid; ammonium phosphate; calcium phosphate; potassium phosphate; sodium phosphate
dicarboxylic acid: cycle
dicentric: chromosome
dichorial: twins
dichorionic diamnionic: placenta
Dick: method; test
Dickens: shunt
Dick test: toxin
dicrotic: notch; pulse; wave
dicumarol: resistance
didactic: analysis
dideoxy: procedure; sequencing
Diels: hydrocarbon
diencephalic: epilepsy; syndrome of infancy
dientamoeba: diarrhea
dietary: amenorrhea; fiber
Dieterle: stain
dietetic: albuminuria; treatment
diethenoid: fatty acid
O-diethylaminoethyl: cellulose
Dietl: crisis
diet quality: index
Dieuaide: diagram
Dieulafoy: erosion; lesion; theory
Di Ferrante: syndrome
difference: limen
differential: diagnosis; display; growth; manometer; stain; stethoscope; thermometer; threshold
differential blood: pressure
differential gene: expression
differential renal function: test
differential spinal: anesthesia

differential ureteral catheterization: test
differential white: blood count
diffuse: abscess; aneurysm; angiokeratoma; choroiditis; ganglion; glomerulonephritis; goiter; hyperkeratosis of palms and soles; leishmaniasis; mastocytosis; panbronchiolitis; peritonitis; phlegmon
diffuse alveolar: damage
diffuse arterial: ectasia
diffuse cutaneous: leishmaniasis; mastocytosis
diffused: reflex
diffuse deep: keratitis
diffuse esophageal: spasm
diffuse idiopathic skeletal: hyperostosis
diffuse infantile familial: sclerosis
diffuse Lewy body: disease
diffuse mesangial: proliferation
diffuse obstructive: emphysema
diffuse small cleaved cell: lymphoma
diffuse unilateral subacute: neuroretinitis
diffuse waxy: spleen
diffusible: stimulant
diffusing: capacity; factor
diffusion: anoxia; coefficient; constant; hypoxia; method; respiration; shell
digastric: branch of facial nerve; fossa; groove; muscle; notch; triangle
DiGeorge: syndrome
digestive: apparatus; enzymes; fever; glycosuria; leukocytosis; system; tract; tube; vacuole
digital: crease; dilatation; fossa; furrow; hearing aid; joints; plethysmograph; pulp; pulp of hand; radiography; reflex; veins; whorl
digital collateral: artery
digital flexion: crease
digital gray: scale
digitalis: tincture; unit
digital subtraction: angiography
digitate: dermatosis; impressions; wart
digitonin: reaction
Di Guglielmo: disease; syndrome
dihydric: alcohol
dihydrogen: phosphate

2,8-dihydroxyadenine: lithiasis
dilantin: gingivitis
dilated: cardiomyopathy; pore
dilation: thrombosis
dilator: muscle; muscle of ileocecal sphincter; muscle of pylorus
dilator pupillae: muscle
dileptic: seizure
dilute: alcohol; phosphoric acid
diluted: acetic acid; hydrochloric acid
dilution: anemia
dimensional: stability
dimidiate: hermaphroditism
Dimmer: keratitis
dimorphic: anemia
dimorphous: leprosy
dimple: sign
dinitrophenylhydrazine: test
dinner: pad
dinoflagellate: toxin
dinucleotide: domain; fold
Diogenes: cup
dioptric: aberration
diovular: twins
DIP: joints
dip: phenomenon
diphasic: complex
diphasic milk: fever
diphenylhydantoin: gingivitis
diphenylmethane: dyes; laxatives
diphtheria: antitoxin; toxin
diphtheria antitoxin: unit
diphtheria toxoid, tetanus toxoid, and pertussis: vaccine
diphtheritic: conjunctivitis; enteritis; membrane; neuropathy; paralysis; ulcer
diphyllobothrium: anemia
diploic: canals; vein
diploid: nucleus
dipolar: buffer; ions
dipole: moment; theory
direct: calorimetry; current; diuretic; embolism; flap; fracture; illumination; image; immunofluorescence; laryngoscopy; lead; method for making inlays; ophthalmoscope; ophthalmoscopy; oxidase; percussion; rays; retainer; retention; technique; transfusion; vision; zoonosis
direct acrylic: restoration
direct bone: impression
direct composite resin: restoration
direct Coombs: test
direct filling: resin

direct fluorescent antibody: test
direct inguinal: hernia
directional: atherectomy; preponderance; weakness
directive: psychotherapy
direct lateral: veins
directly observed: therapy
direct lytic: factor of cobra venom
direct nuclear: division
direct pulp: capping
direct pyramidal: tract
direct reacting: bilirubin
direct resin: restoration
direct vision: spectroscope
direct wet mount: examination
disability-adjusted life: years
disappearing bone: disease
discharging: tubule
Dische: reaction; reagent
Dische-Schwarz: reagent
disciform: degeneration; keratitis
disciform macular: degeneration
disclosing: solution
discoid: lupus erythematosus
discoidal: cleavage
disconjugate: movement of eyes
disconnection: syndrome
discontinuation: test
discontinuous: culture; phase; sterilization
discordant: alternans; alternation
discordant atrioventricular: connections
discordant changes: electrocardiogram
discrete: analyzer; character; smallpox; variable
discrete random: variable
discriminant: analysis; function; stimulus
discrimination: score
disease: determinants
disease modifying antirheumatic: drugs
dish: face
dishpan: fracture
disintegration: constant
disjoined: pyeloplasty
disjunctive: absorption
disk: electrophoresis; herniation; kidney; space; syndrome
disk sensitivity: method
disk-shaped: cataract
dislocation of: lens
dislocation: fracture
disodium: phosphate
disorganized: schizophrenia
disparity: angle

dispensing: tablet
disperse: placenta
dispersed: phase
dispersing: electrode
dispersion: colloid; medium; phase
displacement: analysis; loop; threshold
disproportionate: dwarfism
disproportionating: enzyme
disputed neurogenic thoracic outlet: syndrome
Disse: space
dissecting: aneurysm; cellulitis
dissection: tubercle
disseminated: aspergillosis; choroiditis; coccidioidomycosis; histoplasmosis; lipogranulomatosis; lupus erythematosus; sclerosis; tuberculosis
disseminated cutaneous: gangrene; leishmaniasis
disseminated gonococcal: infection
disseminated intravascular: coagulation
disseminated recurrent: infundibulofolliculitis
dissociated: anesthesia; nystagmus
dissociated horizontal: deviation
dissociated vertical: deviation
dissociation: constant; constant of an acid; constant of a base; constant of water; sensibility
dissociative: anesthesia; disorders; hysteria; reaction
dissociative identity: disorder
distal: caries; centriole; end; ileitis; myopathy; occlusion; part of prostate; part of prostatic urethra; part [TA] of anterior lobe of hypophysis; phalanx of foot; phalanx of hand; surface of tooth; tingling on percussion
distal interphalangeal: joints
distal intestinal obstructive: syndrome
distal medial striate: artery
distal radioulnar: articulation; joint
distal spiral: septum
distal splenorenal: shunt
distal tibiofibular: joint
distance: ceptor
distant: flap
distemper: virus
distention: cyst; ulcer
distilled: water
distortion: aberration

distortion-product otoacoustic: emission
distraction: conus; osteogenesis
distributed: effort
distributing: artery
distribution: coefficient; curve; leukocytosis; volume
distributive: analysis
disulfide: bond; bridge
disuse: atrophy
Dittrich: plugs; stenosis
diurnal: enuresis; periodicity; rhythm
divergence: insufficiency; paresis
divergence excess: exotropia
divergence insufficiency: exotropia
divergent: evolution; squint; strabismus
diverging: meniscus
divers': spectacles
diver's: palsy; paralysis
diverticular: disease
divided: dose; spectacles
diving: goiter; reflex
divisional: block
Dix-Hallpike: maneuver
dizygotic: twins
djenkol: poisoning
dmfs caries: index
DNA: gap; helix; homology; hybridization; polymorphism; virus
DNA-RNA: hybrid
d'Ocagne: nomogram
docking: protein
Döderlein: bacillus
Doerfler-Stewart: test
dog: disease; ear; nose; unit
dog distemper: virus
Dogiel: cells; corpuscle
dogmatic: school
Döhle: bodies; inclusions
dolichoectatic: artery
dolichopellic: pelvis
doll's eye: sign
dolorogenic: zone
dome: cell
dominance: hierarchy
dominant: character; eye; frequency; gene; hemisphere; idea; inheritance; trait
dominant lethal: trait
dominantly inherited Lévi: disease
dominant optic: atrophy
Donath-Landsteiner: phenomenon
Donath-Landsteiner cold: autoantibody
Donders: glaucoma; law; pressure; rings
Donnan: equilibrium

Donné: corpuscle
Donohue: disease; syndrome
donor: insemination
Donovan: bodies
Doose: syndrome
dopa: reaction
Doppler: echocardiography; effect; phenomenon; shift; ultrasonography
Doppler color: flow
Dor: fundoplication; procedure
Dorello: canal
Dorendorf: sign
Dorfman-Chanarin: syndrome
dorsal: artery of clitoris; artery of foot; artery of nose; artery of penis; branch; branches of first and second posterior intercostal artery; branches of the superior intercostal artery; branch of the lumbar artery; branch of the posterior intercostal arteries 3–11; branch of the posterior intercostal veins 4–11; branch of the subcostal artery; branch of the ulnar nerve; column of spinal cord; fascia of foot; fascia of hand; flexure; funiculus; hood; mesocardium; mesogastrium; muscles; nerve of clitoris; nerve of penis; nerve of scapula; nerves of toes; nucleus; nucleus of thalamus; nucleus of trapezoid body; nucleus of vagus; pallidum; pancreas; part of intertransversarii laterales lumborum (muscles); part of pons; plate of neural tube; position; reflex; root of spinal nerve; spine; striatum; surface; surface of digit (of hand or foot); surface of sacrum; surface of scapula; thalamus; tubercle of radius; vein of corpus callosum; veins of clitoris; veins of penis; vertebrae
dorsal accessory olivary: nucleus
dorsal calcaneocuboid: ligament
dorsal callosal: vein
dorsal carpal: branch of radial artery; branch of ulnar artery; ligament; network
dorsal carpal arterial: arch
dorsal carpal tendinous: sheaths
dorsal carpometacarpal: ligaments

dorsal column: stimulation
dorsal cuboideonavicular: ligament
dorsal cuneocuboid: ligament
dorsal cuneonavicular: ligaments
dorsal digital: artery; nerves; nerves of deep fibular nerve; nerves of foot; nerves of hand; nerves of superficial fibular nerve; nerves of ulnar nerve; veins of foot; veins of toes
dorsal hypothalamic: area; region
dorsal intercuneiform: ligaments
dorsal intermediate: sulcus
dorsal interossei (interosseous): muscles of foot; muscles of hand
dorsal interosseous: artery; nerve
dorsalis pedis: artery
dorsal lateral cutaneous: nerve
dorsal lateral geniculate: nucleus
dorsal lingual: branches of lingual artery; vein
dorsal longitudinal: fasciculus
dorsal medial cutaneous: nerve
dorsal median: sulcus
dorsal metacarpal: artery; ligaments; veins
dorsal metatarsal: artery; ligaments; veins
dorsal midbrain: syndrome
dorsal motor: nucleus of vagus
dorsal nasal: artery
dorsal pancreatic: artery
dorsal premammillary: nucleus
dorsal primary: ramus of spinal nerve
dorsal radiocarpal: ligament
dorsal root: ganglion
dorsal sacrococcygeal: muscle
dorsal sacrococcygeus: muscle
dorsal sacroiliac: ligaments
dorsal scapular: artery; nerve; vein
dorsal septal: nucleus
dorsal spinocerebellar: tract
dorsal supraoptic: commissure
dorsal talonavicular: bone
dorsal tarsal: ligaments
dorsal tarsometatarsal: ligaments
dorsal tegmental: decussation

dorsal thoracic: artery; nucleus
dorsal trigeminothalamic: tract
dorsal vagal: nucleus
dorsal venous: arch of foot; network of foot; network of hand
Dorset culture egg: medium
dorsiflexor: compartment of leg
dorsispinal: veins
dorsolateral: fasciculus; nucleus; plate of neural tube; sulcus; tract
dorsomedial: nucleus; nucleus of hypothalamus
dorsomedial hypothalamic: nucleus
dorsosacral: position
dorsum of: hand
dorsum pedis: reflex
dose-response: curve; relationship
dotted: tongue
double: athetosis; bind; bond; chin; consciousness; enterostomy; fracture; helix; hemiplegia; immunodiffusion; intussusception; lip; membrane; pleurisy; pneumonia; product; protrusion; quartan; refraction; salt; stain; tachycardia; tertian; vision
double antibody: immunoassay; method; precipitation
double antibody sandwich: assay
double aortic: arch; stenosis
double back: cross
double blind: experiment; study
double bubble: sign
double-channel: catheter
double compartment: hydrocephalus
double concave: lens
double congenital: athetosis
double contrast: enema
double convex: lens
double displacement: mechanism
double elevator: palsy
double flap: amputation
double (gel) diffusion precipitin: test in one dimension; test in two dimensions
double inlet atrioventricular: connections
double loop: hernia
double-masked: experiment
double minute: chromosomes

double-mouthed: uterus
double outlet right: ventricle
double pedicle: flap
double-point: threshold
double quotidian: fever
double-reciprocal: plot
double ring: sign
double-shock: sound
double-strand: break
double tertian: malaria
double track: sign
doubling: time
doubly: heterozygous
doubly armed: suture
douche: bath
doughnut: pessary
Douglas: abscess; bag; cul-de-sac; fold; line; mechanism; pouch
Douglas spontaneous: evolution
dousing: bath
dovetail stress-broken: abutment
dowager: hump
dowel: graft
Down: syndrome
downbeat: nystagmus
Downey: cell
Downs: analysis
downward: drainage
downy: hair
Doyère: eminence
Doyle: operation
Doyne honeycomb: choroidopathy
Drabkin: reagent
Dragendorff: reagent; test
Dräger: respirometer
drainage: tube
drain-trap: stomach
Draper: law
drawer: sign; test
dream: associations
dreamy: state
drepanocytic: anemia
dressing: forceps
Dressler: beat; syndrome
Dreyer: formula
dried: alum; ferrous sulfate; yeast
dried human: albumin; serum
dried human plasma protein: fraction
drift: movements
Drinker: respirator
drip: phleboclysis; transfusion
drip-suck: irrigation
drooping lily: sign
drop: attack; finger; foot; hand; heart
droplet: infection; nuclei
dropped: beat
drug: abuse; allergy; eruption; fever; pathogenesis;

psychosis; rash; resistance; tetanus

drug-induced: disease; hepatitis; lupus

drug utilization: review

drum: membrane

Drummond: sign

drumstick: appendage

dry: abscess; amputation; beriberi; bronchiectasis; cup; distillation; dressing; drowning; gangrene; hernia; labor; leprosy; nurse; pack; pericarditis; pleurisy; rale; socket; synovitis; tetter; vomiting; weight

dry cutaneous: leishmaniasis

dry eye: syndrome

D-S: test

dual: personality; relationships

dual-cure: resin

Duane: syndrome

Dubin-Johnson: syndrome

DuBois: formula

Dubois: abscesses; disease

Du Bois-Reymond: law

Duboscq: colorimeter

Dubowitz: score

Dubreuil-Chambardel: syndrome

Duchenne: disease; dystrophy; sign

Duchenne-Aran: disease

Duchenne-Erb: paralysis

duckbill: speculum

duck embryo origin: vaccine

duck hepatitis: virus

duck influenza: virus

duck plague: virus

Duckworth: phenomenon

Ducrey: bacillus; test

duct: carcinoma; papilloma

ductal: aneurysm; hyperplasia

ductless: glands

Duddell: membrane

Duffy: antigens

Duhring: disease

Dührssen: incisions

Duke bleeding time: test

Dukes: classification; disease

Dulong-Petit: law

dumb: rabies

dumbbell: ganglioneuroma

Dumdum: fever

dummy: consultand

Dumontpallier: pessary

dumping: syndrome

Duncan: disease; folds; mechanism; placenta; syndrome; ventricle

duodenal: ampulla; branches of anterior superior pancreaticoduodenal artery; branches of posterior superior pancreaticoduodenal artery;

bulb; cap; digestion; diverticulum; fistula; fossae; glands; impression on liver; smear; sphincter

duodenojejunal: angle; flexure; fold; fossa; hernia; junction; recess; sphincter

duodenomesocolic: fold

duodenorenal: ligament

Duplay: disease

duplex: kidney; transmission; ultrasonography; uterus

duplex Doppler: scan

duplication: cyst

duplicity: theory of vision

Dupré: muscle

Dupuytren: amputation; canal; contracture; disease of the foot; fascia; fracture; hydrocele; sign; suture; tourniquet

dural: part of filum terminale; sheath; sheath of optic nerve

dural cavernous sinus: fistula

dural venous: sinuses

Duran-Reynals permeability: factor

Dürck: nodes

Duret: hemorrhage; lesion

Durham: rule; tube

Duroziez: disease; murmur; sign

dust: asthma; cell; corpuscles

Dutton: disease

Dutton relapsing: fever

Duvenhage: virus

Duverney: fissures; gland; muscle

dwarf: pelvis

dwarfed: enamel

Dwyer: osteotomy

dyadic: psychotherapy; symbiosis

dye-dilution: curve

dye disappearance: test

dye exclusion: test

Dyggve-Melchior-Clausen: syndrome

dynamic: aorta; compliance of lung; CT; demography; equilibrium; force; friction; ileus; murmur; posturography; psychiatry; psychology; psychotherapy; refraction; relations; school; splint; viscosity

dynamic computed: tomography

dynein: arm

dysarthria–clumsy hand: syndrome

dysconjugate: gaze

dysembryoplastic neuroepithelial: tumor

dysenteric: diarrhea

dysenteric algid: malaria

dysentery: antitoxin; bacillus

dysfunctional uterine: bleeding

dysgranular: cortex

dysharmonious retinal: correspondence

dyshemopoietic: anemia

dyshidrotic: eczema

dysjunctive: nystagmus

dyskinesia: syndrome

dysmenorrheal: membrane

dysmnesic: syndrome

dysplastic: nevus

dysplastic nevus: syndrome

dysproteinemic: retinopathy

dysspermatogenic: sterility

dysthymic: disorder

dysthyroid: myopathy; orbitopathy

dysthyroidal: infantilism

dystonic: reaction; torticollis

dystrophic: calcification; calcinosis

E

E: rosette; selectin

EAC: rosette

EAC rosette: assay

Eadie-Hofstee: plot

Eagle-Barrett: syndrome

Eagle basal: medium

Eagle minimum essential: medium

EAHF: complex

Eales: disease

ear: bones; canal; crystals; lobe; wax

Earle: solution

Earle L: fibrosarcoma

ear lobe: crease

early: deceleration; discharge; reaction; seizure; syphilis

early diastolic: murmur

early dumping: syndrome

early infantile: autism

early latent: syphilis

early-phase: response

early posttraumatic: epilepsy

early receptor: potential

earth: wax

earthy: water

East African: trypanosomiasis

East African sleeping: sickness

eastern equine: encephalomyelitis

eastern equine encephalomyelitis: virus

eating: disorders; epilepsy

Eaton: agent

Eaton-Lambert: syndrome

EB: virus

Ebbinghaus: test

Eberth: bacillus; lines; perithelium

Ebner: glands; reticulum

Ebola: virus; virus Côte-d'Ivoire; virus Reston; virus Sudan; virus Zaire

Ebola hemorrhagic: fever

Ebstein: anomaly; disease; sign

eccentric: amputation; fixation; hypertrophy; implantation; occlusion; position; relation

ecchymotic: mask

eccrine: acrospiroma; gland; poroma; spiradenoma

ecdysial: glands

ECG: trigger

ecgonine: benzoate

echinococcus: cyst; disease

ECHO: virus

echo: beat; reaction; speech

echocardiographic: differentiation

Eck: fistula

Ecker: fissure

eclamptic: retinopathy

eclipse: blindness; period; phase

ECMO: virus

ecologic: chemistry; study

ecological: ectocrine; system

economic: coefficient

ecotropic: virus

ECSO: virus

ectatic: aneurysm; emphysema

ectatic marginal: degeneration of cornea

ectocervical: smear

ectodermal: cloaca; dysplasia

ectogenic: teratosis

ectopic: beat; decidua; eyelash; hormone; impulse; pacemaker; pinealoma; pregnancy; rhythm; schistosomiasis; tachycardia; teratosis; testis; ureter; ureterocele

ectopic ACTH: syndrome

ectoplacental: cavity

ectotrophoblastic: cavity

ectrodactyly–ectodermal dysplasia–clefting: syndrome

ectromelia: virus

eczematoid: seborrhea

eddy: sounds

Eder-Pustow: bougie

edge: enhancement

edge-to-edge: bite; occlusion

edgewise: appliance

Edinger-Westphal: nucleus

Edlefsen: reagent

Edman: method; reagent

Edridge-Green: lamp

educational: psychology

Edwards: syndrome

EEE: virus

Word Finder

EEG: activation
effective: conjugate; dose; half-life; stroke; temperature
effective osmotic: pressure
effective refractory: period
effective renal blood: flow
effective renal plasma: flow
effective temperature: index
effector: cell
efferent: duct; ductules of testis; fibers; lymphatic; nerve; vessel
efferent glomerular: arteriole
effervescent: lithium citrate; magnesium citrate; magnesium sulfate; potassium citrate; salts; sodium phosphate
effort-induced: thrombosis
egg: albumin; cell; membrane
Egger: line
Eggleston: method
eggshell: calcification
egg shell: nail
egg-white: injury; syndrome
Eglis: glands
ego: analysis; ideal; identity; instincts
ego-dystonic: homosexuality
Egyptian: hematuria; ophthalmia; splenomegaly
Ehlers-Danlos: syndrome
Ehrenritter: ganglion
Ehret: phenomenon
Ehrlich: anemia; phenomenon; postulate; reaction; theory
Ehrlich acid hematoxylin: stain
Ehrlich aniline crystal violet: stain
Ehrlich benzaldehyde: reaction
Ehrlich diazo: reaction; reagent
Ehrlich inner: body
Ehrlich triacid: stain
Ehrlich triple: stain
Ehrlich-Türk: line
Eichhorst: corpuscles; neuritis
Eicken: method
eidetic: image
eighth: nerve
eighth cranial: nerve [CN VIII]
eighth nerve: tumor
Einarson gallocyanin-chrome alum: stain
Einthoven: equation; law; triangle
Einthoven string: galvanometer
Eisenmenger: complex; defect; disease; syndrome; tetralogy
ejaculatory: duct

ejection: click; fraction; murmur; period; sounds
Ejrup: maneuver
Ekbom: syndrome
EKG: trigger
elastic: artery; bandage; bougie; cartilage; cone; fibers; lamella; laminae of arteries; layers of arteries; layers of cornea; ligature; limit; membrane; skin; tissue
elastic band: fixation
elastoid: degeneration
elastotic: degeneration
Elaut: triangle
elbow: bone; jerk; joint; reflex
elbowed: bougie; catheter
elder: abuse
elderly: primigravida
elective: abortion; culture; mutism
Electra: complex
electric: anesthesia; bath; cataract; cautery; chorea; irritability; retinopathy; shock; sleep
electrical: alternans; alternation of heart; axis; diastole; failure; formula; systole
electrical heart: position
electric cardiac: pacemaker
electrocardiographic: complex; wave
electrochemical: gradient
electroconvulsive: therapy
electrode: knife
electrode catheter: ablation
electrodiagnostic: medicine
electroencephalographic: dysrhythmia
electrographic: seizure
electrohydraulic shock wave: lithotripsy
electrolyte: metabolism
electromagnetic: flowmeter; induction; radiation; unit
electromechanical: dissociation; systole
electromotive: force
electromuscular: sensibility
electron: beam; capture; interferometer; interferometry; magneton; micrograph; microscope; microscopy; radiography
electron beam: tomography
electronegative: element
electronic: number; pacemaker
electronic cell: counter
electronic fetal: monitor
electronic pacemaker: load
electron paramagnetic: resonance

electron resonance: absorption
electron spin: resonance
electron transfer: flavin
electron-transport: chain; system
electron transport: particles
electrophonic: effect
electrophrenic: respiration
electropositive: element
electroshock: therapy
electrostatic: bond; unit
electrotherapeutic: sleep
electrotherapeutic sleep: therapy
electrotonic: current; junction; synapse
elementary: bodies; granule; particle
elephant: leg
elephant man's: disease
elephantoid: fever
elevator: disease; muscle of anus; muscle of prostate; muscle of rib; muscle of scapula; muscle of soft palate; muscle of thyroid gland; muscle of upper eyelid; muscle of upper lip; muscle of upper lip and wing of nose
eleventh cranial: nerve [CN XI]
elfin: facies
elfin facies: syndrome
elimination: diet
Ellik: evacuator
Elliot: operation; position
Elliott: law
ellipsoidal: joint
elliptical: amputation; anastomosis; recess of bony labyrinth
elliptocytary: anemia
elliptocytic: anemia
elliptocytotic: anemia
Ellis type 1: glomerulonephritis
Ellis type 2: glomerulonephritis
Ellis-van Creveld: syndrome
Ellsworth-Howard: test
Eloesser: flap; procedure
elongation: factor
Elschnig: pearls; spots
El Tor: vibrio
elusive: ulcer
E-M: syndrome
EMB: agar
Embden: ester
Embden-Meyerhof: pathway
Embden-Meyerhof-Parnas: pathway
embedding: agents
embolic: abscess; gangrene; infarct; pneumonia

emboliform: nucleus
embryo: transfer
embryonal: adenoma; area; carcinoma; inducer; leukemia; medulloepithelioma; rhabdomyosarcoma; tumor; tumor of ciliary body
embryonic: anideus; axis; blastoderm; cataract; cell; circulation; diapause; disk; hemoglobin; membrane; shield
embryopathic: cataract
EMC: virus
emergency: theory
emergency hormonal: contraception
emergent: evolution
emerging: viruses
emery: disks
Emery-Dreifuss muscular: dystrophy
emesis: basin
EMG: biofeedback; examination; syndrome
EMI: scan
emissary: vein
emission: electron
Emmet: needle; operation
emotional: age; amenorrhea; amnesia; attitudes; deprivation; disease; disorder; disturbance; leukocytosis; overlay
empathic: index
emphysematous: cholecystitis; cystitis; gangrene; phlegmon
empiric: risk; treatment
empirical: formula; horopter
empty: sella
empyema: tube
empyemic: scoliosis
emulsifying: wax
emulsion: colloid
enamel: cap; cell; cleavage; cleaver; crypt; cuticle; drop; dysplasia; epithelium; fibers; fissure; germ; hypocalcification; hypoplasia; lamella; layer; ledge; membrane; niche; nodule; organ; pearl; prisms; projection; pulp; rods; tuft; wall
enamel rod: inclination; sheath
enarthrodial: joint
encapsulated: delusion
encephalic: vesicle
encephalithogenic: protein
encephalitis: virus
encephaloclastic: microcephaly

encephalocraniocutaneous: lipomatosis
encephalomyelonic: axis
encephalomyocarditis: virus
encephalotrigeminal: angiomatosis
encephalotrigeminal vascular: syndrome
encounter: group
encu: method
encysted: calculus; pleurisy
end: artery; bud; bulb; cell; organ; oxidation; piece; plate; point; product; stage
endaural: incision
end-cutting: bur
end-diastolic: volume
endemic: disease; funiculitis; goiter; hematuria; hemoptysis; hypertrophy; index; influenza; neuritis; stability; syphilis; typhus
endemic nonbacterial infantile: gastroenteritis
endemic paralytic: vertigo
Endo: agar; medium
endoabdominal: fascia
endobronchial: tube
endocardial: cushions; fibroelastosis; fibrosis; murmur; sclerosis
endocardial cushion: defect
endocervical: smear
endocervical sinus: tumor
endochondral: bone; ossification
endocochlear: potential
endocrine: exophthalmos; glands; hormones; ophthalmopathy; part of pancreas; system
endodermal: canal; cell; cloaca; cyst; pouches
endodermal sinus: tumor
endodontic: stabilizer; treatment
end-of-life: care
endogenic: toxicosis
endogenous: cycle; depression; fibers; hyperglyceridemia; infection; pyrogen
endogenous creatinine: clearance
endolemniscal: nucleus
endolymphatic: duct; hydrops; sac; space
endolymphatic sac: surgery
endolymphatic shunt: operation
endomembrane: system
endometrial: ablation; canal; cyst; hyperplasia; implants; smear
endometrial stromal: sarcoma

endometrioid: carcinoma; tumor
endomyocardial: fibrosis
end-on mattress: suture
endo-osseous: implant
endopeduncular: nucleus
endopelvic: fascia
endoplasmic: reticulum
endorectal pull-through: procedure
endoscopic: biopsy
endoscopic retrograde: cholangiopancreatography
endosseous: implant
endosteal: implant
endoteric: bacterium
endothelial: cell; cyst; leukocyte; myeloma
endothelial-leukocyte adhesion: molecule
endothelial relaxing: factor
endotheliochorial: placenta
endothelio-endothelial: placenta
endothelium-derived relaxing: factor
endothoracic: fascia
endotoxin: shock
endotracheal: anesthesia; intubation; stylet; tube
endovaginal: ultrasonography
endovenous: septum
end-point: measurement; nystagmus
end product: inhibition; repression
endstage: lung
end-systolic: volume
end-tidal: sample
end-to-end: anastomosis; bite; occlusion
energy: metabolism; subtraction
energy-rich: bond; phosphates
Engelmann: disease
Engelmann basal: knobs
engine: reamer
Englisch: sinus
English: lock; position
English sweating: disease
enrichment: culture
ensheathing: callus
ensiform: cartilage; process
ensu: method
enteral: hyperalimentation
enteric: fever; tuberculosis; viruses
enteric coated: tablet
enteric cytopathogenic human orphan: virus
enteric cytopathogenic monkey orphan: virus
enteric cytopathogenic swine orphan: virus
enteric (nervous): plexus
entericoid: fever

enteric orphan: viruses
Enterobius: granuloma
enterochromaffin: cells
enterocutaneous: fistula
enterocyte cobalamin: malabsorption
enteroendocrine: cells
enterogastric: reflex
enterogenous: cyanosis; cyst; methemoglobinemia
enterohemorrhagic: *Escherichia coli*
enterohepatic: circulation
enteroinvasive: *Escherichia coli*
enterokinetic: agent
enteropathic: arthritis
enteropathogenic: *Escherichia coli*
enterotoxigenic: *Escherichia coli*
enterovaginal: fistula
enterovesical: fistula
Entner-Douderoff: pathway
entodermal: cell
entoptic: pulse
entorhinal: area
entrance: block
entrapment: neuropathy
entry: zone
envelope: conformation; flap
environmental: illness; psychology
enzootic: stability
enzootic encephalomyelitis: virus
enzygotic: twins
enzymatic: synthesis
enzyme: analog; antagonist; immunoassay; interconversion; isomerization; kinetics; parameters; regulation; repression
enzyme-catalyzed: ligation
enzyme inhibition: theory of narcosis
enzyme-linked immunosorbent: assay
enzyme-multiplied immunoassay: technique
enzyme-substrate: complex
eosin-methylene blue: agar
eosinopenic: reaction
eosinophil: adenoma; granule
eosinophil cationic: protein
eosinophil chemotactic: factor of anaphylaxis
eosinophilia-myalgia: syndrome
eosinophilic: cellulitis; cystitis; fasciitis; gastritis; gastroenteritis; granuloma; leukemia; leukocyte; leukocytosis; leukopenia; meningitis;

meningoencephalitis; pneumonia; pneumonopathy
eosinophilic endomyocardial: disease
eosinophilic pustular: folliculitis
epactal: bones; ossicles
epamniotic: cavity
eparterial: bronchus
ependymal: cell; cyst; layer; zone
ephemeral: fever
ephemeral fever: virus
epibranchial: placodes
epicanthal: fold
epicranial: aponeurosis; muscle
epicranius: muscle
epicritic: sensibility
epidemic: curve; disease; dropsy; encephalitis; exanthema; hemoglobinuria; hepatitis; hiccup; hysteria; keratoconjunctivitis; myalgia; myositis; nausea; neuromyasthenia; parotiditis; pleurodynia; polyarthritis; roseola; stomatitis; typhus; vertigo; vomiting
epidemic benign dry: pleurisy
epidemic cerebrospinal: meningitis
epidemic diaphragmatic: pleurisy
epidemic gangrenous: proctitis
epidemic gastroenteritis: virus
epidemic hemorrhagic: fever
epidemic keratoconjunctivitis: virus
epidemic myalgia: virus
epidemic myalgic: encephalomyelitis; encephalomyelopathy
epidemic nonbacterial: gastroenteritis
epidemic parotitis: virus
epidemic pleurodynia: virus
epidemic transient diaphragmatic: spasm
epidemiologic: genetics
epidemiological: distribution
epidermal: cyst; ridges
epidermal growth: factor
epidermal growth factor: receptor
epidermal-melanin: unit
epidermal ridge: count
epidermic: cell
epidermic-dermic: nevus
epidermoid: cancer; carcinoma; cyst
epidermolytic: hyperkeratosis

epidural: anesthesia; block; cavity; hematoma; meningitis; space
epifascicular: epineurium
epigastric: angle; fold; fossa; hernia; reflex; region; veins; voice
epiglottic: cartilage; folds; tubercle; vallecula
epihyal: bone; ligament
epikeratophakic: keratoplasty
epilation: dose
epilemmal: ending
epileptic: dementia; seizure; spasm
epileptiform: neuralgia
epileptogenic: zone
epiluminescence: microscopy
epimastical: fever
epimerase deficiency: galactosemia
epimyoepithelial: islands
epinephrine: reversal
epiotic: center
epipapillary: membrane
epipericardial: ridge
epiphrenic: diverticulum
epiphysial: arrest; cartilage; eye; fracture; line; plate
epiphysial aseptic: necrosis
epiploic: appendage; appendix; branches; foramen; tags
epipteric: bone
epiretinal: membrane
episcleral: artery; lamina; layer of fibrous layer of eyeball; space; veins
episodic: hypertension
episodic dyscontrol: syndrome
epistenocardiac: pericarditis
episternal: bone
epithelial: attachment; attachment of Gottlieb; body; cancer; cast; cell; cyst; downgrowth; dysplasia; ectoderm; inlay; lamina; layers; migration; nest; pearl; plug; tissue
epithelial choroid: layer
epithelial membrane: antigen
epithelial myoepithelial: carcinoma
epithelial reticular: cell
epitheliochorial: placenta
epithelioid: cell
epithelioid cell: nevus
epithermal: chemistry; neutron
epitrichial: layer
epituberculous: infiltration
epitympanic: recess; space
epizoic: commensalism
epoxy: resin
epsilon: alcoholism; wave

Epsom: salts
Epstein: disease; pearls; sign; symptom
Epstein-Barr: virus
equal: cleavage
equatorial: cleavage; division; plane; plate; staphyloma
equianalgesic: dose
equilibrium: constant; dialysis
equine: encephalitis; encephalomyelitis; gait; Morbillivirus; rhinoviruses
equine gonadotropin: unit
equiphasic: complex
equivalence: point; zone
equivalent: dose; extract; power; temperature; weight
equivalent form: reliability
equivocal: symptom
Eranko fluorescence: stain
Erb: disease; palsy; paralysis
Erb-Charcot: disease
Erb-Westphal: sign
Erdheim: disease; tumor
Erdmann: reagent
erect: illumination
erectile: tissue
erector: muscle of hair; muscle of spine
erector spinae: muscles
erector-spinal: reflex
ergot: alkaloids; poisoning
ergot alkaloid-associated heart: disease
Erlenmeyer: flask
Erlenmeyer flask: deformity
erogenous: zone
E-rosette: test
erosive: adenomatosis of nipple
erotic: zoophilism
erotomanic: disorder
erroneous: projection
error-prone: repair
error-prone polymerase chain: reaction
eruption: cyst
eruptive: fever; phase; stage; xanthoma
Erwinia **L-:** asparaginase
erythema: dose; threshold
erythematous: syphilid
erythremic: myelosis
erythroblastic: anemia
erythrocyte: indices
erythrocyte adherence: phenomenon; test
erythrocyte fragility: test
erythrocyte maturation: factor
erythrocyte sedimentation: rate
erythrocytic: cycle; series
erythrodysesthesia: syndrome
erythrogenic: toxin
erythroid: cell

erythronormoblastic: anemia
erythropoietic: hormone; porphyria; protoporphyria
Esbach: reagent
escape: beat; conditioning; contraction; impulse; interval; phenomenon; rhythm; training
escape-capture: bigeminy
escape ventricular: contraction
Escherich: sign
Escherichia coli: enterotoxin; RNase I
Esmarch: bandage; tourniquet
esodic: nerve
esophageal: achalasia; arteries; atresia; branches; branches of the inferior thyroid artery; branches of the left gastric artery; branches of the recurrent laryngeal nerve; branches of the thoracic aorta; branches of thoracic ganglia; branches of the vagus nerve; cardiogram; constrictions; dysrhythmia; glands; hiatus; impression on liver; lead; manometry; mucosa; opening; reflux; smear; spasm; speech; varices; veins; web
esophageal (nervous): plexus
esophagogastric: junction; orifice; vestibule
esophagosalivary: reflex
essential: albuminuria; amino acids; anemia; anisocoria; bradycardia; dysmenorrhea; fatty acid; fever; fructosuria; hypertension; nutrients; oils; pentosuria; pruritus; tachycardia; telangiectasia; thrombocytopenia; tremor
essential food: factors
essential progressive: atrophy of iris
Essick cell: bands
Essig: splint
established cell: line
esterified: estrogens
Estes: operation
esthesiodic: system
esthetic: dentistry; surgery
Estlander: flap
estradiol benzoate: unit
estrogen: receptor
estrogenic: hormone
estrogen replacement: therapy
estrone: unit
estrous: cycle
ether: test
ethereal: oil; solution; tincture
ethinyl: estradiol

ethmoid: angle; bone; cells; infundibulum
ethmoid air: cells
ethmoidal: bulla; cells; crest; crest of maxilla; crest of palatine bone; foramen; groove; infundibulum; labyrinth; notch; process of inferior nasal concha; sinuses; veins
ethmoidal-lacrimal: fistula
ethmoidolacrimal: suture
ethmoidomaxillary: suture
ethmovomerine: plate
ethynyl: estradiol
"e"-type: cholinesterase
eucalyptus: gum
euglobulin clot lysis: time
eugnathic: anomaly
Eulenburg: disease
eunuchoid: gigantism; state; voice
eupeptide: bond
euplastic: lymph
European: snakeroot; tarantula; typhus
European bat: Lyssavirus
euroxenous: parasite
eustachian: catheter; cushion; tonsil; tube; tuber; valve
eutectic: alloy; temperature
euthyroid: hypometabolism
euthyroid sick: syndrome
Evans: forceps; syndrome
evidence-based: medicine
evoked: electromyography; potential; response
evoked otoacoustic: emission
evolutionary: fitness
Ewart: procedure; sign
Ewing: sarcoma; sign; tumor
examining: table
exanthematous: disease; fever; typhus
excentric: amputation
excess: lactate
exchange: transfusion
excimer: laser
excision: biopsy; repair
excitable: area; gap
excitation: spectrum; wave
excitatory junction: potential
excitatory postsynaptic: potential
excited: atom; catatonia; state
exciting: cause; electrode; eye
excitor: nerve
excitoreflex: nerve
exclamation point: hair
excretory: duct; duct of seminal gland; duct of seminal vesicle; ducts of lacrimal gland; ductules of lacrimal gland; gland
exercise: bone; imaging; test
exercise-induced: amenorrhea

exercise radionuclide: angiocardiography
exertional: dyspnea; rhabdomyolysis
exfoliation: syndrome
exfoliative: cytology; dermatitis; gastritis; psoriasis
existential: psychiatry; psychology; psychotherapy
exit: block; dose
Exner: plexus
exoccipital: bone
exocelomic: membrane
exocrine: gland; part of pancreas
exocrine pancreatic: insufficiency
exodic: nerve
exoerythrocytic: cycle; stage
exogenic: toxicosis
exogenous: cycle; depression; fibers; hemochromatosis; hyperglyceridemia; ochronosis; pigmentation; pyrogens
exogenous creatinine: clearance
exophthalmic: goiter; ophthalmoplegia
exophthalmos-producing: substance
exoteric: bacterium
expandable: stent
expanded disability status: scale
expansion: arch
expansive: delusion
expectation: neurosis
experiential: aura
experimental: error; group; medicine; method; neurosis; psychology
experimental allergic: encephalitis; encephalomyelitis
experimenter: effects
expiratory: center; dyspnea; resistance; stridor
expiratory reserve: volume
expired: gas
exploratory: drive
exploring: electrode; needle
explosive: decompression; speech
exponential: distribution; growth
exposed: pulp
exposure: dose; keratitis
expressed: mustard oil
expressed skull: fracture
expression: vector
expressive: aphasia
expulsive: pains
exsanguination: transfusion

exsiccated: alum; sodium sulfite
exsiccation: fever
extemporaneous: mixture
extended: clasp; family; mediastinoscopy; pyelotomy; thymectomy
extended family: therapy
extended insulin zinc: suspension
extended radical: mastectomy
extension: bridge; form
extensor: aponeurosis; compartment of arm; compartment of forearm; compartment of leg; compartment of thigh; expansion; muscle; muscle of fingers; muscle of little finger; retinaculum
extensor carpi radialis brevis: muscle
extensor carpi radialis longus: muscle
extensor carpi ulnaris: muscle
extensor digital: expansion
extensor digiti minimi: muscle
extensor digitorum: muscle
extensor digitorum brevis: muscle; muscle of hand
extensor digitorum longus: muscle
extensor hallucis brevis: muscle
extensor hallucis longus: muscle
extensor indicis: muscle
extensor pollicis brevis: muscle
extensor pollicis longus: muscle
external: absorption; aperture of cochlear canaliculus; aperture of vestibular aqueduct; artery of nose; axis of eye; base of skull; branch of superior laryngeal nerve; branch of trunk of accessory nerve; canthus; capsule; conjugate; defibrillator; ear; fistula; fixation; genitalia; hemorrhoids; hydrocephalus; lip of iliac crest; malleolus; matrix; medium; meningitis; naris; nose; opening; opening of cochlear canaliculus; opening of urethra; ophthalmopathy; ophthalmoplegia; os of uterus; pacemaker; phase; pyocephalus; respiration; secretion; sheath of optic nerve; sphincter muscle of

anus; sphincterotomy; squint; strabismus; surface; surface of cochlear duct; surface of cranial base; surface of frontal bone; surface of parietal bone; table of calvaria; traction; urethrotomy; wall of cochlear duct
external acoustic: aperture; foramen; meatus; pore
external anal: sphincter
external arcuate: fibers
external auditory: foramen; meatus
external cardiac: massage
external carotid: artery; nerves
external carotid (nervous): plexus
external cephalic: version
external collateral: ligament of wrist
external conjugate: diameter
external cuneate: nucleus
external dental: epithelium
external exudative: retinopathy
external female genital: organs
external iliac: artery; lymph nodes; vein
external iliac lymphatic: plexus
external inguinal: ring
external intercostal: membrane; muscle
external jugular: vein
external male genital: organs
external malleolar: sign
external mammary: artery
external maxillary: artery; plexus
external medullary: lamina
external nasal: artery; branches of infraorbital nerve; veins
external nuclear: layer of retina
external oblique: muscle; reflex; ridge
external obturator: muscle
external occipital: crest; protuberance
external palatine: vein
external pillar: cells
external pin: fixation; fixation, biphase
external pterygoid: muscle
external pudendal: veins
external respiratory: nerve of Bell
external root: sheath
external salivary: gland
external saphenous: nerve

external semilunar: fibrocartilage
external spermatic: artery; fascia; nerve
external spiral: sulcus
external urethral: orifice; sphincter; sphincter of female; sphincter of male
external urinary: meatus
exterofective: system
extinction: coefficient
Exton: reagent
extra-: systole
extra-abdominal: desmoid
extraamniotic: pregnancy
extra-anatomic: bypass
extracapsular: ankylosis; fracture; ligaments
extracardiac: murmur
extracellular: cholesterolosis; enzyme; fluid; toxin
extracellular fluid: volume
extrachorial: pregnancy
extrachromosomal: DNA; element; gene; inheritance
extracoronal: retainer
extracorporeal: circulation; dialysis; photophoresis
extracorporeal shock wave: lithotripsy
extracranial: arteritis; ganglia; pneumatocele; pneumocele
extracranial-intracranial: bypass
extracting: forceps
extraction: coefficient; ratio
extradural: anesthesia; hematorrhachis; hemorrhage; space
extraembryonic: blastoderm; celom; ectoderm; membrane; mesoderm
extraglomerular: mesangium
extramammary Paget: disease
extramembranous: pregnancy
extramural: practice
extranodal marginal zone: lymphoma
extranuclear: inheritance
extraocular: muscles; part of central retinal artery and vein
extraoral: anchorage
extraoral fracture: appliance
extraperitoneal: fascia; space
extrapineal: pinealoma
extrapleural: pneumothorax
extrapyramidal: disease; dyskinesias; syndrome
extrapyramidal cerebral: palsy
extrapyramidal motor: system
extrapyramidal motor system: disease

extrasaccular: hernia
extrasensory: perception
extrasensory thought:
  transference
extraskeletal: chondroma
extrathyroidal:
  hypermetabolism
extrauterine: pregnancy
extravaginal: torsion
extravasation: cyst
extravascular: fluid
extravesical: reimplantation
extravital: ultraviolet
extremal: quotient
extreme: capsule
extrinsic: asthma; color;
  factor; motivation; muscles;
  muscles of eyeball; proteins;
  sphincter
extrinsic allergic: alveolitis
extrinsic incubation: period
extruded: teeth
exudation: cell; corpuscle;
  cyst
exudative: bronchiolitis;
  choroiditis; drusen;
  glomerulonephritis;
  inflammation; retinitis;
  tuberculosis;
  vitreoretinopathy
exudative discoid and
  lichenoid: dermatitis
exudative retinal: detachment
eye: capsule; cup; drops; lens;
  ointment; reflex; socket;
  speculum; tooth
eyeball compression: reflex
eyeball-heart: reflex
eye-closure: reflex
eye-closure pupil: reaction
eye-ear: plane
eyelash: sign
eyelid: imbrication

F

F: agent; pili; pilus; plasmid;
  thalassemia; waves
F-: actin
f: distribution; wave
FA: virus
FAB: classification
Fab: fragment; piece
Faber: anemia; syndrome
Fabricius: ship
Fabry: disease
face: form; peel; presentation;
  region; validity
face-bow: fork; record
facet: joints; rhizotomy
facial: angle; artery; aspect;
  axis; bones; canal; cleft;
  colliculus; diplegia;
  eminence; height;
  hemiatrophy; hemiatrophy
  of Romberg; hemiplegia;

hillock; index; lymph nodes;
  muscles; myokymia; nerve
  [CN VII]; neuralgia;
  nucleus; palsy; paralysis;
  plane; plexus; profile; reflex;
  root; skeleton; spasm;
  surface of tooth; tic;
  triangle; trophoneurosis;
  vein; vision
facialis: phenomenon
facial motor: nucleus
facial nerve: area
facial recess: approach
facilitated: diffusion; transport
faciodigitogenital: dysplasia
facioscapulohumeral: atrophy
facioscapulohumeral
  muscular: dystrophy
factitial: dermatitis
factitious: disorder; illness by
  proxy; purpura; urticaria
factorial: experiments
facultative: anaerobe;
  heterochromatin; hyperopia;
  parasite; saprophyte
Faden: suture
fading: time
Faget: sign
Fahr: disease
Fahraeus-Lindqvist: effect
Fahrenheit: scale
faith: healing
falciform: cartilage; crest;
  ligament; ligament of liver;
  lobe; margin of saphenous
  opening; process of
  sacrotuberous ligament
falciform retinal: fold
falciparum: fever; malaria
fallen: arches
falling: palate; sickness
falling of the: womb
fallopian: aqueduct; arch;
  canal; hiatus; ligament;
  neuritis; pregnancy; tube
Fallot: tetrad; triad
false: agglutination;
  albuminuria; anemia;
  aneurysm; angina; ankylosis;
  blepharoptosis; branching;
  cast; chordae tendineae;
  conjugate; coxa vara;
  cyanosis; cyst; dextrocardia;
  diphtheria; diverticulum;
  dominance; glottis;
  hellebore; hematuria;
  hermaphroditism;
  hypertrophy; image; joint;
  knots; labor; lumen; macula;
  membrane; mole; neuroma;
  nucleolus; pains; paracusis;
  pelvis; pregnancy;
  projection; ribs; suture;
  thirst; vertebrae; waters
false memory: syndrome
false-negative: reaction

false-positive: reaction
false tendinous: cords
false vocal: cord
familial: aggregation;
  amyloidosis; cancer;
  dysautonomia; emphysema;
  glycinuria; goiter;
  hyperbetalipoproteinemia;
  hyperbetalipoproteinemia
  and
  hyperprebetalipoproteinemia; hypercholesterolemia;
  hypercholesterolemia with
  hyperlipemia;
  hyperchylomicronemia;
  hyperchylomicronemia with
  hyperprebetalipoproteinemia; hyperlipoproteinemia;
  hyperprebetalipoproteinemia; hypertriglyceridemia;
  hypobetalipoproteinemia;
  hypoparathyroidism;
  nephrosis; polyposis coli;
  screening; tremor
familial adenomatous:
  polyposis
familial aminoglycoside:
  ototoxicity
familial amyloid: neuropathy
familial aortic: ectasia
familial aortic ectasia:
  syndrome
familial bipolar mood:
  disorder
familial chylomicronemia:
  syndrome
familial combined:
  hyperlipemia
familial erythrophagocytic:
  lymphohistiocytosis
familial fat-induced:
  hyperlipemia
familial hemophagocytic:
  lymphohistiocytosis
familial high density
  lipoprotein: deficiency
familial hypercholesteremic:
  xanthomatosis
familial hypertrophic:
  cardiomyopathy
familial hypogonadotropic:
  hypogonadism
familial hypophosphatemic:
  rickets
familial hypoplastic: anemia
familial juvenile:
  nephrophthisis
familial lipoprotein lipase:
  inhibitor
familial Mediterranean: fever
familial microcytic: anemia
familial multiple endocrine:
  adenomatosis
familial nonhemolytic:
  jaundice

familial paroxysmal:
  polyserositis;
  rhabdomyolysis
familial partial: lipodystrophy
familial periodic: paralysis
familial
  pseudoinflammatory:
  maculopathy
familial pseudoinflammatory
  macular: degeneration
familial pyridoxine-
  responsive: anemia
familial recurrent:
  polyserositis
familial spinal muscular:
  atrophy
familial white folded:
  dysplasia
family: medicine; physician;
  practice; therapy
famine: dropsy
fan: sign
Fañanás: cell
Fanconi: anemia;
  pancytopenia; syndrome
FAPA: syndrome
far: point; sight
Farabeuf: amputation; triangle
Faraday: constant; laws
far-and-near: suture
Farber: disease; syndrome
Far East hemorrhagic: fever
Far East Russian:
  encephalitis
farmer's: lung; skin
Farnsworth-Munsell color:
  test
far point of: convergence
Farr: laws
Farrant mounting: fluid
Farre: line
Fas: ligand; receptor
fascia: graft
fascial: hernia; sheath of
  eyeball; sheaths of
  extraocular muscles
fascicular: block;
  degeneration; graft; keratitis;
  ophthalmoplegia; sarcoma;
  ulcer
fasciculata: cell
fasciolar: gyrus
fast: smear
fast component of: nystagmus
fastidious: organism
fastigial: nucleus
fastigiobulbar: fibers; tract
fastigiospinal: fibers; tract
fasting: hypoglycemia
fast-neutron radiation:
  therapy
fat: body; body of cheek; body
  of ischioanal fossa; body of
  ischiorectal fossa; body of
  orbit; cell; embolism; graft;
  hernia; indigestion;

metabolism; necrosis; pad; pad of ischioanal fossa; solvents; tide
fatality: rate
fate: map
father: complex
fatigue: fever; fracture; strength
fat-soluble: vitamins
fat-storing: cell
fatty: acid; alcohol; appendices of colon; ascites; atrophy; cast; change; cirrhosis; degeneration; diarrhea; folds of pleura; heart; hernia; infiltration; kidney; layer of subcutaneous tissue; layer of subcutaneous tissue of abdomen; layer of superficial fascia; liver; metamorphosis; oil; phanerosis; series; stool; tissue
fatty acid–binding: protein
fatty acid oxidation: cycle
fatty renal: capsule
faucial: branches of lingual nerve; diphtheria; paralysis; reflex; tonsil
faulty: union
faun tail: nevus
Favre: dystrophy
Favre-Durand-Nicholas: disease
Favre-Racouchot: disease; syndrome
Fazio-Londe: disease
Fc: fragment; piece; receptor
febrile: albuminuria; convulsion; crisis; psychosis; seizure; urine; urticaria
fecal: abscess; concentration; examination; fistula; impaction; incontinence; tumor; vomiting
Fechner-Weber: law
feedback: activation; inhibition; system
feed-forward: activation
feeding: center; tube
fee-for-service: insurance
feeling: tone
Feer: disease
Fehling: reagent; solution
feigned: eruption
Feiss: line
Felty: syndrome
female: catheter; circumcision; gonad; hermaphroditism; homosexuality; prostate; pseudohermaphroditism; sterility; urethra
female external: genitalia
female internal: genitalia

female pattern: alopecia
female urethral: syndrome
femininity: complex
femoral: arch; artery; branch of genitofemoral nerve; canal; fossa; hernia; muscle; nerve; opening; reflex; region; ring; septum; sheath; triangle; vein
femoral (nervous): plexus
femoral nutrient: artery
femoroabdominal: reflex
femoropatellar: joint
femoropopliteal: bypass
femoropopliteal occlusive: disease
fenestrated: capillary; membrane; sheath
fenestration: operation
Fenn: effect
Fenton: reaction
Fenwick-Hunner: ulcer
Ferguson: reflex
Fergusson: incision
fermentation *Lactobacillus casei*: factor
fermentative: dyspepsia
fern: test
Fernandez: reaction
Fernbach: flask
Ferrata: cell
Ferrein: canal; cords; foramen; ligament; pyramid; tube; vasa aberrantia
ferric: alum
ferric and ammonium acetate: solution
ferric chloride: reaction of epinephrine; test
ferruginous: bodies
Ferry: line
Ferry-Porter: law
fertile: period
fertility: agent; factor; ratio; vitamin
fertilization: membrane
fertilized: ovum
festinating: gait
fetal: attitude; bradycardia; circulation; cotyledon; death; distress; dystocia; electrocardiography; erythroblastosis; fracture; gigantism; habitus; hemoglobin; hydrops; inclusion; membrane; movement; ovoid; placenta; souffle; tachycardia; zone
fetal adrenal: cortex
fetal alcohol: syndrome
fetal aspiration: syndrome
fetal death: rate
fetal face: syndrome
fetal growth: restriction
fetal heart: rate
fetal hydantoin: syndrome

fetal scalp: stimulation
fetal trimethadione: syndrome
fetal warfarin: syndrome
fetomaternal: transfusion
fetoplacental: anasarca
Feulgen: cytometry; reaction; stain
fever: blister; therapy
feverish: urine
fiberoptic: gastroscope
fibrillar: baskets
fibrillary: astrocyte; astrocytoma; chorea; contractions; myoclonia; neuroma; waves
fibrillation: threshold
fibrillatory: waves
fibrin: calculus; thrombus
fibrin/fibrinogen degradation: products
fibrinogen-fibrin conversion: syndrome
fibrinoid: degeneration; necrosis
fibrinolytic: purpura
fibrinopurulent: inflammation
fibrinous: adhesion; bronchitis; cast; inflammation; iritis; lymph; pericarditis; pleurisy; polyp
fibrin-stabilizing: factor
fibroblast: interferon
fibrocartilaginous: ring of tympanic membrane
fibrocaseous: peritonitis
fibrocystic: condition of the breast; disease of the pancreas
fibroelastic: membrane of larynx
fibroepithelial: polyp
fibrohyaline: tissue
fibroid: cataract; inflammation; lung; tumor
fibrolamellar liver cell: carcinoma
fibromuscular: dysplasia; hyperplasia
fibromusculocartilagenous: layer of bronchi
fibromyalgia: syndrome
fibrosing: adenomatosis; adenosis; alveolitis; colonopathy; mediastinitis
fibrositic: headache
fibrotic: ophthalmoplegia
fibrous: adhesion; ankylosis; appendix of liver; capsule; capsule of kidney; capsule of liver; capsule of parotid gland; capsule of spleen; capsule of thyroid gland; cavernitis; degeneration; dysplasia of bone; dysplasia of jaws; goiter; hamartoma

of infancy; histiocytoma; joint; layer; layer of eyeball; layer of joint capsule; layer in or on deep aspect of fatty layer of subcutaneous tissue; mediastinitis; membrane of joint capsule; pericarditis; pericardium; pneumonia; polyp; protein; ring; ring of intervertebral disk; sheaths; sheaths of digits of hand; skeleton of heart; tissue; trigones of heart; tubercle; tunic of corpus spongiosum; tunic of eye; union; xanthoma
fibrous articular: capsule
fibrous bacterial: viruses
fibrous cortical: defect
fibrous digital: sheaths of foot; sheaths of hand; sheaths of toes
fibrous tendon: sheath
fibular: artery; compartment of leg; lymph node; margin of foot; node; notch; trochlea of calcaneus; veins
fibular articular: facet of tibia; surface of tibia
fibular collateral: ligament; ligament of ankle
fibularis brevis: muscle
fibularis longus: muscle
fibularis tertius: muscle
fibular nutrient: artery
fibular (peroneal): border of foot
fibular tarsal tendinous: sheaths
Fick: laws of diffusion; method; principle
Ficoll-Hypaque: technique
fictitious: feeding
Fiedler: myocarditis
field: block; carcinogenesis; fever; gradient; lens; survey
field of: consciousness
field block: anesthesia
field emission: tube
Fielding: membrane
Field rapid: stain
Fiessinger-Leroy-Reiter: syndrome
fifth: disease; finger; ventricle
fifth cranial: nerve [CN V]
fifth digit: syndrome
fig: wart
fight or flight: reaction
Figueira: syndrome
figure-of-8: abnormality; bandage; suture
filamentary: keratitis; keratopathy
filament-nonfilament: count
filamentous: bacteriophage; colony

filamentous bacterial: viruses
filament polymorphonuclear: leukocyte
filar: mass; micrometer; substance
filarial: arthritis; funiculitis; hydrocele; periodicity; synovitis
filariform: larva
Filatov: disease; flap; operation; spots
Filatov-Dukes: disease
Filatov-Gillies: flap
filial: generation
filiform: bougie; nucleus; papillae; pulse; wart
fillet: layer
filling: defect
filling internal urethral: orifice
filmless: radiography
filter: paper
filtering: bleb; cicatrix; operation
filtrable: virus
filtrate: factor; nitrogen
filtration: angle; coefficient; fraction; slits; space
fimbriated: fold of inferior surface of tongue
fimbriodentate: sulcus
final: host; impression
Finckh: test
fine: structure; tremor
fine needle: biopsy
finger: agnosia; percussion; phenomenon
finger-nose: test
fingerprint: dystrophy
finger-thumb: reflex
finger-to-finger: test
finishing: bur
Finkelstein: test
Fink-Heimer: stain
Finney: operation; pyloroplasty
fire: ant
first: dentition; finger; messenger; molar; part of duodenum; rib [I]
first arch: syndrome
first cervical: vertebra
first cranial: nerve [CN I]
first cuneiform: bone
first-degree: burn
first degree AV: block
first duodenal: sphincter
first heart: sound
first-order: reaction
first parallel pelvic: plane
first-pass: effect; metabolism
first rank: symptoms
first and second posterior intercostal: arteries
first-set: rejection
first temporal: convolution

first visceral: cleft
Fischer: projection; sign; symptom
Fischer projection: formulas
Fischer projection formulas of: sugars
fish: poison; skin
Fishberg concentration: test
Fisher: syndrome
Fisher exact: test
fish eye: disease
Fishman-Lerner: unit
fish-mouth: meatus
fish-mouth mitral: stenosis
fish-tank: granuloma
fish tapeworm: anemia
fission: fungi; product
fissural: cyst
fissure: bur; caries; sealant; sign
fissured: fracture; tongue
fistula: knife; test
FIT: test
Fitzgerald: factor
Fitz-Hugh and Curtis: syndrome
five-day: fever
five-year survival: rate
fixation: disparity; nystagmus; reaction; suppression
fixational ocular: movement
fixator: muscle
fixed: alkali; alkaloid; bridge; contracture; coupling; dressing; end; idea; macrophage; oil; pupil; torticollis; virus
fixed drug: eruption
fixed partial: denture
fixed-rate: pacemaker
fixed rate pulse: generator
fixing: eye
flaccid: ectropion; membrane; paralysis; part of tympanic membrane
Flack: node
flag: sign
flagellar: agglutinin; antigen
flagellate: diarrhea
flail: chest; joint
flame: arc; cell; figure; photometer; spots
flame emission: spectrophotometry
flammable: anesthetic
flange: contour
flank: bone; incision; position
flap: amputation; operation
flapless: amputation
flapping: tremor
flash: blindness; burn; dispersal; keratoconjunctivitis; method; point
flashing pain: syndrome
flash-lag: effect

flask: closure
flat: affect; bone; chest; condyloma; electroencephalogram; muscle; pelvis; plate; wart
Flatau: law
Flatau-Schilder: disease
flat top: waves
flatulent: dyspepsia
flatus: enema
Flaujeac: factor
flavin: nucleotide
flax-dresser's: disease
flea-bitten: kidney
flea-borne: typhus
Flechsig: areas; fasciculi; tract
Flechsig ground: bundles
fleck: dystrophy of cornea; retina of Kandori
flecked: retina
flecked retina: syndrome
Flegel: disease
Fleisch: pneumotachograph
Fleischer: ring; vortex
Fleischer-Strümpell: ring
Fleischmann: bursa
Fleischner: lines
Fleitmann: test
Flemming: fixative
Flemming triple: stain
Flesch: formula
flesh: fly
fleshy: mole; polyp
Fletcher: factor
flexible: collodion; endoscope; hysteroscope
flexion: crease
flexion-extension: injury
Flexner: bacillus
flexor: compartment of arm; compartment of forearm; compartment of leg; compartment of thigh; muscle; reflex; retinaculum; retinaculum of forearm; retinaculum of lower limb
flexor accessorius: muscle
flexor carpi radialis: muscle
flexor carpi ulnaris: muscle
flexor digiti minimi brevis: muscle of foot; muscle of hand
flexor digitorum brevis: muscle
flexor digitorum longus: muscle
flexor digitorum profundus: muscle
flexor digitorum superficialis: muscle
flexor hallucis brevis: muscle
flexor hallucis longus: muscle
flexor pollicis brevis: muscle
flexor pollicis longus: muscle
flexural: eczema; psoriasis
flick: movements

flicker: fusion; perimetry; photometer
flicker fusion frequency: technique
Flieringa: ring
flight: blindness; nurse
flight of: ideas
flight or fight: response
Flinders Island spotted: fever
Flint: arcade; murmur
flint: disease; glass
flip: angle
flittering: scotoma
floating: cartilage; kidney; organ; patella; ribs [XI–XII]; spleen; villus
floccular: fossa
flocculation: reaction; test
flocculonodular: lobe
Flood: ligament
flood: fever
floor: cell; plate
floppy valve: syndrome
Florence: crystals; flask
Florey: unit
florid oral: papillomatosis
florid osseous: dysplasia
floriform: cataract
Florschütz: formula
floss: silk
flotation: constant; method
Flourens: theory
floury: cornea
flow: cytometry; cytophotometry; diagram; void
Flower: bone
Flower dental: index
flower-spray: ending; organ of Ruffini
flowing: hyperostosis
flow-over: vaporizer
flow-volume: curve
flow-volume loop: studies
fluent: aphasia
fluid: extract; retinopexy; wave
fluid mosaic: model
fluorescein: angiography
fluorescein instillation: test
fluorescein string: test
fluorescence: microscope; microscopy; quenching; spectrum
fluorescence plus Giemsa: stain
fluorescence in situ: hybridization
fluorescent: antibody; screen; stain
fluorescent antibody: technique
fluorescent antinuclear antibody: test
fluorescent in situ: hybridization

fluorescent treponemal antibody-absorption: test
fluoridated: tooth
Flury strain: vaccine
Flury strain rabies: virus
flush: technique
flutter-fibrillation: waves
flux: density; ratio
fluxionary: hyperemia
fly: agaric; blister
flying: blister
flying spot: microscope
Flynn: phenomenon
Flynn-Aird: syndrome
FMD: virus
foam: cells
foam stability: test
foamy: agents; viruses
focal: acrohyperkeratosis; amyloidosis; appendicitis; depth; distance; epilepsy; glomerulonephritis; illumination; infection; interval; necrosis; nephritis; point; reaction; spot
focal condensing: osteitis
focal dermal: hypoplasia
focal embolic: glomerulonephritis
focal epithelial: hyperplasia
focal lymphocytic: thyroiditis
focal metastatic: disease
focal motor: seizure
focal sclerosing: glomerulopathy
focal segmental: glomerulosclerosis
focused: grid
Fogarty: clamp
Fogarty embolectomy: catheter
fogging: retinoscopy
Foix-Alajouanine: myelitis; syndrome
Foix-Cavany-Marie: syndrome
foldable intraocular: lens
fold-back: elements
folded-lung: syndrome
folding: fracture
Foley: catheter
Foley Y-plasty: pyeloplasty
foliate: papillae; papillitis
folic acid: antagonists; conjugate
folic acid deficiency: anemia
Folin: reaction; reagent; test
Folin-Looney: test
folk: medicine
Folli: process
follian: process
follicle-stimulating: hormone; principle
follicular: abscess; adenoma; antrum; carcinoma; conjunctivitis; cyst; cystitis;

gland; goiter; hormone; impetigo; iritis; lymphoma; mange; mucinosis; papule; stigma; syphilid; trachoma; urethritis; vulvitis
follicular epithelial: cell
follicular ovarian: cells
follicular predominantly large cell: lymphoma
follicular predominantly small cleaved cell: lymphoma
Folling: disease
following: bougie
follow-up: study
Foltz: valvule
Fonio: solution
Fontan: operation; procedure
Fontana: canal; spaces; stain
Fontana-Masson silver: stain
food: asthma; ball; fever; impaction; poisoning
foot: bones; plate; plugger; process; yaws
foot-and-mouth: disease
foot-and-mouth disease: virus
foot-and-mouth disease virus: vaccines
football: calf
footling: presentation
foot-pound-second: system; unit
Foot reticulin impregnation: stain
foramen of Bochdalek: hernia
foraminal: herniation; lymph node; node
Forbes: disease
Forbes-Albright: syndrome
forced: alimentation; beat; cycle; duction; feeding; respiration; spirometry
forced expiratory: flow; time; volume
forced grasping: reflex
forced vital: capacity
forceps: delivery
force-velocity: curve
Forchheimer: sign
Fordyce: angiokeratoma; disease; granules; spots
forebrain: eminence; prominence; vesicle
foreign: body; protein; serum
foreign-body: appendicitis
foreign body: granuloma; salpingitis; tumorigenesis
foreign body giant: cell
foreign protein: therapy
Forel: decussation
forensic: dentistry; medicine; odontology; psychiatry; psychology
forequarter: amputation
forest: yaws
Forestier: disease

Formad: kidney
formal: operations
formaldehyde: fixative
formalin: pigment
formalin-ether sedimentation: concentration
formalin-ethyl acetate sedimentation: concentration
formative: cell
formed visual: hallucination
formol: titration
formol-calcium: fixative
formol-gel: test
formol-Müller: fixative
formol-saline: fixative
formol-Zenker: fixative
formyl-methionyl-: tRNA
fornicate: gyrus
Forsius-Eriksson: albinism
Forssman: antibody; antigen; hapten; reaction
Forssman antigen-antibody: reaction
Förster: uveitis
Fort Bragg: fever
fortification: figures; spectrum
fortified: milk
fortified vitamin D: milk
forward: conduction
forward heart: failure
Fosdick-Hansen-Epple: test
Foshay: test
Foster: frame
Foster Kennedy: syndrome
Fothergill: disease; neuralgia; operation; sign
Fouchet: reagent; stain
founder: effect; principle
foundryman's: fever
fountain: decussation; syringe
Four Corners: virus
four-headed: muscle
Fourier: analysis; transfer; transform
Fournier: disease; gangrene
four-tailed: bandage
fourth: disease; finger; toe [IV]; ventricle
fourth cranial: nerve [CN IV]
fourth heart: sound
fourth lumbar: nerve [L4]
fourth parallel pelvic: plane
fourth turbinated: bone
foveated: chest
foveolar: cells of stomach
Foville: fasciculus; syndrome
fowl: typhoid
Fowler: position
Fox-Fordyce: disease
fractional: distillation; dose; sterilization
fractional epidural: anesthesia

fractional spinal: anesthesia
fracture: bed; blister; box; dislocation
Fraenkel: pneumococcus
fragile: site
fragile X: chromosome; syndrome
fragility: test
fragment: reaction
Fraley: syndrome
frame-shift: mutagen; mutation
framework: region
Framingham Heart: Study
Franceschetti: syndrome
Franceschetti-Jadassohn: syndrome
Francke: needle
frank breech: presentation
Frankenhäuser: ganglion
Frankfort: plane
Frankfort horizontal: plane
Frankfort-mandibular incisor: angle
Franklin: disease; spectacles
franklinic: taste
Frank-Starling: curve
Fräntzel: murmur
Fraser: syndrome
Fraser-Lendrum: stain for fibrin
fraternal: twins
Fraunhofer: lines
Frazier: needle
Frazier-Spiller: operation
Fredet-Ramstedt: operation
free: association; border; border of nail; border of ovary; electrophoresis; energy; field; flap; gingiva; graft; macrophage; margin; margin of eyelids; part of lower limb; part of upper limb; radical; tenia; villus; water
free bone: flap
free-floating: anxiety
free-hand: knife
free induction: decay
free mandibular: movements
Freeman-Sheldon: syndrome
free nerve: endings
free thyroxine: index
free water: clearance
freeway: space
freeze: fracture
freezing: point
Frei: test
Freiberg: disease; infarction
Frei-Hoffmann: reaction
Frejka pillow: splint
French: chalk; scale
French-American-British: classification
Frenkel: symptom

Frenkel anterior ocular traumatic: syndrome
frequency: curve; distribution; spectrum
Frerichs: theory
fresh frozen: plasma
Fresnel: lens; prism
Freud: theory
freudian: fixation; psychoanalysis
Freund: adjuvant; anomaly; operation
Freund complete: adjuvant
Freund incomplete: adjuvant
Frey: hairs; syndrome
friction: murmur; rub; sound
frictional: attachment
Fridenberg stigometric card: test
Friderichsen-Waterhouse: syndrome
Friedländer: bacillus; pneumonia; stain for capsules
Friedländer bacillus: pneumonia
Friedman: curve
Friedreich: ataxia; phenomenon; sign
Friend: disease; virus
Friend leukemia: virus
fright: reaction
Froehde: reagent
frog: face
frog leg: position
frog-leg lateral: projection
Fröhlich: dwarfism; syndrome
Frohn: reagent
Froin: syndrome
Froment: sign
frontal: angle of parietal bone; area; artery; aspect; belly of occipitofrontalis muscle; bone; border; border of parietal bone; border of sphenoid bone; branch of middle meningeal artery; branch of superficial temporal artery; cortex; crest; eminence; fontanelle; foramen; forceps; grooves; horn; lobe; lobe of cerebrum; margin; margin of sphenoid; nerve; notch; part of corpus callosum; plane; plate; pole; pole [TA] of cerebrum; process of maxilla; process of zygomatic bone; region of head; section; sinus; squama; suture; triangle; tuber; veins
frontalis: muscle
frontal lobe: epilepsy
frontal sinus: aperture
frontoanterior: position

frontoethmoidal: suture
frontolacrimal: suture
frontomaxillary: suture
frontonasal: duct; process; prominence; suture
fronto-occipital: fasciculus
fronto-orbital: area
frontopolar: artery
frontopontine: fibers; tract
frontoposterior: position
frontosphenoidal: process
frontotemporal: tract
frontotransverse: position
frontozygomatic: suture
front-tap: contraction; reflex
Froriep: ganglion
Frost: suture
frost: itch
frosted: heart
frosted branch: angiitis
frozen: pelvis; section; shoulder
fructokinase: deficiency
fructose: malabsorption
fruit: sugar
fruiting: body
frustration: tolerance
frustration-aggression: hypothesis
FTA-ABS: test
Fuchs: adenoma; coloboma; spur; stomas; syndrome; uveitis
Fuchs black: spot
Fuchs endothelial: dystrophy
Fuchs heterochromic: cyclitis
fuchsin: bodies
fuchsinophil: cell; granule; reaction
fugitive: swelling; wart
fugu: poison
fulcrum: line
fulgurating: migraine
full: denture
fuller's: earth
full liquid: diet
full-thickness: burn; flap; graft
fulminant: hepatitis; hyperpyrexia
fulminating: dysentery; smallpox
fuming: nitric acid; sulfuric acid
functional: albuminuria; anatomy; aphasia; apoplexy; asplenia; autonomy; blindness; castration; congestion; contracture; disease; disorder; dysmenorrhea; dyspepsia; dyspnea; genomics; group; hearing impairment; hypertrophy; illness; murmur; neurosurgery; occlusion; pathology;

pleiotropy; psychosis; sphincter; splint; stricture; visual loss
functional cardiovascular: disease
functional chew-in: record
functional endoscopic sinus: surgery
functional jaw: orthopedics
functional mandibular: movements
functional neck: dissection
functional occlusal: harmony
functional orthodontic: therapy
functional prepubertal castration: syndrome
functional refractory: period
functional residual: air; capacity
functional terminal innervation: ratio
functional vocal: fatigue
fundamental: frequency; tone
fundic: glands
fundiform: ligament of clitoris; ligament of foot; ligament of penis
fundus: reflex
fungating: sore
fungiform: papillae
fungous: foot
fungus: ball
funic: souffle
funicular: graft; hydrocele; myelitis; myelosis; part of ductus deferens; process
funnel: breast; plot
funnel-shaped: pelvis
funny: bone
furcal: nerve
furfurol: reaction
furious: rabies
furnacemen's: cataract
furred: tongue
fused: kidney; silver nitrate; teeth
fusel: oil
fusible: metal
fusiform: aneurysm; cataract; cells of cerebral cortex; gyrus; layer; muscle
fusing: point
fusion: area; beat; energy; temperature (wire method)
fusional: movement
fusion-inferred threshold: test
fusospirochetal: disease; gingivitis; stomatitis
Futcher: line
futile: cycle
Fy: antigens

G

γ: hemolysis
G: antigen; cells; factor; force; proteins; syndrome; unit of streptomycin
G$_{M1}$: gangliosidosis
G$_{M2}$: gangliosidosis
G-: actin; protein
GABA: pathway
Gaboon: ulcer
Gaddum and Schild: test
Gaenslen: sign
Gaffky: scale; table
gag: reflex
Gairdner: disease
Gaisböck: syndrome
gait: apraxia
GAL: virus
galactokinase: deficiency
galactokinase deficiency: galactosemia
galactophorous: canals; ducts
galactopoietic: hormone
galactose: cataract; diabetes
galactose tolerance: test
galactosylceramide: lipoidosis
Galant: reflex
Galassi pupillary: phenomenon
Galeati: glands
Galeazzi: fracture
Galen: anastomosis; nerve
Gall: craniology
gall: bladder; duct
Gallaudet: fascia
Gallavardin: phenomenon
gallbladder: fossa
Gallego differentiating: solution
Gallie: transplant
gallop: rhythm; sound
gallstone: colic; ileus
gallus adenolike: virus
Galton: delta; law; whistle
galtonian: genetics; inheritance; trait
Galtonian-Fisher: genetics
Galton system of classification of: fingerprints
galvanic: cautery; current; nystagmus; threshold
galvanic skin: reaction; reflex; response
galvanocaustic: snare
Gambian: fever; trypanosomiasis
game: theory
gamekeeper's: thumb
gamete intrafallopian: transfer
gametic: nucleus
gametokinetic: hormone
Gamgee: tissue
gamma: alcoholism; angle; camera; cell of pancreas; crystallin; efferent;

encephalography; fibers; knife; loop; radiation; rays
gamma motor: neurons; system
Gamna: disease
Gamna-Favre: bodies
Gamna-Gandy: bodies; nodules
Gandy-Gamna: bodies
Gandy-Nanta: disease
gangliated: cord; nerve
ganglion: cell; cells of dorsal spinal root; cells of retina; ridge
ganglionic: blockade; branches of lingual nerve; branches of lingual nerve to sublingual ganglion; branches of lingual nerve to submandibular ganglion; branches of maxillary nerve; branches of maxillary nerve to pterygopalatine ganglion; branch of internal carotid artery; chain; crest; layer; layer of cerebellar cortex; layer of cerebral cortex; layer of optic nerve; saliva
ganglionic blocking: agent
ganglionic cell: layer of retina
ganglionic motor: neuron
ganglioside: lipidosis
gangrenous: appendicitis; cellulitis; emphysema; pharyngitis; pneumonia; rhinitis; stomatitis
Ganser: commissure; syndrome
Gant: clamp
Gantzer: muscle
Gantzer accessory: bundle
Ganzfeld: stimulation
gap: arthroplasty; junction; phenomenon
gap$_1$: period; phase
gap$_0$: period; phase
gap$_2$: period; phase
garapata: disease
Gardner: syndrome
Gardner-Diamond: syndrome
Gardnerella: vaginitis
gargantuan: mastitis
Gariel: pessary
Garland: triangle
Garré: disease; osteomyelitis
Gartner: canal; cyst; duct
Gärtner: method; tonometer
Gärtner vein: phenomenon
gas: abscess; bacillus; cautery; chromatography; constant; cyst; embolism; gangrene; peritonitis; phlegmon; retinopexy; thermometer
gaseous: mediastinography; pulse
gas gangrene: antitoxin

Gaskell: bridge; clamp
gas-liquid: chromatography
gasserian: ganglion
gastral: mesoderm
gastrea: theory
gastric: analysis; area; arteries; branches of anterior vagal trunk; branches of posterior vagal trunk; bypass; calculus; canal; colic; crisis; diastole; digestion; feeding; fistula; folds; follicles; freezing; glands; hemorrhage; hypersecretion; impression on liver; impression on spleen; indigestion; juice; mucin; mucosa; neurasthenia; pit; plexuses of autonomic system; rugae; smear; stapling; surface of spleen; tetany; ulcer; veins; volvulus
gastric algid: malaria
gastric inhibitory: peptide; polypeptide
gastric lymphoid: nodules
gastric nervous: plexuses
gastrocardiac: syndrome
gastrocnemius: muscle
gastrocolic: fistula; ligament; omentum; reflex
gastrocutaneous: fistula
gastrodiaphragmatic: ligament
gastroduodenal: artery; fistula; lymph nodes; orifice
gastroenteritis: virus type A; virus type B
gastroepiploic: arteries; veins
gastroesophageal: hernia; vestibule
gastroesophageal reflux: disease
gastrogenous: diarrhea
Gastrografin: swallow
gastrohepatic: omentum
gastroileac: reflex
gastrointestinal: fistula; hormone; tract
gastrointestinal autonomic nerve: tumor
gastrointestinal stromal: tumor
gastrojejunal loop obstruction: syndrome
gastrolienal: ligament
gastroomental: arteries
gastropancreatic: folds
gastrophrenic: ligament
gastrosplenic: ligament; omentum
Gatch: bed
gate-control: hypothesis; theory

gated radionuclide: angiocardiography
gating: mechanism
Gaucher: cells; disease
gauge: pressure
gauntlet: bandage
Gauss: sign
gaussian: curve; distribution
gauze: bandage
Gavard: muscle
Gay: glands
gay bowel: syndrome
Gay-Lussac: equation; law
gaze paretic: nystagmus
GB: viruses
G-banding: stain
GC: content
Ge: antigen
Geigel: reflex
Geiger-Müller: counter; tube
gel: diffusion; electrophoresis; filtration; structure
gelastic: seizure
gelatin: sugar
gelatinous: ascites; infiltration; nucleus; polyp; scleritis; substance; tissue; varix
gelatinous bone: marrow
gelatinous droplike corneal: dystrophy
gel diffusion: reactions
gel diffusion precipitin: tests; tests in one dimension; tests in two dimensions
gel filtration: chromatography
Gélineau: syndrome
Gell and Coombs: Classification; reactions
Gellé: test
Gély: suture
geminated: teeth
gemistocytic: astrocyte; astrocytoma; cell; reaction
genal: glands
gender: identity; role
gender dysphoria: syndrome
gender identity: disorders
gene: activation; deletion; duplication; expression; family; flow; frequency; mapping; mosaicism; pool; regulation; therapy
gene dosage: compensation; effect
general: anatomy; anesthesia; anesthetics; bloodletting; hospital; immunity; paresis; peritonitis; physiology; practice; sensation; stimulant; transduction
general adaptation: reaction; syndrome
general duty: nurse
general fertility: rate

generalized: anaphylaxis; chondromalacia; elastolysis; emphysema; epilepsy; gangliosidosis; glycogenosis; lentiginosis; myokymia; paralysis; seizures; tetanus; tuberculosis; vaccinia; xanthelasma
generalized anxiety: disorder
generalized cortical: hyperostosis
generalized epidermolytic: hyperkeratosis
generalized eruptive: histiocytoma
generalized plane: xanthomatosis
generalized pustular: psoriasis of Zambusch
generalized Shwartzman: phenomenon
generalized tonic-clonic: epilepsy; seizure
general somatic afferent: column
general somatic efferent: column
general visceral afferent: column
general visceral efferent: column
generated occlusal: path
generation: effect
generative: empathy
generator: potential
generic: substitution
genesial: cycle
genetic: amplification; association; burden; carrier; code; colonization; compound; counseling; death; determinant; disequilibrium; dominance; drift; engineering; epidemiology; equilibrium; female; fingerprint; fitness; fixation; heterogeneity; homeostasis; isolate; lethal; linkage; load; locus; map; marker; material; model; penetrance; polymorphism; psychology; recombination; testing
genetic human: male
Geneva lens: measure
Gengou: phenomenon
genial: tubercle
genicular: anastomosis; arteries; veins
geniculate: body; ganglion; neuralgia; otalgia; zoster
geniculatus lateralis: nucleus
geniculocalcarine: radiation; tract
genioglossal: muscle
genioglossus: muscle

Word Finder

geniohyoid: muscle
genital: ambiguity; branch of genitofemoral nerve; branch of iliohypogastric nerve; cord; corpuscles; duct; eminence; fold; furrow; gland; ligament; organs; phase; primacy; primordium; ridge; stage; swellings; system; tract; tubercle; wart
genitocrural: nerve
genitofemoral: nerve
genitoinguinal: ligament
genitourinary: apparatus; fistula; surgeon; system
Gennari: band; stria
genomic: clone; DNA; imprinting; library
gentian aniline: water
genucubital: position
genupectoral: position
geographic: choroidopathy; keratitis; stippling of nails; tongue
geographic information: system
geographic retinal: atrophy
geometric: isomer; isomerism; mean; sense
Gerbich: antigen
Gerbode: defect
Gerdy: fibers; fontanelle; ligament; tubercle
Gerdy hyoid: fossa
Gerdy interatrial: loop
Gerhardt: disease; reaction; test for acetoacetic acid; test for urobilin in the urine
Gerhardt-Mitchell: disease
geriatric: medicine; therapy
Gerlach: tonsil; valve; valvula
Gerlach annular: tendon
Gerlier: disease
germ: cell; layer; line; membrane; nucleus; theory; tube
German: measles
German measles: virus
germinal: aplasia; area; cell; center of Flemming; cords; disk; epithelium; localization; mosaicism; pole; rod; streak; vesicle
germinative: layer; layer of nail
Germiston: virus
germ layer: theory
germ tube: test
Gerota: capsule; fascia; method
Gerstmann: syndrome
Gerstmann-Sträussler-Scheinker: syndrome
gestalt: phenomenon; psychology; theory; therapy

gestational: age; diabetes; edema; hypertension; proteinuria; ring; sac
gestational trophoblastic: disease
Gey: solution
ghatti: gum
Gheel: colony
Ghon: complex; focus; tubercle
Ghon primary: lesion
ghost: cell; corpuscle; tooth
ghost cell: glaucoma
ghoul: hand
Giannuzzi: crescents; demilunes
Gianotti-Crosti: syndrome
giant: cell; chromosome; colon; condyloma; drusen; fibroadenoma; hives; hypertrophy of gastric mucosa; melanosome; urticaria
giant axonal: neuropathy
giant cell: aortitis; arteritis; carcinoma; carcinoma of thyroid gland; epulis; fibroma; glioblastoma multiforme; granuloma; hepatitis; myeloma; myocarditis; pneumonia; sarcoma; thyroiditis; tumor of bone; tumor of tendon sheath
giant cell hyaline: angiopathy
giant cell monstrocellular: sarcoma of Zülch
giant follicular: lymphoblastoma; thyroiditis
giant gastric: folds
giant osteoid: osteoma
giant papillary: conjunctivitis
giant pigmented: nevus
Gibb phase: rule
Gibbs: energy of activation; theorem
Gibbs-Donnan: equilibrium
Gibbs free: energy
Gibbs-Helmholtz: equation
Gibney: boot
Gibney fixation: bandage
Gibson: bandage; murmur
Giemsa: stain
Giemsa chromosome banding: stain
Gierke: cells; disease
Gierke respiratory: bundle
Gifford: reflex
gigantiform: cementoma
gigantocellular: glioma; nucleus of medulla oblongata
Gigli: operation; saw
Gilbert: disease; syndrome
Gilchrist: disease
gill: clefts

gill arch: skeleton
Gilles de la Tourette: disease; syndrome
Gillespie: syndrome
Gillette suspensory: ligament
Gilliam: operation
Gillies: operation
Gillmore: needle
Gilmer: wiring
Gil-Vernet: operation
Gimbernat: ligament
ginger: paralysis
gingival: abrasion; abscess; atrophy; clamp; cleft; contour; crest; crevice; curvature; cyst; elephantiasis; embrasure; enlargement; epithelium; festoon; fibromatosis; fistula; flap; fluid; groove; hyperplasia; margin; massage; mucosa; papilla; pocket; proliferation; recession; repositioning; resorption; retraction; septum; space; sulcus; tissues; trough; zone
gingivobuccal: groove; sulcus
gingivodental: ligament
gingivolabial: groove; sulcus
gingivolingual: groove; sulcus
ginglymoid: joint
Giordano-Giovannetti: diet
Giovannetti: diet
Girard: reagent
girdle: anesthesia; pain; sensation
Girdlestone: procedure
Gitelman: syndrome
gitter: cell
glabrous: skin
glacial: acetic acid; phosphoric acid
glairy: mucus
glancing: wound
glandular: branches; branches of facial artery; branches of inferior thyroid artery; branches of submandibular ganglion; cancer; carcinoma; epithelium; fever; lobe of hypophysis; mastitis; plague; substance of prostate; system; tularemia
glandulopreputial: lamella
glanular: hypospadias
Glanzmann: disease; thrombasthenia
glaserian: artery; fissure
Glasgow: sign
glass: body; electrode; factor; rays
glass bead: sterilizer
glass ionomer: cement
glassworker's: cataract
glassy: membrane

Glauber: salt
glaucomatocyclitic: crisis
glaucomatous: cataract; cup; excavation; halo; ring
glaucomatous nerve-fiber bundle: scotoma
Gleason: score
Gleason tumor: grade
Glenn: operation; shunt
Glenner-Lillie: stain for pituitary
glenohumeral: articulation; joint; ligaments
glenoid: cavity; cavity of scapula; fossa; labrum of scapula; ligament; surface
glenoidal: lip
Gley: glands
glia: cells
glial fibrillary acidic: protein
glial limiting: membrane
gliding: joint; occlusion
Glisson: capsule; cirrhosis; sphincter
glitter: cells
global: aphasia; burden of disease; paralysis
globin: insulin
globin zinc: insulin
globoid: cell
globoid cell: leukodystrophy
globosus: nucleus
globular: heart; leukocyte; process; protein; sputum; thrombus
globulomaxillary: cyst
glomerular: capsule; crescent; cyst; layer of olfactory bulb; nephritis; sclerosis
glomerular filtration: rate
glomerulosa: cell
glomiform: glands
glomus: body; tumor
glomus jugulare: tumor
glomus tympanicum: tumor
glossoepiglottic: ligament
glossolabiolaryngeal: paralysis
glossopalatine: arch; fold
glossopalatolabial: paralysis
glossopharyngeal: breathing; nerve [CN IX]; neuralgia; part of superior pharyngeal constrictor; tic
glossopharyngeolabial: paralysis
glossy: skin
glove: anesthesia
gloved-finger: sign
Glover: phenomenon
glover: suture
glucagonlike: peptide
glucagonlike insulinotropic: peptide
glucagonoma: syndrome

glucose-dependent insulinotropic: polypeptide
glucose oxidase: method
glucose oxidase paper strip: test
glucose-6-phosphatase hepatorenal: glycogenosis
glucose-6-phosphate dehydrogenase: deficiency
glucosephosphate isomerase: deficiency
glucose tolerance: factor; test
glucose transport: maximum
glucosidase: inhibitors
α-glucosidase: inhibitor
β-d-glucuronidase: deficiency
glue: ear
Gluge: corpuscles
γ-glutamyl: cycle
glutaraldehyde: fixative
glutathione synthetase: deficiency
gluteal: cleft; crest; fold; furrow; hernia; lines; lymph nodes; reflex; region; ridge; surface of ilium; tuberosity; veins
gluten: ataxia; enteropathy
gluten-free: diet
gluteofemoral: bursa
gluteus maximus: gait; muscle
gluteus medius: bursae; gait; muscle
gluteus minimus: bursa; muscle
glycemic: index
glycerin: suppository
glycerinated: gelatin; tincture
glycerol dehydration: test
glycerophosphate: shuttle
glycine-succinate: cycle
glycogen: cardiomegaly; granule
glycogenic: acanthosis; cardiomegaly
glycogen-storage: disease
glycol: ethers
glycolipid: lipidosis
glycosyl: compound
glycosylated: hemoglobin
glyoxylic acid: cycle
Gm: allotypes; antigens
Gmelin: test
gnathic: index
gnome's: calf
goatpox: virus
goat's milk: anemia
goblet: cell
Godélier: law
Godman: fascia
Godwin: tumor
Goeckerman: treatment
Goethe: bone
Gofman: test
Goggia: sign

gold: alloy; casting; equivalent; inlay; number
Goldblatt: hypertension; kidney; phenomenon
Goldenhar: syndrome
Goldflam: disease
Goldie-Coldman: hypothesis
Goldman: equation
Goldman-Fox: knives
Goldman-Hodgkin-Katz: equation
Goldmann: perimeter
Goldmann applanation: tonometer
Goldmann-Favre: syndrome
gold-myokymia: syndrome
Goldscheider: test
gold sol: test
Goldstein toe: sign
golfer's: skin
golf-hole ureteral: orifice
Golgi: apparatus; body; cells; complex; corpuscle; stain; zone
Golgi epithelial: cell
Golgi internal: reticulum
Golgi-Mazzoni: corpuscle
Golgi osmiobichromate: fixative
Golgi tendon: organ
Golgi type I: neuron
Golgi type II: neuron
Goll: column
Goltz: syndrome
Gombault: triangle
Gomori aldehyde fuchsin: stain
Gomori chrome alum hematoxylin-phloxine: stain
Gomori-Jones periodic acid-methenamine-silver: stain
Gomori methenamine-silver: stain
Gomori nonspecific acid phosphatase: stain
Gomori nonspecific alkaline phosphatase: stain
Gomori one-step trichrome: stain
Gomori silver impregnation: stain
Gompertz: hypothesis; law
gompholic: joint
gonad: dose; nucleus
gonadal: agenesis; aplasia; cords; dose; dysgenesis; hormones; ridge; streak
gonadal steroid-binding: globulin
gonadotrophic: cycle
gonadotropic: hormone
gonadotropin-producing: adenoma
gonadotropin-releasing: factor; hormone

gonococcal: arthritis; conjunctivitis; stomatitis
gonorrheal: conjunctivitis; ophthalmia; rheumatism; salpingitis; urethritis
Good: antigen
good: object
Goodell: dilator; sign
Goodenough draw-a-man: test
goodness of fit: test
Goodpasture: stain; syndrome
Goormaghtigh: cells
goose: flesh
Gopalan: syndrome
Gordon: reflex; sign; symptom
Gordon and Sweet: stain
Gorham: disease; syndrome
Goriaew: rule
Gorlin: cyst; formula; sign; syndrome
Gorlin-Chaudhry-Moss: syndrome
Gorman: syndrome
Gosselin: fracture
Gothic: arch; palate
Gothic arch: tracing
Göthlin: test
Gougerot and Blum: disease
Gougerot-Carteaud: syndrome
Gougerot-Sjögren: disease
Gould: suture
Gouley: catheter
gout: diet
gouty: arthritis; diathesis; pearl; tophus; urine
government: hospital
Gower: sign
Gowers: column; contraction; disease; syndrome; tract
Gr: antigen
graafian: follicle
gracile: fasciculus; habitus; lobule; nucleus; tubercle
gracilespinal: fibers
gracilis: muscle; syndrome
grade I: astrocytoma
grade II: astrocytoma
grade III: astrocytoma
grade IV: astrocytoma
Gradenigo: syndrome
gradient: elution
gradient-recalled: acquisition in the steady state
graduate: nurse
graduated: compress; pipette; tenotomy
Graefe: forceps; knife; operation; sign; spots
Graefenberg: ring
Graffi: virus
graft versus host: disease; reaction
Graham: law

Graham-Cole: test
Graham Little: syndrome
Graham Steell: murmur
grain: alcohol; itch
Gram: iodine; stain
gram: calorie; equivalent
gram-: ion
gram-atomic: weight
Gram-chromotrope: stain
gram-molecular: weight
grand: climacteric; mal; multipara
granddaughter: cyst
grandiose: delusion
grandiose type of paranoid: disorder
grand mal: epilepsy; seizure
Granger: line; projection
Granit: loop
granny: knot
granular: cast; conjunctivitis; cortex; degeneration; foveolae; kidney; layer; layer of cerebellar cortex; layer of cerebellum; layer of epidermis; layers of cerebral cortex; layer of a vesicular ovarian follicle; leukoblast; leukocyte; lids; ophthalmia; pits; pneumonocytes; trachoma; urethritis
granular cell: myoblastoma; tumor
granular corneal: dystrophy
granular endoplasmic: reticulum
granulated: opium
granulation: tissue
granule: cell of connective tissue; cells
granulocyte colony-stimulating: factor
granulocyte-macrophage colony-stimulating: factor
granulocytic: leukemia; sarcoma; series
granulomatous: arteritis; colitis; disease; encephalomyelitis; endophthalmitis; enteritis; inflammation; mastitis; nocardiosis; rosacea
granulosa: cell
granulosa cell: tumor
granulosa lutein: cells
granulovacuolar: degeneration
grape: endings; mole; sugar
graphic: aphasia; formula
graphomotor: aphasia
grasp: reflex
grasping: reflex
grass: bacillus
Grasset: law; phenomenon; sign

Word Finder

Grasset-Gaussel: phenomenon
Gratiolet: fibers; radiation
gratuitous: inducer
Gräupner: method
grave: wax
Graves: disease; ophthalmopathy; orbitopathy
Graves optic: neuropathy
gravid: uterus
gravidic: retinitis; retinopathy
gravitation: abscess
gravitational: ulcer; units
gravity: concentration
Grawitz: basophilia; tumor
gray: cataract; columns; commissure; degeneration; fibers; hepatization; induration; infiltration; layers of superior colliculus; literature; matter; rami communicantes; scale; substance; syndrome; tuber; tubercle; wing
gray-scale: ultrasonography
greaseless: cream
great: foramen; toe I; vein of Galen
great adductor: muscle
great alveolar: cells
great anastomotic: artery
great auricular: nerve
great cardiac: vein
great cerebral: vein; vein of Galen
greater: circulation; cul-de-sac; curvature of stomach; horn of hyoid bone; omentum; pelvis; ring of iris; trochanter; tubercle (of humerus); tuberosity of humerus; wing of sphenoid (bone)
greater alar: cartilage
greater arterial: circle of iris
greater multangular: bone
greater occipital: nerve
greater palatine: artery; canal; foramen; groove; nerve
greater pancreatic: artery
greater pectoral: muscle
greater peritoneal: cavity
greater petrosal: nerve
greater posterior rectus: muscle of head
greater psoas: muscle
greater rhomboid: muscle
greater sciatic: notch
greater splanchnic: nerve
greater superficial petrosal: nerve
greater supraclavicular: fossa
greater tympanic: spine
greater vestibular: gland

greater zygomatic: muscle
greatest: length
great horizontal: fissure
great longitudinal: fissure
great radicular: artery
great saphenous: vein
great sciatic: nerve
great segmental medullary: artery
great superior pancreatic: artery
great-toe: reflex
green: hemoglobin; pus; sickness; soap; sputum; stain; tooth; vision
Greenfield: filter
Greenhow: disease
green monkey: virus
green soap: tincture
greenstick: fracture
green tobacco: sickness
Greig: syndrome
Greig cephalopolysyndactyly: syndrome
grenz: ray; zone
Greville: bath
Grey Turner: sign
grid: ratio
Gridley: stain; stain for fungi
Griesinger: disease; sign
grinding: surface
Grisolle: sign
Gritti: operation
Gritti-Stokes: amputation
Grocco: sign; triangle
grocer: itch
Grocott-Gomori methenamine-silver: stain
Groenouw corneal: dystrophy
Grönblad-Strandberg: syndrome
groove: sign
grooved: tongue
Gross: virus
gross: anatomy; hematuria; lesion
Gross leukemia: virus
gross reproduction: rate
ground: bundles; itch; lamella; state; substance
ground-glass: cytoplasm; pattern
ground itch: anemia
group: agglutination; agglutinin; antigens; dynamics; hospital; immunity; practice; psychotherapy; reaction; test; transfer; translocation
group A: streptococci
group A streptococcal necrotizing: fasciitis
group B: streptococci
Grover: disease
growing: fracture; pains

growing ovarian: follicle
growth: curve; factors; hormone; hormone-inhibiting hormone; hormone-releasing hormone; medium; phase; plate; rate; rate of population; regulators
growth arrest: lines
growth hormone–producing: adenoma
growth hormone-releasing: factor
growth-onset: diabetes
Gruber: cul-de-sac; method; reaction
Gruber-Landzert: fossa
Gruber-Widal: reaction
Grunert: spur
Grunstein-Hogness: assay
Grynfeltt: triangle
gryposis: penis
GTP binding: proteins
guaiac: gum; test
Guama: virus
Guanarito: virus
guanine: cell
guar: gum
Guarnieri: bodies
Guaroa: virus
gubernacular: canal; cord
Gubler: line; paralysis; syndrome; tumor
Gudden: commissure; ganglion
Gudden tegmental: nuclei
Guedel: airway
Guéneau de Mussy: point
Guérin: fold; fracture; glands; sinus; valve
guide: plane; wire
guided tissue: regeneration
Guillain-Barré: reflex; syndrome
guillotine: amputation
guinea corn: yaws
Guldberg-Waage: law
Gulf War: syndrome
Gullstrand: slitlamp
gum: contour; lancet; line; resection; resin
gummatous: abscess; syphilid; ulcer
Gumprecht: shadows
Gunn: dots; phenomenon; pupil; sign; syndrome
Gunn crossing: sign
Gunning: splint
Günning: reaction
gunshot: wound
gunstock: deformity
Günz: ligament
Günzberg: reagent; test
gurgling: rale
Gussenbauer: suture
gustatory: agnosia; anesthesia; aura; bud; cells;

hallucination; hyperesthesia; hyperhidrosis; lemniscus; nucleus; organ; pore; rhinorrhea
gustatory-sudorific: reflex
gustatory sweating: syndrome
gut: glucagon
gut-associated lymphoid: tissue
Guthrie: muscle; test
gutta-percha: cone; points; spreader
guttate: choroidopathy
gutter: dystrophy of cornea; fracture; wound
Guttman: scale
guttural: duct; pulse; rale
Gutzeit: test
Guyon: amputation; canal; isthmus; sign
Guyon tunnel: syndrome
GVH: disease
gym: -diol
gynecoid: obesity; pelvis
gynecophoric: canal
gyrate: atrophy of choroid and retina
gyrochrome: cell
gyromagnetic: ratio

H

H: agglutinin; antigen; band; colony; disk; fields; gene; graft; rays; reflex; shunt; substance
H-2: antigens; complex
H-: meromyosin
HA1: virus
HA2: virus
haarscheibe: tumor
Haase: rule
habenular: commissure; nuclei; sulcus; trigone
habenulointerpeduncular: tract
Haber: syndrome
Haber-Weiss: reaction
habit: chorea; cough; scoliosis; spasm; tic
habitual: abortion
HACEK: group
Haeckel: law
Haeckel gastrea: theory
***Haemophilus influenzae* type B:** vaccine
Haenel: symptom
Haff: disease
Haffkine: vaccine
hafussi: bath
Hagedorn: needle
Hageman: factor
Haglund: deformity; disease
Hahn oxine: reagent
Haidinger: brushes
Hailey-Hailey: disease

hair: bulb; cast; cells; crosses; cycle; disk; follicle; papilla; root; shaft; streams; transplant; whorls
HAIR-AN: syndrome
hairline: fracture
hairpin: loops; vessels
hairy: cells; heart; leukoplakia; mole; tongue
hairy cell: leukemia
Halberstaedter-Prowazek: bodies
Haldane: apparatus; effect; relationship; transformation; tube
Haldane-Priestley: sample
Hale colloidal iron: stain
Hales: piesimeter
half: cystine; hapten
half-: life; time
half amplitude pulse: duration
half axial: view
half-axial: projection
half-chair: form
half-glass: spectacles
half and half: nail
half-value: layer
Hallé: point
Haller: ansa; anulus; arches; cell; circle; cones; habenula; insula; line; plexus; rete; tripod; tunica vasculosa; unguis; vas aberrans
Hallermann-Streiff: syndrome
Hallermann-Streiff-François: syndrome
Haller vascular: tissue
Hallervorden: syndrome
Hallervorden-Spatz: disease; syndrome
Hallgren: syndrome
Hallopeau: disease
hallucinatory: neuralgia
halo: cast; effect; melanoma; nevus; sign; sign of hydrops; traction; vision
halogen: acne
halothane: hepatitis
halothane-ether: azeotrope
Halstead-Reitan: battery
Halsted: law; operation; suture
Ham: test
hamate: bone
Hamburger: phenomenon
Hamilton: pseudophlegmon
Hamilton anxiety rating: scale
Hamilton depression rating: scale
Hamilton-Stewart: formula; method
Hamman: disease; murmur; sign; syndrome
Hamman-Rich: syndrome

Hammarsten: reagent
hammer: finger; nose; toe
Hammerschlag: method
hammock: bandage; ligament
Hammond: disease
Hampton: hump; line; maneuver; technique
hamstring: muscles; tendon
hamular: notch; process of lacrimal bone; process of sphenoid bone
Hancock: amputation
hand: eczema; ratio
hand-and-foot: syndrome
hand-foot: syndrome
hand-foot-and-mouth: disease
hand-foot-and-mouth disease: virus
Hand-Schüller-Christian: disease
Hanes: plot
hanging: drop; septum
hanging-block: culture
hangman's: fracture
Hanhart: syndrome
Hanks: dilators; solution
Hannover: canal
Hanot: cirrhosis
Hansemann: macrophage
Hansen: bacillus; disease
Hantaan: virus
hantavirus pulmonary: syndrome
haphazard: sampling
haploid: set
haploscopic: vision
happy puppet: syndrome
Hapsburg: jaw; lip
hapten: inhibition of precipitation
haptic: hallucination
Harada: disease; syndrome
Harada-Ito: procedure
Harada-Mori filter paper strip: culture
hard: cataract; chancre; corn; drusen; palate; papilloma; paraffin; pulse; rays; soap; sore; tissue; tubercle; ulcer; water
hardened: pelvis
Harden-Young: ester
Harding-Passey: melanoma
hardness: scale
Hardy-Rand-Ritter: test
Hardy-Weinberg: equilibrium; law
hare's: eye
harlequin: fetus; ichthyosis; reaction
harmonic: mean; suture
harmonious retinal: correspondence
Harrington-Flocks: test

Harris: hematoxylin; lines; migraine; syndrome; test
Harrison: groove
Harris and Ray: test
Hartel: technique
Hartman: solution
Hartmann: curette; operation; pouch; solution
Hartnup: disease; syndrome
harvester: ant
Häser: formula
Hashimoto: disease; struma; thyroiditis
Hasner: fold
Hassall: bodies
Hassall concentric: corpuscle
Hassall-Henle: bodies
Hasson: cannula; trocar
hatchet: excavator
hatching: flask
Haudek: niche
Haverhill: fever
haversian: canals; lamella; spaces; system
Hawkins impingement: sign
Hawley: appliance; retainer
Haworth: projection
Haworth conformational formulas of cyclic: sugars
Haworth perspective and conformational: formulas
Haworth perspective formulas of cyclic: sugars
Hawthorne: effect
hay: asthma; bacillus; fever
Hayem: hematoblast; solution
Hayem-Widal: syndrome
Hayflick: limit
Haygarth: nodes
hazard: rate
H and D: curve
He: antigens
Head: areas; lines; zones
head: botflies; cap; cavity; cold; fold; kidney
head: mirror; nurse; presentation; process; tremors
head-bobbing doll: syndrome
head-dropping: test
healed: tuberculosis; ulcer
health: behavior; care; indicator; promotion; psychology
health information: system
health maintenance: organization
health risk: assessment
health status: index
healthy worker: effect
Heaney: operation
hearing: instrument; level; protectors
heart: antigen; arrest; attack; beat; block; failure; hormone; massage; position;

rate; sac; sounds; stroke; tamponade; tones; transplantation
heart chamber: remodeling
heart failure: cell
heart-lung: machine; preparation; transplantation
heart rate: turbulance
heart-shaped: pelvis; uterus
heart valve: prosthesis
heat: apoplexy; capacity; cramps; edema; exhaustion; hyperpyrexia; lamp; prostration; rash; rigor; stroke; treatment; urticaria
heat coagulation: test
heat-curing: resin
Heath-Edwards: grades
heat instability: test
heat-rigor: point
heat shock: proteins
heat-stable: enzyme
heavy: chain; hydrogen; metal; nitrogen; oxygen; water
heavy chain: disease
μ-heavy-chain: disease
γ-heavy-chain: disease
α-heavy-chain: disease
heavy liquid: petrolatum
heavy metal: neuropathy
hebephrenic: dementia; schizophrenia
Heberden: angina; nodes
Hebra: disease; prurigo
Hecht: pneumonia
Heck: disease
hectic: flush
hederiform: ending
Hedström: file
heel: bone; fly; jar; pad; region; spur; tap; tendon
heel-tap: reaction; test
heel-to-knee-to-toe: test
heel-to-shin: test
Heerfordt: disease
Hegar: dilators; sign
Hegglin: anomaly; syndrome
Hehner: number; value
Heidelberger: curve
Heidenhain: crescents; demilunes; law; pouch
Heidenhain azan: stain
Heidenhain iron hematoxylin: stain
height: vertigo
height of: contour
height-length: index
Heilbronner: thigh
Heim-Kreysig: sign
Heimlich: maneuver
Heineke-Mikulicz: pyloroplasty
Heinz: bodies
Heinz body: anemia; test
Heinz-Ehrlich: body
Heister: diverticulum; valve

Word Finder

HeLa: cells
Held: bundle; decussation
helical: CT
helical computed: tomography
helicine: arteries of penis; arteries of the uterus
helicis major: muscle
helicis minor: muscle
helicoid: choroidopathy; ginglymus
helicopod: gait
Helie: bundle
helium: speech
Heller: myotomy; operation; plexus
Hellin: law
HELLP: syndrome
Helly: fixative
helmet: cell
Helmholtz: energy; theory of accommodation; theory of color vision; theory of hearing
Helmholtz axis: ligament
Helmholtz-Gibbs: theory
helminthic: dysentery
helper: cells; virus
Helweg: bundle
Helweg-Larssen: syndrome
Helwig: bundle
hemadsorption: virus type 1; virus type 2
hemadsorption virus: test
hemagglutinating cold: autoantibody
hemagglutination: inhibition; test
hemal: arches; gland; node; spine
hemangiectatic: hypertrophy
hematinic: principle
hematogenetic: calculus
hematogenous: abscess; embolism; jaundice; metastasis; osteitis; pigment
hematoidin: crystals
hematopoietic: gland; system
hematoxylin: bodies
hematoxylin and eosin: stain
hematoxylin-malachite green-basic fuchsin: stain
hematoxylin-phloxine B: stain
hematuric bilious: fever
hemianopic: scotoma; spectacles
hemiazygos: vein
hemibody: radiation
hemic: calculus; distomiasis; murmur
hemifacial: spasm
hemilateral: chorea
hemiplegic: amyotrophy; gait; migraine
hemisulfur: mustard

hemithoracic: duct
hemizona: assay
Hemoccult: test
hemochorial: placenta
hemoclastic: reaction
hemoendothelial: placenta
hemoglobin C: disease
hemoglobin H: disease
hemoglobinuric: fever; nephrosis
hemolymph: gland; node
hemolysin: unit
hemolytic: anemia; anemia of newborn; crisis; disease of newborn; gas; jaundice; splenomegaly; streptococci
α-hemolytic: streptococci
β-hemolytic: streptococci
hemolytic plaque: assay
hemolytic uremic: syndrome
hemophilic: arthritis; joint
hemopoietic: tissue
hemorrhagic: anemia; ascites; bronchitis; colitis; cyst; cystitis; dengue; disease of the newborn; endovasculitis; fever; fever with renal syndrome; gangrene; glaucoma; infarct; iritis; measles; nephritis; pachymeningitis; pericarditis; pian; plague; pleurisy; rickets; scurvy; shock; smallpox
hemorrhagic exudative: erythema
hemorrhoidal: cushions; nerves; plexus; veins; zone
hemostatic: collodion; forceps
HEMPAS: cells
hen-cluck: stertor
Henderson-Hasselbalch: equation
Hendra: virus
Henke: space
Henle: ampulla; ansa; fissures; glands; layer; loop; membrane; reaction; sheath; spine; tubules; warts
Henle fenestrated elastic: membrane
Henle fiber: layer
Henle nervous: layer
Hennebert: sign
Henoch: chorea; purpura
Henoch-Schönlein: purpura; syndrome
Henri-Michaelis-Menten: equation
Henry: law
Henry-Gauer: response
Hensen: canal; cell; disk; duct; knot; line; node; stripe
Hensing: ligament
heparin: complement; unit

hepatic: adenoma; amebiasis; arteries; artery proper; branches of anterior vagal trunk; branches of vagus nerve; capsulitis; colic; coma; cords; cyst; duct; encephalopathy; fistula; flexure; infantilism; insufficiency; laminae; lobule; lymph nodes; porphyria; prominence; segments; steatosis; triad; veins
hepatic intermittent: fever
hepatic (nervous): plexus
hepatic portal: system; vein
hepatitis A: virus
hepatitis-associated: antigen
hepatitis B: vaccine; virus
hepatitis B core: antigen
hepatitis B e: antigen
hepatitis B surface: antigen
hepatitis C: virus
hepatitis D: virus
hepatitis delta: virus
hepatitis E: virus
hepatitis G: virus
hepatocellular: adenoma; carcinoma; jaundice
hepatocolic: ligament
hepatocystic: duct
hepatoduodenal: ligament
hepatoenteric: recess
hepatoerythropoietic: porphyria
hepatoesophageal: ligament
hepatogastric: ligament
hepatogenous: jaundice; pigment
hepatojugular: reflex; reflux
hepatolenticular: degeneration
hepatopancreatic: ampulla; sphincter
hepatophosphorylase deficiency: glycogenosis
hepatopleural: fistula
hepatorenal: ligament; pouch; recess of subhepatic space; syndrome
herald: patch
herd: immunity; instinct
hereditary: amyloidosis; angioedema; chorea; clubbing; coproporphyria; deafness; hearing impairment; hypersegmentation of neutrophils; hyperthyroidism; lymphedema; methemoglobinemia; myokymia; nephritis; photomyoclonus; pyropoikilocytosis; spherocytosis; syphilis

hereditary angioneurotic: edema
hereditary benign: telangiectasia
hereditary cerebellar: ataxia
hereditary deforming: chondrodystrophy
hereditary epithelial: dystrophy
hereditary folate: malabsorption
hereditary fructose: intolerance
hereditary hemorrhagic: telangiectasia; thrombasthenia
hereditary hypertrophic: neuropathy
hereditary hypophosphatemic: rickets
hereditary methemoglobinemic: cyanosis
hereditary multiple: exostoses; trichoepithelioma
hereditary nonpolyposis colorectal: cancer
hereditary opalescent: dentin
hereditary progressive: arthroophthalmopathy
hereditary renal: hypouricuria
hereditary sensory radicular: neuropathy
hereditary spinal: ataxia
heredofamilial: tremor
Hering: test; theory of color vision
Hering-Breuer: reflex
Hering sinus: nerve
Herlitz: syndrome
Hermann: fixative
Hermansky-Pudlak: syndrome
hernia: knife
hernial: aneurysm; sac
herniated: disk
heroin overdose: syndrome
herpes: encephalitis; virus
herpes B: encephalomyelitis
herpes simplex: encephalitis; virus
herpes zoster: virus
herpetic: fever; keratitis; keratoconjunctivitis; meningoencephalitis; ulcer; whitlow
herpetiform: aphthae
Herring: bodies; law
herring-worm: disease
Herrmann: syndrome
Hers: disease
Hershberg: test
Hertwig: sheath
hertzian: experiments
Herxheimer: reaction

herz: hormone
Heschl: gyri
Hess: law; screen; test
Hesselbach: fascia; hernia; ligament; triangle
heterochromic: cyclitis; uveitis
heterocyclic: compound
heterocytotropic: antibody
heterodetic: peptide
heterogametic: embryo
heterogeneic: antigen
heterogeneous: nucleation; radiation; system
heterogeneous nuclear: RNA
heterogenetic: antibody; antigen; parasite
heterogenous: keratoplasty; vaccine
heterogonic life: cycle
heterologous: antiserum; desensitization; graft; insemination; protein; serotype; stimulus; tumor; twins
heteromeric: cell; peptide
heterometabolous: metamorphosis
heterometric: autoregulation
heteronomous: psychotherapy
heteronymous: diplopia; hemianopia; image; parallax
heterophil: antibody; antigen; hemolysin
heterophile: antibody; antigen
heteroplastic: graft
heteropolar: bond
heteropyknotic: chromatin
heterotopic: bones; graft; pregnancy; stimulus
heterotrophic oral gastrointestinal: cyst
heterotropic: pregnancies
heterotype: mitosis
heterotypic: cortex
heterotypical: chromosome
heterovaccine: therapy
heteroxenous: parasite
Heubner: arteritis; artery
Heuser: membrane
hexacanth: embryo
hexaxial reference: system
hexazonium: salts
hexokinase: method
hexon: antigen
hexone: bases
hexose monophosphate: pathway; shunt
Hey: amputation; hernia
Heyer-Pudenz: valve
Hey internal: derangement
Heyns abdominal decompression: apparatus
HFR: strain
HG: factor
hiatal: hernia

Hib: vaccine
hibernating: gland; myocardium
Hickman: catheter
hidden: border of nail; part; part of duodenum
hidden nail: skin
hidebound: disease
hidrotic ectodermal: dysplasia
high: convex; enema; lithotomy; wine
high altitude: chamber
high-calorie: diet
high dose: tolerance
high-dose-rate: brachytherapy
high-egg-passage: vaccine
high endothelial postcapillary: venules
high-energy: compounds; phosphates
high energy phosphate: bond
higher order: conditioning; pregnancy
highest: concha
highest intercostal: artery; vein
highest nuchal: line
highest thoracic: artery
highest turbinated: bone
high-fat: diet
high-fiber: diet
high forceps: delivery
high-frequency: current; hearing impairment; ventilation
high frequency: transduction
high-grade squamous intraepithelial: lesion
high-kV: technique
high lip: line
high molecular weight: kininogen
Highmore: body
high osmolar contrast: agent; medium
high output: failure
high-pass: filter
high-performance liquid: chromatography
high-quality filter: paper
high-resolution: banding
high-resolution computed: tomography
high spinal: anesthesia
high-steppage: gait
Higoumenakia: sign
hilar: dance; lymph nodes; shadow
hilar cell: tumor of ovary
Hill: coefficient; constant; equation; operation; phenomenon; plot; reaction; sign
Hillis-Müller: maneuver
Hill's: criteria of evidence

Hill-Sachs: lesion
Hilton: law; method; sac
Hilton white: line
hilus: cells
hind: kidney
hindbrain: vesicle
hindquarter: amputation
Hines-Brown: test
hinge: axis; joint; movement; position; region
hinged: flap
Hinman: syndrome
Hinton: test
hip: bone; joint; phenomenon
hip-flexion: phenomenon
Hippel: disease
hippocampal: commissure; convolution; fissure; gyrus; sclerosis; sulcus
Hippocratic: nails
hippocratic: school; succussion
hippocratic: face; facies; fingers
hippocratic succussion: sound
Hirschberg: method; test
Hirschfeld: canals
Hirschowitz: syndrome
Hirsch-Peiffer: stain
Hirschsprung: disease
His: band; bundle; copula; line; rule; spindle
His bundle: electrogram
His perivascular: space
Hiss: stain
Histalog: test
histamine: flush; liberators; shock; test
histamine-releasing: factor
histaminic: cephalalgia; headache
His-Tawara: system
histiocytic: lymphoma
histocompatibility: antigen; complex; gene; testing
histoid: leprosy; neoplasm; tumor
histologic: accommodation
histological internal: os of uterus
histoplasmin-latex: test
histotoxic: anoxia
histrionic personality: disorder
hitchhiker: thumb
Hitzig: girdle
HIV: encephalopathy
HIV wasting: syndrome
HL-A: antigens
HLA: complex; typing
HMG CoA-reductase: inhibitors
Ho: antigen
Hoagland: sign
hobnail: cell; liver; tongue

Hoboken: gemmules; nodules; valves
Hoche: bundle; tract
Hodge: pessary
Hodgen: splint
Hodgkin: disease; lymphoma
Hodgkin-Key: murmur
Hodgson: disease
hoe: excavator; scaler
Hofbauer: cell
Hoffa: operation
Hoffman: violet
Hoffmann: duct; phenomenon; reflex; sign
Hoffmann muscular: atrophy
Hofmann: bacillus
Hofmeister: gastrectomy; operation; series
Hofmeister-Pólya: anastomosis
Hogben: number
hog cholera: vaccines; virus
Hogness: box
holandric: gene; inheritance
Holden: line
holiday: syndrome
holiday heart: syndrome
holistic: medicine; psychology
Holl: ligament
Hollander: test
Hollenhorst: plaques
Holliday: junction; structure
hollow: back; bone
Holmes: heart; stain
Holmes-Adie: pupil; syndrome
Holmes-Rahe: questionnaire
Holmgrén-Golgi: canals
Holmgren wool: test
holoblastic: cleavage
holocrine: gland
holoendemic: disease
hologynic: inheritance
holometabolous: metamorphosis
holosystolic: murmur
Holter: monitor
Holthouse: hernia
Holt-Oram: syndrome
Holzknecht: unit
Homans: sign
Home: lobe
home: monitor
home health: nurse
homeometric: autoregulation
homeostatic: equilibrium; lag
homeotic: genes
Homer-Wright: rosettes
homigrade: scale
hominal: physiology
homing: value
homocyclic: compound
homocytotropic: antibody
homodetic: peptide
homogametic: embryo

homogeneous: immersion; nucleation; radiation; system
homogenous: keratoplasty
homogonic life: cycle
homograft: reaction
homolecithal: egg
homologous: antigen; antiserum; chromosomes; desensitization; graft; insemination; proteins; recombination; series; serotype; stimulus; tumor
homologous serum: jaundice
homomeric: peptide
homonymous: diplopia; hemianopia; images; parallax
homoplastic: graft
homosexual: panic
homotypic: cortex
homovanillic acid: test
homozygous: achondroplasia
honey: urine
honeycomb: lung; macula; pattern; ringworm
Hong Kong: foot; influenza; toe
hooded: prepuce
hoof-and-mouth: disease
Hooke: law
hookean: behavior
hooked: bone; bundle of Russell; fasciculus
hook-shaped: cataract
hookworm: anemia; disease
Hoover: signs
Hopkins rod-lens: telescope
Hopmann: papilloma; polyp
horizontal: atrophy; cell of Cajal; cells of retina; fissure of right lung; fissure [TA] of cerebellum; fracture; heart; laryngectomy; osteotomy; overlap; part of duodenum; part of facial canal; planes; plate of palatine bone; resorption; transmission; vertigo
horizontal beam: film
horizontal growth: phase
hormonal: gingivitis
hormone replacement: therapy
Horner: muscle; pupil; syndrome; teeth
Horner-Trantas: dots
horny: cell; layer of epidermis; layer of nail
horsepox: virus
horseradish: peroxidases
horseshoe: fistula; kidney; placenta
Horsley bone: wax
Hortega: cells
Hortega neuroglia: stain

Horton: arteritis; cephalalgia; headache
hospital: fever; formulary; gangrene; nurse; record
hospital-acquired: pneumonia
hospital-based: physician
host: cell
hostile: behavior
hot: abscess; flash; flush; gangrene; nodule; pack; spot
hot salt: sterilizer
Hottentot: tea
hound-dog: facies
Hounsfield: number; unit
hourglass: contraction; head; murmur; pattern; stomach; vertebrae
house: staff; surgeon
housekeeping: genes
housemaid's: knee
Houssay: animal; phenomenon; syndrome
Houston: folds; muscle
Houston-Harris: syndrome
Howard: test
Howell: unit
Howell-Jolly: bodies
Howship: lacunae
Hoyer: anastomoses; canals
HR conduction: time
Hruby: lens
H-shape: vertebrae
H-type: fistula
H-type tracheoesophageal: fistula
Hu: antigens
Hubbard: tank
Hubrecht protochordal: knot
Hückel: rule
Hucker-Conn: stain
Hudson-Ståhli: line
Hueck: ligament
Hueter: maneuver
Hüfner: equation
Huggins: operation
Hughes-Stovin: syndrome
Huguier: canal; circle; sinus
Huhner: test
Hull: triad
human: babesiosis; botfly; communication; ecology; ehrlichiosis; fibrinogen; genetics; herpesvirus 1; herpesvirus 2; herpesvirus 3; herpesvirus 4; herpesvirus 5; herpesvirus 6; herpesvirus 7; herpesvirus 8; insulin; serum; thrombin
human antihemophilic: factor; fraction
human antimouse: antibody
human botfly: myiasis
β-human chorionic: gonadotropin

human chorionic: gonadotropin; somatomammotropin
human chorionic somatomammotropic: hormone
human diploid cell: vaccine
human diploid cell rabies: vaccine
human eosinophilic: enteritis
human fibrin: foam
human gamma: globulin
human glandular: kallikrein 3
human granulocytic: ehrlichiosis
human immunodeficiency: virus; virus-2
humanistic: psychology
human leukocyte: antigens
human measles immune: serum
human menopausal: gonadotropin
human monocytic: ehrlichiosis
human normal: immunoglobulin
human pertussis immune: serum
human placental: lactogen
human plasma protein: fraction
human α₁-protease: inhibitor
human scarlet fever immune: serum
human serum: jaundice
human T-cell lymphoma/leukemia: virus
human T-cell lymphotropic: virus
human T lymphotrophic: virus
humeral: artery; articulation; head
humeral axillary: lymph nodes
humeral nutrient: arteries
humeroradial: articulation; joint
humeroulnar: head of flexor digitorum superficialis muscle; joint
Hummelsheim: operation; procedure
humoral: doctrine; hypercalcemia of benignancy; immunity; pathology; regulator; theory
Humphry: ligament
hunger: contractions; pain; swelling
Hunner: ulcer
Hunt: neuralgia; syndrome
Hunter: canal; glossitis; gubernaculum; ligament;

line; membrane; operation; syndrome
Hunter and Driffield: curve
Hunter-Schreger: bands; lines
Hunter-Thompson: dwarfism
hunting: phenomenon; reaction
Huntington: chorea; disease
Hunt paradoxic: phenomenon
Hurler: disease; syndrome
Hurler-Scheie: syndrome
Hurst: bougies; disease
Hürthle: cell
Hürthle cell: adenoma; carcinoma
Huschke: cartilages; foramen; valve
Huschke auditory: teeth
Hutchinson: facies; freckle; incisors; mask; patch; pupil; teeth; triad
Hutchinson crescentic: notch
Hutchinson-Gilford: disease; syndrome
Hutchison: syndrome
Huxley: layer; membrane; sheath
Huygens: ocular; principle
HV: interval
HVA: test
HV conduction: time
H-Y: antigen
hyaline: bodies; bodies of pituitary; cartilage; cast; degeneration; leukocyte; membrane; thrombus; tubercle
hyaline membrane: disease of the newborn; syndrome
hyalocapsular: ligament
hyaloid: artery; body; canal; fossa; membrane
hyaloideoretinal: degeneration
hybrid: prosthesis
hydatid: cyst; disease; fremitus; polyp; pregnancy; rash; resonance; sand; thrill
hydatidiform: mole
Hyde: disease
hydralazine: syndrome
hydrate: crystal
hydrated: alumina
hydrate microcrystal: theory of anesthesia
hydraulic: conductivity
hydremic: edema
hydride: ion
hydroalcoholic: extract; tincture
hydroelectric: bath
hydrogen: acceptor; bond; carrier; donor; electrode; ion; number; pump; transport
hydrolytic: cleavage

hydrolyzing: enzymes
hydronium: ion
hydrophil: colloid
hydrophilic: ointment; petrolatum
hydrophobic: bond; colloid; interaction
hydropic: degeneration
hydrostatic: dilator; pressure
hydrous: wool fat
17-hydroxycorticosteroid: test
11-hydroxylase: deficiency
21-hydroxylase: deficiency
17-hydroxylase deficiency: syndrome
5-hydroxy tryptamine: antagonists
hygienic laboratory: coefficient
hygroscopic: expansion
hymenal: caruncula
hyobranchial: cleft
hyoepiglottic: ligament
hyoglossal: membrane; muscle
hyoglossus: muscle
hyoid: apparatus; arch; bone
hyomandibular: cleft
Hypaque: enema
hypaque: swallow
hyparterial: bronchi
hyperabduction: syndrome
hyperactive child: syndrome
hyperacute: rejection
hyperacute purulent: conjunctivitis
hyperbaric: anesthesia; chamber; medicine; oxygen; oxygenation
hyperbaric oxygen: therapy
hyperbaric spinal: anesthesia
hypercalcemic: sarcoidosis; uremia
hypercapnic: acidosis
hyperchloremic: acidosis
hyperchromatic: macrocythemia
hyperchromic: effect
hypercyanotic: angina
hyperendemic: disease
hypereosinophilic: syndrome
hyperergic: encephalitis
hyperextension-hyperflexion: injury
hyperfractionated: radiation
hyperfunctional: occlusion
hypergenic: teratosis
hyperglobulinemic: purpura
hyperglycemic-glycogenolytic: factor
hypergonadotropic: eunuchoidism; hypogonadism
hyper-IgM: syndrome
hyperimmune: serum

hyperimmunoglobulin E: syndrome
hyperkalemic periodic: paralysis
hyperkinetic: dysarthria; syndrome
hyperkinetic heart: syndrome
hyperlucent: lung
hypermature: cataract
hypermotor: seizure
hypernatremic: encephalopathy
hyperopic: astigmatism
hyperornithinemia-hyperammonemia-hypercitrullinuria: syndrome
hyperosmolar (hyperglycemic) nonketotic: coma
hyperostotic: spondylosis
hyperplastic: arteriosclerosis; gingivitis; inflammation; osteoarthritis; polyp; pulpitis
hyperprolactinemic: amenorrhea
hyperreactive malarious: splenomegaly
hyperreflexic: bladder
hypersecretion: glaucoma
hypersegmented: neutrophil
hypersensitive: dentin
hypersensitive xiphoid: syndrome
hypersensitivity: angiitis; pneumonitis; reaction; vasculitis
hypertensive: arteriopathy; arteriosclerosis; encephalopathy; retinopathy
hypertensive upper esophageal: sphincter
hyperthyroid: heart
hypertonic: bladder
hypertrophic: arthritis; cardiomyopathy; dystrophy; gastritis; pulpitis; rhinitis; rosacea; scar
hypertrophic cervical: pachymeningitis
hypertrophic hypersecretory: gastropathy
hypertrophic interstitial: neuropathy
hypertrophic pulmonary: osteoarthropathy
hypertrophic pyloric: stenosis
hypervariable: regions
hyperventilation: syndrome; test; tetany
hyperviscosity: syndrome
hypnagogic: hallucination; image
hypnogenic: spot
hypnoid: state

hypnopompic: hallucination; image
hypnotic: psychotherapy; relationship; sleep; state; suggestion
hypobaric spinal: anesthesia
hypobranchial: eminence
hypocalcemic: cataract
hypochondriac: region
hypochondriacal: melancholia; neurosis
hypochondrial: reflex
hypochromic: anemia; effect
hypochromic microcytic: anemia
hypocomplementemic: glomerulonephritis; vasculitis
hypocycloidal: tomography
hypodermic: injection; needle; syringe; tablet
hypoferric: anemia
hypofractionated: radiation
hypogastric: artery; ganglia; nerve; reflex; vein
hypoglossal: canal; eminence; nerve [CN XII]; nucleus; trigone
hypoglycemic: coma
hypogonadotropic: eunuchoidism; hypogonadism
hypohidrotic ectodermal: dysplasia
hypokalemic: nephropathy
hypokalemic periodic: paralysis
hypokinetic: dysarthria
hypometabolic: state; syndrome
hypomotor: seizure
hypoparathyroid: tetany
hypoparathyroidism: syndrome
hypopharyngeal: diverticulum
hypophyseal: cachexia; pouch
hypophyseoportal: system
hypophysial: amenorrhea; cachexia; duct; dwarf; fossa; infantilism; syndrome
hypophysial portal: circulation; system
hypophysioportal: system
hypophysiosphenoidal: syndrome
hypophysiotropic: hormone
hypoplastic: anemia; heart
hypoplastic fetal: chondrodystrophy
hypoplastic left heart: syndrome
hypopyon: ulcer
hyporeninemic: hypoaldosteronism

hypostatic: abscess; congestion; ectasia; pneumonia
hypotensive: anesthesia
hypothalamic: amenorrhea; infundibulum; obesity; obesity with hypogonadism; sulcus
hypothalamocerebellar: fibers
hypothalamohypophysial: tract
hypothalamohypophysial portal: circulation; system
hypothalamospinal: fibers
hypothenar: eminence; fascia; prominence
hypothermic: anesthesia
hypothetical mean: organism; strain
hypothyroid: dwarf; dwarfism; infantilism
hypoventilation: coma
hypovolemic: shock
hypoxanthine guanine phosphoribosyltransferase: deficiency
hypoxemia: test
hypoxia warning: system
hypoxic: hypoxia; nephrosis
hypoxic-hypercarbic: encephalopathy
hypoxic ischemic: encephalopathy
hypsiloid: angle; cartilage; ligament
Hyrtl: anastomosis; foramen; loop; sphincter
Hyrtl epitympanic: recess
hysterical: amblyopia; anesthesia; aphonia; ataxia; blindness; chorea; convulsion; gait; hearing impairment; joint; neurosis; paralysis; personality; polydipsia; pregnancy; psychosis; syncope; torticollis; tremor; vertigo
hysterical personality: disorder

I

I: antigens; band; cell; disk; pili; region
iatrogenic: pneumothorax; transmission
iatromathematical: school
ICAO standard: atmosphere
Iceland: disease; moss
I-cell: disease
ice pick: headache
ichorous: pus
ichthyosiform: erythroderma
icing: heart
iconic: signs

icterohemorrhagic: fever
ICU: psychosis
id: reaction
ideal alveolar: gas
identical: twins
identity: crisis; disorder; matrix
ideokinetic: apraxia
idiodynamic: control
idiographic: approach
idiojunctional: rhythm
idiomuscular: contraction
idionodal: rhythm
idiopathic: aldosteronism; bradycardia; cardiomyopathy; disease; epilepsy; gout; hirsutism; hypercalcemia of infants; hyperlipemia; hypertension; infantilism; megacolon; myocarditis; neuralgia; proctitis; roseola
idiopathic bilateral: vestibulopathy
idiopathic bone: cavity
idiopathic fibrous: mediastinitis; retroperitonitis
idiopathic hypercalcemic: sclerosis of infants
idiopathic hypertrophic: osteoarthropathy
idiopathic hypertrophic subaortic: stenosis
idiopathic interstitial: fibrosis
idiopathic orthostatic: hypotension
idiopathic paroxysmal: rhabdomyolysis
idiopathic pulmonary: fibrosis; hemosiderosis
idiopathic stabbing: headache
idiopathic subglottic: stenosis
idiopathic thrombocytopenic: purpura
idiosyncratic: sensitivity
idiotype: autoantibody
idiotypic: antibody
idiotypic antigenic: determinant
idioventricular: kick; rhythm
IgA: nephropathy
IgM: nephropathy
ileal: arteries; bladder; conduit; intussusception; orifice; papilla; sphincter; ureter; veins
ileoanal: pouch
ileocecal: eminence; fold; intussusception; junction; opening; orifice; valve
ileocecocolic: sphincter
ileocolic: artery; intussusception; lymph nodes; valve; vein
Ilhéus: encephalitis; fever; virus

iliac: arteries; bone; branch of iliolumbar artery; bursa; colon; crest; fascia; fossa; horn; muscle; region; roll; spine; steal; tubercle; tuberosity; veins
iliac (nervous): plexus
iliacosubfascial: fossa; hernia
iliacus: branch of iliolumbar artery
iliacus: muscle
iliacus minor: muscle
iliococcygeal: muscle; raphe
iliococcygeus: muscle
iliocostal: muscle
iliocostalis: muscle
iliocostalis cervicis: muscle
iliocostalis lumborum: muscle
iliocostalis thoracis: muscle
iliofemoral: ligament
iliohypogastric: nerve
ilioinguinal: nerve
iliolumbar: artery; ligament; vein
iliopectineal: arch; bursa; eminence; fascia; fossa; ligament; line
iliopelvic: sphincter
iliopsoas: muscle
iliopubic: eminence; tract
iliosciatic: notch
iliotibial: band; tract
iliotibial band: syndrome
iliotibial band friction: syndrome
iliotrochanteric: ligament
Ilizarov: technique
illegal: abortion
Ilosvay: reagent
image: amplifier; cytometer
imbrication: lines of von Ebner
Imerslünd-Grasbeck: syndrome
Imlach: fat-pad; ring
immature: cataract; granulocyte; neutrophil
immediate: allergy; amputation; auscultation; denture; hypersensitivity; percussion; reaction
immediate hypersensitivity: reaction
immediate insertion: denture
immediate posttraumatic: automatism; convulsion
immersion: bath; foot; lens; microscopy; objective
immobilized: enzyme
immobilizing: antibody
immotile cilia: syndrome
immovable: bandage; joint
immune: adherence; adsorption; agglutination; agglutinin; complex;

deficiency; deviation; hemolysin; hemolysis; inflammation; interferon; opsonin; paralysis; precipitation; protein; reaction; response; serum; suppression; surveillance; system; thrombocytopenia
immune adherence: phenomenon
immune adhesion: test
immune complex: disease; disorder; glomerulonephritis; nephritis
immune electron: microscopy
immune fetal: hydrops
immune response: genes
immune serum: globulin
immune thrombocytopenic: purpura
immunity: deficiency
immunoblastic: lymphadenopathy; lymphoma; sarcoma
immunochemical: assay
immunodeficiency: syndrome
immunofluorescence: method; microscopy
immunofluorescent: stain
immunologic: competence; deficiency; enhancement; mechanism; paralysis; tolerance
immunological: surveillance
immunologically activated: cell
immunologically competent: cell
immunologically privileged: sites
immunologic high dose: tolerance
immunologic pregnancy: test
immunoperoxidase: technique
immunoproliferative: disorders
immunoproliferative small intestinal: disease
immunoradiometric: assay
immunoreactive: insulin
impact: factor; resistance
impacted: fetus; fracture; tooth
impaired glucose: tolerance
impedance: angle; matching; method; plethysmography
imperative: conception
imperfect: fungus; stage; state
imperforate: anus; hymen
impermeable: junction
impetiginous: cheilitis
impingement: sign; syndrome; test
implant: denture

implantation: cone; cyst; theory of the production of endometriosis
implant denture: substructure; superstructure
implanted: suture
implosive: therapy
impression: area; compound; material; tray
impressive: aphasia
impulse control: disorder
impulsive: obsession
impure: flutter
inactivated: serum
inactivated poliovirus: vaccine
inactive: mutant; repressor; tuberculosis
inadequate: personality; stimulus
inanition: fever
inapparent: infection
inappropriate: affect; hormone
inborn: errors of metabolism; reflex
inborn error of: metabolism
inborn lysosomal: disease
incarcerated: hernia; placenta
incarceration: symptom
incarial: bone
incasement: theory
inception: rate
incest: barrier
incidence: density; rate
incident: angle; point; ray
incidental: color; learning; parasite
incipient: abortion; caries
incisal: edge; embrasure; guidance; guide; margin; path; point; rest; surface
incisal guide: angle
incised: wound
incision: biopsy
incisional: hernia
incisive: bone; canals; duct; foramen; fossa; papilla; suture
incisive canal: cyst
incisor: canals; crest; foramen; tooth
inclusion: blennorrhea; bodies; cell; compound; conjunctivitis; cyst; dermoid
inclusion body: disease; encephalitis
inclusion cell: disease
inclusion conjunctivitis: viruses
incomitant: strabismus
incompatible blood transfusion: reaction
incompetent cervical: os
incomplete: abortion; achromatopsia; agglutinin;

alexia; antibody; antigen; ascertainment; cleavage; disinfectant; fistula; fracture; hemianopia; metamorphosis; neurofibromatosis; tetanus

incomplete atrioventricular: block; dissociation

incomplete conjoined: twins

incomplete foot: presentation

incongruent: nystagmus

incongruous: hemianopia

increased markings: emphysema

incremental: lines; lines of von Ebner

incrusted: cystitis

incubation: period

incubative: stage

incubatory: carrier

incudal: fold; fossa

incudiform: uterus

incudomalleolar: articulation; joint

incudostapedial: articulation; joint

indentation: hardness

independent: assortment; variable

independent practice: association

indeterminate: cleavage; leprosy

index: ametropia; case; finger; hypermetropia; myopia

index extensor: muscle

indexical: signs

India ink capsule: stain

Indian: flap; ginger; gum; podophyllum; sickness

Indian podophyllum: resin

Indian tick: typhus

indicator: system; yellow

indicator dilution: method

indicator-dilution: curve

indifference to pain: syndrome

indifferent: cell; electrode; genitalia; gonad; oxide; tissue; water

indirect: agglutination; assay; calorimetry; diuretic; fracture; immunofluorescence; laryngoscopy; lead; method for making inlays; ophthalmoscope; ophthalmoscopy; oxidase; placentography; rays; retainer; retention; technique; test; transfusion; vision

indirect Coombs: test

indirect fluorescent antibody: test

indirect hemagglutination: test

indirect inguinal: hernia

indirect nuclear: division

indirect pulp: capping

indirect pupillary: reaction

indirect reacting: bilirubin

individual: differences; psychology; therapy; tolerance

individuation: field

indocyanine green: angiography

indole: test

indolent: bubo; ulcer

indophenol: method

induced: abortion; apnea; enzyme; fever; fit; hypotension; malaria; mutation; phagocytosis; radioactivity; sensitivity; symptom; trance

induced fit: model

induced psychotic: disorder

inducer: cell

induction: chemotherapy; period

inductive: resistance

indurative: myocarditis

industrial: disease; hygiene; psychiatry; psychology

industrial methylated: spirit

indwelling: catheter

inert: gases

inertia: time

inevitable: abortion

infant: death

infantile: acropustulosis; autism; beriberi; cataract; colic; convulsion; diplegia; dwarfism; eczema; fibrosarcoma; gastroenteritis; hemiplegia; hernia; hypothyroidism; leishmaniasis; myofibromatosis; myxedema; osteomalacia; pellagra; scurvy; sexuality; spasm; tetany

infantile acute hemorrhagic: edema of the skin

infantile celiac: disease

infantile cortical: hyperostosis

infantile digital: fibromatosis

infantile G_{M2}: gangliosidosis

infantile gastroenteritis: virus

infantile, generalized G_{M1}: gangliosidosis

infantile muscular: atrophy

infantile neuroaxonal: dystrophy

infantile neuronal: degeneration

infantile progressive spinal muscular: atrophy

infantile purulent: conjunctivitis

infantile spastic: paraplegia

infant mortality: rate

infected: abortion

infection: calculus; immunity

infection-associated hemophagocytic: syndrome

infection control: nurse

infection-exhaustion: psychosis

infection transmission: parameter

infectious: anemia; disease; endocarditis; granuloma; hepatitis; icterus; jaundice; mononucleosis; myositis; nucleic acid; plasmid; polyneuritis; wart

infectious bronchitis: virus

infectious crystalline: keratopathy

infectious ectromelia: virus

infectious eczematoid: dermatitis

infectious hepatitis: virus

infectious papilloma: virus

infectious porcine encephalomyelitis: virus

infective: embolism; jaundice; thrombus

inferential: statistics

inferior: angle of scapula; belly of omohyoid muscle; border; border of body of pancreas; border of liver; border of lung; border of pancreas; border of spleen; branch; branches of transverse cervical nerve; branch of oculomotor nerve; branch of pubic bone; branch of superior gluteal artery; colliculus; extremity; extremity of kidney; eyelid; fascia of pelvic diaphragm; fascia of urogenital diaphragm; fovea; ganglion of glossopharyngeal nerve; ganglion of vagus nerve; horn; horn of falciform margin of saphenous opening; horn of lateral ventricle; horn of thyroid cartilage; laryngotomy; ligament of epididymis; limb; limb of ansa cervicalis; lobe of (left/right) lung; margin; mediastinum; member; olive; part; part of duodenum; part of lingular vein (of left superior pulmonary vein); part of trapezius (muscle); part of vestibular ganglion; part of vestibulocochlear nerve; pole; pole of kidney; pole of testis; polioencephalitis; recess of omental bursa;

retinaculum of extensor muscles; root of ansa cervicalis; segment; surface of cerebellar hemisphere; surface of petrous part of temporal bone; surface of tongue; tarsus; trunk of brachial plexus; veins of cerebellar hemisphere; vein of vermis; vena cava; wall of orbit; wall of tympanic cavity

inferior aberrant: ductule

inferior accessory: fissure

inferior alveolar: artery; nerve

inferior anal: nerves

inferior anastomotic: vein

inferior articular: facet of atlas; pit of atlas; process; surface of atlas; surface of tibia

inferior basal: vein

inferior calcaneonavicular: ligament

inferior cardiac: vein

inferior carotid: triangle

inferior cerebellar: peduncle

inferior cerebral: surface; veins

inferior cervical: ganglion

inferior cervical cardiac: branches of vagus nerve; nerve

inferior choroid: vein

inferior clunial: nerves

inferior constrictor: muscle of pharynx

inferior costal: facet; pit

inferior dental: arch; artery; branches of inferior dental plexus; canal; foramen; nerve; rami

inferior dental (nervous): plexus

inferior duodenal: flexure; fold; fossa; recess

inferior epigastric: artery; lymph nodes; vein

inferior esophageal: constriction; sphincter

inferior extensor: retinaculum

inferior fibular: retinaculum

inferior frontal: convolution; gyrus; sulcus

inferior gemellus: muscle

inferior gingival: branches of inferior dental plexus

inferior gluteal: artery; nerve; veins

inferior hemiazygos: vein

inferior hemorrhoidal: artery; nerves; plexuses; veins

inferior hypogastric (nervous): plexus

inferior hypophysial: artery

inferior ileocecal: recess
inferior internal parietal: artery
inferiority: complex
inferior labial: artery; branches of mental nerve; branch of facial artery; vein
inferior laryngeal: artery; cavity; nerve; vein
inferior lateral brachial cutaneous: nerve
inferior lateral cutaneous: nerve of arm
inferior lateral genicular: artery
inferior lingual: muscle
inferior lingular: artery; branch of lingular branch of left pulmonary artery
inferior lingular (bronchopulmonary): segment [S V]
inferior lobar: arteries
inferior longitudinal: fasciculus; muscle of tongue; sinus
inferior lumbar: triangle
inferior macular: arteriole; venule
inferior maxillary: nerve
inferior medial genicular: artery
inferior medullary: velum
inferior mesenteric: artery; ganglion; lymph nodes; vein
inferior mesenteric (nervous): plexus
inferior myocardial: infarction
inferior nasal: arteriole of retina; colliculus; concha; venule of retina
inferior nasal retinal: venule
inferior nuchal: line
inferior oblique: muscle of head
inferior oblique: muscle
inferior occipital: gyrus; triangle
inferior occipitofrontal: fasciculus
inferior olivary: complex; nucleus
inferior omental: recess
inferior ophthalmic: vein
inferior orbital: fissure
inferior palpebral: veins
inferior palpebral (arterial): arch
inferior pancreatic: artery
inferior pancreaticoduodenal: artery
inferior parietal: gyrus; lobule
inferior pelvic: aperture

inferior peroneal: retinaculum
inferior petrosal: groove; sinus; sulcus
inferior phrenic: artery; lymph nodes; vein
inferior posterior serratus: muscle
inferior pubic: ligament; ramus
inferior quadrigeminal: brachium
inferior radioulnar: joint
inferior rectal: artery; nerves; veins
inferior rectal (nervous): plexus
inferior rectus: muscle
inferior renal: segment
inferior sagittal: sinus
inferior salivary: nucleus
inferior salivatory: nucleus
inferior segmental: artery of kidney
inferior semilunar: lobule
inferior subtendinous: bursa of biceps femoris
inferior and superior lobar: arteries
inferior suprarenal: artery
inferior tarsal: muscle
inferior temporal: convolution; gyrus; line of parietal bone; sulcus; venule of retina
inferior temporal retinal: arteriole; venule
inferior thalamic: peduncle; radiation
inferior thalamostriate: veins
inferior thoracic: aperture
inferior thyroid: artery; notch; plexus; tubercle; vein
inferior tibiofibular: joint
inferior tracheobronchial: lymph nodes
inferior transverse scapular: ligament
inferior triangle: sign
inferior turbinated: bone
inferior tympanic: artery
inferior ulnar collateral: artery
inferior ventricular: vein
inferior vesical: artery
inferior vesical venous: plexus
inferior vestibular: area; nucleus
inferolateral: margin; margin of cerebral hemisphere; surface of prostate
inferolateral myocardial: infarction
inferomedial: margin of cerebral hemisphere
infertile male: syndrome

infiltration: anesthesia
infinite: distance
inflamed: ulcer
inflammatory: carcinoma; corpuscle; edema; lymph; macrophage; polyp; pseudotumor; rheumatism
inflammatory fibrous: hyperplasia
inflammatory linear verrucous epidermal: nevus
inflammatory papillary: hyperplasia
inflatable: implant; splint
influenza: bacillus; pneumonia; viruses
influenzal virus: pneumonia
influenza virus: vaccines
information: system; theory
informational: RNA
infraauricular deep parotid: lymph nodes
infraauricular subfascial parotid: lymph nodes
infrabony: pocket
infracardiac: bursa
infraclavicular: fossa; infiltrate; part of brachial plexus; triangle
infraclinoid: aneurysm
infracostal: line
infraduodenal: fossa
infraglenoid: tubercle (of scapula); tuberosity
infraglottic: cavity; space
infragranular: layer
infrahyoid: branch of superior thyroid artery; bursa; muscles
infralobar: part of posterior vein (of right superior pulmonary vein)
inframammary: region
infranatant: fluid
infraorbital: artery; canal; foramen; groove; margin; nerve; region; suture
infraorbitomeatal: plane
infrapalpebral: sulcus
infrapatellar: branch of saphenous nerve; fat-pad
infrapatellar fat: body
infrapatellar synovial: fold
infrared: cataract; light; microscope; ray; spectroscopy; spectrum; thermography
infrascapular: artery; region
infrasegmental: part; veins
infraspinatus: bursa; fascia
infraspinatus: muscle
infraspinous: fascia; fossa
infrasternal: angle
infratemporal: approach; crest of greater wing of

sphenoid; fossa; surface of (body of) maxilla; surface of greater wing of sphenoid
infratrochlear: nerve
infundibular: part; recess; stalk; stem; stenosis
infundibuliform: fascia; hymen; sheath
infundibulo-ovarian: ligament
infundibulopelvic: ligament
infusion-aspiration: drainage
Ingelfinger: rule
Ingrassia: process
ingrowing: toenail
ingrown: hairs; nail
inguinal: branches of deep external pudendal arteries; canal; crest; falx; fold; fossa; hernia; ligament; ligament of the kidney; part of ductus deferens; region; triangle; trigone
inguinal aponeurotic: fold
inguinal lymphatic: plexus
inguinocrural: hernia
inguinolabial: hernia
inguinoscrotal: hernia
inguinosuperficial: hernia
inhalation: analgesia; anesthesia; anesthetic; therapy
inherited: character
inherited albumin: variants
inhibiting: antibody
inhibition: factor
inhibitory: fibers; nerve; obsession
inhibitory junction: potential
inhibitory postsynaptic: potential
initial: contact; dose; heat; hematuria; rate; velocity
initiating: agent; codon
initiation: codon; factor; tRNA
injection: flask; mass; molding
injury: potential
inkblot: test
inlay: graft; wax
innate: heat; immunity; reflex
inner: border of iris; layer of eyeball; lip of iliac crest; malleolus; membrane; sheath of optic nerve; stripes of renal medulla; table of skull; zone of renal medulla
inner cell: mass
inner dental: epithelium
innermost intercostal: muscle
inner nuclear: layer
inner plexiform: layer
inner spiral: sulcus
innervation: apraxia
innocent: murmur; tumor

innocent bystander: cell
innominate: artery; bone; fossa; substance; veins
innominate cardiac: veins
inorganic: acid; catalyst; chemistry; compound; diphosphatase; murmur; orthophosphate; phosphate; pyrophosphatase
inorganic dental: cement
inotropic: agents
inquiline: parasite
insect: viruses
insensible: perspiration; thirst
insertion: sequence
insertional: inactivation; mutagenesis
insight: learning
insoluble: soap
inspiratory: capacity; center; stridor
inspiratory reserve: volume
inspired: gas
inspissated bile: syndrome
instantaneous: vector
instantaneous electrical: axis
institutional review: board
instructive: theory
instrumental: amusia; conditioning
insufflation: anesthesia
insular: area; arteries; cortex; gyri; hypothesis; lobe; part; part of middle cerebral artery; sclerosis; veins
insulin: antagonist; injection; lipoatrophy; lipodystrophy; resistance; shock; unit
insulin coma: therapy; treatment
insulin-dependent: diabetes mellitus
insulin hypoglycemia: test
insulinlike: activity
insulinlike growth: factor
insulinopenic: diabetes
insulin receptor: substrate-1
insulin shock: treatment
insulin zinc: suspension
integral: dose; proteins
integrated rate: expression
integumentary: system
intellectual: aura
intelligence: quotient; test
intensification: chemotherapy
intensifying: screen
intensive: care; psychotherapy
intensive care: unit
intention: spasm; tremor
intentional: replantation
intention-to-treat: analysis
interaction process: analysis
interalveolar: pores; septum; space
interannular: segment
interarch: distance

interarticular: fibrocartilage; joints
interarytenoid: fold; notch
interatrial: block; foramen primum; foramen secundum; septum
interatrial conduction: time
interaural: attenuation
interauricular: arc
intercalary: neuron; staphyloma
intercalated: disk; ducts; nucleus
intercapillary: cell; glomerulosclerosis
intercapitular: veins
intercarotid: body; nerve
intercarpal: joints; ligaments
intercartilaginous: part of glottic opening; part of rima glottidis
intercavernous: sinuses
intercellular: bridges; canaliculus; cement; digestion; junctions; lymph
intercellular adhesion: molecule-1
interceptive occlusal: contact
interchondral: articulations; joints
interclavicular: ligament; notch
interclinoid: ligament
intercolumnar: fasciae; fibers; tubercle
intercondylar: eminence; fossa; line of femur; tubercle
intercondyloid: eminence; fossa; notch
intercornual: ligament
intercostal: anesthesia; arteries; ligaments; lymph nodes; membranes; nerves; neuralgia; space; veins
intercostobrachial: nerves
intercostohumeral: nerves
intercrural: fibers of superficial ring; ganglion
intercuneiform: joints; ligaments
intercurrent: disease
intercuspal: position
interdental: canals; caries; papilla; septum; splint
interdigital: folds
interdigitating reticulum: cell
interectopic: interval
interfacial: canals
interfacial surface: tension
interfascial: space
interfascicular: fasciculus
interference: beat; dissociation; microscope
interfoveolar: ligament
interganglionic: branches of sympathetic trunk

intergenic: complementation; suppression
interglobular: dentin; space; space of Owen
intergluteal: cleft
interiliac: lymph nodes
interim: denture
interjudge: reliability
interlaminar: jelly
interlobar: arteries of kidney; artery; duct; surfaces of lung; veins of kidney
interlobular: arteries; arteries of kidney; arteries of liver; duct; ductules; emphysema; pleurisy; septum; veins of kidney; veins of liver
interlocal: additivity
interlocking: gyri
intermaxillary: anchorage; bone; elastic; fixation; relation; segment; suture; traction
intermediary: metabolism; movements; nerve; system
intermediate: abutment; amputation; body of Flemming; branch of hepatic artery proper; bronchus; column; disk; filaments; ganglia; heart; hemorrhage; host; junction; lamella; layer; line of iliac crest; mass; mesoderm; nerve; part; part of adenohypophysis; part of male urethra; part of vestibular bulb; rays; region; trait; uveitis; variable; vein of forearm; zone; zone of iliac crest
intermediate acoustic: stria
intermediate antebrachial: vein
intermediate atrial: branch of left coronary artery; branch of right coronary artery
intermediate basilic: vein
intermediate cephalic: vein
intermediate cervical: septum
intermediate cubital: vein
intermediate cuneiform: bone
intermediate density: lipoprotein
intermediate dorsal cutaneous: nerve
intermediate great: muscle
intermediate hepatic: veins
intermediate hypothalamic: area; region
intermediate lacunar: lymph node; node
intermediate laryngeal: cavity
intermediate lumbar: lymph nodes

intermediate sacral: crest
intermediate supraclavicular: nerve
intermediate temporal: artery; branches of lateral occipital artery
intermediate vastus: muscle
intermediate white: layer [TA] of superior colliculus
intermediolateral: nucleus
intermediolateral cell: column of spinal cord
intermediomedial: nucleus
intermediomedial frontal: branch of callosomarginal artery
intermembrane: space
intermembranous: part of glottic opening; part of rima glottidis
intermenstrual: pain
intermesenteric arterial: anastomoses
intermesenteric (nervous): plexus
intermetacarpal: joints
intermetatarsal: articulations; joints
intermittent: albuminuria; arthralgia; claudication; cramp; hemoglobinuria; hydrarthrosis; hydrosalpinx; malaria; pulse; sterilization
intermittent acute: porphyria
intermittent explosive: disorder
intermittent malarial: fever
intermittent mandatory: ventilation
intermittent positive pressure: breathing; ventilation
intermittent self-: obturation
intermuscular: septum
intermuscular gluteal: bursa
internal: attachment; axis of eye; base of skull; branch of superior laryngeal nerve; branch of trunk of accessory nerve; canthus; capsule; conjugate; decompression; ear; energy; fistula; fixation; hemorrhage; hemorrhoids; hernia; hydrocephalus; lip of iliac crest; malleolus; medicine; meningitis; naris; nostril; ophthalmopathy; ophthalmoplegia; phase; pyocephalus; ramus of accessory nerve; representation; resorption; respiration; sheath of optic nerve; sphincter muscle of anus; squint; strabismus; surface; surface of cranial base; surface of frontal

Word Finder

bone; surface of parietal bone; table of calvaria; traction; urethrotomy

internal acoustic: foramen; meatus; opening; pore

internal adhesive: pericarditis

internal anal: sphincter

internal arcuate: fibers

internal auditory: artery; foramen; meatus; veins

internal capsule: syndrome

internal carotid: artery; nerve

internal carotid (nervous): plexus

internal carotid venous: plexus

internal cephalic: version

internal cerebral: veins

internal collateral: ligament of the wrist

internal conversion: electron

internal female genital: organs

internal iliac: artery; lymph nodes; vein

internal inguinal: ring

internal intercostal: membrane; muscle

internalized: homophobia

internal jugular: vein

internal lacrimal: fistula

internal male genital: organs

internal mammary: artery; plexus

internal maxillary: artery; plexus

internal medullary: lamina

internal nasal: branches

internal oblique: muscle

internal obturator: muscle

internal occipital: crest; protuberance

internal pillar: cells

internal podalic: version

internal pterygoid: muscle

internal pudendal: artery; vein

internal root: sheath

internal salivary: gland

internal saphenous: nerve

internal semilunar: fibrocartilage of knee joint

internal spermatic: artery; fascia

internal spiral: sulcus

internal thoracic: artery; plexus; vein

internal thoracic lymphatic: plexus

internal urethral: opening; orifice; sphincter

internasal: suture

international: unit

International Labour Organization: Classification

international normalized: ratio

international sensitivity: index

internet addiction: disorder

interneuromeric: clefts

internodal: segment

internuclear: ophthalmoplegia

internuncial: neuron

interobserver: error

interocclusal: clearance; distance; gap; record

interocclusal rest: space

interofective: system

interosseous: border; border of fibula; border of radius; border of tibia; border of ulna; bursa of elbow; cartilage; crest; fascia; groove; groove of calcaneus; groove of talus; margin; membrane of forearm; membrane of leg; muscles; nerve of leg

interosseous cubital: bursa

interosseous cuneocuboid: ligament

interosseous cuneometatarsal: ligaments

interosseous metacarpal: ligaments; spaces

interosseous metatarsal: ligaments; spaces

interosseous sacroiliac: ligaments

interosseous talocalcaneal: ligament

interosseous tibiofibular: ligament

interpalpebral: zone

interpapillary: ridges

interparietal: bone; sulcus; suture

interpectoral: lymph nodes

interpeduncular: cistern; fossa; ganglion; nucleus

interpersonal: conflict

interphalangeal: articulations; joints of foot; joints of hand

interpleural: space

interpolated: extrasystole; flap

interposition: arthroplasty

interpositospinal: tract

interpositus: nucleus

interproximal: papilla; space; surface of tooth

interpubic: disk; fibrocartilage

interpulmonary: septum

interradicular: alveoloplasty; septa of maxilla and mandible; space

interrater: reliability

interridge: distance

interrod: enamel

interrupted: respiration; suture

interscalene: triangle

interscapular: gland; hibernoma; reflex

interscapulothoracic: amputation

intersegmental: fasciculi; part of pulmonary vein; veins

intersemilunar: fissure

interseptovalvular: space

intersheath: spaces of optic nerve

intersigmoid: hernia; recess

interspinal: line; muscles; plane

interspinales: muscles

interspinales cervicis: muscles

interspinales lumborum: muscles

interspinales thoracis: muscles

interspinous: ligament; plane

interspongioplastic: substance

intersternebral: joints

interstitial: absorption; brachytherapy; cells; cystitis; deletion; disease; emphysema; fluid; gastritis; gland; growth; hernia; implantation; inflammation; keratitis; lamella; mastitis; myositis; nephritis; neuritis; nuclei of anterior hypothalamus; nucleus; nucleus of Cajal; nucleus of medial longitudinal fasciculus; pattern; pneumonia; pregnancy; therapy; tissue

interstitial amygdaloid: nucleus

interstitial cell: tumor of testis

interstitial cell-stimulating: hormone

interstitial plasma cell: pneumonia

interstitial pulmonary: fibrosis

interstitiospinal: tract

intertarsal: articulations; joints

intertendinous: connections of extensor digitorum

interthalamic: adhesion

intertragic: notch

intertransversarii: muscles

intertransverse: ligament; muscles

intertrochanteric: crest; fracture; line

intertropical: hyphemia

intertubercular: groove; line; plane; sulcus

intertubercular tendon: sheath

intertubular: zone

interureteric: crest; fold

intervaginal subarachnoid: space of optic nerve

interval: gout; operation; scale

intervening: sequence; variable

intervenous: tubercle (of right atrium)

interventional: angiography; radiology

interventricular: foramen; grooves; septum

interventricular septal: branches of left/right coronary artery

intervertebral: cartilage; disk; foramen; ganglion; notch; symphysis; vein

intervillous: lacuna; spaces

interzonal: mesenchyme

intestinal: anastomosis; angina; anthrax; arteries; atresia; calculus; capillariasis; cecum; digestion; emphysema; fistula; follicles; glands; intoxication; juice; lipodystrophy; lymphangiectasis; metaplasia; myiasis; rotation; sand; schistosomiasis; sepsis; stasis; steatorrhea; surface of uterus; villi

intestinal arterial: arcades

intestinal (lymphatic): trunks

in-the-canal: hearing aid

in-the-ear: hearing aid

intra-alveolar: septa

intraaortic: balloon

intra-aortic balloon: counterpulsation

intraaortic balloon: pump

intraarticular: cartilage; fracture; ligament of costal head; ligament of head of rib

intraarticular sternocostal: ligament

intraatrial: block; conduction

intraatrial conduction: time

intrabulbar: fossa

intracanalicular: fibroadenoma

intracapsular: ankylosis; fracture; ligaments

intracapsular temporomandibular joint: arthroplasty

intracardiac: catheter; lead

intracardiac pressure: curve

intracavernous: aneurysm; plexus

intracellular: canaliculus; digestion; enzyme; fluid; toxin; water
intracerebral: hemorrhage
intracorneal: implants
intracoronal: retainer
intracranial: aneurysm; cavity; ganglion; hematoma; hemorrhage; hypotension; part of optic nerve; part of vertebral artery; pneumatocele; pneumocele; pressure
intracranial granulomatous: arteritis
intractable: epilepsy; pain
intraculminate: fissure
intracutaneous: reaction
intracystic: papilloma
intracytoplasmic sperm: injection
intradermal: nevus; test
intraductal: carcinoma; papilloma
intraembryonic: mesoderm
intraepidermal: carcinoma
intraepiploic: hernia
intraepithelial: carcinoma; dyskeratosis; glands
intrafusal: fibers
intragenic: complementation; suppression
intraglandular deep parotid: lymph nodes
intraglandular parotid: lymph nodes
intragracile: sulcus
intrahepatic: cholestasis of pregnancy
intrailiac: hernia
intrajugular: process
intralaminar: nuclei of thalamus; part of intralocular part of optic nerve
intralesional: therapy
intraligamentary: pregnancy
intralobar: part of the posterior vein (of the right superior pulmonary vein)
intralobular: duct
intralocal: additivity
intramaxillary: anchorage
intramedullary: anesthesia; reamer; tractotomy; transfusion
intramembranous: ossification
intramural: hematoma; part of male urethra; practice; pregnancy
intranasal: anesthesia
in-transit: metastasis
intraobserver: error
intraocular: fluid; implant; neuritis; part of optic nerve; pressure

intraoral: anchorage; anesthesia; antrostomy
intraoral fracture: appliance
intraosseous: anesthesia; fixation
intrapapillary: drusen
intraparietal: sulcus; sulcus of Turner
intraparotid: plexus of facial nerve
intrapartum: hemorrhage; period
intrapelvic: hernia
intraperitoneal: pregnancy
intrapersonal: conflict
intrapulmonary: blood vessels; lymph nodes
intrarenal: arteries; reflux
intraretinal: space
intrasegmental: bronchi; part of pulmonary veins; veins
intraspinal: anesthesia
intratendinous: bursa of elbow
intratendinous olecranon: bursa
intrathalamic: fibers
intrathecal: injection
intrathyroid: cartilage
intratracheal: anesthesia; intubation; tube
intrauterine: amputation; contraceptive device; devices; fracture; insemination; pneumonia; transfusion
intrauterine contraceptive: devices
intrauterine growth: retardation
intravagal: glomus
intravaginal: torsion
intravascular: ligature; lymph
intravascular papillary endothelial: hyperplasia
intravenous: anesthesia; anesthetic; bolus; cholangiography; drip; narcosis; pyelography; urography
intravenous regional: anesthesia
intraventricular: block; conduction; hemorrhage; injection
intravital: stain; ultraviolet
intrinsic: asthma; color; deflection; dysmenorrhea; factor; fibers; motivation; muscles; muscles of foot; proteins; reflex; sphincter
intrinsicoid: deflection
intrinsic sympathomimetic: activity
intromittent: organ
introspective: method

intuitive: stage
intumescent: cataract
intussusceptive: growth
inulin: clearance
inundation: fever
InV: allotypes
invaginate: planula
invasive: carcinoma; mole
invasive pituitary: adenoma
inverse: anaphylaxis; symmetry; syntropy
inversed jaw-winking: syndrome
inverse ocular: bobbing
inverse-ratio: ventilation
inverse square: law
inversion: recovery
invert: sugar
inverted: image; papilloma; pelvis; reflex
inverted cone: bur
inverted follicular: keratosis
inverted radial: reflex
investigatory: reflex
investing: cartilage; fascia; layer; layer of cervical fascia; tissues
investment: cast
InV group: antigen
invisible: differentiation; light; spectrum
involuntary: guarding; muscles
involuntary nervous: system
involution: cyst; form
involutional: depression; melancholia
involved: field
iodate: reaction of epinephrine
iodide: acne
iodide transport: defect
iodinated: glycerol
iodinated ^{131}I human serum: albumin
iodinated ^{125}I serum: albumin
iodine: eruption; number; reaction of epinephrine; stain; test; value
iodine-induced: hyperthyroidism
iodized: collodion
iodophil: granule
iodotyrosine deiodinase: defect
ion: channel; pump
ion channel: disorders
ion exchange: chromatography
ion-exchange: resin
ionic: medication; strength
ionization: chamber
ionized: atom
ionizing: radiation
ion-selective: electrodes
ipecac: syrup
ipomea: resin

ipsilateral: reflex
iridescent: virus
iridial: part of retina
iridocorneal: angle
iridocorneal endothelial: syndrome
iridocorneal mesenchymal: dysgenesis
iridopupillary: lamina
IRI/G: ratio
iris: dehiscence; freckles; pits; spatula
Irish: moss
Irish moss: gelatin
iris-nevus: syndrome
iron: hematoxylin; index; line; lung; sulfate
iron-binding: capacity
iron deficiency: anemia
iron-dextran: complex
iron-storage: disease
iron-sulfur: proteins
irradiated vitamin D: milk
irreducible: hernia
irregular: astigmatism; bone; dentin; emphysema; nystagmus; pulse
irresistible: impulse
irreversible: colloid; hydrocolloid; pulpitis; reaction; shock
irritable: breast; colon
irritant contact: dermatitis
irritation: cell; fibroma
Irvine-Gass: syndrome
Isaac: syndrome
Isaac-Merton: syndrome
ischemia-modifying: factors
ischemic: contracture of the left ventricle; hypoxia; lumbago; necrosis; neuropathy
ischemic mitral: regurgitation
ischemic muscular: atrophy
ischemic optic: neuropathy
ischiadic: plexus; spine
ischial: bone; bursa; bursitis; ramus; spine; tuberosity
ischiatic: hernia; notch
ischioanal: fossa
ischiocapsular: ligament
ischiocavernous: muscle
ischiofemoral: ligament
ischiopubic: ramus
ischiorectal: abscess; fat-pad; fossa
Ishihara: test
island: disease; fever; flap
islet: cell; tissue
islet cell: tumor
isoallotypic: determinants
isobaric spinal: anesthesia
isochromic: anemia
isocyclic: compound
isodemographic: map
isodiphasic: complex

isodynamic: law
isoelectric:
electroencephalogram; line;
period; point; zone
isoenzyme: electrophoresis
isogeneic: graft
isogenic: strain
isogenous: chondrocytes; nest
isoimmune neonatal:
thrombocytopenia
isoionic: point
isolated: abutment;
dextrocardia; dyskeratosis
follicularis;
hypoaldosteronism;
proteinuria
isolated explosive: disorder
isolated parietal: endocarditis
isolecithal: egg; ovum
isologous: graft
isomeric: function; transition
isometric: chart; contraction;
exercise; period of cardiac
cycle; relaxation; ruler;
traction
isometric contraction: period
isometric relaxation: period
isomorphic: response
isomorphous: gliosis
isoniazid: neuropathy;
polyneuropathy
isopeptide: bond
isoperistaltic: anastomosis
isophane: insulin
isoplastic: graft
isoprene: rule
isopropanol precipitation:
test
isopycnic: zone
isorhythmic: dissociation
isosbestic: point
isoserum: treatment
isotonic: coefficient;
contraction; exercise;
traction
isotope: clearance
isotropic: disk; lipid
isovolume pressure-flow:
curve
isovolumetric: relaxation
isovolumic: interval; period;
relaxation
Itai-Itai: disease
Italian: flap
ITO: method
Ito: cells; nevus
Ito-Reenstierna: test
^{131}I uptake: test
Ivemark: syndrome
Ivor Lewis: esophagectomy
ivory: exostosis; membrane;
vertebra
Ivy bleeding time: test
Ivy loop: wiring

J

J: chain; point
Jaboulay: amputation;
pyloroplasty
Jaccoud: arthritis; arthropathy
jacket: crown
Jackson: law; membrane; rule;
sign; veil
jacksonian: epilepsy; seizure
Jacobaeus: operation
Jacobson: anastomosis; canal;
cartilage; nerve; organ;
plexus; reflex
Jacquart facial: angle
Jacquemet: recess
Jacquemin: test
Jacques: plexus
Jacquet: erythema
Jadassohn: nevus
Jadassohn-Lewandowski:
syndrome
Jadassohn-Pellizzari:
anetoderma
Jadassohn-Tièche: nevus
Jaeger: test types
Jaffe: reaction; test
Jaffe-Lichtenstein: disease
Jahnke: syndrome
jail: fever
jake: paralysis
jalap: resin
Jamaican vomiting: sickness
James: fibers; tracts
Jamestown Canyon: virus
Janet: test
Janeway: lesion
Jansen: operation
Jansky: classification
Jansky-Bielschowsky: disease
Japan: wax
Japanese B: encephalitis
Japanese B encephalitis:
virus
Japanese river: fever
Japanese spotted: fever
jargon: aphasia
Jarisch-Herxheimer: reaction
Jarman: score
Jarvik artificial: heart
Jatene: procedure
jaw: bone; jerk; joint; reflex;
repositioning; separation;
skeleton
Jaworski: bodies
jaw-winking: phenomenon;
syndrome
jaw-working: reflex
JC: virus
jealous type of paranoid:
disorder
Jeanselme: nodules
Jeghers-Peutz: syndrome
jejunal: arteries
jejunal and ileal: veins

jejunogastric: intussusception
jejunoileal: bypass; shunt
Jellinek: formula
Jendrassik: maneuver
Jenner: stain
Jenner-Kay: unit
Jensen: disease; sarcoma
jerk: finger
jerky: nystagmus; respiration
Jerne: technique
Jerne plaque: assay
Jervell and Lange-Nielsen:
syndrome
Jesuit: tea
jet: injection; injector;
nebulizer
jet ejector: pump
Jeune: syndrome
jeweller: forceps
Jewett: sound
Jewett and Strong: staging
j-g: complex
Jk: antigens
Job: syndrome
Jobbins: antigen
Jobert de Lamballe: fossa;
suture
Jocasta: complex
Jod-Basedow: phenomenon
Joffroy: reflex; sign
Johanson-Blizzard: syndrome
Johnson: method
joint: branches; capsule;
effusion; gamete; mice; oil;
probability; sense
jojoba: oil
Jolles: test
Jolly: bodies; reaction
Jones: criteria; test; transfer
Jones I: test
Jones II: test
Jonnesco: fossa
Jonston: alopecia
Joubert: syndrome
Joule: equivalent
Js: antigen
J-sella: deformity
Judet: view
Judkins: technique
jugal: bone; ligament; point
jugular: bulb; duct; foramen;
fossa; ganglion; gland;
glomus; nerve; notch of
occipital bone; notch of
petrous part of temporal
bone; notch of sternum;
process of occipital bone;
pulse; sinus; tubercle of
occipital bone; veins; wall
of middle ear
jugular foramen: syndrome
jugular lymphatic: plexus;
trunk
jugular venous: arch
jugulodigastric: lymph node;
node

juguloomohyoid: lymph node;
node
jump: flap
jumping: disease; gene
jumping the: bite
**jumping Frenchmen of
Maine:** disease
junction: nevus
junctional: complex; cyst;
epithelium; escape;
extrasystole; rhythm;
tachycardia
Jung: muscle
jungian: psychoanalysis
jungle: fever
jungle yellow: fever
Jüngling: disease
Junin: virus
junk: DNA
Junod: boot
Jurkat: cells
juvenile: angiofibroma;
arrhythmia; arthritis;
carcinoma; cataract; cell;
chorea; cirrhosis; diabetes;
elastoma; hemangiofibroma;
kyphosis; neutrophil;
osteoporosis; papillomatosis;
pattern; pelvis; periodontitis;
polyp; retinoschisis;
xanthogranuloma
juvenile absence: epilepsy
juvenile cerebellar:
astrocytoma
juvenile chronic: arthritis
juvenile hyalin: fibromatosis
juvenile muscular: atrophy
juvenile myoclonic: epilepsy
juvenile-onset: diabetes
juvenile palmo-plantar:
fibromatosis
juvenile plantar: dermatosis
juvenile spinal muscular:
atrophy
juxta-articular: nodules
juxtacolic: artery
juxtacortical: chondroma
juxtacortical osteogenic:
sarcoma
juxtaesophageal: lymph nodes
juxtaglomerular: apparatus;
body; cells; complex;
granules
juxtaglomerular cell: tumor
juxta-intestinal mesenteric:
lymph nodes
juxtamedullary: glomerulus
juxtaphrenic: peak
juxtapupillary: choroiditis
juxtarestiform: body

K

K: antigens; capture; cells;
complex; region; shell; virus
K-: radiation

Word Finder

Krukenberg: amputation; spindle; tumor; veins
Kruse: brush
krypton: laser
KTP: laser
Kufs: disease
Kugel anastomotic: artery
Kugelberg-Welander: disease
Kühne: fiber; methylene blue; phenomenon; plate; spindle
Kuhnt: spaces
Kuhnt-Junius: degeneration
Kulchitsky: cells
Külz: cylinder
Kümmell: spondylitis
Küntscher: nail
Kupffer: cells
Kürsteiner: canals
Kurtzke multiple sclerosis disability: scale
Kurzrok-Ratner: test
Kuskokwim: syndrome
Kussmaul: coma; disease; respiration; sign
Kussmaul-Kien: respiration
Kveim: antigen; test
Kveim-Siltzbach: antigen; test
Kyasanur Forest: disease
Kyasanur Forest disease: virus
kyphoscoliotic: pelvis
kyphotic: pelvis
Kyrle: disease

L

L: chain; doses; form; selectin; shell; unit of streptomycin
L⁺: dose
L-: meromyosin; radiation
L-: serine dehydratase
Laband: syndrome
Labbé: triangle; vein
labeled: atom; thyroxine
labial: arch; bar; branches of mental nerve; commissure; embrasure; flange; gingiva; glands; hernia; occlusion; part of orbicularis oris (muscle); splint; sulcus; swelling; tubercle; veins; vestibule
labile: affect; current; elements; factor; hypertension; pulse
labiodental: sulcus
labiogingival: lamina
labiolingual: appliance; plane
labioscrotal: folds; swellings
labor: curve; pains
laboratory: diagnosis
labored: respiration
Labrador: keratopathy
labyrinthine: apoplexy; artery; fistula; nystagmus; placenta; reflexes; torticollis;

veins; wall of middle ear; wall of tympanic cavity
labyrinthine righting: reflexes
Lac: operon
lacerated: foramen
Lachman: test
laciniate: ligament
lacis: cell
lacquer: cracks
lacrimal: apparatus; artery; bay; bone; border of maxilla; calculus; canaliculus; caruncle; conjunctivitis; fascia; fistula; fold; fossa; gland; groove; hamulus; lake; margin of maxilla; nerve; notch; opening; papilla; part of orbicularis oculi muscle; pathway; process of inferior nasal concha; punctum; reflex; sac; vein
lacrimoconchal: suture
lacrimogustatory: reflex
lacrimomaxillary: suture
La Crosse: virus
lactacid oxygen: debt
β-lactamase: inhibitors
lactase: persistence; restriction
lactate dehydrogenase: virus
lactated Ringer: injection; solution
lactating: adenoma
lactation: amenorrhea; hormone
lactational: mastitis
lacteal: cyst; fistula; vessel
lactic: acidosis
lactic acid: bacillus; fermentation
lactiferous: ampulla; ducts; gland; sinus
lactobacillary: milk
Lactobacillus bulgaricus: factor
Lactobacillus casei: factor
lactogenic: hormone
lacto-ovo-: vegetarian
lactophenol cotton blue: stain
lactose: intolerance
lacunar: abscess; amnesia; ligament; state; tonsillitis
lacunar-molecular: layer
Ladd: band; operation
ladder: splint
Ladd-Franklin: theory
Laënnec: cirrhosis; pearls
Lafora: body; disease
Lafora body: disease
lag: phase
lagophthalmic: keratitis
Lahey: forceps
Lahore: sore
Laimer-Haeckerman: area

Laki-Lorand: factor
laky: blood
Lallemand: bodies
Lallouette: pyramid
lamarckian: theory
Lamaze: method
LAMB: syndrome
Lambda: phage
lambdoid: border of occipital bone; margin of occipital bone; suture
Lambert: law; syndrome
Lambert-Eaton: syndrome
Lambl: excrescences
Lambrinudi: operation
lamellar: bone; cataract; granule; ichthyosis; keratoplasty
lamellated: corpuscles
laminar: flow
laminar cortical: necrosis; sclerosis
laminated: clot; cortex; epithelium; thrombus
laminated epithelial: plug
laminin: receptor
lampbrush: chromosome
Lan: antigen
Lancaster red green: test
Lancefield: classification
Lancisi: sign
land: scurvy
Landau-Kleffner: syndrome
Landolfi: sign
Landouzy-Dejerine: dystrophy
Landouzy-Grasset: law
Landry: paralysis; syndrome
Landry-Guillain-Barré: syndrome
landscape: ecology
Landschutz: tumor
Landsteiner-Donath: test
Landström: muscle
Landzert: fossa
Lane: band; disease; kink
Lange: solution; test
Langenbeck: triangle
Langendorff: method
Langer: arch; lines; muscle
Langerhans: cells; granule; islands
Langerhans cell: histiocytosis
Langer-Saldino: syndrome
Langhans: cells; layer; stria
Langhans-type giant: cells
Langley: granules
Langmuir: trough
language: game; zone
Lannelongue: foramina; ligaments
Lanterman: incisures; segments
lanugo: hair
Lanz: line

L-AP₄: receptor
laparoscopic: cannula; cholecystotomy; knot; nephrectomy; surgery
laparoscopically assisted: surgery
laparoscopic-assisted vaginal: hysterectomy; hysteroscopy
laparoscopic uterosacral nerve: ablation
laparotomy: pad
Lapicque: law
Laplace: forceps; law
Laquer: stain for alcoholic hyalin
larch: turpentine
lardaceous: liver; spleen
large: bowel; calorie; intestine; muscle of helix; pelvis; vein
large cell: carcinoma; lymphoma
large interarch: distance
large pudendal: lip
large saphenous: vein
Larmor: frequency
Laron type: dwarfism
Laroyenne: operation
Larrey: cleft
Larsen: syndrome
larval: conjunctivitis; plague
laryngeal: aditus; aperture; atresia; bursa; cavity; chorea; crisis; diphtheria; epilepsy; glands; granuloma; inlet; mask; mucosa; papillomatosis; part of pharynx; pharynx; polyp; pouch; prominence; reflex; saccule; sinus; stenosis; stridor; syncope; tonsils; veins; ventricle; vertigo; web
laryngeal lymphoid: nodules
laryngopharyngeal: branches of superior cervical ganglion
laryngospastic: reflex
laryngotracheal: diphtheria; diverticulum; groove
laryngotracheoesophageal: cleft
Lasègue: sign; syndrome
laser: corepraxy; iridotomy; microscope; photocoagulator; trabeculoplasty
laser-assisted in situ: keratomileusis
Lash: operation
Lash casein hydrolysate-serum: medium
Lassa: fever; virus
Lassa hemorrhagic: fever
Latarget: nerve; vein

late: cyanosis; deceleration; diastole; reaction; rickets; seizure; syphilis; systole
late apical systolic: murmur
late auditory-evoked: response
late benign: syphilis
late diastolic: murmur
late dumping: syndrome
late latent: syphilis
late luteal phase: dysphoria
late luteal phase dysphoric: disorder
latency: period; phase
latent: allergy; carcinoma; carrier; content; diabetes; empyema; energy; gout; heat; homosexuality; hyperopia; infection; learning; microbism; nystagmus; period; reflex; schizophrenia; stage; syphilis; typhoid; zone
latent adrenocortical: insufficiency
latent membrane: protein
latent rat: virus
late-phase: response
lateral: aberration; angle of eye; angle of scapula; angle of uterus; aperture of fourth ventricle; aspect; border; border of foot; border of forearm; border of humerus; border of kidney; border of nail; border of scapula; branches; branches of artery of tuber cinereum; branches of pontine arteries; branch of posterior rami of spinal nerves; canal; canthus; cartilage of nose; column; column of spinal cord; compartment of leg; condyle; condyle of femur; condyle of tibia; cord of brachial plexus; crus; crus of facial canal; crus of horizontal part of the facial canal; crus of the major alar cartilage of the nose; crus of the superficial inguinal ring; curvature; division of left liver; epicondyle of femur; epicondyle of humerus; excursion; fasciculus proprius; fillet; folds; fossa of brain; funiculus; funiculus of spinal cord; ginglymus; head; hermaphroditism; horn; illumination; incisor; lacunae; lacunae of superior sagittal sinus; lakes; lamina of cartilage of pharyngotympanic (auditory) tube; lemniscus; ligament of

ankle; ligament of bladder; ligament of elbow; ligament of knee; ligament of malleus; ligament of temporomandibular joint; ligament of wrist; limb; lip of linea aspera; lithotomy; malleolus; margin; mass of atlas; mass of ethmoid bone; meniscus; mesoderm; movement; nucleus; nucleus of mammillary body; nucleus of medulla oblongata; nucleus of thalamus; nucleus of trapezoid body; occlusion; part of longitudinal arch of foot; part of middle lobe vein (of right superior pulmonary vein); part of occipital bone; part of posterior cervical intertransversarii (muscles); part of posterior (extensor) compartment of forearm; part of sacrum; part of vaginal fornix; plate; plate of cartilaginous auditory tube; plate of pterygoid process; pole; process of calcaneal tuberosity; process of malleus; process of septal nasal cartilage; process of talus; projection; recess of fourth ventricle; region of abdominal region; region of neck; root of median nerve; root of optic tract; segment; sinus; sulcus; surface; surface of arm; surface of fibula; surface of finger; surface of leg; surface of lower limb; surface of ovary; surface of testis; surface of tibia; surface of toe; surface of zygomatic bone; tubercle (of posterior process) of talus; vein of lateral ventricle; ventricle; vertigo; wall of middle ear; wall of orbit; wall of tympanic cavity; zone
lateral abdominal: region
lateral abdominal/pectoral cutaneous: branches of intercostal nerves
lateral aberrant thyroid: carcinoma
lateral alveolar: abscess
lateral ampullar: nerve
lateral amygdaloid: nucleus
lateral antebrachial cutaneous: nerve
lateral anterior thoracic: nerve
lateral arcuate: ligament

lateral atlantoaxial: joint
lateral atlantoepistrophic: joint
lateral atrial: branch of left coronary artery; branch of right coronary artery; vein
lateral axillary: lymph nodes
lateral basal: branch
lateral basal (bronchopulmonary): segment [S IX]
lateral basal segmental: artery
lateral bicipital: groove
lateral bronchopulmonary: segment S IV
lateral calcaneal: branches of sural nerve
lateral cartilaginous: plate
lateral central palmar: space
lateral cerebellomedullary: cistern
lateral cerebral: fissure; fossa
lateral cervical: nucleus; region
lateral circumflex: artery of thigh
lateral circumflex femoral: artery; veins
lateral collateral: ligament of ankle
lateral condylar: inclination
lateral corticospinal: tract
lateral costal: branch of internal thoracic artery
lateral costotransverse: ligament
lateral cricoarytenoid: muscle
lateral cuneate: nucleus
lateral cuneiform: bone
lateral cutaneous: branch; branches of intercostal nerves; branches of ventral primary ramus of thoracic spinal nerves; nerve of calf; nerve of forearm; nerve of thigh
lateral decubitus: radiograph
lateral direct: veins
lateral dorsal: nucleus
lateral dorsal cutaneous: nerve
lateral epicondylar: crest; ridge
lateral femoral: tuberosity
lateral femoral circumflex: artery
lateral femoral cutaneous: nerve
lateral frontobasal: artery
lateral geniculate: body; nucleus
lateral glossoepiglottic: fold
lateral great: muscle
lateral ground: bundle

lateral habenular: nucleus
lateral humeral: epicondylitis
lateral hypothalamic: area; region
lateral inferior genicular: artery
lateral inferior hepatic: area
lateral inguinal: fossa
lateral jugular: lymph nodes
lateral lacunar: lymph node; node
lateral lingual: swellings
lateral longitudinal: arch of foot; stria
lateral lumbar intertransversarii: muscles
lateral lumbar intertransverse: muscles
lateral lumbocostal: arch
lateral malleolar: arteries; branch (of fibular peroneal artery); facet of talus; ligament; network; surface of talus
lateral malleolar subcutaneous: bursa
lateral malleolus: bursa
lateral mammary: branches; branches of lateral cutaneous branches of intercostal nerves; branches of lateral cutaneous branches of thoracic spinal nerves; branches of lateral thoracic artery
(lateral and medial) palpebral: arteries
(lateral and medial) parietal: arteries
lateral and medial posterior choroidal: branches of posterior cerebral artery
lateral medullary: branches of (intracranial part of) vertebral artery; lamina [TA] of lentiform nucleus; syndrome
lateral midpalmar: space
lateral myocardial: infarction
lateral nasal: artery; branches of anterior ethmoidal nerve; branch of facial artery; fold; process; prominence
lateral oblique: radiograph
lateral occipital: artery; sulcus
lateral occipitotemporal: gyrus
lateral olfactory: gyrus
lateral orbitofrontal: artery
lateral palpebral: commissure; ligament; raphe
lateral parabrachial: nucleus
lateral patellar: retinaculum
lateral pectoral: nerve
lateral pelvic wall: triangle

lateral pericardial: lymph nodes
lateral pericuneate: nucleus
lateral periodontal: abscess; cyst
lateral pharyngeal: space
lateral plantar: artery; nerve
lateral plate: mesoderm
lateral posterior: nucleus
lateral posterior cervical intertransversarii: muscles
lateral preoptic: nucleus
lateral proprius: bundle
lateral pterygoid: muscle; plate
lateral puboprostatic: ligament
lateral pyramidal: fasciculus; tract
lateral ramus: radiograph
lateral raphespinal: tract
lateral rectus: muscle of the head
lateral rectus: muscle
lateral recumbent: position
lateral reticular: nucleus
lateral reticulospinal: tract
lateral sacral: arteries; branches of median sacral artery; crest; veins
lateral sacrococcygeal: ligament
lateral segmental: artery
lateral semicircular: canals
lateral septal: nucleus
lateral skull: radiograph
lateral spinal: sclerosis
lateral spinothalamic: tract
lateral splanchnic: arteries
lateral striate: arteries
lateral superior genicular: artery
lateral superior hepatic: area
lateral superior olivary: nucleus
lateral supraclavicular: nerve
lateral supracondylar: crest; ridge
lateral supraepicondylar: ridge
lateral sural cutaneous: nerve
lateral talocalcaneal: ligament
lateral tarsal: artery
lateral tarsal strip: procedure
lateral temporomandibular: ligament
lateral thalamic: peduncle
lateral thoracic: artery; vein
lateral thyrohyoid: ligament
lateral tuberal: nuclei
lateral umbilical: fold; ligament
lateral vaginal wall: smear
lateral vastus: muscle
lateral venous: lacunae

lateral ventral: hernia
lateral vestibular: nucleus
lateral vestibulospinal: tract
late replicating: chromosome
latex agglutination: test
latex fixation: test
latissimus dorsi: muscle
latitude: film
lattice corneal: dystrophy
latticed: layer
Latzko cesarean: section
laudable: pus
laughing: gas
laughter: reflex
Laugier: hernia
Laumonier: ganglion
Launois-Bensaude: syndrome
Launois-Cléret: syndrome
laurel: fever
Laurence-Moon: syndrome
Laurer: canal
Lauth: canal; ligament
Lavdovsky: nucleoid
Lawrence-Seip: syndrome
lazarine: leprosy
LCAT: deficiency
L-chain: disease; myeloma
LCM: virus
L-D: body
LDH: agent
LDL receptor: disorder
LE: body; cell; factors; phenomenon
Le: antigens
lead: anemia; colic; encephalitis; encephalopathy; gout; line; neuropathy; palsy; paralysis; poisoning; stomatitis
leader: sequences
lead hydroxide: stain
leading: ancestor; edge
lead-pipe: colon; rigidity
leak point: pressure
leapfrog: position
Lear: complex
learned: drive
learning: disability; set; theory
least confusion: circle
least splanchnic: nerve
least squares: estimator
leather-bottle: stomach
Le Bel-van't Hoff: rule
Leber: plexus
Leber hereditary optic: atrophy
Leber idiopathic stellate: neuroretinitis; retinopathy
LE cell: test
Le Chatelier: law; principle
lecithin/sphingomyelin: ratio
LeCompte: maneuver; operation
lectin pathway: molecule
Lederer: anemia
Ledermann: formula

Lee: ganglion
Leede-Rumpel: phenomenon
Leeuwenhoek: canals
leeway: space
Lee-White: method
Le Fort: amputation; osteotomy; sound
Le Fort I: fracture
Le Fort II: fracture
Le Fort III: fracture
Le Fort III craniofacial: dysjunction
left: atrium of heart; auricle; branch; branch of hepatic artery proper; bundle of atrioventricular bundle; crus of atrioventricular bundle; crus of diaphragm; duct of caudate lobe of liver; heart; liver; lobe; lobe of liver; part of liver; ventricle
left anterior descending: artery
(left anterior) lateral hepatic: segment [III]
left atrioventricular: orifice; valve
left auricular: appendage
left axis: deviation
left colic: artery; flexure; lymph nodes; vein
left coronary: artery; vein
left fibrous: trigone (of heart)
left gastric: artery; lymph nodes; vein
left gastroepiploic: artery; lymph nodes; vein
left gastroomental: artery; lymph nodes; vein
left heart: bypass
left hepatic: artery; duct; vein
left inferior pulmonary: vein
left lateral: division of liver
left lumbar: lymph nodes
left main: bronchus
left marginal: artery
left medial: division of liver
(left) medial hepatic: segment [IV]
left ovarian: vein
(left posterior) lateral hepatic: segment III
left pulmonary: artery
(left and right) brachiocephalic: veins
left sagittal: fissure
left-sided: appendicitis
left-sided heart: failure
left superior intercostal: vein
left superior pulmonary: vein
left suprarenal: vein
left testicular: vein
left-to-right: shunt
left triangular: ligament of liver
left umbilical: vein

left ventricular: failure; myomectomy
left-ventricular assist: device
left ventricular ejection: time
left ventricular volume reduction: surgery
leg: phenomenon
Legal: test
legal: blindness; dentistry; medicine
Legendre: sign
Legg-Calvé-Perthes: disease
Legionnaires: disease
Leichtenstern: sign
Leigh: disease
Leiner: disease
Leishman: stain
Leishman chrome: cells
Leishman-Donovan: body
leishmanin: test
Leiter International Performance: Scale
Lejeune: syndrome
Lembert: suture
lemniscal: trigone
lemon: sign
Lendrum phloxine-tartrazine: stain
Lenègre: disease; syndrome
length-breadth: index
lengthening: reaction
length-height: index
Lenhossék: processes
Lennert: classification; lymphoma
Lennox: syndrome
Lennox-Gastaut: syndrome
Lenoir: facet
lens: capsule; pits; placodes; stars; sutures; vesicle
lens-induced: uveitis
lente: insulin
lenticular: ansa; apophysis; astigmatism; bone; capsule; colony; fasciculus; fossa; ganglion; knife; loop; nucleus; papillae; process of incus; syphilid; vesicle
lenticular progressive: disease
lenticulostriate: arteries
lentiform: bone
leonine: facies
LEOPARD: syndrome
leopard: fundus; retina
Leopold: maneuvers
Lepehne-Pickworth: stain
Lepore: thalassemia
lepra: cells
lepromatous: leprosy
lepromin: reaction; test
leprosy: bacillus
leprous: neuropathy
leptomeningeal: carcinoma; carcinomatosis; cyst; fibrosis; space

leptospiral: jaundice
Leri: pleonosteosis; sign
Leriche: operation; syndrome
Leri-Weill: disease; syndrome
Lermoyez: syndrome
Lerner: homeostasis
Lesch-Nyhan: syndrome
Leser-Trélat: sign
Lesser: triangle
lesser: circulation; cul-de-sac; curvature of stomach; horn of hyoid; omentum; pancreas; pelvis; ring of iris
lesser: trochanter; tubercle (of humerus); tuberosity of humerus; wing of sphenoid (bone)
lesser alar: cartilages
lesser arterial: circle of iris
lesser internal cutaneous: nerve
lesser multangular: bone
lesser occipital: nerve
lesser palatine: artery; canals; foramina; nerves
lesser peritoneal: cavity; sac
lesser petrosal: nerve
lesser rhomboid: muscle
lesser sciatic: notch
lesser splanchnic: nerve
lesser superficial petrosal: nerve
lesser supraclavicular: fossa
lesser tympanic: spine
lesser vestibular: glands
lesser zygomatic: muscle
Lesshaft: triangle
let-down: reflex
lethal: coefficient; dose; dwarfism; equivalent; factor; gene; mutation
lethality: rate
lethal midline: granuloma
lethargic: hypnosis
letter: blindness
Letterer-Siwe: disease
leucine: hypoglycemia
leucine-induced: hypoglycemia
leucine-sensitive: hypoglycemia
Leudet: tinnitus
leukemia inhibitory: factor
leukemic: leukemia; myelosis; reticuloendotheliosis; reticulosis; retinitis; retinopathy
leukemic hyperplastic: gingivitis
leukemoid: reaction
leukocyte: cream; inclusions; interferon
leukocyte adherence assay: test
leukocyte adhesion: deficiency

leukocyte bactericidal assay: test
leukocyte common: antigen
leukocytic: pyrogens; sarcoma
leukocytoclastic: vasculitis
leukocytosis-promoting: factor
leukoerythroblastic: anemia
leukopenic: factor; index; leukemia; myelosis
leukotriene receptor: antagonist
Lev: disease; syndrome
Levaditi: stain
levator: cushion; hernia; muscle of thyroid gland; swelling
levator anguli oris: muscle
levator ani: muscle
levatores costarum: muscles
levatores costarum breves: muscles
levatores costarum longi: muscles
levator labii superioris: muscle
levator labii superioris alaeque nasi: muscle
levator palati: muscle
levator palpebrae superioris: muscle
levator prostatae: muscle
levator scapulae: muscle
levator veli palatini: muscle
Levay: antigen
LeVeen: shunt
level-dependent frequency: response
Levey-Jennings: chart
Levin: tube
levoatrio-cardinal: vein
Levret: forceps
Lewis: acid; base
Lewy: bodies
Lewy body: dementia
Leyden: ataxia; crystals; neuritis
Leyden-Möbius muscular: dystrophy
Leydig: cells
Leydig cell: tumor
Lf: dose
Lhermitte: sign
libido: theory
Libman-Sacks: endocarditis; syndrome
Liborius: method
licensed practical: nurse
licensed vocational: nurse
lichen: amyloidosis
lichenoid: amyloidosis; dermatosis; eczema; keratosis
lichen planus-like: keratosis
Lichtheim: sign
lid: reflex

lid-closure: reaction
lid crutch: spectacles
Liddell-Sherrington: reflex
Lieberkühn: follicles; glands
Liebermann-Burchard: reaction; test
Liebermeister: rule
Liebig: theory
lienal: artery
lienophrenic: ligament
lienorenal: ligament
lienteric: diarrhea
Liesegang: rings
Lieutaud: body; triangle; trigone; uvula
life: cycle; instinct; stress; table
life-belt: cataract
life-span: development
Li-Fraumeni cancer: syndrome
ligand-binding: site
ligand-gated: channel
ligase chain: reaction
ligature: wire
light: adaptation; bath; cells of thyroid; chain; difference; metal; micrograph; microscope; reflex; sense; sleep; treatment
light-activated: resin
light-adapted: eye
light chain-related: amyloidosis
light-cured: resin
light differential: threshold
lighthouse: lens
light liquid: petrolatum
light-near: dissociation
lightning: strip
light-touch: palpation
light wire: appliance
ligneous: conjunctivitis; struma; thyroiditis
Likert: scale
Lillie allochrome connective tissue: stain
Lillie azure-eosin: stain
Lillie ferrous iron: stain
Lillie sulfuric acid Nile blue: stain
lilliputian: hallucination
limb: bud; lead; myokymia
limb-girdle muscular: dystrophy
limbic: lobe; system
limb-kinetic: apraxia
lime: water
liminal: stimulus; trait
limit: dextrin; dextrinase
limited neck: dissection
limiting: angle; decision; layers of cornea; membrane of retina; sulcus; sulcus of fourth ventricle; sulcus of Reil

limulus lysate: test
Lindau: disease; tumor
Lindner: bodies
line: angle; pairs; test
linear: acceleration; accelerator; amplification; amputation; atrophy; craniectomy; fracture; phonocardiograph; scleroderma
linear absorption: coefficient
linear energy: transfer
linear epidermal: nevus
linear IgA bullous: disease in children
linear skull: fracture
lined: flap
line spread: function
Lineweaver-Burk: equation; plot
Ling: method
lingual: aponeurosis; arch; artery; bar; bone; branches; branch of facial nerve; crypt; embrasure; flange; follicles; frenulum; gingiva; goiter; gyrus; hemiatrophy; lobe; lymph nodes; mucosa; muscles; nerve; occlusion; papillae; plate; plexus; quinsy; rest; septum; splint; surface of tooth; tonsil; trophoneurosis; vein
lingual-facial-buccal: dyskinesia
lingual gingival: papilla
lingual interdental: papilla
lingual salivary gland: depression
lingular: artery; vein
linguocervical: ridge
linguofacial (arterial): trunk
linguogingival: fissure; groove; ridge
linin: network
lining: cell
linkage: analysis; disequilibrium; group; map; marker
linker: DNA
linking: number
linnaean: system of nomenclature
lion-jaw bone-holding: forceps
lip: pits; reading; reflex; sulcus
lipase: test
lipedematous: alopecia
lipemic: retinopathy
lipid: granulomatosis; histiocytosis; keratopathy; pneumonia
lipid-mobilizing: hormone
lipoatrophic: diabetes
lipogenous: diabetes

lipoid: dermatoarthritis; granuloma; nephrosis; proteinosis; theory of narcosis

lipomatous: hypertrophy; infiltration; polyp

lipomelanic: reticulosis

lipophagic: granuloma

lipophagic intestinal: granulomatosis

lipoprotein: electrophoresis; polymorphism

lipoprotein(a): hyperlipoproteinemia

lipoprotein-associated coagulation: inhibitor

lipotropic: factor; hormone

Lipschütz: cell; ulcer

liquefaction: degeneration

liquefactive: necrosis

liquefied: phenol

liquid: air; extract; glucose; paraffin; petroleum; pitch; scintillator; ventilation

liquid crystal: thermography

liquid human: serum

liquid-liquid: chromatography

Lisch: nodule

Lisfranc: amputation; joints; ligaments; operation; tubercle

Lison-Dunn: stain

lispro: insulin

Lissauer: bundle; column; fasciculus; tract

Lissauer marginal: zone

Lister: dressing; method; tubercle

listeria: meningitis

Listing: law

Listing reduced: eye

Liston: knives; shears

literal: agraphia

lithium: carmine

lithotomy: position

litigious: paranoia

Little: area; disease

little: finger; fossa of the cochlear window; fossa of the oval (vestibular) window; head of humerus; toe [V]

little: ACTH

little league: elbow

Little Leaguer's: elbow

littoral: cell

Littré: glands; hernia

Litzmann: obliquity

live: vaccine

liveborn: infant

livedo: vasculitis

livedoid: dermatitis

live oral poliovirus: vaccine

liver: acinus; breath; bud; flap; palm; spot; starch

liver of: sulfur

liver cell: carcinoma

liver filtrate: factor

liver kidney: syndrome

liver *Lactobacillus casei*: factor

liver-shod: clamp

living: anatomy

L-L: factor

Lloyd: reagent

Lo: dose

load-and-shift: maneuver

loading: dose

lobar: bronchi; pneumonia; sclerosis

Lobo: disease

Lobry de Bruyn-van Ekenstein: transformation

Lobstein: ganglion

lobster-claw: deformity

lobular: carcinoma; carcinoma in situ; glomerulonephritis; neoplasia

lobular capillary: hemangioma

local: anaphylaxis; anemia; anesthesia; anesthetics; asphyxia; bloodletting; death; epilepsy; flap; glomerulonephritis; hormone; immunity; reaction; sign; stimulant; symptom; syncope; tetanus; tic

local anesthetic: reaction

local excitatory: state

localization: agnosia

localization-related: epilepsy

localized: osteitis fibrosa; pemphigoid of Brunsting-Perry; peritonitis; scleroderma

localized nodular: tenosynovitis

localizing: electrode; symptom

lock: finger; stitch

lock-: jaw

lock-and-key: model

Locke: solutions

locked: bite; facets; knee; twins

locked-in: syndrome

Locke-Ringer: solution

locking: suture

Lockwood: ligament

locomotor: ataxia

loculated: empyema

loculated pleural: effusion

loculation: syndrome

locust: gum

lod: method

Loeb: deciduoma

Loeffler: bacillus; methylene blue; stain; syndrome I; syndrome II

Loeffler blood culture: medium

Loeffler caustic: stain

Loevit: cell

Loewenthal: bundle; reaction; tract

Löffler: disease; endocarditis; syndrome

Löffler parietal fibroplastic: endocarditis

Logan: bow

logarithmic: phase; phonocardiograph

logistic: curve; model

Logistic Organ Dysfunction: Score

logit: transformation

lognormal: distribution

Lohlein-Baehr: lesion

Lohmann: reaction

Lombard voice-reflex: test

Lon: protease

Long: coefficient; formula

long: axis; axis of body; bone; chain; crus of incus; gyrus of insula; head; limb of incus; muscle of head; muscle of neck; process of malleus; pulse; root of ciliary ganglion; sight; vinculum

long abductor: muscle of thumb

long-acting thyroid: stimulator

long adductor: muscle

long association: fibers

long axis: view

long buccal: nerve

long central: artery

long-chain 3-hydroxyacyl-CoA dehydrogenase: deficiency

long-chain/very long-chain acyl-CoA dehydrogenase: deficiency

long ciliary: nerve

long cone: technique

long extensor: muscle of great toe; muscle of thumb; muscle of toes

long fibular: muscle

long flexor: muscle of great toe; muscle of thumb; muscle of toes

long incubation: hepatitis

long interspersed: elements

longissimus: muscle

longissimus capitis: muscle

longissimus cervicis: muscle

longissimus thoracis: muscle

longitudinal: aberration; arch of foot; arc of skull; bands of cruciform ligament of atlas; canals of modiolus; dissociation; duct of epoöphoron; fold of duodenum; fracture; layer of

muscle coat of small intestine; layer of muscular coat; layers of muscular tunics; lie; ligaments; method; relaxation; section; sinus; study; sulcus of heart

longitudinal cerebral: fissure

longitudinal oval: pelvis

longitudinal pontine: bundles; fasciculi; fibers

longitudinal vertebral venous: sinus

long-leg: arthropathy

long levatores costarum: muscles

Longmire: operation

long palmar: muscle

long peroneal: muscle

long pitch helicoidal: layer

long plantar: ligament

long posterior ciliary: arteries

long QT: syndromes

long radial extensor: muscle of wrist

long saphenous: nerve; vein

long subscapular: nerve

long-term: memory

long terminal repeat: sequences

long thoracic: artery; nerve; vein

longus capitis: muscle

longus colli: muscle

loop: diuretic; excision; resection; stoma

loop electrocautery excision: procedure

loop electrosurgical excision: procedure

loose: associations; body; cartilage; skin

Looser: lines; zones

lop: ear

Lorain: disease

Lorain-Lévi: dwarfism; infantilism; syndrome

lordotic: albuminuria; pelvis

Lorenz: sign

Lorenzo: oil

Loschmidt: number

loudness discomfort: level

Lou Gehrig: disease

Louis: angle; law

Louis-Bar: syndrome

louping-ill: virus

louse: flies

louse-borne: typhus

Lovén: reflex

Lovibond: angle

Lovibond profile: sign

low: convex; wine

low-calorie: diet

low-density lipoprotein: receptors

Lowe: syndrome

low-egg-passage: vaccine

Löwenberg: canal; forceps; scala
Lowenstein-Jensen: medium
Lowenstein-Jensen culture: medium
Lower: ring; tubercle
lower: airway; extremity; eyelid; jaw; lid; limb; lip; lobe of lung; pole; pole of testis
lower abdominal periosteal: reflex
lower alveolar: point
lower dental: arcade
lower esophageal: sphincter
lower motor: neuron
lower motor neuron: dysarthria; lesion
lower nephron: nephrosis
lower respiratory tract: smear
lower ridge: slope
lower uterine: segment
lower uterine segment cesarean: section
lowest lumbar: arteries
lowest splanchnic: nerve
lowest thyroid: artery
Lowe-Terrey-MacLachlan: syndrome
low-fat: diet
low forceps: delivery
low frequency: transduction
low grade: astrocytoma
low-grade squamous intraepithelial: lesion
low lip: line
low malignant potential: tumor
low molecular weight: kininogen; proteins
Lown-Ganong-Levine: syndrome
low osmolar contrast: agent; medium
low output: failure
low-pass: filter
low purine: diet
low residue: diet
Lowry-Folin: assay
Lowry protein: assay
low salt: diet; syndrome
Lowsley: tractor
low spinal: anesthesia
low-tension: glaucoma
L-phase: variants
Lr: dose
L/S: ratio
Lu: antigens
Lubarsch: crystals
Lublows: diverticulum
lubricating: cream
Luc: operation
Lucas: groove
lucid: interval
Lucio: leprosy

Lucio leprosy: phenomenon
Lucké: virus
Lücke: test
Ludwig: angina; angle; ganglion; labyrinth; nerve; stromuhr
Luer: syringe
Luer-Lok: syringe
luetic: mask
Luft: disease
Luft potassium permanganate: fixative
Lugol iodine: solution
Lukes-Collins: classification
lumbar: appendicitis; arteries; branch of iliolumbar artery; cistern; flexure; ganglia; hernia; lordosis; lymph nodes; myelogram; nephrectomy; nerves [L1–L5]; part of diaphragm; part of spinal cord; puncture; region; rib; segments L1–L5 of spinal cord; segments of spinal cord L1–5; triangle; veins; vertebrae [L1–L5]
lumbar iliocostal: muscle
lumbar interspinal: muscle
lumbar lymphatic: plexus
lumbar (lymphatic): trunks
lumbar (nervous): plexus
lumbar puncture: needle
lumbar quadrate: muscle
lumbar rotator: muscles
lumbar splanchnic: nerves
lumberman's: itch
lumbocostal: ligament; triangle of diaphragm
lumbocostoabdominal: triangle
lumbodorsal: fascia
lumboinguinal: nerve
lumbosacral: angle; enlargement; enlargement of spinal cord; joint
lumbosacral (nerve): trunk
lumbosacral (nervous): plexus
lumbotomy: incision
lumbricals lumbrical: muscles of foot; muscles of hand
luminous: flux; intensity; retinoscope
lumpy: jaw
Luna-Ishak: stain
lunar: periodicity
lunate: bone; fissure; sulcus; surface of acetabulum
Lundh: meal
lung: bud; unit; window
lung fluke: disease
lung volume reduction: surgery
Lunyo: virus

lupoid: hepatitis; leishmaniasis; sycosis; ulcer
lupus: anticoagulant; nephritis
lupus band: test
lupus erythematosus: cell; panniculitis
lupus erythematosus cell: test
lupus-like: syndrome
Luschka: bursa; cartilage; ducts; gland; joints; ligaments; sinus; tonsil
Luschka cystic: glands
Luse: bodies
luteal: cell; phase
luteal phase: defect; deficiency
luteinized unruptured: follicle
luteinizing: hormone; principle
luteinizing hormone/follicle-stimulating hormone-releasing: factor
luteinizing hormone-releasing: factor; hormone
Lutembacher: syndrome
luteoplacental: shift
luting: agent
Lutz-Splendore-Almeida: disease
Luys: body
Lyell: disease; syndrome
Lyme: arthritis; borreliosis; disease
lymph: capillary; cell; circulation; cords; corpuscle; embolism; gland; node; nodule; sacs; scrotum; sinus; space; varix; vessels
lymphadenoid: goiter
lymphadenopathy-associated: virus
lymphangitic: carcinomatosis
lymphatic: angina; duct; edema; fistula; follicles of larynx; follicles of rectum; leukemia; nodule; plexus; ring of cardiac part of stomach; sarcoma; sinus; stroma; system; tissue; valvule; vessels
lymphatic filariasis: granuloma
lymphedematous: keratoderma
lymph node permeability: factor
lymphoblastic: leukemia; lymphoma
lymphocyte: transformation
lymphocyte function associated: antigen
lymphocyte-mediated: cytotoxicity
lymphocytic: adenohypophysitis;

choriomeningitis; hypophysitis; leukemia; leukemoid reaction; leukocytosis; leukopenia; series; thyroiditis
lymphocytic choriomeningitis: virus
lymphocytic interstitial: pneumonia; pneumonitis
lymphocytotoxic: antibodies
lymphoepithelial: cyst
lymphogenous: metastasis
lymphogranuloma venereum: antigen; virus
lymphoid: cell; hemoblast of Pappenheim; hypophysitis; leukemia; nodule; polyp; system
lymphoid interstitial: pneumonia
lymphomatoid: granulomatosis; papulosis; polyposis
lymphoplasmacellular: disorders
lymphoproliferative: syndrome
lymphostatic: verrucosis
Lynch: syndrome
Lyon: hypothesis
lyophilic: colloid
lyophobic: colloid
lyotropic: series
lysinuric protein: intolerance
lysogenic: bacterium; induction; strain
lysosomal: disease
Lyt: antigens

M

M: antigen; band; cell; concentration; line; phase; protein; shell
M2: segment of middle cerebral artery
M$_1$: antigen
MAC: complex
Macchiavello: stain
MacConkey: agar
Macewen: sign; symptom; triangle
Mach: band; effect; line; number
Machado-Guerreiro: test
Machado-Joseph: disease
machinery: murmur
Machupo: virus
Mackay-Marg: tonometer
Mackenrodt: ligament
Mackenzie: amputation; polygraph
Maclagan: test
Maclagan thymol turbidity: test

Macleod: rheumatism; syndrome
MacNeal tetrachrome blood: stain
macroaggregated: albumin
macrobiotic: diet
macrocytic: anemia; anemia of pregnancy; anemia tropical; hyperchromia
macrocytic achylic: anemia
macrofollicular: adenoma
macroglia: cell
macro-Kjeldahl: method
macromolecular: chemistry
macrophage-activating: factor
macrophage colony-stimulating: factor
macrophage inflammatory: protein
macrophage migration inhibition: test
macroscopic: anatomy; sphincter
macular: amyloidosis; area; arteries; atrophy; coloboma; degeneration; drusen; erythema; evasion; fasciculus; leprosy; retinopathy; syphilid
macular corneal: dystrophy
macular retinal: dystrophy
mad cow: disease
Maddox: rod
Madelung: deformity; disease; neck
Mad Hatter: syndrome
Madlener: operation
Madura: boil; foot
Maffucci: syndrome
Magendie: law; spaces
Magendie-Hertwig: sign; syndrome
magenta: tongue
magic: forceps
magical: thinking
Magill: forceps
Magnan: sign
Magnan trombone: movement
magnesia and alumina oral: suspension
magnet: reaction; reflex
magnetic: attraction; field; implant; inertia
magnetic field: gradient
magnetic resonance: angiography; imaging; spectroscopy
magnetogyric: ratio
magnification: angiography; radiography
magnitude: image
Magnus: sign
Mahaim: fibers
Maier: sinus

maintenance: dose
maintenance drug: therapy
Maissiat: band
maize: factor
Majocchi: disease; granulomas
major: agglutinin; amblyoscope; amputation; calices; circulus arteriosus of iris; connector; depression; epilepsy; fissure; forceps; groove; hippocampus; hypnosis; hysteria; operation; surgery; tranquilizer
major alar: cartilage
major arterial: circle of iris
major depressive: disorder
major duodenal: papilla
major histocompatibility: complex
major mood: disorder
major motor: seizure
major salivary: glands
major sublingual: duct
Makeham: hypothesis
Malabar: itch; leprosy
malabsorption: syndrome
Malacarne: pyramid; space
malar: arch; bone; flush; fold; foramen; lymph node; node; point; process
malariae: malaria
malarial: cachexia; crescent; fever; hemoglobinuria; knobs; periodicity; pigment
malarial pigment: stain
Malassez epithelial: rests
malate-aspartate: shuttle
malate-condensing: enzyme
Maldonado-San Jose: stain
male: breast; gonad; hermaphroditism; homosexuality; hypogonadism; pseudohermaphroditism; sterility; urethra
Malecot: catheter
male external: genitalia
male internal: genitalia
male pattern: alopecia; baldness
Malgaigne: amputation; fossa; hernia; luxation; triangle
Malherbe calcifying: epithelioma
malic: enzyme
malignant: anemia; bubo; dysentery; dyskeratosis; endocarditis; exophthalmos; glaucoma; granuloma; hepatoma; histiocytosis; hyperphenylalaninemia; hyperpyrexia; hypertension; hyperthermia; jaundice; lymphadenosis; lymphoma;

malnutrition; melanoma; melanoma in situ; meningioma; myopia; nephrosclerosis; pustule; scleritis; smallpox; stupor; tumor
malignant atrophic: papulosis
malignant carcinoid: syndrome
malignant catarrhal fever: virus
malignant ciliary: epithelioma
malignant external: otitis
malignant fibrous: histiocytoma
malignant lentigo: melanoma
malignant midline: reticulosis
malignant mixed müllerian: tumor
malignant mole: syndrome
malignant tertian: fever; malaria
malignant tertian malarial: parasite
Mall: formula; ridges
mallear: folds; prominence; stripe
malleolar: groove; stria; sulcus
malleolar articular: surface of fibula; surface of tibia
mallet: finger
Mallory: bodies; stain for actinomyces; stain for hemofuchsin
Mallory aniline blue: stain
Mallory collagen: stain
Mallory iodine: stain
Mallory phloxine: stain
Mallory phosphotungstic acid hematoxylin: stain
Mallory trichrome: stain
Mallory triple: stain
Mallory-Weiss: lesion; syndrome; tear
malondialdehyde-modified low-density: lipoprotein
Maloney: bougies
malpighian: bodies; capsule; cell; corpuscles; glands; glomerulus; layer; nodules; pyramid; rete; stigmas; stratum; tubules; tuft; vesicles
malt: liquor; sugar
Malta: fever
maltese: cross
malt-worker's: lung
mamillary: ducts
mamillothalamic: tract
mammary: branches; calculus; ducts; fistula; fold; gland; line; neuralgia; plexus; region; ridge; souffle
mammary cancer: virus of mice

mammary duct: ectasia
mammary tumor: virus of mice
mammillary: arteries; body; line; process of lumbar vertebra; tubercle; tubercle of hypothalamus
mammillotegmental: fasciculus
mammillothalamic: fasciculus
mammosomatotroph cell: adenoma
mammotropic: factor; hormone
managed: care
Manchester: operation; ovoid
Manchurian: fever; typhus
Manchurian hemorrhagic: fever
mandatory minute: ventilation
Mandelin: reagent
mandibular: arch; axis; canal; cartilage; condyle; dentition; disk; foramen; fossa; glide; joint; lymph node; movement; nerve [CN V3]; nodes; notch; process; protraction; reflex; retraction; symphysis; tongue; torus
mandibular dental: arcade
mandibular guide: prosthesis
mandibular hinge: position
mandibuloacral: dysostosis
mandibulofacial: dysostosis; dysplasia
mandibulofacial dysotosis: syndrome
mandibulomaxillary: fixation
mandibulo-oculofacial: syndrome
mango: dermatitis
mangrove: fly
manic: episode; excitement; psychosis
manic-depressive: disorder; illness; psychosis
manifest: content; hyperopia; strabismus; tetany; vector
manifesting: carrier; heterozygote
manna: sugar
Mann-Bollman: fistula
Mannkopf: sign
Mann methyl blue-eosin: stain
mannose-binding: protein
mannose-6-phosphate: receptors
Mann-Williamson: operation; ulcer
Manson: disease; schistosomiasis
Manson eye: worm
Mantel-Haenszel: test

mantle: layer; radiotherapy; sclerosis; zone
mantle cell: lymphoma
Mantoux: pit; test
manual: pelvimetry; ventilation
manual visual: method
manubriosternal: joint; junction; symphysis
map-dot-fingerprint: dystrophy
maple: sugar
maple bark: disease
maple syrup: urine
maple syrup urine: disease
maplike: skull
Marañón: sign; syndrome
marantic: atrophy; edema; endocarditis; thrombosis; thrombus
marasmic: kwashiorkor
marathon group: psychotherapy
marble: bones
marble bone: disease
Marburg: disease; virus
Marburg virus: disease
Marcacci: muscle
march: fracture; hemoglobinuria
Marchand: adrenals; rest
Marchand wandering: cell
Marchant: zone
Marchi: fixative; reaction; stain; tract
Marchiafava-Bignami: disease
Marchiafava-Micheli: anemia; syndrome
Marcille: triangle
Marcus Gunn: phenomenon; pupil; sign; syndrome
Marek disease: virus
Marey: law
Marfan: disease; law; syndrome
margarine: disease
marginal: arcade; artery of colon; blepharitis; branch of cingulate sulcus; branch of parietooccipital sulcus; branch [TA] of cingulate sulcus; crest of tooth; fasciculus; gingivitis; gyrus; integrity of amalgam; keratitis; layer; part of orbicularis oris (muscle); rays; ridge; sinuses of placenta; sphincter; sulcus; tubercle; tubercle (of zygomatic bone); zone
marginal atrial: branch of right coronary artery
marginal mandibular: branch of facial nerve
marginal ring: ulcer of cornea

marginal tentorial: branch of internal carotid artery
marginal zone: lymphoma
marian: lithotomy
Marie: ataxia
Marie-Robinson: syndrome
Marie-Strümpell: disease
marine: pharmacology; soap
Marine-Lenhart: syndrome
Marinesco-Garland: syndrome
Marinesco-Sjögren: syndrome
Marinesco succulent: hand
Marion: disease
Mariotte: bottle; experiment; law
Mariotte blind: spot
marital: counseling; therapy
Marjolin: ulcer
marked fetal: bradycardia
marker: chromosome; enzyme; locus; trait
marker X: syndrome
Markov: process
Marme: reagent
marmoset: virus
Maroteaux-Lamy: syndrome
Marquis: reagent
marriage: therapy
marrow: canal; cell
marrow-lymph: gland
marrow-mesenchyme: connections
Marseilles: fever
marsh: fever; gas
Marshall: method; syndrome; test
Marshall-Marchetti: test
Marshall-Marchetti-Krantz: operation
Marshall oblique: vein
Marshall vestigial: fold
marsupial: notch
Martegiani: area; funnel
Martin: bandage; disease; tube
Martin-Bell: syndrome
Martin-Gruber: anastomosis
Martinotti: cell
Martorell: syndrome
masculine: pelvis; uterus
masculinity-femininity: scale
Masini: sign
masked: epilepsy; gout; hyperthyroidism; virus
masking: dilemma
masking level: difference
masklike: face
Maslow: hierarchy
masochistic: personality
Mason-Pfizer: virus
mason's: lung
MASS: syndrome
mass: hysteria; infection; law; movement; number;

peristalsis; reflex; screening; spectrograph
mass action: principle; theory
mass-action: ratio
Masselon: spectacles
masseter: muscle; reflex
masseteric: artery; fascia; nerve; tuberosity; veins
massive: collapse
massive bowel resection: syndrome
Masson argentaffin: stain
Masson-Fontana ammoniac silver: stain
Masson trichrome: stain
mass sociogenic: illness
mast: cell; leukocyte
mast cell: leukemia
Master: test
master: cast; eye; gland
Master two-step exercise: test
mastery: motive
masticating: cycles; surface
masticator: nerve; space
masticatory: apparatus; diplegia; force; muscles; nucleus; spasm; surface; system
masticatory silent: period
mastoid: abscess; angle of parietal bone; antrum; artery; bone; border of occipital bone; branches of posterior auricular artery; branches of posterior tympanic artery; branch of occipital artery; canaliculus; cells; cortex; empyema; fontanelle; foramen; fossa; groove; lymph nodes; margin of occipital bone; notch; part of the temporal bone; process; process of petrous part of temporal bone; sinuses; wall of middle ear; wall of tympanic cavity
mastoid air: cells
mastoid emissary: vein
mat: burn; gold
matched: groups
maternal: cotyledon; death; dystocia; immunity; inheritance; morbidity; placenta
maternal death: rate
maternal deprivation: syndrome
maternal-fetal: medicine
maternal mortality: ratio
maternity: hospital
mathematical: chaos; determinant; genetics; model
mating: isolate

matrix: band; calculus; metalloproteinase; retainer; vesicles
matrix Gla: protein
mattress: suture
maturation: arrest; factor; index; value
mature: bacteriophage; cataract; neutrophil
mature cell: leukemia
mature ovarian: follicle
maturity-onset: diabetes
maturity onset: diabetes of youth
matutinal: epilepsy
Mauchart: ligaments
Maurer: clefts; dots
Mauriac: syndrome
Mauriceau: maneuver
Mauriceau-Levret: maneuver
Mauthner: sheath; test
maxillary: angle; antrum; artery; dentition; eminence; gland; hiatus; nerve [CN V2]; plexus; process of embryo; process of inferior nasal concha; protraction; sinus; surface of greater wing of sphenoid bone; surface of palatine bone; tuberosity; vein
maxillary dental: arcade
maxillary sinus: radiograph
maxillofacial: prosthetics
maxillomandibular: fixation; record; registration; relation; traction
maximal: dose; stimulus; thymectomy
maximal Histalog: test
maximal permissible: dose
Maxim-Gilbert: sequencing
Maximow: stain for bone marrow
maximum: temperature; velocity
maximum breathing: capacity
maximum intensity: projection
maximum likelihood: estimator
maximum occipital: point
maximum permissible: dose
maximum power: output
maximum tolerated: dose
maximum urea: clearance
maximum voluntary: ventilation
May apple: root
Mayaro: virus
Mayer: pessary; reflex
Mayer hemalum: stain
Mayer mucicarmine: stain
Mayer mucihematein: stain

Mayer-Rokitansky-Küster-Hauser: syndrome
May-Grünwald: stain
May-Hegglin: anomaly
Mayo: bunionectomy; operation; vein
Mayo-Robson: point; position
May-White: syndrome
Mazzoni: corpuscle
Mazzotti: reaction; test
McArdle: disease; syndrome
McArdle-Schmid-Pearson: disease
McBurney: incision; point; sign
McCall culdoplasty: procedure
McCarey-Kaufmann: media
McCarthy: reflexes
McCrea: sound
McCune-Albright: syndrome
McDonald: maneuver
McGoon: technique
McIndoe: operation
McKee: line
McKusick metaphyseal: dysplasia
McMurray: test
McNemar: test
McPhail: test
McRoberts: maneuver
McVay: operation
M:E: ratio
meadow: dermatitis
Meadows: syndrome
meal: worm
mean: calorie; temperature; vector
mean corpuscular: hemoglobin; volume
mean corpuscular hemoglobin: concentration
mean electrical: axis
mean foundation: plane
mean manifest: vector
measles: immunoglobulin; virus
measles convalescent: serum
measles immune: globulin (human)
measles, mumps, and rubella: vaccine
measles virus: vaccine
measured: intelligence
meatal: cartilage; spine
Mecca: balsam
mechanical: abrasion; alternation of the heart; antidote; corepraxy; dysmenorrhea; heart; ileus; intelligence; jaundice; strabismus; vector; ventilation; vertigo
mechanically balanced: occlusion
mechanism-based: inhibitor

mechanistic: school
mechanobullous: disease
mechanoelectric: transduction
Mecke: reagent
Meckel: band; cartilage; cavity; diverticulum; ganglion; ligament; plane; scan; space; syndrome
Meckel-Gruber: syndrome
meconial: colic
meconium: aspiration; ileus; peritonitis; plug
meconium aspiration: syndrome
meconium blockage: syndrome
medial: angle of eye; arteriole of retina; arteriosclerosis; border; border of foot; border of forearm; border of humerus; border of kidney; border of scapula; border of suprarenal gland; border of tibia; branches; branches of artery of tuber cinereum; branches of pontine arteries; branch of posterior branch of spinal nerves; branch of posterior rami of spinal nerves; canthus; compartment of thigh; condyle; condyle of femur; condyle of tibia; cord of brachial plexus; crest of fibula; crus; crus of facial canal; crus of the horizontal part of the facial canal; crus of major alar cartilage of nose; crus of the superficial inguinal ring; eminence; epicondyle of femur; epicondyle of humerus; fillet; head; lamina of cartilage of pharyngotympanic (auditory) tube; lemniscus; ligament of ankle joint; ligament of knee; ligament of talocrural joint; ligament of temporomandibular joint; ligament of wrist; limb; lip of linea aspera; malleolus; margin; meniscus; nuclei of thalamus; nucleus; nucleus of trapezoid body; part of longitudinal arch of foot; part of middle lobe vein (of right superior pulmonary vein); plate of cartilaginous auditory tube; plate of pterygoid process; pole of ovary; process of calcaneal tuberosity; root of median nerve; root of optic tract; rotator; segment; sulcus of crus cerebri; surface; surface

of arytenoid cartilage; surface of cerebral hemisphere; surface of fibula; surface of lung; surface of ovary; surface of testis; surface of tibia; surface of toes; surface of ulna; tubercle (of posterior process) of talus; vein of lateral ventricle; venule of retina; wall of middle ear; wall of orbit; wall of tympanic cavity; zone
medial accessory olivary: nucleus
medial amygdaloid: nucleus
medial antebrachial cutaneous: nerve
medial anterior thoracic: nerve
medial arcuate: ligament
medial atrial: vein
medial basal: branch of pulmonary artery
medial basal bronchopulmonary: segment S VII
medial basal segmental: artery
medial bicipital: groove
medial brachial cutaneous: nerve
medial bronchopulmonary: segment S V
medial calcaneal: branches of tibial nerve
medial canthal: ligament
medial canthic: fold
medial cartilaginous: plate
medial central: nucleus of thalamus
medial cerebral: surface
medial circumflex: artery of thigh
medial circumflex femoral: artery; veins
medial clunial: nerves
medial collateral: artery; ligament of elbow
medial commisural: artery
medial crural cutaneous: branches of saphenous nerve; nerve
medial cuneiform: bone
medial cutaneous: branch of dorsal branch of posterior intercostal arteries; nerve of arm; nerve of forearm; nerve of leg
medial dorsal: nucleus [TA] of thalamus
medial dorsal cutaneous: nerve
medial epicondylar: crest; ridge
medial femoral: tuberosity

medial femoral circumflex: artery
medial forebrain: bundle
medial frontal: gyrus
medial frontobasal: artery
medial geniculate: body; nuclei; nuclei
medial great: muscle
medial habenular: nucleus
medial inferior genicular: artery
medial inguinal: fossa
medial lacunar: lymph node; node
medial longitudinal: arch of foot; bundle; fasciculus; stria
medial lumbar intertransversarii: muscles
medial lumbar intertransverse: muscles
medial lumbocostal: arch
medial magnocellular: nucleus
medial malleolar: arteries; branches (of posterior tibial artery); facet of talus; network
medial malleolar subcutaneous: bursa
medial mammary: branches
medial medullary: branches of vertebral artery; lamina [TA] of lentiform nucleus
medial midpalmar: space
medial nasal: branches of anterior ethmoidal nerve; fold; process; prominence
medial occipital: artery
medial occipitotemporal: gyrus
medial olfactory: gyrus
medial orbitofrontal: artery
medial palpebral: commissure; ligament
medial parabrachial: nucleus
medial patellar: retinaculum
medial pectoral: nerve
medial pericuneate: nucleus
medial plantar: artery; nerve
medial popliteal: nerve
medial posterior cervical intertransversarii: muscles
medial preoptic: nucleus
medial pterygoid: muscle; plate
medial puboprostatic: ligament
medial rectus: muscle
medial reticulospinal: tract
medial segmental: artery
medial septal: nucleus
medial striate: artery
medial superior genicular: artery
medial superior olivary: nucleus

medial supraclavicular: nerve
medial supracondylar: crest; ridge
medial supraepicondylar: ridge
medial sural cutaneous: nerve
medial talocalcaneal: ligament
medial tarsal: arteries
medial umbilical: fold; ligament
medial vastus: muscle
medial ventral: nucleus
medial vestibular: nucleus
medial vestibulospinal: tract
median: aperture of fourth ventricle; artery; bar of Mercier; conjugate; eminence; groove of tongue; laryngotomy; line; lithotomy; nerve; plane; rhinoscopy; section; sternotomy; strumectomy; sulcus of fourth ventricle; sulcus of tongue; vein of forearm; vein of neck
median antebrachial: vein
median anterior maxillary: cyst
median arcuate: ligament
median atlantoaxial: joint
median basilic: vein
median callosal: artery
median cephalic: vein
median commissural: artery
median cricothyroid: ligament
median cubital: vein
median glossoepiglottic: fold
median longitudinal: raphe of tongue
median mandibular: point
median maxillary anterior alveolar: cleft
median palatal: cyst
median palatine: suture
median preoptic: nucleus
median raphe: cyst of the penis
median retruded: relation
median rhomboid: glossitis
median sacral: artery; crest; vein
median thyrohyoid: ligament
median tongue: bud
median umbilical: fold; ligament
mediastinal: arteries; branches; branches of internal thoracic artery; branches of thoracic aorta; emphysema; fibrosis; lipomatosis; part of lung; part of parietal pleura; pleura; pleurisy; space;

surface of lung; veins; window
mediate: auscultation; percussion; transfusion
mediator: complex
medical: anatomy; biophysics; care; diathermy; ethics; examiner; genetics; jurisprudence; model; mycology; pathology; psychology; record; selection; treatment
medical record: linkage
medicinal: charcoal; chemistry; eruption; zinc peroxide
medicinal soft: soap
mediocolic: sphincter
mediodorsal: nucleus
mediopubic: reflex
Mediterranean: fever; lymphoma
Mediterranean erythematous: fever
Mediterranean exanthematous: fever
Mediterranean spotted: fever
medium: artery; vein
medium-chain acyl-CoA dehydrogenase: deficiency
medullary: arteries of brain; callus; carcinoma; carcinoma of breast; carcinoma of thyroid; cavity; center; chemoreceptor; cone; cords; folds; groove; laminae of thalamus; layers of thalamus; membrane; plate; pyramid; pyramidotomy; ray; sarcoma; sheath; space; striae of fourth ventricle; stria of thalamus; substance; teniae; tube
medullary reticulospinal: tract
medullary spinal: arteries
medullary sponge: kidney
medullated nerve: fiber
medullopontine: sulcus
Medusa: head
Meeh: formula
Meeh-Dubois: formula
Mees: lines; stripes
Meesman: dystrophy
megacystic: syndrome
megacystitis-megaureter: syndrome
megacystitis-microcolon-intestinal hypoperistalsis: syndrome
megakaryocyte growth and development: factor
megakaryocytic: leukemia
megaloblastic: anemia
megalocytic: anemia

meibomian: blepharitis; conjunctivitis; cyst; glands; sty
Meige: disease
Meigs: syndrome
Meinicke: test
meiotic: division; drive; phase
Meischer: syndrome
Meissner: corpuscle; plexus
melamine: resin
melanocyte-stimulating: hormone
melanophore-expanding: principle
melanotic: freckle; medulloblastoma; pigment; progonoma
melanotic neuroectodermal: tumor of infancy
melanotropin release-inhibiting: hormone
melanotropin-releasing: factor; hormone
Meleney: gangrene; ulcer
Melkersson-Rosenthal: syndrome
Melnick-Needles: osteodysplasty; syndrome
melon-seed: body
melting: point; temperature; temperature of DNA
Meltzer: law
Meltzer-Lyon: test
membrane: bone; enzyme; potential; rupture; stripping
membrane attack: complex
membrane-coating: granule
membrane expansion: theory
membranoproliferative: glomerulonephritis
membranous: ampulla; ampullae of the semicircular ducts; cataract; cochlea; conjunctivitis; dysmenorrhea; glomerulonephritis; labyrinth; lamina of cartilage of pharyngotympanic (auditory) plate; laryngitis; layer; layer of subcutaneous tissue of abdomen; layer of superficial fascia; layer of superficial fascia of perineum; lipodystrophy; neurocranium; ossification; part of interventricular septum; part of male urethra; part of nasal septum; pharyngitis; septum; urethra; viscerocranium; wall of middle ear; wall of trachea; wall of tympanic cavity
memory: loop; span
memory B: cells
memory T: cells

Menangle: virus
Mendel-Bechterew: reflex
Mendeléeff: law
Mendel first: law
mendelian: character; genetics; inheritance; ratio; trait
Mendel instep: reflex
Mendel second: law
Mendelson: syndrome
Ménétrier: disease; syndrome
Menge: pessary
Mengo: encephalitis; virus
Ménière: disease; syndrome
meningeal: branch of cavernous part of internal carotid artery; branch of cerebral part of internal carotid artery; branches; branch of internal carotid artery; branch of (intracranial part of) vertebral artery; branch of mandibular nerve; branch of maxillary nerve; branch of occipital artery; branch of ophthalmic nerve; branch of spinal nerves; branch of vagus nerve; carcinoma; carcinomatosis; hernia; layer of dura mater; leukemia; neurosyphilis; plexus; veins
meningitic: streak
meningocerebral: cicatrix
meningococcal: meningitis
meningotyphoid: fever
meningovascular: neurosyphilis; syphilis
meniscofemoral: ligaments
meniscus: lens; sign
Menkes: syndrome
menopausal: syndrome
menstrual: age; colic; cycle; edema; leukorrhea; molimina; period; sclerosis
menstrual extraction: abortion
mental: aberration; age; apparatus; artery; branches of mental nerve; branch (of inferior alveolar artery); canal; chronometry; deficiency; disease; disorder; foramen; health; hospital; hygiene; illness; image; impairment; impression; nerve; point; process; protuberance; region; retardation; scotoma; spine; symphysis; tubercle (of mandible)
mentalis: muscle
mentoanterior: position
mentolabial: furrow; sulcus
mentoposterior: position
mentotransverse: position

Word Finder

mercapturic acid: pathway
Mercier: bar; sound; valve
mercurial: diuretics; line; manometer; stomatitis
mercury: arc; poisoning
mercury vapor: lamp
Merendino: technique
Meretoja: syndrome
meridional: aberration; amblyopia; cleavage; fibers of ciliary muscle
Merkel: corpuscle; filtrum ventriculi; fossa; muscle
Merkel cell: tumor
Merkel tactile: cell; disk
mermaid: malformation
meroblastic: cleavage
merocrine: gland
Merrifield: knife; synthesis
Méry: gland
Merzbacher-Pelizaeus: disease
mesangial: cell; nephritis
mesangial proliferative: glomerulonephritis
mesangiocapillary: glomerulonephritis
mesatipellic: pelvis
mesencephalic: flexure; nucleus of trigeminal nerve; tegmentum; tract of trigeminal nerve; veins
mesencephalic corticonuclear: fibers
mesenchymal: cells; epithelium; tissue
mesenteric: adenitis; glands; hernia; lymphadenitis; lymph nodes; portion of small intestine; veins
mesenteric artery: occlusion
mesentericoparietal: fossa; recess
mesenteroaxial: volvulus
mesethmoid: bone
mesh: graft
mesial: angle; caries; displacement; occlusion; surface of tooth
meso: compounds
mesoblastic: nephroma; segment
mesocaval: shunt
mesocolic: lymph nodes; tenia
mesodermal: factor
mesoglial: cells
mesomelic: dwarfism
mesometric: pregnancy
mesonephric: adenocarcinoma; duct; fold; rest; ridge; tissue; tubule
mesonephroid: tumor
mesopic: perimetry
mesothelial: cell
mesovarian: border of ovary; margin of ovary

messenger: RNA
messengerlike: RNA
metabisulfite: test
metabolic: acidosis; alkalosis; calculus; coma; craniopathy; disease; encephalopathy; equivalent; indican; pool
metabolized vitamin D: milk
metabotropic: receptor
metacarpal: bones [I–V]; index; veins
metacarpohypothenar: reflex
metacarpophalangeal: articulations; joints
metacarpothenar: reflex
metacentric: chromosome
metachromatic: bodies; granules; leukodystrophy; stain
metafacial: angle
metaherpetic: keratitis
metahypophysial: diabetes
metal: base; interface
metal fume: fever
metal insert: teeth
metallic: rale
metameric nervous: system
metanephric: blastema; bud; cap; diverticulum; duct; tubule
metanephrogenic: tissue
metaphyseal fibrous cortical: defect
metaphysial: dysostosis; dysplasia
metaplastic: anemia; carcinoma; ossification; polyp
metastasizing: septicemia
metastatic: abscess; calcification; carcinoma; choroiditis; mumps; ophthalmia; pneumonia; retinitis
metastatic carcinoid: syndrome
metatarsal: artery; bones [I–V]; reflex
metatarsal interosseous: ligaments
metatarsophalangeal: articulations; joints
metatropic: dwarfism
Metchnikoff: theory
Metenier: sign
meter: angle
metered-dose: inhaler
meter-kilogram-second: system; unit
methacholine challenge: test
methacrylate: resin
methamphetamine: base
methanol: fixative
methenamine silver: stain
methionine-activating: enzyme

methionine malabsorption: syndrome
methionyl: dipeptidase
methonium: compounds
3-methoxy-4-hydroxymandelic acid: test
methyl: alcohol; mercaptan
methylglucamine: iodipamide
methyl green-pyronin: stain
methylol: riboflavin
metopic: point; suture
metric: system
metroperitoneal: fistula
metrotrophic: test
Meulengracht: diet
Mexican: typhus
Mexican hat: cell; corpuscle
Mexican spotted: fever
Meyenburg: complex; disease
Meyenburg-Altherr-Uehlinger: syndrome
Meyer: cartilages; line; reagent; sinus
Meyer-Archambault: loop
Meyer-Betz: disease; syndrome
Meyerhof oxidation: quotient
Meyer-Overton: rule; theory of narcosis
Meynert: cells; commissure; decussation; layer
MHA-TP: test
MHC: restriction
miasma: theory
Mibelli: angiokeratomas; disease
Michaelis: complex; constant
Michaelis-Gutmann: body
Michaelis-Menten: constant; equation; hypothesis
Michel: malformation; spur
microangiopathic hemolytic: anemia
micro-Astrup: method
microbial: collagenase; genetics; persistence; RNase II; vitamin
micrococcal: endonuclease; nuclease
microcrystalline: cellulose
microcystic: disease of renal medulla
microcystic epithelial: dystrophy
microcytic: anemia
microdrepanocytic: anemia
microelectric: waves
microetching: technique
microfilarial: sheath
microfold: cell
microfollicular: adenoma; goiter
microglandular: adenosis
microglia: cells
microhemagglutination-Treponema pallidum: test

microhematocrit: concentration
microinvasive: carcinoma
micro-Kjeldahl: method
microlecithal: egg
micromelic: dwarfism
micrometastatic: disease
micromyeloblastic: leukemia
microophthalmia transcription factor: gene
microprecipitation: test
microscopic: anatomy; field; hematuria; polyangiitis; section; sphincter
microscopically controlled: surgery
microsphere: method
microsporidian: keratoconjunctivitis
microtubule-associated: proteins
microtubule-organizing: center
microvascular: anastomosis
microvillus inclusion: disease
microwave: therapy
micturating: cystourethrogram
micturition: reflex; syncope
midaxillary: line
midbrain: tegmentum; vesicle
midcarpal: joint
midclavicular: line
middiastolic: murmur
middle: cells; ear; finger; kidney; lobe of prostate; lobe of right lung; mediastinum; pain; phalanges of foot and hand; piece; trunk of brachial plexus
middle atlantoepistrophic: joint
middle axillary: line
middle cardiac: vein
middle carpal: joint
middle cerebellar: peduncle
middle cerebral: artery
middle cervical: fascia; ganglion
middle cervical cardiac: nerve
middle clinoid: process
middle cluneal: nerves
middle colic: artery; lymph nodes; vein
middle collateral: artery
middle constrictor: muscle of pharynx
middle costotransverse: ligament
middle cranial: fossa
middle cuneiform: bone
middle-ear: effusion
middle esophageal: constriction

middle ethmoidal: cells; sinuses
middle ethmoidal air: cells
middle fossa: approach
middle frontal: convolution; gyrus; sulcus
middle genicular: artery
middle glossoepiglottic: fold
middle gray: layer of superior colliculus
middle group of mesenteric: lymph nodes
middle hemorrhoidal: artery; plexuses; veins
middle hepatic: veins
middle latency: response
middle lobar: artery; artery of right lung
middle lobe: branch of right superior pulmonary vein; syndrome; vein
middle macular: arteriole
middle meningeal: artery; branch of maxillary nerve; nerve; veins
middle meningeal artery: groove
middle nasal: concha
middle palmar: space
middle radioulnar: joint
middle rectal: artery; lymph node; node; veins
middle rectal (nervous): plexus
middle sacral: artery
middle sacral lymphatic: plexus
middle scalene: muscle
middle superior alveolar: branch of infraorbital nerve
middle supraclavicular: nerve
middle suprarenal: artery
middle talar articular: surface of calcaneus
middle temporal: artery; branches of lateral occipital artery; branch of insular part of middle cerebral artery; convolution; gyrus; sulcus; vein
middle thyroid: vein
middle transverse rectal: fold
middle turbinated: bone
middle umbilical: fold; ligament
midforceps: delivery
midgastric transverse: sphincter
midget bipolar: cells
midlife: crisis
midline: incision; myelotomy
midline malignant reticulosis: granuloma
midpalmar: space
midsagittal: plane; section

midsigmoid: sphincter
midtarsal: joint
Miescher: elastoma; granuloma; tubes
mignon: lamp
migraine: headache
migraine-related: vestibulopathy
migrating: abscess; teeth
migration: theory
migration inhibition: test
migration-inhibitory: factor
migration inhibitory factor: test
migratory: cell; pneumonia
mika: operation
Mikulicz: aphthae; cells; clamp; disease; drain; operation; syndrome
Mikulicz-Vladimiroff: amputation
mild: silver protein
mild fetal: bradycardia
Miles: operation
miliary: abscess; aneurysm; embolism; fever; pattern; tuberculosis
milieu: therapy
military: medicine
milk of: calcium
milk: anemia; corpuscle; crust; cyst; ducts; factor; fever; gland; line; ridge; scall; sickness; spots; sugar; tetter; tooth
milk-alkali: syndrome
milk-ejection: reflex
milkers': nodes; nodules
milker's nodule: virus
milk let-down: reflex
Milkman: syndrome
milk-ring: test
milky: ascites; urine
mill: fever
Millard-Gubler: syndrome
milled-in: curves; paths
miller: asthma
Miller-Abbott: tube
Miller chemicoparasitic: theory
Millner: needle
Millon: reaction; reagent
Millon clinical multiaxial: inventory
Millon Clinical Multiaxial Inventory: test
Millon-Nasse: test
mill wheel: murmur
Milroy: disease
Milton: disease
MIM: number
mimetic: muscles; paralysis
mimic: genes
Minamata: disease
mind: blindness
mineral: water; wax

miner's: asthma; cramps; disease; elbow; lung; nystagmus
Minerva: jacket
miniature: stomach
miniature scarlet: fever
minicore-multicore: myopathy
minimal: air; dose
minimal alveolar: concentration
minimal amplitude: nystagmus
minimal anesthetic: concentration
minimal brain: dysfunction
minimal-change: disease
minimal-change nephrotic: syndrome
minimal deviation: melanoma
minimal infecting: dose
minimal inhibitory: concentration
minimal lethal: dose
minimally invasive: surgery
minimal reacting: dose
minimum: light; temperature
minimum light: threshold
minimum protein: requirement
mink enteritis: virus
Minnesota Multiphasic Personality: Inventory
Minnesota Multiphasic Personality Inventory: test
minor: agglutinin; amputation; calices; circulus arteriosus of iris; connector; fissure; forceps; groove; hippocampus; hypnosis; hysteria; operation; surgery; tranquilizer
minor alar: cartilage
minor arterial: circle of iris
minor duodenal: papilla
minor histocompatibility: complex
minor motor: seizure
minor salivary: glands
minor sublingual: ducts
Minot-Murphy: diet
minus: lens; strand
minute: output; volume
miostagmin: reaction
Mirchamp: sign
Mirizzi: syndrome
mirror: haploscope; image; speech
mirror image: dextrocardia
mirror-image: cell
misdirection: phenomenon
mismatch: repair
missed: abortion; labor; period
missense: mutation
Mitchell: disease; procedure; treatment

mite: typhus
mite-born: typhus
mitochondrial: biogenesis; chromosome; disorders; gene; matrix; membrane; myopathy; sheath
mitogenic: lectin
mitotic: cycle; division; figure; index; period; rate; spindle
mitral: area; cells; click; commissurotomy; facies; gradient; incompetence; insufficiency; murmur; orifice; regurgitation; stenosis; tap; valve; valvotomy
mitral valve: prolapse
mitral valve prolapse: syndrome
Mitrofanoff: principle
Mitsuda: antigen; reaction
Mitsuo: phenomenon
Mittendorf: dot
mixed: aphasia; astigmatism; beat; chancre; disulfide; esotropia; gland; glioma; glycerides; hearing loss; hyperlipemia; hyperlipidemia; hypoglycemia; infection; leukemia; nerve; paralysis; thrombus; tocopherols concentrate; tumor; tumor of salivary gland; tumor of skin
mixed agglutination: reaction; test
mixed connective-tissue: disease
mixed discrete-continuous random: variable
mixed expired: gas
mixed function: oxygenase
mixed hyperlipoproteinemia familial, type 5: hyperlipidemia
mixed lymphocyte: culture
mixed lymphocyte culture: reaction; test
mixed mesodermal: tumor
Mixter: clamp
Miyagawa: bodies
MLC: test
MM: virus
M-mode: echocardiography
M'Naghten: rule
mnemic: hypothesis; theory
MNSs: antigens
mobile: end; part of nasal septum; spasm
Mobitz: block
Mobitz types of atrioventricular: block
Möbius: sign; syndrome
modal: alteration
model: game

modeling: composition; compound; plastic
moderate: hypothermia
moderator: band; variable
modern: genetics
modified: milk; smallpox
modified acid-fast: stain
modified radical: hysterectomy; mastectomy; mastoidectomy
modified trichrome: stain
modified zinc oxide-eugenol: cement
modifier: gene
modulation transfer: function
Moeller: glossitis
Moeller grass: bacillus
Mogen: clamp
Mohr: pipette; syndrome
Mohrenheim: fossa; space
Mohs: chemosurgery; scale; surgery
Mohs fresh tissue chemosurgery: technique
Mohs micrographic: surgery
moist: gangrene; papule; rale; wart
Mokola: virus
molar: absorptivity; behavior; concentration; glands; mass; pregnancy; tooth; tubercle
molar absorbancy: index
molar absorption: coefficient
molar extinction: coefficient
mold: guide
mole: fraction
molecular: behavior; biology; biophysics; disease; dispersion; distillation; epidemiology; formula; genetics; heat; layer; layer of cerebellar cortex; layer of cerebellum; layer of cerebral cortex; layer of retina; layers of olfactory bulb; mass; movement; pathology; rotation; sieve; weight
molecular dispersed: solution
molecular dissociation: theory
molecular weight: ratio
Molisch: test
Moll: glands
Mollaret: meningitis
molluscum: body; conjunctivitis; corpuscle
molluscum contagiosum: virus
Moloney: test; virus
molybdenum: cofactor
molybdenum target: tube
Monakow: bundle; nucleus; syndrome; tract
Mönckeberg: arteriosclerosis; calcification; degeneration; sclerosis

Mönckeberg medial: calcification
Mondini: dysplasia; hearing impairment
Mondonesi: reflex
Mondor: disease
Monge: disease
mongolian: fold; macula; spot
moniliform: hair
monkey: hand; malaria
monkey B: virus
monkeypox: virus
monoamine: hypothesis
monoamine oxidase: inhibitor
monoamniotic: twins
monobasic: acid; ammonium phosphate; potassium phosphate
monobromated: camphor
monochorial: twins
monochorionic diamnionic: placenta
monochorionic monoamnionic: placenta
monochromatic: aberration; radiation
monoclonal: antibody; gammopathy; gammopathy of undetermined significance; gammopathy of unknown significance; immunoglobulin; peak; protein
monocrotic: pulse
monocular: diplopia; heterochromia; strabismus
monocyte chemoattractant: protein; protein-1
monocyte-derived neutrophil chemotactic: factor
monocytic: angina; leukemia; leukemoid reaction; leukocytosis; leukopenia
monocytoid: cell
Monod-Wyman-Changeux: model
monofixation: syndrome
monohydric: alcohol
monoleptic: fever
monomolecular: reaction
monomorphic: adenoma
mononuclear phagocyte: system
monophasic: complex
monophyletic: theory
monopolar: cautery
monopotassium: phosphate
monorecidive: chancre
monosodium: phosphate
monostotic fibrous: dysplasia
monotonic: sequence
monovalent: antiserum
monovular: twins
monoxenic: culture
monozygotic: twins

Monro: doctrine; foramen; line; sulcus
Monro-Kellie: doctrine
Monro-Richter: line
Monsel: solution
Monson: curve
montan: wax
Monteggia: fracture
Montenegro: test
Montevideo: units
Montgomery: follicles; glands; tubercles
mood: disorders
mood-congruent: hallucination
mood-incongruent: hallucination
mood stabilizing: agent
Moon: molars
moon: face; facies
moon shaped: face
Moore: method
Moore lightning: streaks
Mooren: ulcer
Mooser: bodies
moral: ataxia; treatment
Morand: foot; spur
Moraxella: conjunctivitis
morbid: impulse; obesity; thirst
morbidity: rate
morcellated: nephrectomy
morcellation: operation
Morel: ear
Morgagni: appendix; cartilage; caruncle; cataract; columns; concha; crypts; disease; foramen; fossa; fovea; frenum; globules; humor; hydatid; lacuna; liquor; nodule; prolapse; retinaculum; sinus; spheres; syndrome; tubercle; valves; ventricle
Morgagni-Adams-Stokes: syncope; syndrome
morgagnian: cyst
Morgagni foramen: hernia
Morgan: bacillus; fold
Morison: pouch
Mörner: test
morning: diarrhea; sickness; vomiting
morning after: pill
morning glory: anomaly; syndrome
Moro: reflex
morphine injector's: septicemia
morphogenetic: movement
morphologic: element
Morquio: disease; syndrome
Morquio-Ullrich: disease
mortality: rate
mortar: kidney
mortise: joint

Morton: metatarsalgia; neuralgia; neuroma; plane; syndrome; toe
Morvan: chorea; disease
mosaic: fundus; inheritance; pattern; wart
Moschcowitz: disease; test
Mosenthal: test
Mosler: diabetes; sign
mosquito: clamp; forceps
Moss: tube
moss: starch
Mossman: fever
Mosso: ergograph; sphygmomanometer
mossy: cell; fibers; foot
most comfortable: level
Motais: operation
moth: patch
moth-eaten: alopecia
mother: cell; colony; cyst; liquor; star; surrogate; yaw
mother of: vinegar
motile: leukocyte
motility: test
motility test: medium
motion: sickness
motor: abreaction; agraphia; amusia; aphasia; apraxia; area; ataxia; cell; cortex; decussation; endplate; fibers; image; impersistence; nerve; nerve of face; neuron; nuclei; nucleus of facial nerve; nucleus of trigeminal nerve; nucleus of trigeminus; paralysis; plate; point; root of ciliary ganglion; root of spinal nerve; root of trigeminal nerve; unit; urgency; zone
motor dapsone: neuropathy
motor neuron: disease
motor speech: center
motor system: disease
mottled: enamel; tooth
Motulsky dye reduction: test
Mounier-Kuhn: syndrome
mountain: anemia; balm; disease; sickness
mounting: medium
mouse: cancer; encephalomyelitis; unit
mouse antialopecia: factor
mouse encephalomyelitis: virus
mouse hepatitis: virus
mouse leukemia: viruses
mouse mammary tumor: virus
mouse parotid tumor: virus
mouse poliomyelitis: virus
mousepox: virus
mousetail: pulse
mouse thymic: virus
mouse-tooth: forceps

mouth: breathing; mirror; rehabilitation
mouth-to-mouth: respiration; resuscitation
movable: heart; joint; kidney; pulse; spleen; testis
Mowry colloidal iron: stain
moyamoya: disease
Mozart: ear
MP: joints
MR: angiography
MS-1: hepatitis
MSB trichrome: stain
Mu: antigen
Much: bacillus
Mucha-Habermann: disease; syndrome
mucilaginous: gland
mucin clot: test
mucinogen: granules
mucinoid: degeneration
mucinous: carcinoma
muciparous: gland
Muckle-Wells: syndrome
mucoalbuminous: cells
mucobuccal: fold
mucociliary: clearance
mucociliary clearance: rate
mucocutaneous: junction; leishmaniasis
mucocutaneous lymph node: syndrome
mucoepidermoid: carcinoma; tumor
mucoepithelial: dysplasia
mucoid: adenocarcinoma; colony; degeneration
mucoid impaction of: bronchus
mucoid medial: degeneration
mucomembranous: enteritis
mucoperichondrial: flap
mucoperiosteal: flap
mucopolysaccharide keratin: dystrophy
mucosa-associated lymphoid: tissue
mucosal: folds of gallbladder; graft; tunics; wave
mucosal disease: virus
mucosal relief: radiography
mucoserous: cells
mucous: cast; cell; colitis; cyst; diarrhea; gland; glands of auditory tube; membrane of bronchus; membrane of ductus deferens; membrane of esophagus; membrane of female urethra; membrane of gallbladder; membrane of large intestine; membrane of larynx; membrane of male urethra; membrane of nose; membrane of pharyngotympanic auditory tube; membrane of pharynx;

membranes; membrane of small intestine; membrane of stomach; membrane of tongue; membrane of trachea; membrane of tympanic cavity; membrane of ureter; membrane of urinary bladder; membrane of uterine tube; membrane of vagina; patch; plaque; plug; polyp; rale; sheath of tendon
mucous connective: tissue
mucous neck: cell
mucus: blanket; impaction
mud: bed; fever
Muehrcke: bands; lines; sign
Mueller electronic: tonometer
Mueller-Hinton: agar; medium
muffle: furnace
Muir-Torre: syndrome
mulberry: calculus; molar; ovary; spots
Mulder: test
Mules: operation
mule-spinner's: cancer
mulibrey: nanism
Müller: capsule; duct; fibers; fixative; law; maneuver; muscle; sign; trigone; tubercle
müllerian: adenosarcoma; agenesis
müllerian inhibiting: factor; substance
müllerian regression: factor
Müller radial: cells
multangular: bone
multiaxial: classification; joint
multicentric: reticulohistiocytosis
multicolony-stimulating: factor
multicore: disease
multicuspid: tooth
multidrug: resistance
multienzyme: complex
multifactorial: inheritance
multifidus: muscle
multifocal: choroiditis; lens; osteitis fibrosa
multifocal atrial: tachycardia
multiform: layer; layer [TA] of cerebral cortex
multiformat: camera
multi-infarct: dementia
multilamellar: body
multilaminar primary: follicle
multilocal: genetics
multilocular: cyst; fat
multilocular adipose: tissue
multilocular hydatid: cyst
multimammate: mouse
multinodular: goiter

multinomial: distribution
multinuclear: leukocyte
multipennate: muscle
multiphasic: screening
multiple: alcohol; amputation; anchorage; embolism; exostosis; fission; fracture; myeloma; myelomatosis; myositis; neuritis; parasitism; personality; pregnancy; sclerosis; serositis; stain; sulfatase deficiency; vision
multiple chemical: sensitivity
multiple ego: states
multiple endocrine: adenomatosis; neoplasia; neoplasia 1; neoplasia 2; neoplasia 3; neoplasia 2B; neoplasia, type 1; neoplasia, type 2A
multiple endocrine deficiency: syndrome
multiple endocrine neoplasia: syndrome, type 1; syndrome, type 2A; syndrome, type 2B
multiple epiphyseal: dysplasia
multiple-gated acquisition: scan
multiple glandular deficiency: syndrome
multiple hamartoma: syndrome
multiple idiopathic hemorrhagic: sarcoma
multiple intestinal: polyposis
multiple lentigines: syndrome
multiple marker: screen
multiple mucosal neuroma: syndrome
multiple personality: disorder
multiple puncture tuberculin: test
multiple self-healing squamous: epithelioma
multiple sleep latency: test
multiple symmetric: lipomatosis
multiple system: atrophy
multiplicative: division; growth; model
multipolar: cell; mitosis; neuron
multistage: model
multivalent: vaccine
multivariate: studies
multivesicular: bodies
mummification: necrosis
mummified: pulp
mumps: meningoencephalitis; virus
mumps sensitivity: test
mumps skin test: antigen
mumps virus: vaccine
mumu: fever

Munchausen: syndrome; syndrome by proxy
Münchhausen: syndrome
mung bean: nuclease
municipal: hospital
Munro: abscess; microabscess; point
Munson: sign
mural: cell; endocarditis; pregnancy; thrombosis; thrombus
murine: leukemia; typhus
murine sarcoma: virus
Murphy: button; drip; percussion; sign
Murray Valley: encephalitis; rash
Murray Valley encephalitis: virus
Murutucu: virus
muscarinic: antagonist; receptors
muscle: bundle; curve; epithelium; fascicle; hemoglobin; layer in fatty layer of subcutaneous tissue; plasma; plate; proteins; relaxant; repositioning; resection; serum; sound; spasm; spindle
muscle contraction: headache
muscle phosphorylase: deficiency
muscle-sparing: thoracotomy
muscle-tendon: attachment; junction
muscular: arteries (of ophthalmic artery); artery; asthenopia; atrophy; branches; coat; coat of bronchi; coat of colon; coat of ductus deferens; coat of esophagus; coat of female urethra; coat of gallbladder; coat of intermediate part of male urethra; coat of large intestine; coat of male urethra; coat of pharynx; coat of prostatic urethra; coat of rectum; coat of small intestine; coat of spongy part of male urethra; coat of stomach; coat of trachea; coat of ureter; coat of urinary bladder; coat of uterine tube; coat of uterus; coat of vagina; dystrophy; fascia; fascia of extraocular muscle; fibril; hyperesthesia; incompetence; insufficiency; lacuna; layer; layer of bronchi; layer of colon; layer of ductus deferens; layer of esophagus; layer of female urethra; layer of gallbladder; layer of

intermediate part of (male)
urethra; layer of large
intestine; layer of male
urethra; layer of mucosa;
layer of pharynx; layer of
prostatic urethra; layer of
rectum; layer of renal pelvis;
layer of seminal gland; layer
of small intestine; layer of
spongy (male) urethra; layer
of stomach; layer of trachea;
layer of ureter; layer of
urinary bladder; layer of
uterine tube; layer of vagina;
movement; part of
interventricular septum (of
heart); process of arytenoid
cartilage; pulley; reflex;
rheumatism; sense; space of
retroinguinal compartment;
sphincter supracollicularis;
substance of prostate;
system; tissue; torticollis;
triangle (of neck); trochlea;
trophoneurosis; tunic of
gallbladder; tunics
muscular subaortic: stenosis
musculocutaneous: flap;
nerve; nerve of leg
musculophrenic: artery; veins
musculospiral: groove; nerve;
paralysis
musculotendinous: cuff
musculotubal: canal
mushroom: poisoning
mushroom-worker's: lung
music: blindness
musical: agraphia; alexia;
murmur
musician's: cramp
muskeag: moss
Musset: sign
Mustard: operation; procedure
mustard: gas
mutant: gene
mutation: rate
mutational: frequency
mutilating: keratoderma;
leprosy
mutton-fat keratic:
precipitates
mutual: resistance
mutualistic: symbiosis
MVE: virus
MWC: model
myasthenic: crisis; facies;
reaction; syndrome
mycotic: aneurysm;
endocarditis; keratitis
myelin: body; figure; protein
A1; sheath
myelinated: nerve
myelinated nerve: fiber
myelinic: degeneration
myeloblastic: leukemia

myelocytic: crisis; leukemia;
leukemoid reaction
myelodysplastic: syndrome
myelogenic: sarcoma
myeloid: cell; metaplasia;
sarcoma; series; tissue
myelomonocytic: leukemia
myelophthisic: anemia
myeloproliferative:
syndromes
myenteric: reflex
myenteric (nervous): plexus
mylohyoid: artery; branch (of
inferior alveolar artery);
fossa; groove; line; muscle;
nerve; ridge
mylopharyngeal: part of
superior constrictor muscle
of pharynx; part of superior
pharyngeal constrictor
(muscle) of pharynx
myocardial: bridge;
infarction; insufficiency;
ischemia; rigor mortis
myocardial depressant: factor
myoclonic: seizure
myoclonic astatic: epilepsy
myoclonus: epilepsy
myocutaneous: flap
myodermal: flap
myoelastic: theory
myoepicardial: mantle
myoepithelial: cell
myofascial: syndrome
myofascial pain-dysfunction:
syndrome
myofunctional: therapy
myogenic: potential; tonus
myoid: cells
myomatous: polyp
myometrial arcuate: arteries
myometrial radial: arteries
myoneural: blockade; junction
myopathic: atrophy; facies;
scoliosis
**myophosphorylase
deficiency:** glycogenosis
myopic: astigmatism;
choroidopathy; conus;
crescent; degeneration
myosin: filament
myotatic: contraction;
irritability; reflex
myotonic: cataract;
chondrodystrophy;
dystrophy; response
myotubular: myopathy
myovascular: sphincter
myovenous: sphincter
myxedema: heart; voice
myxedematous: infantilism
myxoid: cyst; degeneration
myxomatosis: virus
myxomembranous: colitis
myxopapillary: ependymoma

N

N: terminus
nabothian: cyst; follicle
nacreous: ichthyosis
Nadi: reaction
Naegeli: syndrome
Naegeli type of monocytic:
leukemia
Naffziger: operation;
syndrome
Nagel: test
Nägele: obliquity; pelvis; rule
Nageotte: cells
nail: bed; extension; fold;
horn; matrix; pits; plate;
pulse; wall
nail-patella: syndrome
**Nair buffered methylene
blue:** stain
Nakanishi: stain
naked: virus
NAME: syndrome
NANB: hepatitis
NANBNC: hepatitis
NANC: neuron
Nance-Insley: syndrome
Nance-Sweeney:
chondrodysplasia
nanoid: enamel
nanukayami: fever
nape: nevus
napkin: rash
narcissistic personality:
disorder
narcoleptic: tetrad
narcotic: blockade; hunger;
reversal
narrow-angle: glaucoma
nasal: arch; atrium; bone;
border of frontal bone;
calculus; capsule; catarrh;
cavity; crest; crest of
horizontal plate of palatine
bone; crest of palatine
process of maxilla; duct;
feeding; foramen; ganglion;
glands; glioma; height;
hemorrhage; index; margin
of frontal bone; meatus;
mucosa; muscle; myiasis;
nerve; notch; part of frontal
bone; part of pharynx;
pharynx; pits; placodes;
point; polyp; process; reflex;
region; ridge; sacs; septum;
spine of frontal bone;
surface of maxilla; surface
of palatine bone; valve;
venules of retina; vestibule
nasalis: muscle
nasal septal: branch of
superior labial branch of
facial artery; cartilage
nasal venous: arch

Nasik: vibrio
nasion-pogonion:
measurement
nasion-postcondylar: plane
nasion soft: tissue
Nasmyth: cuticle; membrane
nasoalveolar: cyst
nasobasilar: line
nasobregmatic: arc
nasociliary: nerve; root of
ciliary ganglion
nasofrontal: vein
nasogastric: tube
nasojugal: fold
nasolabial: cyst; groove;
lymph node; node; sulcus
nasolacrimal: canal; duct
nasomandibular: fixation
nasomaxillary: suture
nasomental: reflex
naso-occipital: arc
nasopalatine: groove; nerve
nasopalatine duct: cyst
nasopharyngeal: carcinoma;
groove; leishmaniasis;
meatus; passage
nasotracheal: intubation; tube
Nasse: law
Natal: sore
natal: cleft; tooth
natiform: skull
native: albumin; protein
natural: antibody; dentition;
dyes; focus of infection;
hemolysin; immunity;
mutation; pigment; products;
selection
natural killer: cells
natural killer cell: leukemia
**natural killer cell
stimulating:** factor
nature-nurture: issue
Nauheim: bath; treatment
Nauta: stain
navicular: abdomen; bone of
hand; fossa of urethra
navicular: bone
navicular articular: surface
of talus
navigator: echo
NBT: test
ND: virus
Nd:YAG: laser
near: drowning; point;
reaction; reflex; sight
nearest neighbor: frequency
near point of: convergence
near-total: thyroidectomy
nebulous: urine
necessary: cause
neck: reflexes; sign
neck-shaft: angle
necrobiotic: xanthogranuloma
necrogenic: wart
necrolytic migratory:
erythema

necrosis: bacillus
necrotic: angina; arachnidism; cirrhosis; cyst; inflammation; pulp
necrotic infectious: conjunctivitis
necrotizing: angiitis; arteriolitis; cellulitis; encephalitis; encephalomyelopathy; encephalopathy; enterocolitis; fasciitis; keratitis; papillitis; scleritis; sialometaplasia
necrotizing hemorrhage: leukomyelitis
necrotizing ulcerative: gingivitis
needle: bath; biopsy; culture; forceps
needle point: tracing
Needles split cast: method
Neer impingement: sign
negative: accommodation; afterimage; anergy; catalyst; chronotropism; control; convergence; cooperativity; electrode; electrotaxis; feedback; image; meniscus; phase; politzerization; pressure; scotoma; stain; symptom; taxis; thermotaxis; transference; valence
negative base: excess
negative end-expiratory: pressure
negatively: inotropic
negative myoclonic: seizure
negative pressure: ventilation
negative strand: virus
Negishi: virus
Negri: bodies; corpuscles
Negro: phenomenon
Neisser: coccus; stain; syringe
Nélaton: catheter; dislocation; fibers; fold; line; sphincter
Nelson: syndrome; tumor
nemaline: myopathy
neonatal: anemia; apoplexy; conjunctivitis; death; diagnosis; hepatitis; herpes; hyperbilirubinemia; hypoglycemia; isoerythrolysis; jaundice; line; lupus; medicine; ring; screening; tetanus; tetany; tooth
neonatal calf diarrhea: virus
neonatal mortality: rate
neoplastic: arachnoiditis; meningitis
neotype: culture; strain
neovascular: glaucoma
nephric: blastema; duct
nephritic: factor; syndrome

nephrogenic: adenoma; cord; diabetes insipidus; tissue
nephronic: loop
nephrostomy: tube
nephrotic: edema; syndrome
nephrotomic: cavity
Neptune: girdle
Néri: sign
Nernst: equation
nerve: avulsion; block; cell; conduction; deafness; decompression; ending; fascicle; fiber; field; force; ganglion; graft; implantation; papilla; plexus; root; stroma; suture; tract; trunk
nerve block: anesthesia
nerve cell: body
nerve conduction: velocity
nerve growth: cone; factor
nerve growth factor: antiserum
nervous: asthenopia; asthma; dyspepsia; indigestion; lobe; part of retina; system; tissue; tunic of eyeball
Nessler: reagent
nested polymerase chain: reaction
net: flux; knot
Netherton: syndrome
nettle: rash
Nettleshop-Falls: albinism
nettling: hairs
Neubauer: artery
Neuberg: ester
Neufeld: reaction
Neufeld capsular: swelling
Neumann: cells; disease; law; sheath
neural: arch of vertebra; axis; canal; crest; cyst; factor; folds; groove; hearing loss; layer of optic part of retina; layer of retina; lobe of hypophysis; part of hypophysis; plate; segment; spine; tube
neural crest: syndrome
neuralgic: amyotrophy
neurasthenic: personality
neurenteric: canal; cysts
neurilemma: cells
neuritic: plaque
neuroaxonal: dystrophy
neurobiotactic: movement
neurocentral: joint; suture; synchondrosis
neurochronaxic: theory
neurocirculatory: asthenia
neurocranial granulomatous: arteritis
neurocutaneous: melanosis; syndrome
neuroectodermal: junction

neuroendocrine: cell
neuroendocrine transducer: cell
neuroepithelial: body; cells; layer of retina
neurofibrillar: network
neurofibrillary: degeneration; tangle
neurogenic: airway; atrophy; bladder; claudication; fracture; tonus
neuroglia: cells
neurohemal: organs
neurohumoral: secretion; transmission
neurohypophysial: hormones
neurolemma: cells
neuroleptic: agent
neuroleptic malignant: syndrome
neurolinguistic: programming
neuromuscular: junction; relaxant; spindle; system
neuromuscular blocking: agents
neuronal: hyperplasia
neuronal ceroid: lipofuscinosis
neuronal intestinal: dysplasia
neuronal migration: abnormality
neuron-specific: enolase
neuroparalytic: keratitis; keratopathy
neuropathic: albuminuria; arthritis; arthropathy; bladder; joint
neuropsychologic: disorder
neurosecretory: cells; substance
neurosomatic: junction
neurotendinous: organ; spindle
neurotic: disorder; excoriation; manifestation
neurotonic: reaction
neurotrophic: atrophy; keratitis
neurotropic: attraction; virus
neurovascular: bundle of Walsh; flap; sheath
Neusser: granules
neutral: axis of straight beam; element; fat; mutation; occlusion; oxide; point; reaction; spirits; stain; zone
neutral buffered formalin: fixative
neutralization: plate; test
neutralizing: antibody
neutral lipid storage: disease
neutron: radiation
neutropenic: angina
neutrophil: granule
neutrophil-activating: factor; protein

neutrophil chemotactant: factor
neutrophilic: leukemia; leukocyte; leukocytosis; leukopenia
neutrophilic eccrine: hidradenitis
nevoid: amentia; elephantiasis; hypertrichosis
nevus: cell; cell, A-type; cell, B-type; cell, C-type
new: combination; growth; methylene blue; mutation
Newcastle: disease
Newcastle disease: virus
Newcomer: fixative
New Hampshire: rule
Newton: disk; law
Newtonian: constant of gravitation
newtonian: aberration; flow; fluid; viscosity
New World: leishmaniasis
new yellow: enzyme
New York: virus
New York Heart Association: classification
Neyman-Pearson statistical: hypothesis
Nezelof: syndrome
Nezelof type of thymic: alymphoplasia
NGF: antiserum
niacin: test
Nick: procedure
nick: translation
nickel: dermatitis
Nickerson-Kveim: test
Nicol: prism
Nicolas-Favre: disease
Nicolle: stain for capsules
Nicolle white: mycetoma
nicotine: stomatitis
nicotinic: receptors
nicotinic acid: maculopathy
nicotinic cholinergic: receptor
nictitating: membrane; spasm
Nieden: syndrome
Niemann: disease; splenomegaly
Niemann-Pick: cell; disease
Niemann-Pick C1: disease
Niewenglowski: rays
night: blindness; hospital; myopia; pain; sight; soil; sweats; vision
nihilistic: delusion
Nikiforoff: method
Nikolsky: sign
nil: disease
nine mile: fever
ninhydrin: reaction
ninhydrin-Schiff: stain for proteins
ninth cranial: nerve [CN IX]
ninth-day: erythema

Word Finder

Nipah: virus
nipple: line; shield
nirvana: principle
Nissen: fundoplication; operation
Nissl: bodies; degeneration; granules; stain; substance
Nitabuch: layer; membrane; stria
niter: paper
nitinol: filter
nitrate: respiration
nitritoid: reaction
nitro: dyes
nitroblue: tetrazolium
nitroblue tetrazolium: test
nitrofurantoin: polyneuropathy
nitrogen: autotrophy; balance; cycle; equivalent; fixation; mustards; narcosis
nitrogenous: equilibrium
nitroid: shock
nitroprusside: test
NK: cells
NMDA: receptor
NNN: medium
Noack: syndrome
Noble: position; stain
noble: element; gases; metal
Noble-Collip: procedure
Nocardia: dacryoliths
nociceptive: reflex
nocifensor: reflex
nocturnal: amblyopia; diarrhea; dyspnea; emission; enuresis; epilepsy; myoclonus; periodicity; vertigo
nodal: bigeminy; bradycardia; fever; plane; point; rhythm; tachycardia; tissue
nodding: spasm
nodose: ganglion; rheumatism
nodoventricular: fibers
nodular: amyloidosis; arteriosclerosis; body; disease; episcleritis; fasciitis; headache; hidradenoma; hyperplasia of prostate; iritis; leprosy; lymphoma; melanoma; mesoneuritis; opacity; panencephalitis; scleritis; sclerosis; syphilid; transformation of the liver; tuberculid; vasculitis
nodular histiocytic: lymphoma
nodular nonsuppurative: panniculitis
nodular non-X: histiocytosis
nodular regenerative: hyperplasia
nodular subepidermal: fibrosis
nodus sinuatrialis: echo

noetic: anxiety
noise: pollution
noise-induced: hearing loss
Nomarski: optics
Nomarski interference: microscopy
nomenclatural: type
nominal: aphasia
nomothetic: approach
nonabsorbable: ligature
nonabsorbable surgical: suture
nonaccommodative: esotropia
nonadrenergic, noncholinergic: neuron
non–A-E: hepatitis
nonan: malaria
nonanatomic: teeth
non-A, non-B: hepatitis
non-A, non-B hepatitis: virus
non-A, non-B, non-C: hepatitis
non-arcon: articulator
nonbacterial thrombotic: endocarditis
nonbacterial verrucous: endocarditis
nonbullous congenital ichthyosiform: erythroderma
nonchromaffin: paraganglioma
nonclassical: phenylketonuria
nonclonogenic: cell
noncohesive: gold
noncommunicating: hydrocele; hydrocephalus
noncompetitive: inhibition
noncomplementary: role
nonconjugative: plasmid
noncontained disk: herniation
nonconvulsive: seizure
noncovalent: bond
non–cycle-specific: agent
nondeciduous: placenta
nondepolarizing: block; relaxant
nondepolarizing neuromuscular blocking: agent
nondiabetic: glycosuria
nondirective: psychotherapy
nonepileptic: seizure
nonessential: amino acids
nonfenestrated: forceps
nonfilament polymorphonuclear: leukocyte
nonfluent: aphasia
nongonococcal: urethritis
nongranular: leukocyte
non-heme iron: protein
non-Hodgkin: lymphoma
nonhomologous: chromosomes
nonhyperglycemic: glycosuria

nonimmune: agglutination; serum
nonimmune fetal: hydrops
noninfiltrating lobular: carcinoma
noninflammatory: edema
non-insulin-dependent: diabetes mellitus
noninvasive positive pressure: ventilation
nonionic: surfactant
nonionic contrast: agent
nonisolated: proteinuria
nonketotic: hyperglycemia; hyperglycinemia
nonlamellar: bone
nonlipid: histiocytosis
nonmedullated: fibers
nonmotile: leukocyte
nonneurogenic neurogenic: bladder
non-newtonian: fluid
nonobstructive: atelectasis; jaundice
nonoccluded: virus
nonorganic: aphonia
nonossifying: fibroma
nonosteogenic: fibroma
nonovulational: menstruation
nonparticipant: observer
nonpedunculated: hydatid
nonpenetrant: trait
nonpenetrating: keratoplasty; wound
nonphasic sinus: arrhythmia
nonpitting: edema
non-PKU: hyperphenylalaninemia
nonplasmatic: compartment
nonpolar: amino acid; compound; solvents
nonprecipitable: antibody
nonprecipitating: antibody
nonprotein: nitrogen
nonrandom: mating
non-rapid eye: movement
nonreactive: depression
nonreassuring fetal: status
nonrebreathing: anesthesia; mask; valve
nonrefractive accommodative: esotropia
nonrenal: azotemia
nonresponder: tolerance
nonrigid: connector
nonsecretory: myeloma
nonsense: codon; mutation; syndrome; triplet
nonseptate: mycelium
nonsexual: generation
nonshivering: thermogenesis
nonspecific: anergy; cholinesterase; protein; system; therapy; urethritis; vaginitis

nonspecific building-related: illnesses
nonsteroidal anti-inflammatory: drugs
nonstress: test
nonsuppressible insulinlike: activity
nonthrombocytopenic: purpura
nontoxic: goiter
nontransmural myocardial: infarction
nontropical: sprue
nontypeable: *Haemophilus influenzae*
nonvenereal: syphilis
nonvital: pulp; tooth
noogenic: neurosis
Noonan: syndrome
NOR-: banding
Nordhausen: sulfuric acid
no reflow: phenomenon
normal: animal; antibody; antithrombin; antitoxin; bite; concentration; distribution; hearing; occlusion; opsonin; ovariotomy; phosphate; serum; solution; tartrate; toxin; values
normal cholesteremic: xanthomatosis
normal electrical: axis
normal horse: serum
normal human: plasma; serum
normal human serum: albumin
normally posed: tooth
normal pressure: hydrocephalus
normal-tension: glaucoma
normochromic: anemia
normocytic: anemia
normoglycemic: glycosuria
normokalemic periodic: paralysis
normospermatogenic: sterility
normotriglyceridemic: abetalipoproteinemia
Norrie: disease
Norris: corpuscles
North American: blastomycosis
Northern blot: analysis
North Queensland tick: fever; typhus
Norton: operation
Norton-Simon: hypothesis
Norwalk: agent; virus
Norway: itch
Norwegian: scabies
Norwood: operation; procedure
nose: drops
nose-bridge-lid: reflex

nose-eye: reflex
nosocomial: gangrene; pneumonia
notched: teeth
note: blindness
Nothnagel: syndrome
no-threshold: concept
notifiable: disease
notochordal: canal; plate; process; sheath
Novy and MacNeal blood: agar
NPH: insulin
nu: body
nuchal: arm; cord; fascia; ligament; plane; rigidity; tubercle
Nuck: diverticulum; hydrocele
nuclear: atom; bag; cataract; chemistry; energy; envelope; factor-κB; family; fusion; hyaloplasm; jaundice; lamina; layers of retina; magneton; matrix; medicine; membrane; ophthalmoplegia; pacemaker; pore; reaction; RNA; sap; sclerosis; spindle; stain
nuclear bag: fiber
nuclear chain: fiber
nuclear-cytoplasmic: ratio
nuclear inclusion: bodies
nuclear magnetic: resonance
nuclear magnetic resonance: imaging; tomography
nuclear Overhauser: effect
nucleate: endonuclease
nucleic acid: base; hybridization; probe
nucleocortical: fibers
nucleolar: chromosome; organizer; zone
nucleolar-nuclear: ratio
nucleolus: organizer
nucleolus organizer: region
nucleoplasmic: index
nucleoside: pair; phosphorylases
nucleotide: deletion; sequence
nude: mouse
Nuel: space
Nuhn: gland
null: cells; hypothesis
null-cell: adenoma
numb chin: syndrome
numerical: aperture; hypertrophy; taxonomy
nummular: dermatitis; eczema; sputum; syphilid
nun's: murmur
nurse: cells
nursemaid's: elbow
nursing bottle: caries
Nussbaum: bracelet
nutmeg: liver

nutrient: agar; arteries of humerus; artery; artery of femur; artery of fibula; artery of radius; artery of the tibia; artery of ulna; canal; enema; foramen; medium; vessel
nutritional: amblyopia; anemia; cirrhosis; dropsy; edema; energy; hemosiderosis; marasmus; polyneuropathy
nutritional macrocytic: anemia
nutritional type cerebellar: atrophy
nutritive: equilibrium
nymphocaruncular: sulcus
nymphohymenal: sulcus
nystagmus: test
nystagmus blockage: syndrome
Nysten: law

O

O: agglutinin; antigen; colony; shell
ω-3: fatty acids
oasthouse urine: disease
oat: cell
oat cell: carcinoma
oatmeal-tomato paste: agar
OAV: syndrome
O'Beirne: sphincter; valve
Ober: test
Obermayer: test
Obermeier: spirillum
Obersteiner-Redlich: line; zone
obesity: index
object: blindness; constancy; glass; libido; relationship
objective: optometer; perimetry; probability; psychology; sign; symptom; synonyms
obligate: aerobe; anaerobe; parasite
oblique: amputation; bandage; bundle of pons; cord of interosseous membrane of forearm; diameter; fibers of muscular layer of stomach; fissure; fissure of lung; fracture; head; illumination; lie; ligament of elbow joint; line; line of mandible; line of thyroid cartilage; muscle of auricle; part of cricothyroid (muscle); projection; ridge; ridge of trapezium; section; sinus of pericardium; vein of left atrium
oblique arytenoid: muscle

oblique auricular: muscle
oblique facial: cleft
oblique pericardial: sinus
oblique pontine: fasciculus
oblique popliteal: ligament
obliquus capitis inferior: muscle
obliquus capitis superior: muscle
obliterative: arachnoiditis; bronchitis; pericarditis
oblong: fovea of arytenoid cartilage; pit of arytenoid cartilage
obsessional: neurosis
obsessive: behavior; personality
obsessive-compulsive: disorder; neurosis; personality
obsessive-compulsive personality: disorder
obstacle: sense
obstetric: conjugate; conjugate of pelvic outlet; hand; palsy; paralysis; position; ultrasound
obstetrical: binder; forceps
obstetric conjugate: diameter
obstructive: appendicitis; dysmenorrhea; hydrocephalus; jaundice; murmur; pneumonia; thrombus; uropathy
obstructive sleep: apnea
obturating: embolism
obturator: appliance; artery; branch of pubic branch of inferior epigastric vein; canal; crest; fascia; foramen; groove; hernia; lymph nodes; membrane; nerve; tubercle; veins
obturator externus: muscle
obturator internus: muscle
occipital: anchorage; angle of parietal bone; artery; aspect; belly of occipitofrontalis muscle; bone; border; border of parietal bone; border of temporal bone; branch; condyle; fontanelle; forceps; groove; gyri; horn; line; lobe; lobe of cerebrum; lymph nodes; margin; margin of temporal bone; neuralgia; neurectomy; neuritis; operculum; part of corpus callosum; plane; plexus; point; pole; pole [TA] of cerebrum; region of head; sinus; somite; stripe; triangle; vein
occipital cerebral: veins
occipital emissary: vein
occipital horn: syndrome

occipitalis: muscle
occipital lobe: epilepsy
occipitoanterior: position
occipitoaxial: ligaments
occipitocollicular: tract
occipitofrontal: diameter; fasciculus; muscle
occipitofrontalis: muscle
occipitomastoid: suture
occipitomental: diameter; projection
occipitopontine: fibers; tract
occipitoposterior: position
occipitotectal: fibers; tract
occipitotemporal: sulcus
occipitothalamic: radiation
occipitotransverse: position
occluded: virus
occluding: frame; ligature; paper; relation
occluding centric relation: record
occlusal: adjustment; analysis; balance; caries; clearance; correction; curvature; disharmony; embrasure; force; form; harmony; imbalance; path; pattern; pivot; plane; position; pressure; radiograph; rest; rim; scheme; surface of tooth; system; table; trauma; wear
occlusal rest: bar
occlusal vertical: dimension
occlusion: rim
occlusive: dressing; ileus; meningitis
occult: bleeding; blood; border of nail; carcinoma; fracture; hydrocephalus
occult choroidal: neovascularization
occult posterior laryngeal: cleft
occupational: disease; therapy
Ochoa: law
ochre: codon; mutation
ochronotic: arthritis
Ochsner: clamp; method
ocular: albinism; albinism 1; albinism 2; albinism 3; albinism with late-onset sensorineural deafness; albinism with sensorineural deafness; bobbing; cone; crisis; cup; dysmetria; flutter; humor; hypertelorism; larva migrans; lens; micrometer; migraine; muscles; myiasis; myopathy; nystagmus; onchocerciasis; paralysis; pemphigoid; prosthesis; rigidity; scoliosis;

sparganosis; tension; torticollis; vertigo; vesicle
ocular cicatricial: pemphigoid
ocular larva migrans: granuloma
ocular motor: apraxia
ocular-mucous membrane: syndrome
oculoauriculovertebral: dysplasia
oculobuccogenital: syndrome
oculocardiac: reflex
oculocephalic: reflex
oculocephalogyric: reflex
oculocerebrorenal: syndrome
oculocutaneous: albinism; syndrome
oculodentodigital: dysplasia
oculodermal: melanosis
oculoencephalic: angiomatosis
oculogravic: illusion
oculogyral: illusion
oculogyric: crises
oculomandibulofacial: syndrome
oculomotor: nerve [CN III]; nucleus; response; root of ciliary ganglion; sulcus of mesencephalon; system
oculopharyngeal: dystrophy; syndrome
oculovagal: reflex
oculovertebral: dysplasia; syndrome
oculovestibulo-auditory: syndrome
odd: chromosome
Oddi: sphincter
Odland: body
odontoblastic: layer; process
odontogenic: cyst; dysplasia; fibroma; keratocyst; myxoma
odontoid: process; process of epistropheus; vertebra
odorant binding: protein
odoriferous: gland
O'Dwyer: tube
oedipal: neurosis; period; phase
Oedipus: complex
Oehl: muscles
Oehler: symptom
OFD: syndrome
official: formula
off label: indication
off-vertical: rotation
Ofuji: disease
Ogilvie: syndrome
Ogino-Knaus: rule
Ogston: line
Ogston-Luc: operation
Oguchi: disease
Ogura: operation
O'Hara: forceps
17-OH-corticoids: test

Ohm: law
Ohngren: line
oil: bath; cyst; embolism; glands; immersion; pneumonia; sugar; tumor; vaccine
oil retention: enema
oily: granuloma
ointment: base
Okazaki: fragment
OKT: cells
Oldfield: syndrome
Old World: leishmaniasis
old yellow: enzyme
olecranon: bursitis; fossa; process; reflex
olfactory: agnosia; angle; area; aura; bulb; bundle; cells; cortex; epithelium; esthesioneuroblastoma; fila; foramen; glands; glomerulus; groove; groove of nasal cavity; hallucination; hyperesthesia; hypesthesia; membrane; mucosa; nerves [CN I]; neuroblastoma; organ; peduncle; pits; placodes; pyramid; region of mucosa of nose; region of nasal mucosa; region of nose; region of tunica mucosa of nose; roots; striae; sulcus; sulcus of nasal cavity; tract; trigone; tubercle
olfactory receptor: cells
oligemic: shock
oligoclonal: band
oligodendroglia: cells
olivary: body; eminence
olive: oil
olive-tipped: catheter
olivocerebellar: tract
olivocochlear: bundle; fibers; tract; tract
olivopontocerebellar: atrophy; degeneration
olivospinal: fibers; tract
Ollier: disease; graft; theory
Ollier-Thiersch: graft
Olmsted: syndrome
olympian: forehead
Ombrédanne: operation
omega-3: fatty acids
omega-: oxidation
omega-oxidation: theory
Omenn: syndrome
omental: appendices; branches; bursa; eminence of pancreas; enterocleisis; flap; foramen; sac; tenia; tuber; tuberosity of liver
Ommaya: reservoir
omnifocal: lens
omoclavicular: triangle
omohyoid: muscle

omotracheal: triangle
omphaloangiopagous: twins
omphalomesenteric: artery; cord; cyst; duct
omphalomesenteric duct: cyst
Omsk hemorrhagic: fever
Omsk hemorrhagic fever: virus
oncocytic: adenoma; carcinoma
oncocytic hepatocellular: tumor
oncofetal: antigens; marker
oncogenic: virus
oncosphere: embryo
oncotic: pressure
Ondine: curse
one-carbon: fragment
one-horned: uterus
onion: bodies
onion bulb: neuropathy
onlay: graft
Onodi: cell
on-off: phenomenon
ontogenic: homeostasis
Onuf: nucleus
o'nyong-nyong: fever; virus
oophoritic: cyst
opacifying: gallstones
opal: codon; mutation
opalescent: dentin
opaline: patch
Opalski: cell
opaque: microscope
open: biopsy; bite; comedo; cordotomy; dislocation; drainage; fracture; hospital; laparoscopy; pneumothorax; reading frame; reduction of fractures; system; tuberculosis; wound
open-angle: glaucoma
open chain: compound
open chest: massage
open circuit: method
open drop: anesthesia
open head: injury
open heart: surgery
opening: axis; contraction; movement; snap
open skull: fracture
opera-glass: hand
operant: behavior; conditioning
operating: microscope; table
operative: dentistry; myxedema
operator: gene
opercular: fold; part
ophryospinal: angle
ophthalmic: artery; hyperthyroidism; nerve [CN V1]; ointment; solutions; veins; vesicle

ophthalmomandibulomelic: dysplasia
ophthalmoplegic: migraine
opiate: receptors
opiate intoxication: syndrome
opioid: antagonists
Opitz BBB: syndrome
Opitz G: syndrome
Oppenheim: disease; reflex; syndrome
opponens: muscle
opponens digiti minimi: muscle
opponens pollicis: muscle
opponent: color
opportunistic: pathogen
opposer: muscle of little finger; muscle of thumb
oppositional: disorder
oppositional defiant: disorder
opsonic: index
optic: activity; agnosia; antipode; ataxia; axis; canal; capsule; chiasm; cup; decussation; density; disk; fissure; foramen; groove; isomerism; layer; nerve [CN II]; neuritis; papilla; part of retina; pit; placodes; radiation; recess; rotation; stalk; tract; vesicle
optical: aberration; illusion; image; iridectomy; keratoplasty; pachymeter
optical righting: reflexes
optic nerve: glioma; head; hypoplasia
optic nerve sheath: decompression; fenestration
opticokinetic: nystagmus
optic rotatory: dispersion
optimum: dose; pH; temperature
optokinetic: nystagmus
O-R: system
oral: biology; cavity; cavity proper; contraceptive; fissure; hygiene; membrane; mucosa; opening; part of pharynx; pathology; pharynx; phase; physiotherapy; plate; primacy; region; shields; smear; stereotypy; surgeon; surgery; teeth; vestibule
oral auditory: method
oral epithelial: nevus
oral (erosive): lichen planus
oral focal: mucinosis
oral lactose tolerance: test
oral poliovirus: vaccine
oral pontine reticular: nucleus
oral submucous: fibrosis
Orbeli: effect

orbicular: bone; ligament; ligament of radius; muscle; muscle of eye; muscle of mouth; process; zone of hip joint

orbicularis: muscle; phenomenon

orbicularis oculi: muscle; reflex

orbicularis oris: muscle

orbicularis pupillary: reflex

orbital: abscess; artery; axis; branches of maxillary nerve; branch of middle meningeal artery; branch of pterygopalatine ganglion; cavity; cellulitis; decompression; eminence of zygomatic bone; exenteration; fasciae; fat-pad; gyri; height; hernia; implant; index; lamina of ethmoid bone; layer of ethmoid bone; margin; margin of eyelids; muscle; nerve; opening; ophthalmoplegia; part of frontal bone; part of lacrimal gland; part of optic nerve; part of orbicularis oculi (muscle); part [TA] of inferior frontal gyrus; plane; plate; plate of ethmoid bone; process of palatine bone; region; rim; septum; sulci; surface; syndrome; tubercle (of zygomatic bone); width

orbital fat: body

orbitalis: muscle

orbitofrontal: artery; cortex

orbitomeatal: line; plane

orbitonasal: index

orcinol: test

ordered: mechanism

ordered on-random off: mechanism

ordinal: scale

orf: virus

organ: culture

organic: acid; catalyst; chemistry; compound; contracture; delusions; disease; evolution; hallucinosis; headache; hearing impairment; murmur; pain; phosphate; principle; stricture; vertigo

organic brain: syndrome

organic dental: cement

organic mental: disorder

organic mood: syndrome

organification: defect

organoid: nevus; tumor

organ-specific: antigen

Oriboca: virus

oriens: layer

Oriental: boil; button; ringworm; schistosomiasis; sore; ulcer

orienting: reflex; response

Ormond: disease

Ornish prevention: diets

Ornish reversal: diet

ornithine: cycle

ornithosis: virus

oroantral: fistula

orodigitofacial: dysostosis

orofacial: fistula

orofaciodigital: syndrome

oronasal: fistula; membrane

oropharyngeal: isthmus; membrane; passage

Oropouche: fever

orotracheal: intubation; tube

Oroya: fever

orphan: disease; drugs; products; receptor; viruses

Orsi-Grocco: method

Orth: fixative; stain

orthodontic: appliance; band; therapy

orthoglycemic: glycosuria

orthognathic: surgery

orthograde: conduction

orthomolecular: psychiatry; therapy

orthopedic: surgery

orthopnea: position

orthopneic: position

orthoscopic: lens; spectacles

orthostatic: albuminuria; hypopiesis; hypotension; proteinuria; tachycardia

orthotopic: graft; ureterocele

Ortolani: maneuver; test

oscillating: vision

oscillatory: potential

Osgood-Schlatter: disease

Osler: disease; node; sign

Osler-Vaquez: disease

osmic acid: fixative

osmolal: clearance

osmotic: diuresis; diuretics; fragility; nephrosis; pressure; shock

osseous: ampulla; cell; labyrinth; lacuna; part of skeletal system; polyp; tissue

osseous hydatid: cyst

osseous spiral: lamina

ossicular: chain; reconstruction

ossific: center

ossification: center

ossifying: cartilage

osteochondrogenic: cell

osteoclast activating: factor

osteocollagenous: fibers

osteogenetic: fibers; layer

osteogenic: cell; sarcoma; tissue

osteoid: osteoma; tissue

osteomalacic: pelvis

osteomyelofibrotic: syndrome

osteopathic: medicine; physician; scoliosis

osteoperiosteal: graft

osteoplastic: amputation; craniotomy; necrotomy; obliteration of the frontal sinus

osteoplastic bone: flap

osteoporotic marrow: defect

osteoprogenitor: cell

osteosclerotic: anemia

ostial: sphincter

ostiomeatal: complex; unit

Ostrum-Furst: syndrome

Ostwald solubility: coefficient

Ot: antigen

Ota: nevus

Othello: syndrome

otic: barotrauma; capsule; ganglion; pits; placodes; vesicle

otitic: abscess; hydrocephalus; meningitis

otoacoustic: emission

otolithic: crisis; membrane; organs

otomandibular: dysostosis; syndrome

otopalatodigital: syndrome

otopharyngeal: tube

otospondylomegaepiphyseal: dysplasia

Otto: disease; pelvis

Ottoson: potential

Ouchterlony: technique; test

outer: border of iris; lip of iliac crest; malleolus; membrane; sheath of optic nerve; stripes of renal medulla; table of skull; zone of renal medulla

outer limiting: layer

outer nuclear: layer

outer plexiform: layer

outer spiral: sulcus

outlet forceps: delivery

outline: form

outpatient: anesthesia

outstanding: ear

oval: area of Flechsig; corpuscle; fasciculus; foramen; foramen of heart; fossa; window

ovale: malaria

ova and parasite: examination

ovarian: amenorrhea; artery; branches of uterine artery; bursa; colic; cortex; cycle; cyst; dysmenorrhea; fimbria; fossa; ligament; pregnancy; varicocele; veins

ovarian (nervous): plexus

ovarian tubular: adenoma

ovarian vein: syndrome

ovarioabdominal: pregnancy

overanxious: disorder

overflow: incontinence; wave

overhanging: restoration

overlap: hybridization

overlay: denture

overproduction: theory

overriding: aorta

overripe: cataract

overt: homosexuality

overvalued: idea

ovo-: vegetarian

ovular: membrane; transmigration

ovulation: inhibitor

ovulational: sclerosis

ovulocyclic: porphyria

Owen: lines

own: controls

Owren: disease

ox: bots; heart

oxalate: calculus

oxazin: dyes

Oxford: unit

oxidase: reaction; test

oxidation-reduction: electrode; indicator; potential; reaction; system

oxidative: deamination; decarboxylation; metabolism; phosphorylation

oxidized: cellulose; glutathione

oxonium: ion

oxygen: capacity; consumption; debt; deficit; effect; electrode; poisoning; tent; therapy; toxicity

oxygen affinity: anoxia; hypoxia

oxygenated: hemoglobin

oxygen deprivation: theory of narcosis

oxygen-derived free: radicals

oxygen utilization: coefficient

oxyntic: cell; gland

oxyphil: adenoma; cell; chromatin; granule

oxyphilic: carcinoma; leukocyte

oxytocin challenge: test

P

π: helix

ψ: factor

P: antigens; cell; elements; enzyme; factor; selectin; substance of Lewis; wave

P1: segment of posterior cerebral artery

P2: segment of posterior cerebral artery

P3: segment of posterior cerebral artery

Word Finder

P4: segment of posterior cerebral artery
PA: interval; projection
Paas: disease
pacchionian: bodies; corpuscles; depressions; glands; granulations
pacemaker: failure; output; potential; sensitivity; syndrome
Pacheco parrot disease: virus
Pachon: method; test
pachydermoperiostosis: syndrome
pacing: catheter
pacinian: corpuscles
packed cell: volume
packed human blood: cells
packing: process
PA conduction: time
Padykula-Herman: stain for myosin ATPase
Pagenstecher: circle
Paget: cells; disease
Paget-Eccleston: stain
pagetoid: cells; reticulosis
Paget-von Schrötter: syndrome
Pahvant Valley: fever; plague
pain: reaction; threshold; tolerance
painful: anesthesia; heel; hematuria; paraplegia; point; toe
painful arc: sign; syndrome
painful-bruising: syndrome
painless: hematuria; jaundice
pain-pleasure: principle
painter's: colic
paired: allosome; associates; beats; organelles
Pajot: maneuver
Palade: granule
palatal: abscess; bar; index; myoclonus; nystagmus; papillomatosis; plate; reflex; seal; shelf; triangle
palate: hook; myograph
palatine: aponeurosis; bone; crest of horizontal process of palatine bone; glands; grooves; papilla; process of maxilla; raphe; ridge; spines; surface of horizontal plate of palatine bone; tonsil; torus; uvula
palatoethmoidal: suture
palatoglossal: arch
palatoglossus: muscle
palatomaxillary: index; suture
palatopharyngeal: arch; muscle; sphincter
palatopharyngeus: muscle
palatouvularis: muscle
palatovaginal: canal; groove

pale: globe; hypertension; infarct; thrombus
paleostriatal: syndrome
Palfyn: sinus
palindromic: DNA; encephalopathy; sequence
palisade: layer
pallesthetic: sensibility
palliative: treatment
pallidal: syndrome
palm: grasp; oil; wax
palmar: aponeurosis; branch of anterior interosseous nerve; branch of median nerve; branch of ulnar nerve; crease; fascia; fibromatosis; flexion; ligaments; ligaments of interphalangeal joints of hand; ligaments of metacarpophalangeal joints; monticuli; plates; psoriasis; reflex; surfaces of fingers; syphilid
palmar carpal: branch of radial artery; branch of ulnar artery; ligament
palmar carpal tendinous: sheaths
palmar carpometacarpal: ligaments
palmar digital: veins
palmar interossei interosseous: muscles
palmar interosseous: artery
palmaris brevis: muscle
palmaris longus: muscle
palmar metacarpal: artery; ligaments; veins
palmar radiocarpal: ligament
palmar ulnocarpal: ligament
palmate: folds of cervical canal
palm-chin: reflex
Palmer acid: test for peptic ulcer
palmin: test
palmomental: reflex
palmoplantar: keratoderma
palpable: rale
palpatory: percussion
palpebral: branches of infratrochlear nerve; conjunctiva; fissure; glands; margins; part of lacrimal gland; part of orbicularis oculi (muscle); raphe; veins
palpebronasal: fold
paludal: fever
pampiniform: body
pampiniform venous: plexus
panacinar: emphysema
pancake: kidney
pancervical: smear
Pancoast: syndrome; tumor

pancreatic: abscess; branches; calculus; cholera; colic; cystoduodenostomy; deoxyribonuclease; diabetes; diarrhea; digestion; diverticula; dornase; duct; encephalopathy; infantilism; islands; islets; juice; lithiasis; lymph nodes; notch; polypeptide; RNase; sphincter; steatorrhea; veins
pancreatic hyperglycemic: hormone
pancreatic (nervous): plexus
pancreaticoduodenal: lymph nodes; transplantation; veins
pancreaticoduodenal arterial: arcades
pancreaticoenteric: recess
pancreaticosplenic: lymph nodes
pancreatogenous: diarrhea
pancreatorenal: syndrome
pancreozymin-secretin: test
Pandy: reaction; test
Paneth granular: cells
panhypopituitary: dwarfism
panic: attack; disorder
panlobular: emphysema
Panner: disease
pannicular: hernia
panniculus carnosus: muscle
panoptic: stain
panoramic: radiograph
panoramic rotating: machine
panoramic x-ray: film
Pansch: fissure
pansystolic: murmur
pantaloon: embolism; hernia
pantoate-activating: enzyme
pantoscopic: spectacles; tilt
pantropic: virus
Panum: area
PAP: technique
Pap: smear; test
Papanicolaou: examination; smear; stain
Papanicolaou smear: test
paper: autoradiography; chromatography; plate
paper mill worker's: disease
Papez: circuit
papillary: adenocarcinoma; adenoma of large intestine; carcinoma; cystadenoma lymphomatosum; ducts; foramina of kidney; hidradenoma; layer; muscle; process of caudate lobe of liver; ridges; stasis; tumor
papillary cystic: adenoma
papillary muscle: dysfunction; syndrome
papilloma: virus
Papillon-Léage and Psaume: syndrome

Papillon-Lefèvre: syndrome
pappataci: fever
pappataci fever: viruses
Pappenheim: stain
Pappenheimer: bodies
papular: acrodermatitis of childhood; dermatitis of pregnancy; fever; mucinosis; scrofuloderma; tuberculid; urticaria
papulonecrotic: tuberculid
papulosquamous: syphilid
papyraceous: scars
paraaortic: bodies
parabasal: body; filament
parabigeminal: nucleus
paraboloid: condenser
parabrachial: nuclei
paracarcinomatous: encephalomyelopathy; myelopathy
paracarmine: stain
paracellular: transport
paracelsian: method
paracentral: artery; branches of callosomarginal artery; branches (of pericallosal artery); fissure; lobule; nucleus of thalamus; scotoma; sulcus
paracentric: inversion
paracervical block: anesthesia
parachordal: cartilage; plate
parachute: deformity; reflex
parachute mitral: valve
paracicatricial: emphysema
paracoccidioidal: granuloma
paracolic: gutters; recesses
paracolon: bacillus
paracyclic: ovulation
paracystic: pouch
paradoxic: pulse
paradoxical: contraction; embolism; incontinence; movement of eyelids; pupil; reflex; respiration; sleep
paradoxical diaphragm: phenomenon
paradoxical extensor: reflex
paradoxical flexor: reflex
paradoxical patellar: reflex
paradoxical pupillary: phenomenon; reflex
paradoxical triceps: reflex
paradoxical vocal cord: movement
paraduodenal: fold; fossa; hernia; recess
paradysentery: bacillus
paraesophageal: hernia
paraffin: cancer; tumor; wax
parafollicular: cells
parafrenal: abscess
paraganglionic: cells
paragenital: tubules
paraglenoid: groove; sulcus

paraglottic: space
Paragonimus: granuloma
Paraguay: tea
parahiatal: hernia
parahippocampal: gyrus
parainfluenza: viruses
parajejunal: fossa
paralemniscal: nucleus
parallax: method; test
parallel: attachment; rays
paraluteal: cell
paralutein: cell
paralytic: dementia; ectropion; ileus; miosis; mydriasis; rabies; scoliosis; strabismus
paralyzing: vertigo
paramammary: lymph nodes
paramastoid: process
paramedial reticular: nucleus
paramedian: arteries; incision; lobule
paramedian pontine: branches of pontine arteries
paramesonephric: duct
parametric: abscess; test
paranasal: sinuses
paraneoplastic: acrokeratosis; encephalomyelopathy; pemphigus; syndrome
paranephric: abscess; body; fat
paraneural: infiltration
paranigral: nucleus
paranoid: disorder; personality; schizophrenia
paranoid personality: disorder
paranuclear: body
parapeduncular: nucleus
paraperitoneal: hernia
parapharyngeal: abscess; space
paraphysial: body; cysts
parapneumonic: effusion
pararectal: fossa; lymph nodes; pouch
parasaccular: hernia
parasagittal: plane; section
paraseptal: cartilage; emphysema
parasinoidal: sinuses
parasite-host: ecosystem
parasitic: chylocele; cyst; disease; granuloma; hemoptysis; leiomyoma; melanoderma; thyroiditis; twin
parasitophorous: vacuole
parasol: insertion
paraspinal: line
parasternal: hernia; line; lymph nodes
parastriate: area; cortex
parasympathetic: ganglia; nerve; part of autonomic

division of peripheral nervous system; root of ciliary ganglion; root of otic ganglion; root of pelvic ganglia; root of pterygopalatine ganglion; root of submandibular ganglion
parasympathetic nervous: system
parasystolic: beat
parataxic: distortion
paratenic: host
paraterminal: body; gyrus
parathyroid: gland; hormone; insufficiency; osteosis; tetany
parathyroid hormonelike: protein
parathyroid hormone-related: peptide; protein
parathyroprival: tetany
paratracheal: lymph node
paratuberculous: lymphadenitis
paratyphoid: bacillus; fever
paraumbilical: veins
paraurethral: ducts; glands
parauterine: lymph nodes
paravaccinia: virus
paravaginal: hysterectomy; lymph nodes
paraventricular: nucleus; nucleus [TA] of hypothalamus
paravertebral: anesthesia; ganglia; gutter; line; triangle
paravesical: fossa; lymph nodes; pouch
paraxial: mesoderm; rays
parchment: heart; skin
parchment right: ventricle
Paré: suture
parenchymal: atelectasis; cell
parenchymatous: cartilage; cell of corpus pineale; degeneration; goiter; hemorrhage; mastitis; neuritis
parent: artery; cell; cyst
parental: generation; rejection
parenteral: absorption; alimentation; hyperalimentation; therapy
parenteric: fever
Parenti-Fraccaro: syndrome
paretic: neurosyphilis
parietal: angle; bone; border; border of frontal bone; border of sphenoid bone; border of squamous part of temporal bone; border of temporal bone; branch; branch of medial occipital artery; branch of middle meningeal artery; branch of

superficial temporal artery; cell; eminence; eye; fistula; foramen; hernia; layer; layer of leptomeninges; layer of serous pericardium; layer of tunica vaginalis of testis; lobe; lobe of cerebrum; lymph nodes; margin; margin of frontal bone; margin of greater wing of sphenoid; nodes; notch; peritoneum; plate; pleura; region; thrombus; tuber; veins; wall
parietal abdominal: fascia
parietal emissary: vein
parietal lobe: epilepsy
parietal pelvic: fascia
parietomastoid: suture
parieto-occipital: branches (of anterior cerebral artery); branch (of posterior cerebral artery)
parietooccipital: artery; fissure; sulcus
parietopontine: fibers; tract
Parinaud: conjunctivitis; ophthalmoplegia; syndrome
Parinaud oculoglandular: syndrome
Paris: line
Park: aneurysm
Parker-Kerr: suture
Parkes Weber: syndrome
Parkinson: disease; facies
Park-Williams: fixative
paroccipital: process
parolfactory: area; sulci
Parona: space
paroophoritic: cyst
parosteal: fasciitis; osteosarcoma
parotid: abscess; bed; branches; bubo; duct; fascia; gland; notch; papilla; plexus of facial nerve; recess; sheath; space; veins
parotideomasseteric: fascia
paroxysmal: hypertension; sleep; tachycardia
paroxysmal cerebral: dysrhythmia
paroxysmal cold: hemoglobinuria
paroxysmal nocturnal: dyspnea; hemoglobinemia; hemoglobinuria
Parrot: disease
parrot: fever; jaw; virus
parrot-beak: nail
Parry: disease
parry: fracture
Parsonage-Turner: syndrome
partial: agglutinin; anencephaly; aneuploidy; anodontia; antigen;

cystectomy; denture; denture, distal extension; enterocele; epilepsy; laryngectomy; lipoatrophy; pressure; sclerectasia; seizure; volume
partial adrenocortical: insufficiency
partial anomalous pulmonary venous: connections
partial breech: extraction
partial cricoid: cleft
partial denture: impression; retention
partial face-sparing: lipodystrophy
partial heart: block
partial ileal: bypass
partial left: ventriculectomy
partial posterior laryngeal: cleft
partial-thickness: burn; graft
partial thromboplastin: time
participant: observer
particulate wear: debris
partition: chromatography; coefficient
parturient: canal
parvilocular: cyst
PAS: stain
Pascal: law
Pascheff: conjunctivitis
Paschen: bodies
Passavant: bar; cushion; pad; ridge
passional: attitudes
passive: agglutination; anaphylaxis; atelectasis; clot; congestion; diffusion; duction; eruption; hemagglutination; hyperemia; immunity; immunization; incontinence; learning; medium; movement; prophylaxis; transference; transport; tremor; vasoconstriction; vasodilation
passive-aggressive: behavior; personality
passive cutaneous: anaphylaxis
passive cutaneous anaphylactic: reaction
passive cutaneous anaphylaxis: test
passive length-tension: curve
Pasteur: effect; pipette; vaccine
Pastia: sign
pastoral: counseling
Patau: syndrome
patch: clamp; test
patchy: atelectasis
Patein: albumin

Word Finder

patellar: anastomosis; fossa of vitreous; ligament; network; reflex; retinaculum; surface of femur
patellar apprehension: sign
patellar tendon: reflex
patelloadductor: reflex
patellofemoral: syndrome
patellofemoral stress: syndrome
patent: ductus arteriosus; medicine; part of umbilical artery
Paterson-Brown-Kelly: syndrome
Paterson-Kelly: syndrome
path: analysis
pathematic: aphasia
pathetic: nerve
pathogenic: occlusion
pathognomonic: symptom
pathologic: absorption; amenorrhea; amputation; calcification; diagnosis; fracture; glycosuria; histology; model; myopia; physiology; proteins; rigidity; sphincter
pathological: anatomy
pathologic retraction: ring
pathologic startle: syndromes
patient-controlled: analgesia; anesthesia
Patois: virus
Paton: lines
Patrick: test
pattern distortion: amblyopia
patterned: alopecia
pattern retinal: dystrophy
pattern-sensitive: epilepsy
Paul: reaction; test
Paul-Bunnell: test
Pauli exclusion: principle
Pauling: theory
Pauling-Corey: helix
pause: signal
Pautrier: abscess; microabscess
pavement: epithelium
Pavlov: method; pouch; reflex; stomach
pavlovian: conditioning
Pavy: disease
Paxton: disease
Payne: operation
Payr: clamp; membrane; sign
PBI: test
PCA: pump
peak: magnitude
peak expiratory: flow
peak flow: rate
Pearl: index
pearl: cyst; moss
pearl-worker's: disease
pear-shaped: area
peat: moss

peccant: humors
pecking: order
Pecquet: cistern; duct; reservoir
pecten: band
pectin: sugar
pectinate: fibers; ligaments of iridocorneal angle; ligaments of iris; line; muscles; zone
pectineal: ligament; line of femur; line of pubis; muscle
pectineus: muscle
pectiniform: septum
pectoral: branch of thoracoacromial artery; fascia; girdle; glands; reflex; region; ridge; veins
pectoral and abdominal anterior cutaneous: branch of intercostal nerves
pectoral axillary: lymph nodes
pectoralis major: muscle
pectoralis minor: muscle
pectorodorsal: muscle
pectorodorsalis: muscle
pedal: system
Pedersen: speculum
pediatric: dentistry; radiology
pedicle: flap; graft
pediculous: blepharitis
pedigree: analysis
peduncular: ansa; loop; veins
pedunculated: hydatid; polyp
pedunculomammillary: fasciculus
pedunculopontine tegmental: nucleus
peeping: testis
peg-and-socket: articulation; joint
pegged: tooth
Pel-Ebstein: disease; fever
Pelger-Huët nuclear: anomaly
peliosis: hepatitis
Pelizaeus-Merzbacher: disease
pellagra-preventing: factor
Pellegrini: disease
Pellegrini-Stieda: disease
pellet: implantation
Pellizzi: syndrome
pellucid: zone
pellucid marginal corneal: degeneration
pelvic: abscess; axis; bone; brim; canal; cavity; cellulitis; diaphragm; exenteration; fascia; ganglia; girdle; hematocele; inclination; index; inlet; kidney; limb; lymph nodes; outlet; part; part of ductus deferens; part of peripheral autonomic plexuses and

ganglia; part of ureter; part of the urogenital sinus; peritonitis; plane of greatest dimensions; plane of inlet; plane of least dimensions; plane of outlet; pole; presentation; promontory; surface of sacrum; version
pelvic inflammatory: disease
pelvic (nervous): plexus
pelvic splanchnic: nerves
pelvirectal: sphincter
pelvivertebral: angle
pelvofemoral muscular: dystrophy
pen: grasp
pencil: tenderness
Pendred: syndrome
pendular: movement; nystagmus
pendulous: abdomen; heart; palate
pendulum: rhythm
penetrant: trait
penetrating: keratoplasty; ulcer; wound
penicillin G: potassium
penile: epispadias; fibromatosis; hypospadias; implant; prosthesis; raphe; urethra
penis: envy
pennate: muscle
penopubic: epispadias
penoscrotal: hypospadias; transposition
Penrose: drain
pension: neurosis
pentagastrin: test
pentavalent gas gangrene: antitoxin
penton: antigen
pentose monophosphate: shunt
pentose phosphate: cycle; pathway
pep: pills
Pepper: syndrome
pepper and salt: fundus
peptic: cell; digestion; gland; ulcer
peptide: antibiotic; bond
peptidyl: leukotrienes
perambulating: ulcer
percept: analysis
perceptive: hearing impairment
perceptual: expansion
percussion: sound; wave
percutaneous: absorption; cholangiography; nephrostomy; stimulation
percutaneous endoscopic: gastrostomy

percutaneous radiofrequency: gangliolysis
percutaneous transhepatic: cholangiography
percutaneous transluminal: angioplasty
percutaneous transluminal coronary: angioplasty
Perez: reflex; sign
perfect: fungus; stage; state
perfectionistic: personality
perforated: layer of sclera; space; ulcer
perforating: abscess; appendicitis; arteries of hand; arteries (of deep femoral artery); arteries (of foot); arteries (of internal thoracic artery); arteries of penis; branch of anterior interosseous artery; branches; branches of internal thoracic artery; branches (of palmar metacarpal arteries); branches (of plantar metatarsal arteries); branch of fibular artery; branch of peroneal artery; fibers; folliculitis; keratoplasty; ulcer of foot; veins; wound
perforating radiate: arteries (of kidney)
performance: intensity; status; test
performic acid: reaction
perfusion: cannula
perhydrase: milk
perialveolar: wiring
periapical: abscess; curettage; cyst; granuloma; osteofibrosis; radiograph; tissue
periapical cemental: dysplasia
periappendiceal: abscess
periaqueductal gray: substance
periarterial: pad; plexus; plexus of anterior cerebral artery; plexus of ascending pharyngeal artery; plexus of choroid artery; plexuses of coronary arteries; plexus of facial artery; plexus of inferior phrenic artery; plexus of inferior thyroid artery; plexus of internal thoracic artery; plexus of lingual artery; plexus of maxillary artery; plexus of middle cerebral artery; plexus of occipital artery; plexus of ophthalmic artery; plexus of popliteal artery;

plexus of posterior auricular artery; plexus of subclavian artery; plexus of superficial temporal artery; plexus of superior thyroid artery; plexus of testicular artery; plexus of thyroid artery; plexus of vertebral artery; sympathectomy

periarterial lymphatic: sheath
periarticular: abscess
pericallosal: artery; cistern
pericanalicular: fibroadenoma
pericapillary: cell
pericardiacophrenic: artery; veins
pericardial: branch of phrenic nerve; branch of thoracic aorta; cavity; decompression; effusion; fremitus; knock; murmur; reflex; rub; symphysis; tap; veins; villi
pericardial friction: sound
pericardioperitoneal: canal
pericardiopleural: membrane
pericardium: fibrosa
pericemental: abscess; attachment
pericentral: fibrosis; scotoma
pericentric: inversion
perichondral: bone
perichoroid: space
perichoroidal: space
periclaustral: lamina
pericolic membrane: syndrome
periconchal: sulcus
pericoronal: abscess; flap
pericorpuscular: synapse
pericytic: venules
peridental: ligament; membrane
peridural: anesthesia
perifornical: nucleus
perimuscular: fibrosis
perihypoglossal: nuclei
periinfarction: block
perilimbal suction: cup
perilunar: dislocation
perilymphatic: duct; fistula; gusher; space
perimortem: delivery
perimuscular: fibrosis
perinatal: death; medicine; mortality; torsion
perinatal mortality: rate
perineal: artery; body; branches of posterior cutaneous nerve of thigh; branches of posterior femoral cutaneous nerve; fascia; flexure of anal canal; flexure of rectum; hernia; hypospadias; lithotomy; membrane; muscles; nerves; raphe; region; section;

spaces; urethrostomy; urethrotomy
perineovaginal: fistula
perinephric: abscess
perineural: infiltration
perineuronal: satellite
perinuclear: cataract; space
periodic: arthralgia; biopolymer; catatonia; disease; edema; fever; filariasis; law; neutropenia; paralysis; peritonitis; polyserositis; system
periodic acid-Schiff: stain
periodic bone: pain
periodic migrainous: neuralgia
periodontal: abscess; anesthesia; atrophy; fiber; file; ligament; membrane; pocket; probe
periodontal ligament: fibers
periolivary: nuclei
periorbital: cellulitis; membrane
periosteal: bone; bud; chondroma; elevator; ganglion; graft; implantation; layer of dura mater; osteosarcoma; reaction; reflex; sarcoma
periotic: bone; cartilage
peripartum: cardiomyopathy
peripeduncular: nucleus
peripharyngeal: space
peripheral: aneurysm; arteriosclerosis; cataract; chemoreceptor; dysostosis; glare; iridectomy; part of nervous system; proteins; resistance; scotoma; seal; tabes; vision
peripheral anterior: synechia
peripheral facial: paralysis
peripheral nervous: system
peripheral ossifying: fibroma
peripheral T-cell: lymphoma, unspecified
peripolar: cell
periportal: cirrhosis; space of Mall
perirectal: abscess
perirenal: fascia; insufflation
perirenal fat: capsule
periscopic: lens; meniscus
perisinusoidal: space
peristatic: hyperemia
peristernal: perichondritis
peristriate: area; cortex
peritarsal: network
perithelial: cell
peritoneal: button; cavity; dialysis; fossae; insufflation; villi
peritoneovenous: shunt
peritonsillar: abscess

peritracheal: glands
peritrigeminal: nucleus
peritubular: dentin; zone
peritubular contractile: cells
perityphlitis: actinomycotica
periungual: fibroma
periureteral: abscess
periurethral: abscess
perivascular: cuffs
perivascular fibrous: capsule
periventricular: fibers; zone
periventricular preoptic: nucleus
perivisceral: cavity
perivitelline: space
Perlia: nucleus
Perls: test
Perls Prussian blue: stain
permanent: callus; cartilage; restoration; stricture; tooth
permanent stained smear: examination
permanent threshold: shift
permeability: coefficient; constant; theory of narcosis; vitamin
permissible exposure: limit
permissive: cell
permissive hypercapnic: ventilation
perna: disease
pernicious: anemia; malaria; vomiting
pernicious anemia type: metarubricyte; prorubricyte; rubriblast
peroneal: artery; bone; border of foot; compartment of leg; lymph node; phenomenon; pulley; retinaculum; trochlea of calcaneus; veins
peroneal anastomotic: ramus
peroneal communicating: branch; nerve
peroneal muscular: atrophy
peroneus brevis: muscle
peroneus longus: muscle
peroneus tertius: muscle
peroral: endoscopy
peroxidase: reaction; stain
perpendicular: fasciculus; plate; plate of ethmoid bone; plate of palatine bone
perpetually growing: tooth
Perrault: syndrome
persecution: complex
persecutory type of paranoid: disorder
Persian Gulf: syndrome
Persian relapsing: fever
persistent: cloaca; tremor; truncus arteriosus
persistent anterior hyperplastic primary: vitreous

persistent atrioventricular: canal
persistent ectopic: pregnancy
persistent frontal: suture
persistent generalized: lymphadenopathy
persistently growing: tooth
persistent müllerian duct: syndrome
persistent posterior hyperplastic primary: vitreous
persistent vegetative: state
personal: equation; motivation; probability; space
personal growth: laboratory
personality: disorder; formation; integration; inventory; profile; test
perspiratory: glands
Perthes: disease; test
Pertik: diverticulum
pertrochanteric: fracture
pertussis: immunoglobulin; syndrome; vaccine
pertussis immune: globulin
pertussis-like: syndrome
Peruvian: tarantula; wart
pervasive developmental: disorder
pervenous: pacemaker
pessary: cell; corpuscle
petechial: angiomas; hemorrhage
Peters: anomaly; ovum
Petit: aponeurosis; canals; hernia; herniotomy; sinus
petit: mal
petite: mutant
Petit lumbar: triangle
petit mal: epilepsy; seizure
Petri: dish
Petri dish: culture
petrooccipital: fissure; joint; synchondrosis
petrosal: bone; branch of middle meningeal artery; foramen; fossa; fossula; ganglion; impression of the pallium; sinus; vein
petrosphenoidal: fissure; syndrome
petrosquamous: fissure; suture
petrotympanic: fissure
petrous: bone; part of internal carotid artery; part of temporal bone; pyramid
Pette-Döring: disease
Petzval: surface
Peutz: syndrome
Peutz-Jeghers: syndrome
Peyer: glands; patches
Peyronie: disease
Peyrot: thorax

Word Finder

Pezzer: catheter
Pfannenstiel: incision
Pfaundler-Hurler: syndrome
Pfeiffer: phenomenon; syndrome
Pflüger: law
Pfuhl: sign
pH: scale; value
phacoanaphylactic: uveitis
phacogenic: glaucoma; uveitis
phacolytic: glaucoma
phacomorphic: glaucoma
phaeomycotic: cyst
phagedenic: ulcer
phagocyte: dysfunction
phagocytic: index; pneumonocyte
phagocytic dysfunction: immunodeficiency
phagocytic dysfunction disorders: immunodeficiency
phakic: eye
phalangeal: cell; joints
Phalen: maneuver
phallic: phase; tubercle
phantom: aneurysm; corpuscle; limb; pregnancy; tumor
phantom limb: pain
pharmaceutical: biology; chemistry
pharmacologic: mediators of anaphylaxis
pharmacologic stress: imaging
pharmacopeial: gel
pharmacoresistent: epilepsy
pharyngeal: arches; branch of the artery of pterygoid canal; branch of the ascending pharyngeal artery; branch of descending palatine artery; branches; branches of recurrent laryngeal nerve; branch of glossopharyngeal nerve; branch of inferior thyroid artery; branch of pterygopalatine ganglion; branch of vagus nerve; bursa; calculus; canal; cartilages; flap; fornix; glands; grooves; hypophysis; isthmus; lacuna; membranes; mucosa; nerve; opening of eustachian tube; opening of pharyngotympanic (auditory) tube; pituitary; pouches; raphe; recess; reflex; ridge; space; tonsil; tubercle (of basilar part of occipital bone); veins
pharyngeal lymphatic: ring
pharyngeal (nervous): plexus
pharyngeal pouch: syndrome

pharyngobasilar: fascia
pharyngobranchial: ducts
pharyngoconjunctival: fever
pharyngoconjunctival fever: virus
pharyngoepiglottic: fold
pharyngoesophageal: constriction; cushions; diverticulum; pads
pharyngomaxillary: space
pharyngonasal: cavity
pharyngopalatine: arch
pharyngotympanic: groove
pharyngotympanic (auditory): tube
phase: image; microscope; rule; shift
phase I: block
phase II: block
phasic: reflex
phasic sinus: arrhythmia
PH conduction: time
phenanthrene: nucleus
phenobarbital: elixir
phenol: coefficient
phenolsulfonphthalein: test
phenotypic: mixing; threshold; value
phentolamine: test
phenylhydrazine: hemolysis
phenylpyruvate: oligophrenia
phenylpyruvic: amentia
phenylthiocarbamoyl: peptide; protein
phi: phenomenon
Phialophore-type: conidiophore
Philadelphia: chromosome; cocktail
philanthropic: hospital
Philip: glands
Philippe: triangle
Philippine hemorrhagic: fever
Phillips: catheter
Phillipson: reflex
philosopher's: stone
phlebotomus: fever
phlebotomus fever: viruses
phlegmonous: abscess; cellulitis; enteritis; erysipelas; gastritis; mastitis; ulcer
phlogiston: theory
phlorizin: diabetes; glycosuria
phlyctenular: conjunctivitis; keratitis; ophthalmia; pannus
PhNCS: protein
phocomelic: dwarfism
phonemic: regression
phonetic: balance
phosphatase: unit
phosphate: diabetes; tetany
phosphogluconate: pathway
phosphohexose isomerase: deficiency

phospholipid: syndrome
phosphor: plate
phosphoroclastic: cleavage; reaction
phosphorylase-rupturing: enzyme
phosphotungstic acid: hematoxylin; stain
phosphureted: hydrogen
photechic: effect
photic: driving; stimulation
photic-sneeze: reflex
photo: cell
photoallergic: sensitivity
photochromic: lens; spectacles
photodynamic: sensitization; therapy
photoelectric: absorption; effect
photogenic: epilepsy
photomultiplier: tube
photon: density
photo-patch: test
photopic: adaptation; eye; vision
photoradiation: therapy
photoreactivating: enzyme
photoreceptor: cells
photorefractive: keratectomy
photosensor: oculography
photostimulable: phosphor
photostress: test
phototherapeutic: keratectomy
phototoxic: sensitivity
phrenic: ampulla; ganglia; nerve; nucleus; pleura; plexus; veins
phrenicoabdominal: branches of phrenic nerve
phrenicoceliac: part of suspensory muscle (ligament) of duodenum
phrenicocolic: ligament
phrenicocostal: sinus
phrenicolienal: ligament
phrenicomediastinal: recess
phrenicopleural: fascia
phrenicosplenic: ligament
phrenic pressure: test
phrenogastric: ligament
phrenopericardial: angle
phrenosplenic: ligament
phrygian: cap
phthinoid: chest
phyllodes: tumor
physaliphorous: cell
physical: age; allergy; anthropology; diagnosis; elasticity of muscle; examination; fitness; half-life; map; medicine; sign; therapy
physician-assisted: suicide
Physick: pouches

physiologic: age; albuminuria; amenorrhea; anatomy; anemia; anisocoria; antidote; chemistry; congestion; cup; dwarfism; elasticity of muscle; equilibrium; excavation; homeostasis; hypertrophy; icterus; incompatibility; jaundice; leukocytosis; occlusion; saline; sclerosis; scotoma; sphincter; tremor; unit; vertigo
physiological: drives
physiologically balanced: occlusion
physiologic dead: space
physiologic rest: position
physiologic retraction: ring
pia: mater encephali; mater spinalis
pial: filament; funnel; part of filum terminale
pial-glial: membrane
pianist's: cramp
piano: percussion
PICC: line
Picchini: syndrome
Pick: atrophy; bodies; bundle; cell; disease; syndrome
picker's: nodules
Pickles: chart
pickwickian: syndrome
pi cone: monochromatism
picrocarmine: stain
picroformol: fixative
picro-Mallory trichrome: stain
picronigrosin: stain
picture: element
picture frame: vertebra
piebald: eyelash; skin
Pierre Robin: syndrome
piezoelectric: effect; transducer
piezogenic pedal: papule
pig: skin
pigeon: breast; chest
pigment: cell; cells of iris; cell of skin; cells of retina; cirrhosis; epithelium; epithelium of optic retina; induration of the lung
pigmentary: cirrhosis; glaucoma; retinopathy; syphilid
pigment dispersion: syndrome
pigmented: ameloblastoma; dermatofibrosarcoma protuberans; epulis; layer of ciliary body; layer of iris; layer of retina; liver; part of retina
pigmented hair epidermal: nevus

pigmented keratic: precipitates
pigmented purpuric lichenoid: dermatosis
pigmented villonodular: synovitis; tenosynovitis
Pignet: formula
pigtail: catheter
pilar: cyst; tumor of scalp
pileous: gland
piliferous: cyst
pillar: cells; cells of Corti
pill-rolling: tremor
pilocytic: astrocytoma
piloid: gliosis
pilomotor: fibers; reflex
pilon: fracture
pilonidal: cyst; fistula; sinus
Piltz: sign
pilular: mass
pin: amalgam; implant
Pinard: maneuver
pincer: nail
pinch: graft
pincushion: distortion
Pindborg: tumor
pineal: body; cells; cyst; eye; gland; habenula; recess; stalk
Pinel: system
ping-pong: bone; fracture; mechanism
pinhole: pupil
pink: disease
pink bread: mold
Pinkus: tumor
pinocytotic: vesicle
Pins: sign; syndrome
pinta: fever
pinworm: vaginitis
PIP: joints
pipe: bone
Piper: forceps
pipe-smoker's: cancer
pipe stem: cirrhosis
pipestem: arteries; fibrosis
piqûre: diabetes
Pirie: bone
piriform: aperture; area; cortex; fossa; muscle; opening; recess; sinus
piriformis: muscle
piriform neuron: layer
Pirogoff: amputation; angle; triangle
Pirquet: index; reaction; test
pisciform: cataract
pisiform: joint
pisiform: bone
pisohamate: ligament
pisometacarpal: ligament
pisotriquetral: joint
pisounciform: ligament
pisouncinate: ligament
pistol-shot: sound
pistol-shot femoral: sound

piston: pulse
pit: caries
pitch: wart
pitch-worker's: cancer
pit and fissure: caries
pithecoid: theory
Pitot: tube
Pitres: area; sign
pitted: keratolysis
pitting: edema
Pittsburgh: pneumonia
Pittsburgh pneumonia: agent
pituitary: adamantinoma; adenoma; ameloblastoma; apoplexy; cachexia; diverticulum; dwarf; dwarfism; dystopia; fossa; gigantism; gland; infantilism; membrane; myxedema; stalk
pituitary gonadotropic: hormone
pituitary growth: hormone
pituitary stalk: section
pivot: joint
pivot shift: test
PJ: interval
P-K: antibodies; test
place: coding; theory
placenta: gonadotropin; protein
placental: barrier; circulation; dysfunction; dystocia; lobes; membrane; plasmodium; polyp; presentation; septa; sign; souffle; thrombosis; transfusion
placental dysfunction: syndrome
placental growth: hormone
placental parasitic: twin
placental site trophoblastic: tumor
placental sulfatase: deficiency
placental transfusion: syndrome
Placido da Costa: disk
plague: bacillus; pneumonia; septicemia; vaccine
plain: film
Planck: constant; theory
plane: joint; suture; wart
planoconcave: lens
planoconvex: lens
plant: agglutinin; antitoxin; casein; indican; RNase; toxin; viruses
plantar: aponeurosis; arch; fascia; fasciitis; fibromatosis; flexion; ligaments; ligaments of interphalangeal joints of foot; ligaments of metatarsophalangeal joints; muscle; reflex; region;

space; surface of foot; surface of toe; syphilid; wart
plantar arterial: arch
plantar calcaneocuboid: ligament
plantar calcaneonavicular: ligament
plantar cuboideonavicular: ligaments
plantar cuneocuboid: ligament
plantar cuneonavicular: ligaments
plantar digital: veins
plantarflexor: compartment of leg
plantar interossei interosseous: muscles
plantaris: muscle
plantar metatarsal: artery; ligaments; veins
plantar muscle: reflex
plantar quadrate: muscle
plantar tarsal: ligaments
plantar tarsometatarsal: ligaments
plantar tendon: sheath of fibularis longus muscle; sheath of peroneus longus muscle
plantar venous: arch; network
plasma: albumin; cell; factor X; fibronectin; layer; membrane; proteins; scalpel; stain; substitute; therapy
plasma accelerator: globulin
plasma cell: balanitis; gingivitis; hepatitis; leukemia; mastitis; myeloma
plasmacrit: test
plasma iodoprotein: disorder
plasmal: reaction
plasma labile: factor
plasma renin: activity
plasma thromboplastin: antecedent; component; factor; factor B
plasmatic: compartment
plasminogen: activator
plasmin prothrombins conversion: factor
plasmocytic: leukemoid reaction
plasmodial: trophoblast
plaster: bandage; splint
plastic: anatomy; bronchitis; corpuscle; cyclitis; induration; iritis; lymph; motor; pleurisy; surgery; teeth
plastic envelope: culture
plastic restoration: material
plastic section: stain
plate: thrombosis
plateau: iris; pulse
Plateau-Talbot: law

platelet: actomyosin; cofactor I; cofactor II; factor 3
platelet-activating: factor
platelet-aggregating: factor
platelet aggregation: test
platelet-derived growth: factor
platelet tissue: factor
platelike: atelectasis
platypellic: pelvis
platypelloid: pelvis
platysma: muscle
play: therapy
Pleasure: curve
pleasure: principle
pledgetted: suture
pleiotropic: gene
pleomorphic: adenoma; lipoma; oligodendroglioma; xanthoastrocytoma
plethysmographic: goggle
pleural: calculus; canal; cavity; cupula; effusion; fluid; fremitus; isthmus; lines; plaque; poudrage; pressure; rale; reaction; recesses; rub; sinuses; space; stripe; tap; villi
pleural friction: rub
pleuritic: pneumonia; rub
pleuroesophageal: line; muscle
pleuroesophageus: muscle
pleuropericardial: canals; fold; hiatus; membrane; murmur
pleuroperitoneal: canal; cavity; fold; hiatus; membrane; shunt
pleuropneumonia-like: organisms
pleurovenous: shunt
plexiform: layer; layer of cerebral cortex; layers of retina; neurofibroma; neuroma
plexogenic pulmonary: arteriopathy
Plimmer: bodies
plugging: instrument
Plummer: disease
Plummer-Vinson: syndrome
plural: pregnancy
pluripotent: cells
plus: lens; strand
PMA: index
pneocardiac: reflex
pneopneic: reflex
pneumatic: bone; dilator; otoscopy; retinopexy; space; tonometer
pneumatic tire: injury
pneumatized: bone
pneumatoenteric: recess
pneumococcal: empyema; polysaccharide; vaccine

pneumococcal/suppurative: keratitis

Pneumocystis carinii: pneumonia

pneumogastric: nerve

pneumogenic: osteoarthropathy

pneumonia: virus of mice

pneumonic: plague

P/O: quotient; ratio

pocketed: calculus

podalic: extraction; version

podiatric: medicine

podophyllum: resin

POEMS: syndrome

point: angle; deletion; epidemic; mutation

pointed: wart

point system: test types

Poirier: gland; line

Poiseuille: law; space

Poiseuille viscosity: coefficient

Poisson: distribution

Poisson-Pearson: formula

Poitou: colic

poker: back; spine

pokeweed: mitogen

Poland: syndrome

polar: amino acid; anemia; body; cataract; cell; compound; fibers; globule; hypogenesis; plates; presentation; ring; solvents; star; zone

polar frontal: artery

polarized: light

polarizing: microscope

polar temporal: artery

pole: ligation

Polenské: number

poliomyelitis: immunoglobulin; vaccines; virus

poliomyelitis immune: globulin (human)

poliovirus: vaccines

polishing: brush

Politzer: bag; method

Politzer luminous: cone

polka: fever

pollen: antigen; extract

Pólya: gastrectomy; operation

polyacrylamide gel: electrophoresis

polyalveolar: lobe

polyamine-methylene: resin

polyaxial: joint

polybasic: acid

polycarboxylate: cement

polychlorinated: biphenyl

polychromatic: cell; radiation

polychromatophil: cell

polychrome: methylene blue

polyclonal: activator; antibody; gammopathy

polycystic: disease of kidneys; kidney; liver; ovary

polycystic liver: disease

polycystic ovary: syndrome

polyendocrine deficiency: syndrome

polyester: resin

polygenic: inheritance

polyhedral: body

polyleptic: fever

polymerase chain: reaction

polymer fume: fever

polymorphic: neuron; reticulosis

polymorphic genetic: marker

polymorphic superficial: keratitis

polymorphocytic: leukemia

polymorphonuclear: leukocyte

polymorphous: layer; perversion

polymorphous light: eruption

polymorphous low-grade: carcinoma of salivary glands

polyol: pathway

polyoma: virus

polyostotic fibrous: dysplasia

polyovular ovarian: follicle

polyoxyethylene: alcohols

polyphenic: gene

polyphyletic: theory

polypoid: adenoma

polypous: endocarditis; gastritis

polysaccharide: sulfate esters

polysaccharide conjugated: vaccine

polysplenia: syndrome

polytene: chromosome

polyuria: test

polyvalent: allergy; antiserum; serum; vaccine

polyzygotic: twins

pomade: acne

Pomeroy: operation

Pompe: disease

pond: fracture

ponderal: index

Ponfick: shadow

pontine: angle; arteries; cistern; flexure; hemorrhage; nuclei; veins

pontine angle: tumor

pontine corticonuclear: fibers

pontine gray: matter

pontobulbar: body; nucleus

pontocerebellar: cistern; fibers; recess

ponto-geniculo-occipital: spike

pontomedullary: groove

pontomesencephalic: vein

pontoreticulospinal: tract

Pool: phenomenon

pooled: serum

Pool-Schlesinger: sign

poorly compliant: bladder

poorly crystalline: hydroxyapatite

poorly differentiated lymphocytic: lymphoma

popliteal: arch; artery; fascia; fossa; groove; line; lymph nodes; muscle; notch; plane of femur; plexus; region; space; surface of femur; vein

popliteal communicating: nerve

popliteal entrapment: syndrome

popliteus: muscle

population: genetics; pyramid

porcelain: gallbladder; inlay

porcine: graft; valve

porcine hemagglutinating encephalomyelitis: virus

porcupine: skin

Porges: method

Porges-Meier: test

porphobilinogen synthase: porphyria

Porro: hysterectomy; operation

portable: radiography

portacaval: anastomoses; shunt

portal: canals; circulation; cirrhosis; fissure; hypertension; lobule of liver; pyemia; system; triad; vein

portal hypophysial: circulation

portal-systemic: anastomoses; encephalopathy

portasystemic: shunt

Porter: fascia

Porter-Silber: chromogens; reaction

Porter-Silber chromogens: test

Portuguese: man-of-war

Portuguese-Azorean: disease

port-wine: mark; stain

Posadas: disease

position: agnosia; effect; sense

positional: cloning; nystagmus; vertigo; vertigo of Bárány

positive: accommodation; afterimage; afterpotential; anergy; chronotropism; control; convergence; cooperativity; electrode; electron; electrotaxis; feedback; meniscus; phase; rays; scotoma; stain; symptom; taxis; thermotaxis; transference; valence

positive contrast: orbitography

positive end-expiratory: pressure

positively: inotropic

positive-negative pressure: breathing

positron emission: tomography

post: dam; implant

postadrenalectomy: syndrome

postanal: dimple; gut

postarsphenamine: jaundice

postauricular: incision

postaxillary: line

postbasic: stare

postcapillary: venules

postcardiotomy: syndrome

postcaval: ureter

postcentral: area; artery; fissure; gyrus; sulcus

postcentral sulcal: artery

postcholecystectomy: syndrome

postcloacal: gut

postcoital: contraception; test

postcommissural: fibers

postcommissurotomy: syndrome

postcommunicating: part of anterior cerebral artery; part of posterior cerebral artery

postconcussion: syndrome

postcostal: anastomosis

post dam: area

postdate: pregnancy

postdiphtheritic: paralysis

postdrive: depression

posterior: aphasia; arch of atlas; asynclitism; belly of digastric muscle; blepharitis; border of eyelids; border of fibula; border of petrous part of temporal bone; border of radius; border of testis; border of ulna; branches; branch of great auricular nerve; branch of inferior pancreaticoduodenal artery; branch of lateral cerebral sulcus; branch of medial antebrachial cutaneous nerve; branch of medial cutaneous nerve of forearm; branch of obturator artery; branch of obturator nerve; branch of recurrent ulnar artery; branch of renal artery; branch of right branch of portal vein; branch of right hepatic duct; branch of right superior pulmonary vein; branch of spinal nerves; branch of superior thyroid artery; branch of ulnar recurrent artery; canaliculus of chorda tympani; cells; centriole;

chamber of eyeball; choroiditis; column; column of spinal cord; commissure; commissure of the larynx; compartment of arm; compartment of forearm; compartment of leg; compartment of thigh; cord of brachial plexus; crus of stapes; curvature; cusp of left atrioventricular valve; cusp of mitral valve; cusp of right atrioventricular valve; cusp of tricuspid valve; divisions of (trunks of) brachial plexus; embryotoxon; extremity of spleen; fascicle of palatopharyngeus muscle; fasciculus proprius; fontanelle; funiculus; horn; layer of rectus sheath; ligament of fibular head; ligament of head of fibula; ligament of incus; ligament of knee; limb of internal capsule; limb of stapes; lip of external os of uterus; liver; lobe of hypophysis; mediastinum; nares; nephrectomy; neuropore; notch of cerebellum; nucleus; nucleus of hypothalamus; nucleus of vagus nerve; occlusion; part; part of anterior commissure of brain; part of the diaphragmatic surface of the liver; part of liver; part of tongue; part of vaginal fornix; pillar of fauces; pillar of fornix; pituitary; pole of eyeball; pole of lens; probability; process of septal cartilage; process of talus; pyramid of the medulla; ramus of lateral cerebral sulcus; ramus of lateral sulcus of cerebrum; ramus of spinal nerve; recess; recess of tympanic membrane; region of arm; region of elbow; region of forearm; region of knee; region of leg; region of neck; region of thigh; region of wrist; rhinoscopy; rhizotomy; root of spinal nerve; scleritis; sclerosis; sclerotomy; segment; sinus of tympanic cavity; staphyloma; surface; surface of arm; surface of arytenoid cartilage; surface of cornea; surface of elbow; surface of eyelids; surface of fibula;

surface of forearm; surface of iris; surface of kidney; surface of leg; surface of lens; surface of lower limb; surface of pancreas; surface of petrous part of temporal bone; surface of prostate; surface of radius; surface of scapula; surface of shaft of humerus; surface of suprarenal gland; surface of thigh; surface of tibia; surface of ulna; symblepharon; synechia; tooth; triangle of neck; tubercle of atlas; tubercle of cervical vertebrae; urethra; urethritis; uveitis; vaginismus; vein of corpus callosum; vein of septum pellucidum; vein(s) of left ventricle; vitrectomy; wall of middle ear; wall of stomach; wall of tympanic cavity; wall of vagina

posterior accessory olivary: nucleus
posterior acoustic: stria
posterior alveolar: artery
posterior ampullar: nerve
posterior antebrachial: nerve; region
posterior antebrachial cutaneous: nerve
posterior anterior jugular: vein
posterior articular: facet of dens; surface of dens
posterior atlanto-occipital: membrane
posterior auricular: artery; groove; nerve; plexus; vein
posterior auricular: muscle
posterior axillary: fold; line; lymph nodes
posterior basal: branch
posterior basal bronchopulmonary: segment S X
posterior basal segmental: artery of left/right lung
posterior brachial: region
posterior brachial cutaneous: nerve
posterior bronchopulmonary: segment S II
posterior cardinal: veins
posterior carpal: region
posterior cecal: artery
posterior central: convolution; gyrus
posterior cerebellar: notch
posterior cerebellomedullary: cistern
posterior cerebral: artery

posterior cervical: region
posterior cervical intertransversarii: muscles
posterior cervical intertransverse: muscles
posterior cervical (nervous): plexus
posterior choroidal: artery
posterior circumflex humeral: artery; vein
posterior clinoid: process
posterior column: cordotomy
posterior communicating: artery
posterior condyloid: foramen
posterior conjunctival: artery
posterior corneal: dystrophy
posterior coronary: plexus
posterior costotransverse: ligament
posterior cranial: fossa
posterior cricoarytenoid: ligament; muscle
posterior cruciate: ligament
posterior crural: region
posterior cubital: region
posterior cutaneous: nerve of arm; nerve of forearm; nerve of thigh
posterior dental: artery
posterior descending coronary: artery
posterior elastic: layer
posterior ethmoidal: artery; cells; nerve
posterior ethmoidal air: cells
posterior external arcuate: fibers
posterior facial: vein
posterior femoral cutaneous: nerve
posterior focal: point
posterior fossa: approach
posterior gastric: artery; branches of posterior vagal trunk
posterior glandular: branch of superior thyroid artery
posterior gray: commissure
posterior hepatic: segment I
posterior humeral circumflex: artery
posterior hypothalamic: area; nucleus; region
posterior inferior cerebellar: artery
posterior inferior cerebellar artery: syndrome
posterior inferior iliac: spine
posterior inferior nasal: branches of greater palatine nerve; nerves
posterior intercondylar: area of tibia
posterior intercostal: arteries 1–2; arteries 3–11; veins

posterior intermediate: groove; sulcus
posterior interosseous: artery; nerve
posterior interpositus: nucleus
posterior interventricular: artery; groove; sulcus
posterior interventricular branch of right coronary: artery
posterior intestinal: portal
posterior intraoccipital: joint; synchondrosis
posterior junction: line
posterior knee: region
posterior labial: arteries; branches of perineal artery; commissure; nerves; veins
posterior labial branches of internal perineal: artery
posterior lacrimal: crest
posterior laryngeal: cleft
posterior lateral nasal: arteries
posterior leukoencephalopathy: syndrome
posterior limiting: lamina of cornea; layer of cornea
posterior longitudinal: bundle; ligament
posterior lunate: lobule
posterior marginal: vein
posterior median: fissure of the medulla oblongata; fissure of spinal cord; line; sulcus of medulla oblongata; sulcus of spinal cord
posterior mediastinal: arteries; lymph nodes
posterior medullary: velum
posterior meningeal: artery
posterior meniscofemoral: ligament
posterior myocardial: infarction
posterior nasal: apertures; spine of horizontal plate of palatine bone
posterior neck: region
posterior occipitoaxial: ligament
posterior palatal: seal
posterior palatal seal: area
posterior palatine: arch; foramina; spine
posterior palpebral: margin
posterior pancreaticoduodenal: artery
posterior paracentral: gyrus
posterior parietal: artery
posterior parolfactory: sulcus
posterior parotid: veins
posterior pelvic: exenteration

posterior perforated: substance

posterior pericallosal: vein

posterior periventricular: nucleus

posterior peroneal: arteries

posterior polymorphous corneal: dystrophy

posterior primary: division

posterior quadrigeminal: body

posterior renal: segment

posterior sacroiliac: ligaments

posterior sacrosciatic: ligament

posterior sagittal: diameter

posterior scalene: muscle

posterior scapular: nerve

posterior scrotal: branches of perineal artery; branch of internal pudendal artery; nerves; veins

posterior segmental: artery; artery (of kidney)

posterior semicircular: canals

posterior septal: artery of nose; branches of sphenopalatine artery; branch of nose

posterior spinal: artery; sclerosis

posterior spinocerebellar: tract

posterior sternoclavicular: ligament

posterior subcapsular: cataract

posterior superior: fissure

posterior superior alveolar: artery; branches of maxillary nerve

posterior superior iliac: spine

posterior superior lateral nasal: branches of maxillary nerve; branches of pterygopalatine ganglion

posterior superior medial nasal: branches of maxillary nerve; branches of pterygopalatine ganglion

posterior supraclavicular: nerve

posterior talar articular: surface (of calcaneus)

posterior talocalcaneal: ligament

posterior talofibular: ligament

posterior talotibial: ligament

posterior tegmental: decussation

posterior temporal: artery; branch of middle cerebral artery

posterior thalamic: radiation

posterior thoracic: nerve; nucleus

posterior tibial: artery; lymph node; muscle; node; veins

posterior tibial recurrent: artery

posterior tibiofibular: ligament

posterior tibiotalar: ligament; part of deltoid ligament; part of medial ligament of ankle joint

posterior tooth: form

posterior transverse temporal: gyrus

posterior trigeminothalamic: tract

posterior tympanic: artery

posterior urethral: valves

posterior vaginal: hernia

posterior vestibular: branch of vestibulocochlear artery

posteroanterior: projection

posterolateral: fissure; fontanelle; groove; nucleus; sulcus; thoracotomy; tract

posterolateral central: arteries

posteromedial: nucleus

posteromedial central: arteries

posteromedial frontal: branch of callosomarginal artery

posteruption: cuticle

postextrasystolic: pause

postextrasystolic T: wave

postganglionic: fibers

postganglionic motor: neuron

postganglionic nerve: fiber

postgastrectomy: syndrome

postglenoid: foramen

posthemiplegic: athetosis; chorea

posthemorrhagic: anemia

posthepatitic: cirrhosis

posthippocampal: fissure

posthypnotic: amnesia; psychosis; suggestion

posthypoglycemic: hyperglycemia

posticus: palsy; paralysis

postinfarction ventricular septal: defect

postinfectious: bradycardia; myelitis; polyneuritis; psychosis

post-kala azar dermal: leishmanoid

postlaminar: part of intraocular part of optic nerve

postlingual: deafness; fissure

post–lumbar puncture: syndrome

postlunate: fissure

postmalaria neurologic: syndrome

post-marketing: surveillance

postmature: infant

postmaturity: syndrome

postmeiotic: phase

postmeningitic: hydrocephalus

postmenopausal: atrophy

postmitotic: phase

postmortem: clot; delivery; examination; hypostasis; livedo; lividity; pustule; rigidity; suggillation; thrombus; tubercle; wart

postmyocardial infarction: pericarditis; syndrome

postnasal: drip

postnatal: life

postnecrotic: cirrhosis

postnormal: occlusion

postobstructive: pneumonia

postoperative: bronchopneumonia; parotiditis; tetany

postoperative pressure: alopecia

postoral: arches

postpalatal: seal

postpalatal seal: area

postpartum: alopecia; amenorrhea; atony; blues; cardiomyopathy; estrus; hemorrhage; hypertension; psychosis; tetanus

postpartum pituitary necrosis: syndrome

postparturient: hemoglobinuria

postperfusion: lung

postpericardiotomy: pericarditis; syndrome

postpharyngeal: space

postphlebitic: syndrome

postprandial: lipemia; pain

postprimary: tuberculosis

postpyloric: sphincter

postpyramidal: fissure

postreduction: phase

postremal: chamber of eyeball

postrenal: albuminuria

postrhinal: fissure

postrubella: syndrome

postsphenoid: bone

poststationary: phase

post–steady: state

post-stenotic: dilation

poststeroid: panniculitis

postsulcal: part of tongue

postsynaptic: membrane

postterm: infant

postthrombotic: syndrome

posttransplant lymphoproliferative: disease

posttraumatic: delirium; dementia; epilepsy; headache; hydrocephalus; neurosis; osteoporosis; pericarditis; psychosis; syndrome

posttraumatic arterial: thrombosis

posttraumatic leptomeningeal: cyst

posttraumatic neck: syndrome

posttraumatic stress: disorder; syndrome

posttussis suction: sound

posttussive: suction

postural: albuminuria; contraction; drainage; hypotension; ischemia; position; reflex; set; syncope; tremor; version; vertigo

postural sway: response

posture: sense

postvaccinal: encephalitis; encephalomyelitis; myelitis

pot: curare

potable: water

Potain: sign

potassium: inhibition

potassium nitrate: paper

potassium sparing: diuretics

potato: nose; tumor of neck

potato dextrose: agar

potential: energy

potential acuity: meter

potentiometric: titration

Pott: abscess; aneurysm; curvature; disease; fracture; gangrene; paralysis; paraplegia

Potter: disease; facies; syndrome; version

Potter-Bucky: diaphragm

Pott puffy: tumor

Potts: anastomosis; clamp; operation

pouch: culture

poultry handler's: disease

poultryman's: itch

Poupart: ligament; line

povidone: iodine

Powassan: encephalitis; virus

powdered: gold; ipecac; opium; stomach

power: failure; injector; point

Pozzi: muscle

P-P: interval

p-p: factor

PQ: interval

PR: enzyme; interval; segment

practical: anatomy; nurse; units

practice: guidelines; parameters

Prader-Willi: syndrome

Prague: maneuver; pelvis
prairie: conjunctivitis; itch
Pratt: dilators; symptom
Prausnitz-Küstner: antibody; reaction
pravastatin: sodium
preanesthetic: medication
preauricular: groove; pit; point; sinus; sulcus
preauricular deep parotid: lymph nodes
preautomatic: pause
preaxillary: line
pre-B: lymphocyte
precancerous: lesion; melanosis of Dubreuilh
precapillary: anastomosis
prececal: lymph nodes
prececocolic: fascia
precentral: area; artery; fissure; gyrus; sulcus
precentral cerebellar: vein
precentral sulcal: artery
precervical: sinus
prechiasmatic: sulcus
prechordal: plate
precipitate: labor
precipitated: calcium carbonate; sulfur
precipitating: antibody; cause
precipitation: curve; test
precipitin: reaction; test
precision: attachment; rest
precocious: pseudopuberty; puberty
precollagenous: fibers
precommissural: bundle; fibers; septum
precommissural septal: area; nucleus
precommunical: segment of anterior cerebral artery; segment of posterior cerebral artery
precommunicating: part of anterior cerebral artery; part of posterior cerebral artery
preconceptual: stage
precordial: electrocardiography; leads
precordial catch: syndrome
precorneal: film
precostal: anastomosis
preculminate: fissure
precuneal: artery; branches (of anterior cerebral artery)
precursory: cartilage
pre-Descemet corneal: dystrophy
predictive: validity; value
predisposing: cause; factors
predorsal: bundle
preejection: period
preepiglottic: space
preexcitation: syndrome
preextraction: record

preferred provider: organization
preformation: theory
prefrontal: area; cortex; leukotomy; lobotomy; veins
preganglionic: fibers
preganglionic motor: neuron
preganglionic nerve: fibers
pregeniculate: nucleus
pregenital: organization; phase
pregnancy: cells; diabetes; gingivitis; hormone; luteoma; tumor
pregnancy-induced: hypertension
pregranulosa: cells
prehyoid: gland
preinfarction: angina; syndrome
preinterparietal: bone
prelaminar: branch of spinal branch of dorsal branch of posterior intercostal artery; part of intraocular part of optic nerve
prelaryngeal: lymph nodes
preliminary: impression
prelingual: deafness
prelogical: mind; thinking
premammary: abscess
premature: alopecia; beat; birth; contact; contraction; delivery; ejaculation; labor; menopause; systole
premature membrane: rupture
premature ovarian: failure
premature senility: syndrome
prematurity: myopia
premaxillary: bone; suture
premeiotic: phase
premenstrual: edema; syndrome; tension
premenstrual dysphoric: disorder
premenstrual salivary: syndrome
premenstrual tension: syndrome
premitotic: phase
premolar: tooth
premotor: area; cortex; syndrome
prenatal: diagnosis; life; screening
prenodular: fissure
Prentice: rule
preoccipital: notch
pre-oedipal: phase
preoperative: record
preoptic: area; region
preoral: gut
prepancreatic: artery
prepapillary: sphincter

prepared: chalk; ipecacuanha; suet
prepared mutton: tallow
prepatellar: bursa; bursitis
prepatent: period
prepericardial: lymph nodes
prepiriform: gyrus
prepontine: cistern
preprostate urethral: sphincter
preprostatic: part of male urethra; sphincter
preputial: calculus; glands; sac
prepyloric: sphincter; vein
prepyramidal: fissure; tract
prerectal: lithotomy
prereduction: phase
prerenal: albuminuria
pre-Rolandic: artery
prerubral: field; nucleus
presacral: anesthesia; fascia; nerve; neurectomy; sympathectomy
presenile: dementia
presenile spontaneous: gangrene
presenting: symptom
preseptal: cellulitis
presomite: embryo
presphenoid: bone
presplenic: fold
pressor: amine; base; fibers; nerve; substance
pressoreceptive: mechanism
pressoreceptor: nerve; reflex; system
pressure: alopecia; amaurosis; anesthesia; atrophy; collapse; dressing; epiphysis; gangrene; palsy; paralysis; plethysmograph; pneumothorax; point; reversal; sense; sore; stasis; ulcer; urticaria; waveform
pressure-controlled: respirator; ventilation
pressure pulse: differentiation
pressure-support: ventilation
pressure-volume: index
pre–steady: state
presternal: notch; region
prestriate: area
presulcal: part of tongue
presumed ocular: histoplasmosis
presumptive: region
presynaptic: membrane
presystolic: gallop; murmur; thrill
pretectal: area; nuclei; region
pretectoolivary: fibers
preterm: infant
preterm membrane: rupture
pretibial: fever; myxedema

pretracheal: fascia; layer of cervical fascia; lymph nodes
preventive: dentistry; dose; medicine; treatment
prevertebral: fascia; ganglia; layer of cervical fascia; lymph nodes; part of vertebral artery
previllous: chorion; embryo
Pribnow: box
Price-Jones: curve
prickle: cell
prickle cell: layer
prickly: heat
primal: repression; scene
primaquine: sensitivity
primary: adhesion; aerodontalgia; alcohol; aldosteronism; amenorrhea; amputation; amyloidosis; anesthetic; atelectasis; bronchus; bubo; carcinoma; cardiomyopathy; caries; cementum; center of ossification; choana; coccidioidomycosis; color; complex; constriction; curvature of vertebral column; dementia; dentin; dentition; deviation; digestion; digit of foot; disease; drives; dysmenorrhea; fissure of cerebellum; gain; gout; hair; hemochromatosis; hemorrhage; hydrocephalus; hyperoxaluria and oxalosis; hyperparathyroidism; hypertension; hyperthyroidism; hypogammaglobulinemia; hypogonadism; impression; irritant; lymphedema; lysosomes; megaureter; mesoderm; metabolism; metabolite; methemoglobinemia; narcissism; neurasthenia; nodule; nondisjunction; oocyte; organizer; palate; pentosuria; point of ossification; process; proteose; pyoderma; radiation; rays; reaction; reinforcement; rejection; screw-worm; sensation; sequestrum; shock; sodium phosphate; spermatocyte; structure; syphilis; telangiectasia; tooth; tuberculosis; union; villus; vitreous
primary adrenocortical: insufficiency
primary amebic: meningoencephalitis

primary atypical: pneumonia
primary biliary: cirrhosis
primary brain: vesicle
primary carnitine: deficiency
primary dental: lamina
primary dried: yeast
primary dye: test
primary egg: membrane
primary embryonic: cell
primary erythroblastic: anemia
primary extrapulmonary: coccidioidomycosis
primary generalized: epilepsy
primary herpetic: gingivostomatitis; stomatitis
primary idiopathic macular: atrophy
primary immune: response
primary interatrial: foramen
primary irritant: dermatitis
primary labial: groove
primary lateral: sclerosis
primary macular: atrophy of skin
primary medical: care
primary myeloid: metaplasia
primary neuroendocrine: carcinoma of the skin
primary neuronal: degeneration
primary ossification: center
primary ovarian: follicle
primary pigmentary: degeneration of retina
primary progressive cerebellar: degeneration
primary pulmonary: lobule
primary refractory: anemia
primary renal: calculus
primary renal tubular: acidosis
primary sclerosing: cholangitis
primary senile: dementia
primary sex: characters
primary skin: graft
primary visual: area; cortex
primer: extension
primitive: aorta; chorion; furrow; groove; gut; knot; meninx; node; palate; pit; ridge; streak
primitive costal: arches
primitive neuroectodermal: tumor
primitive perivisceral: cavity
primitive reticular: cell
primordial: cartilage; cell; cyst; dwarfism; gigantism; kidney
primordial germ: cell
primordial ovarian: follicle
princeps cervicis: artery
princeps pollicis: artery
Princeteau: tubercle

principal: artery of thumb; focus; piece; plane; point
principal olivary: nucleus
principal optic: axis
principal sensory: nucleus of trigeminal nerve; nucleus of the trigeminus
Pringle: disease
Prinzmetal: angina
prion: protein
prior: probability
prism: diopter
prism cover: test
prism vergence: test
prison fever: typhus
private: antigens; blood group; hospital; nurse
private duty: nurse
privet: cough
privileged: site
proacrosomal: granules
proactive: inhibition
probability: curve; sample
probe: gorget; patency; syringe
problem-oriented: record
procentriole: organizer
procerus: muscle
process: schizophrenia
prochordal: plate
procursive: chorea; epilepsy
prodromal: period; stage
prodromic: sign
product: inhibition
productive: inflammation; peritonitis; pleurisy
product-moment: correlation
Profeta: law
proficiency: samples; testing
profile: record
profound: hypothermia
profunda brachii: artery
profunda femoris: artery; vein
progestational: hormone
progesterone: receptor; unit
progesterone challenge: test
programmable: hearing aid
programmed cell: death
progress: curve
progressive: cataract; cleavage; lipodystrophy; processes; staining; vaccinia
progressive bacterial synergistic: gangrene
progressive bulbar: palsy; paralysis
progressive cerebellar: tremor
progressive cerebral: poliodystrophy
progressive choroidal: atrophy
progressive circumscribed cerebral: atrophy

progressive emphysematous: necrosis
progressive familial: scleroderma
progressive hypertrophic: polyneuropathy
progressive infantile spinal muscular: atrophy
progressive multifocal: leukoencephalopathy
progressive muscular: atrophy
progressive outer retinal: necrosis
progressive pigmentary: dermatosis
progressive spinal: amyotrophy
progressive spinal muscular: atrophy
progressive subcortical: encephalopathy
progressive supranuclear: palsy
progressive tapetochoroidal: dystrophy
projectile: vomiting
projection: angiogram; fibers; perimeter; system
projective: identification; test
prolactin: cell; unit
prolactin-inhibiting: factor
prolactin-producing: adenoma
proliferating: pleurisy
proliferating cell nuclear: antigen
proliferating systematized: angioendotheliomatosis
proliferating tricholemmal: cyst
proliferation: cyst; therapy
proliferative: arthritis; bronchiolitis; choroiditis; dermatitis; fasciitis; gingivitis; glomerulonephritis; inflammation; intimitis; myositis; retinopathy
proligerous: disk; membrane
prolonged: pregnancy
prolonged action: tablet
prometaphase: banding
prominent: heel
promontorial common iliac: nodes
promoting: agent
prompt insulin zinc: suspension
pronator: reflex; ridge; tuberosity
pronator: muscle
pronator quadratus: muscle
pronator teres: muscle; syndrome
prone: position

pronephric: duct; tubule
proof: spirit
propagated: thrombus
proparathyroid: hormone
proper: fasciculi; ligament of ovary; membrane of semicircular duct; substance
proper cochlear: artery
properdin: factor B; factor D; system
properitoneal inguinal: hernia
proper palmar digital: arteries; nerves
proper plantar digital: artery; nerves
property: emergence
prophylactic: membrane; odontotomy; treatment
proportional: counter; limit
proportional assist: ventilation
proportionate: dwarfism; infantilism
proprietary: hospital; medicine
proprioceptive: mechanism; reflexes; sensibility
proprioceptive-oculocephalic: reflex
prosecretion: granules
prosector's: tubercle; wart
proserum prothrombin conversion: accelerator
prospective: fate
prostate: gland
prostate-specific: antigen
prostatic: adenoma; branches of inferior vesical artery; branches of middle rectal artery; calculus; catheter; ducts; ductules; fluid; massage; sheath; sinus; urethra; utricle
prostatic intraepithelial: neoplasia
prostatic (nervous): plexus
prostaticovesical venous: plexus
prostatic venous: plexus
prosthetic: dentistry; group; valves
prostomial: mesoderm
protamine zinc: insulin
protease: inhibitor
protection: test
protective: block; colloid; protein; spectacles; zone
protective laryngeal: reflex
protein: factor; fever; malnutrition; metabolism; quotient; shock; synthesis
protein-bound: iodine
protein-bound iodine: test
protein-losing: enteropathy
protein shock: therapy

proteoglycan: aggregate
Proteus: syndrome
prothoracic: glands
prothrombin: accelerator; test; time
prothrombin and proconvertin: test
protochordal: knot
protodiastolic: gallop
proton: pump
proton pump: inhibitor
protopathic: sensibility
protoplasmic: astrocyte; astrocytoma; movement
prototrophic: strains
protozoan: cyst
protruded: disk
protruding: ear; teeth
protrusive: excursion; occlusion; position; record; relation
protrusive jaw: relation
protuberant: abdomen
proud: flesh
Proust: law; space
provisional: callus; cortex; denture; ligature; prosthesis; restoration
provocation: typhoid
provocative: test
provocative Wassermann: test
Prowazek: bodies
Prowazek-Greeff: bodies
proximal: border of nail; caries; centriole; contact; part of prostate; part of prostatic urethra; phalanx of foot; phalanx of hand
proximal deep inguinal: lymph node
proximal femoral focal: deficiency
proximal interphalangeal: joints
proximal medial striate: arteries
proximal myotonic: myopathy
proximal radioulnar: articulation; joint
proximal spiral: septum
proximal splenorenal: shunt
proximal tibiofibular: joint
proximal urethral: sphincter
proximate: cause; principle
prozone: reaction
prune: belly
prune-belly: syndrome
prune-juice: expectoration; sputum
pruritic urticarial: papules and plaques of pregnancy
Prussak: fibers; pouch; space
Prussian blue: stain
PSA: velocity

psalterial: cord
psammoma: bodies
psammomatous: meningioma
pseudo: psychosis
pseudo-: hemianopia
pseudoachondroplastic spondyloepiphysial: dysplasia
pseudoanaphylactic: shock
pseudobulbar: paralysis
pseudocholinesterase: deficiency
pseudochylous: ascites
pseudocoarctation of the: aorta
pseudocowpox: virus
pseudoepitheliomatous: hyperplasia
pseudoexfoliation: syndrome
pseudoexfoliative: glaucoma
pseudofusion: beat
pseudo-Gaucher: cell
pseudo-Graefe: phenomenon; sign
pseudo-Hurler: disease; polydystrophy
pseudohypertrophic muscular: dystrophy
pseudolepromatous: leishmaniasis
pseudolymphocytic choriomeningitis: virus
pseudolysogenic: strain
pseudomembranous: bronchitis; colitis; conjunctivitis; enteritis; enterocolitis; gastritis; inflammation
Pseudomonas: osteomyelitis
pseudomucinous: cyst
pseudoneurogenic: bladder
pseudoneurotic: schizophrenia
pseudoosteomalacic: pelvis
pseudoplastic: fluid
pseudorabies: virus
pseudorheumatoid: nodules
pseudosarcomatous: fasciitis
pseudostratified: epithelium
pseudotubercular: yersiniosis
pseudotubular: degeneration
pseudounipolar: cell; neuron
pseudoxanthoma: cell
psi: factor; phenomenon
psittacosis: virus
psittacosis inclusion: bodies
psoas: abscess; margin
psoas major: muscle
psoas minor: muscle
psoatic: part of iliopsoas fascia
psoriatic: arthritis
psoroptic: acariasis
psychedelic: drug; therapy
psychiatric: nosology

psychic: blindness; contagion; determinism; energy; force; impotence; inertia; overtone; seizure; tic; trauma
psychoanalytic: psychiatry; psychotherapy; situation; therapy
psychocardiac: reflex
psychodysleptic: drug
psychogalvanic: reaction; reflex; response
psychogenic: hearing impairment; pain; polydipsia; purpura; seizure; torticollis; tremor; vomiting
psychogenic nocturnal: polydipsia
psychogenic nocturnal polydipsia: syndrome
psychogenic pain: disorder
psychological: tests
psycholytic: drug
psychomotor: epilepsy; retardation; seizure; tests
psychopathic: personality
psychophysiologic: manifestation
psychosensory: aphasia
psychosexual: development; dysfunction
psychosocial: dwarfism
psychosomatic: disorder; medicine
psychotic: disorder; manifestation
psychotomimetic: drug
psychotropic: agent; drug
PTA: stain
PTC: protein
pterygium: syndrome
pterygoid: branch of maxillary artery; branch of posterior deep temporal artery; canal; chest; depression; fissure; fossa; fovea; hamulus; laminae; nerve; notch; pit; plates; process of sphenoid bone; ridge of sphenoid bone; tubercle; tuberosity (of mandible)
pterygoid venous: plexus
pterygomandibular: ligament; raphe; space
pterygomaxillary: fissure; fossa; notch
pterygomeningeal: artery
pterygopalatine: canal; fossa; ganglion; groove; nerves
pterygopharyngeal: part of superior constrictor muscle of pharynx
pterygospinal: ligament
pterygospinous: ligament; process
ptotic: organ

pubic: angle; arch; arteries; body; bone; branch of inferior epigastric artery; branch of inferior epigastric vein; branch of obturator artery; crest; hair; rami; region; spine; symphysis; tubercle
public: antigens; health; hospital
public health: dentistry; nurse
puboanalis: muscle
pubocapsular: ligament
pubococcygeal: muscle
pubococcygeus: muscle
pubofemoral: ligament
puboperinealis: muscle
puboprostatic: ligament; muscle
puboprostaticus: muscle
puborectal: muscle
puborectalis: muscle
pubourethral: triangle
pubovaginal: muscle; operation
pubovaginalis: muscle
pubovesical: ligament (of female); ligament (of male); muscle
pubovesicalis: muscle
Puchtler-Sweat: stain for basement membranes; stain for hemoglobin and hemosiderin
pudding: opium
puddle: sign
pudendal: anesthesia; canal; cleavage; cleft; hematocele; hernia; nerve; sac; slit; ulcer; veins
pudic: nerve
puerile: respiration
puerperal: eclampsia; fever; hemoglobinemia; mastitis; morbidity; period; psychosis; sepsis; septicemia; tetanus
Puestow: procedure
Pulfrich: phenomenon
pulmonary: acinus; adenomatosis; alveolus; amebiasis; anthrax; arc; area; artery; atresia; bleb; branch of autonomic nervous system; branches of pulmonary nerve plexus; bulla; cavity; circulation; cirrhosis; collapse; cone; conus; distomiasis; edema; embolism; emphysema; encephalopathy; fistula; glomangiosis; glomus; groove; hamartoma; heart; hypertension; hypostasis; incompetence; insufficiency; ligament; lymph nodes;

Word Finder

murmur; orifice;
osteoarthropathy; pleura;
pleurisy; pressure; ridges;
schistosomiasis; siderosis;
sinuses; stenosis; sulcus;
talcosis; toilet; transpiration;
trunk; tuberculosis;
tularemia; valve; veins;
ventilation
pulmonary alveolar:
microlithiasis; proteinosis
pulmonary artery:
anastomosis; aneurysm;
atresia; banding; catheter
pulmonary capillary wedge:
pressure
pulmonary dysmaturity:
syndrome
pulmonary (nervous): plexus
pulmonic: plague;
regurgitation; tularemia;
valve
pulmonocoronary: reflex
pulp: abscess; amputation;
atrophy; calcification;
calculus; canal; cavity;
cavity of crown; chamber;
horn; nodule; polyp;
pressure; stone; test
pulpal: wall
pulpar: cell
pulpit: spectacles
pulpless: tooth
pulsatile: hematoma
pulsatility: index
pulsating: empyema;
metastases; neurasthenia
pulse: curve; deficit;
generator; granuloma;
oximetry; period; pressure;
rate; sequence; therapy;
wave
pulse-chase: experiment
pulsed: laser
pulsed dye: laser
pulsed-field gel:
electrophoresis
pulse-field gel: electrophoresis
pulse height: analyzer
pulseless: disease
pulseless electrical: activity
pulse wave: duration
pulsion: diverticulum
pulvinar: nuclei
pump: failure; lung
pumped: laser
punch: biopsy; grafts
punchdrunk: syndrome
punctate: basophilia; cataract;
hemorrhage; hyalosis;
keratitis; keratoderma;
parotiditis; retinitis
punctuation: codon
puncture: diabetes; wound
pupillary: axis; block; border
of iris; distance; margin of

iris; membrane; reflex; ruff;
zone
pupillary block: glaucoma
pupillary light-near:
dissociation
pupillary-skin: reflex
pupillotonic: pseudotabes
pure: absence; aphasias; color;
culture
pure autonomic: failure
pure random: drift
pure red cell: anemia; aplasia
pure tone: audiogram
pure-tone: audiometer;
average
purified: cotton; ozokerite;
water
purified placental: protein
**purified protein derivative
of:** tuberculin
purine: base; bodies
purine-free: diet
purine-restricted: diet
Purkinje: cells; conduction;
corpuscles; effect; fibers;
figures; images; network;
phenomenon; shift; system
Purkinje cell: layer
Purkinje-Sanson: images
Purmann: method
pursed lips: breathing
purse-string: corepexy;
instrument; suture
Purtscher: disease;
retinopathy
purulent: conjunctivitis;
cyclitis; encephalitis;
inflammation; ophthalmia;
pericarditis; pleurisy;
pneumonia; retinitis;
synovitis
pus: basin; cell; corpuscle;
tube
push-back: procedure
pustular: blepharitis;
melanosis; miliaria;
psoriasis; syphilid
Putnam-Dana: syndrome
putrescent: pulp
putrid: bronchitis
Putti-Platt: operation;
procedure
putty: kidney
Puumala: virus
PVA: fixative
PVM: virus
pyelonephritic: kidney
pyelotubular: reflux
pyelovenous: backflow
pyemic: abscess; embolism
pyloric: antrum; artery; branch
of anterior vagal trunk;
canal; cap; constriction;
glands; incompetence;
insufficiency; lymph nodes;

orifice; part of stomach;
sphincter; stenosis; vein
pylorus-preserving:
pancreaticoduodenectomy
Pym: fever
pyogenic: arthritis; bacterium;
fever; granuloma; infection;
membrane; pachymeningitis;
salpingitis
pyramid: sign
pyramidal: bone; cataract;
cells; eminence; fibers;
fracture; layer; lobe of
thyroid gland; muscle;
muscle of auricle; process of
palatine bone; radiation;
tract; tractotomy
pyramidal auricular: muscle
pyramidal cell: layer
pyramidalis: muscle
pyridoxine: dependency with
seizure
pyriform: apparatus
pyriform aperture: wiring
pyrimidine: base; dimer
pyroligneous: alcohol; spirit;
vinegar
pyrrol: cell
pyrrole: nucleus
pyruvate dehydrogenase:
complex
pyruvate kinase: deficiency
pyruvate oxidation: factor

Q

Q: angle; bands; disks;
enzyme; fever; wave
Q-banding: stain
QR: interval
QRB: interval
QRS: complex; interval
QS$_2$: interval
Q-switched: laser
QT: interval
Q tip: test
quack: medicine
quadrangular: cartilage;
lobule; membrane; space;
therapy
quadrantic: hemianopia;
scotoma
quadrate: ligament; lobe;
lobule; muscle; muscle of
loins; muscle of sole;
muscle of thigh; muscle of
upper lip; part of liver
quadrate pronator: muscle
quadratus: muscle
quadratus femoris: muscle
quadratus lumborum: muscle
quadratus plantae: muscle
quadriceps: muscle of thigh;
reflex
quadriceps femoris: muscle

quadrigeminal: artery; bodies;
cistern; cistern; lamina;
plate; pulse; rhythm
quadrilateral: space
quadripedal extensor: reflex
quadruple: amputation;
rhythm
quail bronchitis: virus
qualitative: alteration;
analysis; trait
quality of: life
quality: control; factor
quality control: chart
Quant: sign
quantal: effect
quantitative: alteration;
analysis; genetics;
hypertrophy; perimetry
quantum: efficiency; limit;
mottle; requirement; theory;
yield
Quaranfil: virus
quarantine: period
quartan: fever; malaria;
parasite
quartz: glass
quasi-continuous wave: laser
quaternary: structure; syphilis
quaternary carbon: atom
Quatrefages: angle
Queckenstedt-Stookey: test
Queensland tick: typhus
quellung: phenomenon;
reaction; test
Quénu hemorrhoidal: plexus
Quénu-Muret: sign
Quick: method; test
quick cure: resin
quick-stop: mutant
quiet: iritis; lung
quiet hip: disease
quilted: suture
**quinacrine chromosome
banding:** stain
Quincke: disease; edema;
pulse; puncture; sign
quinhydrone: electrode
quinine carbacrylic: resin
quinine carbacrylic resin:
test
Quinlan: test
quintan: fever
quisqualate: receptor
quorum: sensing
quotidian: fever; malaria

R

ρ: factor
R: antigen; enzyme; factors;
pili; plasmids; wave
R$_f$: value
rabbit: fever; fibroma
rabbit fibroma: virus
rabbit myxoma: virus
rabbitpox: virus

rabies: immunoglobulin; vaccine; vaccine, Flury strain egg-passage; virus; virus, Flury strain; virus, Kelev strain

rabies immune: globulin (human)

raccoon: eyes

racemic: calcium pantothenate

racemose: aneurysm; gland; hemangioma

rachitic: diet; pelvis; rosary; scoliosis

racial: melanoderma

racket: amputation; nail

racquet: hypha

Radford: nomogram

radial: acceleration; artery; border of forearm; bursa; clubhand; eminence of wrist; fossa of humerus; groove; immunodiffusion; keratotomy; nerve; notch; part of posterior compartment of forearm; phenomenon; pulse; reflex; scar; tuberosity; veins

radial aplasia-thrombocytopenia: syndrome

radial collateral: artery; ligament; ligament of elbow joint; ligament of wrist joint

radial flexor: muscle of wrist

radial growth: phase

radial index: artery

radialis indicis: artery

radial recurrent: artery

radial sclerosing: lesion

radial styloid: tendovaginitis

radial tunnel: syndrome

radiant: energy; heat; intensity; layer

radiate: crown; layer of tympanic membrane; ligament; ligament of head of rib; ligament of wrist

radiate carpal: ligament

radiate sternocostal: ligaments

radiation: anemia; biology; biophysics; burn; caries; cataract; chimera; dermatosis; myelitis; myelopathy; oncologist; oncology; physics; pneumonitis; poisoning; risks; sickness; therapy

radiation weighting: factor

radical: cystectomy; hysterectomy; mastectomy; mastoidectomy; operation for hernia; pericardiectomy

radical neck: dissection

radicular: abscess; cyst; fila; pulp; syndrome

radioactive: atom; constant; cyanocobalamin; equilibrium; iodine; isotope; probe; thyroxine

radioactive iodide uptake: test

radioallergosorbent: test

radiobicipital: reflex

radiocarpal: articulation; joint

radiochemical: purity

radiofrequency: pulse

radiographic: pelvimetry

radiographic parallel line: shadow

radioimmunosorbent: test

radioiodinated serum: albumin

radioisotopic: purity

radiolabeled: thyroxine

radiologic: anatomy; enteroclysis; sphincter

radionuclide: angiocardiography; angiography; cisternography; generator; ventriculography

radionuclide ejection: fraction

radionuclidic: purity

radioperiosteal: reflex

radiopharmaceutical: chemistry; purity; synovectomy

radioreceptor: assay

radiotelemetering: capsule

radiotherapy: localization

radioulnar: disk; syndesmosis

radium: emanation

radium beam: therapy

Raeder paratrigeminal: syndrome

ragpicker's: disease

ragsorter's: disease

Rahe-Holmes social readjustment rating: scale

Rahn-Otis: sample

RAI: test

railroad: nystagmus

rainbow: symptom

Rainey: corpuscles

Raji: cell

Raji cell radioimmune: assay

Ramachandran: plot

Raman: effect; spectrum

Rambourg chromic acid-phosphotungstic acid: stain

Rambourg periodic acid-chromic methenamine-silver: stain

Ramsay Hunt: syndrome

Ramsden: ocular

Ramstedt: operation

Randall: plaques

Randall stone: forceps

random: coil; mating; mechanism; sample; sampling; variable; waves

randomized controlled: trial

random mating: equilibrium

random pattern: flap

Raney: alloy; catalyst; nickel

range of: accommodation; convergence

Ranikhet: disease

ranine: anastomosis; artery; tumor

rank-difference: correlation

Ranke: angle; complex; formula

Rankin: clamp

Rankine: scale

Ransohoff: sign

Ranvier: crosses; disks; plexus; segment

Raoult: law

raphe: nuclei

raphespinal: fibers

rapid: canities; decompression; film changer

rapid eye: movements

rapid eye movement: sleep

rapidly progressive: glomerulonephritis

rapid plasma reagin: test

Rapoport: test

Rapoport-Luebering: shunt

Rappaport: acinus; classification

rare: earths

rare-earth: screen

rare earth: elements; metal

ras: oncogene

Rasmussen: aneurysm; syndrome

raspberry: tongue

Rastelli: operation

rat-bite: disease; fever

rate: constants; equation; meter

Rathke: bundles; diverticulum; pocket; pouch

Rathke cleft: cyst

Rathke pouch: tumor

ratio: scale

rational: formula; therapy

rat mite: dermatitis

Rau: process

Rauber: layer

Rauscher: virus

Rauscher leukemia: virus

Ravius: process

raw: score

ray: fungus; therapeutics

Rayer: disease

Rayleigh: equation; test

Raynaud: disease; phenomenon; sign; syndrome

R-banding: stain

reaction: center; formation; time

reactivation: tuberculosis

reactive: arthritis; astrocyte; cell; changes; depression; hyperemia; schizophrenia

reactive airway: disease

reactive attachment: disorder

reactive perforating: collagenosis

reading-frame-shift: mutation

reaginic: antibody

REAL: classification

real: focus; image

reality: adaptation; principle; testing

real-time: echocardiography; ultrasonography

Réaumur: scale

rebound: phenomenon; tenderness

rebreathing: anesthesia; technique

Rebuck skin window: technique

recall: bias

Récamier: operation

recapitulation: theory

receiver operating: characteristic

receiver operating characteristic: curve

receptive: aphasia

receptor: protein; site

recessive: character; inheritance; trait

reciprocal: anchorage; arm; beat; bigeminy; forces; inhibition; innervation; rhythm; transfusion; translocation

reciprocating: rhythm

reciprocity: law

Recklinghausen: disease of bone

reclotting: phenomenon

recognition: time

recoil: atom; wave

recombinant: DNA; strain; vector

recombinant human: interleukin 11

recombination: fraction

recombinatorial: repair

recommended daily: allowance

reconstructive: mammaplasty; psychotherapy; surgery

record: base; linkage; rim

recovery: score; stroke

recreational: drug

recrudescent: typhus

recrudescent typhus: fever

recruiting: response

rectal: alimentation; ampulla; anesthesia; columns; folds; plexuses; reflex; shelf; sinuses; valves; valvotomy

rectal venous: plexus

rectangular: amputation
rectified: spirit; tar oil; turpentine oil
rectifier: tube
rectocardiac: reflex
rectococcygeal: muscle
rectococcygeus: muscle
rectolabial: fistula
rectolaryngeal: reflex
rectosacral: fascia
rectosigmoid: junction; sphincter
rectourethral: fistula; muscles
rectouterine: fold; muscle; pouch
rectouterinus: muscle
rectovaginal: fistula; septum
rectovaginouterine: pouch
rectovesical: fascia; fistula; fold; muscle; pouch; septum
rectovesicalis: muscle
rectovestibular: fistula
rectovulvar: fistula
rectus: muscle of abdomen; muscle of thigh; sheath
rectus abdominis: muscle
rectus capitis anterior: muscle
rectus capitis lateralis: muscle
rectus capitis posterior major: muscle
rectus capitis posterior minor: muscle
rectus femoris: muscle
recurrence: rate; risk
recurrent: abortion; albuminuria; appendicitis; artery; artery of Heubner; branch of spinal nerves; caries; encephalopathy; fever; hypopyon; jaundice of pregnancy; nerve; polyserositis; stricture
recurrent aphthous: stomatitis; ulcers
recurrent central: retinitis
recurrent corneal: erosion
recurrent herpetic: stomatitis
recurrent interosseous: artery
recurrent laryngeal: nerve
recurrent meningeal: branch of spinal nerves; nerve
recurrent pyogenic: cholangitis
recurrent radial: artery
recurrent respiratory: papillomatosis
recurrent scarring: aphthae
recurrent ulcerative: stomatitis
recurrent ulnar: artery
recurring digital: fibroma of childhood
red: atrophy; corpuscle; degeneration; fever; fibers;

gum; half-moon; hepatization; induration; infarct; lead; muscle; neuralgia; nucleus; oil; precipitate; pulp; pulp of spleen; reflex; sweat; thrombus; tide; vision; wine
red blood: cell
red blood cell: cast
red bone: marrow
red cell: cast
red cell adherence: phenomenon; test
red imported fire: ant
redox: electrode; indicator; potential; system
red oxide of: lead
red pulp: cords
red strawberry: tongue
reduced: eye; glutathione; hematin; hemoglobin
reduced enamel: epithelium
reduced interarch: distance
reducible: hernia
reducing: diet; enzyme; sugar; valve
5α-reductase: inhibitors
reduction: deformity; division; mammaplasty; nucleus; phase
reduction left: ventriculoplasty
reduplicated: cataract
red, white, and blue: sign
Reed: cell
Reed-Frost: model; theory of epidemics
reed instrument: theory
Reed-Sternberg: cell
reedy: nail
re-entrant: mechanism
reentry: phenomenon; theory
Rees-Ecker: fluid
refeeding: gynecomastia
reference: electrode; method; values
referred: pain; sensation
Refetoff: syndrome
reflected: colors; light; ray
reflected inguinal: ligament
reflecting: retinoscope
reflection: coefficient
reflex: angina; arc; asthma; control; cough; dyspepsia; epilepsy; headache; incontinence; inhibition; iridoplegia; ligament; movement; otalgia; symptom; tachycardia; therapy
reflex detrusor: contraction
reflex neurogenic: bladder
reflexogenic: pressosensitivity; zone
reflex sympathetic: dystrophy

reflux: esophagitis; nephropathy; otitis media
refracted: light
refracting: angle of a prism
refractive: amblyopia; ametropia; index; keratoplasty; keratotomy
refractive accommodative: esotropia
refractory: anemia; cast; flask; investment; period; period of electronic pacemaker; rickets; state
refrigeration: anesthesia
Refsum: disease; syndrome
Regaud: fixative
regenerative: polyp
regional: anatomy; anesthesia; enteritis; enterocolitis; hypothermia; lymphadenitis; perfusion
regional granulomatous: lymphadenitis
registered: nurse
regressing atypical: histiocytosis
regression: analysis
regression of the: mean
regressive: staining
regressive-reconstructive: approach
regular: astigmatism; insulin
regular insulin: injection
regulator: gene
regulatory: albuminuria; sequence
regurgitant: fraction; murmur
regurgitation: jaundice
Rehfuss: method
Rehfuss stomach: tube
Reichel-Pólya stomach: procedure
Reichert: cartilage
Reichert cochlear: recess
Reichert-Meissl: number
Reichstein: compound; substance
Reid base: line
Reifenstein: syndrome
Reil: ansa; band; ribbon; triangle
Reinecke: salt
reinfection: tuberculosis
reinforced: anchorage
Reinke: crystalloids; space
Reinsch: test
Reis-Bücklers corneal: dystrophy
Reisseisen: muscles
Reissner: fiber; membrane
Reiter: disease; syndrome; test
relapsing: appendicitis; fever; malaria; perichondritis; polychondritis

relapsing febrile nodular nonsuppurative: panniculitis
relational: threshold
relative: accommodation; dehydration; humidity; immunity; incompetence; leukocytosis; polycythemia; risk; scotoma; sensitivity; specificity; viscosity
relative afferent pupillary: defect
relative biologic: effectiveness
relative molecular: mass
relative refractory: period
relaxation: atelectasis; response; suture; time
release: phenomenon
released: substance
releasing: factors; hormone
reliability: coefficient
relief: area; chamber
relocation: test
REM: syndrome
Remak: fibers; ganglia; plexus; reflex; sign
Remak nuclear: division
REM behavior: disorder
reminiscent: aura
remittent: fever; malaria
remittent malarial: fever
remote: memory
remote afterloading: brachytherapy
removable: bridge
removable partial: denture
renal: adenocarcinoma; agenesis; amyloidosis; artery; ballottement; branch of lesser splanchnic nerve; branch of vagus nerve; calculus; capsulotomy; carcinosarcoma; cast; colic; collar; columns; corpuscle; cortex; diabetes; epistaxis; failure; fascia; ganglia; glycosuria; hematuria; hemorrhage; hypertension; hypoplasia; impression on liver; impression of spleen; infantilism; insufficiency; labyrinth; lobe; medulla; nanism; osteitis fibrosa; osteodystrophy; papilla; pelvis; pyramids; reflex; retinopathy; rickets; segments; sinus; surface of spleen; surface of suprarenal gland; threshold; transplantation; veins
renal cell: carcinoma
renal cortical: adenoma; lobule; scan
renal fibrocystic: osteosis
renal (nervous): plexus
renal papillary: necrosis

renal portal: system
renal-splanchnic: steal
renal-splenic venous: shunt
renal tubular: acidosis
Renaut: body
Rendu-Osler-Weber: syndrome
reniform: pelvis
renin-angiotensin: system
renin-angiotensin-aldosterone: system
renovascular: hypertension
Renpenning: syndrome
Renshaw: cells
REO: virus
reovirus-like: agent
repair: enzyme
reparative: dentin; granuloma
reparative giant cell: granuloma
reperfusion: injury
repetition: rate; time
repetition-compulsion: principle
repetitive: DNA
repetitive strain: disorders
repetitive stress: disorders
replacement: bone; fibrosis; therapy
replica: plating
replication: site
replicative: form; intermediate
reportable: disease
reporting: bias
repressible: enzyme
repressor: gene
reproductive: assimilation; cycle; nucleus; system
required arch: length
resectoscope: electrode; sheath
reserve: air; force
reserve tooth: germ
reservoir: bag; host
resident: physician
residual: abscess; affinity; air; body; body of Regaud; capacity; cleft; cyst; error; inhibition; inhibitor; lumen; ridge; schizophrenia; urine; volume
residual ovary: syndrome
resin: cement
resistance: factors; form; plasmids; pyrometer; thermometer
resistance-inducing: factor
resistance-transfer: factor
resistance-transferring: episomes
resistant ovary: syndrome
resistive: movement
resolution: acuity
resolving: power
resonance: theory of hearing
resonant: frequency

resorcinol: test
resorption: atelectasis; lacunae
respirable: aerosols
respiratory: acidosis; airway; alkalosis; apparatus; arrhythmia; ataxia; bronchioles; burst; capacity; center; chain; coefficient; enzyme; epithelium; failure; frequency; gating; hippus; inhibitor; insufficiency; lobule; metabolism; metal; mucosa; murmur; pause; pigments; poison; pulse; quotient; rate; region of mucosa of nasal cavity; region of tunica mucosa of nose; scleroma; sounds; system; therapy; tract
respiratory dead: space
respiratory distress: syndrome of the newborn; syndrome type II
respiratory enteric orphan: virus
respiratory exchange: ratio
respiratory minute: volume
respiratory syncytial: virus
respirophasic: pain
respondent: behavior; conditioning
response: bias; hierarchy
response-produced: cues
rest: area; bite; body; nitrogen; pain; position; relation; seat
restiform: body; eminence
resting: cell; length; saliva; stage; tremor
resting tidal: volume
resting wandering: cell
rest jaw: relation
restless: legs
restless legs: syndrome
Reston: virus
restorative: dentistry
restorative dental: materials
restored: cycle
restrained: beam
restriction: endonuclease; enzyme; map; methylation; site
restriction fragment length: polymorphism
restriction length: polymorphism
restriction-site: polymorphism
restrictive: cardiomyopathy
restructured: cell
rest vertical: dimension
retained: menstruation; placenta
retained products of: conception
retarded: dentition

rete: cords; cyst of ovary; pegs; ridge
retention: area; cyst; form; groove; jaundice; point; polyp; suture; vomiting
retentive: arm
retentive circumferential clasp: arm
retentive fulcrum: line
reticular: cartilage; cell; degeneration; fibers; formation; lamina; layer of corium; membrane of spinal organ; nuclei of the brainstem; nuclei of medulla oblongata; nuclei of mesencephalon; nuclei of pons; nucleus of thalamus; substance; tissue
reticular activating: system
reticular erythematous: mucinosis
reticularis: cell
reticulated: bone; corpuscle
reticuloendothelial: cell; system
reticulohistiocytic: granuloma
reticulonodular: pattern
reticulospinal: tract
reticulum cell: sarcoma
retinal: adaptation; blood vessels; camera; cones; detachment; disparity; dysplasia; embolism; fold; image; migraine
retinal anlage: tumor
retinoic acid: receptor
retinoid X: receptor
retinol-binding: protein
retractile: testis
retraction: pockets; syndrome
retroactive: inhibition
retroadductor: space
retroauricular: fold; lymph nodes
retrobulbar: abscess; anesthesia; fat; neuritis
retrocalcaneal: bursa
retrocaval: ureter
retrocecal: abscess; lymph nodes; recess
retrocedent: gout
retrochiasmatic: area
retrocochlear: hearing loss
retrocuspid: papilla
retroduodenal: artery; fossa; recess
retroflex: bundle of Meynert; fasciculus
retrogasserian: neurectomy; neurotomy
retrograde: amnesia; aortography; beat; block; cardioplegia; chromatolysis; cystourethrogram; degeneration; ejaculation;

embolism; hernia; intussusception; memory; menstruation; metamorphosis; pyelography; urography
retrograde P: wave
retrograde VA: conduction
retrohyoid: bursa
retroiliac: ureter
retroinguinal: space
retrolental: fibroplasia
retrolenticular: limb of internal capsule; part of internal capsule
retrolentiform: limb of internal capsule
retromammary: mastitis
retromandibular: fossa; process of parotid gland; vein
retromolar: fossa; pad; triangle
retromylohyoid: space
retroperitoneal: fibrosis; hernia; space; veins
retropharyngeal: abscess; lymph nodes; space
retroposterior lateral: nucleus
retropubic: hernia; space
retropyloric: lymph nodes; nodes
retrorectal: lamina of endopelvic fascia; lamina of hypogastric sheath
retrosigmoid: approach
retrospective: falsification
retrosternal: hernia; space
retrotarsal: fold
retroviral: vector
retrozonular: space
retrusive: excursion; occlusion
Rett: syndrome
return: extrasystole
returning: cycle
Retzius: cavity; fibers; gyrus; ligament; space; striae; veins
Reuss: formula; test
Reuss color: tables
reverberating: circuit
Reverdin: graft
reverse: banding; bevel; curve; genetics; mutation; osmosis; transcriptase; transcription
reversed: anaphylaxis; coarctation; peristalsis; shunt
reversed paradoxical: pulse
reversed passive: anaphylaxis
reversed phase: chromatography
reversed Prausnitz-Küstner: reaction
reversed reciprocal: rhythm
reversed-three: sign

Word Finder

reverse Eck: fistula
reverse Kingsley: splint
reverse passive: hemagglutination
reverse pupillary: block
reverse transcriptase polymerase chain: reaction
reverse Trendelenburg: position
reversible: calcinosis; colloid; decortication; hydrocolloid; pulpitis; reaction; shock
Revilliod: sign
Reye: syndrome
Reynolds: number; pentad
Rh: antigens; factor
rhabditiform: larva
rhagiocrine: cell
Rh antigen: incompatibility
Rh blocking: test
$Rh_0(D)$: immunoglobulin
$RH_0(D)$ immune: globulin
rhegmatogenous retinal: detachment
Rheinberg: microscope
Rhese: projection
Rhesus: factor
rhesus: disease
rheumatic: arteritis; carditis; chorea; disease; endocarditis; fever; pericarditis; pneumonia; valvulitis
rheumatic heart: disease
rheumatoid: arteritis; arthritis; disease; factors; nodules; pocket; spondylitis
rhinal: fissure; sulcus
rhizomelic: chondrodysplasia punctata; dwarfism
Rh null: syndrome
rho: factor
Rhodesian: trypanosomiasis
rhombencephalic: isthmus; tegmentum
rhombencephalic gustatory: nucleus
rhombic: grooves; lip
rhomboid: fossa; impression; ligament
rhomboidal: sinus
rhomboid major: muscle
rhomboid minor: muscle
rhonchal: fremitus
rhus: dermatitis
Rhus toxicodendron: antigen
Rhus venenata: antigen
rhythm: method
rhythmic: chorea
rib: spreader
Ribas-Torres: disease
ribbon: arch
ribbon arch: appliance
Ribes: ganglion
riboflavin: deficiency; unit

ribosomal: RNA
ribosome-lamella: complex
Ribot: law of memory
Ricco: law
rice: body; diet; disease; itch; starch
rice-field: fever
rice-Tween: agar
rice-water: stool
Richards-Rundle: syndrome
Richter: hernia; syndrome
Richter-Monro: line
ricin-blocked: antibody
rickettsia: vaccine, attenuated
Rickles: test
Rida: virus
Riddoch: phenomenon
Rideal-Walker: coefficient; method
Ridell: operation
rider's: bone; bursa; leg; muscles
ridge: extension; relation; resorption
riding: embolism
Ridley: circle; sinus
Riedel: disease; lobe; struma; thyroiditis
Rieder: cells; lymphocyte
Rieder cell: leukemia
Riegel: pulse
Rieger: anomaly; syndrome
Riehl: melanosis
Rift Valley: fever
Rift Valley fever: virus
Riga-Fede: disease
right: atrium of heart; auricle; border of heart; branch; branch of hepatic artery proper; branch of portal vein; bundle of atrioventricular bundle; crus of atrioventricular bundle; crus of diaphragm; duct of caudate lobe of liver; heart; liver; lobe; lobe of liver; margin of heart; part of diaphragmatic surface of liver; part of liver; ventricle
right angle: clamp
right anterior lateral hepatic: segment [VI]
right atrial: branch of right coronary artery
right atrioventricular: orifice; valve
right auricular: appendage
right axis: deviation
right colic: artery; flexure; lymph nodes; vein
right coronary: artery
right descending pulmonary: artery
right fibrous: trigone (of heart)

right flexural: artery
right gastric: artery; lymph nodes; vein
right gastroepiploic: artery; lymph nodes; vein
right gastroomental: artery; lymph nodes; vein
right heart: bypass
right hepatic: artery; duct; veins
right inferior pulmonary: vein
righting: reflexes
right lateral: division of liver
(right/left): ventricles of heart
(right and left) fibrous: rings of heart
right or left lateral decubitus: film
right/left pulmonary: surfaces of heart
right lumbar: lymph nodes
right lymphatic: duct
right main: bronchus
right marginal: branch (of right coronary artery)
right medial: division of liver
right ovarian: vein
right parasternal: impulses
(right) posterior lateral hepatic: segment [VII]
(right) posterior medial hepatic: segment [VIII]
right pulmonary: artery
right sagittal: fissure
right splicing: junction
right superior intercostal: vein
right superior pulmonary: vein
right suprarenal: vein
right testicular: vein
right-to-left: shunt
right triangular: ligament of liver
right ventricular: failure; hypoplasia
rigid: connector; dysarthria
Riley-Day: syndrome
Rimini: test
Rindfleisch: cells; folds
ring: abscess; chromosome; compound; enhancement; finger; ligament; pessary; scotoma; syringe; test; ulcer of cornea
ringed: hair
Ringer: injection; lactate; solution
ringlike corneal: dystrophy
ring precipitin: test
ring-shaped: placenta
ring-wall: lesion
ringworm: yaws
Rinne: test

Riolan: anastomosis; arc; arcades; bones; bouquet; muscle
Ripault: sign
ripe: cataract
Ripstein: operation
rise: time
risk: factor
Risley rotary: prism
risorius: muscle
Ritgen: maneuver
Rittenhouse-Manogian: procedure
Ritter opening: tetanus
Ritter-Rollet: phenomenon
ritualistic: behavior
Riva-Rocci: sphygmomanometer
river: blindness
Rivero-Carvallo: effect
Rivers: cocktail
Rivière: salt
Rivinus: canals; ducts; gland; incisure; membrane; notch
RNA: enzyme; virus
RNA tumor: viruses
Ro: spatula
Roach: clasp
Roaf: syndrome
Robert: pelvis
Roberts: syndrome
Robertshaw: tube
Robertson: pupil
robertsonian: translocation
Robin: syndrome
Robinow: dwarfism; syndrome
Robinson: catheter; disease; index
Robison: ester
Robison-Embden: ester
Robison ester: dehydrogenase
ROC: curve
Rochelle: salt
rock: oil
rocket: immunoelectrophoresis
Rocky Mountain spotted: fever
Rocky Mountain spotted fever: vaccine
rod: cell of retina; disks; fiber; granule; monochromatism; myopathy; vision
rodent: ulcer
rod nuclear: cell
roentgen: ray; unit
Roesler-Dressler: infarct
Roger: bruit; disease; murmur; reflex
Roger Anderson pin fixation: appliance
Rogers: sphygmomanometer
Rohr: stria
Röhrer: index

Rokitansky: disease; hernia; pelvis
Rokitansky-Aschoff: sinuses
Rokitansky-Küster-Hauser: syndrome
rolandic: epilepsy
Rolandic sulcal: artery
Rolando: angle; area; cells; column; tubercle
Rolando gelatinous: substance
role: conflict
roll: sulfur; tube
Roller: nucleus
roller: bandage
rollerball: electrode
Rolleston: rule
Rollet: stroma
rolling: circle
roll-tube: culture
Roman: fever
Romaña: sign
Romano-Ward: syndrome
Romanowsky blood: stain
Romberg: disease; sign; syndrome; test; trophoneurosis
Römer: test
Rónne nasal: step
R-on-T: phenomenon
roof: nucleus; plate
room: temperature
root: abscess; amputation; apex; avulsion; canal of tooth; caries; dehiscence; filaments; foramen; pulp; resection; resorption; sheath; tip
root canal: file; orifice; plugger; restoration; spreader; therapy; treatment
root caries: index
root end: cyst; granuloma
root-form: implant
rooting: reflex
rope: burn
Ropes: test
Rorschach: test
rosacea-like: tuberculid
Rosai-Dorfman: disease
rosanilin: dyes
Roscoe-Bunsen: law
Rose: position
rose: cold; spots
rose bengal radioactive (^{131}I): test
Rose-Bradford: kidney
Rose cephalic: tetanus
Rosenbach: law; sign; test
Rosenbach-Gmelin: test
Rosenmüller: fossa; gland; node; recess; valve
Rosenthal: canal; fiber; vein
Rosenthaler-Turk: reagent
Roser-Nélaton: line
rosette: test

rosette-forming: cells
Rose-Waaler: test
Ross: cycle; procedure
Ross-Jones: test
Rossolimo: reflex; sign
Ross River: fever; virus
rostral: lamina; layer; neuropore
rostral transtentorial: herniation
rostrate: pelvis
rotary: joint
rotating: anode
rotating anode: tube
rotation: flap; therapy
rotational: axis; nystagmus
rotator: cuff of shoulder; muscle
rotatores: muscles
rotatores cervicis: muscles
rotatores lumborum: muscles
rotatores thoracis: muscles
rotatory: nystagmus; tic
Rotch: sign
rote: learning
Roth: spots
Rothera nitroprusside: test
Rothmund: syndrome
Rothmund-Thomson: syndrome
Rotor: syndrome
Rouget: bulb; muscle
Rouget-Neumann: sheath
rough: colony; line
rough-surfaced endoplasmic: reticulum
Roughton-Scholander: apparatus; syringe
Rougnon-Heberden: disease
rouleaux: formation
round: bur; eminence; fasciculus; foramen; heart; ligament of elbow joint; ligament of femur; ligament of liver; ligament of uterus; pelvis; window
round cell: sarcoma
rounded: atelectasis
round pronator: muscle
round window: membrane
Rous: sarcoma; tumor
Rous-associated: virus
Rous sarcoma: virus
Roussy-Lévy: disease; syndrome
Roux: method; stain
Roux-en-Y: anastomosis; operation
Rovsing: sign
royal: touch
RPR: test
R-R: interval
Rs: virus
RST: segment
Rubarth disease: virus
rubber: dam; pelvis; tissue

rubber-bulb: syringe
rubber dam: clamp
rubber dam clamp: forceps
rubber-shod: clamp
rubbing: alcohol
rubella: cataract; retinopathy; virus
rubella HI: test
rubella virus: vaccine, live
rubeola: virus
Rubin: test
Rubinstein-Taybi: syndrome
Rubner: laws of growth; test
rubrobulbar: tract
rubroolivary: fibers
rubropontine: tract
rubroreticular: fasciculi; tract
rubrospinal: decussation; tract
ruby: spots
Rud: syndrome
Ruffini: corpuscles
rufous: albinism
rugal: columns of vagina
rugger jersey: vertebra
rum: nose
rumination: disorder
Rummel: tourniquet
Rumpel-Leede: phenomenon; sign; test
runaway: pacemaker
Runeberg: formula
runner's: knee
running: time
runt: disease
runting: syndrome
Runyon: classification
Runyon group I: mycobacteria
Runyon group II: mycobacteria
Runyon group III: mycobacteria
Runyon group IV: mycobacteria
rupial: syphilid
ruptured: aneurysm; disk
rural cutaneous: leishmaniasis
Rushton: bodies
Russell: bodies; effect; sign; syndrome; traction
Russell's: viper
Russell's viper: venom
Russell's viper venom clotting: time
Russian: fly; influenza
Russian autumn: encephalitis
Russian autumn encephalitis: virus
Russian spring-summer: encephalitis (Eastern subtype); encephalitis (Western subtype)
Russian spring-summer encephalitis: virus

Russian tick-borne: encephalitis
Rust: disease; phenomenon
rusty: sputum
Ruysch: membrane; muscle; tube; veins
Ryan: stain
ryanodine: receptor
Rye: classification
Ryle: tube

S

σ: factor
S: antigen; factor; peptide; phase; potential; protein; sign of Golden; unit of streptomycin; wave
S$_7$: gallop
S-A: node
saber: shin; tibia
saber-sheath: trachea
Sabia: virus
Sabin: vaccine
Sabin-Feldman dye: test
sabot: heart
Sabouraud: agar; pastils
Sabouraud dextrose: agar
Sabouraud-Noiré: instrument
saccadic: movement
sacciform: recess of distal radioulnar joint; recess of elbow joint
saccular: aneurysm; bronchiectasis; duct; gland; nerve; recess of bony labyrinth; spot
sacculated: pleurisy
Sachs-Georgi: test
sacral: anesthesia; canal; cornu; crest; flexure; flexure of rectum; foramina; ganglia; hiatus; horn; index; kyphosis; lymph nodes; nerves [S1–S5]; part of spinal cord; plexus; promontory; region; triangle; tuberosity; veins; vertebrae [S1–S5]
sacral splanchnic: nerves
sacral venous: plexus
sacred: bone
sacroanterior: position
sacrococcygeal: disk; joint; junction; teratoma
sacrocolpopexy: procedure
sacrodural: ligament
sacrogenital: folds
sacroiliac: articulation; joint
sacropelvic: surface of ilium
sacroposterior: position
sacrosciatic: notch
sacrospinous: ligament
sacrospinous vaginal vault suspension: procedure
sacrotransverse: position

sacrotuberous: ligament
sacrouterine: fold
sacrovaginal: fold
sacrovesical: fold
saddle: back; embolism; head; joint; nose
saddleback: caterpillar
saddle block: anesthesia
sadomasochistic: relationship
Saemisch: section; ulcer
Saenger: macula; operation; sign
Saethre-Chotzen: syndrome
SAF: fixative
safe: sex
safety: lens; spectacles
sagittal: axis; border of parietal bone; crest; fontanelle; groove; line; plane; section; sulcus; suture; synostosis
sagittal split mandibular: osteotomy
sago: spleen
sagulum: nucleus
Saigon: cinnamon
sail: sound
sailor's: skin
Saint: triad
Saint Anthony: dance
Saint Ignatius: itch
Sakaguchi: reaction
Sakurai-Lisch: nodule
sakushu: fever
salaam: attack; convulsions; spasm
Salah sternal puncture: needle
salicylic acid: collodion
saline: agglutinin; purgative; solution; water
Salinem: fever; infection
Salisbury common cold: viruses
saliva: ejector; pump
salivary: calculus; colic; corpuscle; digestion; duct; fistula; gland; virus
salivary gland: disease; hormone; virus
salivary gland virus: disease
Salk: vaccine
Salla: disease
salmon: patch
Salmonella food: poisoning
salpingopalatine: fold
salpingopharyngeal: fold; muscle
salpingopharyngeus: muscle
salt: action; bridge; depletion; dye; edema; fever; loading; sensitivity; solution; wasting
saltatory: chorea; conduction; evolution; spasm
salt depletion: syndrome
salt-depletion: crisis

salted: plasma; serum
Salter-Harris: classification of epiphysial plate injuries
Salter incremental: lines
salt-losing: defect; nephritis; syndrome
saltpeter: paper
salt water: boils; soap
salvage: chemotherapy; cystectomy; pathway; therapy
Salzmann nodular corneal: degeneration
sampling: bias
Samter: syndrome
Sanarelli: phenomenon
Sanarelli-Shwartzman: phenomenon
Sanchez Salorio: syndrome
sand: bath; bodies; tumor
sandal: foot
sandal strap: dermatitis
sandfly: fever
sandfly fever: viruses
Sandhoff: disease
Sandifer: syndrome
Sandison-Clark: chamber
sandpaper: disks; gallbladder
Sandström: bodies
sandworm: disease
Sanfilippo: syndrome
Sanger: method; reagent
sanguineous: cyst
sanious: pus
San Joaquin: fever
San Joaquin Valley: disease; fever
San Miguel sea lion: virus
Sansom: sign
Sanson: images
Santini booming: sound
Santorini: canal; cartilage; concha; duct; fissures; incisures; labyrinth; muscle; plexus; tubercle; vein
Santorini major: caruncle
Santorini minor: caruncle
Sao Paulo: typhus
São Paulo: fever
saphenous: branch of descending genicular artery; hiatus; nerve; opening; veins
saponification: number
Sappey: fibers; plexus; veins
sarcogenic: cell
sarcoidal: granuloma
sarcomatoid: carcinoma
sarcoplasmic: reticulum
sarcoptic: acariasis; mange
sartorius: bursae; muscle
Sartwell incubation: model
satellite: abscess; cells; cell of skeletal muscle; DNA; metastasis
satellite-rich: heterochromatin
satiety: center

Sattler: veil
Sattler elastic: layer
saturated: color; fat; fatty acid; hydrocarbon; solution
saturation: analysis; index
saturation sound pressure: level
saturnine: colic; encephalopathy; gout
saucer-shaped: cataract
Saundby: test
sausage: fingers
Savage: syndrome
Savage perineal: body
Savary: bougies
Sayre: jacket
Sayre suspension: apparatus; traction
S-BP: line
scabbard: trachea
scabby: mouth
scaffold-associated: regions
scalar: electrocardiogram
scalded mouth: syndrome
scalded skin: syndrome
scalene: hiatus; tubercle; tubercle of Lisfranc
scalenus anterior: muscle; syndrome
scalenus medius: muscle
scalenus minimus: muscle
scalenus posterior: muscle
scalp: contusion; hair; infection; laceration; muscle
scaly: ringworm; tetter
scamping: speech
scanning: speech
scanning electron: microscope
scanning equalization: radiography
Scanzoni: maneuver
Scanzoni second: os
scaphoid: abdomen; bone; fossa; fossa of sphenoid bone; tuberosity
scapular: line; notch; reflex; region
scapulocostal: syndrome
scapulohumeral: atrophy; muscles; reflex
scapulohumeral muscular: dystrophy
scapuloperiosteal: reflex
scar: cancer; cancer of the lungs; carcinoma; emphysema
Scardino vertical flap: pyeloplasty
scarf: bandage; sign
scarification: test
scarlatinal: nephritis
scarlatiniform: erythema
scarlet: fever
scarlet fever: antitoxin

scarlet fever erythrogenic: toxin
Scarpa: fascia; fluid; foramina; ganglion; habenula; hiatus; liquor; membrane; method; sheath; staphyloma; triangle
scarring: alopecia
Scatchard: plot
scattered: radiation
scavenger: cell; receptor
Schacher: ganglion
Schaeffer-Fulton: stain
Schaer: reagent
Schäfer: method
Schaffer: test
Schäffer: reflex
Schamberg: dermatitis; fever
Schapiro: sign
Schardinger: dextrins; enzyme; reaction
Schatzki: ring
Schaudinn: fixative
Schaumann: bodies; lymphogranuloma; syndrome
Schauta vaginal: operation
Schede: method
scheduled: drug
Scheele: green
Scheibe: hearing impairment
Scheibler: reagent
Scheie: syndrome
Scheiner: experiment
Schellong: test
Schellong-Strisower: phenomenon
schematic: eye
Schenck: disease
Scheuermann: disease
Schick: method; test
Schick test: toxin
Schiff: base; reagent
Schiff-Sherrington: phenomenon
Schilder: disease
Schiller: test
Schilling: blood count; index; test
Schilling band: cell
Schilling type of monocytic: leukemia
Schindler: disease
schindyletic: joint
Schiötz: tonometer
Schirmer: test
schistosomal: dermatitis
schistosome: granuloma
schizencephalic: microcephaly
schizo-affective: psychosis
schizoid: personality
schizoid personality: disorder
schizophreniform: disorder
schizotypal: personality
schizotypal personality: disorder

Schlatter: disease
Schlemm: canal
Schlesinger: sign
schlieren: optics
Schmidel: anastomoses
Schmid-Fraccaro: syndrome
Schmidt: diet; syndrome
Schmidt-Lanterman: clefts;
  incisures
Schmidt-Strassburger: diet
Schmidt-Thannhauser:
  method
Schmorl: jaundice; nodule
Schmorl ferric-ferricyanide
  reduction: stain
Schmorl picrothionin: stain
Schneider: carmine
Schneider first rank:
  symptoms
schneiderian: membrane
schneiderian first rank:
  symptoms
Schnitzler: syndrome
Schober: test
Scholander: apparatus
Scholz: disease
Schönbein: test
Schönlein: disease; purpura
Schönlein-Henoch: syndrome
school: nurse; phobia
Schott: treatment
Schreger: lines
Schridde cancer: hairs
Schroeder: operation
Schuchardt: operation
Schüffner: dots; granules
Schüller: disease; ducts;
  phenomenon; syndrome
Schultz: reaction; stain
Schultz-Charlton:
  phenomenon; reaction
Schultz-Dale: reaction
Schultze: cells; fold;
  mechanism; membrane;
  phantom; placenta; sign
Schütz: bundle; law; rule
Schwabach: test
Schwalbe: corpuscle; nucleus;
  ring; spaces
Schwann: cells
Schwann cell: unit
Schwann white: substance
Schwartz: syndrome;
  tractotomy
Schwartz-Jampel: disease
Schweninger: method
Schweninger-Buzzi:
  anetoderma
sciatic: bursa of gluteus
  maximus; foramen; hernia;
  nerve; neuralgia; neuritis;
  plexus; scoliosis; spine
scientific: theory
scimitar: sign
scintigraphic: angiography
scintillating: scotoma

scintillation: camera; counter
scirrhous: carcinoma
scissor: gait
scleral: ectasia; resection;
  rigidity; ring; roll; spur;
  staphyloma; sulcus; veins
scleral buckling: operation
scleral venous: sinus
sclerocorneal: junction
sclerocystic: disease of the
  ovary
sclerosing: adenosis; agent;
  hemangioma; inflammation;
  keratitis; leukoencephalitis;
  mastoiditis; osteitis; therapy
sclerotic: bodies; coat; dentin;
  gastritis; kidney; stomach;
  teeth
sclerotic cemental: mass
scoliotic: pelvis
scombroid: poisoning
scorbutic: anemia
scotopic: adaptation; eye;
  perimetry; vision
Scott: operation
Scott-Wilson: reagent
scout: film; radiograph
scratch: test
screen: defense; memory
screening: audiometry; test
screw: arteries; elevator; joint
screwdriver: teeth
Scribner: shunt
scrivener's: palsy
scrofulous: keratitis; rhinitis
scroll: bones; ear
scrotal: arteries; hernia;
  hypospadias; part of ductus
  deferens; raphe; septum;
  swelling; tongue; veins
scrub: nurse; typhus
Scultetus: bandage; position
scurvy: rickets
sea: louse; scurvy; sickness
seabather's: eruption
sea-blue: histiocyte
sea-blue histiocyte: disease
sea gull: murmur
seal: fingers
sealed jar: technique
seamstress's: cramp
Seashore: test
seasonal affective: disorder
sea urchin: granuloma
sebaceous: adenoma; cyst;
  epithelioma; follicles;
  glands; horn; tubercle
Sebileau: hollow; muscle
seborrheic: blepharitis;
  dermatitis; dermatosis;
  eczema; keratosis; verruca;
  wart
Seckel: dwarfism; syndrome
seclusion of: pupil
second: finger; incisor; law of
  thermodynamics; messenger;

molar; part of duodenum;
  sight; sound; toe [II]; tooth
secondarily generalized
  tonic-clonic: seizure
secondary: adhesion;
  aerodontalgia;
  agammaglobulinemia;
  alcohol; aldosteronism;
  amenorrhea; amputation;
  amyloidosis; anesthetic;
  atelectasis; axis; calcium
  phosphate; carcinoma;
  cardiomyopathy; caries;
  cataract; cementum; center
  of ossification; choana;
  coccidioidomycosis;
  constriction; curvatures of
  vertebral column; dementia;
  dentin; dentition; deviation;
  dextrocardia; digestion;
  disease; drives; drowning;
  dysmenorrhea; elaboration;
  encephalitis; failure; fissure
  [TA] of cerebellum; gain;
  glaucoma; gout;
  hemochromatosis;
  hemorrhage; host;
  hydrocephalus;
  hyperparathyroidism;
  hypertension;
  hyperthyroidism;
  hypogammaglobulinemia;
  hypogonadism;
  hypothyroidism;
  immunodeficiency;
  infection; lysosomes;
  megaureter; mesoderm;
  metabolism; metabolite;
  methemoglobinemia;
  narcissism; nodule;
  nondisjunction; oocyte;
  palate; pellagra; point of
  ossification; process;
  proteose; pyoderma;
  radiation; rays;
  reinforcement; retinitis;
  saturation; screw-worm;
  spermatocyte; structure;
  suture; syphilid; syphilis;
  telangiectasia; thrombus;
  tuberculosis; union; villus;
  vitreous
secondary abdominal:
  pregnancy
secondary adrenocortical:
  insufficiency
secondary antibody:
  deficiency
secondary aortic: area
secondary cartilaginous: joint
secondary dye: test
secondary egg: membrane
secondary generalized:
  epilepsy
secondary immune: response

secondary interatrial:
  foramen
secondary medical: care
secondary myeloid:
  metaplasia
secondary ossification: center
secondary ovarian: follicle
secondary pulmonary: lobule
secondary refractory: anemia
secondary renal: calculus
secondary renal tubular:
  acidosis
secondary sensory: cortex;
  nuclei
secondary sex: characters
secondary spiral: lamina;
  plate
secondary tympanic:
  membrane
secondary visual: area; cortex
secondary X: zone
second cervical: vertebra
second cranial: nerve [CN II]
second cuneiform: bone
second-degree: burn
second degree AV: block
second gas: effect
second heart: sound
second-look: operation
second-order: conditioning
second parallel pelvic: plane
second set: rejection
second signaling: system
second temporal: convolution
second tibial: muscle
Secrétan: syndrome
secretin: test
secretomotor: nerve
secretor: factor
secretory: canaliculus;
  carcinoma; component; cyst;
  duct; granule;
  immunoglobulin;
  immunoglobulin A; nerve;
  otitis media
sectional: impression;
  radiography
sector: echocardiography;
  iridectomy; scan
secular: equilibrium
sedimentary: cataract
sedimentation: coefficient;
  constant; rate; velocity
seed: corn
Seeligmüller: sign
seesaw: murmur; nystagmus
Seessel: pocket; pouch
segmental: anesthesia; arteries
  of kidney; arteries of liver;
  atelectasis; bronchus;
  fracture; glomerulonephritis;
  neuritis; plate; sphincter;
  tubule; zone
segmental alveolar:
  osteotomy

segmental demyelinating: polyneuropathy
segmental medullary: arteries
segmentation: cavity; nucleus
segmented: cell; leukocyte; neutrophil
segmenting: body
segregation: analysis; ratio
Seidel: scotoma; sign
Seidlitz: mixture
Seignette: salt
Seiler: cartilage
Seip: syndrome
Seldinger: technique
selection: coefficient; pressure
selective: angiography; grinding; hypoaldosteronism; immunoglobulin A deficiency; inattention; inhibition; injection; medium; memory; reduction; stain; termination
selective estrogen receptor: modulator
selective norepinephrine reuptake: inhibitor
selective serotonin reuptake: inhibitor
selenium: plate
self-: concept
self-curing: resin
self-limited: disease
self-registering: thermometer
self-retaining: catheter
Selivanoff: test
sellar: diaphragm
Sellick: maneuver
Selters: water
semantic: aphasia
semi-: vegetarian
Semichon acid carmine: stain
semicircular: canals; canals of bony labyrinth; ducts; line; line of Douglas
semi-closed: circle
semiconservative: replication
semidirect: leads
semi-Fowler: position
semihorizontal: heart
semilente: insulin
semilunar: bone; cartilage; cusp; fascia; fasciculus; fibrocartilage; fold; folds of colon; ganglion; hiatus; line; notch; nucleus of Flechsig; valve
semilunar conjunctival: fold
semimembranosus: muscle; reflex
semimembranous: bursa
seminal: capsule; colliculus; duct; fluid; gland; granule; hillock; lake; vesicle
seminal vesical: cyst

seminiferous: epithelium; tubules
seminiferous tubule: dysgenesis
semioval: center
semipennate: muscle
semipermeable: membrane
semipolar: bond
semiprone: position
semispinal: muscle; muscle of head; muscle of neck; muscle of thorax
semispinalis: muscle
semispinalis capitis: muscle
semispinalis cervicis: muscle
semispinalis thoracis: muscle
semisulfur: mustard
semitendinosus: muscle
semivertical: heart
Semliki Forest: virus
Semon-Hering: theory
Semple: vaccine
Sendai: virus
Senear-Usher: disease; syndrome
Seneca: snakeroot
senegal: gum
Sengstaken-Blakemore: tube
senile: amyloidosis; arteriosclerosis; atrophoderma; atrophy; cataract; chorea; degeneration; delirium; dementia; deterioration; dwarfism; emphysema; fibroma; gangrene; halo; hemangioma; involution; keratoderma; keratoma; keratosis; lentigo; melanoderma; memory; nephrosclerosis; osteomalacia; plaque; psychosis; retinoschisis; tremor; vaginitis; wart
senile dental: caries
senile lenticular: myopia
senile sebaceous: hyperplasia
senior: synonym
Sennetsu: fever
Senning: operation
sensation: level; time
sense of: identity
sense: organs; strand
sensible: heat; perspiration; temperature
sensitivity training: group
sensitized: antigen; cell; culture
sensitizing: dose; injection
sensorial: areas
sensorimotor: area; theory
sensorineural: hearing loss
sensory: amblyopia; amusia; aphasia; ataxia; cell; cortex; crossway; decussation of medulla oblongata;

deprivation; epilepsy; ganglion; hearing impairment; image; inattention; nerve; neuron; neuronopathy; nuclei; paralysis; phantom; receptors; root of ciliary ganglion; root of pterygopalatine ganglion; root of spinal nerve; root of sublingual ganglion; root of submandibular ganglion; root of trigeminal nerve; tract; urgency
sensory acuity: level
sensory precipitated: epilepsy
sensory speech: center
sentinal node: biopsy
sentinel: animal; event; gland; lymph node; node; pile; tag
sentinel loop: sign
Seoul: virus
separating: medium; wire
separation: anxiety
separation anxiety: disorder
sepsis: syndrome
septal: area; artery; bone; branches; cartilage; cell; cusp of right atrioventricular valve; cusp of tricuspid valve; gingiva; lines
septal nasal: cartilage
septate: hymen; mycelium; uterus; vagina
septic: abortion; arthritis; endocarditis; fever; infarct; intoxication; phlebitis; pneumonia; retinitis; shock; wound
septicemic: abscess; plague
septofimbrial: nucleus
septomarginal: fasciculus; trabecula; tract
septooptic: dysplasia
sequence: hypothesis; pulse
sequence-tagged: sites
sequence-tagged site (STS): map
sequential: analysis; anastomosis
sequential multichannel: autoanalyzer
sequestration: cyst; dermoid
Sergent white: line
serial: extraction; film changer; interval; passage; radiography; section
serine: carboxypeptidase; hydrolases
serine protease: inhibitors
serofibrinous: inflammation; pleurisy
serologic: pipette
seromucous: cells; gland
serotonin norepinephrine reuptake: inhibitor

serous: cell; coat; coat of peritoneum; cyst; demilunes; diarrhea; gland; hemorrhage; inflammation; iritis; layer of peritoneum; ligament; membrane; meningitis; otitis media; pericardium; pleurisy; retinitis; synovitis; tunic
serpent: ulcer of cornea
serpentine: aneurysm
serpiginous: choroidopathy; keratitis; ulcer
serpiginous corneal: ulcer
serrate: suture
serratus anterior: muscle
serratus posterior inferior: muscle
serratus posterior superior: muscle
Serres: angle; glands
Sertoli: cells; columns
Sertoli-cell-only: syndrome
Sertoli-Leydig cell: tumor
Sertoli-stromal cell: tumor
serum: accelerator; accident; agar; agglutinin; albumin; disease; eruption; hepatitis; nephritis; proteins; rash; reaction; shock; sickness; therapy
serum accelerator: globulin
serumal: calculus
serum hepatitis: virus
serum prothrombin conversion: accelerator
Servetus: circulation
sesamoid: bone; cartilage of cricopharyngeal ligament; cartilage of larynx; cartilages of nose
sessile: hydatid; polyp
set of: idiotopes
seton: operation; wound
setting: expansion
setting sun: sign
seven-day: fever
seventh: sense
seventh cranial: nerve [CN VII]
Sever: disease
severe combined: immunodeficiency
severe postanoxic: encephalopathy
Severinghaus: electrode
severity of: illness
sewer: gas
sex: cell; chromatin; chromosomes; cords; determination; factor; hormones; linkage; object; ratio; reassignment; reversal; role
sex chromosome: imbalance

sex hormone-binding: globulin
sex-influenced: inheritance
sex-limited: inheritance
sex-linked: character; inheritance; locus
sex steroid-binding: globulin
sexual: abuse; deviation; dimorphism; disorders; dwarfism; generation; gland; infantilism; instinct; intercourse; life; neurasthenia; orientation; perversion; potency; reproduction; selection
sexually transmitted: disease
Sézary: cell; erythroderma; syndrome
shadow: cells; corpuscle; nucleus; test
Shaffer-Hartmann: method
shaggy: aorta; chorion; pericardium
shagreen: patch; skin
shake: culture; test
shaken baby: syndrome
shaking: palsy
shallow: breathing
sham: feeding; rage
sham-movement: vertigo
shared: epitope
shared psychotic: disorder
sharp: spoon
Sharpey: fibers
shave: biopsy
Shaver: disease
shaving: cramp
shawl: muscle
shear: flow; rate; stress; thinning
shearing: edge
sheath: ligaments; process of sphenoid bone
sheathed: artery
Sheehan: syndrome
sheep: bots
sheep-pox: virus
shelf: procedure
shell: nail; shock
shellac: base
Shemin: cycle
Shenton: line
Shepherd: fracture
Sherman: unit
Sherman-Bourquin: unit of vitamin B$_2$
Sherman-Munsell: unit
Sherrington: law; phenomenon
sherry: wine
Shibley: sign
shifting: dullness; pacemaker
Shiga: bacillus; toxin
Shiga-Kruse: bacillus
Shigalike: toxin
shilling: scars

shimamushi: disease
shin: bone
shin bone: fever
Shine-Dalgarno: sequence
ship: beriberi; fever
Shipley-Hartford: scale
shipping fever: virus
shipyard: eye
Shirodkar: operation
shivering: thermogenesis
shock: antigen; index; lung; therapy; treatment
shocking: dose
shock wave: lithotripsy
shoddy: fever
Shone: anomaly; complex; syndrome
shop: typhus
Shope: fibroma; papilloma
Shope fibroma: virus
Shope papilloma: virus
short: bone; chain; crus of incus; gyri of insula; head; head of biceps brachii; head of biceps femoris; limb of incus; process of malleus; root of ciliary ganglion; sight; vinculum
short abductor: muscle of thumb
short adductor: muscle
short association: fibers
short-bowel: syndrome
short central: artery
short-chain acyl-CoA dehydrogenase: deficiency
short ciliary: nerve
short circumferential: arteries
shortening: reaction
short extensor: muscle of great toe; muscle of thumb; muscle of toes
short fibular: muscle
short flexor: muscle of great toe; muscle of little finger; muscle of little toe; muscle of thumb; muscle of toes
short gastric: arteries; veins
short increment sensitivity: index
short incubation: hepatitis
short interspersed: elements
short levatores costarum: muscles
short palmar: muscle
short peroneal: muscle
short pitch helicoidal: layer
short posterior ciliary: artery
short radial extensor: muscle of wrist
short saphenous: nerve; vein
short-term: memory
short-term exposure: limit
short TI inversion: recovery
short wave: diathermy
shotgun: prescription

shot-silk: phenomenon; reflex; retina
shotted: suture
shoulder: dystocia; girdle; joint; presentation
shoulder apprehension: sign
shoulder-girdle: syndrome
shoulder-hand: syndrome
Shprintzen: syndrome
Shrapnell: membrane
Shulman: syndrome
shunt: cyanosis; muscle
shut-in: personality
shuttle: vector
Shwachman: syndrome
Shwachman-Diamond: syndrome
Shwartzman: phenomenon; reaction
Shy-Drager: syndrome
SI: units
Siamese: twins
Siberian tick: typhus
sibilant: rale
sibling: rivalry
Sibson: aponeurosis; fascia; groove; muscle
Sibson aortic: vestibule
sicca: complex; syndrome
sick: headache; role
sick building: syndrome
sick euthyroid: syndrome
sickle: cell; form; scotoma
sickle cell: anemia; crisis; dactylitis; disease; hemoglobin; retinopathy; test; trait
sickle cell C: disease
sickle cell-thalassemia: disease
sick sinus: syndrome
side: chain
side-chain: theory
sideroblastic: anemia
sideropenic: dysphagia
siderotic: cataract; nodules
Siegert: sign
Siegle: otoscope
sieve: bone; plate
Siggaard-Andersen: nomogram
sight: blindness
sigma: effect; factor; peptide
sigmoid: arteries; colon; flexure; fossa; groove; kidney; lymph nodes; notch; sinus; sulcus; veins; volvulus
sigmoidovesical: fistula
sign: blindness
signal: lymph node; node; void
signal-processing: circuits
signal recognition: particle
signal-to-noise: ratio
signet: ring

signet ring: cells
signet-ring cell: carcinoma
Signorelli: sign
silastic: band
silent: allele; area; electrode; gallstones; gap; ischemia; mutant; mutation; period
silent myocardial: infarction
silhouette: sign of Felson
silica: granuloma
silicate: cement; restoration
silicone: implant
silicotic: granuloma
silo-filler's: disease; lung
silver: cell; cone; point; poisoning; stain
silver-ammoniac silver: stain
silver-fork: deformity; fracture
silverized: catgut
Silverman-Lilly: pneumotachograph
silver protein: stain
Silver-Russell: dwarfism; syndrome
Silverskiöld: syndrome
silver-tin: alloy
Simbu: virus
simian: crease; fissure; hand; malaria; virus; virus 40
simian hemorrhagic: fever
simian vacuolating: virus No. 40
Simmonds: disease
Simmons citrate: medium
Simon: position; sign
Simonart: bands; ligaments; threads
Simons: disease
simple: absence; anchorage; anisocoria; beam; color; conjunctivitis; crus of semicircular duct; diplopia; dislocation; epithelium; fission; fracture; glaucoma; goiter; heterochromia; hypertrophy; joint; lipids; lobule; lymphangiectasis; mastectomy; mastoidectomy; microscope; myopia; necrosis; obesity; phobia; protein; retinitis; schizophrenia; ulcer; urethritis
simple bone: cyst
simple-central: anisocoria
simple endometrial: hyperplasia
simple hyperopic: astigmatism
simple membranous: limb of semicircular duct
simple myopic: astigmatism
simple partial: seizure
simple pulmonary: eosinophilia

Word Finder

simple skull: fracture
simple squamous: epithelium
Simpson: forceps
Simpson uterine: sound
Sims: position
Sims uterine: sound
simulated: hypertrophy
simultaneous:
  communication; contrast;
  perception
sincipital: presentation
Sindbis: fever; virus
Sinding-Larsen-Johansson:
  syndrome
singer's: nodes; nodules
single: ascertainment; bond;
  immunodiffusion; ventricle
single (gel) diffusion
  precipitin: test in one
  dimension; test in two
  dimensions
single photon emission
  computed: tomography
single-strand: break
single-stranded nucleate:
  endonuclease
singlet: oxygen; state
single vial: fixatives
singular: foramen
Sin Nombre: virus
sinoatrial: block; node
sinoatrial conduction: time
sinoatrial recovery: time
sinoauricular: block
sinoventricular: conduction
sinuatrial: chamber; node
sinuatrial nodal: artery;
  branch of right coronary
  artery
sinuatrial node: artery
sinuatrial (S-A) nodal: branch
  of right coronary artery
sinus: arrest; arrhythmia;
  barotrauma; bradycardia;
  histiocytosis with massive
  lymphadenopathy; nerve of
  Hering; node; pause; reflex;
  rhythm; septum; standstill;
  tachycardia; tubercle
sinus node: artery
sinusoidal: capillary
sinus venosus: syndrome
sinuvertebral: nerves
Sipple: syndrome
Sippy: diet
SISI: test
sister chromatid: exchange
Sistrunk: operation
site-directed: mutagenesis
site specific: mutation
site-specific: recombination
in situ: hybridization
situation: anxiety
situational: psychosis; test
in situ nucleic acid:
  hybridization

sitz: bath
sixth: disease; ventricle
sixth cranial: nerve [CN VI]
sixth venereal: disease
sixth-year: molar
Sjögren: disease; syndrome
Sjögren-Larsson: syndrome
Sjöqvist: tractotomy
skein: cell
skeletal: dysplasias; extension;
  muscle; survey; system;
  traction
skeletal muscle: fibers; tissue
skeleton: hand
Skene: glands; tubules
skew: deviation; distribution;
  form
Skillern: fracture
skim: milk
skin: botflies; dose; flap;
  furrows; graft; grooves;
  ligaments; pore; reaction;
  reflexes; ridges; stones;
  sulci; tag; test; traction
skinbound: disease
skin-muscle: reflexes
Skinner: box
skinnerian: conditioning
skin-puncture: test
skin-pupillary: reflex
skip: areas
skipped: generation
Sklowsky: symptom
Skoda: rale; sign; tympany
skodaic: resonance
skull: fracture
skull base: surgery
slab-off: lens
slaked: lime
slant: culture
slaty: anemia
sleep: apnea; deficit;
  dissociation; drunkenness;
  epilepsy; paralysis; spindle
sleep apnea: syndrome
sleep-induced: apnea
sleeping: sickness
sleep phase delay: syndrome
sleep terror: disorder
sleeve: graft
SLE-like: syndrome
slender: fasciculus; lobule;
  process of malleus
slew: rate
slide: micrometer;
  tracheoplasty
sliding: hernia; hook; lock
sliding esophageal hiatal:
  hernia
sliding filament: hypothesis
sliding hiatal: hernia
sliding oblique: osteotomy
slime: fever
sling: psychrometer
slipped: hernia
slipping: patella; rib

slipping rib: cartilage
slit: lamp; pores
slit ventricle: syndrome
slope: culture
slotted: attachment
sloughing: phagedena; ulcer
slow: combustion; fever; virus
slow channel-blocking: agent
slow component of:
  nystagmus
slow-reacting: factor of
  anaphylaxis; substance
slow virus: disease
SLR: factor
Sluder: neuralgia
sludged: blood
sluggish: layer
slurring: speech
Sly: syndrome
Sm: antigen
small: arteries; bowel; calorie;
  canal of chorda tympani;
  cell; intestine; pancreas;
  pelvis; trochanter; vein
small bowel: enema; series
small cardiac: vein
small cell: carcinoma
small cleaved: cell
small deep petrosal: nerve
smaller: muscle of helix
smaller pectoral: muscle
smaller posterior rectus:
  muscle of head
smaller psoas: muscle
smallest cardiac: veins
smallest scalene: muscle
smallest splanchnic: nerve
small increment sensitivity:
  index
small increment sensitivity
  index: test
small interarch: distance
small lymphocytic: lymphoma
small nuclear: RNA
small plaque: parapsoriasis
smallpox: vaccine; virus
small pudendal: lip
small saphenous: vein
small sciatic: nerve
smear: culture
Smellie: scissors
smelling: salts
smelter's: chills; fever; shakes
Smith: fracture; operation
Smith-Boyce: operation
Smith-Indian: operation
Smith-Lemli-Opitz: syndrome
Smith-Petersen: nail
Smith-Riley: syndrome
Smith-Robinson: operation
smoker's: patches; tongue
smooth: broach; chorion;
  colony; diet; leprosy; muscle
smooth muscle: relaxant;
  tissue
smooth muscular: sphincter

smooth surface: caries
smooth-surfaced
  endoplasmic: reticulum
smudge: cells
S-N: line
S-N-A: angle
snail: fever
snail track: degeneration
snap: finger
snapping: hip; reflex
S-N-B: angle
Sneddon: syndrome
Sneddon-Wilkinson: disease
sneezing: gas
Snell: law
Snellen: sign; test types
sniff: test
snout: reflex
snow: blindness; conjunctivitis
snowball: opacity; sampling
snowman: abnormality
snowshoe hare: virus
snub-nose: dwarfism
S1 nuclease: mapping
Snyder: test
soapsuds: enema
Soave: operation
social: adaptation; control;
  diseases; instinct;
  intelligence; maladjustment;
  medicine; phobia;
  psychiatry; therapy
socialized: medicine
social network: therapy
sociometric: distance
socket: joint
soda: loading
sodium: chromate Cr 51;
  iodide iodine-131;
  methylprednisolone
  succinate; pump
sodium-potassium: pump
sodium-responsive periodic:
  paralysis
Soemmerring: ganglion;
  ligament; muscle; spot
soft: cataract; chancre; corn;
  diet; drusen; palate;
  papilloma; parts; pulse; rays;
  soap; sore; sulfur; tubercle;
  ulcer; wart; water
soft tissue: window
Sohval-Soffer: syndrome
solar: blindness; cheilitis;
  comedo; dermatitis;
  elastosis; energy; fever;
  ganglia; keratosis; lentigo;
  maculopathy; plexus;
  retinopathy; therapy;
  treatment; urticaria
soldier's: patches
sole: nuclei; reflex
soleal: line; part of posterior
  (plantar flexor) compartment
  of leg
sole-plate: ending

sole tap: reflex
soleus: muscle
solid: edema
solid phase: immunoassay
solid-state: detector
solitariospinal: tract
solitary: bundle; fasciculus;
  follicles; glands; nodules of
  intestine; tract
solitary bone: cyst
solitary fibrous: tumor
solitary lymphatic: follicles;
  nodules
solitary osteocartilaginous:
  exostosis
solubility: test
soluble: antigen; ferric
  phosphate; glass; ligature;
  RNA; soap; starch; tartar
soluble gun: cotton
soluble specific: substance
solution: pressure
solvent: drag; ether; inhalation
somatic: agglutinin; antigen;
  arteries; cells; crossing-over;
  death; delusion; layer;
  mesoderm; mitosis;
  mutation; nerve; nucleus;
  reproduction; swallow;
  teniasis
somatic cell: genetics;
  hybridization
somatic motor: neuron; nuclei
somatic mutation: theory of
  cancer
somatic nerve: fibers
somatic sensory: cortex
somatization: disorder
somatoform: disorder; pain
somatosensory: aura
somatosensory evoked:
  potential
somatotropic: hormone
somatotropin release-
  inhibiting: factor; hormone
somatotropin-releasing:
  factor; hormone
somesthetic: area; system
somite: cavity
somitic: mesoderm
somnambulic: epilepsy
somnambulistic: trance
Somogyi: effect; method;
  phenomenon; unit
Sondermann: canal
Songo: fever
sonic: waves
sonomotor: response
sonorous: rale
soot: wart
sorbitol: pathway
sore: mouth; throat
soremouth: virus
Sörensen: scale
Soret: band; phenomenon
Sorsby: syndrome

Sorsby macular: degeneration
SOS: genes; repair
Sotos: syndrome
sound: abatement; field
soundex: code
sound pressure: level
South African tick-bite: fever
South African type: porphyria
South American:
  blastomycosis;
  trypanosomiasis
Southern blot: analysis
Southey: tubes
space: maintainer; medicine;
  myopia; retainer; sense;
  sickness
space adaptation: syndrome
spaced: teeth
spade: fingers; hand
Spallanzani: law
spallation: product
Spanish: influenza
sparing: action; phenomenon
spasmodic: asthma;
  dysmenorrhea; dysphonia;
  laryngitis; stricture; tic;
  torticollis
spasmophilic: diathesis
spastic: anemia; aphonia;
  colon; diplegia; dysarthria;
  dysphonia; ectropion;
  entropion; gait; hemiplegia;
  ileus; miosis; mydriasis;
  paraplegia; speech
spastic flat: foot
spastic spinal: paralysis
spatial: acuity; formula;
  localization; vector;
  vectorcardiography
spatula: needle
speaking: tube
special: anatomy; hospital;
  nurse; sense
specialized: transduction
special somatic afferent:
  column
special visceral efferent:
  column; nuclei
special visceral motor: nuclei
species: tolerance
species-specific: antigen
specific: absorbance; action;
  activity; anergy; antigens;
  antiserum; bactericide;
  cause; cholinesterase;
  compliance; disease; epithet;
  extinction; granules; gravity;
  heat; hemolysin; immunity;
  opsonin; parasite; phobia;
  reaction; serum; therapy;
  transduction; urethritis
specific absorption:
  coefficient
specific active: immunity
specific building-related:
  illnesses

specific capsular: substance
specific dynamic: action
specific immune: globulin
  (human)
specificity: constant
specific optic: rotation
specific passive: immunity
specific soluble:
  polysaccharide; sugar
speck: finger
spectacle: plane
spectral: phonocardiograph;
  sensitivity
specular: glare; image
speculum: forceps
speech: audiogram;
  audiometer; bulb; centers;
  pathology; processor;
  reading
speech awareness: threshold
speech detection: threshold
speech-language: pathologist;
  pathology
speech reception: threshold
Spens: syndrome
sperm: aster; cell; crystal;
  nucleus
spermacytic: seminoma
spermatic: cord; duct;
  filament; fistula; plexus;
  vein
sphagnum: moss
sphenoethmoidal: recess;
  suture; synchondrosis
sphenofrontal: suture
sphenoid: angle; part of
  middle cerebral artery;
  process; process of septal
  nasal cartilage
sphenoid: bone
sphenoidal: angle of parietal
  bone; border of temporal
  bone; conchae; crest; fissure;
  fontanelle; herniation;
  lingula; margin of temporal
  bone; process of palatine
  bone; ridges; rostrum; sinus;
  spine; yoke
sphenoidal emissary: foramen
sphenoidal sinus: aperture
sphenoidal turbinated: bones
sphenomandibular: ligament
sphenomaxillary: fissure;
  fossa; suture
sphenooccipital: joint; suture;
  synchondrosis
spheno-orbital: suture
sphenopalatine: artery;
  foramen; ganglion;
  neuralgia; notch
sphenoparietal: sinus; suture
sphenopetrosal: fissure;
  synchondrosis
sphenosquamous: suture
sphenotic: center; foramen
sphenovomerine: suture

sphenozygomatic: suture
spherical: aberration;
  amalgam; lens; nucleus;
  recess of bony labyrinth
spherical form of: occlusion
spherocylindrical: lens
spherocytic: anemia; jaundice
spheroid: articulation; colony
spheroidal: degeneration; joint
sphincter: muscle; muscle of
  pancreatic duct; muscle of
  pupil; muscle of pylorus;
  muscle of urethra; muscle of
  urinary bladder
sphincter of Oddi:
  dysfunction
sphincteroid: tract of ileum
sphingomyelin: lipidosis
sphygmic: interval
spica: bandage; cast
spider: angioma; cancer; cell;
  finger; hemangioma; mole;
  nevus; pelvis; telangiectasia
Spiegelberg: criteria
Spiegler-Fendt: sarcoid
Spielmeyer acute: swelling
Spielmeyer-Sjögren: disease
Spielmeyer-Stock: disease
Spielmeyer-Vogt: disease
spigelian: hernia
Spigelius: line; lobe
spike: potential
spike and wave: complex
spin: density; echo
spinach: stools
spinal: analgesia; anesthesia;
  anesthetic; apoplexy;
  arachnoid mater; arteries;
  ataxia; block; branches;
  canal; column; concussion;
  cord; curvature;
  decompression; dura mater;
  dysraphism; fusion;
  ganglion; headache;
  induction; instability; lamina
  II; lemniscus; length;
  marrow; muscle; muscle of
  head; muscle of neck;
  muscle of thorax; nerves;
  nucleus of trigeminal nerve;
  nucleus of the trigeminus;
  paralysis; part of accessory
  nerve; part of arachnoid;
  part of deltoid (muscle); part
  of filum terminale; point;
  puncture; pyramidotomy;
  quotient; reflex; root of
  accessory nerve; shock;
  sign; stroke; tap; tract;
  tractotomy; tract of
  trigeminal nerve; veins
spinal accessory: nerve
spinal arachnoid: mater
spinal cord: concussion
spinalis: muscle
spinalis capitis: muscle

Word Finder

spinalis cervicis: muscle
spinalis thoracis: muscle
spinal muscular: atrophy; atrophy, type I; atrophy, type II; atrophy, type III
spinal nerve: plexus
spinal pia: mater
spinal trigeminal: nucleus
spindle: cataract; cell; fiber
spindle cell: carcinoma; lipoma; nevus; sarcoma
spindle-celled: layer
spindle-shaped: muscle
spine: cell; sign
Spinelli: operation
spin-lattice: relaxation
spinning disk: nebulizer
spinoadductor: reflex
spinocerebellar: ataxia; tracts
spinocervical: tract
spinocervicothalamic: tract
spinocuneate: fibers
spinoglenoid: ligament
spinogracile: fibers
spinohypothalamic: fibers
spinomesencephalic: fibers
spinoolivary: fibers; tract; tract
spinoperiaqueductal: fibers
spinoreticular: fibers; tract
spinotectal: fibers; tract
spinothalamic: cordotomy; tract; tractotomy
spinous: layer; process of sphenoid; process of tibia; process of vertebra
spinovestibular: tract
spin-spin: relaxation
spiral: artery; bandage; canal of cochlea; canal of modiolus; crest; crest of cochlear duct; CT; fold of cystic duct; fracture; ganglion of cochlea; groove; hyphae; joint; ligament of cochlea; ligament of cochlear duct; line; membrane; organ; plate; prominence of cochlear duct; septum; suture; tubule; valve of cystic duct; vein of modiolus
spiral bulbar: septum
spiral cochlear: ganglion
spiral computed: tomography
spiral foraminous: tract
spiral modiolar: artery
spiral tip: catheter
spirillum: fever
spirit: lamp; thermometer
spirituous: liquor
spiro-: index
spirochetal: jaundice
spironolactone: test
spiruroid: larva migrans
Spitz: nevus

Spitzer: theory
Spitzka: nucleus
Spitzka marginal: tract; zone
Spix: spine
splanchnesthetic: sensibility
splanchnic: anesthesia; cavity; layer; mesoderm; nerve; wall
spleen: deoxyribonuclease; endonuclease; phosphodiesterases
Splendore-Hoeppli: phenomenon
splenial: gyrus
splenic: anemia; artery; branches of splenic artery; cells; cords; corpuscles; flexure; hilum; index; leukemia; lymph nodes; pulp; recess; sinus; trabeculae; vein
splenic flexure: syndrome
splenic lymph: follicles; nodules
splenic (nervous): plexus
splenic portal: venography
splenius: muscle of head; muscle of neck; muscles
splenius capitis: muscle
splenius cervicis: muscle
splenogonadal: fusion
splenorenal: ligament
splinted: abutment
splinter: hemorrhages
splintered: fracture
split: brain; fat; genes; hand; papules; pelvis; tolerance
split cast: method; mounting
split renal function: test
split-skin: graft
split-thickness: graft
splitting: enzymes
splitting of heart: sounds
split-virus: vaccine
Spondweni: virus
spondyloepiphyseal: dysplasia; dysplasia congenita; dysplasia tarda
spondylolisthetic: pelvis
sponge: biopsy; tent
spongiform: encephalopathy; pustule of Kogoj
spongy: body of penis; bone; degeneration of infancy; layer of female urethra; layer of vagina; part of the male urethra; spot; substance; urethra
spontaneous: abortion; agglutination; amputation; combustion; correction of placenta previa; evolution; fracture; gangrene of newborn; generation; mutation; phagocytosis;

pneumothorax; recovery; remission; version
spontaneous breech: extraction
spontaneous cephalic: delivery
spontaneous membrane: rupture
spoon: nail
sporotrichositic: chancre
sports: medicine
spot: film; map; test for infectious mononucleosis
spot-film: radiography
spotted: fever; sickness
spouse: abuse
sprain: fracture
spreading: depression; factor
Sprengel: deformity
spring: conjunctivitis; finger; lancet; ligament; ophthalmia
spun glass: hair
spur: cell
spur cell: anemia
spurious: ankylosis; cast; meningocele; parasite; pregnancy; torticollis
Spurling: test
sputum: smear
squamocolumnar: junction
squamomastoid: suture
squamoparietal: suture
squamosal: border; border of parietal bone; margin; margin of greater wing of sphenoid
squamotympanic: fissure
squamous: border; border of parietal bone; border of sphenoid bone; cell; margin; metaplasia; metaplasia of amnion; part of frontal bone; part of occipital bone; part of temporal bone; pearl; suture
squamous alveolar: cells
squamous cell: carcinoma; hyperplasia
squamous odontogenic: tumor
square: knot; matrix
square wave: stimuli
squint: hook
squinting: eye
squirrel plague: conjunctivitis
ST: junction; segment
stab: cell; culture; drain; neutrophil; wound
stabilized: baseplate
stabilizing circumferential clasp: arm
stabilizing fulcrum: line
stable: colloid; disease; equilibrium; factor; fracture; isotope
staccato: speech

Stader: splint
Staderini: nucleus
staff: cell
Stafne bone: cyst
staggered spondaic word: test
staghorn: calculus
stagnant: anoxia; hypoxia
stagnation: mastitis
Stahl: ear
staircase: phenomenon
stalked: hydatid
standard: atmosphere; bicarbonate; cell; deviation; pressure; score; solution; substance; temperature; volume
standard error of the: mean
standard error of: difference
standardized mortality: ratio
standard limb: lead
standard serologic: tests for syphilis
standard urea: clearance
standby pulse: generator
standing: test
standing plasma: test
Stanford-Binet intelligence: scale
Stanley cervical: ligaments
Stanley Way: procedure
Stannius: ligature
stapedial: artery; branch of posterior tympanic artery; branch of stylomastoid artery; fold; membrane; reflex
stapedius: muscle
stapes: mobilization
stapes mobilization: operation
staphylococcal: blepharitis; enterotoxin; pneumonia
staphylococcal scalded skin: syndrome
staphylococcus: antitoxin; vaccine
Staphylococcus **food:** poisoning
staphyloopsonic: index
starch: equivalent; glycerite; gum; sugar
starch-iodine: test
Stargardt: disease
Starling: curve; hypothesis; law; reflex
Starr-Edwards: valve
start: codon
starter: tRNA
starting: friction
startle: disease; epilepsy; reaction; reflex
starvation: acidosis; diabetes
stasis: cirrhosis; dermatitis; eczema; ulcer
Stas-Otto: method
state: hospital
state-dependent: learning

static: arthropathy; ataxia; compliance; friction; gangrene; hysteresis; infantilism; perimetry; reflexes; refraction; relation; scoliosis; sense; system; tremor
static bone: cyst
station: test
stationary: anchorage; cataract; phase
statistical: genetics; model; power
statoacoustic: nerve
statoconial: membrane
statokinetic: reflex
statotonic: reflexes
Staub-Traugott: effect; phenomenon
Stauffer: syndrome
steady: state
steady-state: rate; velocity
steady state: approximation
steal: phenomenon
steam-fitter's: asthma
Steele-Richardson-Olszewski: disease; syndrome
Steell: murmur
Steenbock: unit
steeple: skull
steering wheel: injury
Stein: test
Steinberg thumb: sign
Steinert: disease
Stein-Leventhal: syndrome
Steinmann: pin
stellate: abscess; block; cataract; cells of cerebral cortex; cells of liver; fracture; ganglion; hair; ligament; neuroretinitis; reticulum; veins; venules
stellate skull: fracture
Stellwag: sign
stem: bronchus; cell
stem cell: factor; leukemia
Stender: dish
Stenger: test
stenopeic: disk; iridectomy; spectacles
stenosal: murmur
stenosing: tenosynovitis
stenoxous: parasite
Stensen: duct; foramen; plexus; veins
Stent: graft
Stenvers: projection; view
steppage: gait
stercoraceous: vomiting
stercoral: abscess; appendicitis; ulcer
sterculia: gum
stereochemical: formula; isomerism
stereoscopic: acuity; microscope; parallax; vision

stereotactic: brachytherapy; cordotomy; instrument; surgery
stereotaxic: localization; surgery
sterile: abscess; cyst
sterile insect: technique
Stern: posture
sternal: angle; arteries; bar; branches of internal thoracic artery; cartilage; end of clavicle; extremity of clavicle; facet of clavicle; joints; line; line of pleural reflection; membrane; muscle; notch; part of diaphragm; plane; puncture; synchondroses
sternal articular: surface of clavicle
sternalis: muscle
Sternberg: cell; sign
Sternberg-Reed: cell
sternobrachial: reflex
sternochondral: separation
sternochondroscapular: muscle
sternoclavicular: angle; disk; joint; ligaments; muscle
sternocleidomastoid: branches of occipital artery; branch of superior thyroid artery; muscle; region; vein
sternocostal: articulations; head of pectoralis major (muscle); joints; part of pectoralis major muscle; surface of heart; triangle; triangle (of diaphragm)
sternocostalis: muscle
sternohyoid: muscle
sternomanubrial: junction
sternomastoid: artery; muscle
sternopericardial: ligaments
sternothyroid: muscle
steroid: acne; diabetes; fever; hormones; nucleus; ulcer
steroid cell: tumor
steroid metabolic clearance: rate
steroidogenic: diabetes
steroid production: rate
steroid secretory: rate
steroid withdrawal: syndrome
stertorous: breathing; respiration
stethoscopic: phonocardiograph
Stevens-Johnson: syndrome
Stewart: test
Stewart-Hamilton: method
Stewart-Holmes: sign
Stewart-Morel: syndrome
Stewart-Treves: syndrome
stichochrome: cell
Sticker: disease

Stickler: syndrome
sticky-ended: DNA
Stieda: process
Stierlin: sign
stiff: neck; toe
stiff heart: syndrome
stiff man: syndrome
stigmal: plates
Stiles-Crawford: effect
Still: disease; murmur
still: layer
stillbirth: rate
stillborn: infant
Still-Chauffard: syndrome
Stilling: canal; column; nucleus; raphe
Stilling gelatinous: substance
stimulatory: protein 1
stimulus: control; generalization; substitution; threshold
stimulus sensitive: myoclonus
stinging: caterpillar
stippled: epiphysis; tongue
Stirling modification of Gram: stain
stitch: abscess
St. John's: wort
St. Louis encephalitis: virus
Stobo: antigen
stochastic: independence; process
stock: culture; strain; vaccine
Stocker: line
Stockholm: syndrome
stocking: anesthesia
Stoffel: operation
stoichiometric: number
stoker's: cramps
Stokes: amputation; basket; law
Stokes-Adams: disease; syndrome
stomach: ache; drops; pump; reefing; tooth; tube
stomal: ulcer
stomatognathic: system
stone: basket; heart
stone-mason's: disease
Stookey-Scarff: operation
stop: codon
stop-: needle; speculum
stopping: rules
storage: disease; oscilloscope
storiform: neurofibroma
Stout: wiring
stove-pipe: colon
strabismic: amblyopia
straddling: embolism
straight: arteries; conjugate; gyrus; muscle; part of cricothyroid muscle; sinus; tubule; tubule of testis; venules of kidney
straight back: syndrome
straight seminiferous: tubule

strain: fracture; gauge
strangulated: hernia
strap: cell; muscles
Strassburg: test
Strassman: phenomenon
stratified: epithelium; sample; thrombus
stratified ciliated columnar: epithelium
stratified squamous: epithelium
stratiform: fibrocartilage
Straus: reaction; sign
straw: itch
strawberry: birthmark; cervix; gallbladder; hemangioma; mark; nevus; tongue
streak: culture; gonad; hyperostosis
streaming: movement
street: drug; virus
Streeter: bands
strength-duration: curve
streptococcal: empyema; fibrinolysin; pneumonia
streptococcal toxic shock: syndrome
streptococcus erythrogenic: toxin
Streptococcus M: antigen
streptomycin: units
stress: echocardiography; fibers; fracture; immunity; inoculation; reaction; test; ulcer
stress-bearing: area
stress-broken: connector; joint
stress-strain: curve
stress urinary: incontinence
stretch: marks; receptors; reflex
striate: area; atrophy of skin; body; cortex; keratopathy; veins
striated: border; duct; membrane; muscle
striated muscular: sphincter
striatonigral: fibers
string: sign; test
stringed instrument: theory
stringent: factor; response
strionigral: fibers
stripped: atom
stripper's: asthma
stroboscopic: disk; microscope
Stroganoff: method
stroke: output; volume
stroke work: index
stroma: plexus
stromal: hyperthecosis
stromal corneal: dystrophy
strong: silver protein
Strong vocational interest: test

Word Finder

structural: color; formula; gene; interface; isomerism; pleiotropy

structure: proteins

structured: abstract; noise

Strümpell: disease; phenomenon; reflex

Strümpell-Marie: disease

struvite: calculus

Stryker: frame; saw

Stryker-Halbeisen: syndrome

Stuart: factor

stuck: finger

student: nurse

Student's *t*: test

stump: cancer; hallucination; neuralgia

stunned: myocardium

stuporous: catatonia

Sturge-Kalischer-Weber: syndrome

Sturge-Weber: disease; syndrome

Sturm: conoid; interval

Sturmdorf: operation

stuttering: urination

styloauricular: muscle

styloglossus: muscle

stylohyoid: branch of facial nerve; ligament; muscle

styloid: cornu; process of fibula; process of radius; process of temporal bone; process of third metacarpal bone; process of ulna; prominence

stylomandibular: ligament

stylomastoid: artery; foramen; vein

stylomaxillary: ligament

stylopharyngeal: branch of glossopharyngeal nerve; muscle

stylopharyngeus: muscle

styloradial: reflex

stylus: tracing

"s"-type: cholinesterase

styptic: collodion; colloid; cotton

Stypven time: test

subacromial: bursa; bursitis

subacute: glomerulonephritis; hepatitis; inflammation; nephritis; rheumatism

subacute bacterial: endocarditis

subacute combined: degeneration of the spinal cord

subacute granulomatous: thyroiditis

subacute inclusion body: encephalitis

subacute lymphocyte: thyroiditis

subacute migratory: panniculitis

subacute necrotizing: encephalomyelopathy; myelitis

subacute sclerosing: leukoencephalitis; panencephalitis

subacute spongiform: encephalopathy

subadventitial: fibrosis

subanconeus: muscle

subaortic: lymph nodes; stenosis

subapical: segment

subarachnoid: anesthesia; cavity; cisterns; hemorrhage; space

subarcuate: fossa

subareolar duct: papillomatosis

subastragalar: amputation

subcaeruleus: nucleus

subcallosal: area; fasciculus; gyrus

subcapital: fracture

subcapsular: cataract

subcecal: fossa

subchorial: lake; space

subclavian: artery; duct; groove; loop; muscle; nerve; plexus; steal; sulcus; triangle; vein

subclavian lymphatic: trunk

subclavian steal: syndrome

subclavius: muscle

subclinical: coccidioidomycosis; diabetes; seizure

subcommissural: organ

subconscious: memory; mind

subcoracoid: bursa

subcoracoid-pectoralis minor tendon: syndrome

subcorneal pustular: dermatitis; dermatosis

subcoronal: hypospadias

subcortical arteriosclerotic: encephalopathy

subcostal: angle; arch; artery; groove; line; muscle; nerve; plane

subcrepitant: rale

subcrestal: pocket

subcrural: muscle

subcuneiform: nucleus

subcutaneous: bursa of the laryngeal prominence; bursa of lateral malleolus; bursa of medial malleolus; bursa of teres major; bursa of tibial tuberosity; bursa of tuberosity of tibia; emphysema; flap; implantation; mastectomy; myiasis; operation; part of

external anal sphincter; phycomycosis; portion of external anal sphincter; ring; tenotomy; tissue; tissue of penis; tissue of perineum; transfusion; veins of abdomen; wound

subcutaneous acromial: bursa

subcutaneous calcaneal: bursa

subcutaneous fat: necrosis of newborn

subcutaneous infrapatellar: bursa

subcutaneous olecranon: bursa

subcutaneous prepatellar: bursa

subcuticular: suture

subdeltoid: bursa; bursitis

subdiaphragmatic: abscess; pyopneumothorax

subdigastric: node

subdural: cavity; cleavage; cleft; hematoma; hematorrhachis; hemorrhage; hygroma; space

subendocardial: branches of atrioventricular bundles; layer

subendocardial conducting: system of heart

subendocardial myocardial: infarction

subendothelial: layer

subependymal giant cell: astrocytoma

subepidermal: abscess

subfalcial: herniation

subfascial prepatellar: bursa

subfornical: organ

subgaleal: emphysema; hemorrhage

subgerminal: cavity

subgingival: calculus; curettage; space

subhepatic: abscess; recess; space

subhyoid: bursa

subhypoglossal: nucleus

subinguinal: fossa; triangle

subjective: fremitus; insomnia; probability; psychology; sign; symptom; synonyms; vision

sublenticular: limb of internal capsule; part of internal capsule

sublentiform: limb of internal capsule

subleukemic: leukemia

sublimed: sulfur

subliminal: self; stimulus; thirst

sublingual: artery; bursa; caruncula; crescent; cyst;

fold; fossa; ganglion; gland; medication; nerve; pit; tablet; vein

submammary: mastitis

submandibular: duct; fossa; ganglion; gland; lymph nodes; triangle

submaxillary: duct; fossa; ganglion; gland; triangle

submental: artery; lymph nodes; triangle; vein

submental vertex: projection; radiograph

submentovertex: radiograph

submentovertical: projection

submerged: tonsil

submetacentric: chromosome

submitochondrial: particles

submucosal: implant

submucosal (nervous): plexus

submucous laryngeal: cleft

subnasal: point

subneural: apparatus

suboccipital: decompression; muscles; nerve; neuralgia; neuritis; part of vertebral artery; region; triangle

suboccipital venous: plexus

suboccipitobregmatic: diameter

suboccluding: ligature

subocclusal: surface

subpapillary: layer; network

subparabrachial: nucleus [TA]

subparietal: sulcus

subpellicular: fibril; microtubule

subperiodic: periodicity

subperiosteal: abscess; amputation; fracture; implant

subperitoneal: appendicitis; fascia

subphrenic: abscess; recesses; space

subplasmalemmal dense: zone

subpopliteal: recess

subpubic: angle

subpulmonic: effusion

subpyloric: lymph nodes; node

subquadricipital: muscle

subsartorial: canal; fascia

subscapular: artery; branches of axillary artery; bursa; fossa; muscle; nerves

subscapular axillary: lymph nodes

subscapularis: muscle

subsegmental: atelectasis

subseptate: uterus

subserous: layer

subserous (nervous): plexus

subsidiary atrial: pacemaker

subsistence: diet
substance: abuse; dependence
substance abuse: disorders
substance dependence: disorder
substance-induced organic mental: disorders
substernal: angle; goiter
substituted: amide
substitution: product; therapy; transfusion
substitutive: therapy
substrate: cycle; inhibition; specificity
substrate-level: phosphorylation
subsuperior: segment
subsurface: cisterna
subtalar: joint
subtemporal: decompression
subtendinous: bursae of gastrocnemius (muscle); bursa of iliacus; bursa of infraspinatus; bursa of latissimus dorsi; bursa of sartorius; bursa of subscapularis; bursa of tibialis anterior; bursa of trapezius; bursa of triceps brachii
subtendinous iliac: bursa
subtendinous prepatellar: bursa
subthalamic: fasciculus; nucleus
subthreshold: stimulus
subtotal: hysterectomy; thyroidectomy
subungual: abscess; exostosis; melanoma
subunit: vaccine
subvalvar: stenosis
subvalvular aortic: stenosis
subvocal: speech
succedaneous: dentition; tooth
succenturiate: placenta
successional: lamina
successive: contrast
succinic acid: cycle
succussion: sound
sucking: blister; cushion; louse; pad
sucking chest: wound
suckling: reflex
Sucquet: anastomoses; canals
Sucquet-Hoyer: anastomoses; canals
sucrose hemolysis: test
suction: cup; curettage; drainage; ophthalmodynamometer; plate
Sudan: virus
sudanophobic: zone
sudden: deafness; death

sudden infant death: syndrome
Sudeck: atrophy; syndrome
Sudeck critical: point
sudomotor: fibers; nerves
sudoriferous: abscess; cyst; duct; glands
sufficient: cause
suffocating: gas
suffocative: goiter
sugar: alcohol; cataract; ester; tumor
sugar-coated: spleen
suggestive: psychotherapy; therapeutics
Sugiura: procedure
suicide: gesture; inhibitor; substrate
suid: herpesvirus
sulcal: artery
sulcomarginal: tract
sulcular: epithelium; fluid
sulcus: test
sulfate: respiration; water
sulfatide: lipidosis
sulfhydryl: reagent
sulfonium: ion
sulfosalicylic acid turbidity: test
sulfur: autotrophy; mustard; water
sulfurated: lime; potash
sulfureted: hydrogen
Sulkowitch: reagent
Sulzberger-Garbe: disease; syndrome
summating: potentials
summation: beat; gallop
summer: asthma; diarrhea; itch; prurigo; rash
Sumner: sign
sump: drain; syndrome
sun: stroke
sunflower: cataract
sun protection: factor
superciliary: arch; ridge
superconducting: magnet
superfatted: soap
superficial: angioma; branch; branch of the lateral plantar nerve; branch of medial circumflex femoral artery; branch of the medial plantar artery; branch of the radial nerve; branch of the superior gluteal artery; branch of the transverse cervical artery; branch of the ulnar nerve; burn; cleavage; ectoderm; fascia; fascia of penis; fascia of perineum; fascia of scrotum; head of flexor pollicis brevis; implantation; lamina; layer; layer of deep cervical fascia; layer of the levator palpebrae superioris;

layer of temporal fascia; part of anterior (flexor) compartment of forearm; part of external anal sphincter; part of masseter muscle; part of parotid gland; part of posterior (plantar flexor) compartment of leg; reflex; vein
superficial back: muscles
superficial brachial: artery
superficial cardiac (nervous): plexus
superficial cerebral: veins
superficial cervical: artery; nerve
superficial circumflex iliac: artery; vein
(superficial and deep) external pudendal: arteries
superficial dorsal: veins of clitoris; veins of penis
superficial dorsal sacrococcygeal: ligament
superficial epigastric: artery; vein
superficial fibular: nerve
superficial flexor: muscle of fingers
superficial gray: layer [TA] of superior colliculus
superficial inguinal: lymph nodes; pouch; ring
superficial investing: fascia of perineum
superficial lateral cervical: lymph nodes
superficial linear: keratitis
superficial lingual: muscle
superficial lymph: vessel
superficial middle cerebral: vein
superficial palmar: artery; branch of radial artery
superficial palmar (arterial): arch
superficial palmar venous: arch
superficial parotid: lymph nodes
superficial perineal: pouch; space
superficial peroneal: nerve
superficial posterior sacrococcygeal: ligament
superficial punctate: keratitis
superficial pustular: perifolliculitis
superficial spreading: melanoma
superficial temporal: artery; branch of auriculotemporal nerve; plexus; veins
superficial transverse: muscle of perineum

superficial transverse metacarpal: ligament
superficial transverse metatarsal: ligament
superficial transverse perineal: muscle
superficial volar: artery
superimposed: eclampsia; preeclampsia
superior: angle of scapula; aspect; belly of omohyoid muscle; border; border of body of pancreas; border of pancreas; border of petrous part of temporal bone; border of scapula; border of spleen; border of suprarenal gland; branch; branch of the oculomotor nerve; branch of the pubic bone; branch of the right and left inferior pulmonary veins; branch of the superior gluteal artery; branch of the transverse cervical nerve; bursa of biceps femoris; cistern; colliculus; extremity; extremity of kidney; eyelid; facet of trochlear of talus; fascia of pelvic diaphragm; fovea; ganglion of glossopharyngeal nerve; ganglion of vagus nerve; horn of falciform margin of saphenous opening; horn of thyroid cartilage; laryngotomy; ligament of epididymis; ligament of incus; ligament of malleus; limb; limb of ansa cervicalis; lobe of (right/left) lung; margin of cerebral hemisphere; mediastinum; member; olive; paraplegia; part of diaphragmatic surface of liver; part of duodenum; part of lingual vein (of left superior pulmonary vein); part of vestibular ganglion; part of vestibulocochlear nerve; pole; pole of kidney; pole of testis; polioencephalitis; recess of lesser peritoneal sac; recess of omental bursa; recess of tympanic membrane; retinaculum of extensor muscles; root of ansa cervicalis; segment; surface of cerebellar hemisphere; surface of talus; tarsus; trunk of brachial plexus; veins of cerebellar hemisphere; vein of vermis; vena cava; wall of orbit
superior aberrant: ductule

superior alveolar: nerves
superior anastomotic: vein
superior articular: facet of atlas; pit of atlas; process; process of sacrum; surface of atlas; surface of tibia
superior auricular: muscle
superior azygoesophageal: recess
superior basal: vein
superior carotid: triangle
superior central tegmental: nucleus
superior cerebellar: artery; peduncle
superior cerebellar artery: syndrome
superior cerebral: veins
superior cervical: ganglion
superior cervical cardiac: branches of vagus nerve; nerve
superior choroid: vein
superior clunial: nerves
superior costal: facet; pit
superior costotransverse: ligament
superior dental: arch; branches of superior dental plexus; nerves; rami
superior dental (nervous): plexus
superior duodenal: flexure; fold; fossa; recess
superior epigastric: artery; veins
superior esophageal: sphincter
superior extensor: retinaculum
superior fibular: retinaculum
superior frontal: convolution; gyrus; sulcus
superior gastric: lymph nodes
superior gemellus: muscle
superior gingival: branches of superior dental plexus
superior gluteal: artery; nerve; veins
superior hemorrhagic: polioencephalitis
superior hemorrhoidal: artery; plexus; vein
superior hypogastric (nervous): plexus
superior hypophysial: artery
superior ileocecal: recess
superior intercostal: artery; vein
superior internal parietal: artery
superiority: complex
superior labial: artery; branches of infraorbital nerve; branch of facial artery; vein

superior laryngeal: artery; cavity; nerve; vein
superior lateral brachial cutaneous: nerve
superior lateral genicular: artery
superior limbic: keratoconjunctivitis
superior lingular: artery; branch of lingular branch of superior lobar left pulmonary artery
superior lingular bronchopulmonary: segment S IV
superior lobar: arteries
superior longitudinal: fasciculus; muscle of tongue; sinus; sulcus
superior macular: arteriole; venule
superior maxillary: nerve
superior medial genicular: artery
superior medullary: velum
superior mesenteric: artery; ganglion; lymph nodes; vein
superior mesenteric artery: syndrome
superior mesenteric (nervous): plexus
superior nasal: concha; venule of retina
superior nasal retinal: arteriole; venule
superior nuchal: line
superior oblique: muscle; muscle of head
superior occipital: gyrus; sulcus
superior occipitofrontal: fasciculus
superior olivary: complex; nucleus
superior omental: recess
superior ophthalmic: vein
superior orbital: fissure
superior palpebral: veins
superior palpebral (arterial): arch
superior parietal: gyrus; lobule
superior pelvic: aperture
superior peroneal: retinaculum
superior petrosal: sinus; sulcus
superior pharyngeal constrictor: muscle
superior phrenic: artery; lymph nodes; veins
superior posterior serratus: muscle
superior pubic: ligament; ramus

superior pulmonary sulcus: tumor
superior quadrigeminal: brachium
superior radioulnar: joint
superior rectal: artery; lymph nodes; vein
superior rectal (nervous): plexus
superior rectus: muscle
superior renal: segment
superior sagittal: sinus
superior salivary: nucleus
superior salivatory: nucleus
superior segmental: artery; artery of kidney
superior semilunar: lobule
superior suprarenal: arteries
superior tarsal: muscle
superior temporal: convolution; fissure; gyrus; line of parietal bone; sulcus; venule of retina
superior temporal retinal: arteriole; venule
superior thalamostriate: vein
superior thoracic: aperture; artery
superior thyroid: artery; notch; plexus; tubercle; vein
superior tibial: articulation
superior tibiofibular: joint
superior tracheobronchial: lymph nodes
superior transverse scapular: ligament
superior triangle: sign
superior turbinated: bone
superior tympanic: artery
superior ulnar collateral: artery
superior vena cava: syndrome
superior vermian: branch (of superior cerebellar artery)
superior vesical: artery
superior vestibular: area; nucleus
supernatant: fluid
supernormal: conduction
supernormal recovery: phase
supernumerary: breast; kidney; mamma; organs; placenta
superolateral: face of cerebral hemisphere; surface of cerebrum
superolateral cerebral: surface
superomedial: margin
supersaturated: solution
supersonic: rays; waves
supertraction: conus
supination: reflex
supinator: crest (of ulna); jerk; muscle; reflex
supine: position

supine hypotensive: syndrome
supplemental: air; groove; lobe; ridge
supplementary: menstruation
supplementary motor: cortex
supplementary motor area: epilepsy
support: medium
supporting: area; cell; reactions; reflexes
supportive: psychotherapy
suppressed: menstruation
suppression: amblyopia
suppressor: cells; mutation; tRNA
suppressor-sensitive: mutant
suppurative: appendicitis; arthritis; cerebritis; choroiditis; encephalitis; gingivitis; hepatitis; hyalitis; inflammation; mastitis; necrosis; nephritis; periodontitis; pleurisy; pneumonia; pulpitis; synovitis
supra-acetabular: groove
supraacetabular: sulcus
supra-arytenoid: cartilage
supra-auricular: point
supracallosal: gyrus
supracervical: hysterectomy
suprachiasmatic: artery; nucleus
suprachoroid: lamina of sclera; layer
supraclavicular: lymph nodes; muscle; part of brachial plexus; triangle
supraclinoid: aneurysm
supracollicular: sphincter
supracondylar: fracture; process of humerus
supracrestal: line; plane
supracristal: plane
supraduodenal: artery
supraepicondylar: process
supragingival: calculus
supraglenoid: tubercle (of scapula)
supraglottic: laryngectomy
suprahepatic: spaces
suprahisian: block
suprahyoid: branch of lingual artery; gland; muscles
suprainterparietal: bone
supralemniscal: nucleus
supramammillary: nucleus
supramarginal: convolution; gyrus
supramastoid: crest; fossa
supramaximal: stimulus
suprameatal: pit; spine; triangle
supranasal: point
supranormal: conduction; excitability

supranuclear: lesion; paralysis
supraoptic: artery; nucleus; nucleus [TA] of hypothalamus; recess
supraopticohypophysial: tract
supraorbital: arch; artery; foramen; margin; nerve; neuralgia; notch; point; reflex; ridge; vein
supraorbitomeatal: plane
suprapatellar: bursa; reflex
supraperiosteal: implant
suprapineal: recess
suprapleural: membrane
suprapubic: cystotomy; lithotomy
suprapyloric: lymph node; node
suprarenal: body; capsule; cortex; gland; impression on liver; medulla; veins
suprarenal (nervous): plexus
suprascapular: artery; ligament; nerve; notch; vein
suprasellar: cyst
supraspinalis: muscle
supraspinatus: muscle; syndrome
supraspinous: fossa; ligament; muscle
suprasternal: bones; notch; plane; pulsation; space
suprastyloid: crest of radius
supratonsillar: fossa; recess
supratragic: tubercle
supratrochlear: artery; nerve; veins
supraumbilical: reflex
supravaginal: part of cervix
supravalvar: stenosis
supravalvar aortic stenosis: syndrome
supravalvar aortic stenosis-infantile hypercalcemia: syndrome
supravalvular: stenosis
supraventricular: crest; extrasystole; tachycardia
supravesical: fossa
supravital: stain
supreme: concha
supreme intercostal: artery; vein
supreme nasal: concha
supreme turbinated: bone
sural: arteries; nerve; region
sural communicating: branch of common fibular nerve; branch of common peroneal nerve
surdocardiac: syndrome
surface: anatomy; catalysis; coil; epithelium; microscopy; tension; thermometer

surface mucous: cells of stomach
surface tension: theory of narcosis
surface thalamic: veins
surfactant-specific: proteins
surgeon's: knot
surgical: abdomen; anatomy; anesthesia; appliance; diathermy; emphysema; eruption; erysipelas; ligation; maggot; microscope; neck of humerus; orthodontics; pathology; prosthesis; rod; silk; splint; template
surgical ciliated: cyst
surging: faradism
surrogate: mother
survey: line
survival: analysis; time
susceptibility: cassette; testing
suspended: animation
suspension: colloid; laryngoscopy; stability
suspensory: bandage; ligament of axilla; ligament of clitoris; ligament of duodenum; ligament of esophagus; ligament of eyeball; ligament of gonad; ligament of lens; ligament of ovary; ligament of penis; ligaments of breast; ligaments of Cooper; ligament of testis; ligament of thyroid gland; muscle of duodenum; retinaculum of breast
sustained: pulse
sustained action: tablet
sustentacular: cell; fibers of retina
Sutton: disease; nevus; ulcer
sutural: bones; cataract; ligament
suture: abscess; joint; ligature
Suzanne: gland
SV40-adenovirus: hybrid
Svedberg: equation; unit
Sw^a: antigen
swallow: syncope
swallowing: reflex; threshold
swamp: itch
Swan-Ganz: catheter
Swann: antigens
swan-neck: deformity
sweat: duct; glands; pore; test
sweat gland: carcinoma
sweating: test
sweaty feet: syndrome
Swedish: gymnastics; movements
Sweet: disease
sweet: balm; precipitate
sweet birch: oil

Swift: disease
swim: bladder
swimmer's: ear; itch
swimming pool: conjunctivitis; granuloma
swine: erysipelas; influenza
swine encephalitis: virus
swine fever: virus
swineherd's: disease
swine influenza: viruses
swinepox: virus
swine vesicular: disease
swinging light: test
Swiss cheese: endometrium
Swiss mouse leukemia: virus
Swiss type: agammaglobulinemia
switching: site
swollen belly: disease; syndrome
Swyer: syndrome
Swyer-James: syndrome
Swyer-James-MacLeod: syndrome
Sydenham: chorea; disease
Sydney: crease; line
syllabic: speech
sylvatic: plague
Sylvest: disease
Sylvian: cistern
sylvian: angle; aqueduct; fissure; line; point; valve; ventricle
symbiotic fermentation: phenomenon
Syme: amputation; operation
Symington anococcygeal: body
Symmers clay pipestem: fibrosis
symmetric: adenolipomatosis; asphyxia; disulfide
symmetrical: gangrene
symmetric distal: neuropathy
symmetric fetal growth: restriction
sympathetic: agent; amine; blockade; branch to submandibular ganglion; ganglia; heterochromia; hormone; hypertonia; imbalance; iridoplegia; iritis; nerve; ophthalmia; part of autonomic division of peripheral nervous system; plexuses; root of ciliary ganglion; root of otic ganglion; root of pterygopalatine ganglion; root of sublingual ganglion; root of submandibular ganglion; saliva; segment; symptom; trunk; uveitis
sympathetic formative: cell
sympathetic nervous: system
sympathetic reflex: dystrophy

sympathicotropic: cells
sympathizing: eye
sympathochromaffin: cell
sympathomimetic: amine
symphysial: surface of pubis
symphysic: teratosis
symptom: complex; formation; group; score; substitution
symptomatic: epilepsy; erythema; fever; headache; nanism; neuralgia; porphyria; pruritus; reaction; tetany; torticollis; treatment; varicocele
symptomatic myeloid: metaplasia
Syms: tractor
synaptic: boutons; cleft; conduction; endings; phase; resistance; terminals; trough; vesicles
synaptinemal: complex
synaptonemal: complex
synarthrodial: joint
synchondrodial: joint
synchronic: study
synchronized intermittent mandatory: ventilation
synchronous: reflex
syncytial: bud; knot; sprout; trophoblast
syndesmodial: joint
synergic: control
synergistic: effect; muscles
syngeneic: graft
synovial: bursa; cell; chondromatosis; crypt; cyst; fluid; fold; frena; frenula; fringe; hernia; joint; joints of free lower limb; joints of free upper limb; joints of thorax; ligament; membrane; mesenchyme; osteochondromatosis; sarcoma; sheath; sheaths of digits of foot; sheaths of digits of hand; sheaths of toes; tufts; villi
synovial tendon: sheath
synovial trochlear: bursa
syntactical: aphasia
synthesis: period
synthetic: chemistry; dyes
synthetic sentence: identification
syntonic: personality
syphilitic: aneurysm; aortitis; cirrhosis; fever; leukoderma; meningoencephalitis; nephritis; osteochondritis; roseola; teeth; ulcer
Syriac: ulcer
syringomyelic: dissociation; hemorrhage

Word Finder

systematic: anatomy; bacteriology; desensitization
systematized: delusion; nevus
systemic: anaphylaxis; anatomy; blastomycosis; chondromalacia; circulation; heart; hyalinosis; lupus erythematosus; mastocytosis; myelitis; poisoning; scleroderma; sclerosis
systemic autoimmune: diseases
systemic capillary leak: syndrome
systemic febrile: diseases
systemic vascular: resistance
systemic venous: hypertension
systolic: bruit; click; gallop; gradient; honk; murmur; pressure; shock; thrill; whoop
systolic/diastolic: ratio
systolic gallop: rhythm
systolic time: intervals

T

T: agglutinogen; antigens; cell; enzyme; fiber; group; lymphocyte; myelotomy; system; tube; tubule; wave
Tγ: cells
Tμ: cells
T-: bandage; binder
t: distribution; test
T.A.B.: vaccine
tabby cat: striation
tabetic: arthropathy; crisis; cuirass; dissociation; neurosyphilis
table: salt
Tac: antigen
Tacaribe: complex of viruses; virus
tachybradycardia: syndrome
tachycardia: window
tachycardia-bradycardia: syndrome
tactile: agnosia; anesthesia; cell; corpuscle; disk; elevations; fremitus; hallucination; hyperesthesia; image; meniscus; organ; papilla; sense
Tactual Performance: Test
tadpole-shaped: pupil
Taenzer: stain
tagged: atom
Tahyna: virus
tail: bone; bud; fold; sheath; vertebrae
tailor's: cramp; muscle
Tait: law
Taiwan Dobrava-Belgrade: virus
Takahara: disease

Takayama: stain
Takayasu: arteritis; disease; syndrome
talar: sulcus
talar articular: surfaces of calcaneus
talc: operation
Tallerman: treatment
tallow: soap
talocalcaneal: joint; ligament
talocalcaneal interosseous: ligament
talocalcaneonavicular: joint
talocrural: articulation; joint
talon: cusp
talonavicular: joint; ligament
tambour: sound
tamed: iodine
Tamm-Horsfall: mucoprotein; protein
tangent: screen
tangential: wound
tangible body: macrophage
Tangier: disease
tank: respirator
tanned red: cells
Tanner: stage
Tanner growth: chart
tanner's: ulcer
tannic acid: glycerite
tantalum: bronchography
tapered: bougie
tapetoretinal: degeneration
Tapia: syndrome
tapir: mouth
Taq: polymerase
tar: acne; camphor; keratosis
Tardieu: ecchymoses; petechiae; spots
tardive: cyanosis; dyskinesia
target: behavior; cell; gland; organ; patient; response
target cell: anemia
Tarin: space; tenia; valve
Tarlov: cyst
Tarnier: forceps
tarry: cyst
tarsal: arch; bones; canal; cartilage; cyst; fold; glands; joints; ligaments; plates; sinus
tarsal interosseous: ligaments
tarsal tunnel: syndrome
tarsoepiphyseal: aclasis
tarsometatarsal: joints; ligaments
tarsophalangeal: reflex
tarsotibial: amputation
tart: cell
tartrated: antimony
taste: blindness; bud; bulb; cells; corpuscle; deficiency; hairs; pore; ridge
TATA: box
Taussig-Bing: disease; syndrome

tautomeric: fibers
Tawara: node
Tay cherry-red: spot
Taylor: apparatus; disease; splint
Taylor back: brace
Tay-Sachs: disease
99mTc: pyrophosphate
T cell antigen: receptors
T-cell growth: factor; factor-1; factor-2
T-cell–rich, B-cell: lymphoma
T cytotoxic: cells
T-dependent: antigen
TDTH: cells
T-E: fistula
teacher's: nodes
teaching: hospital
TEAE-: cellulose
tear: film; gas; sac; stone
technical: error
tectal: plate; stria
tectobulbar: tract
tectonic: keratoplasty
tectoolivary: fibers
tectopontine: fibers; tract
tectoreticular: fibers
tectorial: membrane of cochlear duct; membrane (of median atlantoaxial joint)
tectospinal: decussation; tract
tegmental: decussations; fields of Forel; nuclei; root of tympanic cavity; syndrome; wall of middle ear; wall of tympanic cavity
Teichmann: crystals
telangiectatic: angioma; angiomatosis; cancer; fibroma; glioma; lipoma; wart
telangiectatic osteogenic: sarcoma
telencephalic: flexure; vesicle
telephone: ear; theory
teleradium: therapy
telescopic: denture; spectacles
television: microscope
TeLinde: operation
telocentric: chromosome
telogen: effluvium
telolecithal: egg; ovum
telomeric R-banding: stain
temperate: bacteriophage; virus
temperature: coefficient; sense; spot
temperature-compensated: vaporizer
temperature-sensitive: mutant
template: RNA
temporal: aponeurosis; apophysis; arteritis; bone; branch of facial nerve; canal; cortex; crest of mandible; dispersion; fascia;

fossa; horn; line; line of frontal bone; lobe; muscle; plane; pole; pole [TA] of cerebrum; process of zygomatic bone; region of head; ridge; squama; surface; veins; venules of retina
temporalis: muscle
temporal lobe: epilepsy
temporary: base; callus; cartilage; denture; memory; parasite; restoration; stricture; tooth
temporary threshold: shift
temporofrontal: tract
temporomandibular: arthrosis; articulation; joint; ligament; nerve; syndrome
temporomandibular articular: disk
temporomandibular joint: dysfunction
temporomandibular joint pain-dysfunction: syndrome
temporomaxillary: vein
temporoparietal: muscle
temporoparietalis: muscle
temporopontine: fibers; tract
temporozygomatic: suture
tenaculum: forceps
tender: lines; points; zones
tendinous: arch; arch of levator ani muscle; arch of pelvic fascia; arch of soleus muscle; chiasm of the digital tendons; cords; inscription; intersection; intersections of rectus abdominis; opening; sheath of abductor pollicis longus and extensor pollicis brevis muscles; sheath of extensor carpi radialis muscles; sheath of extensor carpi ulnaris muscle; sheath of extensor digiti minimi muscle; sheath of extensor digitorum and extensor indicis muscles; sheath of extensor digitorum longus muscle of foot; sheath of extensor hallucis longus muscle; sheath of extensor pollicis longus muscle; sheath of flexor carpi radialis muscle; sheath of flexor digitorum longus muscle (of foot); sheath of flexor hallucis longus muscle; sheath of flexor pollicis longus muscle; sheath of superior oblique muscle; sheath of tibialis anterior muscle; sheath of tibialis posterior muscle; spot; synovitis; xanthoma

tendo Achillis: reflex
tendon: advancement; bundle; cells; graft; recession; reflex; suture; transplantation
tendon sheath: syndrome
ten Horn: sign
tennis: elbow; leg; thumb
Tenon: capsule; space
tense: part of the tympanic membrane; pulse
tensile: strength; stress
tension: curve; headache; lines; pneumopericardium; pneumothorax; suture
tension-type: headache
tensor: muscle of fascia lata; muscle of soft palate; muscle) of tympanic membrane
tensor fasciae latae: muscle
tensor tarsi: muscle
tensor tympani: muscle; reflex
tensor veli palati: muscle
tenth cranial: nerve [CN X]
tentorial: angle; nerve; notch; sinus; surface
tentorial basal: branch of internal carotid artery
tentorial marginal: branch of cavernous part of internal carotid artery
teratoid: tumor
teratomatous: cyst
teres major: muscle
teres minor: muscle
term: infant
terminal: artery; bar; boutons; branches of middle cerebral artery; bronchiole; cisternae; crest; deletion; disinfection; endocarditis; filum; ganglion; hair; hematuria; ileus; infection; leukocytosis; line; nerve; notch of auricle; nucleus; oxidase; oxidation; part; plate; pneumonia; redundancy; sinus; stria; sulcus; sulcus of tongue; thread; transferases; vein; ventricle; web
terminal addition: enzyme
terminal deoxynucleotidyl: transferase
terminal duct: carcinoma
terminal hinge: position
terminal jaw relation: record
terminal nerve: corpuscles
terminal respiratory: unit
termination: codon; factor; sequence; signal
terminoterminal: anastomosis
ternary: complex
Terrien: valve

Terrien marginal: degeneration
territorial: matrix
Terry: nails; syndrome
Terson: glands; syndrome
tertian: fever; malaria; parasite
tertiary: alcohol; amyl alcohol; calcium phosphate; cortex; dentin; structure; syphilid; syphilis; villus; vitreous
tertiary egg: membrane
tertiary medical: care
Teschen disease: virus
Tesla: current
tessellated: fundus
Tessier: classification
test: cross; injection; meal; object; profile; solution; tube; type
test handle: instrument
testicular: appendage; artery; cord; duct; dysgenesis; feminization; implant; plexus; prosthesis; veins
testicular feminization: syndrome
testis: cords; ectopia
testis-determining: factor
testosterone-estrogen-binding: globulin
test-retest: reliability
test-tube: baby
tetanic: contraction; convulsion
tetanus: antitoxin; immunoglobulin; toxin; vaccine
tetanus antitoxin: unit
tetanus and gas gangrene: antitoxins
tetanus immune: globulin
tetanus-perfringens: antitoxin
tetany: cataract
Tete: viruses
tethered cord: syndrome
tetracyclic: antidepressant
tetracyclic steroid: nucleus
tetraethyl: poisoning
tetramethyl: acridine
tetrazonium: salts
Teutleben: ligament
Texas: snakeroot
text: blindness
TGE: virus
Thal: procedure
thalamic: fasciculus; syndrome; tenia
thalamic gustatory: nucleus
thalamocortical: fibers
thalamostriate: veins
thallium: poisoning
thanatophoric: dwarfism
Thane: method
Thayer-Martin: agar; medium

thebesian: circulation; foramina; valve; veins
theca: cells of stomach
theca cell: tumor
theca interna: cone
thecal: abscess; whitlow
theca lutein: cell
Theden: method
Theile: canal; glands; muscle
Theiler: virus
Theiler mouse encephalomyelitis: virus
Theiler original: virus
T helper: cells
T helper subset 1: cells
T helper subset 2: cells
thematic: paralogia; paraphasia
thematic apperception: test
thenar: eminence; prominence; space
Theobald Smith: phenomenon
therapeutic: abortion; anesthesia; angiography; community; crisis; dose; electrode; fever; group; incompatibility; index; iridectomy; malaria; nihilism; optimism; pessimism; pneumothorax; radiology; range; ratio
thermal: anesthesia; artifact; burn; capacity; sense; spectrum
thermic: fever
thermo-: stromuhr
thermodynamic: potential; theory of narcosis
thermoelectric: pile
thermogenic: action
thermolabile: opsonin
thermoluminescence: dosimetry
thermoprecipitin: reaction
thermostable: enzyme; opsonin
thermostable opsonin: test
theta: antigen; rhythm; wave
Thezac-Porsmeur: method
thiamin chloride: unit
thiamin hydrochloride: unit
thiazide: diabetes
thiazin: dyes
thick: filament; skin
Thiemann: disease; syndrome
Thiersch: canaliculi; graft
thigh: bone; joint
thin: filament; section; skin
thin-layer: chromatography; electrophoresis; immunoassay
thiochrome: method
thioclastic: cleavage
thiocyanogen: number; value
thioflavine T: stain
thiol: enzyme; ester

third: corpuscle; disease; eyelid; finger; molar; ovary; part of duodenum; sound; spacing; toe [III]; tonsil; trochanter; ventricle; ventriculostomy
third cranial: nerve [CN III]
third cuneiform: bone
third-degree: burn
third degree AV: block
third and fourth pharyngeal pouch: syndrome
third heart: sound
third occipital: nerve
third parallel pelvic: plane
third peroneal: muscle
third temporal: convolution
third-year molar: tooth
thirst: fever
Thiry: fistula
Thiry-Vella: fistula
thixotropic: fluid
Thoma: ampulla; fixative; laws
Thomas: splint
Thompson: ligament; test
Thomsen: disease
Thomson: sign
thoracic: aorta; axis; cage; cavity; compliance; constriction of esophagus; duct; fistula; ganglia; girdle; glands; goiter; index; inlet; kidney; kyphosis; limb; lymph nodes; nerves [T1–T12]; outlet; part of aorta; part of esophagus; part of iliocostalis lumborum (muscle); part of peripheral autonomic plexuses and ganglia; part of spinal cord; part of thoracic duct; part of trachea; respiration; skeleton; spine; splenosis; stomach; veins; vertebrae [T1–T12]; wall
thoracic aortic (nervous): plexus
thoracic cardiac: branches of thoracic ganglia; branches of vagus nerve; nerves
thoracic interspinal: muscle
thoracic interspinales: muscles
thoracic intertransversarii: muscles
thoracic intertransverse: muscles
thoracic longissimus: muscle
thoracic outlet: syndrome
thoracic-pelvic-phalangeal: dystrophy
thoracic pulmonary: branches of thoracic ganglia
thoracic rotator: muscles

thoracic splanchnic: ganglion; nerves

thoracoabdominal: ectopia cordis; nerves

thoracoacromial: artery; trunk; vein

thoracoappendicular: muscles

thoracodorsal: artery; nerve

thoracoepigastric: vein

thoracolumbar: aponeurosis; fascia; system

thoracolumbar nervous: system

thoracolumbosacral: orthosis

thoracoscopic: surgery

thoracostomy: tube

thorium: emanation

Thormählen: test

Thorn: syndrome; test

thorn apple: crystals

thought: disorder

thought process: disorder

threaded: implant

thready: pulse

threatened: abortion

three-chambered: heart

three-cornered: bone

three-day: fever; measles

three-dimensional: record

three-glass: test

three-headed: muscle

three-incision: esophagectomy

thresher's: lung

threshold: body; differential; pads of anal canal; percussion; shift; stimulus; substance; trait

threshold limit: value

thrombin: time

thrombocytic: series

thrombocytopenia-absent radius: syndrome

thrombocytopenic: purpura

thrombolytic: therapy

thrombopathic: syndrome

thrombopenic: purpura

thrombospondin-related adhesive: protein

thrombotic: gangrene; hydrocephalus; infarct; microangiopathy

thrombotic thrombocytopenic: purpura

through: drainage

through-and-through myocardial: infarction

through transfer: imaging

thrush: fungus

thumb: forceps; lancet; reflex

thunderclap: headache

Thygeson: disease

thyme: camphor

thymic: abscesses; agenesis; alymphoplasia; branches of

internal thoracic artery; corpuscle; hypoplasia; veins

thymic lymphopoietic: factor

thymine: dimer

thymol turbidity: test

thymus: gland; treatment

thymus-dependent: zone

thymus-independent: antigen

thyroarytenoid: muscle

thyrocardiac: disease

thyrocervical (arterial): trunk

thyroepiglottic: ligament; muscle; part of thyroarytenoid (muscle)

thyroglossal: duct

thyroglossal duct: cyst

thyrohyoid: branch of ansa cervicalis; membrane; muscle

thyrohypophysial: syndrome

thyroid: axis; body; bruit; cartilage; colloid; diverticulum; eminence; foramen; gland; insufficiency; lymph nodes; storm; therapy; toxicosis; veins

thyroid articular: surface of cricoid (cartilage)

thyroid ima: artery

thyroid-stimulating: hormone; immunoglobulins

thyroid-stimulating hormone-releasing: factor

thyroid-stimulating hormone stimulation: test

thyroid suppression: test

thyrolingual: duct

thyropharyngeal: part of inferior constrictor muscle of pharynx; part of inferior pharyngeal constrictor (muscle) of pharynx

thyrotoxic: coma; crisis; encephalopathy; myopathy; serum

thyrotoxic heart: disease

thyrotropic: hormone

thyrotropin: resistance

thyrotropin-producing: adenoma

thyrotropin-releasing: factor; hormone

thyrotropin-releasing hormone stimulation: test

thyroxine-binding: globulin; prealbumin; protein

tibial: border of foot; crest; nerve; phenomenon; tuberosity

tibial collateral: ligament; ligament of ankle joint

tibial communicating: nerve

tibial intertendinous: bursa

tibialis anterior: muscle

tibialis posterior: muscle

tibial nutrient: artery

tibial tarsal tendinous: sheaths

tibiocalcaneal: ligament; part of deltoid ligament; part of medial ligament of ankle joint

tibiofemoral: index

tibiofibular: articulation; joint; ligament; syndesmosis

tibionavicular: ligament; part of deltoid ligament; part of medial ligament of ankle joint

tibiotalar: part of medial ligament of ankle joint

tick: paralysis; typhus

tick-borne: encephalitis (Central European subtype); encephalitis (Eastern subtype); virus

tick-borne encephalitis: virus

tic-tac: rhythm; sounds

tidal: air; drainage; volume; wave

Tiedemann: gland; nerve

tie-over: dressing

Tietz: syndrome

Tietze: syndrome

tiger: heart

tight: junction

tigroid: bodies; fundus; retina; striation; substance

tilt: table; test

tilting disk: valve

tilting disk valve: prosthesis

time: constant; marker; sense

time-compensated: gain

time compensation: gain

time-gain: compensation

time-lapse: microscopy

Time-Line: therapy

time-varied: gain

time-varied gain: control

tine: test

Tinel: sign

tinted: vision

tinted denture: base

tip: links

Tiselius: apparatus

Tiselius electrophoresis: cell

Tissot: spirometer

tissue: basophil; culture; displaceability; displacement; factor; fluid; hormones; lymph; molding; registration; respiration; tension; valve

tissue-bearing: area

tissue culture infectious: dose

tissue plasminogen: activator

tissue-specific: antigen

tissue thromboplastin inhibition: time

tissue weighting: factor

titratable acidity: test

Tizzoni: stain

Tj: antigen

TMJ: syndrome

TNM: staging

TO: virus

toad: skin

to-and-fro: anesthesia; murmur; sound

toasted: shins

tobacco: heart

tobacco-alcohol: amblyopia

Tobia: fever

Tobruk: splint

Tod: muscle

Todaro: tendon

Todd: paralysis; unit

toddler's: diarrhea; fracture

Todd postepileptic: paralysis

toe: clonus; itch; phenomenon

toilet: training

Toison: stain

Tokelau: ringworm

Toker: cell

tolbutamide: test

Toldt: fascia; membrane

tolerance: dose; limits

Tolosa-Hunt: syndrome

Tolu: balsam

toluidine blue: stain

Toma: sign

Tomes: fibers; processes

Tomes granular: layer

Tommaselli: disease

tone: color

tone decay: test

tongue: bone; depressor; phenomenon

tonic: contraction; control; convulsion; epilepsy; pupil; reflex; seizure

tonic-clonic: seizure

tonsillar: branches of glossopharyngeal nerve; branches of lesser palatine nerves; branch of the facial artery; calculus; crypt; fossa; fossulae; herniation; ring

tonsillolingual: sulcus

tooth: abrasion; avulsion; bud; cement; form; germ; ligation; plane; polyp; pulp; sac; socket; transplantation

tooth-and-nail: syndrome

tooth-borne: base

toothed: vertebra

toper's: nose

Töpfer: test

tophaceous: gout

topical: anesthesia; anesthetic

Topinard: line

Topinard facial: angle

Topografov: virus

topographic: anatomy

Topolanski: sign

toppling: gait

TORCH: syndrome

Torek: operation
toric: lens
Torkildsen: shunt
tornado: epilepsy
Tornwaldt: abscess; cyst; disease; syndrome
Toronto: formula for pulmonary artery banding
Torre: syndrome
torsion: disease of childhood; dystonia; fracture; neurosis
torsional: deformity
torsive: occlusion
Torsten Sjögren: syndrome
torus: fracture
total: acidity; aphasia; ascertainment; cataract; cleavage; communication; cystectomy; elasticity of muscle; energy; hematuria; hyperopia; keratoplasty; mastectomy; necrosis; placenta previa; sclerectasia; synechia; transfusion
total anomalous pulmonary venous: return
total body: hypothermia; water
total breech: extraction
total catecholamine: test
total cell: count
total cricoid: cleft
total end-diastolic: diameter
total end-systolic: diameter
total joint: arthroplasty
total lung: capacity
total parenteral: nutrition
total pelvic: exenteration
total peripheral: resistance
total push: therapy
total refractory: period
total spinal: anesthesia
totipotent: cell
totipotential: protoplasm
touch: cell; corpuscle
toughened: silver nitrate
Toupet: fundoplication
Tourette: disease; syndrome
Tournay: phenomenon; sign
tourniquet: poditis; test
Tourtual: membrane; sinus
Touton giant: cell
Tovell: tube
Towne: projection; view
Towne projection: radiograph
toxemic: jaundice; retinopathy of pregnancy
toxic: amaurosis; amblyopia; anemia; cataract; cirrhosis; cyanosis; delirium; dementia; equivalent; goiter; hemoglobinuria; hydrocephalus; megacolon; myocarditis; nephrosis; neuritis; psychosis;

retinopathy; shock; tetanus; unit
toxic epidermal: necrolysis
toxicogenic: conjunctivitis
toxic shock: syndrome
toxin: unit
Toynbee: corpuscles; muscle; tube
TPHA: test
TPI: test
Tr^a: antigen
trabecular: bone; carcinoma; meshwork; network; reticulum; tissue of sclera; zone
trabeculated: bladder
trace: conditioning; elements; nutrient
trace conditioned: reflex
tracheal: bifurcation; branches; carina; cartilages; fenestration; glands; intubation; lymph nodes; mucosa; ring; triangle; tube; tug; ulceration; veins
tracheal breath: sounds
trachealis: muscle
tracheal wall: stripe
trachelobregmatic: diameter
tracheloclavicular: muscle
tracheobronchial: diverticulum; dyskinesia; groove
tracheoesophageal: fistula; puncture; shunt; speech
tracheostomy: tube
tracheotomy: hook; tube
trachoma: bodies; glands; virus
trachomatous: conjunctivitis; keratitis; pannus
traction: alopecia; atrophy; diverticulum; epiphysis
tragal: lamina
tragicus: muscle
trained: reflex
training: analysis; group
train-of-four: stimulus
trainwheel: rhythm
tram: lines
trance: coma
trans: phase
transactional: analysis; psychotherapy
transaxial: plane
transcapsular gray: bridges
transcellular: fluids; transport; water
transcendental: anatomy
transcervical: fracture; thymectomy
transcochlear: approach
transcondylar: fracture
transcortical: aphasia; apraxia
transcranial: radiograph

transcription-based chain: reaction
transducer: cell
transduodenal: sphincterotomy
transesophageal: echocardiography
transfer: coping; factor; genes; imaging; RNA
transferase deficiency: galactosemia
transference: neurosis
transferred: ophthalmia
transferring: enzymes
transfixion: suture
transformation: constant; zone
transformed: lymphocyte
transforming: agent; factor; gene
transforming growth: factor α; factor β; factors
transfusion: hepatitis; nephritis
transgenic: mice
trans-Golgi: reticulum
transhiatal: esophagectomy
transient: agammaglobulinemia; albuminuria; equilibrium; erythroblastopenia of childhood; hypogammaglobulinemia of infancy; myopia; retinopathy; tachypnea of the newborn
transient acantholytic: dermatosis
transient evoked otoacoustic: emission
transient global: amnesia
transient ischemic: attack
transition: electron; mutation
transitional: cell; convolution; denture; epithelium; gyrus; leukocyte; object; zone; zone of lips
transitional cell: carcinoma; papilloma
transjugular intrahepatic portosystemic: shunt
translabyrinthine: approach
translatory: movement
translocation: carrier; chromosome
translumbar: aortography
transmeatal: incision
transmembrane: potential
transmethylation: factor
transmissible: plasmid
transmissible gastroenteritis: virus of swine
transmitted: light
transmural: pressure
transmural myocardial: infarction

transnasal fiberoptic: laryngoscopy
transneuronal: atrophy
transnexus: channel
transorbital: leukotomy; lobotomy
transosseous: venography
transovarial: transmission
transparent: dentin; septum; ulcer of the cornea
transplantation: antigen; genetics
transplant lung: syndrome
transporionic: axis
transport: antibiotic; host; maximum; medium; number
transposable: element
transpulmonary: pressure
transpyloric: plane
transseptal: fibers; orchiopexy
transsexual: surgery
transstadial: transmission
transsynaptic: chromatolysis; degeneration
transtentorial: herniation
transthoracic: echocardiography; esophagectomy; pacemaker; pressure
transureteroureteral: anastomosis
transurethral: resection
transurethral resection: syndrome
transvaginal: scanning
transversalis: fascia
transversarial: part of vertebral artery
transverse: amputation; arch of foot; artery of neck; branch of lateral femoral circumflex artery; colon; crest; crest of internal acoustic meatus; diameter; disk; ductules of epoöphoron; fasciculi; fissure of cerebellum; fissure of the right lung; folds of rectum; foramen; fornix; fracture; head; hermaphroditism; lie; ligament of acetabulum; ligament of the atlas; ligament of elbow; ligament of knee; ligament of leg; ligament of pelvis; ligament of perineum; muscle of abdomen; muscle of auricle; muscle of chin; muscle of nape; muscle of thorax; muscle of tongue; myelitis; nerve of neck; part of iliofemoral ligament; part of left branch of portal vein; part of nasalis muscle; part of trapezius (muscle); plane;

Word Finder

presentation; process of vertebra; relaxation; ridge; ridges of sacrum; section; septum; sinus; sinus of pericardium; thoracosternotomy; vein of face; vein of scapula; veins of neck; velum

transverse abdominal: incision

transverse acetabular: ligament

transverse anthelicine: groove

transverse arytenoid: muscle

transverse atlantal: ligament

transverse auricular: muscle

transverse carpal: ligament

transverse cerebral: fissure

transverse cervical: artery; ligament; nerve; veins

transverse costal: facet

transverse crural: ligament

transverse facial: artery; fracture; vein

transverse genicular: ligament

transverse horizontal: axis

transverse humeral: ligament

transverse intermesocolic: fossa

transverse metacarpal: ligament

transverse metatarsal: ligament

transverse nasal: groove

transverse occipital: sulcus

transverse oval: pelvis

transverse palatine: fold; ridge; suture

transverse pancreatic: artery

transverse pericardial: sinus

transverse perineal: ligament

transverse pontine: fibers

transverse rhombencephalic: flexure

transverse scapular: artery

transverse tarsal: articulation; joint

transverse temporal: convolutions; gyri; sulcus

transverse tibiofibular: ligament

transverse vesical: fold

transversion: mutation

transversospinal: muscle

transversospinales: muscles

transversovertical: index

transversus abdominis: muscle

transversus menti: muscle

transversus nuchae: muscle

transversus thoracis: muscle

Trantas: dots

trapezium: bone

trapezius: muscle

trapezoid: body; bone; ligament; line; ridge

Trapp: formula

Trapp-Häser: formula

Traube: bruit; corpuscle; dyspnea; plugs; sign

Traube double: tone

Traube-Hering: curves; waves

Traube semilunar: space

traumatic: alopecia; amenorrhea; amnesia; amputation; anemia; anesthesia; aneurysm; asphyxia; cataract; dermatitis; encephalopathy; fever; herpes; meningocele; neurasthenia; neuritis; neuroma; neurosis; occlusion; orchitis; pneumothorax; psychosis; retinopathy; tetanus

traumatic bone: cyst

traumatic cervical: discopathy

traumatic progressive: encephalopathy

traumatogenic: occlusion

Trautmann triangular: space

traveler's: diarrhea

traveling wave: theory

Treacher Collins: syndrome

treatment: denture

treble: increase at low levels

trefoil: polypeptide; tendon

Treitz: arch; fascia; fossa; hernia; ligament; muscle

Trélat: stools

tremulous: iris

trench: fever; foot; hand; lung; mouth

Trendelenburg: gait; operation; position; radiograph; sign; symptom; test

trephine: biopsy

treponema-immobilizing: antibody

treponemal: antibody

Treponema pallidum **hemagglutination:** test

Treponema pallidum **immobilization:** reaction; test

Tresilian: sign

Treves: fold

Trevor: disease

triad: asthma

triadic: symbiosis

trial: base; case; denture; frame; lenses

trial of: labor after cesarean section

triangular: bandage; bone; cartilage; crest; disk of wrist; fascia; fold; fossa of

auricle; fovea of arytenoid cartilage; lamella; ligament; ligaments of liver; muscle; nucleus; nucleus of septum; part; pit of arytenoid cartilage; recess; ridge; uterus

triaxial reference: system

triazolopyridine: antidepressant

tribasic: calcium phosphate; magnesium phosphate

tribasilar: synostosis

TRIC: agents

tricarboxylic acid: cycle

triceps: bursa; muscle; muscle of arm; muscle of calf; muscle of hip; reflex

triceps brachii: muscle

triceps coxae: muscle

triceps surae: muscle; reflex

trichilemmal: cyst

trichinosis: granuloma

trichorhinophalangeal: syndrome

trichrome: stain

tricorn: protease

tricuspid: area; atresia; incompetence; insufficiency; murmur; orifice; stenosis; tooth; valve

tricyclic: antidepressant

trident: hand

O-(triethylaminoethyl): cellulose

trifacial: nerve; neuralgia

trifid: stomach

trifocal: lens

trigeminal: cave; cavity; crest; decompression; ganglion; impression; lemniscus; nerve [CN V]; neuralgia; pulse; rhizotomy; rhythm; tractotomy; tubercle

trigeminofacial: reflex

trigeminospinal: tract

trigeminothalamic: tract

trigger: area; finger; point; zone

triggered: activity

trihydric: alcohol

triiodothyronine: toxicosis

triiodothyronine uptake: test

triketohydrindene: reaction

trilaminar: blastoderm

trimalleolar: fracture

triphammer: pulse

triphenylmethane: dyes

triphyllomatous: teratoma

Tripier: amputation

triplant: implant

triple: arthrodesis; bond; helix; phosphate; point; quartan; response; rhythm; screen; vision

triple A: syndrome

triple repeat: disorders

triple symptom: complex

triplet: oxygen; state

triple X: syndrome

tripod: fracture

triquetrous: cartilage

triquetrum: bone

trisodium: phosphate

trisomy 8: syndrome

trisomy 13: syndrome

trisomy 18: syndrome

trisomy 20: syndrome

trisomy 21: syndrome

trisomy C: syndrome

trisomy D: syndrome

trispiral: tomography

tritiated: thymidine

triticeal: cartilage

triton: tumor

trochanter: reflex

trochanteric: bursa; bursae of gluteus medius; bursae of gluteus minimus; crest; fossa; syndrome

trochlear: fossa; fovea; nerve [CN IV]; notch; nucleus; pit; process; spine

trochlear synovial: bursa

trochoid: articulation; joint

Troisier: ganglion; node

Trolard: vein

Tröltsch: corpuscles; pockets; recesses

Trömner: reflex

trophic: changes; gangrene; nucleus; syndrome; ulcer

trophoblast: interferon

trophoblastic: lacuna; operculum

trophoneurotic: atrophy; leprosy

trophotropic: zone of Hess

tropic: hormones

tropical: abscess; acne; anemia; boil; bubo; diarrhea; diseases; eczema; eosinophilia; lichen; mask; measles; medicine; myositis; pyomyositis; sore; splenomegaly; sprue; typhus; ulcer

tropical splenomegaly: syndrome

trough: sign

Trousseau: point; sign; spot; syndrome

Trousseau-Lallemand: bodies

true: aneurysm; ankylosis; cementoma; cholinesterase; conjugate; diverticulum; dwarfism; glottis; hermaphroditism; hypertrophy; knot; lumen; muscles of back; pelvis; ribs [I–VII]; thirst; vertebra

true neurogenic thoracic outlet: syndrome
true precocious: puberty
true vocal: cord
truncate: ascertainment
Trunecek: sign
Trusler: rule for pulmonary artery banding
truth: serum
trypanosome: fever; stage
trypsin: inhibitor
α_1-trypsin: inhibitor
trypsin G-banding: stain
tsutsugamushi: disease; fever
tubal: abortion; branch; branch of ovarian artery; branch of the tympanic plexus; branch of the uterine artery; cartilage; colic; dysmenorrhea; extremity of ovary; glands of pharyngotympanic tube; infantilism; ligation; pregnancy; prominence; tonsil
tubal air: cells (of pharyngotympanic tube)
tube: cast; curare; tooth
tubed: flap
tubed pedicle: flap
tuberal: nuclei
tubercle: bacillus
tuberculin: test
tuberculin-type: hypersensitivity
tuberculoid: leprosy; rosacea
tuberculoopsonic: index
tuberculosis: lymphadenitis; vaccine
tuberculous: bronchopneumonia; enteritis; lymphadenitis; meningitis; nephritis; pericarditis; peritonitis; rheumatism; spondylitis; wart
tuberoinfundibular: tract
tuberomammillary: nucleus
tuberosity: reduction
tuberous: root; sclerosis
Tübinger: perimeter
tuboabdominal: pregnancy
tubo-ovarian: varicocele
tuboovarian: abscess; pregnancy
tuboreticular: structure
tubotympanic: canal; recess
tubouterine: pregnancy
tubular: adenoma; aneurysm; carcinoma; cyst; forceps; gland; maximum; respiration; vision
tubular excretory: mass
tubuloacinar: gland
tubuloalveolar: gland
tubuloglomerular: feedback
tubulointerstitial: nephritis

Tucker-McLean: forceps
tuffstone: body
tufted: cell; phalanx
tularemic: chancre; conjunctivitis; pneumonia
Tullio: phenomenon
Tulp: valve
tumbu dermal: myiasis
tumescent: liposuction
tumor: antigens; blush; embolism; marker; stage; virus
tumoral: calcinosis
tumor angiogenic: factor
tumor-associated: antigen
tumor-infiltrating: lymphocytes
tumor lysis: syndrome
tumor necrosis: factor; factor-α; factor-β
tumor-specific transplantation: antigens
tumor suppressor: gene
tungsten arc: lamp
tuning: curve; fork
tunnel: cells; disease; vision
Tuohy: needle
T_3 uptake: test
TUR: syndrome
turban: tumor
turbinal: varix
turbinated: body; bones; crest
Türck: bundle; column; degeneration; tract
Turcot: syndrome
Türk: cell; leukocyte
turkey gobbler: neck
Turkish: saddle
Turlock: virus
Turner: sulcus; syndrome; tooth
turnover: number
turpentine: enema; poisoning
tussive: fremitus; syncope
Tuttle: proctoscope
Tweed: triangle
Tweed edgewise: treatment
twelfth cranial: nerve [CN XII]
twelfth-year: molar
twenty-nail: dystrophy
twiddler's: syndrome
twilight: sleep; state; vision
twin: cone; crystal; helix; method; placenta; pregnancy
twin reversed arterial perfusion: sequence
twin-twin: transfusion
twist: form
twisted: hairs
two-bellied: muscle
two-carbon: fragment
two-dimensional: chromatography; echocardiography; immunoelectrophoresis

two-dimension–three-dimension: phenomenon
two-glass: test
two-headed: muscle
Twort: phenomenon
Twort-d'Herelle: phenomenon
two-step exercise: test
two-tail: test
two-way: catheter
tying: forceps
tympanic: antrum; aperture of canaliculus for chorda tympani; attic; body; bone; canal; canaliculus; cavity; cells; enlargement; ganglion; gland; groove; incisure; intumescence; labium of limbus of spiral lamina; lamella (of osseous spiral lamina); lip of limbus of spiral lamina; lip of spiral limbus; membrane; nerve; notch; opening of canaliculus for chorda tympani; opening of eustachian tube; opening of pharyngotympanic (auditory) tube; part of temporal bone; plate of temporal bone; promontory; ring; scute; sinus; sulcus; surface of cochlear duct; veins; wall of cochlear duct
tympanic air: cells
tympanic (nervous): plexus
tympanitic: resonance
tympanohyal: bone
tympanomastoid: fissure; suture
tympanosquamous: fissure
tympanostapedial: junction; syndesmosis
tympanostomy: tube
Tyndall: effect; phenomenon
type: culture; species; strain
type 1: dextrocardia; glycogenosis
type 2: dextrocardia; glycogenosis
type 3: dextrocardia; glycogenosis
type 4: dextrocardia; glycogenosis
type 5: glycogenosis
type 6: glycogenosis
type 7: glycogenosis
type A: behavior; personality
type B: behavior
Type 1 choroidal: neovascularization
Type 2 choroidal: neovascularization
Type 1 G_{M1}: gangliosidosis
Type I: osteogenesis imperfecta

type I: acrocephalosyndactyly; cells; collagen; diabetes; diabetes mellitus; dip; error; interferon
Type IA: achondrogenesis
Type IB: achondrogenesis
type I familial: hyperlipoproteinemia
type IH: mucopolysaccharidosis
type I H/S: mucopolysaccharidosis
Type II: achondrogenesis; osteogenesis imperfecta
type II: acrocephalosyndactyly; cells; collagen; diabetes; dip; error; interferon; mucopolysaccharidosis
type II familial: hyperlipoproteinemia
Type III: osteogenesis imperfecta
type III: acrocephalosyndactyly; collagen; mucopolysaccharidosis
type III familial: hyperlipoproteinemia
type III hypersensitivity: reaction
type III punctate palmoplantar: keratoderma
type IS: mucopolysaccharidosis
Type IV: osteogenesis imperfecta
type IV: collagen
type IVA, B: mucopolysaccharidosis
type IV familial: hyperlipoproteinemia
type V: acrocephalosyndactyly; mucopolysaccharidosis
type V familial: hyperlipoproteinemia
type VI: mucopolysaccharidosis
type VII: mucopolysaccharidosis
typhoid: bacillus; bacteriophage; cholera; fever; pleurisy; pneumonia; septicemia; vaccine
typhoid-paratyphoid A and B: vaccine
typhus: vaccine
typical: achromatopsia; drusen; pseudocholinesterase
typical antipsychotic: agent
typist's: cramp
Tyrode: solution
Tyrrell: fascia
TY1-S-33: medium
TYSGM-9: medium

Word Finder

Tyson: glands
Tzanck: cells; test

U

U: wave
ubiquitin-protease: pathway
Uffelmann: reagent
Uhl: anomaly
Uhthoff: sign; symptom; syndrome
ulcerating: granuloma of pudenda
ulcerative: colitis; pharyngitis; stomatitis
ulceromembranous: gingivitis; pharyngitis
Ullmann: line; syndrome
ulnar: artery; border of forearm; branch of medial antebrachial cutaneous nerve; bursa; clubhand; eminence of wrist; head; margin of forearm; nerve; notch; reflex; veins
ulnar collateral: ligament; ligament of elbow joint; ligament of wrist joint
ulnar communicating: branch of superficial radial nerve
ulnar extensor: muscle of wrist
ulnar flexor: muscle of wrist
ulnar recurrent: artery
ultimate: principle; strength
ultimobranchial: body; pouch
ultra-: microscope
ultradian: rhythm
ultrafast Pap: stain
ultrafiltration: coefficient; hemodialyzer
ultralente: insulin
ultrashortwave: diathermy
ultrasonic: cardiography; cephalometry; cleaning; lithotripsy; microscope; nebulizer; rays; scaler; therapy; waves
ultrasonic egg: recovery
ultrasound: cardiography; transducer
ultrastructural: anatomy
ultraviolet: index; keratoconjunctivitis; lamp; microscope; rays; spectrum
ultropaque: method
Ulysses: syndrome
umber: codon; mutation
umbilical: artery; cord; cyst; duct; fascia; fissure; fistula; fossa; fungus; granuloma; hernia; notch; part of left branch of portal vein; region; ring; souffle; vein; vesicle
umbilical prevesical: fascia

umbilicated: cataract
umbilicomammillary: triangle
umbilicovesical: fascia
Umbre: virus
unarmed: rostellum
unavoidable: hemorrhage
unbalanced: translocation
uncal: artery; herniation
unciform: bone; fasciculus
uncinate: attack; bundle of Russell; epilepsy; fasciculus of cerebellum; fasciculus of Russell; fit; gyrus; pancreas; process of cervical vertebra; process of ethmoid bone; process of first thoracic vertebra; process of pancreas
uncombable hair: syndrome
uncomfortable: level
uncompensated: acidosis; alkalosis
uncompetitive: inhibition; inhibitor
unconditioned: reflex; response; stimulus
unconjugated: bilirubin
unconscious: homosexuality
uncoupling: factors
uncovertebral: joints
uncrossed: diplopia
uncus: band of Giacomini
undercut: gauge
undermining: ulcer
Underwood: disease
undescended: testis
undetermined: nitrogen
undifferentiated: cell
undifferentiated cell: adenoma
undifferentiated type: fevers
undulant: fever
undulating: fever; membrane; pulse
unequal: cleavage; pulse
unequal retinal: image
unerupted: tooth
unesterified free: fatty acid
uneven: crossing-over
unformed visual: hallucination
ungual: phalanx; tuberosity
uniaxial: joint
unicameral: cyst
unicameral bone: cyst
unicanalicular: sphincter
unicellular: gland; sclerosis
unicorn: uterus
unidentified: reading frame
unidirectional: block; flux; replication
unilaminar primary: follicle
unilateral: anesthesia; hemianopia; hermaphroditism
unilateral hyperlucent: lung
unilateral lobar: emphysema

unilocular: cyst; fat; joint
unilocular hydatid: cyst
unimolecular: reaction
uninducible: mutant
uninhibited neurogenic: bladder
uninterrupted: suture
uniovular: twins
unipennate: muscle
unipolar: cell; electrocardiogram; leads; neuron
unit: character; fibrils; membrane
unit of: convergence
uniting: canal; cartilage; duct
univalent: antibody
univentricular: connections; heart
universal: antidote; appliance; donor; infantilism; solvent
unmodified zinc oxide-eugenol: cement
unmyelinated: fibers; nerve
Unna: disease; mark; nevus; stain
Unna-Pappenheim: stain
Unna-Taenzer: stain
Unna-Thost: syndrome
unpaired: allosome; chromosome
unpaired thyroid venous: plexus
unresolved: pneumonia
unroofed coronary sinus: syndrome
unsaturated: alcohols; fat; fatty acid
unsharp: masking
unstable: angina; bladder; colloid; equilibrium; fracture; hemoglobins; lie
unstable hemoglobin hemolytic: anemia
unstrained jaw: relation
unstriated: muscle
unsystematized: delusion
ununited: fracture
Unverricht: disease
unwinding: proteins
upbeat: nystagmus
upper: airway; extremity; extremity of fibula; eyelid; jaw; lid; limb; lip; lobe of lung; pole; pole of testis
upper abdominal periosteal: reflex
upper dental: arcade
upper esophageal: constriction
upper GI: series
upper jaw: bone
upper lateral cutaneous: nerve of arm
upper motor: neuron
upper motor neuron: lesion

upper subscapular: nerve
upper thoracic splanchnic: nerves
upper uterine: segment
up promoter: mutation
upregulation/downregulation: hypothesis
ur-: defenses
urachal: cyst; fistula; fold; ligament
uracil: mustard
uranium: nephritis
uranyl acetate: stain
Urbach-Wiethe: disease
Urban: operation
urban: typhus
urban cutaneous: leishmaniasis
urea: clearance; cycle; frost; nitrogen
urea clearance: test
urease: test
urecholine supersensitivity: test
uremic: breath; colitis; coma; lung; pericarditis; pneumonia; pneumonitis; polyneuropathy
ureteral: branches; colic; ectopia; meatus; opening; reimplantation
ureteric: branches; branches of the inferior suprarenal artery; branches of the ovarian artery; branches of the patent part of umbilical artery; branches of the renal artery; branches of the testicular artery; bud; dysmenorrhea; fold; orifice; pelvis
ureteric (nervous): plexus
ureterocutaneous: fistula
ureteroileal: anastomosis
ureteropelvic: junction
ureteropelvic junction: obstruction
ureterorenal: reflux
ureterosigmoid: anastomosis
ureteroureteral: anastomosis
ureterovaginal: fistula
ureterovesical: junction; obstruction
urethral: artery; calculus; carina of vagina; caruncle; crest; crest of female; crest of male; dilation; diverticulum; fever; glands; glands of female; glands of male; groove; hematuria; lacuna; openings; papilla; plate; stricture; surface of penis; syndrome; valves
urethral pressure: profile

urethrocutaneous: fistula
urethrovaginal: fistula; sphincter
urethrovesical: angle
urge: incontinence
uric acid: infarct
uricolytic: index
urinary: apparatus; bladder; calculus; casts; cyst; fever; fistula; nitrogen; organs; reflex; sand; schistosomiasis; smear; stuttering; system; tract
urinary concentration: test
urinary exertional: incontinence
urinary tract: infection
uriniferous: tubule
urogenital: apparatus; cleft; diaphragm; fistula; membrane; mesentery; peritoneum; region; ridge; septum; sinus; system; triangle
urogenital sinus: anomaly
uropoietic: system
urorectal: fold; membrane; septum
urothelial: carcinoma; papilloma
urticarial: fever; vasculitis
u-score: method
Usher: syndrome
USP: unit
usual interstitial: pneumonia of Liebow
uterine: appendages; artery; atony; calculus; cavity; colic; contraction; dysmenorrhea; extremity of ovary; glands; horn; inertia; insufficiency; milk; opening of uterine tubes; ostium of uterine tubes; part of uterine tube; pregnancy; sinus; sinusoid; souffle; tetanus; tube; tympanites; veins
uterine venous: plexus
uteroabdominal: pregnancy
uteroepichorial: membrane
utero-ovarian: varicocele
uteroperitoneal: fistula
uteroplacental: apoplexy; sinuses
uterovaginal: canal
uterovaginal (nervous): plexus
uterovesical: fold; ligament; pouch
utilization: time
utricular: cyst; duct; nerve; recess of bony labyrinth; recess of membranous labyrinth; reflexes; spot
utriculoampullar: nerve
utriculosaccular: duct

uveal: part of trabecular reticulum; part of trabecular tissue of sclera; staphyloma; tract
uveocutaneous: syndrome
uveoencephalitic: syndrome
uveomeningitis: syndrome
uveoparotid: fever
uviol: lamp
uvular: muscle
Uzbekistan hemorrhagic: fever

V

V: antigen; gene; lead; wave
V-2: carcinoma
vaccine: bodies; lymph; virus
vaccinia: virus
vaccinoid: reaction
VACTERL: syndrome
vacuolar: degeneration; nephrosis
vacuolating: virus
vacuum: aspirator; casting; desiccator; extractor; flask; headache; investing; tube
vacuum disk: phenomenon
vacuum pack: technique
vagabond's: disease
vagal: attack; bradycardia; part of accessory nerve
vagal nerve: stimulation
vagal (nerve): trigone; trunk
vagi: eminentia
vaginal: artery; atresia; celiotomy; columns; cuff; dysmenorrhea; fornix; gland; hysterectomy; hysterotomy; introitus; laceration; lithotomy; mucosa; myomectomy; nerves; opening; orifice; part of cervix; pool; process; process of peritoneum; process of sphenoid bone; process of testis; rugae; smear
vaginal cornification: test
vaginal intraepithelial: neoplasia
vaginal mucification: test
vaginal synovial: membrane
vaginal venous: plexus
vagovagal: reflex
vagrant's: disease
vagus: area; nerve [CN X]; pulse
valence: electron
Valentin: corpuscles; ganglion; nerve
Valentine: position; test
vallate: papillae
vallecular: dysphagia
Valleix: points
valley: fever

Valsalva: antrum; ligaments; maneuver; muscle; sinus; test
valvotomy: knife
valvular: endocarditis; incompetence; insufficiency; prolapse; regurgitation; sclerosis; thrombus
vampire: bat
van Bogaert: encephalitis
van Buchem: syndrome
van Buren: disease; sound
van Deen: test
van den Bergh: test
van der Hoeve: syndrome
van der Velden: test
van der Waals: forces
van Ermengen: stain
van Gieson: stain
van Helmont: mirror
van Horne: canal
vanillylmandelic acid: test
vanished testis: syndrome
vanishing: cream; lung
vanishing lung: syndrome
Van Lohuizen: syndrome
Van Slyke: apparatus; formula
van't Hoff: equation; law; theory
vapor: density; pressure
Vaquez: disease
variable: coupling; deceleration; region
variance: ratio
variant: angina pectoris; hemoglobin
varicella: encephalitis
varicella-zoster: virus
varicose: aneurysm; bronchiectasis; eczema; ulcer; veins
variegate: porphyria
variola: virus
Varolius: sphincter
vascular: bud; cataract; circle; circle of optic nerve; cones; dementia; dentin; fold of the cecum; gland; headache; keratitis; lacuna; lamina of choroid; layer; layer of choroid coat of eye; layer of eyeball; layer of testis; leiomyoma; meninx; murmur; nerves; organ of lamina terminalis; papillae; pedicle; plexus; polyp; ring; sclerosis; sheaths; space of retroinguinal compartment; spider; spur; stripe; system; tunic of eye; zone
vasculocardiac: syndrome of hyperserotonemia
vasculogenic: impotence
vasoactive: amine
vasoactive intestinal: peptide; polypeptide

vasodepressor: substance; syncope
vasoformative: cell
vasogenic: shock
vasomotor: angina; ataxia; center; epilepsy; fibers; imbalance; nerve; paralysis; rhinitis
vasoocclusive: crisis
vasopressin-resistant: diabetes
vasopressor: reflex
vasovagal: attack; epilepsy; syncope; syndrome
vastoadductor: fascia
vastus intermedius: muscle
vastus lateralis: muscle
vastus medialis: muscle
VATER: complex
Vater: corpuscles; fold
Vater-Pacini: corpuscles
VCE: smear
VDRL: test
vector: loop
vector-borne: infection
VEE: virus
vegetable: alkali; base; calomel; charcoal; gelatin; sulfur; wax
vegetal: pole
vegetative: bacteriophage; endocarditis; life; reproduction; stage; state
vegetative nervous: system
veil: cell
veiled: cells; puff
veiling: glare
vein: stone; stripper
Vel: antigen
velamentous: insertion
veldt: sore
Vella: fistula
vellus: hair
velocardiofacial: syndrome
velocity: coefficient; constants
velopharyngeal: closure; insufficiency; seal; sphincter
Velpeau: bandage; canal; fossa; hernia
velvet: ant
Ven: antigen
vena cava: filter
vena caval: foramen
venereal: bubo; disease; lymphogranuloma; sore; ulcer; wart
Venezuelan equine: encephalomyelitis
Venezuelan equine encephalomyelitis: virus
Venezuelan hemorrhagic: fever
Venice: turpentine
Venn: diagram
venocaval: filter
venom: hemolysis

Word Finder

venoocclusive: disease of the liver
venorespiratory: reflex
venous: angioma; angle; artery; blood; capillary; circle of mammary gland; congestion; embolism; foramen; gangrene; grooves; heart; hum; hyperemia; insufficiency; lakes; ligament; malformation; murmur; plexus; plexus of bladder; plexus of canal of hypoglossal nerve; plexus of foramen ovale; pulse; return; segments of the kidney; sinuses; sinus of sclera; star; stasis; ulcer; valve
venous occlusion: plethysmography
venous-stasis: retinopathy
ventilation: meter
ventilation-perfusion: scan
ventilation/perfusion: ratio
ventilatory: compliance
ventral: aortas; border; branch; decubitus; funiculus; glands; hernia; horn; mesocardium; mesogastrium; nuclei of thalamus; nucleus of trapezoid body; pallidum; pancreas; part of intertransversarii laterales lumborum (muscles); part of pons; plate; plate of neural tube; rami of cervical nerves; rami of lumbar nerves; rami of sacral nerves; rami of thoracic nerves; ramus of spinal nerve; root of spinal nerve; striatum; surface of digit; thalamus
ventral acoustic: stria
ventral anterior: nucleus [TA] of thalamus
ventral apron: prepuce
ventral intermediate: nucleus [TA] of thalamus
ventral lateral: nucleus of thalamus
ventral lateral geniculate: nucleus
ventral posterior: nucleus of thalamus
ventral posterior intermediate: nucleus of thalamus
ventral posterolateral: nucleus [TA] of thalamus
ventral posteromedial: nucleus [TA] of thalamus
ventral premammillary: nucleus

ventral primary: rami of cervical spinal nerves; rami of lumbar spinal nerves; rami of sacral spinal nerves; rami of thoracic spinal nerves; ramus of spinal nerve
ventral principal: nucleus
ventral raphespinal: tract
ventral sacrococcygeal: ligament; muscle
ventral sacrococcygeus: muscle
ventral sacroiliac: ligaments
ventral spinocerebellar: tract
ventral spinothalamic: tract
ventral splanchnic: arteries
ventral tegmental: decussation
ventral thalamic: peduncle
ventral tier thalamic: nuclei
ventral trigeminothalamic: tract
ventral white: column; commissure
ventricular: aberration; afterload; aneurysm; arteries; band of larynx; bigeminy; bradycardia; capture; complex; conduction; diastole; diverticulum; escape; extrasystole; fibrillation; fluid; flutter; fold; gradient; layer; ligament; loop; plateau; preexcitation; preload; rhythm; septum; standstill; systole; tachycardia; trigone
ventricular assist: device
ventricular filling: pressure
ventricular fusion: beat
ventricular inhibited pulse: generator
ventricular late: potential
ventricular reduction: surgery
ventricular septal: defect
ventricular synchronous pulse: generator
ventricular triggered pulse: generator
ventriculoatrial: conduction
ventriculoradial: dysplasia
ventrobasal: complex; nuclei (complex)
ventrolateral: nucleus; sulcus
ventromedial: nucleus; nucleus of hypothalamus
Venturi: effect; meter; tube
verbal: agraphia; apraxia; autopsy
Veress: needle
Verga: ventricle
Verheyen: stars
Verhoeff elastic tissue: stain

vermian: fossa
vermicular: colic; movement; pulse
vermiform: appendage; appendix; process
vermilion: border; zone
verminous: abscess; appendicitis; ileus
vernal: catarrh; conjunctivitis; encephalitis; keratoconjunctivitis
Verner-Morrison: syndrome
Vernet: syndrome
Verneuil: neuroma
Vernier: acuity
vero: cytotoxin
Verocay: bodies
verrucous: carcinoma; hemangioma; hyperplasia; nevus; scrofuloderma; vegetations; xanthoma
versive: seizure
vertebral: arch; artery; body; border of scapula; canal; column; foramen; formula; fusion; ganglion; groove; line of pleural reflection; nerve; notch; part of the costal surface of the lungs; part of diaphragm; plexus; polyarthritis; pulp; region; ribs; vein; venography
vertebral-basilar: system
vertebral epidural: space
vertebral venous: plexus; system
vertebrate: hormones
vertebrated: catheter; probe
vertebroarterial: foramen
vertebrochondral: ribs
vertebrocostal: trigone
vertebromediastinal: recess
vertebropelvic: ligaments
vertebrosternal: ribs
vertex: presentation
vertical: aspect; axis; crest of internal acoustic meatus; dimension; elastic; heart; hymen; illumination; index; muscle of tongue; nystagmus; opening; osteotomy; overlap; parallax; plate; strabismus; transmission; vertigo
vertical banded: gastroplasty
vertical growth: phase
vertical retraction: syndrome
verticosubmental: view
Vesalius: bone; foramen; vein
vesical: calculus; diverticulum; fistula; gland; hematuria; lithotomy; reflex; surface of uterus; triangle; veins
vesicalis: anus
vesical (nervous): plexus
vesicating: gas

vesicle: hernia
vesicocolic: fistula
vesicocutaneous: fistula
vesicointestinal: fistula
vesicoumbilical: ligament
vesicoureteral: reflux; valve
vesicourethral: canal
vesicouterine: fistula; ligament; pouch
vesicovaginal: fistula
vesicovaginorectal: fistula
vesicular: appendages of epoophoron; appendices of uterine tube; follicle; keratitis; keratopathy; mole; murmur; rale; resonance; respiration; rickettsiosis; stomatitis; transport
vesicular breath: sounds
vesicular exanthema of swine: virus
vesicular ovarian: follicle
vesicular stomatitis: virus
vesicular venous: plexus
vesiculocavernous: respiration
vesiculotympanitic: resonance
Vesling: line
vestibular: anus; apparatus; aqueduct; area; branches of labyrinthine artery; canal; cecum of the cochlear duct; crest; fissure of cochlea; fold; fossa; ganglion; glands; labium of limbus of spiral lamina; labyrinth; lamella (of osseous spiral lamina); ligament; lip of limbus of spiral lamina; lip of spiral limbus; membrane; nerve; neurectomy; neuronitis; nuclei; nystagmus; organ; part of vestibulocochlear nerve; root; root of vestibulocochlear nerve; schwannoma; screen; surface of cochlear duct; surface of tooth; wall of cochlear duct; window
vestibular blind: sac
vestibular hair: cells
vestibulocerebellar: ataxia
vestibulocochlear: artery; nerve [CN VIII]; nuclei; organ
vestibulo-equilibratory: control
vestibuloocular: reflex
vestibulospinal: reflex; tracts
vestigial: fold; muscle; organ
Veterans Administration: hospital
veterinary: medicine
Vi: antibody; antigen
viable cell: count
vibrating: line

vibration: syndrome; tolerance

vibratory: massage; sensibility; urticaria

vicarious: hypertrophy; menstruation

vicious: cicatrix; circle; union

Vicq d'Azyr: bundle; centrum semiovale; foramen

Vidal: disease

video: fluoroscopy

video-assisted thoracic: surgery

vidian: artery; canal; nerve; vein

Vierra: sign

Vieth-Müller: circle

Vieussens: ansa; anulus; centrum; foramina; ganglia; isthmus; limbus; loop; ring; valve; veins; ventricle

view: box

villous: adenoma; atrophy; carcinoma; papilloma; placenta; tenosynovitis; tumor

Vinca: alkaloids

Vincent: angina; bacillus; disease; infection; spirillum; tonsillitis

Vincent white: mycetoma

Vineberg: procedure

vinegar: eel

vinous: liquor

violinist's: cramp

Vipond: sign

viral: cystitis; dysentery; encephalomyelitis; envelope; gastroenteritis; hemagglutination; hepatitis; hepatitis type A; hepatitis type B; hepatitis type C; hepatitis type D; hepatitis type E; load; neutralization; pericarditis; probe; strand; therapy; tropism; wart

viral hemorrhagic: fever

viral hemorrhagic fever: virus

Virchow: angle; cells; corpuscles; crystals; disease; law; node; psammoma

Virchow-Hassall: bodies

Virchow-Holder: angle

Virchow-Robin: space

virgin: generation; silk

virginal: membrane

Virginia: snakeroot

viridans: hemolysis; streptococci

virile: member

virtual: endoscopy; focus; image

virulent: bacteriophage; bubo

virulent phage: mutant

virus: blockade; hepatitis; keratoconjunctivitis

virus A: hepatitis

virus-associated hemophagocytic: syndrome

virus B: hepatitis

virus C: hepatitis

virus-transformed: cell

virus X: disease

visceral: anesthesia; arches; brain; cavity; cleft; crises; disorder; epilepsy; fascia; inversion; larva migrans; layer; layer of serous pericardium; layer of tunica vaginalis of testis; leishmaniasis; lymph nodes; lymph nodes of abdomen; mesoderm; muscle; nerve; nodes; nuclei of oculomotor nerve; pericardium; peritoneum; plate; pleura; pleurisy; sense; skeleton; surface of liver; surface of the spleen; swallow

visceral disease: virus

visceral motor: fibers; neuron; system

visceral nervous: system

visceral pelvic: fascia

visceral traction: reflex

viscerogenic: reflex

visceromotor: reflex

viscerosensory: reflex

viscerotrophic: reflex

viscoelastic: retardation

visibility: acuity

visible: spectrum

visiting: nurse

visna: virus

visual: acuity; agnosia; angle; aphasia; area; aura; axis; blackout; cortex; cycle; efficiency; extinction; field; image; inattention; inspection with acetic acid; organ; pathway; pigments; projection; purple; threshold; vertigo; violet; yellow

visual evoked: potential

visual-kinetic: dissociation

visual orbicularis: reflex

visual receptor: cells

visual-spatial: agnosia

vita: glass

vital: capacity; center; force; index; knot; node; pulp; signs; spirits; stain; statistics; tooth; tripod

vitality: test

vitamin A: unit

vitamin B$_{12}$: neuropathy

vitamin B$_2$: unit

vitamin B$_6$: unit

vitamin B$_1$ hydrochloride: unit

vitamin C: test; unit

vitamin D: milk; unit

vitamin D–binding: protein

vitamin D-resistant: rickets

vitamin E: unit

vitamin K: unit

vitelliform: degeneration

vitelliform retinal: dystrophy

vitelline: artery; cord; duct; fistula; membrane; pole; reservoir; sac; vein; vessels

vitelliruptive: degeneration

vitellointestinal: cyst

vitiated: air

vitiliginous: choroiditis

vitreoretinal choroidopathy: syndrome

vitreoretinal traction: syndrome

vitreotapetoretinal: dystrophy

vitreous: body; camera; cell; chamber; chamber of eye; detachment; hernia; humor; lamella; membrane; table

in vitro: fertilization

vivax: fever; malaria

in vivo: fertilization

Vladimiroff-Mikulicz: amputation

VMA: test

vocal: amusia; cord; fold; fremitus; ligament; muscle; process; process of arytenoid cartilage; resonance; shelf; spectrum; tract

vocal cord: nodules

vocalis: muscle

Vogel: law

Voges-Proskauer: reaction

Vogt: angle; syndrome

Vogt-Koyanagi: syndrome

Vogt-Spielmeyer: disease

Vohwinkel: syndrome

voice fatigue: syndrome

voiding: cystogram; cystourethrogram

voiding flow: rate

voiding internal urethral: orifice

volar carpal: ligament

volar interosseous: artery; nerve

volatile: anesthetic; mustard oil; oil

volatile fatty acid: number

Volhard: test

volitional: tremor

Volkmann: canals; cheilitis; contracture; spoon

Vollmer: test

Volpe-Manhold: Index

voltage-gated: channel

voltaic: taste

Voltolini: disease

volume: element; index; substitute; unit

volume-controlled: respirator

volume-displacement: plethysmograph

volume-time: curve

volumetric: analysis; flask; solution

voluntary: dehydration; guarding; hospital; muscle; mutism; nystagmus

volutin: granules

vomeral: groove; sulcus

vomerine: canal; cartilage; crest of choana; groove

vomerobasilar: canal

vomeronasal: cartilage; organ

vomerorostral: canal

vomerovaginal: canal; groove

vomiting: gas; reflex

von Economo: disease

von Gierke: disease

von Graefe: sign

von Hippel: disease

von Hippel-Lindau: syndrome

von Kossa: stain

von Recklinghausen: disease

von Spee: curve

von Willebrand: disease; factor

Voorhoeve: disease

vortex: veins

vortex corneal: dystrophy

vorticose: veins

Vossius lenticular: ring

V-pattern: esotropia; exotropia

VS: virus

V-shaped: area of esophagus

vulnerable: period; phase

vulnerable child: syndrome

Vulpian: atrophy

vulsella: forceps

vulvar: dystrophy; slit

vulvar intraepithelial: neoplasia

vulvovaginal: cystectomy; gland

Vw: antigen

V-Y: flap

W

W: chromosome; factor; rays

W-: arch

"w": hernia

Waardenburg: syndrome

Wachendorf: membrane

Wachstein-Meissel: stain for calcium-magnesium-ATPase

Wada: test

waddingtonian: homeostasis

waddling: gait

Wagner: disease; syndrome

WAGR: syndrome

waist-hip: ratio

waiter's: cramp

Walcher: position
Waldenström: macroglobulinemia; purpura; syndrome; test
Waldeyer: fossae; glands; sheath; space; tract
Waldeyer throat: ring
Waldeyer zonal: layer
Walker: chart; tractotomy
walking: typhoid
walk-through: angina
Wallenberg: syndrome
wallerian: degeneration; law
wallet: stomach
wall-eyed bilateral internuclear: ophthalmoplegia
Walsh: procedure
Walthard cell: rest
Walther: canals; dilator; ducts; ganglion; plexus
wandering: abscess; cell; erysipelas; goiter; kidney; liver; organ; pacemaker; pneumonia
Wang: test
Wangensteen: drainage; suction; tube
war: neurosis
warble: botfly; fly
Warburg: apparatus; theory
Warburg-Dickens-Horecker: shunt
Warburg-Lipmann-Dickens-Horecker: shunt
Warburg old yellow: enzyme
Warburg respiratory: enzyme
Ward: triangle
Ward-Romano: syndrome
Wardrop: disease; method
warehouseman's: itch
warm: agglutinins; autoantibody
warm-blooded: animal
warm-cold: hemolysin
warmup: phenomenon
Warren: shunt
Wartenberg: symptom
Warthin: tumor
Warthin-Finkeldey: cells
Warthin-Starry silver: stain
warty: dyskeratoma; horn
wash-: bottle
washed: sulfur
washed field: technique
washerwoman's: itch
washing: soda
washout: cannula; test
Wasmann: glands
wasserhelle: cell
Wassermann: antibody; reaction; test
wasted: ventilation
wasting: disease; syndrome
watchmaker's: cramp

water: aspirator; bath; bed; canker; depletion; diuresis; dressing; gas; glass; intoxication; itch; sore
water-clear: cell of parathyroid
water-drinking: test
water-hammer: pulse
Waterhouse-Friderichsen: syndrome
watering-can: perineum; scrotum
Waters: operation; projection; view
watershed: infarction
water-soluble: chlorophyll derivatives
Waterston: operation; shunt
Waters view: radiograph
water-trap: stomach
water wheel: murmur
waterwheel: sound
water-whistle: sound
watery: eye
Watson-Crick: helix
Watson-Schwartz: test
wave: analyzer; form; number
wax: acid; alcohol; expansion; form; pattern
wax model: denture
wax-tipped: bougie
waxy: cast; degeneration; fingers; kidney; liver; spleen
WDHA: syndrome
wear-and-tear: pigment
weaver's: cough
web: eye
Webb: antigen
webbed: fingers; neck; penis; toes
Weber: glands; law; organ; paradox; point; sign; stain; syndrome; test for hearing; triangle
Weber-Christian: disease
Weber-Cockayne: syndrome
Weber-Fechner: law
Webster: test
Wechsler-Bellevue: scale
Wechsler intelligence: scales
weddellite: calculus
Wedensky: effect; facilitation; inhibition
wedge: biopsy; bone; pressure; resection; spirometer
wedge-and-groove: joint; suture
wedge-shaped: fasciculus; tubercle
WEE: virus
weekend: hospital
Weeks: bacillus
weeping: eczema
Wegener: granulomatosis
Wegner: disease; line
Weibel-Palade: bodies

Weichselbaum: coccus
Weidel: reaction
Weigert: law; stain for actinomyces; stain for elastin; stain for fibrin; stain for myelin; stain for neuroglia
Weigert-Gram: stain
Weigert iodine: solution
Weigert iron hematoxylin: stain
weight: sense
Weil: disease
Weil basal: layer; zone
Weil-Felix: reaction; test
Weill-Marchesani: syndrome
Weinberg: reaction
Weingrow: reflex
Weir: operation
Weir Mitchell: disease; treatment
Weisbach: angle
Weiss: sign
Weitbrecht: cartilage; cord; fibers; foramen; ligament
Welch: bacillus
Welcker: angle
welder's: conjunctivitis; lung
well: counter
well-differentiated lymphocytic: lymphoma
Wells: syndrome
Wenckebach: block; period; phenomenon
Wenzel: ventricle
Wepfer: glands
Werdnig-Hoffmann: disease
Werdnig-Hoffmann muscular: atrophy
Werlhof: disease
Wermer: syndrome
Wernekinck: commissure; decussation
Werner: syndrome; test
Wernicke: aphasia; area; center; disease; encephalopathy; field; radiation; reaction; region; sign; syndrome; zone
Wernicke-Korsakoff: encephalopathy; syndrome
Wertheim: operation
Werther: disease
Wesselsbron: disease; fever
Wesselsbron disease: virus
West: syndrome
West African: fever; trypanosomiasis
West African sleeping: sickness
Westberg: space
Westergren: method
Westermark: sign
Western blot: analysis
western equine: encephalomyelitis

western equine encephalomyelitis: virus
West Indian: smallpox
West Nile: fever; virus
West Nile encephalitis: virus
Westphal-Piltz: phenomenon
Westphal pupillary: reflex
wet: beriberi; compress; cup; dream; gangrene; lung; nurse; pack; pleurisy; shock; tetter
wet cutaneous: leishmaniasis
wet and dry bulb: thermometer
wettable: sulfur
wet-technique: liposuction
wet-to-dry: dressing
Wetzel: grid
Wever-Bray: phenomenon
Weyers-Thier: syndrome
whale: fingers
Wharton: duct; jelly
wheal-and-erythema: reaction
wheal-and-flare: reaction
wheat: germ; gum
Wheatstone: bridge
Wheeler: method
Wheeler-Johnson: test
whetstone: crystals
whewellite: calculus
whey: alum; protein
whiff: test
whip: bougie
whiplash: injury; retinopathy
Whipple: disease; operation
whispered: bronchophony; pectoriloquy
whistle-tip: catheter
whistling: deformity; rale
whistling face: syndrome
Whitaker: test
white: arsenic; beeswax; bile; commissure; corpuscle; fat; fiber; fingers; forelock; gangrene; infarct; lead; line; line of anal canal; line of Toldt; matter; muscle; mustard; noise; petrolatum; piedra; pine; pitch; pulp; pulp of spleen; rami communicantes; reaction; spot; substance; thrombus; turpentine; wax; yolk
white blood: cell
white blood cell: cast
white cell: cast
whitegraft: reaction
Whitehead: deformity; operation
white limbal: girdle of Vogt
white mercuric: precipitate
white-out: syndrome
white pupillary: reflex
white soft: paraffin
white sponge: nevus
white spot: disease

Whitman: frame
Whitmore: bacillus; disease
Whitnall: tubercle
whole: blood
whole-body: counter
whole-body titration: curve
whooping: cough
whooping-cough: vaccine
whorled: enamel
WI-38: cells
Wickham: striae
Widal: reaction; syndrome
wide: plane; spectrum
wide dynamic range: compression
wide field: ocular
wide-latitude: film
Wigand: maneuver
Wilbrand: knee
wild: ginger; mandrake; tobacco; type; yeast
Wilde: cords; triangle
Wilder: diet; sign; stain for reticulum
Wildermuth: ear
Wildervanck: syndrome
wildfire: rash
wild-type: strain
Wilhelmy: balance
Wilkie: disease
Willett: forceps
Williams: factor; stain; syndrome
Williams-Beuren: syndrome
Willis: centrum nervosum; cords; pancreas; paracusis; pouch
Williston: law
Wilms: tumor
Wilson: disease; lichen; method; muscle
Wilson-Mikity: syndrome
Windigo: psychosis
window: level; width
wine: spirit
wing: cell; plate
wing-beating: tremor
winged: catheter; scapula
Winiwarter-Buerger: disease
wink: reflex
winking: spasm
Winkler: disease
Winslow: ligament; pancreas; stars
winter: eczema; itch; sleep
Winterbottom: sign
Winternitz: sound
Wintersteiner: compound F; rosettes
wire: arch; splint
wire-loop: lesion
Wirsung: canal; duct
wiry: pulse
wisdom: tooth
Wiskott-Aldrich: syndrome
Wissler: syndrome

Wistar: rats
witch's: milk
withdrawal: reflex; symptoms; syndrome
wobble: base; hypothesis
Wohlfart-Kugelberg-Welander: disease
Wolfe: graft
Wolfe-Krause: graft
Wolff: law
Wolff-Chaikoff: block; effect
wolffian: body; cyst; duct; rest; ridge; tubules
wolffian duct: carcinoma
Wolff-Parkinson-White: syndrome
Wölfler: gland
Wolf-Orton: bodies
Wolfram: syndrome
Wolfring: glands
Wollaston: doublet; theory
Wolman: disease; xanthomatosis
Wood: glass; lamp; light; units
wood: charcoal; naphtha; spirit; sugar; vinegar
woodcutter's: encephalitis
wooden: resonance
wooden-shoe: heart
wool: wax
Woolf-Lineweaver-Burk: plot
woolly: hair
woolly hair: nevus
Woolner: tip
woolsorter's: disease; pneumonia
word: deafness
Woringer-Kolopp: disease
working: bite; contacts; occlusion; side
working occlusal: surfaces
working side: condyle
worm: abscess
wormian: bones
Wormley: test
Worth: amblyoscope
Woulfe: bottle
wound: botulism; clip; dehiscence; fever; myiasis
woven: bone
Wr^a: antigen
Wright: antigens; respirometer; stain; syndrome; version
wrinkler: muscle of eyebrow
Wrisberg: cartilage; ganglia; ligament; nerve; tubercle
wrist: clonus; joint; sign
wrist clonus: reflex
wrist-hand: orthosis
writer's: cramp
writhing: number
writing: hand
wrought: wire
wry: neck
Wurster: reagent; test

Wyburn-Mason: syndrome

X

χ^2**:** test
X: body; disease; inactivation; zone
X-: strabismus
x: wave
x-: ray
xanthene: dyes
xanthogranulomatous: cholecystitis; pyelonephritis
xanthoprotein: reaction
xenic: culture
xenogeneic: graft
xenon-arc: photocoagulator
xenotropic: virus
xerotic: degeneration; keratitis
Xg: antigen
xiphisternal: joint
xiphisternal crunching: sound
xiphocostal: angle
xiphoid: cartilage; process
X-linked: agammaglobulinemia; gene; hypogammaglobulinemia; hypogammaglobulinemia with growth hormone deficiency; ichthyosis; inheritance; locus
X-linked lymphoproliferative: disease; syndrome
X-linked recessive bulbospinal: neuronopathy
XO: female; syndrome
X-pattern: esotropia; exotropia
x-ray: dosimetry; generator; microscope; therapy; tube
XX: male
XXX: female
XXY: male; syndrome
xylose: test
xylostyptic: ether
XYY: male; syndrome

Y

Y: body; cartilage
Y-: axis
y: wave
y-: angle
Yaba: virus
Yaba monkey: virus
Yangtze: edema
Yangtze Valley: fever
yeast: fungus; RNase
yeast artificial: chromosomes
yeast extract: agar
yellow: atrophy of the liver; body; cartilage; corallin; disease; enzyme; fever; fibers; hepatization;

ligament; mercury iodide; nail; precipitate; skin; spot; vision; wax; yolk
yellow bone: marrow
yellow fever: vaccine; virus
yellow nail: syndrome
yellow soft: paraffin
yield: strength; stress
Y-linked: gene; inheritance; locus
yoke: bone
yolk: cells; cleavage; membrane; sac; stalk
yolk sac: carcinoma; tumor
Yorke autolytic: reaction
Young: modulus; rule; syndrome
Young-Helmholtz: theory of color vision
Young prostatic: tractor
Y-shaped: ligament
Yt^a: antigen
Yvon: test

Z

Z: band; disk; filament; gene; line
Z-: DNA; protein
Zaffaroni: system
Zaglas: ligament
Zahn: infarct
Zaire: virus
Zambesi: ulcer
Zappert counting: chamber
Zarit burden: interview
Zavanelli: maneuver
zebra: body
Zeeman: effect
Zeis: glands
zeisian: sty
Zellweger: syndrome
Zenker: degeneration; diverticulum; fixative; paralysis
zero: gravity
zero degree: teeth
zero end-expiratory: pressure
zero-order: reaction
zero time-binding: DNA
zeta: potential
zeta sedimentation: ratio
Ziehen-Oppenheim: disease
Ziehl: stain
Ziehl-Neelsen: stain
Ziemann: dots; stippling
Zieve: syndrome
Zika: fever; virus
Zimmerlin: atrophy
Zimmermann: corpuscle; granule; reaction; test
Zimmermann elementary: particle
zinc: colic; finger; gelatin
zinc fume: fever
zinc phosphate: cement

zinc sulfate flotation: concentration

zinc sulfate flotation centrifugation: method

Zinn: artery; corona; ligament; membrane; ring; tendon; zonule

Zinn vascular: circle

zirconium: granuloma

Zivert: syndrome

Zollinger-Ellison: syndrome; tumor

Zöllner: lines

zonal: necrosis

zonary: placenta

zone: centrifugation

zonular: band; cataract; fibers; layer; scotoma; spaces

zoo blot: analysis

Zoon: erythroplasia

zoonotic: infection; potential

zoonotic cutaneous: leishmaniasis

zooplastic: graft

zoster: encephalomyelitis

zoster immune: globulin

Zsigmondy: test

Z-tract: injection

Zubrod: scale

Zuckerkandl: bodies; convolution; fascia

zwitter: hypothesis

zwitterionic: buffer; detergent; surfactant

zygal: fissure

zygapophysial: joints

zygomatic: arch; bone; border of greater wing of sphenoid bone; branches of facial nerve; diameter; fossa; margin of greater wing of sphenoid bone; nerve; process of frontal bone; process of maxilla; process of temporal bone; region

zygomaticoauricular: index

zygomaticofacial: branch of zygomatic nerve; foramen

zygomaticomaxillary: suture

zygomatico-orbital: artery; foramen

zygomaticotemporal: branch of zygomatic nerve; foramen; suture

zygomaticus major: muscle

zygomaticus minor: muscle

zygomaxillary: point

zymogen: granule

zymogenic: cell

zymoplastic: substance

zymotic: papilloma

ZZ: genotype

α **1.** First letter of the Greek alphabet, alpha; used as a classifier in the nomenclature of many sciences. **2.** Symbol for Bunsen solubility *coefficient*. **3.** In chemistry, denotes the first in a series, a position immediately adjacent to a carboxyl group, the first of a series of closely related compounds, an aromatic substituent on an aliphatic chain, or the direction of a chemical bond away from the viewer. **4.** Abbreviation for alpha *particle*. **5.** In chemistry, symbol for angle of optic *rotation*; degree of dissociation. For terms beginning with this prefix, see the specific term.

[α] Symbol for specific optic *rotation*.

α₁PI Abbreviation for human α_1-protease *inhibitor*.

A 1. Abbreviation for ampere; adenine; alanine. **2.** As a subscript, refers to alveolar *gas*. **3.** Symbol (usually capitalized italic) for absorbance. **4.** Symbol for adenosine or adenylic acid in polynucleotides; alanine or alanyl in polypeptides; first substrate in a multisubstrate enzyme-catalyzed reaction.

Å Symbol for angstrom.

°A Symbol for degree absolute; replaced by K (kelvin).

A⁻ Symbol for anion.

A. Symbol for absorbance; Helmholtz *energy*.

a 1. Abbreviation for total *acidity*; ante; area; asymmetric; auris; artery; arteria [TA]. **2.** Symbol for atto-. **3.** As a subscript, refers to systemic arterial blood.

a Symbol for specific absorption *coefficient*; abbreviation for absorptivity.

⌂**a-, an-.** Not, without, -less; equivalent to L. in- and E. un-. [G. not, un-, usually *an-* before a vowel]

AA, aa Abbreviation for amino acid; aminoacyl.

aa. Abbreviation for arteries [TA], arteriae [TA].

āā. Abbreviation for G. *ana*, of each; used in prescription writing following the name of two or more ingredients.

AAA Abbreviation for abdominal aortic aneurysm; commonly, procedure for surgical correction of an AAA.

Aad Abbreviation for α-aminoadipic acid.

AAF Abbreviation for 2-acetylaminofluorene; 2-acetamidofluorene.

Aagenaes, O., Norwegian physician. SEE Aagenaes *syndrome*.

AAMC Abbreviation for Association of American Medical Colleges.

AAR Abbreviation for antigen-antibody *reaction*.

Aaron, Charles D., U.S. physician, 1866–1951. SEE A. *sign*.

Aarskog, Dagfinn J., Norwegian pediatrician, *1928. SEE A.-Scott *syndrome*.

AASH Abbreviation for adrenal androgen-stimulating *hormone*.

AAV Abbreviation for adeno-associated *virus*.

Ab Abbreviation for antibody.

⌂**ab-, abs-. 1.** From, away from, off. **2.** Prefix applied to electrical units in the CGS-electromagnetic system to distinguish them from units in the CGS-electrostatic system (prefix stat-) and those in the metric system or SI (no prefix). [L. *ab*, from, usually *abs-* before c, q, and t; often *a-* before m, p, or v]

Abadie, Joseph Louis Irénée Jean, French neurosurgeon, 1873–1946. SEE A. *sign* of tabes dorsalis.

ab·am·pere (ab-am′pēr). Electromagnetic unit of current equal to 10 absolute amperes; a current that exerts a force of 2π dynes on a unit magnetic pole at the center of a circle of wire 1 cm in radius.

abap·i·cal (ă-bap′i-kăl). Opposite the apex.

abar·og·no·sis (ă-bar′og-nō′sis). Loss of ability to appreciate the weight of objects held in the hand, or to differentiate objects of different weights. When the primary senses are intact, caused by a lesion of the contralateral parietal lobe. [G. *a-* priv. + *baros*, weight, + *gnōsis*, knowledge]

aba·sia (ă-bā′zē-ă). Inability to walk. SEE gait. [G. *a-* priv. + *basis*, step]

atactic a., ataxic a., difficulty in walking due to ataxia of the legs.

aba·si·a-asta·si·a. SEE astasia-abasia.

aba·sic (ă-bā′sik). **1.** Affected by, or associated with, abasia. **2.** Refers to loss of pyrimidine sites in DNA. SYN abatic.

abate·ment (ă-bāt′ment). **1.** A diminution or easing. **2.** Reduction, ultimately elimination, of public health nuisances such as smoke, loud noise. [abate, fr. M.E. *abaten*, fr. O.Fr. *abattre*, to beat down, fr. L. L. *batto*, to beat, + -ment]

sound a., generic term for any measures to reduce environmental noise.

abatic (ă-bat′ik). SYN abasic.

ab·ax·i·al, ab·ax·ile (ab-ak′sē-ăl, -ak′sīl). **1.** Lying outside the axis of any body or part. **2.** Situated at the opposite extremity of the axis of a part.

Abbe, Robert W., U.S. surgeon, 1851–1928. SEE A. *flap*.

Abbé, Ernst K., German physicist, 1840–1905. SEE A. *condenser*.

Abbott, W. Osler, U.S. physician, 1902–1943. SEE A. *tube*; Miller-A. *tube*.

Abbott, Alexander C., U.S. bacteriologist, 1860–1935. SEE A. *stain* for spores.

Abbott ar·tery. See under artery.

abciximab. Monoclonal antibody with antithrombotic properties used for the prevention and treatment of arterial occlusive disorders.

ab·cou·lomb (ab-koo-lom′). A unit of electrical charge equal to 10 coulombs. The charge that passes over a given surface in 1 sec if a current of 1 abampere is flowing across the surface. [ab + coulomb]

🔲**ab·do·men** (ab-dō′men, ab′dō-men) [TA]. The part of the trunk that lies between the thorax and the pelvis. The a. does not include the vertebral region posteriorly but is considered by some anatomists to include the pelvis (abdominopelvic cavity). It includes the greater part of the abdominal cavity (cavitas abdominis [TA]), and is divided by arbitrary planes into nine regions. SEE ALSO abdominal *regions*, under *region*. SYN venter (1) [TA]. [L. *abdomen*, etym. uncertain]

acute a., any serious acute intra-abdominal condition (such as appendicitis) attended by pain, tenderness, and muscular rigidity, and for which emergency surgery must be considered. SYN surgical a.

carinate a., a sloping of the sides with prominence of the central line of the a.

navicular a., SYN scaphoid a.

a. obsti′pum, rarely used term for deformity of the a. due to congenitally short rectus muscles.

pendulous a., an a. with greatly relaxed muscular walls that sag down over the pubic region.

protuberant a., unusual or prominent convexity of the a., due to excessive subcutaneous fat, poor muscle tone, or an increase in intraabdominal content.

scaphoid a., a condition in which the anterior abdominal wall is sunken and presents a concave rather than a convex contour. SYN navicular a.

surgical a., SYN acute a.

ab·dom·i·nal (ab-dom′i-năl). Relating to the abdomen.

⌂**abdomino-, abdomin-.** The abdomen, abdominal. [L. *abdomen*, *abdominis*]

⌂ **Combining Forms**	☆ **Official alternate Terminologia Anatomica term**
🔲 **Indicates term is illustrated, see Illustration Index**	
SYN Synonym	**[MIM] Mendelian Inheritance in Man**
Cf. Compare	**C.I. Colour Index**
[NA] Nomina Anatomica	
[TA] Terminologia Anatomica	**High Profile Term**

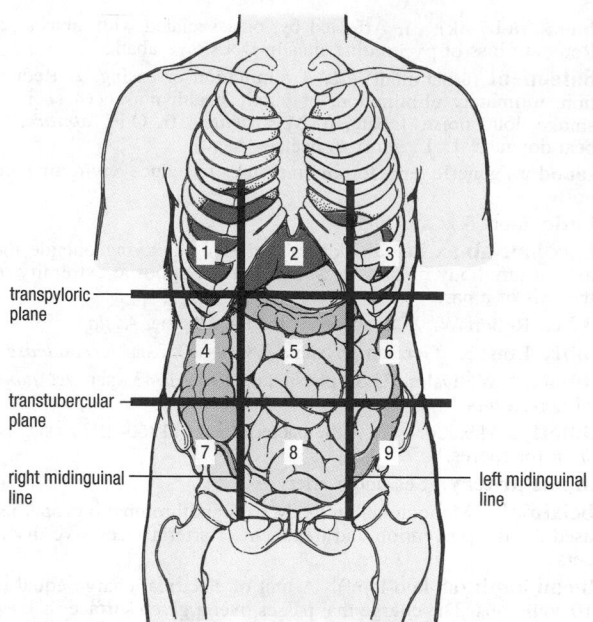

abdominal regions: (1) right hypochondriac, (2) epigastric, (3) left hypochondriac, (4) right lateral (lumbar), (5) umbilical, (6) left lateral (lumbar), (7) right iliac, (8) hypogastric (suprapubic), (9) left iliac

ab·dom·i·no·cen·te·sis (ab-dom′i-nō-sen-tē′sis). Paracentesis of the abdomen. [abdomino- + G. *kentēsis,* puncture]

ab·dom·i·no·cy·e·sis (ab-dom′i-nō-sī-ē′sis). **1.** SYN abdominal *pregnancy.* **2.** SYN secondary abdominal *pregnancy.* [abdomino- + G. *kyēsis,* pregnancy]

ab·dom·i·no·cys·tic (ab-dom-i-nō-sis′tik). SYN abdominovesical. [abdomino- + G. *kystis,* bladder]

ab·dom·i·no·gen·i·tal (ab-dom′i-nō-gen′i-tăl). Relating to the abdomen and the genital organs.

ab·dom·i·no·hys·ter·ec·to·my (ab-dom′i-nō-his-ter-ek′tō-mē). SYN abdominal *hysterectomy.*

ab·dom·i·no·hys·ter·ot·o·my (ab-dom′i-nō-his-ter-ot′ō-mē). SYN abdominal *hysterotomy.*

ab·dom·i·no·pel·vic (ab-dom′i-nō-pel′vik). Relating to the abdomen and pelvis, especially the combined abdominal and pelvic cavities.

ab·dom·i·no·per·i·ne·al (ab-dom′i-nō-păr-i-nē′ăl). Relating to both abdomen and perineum, as in abdominoperineal resection of the rectum.

ab·dom·i·no·plas·ty (ab-dom′i-nō-plas-tē). An operation performed on the abdominal wall for cosmetic purposes. [abdomino- + G. *plastos,* formed]

ab·dom·i·nos·co·py (ab-dom-i-nos′kŏ-pē). SYN laparoscopy. [abdomino- + G. *skopeō,* to examine]

ab·dom·i·no·scro·tal (ab-dom′i-nō-skrō′tăl). Relating to the abdomen and the scrotum.

ab·dom·i·no·tho·rac·ic (ab-dom′i-nō-thō-ras′ik). Relating to both abdomen and thorax.

ab·dom·i·no·vag·i·nal (ab-dom′i-nō-vag′i-năl). Relating to both abdomen and vagina.

ab·dom·i·no·ves·i·cal (ab-dom′i-nō-ves′i-kăl). Relating to the abdomen and urinary bladder, or to the abdomen and gallbladder. SYN abdominocystic.

ab·duce (ab-doos′). SYN abduct.

ab·du·cens (ab-doo′senz). SYN abducent. [L.]
   a. oc′uli, SYN lateral rectus (*muscle*).

ab·du·cent (ab-doo′sent). **1.** Abducting; drawing away, especially

away from the median plane. **2.** SYN abducent *nerve* [CN VI]. SYN abducens. [L. *abducens*]

ab·duct (ab-dŭkt′). To move away from the median plane. SYN abduce.

ab·duc·tion (ab-dŭk′shŭn). **1.** Movement of a body part away from the median plane (of the body, in the case of limbs; of the hand or foot, in the case of digits). **2.** Monocular rotation (duction) of the eye toward the temple. **3.** A position resulting from such movement. Cf. adduction. [L. *abductio*]

ab·duc·tor (ab-dŭk′ter, -tōr). SYN abductor (*muscle*).

Abegg, Richard, Danish chemist, 1869–1910. SEE A. *rule.*

Abell-Kendall meth·od. See under method.

Abelson, Herbert T., U.S. pediatrician, *1941. SEE A. murine leukemia *virus.*

ab·em·bry·on·ic (ab′em-brē-on′ik). The area of the blastocyst opposite the region where the embryo is formed. [L. *ab,* from, + embryonic]

ab·en·ter·ic (ab-en-ter′ik). A rarely used term meaning away from the intestine, said of a morbid process occurring elsewhere that would normally occur in the intestine. [L. *ab,* from, + G. *enteron,* intestine]

Abernethy, John, British surgeon and anatomist, 1764–1831. SEE A. *fascia.*

ab·er·rant (ab-er′ant). **1.** Differing from the normal; in botany or zoology, said of certain atypical individuals in a species. **2.** Wandering off; said of certain ducts, vessels, or nerves deviating from the normal course or pattern. **3.** SYN ectopic (1). [L. *aberrans*]

ab·er·ra·tion (ab-er-ā′shŭn). **1.** Deviating from the normal course or pattern. **2.** Deviant development or growth. SEE ALSO chromosome. [L. *aberratio*]
   chromatic a., the difference in focus or magnification of an image arising because of a difference in the refraction of different wavelengths composing white light. SYN chromatism (2), color a., newtonian a.
   chromosome a., any deviation from the normal number or morphology of chromosomes; also the phenotypic consequences thereof.

frequent numerical chromosome aberrations	
	Chromosome Count
autosomal trisomy G (Down syndrome)	
1 extra chromosome 21	
a) extra chromosome normal	47
with mosaicism	46/47
b) translocation G/G extra chromosome, fused	46
with chromosome 21 or 22	
c) translocation D/G extra chromosome, fused with a	46
chromosome of the D group	
trisomy D (Patau syndrome) 1 extra D1, chromosome (no. 13)	47
trisomy E (Edward syndrome) 1 extra chromosome 18	47
sex chromosomes monosomy X-XO (Turner syndrome) 1 X-chromosome is missing, female phenotype	45 (Ø)
trisomy XXX 1 extra X chromosome, female phenotype	47 (++)
trisomy XXY 1 extra X chromosome, male phenotype (Klinefelter syndrome)	47 (+)
1 extra Y chromosome, usually male phenotype	47 (Ø)
tetrasomies (XXXY, XXYY) and pentasomies are rarely observed	

color a., SYN chromatic a.

coma a., (1) the distortion of image formation created when a bundle of light rays enters an optical system not parallel to the optic axis. (2) in botany, any tuft, as the hairs on a seed, or the greenery on a radish or a pineapple. SYN coma (3). [G. *komē*, hair, foliage]

curvature a., lack of spatial correspondence causing the image of a straight extended object to appear curved.

dioptric a., SYN spherical a.

distortion a., the faulty formation of an image arising because the magnification of the peripheral part of an object is different from that of the central part when viewed through a lens. SEE ALSO Petzval *surface*.

lateral a., in spherical a., the distance between paraxial focus of central rays on the optic axis.

longitudinal a., in spherical a., the distance separating the focus of paraxial and peripheral rays on the optic axis.

mental a., disturbed thought or behavior that connotes a psychological or psychiatric impairment. SEE delusion.

meridional a., an a. produced in the plane of a single meridian of a lens.

monochromatic a., a defect in an optical image arising because of the nature of lenses; the main types are spherical, coma, curvature, and distortion a., and astigmatism of oblique pencils.

newtonian a., SYN chromatic a.

optical a., failure of rays from a point source to form a perfect image after traversing an optical system.

spherical a., a monochromatic a. occurring in refraction at a spherical surface in which the paraxial and peripheral rays focus along the axis at different points. SYN dioptric a.

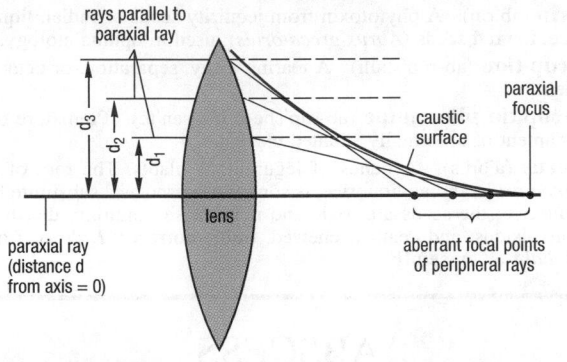

aberration (spherical)

ventricular a., SYN aberrant ventricular *conduction*.

ab·er·rom·e·ter (ab-er-rom′ĕ-ter). An instrument for measuring optical aberration or any error in experimentation. [L. *aberratio,* aberration, + G. *metron,* measure]

abe·ta·lip·o·pro·tein·e·mia (ā-bā′tă-lip′ō-prō′tēn-ē′mē-ă) [MIM*200100]. A disorder characterized by an absence of low-density beta-lipoprotein, presence of acanthocytes in blood, retinal pigmentary degeneration, malabsorption, engorgement of upper intestinal absorptive cells with dietary triglycerides, and neuromuscular abnormalities; autosomal recessive inheritance, caused by mutation in the gene encoding microsomal triglyceride transfer protein (MTP) on chromosome 4q. SYN Bassen-Kornzweig syndrome. [G. *a-,* priv., + β, + lipoprotein + *-emia,* blood]

normotriglyceridemic a., a. with normal levels of triglycerides. This inherited disorder (possibly autosomal recessive) is probably due to the absence of apolipoprotein B-100.

abey·ance (ă-bā′ans). A state of temporary abolition of function. [fr. O. Fr.]

ab·far·ad (ab-far′ad). Electromagnetic unit of capacity equal to 10^9 farads.

ABG Abbreviation for arterial blood gas. SEE blood *gases,* under *gas.*

ab·hen·ry (ab-hen′rē). Electromagnetic unit of inductance equal to 10^{-9} henry.

abil·i·ty (ă-bil′i-tē). The physical, mental, or legal competence to function. [L. *habilitas,* aptitude]

abi·ot·ic (ā-bī-ot′ik). **1.** Incompatible with life. **2.** Without life.

ab·i·ot·ro·phy (ab-ē-ot′rō-fē). An age-dependent manifestation of a genetically determined trait. [G. *a-* priv. + *bios,* life, + *trophē,* nourishment]

ab·ir·ri·ta·tion (ab-ir-i-tā′shŭn). Obsolete term for diminution or abolition of irritability in a part. [L. *ab,* from, + *irrito,* pp. *-atus,* to irritate]

abl An oncogene found in the Abelson strain of mouse leukemia virus and involved in the Philadelphia chromosome translocation in chronic granulocytic leukemia.

ablas·te·mic (ā-blas-tem′ik). Not germinal or blastemic. [G. *a-* priv. + *blastēma,* sprout]

ablas·tin (ă-blas′tin). An antibody that seems to inhibit reproduction of trypanosomes; found in rats infected with *Trypanosoma lewisi.* [G. *a-* priv. + *blastos,* germ]

ab·late (ab-lāt′). To remove, or to destroy the function of. [L. *aufero,* pp. *ab- latus,* to take away]

ab·la·tion (ab-lā′shun). Removal of a body part or the destruction of its function, as by a surgical procedure, morbid process, or noxious substance. [L. see ablate]

electrode catheter a., a method of ablating the site of origin of arrhythmias whereby high-energy electrical current is delivered by intravascular catheters.

endometrial a., therapeutic selective endometrial destruction.

laparoscopic uterosacral nerve a., laparoscopic transection via laser (usually KTP or argon) of the uterosacral nerves for the treatment of primary dysmenorrhea.

ableph·a·ria (ā-blef-ar′ē-ă). Congenital absence of the eyelids. SEE ALSO cryptophthalmus, microblepharon. [G. *a-* priv. + *blepharon,* eyelid]

ab·lu·ent (ab′loo-ent). **1.** Cleansing. **2.** Anything with cleansing properties. [L. *abluens,* fr. *ab-luo,* to wash off]

ab·lu·tion (ab-loo′shŭn). An act of washing or bathing. [L. *ablutio,* washing off, cleansing]

ab·ner·val (ab-ner′văl). Away from a nerve; denoting specifically a current of electricity passing through a muscular fiber in a direction away from the point of entrance of the nerve fiber. SYN abneural (1).

ab·neu·ral (ab-noor′ăl). **1.** SYN abnerval. **2.** Away from the neural axis. [L. *ab,* away from, + G. *neuron,* nerve]

ab·nor·mal (ab-nōr′măl). Not normal; differing in any way from the usual state, structure, condition, or rule.

ab·nor·mal·i·ty (ab-nōr-mal′i-tē). **1.** The state or quality of being abnormal. **2.** An anomaly, deformity, malformation, impairment, or dysfunction.

figure-of-8 a., a radiographic appearance associated with total anomalous drainage of the pulmonary venous circulation into enlarged right and anomalous left superior venae cavae, that produces a globular density above the heart; the silhouette suggests the figure 8; e.g., TAPVR. SEE ALSO anomalous pulmonary venous *connections,* total or partial, under *connection.* SYN snowman a.

neuronal migration a., SYN cortical *dysplasia.*

snowman a., SYN figure-of-8 a.

ABO blood group. See Blood Groups appendix.

ab·ohm (ab′ōm). Electromagnetic unit of resistance equal to 10^{-9} ohm.

ab·o·rad, ab·o·ral (ab-ō′rad, -răl). In a direction away from the mouth; opposite of orad. [L. *ab,* from, + *os* (*or-*), mouth]

abort (ă-bōrt′). **1.** To give birth to an embryo or fetus before it is viable. SEE ALSO miscarry. **2.** To remove products of conception prematurely to destroy the offspring. **3.** To arrest a disease in its earliest stages. [L. *aborior,* to fail at onset]

a·bor·ti·cide (ah-bor′tī-sīd). SYN abortifacient (1). [L. *flabboriri,* to miscarry + *cadere,* to kill.]

abor·tient (ă-bōr′shent). SYN abortifacient (1).

abor·ti·fa·cient (ă-bōr-ti-fā′shent). **1.** Producing abortion. SYN aborticide, abortient, abortigenic, abortive (3). **2.** An agent that produces abortion. [L. *abortus,* abortion, + *facio,* to make]

abor·ti·gen·ic (ă-bōr-ti-jen′ik). SYN abortifacient (1). [L. *abortus,* abortion, + *genesis,* production]

abor·tion (ă-bōr′shŭn). **1.** Expulsion from the uterus of an embryo or fetus prior to the stage of viability (20 weeks' gestation or fetal weight <500 g). A distinction made between a. and premature birth: premature infants are those born after the stage of viability but prior to 37 weeks. A. may be either spontaneous (occurring from natural causes) or induced (artificial or therapeutic). **2.** The arrest of any action or process before its normal completion.

ampullar a., a. resulting from pregnancy in the ampulla of the fallopian tube.

complete a., (1) the complete expulsion or extraction from its mother of a fetus or embryo; **(2)** complete expulsion of any other product of gestation. (e.g., blighted ovum).

criminal a., termination of pregnancy in violation of law. SYN illegal a.

elective a., an a. without medical justification but done in a legal way, as in the United States.

habitual a., SYN recurrent a.

illegal a., SYN criminal a.

incomplete a., a. in which part of the products of conception have been passed but part (usually the placenta) remains in the uterus.

induced a., a. brought on purposely by drugs or mechanical means.

inevitable a., a. characterized by rupture of the membranes or the cervical dilation in a previable pregnancy in the presence of vaginal bleeding and uterine contractions.

infected a., a septic complication of an a.

menstrual extraction a., a technique for aspiration of early products of conception from the uterus a few days after the first missed menstrual period.

missed a., a. in which the fetus dies *in utero* but the product of conception is retained *in utero* for two months or longer.

recurrent a., the loss of 3 or more sequential pregnancies before 20 weeks of gestation. SYN habitual a.

septic a., an infectious a. complicated by fever, endometritis, and parametritis.

spontaneous a., a. that has not been artificially induced. SYN miscarriage.

therapeutic a., a. induced because of the mother's physical or mental health, or to prevent birth of a deformed child or a child resulting from rape.

threatened a., cramplike pains and slight show of blood that may or may not be followed by the expulsion of the fetus during the first 20 weeks of pregnancy.

tubal a., rupture of an oviduct, the seat of ectopic pregnancy, or extrusion of the product of conception through the fimbriated end of the oviduct; aborted ectopic pregnancy, the pregnancy having originated in a fallopian tube. SYN aborted ectopic pregnancy.

abor·tion·ist (ă-bōr′shŭn-ist). One who interrupts a pregnancy.

abor·tive (ă-bōr′tiv). **1.** Not reaching completion; e.g., said of an attack of a disease subsiding before it has fully developed or completed its course. **2.** SYN rudimentary. **3.** SYN abortifacient (1). [L. *abortivus*]

abor·tus (ă-bōr′tŭs). Any product (or all products) of an abortion. [L.]

abou·lia (ă-boo′lē-ă). SYN abulia.

ABP Abbreviation for androgen binding *protein.*

ABPA Abbreviation for allergic bronchopulmonary aspergillosis.

ABR Abbreviation for auditory brainstem *response.* SEE auditory brainstem *response.*

abra·chia (ă-brā′kē-ă). Congenital absence of arms. SEE amelia. [G. *a-* priv. + *brachiōn,* arm]

abra·chi·o·ceph·a·ly, abra·chi·o·ce·pha·lia (ă-brā′kē-ō-sef′ă-lē, -se-fā′lē-ă). Congenital absence of arms and head. SYN acephalobrachia. [G. *a-* priv. + *brachiōn,* arm, + *kephalē,* head]

abrade (ă-brād′). **1.** To wear away by mechanical action. **2.** To scrape away part or all of the surface layer from a part. [L. *ab-rado,* pp. *-rasus,* to scrape off]

Abrahams, Robert, U.S. physician, 1861–1935. SEE A. *sign.*

Abrams, Albert, U.S. physician, 1863–1924. SEE A. heart *reflex.*

abra·sion (ă-brā′zhŭn). **1.** An excoriation, or circumscribed removal of the superficial layers of skin or mucous membrane. SYN abraded wound. **2.** A scraping away of a portion of the surface. **3.** In dentistry, the pathological grinding or wearing away of tooth substance by incorrect tooth-brushing methods, foreign objects, bruxism, or similar causes. SYN grinding. Cf. attrition. [see abrade]

brush burn a., SEE brush *burn.*

gingival a., a lesion of the gingiva resulting from mechanical removal of a portion of the surface epithelium.

tooth a., loss or wearing away of tooth structure caused by the abrasive characteristics of substances other than foods.

abra·sive (a-brā′siv). **1.** Causing abrasion. **2.** Any material used to produce abrasions. **3.** A substance used in dentistry for abrading, grinding, or polishing.

abra·sive·ness (ă-brā′siv-nes). **1.** That property of a substance that causes surface wear by friction. **2.** The quality of being able to scratch or wear away another material.

ab·re·act (ab-rē-akt′). **1.** To show strong emotion while reliving a previous traumatic experience. **2.** To discharge or release repressed emotion.

ab·re·ac·tion (ab-rē-ak′shŭn). In freudian psychoanalysis, an episode of emotional release or catharsis associated with the bringing into conscious recollection previously repressed unpleasant experiences.

motor a., the release of an unconscious thought, idea, or impulse through motor or muscular expression.

abrin (ab′rin). A phytotoxin from jequirity seeds or Indian liquorice, the red seeds (*Abrus precatorius*); used in ophthalmology.

abrup·tion (ab-rŭp′shŭn). A tearing away, separation, or detachment.

ab·rup·tio pla·cen·tae (ab-rŭp′shē-ō pla-sen′tē). Premature detachment of a normally situated placenta.

Ab·rus (ā′brŭs). A genus of leguminous plants. The root of *A. precatorius,* Indian liquorice, is sometimes used as a substitute for liquorice; the seeds are toxic and may cause vomiting, diarrhea, convulsions, and death if chewed. [more correctly *Habrus,* from G. *habros,* graceful]

ABSCESS

ab·scess (ab′ses). **1.** A circumscribed collection of purulent exudate frequently associated with swelling and other signs of inflammation. **2.** A cavity formed by liquefactive necrosis within solid tissue. [L. *abscessus,* a going away]

acute a., a recently formed a. with little or no fibrosis in the wall of the cavity. SYN hot a.

alveolar a., an a. situated within the alveolar process of the jaws, most often caused by extension of infection from an adjacent nonvital tooth. SYN dental a., dentoalveolar a., root a.

amebic a., an area of liquefaction necrosis of the liver or other organ containing amebae, often following amebic dysentery. SYN tropical a.

apical a., SYN periapical a.

apical periodontal a., SYN periapical a.

appendiceal a., an intraperitoneal a., usually in the right iliac fossa, resulting from extension of infection in acute appendicitis, especially with perforation of the appendix. SYN periappendiceal a.

Bartholin a., an a. of the vulvovaginal gland.

Bezold a., an a. deep to the superior part of the sternocleidomastoid muscle due to suppurative destruction of the mastoid tip cells in mastoiditis.

bicameral a., an a. with two separate cavities or chambers.

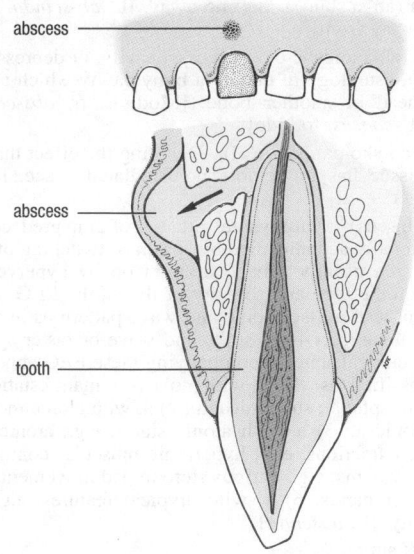

alveolar abscess

bone a., suppuration within the medullary cavity (osteomyelitis), cortex, or periosteum of bone.

Brodie a., a chronic a. of bone surrounded by dense fibrous tissue and sclerotic bone.

bursal a., suppuration within a bursa.

caseous a., an a. containing white solid or semisolid material of cheeselike consistency; usually tuberculous. SEE ALSO cheesy a.

cheesy a., an a. that contains necrotic tissue with a cheeselike consistency; typically seen in tuberculosis. SEE ALSO caseous a.

cholangitic a. (kō-lan-jī′-tik), a focal area of pus formation in the liver resulting from infection arising in the biliary tract.

chronic a., a long-standing collection of pus surrounded by fibrous tissue.

cold a., an a. without heat or other usual signs of inflammation;

crypt a.'s, a.'s in crypts of Lieberkühn of the large intestinal mucosa; a characteristic feature of ulcerative colitis.

dental a., dentoalveolar a., SYN alveolar a.

diffuse a., a collection of pus not circumscribed by a well-defined capsule.

Douglas a., suppuration in Douglas pouch.

dry a., the remains of an a. after the pus is absorbed.

Dubois a.'s, small cysts of the thymus containing polymorphonuclear leukocytes but lined by squamous epithelium; reported in congenital syphilis but also found in the absence of syphilis. SYN Dubois disease, thymic a.'s.

embolic a., an a. arising distal to the point of arrest of a septic embolus.

fecal a., SYN stercoral a.

follicular a., an a. in a hair, tonsillar, or other follicle.

gas a., an a. containing gas. Frequently caused by gas-forming organisms such as *Enterobacter aerogenes* or *Escherichia coli*.

gingival a., an a. confined to the gingival soft tissue. SYN gumboil, parulis.

gravitation a., SYN perforating a.

gummatous a., an a. due to the softening and breaking down of a gumma, especially in bone.

hematogenous a., an a. caused by blood-borne organisms.

hot a., SYN acute a.

hypostatic a., SYN perforating a.

ischiorectal a., an a. involving the ischiorectal fossa.

lateral alveolar a., an alveolar a. located along the lateral root surface of a tooth. SYN pericemental a.

lateral periodontal a., an a. that forms at the depth of a periodon-

tal pocket due to multiplication of pyogenic microorganisms or the presence of foreign material.

mastoid a., an a. due to coalescence of the mastoid air cells in mastoiditis.

metastatic a., a secondary a. formed, at a distance from the primary focus, as a result of the transportation of pyogenic bacteria by the lymph or bloodstream.

migrating a., SYN perforating a.

miliary a., one of a number of minute collections of pus, widely disseminated throughout an area or the whole body.

Munro a., SYN Munro *microabscess*.

orbital a., a collection of pus between the orbital periosteum and the lamina papyracea; frequently an extension of purulent infection of the paranasal sinuses, usually the ethmoids.

otitic a., a brain a., usually involving the temporal lobe or cerebellar hemisphere, secondary to suppuration of the middle ear.

palatal a., (1) a lateral periodontal a. associated with the lingual surface of a maxillary tooth; (2) an alveolar a. that has eroded the cortical plate, allowing extension into the palatal soft tissues.

pancreatic a., an a. in the pancreatic or peripancreatic area usually related to pancreatitis.

parafrenal a., an a. that occurs on either side of the frenum of the penis.

parametric a., parametritic a., an a. in the connective tissue of the broad ligament of the uterus.

paranephric a., an a. in the region of the kidney, outside the renal fascia.

parapharyngeal a., an a. lying lateral to the pharynx.

parotid a., suppuration in the parotid gland; an often rapidly progressing complication of parotitis.

Pautrier a., SYN Pautrier *microabscess*.

pelvic a., an a. in the pelvic peritoneal cavity, developing as a complication of diffuse peritonitis or of localized peritonitis associated with abdominal or pelvic inflammatory disease, such as salpingitis; the pus frequently collects in the rectovesical or rectouterine pouch.

perforating a., an a. that breaks down tissue barriers to enter adjacent areas. SYN gravitation a., hypostatic a., migrating a., wandering a.

periapical a., an alveolar a. localized around the apex of a tooth root. SYN apical a., apical periodontal a.

periappendiceal a., SYN appendiceal a.

periarticular a., an a. surrounding a joint, but not necessarily involving it.

pericemental a., SYN lateral alveolar a.

pericoronal a., an a. developing in the inflamed dental follicular tissue overlying the crown of a partially erupted tooth.

perinephric a., an a. within Gerota fascia but outside the renal capsule.

periodontal a., an alveolar a. or a lateral periodontal a.

perirectal a., an a. in connective tissue adjacent to the rectum or anus.

peritonsillar a., extension of tonsillar infection beyond the tonsillar capsule with abscess formation between the capsule and the musculature of the tonsillar fossa.

periureteral a., an a. surrounding the ureter.

periurethral a., an a. involving the tissues around the urethra, particularly the corpus spongiosum.

phlegmonous a., circumscribed suppuration characterized by intense surrounding inflammatory reaction that produces induration and thickening of the affected area.

Pott a., tuberculous a. of the spine.

premammary a., an a. in the subcutaneous tissue covering the mammary gland.

psoas a., an a., usually tuberculous, originating in tuberculous spondylitis and extending through the iliopsoas muscle to the inguinal region.

pulp a., an a. involving the soft tissue within the pulp chamber of a tooth, usually a sequela of caries or less frequently of trauma.

pyemic a., a hematogenous a. resulting from pyemia, septicemia, or bacteremia. SYN septicemic a.

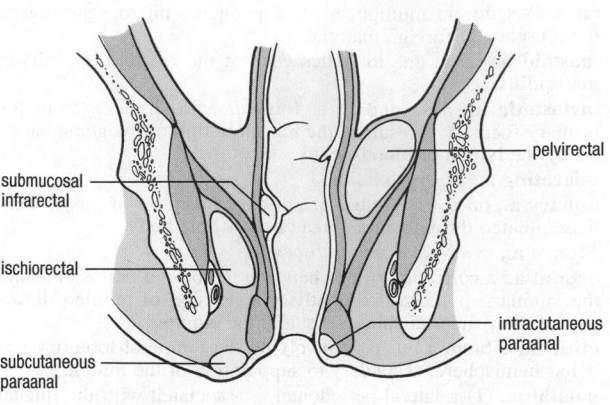

perirectal abscesses

radicular a., alveolar a., an a. around a tooth root.

residual a., an a. recurring at the site of a former a. resulting from persistence of microbes and pus.

retrobulbar a., an a. posterior to the globe of the eye.

retrocecal a., an a. located posterior to the cecum, usually resulting from perforation of a retrocecal appendix.

retropharyngeal a., an a. arising, usually, in retropharyngeal lymph nodes, most commonly in infants.

ring a., an acute purulent inflammation of the corneal periphery in which a necrotic area is surrounded by an annular girdle of leukocytic infiltration.

root a., SYN alveolar a.

satellite a., an a. closely associated with a primary a.

septicemic a., SYN pyemic a.

stellate a., a star-shaped necrotic area surrounded by histiocytes, seen within swollen lymph nodes in lymphogranuloma venereum and cat scratch fever.

stercoral a., a collection of pus and feces. SYN fecal a.

sterile a., (1) an a. whose contents are not caused by pyogenic bacteria. **(2)** an a. that when aspirated or cultured does not grow bacteria.

stitch a., SYN suture a.

subdiaphragmatic a., SYN subphrenic a.

subepidermal a., a microscopic a. located in the dermis just beneath the epidermis.

subhepatic a., an a. located immediately beneath the liver.

subperiosteal a., an a. between the periosteum and cortical plate of the bone.

subphrenic a., an a. directly beneath the diaphragm. SYN subdiaphragmatic a.

subungual a., suppuration extending beneath a fingernail or toenail, usually from a paronychia.

sudoriferous a., a collection of pus in a sweat gland.

suture a., a purulent exudate surrounding a stitch, particularly a corneal stitch. SYN stitch a.

thymic a.'s, SYN Dubois a.'s.

Tornwaldt a., chronic infection of the pharyngeal bursa. SEE ALSO Tornwaldt *syndrome.*

tropical a., SYN amebic a.

tuboovarian a., a large a. involving a uterine tube and an adherent ovary, resulting from extension of purulent inflammation of the tube.

verminous a., SYN worm a.

wandering a., SYN perforating a.

worm a., a. due to parasitic worms or in which worms are found. SYN verminous a.

ab·scis·sa (ab-sis′ă). In a plane cartesian coordinate system, the horizontal axis (*x*). Cf. ordinate. [L. *ab-scindo,* pp. *-scissus,* to cut away from]

ab·scis·sion (ab-si′shŭn). Cutting away. [L. *ab-scindo,* pp. *-scissus,* to cut away from]

ab·scon·sio (ab-skon′shē-ō). A recess, cavity, or depression; used especially in osteology to denote a bony cavity which accommodates the head of another bone. [Mod. L. fr. *abs-condo,* pp. *-conditus* or *-consus,* to hide]

ab·sco·pal (ab-skō′păl, -skop′ăl). Denoting the effect that irradiation of a tissue has on remote nonirradiated tissue. [ab- + G. *skopos,* target, + -al]

ab·sence (ab′sens). Paroxysmal attacks of impaired consciousness, occasionally accompanied by spasm or twitching of cephalic muscles, which usually can be brought on by hyperventilation; depending on the type and severity of the a., the EEG may show an abrupt onset of a 3-sec spike and wave pattern as in simple a., or in atypical cases, a 4-sec spike and wave or faster spike complexes. The clinical states accompanying these EEG abnormalities may be classified as: 1) a. with no overt manifestations, e.g., simple a.; epileptic a.; subclinical a.; 2) a. with clonic movements, e.g., myoclonic a.; 3) a. with atonic states, e.g., atonic a.; 4) a. with tonic contractions, e.g., hypertonic muscular contraction; 5) a. with automatisms, e.g., various stereotyped movements, usually of the face or hands; 6) a. with atypical features, e.g., bizarre motor activity. [L. *absentia*]

pure a., SYN simple a.

simple a., a brief clouding of consciousness accompanied by the abrupt onset of 3-sec spikes and waves on EEG. SYN pure a.

abs. feb. Abbreviation for L. *absente febre,* when fever is absent.

Ab·sid·ia (ab-sid′ē-ă). A genus of fungi (family Mucoraceae) commonly found in nature. Thermophilic species survive in compost piles at temperatures exceeding 45°C and may cause mucormycosis (zygomycosis) in humans.

ab·sinthe (ab′sinth). A liqueur consisting of an alcoholic extract of absinthium and other bitter herbs.

ab·sin·thin (ab′sin-thin). A bitter principle, $C_{30}H_{40}O_8$, obtained from absinthium.

ab·sin·thi·um (ab-sin′thē-ŭm). The dried leaves and tops of *Artemisia absinthium* (family Compositae). The infusion is now seldom used, but it has been used as a tonic; in large or frequently repeated doses it produces headache, trembling, and epileptiform convulsions. SYN wormwood. [L., fr. G. *apsinthion*]

ab·sin·thol (ab-sin′thawl). SYN thujone.

ab·so·lute (ab′sō-loot). Unconditional; unlimited; uncombined; undiluted (as in case of alcohol); certain. [L. *absolutus,* complete, pp. of *ab-solvo,* to loosen from]

ab·sorb (ab-sōrb′). **1.** To take in by absorption. **2.** To reduce the intensity of transmitted light. [L. *ab-sorbeo,* pp. *-sorptus,* to suck in]

ab·sor·bance (*A*, A) (ab-sōr′bans). In spectrophotometry, log of the ratio of the radiant power of the incident radiation to the radiant power of the transmitted radiation. SYN absorbancy, absorbency, extinction (2), optic density.

specific a., a. per unit of concentration. SEE specific absorption *coefficient.*

ab·sor·ban·cy (ab-sōr′ban-sē). SYN absorbance.

ab·sor·be·fa·cient (ab-sōr-bĕ-fā′shŭnt). **1.** Causing absorption. **2.** Any substance possessing such quality. [L. *ab-sorbeo,* to suck in, + *facio,* to make]

ab·sorb·en·cy (ab-sōr′ben-sē). SYN absorbance.

ab·sor·bent (ab-sōr′bent). **1.** Having the power to absorb, soak up, or take into itself a gas, liquid, light rays, or heat. SYN absorptive, bibulous. **2.** Any substance possessing such power. **3.** Material (usually caustic) for removal of carbon dioxide from circuits in which rebreathing occurs; e.g., anesthesia and basal metabolism equipment.

ab·sorb·er head (ab-sōr′ber hed). Portion of a rebreathing anesthesia circuit that contains carbon dioxide absorbent; often referred to as a canister.

ab·sorp·tion (ab-sōrp′shŭn). **1.** The taking in, incorporation, or reception of gases, liquids, light, or heat. Cf. adsorption. **2.** In radiology, the uptake of energy from radiation by the tissue or

ac

medium through which it passes. SEE half-value *layer*, photoelectric *effect*, attenuation. [L. *absorptio*, fr. *absorbeo*, to swallow]

cutaneous a., SYN percutaneous a.

disjunctive a., a. of living tissue in immediate relation with a necrosed part, producing a line of demarcation.

electron resonance a., SEE electron spin *resonance*.

external a., the a. of substances through skin, mucocutaneous surfaces, or mucous membranes.

interstitial a., the removal of water or of substances in the interstitial fluid by the lymphatics.

parenteral a., a. by any route other than the alimentary tract.

pathologic a., parenteral a. of any excremental or pathologic material into the bloodstream, e.g., pus, urine, bile, etc.

percutaneous a., the a. of drugs, allergens, and other substances through unbroken skin. The corneal layer of epidermis is the principal barrier. SYN cutaneous a.

photoelectric a., interaction of a gamma photon with matter in which the incident photon is completely absorbed, giving up all its energy by displacing and accelerating an inner shell electron. SEE ALSO photoelectric *effect*.

ab·sorp·tive (ab-sōrp′tiv). SYN absorbent (1).

ab·sorp·tiv·i·ty (*a*) (ab-sōrp-tiv′i-tē). **1.** SYN specific absorption *coefficient*. **2.** SYN molar absorption *coefficient*. **3.** The ability of a material to absorb electromagnetic radiation.

molar a., SYN molar absorption *coefficient*.

ab·sti·nence (ab′sti-nens). Refraining from the use of certain articles of diet, alcoholic beverages, illegal drugs, or from sexual intercourse. [L. *abs-tineo*, to hold back, fr. *teneo*, to hold]

ab·stract (ab′strakt). **1.** A preparation made by evaporating a fluid extract to a powder and triturating with milk sugar. **2.** A condensation or summary of a scientific or literary article or address. [L. *ab-straho*, pp. *-tractus*, to draw away]

structured a., summary description of a published paper, in which information about the study reported in the paper is set out in a systematic, stylized form under headings such as aims, methods, main outcome measures, results, conclusions.

ab·strac·tion (ab-strak′shŭn). **1.** Distillation or separation of the volatile constituents of a substance. **2.** Exclusive mental concentration. **3.** The making of an abstract from the crude drug. **4.** Malocclusion in which the teeth or associated structures are lower than their normal occlusal plane. SEE ALSO odontoptosis. **5.** The process of selecting a certain aspect of a concept from the whole. [L. *abs-traho*, pp. *-tractus*, to draw away]

ab·stric·tion (ab-strik′shŭn). In fungi, the formation of asexual spores by cutting off portions of the sporophore through the growth of dividing partitions. [L. *ab-*, from, + *strictura*, a contraction]

ab·ter·mi·nal (ab-ter′mi-năl). In a direction away from the end and toward the center; denoting the course of an electrical current in a muscle. [L. *ab*, from, + *terminus*, end]

γ-Abu Abbreviation for γ-aminobutyric acid.

abu·lia (ă-boo′lē-ă). **1.** Loss or impairment of the ability to perform voluntary actions or to make decisions. **2.** Reduction in speech, movement, thought, and emotional reaction; a common result of bilateral frontal lobe disease. SYN aboulia. [G. *a-* priv. + *boulē*, will]

abu·lic (ă-boo′lik). Relating to, or suffering from, abulia.

a·bun·dance (a-bŭn′dans). The average number of types of macromolecules (e.g., mRNAs) per cell.

abuse (ă-būs′). **1.** Misuse, wrong use, especially excessive use, of anything. **2.** Injurious, harmful, or offensive treatment, as in child a. or sexual a.

child a., the psychological, emotional, and sexual a. of a child, typically by a parent, stepparent, or parent surrogate. SEE domestic violence.

drug a., habitual use of drugs not needed for therapeutic purposes, such as solely to alter one's mood, affect, or state of consciousness, or to affect a body function unnecessarily (as in laxative a.); nontherapeutic use of drugs.

elder a., the physical or emotional a., including financial exploita-

tion, of an elderly person, by one or more of the individual's children, nursing home caregivers, or others.

sexual a., SEE domestic violence.

spouse a., spousal a., SEE domestic violence.

substance a., maladaptive pattern of use of a drug, alcohol, or other chemical agent that may lead to social, occupational, psychological, or physical problems.

abut·ment (ă-bŭt′ment). In dentistry, a natural tooth or implanted tooth substitute, used for the support or anchorage of a fixed or removable prosthesis.

auxiliary a., a tooth other than the one supporting the direct retainer, assisting in the overall support of a removable partial denture.

ball and socket a., an a. connected to a fixed partial denture by a ball and socket-shaped nonrigid connector.

dovetail stress-broken a., an a. connected to a fixed partial denture by a nonrigid connector that is trapezoidal in cross-section.

intermediate a., a natural tooth, or an implanted tooth substitute, without other natural teeth in proximal contact, used along with the mesial and distal a.'s to support a prosthesis; often called a "pier."

isolated a., a lone-standing tooth, or root, used as an a. with edentulous areas mesial and distal to it.

splinted a., the joining of two or more teeth into a rigid unit by means of fixed restorations to form a single a. with multiple roots.

ABVD Abbreviation for a chemotherapy regimen of Adriamycin (doxorubicin), bleomycin, vinblastine, and dacarbazine; used to treat neoplastic diseases, such as Hodgkin lymphoma.

ab·volt (ab′vōlt). The CGS electromagnetic unit of difference of potential equal to 10^{-8} V. The potential difference between two points such that 1 erg of work will be done when 1 abcoulomb of charge moves from point to point.

ab·zyme (ab′zīm). SYN catalytic *antibody*. [*antibody* + en*zyme*]

AC Abbreviation for alternating *current*.

Ac Symbol for actinium; acetyl.

aC Symbol for arabinosylcytosine.

a.c. Abbreviation for L. *ante cibum*, before a meal or *ante cibos*, before meals.

AC/A Abbreviation for accommodative convergence-accommodation *ratio*.

aca·cia (ă-kā′shē-ă). The dried gummy exudation from *Acacia senegal* and other species of *A.* (family Leguminosae), prepared as a mucilage and syrup; used as an emollient, demulcent excipient, and suspending agent in pharmaceuticals and foods; formerly used as a transfusion fluid. SYN gum arabic. [G. *akakia*]

acal·cu·lia (ā′kal-kū′lē-a). A form of aphasia characterized by the inability to perform simple mathematical problems; found with lesions of various areas of the cerebral hemispheres, and often an early sign of dementia. [G. *a-* priv. + L. *calculo*, to reckon]

acamp·sia (ă-kamp′sē-ă). Rarely used term for stiffening or rigidity of a joint for any reason. [G. *a-* priv. + *kamptō*, to bend]

♻**acanth-.** SEE acantho-.

acan·tha (ă-kan′thă). **1.** A spine or spinous process. **2.** The spinous process of a vertebra. [G. *akantha*, a thorn]

acan·tha·me·bi·a·sis (ă-kan′thă-mē-bī′ă-sis). Infection by free-living soil and water amebae of the genus *Acanthamoeba* that may result in a necrotizing dermal or tissue invasion, a fulminating and usually fatal primary amebic meningoencephalitis, or a subacute or chronic granulomatous amebic encephalitis.

ℹ*Acan·tha·moe·ba* (ă-kan-thă-mē′bă). A genus of free-living ameba (family Acanthamoebidae, order Amoebida) found in and characterized by the presence of acanthopodia. Human infection includes invasion of skin or colonization following injury, corneal invasion and colonization, and possibly lung or genitourinary tract colonization; a few cases of brain or CNS invasion have occurred, but not solely by the olfactory epithelium route of entry as with the more virulent infections caused by *Naegleria fowleri*. Species responsible are chiefly *A. culbertsoni*, but cases have been reported involving *A. castellanii*, *A. polyphaga*, and *A. astronyxis*, though most cases have been chronic rather than fulminating and rapidly fatal as with *Naegleria fowleri* infection. [G. *akantha,* thorn, spine, + Mod. L. *amoeba,* fr. G. *amoibē,* change]

ac·an·thel·la (ă-kan-thel′ă). An intermediate larva stage of Acanthocephala, formed within the arthropod host; a preinfective, nonencysted stage leading to the infective cystacanth. [G. *akantha,* thorn, spine]

acan·thes·the·sia (ă-kan-thes-thē′zē-ă). Paresthesia of a pinprick. [G. *akantha,* thorn, + *aisthēsis,* sensation]

Acan·thia lec·tu·lar·ia (ă-kan′thē-ă lek-tū-lār′ē-ă). Early name for *Cimex lectularius.* [G. *akantha,* thorn, prickle; L. *lectus,* a bed]

acan·thi·on (ă-kan′thē-on). The tip of the anterior nasal spine. SYN akanthion. [G. *akantha,* thorn]

△**acantho-.** A spinous process; spiny, thorny. [G. *akantha,* a thorn, the backbone, the spine, fr. *akē,* a point, + *anthos,* a flower]

Acan·tho·ceph·a·la (ă-kan-thō-sef′ă-lă). The thorny-headed worms, a phylum (formerly considered a class) of obligatory parasites without an alimentary canal, characterized by an anterior introvertible spiny proboscis. They superficially resemble nematodes but are cestode like in other traits, and hence are grouped as a distinctive phylum of helminths. In the adult stage they are parasites of vertebrate animals, mostly fish and amphibians; the larval stage is passed in invertebrates, chiefly crustaceans and insects. [acantho- + G. *kephalē,* head]

acan·tho·ceph·a·li·a·sis (ă-kan′thō-sef-ă-lī′ă-sis). An illness caused by infection with a species of Acanthocephala.

Acan·tho·chei·lo·ne·ma (ă-kan′thō-kī-lō-nē′mă). A genus of filarial worms parasitic in man, now considered part of the genus *Mansonella.* [acantho- + G. *cheilos,* lip, + *nēma,* thread]

acan·tho·cyte (ă-kan′thō-sīt). An erythrocyte characterized by multiple spiny cytoplasmic projections, as in acanthocytosis. [acantho- + G. *kytos,* cell]

acan·tho·cy·to·sis (ă-kan′thō-sī-tō′sis). A rare condition in which the majority of erythrocytes are acanthocytes; a regular feature of abetalipoproteinemia; also sometimes present in severe hepatocellular disease. SYN acanthrocytosis.

acan·thoid (ă-kan′thoyd). Spine-shaped.

ac·an·thol·y·sis (ak-an-thol′i-sis). Separation of individual epidermal keratinocytes from their neighbor, as in conditions such as pemphigus vulgaris and Darier disease. [acantho- + G. *lysis,* loosening]

ac·an·tho·ma (ak-an-thō′mă). A tumor formed by proliferation of epithelial squamous cells. SEE ALSO keratoacanthoma. [acantho- + G. *-oma,* tumor]

clear cell a., a small sharply demarcated benign epidermal tumor of a leg or arm with acanthosis and accumulation of glycogen in keratinocytes having pale-staining cytoplasm.

acan·tho·po·dia (ă-kan-thō-pō′dē-ă). Toothlike pseudopodia observed in some amebae, typically in members of the genus *Acanthamoeba.* [acantho- + G. *pous, podos,* foot]

acan·thor (ă-kan′thōr). The spindle-shaped embryo, with rostellar hooks and body spines, formed within the egg shell of Acanthocephala; this stage burrows into the body cavity of its first intermediate host, usually a crustacean in aquatic cycles, or insects in terrestrial cycles. [G. *akantha,* thorn or spine]

ac·an·tho·sis (ak-an-thō′sis). An increase in the thickness of the stratum spinosum of the epidermis. [acantho- + G. *-osis,* condition]

glycogenic a., elevated gray-white plaques of distal esophageal or vaginal mucosa, with epithelium thickened by proliferation of large glycogen-filled squamous cells.

ⓘ**a. ni′gricans,** an eruption of velvet warty benign growths and hyperpigmentation occurring in the skin of the axillae, neck, anogenital area, and groin; in adults, may be associated with internal malignancy, endocrine disorders, or obesity; a benign hereditary type occurs in children. SEE ALSO pseudoacanthosis nigricans. [L. fr. *niger,* black]

ac·an·thot·ic (ak-an-thot′ik). Pertaining to or characteristic of acanthosis.

acan·thro·cyte (a-kan′thrō-sīt). Obsolete term for acanthocyte.

acan·thro·cy·to·sis (ă-kan′thrō-sī-tō′sis). Obsolete term for acanthocytosis. SYN acanthocytosis.

acap·nia (ă-kap′nē-ă). Absence of carbon dioxide in the blood; sometimes used erroneously for hypocapnia. [G. *a-* priv. + *kapnos,* smoke]

acarbose (ā-kar′bōs). An oligosaccharide alpha-glucosidase inhibitor; adjunctive therapy in type 2 diabetes mellitus to blunt postprandial hyperglycemia.

acar·dia (ā-kar′dē-ă). Congenital absence of the heart; a condition sometimes occurring in one member of monozygotic twins or in one member of conjoined twins when pair partner monopolizes the placental blood supply; can also occur in triplet pregnancies. [G. *a-* priv. + *kardia,* heart]

acar·di·ac (ā-car′dē-ak). Without a heart.

acar·di·us (ă-kar′dē-ŭs). A twin without a heart that remains viable by using the placental circulation of its mate.

a. aceph′alus, acephalocardius; an acardiac conceptus in which the head and thoracic organs are absent; ribs and vertebrae may be present, and upper limbs are either absent or defective.

a. amor′phus, a shapeless product of conception covered by skin and hair.

a. an′ceps, an acardiac fetus with partly developed head and deformed face, trunk, and limbs.

ac·a·ri·a·sis (ak-ar-ī′ă-sis). Any disease caused by mites, usually a skin infestation. SEE mange.

psoroptic a., infestation of mammalian skin with *Psoroptes* mites.

sarcoptic a., infestation of skin with *Sarcoptes scabiei.* SEE scabies (1).

acar·i·cide (ă-kar′i-sīd). An agent that kills acarines; commonly used to denote chemicals that kill ticks. [Mod. L. *acarus,* a mite, fr. G. *akari* + L. *caedo,* to cut, kill]

ⓘ**ac·a·rid** (ak′ă-rid). A general term for a member of the family Acaridae or for a mite. SYN acaridan. [G. *akari,* mite]

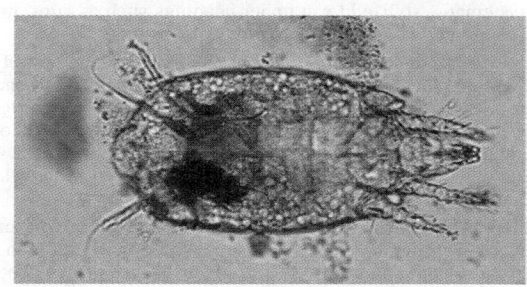

acarid (mite)

Acar·i·dae (ă-kar′i-dē). A family of the order Acarina, a large group of exceptionally small mites, usually 0.5 mm or less, abundant in dried fruits and meats, grain, meal, and flour; frequently a cause of severe dermatitis among persons hypersensitized by frequent handling of infested products.

acar·i·dan (ă-kar′i-dan). SYN acarid.

Ac·a·ri·na (ak-ă-rī′nă). An order of Arachnida that includes the mites and ticks. [G. *akari,* a mite]

ac·a·rine (ak′ă-rīn). A member of the order Acarina.

ac·a·ro·der·ma·ti·tis (ak′ă-rō-der-mă-tī′tis). A skin inflammation or eruption produced by a mite. [G. *akari,* mite, + *derma* (*dermat-*), skin]

a. urticarioi′des, infestation with the grain itch mite, *Pyemotes ventricosus.* SEE grain *itch.*

ac·a·roid (ak′ă-royd). Resembling a mite. [G. *akari,* mite, + *eidos,* resemblance]

ac·a·rol·o·gy (ak-ă-rol′ō-jē). The study of acarine parasites, the ticks and mites, and the diseases they transmit. [G. *akari,* mite, + *logos,* study]

ac·a·ro·pho·bia (ak′ă-rō-fō′bē-ă). Morbid fear of small parasites, small particles, or of itching. [G. *akari,* mite, + *phobos,* fear]

Ac·a·rus (ak'ă-rŭs). A genus of mites of the family Acaridae. [G. *akari*, mite]

A. bala'tus, a tropical species of mite that causes a particularly severe type of scabies-like irritation.

A. folliculo'rum, SYN *Demodex folliculorum.*

A. galli'nae, SYN *Dermanyssus gallinae.*

A. horde'i, the barley mite, a species that penetrates beneath the skin.

A. rhizoglyp'ticus hyacin'thi, a species of mite that develops in spoiled onions and may cause dermatitis.

A. scabe'i, former term for *Sarcoptes scabiei.*

acar·y·ote (ă-kar'ē-ōt). SYN akaryocyte.

acat·a·la·se·mia [MIM*115500]. SYN acatalasia.

acat·a·la·sia (ā-kat-ă-lā'zē-ă) [MIM*115500]. Absence or deficiency of catalase from blood and tissues, often manifested by recurrent infection or ulceration of the gums and related oral structures and caused by mutations in the catalase gene (CAT) on 11p. Homozygotes may have complete absence (Japanese variety) or very low levels (Swiss variety) of catalase; heterozygotes have reduced catalase levels (hypocatalasia), which overlap with the normal range. SYN acatalasemia, Takahara disease.

ac·a·thec·tic (ak-ă-thek'tik). Rarely used term relating to acathexia.

ac·a·thex·ia (ak-ă-thek'sē-ă). Rarely used term for an abnormal release of secretions. [G. *a-* priv. + *kathexis*, retention]

ac·a·thex·is (ak-ă-thek'sis). Rarely used term for a mental disorder in which certain objects or ideas fail to arouse an emotional response in the individual. [G. *a-* priv. + *kathexis*, retention]

aca·thi·sia (ak-ă-thiz'ē-ă). SYN akathisia.

acau·dal, acau·date (ă-kaw'dăl, ă-kaw'dāt). Having no tail. [G. *a-* priv. + L. *cauda*, tail]

ACC Abbreviation for anodal closure *contraction.*

ac·cel·er·ans (ak-sel'er-anz). 1. Accelerating. 2. Obsolete term for an accelerator (sympathetic) nerve to the heart. [L. accelerator]

ac·cel·er·ant (ak-sel'er-ant). SYN accelerator (3).

ac·cel·er·a·tion (ak-sel-er-ā'shŭn). 1. The act of accelerating. 2. The rate of increase in velocity per unit of time; commonly expressed in *g* units; also expressed in centimeters or feet per second squared. 3. The rate of increasing deviation from a rectilinear course. SEE radial a. [see accelerator]

angular a., the rate of change of angular velocity; e.g., when a centrifuge rotor is speeding up, or when there is a simultaneous change in velocity and direction, as in an aircraft in a tight spin.

linear a., the rate of change of velocity without a change in direction; e.g., when the speed of an aircraft increases while flying a straight pathway.

radial a., the centripetal a. of a particle or vehicle moving along a curved path at a constant velocity; e.g., turning a curve in an automobile, pulling out of a dive, or performing a loop maneuver in an aircraft. In aviation, a. varies directly with the square of the air speed and inversely with the radius of the turn ($a = V^2/r$, where V is air speed and r is radius of turn).

ac·cel·er·a·tor (ak-sel'er-ā-ter). 1. Anything that increases rapidity of action or function. 2. In physiology, a nerve, muscle, or substance that quickens movement or response. 3. A catalytic agent used to hasten a chemical reaction. SYN accelerant. 4. In nuclear physics, a device that accelerates charged particles (e.g., protons) to high speed in order to produce nuclear reactions in a target, for the study of subatomic structure or for the production of radionuclides or for radiation therapy. [L. *accelerans*, pres. p. of *ac-celero*, to hasten, fr. *celer*, swift]

linear a. (LINAC), a device imparting high velocity and energy to atomic and subatomic particles; an important device for radiation therapy.

proserum prothrombin conversion a. (PPCA), obsolete term for factor VIII.

prothrombin a., obsolete term for factor V.

serum a., obsolete term for factor VII.

serum prothrombin conversion a. (SPCA), obsolete term for factor VII.

ac·cel·er·in (ak-sel'er-in). Obsolete term for what was once considered an intermediary product of coagulation but is no longer thought to exist.

ac·cel·er·om·e·ter (ak-sel-er-om'ĕ-ter). An instrument for measuring the rate of change of velocity per unit of time.

ac·cen·tu·a·tor (ak-sent'ū-ā-ter). A substance, such as aniline, the presence of which allows a combination between a tissue or histologic element and a stain that might otherwise be impossible. [L. *accentus*, accent, fr. *cano*, to sing]

ac·cep·tor (ak-sep'ter). 1. A compound that will take up a chemical group (e.g., an amine group, a methyl group, a carbamoyl group) from another compound (the donor); under the action of alanine transaminase, L-glutamic acid is an amine donor while pyruvic acid is an amine a. 2. A receptor that binds a hormone. [L. *ac-cipio*, pp. *-ceptus*, to accept]

hydrogen a., SYN hydrogen *carrier.*

ac·cès per·ni·ci·eux (ak-sā' per-ni-syu'). A series of severe attacks of falciparum malaria, sometimes occurring in apparently mild cases; roughly classified as cerebral and algid. [Fr., pernicious attacks or symptoms]

ac·cess (ak'ses). A way or means of approach or admittance. In dentistry: 1. The space required for visualization and for manipulation of instruments to remove decay and prepare a tooth for restoration. 2. The opening in the crown of a tooth required to allow adequate admittance to the pulp space to clean, shape, and seal the root canal(s). SYN access opening. [L. *accessus*]

ac·ces·so·ri·us (ak-ses-ō'rē-ŭs). SYN accessory. [L.]

a. willis'ii, SYN accessory *nerve* [CN XI].

ac·ces·so·ry (ak-ses'ō-rē). In anatomy, denoting certain muscles, nerves, glands, etc. that are auxiliary or supernumerary to some similar, generally more important thing. SYN accessorius. [L. *accessorius*, fr. *ac-cedo*, pp. *-cessus*, to move toward]

ac·ci·dent (ak'si-dent). An unplanned or unintended but sometimes predictable event leading to injury, e.g., in traffic, industry, or a domestic setting, or such an event developing in the course of a disease. [L. *ac-cido*, to happen]

cardiac a., sudden cardiac catastrophe, such as may result from coronary occlusion.

cerebrovascular a. (CVA), an imprecise term for cerebral stroke.

serum a., anaphylactic shock resulting from injection of serum of a different species for therapeutic purposes. SEE ALSO serum *sickness.*

ac·ci·dent-prone. 1. Having a greater number of accidents than would be expected of the average person in similar circumstances. 2. Having personality characteristics predisposing one to accidents.

ac·cli·ma·tion (ak-li-mā'shŭn). SYN acclimatization.

ac·cli·ma·ti·za·tion (ă-klī'mă-ti-zā'shŭn). Physiological adjustment of an individual to a different climate, especially to a change in environmental temperature or altitude. SYN acclimation.

ac·com·mo·da·tion (ă-kom'ŏ-dā'shŭn). 1. The act or state of adjustment or adaptation. 2. In sensorimotor theory, the alteration of schemata or cognitive expectations to conform with experience. [L. *ac-commodo*, pp. *-atus*, to adapt, fr. *modus*, a measure]

amplitude of a., the difference in refractivity of the eye at rest and when fully accommodated.

a. of eye, the increase in thickness and convexity of the eye's lens in response to ciliary muscle contraction in order to focus the image of an external object on the retina.

histologic a., change in shape of cells to meet altered physical conditions, as the flattening of cuboidal cells in cysts as a result of pressure. SYN pseudometaplasia.

negative a., the decrease of a. that occurs when shifting from near vision to distance vision.

a. of nerve, the property of a nerve by which it adjusts to a slowly increasing strength of stimulus, so that its threshold of excitation is greater than it would be were the stimulus strength to have risen more rapidly.

positive a., increased refractivity of the eye that occurs when shifting from the distance to a near object.

range of a., the distance between an object viewed with minimal

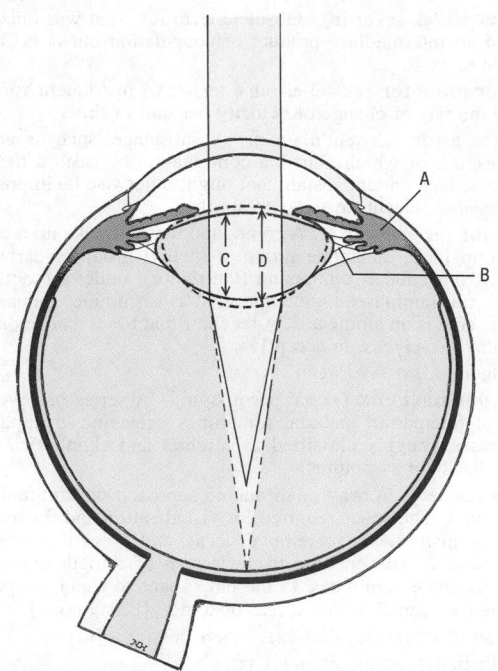

accommodation: (A) ciliary muscle, (B) suspensory ligaments, (C) lens focuses image in front of retina; image is blurred, (D) lens accommodates to focus on retina, image is sharp

refractivity of the eye and one viewed with maximal accommodation.

relative a., quantity of a. required for single binocular vision for any specified distance, or for any particular degree of convergence.

ac·com·mo·da·tive (ă-kom′ŏ-dā-tiv). Relating to accommodation.

ac·com·plice (ă-kom′plis). A bacterium that accompanies the main infecting agent in a mixed infection and that influences the virulence of the main organism. [M.E., fr. O.Fr., fr. L. *comples,* closely connected]

ac·couche·ment (a-koosh-mawn′). Childbirth, particularly parturition. SEE ALSO birth. [Fr. from *coucher,* to lie down]

a. forcé (fōr-sā′), forced, artificially hastened delivery, by means of forceps, version, etc.; originally applied to rapid dilation of the cervix with the hands, with version and forcible extraction of the fetus.

ac·cou·cheur (a-koo-sher′). Obsolete term for obstetrician.

ac·cre·men·ti·tion (ak′rē-men-tish′ŭn). **1.** Reproduction by budding or germination. **2.** SYN accretion (1). [L. *accresco,* pp. -*cretus,* to increase]

ac·cre·tio cor·dis (ă-krē′shē-ō kōr′dis). Adhesion of the pericardium to adjacent extracardiac structures.

ac·cre·tion (ă-krē′shŭn). **1.** Increase by addition to the periphery of material of the same nature as that already present; e.g., the manner of growth of crystals. SYN accrementition (2). **2.** In dentistry, foreign material (usually plaque or calculus) collecting on the surface of a tooth or in a cavity. **3.** A growing together. [L. *accretio,* fr. *ad,* to, + *crescere,* to grow]

ac·cro·chage (ak-rō-shahj′). Intermittent synchronization of two different rhythms of the heart with one influencing the behavior of the other when neither is dominant; seen in cases of atrioventricular dissociation when an atrial beat falls shortly after a ventricular beat, the latter causing the atrial beat to occur sooner than expected. [Fr. hooking, hitching]

ac·cur·a·cy (ak′kū-ră-sē). The degree to which a measurement, or an estimate based on measurements, represents the true value of the attribute that is being measured. In the laboratory, a. of a test

is determined when possible by comparing results from the test in question with results generated using reference standards or an established reference method.

ACD Abbreviation for acid-citrate-dextrose.

ACE Abbreviation for angiotensin-converting *enzyme.*

ac·e·bu·to·lol (as-ĕ-bū′tō-lol). A β-adrenergic blocking agent.

acec·li·dine (a-sek′li-dēn). A cholinergic drug used for topical therapy of glaucoma.

ac·e·dap·sone (as-ĕ-dap′sōn). A derivative of dapsone with a longer duration of action; used to enhance the malaria chemoprophylaxis of quinine or of a combination of chloroquine-primaquine, and believed to act by interference with the utilization of folic acid.

ace·dia (ă-sē-dē′-ă). Obsolete term for a mental syndrome, the chief features of which are listlessness, carelessness, apathy, and melancholia.

acef·yl·line pi·per·a·zine (ă-sef′i-lēn). A diuretic and smooth muscle relaxant.

ACEI Abbreviation for angiotensin-converting enzyme *inhibitors,* under *inhibitor.*

acel·lu·lar (ā-sel′ū-lăr). **1.** Devoid of cells. SYN noncellular (2). **2.** A term applied to unicellular organisms that do not become multicellular and are complete within a single cell unit; frequently applied to protozoans to emphasize their complete organization within a single cell. [G. *a-* priv. + L. *cellula,* a small chamber]

ace·lom (ā-sē′lom). Absence of a true celom or body cavity lined with mesothelium; typically found in Platyhelminthes (flatworms), which have a syncytial mass of parenchymal cells instead of a true body cavity. [G. *a-* priv. + *koilōma,* hollow (celom)]

ace·lo·mate, ace·lo·ma·tous (ā-sē′lō-māt, ā-sē-lō′mă-tŭs). Not having a celom or body cavity.

acen·o·cou·ma·rin (ă-sē-nō-koo′mă-rin). SYN acenocoumarol.

acen·o·cou·ma·rol (ă-sē-nō-koo′mă-rol). An orally effective synthetic anticoagulant of the coumarin type, with similar actions. SYN acenocoumarin, nicoumalone.

acen·tric (ā-sen′trik). Lacking a center; in cytogenetics, denoting a chromosome fragment without a centromere. [G. *a-* priv. + *kentron,* center]

ace·pha·lia, aceph·a·lism (ā-se-fā′lē-ă, ā-sef′ă-lizm). **1.** SYN acephaly. **2.** SYN acephalus.

aceph·a·line (ă-sef′ă-līn). Denoting members of the protozoan suborder Acephalina (order Eugregarinida), characterized by simple noncompartmentalized bodies, that parasitize invertebrates.

aceph·a·lo·bra·chia (ā-sef′ă-lō-brā′kē-ă). SYN abrachiocephaly. [G. *a-* priv. + *kephalē,* head, + *brachiōn,* arm]

aceph·a·lo·car·dia (ā-sef′ă-lō-kar′dē-ă). Absence of head and heart as seen in a parasitic twin. [G. *a-* priv. + *kephalē,* head, + *kardia,* heart]

aceph·a·lo·chei·ria, aceph·a·lo·chi·ria (ā-sef′ă-lō-kī′rē-ă). Congenital absence of head and hands. [G. *a-* priv. + *kephalē,* head, + *cheir,* hand]

aceph·a·lo·cyst (ă-sef′ă-lō-sist). A hydatid cyst with no daughter cyst; a sterile hydatid, so called because it fails to develop scoleces (tapeworm heads). [G. *a-* priv. + *kephalē,* head, + *kystis,* bladder]

aceph·a·lo·gas·ter·ia (ā-sef′ă-lō-gas-tēr′ē-ă). Congenital absence of head, thorax, and abdomen as seen in a parasitic twin with pelvis and legs only.

aceph·a·lo·po·dia (ā-sef′ă-lō-pō′dē-ă). Congenital absence of head and feet. [G. *a-* priv. + *kephalē,* head, + *pous,* foot]

aceph·a·lor·rha·chia (ā-sef′ă-lō-rāk′ē-ă). Congenital absence of head and vertebral column. [G. *a-* priv. + *kephalē,* head, + *rhachis,* spine]

aceph·a·lo·tho·ra·cia (ā-sef′ă-lō-thōr-asē-ă). Congenital absence of head and thorax. [G. *a-* priv. + *kephalē,* head, + *thorax,* chest]

aceph·a·lous (ā-sef′ă-lŭs). Headless.

aceph·a·lus (ā-sef′ă-lŭs). A headless fetus. SYN acephalia (2), acephalism. [G. *a-* priv. + *kephalē,* head]

ac

a. acormus (ă-kōr′mus), condition in which a head without a body is attached to the placenta by an umbilical cord.

a. dibra′chius, a fetus lacking a head but having two recognizably developed upper limbs.

a. di′pus, a fetus lacking a head but showing two recognizably developed lower limbs.

a. monobra′chius, a fetus lacking a head and showing only one recognizable upper limb.

a. mon′opus, a fetus lacking a head and with fusion of the lower extremities so extreme that only a single foot is recognizable.

a. sym′pus, a fetus lacking a head and showing fusion of the lower limbs.

aceph·a·ly (ă-sef′ă-lē). Congenital absence of the head. SYN acephalia (1), acephalism. [G. *a-* priv. + *kephalē,* head]

ace·ro·la (ă-sĕ-rō-lă). Fruit of a bushy tree that grows in Central and South America and Puerto Rico. The berry is the richest known source of vitamin C (ascorbic acid).

acer·vu·lus (ă-ser′vū-lŭs). SYN *corpora* arenacea, under *corpus.* [Mod. L. dim. of L. *acervus,* a heap]

aces·to·ma (ă-ses-tō′mă). Exuberant granulations that form a cicatrix. [G. *akestos,* curable, + *-ōma,* tumor]

ace·sul·fame (ă-sē-sul-fām). A synthetic, noncaloric sweetener similar to saccharin.

△**acet-, aceto-.** Combining forms denoting the two-carbon fragment of acetic acid.

ac·e·tab·u·la (as-ĕ-tab′ū-lă). Plural of acetabulum.

ac·e·tab·u·lar (as-ĕ-tab′ū-lăr). Relating to the acetabulum.

ac·e·tab·u·lec·to·my (as′ĕ-tab-ū-lek′tō-mē). Excision of the acetabulum. [acetabulum + G. *ektomē,* excision]

ac·e·tab·u·lo·plas·ty (as-ĕ-tab′ū-lō-plas-tē). Any operation aimed at restoring the acetabulum to as near a normal state as possible. [acetabulum + G. *plastos,* formed]

ac·e·tab·u·lum, pl. **ac·e·tab·u·la** (as-ĕ-tab′ū-lŭm, -lă) [TA]. A cup-shaped depression on the external surface of the hip bone, with which the head of the femur articulates. SYN cotyle (2), cotyloid cavity. [L. a shallow vinegar vessel or cup]

ac·e·tal (as′e-tal). Product of the addition of 2 mol of alcohol to one of an aldehyde, thus: $RCHO + 2R'OH \rightarrow RCH(OR')_2 + H_2O$; in mixed acetals (e.g., glycosides), two different alcohols are bound to the original aldehyde group. SEE ALSO hemiacetal, hemiketal, ketal.

a. phosphatide, older trivial name for alk-1-enylglycerophospholipid.

ac·et·al·de·hyde (as-e-tal′dĕ-hīd). An intermediate in yeast fermentation of carbohydrate and in alcohol metabolism. It is a central agent for the toxic effects of ethanol. SYN acetic aldehyde, ethanal.

activated a., the activated form of acetaldehyde that is formed during the decarboxylation of active pyruvate. Formed in alcohol fermentation and in carbohydrate metabolism. SYN α-hydroxyethylthiamin pyrophosphate.

acet·a·mide (as-et-am′īd, ă-set′ă-mīd). CH_3CONH_2; used in biomedical research. SYN acetic amide.

2-ac·et·am·i·do·flu·o·rene (AAF) (as′et-am′i-dō-flōr′ēn). SYN 2-acetylaminofluorene.

ac·et·a·min·o·phen (as-et-ă-mē′nō-fen). An antipyretic and analgesic, with potency similar to aspirin. SYN paracetamol.

ac·e·tam·in·o·sal·ol (as-ĕ-tam′in-ō-sal′ol). Used as an analgesic, antipyretic, and intestinal antiseptic. SYN phenetsal.

ac·et·ar·sol (as-ĕ-tar′sol). SYN acetarsone.

ac·et·ar·sone (as-ĕ-tar′sōn). Used in the treatment of amebiasis, and as a local application in Vincent angina and in trichomoniasis vaginitis. The diethylamine salt is used as an antisyphilitic. SYN acetarsol.

ac·e·tate (as′e-tāt). A salt or ester of acetic acid.

active a., SYN acetyl-CoA.

a. kinase [EC 2.7.2.1], a phosphotransferase forming acetyl phosphate and ADP from ATP and acetate. An important enzyme in the formation of "high-energy" phosphate in certain microorganisms. SYN acetokinase.

a. thiokinase, SYN *acetyl-CoA* ligase.

ac·e·tate-CoA ligase. SYN *acetyl-CoA* ligase.

acet·a·zol·a·mide (as′e-tă-zol′ă-mīd). The heterocyclic sulfonamide, 5-acetylamido-1,3,4-thiadiazole-2-sulfonamide, which inhibits the action of carbonic anhydrase in the kidney, increasing the urinary excretion of sodium, potassium, and bicarbonate, reducing excretion of ammonium, raising the pH of the urine, and lowering the pH of the blood; used in respiratory acidosis for diuresis and to stimulate respiratory drive, in glaucoma to reduce intraocular pressure, and in epilepsy. A. sodium has the same actions and uses as a., but is more soluble and thus more suitable for parenteral administration.

acet·e·nyl (a-sē′ten-il). SYN ethynyl.

ace·tic (a-sē′tik, -set′ik). **1.** Denoting the presence of the two-carbon fragment of acetic acid. **2.** Relating to vinegar; sour. [L. *acetum,* vinegar]

ace·tic ac·id. A product of the oxidation of ethanol and of the destructive distillation of wood; used locally as a counterirritant and occasionally internally, and also as a reagent; contained in vinegars. SYN ethanoic acid.

diluted a. a., contains 6% w/v of a. a.

glacial a. a., contains 99% absolute a. a.; a caustic for removal of corns and warts.

ace·tic al·de·hyde. SYN acetaldehyde.

ace·tic am·ide. SYN acetamide.

ace·ti·co·cep·tor (a-sē′ti-kō-sep′tōr). A side chain of molecules with a special affinity for the acetic acid radical. [L. *acetum,* vinegar, + *capio,* to take]

ace·ti·fy (ă-set′i-fī). To cause acetic fermentation; to make vinegar or become vinegar. [L. *acetum,* vinegar, + *facio,* to make; or *fieri,* to be made, to become]

ace·tim·e·ter (as-ĕ-tim′ĕ-ter). An apparatus for determining the content of acetic acid in vinegar or other fluid. SYN acetometer. [L. *acetum,* vinegar, + G. *metron,* measure]

△**aceto-.** SEE acet-.

ac·e·to·ac·e·tate (as′e-tō-as′e-tāt). A salt or ion of acetoacetic acid. A ketone body formed in ketogenesis. SYN diacetate (1).

a. decarboxylase [EC 4.1.1.4], a carboxy-lyase cleaving CO_2 from a. to form acetone.

ac·e·to·a·ce·tic ac·id (as′e-tō-a-sē′tik). One of the ketone bodies, formed in excess and appearing in the urine in starvation or diabetes.

ac·e·to·a·ce·tyl-CoA (as′e-tō-a-sē′til). Intermediate in the oxidation of fatty acids and in the formation of ketone bodies; also formed from two molecules of acetyl-CoA; major role in condensation with acetyl-CoA to form the important β-hydroxy-β-methylglutaryl-CoA. SYN acetoacetyl-coenzyme A.

a.-CoA reductase [EC 1.1.1.36], an oxidoreductase catalyzing interconversion of a 3-oxoacyl-CoA and NADPH, and the corresponding D-3-hydroxyacyl-CoA, and NADP⁺. A step in fatty acid synthesis.

a.-CoA thiolase, SYN *acetyl-CoA* acetyltransferase.

ac·e·to·a·ce·tyl-co·en·zyme A (as′e-tō-as′e-til-kō-en′zīm). SYN acetoacetyl-CoA.

ac·e·to·a·ce·tyl-suc·cin·ic thi·o·phor·ase (as′e-tō-as′e-til-sŭk-sin′ik). SYN 3-oxoacid-CoA transferase.

ac·e·to·hex·am·ide (as-ĕ-tō-heks′ă-mīd). An oral hypoglycemic agent that stimulates pancreatic insulin secretion; most useful therapeutically in mild cases of non-insulin-dependent diabetes mellitus.

ac·e·to·hy·drox·a·mic ac·id (as′e-tō-hī-drok′să-mik). An inhibitor of urease, used as adjunctive therapy in chronic urea-splitting urinary infections.

acet·o·in (as-et′-ō-in). A condensation product of two molecules of acetaldehyde.

ac·e·to·ki·nase (as′e-tō-kī′nās). SYN *acetate* kinase.

ac·e·tol (as′e-tol). Obsolete term for 1-hydroxy-2-propanone, or hydroxyacetone; also used as a proprietary name for certain commercial items.

α·ac·e·to·lac·tic ac·id (as'e-tō-lak'tik). An intermediate in pyruvic acid catabolism and valine biosynthesis.

ac·e·tol·y·sis (as-e-tol'i-sis). Decomposition of an organic compound with the addition of the elements of acetic acid at the point of decomposition; analogous to hydrolysis and phosphorolysis.

ac·e·to·me·naph·thone (as'ĕ-tō-me-naf'thōn). SYN menadiol diacetate.

ac·e·tom·e·ter (as-ĕ-tom'ĕ-ter). SYN acetimeter.

ac·e·tone (as'e-tōn). A colorless, volatile, flammable liquid; extremely small amounts are found in normal urine, but larger quantities occur in urine and blood of diabetic persons, sometimes imparting an ethereal odor to the urine and breath. It is one of the ketone bodies. The synthetic is used as a solvent in some pharmaceutical and commercial preparations. SYN dimethyl ketone.

ac·e·ton·e·mia (as'ĕ-tō-nē'mē-ă). The presence of acetone or acetone bodies in relatively large amounts in the blood, manifested at first by erethism, and later by a progressive depression. [acetone + G. *haima,* blood]

ac·e·to·ne·mic (as'ĕ-tō-nē'mik). Relating to or caused by acetonemia.

ac·e·to·ni·trile (as'e-tō-nī'tril). Methyl cyanide; a colorless fluid of aromatic odor, soluble in water and alcohol.

ac·e·to·nu·ria (as'e-tō-noor'ē-ă). Excretion in the urine of large amounts of acetone, an indication of incomplete oxidation of large amounts of lipids; commonly occurs in diabetic acidosis. [acetone + G. *ouron,* urine]

ac·e·to·phen·a·zine ma·le·ate (as-ĕ-tō-fē'nă-zēn mal'ē-āt). A phenothiazine tranquilizer.

ac·e·to·phe·net·i·din (as'ĕ-tō-fe-net'i-din). SYN phenacetin.

ac·e·to·sul·fone so·di·um (as'ĕ-tō-sŭl'fōn). A leprostatic administered orally.

ace·tous (as'e-tŭs). Relating to vinegar; sour-tasting.

ac·e·to·whit·en·ing (ă-sē'tō- hwīt'en-ing). Blanching of skin or mucous membranes after application of 3–5% acetic acid solution, a sign of increased cellular protein and increased nuclear density; used particularly on genital skin and mucous membranes, including the uterine cervix, to identify zones of squamous cell change for biopsy and *condyloma* acuminatum for treatment. SYN visual inspection with acetic acid. [acetic acid + whitening]

ac·e·tri·zo·ate so·di·um (as-ĕ-trī-zō'āt). Salt of 3-acetamido-2,4,6-triiobenzoic acid, a formerly used water-soluble radiographic contrast medium.

ace·tum, pl. **ace·ta** (ă-sē'tŭm, -tă). SYN vinegar. [L. *vinum acetum,* soured wine, vinegar]

acet·u·rate (ă-set'ū-rāt). USAN-approved contraction for *N*-acetylglycinate, CH₃CONHCH₂COO⁻.

ace·tyl (Ac) (as'e-til). CH₃CO–; an acetic acid molecule from which the hydroxyl group has been removed.

a. chloride, a colorless liquid used as a reagent; also corrosive, causing severe burns because of hydrolysis to HCl.

a. phosphate, a "high-energy" phosphate that acts as an acetate donor in the metabolism of various bacteria.

a. transacylase, SYN ACP-acetyltransferase.

ace·tyl·ad·e·nyl·ate (as'e-til-ă-den'il-āt). Mixed anhydride between the carboxyl group of acetic acid and the phosphoric residue of adenosine 5'-monophosphoric acid.

2-ace·tylami·no·flu·o·rene (AAF) (as'e-til-am'i-nō-flōr'ēn). A potent carcinogenic compound. SYN 2-acetamidofluorene.

acet·y·lase (a-set'il-ās). Any enzyme catalyzing acetylation or deacetylation, as in the formation of *N*-acetylglutamate from glutamate plus acetyl-CoA, or the reverse; a.'s are usually called acetyltransferases.

N-ace·tyl·as·par·tate (as'-ē-til-as-par'tāt). An acetylated derivative of aspartate found in the brain. Used as a marker in brain NMR and in neuroimaging.

acet·y·la·tion (a-set-i-lā'shŭn). Formation of an acetyl derivative.

ace·tyl·car·bro·mal (ă-sē'til-kar-brō'măl). A sedative replaced by benzodiazepines and newer drugs.

***O*-ace·tyl·car·ni·tine** (as-e-til-kar'ni-tēn). The acetyl derivative of carnitine formed by carnitine acetyltransferase. Facilitates ace-

tyl transport into the mitochondria and is an important fuel source for sperm.

ace·tyl·cho·line (ACH, Ach) (as-e-til-kō'lēn). The acetic ester of choline, the neurotransmitter substance at cholinergic synapses, which causes cardiac inhibition, vasodilation, gastrointestinal peristalsis, and other parasympathetic effects. It is liberated from preganglionic and postganglionic endings of parasympathetic fibers and from preganglionic fibers of the sympathetic as a result of nerve injuries, whereupon it acts as a transmitter on the effector organ; it is hydrolyzed rapidly into choline and acetic acid by acetylcholinesterase in the tissues and by pseudocholinesterase in the blood.

a. chloride, a miotic, administered as an ophthalmic solution for parasympathomimetic effect; used in cataract surgery.

ace·tyl·cho·lin·es·ter·ase (as'e-til-kō-lin-es'ter-ās). The cholinesterases that hydrolyze acetylcholine to acetate and choline within the central nervous system and at peripheral neuroeffector junctions (e.g., motor endplates and autonomic ganglia). SYN choline esterase I, "e"-type cholinesterase, specific cholinesterase, true cholinesterase.

ace·tyl-CoA. Condensation product of coenzyme A and acetic acid, symbolized as CoAS~COCH₃; intermediate in transfer of two-carbon fragment, notably in its entrance into the tricarboxylic acid cycle and in fatty acid synthesis. SYN acetyl-coenzyme A, active acetate.

a.-CoA acetyltransferase, an acetyltransferase forming acetoacetyl-CoA from two molecules of a.-CoA, releasing one CoA. A key step in ketogenesis and sterol synthesis. SYN acetoacetyl-CoA thiolase, a.-CoA thiolase, thiolase.

a.-CoA acylase, SYN a.-CoA hydrolase.

a.-CoA acyltransferase, an enzyme catalyzing the thioclastic cleavage by coenzyme A of β-ketoacyl-CoA, forming an acyl-CoA with a carbon chain shorter by two atoms, the missing two atoms appearing as a.-CoA. A step in fatty acid degradation. SEE ALSO a.-CoA acetyltransferase. SYN 3-ketoacyl-CoA thiolase, β-ketothiolase.

a.-CoA carboxylase, a ligase that catalyzes the reaction of a.-CoA, CO₂, H₂O, and ATP, with a divalent cation as catalyst and covalently bound biotin, to form malonyl-CoA, ADP, and Pᵢ (or the reverse decarboxylase); *N*-carboxybiotin is an intermediate. A crucial enzyme in fatty acid synthesis.

a.-CoA deacylase, SYN a.-CoA hydrolase.

a.-CoA:α-glucosaminide acetyltransferase, an enzyme involved in the synthesis of certain carbohydrate moieties on proteins. A deficiency of this enzyme leads to mucopolysaccharidosis type III C.

a.-CoA hydrolase, a hydrolase that cleaves acetate and coenzyme A from a.-CoA. SYN a.-CoA acylase, a.-CoA deacylase.

a.-CoA ligase, a ligase that catalyzes the reaction of acetate and CoA and ATP to form AMP, pyrophosphate, and a.-CoA. A key step in the activation of acetate. SYN acetate thiokinase, acetate-CoA ligase, acetyl-activating enzyme, a.-CoA synthetase.

a.-CoA synthetase, SYN a.-CoA ligase.

a.-CoA thiolase, SYN a.-CoA acetyltransferase.

ace·tyl-co·en·zyme A (as'e-til-kō-en'zīm). SYN acetyl-CoA.

ace·tyl·cys·te·ine (as'ĕ-til-sis'tē-in). A mucolytic agent that reduces the viscosity of mucous secretions; used to prevent liver injury produced by acetaminophen toxicity.

ace·tyl·dig·i·tox·in (ă-sē'til-dij-i-tok'sin). The α-acetyl ester of digitoxin derived from lanatoside A, having the same actions and uses as digitoxin, but more rapid onset and shorter duration of action.

ace·tyl·di·gox·in (ă-sē'til-dī-jok'sin). A digitalis glycoside with properties similar to those of digoxin; derived from digilanide C.

α-N-ace·tyl·ga·lac·to·sam·in·id·ase (as'ē-til-gal-ăk-tōs-a-min-i-dās). An enzyme that hydrolyzes 2-acetamido-2-deoxy-α-D-galactosides to the alcohol and free 2-acetamido-2-deoxy-D-galactose. A deficiency of this enzyme will result in Schindler disease.

N-ace·tyl·glu·co·sam·ine (as'ē-til-glu-cōs'a-mēn). An acetylated amino sugar that is an important moiety of glycoproteins.

α-N-ace·tyl·glu·co·sam·in·id·ase (as'ē-til-glu-cōs-a-min-i-dās). An enzyme that hydrolyzes glycosides of *N*-acetylglucosamine producing the alcohol and *N*-acetylglucosamine. A deficiency of this enzyme results in mucopolysaccharidosis III B.

N-ace·tyl·glu·ta·mate (NAG) (ă-sē′til-gloo′tă-māt). The salt of *N*-acetylglutamic acid. An activator of carbamoyl phosphate synthetase I during urea synthesis; this amino acid causes a configurational change in the enzyme, increasing the activity of that enzyme. The inability to synthesize acetylglutamate results in a defect in urea biosynthesis.

ace·tyl·meth·a·dol (as′ĕ-til-meth-ă-dol). An opioid analgesic which exists in 4 different optical isomers. The *l* isomers are active and *l*-acetylmethadol (LAM) has a long duration of action and has been tried as a substitute for methadone in methadone maintenance programs and in programs where methadone is to be withdrawn, as in physical dependence of the morphine type.

N-ace·tyl·neu·ra·min·ic ac·id (NeuAc) (as′ē-til-nur-a-min′ik-as′id). The most common form of sialic acid in mammals.

ace·tyl·or·ni·thine de·a·cet·yl·ase (as′e-til-ōr′ni-thēn) [EC 3.5.1.16]. An enzyme catalyzing the hydrolysis of N^2-acetyl-L-ornithine to L-ornithine and acetate.

3-ace·tyl·pyr·i·dine (as′e-til-pir′i-dēn). An antimetabolite of nicotinamide that produces symptoms of nicotinamide deficiency in mice; a neurotoxin that damages hypothalamus, brainstem, and basal ganglia.

ace·tyl·sal·i·cyl·ic ac·id (as′ĕ-til-sal-i-sil′ik). SYN aspirin.

N^4-ace·tyl·sul·fa·nil·a·mide (as′e-til-sŭl-fă-nil′ă-mīd). An intermediate in the synthesis of sulfanilamide; formed in animal bodies by acetylation of sulfanilamide. SYN *p*-sulfamylacetanilide.

N^1-ace·tyl·sul·fa·nil·a·mide. An antibacterial sulfa drug used topically and in the eye.

ace·tyl sul·fi·sox·a·zole. A derivative of sulfisoxazole with the same actions and uses; an antibacterial sulfa drug.

ace·tyl·tan·nic ac·id (as′ĕ-til-tan′ik). An astringent formerly used for treatment of diarrhea. SYN diacetyltannic acid, tannylacetate.

ace·tyl·trans·fer·ase (as′e-til-trans′fer-ās). Any enzyme transferring acetyl groups from one compound to another. SEE ALSO *ace-tyl-CoA* acetyltransferase, *choline* acetyltransferase, dihydrolipoamide *S*-acetyltransferase. SYN transacetylase.

AcG, ac-g Abbreviation for accelerator *globulin*.

ACH, Ach Abbreviation for acetylcholine.

Ach SEE ACH.

acha·la·sia (ak-ă-lā′-zē-ă). Failure to relax; referring especially to visceral openings such as the pylorus, cardia, or any other sphincter muscles. [G. *a*- priv. + *chalasis*, a slackening]

    a. of the cardia, SYN esophageal a.

    cricopharyngeal a., functional obstruction at the level of the upper esophageal sphincter due to failure of relaxation of the cricopharyngeal muscles; often associated with a pharyngoesophageal *diverticulum*. SYN a. of the upper sphincter, hypertensive upper esophageal sphincter.

    esophageal a., failure of normal relaxation of the lower esophageal sphincter associated with uncoordinated contractions of the thoracic esophagus, resulting in functional obstruction and difficulty swallowing. SYN a. of the cardia, cardiospasm.

    a. of the upper sphincter, SYN cricopharyngeal a.

Achard, Émile C., French physician, 1860–1941. SEE A. *syndrome;* A.-Thiers *syndrome*.

ache (āk). A dull, poorly localized pain, usually one of less than severe intensity.

    bone a., a dull pain in one or more bones, often severe; an extreme variety occurs in dengue.

    stomach a., pain in the abdomen, usually arising in the stomach or intestine. SYN gastralgia, gastrodynia.

achei·lia (ă-kī′lē-ă). Congenital absence of the lips. [G. *a*- priv. + *cheilos*, lip]

achei·lous, achi·lous (ă-kī′lŭs). Characterized by or relating to acheilia.

achei·ria (ă-kī′rē-ă). **1.** Congenital absence of one or both hands. **2.** Anesthesia in, with loss of the sense of possession of, one or both hands. **3.** A form of dyscheiria in which the patient is unable

to tell on which side of the body a stimulus has been applied. [G. *a*- priv. + *cheir,* hand]

achei·rop·o·dy, achi·rop·o·dy (ă-kī-rop′ō-dē, ă-kī-rop′ō-dē) [MIM*200500]. Congenital absence of the hands and feet; autosomal recessive inheritance. [G. *a*- priv. + *cheir,* hand, + *podos,* foot]

achei·rous, achi·rous (ă-kī′rŭs). Characterized by or relating to acheiria (1).

Achenbach, Walter, 20th century German internist. SEE A. *syndrome*.

Achilles, Mythical Greek warrior, vulnerable only in the heel. SEE A. *bursa, reflex, tendon*.

achil·lo·bur·si·tis (ă-kil′ō-ber-sī′tis). Inflammation of a bursa in proximity to the tendo calcaneus. SYN retrocalcaneobursitis.

achil·lo·ten·ot·o·my (ă-kil′ō-ten-ot′ō-mē). Cutting the Achilles tendon. [Achilles (tendon) + G. *tenōn,* tendon, + *tomē,* a cutting]

achi·ral (ā-kī′răl). Not chiral; denoting an absence of chirality. [G. *a*- priv. + *cheir,* hand]

achlor·hy·dria (ā-klōr-hī′drē-ă). Absence of hydrochloric acid from the gastric juice. [G. *a*- priv. + chlorhydric (acid)]

achlor·o·phyl·lous (ā-klōr-ŏf′ĭ-lŭs). Without chlorophyll, as in fungi.

Acho·le·plas·ma, pl. **Acho·le·plas·ma·ta** (ă-kō-lē-plas′mă, mah-tă). A genus of bacteria (order Mycoplasmatales) that have characteristics identical to those of the species in the genus *Mycoplasma,* with the exception that the acholeplasmas do not require sterol for growth; saprophytic and parasitic species occur. The type species is *A. laidlawii.*

    A. axan′thum, a species originally found in a murine leukemia cell line; ecology bovine, porcine, botanical.

    A. laidla′wii, a species that occurs as a saprophyte in sewage, manure, humus, and soil; type species of the genus *A.* SYN *Mycoplasma laidlawii.*

acho·lia (ă-kō′lē-ă). Suppressed or absent secretion of bile. [G. *a*- priv. + *cholē,* bile]

achol·ic (ă-kol′ik). Without bile, as in a. (pale) stools.

achol·u·ria (ā-kō-loo′rē-ă). Absence of bile pigments from the urine in certain cases of jaundice. [G. *a*- priv. + *cholē,* bile, + *ouron,* urine]

achol·u·ric (ā-kō-loo′rik). Without bile in the urine.

achon·dro·gen·e·sis (ā-kon-drō-jen′ĕ-sis). Neonatal lethal dwarfism characterized by severe bone dysplasia of all four limbs, micromelia, enlarged skull, and a short trunk with delayed or absent ossification of the lower spine and pubic bones. There are various types. [G. *a*- priv. + *chondros,* cartilage, + *genesis,* origin]

    Type IA a. [MIM*200600], a. with hypervascular cartilage and hypercellular bone; uncertain inheritance pattern. SYN Houston-Harris syndrome.

    Type IB a. [MIM*600972], a. with severely disorganized intra-cartilaginous ossification; autosomal recessive inheritance, caused by mutation in the diastrophic dysplasia sulfate transporter gene (DTDST) on chromosome 5q. SYN Parenti-Fraccaro syndrome.

    Type II a. [MIM*200610], a. with autosomal dominant inheritance, caused by mutation in the collagen type II gene (COL2A1) on chromosome 12q. SYN Langer-Saldino syndrome.

achon·dro·pla·sia (ā-kon-drō-plā′zē-ă) [MIM*100800 *134934]. This chondrodystrophy, characterized by an abnormality in conversion of cartilage to bone, is the most common form of short-limb dwarfisim; characterized by short stature with rhizomelic shortening of the limbs, large head with frontal bossing and midface hypoplasia, exaggerated lumbar lordosis, limitation of elbow extension, genu varum, trident hand, characteristic radiographic skeletal findings, and neurologic symptoms complicating hydrocephalus and spinal canal stenosis. Autosomal dominant inheritance with most cases sporadic, caused by mutation in the fibroblast growth factor receptor 3 gene (FGFR3) on chromosome 4p. [G. *a*- priv. + *chondros,* cartilage, + *plasis,* a molding]

    homozygous a., severe a. caused by inheritance of two a. alleles, one from each parent; usually fatal in the first year of life.

achon·dro·plas·tic (ā-kon-drō-plas′tik). Relating to or characterized by achondroplasia.

achor·date, achor·dal (ā-kōr'dāt, ā-kōr'dăl). Referring to animal forms below the Chordata that do not develop a notochord or chorda.

acho·re·sis (ă-kō-rē'sis). Permanent contraction of a hollow viscus, such as the stomach or bladder, whereby its capacity is reduced. [G. *a-* priv. + *chōreō,* to make room, fr. *chōros,* space]

Acho·ri·on (ă-kō'rē-on). Former name for dermatophytes now placed in the genus *Trichophyton* or *Microsporum.* [G. *achōr,* dandruff]

achro·a·cyte (ă-krō'ă-sīt). A colorless cell. [G. *a-* priv. + *chroa,* color, + *kytos,* a hollow (cell)]

ach·ro·dex·trin (ak-rō-deks'trin). SYN achroodextrin. [G. *a-* priv. + *chrōma,* color, + dextrin]

achro·ma·cyte (ă-krō'mă-sīt). SYN achromocyte.

ach·ro·ma·sia (ak-rō-mā'sē-ă). **1.** Pallor associated with hippocratic facies, emaciation, and weakness, often heralding a moribund state. SYN cachectic pallor. **2.** SYN achromia. [G. *achrōmos,* colorless]

achro·mat (ă-krō'măt). A person exhibiting achromatopsia. [G. *a-* priv. + *chrōma,* color]

ach·ro·mat·ic (ak-rō-mat'ik). **1.** Colorless. **2.** Not staining readily. **3.** Refracting light without chromatic aberration. [G. *a-* priv. + *chrōma,* color]

achro·ma·tin (ă-krō'mă-tin). The weakly staining components of the nucleus, such as the nuclear sap and euchromatin.

achro·ma·tin·ic (ă-krō-mă-tin'ik). Relating to or containing achromatin.

achro·ma·tism (ă-krō'mă-tizm). **1.** The quality of being achromatic. **2.** The annulment of chromatic aberration by combining glasses of different refractive indexes and different dispersion.

achro·mat·o·cyte (ā-krō-mat'ō-sīt). SYN achromocyte.

achro·ma·tol·y·sis (ă-krō-mă-tol'i-sis). Dissolution of the achromatin of a cell or of its nucleus. SYN karyoplasmolysis.

achro·mat·o·phil (ă-krō-mat'ō-fil). **1.** Not being colored by the histologic or bacteriologic stains. SYN achromophilic, achromophilous. **2.** A cell or tissue that cannot be stained in the usual way. SYN achromophil. [G. *a-* priv. + *chrōma,* color, + *philos,* fond]

achro·mat·o·phil·ia (ă-krō'mat-ō-fil'ē-ă). A condition of being refractory to staining processes.

achro·ma·top·sia, achro·ma·top·sy (ă-krō-mă-top'sē-ă, ă-krō'mă-top-sē) [MIM*216900]. This is the compete form of a., characterized by severe deficiency of color perception, associated with nystagmus, photophobia, reduced visual acuity, and "day blindness"; autosomal recessive inheritance, caused by mutation in the cone photoreceptor cGMP-gated cation channel, alpha-subunit 3 gene (CNGA3) on chromosome 2q. SYN achromatic vision, monochromasia, monochromasy, monochromatism (2). [G. *a-* priv. + *chrōma,* color, + *opsis,* vision]

atypical a., incomplete a. with normal visual acuity and no nystagmus. Cf. dyschromatopsia.

complete a., a. with absent color vision, nystagmus, reduced visual acuity, and light aversion. SYN rod monochromatism, typical a.

incomplete a. [MIM*200930], impaired but not absent color vision with less severely reduced visual acuity than in complete a., associated with photophobia and nystagmus; autosomal recessive inheritance. An autosomal dominant [MIM*180020] form and several X-linked [MIM*304020, MIM*300085, and MIM*303700] forms exist.

typical a., SYN complete a.

achro·ma·to·sis (ă-krō-mă-tō'sis). SYN achromia. [G. *a-* priv. + *chrōma,* color]

achro·ma·tous (ă-krō'mă-tŭs). Colorless.

achro·ma·tu·ria (ă-krō-mă-too'rē-ă). The passage of colorless or very pale urine. [G. *a-* priv. + *chrōma,* color, + *ouron,* urine]

achro·mia (ă-krō'mē-ă). **1.** Hypopigmentation; absence or loss of natural pigmentation of the skin and iris; may be congenital or acquired. SEE ALSO depigmentation. **2.** Lack of capacity to accept stains in cells or tissue. SYN achromasia (2), achromatosis. [G. *a-* priv. + *chrōma,* color]

a. parasit'ica, a phase of lessening or absence of pigmentation in cutaneous lesions, caused by the fungus *Malassezia furfur.* SEE ALSO *tinea* versicolor.

achro·mic (ā-krō'mik). Colorless.

Achromobacter (a'krō-mō-bak'ter). A Gram-negative bacterial genus of uncertain clinical significance, closely related to members of the *Alcaligenes* and *Ochrobactrum* species.

achro·mo·cyte (ă-krō'mō-sīt). A hypochromic, crescent-shaped erythrocyte, probably resulting from artifactual rupture of a red cell with loss of hemoglobin. SYN achromacyte, achromatocyte, ghost corpuscle, phantom corpuscle, Ponfick shadow, shadow corpuscle, shadow (3), Traube corpuscle. [G. *a-* priv. + *chrōma,* color, + *kytos,* hollow (cell)]

achro·mo·phil (ă-krō'mō-fil). SYN achromatophil.

achro·mo·phil·ic, achro·moph·i·lous (ā-krō-mō-fil'ik, ā-krō-mof'i-lŭs). SYN achromatophil (1).

achro·mo·trich·ia (ă-krō-mō-trik'ē-ă). Absence or loss of pigment in the hair. SEE ALSO canities. [G. *a-* priv. + *chrōma,* color, + *thrix,* hair]

ach·ro·o·dex·trin (ak-rō'ō-deks'trin). Dextrin of low molecular weight, formed from starch in a stage of the digestion of the latter by amylase; it gives no color reaction with iodine. Cf. amylodextrin, erythrodextrin. SYN achrodextrin. [G. *achromos,* uncolored, + dextrin]

achy·lia (ă-kī'lē-ă). **1.** Absence of gastric juice or other digestive secretions. **2.** Absence of chyle. [G. *a-* priv. + *chylos,* juice]

a. gas'trica, diminished or abolished secretion of gastric juice associated with atrophy of the mucous membrane of the stomach.

a. pancreat'ica, deficiency or absence of pancreatic secretion, usually resulting in fatty stools, emaciation, and impaired nutrition.

achy·lous (ă-kī'lŭs). **1.** Lacking in gastric juice or other digestive secretions. **2.** Having no chyle. [G. *achylos,* without juice]

acic·u·lar (ă-sik'ū-lar). Needle-shaped or needle-pointed; applied particularly to leaves and crystals. [L. *acicular,* small pin]

ac·id (as'id). **1.** A compound yielding a hydrogen ion in a polar solvent (e.g., in water); a.'s form salts by replacing all or part of the ionizable hydrogen with an electropositive element or radical. **2.** In popular language, any chemical compound that has a sour taste (given by the hydrogen ion). **3.** Sour; sharp to the taste. **4.** Relating to a.; giving an a. reaction. For individual acids, see specific names. [L. *acidus,* sour]

bile a.'s, steroid a.'s found in bile; e.g., taurocholic and glycocholic a.'s, used therapeutically when biliary secretion is inadequate and for biliary colic. Their physiologic roles include fat emulsification. Their synthesis is reduced in disorders of the peroxisomes.

Brónsted a., an a. that is a proton donor.

conjugate a., the protonated compound of two compounds that differ in structure only by the presence of the labile proton.

dibasic a., an a. containing two ionizable atoms of hydrogen in the molecule. SEE acid (1).

fatty a., SEE fatty acid.

inorganic a., an a. made up of molecules not containing organic radicals; e.g., HCl, H_2SO_4, H_3PO_4.

Lewis a., an a. that is an electron pair acceptor.

monobasic a., an a. containing one ionizable atom of hydrogen in the molecule. SEE acid (1).

organic a., an a. made up of molecules containing organic radicals; e.g., acetic a., citric a., which contain the ionizable –COOH group.

polybasic a., an a. containing more than three ionizable atoms of hydrogen in the molecule. SEE acid (1).

wax a., a long-chain monocarboxylic a. with an even number of carbons, often found esterified in waxes (e.g., lauric acid).

ac·id-cit·rate-dex·trose (ACD). A citrate anticoagulant used for the collection and preservation of whole blood. It has largely been replaced by newer anticoagulants (CPD, Adsol) that allow for longer shelf life for blood and blood products.

ac·i·de·mia (as-i-dē'mē-ă). An increase in the H-ion concentration of the blood or a fall below normal in pH. Individual types of

a. are listed by specific name, e.g., isovalericacidemia, aminoacidemia, etc. [acid + G. *haima,* blood]

ac·id-fast (as'id-fast). Denoting bacteria that are not decolorized by acid-alcohol after having been stained with dyes such as basic fuchsin; e.g., the mycobacteria and nocardiae.

acid·i·fy (a-sid'i-fī). **1.** To render acid. **2.** To become acid.

acid·i·ty (a-sid'i-tē). **1.** The state of being acid. **2.** The acid content of a fluid.

> **total a. (a),** an obsolete expression of gastric a., the a. being determined by titration with sodium hydroxide, using phenolphthalein as indicator.

ac·i·do·phil, ac·i·do·phile (ă-sid'ō-fil, ă-sid'ō-fīl). **1.** One of the acid-staining cells of the anterior pituitary. **2.** A microorganism that grows well in a highly acid medium. [acid + G. *philos,* fond]

ac·i·do·phil·ic (as'i-dō-fil'ik, ă-sid'ō-fil-ik). Having an affinity for acid dyes; denoting a cell or tissue element that stains with an acid dye, such as eosin. SYN oxychromatic.

ac·i·do·sis (as-i-dō'sis). A pathologic state characterized by an increase in the concentration of hydrogen ions in the arterial blood above the normal level, 40 nmol/L, or pH 7.4; may be caused by an accumulation of carbon dioxide or acidic products of metabolism, or by a decrease in the concentration of alkaline compounds. [acid + G. *-ōsis,* condition]

> **carbon dioxide a.,** SYN respiratory a.

> **compensated a.,** an a. in which the pH of body fluids is normal; compensation is achieved by respiratory or renal mechanisms.

> **compensated respiratory a.,** retention of bicarbonate by the renal tubules to minimize the effect on the pH of the blood of retention of carbon dioxide by the lungs, such as occurs with hypoventilation.

> **diabetic a.,** a type of metabolic a. caused by accumulation of ketone bodies in diabetes mellitus.

> **hypercapnic a.,** SYN respiratory a.

> **hyperchloremic a.,** SYN renal tubular a.

> **lactic a.,** a type of metabolic a. caused by accumulation of lactic acid due to tissue hypoxia, drug effect, or unknown etiology.

> **metabolic a.,** decreased pH and bicarbonate concentration in the body fluids caused either by the accumulation of acids or by abnormal losses of fixed base from the body, as in diarrhea or renal disease.

> **primary renal tubular a.,** a metabolic defect in the mechanism of urinary acidification that may be either the transient type, with onset in infancy, or the persistent type, with onset in childhood or adult years; both types are familial.

> **renal tubular a.,** a clinical syndrome characterized by decreased ability to acidify urine, and by low plasma bicarbonate and high plasma chloride concentrations, often with hypokalemia; often complicated by osteomalacia, nephrocalcinosis, or renal calculi. SEE ALSO primary renal tubular a., secondary renal tubular a. SYN hyperchloremic a.

> **respiratory a.,** a. caused by retention of carbon dioxide; due to inadequate pulmonary ventilation or hypoventilation, with decrease in blood pH unless compensated by renal retention of bicarbonate. SYN carbon dioxide a., hypercapnic a.

> **secondary renal tubular a.,** renal tubular a. that may occur as a complication of hypercalcemic states, hyperglobulinemic disorders, and in some other chronic renal conditions; a regular component of De Toni-Fanconi syndrome.

> **starvation a.,** ketoacidosis resulting from lack of food intake, leading to fat catabolism to provide energy, releasing acidic ketone bodies.

> **uncompensated a.,** an a. in which the pH of body fluids is subnormal, because restoration of normal acid-base balance is not possible or has not yet been achieved.

ac·i·dot·ic (as-i-dot'ik). Pertaining to or indicating acidosis.

ac·id red 87. SYN *eosin* y.

ac·id red 91. SYN *eosin* B.

ac·i·du·ria (as-i-doo'rē-ă). **1.** Excretion of an acid urine. **2.** Excretion of an abnormal amount of any specified acid. Individual types of a. are prefixed by the specific acid; e.g., aminoaciduria, ketoaciduria. [acid + G. *ouron,* urine]

argininosuccinic a. [MIM*207900], an autosomal-recessive disorder characterized by excessive urinary excretion of argininosuccinic acid, epilepsy, ataxia, mental retardation, liver disease, and friable, tufted hair; presumed to be the consequence of a deficiency of an enzyme responsible for splitting argininosuccinic acid to arginine and fumaric acid. SYN arginosuccinate lyase deficiency.

ac·i·du·ric (as-i-doo'rik). Pertaining to bacteria that tolerate an acid environment. [acid + L. *duro,* to endure]

ac·i·nar (as'i-nar). Pertaining to the acinus. SYN acinic.

Ac·i·ne·to·bac·ter (as-i-nē'tō-bak'ter). A genus of nonmotile, aerobic bacteria (family Moraxellaceae) containing Gram-negative or -variable coccoid or short rods, or cocci, often occurring in pairs. Spores are not produced. These bacteria grow on ordinary media without the addition of serum. They are oxidase-negative and catalase-positive; carbohydrates are oxidized or not attacked at all, and arginine dihydrolase is not produced. They are a frequent cause of nosocomial infections; often resistant to many antibiotics, they can also cause severe primary infections in immunocompromised people. The type species is *A. calcoaceticus.* SYN *Lingelsheimia.*

> *A. calcoacet'icus,* a species of bacteria originally found in a quinate enrichment; strains of this organism previously identified as *Bacterium anitratum* were found in the genitourinary tract; it is the type species of the genus *A.* SYN *Lingelsheimia anitrata.*

ac·i·ni (as'i-nī). Plural of acinus.

acin·ic (a-sin'ik). SYN acinar.

acin·i·form (a-sin'i-fŏrm). SYN acinous. [L. *acinus,* grape, + *forma,* shape]

ac·i·nose (as'i-nōs). SYN acinous.

ac·i·nous (as'i-nŭs). Resembling an acinus or grape-shaped structure. SYN aciniform, acinose.

■ **ac·i·nus,** gen. and pl. **ac·i·ni** (as'i-nŭs, -nī). One of the minute grape-shaped secretory portions of an acinous gland. Some authorities use the terms a. and alveolus interchangeably, whereas others differentiate them by the constricted openings of the a. into the excretory duct. [L. berry, grape]

> **liver a.,** a functional unit of the liver, comprising all of the liver parenchyma supplied by a terminal branch of the portal vein and hepatic artery; typically involves segments of two lobules lying between two terminal hepatic venules. SYN Rappaport a.

> **pulmonary a.,** that part of the airway consisting of a respiratory bronchiole and all of its branches. SYN primary pulmonary lobule, respiratory lobule.

> **Rappaport a.,** SYN liver a.

a·clas·ia (ă-klā'zē-ă). SYN aclasis.

ac·la·sis (ak'lă-sis). A state of continuity between normal and abnormal tissue. SYN aclasia. [G. *a-* priv. + *klasis,* a breaking away, a fragment]

> **tarsoepiphyseal a.** (tăr'-sō-ep'ĭ-fiz'e- al), epiphysealis hemimelica, affects ankles and knees, leading to limitation of motion. SYN Trevor disease.

ac·me (ak'mē). The period of greatest intensity of any symptom, sign, or process. [G. *akmē,* the highest point]

ac·ne (ak'nē). An inflammatory follicular, papular, and pustular eruption involving the pilosebaceous apparatus. SEE ALSO a. vulgaris. [probably a corruption (or copyist's error) of G. *akmē,* point of efflorescence]

> **a. artificia'lis,** a. produced by external irritants, such as tar (chloracne), or drugs internally administered, such as iodides or bromides. SYN a. venenata.

> **bromide a.,** follicular eruption on face, trunk, and extremities, due to bromide ingestion. SEE ALSO bromoderma.

> **a. cachectico'rum,** a. occurring in persons who have a debilitating constitutional disease; characterized by large, soft, purulent, ulcerative, cystic, and scarred lesions.

> **a. cilia'ris,** follicular papules and pustules on the free edges of the eyelids.

> ■ **a. congloba'ta,** severe cystic a., characterized by cystic lesions, abscesses, communicating sinuses, and thickened, nodular scars; usually sparing the face.

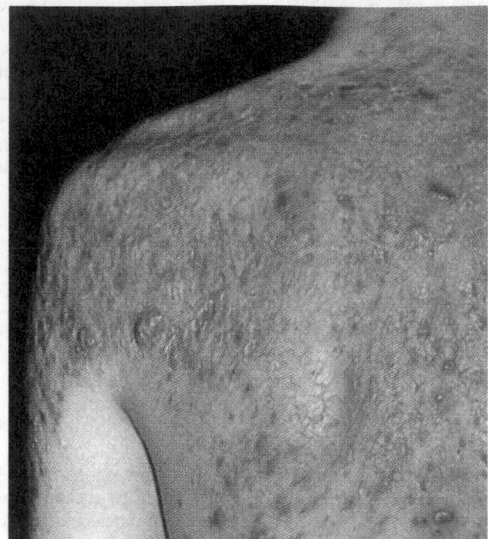

acne conglobata

a. cosmet'ica, low-grade, non-inflammatory acne lesions from repeated application of comedogenic agents in cosmetics.

cystic a., severe a. in which the predominant lesions are follicular cysts which rupture and scar.

a. fulminans (ak'nē ful'mi-nanz), severe scarring a. associated with fever, polyarthralgia, crusted ulcerative lesions, weight loss, and anemia. [*fulmen, fulminis,* thunder, lightning]

a. genera'lis, a. lesions involving the face, chest, and back.

halogen a., an acneform eruption caused by bromides or iodides.

a. hypertroph'ica, a. vulgaris in which the lesions, on healing, leave hypertrophic scars.

iodide a., a follicular eruption on the face, trunk, and extremities, due to injection or ingestion of iodide in a hypersensitive individual. SEE ALSO iododerma.

a. medicamento'sa, a. caused or exacerbated by drugs, e.g., lithium, halogens, or steroids.

a. necrotica miliaris, SYN a. varioliformis.

a. neonato'rum, a condition in newborn male infants, characterized by papules, pustules, and comedones on forehead and cheeks, usually resolving in a few months.

pomade a., a form of a. caused by repeated application of hair creams containing oils that block release of sebum from hair follicles; most commonly seen on forehead and temples in young African Americans.

a. puncta'ta, a. with black open comedones.

a. pustulo'sa, a. vulgaris in which pustular lesions predominate.

a. rosa'cea, SYN rosacea.

steroid a., folliculitis or follicular hyperkeratosis resulting from topical or oral administration of steroids.

tar a., SYN chloracne.

tropical a., a severe type of a. of the entire trunk, shoulders, upper arms, buttocks, and thighs; occurs in hot, humid climates.

a. variolifor'mis, a pyogenic infection involving follicles occurring chiefly on the forehead and temples; involution of the umbilicated and crusting lesions is followed by scar formation. SYN a. necrotica miliaris.

a. venena'ta, SYN a. artificialis.

a. vulga'ris, an eruption, predominantly of the face, upper back, and chest, composed of comedones, cysts, papules, and pustules on an inflammatory base; the condition occurs in a majority of people during puberty and adolescence, due to androgenic stimulation of sebum secretion, with plugging of follicles by keratinization, associated with proliferation of *Propionibacterium acnes.* Follicular suppuration may lead to scarring. Topical treatments include tretinoin, benzoyl peroxide, and antibiotics. Sunlight, sys-

temic antibiotics, and oral 13-*cis*-retinoic acid (except in pregnancy) are also effective. SEE ALSO acne.

ac·ne·form (ak'nē-fōrm). Resembling acne. SYN acneiform.

ac·ne·i·form (ak-nē'i-fōrm). SYN acneform.

ac·ne·mia, ak·ne·mia (ak-nē'mē-ă). **1.** Congenital absence of legs. **2.** Atrophy of the muscles of the calves of the legs. [G. *a*-priv. + *knēmē,* leg]

ACNM. Abbreviation for American College of Nuclear Medicine.

ACNP. Abbreviation for American College of Nuclear Physicians.

ac·o·kan·thera (ak-ō-kan'ther-ă). Juice from the leaves and stems of *Acokanthera ouabaio* (family Apocynaceae), a South African arrow poison containing ouabain. [G. *akōkē,* a point, + *anthēros,* blooming]

aco·lous (ak'ō-lŭs). Without limbs. [G. *a*- priv. + *kōlon,* limb]

acon·i·tase (ă-kon'i-tās). SYN aconitate hydratase.

acon·i·tate hy·dra·tase (ă-kon'i-tāt). An iron-containing enzyme catalyzing the dehydration of citric acid to *cis*-aconitic acid, a reaction of significance in the tricarboxylic acid cycle. SYN aconitase.

ac·o·nite (ak'ō-nīt). The dried root of *Aconitum napellus* (family Ranunculaceae), monkshood or wolfsbane; a powerful and rapid-acting poison formerly used as an antipyretic, diuretic, diaphoretic, anodyne, cardiac and respiratory depressant, and externally as an analgesic.

***cis*-ac·o·nit·ic ac·id** (ak-ō-nit'ik). Dehydration product of citric acid; an enzyme-bound intermediate in the tricarboxylic acid cycle.

acon·i·tine (a-kon'i-tēn). The exceedingly poisonous active principle (diterpene alkaloid) of *Aconitum* sp. and *Delphinium* sp., formerly used as a cardiac sedative and applied externally for neuralgia.

aco·rea (ă-kō'rē-ă). Congenital absence of the pupil of the eye. [G. *a*- priv. + *korē,* pupil]

Acosta, Joseph (José) de, Spanish Jesuit missionary, 1539–1600. SEE A. *disease.*

acous·tic (ă-koos'tik). Pertaining to sound, e.g., acoustic meatus, acoustic nerve. [Gr. *akoustikos*]

acous·ti·co·pho·bia (ă-koos'ti-kō-fō'bē-ă). Morbid fear of sounds. [G. *akoustikos,* acoustic, + *phobos,* fear]

acous·tics (ă-koos'tiks). The science concerned with sound. [G. *akoustikos,* relating to sound]

ACP Abbreviation for acyl carrier *protein*; American College of Physicians.

ACP-ace·tyl·trans·fer·ase. Enzyme transferring acetyl from acetyl-CoA to ACP and releasing CoA to begin fatty acid synthesis. SYN acetyl transacylase.

ACP-mal·o·nyl·trans·fer·ase. An enzyme transferring malonyl from malonyl-CoA to ACP and releasing free CoA; a key step in fatty acid synthesis. SYN malonyl transacylase.

ACPS Abbreviation for acrocephalosyndactyly.

ac·quired (ă-kwīrd'). Denoting a disease, predisposition, abnormality, that is not inherited. [L. *ac-quiro (adq-),* to obtain, fr. *quaero,* to seek]

ac·qui·si·tion (ak-wi-zish'ŭn). In psychology, the empiric demonstration of an increase in the strength of the conditioned response in successive trials of pairing the conditioned and unconditioned stimuli.

gradient-recalled a. in the steady state, a type of gradient echo sequence with free induction decay sampling in magnetic resonance imaging; also called "fast imaging with steady-state precession." This family of sequences is faster than spin echo techniques, and is used for magnetic resonance angiography and cardiac imaging.

ACR Abbreviation for American College of Radiology.

ac·ral (ak'răl). Relating to or affecting the peripheral parts, e.g., limbs, fingers, ears, etc. [G. *akron,* extremity]

Acra·nia (ă-krā'nē-ă). A group of the phylum Chordata whose members possess a notochord, gill slits, and nerve cord but no vertebrae, ribs, or skull; e.g., *Amphioxus,* tunicates, and acorn worms. [G. *a-* priv. + *kranion,* skull]

acra·nia (ā-krā′nē-ă). Complete or partial absence of a skull; associated with anencephaly. [G. *a-* priv. + *kranion,* skull]

acra·ni·al (ā-krā′nē-ăl). Having no cranium; relating to acrania or an acranius.

acra·ni·us. A malformed fetus exhibiting acrania.

Acrel, Olaf, Swedish surgeon, 1717–1806. SEE A. *ganglion.*

Ac·re·mo·ni·um (ak-rĕ-mō′nē-ŭm). A genus of fungi (family Moniliaceae, order Moniliales) that causes eumycotic mycetoma; three species, *A. falciforme, A. kiliense,* and *A. recifei,* produce whitish to yellow grains in the tissues. Produces keratomycosis, occasionally other infections, and the antibiotic cephalosporin.

ac·ri·bom·e·ter (ak-ri-bom′ĕ-ter). An instrument for measuring very minute objects. [G. *akribēs,* exact, + *metron,* measure]

ac·rid (ak′rid). Sharp, pungent, biting, or irritating. [L. *acer* (*acr*-), pungent]

ac·ri·dine (ak′ri-dēn). 10-Azaanthracene; a dye, dye intermediate, and antiseptic precursor (9-aminoacridine, acriflavine, proflavine hemisulfate) derived from coal tar and irritating to skin and mucous membranes. SYN dibenzopyridine.
  tetramethyl a., SYN acridine orange.

ac·ri·dine or·ange [C.I. 46005]. 3,6-bis(dimethylamino)acridine hydrochloride; a basic fluorescent dye useful as a metachromatic stain for nucleic acids; also used in screening cervical smears for abnormal and malignant cells, where unusual amounts of DNA and RNA occur during proliferation and in tumors (DNA fluoresces yellow to green; RNA fluoresces orange to red). SYN tetramethyl acridine.

ac·ri·dine yel·low. A faintly yellow solution with strong bluishviolet fluorescence; used as a topical antiseptic and as a fluorescent stain in histology. SYN 5-aminoacridine hydrochloride, 9-aminoacridine hydrochloride.

ac·ri·fla·vine (ak-ri-flā′vin) [C.I. 46000]. An acridine dye, a mixture of 3,6-diamino-10-methylacridinium chloride and 3,6-diaminoacridine; formerly used as a topical and urinary antiseptic, and used as one of Kasten fluorescent Schiff reagents to reveal polysaccharides and DNA.

ac·ri·mo·nia (ak-ri-mō′nē-ă). In ancient humoral pathology, a sharp, pungent, disease-provoking humor. [L. pungency]

ac·ri·mo·ny (ak′rĭ-mō-nē). The quality of being intensely irritant, biting, or pungent. [L. *acrimonia,* pungency]

ac·ri·nol (ak′ri-nol). SYN ethacridine lactate.

ac·ri·sor·cin (ak-ri-sōr′sin). A synthetic topical antifungal agent.

acrit·i·cal (ă-krit′i-kăl, ā-). Rarely used term for: **1.** Not critical; marked by no crisis; denoting diseases terminating by lysis. **2.** Indeterminate, especially concerning prognosis. [G. *a-* priv. + *kritikos,* critical]

♻**acro-.** Combining form meaning: **1.** Extremity, tip, end, peak, topmost. **2.** Extreme. [G. *akron,* highest point, extremity; *akros,* topmost, outermost, inmost, extreme, tip]

ac·ro·ag·no·sis (ak′rō-ag-nō′sis). Loss or impairment of the sensory recognition of a limb. Absence of acrognosis.

ac·ro·an·es·the·sia (ak′rō-an-es-thē′zē-ă). Anesthesia of one or more of the extremities. [acro- + G. *an-* priv. + *aisthēsis* sensation]

ac·ro·ar·thri·tis (ak′rō-arth-rī′tis). Inflammation of the joints of the hands or feet. [acro- + G. *arthron,* joint, + *-itis*]

ac·ro·as·phyx·ia (ak′rō-as-fik′sē-ă). Impaired digital circulation, possibly a mild form of Raynaud disease, marked by a purplish or waxy white color of the fingers, with subnormal local temperature and paresthesia. SYN dead fingers, waxy fingers. [acro- + G. *asphyxia,* stoppage of the pulse]

ac·ro·a·tax·ia (ak′rō-ă-tak′sē-ă). Ataxia affecting the distal portion of the extremities, i.e., hands and fingers, feet, and toes. Cf. proximoataxia. [acro- + ataxia]

ac·ro·blast (ak′rō-blast). Component of the developing spermatid composed of numerous Golgi elements; it contains the proacrosomal granules. [acro- + G. *blastos,* germ]

ac·ro·brach·y·ceph·a·ly (ak′rō-brak-i-sef′ă-lē). Type of cranio-

synostosis with premature closure of the coronal suture, resulting in abnormally short anteroposterior diameter of the skull. [acro- + G. *brachys,* short, + *kephalē,* head]

ac·ro·cen·tric (ak-rō-sen′trik). Having the centromere close to one end; said of normal chromosomes 13–15 and 21–22. [acro- + G. *kentron,* center]

ac·ro·ce·pha·lia (ak-rō-se-fā′lē-ă). SYN oxycephaly.

ac·ro·ce·phal·ic (ak-rō-se-fal′ik). SYN oxycephalic.

ac·ro·ceph·a·lo·pol·y·syn·dac·ty·ly (ak′rō-sef′ă-lō-pol′ē-sin-dak′tĭ-lē). A group of congenital syndromes characterized by abnormal skull shape due to craniosynostosis, brachydactyly, syndactyly, and preaxial polydactyly of hands and/or feet; mental retardation is a variable feature. There are several autosomal recessive syndromes [MIM*201000, MIM*201020, and MIM*272350] and one autosomal dominant form [MIM*101600]. A former classification of a., type I to type IV, is now considered obsolete.

ac·ro·ceph·a·lo·syn·dac·ty·ly (ACPS) (ak′rō-sef′ă-lō-sin-dak′ti-lē). A group of congenital syndromes characterized by craniosynostosis with abnormal head shape and cutaneous and/or bony syndactyly. There are several types with most types inherited as autosomal dominant. The phenotypes of types II and IV are not well defined. [acrocephaly + G. *syn,* together, + *daktylos,* finger]
  type I a., SYN Apert *syndrome.*
  type II a., SYN Vogt cephalodactyly.
  type III a., SYN Saethre-Chotzen *syndrome.*
  type V a., SYN Pfeiffer *syndrome.*

ac·ro·ceph·a·lous (ak-rō-sef′ă-lŭs). SYN oxycephalic.

ac·ro·ceph·a·ly (ak′rō-sef′ă-lē). SYN oxycephaly. [acro- + G. *kephalē,* head]

ac·ro·chor·don (ak-rō-kōr′don). SYN skin *tag.* [acro- + G. *chordē,* cord]

ac·ro·ci·ne·sia, ac·ro·ci·ne·sis (ak′rō-si-nē′zē-ă, -ē′sis). Excessive movement. SYN acrokinesia. [acro- + G. *kinēsis,* movement]

ac·ro·con·trac·ture (ak′rō-kon-trak′choor). Contracture of the joints of the hands or feet.

ac·ro·cy·a·no·sis (ak′rō-sī-ă-nō′sis). A circulatory disorder in which the hands, and less commonly the feet, are persistently cold and blue; some forms are related to Raynaud phenomenon. SYN Crocq disease, Raynaud sign. [acro- + G. *kyanos,* blue, + *-osis,* condition]

ac·ro·cy·a·not·ic (ak′rō-sī-ă-not′ik). Characterized by acrocyanosis.

ac·ro·der·ma·ti·tis (ak′rō-der-mă-tī′tis). Inflammation of the skin of the extremities. [acro- + G. *derma,* skin, + *-itis,* inflammation]
  📖**a. chron′ica atroph′icans,** a gradually progressive late skin manifestation of Lyme disease, appearing first on the feet, hands, elbows or knees, and composed of indurated, erythematous plaques that become atrophic, giving a tissue-paper appearance of the involved sites.
  a. contin′ua, SYN *pustulosis* palmaris et plantaris.
  a. enteropath′ica [MIM*201100], a progressive hereditary defect of zinc metabolism in young children (onset 3 weeks to 18 months), often manifests first as a blistering, oozing, and crusting eruption on an extremity or around one of the orifices of the body, followed by loss of hair and diarrhea or other gastrointestinal disturbances; relieved by lifelong oral zinc supplementation; autosomal recessive trait.
  papular a. of childhood, SYN Gianotti-Crosti *syndrome.*
  a. per′stans, SYN *pustulosis* palmaris et plantaris.

ac·ro·der·ma·to·sis (ak′rō-der-mă-tō′sis). Any cutaneous affection involving the more distal portions of the extremities. [acro- + G. *derma,* skin, + *-osis,* condition]

ac·ro·dont (ak′rō-dont). Tooth attachment in some lower vertebrates (mainly fish) in which the teeth rest on the edge of the jaw bone rather than in sockets or alveoli. [acro- + G. *odous,* tooth]

ac·ro·dyn·ia (ak-rō-din′ē-ă). **1.** Pain in peripheral or acral parts of the body. **2.** A syndrome caused almost exclusively in the past by mercury poisoning: in children, characterized by erythema of the extremities, chest, and nose, gastrointestinal symptoms and by

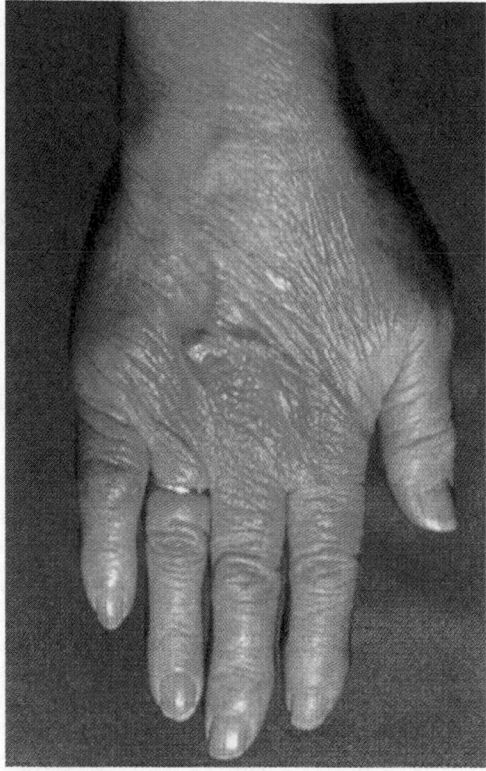

acrodermatitis chronica atrophicans

polyneuritis (in Japan); in adults, characterized by anorexia, photophobia, sweating, and tachycardia. SYN acrodynic erythema, dermatopolyneuritis, erythredema, Feer disease, pink disease. [acro- + G. *odynē,* pain]

ac·ro·dys·es·the·sia (ak′rō-dis-es-thē′zē-ă). Abnormal and unpleasant sensations in the peripheral portions of the extremities. [acro- + dysesthesia]

ac·ro·dys·os·to·sis (ak′rō-dis-os-tō′sis) [MIM*101800]. A disorder in which the hands and feet are short with stubby fingers and toes. Growth retardation is progressive. Mental retardation and marked nasal hypoplasia are also present; autosomal dominant inheritance. [acro- + dysostosis]

ac·ro·es·the·sia (ak′ro-es-thē′zē-ă). **1.** An extreme degree of hyperesthesia. **2.** Hyperesthesia of one or more of the extremities. [acro- + G. *aisthēsis,* sensation]

acrog·e·nous (ak-roj′ĕ-nŭs). Denoting conidia of fungi produced by the conidiogenous cell at the tip of a conidiophore. [acro- + G. *genos,* birth]

ac·ro·ger·ia (ak-rō-jēr′ē-ă) [MIM*201200]. Reduction or loss of subcutaneous fat and collagen of the hands and feet, giving the appearance of premature aging. [acro- + G. *gerōn,* old]

ac·rog·no·sis (ak-rog-nō′sis). Cenesthesia, or normal sensory perception, of the extremities. [acro- + G. *gnōsis,* knowledge]

ac·ro·hy·per·hi·dro·sis (ak′rō-hī′per-hī-drō′sis). Hyperhidrosis of the hands and feet.

acrohyperkeratosis.

focal acrohyperkeratosis, SYN acrokeratoelastoidosis.

ac·ro·ker·a·to·e·las·toi·do·sis (ak′rō-ker′ă-tō-ē-las-toy-dō′sis) [MIM*101850]. An autosomal dominant papular keratosis of the palms and soles, with disorganization of dermal elastic fibers; a similar, but acquired, condition may result from actinic damage of the hands. SEE ALSO keratoelastoidosis. SYN focal acrohyperkeratosis, type III punctate palmoplantar keratoderma. [acro + G. *keras,* horn, + *elastos,* beaten, + *eidos,* resemblance, + *-ōsis,* condition]

ac·ro·ker·a·to·sis (ak′rō-ker-ă-tō′sis). Overgrowth of the horny layer of the skin, usually nodular configurations, of the dorsum of the fingers and toes, and occasionally on the rim of the ear and tip of the nose. [acro- + G. *keras,* horn, + *-osis,* condition]

paraneoplastic a., a rare nail dystrophy with acral erythema and scaling associated with upper respiratory or upper alimentary cancer. SYN Bazex syndrome.

ac·ro·ki·ne·sia (ak′rō-ki-nē′zē-ă). SYN acrocinesia.

ac·ro·me·ga·lia (ak′rō-mĕ-gā′lē-ă). SYN acromegaly.

ac·ro·me·gal·ic (ak′rō-mĕ-gal′ik). Pertaining to or characterized by acromegaly.

ac·ro·meg·a·lo·gi·gan·tism (ak′rō-meg′ă-lō-jī′gan-tizm). Gigantism in which the facial features, disproportionate enlargement of the extremities, and other signs of acromegaly are prominent. [acro- + G. *megas,* great, + *gigas,* giant]

ac·ro·meg·a·loid·ism (ak-rō-meg′ă-loyd-izm). Rarely used term for a condition in which body proportions resemble those of acromegaly.

ac·ro·meg·a·ly (ak-rō-meg′ă-lē). A disorder marked by progressive enlargement of peripheral parts of the body, especially the head, face, hands, and feet, due to excessive secretion of somatotropin; organomegaly and metabolic disorders occur; diabetes mellitus may develop. SYN acromegalia. [acro- + G. *megas,* large]

ac·ro·mel·al·gia (ak-rō-mel-al′jē-ă). SEE erythromelalgia. [acro- + G. *melos,* limb, + *algos,* pain]

acromelia (ak-rō-mez-ō-mē′lē-ă). SYN acromesomelia.

ac·ro·mel·ic (ak-rō-mel′ik). Affecting the terminal part of a limb. [acro- + G. *melos,* limb]

ac·ro·mes·o·me·lia (ak-rō-mē-sō-mē′lē-ă). SYN acromesomelic *dwarfism.* SYN acromelia. [acro- + G. *melos,* limb, + *ia,* condition]

ac·ro·met·a·gen·e·sis (ak′rō-met-ă-jen′ĕ-sis). Abnormal growth of the extremities resulting in malformation. [acro- + G. *meta,* beyond, + *genesis,* origin]

acro·mi·al (ă-krō′mē-ăl). Relating to the acromion.

ac·ro·mic·ria (ak-rō-mik′rē-ă, ak-rō-mī′krē-ă). The antithesis of acromegaly; a condition in which the bones of the face and extremities are small and delicate; possibly due to a deficiency of somatotropin. [acro- + G. *mikros,* small]

acro·mi·o·cla·vic·u·lar (ă-krō′mē-ō-kla-vik′ū-lăr). Relating to the acromion and the clavicle; denoting the articulation and ligaments between the clavicle and the acromion of the scapula. SYN scapuloclavicular (1).

acro·mi·o·cor·a·coid (ă-krō-mē-ō-kōr′ă-koyd). SYN coracoacromial.

acro·mi·o·hu·mer·al (ă-krō′mē-ō-hū′mer-ăl). Relating to the acromion and the humerus.

acro·mi·on (ă-krō′mē-on) [TA]. The lateral end of the spine of the scapula which projects as a broad flattened process overhanging the glenoid fossa; it articulates with the clavicle and gives attachment to part of the deltoid and trapezius muscles. Its lateral border is a palpable landmark ("the point of the shoulder"). SYN acromial process. [G. *akrōmion,* fr. *akron,* tip, + *ōmos,* shoulder]

acromioplasty (ă-krō′mē-ō-plas-ty). A surgical reshaping of the acromion, frequently performed to remedy compression of the supraspinatus portion of the rotator cuff of the shoulder joint between the acromion and the greater tubercle of the humerus.

acro·mi·o·scap·u·lar (ă-krō′mē-ō-skap′ū-lăr). Relating to both the acromion and body of the scapula.

acro·mi·o·tho·rac·ic (ă-krō′mē-ō-thō-ras′ik). SYN thoracoacromial.

a·crom·pha·lus (ak-rom′fal-ŭs). Abnormal projection of the umbilicus. [acro- + G. *omphalos,* umbilicus]

ac·ro·my·o·to·nia (ak′rō-mī-ō-tō′nē-ă). Myotonia affecting the extremities only, resulting in spastic deformity of the hand or foot. SYN acromyotonus. [acro- + G. *mys,* muscle, + *tonos,* tension]

ac·ro·my·ot·o·nus (ak-rō-mī-ot′ō-nŭs). SYN acromyotonia.

ac·ro·os·te·ol·y·sis (ak′rō-os-tē-ol′i-sis) [MIM*102500]. Congenital condition manifested by palmar and plantar ulcerating lesions with osteolysis involving distal phalanges of the fingers and toes. Acquired a. has been reported in workers exposed to vinyl chloride. There is an autosomal disorder, Cheney syndrome [MIM*102500], in which this finding is combined with wormian bones, hypoplasia of the mandibular rami, and basilar osteoporosis. SEE ALSO Cheney *syndrome*. [acro- + G. *osteon*, bone, + *lysis*, loosening]

ac·ro·pachy (ak′rō-pak-ē, ă-krop′ă-kē) [MIM*119900]. SYN hereditary *clubbing*. [acro- + G. *pachys*, thick]

ac·ro·pach·y·der·ma (ak′rō-pak-i-der′mă). SYN pachydermoperiostosis. [acro- + G. *pachys*, thick, + *derma*, skin]

ac·ro·par·es·the·sia (ak′rō-par-es-thēs′ē-a). **1.** Paresthesia of one or more of the extremities. **2.** Nocturnal paresthesia involving the hands, most often of middle-aged women; formerly attributed to a lesion in the thoracic outlet, but now known to be a classic symptom of carpal tunnel syndrome. [acro- + paresthesia]

acrop·e·tal (ă-krop′ĕ-tăl). **1.** In a direction toward the summit. **2.** Produced successively toward the apex, with the youngest conidium formed at the tip and the oldest at the base of a chain of conidia; pertaining to asexual spore production in fungi by successive budding of the distal spore in a spore chain. [acro- + L. *peto*, to seek]

ac·ro·pho·bia (ak-rō-fō′bē-ă). Morbid fear of heights. [acro- + G. *phobos*, fear]

ac·ro·pig·men·ta·tion (ak′rō-pig-men-tā′shŭn). Punctate and reticulate hyperpigmentation of the dorsal surfaces of the fingers and toes beginning in early childhood and usually increasing with age; more common in Asian persons of dark complexion.

ac·ro·pleu·rog·e·nous (ak′rō-ploo-roj′ĕ-nŭs). Denoting spores developing at the tip and along the sides of fungal hyphae.

ac·ro·pus·tu·lo·sis (ak′rō-pŭs-tū-lō′sis). Pustular eruptions of the hands and feet, often a form of psoriasis. [acro- + pustulosis]

infantile a., a cyclically recurrent vesicopustular and crusting pruritic eruption, usually in black children, appearing soon after birth to 10 months; remission occurs at about 2 years of age.

ac·ro·scle·ro·der·ma (ak′rō-sklēr-ō-der′mă). SYN acrosclerosis. [acro- + G. *sklēros*, hard, + *derma*, skin]

ac·ro·scle·ro·sis (ak′rō-sklĕ-rō′sis). Stiffness and tightness of the skin of the fingers, with atrophy of the soft tissue and osteoporosis of the distal phalanges of the hands and feet; a limited form of progressive systemic sclerosis occurring with Raynaud phenomenon and scleroderma of the forearms. SEE CREST *syndrome*. SYN acroscleroderma, sclerodactyly, sclerodactylia.

ac·ro·sin (ak′rō-sin). A serine proteinase in spermatozoa similar in specificity to trypsin.

ac·ro·some (ak′rō-sōm). A caplike organelle or saccule derived from the golgi that surrounds the anterior two-thirds of the nucleus of a sperm cell. Within this cap are enzymes that are thought to facilitate entry of the sperm through the zona pellucida. [acro- + G. *soma*, body]

ac·ro·so·min (ak-rō-sō′min). A lipoglycoprotein complex present in the acrosomal cap.

ac·ro·spi·ro·ma (ak′rō-spī-rō′mă). A tumor of the distal dermal segment of a sweat gland. [scro- + G. *speira*, coil, + -oma, tumor]

eccrine a., SYN clear cell *hidradenoma.*

ac·ro·ter·ic (ak-rō-ter′ik). Relating to the extreme peripheral or apical parts, such as the tips of fingers and toes, the end of the nose. [G. *akrōterion*, the topmost point]

Ac·ro·the·ca (ak-rō-thē′kă). Former name for species now placed in the genus *Rhinocladiella* or *Fonsecaea*. [see acrotheca]

ac·ro·the·ca (ak-rō-thē′kă). In fungi, a type of spore formation characteristic of the genus *Fonsecaea*, in which conidia are formed along the ends and sides of irregular club-shaped conidiophores. [acro- + G. *thēkē*, box, case]

acrot·ic (ă-krot′ik). **1.** Marked by great weakness or absence of the pulse; pulseless. [G. *a-* priv. + *krotos*, a striking] **2.** Obsolete term relating to the surface of the body, especially the cutaneous glands. [G. *akrotēs*, extremity]

ac·ro·tism (ak′rō-tizm). Absence or imperceptibility of the pulse. [G. *a-* priv. + *krotos*, a striking]

ac·ro·troph·o·dyn·ia (ak′rō-trōf′ō-din′ē-a). Pain, paresthesia,

sensory loss, and trophic changes affecting the distal extremities, usually the feet, that can follow prolonged exposure of the limbs to cold and moisture. [acro- + G. *trophē,* nourishment, + *odynē,* pain]

ac·ro·troph·o·neu·ro·sis (ak′rō-trof′ō-noo-rō′sis). Trophoneurosis of one or more of the extremities. [acro- + G. *trophē,* nourishment, + *neuron,* nerve, + *-osis,* condition]

a·cryl·ate (ă′kril-āt). A salt or ester of acrylic acid.

acryl·ic (ă-kril′ik). Denoting certain synthetic plastic resins derived from a. acid. SEE ALSO acrylic *resin.*

acryl·ic ac·ids. A series of unsaturated aliphatic acids of the general formula $R=CH-COOH$; the prototype, acrylic acid ($R = CH_2$) or 2-propenoic acid, is derived from propionic acid by reduction or from glycerol by dehydration.

ACT Abbreviation for activated clotting *time.*

ACTH Abbreviation for adrenocorticotropic *hormone.*

big ACTH, a form of ACTH, produced by certain tumors, which is a larger and more acidic peptide molecule than little ACTH, but is not immunochemically distinguishable from it and does not exert any of the biologic effects characteristic of ACTH; proteolytic digestion of big ACTH yields hormonally active little ACTH.

little ACTH, a term coined to denote the conventional ACTH molecule when contrasted with big ACTH.

ac·tin (ak′tin). One of the protein components into which actomyosin can be split; it can exist in a fibrous form (F-actin) or a globular form (G-actin).

F-a., the association of G-a. subunits into a fibrous (F) protein caused by an increase in salt concentration; the conversion of G-a. to F-a. is catalyzed by small concentrations of magnesium ion, is reversible, and is accompanied by the conversion of the bound ATP molecule to ADP and the conversion of one reactive -thiol group to an unreactive form.

G-a., the globular (G) subunits of the a. molecule, having a molecular weight 42 kd and containing one molecule of ATP; it is soluble in dilute salt, polymerizing to F-a. when the ionic strength is increased.

act·ing out. An overt act or set of actions that provides an emotional outlet for the expression of emotional conflicts (usually unconscious).

ac·tin·ic (ak-tin′ik). Relating to the chemically active rays of the electromagnetic spectrum. [G. *aktis (aktin-),* a ray]

ac·tin·ides (ak′tin-īdz). Those elements with atomic numbers 89 to 103, corresponding to the lanthanides in the Periodic Table. SYN actinide elements. [*actinium,* first element of the series]

α-**ac·tin·in** (ak-tin′in). An F-actin binding protein in vertebrate cells that cross-links actin filaments into regular parallel arrays. It is found in both the Z line and the I band.

ac·tin·i·um (Ac) (ak-tin′ē-ŭm). An element, atomic no. 89, atomic wt. 227.05; it possesses no stable isotopes and exists in nature only as a disintegration product of uranium and thorium. [G. *aktis,* a ray]

actino-. Combining form meaning a ray, as of light; applied to any form of radiation or to any structure with radiating parts. SEE ALSO radio-. [G. *aktis, aktinos,* a ray of light, a beam.]

ac·ti·no·bac·il·lo·sis (ak′tin-ō-bas-i-lō′sis). A disease of cattle and swine, occasionally reported in humans, caused by the bacterium *Actinobacillus lignieresii*. It affects the soft tissues, often the tongue and cervical lymph nodes, where granulomatous swellings are formed that eventually break down to form abscesses.

Ac·ti·no·ba·cil·lus (ak′tin-ō-bă-sil′lŭs). A genus of very small, nonmotile, nonsporeforming, aerobic, facultatively anaerobic bacteria containing Gram-negative rods interspersed with coccal elements. The metabolism of these bacteria is fermentative. They are pathogenic to animals. The type species is *A. lignieresii*. [actino- + L. *bacillus,* a little rod]

A. actinomycetemcom′itans, a species of doubtful taxonomic position; frequently associated with human periodontal disease as well as subacute and chronic endocarditis; occurs with actinomycetes in actinomycotic lesions. SYN *Haemophilus actinomycetemcomitans.*

A. lignieres′ii, a species producing infections of the upper alimentary tract and mouth in cattle and swine (actinobacillosis) and suppurative lesions in the skin and lungs of sheep; it is the type species of its genus.

ac·ti·no·he·ma·tin (ak′ti-nō-hē′mă-tin). A red respiratory pigment found in certain forms of *Actinia* (sea anemones). [actino- + G. *haima,* blood]

Ac·ti·no·ma·du·ra (ak′ti-nō-ma-dū′-ră). A genus of aerobic Gram-positive, branching, nonacidfast filamentous bacteria; it may form aerial hyphae and may contain chains of up to 15 spores. [actino- + *Madura,* India]

A. africa′na, a bacterial species found in cases of mycetoma of the foot in Africa.

A. latina, a species of bacteria associated with mycetoma in South America.

A. madurae, an aerobic actinomycete; a cause of actinomycetoma.

A. pelliertieri, SEE *A. latina.*

ac·ti·no·my·ce·li·al (ak′ti-nō-mī-sē′lē-ăl). Relating to the mycelium-like filaments of the Actinomycetales.

Ac·ti·no·my·ces (ak′ti-nō-mī′sēz). A genus of slow-growing, nonmotile, nonsporeforming, anaerobic to facultatively anaerobic bacteria (family Actinomycetaceae) containing Gram-positive, irregularly staining filaments; diphtheroid cells may be predominant. They exhibit true branching while forming mycelial type colonies. Most of the species produce a filamentous microcolony. The metabolism of these chemoheterotrophs is fermentative; the products of glucose fermentation include acetic, formic, lactic, and succinic acids but not propionic acid. A. may have characteristic sulfur granules in purulent drainage. These organisms are pathogenic for humans and other animals and can cause chronic suppurative infection in humans. Over 16 species have been described; type species is *A. bovis.* [actino- + G. *mykēs,* fungus]

A. bo′vis, a species of bacteria causing actinomycosis in cattle; infection in humans is not established; it is the type species of its genus.

A. israe′lii, the most common species of actinomyces causing human actinomycosis and, occasionally, infections in cattle.

A. naeslun′dii, a species whose natural habitat is the oral cavity; human infections occur and it produces periodontal destruction in some species of animals.

A. odontoly′ticus, a species whose normal habitat is the human oral cavity; it has been isolated from deep dental caries.

A. visco′sus, a species that has been isolated from the oral cavity of humans and some species of other animals; it produces periodontal disease in animals and has been isolated from human dental calculus and root surface caries.

Ac·ti·no·my·ce·ta·ce·ae (ak′ti-nō-mī′sē-tā′sē-ē). A family of nonsporeforming, nonmotile, ordinarily facultatively anaerobic (some species are aerobic and others are anaerobic) bacteria (order Actinomycetales) containing Gram-positive, nonacidfast, predominantly diphtheroid cells which tend to form branched filaments in tissue or in some stages of cultural development; the filaments readily fragment, producing diphtheroid or coccoid forms. The metabolism of these chemoheterotrophic bacteria is fermentative. This family contains the genera *Actinomyces* (type genus), *Arachnia, Bacterionema, Bifidobacterium,* and *Rothia.*

Ac·ti·no·my·ce·ta·les (ak′ti-nō-mī′sē-tā′lēz). An order of bacteria consisting of moldlike, rod-shaped, clubbed or filamentous forms with decided tendency to true branching, without endospores, but sometimes developing conidia; it includes the families Mycobacteriaceae, Actinomycetaceae, and Nocardiaceae.

ac·ti·no·my·cetes (ak′ti-nō-mī-sē′tēz). A term used to refer to members of the genus *Actinomyces;* sometimes improperly used to refer to any member of the family Actinomycetaceae or order Actinomycetales.

actinomycetoma (ak′tin-ō-mī-set-ō′ma). Mycetoma caused by higher bacteria. Cf. eumycetoma.

ac·ti·no·my·cin (ak′tin-ō-mī′sin). A group of peptide antibiotic agents, isolated from several species of *Streptomyces* (originally *Actinomyces*), that are active against Gram-positive bacteria, fungi, and neoplasms. A.'s are chromopeptides, most containing the chromophore actinocin, and are derivatives of phenoxazine that differ in their amino acids and their sequence in the peptide chains; they form complexes with DNA and therefore inhibit RNA synthesis, primarily the ribosomal type.

a. A, the first of the a.'s isolated in crystalline form.

a. C, SYN cactinomycin.

a. D, SYN dactinomycin.

a. F₁, KS4; produced by actinomycin C-elaborating strains of *Streptomyces chrysomallus;* used as an antineoplastic agent.

ac·ti·no·my·co·sis (ak′ti-nō-mī-kō′sis). A disease primarily of cattle and humans caused by the bacterium *Actinomyces bovis* in cattle and by *A. israelii* and *Arachnia propionica* in humans. These actinomycetes are part of the normal bacterial flora of the mouth and pharynx, but when introduced into tissue they may produce chronic destructive abscesses or granulomas that eventually discharge a viscid pus containing minute yellowish granules (sulfur granules). In humans, the disease commonly affects the cervicofacial area, abdomen, or thorax; in cattle, the lesion is commonly found in the mandible. SYN actinophytosis (1), lumpy jaw. [actino- + G. *mykēs,* fungus, + *-osis,* condition]

ac·ti·no·my·cot·ic (ak′ti-nō-mī-kot′ik). Relating to actinomycosis.

Ac·ti·no·myx·id·ia (ak′ti-nō-mik-sid′ē-ă). A sporozoan order having a double cellular envelope, three polar capsules, and eight spores; parasitic chiefly in segmented worms, such as the common earthworm. [actino- + G. *myxa,* mucus]

ac·tin·o·phage (ak-tin′ō-fāj). A virus specific for actinomycetes. [actino(myces) + G. *phagō,* to eat]

ac·ti·no·phy·to·sis (ak′ti-nō-fī-tō′sis). **1.** SYN actinomycosis. **2.** SYN botryomycosis.

Ac·ti·no·po·da (ak-ti-nop′ō-dă). A class of Sarcodina having slender pseudopodia with a central axial filament. [actino- + G. *pous,* foot]

ac·tin·o·sin (ak-tin′ō-sin). A phenoxazone derivative that is the chromophore of the actinomycins.

ac·ti·no·ther·a·py (ak′ti-nō-thār′ă-pē). In dermatology, sunlight or ultraviolet light therapy.

ac·tion (ak′shŭn). **1.** The performance of any of the vital functions, the manner of such performance, or the result of the same. **2.** The exertion of any force or power, physical, chemical, or mental. [L. *actio,* from *ago,* pp. *actus,* to do]

ball valve a., intermittent blockage of a tube or outlet of a cavity by some object or material that permits passage in one direction but not in the other.

calorigenic a., increase of heat production of the body, as by the thyroid hormone. SYN thermogenic a.

cumulative a., SYN cumulative *effect.*

salt a., any physicochemical effect produced by hypertonic concentrations of osmotically active electrolytes.

sparing a., the manner in which a nonessential nutritive component, by its presence in the diet, lowers the dietary requirement for an essential component; thus, nonessential L-cysteine spares essential L-methionine and nonessential L-tyrosine spares essential L-phenylalanine. SYN sparing phenomenon.

specific a., the a. of a drug or a method of treatment which has a direct and especially curative effect upon a disease, e.g., the a. of vitamin B₁₂ in pernicious anemia.

specific dynamic a. (SDA), increase of heat production caused by the ingestion of food, especially of protein.

thermogenic a., SYN calorigenic a.

ac·ti·vate (ak′ti-vāt). **1.** To render active. **2.** To make radioactive.

ac·ti·va·tion (ak-ti-vā′shŭn). **1.** The act of rendering active. **2.** An increase in the energy content of an atom or molecule, through the raising of temperature, absorption of light photons, etc., which renders that atom or molecule more reactive. **3.** Techniques of stimulating the brain by light, sound, electricity, or chemical agents, in order to elicit abnormal activity in the electroencephalogram. **4.** Stimulation of peripheral nerve fibers to the point that action potentials are initiated. **5.** Stimulation of cell division in an ovum by fertilization or by artificial means. **6.** The act of making radioactive. SEE ALSO cross-section.

amino acid a., the formation of the amino acyl adenylate derivative (e.g., during protein biosynthesis).

EEG a., the low voltage, fast pattern of attentive wakefulness.

feedback a., inhibitory or antiinhibitory a. on an enzyme by an end product of a biochemical pathway in which that enzyme plays a part. For example, the activation of factors VIII and V by thrombin during blood clotting.

feed-forward a., the a. or stimulation of an enzyme by a precursor of the substrate of that enzyme.

gene a., the process of a. of a gene so that it is expressed at a particular time. This process is crucial in growth and development.

ac·ti·va·tor (ak'ti-vā-tōr). **1.** A substance that renders another substance, or catalyst, active, or that accelerates a process or reaction. **2.** The fragment, produced by chemical cleavage of a proactivator, that induces the enzymic activity of another substance. **3.** An apparatus for making substances radioactive; e.g., neutron generator, cyclotron. **4.** A removable type of myofunctional orthodontic appliance that acts as a passive transmitter of force, produced by the function of the activated muscles, to the teeth and alveolar process that are in contact with it. **5.** a protein that binds to a DNA sequence before RNA polymerase transcription.

catabolite gene a. (CGA), SYN catabolite (gene) activator *protein.*

plasminogen a., a proteinase converting plasminogen to plasmin by cleavage of a single (usually Arg-Val) bond in the former. SYN urokinase.

polyclonal a. (pol-ē-klō'năl), a substance that will activate T cells, B cells, or both regardless of their specificities.

tissue plasminogen a. (TPA, tPA), (1) a naturally occurring thrombolytic serine protease that catalyzes the conversion of plasminogen to plasmin; (2) a genetically engineered protein used as a thrombolytic agent in myocardial infarction, stroke, and peripheral vascular thrombosis.

> TPA is a single-chain glycoprotein with a molecular weight of about 70 kD. Produced by endothelial cells at sites of vascular injury, it modulates thrombogenesis by converting fibrin-bound plasminogen to plasmin, cleaving the arginine-valine bond in the 560–561 position of plasminogen. As a result, fibrin strands in a clot are chemically degraded and platelet adhesion and aggregation are inhibited. TPA has little effect on plasminogen in the absence of fibrin, and its release does not significantly reduce systemic concentrations of fibrinogen. Alteplase, a synthetic TPA produced by recombinant DNA technology, improves outcome when administered intravenously in acute myocardial infarction and in selected cases of stroke and peripheral ischemia due to thrombosis. It has a circulating half-life of only 4–6 minutes, but persists in clots up to 7 hours. SEE thrombolytic therapy.

ac·tiv·in (ak'ti-vin). Placental hormone that reaches maximum levels in maternal serum during labor. [active + -in]

ac·tiv·i·ty (ak-tiv'i-tē). **1.** In electroencephalography, the presence of neurogenic electrical energy. **2.** In physical chemistry, an ideal concentration for which the law of mass action will apply perfectly; the ratio of the a. to the true concentration is the a. coefficient (γ), which becomes 1.00 at infinite dilution. **3.** For enzymes, the amount of substrate consumed (or product formed) in a given time under given conditions; turnover *number.* **4.** The number of nuclear transformations (disintegrations) in a given quantity of a material per unit time. Units: curie (Ci), millicurie (mCi), becquerel (Bq), megabecquerel (MBq). SEE ALSO radioactivity.

blocking a., repression or elimination of electrical activity in the brain by the arrival of a sensory stimulus.

insulinlike a. (ILA), a measure of substances, usually in plasma, that exert biologic effects similar to those of insulin in various bioassays; sometimes used as a measure of plasma insulin concentrations; always gives higher values than immunochemical techniques for the measurement of insulin.

intrinsic sympathomimetic a. (ISA), the property of a drug that causes activation of adrenergic receptors so as to produce effects similar to stimulation of the sympathetic nervous system.

nonsuppressible insulinlike a. (NSILA), plasma insulinlike a. not suppressed by antibodies to insulin and mostly present after pancreatectomy. Nonsuppressible insulinlike a. is mostly the action of polypeptide insulinlike growth factors IGF-I and IGF-II.

optic a., the ability of a compound in solution (one possessing no plane of symmetry, usually because of the presence of one or more asymmetric carbon atoms) to rotate the plane of polarized light.

plasma renin a. (PRA), estimation of renin in plasma by measuring the rate of formation of angiotensin I or II.

pulseless electrical a. (PEA), SYN electromechanical *dissociation.*

specific a., (1) radioactivity per unit mass of the stated element or compound; (2) for an enzyme, the amount of substrate consumed (or product formed) in a given time under given conditions per milligram of protein; (3) a. per unit mass of the stated radionuclide.

triggered a., one or a series of spontaneously generated heartbeats originating from an action potential that produces an afterdepolarization which reaches activation threshold.

ac·to·my·o·sin (ak'-tō-mī'ō-sin). A protein complex composed of actin and myosin; it is the essential contractile substance of muscle fiber, active with MgATP.

platelet a., the contractile protein of platelets, responsible for clot retraction, platelet aggregation, and release of ADP and other biologic amines essential to platelet function. SYN thrombosthenin.

Ac·u·a·ria spi·ra·lis (ak-ū-ā'rē-ă spī-rā'lis). A nematode parasite in the proventriculus and esophagus, and sometimes the intestine, of chickens, turkeys, pheasants, and other birds. [L. *acus,* needle; Mod. L. *spiralis,* spiral]

acu·i·ty (ă-kū'i-tē). **1.** Sharpness, clearness, distinctness. **2.** Severity. [thr. Fr., fr. L. *acuo,* pp. *acutus,* sharpen]

absolute intensity threshold a., the minimal light that can be seen.

resolution a., detection of a target having two or more parts, often measured by using the Snellen test types; indicated by two numbers: the first represents the distance at which an individual sees the test types (usually 6 m or 20 ft), and the second, the distance at which the test types subtend an angle of 5 min.; e.g., vision of 6/9 indicates a test distance of 6 m and recognition of symbols that subtend an angle of 5 min. at a distance of 9 m. SYN visual a.

spatial a., detection of the shape of a test object; e.g., perceiving polygons of the same size but with different numbers of sides.

stereoscopic a., the detection of differences in distance by superimposition of slightly different retinal images into a single image to the brain.

Vernier a., detection of displacement of a portion of a line.

visibility a., recognition of an object on a background of different character.

visual a. (V), SYN resolution a.

acu·le·ate (ă-kū'lē-āt). Pointed; covered with sharp spines. [L. *aculeatus,* pointed, fr. *acus,* needle]

acu·men·tin (ak-ū-men'tin). A neutrophil and macrophage motility protein that links to the actin molecule to control filament length.

acu·mi·nate (ă-kū'mi-nāt). Pointed; tapering to a point. [L. *acumino,* pp. -*atus,* to sharpen]

ac·u·ol·o·gy (ak-ū-ol'ō-jē). The study of the use of needles for therapeutic purposes, as in acupuncture. [L. *acus,* needle, + G. *logos,* study]

a·cu·pres·sure. Application of pressure in sites used for acupuncture with therapeutic intent.

ac·u·punc·ture (ak-ū-punk'choor). Puncture with long, fine needles: **1.** An ancient Asian system of therapy. **2.** More recently, acupuncture *anesthesia* or analgesia. [L. *acus,* needle, + puncture]

acu·sis (ă-kū'sis). The ability to perceive sound normally. SYN normal hearing. [G. *akousis,* hearing]

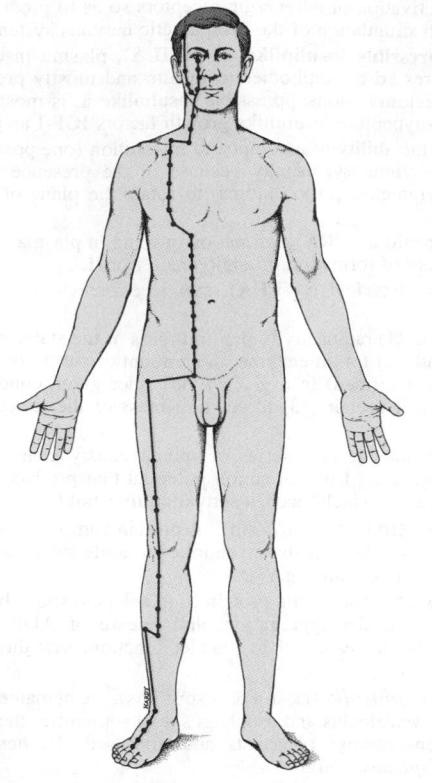

acupuncture (stomach meridian)

acute (ă-kūt′). **1.** Referring to a health effect, usually of rapid onset, brief, not prolonged; sometimes loosely used to mean severe. **2.** Referring to exposure, brief, intense, short-term; sometimes specifically referring to brief exposure of high intensity. [L. *acutus,* sharp]

acy·a·not·ic (ă-sī-ă-not′ik). Characterized by absence of cyanosis.

acy·clic (ā-sī′klik). Not cyclic; denoting especially an a. compound.

acy·clo·guan·o·sine (ā-sī-klō-gwan′ō-sēn). SYN acyclovir.

acy·clo·vir (ā-sī′klō-vir). A synthetic acyclic purine nucleoside analog used as an antiviral agent in the treatment of genital herpes; the sodium salt is used for parenteral therapy. SYN acycloguanosine.

ac·yl (as′il). An organic radical derived from an organic acid by the removal of the carboxylic hydroxyl group.

ac·yl-ACP de·hy·dro·gen·ase, ac·yl-ACP re·duc·tase. SYN enoyl-ACP reductase (NADPH).

ac·yl·ad·e·nyl·ate (as′il-ă-den′il-āt). A compound in which an acyl group is combined with AMP by elimination of H_2O between the OHs of a carboxyl group and of the phosphate residue of AMP, usually initially in the form of ATP and eliminating inorganic pyrophosphate in the condensation.

***n*-ac·yl·a·mi·no ac·id** (as-il-am′i-nō). An amino acid that has an acyl group attached to its N, as in hippuric acid (*N*-benzoylglycine) or phenaceturic acid.

ac·yl·a·tion (as-i-lā′shŭn). Introduction of an acyl radical into an organic compound or formation of such a radical within an organic compound.

a·cyl·car·ni·tine (as′il-kar′ni-tēn). Condensation product of a carboxylic acid and carnitine. The transport form for a fatty acid crossing the inner mitochondrial membrane.

ac·yl-CoA. Condensation product of a carboxylic acid and coenzyme A; metabolic intermediate of importance, notably in the oxidation and synthesis of fat. SYN acyl-coenzyme A.

a.-CoA dehydrogenase (NADPH), enzyme catalyzing the re-

versible reduction of enoyl-CoA derivatives of chain length 4–16, with NADPH as the hydrogen donor, forming a.-CoA and NADP+. SYN enoyl-CoA reductase.

a.-CoA synthetase, (1) general term for enzymes (EC 6.2.1.x) that form a.-CoA, now called ligases; **(2)** specifically, long-chain fatty acid–CoA ligase.

ac·yl-co·en·zyme A (as′il-kō-en′zīm). SYN acyl-CoA.

1-ac·yl·gly·ce·rol-3-phos·phate ac·yl·trans·fer·ase. SEE *lysophosphatidic acid* acyltransferase.

ac·yl-mal·o·nyl-ACP syn·thase. SYN 3-oxoacyl-ACP synthase.

ac·yl·mer·cap·tan (as′il-mer-kap′tan). SYN thioester.

***N*-ac·yl·sphin·go·sine** (as-il-sfing′gō-sēn). A condensation product of an organic acid with sphingosine at the amino group of the latter compound.

ac·yl·trans·fer·as·es (as-il-trans′fer-ă-sez) [EC 2.3.x.x]. Enzymes catalyzing the transfer of an acyl group from an acyl-CoA to various acceptors. SYN transacylases.

acys·tia (ā-sis′tē-ă). Congenital absence of the urinary bladder. [G. *a-* priv. + *kystis,* bladder]

A.D. Abbreviation for *auris dexter* [L.], right ear.

ad-. Prefix denoting increase, adherence, to, toward; near; very. [L. *ad,* to, toward;]

-ad. In anatomical nomenclature, -ward; toward or in the direction of the part indicated by the main portion of the word. [L. *ad,* to]

ADA Abbreviation for American Dental Association.

ad·a·cr·ya (a-dak′rē-ă). Absence of tears; tearlessness. [G. *a-* priv. + *dakryon,* tear, + -ia]

adac·ty·lous (ā-dak′tǐ-lŭs). Without fingers or toes.

Adair-Koshland-Némethy-Filmer mod·el (AKNF). See under model.

ad·a·man·tine (ad-ă-man′tēn). Exceedingly hard; formerly used in reference to the enamel of the teeth. [G. *adamantinos,* very hard]

adamantinoma.

a. of long bones, a rare tumor of limb bones, usually the tibia, that microscopically resembles an ameloblastoma; the histogenesis is uncertain.

pituitary a., SYN craniopharyngioma.

Adamkiewicz, Albert, Polish pathologist, 1850–1921. SEE *artery* of Adamkiewicz.

Adams, Sir William, British surgeon, 1760–1829.

Adams, Robert, Irish physician, 1791–1875. SEE A.-Stokes *disease;* Stokes-A. *disease;* A.-Stokes *syncope, syndrome;* Stokes-A. *syndrome;* Morgagni-A.-Stokes *syndrome.*

Adam's ap·ple. SYN laryngeal *prominence.*

ad·am·site (DM) (ad′ăm-sīt). A vomiting agent that has been used in military training and in riot control. [Roger *Adams,* Am. chemist]

Adanson, Michel, French naturalist, 1727–1806. SEE adansonian *classification.*

ad·ap·ta·tion (ad-ap-tā′shŭn). **1.** Preferential survival of members of a species because of a phenotype that gives them an enhanced capacity to withstand the environment including the ecology. **2.** An advantageous change in function or constitution of an organ or tissue to meet new conditions. **3.** Adjustment of the sensitivity of the retina to light intensity. **4.** A property of certain sensory receptors that modifies the response to repeated or continued stimuli at constant intensity. **5.** The fitting, condensing, or contouring of a restorative material, foil, or shell to a tooth or cast so as to be in close contact. **6.** The dynamic process wherein the thoughts, feelings, behavior, and biophysiologic mechanisms of the individual continually change to adjust to a constantly changing environment. SYN adjustment (2). **7.** A homeostatic response. [L. *ad-apto,* pp. -*atus,* to adjust]

dark a., the visual adjustment occurring under reduced illumination in which the retinal sensitivity to light is increased. SEE ALSO dark-adapted *eye,* Purkinje *shift.* SYN scotopic a.

light a., the visual adjustment occurring under increased illumination in which the retinal sensitivity to light is reduced. SEE ALSO light-adapted *eye,* Purkinje *shift.* SYN photopic a.

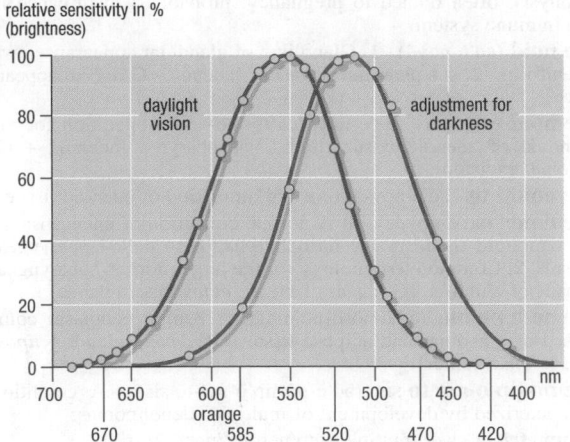

relative sensitivity in %
(brightness)

daylight vision — adjustment for darkness

| 670 red | 585 yellow | 520 green | 470 blue | 420 violet |

orange

dark and light adaptation: brightness of the colors during daytime and twilight

photopic a., SYN light a.

reality a., the ability to adjust to the world as it exists.

retinal a., adjustment to degree of illumination.

scotopic a., SYN dark a.

social a., adjustment to living in accordance with interpersonal, social, and cultural norms.

adapt·er, adap·tor (a-dap′ter, -tōr). **1.** A connecting part, joining two pieces of apparatus. **2.** A converter of electric current to a desired form.

ad·ap·tom·e·ter (ad-ap-tom′ĕ-ter). A device for determining the course of retinal dark adaptation and for measuring the minimum light threshold.

ad·ax·i·al (ad-ak′sē-ăl). Toward an axis, or on one or other side of an axis.

ADC Abbreviation for AIDS dementia *complex.*

ADCC Abbreviation for antibody-dependent cell-mediated *cytotoxicity.*

add. Abbreviation for L. *adde,* add; L. *addantur,* let them be added; *addendus,* to be added; and *addendo,* by adding.

ad·der. Common name for many members of the family Viperidae (the vipers), applied to several genera, although true a.'s are of the genus *Vipera.* [M.E. *naddre,* fr. O.E. *næedre*]

ad·dict (ad′ikt). A person who is habituated to a substance or practice, especially one considered harmful or illegal.

ad·dic·tion (ă-dik′shŭn). Habitual psychological and physiologic dependence on a substance or practice that is beyond voluntary control. [L. *ad-dico,* pp. *-dictus,* consent, fr. *ad-* + *dico,* to say]

alcohol a., SYN alcoholism.

Addis, Thomas, U.S. internist, 1881–1949. SEE A. *count.*

Addison, Thomas, English physician, 1793–1860. SEE A. *anemia; disease;* addisonian *anemia;* addisonian *crisis;* A.-Biermer *disease.*

Addison, Christopher, English anatomist, 1869–1951. SEE A. clinical *planes,* under *plane.*

ad·di·so·ni·an (ad-i-sō′nē-an). Relating to or described by Thomas Addison; used in relation to pernicious *anemia* or the various features of Addison disease.

ad·di·tive (ad′i-tiv). **1.** A substance not naturally a part of a material (e.g., food) but deliberately added to fulfill some specific purpose (e.g., preservation). **2.** Tending to add or be added; denoting addition. **3.** In metrical studies (e.g., genetics, epidemiology, physiology, statistics), having the property that the total combined effect of two or more factors equals the sum of their individual effects in isolation. Cf. synergism.

ad·di·tiv·i·ty (ad-i-tiv′i-tē). The quality or state of being additive.

causal a., the relationship between two or more causal compo-

nents such that their combined effect is the algebraic sum of their individual effects.

interlocal a., the relationship among quantitative effects of different genetic loci such that their joint effect is equal to the sum of their individual effects; an absence of epistasis or interaction.

intralocal a., the relationship between alleles such that the quantifiable phenotype of the heterozygote is at the midpoint between those for the two homozygotes; an absence of dominance.

ad·dres·sin (ad-res′in). A molecule on the surface of a cell that serves as a homing device to direct another molecule to a specific location. [address, fr. O.Fr. *adresser,* to direct, fr. L.L. *addirectiare,* fr. L. *ad,* to, + *directus,* straight, direct, + -in]

ad·du·cent (ă-doo′sent). Bringing toward; adducting. [L. *adducens,* pres. p. of *ad-duco,* to bring]

ad·du·cin (ă-doo′sen). A protein that binds to spectrin and actin and links the spectrin assembly.

ad·duct (a-dŭkt′). **1.** To draw toward the median plane. **2.** An addition product, or complex, or one part of the same. [L. *ad-duco,* pp. *-ductus,* to bring toward]

ad·duc·tion (ă-dŭk′shŭn). **1.** Movement of a body part toward the median plane (of the body, in the case of limbs; of the hand or foot, in the case of digits). **2.** Monocular rotation (duction) of the eye toward the nose. **3.** A position resulting from such movement. Cf. abduction.

ad·duc·tor (ă-dŭk′ter, tōr). SYN adductor *muscle.*

Ade Abbreviation for adenine.

ade·lo·mor·phous (ă-del-ō-mōr′fŭs). Of not clearly defined form. In the past this term was applied to certain cells of the gastric glands. [G. *adēlos,* uncertain, not clear, + *morphē,* shape]

aden-. SEE adeno-.

ad·e·nal·gia (ad-ĕ-nal′jē-ă). Rarely used term for pain in a gland. [aden- + G. *algos,* pain]

aden·dric (ā-den′drik). SYN adendritic.

aden·drit·ic (ā-den-drit′ik). Without dendrites. SYN adendric. [G., *a-* priv. + *dendron,* tree]

ad·e·nec·to·my (ad-ĕ-nek′tō-mē). Excision of a gland. [aden- + G. *ektomē,* excision]

ad·e·nec·to·pia (ad′ĕ-nek-tō′pē-ă). Presence of a gland other than in its normal anatomical position. [aden- + G. *ek,* out of, + *topos,* place]

ad·e·nem·phrax·is (ad′ĕ-nem-frak′sis). Rarely used term for an obstruction to the discharge of a glandular secretion. [aden- + G. *emphraxis,* stoppage]

aden·i·form (ă-den′i-fōrm). SYN adenoid (1).

ad·e·nine (A, Ade) (ad′ĕ-nēn). One of the two major purines (the other being guanine) found in both RNA and DNA, and also in various free nucleotides of importance to the body, such as AMP (adenylic acid), ATP, NAD$^+$ and NADP$^+$, and FAD; in all these smaller compounds, a. is condensed with ribose at nitrogen-9, forming adenosine. For structure, see adenylic acid. SYN 6-aminopurine.

a. arabinoside, misnomer for arabinosyladenine.

a. deaminase, an enzyme that catalyzes the hydrolysis of a. to ammonia and hypoxanthine. A part of purine degradation.

a. deoxyribonucleotide, SYN deoxyadenylic acid.

a. nucleotide, SYN adenylic acid.

a. phosphoribosyltransferase, an enzyme that catalyzes the reaction of a. with 5-phospho-α-D-ribose 1-diphosphate (PRPP) to form AMP and pyrophosphate. An important step in purine salvage. A deficiency of this enzyme can lead to 2,8-dihydroxyadenine lithiasis.

a. sulfate, a. conjugated with sulfuric acid; used to stimulate leukocyte production in agranulocytosis.

ad·e·ni·tis (ad-ĕ-nī′tis). Inflammation of a lymph node or of a gland. [aden- + G. *-itis,* inflammation]

mesenteric a., an illness with abdominal pain and fever due to enlargement and inflammation of the mesenteric lymph nodes; often mistaken for appendicitis. SYN mesenteric lymphadenitis.

ad·e·ni·za·tion (ad-ĕ-nī-zā′shŭn). Conversion into glandlike structure.

⌂**adeno-, aden-.** Combining forms denoting gland, glandular; corresponds to L. glandul-, glandi-. [G. *adēn, adenos* a gland]

ad·e·no·ac·an·tho·ma (ad'ĕ-nō-ak-an-thō'mă). A malignant neoplasm consisting chiefly of glandular epithelium (adenocarcinoma), usually well differentiated, with foci of squamous (or epidermoid) neoplastic cells.

ad·e·no·am·e·lo·blas·to·ma (ad'ĕ-nō-am'el-ō-blast-ō'mă). SYN adenomatoid odontogenic *tumor.*

ad·e·no·blast (ad'ĕ-nō-blast). A proliferating embryonic cell with the potential to form glandular parenchyma. [adeno- + G. *blastos,* germ]

ad·e·no·car·ci·no·ma (ad'ĕ-nō-kar-si-nō'mă). A malignant neoplasm of epithelial cells in glandular or glandlike pattern. SYN glandular cancer, glandular carcinoma.

    acinic cell a., an a. arising from secreting cells of a racemose gland, particularly the salivary glands. SYN acinar carcinoma, acinic cell carcinoma.

    alveolar a., a. of the lung in which tumor cells form structures resembling alveoli.

    a. in Barrett esophagus, an a. arising in the esophagus that has become lined with columnar cells (Barrett mucosa).

    bronchiolar a., SYN alveolar cell *carcinoma.*

    bronchioloalveolar a., SYN alveolar cell *carcinoma.*

    clear cell a., (1) a histologic type of renal a.; (2) a histologic type of a. occurring chiefly in the male and female genitourinary tracts that is characterized by distinctive hobnail cell growth of neoplastic cells in sheets, papillae, and coalescing glands.

    mesonephric a., SYN mesonephroma.

    mucoid a., sometimes applied to mucinous carcinoma, or a. containing mucin secreting neoplastic cells.

    papillary a., an a. containing fingerlike processes of vascular connective tissue covered by neoplastic epithelium, projecting into cysts or the cavity of glands or follicles; occurs most frequently in the ovary and thyroid gland.

    renal a., an a. arising in the renal parenchyma, usually occurring in middle-aged or older people of either sex (although more common in males). SYN clear cell carcinoma of kidney, renal cell carcinoma.

    a. in si'tu, a noninvasive abnormal proliferation of glands believed to precede the appearance of invasive adenocarcinoma; reported in the endometrium, breast, large intestine, cervix, and other sites.

ad·e·no·cys·to·ma (ad'ĕ-nō-sis-tō'mă). Adenoma in which the neoplastic glandular epithelium forms cysts.

ad·e·no·cyte (ad'ĕ-nō-sīt). A secretory cell of a gland. [adeno- + G. *kytos,* a hollow (cell)]

ad·e·no·di·as·ta·sis (ad'ĕ-nō-dī-as'tă-sis). Separation or ectopia of glands or glandular tissue from their usual anatomical sites, e.g., pancreatic glands in the wall of the small intestine, gastric glands in the wall of the esophagus. [adeno- + G. *diastasis,* a separation]

ad·e·no·dyn·ia (ad'ĕ-nō-din'ē-ă). Rarely used term for adenalgia. [adeno- + G. *odynē,* pain]

ad·e·no·fi·bro·ma (ad'ĕ-nō-fī-brō'mă). A benign neoplasm composed of glandular and fibrous tissues, with a relatively large proportion of glands.

ad·e·no·fi·bro·sis (ad'ĕ-nō-fī-brō'sis). SYN sclerosing *adenosis.*

ad·e·nog·en·ous (ad-ĕ-noj'en-ŭs). Having an origin from glandular tissue.

ad·e·no·hy·po·phy·si·al (ad'ĕ-nō-hī-pō-fiz'ē-ăl). Relating to the adenohypophysis.

ad·e·no·hy·poph·y·sis (ad'ĕ-nō-hī-pof'i-sis) [TA]. The anterior pituitary gland; it consists of the distal part, intermediate part, and infundibular part. SEE ALSO pituitary *gland.* SYN lobus anterior hypophyseos [TA], anterior lobe of hypophysis✩, glandular lobe of hypophysis, lobus glandularis hypophyseos.

ad·e·no·hy·poph·y·si·tis (ad'ĕ-nō-hī-pof-ĭ-sī'tis). Inflammatory and fibrotic reaction affecting the anterior pituitary gland, often related to pregnancy.

    lymphocytic a., a diffuse lymphocytic infiltration of the adenohy-

pophysis, often related to pregnancy; probably a disturbance in the immune system.

ad·e·noid (ad'ĕ-noyd). **1.** Glandlike; of glandular appearance. SYN adeniform. **2.** SEE pharyngeal *tonsil.* [adeno- + G. *eidos,* appearance]

ad·e·noid·ec·to·my (ad'ĕ-noy-dek'tō-mē). An operation for the removal of adenoid tissue in the nasopharynx. [adenoid + G. *ektomē,* excision]

ad·e·noid·i·tis (ad'ĕ-noy-dī'tis). Inflammation of adenoid tissue.

ad·e·noids (ad'ĕ-noydz). **1.** A normal collection of unencapsulated lymphoid tissue in the nasopharynx. Also called pharyngeal tonsils. **2.** Common terminology for the large (normal) pharyngeal tonsils of children. [G. *adēn,* gland, + *-eidos,* resemblance]

ad·e·no·li·po·ma (ad'ĕ-nō-li-pō'mă). A benign neoplasm composed of glandular and adipose tissues. [G. *adēn,* gland, + *lipos,* fat, + *-oma,* tumor]

ad·e·no·lip·o·ma·to·sis (ad'ĕ-nō-lip'ō-mă-tō'sis). A condition characterized by development of multiple adenolipomas.

    symmetric a., SYN multiple symmetric *lipomatosis.*

ad·e·no·lym·pho·cele (ad'ĕ-nō-lim'fō-sēl). Cystic dilation of a lymph node following obstruction of the efferent lymphatic vessels. [adeno- + L. *lympha,* spring water, + G. *kēlē,* tumor]

ad·e·no·lym·pho·ma (ad'ĕ-nō-lim-fō'mă). Obsolete term for a benign glandular tumor usually arising in the parotid gland and composed of two rows of eosinophilic epithelial cells, which are often cystic and papillary, together with a lymphoid stroma. SYN papillary cystadenoma lymphomatosum, Warthin tumor.

ad·e·no·ma (ad-ĕ-nō'mă). A benign epithelial neoplasm in which the tumor cells form glands or glandlike structures; usually well circumscribed, tending to compress rather than infiltrate or invade adjacent tissue. [adeno- + G. *-oma,* tumor]

    acidophil a., a tumor of the adenohypophysis in which cell cytoplasm stains with acid dyes; often growth hormone–producing. SYN eosinophil a.

    ACTH-producing a., a pituitary tumor composed of corticotrophs that produce ACTH, often a basophilic adenoma; may give rise to Cushing disease or Nelson syndrome.

    adnexal a., an a. arising in, or forming structures resembling, skin appendages.

    adrenocortical a., a benign tumor of adrenal cortical cells; small unencapuslated nodules of adrenal cortex are probably localized areas of hyperplasia rather than a.'s; true a.'s are rare and may be symptomless or associated with Cushing syndrome or primary aldosteronism.

    apocrine a., SYN papillary *hidradenoma.*

    basal cell a., a benign tumor of major or minor salivary glands or other organs composed of small cells showing peripheral palisading.

    basophil a., a tumor of the adenohypophysis in which the cell cytoplasm stains with basic dyes, often ACTH-producing.

    bronchial a., obsolete term once used to encompass carcinoid tumors, mucoepidermoid *carcinoma,* and adenoid cystic *carcinoma.* Cf. bronchial mucous gland a.

    bronchial mucous gland a., a rare benign tumor arising from the mucous glands of bronchial mucosa.

    canalicular a. (ca-na-lik'oo-lar), a variant of monomorphic a. composed of double rows of epithelial cells in long cords.

    chromophobe a., chromophobic a., a tumor of the adenohypophysis whose cells do not stain with either acid or basic dyes.

    colloid a., a follicular a. of the thyroid, composed of large follicles containing colloid. SYN macrofollicular a.

    embryonal a., a benign neoplasm in which the glandular epithelial elements are not fully differentiated, resembling immature tissue observed in embryonic development.

    eosinophil a., SYN acidophil a.

    follicular a., an a. of the thyroid with a simple glandular pattern.

    Fuchs a., a benign epithelial tumor of the nonpigmented epithelium of the ciliary body, rarely exceeding 1 mm in diameter.

    gonadotropin-producing a., a rare type of pituitary a. that produces FSH and LH; its cells can be identified only by immunochemical techniques.

growth hormone–producing a., an a. that produces the clinical picture of gigantism or acromegaly, although a third of the cells have no granules or are a mixture of acidophils and chromophobes; some tumors may secrete both growth hormone and prolactin; often an acidophil or eosinophil adenoma.

hepatic a., a benign tumor of the liver, usually occurring in women during the reproductive years in association with lengthy oral contraceptive use. The tumor is usually solitary, subcapsular, and large, composed of cords of hepatocytes with portal triads. SYN hepatocellular a.

hepatocellular a., SYN hepatic a.

Hürthle cell a., an uncommon type of thyroid tumor characterized by abundant eosinophilic cytoplasm containing numerous mitochondria. Often malignant with widespread metastases; rarely takes up radioiodine. SEE ALSO Hürthle cell *carcinoma.* SYN oncocytic a.

invasive pituitary a., extensive infiltrates of the dura, bone, and sinuses.

lactating a., an uncommon a. of the breast composed of tubuloacinar structures with pronounced secretory changes such as seen in pregnancy and lactation.

macrofollicular a., SYN colloid a.

mammosomatotroph cell a., a rare prolactin- and growth hormone–producing pituitary a. composed of ultrastructurally monomorphic cells with both somatotrophic and lactotrophic differentiation.

microfollicular a., a fetal a. of the thyroid composed of very small follicles and solid alveolar groups of thyroid epithelial cells.

monomorphic a., a benign ductal neoplasm of the salivary glands, with a uniform epithelial pattern and lacking the chondromyxoid stroma of a pleomorphic a.

nephrogenic a., a benign tumor of the urinary bladder or urothelial mucosa, composed of glandular structures resembling renal tubules.

a. of nipple, SYN subareolar duct *papillomatosis.*

null-cell a., an a. of the hypophysis composed of cells for which there is no overt evidence of hormone production, but which usually produces hypopituitarism and visual disturbances by compression of adjacent structures; approximately one third of these tumors have cells with abundant mitochondria (oncocytes) that are somewhat larger than the monocytic null cells. SYN undifferentiated cell a.

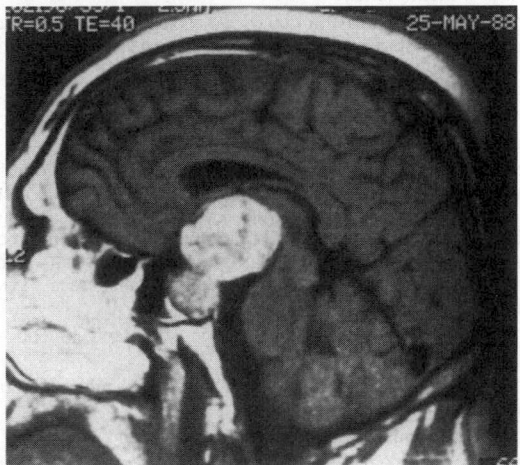

adenoma of the hypophysis: magnetic resonance image, after injection of contrast medium

oncocytic a., SYN Hürthle cell a.

oxyphil a., SYN oncocytoma.

papillary cystic a., an a. in which the lumens of the acini are frequently distended by fluid, and the neoplastic epithelial elements tend to form irregular, fingerlike projections.

papillary a. of large intestine, SYN villous a.

pituitary a., a benign neoplasm of the pituitary generally arising in the adenohypophysis.

pleomorphic a., SYN mixed *tumor* of salivary gland.

polypoid a., SYN adenomatous *polyp.*

prolactin-producing a., a pituitary adenoma composed of prolactin-producing cells; it gives rise to symptoms of nonpuerperal amenorrhea and galactorrhea (Forbes-Albright syndrome) in women and to impotence in men. SYN prolactinoma.

prostatic a., the growth in benign prostatic hyperplasia.

renal cortical a., an a., usually small, sometimes found in the renal cortex incidentally at autopsy and derived from renal tubular tissue.

sebaceous a., a benign neoplasm of sebaceous tissue, with a predominance of mature secretory sebaceous cells. Cf. a. sebaceum.

a. seba′ceum, archaic misnomer for a hamartoma occurring on the face, composed of fibrovascular tissue and appearing as an aggregation of red or yellow papules that may be associated with tuberous sclerosis; sebaceous glands may be present but are not increased. Cf. sebaceous a. SYN Pringle disease.

thyrotropin-producing a., a rare pituitary adenoma usually associated with hypo- or hyperthyroidism.

tubular a., (1) a benign neoplasm composed of epithelial tissue resembling a tubular gland. **(2)** dysplastic polyp of the colonic mucosa which is considered a potential precursor of adenocarcinoma.

undifferentiated cell a., SYN null-cell a.

villous a., frequently appears as a solitary, sessile, often large, tumor of colonic mucosa, although it can occur anywhere through the GI tract; composed of mucinous epithelium covering delicate vascular projections; malignant change occurs frequently; hypersecretion occurs rarely. Also known as adenoma. SYN papillary a. of large intestine.

ad·e·no·ma·toid (ad-ĕ-nō′mă-toyd). Resembling an adenoma.

ad·e·no·ma·to·sis (ad′ĕ-nō-mă-tō′sis). A condition characterized by multiple glandular overgrowths.

erosive a. of nipple, SYN subareolar duct *papillomatosis.*

familial multiple endocrine a. [MIM*131100], SYN multiple endocrine *neoplasia.*

fibrosing a., SYN sclerosing *adenosis.*

multiple endocrine a., SYN multiple endocrine *neoplasia.*

pulmonary a., a neoplastic disease in which the alveoli and distal bronchi are filled with mucus and mucus-secreting columnar epithelial cells; characterized by abundant, extremely tenacious sputum, chills, fever, cough, dyspnea, and pleuritic pain.

ad·e·nom·a·tous (ad-ĕ-nō′mă-tŭs). Relating to an adenoma, and to some types of glandular hyperplasia.

ad·e·no·meg·a·ly (ad′ē-nō-meg′ă-lē). Enlargement of a gland. [adeno- + G. *megas,* large]

ad·e·no·mere (ad′ĕ-nō-mēr). Structural unit in the parenchyma of a developing gland which becomes the functional portion of the organ. [adeno- + G. *meros,* part]

ad·e·no·my·o·ma (ad′ĕ-nō-mī-ō′mă). A benign neoplasm of muscle (usually smooth muscle) with glandular elements; occurs most frequently in uterus and uterine ligaments. [G. *adēn,* gland, + *mys,* muscle, + -*oma,* tumor]

ad·e·no·my·o·sis (ad′ĕ-nō-mī-ō′sis). The ectopic occurrence or diffuse implantation of adenomatous tissue in muscle (usually smooth muscle). [G. *adēn,* gland, + *mys,* muscle, + -*osis* condition]

a. u′teri, a benign invasion of myometrium by endometrial tissue.

ad·e·nop·a·thy (ad-ĕ-nop′ă-thē). Swelling or morbid enlargement of the lymph nodes. [adeno- + G. *pathos,* suffering]

ad·e·no·phleg·mon (ad′ĕ-nō-fleg′mon). Acute inflammation of a gland and the adjacent connective tissue. [adeno- + G. *phlegmonē,* inflammation]

Ad·e·no·pho·ra·si·da (ad′ĕ-nō-fō-ras′i-dă). A class of nematodes lacking lateral canals opening into the excretory system and phasmids, with few or no caudal papillae, eggs unsegmented, and with polar plugs or hatching *in utero.* It includes the genera

Trichuris, Capillaria, and *Trichinella* among important parasites of humans and domestic animals. SEE ALSO Secernentasida. SYN Adenophorea, Aphasmidia. [G. *adēn,* gland, + *phōr,* thief]

Ad·e·no·pho·rea (ad′ĕ-nō-fō′rē-ă). SYN Adenophorasida.

ad·e·no·sal·pin·gi·tis (ad′ĕ-nō-sal-pin-jī′tis). SYN *salpingitis* isthmica nodosa.

▓ **ad·e·no·sar·co·ma** (ad′ĕ-nō-sar-kō′mă). A malignant neoplasm arising simultaneously or consecutively in mesodermal tissue and glandular epithelium of the same part.

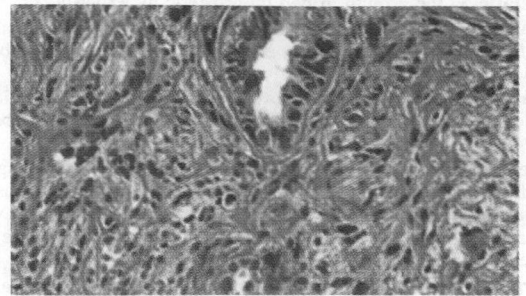

müllerian adenosarcoma of the uterus: histologic preparation showing malignant components of both epithelial and mesenchymal origin

müllerian a., a tumor of the uterus or ovaries, of low-grade malignancy, composed of benign-appearing glands and a sarcomatous stroma.

ad·e·nose (ad′ĕ-nōs). Relating to a gland or like a gland.

aden·o·sine (Ado) (ă-den′ō-sēn). **1.** A condensation product of adenine and D-ribose; a nucleoside found among the hydrolysis products of all nucleic acids and of the various adenine nucleotides. A. accumulates in severe combined immunodeficiency disease. **2.** A potent coronary vasodilator used in place of exercise for radionuclide myocardial perfusion studies. SYN 9-β-D-ribofuranosyladenine.

a. cyclic phosphate, SEE adenosine 3′,5′-cyclic monophosphate.

a. deaminase, an enzyme found in mammalian tissues, capable of catalyzing the deamination of adenosine, forming inosine and ammonia. A deficiency of a. can lead to one form of severe combined immunodeficiency disease.

a. diphosphate, SEE adenosine 5′-diphosphate.

a. kinase, enzyme catalyzing the transfer of a phosphate group from MgATP to adenosine, forming MgADP and AMP. An important step in nucleoside salvage.

a. monophosphate (AMP), specifically, adenosine-5′-monophosphate. SEE adenylic acid.

a. nucleosidase, an enzyme hydrolyzing adenosine to adenine and D-ribose.

a. phosphate, specifically, adenosine 3′- or 5′-phosphate. SEE adenylic acid.

a. tetraphosphate, a condensation product of adenosine with tetraphosphoric acid at the 5′ position.

a. triphosphate, SYN adenosine 5′-triphosphate.

aden·o·sine 3′,5′-cy·clic mono·phos·phate (cAMP). An activator of phosphorylase kinase and an effector of other enzymes, formed in muscle from ATP by adenylate cyclase and broken down to 5′-AMP by a phosphodiesterase; the first compound referred to as a "second messenger." It is a metabolic regulator. A related compound (2′,3′) is also known. SYN cyclic adenylic acid, cyclic AMP, cyclic phosphate.

aden·o·sine 3′,5′-cy·clic phos·phate phos·pho·di·es·ter·ase. An enzyme that catalyzes the hydrolysis of adenosine 3′,5′-cyclic phosphate forming 5′-AMP. A crucial step in the regulation of cellular adenosine 3′,5′-cyclic phosphate levels. Inhibited by caffeine. SYN cAMP phosphodiesterase.

aden·o·sine 5′-di·phos·phate (ADP). A condensation product of adenosine with pyrophosphoric acid, formed from ATP by the hydrolysis of the terminal phosphate group of the latter compound.

aden·o·sine 3′-phos·phate. 3′-Adenylic acid. SEE adenylic acid.

aden·o·sine 5′-phos·phate. 5′-Adenylic acid. SEE adenylic acid.

aden·o·sine 3′-phos·phate 5′-phos·pho·sul·fate (PAPS). An intermediate in the formation of urinary ethereal sulfates, notable for containing a "high-energy" sulfate bond; the 3′-OH of adenosine is replaced by $-OPO_3H_2$, the 5′-OH by $-OP(O_2H)-OSO_3H$. SYN active sulfate.

ad·e·no·sine 5′-phos·pho·sul·fate (APS). An intermediate in the formation of PAPS (active sulfate).

adenosine 5′-phosphosulfate kinase, the enzyme that catalyzes the formation of active sulfate from adenosine 5′-phosphosulfate and ATP.

ad·e·no·sine tri·phos·pha·tase (ATPase) (a-den′ō-sēn-trī-fos′fă-tās). An enzyme that catalyzes the release of the terminal phosphate group of adenosine 5′-triphosphate; visualized cytochemically in various cell membranes, mitochondria, and in the A band of striated muscle sarcomeres associated with myosin.

aden·o·sine 5′-tri·phos·phate (ATP). Adenosine (5)pyrophosphate; adenosine with triphosphoric acid esterified at its 5′ position; immediate precursors of adenine nucleotides in RNA. The primary energy currency of a cell. SYN adenosine triphosphate.

ad·e·no·sis (ad-ĕ-nō′sis). **1.** A rarely used term for a more or less generalized glandular disease. **2.** Glandular tissue in one or more sites in which it is not usually found.

blunt duct a., a. of the breast in which the ducts are enlarged but not increased in number.

fibrosing a., SYN sclerosing a.

microglandular a., a. of the breast in which irregular clusters of small tubules are present in adipose or fibrous tissues, resembling tubular carcinoma but lacking stromal fibroblastic proliferation.

sclerosing a., a nodular, benign breast lesion occurring most frequently in relatively young women and consisting of hyperplastic distorted lobules of acinar tissue with increased collagenous stroma; the changes may be difficult to distinguish microscopically from carcinoma. Also, a benign nodular microscopic lesion of the prostate consisting of acimar tissue with increased stroma; the basal cell layer shows characteristic smooth muscle metaplasia. SYN adenofibrosis, fibrosing adenomatosis, fibrosing a.

aden·o·syl (a-den′ō-sil). The radical of adenosine minus an H or OH from one of the ribosyl OH groups, usually the 5′, e.g., *S*-adenosyl-L-methionine.

ad·e·no·sylco·bal·a·min (a-den′ō-sil-kō-bal′ă-min). A derivative of vitamin B_{12}. Its impaired biosynthesis can lead to methylmalonic acidemia.

***S*-aden·o·syl-L-ho·mo·cys·te·ine** (a-den′ō-sil-hō-mō-sis′te-ēn). The compound formed by the demethylation of *S*-adenosyl-L-methionine.

***S*-aden·o·syl-L-me·thi·o·nine (SAM, AdoMet)** (a-den′ō-sil-me-thī′ō-nēn). Condensation product of adenosine and L-methionine involving replacement of the $-OPO_3H_2$ of adenylic acid by $-S^+(CH_3)CH_2CH_2CH(NH_3^+)CO_2$ of methionine; a sulfonium compound bearing a methyl group that is transferred in transmethylation reactions. SEE ALSO *methionine* adenosyltransferase. SYN active methionine.

ad·e·not·o·my (ad-ĕ-not′ō-mē). Incision of a gland. [adeno- + G. *tomē,* a cutting]

ad·e·no·ton·sil·lec·to·my (ad′ĕ-nō-ton-si-lek′tō-mē). Operative removal of tonsils and adenoids.

ad·e·nous (ad′ĕ-nŭs). Rarely used term for adenose.

Ad·e·no·vi·ri·dae (ad′ĕ-nō-vir′i-dē). A family of double-stranded DNA viruses, commonly known as adenoviruses, that develop in the nuclei of infected cells in mammals and birds. The virion is 70 to 90 nm in diameter, naked, and ether-resistant; the capsids are icosahedral and composed of 252 capsomeres. The family includes two genera, Mastadenovirus and Aviadenovirus.

ad·e·no·vi·rus (ad′ĕ-nō-vī′rŭs). Adenoidal-pharyngeal-conjunctival or A-P-C virus; any virus of the family Adenoviridae. More than 40 types are known to infect humans causing upper respiratory symptoms, acute respiratory disease, conjunctivitis, gastroenteritis, hemorrhagic cystitis, and serious infections in neonates. SYN A-P-C virus, adenoidal-pharyngeal-conjunctival virus. [G. *adēn,* gland, + virus]

canine a. 1, a virus causing infectious canine hepatitis in dogs. SYN Rubarth disease virus.

ad·e·nyl (ad′e-nil). The radical or ion of adenine; often used for adenylyl, as in adenylosuccinic acid.

aden·y·late (a-den′i-lāt). Salt or ester of adenylic acid.

a. cyclase, an enzyme acting on ATP to form 3′,5′-cyclic AMP plus pyrophosphate. A crucial step in the regulation and formation of second messengers. SYN 3′,5′-cyclic AMP synthetase.

a. kinase, adenylic acid kinase; a phosphotransferase that catalyzes the reversible phosphorylation of a molecule of ADP by MgADP, yielding MgATP and AMP. SYN adenylic acid kinase, myokinase.

ad·e·nyl cy·clase (ad′e-nil sī′klās). An enzyme that converts adenosine monophosphate to cyclic adenosine monophosphate, an intracellular second messenger of neural and hormonal activation.

ad·e·nyl·ic ac·id (ad-e-nil′ik). A condensation product of adenosine and phosphoric acid; a nucleotide found among the hydrolysis products of all nucleic acids. 3′-Adenylic acid (adenosine 3′-monophosphate) and 5′-adenylic acid (adenosine 5′-monophosphate [AMP]) differ in the place of attachment of the phosphoric acid to the D-ribose; deoxyadenylic acid differs in having H instead of OH at the 2′ position of D-ribose. SEE ALSO AMP. SYN adenine nucleotide.

cyclic a. a., SYN adenosine 3′,5′-cyclic monophosphate.

a. a. deaminase, SYN AMP deaminase.

a. a. kinase, SYN *adenylate* kinase.

ad·e·nyl·o·suc·ci·nase (ad′e-nil-ō-sŭk′sin-ās). SYN adenylosuccinate lyase.

ad·e·nyl·o·suc·ci·nate ly·ase (ad′e-nil-ō-sŭk′sin-āt). Adenylylsuccinate lyase; an enzyme catalyzing the nonhydrolytic cleavage of adenylosuccinic acid producing AMP and fumarate and also of 4-(*N*-succinocarboxamido)-5-aminoimidazole nucleotide to yield fumarate and aminoimidazole carboxamide ribosyl-5-phosphate. Both are steps in purine nucleotide biosynthesis. SYN adenylosuccinase, adenylylsuccinate lyase.

ad·e·nyl·o·suc·ci·nate syn·thase. A ligase catalyzing the formation of adenylosuccinate, GDP, and P_i from inosinic acid, aspartate, and GTP. An important enzyme in purine nucleotide biosynthesis. SYN adenylylsuccinate synthase, IMP-aspartate ligase.

ad·e·nyl·o·suc·cin·ic ac·id (sAMP) (ad′e-nil-ō-sŭk′sin-ik). A condensation product of aspartic acid and inosine 5′-monophosphate; an intermediate in the biosynthesis of adenylic acid. Formally, it is adenylic acid with succinic acid replacing an H of the NH_2 group, forming a C–N. SYN adenylylsuccinic acid, *N*-succinyladenylic acid.

aden·y·lyl (a-den′i-lil). The radical of adenylic acid minus an OH from the phosphoric group; often shortened to adenyl in compound names, such as adenylosuccinic acid.

a. cyclase, former name for *adenylate* cyclase.

aden·y·lyl·o·suc·ci·nate ly·ase (a-den′i-lil-ō-sŭk′sin-āt). SYN adenylosuccinate lyase.

aden·y·lyl·o·suc·ci·nate syn·thase. SYN adenylosuccinate synthase.

aden·y·lyl·o·suc·cin·ic ac·id (a-den′i-lil-ō-sŭk′sin-ik). SYN adenylosuccinic acid.

aden·y·lyl·sul·fate ki·nase. SEE *adenosine 5′-phosphosulfate* kinase.

a·deps, gen. **adi·pis, adi·pes** (ad′eps, ad′i-pis, -pēz). 1. Denoting fat or adipose tissue. 2. The rendered fat of swine, lard, used in the preparation of ointments. SYN lard. SEE ALSO a. lanae. [L. lard, fat]

a. lanae, the greasy substance obtained from the wool of the sheep *Ovis aries* (family Bovidae). Used as an emollient base for creams and ointments. SYN hydrous wool fat, lanolin, wool wax. [L. fat of wool]

a. re′nis, obsolete term for the layer of adipose tissue ("fatty capsule") surrounding the kidney (perirenal fat).

ader·mia (ā-der′mē-ă). Congenital defect of absence of skin. [G. *a*- priv. + *derma,* skin]

ADH Abbreviation for antidiuretic *hormone;* alcohol dehydrogenase.

ad·her·ence (ad-hēr′ens). 1. The act or quality of sticking to something. SEE ALSO adhesion. 2. The extent to which a patient continues an agreed-upon mode of treatment without close supervision. Cf. compliance (2), maintenance. [L. *adhaereo,* to stick to]

immune a., the binding of cells via antigen-antibody complexes that have triggered complement fixation; adherence is to appropriate complement receptors.

ad·he·sins (ad-hē′zins). Microbial surface antigens that frequently exist in the form of filamentous projections (pili or fimbriae) and bind to specific receptors on epithelial cell membranes; usually classified according to their ability to induce agglutination of erythrocytes from various species, their differential attachment to epithelial cells of various origins, or their susceptibility to reversal of such binding activities in the presence of mannose. [L. *adhaereo,* pp. *ad-haesum,* to stick to, + -in]

ad·he·sio, pl. **ad·he·si·o·nes** (ad-hē′zē-ō, ad-hē-zē-ō′nēz) [TA]. SYN adhesion (1). [L.]

a. interthalam′ica [TA], SYN interthalamic *adhesion.*

ad·hes·i·ol·y·sis (ad-hēz-ē-ol′ō-sis). Severing of adhesive band(s); done by laparoscopy or laparotomy. [adhesion + lysis]

ad·he·sion (ad-hē′zhŭn) [TA]. 1. The process of adhering or uniting of two surfaces or parts, especially the union of the opposing surfaces of a wound. SYN adhesio [TA], conglutination (1). 2. In the pleural cavity and peritoneal cavity, inflammatory bands that connect opposing serous surfaces. 3. Physical attraction of unlike molecules for one another. 4. Molecular attraction existing between the surfaces of bodies in contact. [L. *adhaesio,,* fr. *adhaereo,* to stick to]

amnionic a.'s, SYN amnionic *band.*

fibrinous a., (1) an a. that consists of fine threads of fibrin resulting from an exudate of plasma or lymph, or an extravasation of blood. (2) multiple fine or thin threads of fibrin.

fibrous a., strong fibrous strands resulting from the organization of fibrinous a.'s, often after previous operative procedure; commonly seen in patients with mechanical bowel obstruction.

interthalamic a. [TA], the variable connection between the two thalamic masses across the third ventricle; absent in about 20% of human brains. SYN adhesio interthalamica [TA], massa intermedia★, commissura cinerea, commissura grisea (1), intermediate mass.

primary a., SYN *healing* by first intention.

secondary a., SYN *healing* by second intention.

ad·he·si·ot·o·my (ad-hē-sē-ot′ō-mē). Surgical section or lysis of adhesions.

ad·he·sive (ad-hē′siv). 1. Relating to, or having the characteristics of, an adhesion. 2. Any material that adheres to a surface or causes adherence between surfaces.

adhib. Abbreviation for L. *adhibendus,* to be administered.

a·di·a·ba·tic (ā-dē-ă-bă′tik). Referring to a thermodynamic process in which there is no gain or loss of heat between the system and its surroundings. [G. *adiabatos,* impassable, fr. *a* priv. + *diabainō,* to go through]

ad·i·ad·o·cho·ci·ne·sia, ad·i·ad·o·cho·ci·ne·sis (ă-dī′ă-dō-kō-si-nē′sē-ă, -sis). SYN adiadochokinesis. [G. *a*-priv. + *diadochos,* successive, + *kinēsis,* movement]

ad·i·ad·o·cho·ki·ne·sis (ă-dī′ă-dō-kō-kin-ē′sis). Inability to perform rapid alternating movements. One of the clinical manifestations of cerebellar dysfunction. SEE ALSO dysdiadochokinesia. Cf. diadochokinesia. SYN adiadochocinesia, adiadochocinesis, dysdiadochokinesis. [G. *a*- priv. + *diadochos,* successive, + *kinēsis,* movement]

adi·a·pho·re·sis (ā′dī-ă-fō-rē′sis). SYN anhidrosis. [G. *a*- priv. + *diaphorēsis,* perspiration]

adi·a·pho·ret·ic (ā-dī′ă-fō-ret′ik). SYN anhidrotic.

adi·a·pho·ria (ă-dī-ă-fō′rē-ă). Failure to respond to stimulation after a series of previously applied stimuli. [G. *a-* priv. + *dia,* through, + *phoros,* bearing]

adi·a·spi·ro·my·co·sis (ā'dē-ă-spī'rō-mī-kō'sis). A rare pulmonary mycosis of humans and of rodents and other animals that dig in soil or are aquatic, caused by the fungus *Emmonsia parva var. crescens.*

adi·a·spore (a'dē-ă-spōr). A fungus spore which, when growing in the lungs of an animal or incubated in vitro at elevated temperatures, increases greatly in size without eventual reproduction or replication. [G. *a-* priv. + *dia,* through, + *sporos,* seed]

adi·as·to·le (ă-dī-as'tō-lē). Absence or imperceptibility of the diastolic movement of the heart; diastolic ventricular functional abnormality. Mostly European usage. [G. *a-* priv. + *diastolē,* dilation]

adi·a·ther·man·cy (ă-dī-ă-ther'man-sē). Impermeability to heat. [G. *dia-thermainō,* to warm through, fr. *a-* priv. + *dia,* through, + *thermē,* heat]

Adie, William J., Australian physician, 1886–1935. SEE A. *pupil, syndrome;* Holmes-Adie *pupil;* Holmes-Adie *syndrome.*

ad·i·em·or·rhy·sis (ad'i-em-ōr'i-sis). Arrest of the capillary circulation. [G. *a-* priv. + *dia,* through, + *haima,* blood, + *rhysis,* a flowing]

Adin·i·da (ă-din'i-dă). A suborder of dinoflagellates, in which the flagella are free and do not lie in furrows. [G. *a-* priv. + *diēn,* a whirling]

⌂**adip-, adipo-.** Fat, fatty. Corresponds to G. lip-, lipo-. SEE ALSO lipo-. [L. *adeps, adipis,* soft animal fat, lard, grease; fatty tissue; obesity; akin to G. *aleipha,* unguent, anointing-oil, oil, fat, pitch, resin; *lipos,* animal fat, lard, tallow, vegetable oil]

adiph·e·nine hy·dro·chlo·ride (ă-dif'e-nen). A spasmolytic agent used to decrease spasm of the biliary tract, gastrointestinal tract, uterus, and ureter.

adip·ic ac·id (ă-dip'ik). Hexanedioic acid; the dicarboxylic acid, $HOOC(CH_2)_4COOH.$

Ad·i·pi·o·done. SYN iodipamide.

⌂**adipo-.** SEE adip-.

ad·i·po·cel·lu·lar (ad'i-pō-sel'ū-lăr). Relating to both fatty and cellular tissues, or to connective tissue with many fat cells.

ad·i·po·cer·a·tous (ad-i-pō-ser'ă-tŭs). Relating to adipocere. SYN lipoceratous.

ad·i·po·cere (ad'i-pō-sēr). A fatty substance of waxy consistency into which dead animal tissues (as those of a corpse) are sometimes converted when kept from the air under certain favoring conditions of temperature. SYN grave wax, lipocere. [adipo- + L. *cera,* wax]

ad·i·po·cyte (ad'i-pō-sīt). SYN fat *cell.*

ad·i·po·gen·e·sis (ad'i-pō-jen'ĕ-sis). SYN lipogenesis.

ad·i·po·gen·ic, ad·i·pog·e·nous (ad'i-pō-jen'ik, ad-i-poj'ĕ-nŭs). SYN lipogenic.

ad·i·poid (ad'i-poyd). SYN lipoid. [adipo- + G. *eidos,* resemblance]

ad·i·po·ki·net·ic (ad'i-pō-ki-net'ik). Denoting a substance or factor that causes mobilization of stored lipid. [adipo- + G. *kinēsis,* movement]

ad·i·po·ki·nin (ad-i-pō-kī'nin). An anterior pituitary hormone that causes mobilization of fat from adipose tissue. SYN adipokinetic hormone.

ad·i·pom·e·ter (ad-i-pom'ĕ-ter). An instrument for determining the thickness of the skin. [adipo- + G. *metron,* measure]

ad·i·po·ne·cro·sis (ad'i-pō-ne-krō'sis). Rarely used term referring to necrosis of fat, as in hemorrhagic pancreatitis.

ad·i·po·sal·gia (ad'i-pō-sal'jē-ă). Condition in which painful areas of subcutaneous fat develop. [adipo- + G. *algos,* pain]

ad·i·pose (ad'i-pōs). Denoting fat.

ad·i·po·sis (ad-i-pō'sis). Excessive local or general accumulation of fat in the body. SYN lipomatosis, liposis (1), steatosis (1). [adipo- + G. *-osis,* condition]

a. cerebra'lis, obesity resulting from intracranial disease, most commonly of the hypothalamus, resulting in hyperphagia.

a. doloro'sa, a condition characterized by a deposit of symmetri-

cal nodular or pendulous masses of fat in various regions of the body, with discomfort or pain. SYN Anders disease, Dercum disease, lipomatosis neurotica.

a. or'chica, SYN adiposogenital *dystrophy.*

a. tubero'sa sim'plex, a condition resembling a. dolorosa, in which the fat occurs in small, nodular masses, which are sensitive to touch and may be spontaneously painful, on the abdomen or on the extremities.

a. universa'lis, excessive deposition of fat throughout all parts of the body, including the viscera.

ad·i·pos·i·ty (ad-i-pos'i-tē). **1.** SYN obesity. **2.** Excessive accumulation of lipids in a site or organ.

ad·i·po·su·ria (ad'i-pō-soo'rē-ă). SYN lipuria. [adipo- + G. *ouron,* urine]

adip·sia, adip·sy (ă-dip'sē-ă, -dip'sē). Absence of thirst or the lack of desire to drink. [G. *a-* priv. + *dipsa,* thirst]

ad·i·tus (ad'i-tŭs) [TA]. SYN aperture, inlet. [L. access, fr. *ad-eo,* pp. *-itus,* go to]

a. ad an'trum [TA], SYN a. to mastoid antrum.

a. ad antrum mastoideum [TA], SYN a. to mastoid antrum.

a. ad aqueduc'tum cer'ebri, SYN *opening* of aqueduct of midbrain.

a. ad infundib'ulum [TA], SYN infundibular *recess.*

a. ad sac'cum peritone'i mino'rem, SYN omental *foramen.*

a. glot'tidis infe'rior, SYN infraglottic *cavity.*

a. glot'tidis supe'rior, SYN intermediate laryngeal *cavity.*

laryngeal a. [TA], SYN laryngeal *inlet.*

a. laryn'gis [TA], SYN laryngeal *inlet.*

a. to mastoid antrum [TA], the orifice leading from the epitympanic recess to the mastoid antrum. SYN a. ad antrum mastoideum [TA], a. ad antrum [TA], aperture of mastoid antrum.

a. or'bitae [TA], SYN orbital *opening.*

a. pel'vis, SYN pelvic *inlet.*

ad·just·ment (ă-jŭst'ment). **1.** In dentistry, any modification made upon a fixed or removable prosthesis during or after its insertion to perfect its adaptation and function. **2.** SYN adaptation (6). **3.** A summarizing procedure for a statistical measure in which the effects of differences in composition of the populations being compared have been minimized by statistical methods.

occlusal a., modification of the occluding and incising surfaces of teeth to develop harmonious relationships between these surfaces.

ad·ju·vant (ad'joo-vănt). **1.** A substance added to a drug product formulation that affects the action of the active ingredient in a predictable way. **2.** In immunology, a vehicle used to enhance antigenicity; e.g., a suspension of minerals (alum, aluminum hydroxide, or phosphate) on which antigen is adsorbed; or water-in-oil emulsion in which antigen solution is emulsified in mineral oil (Freund incomplete a.), sometimes with the inclusion of killed mycobacteria (Freund's complete a.) to further enhance antigenicity (inhibits degradation of antigen and/or causes influx of macrophages). **3.** Additional therapy given to enhance or extend primary therapy's effect, as in chemotherapy's addition to a surgical regimen. **4.** A treatment added to a curative treatment to prevent recurrence of clinical cancer from microscopic residual disease. [L. *ad-juvo,* pres. p. *-juvans,* to give aid to]

Freund a., SEE adjuvant.

Freund complete a., water-in-oil emulsion of antigen, to which killed mycobacteria or tuberculosis bacteria are added.

Freund incomplete a., water-in-oil emulsion of antigen, without mycobacteria.

ADL. Abbreviation for activities of daily living. SEE activities of daily living *scale.*

Adler, Alfred, Austrian psychiatrist, 1870–1937. SEE adlerian *psychology;* adlerian *psychoanalysis.*

Adler, Oscar, German physician, 1879–1932. SEE A. *test.*

ad·le·ri·an (ad-ler'ē-an). Relating to or described by Alfred Adler.

ad lib Abbreviation for L. *ad libitum,* freely, as desired.

adm. SEE admov.

ad·me·di·al, ad·me·di·an (ad-mē′dē-ăl, -dē-an). Toward or near the median plane.

ad·mi·nic·u·lum, pl. **ad·mi·nic·u·la** (ad-mi-nik′ū-lŭm, -ū-lă). That which gives support to a part. [L. a hand-rest, prop, fr. *ad + manus,* hand]
a. lin′eae al′bae, a triangular fibrous expansion, sometimes containing a few muscular fibers, passing from the superior pubic ligament to the posterior surface of the linea alba.

ad·mit·tance (ad-mit′ans). SYN immittance.

admov. Abbreviation for L. *admove,* apply.

ad·ner·val (ad-ner′văl). SYN adneural.

ad·neu·ral (ad-noor′ăl). 1. Lying near a nerve. 2. In the direction of a nerve; said of an electric current passing through muscular tissue toward the point of entrance of the nerve. SYN adnerval.

ad·nexa, sing. **ad·nex·um** (ad-nek′să, -sŭm). SYN accessory *structures,* under *structure.* SEE ALSO appendage. [L. connected parts]
a. o′culi, SYN accessory visual *structures,* under *structure.*
a. u′teri, SYN uterine *appendages,* under *appendage.*

ad·nex·al (ad-nek′săl). Relating to the adnexa. SYN annexal.

ad·nex·ec·to·my (ad-nek-sek′tō-mē). 1. Excision of any adnexa. 2. In gynecology, excision of the fallopian tube and ovary if unilateral and excision of both tubes and ovaries (adnexa uteri) if bilateral.

ad·nex·i·tis (ad-neks-ī′tis). Inflammation of the adnexa uteri. [L. *annexa,* adnexa, + *-itis,* inflammation]

ad·nex·o·pexy (ad-neks′ō-pek-sē). Operation for suspension of the fallopian tube and ovary; usually, oophoropexy is accomplished without suspension of the tube. [L. *annexa,* adnexa, + G. *pēxis,* fixation]

Ado Symbol for adenosine.

ad·o·les·cence (ad-ō-les′ens). The period of life beginning with puberty and ending with completed growth and physical maturity. [L. *adolescentia*]

ad·o·les·cent (ad-ō-les′ent). 1. Pertaining to adolescence. 2. An individual in that stage of development.

AdoMet Abbreviation for *S*-adenosyl-L-methionine.

adon·is (a-don′is). Medicinal herb obtained from *Adonis vernalis* (family Ranunculaceae), grown in Eastern Europe and used there in the treatment of congestive heart failure. Contains strophanthidin and related cardiotonic glycosides. SYN false hellebore. [G. *Adōnis,* mythical figure, fr. Phoenicial *adon,* lord]

adon·i·tol (ă-don′i-tol). SYN ribitol.

ADP Abbreviation for adenosine 5′-diphosphate.

ADPase. SYN apyrase.

△**adren-.** SEE adreno-.

ad·re·nal (ă-drē′năl). 1. Near or upon the kidney; denoting the suprarenal (adrenal) gland. 2. A suprarenal gland or separate tissue or product thereof. SEE ALSO suprarenal. [L. *ad,* to, + *ren,* kidney]
accessory a., an island of a. cortical tissue separate from the adrenal gland, usually found in the retroperitoneal tissues, kidney, or genital organs. SYN adrenal rest.
Marchand a.'s, small collections of accessory a. tissue in the broad ligament of the uterus or in the testes. SYN Marchand rest.

ad·re·nal·ec·to·my (ă-drē-năl-ek′tō-mē). Removal of one or both adrenal glands. [adrenal + G. *ektomē,* excision]

adren·a·line (ă-dren′ă-lin). SYN epinephrine.
a. oxidase, SYN *amine* oxidase (flavin-containing).

ad·re·nal·ism. SYN hypercorticoidism.

adre·nal·i·tis (ă-drē-năl-ī′tis). Inflammation of the adrenal gland.

adren·a·lone (ă-dren′ă-lōn). Precursor of epinephrine in some manufacturing processes; a topical adrenergic agent in ophthalmology.

adre·na·lop·a·thy (ă-drē-nă-lop′ă-thē). Any pathologic condition of the adrenal glands. SYN adrenopathy. [adrenal + G. *pathos,* suffering]

ad·ren·ar·che (ad′ren-ar-kē). 1. Axillary and pubic hair growth during puberty induced by hyperactivity of the adrenal cortex. 2.

Physiologic change at puberty caused by adrenocortical secretion of androgenic hormones or precursors of them. [adren- + G. *archē,* beginning]

ad·re·ner·gic (ad-rĕ-ner′jik). 1. Relating to nerve cells or fibers of the autonomic nervous system that employ norepinephrine as their neurotransmitter. Cf. cholinergic. 2. Relating to drugs that mimic the actions of the sympathetic nervous system. SEE α-adrenergic *receptors,* under *receptor,* β-adrenergic *receptors,* under *receptor.* [adren- + G. *ergon,* work]

adren·ic (ă-drē′nik). Relating to the suprarenal gland.

△**adreno-, adrenal-, adren-.** Relating to the adrenal gland. [L. *ad,* to, near, + *ren,* kidney, + -o- + *-alis,* pertaining to]

adre·no·cep·tive (ă-dren-ō-sep′tiv). Referring to chemical sites in effectors with which the adrenergic mediator unites. Cf. cholinoceptive.

adre·no·cep·tor (ă-drē′sep′tor). SYN adrenergic *receptors,* under *receptor.*

adre·no·cor·ti·cal (ă-drē-nō-kōr′ti-kăl). Pertaining to suprarenal cortex.

adre·no·cor·ti·coid (ă-drē-nō-kor′ti-koid). SYN corticosteroid.

adre·no·cor·ti·co·mi·met·ic (ă-drē′nō-kōr′ti-kō-mi-met′ik). Mimicking or producing effects similar to adrenocortical function. [adrenal + cortex + G. *mimētikos,* imitating]

adre·no·cor·ti·co·tro·pic, adre·no·cor·ti·co·tro·phic (ă-drē′nō-kōr′ti-kō-trō′pik, -trō′fik). Stimulating growth of the adrenal cortex or secretion of its hormones. SYN adrenotropic, adrenotrophic. [adrenal cortex + G. *trophē,* nurture; *tropē,* a turning]

adre·no·cor·ti·co·tro·pin (ă-drē′nō-kōr-ti-kō-trō′pin). SYN adrenocorticotropic *hormone.*

adre·no·gen·ic, adre·nog·e·nous (ă-drē-nō-jen′ik, a-drē-noj′ē-nŭs). Of adrenal origin. [adreno- + G. *-gen,* producing]

adre·no·leu·ko·dys·tro·phy (ALD) (ă-drē′nō-loo-kō-dis′trō-fē) [MIM*300100]. An X-linked recessive disorder affecting young males, characterized by chronic adrenocortical insufficiency, skin hyperpigmentation, progressive dementia, spastic paralysis, and other intellectual and neurologic disturbances; due to myelin degeneration in the white matter of the brain. The causative gene maps to Xq and encodes a. protein (ALDP), an ATP-binding transporter located in the peroxisomal membrane.

adre·no·lyt·ic (ă-dren-ō-lit′ik). Denoting antagonism to or inhibition or blockade of the action of epinephrine, norepinephrine, and related sympathomimetics. SEE ALSO adrenergic blocking *agent.* [adreno- + G. *lysis,* loosening, dissolution]

adre·no·meg·a·ly (ă-drē-nō-meg′ă-lē). Enlargement of one or both adrenal glands. [adreno- + G. *megas,* big]

adre·no·mi·met·ic (ă-drē′nō-mi-met′ik). Having an action similar to that of the compounds epinephrine and norepinephrine, which are liberated from the adrenal medulla and adrenergic nerves; term proposed to replace the less accurate term, sympathomimetic. Cf. adrenergic, cholinomimetic. [adreno- + G. *mimētikos,* imitative]

adre·no·my·e·lo·neu·rop·a·thy (ad-rē′nō-mī′e-lō-noo-rop′a-thē). A disorder of adult males, consisting of long-standing adrenal insufficiency, hypogonadism, progressive myelopathy, peripheral neuropathy, and sphincter disturbances; considered a variant of adrenoleukodystrophy. [adreno- + G. *myelos,* medulla, + *neuron,* nerve, + *pathos,* suffering]

adre·nop·a·thy (ă-drē-nop′ă-thē). SYN adrenalopathy.

adrenopause. Decrease in function of adrenal glands with increasing age, analogous to menopause.

adre·no·pri·val (ă-drē-nō-prī′văl). Rarely used term indicating a loss of adrenal function, as a result of either disease or surgical excision. [adreno- + L. *privo,* to deprive]

adre·no·re·ac·tive (ă-drē′nō-rē-ak′tiv). Responding to the catecholamines.

adre·no·re·cep·tors (ă-drē′nō-rē-sep′terz). SYN adrenergic *receptors,* under *receptor.*

adre·nos·ter·one (a-drē-nos′ter-ōn). An androgen isolated from the adrenal cortex. SYN andrenosterone.

adre·no·tox·in (ă-drē-nō-tok′sin). A substance toxic for the adrenal glands. [adreno- + toxin]

adre·no·tro·pic, adre·no·tro·phic (ă-drē-nō-trō'pik, -trō'fik). SYN adrenocorticotropic.

adre·no·tro·pin (ă-drē-nō-trō'pin). SYN adrenocorticotropic *hormone.*

adri·a·my·cin (ā'drē-ă-mī'sin). SYN doxorubicin.

ad sat Abbreviation for L. *ad saturatum,* to saturation.

Adson, Alfred W., U.S. neurosurgeon, 1887–1951. SEE A. *test, forceps, maneuver;* Brown-A. *forceps.*

ad·sorb (ad-sōrb'). To take up by adsorption. [L. *ad,* to, + *sorbeo,* to suck in]

ad·sorb·ate (ad-sōr'bāt). Any substance adsorbed.

ad·sorb·ent (ad-sōr'bent). **1.** A substance that adsorbs, i.e., a solid substance endowed with the property of attaching other substances to its surface without any covalent bonding, e.g., activated charcoal. **2.** An antigen or antibody used in immune adsorption.

ad·sorp·tion (ad-sōrp'shŭn). The property of a solid substance to attract and hold to its surface a gas, liquid, or a substance in solution or in suspension. For example, condensation of a gas onto a surface. Cf. absorption. [L. *ad,* to, + *sorbeo,* to suck up]

immune a., **(1)** removal of antibody (agglutinin or precipitin) from antiserum by use of specific antigen; after aggregation has occurred, the antigen-antibody complex is separated either by centrifugation or by filtration; **(2)** removal of antigen by specific antiserum in a similar manner.

ad·ster·nal (ad-ster'năl). Near or upon the sternum.

ad·ter·mi·nal (ad-ter'mi-năl). In a direction toward the nerve endings, muscular insertions, or the extremity of any structure.

adult (ă-dŭlt'). **1.** Fully grown and physically mature. **2.** A fully grown and mature individual. [L. *adultus,* grown up fr. *adolesco,* to grow up]

adul·ter·ant (ă-dŭl'ter-ănt). An impurity; an additive that is considered to have an undesirable effect or to dilute the active material so as to reduce its therapeutic or monetary value.

adul·ter·a·tion (ă-dŭl-ter-ā'shŭn). The alteration of any substance by the deliberate addition of a component not ordinarily part of that substance; usually used to imply that the substance is debased as a result.

adul·to·mor·phism (ă-dŭl-tō-mōr'fizm). Interpretation of children's behavior in adult terms.

adv. Abbreviation for L. *adversum,* against.

ad·vance (ad-vans'). To move forward. [Fr. *avancer,* to set forward]

ad·vanced life sup·port. Definitive emergency medical care that may include defibrillation, airway management, and use of drugs and medications. Cf. basic life support.

ad·vance·ment (ad-vans'ment). Surgical procedure in which an attachment is partially severed or released so that tissue may be moved to a more distal point.

capsular a., surgical reattachment of the anterior portion of Tenon capsule.

tendon a., excision of the tendon of an eye muscle and attachment of it to a more anterior location on the globe.

ad·ven·ti·tia (ad-ven-tish'ă). The outermost connective tissue covering of any organ, vessel, or other structure not covered by a serosa; instead, the covering is properly derived from without (i.e., from the surrounding connective tissue) and does not form an integral part of such organ or structure. Terminologia Anatomica [TA] lists adventitia (tunica adventitia) of the following organs: ductus deferens, esophagus, renal pelvis, seminal glands, and ureters. SYN membrana adventitia (1), tunica adventitia. [L. *adventicius,* coming from abroad, foreign, fr. *ad,* to + *venio,* to come]

ad·ven·ti·tial (ad-ven-tish'ăl). Relating to the outer coat or adventitia of a blood vessel or other structure. SYN adventitious (3).

ad·ven·ti·tious (ad-ven-tish'ŭs). **1.** Arising from an external source or occurring in an unusual place or manner. SEE ALSO extrinsic. **2.** Occurring accidentally or spontaneously, as opposed to natural causes or hereditary. **3.** SYN adventitial.

ady·nam·ia (ā-dī-nam'ē-ă, ad-i-nā'mē-ă). **1.** SYN asthenia. **2.**

Lack of motor activity or strength. **3.** Obsolete term for paralytic *ileus* of the intestine. [G. *a-* priv. + *dynamis,* power]

a. episodica hereditaria, hyperkalemic periodic *paralysis,* without myotonia. See entries under paralysis..

ady·nam·ic (ă-dī-nam'ik). Relating to adynamia.

△**ae-.** For words so beginning and not found here, see under e-.

Aeby, Christopher T., Swiss anatomist, 1835–1885. SEE A. *plane.*

Aedes (ā-ē'dēz). A widespread genus of small mosquitoes frequently found in tropical and subtropical regions. [G. *aēdēs,* unpleasant, unfriendly]

A. aegyp'ti, the yellow fever mosquito, a species that is also the vector of the pathogen of dengue; characterized by white lyre-shaped markings on the thorax.

A. albopic'tus, species that is an important vector of dengue viruses widespread in the Pacific basin.

A. atlanticus, mosquitoes in the family Culicidae known to transmit viruses that cause dengue, yellow fever, and encephalitis.

A. cabal'lus, species that is an important vector of Rift Valley fever in Africa.

A. dorsalis, mosquito species that is a secondary or suspected vector of Western equine encephalitis.

A. leucocelae'nus, species that transmits yellow fever in South America.

A. melanimon, mosquito species that is a vector of Western equine encephalitis and California group encephalitis.

A. mitchellae, mosquito species that is a secondary or suspected vector of Eastern equine encephalitis.

A. nigromaculis, mosquito species that is a secondary or suspected vector of Western equine encephalitis and California group encephalitis.

A. polynesien'sis, species that is an important vector of filariasis and dengue in the Polynesian region.

A. sollic'itans, a common salt-marsh mosquito species and vector of eastern equine encephalomyelitis on the Atlantic and Gulf coasts of the United States.

A. taeniorhynchus, mosquito species that is a vector of Venezuelan equine encephalitis and a secondary or suspected vector of California group encephalitis.

A. triseriatus, mosquito species that is a vector of California group encephalitis.

A. trivittatus, mosquito species that is a vector of California group encephalitis.

A. variegat'us, a species that is a vector of filarial parasites in the Pacific Islands (Gilbert and Ellice group).

A. vexans, mosquito species that is a vector of California group encephalitis and a secondary or suspected vector of Eastern equine encephalitis.

Aelu·ro·stron·gy·lus (ē'loor-ō-stron'jī-lŭs). A common genus of lungworm in cats; land snails and slugs serve as intermediate hosts and snail-eating animals can serve as transport hosts. [G. *ailuros,* cat, + Mod. L., fr. G. *strongylus,* round]

ae·quo·rin (ē'kwō-rin). A luminescent protein isolated from the jellyfish *Aequorea* which emits blue light in the presence of even minute amounts of calcium ion; injected intracellularly, it is used to measure free calcium ion transients within cells. SEE ALSO fura-2, quin-2.

△**aer-, aero-.** The air, a gas; aerial, gassy. [G. *aēr* (L. *aer*), air]

aer·ate (ār'āte). **1.** To supply (blood) with oxygen. **2.** To expose to the circulation of air for purification. **3.** To supply or charge (liquid) with a gas, especially carbon dioxide.

aer·en·do·car·dia (ār-en-dō-kar'dē-ă). Presence of undissolved air in the blood within the heart. [aer- + G. *endon,* within, + *kardia,* heart]

△**aero-.** SEE aer-.

Aer·o·bac·ter (ār-ō-bak'ter). SEE *Enterobacter.* [aero- + G. *baktērion,* a small staff]

aer·obe (ār'ōb). **1.** An organism that can live and grow in the presence of oxygen. **2.** An organism that can use oxygen as a final electron acceptor in a respiratory chain. [aero- + G. *bios,* life]

obligate a., an organism which cannot live or grow in the absence of oxygen.

aer·o·bic (ār-ō′bik). **1.** Living in air. **2.** Relating to an aerobe. SYN aerophilic, aerophilous.

aer·o·bi·ol·o·gy (ār′ō-bī-ol′ō-jē). The study of atmospheric constituents, living and nonliving, of biological significance, e.g., airborne spores, pathogenic bacteria, allergenic substances, pollutants.

aer·o·bi·o·scope (ar-ō-bī′ō-skōp). An apparatus for determining the bacterial content of the air. [aero- + G. *bios,* life, + *skopeō,* to view]

aer·o·bi·o·sis (ār-ō-bī-ō′sis). Existence in an atmosphere containing oxygen. [aero- + G. *biōsis,* mode of living]

aer·o·bi·ot·ic (ār-ō-bī-ot′ik). Relating to aerobiosis.

aer·o·cele (ār′ō-sēl). Distention of a small natural cavity with gas. [aero- + G. *kēlē,* tumor]

Aer·o·coc·cus (ār-ō-kok′ŭs). A genus of aerobic Gram-positive cocci occurring as airborne saprophytes; they produce α-hemolysis on blood agar and grow in the presence of 40% bile. *A. viridans,* the type species, is commonly recovered as part of the normal skin flora; it has low pathogenicity, but has been reported as a rare cause of endocarditis. [aero- + G. *kokkos,* berry]

aer·o·col·pos (ār-ō-kol′pos). Obsolete term for distention of the vagina with gas. [aero- + G. *kolpos,* lap, hollow]

aer·o·der·mec·ta·sia (ār′ō-der-mek-tā′zē-ă). SYN subcutaneous *emphysema.* [aero- + G. *derma,* skin, + *ektasis,* a stretching out]

aer·o·don·tal·gia (ār′ō-don-tal′jē-ă). Dental pain caused by either increased or reduced atmospheric pressure. SYN aero-odontalgia, aero-odontodynia. [aero- + G. *odous,* tooth, + *algos,* pain]

primary a., dental pain associated with expansion of trapped gases within a tooth, as under a filling or in an infected pulp.

secondary a., pain referred to the dental area from an area of aerosinusitis.

aer·o·don·tia (ār-ō-don′shē-ă). The science of the effect of either increased or reduced atmospheric pressure on the teeth. [aero- + G. *odous,* tooth]

aer·o·dy·nam·ics (ār′ō-dī-nam′iks). The study of air and other gases in motion, the forces that set them in motion, and the results of such motion. [aero- + G. *dynamis,* force]

aer·o·dy·nam·ic size. In aerosols, the particle size with unit density that best represents the aerodynamic behavior of a particle.

aer·o·gas·tria (ār-ō-gas′trē-ă). Distention of the stomach with gas.

blocked a., retention of gas in the stomach due to spasm of the sphincteric region of the lower esophagus which prevents belching.

aer·o·gen (ār′ō-jen). A gas-forming microorganism.

aer·o·gen·e·sis (ār-ō-jen′ě-sis). Production of gas, as by a microorganism. [aero- + G. *genesis,* origin]

aer·o·gen·ic, aer·og·e·nous (ār-ō-jen′ik, -oj′ě-nŭs). Gas-forming.

aer·o·med·i·cine (ār-ō-med′i-sin). SYN aviation *medicine.*

aer·o·mo·nad (ār-ō-mō′nad). A vernacular term used to refer to any member of the genus *Aeromonas.*

Aer·o·mo·nas (ār-ō-mō′nas). A genus of Gram-negative, oxidase-positive, aerobic, facultatively anaerobic bacteria (family Vibrionaceae) containing rod-shaped to coccoid cells; motile cells ordinarily possess a single, polar flagellum; some species are nonmotile. The metabolism of these organisms is both respiratory and fermentative; nutritional requirements are not stringent. These bacteria are found in water and sewage; some are pathogenic to fresh water and marine animals, and to humans. The type species is *A. hydrophila.*

A. hydroph′ila, a species that causes cellulitis, wound infections, acute diarrhea (waterborne and shellfish-associated), septicemia, and urinary tract infections in humans. Also causes red leg disease of frogs. The type species of *Aeromonas.*

aer·o·o·don·tal·gia (ār′ō-ō-don-tal′jē-ă). SYN aerodontalgia.

aer·o·o·don·to·dyn·ia (ār′ō-ō-don-tō-din′ē-ă). SYN aerodontalgia.

aer·o·pause (ār′ō-pawz). An upper region of the atmosphere, between the stratosphere and outer space, in which gas particles are so sparse as to provide almost no support for man's physiologic requirements or for vehicles that require air for burning fuel.

aer·o·pha·gia, aer·oph·a·gy (ār-ō-fā′jē-ă, -of′ă-jē). An abnormal swallowing of air as seen in crib-biting and wind-sucking. SYN pneumophagia. [aero- + G. *phagō,* to eat]

aer·o·phil, aer·o·phile (ār′ō-fil, -fīl). **1.** Air-loving. **2.** An aerobic organism (aerobe), especially an obligate aerobe. [aero- + G. *philos,* fond]

aer·o·phil·ic, aer·oph·i·lous (ār-ō-fil′ik, ār-of′i-lŭs). SYN aerobic.

aer·o·pho·bia (ār-ō-fō′bē-ă). Morbid dread of fresh air or of air in motion. [aero- + G. *phobos,* fear]

aer·o·pi·e·so·ther·a·py (ār′ō-pī-ē′sō-thār′ă-pē). Treatment of disease by compressed (or rarified) air. [aero- + G. *piesis,* pressure, + *therapeia,* medical treatment]

aer·o·plank·ton (ār-ō-plank′tŏn). An organism or a substance carried by air, e.g., bacterium, pollen, grain. [aero- + G. *planktos,* ntr. *-on,* wandering]

aer·o·si·al·oph·a·gy (ār′ō-sī-al-of′ă-jē). SYN sialoaerophagy.

aer·o·si·nus·i·tis (ār-ō-sī-nŭ-sī′tis). SYN barosinusitis.

aer·o·sis (ār-ō′sis). Generation of gas in the tissues. [aero- + G. *-osis,* condition]

■ **aer·o·sol** (ār′ō-sol). **1.** Liquid or particulate matter dispersed in air, gas, or vapor in the form of a fine mist for therapeutic, insecticidal, or other purposes. **2.** A product that is packaged under pressure and contains therapeutically or chemically active ingredients intended for topical application, inhalation, or introduction into body orifices. [aero- + solution]

aerosol therapy		
(Relationship between particle size, target area, and mode of transport.)		
particle size	**target area**	**mode of transport**
< 1 μm	particles are exhaled	remain in gaseous state
1–5 μm	peripheral bronchial passages	particles form a sediment
5–10 μm	upper respiratory passages and central bronchial passages	particles rebound
> 10 μm	upper respiratory passages	

respirable a.'s, a.'s with an aerodynamic size under 10 μm.

aer·o·sol·i·za·tion (ār-ō-sol-i-zā′shŭn). Dispersion in air of a liquid material or a solution in the form of a fine mist, usually for therapeutic purposes, especially to the respiratory passages.

aer·o·ther·a·peu·tics, aer·o·ther·a·py (ār′ō-thār-ă-pū′tiks, -thār′ă-pē). Treatment of disease by fresh air, by air of different degrees of pressure or rarity, or by air medicated in various ways.

aer·o·ti·tis me·dia (ār-ō-tī′tis mē′dē-ă). SYN barotitis media. [aero- + G. *ous,* ear, + *-itis,* inflammation]

aer·o·ton·om·e·ter (ār′ō-ton-om′ě-ter). **1.** An instrument for estimating the tension or pressure of a gas. **2.** SYN tonometer (2). [aero- + G. *tonos,* tension, + *metron,* measure]

aes·cu·la·pi·an (es-kū-lā′pē-an). Relating to Aesculapius, the art of medicine, or a medical practitioner. SYN esculapian. [L. *Aesculapius,* G. *Asklēpios,* the god of medicine]

aes·cu·lin (es′kū-lin). SYN esculin.

aes·ti·val (es′ti-văl). SYN estival.

AFB 1. Abbreviation for acid-fast bacillus. SEE acid-fast. **2.** Abbreviation for aortofemoral bypass (vascular prosthetic surgery), the surgical procedure or its result.

afe·brile (ā-feb′ril). Without fever, denoting apyrexia; having a normal body temperature. SYN apyretic, apyrexial.

afe·tal (ă-fē′tăl). Without relation to a fetus or intrauterine life.

af·fect (af′fekt). The emotional feeling, tone, and mood attached to a thought, including its external manifestations. [L. *affectus,* state of mind, fr. *afficio,* to have influence on]

blunted a., a disturbance in mood seen in schizophrenic patients manifested by shallowness and a severe reduction in the expression of feeling.

flat a., absence of or diminution in the amount of emotional tone or outward emotional reaction typically shown by others or oneself under similar circumstances; a milder form is termed blunted a.

inappropriate a., emotional tone or outward emotional reaction out of harmony with the idea, object, or thought accompanying it.

labile a., rapid shifts in outward emotional expressions; often associated with organic brain syndromes such as intoxication.

af·fect dis·play. Facial expressions, postures, and gestures indicating emotional states.

af·fec·tion (ă-fek′shŭn). **1.** A moderate feeling of tenderness, caring, or love. **2.** An abnormal condition of body or mind. [L. *affectio,* fr. *af-ficio,* to affect, influence]

af·fec·tive (af-fek′tiv). Pertaining to mood, emotion, feeling, sensibility, or a mental state.

af·fec·tiv·i·ty (af-fek-tiv′i-tē). SYN feeling *tone.*

af·fec·to·mo·tor (af′fek-tō-mō′ter). Pertaining to muscular manifestations associated with affective tone.

af·fer·ent (af′er-ent). Inflowing; conducting toward a center, denoting certain arteries, veins, lymphatics, and nerves. Opposite of efferent. SYN centripetal (1), esodic. [L. *afferens,* fr. *af-fero,* to bring to]

af·fin·i·ty (ă-fin′i-tē). **1.** In chemistry, the force that impels certain atoms to bind to or unite with certain others to form complexes or compounds; chemical attraction. **2.** Selective staining of a tissue by a dye or the selective uptake of a dye, chemical, or other substance by a tissue. [L. *affinis,* neighboring, fr. *ad,* to, + *finis,* end, boundary]

residual a., secondary forces that enable apparently saturated atoms, ions, or molecules to attract other atoms or groups, causing such phenomena as complex formation, hydration, adsorption, etc.

af·fi·nous (af′i-nŭs). Pertaining to a marriage in which the partners are related, not by consanguinity, but through another marriage. [L. *affinis,* related by marriage, fr. *ad,* to + *finis,* limit]

af·fir·ma·tion (af-fer-mā′shŭn). The stage in autosuggestion in which one exhibits a positive reactive tendency. [L. *affirmatio,* fr. affirm, to make strong, fr *firmus,* strong]

af·fu·sion (ă-fū′zhŭn). Pouring of water upon the body or any of its parts for therapeutic purposes. [L. *af- fundo,* to pour into]

AFH Abbreviation for anterior facial *height.*

afi·bril·lar (ā-fī′bri-lăr). Denoting a biological structure that does not contain fibrils.

afi·brin·o·gen·e·mia (ā-fī′brin-ō-jĕ-nē′mē-ă). The absence of fibrinogen in the plasma. SEE ALSO hypofibrinogenemia.

congenital a. [MIM*202400], a rare disorder of blood coagulation in which little or no fibrinogen can be found in plasma because of a mutant form in one of the three fibrinogen loci. Leads to defective platelet aggregation; autosomal recessive inheritance.

Afipia (ă-fip′ē-ă). A genus of Gram-negative, oxidase-positive, motile, nonfermenting bacteria that have been placed in the class Proteobacteria. They are morphologically variable, appearing as rods or filaments that may stain poorly. Over 10 species have been identified; originally reported to be the agent of catscratch disease, their current pathogenic role remains uncertain. The type strain is *A. felis.*

af·la·tox·i·co·sis (af′la-toks-ē-cō′sis). A disease caused by ingestion of aflatoxin.

af·la·tox·in (af′lă-tok′sin). Toxic metabolites of some *Aspergillus* strains including the fungi *Aspergillus flavus, Aspergillus parasiticus,* and *Aspergillus oryzae.* They may play a role in the etiology of primary cancer of the liver in humans and produce disease in animals eating peanut meal and other feed contaminated by these fungi.

AFORMED SEE AFORMED *phenomenon.*

AFP Abbreviation for α-*fetoproteins.* SEE fetoproteins.

af·ter·birth (af′ter-berth). The placenta and membranes that are extruded from the uterus after birth. SYN secundina, secundines.

af·ter·care (af′ter-kār). **1.** The care and treatment of a patient after an operation,delivery, or convalescence from an illness. **2.** Following psychiatric hospitalization, a continuing program of rehabilitation designed to reinforce the effects of the therapy; may include partial hospitalization, day hospital, or outpatient treatment.

af·ter·chrom·ing (af′ter-krōm′ing). Additional treatment of a tissue specimen with chromate or a metal mordant to impart special staining properties. SYN postchroming.

af·ter·con·trac·tion (af′ter-kon-trak′shŭn). A muscular contraction persisting a noticeable time after the stimulus has ceased.

af·ter·cur·rent (af′ter-kŭr-ent). An electrical current induced in a muscle upon the termination of a constant current that has been passed through it.

af·ter·dis·charge (af-ter-dis′charj). Persistence of response of muscle or neural elements after cessation of stimulation. Myotonia is a clinical manifestation of prolonged muscle a.

af·ter·ef·fect (af′ter-ĕ-fekt′). A physical, physiologic, psychologic, or emotional effect that continues after removal of the stimulus. SEE flashback.

af·ter·gild·ing (af′ter-gild′ing). The treatment of a fixed and hardened histologic specimen of nervous tissue with gold salts.

af·ter·im·age (af′ter-im′ij). Persistence of a visual response after cessation of the stimulus. SYN accidental image, negative image.

negative a., a. in which the lightness relationship is reversed; if chromatic, it appears in complementary color.

positive a., a. in which the lightness relationship is the same as the original one; if chromatic, it appears in the same color.

af·ter·im·pres·sion (af′ter-im-presh′ŭn). SYN aftersensation.

af·ter·load (af′ter-lōd). **1.** The arrangement of a muscle so that, in shortening, it lifts a weight from an adjustable support or otherwise does work against a constant opposing force to which it is not exposed at rest. **2.** The load or force thus encountered in shortening.

ventricular a., formerly and erroneously, the arterial pressure or some other measure of the force that a ventricle must overcome while it contracts during ejection, contributed to by aortic or pulmonic artery impedance, peripheral vascular resistance, and mass and viscosity of blood; now, more rigorously expressed in terms of the wall stress, i.e., the tension per unit cross-sectional area in the ventricular muscle fibers (calculated by an expansion of Laplace law using pressure, internal radius, and wall thickness) that is required to produce the intracavitary pressure required during ejection.

af·ter·move·ment (af′ter-moov′ment). Involuntary arm abduction that follows sustained isometric contraction of the deltoid and supraspinatus muscles (usually performed by pushing the upper extremity forcibly and against an immovable vertical surface while standing closely beside it). SYN Kohnstamm phenomenon.

af·ter·pains (af′ter-pānz). Painful cramplike contractions of the uterus occurring after childbirth.

af·ter·per·cep·tion (af′ter-per-sep′shŭn). SYN aftersensation.

af·ter·po·ten·tial (af′ter-pō-ten′shăl). The small change in electrical potential in a stimulated nerve that follows the main, or spike, potential; it consists of an initial negative deflection followed by a positive deflection in the oscillograph record.

diastolic a., in the heart, a transmembrane potential change following repolarization, which may reach threshold magnitude and cause a rhythm disturbance; often recorded in poisoning, as by digitalis overdosage.

positive a., a spontaneous or inducible increase in transmembrane potential of a cardiac or nerve cell following the completion of repolarization. In the heart, this usually corresponds temporal to the electrocardiographic U wave.

af·ter·sen·sa·tion (af′ter-sen-sā′shŭn). Subjective persistence of sensation after cessation of stimulus. SYN afterimpression, afterperception.

ag

af·ter·sound (af′ter-sownd). Subjective persistence of an auditory sensation after the stimulus stops.

af·ter·taste (af′ter-tāst). Subjective persistence of a gustatory sensation after contact with the stimulating substance has ceased.

af·ter·touch (af′ter-tŭch). Subjective persistence of tactile sensation after cessation of the stimulus; a form of aftersensation.

af·to·sa (af-tō′să). SYN foot-and-mouth *disease*. [Sp. *fiebre aftosa*, aphthous fever]

Ag 1. Symbol for silver (argentum). **2.** Abbreviation for antigen.

ag·a·lac·tia (ă-gal-ak′shē-ă). Absence of milk in the breasts after childbirth. SYN agalactosis. [G. *a-* priv. + *gala* (*galakt-*), milk]

aga·lac·tor·rhea (ā-ga-lak-tō-rē′ă). Absence of the secretion or flow of breast milk. [G. *a-* priv. + *gala*, milk, + *rhoia*, a flow]

ag·a·lac·to·sis (ă-gal-ak-tō′sis). SYN agalactia.

ag·a·lac·tous (ă-gal-ak′tŭs). Relating to agalactia, or to the diminution or absence of breast milk.

ag·a·mete (ā-gam′ēt, ag′a-mēt). A protozoan organism produced by asexual multiple fission. SEE ALSO schizogony. [G. *a-* priv. + *gametēs*, husband]

agam·ic (ā-gam′ik). Denoting nonsexual reproduction, as by fission, budding, etc. SYN agamous.

agam·ma·glob·u·lin·e·mia (ā-gam′ă-glob′ū-li-nē′mē-ă). Absence of, or extremely low levels of, the gamma fraction of serum globulin; sometimes used loosely to denote absence of immunoglobulins in general. SEE ALSO hypogammaglobulinemia.

acquired a., SYN common variable *immunodeficiency.*

Bruton a., an X-linked condition, with hypo- or agammaglobulinemia; the immune deficiency becomes apparent as maternally transmitted immunoglobulin levels decline in early infancy. SYN X-linked a.

secondary a., SYN secondary *immunodeficiency.*

Swiss type a., SYN severe combined *immunodeficiency.*

transient a., SYN transient *hypogammaglobulinemia* of infancy.

X-linked a., SYN Bruton a.

agam·o·cy·tog·e·ny (ā-gam′ō-sī-toj′ĕ-nē). SYN schizogony. [G. *agamos*, unmarried, + *kytos*, cell, + *genesis*, becoming]

Agam·o·fi·lar·ia (ă-gam′ō-fī-lā′rē-ă). A name given to immature filarial forms, the genera of the adult forms being undetermined. [G. *agamos*, unmarried, + L. *filum*, thread]

ag·a·mo·gen·e·sis (ag′ă-mō-jen′ĕ-sis, ā-gam-ō-). SYN asexual *reproduction.* [G. *agamos*, unmarried, + *genesis*, production]

ag·a·mo·ge·net·ic (ag′ă-mō-jĕ-net′ik, -ā-gam-ō-). Indicating asexual reproduction.

ag·a·mog·o·ny (ag-ă-mog′ō-nē). SYN asexual *reproduction.* [G. *agamos*, unmarried, + *gonos*, offspring]

Ag·a·mo·mer·mis cu·li·cis (ag-ă-mō-mer′mis kū′li-kis). A species of nematode parasitic in the mosquito; a few cases have been recorded in humans, usually larval worms found emerging from body openings, presumably after ingestion of infected insects or application of moist earth bearing free-living larval stages. [G. *agamos*, unmarried, + Mod. L., fr. G. *mermis*, cord; L. *culex*, gnat]

ag·a·mont (ag′ă-mont). SYN schizont. [G. *agamos*, unmarried, + *ōn* (*ont-*), being]

ag·a·mous (ag′ă-mŭs). SYN agamic. [G. *agamos*, unmarried]

agan·gli·on·ic (ā-gang-glē-on′ik). Without ganglia.

agan·gli·o·no·sis (ā-gang′glē-ō-nō′sis). The state of being without ganglia; e.g., absence of ganglion cells from the myenteric plexus as a characteristic of congenital megacolon. [G. ā- priv. + ganglion + *-osis*, condition]

agap·ism (ah′gahp-izm). The doctrine that exalts nonsexual (brotherly) love. [G. *agapē*, brotherly love]

agar (ah′gar, ā′gar). A complex polysaccharide (a sulfated galactan) derived from seaweed (various red algae); used as a solidifying agent in culture media; it has the valuable property of melting at 100°C, but not solidifying until 49°C. [Bengalese]

bile salt a., an a. medium containing lactose, peptone, sodium taurocholate, and neutral red, for the growth and isolation of Gram-negative rods.

birdseed a., media prepared from *Guizottia abyssinica* seeds used in culturing and in the presumptive diagnosis of *Cryptococcus neoformans.*

blood a., a mixture of blood, usually sheep or horse, and an agar-based medium used for the cultivation of many medically important microorganisms.

Bordet-Gengou potato blood a., glycerine-potato a. with 25% of blood, used for the isolation of *Bordetella pertussis.*

brain-heart infusion a., a medium used for the isolation of fastidious microorganisms, especially fungi.

chocolate a., blood a. heated until the blood becomes brown or chocolate in color, used especially to isolate *Haemophilus* or *Neisseria* and other species for which unheated blood is inhibitory.

cholera a., an alkaline a. medium for cultivating *Vibrio cholerae.*

cornmeal a., a culture medium that is low in nutrients, used extensively in the study of yeastlike and filamentous fungi; it suppresses vegetative growth while stimulating sporulation of many species, and is widely used for producing the distinctive chlamydospores of *Candida albicans.*

Czapek solution a., a culture medium used for the cultivation of fungus species and for identification of *Aspergillus* and *Penicillium* species. SYN Czapek-Dox medium.

EMB a., SYN eosin-methylene blue a.

Endo a., a medium containing peptone, lactose, dipotassium phosphate, a., sodium sulfite, basic fuchsin, and distilled water; originally developed for the isolation of *Salmonella typhi*, this medium is now most useful in the bacteriological examination of water; coliform organisms ferment the lactose, and their colonies become red and color the surrounding medium; non-lactose-fermenting organisms produce clear, colorless colonies against the faint pink background of the medium. SYN Endo medium.

eosin-methylene blue a., a. composed of peptone, lactose, and sucrose and containing eosin and methylene blue, used to distinguish between lactose-fermenting and non–lactose-fermenting Gram-negative bacteria. *Echerichia sp.* show a characteristic sheen. SYN EMB a.

MacConkey a., medium containing peptone, lactose, bile salts, neutral red, and crystal violet, used to identify Gram-negative bacilli and characterize them according to their status as lactose fermenters. Fermenters appear as pink colonies while nonfermenters are colorless.

Mueller-Hinton a., medium containing beef infusion, peptone, and starch used primarily for the disk-agar diffusion method for antimicrobial susceptibility testing.

Novy and MacNeal blood a., a nutrient a. containing two volumes of defibrinated rabbit's blood; suitable for the cultivation of a number of trypanosomes.

nutrient a., a simple solid medium containing beef extract, peptone, agar, and water; used for growing many common heterotrophic bacteria.

oatmeal-tomato paste a., a special culture medium for the production of ascospore formation in the dermatophytes.

potato dextrose a., a culture medium used extensively for the cultivation of fungi; especially good for development of conidia and other sporulating forms by which an organism is identified microscopically.

rice-Tween a., a useful medium for the development of the chlamydospores in *Candida albicans* and for preparation of slide cultures for other forms of sporulation in other fungal species.

Sabouraud a., a culture medium for fungi containing neopeptone or polypeptone a. and glucose, with final pH 5.6; it is the standard, most universally used medium in mycology and is the international reference. Modified Sabouraud a. (Emmons modification) with neutral pH and less glucose is better for pigment development in the colonies.

Sabouraud dextrose a., a dextrose peptone medium that supports the growth of most pathogenic fungi.

serum a., an enriched medium for cultivation of fastidious organisms; prepared by adding sterile serum to melted a.

Thayer-Martin a., a Mueller-Hinton a. with 5% heat-hemolyzed sheep blood and antibiotics, used for transport and primary isolation of *Neisseria gonorrhoeae* and *Neisseria meningitidis*. SYN Thayer-Martin medium.

yeast extract a., a medium used to induce sporulation and reduce vegetative growth in the cultivation of fungi.

agar·ic (ă-gar′ik). The dried fruit body of *Polyporus officinalis* (family Polyporaceae), occurring in the form of brownish or whitish light masses, which contains agaric acid. SYN amadou. [G. *agarikon,* a kind of fungus]

deadly a. a., SYN *Amanita phalloides*.

fly a. a., SYN *Amanita muscaria*.

agar·ic ac·id (ă-gar′ik). Obtained from agaric and responsible for the anhidrotic action of the mushroom; used as an anhidrotic agent.

Agar·i·cus (ă-gar′i-kŭs). A large genus of mushrooms of which many are edible and others poisonous. [L. *agaricum,* fr. G. *agarikon,* a tree fungus]

agar·o·pec·tin (ag′ă-rō-pek′tin). A polysaccharide found in agar preparations consisting of D-galactose linked β1,3 glycosidically. Some of the galactosyl units are sulfated.

ag·a·rose (ag′ă-rōs). The neutral linear polysaccharide fraction found in agar preparations, generally composed of D-galactose and altered 3,6-anhydrogalactose residues; used in chromatography and electrophoresis.

agas·tric (ă-gas′trik). Without stomach or digestive tract. [G. *a*-priv. + *gastēr,* belly]

agas·tro·neu·ria (ă-gas-trō-noor′ē-ă). Lessened nervous control of the stomach. [G. *a*- priv. + *gastēr,* belly, + *neuron,* nerve]

AGC Abbreviation for automatic gain *control*.

age (āj). **1.** The period that has elapsed since birth. **2.** One of the periods into which human life is divided, distinguished by physical evolution, equilibrium, and involution; e.g., the seven a.'s of mankind are: infancy, childhood, adolescence, maturity, middle life, senescence, and senility. **3.** To grow old; to gradually develop changes in structure that are not due to preventable disease or trauma and that are associated with decreased functional capacity and an increased probability of death. **4.** To cause artificially the appearance characteristic of one who has lived long or of a thing that has existed for a long time. **5.** In dentistry, to heat an alloy for amalgam so as to make it set more slowly, increase strength, reduce flow, and have a stable shelf life; aging occurs by relieving internal strains. [F. *âge,* L. *aetas*]

achievement a., the relationship between the chronologic age and the age of achievement, as established by standard achievement tests.

anatomical a., a. in terms of structure rather than of function or of passage of time. SYN physical a.

basal a., highest mental a. level of the Stanford-Binet intelligence scale at which all items are passed.

Binet a., the a. of the normal child with whose intelligence (as measured by the Stanford-Binet scale) the intelligence of the abnormal child corresponds (the profoundly retarded individual functions like a child of 1–2 years; the moderately to severely retarded, 3–7 years; the borderline to mildly retarded, 8–12 years).

bone a., stage of development of bone (in years) as adjudged by radiography, in contrast to chronologic age.

childbearing a., the period in a woman's life between puberty and menopause.

chronologic a. (CA), a. expressed in years and months; used as a measurement against which to evaluate a child's mental a. in computing the Stanford-Binet intelligence quotient.

developmental a., (1) a. estimated by anatomic development since fertilization; **(2) (DA),** a. of an individual estimated from the degree of anatomic, physiologic, mental, and emotional maturation.

emotional a., a measure of emotional maturity by comparison with average emotional development.

gestational a., (1) in embryology, the a. of a conceptus expressed in elapsed time since conception; **(2)** in obstetrics, the developmental a. of a fetus, usually based on the presumed first day of the last normal menstrual period.

menstrual a., a. of the conceptus computed from the start of the mother's last menstrual period.

mental a. (MA), a measure, expressed in years and months, of a child's intelligence relative to age norms as determined by testing with the Stanford-Binet intelligence scale.

physical a., SYN anatomical a.

physiologic a., a. estimated in terms of function.

agen·e·sis (ā-jen′ĕ-sis). Absence or failure of formation of any part. [G. *a*- priv. + *genesis,* production]

gonadal a., absence of one or both gonads.

müllerian a., SYN Mayer-Rokitansky-Küster-Hauser *syndrome*.

renal a., absence of one or both kidneys, most commonly unilateral with absence of the ipsilateral paramesonephric duct and its derivatives; renal function is normal as long as the remaining kidney is intact; bilateral or complete renal a. is associated with Potter facies and neonatal death.

thymic a., absence of the thymus, which may be associated with parathyroid a. in DiGeorge syndrome.

agen·i·tal·ism (ā-jen′i-tal-izm). Congenital absence of genitalia.

agen·o·so·mia (ā-gen-ō-sō′mē-ă). Markedly defective formation or absence of the genitalia; usually accompanied by protrusion of the abdominal viscera through an incomplete abdominal wall. [G. *a*- priv. + *genos,* sex, + *soma,* body]

agent (ā′jent). **1.** An active force or substance capable of producing an effect. For agents not listed here, see the specific name. **2.** A disease, a factor such as a microorganism, chemical substance, or a form of radiation the presence or absence of which (as in deficiency diseases) results in disease or more advanced disease. [L. *ago,* pres. p. *agens* (*agent-*), to perform]

adrenergic blocking a., a compound that selectively blocks or inhibits responses to sympathetic adrenergic nerve activity (sympatholytic a.) and to epinephrine, norepinephrine, and other adrenergic amines (adrenolytic a.); two distinct classes exist, alpha- and beta-adrenergic receptor blocking a.'s.

α-adrenergic blocking a., a class of drugs that compete with α-adrenergic agonists for available receptor sites: some compete for both α_1 and α_2 receptors (e.g., phentolamine, dibenzyline) while others are primarily either α_1 (e.g., prazosin, terazosin) or α_2 receptor blocking agents (e.g., yohimbine). SYN α-adrenoceptor antagonist, alpha-blocker.

β-adrenergic blocking a., a class of drugs that compete with β-adrenergic agonists for available receptor sites; some compete for both β_1 and β_2 receptors (e.g., propranolol) while others are primarily either β_1 (e.g., metoprolol) or β_2 blockers; used in the treatment of a variety of cardiovascular diseases where β-adrenergic blockade is desirable. SYN β-adrenergic receptor blocking a., β-adrenoreceptor antagonist, beta-blocker.

adrenergic neuronal blocking a., a drug that prevents the release of norepinephrine from sympathetic nerve terminals (e.g., guanethidine); it does not inhibit the responses of the adrenergic receptors to circulating epinephrine, norepinephrine, and other adrenergic amines.

β-adrenergic receptor blocking a., SYN β-adrenergic blocking a.

alkylating a., a drug or chemical that, via the formation of covalent bonds, forms a derivatized tissue constituent permanently containing part of the drug or chemical compound; frequently carcinogenic and mutagenic, but often used in the chemotherapy of cancer (e.g., nitrogen mustards and carmustine).

antianxiety a., a functional category of drugs useful in the treatment of anxiety and able to reduce anxiety at doses that do not cause excessive sedation. The majority of commonly used drugs falling into this category are benzodiazepines, which act at the γ-aminobutyric acid (GABA) receptor sites. Historically, barbiturates were the main agents in this category; a newer category, which acts at serotonin (5-HT$_{1A}$) receptor sites, is currently represented by buspirone. SYN anxiolytic (1), minor tranquilizer.

antidyskinetic a., a functional category of drugs with anticholinergic action, used to treat Parkinson disease and some of the acute movement disorders that may be caused by antipsychotic a.'s.

antifoaming a.'s, chemicals that lower surface tension (hence production of foam), used in laboratory evaporations, and also administered with oxygen to relieve the respiratory obstruction aggravated by the foam of edema fluid in pulmonary edema (pulmonary surfactant).

antipsychotic a., a functional category of neuroleptic drugs that are helpful in the treatment of psychosis and have a capacity to ameliorate thought disorders. SYN antipsychotic (1), major tranquilizer.

atypical antipsychotic a., a functional category of newer antipsychotic drugs thought to exert their action predominantly via serotonergic blockade.

bacteriostatic a., SYN bacteriostat.

Bittner a., SYN mammary tumor *virus* of mice.

blister a.,

blocking a., a class of drugs that inhibit (block) a biologic activity or process, such as axonal conduction or transmission, access to a receptor, or movement of ions across a cell membrane; frequently called "blockers."

calcium channel-blocking a., a class of drugs that have the ability to inhibit movement of calcium ions across the cell membrane; of particular value in the treatment of cardiovascular disorders because of pharmacologic effects such as depression of mechanical contraction of cardiac and smooth muscle and of both impulse formation and conduction velocity (e.g., verapamil, nifedipine). SYN calcium antagonist, slow channel-blocking a.

chimpanzee coryza a. (CCA), SYN respiratory syncytial *virus*.

cholinergic a., an a. that mimics the action of acetylcholine or of the parasympathetic nervous system (e.g., methacholine).

contrast a., SYN contrast *medium*.

cycle-specific a., an a. that has effect in only one part of the cell cycle (S phase) or only when the cell is in a specific part of the cell cycle.

delta a., SYN hepatitis D *virus*.

Eaton a., SYN *Mycoplasma pneumoniae*.

embedding a.'s, materials such as celloidin, paraffin, etc. in which specimens of tissue are set before being cut into sections for microscopic examination.

enterokinetic a., an a. used to relieve intestinal atony.

F a., obsolete term for F *plasmid*.

fertility a., obsolete term for F *plasmid*.

foamy a.'s, SYN foamy *viruses*, under *virus*.

ganglionic blocking a., an a. that impairs the passage of impulses in autonomic ganglia (e.g., tetraethylammonium, trimethaphan).

high osmolar contrast a., ionic water-soluble iodinated contrast medium. SYN high osmolar contrast medium.

initiating a., SEE initiation.

inotropic a.'s, drugs that increase the force of contraction of cardiac muscle; examples include digitalis glycosides, amrinone, and epinephrine.

LDH a., SYN lactate dehydrogenase *virus*.

low osmolar contrast a. (LOCA), nonionic water-soluble radiographic contrast material. SYN low osmolar contrast medium, nonionic contrast a.

luting a., a fastening material or cement; e.g., plaster or wax to hold casts to an articulator, or material to hold crowns to teeth.

mood stabilizing a., a functional category of drugs used to normalize mood, particularly by dampening mood swings (e.g., lithium and some anticonvulsants such as carbamazepine and valproic acid).

neuroleptic a., SYN neuroleptic.

neuromuscular blocking a.'s, a group of drugs that prevent motor nerve endings from exciting skeletal muscle. They act either by competing for the neurotransmitter, acetylcholine (like D-tubocurarine, mivacurium, and pancuronium), or by first stimulating the postjunctional muscle membrane and subsequently desensitizing the muscle endplates to the acetylcholine (like succinylcholine or decamethonium); used in surgery to produce paralysis and facilitate manipulation of muscles.

non–cycle-specific a., a. that has effect regardless of where the cell is in its division cycle.

nondepolarizing neuromuscular blocking a., a compound that paralyzes skeletal muscle primarily by inhibiting transmission of nerve impulses at the neuromuscular junction rather than by af-

fecting the membrane potention of motor endplate or muscle fibers (e.g., curare, gallamine, vecuronium).

nonionic contrast a., SYN low osmolar contrast a.

Norwalk a., a strain of epidemic gastroenteritis virus that belongs to the calciviruses. [*Norwalk,* Ohio, where first implicated in disease]

Pittsburgh pneumonia a., SYN *Legionella micdadei*.

promoting a., SEE promotion.

psychotropic a., a chemical compound that influences the human psyche.

reovirus-like a., SYN rotavirus.

sclerosing a., a compound that acts by irritation of the veinous intimal epithelium; used in the treatment of varicose veins.

slow channel-blocking a., SYN calcium channel-blocking a.

sympathetic a., SEE sympathomimetic *amine*.

transforming a., (1) SYN mitogen; (2) virus that can transform cells.

TRIC a.'s, strains of *Chlamydia trachomatis* that cause *t*rachoma and *i*nclusion *c*onjunctivitis a.'s SEE *Chlamydia trachomatis*.

typical antipsychotic a., a functional category of older antipsychotic drugs thought to exert their action predominantly via dopaminergic blockade.

Agent Orange. An herbicide and defoliant, consisting of (2,4,5-trichlorophenoxy)acetic acid, (2,4-dichlorophenoxy) acetic acid, and dioxin, that was widely used in the Vietnam War; it has been shown to possess residual post-exposure carcinogenic and teratogenic properties in humans.

age·ra·sia (ă-jer-ā′zē-ă). An appearance of youth in old age. [G. *agērasia,* eternal youth, fr. *a*- priv. + *gēras,* old age]

ageu·sia (ă-goo′sē-ă). Loss or absence of the sense of taste. It may be: 1) general to all tastants (total), partial to some tastants, or specific to one or more tastants; 2) due to transport disorders (in access to the interior of the taste bud) or sensorineural disorders (affecting the gustatory sensory cells or nerves or the central gustatory neural pathways); or 3) hereditary or acquired. SYN ageustia, gustatory anesthesia. [G. *a*- priv. + *geusis,* taste]

ageus·tia (ă-goos′tē-ă). SYN ageusia.

ag·ger, pl. **ag·ger·es** (aj′er, -ēz; ag′er) [TA]. An eminence, projection, or shallow ridge. [L. mound]

a. na′si [TA], an elevation on the lateral wall of the nasal cavity lying between the atrium of the middle meatus and the olfactory sulcus; it is formed by the mucous membrane covering the base of the ethmoidal crest of the maxilla. SYN nasal ridge.

a. perpendicula′ris, SYN *eminence* of triangular fossa of auricle.

a. val′vae ve′nae, SYN *prominence* of venous valvular sinus.

ag·glom·er·ate, ag·glom·er·at·ed (ă-glom′er-āt). SYN aggregated. [L. *ag-glomero,* to wind into a ball; from *ad,* to, + *glomus,* a ball]

ag·glom·er·a·tion (ă-glom-er-ā′shŭn). SYN aggregation.

ag·glu·ti·nant (ă-gloo′ti-nant). A substance that holds parts together or causes agglutination. [L. *ad,* to + *gluten,* glue]

ag·glu·ti·nate (ă-gloo′ti-nāt). To accomplish, or be subjected to, agglutination.

ag·glu·ti·na·tion (ă-gloo-ti-nā′shŭn). **1.** The process by which suspended bacteria, cells, or other particles are caused to adhere and form into clumps; similar to precipitation, but the particles are larger and are in suspension rather than being in solution. For specific a. reactions in the various blood groups, see Blood Groups appendix. **2.** Adhesion of the surfaces of a wound. **3.** The process of adhering. [L. *ad,* to, + *gluten,* glue]

acid a., the clumping together of certain microorganisms at high hydrogen ion concentration.

bacteriogenic a., the clumping of cells as a result of effects of bacteria or their products.

cold a., a. of red blood cells by their own serum (see autoagglutination), or by any other serum when the blood is cooled below body temperature, but most pronounced below 25°C; the phenomenon results from cold agglutinins; may be seen occasionally in the blood of apparently normal persons or as a pathologic finding in patients with primary atypical pneumonia, infectious mononucleosis, and other viral diseases, certain protozoan infections, or lymphoproliferative neoplasms. SEE autoagglutination.

cross a., SYN group a.

false a., SYN pseudoagglutination (1).

group a., a. by antibodies specific for minor (group) antigens common to several microorganisms, each of which possesses its own major specific antigen. SYN cross a.

immune a., a. caused by antibody (agglutinin) that is specific for the suspended microorganism, cell, or for an antigen that has been coated on a particle of suitable size.

indirect a., SYN passive a.

nonimmune a., (1) a. caused by a lectin having a degree of specificity for a particular sugar, the mechanism of which is not understood; (2) a. that results from nonspecific factors, as in the case of acid a. or spontaneous a.

passive a., a. of particles that have been coated with soluble antigen, by antiserum specific for the adsorbed antigen. SYN indirect a.

spontaneous a., nonspecific clumping of organisms in saline related to lack of polar groups in electrolyte solution.

ag·glu·ti·na·tive (ă-gloo'ti-nă-tiv). Causing, or able to cause, agglutination.

ag·glu·ti·nin (ă-gloo'ti-nin). **1.** An antibody that causes clumping or agglutination of the bacteria or other cells that either stimulated the formation of the a., or contain immunologically similar, reactive antigen. SYN agglutinating antibody, immune a. **2.** A substance, other than a specific agglutinating antibody, that causes organic particles to agglutinate, e.g., plant a.

blood group a.'s, see Blood Groups appendix.

chief a., SYN major a.

cold a., an antibody which reacts more efficiently at temperatures below 37°C.

cross-reacting a., SYN group a.

flagellar a., SYN H a. (1).

group a., an immune a. specific for a "shared" or common antigen. SYN cross-reacting a.

H a., (1) an a. that is formed as the result of stimulation by, and which reacts with, the thermolabile antigen(s) in the flagella of motile strains of microorganisms; SYN flagellar a. (2) see ABO blood group, Blood Groups appendix.

immune a., SYN agglutinin (1).

incomplete a. (ă-gloo'ti-nin), antibody that binds to antigen but does not induce agglutination. These antibodies are usually of the IgG class and are referred to as incomplete antibody.

major a., immune a. present in greatest quantity in an antiserum and evoked by the most dominant of a mosaic of antigens. SYN chief a.

minor a., immune a. present in an antiserum in lesser concentration than the major a. SYN partial a.

O a., (1) an a. that is formed as the result of stimulation by, and that reacts with, the relatively thermostable antigen(s) that are part of the cell wall of certain microorganisms; SYN somatic a. (2) see ABO blood group, Blood Groups appendix.

partial a., SYN minor a.

plant a., a lectin.

saline a., an antibody that causes agglutination of erythrocytes when they are suspended either in saline or in a protein medium. SYN complete antibody.

somatic a., SYN O a. (1).

warm a.'s, an a. that is more reactive at 37°C than at lower temperatures.

ag·glu·tin·o·gen (ă-gloo-tin'ō-jen). An antigenic substance that stimulates the formation of specific agglutinin, which can cause agglutination of cells that contain the antigen or particles coated with the antigen. SYN agglutogen. [agglutinin + G. -gen, production]

blood group a.'s, see Blood Groups appendix.

T a., obsolete term for an a. formed from a latent receptor on human red cells by the action of an enzyme in cultures of certain bacteria.

ag·glu·tin·o·gen·ic (ă-gloo'tin-ō-jen'ik). Capable of causing the production of an agglutinin. SYN agglutogenic.

ag·glu·tin·o·phil·ic (ă-gloo'tin-ō-fil'ik). Readily undergoing pronounced agglutination. [agglutination + G. phileō, to love]

ag·glu·to·gen (ă-gloo'tō-jen). SYN agglutinogen.

ag·glu·to·gen·ic (ă-gloo-tō-jen'ik). SYN agglutinogenic.

ag·gre·can (ag'gre-kan). Candidate gene for otosclerosis located at 15q25 to q26.

ag·gre·gate (ag'rĕ-gāt). **1.** To unite or come together in a mass or cluster. **2.** The total of individual units making up a mass or cluster. [L. ag-grego, pp. -atus, to add to, fr. grex (greg-), a flock]

proteoglycan a., a large a.'s of proteoglycans noncovalently bound to a long molecule of hyaluronic acid; involved in cross-linking the collagen fibrils of cartilage matrix.

ag·gre·gat·ed (ag'rĕ-gā-ted). Collected together, thereby forming a cluster, clump, or mass of individual units. SYN agglomerate, agglomerated, agminate, agminated.

ag·gre·ga·tion (ag-rĕ-gā'shŭn). A crowded mass of independent but similar units; a cluster. SYN agglomeration.

familial a., occurrence of a trait in more members of a family than can be readily accounted for by chance; presumptive but not cogent evidence of the operation of genetic factors.

ag·gre·gom·e·ter (ag-rē-gom'ĕ-ter). An instrument for measuring platelet aggregation by monitoring over time the changes in optic density of a platelet suspension treated with aggregating agents such as ADP, collagen, epinephrine, etc.

ag·gres·sin (ă-gres'in). A substance of microbial origin postulated to inhibit the resistance mechanisms of the host. [L. agressor, an assailant, fr. ad-gredio, pp. -gressus, to attack]

ag·gres·sion (ă-gresh'ŭn). A domineering, forceful, or assaultive verbal or physical action toward another person as the motor component of the affects of anger, hostility, or rage. [L. aggressio, fr. aggredior, to accost, attack]

ag·gres·sive (ă-gres'iv). **1.** Denoting aggression. **2.** Denoting a competitive forcefulness or invasiveness, as of a behavioral pattern, a pathogenic organism, or a disease process.

ag·ing (ā'jing). **1.** The process of growing old, especially by failure of replacement of cells in sufficient number to maintain full functional capacity; particularly affects cells (e.g., neurons) incapable of mitotic division. **2.** The gradual deterioration of a mature organism resulting from time-dependent, irreversible changes in structure that are intrinsic to the particular species, and that eventually lead to decreased ability to cope with the stresses of the environment, thereby increasing the probability of death. **3.** In the cardiovascular system, the progressive replacement of functional cell types by fibrous connective tissue. **4.** A demographic term, meaning an increase over time in the proportion of older persons in the population.

clonal a., the deterioration in successive generations of a clone; thus paramecia and other simple forms, if allowed to reproduce asexually for a number of generations, invariably undergo deterioration, the characters of each group of descendants progressively departing from those of the original sexually produced ancestor.

ag·i·to·la·lia (aj'i-tō-lā'lē-ă). SYN agitophasia.

ag·i·to·pha·sia (aj'i-tō-fā'zē-ă). Abnormally rapid speech in which words are imperfectly spoken or dropped out of a sentence. SYN agitolalia. [L. agito, to hurry, + G. phasis, speech]

aglo·mer·u·lar (ă-glō-mer'ū-lăr). Having no glomeruli; said especially of a kidney in which the glomeruli have been destroyed, or kidneys of certain fish, e.g., toad fish, that possess tubules but no glomeruli.

aglos·sia (ă-glos'ē-ă). Congenital absence of the tongue. [G. a- priv. + glōssa, tongue]

aglos·so·sto·mia (ā-glos-ō-stō'mē-ă). Congenital absence of the tongue, with a malformed (usually closed) mouth. [G. a- priv. + glōssa, tongue, + stoma, mouth]

aglu·con (ă-gloo'kon). The portion of a glucoside other than the glucose. [G. a- priv. + glucose + -on]

ag·lu·ti·tion (ā-gloo-tish'ŭn). Inability to swallow. SEE ALSO dysphagia.

agly·ca, sing. **agly·con** (ā-glī'kon).

agly·con, a·gly·cone, pl. **agly·ca** (ā-glī′kon). The noncarbohydrate portion of a glycoside (e.g., digoxigenin). [G. *a-* priv. + *glykys,* sweet]

a·gly·cone. SEE aglycon.

agly·cos·u·ria (ā-glī-kō-soo′rē-ă). Absence of carbohydrate in the urine.

agly·cos·u·ric (ă-glī-kō-soo′rik). Relating to aglycosuria.

ag·men, pl. **ag·mina** (ag′men, ag′min-ă). Obsolete term for aggregation. [L. a multitude]

a. peyerian′um, SYN aggregated lymphoid *nodules* of small intestine, under *nodule.*

ag·mi·nate, ag·mi·nat·ed (ag′mi-nāt, ag′mi-nā-ted). SYN aggregated. [L. *agmen,* a multitude]

ag·na·thia (ăg-nā′thē-ă). Congenital absence of the lower jaw, usually accompanied by approximation of the ears. SEE ALSO otocephaly, synotia. [G. *a-* priv. + *gnathos,* jaw]

ag·na·thous (ăg′nā-thŭs). Relating to agnathia.

ag·nea (ag-nē′ă). SYN agnosia. [G. *agnoia,* want of perception]

ag·no·gen·ic (ag-nō-jen′ik). SYN idiopathic. [G. *a-* priv. + *gnosis,* knowledge, + *genesis,* origin]

ag·no·sia (ag-nō′zē-ă). Impairment of ability to recognize, or comprehend the meaning of, various sensory stimuli, not attributable to disorders of the primary receptors or general intellect; a.'s are receptive defects caused by lesions in various portions of the cerebrum. SYN agnea. [G. ignorance; from *a-* priv. + *gnōsis,* knowledge]

auditory a., inability to recognize sounds, words, or music; caused by a lesion of the auditory cortex of the temporal lobe.

color a., inability to name or identify specific colors by sight; caused by lesions of the dominant occipital and temporal lobes.

finger a., inability to name or recognize individual fingers, of one's own or of other persons; most often caused by lesion of or near the angular gyrus of the dominant hemisphere.

gustatory a., inability to classify or identify a tastant, even though the ability to distinguish between or recognize tastants may be normal; may be general, partial, or specific.

localization a., inability to recognize the area where the skin is touched.

olfactory a., inability to classify or identify an odorant, although the ability to distinguish between or recognize odorants may be normal; may be general, partial, or specific.

optic a., SYN visual a.

position a., failure to recognize the posture of an extremity.

tactile a., inability to recognize objects by touch, in the presence of intact cutaneous and proprioceptive hand sensation; caused by a lesion in the contralateral parietal lobe. SYN astereognosis, stereoagnosis, stereoanesthesia.

visual a., inability to recognize objects by sight; usually caused by bilateral parieto-occipital lesions. SYN optic a.

visual-spatial a., inability to localize objects or to appreciate distance, motion, and spatial relationships; caused by lesion in the occipital lobe. Cf. simultanagnosia.

△**-agogue, -agog.** Leading, promoting, stimulating; a promoter or stimulant of. [G. *agōgos,* leading forth, fr. *agō,* to lead]

agom·phi·ous (ă-gom′-fē-us). SYN anodontia.

agom·pho·sis, agom·phi·a·sis (ag-om-fō′sis, fī′ă-sis). SYN anodontia. [G. *a-* priv. + *gomphos,* peg, bolt]

ago·nad·al (ā-gon′ă-dăl). Denoting the absence of gonads.

ag·o·nal (ag′on-ăl). Relating to the process of dying or the moment of death, so called because of the former erroneous notion that dying is a painful process.

ag·o·nist (ag′on-ist). **1.** Denoting a muscle in a state of contraction, with reference to its opposing muscle, or antagonist. **2.** A drug capable of combining with receptors to initiate drug actions; it possesses affinity and intrinsic activity. [G. *agōn,* a contest]

ag·o·ny (ag′ŏ-nē). Intense pain or anguish of body or mind. [G. *agōn,* a struggle, trial]

ag·o·ra·pho·bia (ag′ŏr-ă-fō′bē-ă). A mental disorder characterized by an irrational fear of leaving the familiar setting of home, or venturing into the open, so pervasive that a large number of external life situations are entered into reluctantly or are avoided; often associated with panic attacks. [G. *agora,* marketplace, + *phobos,* fear]

agor·a·pho·bic (ă-gōr-ă-fō′bik). Relating to or characteristic of agoraphobia.

agou·ti (ah-gu′tē). SYN *Dasyprocta.* [Fr., fr. native Indian]

△**-agra.** Sudden onslaught of acute pain. [G. *agra,* a hunting, a catching, a trap]

agraffe (ă-graf′). An appliance for clamping together the edges of a wound, used in lieu of sutures. [Fr. *agrafe,* a hook, clasp]

ag·ram·mat·i·ca (ag-ră-mat′i-kă). SYN agrammatism.

agram·ma·tism (ā-gram′a-tizm). A form of aphasia characterized by an inability to construct a grammatical sentence, and the use of unintelligible or incorrect words; caused by a lesion in the dominant temporal lobe. SYN agrammatica, agrammatologia, jargon aphasia.

agram·ma·to·lo·gia (ă-gram′mă-tō-lō′jē-ă). SYN agrammatism.

agran·u·lo·cyte (ă-gran′ū-lō-sīt). A nongranular leukocyte. [G. *a-* priv. + L. *granulum,* granule, + G. *kytos,* cell]

agran·u·lo·cy·to·sis (ă-gran′ū-lō-sī-tō′sis). An acute condition characterized by pronounced leukopenia with great reduction in the number of polymorphonuclear leukocytes (frequently less than 500 granulocytes/mm^3); infected ulcers are likely to develop in the throat, intestinal tract, and other mucous membranes, as well as in the skin. SYN agranulocytic angina, angina lymphomatosa, neutropenic angina.

agran·u·lo·plas·tic (ă-gran′ū-lō-plas′tik). Capable of forming nongranular cells, and incapable of forming granular cells. [G. *a-* priv. + L. *granulum,* granule, + G. *plastikos,* formative]

agraph·ia (ă-graf′ē-ă). Inability to write properly in the absence of abnormalities of the limb; often accompanies aphasia and alexia; caused by lesions in various portions of the cerebrum, especially those in or near the angular gyrus. SYN graphic aphasia, graphomotor aphasia. [G. *a-* priv. + *graphō,* to write]

absolute a., a. in which not even unconnected letters can be written. SYN atactic a., literal a.

acoustic a., inability to write from dictation.

amnemonic a., a. in which letters and words can be written, but not connected sentences.

atactic a., SYN absolute a.

constructional a., an a. in which letters and words can be written correctly, but not arranged appropriately on the writing surface.

literal a., SYN absolute a.

motor a., a. due to muscular incoordination.

musical a., an inability to write musical notation.

verbal a., a. in which single letters can be written, but not words.

agraph·ic (ă-graf′ik). Relating to or marked by agraphia.

agre·tope (ag-rē′tōp). That part of a processed antigen that binds to the major histocompatibility complex molecule.

ague (ā′goo). **1.** Archaic term for malarial fever. **2.** A chill. [Fr. *aigu,* acute]

brass founder's a., SYN brass founder's *fever.*

AGUS Acronym for atypical glandular *cells* of undetermined significance, under *cell.* SEE ALSO Bethesda *system.*

ag·yi·o·pho·bia (aj′ē-ō-fō′bē-ă). A form of agoraphobia characterized by a morbid fear of being in the street. [G. *agyia,* street, + *phobos,* fear]

agy·ria (ā-jī′rē-ă). Congenital lack or underdevelopment of the convolutional pattern of the cerebral cortex. SYN lissencephalia, lissencephaly. [G. *a-* priv. + *gyros,* circle]

ahaus·tral (ā-hos′trăl). Lacking haustra, smooth; describing the appearance of the colon on radiographs of a barium enema in ulcerative colitis. [G. *a-* priv. + haustra]

AHF Abbreviation for antihemophilic *factor* A.

AHG Abbreviation for antihemophilic *globulin.*

aHyl Symbol for allohydroxylysine.

ahy·log·no·sia (ā-hī-log-nō′sē-ă). Inability to recognize differences of density, weight, and coarseness. [G. *a-* priv. + *hylē,* matter, + *gnōsis,* recognition]

clinical diagnosis of HIV-infected individuals

CD4+ T-cell count	clinical categories*		
	(A)	(B)	(C)
(1) ≥500 / μl	A1	B1	C2
(2) 200—499 / μl	A2	B2	C2
(3) <200 / μl	A3	B3	C3

category A

asymptomatic: no symptoms at the time of HIV infection

acute infection: mononucleosis-like illness lasting a few weeks at the time of infection

persistent generalized lymphadenopathy: lymph node enlargement persisting for 3 or more months with no evidence of infection

category B

bacillary angiomatosis

candidiasis, oropharyngeal (thrush)

candidiasis, vulvovaginal: persistent, frequent, or poorly responsive to therapy

cervical dysplasia (moderate or severe)/cervical carcinoma in situ

constitutional symptoms such as fever or diarrhea lasting ≥ 1 month

hairy leukoplakia, oral

herpes zoster (shingles) involving at least two distinct episodes or more than one dermatome

idiopathic thrombocytopenic purpura

listeriosis

pelvic inflammatory disease, particularly by tuboovarian abscess

peripheral neuropathy

category C

candidiasis of bronchi, trachea, or lungs

candidiasis, esophageal

cervical cancer (invasive)

coccidioidomycosis, disseminated or extrapulmonary

cryptococcosis, extrapulmonary

cryptosporidiosis, chronic intestinal (> 1 month's duration)

cytomegalovirus disease (other than liver, spleen, or nodes)

cytomegalovirus retinitis (with loss of vision)

encephalopathy, HIV-related

herpes simplex: chronic ulcer(s) (> 1 month's duration) or bronchitis, pneumonitis, or esophagitis

histoplasmosis, disseminated or extrapulmonary

isosporiasis, disseminated or extrapulmonary

Kaposi sarcoma

lymphoma, Burkitt-type

lymphoma, immunoblastic

Mycobacterium avium complex or *M. kansasii*, disseminated or extrapulmonary

Mycobacterium, other species, disseminated or extrapulmonary

Pneumocystis carinii pneumonia

progressive multifocal leukoencephalopathy

Salmonella septicemia (recurrent)

toxoplasmosis of brain

wasting syndrome due to HIV

Aicardi, J. Dennis, 20th century French neurologist. SEE A. *syndrome.*

aich·mo·pho·bia (īk-mō-fō′bē-ă). Morbid fear of being touched by the finger or any slender pointed object. [G. *aichmē,* a point, + *phobos,* fear]

AID Abbreviation for donor of heterologous (artificial) insemination.

programmable hearing aid, multichannel hearing aid that can use more than one level-dependent frequency response strategy.

△**aidoi-, aidoio-.** The genitals; corresponds to L. pudend-. [G. *aidoia,* shameful things, the genitals]

AIDS (ādz). A deficiency of cellular immunity induced by infection with the human immunodeficiency virus (HIV-1) and characterized by opportunistic diseases, including *Pneumocystis carinii* pneumonia, Kaposi sarcoma, oral hairy leukoplakia, cytomegalovirus disease, tuberculosis, *Mycobacterium avium* complex (MAC) disease, candidal esophagitis, cryptosporidiosis, isosporiasis, cryptococcosis, non-Hodgkin lymphoma, progressive multifocal leukoencephalopathy (PML), herpes zoster, and lymphoma. HIV is transmitted from person to person in cell-rich body fluids (notably blood and semen) through sexual contact, sharing of contaminated needles (as by IV drug abusers), or other contact with contaminated blood (as in accidental needle sticks among health care workers). The primary targets of HIV are cells with the CD4 surface protein, including principally helper T lymphocytes. Antibody to HIV, which appears in the serum 6 weeks to 6 months after infection, serves as a reliable diagnostic marker but does not bind or inactivate HIV. Gradual decline in the CD4 lymphocyte count, typically occurring over a period of 10–12 years, culminates in loss of ability to resist opportunistic infections; the appearance of one or more of these defines the onset of AIDS. In some patients, generalized lymphadenopathy, fever, weight loss, dementia, and chronic diarrhea are associated with early stages of the disease. AIDS is uniformly lethal, most patients dying of one or more opportunistic infections or their complications within 2–5 years of the onset of symptoms. In the U.S., AIDS is the leading cause of death among men 25–44, and the fourth leading cause among women in the same age group. During the past 5 years, the mortality of the disease and rates of perinatal transmission have declined substantially, as has transmission among homosexual men and intravenous drug users. Meanwhile heterosexual transmission and case rates among blacks and Hispanics have increased. Some 50 million people are estimated to be infected worldwide, with the highest incidence in some Central and East African countries, where as many as 25% of the adult population may be HIV-positive. Besides prophylaxis against opportunistic infection, standard therapy of HIV infection includes use of nucleoside analogs (didanoxine, lamivudine, ribavirin, stavudine, zidovudine), nonnucleoside reverse transcriptase inhibitors (delavirine, efavirenz, nevirapine), and protease inhibitors (crixivan, indinavir, ritonavir, saquinavir). SEE ALSO human immunodeficiency *virus.* SYN acquired immunodeficiency syndrome. [acronym, *acquired immunodeficiency syndrome*]

The development of effective antiretroviral agents (reverse transcriptase inhibitors and protease inhibitors) and of quantitative plasma HIV RNA assays that can monitor progression of disease and response to treatment has shifted the goal of management in AIDS from prophylaxis and treatment of opportunistic infections to achievement of remission through suppressive therapy. Immune compromise is monitored by serial CD4 counts; viral replication, by plasma HIV RNA assay (viral load). Indications for starting antiretroviral therapy are the appearance of symptoms of opportunistic infection, decline of the CD4 count below 500/mm$_3$, or viral load exceeding 5000 copies/mL. Protease inhibitors have been shown to be highly effective antiretroviral agents, and standard treatment regimens combining 2 reverse transcriptase inhibitors with 1 protease inhibitor ("triple therapy") have clearly demonstrated superiority over monotherapy. However, these drugs are expensive; in 1999 the annual cost of therapy and monitoring exceeded $10,000. Regimens are often complex, with varying requirements for fasting and timing of doses, and adverse effects and drug interactions are common. Protease inhibitors have been associated with elevation of cholesterol and triglycerides, insulin resistance, and disfiguring lipodystrophy. Strains of HIV resistant to all available protease inhibitors have appeared. The rationale for current AIDS regimens is an effort to eradicate HIV infection by inhibiting spread of virus to new cells until all infected cells have died. However, no one has ever been cured of AIDS. A small number of resting CD4 memory cells in treated patients with undetectable plasma HIV RNA levels harbor HIV proviral DNA capable of replication, and these cells may survive for months or years. Macrophages and CNS neurons may serve as an anatomic sanctuary for HIV to which antiretroviral drugs cannot penetrate in adequate concentration. When antiretroviral therapy is initiated early, CD4 helper cell counts rise, CD4 cell activity is preserved, and HIV RNA levels may remain undetectable for long periods. However, in about 50% of patients with advanced disease, even multidrug regimens fail to suppress plasma viral RNA to undetectable levels. Many treatment failures result from poor compliance with multidrug regimens. One-fourth of patients queried admit to allowing themselves occasional "drug holidays." Failure of one therapeutic regimen often precludes success with others because of the high degree of cross-resistance among antiretroviral drugs. After failure of an initial regimen, genotypic testing can be used to identify mutations in the HIV genome that confer resistance to one or more classes of HIV drugs. In a significant number of patients, opportunistic infections continue despite restoration of CD4 counts, probably because some T-cell subpopulations have been annihilated by HIV infection and are not recoverable even after viral suppression. Hence prophylaxis against opportunistic infections remains an essential component of the management of HIV disease. Moreover, even HIV-infected persons with undetectable viral loads must still be considered infectious. Evolving standards of treatment in HIV disease include aggressive therapy of the acute phase of infection and prophylactic administration of antiretroviral therapy after accidental needlestick or sexual assault. Efforts to develop a vaccine against HIV have been hampered by the unique properties of the virus and the long incubation period of AIDS. A bivalent vaccine that elicits antibody to the outer shell protein of HIV is in Phase III trials. Many authorities believe that an effective vaccine must also stimulate cell-mediated immunity.

AIH Abbreviation for homologous (artificial) insemination.

AILD Abbreviation for angioimmunoblastic *lymphadenopathy* with dysproteinemia.

aIle Abbreviation for alloisoleucine.

ai·lu·ro·pho·bia (ī′loo-rō-fō′bē-ă, ā′lu-). Morbid fear of or aversion to cats. [G. *ailouros*, cat, + *phobos*, fear]

ai·nhum (ī′ŭm). An acquired slowly progressive painful fibrous constriction that develops in the digitoplantar fold, usually of the little toe, gradually resulting in spontaneous amputation of the toe; most commonly affects black males in the tropics. [fr. Af. (Lagos), to saw]

AIR Abbreviation for 5-aminoimidazole ribose 5′-phosphate and 5-aminoimidazole ribotide.

air (ār). **1.** A mixture of odorless gases found in the atmosphere in the following approximate percentages by volume after water vapor has been removed: oxygen, 20.95; nitrogen, 78.08; argon 0.93; carbon dioxide, 0.03; other gases, 0.01. Formerly used to mean any respiratory gas, regardless of its composition. **2.** SYN ventilate. [G. *aēr*; L. *aer*]

alveolar a., SYN alveolar *gas*.

complemental a., SYN inspiratory reserve *volume*.

complementary a., SYN inspiratory *capacity*.

functional residual a., SYN functional residual *capacity*.

a. hunger, extremely deep ventilation such as occurs in patients with acidosis attempting to increase ventilation of alveoli and exhale more carbon dioxide. SEE ALSO Kussmaul *respiration*.

liquid a., a. that, by means of intense cold and pressure, has been liquefied.

minimal a., the volume of gas that remains in the lungs and cannot be expelled after they have been removed from the body, or after the chest has been opened.

reserve a., SYN expiratory reserve *volume*.

residual a., SYN residual *volume*.

supplemental a., SYN expiratory reserve *volume*.

tidal a., SYN tidal *volume*.

vitiated a., a. containing a reduced percentage of oxygen.

Aird, Robert B., U.S. neurologist, *1903. SEE Flynn-A. *syndrome*.

air·sick·ness. A condition resembling seasickness or other forms of motion sickness occurring in airplane or space flight as a result of erratic and continuous stimuli of the inner ear.

air·space (ār′spās). Pertaining to the portion of the lung distal to the conducting airways or bronchi; alveolar.

air·trap·ping (ār-trap′ing). Slow or incomplete emptying of gas from all or part of a lung on expiration; implies obstruction of regional airways or emphysema.

air·way (ār′wā). **1.** Any part of the respiratory tract through which air passes during breathing. **2.** In anesthesia or resuscitation, a device for correcting obstruction to breathing, especially an oropharyngeal and nasopharyngeal a., endotracheal a., or tracheotomy tube.

anatomic a., SYN anatomic dead *space*.

conducting a., the a. from the nasal cavity to a terminal bronchiole.

Guedel a., oropharyngeal a. used to ensure airway patency during general anesthesia.

lower a., the portion of the respiratory tract that extends from the subglottis to and including the terminal bronchioles.

neurogenic a., upper-airway obstruction due to abnormal muscle tone in the upper a.; found in patients with severe developmental delay or brain injury, and especially in those with spastic quadriplegia.

respiratory a., that part of the a. where interchange of gases occurs; it includes respiratory bronchioles, alveolar ducts, sacs, and alveoli.

upper a., the portion of the respiratory tract that extends from the nares or mouth to and including the larynx.

Ajel·lo·my·ces cap·su·la·tum (ah-jě-lō-mī′sēz kap-soo-lā′tŭm). The ascomycetous (perfect, sexual, teleomorph) state of *Histoplasma capsulatum*. SYN Emmonsiella capsulata.

Ajel·lo·my·ces der·ma·tit·i·dis (ah-jě-lō-mī′sēz der-mă-tit′i-

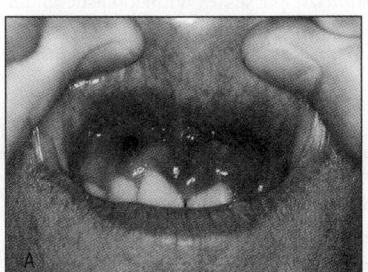
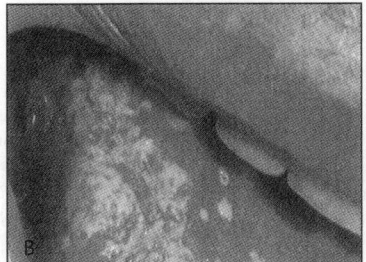
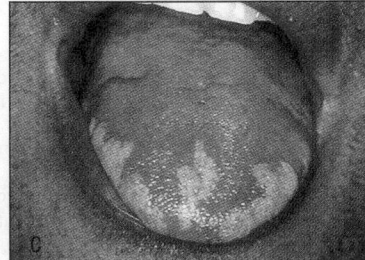

AIDS: oral lesions associated with AIDS: (A) Kaposi's sarcoma, (B) thrush (due to *Candida albicans*), (C) hairy leukoplakia

dis). The perfect (teleomorph) state of the fungus *Blastomyces dermatitidis;* the (+) and (-) mating types cause disease with equal frequency. This sexual state is placed in the family Gymnoascaceae.

aj·ma·line (aj′mă-lēn). An indole alkaloid from the roots of *Rauwolfia serpentina*, related to reserpine, serpentine, and yohimbine; has been used for treatment of hypertension and as a tranquilizer or sedative.

aj·o·wan oil (aj′ō-wan). A volatile oil distilled from the fruit of *Carum copticum*, one of the sources of thymol; a carminative, aromatic, and expectorant. SYN ptychotis oil.

akan·thi·on (ă-kan′thē-on). SYN acanthion.

akar·y·o·cyte (ā-kar′ē-ō-sīt). A cell without a nucleus (karyon), such as the erythrocyte. SYN acaryote, akaryote. [G. *a*- priv. + *karyon*, kernel, + *kytos,* a hollow (cell)]

akar·y·ote (ā-kar′ē-ōt). SYN akaryocyte. [G. *a*- priv. + *karyon*, kernel]

a·ka·thi·sia (ak-ă-thiz′ē-ă). A syndrome characterized by an inability to remain in a sitting posture, with motor restlessness and a feeling of muscular quivering; may appear as a side effect of antipsychotic and neuroleptic medication. SYN acathisia. [G. *a*- priv. + *kathisis,* a sitting]

akem·be (ă-kem′bē). SYN onyalai.

Åkerlund, A. Olof, Swedish radiologist, 1885–1958. SEE A. *deformity*.

aki·ne·sia (ā-ki-nē′sē-ă, ā-kī-). **1.** Absence or loss of the power of voluntary movement, due to an extrapyramidal disorder. **2.** Obsolete term denoting the postsystolic interval of rest of the heart. **3.** A neurosis accompanied by paretic symptoms. SYN akinesis. [G. *a*- priv. + *kinēsis,* movement]

a. al′gera, a condition marked by severe generalized pain produced by any movement; often of psychogenic origin. [G. *algos,* pain]

a. amnes′tica, loss of muscular power from disuse.

aki·ne·sic (ā-ki-nē′sik, ā-kī-). SYN akinetic.

aki·ne·sis (ā-ki-nē′sis, ā-kī-). SYN akinesia.

akin·es·the·sia (ā-kin′es-thē′zē-ă). Inability to perceive movement or position. Absence of the sense of perception of movement or of the muscular sense. [G. *a*- priv. + *kinēsis,* motion, + *aisthēsis,* sensation]

aki·net·ic (ā-ki-net′ik, -kī-net′ik). Relating to or suffering from akinesia. SYN akinesic.

aki·ya·mi (ah-kē-yah′mē). SYN hasamiyami.

ak·lo·mide (ak′lō-mīd). A coccidiostat used in veterinary practice.

ak·ne·mia. SEE acnemia.

AKNF Abbreviation for Adair-Koshland-Némethy-Filmer *model*.

Al Symbol for aluminum.

ALA Abbreviation for δ-aminolevulinic acid.

Ala Symbol for alanine or its mono- or diradical.

ala, gen. and pl. **alae** (ā′lă, ā′lē). **1** [TA]. SYN wing. **2.** Pronounced, longitudinal cuticular ridges in nematodes, usually found in larval stages (*Ascaris lumbricoides*), although occasionally present in adult worm (*Enterobius vermicularis*). [L. wing]

a. au′ris, SYN auricle (1).

a. cerebel′li, SYN *wing* of central lobule.

a. cine′rea, SYN vagal (nerve) *trigone*.

a. cris′tae gal′li [TA], SYN a. of crista galli.

a. of crista galli [TA], a small lateral expansion of the ethmoid bone from the front of the crista galli on each side that articulates with the frontal bone and forms the foramen cecum. SYN a. cristae galli [TA], alar process, wing of crista galli.

a. of ilium [TA], the upper flaring portion of the ilium. SYN a. ossis ilii [TA], wing of ilium✩.

alae lin′gulae cerebel′li, SYN *lingula* of cerebellum.

a. lob′ulis centra′lis [TA], SYN *wing* of central lobule.

a. ma′jor os′sis sphenoida′lis [TA], SYN greater *wing* of sphenoid (bone).

a. mi′nor os′sis sphenoida′lis [TA], SYN lesser *wing* of sphenoid (bone).

a. na′si [TA], SYN a. of nose.

a. of nose [TA], the outer, more or less flaring, wall of each nostril. SYN a. nasi [TA], pinna nasi, wing of nose.

a. orbitalis, SYN lesser *wing* of sphenoid (bone).

a. os′sis il′ii [TA], SYN a. of ilium.

a. sacra′lis [TA], SYN a. of sacrum.

a. of sacrum [TA], the upper surface of the lateral part of the sacrum adjacent to the body. SYN a. sacralis [TA], wing of sacrum✩.

a. tempora′lis, SYN greater *wing* of sphenoid (bone).

a. of vomer [TA], an everted lip on either side of the upper border of the vomer, between which fits the rostrum of the sphenoid bone. SYN a. vomeris [TA], wing of vomer.

a. vo′meris [TA], SYN a. of vomer.

alacrima (ā-lak′rē-ma). Deficiency of tear secretion. [G. *a*- priv. + L. *lacrima,* tear]

Alagille, Daniel, French physician, *1925. SEE Alagille *syndrome*.

Alajouanine, Théophile, French neurologist, 1890–1980. SEE Foix-Alajouanine *myelitis;* Foix-Alajouanine *syndrome*.

ala·lia (ă-la′lē-ă). Mutism; inability to speak. SEE aphonia. [G. *a*- priv. + *lalia,* talking]

alal·ic (ă-lal′ik). Relating to alalia.

al·a·nine (A, Ala) (al′ă-nēn). 2-Aminopropionic acid; α-amino-propionic acid; the L-stereoisomer is one of the amino acids widely occurring in proteins.

β-al·a·nine. 3-Aminopropionic acid or β-aminopropionic acid; a decarboxylation production of aspartic acid. Found in brain, in carnosine, and in coenzyme A.

al·a·nine ami·no·trans·fer·ase (ALT). An enzyme transferring amino groups from L-alanine to 2-ketoglutarate, or the reverse (from L-glutamate to pyruvate); there is a D-alanine transaminase that effects the same reaction, but using D-alanine and D-glutamate. Serum concentration is increased in viral hepatitis and myocardial infarction. SYN alanine transaminase, glutamic-pyruvic transaminase, serum glutamic-pyruvic transaminase.

al·a·nine-gly·ox·y·late ami·no·trans·fer·ase. An enzyme that reversibly catalyzes the transfer of an amino group of L-alanine to glyoxylate, thus producing pyruvate and glycine. An inherited disorder that results in an alteration of a.-g. a. activity is associated with primary hyperoxaluria type I.

al·a·nine-ox·o·mal·o·nate ami·no·trans·fer·ase. An enzyme that accomplishes the reversible transfer of the amino groups from L-alanine to oxomalonate, an action similar to that of alanine aminotransferase, producing pyruvate and aminomalonate.

β-ala·nine-py·ru·vate ami·no·trans·fer·ase. An enzyme that reversibly transfers the amino group of β-alanine to pyruvate, thus producing L-alanine and malonate semialdehyde. A deficiency of this enzyme is believed to be the cause of hyper-β-alaninemia.

al·a·nine rac·e·mase. An enzyme, requiring pyridoxal phosphate as coenzyme, that catalyzes the reversible racemization of L-alanine to D-alanine; found in various microorganisms, where it plays a role in the biosynthesis of the D-amino acids present in the capsular proteins.

al·a·nine trans·am·i·nase. SYN alanine aminotransferase.

alan·o·sine (ă-lan′ō-sēn). An antibiotic substance produced by *Streptomyces alanosinicus;* possesses antineoplastic and antiviral activity.

Alanson, Edward, British surgeon, 1747–1823. SEE A. *amputation*.

alan·tin (ă-lan′tin). SYN inulin.

al·an·tol (al′an-tol). A yellowish liquid obtained by distillation from the root of *Inula helenium* or elecampane; used internally as an irritating tonic and externally as a mild rubefacient. SYN inulol.

al·ant starch (ă-lant′). SYN inulin.

al·a·nyl (al′ă-nil). The acyl radical of alanine.

alar (ā′lăr). **1.** Relating to a wing; winged. **2.** SYN axillary. **3.** Relating to the wings (ala) of such structures as the nose, sphenoid, sacrum, etc.

ALARA. Acronym for a philosophy of use of radiation based on using dosages *as low as reasonably achievable* to attain the desired diagnostic, therapeutic, or other goal.

alar·mone (ă-lar′mōn). A biochemical whose synthesis increases under certain stress conditions (for example, a nutritional deficiency affecting certain enzymes). [*alar*m + *-mone*]

alas·trim (ă-las′trim). A mild form of smallpox caused by a less virulent strain of the virus. SYN Cuban itch, Kaffir pox, milkpox, pseudosmallpox, pseudovariola, variola minor, West Indian smallpox, whitepox. [Pg. *alastrar,* to scatter over]

al·ba (al′bă). SYN white *matter.* [fem. of L. *albus,* white]

Albarran y Dominguez, Joaquin, Cuban urologist, 1860–1912. SEE Albarran *glands,* under *gland;* Albarran *test;* A. *tubules,* under *tubule.*

al·be·do (al-bē′dō). A white area of the retina due to edema or infarction. [L. whiteness]

Albers-Schönberg, Heinrich E., German radiologist, 1865–1921. SEE Albers-Schönberg *disease.*

Albert, Eduard, Austrian surgeon, 1841–1900. SEE A. *suture.*

Albert, Henry, U.S. physician, 1878–1930. SEE A. *stain.*

al·bi·cans, pl. **al·bi·can·tia** (al′bi-kanz, -kan′tē-ă). **1.** SYN white. **2.** SYN *corpus* albicans. [L.]

al·bi·du·ria (al-bi-doo′rē-ă). The passing of pale or white urine of low specific gravity, as in chyluria. SYN albinuria. [L. *albidus,* whitish, + G. *ouron,* urine]

al·bi·dus (al′bi-dŭs). White, whitish. [L.]

Albini, Giuseppe, Italian physiologist, 1827–1911. SEE A. *nodules,* under *nodule.*

al·bi·nism (al′bi-nizm). A group of inherited (usually autosomal recessive) disorders with deficiency or absence of pigment in the skin, hair, and eyes, or eyes only, due to an abnormality in production of melanin. SEE ocular a., piebaldism. [albino + ism]

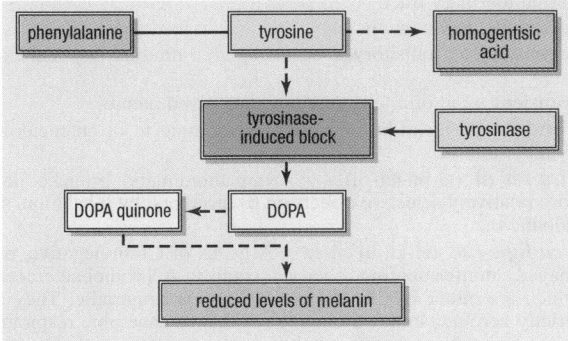

albinism: chart showing effects of tyrosinase on melanin production

Åland Island a., SYN ocular a. 2.

cutaneous a. [MIM*126070], SYN piebaldism.

Forsius-Eriksson a., SYN ocular a. 2.

Nettleshop-Falls a., SYN ocular a. 1.

ocular a. [MIM*300650 & *300700], absence of pigment chiefly in the iris, choroid, and retinal epithelium.

ocular a. 1 [MIM*300500], type of ocular a. characterized by depigmentation of the fundus and prominent choroidal vessels, nystagmus, and titubation; vision is usually impaired; caused by mutation in the OA1 gene on chromosome Xp; X-linked inheritance. SYN Nettleshop-Falls a.

ocular a. 2 [MIM*300600], type of ocular a. characterized by hypoplasia of the fovea, marked impairment of vision, nystagmus, myopia, astigmatism, and protanomalous color blindness, in addition to a. of the fundus. SYN Åland Island a., Forsius-Eriksson a.

ocular a. 3 [MIM*203310], type of ocular a. characterized by impaired vision, translucent irides, congenital nystagmus, photophobia, albinotic fundi with hyperplasia of the fovea, and strabismus; caused by mutation in the pinkeye gene (P) on 6q; autosomal recessive inheritance.

ocular a. with late-onset sensorineural deafness [MIM* 300650], x-linked inheritance.

ocular a. with sensorineural deafness [MIM*103470], Waardenburg *syndrome,* type II.. SEE Waardenburg *syndrome.*

oculocutaneous a., a disorder characterized by deficiency of pigment in skin, hair, and eyes, photophobia, nystagmus, and decreased visual acuity; there are two groups: tyrosinase-negative [MIM*203100] in which there is absence of tyrosinase, and tyrosinase-positive [MIM*203200] in which normal tyrosinase cannot enter pigment cells; the compound heterozygote is normal so the two forms are not allelic. There are several forms of autosomal recessive inheritance: type IA is characterized by absence of tyrosinase with life-long complete absence of melanin, marked photophobia, and nystagmus, caused by mutation in the tyrosinase gene (TYR) on chromosome 11q. Type II has normal tyrosinase activity and is the most common; hair darkens and nevi and freckles develop; caused by mutation in the oculocutaneous abinism gene (OCA2) on 15q. Type III is characterized by absent tyrosinase but pigmentation of the iris in the first decade; caused by mutation in the tyrosine-related protein-1gene (TYRP1) on 9p. Type IV is found in Africans with normal tyrosinase and type V is associated with red hair. Type VI is synonymous to Hermansky-Pudlak syndrome [MIM*203300], with low to absent tyrosinase and hemorrhage due to platelet deficiency, caused by mutation in the Hermansky-Pudlak gene (HPS) on 10q.

rufous a., SYN xanthism.

al·bi·no (al-bī′nō). An individual with albinism. [Pg., little white one, fr. *albo,* white, fr. L. *albus* + *-ino,* dim. suffix]

al·bi·not·ic (al-bi-not′ik). Pertaining to albinism.

al·bi·nu·ria (al-bi-noo′rē-ă). SYN albiduria.

Albinus (Weiss), Bernhard S., German anatomist and surgeon, 1697–1770. SEE A. *muscle.*

al·bo·ci·ne·re·ous (al-bō-si-nē′rē-ŭs). Relating to both the white and the gray matter of the brain or spinal cord. [L. *albus,* white, + *cinereus,* ashen, fr. *cinis* (*ciner-*), ashes]

Albrecht, Karl M.P., German anatomist, 1851–1894. SEE A. *bone.*

Albright, Fuller, U.S. physician, 1900–1969. SEE A. *disease, syndrome,* hereditary *osteodystrophy;* Forbes-A. *syndrome;* Mc-Cune-A. *syndrome.*

al·bu·gin·ea (al-bū-jin′ē-ă). A white fibrous tissue layer, such as the tunica albuginea. SEE *tunica* albuginea, *tunica* albuginea of corpus spongiosum, *tunica* albuginea of corpora cavernosa, *tunica* albuginea oculi, *tunica* albuginea of testis. [L. *albugineus,* fr. *albugo,* white spot]

al·bu·gin·e·ot·o·my (al-bū-jin-ē-ot′ō-mē). Incision into any tunica albuginea. [albuginea + G. *tomē,* cutting]

al·bu·gin·e·ous (al-bū-jin′ē-ŭs). **1.** Resembling boiled white of egg. **2.** Relating to any tunica albuginea. [L. *albugineus,* fr. *albugo,* white spot]

al·bu·men (al-bū′men). SYN ovalbumin. [see albumin]

al·bu·min (al-bū′min). A type of simple protein, varieties of which are widely distributed throughout the tissues and fluids of plants and animals; a. is soluble in pure water, precipitable from solution by strong acids, and coagulable by heat in acid or neutral solution. [L. *albumen* (*-min-*), the white of egg]

a. A, the normal or common type of human serum a.

acetosoluble a., SYN Patein a.

a. B, SEE inherited albumin *variants,* under *variant.*

Bence Jones a., SEE Bence Jones *proteins,* under *protein.*

blood a., SYN serum a.

bovine serum a. (BSA), a source of a. commonly used in in vitro biologic studies.

dried human a., SYN normal human serum a.

egg a., SYN ovalbumin.

a. Ghent, SEE inherited albumin *variants,* under *variant.*

iodinated ^{131}**I human serum a.,** a sterile, buffered, isotonic solution prepared to contain not less than 10 mg of radioiodinated normal human serum a. per ml, and adjusted to provide not more than 1 mCi of radioactivity per ml; used as a diagnostic aid in the measurement of blood volume and cardiac output.

iodinated ^{125}**I serum a.,** a sterile, buffered, isotonic solution prepared to contain not less than 10 mg of radioiodinated normal human serum albumin per ml, and adjusted to provide not more than 1 mCi of radioactivity per ml; used as a diagnostic aid in determining blood volume and cardiac output. SYN radioiodinated serum a.

macroaggregated a. (MAA), conglomerates of human serum a. in a suspension; usually refers to particles 10 to 50 μm in size; used as a tagged agent for lung scintigraphy.

a. Mexico, SEE inherited albumin *variants,* under *variant.*

a. Naskapi, SEE inherited albumin *variants,* under *variant.*

native a., a. existing in its natural state, the two principal forms being serum a. and egg a.; it is soluble in water and not precipitated by diluted acids.

normal human serum a., a sterile preparation of serum a. obtained by fractionating blood plasma proteins from healthy persons; used as a transfusion material and to treat edema due to hypoproteinemia. SYN dried human a.

Patein a., a substance resembling serum a., but soluble in acetic acid. SYN acetosoluble a.

plasma a., SYN serum a.

radioiodinated serum a. (RISA), SYN iodinated ^{125}I serum a.

a. Reading, SEE inherited albumin *variants,* under *variant.*

serum a., the principal protein in plasma, present in blood plasma and in serous fluids. Participates in fatty acid transport and helps regulate the osmotic pressure of blood. It will also bind hormones, bilirubin, and drugs. SYN blood a., plasma a., seralbumin.

a. tannate, an astringent powder obtained by the action of tannic acid on a.; contains about 50% tannic acid; used as an astringent disinfectant in diarrhea and as a dusting powder.

al·bu·min·ate (al-bū′min-āt). The product of the reaction between native albumin and dilute acids or dilute bases, thereby resulting in acid a.'s or alkali a.'s; both types are characterized by solubility in dilute acid or alkali, and relative insolubility in water, dilute solutions of salts, and alcohol.

al·bu·mi·na·tu·ria (al-bū′mi-nă-too′rē-ă). The presence of an abnormally large quantity of albuminates in the urine when voided. [albuminate + G. *ouron,* urine]

al·bu·min·if·er·ous (al-bū-min-if′er-ŭs). Producing albumin. [albumin + L. *fero,* to bear]

al·bu·min·ip·ar·ous (al-bū-min-ip′ăr-ŭs). Forming albumin. [albumin + L. *pario,* to bring forth]

al·bu·min·og·e·nous (al-bū-min-oj′en-ŭs). Producing or forming albumin.

al·bu·mi·noid (al-bū′min-oyd). **1.** Resembling albumin. **2.** Any protein. **3.** A simple type of protein, insoluble in neutral solvents, present in horny and cartilaginous tissues and in the lens of the eye; e.g., keratin, elastin, collagen. SYN glutinoid, scleroprotein.

al·bu·mi·nol·y·sis (al-bū-min-ol′i-sis). Proteolysis; often, specifically the proteolysis of albumins. [albumin + G. *lysis,* dissolution]

al·bu·mi·nop·ty·sis (al-bū-mi-nop′ti-sis). Albuminous expectoration. [albumin + G. *ptysis,* a spitting]

al·bu·mi·nor·rhea (al-bū-min-ō-rē′ă). SYN albuminuria. [albumin + G. *rhoia,* a flow]

al·bu·min·ous (al-bū′min-ŭs). Relating to, containing, or consisting of albumin.

al·bu·min·ur·ia (al-bū-mi-noo′rē-ă). Presence of protein in urine, chiefly albumin but also globulin; usually indicative of disease, but sometimes resulting from a temporary or transient dysfunction. SYN albuminorrhea, proteinuria (2). [albumin + G. *ouron,* urine]

adolescent a., functional a. occurring at about the time of puberty; it is usually cyclic or orthostatic a.

adventitious a., a. resulting from the presence of blood escaping somewhere in the urinary tract, of chyle, or of some other albuminous fluid, not caused by filtration of albumin from the blood through the kidneys. SYN false a.

a. of athletes, a form of functional a. following excessive muscular exertion.

Bamberger a., obsolete term for hematogenous a. that is sometimes observed during the later phases of advanced anemia.

benign a., a collective term for types that are not the result of pathologic changes in the kidneys. SYN essential a.

cardiac a., a. caused by congestive heart failure.

colliquative a., an a. that is at first slight in degree, but unexpectedly becomes greatly increased during convalescence from highly febrile disease, e.g., typhoid fever.

cyclic a., a functional a. sometimes observed intermittently in cycles of 12–36 hours' duration, chiefly in younger persons; the degree of a. is usually slight. SYN recurrent a.

dietetic a., the excretion of protein in the urine following the ingestion of certain foods.

essential a., SYN benign a.

false a., SYN adventitious a.

febrile a., a. associated with fever.

functional a., a collective term denoting types of benign a. that are associated with physical exertion or other conditions in which there are physiologic changes such as during pregnancy or adolescence. SYN physiologic a. (2).

intermittent a., functional a. occurring at intervals, such as cyclic a. or a. of athletes.

lordotic a., so-called on the theory that the a. results from pressure due to lordosis in the lumbar spine.

neuropathic a., a. associated with epilepsy or other convulsive disorders, trauma to the brain, and cerebral hemorrhage.

orthostatic a., the appearance of albumin in the urine when the patient is erect and its disappearance when recumbent. SYN orthostatic proteinuria, postural proteinuria, postural a.

physiologic a., (1) presence of slight traces of protein in otherwise normal urine; **(2)** SYN functional a.

postrenal a., a. caused by disease distal to the kidney.

postural a., SYN orthostatic a.

prerenal a., a. caused by disease other than disease of the kidney or genitourinary tract.

recurrent a., SYN cyclic a.

regulatory a., transitory a. occurring after unusual physical exertion.

transient a., a. of a temporary or short-lived nature.

al·bu·min·ur·ic (al-bū-mi-noo′rik). Relating to or characterized by albuminuria.

al·bu·ter·ol (al-bū′ter-ol). A sympathomimetic bronchodilator with relatively selective effects on β_2 receptors, by inhalation. SYN salbutamol.

Al·ca·lig·e·nes (al-kā-lij′en-ēz). A genus of Gram-negative, rod-shaped, nonfermenting bacteria (family Achromobacteraceae) which are either motile and peritrichous or nonmotile. They are strictly aerobic; some strains are capable of anaerobic respiration in the presence of nitrate or nitrite; their metabolism is respiratory, never fermentative; they do not use carbohydrates. Found mostly in the intestinal canal, decaying materials, dairy products, water, and soil; they can be isolated from human respiratory and gastrointestinal tracts and wounds in hospitalized patients with compromised immune systems; occasionally the cause of opportunistic infections, including nosocomial septicemia. Type species is *A. faecalis.* [alkali + G. *-gen,* producing]

al·cap·ton (al-kap′tŏn). SYN homogentisic acid.

al·cap·ton·u·ria, al·kap·ton·u·ria (al-kap-tō-noo′rē-ă) [MIM* 203500]. Excretion of homogentisic acid (alkapton) in the urine due to congenital lack of the enzyme homogentisate 1,2-dioxygenase, which mediates an essential step in the catabolism of phenylalanine and tyrosine; urine turns dark if allowed to stand or is alkalinized (a result of formation of polymerization products of homogentisic acid); frequently occurs throughout relatively long periods or may recur and subside at irregular intervals; arthritis and ochronosis are late complications; autosomal recessive inheritance; caused by mutation in the homogentisate 1,2-dioxygenase gene (HGD) on chromosome 3q. [alkapton + G. *ouron,* urine]

al·cap·ton·ur·ic, al·kap·to·nur·ic (al-kap-tō-noo-rik;). **1.** Relating to alcaptonuria. **2.** A person with alcaptonuria.

Al·ci·an blue (al′sē-an) [C.I. 74240]. A complex phthalocyanin dye used as a stain to distinguish sulfomucins from sialomucins and uronic acid mucins, to demonstrate sulfated polysaccharides, and to detect glycoproteins in electrophoresis; often used in combination with PAS or aldehyde fuchsin.

al·clo·fe·nac (al-klō'fĕ-nak). An anti-inflammatory agent.

al·clo·met·a·sone (al-klō-met'ă-sōn). A potent corticosteroid used as the 17,21-dipropionate in topical therapy for psoriasis and other deep-seated dermatoses.

Alcock, Benjamin, Irish anatomist, 1801–?. SEE A. *canal.*

al·co·gel (al'kō-jel). A hydrogel, with alcohol instead of water as the dispersion medium.

al·co·hol (al'kō-hol). **1.** One of a series of organic chemical compounds in which a hydrogen (H) attached to carbon is replaced by a hydroxyl (OH); a.'s react with acids to form esters and with alkali metals to form alcoholates. For individual a.'s not listed here, see specific name. **2.** CH_3CH_2OH; made from sugar, starch, and other carbohydrates by fermentation with yeast, and synthetically from ethylene or acetylene. It has been used in beverages and as a solvent, vehicle, and preservative; medicinally, it is used externally as a rubefacient, coolant, and disinfectant, and has been used internally as an analgesic, stomachic, sedative, and antipyretic. SYN ethanol, ethyl alcohol, grain a., rectified spirit, wine spirit. **3.** The azeotropic mixture of CH_3CH_2OH and water (92.3% by weight of ethanol at 15.56°C). [Ar. *al,* the, + *kohl,* fine antimonial powder, the term being applied first to a fine powder, then to anything impalpable (spirit)]

absolute a., (1) 100% a., water having been removed; SYN anhydrous a. **(2)** a. with a minimum admixture of water, at most 1%. SYN dehydrated a.

acid a., ethyl a. (70%) containing 1% hydrochloric acid.

anhydrous a., SYN absolute a. (1).

bile a., one of a group of polyhydroxylated a.'s derived from cholestane.

dehydrated a., SYN absolute a. (2).

denatured a., ethyl a. rendered unfit for consumption as a beverage by the addition of one or several chemicals for commercial purposes (e.g., methanol, aldehol, sucrose octa-acetate). SYN industrial methylated spirit, methylated spirit.

dihydric a., a. containing two OH groups in its molecule; e.g., ethylene glycol.

dilute a., an a. in water mixtures of various concentrations, e.g., 90, 80, 70, 60, 50, 45, 25, and 20% v/v of C_2H_5OH.

fatty a., a long chain a., analogous to the fatty acids, of which the fatty a. may be viewed as a reduction product; e.g., octadecanol from stearic acid. It is often found esterified in waxes. SYN wax a.

grain a., SYN alcohol (2).

methyl a., CH_3OH; a flammable, toxic, mobile liquid, used as an industrial solvent, antifreeze, and in chemical manufacture; ingestion may result in severe acidosis, visual impairment, and other effects on the central nervous system. SYN carbinol, methanol, pyroligneous a., pyroligneous spirit, pyroxylic spirit, wood alcohol, wood naphtha, wood spirit.

monohydric a., an a. containing one OH group.

multiple a., an a. containing more than one OH group.

polyoxyethylene a.'s, used as emulsifying and wetting agents, antistats, solubilizers, defoamers, and other industrial applications. Laureth 9 as spermaticide; pharmaceutic aid (surfactant).

primary a., an a. characterized by the univalent radical, –CH_2OH.

pyroligneous a., SYN methyl a.

rubbing a., an alcoholic mixture intended for external use; it usually contains 70% by volume of absolute a. or isopropyl a.; the remainder consists of water, denaturants (with and without coal tar colors), and perfume oils; used as a rubefacient for muscle and joint aches and pains.

secondary a., an a. characterized by the bivalent atom group,

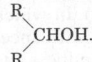

sugar a., SEE sugar alcohol.

tertiary a., an a. characterized by the trivalent atom group,

$$R$$
$$|$$
$$R—COH.$$
$$|$$
$$R$$

trihydric a., an a. containing three OH groups; e.g., glycerol.

unsaturated a.'s, those a.'s whose carbon chains contain one or more double or triple bonds.

wax a., SYN fatty a.

al·co·hol ac·ids. A group of compounds that contain both the carboxyl and hydroxy radicals; e.g., glycolic acid.

al·co·hol·ate (al-kō-hol'āt). **1.** A tincture or other preparation containing alcohol. **2.** A chemical compound in which the hydrogen in the OH group of an alcohol is replaced by an alkali metal; e.g., sodium methylate, CH_3ONa.

al·co·hol de·hy·dro·gen·ase (ADH). An oxidoreductase that reversibly converts an alcohol to an aldehyde (or ketone) with NAD^+ as the H acceptor. For example, ethanol + NAD^+ ↔ acetaldehyde + NADH. SEE ALSO alcohol dehydrogenase (acceptor), alcohol dehydrogenase ($NADP^+$).

al·co·hol de·hy·dro·gen·ase (ac·cep·tor). An oxidoreductase that reversibly converts primary alcohols to aldehydes with an H acceptor other than $NADP^+$.

al·co·hol de·hy·dro·gen·ase ($NADP^+$). An oxidoreductase reversibly converting alcohols to aldehydes (or ketones) with $NAD(P)^+$ as H acceptor. SYN aldehyde reductase.

al·co·hol·ic (al-kō-hol'ik). **1.** Relating to, containing, or produced by alcohol. **2.** One who suffers from alcoholism. **3.** One who abuses or is dependent upon alcohol.

al·co·hol·ism (al'kō-hol-izm). Chronic alcohol abuse, dependence, or addiction; chronic excessive drinking of alcoholic beverages resulting in impairment of health and/or social or occupational functioning, and increasing adaptation to the effects of alcohol requiring increasing doses to achieve and sustain a desired effect; specific signs and symptoms of withdrawal usually are shown upon sudden cessation of such drinking. SYN alcohol addiction.

acute a., a temporary deterioration in mental function, accompanied by muscular incoordination and paresis, induced by the rapid ingestion of alcoholic beverages. SYN intoxication (2).

chronic a., a pathologic condition, affecting chiefly the nervous and gastroenteric systems, associated with impairment in social and occupational functioning, caused by the habitual use of alcoholic beverages in toxic amounts.

al·co·hol·i·za·tion (al'kō-hol-i-zā'shŭn). Permeation or saturation with alcohol.

al·co·hol·o·pho·bia (al'kō-hol-ō-fō'bē-ă). Morbid fear of alcohol, or of becoming an alcoholic. [alcohol + G. *phobos,* fear]

al·co·hol·y·sis (al-kō-hol'i-sis). Splitting of a chemical bond with the addition of the elements of alcohol at the point of splitting. [alcohol + G. *lysis,* dissolution]

al·cur·o·ni·um chlo·ride (al-kūr-ō'nē-ŭm). A skeletal muscle relaxant active as a nondepolarizing neuromuscular blocking agent, resembling curare.

ALD Abbreviation for adrenoleukodystrophy.

al·da·di·ene (al-dă-dī'ēn). A metabolite of spironolactone that contains double bonds between C-4 and C-5 and between C-6 and C-7; formed upon removal of the 7α-acetylthiol side chain from spironolactone and as potent a diuretic as the parent compound.

al·dar·ic ac·id (al'dar-ik). One of a group of sugar acids characterized by the formula HOOC–$(CHOH)_n$–COOH; e.g., saccharic acid.

al·de·hol (al'dĕ-hol). An oxidation product of kerosene; used for denaturing ethyl alcohol.

al·de·hyde (al'dĕ-hīd). A compound containing the radical –CH= O, reducible to an alcohol (CH_2OH), oxidizable to a carboxylic acid (COOH); e.g., acetaldehyde.

activated glycol aldehyde, 2-(1,2-dihydroxyethyl)thiamin pyrophosphate; an intermediate in carbohydrate metabolism and in transketolization.

active a., any aldehyde derivative of thiamin pyrophosphate.

angular a., the a. group attached to carbon 13 (between rings C and D) of the steroid nucleus in aldosterone.

a. reductase, SYN alcohol dehydrogenase (NADP⁺).

al·de·hyde de·hy·dro·gen·ase (ac·yl·at·ing). An oxidoreductase converting an aldehyde and CoA to acyl-CoA with NAD⁺ as H acceptor.

al·de·hyde de·hy·dro·gen·ase (NAD⁺). An oxidoreductase reversibly converting aldehydes to acids with NADP⁺ as H acceptor.

al·de·hyde de·hy·dro·gen·ase (NAD(P)⁺). An oxidoreductase reversibly converting aldehydes to acids with NAD⁺ or NADP⁺ as H acceptor.

al·de·hyde-ly·as·es [EC 4.1.2.x]. Enzymes catalyzing the reversal of an aldol condensation.

Alder, Albert von. SEE A. *anomaly, bodies,* under *body.*

al·dim·ine (al′dĕ-mēn). SYN Schiff *base.*

al·di·tol (al′di-tol). The polyalcohol derived by reduction of an aldose; e.g., sorbitol. SEE ALSO *aldose* reductase.

al·do·bi·u·ron·ic ac·id (al′dō-bī-ū-ron′ik). Condensation products of an aldose and a uronic acid; such groupings occur among the components of various mucopolysaccharides, notably hyaluronic acid.

al·do·cor·tin (al′dō-kōr′tin). SYN aldosterone.

al·do·hex·ose (al-dō-heks′ōs). A 6-carbon sugar characterized by the (potential) presence of an aldehyde group in the molecule; e.g., glucose, galactose.

al·do·ke·to·mu·tase (al′dō-kē-tō-mū′tās). SYN lactoylglutathione lyase.

al·dol (al′dōl). SEE aldol *condensation.*

al·dol·ase (al′dō-lās). **1.** Generic term for aldehyde-lyase. **2.** Name sometimes applied to fructose-bisphosphate aldolase.

al·don·ic ac·ids (al-don′ik). Monosaccharide derivatives in which the aldehyde group has been oxidized to a carboxyl group. They may form lactones (e.g., galactonic acid). SYN glyconic acids.

al·do·pen·tose (al-dō-pen′tōs). A monosaccharide with five carbon atoms, of which one is a (potential) aldehyde group; e.g., ribose.

al·dose (al′dōs). A monosaccharide potentially containing the characteristic group of the aldehydes, –CHO; a polyhydroxyaldehyde.

a. mutarotase, SYN aldose 1-epimerase.

a. reductase, polyol dehydrogenase (NADP⁺); an oxidoreductase that reversibly converts aldoses to alditols (e.g., glucose to sorbitol) with NADPH as hydrogen donor. An important step in the metabolism of sorbitol and in the formation of diabetic cataracts. SEE ALSO D-sorbitol-6-phosphate dehydrogenase.

al·dose 1-ep·i·mer·ase. An enzyme catalyzing the reversible interconversion of α- and β-aldoses (e.g., α- and β-D-glucose); also acts on L-arabinose, D-xylose, D-galactose, maltose, and lactose. SYN aldose mutarotase, mutarotase.

al·do·side (al′dō-sīd). A glucoside in which the sugar moiety is an aldose.

al·dos·ter·one (al-dos′ter-ōn). A mineralocorticoid hormone produced by the zona glomerulosa of the adrenal cortex; its major action is to facilitate potassium exchange for sodium in the distal renal tubule, causing sodium reabsorption and potassium and hydrogen loss; the principal mineralocorticoid. It exists in equilibrium with the aldehyde form. SYN aldocortin.

al·do·ste·ron·ism (al-dos′ter-on-izm). A disorder caused by excessive secretion of aldosterone. SYN hyperaldosteronism.

idiopathic a., SYN primary a.

primary a., an adrenocortical disorder caused by excessive secretion of aldosterone and characterized by headaches, nocturia, polyuria, fatigue, hypertension, potassium depletion, hypokalemic alkalosis, hypervolemia, and decreased plasma renin activity; may be associated with small benign adrenocortical adenomas. SYN Conn syndrome, idiopathic a.

secondary a., a. resulting not from a defect intrinsic to the adrenal cortex but from a stimulation of hormonal secretion

caused by extra-adrenal disorders; associated with increased plasma renin activity and occurs in heart failure, nephrotic syndrome, cirrhosis, and hypoproteinemia.

al·do·ste·ron·o·gen·e·sis (al-dos′ter-on-ō-jen′ĕ-sis). Formation of the hormone, aldosterone. [aldosterone + G. *genesis,* production]

al·do·tet·rose (al-dō-tet′rōs). A four-carbon aldose; e.g., threose, erythrose.

al·do·tri·ose (al-dō-trī′os). A three-carbon aldose; e.g., D- or L-glyceraldehyde.

al·dox·ime (al-doks′ēm). A compound derived by the reaction of an aldose with hydroxylamine, thus containing the a. group –HC= NOH.

Aldrich, Robert Anderson, U.S. pediatrician, *1917. SEE A. *syndrome;* Wiskott-Aldrich *syndrome.*

al·drin (al′drĭn). A volatile chlorinated hydrocarbon used as an insecticide; if absorbed through the skin, it causes toxic symptoms consisting of irritability followed by depression.

alec·i·thal (ă-les′i-thal). Without yolk; denoting ova with little or no deutoplasm. [G. *a-* priv. + *lekithos,* yolk]

Alec·to·ro·bi·us ta·la·je (ă-lek-tōr-ō′bē-ŭs tă-lā′jē). An insect, commonly found in Mexico and South America, whose bites, like those of the bedbug, may suppurate.

alem·mal (ă-lem′ăl). Denoting a nerve fiber lacking a neurolemma. [G. *a-* priv. + *lemma,* husk]

aleu·ke·mia (ă-loo-kē′mē-ă). **1.** Literally, a lack of leukocytes in the blood. The term is generally used to indicate varieties of leukemic disease in which the white blood cell count in circulating blood is normal or even less than normal (i.e., no leukocytosis), but a few young leukocytes are observed; sometimes used more restrictedly for unusual instances of leukemia with no leukocytosis and no young forms in the blood. **2.** Leukemic changes in bone marrow associated with a subnormal number of leukocytes in the blood. SEE ALSO subleukemic *leukemia.* [G. *a-* priv. + *leukos,* white, + *haima,* blood]

aleu·ke·mic (ă-loo-kē′mik). Pertaining to aleukemia.

aleu·ke·moid (ā-loo-kē′moyd). Resembling aleukemia symptomatically.

aleu·kia (ā-loo′kē-ă). **1.** Absence or extremely decreased number of leukocytes in the circulating blood; sometimes also termed aleukemic myelosis. **2.** Obsolete name for thrombocytopenia. [G. *a-* priv. + *leukos,* white]

aleu·ko·cyt·ic (ā-loo-kō-sit′ik). Manifesting absence or extremely reduced numbers of leukocytes in blood or lesions.

aleu·ko·cy·to·sis (ā-loo-kō-sī-tō′sis). Absence or great reduction (relative or absolute) of the number of white blood cells in the circulating blood (i.e., an advanced degree of leukopenia), or the lack of leukocytes in an anatomical lesion. [G. *a-* priv. + *leukos,* white, + *kytos,* a hollow (cell)]

aleu·ri·o·co·nid·i·um (ă-loo′rē-ō-kŏ-nid′ē-ŭm). A conidium developed from the blown-out end of conidiogenous cells or hyphal branches, and released by rupture below the base of attachment. SYN aleuriospore. [G. *aleuron,* flour, + conidium]

aleu·ri·o·spore (ă-loo′rē-ō-spōr). SYN aleurioconidium.

al·eu·ron (al′oo-rōn). Protein granules in the endosperm of seeds, supposed to contain the vitamins of edible seeds and grains. [G. flour]

aleu·ro·nate (ă-loo′rō-nāt). Protein from the aleuron layer (endosperm) of cereal grains; used to make bread for diabetics.

aleu·ro·noid (ă-loo′rō-noyd). Resembling flour.

Alexander, Gustav, Austrian otolaryngologist, 1873–1932. SEE A. *hearing impairment.*

Alexander, W. Stewart, 20th century New Zealand pathologist. SEE A. *disease.*

alex·ia (ă-lek′sē-ă). An inability to comprehend the meaning of written or printed words and sentences, caused by a cerebral lesion. Also called **optical a., sensory a.,** or **visual a.,** in distinction to **motor a.** (anarthria), in which there is loss of the power to read aloud although the significance of what is written or printed is understood. SYN text blindness, word blindness, visual aphasia (1). [G. *a-* priv. + *lexis,* a word or phrase]

incomplete a., SYN dyslexia.

musical a., loss of the power to read musical notation. SYN music blindness, note blindness.

alex·ic (ă-lek'sik). Pertaining to alexia.

alex·in (ă-lek'sin). Obsolete term for the bactericidal substances of cell-free serum, the activity of which is destroyed by heating at 56°C; applied by Bordet to the heat-labile substance normally present in serum and distinct from the sensitizing substance (antibody) produced by infection or immunization. In this sense it is synonymous with complement. [G. *alexō,* to ward off]

alex·i·thy·mia (ă-lek-si-thī'mē-ă). Difficulty in recognizing and describing one's emotions, defining them in terms of somatic sensations or behavioral reactions. [G. *a-* priv. + *lexis,* word, + *-thymia,* feelings, passion]

al·fa·cal·ci·dol (al-fă-kal'si-dol). A derivative of vitamin D used in the treatment of hypoparathyroidism, vitamin D-dependent rickets, and rickets associated with malabsorption syndromes.

al·fen·ta·nil hy·dro·chlo·ride (al-fen'tă-nil). A very potent, short-acting narcotic agonist analgesic used as an anesthetic or as an adjunct in the maintenance of general anesthesia.

ALG Abbreviation for antilymphocyte *globulin.*

al·gae (al'jē). A division of eukaryotic, photosynthetic, nonflowering organisms that includes many seaweeds. [pl. of L. *alga,* seaweed]

blue-green a., former name for the blue-green bacteria, now classified as Cyanobacteria.

al·gal (al'găl). Resembling or pertaining to algae.

al·ga·ro·ba (al-gă-rō'bă). Ground meal of the fruit of *Ceratonia siliqua;* used as an adsorbent-demulcent in the treatment of diarrhea. SYN carob flour, locust gum.

△**alge-, algesi-, algio-, algo-.** Pain; corresponds to L. dolor-. [G. *algos,* a pain]

al·ge·fa·cient (al-jē-fā'shent). An agent that has a cooling action. [L. *algeo,* to be cold, + *facio,* pr. pl. *-iens,* to make]

△**algesi-.** SEE alge-.

al·ge·sia (al-jē'zē-ă). SYN algesthesia. [G. *algēsis,* a sense of pain]

al·ge·sic (al-jēz-ik). **1.** Painful; related to or causing pain. **2.** Relating to hypersensitivity to pain. SYN algetic.

al·ge·si·chro·nom·e·ter (al-jē'zē-krō-nom'ĕ-ter). An instrument for recording the time required for the perception of a painful stimulus. [G. *algēsis,* sense of pain, + *chronos,* time, + *metron,* measure]

al·ge·sim·e·ter (al-jē-sim'ĕ-ter). SYN algesiometer.

al·ge·si·o·gen·ic (al-jē'zē-ō-jen'ik). Pain-producing. SYN algogenic. [G. *algēsis,* sense of pain, + *-gen,* production]

al·ge·si·om·e·ter (al-jē-zē-om'ĕ-ter). An instrument for measuring the degree of sensitivity to a painful stimulus. SYN algesimeter, algometer. [G. *algēsis,* sense of pain, + *metron,* measure]

al·ges·the·sia (al-jes-thē'zē-ă). **1.** The appreciation of pain. **2.** Hypersensitivity to pain. SYN algesia, algesthesis. [G. *algos,* pain, + *aisthēsis,* sensation]

al·ges·the·sis (al-jes-thē'sis). SYN algesthesia.

al·ges·tone ac·e·to·phe·nide (al-jes'tōn ă-sē-tō-fē'nīd). A progestogen with contraceptive properties. SYN alphasone acetophenide.

al·get·ic (al-jet'ik). SYN algesic.

△**-algia.** Pain, painful condition. [G. *algos,* a pain]

al·gi·cide (al'ji-sīd). An agent active against algae. [algae, + L. *caedo,* to kill]

al·gid (al'jid). Chilly, cold. [L. *algidus,* cold]

al·gin (al'jin). A carbohydrate product from a seaweed, *Macrocystis pyrifera;* used as a gel in pharmaceutical preparations. SYN sodium alginate.

al·gi·nate (al'ji-nāt). An irreversible hydrocolloid consisting of salts of alginic acid, a colloidal acid polysaccharide obtained from seaweed and composed of mannuronic acid residues; used in dental impression materials.

△**algio-.** SEE alge-.

al·gi·o·mo·tor (al-jē-ō-mō'tōr). Causing painful muscular contractions. SYN algiomuscular. [algio- + L. *motor,* mover]

al·gi·o·mus·cu·lar (al'jē-ō-mŭs'kū-lăr). SYN algiomotor.

al·gi·o·vas·cu·lar (al'jē-ō-vas'kū-lăr). SYN algovascular.

△**algo-.** SEE alge-.

al·go·dys·tro·phy (al-gō-dis'trō-fē). A painful local disturbance of growth, particularly due to focal aseptic necrosis of bone and cartilage. [algo- + G. *dys-,* bad, + *trophē,* nourishment]

al·go·gen·e·sis, al·go·ge·ne·sia (al-gō-jen'ĕ-sis, -jĕ-nē'zē-ă). The production or origin of pain. [algo- + G. *genesis,* origin]

al·go·gen·ic (al-gō-jen'ik). SYN algesiogenic.

al·go·lag·nia (al-gō-lag'nē-ă). Obsolete term for algophilia. [algo- + G. *lagneia,* lust]

al·gol·o·gy (al-gōlō-jē). **1.** The study of pain. [G. *algos,*pain, + -logy] **2.** The scientific study of algae.

al·gom·e·ter (al-gom'ĕ-ter). SYN algesiometer. [algo- + G. *metron,* measure]

al·gom·e·try (al-gom'ĕ-trē). The process of measuring pain.

al·go·phil·ia (al-gō-fil'ē-ă). Form of sexual perversion in which the infliction or the experiencing of pain increases the pleasure of the sexual act or causes sexual pleasure independent of the act; includes both sadism and masochism. [algo- + G. *phileō,* to love]

al·go·pho·bia (al-gō-fō'bē-ă). Abnormal fear of or sensitiveness to pain. [algo- + G. *phobos,* fear]

al·go·rithm (al'gō-rithm). A systematic process consisting of an ordered sequence of steps, each step depending on the outcome of the previous one. In clinical medicine, a step-by-step protocol for management of a health care problem; in computed tomography, the formulas used for calculation of the final image from the transmitted x-ray data. [Mediev. L. *algorismus,* after Muhammad ibn-Musa *al-Khwarizmi,* Arabian mathematician, + G. *arithmos,* number]

al·gos·co·py (al-gos'kŏ-pē). SYN cryoscopy. [L. *algor,* cold, + G. *skopeō,* to view]

al·go·spasm (al'gō-spazm). Spasm produced by pain. [G. *algos,* pain, + *spasmos,* convulsion]

al·go·vas·cu·lar (al-gō-vas'kū-lăr). Relating to changes in the lumen of the blood vessels occurring under the influence of pain. SYN algiovascular. [G. *algos,* pain]

al·i·ble (al'i-bl). SYN nutritive. [L. *alibilis,* nutritive, fr. *alo,* to nourish]

al·i·cy·clic (al-i-sik'lik). Denoting an alicyclic compound.

alien·a·tion (ā-lē-en-ā'shŭn). A condition characterized by lack of meaningful relationships with others, sometimes resulting in depersonalization and estrangement from others. [L. *alieno,* pp. *-atus,* to make strange]

ali·e·nia (ā-li-ē'nē-ă). Congenital absence of the spleen. [G. *a-* priv. + L. *lien,* spleen]

al·i·form (al'i-fōrm). Wing-shaped. [L. *ala,* + *forma,* shape]

align·ment (ă-līn'ment). **1.** The longitudinal position of a bone or limb. **2.** The act of bringing into line. **3.** In dentistry, the arrangement of the teeth in relation to the supporting structures and the adjacent and opposing dentitions. SYN alinement. [Fr. *aligner,* to line up, fr. L. *linea,* line]

al·i·ment (al'i-ment). **1.** SYN nourishment. **2.** In sensorimotor theory, that which is assimilated to a schema; analogous to a stimulus. [L. *alo,* to nourish]

al·i·men·ta·ry (al-i-men'ter-ē). Relating to food or nutrition. [L. *alimentarius,* fr. *alimentum,* nourishment]

al·i·men·ta·tion (al-i-men-tā'shŭn). Providing nourishment. SEE ALSO feeding.

forced a., SYN forced *feeding.*

parenteral a., providing nourishment intravenously.

rectal a., nourishment provided by retention enemas.

al·i·na·sal (al'i-nā'săl). Relating to the wings of the nose (alae nasi), or flaring portions of the nostrils. [L. *ala,* + *nasus,* nose]

aline·ment (ă-līn'ment). SYN alignment.

al·in·jec·tion (al'in-jek'shŭn). Injection of alcohol for hardening and preserving pathologic and histologic specimens.

al·i·phat·ic (al-i-fat'ik). Denoting the acyclic carbon compounds, most of which belong to the fatty acid series. [G. *aleiphar* (*aleiphat-*), fat, oil]

a. acids, the acids of nonaromatic hydrocarbons (e.g., acetic, propionic, butyric acids); the so-called fatty acids of the formula R–COOH, where R is a nonaromatic (aliphatic) hydrocarbon.

ali·poid (ā-lip'oyd). Characterized by absence of lipoids. [G. *a-* priv. + *lipoidēs,* resembling fat]

alip·o·tro·pic (ā'lip-ō-trōp'ik). Having no effect upon fat metabolism, or upon the movement of fat to the liver. [G. *a-* priv. + *lipos,* fat, + *tropos,* a turning]

al·i·quot (al'i-kwot). In chemistry and immunology, pertaining to a portion of the whole; loosely, any one of two or more samples of something, of the same volume or weight. [L. a few, several]

al·i·sphe·noid (al-i-sfē'noyd). Relating to the greater wing of the sphenoid bone. [L. *ala,* + *sphēn,* wedge]

aliz·a·rin (ă-liz'ă-rin) [C.I. 58000]. 1,2-Dihydroxyanthraquinone; a red dye that occurs in the root of madder (*Rubia tinctorum* and other *Rubiaceae*) in glucose combination (ruberythric acid) as orange needles, slightly soluble in water; used by the ancients as a dye. Now made synthetically from anthracene and used in the manufacture of dyes, e.g., a. blue, a. orange, "Turkey red." As an indicator, it is yellow below pH 5.5 and red above pH 6.8; other modified a.'s have other colors and change color at other pH values.

a. cyanin [C.I. 58610], disulfonate of hexahydroxyanthraquinone; an acid dye used as a nuclear stain after mordanting and as a fluorochrome in ultraviolet microscopy.

a. purpurin, SYN purpurin (2).

a. red S [C.I. 58005], sodium *a.* sulfonate; used as a stain for calcium in bone (calcium appears red-orange, magnesium, aluminum, and barium are varying shades of red), in the determination of fluorine; as a pH indicator it changes from yellow to purple between pH 3.7 and 5.2.

al·ka·di·ene (al-kă-dī'ēn). An acyclic hydrocarbon (alkane) containing two double bonds.

al·ka·le·mia (al-kă-lē'mē-ă). A decrease in H-ion concentration of the blood or a rise in pH. [alkali + G. *haima,* blood]

al·ka·li, pl. **alkalies** (al'kă-lī). **1.** A strongly basic substance yielding hydroxide ions (OH⁻ in solution); e.g., sodium hydroxide, potassium hydroxide. **2.** SYN base (3). **3.** SYN alkali metal. [Ar., *al,* the, + *qalīy,* soda ash]

caustic a., a highly ionized (in solution) alkali; e.g., NaOH.

fixed a., any a. other than a weakly ionized one, like ammonia.

vegetable a., a mixture of potassium hydroxide and carbonate.

al·ka·line (al'kă-līn). Relating to or having the reaction of an alkali.

al·ka·lin·i·ty (al-kă-lin'i-tē). The state of being alkaline.

al·ka·lin·i·za·tion (al'kă-lin-i-zā'shŭn). SYN alkalization.

al·ka·li·nu·ria (al'kă-li-noo'rē-ă). The passage of alkaline urine. SYN alkaluria. [alkaline + G. *ouron,* urine]

al·ka·li·ther·a·py (al'kă-lī-thār'ă-pē). Therapeutic use of alkali for local or systemic effect.

al·ka·li·za·tion (al'kal-i-zā'shŭn). The process of rendering alkaline. SYN alkalinization.

al·ka·liz·er (al'kă-līz-er). An agent that neutralizes acids or renders a solution alkaline.

al·ka·loid (al'kă-loyd). Originally, any one of hundreds of plant and fungal products distinguished by alkaline (basic) reactions, but now restricted to heterocyclic nitrogen-containing and often complex structures possessing pharmacologic activity; their trivial names usually end in -ine (e.g., morphine, atropine, colchicine). A.'s are synthesized by plants and are found in the leaf, bark, seed, or other parts, usually constituting the active principle of the crude drug; they are a loosely defined group, but may be classified according to the chemical structure of their main nucleus. For medicinal purposes, due to improved water solubility, the salts of a.'s (e.g., morphine sulfate, codeine phosphate) are usually used. see also individual a. or a. class. SYN vegetable base.

ergot a.'s (er'got), any of a large number of a.'s obtained from the ergot fungus *Claviceps purpurea* or semisynthetically derived;

examples include ergotamine, ergonovine, dihydroergotamine, lysergic acid diethylamide (LSD), methysergide.

fixed a., a nonvolatile a.

Vinca a.'s, a.'s such as vincristine and vinblastine (antitumor agents) extracted from the periwinkle plant. SYN Catharanthus alkaloids.

al·ka·lo·sis (al-kă-lō'sis). A state characterized by a decrease in the hydrogen ion concentration of arterial blood below normal level, 40 nmol/L, or pH 7.4. The condition may be caused by an increase in the concentration of alkaline compounds, or by a decrease in the concentration of acidic compounds or carbon dioxide.

acapnial a., SYN respiratory a.

compensated a., a. in which there is a change in bicarbonate but the pH of body fluids approaches normal; respiratory a. may be compensated by increased production of metabolic acids or increased renal excretion of bicarbonate; metabolic a. is rarely compensated by hypoventilation.

compensated metabolic a., retention of acid, primarily carbon dioxide by the lung and acid ions by the renal tubules, to reduce the effect on the pH of the blood of excess alkali produced by ingestion or metabolism of alkali-producing substances.

compensated respiratory a., increased excretion of acid ions by the kidney to minimize the effect on the pH of the blood of excessive loss of carbon dioxide via the lungs, such as occurs with hyperventilation.

metabolic a., an a. associated with an increased arterial plasma bicarbonate concentration, possibly resulting from an excessive intake of alkaline materials or an excessive loss of acid in the urine or through persistent vomiting; the base excess and standard bicarbonate are both elevated. SEE ALSO compensated a.

respiratory a., a. resulting from abnormal loss of CO_2 produced by hyperventilation, either active or passive, with concomitant reduction in arterial plasma bicarbonate concentration. SEE ALSO compensated a. SYN acapnial a.

uncompensated a., a. in which the pH of body fluids is elevated because of lack of the compensatory mechanisms of compensated a.

al·ka·lot·ic (al-kă-lot'ik). Relating to alkalosis.

al·ka·lu·ria (al-kă-loo'rē-ă). SYN alkalinuria.

al·kane (al'kān). The general term for a saturated acyclic hydrocarbon; e.g., propane, butane.

al·ka·net (al'kă-net) [C.I. 75530, 75520]. The root of an herb, *Alkanna,* or *Anchusa tinctoria* (family Boraginaceae), that yields red dyes alkannan and alkannin; used as a coloring agent; also used, combined with tannin, as an astringent.

al·kan·nan (al'kă-nan) [C.I. 75520]. A minor red dye component derived from alkanet.

al·kan·nin (al'kă-nin) [C.I. 75530]. The major red dye derived from alkanet; used as an astringent, and in cosmetics and foods; can be used as an indicator: red at pH 6.8, changing to purple at pH 8.8 and blue at pH 10.0; also used as a fat stain. SYN anchusin.

al·kap·ton (al-kap'tŏn). SYN homogentisic acid. [Boedeker's coinage fr. alkali + L + G. *kaptō,* to suck up greedily]

al·ka·tri·ene (al-kă-trī'ēn). An acyclic hydrocarbon containing three double bonds; e.g., 2,4,6-octatriene, CH₃–CH=CH–CH= CH–CH=CH–CH₃.

al·ka·ver·vir (al-kă-ver'vir). A mixture of alkaloids obtained by the selective extraction of *Veratrum viride* with various organic solvents; used orally or parenterally as a hypotensive agent.

al·kene (al'kēn). An acyclic hydrocarbon containing one or more double bonds; e.g., ethene, propene. SYN olefin.

al·ke·nyl (al'ken-il). The radical of an alkene.

alk-1-en·yl. The radical of an alkene in which the double bond indicated by "en(e)" is between carbons 1 and 2 (carbon 1 being the radical or "yl" carbon), i.e., R–CH=CH–; sometimes expressed as alk-1-en-1-yl.

alk-1-en·yl·glyc·er·o·phos·pho·lip·id. A phosphatidate in which at least one of the radicals attached to the glycerol is an alk-1-enyl rather than the usual acyl radical (i.e., is derived from an aldehyde rather than an acid, hence the older trivial names phosphatidal and acetal phosphatid(at)e); "plasmenic acid" has been proposed as a name for such phosphatidates.

al·kide (al′kīd). SYN alkyl (2).

al·kyl (al′kil). **1.** A hydrocarbon radical of the general formula C_nH_{2n+1}. **2.** A compound, such as tetraethyl lead, in which a metal is combined with alkyl radicals. SYN alkide.

arylated a., SYN aralkyl.

al·kyl·a·mine (al-kil′ă-mēn). An alkane containing an –NH_2 group in place of one H atom; e.g., ethylamine.

al·kyl·a·tion (al′ki-lā′shŭn). Substitution of an alkyl radical for a hydrogen atom; e.g., introduction of a side chain into an aromatic compound.

ALL Abbreviation for acute lymphocytic leukemia.

al·la·ches·the·sia (al′ă-kes-thē′zē-ă). A condition in which a tactile sensation is referred to a point other than to that to which the stimulus is applied. SEE ALSO allochiria. [G. *allachē,* elsewhere, + *aisthēsis,* sensation]

⊘**allanto-, allant-.** Allantois; allantoid; sausage. [G. *allas, allantos,* sausage]

al·lan·to·ate de·im·i·nase. An enzyme that catalyzes the conversion of allantoic acid to ureidoglycine, NH_3, and CO_2.

al·lan·to·cho·ri·on (ă-lan-tō-kōr′ē-on). Extraembryonic membrane formed by the fusion of the allantois and chorion.

al·lan·to·gen·e·sis (ă-lan-tō-jen′ĕ-sis). Formation and development of the allantois. [allanto- + G. *genesis,* origin]

al·lan·to·ic (ă-lan-tō′ik). Relating to the allantois.

al·lan·to·ic ac·id (ă-lan-tō′ik as′id). Diureidoacetic acid; a degradation product of allantoin. An important source of nitrogen in plants.

al·lan·toid (ă-lan′toyd). **1.** Sausage-shaped. **2.** Relating to, or resembling, the allantois. [allanto- + G. *eidos,* appearance]

al·lan·toid·o·an·gi·op·a·gus (ă-lan-toyd′ō-an-jē-op′ă-gŭs). SYN omphaloangiopagus. SEE allantoidoangiopagous *twins,* under *twin.* [allantoid + G. *angeion,* vessel, + *pagos,* fastened]

al·lan·to·in (ă-lan′tō-in). A substance present in allantoic fluid, fetal urine, and elsewhere; also an oxidation product of uric acid and the end product of purine metabolism in animals other than humans and the other primates. SYN 3-ureidohydantoin, cordianine, glyoxyldiureide.

al·lan·to·in·ase (ă-lan-tō′i-nās). An enzyme (an amidohydrolase) that catalyzes the hydrolysis of allantoin to allantoic acid.

al·lan·to·in·u·ria (ă-lan′tō-in-ū′rē-ă). The urinary excretion of allantoin; normal in most mammals, abnormal in humans. [allantoin + G. *ouron,* urine]

al·lan·to·is (ă-lan′tō-is). A fetal membrane developing from the hindgut (or yolk sac, in humans). In humans it is vestigial; externally, in mammals, it contributes to the formation of the umbilical cord and placenta; in birds and reptiles, it lies close beneath the porous shell and serves as an organ of respiration. SYN allantoid membrane. [allanto- + G. *eidos,* appearance]

al·lax·is (ă-laks′is). SYN metamorphosis. [G. *allattein,* to alter]

al·lele (ă-lēl′). Any one of a series of two or more different genes that may occupy the same locus on a specific chromosome. As autosomal chromosomes are paired, each autosomal gene is represented twice in normal somatic cells. If the same a. occupies both units of the locus, the individual or cell is homozygous for this a. If the a.'s are different, the individual or cell is heterozygous for both a.'s. SEE DNA markers. SEE ALSO *dominance* of traits. SYN allelomorph. [G. *allēlōn,* reciprocally]

codominant a., SEE codominant.

silent a., SYN amorph.

al·le·lic (ă-lē′lik). Relating to an allele. SYN allelomorphic.

al·lel·ism (al′ē-lizm). The state held in common by alleles. SYN allelomorphism.

al·le·lo·ca·tal·y·sis (ă-lē′lō-kă-tal′i-sis). Self-stimulation of growth in a bacterial culture by addition of similar cells. [G. *allēlōn,* mutually, reciprocally, + *catalytikos,* able to dissolve]

al·le·lo·cat·a·lyt·ic (ă-lē′lō-kat-ă-lit′ik). Mutually catalytic; denoting two substances each of which is decomposed in the presence of the other.

al·le·lo·chem·i·cals (ă-lē′lō-kem′i-kălz). Signal substances between individuals of different species. Cf. pheromones. [G. *allēlōn,* reciprocally, + chemical]

al·le·lo·morph (ă-lē′lō-mōrf). SYN allele. [G. *allēlōn,* reciprocally, + *morphē,* shape]

al·le·lo·mor·phic (ă-lē-lō-mōr′fik). SYN allelic.

al·le·lo·mor·phism (ă-lē-lō-mōr′fizm). SYN allelism.

al·le·lo·tax·is, al·le·lo·taxy (ă-lēl-ō-taks′is, -taks′ē). Development of an organ from a number of embryonal structures or tissues. [G. *allēlōn,* reciprocally, + *taxis,* an arranging]

Allen, Alfred Henry, U.S. chemist, 1846–1904. SEE A. *test.*

Allen, Edgar Van Nuys, U.S. physician, 1900–1961. SEE A. *test.*

Allen, Edgar, U.S. endocrinologist, 1892–1943. SEE A.-Doisy *test, unit.*

Allen, Willard Myron, U.S. gynecologist, *1904. SEE Corner-A. *test, unit;* A.-Masters *syndrome.*

al·ler·gen (al′er-jen). Term for an antigen that induces an allergic or hypersensitive response. [allergy + G. -*gen,* producing]

al·ler·gen·ic (al-er-jen′ik). SYN antigenic.

al·ler·gic (ă-ler′jik). Relating to any response stimulated by an allergen.

al·ler·gic sa·lute. A characteristic wiping or rubbing of the nose with a transverse or upward movement of the hand, as seen in children with allergic rhinitis.

al·ler·gist (al′er-jist). One who specializes in the treatment of allergies.

al·ler·gi·za·tion (al′er-ji-zā′shŭn). Active sensitization as a result of allergens being naturally or artificially brought into contact with susceptible tissues; the procedure of being allergized.

al·ler·gized (al′er-jīzd). Specifically altered in reactivity; rendered capable of exhibiting one or another aspect of allergy.

al·ler·gol·ogy (al-er-gol′ō-gē). The science concerned with allergic conditions.

al·ler·go·sis (al′er-gō′sis). Any abnormal condition characterized by allergy. [allergy + G. -*osis,* condition]

⊞al·ler·gy (al′er-jē). **1.** Hypersensitivity caused by exposure to a particular antigen (allergen) resulting in a marked increase in reactivity to that antigen upon subsequent exposure, sometimes resulting in harmful immunologic consequences. SYN acquired sensitivity, induced sensitivity. SEE ALSO allergic *reaction,* anaphylaxis, immune. **2.** That branch of medicine concerned with the study, diagnosis, and treatment of allergic manifestations. **3.** An acquired hypersensitivity to certain drugs and biologic materials. [G. *allos,* other, + *ergon,* work]

food allergies	
percentage distribution of foods implicated in 600 cases of food allergy	
food	**%**
cow's milk	42.0
hen's eggs	
egg white	14.5
egg yolk	9.0
white and yolk	9.7
fish	11.0
citrus fruit	4.5
legumes	2.5
meat	2.8
vegetables	1.0
onions	1.0
other (nuts, chocolate)	2.0

atopic a., SEE atopy.

bacterial a., (1) type I hypersensitivity allergic reaction caused by bacterial allergens; **(2)** the delayed type of skin test (type IV hypersensitivity reaction), so-called because of its early association with bacterial antigens (e.g., the tuberculin test).

cold a., physical symptoms produced by hypersensitivity to cold.

contact a., SYN allergic contact *dermatitis.*

delayed a., a type IV hypersensitivity allergic reaction; so called because in a sensitized subject the reaction becomes evident hours after contact with the allergen (antigen), reaches its peak after 24–48 hours, then recedes slowly. Associated with cell-mediated responses. SEE ALSO delayed *reaction;* Cf. immediate a.

drug a., sensitivity (hypersensitivity) to a drug or other chemical.

immediate a., a type I hypersensitivity allergic reaction; so called because in a sensitized subject the reaction becomes evident usually within minutes after contact with the allergen (antigen), reaches its peak within an hour or so, then rapidly recedes. SEE ALSO immediate *reaction,* anaphylaxis; Cf. delayed a.

latent a., a. that causes no signs or symptoms but can be revealed by means of certain immunologic tests with specific allergens.

physical a., excessive response to factors in the environment such as heat or cold.

polyvalent a., allergic response manifested simultaneously for several or numerous specific allergens.

Al·les·che·ria boy·dii (al-es-kē′rē-ă boy′dē-ī). Former name for *Pseudallescheria boydii.* Anamorph is *Scedosporium apiosperman.*

al·les·the·sia (al-es-thē′zē-ă). SYN allochiria. [G. *allos,* other, + *aisthēsis,* sensation]

al·le·thrins (al′ĕ-thrinz). Allethrolone esters of chrysanthemummonocarboxylic acids and synthetic analogs of pyrethrins, which are pyrethrolone esters of the same acids; viscous liquids, insoluble in water, that can be absorbed by lungs, skin, and mucous membranes and may cause liver and kidney injury, with lung congestion; used as an insecticide.

al·leth·ro·lone (ă-leth′rō-lōn). An analog of pyrethrolone (2-propenyl replacing the 2,4-pentadienyl group) used in allethrins.

al·lied health pro·fes·sion·al. An individual trained to perform services in the care of patients other than a physician or registered nurse; includes a variety of therapy technicians (e.g., pulmonary), radiology technicians, physical therapists, etc.

al·li·ga·tion (al-i-gā′shŭn). A rule of mixtures whereby 1) the cost of a mixture may be determined, given the proportions and prices of the several ingredients; or 2) in pharmacy, the relative amounts of solutions of different percentages which must be taken to form a mixture of a given strength. [L. *alligatio,* fr. *al-ligo* (*adl-*), pp. *-atus,* to bind to]

Allis, Oscar Huntington, U.S. surgeon, 1836–1921. SEE A. *forceps.*

al·lit·er·a·tion (ă-lit-er-ā′shŭn). In psychiatry, a speech disturbance in which words commencing with the same sounds, usually consonants, are notably frequent. [Fr. *allitération,* fr. L. *ad,* to, + *littera,* letter of alphabet]

al·li·um (al′ē-ŭm). *Allium sativum* (family Liliaceae), whose bulb contains up to 0.9% of volatile irritating oil with antiseptic action; has been used as a diaphoretic, diuretic, and expectorant. SYN garlic. [L.]

all or none. SEE Bowditch *law.*

allo-. **1.** Other; differing from the normal or usual. **2.** Chemical prefix formerly used with an amino acid whose side chain contains an asymmetric carbon; for example, the alloisoleucines and allothreonines. [G. *allos,* other]

al·lo·al·bu·mi·ne·mia (al′ō-al-bū′mi-nē′mē-ă) [MIM*103600]. The autosomal dominant condition of having serum albumin of a variant type that differs in mobility on electrophoresis from the usual type A; individuals are heterozygous or homozygous for one of the alleles for variant albumin types, a genetic polymorphism without known clinical significance. SEE ALSO inherited albumin *variants,* under *variant.* [allo- + albumin + G. *haima,* blood, + *-ia*]

al·lo·an·ti·body (al-ō-an′ti-bod-ē). An antibody specific for an alloantigen.

al·lo·an·ti·gen (al-ō-an′ti-jen). An antigen that occurs in some, but not in other members of the same species.

al·lo·bar·bi·tal (al-ō-bar′bi-tal). A hypnotic with an intermediate to long duration of action.

al·lo·cen·tric (al-ō-sen′trik). Characterized by or denoting inter-est centered in other persons rather than in one's self. Cf. egocentric. SYN heterocentric (2). [allo- + G. *kentron,* center]

al·lo·chi·ria, al·lo·chei·ria (al′-ō-kī′rē-ă, al-ō-kī′rē-ă). A form of allachesthesia in which the sensation of a stimulus in one limb is referred to the contralateral limb. SYN allesthesia, alloesthesia, Bamberger sign (2). [allo- + G. *cheir,* hand]

al·lo·cho·les·ter·ol (al-ō-kō-les′ter-ol). An isomer of cholesterol, differing in the position of the one double bond. SYN coprostenol.

al·lo·chro·ic (al-ō-krō′ik). Changed or changeable in color; relating to allochroism.

al·lo·chro·ism (al-ō-krō′izm). A change or changeableness in color. [allo- + G. *chrōa,* color]

al·lo·cor·tex (al′ō-kōr′teks) [TA]. O. Vogt term denoting several regions of the cerebral cortex, in particular the olfactory cortex and the hippocampus, characterized by fewer cell layers than the isocortex; SEE ALSO cerebral *cortex.* SYN heterotypic cortex. [allo- + L. *cortex,* bark (cortex)]

α-al·lo·cor·tol (al-ō-kōr′tol). The 5α enantiomer of α-cortol; a metabolite of hydroxycortisone found in the urine.

β-al·lo·cor·tol. The 20β isomer of α-allocortol and 5α enantiomer of β-cortol; a metabolite of hydrocortisone found in urine.

α-al·lo·cor·to·lone (al-ō-kōr′tō-lōn). The 5α enantiomer of α-cortolone; a metabolite of hydrocortisone found in urine.

β-al·lo·cor·to·lone. The 20β isomer of α-allocortolone and 5α enantiomer of β-cortolone; a metabolite of hydrocortisone found in urine.

al·lo·de·ox·y·cho·lic ac·id (al-ō-dē-oks′e-ko′lik). One of the bile acids.

al·lo·dip·loid (al-ō-dip′loyd). SEE alloploid.

al·lo·dyn·ia (al-ō-din′ē-ă). Condition in which ordinarily nonpainful stimuli evoke pain. [allo- + G. *odynē,* pain]

al·lo·er·o·tism (al-ō-ār′ō-tizm). Sexual attraction toward another person. [allo- + G. *erōs,* love]

al·lo·es·the·sia (al-ō-es-thē′zē-ă). SYN allochiria.

al·log·a·my (al-og′ă-mē). Fertilization of the ova of one individual by the spermatozoa of another. Cf. autogamy. [allo- + G. *gamos,* marriage]

al·lo·gen·ic, al·lo·ge·ne·ic (al-ō-jen′ik, -jĕ-nē′ik). Used in transplantation biology. It pertains to different gene constitutions within the same species; antigenically distinct.

al·lo·go·tro·phia (al′ō-gō-trō′fē-ă). Growth or nourishment of one part or tissue at the expense of another part of the body. [allo- + G. *trophē,* nourishment]

al·lo·graft (al′ō-graft). A graft transplanted between genetically nonidentical individuals of the same species. SYN allogeneic graft, homograft, homologous graft, homoplastic graft.

al·lo·group (al′ō-groop). A term formerly used to denote a haplotype composed of closely linked allotypic markers.

al·lo·hex·a·ploid (al-ō-heks′ă-ployd). SEE alloploid.

allohy·drox·y·ly·sine (aHyl) (ă-lō-hī-drok-sē-lī-sēn). 5-allohydroxylysine; a stereoisomer of 5-hydroxylysine; D-a is the diastereoisomer of D-5-hydroxylysine.

alloimmune (al′ō-im-oon′). Immune to an allogenic antigen. [allo- + immune]

al·lo·i·so·leu·cine (aIle) (ă-lō-ī-sō-loo′sēn). A stereoisomer of isoleucine; D-a. is the diastereoisomer of D-isoleucine.

al·lo·i·so·mer (al-ō-ī′sŏm-er). A geometric isomer.

al·lo·ker·a·to·plas·ty (al-ō-ker′ă-tō-plas-tē). Replacement of opaque corneal tissue with a transparent prosthesis, usually plastic.

al·lo·ki·ne·sis (al-ō-ki-nē′sis, -kī-nē′sis). Passive or reflex movement; nonvoluntary movement. [allo- + G. *kinēsis,* movement]

al·lo·lac·tose (ă-lō-lăk′tōs). A sugar, isomeric with lactose, that is the true inducer of the *lac* operon.

al·lo·la·lia (al-ō-lā′lē-ă). Any speech defect, especially one caused by a cerebral disorder. [allo- + G. *lalia,* talking]

al·lom·er·ism (ă-lom′er-izm). The state of differing in chemical composition but having the same crystalline form. [allo- + G. *meros,* part]

al·lom·e·tron (al-ō-me′tron). An evolutionary change in form or proportion of organic beings. [allo- + G. *metron,* measure]

al·lo·mones (ă-lō-mōn). A pheromone that induces a behavioral or physiologic change in a member of another species that is of benefit to the producer. Cf. kairomones, pheromones. [G. *allos,* other, + -mone]

al·lo·mor·phism (al-ō-mōr′fizm). **1.** Change of shape in cells due to mechanical causes, such as flattening from pressure, or to progressive metaplasia, such as the change of bile duct cells into liver cells. **2.** The state of being similar in chemical composition but differing in form (especially crystalline). [allo- + G. *morphē,* form]

al·longe·ment (al-onzh′-maw). Rarely used term for lengthening of a structure during an operation by appropriate incisions. [Fr. elongation]

al·lo·path (al′ō-path). **1.** A traditional medical physician, as distinguished from eclectic or homeopathic practitioners. **2.** One who is a practitioner of allopathy. SYN allopathist.

al·lo·path·ic (al-ō-path′ik). Relating to allopathy.

al·lop·a·thist (al-op′ă-thist). SYN allopath.

al·lop·a·thy (al-op′ă-thē). Regular medicine, the traditional form of medical practice. Cf. homeopathy. SYN heteropathy (2), substitutive therapy. [allo- + G. *pathos,* suffering]

al·lo·pen·ta·ploid (al-ō-pent′ă-ployd). SEE alloploid.

al·lo·phan·ic ac·id (al-ō-fan′ik). Urea carbonic acid; its amide is biuret (allophanamide). SYN carbamoylcarbamic acid, *N*-carboxyurea.

al·loph·a·sis (al-of′ă-sis). Speech that is incoherent, disordered. [allo- + G. *phasis,* speech]

al·lo·phe·nic (al-ō-fē′nik). Pertaining to an animal produced by combining blastomeres of different genotypes (i.e., from different pairs of parents). SEE ALSO mosaic. [allo- + G. *phainō,* to appear, + -ic]

al·lo·phore (al′ō-fōr). SYN erythrophore.

al·loph·thal·mia (al-of-thal′mē-ă). SYN heterophthalmus.

al·lo·pla·sia (al-ō-plā′zē-ă). SYN heteroplasia. [allo- + G. *plasis,* a molding]

al·lo·plast (al′ō-plast). An inert material used to construct, reconstruct, or augment tissue. [allo- + G. *plastos,* formed]

al·lo·plas·ty (al′ō-plas-tē). Repair of defects by allotransplantation.

al·lo·ploid (al′ō-ployd). Relating to a hybrid individual or cell with two or more sets of chromosomes derived from two different ancestral species; depending on the number of multiples of haploid sets, a.'s are referred to as allodiploids, allotriploids, allotetraploids, allopentaploids, allohexaploids, etc. SEE ALSO heterokaryon. [allo- + -ploid]

al·lo·ploi·dy (al-ō-ploy′dē). The condition of being alloploid.

al·lo·pol·y·ploid (al-ō-pol′i-ployd). An alloploid having three or more haploid sets of chromosomes. [allo- + polyploid]

al·lo·pol·y·ploi·dy (al-ō-pol′i-ploy-dē). The condition of being allopolyploid.

al·lo·preg·nane (al-ō-preg′nān). Original name for 5α-pregnane. SEE pregnane.

α-al·lo·preg·nane·di·ol (al′ō-preg-nān-dī′ol). 5α-Pregnane-3α,20α-diol; a metabolite of progesterone and adrenocortical hormones, found in urine.

β-al·lo·preg·nane·di·ol. The 5α-pregnane-3β,20α(and β)-diols; both are metabolites of progesterone and adrenocortical hormones; found in urine.

al·lo·psy·chic (al-ō-sī′kik). Denoting the mental processes in their relation to the outer world. [allo- + G. *psychē,* mind]

al·lo·pu·ri·nol (al-ō-pū′ri-nol). Inhibitor of xanthine oxidase to inhibit uric acid formation; used in the treatment of gout and to retard the rapid metabolic degradation of 6-mercaptopurine.

al·lo·rhyth·mia (al-ŏ-rith′mē-ă). An irregularity in the cardiac rhythm that repeats itself any number of times. [allo- + G. *rhythmos,* rhythm]

al·lo·rhyth·mic (al-ō-rith′mik). Relating to or characterized by allorhythmia.

al·lose (al′ōs). $C_6H_{12}O_6$; an aldohexose. D-A. is epimeric with D-glucose.

al·lo·sen·si·ti·za·tion (al′ō-sen′si-ti-zā-shun). Exposure to an alloantigen that induces immunologic memory cells.

al·lo·some (al′ō-sōm). Obsolete term for one of the chromosomes differing in appearance or behavior from the autosomes and sometimes unequally distributed among the germ cells. [allo- + G. *sōma, body*]

paired a., SYN diplosome.

unpaired a., SYN accessory *chromosome.*

al·lo·ste·ric (al-ō-stār′ik). Pertaining to or characterized by allosterism.

al·lo·ster·ism, al·lo·ste·ry (ă-los′ter-izm, -los′ter-ē). The influencing of an enzyme activity, or the binding of a ligand to a protein, by a change in the conformation of the protein, brought about by the binding of a substrate or other effector at a site (allosteric site) other than the active site of the protein. Cf. cooperativity, hysteresis.

al·lo·tet·ra·ploid (al-ō-tet′ră-ployd). SEE alloploid. [allo- + tetraploid]

al·lo·therm (al′ō-therm). SYN poikilotherm. [allo- + G. *thermē,* heat]

al·lo·thre·o·nines (aThr) (al-o-thrē′ō-nēnz). Two of the four diastereoisomers of threonine, differing from the L- and D-threonines in the configuration of the hydroxyl group in the side chain.

al·lo·tope (al′ō-tōp). The antigenic determinant on the constant or nonvariable region of an allotype. [allo- + -tope]

al·lo·to·pia (al-ō-tō′pē-ă). SYN dystopia. [allo- + G. *topos,* place]

al·lo·trans·plan·ta·tion (al′ō-tranz-plan-ta′shŭn). Transplantation of an allograft. SYN homotransplantation.

al·lot·ri·o·don·tia (al-ot′rē-ō-don′shē-ă). **1.** Growth of a tooth in some abnormal location. **2.** Transplantation of teeth. [G. *allotrios,* foreign, + *odous* (*odont-*), tooth]

al·lot·ri·os·mia (al-ot-rē-oz′mē-ă). Incorrect recognition of odors. SYN heterosmia. [G. *allotrios,* foreign, + *osmē,* smell]

al·lo·trip·loid (al-ō-trip′loyd). SEE alloploid. [allo + triploid]

al·lo·trope (al′ō-trōp). An element in one of the allotropic forms that it may assume. [allo- + G. *tropos,* a turning]

al·lo·tro·phic (al-o-trō′fik). Having an altered nutritive value. [allo- + G. *trophē,* nourishment]

al·lo·tro·pic (al-ō-trop′ik). **1.** Relating to allotropism. **2.** Denoting a type of personality characterized by a preoccupation with the reactions of others.

al·lot·ro·pism, al·lot·ro·py (ă-lot′rō-pizm, -lot′rō-pē). The existence of certain elements, in several forms differing in physical properties; e.g., carbon black, graphite, and diamond are all pure carbon. [allo- + G. *tropos,* a turning]

al·lo·type (al′ō-tīp). Any one of the genetically determined antigenic differences within a given class of immunoglobulin that occur among members of the same species. SEE ALSO antibody. SYN allotypic marker. [allo- + G. *typos,* model]

Gm a.'s, (ăl′lō-tīps), refers to human immunoglobulin gamma heavy chains that express different Gm allotypic determinants (antigens). Each of the 25 different Gm a.'s is the product of genes within the constant regions of the human gamma heavy chain.

InV a.'s, (ăl′lō-tīps), SYN Km a.'s.

Km a.'s, (ăl′lō-tīp), refers to human kappa immunoglobulin light chains that express different Km allotypic determinants (antigens). SYN InV a.'s.

al·lo·typ·ic (al-ō-tip′ik). Pertaining to an allotype.

al·low·ance (a′lau-antz). **1.** Permission. **2.** A portion allotted.

recommended daily a. (RDA), the amount of daily nutrient intake judged to be adequate for the maintenance of good nutrition in an average adult.

al·lox·an (ă-loks′-an). An oxidation product of uric acid, 2,4,5,6-pyrimidinetetrone; administration to experimental animals causes hypoglycemia due to insulin liberation, followed by hyperglycemia due to destruction of the islets of Langerhans (alloxan diabetes).

al·lox·an·tin (ă-loks′an-tin). A condensation product of two molecules of alloxan, formed in the presence of reducing agents; a diabetogenic. SYN uroxin.

al·lox·u·re·mia (al-oks-ū-rē′mē-ă, al-ok-soo-rē′mē-ă). The presence of purine bases in the blood. [alloxan + G. *haima,* blood]

al·lox·u·ria (al-oks-ū′rē-ă, al-ok-soo′rē-ă). The presence of purine bodies in the urine. [alloxan + G. *ouron,* urine]

al·loy (al′oy). A substance composed of a mixture of two or more metals.

chrome-cobalt a.'s, a.'s of cobalt and chromium containing molybdenum and/or tungsten plus trace elements; used in dentistry for denture bases and frameworks, and other structures.

eutectic a., an a., generally brittle and subject to tarnish and corrosion, with a fusion temperature lower than that of any of its components; used in dentistry mainly in solders.

gold a., an a. whose principal ingredient is gold, usually contains copper or platinum and silver; used in dentistry for restorations requiring considerable strength.

Raney a., an a. of Ni and Al in equal proportions, used in the preparation of Raney Nickel.

silver-tin a., any a. of silver and tin; commonly 3 parts Ag and 1 part Sn, forming Ag_3Sn, the chief intermetallic compound in dental amalgam.

all-*trans*-ret·i·nal. The orange retinaldehyde resulting from the action of light on the rhodopsin of the retina, which converts the 11-*cis*-retinal component of the rhodopsin to all-*trans*-retinal plus opsin. SYN *trans*-retinal, visual yellow.

all·spice oil (awl′spīs). SYN *pimenta* oil.

al·lyl (al′il). The monovalent radical, CH_2=$CHCH_2$–.

a. alcohol, a colorless liquid of pungent odor used in making resins and plasticizers; highly irritating to mucous membranes and readily absorbed, causing depression and coma. SYN vinyl carbinol.

a. cyanide, found in some mustard oils.

a. isothiocyanate, obtained from *Brassica nigra* by the action of water on sinigrin and myrosin or produced synthetically; a vesicant, used in 10% solution in 50% alcohol as a counterirritant in neuralgia. Gives mustard its characteristic flavor and aroma. SEE ALSO mustard oil. SYN volatile mustard oil.

a. sulfide, a constituent of garlic oil used in the manufacture of flavors.

al·lyl·a·mine (al-il-am′ēn). A colorless liquid derived from crude oil of mustard and used in the pharmaceutical industry, e.g., in the manufacture of mercurial diuretics.

al·lyl·es·tre·nol (al-il-es′trĕ-nol). A progestational agent.

al·lyl·mer·cap·to·meth·yl·pen·i·cil·lin (al′il-mer-kap′tō-meth′il-pen-i-sil′in). SYN *penicillin* O.

***N*-al·lyl·nor·mor·phine** (al′il-nor-mor′fēn). SYN nalorphine.

al·ly·sines (al′i-sēnz). Two or more six-carbon α-amino acids connected by a carbon-carbon bond; constituents of connective tissue and other structural elements. SEE ALSO desmin.

Almeida, Floriano Paulo de, Brazilian physician, *1898. SEE A. *disease;* Lutz-Splendore-A. *disease.*

Almén, August Teodor, Swedish physiologist, 1833–1903. SEE A. *test* for blood.

al·mond oil (aw′mŭnd, awl′mŭnd). A fixed oil expressed from sweet almonds, the kernels of varieties of *Prunus amygdalus;* used in ointments.

bitter almond a. o., a volatile oil from the dried ripe kernels of bitter almonds and from other kernels containing amygdalin; it contains between 2 and 4% of hydrocyanic acid and 95% of benzaldehyde.

al·oe (al′ō). **1.** The dried juice from the leaves of plants of the genus *Aloe* (family Liliaceae), from which are derived aloin, resin, emodin, and volatile oils. **2.** The dried juice from the leaves of *Aloe perryi* (socotrine a.'s), of *A. barbadensis* (Barbados and Curaçao a.'s), or of *A. capensis* (Cape a.'s); used as a purgative; used topically in cosmetics where it has no demonstrated value.

al·oe-em·o·din (al′ō-em′ō-din). The trimethyl ether of emodin; used as a laxative. SEE aloin, emodin. SYN rhabarberone.

al·o·e·tin (al-ō-ē′tin). SYN aloin.

alo·gia (ă-lō′jē-ă). **1.** SYN aphasia. **2.** Inability to speak due to mental deficiency or an episode of dementia. [G. *a-* priv. + *logos,* speech]

al·o·in (al′ō-in). A yellow crystalline principle made up of aloe-emodin and glucose, obtained from aloe; used as a laxative. SYN aloetin, barbaloin.

al·o·pe·cia (al-ō-pē′shē-ă). Absence or loss of hair. SYN baldness, calvities, pelade. [G. *alōpekia,* a disease like fox mange, fr. *alōpēx,* a fox]

a. adnata, underdevelopment of the lashes. SEE ALSO a. congenitalis, milphosis. SYN madarosis (2).

androgenic a., gradual decrease of scalp hair density in adults with transformation of terminal to vellus hairs, which become lost as a result of familial increased susceptibility of hair follicles to androgen secretion following puberty. Two areas of the scalp are commonly affected in men; when it occurs in females it is associated with other evidence of excessive androgen activity, such as hirsutism. Autosomal dominant inheritance. SEE female pattern a., male pattern a. SYN common baldness.

a. area′ta [MIM*104000], a common condition of undetermined etiology characterized by circumscribed, nonscarring, usually asymmetrical areas of baldness on the scalp, eyebrows, and bearded portion of the face. Hairy skin anywhere on the body may be affected; occasionally follows autosomal dominant inheritance. Peribulbar lymphocytic infiltration and association with autoimmune disorders suggest an autoimmune etiology. Slow enlargement with eventual regrowth within 1 year is common, but relapse is frequent and progression to a. totalis may occur, especially with childhood onset.

a. cap′itis tota′lis, SYN a. totalis.

cicatricial a., SYN scarring a. [L. *cicatrix, cicatricis,* scar + suffix *-al,* characterized by]

a. congenita′lis, absence of all hair at birth. May be associated with psychomotor epilepsy [MIM*104130]; autosomal dominant or X-linked [MIM*300042] inheritance. SYN congenital baldness, hypotrichiasis (2).

congenital sutural a., obsolete term for *dyscephalia* mandibulo-oculofacialis.

female pattern a., diffuse partial hair loss in the centroparietal area of the scalp, with preservation of the frontal and temporal hairlines; the most frequent type of androgenic a. in women.

a. heredita′ria, SYN male pattern a.

a. leproti′ca, thinning or total loss of the lateral third of the eyebrows, eyelashes, and body hairs, seen in leprosy; loss of scalp hair is rare.

a. limina′ris fronta′lis, SYN a. marginalis.

lipedematous a., a. with itching, soreness, or tenderness of the scalp in black women; the scalp is thickened and soft, subcutaneous fat is increased, and the hair is sparse and short.

male pattern a. [MIM*109200], the most common form of androgenic a., seen in men as receding frontal and bilateral triangular temple hairlines, and a balding patch on the vertex, which may progress to complete a.; inheritance is autosomal dominant in males, recessive in females. SYN a. hereditaria, male pattern baldness, patterned a.

a. margina′lis, hair loss at the hairline, a condition most commonly seen in blacks; commonly transient and caused by chronic traction, although long-continued traction may cause permanent a. SYN a. liminaris frontalis.

a. medicamento′sa, diffuse hair loss, most notably of the scalp, caused by administration of various types of drugs.

moth-eaten a., patchy hair loss of parietal and occipital regions of the scalp, characteristic of secondary syphilis.

a. mucino′sa, follicular mucinosis with a. appearing in areas of erythema and edema in the bearded portion of the face or in the scalp.

patterned a., SYN male pattern a.

postoperative pressure a., SYN pressure a.

postpartum a., temporary diffuse telogen loss of scalp hair at the termination of pregnancy.

al

premature a., a. prematu′ra, male pattern baldness appearing at an unusually early age.

a. preseni′lis, ordinary or common baldness occurring in early or middle life without any apparent disease of the scalp.

pressure a., loss of hair over a circumscribed area usually on the posterior scalp, resulting from the continuous pressure on the occiput in a lengthy operative procedure, or unconsciousness following a drug overdose. SYN postoperative pressure a.

scarring a., a. in which hair follicles are irreversibly destroyed by scarring processes including trauma, burns, lupus erythematosus, lichen planopilaris, scleroderma, folliculitis decalvans, or of uncertain cause (pseudopelade). SYN cicatricial a.

a. seni′lis, the normal loss of scalp hair in old age.

a. symptomat′ica, a. occurring in the course of various constitutional or local diseases, or following prolonged febrile illness.

a. syphilit′ica, moth-eaten a. of secondary syphilis.

a. tota′lis, total loss of hair of the scalp either within a very short period of time or from progression of localized a., especially a. areata. Cf. a. universalis. SYN a. capitis totalis.

a. tox′ica, hair loss attributed to febrile illness.

traction a., circumscribed or diffuse loss of hair resulting from repetitive traction on the hair by pulling or twisting; also occurs after excessive application of hair "softeners" such as permanent wave solutions or hot combs. A. marginalis is a form of traction a. SYN traumatic a.

traumatic a., SYN traction a.

a. triangularis (trī′ang-oo-la-ris), bilateral receding temporal hair lines in male pattern a.

a. triangula′ris congenita′lis, a congenital triangular patch of baldness on the frontal or temporal region of the scalp.

a. universa′lis, total loss of hair from all parts of the body. Cf. a. totalis.

al·o·pe·cic (al-ō-pē′sik). Relating to alopecia.

Alpers, Bernard J., U.S. neurologist, 1900–1981. SEE A. *disease*.

al·pha (al′fă). First letter of the Greek alphabet, α.

al·pha am·y·lase. A starch-splitting enzyme obtained from a nonpathogenic bacterium of the *Bacillus subtilis* class, used in the treatment of inflammatory conditions and edema of soft tissues associated with traumatic injury; its therapeutic usefulness has not been fully established and its mode of action is not known.

al·pha-block·er (al′fă-blok′er). SYN α-adrenergic blocking *agent*.

al·pha·di·one (al-fă-dī′ōn). An intravenous anesthetic containing two steroids, alfaxalone, and alfadolone acetate, dissolved in 20% polyoxyethylated castor oil.

Al·pha·her·pes·vir·inae (al′fa-her′pēz-vir′i-nē). A subfamily of Herpesviridae containing Simplexvirus and Varicellavirus.

al·pha·pro·dine (al-fă-prō′dēn). A narcotic analgesic related to meperidine; physical and psychic dependence may develop.

al·pha·sone ac·e·to·phe·nide (al′fă-sōn). SYN algestone acetophenide.

Al·pha·vi·rus (al′fă-vī-rŭs). One of the genera of the family Togaviridae that was formerly classified as part of the "group A" arboviruses and includes the viruses that cause eastern equine, western equine, and Venezuelan encephalitis.

al·pi·dem (al-pī′dem). A benzodiazepine anxiolytic/sedative/hypnotic.

Alport, Arthur Cecil, South African physician, 1880–1959. SEE A. *syndrome.*

al·praz·o·lam (al-praz′ō-lam). A benzodiazepine minor tranquilizer used for management of anxiety disorders and panic attack; abuse may lead to habituation or addiction.

al·pren·o·lol hy·dro·chlo·ride (al-pren′ō-lol). The hydrochloride salt of 1-(*o*-allylphenoxy)-3-(isopropylamino)propan-2-ol; β-receptor blocking agent, used for the treatment of cardiac arrhythmias.

al·pros·ta·dil (al-pros′tă-dil). A vasodilator used for palliative therapy to temporarily maintain patency of the ductus arteriosus in neonates with congenital heart defects. SYN prostaglandin E₁.

ALS Abbreviation for amyotrophic lateral *sclerosis*; antilymphocyte *serum.*

al·ser·ox·y·lon (al′ser-ok′si-lon). A fat-soluble alkaloidal fraction extracted from the root of *Rauwolfia serpentina*, containing reserpine and other nonadrenolytic amorphous alkaloids; used as a sedative in psychoses, in mild hypertension, and as an adjunct to more potent hypotensive drugs.

Alström, Carl-Henry, Swedish geneticist, *1907. SEE A. *syndrome.*

ALT Abbreviation for alanine aminotransferase.

Altemeier, William A., 20th century U.S. surgeon. SEE A. *operation.*

al·ter·a·tion (awl-ter-ā′shŭn). **1.** A change. **2.** A changing; a making different.

modal a., in electric irritability, a change in the mode of response of degenerated muscle to electric stimulation, the contraction being sluggish instead of quick.

qualitative a., in electric irritability, a change in which the muscle contracts as readily on application of the anode as on that of the cathode.

quantitative a., in electric irritability, a gradual loss of contractility in a muscle in response to static, faradic, and galvanic currents successively.

al·ter·e·go·ism (awl-ter-ē′gō-izm). Identification with people of similar personality to one's own.

al·ter·nans (awl-ter′nanz). Alternating; often used substantively for alternation of the heart, either electrical or mechanical. Alternating; used as a noun in the sense of *pulsus* alternans. [L.]

auditory a., SYN auscultatory a.

auscultatory a., alternation in the intensity of heart sounds or murmurs in the presence of a regular cardiac rhythm as a result of mechanical alternation of the heart. SYN auditory a.

concordant a., simultaneous occurrence of right ventricular and pulmonary artery a. with left ventricular and peripheral pulsus a.

cycle length a., a succession of long and short diastolic intervals.

discordant a., presence of right ventricular and pulmonary artery a. with peripheral pulsus a., but with the strong beat of the right ventricle coinciding with the weak beat of the left and vice versa.

electrical a., electrical alternation of the heart.

Al·ter·nar·ia (al-ter-nā′rē-ă). A genus of fungi easily isolated from air and considered to be a common laboratory contaminant and an allergen; occasionally pathogenic in humans.

al·ter·na·tion (awl-ter-nā′shŭn). The occurrence of two things or phases in succession and recurrently; used interchangeably with alternans.

cardiac a., the occurrence of any cardiac phenomenon every other beat.

concordant a., a. in either the mechanical or electrical activity of the heart, occurring in both systemic and pulmonary circulations.

discordant a., a. in cardiac activities of either the systemic or the pulmonary circulation, but not of both, or in both but oppositely directed in each.

electrical a. of heart, a disorder in which the ventricular or atrial complexes or both are regular in time but of alternating pattern; detected by electrocardiography. The P, PR segment, QRS, T, QRS-T, or P-QRST alternate singly or in combination.

a. of generations, a succession of generations of individuals like and unlike the original parents, or an a. of sexual and nonsexual generations.

mechanical a. of the heart, disorder in which contractions of the heart are regular but are alternately stronger and weaker.

al·ter·na·tor (awl′ter-nā-ter). Mechanical apparatus with movable transparent racks to which a large number of radiographs can be attached, to enable selection and viewing in front of a stationary bank of lights. [L. *alterno*, to do by turns, fr. *alter*, either of two]

al·ter·noc·u·lar (awl-ter-nok′ū-lăr). Denoting the use of each eye separately instead of binocularly. [L. *alternus*, by turns, + ocular]

Al·te·ro·mo·nas. A genus of Gram-negative bacteria with curved rods, and motile by means of a single polar flagellum; require a seawater base for growth; a cause of spoilage of poultry.

A. putrefa′ciens, a marine species of bacteria implicated as a cause of fish spoilage but rarely as a human pathogen.

al·thea (al-thē′ă). Derived from *Althaea officinalis*, a perennial herb which is found wild in moist places in Europe. Contains a high proportion of starches, pectin, and sugars; used as a flavor and demulcent. SYN marshmallow root. [L., fr. G. *althaia*, marshmallow]

Altherr, Franz. SEE Meyenburg-A.-Uehlinger *syndrome*.

alt. hor. Abbreviation for L. *alternis horis*, every other hour.

al·ti·tu·di·nal (al-ti-too′di-năl). Relating to vertical relationships; e.g., a. hemianopsia.

Altmann, Richard, German histologist, 1852–1900. SEE A. *fixative, granule,* anilin-acid fuchsin *stain, theory;* A.-Gersh *method.*

al·trose (al′trōs). An aldohexose isomeric with glucose, tallose, allose, etc. D-A. is epimeric with D-mannose.

al·um (al′ŭm). A double sulfate of aluminum and of an alkaline earth element or ammonium; chemically, an a. is any one of the markedly astringent double salts formed by a combination of a sulfate of aluminum, iron, manganese, chromium, or gallium with a sulfate of lithium, sodium, potassium, ammonium, cesium, or rubidium; used locally as styptics. [L. *alumen*]

    burnt a., SYN dried a.

    cake a., SYN *aluminum* sulfate octadecahydrate.

    chrome a., the sulfate of chromium and potassium; used as a mordant in histologic staining.

    dried a., a. deprived of its water of crystallization by heat; an astringent dusting powder. SYN burnt a.

    exsiccated a., a. heated to complete dryness; a local astringent.

    ferric a., SYN *ferric* ammonium sulfate.

    whey a., an astringent and styptic preparation made by boiling a. (1 oz.) in milk (10 oz.).

al·um·he·ma·tox·y·lin (al′ŭm-hē-mă-tok′si-lin). A purple nuclear stain used in histology; a mixture of an aqueous solution of ammonium alum and an alcoholic solution of hematoxylin which is ripened or oxidized to hematein.

alu·mi·na (ă-loo′mi-nă). SYN *aluminum* oxide.

    hydrated a., SYN *aluminum* hydroxide.

alu·mi·nat·ed (ă-loo′mi-nā-ted). Containing alum.

alu·mi·non (ă-loo′min-on). The ammonium salt of aurintricarboxylic acid, so-called because of its usefulness in the detection of aluminum in biologic material, foods, etc.

alu·mi·no·sis (ă-loo-min-ō′sis). A pneumoconiosis caused by inhalation of aluminum particles into the lungs.

alu·mi·num (Al) (ă-loo′min-ŭm). A white silvery metal of very light weight; atomic no. 13, atomic wt. 26.981539. Many salts and compounds are used in medicine and dentistry. [L. *alumen,* alum]

    a. acetate, used as a disinfectant by embalmers; proposed as desiccant and deodorant powder for eczema and chronic skin ulcers.

    a. acetotartrate, basic aluminum acetate (70%) and tartaric acid (30%); antiseptic.

    a. acetylsalicylate, SYN a. aspirin.

    a. ammonium sulfate, an astringent.

    a. aspirin, an analgesic and antipyretic. SYN a. acetylsalicylate.

    a. bismuth oxide, SYN *bismuth* aluminate.

    a. carbonate, basic, an a. hydroxide-carbonate complex consisting of white lumps, insoluble in water; aqueous suspensions bind phosphorus in the intestine and lower serum inorganic phosphorus resulting in an increase in reabsorption of phosphorus by renal tubules and reduction of urinary excretion of phosphorus; it reduces formation of phosphatic urinary calculi and gastric acidity.

    a. chlorate nonahydrate, an antiseptic. SYN mallebrin.

    a. chloride hexahydrate, used as an astringent or antiseptic in solution.

    a. diacetate, SYN a. subacetate.

    a. hydrate, SYN a. hydroxide.

    a. hydroxide, an astringent dusting powder; also used internally as a mild astringent antacid. SYN a. hydrate, hydrated alumina.

    a. hydroxide gel, a suspension containing Al_2O_3, mainly in the form of a. hydroxide, used as an antacid; a dried form, with the same use, is obtained by drying the product of interaction in aqueous solution of an a. salt with ammonium or sodium carbonate.

    a. hydroxychloride, an antiperspirant.

    a. magnesium silicate, SYN *magnesium* aluminum silicate.

    a. monostearate, a compound of a. with a mixture of solid organic acids obtained from fats, and consisting chiefly of a. monostearate and a. monopalmitate; used as a suspending medium in pharmaceutical preparations.

    a. nicotinate, a lipid-lowering agent with peripheral vasodilator action.

    a. oleate, used as an ointment in certain cutaneous affections and in burns.

    a. oxide, used as an abrasive, as a refractory, and in chromatography. SYN alumina.

    a. penicillin, SEE aluminum *penicillin.*

    a. phenolsulfonate, antiseptic and astringent for local application, usually for cutaneous ulcers.

    a. phosphate, an infusible powder, insoluble in water but soluble in alkali hydroxides, used for dental cements with calcium sulfate and sodium silicate.

    a. phosphate gel, an aqueous suspension of between 4.0 and 5.0% of a. phosphate; used as an antacid.

    a. potassium sulfate, an astringent and styptic; also used in veterinary medicine for ulcerative stomatitis, leukorrhea, and conjunctivitis. SYN potassium alum.

    a. salicylate, basic, used in the treatment of ozena and pharyngitis.

    a. salicylate, basic, soluble, used in solution as a spray for diseases of the upper air passages.

    a. silicate, SYN kaolin.

    a. subacetate, used in solution (as in Burow solution) as an astringent, as an ingredient in mouthwashes, and in embalming fluids. SYN a. diacetate.

    a. sulfate octadecahydrate, astringent detergent for skin ulcers. SYN cake alum.

alu·mi·num group. Aluminum, boron, gallium, indium, and thallium.

al·vei (al′vē-ī). Plural of alveus.

al·ve·o·al·gia (al′vē-ō-al′jē-ă). A postoperative complication of tooth extraction in which the blood clot in the socket disintegrates, resulting in focal osteomyelitis and severe pain. SYN alveolalgia, alveolar osteitis, dry socket. [alveolus + G. *algos,* pain]

al·ve·o·lal·gia (al′vē-ō-lal′jē-ă). SYN alveoalgia.

al·ve·o·lar (al-vē′ō-lăr). Relating to an alveolus.

al·ve·o·late (al-vē′ō-lāt). Pitted like a honeycomb. [L. *alveolus,* dim. of *alveus,* trough, hollow sac, cavity]

al·ve·o·lec·to·my (al′vē-ō-lek′tō-mē). Surgical excision of a portion of the dentoalveolar process, for recontouring of the alveolar ridge at the time of tooth removal to facilitate a dental prosthesis. [alveolus + G. *ektomē,* excision]

al·ve·o·li (al-vē′ō-lī). Plural of alveolus.

al·ve·o·lin·gual (al′vē-o-ling′gwăl). SYN alveololingual.

al·ve·o·li·tis (al′vē-ō-lī′tis). **1.** Inflammation of lung alveoli. **2.** Inflammation of a tooth socket.

    acute pulmonary a., acute inflammation involving exudate into the pulmonary alveoli and impaired gas exchange such as occurs in a host of interstitial lung diseases, including diffuse alveolar damage, drug-induced lung disease, and acute immunologic injury.

    chronic fibrosing a., SYN idiopathic pulmonary *fibrosis.*

    cryptogenic fibrosing a., SYN idiopathic pulmonary *fibrosis.*

    extrinsic allergic a., pneumoconiosis resulting from hypersensitivity due to repeated inhalation of organic dust, usually specified according to occupational exposure; in the acute form, respiratory symptoms and fever start several hours after exposure to the dust; in the chronic form, there is eventual diffuse pulmonary fibrosis after exposure over several years.

    fibrosing a., SYN idiopathic pulmonary *fibrosis.*

alveolo-. An alveolus, the alveolar process; alveolar. [L. *alveolus,* a concave vessel, a bowl, a basin, fr. *alveus,* a trough, + *-olus,* small, little; akin to *alvus,* the belly, the womb]

al·ve·o·lo·cla·sia (al-vē-ō-lō-klā′zē-ă). Destruction of the alveolus. [alveolo- + G. *klasis,* breaking]

al·ve·o·lo·den·tal (al-vē-ō-lō-den′tăl). Relating to the alveoli and the teeth.

al·ve·o·lo·la·bi·al (al-vē-ō-lō-lā′bē-ăl). Relating to the labial or vestibular (outer) surface of the alveolar processes of the upper or lower jaw.

al·ve·o·lo·la·bi·a·lis (al-vē-ō-lō-lā-bē-ā′lis). Relating to the alveololabial groove or region. [L.]

al·ve·o·lo·lin·gual (al-vē-ō-lō-ling′gwăl). Relating to the lingual (inner) surface of the alveolar process of the lower jaw. SYN alveolingual.

al·ve·o·lo·pal·a·tal (al-vē-ō-lō-pal′ă-tăl). Relating to the palatal surface of the alveolar process of the upper jaw.

al·ve·o·lo·plas·ty (al-vē′ō-lō-plas-tē). Surgical preparation of the alveolar ridges for the reception of dentures; shaping and smoothing of socket margins after extraction of teeth with subsequent suturing to insure optimal healing. SYN alveoplasty. [alveolo- + G. *plassō,* to form]

interradicular a., intraseptal a., removal of the interradicular bone and collapsing of the cortical plates to a more desirable alveolar contour.

al·ve·o·los·chi·sis (al-vē-ō-lō-los′ki-sis). A cleft of the alveolar process. [alveolo- + G. *schisis,* cleaving]

al·ve·o·lot·o·my (al-vē-ō-lot′ō-mē). Surgical opening into a dental alveolus to allow drainage of pus from a periapical or other intraosseous abscess. [alveolo- + G. *tomē,* incision]

al·ve·o·lus, gen. and pl. **al·ve·o·li** (al-vē′ō-lŭs, -ō-lī) [NA]. A small cell, cavity, or socket. **1.** SYN pulmonary a. **2.** One of the terminal secretory portions of an alveolar or racemose gland. **3.** One of the honeycomb pits in the wall of the stomach. **4.** SYN tooth *socket.* [L. dim. of *alveus,* trough, hollow sac, cavity]

a. dentalis, pl. **alveoli dentales** [TA], SYN tooth *socket.*

🄸**pulmonary a.,** a thin-walled saclike terminal dilation of the respiratory bronchioles, alveolar ducts, and alveolar sacs across which gas exchange occurs between alveolar air and the pulmonary capillaries. SYN alveolus (1) [NA], air cells (1), air vesicles, alveoli pulmonis, bronchic cells.

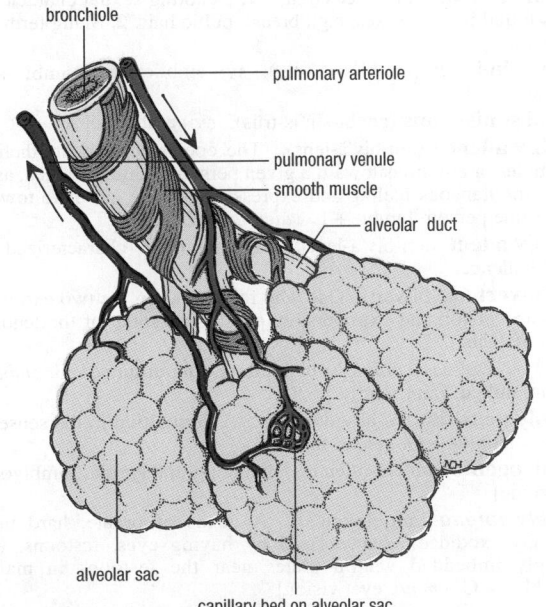

bronchiole
pulmonary arteriole
pulmonary venule
smooth muscle
alveolar duct
alveolar sac
capillary bed on alveolar sac

pulmonary alveoli

alveoli pulmo′nis, SYN pulmonary a.

al·ve·o·plas·ty (al′vē-ō-plas-tē). SYN alveoloplasty.

al·ve·us, pl. **al·vei** (al′vē-ŭs, -vē-ī). A channel or trough. [L. tray, trough, cavity, fr. *alvus,* belly]

a. hippocam′pi [TA], SYN a. of hippocampus.

a. of hippocampus [TA], a thin white band of fornix fibers covering the ventricular surface of the hippocampus. SYN a. hippocampi [TA].

a. urogenita′lis, obsolete term for prostatic *utricle.*

ALW Abbreviation for arch-loop-whorl *system.*

alym·phia (ă-lim′fē-ă). Absence or deficiency of lymph. [G. *a-* priv + lymph +-ia]

alym·pho·cy·to·sis (ă-lim′fō-sī-tō′sis). Absence or great reduction of lymphocytes.

alym·pho·pla·sia (ă-lim-fō-plā′zē-ă). Lack of development or hypoplasia of lymphoid tissue.

Nezelof type of thymic a., cellular immunodeficiency with failure of development of T cells and T-cell function.

thymic a., hypoplasia with absence of Hassall corpuscles and deficiency of lymphocytes in the thymus and usually in lymph nodes, spleen, and gastrointestinal tract resulting in severe combined immunodeficiency. SEE ALSO *immunodeficiency* with hypoparathyroidism.

Alzheimer, Alois, German neurologist, 1864–1915. SEE A. *dementia, disease, sclerosis.*

al·zyme (al′zīm). Union of antibody and enzyme to form a hybrid catalytic molecule.

Am Symbol for americium.

am Abbreviation for ammeter.

AMA. Abbreviation for American Medical Association.

am·a·crine (am′ă-krin). **1.** A cell or structure lacking a long, fibrous process. **2.** Denoting such a cell or structure. SEE ALSO amacrine *cell.* [G. *a-* priv. + *makros,* long, + *is (in-),* fiber]

am·a·dou (ahm′ah-doo). SYN agaric. [Fr.]

amal·gam (ă-mal′gam). An alloy of an element or a metal with mercury. In dentistry, primarily of two types: silver-tin alloy, containing small amounts of copper, zinc and perhaps other metals, and a second type containing more copper (12 to 30% by weight); they are used for restoring teeth and making dies. [G. *malagma,* a soft mass]

pin a., an a. restoration held in place largely by small metal rods protruding from holes drilled into tooth structure.

spherical a., an alloy for dental a. composed of spherical particles instead of filings.

amal·ga·mate (ă-mal′gă-māt). To make an amalgam.

amal·ga·ma·tion (ă-mal-gă-mā′shŭn). The process of combining mercury with a metal or an alloy to form a new alloy.

amal·ga·ma·tor (ă-mal′gă-mā-tŏr). A device for combining mercury with a metal or an alloy to form a new alloy.

Am·a·ni·ta (am-ă-nī′tă). A genus of fungi, many members of which are highly poisonous. [G. *amanitai,* fungi]

🄸*A. musca′ria,* a toxic species of mushroom with yellow to red pileus and white gills; it contains muscarine, a cholinomimetic, which produces psychosislike states and other symptoms. SYN fly agaric.

A. phalloi′des, a species containing poisonous principles, including phalloidin and amanitin, that cause gastroenteritis, hepatic necrosis, and renal necrosis. SYN deadly agaric.

α**-am·a·ni·tin** (am-ă-nī′tin). A highly toxic, heat-stable bicyclic oligopeptide in *Amanita phalloides.* It inhibits transcription by certain RNA polymerases.

aman·ta·dine hy·dro·chlo·ride (ă-man′tă-dēn). An antiviral agent used for influenza; also used to treat parkinsonism where it increases dopamine release and reduces its reuptake into dopaminergic nerve terminals of substantia nigra neurons.

am·a·ra (ă-mah′ră). SYN bitters (2). [neut. pl. of L. *amarus,* bitter]

am·a·ranth, am·a·ran·thum (am′ă-ranth, am-ă-ran′thŭm) [C.I. 16185]. An azo dye; a soluble reddish brown powder, the color turning to magenta red in solution; used as a food, pharmaceuti-

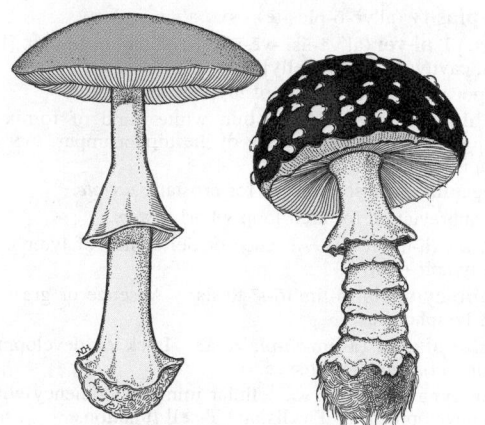

Amanita phalloides (left) and *Amanita muscaria* (right)

cal, and cosmetic coloring agent, and occasionally in histology. [G. *amaranthon,* a never-fading flower]

am·a·rine (am′ă-rin). A name applied to various bitter principles derived from plants, especially to a poisonous substance, 2,4,5-triphenylimidazoline, obtained from oil of bitter almond. [L. *amarus,* bitter]

am·a·roid (am′ă-royd). A bitter extractive that does not belong to the class of glycosides, alkaloids, or any of the known proximate principles of plants. [L. *amarus,* bitter, + G. *eidos,* like]

am·a·roi·dal (am-ă-roy′dăl). Resembling bitters; having a slightly bitter taste.

ama·rum (ă-mah′rŭm). One of a class of vegetable drugs of bitter taste, such as gentian and quassia, used as appetizers and tonics. [neut. of L. *amarus,* bitter]

amas·tia (ă-mas′tē-ă). Absence of the breasts. [G. *a-* priv. + *mastos,* breast]

amas·ti·gote (ă-mas′ti-gōt). SYN Leishman-Donovan *body.* [G. *a-* priv. + *mastix,* whip]

am·a·tho·pho·bia (ă-math-ō-fō′bē-ă). Morbid dread of dust or dirt. [G. *amathos,* dust, + *phobos,* fear]

am·a·tox·in (am-a-tok′sin). One of a group of bicyclic octapeptides from death-cap fungus and deadly agaric (*Amanita phalloides*).

am·au·ro·sis (am-aw-rō′sis). Blindness, especially that occurring without apparent change in the eye itself, as from a brain lesion. [G. *amauros,* dark, obscure, + *-osis,* condition]

a. congen′ita of Leber [MIM*204000 & MIM*204100], a disorder of cone-rod abiotrophy causing blindness or severely reduced vision at birth; autosomal recessive inheritance with at least 3 different loci. Type I is caused by mutation in the gene for retinal guanylate cyclase (GUC2D) on chromosome 17p, type II by mutation in the gene for retinal pigment epithelium-specific 65-kD protein (RPE65) on 1p, and type III by mutation in the gene for photoreceptor-specific homeobox gene CRX on 19q.

a. fu′gax, a transient blindness that may result from a transient ischemia due to carotid artery insufficiency, retinal artery embolus, or to centrifugal force (visual blackout in flight).

pressure a., loss of vision occurring a few seconds after intraocular pressure exceeds systolic pressure of retinal arteries.

toxic a., blindness due to optic neuritis caused by methyl alcohol, lead, arsenic, quinine, or other poisons.

am·au·rot·ic (am-aw-rot′ik). Relating to or suffering from amaurosis.

amax·o·pho·bia (ă-mak-sō-fō′bē-ă). Rarely used term for morbid fear of, or of riding in, a vehicle. [G. *amaxa, hamaxa,* a carriage, + *phobos,* fear]

am·ba·geu·sia (am-bă-goo′sē-ă). Loss of taste from both sides of the tongue. [L. *ambo,* both, + G. *a-* priv. + *geusis,* taste]

am·be·no·ni·um chlo·ride (am-bē-nō′nē-ŭm). A cholinesterase

inhibitor similar to neostigmine in actions; used chiefly in the management of myasthenia gravis and occasionally for intestinal and urinary tract obstruction.

AMBER (am′ber) Acronym for advanced multiple-beam equalization *radiography.*

am·ber (am′ber). **1.** A hard, dark yellow to tan, fossilized resin derived from pine trees. **2.** SEE amber *codon.* [Ar. *anbar*]

Amberg, Emil, U.S. otologist, 1868–1948. SEE A. lateral sinus *line.*

am·ber·gris (am′ber-gris). A grayish pathologic secretion from the intestine of the sperm whale that occurs as a flammable waxy mass (melting point about 60°C), insoluble in water; contains cholesterol and benzoic acid, and is used as a base for perfume. [Mod. L. *ambra grisea,* gray amber]

♲ambi-. Around; on all (both) sides; both, double; corresponds to G. amphi-. SEE ALSO ambo-. [L., around, about, akin to *ambo,* both]

am·bi·dex·ter·i·ty (am-bi-deks-ter′i-tē). The ability to use both hands with equal ease. SYN ambidextrism.

am·bi·dex·trism (am-bi-deks′trizm). SYN ambidexterity.

am·bi·dex·trous (am-bi-deks′trŭs). Having equal facility in the use of both hands.

am·bi·ent (am′bē-ent). Surrounding, encompassing; pertaining to the environment in which an organism or apparatus functions. [L. *ambiens,* going around]

am·bi·gu·i·ty (am-bi-goo′ĭ-tē). Condition of being ambiguous; uncertainty.

genital a., incomplete development of fetal genitalia as a result of excessive androgen action on a female fetus or inadequate amounts of androgen in a male fetus. SYN ambiguous external genitalia, ambiguous genitalia.

am·big·u·ous (am-big′ū-ŭs). **1.** Having more than one interpretation. **2.** In anatomy, wandering; having more than one direction. **3.** In neuroanatomy, applied to a nucleus (nucleus ambiguus) supplying special visceral efferent fibers to vagus and glossopharyngeal nerves. [L. *ambiguus,* fr. *ambigo,* to wander]

am·bi·lat·er·al (am-bi-lat′er-ăl). Relating to both sides. [ambi- + L. *latus,* side]

am·bi·le·vous (am-bi-lē′vŭs). Awkwardness in the use of both hands. SYN ambisinister, ambisinistrous. [ambi- + L. *laevus,* left]

am·bi·sex·u·al (am-bi-seks′ū-ăl). **1.** Denoting sexual characteristics found in both sexes, e.g., breast, pubic hair. **2.** Slang term for bisexual.

am·bi·sin·is·ter (am-bi-sin′is-ter). SYN ambilevous. [ambi- + L. *sinister,* left]

am·bi·si·nis·trous (am′bi-sin′is-trŭs). SYN ambilevous.

am·biv·a·lence (am-biv′ă-lens). The coexistence of antithetical attitudes or emotions toward a given person or thing, or idea, as in the simultaneous feeling and expression of love and hate toward the same person. [ambi- + L. *valentia,* strength]

am·biv·a·lent (am-biv′ă-lent). Relating to or characterized by ambivalence.

am·bi·vert (am′bi-vert). One who falls between the two extremes of introversion and extroversion, possessing some of the tendencies of each.

♲ambly-. Dullness, dimness; blunt, dull, dim, dimmed. [G. *amblys,* blunt, dulled; faint, dim]

am·bly·geus·tia (am-bli-goos′tē-ă). A diminution in the sense of taste. [ambly- + G. *geusis,* taste]

amblyogenic (am′blē-ō-jen′ic). Inducing amblyopia. [amblyopia + -genic]

Am·bly·om·ma (am-blē-om′ă). A genus of ornate, hard ticks (family Ixodidae) characterized by having eyes, festoons, and deeply imbedded ventral plates near the festoons in males. [ambly- + G. *omma,* eye, vision]

A. america′num, the Lone Star tick, a species that is an important pest and vector of Rocky Mountain spotted fever, found primarily in the southern United States and northern Mexico; it occurs on dogs and many other hosts, including domestic animals, birds, and humans, whom it bites in larval, nymphal, and adult stages.

A. cajennen'se, the Cayenne tick, a species that is an important pest in southern Texas, Central and South America, and the larger Caribbean islands, and a vector of Rocky Mountain spotted fever in Mexico and Central and South America; all stages attack humans and many species of domestic and wild animals.

A. hebrae'um, the South African bont tick, an important vector of heartwater in southern Africa.

A. macula'tum, the Gulf Coast tick, a species that is a pest of livestock in the southeastern United States.

A. variega'tum, the tropical bont tick, a serious pest of domestic livestock and an important vector of heartwater in Africa and the Caribbean; it is closely associated with the development of severe clinical dermatophilosis in cattle in the Caribbean.

am·bly·o·pia (am-blē-ō′pē-ă). Poor vision caused by abnormal development of visual areas of the brain in response to abnormal visual stimulation during early development. [G. *amblyōpia,* dimness of vision, fr. *amblys* dull, + *ōps,* eye]

anisometropic a., a suppression of central vision due to an unequal refractive error (anisometropia) of at least two diopters. This induces a sufficient difference in image size (aniseikonia) that the two images cannot be fused. In order to avoid confusion, the blurrier image is suppressed. SYN refractive a.

deprivation a., SYN sensory a.

a. ex anop′sia, SYN suppression a.

hysterical a., functional visual loss.

meridional a., a. due to an uncorrected, large astigmatism during the amblyogenic *period* of visual development.

nocturnal a., SYN nyctalopia.

nutritional a., a. resulting from lack of vitamin B–complex constituents.

pattern distortion a., a. due to a blurred retinal image during the amblyogenic *period* of visual development.

refractive a., SYN anisometropic a.

sensory a., a suppression of central vision in an eye due to poor image formation; e.g., by a corneal scar, a cataract, or a droopy eyelid. SYN deprivation a.

strabismic a., a suppression of central vision due to the two eyes pointing in different directions. The two scenes cannot be fused into a single image, so, to avoid confusion, one of the images is suppressed.

suppression a., suppression of the central vision in one eye when the images from the two eyes are so different that they cannot be fused into one. This may be due to: 1) faulty image formation (sensory a.); 2) a large difference in refraction between the two eyes (anisometropic a.); or 3) the two eyes pointing in different directions (strabismic a.). Most suppression a. can be reversed if appropriately treated before age 6 years. SYN a. ex anopsia.

tobacco-alcohol a., an acquired optic neuropathy particularly involving the maculopapillary bundle nerve fibers associated with excessive alcohol and tobacco consumption.

toxic a., SEE toxic *amaurosis.*

am·bly·o·pic (am-blē-ō′pik). Relating to, or suffering from, amblyopia.

am·bly·o·scope (am′blē-ō-skōp). A reflecting stereoscope used to evaluate or simulate binocular vision. SEE ALSO haploscope. [amblyopia + G. *skopeō,* to view]

major a., an a. in which intensity of illumination as well as targets may be varied.

Worth a., the original a.; a hand-held a. consisting of angled tubes that can be swiveled to any degree of convergence or divergence.

△**ambo-.** Around; on all (both) sides; corresponds to G. ampho-. SEE ALSO ambi-. [L. *ambo,* both]

am·bo·cep·tor (am′bō-sep-tŏr). Ehrlich term for his concept, now obsolete, of the structure of complement-fixing antibody; now used chiefly to denote the anti-sheep erythrocyte antibody used in the hemolytic system of complement-fixation tests. [ambo- + L. *capio,* to take]

am·bo·mal·le·al (am-bō-mal′ē-ăl). SYN incudomalleal.

am·bro·sin (am-brō′sin). A principle in ragweed related to absinthin.

am·bu·cet·a·mide (am-bū-set′ă-mīd). An intestinal antispasmodic.

am·bu·lance (am′bū-lans). A vehicle used to transport sick or injured persons to a treatment facility. [Fr., fr. *(hôpital) ambulant,* mobile hospital]

am·bu·la·to·ry, am·bu·lant (am′bū-lă-tōr-ē, am′bū-lant). Walking about or able to walk about; denoting a patient who is not confined to bed or hospital as a result of disease or surgery. [L. *ambulans,* walking]

am·bu·phyl·line (am-bū′fi-lin). A diuretic and bronchodilator.

am·cin·o·nide (am-sin′ō-nid). A glucocorticoid used topically in the treatment of dermatoses.

▣**ame·ba,** pl. **ame·bae, ame·bas** (ă-mē′bă, -bē, -băz). Common name for *Amoeba* and similar naked, lobose, sarcodine protozoa.

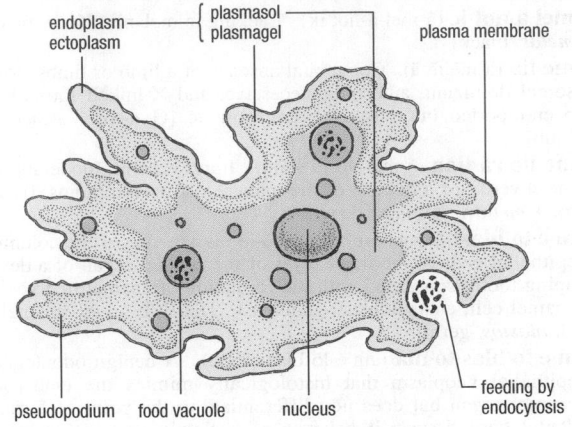

ameba

ame·ba·cide (ă-mē′bă-sīd). SYN amebicide.

ame·ba·ism (ă-mē′bă-izm). **1.** SYN ameboidism (1). **2.** SYN ameboididity.

am·e·bi·a·sis (ă-mē-bī′ă-sis). Infection with the protozoon *Entamoeba histolytica.* [ameba + G. *-iasis,* condition]

canine a., infection of dogs with *Entamoeba histolytica* acquired from humans; dogs are seldom cyst passers, and therefore are not a reservoir for human infection.

a. cu′tis, cutaneous a., appearing usually as an extension of underlying infection (e.g., perianal or colostomy site or over a liver abscess).

hepatic a., infection of the liver with *Entamoeba histolytica;* may occur with or without antecedent amebic dysentery.

pulmonary a., infection of the lung by amebae; usually indicates extension of *Entamoeba histolytica* infection from abscess of liver, penetrating through the diaphragm into the lung.

ame·bic (ă-mē′bik). Relating to, resembling, or caused by amebas.

ame·bi·ci·dal (ă-mē-bi-sī′dăl). Destructive to amebas.

ame·bi·cide (ă-mē′bi-sīd). Any agent that causes the destruction of amebas. SYN amebacide. [ameba + L. *caedo,* to kill]

ame·bi·form (ă-mē′bi-fōrm). Of the shape or appearance of an ameba. [ameba + L. *forma,* shape]

am·e·bi·o·sis (ă-mē-bī-ō′sis). Obsolete term for amebiasis.

ame·bism (ă-mē′bizm). Obsolete term for amebiasis.

ame·bo·cyte (ă-mē′bō-sīt). **1.** A wandering cell found in invertebrates. **2.** Obsolete term for leukocyte. **3.** An in vitro tissue culture leukocyte. [ameba, + *kytos,* cell]

ame·boid (ă-mē′boyd). **1.** Resembling an ameba in appearance or characteristics. **2.** Of irregular outline with peripheral projections; denoting the outline of a form of colony in plate culture. [ameba + G. *eidos,* appearance]

ame·boi·did·i·ty (ă-mē-boy-did′i-tē). The power of locomotion after the manner of an ameboid cell. SYN amebaism (2).

ame·boid·ism (ă-mē′boyd-izm). **1.** The performance of movements similar to those of an ameba. SYN amebaism (1). **2.** Denoting a condition sometimes seen in certain nerve cells.

am·e·bo·ma (ă-mē-bō′mă). A nodular, tumorlike focus of proliferative inflammation sometimes developing in chronic amebiasis, especially in the wall of the colon. SYN amebic granuloma. [ameba + G. -oma, tumor]

ame·bu·la, pl. **ame·bu·lae** (ă-mē′bū-lă, -lē). Term applied to the excysted young amebas of Entamoeba species that emerge from the cyst in the human or vertebrate gut and their immediate progeny, usually totalling eight, prior to their localization in the large intestine. [fr. G. amoibē, a change, alteration]

ame·bule (ă-mē′būl). A minute ameba.

am·e·bu·ria (am-ē-bū′rē-ă). The presence of amebas in the urine. [ameba + G. ouron, urine]

amel·a·not·ic (ă-mel-ă-not′ik). Lacking in melanin. [G. a- priv. + melas, black]

ame·lia (ă-mē′lē-ă). Congenital absence of a limb or limbs. Autosomal dominant, autosomal recessive, and X-linked forms have been reported, but most cases are sporadic. [G. a- priv. + melos, a limb]

ame·lio·ra·tion (ă-mēl-yō-rā′shŭn). Improvement; moderation in the severity of a disease or the intensity of its symptoms. [L. ad, to, + melioro, to make better]

am·e·lo·blast (ă-mel′ō-blast, am-ĕ-lō′blast). One of the columnar epithelial cells of the inner layer of the enamel organ of a developing tooth, concerned with the formation of enamel matrix. SYN enamel cell, enameloblast, ganoblast. [Early E. amel, enamel, + G. blastos, germ]

am·e·lo·blas·to·ma (am′ĕ-lō-blas-tō′mă). A benign odontogenic epithelial neoplasm that histologically mimics the embryonal enamel organ but does not differentiate to the point of forming dental hard tissues; it behaves as a slowly growing expansile radiolucent tumor, occurs most commonly in the posterior regions of the mandible, and has a marked tendency to recur if inadequately excised. [ameloblast + G. -oma, tumor]

pigmented a., SYN melanotic neuroectodermal tumor of infancy.

pituitary a., SYN craniopharyngioma.

am·e·lo·den·tin·al (am′ĕ-lō-den′ti-năl). SYN dentinoenamel.

am·e·lo·gen·e·sis (am′ĕ-lō-jen′ĕ-sis). The deposition and maturation of enamel. SYN enamelogenesis.

a. imperfec′ta, a group of hereditary ectodermal disorders in which the enamel is defective in structure or deficient in quantity. Three major groups are recognized: hypoplastic types, with defective enamel matrix deposition but normal mineralization; hypomineralization types, with normal matrix but defective mineralization; and hypomaturation type, in which the enamel crystallites remain immature. The several types may be inherited as autosomal dominant [MIM*104500, 104510, 104530], recessive [MIM*204650, 204690, 204700] or X-linked [MIM*301100, 301200, 301201]. SYN enamel dysplasia, enamelogenesis imperfecta.

a·mel·o·gen·ins (am′el-ō-jen′inz). A class of proteins that form much of the organic matrix during the early development of tooth enamel. [amelogenesis + -in]

ame·nia (ă-mē′nē-ă). Rarely used term for amenorrhea. [G. a- priv. + mēn, month]

amen·or·rhea (ă-men-ō-rē′ă). Absence or abnormal cessation of the menses. [G. a- priv. + mēn, month, + rhoia, flow]

dietary a., loss of menstrual function due to severe weight loss or gain.

emotional a., a. caused by a strong emotional disturbance, e.g., fright, grief.

exercise-induced a., temporary cessation of menstrual function due to strenuous, daily exercise, as in jogging, increased endorphins inhibiting hypothalamic function.

hyperprolactinemic a., a. associated with abnormally high levels of serum prolactin; may be accompanied by unphysiological lactation.

hypophysial a., a. due to inadequate gonadotrophic secretions by the anterior lobe of the hypophysis.

hypothalamic a., secondary a. arising from defective hypothalamic stimulation of the anterior lobe of the pituitary.

lactation a., physiological suppression of menses while nursing.

ovarian a., a. due to deficiency of estrogenic hormone production by ovary. often referred to menopause if permanent.

pathologic a., a. due to organic disease, either uterine or other, e.g., ovarian or pituitary failure.

physiologic a., a. of pregnancy or the menopause, not associated with an organic disorder.

postpartum a., permanent a. following childbirth resulting from Sheehan syndrome. SEE Sheehan syndrome.

primary a., a. in which the menses have never occurred.

secondary a., a. in which the menses appeared at puberty but subsequently ceased.

traumatic a., absence of menses because of endometrial scarring or cervical stenosis resulting from injury or disease. SYN Asherman syndrome.

amen·or·rhe·al, amen·or·rhe·ic (ă-men-ō-rē′ăl, -rē′ik). Relating to, accompanied by, or due to amenorrhea.

amen·tia (ă-men′shē-ă). **1.** SYN mental retardation. **2.** SYN dementia. [L. madness, fr. ab, from, + mens, mind]

nevoid a., SYN Brushfield-Wyatt disease.

phenylpyruvic a., a. accompanied by the appearance of phenylpyruvate in the urine.

amen·ti·al (ă-men′shē-al). Pertaining to amentia.

Amer·i·can Law In·sti·tute for·mu·la·tion. Used in certain jurisdictions to determine criminal responsibility in legal proceedings. SEE criminal insanity.

Amer·i·can Law In·sti·tute rule. See under rule.

American National Standards Institute (ANSI). Organization that sets standards for physical measures in the United States.

Amer·i·can Red Cross. The national Red Cross society of the United States, established by Congress to assist in caring for the sick and wounded, serving as a communications link between members of the U.S. armed forces and their families, conducting disaster relief and prevention programs, and furnishing other humanitarian services, the largest of which is a network of regional blood centers providing blood and blood products.

am·er·i·ci·um (Am) (am′ĕ-ris′ē-ŭm). An element obtained by the bombardment of uranium with neutrons or β decay of plutoniums 241, 242, and 243; atomic no. 95; atomic weight 243.06. ^{241}Am (half-life of 432.2 years) has been used in the diagnosis of bone disorders. ^{243}Am has a half-life of 7370 years. [the Americas]

am·er·ism (am′er-izm). The condition or quality of not dividing into parts, segments, or merozoites. [G. a- priv. + meros, part]

am·er·is·tic (am-ĕ-ris′tik). Endowed with amerism; not dividing into parts or segments.

Ames, Bruce N., U.S. molecular geneticist, *1928. SEE A. assay, test.

am·e·thop·ter·in (ă-meth-ō-ter′in, am-ĕ-thop′tĕ-rin). SYN methotrexate.

ame·tria (ă-mē′trē-ă). Congenital absence of the uterus; the genetics is obscure. [G. a- priv. + mētra, uterus]

ame·tri·o·din·ic ac·id (ă′mĕ-trī-ō-din′ik). SYN iodamide.

am·e·tro·pia (am-ĕ-trō′pē-ă). The optic condition in which there is an error of refraction so that with the eye at rest the retina is not in conjugate focus with light rays from distant objects, i.e., only less distant objects are focused on the retina. [G. ametros, disproportionate, fr. a- priv. + metron, measure, + ōps, eye]

axial a., that resulting from a shortening or lengthening of the eyeball on the optic axis, causing hyperopia or myopia, respectively.

index a., that resulting from alteration in the refractive index of the lens of the eye. SYN refractive a.

refractive a., SYN index a.

am·e·tro·pic (am-ĕ-trō′pik). Relating to, or suffering from, ametropia.

am·i·an·ta·ceous (am′i-an-tā′shŭs). Asbestos-like; describing thin plates of inflammatory crusting of a cutaneous lesion. [G. *amiantus*, asbestos]

am·i·an·thoid (am-i-an'thoyd). Having a crystalline appearance like asbestos. SYN asbestoid. [G. *amianthus*, asbestos]

⊘**-amic.** Chemical suffix denoting the replacement of one COOH group of a dicarboxylic acid by a carboxamide group (–CONH₂); applied only to trivial names (e.g., succinamic acid).

ami·cro·bic (ā-mī-krō'bik). Not microbic; not related to or caused by microorganisms.

ami·cro·scop·ic (ā'mī-krō-skop'ik). SYN submicroscopic.

am·i·dase (am'i-dās). An enzyme that catalyzes the hydrolysis of monocarboxylic amides to free acid plus NH₃; ω-a. acts on amides such as α-ketoglutaramic acid and α-ketosuccinamic acid.

am·i·das·es. SYN amidohydrolases.

am·ide (am'īd, am'id). A substance formally derived from ammonia through the substitution of one or more of the hydrogen atoms by acyl groups, R–CO–NH₂, or from a carboxylic acid by replacement of a carboxylic OH by NH₂. Replacement of one hydrogen atom constitutes a **primary a.**; that of two hydrogen atoms, a **secondary a.**; and that of three atoms, a **tertiary a.**.

substituted a., a secondary or tertiary a.; peptide linkages are substituted a.'s.

am·i·dine (am'i-din). The monovalent radical —C(NH)-NH₂.

am·i·di·no·hy·dro·las·es (am'i-din-ō-hī'drō-lās-ez) [EC 3.5.3.x]. Enzymes cleaving linear amidines; e.g., arginase, creatinase.

am·i·din·o·trans·fer·as·es (am'i-din-ō-trans'fer-ās-ez) [EC 2.1.4.x]. Enzymes catalyzing a transamidination reaction (e.g., glycine amidinotransferase). SYN transamidinases.

⊘**amido-.** Prefix denoting the amide radical, R–CO–NH– or R–SO₂–NH–, etc. [am(monia) + -id(e) + -o-]

ami·do black 10B (am'i-dō) [C.I. 20470]. An acid diazo dye, C₁₂H₁₄N₆O₉S₂Na₂, used as a connective tissue stain, for staining protein in paper chromatography, and in electrophoresis.

ami·do·hy·dro·las·es (am'i-dō-hī'drō-lā-sez) [EC 3.5.1.x and 3.5.2.x]. Enzymes hydrolyzing C–N bonds of amides and cyclic amides; e.g., asparaginase, barbiturase, urease, amidase. SYN amidases, deamidases, deamidizing enzymes.

ami·do·naph·thol red (am'i-dō-naf'thol) [C.I. 18050]. An azo dye, C₁₈H₁₃N₃S₂Na₂, used in light and fluorescence microscopy as a real acid counterstain. SYN azophloxin.

ami·do·py·rine (am-i-dō-pī'rēn). SYN aminopyrine.

Am·i·dos·to·mum an·ser·is (am-i-dos'tō-mŭm an'ser-is). A species of bloodsucking nematodes, similar to those of the genus *Trichostrongylus*, that parasitizes the gizzard and sometimes also the proventriculus and esophagus of domestic and wild ducks and geese; it causes heavy mortality in young birds. [amido- + G. *stoma*, mouth, + L. *anser*, goose]

am·i·dox·imes (am-i-doks'īmz, -dok'sēmz). The oximes of amides with the general formula, R–C(NH₂)–NOH. SYN amide oximes.

am·i·dox·yl (am-i-dok'sil). The radical of an amide oxime (amidoxime), the terminal H (of the NOH) having been lost.

am·i·ka·cin sul·fate (am-i-kā'sin). An aminoglycoside antibiotic agent with antimicrobial activity similar to that of kanamycin; also effective against *Pseudomonas aeruginosa*.

amil·o·ride hy·dro·chlo·ride (ă-mil'ō-rīd). A nonsteroidal compound exerting an effect similar to that of an aldosterone inhibitor, i.e., urinary sodium excretion is enhanced and potassium excretion is reduced; a potassium sparing diuretic.

amim·ia (ā-mim'ē-a). **1.** Inability to express ideas by nonverbal communication, such as gestures or signs. **2.** Asymbolia; the inability to comprehend the meaning of gestures, signs, symbols, or pantomime. [G. *a-* priv. + *minos*, a mimic]

am·i·nac·rine hy·dro·chlo·ride (am'i-nak'rin). Bactericidal agent for external use. SEE ALSO acridine yellow. SYN 5-aminoacridine hydrochloride, 9-aminoacridine hydrochloride.

am·i·nate (am'i-nāt). To combine with ammonia.

am·i·na·tion (ă-me-nā'shŭn). The introduction of an amine moiety into a compound.

amine (ă-mēn', am'in). A substance formally derived from ammonia by the replacement of one or more of the hydrogen atoms by hydrocarbon or other radicals. The substitution of one hydrogen atom constitutes a **primary a.**, e.g., NH₂CH₃; that of two atoms, a **secondary a.**, e.g., NH(CH₃)₂; that of three atoms, a **tertiary a.**, e.g., N(CH₃)₃; and that of four atoms, a **quaternary ammonium ion**, e.g., ⁺N(CH₃)₄, a positively charged ion isolated only in association with a negative ion. The a.'s form salts with acids.

adrenergic a., SYN sympathomimetic a.

adrenomimetic a., SYN sympathomimetic a.

biogenic a.'s, a class of compounds, each containing an a. group, produced by a living organism. This class normally does not include amino acids.

a. oxidase (copper-containing), an oxidoreductase containing copper, and perhaps pyridoxal phosphate, and carrying out the same reaction as a. oxidase (flavin-containing). SYN diamine oxidase, histaminase.

a. oxidase (flavin-containing), an oxidoreductase containing flavin and oxidizing amines with the aid of O₂ and water to aldehydes or ketones with the release of NH₃ and H₂O₂. Acted upon by antidepressants. SYN adrenaline oxidase, diamine oxidase, monoamine oxidase, tyraminase, tyramine oxidase.

pressor a., SYN pressor *base*.

sympathetic a., SYN sympathomimetic a.

sympathomimetic a., an agent that evokes responses similar to those produced by adrenergic nerve activity (e.g., epinephrine, ephedrine, isoproterenol). SYN adrenergic a., adrenomimetic a., sympathetic a.

vasoactive a., a substance, such as histamine or serotonin, that contains amino groups and is pharmacologically characterized by its action on the blood vessels (altering vascular caliber or permeability).

am·in·er·gic (ă-mēn'er-gik). Relating to nerve cells or fibers.

⊘**amino-.** Prefix denoting a compound containing the radical, –NH₂. [am(monia) + in(e) + -o-]

ami·no ac·id (AA, aa) (ă-mē'nō). An organic acid in which one of the hydrogen atoms on a carbon atom has been replaced by NH₂. Usually refers to an aminocarboxylic acid. However, taurine is also an a. a. SEE ALSO α-amino acid.

acidic a. a., an a. a. with a second acid moiety, e.g., glutamic acid, aspartic acid, cysteic acid.

activated a. a., SYN aminoacyl adenylate.

basic a. a., an a. a. containing a second basic group (usually an amino group); e.g., lysine, arginine, ornithine. SYN dibasic a. a.

a. a. dehydrogenases, enzymes catalyzing the oxidative deamination of amino acids to the corresponding OXO (keto) acids; two relatively nonspecific varieties exist, L and D, for which L-amino acids and D-amino acids are the respective substrates; the products include NH₃ and a reduced hydrogen acceptor (NADH in the L case); a. a. dehydrogenases of greater specificity exist (e.g., glycine dehydrogenase). Cf. a. a. oxidases.

dibasic a. a., SYN basic a. a.

essential a. a.'s, α-amino acids nutritionally required by an organism and which must be supplied in its diet (i.e., cannot be synthesized by the organism) either as free a. a. or in proteins.

nonessential a. a.'s, those a. a.'s that may be synthesized by an organism and are thus not required as such in its diet.

nonpolar a. a., an α-a. a. in which the functional group attached to the α-carbon (i.e., R in RCH(NH₂)COOH) has hydrophobic properties; e.g., valine, leucine, α-aminobutyrate.

a. a. oxidases, flavoenzymes oxidizing, with O₂ and H₂O, either L- or D-amino acids specifically, to the corresponding 2-keto acids, NH₃ and H₂O₂. Cf. a. a. dehydrogenases, yellow *enzyme*.

polar a. a., an α-a. a. in which the functional group attached to the α-carbon (i.e., R in RCH(NH₂)COOH) has hydrophilic properties; e.g., serine, cysteine, homocysteine.

α-ami·no ac·id. Typically, an amino acid of the general formula R–CHNH₂–COOH (i.e., the NH₂ in the α position). The L forms of these are the hydrolysis products of proteins. In rarer usages, this class of molecules also includes α-amino phosphoric acids and α-aminosulfonic acids.

ami·no·ac·i·de·mia (ă-mē'nō-as-i-dē'mē-ă, am'i-nō-). The presence of excessive amounts of specific amino acids in the blood. [amino acid + G. *haima*, blood]

ami·no·ac·id-tRNA li·gas·es. Recommended name for amino-acyl-tRNA synthetases, e.g., tyrosine-tRNA ligase for tyrosyl-tRNA synthetase.

ami·no·ac·i·du·ria (am′i-nō-as-i-doo′rē-ă). Excretion of amino acids in the urine, especially in excessive amounts. SYN hyperaminoaciduria. [amino acid + G. *ouron*, urine]

hyperbasic aminoaciduria, an inherited disorder associated with a deficiency of a dibasic amino acid transport. Individuals do not typically display protein intolerance. Cf. lysinuric protein *intolerance.*

9-ami·no·ac·ri·dine (ă-mē-nō-ak′ri-dēn). One of the acridine group of antiseptics (flavins); highly fluorescent in solution; used topically as an antiseptic.

5-ami·no·ac·ri·dine hy·dro·chlo·ride, 9-ami·no·ac·ri·dine hy·dro·chlo·ride. SYN acridine yellow, aminacrine hydrochloride.

ami·no·ac·yl (AA, aa) (ă-mē′nō-as′il). The radical formed from an amino acid by removal of OH from a COOH group.

ami·no·ac·yl a·den·y·late (ă-mē′nō-as-il-ă-den′i-lāt). The product formed by the condensation of the acyl radical of an amino acid and adenosine 5′-monophosphate (originally in the form of adenosine 5′-triphosphate, with elimination of a pyrophosphoric group). Formed in the first step of protein biosynthesis. SYN activated amino acid.

ami·no·ac·yl·ase (ă-mē′nō-as′i-lās). An enzyme catalyzing hydrolysis of a wide variety of *N*-acyl amino acids to the corresponding amino acid and an acid anion. SYN hippuricase, histozyme.

ami·no·ac·yl-tRNA. Generic term for those compounds in which amino acids are esterfied through their COOH groups to the 3′- (or 2′-) OH's of the terminal adenosine residues of transfer RNA's (e.g., alanyl-tRNA, glycyl-tRNA); each compound involves one, or a small number, of tRNA's of specific chemical structure. Used in protein biosynthesis.

a.-tRNA ligases, SYN a.-tRNA synthetases.

a.-tRNA synthetases, enzymes catalyzing the formation of a specific a.-tRNA from an amino acid and adenosine 5′-triphosphate with the concomitant formation of adenosine 5′-monophosphate and pyrophosphate. SYN amino acid activating enzyme, a.-tRNA ligases.

ami·no·a·dip·ic δ-sem·i·al·de·hyde syn·thase. A bifunctional enzyme used in lysine degradation; it has a lysine:α-ketoglutarate reductase activity as well as a saccharopine dehydrogenase activity. A deficiency of this enzyme results in familial hyperlysinemia.

α-ami·no·a·dip·ic ac·id (Aad) (ă-mē′nō-ă-dip′ik). 2-amino-1,6-hexanedioic acid; an intermediate of lysine biosynthesis in higher fungi and bacteria, but not in algae and higher plants. Also found in the degradation of lysine in mammals.

ami·no·ben·zene (ă-mē′nō-ben′zēn). SYN aniline.

o-**ami·no·ben·zo·ic ac·id** (ă-mē′nō-ben-zō′ik). SYN anthranilic acid.

p-**ami·no·ben·zo·ic ac·id (PABA).** A factor in the vitamin B complex, a part of all folic acids and required for its formation; neutralizes the bacteriostatic effects of the sulfonamides since it furnishes an essential growth factor for bacteria, with the utilization of which the sulfonamides interfere; used as an ultraviolet screen in lotions and creams. It is produced in a test of pancreatic function. SYN paraaminobenzoic acid, vitamin B$_x$.

D(-)-**α-ami·no·ben·zyl·pen·i·cil·lin** (ă-mē-nō-ben′zil-pen-i-sil′in). SYN ampicillin.

γ-ami·no·bu·tyr·ic ac·id (GABA, γ-Abu) (ă-mē′nō-bū-tēr′ik). 4-Aminobutyric acid; a constituent of the central nervous system; quantitatively the principal inhibitory neurotransmitter. Used in the treatment of a number of disorders (e.g., epilepsy).

δ-ami·no·bu·tyr·ic ac·id amino transferase. An enzyme catalyzing the reversible transfer of an amino group from δ-aminobutyric acid to 2-oxoglutarate, thus forming a L-glutamic acid and succinate semialdehyde. An important step in the catabolism of δ-aminobutyric acid.

ami·no·ca·pro·ic ac·id (ă-mē′nō-că-prō′ik). An antifibrinolytic agent, used to prevent bleeding in hemophilia, and after heart and prostate surgery when plasminogen or urokinase may be activated.

am·i·no·car·bon·yl (am-i-nō-kar′bon-il). SYN carboxamide.

ami·no·cit·ric ac·id (ă-mē′no-sit′rik). Found in acid hydrolysates of ribonucleoprotein in human spleen.

2-ami·no-2-de·oxy-D-ga·lac·tose. SEE galactosamine.

ami·no·glu·teth·i·mide (ă-mē′nō-gloo-teth′i-mīd). An aromatase inhibitor used in the treatment of breast cancer; blocks the synthesis of estrogen; formerly tried as an anticonvulsant but no longer used for that purpose.

am·i·no·gly·co·side (am′i-nō-glī′kō-sīd). Any one of a group of bacteriocidal antibiotics derived from species of *Streptomyces* or *Micromonosporum* and characterized by two or more amino sugars joined by a glycoside linkage to a central hexose; a.'s act by causing misreading and inhibition of protein synthesis on bacterial ribosomes and are effective against aerobic Gram-negative bacilli and *Mycobacterium tuberculosis*. Some commonly used a.'s are streptomycin, neomycin, and gentamycin.

p-**ami·no·hip·pu·ric ac·id (PAH)** (ă-mē′nō-hi-pūr′ik). Used in renal function tests to measure renal plasma flow; actively secreted (and filtered) by the kidney.

p.-a. a. synthase, an enzyme in the liver that catalyzes the synthesis of *p*-aminohippuric acid from *p*-aminobenzoic acid (or the CoA derivative) and glycine. It may be identical with glycine acyltransferase.

5-ami·no·im·id·az·ole ri·bose 5′-phos·phate (AIR) (ă-mē′nō-im-id-āz′ōl). An intermediate in the biosynthesis of purines. SYN 5-aminoimidazole ribotide.

5-ami·no·im·id·az·ole ri·bo·tide (AIR) (ă-mē′n′o-im-id-āz′ōl). SYN 5-aminoimidazole ribose 5′-phosphate.

5-ami·no·im·id·az·ole-4-*N*-suc·ci·no·car·box·am·ide ri·bo·nu·cle·o·tide (ă-mē′nō-im-id-āz′ōl). An intermediate in purine biosynthesis.

β-ami·no·iso·bu·ty·rate:py·ru·vate ami·no·trans·fer·ase. β-Aminosiobutyrate:pyruvate transaminase; an enzyme that catalyzes the reversible transfer of an amino group from β-aminoisobutyrate to pyruvate, producing L-alanine and methylmalonate semialdehyde, a step in valine degradation. A deficiency of this enzyme results in hyper-β-aminoisobutyric aciduria.

α-ami·no·i·so·bu·tyr·ic ac·id (ă-mē′nō-ī-sō-bū-tēr′ik). 2-amino-2-methylpropionic acid; a synthetic amino acid useful in the study of amino acid transport across cell membranes and in the study of cytokine effects; it is not metabolized by the cell.

β-ami·no·i·so·bu·tyr·ic ac·id. 3-Amino-2-methylpropionic acid; an end product of thymine catabolism; high urinary levels (200–300 mg/day) have been noted in some individuals, either from some disease process or following a genetic pattern.

α-ami·no-β-ke·to·a·dip·ic ac·id. An intermediate of porphobilinogen synthesis formed by δ-aminolevulinic acid synthase from succinyl-CoA and glycine; it rapidly decarboxylates to δ-aminolevulinic acid.

δ-ami·no·lev·u·li·nate de·hy·dra·tase (ă-mē′nō-lev-ū-lin′āt). SYN *porphobilinogen* synthase.

δ-ami·no·lev·u·lin·ic ac·id (ALA) (ă-mē′nō-lev-ū-lin′ik). An acid formed by δ-aminolevulinate synthase from glycine and succinyl-coenzyme A; a precursor of porphobilinogen, hence an important intermediate in the biosynthesis of heme. ALA levels are elevated in cases of lead poisoning.

δ-aminolevulinic acid synthase, an enzyme that catalyzes the reaction of succinyl-CoA with glycine to form δ-aminolevulinic acid, coenzyme A, and CO_2. The committed step in porphyrin biosynthesis.

am·i·nol·y·sis (am-i-nol′i-sis). Replacement of a halogen in an alkyl or aryl molecule by an amine radical, with elimination of hydrogen halide.

ami·no·met·ra·dine (ă-mē′nō-met′ră-dēn). SYN aminometramide.

ami·no·met·ra·mide (ă-mē′nō-met′ră-mīd). Synthetic uracil derivative; an orally effective diuretic that is believed to act by inhibiting the reabsorption of sodium by the renal tubules; used in the treatment of edema due to congestive heart failure, liver disease, pregnancy, and certain drugs. SYN aminometradine.

6-ami·no·pen·i·cil·lan·ic ac·id (6-APS) (ă-mē′nō-pen-i-sil-ăn′ ik). An important precursor in the synthesis of penicillin derivatives. By itself, it has no antibiotic activity. For structure, see under penicillin in which R = H. SYN penicin.

ami·no·pen·i·cil·lins (ă-mē′nō-pen-i-sil′inz). A class of penicillin-like antibiotics that chemically contain an amine group; this class includes ampicillin and amoxicillin; used in upper respiratory infections, urinary tract infections, meningitis, *Salmonella* infections.

ami·no·pep·ti·dase (cy·to·sol). An enzyme of broad specificity, containing zinc, and catalyzing the hydrolysis of the N-terminal amino acid of a peptide (i.e., an exopeptidase).

ami·no·pep·ti·dase (mi·cro·som·al). An aminopeptidase of broad specificity, but preferring alanine and discriminating against proline.

ami·no·pep·ti·das·es (ă-mē′nō-pep′ti-dās-ez) [EC 3.4.11.x]. Enzymes catalyzing the breakdown of a peptide, removing the amino acid at the amino end of the chain (i.e., an exopeptidase); found in intestinal secretions.

ami·no·phen·a·zone (ă-mē-nō-fen′ă-zōn). SYN aminopyrine.

ami·no·phyl·line (ă-mē-nō-fil′in, am-i-nof′i-lin, -ēn). A solubilized form of theophylline; a diuretic, vasodilator, and cardiac stimulant; also used as a bronchodilator in asthma and in veterinary medicine. SYN theophylline ethylenediamine.

ami·no·pro·ma·zine (ă-mē-nō-prō′mă-zēn). An intestinal antispasmodic.

ami·no·pro·pi·on·ic ac·id (ă-mē′nō-prō-pē-on′ik). SEE alanine.

p-ami·no·pro·pi·o·phe·none (PAPP) (ă-mē′nō-prō-pē-ō-fē′ nōn). An antidote for cyanide poisoning.

am·i·nop·ter·in (am-i-nop′ter-in). A folic acid antagonist formerly used in the treatment of acute leukemia and other neoplastic diseases.

6-ami·no·pu·rine (ă-mē′nō-pūr′ēn). SYN adenine.

4-ami·no·pyr·i·dine (am-i-nō-pir′i-dēn). An antagonist of nondepolarizing neuromuscular blockade; devoid of muscarinic side-effects but associated with central nervous system stimulation.

ami·no·py·rine (am′i-nō-pī′rēn). Formerly widely used as an antipyretic and analgesic in rheumatism, neuritis, and common colds; may cause leukocytopenia; used to measure total body water. SYN amidopyrine, aminophenazone, dipyrine.

amin·o·rex (ă-min′ō-reks). A sympathomimetic appetite suppressant.

p-ami·no·sal·i·cyl·ic ac·id (PAS, PASA) (am′i-nō-sal-i-sil′ik). A bacteriostatic agent against tubercle bacilli, used as a second-line agent; potassium, sodium, and calcium salts have the same use.

ami·no·ter·mi·nal (ă-mē′nō-ter′min-ăl). The α-NH$_2$ group or the aminoacyl residue containing it at one end of a peptide or protein (usually at left as written). SYN NH$_2$-terminal.

ami·no·trans·fer·as·es (ă-mē′nō-trans′fer-ās-ez) [EC 2.6.1.x]. Enzymes transferring amino groups between an amino acid to (usually) a 2-keto acid; e.g., L-alanine and 2-ketoglutarate. Often, the amino acid is an α-amino acid. SYN transaminases.

ami·no·tri·a·zole (ă-mē′i-nō-trī′ă-zol). An effective weed killer that also possesses some antithyroid activity. SYN amitrole.

ami·no·tri·pep·tid·ase (ă-mē′nō-trī-pep′tă-dās). An intestinal peptidase that acts on tripeptides, releasing an amino acid and a dipeptide.

ami·i·nu·ria (am-i-noo′rē-ă). Excretion of amines in the urine. [amine + G. *ouron*, urine]

ami·o·da·rone hy·dro·chlo·ride (ă-mē′ō-dă-rōn). An antiarrhythmic agent used in control of ventricular and supraventricular arrhythmias. Can cause significant and distinctive pulmonary toxicity.

am·i·thi·o·zone (am-i-thī′ō-zōn). A leprostatic agent. SYN thiacetazone.

ami·to·sis (am-i-tō′sis). Direct division of the nucleus and cell,

without the complicated changes in the nucleus that occur in the ordinary process of cell reproduction. SYN direct nuclear division, Remak nuclear division. [G. *a-* priv. + mitosis]

ami·tot·ic (am-i-tot′ik). Relating to or marked by amitosis.

am·i·trip·ty·line hy·dro·chlo·ride (am-i-trip′ti-lēn). Chemically and pharmacologically related to imipramine hydrochloride; an antidepressant agent with mild tranquilizing properties, used in the treatment of mental depression and in the depressive phase of manic-depressive states; sometimes used in the treatment of sleep disorders and neurogenic pain syndromes.

am·i·trole (am′i-trōl). SYN aminotriazole.

am·lo·dip·ine (am-lō′dī-pēn). A calcium-blocking drug of the dihydropyridine series; belongs to the same class of agents as nifedipine.

am·me·ter (am) (am′mē-ter). An instrument for measuring strength of electric current in amperes.

Ammon, Friedrich A. von, German ophthalmologist and pathologist, 1799–1861. SEE A. *fissure, prominence.*

Ammon, Greek name of Egyptian god, Amun. SEE A. *horn.*

am·mo·ne·mia, am·mo·ni·e·mia (am-ō-nē′mē-ă). The presence of ammonia or some of its compounds in the blood, thought to be formed from the decomposition of urea; it usually results in subnormal temperature, weak pulse, gastroenteric symptoms, and coma. SYN hyperammonemia. [ammonia + G. *haima*, blood]

am·mo·nia (ă-mō′nē-ă). A colorless volatile gas, NH$_3$, very soluble in water, capable of forming the weak base, NH$_4^+$OH$^-$, which combines with acids to form ammonium compounds. [fr. L. *sal ammoniacus*, salt of Amen (G. *Ammōn*), obtained near a temple of Amen in Libya]

am·mo·ni·ac (ă-mō′nē-ak). A gum resin from a plant of western Asia, *Dorema ammoniacum* (family Umbelliferae); used internally as a stimulant and expectorant, and externally as a counterirritant plaster.

am·mo·ni·a·cal (ă-mō′nī′ă-kl). Relating to ammonia.

am·mo·nia-ly·as·es. Enzymes removing ammonia or an amino compound nonhydrolytically (hence lyases, EC class 4), by rupture of a C–N bond leaving a double bond (EC subgroup 4.3); e.g., aspartate ammonia-lyase (aspartase).

am·mo·ni·at·ed (ă-mō′nē-āt-ed). Containing or combined with ammonia.

△**ammonio-.** Combining form indicating an ammonium group; e.g., trimethylammonioethanol (choline).

am·mo·ni·um (ă-mō′nē-ŭm). The ion, NH$_4^+$, formed by combination of NH$_3$ and H$^+$ (the pK_a value is 9.24); behaves as a univalent metal in forming ammonium compounds.

a. benzoate, has been used as a stimulant, diuretic, urinary antiseptic, and antirheumatic.

a. carbonate, (NH$_4$)$_2$CO$_3$; a cardiac and respiratory stimulant and carminative expectorant.

a. chloride, NH$_4$Cl; a stimulant expectorant and cholagogue; used to relieve alkalosis and to promote lead excretion; a urinary acidifier. SYN sal ammoniac.

dibasic a. phosphate, (NH$_4$)$_2$HPO$_4$; used for fireproofing, in baking powder, and as an antirheumatic.

a. ferric sulfate, SYN *ferric* ammonium sulfate.

a. ichthosulfonate, SYN ichthammol.

a. iodide, NH$_4$I; an expectorant.

a. mandelate, mandelic acid ammonium salt; a urinary antiseptic.

a. molybdate, used in electron microscopy as a negative stain, and as a reagent for alkaloids and other substances.

monobasic a. phosphate, used in baking powder.

a. nitrate, used in making nitrous oxide gas, in freezing mixtures, matches, and fertilizers; also used in veterinary medicine.

am·mo·ni·u·ria (ă-mō-nē-ū′rē-ă). Excretion of urine that contains an excessive amount of ammonia. SYN ammoniacal urine. [ammonia + G. *ouron*, urine]

am·mo·nol·y·sis (ă-mō-nol′i-sis). The breaking of a chemical bond with the addition of the elements of ammonia (NH$_2$ and H) at the point of breakage. [ammonia + G. *lysis*, dissolution]

am·mo·no·tel·ia (ă-mōn-ō-tēl′-e-ă). The process or type of nitro-

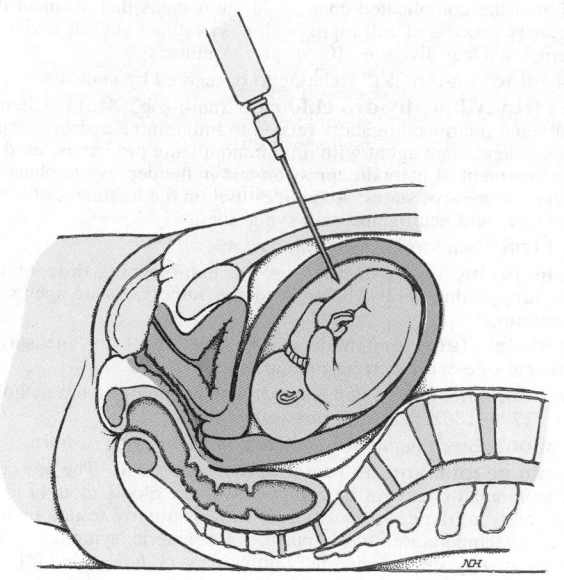

amniocentesis

gen excretion in which ammonia and ammonium ions are the primary form by which nitrogen is excreted from an organism. [ammonia + G. *telos*, end, outcome, + -ia]

am·mo·no·tel·ic (ă-mōn-ō-tēl'ik). Having the property of ammonotelism.

am·mo·no·tel·ism (ă-mōn-ō-tēl'izm). The excretion of ammonia and ammonium ions. Cf. ammonotelia.

am·ne·sia (am-nē'zē-ă). A disturbance in the memory of information stored in long-term memory, in contrast to short-term memory, manifested by total or partial inability to recall past experiences. [G. *amnēsia*, forgetfulness]

anterograde a., a. in reference to events occurring after the trauma or disease that caused the condition.

emotional a., psychological etiology of forgetting or repression of emotion.

lacunar a., localized a., a. in reference to isolated events.

posthypnotic a., selective forgetting, after a hypnotic state, of events occurring during hypnosis or of information stored in long-term memory, such as one's name, address, and names of relatives.

retrograde a., a. in reference to events that occurred before the trauma or disease that caused the condition.

transient global a., a memory disorder seen in middle aged and elderly persons characterized by an episode of a. and bewilderment that persists for several hours; during the episode the patient has a memory defect for present and recent past events, but is fully alert, oriented, capable of high-level intellectual activity, and has a normal neurological examination. Typically, these amnesic episodes occur spontaneously, and most patients experience only one; of uncertain etiology—probably ischemic, but not due to atherosclerosis.

traumatic a., the loss or disturbance of memory following an insult or injury to the brain of the type that accompanies a head injury, or excessive use of alcohol, or following the cessation of alcohol ingestion or other psychoactive drugs; or loss or disturbance of memory of the type seen in hysteria and other forms of dissociative disorders.

am·ne·si·ac (am-nē'sē-ak). One suffering from amnesia.

am·ne·sic (am-nē'sik). Relating to or characterized by amnesia. SYN amnestic (1).

am·nes·tic (am-nes'tik). 1. SYN amnesic. 2. An agent causing amnesia.

amnio-. The amnion. [G. *amnion*]

am·ni·o·cele (am'-nē-ō-sēl). SYN omphalocele.

am·ni·o·cen·te·sis (am'nē-ō-sen-tē'sis). Transabdominal aspiration of fluid from the amniotic sac. [amnio- + G. *kentēsis*, puncture]

am·ni·o·cho·ri·al, am·ni·o·cho·ri·on·ic (am'nē-ō-kōr'ē-ăl, -kōr-ē-on'ik). Relating to both amnion and chorion.

am·ni·o·gen·e·sis (am'nē-ō-jen'ĕ-sis). Formation of the amnion. [amnio- + G. *genesis*, production]

am·ni·og·ra·phy (am-nē-og'ră-fē). Radiography of the amniotic sac after the injection of radiopaque, water-soluble solution into the sac, which outlines the umbilical cord, the placenta, and the soft tissues of the fetal body; an obsolete technique. SEE ALSO fetography. [amnio- + G. *graphō*, to write]

am·ni·o·hook (am'nē-ō-hook'). Instrument designed to tear a hole in the amnionic sac without injuring the fetus.

amnioinfusion (am'nē-ō-in-fyu'zhun). Infusion of warmed saline through an intrauterine catheter during labor, for umbilical cord compromise due to low volume of amnionic fluid, or for thick meconium in labor.

am·ni·o·ma (am-nē-ō'mă). Broad flat mass on the skin resulting from antenatal adhesion of the amnion. [amnio- + G. *-oma*, tumor]

am·ni·on (am'nē-on). Innermost of the extraembryonic membranes enveloping the embryo in utero and containing the amniotic fluid; it consists of an internal embryonic layer with its ectodermal component, and an external somatic mesodermal component; in the later stages of pregnancy the amnion expands to come in contact with and partially fuse to the inner wall of the chorionic vesicle; derived from the trophoblast cells. SYN amnionic sac. [G. the membrane around the fetus, fr. *amnios*, lamb]

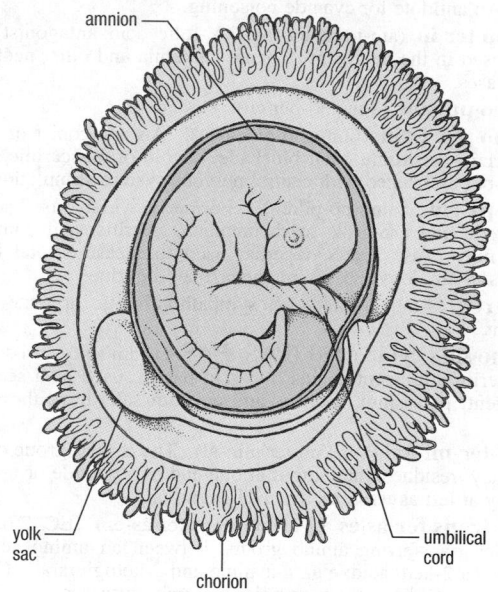

amnion and related structures: showing 5-week embryo

a. nodo'sum, nodules in the a. that consist of typical stratified squamous epithelium. SYN squamous metaplasia of amnion.

am·ni·on·ic (am-nē-on'ik). Relating to the amnion. SYN amniotic.

am·ni·o·ni·tis (am'nē-ō-nī'tis). Inflammation resulting from infection of the amniotic sac, which, in turn, commonly results from premature rupture of the membranes (a condition often associated with neonatal infection). [amnion + G. *-itis*, inflammation]

am·ni·or·rhea (am-nē-ō-rē'ă). Escape of amniotic fluid. [amnio- + G. *rhoia*, flow]

am·ni·or·rhex·is (am-nē-ō-rek'sis). Rupture of the amniotic membrane. [amnio- + G. *rhēxis*, rupture]

am·ni·o·scope (am'nē-ō-skōp). An endoscope for studying amniotic fluid through the intact amniotic sac.

am·ni·os·co·py (am-nē-os'kō-pē). Examination of the amniotic fluid in the lowest part of the amniotic sac by means of an endoscope introduced through the cervical canal. [amnio- + G. *skopeō,* to view]

Am·ni·o·ta (am'nē-ō'tă). A group of vertebrates whose embryos are enclosed in an amnion; it includes all the reptiles, birds, and mammals.

am·ni·ot·ic (am-nē-ot'ik). SYN amnionic.

am·ni·o·tome (am'nē-ō-tōm). An instrument for puncturing the fetal membranes. [amnio- + G. *tomē,* cutting]

am·ni·ot·o·my (am-nē-ot'ō-mē). Artificial rupture of the fetal membranes as a means of inducing or expediting labor.

am·o·bar·bi·tal (am-ō-bar'bi-tahl). A central nervous system depressant with an intermediate duration of action; also used as the sodium salt.

A-mode. In diagnostic ultrasound, a one-dimensional presentation of a reflected sound wave in which echo amplitude (A) is displayed along the vertical axis and echo delay (depth) along the horizontal axis; the echo information results from tissue interfaces along a single line in the direction of the sound beam.

am·o·di·a·quine hy·dro·chlo·ride (am-ō-dī'ă-kwīn). An antimalarial drug, also used in the treatment of amebic hepatitis; large doses may result in sialorrhea, nausea, vomiting, diarrhea, insomnia, palpitations, spasticity, and possibly convulsions.

△**amoeb-.** Ameba, *Amoeba.*

🔲*Amoe·ba* (ă-mē'bă). A genus of naked, lobose, pseudopod-forming protozoa of the class Sarcodina (or Rhizopoda), that are abundant soil-dwellers, especially in rich organic debris, and are also commonly found as parasites. The typical amebic parasites of humans are now placed in the genera *Entamoeba, Endolimax,* and *Iodamoeba.* SEE ALSO *Naegleria.* [Mod. L. fr. G. *amoibē* change]

A. bucca'lis, former name for *Entamoeba gingivalis.*

A. co'li, old, incorrect name *Entamoeba coli.*

A. denta'lis, former name for *Entamoeba gingivalis.*

A. dysenter'iae, old, incorrect name for *Entamoeba histolytica.*

A. histolyt'ica, old, incorrect name for *Entamoeba histolytica.*

A. pro'teus, an abundant, nonparasitic species, remarkable for the number and varied shapes of its pseudopodia.

amoebapore (ă-mē'ba-pōr). An active peptide released from *Entamoeba histolytica* that can insert ion channels into liposomes and possesses cytolytic and bactericidal activities. [amoeba + G. *poros,* passageway]

Amoe·bo·tae·nia (ă-mē'bō-tē'nē-ă). A genus of small intestinal tapeworms of birds, seldom possessing more than 30 segments. *A. cuneata* (*A. sphenoides*) is a species common in domestic fowl; its cysticercoid is developed in earthworms. [amoeb- + L. fr. G. *tainia,* band, tape, a tapeworm]

amok (ă-mok'). **1.** A culture-bound mental disorder originally observed in Malaya in which the subject becomes dangerously maniacal ("running amok"). **2.** Colloquialism denoting maniacal, wild, or uncontrolled behavior threatening injury to others. SYN amuck. [Mayal, *amoq,* engaged in battle]

amorph (ā'mōrf). An allele that has no phenotypically recognizable product and therefore its existence can be inferred on molecular evidence only, depending on the subtlety of the means of detection available. SYN silent allele. [G. *a-* neg. + *morphē,* form, shape]

amor·phag·no·sia (ă-mōr-fag-nō'sē-ă). Inability to recognize the size and shape of objects. [G. *a-* priv. + *morphē,* shape, + *gnōsis,* recognition]

amor·phia, amor·phism (ă-mōr'fē-ă, -fizm). Condition of being amorphous (1). [G. *a-* priv. + *morphē,* form]

amor·pho·syn·the·sis (ă-mōr'fō-sin'thĕ-sis). Disorder of recognition of the right side of the body in spatial relationships, caused by a lesion of the left parietal lobe. [G. *a-* priv. + *morphē,* form, + synthesis]

amor·phous (ă-mōr'fŭs). **1.** Without definite shape or visible differentiation in structure. **2.** Not crystallized.

amor·phus (ă-mōr'fŭs). A malformed fetus with rudimentary head, limbs, and heart. [G. *ā-* priv. + *morphē,* form, shape]

amox·a·pine (ă-mok'să-pēn). A tricyclic antidepressant/anti-psychotic drug; overdose can produce seizures.

amox·i·cil·lin (ă-mok-si-sil'in). A semisynthetic penicillin antibiotic with an antimicrobial spectrum similar to that of ampicillin.

AMP Abbreviation for *adenosine* monophosphate; specifically, the 5'-monophosphate unless modified by a numerical prefix. SEE adenylic acid.

AMP de·am·i·nase. An enzyme hydrolyzing adenylic acid to inosinic acid and NH_3. A deficiency of AMP d. in muscles can lead to excess fatigue following exercise. SYN adenylic acid deaminase.

am·per·age (am'pēr-ij). Strength of electric current. SEE ampere.

Ampère, André-Marie, French physicist, 1775–1836. SEE ampere; statampere; A. *postulate.*

am·pere (A) (am-pēr). The practical unit of electrical current; the absolute, practical a. originally was defined as having the value of $^1/_{10}$ of the electromagnetic unit (see abampere and coulomb). Present definitions are: **1.** The practical unit of electrical current; the absolute, practical a. originally was defined as having the value of $^1/_{10}$ of the electromagnetic unit (see abampere and coulomb). **2.** Legal definition: the current that, flowing for 1 second, will deposit 1.118 mg of silver from silver nitrate solution. **3.** Scientific (SI) definition: the current that, if maintained in two straight parallel conductors of infinite length and of negligible circular cross-sections and placed 1 m apart in a vacuum, produces between them a force of 2×10^{-7} N/m of length. [A. *Ampère*]

am·per·om·e·try (am-pĕ-rom'ĕ-trē). Determination of any analyte concentration by measurement of the current generated in a suitable chemical reaction.

△**amph-.** SEE amphi-, ampho-.

am·phe·clex·is (am-fĕ-klek'-sis). Reciprocal sexual selection, i.e., by both male and female. [G. *amphi,* two-sided, + *eklexis,* selection]

am·phet·a·mine (am-fet'ă-mēn). Closely related in its structure and action to ephedrine and other sympathomimetic amines. A psychostimulant substance that can be abused.

a. (4-chlorophenoxy)acetate, same actions and uses as a. sulfate.

a. phosphate, same actions and uses as a. sulfate.

a. sulfate, exerts less vasopressor, cardiac, and bronchial effect than ephedrine, but has a greater central nervous stimulating effect, decreasing the sensation of fatigue; used in the treatment of narcolepsy and certain types of paralysis agitans, and to reduce appetite (temporarily (1–2 weeks) in obesity.

*d-***am·phet·a·mine phos·phate.** SYN dextroamphetamine phosphate.

*d-***am·phet·a·mine sul·fate.** SYN dextroamphetamine sulfate.

△**amphi-.** On both sides, surrounding, double; corresponds to L. *ambi-.* [G. *amphi, amphi-,* on both sides, about, around]

am·phi·ar·thro·di·al (am'fi-ar-thrō'dē-ăl). Relating to a symphysis (1) (amphiarthrosis).

am·phi·ar·thro·sis (am'fi-ar-thrō'sis). SYN symphysis (1). [amphi- + G. *arthrōsis,* joint]

am·phi·as·ter (am-fi-as'ter). The double-star figure formed by the two astrospheres and their connecting spindle fibers during mitosis. SYN diaster. [amphi- + G. *astēr,* star]

am·phi·bol·ic (am'fi-bol'ik). Referring to reactions or biologic pathways that serve in both biosynthesis and degradation (i.e., anabolism and catabolism). [amphi- + metabolic]

am·phi·ce·lous (am-fi-sē'lŭs). Concave at each end, as the body of a vertebra of a fish. [amphi- + G. *koilos,* hollow]

am·phi·cen·tric (am-fi-sen'trik). Centering at both ends, said of a rete mirabile that begins by the vessel breaking up into a number of branches and ends by the branches joining again to form the same vessel. [amphi- + G. *kentron,* center]

am·phi·chro·ic (am-fi-krō'ik). SYN amphichromatic.

am·phi·chro·mat·ic (am'fi-krō-mat'ik). Having the property of exhibiting either of two colors; e.g., litmus, an a. pigment that is red in acids and blue in alkalis. SYN amphichroic. [amphi- + G. *chrōma*, color]

am·phi·cyte (am'fi-sīt). One of the cells located around the bodies of the cerebrospinal and sympathetic ganglionic neurons. SYN capsule cell. [amphi- + G. *kytos*, cell]

am·phid (am'fid). In the nervous system of nematodes, a pair of laterally placed minute receptor organs in the cephalic or cervical region. [amphi- + -id]

am·phi·dip·loid (am'fi-dip'loid). Having a complete diploid chromosome set from each parent strain. [*amphi* + diploid]

am·phi·kar·y·on (am'fē-kar'ē-on). A diploid nucleus containing two haploid sets of chromosomes. [amphi- + G. *karyon*, kernel]

am·phi·leu·ke·mic (am'fi-loo-kē'mik). Denoting a leukemic condition that corresponds in degree to the changes in the organ or tissue.

Am·phim·er·us (am-fim'er-ŭs). A genus of opisthorchid trematodes found in the bile ducts of mammals, birds, and reptiles; probably transmitted by fish. [amphi- + G. *meros*, segment]

am·phi·mi·crobe (am'fi-mī'krōb). A microorganism that is either aerobic or anaerobic, according to the environment.

am·phi·mic·tic (am'fi-mik'tik). The ability to freely interbreed and produce fertile offspring. [amphi + G. *miktos*, joined, mated, fr. *mignumi*, to mix, mae, + -ia]

am·phi·mix·is (am-fi-mik'sis). 1. Union of the paternal and maternal chromatin after impregnation of the ovum. 2. In psychoanalysis, a combination of genital and anal eroticism. [amphi- + G. *mixis*, mingling]

am·phi·nu·cle·o·lus (am'fi-noo-klē'ō-lŭs). A double nucleolus having both basophilic and oxyphilic components. [amphi- + L. *nucleolus*, dim. of *nucleus*, kernel]

am·phi·ons (am'fi-ons). SYN dipolar *ions*, under *ion*.

Am·phi·ox·us (am-fē-ok'sŭs). A genus of small, translucent, fishlike chordates found in warm marine waters. Members are structurally similar to vertebrates in having a notochord, gills, digestive tract, and nerve cord, but they lack paired fins, vertebrae, ribs, or a skull. [amphi- + G. *oxys*, sharp]

am·phi·path·ic (am-fē-path'ik). Denoting a molecule, such as comprises detergents or wetting agents, that contains groups with characteristically different properties, e.g., both hydrophilic and hydrophobic properties. SYN amphiphilic, amphiphobic. [amphi- + G. *pathos*, feeling]

am·phi·phil·ic (am-fē-fil'ik). SYN amphipathic. [amphi- + G. *philos*, fond]

am·phi·pho·bic (am-fē-fōb'ik). SYN amphipathic. [amphi- + G. *phobos*, fear]

am·phis·tome (am-fis'tōm). A common name for any trematode of the genus *Paramphistomum*. [amphi- + G. *stoma*, mouth]

am·phit·ri·chate, am·phit·ri·chous (am-fit'ri-kāt, am-fit'ri-kŭs). Having a flagellum or flagella at both extremities of a microbial cell; denoting certain microorganisms. [amphi- + G. *thrix*, hair]

am·phit·y·py (am-fit'i-pē). Exhibition of the properties characteristic of two types.

am·phix·en·o·sis (am-fiks-en-ō'sis). A zoonosis maintained in nature by humans and lower animals, e.g., certain staphylococcoses. Cf. anthropozoonosis, zooanthroponosis. [amphi- + G. *xenos*, stranger, + G. *-osis*, condition]

⌂**ampho-**. On both sides, surrounding, double. [G. *amphō*, both]

am·pho·chro·mat·o·phil, am·pho·chro·mat·o·phile (am'fō-krō-mat'ō-fil, -ō-fīl). SYN amphophil (2).

am·pho·chro·mo·phil, am·pho·chro·mo·phile (am-fō-krō'mō-fil, -fīl). SYN amphophil. [ampho- + G. *chrōma*, color, + *philos*, fond]

am·pho·cyte (am'fō-sīt). SYN amphophil (2).

am·pho·lyte (am'fō-līt). SYN amphoteric *electrolyte*.

am·pho·my·cin (am-fō-mī'sin). An antibiotic substance produced by *Streptomyces canus;* used topically for skin infections.

am·pho·phil, am·pho·phile (am'fō-fil, -fīl). 1. Having an affinity both for acid and for basic dyes. SYN amphophilic, amphophilous. 2. A cell that stains readily with either acid or basic dyes.

SYN amphochromatophil, amphochromatophile, amphocyte. SYN amphochromophil, amphochromophile. [ampho- + G. *philos*, fond]

am·pho·phil·ic, am·phoph·i·lous (am-fō-fil'ik, am-fof'i-lŭs). SYN amphophil (1).

am·phor·ic (am-fōr'ik). Denoting the sound heard in percussion and auscultation, resembling the noise made by blowing across the mouth of a bottle. [G. *amphora*, a jar]

am·pho·ril·o·quy (am-fō-ril'ō-kwē). Presence of amphoric voice. [G. *amphora*, a jar, + *loquor*, to speak]

am·phor·oph·o·ny (am-fŏ-rof'ō-nē). SYN amphoric *voice*. [G. *amphora*, a jar, + *phōnē*, voice]

am·pho·ter·ic (am-fō-tār'ik). Having two opposite characteristics, especially having the capacity of reacting as either an acid or a base; e.g., $Al(OH)_3 \equiv H_3AlO_3$ or an amino acid. [G. *amphoteroi* (pl.), both, fr. *amphō*, both]

am·pho·ter·i·cin, am·pho·ter·i·cin B (am-fō-tār'i-sin). $C_{46}H_{73}NO_{20}$; an amphoteric polyene antibiotic prepared from *Streptomyces nodosus* and available as the sodium deoxycholate complex; also a nephrotoxic antifungal agent used extensively in the treatment of systemic mycoses.

am·pi·cil·lin (am-pi-si'lin). An acid-stable semisynthetic penicillin derived from 6-aminopenicillanic acid; it has a broader spectrum of antimicrobial action than penicillin G, inhibits the growth of Gram-positive and Gram-negative bacteria, and is not resistant to penicillinase; also available as a. sodium and a. trihydrate. SYN D(-)-α-aminobenzylpenicillin.

ampl. Abbreviation for L. *amplus*, large.

am·plex·us (am-plek'sŭs). The pairing of male and female at the time that eggs and sperm are discharged simultaneously in those species, such as frogs, in which fertilization occurs externally. [L. an embrace, fr. *amplector*, pp. *-plexus*, to wind around]

am·pli·fi·ca·tion (am'pli-fi-kā'shŭn). The process of making larger, as in increasing an auditory or visual stimulus to enhance its perception. [L. *amplificatio*, an enlarging]

genetic a., a process for producing an increase in pertinent genetic material, particularly for increasing the proportion of plasmid DNA to that of bacterial DNA. Includes the production of extrachromosomal copies of the genes for RNA. This process is usually seen in malignant cells in humans.

linear a., a hearing aid circuit in which all frequencies receive equivalent amplification.

am·pli·fi·er. 1. A device that increases the magnification of a microscope. 2. An electronic apparatus that increases the strength of input signals.

image amplifier, a device for converting a low light level fluoroscopic image to one that can be seen by the eye in a lighted environment; usually consists of an electronic light amplifier chained to a television tube. SYN image intensifier.

am·pli·tude (am'pli-tood). Largeness; extent; breadth or range. [L. *amplitudo*, fr. *amplus*, large]

a. of pulse, SEE average pulse *magnitude*, peak *magnitude*.

am·poule (am'pul). SYN ampule.

am·pro·tro·pine phos·phate (am'prō-trō'pēn). An antispasmodic, similar in action to atropine.

am·pule, am·pul (am'pool). A hermetically sealed container, usually made of glass, containing a sterile medicinal solution, or powder to be made up in solution, to be used for subcutaneous, intramuscular, or intravenous injection. SYN ampoule. [L. *ampulla*]

am·pul·la, gen. and pl. **am·pul·lae** (am-pul'lă, -ē) [TA]. A saccular dilation of a canal or duct. [L. a two-handled bottle]

biliaropancreatic a., ✩official alternate term for hepatopancreatic a.

a. biliaropancreatica, ✩official alternate term for hepatopancreatic a.

bony ampullae of semicircular canals [TA], a circumscribed dilation of one extremity of each of the three bony semicircular canals, anterior, posterior, and lateral; each contains a membranous a. of the semicircular ducts. SYN ampullae osseae canalium semicircularium [TA], osseous a.

a. canalic′uli lacrima′lis [TA], SYN a. of lacrimal canaliculus.

a. chy′li, SYN *cisterna* chyli.

a. of ductus deferens [TA], the dilation of the ductus deferens at the base of the bladder where it approaches its contralateral partner just before it is joined by the duct of the seminal vesicle to form the ejaculatory duct. SYN a. ductus deferentis [TA], Henle a.

a. duc′tus deferen′tis [TA], SYN a. of ductus deferens.

a. duc′tus lacrima′lis, incorrect term for a. of lacrimal canaliculus.

duodenal a., (1) SYN a. of duodenum; **(2)** SYN hepatopancreatic a.

a. duode′ni [TA], SYN a. of duodenum.

a. of duodenum [TA], the dilated portion of the superior part of the duodenum. SEE ALSO duodenal *cap.* SEE ALSO a. duodeni [TA], bulbus duodeni✫, duodenal a. (1).

a. of gallbladder, SYN Hartmann *pouch.*

Henle a., SYN a. of ductus deferens.

hepatopancreatic a. [TA], the dilation within the major duodenal papilla that normally receives both the (common) bile duct and the main pancreatic duct. SYN a. hepatopancreatica [TA], a. biliaropancreatica✫, biliaropancreatic a.✫, a. of Vater, duodenal a. (2).

a. hepat′opancreat′ica [TA], SYN hepatopancreatic a.

a. of lacrimal canaliculus [TA], a slight dilation at the angle of the lacrimal canaliculus immediately beyond the lacrimal punctum. SYN a. canaliculi lacrimalis [TA].

a. lactif′era, SYN lactiferous *sinus.*

lactiferous a., SYN lactiferous *sinus.*

a. of lactiferous duct, SYN lactiferous *sinus.*

a. membrana′cea, pl. **ampullae membrana′ceae ductuum semicircularium** [TA], SYN membranous ampullae of the semicircular ducts.

membranous a., SYN membranous ampullae of the semicircular ducts.

membranous ampullae of the semicircular ducts [TA], a nearly spherical enlargement of one end of each of the three semicircular ducts, anterior, posterior, and lateral, where they connect with the utricle. Each contains a neuroepithelial crista ampullaris. SYN a. membranacea [TA], membranous a.

a. of milk duct, SYN lactiferous *sinus.*

ampullae osseae canalium semicircularium [TA], SYN bony ampullae of semicircular canals.

osseous a., SYN bony ampullae of semicircular canals.

phrenic a., a physiologic localized dilatation of the distal esophagus, commonly demonstrated by esophagography.

rectal a. [TA], a dilated portion of the rectum just above the pelvic diaphragm and proximal to the anal canal. SYN a. recti [TA], a. of rectum.

a. rec′ti [TA], SYN rectal a.

a. of rectum, SYN rectal a.

Thoma a., a dilation of the arterial capillary beyond the sheathed artery of the spleen.

a. tu′bae uteri′nae [TA], SYN a. of uterine tube.

a. of uterine tube [TA], the wide portion of the uterine (fallopian) tube near the fimbriated extremity; it has a complexly folded mucosa with a columnar epithelium of mostly ciliated cells between which are secretory cells. SYN a. tubae uterinae [TA].

a. of Vater, SYN hepatopancreatic a.

am·pul·lar (am-pul′ăr). Relating in any sense to an ampulla.

am·pul·li·tis (am-pul-lī′tis). Inflammation of any ampulla, especially of the dilated extremity of the vas deferens or of the ampulla of Vater. [ampulla + G. *itis,* inflammation]

am·pul·lu·la (am-pul′oo-lă). A circumscribed dilation of any minute lymphatic or blood vessel or duct. [Mod. L. dim. of L. *ampulla*]

AMPUTATION

▣**am·pu·ta·tion** (am-pū-tā′shŭn). **1.** The cutting off of a limb or part of a limb, the breast, or other projecting part. **2.** In dentistry, removal of the root of a tooth, or of the pulp, or of a nerve root or ganglion; a modifying adjective is therefore used (pulp a.; root a.). [L. *amputatio,* fr. *am-puto,* pp. *-atus,* to cut around, prune]

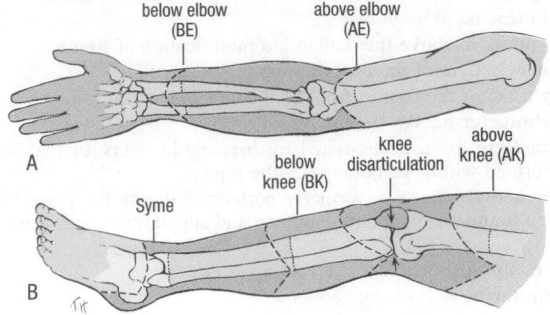

amputation: (A) levels of upper extremity, (B) levels of lower extremity

A-E a., acronym for *a*bove-the-*e*lbow a.

A-K a., acronym for *a*bove-the-*k*nee a.

Alanson a., a circular a., the stump shaped like a cone.

amnionic a., SYN congenital a.

aperiosteal a., a. with removal of periosteum from bone at the site of a.

B-E a., acronym for *b*elow-the-*e*lbow a.

Bier a., osteoplastic a. of tibia and fibula.

B-K a., acronym for *b*elow-the-*k*nee a.

bloodless a., a. in which, by means of a tourniquet, the escape of blood from the cut surfaces is minimal. SYN dry a.

Callander a., tenontoplastic a. through the femur at the knee. SYN knee disarticulation a.

Carden a., transcondylar a. of the leg, the femur is sawed through the condyles just above the articular surface.

central a., a. in which the flaps are so united that the cicatrix runs across the end of the stump.

cervical a., a. of the uterine cervix.

Chopart a., a. through the midtarsal joint; i.e., between the tarsal navicular and the calcaneocuboid joints.

cinematic a., SYN cineplastic a.

cineplastic a., a method of a. of an extremity whereby the muscles and tendons are so arranged in the stump that they are able to execute independent movements and to communicate motion to a specially constructed prosthetic apparatus. SYN cinematic a., cineplastics, kineplastic a.

circular a., a. performed by a circular incision through the skin, the muscles being similarly divided higher up, and the bone higher still. SYN guillotine a., linear a.

congenital a. [MIM*217100], a. produced *in utero;* attributed to the pressure of constricting bands (amniotic). SEE ALSO amputation (1). SYN amnionic a., intrauterine a., spontaneous a. (1).

a. in continuity, a. through a segment of a limb, not at a joint.

double flap a., a. in which a flap is cut from the soft parts on either side of the limb.

dry a., SYN bloodless a.

Dupuytren a., a. of the arm at the shoulder joint.

eccentric a., a. with the scar of the stump off-center. SYN excentric a.

elliptical a., circular a. in which the sweep of the knife is not exactly vertical to the axis of the limb, the outline of the cut surface being therefore elliptical.

excentric a., SYN eccentric a.

Farabeuf a., (1) a. of the leg, the flap being large and on the outer side; (2) a. of the foot; disarticulation of the foot through the subtalar joint and the talo-navicular joint.

flap a., an a. in which flaps of the muscular and cutaneous tissues are made to cover the end of the bone. SYN flap operation (1).

flapless a., an a. without any tissue to cover the stump

forequarter a., amputation of the arm with removal of the scapula and a portion of the clavicle. SYN interscapulothoracic a.

Gritti-Stokes a., supracondylar a. of the femur, the patella being preserved and applied to the end of the bone, its articular cartilage being removed so as to obtain union. SYN Gritti operation.

guillotine a., SYN circular a.

Guyon a., a. above the malleoli, a modification of Syme a.

Hancock a., a. of the foot through the astragalus.

Hey a., a. of the foot in front of the tarsometatarsal joint.

hindquarter a., SYN hemipelvectomy.

immediate a., a. necessitated by irreparable injury to the limb, performed within 12 hours after the injury.

intermediate a., an a. formerly performed during the period between trauma or incipient gangrene and suppuration. SYN primary a.

interscapulothoracic a., SYN forequarter a.

intrauterine a., SYN congenital a.

Jaboulay a., SYN hemipelvectomy.

kineplastic a., SYN cineplastic a.

Kirk a., a. at the lower end of the femur, using the tendon of the quadriceps extensor to cover the end of the bone.

knee disarticulation a., SYN Callander a.

Krukenberg a., a cineplastic a. at the carpus with the distal end of the forearm used to create a forklike stump between radius and ulna; especially valuable in the blind because the stump has proprioception.

Le Fort a., a modification of Pirogoff a.; the calcaneus is sawed through horizontally instead of vertically so that the patient steps on the same part of the heel as before.

linear a., SYN circular a.

Lisfranc a., a. of the foot at the tarsometatarsal joint, the sole being preserved to make the flap. SYN Lisfranc operation.

Mackenzie a., a modification of Syme a. at the ankle joint, the flap being taken from the inner side.

major a., a. of the lower or upper extremity above the ankle or the wrist, respectively.

Malgaigne a., SYN subastragalar a.

Mikulicz-Vladimiroff a., an osteoplastic resection of the foot in which the talus and calcaneus are excised, the anterior row of tarsal bones being united to the lower end of the tibia, the articular surfaces of both being removed; the lower end of the stump is therefore the anterior portion of the foot, the patient walking thereafter on tiptoe. SYN Vladimiroff-Mikulicz a.

minor a., a. of a hand or foot or any parts of either.

multiple a., a. of two or more limbs or parts of limbs performed at the same operation.

oblique a., a. in which the line of section through an extremity is at other than a right angle; this yields an oval appearance to the cut surface (hence sometimes, though rarely, referred to as an oval a.).

osteoplastic a., an a., e.g., through the tarsus, in which the cut surface of another bone is brought in apposition with the one primarily divided so that the two unite, thus giving a better stump.

pathologic a., a. necessitated by cancer or other disease of the limb and not by an injury.

Pirogoff a., a. of the foot; the lower articular surfaces of the tibia and fibula are sawed through and the ends covered with a portion of the os calcis which has also been sawed through from above posteriorly downward and forward.

primary a., SYN intermediate a.

pulp a., SYN pulpotomy.

quadruple a., a. of both arms and both legs.

racket a., a circular or slightly oval a., in which a long incision is made in the axis of the limb.

rectangular a., a. in which the flaps are fashioned in the shape of a rectangle.

root a., surgical removal of one or more roots of a multirooted tooth, the remaining root canal(s) usually being treated endodontically. SYN radectomy, radiectomy, radisectomy.

secondary a., a. performed some time after a previous a. that has failed to heal satisfactorily.

spontaneous a., (1) SYN congenital a; (2) a. as the result of a pathologic process rather than external trauma.

Stokes a., a modification of the Gritti-Stokes a. in that the line of section of the femur is slightly higher.

subastragalar a., a. of the foot in which only the astragalus is retained. SYN Malgaigne a.

subperiosteal a., a. in which the periosteum is stripped back from the bone and replaced afterward, forming a periosteal flap over the cut end.

Syme a., a. of the foot at the ankle joint, the malleoli being sawed off, and a flap being made with the soft parts of the heel. SYN Syme operation.

tarsotibial a., a. through the ankle joint.

transverse a., a. in which the line of section through the extremity is at right angles to the long axis.

traumatic a., a. resulting from accidental or nonsurgical injury; may be complete or incomplete.

Tripier a., a modification of Chopart a., in that a part of the calcaneus is also removed.

Vladimiroff-Mikulicz a., SYN Mikulicz-Vladimiroff a.

---

am·pu·tee (am′pū-tē). A person with an amputated limb or part of limb.

am·ri·none lac·tate (am′ri-nōn). A phosphodiesterase inhibitor with inotropic and vasodilator activity, used in management of congestive heart failure.

Amsler, Marc, Swiss ophthalmologist, 1891–1968. SEE A. *chart;* Amsler *grid;* A. *test.*

amu Abbreviation for atomic mass *unit.*

amuck (ă-mŭk′). SYN amok (2).

amu·sia (ă-mū′zē-ă). A form of aphasia characterized by an inability to produce or recognize music. [G. *a-* priv. + *mousa,* music]

instrumental a., loss of ability to play a musical instrument.

motor a., inability to produce music.

sensory a., inability to interpret or appreciate musical sounds.

vocal a., the inability to sing, although speech is intact.

Amussat, Jean Z., French surgeon, 1796–1856. SEE A. *valve, valvula.*

am·y·cho·pho·bia (am′ī-kō-fō′bē-ă). Morbid fear of being scratched. [G. *amychē,* a scratch, + *phobos,* fear]

Am·y·co·la·top·sis (am-ē-kō-la-top′sis). A genus of Gram-positive, filamentous bacteria, defined as a separate genus in 1986, that tends to break up into square fragments; recovered from soil and vegetable matter; *A.* is rare human pathogen that has been recovered from various clinical specimens, including spinal fluid. The type species is *A. orientalis.*

A. orienta′lis subsp. *lu′rida,* a bacterial species that produces ristocetin.

amy·el·en·ce·pha·lia (ă-mī′el-en-sĕ-fā′lē-ă). Congenital absence of both brain and spinal cord. [G. *a-* priv. + *myelos,* marrow, + *enkephalos,* brain]

amy·el·en·ce·phal·ic, amy·el·en·ceph·a·lous (ă-mī′el-en-se-fal′ik, -sef′ă-lŭs). Denoting or characteristic of amyelencephalia.

amy·e·lia (ă-mī-ē′lē-ă). Congenital absence of the spinal cord, found in association with anencephaly. [G. *a-* priv. + *myelos,* marrow]

amy·el·ic (ă-mī-ē′lik). SYN amyelous.

amy·e·li·nat·ed (ă-mī′e-li-nā′ted). SYN unmyelinated.

amy·e·li·na·tion (ă-mī′ĕ-li-nā′shŭn). Failure of formation of myelin sheath of a nerve.

amy·e·lin·ic (ă-mī′ĕ-lin′ik). SYN unmyelinated.

amy·e·lo·ic, amy·e·lon·ic (ă-mī-ĕ-lō′ik, ă-mī-ĕ-lon′ik). **1.** SYN amyelous. **2.** In hematology, sometimes used to indicate the absence of bone marrow or the lack of functional participation of bone marrow in hemopoiesis. [G. *a-* priv. + *myelos,* marrow]

amy·e·lous (ă-mī′ĕ-lŭs). Without spinal cord. SYN amyelic, amyeloic (1), amyelonic.

amyg·da·la, gen. and pl. **amyg·da·lae** (ă-mig′dă-lă, -lē). **1.** Term for the lymphatic tonsils (pharyngeal, palatine, lingual, laryngeal, and tubal). **2.** General term describing a nucleus in the temporal lobe, amygdaloid body. [L. fr. G. *amygdalē,* almond; in Mediev. & Mod. L., a tonsil]

a. cerebel′li, obsolete term for cerebellar *tonsil.*

amyg·da·lase (ă-mig′dă-lās). SYN β-glucosidase.

amyg·da·lin (ă-mig′dă-lin). A cyanogenic glucoside present in almonds and seeds of other plants of the family Rosaceae; the principal component of laetrile. Emulsin splits a. into benzaldehyde, D-glucose, and hydrocyanic acid. SYN amygdaloside. [G. *amygdala,* almond, + -*in*]

amyg·da·line (ă-mig′dă-līn). **1.** Relating to an almond. **2** [TA] Relating to a tonsil, or to the brain structure called amygdala or amygdaloid complex [TA]. **3.** SYN tonsillar.

amyg·da·loid (ă-mig′dă-loyd). Resembling an almond or a tonsil. [amygdala + G. *eidos,* appearance]

a·myg·dal·ose (ă-mig′dal-ōs). SYN gentiobiose.

amyg·da·lo·side (ă-mig′dă-lō-sīd). SYN amygdalin.

am·yl (ă′mil). The radical formed from a pentane, C_5H_{12}, by removal of one H. Several isomeric forms exist, the more important being $CH_3CH_2CH_2CH_2CH_2-$ (amyl or pentyl); $(CH_3)_2CHCH_2CH_2-$ (isoamyl or isopentyl); $CH_3CH_2CH_2CH-(CH)_3-$ and $(CH_3CH_2)_2CH-$ (secondary amyl or pentyl); and $CH_3CH_2C(CH_3)_2-$ (tertiary amyl or pentyl). SYN pentyl (1).

a. alcohol, used as a solvent for varnishes and oils; highly toxic, with irritating vapors. SEE ALSO fusel *oil.*

a. hydrate, SYN *amylene* hydrate.

a. nitrite, a vasodilator used in angina pectoris and cyanide poisoning.

tertiary a. alcohol, SYN *amylene* hydrate.

a. valerate, used as a sedative; formerly used in the treatment of gallstones because of its solvent action on cholesterol. SYN apple oil.

△**amyl-. 1.** SEE amylo-. **2.** Pentyl- SEE amyl.

am·y·la·ceous (am′i-lā′shŭs). Starchy.

am·y·lase (am′il-ās). One of a group of amylolytic enzymes that cleave starch, glycogen, and related 1,4-α-glucans.

α-am·y·lase. A glucanohydrolase yielding α-glucose and maltose in a random manner from 1,4-α-glucans. An amylase that has been used clinically as a digestive aid. SYN glycogenase, ptyalin, Taka-diastase.

β-am·y·lase. A glucanohydrolase yielding β-maltose units from the nonreducing ends of 1,4-α-glucans. An exoamylase. SYN glycogenase, saccharogen amylase.

γ-am·y·lase. SYN exo-1,4-α-D-glucosidase.

am·y·la·su·ria (am·y·lā-soo′rē-ă). The excretion of amylase (sometimes termed diastase) in the urine, especially increased amounts likely in acute pancreatitis. SYN diastasuria.

am·y·le·mia (am-i-lē′mē-ă). The hypothetical presence of starch in the circulating blood. [amylo- + G. *haima,* blood]

am·yl·ene (am′i-lēn). A flammable liquid hydrocarbon formed by the decomposition of amyl alcohol; has anesthetic properties but undesirable side actions. SYN trimethylethylene.

a. chloral, a hypnotic.

a. hydrate, an obsolete hypnotic used as a solvent for tribromoethanol. SYN amyl hydrate, tertiary amyl alcohol.

am·y·lin (am′i-lin). The cellulose of starch; the insoluble envelope of starch grains.

△**amylo-.** Starch; of polysaccharide nature or origin. [G. *amylon,* unmilled; starch, fr. *a-* + *mylē,* a mill]

am·y·lo·dex·trin (am-i-lō-deks′trin). End product of hydrolysis of amylopectin by β-amylase; further hydrolysis requires amylo-1,6-glucosidase, which attacks the branch points. Identified by its color reaction with iodine (a. turns blue). Cf. achroodextrin, erythrodextrin.

am·y·lo·gen·e·sis (am-i-lō-jen′ĕ-sis). Biosynthesis of starch. [amylo- + G. *genesis,* production]

am·y·lo·gen·ic (am-i-lō-jen′ik). Relating to amylogenesis.

am·y·lo-1,4:1,6-glu·can·trans·fer·ase. SYN 1,4-α-D-glucan-branching enzyme.

am·y·lo·glu·co·si·dase (am-i-lō-gloo′kō-si-dās). SYN exo-1,4-α-D-glucosidase.

am·y·lo-1,6-glu·co·si·dase. An enzyme hydrolyzing α-D-1,6 links (branch points) in chains of 1,4-linked α-D-glucose residues, hence the term debranching enzyme or factor; deficiency causes type III glycogenosis. SYN dextrin 6-α-D-glucosidase.

am·y·loid (am′i-loyd). **1.** Any of a group of chemically diverse proteins that appears microscopically homogeneous, but is composed of linear nonbranching aggregated fibrils arranged in sheets when seen under the electron microscope; it stains dark brown with iodine, produces a characteristic green birefringence in polarized light after staining with Congo red, is metachromatic with either methyl violet (pink-red) or crystal violet (purple-red), and fluoresces yellow after thioflavine T staining; a. occurs characteristically as pathologic extracellular deposits (amyloidosis), especially in association with reticuloendothelial tissue; the chemical nature of the proteinaceous fibrils is dependent upon the underlying disease process. **2.** Resembling or containing starch. [amylo- + G. *eidos,* resemblance]

amyloidoma (am′il-oyd-ō′ma). A tumor within which amyloid is produced. [amyloid + G. -*oma,* tumor]

am·y·loi·do·sis (am′i-loy-dō′sis). **1.** A disease characterized by extracellular accumulation of amyloid in various organs and tissues of the body; may be local or generalized; may be primary or secondary. **2.** The process of deposition of amyloid protein. [amyloid + G. -*osis,* condition]

a. of aging, characterized by deposition of Congo-red staining material, derived from a variety of proteins, especially in nervous tissue, myocardium and pancreas. Associated with Alzheimer syndrome; intractable congestive heart failure may result.

chronic amyloidosis, a. of long duration.

a. cu′tis, SYN lichenoid a.

familial a., SYN familial amyloid *neuropathy.*

focal a., SYN nodular a.

hereditary a., SYN familial amyloid *neuropathy.*

lichen a., SYN lichenoid a.

lichenoid a. (līk′en-oyd), localized cutaneous a. with pruritic brownish-red papules, often scaling, most commonly on the lower legs in middle age, due to amyloid infiltration of the papillary dermis. SYN a. cutis, lichen a. [G. *leichēn,* lichen, a lichen-like eruption + *eidos,* resemblance]

light chain-related a., the most common form of primary a. in which the fibrillar amyloid deposits are derived from the amino terminal variable region of the light chains of immunoglobulin; seen in B-lymphocyte and plasma-cell dyscrasias (especially multiple myeloma) and other forms of gammopathy.

macular a., a localized form of a. cutis characterized by pruritic symmetrical brown reticulated macules, especially on the upper back; microscopically, amyloid is deposited as small subepidermal globules.

a. of multiple myeloma, foci of a. in mesenchymal tissues of some persons with multiple myeloma; no direct relation between amyloid and Bence Jones protein is conclusively known.

nodular a., a localized form of a. in which amyloid occurs as hard masses or nodules beneath the skin or mucous membranes, e.g., in the larynx, often with local plasma cell infiltration; may be associated with plasma cell dyscrasia or systemic a. SYN amyloid tumor, focal a.

primary a., several forms of a. are known, following autosomal dominant [MIM *104750, *105120, *105150, *105200, *105210, *105250] recessive [MIM 204850 and *204900], and X-linked [MIM 301220] inheritance and not associated with other recognized disease. Tends to involve diffusely the arterial walls and mesenchymal tissues in the tongue, lungs, intestinal tract, skin, skeletal muscle, and myocardium, interfering with vital functions;

the amyloid frequently does not manifest the usual affinity for Congo red, and sometimes provokes a foreign-body type of inflammatory reaction in the adjacent tissue.

renal a., renal deposits of amyloid, especially in glomerular capillary walls, which may cause albuminuria and the nephrotic syndrome. SYN amyloid nephrosis (1).

secondary a., a. occurring in association with another chronic inflammatory disease; organs chiefly involved are the liver, spleen, and kidneys, and the adrenal glands less frequently.

senile a., a common form of a. in very old people, usually mild and limited to the heart or seminal vesicles. SEE ALSO a. of aging.

am·y·lol·y·sis (am-i-lol′i-sis). Hydrolysis of starch into soluble products. [amylo- + G. *lysis,* dissolution]

am·y·lo·lyt·ic (am-i-lō-lit′ik). Relating to amylolysis.

am·y·lo·malt·ase (am-i-lō-mal′tās). SYN 4-α-D-glucanotransferase.

am·y·lo·pec·tin (am-i-lō-pek′tin). A branched-chain polyglucose (glucan) in starch containing both 1,4 and 1,6 linkages. Cf. amylose.

am·y·lo·pec·tin 6-glu·can·o·hy·dro·lase. Former name for α-dextrin endo-1,6-α-glucosidase.

am·y·lo·pec·tin 1,6-glu·co·si·dase. Former name for an enzyme now known to be at least two enzymes, α-dextrin endoglucanohydrolase and isoamylase.

am·y·lo·pec·tin·o·sis (am′i-lō-pek-tin-ō′sis). SEE type 4 *glycogenosis.* [amylopectin + G. *-osis,* condition]

am·y·lo·pha·gia (am′i-lō-fā′jē-ă). A morbid craving for starch. SYN starch-eating. [amylo- + G. *phagō,* to eat]

am·y·lo·plast (am′i-lō-plast). A granule in the protoplasm of a plant cell that is the center of a starch-forming process. SYN amylogenic body. [amylo- + G. *plastos,* formed]

am·y·lo·psin (am-il-op′sin). The amylase of pancreatic juice.

am·y·lor·rhea (am′i-lō-rē′ă). Passage of undigested starch in the stools, implying a deficiency of amylase activity in the intestine. [amylo- + G. *rhoia,* flow]

am·y·lose (am′i-lōs). An unbranched polyglucose (glucan) in starch, similar to cellulose, containing α(1→4) linkages. Cf. amylopectin.

am·y·lo·su·ria (am′i-lō-soo′rē-ă). Excretion of starch in the urine. SYN amyluria.

am·y·lo-(1,4→1,6)-trans·glu·co·si·dase, am·y·lo-(1,4→1,6)-trans·glu·co·syl·ase. SYN 1,4-α-D-glucan-branching enzyme.

am·y·lum (am′i-lŭm). SYN starch.

am·y·lu·ria (am-i-loo′rē-ă). SYN amylosuria.

amy·o·es·the·sia, amy·o·es·the·sis (ă-mī′ō-es-thē′zē-ă, -thē′sis). Absence of muscle sensation. [G. *a-* priv. + *mys,* muscle, + *aisthēsis,* perception]

amy·o·pla·sia (ă-mī-ō-plā′zē-ă). Deficient formation of muscle tissue and deficient muscle growth. [G. *a-* priv. + *mys,* muscle, + *plasis,* a molding]

a. congen′ita, SYN *arthrogryposis* multiplex congenita.

amy·o·sta·sia (ă-mī-ō-stā′zē-ă). Difficulty in standing, due to muscular tremor or incoordination. [G. *a-* priv. + *mys,* muscle, + *stasis,* standing]

amy·o·stat·ic (ă-mī-ō-stat′ik). Showing muscular tremors.

amy·os·the·nia (ă-mī′os-thē′nē-ă). Muscular weakness. [G. *a-* priv. + *mys,* muscle, + *sthenos,* strength]

amy·os·then·ic (ă-mī-os-then′ik). Relating to or causing muscular weakness.

amy·o·taxy, amy·o·tax·ia (ă-mī′ō-tak-sē, ă-mī-ō-tak′sē-ă). Muscular ataxia. [G. *a-* priv. + *mys,* muscle, + *taxis,* order]

amy·o·to·nia (ă-mī-ō-tō′nē-ă). Generalized absence of muscle tone, usually associated with flabby musculature and an increased range of passive movement at joints. [G. *a-* priv. + *mys,* muscle, + *tonos,* tone]

a. congen′ita, an indefinite term for a number of congenital neuromuscular disorders that cause generalized loss of muscle tone, and sometimes weakness, in infants and young children; most of these disorders have a benign course. SYN congenital atonic pseu-

doparalysis, myatonia congenita, Oppenheim disease, Oppenheim syndrome.

amy·o·tro·phia (ă-mī-ō-trō′fē-ă). SYN amyotrophy.

amy·o·tro·phic (ă-mī-ō-trō′fik). Relating to muscular atrophy.

amy·ot·ro·phy (ă-mī-ot′rō-fē). Muscular wasting or atrophy. SYN amyotrophia. [G. *a-* priv. + *mys,* muscle, + *trophē,* nourishment]

diabetic a., a type of diabetic neuropathy that primarily affects elderly patients with diabetes mellitus; clinically characterized by unilateral or bilateral anterior thigh pain, weakness, and atrophy; of abrupt or gradual onset and, when bilateral, of simultaneous or sequential onset, and usually asymmetrical; one type of diabetic polyradiculopathy. Sometimes referred to, erroneously, as diabetic femoral neuropathy.

hemiplegic a., muscular atrophy seen in hemiplegic limbs.

neuralgic a., a neurological disorder, of unknown cause, characterized by the sudden onset of severe pain, usually about the shoulder and often beginning at night, soon followed by weakness and wasting of various forequarter muscles, particularly shoulder girdle muscles; both sporadic and familial in occurrence with the former much more common; often preceded by some antecedent event, such as an upper respiratory infection, hospitalization, vaccination, or nonspecific trauma; usually attributed to a brachial plexus lesion, because the nerve fibers involved are most often derived from the upper trunk, but actually multiple proximal mononeuropathies. SYN acute brachial radiculitis, brachial neuritis, brachial plexitis, brachial plexus neuropathy, Parsonage-Turner syndrome, shoulder-girdle syndrome.

progressive spinal a., SYN amyotrophic lateral *sclerosis.*

am·y·ous (am′ē-ŭs). Lacking in muscular tissue, or in muscular strength. [G. *a-* priv. + *mys,* muscle]

amyx·or·rhea (ă-mik-sō-rē′ă). Absence of the normal secretion of mucus. [G. *a-* priv. + *myxa,* mucus, + *rhoia,* flow]

△**an-.** SEE a-.

ANA. Abbreviation for antinuclear *antibody*; American Nurses Association.

△**ana-.** Up, again, back; sometimes *an-* before a vowel; corresponds to L. sursum-; CAUTION: an- before a vowel usually stands for a- meaning not; sometimes ana- becomes am- before p, b, or ph. [G. *ana,* up]

An·a·bae·na (an-ă-bē′nă). A genus of Cyanobacteria found in fresh water that can cause odor in water supplies; although not invasive pathogens, they produce potent saxitoxinlike neurotoxins that can poison farm animals ingesting heavily infected pond water.

an·a·bi·o·sis (an′ă-bī-ō′sis). Resuscitation after apparent death. [G. a reviving, fr. *ana,* again, + *biōsis,* life]

an·a·bi·ot·ic (an′ă-bī-ot′ik). 1. Resuscitating or restorative. 2. A revivifying remedy; a powerful stimulant. [ana- + G. *bios,* life]

an·a·bol·ic (an-ă-bol′ik). Relating to or promoting anabolism.

anab·o·lism (ă-nab′ō-lizm). 1. The building up in the body of complex chemical compounds from smaller simpler compounds (e.g., proteins from amino acids), usually with the use of energy. Cf. catabolism, metabolism. 2. The sum of synthetic metabolic reactions. [G. *anabolē,* a raising up]

anab·o·lite (ă-nab′ō-līt). Any substance formed as a result of anabolic processes.

an·a·camp·tom·e·ter (an-ă-kamp-tom′ĕ-ter). Instrument for measuring the intensity of the deep reflexes. [G. *anakampsis,* a bending back, reflection, + *metron,* measure]

an·a·cat·es·the·sia (an′ă-kat′es-thē′zē-ă). A hovering sensation. [G. *ana,* up, + *kata,* down, + *aisthēsis,* sensation]

an·a·cid·i·ty (an-ă-sid′i-tē). Absence of acidity; used especially to denote absence of hydrochloric acid in the gastric juice.

anac·la·sis (ă-nak′lă-sis). 1. Reflection of light or sound. 2. Refraction of the ocular media. [G. a bending back, reflection]

an·a·clit·ic (an-ă-klit′ik). Leaning or depending upon; in psychoanalysis, relating to the dependence of the infant on the mother or mother substitute. SEE anaclitic *depression.* [G. *ana,* toward, + *klinō,* to lean]

an·a·crot·ic (an-ă-krot′ik). Referring to the upstroke or ascending limb of the arterial pulse tracing; an abbreviated form for anadicrotic, twice beating on the upstroke. SYN anadicrotic.

anac·ro·tism (ă-nak′rō-tizm). Peculiarity of the pulse wave. SEE anacrotic *pulse.* SYN anadicrotism. [G. *ana,* up, + *krotos,* a beat]

an·a·cu·sis (an′ă-koo′sis). Total loss or absence of the ability to perceive sound as such. SYN anakusis. [G. *an-* priv. + *akousis,* hearing]

an·a·de·nia (an-ă-dē′nē-ă). Obsolete term for absence of glands or abeyance of glandular function. [G. *an-* priv. + *adēn,* gland]
  a. ventric′uli, absence of glands from the stomach.

an·a·di·crot·ic (an-ă-dī-krot′ik). SYN anacrotic.

an·a·di·cro·tism (an-ă-dik′rō-tizm). SYN anacrotism. [G. *ana,* up, + *di-krotos,* double beating]

an·a·did·y·mus (an-ă-did′i-mŭs). SYN *duplicitas* posterior. [G. *ana,* up, + *didymos,* twin]

an·a·dip·sia (an-ă-dip′sē-ă). Rarely used term for extreme thirst. SEE ALSO polydipsia. [G. *ana,* intensive, + *dipsa,* thirst]

an·ad·re·nal·ism (an-ă-drē′năl-izm). Complete lack of adrenal function.

an·a·dro·mous (an-a-drō′mus). Migrating from ocean water to fresh water to spawn; some such fish harbor human pathogens. SEE ALSO catadromous.

an·aer·obe (an′ār-ōb, an-ār′ōb). A microorganism that can live and grow in the absence of oxygen. [G. *an-* priv. + *aēr,* air, + *bios,* life]
  facultative a., an a. that either grows in the presence of air or under conditions of reduced oxygen tension.
  obligate a., an a. that will grow only in the absence of free oxygen.

an·aer·o·bic (an-ār-ō′bik). Relating to an anaerobe; living without oxygen.

an·aer·o·bi·o·sis (an-ār-ō-bī-ō′sis). Existence in an oxygen-free atmosphere. [G. *an-* priv. + *aēr,* air, + *biōsis,* way of living]

An·aer·o·bo·plasma (an-ār-ō′bō-plaz′ma). An order in the class Molicutes that is oxygen-sensitive. A role in human disease has not been defined.

an·aer·o·gen·ic (an-ār-ō-jen′ik). Not producing gas. [G. *an-* priv. + *aēr,* air, + *-gen,* producing]

an·aer·o·phyte (an-ār′ō-fīt). 1. A plant that grows without air. 2. An anaerobic bacterium. [G. *an-* priv. + *aēr,* air, + *phyton,* plant]

an·aer·o·plas·ty (an-ār′ō-plas-tē). Treatment of wounds by exclusion of air. [G. *an-* not + *aēr,* air, + *plastos,* formed]

an·a·gen (an′ă-jen). Growth phase of the hair cycle, lasting about 3–6 years in human scalp hair. [G. *ana,* up, + *-gen,* producing]

an·a·gen·e·sis (an-ă-jen′ĕ-sis). 1. Repair of tissue. 2. Regeneration of lost parts. [G. *ana,* up, + *genesis,* production]

an·a·ge·net·ic (an′ă-jĕ-net′ik). Pertaining to anagenesis.

an·a·ges·tone ac·e·tate (an-ă-jes′tōn). A progestational agent.

Anagnostakis, Andreas, Cretan ophthalmologist, 1826–1897.

an·a·go·gy (an-ă-gō′jē). A rarely used term for psychic content of an idealistic or spiritual nature. [G. *anagōgē,* fr. *an-* ago, to lead up]

an·a·kat·a·did·y·mus, an·a·cat·a·did·y·mus (an′ă-kat-ă-did′i-mŭs). Conjoined twins united in the middle but separated above and below. SYN dicephalus dipygus. [G. *ana,* up, + *kata,* down, + *didymos,* twin]

an·á·khré (an-ah-krā′). SYN goundou. [Fr. fr. Af. native term meaning "big nose"]

an·ak·me·sis (an-ak′mē-sis). Arrest of maturation of leukocytes in their production centers, thereby resulting in greater numbers of young forms and progressively smaller proportions of mature granular cells in the bone marrow, as observed in agranulocytosis. [G. *an-* priv. + *akmēnos,* full grown, fr. *akmē,* highest point]

an·a·ku·sis (an-ă-koo′sis). SYN anacusis.

anal (ā′năl). Relating to the anus.

an·al·bu·mi·ne·mia (an′al-boo-mi-nē′mē-ă). Absence of albumin from the serum. [G. *an-* priv. + albumin + G. *haima,* blood]

an·a·lep·tic (an-ă-lep′tik). 1. Strengthening, stimulating, or invigorating. 2. A restorative remedy. 3. A central nervous system stimulant, particularly used to denote agents that reverse depressed central nervous system function. [G. *analēptikos,* restorative]

an·al·ge·sia (an-ăl-jē′zē-ă, an-ăl-jēprime;z-ă). A neurologic or pharmacologic state in which painful stimuli are so moderated that, though still perceived, they are no longer painful. Cf. anesthesia. [G. insensibility, fr. *an-* priv. + *algēsis,* sensation of pain]
  conduction a., SYN regional *anesthesia.*
  inhalation a., a. produced by inhalation of a central nervous system depressant gas (especially nitrous oxide) or vapor.
  patient-controlled a. (PCA), a method for control of pain based upon a pump for the constant intravenous or, less frequently, epidural infusion of a dilute narcotic solution that includes a mechanism for the self-administration at predetermined intervals of a predetermined amount of the narcotic solution should the infusion fail to relieve pain. SYN outpatient anesthesia, patient-controlled anesthesia.
  spinal a., euphemism for spinal *anesthesia.*

an·al·ge·sic (an-ăl-jē′zik). 1. A compound capable of producing analgesia, i.e., one that relieves pain by altering perception of nociceptive stimuli without producing anesthesia or loss of consciousness. SYN analgetic (1). 2. Characterized by reduced response to painful stimuli. SYN antalgic.

an·al·ge·sim·e·ter (an′ăl-jē-zim′i-ter). A device for eliciting painful stimuli in order to measure pain under experimental conditions. [analgesia + G. *metron,* measure]

an·al·get·ic (an-ăl-jet′ik). 1. SYN analgesic (1). 2. Associated with decreased pain perception.

anal·i·ty (ā-nal′i-tē). Referring to the psychic organization derived from, and characteristic of, the freudian anal period of psychosexual development.

an·al·ler·gic (an-ă-ler′jik). Not allergic.

an·a·log (an′ă-log). 1. One of two organs or parts in different species of animals or plants that differ in structure or development but are similar in function. 2. A compound that resembles another in structure but is not necessarily an isomer (e.g., 5-fluorouracil is an analog of thymine); a.'s are often used to block enzymatic reactions by combining with enzymes (e.g., isopropyl thiogalactoside vs. lactose). SYN analogue. [G. *analogos,* proportionate]
  enzyme a., SYN synzyme.

anal·o·gous (ă-nal′ō-gŭs). Possessing a functional resemblance, but having a different origin or structure.

an·a·logue (an′ă-log). SYN analog.

an·al·pha·lip·o·pro·tein·e·mia (an-al′fă-lip′ō-prō′tēn-ē′mē-ă) [MIM*205400]. High-density lipoprotein deficiency; a heritable disorder of lipid metabolism characterized by almost complete absence from plasma of high density lipoproteins, and by storage of cholesterol esters in foam cells, tonsillar enlargement, an orange or yellow-gray color of the pharyngeal and rectal mucosa, hepatosplenomegaly, lymph node enlargement, corneal opacity, and peripheral neuropathy; autosomal recessive inheritance. SYN familial high density lipoprotein deficiency, Tangier disease. [G. *an-,* priv., + *alpha,* α, + lipoprotein + *-emia,* blood]

anal·y·sand (ă-nal′i-sand). In psychoanalysis, the person being analyzed. [analysis + L. *-andus,* gerundive ending]

anal·y·sis, pl. **anal·y·ses** (ă-nal′i-sis, -sēz). 1. The breaking up of a chemical compound or mixture into simpler elements; a process by which the composition of a substance is determined. 2. The examination and study of a whole in terms of the parts composing it. 3. SEE psychoanalysis. [G. a breaking up, fr. *ana,* up, + *lysis,* a loosening]
  accumulation a., a technique in which an intermediate of a metabolic pathway accumulates due to selective inhibition of a particular step in that pathway or in a mutant that is deficient in a certain step. The intermediate is then isolated, analyzed, and identified.
  activation a., the identification and quantification of unknown elements from their characteristic emissions and decay constants after they have been made radioactive by exposure to neutron or charged particle radiation.
  amino acid a., (1) determination and identification of amino acid content of a macromolecule; (2) identification of a specific amino acid in macromolecules, often a mutated protein; (3) identification

and quantitation of amino acid content in blood plasma or urine; a key diagnostic aid.

bite a., SYN occlusal a.

blood gas a., the direct electrode measurement of the partial pressure of oxygen and carbon dioxide in the blood.

bradykinetic a., the a. of a movement by means of slow cinematography.

breath a., SYN breath *test*.

cephalometric a., a study of the skeletal and dental relationships used in orthodontic case a.

character a., a. of the defenses and personality traits that characterize an individual.

cluster a., a set of statistical methods used to group variables or observations into strongly interrelated subgroups.

content a., any of a variety of techniques for classification and study of the verbal products of normal or of psychologically disabled individuals.

decision a., a derivative of operations research and game theory that involves identifying all available choices and the potential outcomes of each, in a series of decisions that have to be made about patient care—diagnostic procedures, therapeutic regimens, prognostic expectations; the range of choices can be plotted on a decision tree.

didactic a., SYN training a.

discriminant a., a statistical analytic technique used with discrete dependent variables, concerned with separating sets of observed values and allocating new values; an alternative to regression analysis.

displacement a., SYN competitive binding *assay*.

distributive a., the a. of information gained about the patient and its distribution by the physician, as indicated by the patient's complaint and symptoms.

Downs a., a series of cephalometric criteria used as an aid in orthodontic diagnosis.

ego a., psychoanalytic study of the ways in which the ego deals with intrapsychic conflicts.

Fourier a., a mathematical approximation of a function as the sum of periodic functions (sine and/or cosine waves) of different frequencies; a method of converting a function of time or space into a function of frequency; used in reconstruction of images in computed tomography and magnetic resonance imaging in radiology and in analysis of any kind of signal for its frequency content. SYN Fourier transfer, Fourier transform.

gastric a., measurement of pH and acid output of stomach contents; basal acid output can be determined by collecting the overnight gastric secretion or by a 1-hr collection; maximal acid output is determined following injection of histamine; output is measured by titration with a strong base.

intention-to-treat a., method of analyzing results of a randomized controlled trial that includes in the a. all the cases that should have received a treatment regimen but for whatever reason did not do so. All cases allocated to each arm of the trial are analyzed together as representing that treatment arm, whether or not they received or completed the prescribed regimen.

interaction process a., in psychology, a. of small group behavior in terms of 12 specific categories, e.g., solidarity, tension release, agreement.

Kaplan-Meier a., a method of calculating survival of a patient population in which the increments are the actual survival times of the patients.

linkage a., the assessment of the linkage relationship between two loci by the examination of data in pedigrees. The classical concern is with estimating recombination fractions and (because of its elasticity, efficiency, and other optimal properties) the preferred method is maximum likelihood estimation. However, there are other more modern concerns, notably determining the order of loci, testing for additive and interactive properties in the mapping function, and reconciling the pedigree data with evidence from other methods (e.g., cytogenetics, in situ hybridization studies, etc.).

Northern blot a., a procedure similar to the Southern blot a., used to separate and identify RNA fragments; typically via transferring (blotting) RNA fragments from an agarose gel to a nitrocellulose filter followed by detection with a suitable probe. [coined to distinguish it from eponymic Southern blot a.]

occlusal a., a study of the relations of the occlusal surfaces of opposing teeth and their effect upon related structures. SYN bite a.

path a., a mode of a. involving assumptions about the direction of causal relationships among linked sequences and configurations of variables.

pedigree a., the formal study of the pattern of a trait in a pedigree to determine such properties as its mode of inheritance, age of onset, and variability in phenotype.

percept a., psychologic survey of an individual's personality using Rorschach series of inkblots.

qualitative a., determination of the nature, as opposed to the quantity, of each of the elements composing a substance.

quantitative a., determination of the amount, as well as the nature, of each of the elements composing a substance.

regression a., the statistical method of finding the "best" mathematical model to describe one variable as a function of another.

saturation a., SYN competitive binding *assay*.

segregation a., in genetics, the enumeration of progeny according to distinct and mutually exclusive phenotypes; used as a test of a putative pattern of inheritance, e.g., mendelian, dominant autosomal, epistatic, age-dependent.

sequential a., a statistical method that allows an experiment to be ended as soon as a result of desired precision is obtained.

Southern blot a., a procedure to separate and identify DNA sequences; DNA fragments are separated by electrophoresis on an agarose gel, transferred (blotted) onto a nitrocellulose or nylon membrane, and hybridized with complementary (labeled) nucleic acid probes.

survival a., a class of statistical procedures for estimating survival rates and making inferences about effects of treatment, prognostic factors, etc.

training a., psychoanalytic treatment for the purpose of training of an analytic candidate carried out under the official auspices of a psychoanalytic training institute. SYN didactic a.

transactional a., a psychotherapy system, used in both individual and group treatment, involving a systematic understanding of the qualities of interpersonal interactions in the treatment sessions; includes four components: 1) structural analysis of intrapsychic phenomena; 2) transactional a. proper, determination of the currently dominant ego state (parent, child, or adult) of each participant; 3) game analysis, identification of the games played in their interactions and of the gratifications provided; 4) script analysis, uncovering of the causes of the patient's emotional problems.

a. of variance (ANOVA), a statistical technique that isolates and assesses the contribution of categorical independent variables to variation in the mean of a continuous dependent variable.

volumetric a., quantitative a. by the addition of graduated amounts of a standard test solution to a solution of a known amount of the substance analyzed, until the reaction is just at an end; depends upon the stoichiometric nature of the reaction between the test solution and the unknown.

Western blot a., a procedure in which proteins separated by electrophoresis in polyacrylamide gels are transferred (blotted) onto nitrocellulose or nylon membranes and identified by specific complexing with antibodies that are either pre- or posttagged with a labeled secondary protein. SEE ALSO immunoblot. SYN Western blot, Western blotting. [coined to distinguish it from eponymic Southern blot a.]

zoo blot a., a procedure using Southern blot a. to test the ability of a nucleic acid probe from one species to hybridize with the DNA fragment of another species.

an·a·lyst (an'ă-list). **1.** One who makes analytic determinations. **2.** Short term for psychoanalyst.

an·a·lyte (an'ă-līt). Any material or chemical substance subjected to analysis.

an·a·lyt·ic, an·a·lyt·i·cal (an-ă-lit'-ik, -i-kăl). **1.** Relating to analysis. **2.** Relating to psychoanalysis.

an·a·lyz·er, an·a·lyz·or (an'ă-līz-er, -ŏr). **1.** Any instrument that performs an analysis. **2.** The prism in a polariscope by means of which the polarized light is examined. **3.** The neural basis of the conditioned reflex; includes all of the sensory side of the reflex arc and its central connections. **4.** A device that electronically determines the frequency and amplitude of a particular channel of an electroencephalogram.

batch a., a discrete automated chemical a. in which the instrument system sequentially performs a single test on each of a group of samples.

centrifugal fast a., an automatic spectrophotometer that uses centrifugal force to mix samples and reagents, and propels the reactants at high speed in view of a detector that makes multiple absorbance readings.

continuous flow a., an automated chemical a. in which the samples and reagents are pumped continuously through a system of modules interconnected by tubing.

discrete a., an automated chemical a. in which the instrument performs tests on samples that are kept in discrete containers in contrast to a continuous flow analyzer.

kinetic a., an instrument that measures the rate of change in a chemical substance; used mainly for enzyme measurement.

pulse height a., electronic circuitry that determines the energy of scintillations recorded by a detector, allowing use of a discriminator to select for photons of a specific type.

wave a., an apparatus that assesses a complex mixture of wave forms by separating out their component frequencies and displaying their distribution.

an·am·ne·sis (an-am-nē′sis). **1.** The act of remembering. **2.** The medical or developmental history of a patient. [G. *anamnēsis,* recollection]

an·am·nes·tic (an-am-nes′tik). **1.** Assisting the memory. SYN mnemonic. **2.** Relating to the medical history of a patient.

an·am·ni·on·ic, an·am·ni·ot·ic (an-am-nē-on′ik, -ot′ik). Without an amnion.

An·am·ni·o·ta (an-am-nē-ō′tă). A group of vertebrates whose embryos are not enclosed in an amnion; it includes the cyclostomes, fish, and amphibians.

ana·morph. A somatic or reproductive structure that originates without nuclear recombination (asexual reproduction); the imperfect part of the life cycle of fungi. [G. *ana,* up, + *morphē,* form]

an·a·mor·pho·sis (an′ă-mōr-fō′sis). **1.** In phylogeny, a progressive series of changes in the evolution of a group of animals or plants. **2.** In optics, the process of correcting a distorted image with a curved mirror. [G. *ana,* up, + *morphē,* form]

an·an·a·sta·sia (an′an-ă-stā′zē-ă). Inability to stand up. [G. *a-* priv. + *anastasis,* stand up]

an·an·casm (an′an-kazm). Any form of repetitious stereotyped behavior which, if prevented, results in anxiety. [G. *anankasma,* compulsion]

an·an·cas·tia (an-an-kas′tē-ă). An obsession in which a person feels forced to act or think against her or his will. [G. *anankastos,* compelled]

an·an·cas·tic (an-an-kas′tik). Pertaining to anancasm or anancastia.

an·an·dria (an-an′drē-ă). Absence of masculinity. [G. want of manhood, fr. *an-* priv. + *anēr-* (*andr-*), man]

an·an·gi·o·pla·sia (an-an′jē-ō-pla′zē-ă). Imperfect vascularization of a part due to nonformation of vessels, or vessels with inadequate caliber. [G. *an-* priv. + *angeion,* vessel, + *plastos,* formed]

an·an·gi·o·plas·tic (an-an′jē-ō-plas′tik). Relating to, characterized by, or due to anangioplasia.

ANAP Abbreviation for anionic neutrophil-activating *peptide.*

an·a·phase (an′ă-fāz). The stage of mitosis or meiosis in which the chromosomes move from the equatorial plate toward the poles of the cell. In mitosis a full set of daughter chromosomes (46 in humans) moves toward each pole. In the first division of meiosis one member of each homologous pair (23 in humans), consisting of two chromatids united at the centromere, moves toward each pole. In the second division of meiosis the centromere divides, and the two chromatids separate with one moving to each pole. [G. *ana,* up, + *phasis,* appearance]

an·a·phia (an-ā′fē-ă, an-af′ē-ă). Absence of the sense of touch. SYN anhaphia. [G. *an-* priv. + *haphē,* touch]

an·a·pho·re·sis (an′ă-fō-rē′sis). Movement of negatively charged particles (anions) in a solution or suspension toward the anode in electrophoresis. Cf. cataphoresis. [G. *ana,* up + *phorēsis,* a being borne]

an·aph·o·ret·ic (an′ă-fō-ret′ik). Relating to anaphoresis (1).

an·aph·ro·di·si·ac (an′af-rō-diz′ē-ak). **1.** Relating to anaphrodisia. **2.** Repressing or destroying sexual desire. **3.** An agent that lessens or abolishes sexual desire. SYN antaphrodisiac, antaphroditic (1). [G. *an-* priv. + *aphrodisia,* sexual pleasure]

an·a·phy·lac·tic (an′ă-fī-lak′tik). Relating to anaphylaxis; manifesting extremely great sensitivity to foreign protein or other material.

an·a·phy·lac·to·gen (an′ă-fī-lak′tō-jen). A substance (antigen) capable of rendering an individual susceptible to anaphylaxis; a substance (antigen) that will cause an anaphylactic reaction in such a sensitized individual.

an·a·phy·lac·to·gen·e·sis (an′ă-fī-lak-tō-jen′ĕ-sis). The production of anaphylaxis.

an·a·phy·lac·to·gen·ic (an′ă-fī-lak-tō-jen′ik). Producing anaphylaxis; pertaining to substances (antigens) that result in an individual becoming susceptible to anaphylaxis.

an·a·phy·lac·toid (an′ă-fī-lak′toyd). Resembling anaphylaxis. SYN pseudoanaphylactic. [anaphylaxis + G. *eidos,* resemblance]

an·a·phyl·a·tox·in (an′ă-fil-ă-tok′sin). Low molecular weight substances generated by the activation of complement; the biologically active complement components are derived from C3, C4, and C5 and lead to increased vascular permeability as a result of the degranulation of primarily mast cells; release of mediators of immediate hypersensitivity (Type I), i.e., histamine, follows mast cell degranulation. SYN anaphylotoxin. [anaphylaxis + toxin]

an·a·phyl·a·tox·in in·ac·ti·va·tor. An α-globulin (MW 300,000) which destroys the activity of the anaphylatoxic complement fragments. SEE anaphylatoxin.

an·a·phy·lax·is (an′ă-fī-lak′sis). An induced systemic or generalized sensitivity; at times the term a. is used for anaphylactic shock. The term is commonly used to denote the immediate, transient kind of immunologic (allergic) reaction characterized by contraction of smooth muscle and dilation of capillaries due to release of pharmacologically active substances (histamine, bradykinin, serotonin, and slow-reacting substances), classically initiated by the combination of antigen (allergen) with mast-cell–fixed, cytophilic antibody (chiefly IgE); the reaction can be initiated, also, by relatively large quantities of serum aggregates (antigen-antibody complexes, and others) that seemingly activate complement leading to production of anaphylatoxins. SYN anaphylactic reaction. [G. *ana,* away from, back from, + *phylaxis,* protection]

active a., reaction following inoculation of antigen in a subject previously sensitized to the specific antigen, in contrast to passive a.

aggregate a., an anaphylactic reaction initiated by the formation of antigen-antibody complexes that activate complement.

antiserum a., SYN passive a.

chronic a., SYN *enteritis* anaphylactica.

generalized a., the immediate response, involving smooth muscles and capillaries throughout the body of a sensitized individual, that follows intravenous (and occasionally intracutaneous) injection of antigen (allergen). SEE ALSO anaphylactic *shock.* SYN systemic a.

inverse a., anaphylactic shock in an animal (e.g., guinea pig) whose tissues contain Forssman antigen, resulting from an intravenous injection of serum that contains Forssman antibody.

local a., the immediate, transient kind of response that follows the injection of antigen (allergen) into the skin of a sensitized individual and is limited to the area surrounding the site of inoculation. SEE ALSO skin *test.*

passive a., a reaction resulting from inoculation of antigen in an animal previously inoculated intravenously with specific antiserum from another animal, a latent period being required between the two inoculations. SYN antiserum a.

passive cutaneous a. (PCA), a reaction that occurs in the guinea pig when antiserum is injected into the skin and, 6–24 hours later, specific antigen and a dye such as Pontamine blue or Evans blue are inoculated intravenously; the size of the blue areas at the sites of the antibody injections is a measure of the degree of altered permeability to dye-bound albumin.

reversed a., SYN reversed passive a.

reversed passive a., an anaphylactic reaction induced in an animal injected with a specific antigen, which will bind to reactive tissue, and then, after a latent period, with serum from another animal previously sensitized to the identical antigen. SYN reversed a.

systemic a., SYN generalized a.

an·a·phyl·o·tox·in (an′ă-fil-ō-tok′sin). SYN anaphylatoxin.

an·a·pla·sia (an-ă-plā′sē-ă). Loss of structural differentiation, especially as seen in most, but not all, malignant neoplasms. SYN dedifferentiation (2). [G. *ana*, again, + *plasis*, a molding]

an·a·plas·tic (an-ă-plas′tik). **1.** Relating to anaplasty. **2.** Characterized by or pertaining to anaplasia. **3.** Growing without form or structure.

an·a·plas·to·lo·gy (an′ă-plas-tol′ō-jē). Application of prosthetic materials for construction and/or reconstruction of a missing body part. [G. *ana*, again, + *plastos*, formed]

an·a·ple·ro·sis (an′ă-pler-ō′sis). The process of replenishment of depleted metabolic cycle or pathway intermediates; most commonly referring to the tricarboxylic acid cycle. [G. filling up, fr. *ana-*, up, + *plerosis*, filling, fr. *pleroō*, to fill]

an·a·ple·rot·ic (an′ă-pler-ŏ′tik). Referring to reactions or pathways that contribute to anaplerosis.

an·a·poph·y·sis (an-ă-pof′i-sis). An accessory spinal process of a vertebra, found especially in the thoracic or lumbar vertebrae. [G. *ana*, back, + *apophysis*, offshoot]

anap·tic (ă-nap′tik). Relating to anaphia.

an·a·rith·mia (an-ă-rith′mē-ă). Aphasia characterized by an inability to count or use numbers. [G. *an-* priv. + *arithmos*, number]

an·ar·thria (an-ar′thrē-a). Loss of the power of articulate speech. SEE ALSO aphasia, alexia, dysarthria. [G. fr. *an-anthos*, without joints; (of sound) inarticulate]

an·a·sar·ca (an-ă-sar′kă). A generalized infiltration of edema fluid into subcutaneous connective tissue. SYN hydrosarca. [G. *ana*, through, + *sarx* (*sark-*), flesh]

    fetoplacental a., edema of fetus and placenta as found in fetal hydrops.

an·a·sar·cous (an-ă-sar′kŭs). Characterized by anasarca.

an·a·stig·mat·ic (an′as-tig-mat′ik). Not astigmatic.

an·as·tig·mats. **1.** Lenses in which astigmatism is corrected. **2.** Lenses in which both astigmatism and field curvature are corrected.

an·as·to·le (an-as′tō-lē). Obsolete term for the gaping of a wound. [G. *anastolē*, the laying bare of a wound]

anas·to·mose (ă-nas′tō-mōs). **1.** To open one structure into another directly or by connecting channels, said of blood vessels, lymphatics, and hollow viscera; also incorrectly applied to nerves. **2.** To unite by means of an anastomosis, or connection between formerly separate structures.

⌶anas·to·mo·sis, pl. **anas·to·mo·ses** (ă-nas′tō-mō′sis, -sez). **1.** A natural communication, direct or indirect, between two blood vessels or other tubular structures. SEE communication. **2.** An operative union of two structures (e.g., vessels, ureters, nerves). **3.** An opening created by surgery, trauma, or disease between two or more normally separate spaces or organs. [G. *anastomōsis,* from *anastomoō,* to furnish with a mouth]

    acromial a. of the thoracoacromial artery [TA], a vascular network between the acromion and the skin of the shoulder, formed by anastomoses of the acromial branch of the suprascapular artery with the acromial branch of the thoracoacromial artery. SYN rete acromiale arteriae thoracoacromialis [TA], acromial arterial network, acromial plexus.

    arteriolovenular a. [TA], vessels through which blood is shunted from arterioles to venules without passing through the capillaries. The term "arteriovenous a." is widely used, but not preferred,

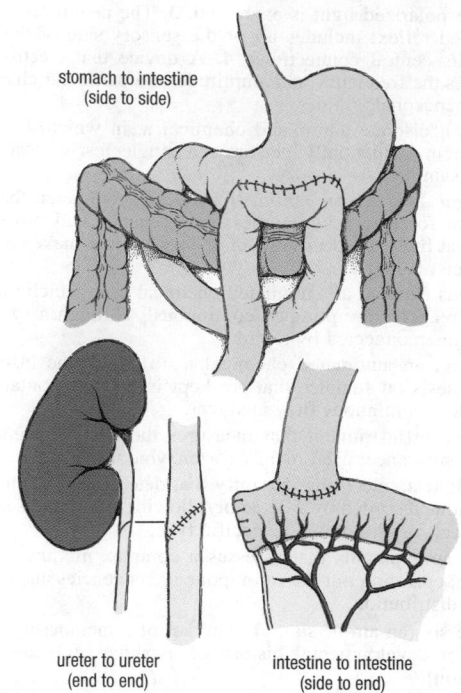

stomach to intestine
(side to side)

ureter to ureter
(end to end)

intestine to intestine
(side to end)

surgical anastomoses

since the connection is between arterioles and venules rather than arteries and veins. SYN a. arteriolovenularis☆, a. arteriovenosa, arteriovenous a.

    a. arteriolovenularis, ☆official alternate term for arteriolovenular a.

    a. arterioveno′sa, SYN arteriolovenular a.

    arteriovenous a. (ava), SYN arteriolovenular a.

    Béclard a., SYN ranine a.

    bevelled a., a. performed after cutting each of the structures to be joined in an oblique fashion.

    Billroth I a., reestablishment of intestinal continuity by a gastroduodenostomy. SEE ALSO Billroth *operation* I.

    Billroth II a., reestablishment of intestinal continuity by a loop gastrojejunostomy. SEE ALSO Billroth *operation* II.

    Braun a., after a loop gastroenterostomy, a. between afferent and efferent loops of jejunum.

    calcaneal a. [TA], a superficial network over the calcaneus, formed by branches of the peroneal and posterior tibial arteries and twigs from the malleolar retia. SYN rete calcaneum [TA], calcaneal arterial network.

    cavopulmonary a., a means of palliating cyanotic heart disease by anastomosing the right pulmonary artery to the superior vena cava. SYN cavopulmonary shunt, Glenn shunt.

    Clado a., a. in the right suspensory ligament of the ovary between the appendicular and ovarian arteries.

    conjoined a., the joining together of two small blood vessels by side-to-side elliptical a. to create a single larger stoma for subsequent end-to-end a.

    cruciate a., crucial a., a four-way a. between branches of the first perforating branch of the deep femoral, inferior gluteal, and medial and lateral circumflex femoral arteries, located posterior to the upper part of the femur. Formerly described as common, investigations show it rarely occurs in the four-way "cross" pattern.

    cubital a. [TA], vascular networks in the region of the elbow, composed of anastomoses between branches of the radial and middle collateral, superior and inferior ulnar collateral, radial recurrent, interosseous recurrent, and recurrent ulnar arteries. SYN rete articulare cubiti [TA], articular vascular network of elbow.

    Damus-Stancel-Kaye a., SYN Damus-Kaye-Stancel *procedure*.

elliptical a., a modification of direct a. whereby one or both tubular structures are spatulated beforehand, thus creating an ellipse of greater cross-sectional as well as circumferential dimension than would be possible with a bevelled or circular a.

end-to-end a., a. performed after cutting each structure to be joined in a plane perpendicular to the ultimate flow through the structures.

Galen a., SYN communicating *branch* of internal laryngeal nerve with recurrent laryngeal nerve.

genicular a. [TA], an arterial network over the front and sides of the knee, formed by branches of the descending genicular artery, of the five genicular arteries from the popliteal, of the anterior tibial recurrent, and of the fibular circumflex branches of the posterior tibial. SYN rete articulare genus [TA], articular vascular network of knee.

Hofmeister-Pólya a., SEE Hofmeister *operation*, Pólya *operation*.

Hoyer anastomoses, SYN Sucquet-Hoyer *canals*, under *canal*.

Hyrtl a., SYN Hyrtl *loop*.

intermesenteric arterial anastomoses, SYN intestinal arterial *arcades*, under *arcade*.

intestinal a., SYN enteroenterostomy.

isoperistaltic a., an a. allowing flow of contents in the same and normal direction.

Jacobson a., a portion of the tympanic plexus.

Martin-Gruber a., a nerve anomaly in the forearm, consisting of a median to ulnar nerve communication; Also referred to as a median-to-ulnar crossover.

microvascular a., a. of very small blood vessels performed under a surgical microscope.

patellar a. [TA], the superficial portion of the articular vascular network of the knee. SYN rete patellare [TA], patellar network.

portacaval anastomoses, SYN portal-systemic anastomoses.

portal-systemic anastomoses, (1) naturally-occurring venous communications between tributaries of the portal venous system and tributaries of the systemic venous system. The major portal-systemic anastomoses include: 1) esophageal branches of left gastric vein with esophageal veins, 2) superior rectal vein with middle and inferior rectal veins, 3) paraumbilical veins with subcutaneous veins of anterior abdominal wall, 4) retroperitoneal veins with venous branches of veins of the colon and bare area of the liver, and 5) a patent ductus venosus connecting left branch of portal vein to inferior vena cava (rare). These anastomoses are important clinically, providing collateral circulation during portal obstruction or hypertension, although they may become varicose; SEE *caput* medusae, esophageal *varices*, under *varix*, hemorrhoids; **(2)** surgically-created communications between the portal vein and the inferior vena cava or their tributaries, to relieve portal hypertension. SYN portacaval anastomoses.

postcostal a., longitudinal a. of intersegmental arteries giving rise to the vertebral artery.

Potts a., SYN Potts *operation*.

precapillary a., an a. between arterioles just before they become capillaries.

precostal a. (prē-kos′-tal), longitudinal a. of intersegmental arteries in the embryo that gives rise to the thyrocervical and costocervical trunks.

pulmonary artery a., a. of the pulmonary artery; 40–50% are associated with congenital heart defects.

ranine a., an a. between the right and the left end-branch of the deep lingual artery. SYN arcus raninus, Béclard a.

Riolan a., the specific portion of the marginal artery of the colon connecting the middle and left colic arteries. SYN Riolan arc (3).

Roux-en-Y a., a. of the distal end of the divided jejunum to the stomach, bile duct, or another structure, with implantation of the proximal end into the side of the jejunum at a suitable distance (usually greater than 40 cm) below the first a., the bowel then forming a Y-shaped pattern.

Schmidel anastomoses, abnormal channels of communication between the caval and portal venous systems.

sequential a., two or more anastomoses fashioned from a single conduit, e.g., two or more coronary arteries from a single vein graft or mammary artery.

Sucquet anastomoses, SYN Sucquet-Hoyer *canals,* under *canal.*

Sucquet-Hoyer anastomoses, SYN Sucquet-Hoyer *canals,* under *canal.*

terminoterminal a., an operation by which the central end of an artery is connected with the peripheral end of the corresponding vein, and the peripheral end of the artery with the central end of the vein.

transureteroureteral a., SYN transureteroureterostomy.

ureteroileal a., a. between the ureter and an isolated segment of ileum. SEE ALSO Bricker *operation*.

ureterosigmoid a., a. between the ureter and a segment or entire sigmoid colon. SEE ALSO ureterosigmoidostomy.

ureteroureteral a., a. from one part of a ureter to another part of the same ureter.

anas·to·mot·ic (a-nas-tō-mot′ik). Pertaining to an anastomosis.

an·as·tral (an-as′trăl). Lacking an astrosphere.

an·a·tom·i·cal (an′ă-tom′i-kăl). **1.** Relating to anatomy. **2.** SYN structural. **3.** Denoting a strictly morphological feature distinct from its physiological or surgical considerations, e.g., anatomical neck of humerus, anatomical dead space, anatomical lobulation of the liver.

an·a·tom·i·co·med·i·cal (an-ă-tom′i-kō-med′i-kăl). Referring to both medicine and anatomy.

an·a·tom·i·co·path·o·log·ic (an-ă-tom′i-kō-path-ŏ-loj′i-kăl). Relating to anatomical pathology.

an·a·tom·i·co·sur·gi·cal (an-ă-tom′i-kō-ser′ji-kăl). Relating to surgical anatomy.

an·a·tom·ic snuff·box (snŭf′boks). A hollow seen on the radial aspect of the wrist when the thumb is extended fully; it is bounded by the prominences of the tendon of the extensor pollicis longus posteriorly and of the tendons of the extensor pollicis brevis and abductor pollicis longus anteriorly. The radial artery crosses the floor which is formed by the scaphoid and the trapezium bones. SYN tabatière anatomique.

anat·o·mist (ă-nat′ŏ-mist). A specialist in the science of anatomy.

anat·o·my (ă-nat′ŏ-mē) [TA]. **1.** The morphologic structure of an organism. **2.** The science of the morphology or structure of organisms. **3.** SYN dissection. **4.** A work describing the form and structure of an organism and its various parts. [G. *anatomē,* dissection, from *ana,* apart, + *tomē,* a cutting]

applied a., SYN clinical a.

artificial a., the manufacture of models of anatomic structures, or the study of a. from such models.

artistic a., the study of a. for artistic purposes, as applied to painting, drawing, or sculpture.

clastic a., the construction or study of models in layers which can be removed one after the other to show the structure of the organism and/or organ. SYN plastic a.

clinical a., the practical application of anatomical knowledge to diagnosis and treatment. SYN applied a.

comparative a., the comparative study of animal structure with regard to homologous organs or parts.

dental a., that branch of gross a. concerned with the morphology of teeth, their location, position, and relationships.

descriptive a., a description of, especially a treatise describing, physical structure, more particularly that of man. SYN systematic a.

developmental a., a. of the structural changes of an individual from fertilization to adulthood; includes embryology, fetology, and postnatal development.

functional a., a. studied in its relation to function. SYN morphophysiology, physiologic a.

general a., the study of gross and microscopic structures as well as of the composition of the body, its tissues and fluids.

gross a., general a., so far as it can be studied without the use of the microscope; commonly used to denote the study of a. by dissection of a cadaver. SEE practical a. SYN macroscopic a.

living a., the study of a. in the living individual by inspection.

macroscopic a., SYN gross a.

medical a., a. in its bearing upon the diagnosis and treatment of diseases.

microscopic a., the branch of a. in which the structure of cells, tissues, and organs is studied with the light microscope. SEE histology.

pathological a., SYN anatomic *pathology.*

physiologic a., SYN functional a.

plastic a., SYN clastic a.

practical a., a. studied by means of dissection. SEE gross a.

radiologic a., the study of bodily structure using radiographs and other imaging methods.

regional a., an approach to anatomic study based on regions, parts, or divisions of the body (e.g., the foot or the inguinal region), emphasizing the relationships of various systemic structures (e.g., muscles, nerves, and arteries) within that area; distinguished from systemic a. SYN topographic a., topology (1).

special a., the a. of certain definite organs or groups of organs involved in the performance of special functions; descriptive a. dealing with the separate systems.

surface a., the study of the configuration of the surface of the body, especially in its relation to deeper parts.

surgical a., applied a. in reference to surgical diagnosis, dissection, or treatment.

systematic a., SYN descriptive a.

systemic a., a. of the systems of the body; an approach to anatomical study organized by organ systems, e.g., the cardiovascular system, emphasizing an overview of the system throughout the body; distinguished from regional a.

topographic a., SYN regional a.

transcendental a., the theories and deductions based upon the morphology of the organs and individual parts of the body.

ultrastructural a., the ultramicroscopic study of structures too small to be seen with a light microscope.

anat·o·pism (ă-nat′ō-pizm). Failure to conform to the cultural pattern. [G. *ana,* backward, + *topos,* place]

an·a·tox·ic (an-ă-tok′sik). Pertaining to the characteristic properties of anatoxin (toxoid).

an·a·tox·in (an-ă-tok′sin). SYN toxoid.

an·a·tri·crot·ic (an′ă-trī-krot′ik). Characterized by anatricrotism; denoting a sphygmographic tracing with three waves on the ascending limb.

an·a·tric·ro·tism (an′ă-trik′rō-tizm). A condition of the pulse manifested by a triple beat on the ascending limb of the sphygmographic tracing. [G. *ana,* up, + *tri-,* thrice, *krotos,* beating]

an·a·trip·sis (an-ă-trip′sis). Therapeutic use of rubbing or friction with or without simultaneous application of a medicament. [G. a rubbing, fr. *anatribō,* fr. *ana,* intensive, + *tribō,* to rub]

an·a·trip·tic (an-ă-trip′tik). 1. Pertaining to anatripsis. 2. A remedy to be applied by friction or rubbing.

an·ax·on, an·ax·one (an-aks′on, -aks′ōn). Having no axon; denoting certain nerve cells first described by S. Ramón y Cajal as amacrine cells in the retina, and later discovered in several brain regions. [G. *an-* priv. + *axōn,* axis]

an·a·zo·tu·ria (an′az-ō-too′rē-ă). A deficiency or lack of nitrogenous metabolic products excreted in the urine; pertains especially to unusually small quantities of urea in the urine. [G. *an-* priv. + azoturia]

ANCA Abbreviation for antineutrophil cytoplasmic *antibodies,* under *antibody.*

AnCC Abbreviation for anodal closure *contraction.*

an·ces·tor. A person in the direct line of descent from which a subject of interest is derived (parents, grandparents, etc.; but no collaterals or descendants).

leading ancestor, in genetic counseling given to a consultand unaffected by but possibly a carrier or a latent subject of the disease; the most recent ancestor in the direct line of descent known to have had the affected gene in question.

an·chor·age (ang′kōr-ij). 1. Operative fixation of loose or prolapsed abdominal or pelvic organs. 2. The part to which anything is fastened. In dentistry, a tooth or an implanted tooth substitute

with which a fixed or removable partial denture, crown, or restoration is retained. 3. The nature and degree of resistance to displacement offered by an anatomical unit when used for the purpose of effecting tooth movement. [L. *ancora,* fr. G. *ankyra,* anchor]

cervical a., a. in which the back of the neck is used for resistance by means of a cervical strap.

extraoral a., a. in which the resistance unit is outside the oral cavity; e.g., cranial, occipital, or cervical a.

intermaxillary a., a. in which the units in one jaw are used to effect tooth movement in the other jaw.

intramaxillary a., a. in which the resistance units are all situated within the same jaw.

intraoral a., a. in which the resistance units are all located within the oral cavity.

multiple a., a. in which more than one type of resistance unit is utilized. SYN reinforced a.

occipital a., a. in which the top and back of the head are used for resistance by means of a headgear.

reciprocal a., a. in which the movement of one or more teeth is balanced against the movement of one or more opposing teeth.

reinforced a., SYN multiple a.

simple a., a. in which the resistance to the movement of one or more teeth comes solely from resistance to tipping movement of the a. unit.

stationary a., a. in which the resistance to the movement of one or more teeth comes from the resistance to bodily movement of the a. unit; a questionable concept since the selected teeth remain only relatively stable.

an·chor·in (ang′kōr-in). SYN ankyrin. [anchor + -in]

an·chu·sin (an′koo-sin). SYN alkannin.

an·cil·lary (an′si-lār-ē). Auxiliary, accessory, or secondary. [L. *ancillaris,* relating to a maidservant]

an·cip·i·tal, an·cip·i·tate, an·cip·i·tous (an-sip′i-tăl, -i-tāt, -itŭs). Two-headed; two-edged. [L. *anceps,* two-headed]

an·con (ang′kŏn). SYN elbow (2). [G. *ankon,* elbow]

an·co·nad (ang′kō-nad). Toward the elbow. [G. *ankōn,* elbow, + L. *ad,* to]

an·co·nal, an·co·ne·al (ang′kŏ-năl, ang-kō′nē-ăl). 1. Relating to the elbow (ancon). 2. Relating to the anconeus muscle.

an·co·ne·us (ang-kō′nē-ŭs). SYN anconeus *muscle.* [L.]

an·co·noid (ang′kō-noyd). Resembling the elbow.

an·crod (an′krod). A fraction obtained from the venom of the pit viper, *Angkistrodon rhodostoma,* which contains a fibrinogen-splitting enzyme; produces hypofibrinogenemia and diminution of both whole blood and plasma viscosity for improvement of the rheologic properties of blood, and is used in treatment of chronic peripheral vascular disease.

△**ancylo-.** SEE ankylo-.

An·cy·los·to·ma (an-si-los′tō-mă, an-ki-). A genus of Nematoda, the Old World hookworm, the members of which are parasitic in the duodenum. They attach themselves to villi in the mucous membrane, suck blood, and may cause a state of anemia, especially in cases of malnutrition. The eggs are passed with the feces, and the larvae develop in moist soil to become infectious third-stage (filariform) larvae that enter the human body through the skin and possibly in drinking water; they migrate by the bloodstream to lung alveoli, are carried to bronchi and trachea, swallowed, and passed to the intestine, where they mature. SEE ALSO ancylostomiasis, *Necator.* SYN *Ankylostoma* (1). [G. *ankylos,* curved, hooked, + *stoma,* mouth]

A. brazilien′se, a species characterized by one pair of ventral buccal teeth, normally an intestinal parasite of dogs and cats but also found in humans as a cause of human cutaneous larva migrans.

A. cani′num, a species possessing three pairs of ventral teeth in the oral cavity; common in dogs, but also occurring in human skin as a cause of cutaneous larva migrans.

A. ceylan′icum, species found in the civet cat of Ceylon; rarely, reported from humans as an intestinal parasite in Southeast Asia.

A. duodena′le, the Old World hookworm of humans, a species widespread in temperate areas, in contrast to the more tropical distribution of the New World hookworm, *Necator americanus*, that is the only hookworm found in the U.S.

A. tubaeforme, a nematode species found in the cat; cutaneous larva migrans seen in humans.

an·cy·lo·sto·mat·ic (an'si-lō-stō-mat'ik, an'ki-). Referring to hookworms of the genus *Ancylostoma*.

an·cy·lo·sto·mi·a·sis (an'si-lō-stō-mī'ă-sis, an'ki-). Hookworm disease caused by *Ancylostoma duodenale* and characterized by eosinophilia, anemia, emaciation, dyspepsia, and, in children with severe chronic infections, swelling of the abdomen with mental and physical maldevelopment. SYN ankylostomiasis, intertropical hyphemia, tropical hyphemia, miner's disease (1), tunnel disease, uncinariasis.

cutaneous a., SYN cutaneous *larva migrans.*

an·cy·roid (an'si-royd). Shaped like the fluke of an anchor; denoting the cornua of the lateral ventricles of the brain and the coracoid process of the scapula. SYN ankyroid. [G. *ankyra*, anchor, + *eidos*, resemblance]

Andernach, Johann W. (Guenther von Andernach), German physician, 1505–1574. SEE A. *ossicles*, under *ossicle*.

Anders, James Meschter, U.S. physician, 1854–1936. SEE A. *disease*.

Andersch, Carolus Samuel, German anatomist, 1732–1777. SEE A. *ganglion, nerve*.

Andersen, Dorothy Hansine, U.S. pediatrician, 1901–1963. SEE A. *disease*.

Anderson, Evelyn, U.S. physician, *1899. SEE A.-Collip *test*.

Anderson, Roger, U.S. surgeon, 1891–1971. SEE A. *splint;* Roger A. pin fixation *appliance*.

Anderson, James C., British urologist, *1899.

an·di·ra (an-dī'ră). The bark of *Andira inermis*, a leguminous tree of tropical America, used as an emetic, purgative, and anthelmintic. SYN cabbage tree, worm bark. [West Indian native name]

Andral, Gabriel, French physician, 1797–1876. SEE A. *decubitus*.

an·dre·nos·ter·one (an-drĕ-nos'ter-ōn). SYN adrenosterone.

an·dri·at·rics, an·dri·a·try (an-dri-at'riks, -drī'ă-trē). Medical science relating to diseases of male genital organs and of men in general. [G. *anēr*, a man, + *iatreia*, medical treatment]

⌂**andro-.** Masculine. [G. *anēr, andros*, a male human being]

an·dro·gen (an'drō-jen). Generic term for an agent, usually a hormone (e.g., androsterone, testosterone), that stimulates activity of the accessory male sex organs, encourages development of male sex characteristics, or prevents changes in the latter that follow castration; natural a.'s are steroids, derivatives of androstane. SYN testoid (2).

adrenal a., any androgenic hormone of adrenocortical origin; e.g., dehydroepiandrosterone (and its sulfate), androstenedione, 11β-hydroxyandrostenedione.

an·dro·gen·e·sis (an-drō-jen'ĕ-sis). Development in the presence of paternal chromosomes only. [andro- + G. *genesis,* production]

an·dro·gen·ic (an-drō-jen'ik). Relating to an androgen; having a masculinizing effect. SYN testoid (1).

an·drog·e·nous (an-droj'ĕ-nŭs). Giving birth to males.

an·drog·y·nism (an-droj'i-nizm). SYN female *pseudohermaphroditism.*

an·drog·y·noid (an-droj'i-noyd). A male resembling a female, or possessing female features. [andro- + G. *gynē*, woman, + *eidos,* resemblance]

an·drog·y·nous (an-droj'i-nŭs). Pertaining to androgyny.

an·drog·y·ny (an-droj'i-nē). **1.** SYN female *pseudohermaphroditism.* **2.** Having both masculine and feminine characteristics, as in attitudes and behaviors that contain features of stereotyped, culturally sanctioned sexual roles of both male and female. [andro- + G. *gynē,* woman]

an·droid (an'droyd). SYN andromorphous. [andro- + G. *eidos,* resemblance]

an·drol·o·gy (an-drol'ō-jē). The branch of medicine concerned with diseases peculiar to the male sex, particularly infertility and sexual dysfunction. [andro- + G. *logos,* treatise]

an·drom·e·do·tox·in (an-drom'ĕ-dō-tok'sin). A strongly emetic active principle obtained from several species of *Andromeda* and *Rhododendron* (family Ericaceae); it is a cardiac poison, first stimulating and then paralyzing the vagus; it also paralyzes the motor nerve ends in striated muscle.

an·dro·mor·phous (an-drō-mōr'fŭs). Having a male form or habitus. SYN android. [andro- + G. *morphē,* form]

an·drop·a·thy (an-drop'ă-thē). Any disease, such as prostatitis, peculiar to the male sex. [andro- + G. *pathos,* suffering]

andropause. A postulated decrease in function of male gonads with increasing age, analogous to menopause.

an·dro·pho·bia (an-drō-fō'bē-ă). Morbid fear of men, or of the male sex. [andro- + G. *phobos,* fear]

an·dro·stane (an'drō-stān). The parent hydrocarbon of the androgenic steroids. For structure, see steroids.

an·dro·stane·di·ol (an-drō-stān'dī-ol). 5α-Androstane-3β,17β-diol; a steroid metabolite, of which 5β isomers are also known.

an·dro·stane·di·one (an-drō-stān'dī-ōn). 5α-Androstane-3,17-dione; a steroid metabolite, of which the 5β isomer is also known. It is a precursor of both testosterone and estrone. It is secreted by the adrenals.

an·dro·stene (an'drō-stēn). Androstane with an unsaturated (i.e., –CH=CH–) bond in the molecule.

an·dro·stene·di·ol (an-drō-stēn'dī-ol). 5-Androsten-3β,17β-diol; a steroid metabolite differing from androstanediol by possessing a double bond between C-5 and C-6.

an·dro·stene·di·one (an-drō-stēn'dī-ōn). 4-Androstene-3,17-dione; androstanedione with a double bond between C-4 and C-5; an androgenic steroid of weaker biological potency than testosterone; secreted by the testis, ovary, and adrenal cortex.

androstenol. A substance that is a postulated pheromone; it is found in male sweat where it is oxidized to androstenone. In tests, women like the dry musky smell of androstenol, but find androstenone to have a chemical, urinelike odor that is unpleasant; however, ovulating women react neutrally.

an·dro·sten·o·lone (an-drō-stēn-ō-lōn). SYN dehydro-3-epiandrosterone.

an·dros·ter·one (an-dros'ter-ōn). *cis*-Androsterone; 3α-hydroxy-5α-androstan-17-one; a steroid metabolite, found in male urine, having weak androgenic potency. Formed in testes from progesterone.

an·ec·dot·al (ă-nek'dō-tal). Report of clinical experiences based in individual cases, rather than an organized investigation with appropriate controls, etc. [G. *anekdota,* unpublished items, fr. *an-* priv + *ekidomi,* to publish]

an·e·cho·ic (an-ĕ-kō'ik). The property of being echo-free or appearing without echoes on a sonographic image; a cyst filled with clear fluid appears anechoic. SEE transonic. SYN echo-free. [G. *an-* priv. + echo + ic]

Anel, Dominique, French surgeon, 1679–1725. SEE A. *method*.

an·e·lec·tro·ton·ic (an-ē-lek-trō-ton'ik). Relating to anelectrotonus.

an·e·lec·trot·o·nus (an'ē-lek-trot'ō-nŭs). Changes in excitability and conductivity in a nerve or muscle cell in the neighborhood of the anode during the passage of a constant electric current. [anelectrode + G. *tonos,* tension]

ANEMIA

ane·mia (ă-nē'mē-ă). Any condition in which the number of red blood cells per mm³, the amount of hemoglobin in 100 ml of blood, and/or the volume of packed red blood cells per 100 ml of blood are less than normal; clinically, generally pertaining to the concentration of oxygen-transporting material in a designated volume of blood, in contrast to total quantities as in oligocythemia, oligochromemia, and oligemia. A. is frequently manifested by pallor of the skin and mucous membranes, shortness of breath, palpitations of the heart, soft systolic murmurs, lethargy, and fatigability. [G. *anaimia*, fr. *an-* priv. + *haima*, blood]

achlorhydric a., a form of chronic hypochromic microcytic a. associated with achlorhydria or achylia gastrica; observed most frequently in women in the third to fifth decades. SYN Faber a., Faber syndrome.

achrestic a., a form of chronic progressive macrocytic a. that can be fatal in which the changes in bone marrow and circulating blood closely resemble those of pernicious a., but in which there is only transient or no response to therapy with vitamin B_{12}; glossitis, gastrointestinal disturbances, central nervous system disease, and pyrexia are not observed, and there is only little bleeding or hemolysis. [G. *a-* priv. + *chrēsis*, a using]

acquired hemolytic a., nonhereditary acute or chronic a. associated with or caused by extracorpuscular factors, e.g., certain infectious agents, chemicals (including autoantibodies or therapeutic agents), burns, toxic materials from higher plant and animal forms (including snake venoms).

Addison a., SYN pernicious a.

addisonian a., SYN pernicious a.

angiopathic hemolytic a., a rare postpartum a. of unknown etiology with uremia and nephrosclerosis; may be a rare complication following use of contraceptive steroids.

aplastic a., a. characterized by a greatly decreased formation of erythrocytes and hemoglobin, usually associated with pronounced granulocytopenia and thrombocytopenia, as a result of hypoplastic or aplastic bone marrow. SYN a. gravis, Ehrlich a.

asiderotic a., SYN chlorosis.

autoimmune hemolytic a., **(1)** cold-antibody type, caused by hemagglutinating antibody (usually IgM class) maximally active at 4°C; and resulting from severe hemolysis in cold hemagglutinin disease; **(2)** warm-antibody type (which is the most common), acquired hemolytic a. due to serum autoantibodies (usually IgG class), maximally active at 37°C, that react with the patient's red blood cells; it varies in severity, occurs in all age groups of both sexes, and may be idiopathic or secondary to neoplastic, autoimmune, or other disease.

Bartonella a., a. occurring in infection with *Bartonella bacilliformis* and characterized by an acute febrile a. of rapid onset and high mortality. Occurs in central Andean mountains of northern South America; vector is phlebotomine sandfly, *Lutzomyia*.

Belgian Congo a., SYN kasai.

Biermer a., SYN pernicious a.

brickmaker's a., a. associated with hookworm disease.

chlorotic a., SYN chlorosis.

congenital a., SYN *erythroblastosis* fetalis.

congenital aplastic a., SYN Fanconi a.

congenital dyserythropoietic a., a group of a.'s characterized by ineffective erythropoiesis, bone marrow erythroblastic multinuclearity, and secondary hemochromatosis. Three types are described: **type I** [MIM224120], macrocytic, megaloblastic a. with erythroblastic internuclear chromatin bridges; **type II**, [MIM*224100], normoblastic a. with multinucleated erythroblasts; **type III**, macrocytic a. with erythroblastic multinuclearity and gigantoblasts [MIM*105600]. Both types I and II are autosomal recessively inherited, type III is of autosomal dominant inheritance.

congenital hemolytic a., accelerated destruction of red blood cells due to an inherited defect, such as in the membrane in hereditary spherocytosis.

congenital hypoplastic a. [MIM*205900], a macrocytic a. resulting from congenital hypoplasia of the bone marrow, which is grossly deficient in erythroid precursors while other elements are normal; a. is progressive and severe, but leukocyte and platelet counts are normal or slightly reduced; survival of transfused erythrocytes is normal; minor congenital anomalies are found in some patients. Both autosomal dominant and recessive forms have been described, caused by mutation in the gene encoding ribosomal protein S19 (RBS19) on chromosomal 19q. SYN congenital nonregenerative a., Diamond-Blackfan a., Diamond-Blackfan syndrome, erythrogenesis imperfecta, familial hypoplastic a., pure red cell a.

congenital nonregenerative a., SYN congenital hypoplastic a.

Cooley a., SYN *thalassemia* major.

cow milk a., a. occurring in infants fed cow milk without iron supplementation, attributed to digestive tract allergic reaction leading to blood loss and hence iron deficiency.

deficiency a., SYN nutritional a.

Diamond-Blackfan a., SYN congenital hypoplastic a.

dilution a., SYN hydremia.

dimorphic a., a. in which two distinct forms of red cells are circulating.

diphyllobothrium a., a rare form of macrocytic a. associated with *Diphyllobothrium latum* infection, especially in Finland. SYN fish tapeworm a.

drepanocytic a., SYN sickle cell a.

dyshemopoietic a., any a. resulting from defective function of the bone marrow.

Ehrlich a., SYN aplastic a.

elliptocytary a. (ē-lip′tō-sī′tar-ē), a. with elliptocytosis; a heterogeneous group of inherited a.'s having in common elliptical red cells on blood smear. The defect may reside in dysfunction or deficiency of proteins of the red cell membrane skeleton. SYN elliptocytotic a.

elliptocytotic a. (ē-lip′tō-sī-tot′ik), SYN elliptocytary a.

erythroblastic a., a. characterized by the presence of large numbers of nucleated red cells (normoblasts and erythroblasts) in the peripheral blood. Seen in newborns with hemolytic a., due to isoimmunization, such as that caused by Rh or ABO incompatibility. SEE ALSO *erythroblastosis* fetalis. SYN erythronormoblastic a.

erythronormoblastic a. (ĕ-rith′rō-nōr′mō-blast- ik), SYN erythroblastic a.

essential a., obsolete term for pernicious a.; also used formerly for any type of a. of unknown mechanism.

Faber a., SYN achlorhydric a.

false a., SYN pseudoanemia.

familial hypoplastic a., SYN congenital hypoplastic a.

familial microcytic a. [MIM*206200], a rare type of autosomal recessive hypochromic microcytic a. associated with a defect of iron metabolism characterized by high serum iron, hepatic iron deposits, and absence of stainable bone marrow iron stores.

familial pyridoxine-responsive a. [MIM*206000], a rare autosomal recessive hereditary hypochromic a.; responsive to pyridoxine.

Fanconi a., a type of idiopathic refractory a. characterized by pancytopenia, hypoplasia of the bone marrow, and congenital anomalies, occurring in members of the same family (an autosomal recessive trait in at least five nonallelic types [MIM*227650, 227660, 227645, 227646, 600901]); the a. is normocytic or slightly macrocytic, macrocytes and target cells may be found in the circulating blood, and the leukopenia usually is due to neutropenia. Congenital anomalies include short stature; microcephaly; hypogenitalism; strabismus; anomalies of the thumbs, radii, and kidneys and urinary tract; mental retardation; and microphthalmia. SYN congenital aplastic a., congenital pancytopenia, Fanconi pancytopenia, Fanconi syndrome (1).

fish tapeworm a., SYN diphyllobothrium a.

folic acid deficiency a., a. due to deficiency of folic acid, characterized by large-sized red blood cells (macrocytosis) and presence of large nuclei in erythroid precursor cells (megaloblasts) in the bone marrow.

goat's milk a., nutritional a. in infants maintained chiefly with goat's milk, which is relatively poor in iron content.

a. gra′vis, SYN aplastic a.

ground itch a., a. associated with hookworm disease.

Heinz body a., SEE unstable hemoglobin hemolytic a.

hemolytic a., any a. resulting from an increased rate of erythrocyte destruction.

hemolytic a. of newborn, SYN *erythroblastosis* fetalis.

hemorrhagic a., a. resulting directly from loss of blood.

hookworm a., a. associated with heavy infestation by *Ancylostoma duodenale* or *Necator americanus*.

hypochromic a., a. characterized by a decrease in the ratio of the weight of hemoglobin to the volume of the erythrocyte, i.e., the mean corpuscular hemoglobin concentration is less than normal; the individual cells contain less hemoglobin than they do under optimal conditions and stain more faintly.

hypochromic microcytic a., a. due to iron deficiency or thalassemia, and characterized by lower than normal mean corpuscular volume, mean corpuscular hemoglobin, and mean corpuscular hemoglobin concentration.

hypoferric a., SYN iron deficiency a.

hypoplastic a., progressive nonregenerative a. resulting from greatly depressed, inadequately functioning bone marrow; as the process persists, aplastic a. may occur.

infectious a., a. developing as a complication of infection; probably results from depressed formation and short survival of erythrocytes and abnormal iron metabolism.

iron deficiency a., hypochromic microcytic a. characterized by low serum iron, increased serum iron-binding capacity, decreased serum ferritin, and decreased marrow iron stores. SYN hypoferric a.

isochromic a., SYN normochromic a.

lead a., a. associated with poisoning from lead; thought to result from a defect in synthesis of hemoglobin based on the failure of iron being combined in the porphyrin ring.

leukoerythroblastic a., SYN leukoerythroblastosis.

local a., a. resulting from a decreased supply of blood to a part, as in the occlusion of a vessel.

macrocytic a., any a. in which the average size of circulating erythrocytes is greater than normal, i.e., the mean corpuscular volume is 94 cu μm^3 or more (normal range, 82–92 cu μm^3), including such syndromes as pernicious a., sprue, celiac disease, macrocytic a. of pregnancy, a. of diphyllobothriasis, and others. SYN megalocytic a.

macrocytic achylic a., SYN pernicious a.

macrocytic a. of pregnancy, an a. occurring in pregnancy, related to folate deficiency and characterized by a low level of hemoglobin and a reduced number of erythrocytes, which are larger than normal (macrocytes).

macrocytic a. tropical, the macrocytic, megaloblastic a. of tropical sprue.

malignant a., SYN pernicious a.

Marchiafava-Micheli a., SYN paroxysmal nocturnal *hemoglobinuria.*

megaloblastic a., any a. in which there is a predominant number of megaloblastic erythroblasts, and relatively few normoblasts, among the hyperplastic erythroid cells in the bone marrow (as in pernicious a.).

megalocytic a., SYN macrocytic a.

metaplastic a., pernicious a. in which the various formed elements in the blood are changed, e.g., multisegmented, unusually large neutrophils (macropolycytes), immature myeloid cells, bizarre platelets.

microangiopathic hemolytic a., hemolysis due to intravascular fragmentation of red blood cells; may be due to microcirculatory lesions or the insertion of cardiac or intravascular prosthetic devices.

⊞**microcytic a.,** any a. in which the average size of circulating erythrocytes is smaller than normal, i.e., the mean corpuscular volume is 80 cu μm or less (normal range, 82–92 cu μm).

microdrepanocytic a., SYN sickle cell-thalassemia *disease.*

milk a., a type of hypochromic microcytic a., resulting from deficiency of iron, occurring in infants maintained on a milk diet for too long a time.

mountain a., term sometimes used for mountain sickness.

myelophthisic a., myelopathic a., SYN leukoerythroblastosis.

neonatal a., SYN *erythroblastosis* fetalis.

a. neonato′rum, SYN *erythroblastosis* fetalis.

normochromic a., any a. in which the concentration of hemoglobin in the erythrocytes is within the normal range, i.e., the mean corpuscular hemoglobin concentration is from 32 to 36%. SYN isochromic a.

normocytic a., any a. in which the erythrocytes are normal in size, i.e., the mean corpuscular volume ranges from 82 to 92 cu μm.

nutritional a., any a. resulting from a dietary deficiency of materials essential to red blood cell formation, e.g., iron, vitamins (especially folic acid), protein. SYN deficiency a.

nutritional macrocytic a., macrocytic, megaloblastic anemia due to deficiency of either folate or vitamin B12.

osteosclerotic a., a. due to compromise of erythropoiesis due to osteosclerosis.

⊞**pernicious a.** [MIM*361000], a chronic progressive a. of older adults (occurring more frequently during the fifth and later decades, rarely prior to 30 years of age), due to failure of absorption of vitamin B_{12}, usually resulting from a defect of the stomach accompanied by mucosal atrophy and associated with lack of secretion of "intrinsic" factor; characterized by numbness and tingling, weakness, and a sore smooth tongue, as well as dyspnea after slight exertion, faintness, pallor of the skin and mucous membranes, anorexia, diarrhea, loss of weight, and fever; laboratory studies usually reveal greatly decreased red blood cell counts, low levels of hemoglobin, numerous characteristically oval shaped macrocytic erythrocytes (color index greater than normal, but not truly hyperchromic), and hypo- or achlorhydria, in association with a predominant number of megaloblasts and relatively few normoblasts in the bone marrow; the leukocyte count in peripheral blood may be less than normal, with relative lymphocytosis and hypersegmented neutrophils; a low level of vitamin B_{12} is found in peripheral red blood cells; administration of vitamin B_{12} results in a characteristic reticulocyte response, relief from symptoms, and an increase in erythrocytes, provided that pernicious a. is not complicated by another disease; the condition is not actually "pernicious," as it was prior to the availability of therapy with vitamin B_{12}. At least two autosomal recessive forms are known. In one there is a defect of intrinsic factor [MIM*26100] and in the other a defective absorption of vitamin B_{12} from the intestine [MIM*261100]. SYN Addison a., Addison-Biermer disease, addisonian a., Biermer a., Biermer disease, macrocytic achylic a., malignant a.

physiologic a., an obsolete term for apparent a. caused by increased fluid volume of the blood (overhydration).

polar a., a form of a. sometimes observed in natives of temperate climates when they migrate to the Arctic or Antarctic regions.

posthemorrhagic a., an acute a. caused by fairly sudden and rapid loss of blood, as by traumatic laceration of a relatively large vessel, erosion of an artery in a duodenal ulcer, or hemorrhage in an ectopic pregnancy. SYN traumatic a.

primary erythroblastic a., SYN *thalassemia* major.

primary refractory a., any of a group of anemic conditions in which there is persistent, frequently advanced a. that is not successfully treated by any means except blood transfusions, and that is not associated with another primary disease.

pure red cell a., SYN congenital hypoplastic a.

radiation a., hypoplastic a. sometimes occurring after high-level acute or low-level chronic exposure to ionizing radiation.

refractory a., progressive a. unresponsive to therapy other than transfusion. SEE primary refractory a., secondary refractory a.

scorbutic a., a. occurring in patients with scurvy, usually due to coincident nutritional deficiency; e.g., the "megaloblastic a. of scurvy" is due to concomitant folic acid deficiency.

secondary refractory a., any persistent a. that is successfully treated only by blood transfusions, and that is associated with another condition.

⊞**sickle cell a.** [MIM*141900], an autosomal recessive a. characterized by crescent- or sickle-shaped erythrocytes and accelerated hemolysis, due to substitution of a single amino acid (valine for glutamic acid) in the sixth position of the β-chain of hemoglobin the gene of which is on chromosome 11; affected homozygotes have 85–95% Hb S and severe anemia, while heterozygotes (said to have sickle cell trait) have 40–45% Hb S, the rest being normal Hb A; low oxygen tension causes polymerization of the abnormal β-chains, thus distorting the shape of the red blood cells to the sickle form. Homozygotes develop "crisis" episodes of severe pain due to microvascular occlusions, bone infarcts, leg ulcers, and atrophy of the spleen associated with increased susceptibility to bacterial infections, especially streptococcal pneumonia. Occurs most commonly in individuals of African descent. SYN drepanocytic a., sickle cell disease, vasoocclusive crisis.

sideroblastic a., sideroachrestic a., refractory a. characterized by the presence of sideroblasts in the bone marrow.

slaty a., an ash-gray pallor in poisoning from acetanilide or silver (argyria).

spastic a., local a. resulting from nontransitory intrinsic contraction of the arterial vessels supplying the affected region.

spherocytic a., SYN hereditary *spherocytosis.*

splenic a., SYN Banti *syndrome.*

spur cell a., a. in which the red cells have a spiculated appearance and are destroyed prematurely, predominantly in the spleen; may be seen in patients with severe liver disease as a result of an abnormality in the cholesterol content of the red cell membrane.

target cell a., any a. with a conspicuous number of target cells in the peripheral blood; characteristic of the thalassemias and also found in several hemoglobinopathies.

toxic a., any a. resulting from the destructive effects of a chemical, metabolic poison, bacterial toxin, venom, and similar materials.

traumatic a., SYN posthemorrhagic a.

tropical a., various syndromes frequently observed in persons in tropical climates, usually resulting from nutritional deficiencies or hookworm or other parasitic diseases.

unstable hemoglobin hemolytic a., a congenital hemolytic a., due to autosomal inheritance of one of many unstable hemoglobins. The a. is of variable severity and characterized by the presence in vivo or in vitro of Heinz bodies.

ane·mic (ă-nē′mik). Pertaining to or manifesting the various features of anemia.

an·e·mom·e·ter (an-ĕ-mom′ĕ-ter). An instrument for measuring the velocity of air flow. [G. *anemos,* wind, + *metron,* measure]

a·nem·o·nol (ă-nem′ŏ-nol). A volatile oil, possessing markedly toxic properties, obtained from plants of the genus *Anemone.*

an·e·mo·pho·bia (an′ĕ-mō-fō′bē-ă). Morbid fear of wind. [G. *anemos,* wind, + *phobos,* fear]

an·e·mot·ro·phy (an-ĕ-mot′rō-fē). Lack of substances essential to the formation of blood, thereby resulting in hypoplastic anemia. [G. *an-* priv. + *haima,* blood, + *trophē,* nourishment]

an·en·ce·pha·lia (an′en-se-fā′lē-ă). SYN anencephaly.

an·en·ce·phal·ic (an-en-se-fal′ik). Relating to anencephaly. SYN anencephalous.

an·en·ceph·a·lous (an-en-sef′ă-lŭs). SYN anencephalic.

an·en·ceph·a·ly (an′en-sef′ă-lē). Congenital defective development of the brain, with absence of the bones of the cranial vault and absent or rudimentary cerebral and cerebellar hemispheres, brainstem, and basal ganglia. SYN anencephalia. [G. *an-* priv. + *enkephalos,* brain]

partial a., SYN hemicephalia.

an·en·ter·ous (an-en′ter-ŭs). Having no intestine; denoting certain parasites, such as tapeworms. [G. *an-* priv. + *entera,* intestines]

an·en·zy·mia (an-en-zī′mē-ă). Congenital absence of an enzyme.

aneph·ric (ă-nef′rik). Lacking kidneys. [*a-* priv. + G. *nephros,* kidney]

an·ep·i·plo·ic (an-ep-i-plō′ik). Lacking an omentum (epiploon).

an·er·gia (an-er′jē-ă). SYN anergy (2).

an·er·gic (an-er′jik). Relating to, or marked by, anergy.

an·er·gy (an′er-jē). **1.** Absence of ability to generate a sensitivity reaction to substances expected to be antigenic (immunogenic, allergenic) in that individual. **2.** Lack of energy. SYN anergia. [G. *an-* priv. + *energeia,* energy, from *ergon,* work]

negative a., a reduction of the normal or usual immunologic responses because of unrelated intervening disease. SYN nonspecific a.

nonspecific a., SYN negative a.

positive a., a reduction of the normal or usual immunologic response resulting from a reaction to a specific allergen. SYN specific a.

specific a., SYN positive a.

an·er·oid (an′er-oyd). Without fluid; denoting a form of barometer without mercury, in which the varying air pressure is indicated by a pointer governed by the movement of the elastic wall of an evacuated chamber. Also used to denote a mercury-free pressure gauge used with some sphygmomanometers. [G. *a-* priv. + *nēros,* wet, + *eidos,* form]

an·e·ryth·ro·pla·sia (an′ĕ-rith-rō-plā′zē-ă). A condition in which there is no formation of red blood cells. [G. *an-* priv. + erythro-(cyte) + G. *plasis,* a molding]

an·e·ryth·ro·plas·tic (an′ĕ-rith-rō-plas′tik). Pertaining to or characterized by anerythroplasia.

an·e·ryth·ro·re·gen·er·a·tive (an-ĕ-rith′thrō-rē-jen′er-ă-tiv). Pertaining to or characterized by lack of regeneration of red blood cells.

an·es·the·ci·ne·sia (an-es′thē-si-nē′zē-ă). SYN anesthekinesia.

an·es·the·ki·ne·sia (an-es′thē-ki-nē′zē-ă). Combined sensory and motor paralysis. SYN anesthecinesia. [G. *an-* priv. + *aisthēsis,* sensation, + *kinēsis,* movement]

ANESTHESIA

an·es·the·sia (an′es-thē′zē-ă). **1.** Loss of sensation resulting from pharmacologic depression of nerve function or from neurologic dysfunction. **2.** Broad term for anesthesiology as a clinical specialty. [G. *anaisthēsia,* fr. *an-* priv. + *aisthēsis,* sensation]

acupuncture a., percutaneous insertion of, and stimulation by, needles placed in critical areas of the body to produce loss of sensation in another area.

ambulatory a., a. provided on an outpatient basis.

axillary a., loss of sensation in the distal two-thirds of the upper extremity following injection of a local anesthetic solution about the nerve trunks in the axilla.

balanced a., a technique of general a. based on the concept that administration of a mixture of small amounts of several neuronal depressants summates the advantages, but not the disadvantages of, the individual components of the mixture.

basal a., parenteral administration of one or more sedatives to produce a state of depressed consciousness short of a general a.

block a., SYN conduction a.

brachial a., anesthetization of an upper extremity by injection of local anesthetic solution about the brachial plexus.

caudal a., regional a. by injection of local anesthetic solution into the epidural space via the sacral hiatus.

cervical a., regional a. of the neck by injection of a local anesthetic solution about the cervical nerves or into the cervical epidural space.

circle absorption a., inhalation a. in which a circuit with carbon dioxide absorbent is used for complete (closed) or partial (semi-closed) rebreathing of exhaled gases.

closed a., inhalation a. in which there is total rebreathing of all exhaled gases, except carbon dioxide which is absorbed; gas flow into the anesthetic circuit consists only of oxygen, in amounts equal to the patient's metabolic consumption, plus small amounts of other gases (e.g., nitrous oxide) that undergo continued uptake by and distribution in the patient.

compression a., SYN pressure a.

conduction a., regional a. in which local anesthetic solution is injected about nerves to inhibit nerve transmission; includes spinal, epidural, nerve block, and field block a., but not local or topical a. SYN block a.

continuous epidural a., insertion of a catheter into the lumbar or caudal epidural space for the repeated injection of local anesthetic solutions as a means of prolonging duration of anesthesia. SYN fractional epidural a.

continuous spinal a., insertion of a catheter into the spinal subarachnoid space and leaving it in situ to permit serial intermittent injection of local anesthetic solution for prolonged spinal a. SYN fractional spinal a.

crossed a., a. of one side of the head and the other side of the body due to a brainstem lesion.

dental a., general, conduction, local, or topical a. for operations upon the teeth, gingivae, or associated structures.

diagnostic a., a. induced for evaluation of the mechanism responsible for a painful condition.

differential spinal a., a form of diagnostic spinal a. producing blockade of different types of nerves in the subarachnoid space, based upon their differences in sensitivity to local anesthetics; also observed during surgical spinal a.

dissociated a., loss of some types of sensation with persistence of others; most often used in context of nerve blocks, wherein a loss of sensation for pain and temperature occurs without loss of tactile sense.

dissociative a., a form of general a., but not necessarily complete unconsciousness, characterized by catalepsy, catatonia, and amnesia, especially that produced by phenylcyclohexylamine compounds, including ketamine.

a. doloro′sa, severe spontaneous pain occurring in an anesthetic area. SYN painful a.

electric a., a., usually general a., produced by application of an electrical current.

endotracheal a., inhalation a. technique in which anesthetic and respiratory gases pass through a tube placed in the trachea via the mouth or nose. SYN intratracheal a.

epidural a., regional a. produced by injection of local anesthetic solution into the peridural space. SYN peridural a.

extradural a., anesthetization, by local anesthetics, of nerves near the spinal canal external to the dura mater; often refers to epidural a., but may include paravertebral a.

field block a., conduction a. in which small nerves are not anesthetized individually, as in nerve block a., but instead are blocked *en masse* by local anesthetic solution injected to form a barrier proximal to the operative site.

fractional epidural a., SYN continuous epidural a.

fractional spinal a., SYN continuous spinal a.

general a., loss of ability to perceive pain associated with loss of consciousness produced by intravenous or inhalation anesthetic agents.

girdle a., a. distributed as a band encircling the trunk.

glove a., loss of sensation in the distal upper extremity, i.e., the hand and fingers.

gustatory a., SYN ageusia.

high spinal a., spinal a. in which the level of sensory denervation extends to the second or third thoracic dermatome.

hyperbaric a., inhalation of depressant gases or vapors at pressures greater than 1 atmosphere, especially as a means of producing general a. with agents too weak to produce a. at 1 atmosphere.

hyperbaric spinal a., spinal a. in which spread of local anesthetic solution in the subarachnoid space is controlled by adjusting the position of the patient when the density of local anesthetic is made greater than the density of cerebrospinal fluid (i.e., hyperbaric) by the addition of glucose.

hypobaric spinal a., spinal a. in which spread of local anesthetic solution in the subarachnoid space is controlled by adjusting the position of the patient when the density of the local anesthetic solution is made less than the density of cerebrospinal fluid (i.e., hypobaric) by the addition of distilled water.

hypotensive a., a. in which arterial hypotension is deliberately induced as a means of decreasing operative blood loss.

hypothermic a., general a. administered in conjunction with artificial lowering of body temperature.

hysterical a., a. as a manifestation of hysteria, usually involving the surface areas of the body not conforming to neuroanatomic distribution.

infiltration a., a. produced by injection of local anesthetic solution directly into an area that is painful or about to be operated upon.

inhalation a., general a. resulting from breathing of anesthetic gases or vapors.

insufflation a., maintenance of inhalation a. by delivery of anesthetic gases or vapors directly to the airway of a spontaneously breathing patient.

intercostal a., regional a. produced by injection of local anesthetic solution about intercostal nerves.

intramedullary a., rarely used method of general a. by injection of intravenous anesthetic agent(s) into the medullary canal of long bones. SYN intraosseous a.

intranasal a., (1) insufflation a. in which an inhalation anesthetic is added to inhaled air passing through the nose or nasopharynx; (2) a. of nasal passages by infiltration and topical application of local anesthetic solution to nasal mucosa.

intraoral a., (1) insufflation a. in which an inhalation anesthetic is added to inhaled air passing through the mouth; (2) regional a. of the mouth and associated structures when local anesthetic solutions are used by topical application to oral mucosa, by local infiltration, or as nerve blocks.

intraosseous a., SYN intramedullary a.

intraspinal a., inaccurate synonym for spinal a.; local anesthetic solutions are not injected into the spinal cord.

intratracheal a., SYN endotracheal a.

intravenous a., general a. produced by injection of central nervous system depressants into the venous circulation.

intravenous regional a., regional a. by intravenous injection of local anesthetic solution distal to an occlusive tourniquet in an extremity previously exsanguinated by pressure or gravity. SYN Bier method (1).

isobaric spinal a., spinal a. of same density as cerebrospinal fluid so that the level of a. is not influenced by a change in the position of the patient.

local a., a general term referring to topical, infiltration, field block, or nerve block a. but usually not to spinal or epidural a. SEE ALSO local *anesthetics*, under *anesthetic*.

low spinal a., spinal a. in which the level of sensory denervation extends to the tenth or eleventh thoracic dermatome.

nerve block a., conduction a. in which local anesthetic solution is injected about nerves, nerve trunks, or nerve plexuses.

nonrebreathing a., a technique for inhalation a. in which valves exhaust all exhaled air from the circuit.

open drop a., inhalation a. by vaporization of a liquid anesthetic placed drop by drop on a gauze mask covering the mouth and nose.

outpatient a., SYN patient-controlled *analgesia*.

painful a., SYN a. dolorosa.

paracervical block a., regional a. of the cervix uteri by injection of local anesthetic solution into tissues adjacent to the cervix.

paravertebral a., (1) a. by injection of local anesthetic solution about nerves as they exit from the vertebral canal; (2) combined presynaptic, postsynaptic, and ganglionic sympathetic block by injection of local anesthetic solution about paravertebral sympathetic chains.

patient-controlled a. (PCA), SYN patient-controlled *analgesia*.

peridural a., SYN epidural a.

periodontal a., a. of the periodontal ligament, produced by injection of a local anesthetic drug.

presacral a., injection of local anesthetic solution anterior to the sacrum, to block nerves as they exit from the sacral foramina.

pressure a., loss of sensation produced by pressure applied to a nerve. SYN compression a.

pudendal a., local a. produced by blocking the pudendal nerves near the spinal processes of the ischium; used in obstetrics.

rebreathing a., a technique for inhalation a. in which a portion or all of the gases that are exhaled are subsequently inhaled after carbon dioxide has been absorbed.

rectal a., general a. produced by instillation into the rectum of a solution containing a central nervous system depressant.

refrigeration a., SYN cryoanesthesia.

ℹ️ **regional a.,** use of local anesthetic solution(s) to produce circumscribed areas of loss of sensation; a generic term including conduction, nerve block, spinal, epidural, field block, infiltration, and topical a. SYN conduction analgesia.

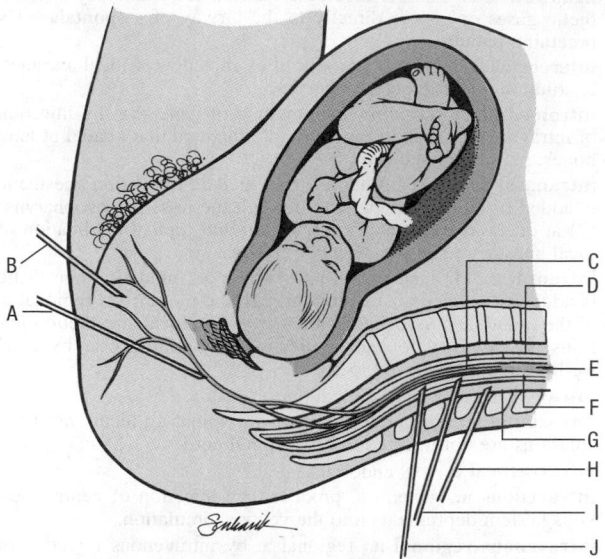

regional anesthesia for childbirth: sites of injection; (A) pudendal block, (B) local infiltration of perineum, (C) pia mater, (D) dura mater, (E) spinal cord, (F) subarachnoid space, (G) epidural space, (H) lumbar epidural block, (I) low spinal block, (J) saddle block

retrobulbar a., injection of a local anesthetic behind the eye to produce sensory denervation of the eye.

sacral a., regional a. limited to those areas innervated by sacral sensory nerves.

saddle block a., a form of spinal a. limited in area to the buttocks, perineum, and inner surfaces of the thighs.

segmental a., loss of sensation limited to an area supplied by one or more spinal nerve roots.

spinal a., (1) loss of sensation produced by injection of local anesthetic solution(s) into the spinal subarachnoid space; SYN subarachnoid a. (2) loss of sensation produced by disease of the spinal cord.

splanchnic a., loss of sensation in areas of the visceral peritoneum innervated by the splanchnic nerves. SYN visceral a.

stocking a., loss of sensation in the distal lower extremity, i.e., the foot and toes.

subarachnoid a., SYN spinal a. (1).

surgical a., (1) any a. administered for the purpose of permitting performance of an operative procedure, as differentiated from obstetrical, diagnostic, and therapeutic a.; (2) loss of sensation with muscle relaxation adequate for an operative procedure.

tactile a., loss or impairment of the sense of touch.

therapeutic a., administration of an anesthetic as a means of treatment.

thermal a., thermic a., loss of temperature appreciation.

to-and-fro a., a. using of a valveless closed a. circuit in which respired gases pass back and forth through a carbon dioxide absorbent interposed between patient and respiratory reservoir bag.

topical a., superficial loss of sensation in conjunctiva, mucous membranes or skin, produced by direct application of local anesthetic solutions, ointments, or jellies.

total spinal a., spinal a. extensive enough to produce loss of sensation in all extracranial sensory roots.

traumatic a., loss of sensation resulting from nerve injury.

unilateral a., SYN hemianesthesia.

visceral a., SYN splanchnic a.

---

an·es·the·si·ol·o·gist (an′es-thē-zē-ol′ō-jist). **1.** A physician specializing solely in anesthesiology and related areas. **2.** An individual with a doctorate degree who is board-certified and legally qualified to administer anesthetics and related techniques. Cf. anesthetist.

an·es·the·si·ol·o·gy (an′es-thē-zē-ol′ō-jē). The medical specialty concerned with the pharmacological, physiological, and clinical basis of anesthesia and related fields, including resuscitation, intensive respiratory care, and acute and chronic pain. [anesthesia + G. *logos,* treatise]

an·es·thet·ic (an-es-thet′ik). **1.** A compound that reversibly depresses neuronal function, producing loss of ability to perceive pain and/or other sensations. **2.** Collective designation for anesthetizing agents administered to an individual at a particular time. **3.** Characterized by loss of sensation or capable of producing loss of sensation. **4.** Associated with or due to the state of anesthesia.

flammable a., an inhalation a. that supports combustion and forms explosive mixtures with oxidizing gases.

general a.'s, drugs used either by the intravenous route or by inhalation that render the subject unconscious and incapable of perceiving pain as might otherwise occur in surgery.

inhalation a., a gas or a liquid with sufficient vapor pressure to produce general anesthesia when breathed.

intravenous a., a compound that produces anesthesia when injected intravenously.

local a.'s, drugs used for the interruption of the nerve transmission of pain sensations. They act at the site of application to prevent perception of pain; examples include procaine and lidocaine.

primary a., the compound that contributes most to loss of sensation when a mixture of anesthetics is administered.

secondary a., a compound that contributes to, but is not primarily responsible for, loss of sensation when two or more anesthetics are simultaneously administered.

spinal a., a local anesthetic agent producing loss of sensation when injected into the subarachnoid space.

topical a., a local a. preparation suitable for anesthetizing skin surfaces or mucous membranes. Can be used in the form of ointments, creams, jellies, sprays, or solutions.

volatile a., a liquid a. that at room temperature volatilizes to a vapor which when inhaled is capable of producing general anesthesia. SEE ALSO anesthetic *vapor.*

anes·the·tist (ă-nes′thĕ-tist). One who administers an anesthetic, whether an anesthesiologist, a physician who is not an anesthesiologist, a nurse a., or an anesthesia assistant.

anes·the·ti·za·tion (ă-nes′thĕ-ti-zā′shun). The act of producing loss of sensation.

anes·the·tize (ă-nes′thĕ-tīz). To produce loss of sensation.

an·es·trous (an-es′trŭs). Relating to the anestrus.

a·nes·trum (an-es′trŭm). The period between two estrus cycles [G. *an-* priv. + *oistros,* estrus]

an·es·trus (an-es′trŭs). The period of sexual quiescence between the estrus cycles of mammals; may be: 1) a prolonged period in monestrous animals (dogs) or seasonally polyestrous animals (sheep), or 2) a prolonged period of failure of estrus in mature nonpregnant, polyestrous animals. [G. *a-* priv. + *oistros,* a gadfly, mad desire (estrus)]

ane·tho·path (ă-nē′thō-path). A morally uninhibited person. [*an-* priv. + *ethos,* custom, + *pathos,* suffering]

an·e·to·der·ma (an-ě-tō-der′mă). Atrophoderma in which the skin becomes baglike and wrinkled or depressed, with loss of dermal elasticity. SYN atrophia maculosa varioliformis cutis, atrophoderma maculatum, macular atrophy, primary idiopathic macular atrophy, primary macular atrophy of skin. [G. *anetos,* relaxed, + *derma,* skin]

Jadassohn-Pellizzari a., cutaneous atrophy preceded by inflammatory erythematous or urticarial lesions of the trunk and upper portions of the extremities, and enlarging to 2–3 cm before undergoing involution.

Schweninger-Buzzi a., sudden appearance of permanent, noninflamatory bluish-white balloon-like lesions, soft and readily indented, chiefly on the trunk of women.

an·eu·ploid (an′ū-ployd). Having an abnormal number of chromosomes not an exact multiple of the haploid number, as contrasted with abnormal numbers of complete haploid sets of chromosomes, such as diploid, triploid, etc. [G. *an-* priv. + euploid]

an·eu·ploi·dy (an′ū-ploy-dē). State of being aneuploid.

partial a., a type of mosaicism in which some cells have a normal number of chromosomes and some have an abnormal number.

an·eu·rine (an′ū-rēn). SYN thiamin.

a. hydrochloride, SYN *thiamin* hydrochloride.

a. pyrophosphate, SYN *thiamin* pyrophosphate.

aneu·ro·lem·mic (ă-noo-rō-lem′ik). Without a neurolemma.

an·eu·rysm (an′ū-rizm). **1.** Circumscribed dilation of an artery or a cardiac chamber, a direct communication with the lumen, usually due to an acquired or congenital weakness of the wall of the artery or chamber. **2.** Circumscribed dilation of a cardiac chamber usually due to an acquired or congenital weakness of the wall of the heart. [G. *aneurysma* (*-mat-*), a dilation, fr. *eurys,* wide]

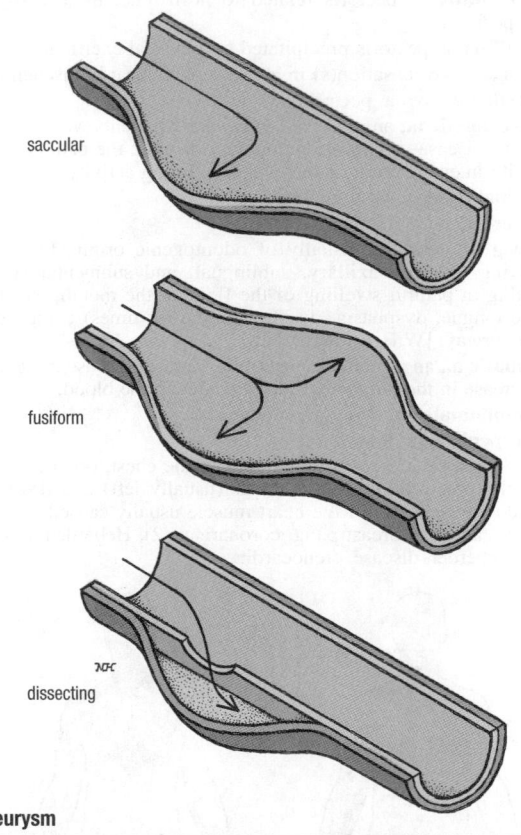

saccular

fusiform

dissecting

aneurysm

ampullary a., SYN saccular a.

a. by anastomosis, a mass of dilated anastomosing vessels that produce a pulsating tumor usually in a superficial position.

aortic a., diffuse or circumscribed dilation of a portion of the aorta (e.g., abdominal aortic a., aortic arch a. SEE ALSO dissecting a.

aortic sinus a., abnormal dilation of one or more of the three aortic sinuses situated behind the three aortic valve cusps.

arteriosclerotic a., SYN atherosclerotic a.

arteriovenous a., (**1**) a dilated arteriovenous shunt; (**2**) communication between an artery and a vein, usually congenital or associated with atherosclerotic changes; more appropriately termed arteriovenous fistula or arteriovenous malformation.

atherosclerotic a., the most common type of a., occurring in the abdominal aorta and other large arteries, primarily in the elderly. Often associated with atherosclerotic changes in blood vessels in other parts of the body. SYN arteriosclerotic a.

axial a., an a. involving the entire circumference of a blood vessel.

benign bone a., obsolete term for aneurysmal bone *cyst.*

Bérard a., an arteriovenous a. in the tissues outside the injured vein.

berry a., a small saccular a. of a cerebral artery that resembles a berry. Such a.'s can rupture causing a subarachnoid hemorrhage.

cardiac a., SYN ventricular a.

Charcot-Bouchard a., SYN miliary a.

cirsoid a., dilation of a group of blood vessels owing to congenital malformation with arteriovenous shunting. SYN cirsoid varix, racemose a., racemose hemangioma.

compound a., an a. in which some of the coats of the artery are ruptured, others intact.

congenital cerebral a., localized dilation of a cerebral vessel; usually a berry a.

consecutive a., two or more a.'s along the path of blood flow.

coronary artery a., a. of the coronary artery, rarely congenital, usually due to atherosclerosis, inflammatory processes, or a coronary fistula.

cylindroid a., SYN tubular a.

diffuse a., an a. that has enlarged and spread to the surrounding tissues as a consequence of rupture of its walls.

dissecting a., condition resulting when blood passes from the true lumen of an artery into a false lumen within the arterial wall; layers of the wall are effectively split; most often due to necrosis of the medial layer, as in Marfan *syndrome* and with tear originating in the ascending (type A) or descending (type B) thoracic aorta or occasionally in smaller arteries such as the carotids; the false *lumen* may thrombose, rupture, re-enter the true *lumen* downstream, and/or shear off vital arterial branches; more properly termed aortic dissection rather than aneurysm since the process is not transmural. SEE ALSO aortic *dissection.*

ductal a., a. of the patent ductus arteriosus, occurs either in infants or adults. SYN ductus diverticulum.

ectatic a., an a. in which all the coats of the artery, though stretched, are unruptured.

false a., SYN pseudoaneurysm.

fusiform a., an elongated spindle-shaped dilation of an artery.

hernial a., the protrusion of the stretched inner coats of an artery through a defect in the adventitia.

infraclinoid a., an intracranial a. occurring below the level of the anterior clinoid process of the sphenoid bone.

intracavernous a., an a. of the carotid artery within the cavernous sinus.

intracranial a., any a. located within the cranium.

miliary a., dilation in the diameter of small arteries and arterioles secondary to lipohyalinosis from long-standing hypertension; associated with intracerebral hematomas. SYN Charcot-Bouchard a.

mural aneurysm, SYN ventricular a.

mycotic a., an a. caused by the growth of fungi or bacteria within the vascular wall, usually following impaction of a septic embolus.

Park a., an arteriovenous a. in which the brachial artery communicates with the brachial and median basilic veins.

peripheral a., (**1**) a saclike a. springing from one side of an artery; (**2**) an a. of one of the smaller branches of an artery.

phantom a., a palpable pulsating aorta, mistaken by novices for an a.

Pott a., SYN aneurysmal *varix.*

pulmonary artery a., a. of the pulmonary artery; may be secondary to congenital valvular or infundibular stenosis; some are mycotic a.'s (q.v.).

racemose a., SYN cirsoid a.

Rasmussen a., aneurysmal dilation of a branch of a pulmonary artery in a tuberculous cavity, rupture of which may cause serious hemoptysis.

a. of the right ventricle or right ventricular outflow patch, a. occurring after right ventriculotomy; the a. may either be a false or a true a.

ruptured a., an a. that is hemorrhaging into its wall or surrounding tissues.

saccular a., sacculated a., a saclike bulging on one side of an artery. SYN ampullary a.

serpentine a., dilation and tortuosity of an artery, sometimes affecting the temporal, splenic, or iliac arteries in the elderly.

a. of sinus of Valsalva, a congenital thin-walled out pouching with an entirely intracardiac course, usually in the right or noncoronary sinus, that may rupture into the right, or rarely, the left heart chambers to form an aortocardiac fistula.

supraclinoid a., an intracranial a. located immediately above the anterior clinoid process of the sphenoid bone.

syphilitic a., an a., usually involving the thoracic aorta, resulting from tertiary syphilitic aortitis.

traumatic a., an a. resulting from physical damage to the wall of an artery; usually a false a. or arteriovenous a.

true a., localized dilation of an artery with an expanded lumen lined by stretched remnants of the arterial wall.

tubular a., the uniform dilation of an artery along a considerable distance. SYN cylindroid a.

varicose a., a blood-containing sac, communicating with both an artery and a vein.

ventricular a., thinning, stretching, and bulging of a weakened ventricular wall, usually as a result of myocardial infarction; rarely postinflammatory or congenital. SYN cardiac a., mural aneurysm.

a. of the ventricular portion of the membranous septum, an a. that bulges toward the right in systole, often consisting of the anterior leaflet of the tricuspid valve.

an·eu·rys·mal, an·eu·rys·mat·ic (an-ū-riz′măl, -riz-mat′ik). Relating to an aneurysm.

an·eu·rys·mec·to·my (an-ū-riz-mek′tō-mē). Excision of an aneurysm. [aneurysm + G. *ektomē,* excision]

an·eu·rys·mo·plas·ty (an-ū-riz′mō-plas-tē). Repair of an aneurysm by opening the sac and suturing its walls to restore the normal dimension to the lumen of the artery. SEE ALSO aneurysmorrhaphy. SYN endoaneurysmoplasty, endoaneurysmorrhaphy. [aneurysm + G. *plastos,* formed]

an·eu·rys·mor·rha·phy (an′ū-riz-mōr′ă-fē). Closure by suture of the sac of an aneurysm to restore the normal lumen dimensions. [aneurysm + G. *rhaphē,* suture]

an·eu·rys·mot·o·my (an′ū-riz-mot′ō-mē). Incision into the sac of an aneurysm. [aneurysm + G. *tomē,* incision]

ANF Abbreviation for antinuclear *factor;* atrial natriuretic *factor.*

⌂**angei-.** SEE angio-.

an·gel·i·ca root (an-jel′i-kă). The root of *Angelica archangelica* (family Umbelliferae); a tonic and stimulant that may cause nausea; used as a carminative, diuretic, and externally as a counterirritant.

Angelucci, Arnaldo, Italian ophthalmologist, 1854–1934. SEE A. *syndrome.*

Anger, Hal, U.S. electrical engineer, *1920. SEE A. *camera.*

⌂**angi-.** SEE angio-.

an·gi·ec·ta·sia, an·gi·ec·ta·sis (an-jē-ek-tā′zē-ă, -ek′tă-sis). Dilation of a lymphatic or blood vessel. [angio- + G. *ektasis,* a stretching]

congenital dysplastic a., SYN Klippel-Trenaunay-Weber *syndrome.*

an·gi·ec·tat·ic (an-jē-ek-tat′ik). Marked by the presence of dilated blood vessels. [angio- + G. *ektatos,* capable of extension]

an·gi·ec·to·pia (an-jē-ek-tō′pē-ă). Abnormal location of a blood vessel. SYN angioplany. [angio- + G. *ektopos,* out of place]

an·gi·i·tis, an·gi·tis (an-jē-ī′tis, an-jī′tis). Inflammation of a blood vessel (arteritis, phlebitis) or lymphatic vessel (lymphangitis). SYN vasculitis. [angio- + G. *-itis,* inflammation]

allergic granulomatous a., SYN Churg-Strauss *syndrome.*

consecutive a., a. caused by extension of the inflammatory process from the surrounding tissues.

frosted branch a., a. characterized by inflammation of blood vessels with sheathing giving the appearance of branches on a tree.

hypersensitivity a., an inflammatory reaction in a blood vessel, the result of a specific reaction to an antigenic (allergic) substance or other agents to which the individual expresses unusual vascular sensitization.

necrotizing a., inflammatory reaction of blood vessels resulting in fibrinoid necrosis of tissue, especially of the blood vessel wall.

an·gi·na (an′ji-nă, an-jī′nă). **1.** A severe, often constricting pain, usually referring to a. pectoris. **2.** Old term for a sore throat from any cause. [L. quinsy]

abdominal a., a. abdom′inis, intermittent abdominal pain, frequently occurring at a fixed time after eating, caused by inadequacy of the mesenteric circulation from arteriosclerosis or other arterial disease. SYN intestinal a.

agranulocytic a., SYN agranulocytosis.

crescendo a., a. pectoris that occurs with increasing frequency, intensity, or duration.

a. cru′ris, intermittent claudication of the leg.

a. decu′bitus, a. pectoris related to horizontal, usually supine, body position.

a. of effort, a. pectoris precipitated by physical exertion.

false a., a.-like sensation(s) in absence of myocardial ischemia.

Heberden a., SYN a. pectoris.

hypercyanotic a., anginal pain in cyanotic patients with congenital heart disease or chronic pulmonary disease, the pain developing with intensification of the cyanosis during activity.

intestinal a., SYN abdominal a.

a. inver′sa, SYN Prinzmetal a.

Ludwig a., cellulitis, usually of odontogenic origin, bilaterally involving the submaxillary, sublingual, and submental spaces, resulting in painful swelling of the floor of the mouth, elevation of the tongue, dysphasia, dysphonia, and (at times) compromise of the airway. [W.F. Ludwig]

lymphatic a., an affection resembling Vincent disease marked by an increase in the number of lymphocytes in the blood.

a. lymphomato′sa, SYN agranulocytosis.

neutropenic a., SYN agranulocytosis.

▣**a. pec′toris,** severe constricting pain in the chest, often radiating from the precordium to a shoulder (usually left) and down the arm, due to ischemia of the heart muscle usually caused by coronary disease. SYN breast pang, coronarism (2), Heberden a., Rougnon-Heberden disease, stenocardia.

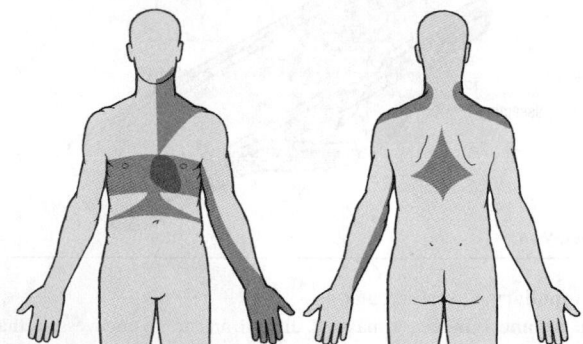

angina pectoris: zones of pain

a. pec′toris decu′bitus, anginal pain developing while the subject is recumbent.

a. pec′toris si′ne dolor′e, SYN Gairdner *disease.*

a. pec′toris vasomoto′ria, a. pectoris in which the breast pain is comparatively slight, but pallor followed by cyanosis, and coldness and numbness of the extremities, are marked. SYN a. spuria, a. vasomotoria, pseudangina, pseudoangina, reflex a., vasomotor a.

preinfarction a., obsolete term for unstable a., including crescendo a.

Prinzmetal a., a form of a. pectoris, characterized by pain that is not precipitated by cardiac work, is of longer duration, is usually more severe, and is associated with unusual electrocardiographic manifestations including elevated ST segments in leads that are ordinarily depressed in typical a., and usually without reciprocal ST changes; occurring at night in bed. SYN a. inversa, variant a. pectoris.

reflex a., SYN a. pectoris vasomotoria.

a. si′ne do′lore, symptoms of coronary insufficiency occurring without pain.

a. spu′ria, SYN a. pectoris vasomotoria.

unstable a., (1) a. pectoris characterized by pain in the chest of coronary origin occurring in response to progressively less exercise or fewer other stimuli than ordinarily required to produce a.; often leading to myocardial infarction, if untreated. **(2)** a. that has not achieved a constant or reproducible pattern in 30 or 60 days.

variant a. pectoris, SYN Prinzmetal a.

vasomotor a., SYN a. pectoris vasomotoria.

a. vasomotor′ia, SYN a. pectoris vasomotoria.

Vincent a., an ulcerative infection of the oral soft tissues including the tonsils and pharynx caused by fusiform and spirochetal organisms; it is usually associated with necrotizing ulcerative gingivitis and may progress to noma. Death from suffocation or sepsis may occur.

walk-through a., a circumstance in which despite continuing activity, such as walking, the pain of a. pectoris diminishes or disappears.

an·gi·nal (an′ji-năl, an-jī′). Relating to angina in any sense.

an·gi·ni·form (an-jin′i-fōrm). Resembling angina.

an·gi·noid (an′jin-oid). Rarely used term for resembling an angina, especially angina pectoris.

an·gin·o·pho·bia (an′ji-nō-fō′bē-ă). Extreme fear of an attack of angina pectoris. [angina + G. *phobos,* fear]

an·gi·nose, an·gi·nous (an′ji-nōs, -ji-nŭs). Rarely used term for relating to any angina.

△**angio-, angi-.** Blood or lymph vessels; a covering, an enclosure; corresponds to L. vas-, vaso-, vasculo-. [G. *angeion,* a vessel or cavity of the body, fr. *angos,* a vessel, vat, bucket, + *-eion,* small, little]

an·gi·o·ar·chi·tec·ture (an′jē-ō-ar′ki-tek-choor). **1.** The arrangement and distribution of the blood vessels of any organ. **2.** The vascular framework of an organ or tissue.

an·gi·o·blast (an′jē-ō-blast). **1.** A cell taking part in blood vessel formation. SYN vasoformative cell. **2.** Primordial mesenchymal tissue from which embryonic blood cells and vascular endothelium are differentiated. SYN angioderm. [angio- + G. *blastos,* germ]

an·gi·o·blas·to·ma (an′jē-ō-blas-tō′mă). SYN hemangioblastoma.

a. of Nakagawa, SYN acquired tufted *angioma.*

an·gi·o·car·di·og·ra·phy (an′jē-ō-kar-dē-og′ră-fē). X-ray imaging of the heart and great vessels made visible by injection of a radiopaque solution. SEE coronary *angiography.* SYN cardioangiography. [angio- + G. *kardia,* heart, + *graphō,* to write]

exercise radionuclide a., radionuclide a. while patient is performing exercise, such as on a treadmill or bicycle.

gated radionuclide a., radionuclide a. using cardiac gating to combine images from several cardiac cycles to improve the quality of the images of separate phases (e.g., systole and diastole).

radionuclide a., the display, by means of a stationary scintillation camera device, of the passage of a bolus of a rapidly injected radiopharmaceutical through the heart. SYN radionuclide ventriculography.

an·gi·o·car·di·o·ki·net·ic, an·gi·o·car·di·o·ci·net·ic (an′jē-ō-kar′dē-ō-ki-net′ik, -dē-ō-si-net′ik). Causing dilation or contraction in the heart and blood vessels. [angio- + G. *kardia,* heart, + *kinēsis,* movement]

an·gi·o·car·di·op·a·thy (an′jē-ō-kar-dē-op′ă-thē). Disease af-

fecting both heart and blood vessels. [angio- + G. *kardia,* heart, + *pathos,* disease]

an·gi·o·cho·li·tis (an′jē-ō-kō-lī′tis). SYN cholangitis.

an·gi·o·cyst (an′jē-ō-sist). A small vesicular aggregation of embryonic mesodermal cells that may give rise to vascular endothelium and blood cells.

an·gi·o·derm (an′jē-ō-derm). SYN angioblast (2).

an·gi·o·dys·pla·sia (an′jē-ō-dis-plā′zē-ă). Degenerative or congenital structural abnormality of the normally distributed vasculature.

an·gi·o·dys·tro·phy, an·gi·o·dys·tro·phia (an′jē-ō-dis′trō-fē, -dis-trō′fē-ă). Defective formation or growth associated with marked vascular changes. [angio- + G. *dys-,* bad, + *trophē,* nourishment]

an·gi·o·e·de·ma (an′jē-ō-ĕ-dē′mă). Recurrent large circumscribed areas of subcutaneous or mucosal edema of sudden onset, usually disappearing within 24 hours; seen mainly in young women, frequently as an allergic reaction to foods or drugs. SYN angioneurotic edema, giant hives, giant urticaria, periodic edema.

hereditary a., an inherited, autosomal dominant disease characterized by episodic appearance of brawny nonpitting edema, most often affecting the extremities but can involve any part of the body, including mucosal surfaces such as those of the intestine (causing abdominal pain) or respiratory tract (causing asphyxia, which can require intubation to avoid fatal outcome). Associated with deficiency of inhibitor of first component of complement pathway (C1). Emergency treatment with epinephrine, long-term treatment with a variety of agents is effective.

an·gi·o·el·e·phan·ti·a·sis (an′jē-ō-el′ĕ-fan-tī′ă-sis). Extensive increase in vascularity of the subcutaneous tissue, producing great thickening simulating large, diffuse angioma formation.

an·gi·o·en·do·the·li·o·ma·to·sis (an′jē-ō-en-dō-thē′lē-ō-mă-tō′sis). Proliferation of endothelial cells within blood vessels.

proliferating systematized a., a rare generalized cutaneous and visceral intracapillary proliferation of endothelial cells, with vascular thrombosis and obstruction. The condition has been divided into a benign reactive type and a rapidly fatal neoplastic type; however, most of the latter cases have been shown to be intravascular large-cell lymphomas.

an·gi·o·fi·bro·li·po·ma (an′jē-ō-fī′brō-li-pō′mă). A neoplasm composed of fibroblasts, capillaries, and adipose tissue. SYN angiolipofibroma.

an·gi·o·fi·bro·ma (an′jē-ō-fī-brō′mă). SYN telangiectatic *fibroma.*

juvenile a., a markedly vascular fibrous tumor occurring in the nasopharynx of males, usually in the second decade of life; epistaxis and local invasion may result, but spontaneous regression may occur after sexual maturity. SYN juvenile hemangiofibroma.

an·gi·o·fi·bro·sis (an′jē-ō-fī-brō′sis). Fibrosis of the walls of blood vessels.

an·gi·o·gen·e·sis (an′jē-ō-jen′ĕ-sis). Development of new blood vessels. [angio- + G. *genesis,* production]

an·gi·o·gen·ic (an′jē-ō-jen′ik). **1.** Relating to angiogenesis. **2.** Of vascular origin.

an·gi·o·gli·o·ma (an′jē-ō-glī-ō′mă). A mixed glioma and angioma.

an·gi·o·gli·o·ma·to·sis (an′jē-ō-glī′ō-mă-tō′sis). Occurrence of multiple areas of proliferating capillaries and neuroglia or a condition of multiple angiogliomas.

an·gi·o·gli·o·sis (an′jē-ō-glī-ō′sis). Glial scarring about a blood vessel or a condition of multiple angiogliomas.

an·gi·o·gram (an′jē-ō-gram). Radiograph obtained by angiography. [angio- + G. *gramma,* a writing]

projection a., a digital a., such as in computed tomography or magnetic resonance imaging, reconstructed by computer to appear as does a radiographic a.

an·gi·o·graph·ic (an-jē-ō-graf′ik). Relating to or using angiography.

▯**an·gi·og·ra·phy** (an-jē-og′ră-fē). Radiography of vessels after the injection of a radiopaque contrast material; usually requires percutaneous insertion of a radiopaque catheter and positioning under fluoroscopic control. SEE ALSO arteriography, venography. [angio- + G. *graphō,* to write]

biplane a., synchronous a. in two planes at right angles to each other or in two orthogonal planes.

cerebral a., radiographic visualization of the blood vessels supplying the brain, including their extracranial portions; the injection of contrast medium may be made percutaneously, by open exposure and puncture of the carotid artery or by catheterization after introduction of the catheter at a distant site. SYN cerebral arteriography.

coronary a., imaging of the circulation of the myocardium by injection of contrast medium, usually by selective catheterization of each coronary artery, formerly by nonselective injection at the root of the aorta.

digital subtraction a. (DSA), computer-assisted radiographic a. permitting visualization of vascular structures without superimposed bone and soft tissue densities; subtraction of images made before and after contrast injection removes structures not enhanced by the contrast medium. Other image processing can be performed. Contrast material may be injected intravenously or in a lower-than-usual amount intraarterially.

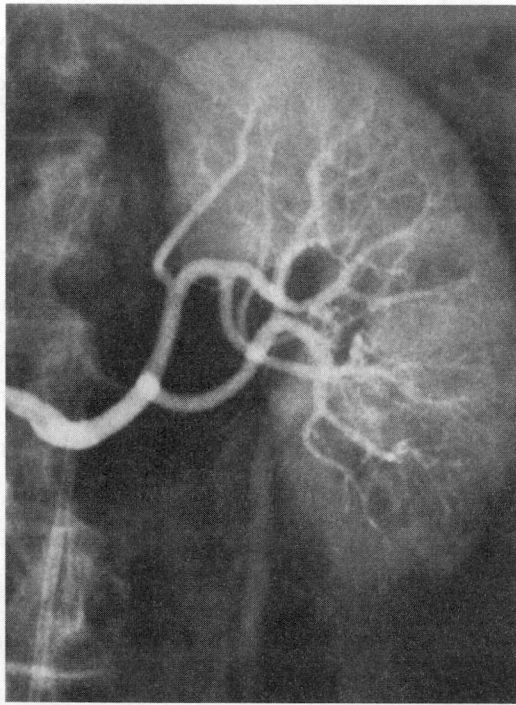

renal angiography

fluorescein a., photographic visualization of the passage of fluorescein through intraocular vessels after intravenous injection.

indocyanine green a., a test for studying choroidal vasculature by which indocyanine green dye, which absorbs infrared light at 805 nm and emits at 835 nm, is injected intravenously and photographed as it flows through the retinal and choroidal vessels.

interventional a., SYN angioplasty.

magnetic resonance a., SYN MR a.

magnification a., enhanced imaging of small blood vessels using an increased distance from subject to film, as in magnification radiography.

MR a. (MRA), imaging of blood vessels using special magnetic resonance (MR) sequences that enhance the signal of flowing blood and suppress that from other tissues. SYN magnetic resonance a.

radionuclide a., scintillation camera imaging of tissue perfusion by intravascular injection of a radioactive pharmaceutical. SEE ALSO radionuclide *angiocardiography.* SYN scintigraphic a.

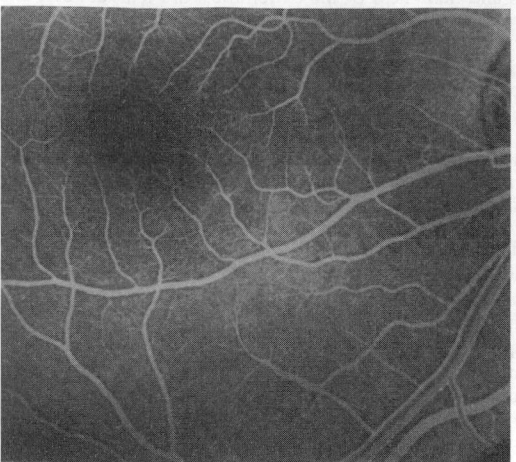

fluorescein angiography: fluorescein angiogram (early venous phase; the filling of the retinal capillary system is apparent)

scintigraphic a., SYN radionuclide a.

selective a., a. in which visualization is improved by concentrating the contrast medium in the region to be studied by injection through a catheter positioned in a regional artery, e.g., coronary a.

therapeutic a., use of angiographic catheters that have been modified to reduce or increase regional blood flow, or to deliver medicinal agents; interventional a. SEE angioplasty, balloon *catheter,* interventional a.

an·gi·o·hy·a·li·no·sis (an'jē-ō-hī'ă-li-nō'sis). Hyaline degeneration of the walls of the blood vessels. [angio- + G. *hyalos,* glass, + *-osis,* condition]

an·gi·o·hy·per·to·nia (an'jē-ō-hī-per-tō'nē-ă). SYN vasospasm. [angio- + G. *hyper,* over, + *tonos,* tension]

an·gi·o·hy·po·to·nia (an'jē-ō-hī-pō-tō'nē-ă). SYN vasoparalysis. [angio- + G. *hypo,* under, + *tonos,* tension]

an·gi·oid (an'jē-oyd). Resembling blood vessels; an arborizing pattern. [angio- + G. *eidos,* resemblance]

an·gi·o·in·va·sive (an'jē-ō-in-vā'siv). Denoting a neoplasm or other pathologic condition capable of entering the vascular bed.

an·gi·o·ker·a·to·ma (an'jē-ō-ker-ă-tō'mă). A superficial intradermal capillary acquired telangiectasis, over which there is a wartlike hyperkeratosis and acanthosis. SYN keratoangioma, telangiectasia verrucosa, telangiectatic wart. [angio- + G. *keras,* horn, + *-ōma,* tumor]

diffuse a., SYN Fabry *disease.*

Fordyce a., asymptomatic vascular papules of the scrotum, appearing in adults.

Mibelli a.'s, telangiectatic small papules of the extremities, common in adolescent girls.

an·gi·o·ker·a·to·sis (an'jē-ō-ker-ă-tō'sis). The occurrence of multiple angiokeratomas.

an·gi·o·lei·o·my·o·ma (an'jē-ō-lī'ō-mī-ō'mă). SYN vascular *leiomyoma.*

an·gi·o·lip·o·fi·bro·ma (an'jē-ō-lip'ō-fī-brō'mă). SYN angiofibrolipoma.

an·gi·o·li·po·ma (an'jē-ō-li-pō'mă). A lipoma that contains an unusually large number, or foci of proliferated, neoplasticlike, frequently dilated vascular channels. SYN lipoma cavernosum, telangiectatic lipoma.

an·gi·o·lith (an'jē-ō-lith). An arteriolith or a phlebolith. [angio- + G. *lithos,* stone]

an·gi·o·lith·ic (an'jē-ō-lith'ik). Relating to an angiolith.

an·gi·o·lo·gia (an'jē-ō-lō'jē-ă). SYN angiology. [angio- + G. *logos,* treatise, discourse]

an·gi·ol·o·gy (an-jē-ol'ō-jē). The science concerned with the blood vessels and lymphatics in all their relations. SYN angiologia. [angio- + G. *logos,* treatise, discourse]

an·gi·ol·y·sis (an-jē-ol'i-sis). Obliteration of a blood vessel, such as occurs in the newborn infant after tying of the umbilical cord. [angio- + G. *lysis,* destruction]

an·gi·o·ma (an-jē-ō'mă). A swelling or tumor due to proliferation, with or without dilation, of the blood vessels (hemangioma) or lymphatics (lymphangioma). [angio- + G. *-ōma,* tumor]

acquired tufted a., enlarging erythematous macules and plaques in children and adults, composed microscopically of lobules of capillaries and spindle cells that project into thin-walled venular dermal clefts. SYN angioblastoma of Nakagawa.

capillary a., SYN capillary *hemangioma.*

cavernous a., vascular malformation composed of sinusoidal vessels without a large feeding artery; can be multiple, especially if inherited as an autosomal dominant trait. SYN nevus cavernosus.

cherry a., SYN senile *hemangioma.*

petechial a.'s, multiple lesions resembling petechiae but due to dilation of capillary walls; they are obliterated by pressure.

a. serpigino'sum, the presence of rings of red dots on the skin, especially in female children, which tend to widen peripherally, due to dilation of superficial capillaries. SYN essential telangiectasia (2), primary telangiectasia.

spider a., a telangiectatic arteriole in the skin with radiating capillary branches simulating the legs of a spider; characteristic, but not pathognomonic, of parenchymatous liver disease; also seen in pregnancy, often disappearing after delivery, and at times in normal persons. SYN arterial spider, nevus araneus, spider hemangioma, spider nevus, spider telangiectasia, vascular spider.

superficial a., SYN capillary *hemangioma.*

telangiectatic a., a. composed of dilated vessels.

a. veno'sum racemo'sum, tortuous swelling caused by varicosities of superficial veins.

venous a., vascular anomaly composed of anomalous veins. SYN venous malformation.

an·gi·o·ma·toid (an-jē-ō'mă-toyd). Resembling a tumor of vascular origin.

an·gi·o·ma·to·sis (an'jē-ō-mă-tō'sis). A condition characterized by multiple angiomas.

bacillary a., (1) an infection of immunocompromised patients by a newly recognized Rickettsial species *Rochalimaea henselae,* characterized by fever and granulomatous cutaneous nodules, and peliosis hepatis in some cases. Skin biopsy shows vascular proliferation and infiltration of vessel walls by neutrophils and clumps of organisms seen with Warthin-Starry silver staining. **(2)** infectious disease characterized by fever and granulomatous cutaneous lesions. There are two forms. In one, associated with *Bartonella henselae* cat bites and scratches are predisposing; lymph nodes and viscera may be involved, and bacillary peliosis of liver and spleen can occur. A separate form, associated with *B. quintana,* is linked with conditions of poor hygiene (louse infestation, low income, poor or no housing); subcutaneous and bone lesions are more predominant.

cephalotrigeminal a., SYN Sturge-Weber *syndrome.*

cerebroretinal a., SYN von Hippel-Lindau *syndrome.*

congenital dysplastic a. [MIM*185300 & MIM149000], autosomal dominant a. in which there is dysplasia of the underlying tissues, sometimes with overgrowth of bone (Klippel-Trenaunay-Weber syndrome), or encephalotrigeminal a. (Sturge-Weber syndrome) in which there is an angioma in the distribution of one or more branches of the trigeminal nerve, with vascular anomalies and calcification of the cerebral cortex.

cutaneomeningospinal a., SYN Cobb *syndrome.*

encephalotrigeminal a., SYN Sturge-Weber *syndrome.*

oculoencephalic a. [MIM*185300], a forme fruste of Sturge-Weber syndrome, consisting of angiomas of the choroid and meninges only; probable autosomal dominant inheritance.

telangiectatic a., disseminated capillary and venous vascular malformations of the cerebral hemispheres and leptomeninges, occurring in Sturge-Weber syndrome.

an·gi·o·ma·tous (an-jē-ō'mă-tŭs). Relating to or resembling an angioma.

an·gi·o·meg·a·ly (an'jē-ō-meg'ă-lē). Enlargement of blood vessels or lymphatics. [angio- + G. *megas,* large]

an·gi·o·my·o·car·di·ac (an'jē-ō-mī'ō-kar'dē-ak). Relating to the blood vessels and the cardiac muscle. [angio- + G. *mys,* muscle, + *kardia,* heart]

an·gi·o·my·o·fi·bro·ma (an'jē-ō-mī'ō-fī-brō'mă). SYN vascular *leiomyoma.*

an·gi·o·my·o·li·po·ma (an'jē-ō-mī'ō-li-pō'mă). A benign neoplasm of adipose tissue (lipoma) in which muscle cells and vascular structures are fairly conspicuous; most commonly a renal tumor containing smooth muscle, often associated with tuberous sclerosis. [angio- + G. *mys,* muscle, + *lipos,* fat, + *-oma,* tumor]

an·gi·o·my·o·ma (an'jē-ō-mī-ō'mă). SYN vascular *leiomyoma.* [angio- + G. *mys,* muscle, + *-ōma,* tumor]

an·gi·o·my·op·a·thy (an'jē-ō-mī-op'ă-thē). Any disease of blood vessels involving the muscular layer. [angio- + G. *mys,* muscle, + *pathos,* suffering]

an·gi·o·my·o·sar·co·ma (an'jē-ō-mī'ō-sar-kō'mă). A myosarcoma that has an unusually large number of proliferated, frequently dilated, vascular channels.

an·gi·o·myx·o·ma (an'jē-ō-miks-ō'mă). A myxoma in which there is an unusually large number of vascular structures.

aggressive a., locally invasive, but nonmetastasizing tumor of genital organs in young women.

an·gi·o·neu·rec·to·my (an'jē-ō-noo-rek'tō-mē). Excision of the vessels and nerves of a part. [angio- + G. *neuron,* nerve, + *ektomē,* excision]

an·gi·o·neu·rop·a·thy (an'jē-ō-noo-rop'ă-thē). A vascular disorder attributed to an abnormality of the autonomic nervous system fibers supplying the blood vessels (i.e., the vasomotor system).

an·gi·o·neu·rot·ic (an'jē-ō-noo-rot'ik). Relating to angioneuroses.

an·gi·o·neu·rot·o·my (an'jē-ō-noo-rot'ō-mē). Division of both nerves and vessels of a part. [angio- + G. *neuron,* nerve, + *tomē,* a cutting]

an·gi·o·pa·ral·y·sis (an'jē-ō-pă-ral'i-sis). SYN vasoparalysis.

an·gi·o·pa·re·sis (an'jē-ō-pă-rē'sis, -par'ĕ-sis). SYN vasoparesis.

an·gi·o·path·ic (an'jē-ō-path'ik). Relating to angiopathy.

an·gi·op·a·thy (an-jē-op'ă-thē). Any disease of the blood vessels or lymphatics. SYN angiosis. [angio- + G. *pathos,* suffering]

amyloid a., deposition of acellular hyaline material in small arteries and arterioles of the leptomeninges and cerebral cortex in the elderly with resulting predilection for recurrent lobar intraparenchymal hematomas.

cerebral amyloid a., a pathologic condition of small cerebral vessels characterized by deposits of amyloid in the vessel walls, which may lead to infarcts or hemorrhage; may also occur in Alzheimer disease or Down syndrome. SEE ALSO congophilic a.

congophilic a., a condition of blood vessels characterized by deposits in the vessel walls of a substance, usually amyloid, that take a Congo red stain. SEE ALSO cerebral amyloid a.

giant cell hyaline a., an inflammatory infiltrate containing foreign body giant cells and eosinophilic material. Fragments of foreign material resembling vegetable matter may be included. SYN pulse granuloma.

an·gi·o·phac·o·ma·to·sis, an·gi·o·phak·o·ma·to·sis (an'jē-ō-fak'ō-mă-tō'sis). The angiomatous phacomatoses e.g., von Hippel-Lindau disease and the Sturge-Weber *syndrome.*

an·gi·o·pla·ny (an'jē-ō-plā-nē). SYN angiectopia. [angio- + G. *planē,* a wandering]

an·gi·o·plas·ty (an'jē-ō-plas-tē). Reconstitution or recanalization of a blood vessel; may involve balloon dilation, mechanical stripping of intima, forceful injection of fibrinolytics, or placement of a stent. SYN interventional angiography. [angio- + G. *plastos,* formed, shaped]

percutaneous transluminal a. (PTA), an operation for enlarging a narrowed vascular lumen by inflating and withdrawing through the stenotic region a balloon on the tip of an angiographic catheter; may include positioning of an intravascular endoluminal stent.

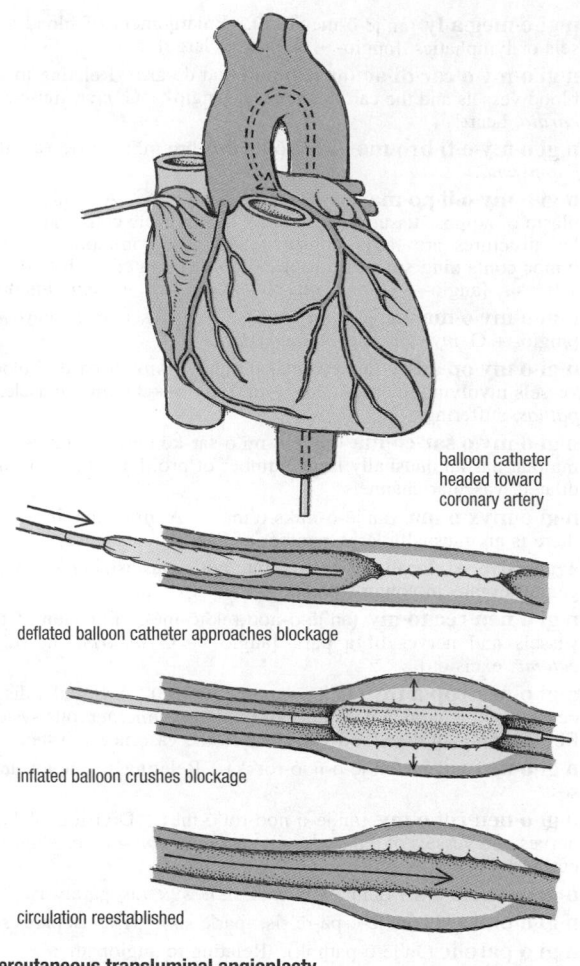

balloon catheter
headed toward
coronary artery

deflated balloon catheter approaches blockage

inflated balloon crushes blockage

circulation reestablished

percutaneous transluminal angioplasty

percutaneous transluminal coronary a. (PTCA), an operation for enlarging a narrowed vascular lumen by inflating and withdrawing through the stenotic region a balloon on the tip of an angiographic catheter.

PTCA is a minimally invasive surgical procedure for the treatment of coronary atherosclerosis. A balloon-tipped catheter is inserted percutaneously into the arterial circulation, advanced to the aortic root, and directed with a flexible guide wire to the site of coronary stenosis. Once positioned within the narrowed arterial segment, the balloon is inflated so as to stretch the lumen, fracture the obstructing plaque, or both. Balloon angioplasty is considered successful when there is more than a 20% increase in the caliber of the stenotic artery and restoration of at least 50% of normal patency, without acute complications. The procedure has approximately a 90% immediate success rate. It offers advantages in symptom improvement and exercise tolerance when compared to medical therapy, particularly in the short term, and is less hazardous and has a shorter recovery period than coronary artery bypass grafting (CABG). Operative mortality is about 2%. There is a 1–3% risk of nonfatal acute myocardial infarction during the procedure and a 1–3% risk that emergency CABG will be required. Hence the procedure is contraindicated unless a bypass team is immediately available. It is also contraindicated in patients without demonstrated significant vascular obstruction, as well as in those with severe multivessel disease or more than 50% stenosis of the left main coronary artery. Despite the advantages of

PTCA, 30–50% of patients require repeat balloon angioplasty or CABG for restenosis within 6 months. Insertion of a stainless steel stent at the time of balloon angioplasty to maintain arterial patency has improved initial success and reduced the 6-month restenosis rate. High-dose verapamil has also been associated with lower restenosis rates.

an·gi·o·poi·e·sis (an'jē-ō-poy-ē'sis). Formation of blood or lymphatic vessels. SYN vasifaction, vasoformation. [angio- + G. *poiesis,* making]

an·gi·o·poi·et·ic (an'jē-ō-poy-et'ik). Relating to angiopoiesis. SYN vasifactive, vasofactive, vasoformative.

an·gi·or·rha·phy (an-jē-ōr'ă-fē). Suture repair of any vessel, especially of a blood vessel. [angio- + G. *rhaphē,* a seam]

an·gi·o·sar·co·ma (an'jē-ō-sar-kō'mă). A rare malignant neoplasm occurring most often in soft tissues, and believed to originate from the endothelial cells of blood vessels; microscopically composed of spindle-shaped cells, some of which line small spaces resembling vascular clefts.

an·gi·o·scope (an'jē-ō-skōp). A modified microscope for studying the capillary vessels and a scope used for viewing larger vessels. [angio- + G. *skopeō,* to view]

an·gi·os·co·py (an-jē-os'kō-pē). **1.** Visualization with a microscope of the passage of substances (e.g., contrast media, radiopaque agents) through capillaries after intravenous injection. **2.** Visualization of the interior of blood vessels, especially the pulmonary arteries, using a fiberoptic catheter inserted through a peripheral artery. [angio- + G. *skopeō,* to view]

an·gi·o·sco·to·ma (an'jē-ō-skō-tō'mă). Ribbon-shaped defect of the visual fields caused by the retinal vessels overlying photoreceptors. [angio- + G. *skotōma,* dizziness, vertigo]

an·gi·o·sco·tom·e·try (an'jē-ō-skō-tom'ĕ-trē). The measurement or projection of the angioscotoma pattern.

an·gi·o·sis (an-jē-ō'sis). SYN angiopathy.

angiosome. Composite anatomic vascular territories of skin and underlying muscles, tendons, nerves, and bones, based on segmental or distributing arteries.

an·gi·o·spasm (an'jē-ō-spazm). SYN vasospasm.

an·gi·o·spas·tic (an'jē-ō-spas'tik). SYN vasospastic.

an·gi·o·ste·no·sis (an'jē-ō-stĕ-nō'sis). Narrowing of one or more blood vessels. [angio- + G. *stenōsis,* a narrowing]

an·gi·o·stron·gy·lo·sis (an'jē-ō-stron-ji-lō'sis). Infection of animals and humans with nematodes of the genus *Angiostrongylus.* SYN eosinophilic meningitis.

An·gi·o·stron·gy·lus (an'jē-ō-stron'jĭ-lŭs). A genus of metastrongyle nematodes parasitic in respiratory or circulatory systems of rodents, carnivores, and marsupials. SYN *Parastrongylus.* [G. *angeion,* vessel, + *strongylos,* round]

A. cantonen'sis, lungworm of rodents, a species transmitted by infected mollusks ingested by rodents; larvae develop in the brain and migrate to lungs, where the adult worms are found; thought to cause eosinophilic encephalomeningitis in humans in the Pacific basin; larvae have been removed from cerebrospinal fluid and the anterior chamber of the eye from persons in Thailand who had eaten raw snails.

A. costaricen'sis, a nematode parasite of rats and other rodents in Central America, recently found to infect humans, where they locate in the mesenteric arteries; infective third-stage larvae have been found in the slug, *Vaginulus plebeius.* SYN *Morerastrongylus costaricensis.*

A. malaysien'sis, species of *A.* found in Malaysia, a common rodent parasite similar to *A. cantonensis* and an actual or potential agent of eosinophilic meningitis in that region.

an·gi·o·te·lec·ta·sis, an·gi·o·tel·ec·ta·sia (an'jē-ō-tĕ-lek'tă-sis, -tel'ek-tā'sē-ă). SYN telangiectasia. [angio- + G. *telos,* end, + *ektasis,* a stretching out]

an·gi·o·ten·sin (an-jē-ō-ten'sin). A family of peptides of known and similar sequence, with vasoconstrictive activity, produced by enzymatic action of renin upon angiotensinogen. SEE angiotensin I, angiotensin II, angiotensin III.

an·gi·o·ten·sin I. A decapeptide of slightly variable sequence, depending on the animal source, formed from the tetradecapeptide angiotensinogen by the removal of four amino acid residues, a reaction catalyzed by renin; a peptidase cleaves off a dipeptide (histidylleucine) to yield angiotensin II, the physiologically active form.

an·gi·o·ten·sin II. A vasoactive octapeptide produced by the action of angiotensin-converting enzyme on angiotensin I; produces stimulation of vascular smooth muscle, promotes aldosterone production, and stimulates the sympathetic nervous system.

an·gi·o·ten·sin III. A vasoactive heptapeptide less potent than angiotensin II on vascular smooth muscle but approximately equally active in promoting aldosterone secretion.

an·gi·o·ten·sin am·ide. A synthetic substance closely related to the naturally occurring angiotensin II; a potent vasopressor agent useful in the management of certain types of shock and circulatory collapse.

an·gi·o·ten·sin·ase (an-jē-ō-ten′sin-ās). Former name for the enzyme responsible for converting angiotensin I to II; now applied to the enzyme that degrades angiotensin II. It hydrolyzes a peptide bond between a tyrosyl and an isoleucyl residue.

an·gi·o·ten·sin·o·gen (an′jē-ō-ten-sin′ō-jen). The substrate for renin whereupon through enzymatic action angiotensin I is liberated; an abundant α_2-globulin that circulates in the blood plasma. SYN angiotensin precursor.

an·gi·o·ten·sin·o·gen·ase (an′jē-ō-ten-sin′ō-jen-ās). SYN renin.

an·gi·o·ten·sin pre·cur·sor. SYN angiotensinogen.

an·gi·ot·o·my (an-jē-ot′ō-mē). Sectioning of a blood vessel, or the creation of an opening into a vessel prior to its repair. [angio- + G. *tomē*, cutting]

Angle, Edward Hartley, U.S. orthodontist, 1855–1930. SEE A. *classification* of malocclusion.

ANGLE

an·gle (θ) (ang′gl) [TA]. The meeting point of two lines or planes; the figure formed by the junction of two lines or planes; the space bounded on two sides by lines or planes that meet. For a.'s not listed below, see the descriptive term; e.g., axioincisal, distobuccal, labiogingival, linguogingival (2), mesiogingival, proximobuccal, etc. SYN angulus [TA]. [L. *angulus*]

acromial a. [TA], the prominent angle at the junction of the posterior and lateral borders of the acromion. SYN angulus acromii [TA].

acute a., any a. less than 90°.

adjacent a., an a. with a line in common with another a.

alpha a., (1) the a. between the visual and optic axes as they cross at the nodal point of the eye; (2) the a. between the visual line and the major axis of the corneal ellipse.

alveolar a., the a. between the horizontal plane and a line connecting the base of the nasal spine and the middle point of the projection of the alveolus of the maxilla.

anorectal a., SYN anorectal *flexure*.

a. of antetorsion, SYN a. of anteversion.

a. of anteversion, the a. formed by a line drawn through the center of the long axis of the neck of the femur meeting a line drawn in the transverse axis of the condyles, when the bone is viewed from above, looking straight down from above the head of the femur; used to illustrate the normal degree of anteversion about 12° of the neck of the femur, which may be increased or decreased in some diseases. SYN a. of antetorsion.

a. of aperture, the a. formed by lines drawn from the ends of the diameter of a lens to its point of focus. SEE ALSO angular *aperture*.

apical a., the a. between two plane surfaces of a prism. SYN refracting a. of a prism.

axial a., an a. formed by two surfaces of a body, the line of union of which is parallel with its axis; the axial a.'s of a tooth are the

distobuccal, distolabial, distolingual, mesiobuccal, mesiolabial, and mesiolingual.

basilar a., an a. formed by the intersection at the basion of lines coming from the nasal spine and the nasal point.

Bennett a., the a. formed by the sagittal plane and the path of the advancing condyle during lateral mandibular movement as viewed in the horizontal plane.

beta a., the a. formed by a line connecting the bregma and hormion meeting the radius fixus.

biorbital a., an a. formed by the meeting of the axes of the orbits.

Broca a.'s, (1) SYN Broca basilar a; (2) SYN Broca facial a; (3) SYN occipital a. of parietal bone (1).

Broca basilar a., the a. formed at the basion of lines drawn from the nasion and the alveolar point. SYN Broca a.'s (1).

Broca facial a., the a. formed by the intersection at the biauricular axis of lines drawn from the supraorbital point and the alveolar point. SYN Broca a.'s (2).

buccal a.'s, a.'s formed by the buccal surface of a tooth joining the other surfaces.

bucco-occlusal a., the line of junction of the buccal and occlusal surfaces of a tooth.

cardiodiaphragmatic a., SYN cardiophrenic a.

cardiohepatic a., the a. formed by the upper border of the liver and the right border of the heart, especially as defined by percussion. SYN cardiohepatic triangle.

cardiophrenic a., the a. between the heart and the diaphragm at either lateral end of the cardiac projection on imaging (usually the chest x-ray film). The right cardiophrenic a. is normally indistinguishable from the cardiohepatic a. radiographically. SYN cardiodiaphragmatic a., phrenopericardial a.

carrying a., the a. made by the axes of the arm and the forearm, with the elbow in full extension.

cavity line a., in dentistry, the a. formed by two walls of a cavity, e.g., a tooth cavity, meeting along a line.

cavosurface a., the a. formed by the junction of a cavity wall and the surface of the tooth.

cephalic a., one of several a.'s formed by the intersection of two lines passing through certain points of the face or cranium.

cephalomedullary a., the a. made by the junction of the cerebrum and the brainstem.

cerebellopontile a., SYN cerebellopontine a.

cerebellopontine a., the a. formed at the junction of the cerebellum, pons, and medulla; the most common tumor found in this location is the acoustic neuroma. SYN angulus pontocerebellaris [TA], cerebellopontile a., pontine a., pontocerebellar recess.

costal a., SYN a. of rib.

costophrenic a., the a. between the costal and diaphragmatic parietal pleura as they meet at the costodiaphragmatic line of pleura reflection. Used as a synonym in radiology to identify the costodiaphragmatic recess. SEE ALSO costodiaphragmatic *recess.*

costovertebral a., the acute a. formed between either twelfth rib and the vertebral column.

costoxiphoid a., the a. formed between the right or left costal arch and the long axis of the xiphoid process (usually identical to the midline); it is one half of the infrasternal a. SEE ALSO infrasternal a. SYN xiphocostal a.

craniofacial a., the a. formed by the basifacial and basicranial axes at the midpoint of the sphenoethmoidal suture.

critical a., the a. of incidence at which a ray of light, in passing between two media, changes from refraction to total reflection. SYN limiting a.

cusp a., (1) the a. made by the slopes of a cusp with the plane which passes through the tip of the cusp and which is perpendicular to a line bisecting the cusp, measured mesiodistally or buccolingually; (2) the a. made by the slopes of a cusp with a perpendicular line bisecting the cusp, measured mesiodistally or buccolingually; (3) one-half of the included a. between the buccal and lingual or mesial and distal cusp inclines.

Daubenton a., SYN occipital a. of parietal bone (2).

a. of declination, obsolete term for a. of anteversion.

a. of deviation, (1) in a prism, the sum of the a.'s of incidence and emergence minus the apical a. of a prism; **(2)** in optics, a. of refraction; **(3)** in strabismus, a. of anomaly.

disparity a., the difference in position of images on the retina, still permitting fusion.

duodenojejunal a., SYN duodenojejunal *flexure*.

a. of eccentricity, in strabismus, the a. between the line of fixation and the line of normal foveal fixation.

a. of emergence, the a. formed by a light ray emerging from the second surface of a prism and a line parallel to the incident ray. Cf. a. of deviation.

epigastric a., the a. formed by the xiphoid process with the body of the sternum.

ethmoid a., the a. made by the plane of the cribriform plate of the ethmoid bone extended to meet the basicranial axis.

facial a., **(1)** any of several variously named and variously defined anatomic a.'s that have been used to quantify facial protrusion; **(2)** in dentistry, the a. formed by the intersection of the orbitomeatal (Frankfort) plane with the nasion-pogonion line (inner lower a.), which establishes the anteroposterior relation of the mandible to the upper face at the orbitomeatal plane. SYN Frankfort-mandibular incisor a.

a. of femoral torsion, the a. formed between the longitudinal axis of the head and neck of the femur proximally and the transverse axis of the femoral condyles distally, when the femur is viewed along the axis of its shaft; normally, this a. is approximately 15° in adults, but is considerably greater in infancy.

filtration a., SYN iridocorneal a.

flip a., in a magnetic resonance imaging pulse sequence, the deviation toward transverse plane of the average axis of the protons induced by radiofrequency signals; low angles are used in rapid or bright blood imaging sequences.

Frankfort-mandibular incisor a., SYN facial a. (2).

frontal a. of parietal bone [TA], the anterior superior a. of the parietal bone. SYN angulus frontalis ossis parietalis [TA].

a. of Fuchs, a crevice between the ciliary and pupillary zones of the iris formed by atrophy of superficial layers of the iris in the pupillary zone.

gamma a., the a. formed between a line joining the fixation point to the center of the eye and the optic axis.

hypsiloid a., SYN y-a.

impedance a., a term expressing the ratio of electric resistance to electric capacitance (ohms to microfarads) in the tissues of the body or any other substance.

a. of incidence, **(1)** the a. that a ray entering a refracting medium makes with a line drawn perpendicular to the surface of this medium; **(2)** the a. that a ray striking a reflecting surface makes with a line perpendicular to this surface. SYN incident a.

incident a., SYN a. of incidence.

incisal guide a., the a. formed with the horizontal plane by drawing a line in the sagittal plane between incisal edges of the maxillary and mandibular central incisors when the teeth are in centric occlusion.

a. of inclination, the a. formed by the meeting of a line drawn through the shaft of a long bone with one passing through the long axis of its femoral neck; normally refers to the femur and humerus. SYN neck-shaft a.

inferior a. of scapula [TA], the acute a. formed by junction of the medial and lateral borders of the scapula. SYN angulus inferior scapulae [TA].

infrasternal a. [TA], the a. between the lower borders of the costal cartilages of the two sides as they approach the sternum. SYN angulus infrasternalis [TA], subcostal a.☆, subcostal arch☆, substernal a.

iridocorneal a. [TA], the acute a. between the iris and the cornea at the periphery of the anterior chamber of the eye. SYN angulus iridocornealis [TA], a. of iris, angulus iridis, filtration a.

a. of iris, SYN iridocorneal a.

Jacquart facial a., a facial a. with the intersection always at the nasal spine point; additional variation uses the supraorbital point instead of the glabella, and this latter version is also known as ophryospinal facial a. or Topinard facial a.

a. of jaw, SYN a. of mandible.

kappa a., the a. between the pupillary axis and the visual axis; it is positive when the pupillary axis is nasal to the visual axis, and negative when the pupillary axis is temporal to the visual axis.

lateral a. of eye [TA], the a. formed by the junction of the lateral parts of the upper and lower eyelids. SYN angulus oculi lateralis [TA], angulus oculi temporalis, external canthus, lateral canthus.

lateral a. of scapula [TA], the blunt, concave head of the scapula forming the glenoid cavity at the junction of the superior and lateral borders of the bone. SYN angulus lateralis scapulae [TA].

lateral a. of uterus, the upper part of the side of the uterus at the point of its junction with the uterine tube.

limiting a., SYN critical a.

line a., in dentistry, the junction of two surfaces of the crown of a tooth, or of a tooth cavity (cavity line a.).

Louis a., SYN sternal a.

Lovibond a., the a. made at the meeting of the proximal nail fold and the nail plate when viewed from the radial aspect; normally, less than 180° but exceeding this in clubbing of the fingers. SYN Lovibond profile sign.

Ludwig a., SYN sternal a.

lumbosacral a., the a. between the long axis of the lumbar part of the vertebral column and that of the sacrum.

a. of mandible [TA], the a. formed by the lower margin of the body and the posterior margin of the ramus of the mandible. SYN angulus mandibulae [TA], a. of jaw.

mastoid a. of parietal bone [TA], the posteroinferior point of the parietal bone. SYN angulus mastoideus ossis parietalis [TA].

maxillary a., the a. formed by a line drawn from the ophryon and another from the point of the mandible and meeting at the contact between the upper and lower incisor teeth.

medial a. of eye [TA], the a. formed by the union of the upper and lower eyelids medially. SYN angulus oculi medialis [TA], angulus oculi nasalis, internal canthus, medial canthus.

mesial a., the a. formed by the meeting of the mesial with the labial (or buccal) or lingual surface of a tooth.

metafacial a., the a. between the pterygoid processes and the base of the skull. SYN Serres a.

meter a., the amount of convergence required to view binocularly an object 1 m distant and exerting 1 diopter of accommodation. SYN unit of ocular convergence.

a. of mouth [TA], the lateral limit of the oral fissure. SEE ALSO labial *commissure*. SYN angulus oris [TA].

neck-shaft a., SYN a. of inclination.

occipital a. of parietal bone [TA], **(1)** the posterior superior angle of the parietal bone; SYN Broca a.'s (3). **(2)** an a. formed by the junction, at the opisthion, of lines coming from the basion and from the projection in the median plane of the lower border of the orbits. SYN angulus occipitalis ossis parietalis [TA], Daubenton a. SEE ALSO Daubenton *line*, Daubenton *plane*.

olfactory a., the a. formed by the plane of the lamina cribrosa and the basicranial axis.

ophryospinal a., SEE Jacquart facial a.

parietal a., an a. formed by the meeting of the prolongation of two lines tangential to the most prominent part of the zygomatic arch and to the parietofrontal suture on each side; when the lines remain parallel the a. is zero; when they diverge it is negative. SYN Quatrefages a.

pelvivertebral a., the a. made by the pelvis as defined by the plane of the superior pelvic aperture with the general axis of the trunk or vertebral column. SEE ALSO pelvic *inclination*.

phrenopericardial a., SYN cardiophrenic a.

Pirogoff a., SYN venous a. (1).

point a., the junction of three surfaces of the crown of a tooth, or of the walls of a cavity.

a. of polarization, the a. of incidence at which the reflected light is all polarized.

pontine a., SYN cerebellopontine a.

pubic a., SYN subpubic a.

Q a., the a. formed by lines representing the pull of the quadriceps muscle and the axis of the patellar tendon.

Quatrefages a., SYN parietal a.

Ranke a., the a. formed by the horizontal plane of the head and a line passing from the center of the margin of the alveolar arch of the maxilla, below the nasal spine to the center of the frontonasal suture. [J. Ranke]

a. of reflection, the a. that a ray reflected from a surface makes with a line drawn perpendicular to this surface; it is equal to the a. of incidence (2).

refracting a. of a prism, SYN apical a.

a. of refraction, the a. that a ray leaving a refracting medium makes with a line drawn perpendicular to the surface of this medium.

a. of retroversion, the a. formed by a line drawn through the center of the longitudinal axis of the neck and head of the humerus meeting a line drawn along the transverse axis of the condyles, when the base is viewed from above, looking straight down from above the head of the humerus; the normal a. of retroversion of the humerus is between 20° and 40°.

a. of rib [TA], the rather abrupt change in curvature of the body of a rib posteriorly, such that the neck and head of the rib are directed upward. SYN angulus costae [TA], costal a.

Rolando a., the a. which the fissure of Rolando (central sulcus) makes with the midplane.

Serres a., SYN metafacial a.

S-N-A a., in cephalometrics, an a. measuring the anteroposterior relationship of the maxillary basal arch on the anterior cranial base; it shows the degree of maxillary prognathism. SEE ALSO subspinale. [sella-nasion-subspinale (or point *A*)]

S-N-B a., an a. showing the anterior limit of the mandibular basal arch in relation to the anterior cranial base. SEE ALSO supramentale. [sella-nasion-supramentale (or point *B*)]

sphenoid a., sphenoidal a., (1) a. formed by the intersection at the top of the sella turcica (dorsum sellae), of lines coming from the nasal point and from the tip of the rostrum of the sphenoid; **(2)** SYN sphenoidal a. of parietal bone.

sphenoidal a. of parietal bone [TA], the anterior inferior a. of the parietal bone. SYN angulus sphenoidalis ossis parietalis [TA], sphenoid a. (2), sphenoidal a., Welcker a.

sternal a. [TA], the a. between the manubrium and the body of the sternum at the manubriosternal junction. Marks the level of the second costal cartilage (rib) for counting ribs or intercostal spaces. Denotes level of aortic arch, bifurcation of trachea, and T4/T5 intervertebral disc. SYN angulus sterni [TA], Louis a., Ludwig a., manubriosternal junction.

sternoclavicular a., the a. formed by the junction of the clavicle with the sternum.

subcostal a., ✫official alternate term for infrasternal a.

subpubic a. [TA], the a. formed between the inferior rami of the pubic bones. In the female, the a. approximates that a. between the widely extended thumb and index finger (90°); in the male, it approximates the a. between the widely abducted index and middle fingers (60°). SEE ALSO pubic *arch*. SYN angulus subpubicus [TA], pubic a.

substernal a., SYN infrasternal a.

superior a. of scapula [TA], formerly named the medial angle, it lies at the junction of the superior and medial borders of the bone. SYN angulus superior scapulae [TA].

sylvian a., the a. formed by the sylvian line and a line perpendicular to the horizontal plane tangential to the highest point of the hemisphere.

tentorial a., the a. made by the plane of the tentorium and the basicranial axis.

Topinard facial a., SEE Jacquart facial a.

a. of torsion, the amount of rotation of a long bone along its axis or between two axes, measured in degrees; when this a. is oriented anteriorly, it is referred to as the a. of anteversion and most commonly describes the femur; when this a. is oriented posteriorly, it is the a. of retroversion and most commonly describes the humerus.

urethrovesical a., the a. between the female urethra and the posterior vesical wall, normally about 90°; narrowing of this angle in cystocele predisposes to stress incontinence.

■**venous a., (1)** the junction of the internal jugular and subclavian veins, toward which converge the external and the anterior jugular and the vertebral veins, the thoracic duct in the left a. and the right lymphatic duct in the right a.; SYN Pirogoff a. **(2)** in neuroradiology, the a. of union of the superior thalamostriate vein (vena terminalis) with the internal cerebral vein, usually closely behind the interventricular foramen (of Monro).

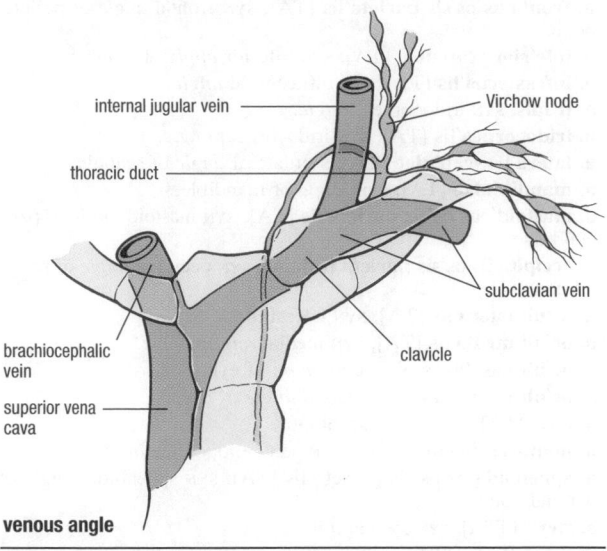

internal jugular vein — Virchow node

thoracic duct —

— subclavian vein

brachiocephalic vein

— clavicle

superior vena cava

venous angle

Virchow a., an a. formed by the meeting of a line drawn from the middle of the nasofrontal suture to the base of the anterior nasal spine with a line drawn from this last point to the center of the external auditory meatus. SYN Virchow-Holder a.

Virchow-Holder a., SYN Virchow a.

visual a., the a. formed at the retina by the meeting of lines drawn from the periphery of the object seen.

Vogt a., a craniometric a. formed by the nasobasilar and alveolonasal lines. [K. Vogt]

Weisbach a., a craniometric a. formed by the junction, at the alveolar point, of lines passing from the basion and from the middle of the frontonasal suture.

Welcker a., SYN sphenoidal a. of parietal bone.

xiphocostal a., SYN costoxiphoid a.

y-a., in craniometry, the a. at the inion formed by lines drawn from the hormion and the lambda. SYN hypsiloid a.

an·gor (ang′gōr). Rarely used term for extreme distress or mental anguish. [L. quinsy, anguish]

a. an′imi, the sense of being in the act of dying, differing from the fear of death or the desire for death; a symptom that may occur with angina pectoris and occasionally in diseases of the medulla. SYN a. pectoris (2).

a. pec′toris, (1) SYN Gairdner *disease*; **(2)** SYN a. animi.

Ångström, Anders J., Swedish physicist, 1814–1874. SEE angstrom; A. *law*, *unit*, *scale*.

ang·strom (Å) (ang′strŏm). A unit of wavelength, 10^{-10} m, roughly the diameter of an atom; equivalent to 0.1 nm. [AJ Ångström]

An·guil·lu·la (ang-gwil′loo-lă). Old name for a genus of free-living nematodes. SEE *Turbatrix*. [Mod. L. dim. of L. *anguilla*, eel]

an·gu·la·tion (ang′goo-lā′shŭn). **1.** Formation of an angle; an abnormal angle or bend in an organ. **2.** In orthopaedics, a method of describing the alignment of long bones that have been affected by injury or disease; can be described in both anteroposterior and lateral planes.

apex anterior a., a. in the lateral plane in which the apex of the angle is directed anteriorly.

apex posterior a., a. in the lateral plane in which the apex of the angle is directed posteriorly.

an·gu·lus, gen. and pl. **an·gu·li** (ang'gū-lŭs, -lī) [TA]. SYN angle. [L.]

  a. acromii [TA], SYN acromial *angle.*

  a. cos'tae [TA], SYN *angle* of rib.

  a. fronta'lis os'sis parieta'lis [TA], SYN frontal *angle* of parietal bone.

  a. infe'rior scap'ulae [TA], SYN inferior *angle* of scapula.

  a. infrasterna'lis [TA], SYN infrasternal *angle.*

  a. ir'idis, SYN iridocorneal *angle.*

  a. iridocornea'lis [TA], SYN iridocorneal *angle.*

  a. latera'lis scap'ulae [TA], SYN lateral *angle* of scapula.

  a. mandib'ulae [TA], SYN *angle* of mandible.

  a. mastoid'eus os'sis parieta'lis [TA], SYN mastoid *angle* of parietal bone.

  a. occipita'lis os'sis parieta'lis [TA], SYN occipital *angle* of parietal bone (2).

  a. oc'uli latera'lis [TA], SYN lateral *angle* of eye.

  a. oc'uli media'lis [TA], SYN medial *angle* of eye.

  a. oc'uli nasa'lis, SYN medial *angle* of eye.

  a. oc'uli temporalis, SYN lateral *angle* of eye.

  a. o'ris [TA], SYN *angle* of mouth.

  a. pontocerebellaris [TA], SYN cerebellopontine *angle.*

  a. sphenoida'lis os'sis parieta'lis [TA], SYN sphenoidal *angle* of parietal bone.

  a. ster'ni [TA], SYN sternal *angle.*

  a. subpu'bicus [TA], SYN subpubic *angle.*

  a. supe'rior scap'ulae [TA], SYN superior *angle* of scapula.

an·haph·ia (an-haf'ē-ă). SYN anaphia.

an·he·do·nia (an-hē-dō'nē-ă). Absence of pleasure from the performance of acts that would ordinarily be pleasurable. [G. *an-* priv. + *hedonē,* pleasure]

an·hi·dro·sis (an-hī-drō'sis). Absence of sweat glands or absence of sweating, e.g., due to anticholinergic drugs. SYN adiaphoresis. [G. *an-* priv. + *hidrōs,* sweat]

an·hi·drot·ic (an-hī-drot'ik). **1.** Relating to, or characterized by, anhidrosis. **2.** SYN antiperspirant (2). **3.** Denoting a reduction or absence of sweat glands, characteristic of congenital ectodermal defect and anhidrotic ectodermal dysplasia. SYN adiaphoretic.

an·his·tic, an·his·tous (an-his'tik, -tŭs). Without apparent structure. [G. *an-* priv. + *histos,* web]

an·hy·drase (an-hī'drās). An enzyme that catalyzes the removal of water from a compound; most such enzymes are now known as hydrases, hydro-lyases, or dehydratases.

  carbonic a., a zinc-containing enzyme that catalyzes the interconversion of CO_2 with HCO_3^- and H^+. There are at least seven human isozymes that appear predominantly in red blood cells, secretory tissues, muscle, etc. A deficiency of carbonic a. II can result in osteopetrosis and metabolic acidosis. The inhibition of carbonic a. IV and possibly carbonic a. II by sulfonamides is a current therapy in the treatment of glaucoma. SYN carbonate dehydratase, carbonate hydro-lyase.

an·hy·dra·tion (an-hī-drā'shŭn). SYN dehydration (1).

an·hy·dride (an-hī'drīd). An oxide that can combine with water to form an acid or that is derived from an acid by the abstraction of water.

△**anhydro-.** Chemical prefix denoting the removal of water. Cf. pyro- (2). [G. *an-* priv., + *hydōr,* water]

3,6-an·hy·dro·ga·lac·tose (an-hī'drō-gă-lak'tōs). A galactose derivative found in a number of polysaccharides (e.g., agarose).

an·hy·dro·gi·tal·in (an-hī'drō-jit'ă-lin). SYN gitoxin.

an·hy·dro·leu·cov·o·rin (an-hī'drō-loo-kō-vōr'in). An intermediate formed in the folic acid-catalyzed glycine-serine interconversion. SYN N^5,N^{10}-methenyltetrahydrofolic acid.

an·hy·dro·sug·ars (an-hī'drō-shug-ărz). Sugars from which one or more molecules of water, other than water of crystallization, have been eliminated. SYN dehydrosugars.

an·hy·drous (an-hī'drŭs). Containing no water, especially water of crystallization.

a·ni·a·cin·am·i·do·sis (ă-nī'ă-sin-am-i-dō'sis). Rarely used term for deficiency of niacinamide which may be associated with pellagra. [G. *a-* priv. + niacinamide + -*osis,* condition]

a·ni·a·cin·o·sis (ă-nī'ă-sin-ō'sis). Rarely used term for aniacinamidosis. [G. *a-* oruv. + niacin + -*osis* condition]

an·ic·ter·ic (an-ik-ter'ik). Not icteric.

an·id·e·an (an-id'ē-an). Shapeless; denoting a formless mass of tissue. SYN anidous. [see anideus]

an·id·e·us (an-id'ē-ŭs). A parasitic fetus consisting of a poorly differentiated mass of tissue with slight indications of parts. SEE ALSO *holoacardius* amorphus. [G. *an-* priv. + *eidos,* shape]

  embryonic a., a blastoderm without axial organization.

an·i·dous (an-ī'dŭs). SYN anidean.

an·i·ler·i·dine (an-i-ler'i-dēn). Analgesic agent related chemically and pharmacologically to meperidine hydrochloride; used for relief of moderate to severe pain; also mildly antihistaminic and spasmolytic; addiction liability is equivalent to that of morphine.

an·i·lide (an'i-lid). An *N*-acyl aniline; e.g., acetanilide.

ani·linc·tion, ani·linc·tus (ā-ni-lingk'shŭn, -lingk'tŭs). SYN anilingus.

an·i·line (an'i-lin, -lēn). $C_6H_5(NH_2)$; an oily, colorless or brownish liquid, of aromatic odor and acrid taste, that is the parent substance of many synthetic dyes; derived from benzene by the substitution of the group —NH_2 for one of the hydrogen unatoms. A. is highly toxic, may cause industrial poisoning, and may be carcinogenic. SYN aminobenzene, benzeneamine, phenylamine. [Ar. *an-nil,* indigo]

an·i·line blue [C.I. 42755]. A mixture of sulfonated triphenylmethane dyes used widely as a connective tissue stain and counterstain.

ani·lin·gus (ā-ni-ling'gŭs). Sexual stimulation by licking or kissing the anus; a type of oral-genital sexual activity. SYN anilinction, anilinctus. [L. *anus,* + *lingo,* to lick]

an·i·lin·ism (an'i-lin-izm). SYN anilism.

an·i·li·no·phil, an·i·li·no·phile (an-i-lin'ō-fil, -fīl). Denoting a cell or histologic structure that stains readily with an aniline dye. SYN anilinophilous. [aniline + G. *philos,* fond]

an·i·li·noph·i·lous (an-i-li-nof'ĭ-lŭs). SYN anilinophil.

an·il·ism (an'i-lizm). Chronic aniline poisoning characterized by gastric and cardiac weakness, vertigo, muscular depression, intermittent pulse, and cyanosis. SYN anilinism.

an·i·ma (an'i-mă). **1.** The soul or spirit. SEE animus (4). **2.** In jungian psychology, the inner self, in contrast to persona; a female archetype in a man. Cf. animus (5). [L. breath, soul]

an·i·mal (an'i-măl). **1.** A living, sentient organism that has membranous cell walls, requires oxygen and organic foods, and is capable of voluntary movement, as distinguished from a plant or mineral. **2.** One of the lower a. organisms as distinguished from humans. [L.]

  cold-blooded a., SYN poikilotherm.

  control a., in research, an a. submitted to the same conditions as the others used for the experiment, but with the crucial factor (such as the injection of antitoxin, the administration of a drug, etc.) omitted. SEE ALSO control, control *experiment.*

  conventional a., an a. colonized by the burden of resident microorganisms normally associated with its particular species.

  Houssay a., an a. that has been pancreatectomized and hypophysectomized. Named after the discoverer of the principle that a.'s are more sensitive to insulin after removal of the pituitary, and that after this operation the intensity of diabetes in depancreatized a.'s is diminished.

  normal a., in research, an experimental a. that has neither suffered an attack of a particular disease nor received an injection of a specific microorganism or its toxin.

  sentinel a., an a. deliberately placed in a particular environment to detect the presence of an infectious agent, such as a virus.

  warm-blooded a., SYN homeotherm.

an·i·mal black. SYN animal *charcoal.*

an·i·mal·cule (an-i-mal′kūl). Term used by believers in the pre-formation theory to designate the supposed miniature body contained in a gamete. SEE homunculus. [Mod. L. *animalculum,* dim. of L. *animal,* a living being]

an·i·ma·tion (an-i-mā′shŭn). **1.** The state of being alive. **2.** Liveliness; high spirits. [L. *animo,* pp. *-atus,* to make alive; *anima,* breath, soul]

suspended a., a temporary state resembling death, with cessation of respiration; may also refer to certain forms of hibernation in animals or to endospore formation by some bacteria.

an·i·mat·ism (an′i-mă-tizm). Attribution of mental or spiritual qualities to both living beings and nonliving things. SEE ALSO animism.

an·i·mism (an′i-mizm). The view that all things in nature, both animate and inanimate, contain a spirit or soul; held by primitive peoples and young children. SEE ALSO animatism. [L. *anima,* soul]

an·i·mus (an′i-mŭs). **1.** An animating or energizing spirit. **2.** Intention to do something; disposition. **3.** In psychiatry, a spirit of active hostility or grudge. **4.** The ideal image toward which a person strives. **5.** In jungian psychology, a male archetype in a woman. Cf. anima (2). [L. *animus,* breath, rational soul in man, will]

an·i·on (A⁻) (an′ī-on). An ion that carries a negative charge, going therefore to the positively charged anode; in salts, acid radicals are a.'s.

an·i·on ex·change. The process by which an anion in a mobile (liquid) phase exchanges with another anion previously bound to a solid, positively charged phase, the latter being an anion exchanger. It takes place when Cl^- is exchanged for OH^- in desalting. The reaction is Cl^- (in solution) + (OH^- on anion exchanger⁺) → (Cl^- on anion exchanger) + OH^- (in solution); combined with cation exchange, NaCl is removed from solution. Anion exchange may also be used chromatographically, to separate anions, and medicinally, to remove an anion (e.g., Cl^-) from gastric contents or bile acids in the intestine.

an·i·on ex·chang·er. An insoluble solid, usually a polystyrene or a polysaccharide, with cation groups (e.g., $-NR_3^+$ or $-NR_2H^+$), which can attract and hold anions that pass by in a moving solution in exchange for anions previously held.

an·i·on·ic (an-ī-on′ik). Referring to a negatively charged ion.

an·i·on·ot·ro·py (an′-ī-on-ot′rō-pē). The migration of a negative ion in tautomeric changes.

an·i·rid·ia (an-i-rid′ē-ă) [MIM*106200]. Absence of the iris; when congenital, a rudimentary iris root is usually present. About 60% of cases are inherited as autosomal dominant, although somewhat irregularly manifested. Cf. irideremia. [G. *an-* priv. + irid- + -ia]

an·i·sa·ki·a·sis (an′i-să-kī′ă-sis). Infection of the intestinal wall by larvae of *Anisakis marina* and other genera of anisakid nematodes (*Contracaecum, Phocanema*), characterized by intestinal eosinophilic granuloma and symptoms like those of peptic ulcer or tumor. SYN herring-worm disease. [G. *anisos,* unequal, + *akis,* a point, + *-iasis,* condition]

an·i·sa·kid (an-i-sā′kid). Common name for nematodes of the family Anisakidae.

An·i·sa·ki·dae (an-i-sā′ki-dē). Family of large nematode worms (superfamily Heterocheilidae) found in the stomach and intestines of fish-eating birds and marine mammals, infection being acquired from marine fish; human cases of anisakiasis have been reported from Japan. SEE ALSO *Anisakis.*

An·i·sa·kis (an-i-sā′kis). Genus of nematodes (family Anisakidae) that includes many common parasites of marine fish-eating birds and marine mammals. [G. *anisos,* unequal, + *akis,* a point]

an·is·ate (an′ī-sāt). A salt of anisic acid, usually possessing antiseptic properties.

an·ise (an′is). The fruit of *Pimpinellla anisum* (family Umbelliferae); an aromatic and carminative resembling fennel.

an·is·ei·ko·nia (an′ī-sī-kō′nē-ă). An ocular condition in which the image of an object in one eye differs in size or shape from the image of the same object in the fellow eye. SYN unequal retinal image. [G. *anisos,* unequal, + *eikōn,* an image]

anis·ic (an-is′ik). Relating to anise.

anis·ic ac·id (an-is′ik). A crystalline volatile acid obtained from anise; its compounds are the antiseptic anisates. SYN 4-methoxybenzoic acid.

an·i·sin·di·one (an′i-sin-dī′ōn). An anticoagulant with pharmacologic actions similar to those of phenindone and bishydroxycoumarin.

aniso-. Unequal, dissimilar, unlike. [G. *anisos,* unequal, fr. *an-,* not, + *isos,* equal]

an·i·so·ac·com·mo·da·tion (an-ī′sō-ă-kom-ō-dā′shŭn). Variation between the two eyes in accommodation capacity. [aniso- + L. *accommodo,* to adapt]

an·i·so·chro·ma·sia (an-ī′sō-krō-mā′zē-ă). The unequal distribution of hemoglobin in the red blood cells, such that the periphery is pigmented and the central region is virtually colorless, as observed in films of blood from persons with certain forms of anemia caused by deficiency of iron; normal red blood cells show mild a. because of their biconcave shape. [aniso- + G. *chrōma,* color]

an·i·so·chro·mat·ic (an-ī′sō-krō-mat′ik). Not uniformly of one color.

an·i·so·co·ria (an-ī-sō-kō′rē-ă). A condition in which the two pupils are not of equal size. [aniso- + G. *korē,* pupil]

essential a., SYN simple a.

physiologic a., SYN simple a.

simple a., a common (20% of normals) benign inequality of the pupils that may change from one hour to the next. SYN essential a., physiologic a., simple-central a.

simple-central a., SYN simple a.

an·i·so·cy·to·sis (an-ī′sō-sī-tō′sis). Considerable variation in the size of cells that are normally uniform, especially with reference to red blood cells. [aniso- + G. *kytos,* cell, + *-osis,* condition]

an·i·so·dac·ty·lous (an-ī′sō-dak′ti-lŭs). Relating to anisodactyly.

an·i·so·dac·ty·ly (an-ī′sō-dak′ti-lē). Unequal length in corresponding fingers. [aniso- + G. *daktylon,* finger]

an·i·sog·a·my (an′-i-sog′ă-mē). Fusion of two gametes unequal in size or form; fertilization as distinguished from isogamy or conjugation. [aniso- + G. *gamos,* marriage]

an·i·sog·na·thous (an-i-sog′nă-thŭs). Having jaws of unequal size, the upper being wider than the lower. [aniso- + G. *gnathos,* jaw]

an·i·so·kar·y·o·sis (an-ī′sō-kar-ē-ō′sis). Variation in size of nuclei, greater than the normal range for a tissue. [aniso- + G. *karyon,* nut (nucleus), + *-osis,* condition]

an·is·ole (an′i-sōl). Obtained from anisic acid; used in perfumery.

an·i·so·mas·tia (an-i-sō-mas′tē-ă). Breasts of unequal size. [aniso- + G. *mastos,* breast]

an·i·so·me·lia (an-i-sō-mē′lē-ă). A condition of inequality between two paired limbs. [aniso- + G. *melos,* limb]

an·i·so·me·tro·pia (an-ī′sō-me-trō′pē-ă). A difference in the refractive power of the two eyes. [aniso- + G. *metron,* measure, + *ōps,* sight]

an·i·so·me·tro·pic (an-ī′sō-me-trop′ik). **1.** Relating to anisometropia. **2.** Having eyes of unequal refractive power.

an·i·so·pi·e·sis (an-ī-sō-pī-ē′sis). Unequal arterial blood pressure on the two sides of the body. [aniso- + G. *piesis,* pressure]

an·i·sor·rhyth·mia (an-ī-sō-ridth′mē-ă). Irregular action of the heart, or absence of synchronism in the rate of atria and ventricles. [aniso- + G. *rhythmos,* rhythm]

an·i·so·sphyg·mia (an-ī-sō-sfig′mē-ă). Difference in volume, force, or time of the pulse in the corresponding arteries on two sides of the body, e.g., the two radials, or femorals. [aniso- + G. *sphygmos,* pulse]

an·i·sos·then·ic (an-ī-sos-then′ik). Of unequal strength; denoting two muscles or groups of muscles that are either paired or are antagonists. [aniso- + G. *sthenos,* strength]

an·i·so·ton·ic (an-ī-sō-ton′ik). Not having equal tension; having unequal osmotic pressure. [aniso- + G. *tonus,* tension]

an·i·so·tro·pic (an-ī-sō-trop′ik). Not having properties that are the same in all directions. [aniso- + G. *tropos,* a turning]

an·i·so·tro·pine meth·yl·bro·mide (an′i-sō-trō′pēn). An anticholinergic and intestinal antispasmodic.

Anitschkow, Nikolai, Russian pathologist, 1885–1964. SEE A. *cell, myocyte.*

an·kle (ang′kl). 1. SYN ankle *joint.* 2. The region of the a. joint. 3. SYN talus.

ankylo-. Bent, crooked, stiff, fused, fixed, closed. SEE ALSO ancylo-. [G. *ankylos,* bent, crooked; *ankylōsis,* stiffening of the joints, fr. *ankos,* a bend, a hollow]

an·ky·lo·bleph·a·ron (ang′ki-lō-blef′ă-ron). Congenital or acquired adhesion of the upper and lower eyelid by bands of tissue. SYN blepharocoloboma, filiform adnatum. [ankylo- + G. *blepharon,* eyelid]

an·ky·lo·dac·ty·ly, an·ky·lo·dac·tyl·ia (ang′ki-lō-dak′ti-lē, -dak-til′ē-ă). Adhesion between two or more fingers or toes. SEE ALSO syndactyly. [ankylo- + G. *daktylos,* finger]

an·ky·lo·glos·sia (ang′ki-lō-glos′ē-ă) [MIM 106280]. Partial or complete fusion of the tongue to the floor of the mouth; abnormal shortness of the frenulum linguae. SYN tongue-tie. [ankylo- + G. *glōssa,* tongue]

an·ky·lo·me·le (ang′ki-lō-mē′lē). A curved or bent probe. [ankylo- + G. *mēlē,* probe]

an·ky·losed (ang′ki-lōst). Stiffened; bound by adhesions; denoting a joint in a state of ankylosis.

an·ky·lo·sis (ang′ki-lō′sis). Stiffening or fixation of a joint as the result of a disease process, with fibrous or bony union across the joint. [G. *ankylōsis,* stiffening of a joint]

   artificial a., SYN arthrodesis.

   bony a., SYN synostosis.

   dental a., bony union of the radicular surface of a tooth to the surrounding alveolar bone in an area of previous partial root resorption.

   extracapsular a., stiffness of a joint due to induration or heterotopic ossification of the surrounding tissues. SYN spurious a.

   false a., SYN fibrous a.

   fibrous a., stiffening of a joint due to the presence of fibrous bands between and about the bones forming the joint. SYN false a., pseudankylosis.

   intracapsular a., stiffness of a joint due to the presence of bony or fibrous adhesions between the articular surfaces of the joint.

   spurious a., SYN extracapsular a.

   true a., SYN synostosis.

An·ky·los·to·ma (ang-ki-los′tō-mă). 1. SYN *Ancylostoma.* 2. SYN trismus. [ankylo- + G. *stoma,* mouth]

an·ky·lo·sto·mi·a·sis (ang′ki-lō-stō-mī′ă-sis). SYN ancylostomiasis.

an·ky·lot·ic (ang-ki-lot′ik). Characterized by or pertaining to ankylosis.

an·ky·rin (ang′ki-rin). An erythrocyte membranal protein that binds spectrin. A deficiency in ankyrin may lead to a type of hereditary spherocytosis. SYN anchorin, syndein. [G. *ankyra,* anchor, + -in]

an·ky·roid (an′ki-royd). SYN ancyroid.

an·la·ge, pl. **an·la·gen** (ahn′lah-ge, -gen). 1. SYN primordium. 2. In psychoanalysis, genetic predisposition to a given trait or personality characteristic. [Ger. plan, outline]

an·neal (an-nēl′). 1. To soften or temper a metal by controlled heating and cooling; the process makes a metal more easily adapted, bent, or swaged, and less brittle. 2. In dentistry, to heat gold leaf preparatory to its insertion into a cavity, in order to remove adsorbed gases and other contaminants. 3. The pairing of complementary single strands of DNA; or of DNA-RNA. 4. The attachment of the ends of two macromolecules; e.g., two microtubules annealing to form one longer microtubule. 5. In molecular biology, annealing is a process in which short sections of single-stranded DNA from one source are bound to a filter and incubated with single-stranded, radioactively conjugated DNA from a second source. Where the two sets of DNA possess complementa-

ry sequences of nucleotides, bonding occurs. The degree of relatedness (homology) of the two sets of DNA is then estimated according to the radioactivity level of the filter. This technique plays a central role in the classification of bacteria and viruses. SYN nucleic acid hybridization. [A.S. *anaelan,* to burn]

an·nec·tent (a-nek′tent). Connected with; joined. [L. *an-necto,* pres. p. *-nectere,* pp. *-nexus,* to join to]

An·nel·i·da (an′ně-lī′dă). A phylum that includes the segmented or true worms, such as the earthworm.

an·ne·lids (an′ně-lids). Common name for members of the phylum Annelida.

an·nel·ide (an′ě-līd). A conidiogenous cell that produces conidia in succession, each leaving a ringlike collar on the cell wall when released. [Fr. *annelide,* fr. L. *anellus,* a ring]

an·nel·lo·co·nid·i·um (an′ě-lō-kŏ-nid′ē-um). A conidium produced by an annellide.

an·nexa (a-nek′să). SYN accessory *structures,* under *structure.*

an·nex·al (a-neks-ăl). SYN adnexal.

an·nex·ins (a-nek′sinz). A family of at least 13 Ca²⁺-dependent phospholipid-binding proteins that may act as mediators of intracellular calcium signals.

an·not·to (ă-not′ō). Coloring matter extracted from the seeds of *Bixa orellana;* contains bixin and several other yellow to orange-red pigments; used for coloring butter, margarine, cheese, and oils.

an·nu·lar (an′ū-lăr). SYN anular. [L. *anulus,* ring]

an·nu·lo·plasty (an′ū-lō-plas-tē). Reconstruction of the ring (or annulus) of a cardiac valve. [L. *anulus,* ring, + G. *plastos,* formed]

an·nu·lor·rha·phy (an-ū-lōr′ă-fē). Closure of a hernial ring by suture. [L. *anulus,* ring, + G. *rhaphē,* seam]

an·nu·lus (an′ū-lŭs). SYN ring.

AnOC Abbreviation for anodal opening *contraction.*

an·o·chro·ma·sia (an′ō-krō-mā′zē-ă). 1. Failure of cells or other elements of tissue to be colored in the usual manner when treated with a stain (or stains). 2. Accumulation of hemoglobin in the peripheral zone of erythrocytes, thereby resulting in a pale, virtually colorless central portion. [G. *anō,* upward, + *chrōma,* color]

ano·ci·as·so·ci·a·tion (ă-nō′sē-ă-sō-sē-ā′shŭn). Theory that afferent stimuli, especially pain, contribute to the development of surgical shock, and, as a corollary, that conduction anesthesia at the surgical field and presurgical sedation protect against shock. [G. *a-* priv. + L. *noceo,* to injure, + association]

ano·coc·cyg·e·al (a-nō-kok-sij′ē-ăl). Relating to both anus and coccyx.

anod·al (an-ōd′ăl). Of, pertaining to, or emanating from an anode. SYN anodic.

an·ode (an′ōd). 1. The positive pole of a galvanic battery or the electrode connected with it; an electrode toward which negatively charged ions (anions) migrate; a positively charged electrode. Cf. cathode. 2. The portion, usually made of tungsten, of an x-ray tube from which x-rays are released by bombardment by cathode rays (electrons). SYN positive electrode. [G. *anodos,* a way up, fr. *ana,* up, + *hodos,* a way]

   rotating a., in diagnostic radiography, a mushroom-shaped anode in modern x-ray tubes that rotates rapidly to avoid local heat buildup from electron impact during x-ray generation.

an·o·derm (ā′nō-derm). Lining of the anal canal immediately inferior to the dentate line and extending for about 1.5 cm to the anal verge; it is devoid of hair and sebaceous and sweat glands, and so is not true skin, although it is squamous epithelium; it is pale, smooth, thin, and delicate, and shiny when stretched; it is especially vulnerable to abrasion (as from rough toilet paper), chemical irritants (soaps), and is well provided with tactile and nociceptive (pain, itch) endings innervated by the inferior rectal (pudendal) nerve.

an·od·ic (an-ōd′ik). SYN anodal.

an·o·don·tia (an-ō-don′shē-ă). Congenital absence of the teeth; developmental, not due to extraction or impaction. SYN agomphious, agomphosis, agomphiasis. [G. *an-* priv. + *odous,* tooth]

   partial a., SYN hypodontia.

an·o·dont·ism (an-ō-dont'izm). Congenital absence of tooth germ development.

an·o·dyne (an'ō-dīn). A compound less potent than an anesthetic or a narcotic but capable of relieving pain. [G. *an-* priv. + *odynē,* pain]

an·o·et·ic (an-ō-et'ik). Lacking the power of comprehension, as in severe and profound levels of mental retardation. [G. *anoēsia,* from *a-* priv. + *noos,* perception]

ano·gen·i·tal (ā'nō-jen'ĭ-tăl). Relating in any way to both the anal and the genital regions.

anom·a·lad (ă-nom'ă-lad). A malformation together with its subsequently derived structural changes. [see anomaly]

anom·a·lo·scope (ă-nom'ă-lō-skōp). An instrument used to diagnose abnormalities of color perception in which one-half of a field of color is matched by mixing two other colors. [G. *anōmalos,* irregular, + *skopeō,* to examine]

anom·a·ly (ă-nom'ă-lē). Deviation from the average or norm; anything that is structurally unusual or irregular or contrary to a general rule. Congenital defects are an example of the definition of anomaly. [G. *anōmalia,* irregularity]
Alder a., coarse azurophilic granulation of leukocytes, especially granulocytes, which may be associated with gargoylism and Morquio *syndrome.*
Aristotle a., when a small object is held between the first and second fingers crossed in such a way that it touches or presses upon skin surfaces that ordinarily are not pressed upon simultaneously by a single object, it is perceived falsely as two.
Chédiak-Steinbrinck-Higashi a., SYN Chédiak-Higashi *syndrome.*
developmental a., an a. established during intrauterine life; a congenital a.
Ebstein a., congenital downward displacement of the tricuspid valve into the right ventricle. SYN Ebstein disease.
eugnathic a., SYN eugnathia.
Freund a., a narrowing of the upper aperture of the thorax by shortening of the first rib and its cartilage; formerly believed to predispose to tuberculosis because of defective expansion of the lung apex.
Hegglin a., a disorder in which neutrophils and eosinophils contain basophilic structures known as Döhle or Amato bodies and in which there is faulty maturation of platelets, with thrombocytopenia; autosomal dominant inheritance. SYN May-Hegglin a.
May-Hegglin a., SYN Hegglin a.
morning glory a., congenital a. of the optic disk in which the nerve head is funnel-shaped, with a dot of white tissue at the end of the excavation, and is surrounded by an elevated pigmented annulus; the retinal vessels seen are multiple narrow bands at the edge of the disk.
Pelger-Huët nuclear a. [MIM*169400], congenital inhibition of lobulation in the nuclei of neutrophilic leukocytes; most cells present band or bilobulate appearance, and only an occasional cell is trilobed; it is not associated with disease, but may be confused with leukocyte "shift to left"; autosomal dominant inheritance.
Peters a., SYN anterior chamber cleavage *syndrome.*
Rieger a., iridocorneal mesochymal dysgenesis.
Shone a., coarctation of the aorta, subaortic stenosis, and stenosing ring of the left atrium found in association with a parachute mitral valve.
Uhl a., right ventricular myocardial aplasia, causing a dilated, thin-walled right ventricle without murmurs; death results in early childhood. SYN parchment right ventricle.
urogenital sinus a., SYN hypospadias.

an·o·mer (an'ō-mer). One of two sugar molecules that are epimeric at the hemiacetal or hemiketal carbon atom (carbon-1 in aldoses, carbon-2 in most ketoses); e.g., α-D-glucose and β-D-glucose. SEE ALSO sugars. Cf. epimer.

ano·mia (ă-nō'mē-ă). SYN nominal *aphasia.* [G. *a-* priv. + *ōnoma,* name]

an·o·mie (an'ō-mē). **1.** Lawlessness; absence or weakening of social norms or values, with corresponding erosion of social cohesion. **2.** In psychiatry, absence or weakening of individual norms or values; characterized by anxiety, isolation, and personal disorientation. [Fr., fr. G. *anomia,* lawlessness]

an·o·nych·ia, an·o·ny·cho·sis (an-ō-nik'ē-ă, an-ō-nī-kō'sis). Absence of the nails. [G. *an-* priv. + *onyx* (*onych-*), nail]

anon·y·ma (ă-non'i-mă). SYN innominate. [G. *an-* priv. + *onyma,* name]

Anoph·e·les (ă-nof'ĕ-lēz). A genus of mosquitoes (family Culicidae, subfamily Anophelinae). The sporogenous cycle of the malarial parasite is passed in the body cavity of female mosquitoes of certain species of this genus; a few selected vectors (from among over 90 species) are listed below. [G. *anōphelēs,* useless, harmful, fr. *an-* priv. + *ōpheleō,* to be of use]
A. aconitus, mosquito species that is a vector of malaria in Indonesia, Thailand, and Cambodia.
A. albima'nus, a species having white hind feet, a common carrier of the malaria parasite in the West Indies and Central America.
A. albitar'sus, a South American species that transmits malaria.
A. annularis, mosquito species that is an incidental vector of malaria in India.
A. annulipes, mosquito species that is a vector of malaria in Australia.
A. aquasalis, mosquito species that is a vector of malaria in the lesser Antilles, Trinidad, and Brazil.
A. arabiensis, mosquito species that is a principal vector of malaria in arid or montane areas across sub-Saharan Africa to Kenya and the Sudan.
A. aztecus, mosquito species that is a vector of malaria at higher elevations in Mexico.
A. balabacen'sis, a vector species in Southeast Asia, Burma, and India.
A. barbirostris, mosquito species that is a vector of malaria in Indonesia and the Malay Peninsula.
A. bellator, mosquito species that is a vector of malaria in Trinidad and Brazil.
A. brunnipes, mosquito species that is an incidental vector of malaria throughout tropical Africa.
A. campestris, mosquito species that is a vector of malaria in Malaysia.
A. crucians, mosquito species that is a secondary or suspected vector of malaria, Venezuelan equine encephalitis, and Eastern equine encephalitis within the United States.
A. cruzi, mosquito species that is a vector of malaria in Brazil.
A. culicifa'cies, mosquito species that is a common malaria vector in India and Sri Lanka, China, and elsewhere in the Orient.
A. darling'i, a South American species, an important carrier of the malarial parasite.
A. flavirostris, mosquito species that is an important vector of malaria in the Philippines, Java, and northern Celebes.
A. fluviatil'is, a species that is an important vector in India and Pakistan.
A. freebor'ni, mosquito species that is a vector in the western U.S. (although endemic cases are no longer present).
A. funes'tus, an important African mosquito species that transmits malaria.
A. gam'biae, an African mosquito species that is a most important vector of malaria.
A. jeyporien'sis, mosquito species that is a vector of malaria in south China.
A. karwa'ri, mosquito species that is a vector of malaria in New Guinea.
A. kwei'yangen'sis, mosquito species that is an important vector of malaria in Szechuan province in China.
A. labranch'iae, mosquito species that is an important vector of malaria wherever found in the Palearctic region.
A. les'teri, mosquito species that is an important vector of malaria in the lower Yangtze Valley in China.
A. leucosphy'rus, mosquito species that is an important vector of malaria in Borneo.
A. macula'tus, mosquito species that is a vector in Malaysia and Indonesia.
A. maculipen'nis, the type species of this genus; its wings are

marked by spots formed of collections of scales; one of the most widely spread species active in the dissemination of malaria (formerly an important vector in continental Europe).

A. mes'seae, mosquito species that is a vector of malaria in parts of Hungary and eastern Romania.

A. min'imus, mosquito species that is an important vector of malaria wherever found throughout the Orient.

A. pseudopunctipen'nis, a South American vector mosquito species.

A. quadrimacula'tus, mosquito species that was formerly an important carrier of malaria in the southern United States.

A. stephen'si, a widespread mosquito species that is an important vector of malaria in Asia.

A. sundai'cus, mosquito species that is an important vector in the Orient and Southeast Asia.

A. superpic'tus, mosquito species that is an important vector in the Mediterranean region, Middle East, and southern Asia.

anoph·e·li·cide (ă-nof'ĕ-li-sīd). An agent that destroys the *Anopheles* mosquito.

anoph·e·li·fuge (ă-nof'ĕ-li-fooj). An agent that drives away or prevents the bite of *Anopheles* mosquitoes.

Anoph·e·li·nae (an-of-ĕ-lī'nē). A subfamily of the mosquitoes (Culicidae) consisting of several genera, including *Anopheles.*

anoph·e·line (ă-nof'ĕ-līn). Referring to the *Anopheles* mosquito.

Anophe·li·ni (ă-nof-ĕ-lī-nī). The tribe of mosquitoes (family Culicidae) that includes the genus *Anopheles.* [G. *anôphelēs,* useless, troublesome]

anoph·e·lism (ă-nof'ĕ-lizm). The habitual presence in any region of *Anopheles* mosquitoes.

an·oph·thal·mia (an-of-thal'mē-ă). Congenital absence of all tissues of the eyes. SYN anophthalmos. [G. *an-* priv. + *ophthalmos,* eye]

anophthalmos. SYN anophthalmia.

ano·plas·ty (ā'nō-plas-tē). Reconstruction of the anus often using advancement flaps. [L. *anus* + G. *plastos,* formed]

An·op·lo·ceph·a·la (an-op'lō-sef'ă-lă). A genus of large tapeworms (family Anoplocephalidae) with strong linear segmentation, numerous scattered testes, and eggs with a pyriform apparatus; they are parasitic in herbivores, with terrestrial mites serving as intermediate hosts. [G. *anoplos,* unarmed, + *kephalē,* head]

A. perfolia'ta, a cosmopolitan species of the horse, donkey, mule, and zebra; cysticercoid larvae are found in arthropods. SYN *Taenia equina, Taenia quadrilobata.*

An·o·plu·ra (an-ō-ploo'ră). The order of insects that includes the bloodsucking lice of mammals, with some 450 species arranged in 6 families, of which 4 contain species of medical or veterinary importance: *Haematopinus, Linognathus,* and *Solenopotes* of domestic mammals, and the human sucking lice *Pediculus humanus.* [G. *anoplos,* unarmed, + *oura,* tail]

an·or·chia (an-ōr'kē-ă). SYN anorchism.

an·or·chism (an-ōr'kizm). Absence of the testes; may be congenital or acquired. SYN anorchia. [G. *an-* priv. + *orchis,* testicle]

ano·rec·tal (ā'nō-rek'tăl). Relating to both anus and rectum.

an·o·rec·tic, an·o·ret·ic (an-ō-rek'tic, -ret'ik). **1.** Relating to, characteristic of, or suffering from anorexia, especially anorexia nervosa. **2.** An agent that causes anorexia. SYN anorexic.

an·o·rex·ia (an-ō-rek'sē-ă). Diminished appetite; aversion to food. [G. fr. *an-* priv. + *orexis,* appetite]

a. nervo'sa, a mental disorder manifested by extreme fear of becoming obese and an aversion to food, usually occurring in young women and often resulting in life-threatening weight loss, accompanied by a disturbance in body image, hyperactivity, and amenorrhea.

an·o·rex·i·ant (an-ō-rek'sē-ănt). A drug ("diet pills"), process, or event that leads to anorexia.

an·o·rex·ic (an-ō-rek'sik). SYN anorectic.

an·o·rex·i·gen·ic (an'ō-rek-si-jen'ik). Promoting or causing anorexia.

an·or·gas·my, an·or·gas·mia (an-ōr-gaz'mē, -gaz'mē-ă). Failure to experience an orgasm; may be biogenic (secondary to a physical disorder or medication), psychogenic (secondary to psychological or situational factors), or a combination of the two. [G. *an-* priv. + orgasm + *-ia*]

ano·scope (ā'nō-skōp). A short speculum for examining the anal canal and lower rectum.

Bacon a., an instrument resembling a rectal speculum, with a long slit on one side and an light source opposite.

ano·sig·moid·os·co·py (ā'nō-sig-moy-dos'-kŏ-pē). Endoscopy of the anus, rectum and sigmoid colon.

an·os·mia (an-oz'mē-ă). Loss or absense of the sense of smell. It may be: 1, general to all odorants (total), partial to some odorants, or specific to one or more odorants; 2, due to transport disorders (in nasal obstruction) or sensorineural disorders (affecting the olfactory neuroepithelium or the central olfactory neural pathways); or 3, hereditary or acquired. [G. *an-* priv. + *osmē,* sense of smell]

an·os·mic (an-oz'mik). Relating to anosmia.

ano·so·di·a·pho·ria (ă-nō'sō-dī-ă-fōr'ē-ă). Indifference, real or assumed, regarding the presence of disease, specifically of paralysis. [G. *a-* priv. + *nosos,* disease, + *diaphora,* difference]

ano·sog·no·sia (ă-nō'sog-nō'sē-ă). Ignorance of the presence of disease, specifically of paralysis. Most often seen in patients with non-dominant parietal lobe lesions, who deny their hemiparesis. [G. *a-* priv. + *nosos,* disease, + *gnōsis,* knowledge]

ano·sog·no·sic (ă-nō-sog-nō'sik). Relating to anosognosia.

ano·spi·nal (ā'nō-spī'năl). Relating to the anus and the spinal cord.

an·os·te·o·pla·sia (an-os'tē-ō-plā'zē-ă). Failure of bone formation. [G. *an-* priv. + *osteon,* bone, + *plassō,* to form]

an·os·to·sis (an-os-tō'sis). Failure of ossification. [G. *an-* priv. + *osteon,* bone]

an·o·tia (an-ō'shē-ă). Congenital absence of one or both auricles of the ears. [G. *an-* priv. + *ous,* ear]

ANOVA Acronym for *analysis* of variance.

ano·ves·i·cal (ā'nō-ves'i-kăl). Relating in any way to both anus and urinary bladder.

an·ov·u·lar (an-ov'ū-lăr). SYN anovulatory.

an·ov·u·la·tion (an-ov-ū-lā'shŭn). Suspension or cessation of ovulation.

an·ov·u·la·to·ry (an-ov'ū-lă-tōr-ē). Absence of the development of a mature graafian follicle and/or the discharge of the ovum during a menstrual cycle. SYN anovular.

an·ox·e·mia (an-ok-sē'mē-ă). Absence of oxygen in arterial blood; formerly often used to include moderate decrease in oxygen now properly distinguished as hypoxemia. [G. *an-* priv. + oxygen + G. *haima,* blood]

an·ox·ia (an-ok'sē-ă). Absence or almost complete absence of oxygen from inspired gases, arterial blood, or tissues; to be differentiated from hypoxia. [G. *an-* priv. + oxygen]

anemic a., a term formerly considered synonymous with anemic hypoxia, but now reserved for extremely severe cases in which oxygen and functional erythrocyte volume are almost completely lacking.

anoxic a., a term formerly considered synonymous with hypoxic hypoxia, but now reserved for extremely severe cases in which oxygen is almost completely lacking.

diffusion a., diffusion hypoxia severe enough to result in the absence of oxygen in alveolar gas.

histotoxic a., poisoning of the respiratory enzyme systems of the tissues, as in the inhibition of cytochrome oxidase by cyanides; owing to the inability of tissue cells to utilize oxygen, its tension in arterial and capillary blood is usually greater than normal.

a. neonator'um, any a. observed in newborn infants.

oxygen affinity a., a. due to inability of hemoglobin to release oxygen.

stagnant a., stagnant hypoxia severe enough to result in the absence of oxygen in tissues.

an·ox·ic (an-ok'sik). Denoting or characteristic of anoxia.

ANP Abbreviation for atrial natriuretic *peptide.*

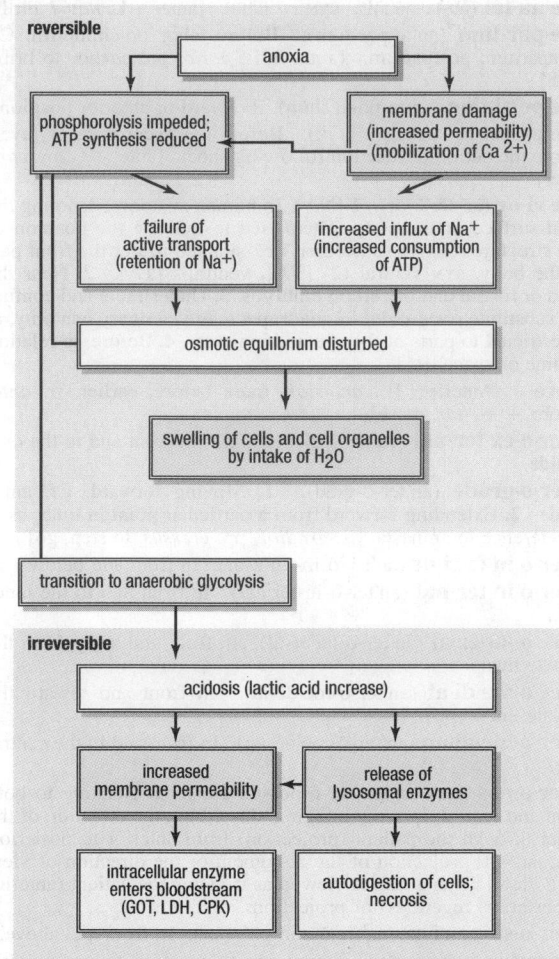

anoxia: pathogenesis of anoxic cell destruction; ATP, adenosine 5'-triphosphate; GOT, glutamic-oxaloacetic transaminase; LDH, lactate dehydrogenase; CPK, creatine phosphokinase

Anrep, G.V., 20th century Lebanese physiologist in Britain. SEE A. *phenomenon*.

ANS Abbreviation for anterior nasal *spine*; autonomic nervous *system*.

an·sa, gen. and pl. **an·sae** (an'să, -sē) [TA]. Any anatomical structure in the form of a loop or an arc. SEE ALSO loop. [L. loop, handle]

a. cervica'lis [TA], a loop in the cervical plexus consisting of fibers from the first three cervical nerves. Fibers from a loop between the C1 and C2 spinal nerves accompany the hypoglossal nerve for a short distance, leaving it as the superior root of the a. cervicalis. Fibers from a loop between the C2 and C3 spinal nerves form the inferior root of the a. cervicalis. Most commonly, the roots merge, forming the a. cervicalis, which gives rise to branches innervating infrahyoid muscles. SYN cervical loop, loop of hypoglossal nerve.

Haller a., SYN communicating *branch* of facial nerve with glossopharyngeal nerve.

Henle a., SYN nephronic *loop*.

a. hypoglos'si, obsolete term for a. cervicalis.

lenticular a., SYN lenticular *loop*.

a. lenticula'ris [TA], SYN lenticular *loop*.

ansae nervo'rum spina'lium, SYN *loops* of spinal nerves, under *loop*.

peduncular a., SYN a. peduncularis.

a. peduncula'ris [TA], a complex fiber bundle curving around the medial edge of the internal capsule and connecting the anterior part of the temporal lobe (temporal cortex), amygdala, and olfactory cortex with the mediodorsal nucleus of the thalamus; it enters the thalamus as a component of the inferior thalamic peduncle which also contains a major part of the fibers connecting the mediodorsal nucleus to the orbitofrontal cortex. SYN peduncular a., peduncular loop, Reil a.

Reil a., SYN a. peduncularis.

a. sacra'lis, a nerve cord connecting one or both of the sympathetic nerve trunks with the ganglion impar.

a. subcla'via [TA], a nerve cord connecting the middle cervical and inferior cervical or stellate sympathetic ganglia, forming a loop around the subclavian artery. SYN subclavian loop, Vieussens a., Vieussens loop.

Vieussens a., SYN a. subclavia.

an·sate (an'sāt). SYN ansiform.

an·ser·ine. 1 (an'ser-īn). Resembling or characteristic of a goose. SEE *cutis* anserina, *pes* anserinus. 2 (an'ser-ēn). N^a-(β-Alanyl)-π-methyl-L-histidine; present in muscle and brain. SYN N-methylcarnosine. [L. *anserinus,* fr. *anser,* goose]

ANSI Abbreviation for American National Standards Institute.

an·si·form (an'si-fōrm). In the shape of a loop or arc. SYN ansate. [L. *ansa,* handle, + *forma,* shape]

an·sot·o·my (an-sot'ō-mē). 1. Surgical division of a loop, usually a constricting loop. 2. Section of the ansa lenticularis for treatment of striatal syndromes. [L. *ansa,* handle + G. *tomē,* cutting]

△**ant-.** SEE anti-.

ant. One of the most numerous insects (order Hymenoptera), characterized by an extraordinary development of colonial dwelling and caste specialization.

black imported fire a., SYN *Solenopsis richteri.*

fire a., any of several species in the genus *Solenopsis* whose bite causes a fiery, burning sensation and sometimes severe allergic reactions. SEE ALSO solenopsin A.

harvester a., SYN *Pogonomyrmex.*

red imported fire a., SYN *Solenopsis invicta.*

velvet a., a wingless mutilid wasp (family Mutilidae, order Hymenoptera) known for its venomous sting.

ant·ac·id (ant-as'id). 1. Neutralizing an acid. 2. Any agent that reduces or neutralizes acidity, as of the gastric juice or any other secretion (e.g., calcium carbonate, magnesium hydroxide). SYN antiacid.

an·tag·o·nism (an-tag'on-izm). 1. Denoting mutual opposition in action between structures, agents, diseases, or physiologic processes. Cf. synergism. 2. The situation in which the combined effect of two or more factors is smaller than the solitary effect of any one of the factors. SYN mutual resistance. [G. *antagōnisma,* from *anti,* against, + *agōnizomai,* to fight, fr. *agōn,* a contest]

bacterial a., the inhibition of one bacterium by another.

an·tag·o·nist (an-tag'ŏ-nist). Something opposing or resisting the action of another; certain structures, agents, diseases, or physiologic processes that tend to neutralize or impede the action or effect of others. Cf. synergist.

α-adrenoceptor a., SYN α-adrenergic blocking *agent*.

β-adrenoreceptor a., SYN β-adrenergic blocking *agent*.

aldosterone a., an agent that opposes the action of the adrenal hormone aldosterone on renal tubular mineralocorticoid retention; these agents, e.g., spironolactone, are useful in treating the hypertension of primary hyperaldosteronism, or the sodium retention of secondary hyperaldosteronism.

associated a., one of two muscles or groups of muscles which pull in nearly opposite directions, but which, when acting together, move the part in a path between their diverging lines of action.

calcium a., SYN calcium channel-blocking *agent*.

competitive a., an antimetabolite.

enzyme a., an antimetabolite or inhibitor of enzyme action.

folic acid a.'s, modified pterins, such as aminopterin and methotrexate, that interfere with the action of folic acid and thus produce the symptoms of folic acid deficiency; have been used in cancer chemotherapy and inflammatory disorders.

5-hydroxy tryptamine a.'s, agents that block serotonin receptors and hence interfere with the biological actions of serotonin (5-HT).

insulin a., substances in the β- and γ-globulin or β₁-lipoprotein fractions of serum that may induce a functional insulin deficiency; may include nonprecipitating antibodies against nonhuman insulin.

leukotriene receptor a., a class of agents, of which zileuton, montelukast, zafirlukast are the best known, used in the prophylactic and chronic treatment of asthma in older children and adults; these drugs are not bronchodilators in themselves, but act by interfering with the leukotriene-mediated inflammatory process present in asthma.

muscarinic a., drugs that bind with muscarinic cholinergic receptors but do not activate them, thus preventing access to acetylcholine; examples include atropine, scopolamine, propantheline, and pirenzepine.

opioid a.'s, agents such as naloxone and naltrexone that have high affinity for opiate receptors but do not activate these receptors. These drugs block the effects of exogenously administered opioids such as morphine, heroin, meperidine, and methadone, or of endogenously released endorphins and enkephalins.

ant·al·ge·sia (ant-al-jē′zē-ă). Rarely used term for lowering of a previous elevation in pain threshold. [anti- + G. *algēsis,* sense of pain]

ant·al·gic (ant-al′jik). SYN analgesic (2).

ant·al·ka·line (ant-al′kă-līn). Reducing or neutralizing alkalinity.

ant·aph·ro·di·si·ac (ant′af-rō-diz′ē-ak). SYN anaphrodisiac.

ant·aph·ro·dit·ic (ant′af-rō-dit′ik). **1.** SYN anaphrodisiac. **2.** SYN antivenereal.

ant·ar·thrit·ic (ant′ar-thrit′ik). Rarely used term for: SYN antiarthritic.

ant·as·then·ic (ant-as-then′ik). **1.** Strengthening or invigorating. **2.** An agent possessing such qualities. [anti- + G. *astheneia,* weakness]

ant·asth·mat·ic (ant-az-mat′ik). SYN antiasthmatic.

ant·a·tro·phic (ant-ă-trof′ik). **1.** Preventing or curing atrophy. **2.** An agent that promotes the restoration of atrophied structures.

an·taz·o·line hy·dro·chlo·ride (an-taz′ŏ-lēn). A histamine-antagonizing agent used in treating allergy; also available as a. h. phosphate. SYN phenazoline hydrochloride.

△**ante-.** Before, in front of (in time or place or order). SEE ALSO pre-, pro- (1). [L. *ante,* before, in front of]

an·te·brach·i·al (an′te-brā′kē-ăl). Relating to the forearm.

an·te·bra·chi·um (an-te-brā′kē-ŭm) [TA]. SYN forearm. [ante- + L. *brachium,* arm]

an·te·car·di·um (an-te-kar′dē-ŭm). SYN precordia.

an·te·ced·ent (an-te-sē′dent). A precursor. [L. *antecedo,* to go before]

plasma thromboplastin a. (PTA), SYN *factor* XI.

an·te ci·bum (an′tē sī′bŭm). Before a meal. The plural is ante cibos, before meals. [L.]

an·te·cu·bi·tal (an-te-kū′bi-tăl). In front of the elbow. [ante- + L. *cubitum,* elbow]

an·te·fe·brile (an-te-feb′ril). Rarely used term for antepyretic. [ante- + L. *febris,* fever]

an·te·flex (an′te-fleks). To bend anteriorly (forward) or cause to bend anteriorly. [ante- + L. *flecto,* pp. *flexus,* to bend]

an·te·flex·ion (an-te-flek′shŭn). A bending forward; a sharp forward curve or angulation; denoting especially the normal forward bend in the uterus at the junction of corpus and cervix uteri.

a. of iris, rarely used term for an iris that is, in part, folded forward after a severe iridodialysis so that the pigmented layer faces forward.

an·te·grade (an′tĕ-grād). In the direction of normal movement, as in blood flow or peristalsis. [ante- + L. *gradior,* to walk]

an·te·mor·tem (an′te-mōr-tem). Before death. Cf. postmortem. [ante- + L. *mors* (*mort-*), death]

an·te·na·tal (an-te-nā′tăl). SYN prenatal. [ante- + L. *natus,* birth]

an·te·par·tum (an′te-par-tŭm). Before labor or childbirth. Cf. intrapartum, postpartum. [ante- + L. *pario,* pp. *partus,* to bring forth]

an·te·po·si·tion (an′te-pō-si′shŭn). Forward or anterior position.

an·te·py·ret·ic (an′te-pī-ret′ik). Before the occurrence of fever; before the period of reaction following shock. [ante- + G. *pyretos,* fever]

▣**an·te·ri·or** (an-tēr′ē-ōr). **1** [NA]. In human anatomy, denoting the front surface of the body; often used to indicate the position of one structure relative to another, i.e., situated nearer the front part of the body. SYN ventral (2) [TA], ventralis [TA]. **2.** Near the head or rostral end of certain embryos. **3.** Undesirable and confusing substitute for *cranial* in quadrupeds. In veterinary anatomy, a. is restricted to parts of the eye and inner ear. **4.** Before, in relation to time or space. [L.]

△**antero-.** Anterior. [L. *anterior,* more before, earlier, fr. *ante,* before, + -r- *-ior,* more]

an·ter·o·ex·ter·nal (an′ter-ō-eks-ter′năl). In front and to the outer side.

an·ter·o·grade (an′ter-ō-grād). **1.** Moving forward. Cf. antegrade. **2.** Extending forward from a particular point in time; used in reference to amnesia. [L. *gradior,* pp. *gressus,* to step, go]

an·ter·o·in·fe·ri·or (an′ter-ō-in-fēr′ē-ōr). In front and below.

an·ter·o·in·ter·nal (an′ter-ō-in-ter′năl). In front and to the inner side.

an·ter·o·lat·er·al (an′ter-ō-lat′er-ăl). In front and away from the middle line.

an·ter·o·me·di·al (an′ter-ō-mē′dē-ăl). In front and toward the middle line.

an·ter·o·me·di·an (an′ter-ō-mē′dē-an). In front and in the central line.

an·ter·o·pos·te·ri·or (an′ter-ō-pos-tēr-ē-er). **1.** Relating to both front and rear. **2.** In x-ray imaging, describing the direction of the beam through the patient (projection) from anterior to posterior, e.g., an A-P projection of the abdomen; or the direction of view (A-P view) when a film is viewed as if facing the patient (anterior to posterior) regardless of projection.

an·ter·o·su·pe·ri·or (an′ter-ō-soo-pē′rē-er). In front and above.

ant·e·rot·ic (ant-er-ot′ik). Pertaining to an effort to avoid erotic feelings. [anti- + G. *erōtikos,* pertaining to love]

an·te·sys·to·le (an-te-sis′tō-lē). Premature activation of the ventricle responsible for the pre-excitation syndrome of the Wolff-Parkinson-White or Lown-Ganong-Levine types.

an·te·ver·sion (an-te-ver′shŭn). Turning forward, inclining forward as a whole without bending. [ante- + Mediev. L. *versio,* a turning]

an·te·vert·ed (an-te-vert′ed). Tilted forward; in a position of anteversion.

ant·hel·ix (ant′hē-liks, an′thē-liks). SYN antihelix. [anti- + G. *helix,* coil]

ant·hel·min·thic (ant-hel-min′thik). SYN anthelmintic (1).

ant·hel·min·tic (ant-hel-min′tik, an-thel-). **1.** An agent that destroys or expels intestinal worms. SYN anthelminthic, antihelminthic, helminthagogue, helminthic (2), helmintic (2), vermifuge. **2.** Having the power to destroy or expel intestinal worms. SYN vermifugal. [anti- + G. *helmins,* worm]

an·the·lone (an′thĕ-lōn). SYN urogastrone.

a. E, SYN enterogastrone.

a. U, SYN urogastrone.

an·ther·id·i·um (an′ther-id′e-um). The male gametangium produced in the teleomorph part of the life cycle of fungi. [Mod. L. *anthera,* flower, fr. G *antheros,* blooming, fr. *antheo,* to bloom, + dim. suffix *-idium,* fr. G. *-idion*]

an·thi·o·li·mine (an-thī-ō′li-mēn). Used in the treatment of filariasis and schistosomiasis.

an·tho·cy·a·nins (an-thō-sī′ă-ninz). A group of floral pigments, existing as glycosides in combination with glucose or cellobiose molecules, that range from red to blue and are often pH dependent; soluble in water and alcohol but not in ether. A. are

an

divided into derivatives of pelargonidin, cyanidins, and delphinidins. Some have been used as hematoxylin substitutes. [G. *anthos,* flower, + *kyanos,* a blue substance]

An·tho·my·ia (an-thō-mī′yă). A genus of muscoid flies similar in appearance to the common housefly. [G. *anthos,* flower, + *myia,* fly]

A. canicula′ris, a small black horsefly, the larvae of which have been reported as accidental parasites in the intestine of humans, being hatched there from the ingested eggs; symptoms of gastroenteric irritation may be caused by it; adults may transport eggs of the tropical warble fly or botfly to humans, *Dermatobia hominis,* a cause of myiasis.

an·thra·ce·mia (an-thră-sē′mē-ă). The presence of *Bacillus anthracis* in the circulating blood, usually resulting from previously developed anthrax of the skin or lungs. SYN anthrax septicemia.

an·thra·cene (an′thră-sēn). **1.** A hydrocarbon obtained from coal tar; it oxidizes to anthraquinone, which is converted to alizarin dyes. SYN anthracin. **2.** A compound containing a. (1) as a part of its structure. [G. *anthrax,* coal]

an·thrac·ic (an-thras′ik). Relating to anthrax.

an·thra·cin (an′thră-sin). SYN anthracene (1).

⟁**anthraco-** (an′thră-kō-). Coal; carbon; carbuncle; corresponds to L. carb-, carbo-. [G. *anthrax, anthrakos,* charcoal, a live coal; a carbuncle, a pustule]

an·thra·co·sil·i·co·sis (an′thră-kō-sil′i-kō′sis). Pneumoconiosis from accumulation of carbon and silica in the lungs from inhaled coal dust; the silica content produces fibrous nodules. SYN coal worker's pneumoconiosis. [anthraco- + silicosis]

an·thra·co·sis (an-thră-kō′sis). Pneumoconiosis from accumulation of carbon from inhaled smoke or coal dust in the lungs. SEE ALSO pneumomelanosis. SYN collier lung, miner's lung (1). [anthraco- + G. *-osis,* condition]

an·thra·cot·ic (an-thră-kot′ik). Characterized by anthracosis.

anthracycline (an-thra-sīk′lin, -lēn). Anticancer agent consisting of 3 moieties: a pigmented aglycone, an amino sugar, and a lateral chain. Examples are doxorubicin, daunorubicin, and daunomycin.

an·thra·lin (an′thră-lin). Used as a substitute for chrysarobin in ointment for treatment of psoriasis and ringworm infestation. SYN dithranol.

an·thra·mu·cin (an-thră-mū′sin). A neutralizing material from the capsule of *Bacillus anthracis* that neutralizes serum and tissue antimicrobial action.

an·thra·nil·ic ac·id (an-thră-nil′ik). One of the products of tryptophan catabolism. SYN *o*-aminobenzoic acid.

an·thra·nil·o·yl (an-thră-nil′ō-il). The acyl radical of anthranilic acid.

an·thra·pur·pu·rin (an′thră-poor′poo-rin). $C_{14}H_8O_5$; 1,2,7-Trihydroxyanthraquinone; a purple dye used in histology as a reagent for calcium, although the specificity has been questioned.

9,10-an·thra·qui·none (an′thrǎ-kwi′nōn). **1.** The basis of natural cathartic principles in plants; used as a reagent. **2.** A compound containing 9,10-anthraquinone (1) as a part of its structure; this class of compound comprises the largest group of naturally occurring quinones.

an·thrax (an′thraks). **1.** A disease in humans caused by infection by cutaneous anthrax (q.v.) followed by septicemia with the bacterium *Bacillus anthracis* from infected animals through skin; marked by hemorrhage and serous effusions in various organs and body cavities and by symptoms of extreme prostration. Rarely, infection is airborne, causing rapidly fatal pneumonia. This is the most severe form. **2.** An infectious disease of animals, especially herbivores, due to presence in the blood of *Bacillus anthracis.* SYN charbon. [G. *anthrax (anthrak-),* charcoal, coal, a carbuncle]

cerebral a., a form of a., associated with pulmonary or intestinal a., in which the specific bacilli invade the capillaries of the brain causing violent delirium; frequently associated with hemorrhagic meningitis.

cutaneous a., the skin of *B. anthracis* infection characteristic lesion that begins as a papule and soon becomes a vesicle and breaks, discharging a bloody serum; the seat of this vesicle, in about 36 hours, becomes a bluish black necrotic mass; constitu-

tional symptoms of septicemia are severe: high fever, vomiting, profuse sweating, and extreme prostration; the infection is often fatal. SYN malignant pustule.

intestinal a., a usually fatal form of a. marked by chill, high fever, pain in the head, back, and extremities, vomiting, bloody diarrhea, cardiovascular collapse, and frequently hemorrhages from the mucous membranes and in the skin (petechiae). SEE ALSO *mycosis* intestinalis.

pulmonary a., a form of a. acquired by inhalation of dust containing *Bacillus anthracis;* there is an initial chill followed by pain in the back and legs, rapid respiration, dyspnea, cough, fever, rapid pulse, and extreme cardiovascular collapse. SYN ragpicker's disease, ragsorter's disease, woolsorter's disease, woolsorter's pneumonia.

an·throne (an′thrōn). 9,10-Dihydro-9-oxoanthracene; a reagent used in the detection of carbohydrates.

⟁**anthropo-.** Human. [G. *anthrōpos,* a human being (of either sex)]

an·thro·po·bi·ol·o·gy (an′thrō-pō-bī-ol′ō-jē). The study of the biologic relationships of humans as a species.

an·thro·po·cen·tric (an′thrō-pō-sen′trik). With a human bias; under the assumption that humans are the central fact of the universe. [anthropo- + G. *kentron,* center]

an·thro·po·gen·e·sis (an′thrō-pō-jen′ĕ-sis). SYN anthropogeny.

an·thro·po·gen·ic, an·thro·po·ge·net·ic (an′thrō-pō-jen′ik, -jĕ-net′ik). Relating to anthropogeny.

an·thro·pog·e·ny (an-thrō-poj′ĕ-nē). The origin and development of man, both individual and racial. SYN anthropogenesis, anthropogony. [anthropo- + G. *genesis,* origin]

an·thro·pog·o·ny (an-thrō-poj′ō-nē). SYN anthropogeny.

an·thro·pog·ra·phy (an-thrō-pog′ră-fē). The geographical distribution of the varieties of human beings. [anthropo- + G. *graphō,* to write]

an·thro·poid (an′thrō-poyd). **1.** Resembling humans in structure and form. **2.** One of the monkeys resembling humans; an ape. [G. *anthrōpo-eidēs,* man-like]

An·thro·poi·dea (an′thrō-pō-id′ē-ă). A suborder of the mammalian order Primates, that comprises the families Cebidae (New World monkeys), Callithricidae (marmosets), Cercopithecidae (Old World monkeys), Pongidae (gibbons, gorillas, chimpanzees, and orangutans), and Hominidae (humans).

an·thro·pol·o·gy (an-thrō-pol′ō-jē). The branch of science concerned with origin and development of humans in all their physical, social, and cultural relationships. [anthropo- + G. *logos,* treatise]

applied a., a fusion of modern cultural a. and some aspects of sociology in the study of literate peoples in their cultures and deriving applications therefrom.

criminal a., a. in relation to the physical and mental characteristics, heredity, and social relations of the criminal. SEE ALSO criminology.

cultural a., study of all aspects of culture resulting from human behavior, including, among others, speech and language, systems of thought, social systems, and the artifacts produced by a culture.

physical a., the study of the physical attributes of human beings.

an·thro·pom·e·ter (an-thrō-pom′ĕ-ter). An instrument for measuring various dimensions of the human body.

an·thro·po·met·ric (an-thrō-pō-met′rik). Relating to anthropometry.

an·thro·pom·e·try (an-thrō-pom′ĕ-trē). The branch of anthropology concerned with comparative measurements of the human body. [anthropo- + G. *metron,* measure]

an·thro·po·mor·phism (an′thrō-pō-mōr′fizm). Ascription of human shape or qualities to nonhuman creatures or inanimate objects. Cf. theriomorphism. [anthropo- + G. *morphē,* form]

an·thro·pon·o·my (an-thrō-pon′ō-mē). The study of the laws governing the development of the human species and the relation to the environment. [anthropo- + G. *nomos,* law]

an·thro·pop·a·thy (an-thrō-pop′ă-thē). Attribution of human feelings to nonhumans, e.g., to gods or lower animals. [anthropo- + G. *pathos,* suffering]

an·thro·po·phil·ic (an'thrō-pō-fil'ik). Human-seeking or human-preferring, especially with reference to: 1) bloodsucking arthropods, denoting the preference of a parasite for the human host as a source of blood or tissues over an animal host; and 2) dermatophytic fungi which grow preferentially on humans rather than other animals. [anthropo- + G. *phileō*, to love]

an·thro·po·pho·bia (an'thrō-pō-fō'bē-ă). Morbid aversion to or dread of human companionship. [anthropo- + G. *phobos*, fear]

an·thro·pos·co·py (an'thrō-pos'kŏ-pē). Judging body type and build by inspection. [anthropo- + G. *skopeō*, to view]

an·thro·po·so·ma·tol·o·gy (an'thrō-pō'sō-mă-tol'ō-jē). That part of anthropology concerned with the human body, e.g., anatomy, physiology, or pathology. [anthropo- + G. *sōma*, body, + *logos*, study]

an·thro·po·zo·o·no·sis (an'thrō-pō-zō'ō-nō'sis). A zoonosis maintained in nature by animals and transmissible to humans; e.g., rabies, brucellosis. Cf. zooanthroponosis, amphixenosis. [anthropo- + G. *zōon*, animal, + *nosos*, disease]

⚠**anti-**. **1.** Against, opposing or, in relation to symptoms and diseases, curative. **2.** Prefix denoting an antibody (immunoglobulin) specific for the thing indicated; e.g., antitoxin (antibody specific for a toxin). [G. *anti,* against, opposite, instead of]

an·ti·ac·id (an-tē-as'id). SYN antacid.

an·ti·ad·ren·er·gic (an'tē-ad-rĕ-ner'jik). Antagonistic to the action of sympathetic or other adrenergic nerve fibers. SEE ALSO sympatholytic.

an·ti·ag·glu·ti·nin (an'tē-ă-gloo'ti-nin). A specific antibody that inhibits or destroys the action of an agglutinin.

an·ti·a·lex·in (an'tē-ă-lek'sin). SYN anticomplement.

an·ti·al·ler·gic (an'tē-ă-ler'jik). Relating to any agent or measure that prevents, inhibits, or alleviates an allergic reaction.

an·ti·an·a·phy·lax·is (an'tē-an'ă-fī-lak'sis). SYN desensitization (1).

an·ti·an·dro·gen (an-tē-an'drō-jen). Any substance capable of preventing full expression of the biologic effects of androgenic hormones on responsive tissues, either by producing antagonistic effects on the target tissue, as estrogens do, or by merely inhibiting androgenic effects, such as by competing for binding sites at the cell surface.

an·ti·a·ne·mic (an'tē-ă-nē'mik). Pertaining to factors or substances that prevent or correct anemic conditions.

an·ti·an·ti·body (an'tē-an'tē-bod-ē). Antibody specific for another antibody.

an·ti·an·ti·tox·in (an'tē-an-tē-tok'sin). An antiantibody that inhibits or counteracts the effects of an antitoxin.

an·ti·a·rach·nol·y·sin (an-tē-ar-ak-nol'i-sin). An antivenin counteracting the poison (lysin) of a spider. [anti- + G. *arachnē*, spider, + lysin]

an·ti·ar·rhyth·mic (an'tē-ă-rith'mik). Combating an arrhythmia. SYN antidysrhythmic.

an·ti·ar·thrit·ic (an'tē-ar-thrit'ik). **1.** Relieving arthritis. **2.** A remedy for arthritis. SYN antarthritic.

an·ti·asth·mat·ic (an'tē-az-mat'ik). **1.** Tending to relieve or prevent asthma. **2.** An agent that prevents or aborts an asthmatic attack. SYN antasthmatic.

an·ti·au·tol·y·sin (an'tē-aw-tol'i-sin). An antibody that inhibits or neutralizes the activity of an autolysin.

an·ti·bac·te·ri·al (an'tē-bak-tēr'ē-ăl). Destructive to or preventing the growth of bacteria.

an·ti·bech·ic (an-tē-bek'ik). SYN antitussive. [anti- + G. *bēx* (*bēch*-), cough]

an·ti·bi·ont (an-tē-bī'ont). A microorganism producing antimicrobial substance.

an·ti·bi·o·sis (an'tē-bī-ō'sis). **1.** An association of two organisms that is detrimental to one of them, in contrast to probiosis. **2.** Production of an antibiotic by bacteria or other organisms inhibitory to other living things, especially among soil microbes. [anti- + G. *biōsis,* life]

an·ti·bi·ot·ic (an'tē-bī-ot'ik). **1.** Relating to antibiosis. **2.** Prejudicial to life. **3.** A soluble substance derived from a mold or bacteri-

um that inhibits the growth of other microorganisms. **4.** Relating to such an action.

antibiotic groups
aminoglycosides
(e.g., streptomycin, gentamicin, sisomicin, tobramycin, amicacin)
ansamycins
(e.g., rifamycin)
antimycotics
polyenes
(e.g., nystatin, pimaricin, amphotericin B, pecilocin)
benzofuran derivatives
(griseofulvin)
β–lactam antibiotics
penicillins
(penicillin G and its derivatives, oral penicillins, penicillinase-fixed penicillins, broad-spectrum penicillins, penicillins active against *Proteus* and *Pseudomonas*)
cephalosporins
(e.g., cephalothin, cephaloridine, cephalexin, cefazolin, cefotaxime)
chloramphenicol group
(chloramphenicol, thiamphenicol, azidamphenicol)
Imidazole
fluconazole, itraconazole
linosamides
(lincomycin, clindamycin)
macrolides
(e.g., azithromycin, erythromycin, oleandomycin, spiramycin, clarithromycin)
peptides, peptolides, polypeptides
(e.g., polymyxin B and E, bacitracin, tyrothricin, capreomycin, vancomycin)
quinolones
(nalidixic acid, ofloxacin, ciprofloxacin, norfloxin)
tetracyclines
(e.g., tetracycline, oxytetracycline, minocycline, doxycycline)
other antibiotics
(phosphomycin, fusidic acid)

broad-spectrum a., an a. having a wide range of activity against both Gram-positive and Gram-negative organisms.

peptide a., a. composed of peptides; the antibacterial action is based on the physical disruption of cell membranes.

transport a., a substance that makes biomembranes permeable to certain ions.

an·ti·bi·ot·ic·re·sis·tant. Indicating microorganisms that continue to multiply although exposed to antibiotic agents.

an·ti·bi·o·tin (an-tē-bī'ō-tin). SYN avidin.

an·ti·blen·nor·rhag·ic (an'tē-blen-ō-raj'ik). Rarely used term for: **1.** Preventive or curative of a mucous discharge (blennorrhagia). **2.** A remedy possessing such properties.

ANTIBODY

▯**an·ti·body (Ab)** (an'tē-bod-ē). An immunoglobulin molecule produced by B lymphoid cells with a specific amino acid sequence evoked in humans or other animals by an antigen (immunogen). These molecules are characterized by reacting specifically with the antigen in some demonstrable way, antibody and antigen each being defined in terms of the other. A.'s may also exist naturally, without being present as a result of the stimulus provided by the introduction of an antigen; a.'s are found in the blood and body fluids, although the basic structure of the molecule consists of two light and two heavy chains, a.'s may also be found as dimers, trimers, or pentamers. SEE ALSO immunoglobulin. SYN immune protein, protective protein, sensitizer (2).

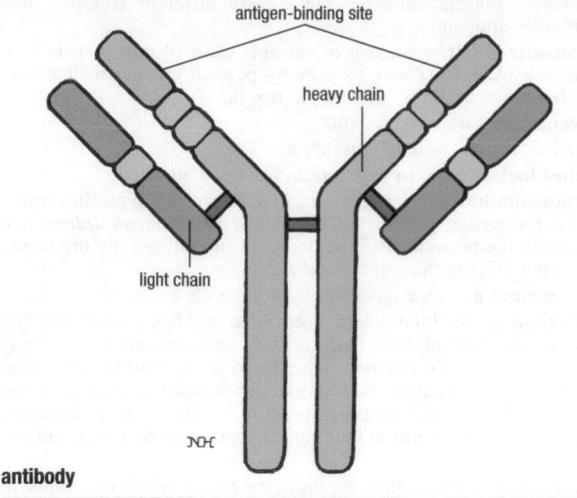

antibody

affinity a., the strength of binding between an antibody and an antigen. This interaction is reversible.

agglutinating a., SYN agglutinin (1).

anaphylactic a., SYN cytotropic a.

anti–basement membrane a., autoantibodies to renal glomerular basement membrane antigens.

anticardiolipin a.'s, a.'s directed against cardiolipid, a phosphorylated polysaccharide ester of fatty acids found in cell membranes. Associated with immune-mediated illnesses, syphilis, and strokes; thought to be from a hypercoagulable state.

antiidiotype a., an antiantibody, the activity of which is directed specifically against the antigenic determinants (idiotope) of a particular immunoglobulin (antibody) molecule. SYN idiotypic a.

anti-MAG a., a specific a. against myelin-associated glycoprotein; the most important of the specific a.'s against myelin so far identified, present in the majority of patients with IgM-associated polyneuropathies.

antineutrophil cytoplasmic a., an autoantibody to cytoplasmic constituents of monocytes and neutrophils found in patients with vasculitis.

antineutrophil cytoplasmic a.'s (ANCA), autoantibodies found in some autoimmune diseases, recognized by their reactivity with cytoplasmic antigens in neutrophils; two groups are recognized: c-ANCA, reacting with proteinase 3, is found in polyangiitis and Churg-Strauss syndrome; p-ANCA, reacting with myeloperoxidase is found in Wegener granulomatosis.

antinuclear a. (ANA), an a. showing an affinity for nuclear antigens including DNA and found in the serum of a high proportion of patients with systemic lupus erythematosus, rheumatoid arthritis, and certain collagen diseases, in some of their healthy relatives; also in about 1% of normal individuals.

antiphospholipid a.'s, a.'s directed against phosphorylated polysaccharide esters of fatty acids, includes lupus anticoagulant, VDRL, and anticardiolipin a.'s. Associated with immune-mediated illnesses, syphilis, and stroke; thought to be from a hypercoagulable disorder.

antithyroglobulin a., a. to thyroglobulin.

avidity a., the sum total of the functional binding strength between a polyvalent and its a. antigen. The total binding strength represents the sum strength of all the affinity bonds.

bivalent a., a. that causes a visible reaction with specific antigen as in agglutination, precipitation, and so on; so-called because according to the "lattice theory" aggregation occurs when the antibody molecule has two or more binding sites that can cross-link one antigen particle to another; probably a characteristic of the class of immunoglobulin.

blocking a., (1) a. which, in certain concentrations, does not cause precipitation after combining with specific antigen, and which, in this combined state, "blocks" activity of additional a. added to increase the concentration to a level at which precipitation would ordinarily occur; **(2)** the IgG class of immunoglobulin which combines specifically with an atopic allergen but does not elicit a type I allergic reaction, the combined IgG a. "blocking" available IgE class (reaginic) a. activity.

blood group a.'s, see Blood Groups appendix.

catalytic a., an a. that has been altered to give it a catalytic activity. SYN abzyme.

cell-bound a., a term used for a. on the surface of cells that may be bound either through antigen combining sites or other sites such as the Fc region.

CF a., SYN complement-fixing a.

chimeric a.'s, a. that may have the FAB fragment from one species fused with FC fragment from another species.

cold a., SEE cold *agglutinin.*

cold-reactive a., SEE cold *agglutinin.*

complement-fixing a., a. that combines with antigen leading to the binding and activation of complement, which may result in cell lysis. SYN CF a.

complete a., SYN saline *agglutinin.*

cross-reacting a., (1) a. specific for an epitope shared by members of a group, i.e., those with identical functional epitopes; **(2)** a. for antigens that have functional groups of similar, but not identical, chemical structure.

cytophilic a., SYN cytotropic a.

cytotropic a., a. that has an affinity for certain kinds of cells, in addition to and unrelated to its specific affinity for the antigen that induced it, because of the properties of the Fc portion of the heavy chain. SEE ALSO heterocytotropic a., homocytotropic a., cytotropic antibody *test.* SYN anaphylactic a., cytophilic a.

fluorescent a., an immunoglobulin (antibody) to which a fluorescent dye has been attached.

Forssman a., a heterogenetic a. specific for the Forssman group of heterogenetic antigens. SYN heterophil a., heterophile a.

heterocytotropic a., a cytotropic a. (chiefly of the IgG class) similar in activity to homocytotropic a., but having an affinity for cells of a different species rather than for cells of the same or a closely related species.

heterogenetic a., an a. that reacts to a heterogenetic antigen.

heterophil a., SYN Forssman a.

heterophile a., SYN Forssman a.

homocytotropic a., a. usually of the IgE class that has an affinity for tissues (notably mast cells) of the same or a closely related species and that, upon combining with specific antigen, triggers the release of pharmacologic mediators of anaphylaxis from the cells to which it is attached; the tropism seems to be dependent upon the Fc portion of the antibody molecule; in anaphylaxis in the guinea pig, the homocytotropic a. involved is of the γG class. SYN reagin (4), reaginic a.

human antimouse a. (HAMA), a. produced after exposure to mouse proteins.

idiotypic a., an a. that binds to an idiotope of another a. SYN antiidiotype a.

immobilizing a., SYN treponema-immobilizing a.

incomplete a., (1) SYN univalent a; **(2)** nonagglutinating.

inhibiting a., SYN univalent a.

lymphocytotoxic a.'s, a.'s specific for antigens of lymphocytes and which, upon combining with the antigens, induce cellular damage or death.

monoclonal a. (MAB, MoAb), an a. produced by a clone or genetically homogeneous population of fused hybrid cells, i.e., hybridoma; hybrid cells are cloned to establish cell lines producing a specific a. that is chemically and immunologically homogeneous.

The technique for producing monoclonal antibodies, invented in 1975 by molecular biologists Cesar Milstein and Georges Kohler, has become a mainstay of immunologic research and medical diagnosis. MoAbs serve as experimental probes in cell biology, biochemistry, and parasitology, and are used in purification of biologic substances and certain drugs (e.g., interferons). Because of their high specificity in binding to target antigens, they provide far more accurate assays than conventional antiserum. Tagged with radionuclides, they have been employed to deliver radiation doses directly to cancerous tissues.

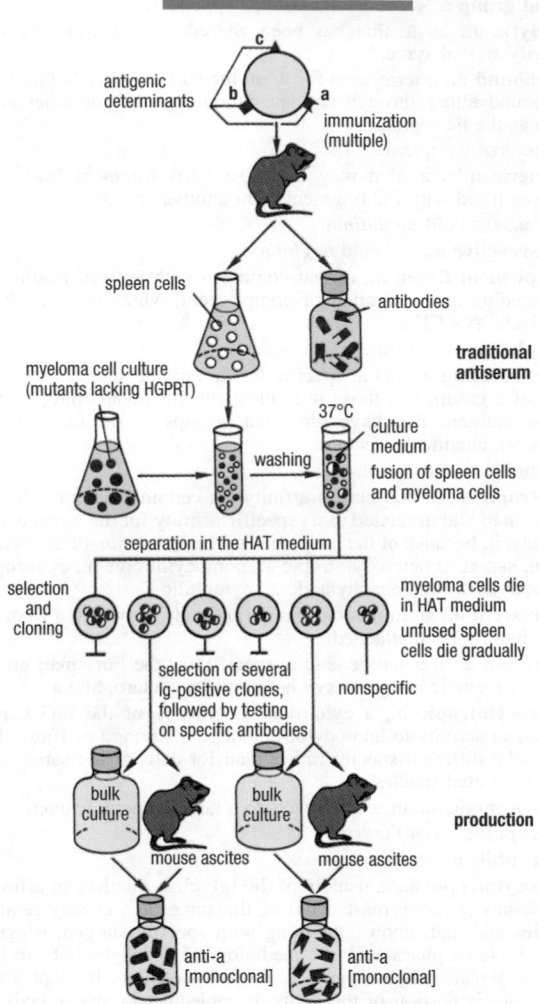

HGPRT = hypoxanthine-guanosine-phosphoribosyl transferase
HAT = hypoxanthine, aminopterin, and thymidine

monoclonal antibodies: preparation

natural a., SYN normal a.

neutralizing a., a form of a. that reacts with an infectious agent (usually a virus) and destroys or inhibits its infectivity and virulence; may be demonstrated by means of mixing serum with the suspension of infectious agent, and then injecting the mixture into animals or cell cultures that are susceptible to the agent in question.

nonprecipitable a., SYN nonprecipitating a.

nonprecipitating a., a. that, under conditions normally employed in precipitin tests, is refractory to precipitation by specific a., demonstrable when antigen is added serially in small amounts; nonprecipitating a. will precipitate under special conditions such as addition of complement. SYN nonprecipitable a.

normal a., a. demonstrable in the serum or plasma of various persons or animals not known to have been stimulated by specific antigen, either artificially or as the result of naturally occurring contact. SYN natural a.

P-K a.'s, igE a.'s involved in the Prausnitz-Kustner reaction.

polyclonal a. (pol-ē-klō'năl), a. that is derived from different clones of plasma cells but reacts with different epitopes of a particular antigen.

Prausnitz-Küstner a., one of the IgE class of a.'s first demonstrated by Prausnitz and Küstner by passive transfer to the skin. SEE homocytotropic a. SYN atopic reagin.

precipitating a., SYN precipitin.

reaginic a., SYN homocytotropic a.

ricin-blocked a., a. to which ricin has been attached.

treponema-immobilizing a., a., evoked during syphilitic infections, possessing specific affinity for *Treponema pallidum*, and which in the presence of complement immobilizes the organism. SYN immobilizing a., treponemal a.

treponemal a., SYN treponema-immobilizing a.

univalent a., an "incomplete" form of a. that has a single binding site; in the case of Rh+ erythrocytes, such an anti-Rh antibody may coat the cells but not cause them to agglutinate in saline; however, agglutination does occur when such coated cells are suspended in serum or other protein media, such as albumin, therefore called serum agglutinin. SYN incomplete a. (1), inhibiting a.

Vi a., a form of a. that agglutinates highly virulent strains of *Salmonella typhi*, i.e., cells with Vi antigen; such bacteria are not agglutinable with O antiserum until the Vi antigen is destroyed. SEE Vi *antigen*.

Wassermann a., a nonspecific a., evoked during syphilitic infections, that combines with cardiolipin in the presence of lecithin and cholesterol; it is distinct from the treponema-immobilizing a.

an·ti·bra·chi·al (an-tē-brā'kē-ăl). Incorrect spelling of antebrachial.

an·ti·bra·chi·um (an-tē-brā'kē-ŭm). Incorrect spelling of antebrachium.

an·ti·bro·mic (an-tē-brō'mik). **1.** Deodorizing. **2.** A deodorizer. [anti- + G. *brōmos*, smell]

an·ti·cal·cu·lous (an-tē-kal'kū-lŭs). SYN antilithic.

an·ti·car·i·ous (an'tē-kār'ē-ŭs). Preventing or inhibiting caries.

an·ti·ca·thex·is (an'tē-kă-thek'sis). In psychoanalysis, the shifting of an emotional charge to an impulse or action of an opposite character; e.g., unconscious hatred expressed as conscious love. SYN counterinvestment.

an·ti·ceph·a·lal·gic (an'tē-sef-ă-lal'jik). Headache-relieving or preventing.

an·ti·chol·a·gogue (an-tē-kol'ă-gog). Rarely used term for an agent or process that reduces or suspends the flow of bile.

an·ti·cho·lin·er·gic (an'tē-kol-i-ner'jik). Antagonistic to the action of parasympathetic or other cholinergic nerve fibers (e.g., atropine).

an·ti·cho·lin·es·ter·ase (an'tē-kō-lin-es'ter-ās). One of the drugs that inhibit or inactivate acetylcholinesterase, either reversibly (e.g., physostigmine) or irreversibly (e.g., tetraethyl pyrophosphate).

α_1**-an·ti·chy·mo·tryp·sin** (an'ti-kī'mō-trip-sin). An inhibitor protein of the digestive protease, chymotrypsin.

an·tic·i·pate (an-tis'i-pāt). To come before the appointed time; said of a periodic symptom or disease, such as a malarial paroxysm, when it recurs at progressively shorter intervals. [L. *anticipo*, pp. *-cipatus*, to anticipate, fr. *anti* (old form of *ante*), before, + *capio*, to take]

an·tic·i·pa·tion (an-tis-i-pā'shŭn). **1.** Appearance before the appointed time of a periodic symptom or sign. **2.** Progressively earlier age of manifestation of a hereditary disease in successive generations; may be factitious (because of heightened awareness to early signs of the disease or because they are more conspicuous in the young) or authentic (because of progressive loss of epistatic and modifier genes by recombination and segregation, or because of expansion of unstable alleles in successive generations). **3.** An increase in the severity of a phenotype in successive generations of a family, often associated with an increase in the number of trinucleotide repeats in a causative gene (e.g., fragile X syndrome, myotonic dystrophy, Huntington disease).

an·ti·cli·nal (an-tē-klī′năl). Inclined in opposite directions, as two sides of a pyramid. [anti- + G. *klinō*, to incline]

an·tic·ne·mi·on (an-tik-nē′mē-on). SYN anterior *border* of tibia. [G. *antiknēmion*]

an·ti·co·ag·u·lant (an′tē-kō-ag′ū-lant). **1.** Preventing coagulation. **2.** An agent having such action (e.g., warfarin).

lupus a., antiphospholipid antibody causing elevation in partial thromboplastin time; associated with venous and arterial thrombosis.

an·ti·co·don (an-tē-kō′don). The trinucleotide sequence complementary to a codon found in one loop of a tRNA molecule; e.g., if a codon is A–G–C, its anticodon is U (or T)–C–G. The complementarity principle arises from Watson-Crick base-pairing, in which A is complementary to U (or T) and G is complementary to C. Sometimes called "nodoc."

an·ti·com·ple·ment (an-tē-kom′plĕ-ment). A substance that combines with a complement component and neutralizes its action by preventing its union with an antibody. SYN antialexin.

an·ti·com·ple·men·ta·ry (an′tē-kom-plĕ-men′tă-rē). Denoting a substance possessing the power of diminishing or abolishing the action of a complement.

an·ti·con·ta·gious (an′tē-kon-tā′jŭs). Preventing contagion.

an·ti·con·vul·sant (an′tē-kon-vŭl′sant). **1.** Preventing or arresting seizures. **2.** An agent having such action. SYN anticonvulsive, antiepileptic.

an·ti·con·vul·sive (an′tē-kon-vŭl′siv). SYN anticonvulsant.

an·ti·cu·ra·re (an-tē-koo-ră′-rē). A drug property referring to the capacity to reverse the muscle paralysis produced by *d*-tubocurarine and other curarelike neuromuscular blocking drugs. Examples include neostigmine, pyridostigmine, and edrophonium.

an·ti·cus (an-tī′kŭs). A term in anatomic nomenclature to designate a muscle or other structure which of all similar structures is nearest the front or ventral surface. Nomina Anatomica uses "anterior" in place of this term. [L. in the very front, fr. *ante*, before]

an·ti·cy·to·tox·in (an′tē-sī-tō-tok′sin). A specific antibody that inhibits or destroys the activity of a cytotoxin.

an·ti·de·pres·sant (an′tē-dē-pres′ănt). **1.** Counteracting depression. **2.** An agent used in treating depression.

tetracyclic a., a class of a.'s similar to the tricyclic a.'s and also related to the phenothiazine antipsychotics; e.g., maprotiline.

triazolopyridine a., a class of a.'s structurally and pharmacologically unrelated to other a.'s; clinical effectiveness appears to be equivalent to the tricyclic a.'s, but with less anticholinergic side effects; e.g., trazodone.

tricyclic a., a chemical group of a. drugs that share a 3-ringed nucleus; e.g., amitriptyline, imipramine, desipramine, and nortriptyline.

an·ti·di·a·bet·ic (an′tē-dī-ă-bet′ik). Counteracting diabetes; denoting an agent that lowers blood sugar (e.g., tolbutamide, insulin).

an·ti·di·ar·rhe·al, an·ti·di·ar·rhet·ic (an′tē-dī-ă-re′ăl, -dī-ă-ret′ik). **1.** Having the property of opposing or correcting diarrhea. **2.** An agent having such action (e.g., loperamide).

an·ti·di·u·re·sis (an′tē-dī-ū-rē′sis). Reduction of urinary volume.

an·ti·di·u·ret·ic (an′tē-dī-ū-ret′ik). An agent that reduces the output of urine.

an·ti·dot·al (an-tē-dō′tăl). Relating to or acting as an antidote.

an·ti·dote (an′tē-dōt). An agent that neutralizes a poison or counteracts its effects. [G. *antidotos,* fr. *anti,* against, + *dotos,* what is given, fr. *didōmi,* to give]

chemical a., a substance that unites with a poison to form an innocuous chemical compound.

mechanical a., a substance that prevents the absorption of a poison.

physiologic a., an agent that produces systemic effects contrary to those of a given poison.

universal a., a dated mixture of 2 parts activated charcoal, 1 part tannic acid, and 1 part magnesium oxide intended to be adminis-

tered to patients who consumed poison. The mixture is ineffective and no longer used; activated charcoal is useful.

an·ti·drom·ic (an-tē-drom′ik). Denoting the propagation of an impulse along a conduction system (e.g., nerve fiber) in the direction opposite to which it normally travels.

an·ti·dys·en·ter·ic (an′tē-dis-en-ter′ik). Relieving or preventing dysentery.

an·ti·dys·rhyth·mic (an′tē-dis-rith′mik). SYN antiarrhythmic.

an·ti·dys·u·ric (an′tē-dis-ū′rik). Preventing or relieving strangury or distress in urination.

an·ti·e·met·ic (an′tē-ĕ-met′ik). **1.** Preventing or arresting vomiting. **2.** A remedy that tends to control nausea and vomiting. [anti- + G. *emetikos,* emetic]

an·ti·e·ner·gic (an′tē-en-er′jik). Acting against or in opposition. [anti- + G. *energos,* active]

an·ti·en·zyme (an-tē-en′zīm). An agent or principle that retards, inhibits, or destroys the activity of an enzyme; may be an inhibitory enzyme or an antibody to an enzyme (e.g., serum antitrypsin).

an·ti·ep·i·lep·tic (an′tē-ep-i-lep′tik). SYN anticonvulsant.

an·ti·es·tro·gen (an′tē-es′trō-jen). Any substance capable of preventing full expression of the biological effects of estrogenic hormones on responsive tissues, either by producing antagonistic effects on the target tissue, as androgens and progestogens do, or by competing with estrogens at estrogen receptors at the cellular level (e.g., tamoxifen).

an·ti·fe·brile (an-tē-fē′brīl, -feb′ril). SYN antipyretic (1). [anti- + L. *febris,* fever]

an·ti·fi·bril·la·tory (an′tē-fī′bri-lă-tōr-ē). Any measure or medication that tends to suppress fibrillary arrhythmias (atrial fibrillation, ventricular fibrillation).

an·ti·fi·bri·nol·y·sin (an′tē-fī-bri-nol′i-sin). SYN antiplasmin.

an·ti·fi·bri·no·lyt·ic (an′tē-fī-brin-ō-lit′ik). Denoting a substance that decreases the breakdown of fibrin; e.g., aminocaproic acid.

an·ti·fo·lic (an-tē-fō′lik). **1.** Antagonistic to the action of folic acid. **2.** Any agent with this effect. SEE ALSO folic acid *antagonists,* under *antagonist.*

an·ti·fun·gal (an-tē-fŭng′ăl). SYN antimycotic.

an·ti-G. In the strict sense, a term that means "antigravity" but, as commonly used, an adjectival term that implies protection against the effects of gravity (e.g., anti-G *suit*).

ANTIGEN

an·ti·gen (Ag) (an′ti-jen). Any substance that, as a result of coming in contact with appropriate cells, induces a state of sensitivity and/or immune responsiveness after a latent period (days to weeks) and that reacts in a demonstrable way with antibodies and/or immune cells of the sensitized subject in vivo or in vitro. Modern usage tends to retain the broad meaning of a., employing the terms "antigenic determinant" or "determinant group" for the particular chemical group of a molecule that confers antigenic specificity. SEE ALSO hapten. SYN immunogen. [anti(body) + G. *-gen,* producing]

ABO a.'s, see ABO blood group, Blood Groups appendix.

acetone-insoluble a., SYN cardiolipin.

allogeneic a. (al′ō-jĕ-ne′ik), genetic variations of the same a.'s within a given species.

Am a.'s, allotypic determinants (antigens) on the heavy chain of human IgA molecules.

Au a., (1) see Auberger blood group, Blood Groups appendix; (2) SYN Australia a.

Aus a., SYN Australia a.

Australia a., so-called because it was first recognized in an Australian aborigine, but now known to be subunits of the hepatitis B virus surface antigen. SYN Au a. (2), Aus a.

Be^a a.'s, see low frequency blood groups, Blood Groups appendix. SYN Becker a.

Becker a., SYN Be^a a.'s.

Bi a., see low frequency blood groups, Blood Groups appendix. SYN Bile a.

Bile a., SYN Bi a.

blood group a., generic term for any inherited antigen found on the surface of erythrocytes that determines a blood grouping reaction with specific antiserum; a.'s of the ABO and Lewis blood groups may be found also in saliva and other body fluids; the genes controlling development of blood group a.'s vary in frequency in different population and ethnic groups. See also Blood Groups appendix. SYN blood group substance.

By a., see low frequency blood groups, Blood Groups appendix.

CA-125 a., tumor marker elevated in 85% of women with advanced ovarian cancer. SEE ALSO cancer antigen 125 *test.*

CA-15-3 a., a. present in some patients with breast cancer.

CA-19-9 a., tumor a. present in cholangiocarcinomas and pancreatic carcinomas.

capsular a., that found only in the capsules of certain microorganisms; e.g., the specific polysaccharides of various types of pneumococci.

carcinoembryonic a. (CEA), a glycoprotein constituent of the glycocalyx of embryonic endodermal epithelium, which may be elevated in the serum of some patients with colon and certain other cancers and in serum of chronic tobacco smokers.

Casoni a., skin-test a. composed of sterile hydatid fluid; used in test for hydatid disease.

C carbohydrate a., an antigen found in the cell wall of *Streptococcus* species and denotes different strains. SEE β-hemolytic *streptococci,* under *streptococcus.*

CDE a.'s, see Rh blood group, Blood Groups appendix.

cholesterinized a., cardiolipin to which cholesterol has been added.

Chr^a a.'s, see low frequency blood groups, Blood Groups appendix.

class I a.'s, cell-membrane–bound glycoproteins found on most nucleated cells that are coded by genes of the major histocompatibility complex.

class II a.'s, a cell membrane glycoprotein encoded by genes of the major histocompatibility complex. These antigens are distributed on a.-presenting cells such as macrophages, B cells, and dendritic cells.

class III a.'s, non–cell-membrane molecules that are encoded by the S region of the major histocompatibility complex. These a.'s are not involved in determining histocompatibility and include the complement proteins as well as certain cytokine genes i.e., tumor necrosis factors α and β.

cluster of differentiation (CD) a., an antigen (marker) on the surface of a cell, usually a lymphocyte.

common a., cross-reacting a. (epitope); a common a. that occurs in two or more different molecules or organisms.

complete a., any a. capable of stimulating the formation of antibody with which it reacts in vivo or in vitro, as distinguished from incomplete a. (hapten).

conjugated a., SYN conjugated *hapten.*

D a., one of 6 antigens that compose the Rh locus. Antibody induced by D antigen is the most frequent cause of hemolytic disease of the newborn.

delta a., SYN hepatitis D *virus.*

Dharmendra a., a chloroform-ether extracted suspension of *Mycobacterium leprae;* used to produce the Fernandez reaction in a lepromin test.

Di a., see Diego blood group, Blood Groups appendix.

Duffy a.'s, see Duffy blood group, Blood Groups appendix.

epithelial membrane a. (EMA), a heavily glycosylated, 70 kd protein complex, first isolated in human milk fat globulin; this a. is present in a variety of glandular epithelia, especially in breast carcinoma cells, but may also be seen in cultured fibroblasts, lymphoid cells, and some stromal cells. Immunohistochemical staining may be used as a diagnostic aid in tissue diagnosis.

flagellar a., the heat-labile a.'s associated with bacterial flagella, in contrast to somatic a. SEE ALSO H a.

Forssman a., a type of heterogenetic a. found in dogs, horses, sheep, cats, turtles, eggs of some fish, in certain bacteria (e.g., some strains of enteric organisms and pneumococci), and varieties of corn; usually found in the tissues and organs (not in blood), but is present in sheep erythrocytes, though not in this animal's tissues; with the exception of guinea pigs and hamsters, Forssman a. is not found in rodents, or in frogs, hogs, and most primates; the antibody that develops in infectious mononucleosis of humans reacts specifically with the Forssman. a.

Fy a.'s, see Duffy blood group, Blood Groups appendix.

G a., an antigenic glycoprotein frequently associated with viral surfaces. [Ger. *gebundenes,* bound]

Ge a., see high frequency blood groups, Blood Groups appendix.

Gerbich a., glycophorin C. SEE glycophorins.

Gm a.'s, allotypic determinants (antigens) that are present on the heavy chain of immunoglobulin G. There are 25 different determinants present throughout the human population.

Good a., see low frequency blood groups, Blood Groups appendix.

Gr a., SYN Vw a; See Vw a. under MNSs blood group in Blood Groups appendix.

group a.'s, a.'s that are present on different organisms.

H a., **(1)** the a. in the flagella of motile bacteria; important in serologic classification of enteric bacteria. SEE ALSO O a. (1); **(2)** the chemical precursor of a.'s of the ABO blood group locus.

H-2 a.'s, a.'s that are coded by the H-2 complex of genes in mice and are involved in self/nonself recognition.

He a.'s, see MNSs blood group, Blood Groups appendix. SYN Hu a.'s.

heart a., SYN cardiolipin.

hepatitis-associated a. (HAA), a term used for the surface a. of hepatitis B virus before its nature was established. SEE hepatitis B surface a.

hepatitis B core a. (HB$_c$Ab, HB$_c$Ag), the a. found in the core of the Dane particle (which is the complete virus) and also in hepatocyte nuclei in hepatitis B infections.

hepatitis B e a. (HB$_e$Ab, HBe, HB$_e$Ag), an a., or group of a.'s, associated with hepatitis B infection and distinct from the surface a. (HB$_s$Ag) and the core a. (HB$_c$Ag); it is associated with the viral nucleocapsid. Its presence indicates that the virus is replicating and the individual is potentially infectious.

hepatitis B surface a. (HB$_s$Ab, HB$_s$Ag), a. of the small (20 nm) spherical and filamentous forms of hepatitis B a., and a surface a. of the larger (42 nm) Dane particle (complete infectious hepatitis B virus). SEE ALSO hepatitis B core a., hepatitis B e a.

heterogeneic a., SEE heterophile a.

heterogenetic a., SYN heterophile a.

heterophil a., SYN heterophile a.

heterophile a., **(1)** an a. or antigenic determinant that is found in different tissues in more than one species. **(2)** an a. that is possessed by a variety of different phylogenetically unrelated species; e.g., the various organ- or tissue-specific a.'s, the α- and β-crystalline protein of the lens of the eye, and Forssman a. SYN heterogenetic a., heterophil a.

hexon a., viral subunit. SEE hexon.

histocompatibility a., an a. on the surface of nucleated cells, particularly leucocytes and thrombocytes. SEE ALSO H-2 a.'s. SYN transplantation a.

HL-A a.'s, now obsolete, this was the original designation for *human leukocyte histocompatibility a.'s. The HLA histocompatibility system in humans is composed of MHC classes I, II, III. SEE major histocompatibility *complex.*

Ho a., see low frequency blood groups, Blood Groups appendix.

homologous a., the specific a. that generates the formation of an antibody that in turn can react with that antigen.

Hu a.'s, SYN He a.'s.

human leukocyte a.'s (HLA) [MIM*142560], system designation for the gene products of at least four linked loci (A, B, C, and D) and a number of subloci on the sixth human chromosome that

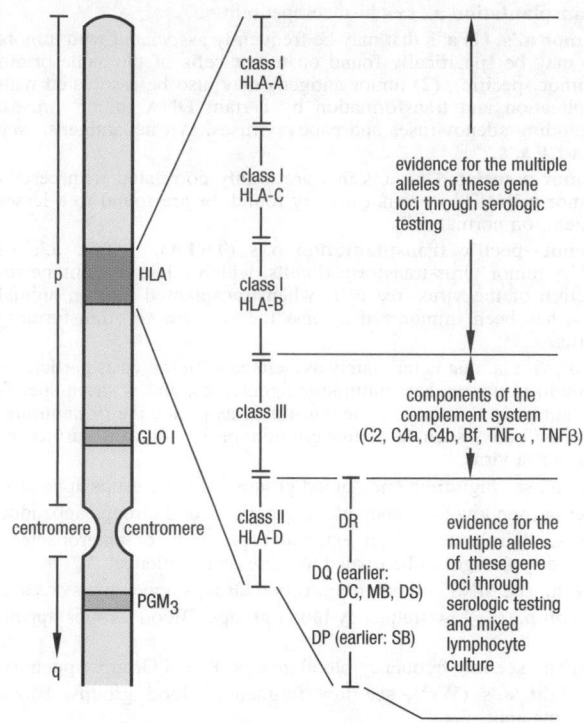

HLA system (chromosome 6)

---

have been shown to have a strong influence on human allotransplantation, transfusions in refractory patients, and certain disease associations; more than 50 alleles are recognized, most of which are at loci HLA-A and HLA-B; autosomal dominant inheritance.

H-Y a., an a. factor, dependent on the Y chromosome, responsible for the differentiation of the human embryo into the male phenotype by inducing the initially bipotential embryonic gonad to develop into a testis; in the absence of this a., the indifferent gonad develops into an ovary. There are at least two loci involved, an autosomal gene that generates the a. [MIM*143170] and one that makes the receptor [MIM*143150].

I a.'s, see I blood group, Blood Groups appendix.

incomplete a., SYN hapten.

InV group a., SYN Km a.

Jk a.'s, see Kidd blood group, Blood Groups appendix.

Jobbins a., see low frequency blood groups, Blood Groups appendix.

Js a., see Sutter Blood Group, Blood Groups appendix.

K a.'s, see Kell blood group, Blood Groups appendix.

Km a., allotypic a.'s that are present on human kappa immunoglobulin light chains. SYN InV group a.

Kveim a., a saline suspension of human sarcoid tissue prepared from the spleen of an individual with active sarcoidosis; used in the Kveim test. SYN Kveim-Siltzbach a.

Kveim-Siltzbach a., SYN Kveim a.

Lan a., see high frequency blood groups, Blood Groups appendix.

Le a.'s, see Lewis blood group, Blood Groups appendix.

leukocyte common a. (loo′kō-sīt), family of glycoproteins found on most leukocytes and absent from other cell types. These cell surface a.'s can comprise up to 10% of the membrane proteins.

Levay a., see low frequency blood groups, Blood Groups appendix.

Lu a.'s, see Lutheran blood group, Blood Groups appendix.

lymphocyte function associated a. (**LFA**) (limf′ō-sit), a member of the integrin family that is expressed on all leukocytes and binds to ICAM-1 and ICAM-2 on a variety of cells.

lymphogranuloma venereum a., a sterile preparation of inacti-

---

vated chlamydiae grown in the yolk sac of domestic fowl and used as an a. in the Frei *test.*

Lyt a.'s, a group of alloantigens that are present on either T or B murine lymphocytes, e.g., Lyt 2,3 is equivalent to human CD8.

M a., an antigen found in the cell of *Streptococcus pyogenes;* associated with virulence. SEE β-hemolytic *streptococci,* under *streptococcus.*

M_1 a., M^g a., M^c a., M_2 a., see MNSs blood group, Blood Groups appendix.

Mitsuda a., an autoclaved suspension of human tissue naturally infected with *Mycobacterium leprae;* used to produce the Mitsuda reaction in a lepromin test.

MNSs a.'s, see MNSs blood group, Blood Groups appendix.

Mu a., see MNS blood group, Blood Groups appendix.

mumps skin test a., a sterile suspension of killed mumps virus in isotonic sodium chloride solution, used to determine susceptibility to mumps or to confirm previous exposure.

O a., (1) somatic a. of enteric Gram-negative bacteria. External part of cell wall lipopolysaccharide; SEE ALSO H a. (1); **(2)** see ABO blood group, Blood Groups appendix.

oncofetal a.'s, tumor-associated a.'s present in fetal tissue and some malignant tumors but not in normal adult tissue, including α-fetoprotein.

organ-specific a., a heterogenetic antigen with organ specificity; e.g., in addition to species-specific a., kidney of one species contains a. that is identical to that in kidney of other species. SYN tissue-specific a.

Ot a., see low frequency blood groups, Blood Groups appendix.

P a.'s, see P blood group, Blood Groups appendix.

partial a., SYN hapten.

penton a., SEE penton.

pollen a., an extract of the antigenic protein from the pollen of plants; i.e., pollen allergen, used in the diagnosis and prevention of hay fever.

private a.'s, see low frequency blood groups, Blood Groups appendix.

proliferating cell nuclear a., a nuclear nonhistone protein with a molecular weight of 36 kd that plays a role in the initiation of cell proliferation by augmenting DNA polymerase; stains for proliferating cell nuclear a. in tumors correlate with grade and mitotic activity.

---

prostate-specific a. (PSA), a single-chain, 31-kDa glycoprotein with 240 amino acid residues and 4 carbohydrate side-chains; a kallikrein protease produced by prostatic epithelial cells and normally found in seminal fluid and circulating blood. Elevations of serum PSA are highly organ-specific but occur in both cancer (adenocarcinoma) and benign disease (benign prostatic hyperplasia, prostatitis). A significant number of patients with organ-confined cancer have normal PSA values. SYN human glandular kallikrein 3.

Levels of PSA below 4 ng/dL are considered normal, while levels above 10 ng/dL are strongly indicative of prostatic carcinoma. Approximately 30% of patients with PSA levels between these limits will have prostate cancer detectable by biopsy within 1 year. Measurement of both free PSA and PSA that is complexed with the protease inhibitor α-1 antichymotrypsin (PSA-ACT) enhances the sensitivity of testing for carcinoma in men with total PSA levels between 4 and 10 ng/dL. The percentage of free PSA is lower in the serum of men with prostate cancer than in patients with normal prostates or benign disease. A level of free PSA that is 25% or more of total PSA in a patient with a palpably benign gland effectively rules out the need for prostatic biopsy when total PSA is below 10 ng/dL. A free PSA of 15% or less strongly suggests carcinoma. A level of 20% or more may be seen in adenocarcinoma when the prostate is enlarged. During the 1980s the increased use of PSA screening led to an apparent shift in the incidence of prostatic carcinoma, with proportionately more diagnoses in men under 70 and fewer in men over 70, and also a higher incidence of early or prostate-confined disease. This shift peaked in 1992; incidence statistics have now nearly returned to pre–PSA-screening levels. Prostatic cancer mortality has declined substantially since 1990. Many observers attribute this decline to the ability of PSA screening to detect cancer at a curable stage. However, the use of PSA testing as well as other diagnostic maneuvers to screen asymptomatic elderly men for prostate cancer is controversial, since most men with prostate cancer do not die of it, and to many observers the consequences of aggressive treatment, which may include urinary incontinence and impotence, seem worse than the disease.

public a.'s, see high frequency blood groups, Blood Groups appendix.

R a., SEE β-hemolytic *streptococci*, under *streptococcus*.

Rh a.'s, see Rh blood group, Blood Groups appendix.

Rhus toxicodendron a., an extract of fresh leaves of poison ivy, with 0.4% of procaine hydrochloride; used by intradermal injection to determine sensitiveness to the poison of *Rhus toxicodendron.*

Rhus venenata a., an extract of fresh leaves of poison sumac; used to determine sensitiveness to the plant or to relieve the dermatitis caused by contact with its leaves.

S a., SYN soluble a.

sensitized a., the complex formed when a. combines with specific antibody; so called because the a., by the mediation of antibody, is rendered sensitive to the action of complement.

shock a., an a. capable of producing anaphylactic shock in an animal that has been sensitized to it.

Sm a., see high frequency blood groups, Blood Groups appendix.

soluble a., viral a. that remains in solution after the particles of virus have been removed by means of centrifugation; in the case of the influenza viruses, it is the internal helical structure, free of the external envelope. SYN S a.

somatic a., an a. located in the cell wall of a bacterium in contrast to one in the flagella (flagellar a.) or in a capsule (capsular a.).

species-specific a., antigenic components in the tissues and fluids of members of a species of animal, by means of which various species may be immunologically distinguished; e.g., serum albumin of horses is immunologically different from that of man, dogs, sheep, and so on.

specific a.'s, a.'s that characterize a single genus of microorganisms.

Stobo a., see low frequency blood groups, Blood Groups appendix.

Streptococcus M a., the somatic a. associated with virulence and type specificity of group A streptococci. It is antiphagocytic and there are more than 80 different types. SYN M protein (1).

Sw^a a., see low frequency blood groups, Blood Groups appendix.

Swann a.'s, see low frequency blood groups, Blood Groups appendix.

T a.'s, tumor antigens associated wtih replication and transformation by certain DNA tumor viruses, including adenoviruses and papovaviruses. SEE ALSO β-hemolytic *streptococci*, under *streptococcus*, tumor a.'s.

Tac a., an antigenic determinant of the human interleukin 2 receptor that is identified by a murine monoclonal antibody, anti-Tac. Binding of this antigen with antibodies to TAC prevents the proliferation of T cells, which is normally stimulated by binding interleukin-2.

T-dependent a., an a. that requires T helper cells in addition to appropriate B cells. Most a.'s are T-dependent.

theta a. (thā′tă), a surface glycoprotein that is present on thymocytes and mature T cells of mice and rats.

thymus-independent a., an a. that does not require T helper cell activation in order for the host's B cells to be stimulated. Repeating polymers such as polysaccharides are examples of T-independent a.'s.

tissue-specific a., SYN organ-specific a.

Tj a., see P blood group, Blood Groups appendix.

Tr^a a., see low-frequency blood groups, Blood Groups appendix.

transplantation a., SYN histocompatibility a.

tumor a.'s, (1) a.'s that may be frequently associated with tumors or may be specifically found on tumor cells of the same origin (tumor specific); **(2)** tumor antigens may also be associated with replication and transformation by certain DNA tumor viruses, including adenoviruses and papovaviruses. SYN neoantigens. SEE ALSO T a.'s.

tumor-associated a., a.'s that are highly correlated with certain tumor cells. They are not usually found, or are found to a lesser extent, on normal cells.

tumor-specific transplantation a.'s (TSTA), surface a.'s of DNA tumor virus-transformed cells, which elicit an immune rejection of the virus-free cells when transplanted into an animal that has been immunized against the specific cell-transforming virus.

V a., viral a. that is intimately associated with the virus particle, is protein in nature, has multiple antigenicities, and is strain-specific; antibody to such a. is demonstrable as protective or neutralizing antibody, such as hemagglutinin projections on surface of influenza virus.

Vel a., see high frequency blood groups, Blood Groups appendix.

Ven a., see low frequency blood groups, Blood Groups appendix.

Vi a., "virulence a.," an external capsular a. of enterobacteria formerly thought to be related to increased virulence.

Vw a., see MNSs blood group, Blood Groups appendix. SYN Gr a.

Webb a., see low frequency blood groups, Blood Groups appendix.

Wr^a a., see low frequency blood groups, Blood Groups appendix.

Wright a.'s (Wr^a), see low frequency blood groups, Blood Groups appendix.

Xg a., see Xg blood group, Blood Groups appendix.

Yt^a a., see high frequency blood groups, Blood Groups appendix.

an·ti·ge·ne·mia (an′ti-jĕ-nē′mē-ă). Persistence of antigen in circulating blood; e.g., HB_s-antigenemia (presence of hepatitis B virus surface antigen in blood serum). [antigen + G. *haima,* blood]

an·ti·gen·ic (an-ti-jen′ik). Having the properties of an antigen (allergen). SYN allergenic, immunogenic.

an·ti·ge·nic·i·ty (an′ti-jĕ-nis′i-tē). The state or property of being antigenic. SYN immunogenicity.

anti·gen·ome. The complementary positive RNA strand on which is made the negative-strand genome of viruses.

an·ti·gon·or·rhe·ic (an′tē-gon-ō-rē′ik). Curative of gonorrhea.

an·ti·grav·i·ty (an-tē-grav′i-tē). SEE anti-G.

an·ti·HB_e. Antibody to the hepatitis B e *antigen* (HB_eAg).

an·ti·HB_c. Antibody to the hepatitis B core *antigen* (HB_cAg).

an·ti·HB_s. Antibody to the hepatitis B surface *antigen* (HB_sAg).

an·ti·he·lix (an-tē-hē′liks) [TA]. An elevated ridge of cartilage anterior and roughly parallel to the posterior portion of the helix of the external ear. SYN anthelix.

an·ti·helminthic (an′tē-hel-minth′ik). SYN anthelmintic (1).

an·ti·hem·ag·glu·ti·nin (an′tē-hē-mă-gloo′ti-nin, an′tē-hem-ă-). A substance (including antibody) that inhibits or prevents hemagglutination.

an·ti·he·mo·ly·sin (an′tē-hē-mol′i-sin, an′tē-hem-ol′-). A substance (including antibody) that inhibits or prevents the effects of hemolysin.

an·ti·he·mo·lyt·ic (an′tē-hē-mō-lit′ik, an′tē-hem-ō-). Preventing hemolysis.

an·ti·hem·or·rhag·ic (an′tē-hem-ō-rāj′ik). Arresting hemorrhage. SYN hemostatic (2).

an·ti·his·ta·mines (an-tē-his′tă-mēnz). Drugs having an action antagonistic to that of histamine on either H₁ or H₂ receptors; H₁ type a. are used in the treatment of allergy symptoms; whereas H₂ type a. reduce gastric acidity in ulcer disease and gastroesophageal reflux.

an·ti·his·ta·min·ic (an′tē-his-tă-min′ik). **1.** Tending to neutralize or antagonize the action of histamine or to inhibit its production in the body. **2.** An agent having such an effect can be used to relieve the symptoms of allergy or hyperacidity.

an·ti·hor·mones (an-tē-hōr′mōnz). Substances demonstrable in serum that inhibit or prevent the usual effects of certain hormones, e.g., specific antibodies.

an·ti·hy·drop·ic (an′tē-hī-drop′ik). **1.** Relieving edema (dropsy). **2.** An agent that mobilizes accumulated fluids.

an·ti·hy·per·ten·sive (an′tē-hī-per-ten′siv). Indicating a drug or mode of treatment that reduces the blood pressure of hypertensive individuals.

an·ti·hyp·not·ic (an′tē-hip-not′ik). **1.** Preventing or tending to prevent sleep. **2.** An arousing agent, or one antagonistic to sleep.

an·ti·hy·po·ten·sive (an′tē-hī′pō-ten′siv). Any measure or medication that tends to raise reduced blood pressure.

an·ti·ic·ter·ic (an′tē-ik-ter′ik). Rarely used term for preventing or curing icterus (jaundice).

an·ti·in·flam·ma·to·ry (an′tē-in-flam′ă-tō-rē). Reducing inflammation by acting on body responses, without directly antagonizing the causative agent; denoting agents such as glucocorticoids and aspirin.

an·ti·-in·su·lin. A factor, usually an antibody, which antagonizes the action of insulin.

an·ti·ke·to·gen·e·sis (an′tē-kē-tō-jen′ĕ-sis). Prevention or reduction of ketosis either by decreased production or increased utilization of ketone bodies.

an·ti·ke·to·gen·ic (an′tē-kē-tō-jen′ik). Inhibiting the formation of ketone bodies, or accelerating their utilization.

an·ti·leu·koc·i·din (an′tē-loo-kos′i-din, loo-kō-sī′din). **1.** A substance that inhibits or prevents the effects of leukocidin. **2.** A leukocidin-specific antibody.

an·ti·leu·ko·tox·in (an′tē-loo-kō-tok′sin). A substance (including antibody) that inhibits or prevents the effects of leukocytoxin; frequently regarded as synonymous with antileukocidin.

an·ti·leu·ko·tri·ene (an-tē-loo-ko-trī-′ēn). A drug that prevents or alleviates bronchoconstriction in asthma by blocking the production or action of naturally occurring leukotrienes; may also be useful in psoriasis.

> In 1940 a naturally occurring mediator of asthmatic bronchoconstriction, distinct from histamine and with a longer duration of action, was isolated and named slow-reacting substance of anaphylaxis (SRS-A). Analysis has shown this agent to consist of three cysteinyl leukotrienes, called C4, D4, and E4. The last-named substance, of which the others are precursors, is the most potent. Leukotrienes are eicosanoids derived from arachidonic acid, which is present in cell membranes. The cysteinyl leukotrienes, which are elaborated by bronchopulmonary mast cells, eosinophils, and probably alveolar macrophages, have been shown to mediate bronchoconstriction induced by exercise, hyperventilation in cold air, aspirin, and inhaled allergens; they act by stimulating a specific receptor, known as cysteinyl leukotriene receptor type 1 (CysLT1). Antileukotrienes with clinical usefulness in asthma include zileuton, which inhibits 5-lipoxygenase, an enzyme critical in the biosynthesis of leukotrienes, and leukotriene receptor antagonists (cinalukast, montelukast, zafirlukast, and others). Antileukotrienes reverse bronchoconstriction in asthma to a lesser degree than β_2-adrenergic agonists, but their effects are additive to those of the latter agents. In chronic asthma, antileukotrienes improve peak flow and FEV_1 and reduce the frequency and severity of acute asthmatic attacks, the need for β_2-agonists, and the need for corticosteroid rescue. They are particularly effective in the prophylaxis of exercise- and aspirin-induced asthma; in contrast, many persons with allergic asthma show little or no response. Antileukotrienes are not indicated in the treatment of an acute asthmatic attack or in mild, intermittent asthma controlled adequately with occasional use of inhaled β_2-agonists. They have not been recommended as a substitute for inhaled corticosteroid in prophylaxis of asthma. An antagonist of the leukotriene LTB4 receptor in

skin cells has shown promise in the treatment of psoriasis. Antileukotrienes are administered orally or by inhalation. Both onset and waning of clinical effects are gradual. Side effects are minimal, but drug interactions may occur because of interference with cytochrome P-450 enzymes. Rare transitory elevations of hepatic aminotransferase have been reported with some agents.

an·ti·lew·is·ite (an-tē-loo′i-sīt). SYN dimercaprol.

an·ti·lip·o·tro·pic (an′tē-lip-ō-trop′ik). Pertaining to substances depressing choline synthesis (e.g., by competing for methyl groups) and thus enhancing dietary fatty liver.

an·ti·lith·ic (an-tē-lith′ik). **1.** Preventing the formation of calculi or promoting their dissolution. **2.** An agent so acting. SYN anticalculous. [anti- + G. *lithos,* stone]

an·ti·lo·bi·um (an-tē-lō′bē-ŭm). SYN tragus (1). [L., fr. G. *antilobion*]

an·ti·lu·te·o·gen·ic (an′tē-loo-tē-ō-jen′ik). Inhibiting the growth or hastening involution of the corpus luteum.

an·ti·ly·sin (an-tē-lī′sin). An antibody that inhibits or prevents the effects of lysin.

an·ti·ma·lar·i·al (an′tē-mă-lā′rē-ăl). **1.** Preventing or curing malaria. **2.** A chemotherapeutic agent that inhibits or destroys malarial parasites.

an·ti·mere (an′ti-mēr). **1.** A segment of an animal body formed by planes cutting the axis of the body at right angles. **2.** One of the symmetrical parts of a bilateral organism. **3.** The right or left half of the body. [anti- + G. *meros,* a part]

an·ti·mes·en·ter·ic (an′tē-mez′en-ter′ik). Pertaining to the part of the intestine that lies opposite the mesenteric attachment.

an·ti·me·tab·o·lite (an′tē-me-tab′ō-līt). A substance that competes with, replaces, or antagonizes a particular metabolite; e.g., ethionine is an a. of methionine.

an·ti·me·tro·pia (an′tē-me-trō′pē-ă). A form of anisometropia in which one eye is myopic and the other hypermetropic. [anti- + G. *metron,* measure, + *ōps,* eye]

an·ti·mi·cro·bi·al (an′tē-mī-krō′bē-ăl). Tending to destroy microbes, to prevent their multiplication or growth, or to prevent their pathogenic action.

an·ti·mi·tot·ic (an′tē-mī-tot′ik). **1.** Having an arresting action upon mitosis. **2.** A drug having such an effect; e.g., a folic acid antagonist that is used in leukemia to inhibit the multiplication of white cells.

an·ti·mon·gol·oid (an-tē-mon′gō-loyd). The condition in which the lateral portion of the palpebral fissure is lower than the medial portion.

an·ti·mo·nid (an-tē-mō′nid). A chemical compound containing antimony in union with a more positive element; e.g., sodium a., Na_3Sb.

an·ti·mo·nous ox·ide (an-ti-mō′nŭs). SYN *antimony* trioxide.

an·ti·mo·ny (Sb) (an′-ti-mō-nē). A metallic element, atomic no. 51, atomic wt. 121.757, valences 0, −3, +3, +5; used in alloys; toxic and irritating to the skin and mucous membranes. SYN stibium. [G. *anti* + *monos,* not found alone]

a. chloride, SYN a. trichloride.

a. dimercaptosuccinate, an antiparasitic effective against *Schistosoma mansoni* and *S. haematobium.* SYN stibocaptate.

a. oxide, SYN a. trioxide.

a. potassium tartrate, a compound used as an expectorant and in the treatment of schistosomiasis japonicum, although it is extremely toxic and must be administered very slowly intravenously; common toxic manifestations are phlebitis, tachycardia, and hypotension; sudden deaths have been reported, chiefly from circulatory collapse. SYN potassium antimonyltartrate, tartar emetic, tartrated a.

a. sodium gluconate, SYN stibogluconate *sodium* (1).

a. sodium tartrate, used in the treatment of schistosomiasis, and as an emetic. SYN sodium antimonyl tartrate.

a. sodium thioglycollate, a compound of a. trioxide and thioglycolic acid, used for tropical parasites.

tartrated a., SYN a. potassium tartrate.

a. thioglycollamide, the triamide of a. thioglycolic acid; used in the treatment of trypanosomiasis, kala azar, and filariasis.

a. trichloride, combines with vitamin A to form a blue compound and with β-carotene to form a green one, as a method for assay of these substances; also used externally as a caustic. SYN a. chloride.

a. trioxide, used technically in paints and flame-proofing; also formerly used as an expectorant and emetic. SYN antimonous oxide, a. oxide, flowers of antimony.

an·ti·mo·nyl (an-tim′ō-nil). The univalent radical, SbO–, of antimony.

an·ti·mus·ca·rin·ic (an′tē-mŭs′kă-rin′ik). Inhibiting or preventing the actions of muscarine and muscarinelike agents, or the effects of parasympathetic stimulation at the neuroeffector junction (e.g., atropine).

an·ti·mu·ta·gen (an-tē-mū′tă-jen). A factor that reduces or interferes with the mutagenic actions or effects of a substance.

an·ti·mu·ta·gen·ic (an′tē-mū-tă-jen′ik). Pertaining to or characteristic of an antimutagen.

an·ti·my·as·then·ic (an′tē-mī′as-then′ik). Tending toward the correction of the symptoms of myasthenia gravis, e.g., as in the action of neostigmine.

an·ti·my·cot·ic (an′-tē-mī-kot′ik). Antagonistic to fungi. SYN antifungal. [anti- + G. *mykēs,* fungus]

an·ti·nau·se·ant (an-tē-naw′sē-ănt). Having an action to prevent nausea.

an·ti·ne·o·plas·tic (an′tē-nē-ō-plas′tik). Preventing the development, maturation, or spread of neoplastic cells.

anti·neo·plas·tons (an-tē-nē-ō-plas′-tonz). Mixtures of various chemicals such as amino acids and peptides, with theoretical support as natural defense aids against cancer and various other diseases.

an·ti·neu·ro·tox·in (an′tē-noo-rō-tok′sin). An antibody to a neurotoxin.

an·tin·i·ad (an-tin′ē-ad). Toward the antinion.

an·tin·i·al (an-tin′ē-ăl). Relating to the antinion.

an·tin·i·on (an-tin′ē-on). The space between the eyebrows; the point on the skull opposite the inion. SEE ALSO glabella. [anti- + G. *inion,* nape of the neck]

an·tin·o·my (an-tin′ō-mē). A contradiction between two principles, each of which is considered true. [anti- + G. *nomos,* law]

an·ti·nu·cle·ar (an-tē-noo′klē-er). Having an affinity for or reacting with the cell nucleus.

an·ti·o·don·tal·gic (an′tē-ō-don-tăl-jik). **1.** Relieving toothache. **2.** A toothache remedy. [anti- + G. *odous,* tooth, + *algos,* pain]

antioncogene. SYN tumor suppressor *gene.*

an·ti·ox·i·dant (an-tē-oks′ĭ-dant). An agent that inhibits oxidation; any of numerous chemical substances, including certain natural body products and nutrients, that can neutralize the oxidant effect of free radicals and other substances.

Free radicals, formed in the course of normal cellular respiration and metabolism, and more abundantly under the influence of certain environmental chemicals and sunlight, have been implicated in the causation of various types of tissue damage, particularly those involved in atherosclerosis, the aging process, and the development of cancer. A free radical is any atom or molecule that has 1 or more unpaired electrons and is therefore highly reactive, seeking to acquire electrons from other substances. Free radicals are normally scavenged from tissues by the antioxidant enzymes superoxide dismutase and glutathione peroxidase. Ubidecarenone (coenzyme Q10) is also thought to act as an antioxidant in mitochondrial respiration reactions. In addition, a number of nutrient substances, vitamins, and minerals have been shown to contribute to antioxidant functions, generally by serving as co-factors or co-enzymes. These include selenium, β-carotene, and vitamins C and E. It has been postulated that an imbalance between the production of free radicals and natural antioxidant processes may be a major causative factor in aging and in many chronic and degenerative disorders, and some have speculated that antioxidant nutrients may have a role in disease prevention. Oxidation of LDL cholesterol does indeed seem to be responsible for foam cell formation in the genesis of atherosclerotic plaques. In addition, free radicals have been shown to damage DNA in ways that can culminate in malignant change. But oxidation also occurs in many beneficial processes, including chemotaxis of cells with immunological functions, phagocytosis, clotting mechanisms, and apoptosis. Moreover, antioxidants do not exert their effects in only one way, but can act during initiation or propagation of reactions at a variety of intracellular and extracellular sites, and in some circumstances can be pro-oxidant. Claims that vitamins and other nutrients, when taken in massive doses, can prevent heart attack or cancer or retard aging are not based on scientific evidence. Although a high intake of antioxidant nutrients from food sources appears to offer some health advantages, there is at present no unequivocal evidence that any antioxidant nutrient, when taken in excess of normal dietary amounts, has value in the prevention or treatment of cardiovascular disease, cancer, or any other abnormal process except such as may be associated with frank nutritional or vitamin deficiency. In fact, although naturally occurring antioxidant nutrients are vital dietary components, they can cause adverse effects when large amounts are taken for prolonged periods. A controlled trial of β-carotene and retinol not only failed to show any benefit but was aborted when statistics showed large increases in the risk of death from lung cancer and cardiovascular disease.

an·ti·pain (an′tē-pā-in). A peptide that inhibits the proteolytic enzymes, papain, trypsin, and plasmin. [anti- + pa*pain*]

an·ti·par·al·lel (an-tē-par′ă-lel). Denoting molecules that are parallel but have opposite directional polarity; e.g., the two strands of a DNA double helix.

an·ti·par·a·sit·ic (an′tē-par-ă-sit′ik). Destructive to parasites.

an·ti·pe·dic·u·lar (an′tē-pe-dik′ū-lăr). Destructive to lice.

an·ti·pe·dic·u·lot·ic (an′tē-pe-dik-ū-lot′ik). Effective in the treatment of pediculosis, especially denoting such an agent.

an·ti·pe·ri·od·ic (an′tē-pēr-ē-od′ik). Preventing the regular recurrence of a disease (e.g., malaria) or a symptom.

an·ti·per·i·stal·sis (an′tē-per-i-stal′sis). SYN reversed *peristalsis.*

an·ti·per·i·stal·tic (an′tē-per-i-stal′tik). **1.** Relating to antiperistalsis. **2.** Impeding or arresting peristalsis.

an·ti·per·spi·rant (an-tē-per′spi-rant). **1.** Having an inhibitory action upon the secretion of sweat. **2.** An agent having such an action (e.g., aluminum chloride). SYN anhidrotic (2).

an·ti·phag·o·cyt·ic (an′tē-fag-ō-sit′-ik). Impeding or preventing the action of the phagocytes.

an·ti·phlo·gis·tic (an′tē-flō-jis′tik). **1.** Older term denoting preventing or relieving inflammation. **2.** An agent that reduces inflammation. SYN antipyrotic (1). [anti- + G. *phogistos,* burnt up]

an·ti·pho·bic (an-tē-fō′bik). A mechanism or drug designed to control phobias.

an·ti·plas·min (an-tē-plaz′min). A substance that inhibits or prevents the effects of plasmin; found in plasma and some tissues, especially the spleen and liver. SYN antifibrinolysin.

an·ti·plate·let (an-tē-plāt′let). A substance that manifests a lytic or agglutinative action on the blood platelets, thereby inhibiting or destroying the effects of the latter.

an·ti·pneu·mo·coc·cic (an′tē-noo-mō-kok′sik). Destructive to, or repressing the growth of, the pneumococcus (e.g., penicillin).

an·tip·o·dal (an-tip′ō-dăl). Denoting opposite positions; positioned at opposite sides of a cell or other body.

an·ti·pode (an′ti-pōd). That which is diametrically opposite. [G. *antipous,* with the feet opposite]

optic a., SYN enantiomer.

an·ti·port (an′tē-pōrt). The coupled transport of two different molecules or ions through a membrane in opposite directions by a common carrier mechanism (antiporter). Cf. symport, uniport. [anti- + L. *porto,* to carry]

an·ti·por·ter (an'tē-pōr-ter). A protein responsible for mediating the transport of two different molecules or ions simultaneously in opposite directions through a membrane.

an·ti·pre·cip·i·tin (an'tē-prē-sip'i-tin). A specific antibody that inhibits or prevents the effects of a precipitin.

an·ti·pro·ges·tin (an'tē-prō-jes'tin). A substance that inhibits progesterone formation, that interferes with its carriage or stability in the blood, or that reduces its uptake by, or effects on, target organs (e.g., RU-486).

an·ti·pro·throm·bin (an'tē-prō-throm'bin). An anticoagulant that inhibits or prevents the conversion of prothrombin into thrombin; examples are heparin, which is present in various tissues (especially in liver), and dicoumarin, which is isolated from partially decomposed sweet clover.

an·ti·pru·rit·ic (an'tē-proo-rit'ik). **1.** Preventing or relieving itching. **2.** An agent that relieves itching.

an·ti·psy·chot·ic (an'tē-sī-kot'ik). **1.** SYN antipsychotic *agent.* **2.** Denoting the actions of such an agent (e.g., chlorpromazine).

an·ti·pu·rine (an'tē-pūr'ēn). An analog of the purines and purine nucleotides that acts as an antimetabolite.

an·ti·py·o·gen·ic (an'tē-pī-ō-jen'ik). Preventing suppuration. [anti- + G. *pyon,* pus, + -*gen,* production]

an·ti·py·re·sis (an'tē-pī-rē'sis). Symptomatic treatment of fever rather than of the underlying disease.

an·ti·py·ret·ic (an'tē-pī-ret'ik). **1.** Reducing fever. SYN antifebrile, febrifugal. **2.** An agent that reduces fever (e.g., acetaminophen, aspirin). SYN febrifuge. [anti- + G. *pyretos,* fever]

an·ti·py·rim·i·dine (an'tē-pir-im'i-dēn). An analog of the pyrimidines and pyrimidine nucleotides that acts as an antimetabolite.

an·ti·py·rine (an-tē-pī'rin, -pī'rēn). An obsolescent analgesic and antipyretic.

  a. acetylsalicylate, a compound of a. and aspirin; an antirheumatic and analgesic.

  a. salicylacetate, an analgesic, antirheumatic, and antipyretic.

  a. salicylate, an analgesic and antipyretic; formerly used in dysmenorrhea, influenza, and acute rhinitis in the early stages.

an·ti·py·rot·ic (an'tē-pī-rot'ik). **1.** SYN antiphlogistic. **2.** Relieving the pain and promoting the healing of superficial burns. **3.** A topical application for burns. [anti- + G. *pyrōtikos,* burning, inflaming]

an·ti·ra·chit·ic (an'tē-ră-kit'ik). Promoting the cure of rickets or preventing its development (e.g., vitamin D preparations).

an·ti·rheu·mat·ic (an'tē-roo-mat'ik). **1.** Denoting an agent that suppresses manifestations of rheumatic disease; usually applied to antiinflammatory agents or agents that are capable of delaying progression of the basic disease process in inflammatory arthritis. **2.** An agent possessing such properties (e.g., gold compounds).

an·ti·ri·cin (an-tē-rī'sin). An antibody or antitoxin that inhibits or prevents the effects of ricin.

an·ti·ru·mi·nant (an-tē-roo'mi-nănt). Denoting a method to 1) control regurgitation of food or 2) break a compulsive trend of thought. [anti- + L. *rumino,* to chew the cud, fr. *rumen,* throat]

an·ti-S. See MNS blood group, Blood Groups appendix.

an·ti·scor·bu·tic (an'tē-skōr-bū'tik). **1.** Preventive or curative of scurvy (scorbutus). **2.** A treatment for scurvy (e.g., vitamin C).

an·ti·seb·or·rhe·ic (an'tē-seb-ō-rē'ik). **1.** Preventing or relieving excessive secretion of sebum; preventing or relieving seborrheic dermatitis. **2.** An agent having such actions.

an·ti·se·cre·to·ry (an'tē-sē-krē'tō-rī). Inhibitory to secretion, said of certain drugs that reduce or suppress gastric secretion (e.g., ranitidine, omeprazole).

an·ti·sense (an'tē-sens). SEE antisense DNA, antisense RNA.

an·ti·sep·sis (an-tē-sep'sis). Prevention of infection by inhibiting the growth of infectious agents. SEE ALSO disinfection. [anti- + G. *sēpsis,* putrefaction]

an·ti·sep·tic (an-tē-sep'tik). **1.** Relating to antisepsis. **2.** An agent or substance capable of effecting antisepsis.

an·ti·se·rum (an-tē-sē'rŭm). Serum that contains demonstrable

antibody or antibodies specific for one (monovalent or specific a.) or more (polyvalent a.) antigens; may be prepared from the blood of animals inoculated with an antigenic material or from the blood of animals and persons that have been stimulated by natural contact with an antigen (as in those who recover from an attack of disease). SYN immune serum.

  blood group a.'s, see Blood Groups appendix.

  heterologous a., an a. that reacts with (e.g., agglutinates) certain microorganisms or other complexes of antigens, even though the a. was produced by means of stimulation with a different microorganism or antigenic material. SEE ALSO homologous a.

  homologous a., an a. in which there is complete correspondence between the content of antibodies and the antigenic material used for producing the a.

  monovalent a., SEE antiserum.

  nerve growth factor a., an a. containing antibodies against nerve growth factor; when injected into newborn animals the majority of sympathetic ganglion cells are permanently destroyed, resulting in hypoinnervation of peripheral tissues. SYN NGF a.

  NGF a., SYN nerve growth factor a.

  polyvalent a., SEE antiserum.

  specific a., SEE antiserum.

an·ti·shock gar·ment. SEE military antishock trousers, pneumatic antishock *garment.*

an·ti·si·al·a·gogue (an-tē-sī-al'ă-gog). An agent that diminishes or arrests the flow of saliva (e.g., atropine). [anti- + G. *sialon,* saliva, + *agōgos,* drawing forth]

an·ti·si·der·ic (an-tē-sid'er-ik). Counteracting the physiological action of iron, probably by chelating or precipitation. [anti- + G. *sideros,* iron]

an·ti·so·cial (an-tē-sō'shŭl). Opposed to the rights of individuals or to the legal norms of society; e.g., the antisocial personality, the psychopath. Cf. asocial.

an·ti·spas·mod·ic (an'tē-spaz-mod'ik). **1.** Preventing or alleviating muscle spasms (cramps). **2.** An agent that quiets spasm.

an·ti·staph·y·lo·coc·cic (an'tē-staf'i-lō-kok'sik). Antagonistic to staphylococci or their toxins.

an·ti·staph·y·lol·y·sin (an'tē-staf-i-lol'i-sin). A substance that antagonizes or neutralizes the action of staphylolysin.

an·ti·ste·ap·sin (an'tē-stē-ap'sin). An antibody counteracting the action of triacylglycerol lipase (steapsin).

an·ti·strep·to·coc·cic (an'tē-strep-tō-kok'sik). Destructive to streptococci or antagonistic to their toxins.

an·ti·strep·to·ki·nase (an'tē-strep-tō-kī'nāz). An antibody that inhibits or prevents the dissolution of fibrin by streptokinase.

an·ti·strep·tol·y·sin (an'tē-strep-tol'i-sin). An antibody that inhibits or prevents the effects of streptolysin O elaborated by group A streptococci; the amount of a. in the serum is frequently increased during and after streptococcal disease, and comparative titers may be a diagnostic and prognostic aid.

an·ti·tac (an'-tē-tak). Monoclonal antibody that recognizes the alpha chain of the IL-2 receptor.

anti·ter·min·a·tion. A state of bacterial RNA polymerase wherein it is resistant to pause, arrest, or termination signals. SEE ALSO hesitant, overdrive.

an·ti·te·tan·ic (an'tē-te-tan'ik). Preventing or alleviating muscular contraction.

an·ti·the·nar (an-tē-thē'nar). SYN hypothenar *eminence.*

an·ti·throm·bin (an-tē-throm'bin). Any substance that inhibits or prevents the effects of thrombin in such a manner that blood does not coagulate. A deficiency of a. results in impaired inhibition of coagulation factors IIa, IXa, and Xa in plasma, causing recurrent thrombosis.

  a. III, a plasma α_2-globulin process that inhibits thrombin and has anticoagulant activities. Deficiency [MIM*107300] is commonly inherited as an autosomal dominant trait, caused by mutation in antithrombin III gene (AT_3) or chromosome 1q; this is one of the few known mendelizing disorders from which thrombotic disease occurs.

  normal a., an a. naturally occurring in blood and certain tissues under normal conditions in contrast to abnormal states or a. from other sources.

an·ti·thy·roid (an-tē-thī′royd). Relating to an agent that suppresses thyroid function (e.g., propylthiouracil).

an·ti·ton·ic (an-tē-ton′ik). Diminishing muscular or vascular tonus.

an·ti·tox·ic (an-tē-tok′sik). Neutralizing the action of a poison; specifically, relating to an antitoxin. SEE ALSO antidotal.

an·ti·tox·i·gen (an-tē-toks′i-jen). SYN antitoxinogen.

an·ti·tox·in (an-tē-tok′sin). Antibody formed in response to antigenic poisonous substances of biologic origin, such as bacterial exotoxins (e.g., those elaborated by *Clostridium tetani* or *Corynebacterium diphtheriae*), phytotoxins, and zootoxins; in general usage, a. refers to whole, or globulin fraction of, serum from persons or animals (usually horses) immunized by injections of the specific toxoid. A. neutralizes the pharmacologic effects of its specific toxin in vitro, and also in vivo if the toxin is not already fixed to the tissue cells. [anti- + G. *toxikon,* poison]

bivalent gas gangrene a., a. specific for the toxins of *Clostridium perfringens* and *C. septicum.*

bothropic a., a. specific for the venom of pit vipers of the genus *Bothrops* (*Bothrophora*) of the family Crotalidae. SYN Bothrops a.

Bothrops a., SYN bothropic a.

botulinum a., SYN botulism a.

botulism a., a. specific for a toxin of one or another strain of *Clostridium botulinum.* SYN botulinum a.

bovine a., a. prepared from cattle instead of horses, used in the treatment of persons who are sensitive to horse serum; the cattle are immunized against the toxin for which specific a. is desired.

Crotalus a., a. specific for venom of rattlesnakes (*Crotalus* species).

despeciated a., an antitoxic serum treated in an appropriate manner to alter the species-specific protein, so that a person sensitized to the animal protein is not likely to have a serious reaction when the a. is administered.

diphtheria a., a. specific for the toxin of *Corynebacterium diphtheriae.*

dysentery a., a. specific for the neurotoxin of *Shigella dysenteriae.*

gas gangrene a., a. specific for the toxin of one or more species of *Clostridium* that cause gas gangrene and associated toxemia, especially *C. perfringens, C. novyi, C. histolyticum,* and commercially available preparations are usually polyvalent, i.e., contain a. for two or more species. SYN pentavalent gas gangrene a.

normal a., serum that is capable of neutralizing an equivalent quantity of a normal toxin solution.

pentavalent gas gangrene a., SYN gas gangrene a.

plant a., a. specific for a phytotoxin.

scarlet fever a., a. specific for the erythrogenic toxin of certain strains of group A β-hemolytic streptococci.

staphylococcus a., a serum containing antitoxic globulins or their derivatives that specifically neutralize the lethal, skin-necrosing, and hemolytic properties of the α-toxin of *Staphylococcus aureus.*

tetanus a., a. specific for the toxin of *Clostridium tetani.*

tetanus and gas gangrene a.'s, a mixture of antibodies obtained from animals immunized against the toxins of *Clostridium tetani, C. perfringens,* and *C. septicum.*

tetanus-perfringens a., an a. prepared from animals immunized against the toxins of *Clostridium tetani* and *C. perfringens* (*C. welchii*).

an·ti·tox·in·o·gen (an′tē-tok-sin′ō-jen). Any antigen that stimulates the formation of antitoxin in an animal or person, i.e., a toxin or a toxoid. SYN antitoxigen. [antitoxin + G. *-gen,* producing]

an·ti·trag·i·cus (an′tē-traj′i-kŭs). SEE antitragicus (*muscle*).

an·ti·tra·go·hel·i·cine (an′tē-trā′gō-hel′i-sēn). SEE antitragohelicine *fissure.*

an·ti·tra·gus (an-tē-trā′gŭs) [TA]. A projection of the cartilage of the auricle, in front of the tail of the helix, just above the lobule, and posterior to the tragus from which it is separated by the intertragic notch. [G. *anti-tragos,* the eminence of the external ear, fr. *anti,* opposite, + *tragos,* a goat, the tragus]

an·ti·trep·o·ne·mal (an′tē-trep-ō-nē′măl). SYN treponemicidal.

an·ti·tris·mus (an-tē-triz′mŭs). A condition of tonic muscular spasm that prevents closing.

an·ti·trope (an′ti-trōp). An organ or appendage that forms a symmetrically reversed pair with another of the same type, e.g., the right and left legs of a vertebrate. [anti- + G. *tropē,* a turn]

an·ti·tro·pic (an-tē-trō′pik). Similar, bilaterally symmetrical, but in an opposite location (as in a mirror image), e.g., the right thumb in relation to the left thumb.

an·ti·tryp·sic (an-tē-trip′sik). SYN antitryptic.

an·ti·tryp·sin (an-tē-trip′sin). A substance that inhibits or prevents the action of trypsin.

α₁-a., A glycoprotein that is the major protease inhibitor of human serum, is synthesized in the liver, and is genetically polymorphic due to the presence of 25 alleles; individuals appropriately homozygous are deficient in α₁-trypsin and are predisposed to pulmonary emphysema and juvenile hepatic cirrhosis because of alterations in the amino acid and sialic acid components of the glycoprotein. The concentration of a. rises in response to injury or infection. A. also inhibits thrombin and elastase. SYN α₁-trypsin inhibitor, human α₁-protease inhibitor.

an·ti·tryp·tic (an-tē-trip′tik). Possessing properties of antitrypsin. SYN antitrypsic.

an·ti·tu·mor·i·gen·e·sis (an′tē-too-mōr-i-jen′ĕ-sis). Inhibition of the development of a neoplasm.

an·ti·tus·sive (an-tē-tŭs′iv). 1. Relieving cough. 2. A cough remedy (e.g., codeine). SYN antibechic. [anti- + L. *tussis,* cough]

an·ti·ty·phoid (an-tē-tī′foyd). Preventive or curative of typhoid fever.

an·ti·ve·nene (an-tē-vĕ-nēn′). SYN antivenin.

an·ti·ve·ne·re·al (an′tē-ve-nē′rē-ăl). Rarely used term for preventive or curative of venereal diseases. SYN antaphroditic (2).

an·ti·ven·in (an-tē-ven′in). An antitoxin specific for an animal or insect venom. SYN antivenene. [anti- + L. *venenum,* poison]

an·ti·vi·ral (an-tē-vī′răl). Opposing a virus; interfering with its replication; weakening or abolishing its action (e.g., zidovudine, acyclovir).

an·ti·vi·ta·min (an-tē-vī′tă-min). A substance that prevents a vitamin from exerting its typical biological effects. Most a.'s have chemical structures like those of vitamins (e.g., pyridoxine and its a., deoxypyridoxine) and appear to function as competitive antagonists; some a.'s produce effects, in addition, that are unrelated to vitamin antagonism.

an·ti·viv·i·sec·tion (an′tē-viv-i-sek′shŭn). Opposition to the use of living animals for experimentation. SEE vivisection.

an·ti·xe·roph·thal·mic (an′tē-zē-rof-thal′mik). Denoting agents (vitamin A and retinoic acid) that inhibit pathologic drying of the conjunctiva (xerophthalmia). [anti- + G. *xēros,* dry, + *ophthalmos,* eye]

an·ti·xe·rot·ic (an′tē-zē-rot′ik). Preventing xerosis.

Anton, Gabriel, German neuropsychiatrist, 1858–1933. SEE A. *syndrome.*

Antoni, Nils R., Swedish neurologist, 1887–1968. SEE A. type A *neurilemoma,* type B *neurilemoma.*

an·tra (an′tră). Plural of antrum.

an·tral (an′trăl). Relating to an antrum.

an·trec·to·my (an-trek′tō-mē). Removal of a portion of the walls of the maxillary antrum. Removal of the antrum (distal half) of the stomach; often combined with bilateral excision of portions of vagus nerve trunks (vagectomy) in treatment of peptic ulcer. Reconstruction of the continuity of the alimentary tract can be by a gastroduodenostomy (Billroth I) or a loop gastrojejunostomy (Billroth II). [antrum + G. *ektomē,* excision]

⬡**antro-.** An antrum. [L. *antrum,* from G. *antron,* a cave]

an·tro·na·sal (an-trō-nā′săl). Relating to a maxillary sinus and the corresponding nasal cavity.

an·tro·phose (an′trō-fōz). A subjective sensation of light or color originating in the visual centers of the brain. SEE ALSO phosphene. [antro- + G. *phos,* light]

an·tro·py·lo·ric (an′trō-pī-lōr′ik). Related to or affecting the pyloric antrum.

an·tro·scope (an′trō-skōp). An instrument to aid in the visual examination of any cavity, particularly the antrum of Highmore (maxillary sinus). [antro- + G. *skopeō,* to view]

an·tros·co·py (an-tros′cō-pē). Examination of any cavity, especially of the antrum of Highmore (maxillary sinus), by means of an antroscope.

an·tros·to·my (an-tros′tō-mē). Formation of a permanent opening into any antrum (maxillary sinus). [antro- + G. *stoma,* mouth]
   intraoral a., SYN Caldwell-Luc *operation.*

an·trot·o·my (an-trot′ō-mē). Incision through the wall of any antrum. [antro- + G. *tomē,* incision]

an·tro·to·nia (an-trō-tō′nē-ă). Tonus of the muscular walls of an antrum, such as that of the stomach.

an·tro·tym·pan·ic (an′trō-tim-pan′ik). Relating to the mastoid antrum and the tympanic cavity.

an·trum, gen. **an·tri,** pl. **an·tra** (an′trŭm, -trī, -tră) [TA]. **1.** Any nearly closed cavity, particularly one with bony walls. **2.** SYN pyloric a. [L. fr. G. *antron,* a cave]
   a. au′ris, SYN external acoustic *meatus.*
   cardiac a., a dilation that occasionally occurs in the abdominal part of esophagus. SEE ALSO abdominal *part* of esophagus. SYN a. cardiacum, forestomach.
   a. cardi′acum, SYN cardiac a.
   antra ethmoida′lia, SYN ethmoid *cells,* under *cell.*
   follicular a., the cavity of an ovarian follicle filled with liquor folliculi.
   a. of Highmore, SYN maxillary *sinus.*
   mastoid a. [TA], a cavity in the petrous portion of the temporal bone, communicating posteriorly with the mastoid cells and anteriorly with the epitympanic recess of the middle ear via the aperture of the mastoid a. SYN a. mastoideum [TA], tympanic a., Valsalva a.
   a. mastoid′eum [TA], SYN mastoid a.
   maxillary a., SYN maxillary *sinus.*
   pyloric a. [TA], the initial portion of the pyloric part of the stomach, which may temporarily become partially or completely shut off from the remainder of the stomach during digestion by peristaltic contraction of the prepyloric "sphincter"; it is sometimes demarcated from the second part of the pyloric part of the stomach (pyloric canal) by a slight groove. SYN a. pyloricum [TA], antrum (2) [TA], lesser cul-de-sac.
   a. pylor′icum [TA], SYN pyloric a.
   tympanic a., SYN mastoid a.
   Valsalva a., SYN mastoid a.

ANTU Abbreviation for α-naphthylthiourea.

Antyllus, Greek physician, *ca.* 150 A.D. SEE A. *method.*

ANUG Abbreviation for acute necrotizing ulcerative *gingivitis.*

an·u·lar (an′ū-lar). Ring-shaped. SYN annular.

an·u·lus, pl. **an·u·li** (an′ū-lŭs, -lī) [TA]. SYN ring (1). [L.]
   a. abdomina′lis, SYN deep inguinal *ring.*
   a. cilia′ris, SYN ciliary *body.*
   a. conjuncti′vae [TA], SYN conjunctival *ring.*
   a. femora′lis [TA], SYN femoral *ring.*
   a. fibrocartilagin′eus membra′nae tympa′ni [TA], SYN fibrocartilaginous *ring* of tympanic membrane.
   a. fibro′sus [TA], **(1)** SYN (right and left) fibrous *rings* of heart, under *ring*; **(2)** SYN a. fibrosus of intervertebral disk.
   a. fibro′sus dexter/sinister cordis, SYN (right and left) fibrous *rings* of heart, under *ring.*
   a. fibro′sus dis′ci intervertebra′lis [TA], SYN a. fibrosus of intervertebral disk.
   a. fibrosus of intervertebral disk [TA], the ring of fibrocartilage and fibrous tissue forming the circumference of the intervertebral disk; surrounds the nucleus pulposus, which is prone to herniation when the a. fibrosus is compromised. SYN a. fibrosus disci intervertebralis [TA], a. fibrosus (2) [TA], fibrous ring of intervertebral disk, fibrous ring (2).

a. of fibrous sheath, SYN anular *part* of fibrous digital sheath of digits of hand and foot.
Haller a., SYN Haller *insula.*
a. hemorrhoida′lis, SYN hemorrhoidal *zone.*
a. inguina′lis profun′dus [TA], SYN deep inguinal *ring.*
a. inguina′lis superficia′lis, SYN superficial inguinal *ring.*
a. ir′idis [TA], SYN *border* of iris.
a. iridis major [TA], SYN outer *border* of iris.
a. iridis minor [TA], SYN inner *border* of iris.
a. lymphat′icus car′diae [TA], SYN *lymph nodes* around cardia of stomach, under *lymph node.*
a. lymphoideus pharyngis [TA], SYN pharyngeal lymphatic *ring.*
a. ova′lis, SYN *limbus* fossae ovalis.
a. tendin′eus commu′nis, SYN common tendinous *ring* of extraocular muscles.
a. tympan′icus, SYN tympanic *ring.*
a. umbilica′lis, SYN umbilical *ring.*
a. urethra′lis, SYN internal urethral *sphincter.*
Vieussens a., SYN *limbus* fossae ovalis.
a. of Zinn, SYN common tendinous *ring* of extraocular muscles.

an·u·ria (an-ū′rē-ă). Absence of urine formation.
an·u·ric (an-ūr′ik). Relating to anuria.
anus, gen. and pl. **ani** (ā′nŭs, -nī) [TA]. The lower opening of the digestive tract, lying in the cleft between the buttocks, through which fecal matter is extruded. SYN anal orifice. [L.]
   Bartholin a., SYN *opening* of aqueduct of midbrain.
   a. cer′ebri, obsolete term for *opening* of aqueduct of midbrain.
   imperforate a., SYN anal *atresia.*
   a. vesica′lis, rectal emptying into the urinary bladder.
   vesicalis a. (ve-sī′kal-is), imperforate a. with urinary bladder opening into the a.
   vestibular a., vulvovaginal a., a congenital malformation in which the a. is imperforate but the rectum opens into the vagina just above the vulva.
an·vil. SYN incus.
anx·i·e·ty (ang-zī′ĕ-tē). **1.** Fear or apprehension or dread of impending danger and accompanied by restlessness, tension, tachycardia, and dyspnea unattached to a clearly identifiable stimulus. **2.** In experimental psychology, a drive or motivational state learned from and thereafter associated with previously neutral cues. [L. *anxietas,* anxiety, fr. *anxius,* distressed, fr. *ango,* to press tight, to torment]
   a. attack, an acute episode of anxiety.
   castration a., SYN castration *complex.*
   free-floating a., in psychoanalysis, a pervasive unrealistic expectation unattached to a clearly formulated concept or object of fear; observed particularly in a. neurosis and may be seen in some cases of latent schizophrenia.
   noetic a., in existential psychotherapy, a. caused by confusion or loss of meaning in life.
   separation a., a child's apprehension or fear associated with removal from or loss of a parent or significant other.
   situation a., a. related to current life problems.
anx·i·o·lyt·ic (ang′zē-ō-lit′ik). **1.** SYN antianxiety *agent.* **2.** Denoting the actions of such an agent (e.g., diazepam). [anxiety + G. *lysis,* a dissolution or loosening]
AOC Abbreviation for anodal opening *contraction.*
Aon·cho·the·ca (ā-on-kō-the′ka). One of three trichurid nematode genera, commonly referred to as *Capillaria.*
aor·ta, gen. and pl. **aor·tae** (ā-ōr′tă, ā-ōr′tē) [TA]. A large artery of the elastic type that is the main trunk of the systemic arterial system, arising from the base of the left ventricle and ending at the left side of the body of the fourth lumbar vertebra by dividing to form the right and left common iliac arteries. The a. is subdivided into: ascending a.; aortic arch; and descending a., which is in turn, divided into the thoracic a. and the abdominal a. SYN arteria aorta. [Mod. L. fr. G. *aortē,* from *aeirō,* to lift up]
   abdominal a. [TA], the part of the descending a. that supplies structures below the diaphragm. SYN pars abdominalis aortae [TA], a. abdominalis☆, abdominal part of aorta.

a. abdomina′lis, ☆official alternate term for abdominal a.

a. angus′ta, congenital narrowness of a.

a. ascen′dens, ☆official alternate term for ascending a.

ascending a. [TA], the part of the a. prior to the aortic arch from which arise the coronary arteries. SYN pars ascendens aortae [TA], a. ascendens☆, ascending part of aorta.

buckled a., SYN pseudocoarctation.

a. descen′dens, ☆official alternate term for descending a.

descending a. [TA], a part of the a., further divided into the thoracic a. and the abdominal a. SYN pars descendens aortae [TA], a. descendens☆, descending part of aorta.

dynamic a., abnormally marked pulsations of a.

kinked a., SYN pseudocoarctation.

overriding a., a congenitally malpositioned a. whose origin straddles the ventricular septum and so receives ejected blood from the right ventricle as well as from the left; it is found especially in tetralogy of Fallot.

primitive a., the paired aortic primordia in young embryos.

pseudocoarctation of the a., a rare abnormality of the arch of the a. that constricts that vessel but is not a true coarctation in that there is no significant encroachment on the lumen.

shaggy a., a colloquial but fitting description for severe arterial degeneration of the aorta, the surface of which is extremely friable and likely to cause atheroembolism.

thoracic a. [TA], the part of the descending a. that supplies structures as far down as the diaphragm. SYN pars thoracica aortae [TA], a. thoracica☆, thoracic part of aorta.

a. thorac′ica, ☆official alternate term for thoracic a.

ventral aortas, the paired vessels ventral to the pharynx, which give rise to the aortic arches.

aor·tal (ā-ōr′tăl). SYN aortic.

aor·tal·gia (ā-ōr-tal′jē-ă). Pain assumed to be due to aneurysm or other pathologic conditions of the aorta. [aorta + G. *algos,* pain]

aor·tarc·tia (ā-ōr-tark′shē-ă). SYN aortostenosis. [aorta + L. *arcto,* properly *arto,* to narrow]

aor·tar·tia (ā-ōr-tar′shē-ă). SYN aortostenosis.

aor·tec·ta·sis, aor·tec·ta·sia (ā-ōr-tek′tă-sis, -tek-tā′zē-ă). Dilation of aorta. [aorta + G. *ektasis,* a stretching]

aor·tec·to·my (ā-ōr-tek′tō-mē). Excision of a portion of the aorta. [aorta + G. *ektomē,* excision]

aor·tic (ā-ōr′tik). Relating to the aorta or the a. orifice of the left ventricle of the heart. SYN aortal.

aor·tic cur·tain. An intertrigonal sheet of fibrous tissue between the aortic annulus and the anterior leaflet of the mitral valve.

aor·ti·co·re·nal (ā-ōr′ti-kō-rē′năl). Related to the aorta and kidney, specifically the ganglion aorticorenale.

aor·ti·tis (ā-ōr-tī′tis). Inflammation of the aorta.

giant cell a., giant cell arteritis involving the aorta.

syphilitic a., a common manifestation of tertiary syphilis, involving the thoracic aorta, where destruction of elastic tissue in the media results in dilation and aneurysm formation.

aor·to·cor·o·nary (ā-ōr′tō-kōr′ō-nār-ē). Relating to the aorta and the coronary arteries.

aor·to·gram (ā-ōr′tō-gram). The image or set of images resulting from aortography.

aor·tog·ra·phy (ā-ōr-tog′ră-fē). **1.** Radiographic imaging of the aorta and its branches, or a portion of the aorta, by injection of contrast medium. **2.** Imaging of the aorta by ultrasound or magnetic resonance. [aorta + G. *graphō,* to write]

retrograde a., a. by the injection of contrast medium into the aorta through one of its branches, e.g., the brachial artery, in a direction against normal arterial blood flow.

translumbar a., early method of a. by injection into the abdominal aorta through a needle just below the twelfth rib and four fingerbreadths to the left of the spinous process of the vertebra.

aor·top·a·thy (ā-ōr-top′ă-thē). Disease affecting the aorta. [aorta + G. *pathos,* suffering]

aor·to·pex·y. A surgical procedure used to treat tracheomalacia or tracheal compression.

aor·to·plas·ty (ā-ōr′tō-plas′tē). A procedure for surgical repair of the aorta.

aor·top·to·sia, aor·top·to·sis (ā-ōr-top-tō′zē-ă, -top-tō′sis). A sinking down of the abdominal aorta in splanchnoptosia. [aorta + G. *ptōsis,* a failing]

aor·tor·rha·phy (ā-ōr-tōr′ă-fē). Suture of the aorta. [aorta + G. *rhaphē,* seam]

aor·to·scle·ro·sis (ā-ōr′tō-skler-ō′sis). Arteriosclerosis of the aorta.

aor·to·ste·no·sis (ā-ōr-tō-stĕ-nō′sis). Narrowing of the aorta. SYN aortarctia, aortartia. [aorta + G. *stenōsis,* a narrowing]

aor·tot·o·my (ā-ōr-tot′ō-mē). Incision of the aorta. [aorta + G. *tomē,* a cutting]

AP Abbreviation for *area* postrema.

APA Abbreviation for antipernicious anemia *factor.*

apall·es·the·sia (ă-pal-es-thē′zē-ă). SYN pallanesthesia. [G. *a*-priv. + *pallo,* to tremble, quiver, + *aisthēsis,* feeling]

apal·lic (ă-pal′ik). SYN apallic state. [G. *a*- priv. + L. *pallium,* brain mantle (cerebral cortex)]

apan·cre·at·ic (ā-pan-krē-at′ik). Without a pancreas.

apar·a·lyt·ic (ā-par′ă-lit′ik). Without paralysis; not causing paralysis.

apar·a·thy·re·o·sis (ă-par-ă-thī′rē-ō- sis). hypoparathyroidism, especially that caused by removal of the parathyroid glands. [G. *a*- priv. + parathyroid + *-osis,* condition]

apar·a·thy·roid·ism (ā-par-ă-thī′royd-izm). Congenital absence, deficiency, or surgical removal of the parathyroid glands.

apa·reu·nia (ā-par-ū′nē-ă). Absence or impossibility of coitus. [G. *a*- priv. + *para,* alongside, + *eunē,* bed]

ap·a·thet·ic (ap-ă-thet′ik). Exhibiting apathy; indifferent.

ap·a·thism (ap′ă-thizm). A sluggishness of reaction.

ap·a·thy (ap′ă-thē). Indifference; absence of interest in the environment. Often one of the earliest signs of cerebral disease. [G. *apatheia,* fr. *a*- priv. + *pathos,* suffering]

ap·a·tite (ap′ă-tīt). **1.** Generic name for a class of minerals with compositions that are variants of the formula D_5T_3M, where D is a divalent cation, T is a trivalent tetrahedral compound ion, and M is a monovalent anion; calcium phosphate a.'s are important mineral constituents of bones and teeth. SEE hydroxyapatite. **2.** $Ca_5(PO_4)_3(OH,F,Cl)$.

APC Acronym for *a*cetylsalicylic acid, *p*henacetin, and *c*affeine combined as a formerly widely used antipyretic and analgesic; antigen-presenting *cells,* under *cell.*

A-P-C 1. Abbreviation for adenoidal-pharyngeal-conjunctival. **2.** Antigen-presenting cell.

apel·lous (ă-pel′ŭs). **1.** Without skin. **2.** Without foreskin; circumcised. [G. *a*- priv + L. *pellis,* skin]

ap·en·ter·ic (ap-en-ter′ik). An obsolete term for abenteric. [G. *apo,* from, + *enteron,* intestine]

apep·sin·ia (ā-pep-sin′ē-ă). Rarely used term for lack of pepsin in the gastric juice.

ape·ri·od·ic (ā-pēr-ē-od′ik). Not occurring periodically.

aper·i·stal·sis (ā′per-i-stal′sis). Absence of peristalsis.

aper·i·tive (ă-per′i-tiv). Stimulating the appetite. [Fr. *apéritif,* from L. *aperio,* to open]

Apert, Eugène, French pediatrician, 1868–1940. SEE A. *syndrome.*

aper·to·gnath·ia (ă-per-tō-nath′ē-ă). An open bite deformity, a type of malocclusion characterized by premature posterior occlusion and absence of anterior occlusion. SYN open bite (2). [L. *apertus,* open, + G. *gnathos,* jaw]

ap·er·tom·e·ter (ap-er-tom′ē-ter). Instrument for measuring the angular aperture of a microscope objective.

ap·er·tu·ra, pl. **ap·er·tu·rae** (ap-er-too′ră, -rē) [TA]. SYN aperture. [L. fr. *aperio,* pp. *apertus,* to open]

a. aqueductus cerebri, ☆official alternate term for *opening* of aqueduct of midbrain.

a. aqueductus mesencephali [TA], SYN *opening* of aqueduct of midbrain.

a. canalic′uli coch′leae, SYN external *opening* of cochlear canalic-ulus.

a. canaliculi vestib′uli, SYN *opening* of vestibular canaliculus.

a. latera′lis ventric′uli quar′ti [TA], SYN lateral *aperture* of fourth ventricle.

a. media′na ventric′uli quar′ti [TA], SYN median *aperture* of fourth ventricle.

a. pel′vis infe′rior [TA], SYN pelvic *outlet*.

a. pel′vis mino′ris, SYN pelvic *outlet*.

a. pel′vis supe′rior [TA], SYN pelvic *inlet*.

a. pirifor′mis [TA], SYN piriform *aperture*.

a. si′nus fronta′lis [TA], SYN *opening* of frontal sinus.

a. si′nus sphenoidal′is [TA], SYN *opening* of the sphenoidal sinus.

a. thora′cis infe′rior [TA], SYN inferior thoracic *aperture*.

a. thora′cis supe′rior [TA], SYN superior thoracic *aperture*.

a. tympan′ica canalic′uli chor′dae tym′pani [TA], SYN tympanic *aperture* of caniculus for chorda tympani.

ap·er·ture (ap′er-choor) [TA]. **1.** An inlet or entrance to a cavity or channel. in anatomy, an open gap or hole. SEE ALSO fossa, ostium, orifice, pore. **2.** The diameter of the objective of a microscope. SYN aditus [TA], apertura [TA]. [L. *apertura,* an opening]

angular a., the angle, in air, of light that passes from the object to the ends of the diameter of the front lens of the microscope objective.

external acoustic a., ☆official alternate term for external acous-tic *pore*.

external a. of cochlear canaliculus, SYN external *opening* of cochlear canaliculus.

external a. of vestibular aqueduct, SYN *opening* of vestibular canaliculus.

frontal sinus a., SYN *opening* of frontal sinus.

inferior pelvic a., SYN pelvic *outlet*.

inferior thoracic a. [TA], the inferior boundary of the bony thorax composed of the twelfth thoracic vertebra and the lower margins of the rib cage and sternum. SYN apertura thoracis inferior [TA], thoracic outlet (1).

laryngeal a., SYN laryngeal *inlet*.

lateral a. of fourth ventricle [TA], one of the two lateral open-ings of the fourth ventricle into the subarachnoid space (the lateral cerebellomedullary cistern) at the cerebellopontine angle. SYN ap-ertura lateralis ventriculi quarti [TA], foramen lateralis ventriculi quarti, foramen of Key-Retzius, foramen of Luschka, foramen of Retzius.

a. of mastoid antrum, SYN *aditus* to mastoid antrum.

median a. of fourth ventricle [TA], the large midline opening in the posterior inferior part of the roof of the fourth ventricle, connecting the ventricle with the posterior cerebellomedullary cistern. SYN apertura mediana ventriculi quarti [TA], arachnoid foramen, foramen of Magendie.

numerical a. (N.A.), defined by the formula *n* sine *a*, where *n* is the refractive index of the medium between the object and objec-tive lens and *a* is the angle between the central and the marginal ray entering the objective.

a. of orbit, SYN orbital *opening*.

piriform a. [TA], the anterior nasal opening in the skull. SYN apertura piriformis [TA], piriform opening.

posterior nasal a.'s, ☆official alternate term for choanae.

sphenoidal sinus a., SYN *opening* of the sphenoidal sinus.

superior pelvic a., SYN pelvic *inlet*.

superior thoracic a. [TA], the upper boundary of the bony thorax composed of the first thoracic vertebra and the upper margins of the first ribs and manubrium of the sternum. Note: clinicians refer to the superior thoracic aperture as the "thoracic outlet." as in "thoracic outlet syndrome." SYN apertura thoracis superior [TA], thoracic inlet, thoracic outlet (2).

tympanic a. of canaliculus for chorda tympani [TA], the small canal opening found lateral to the pyramidal eminence in the posterior wall of the middle ear cavity from which the chorda tympani nerve emerges to pass anteriorly between the ossicles accompanied by a branch of the stylomastoid artery. SYN apertura tympanica canaliculi chordae tympani [TA], tympanic opening of canaliculus for chorda tympani.

apex, gen. **ap·i·cis,** pl. **ap·i·ces** (ā′peks, ap′i-sis, ap′i-sēs) [TA]. The extremity of a conical or pyramidal structure, such as the heart or the lung. [L. summit or tip]

a. of arytenoid cartilage [TA], the pointed upper end of the cartilage that supports the corniculate cartilage and the aryepiglot-tic fold. SYN a. cartilaginis arytenoideae [TA].

a. of auricle [TA], a point projecting upward and posteriorly from the free outcurved margin of the helix a little posterior to its upper end. SYN a. auriculae [TA], tip of ear ☆, a. satyri, tip of auricle, Woolner tip.

a. auric′ulae, SYN a. of auricle.

a. cap′itis fib′ulae [TA], SYN a. of head of fibula.

a. cartila′ginis arytenoi′deae [TA], SYN a. of arytenoid cartilage.

a. cor′dis [TA], SYN a. of heart.

a. cor′nus posterio′ris [TA], SYN a. of posterior horn.

a. cus′pidis den′tis [TA], SYN a. of cusp of tooth.

a. of cusp of tooth [TA], the tip of the peaklike projections from the crown of a tooth. SYN a. cuspidis dentis [TA].

a. of dens [TA], the tip of the dens of the axis to which is attached the apical ligament of the dens. SYN a. dentis [TA].

a. den′tis [TA], SYN a. of dens.

a. of head of fibula [TA], the pointed upper end of the fibular head to which is attached the arcuate popliteal ligament and part of the biceps femoris tendon. SYN a. capitis fibulae [TA], styloid process of fibula.

a. of heart [TA], the blunt extremity of the heart formed by the left ventricle. SEE apex *beat*. SYN a. cordis [TA], vertex cordis.

a. lin′guae [TA], SYN a. of tongue.

a. of lung [TA], the rounded, upper extremity of each lung that extends into the cupula of the pleura. SYN a. pulmonis [TA].

a. na′si [TA], SYN a. of nose.

a. of nose [TA], anteriormost pointed end of external nose. SYN a. nasi [TA], tip of nose ☆.

a. of orbit, the posterior part of the orbit into which the optic canal opens; forms the tip of the pyramidal space.

a. os′sis sa′cri [TA], SYN a. of sacrum.

a. par′tis petro′sae ossis temporalis [TA], SYN a. of petrous part of temporal bone.

a. of patella [TA], the pointed inferior end of the patella from which the ligamentum patellae passes to insert on the tibial tuber-osity. SYN a. patellae [TA].

a. patel′lae [TA], SYN a. of patella.

a. of petrous part of temporal bone [TA], the irregular antero-medial extremity of the petrous part on which the anterior end of the carotid canal opens. SYN a. partis petrosae ossis temporalis [TA].

a. of posterior horn [TA], the pointed extremity of each posterior gray column or cornu of the spinal cord. SYN a. cornus posterioris [TA], tip of posterior horn.

a. pro′statae [TA], SYN a. of prostate.

a. of prostate [TA], the lowermost part of the prostate, situated above the urogenital diaphragm. SYN a. prostatae [TA].

a. pulmo′nis [TA], SYN a. of lung.

a. rad′icis den′tis [TA], SYN root a.

root a. [TA], the tip of a tooth root, that part farthest from the incisal or occlusal side. SYN a. radicis dentis [TA], root tip, tip of tooth root.

a. of sacrum [TA], the tapering lower end of the sacrum that articulates with the coccyx. SYN a. ossis sacri [TA].

a. sat′yri, SYN a. of auricle.

a. of tongue [TA], the anterior extreme of the tongue which can be made pointed for sensing or probing and which rests against the lingual aspect of the incisor teeth. SYN a. linguae [TA], tip of tongue ☆.

a. of (urinary) bladder [TA], the junction of the superior and anteroinferior surfaces of the bladder, continuous above with the median umbilical ligament. SYN a. vesicae.

a. vesi′cae, SYN a. of (urinary) bladder.

apex·car·di·o·gram (ā-peks-kar'dē-ō-gram). Graphic recording of the movements of the chest wall produced by the apex beat of the heart.

apex·car·di·og·ra·phy (ā'peks-kar'dē-og-ră-fē). Noninvasive graphic recording of cardiac pulsations from the region of the apex, usually of the left ventricle, and resembling the ventricular pressure curve.

apex·i·fi·ca·tion (ā-pek'si-fi-kā'shŭn). Induced tooth root development or closure of the root apex by hard tissue deposition.

apex·i·graph (ā-pek'si-graf). A device for determining the size and position of the apex of a tooth root. [apex + G. *graphō*, to write]

APF Abbreviation for animal protein *factor*.

Apgar, Virginia, U.S. anesthesiologist, 1909–1974. SEE A. *score*.

apha·gia (ă-fā'jē-ă). Inability to eat. [G. *a-* priv. + *phagō*, to eat]

apha·kia (ă-fā'kē-ă). Absence of the lens of the eye. [G. *a-* priv. + *phakos,* lentil, anything shaped like a lentil]

apha·lan·gia (ā-fă-lan'jē-ă). Congenital absence of a digit, or more specifically, absence of one or more of the long bones (phalanges) of a finger or toe. [G. *a-* priv. + phalanx]

apha·sia (ă-fā'zē-ă). Impaired or absent comprehension or production of, or communication by, speech, writing, or signs, due to an acquired lesion of the dominant cerebral hemisphere. SYN alogia (1). [G. speechlessness, fr. *a-* priv. + *phasis,* speech]

acoustic a., SYN auditory a.

acquired epileptic a., SYN Landau-Kleffner *syndrome.*

amnestic a., amnesic a., SYN nominal a.

anomic a., SYN nominal a.

anterior a., SYN motor a.

associative a., SYN conduction a.

ataxic a., SYN motor a.

auditory a., an impairment in comprehension of the auditory forms of language and communication, including the ability to write from dictation in the presence of normal hearing. Spontaneous speech, reading, and writing are not affected. SYN acoustic a., word deafness.

Broca a., SYN motor a.

conduction a., a form of a. in which the patient understands spoken and written words, is aware of his deficit, and can speak and write, but skips or repeats words, or substitutes one word for another (paraphasia); word repetition is severely impaired. The responsible lesion is in the associate tracts connecting the various language centers. SYN associative a.

crossed a., a. in a right-handed person due to a solely right cerebral lesion.

expressive a., SYN motor a.

fluent a., SYN sensory a.

functional a., nonorganic a. related to conversion hysteria.

global a., in which all aspects of speech and communication are severely impaired. At best, patients can understand or speak only a few words or phrases; they cannot read or write. SYN mixed a., total a.

graphic a., SYN agraphia.

graphomotor a., SYN agraphia.

impressive a., SYN sensory a.

jargon a., SYN agrammatism.

mixed a., SYN global a.

motor a., a type of a. in which there is a deficit in speech production or language output, often accompanied by a deficit in communicating by writing, signs, etc. The patient is aware of the impairment. SYN anterior a., ataxic a., Broca a., expressive a., nonfluent a.

nominal a., an a. in which the principal deficit is difficulty in naming persons and objects seen, heard, or felt; due to lesions in various portions of the language area. SYN amnestic a., amnesic a., anomia, anomic a.

nonfluent a., SYN motor a.

pathematic a., mutism related to anger or strong emotions.

posterior a., SYN sensory a.

psychosensory a., SYN sensory a.

pure a.'s, rare a.'s affecting only one type of communication, e.g., reading, while related communication forms such as writing, auditory comprehension, etc. remain intact.

receptive a., SYN sensory a.

semantic a., a. in which objects are correctly named; there is little disturbance in the articulation of words; individual words are understood, but the broader meaning of what is heard cannot be grasped.

sensory a., a. in which there is impairment in the comprehension of spoken and written words, associated with effortless, articulated, but paraphrastic, speech and writing; malformed words, substitute words, and neologisms are characteristic. When severe, and speech is incomprehensible, it is called jargon a. The patient often appears unaware of the deficit. SYN fluent a., impressive a., posterior a., psychosensory a., receptive a., Wernicke a.

syntactical a., a. in which the words are fairly well pronounced but are spoken in short phrases or poorly constructed sentences without articles, prepositions, or conjunctions.

total a., SYN global a.

transcortical a., an a. in which the unaffected motor and sensory language areas are isolated from the rest of the hemispheric cortex. Subdivided into transcortical sensory and transcortical motor a.'s.

visual a., (1) SYN alexia; (2) improperly used as a synonym for anomia.

Wernicke a., SYN sensory a.

apha·si·ac, apha·sic (ă-fā'zē-ak, ă-fā'sik). Relating to or suffering from aphasia.

apha·si·ol·o·gist (ă-fā'zē-ol'ŏ-gist). A specialist who deals with speech disorders caused by dysfunction of the language areas of the brain.

apha·si·ol·o·gy (ă-fā'zē-ol'ŏ-gē). The science of speech disorders caused by dysfunction of the cerebral language areas.

aphas·mid (ā-faz'mid). 1. Lacking phasmids, as seen in nematodes of the class Adenophorasida (Aphasmidia). 2. Common name for a member of the class Aphasmidia, now Adenophorasida.

Aphas·mid·ia (ā-faz-mid'ē-ă). SYN Adenophorasida.

aph·e·li·ot·ro·pism (ap-hē-lē-ot'rō-pizm). Negative heliotaxis. [G. *apo,* away, + *helios,* sun, + *tropein,* to turn]

apher·e·sis (ā-fer-ē'sis). Infusion of a patient's own blood from which certain cellular or fluid elements (plasma, leukocytes, platelets, etc.) have been removed. [G. *aphairesis,* withdrawal]

aphil·op·o·ny (ā-fil-op'ō-nē). Obsolete term for an aversion, or lack of desire, to work. [G. *a-* priv. + *philō,* to like, + *ponos,* work]

apho·nia (ă-fō'nē-ă). Loss of the voice as a result of disease or injury to the larynx. [G. *a-* priv. + *phōnē,* voice]

hysterical a., loss of voice for psychogenic reasons, as in some varieties of hysteria. SYN nonorganic a.

nonorganic a., SYN hysterical a.

a. paralyt'ica, a. due to paralysis of the vocal cords.

spastic a., a. caused by spasmodic contraction of the laryngeal adductor muscles provoked by attempted phonation.

aphon·ic (ă-fon'ik). Relating to aphonia. SYN aphonous.

aph·o·nous (af'ō-nŭs). SYN aphonic.

apho·tes·the·sia (ă-fō-tes-thē'zē-ă). Decreased sensitivity of the retina to light caused by excessive exposure to sunlight. [G. *a-* priv. + *phōs,* light, + *aisthēsis,* perception]

aphra·sia (ă-frā'zē-ă). Inability to speak, from any cause. [G. *a-* priv. + *phrasis,* speaking]

aph·ro·di·sia (af-rō-diz'ē-ă). Sexual desire, especially when excessive. [G. *aphrodisios,* relating to Aphrodite]

aph·ro·di·si·ac (af-rō-diz'ē-ak). 1. Increasing sexual desire. 2. Anything that arouses or increases sexual desire.

aph·ro·di·si·o·ma·nia (af-rō-diz'ē-ō-mā'nē-ă). Abnormal and excessive erotic interest. [G. *aphrodisia,* sexual pleasures, + *mania,* insanity]

aph·tha, pl. **aph·thae** (af'thă, af'thē). 1. In the singular, a small ulcer on a mucous membrane. 2. In the plural, stomatitis charactized by intermittent episodes of painful oral ulcers of unknown etiology that are covered by gray exudate, are surrounded by an erythematous halo, and range from several millimeters to 2 cm in diameter; they are limited to oral mucous membranes that are not bound to periosteum, occur as solitary or multiple lesions, and heal spontaneously in 1–2 weeks. SYN aphthae minor, aphthous stomatitis, canker sores, recurrent aphthous stomatitis, recurrent aphthous ulcers, recurrent ulcerative stomatitis, ulcerative stomatitis. [G. ulceration]

Bednar aphthae, traumatic ulcers located bilaterally on either side of the midpalatal raphe in infants.

herpetiform aphthae, a variant of oral aphthae, of unknown etiology, characterized by up to several dozen ulcers, 2–3 mm in diameter, organized in a clustered herpetiform distribution.

aphthae ma′jor, a severe form of aphthae characterized by unusually numerous, large, deep, and frequent ulcers; healing may take as long as 6 weeks and results in scarring. SYN Mikulicz aphthae, periadenitis mucosa necrotica recurrens, recurrent scarring aphthae, Sutton disease.

Mikulicz aphthae, SYN aphthae major.

aphthae mi′nor, SYN aphtha (2).

recurrent scarring aphthae, SYN aphthae major.

aph·thoid (af′thoyd). Resembling aphthae.

aph·tho·sis (af-thō′sis). Any condition characterized by the presence of aphthae.

aph·thous (af′thŭs). Characterized by or relating to aphthae or aphthosis.

Aph·tho·vi·rus (af′thō-vī′rus). A genus in the family Picornaviridae associated with foot and mouth disease of cattle.

aphy·lac·tic (ā-fī-lak′tik). Obsolete term for pertaining to or characterized by aphylaxis.

aphy·lax·is (ā-fī-lak′sis). Obsolete term for lack of protection against disease. SYN nonimmunity. [G. *a-* priv. + *phylaxis,* a guarding]

ap·i·cal (ap′i-kăl) [TA]. **1.** Relating to the apex or tip of a pyramidal or pointed structure. **2.** Situated nearer to the apex of a structure in relation to a specific reference point; opposite of basal. SYN apicalis [TA].

ap·i·ca·lis (ap-i-kā′lis) [TA]. SYN apical, apical. [L.]

ap·i·cec·to·my (ap-i-sek′tō-mē). **1.** Opening and exenteration of air cells in the apex of the petrous part of the temporal bone. **2.** In dental surgery, an obsolete synonym for apicoectomy. [L. *apex,* summit or tip, + G. *ektomē,* excision]

apic·e·ot·o·my (ă-pis-ē-ot′ō-mē). SYN apicotomy.

ap·i·ces (ap′i-sēs). Plural of apex.

♻**apico-.** An apex; apical [L. *apex, apicis,* a summit or a tip + -o-]

ap·i·co·ec·to·my (ap′i-kō-ek′tō-mē). Surgical removal of a tooth root apex. SYN root resection. [apico- + G. *ektomē,* tooth excision]

ap·i·co·lo·ca·tor (ap′i-kō-lō′kā-tŏr). A device for locating the root apex of a tooth.

ap·i·col·y·sis (ap-i-kol′i-sis). Surgical collapse of the upper portion of the lung by the operative detachment of the parietal pleura allowing inferomedial displacement of the pulmonary apex. [apico- + G. *lysis,* destruction]

Api·com·plexa (ap-i-kom-plek′să). A phylum of the subkingdom Protozoa, which includes the class Sporozoea and the subclasses Coccidia and Piroplasmia, and is characterized by the presence of an apical complex. [L. *apex,* pl. *apicis,* tip, summit, + *complexus,* woven together]

ap·i·co·stome (ap′i-kō-stōm). The trocar and cannula used in apicostomy.

ap·i·cos·to·my (ap-i-kos′tō-mē). An operation in which the labial or buccal alveolar plate is perforated with a trocar and cannula; done to reach the root apex and to take bacterial cultures from this area. [apico- + G. *stoma,* mouth]

ap·i·cot·o·my (ap-i-kot′ō-mē). Incision into an apical structure. SYN apiceotomy. [apico- + G. *tomē,* a cutting]

apic·u·late (ă-pik′ū-lāt). Terminated abruptly by a small point. [L. *apiculus,* a tip or point]

apic·u·lus (ă-pik′ū-lŭs). A short, sharp projection on one end of a fungus spore at the point of attachment, or on the wall, of a hypha or condiophore. [L.]

ap·i·cu·ret·tage (ap-i-kū′rĕ-tahzh). Apical curettage after removal of an infected tooth.

apin·e·al·ism (ā-pin′ē-al-izm). Acquired absence of the pineal gland.

api·pho·bia (ā-pi-fō′bē-ă). Morbid fear of bees. SYN melissophobia. [L. *apis,* bee, + G. *phobos,* fear]

api·tu·i·tar·ism (ā-pi-too′i-tār-izm). Total lack of functional pituitary tissue; may be iatrogenic (e.g., as a consequence of hypophysectomy) or the result of a spontaneous disease process.

apla·cen·tal (ā-pla-sen′tăl). Without a placenta; denoting the monotremes (which lay eggs and have no placenta) and the marsupials (which have a transitory simple yolk-sac placenta).

ap·la·nat·ic (ap-la-nat′ik). Pertaining to aplanatism, or to an aplanatic lens.

aplan·a·tism (ă-plan′ă-tizm). Freedom from spherical aberration; said of a lens. [G. *a-* priv. + *planētos,* wandering]

apla·sia (ā-plā′zē-ă). **1.** Defective development or congenital absence of an organ or tissue. **2.** In hematology, incomplete, retarded, or defective development, or cessation of the usual regenerative process. [G. *a-* priv. + *plasis,* a molding]

congenital a. of thymus, SYN DiGeorge *syndrome.*

a. cu′tis congen′ita [MIM*107600, *207700, *207730], congenital absence or deficiency of a localized area of skin, with the base of the defect covered by a thin translucent membrane; most often a single area near the vertex of the scalp, but may occur in other areas; underlying structures may also be affected; autosomal inheritance, either dominant or recessive.

germinal a., SYN seminiferous tubule *dysgenesis.*

gonadal a., congenital absence of essentially all gonadal tissue; the external genitalia and genital ducts are female, but if interstitial cells of Leydig are present, the external genitalia are commonly ambiguous and the genital ducts are female. SEE ALSO gonadal *dysgenesis,* gonadal *agenesis;* Cf. Klinefelter *syndrome,* Turner *syndrome.*

pure red cell a., a transitory arrest of red blood cell production which may occur in the course of a hemolytic anemia, often preceded by infection, or as a complication of certain drugs; if the arrest persists, severe anemia may result. SEE ALSO congenital hypoplastic *anemia.*

aplas·tic (ā-plas′tik, ă-). Pertaining to aplasia, or conditions characterized by defective regeneration, as in a. anemia.

apleu·ria (ā-ploor′ē-ă). Congenital absence of one or more ribs; usually associated with absent transverse process or processes. [*a-* priv. + G. *pleura,* rib]

ap·nea (ap′nē-ă). Absence of breathing. [G. *apnoia,* want of breath]

central a., a. as the result of medullary depression which inhibits respiratory movement.

deglutition a., inhibition of breathing during swallowing.

induced a., intentional respiratory arrest during general anesthesia produced by hypocapnia, a muscle relaxant drug, respiratory center depression, or sudden cessation of controlled respiration.

obstructive sleep a., a disorder, first described in 1965, characterized by recurrent interruptions of breathing during sleep due to temporary obstruction of the airway by lax, excessively bulky, or malformed pharyngeal tissues (soft palate, uvula, and sometimes tonsils), with resultant hypoxemia and chronic lethargy.

Symptoms of obstructive sleep apnea are loud snoring, recurrent apneic episodes during sleep followed by gasping inspiration with partial or complete arousal, nocturnal restlessness, and daytime sleepiness. Apneic episodes last 10–120 seconds and may be accompanied by sinus bradycardia or atrioventricular block. The cumulative effect of recurrent spells of apnea is hypoxemia and shallow, nonrefreshing sleep, which may lead to excessive drowsiness, personality change, impairment of intellectual function, and heightened tendency to accidents during waking hours. However, evidence establishing obstructive sleep apnea as an independent risk factor for motor vehicle accidents, heart attack, stroke, and sudden death is weak. About 15% of persons with this disorder develop sustained pulmonary hypertension. Obstructive sleep apnea affects about 4% of men and 2% percent of women between the ages of 30 and 60. Obesity, hypothyroidism, cigarette smoking, alcohol, and some hypnotics (particularly benzodiazepines) predispose to this disorder, and its incidence increases with advancing age. Diagnosis is confirmed by polysomnography (continuous measurement of airflow, respiratory activity, chin electromyography, ECG, EEG, electrooculogram, and arterial oxygen saturation during sleep) and by evaluation of the shape and size of the upper respiratory tract. Weight loss, smoking cessation, and avoidance of benzodiazepine hypnotics are advised for all patients. A mandibular advancement appliance worn inside the mouth at night reduces symptoms in some patients. An effective if somewhat cumbrous treatment is the nightly use of continuous positive airway pressure, which provides a steady flow of room air at low pressure through the nose to overcome intermittent upper respiratory obstruction. Selected patients benefit from surgical procedures such as uvulopalatopharyngoplasty (trimming and reshaping of the uvula and soft palate), which can be performed by laser or radiofrequency ablation under local anesthesia, and mandibular osteotomy with genioglossus muscle advancement.

sleep a., central and/or peripheral a. during sleep, associated with frequent awakening and often with daytime sleepiness. Cf. sleep-induced a.

sleep-induced a., a. resulting from failure of the respiratory center to stimulate adequate respiration during sleep; divided into respiratory pause (cessation of air flow for less than 10 seconds) and apneic pause (cessation of air flow greater than 10 seconds).

ap·ne·ic (ap′nē-ik). Related to or suffering from apnea.

a·pneu·mia (a-pnoo′mē-ă). Congenital absence of the lungs. [G. a- priv. + pneumōn, lung]

ap·neu·sis (ap-noo′sis). An abnormal respiratory pattern consisting of a pause at full inspiration; a prolonged inspiratory cramp caused by a lesion at the mid or caudal pontine level of the brainstem. [G. a- priv. + pneusis, a breathing, fr. pneō, to breathe]

apo Abbreviation for apoenzyme; apolipoprotein.

△**apo-.** Combining form usually meaning separated from or derived from. [G. apo, away from, off; apo- becomes ap-, especially before a vowel or h]

ap·o·bi·o·sis (ap-ō-bī-ō′sis). Death, especially local death of a part of the organism. [G. death, fr. apo, from, + biōsis, life]

ap·o·crine (ap′ō-krin). Denoting a mechanism of glandular secretion in which the apical portion of secretory cells is shed and incorporated into the secretion. SEE ALSO apocrine gland. [G. apo-krinō, to separate]

ap·o·crus·tic (ap-ō-krŭs′tik). 1. Astringent and repellent. 2. An agent with such action. [G. apokroustikos, able to beat off, fr. apo, off, + krouō, to strike]

a·po·dal (ā-pō′dal). Relating to apodia. SYN apodous. [G. a- priv. + pous, foot]

apo·dia (ā-pō′dē-ă). Congenital absence of feet. SYN apody. [G. a- priv. + pous, foot]

ap·o·dous (ap′ō-dŭs). SYN apodal.

ap·o·dy (ap′ō-dē). SYN apodia.

ap·o·en·zyme (apo) (ap′ō-en-zīm). The protein portion of an enzyme as contrasted with the nonprotein portion, coenzyme, or prosthetic portion (if present in the intact protein).

ap·o·fer·ri·tin (ap-ō-fer′i-tin). A protein in the intestinal wall that combines with a ferric hydroxide-phosphate compound to form ferritin, the first stage in the absorption of iron.

ap·o·gam·ia, apog·a·my (ap-ō-gam′ē-ă, ă-pog′ă-mē). SYN parthenogenesis. [G. apo, away, + gameō, to wed]

apo·gee. The peak of severity of the clinical manifestations of an illness. [Fr., fr. Mod. L. apogaeum, fr. G. apogaios, far from the earth, fr. apo, + gaia, earth]

ap·o·in·duc·er (ā′pō-in-doos′er). A protein that binds to DNA to switch on transcription.

apo-2L. SYN TRAIL.

apo·lar (ā-pō′lăr). 1. Without poles; denoting specifically embryonic nerve cells (neuroblasts) that have not yet begun to sprout processes. 2. SYN hydrophobic (2).

ap·o·lip·o·pro·tein (apo) (ap′ō-lip-ō-prō′tēn). The protein component of any lipoprotein complexes that is a normal constituent of plasma chylomicrons, HDL, LDL, and VLDL in humans.

a. A-I, an a. found in HDL and chylomicrons. It is an activator of LCAT and a ligand for the HDL receptor. A deficiency of this a. has been associated with low HDL levels and with Tangier disease.

a. A-II, an a. found in HDL and chylomicrons. It stabilizes HDL.

a. A-IV, an a. secreted with chylomicrons and also found in HDL. It participates in the catabolism of chylomicrons and VLDL. It is also required for activation of lipoprotein lipase.

a. B, a.'s found in chylomicrons, LDL, VLDL, and IDL. Elevated in the plasma of individuals with familial hyperlipoproteinemia.

a. B-100, an a. found in LDL, VLDL, and IDL. The ligand for the LDL receptor; absent in certain types of abetalipoproteinemia.

a. B-48, an a. found in chylomicrons and chylomicron remnants. Retained in intestine of individuals with chylomicron retention disease.

a. C-I, an a. found in VLDL and chylomicrons. It modulates the interaction of a. E with VLDL.

a. C-II, an a. found in VLDL, HDL, and chylomicrons; an activator of lipoprotein lipase; a deficiency will result in accumulation of chylomicrons and triacylglycerols.

a. C-III, an a. found in VLDL, HDL, and chylomicrons. It inhibits a number of lipases.

a. D, an a. found in HDL. It forms a complex with LCAT and appears to be involved in the transport of bilin.

a. E, an a. found in VLDL, HDL, chylomicrons, and chylomicron remnants. Elevated in individuals with type III hyperlipoproteinemia. It has an important role in cholesterol transport.

ap·o·mix·ia (ap-ō-mik′sē-ă). SYN parthenogenesis. [G. apo, from, + mixis, a mingling]

ap·o·mor·phine hy·dro·chlo·ride (ap-ō-mōr′fēn). A derivative of morphine used as an emetic by the parenteral route of administration.

ap·o·neu·rec·to·my (ap′ō-noo-rek′tō-mē). Excision of an aponeurosis. [aponeurosis + G. ektomē, excision]

ap·o·neu·ror·rha·phy (ap′ō-noo-rōr′ă-fē). SYN fasciorrhaphy. [aponeurosis + G. rhaphē, suture]

ap·o·neu·ro·sis, pl. **ap·o·neu·ro·ses** (ap′ō-noo-rō′sis, -sēz) [TA]. A fibrous sheet or flat, expanded tendon, giving attachment to muscular fibers and serving as the means of origin or insertion of a flat muscle; it sometimes also performs the office of a fascia for other muscles. [G. the end of the muscle where it becomes tendon, fr. apo, from, + neuron, sinew]

bicipital a., a. bicipita′lis [TA], radiating fibers from the tendon of insertion of the biceps that form a triangular band passing obliquely across the hollow of the elbow to the ulnar side and becoming merged into the deep fascia of the forearm, thus providing the muscle with an indirect attachment to the subcutaneous border of the ulna. Formerly called "grace Dieu" fascia, it serves to protect the brachial artery and median nerve during phlebotomy of median cubital vein. SYN a. musculi bicipitis brachii [TA], lacertus fibrosus✯, bicipital fascia, semilunar fascia.

Denonvilliers a., SYN rectovesical septum.

epicranial a. [TA], the aponeurosis or intermediate tendon connecting the frontal belly and occipital belly of the occipitofrontalis muscle to form—with the temporoparietalis— the epicranius. SYN galea aponeurotica [TA], a. epicranialis✯, galea (2).

a. epicrania′lis, ✯official alternate term for epicranial a.

extensor a., SYN extensor digital expansion.

a. of external oblique muscle, broad, flat tendinous portion of the external abdominal oblique muscle. The fleshy fibers of the muscle end in the a. along a line descending vertically from the costochondral joint of the ninth rib then turning laterally just below the level of the umbilicus toward the anterior superior iliac spine. The fibers of the aponeurosis run medially and inferiorly, contributing to the anterior wall of the sheath of the rectus abdominis muscle and decussating with those of the contralateral a. at the median linea alba. Inferomedially, the a. is attached to the upper border of the pubic symphysis, the pubic crest and pubic tubercle. Between the anterior superior iliac spine and the pubic tubercle, it is thickened and turned under, forming the inguinal ligaments. The portion of the a. attached to the pubic bone forms the superficial inguinal ring by splitting into medial and lateral crura. SEE ALSO external spermatic *fascia*, inguinal *ligament*, lacunar *ligament*, pectineal *ligament*, reflected inguinal *ligament*, superficial inguinal *ring*, rectus *sheath*.

a. of insertion, a tendinous sheet serving for the insertion of a broad muscle.

a. of internal oblique muscle, broad, flat tendinous portion of the internal abdominal oblique muscle. The fleshy fibers of the muscle end in the a. lateral to the semilunar line. The uppermost portion of the a. is attached to the outer surfaces and lower borders of the seventh to ninth costal cartilages. Of the portion extending between the costoxiphoid margin and the pubis, the upper two-thirds splits into anterior and posterior laminae at the lateral border of the rectus abdominis muscle to contribute to both the anterior and posterior walls of the sheath of the rectus abdominis muscle as they extend to the midline linea alba. The lower third of the a. does not split but joins the aponeuroses of the external abdominal oblique and transversus abdominis muscles to form the anterior wall of the sheath of the rectus abdominis muscle. The fibers of the portion of the a. contributing to the rectus sheath decussate with those of the contralateral a. in the linea alba. The lowermost portion of the a. blends with the a. of the transversus abdominis muscle to form the conjoint tendon, attaching to the pubic crest and often the pecten pubis, thus forming the posterior wall of the inguinal canal at the superficial inguinal ring. SEE ALSO cremasteric *fascia*, inguinal *falx*, rectus *sheath*.

a. of investment, a fibrous membrane covering and keeping in place a muscle or group of muscles.

a. lin′guae [TA], SYN lingual a.

lingual a. [TA], the thickened lamina propria of the tongue to which the lingual muscles attach. SYN a. linguae [TA].

a. mus′culi bicip′itis bra′chii [TA], SYN bicipital a.

a. of origin, a tendinous expansion serving as the attachment of origin of a broad muscle.

a. palati′na [TA], SYN palatine a.

palatine a. [TA], the expanded tendons of the tensor veli palatini muscles in the anterior two-thirds of the soft palate to which the other palatine muscles attach. SYN a. palatina [TA].

palmar a. [TA], the thickened, central portion of the fascia ensheathing the hand; it radiates toward the bases of the fingers from the tendon of the palmaris longus muscle. SEE ALSO palmar *fascia*. SYN a. palmaris [TA], Dupuytren fascia.

a. palma′ris [TA], SYN palmar a.

Petit a., the posterior layer of the broad ligament of the uterus. [P. Petit]

a. pharyn′gea, SYN pharyngobasilar *fascia*.

plantar a. [TA], the very thick, central portion of the fascia investing the plantar muscles; it radiates toward the toes from the medial process of the calcaneal tuberosity and gives attachment to the short flexor muscle of the toes. SEE ALSO plantar *fascia*. SYN a. plantaris [TA].

a. planta′ris [TA], SYN plantar a.

Sibson a., SYN suprapleural *membrane*.

temporal a., SYN temporal *fascia*.

thoracolumbar a., SYN thoracolumbar *fascia*.

a. of vastus muscles, SEE patellar *retinaculum*, medial patellar *retinaculum*, lateral patellar *retinaculum*.

ap·o·neu·ro·si·tis (ap′ō-noo-rō-sī′tis). Inflammation of an aponeurosis.

ap·o·neu·rot·ic (ap′ō-noo-rot′ik). Relating to an aponeurosis.

ap·o·neu·ro·tome (ap-ō-noo′rō-tōm). Obsolete. Instrument for dividing an aponeurosis. [aponeurosis + G. *tomē*, a cutting]

ap·o·neu·rot·o·my (ap′ō-noo-rot′ō-mē). Incision of an aponeurosis.

ap·o·phy·lax·is (ap′ō-fī-lak′sis). Obsolete term for a diminution of the phylactic power of the body fluids, as sometimes observed in the negative phase of therapy with immunizing agents.

apoph·y·sary (ă-pof′i-sā-rē). SYN apophysial.

ap·o·phys·i·al, apoph·y·se·al (ă-pō-fiz′ē-ăl). Relating to or resembling an apophysis. SYN apophysary.

apoph·y·sis, pl. **apoph·y·ses** (ă-pof′i-sis, -sēz) [TA]. An outgrowth or projection, especially one from a bone. A bony process or outgrowth that lacks an independent center of ossification. [G. an offshoot]

basilar a., SYN basilar *part* of occipital bone.

a. con′chae, SYN *eminence* of concha.

a. hel′icis, SYN *spine* of helix.

lenticular a., SYN lenticular *process* of incus.

temporal a., SYN mastoid *process*.

apoph·y·si·tis (ă-pof-i-sī′tis). Inflammation of any apophysis.

calcaneal a., SYN Sever *disease*.

a. tibia′lis adolescen′tium, SYN Osgood-Schlatter *disease*.

Apophysomyces (ap-ō-fiz-ō-mī′sēz). A genus of fungi in the family Mucoraceae; a cause of mucormycosis.

ap·o·plas·mia (ap-ō-plaz′mē-ă). Obsolete term for a decrease in the amount of blood plasma.

ap·o·plec·tic (ap-ŏ-plek′tik). Relating to, suffering from, or predisposed to apoplexy.

ap·o·plec·ti·form (ap-ŏ-plek′ti-fōrm). Resembling apoplexy.

ap·o·plexy (ap′ŏ-plek-sē). SYN stroke (1). [G. *apoplēxia*]

abdominal a., mesenteric hemorrhage, thrombosis, or embolus involving the mesenteric or abdominal blood vessels.

adrenal a., hemorrhage into the adrenal glands or thrombosis of the adrenal veins, followed by acute adrenal insufficiency, occurring in the Waterhouse-Friderichsen syndrome.

bulbar a., a. due to vascular lesion in the brainstem.

functional a., a condition simulating a. without any cerebral lesion; a form of conversion hysteria.

heat a., (1) SYN heatstroke; **(2)** SYN ardent *fever*.

labyrinthine a., a clinical syndrome manifested as a single, abrupt attack of severe vertigo, nausea, and vomiting, with permanent loss of labyrinthine function on one side, but without associated hearing loss or tinnitus. Attributed to occlusion of the labyrinthine branch of the internal auditory artery.

neonatal a., intracranial hemorrhage in newborn children.

pituitary a., the sudden onset of visual loss, ophthalmoplegia, and meningeal pain due to infarction of a a. adenoma, producing compression of chiasm and cavernous sinus and some subarachnoid hemorrhage.

spinal a., stroke involving the spinal cord.

uteroplacental a., SYN Couvelaire *uterus*.

ap·o·pro·tein (ap-ō-prō′tēn). A polypeptide chain (protein) not yet complexed with the prosthetic group that is necessary to form the active holoprotein.

ap·o·pto·sis (ap′op-tō′sis, ap′ō-tō′sis). Programmed cell death; deletion of individual cells by fragmentation into membrane-bound particles, which are phagocytized by other cells. SYN programmed cell death. [G. a falling or dropping off, fr. *apo*, off, + *ptosis*, a falling]

> Whereas some cells (e.g., cardiac and skeletal muscle fibers, CNS neurons) last a lifetime, others (e.g., epithelial and glandular cells, erythrocytes) have limited life-spans, at the end of which they are genetically programmed to self-destruct, usually to be replaced by others formed by mitosis from surviving cells. Cells in tissue cultures spontaneously undergo apoptosis after about 50 cell divisions. In contrast to cell death caused by injury, infection, or circulatory impairment, apoptosis elicits no inflammatory response in adjacent cells and tissues. Features of apopto-

sis detectable by histologic and histochemical methods include cell shrinkage, due chiefly to dehydration; increased membrane permeability, with a rise in intracellular calcium and a fall in pH; endonucleolysis (fragmentation of nuclear DNA); and ultimately formation of apoptotic bodies, which are absorbed and removed by macrophages. Besides being due to genetic programming, apoptosis can be induced by injury to cellular DNA, as by irradiation and some cytotoxic agents used to treat cancer. It can be suppressed by naturally occurring factors (e.g., cytokines) and by some drugs (e.g., protease inhibitors). Apoptosis typically does not occur in malignant cells. Such cells therefore escape the destiny of their nonmalignant precursor cells and are said to be immortal. Immortalization can occur in various ways. The bcl-2 gene, present in many cancers, directs the production of an enzyme that blocks apoptosis and immortalizes affected cells. Injury to DNA normally triggers apoptosis by activating the p53 tumor suppressor gene, which is missing or mutated in about one-half of all human cancers. Cells that lack this gene can survive chemotherapy and irradiation intended to destroy cancer cells. Failure of apoptosis to occur is also involved in some degenerative diseases, including lupus erythematosus, and may be responsible for cellular damage caused by certain viruses, including HIV.

ap·o·re·pres·sor (ap′ō-rē-pres′er). A regulatory protein which, when combined with another corepressor, undergoes allosteric transformation, allowing it to combine with an operator locus and inhibit transcription of certain genes.

ap·o·some (ap′ō-sōm). A cytoplasmic inclusion produced by the cell itself. [G. *apo*, from, + *sōma*, body]

ap·o·stax·is (ap-ō-staks′is). Slight hemorrhage, or bleeding by drops. [G. a trickling down]

apos·thia (ă-pos′thē-ă). Congenital absence of the prepuce. [G. *a*-priv. + *posthē*, foreskin]

ap·o·stilb (ap′ō-stilb). A unit of brightness equal to 0.1 millilambert. [G. *apo*, from + *stilbē*, lamp]

ap·o·tha·na·sia (ap′-ō-thă-nā′zē-ă). Postponement of death; prolongation of life, as opposed to euthanasia. [G. *apo*, away, + *thanatos*, death]

apoth·e·cary (ă-poth′ĕ-kār-ē). Obsolescent term for pharmacist or druggist. [G. *apothēkē*, a barn, storehouse, fr. *apo*, from, + *thēkē*, a box]

ap·o·them, ap·o·theme (ap′ō-them, ap′ō-thēm). A precipitate caused by long boiling of a vegetable infusion or by its exposure to air. [G. *apo*, from, + *thema*, something set down, fr. *tithēmi*, to place]

ap·ox·e·sis (ap-ok-sē′sis). SYN subgingival *curettage*. [G. *apo*, away, + *xeein*, to scrape]

ap·o·zem, apoz·e·ma (ap′ō-zem, ap-oz′ē-mă). SYN decoction. [apo- + G. *zema*, something boiled]

ap·pa·ra·tus (ap-ă-rā′tŭs). 1. A collection of instruments adapted for a special purpose. 2. An instrument made up of several parts. 3 [TA]. A group or system of glands, ducts, blood vessels, muscles, or other anatomic structures involved in the performance of some function. SEE ALSO system. [L. equipment. fr. *ap-paro*, pp. -*atus*, to prepare]

accessory visual a., SYN accessory visual *structures*, under *structure*.

achromatic a., the nonstaining asters and spindle fibers in a dividing cell.

alimentary a., SYN alimentary *system*.

attachment a., the tissues that attach the tooth to the alveolar process: cementum, periodontal membrane, and alveolar bone.

Barcroft-Warburg a., SYN Warburg a.

Beckmann a., a. for the accurate measurement of melting points and boiling points in connection with molecular weight determinations.

Benedict-Roth a., a device employed to measure the amount of oxygen utilized in quiet breathing in the basal state for the estima-

tion of the basal metabolic rate; the subject rebreathes oxygen through soda lime from a recording spirometer.

branchial a., the aggregate of the pharyngeal arches, pouches, clefts, and membranes seen in the developing embryo of vertebrates.

central a., the centrosome and centrosphere.

chromatic a., the deeply staining mass of chromosomes in a dividing cell.

chromidial a., the aggregate of extranuclear network, irregular strands, and masses of basophilic staining material permeating the protoplasm of the cell. SEE ALSO ribosome, endoplasmic *reticulum*.

dental a., SYN masticatory *system*.

digestive a., SYN alimentary *system*.

a. digesto′rius, SYN alimentary *system*.

genitourinary a., SYN urogenital *system*.

Golgi a., a membranous system of cisternae and vesicles located between the nucleus and the secretory pole or surface of a cell; concerned with the investment and intracellular transport of membrane-bounded secretory proteins, and the synthesis of polysaccharides and glycoproteins. SYN dictyosome, Golgi body, Golgi complex, Golgi internal reticulum, Holmgrén-Golgi canals.

Haldane a., a device used for the analysis of respiratory gases.

hyoid a., veterinary anatomy term for hyoid bones, a modified portion of the ancestral branchial skeleton consisting of an articulated chain of bones extending from the mastoid region of the skull on each side to the base of the tongue; in humans, it is reduced to a single bone, os hyoideum; in a typical mammal (the dog), it consists of a tympanohyoid cartilage attached to the skull, followed by the stylohyoid, epihyoid, keratohyoid, basihyoid, and thyrohyoid bones. SYN a. hyoideus.

a. hyoi′deus, SYN hyoid a.

juxtaglomerular a., SYN juxtaglomerular *complex*.

Kirschner a., SYN Kirschner *wire*.

Kjeldahl a., an a. for distilling ammonia arising from acid decomposition of an organic compound; used in nitrogen analysis.

lacrimal a. [TA], consisting of the lacrimal gland, the lacrimal lake, the lacrimal canaliculi, the lacrimal sac, and the nasolacrimal duct. SYN a. lacrimalis [TA].

a. lacrima′lis [TA], SYN lacrimal a.

a. ligamento′sus col′li, SYN *ligamentum* nuchae.

a. ligamento′sus weitbrecht′i, SYN tectorial *membrane* (of median atlantoaxial joint).

masticatory a., (1) SYN masticatory *system*; **(2)** SYN stomatognathic *system*.

mental a., mental structure consisting of thoughts, feelings, cognitions, and memories; in psychoanalysis, the topographic structure of the mind.

pyriform a., a pear-shaped structure within the eggshell of certain tapeworms (family Anoplocephalidae), of uncertain function.

a. respirato′rius, SYN respiratory *system*.

respiratory a., SYN respiratory *system*.

Roughton-Scholander a., a syringe-like device for analyzing the respiratory gases in a small sample of blood. SYN Roughton-Scholander syringe.

Scholander a., a device used for determining the oxygen and carbon dioxide percentage in 0.5 ml of a respiratory gas.

subneural a., modified sarcoplasm in a motor end-plate.

a. suspenso′rius len′tis, SYN ciliary *zonule*.

Taylor a., SYN Taylor back *brace*.

Tiselius a., an a. for separating proteins in solution by electrophoresis and thus for determining the isoelectric point, molecular weight, and related physical properties; the direction and rate of migration of the protein and the characteristics of the boundary phase between the protein solution and the supernatant salt solution are recorded by photography of the changes in refractive index at the boundary.

urinary a., SYN urinary *system*.

urogenital a., SYN urogenital *system*.

a. urogenita′lis, SYN urogenital *system*.

Van Slyke a., an a. for determining the amounts of respiratory gases in the blood.

vestibular a., the receptor organ of the vestibular portion of the 8th cranial nerve, consisting of the three semicircular canals and the otolith, located within the petrous portion of the temporal bone of the skull.

Warburg a., an a. for measuring the oxygen consumption of incubated tissue slices by manometric measurement of changes in gas pressure produced by oxygen absorption in an enclosed flask. SYN Barcroft-Warburg a.

ap·par·ent (ă-păr′ent). **1.** Manifest; obvious; evident; e.g., a clinically a. infection. **2.** Frequently used (confusingly) to mean "seeming to be," ostensible, pseudo-. [L. *apparens,* visible, fr. *appareo,* to come in sight]

ap·pend·age (ă-pen′dij). Any part, subordinate in function or size, attached to a main structure. SEE ALSO accessory *structures,* under *structure.* SYN appendix (1). [L. *appendix*]
  atrial a., SYN *auricles* (of atria), under *auricle.*
  auricular a., (1) SYN right *auricle;* **(2)** a small congenital skin tag usually located anterior to the tragus of the ear, often called a skin tag; more often unilateral than bilateral.
  drumstick a., an a. of the nucleus that represents the inactive heterochromatic X chromosome seen in 3% of the neutrophil leukocytes of human females. SEE sex *chromatin,* lyonization.
  epiploic a., SYN omental *appendices,* under *appendix.*
  a.'s of eye, accessory visual *structures,* under *structure.*
  a.'s of the fetus, amnion, yolk sac, and the fetal (chorionic) part of the placenta together with the umbilical cord.
  left auricular a., SYN left *auricle.*
  right auricular a., SYN right *auricle.*
  a.'s of skin, the hairs, nails, and sweat, sebaceous, and mammary glands.
  testicular a., SYN *appendix* of testis.
  uterine a.'s, the ovaries, uterine (fallopian) tubes, and associated ligaments. SYN adnexa uteri.
  vermiform a., SYN appendix (2).
  vesicular a.'s of epoophoron [TA], a small fluid-filled cyst attached by a slender stalk to the fimbriated end of the uterine tube; a vestigial remnant of the embryonic mesonephric duct. SYN appendix vesiculosa [TA], Morgagni hydatid, morgagnian cyst, stalked hydatid, vesicular appendices of uterine tube.

ap·pen·dal·gia (ap-pen-dal′jē-ă). Obsolete term for pain in the right lower quadrant of the abdomen in the region of the vermiform appendix. [appendix + G. *algos,* pain]

ap·pen·dec·to·my (ap-pen-dek′tō-mē). Surgical removal of the vermiform appendix. SYN appendicectomy. [appendix + G. *ektomē,* excision]
  auricular a., excision of the auricular appendix of an atrium, usually the left.

ap·pen·di·cal (ă-pen′di-kăl). SYN appendiceal.

ap·pen·dic·e·al (ă-pen-dis′ē-ăl). Relating to an appendix. SYN appendical.

ap·pen·di·cec·ta·sis (ap-pen-di-sek′tă-sis). Ectasia of the appendix.

ap·pen·di·cec·to·my (ap-pen-di-sek′tō-mē). SYN appendectomy.

ap·pen·di·cism (ă-pen′di-sizm). Rarely used term for any chronic disease of the vermiform appendix, or a symptomatic uneasiness in that area.

ap·pen·di·ci·tis (ă-pen-di-sī′tis). Inflammation of the vermiform appendix. [appendix + G. *-itis,* inflammation]
  actinomycotic a., chronic suppurative a. due to infection by *Actinomyces israelii.*
  acute a., acute inflammation of the appendix, usually due to bacterial infection, which may be precipitated by obstruction of the lumen by a fecalith; variable symptoms often consisting of periumbilical colicky pain and vomiting may be followed by fever, leukocytosis, persistent pain, and signs of peritoneal inflammation in the right lower quadrant of the abdomen; perforation or abscess formation is a frequent complication of delayed surgical intervention.
  bilharzial a., a. caused by the deposition of the eggs of the blood fluke, *Schistosoma mansoni,* in the vermiform appendix.
  chronic a., fibrous adhesions, scarring, or deformity of the appen-

dix following subsidence of acute a.; fibrous obliteration of the distal lumen is not abnormal in older persons; term frequently used to refer to repeated mild attacks of acute a.
  focal a., acute a. involving only part of the appendix, sometimes at the site of, or distal to, an obstruction of the lumen.
  foreign-body a., a. caused by obstruction of the lumen of the appendix by a foreign substance, such as a particulate foreign body.
  gangrenous a., acute a. with necrosis of the wall of the appendix, most commonly developing in obstructive a. and frequently causing perforation and acute peritonitis.
  left-sided a., a. occurring on the left side of the abdomen, usually the left-lower quadrant, due to abnormal rotation of the gut (such as situs inversus).
  lumbar a., acute a. in a retrodisplaced appendix in the lumbar region.
  obstructive a., acute a. due to infection of retained secretion behind an obstruction of the lumen by a fecalith or some other cause, including carcinoma of the cecum.
  perforating a., inflammation of the appendix leading to perforation of the wall of the appendix into the peritoneal cavity, resulting in peritonitis.
  recurrent a., repeated episodes of right lower quadrant abdominal pain attributed to recurrence of inflammation of the appendix in an individual who did not have an appendectomy for prior episodes. SYN relapsing a.
  relapsing a., SYN recurrent a.
  stercoral a., a. following a lodgment of fecal material in the appendix.
  subperitoneal a., a. of a subperitoneally displaced appendix.
  suppurative a., acute a. with purulent exudate in the lumen and wall of the appendix.
  verminous a., a. caused by obstruction or response to the presence of parasitic worms such as *Ascaris lumbricoides, Strongyloides stercoralis,* or the pinworm *Enterobius vermicularis.*

⌂**appendico-.** An appendix, usually the vermiform appendix. [L. *appendix, appendicis* an appendage, fr. *appendo,* to hang something onto something, fr. *ad-, ap-,* to, onto, + *pendo,* to hang, + *-o-*]

ap·pen·di·co·cele (ă-pen′di-kō-sēl). The vermiform appendix in a hernial sac. [appendico- + G. *kēlē,* hernia]

ap·pen·di·co·lith (ă-pen′di-kō-lith). A calcified concretion in the appendix visible on an abdominal radiograph; considered diagnostic of appendicitis in the acute abdomen. [appendico- + G. *lithos,* stone]

ap·pen·di·co·li·thi·a·sis (ă-pen′di-kō-li-thī′ă-sis). The presence of concretions in the vermiform appendix. [appendico- + G. *lithos,* stone]

ap·pen·di·col·y·sis (ă-pen-di-kol′i-sis). An operation for freeing the appendix from adhesions. [appendico- + G. *lysis,* a loosening]

ap·pen·di·cos·to·my (ă-pen-di-kos′tō-mē). An operation for opening into the intestine through the tip of the vermiform appendix, previously attached to the anterior abdominal wall. [appendico- + G. *stoma,* mouth]

ap·pen·di·co·ves·i·cos·to·my (ă-pen-di-ko′ves′ĭ-kos-tō-mē). Use of an isolated appendix on a vascularized pedicle as a catheterizable route of access to the bladder from the skin. SEE ALSO Mitrofanoff *principle.* [eppendico- + L. *vesica,* bladder, + G. *stoma,* mouth]

ap·pen·dic·u·lar (ap′en-dik′ū-lăr). **1.** Relating to an appendix or appendage. **2.** Relating to the limbs, as opposed to axial, which refers to the trunk and head.

ap·pen·dix, gen. **ap·pen·di·cis,** pl. **ap·pen·di·ces** (ă-pen′diks, -di-sis, -di-sēs). **1.** SYN appendage. **2** [TA]. A wormlike intestinal diverticulum extending from the blind end of the cecum; it varies in length and ends in a blind extremity. SYN a. vermiformis [TA], a. ceci, processus vermiformis, vermiform appendage, vermiform a., vermiform process, vermix. [L. appendage, fr. *ap-pendo,* to hang something on]
  appendices adiposae coli, ✶official alternate term for omental appendices.

auricular a., SYN *auricles* (of atria), under *auricle*.

a. ce′ci, SYN appendix (2).

a. epididym′idis [TA], SYN a. of epididymidis.

a. of epididymidis [TA], a small pedunculated body often attached to the head of the epididymis which is a vestige of the embryonic mesonephric duct. SYN a. epididymidis [TA], pedunculated hydatid.

epiploic a., SYN omental appendices.

a. epiplo′ica, pl. **appen′dices epiplo′icae,** SYN omental appendices.

fatty appendices of colon, ✩official alternate term for omental appendices.

a. fibro′sa hep′atis [TA], SYN fibrous a. of liver.

fibrous a. of liver [TA], a fibrous process, into which the tip of the left lobe of the liver may taper out, that passes with the left triangular ligament to be attached to the diaphragm. SYN a. fibrosa hepatis [TA].

Morgagni a., SYN pyramidal *lobe* of thyroid gland.

omental appendices [TA], one of a number of little processes or sacs of peritoneum filled with adipose tissue and projecting from the serous coat of the large intestine, except the rectum; they are most evident on the transverse and sigmoid colon, being most numerous along the free tenia. SYN appendices omentales [TA], appendices adiposae coli✩, fatty appendices of colon✩, a. epiploica, epiploic appendage, epiploic a., epiploic tags.

appendices omentales [TA], SYN omental appendices.

a. tes′tis [TA], SYN a. of testis.

a. of the testis, SYN a. of testis.

a. of testis [TA], a vesicular nonpedunculated structure attached to the cephalic pole of the testis; a vestige of the cephalic end of the paramesonephric (müllerian) duct. SYN a. testis [TA], a. of the testis, nonpedunculated hydatid, ovarium masculinum, sessile hydatid, testicular appendage.

a. ventric′uli laryn′gis, SYN laryngeal *saccule*.

vermiform a., SYN appendix (2).

a. vermifor′mis [TA], SYN appendix (2).

vesicular appendices of uterine tube, SYN vesicular *appendages* of epoophoron, under *appendage*.

a. vesiculo′sa, pl. **appen′dices vesiculo′sae** [TA], SYN vesicular *appendages* of epoophoron, under *appendage*.

ap·per·cep·tion (ap-er-sep′shŭn). **1.** The final stage of attentive perception in which something is clearly apprehended and thus is relatively prominent in awareness; the full apprehension of any psychic content. **2.** The process of referring the perception of ideas to one's own personality. [L. *ad,* to, + *per- cipio,* pp. *-ceptus,* to take wholly, perceive]

ap·per·cep·tive (ap-er-sep′tiv). Relating to, involved in, or capable of apperception.

ap·per·son·a·tion, ap·per·son·i·fi·ca·tion (ă-per′sŏ-nā′shŭn, ap-er-son′i-fi-kā′shŭn). A delusion in which one assumes the character of another person.

ap·pe·stat (ap′e-stat). The mechanism in the brain (possibly in the hypothalamus) concerned with the appetite and control of food intake. [appetite + G. *statos,* standing]

ap·pe·tite (ap′ĕ-tīt). A desire or motive derived from a biologic or psychological need for food, water, sex, or affection; a desire or longing to satisfy any conscious physical or mental need. SYN orexia (2). [L. *ad-peto,* pp. *-petitus,* to seek after, desire]

ap·pla·na·tion (ap′lan-ā′shŭn). In tonometry, the flattening of the cornea by pressure. Intraocular pressure is directly proportional to external pressure, and inversely proportional to the area flattened. SEE ALSO applanation *tonometer.* [L. *ad,* toward, + *planum,* plane]

ap·pla·nom·e·try (ap-lan-om′ĕ-trē). Use of an applanation tonometer.

ap·ple oil. SYN *amyl* valerate.

ap·pli·ance (ă-plī′ans). A device used to improve function of a part, or for therapeutic purposes. [fr, O. Fr. *aplier,* to apply, fr. L. *applico,* to fold together]

craniofacial a., a device used to immobilize and/or reduce mandibular or midfacial fractures. SEE ALSO fixation.

edgewise a., a fixed, multibanded orthodontic a. using an attachment bracket the slot of which receives a rectangular archwire horizontally, which gives precise control of tooth movement in all three planes of space.

extraoral fracture a., a device used for extraoral reduction and fixation of maxillary or mandibular fractures, in which pins, clamps, or screws interjoined with metal or acrylic connectors are used to align the fractured segments. SEE ALSO external pin *fixation.*

Hawley a., SYN Hawley *retainer.*

intraoral fracture a., a metal or acrylic device attached to the teeth with wire or cement; used to immobilize fractures of the maxilla and mandible.

labiolingual a., an orthodontic a. that consists of a maxillary labial arch wire and a mandibular lingual arch wire.

light wire a., an orthodontic a. utilizing small gauge labial wires with expansion and contraction loops formed into it and attached to bands fitted to individual teeth; sometimes called Begg light wire differential force technique.

obturator a., an a. used to obliterate congenital or acquired defects of the palate and surrounding structures, usually made of acrylic or rubber.

orthodontic a., a mechanism for the application of force to the teeth and their supporting tissues to produce changes in the relationship of the teeth and/or the related osseous structures.

ribbon arch a., an a. consisting of a rectangular wire inserted into a specially designed bracket attached to the labial and buccal surfaces of the teeth.

Roger Anderson pin fixation a., an a. used in extraoral fixation of mandibular fractures and prognathic corrections in which pins placed in the bone segments are joined by metal connecting rods. SEE ALSO external pin *fixation.*

surgical a., a metal or plastic a. constructed prior to an operation and used to immobilize or support tissue during the postoperative phase.

universal a., a combination of the edgewise and ribbon arch a. techniques, affording precise control of individual teeth in all planes of space.

applicand. Abbreviation for *applicandus,* to be applied. [L.]

ap·pli·ca·tor (ap′li-kā-tōr). A slender rod of wood, flexible metal, or synthetic material, at one end of which is attached a pledget of cotton or other substance for making local applications to any accessible surface. [L. *ap-plico,* to attach to]

ap·po·si·tion (ap-ō-zish′ŭn). **1.** The placing in contact of two substances. **2.** The condition of being placed or fitted together. **3.** The relationship of fracture fragments to one another. **4.** The process of thickening of the cell wall. [L. *ap-pono,* pp. *-positus,* to place at or to]

bayonet a., relationship of two fracture fragments that lie next to each other rather than in end-to-end contact.

ap·proach (ă-prōch′). **1.** In psychiatry, a term used to describe how interpersonal relationships are negotiated. **2.** The path or method used to expose the operative field during an operation. [M.E., fr. O. Fr., fr L.L. *appropio,* to come nearer, fr. *ad,* to + *propius,* nearer]

facial recess a., a surgical a. to the middle ear from the mastoid through the recess lateral to the facial nerve canal.

idiographic a., the comprehensive study of an individual as a basis for understanding human behavior in general.

infratemporal a., surgical a. to the base of the skull and its contents from inferior to the temporal bone.

middle fossa a., surgical a. to the cerebellopontine angle through that portion of the floor of the middle cranial fossa that is the anterior surface of the petrous pyramid of the temporal bone.

nomothetic a., a frame of psychologic reference that attempts to provide norms and general principles of behavior by the study of groups.

posterior fossa a., surgical a. to the cerebellopontine angle through the mastoid process of the temporal bone.

regressive-reconstructive a., a form of psychotherapy in which regression, in order to resurrect some original psychic trauma, is an integral part of the treatment.

retrosigmoid a., a surgical a. to the cerebellopontine angle through the occipital bone posterior to the sigmoid sinus.

transcochlear a., a surgical a. to the internal auditory canal through the cochlea.

translabyrinthine a., surgical a. to the cerebellopontine angle through the inner ear.

ap·prox·i·mate (ă-prok′si-māt). To bring close together. In dentistry: **1.** Proximate, denoting the contact surfaces, either mesial or distal, of two adjacent teeth. **2.** Close together; denoting the teeth in the human jaw, as distinguished from the separated teeth in certain of the lower animals. [L. *ad,* to, + *proximus,* nearest]

ap·prox·i·ma·tion (ă-prok-si-mā′shŭn). In surgery, bringing tissue edges into desired apposition for suturing.

steady state a., an assumption in the derivation of an enzyme rate expression in which the rate of change of the concentration of any enzyme species is zero or much smaller than d[P]/dt.

APR Abbreviation for abdominoperineal *resection.*

aprac·tag·no·sia (ā-prak-tag-nō′sē-ă). SYN constructional *apraxia.* [G. *a-* priv. + *praktea,* things to be done, + *gnōsis,* recognition]

aprac·tic (ā-prak′tik). SYN apraxic.

aprag·ma·tism (ā-prag′mă-tizm). An interest in theory or dogmatism rather than in practical results. [G. *a-* priv. + pragmatism]

aprax·ia (ă-prak′sē-ă). **1.** A disorder of voluntary movement, consisting of impairment in the performance of skilled or purposeful movements, notwithstanding the preservation of comprehension, muscular power, sensibility, and coordination in general; due to acquired cerebral disease. **2.** A psychomotor defect in which the proper use of an object can not be carried out although the object can be named and its uses described. [G. *a-* priv. + *prattō,* to do]

constructional a., a. manifested as an impairment in activity such as building, assembling, and drawings; caused by parietal lobe lesions. SYN apractagnosia.

cortical a., SYN motor a.

gait a., a. for walking, accompanied by inability to make walking movements with the legs.

ideokinetic a., ideomotor a., a form of a. in which simple acts are incapable of being performed, presumably because the connections between the cortical centers that control volition and the motor cortex are interrupted. SYN transcortical a.

innervation a., SYN motor a.

limb-kinetic a., SYN motor a.

motor a., an inability to make movements or to use objects for the purpose intended. SYN cortical a., innervation a., limb-kinetic a.

ocular motor a., a congenital inability to initiate horizontal saccades. Children with this condition often use head thrusts to move their eyes to the left and right.

transcortical a., SYN ideokinetic a.

verbal a., a speech disorder in which phonemic substitutions are constantly used for the desired syllable or word.

aprax·ic (ă-prak′sik). Marked by or pertaining to apraxia. SYN apractic.

ap·ri·cot ker·nel oil (ā′pri-kot). SEE persic oil.

aproc·tia (ā-prok′shē-ă). Congenital absence or imperforation of the anus. [G. *a-* priv. + *prōktos,* anus]

ap·ro·fen, ap·ro·fene, ap·ro·phen (ap′rō-fen, ap′rō-fēn, ap′rō-fen). Analgesic and antispasmodic.

apros·o·dy (ă-pros′ō-dē). Absence, in speech, of the normal pitch, rhythm, and variations in stress. [G. *a-* priv. + *prosōdia,* voice modulation]

ap·ro·so·pia (ap-rō-sō′pē-ă). Congenital absence of the greater part or all of the face, usually associated with other malformations. [G. *a-* priv. + *prosōpon,* face]

apro·ti·nin (ā-prō′ti-nin). A protease and kallikrein inhibitor obtained from animal organs; a polypeptide with a molecular weight of about 6000. May be useful in the treatment of pancreatitis and in preventing bleeding after surgery involving cardiopulmonary bypass.

APS Abbreviation for adenosine 5′-phosphosulfate.

6-APS Abbreviation for 6-aminopenicillanic acid.

aPTT Abbreviation for activated partial thromboplastin *time.*

APUD Proposed designation for a group of cells in different organs secreting polypeptide hormones or neurotransmitters. Cells in this group have certain biochemical characteristics in common, the first letters of which form the name: they contain amines, such as catecholamine and 5-hydroxytryptamine, take up precursors of these amines in vivo, and contain amino-acid decarboxylase. [*amine* precursor *uptake, decarboxylase*]

apu·rin·ic ac·id (a-pū-rin′ik). DNA from which the purine bases have been removed by mild acid treatment.

apyk·no·mor·phous (ă-pik-nō-mōr′fŭs). Denoting a cell or other structure that does not stain deeply because the stainable or chromophil material is not closely aggregated. [G. *a-* priv. + *pyknos,* thick, + *morphē,* shape, form]

ap·y·rase (ă-pī′rās). An enzyme catalyzing hydrolytic removal of two orthophosphate residues from adenosine 5′-triphosphate to yield adenosine 5′-monophosphate; i.e., ATP + 2H₂O → AMP + 2P_i. SYN ADPase, ATP-diphosphatase.

apy·ret·ic (ă-pī-ret′ik). SYN afebrile.

apy·rex·ia (ā-pī-rek′sē-ă). Absence of fever. [G. *a-* priv. + *pyrexis,* fever]

apy·rex·i·al (ā-pī-rek′sē-ăl). SYN afebrile.

apy·rim·i·din·ic ac·id (ă-pī′rim-i-din′ik). DNA from which the pyrimidine bases have been removed by chemical treatment (e.g., exposure to hydrazine).

aq. Abbreviation for L. *aqua,* water.

aq. bull. Abbreviation for L. *aqua bulliens,* boiling water.

aq. dest. Abbreviation for L. *aqua destillata,* distilled water.

aq. ferv. Abbreviation for L. *aqua fervens,* hot water.

aq. frig. Abbreviation for L. *aqua frigida,* cold water.

aq·ua, gen. and pl. **aq·uae** (ak′wă, ah′kwah). H₂O. Pharmaceutical waters, aquae, are aqueous solutions of volatile substances (e.g., rose water). Pharmaceutical solutions, liquors, are aqueous solutions of nonvolatile substances. SEE water (3), solution (3). [L.]

a. re′gia, a. rega′lis, SYN nitrohydrochloric acid. [L. royal water, so called from its power to dissolve gold]

aq·ua·co·bal·a·min (ak′wă-kō-bal′ă-min). Vitamin B₁₂ₐ (tautomeric with B₁₂ᵦ); a cobalamin derivative in which the sixth coordinate bond of the cobaltic ion is attached to a water molecule. SEE ALSO *vitamin* B₁₂. SYN aquocobalamin.

aq·ua·pho·bia (ak-wă-fō′bē-ă). Morbid fear of water. [L. *aqua,* water, + G. *phobos,* fear]

aq·ua·punc·ture (ak-wă-pŭnk′chūr). Rarely used term for a hypodermic injection of water. [L. *aqua,* water, + *punctura,* puncture]

Aq·ua·spi·ril·lum (ah-kwah-spī-ril′ŭm). A genus of motile, nonsporeforming, aerobic bacteria (family Spirillaceae) containing Gram-negative, rigid, helical or helically curved cells that are 0.2–1.5 μm in diameter. Motile cells contain fascicles of flagella at one or both poles. Some species can grow anaerobically with nitrate instead of oxygen as the terminal electron acceptor. These organisms are chemoorganotrophic, possessing a strictly respiratory metabolism. They do not ferment carbohydrates; a few species can oxidize a limited variety of carbohydrates. The habitat of these organisms is fresh water. The type species is *A. serpens.* [L. *aqua,* water, + *spirillum,* coil]

aquat·ic (ă-kwat′ik). **1.** Of or pertaining to water. **2.** Denoting an organism that lives in water.

aq·ue·duct (ak′we-dŭkt). A conduit or canal. SYN aqueductus. [L. *aquaeductus*]

cerebral a., an ependyma-lined canal in the mesencephalon about 20 mm long, connecting the third to the fourth ventricle. SYN aqueductus mesencephali [TA], aqueductus cerebri☆, a. of cerebrum, aqueductus sylvii, iter a tertio ad quartum ventriculum, sylvian a.

a. of cerebrum, SYN cerebral a.

cochlear a. [TA], a fine canal in the temporal bone, opening superior to the tympanic canaliculus, connecting the perilymphatic space of the cochlea with the subarachnoid space. SYN aqueductus cochleae [TA], ductus perilymphaticus, perilymphatic duct.

Cotunnius a., SYN vestibular a.

fallopian a., SYN facial *canal.*

sylvian a., SYN cerebral a.

vestibular a. [TA], a bony canal running from the vestibule and opening on the posterior surface of the petrous portion of the temporal bone, giving passage to the endolymphatic duct and a small vein. SYN aqueductus vestibuli [TA], aqueductus cotunnii, Cotunnius a., Cotunnius canal.

aq·ue·duc·tus (ak-we-dŭk′tŭs). SYN aqueduct. [L. fr. *aqua,* water, + *ductus,* a leading, fr. *duco,* pp. *ductus,* to lead]

a. cer′ebri, [offalt] ⭑ official alternate term for cerebral *aqueduct.*

a. coch′leae [TA], SYN cochlear *aqueduct.*

a. cotun′nii, SYN vestibular *aqueduct.*

a. fallo′pii, SYN facial *canal.*

a. mesencephali [TA], SYN cerebral *aqueduct.*

a. syl′vii, SYN cerebral *aqueduct.*

a. vestib′uli [TA], [NA] SYN vestibular *aqueduct.*

aque·ous (ak′wē-ŭs, ā′kwē-ŭs). Watery; of, like, or containing water.

aquip·ar·ous (ă-kwip′er-ŭs). Secreting or excreting a watery fluid. [L. *aqua,* water, + *pario,* to bring forth]

aq·uo·co·bal·a·min (ak′wō-kō-bal′ă-min). SYN aquacobalamin.

aq·uo·i·on (ak′wō-ī′on). A hydrated ion; an ion containing one or more water molecules; e.g., $Cu(H_2O)_4^{2+}$.

aquos·i·ty (ă-kwos′i-tē). **1.** The state of being watery. **2.** Moisture.

Ar Symbol for argon.

Ara Symbol for arabinose, or its mono- or diradical.

△**ara-.** Prefix for arabinose or arabinosyl.

△**arab-.** Gum arabic; similar gummy substances. [G. *Araps, Arabos,* an Arab]

ar·a·ban (a′ră-ban). A polysaccharide that yields arabinose on hydrolysis; a constituent of some pectins.

ar·a·bic (a′ră-bik). Relating to or derived from various species of *Acacia* having a gummy or resinous exudate.

ar·a·bic ac·id. SYN arabin.

ar·a·bin (a′ră-bin). A carbohydrate gum, hydrolyzing to D-arabinose and hexoses, found naturally in union with calcium, potassium, and magnesium ions, when it is called gum arabic. SYN arabic acid.

ar·a·bi·no·a·den·o·sine (a′ră-bin-ō-ah-den′ō-sēn). SYN arabinosyladenine.

ar·a·bi·no·cy·ti·dine (a′ră-bin-ō-sī′ti-dēn). SYN arabinosylcytosine.

ara·bin·o·fur·a·no·syl·ad·e·nine (a′ră-bin-ō-foor′ă-nō-sil-ad′ě-nēn). An arabinoside that has antiviral activity.

ar·a·bi·no·fu·ra·no·syl·cy·to·sine (a′ră-bin-ō-foor′ă-nō-sil-sī′tō-sēn). SYN arabinosylcytosine.

arab·i·nose (Ara) (ă-rab′i-nōs, a′ră-bin-ōs). A pentose; both of its enantiomers are widely distributed in plants, usually in complex polysaccharides; used in culture media. D-A. is an epimer of D-ribose. [arabin + -ose (1)]

a. 5-phosphate, a phosphorylated a. that is an intermediate in the pentose phosphate pathway.

a. 5-phosphate 2-epimerase, an enzyme in the pentose phosphate pathway that reversibly interconverts a. and ribose 5-phosphate.

ar·a·bi·no·side (ă-rab′i-nō-sīd). A ribonucleoside in which the sugar moiety is arabinose. It often has antibiotic activity.

arab·i·no·sis (ă-rab-i-nō′sis). Disordered metabolism of arabinose.

ar·a·bi·no·su·ria (ă-rab′i-nō-soo′rē-ă). Excretion of arabinose in the urine.

ar·a·bi·no·syl·ad·e·nine (a′ră-bin-ō-sil-a′den-ēn). Used for herpes simplex corneae and vaccinial keratitis. SYN arabinoadenosine.

ar·a·bi·no·syl·cy·to·sine (aC, araC) (a′ră-bin-ō-sil-sī′tō-sēn). A compound of arabinose and cytosine, analogous to

ribosylcytosine (cytidine), that inhibits the biosynthesis of DNA; used as a chemotherapeutic agent because of antiviral and tumor-growth-inhibiting properties. SYN arabinocytidine, arabinofuranosylcytosine, cytarabine.

arab·i·tol (ă-rab′i-tol). A sugar alcohol obtained from the reduction of arabinose.

AraC. Abbreviation for *cytosine* arabinoside.

araC Symbol for arabinosylcytosine.

arach·ic ac·id (ă-rak′ik). SYN arachidic acid.

ar·a·chid·ic ac·id (a-ră-kid′ik). A fatty acid contained in peanut oil, butter, and other fats. SYN arachic acid, *n*-eicosanoic acid, *n*-icosanoic acid. [*Arachis,* fr. G. *arakis,* leguminous weed]

ar·a·chi·don·ic ac·id (ă-rak-i-don′ik). 5,8,11,14-Eicosatetraenoic (icosatetraenoic) acid; an unsaturated fatty acid, usually essential in nutrition; the biological precursor of the prostaglandins, the thromboxanes, and the leukotrienes (collectively known as eicosanoids).

ar·a·chi·don·ic ac·id cas·cade. Eicosanoid synthetic pathway.

ar·a·chis oil (ar′ă-kis). SYN peanut oil.

arach·ne·pho·bia (ă-rak-nē-fō′bē-ă). Morbid fear of spiders. SYN arachnophobia. [G. *arachne,* spider, + *phobos,* fear]

Arach·nia (ă-rak′nē-ă). A genus of nonmotile, nonsporeforming, facultatively anaerobic bacteria (family Actinomycetaceae) containing Gram-positive, non–acid-fast, branched, diphtheroid rods (0.2–0.3 by 3.0–5.0 μm and longer). These organisms produce filamentous microcolonies. Their metabolism is fermentative. Primarily propionic and acetic acids are produced from glucose. Catalase is not produced. The cell wall contains diaminopimelic acid but not arabinose. These organisms are pathogenic for humans, causing lacrimal canaliculitis and typical actinomycosis. The type species is *A. propionica.*

A. propio′nica, a species causing lacrimal canaliculitis and typical actinomycosis; it is the type species of the genus *A.* SYN *Propionibacterium propionicus.*

Arach·ni·da (ă-rak′ni-dă). A class of arthropods in the subphylum Chelicerata, consisting of spiders, scorpions, harvestmen, mites, ticks, and allies. [G. *arachnē,* spider]

arach·nid·ism (ă-rak′ni-dizm). Systemic poisoning following the bite of a spider (especially of the black widow).

necrotic a., a. caused by spiders belonging to the genus *Loxosceles;* cutaneous necrosis develops at the bite site, with slow healing and possible disfigurement.

arach·no·dac·ty·ly (ă-rak-nō-dak′ti-lē). A condition in which the hands and fingers, and often the feet and toes, are abnormally long and slender; a characteristic of Marfan syndrome [MIM*154700], Achard syndrome [MIM*100700], the MASS syndrome [MIM*157700], and kindred hereditary disorders of connective tissue. SYN spider finger. [G. *arachnē,* spider, + *daktylos,* finger]

arach·noid (ă-rak′noyd). SYN a. mater. [G. *arachnē,* spider, cobweb, + *eidos,* resemblance]

a. of brain, SYN cranial a. mater.

cranial a. mater [TA], that portion of the a. that lies within the cranial cavity and surrounds the brain and the cranial portion of the subarachnoid space. In several sites it is relatively widely separated from the pia mater, creating the cranial subarachnoid cisterns. SEE ALSO a. mater. SYN arachnoidea mater cranialis [TA], arachnoidea mater encephali⭑, a. mater cranialis, a. mater encephali, a. of brain, cerebral part of arachnoid.

a. mater [TA], A delicate fibrous membrane forming the middle of the three coverings of the central nervous system. In life the a. (specifically the arachnoid barrier cell layer) is tenuously attached to the externally adjacent dura mater (specifically the dural border cells) and there is no naturally occurring space at the dura-arachnoid interface. Thus in a spinal puncture dura mater and a. are penetrated simultaneously as if a single layer. Separation of the a. mater from the dura mater (usually through the dural border cell layer) may result from traumatic or pathologic processes creating what is commonly, but incorrectly, called a subdural hematoma. The a. mater is named for the delicate, spider weblike filaments that extend from its deep surface, through the CSF of the subarachnoid space, to the pia mater. SEE ALSO leptomeninx. SYN arachnoidea mater, arachnoides [TA], arachnoid membrane, arachnoid, parietal layer of leptomeninges.

a. mater crania·lis, SYN cranial a. mater.

a. mater enceph·ali, SYN cranial a. mater.

a. mater and pia mater,

a. of spinal cord, SYN spinal a. mater.

spinal a. mater [TA], that portion of the a. that lies within the vertebral canal and surrounds the spinal cord and the vertebral portion of the subarachnoid space. It extends from the foramen magnum above to the S2 vertebral level. Since the spinal cord ends at the L2 vertebral level, a wide separation occurs between the a. and pia mater, the lumbar cistern, filled with cerebrospinal fluid in which the cauda equina is suspended. SYN arachnoidea mater spinalis [TA], a. of spinal cord, a. spinalis, spinal part of arachnoid.

a. spina·lis, SYN spinal a. mater.

ar·ach·noi·dal (ă-rak-noy′dăl). Relating to the arachnoid membrane, or arachnoidea.

ar·ach·noi·dea mater, ar·ach·noi·des (ă-rak-noyd′ē-ă, -dēz) [TA]. SYN *arachnoid* mater. [Mod. L. *arachnoideus* fr. G. *arach-nē,* spider, + *eidos,* resemblance]

a.'s spinalis [TA], SYN spinal *arachnoid* mater.

arach·noi·di·tis (ă-rak-noy-dī′tis). Inflammation of the arachnoid membrane often with involvement of the subjacent subarachnoid space. SEE ALSO leptomeningitis. [arachnoidea + *-itis,* inflammation]

adhesive a., thickening of the leptomeninges, sometimes with obliteration of the subarachnoid space; commonly related to acute or chronic leptomeningitis of bacterial or chemical origin. SEE ALSO leptomeningeal *fibrosis.* SYN obliterative a.

neoplastic a., SYN neoplastic *meningitis.*

obliterative a., SYN adhesive a.

arach·no·ly·sin (ă-rak-nol′i-sin). A hemolytic substance in the venom of certain spiders.

arach·no·pho·bia (ă-rak-nō-fō′bē-ă). SYN arachnephobia.

ar·al·kyl (ă-ral′kil). A radical in which an aryl group is substituted for a hydrogen atom of an alkyl group; e.g., $C_6H_5CH_2–$. SYN arylated alkyl.

Aran, François A., French physician, 1817–1861. SEE A.-Duchenne *disease;* Duchenne-A. *disease.*

arane·ism (ă-rān′ism). Rarely used term for arachnidism.

Arantius, (Aranzio), Giulio C., Italian anatomist and physician, 1530–1589. SEE A. *ligament, nodule, ventricle; corpus* arantii; *ductus* venosus arantii.

ara·phia (ă-rā′fē-ă). SYN holorachischisis. [G. *a-* priv. + *rhaphē,* a seam]

ar·bor, pl. **ar·bo·res** (ar′bōr, ar-bō′rēz). In anatomy, a treelike structure with branchings. [L. tree]

a. vi′tae [TA], the arborescent appearance of gray and white matter in sagittal sections of the cerebellum.

a. vi′tae u′teri, SYN palmate *folds* of cervical canal, under *fold.*

ar·bo·res·cent (ar-bō-res′ent). SYN dendriform.

ar·bo·ri·za·tion (ar′bōr-i-zā′shŭn). **1.** The terminal branching of nerve fibers or blood vessels in a branching treelike pattern. **2.** The branched pattern formed under certain conditions by a dried smear of cervical mucus.

ar·bo·rize (ar′bōr-īz). To spread in a treelike branching pattern.

ar·bo·roid (ar′bōr-oyd). Denoting a colony of protozoa, each of which remains attached to another cell or to the main stem at one point, forming a branching or dendritic figure. [L. *arbor,* tree, + G. *eidos,* resemblance]

ar·bor·vi·rus (ar′bōr-vī′rŭs). Obsolete term for arbovirus.

ar·bo·vi·rus (ar′bō-vī′rŭs). An old name for a large, heterogeneous group of RNA viruses. There are over 500 species, which are distributed among several families (Togaviridae, Flaviviridae, Bunyaviridae, Arenaviridae, Rhabdoviridae, Reoviridae), and which have been recovered from arthropods, bats, and rodents; most, but not all, are arthropod-borne. These taxonomically diverse animal viruses are unified by an epidemiologic concept, i.e., transmission between vertebrate hosts by blood-feeding (hema-

tophagous) arthropod vectors, such as mosquitoes, ticks, sandflies, and midges.. Although about 100 species can infect humans, in most instances diseases produced by these viruses are of a very mild nature and difficult to distinguish from illnesses caused by viruses of other taxonomic groups. Apparent infections may be separated into several clinical syndromes: undifferentiated type fevers (systemic febrile disease), hepatitis, hemorrhagic fevers, and encephalitides. [*ar,* arthropod, + *bo,* borne, + virus]

ARC Abbreviation for AIDS-related *complex.*

arc (ark). **1.** A curved line or segment of a circle. **2.** Continuous luminous passage of an electric current in a gas or vacuum between two or more separated carbon or other electrodes. [L. *arcus,* a bow]

auricular a., binauricular a., a line carried over the cranium from the center of one external auditory meatus to that of the other. SYN interauricular a.

bregmatolambdoid a., the line running along the sagittal suture from the bregma to the apex of the lambdoid suture.

crater a., an a. of a direct current that forms a pitlike excavation at the positive pole.

flame a., an a. between two impregnated electrodes that causes volatilization of the core with resultant flame.

interauricular a., SYN auricular a.

longitudinal a. of skull, the line carried over the skull in the midline from the nasion to the opisthion.

mercury a., an electric discharge through mercury vapor between electrodes, one of which is usually mercury; provides a rich source of therapeutic ultraviolet rays; the containing tube is usually quartz; may also be glass with a fluorite window.

nasobregmatic a., a line running through the midline of the forehead from the nasion to the bregma.

naso-occipital a., the a. in the midline from the root of the nose to the inferior limit of the external occipital protuberance.

pulmonary a., radiographically displayed contour of main pulmonary artery on frontal chest radiograph.

🔲 **reflex a.,** the route followed by nerve impulses in the production of a reflex act, from the peripheral receptor organ through the afferent nerve to the central nervous system synapse and then through the efferent nerve to the effector organ.

Riolan a., (1) SYN intestinal arterial *arcades,* under *arcade;* **(2)** SYN marginal *artery* of colon; SEE ALSO Riolan *anastomosis;* **(3)** SYN Riolan *anastomosis.*

ar·cade (ar-kād). An anatomic structure or structures (especially a blood vessel) taking the form of a series of arches. [L. *arcus,* arc, bow]

anomalous mitral a., short chordae tendineae extending from both papillary muscles to the central portion of the anterior leaflet of the mitral valve and resulting in stenosis or incompetence of the valve.

arterial a.'s, a series of anastomosing arterial arches, as the intestinal arterial a.'s between the branches of the jejunal and ileal arteries in the mesentery and the pancreaticoduodenal arteries on the head of the pancreas.

Flint a., a series of vascular arches at the bases of the pyramids of the kidney.

intestinal arterial a.'s, the series of arterial arches formed in the mesentery by anastomoses between adjacent jejunal and ileal arteries and from which vasa recta arise. The arterial a.'s of the ileum are shorter and more complex than those of the jejunum. SEE ALSO arterial *arches* of ileum, under *arch,* arterial *arches* of jejunum, under *arch,* marginal *artery* of colon. SYN intermesenteric arterial anastomoses, Riolan arc (1), Riolan a.'s.

lower dental a., ☆official alternate term for mandibular dental a.

mandibular dental a. [TA], the teeth supported by the alveolar part of the mandible, whether the 10 deciduous teeth or the 16 permanent teeth. SYN arcus dentalis inferior☆, lower dental a.☆, inferior dental arch, mandibular dentition.

marginal a., ☆official alternate term for marginal *artery* of colon.

maxillary dental a. [TA], the teeth supported by the alveolar process of the two maxillae, whether the 10 deciduous teeth or the 16 permanent teeth. SYN arcus dentalis maxillaris [TA], arcus dentalis superior⋆, upper dental a.⋆, maxillary dentition, superior dental arch.

pancreaticoduodenal arterial a.'s, anastomoses between the anterior and posterior pancreaticoduodenal arteries (from the gastroduodenal artery) and the anterior and posterior inferior pancreaticoduodenal arteries (from the superior mesenteric artery) on the anterior and posterior aspects of the head of the pancreas and the duodenum, supplying both structures.

Riolan a.'s, SYN intestinal arterial a.'s; SEE ALSO Riolan *anastomosis.*

upper dental a., ⋆official alternate term for maxillary dental a.

Ar·can·o·bac·te·ri·um (ar-kā′nō-bac-tēr′ē-um). A genus of nonmotile, facultatively anaerobic bacteria containing Gram-positive slender irregular rods, sometimes showing clubbed ends that may be in V formation with no filaments. These organisms are obligate parasites of the pharynx in farm animals and humans, occasionally causing lesions on the pharynx or skin. The type species is *A. haemolyticum.*

A. haemolyticum, a species that causes pharyngitis and chronic skin ulcers in humans as well as farm animals.

ar·cate (ar′kāt). SYN arcuate.

ARCH

arch [TA]. Any structure resembling a bent bow or an arch; an arc. In anatomy, any vaulted or archlike structure. SEE arcus. SYN arcus [TA]. [thru O. Fr. fr. L. *arcus,* bow]

abdominothoracic a., a bell-shaped line defined by the lower end of the sternum and the costal a.'s on each side, constituting a boundary line between the anterolateral portions of the thoracic and abdominal walls.

alveolar a. of mandible [TA], the free margin of the alveolar process of the mandible. SYN arcus alveolaris mandibulae [TA], limbus alveolaris (1).

alveolar a. of maxilla [TA], the free border of the alveolar process of the maxilla. SYN arcus alveolaris maxillae [TA], limbus alveolaris (2).

anterior a. of atlas [TA], an arch that connects the lateral masses of the atlas anteriorly and articulates with the anterior articular facet of the dens of the axis. SYN arcus anterior atlantis [TA].

anterior palatine a., SYN palatoglossal a.

a. of the aorta, SYN aortic a. (1).

aortic a., (1) the curved portion between the ascending and descending parts of the aorta; it begins as a continuation of the ascending aorta posterior to the sternal angle, runs posteriorly and slightly to the left as it passes over the root of the left lung, and becomes the descending aorta as it reaches and begins to course along the vertebral column; it gives rise to the brachiocephalic trunk, the left common carotid and left subclavian arteries; SYN a. of the aorta. **(2)** any member of the several pairs of arterial channels encircling the embryonic pharynx in the mesenchyme of the brachial a.'s; there are potentially six pairs, but in mammals the fifth pair is poorly developed or absent. The first and second pairs are functional only in very young embryos; the third pair is involved in the formation of the carotids; the fourth a. on the left is incorporated in the a. of the aorta; the sixth pair forms the proximal part of the pulmonary arteries. SYN arcus aortae.

aortic a.'s, a series of arterial channels encircling the embryonic pharynx in the mesenchyme of the branchial a.'s; there are potentially six pairs, but in mammals the fifth pair is poorly developed or absent. The first and second pairs are functional only in very young embryos; the third pair is involved in the formation of the carotids; the fourth a. on the left is incorporated in the a. of the aorta; the sixth pair forms the proximal part of the pulmonary arteries.

arterial a.'s of colon, anastomoses between adjacent branches of the colic arteries that form a.'s in the mesocolon from which the walls of the colon are supplied. When these form a continuous paracolic artery, it is referred to as the marginal artery of the colon. SEE marginal *artery* of colon.

arterial a.'s of ileum, a.'s formed in the mesentery by branches of the superior mesenteric artery from which vessels (*vasa* recta, under *vas*) arise to supply the wall of the ileum. SEE ALSO intestinal arterial *arcades,* under *arcade.*

arterial a.'s of jejunum, a.'s formed in the mesentery by branches of the superior mesenteric artery from which vessels (*vasa* recta, under *vas*) arise to supply the walls of the jejunum. SEE ALSO intestinal arterial *arcades,* under *arcade.*

arterial a. of lower eyelid, SYN inferior palpebral (arterial) a.

arterial a. of upper eyelid, SYN superior palpebral (arterial) a.

axillary a., SYN pectorodorsalis *muscle.*

branchial a.'s, typically, 6 a.'s in vertebrates; in the lower vertebrates, they bear gills; in the higher vertebrates, they appear transiently and give rise to specialized structures in the head and neck. SYN pharyngeal a.'s, visceral a.'s.

carpal a.'s, two anastomotic arterial twigs running transversely across the wrist: the *palmar* or *anterior* lies in front of the carpus, being formed by palmar carpal branches of the radial and ulnar arteries; the *dorsal* or *posterior* lies on the dorsal surface of the carpus, being formed by the dorsal carpal branches of the radial and ulnar arteries.

coracoacromial a., a protective a. formed by the smooth inferior aspect of the acromion and the coracoid process of the scapula with the coracoacromial ligament spanning between them. This

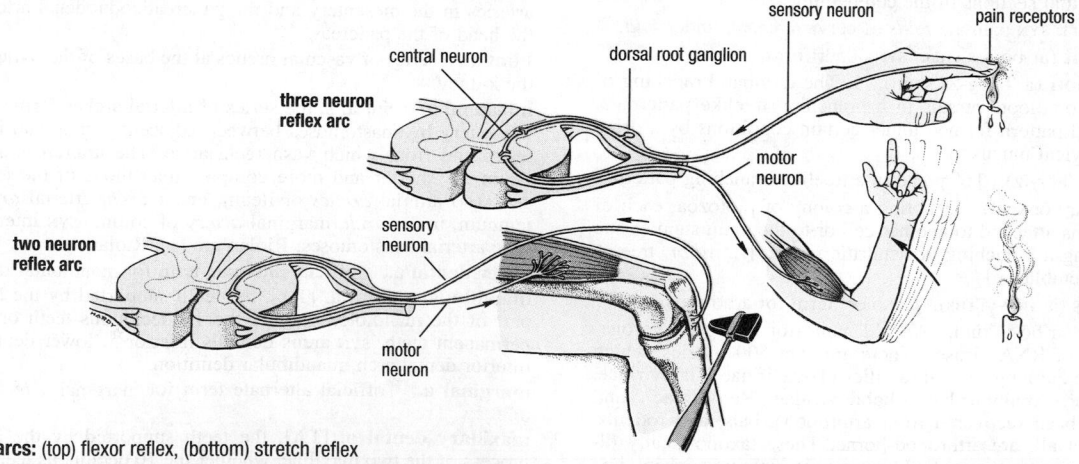

reflex arcs: (top) flexor reflex, (bottom) stretch reflex

osseoligamentous structure overlies the head of the humerus, preventing its upward displacement from the glenoid fossa.

Corti a., the a. formed by the junction of the heads of Corti inner and outer pillar cells.

cortical a.'s of kidney, the portions of renal substance (cortex) intervening between the bases of the pyramids and the capsule of the kidney.

costal a., ☆official alternate term for costal *margin.*

a. of cricoid cartilage [TA], the narrow part of the cartilage that encircles the air passage anterior to the lamina. SYN arcus cartilaginis cricoideae [TA].

crural a., SYN inguinal *ligament.*

deep crural a., SYN iliopubic *tract.*

deep palmar (arterial) a. [TA], the arterial arch located deep to the long flexor tendons in the hand. It is formed by the terminal part of the radial artery in conjunction with the deep palmar branch of the ulnar artery. The a. gives rise to palmar metacarpal and princeps pollicis arteries. SYN arcus palmaris profundus, arcus volaris profundus.

deep palmar venous a. [TA], the venous arch that accompanies the deep palmar arterial arch; it usually consists of paired venae comitantes. SYN arcus venosus palmaris profundus [TA].

dental a., the curved composite structure of the natural dentition and the residual ridge, or the remains thereof after the loss of some or all of the natural teeth.

dorsal carpal arterial a. [TA], a vascular network over the dorsal surface of the carpal joints, formed by anastomoses of branches of the anterior and posterior interosseous, and dorsal carpal branches of the radial and ulnar arteries. SYN rete carpale dorsale [TA], dorsal carpal network, rete carpi posterius.

dorsal venous a. of foot [TA], the arch in the subcutaneous tissue of the dorsum of the foot formed by the dorsal and digital veins; it unites medially with the dorsal vein of the great toe to form the great saphenous vein, and laterally with the dorsal vein of the little toe to form the small saphenous. SYN arcus venosus dorsalis pedis [TA].

double aortic a., congenital malformation of the aorta that splits and has a right and a left a. instead of a single a.

expansion a., an orthodontic appliance that moves the dental structures distally, bucally, or labially, creating increased molar to molar width and arch length.

fallen a.'s, a breaking down of the a.'s of the foot, either longitudinal, transverse, or both; the resulting deformity is flat (longitudinal) or splay (transverse) foot, or both.

fallopian a., SYN inguinal *ligament.*

femoral a., SYN inguinal *ligament.*

a.'s of the foot, SEE longitudinal a. of foot, plantar a.

glossopalatine a., SYN palatoglossal a.

Gothic a., SYN needle point *tracing.*

Haller a.'s, SEE lateral arcuate *ligament,* medial arcuate *ligament.*

hemal a.'s, (1) the a.'s that collectively comprise the thoracic cage, each consisting of a vertebra (body, pedicle, and transverse processes), the corresponding pair of ribs and their articular cartilages, and the portion of the sternum to which they attach. **(2)** three or four V-shaped bones located ventral to the bodies of the third to sixth coccygeal vertebrae; they represent intercentra and usually enclose the ventral caudal artery and vein.

hyoid a., the second visceral, or branchial, a; the second postoral a. in the branchial a. series.

iliopectineal a. [TA], a thickened band of fused iliac and psoas fascia passing from the posterior aspect of the inguinal ligament anteriorly across the front of the femoral nerve to attach to the iliopectineal eminence of the hip bone posteriorly. The iliopectineal a. thus forms a septum which subdivides the space deep to the inguinal ligament into a lateral muscular lacunae and a medial vascular lacunae. When a psoas minor muscle is present, its tendon of insertion blends with the iliopectineal a. SYN arcus iliopectineus [TA], iliopectineal ligament, ligamentum iliopectineale.

inferior dental a., SYN mandibular dental *arcade.* SYN arcus dentalis mandibularis [TA].

inferior palpebral (arterial) a. [TA], formed by the medial palpebral artery, which communicates with a branch of the lacrimal artery along the tarsal margin. SYN arcus palpebralis inferior [TA], arterial a. of lower eyelid.

jugular venous a. [TA], a connecting vein between the two anterior jugular veins in the suprasternal space. SYN arcus venosus juguli [TA].

labial a., an orthodontic a. wire that approximates the labial surfaces of the teeth.

Langer a., SYN pectorodorsalis *muscle.*

lateral longitudinal a. of foot, formed by calcaneus, cuboid, and two lateral metatarsals; the combined a. is supported normally by ligaments, intrinsic muscles, and the tendons of extrinsic muscles of the foot. SYN arcus pedis longitudinalis pars lateralis.

lateral lumbocostal a., SYN lateral arcuate *ligament.*

lingual a., an orthodontic a. wire that approximates the lingual surfaces of the teeth.

longitudinal a. of foot, SEE medial longitudinal a. of foot, lateral longitudinal a. of foot. SYN arcus pedis longitudinalis.

malar a., SYN zygomatic a.

mandibular a., the first postoral a. in the branchial a. series. SYN mandibular process.

medial longitudinal a. of foot, formed by the calcaneus, talus, navicular, three cuneiform bones, and the three medial metatarsals. SYN arcus pedis longitudinalis pars medialis.

medial lumbocostal a., SYN medial arcuate *ligament.*

nasal a., bridge of the nose, the upward arching roof of the piriform aperture formed by the nasal processes of the maxilla of each side and the nasal bones between them. Eyeglasses rest centrally on various portions of this a.

nasal venous a., an a. formed at the root of the nose by the two supratrochlear veins connected by a transverse vein.

neural a. of vertebra, SYN vertebral a.

a. of the palate, the vaulted roof of the mouth.

palatoglossal a. [TA], one of a pair of ridges or folds of mucous membrane passing from the soft palate to the side of the tongue; it encloses the palatoglossus muscle and forms the anterior margin of the tonsillar fossa. Also demarcates the oral cavity from the isthmus of fauces. SYN arcus palatoglossus [TA], anterior pillar of fauces☆, plica anterior faucium☆, anterior palatine a., arcus glossopalatinus, glossopalatine a., glossopalatine fold.

palatopharyngeal a. [TA], one of a pair of ridges or folds of mucous membrane that pass downward from the posterior margin of the soft palate to the lateral wall of the pharynx. It encloses the palatopharyngeus muscle and forms the posterior margin of the tonsillar fossa. It also demarcates the isthmus of fauces from the oropharynx. SYN arcus palatopharyngeus [TA], plica posterior faucium☆, posterior pillar of fauces☆, pharyngopalatine a., posterior palatine a.

pharyngeal a.'s, SYN branchial a.'s.

pharyngopalatine a., SYN palatopharyngeal a.

plantar a., SYN deep plantar (arterial) *arch.*

plantar arterial a., SYN deep plantar (arterial) *arch.*

plantar venous a. [TA], the arch formed by the plantar digital veins from the toes, which accompanies the plantar arterial arch. SYN arcus venosus plantaris [TA].

popliteal a., SYN arcuate popliteal *ligament.*

posterior a. of atlas [TA], the posterior arch of the atlas that connects the lateral masses of the atlas posteriorly, forming the posterior wall of the vertebral canal at this level. SYN arcus posterior atlantis [TA].

posterior palatine a., SYN palatopharyngeal a.

postoral a.'s, the series of branchial a.'s caudal to the mouth; the first is the mandibular, the second is the hyoid; caudal to the hyoid, the a.'s are unnamed, and designated only by their postoral number.

primitive costal a.'s, a.'s formed in the thoracic region of the vertebral column in the embryo from the costal processes or costal elements which give rise to the ribs.

pubic a. [TA], the arch formed by the symphysis, bodies, and inferior rami of the pubic bones. SEE ALSO subpubic *angle.* SYN arcus pubis [TA].

ribbon a., a thin, ribbon-shaped, rectangular orthodontic a. wire applied to the dental a.'s so that its widest dimension is parallel to the labial or buccal surfaces of the teeth.

subcostal a., ☆official alternate term for infrasternal *angle.*

superciliary a. [TA], a fullness extending laterally from the glabella on either side, above the orbital margin of the frontal bone. SYN arcus superciliaris [TA], superciliary ridge.

superficial palmar (arterial) a. [TA], the arterial arch in the hand located superficial to the long flexor tendons approximately at the level of a line extrapolated across the palm from the distal side of the outstretched thumb. It is formed principally by the termination of the superficial ulnar artery and is usually completed by a communication with the superficial palmar branch of the radial artery. The a. gives rise to the common palmar digital arteries. SYN arcus palmaris superficialis [TA], arcus volaris superficialis.

superficial palmar venous a. [TA], the venous arch accompanying the superficial palmar arterial arch; it consists usually of paired venae comitantes and is drained by the superficial ulnar and radial veins. SYN arcus venosus palmaris superficialis [TA].

superior dental a., SYN maxillary dental *arcade.*

superior palpebral (arterial) a. [TA], formed by communicating branches of the medial and lateral palpebral arteries. Often two arches are present, one located near the free border of the tarsal plate, the other along the upper border of the tarsus. SYN arcus palpebralis superior [TA], arterial a. of upper eyelid.

supraorbital a., SYN supraorbital *margin.*

tarsal a., SEE inferior palpebral (arterial) a., superior palpebral (arterial) a.

tendinous a. [TA], **(1)** a white, fibrous band attached to bone and/or muscle, arching over and thus protecting neurovascular elements passing beneath it from injurious compression; **(2)** a linear thickening of the deep fascia of a muscle which provides attachment for ligaments and/or muscle fibers. SYN arcus tendineus [TA].

tendinous a. of levator ani muscle [TA], a thickened portion of the obturator fascia that extends in an arching line from the pubis posteriorly to the ischial spine and gives origin to part of the levator ani muscle. SYN arcus tendineus musculi levatoris ani [TA], arcus tendineus of obturator fascia, arcus tendineus of pelvic diaphragm.

tendinous a. of pelvic fascia [TA], a linear thickening of the superior fascia of the pelvic diaphragm extending posteriorly from the body of the pubis alongside the bladder (and vagina in the female) and giving attachment to the supporting ligaments of the pelvic viscera. SYN arcus tendineus fasciae pelvis [TA].

tendinous a. of soleus muscle [TA], a tendinous arch stretching over—and defining the termination of—the popliteal vessels between the tibia and fibula, which gives origin to the central portion of the soleus muscle. SYN arcus tendineus musculi solei [TA].

a. of thoracic duct [TA], terminal portion of thoracic duct that turns abruptly to the left, usually at the C7 vertebral level, to enter the superolateral aspect of the junction of the left subclavian and internal jugular veins. SEE ALSO thoracic *duct.* SYN arcus ductus thoracici [TA].

transverse a. of foot, the arch formed by the proximal parts of the metatarsal bones, the three cuneiform bones, and the cuboid. SYN arcus pedis transversalis.

Treitz a., SYN paraduodenal *fold.*

vertebral a. [TA], the posterior projection from the body of a vertebra that encloses the vertebral foramen; it consists of paired pedicles and laminae; the spinous, transverse, and articular processes arise from the arch. In aggregate, the venous a.'s—and the ligamenta flava that unite them—form the posterior wall of the vertebral (spinal) canal. SYN arcus vertebrae [TA], neural a. of vertebra.

visceral a.'s, SYN branchial a.'s.

W-a., a fixed maxillary expansion device attached to the lingual part of the molars, with either bilateral or unilateral extension arms.

wire a., a wire conforming to the dental a.; used to restore the normal curve to the denture.

zygomatic a. [TA], the arch formed by the temporal process of the zygomatic bone that joins the zygomatic process of the temporal bone. SYN arcus zygomaticus [TA], cheek bone (2), malar a., zygoma (2).

△**arch-, arche-, archi-.** Combining forms meaning primitive or ancestral; also first, chief, extreme. [G. *archē,* origin, beginning, + -o-]

ar·chae·o·cer·e·bel·lum (ar′kē-ō-ser′ĕ-bel′lŭm). SYN archicerebellum. [G. *archaios,* ancient, + cerebellum]

ar·chae·us (ar-kē′ŭs). Term first used by Valentine and later by Paracelsus and van Helmont to denote a spirit that presided over and governed bodily processes. SYN archeus. [L. fr. G. *archaios,* chief, leader]

ar·cha·ic (ar-kā′ik). Ancient; old; in jungian psychology, denoting the ancestral past of mental processes. [G. *archaikos,* ancient]

Archambault, LaSalle, U.S. neurologist, 1879–1940. SEE Meyer-A. *loop.*

△**arche-.** SEE arch-.

arch·en·ter·on (ark-en′ter-on). SYN primitive *gut.* [G. *archē,* beginning, + *enteron,* intestine]

ar·che·o·cer·e·bel·lum (ar-kē-ō-ser′-ĕ-bel′ lŭm). SYN vestibulocerebellum.

ar·che·o·ki·net·ic (ar-kē-ō-ki-net′ik). Denoting a low and primitive type of motor nerve mechanism, such as is found in the peripheral and the ganglionic nervous systems. Cf. neokinetic, paleokinetic. [G. *archaios,* ancient, + *kinētikos,* relating to movement]

ar·che·type (ar′kē-tīp). **1.** A primitive structural plan from which various modifications have evolved. **2.** In jungian psychology, structural manifestation of the collective unconscious. SYN imago (2). [G. *archetypos,* pattern, model, fr. *archē,* beginning, + *typtō,* to stamp out]

ar·che·us (ar-kē′ŭs). SYN archaeus.

△**archi-.** SEE arch-.

ar·chi·cer·e·bel·lum (ar′ki-ser-ĕ-bel′ŭm) [TA]. The small, phylogenetically oldest portion of the cerebellum, sometimes called vestibulocerebellum because its afferents arise primarily from the vestibular ganglion and nuclei; in mammals, it is represented by four subdivisions of the cerebellum: nodulus, uvula vermis, flocculus, and lingula of cerebellum. SYN archaeocerebellum. [archi- + L. *cerebellum*]

ar·chi·cor·tex (ar′ki-kōr′teks) [TA]. **1.** Typically, the phylogenetically older parts of the cerebral cortex. **2.** More specifically, the cortex forming the hippocampus. SEE ALSO allocortex, cerebral *cortex.* SYN archipallium. [archi- + L. *cortex*]

ar·chil (ar′kil) [old C.I. 1242]. A violet dye from the lichens *Rocella tinctoria* and *R. fuciformis.* SYN orchella, orchil, roccellin.

ar·chin (ar′kin). SYN emodin.

ar·chi·pal·li·um (ar-ki-pal′ē-ŭm). SYN archicortex. [archi- + L. *pallium*]

ar·chi·tec·ton·ics (ar-ki-tek-ton′iks). SYN cytoarchitecture.

arch·wire (arch′wīr). A device consisting of a wire conforming to the alveolar or dental arch, used as an anchorage in correcting irregularities in the position of the teeth. SYN arch wire.

ar·ci·form (ar′si-fōrm). SYN arcuate.

Ar·co·bac·ter (ar-kō-bak′ter). A genus of bacteria in the family Campylobacteraceae that are Gram-negative, aerotolerant, and able to grow at 15° C. The type strain is *Arcobacter butzleri.*

A. butzleri, a bacterial species of *Arcobacter* found in poultry and meat; has been associated with diarrheal and systemic diseases in humans.

arc·ta·tion (ark-tā′shŭn). A narrowing, contraction, stricture, or coarctation. [L. *arto* (improp. *arcto*), pp. *-atus,* to tighten]

ar·cu·al (ar′kū-ăl). Relating to an arch.

ar·cu·ate (ar′kū-āt). Denoting a form that is arched or has the shape of a bow. SYN arcate, arciform. [L. *arcuatus,* bowed]

ar·cu·a·tion (ar-kū-ā′shŭn). A bending or curvature.

ARCUS

ar·cus (ar'kŭs) [TA]. SYN arch. [L. a bow]
  a. adipo'sus, SYN a. senilis.
  a. alveola'ris mandib'ulae [TA], SYN alveolar *arch* of mandible.
  a. alveola'ris maxil'lae [TA], SYN alveolar *arch* of maxilla.
  a. ante'rior atlan'tis [TA], SYN anterior *arch* of atlas.
  a. aor'tae, SYN aortic *arch* (2).
  a. cartila'ginis cricoi'deae [TA], SYN *arch* of cricoid cartilage.
  a. cornea'lis, SYN a. senilis.
  a. costa'lis [TA], SYN costal *margin*.
  a. costa'rum, SYN costal *margin*.
  a. denta'lis infe'rior, ⋆official alternate term for mandibular dental *arcade*.
  a. dentalis mandibularis [TA], SYN inferior dental *arch*.
  a. dentalis maxillaris [TA], SYN maxillary dental *arcade*.
  a. denta'lis supe'rior, ⋆official alternate term for maxillary dental *arcade*.
  a. ductus thoracici [TA], SYN *arch* of thoracic duct.
  a. glossopalati'nus, SYN palatoglossal *arch*.
  a. iliopectin'eus [TA], SYN iliopectineal *arch*.
  a. inguina'lis, ⋆official alternate term for inguinal *ligament*.
  a. juveni'lis, SYN a. senilis.
  a. lipoi'des, SYN a. senilis.
  a. lumbocosta'lis latera'lis, SYN lateral arcuate *ligament*.
  a. lumbocosta'lis media'lis, SYN medial arcuate *ligament*.
  a. marginalis coli, ⋆official alternate term for marginal *artery* of colon.
  a. palati'ni, SEE palatoglossal *arch*, palatopharyngeal *arch*.
  a. palatoglos'sus [TA], SYN palatoglossal *arch*.
  a. palatopharyn'geus [TA], SYN palatopharyngeal *arch*.
  a. palma'ris profun'dus, SYN deep palmar (arterial) *arch*.
  a. palma'ris superficia'lis [TA], SYN superficial palmar (arterial) *arch*.
  a. palpebra'lis infe'rior [TA], SYN inferior palpebral (arterial) *arch*.
  a. palpebra'lis supe'rior [TA], SYN superior palpebral (arterial) *arch*.
  a. pe'dis longitudina'lis, SYN longitudinal *arch* of foot.
  a. pe'dis longitudina'lis pars lateralis, SYN lateral longitudinal *arch* of foot.
  a. pe'dis longitudina'lis pars medialis, SYN medial longitudinal *arch* of foot.
  a. pe'dis transversa'lis, SYN transverse *arch* of foot.
  a. plantaris profundus, SYN deep plantar (arterial) *arch*.
  a. poste'rior atlan'tis [TA], SYN posterior *arch* of atlas.
  a. pu'bis [TA], SYN pubic *arch*.
  a. rani'nus, SYN ranine *anastomosis*.
  a. seni'lis, an opaque, grayish ring at the periphery of the cornea just within the sclerocorneal junction, of frequent occurrence in the aged; it results from a deposit of fatty granules in, or hyaline degeneration of, the lamellae and cells of the cornea. SYN anterior embryotoxon, a. adiposus, a. cornealis, a. juvenilis, a. lipoides, gerontoxon, linea corneae senilis, lipoidosis corneae.
  a. supercilia'ris [TA], SYN superciliary *arch*.
  a. tar'seus, SEE inferior palpebral (arterial) *arch*, superior palpebral (arterial) *arch*.
  a. tendin'eus [TA], SYN tendinous *arch*.
  a. tendin'eus fas'ciae pel'vis [TA], SYN tendinous *arch* of pelvic fascia.
  a. tendin'eus mus'culi levato'ris ani [TA], SYN tendinous *arch* of levator ani muscle.
  a. tendin'eus mus'culi so'lei [TA], SYN tendinous *arch* of soleus muscle.
  a. tendineus of obturator fascia, SYN tendinous *arch* of levator ani muscle.
  a. tendineus of pelvic diaphragm, SYN tendinous *arch* of levator ani muscle.
  a. un'guium, SYN *lunule* of nail.
  a. veno'sus dorsa'lis pe'dis [TA], SYN dorsal venous *arch* of foot.
  a. veno'sus jug'uli [TA], SYN jugular venous *arch*.
  a. veno'sus palma'ris profun'dus [TA], SYN deep palmar venous *arch*.
  a. veno'sus palma'ris superficia'lis [TA], SYN superficial palmar venous *arch*.
  a. veno'sus planta'ris [TA], SYN plantar venous *arch*.
  a. ver'tebrae [TA], SYN vertebral *arch*; SEE ALSO hemal *arches*, under *arch*.
  a. vola'ris profun'dus, SYN deep palmar (arterial) *arch*.
  a. vola'ris superficia'lis, SYN superficial palmar (arterial) *arch*.
  a. zygomat'icus [TA], SYN zygomatic *arch*.

ar·dor (ar'dōr). Old term for a hot or burning sensation. [L. fire, heat]

ⓘARDS Abbreviation for adult respiratory distress *syndrome*.

AREA

ar·ea (a), pl. **ar·e·ae** (ār'ē-ă, -ē). **1** [TA]. Any circumscribed surface or space. **2.** All of the part supplied by a given artery or nerve. **3.** A part of an organ having a special function, as the motor a. of the brain. SEE ALSO regio, region, space, spatium, zone. [L. a courtyard]
  acoustic a., the floor of the lateral recess of the fourth ventricle, extending medially to the limiting sulcus and overlying the cochlear and vestibular nuclei of the rhombencephalon. SYN a. vestibularis [TA], a. acustica.
  a. acu'stica, SYN acoustic a.
  amygdaloclaustral a. [TA], that region in the temporal lobe where lateral portions of the amygdaloid nucleus are in close apposition to, or fuse with, ventral aspects of the claustrum. SYN a. amygdaloclaustralis [TA].
  a. amygdaloclaustralis [TA], SYN amygdaloclaustral a.
  a. amygdaloidea anterior [TA], SYN anterior amygdaloid a.
  amygdalopiriform transition a. [TA], the area where the groups of cells forming the amygdaloid nucleus are closely adjacent to the piriform cortex. SYN a. transitionis amygdalopiriformis [TA].
  anterior amygdaloid a. [TA], the most rostral portion of the amygdaloid complex composed of scattered cells representing a transition into the more distinctly organized divisions of the amygdala. SYN a. amygdaloidea anterior [TA].
  anterior hypothalamic a., the rostral portion of the hypothalamus located generally internal to the region of the optic chiasm; contains the following nuclei: anterior hypothalamic nucleus [TA] (nucleus anterior hypothalami [TA]), anterior periventricular nucleus [TA] (nucleus periventricularis ventralis [TA], interstitial nuclei of anterior hypothalamus [TA] (nuclei interstitiales hypothalami anteriores [TA]), lateral preoptic nucleus [TA] (nucleus preopticus lateralis [TA]), medial preoptic nucleus [TA] (nucleus preopticus medialis [TA]), median preoptic nucleus [TA] (nucleus preopticus medianus [TA]), paraventricular nucleus [TA] (nucleus paraventricularis hypothalami [TA]), periventricular preoptic nucleus [TA] (nucleus preopticus periventricularis [TA]), suprachiasmatic nucleus [TA] (nucleus suprachiasmaticus [TA]) and the supraoptic nucleus [TA] (nucleus supraopticus [TA]). The latter cell group consists of dorsomedial, ventromedial, and dorsolateral parts. SEE ALSO hypothalamus. SYN a. hypothalamica rostralis [TA], anterior hypothalamic region⋆.
  anterior intercondylar a. of tibia [TA], the broad depressed a. between the tibial condyles anteriorly to which attach the anterior

ends of the menisci and the anterior cruciate ligament. SYN a. intercondylaris anterior tibiae [TA].

aortic a. (of auscultation), the region of the chest wall over the second right costal cartilage, where sounds produced at the aortic orifice are often best heard.

apical a., the a. about the root end of a tooth.

association areas, SYN association *cortex*.

auditory a., SYN auditory *cortex*.

bare a. of liver [TA], the a. on the posterosuperior (diaphragmatic) surface of the liver, bordered by the coronary ligament but itself devoid of peritoneum, so that the diaphragm and liver lie in direct contact and are adherent to each other. not covered by peritoneum. SYN a. nuda hepatis [TA].

bare a. of stomach, the part of posterior surface of the fundus of the stomach between the two diverging layers of the gastrophrenic ligament, that is not covered by peritoneum.

basal seat a., that portion of the oral structures which is available to support a denture.

Broca a., SYN Broca *center*.

Broca parolfactory a., SYN parolfactory a.

Brodmann areas, areas of the cerebral cortex mapped out on the basis of the cortical cytoarchitectural patterns. SEE cerebral *cortex*.

a. of cardiac dullness, a triangular a. determined by percussion of the front of the chest; it corresponds to the part of the heart that is not covered by lung tissue.

catchment a., a term relating to community mental health center which delimits the geographic area surrounding each center, and thus the population of individuals who qualify for mental health services provided by each center.

a. centra′lis, SYN *macula* of retina.

a. coch′leae [TA], SYN cochlear a.

cochlear a. [TA], the a. inferior to the transverse crest of the fundus of the internal acoustic meatus through which the filaments of the cochlear nerve pass to enter the cochlea; forms the base of the conical modiolus about which the cochlear canal spirals. SEE *base* of modiolus of cochlea. SYN a. cochleae [TA].

Cohnheim a., a polygonal mosaic-like figure formed by a group of myofibrils, as seen in the cross-section of a skeletal muscle fiber examined under the microscope; a shrinkage artifact of fixation. SYN Cohnheim field.

contact a., that part of the proximal surface of a tooth which touches the adjacent tooth mesially or distally. SYN contact point, point of proximal contact.

cribriform a. of the renal papilla [TA], the apex of a renal papilla pierced by 10–22 openings of the papillary ducts, the foramina papillaria. SYN a. cribrosa papillae renalis [TA].

a. cribro′sa papillae renalis [TA], SYN cribriform a. of the renal papilla.

denture-bearing a., SYN denture foundation a.

denture foundation a., that portion of the basal seat which supports the complete or partial denture base under occlusal load. SYN basal seat, denture-bearing a., denture-supporting a., stress-bearing a. (1), supporting a. (2), tissue-bearing a.

denture-supporting a., SYN denture foundation a.

dermatomic a., SYN dermatome (3).

dorsal hypothalamic a. [TA], a relatively small region of the hypothalamus located ventral to the hypothalamic sulcus; contains the following nuclei: portions of the dorsomedial nucleus [TA] (nucleus dorsomedialis [TA]), endopeduncular nucleus [TA]) (nucleus endopeduncularis [TA]) and portions of the nucleus of the ansa lenticularis (nucleus ansae lenticularis [TA]). SEE ALSO hypothalamus. SYN a. hypothalamica dorsalis [TA], dorsal hypothalamic region✩.

embryonal a., embryonic a., the a. of the blastoderm on either side of, and immediately cephalic to, the primitive streak where the component cell layers have become thickened.

entorhinal a., brodmann a. 28, a cytoarchitecturally well-defined a. of multilaminate cerebral cortex on the medial aspect of the parahippocampal gyrus, immediately caudal to the olfactory cortex of the uncus; the a. is the origin of the major fiber system afferent to the hippocampus, the so-called perforant pathway.

excitable a., SYN motor *cortex*.

facial nerve a. [TA], the a. of the fundus of the internal acoustic meatus superior to the transverse crest through which the facial nerve passes to enter the facial canal. SYN a. nervi facialis [TA].

Flechsig areas, three divisions (anterior, lateral, posterior) of each lateral half of the medulla as seen on transverse section, marked off by the root fibers of the hypoglossal and vagus nerves.

frontal a., SYN frontal *cortex*.

fronto-orbital a., SYN orbitofrontal *cortex*.

fusion a., SYN Panum a.

gastric a. [TA], one of a number of small polygonal areas, 1–6 mm in diameter, separated by linear depressions on the surface of the mucous membrane of the stomach; they contain the gastric pits, with several gastric glands opening into each pit. SYN a. gastrica [TA].

a. gas′trica [TA], SYN gastric a.

germinal a., a. germinati′va, the place in the blastoderm where the embryo begins to be formed. SYN germinal *disk*.

Head areas, areas of skin exhibiting reflex hyperesthesia and hyperalgesia due to visceral disease.

a. hypothalamica dorsalis [TA], SYN dorsal hypothalamic a.

a. hypothalamica intermedia, SYN intermediate hypothalamic a.

a. hypothalamica lateralis [TA], SYN lateral hypothalamic a.

a. hypothalamica posterior [TA], SYN posterior hypothalamic a.

a. hypothalamica rostralis [TA], SYN anterior hypothalamic a.

impression a., in dentistry, that surface which is recorded in an impression.

inferior vestibular a. [TA], the a. of the fundus of the internal acoustic meatus inferior to the transverse crest through which the inferior portion of the vestibular (saccular) nerve passes. SYN a. vestibularis inferior [TA].

insular a., SYN insula (1).

a. intercondyla′ris ante′rior tibiae [TA], SYN anterior intercondylar a. of tibia.

a. intercondyla′ris poste′rior tibiae [TA], SYN posterior intercondylar a. of tibia.

intermediate hypothalamic a. [TA], the portion of the hypothalamus located generally internal to the region of the infundibulum; contains the following nuclei; dorsal nucleus [TA] (nucleus dorsalis hypothalami [TA]), parts of the dorsomedial nucleus [TA] (nucleus dorsomedialis [TA]), arcuate nucleus [TA] (nucleus arcuatus [TA]), posterior periventricular nucleus [TA] (nucleus periventricularis posterior [TA]), retrochiasmatic area [TA] (area retrochiasmatica [TA]), lateral tuberal nuclei [TA] (nuclei tuberales laterales [TA]), and the ventromedial nucleus [TA] (nucleus ventromedialis hypothalami [TA]). SEE ALSO hypothalamus. SYN intermediate hypothalamic region✩, a. hypothalamica intermedia.

Kiesselbach a., an a. on the anterior portion of the nasal septum rich in capillaries (Kiesselbach plexus) and often the seat of epistaxis. SYN Little a.

a. of Laimer, a triangular (or V-shaped) a. on the posterior aspect of the proximal esophagus, with its apex directed inferiorly in the midline and the cricopharyngeus muscle forming its base, which is an a. of weakness due to a near absence of longitudinal muscle; potential site of herniation of pharyngeal or esophageal mucosa. SYN Laimer-Haeckerman a., V-shaped a. of esophagus.

Laimer-Haeckerman a., SYN a. of Laimer.

lateral hypothalamic a. [TA], the portion of the hypothalamus located generally lateral to a rosterocaudal line drawn through the column of the fornix and the mammillothalamic tract; contains fibers collectively comprising the medial forebrain bundle [TA] and the following nuclei: portions of the preoptic area [TA] (area preoptica [TA]), portions of the lateral tuberal nuclei [TA] (nuclei tuberales laterales [TA]), the perifornical nucleus [TA] (nucleus perifornicalis [TA]), and the tuberomammillary nucleus [TA] (nucleus tuberomammillaris [TA]). SEE ALSO hypothalamus. SYN a. hypothalamica lateralis [TA].

lateral inferior hepatic a. [TA], SYN (left anterior) lateral hepatic *segment* [III].

lateral superior hepatic a. [TA], SYN (left posterior) lateral hepatic *segment* III.

Little a., SYN Kiesselbach a.

macular a., SYN *macula* of retina.

Martegiani a., SYN Martegiani *funnel.*

mitral a., the region of the chest over the apex of the heart, where the sounds, normal or pathologic, produced at the mitral valves are usually heard most distinctly.

motor a., SYN motor *cortex.*

a. ner'vi facia'lis [TA], SYN facial nerve a.

a. nu'da hep'atis [TA], SYN bare a. of liver.

olfactory a., SYN anterior perforated *substance.*

oval a. of Flechsig, SEE semilunar *fasciculus.*

Panum a., a. in space surrounding the empirical horopter where single binocular vision is observed despite stimulation of noncorresponding retinal points. SYN fusion a.

parastriate a., SEE visual *cortex.*

a. parolfacto'ria [TA], SYN parolfactory a.

parolfactory a. [TA], a small region of cerebral cortex on the medial surface of the frontal lobe, formed by the junction of the straight gyrus with the cingulate gyrus, demarcated from the subcallosal gyrus by the posterior parolfactory sulcus. SYN a. parolfactoria [TA], Broca parolfactory a.

pear-shaped a., SYN retromolar *pad.*

peristriate a., SEE visual *cortex.*

piriform a., SYN piriform *cortex.*

Pitres a., prefrontal cortex of the cerebral hemisphere. SEE frontal *cortex.*

postcentral a., the cortex of the postcentral gyrus.

post dam a., SYN posterior palatal seal a.

posterior hypothalamic a. [TA], the portion of the hypothalamus located generally inside the region of the mammillary bodies; contains the following nuclei: dorsal premammillary nucleus [TA] (nucleus premammillaris dorsalis [TA]), lateral nucleuus of mammillary body [TA] (nucleus mammillaris medialis [TA]), supramammillary nucleus [TA] (nucleus supramammillaris [TA], and the ventral premammillary nucleus [TA] (nucleus premammillaris ventralis [TA]). The posterior nucleus of hypothalamus [TA] is located at the interface of intermediate and posterior hypothalamic areas and is sometimes considered a part of the latter. SEE ALSO hypothalamus, posterior hypothalamic *region.* SYN a. hypothalamica posterior [TA].

posterior intercondylar a. of tibia [TA], the deep notch between the tibial condyles posteriorly to which attaches the posterior cruciate ligament. SYN a. intercondylaris posterior tibiae [TA].

posterior palatal seal a., the soft tissues along the junction of the hard and soft palates on which pressure within the physiologic limits of the tissues can be applied by a denture to aid in the retention of the denture. SYN post dam a., postpalatal seal a.

postpalatal seal a., SYN posterior palatal seal a.

a. postre'ma (AP) [TA], a small, elevated a. in the lateral wall of the inferior recess of the fourth ventricle; one of the few loci in the brain where the blood-brain barrier is lacking; a chemoreceptor area associated with vomiting.

precentral a., the cortex of the precentral gyrus.

precommissural septal a., SYN subcallosal *gyrus.*

prefrontal a., SEE frontal *cortex.*

premotor a., SYN premotor *cortex.*

preoptic a. [TA], SYN preoptic *region.*

a. preoptica [TA], SYN preoptic *region.*

prestriate a., SEE visual *cortex.*

pretectal a. [TA], a narrow, transversely oriented rostral zone of the mesencephalic tectum, bounded caudally by the superior colliculus, rostrally by the habenular trigone, and laterally by the pulvinar thalami; the pretectal a. contains several nuclei that receive fibers from the optic tract; it has bilateral efferent connections with the Edinger-Westphal nucleus of the oculomotor nuclear complex by way of which it mediates the pupillary light reflex. SYN pretectal region, pretectum.

primary visual a., SEE visual *cortex.*

pulmonary a., the region of the chest at the second left intercostal space, where sounds produced at the pulmonary valve of the right ventricle are heard most distinctly.

relief a., in dentistry, the portion of the denture-bearing a. over which the denture base is altered to reduce functional pressure.

rest a., the portion of a tooth structure or of a restoration in a tooth that is prepared to receive the positive seating of the metallic occlusal, incisal, lingual, or cingulum rest of a removable prosthesis. SYN rest seat.

retention a., an a. of a tooth provided during its preparation for restoration that will aid in holding the restoration in place. SEE ALSO retention *groove,* retention *point.*

retrochiasmatic a. [TA], SEE intermediate hypothalamic a. SYN a. retrochiasmatica [TA].

a. retrochiasmatica [TA], SYN retrochiasmatic a; SEE intermediate hypothalamic a.

Rolando a., SYN motor *cortex.*

secondary aortic a., region of the chest at the mid-left sternal bases where aortic diastolic murmurs are often best heard.

secondary visual a., SEE visual *cortex.*

sensorial areas, sensory areas, SEE cerebral *cortex.*

sensorimotor a., the precentral gyrus [TA] and postcentral gyrus [TA] of the cerebral cortex.

septal a. [TA], the region of the cerebral hemisphere that stretches as a thin sheet of brain tissue between the fornix bundle and the ventral surface of the corpus callosum, forming the medial wall of the lateral ventricle's frontal horn; it extends ventrally through the narrow interval between the anterior commissure and the rostrum of corpus collosum as the precommissural septum or subcallosal gyrus, which is continuous caudally with the preoptic a. and hypothalamus, as well as more laterally with the innominate substance; its major functional connections are with the hippocampus and hypothalamus. It is composed of a dorsal septal nucleus [TA], lateral septal nucleus [TA], medial septal nucleus [TA], septofimbrial nucleus [TA], and triangular nucleus of septum [TA]. The subformical organ [TA] is also found in this a.

silent a., any a. of the cerebrum or cerebellum in which lesions cause no definite sensory or motor symptoms.

skip areas, subsidiary segments of diseased intestine or colon in regional enteritis or Crohn colitis, separated from the region of major involvement.

somesthetic a., SYN somatic sensory *cortex.*

stress-bearing a., (1) SYN denture foundation a; **(2)** surfaces of oral structures that resist forces, strains, or pressures brought upon them during function.

striate a., SEE visual *cortex.*

a. subcallo'sa [TA], SYN subcallosal *gyrus.*

subcallosal a. [TA], SYN subcallosal *gyrus.*

superior vestibular a. [TA], the a. in the fundus of the internal acoustic meatus superior to the transverse crest through which the superior part of the vestibular (utriculoampullary) nerve passes to reach the macula utriculus and the ampullae of the anterior and lateral semicircular ducts. SYN a. vestibularis superior [TA].

supporting a., (1) those areas of the maxillary and mandibular edentulous ridges which are considered best suited to carry the forces of mastication when the dentures are in function; **(2)** SYN denture foundation a.

tissue-bearing a., SYN denture foundation a.

a. transitionis amygdalopiriformis [TA], SYN amygdalopiriform transition a.

tricuspid a., the region of the chest wall over the lower part of the body of the sternum, where the sounds produced at the tricuspid valve are heard most distinctly.

trigger a., SYN trigger *point.*

vagus a., a portion of the floor of the fourth ventricle overlying the vagoglossopharyngeal nuclei.

vestibular a. [TA], the area in the floor of the fourth ventricle lateral to the sulcus limitans [TA] and medial to the restiform body [TA] that overlies the vestibular nuclei and portions of the cochlear nuclei. SEE ALSO inferior vestibular a., superior vestibular a.

a. vestibularis [TA], SYN acoustic a.

a. vestibula'ris infe'rior [TA], SYN inferior vestibular a.

a. vestibula'ris supe'rior [TA], SYN superior vestibular a.

visual a., SYN visual *cortex.*

V-shaped a. of esophagus, SYN a. of Laimer.

Wernicke a., SYN Wernicke *center.*

---

ar·e·a·tus, ar·e·a·ta (ā-rē-ā'tŭs, -tă). Occurring in patches or circumscribed areas. [L.]

Are·ca (ar'ĕ-kă). A genus of palms of India and the Malay Archipelago. A species, *A. catechu,* furnishes a. nuts, or betel nuts, which contain arecoline and 15% red tannin, are chewed in the East Indies, and have an anthelmintic and stimulant action. SEE ALSO betel nut. [Malay]

arec·ai·dine (ă-rek'ā-dēn). A crystalline alkaloid resembling betaine, derived from the betel nut. SYN arecaine.

are·caine (ar'e-kān). SYN arecaidine.

arec·o·line (ă-rek'ō-lēn). A colorless oily alkaloid from the betel nut.

are·flex·ia (ā-rē-flek'sē-ă). Absence of reflexes.

detrusor a., a failure of the detrusor muscle to have a reflex contraction even though the bladder has reached or exceeded its capacity.

ar·e·na·ceous (ar-ĕ-nā'shŭs). Sandy; of sandlike consistency. [L. *arena,* sand]

Are·na·vi·ri·dae (ă-rē-nă-vir'i-dē). A family of over 15 RNA viruses, many of which are natural parasites of rodents, that includes lymphocytic choriomeningitis virus, Lassa virus, and the Tacaribe virus complex. The virions are 50–300 nm (average 100 nm) in diameter, enveloped, ether-sensitive, and contain 2 single-stranded RNA molecules (molecular weight $3–5 \times 10^6$); they also contain electron-dense, RNA-containing granules (20 to 30 nm in diameter) that resemble ribosomes, with an electron-microscopic appearance of sandiness. [L. *arena (harena),* sand]

Are·na·vi·rus (ă-rē'nă-vī'rŭs). A genus in the family Arenaviridae that is associated with lymphocytic choriomeningitis and a number of hemorrhagic fevers.

are·o·la, pl. **are·o·lae** (ă-rē'ō-lă, -lē). **1** [NA]. Any small area. **2.** One of the spaces or interstices in areolar tissue. **3.** SYN a. of breast. **4.** A pigmented, depigmented, or erythematous zone surrounding a papule, pustule, wheal, or cutaneous neoplasm. SYN halo (3). [L. dim. of *area*]

a. of breast [TA], a circular pigmented area surrounding the nipple (papilla mammae); its surface is dotted with little projections due to the presence of areolar glands beneath. SYN a. mammae [TA], a. of nipple, a. papillaris, areola (3).

a. mam'mae [TA], SYN a. of breast.

a. of nipple, SYN a. of breast.

a. papilla'ris, SYN a. of breast.

a. umbilicus, a pigmented ring around the umbilicus in the pregnant woman.

are·o·lar (ă-rē'ō-lăr). Relating to an areola.

ar·e·om·e·ter (ar-ē-om'ĕ-ter). SYN hydrometer. [G. *araios,* thin, + G. *metron,* measure]

Arg Symbol for arginine or its mono- or diradical.

Argas. A genus of soft ticks of the family Argasidae, some species of which usually infest birds but may attack humans.

A. reflex'us, the pigeon tick, a species that may cause a cutaneous inflammatory lesion in humans.

ar·ga·sid (ar-gas'id). Common name for members of the family Argasidae.

Argas·i·dae (ar-gas'i-dē). Family of ticks (superfamily Ixodoidea, order Acarina), the soft ticks, so called because of their wrinkled, leathery, tuberculated appearance that fills out when the tick is engorged with blood. A. contains 4 genera: *Argas, Ornithodoros, Otobius,* and *Antricola;* argasid ticks, chiefly species of *Ornithodoros,* harbor and transmit spirochetes of the genus *Borrelia* that cause relapsing fever in birds and mammals.

ar·gen·taf·fin, ar·gen·taf·fine (ar-jen'tă-fin, -fēn). Pertaining to cells or tissue elements that reduce silver ions in solution, thereby becoming stained brown or black. [L. *argentum,* silver, + *affinitas,* affinity]

ar·gen·ta·tion (ar-jen-tā'shŭn). Impregnation with a silver salt. SEE ALSO argyria. [L. *argentum,* silver]

ar·gen·tic (ar-jen'tik). **1.** Relating to silver. SYN argyric (1). **2.** Denoting a chemical compound containing silver as the rare dication (Ag^{2+}).

ar·gen·tine (ar'jen-tēn). Relating to, resembling, or containing silver.

ar·gen·to·phil, ar·gen·to·phile (ar-jen'tō-fil, -fīl). SYN argyrophil.

ar·gen·tous (ar-jen'tŭs). Denoting a chemical compound containing silver as a singly charged (Ag^+) ion. The vast majority of silver compounds contain the a. ion; where the ionic state of silver is not specifically stated, as in silver nitrate, the a. state is assumed.

ar·gen·tum, gen. **ar·gen·ti** (ar-jen'tŭm, -jen'tī). SYN silver. [L.]

ar·gi·nase (ar'ji-nās). An enzyme of the liver that catalyzes the hydrolysis of L-arginine to L-ornithine and urea; a key enzyme of the urea cycle. A deficiency of a. leads to arginemia. SYN canavanase.

ar·gi·nine (Arg) (ar'ji-nēn). 2-Amino-5-guanidinopentanoic acid; one of the amino acids occurring among the hydrolysis products of proteins, particularly abundant in the basic proteins such as histones and protamines. A dibasic amino acid.

a. deiminase, an enzyme catalyzing the hydrolytic deamination of L-a. to L-citrulline and ammonia. Cf. *nitric oxide* synthase.

a. glutamate, a compound composed of arginine and glutamic acid, given intravenously to detoxify ammonia; used in the treatment of ammoniemia resulting from liver dysfunction.

a. hydrochloride, a form of a. used for intravenous administration as an adjunct in the treatment of encephalopathies associated with liver diseases and ammoniacal azotemia.

a. phosphate, SYN phosphoarginine.

ar·gi·ni·no·suc·ci·nase (ar'ji-ni-nō-sŭk'si-nās). SYN argininosuccinate lyase.

ar·gi·ni·no·suc·ci·nate ly·ase (ar'ji-ni-nō-sŭk'si-nāt). An enzyme cleaving L-argininosuccinate nonhydrolytically to L-arginine and fumarate; a deficiency of this enzyme leads to argininosuccinoaciduria; a key step in the urea cycle. SYN argininosuccinase.

ar·gi·ni·no·suc·cin·ic ac·id (ar'ji-ni-nō-sŭk-sin'ik). Formed as an intermediate in the conversion of L-citrulline to L-arginine in the urea cycle.

ar·gi·ni·no·suc·cin·ic·ac·i·du·ria (ar-ji-nin'ō-sŭk-sin'ik-as-i-doo'rē-ă) [MIM*207900]. A disorder of urea cycle due to a deficiency of argininosuccinate lyase; characterized by physical and mental retardation, epilepsy, ataxia, liver disease, friable, tufted hair, and excessive urinary excretion of argininosuccinic acid. Autosomal recessive inheritance, caused by mutation in argininosuccinate lyase gene (ASL) on chromosome 7q.

ar·gin·yl (ar'jin-il). The aminoacyl radical of arginine.

ar·gi·pres·sin (ar-ji-pres'in). SYN arginine *vasopressin.*

ar·gon (Ar) (ar'gon). A gaseous element, atomic no. 18, atomic wt. 39.948, present in the dry atmosphere in the proportion of about 0.94%; one of the noble gases. [G. ntr. of *argos,* lazy, inactive, fr. *a-* priv. + *ergon,* work]

Argyll Robertson. Douglas, Scottish ophthalmologist, 1837–1909.

ar·gyr·ia (ar-jir'ē-ă, -jī'rē-ă). A slate-gray or bluish discoloration of the skin and deep tissues, due to the deposit of insoluble albuminate of silver, occurring after the medicinal administration for a long period of a soluble silver salt; formerly fairly common from use of proprietary preparations of silver-containing materials in the nose and sinuses. SYN argyrism, silver poisoning. [G. *argyros,* silver]

ar·gyr·ic (ar-jir'ik). **1.** SYN argentic (1). **2.** Relating to argyria.

ar·gy·rism (ar'ji-rizm). SYN argyria.

ar·gy·rol. SYN mild *silver* protein.

ar·gyr·o·phil, ar·gyr·o·phile (ar-jī'rō-fil, -fīl). Pertaining to tissue elements that are capable of impregnation with silver ions and being made visible after an external reducing agent is used. SYN argentophil, argentophile. [G. *argyros,* silver, + *philos,* fond]

arhin·ia (ă-rĭn′ē-ă). Congenital absence of the nose. SYN arrhinia.

Arias-Stella, Javier, Peruvian pathologist, *1924. SEE Arias-Stella *effect;* Arias-Stella *phenomenon;* Arias-Stella *reaction.*

ari·bo·fla·vin·o·sis (ă-rī′bō-flā-vi-nō′sis). Properly hyporiboflavinosis: a nutritional condition produced by a deficiency of riboflavin in the diet, characterized by cheilosis and magenta tongue and usually associated with other manifestations of B vitamin deficiency.

aris·to·loch·ic ac·id (ă-ris-tō-lō′kik). An aromatic bitter derived from plants of the genus *Aristolochia.*

ar·is·to·te·lian (ar′is-tō-tē′lē-ăn, ar′i-stŏ-tēl′yan). Attributed to or described by Aristotle.

Aristotle. Of Stagira, Greek philosopher and scientist, 384–322 B.C. SEE Aristotle *anomaly,* aristotelian *method.*

arith·mo·ma·nia (ă-rith-mō-mā′nē-ă). A morbid impulse to count. [G. *arithmeō,* to count, fr. *arithmos,* number, + *mania,* madness]

A·ri·zo·na (ar′i-zō′nă). Former name for *Salmonella enterica,* subspecies *arizonae.*

A. hinshawii, former name for *Salmonella enterica* subsp. *arizonae.*

Arlt, Carl Ferdinand von, Austrian ophthalmologist, 1812–1887. SEE A. *operation, sinus.*

arm [TA]. **1.** Arm, specifically the segment of the upper limb between the shoulder and the elbow; commonly used to mean the whole superior limb. SYN brachium (1) [TA], brachio-. **2.** An anatomic extension resembling an a. **3.** A specifically shaped and positioned extension of a removable partial denture framework. **4.** One set of cases or persons in an epidemiologic study, especially a randomized controlled trial, in which comparisons or contrasts are being made between sets. [L. *armus,* forequarter of an animal; G. *harmos,* a shoulder joint]

bar clasp a., a clasp a. which has its origin in the denture base or major connector; it consists of the a. which traverses but does not contact the gingival structures, and a terminal end which approaches its contact with the tooth in a gingivo-occlusal direction.

brawny a., a swollen arm caused by lymphedema, can be seen after ipsilateral radical mastectomy.

circumferential clasp a., a clasp a. which has its origin in a minor connector and which follows the contour of the tooth approximately in a plane perpendicular to the path of insertion of the partial denture.

clasp a., a portion of a clasp of a removable partial denture which projects from the clasp body and helps retain the partial denture in position in the mouth. SEE clasp (2).

dynein a., a structure extending clockwise from one tubule of each of the 9 doublet microtubules toward the adjacent doublet seen in the axoneme of cilia or flagella (including human sperm tails); congenital absence of dynein, reflected structurally by absence of dynein a.'s, can account for symptoms seen in Kartagener syndrome, an immotile cilia syndrome.

nuchal a., situation in vaginal breech delivery during which one or both arms are found around the back of the neck, interfering with delivery.

reciprocal a., a clasp a. or other extension used on a removable partial denture to oppose the action of some other part or parts of the appliance.

retentive a., retention a., a flexible segment of a removable partial denture that engages an undercut on an abutment and is designed to retain the denture.

retentive circumferential clasp a., an a. that is flexible and engages the infrabulge at the terminal end of the a.

stabilizing circumferential clasp a., an a. that is relatively rigid and embraces the height of contour of the tooth.

ar·ma·men·tar·i·um (ar′mă-men-tār′ē-ŭm). All the therapeutic means available to the health practitioner for professional practice. [L. an arsenal, fr. *armamenta,* implements, tackle, fr. *arma,* armor, arms]

Armanni, Luciano, Italian pathologist, 1839–1903. SEE A.-Ebstein *kidney, change.*

ar·mar·i·um (ar-mar′ē-ŭm). Rarely used term for the physician's

library, as part of her or his armamentarium. [L. a closet, chest, fr. *arma,* armor]

Ar·mil·li·fer (ar-mil′i-fer). A genus of Pentastomida (order Porocephalida, family Porocephalidae); adults are found in the lungs of reptiles and the young in many mammals, including humans. [O. Fr. *armille,* fr. L. *armilla,* a bracelet]

A. armilla′tus, species occurring in the python, the larva or nymph being occasionally found in humans. SYN *Porocephalus armillatus.*

Armitage, Peter, British statistician, (1924-). SEE A.-Doll *model.*

arm·pit. SYN axilla.

Armstrong, Arthur Riley, Canadian physician, *1904. SEE King-A. *unit.*

Armstrong, Henry E., British physician.

ARN Acronym for acute retinal *necrosis.*

Arndt, Rudolph G., German psychiatrist, 1835–1900. SEE A. *law.*

Arneth, Joseph, German physician, 1873–1956. SEE A. *classification, count, formula, index, stages,* under *stage.*

ar·ni·ca (ar′ni-kă). The dried flower heads of *Arnica montana* (family Compositae); Obsolete cardiac sedative seldom given internally; used externally for sprains and bruises; formerly widely used as a counterirritant liniment. SYN leopard's bane. [Mod. L.]

Arnold, Julius, German pathologist, 1835–1915. SEE A. *bodies,* under *body;* A.-Chiari *deformity, malformation, syndrome.*

Arnold, Friedrich, German anatomist, 1803–1890. SEE A. *bundle, canal, ganglion, nerve, tract; foramen* of A.

ar·o·mat·ic (ar-ō-mat′ik). **1.** Having an agreeable, somewhat pungent, spicy odor. **2.** One of a group of vegetable drugs having a fragrant odor and slightly stimulant properties. **3.** SEE aromatic *compound.* [G. *arōmatikos,* fr. *arōma,* spice, sweet herb]

ar·o·mat·ic D-amino ac·id de·car·box·yl·ase. An enzyme that catalyzes the decarboxylation of L-dopa to dopamine, of L-tryptophan to tryptamine, and of L-hydroxytryptophan to serotonin; important in the biosynthetic pathway of catecholamines and melanin. SYN dopa decarboxylase, hydroxytryptophan decarboxylase, tryptophan decarboxylase.

arotinoid (ă-rot′in-oyd). A synthetic polyaromatic retinoid derivative of vitamin A. SEE ALSO retinoid, retinoic acid. [*aromatic* + re*tinoid*]

ar·o·yl (a′rō-il). The radical of an aromatic acid (e.g., benzoyl); analogous to acyl, the more general term.

ar·rack (a-rak′). A strong alcoholic liquor distilled from dates, rice, sap of the coconut palm, and other substances. [Ar. sweet juice]

ar·rec·tor, pl. **ar·rec·to·res** (ă-rek′tōr, ă-rek-tō′rēz). SYN erector. [L. that which raises, fr. *ar-rigo,* pp. *-rectus,* to raise up]

ar·rest (ă-rest′). **1.** To stop, check, or restrain. **2.** A stoppage; interference with, or checking of, the regular course of a disease, a symptom, or the performance of a function. **3.** Inhibition of a developmental process, usually at the ultimate stage of development; premature a. may lead to a congenital abnormality. [O. Fr. *arester,* fr. LL. *adresto,* to stop behind]

cardiac a. (CA), complete cessation of cardiac activity either electric, mechanical, or both; may be purposely induced for therapeutic reasons. SYN heart a.

cardioplegic a., temporary intentional stoppage of electrical and mechanical cardiac activity, usually by potassium-containing solutions, used to protect heart muscle by decreasing its metabolic demand during open-heart surgery with cardiopulmonary *bypass.*

cardiopulmonary a., an a. resulting in absence of cardiac and pulmonary activity.

circulatory a., **(1)** cessation of the circulation of blood as a result of ventricular standstill or fibrillation. **(2)** intentional cessation of circulation by temporarily stopping cardiopulmonary bypass flow during certain thoracic aortic operations; used with intentional profound total-body hypothermia to protect vital organs.

deep hypothermic a., stoppage of electrical and mechanical cardiac activity that occurs when the heart is cooled.

epiphysial a., early and premature fusion between epiphysis and diaphysis.

heart a., SYN cardiac a.

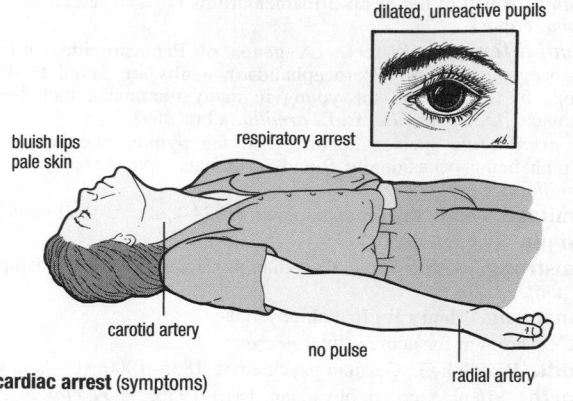

dilated, unreactive pupils

respiratory arrest

bluish lips
pale skin

carotid artery

no pulse

radial artery

cardiac arrest (symptoms)

a. of labor, absence of progress of active labor (as defined by cervical dilation and descent of the presenting part) for 2 hr or longer.

maturation a., cessation of complete differentiation of cells at an immature stage; in spermatogenic maturation a., the seminiferous tubules contain spermatocytes, but no spermatozoa develop.

sinus a., cessation of sinus activity; the ventricles may continue to beat under ectopic atrial, A-V junctional, or idioventricular control. SEE ALSO sinus *standstill*, atrial *standstill*.

ar·rhaph·i·a. SYN *status* dysraphicus.

ar·rhen·ic (ă-ren′ik). Relating to arsenic. [G. *arrhenikon* (var.), arsenic]

Arrhenius, Svante, Swedish chemist and Nobel laureate, 1859–1927. SEE A. *doctrine, equation, law;* A.-Madsen *theory.*

ar·rhe·no·blas·to·ma (ă-rē′nō-blas-tō′mă). SYN Sertoli-Leydig cell *tumor.* [G. *arrhēn,* male, + *blastos,* germ, + *-ōma,* tumor]

ar·rhin·en·ceph·a·ly, ar·rhin·en·ce·pha·lia, a·rhin·en·ceph·aly (ā-rīn-en-sef′ă-lē, -se-fā′lē-ă). Congenital absence or rudimentary state of the rhinencephalon, or olfactory lobe of the brain, on one or both sides, with a corresponding lack of development of the external olfactory organs. [G. *a-* priv. + *rhis* (rhin-), nose, + *enkephalos,* brain]

ar·rhin·ia (ā-rīn′ē-ă). SYN arhinia. [G. *a-* priv. + *rhis* (rhin-), nose]

ar·rhyth·mia (ă-rith′mē-ă). Loss or abnormality of rhythm; denoting especially an irregularity of the heartbeat. See also entries under rhythm. Cf. dysrhythmia. [G. *a-* priv. + *rhythmos,* rhythm]

cardiac a., SEE cardiac *dysrhythmia.*

continuous a., obsolete term for atrial *fibrillation.*

juvenile a., SYN sinus a.

nonphasic sinus a., sinus a. in which variations in rhythm are not related to the phases of respiration.

phasic sinus a., sinus a. in which the irregularity is related to the phases of respiration, the rate being faster in inspiration and slower in expiration.

respiratory a., phasic sinus a. or any other rhythm fluctuation induced by respiratory fluctuation.

sinus a., rhythmic, repetitive irregularity of the heartbeat, the heart being under the control of its normal pacemaker, the sinoatrial node. SYN juvenile a.

ar·rhyth·mic (ă-ridh′mik, ā-). Marked by loss of rhythm; pertaining to arrhythmia.

ar·rhyth·mo·gen·ic (ă-ridh-mō-jen′ik). Capable of inducing cardiac arrhythmias. [G. *a-* priv. + *rhythmos,* rhythm, + *-gen,* production]

ar·row·root (ar′ō-root). The rhizome of *Maranta arundinacea,* a plant of tropical America, which is the source of a form of starch formerly used as a dietary supplement.

Arruga, Count Hermenegildo, Spanish ophthalmologist, 1886–1972. SEE A. *forceps.*

ar·sa·ce·tin (ar-să-sē′tin). Formerly used as an antisyphilitic agent.

ar·sen·a·mide (ar-sen′ă-mīd). Used in the treatment of filariasis.

ar·se·nate (ar′sĕ-nāt). A salt of arsenic acid.

ar·sen·i·a·sis (ar-sen-ī′ă-sis). Chronic arsenical poisoning. SYN arsenicalism.

ar·se·nic (ar-sen′ik). Denoting the element arsenic or one of its compounds, especially arsenic acid.

ar·se·nic (As) (ar′sĕ-nik). A metallic element, atomic no. 33, atomic wt. 74.92159; forms a number of poisonous compounds, some of which are used in medicine. SYN arsenium, ratsbane. [L. *arsenicum,* G. *arsenikon,* fr. Pers. *zarnik*]

a. acid, the hydrate of arsenic oxide or arsenic pentoxide which forms arsenates with certain bases.

a. trihydride, SYN arsine.

a. trioxide, As_2O_3; dissolves in water to give arsenous acid, H_3AsO_3; used in the treatment of skin diseases and malaria, and as a tonic; also used externally as a caustic. SYN arsenous oxide, white a.

white a., SYN a. trioxide.

ar·sen·i·cal (ar-sen′i-kăl). **1.** A drug or agent, the effect of which depends on its arsenic content. **2.** Denoting or containing arsenic.

ar·sen·i·cal·ism (ar-sen′i-kăl-izm). SYN arseniasis.

ar·se·nic-fast. Resistant to the poisonous action of arsenic; denoting especially spirochetes and other protozoan parasites, which acquire resistance after repeated administration of the drug.

ar·se·nide (ar′sĕ-nīd). A compound of arsenic with a metal or other positively charged atoms or groups in which the arsenic is not bound to any atoms of oxygen. SYN arseniuret.

ar·se·ni·ous (ar-sēn′ē-ŭs). Arsenic (adj.).

ar·se·ni·um (ar-sē′nē-ŭm). SYN arsenic.

ar·sen·iu·ret (ar-se′nū-ret). SYN arsenide.

ar·se·no·ther·a·py (ar′sen-ō-thār′ă-pē). Therapeutic treatment with arsenic.

ar·se·nous (ar′-sen-ŭs). **1.** Denoting a compound of arsenic with a valence of +3. **2.** Arsenic (adj.).

ar·se·nous ac·id. SEE *arsenic* trioxide.

ar·se·nous hy·dride. SYN arsine.

ar·se·nous ox·ide. SYN *arsenic* trioxide.

ar·se·nox·i·des (ar-sĕ-nok′i-dēs). Oxidation products in the body of arsphenamines; believed to be the agents active against spirochetes.

ar·sine (ar′sēn). A cell and blood poison, many organic derivatives of which have been used in chemical warfare. SYN arsenic trihydride, arseniureted hydrogen, arsenous hydride.

ar·son·ic ac·id (ar-son′ik). A derivative of arsenic acid by replacement of a hydroxyl group by an organic radical.

ar·so·ni·um (ar-son′ē-ŭm). The positively charged ion, AsH_4^+; analogous to the ammonium ion, NH_4^+.

ars·phen·a·mine (ars-fen′ă-min). Formerly used in the treatment of syphilis, yaws, and some other diseases of protozoan origin, after neutralization with NaOH. The synthesis of a. in 1907 and the demonstration of its usefulness as a therapeutic agent by Paul Ehrlich and co-workers (1909) marked the beginning of chemotherapy. SYN phenarsenamine.

ars·thi·nol (ars′thī-nol). An amebicide.

ar·te·fact (ar′tĕ-fakt). SEE artifact.

artemether (ar-tem′ĕ-ther). Semisynthetic derivative of artemisinin used in the treatment of cerebral malaria.

Artemisia annua. a plant in the family Compositae from which an antimalarial and antischistosomal drug is produced.

artemisinin (ar-te-mis′in-in). A sesquiterpene antimalarial and antischistosomal drug derived from *Artemisia annua;* a. is a potent and rapidly acting blood schizontocide that has been reported to be very useful in the treatment of cerebral malaria; active against chloroquine-resistant *P. falciparum* and chloroquine-sensitive *P. falciparum* and *P. vivax.*

ar·te·re·nol (ar′ter-ĕ-nol). The hydrochloride salt of norepinephrine. SEE norepinephrine.

arteri-. SEE arterio-.

ARTERIA

ar·te·ria (a), gen. and pl. **ar·te·ri·ae (aa)** (ar-tēr′ē-ă, ar-tēr′ĭ-e) [TA]. SYN artery. SEE ALSO branch. [L. from G. *artēria,* the windpipe, later an artery as distinct from a vein]

a. acetab′uli, SYN acetabular *branch.*

arteriae alveola′res superio′res anterio′res [TA], SYN anterior superior alveolar *arteries,* under *artery.*

a. alveola′ris infe′rior [TA], SYN inferior alveolar *artery.*

a. alveola′ris supe′rior poste′rior [TA], SYN posterior superior alveolar *artery.*

a. anastomot′ica auricula′ris mag′na, SYN atrial anastomotic *branch* of circumflex branch of left coronary artery.

a. anastomot′ica mag′na, (1) SYN inferior ulnar collateral *artery;* **(2)** SYN descending genicular *artery.*

a. angula′ris [TA], SYN *branch* to angular gyrus.

a. aorta, SYN aorta.

a. appendicula′ris [TA], SYN appendicular *artery.*

arte′riae arcua′tae renis [TA], SYN arcuate *arteries* of kidney, under *artery.*

a. arcua′ta (pedis) [TA], SYN arcuate *artery* (of foot) (inconstant).

a. articula′ris az′ygos, SYN middle genicular *artery.*

a. ascen′dens [TA], **(1)** SYN colic *branch* of ileocolic artery; **(2)** SYN ascending *artery* (2).

arteriae atria′les, SYN atrial *arteries,* under *artery.*

a. auditi′va inter′na, SYN labyrinthine *artery.*

a. auricula′ris poste′rior [TA], SYN posterior auricular *artery.*

a. auricula′ris profun′da [TA], SYN deep auricular *artery.*

a. axilla′ris [TA], SYN axillary *artery.*

a. basila′ris [TA], SYN basilar *artery.*

a. brachia′lis [TA], SYN brachial *artery.*

a. brachia′lis superficia′lis [TA], SYN superficial brachial *artery.*

a. bucca′lis [TA], SYN buccal *artery.*

a. bul′bi pe′nis [TA], SYN *artery* of bulb of penis.

a. bul′bi ure′thrae, SYN *artery* of bulb of penis.

a. bulbi vaginae, SYN *artery* of bulb of vestibule.

a. bul′bi vestib′uli [TA], SYN *artery* of bulb of vestibule.

a. calcari′na, SYN calcarine *branch* of medial occipital artery.

a. callosa mediana [TA], SYN median callosal *artery.*

a. callo′somargina′lis [TA], SYN callosomarginal *artery.*

a. cana′lis pterygoid′ei [TA], SYN *artery* of pterygoid canal.

arte′riae carot′icotympan′icae (arteriae carotidis internae) [TA], SYN caroticotympanic *arteries* (of internal carotid artery), under *artery.*

a. carot′is commu′nis [TA], SYN common carotid *artery.*

a. carot′is exter′na [TA], SYN external carotid *artery.*

a. carot′is inter′na [TA], SYN internal carotid *artery.*

a. cau′dae pancrea′tis [TA], SYN *artery* to tail of pancreas.

a. ceca′lis ante′rior [TA], SYN anterior cecal *artery.*

a. ceca′lis poste′rior [TA], SYN posterior cecal *artery.*

a. celi′aca, SYN celiac (arterial) *trunk.*

arte′riae centra′les anterolatera′les [TA], SYN anterolateral central *arteries,* under *artery.*

arte′riae centra′les anteromedia′les [TA], SYN anteromedial central *arteries,* under *artery.*

arte′riae centra′les posterolatera′les [TA], SYN posterolateral central *arteries,* under *artery.*

arte′riae centra′les posteromedia′les [TA], SYN posteromedial central *arteries,* under *artery.*

a. centra′lis brev′is, SYN proximal medial striate *arteries,* under *artery.*

a. centra′lis ret′inae [TA], SYN central retinal *artery.*

a. cer′ebri ante′rior [TA], SYN anterior cerebral *artery.*

a. cer′ebri me′dia [TA], SYN middle cerebral *artery.*

a. cer′ebri poste′rior [TA], SYN posterior cerebral *artery.*

a. cervica′lis ascen′dens [TA], SYN ascending cervical *artery.*

a. cervica′lis profun′da [TA], SYN deep cervical *artery.*

a. cervica′lis superficia′lis, SYN superficial cervical *artery;* SEE ALSO superficial *branch* of the transverse cervical artery.

a. cervicovagina′lis, SYN cervicovaginal *artery.*

a. choroi′dea ante′rior [TA], SYN anterior choroidal *artery.*

a. choroi′dea poste′rior, SYN posterior choroidal *artery.*

arteriae cilia′res anterio′res, SYN anterior ciliary *arteries,* under *artery.*

arteriae cilia′res posterio′res lon′gae, SYN long posterior ciliary *arteries,* under *artery.*

a. cilia′ris poste′rior bre′vis [TA], SYN short posterior ciliary *artery.*

arteriae circumferentiales brevis [TA], SYN short circumferential *arteries,* under *artery.*

a. circumflex′a fem′oris latera′lis [TA], SYN lateral circumflex femoral *artery.*

a. circumflex′a fem′oris media′lis [TA], SYN medial circumflex femoral *artery.*

a. circumflex′a hu′meri ante′rior [TA], SYN anterior circumflex humeral *artery.*

a. circumflex′a hu′meri poste′rior [TA], SYN posterior circumflex humeral *artery.*

a. circumflex′a ili′aca profun′da [TA], SYN deep circumflex iliac *artery.*

a. circumflex′a ili′aca superficia′lis [TA], SYN superficial circumflex iliac *artery.*

a. circumflex′a scap′ulae [TA], SYN circumflex scapular *artery.*

a. cochlearis communis [TA], SYN common cochlear *artery.*

a. cochlearis propria [TA], SYN proper cochlear *artery.*

a. col′ica dex′tra [TA], SYN right colic *artery.*

a. col′ica me′dia [TA], SYN middle colic *artery.*

a. col′ica sinis′tra [TA], SYN left colic *artery.*

a. collatera′lis me′dia [TA], SYN middle collateral *artery.*

a. collatera′lis radia′lis [TA], SYN radial collateral *artery.*

a. collatera′lis ulna′ris infe′rior [TA], SYN inferior ulnar collateral *artery.*

a. collatera′lis ulna′ris supe′rior [TA], SYN superior ulnar collateral *artery.*

a. collicularis [TA], SYN collicular *artery.*

a. co′mes ner′vi phren′ici, SYN pericardiacophrenic *artery.*

a. com′itans ner′vi ischiad′ici [TA], SYN *artery* to sciatic nerve.

a. co′mitans ner′vi media′ni [TA], SYN median *artery.*

a. commissuralis mediana [TA], SYN median commissural *artery.*

a. commu′nicans ante′rior [TA], SYN anterior communicating *artery.*

a. commu′nicans poste′rior [TA], SYN posterior communicating *artery.*

a. conjunctiva′lis ante′rior [TA], SYN anterior conjunctival *artery.*

a. conjunctiva′lis poste′rior [TA], SYN posterior conjunctival *artery.*

a. corona′ria dex′tra [TA], SYN right coronary *artery.*

a. corona′ria sinis′tra [TA], SYN left coronary *artery.*

arteriae corticales radiatae [TA], SYN cortical radiate *arteries,* under *artery.*

a. cremaster′ica [TA], SYN cremasteric *artery.*

a. cys′tica [TA], SYN cystic *artery.*

a. deferentia′lis, SYN *artery* to ductus deferens.

a. descen′dens ge′nus [TA], SYN descending genicular *artery.*

arteriae digitales palmares propriae [TA], SYN proper palmar digital *arteries,* under *artery.*

arteriae digita′les planta′res pro′priae, SYN proper plantar digital *artery.*

a. digita′lis dorsa′lis [TA], SYN dorsal digital *artery.*

a. digita′lis palma′ris commu′nis [TA], SYN common palmar digital *artery.*

a. digita′lis palma′ris pro′pria, SYN proper palmar digital *arteries,* under *artery.*

a. digita′lis planta′ris commu′nis [TA], SYN common plantar digital *artery.*

a. digitalis plantaris propria [TA], SYN proper plantar digital *artery.*

a. dorsa′lis clitor′idis [TA], SYN dorsal *artery* of clitoris.

a. dorsa′lis na′si [TA], SYN dorsal nasal *artery.*

a. dorsa′lis pe′dis [TA], SYN dorsalis pedis *artery.*

a. dorsa′lis pe′nis [TA], SYN dorsal *artery* of penis.

a. dorsa′lis scap′ulae [TA], SYN dorsal scapular *artery.*

a. duc′tus deferen′tis, SYN *artery* to ductus deferens.

arteriae encephali [TA], SYN *arteries* of brain, under *artery.*

a. epigas′trica infe′rior [TA], SYN inferior epigastric *artery.*

a. epigas′trica superficia′lis [TA], SYN superficial epigastric *artery.*

a. epigas′trica supe′rior [TA], SYN superior epigastric *artery.*

a. episclera′lis [TA], SYN episcleral *artery.*

a. ethmoida′lis ante′rior [TA], SYN anterior ethmoidal *artery.*

a. ethmoida′lis poste′rior [TA], SYN posterior ethmoidal *artery.*

a. facia′lis [TA], SYN facial *artery.*

a. femora′lis [TA], SYN femoral *artery.*

a. fibula′ris [TA], SYN fibular *artery.*

a. flexurae dextrae [TA], SYN right flexural *artery.*

a. fronta′lis, SYN supratrochlear *artery.*

a. frontobasa′lis latera′lis [TA], SYN lateral frontobasal *artery.*

a. frontobasa′lis media′lis [TA], SYN medial frontobasal *artery.*

a. gas′trica dex′tra [TA], SYN right gastric *artery.*

arte′riae gas′tricae bre′ves [TA], SYN short gastric *arteries,* under *artery.*

a. gastrica posterior [TA], SYN posterior gastric *artery.*

a. gas′trica sinis′tra [TA], SYN left gastric *artery.*

a. gastroduodena′lis [TA], SYN gastroduodenal *artery.*

a. gastroepiplo′ica dex′tra, SYN right gastroomental *artery.*

arteriae gastroepiploicae, ⋆official alternate term for gastroomental *arteries,* under *artery.*

a. gastroepiplo′ica sinis′tra, SYN left gastroomental *artery.*

arteriae gastro-omentales [TA], SYN gastroomental *arteries,* under *artery.*

a. gastroomenta′lis dex′tra [TA], SYN right gastroomental *artery.*

a. gastroomenta′lis sinis′tra [TA], SYN left gastroomental *artery.*

a. ge′nus infe′rior latera′lis, SYN inferior lateral genicular *artery.*

a. ge′nus infe′rior media′lis, SYN inferior medial genicular *artery.*

a. ge′nus me′dia, SYN middle genicular *artery.*

a. glu′tea infe′rior [TA], SYN inferior gluteal *artery.*

a. glu′tea supe′rior [TA], SYN superior gluteal *artery.*

a. gy′ri angula′ris [TA], SYN *branch* to angular gyrus.

arteriae helicinae penis [TA], SYN helicine *arteries* of penis, under *artery.*

arteriae helicinae uteri [TA], SYN helicine *arteries* of the uterus, under *artery.*

a. hepat′ica commu′nis [TA], SYN common hepatic *artery.*

a. hepat′ica pro′pria, SYN hepatic *artery* proper.

a. hyaloi′dea [TA], SYN hyaloid *artery.*

a. hypogas′trica, SYN internal iliac *artery.*

a. hypophysia′lis infe′rior [TA], SYN inferior hypophysial *artery.*

a. hypophysia′lis supe′rior [TA], SYN superior hypophysial *artery.*

arte′riae ilea′les [TA], SYN ileal *arteries,* under *artery.*

a. ileocol′ica [TA], SYN ileocolic *artery.*

a. ili′aca commu′nis [TA], SYN common iliac *artery.*

a. ili′aca exter′na [TA], SYN external iliac *artery.*

a. ili′aca inter′na [TA], SYN internal iliac *artery.*

a. iliolumba′lis [TA], SYN iliolumbar *artery.*

a. infe′rior ante′rior cerebel′li [TA], SYN anterior inferior cerebellar *artery.*

a. inferior lateralis genus [TA], SYN inferior lateral genicular *artery.*

a. inferior medialis genus [TA], SYN inferior medial genicular *artery.*

a. infe′rior poste′rior cerebel′li [TA], SYN posterior inferior cerebellar *artery.*

a. infraorbita′lis [TA], SYN infraorbital *artery.*

arte′riae insula′res [TA], SYN insular *arteries,* under *artery.*

arte′riae intercosta′les posterio′res I et II, SYN first and second posterior intercostal *arteries,* under *artery.*

arteriae intercosta′les poste′riores III-XI [TA], SYN posterior intercostal *arteries* 3–11, under *artery.*

arteriae intercostales posteriores prima et secunda [TA],

a. intercosta′lis supre′ma [TA], SYN supreme intercostal *artery.*

arte′riae interloba′res re′nis [TA], SYN interlobar *arteries* of kidney, under *artery.*

arteriae interlobula′res [TA], SYN interlobular *arteries,* under *artery.*

a. interlobula′res (hepatis), SYN interlobular *arteries* of liver, under *artery.*

a. interlobula′res (renis), SYN cortical radiate *arteries,* under *artery.*

a. intermesenter′ica, SYN ascending *artery* (2).

a. interos′sea ante′rior [TA], SYN anterior interosseous *artery.*

a. interos′sea commu′nis [TA], SYN common interosseous *artery.*

a. interos′sea poste′rior [TA], SYN posterior interosseous *artery.*

a. interos′sea recur′rens [TA], SYN recurrent interosseous *artery.*

a. interos′sea vola′ris, SYN anterior interosseous *artery.*

arte′riae intestina′les, SEE ileal *arteries,* under *artery,* jejunal *arteries,* under *artery.*

arteriae intrarenales [TA], SYN intrarenal *arteries,* under *artery.*

a. ischiad′ica, a. ischiat′ica, SYN inferior gluteal *artery.*

arteriae jejuna′les [TA], SYN jejunal *arteries,* under *artery.*

a. juxtacolica, ⋆official alternate term for marginal *artery* of colon.

arte′riae labia′les anterio′res, SYN anterior labial *branches* of deep external pudendal artery, under *branch.*

a. labia′lis infe′rior, SYN inferior labial *branch* of facial artery.

a. labia′lis supe′rior, SYN superior labial *branch* of facial artery.

a. labyrin′thi [TA], SYN labyrinthine *artery.*

a. lacrima′lis [TA], SYN lacrimal *artery.*

a. laryn′gea infe′rior [TA], SYN inferior laryngeal *artery.*

a. laryn′gea supe′rior [TA], SYN superior laryngeal *artery.*

a. liena′lis, ⋆official alternate term for splenic *artery.*

a. ligamen′ti tere′tis u′teri, SYN *artery* of round ligament of uterus.

a. lingua′lis [TA], SYN lingual *artery.*

a. lingularis [TA], SEE left pulmonary *artery.*

a. lingularis inferior [TA], SYN inferior lingular *artery;* SEE left pulmonary *artery.*

a. lingularis superior [TA], SYN superior lingular *artery;* SEE left pulmonary *artery.*

arteriae lobares inferiores [TA], SEE left pulmonary *artery,* right pulmonary *artery.*

arteriae lobares inferior et superior [TA], SEE left pulmonary *artery,* right pulmonary *artery.*

arteriae lobares superiores [TA], SEE left pulmonary *artery,* right pulmonary *artery.*

a. lobaris media [TA], SEE left pulmonary *artery,* right pulmonary *artery.*

a. lobaris media pulmonis dextri [TA], SEE right pulmonary *artery.*

a. lo′bi cauda′ti [TA], SYN *artery* of caudate lobe.

arteriae lumba′les [TA], SYN lumbar *arteries,* under *artery.*

arteriae lumba′les i′mae [TA], SYN lowest lumbar *arteries,* under *artery.*

a. luso′ria, an aberrant right subclavian artery arising from the descending aorta; it passes posterior to the esophagus, often producing dysphagia.

arte′riae malleola′res posterio′res latera′les, SYN lateral malleolar *branch* (of fibular peroneal artery).

arte′riae malleola′res posterio′res media′les, SYN medial malleolar *branches* (of posterior tibial artery), under *branch*.

a. malleola′ris ante′rior latera′lis [TA], SYN anterior lateral malleolar *artery*.

a. malleola′ris ante′rior media′lis [TA], SYN anterior medial malleolar *artery*.

a. mamma′ria inter′na, SYN internal thoracic *artery*.

arteriae mammillares [TA], SYN mammillary *arteries*, under *artery*.

a. marginalis coli [TA], SYN marginal *artery* of colon.

a. masseter′ica [TA], SYN masseteric *artery*.

a. maxilla′ris [TA], SYN maxillary *artery*.

a. maxilla′ris exter′na, SYN facial *artery*.

a. media genus [TA], SYN middle genicular *artery*.

a. media′na, SYN median *artery*.

arteriae medullares segmentales [TA], SYN segmental medullary *arteries*, under *artery*.

arteriae membri inferioris [TA], SYN *arteries* of lower limb, under *artery*.

arteriae membri superioris [TA], SYN *arteries* of upper limb, under *artery*.

a. menin′gea ante′rior [TA], SYN anterior meningeal *branch* (of anterior ethmoidal artery).

a. menin′gea me′dia [TA], SYN middle meningeal *artery*.

a. menin′gea poste′rior [TA], SYN posterior meningeal *artery*.

a. menta′lis, SYN mental *branch* (of inferior alveolar artery).

a. mesenter′ica infe′rior [TA], SYN inferior mesenteric *artery*.

a. mesenter′ica supe′rior [TA], SYN superior mesenteric *artery*.

a. metacarpa′lis dorsa′lis [TA], SYN dorsal metacarpal *artery*.

a. metacarpa′lis palma′ris [TA], SYN palmar metacarpal *artery*.

a. metatarsa′lis [TA], SYN metatarsal *artery*.

a. metatarsa′lis dorsa′lis [TA], SYN dorsal metatarsal *artery*.

a. metatarsa′lis planta′ris [TA], SYN plantar metatarsal *artery*.

arteriae musculares (arteriae ophthalmicae) [TA], SYN muscular *arteries* (of ophthalmic artery), under *artery*.

a. musculophren′ica [TA], SYN musculophrenic *artery*.

arte′riae nasa′les posterio′res latera′les [TA], SYN posterior lateral nasal *arteries*, under *artery*.

a. nasa′lis poste′rior sep′ti, SYN posterior septal *branch* of nose.

a. na′si exter′na, SYN dorsal nasal *artery*.

arteriae nervo′rum, arteries to nerves.

a. nutri′cia [TA], SYN nutrient *artery*.

a. nutriciae femoris [TA], SYN nutrient *artery* of femur.

arte′riae nutri′ciae hu′meri [TA], SYN humeral nutrient *arteries*, under *artery*.

a. nutricia tibiae [TA], SYN tibial nutrient *artery*.

a. nutricia ulnae [TA], SYN nutrient *artery* of ulna.

a. nutriens femoris, ✶official alternate term for nutrient *artery* of femur.

a. nu′triens fib′ulae, ✶official alternate term for fibular nutrient *artery*.

a. nutriens humeri, ✶official alternate term for nutrient *arteries* of humerus, under *artery*.

a. nutriens radii, ✶official alternate term for nutrient *artery* of radius.

a. nutriens tibiae, ✶official alternate term for tibial nutrient *artery*.

a. nu′triens tibia′lis, SYN tibial nutrient *artery*.

a. nutriens ulnae, ✶official alternate term for nutrient *artery* of ulna.

a. obturato′ria [TA], SYN obturator *artery*.

a. obturato′ria accesso′ria [TA], SYN accessory obturator *artery*.

a. occipita′lis [TA], SYN occipital *artery*.

a. occipita′lis latera′lis [TA], SYN lateral occipital *artery*.

a. occipita′lis media′lis [TA], SYN medial occipital *artery*.

a. ophthal′mica [TA], SYN ophthalmic *artery*.

a. orbitofronta′lis latera′lis, ✶official alternate term for lateral frontobasal *artery*.

a. orbitofronta′lis media′lis, ✶official alternate term for medial frontobasal *artery*.

a. ova′rica [TA], SYN ovarian *artery*.

a. palati′na ascen′dens [TA], SYN ascending palatine *artery*.

a. palati′na descen′dens [TA], SYN descending palatine *artery*.

a. palati′na ma′jor [TA], SYN greater palatine *artery*.

a. palati′na mi′nor [TA], SYN lesser palatine *artery*.

arte′riae palpebra′les (laterales et mediales) [TA], SYN (lateral and medial) palpebral *arteries*, under *artery*.

a. pancreat′ica dorsa′lis [TA], SYN dorsal pancreatic *artery*.

a. pancreat′ica infe′rior [TA], SYN inferior pancreatic *artery*.

a. pancreat′ica mag′na, SYN greater pancreatic *artery*.

a. pancreat′icoduodena′lis infe′rior [TA], SYN inferior pancreaticoduodenal *artery*.

a. pancreat′icoduodena′lis supe′rior (anterior et posterior), SYN (anterior and posterior) superior pancreaticoduodenal *artery*.

a. paracentra′lis, SYN paracentral *branches* (of pericallosal artery), under *branch*.

a. parieta′lis anterior [TA], SYN anterior parietal *artery*.

arte′riae parieta′les (laterales et mediales) [TA], SYN (lateral and medial) parietal *arteries*, under *artery*.

a. parieta′lis posterior [TA], SYN posterior parietal *artery*.

arteriae pari′eto-occipita′les, SYN parieto-occipital *branches* (of anterior cerebral artery), under *branch*.

arteriae perforantes anteriores [TA], SYN anterior perforating *arteries*, under *artery*.

arte′riae perforan′tes arteriae profundae femoris [TA], SYN perforating *arteries* (of deep femoral artery), under *artery*.

arteriae perforantes penis [TA], SYN perforating *arteries* of penis, under *artery*.

arteriae perforantes radiatae (renis) [TA], SYN perforating radiate *arteries* (of kidney), under *artery*.

a. pericallo′sa [TA], SYN pericallosal *artery*.

a. pericardiacophren′ica [TA], SYN pericardiacophrenic *artery*.

a. perinea′lis [TA], SYN perineal *artery*.

a. perone′a, ✶official alternate term for fibular *artery*.

a. pharyn′gea ascen′dens [TA], SYN ascending pharyngeal *artery*.

a. phren′ica infe′rior [TA], SYN inferior phrenic *artery*.

a. phren′ica supe′rior [TA], SYN superior phrenic *artery*.

a. planta′ris latera′lis [TA], SYN lateral plantar *artery*.

a. planta′ris media′lis [TA], SYN medial plantar *artery*.

a. plantaris profunda arteriae dorsalis pedis [TA], SYN deep plantar *artery*.

a. plantaris profundus, SYN deep plantar *branch* of dorsalis pedis artery.

a. polaris frontalis [TA], SYN polar frontal *artery*.

a. polaris temporalis [TA], SYN polar temporal *artery*.

arte′riae pon′tis [TA], SYN pontine *arteries*, under *artery*.

a. poplit′ea [TA], SYN popliteal *artery*.

a. precunea′lis, SYN precuneal *branches* (of anterior cerebral artery), under *branch*.

a. prepancreatica [TA], SYN prepancreatic *artery*.

a. prin′ceps pol′licis [TA], SYN princeps pollicis *artery*.

a. profun′da bra′chii [TA], SYN profunda brachii *artery*.

a. profun′da clitor′idis [TA], SYN deep *artery* of clitoris.

a. profun′da fem′oris, SYN deep *artery* of thigh.

a. profun′da lin′guae [TA], SYN deep lingual *artery*.

a. profun′da pe′nis [TA], SYN deep *artery* of penis.

a. pterygomeningealis [TA], SYN pterygomeningeal *artery*.

arte′riae puden′dae exter′nae [TA], SYN (superficial and deep) external pudendal *arteries*, under *artery*.

a. puden′da inter′na [TA], SYN internal pudendal *artery*.

a. pulmona′lis, SYN pulmonary *trunk*.

a. pulmona′lis dex′tra [TA], SYN right pulmonary *artery*.

a. pulmona′lis sinis′tra [TA], SYN left pulmonary *artery*.

a. quadrigeminalis, ⭐official alternate term for collicular *artery*.

a. radia'lis [TA], SYN radial *artery*.

a. radia'lis in'dicis [TA], SYN radialis indicis *artery*.

arteriae radiculares (anterior et posterior), SYN (anterior and posterior) radicular *arteries*, under *artery*.

a. radicula'ris mag'na, SYN great segmental medullary *artery*.

a. radii nutricia [TA], SYN nutrient *artery* of radius.

a. rani'na, SYN deep lingual *artery*.

a. recta'lis infe'rior [TA], SYN inferior rectal *artery*.

a. recta'lis me'dia [TA], SYN middle rectal *artery*.

a. recta'lis supe'rior [TA], SYN superior rectal *artery*.

a. recur'rens, SYN medial striate *artery*.

a. recur'rens radia'lis [TA], SYN radial recurrent *artery*.

a. recur'rens tibia'lis ante'rior [TA], SYN anterior tibial recurrent *artery*.

a. recur'rens tibia'lis poste'rior [TA], SYN posterior tibial recurrent *artery*.

a. recur'rens ulna'ris [TA], SYN ulnar recurrent *artery*.

a. rena'lis [TA], SYN renal *artery*.

arte'riae re'nis [TA], SYN segmental *arteries* of kidney, under *artery*.

a. ret'inae centra'lis, SYN central retinal *artery*.

a. retroduodena'lis [TA], SYN retroduodenal *artery*.

arteriae sacra'les latera'les, SYN lateral sacral *arteries*, under *artery*.

a. sacra'lis media'na [TA], SYN median sacral *artery*.

a. scapula'ris descen'dens, SYN dorsal scapular *artery*.

a. scapula'ris dorsa'lis, SYN dorsal scapular *artery*.

a. segmentalis anterior [TA], SEE left pulmonary *artery*, right pulmonary *artery*.

a. segmentalis apicalis [TA], SEE left pulmonary *artery*, right pulmonary *artery*.

a. segmentalis basalis anterior [TA], SYN anterior basal segmental *artery*.

a. segmentalis basalis lateralis [TA], SYN lateral basal segmental *artery*.

a. segmentalis basalis medialis [TA], SYN medial basal segmental *artery*.

a. segmentalis lateralis [TA], SYN lateral basal segmental *artery*; SEE left pulmonary *artery*, right pulmonary *artery*.

a. segmentalis medialis [TA], SYN medial basal segmental *artery*; SEE left pulmonary *artery*, right pulmonary *artery*.

a. segmentalis posterior [TA], SEE left pulmonary *artery*, right pulmonary *artery*.

a. segmentalis superior [TA], SEE left pulmonary *artery*, right pulmonary *artery*.

a. segmen'ti anterio'ris inferio'ris re'nis [TA], SEE segmental *arteries* of kidney, under *artery*.

a. segmen'ti anterio'ris superio'ris re'nis [TA], SEE segmental *arteries* of kidney, under *artery*.

arteriae segmenti hepaticae, SYN segmental *arteries* of liver, under *artery*.

a. segmen'ti inferio'ris re'nis [TA], SEE segmental *arteries* of kidney, under *artery*.

a. segmen'ti posterio'ris re'nis [TA], SEE segmental *arteries* of kidney, under *artery*.

a. segmen'ti superio'ris re'nis [TA], SEE segmental *arteries* of kidney, under *artery*.

arte'riae sigmoi'deae [TA], SYN sigmoid *arteries*, under *artery*.

a. spermat'ica inter'na, SYN testicular *artery*.

a. sphe'nopalati'na [TA], SYN sphenopalatine *artery*.

a. spina'lis ante'rior [TA], SYN anterior spinal *artery*.

a. spina'lis poste'rior [TA], SYN posterior spinal *artery*.

a. sple'nica [TA], SYN splenic *artery*.

a. striata medialis distalis [TA], SYN medial striate *artery*.

a. stylomastoi'dea [TA], SYN stylomastoid *artery*.

a. subcla'via [TA], SYN subclavian *artery*.

a. subcosta'lis [TA], SYN subcostal *artery*.

a. sublingua'lis [TA], SYN sublingual *artery*.

a. submenta'lis [TA], SYN submental *artery*.

a. subscapula'ris [TA], SYN subscapular *artery*.

a. sul'ci centra'lis [TA], SYN *artery* of central sulcus.

a. sul'ci postcentra'lis [TA], SYN *artery* of postcentral sulcus.

a. sul'ci precentra'lis [TA], SYN *artery* of precentral sulcus.

a. supe'rior cerebel'li [TA], SYN superior cerebellar *artery*.

a. supe'rior latera'lis ge'nus [TA], SYN superior lateral genicular *artery*.

a. supe'rior media'lis ge'nus [TA], SYN superior medial genicular *artery*.

a. suprachiasmatica [TA], SYN suprachiasmatic *artery*.

a. supraduodena'lis [TA], SYN supraduodenal *artery*.

a. supraoptica [TA], SYN supraoptic *artery*.

a. supraorbita'lis [TA], SYN supraorbital *artery*.

arteriae suprarena'les supe'riores [TA], SYN superior suprarenal *arteries*, under *artery*.

a. suprarena'lis infe'rior [TA], SYN inferior suprarenal *artery*.

a. suprarena'lis me'dia [TA], SYN middle suprarenal *artery*.

a. suprascapula'ris [TA], SYN suprascapular *artery*.

a. supratrochlea'ris [TA], SYN supratrochlear *artery*.

arteriae sura'les [TA], SYN sural *arteries*, under *artery*.

a. tar'sea latera'lis [TA], SYN lateral tarsal *artery*.

a. tar'sea media'lis [TA], SYN medial tarsal *arteries*, under *artery*.

a. tempora'lis ante'rior, SYN anterior temporal *branch*.

a. tempora'lis interme'dia, SYN middle temporal *branch* of insular part of middle cerebral artery.

a. tempora'lis media [TA], SYN middle temporal *artery*.

a. tempora'lis poste'rior, SYN posterior temporal *branch* of middle cerebral artery.

a. tempora'lis profun'da [TA], SYN deep temporal *artery*.

a. tempora'lis superficia'lis [TA], SYN superficial temporal *artery*.

a. testicula'ris [TA], SYN testicular *artery*.

arte'riae thalamostria'tae anterolatera'les, SYN anterolateral central *arteries*, under *artery*.

arte'riae thalamostria'tae anteromedia'les, SYN anteromedial central *arteries*, under *artery*.

a. thora'cica inter'na [TA], SYN internal thoracic *artery*.

a. thora'cica latera'lis [TA], SYN lateral thoracic *artery*.

a. thora'cica supe'rior [TA], SYN superior thoracic *artery*.

a. thoracoacromia'lis [TA], SYN thoracoacromial *artery*.

a. thoracodorsa'lis [TA], SYN thoracodorsal *artery*.

a. thyroi'dea i'ma [TA], SYN thyroid ima *artery*.

a. thyroi'dea infe'rior [TA], SYN inferior thyroid *artery*.

a. thyroi'dea supe'rior [TA], SYN superior thyroid *artery*.

a. tibia'lis ante'rior [TA], SYN anterior tibial *artery*.

a. tibia'lis poste'rior [TA], SYN posterior tibial *artery*.

a. transver'sa cer'vicis, ⭐official alternate term for transverse cervical *artery*.

a. transver'sa col'li [TA], SYN transverse cervical *artery*.

a. transver'sa facie'i [TA], SYN transverse facial *artery*.

a. tuberis cinerei [TA], SYN *artery* of tuber cinereum.

a. tympan'ica ante'rior [TA], SYN anterior tympanic *artery*.

a. tympan'ica infe'rior [TA], SYN inferior tympanic *artery*.

a. tympan'ica poste'rior [TA], SYN posterior tympanic *artery*.

a. tympan'ica supe'rior [TA], SYN superior tympanic *artery*.

a. ulna'ris [TA], SYN ulnar *artery*.

a. umbilica'lis [TA], SYN umbilical *artery*.

a. uncalis [TA], SYN uncal *artery*.

a. urethra'lis [TA], SYN urethral *artery*.

a. uteri'na [TA], SYN uterine *artery*.

a. vagina'lis [TA], SYN vaginal *artery*.

arte'riae ventricula'res [TA], SYN ventricular *arteries*, under *artery*.

a. vertebra'lis [TA], SYN vertebral *artery*.

a. vesica'lis infe'rior [TA], SYN inferior vesical *artery*.

a. vesica'lis supe'rior [TA], SYN superior vesical *artery*.

a. vestibularis anterior [TA], SYN anterior vestibular *artery*.

a. vestibuli, ☆official alternate term for anterior vestibular *artery.*
a. vestibulocochlearis [TA], SYN vestibulocochlear *artery.*
a. vitelli′na, SYN vitelline *artery.*
a. vola′ris ind′icis radia′lis, SYN radialis indicis *artery.*
a. zygomat′ico-orbita′lis [TA], SYN zygomatico-orbital *artery.*

ar·te·ri·al (ar-tē′rē-ăl). Relating to one or more arteries or to the entire system of arteries.
ar·te·ri·al·i·za·tion (ar-tē′rē-ăl-ī-zā′shŭn). **1.** Making or becoming arterial. **2.** Aeration or oxygenation of the blood whereby it is changed in character from venous to arterial. **3.** SYN vascularization. **4.** Conversion of a venous structure to function as an artery.
ar·te·ri·ec·ta·sis, ar·te·ri·ec·ta·sia (ar-tēr-ē-ek′tă-sis, -ek-tā′zē-ă). Obsolete term for vasodilation of the arteries. [L. *arteria,* artery, + G. *ektasis,* distention]
ar·te·ri·ec·to·my (ar-tēr-ē-ek′tō-mē). Excision of part of an artery. [L. *arteria,* artery, + G. *ektomē,* excision]
△**arterio-, arteri-.** Artery. [L. *arteria,* fr. G. *artēria,* a windpipe, an artery]
ar·te·ri·o·at·o·ny (ar-tēr′ē-ō-at′ō-nē). An abnormally relaxed state of the arterial walls. [arterio- + G. *atonia,* atony]
ar·te·ri·o·cap·il·lary (ar-tēr′ē-ō-cap′i-lār-ē). Relating to both arteries and capillaries.
ar·te·ri·o·gram (ar-tēr′ē-ō-gram). Radiographic demonstration of an artery after injection of contrast medium into it. [arterio- + G. *gramma,* something written]
ar·te·ri·o·graph·ic (ar-tēr′ē-ō-graf′ik). Relating to or utilizing arteriography.
▪**ar·te·ri·og·ra·phy** (ar-tēr-ē-og′ră-fē). Demonstration of an artery or arteries by x-ray imaging after injection of a radiopaque contrast medium. [arterio- + G. *graphō,* to write]

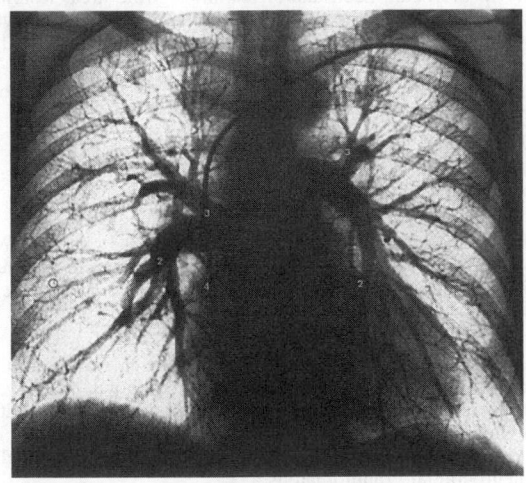

arteriography: normal study of the pulmonary arteries

bronchial a., radiography of bronchial arteries by selective injection of the intercostal arteries from which they arise.
cerebral a., SYN cerebral *angiography.*
ar·te·ri·o·la, pl. **ar·te·ri·o·lae** (ar-tēr-ē-ō′lă, -ō′lē) [TA]. SYN arteriole. [Mod. L. dim. of *arteria,* artery]
a. glomerula′ris af′ferens [TA], SYN afferent glomerular *arteriole.*
a. glomerula′ris ef′ferens [TA], SYN efferent glomerular *arteriole.*
a. maculae medius [TA],
a. macula′ris infe′rior [TA], SYN inferior macular *arteriole.*
a. macula′ris supe′rior [TA], SYN superior macular *arteriole.*
a. media′lis ret′inae [TA], SYN middle macular *arteriole.*
a. nasa′lis ret′inae infe′rior [TA], SYN inferior nasal *arteriole* of retina.

a. nasa′lis ret′inae supe′rior [TA], SYN superior nasal retinal *arteriole.*
arteriolae rectae [TA], SYN *vasa* recta renis, under *vas.*
a. tempora′lis ret′inae infe′rior [TA], SYN inferior temporal retinal *arteriole.*
a. tempora′lis ret′inae supe′rior [TA], SYN superior temporal retinal *arteriole.*
ar·te·ri·o·lar (ar-ter-ē-ō′lăr). Of or pertaining to an arteriole or the arterioles collectively.
▪**ar·te·ri·ole** (ar-tēr′ē-ōl) [TA]. A minute artery with a tunica media comprising only one or two layers of smooth muscle cells; a terminal artery continuous with the capillary network. SYN arteriola [TA].

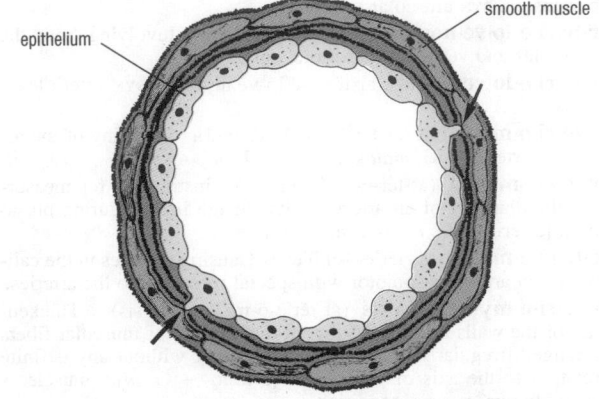

epithelium   smooth muscle

arteriole: arrows show points of contact between epithelium and smooth muscle

afferent glomerular a. [TA], a branch of an interlobular artery of the kidney that conveys blood to the glomerulus. SYN arteriola glomerularis afferens [TA], afferent vessel (2), vas afferens.
capillary a., a minute artery that terminates in a capillary.
efferent glomerular a. [TA], the vessel that carries blood from the glomerular capillary network to the capillary bed of the proximal convoluted tubule; collectively, these vessels constitute the renal portal system. SYN arteriola glomerularis efferens [TA], efferent vessel, vas efferens (2).
inferior macular a. [TA], *origin,* central artery of retina; *distribution,* inferior part of macula. SYN arteriola macularis inferior [TA].
inferior nasal a. of retina [TA], the branch of the central artery of the retina that supplies the lower medial, or nasal, part of the retina. SYN arteriola nasalis retinae inferior [TA].
inferior temporal retinal a. [TA], the branch of the central artery of the retina that passes laterally below the macula to supply the lower lateral or temporal part of the retina. SYN arteriola temporalis retinae inferior [TA].
medial a. of retina, SYN middle macular a.
middle macular a. [TA], an arteriole supplying the part of the retina between the optic disk and the macula. SYN arteriola medialis retinae [TA], medial a. of retina.
superior macular a. [TA], *origin,* central artery of retina; *distribution,* upper part of macula. SYN arteriola macularis superior [TA].
superior nasal retinal a. [TA], the branch of the central artery of the retina that passes to the upper medial, or nasal, part of the retina. SYN arteriola nasalis retinae superior [TA].
superior temporal retinal a. [TA], the branch of the central artery of the retina that passes laterally above the macula to supply the upper lateral or temporal part of the retina. SYN arteriola temporalis retinae superior [TA].
ar·te·ri·o·lith (ar-tēr′ē-ō-lith). A calcareous deposit in an arterial wall or thrombus. [L. *arteria,* artery, + G. *lithos,* a stone]

ar·ter·i·o·li·tis (ar-tēr′ē-ō-lī′tis). Inflammation of the wall of the arterioles. [L. *arteriola,* arteriole, + G. *-itis,* inflammation]

necrotizing a., necrosis in the media of arterioles, characteristic of malignant hypertension. SYN arteriolonecrosis.

△**arteriolo-.** The arterioles. [Modern L. *arteriola,* arteriole]

ar·te·ri·ol·o·gy (ar-tēr′ē-ol′ō-jē). The anatomy of the arteries: usually associated with the study of the other vessels under the name angiology. [L. *arteria,* artery, + G. *logos,* study]

ar·te·ri·o·lo·ne·cro·sis (ar-tēr-ē-ō′lō-nĕ-krō′sis). SYN necrotizing *arteriolitis.* [L. *arteriola,* arteriole, + G. *nekrōsis,* a killing]

ar·te·ri·o·lo·neph·ro·scle·ro·sis (ar-tēr-ē-ō′lō-nef′rō-skler-ō′sis). SYN arteriolar *nephrosclerosis.*

ar·te·ri·o·lo·scle·ro·sis (ar-tēr-ē-ō′lō-skler-ō′sis). Arteriosclerosis affecting mainly the arterioles, seen especially in chronic hypertension. SYN arteriolar sclerosis.

ar·te·ri·o·lo·ve·nous (ar-tēr-ē-ō′lō-vē′nŭs). Involving both the arterioles and veins. SYN arteriolovenular.

ar·te·ri·o·lo·ven·u·lar (ar-tēr-ē-ō′lō-vē′nū-lăr). SYN arteriolovenous.

ar·te·ri·o·ma·la·cia (ar-tēr′ē-ō-mă-lā′shē-ă). Softening of the arteries. [arterio- + G. *malakia,* softness]

ar·te·ri·om·e·ter (ar-tēr-ē-om′ĕ-ter). An instrument for measuring the diameter of an artery, or its change in size during pulsation. [arterio- + G. *metron,* measure]

ar·te·ri·o·mo·tor (ar-tēr′ē-ō-mō′ter). Causing changes in the caliber of an artery; vasomotor with special reference to the arteries.

ar·te·ri·o·my·o·ma·to·sis (ar-tēr′ē-ō-mī′ō-mă-tō′sis). Thickening of the walls of an artery by an overgrowth of muscular fibers arranged irregularly, intersecting each other without any definite relation to the axis of the vessel. [arterio- + G. *mys,* muscle, + *-oma,* tumor, + *-osis,* condition]

ar·te·ri·o·neph·ro·scle·ro·sis (ar-tēr′ē-ō-nef′rō-skler-ō′sis). SYN arterial *nephrosclerosis.*

ar·te·ri·o·pal·mus (ar-tēr′ē-ō-pal′mŭs). Subjective sensation of throbbing of an artery. [arterio- + G. *palmos,* throbbing]

ar·te·ri·op·a·thy (ar-tēr-ē-op′ă-thē). Any disease of the arteries. [arterio- + G. *pathos,* suffering]

hypertensive a., arterial degeneration resulting from hypertension.

plexogenic pulmonary a., SYN Ayerza *syndrome.*

ar·te·ri·o·pla·nia (ar-tēr′ē-ō-plā′nē-ă). Presence of an anomaly in the course of an artery. [arterio- + G. *planē,* a straying]

ar·te·ri·o·plas·ty (ar-tēr′ē-ō-plas-tē). Any operation for the reconstruction of the wall of an artery. [arterio- + G. *plastos,* formed]

ar·te·ri·o·pres·sor (ar-tēr′ē-ō-pres′ser). Causing increased arterial blood pressure.

ar·te·ri·or·rha·phy (ar-tēr-ē-ōr′ă-fē). Suture of an artery. [arterio- + G. *rhaphē,* seam]

ar·te·ri·or·rhex·is (ar-tēr′ē-ō-rek′sis). Rupture of an artery. [arterio- + G. *rhēxis,* rupture]

ar·te·ri·o·scle·ro·sis (ar-tēr′ē-ō-skler-ō′sis). Hardening of the arteries; types generally recognized are: atherosclerosis, Mönckeberg a., and arteriolosclerosis. SYN arterial sclerosis, vascular sclerosis. [arterio- + G. *sklērōsis,* hardness]

coronary a., degenerative and metabolic changes of the walls of the coronary arteries usually beginning with atheroma of the intima and preceding to involve the media; also, calcified lesions known as Mönckeberg a.

hyperplastic a., hyperplasia of the intima and internal elastic layer and hypertrophy of the media independent of atheromatous lesions.

hypertensive a., progressive increase in muscle and elastic tissue of arterial walls, resulting from hypertension; in longstanding hypertension, elastic tissue forms numerous concentric layers in the intima and there is replacement of muscle by collagen fibers and hyaline thickening of the intima of arterioles; such changes can develop with increasing age in the absence of hypertension and may then be referred to as senile a.

medial a., SYN Mönckeberg a.

Mönckeberg a., arterial sclerosis involving the peripheral arteries, especially of the legs of older people, with deposition of calcium in the medial coat (pipestem arteries) but with little or no encroachment on the lumen. SYN medial a., Mönckeberg calcification, Mönckeberg degeneration, Mönckeberg medial calcification, Mönckeberg sclerosis.

nodular a., atheromas occurring in the arterial intima as discrete tumors.

a. oblit′erans, a. producing narrowing and occlusion of the arterial lumen.

peripheral a., a. in any of the vessels beyond the aorta; most often refers to the lower extremities.

senile a., a. similar to hypertensive a., but as a result of advanced age rather than hypertension.

ar·te·ri·o·scle·rot·ic (ar-tēr′ē-ō-skler-ot′ik). Relating to or affected by arteriosclerosis.

ar·te·ri·o·spasm (ar-tēr′ē-ō-spazm). Spasm of an artery or arteries.

ar·te·ri·o·ste·no·sis (ar-tēr′ē-ō-stĕ-nō′sis). Narrowing of the caliber of an artery, either temporary, through vasoconstriction, or permanent, through arteriosclerosis. [arterio- + G. *stenōsis,* a narrowing]

ar·te·ri·ot·o·my (ar-tēr-ē-ot′ō-mē). Any surgical incision into the lumen of an artery, e.g., to remove an embolus. [arterio- + G. *tomē,* incision]

ar·te·ri·o·ve·nous (AV) (ar-tēr′ē-ō-vē′nŭs). Relating to both an artery and a vein or to both arteries and veins in general; both arterial and venous, as an "AV anastomosis."

ar·te·ri·tis (ar-ter-ī′tis). Inflammation or infection involving an artery or arteries. [L. *arteria,* artery, + G. *-itis,* inflammation]

brachiocephalic a., giant-cell a. seen in older adults; characterized by inflammatory lesions in medium sized arteries, most commonly in the head, neck and/or shoulder girdle area; lesions include fragmented elastin, macrophages, and giant cells. Erythrocyte sedimentation rate is usually markedly elevated. Visual loss can occur.

coronary a., inflammation of any or all of the layers of coronary artery walls.

cranial a., SYN temporal a.

extracranial a., SYN temporal a.

giant cell a., SYN temporal a.

granulomatous a., SYN temporal a.

Heubner a., inflammation of arteries within the circle of Willis secondary to chronic basal meningitis from tubercle bacillus or particular fungi such as *Cryptococcus, Histoplasma,* or *Coccidioides.*

Horton a., SYN temporal a.

intracranial granulomatous a., a small vessel, giant cell a. that affects only intracranial blood vessels, of unknown etiology, and with diverse clinical manifestations, including those seen with an involving cerebral tumor, and with a low grade meningitis, leading to infarction of one portion of the cerebrum or cerebellum. SYN neurocranial granulomatous a.

neurocranial granulomatous a., SYN intracranial granulomatous a.

a. nodo′sa, SYN *polyarteritis* nodosa.

a. oblit′erans, obliterating a., SYN *endarteritis* obliterans.

rheumatic a., a. due to rheumatic fever; Aschoff bodies are frequently found in the adventitia of small arteries, especially in the myocardium, and may lead to fibrosis and constriction of the lumens.

rheumatoid a., a. associated with rheumatoid arthritis; aortitis with aortic valve incompetence accompanying ankylosing spondylitis may be related.

Takayasu a., a progressive obliterative arteritis of unknown origin involving chronic inflammation of the aortic arch with fibrosis and marked luminal narrowing that affects the aorta and its branches, often with complete or near complete occlusion of segments of the aorta; more common in females. SEE ALSO aortic arch *syndrome.* SYN pulseless disease, Takayasu disease, Takayasu syndrome.

ar

temporal a., a subacute, granulomatous a. involving the external carotid arteries, especially the temporal artery; occurs in elderly persons and may be manifested by constitutional symptoms, particularly severe headache, and sometimes sudden unilateral blindness. Shares many of the symptoms of *polymyalgia* rheumatica. SYN cranial a., extracranial a., giant cell a., granulomatous a., Horton a.

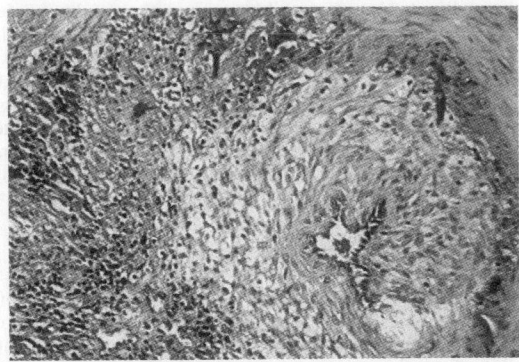

temporal arteritis (giant cell arteritis): cross-section showing infiltration of tunica media by a granulomatous process, with giant-cell formation and marked narrowing of lumen

ARTERY

ar·tery (a) (ar'ter-ē) [TA]. A relatively thick-walled, muscular, pulsating blood vessel conveying blood away from the heart. With the exception of the pulmonary and umbilical a.'s, the a.'s contain red or oxygenated blood. At the major a.'s, the arterial branches are listed separately following the designation *branches*. SYN arteria [TA]. [L. *arteria,* fr. G. *artēria*]

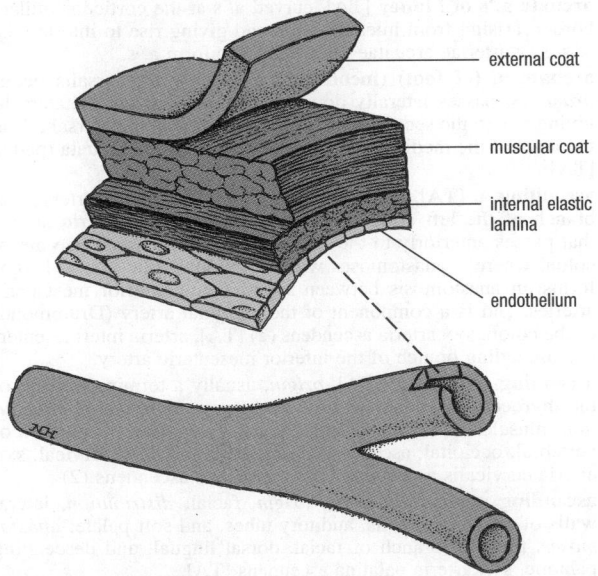

external coat

muscular coat

internal elastic lamina

endothelium

artery: showing layers of wall

Abbott a., an anomalous a. arising from the posteromedial proximal descending aorta, important during coarctation repair.

aberrant a., a. having an unusual origin or course.

aberrant obturator a. [TA], SEE pubic *branch* of inferior epigastric artery.

accessory meningeal a., SYN pterygomeningeal a.

accessory obturator a. [TA], term applied to the anastomosis of the pubic branch of the inferior epigastric a. with the pubic branch of the obturator a. when it contributes a significant supply through the obturator canal. SYN arteria obturatoria accessoria [TA], ramus obturatorius arteriae epigastricae inferioris.

acetabular a., SYN acetabular *branch.*

acromial a., SYN acromial *branch* of thoracoacromial artery.

acromiothoracic a., SYN thoracoacromial a.

a. of Adamkiewicz, SYN great segmental medullary a.

alar a. of nose, a branch of the angular a. that supplies the ala of the nose.

angular a. [TA], (1) the terminal branch of the facial a.; *distribution,* muscles and skin of side of nose; *anastomoses,* lateral nasal, and dorsal artery of nose and palpebrals from the ophthalmic a., thereby providing an external-internal carotid arterial anastomosis; (2) SYN *branch* to angular gyrus.

a. of angular gyrus, SYN *branch* to angular gyrus.

anterior basal segmental a. [TA], anterior basal branch of superior basal veins of the lower right and left lobes of left and right lungs. SYN arteria segmentalis basalis anterior [TA], anterior basal branch, ramus basalis anterior.

anterior cecal a. [TA], *origin,* ileocolic artery; *distribution,* anterior region of cecum. SYN arteria cecalis anterior [TA].

anterior cerebral a. [TA], one of the two terminal branches (with middle cerebral a. of the internal carotid; it passes anteriorly, loops around the genu of the corpus callosum, then posteriorly in the interhemispheric fissure along with its fellow of the opposite side, the two being joined by the anterior communicating a. [TA]; for descriptive purposes, it is divided into two parts: the precommunicating part [TA] (A_1 segment of clinical terminology), which gives rise to the anteromedial central a.'s [TA], which consist of proximal medial striate a.'s [TA], the supraoptic a. [TA], anterior perforating a.'s [TA] and preoptic arteries [TA] and a postcommunical part [TA], (A_2 segment), which gives rise to a distal medial striate a. [TA], medial frontobasal artery [TA], polar frontal a. [TA], and two large terminal branches: the pericallosal artery [TA] and the callosomarginal artery [TA]. The latter two have branches that serve specific regions of cortex. SYN arteria cerebri anterior [TA].

anterior choroidal a. [TA], *origin,* internal carotid or (rarely) middle cerebral artery; *distribution,* named branches [TA] to choroid plexus of lateral and third ventricles, optic chiasm and tract, internal capsule (genu, posterior limb, retrolentiform limb), lateral geniculate body, globus pallidus, tail of caudate nucleus, hippocampus, amygdaloid body, tuber cinereum, hypothalamic nuclei, thalamic nuclei, substantia nigra, red nucleus, and crus cerebri. SYN arteria choroidea anterior [TA].

anterior ciliary a.'s, one of several a.'s derived from muscular branches of the ophthalmic that perforate the anterior part of the sclera and anastomose with posterior ciliary a.'s. SYN arteriae ciliares anteriores.

anterior circumflex humeral a. [TA], *origin,* axillary; *distribution,* shoulder joint and biceps muscle; *anastomoses,* posterior circumflex humeral a. SYN arteria circumflexa humeri anterior [TA], anterior humeral circumflex a.

anterior communicating a. [TA], a short vessel joining the two anterior cerebral a.'s and completing the cerebral arterial circle (circle of Willis) anteriorly. SYN arteria communicans anterior [TA].

anterior conjunctival a. [TA], one of a number of small branches of the anterior ciliary a.'s that supplies the conjunctiva. SYN arteria conjunctivalis anterior [TA], conjunctival a.'s.

anterior ethmoidal a. [TA], *origin,* ophthalmic; *distribution,* cerebral membranes in anterior cranial fossa, anterior ethmoidal cells, frontal sinus, anterior upper part of nasal mucous membrane, skin of dorsum of nose. SYN arteria ethmoidalis anterior [TA].

anterior humeral circumflex a., SYN anterior circumflex humeral a.

anterior inferior cerebellar a. [TA], *origin*, basilar; *distribution*, lower surface of lateral lobes of cerebellum, choroid plexus in cerebellopontine angle; *anastomoses*, posterior inferior cerebellar; usual source of labyrinthine artery. SYN arteria inferior anterior cerebelli [TA].

anterior inferior segmental a. of kidney [TA], *origin*, anterior branch of renal. SEE segmental a.'s of kidney. SYN a. of anterior inferior segment of kidney.

a. of anterior inferior segment of kidney, SYN anterior inferior segmental a. of kidney.

anterior intercostal a.'s, SYN anterior intercostal *branches* of internal thoracic artery, under *branch*.

anterior interosseous a. [TA], *origin*, common interosseous; *distribution*, deep parts of the forearm anteriorly; *anastomoses*, posterior interosseous. SYN arteria interossea anterior [TA], arteria interossea volaris, volar interosseous a.

anterior interventricular a., SYN anterior interventricular *branch* of left coronary artery.

anterior labial a.'s, SYN anterior labial *branches* of deep external pudendal artery, under *branch*.

anterior lateral malleolar a. [TA], *origin*, anterior tibial; *distribution*, ankle joint; *anastomoses*, peroneal, lateral tarsal. SYN arteria malleolaris anterior lateralis [TA].

anterior medial malleolar a. [TA], *origin*, anterior tibial; *distribution*, ankle joint and neighboring integument; *anastomoses*, branches of posterior tibial. SYN arteria malleolaris anterior medialis [TA].

anterior mediastinal a.'s, SYN mediastinal *branches* of internal thoracic artery, under *branch*.

anterior meningeal a., SYN anterior meningeal *branch* (of anterior ethmoidal artery).

anterior parietal a. [TA], one of the terminal branches of the insular part of the middle cerebral a., distributed to the anterior part of the parietal lobe. SYN arteria parietalis anterior [TA].

anterior perforating a.'s [TA], *origin*: as part of the anteromedial central a.'s arising from the precommunicating part (A1 segment) of the anterior cerebral a.; enters the anterior perforated substance of the cranial base. SYN arteriae perforantes anteriores [TA].

anterior peroneal a., SEE perforating *branches*, under *branch*.

(anterior and posterior) radicular a.'s, branches of spinal a.'s distributed to the dorsal and ventral roots of spinal nerves and their coverings. SEE spinal a.'s, segmental medullary a.'s. SYN arteriae radiculares (anterior et posterior).

(anterior and posterior) superior pancreaticoduodenal a., *origin*, gastroduodenal; one of two a.'s, anterior and superior; *distribution*, head of pancreas, duodenum, common bile duct; *anastomoses*, inferior pancreaticoduodenal, splenic. SYN arteria pancreaticoduodenalis superior (anterior et posterior).

anterior segmental a., SEE left pulmonary a., right pulmonary a.

anterior spinal a. [TA], *origin*, intracranial part of vertebral; *distribution*, anteromedial spinal cord and adjacent pia mater; *anastomoses*, spinal of intercostal and lumbar arteries. SYN arteria spinalis anterior [TA].

anterior superior alveolar a.'s [TA], *origin*, infraorbital artery within intraorbital canal; *distribution*, via anterior alveolar canals to upper incisors and canine teeth, mucous membrane of maxillary sinus. SYN arteriae alveolares superiores anteriores [TA], anterior superior dental a.'s.

anterior superior dental a.'s, SYN anterior superior alveolar a.'s.

anterior superior segmental a. of kidney [TA], *origin*, anterior branch of renal. SEE segmental a.'s of kidney. SYN a. of anterior superior segment of kidney.

a. of anterior superior segment of kidney, SYN anterior superior segmental a. of kidney.

anterior temporal a., SYN anterior temporal *branch*.

anterior tibial a., *origin*, popliteal; *branches*, posterior and anterior tibial recurrent, lateral and medial anterior malleolar, dorsalis pedis, lateral tarsal, medial tarsal, arcuate, dorsal metatarsal, and dorsal digital. SYN arteria tibialis anterior [TA].

anterior tibial recurrent a. [TA], a branch of the anterior tibial a. that ascends to supply the front and sides of the knee joint, thus contributing to the articular network of the knee. SYN arteria recurrens tibialis anterior [TA].

anterior tympanic a. [TA], *origin*, first (retromandibular) part of the maxillary; *distribution*, middle ear; *anastomoses*, tympanic branches of internal carotid and ascending pharyngeal and stylomastoid. SYN arteria tympanica anterior [TA], glaserian a.

anterior vestibular a., *origin*: as a terminal branch, with the common cochlear a., of the labyrinthine a.; *branch*: vestibulocochlear a.; *distribution*: to vestibular ganglion, utricle and (especially the ampullae of the) lateral and posterior semicircular ducts. SYN arteria vestibularis anterior [TA], arteria vestibuli ✶.

anterolateral central a.'s [TA], numerous small branches from the sphenoidal part of the middle cerebral a.'s supplying the lateral and anterior parts of the corpus striatum. SYN arteriae centrales anterolaterales [TA], lenticulostriate a.'s (1) ✶, anterolateral striate a.'s, anterolateral thalamostriate a.'s, arteriae thalamostriatae anterolaterales, a.'s of cerebral hemorrhage, lateral striate a.'s.

anterolateral striate a.'s, SYN anterolateral central a.'s.

anterolateral thalamostriate a.'s, SYN anterolateral central a.'s.

anteromedial central a.'s [TA], several small branches of the precommunical part (A1 segment) of the anterior cerebral a. or of the anterior communicating a.; they are distributed to the anteromedial part of the corpus striatum part of the thalamus. SYN arteriae centrales anteromediales [TA], anteromedial thalamostriate a.'s, arteriae thalamostriatae anteromediales.

anteromedial thalamostriate a.'s, SYN anteromedial central a.'s.

apical segmental a. [TA], SEE left pulmonary a., right pulmonary a.

apical segmental a. of superior lobar artery of right lung [TA], branch (of the inferior lobar branch) of the right pulmonary a. serving the apical segment of the inferior lobe of the right lung. SYN apical branch of inferior lobar branch of right pulmonary artery ✶, ramus apicalis lobi inferioris arteriae pulmonalis dextrae ✶.

apicoposterior a., a pulmonary a. branch to the apicoposterior segment left of the upper lobe.

appendicular a. [TA], the branch of the ileocolic a. that descends posterior to the terminal ileum in the mesoappendix to supply the vermiform appendix. SYN arteria appendicularis [TA].

arciform a.'s, SYN arcuate a.'s of kidney.

arcuate a.'s of kidney [TA], curved a.'s at the corticomedullary border, arising from interlobar a.'s and giving rise to interlobular a.'s. SYN arteriae arcuatae renis [TA], arciform a.'s.

arcuate a. (of foot) (inconstant) [TA], *origin*, dorsalis pedis; *branches*, passes laterally dorsal to the bases of the metatarsals, giving rise to the second, third, and fourth dorsal metatarsal a.'s at the level of the medial cuneiform bone. SYN arteria arcuata (pedis) [TA].

ascending a. [TA], **(1)** SYN colic *branch* of ileocolic artery; **(2)** branch of the left colic artery (from inferior mesenteric artery) that passes anteriorly to the left kidney into the transverse mesocolon, where it anastomoses with the middle colic artery. It thus forms an anastomosis between superior and inferior mesenteric arteries, and is a component of the marginal artery (Drummond) of the colon. SYN arteria ascendens (2) [TA], arteria intermesenterica, ascending branch of the inferior mesenteric artery.

ascending cervical a. [TA], *origin*, usually a terminal branch of the thyrocervical trunk (along with interior thyroid a.); *distribution*, muscles of neck and spinal cord; *anastomoses*, branches of vertebral, occipital, ascending pharyngeal, and deep cervical. SYN arteria cervicalis ascendens [TA], cervicalis ascendens (2).

ascending palatine a. [TA], *origin*, facial; *distribution*, lateral walls of pharynx, tonsils, auditory tubes, and soft palate; *anastomoses*, tonsillar branch of facial, dorsal lingual, and descending palatine. SYN arteria palatina ascendens [TA].

ascending pharyngeal a. [TA], *origin*, external carotid; *distribution*, wall of pharynx and soft palate, posterior cranial fossa. SYN arteria pharyngea ascendens [TA].

atrial a.'s, branches of the right and left coronary a.'s distributed to the muscle of the atria. SYN arteriae atriales.

a. to atrioventricular node, SYN atrioventricular nodal *branch*.

axillary a. [TA], the continuation of the subclavian a. after crossing the first rib to enter the axilla; becomes the brachial a. upon passing the inferior border of the teres major muscle. It is accompanied by the cords of the brachial plexus and is enclosed with them and the axillary vein in the axillary sheath as it traverses the axilla. The parts of the axillary a. are described: proximal, posterior, and distal to the pectoralis minor muscle. Branches: first part—superior thoracic a.; second part—thoracoacromial arterial trunk, lateral thoracic a.; third part—subscapular a., anterior and posterior humeral circumflex a.'s. SYN arteria axillaris [TA].

azygos a. of vagina, one of two a.'s that run longitudinally in the midline on the anterior and posterior aspects of the vagina; they take origin from the uterine a.

basilar a. [TA], formed by union of the intracranial portions of the two vertebral a.'s; runs along the clivus in the pontine cistern of the subarachnoid space from the lower to the upper border of the pons, where it bifurcates into the two posterior cerebral arteries; *branches,* anterior inferior cerebellar artery [TA], pontine arteries [TA], mesencephalic arteries [TA], superior cerebellar artery [TA], and posterior cerebral artery [TA]. SYN arteria basilaris [TA].

brachial a. [TA], *origin,* is a continuation of the axillary beginning at the inferior border of the teres major muscle; *branches,* deep brachial, superior ulnar collateral, inferior ulnar collateral, muscular, and nutrient; terminates in the cubital fossa (elbow level) by bifurcating into radial and ulnar a.'s. SYN arteria brachialis [TA], humeral a.

a.'s of brain [TA], a.'s and arterial branches supplying the brain; they are derived from the cerebral arterial circle and the anterior choroidal a. SYN arteriae encephali [TA].

bronchial a.'s, SYN bronchial *branches* of thoracic aorta, under *branch.*

buccal a., buccinator a. [TA], *origin,* maxillary; *distribution,* buccinator muscle, skin, and mucous membrane of cheek; *anastomoses,* buccal branch of facial. SYN arteria buccalis [TA].

buckled innominate a., elongation of the innominate a. manifest as a pulsating mass in the right supraclavicular space and as a radiographic appearance mimicking an aneurysm or tumor of the apex of the right lung or superior mediastinum.

a. of bulb of penis [TA], a branch of the internal pudendal a. that supplies the bulb of the penis including the bulbar urethra. SYN arteria bulbi penis [TA], arteria bulbi urethrae.

a. of bulb of vestibule [TA], the branch of the internal pudendal a. in the female that supplies the bulb of the vestibule. SYN arteria bulbi vestibuli [TA], arteria bulbi vaginae.

calcaneal a.'s, SYN calcaneal *branches,* under *branch.*

calcarine a., SYN calcarine *branch* of medial occipital artery.

a. of calf, SYN sural a.'s.

callosomarginal a. [TA], the second branch of the pericallosal artery running in the cingulate sulcus and sending branches to supply part of the medial and superolateral surfaces of the cerebral hemisphere. SYN arteria callosomarginalis [TA].

caroticotympanic a.'s (of internal carotid artery) [TA], small branches from the petrous part of the internal carotid artery supplying the tympanic cavity; anastomose with the anterior tympanic and maxillary arteries. SYN arteriae caroticotympanicae (arteriae carotidis internae) [TA], rami caroticotympanici.

carotid a.'s, SEE common carotid a., external carotid a., internal carotid a.

carpal a., a.'s related to and supplying the wrist joint. SEE dorsal carpal *branch* of radial artery, dorsal carpal *branch* of ulnar artery, palmar carpal *branch* of radial artery, palmar carpal *branch* of ulnar artery.

caudal pancreatic a., SYN a. to tail of pancreas.

a. of caudate lobe [TA], *origin,* left branch of proper hepatic; *distribution,* caudate lobe of the liver. SYN arteria lobi caudati [TA].

cavernous a.'s, SYN cavernous *branch* of cavernous part of internal carotid artery.

cecal a.'s, SEE anterior cecal a., posterior cecal a.

celiac a., SYN celiac (arterial) *trunk.*

central a., SYN a. of central sulcus.

central a. of retina, SYN central retinal a.

central retinal a. [TA], a branch of the ophthalmic a. that penetrates the optic nerve 1 cm behind the eye (extraocular part) to enter the eye (intraocular part) at the optic papilla in the retina; it divides into superior and inferior temporal and nasal branches. SYN arteria centralis retinae [TA], arteria retinae centralis, central a. of retina, Zinn a.

central sulcal a., SYN a. of central sulcus.

a. of central sulcus [TA], a branch of the terminal part of the middle cerebral a. distributed to the cortex on either side of the central sulcus. SYN arteria sulci centralis [TA], central a., central sulcal a., Rolandic sulcal a.

cerebellar a.'s, an artery related to and supplying the cerebellum. SEE anterior inferior cerebellar a., posterior inferior cerebellar a., superior cerebellar a.

cerebral a.'s, a.'s related to and supplying the cerebral cortex. SEE anterior cerebral a., middle cerebral a., posterior cerebral a.

a.'s of cerebral hemorrhage, SYN anterolateral central a.'s.

cervicovaginal a., an anastomotic communication between the uterine a. and the vaginal a.; it courses along the lateral aspect of the cervix and vagina. SYN arteria cervicovaginalis.

Charcot a., SYN lenticulostriate a.'s (2).

chief a. of thumb, SYN princeps pollicis a.

circumflex femoral a.'s, SEE lateral circumflex femoral a., medial circumflex femoral a.

circumflex fibular a., SYN circumflex fibular *branch* (of posterior tibial artery).

circumflex humeral a.'s, SEE anterior circumflex humeral a., posterior circumflex humeral a.

circumflex iliac a.'s, SEE deep circumflex iliac a., superficial circumflex iliac a.

circumflex scapular a. [TA], *origin,* terminal branch (with thoracodorsal a.) of the subscapular; *distribution,* muscles of shoulder and scapular region; *anastomoses,* branches of suprascapular and transverse cervical. SYN arteria circumflexa scapulae [TA].

coiled a. of the uterus, SYN spiral a.

colic a.'s, a.'s supplying the colon. SEE left colic a., middle colic a., right colic a.

collateral a., (1) one that runs parallel with a nerve or other structure; (2) one through which a collateral circulation is established. SEE articular vascular *network.*

collateral digital a., SYN proper palmar digital a.'s.

collicular a. [TA], *origin,* precommunicating part (P1 segment) of posterior cerebral a.; *distribution:* to superior and inferior colliculi (corpora quadrigemina) of tectum of midbrain. SYN arteria collicularis [TA], arteria quadrigeminalis✩, quadrigeminal a.✩.

comitant a. of median nerve, SYN median a.

common carotid a. [TA], *origin,* right from brachiocephalic, left from arch of aorta; runs upward in the neck and divides opposite upper border of thyroid cartilage (C-4 vertebral level) into *terminal branches,* external and internal carotid. SYN arteria carotis communis [TA].

common cochlear a. [TA], *origin:* as a terminal branch, with the anterior vestibular a., of the labyrinthine a.; *distribution:* runs in the cochlear axis of modiolus serving the spiral ganglia; sends the proper cochlear a. to the cochlear duct and supplies the apical two turns of the spiral modiolar a. SYN arteria cochlearis communis [TA].

common hepatic a. [TA], *origin,* celiac; *branches,* right gastric, gastroduodenal, and proper hepatic. SYN arteria hepatica communis [TA].

common iliac a. [TA], one of two terminal branches of the abdominal aorta; anterior to the sacroiliac joint at the level of the sacral promontory, it bifurcates to form the internal iliac and the external iliac. SYN arteria iliaca communis [TA].

common interosseous a. [TA], *origin,* ulnar; *branches,* anterior and posterior interosseous. SYN arteria interossea communis [TA].

common palmar digital a. [TA], one of three a.'s arising from the superficial palmar arch and running to the interdigital clefts where each divides into two proper palmar digital arteries. SYN arteria digitalis palmaris communis [TA].

common plantar digital a. [TA], one of four a.'s arising from a superficial plantar arch, when present as a variation. They unite with the plantar metatarsal a.'s distal to the perforating branches. SYN arteria digitalis plantaris communis [TA].

communicating a., an a. that connects two larger a.'s. SEE anterior communicating a., posterior communicating a.

companion a. to sciatic nerve, SYN a. to sciatic nerve.

conjunctival a.'s, SYN anterior conjunctival a., posterior conjunctival a.

ⓘ**coronary a.,** (1) SEE right coronary a., left coronary a.; (2) SYN left gastric a.

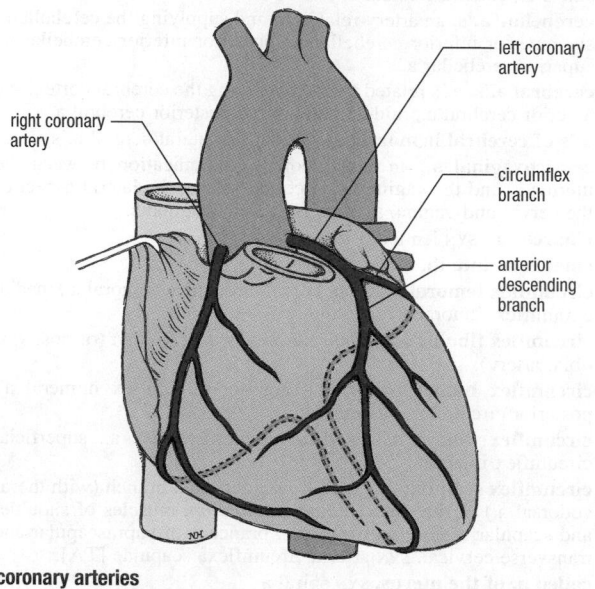

left coronary artery

right coronary artery

circumflex branch

anterior descending branch

coronary arteries

cortical a.'s, branches of the anterior, middle, and posterior cerebral a.'s that supply the cerebral cortex.

cortical radiate a.'s [TA], the branches of the arcuate a.'s of the kidney radiating outward through the renal columns and cortex and supplying the glomeruli. SYN arteriae corticales radiatae [TA], arteria interlobulares (renis), interlobular a.'s of kidney.

costocervical a., SYN costocervical (arterial) *trunk.*

cremasteric a. [TA], *origin,* inferior epigastric; *distribution,* coverings of spermatic cord; *anastomoses,* external pudendal, spermatic, and perineal a. SYN arteria cremasterica [TA], external spermatic a.

cricothyroid a., SYN cricothyroid *branch* of superior thyroid artery.

cystic a. [TA], *origin,* right branch of hepatic; *distribution,* gall bladder and visceral surface of the liver. SYN arteria cystica [TA].

deep a. of arm, ✲official alternate term for profunda brachii a.

deep auricular a. [TA], *origin,* first part of maxillary; *distribution,* articulation of jaw, parotid gland, and external acoustic meatus and external tympanic membrane; *anastomoses,* auricular branches of superficial temporal and posterior auricular. SYN arteria auricularis profunda [TA].

deep brachial a., SYN profunda brachii a.

deep cervical a. [TA], *origin,* terminal branch of costocervical trunk (along with superior intercostal artery); *distribution,* posterior deep muscles of neck; *anastomoses,* branches of occipital, ascending cervical, and vertebral. SYN arteria cervicalis profunda [TA].

deep circumflex iliac a. [TA], *origin,* external iliac; *distribution,* muscles and skin of lower abdomen, sartorius and tensor fasciae latae; *anastomoses,* lumbar, inferior epigastric, superior gluteal, iliolumbar, and superficial circumflex iliac. SYN arteria circumflexa iliaca profunda [TA].

deep a. of clitoris [TA], the deep terminal branch of the internal pudendal artery in the female; it supplies the crus of the clitoris. SYN arteria profunda clitoridis [TA].

deep epigastric a., SYN inferior epigastric a.

deep lingual a. [TA], termination of lingual artery, *distribution,* muscles and mucous membrane of under surface of tongue. SYN arteria profunda linguae [TA], arteria ranina, deep a. of tongue, ranine a.

deep a. of penis [TA], *origin,* terminal branch (with dorsal a. of penis) of the internal pudendal artery; *distribution,* corpus cavernosum of the penis via capillary beds and via helicine arteries and arteriovenous anastomoses to produce erection. SYN arteria profunda penis [TA].

deep plantar a. [TA], deep plantar branch of arcuate a. or its first metatarsal a. branch that penetrates the foot between first and second metatarsal bones to anastomose with the termination of the plantar arterial arch. SYN arteria plantaris profunda arteriae dorsalis pedis [TA], deep plantar branch of dorsalis pedis artery, ramus plantaris profundus arteriae dorsalis pedis.

deep temporal a., deep temporal artery, two in number, anterior and posterior; *origin,* maxillary; *distribution,* temporal muscle and periosteum, bone and diploe of temporal fossa; *anastomoses,* branches of superficial temporal, lacrimal, and middle meningeal. SYN arteria temporalis profunda [TA].

deep a. of thigh [TA], *origin,* femoral; *branches,* lateral circumflex femoral, medial circumflex femoral, terminating in three or four perforating a.'s. SYN arteria profunda femoris, profunda femoris a.

deep a. of tongue, SYN deep lingual a.

deferential a., SYN a. to ductus deferens.

descending genicular a. [TA], *origin,* femoral, in adductor canal; *distribution,* penetrates vastoadductor fascia to supply knee joint and adjacent parts; *anastomoses,* medial superior genicular, medial inferior genicular, lateral superior genicular, lateral inferior genicular and anterior tibial recurrent a.'s, i.e., articular network of knee. SYN arteria descendens genus [TA], arteria anastomotica magna (2), descending a. of knee, great anastomotic a. (2).

descending a. of knee, SYN descending genicular a.

descending palatine a. [TA], *origin,* maxillary; *distribution,* soft palate, gums, and bones and mucous membrane of hard palate; *anastomoses,* sphenopalatine, ascending palatine, ascending pharyngeal, and tonsillar branches of facial. SYN arteria palatina descendens [TA].

descending scapular a., SYN dorsal scapular a.

digital collateral a., SYN proper palmar digital a.'s.

distal medial striate a. [TA], SYN medial striate a.

distributing a., SYN muscular a.

dolichoectatic a., a distorted, dilated, and elongated artery that may compress adjacent neural structures.

dorsal a. of clitoris [TA], one of the two terminal branches of the internal pudendal a. in the female, the other being the deep a. of the clitoris. SYN arteria dorsalis clitoridis [TA].

dorsal digital a. [TA], one of the collateral digital branches of the dorsal metatarsal arteries in the foot, and/or of the dorsal metacarpal arteries in the hand. SYN arteria digitalis dorsalis [TA].

dorsal a. of foot, SYN dorsalis pedis a.

dorsal interosseous a., SYN posterior interosseous a.

dorsalis pedis a. [TA], continuation of anterior tibial artery after crossing ankle; *branches,* lateral tarsal, arcuate, dorsal metatarsal; a continuation of the anterior tibial; *anastomoses,* with the lateral plantar to form the plantar arch. SYN arteria dorsalis pedis [TA], dorsal a. of foot.

dorsal metacarpal a. [TA], one of four a.'s taking origin from the dorsal carpal arch and running on the posterior aspect of the interosseous muscles of the hand. SYN arteria metacarpalis dorsalis [TA].

dorsal metatarsal a. [TA], one of four a.'s arising from the dorsalis pedis (I) and arcuate (II–IV) a.'s and running on the dorsum of the interosseous muscles of the foot. SYN arteria metatarsalis dorsalis [TA].

dorsal nasal a. [TA], *origin,* ophthalmic; external artery of the nose; *distribution,* skin of side of root of nose; *anastomoses,* angular a. SYN arteria dorsalis nasi [TA], external nasal a.☆, arteria nasi externa, dorsal a. of nose, external a. of nose.

dorsal a. of nose, SYN dorsal nasal a.

dorsal pancreatic a. [TA], *origin*, splenic; *distribution*, head and body of pancreas; *anastomoses*, superior pancreaticoduodenal. SYN arteria pancreatica dorsalis [TA], great superior pancreatic a.

dorsal a. of penis [TA], the dorsal terminal branch of the internal pudendal artery in the male. SYN arteria dorsalis penis [TA].

dorsal scapular a. [TA], *origin*, inconstant: subclavian (when this term is preferred) or as the deep branch of the transverse cervical; *distribution*, passes deep to the rhomboid muscles, supplying them and other muscles and skin along the vertebral border of the scapula; *anastomoses*, suprascapular and scapular circumflex. SYN arteria dorsalis scapulae [TA], rami profundi arteriae transversae cervicis [TA], ramus profundus arteriae transversae colli [TA], arteria scapularis descendens, arteria scapularis dorsalis, deep branch of the transverse cervical artery, descending scapular a., ramus profundus arteriae scapularis descendentis.

dorsal thoracic a., SYN thoracodorsal a.

a. of Drummond, SYN marginal a. of colon.

a. to ductus deferens [TA], *origin*, anterior division of internal iliac, or sometimes superior vesical; *distribution*, ductus deferens, seminal vesicles, testicle, ureter; *anastomoses*, testicular, cremasteric a.'s. SYN a. to vas deferens☆, arteria deferentialis, arteria ductus deferentis, deferential a.

elastic a., a large a., such as the aorta or pulmonary a., which has many elastic lamella in its tunica media.

end a., an a. with insufficient anastomoses to maintain viability of the tissue supplied if occlusion of the a. occurs. SYN terminal a.

episcleral a. [TA], one of many small branches of the anterior ciliary a.'s that arise as they perforate the sclera near the corneoscleral junction, and course on the sclera. SYN arteria episcleralis [TA].

esophageal a.'s, esophageal branches of the following: 1) inferior thyroid a.; 2) left gastric a.; 3) thoracic aorta.

external carotid a. [TA], *origin*, common carotid at C-4 vertebral level; *branches*, superior thyroid, lingual, facial, occipital, posterior auricular, ascending pharyngeal, and *terminal branches*, maxillary and superficial temporal at level of neck of mandible. SYN arteria carotis externa [TA].

external iliac a. [TA], *origin*, common iliac; *branches*, inferior epigastric, deep circumflex iliac; becomes the femoral at the inguinal ligament. SYN arteria iliaca externa [TA].

external mammary a., SYN lateral thoracic a.

external maxillary a., SYN facial a.

external nasal a., ☆official alternate term for dorsal nasal a.

external a. of nose, SYN dorsal nasal a.

external spermatic a., SYN cremasteric a.

facial a. [TA], *origin*, external carotid; *branches*, ascending palatine, tonsillar and glandular branches, submental, inferior labial, superior labial, masseteric, buccal, lateral nasal branches, and angular. SYN arteria facialis [TA], arteria maxillaris externa, external maxillary a.

femoral a. [TA], *origin*, continuation of external iliac, beginning at inguinal ligament; *branches*, external pudendal, superficial epigastric, superficial circumflex iliac, profunda femoris, descending genicular, terminating as the popliteal a. as it passes through the adductor hiatus to enter the popliteal space. SYN arteria femoralis [TA].

femoral nutrient a. [TA], one of two a.'s, superior and inferior, arising from the first and third perforating a.'s, respectively (sometimes second and fourth). SYN nutrient a. of femur.

fibular a. [TA], *origin*, posterior tibial; *distribution*, soleus, tibialis posterior, flexor longus hallucis, peroneal muscles, inferior tibiofibular articulation, and ankle joint; *anastomoses*, anterior lateral malleolar, lateral tarsal, lateral plantar, dorsalis pedis. SYN arteria fibularis [TA], arteria peronea☆, peroneal a.☆.

fibular nutrient a. [TA], *origin*, fibular (peroneal); *distribution*, fibula. SYN arteria nutriens fibulae☆, nutrient a. of fibula.

first and second posterior intercostal a.'s [TA], terminal branches of the superior intercostal a. (from costocervical trunk) supplying upper two intercostal spaces. SYN arteriae intercostales posteriores I et II, posterior intercostal a.'s 1–2.

frontal a., SYN supratrochlear a.

frontopolar a. [TA], SYN polar frontal a.

gastric a.'s, a.'s supplying the stomach along the lesser curvature. SEE left gastric a., right gastric a.

gastroduodenal a. [TA], *origin*, hepatic; terminal *branches*, right gastroepiploic, superior pancreaticoduodenal. SYN arteria gastroduodenalis [TA].

gastroepiploic a.'s, ☆official alternate term for gastroomental a.'s; SEE left gastroomental a., right gastroomental a.

gastroomental a.'s [TA], a.'s that supply the stomach and greater omentum as they course along the greater curvature of the stomach. SYN arteriae gastro-omentales [TA], arteriae gastroepiploicae☆, gastroepiploic a.'s☆.

genicular a.'s, a.'s contributing to the articular network of the knee. SEE descending genicular a., inferior lateral genicular a., inferior medial genicular a., middle genicular a., superior lateral genicular a., superior medial genicular a.

glaserian a., SYN anterior tympanic a.

great anastomotic a., (1) SYN inferior ulnar collateral a; (2) SYN descending genicular a; (3) SYN great segmental medullary a.

greater palatine a. [TA], anterior branch of descending palatine artery, supplying the gums and mucous membrane of the hard palate. SYN arteria palatina major [TA].

greater pancreatic a. [TA], *origin*, splenic; *distribution*, tail of pancreas; *anastomoses*, inferior pancreatic a. and a.'s of pancreatic tail. SYN arteria pancreatica magna.

great radicular a., SYN great segmental medullary a.

great segmental medullary a., largest of the medullary a.'s that supply the spinal cord by anastomosing with the anterior (longitudinal) spinal a.; it arises from a lower intercostal or upper lumbar a. (on the left side about 65% of the time) supplying most of the blood to the lower two-thirds of the anterior spinal a. SEE medullary a.'s of brain. SYN arteria radicularis magna, a. of Adamkiewicz, great anastomotic a. (3), great radicular a.

great superior pancreatic a., SYN dorsal pancreatic a.

helicine a.'s of penis [TA], the coiled terminal branches of the deep and dorsal arteries of the penis. Parasympathetic stimulation causes them to uncoil, allowing blood at arterial pressure to fill the cavernous tissue causing erection. SYN arteriae helicinae penis [TA].

helicine a.'s of the uterus [TA], the coiled terminal branches of the uterine a. in the uterine musculature (myometrium). SYN arteriae helicinae uteri [TA].

hepatic a.'s, a.'s involved in supplying blood to the liver. SEE common hepatic a., hepatic a. proper, left *branch* of hepatic artery proper, right *branch* of hepatic artery proper.

hepatic a. proper [TA], *origin*, common hepatic; *branches*, right and left hepatic. SYN arteria hepatica propria.

Heubner a., SYN medial striate a.

a. of Heubner, SYN medial striate a.

highest intercostal a., SYN supreme intercostal a.

highest thoracic a., SYN superior thoracic a.

humeral a., SYN brachial a.

humeral nutrient a.'s [TA], *origin*, deep brachial; *distribution*, the medullary cavity of the humerus. SYN arteriae nutriciae humeri [TA], nutrient a.'s of humerus.

hyaloid a., the terminal branch of the primitive ophthalmic artery, which forms in the embryo an extensive ramification in the primary vitreous and a vascular tunic around the lens; by 8½ months, these vessels have atrophied almost completely, but a few persistent remnants are evident entoptically as muscae volitantes. SYN arteria hyaloidea [TA].

hypogastric a., SYN internal iliac a.

ileal a.'s [TA], *origin*, superior mesenteric; *distribution*, ileum; *anastomoses*, other branches of superior mesenteric. SYN arteriae ileales [TA].

ileocolic a. [TA], *origin*, superior mesenteric, often by a common trunk with the right colic; *distribution*, terminal part of ileum, cecum, vermiform appendix, and ascending colon; *anastomoses*, right colic and ileal. SYN arteria ileocolica [TA].

iliac a.'s, a.'s related to the ilium. SEE common iliac a., deep circumflex iliac a., external iliac a., internal iliac a., superficial circumflex iliac a.

iliolumbar a. [TA], *origin*, internal iliac; *distribution*, pelvic muscles and bones; *anastomoses*, deep circumflex iliac, lumbar. SYN arteria iliolumbalis [TA].

inferior alveolar a. [TA], *origin*, 1st part of maxillary a.; *distribution*, through mandibular foramen/canal to lower teeth and chin; *branches*, a. to mylohyoid, mental a., dental a.'s. SYN arteria alveolaris inferior [TA], inferior dental a.

inferior dental a., SYN inferior alveolar a.

inferior epigastric a. [TA], *origin*, external iliac; *branches*, cremasteric, muscular and pubic; *anastomoses*, superior epigastric, obturator. With overlying peritoneum, forms lateral umbilical ligament and forms a basis for distinguishing types of inguinal herniae: direct hernias pass medial to the a.; indirect hernias pass laterally. SYN arteria epigastrica inferior [TA], deep epigastric a.

inferior gluteal a. [TA], *origin*, internal iliac; *distribution*, hip joint and gluteal region; *anastomoses*, branches of internal pudendal, lateral sacral, superior gluteal, obturator, medial and lateral circumflex femoral. SYN arteria glutea inferior [TA], arteria ischiadica, arteria ischiatica.

inferior hemorrhoidal a., SYN inferior rectal a.

inferior hypophysial a. [TA], a small branch of the cavernous part of the internal carotid to the hypophysis. SYN arteria hypophysialis inferior [TA].

inferior internal parietal a., SYN precuneal branches (of anterior cerebral artery), under branch.

inferior labial a., SYN inferior labial branch of facial artery.

inferior laryngeal a. [TA], *origin*, inferior thyroid; *distribution*, muscles and mucous membrane of larynx; *anastomoses*, superior laryngeal. SYN arteria laryngea inferior [TA].

inferior lateral genicular a. [TA], *origin*, popliteal; *distribution*, knee joint; *anastomoses*, lateral superior genicular and anterior tibial recurrent (and posterior); i.e., articular vascular *network* of knee. SYN arteria inferior lateralis genus [TA], arteria genus inferior lateralis, lateral inferior genicular a.

inferior lingular a. [TA], branch (of the lingular branch) of the left pulmonary a. serving the inferior lingular segment of the superior lobe of the left lung. SEE left pulmonary a. SYN arteria lingularis inferior [TA], inferior lingular branch of lingular branch of left pulmonary artery, ramus lingularis inferior.

inferior lobar a.'s [TA], SEE left pulmonary a., right pulmonary a.

inferior medial genicular a. [TA], *origin*, popliteal; *distribution*, knee joint; *anastomoses*, anterior and posterior tibial recurrent and medial superior genicular, i.e., articular vascular *network* of knee. SYN arteria inferior medialis genus [TA], arteria genus inferior medialis, medial inferior genicular a.

inferior mesenteric a. [TA], *origin*, abdominal aorta; *branches*, left colic, sigmoid, superior rectal; *anastomoses*, middle colic and middle rectal. SYN arteria mesenterica inferior [TA].

inferior pancreatic a. [TA], *origin*, dorsal pancreatic; *distribution*, body and tail of pancreas; *anastomoses*, great pancreatic a. SYN arteria pancreatica inferior [TA], transverse pancreatic a.

inferior pancreaticoduodenal a. [TA], *origin*, superior mesenteric; one of two arteries, anterior and posterior; *distribution*, head of pancreas, duodenum; *anastomoses*, superior pancreaticoduodenal. SYN arteria pancreaticoduodenalis inferior [TA].

inferior phrenic a. [TA], *origin*, the first paired branch from the abdominal aorta inferior to the diaphragm; *distribution*, diaphragm; *anastomoses*, superior phrenic, internal thoracic, and musculophrenic. SYN arteria phrenica inferior [TA].

inferior rectal a. [TA], *origin*, internal pudendal; *distribution*, anal canal, muscles and skin of the anal region, and skin of the buttock; *anastomoses*, middle rectal, perineal, and gluteal. SYN arteria rectalis inferior [TA], inferior hemorrhoidal a.

inferior segmental a. of kidney [TA], *origin*, anterior branch of renal. SEE segmental a.'s of kidney. SYN a. of inferior segment of kidney.

a. of inferior segment of kidney, SYN inferior segmental a. of kidney.

inferior and superior lobar a.'s [TA], SEE left pulmonary a., right pulmonary a.

inferior suprarenal a. [TA], *origin*, renal; *distribution*, suprarenal gland. SYN arteria suprarenalis inferior [TA].

inferior thyroid a. [TA], *origin*, terminal branch of thyrocervical trunk (with ascending cervical artery); *branches*, inferior laryngeal, and muscular, esophageal, and tracheal. SYN arteria thyroidea inferior [TA].

inferior tympanic a. [TA], *origin*, ascending pharyngeal; *distribution*, middle ear; *anastomoses*, tympanic branches of other arteries. SYN arteria tympanica inferior [TA].

inferior ulnar collateral a. [TA], *origin*, brachial; *distribution*, arm muscles at back of elbow; *anastomoses*, anterior and posterior ulnar recurrent, superior ulnar collateral, profunda brachii, and recurrent interosseous, as part of the articular network of the elbow. SYN arteria collateralis ulnaris inferior [TA], arteria anastomotica magna (1), great anastomotic a. (1).

inferior vesical a. [TA], *origin*, internal iliac; *distribution*, base of bladder, ureter, and (in the male) seminal vesicles, ductus deferens, and prostate; *anastomoses*, middle rectal, and other vesical branches. SYN arteria vesicalis inferior [TA].

infraorbital a. [TA], *origin*, third part of maxillary; *distribution*, upper canine and incisor teeth, inferior rectus and inferior oblique muscles, lower eyelid, lacrimal sac, maxillary sinus, and upper lip; *anastomoses*, branches of ophthalmic, facial, superior labial, transverse facial, and buccal. SYN arteria infraorbitalis [TA].

infrascapular a., a small branch of the circumflex scapular a.

innominate a., obsolete term for brachiocephalic (arterial) *trunk*.

insular a.'s [TA], branches from the insular part (M2 segment) of the middle cerebral artery distributed to the cortex of the insula. SYN arteriae insulares [TA].

intercostal a.'s, a.'s that course in the thoracic wall between ribs. SEE anterior intercostal *branches* of internal thoracic artery, under *branch*, first and second posterior intercostal a.'s, posterior intercostal a.'s 3–11, supreme intercostal a.

interlobar a., the right descending pulmonary a., which is contiguous with and perfuses the right middle and lower lobes.

interlobar a.'s of kidney [TA], the branches of the segmental a.'s of the kidney; they run between the renal lobes and give rise to the arcuate arteries. SYN arteriae interlobares renis [TA].

interlobular a.'s [TA], a.'s that pass between lobules of an organ. SEE interlobular a.'s of liver, cortical radiate a.'s. SYN arteriae interlobulares [TA].

interlobular a.'s of kidney, SYN cortical radiate a.'s.

interlobular a.'s of liver, the many terminal branches of the hepatic a. passing between hepatic lobules. SYN arteriae interlobulares (hepatis).

intermediate temporal a., SYN middle temporal branch of insular part of middle cerebral artery.

internal auditory a., SYN labyrinthine a.

internal carotid a. [TA], arises from the common carotid opposite upper border of thyroid cartilage (C-4 vertebral level) and terminates in the middle cranial fossa by dividing into the anterior and middle cerebral arteries; for descriptive purposes it is divided into four parts: cervical, petrous, cavernous, and cerebral. SYN arteria carotis interna [TA].

internal iliac a. [TA], *origin*, common iliac; *branches*, iliolumbar, lateral sacral, obturator, superior gluteal, inferior gluteal, umbilical, superior vesical, inferior vesical, middle rectal, and internal pudendal. SYN arteria iliaca interna [TA], arteria hypogastrica, hypogastric a.

internal mammary a., SYN internal thoracic a.

internal maxillary a., SYN maxillary a.

internal pudendal a. [TA], *origin*, internal iliac; *branches*, inferior rectal, perineal, posterior scrotal (or labial), urethral, artery of bulb of penis (or of vestibule), deep artery of penis (or clitoris), dorsal artery of penis (or clitoris). SYN arteria pudenda interna [TA].

internal spermatic a., SYN testicular a.

internal thoracic a. [TA], *origin*, subclavian; *branches*, pericardiacophrenic, anterior intercostal, sternal, mediastinal, thymic, bronchial, muscular, and perforating branches, and bifurcates into the musculophrenic and superior epigastric. SYN arteria thoracica interna [TA], arteria mammaria interna, internal mammary a.

intestinal a.'s, SEE ileal a.'s, jejunal a.'s.

intrarenal a.'s [TA], a.'s and arterial branches distributed within the kidney; arise as branches and derivatives of the segmental a.'s of kidney. SYN arteriae intrarenales [TA].

jejunal a.'s [TA], *origin*, superior mesenteric; *distribution*, jejunum; *anastomoses*, by a series of arches with each other and with ileal arteries. SYN arteriae jejunales [TA].

juxtacolic a., ⚹official alternate term for marginal a. of colon.

a.'s of kidney, SYN segmental a.'s of kidney.

Kugel anastomotic a., SYN atrial anastomotic *branch* of circumflex branch of left coronary artery.

a. of labyrinth, SYN labyrinthine a.

labyrinthine a. [TA], internal acoustic meatal branch; a branch of the basilar artery that enters the labyrinth through the internal acoustic meatus. SYN arteria labyrinthi [TA], arteria auditiva interna, a. of labyrinth, internal auditory a., ramus meatus acustici interni.

lacrimal a. [TA], *origin*, ophthalmic; *distribution*, lacrimal gland, lateral and superior rectus muscles, superior eyelid, forehead, and temporal fossa. SYN arteria lacrimalis [TA].

lateral basal segmental a. [TA], lateral basal branch of the following: 1) basal part of inferior lobar branch of right pulmonary a.; 2) basal part of inferior lobar branch of left pulmonary a. SYN arteria segmentalis basalis lateralis [TA], arteria segmentalis lateralis [TA], lateral basal branch, ramus basalis lateralis.

lateral circumflex femoral a. [TA], *origin*, profunda femoris; *distribution*, hip joint, thigh muscles; *anastomoses*, medial circumflex femoral, inferior gluteal, superior gluteal. SYN arteria circumflexa femoris lateralis [TA], lateral circumflex a. of thigh, lateral femoral circumflex a.

lateral circumflex a. of thigh, SYN lateral circumflex femoral a.

lateral femoral circumflex a., SYN lateral circumflex femoral a.

lateral frontobasal a. [TA], a branch of the insular part of the middle cerebral a. distributed to the cortex of the lateral, inferior part of the frontal lobe. SYN arteria frontobasalis lateralis [TA], arteria orbitofrontalis lateralis⚹, lateral orbitofrontal a.⚹.

lateral inferior genicular a., SYN inferior lateral genicular a.

lateral malleolar a.'s, SYN lateral malleolar *branch* (of fibular peroneal artery).

(lateral and medial) palpebral a.'s [TA], branches of the ophthalmic supplying the upper and lower eyelids, consisting of two sets, lateral and medial. SYN arteriae palpebrales (laterales et mediales) [TA].

(lateral and medial) parietal a.'s [TA], branches of the terminal part of the middle cerebral a., divided into two branches: anterior parietal a. and posterior parietal a. SYN arteriae parietales (laterales et mediales) [TA].

lateral nasal a., SYN lateral nasal *branch* of facial artery.

lateral occipital a. [TA], one of the terminal branches of the posterior cerebral artery; it supplies medial and ventral portions of the temporal lobe via anterior, intermediate, medial, and posterior temporal branches; can be called the P3 segment of the posterior cerebral artery. SYN arteria occipitalis lateralis [TA], P3 segment of posterior cerebral artery [TA], segmentum P3 arteriae cerebri posterioris [TA].

lateral orbitofrontal a., ⚹official alternate term for lateral frontobasal a.

lateral plantar a. [TA], larger of the two terminal branches of the posterior tibial a.; *distribution*, forms the plantar arch and through it supplies the sole of the foot and plantar surfaces of the toes; *anastomoses*, medial plantar, dorsalis pedis. SYN arteria plantaris lateralis [TA].

lateral sacral a.'s [TA], usually one of two a.'s that arise from the internal iliac a. or its branches; they supply muscles and skin in the neighborhood and send branches into the sacral canal, supplying radicular and spinal a.'s, and continuing on to the skin and subcutaneous tissues overlying the sacrum. SYN arteriae sacrales laterales.

lateral segmental a. [TA], SEE left pulmonary a., right pulmonary a.

lateral splanchnic a.'s, a.'s that arise in the embryo from the dorsal aorta to supply the mesonephros, testis or ovary, and adrenal gland.

lateral striate a.'s, SYN anterolateral central a.'s.

lateral superior genicular a., SYN superior lateral genicular a.

lateral tarsal a. [TA], *origin*, dorsalis pedis a.; *distribution*, tarsal joints and extensor digitorum brevis muscle; *anastomoses*, arcuate, peroneal, lateral plantar, anterior lateral malleolar. SYN arteria tarsea lateralis [TA].

lateral thoracic a. [TA], *origin*, third part of axillary; *distribution*, passes around lateral border of pectoral muscles, supplying them and other muscles of chest and mammary gland. SYN arteria thoracica lateralis [TA], external mammary a., long thoracic a.

left anterior descending a., SYN anterior interventricular *branch* of left coronary artery.

left colic a. [TA], *origin*, inferior mesenteric; *distribution*, descending colon and splenic flexure; *anastomoses*, middle colic, sigmoid. SYN arteria colica sinistra [TA].

left coronary a. [TA], *origin*, left aortic sinus; *distribution*, it divides into two major branches, an anterior interventricular which descends in the anterior interventricular sulcus, and a circumflex branch which passes to the diaphragmatic surface of the left ventricle; gives atrial, ventricular, and atrioventricular branches. SYN arteria coronaria sinistra [TA].

left gastric a. [TA], *origin*, celiac; *distribution*, cardia of stomach at lesser curvature, abdominal part of the esophagus, and, frequently, a portion of the left lobe of the liver via an aberrant left hepatic branch; *anastomoses*, esophageal, right gastric. SYN arteria gastrica sinistra [TA], coronary a. (2).

left gastroepiploic a., SYN left gastroomental a.

left gastroomental a. [TA], *origin*, splenic; *distribution*, greater curvature of stomach and greater omentum; *anastomoses*, right gastroepiploic and short gastric a.'s. SYN arteria gastroomentalis sinistra [TA], arteria gastroepiploica sinistra, left gastroepiploic a.

left hepatic a., SYN left *branch* of hepatic artery proper.

left marginal a. [TA], a large ventricular branch of the circumflex branch of the left coronary a. that courses along the center of the left pulmonary surface (obtuse margin) of the heart, usually to the apex. SYN ramus marginalis sinister arteriae coronariae sinistrae [TA].

left pulmonary a. [TA], the shorter of the two terminal branches of the pulmonary trunk; it pierces the pericardium to enter the hilum of the left lung. Branches ramify and are distributed with the segmental and subsegmental bronchi; frequent variations occur. *Typical branches:* of the superior lobar a.'s [TA] (*arteriae lobares superiores*, under *arteria* [TA]) are the apical segmental a. [TA] (*arteria* segmentalis apicalis [TA]), anterior segmental a. [TA] (*arteria* segmentalis anterior [TA]), and posterior segmental a. [TA] (*arteria* segmentalis posterior [TA]), with the latter two having ascending and descending branches [TA] (rami ascendens et descendens [TA]); of the lingular a. [TA] (*arteria* lingularis [TA]) are the superior lingular a. [TA] (*arteria* lingularis superior [TA]) and inferior lingular a. [TA] (*arteria* lingularis inferior [TA]); and of the inferior lobar a.'s [TA] (*arteriae* lobares inferiores, under *arteria* [TA]) are the superior segmental a. [TA] (*arteria* segmentalis superior [TA]) and a basal part [TA] (pars basalis [TA]) giving rise to anterior, posterior, lateral, and medial basal segmental arteries [TA] (arteriae segmentales basales anterior, posterior, lateralis et medialis [TA]). SYN arteria pulmonalis sinistra [TA].

lenticulostriate a.'s, (1) ⚹official alternate term for anterolateral central a.'s; **(2)** any one of a variety of small a.'s entering the base of the brain through the anterior perforated substance and supplying the striatum, globus pallidus, and internal capsule; most of these perforating a.'s are branches of the M_1 segment (clinical terminology) of the middle cerebral and (rarely) of the anterior choroidal a. SYN Charcot a.

lesser palatine a. [TA], one of several posterior branches of the descending palatine in the greater palatine canal, distributed to the soft palate and tonsil. SYN arteria palatina minor [TA].

lienal a., SYN splenic a.

lingual a. [TA], *origin*, external carotid; *distribution*, runs along under surface of tongue, terminates as deep lingual a.; *branches*, suprahyoid and dorsal lingual branches and sublingual artery. SYN arteria lingualis [TA].

lingular a. [TA], SEE left pulmonary a.

long central a., SYN medial striate a.

long posterior ciliary a.'s [TA], one of two branches of the ophthalmic running forward between the sclerotic and choroid coats to the iris, at the outer and inner margins of which they form by anastomosis two circles. SYN arteriae ciliares posteriores longae.

long thoracic a., SYN lateral thoracic a.

a.'s of lower limb [TA], a.'s that supply the lower limb, all of which are derivatives of the external iliac. SYN arteriae membri inferioris [TA].

lowest lumbar a.'s [TA], *origin*, middle sacral; *distribution*, sacrum and iliac muscle; *anastomosis*, deep circumflex iliac artery. SYN arteriae lumbales imae [TA].

lowest thyroid a., SYN thyroid ima a.

lumbar a.'s [TA], *origin*, abdominal aorta; one of four or five pairs; *distribution*, lumbar vertebrae, muscles of back, abdominal wall; *anastomoses*, intercostal, subcostal, superior and inferior epigastric, deep circumflex iliac, and iliolumbar. SYN arteriae lumbales [TA].

macular a.'s, SEE inferior macular *arteriole*, superior macular *arteriole*.

mammillary a.'s [TA], *origin*: posterior communicating artery; *distribution*: to mammillary bodies of hypothalamus. SYN arteriae mammillares [TA].

marginal a. of colon [TA], a. formed by anastomoses between the right and left colic a.'s; it passes downward from the left colic flexure to the aboral end of the pelvic colon. SYN arteria marginalis coli [TA], arcus marginalis coli⋆, arteria juxtacolica⋆, juxtacolic a.⋆, marginal arcade⋆, a. of Drummond, Riolan arc (2).

masseteric a. [TA], *origin*, second (infratemporal) part of maxillary; *distribution*, masseter muscle via mandibular notch, temporomandibular joint; *anastomoses*, branches of transverse facial and masseteric branches of facial. SYN arteria masseterica [TA].

mastoid a., SYN mastoid *branch* of occipital artery.

maxillary a. [TA], *origin*, external carotid; *branches*, first (retromandibular) part: deep auricular, anterior tympanic; second (infratemporal part: middle meningeal, inferior alveolar, masseteric, deep temporal, buccal; third (pterygopalatine) part: posterior superior alveolar, infraorbital, descending palatine, artery of pterygoid canal, sphenopalatine. SYN arteria maxillaris [TA], internal maxillary a.

medial basal segmental a. [TA], arises from the basal part of inferior lobar a.'s of the left and right lungs. SYN arteria segmentalis basalis medialis [TA], arteria segmentalis medialis [TA], medial basal branch of pulmonary artery, ramus basalis medialis.

medial circumflex femoral a. [TA], *origin*, profunda femoris; *distribution*, hip joint, muscles of thigh; *anastomoses*, inferior gluteal, superior gluteal, lateral circumflex femoral. SYN arteria circumflexa femoris medialis [TA], medial circumflex a. of thigh, medial femoral circumflex a.

medial circumflex a. of thigh, SYN medial circumflex femoral a.

medial collateral a. [TA], SYN middle collateral a.

medial commisural a. [TA], *origin*: anterior communicating a.; *distribution*: to supraoptic commissure, optic chiasm.

medial femoral circumflex a., SYN medial circumflex femoral a.

medial frontobasal a. [TA], the first branch of the postcommunicating part (A2 segment) of the anterior cerebral a. (pericallosal a.); it supplies the medial half of the inferior surface of the frontal cortex. SYN arteria frontobasalis medialis [TA], arteria orbitofrontalis medialis⋆, medial orbitofrontal a.⋆, orbital a.

medial inferior genicular a., SYN inferior medial genicular a.

medial malleolar a.'s, SYN medial malleolar *branches* (of posterior tibial artery), under *branch*.

medial occipital a. [TA], one of the terminal branches of the posterior cerebral a.; it is distributed to the corpus callosum, medial aspects of the caudal aspect of the parietal lobe, and medial occipital lobe including the visual cortex by named branches that include the dorsal branch to the corpus callosum, parietal branch, parietooccipital branch, occipitotemporal branch, and calcarine branch; can be called the P4 segment of the posterior cerebral artery. SYN arteria occipitalis medialis [TA], P4 segment of posterior cerebral artery⋆, segmentum P1 arteriae cerebri posterioris⋆, segmentum P4 arteriae cerebri posterioris⋆.

medial orbitofrontal a., ⋆official alternate term for medial frontobasal a.

medial plantar a. [TA], one of the terminal branches of the posterior tibial; *distribution*, medial side of the sole of the foot; *anastomoses*, dorsalis pedis, lateral plantar. SYN arteria plantaris medialis [TA].

medial segmental a. [TA], SEE left pulmonary a., right pulmonary a.

medial striate a., arises at or just distal to the anterior communicating a. [TA]; *distribution*: anterior caudate and putamen and anterior limb of internal capsule. SEE distal medial striate a., proximal medial striate a.'s. SYN arteria striata medialis distalis [TA], distal medial striate a. [TA], arteria recurrens, a. of Heubner, Heubner a., long central a., recurrent a. of Heubner, recurrent a. (2).

medial superior genicular a., SYN superior medial genicular a.

medial tarsal a.'s [TA], two small branches of the dorsalis pedis a.; *distribution*, to inner margin of foot. SYN arteria tarsea medialis [TA].

median a. [TA], *origin*, anterior interosseous; *distribution*, accompanies median nerve to palm; *anastomoses*, branches of superficial palmar arch. SYN arteria comitans nervi mediani [TA], arteria mediana, comitant a. of median nerve.

median callosal a. [TA], *origin*: anterior communicating a.; *distribution*: terminal lamina and rostrum of corpus callosum. SYN arteria callosa mediana [TA].

median commissural a. [TA], *origin*: anterior communicating a.; *distribution*: to supraoptic commissure and optic chiasm. SYN arteria commissuralis mediana [TA].

median sacral a. [TA], *origin*, posterior aspect of abdominal aorta just above the bifurcation; *distribution*, lower lumbar vertebrae, sacrum, and coccyx; *anastomoses*, lateral sacral, superior and middle rectal. SYN arteria sacralis mediana [TA], middle sacral a.

mediastinal a.'s, SYN mediastinal *branches*, under *branch*.

medium a., SYN muscular a.

medullary a.'s of brain, branches of the cortical a.'s which penetrate to and supply the white matter of the cerebrum.

medullary spinal a.'s, SYN segmental medullary a.'s.

mental a., SYN mental *branch* (of inferior alveolar artery).

metatarsal a. [TA], one of four dorsal or four plantar a.'s coursing in relation to the metatarsal bones, each dividing distally into a medial and a lateral digital a., serving the dorsal or plantar aspects of adjacent sides of two toes. SEE dorsal metatarsal a., plantar metatarsal a. SYN arteria metatarsalis [TA].

middle cerebral a. [TA], one of the two large terminal branches (with anterior cerebral a.) of the internal carotid artery; it passes laterally around the pole of the temporal lobe, then posteriorly in the depth of the lateral cerebral fissure; for descriptive purposes it is divided into three parts: 1) the sphenoidal part (M_1 segment of clinical terminology), supplying perforating branches to the internal capsule, thalamus, and striate body; 2) the insular part, supplying branches to the insula and adjacent cortical areas; and 3) the terminal part or cortical part, supplying a large part of the central cortical convexity (the latter two collectively forming M_2 segment). SYN arteria cerebri media [TA].

middle colic a. [TA], *origin*, superior mesenteric; *distribution*, transverse colon; *anastomoses*, right and left colic. SYN arteria colica media [TA].

middle collateral a., the posterior terminal branch of the profunda brachii, anastomosing with the arteries which form the articular network of the elbow. SYN arteria collateralis media [TA], medial collateral a. [TA].

middle genicular a. [TA], *origin*, popliteal; *distribution*, synovial membrane and cruciate ligaments of knee joint. SYN arteria media genus [TA], arteria articularis azygos, arteria genus media.

middle hemorrhoidal a., SYN middle rectal a.

middle lobar a. [TA], SEE left pulmonary a., right pulmonary a.

middle lobar a. of right lung [TA], SEE right pulmonary a.

middle meningeal a. [TA], *origin*, maxillary; *branches*, petrosal, superior tympanic, frontal and parietal; *distribution*, to parts mentioned and through terminal branches to anterior and middle cranial fossae; *anastomoses*, meningeal branches of occipital, ascending pharyngeal, ophthalmic and lacrimal, stylomastoid, accessory meningeal branch of maxillary, and deep temporal. SYN arteria meningea media [TA].

middle rectal a. [TA], *origin*, internal iliac; *distribution*, middle portion of rectum; *anastomoses*, inferior rectal and superior rectal. Because the latter is a tributary of the portal system, this is a portosystemic or portocaval anastomosis. SYN arteria rectalis media [TA], middle hemorrhoidal a.

middle sacral a., SYN median sacral a.

middle suprarenal a. [TA], *origin*, aorta; *distribution*, suprarenal gland. SYN arteria suprarenalis media [TA].

middle temporal a. [TA], *origin*, superficial temporal; *distribution*, temporal fascia and muscle; *anastomoses*, branches of maxillary. SEE ALSO middle temporal *branch* of insular part of middle cerebral artery, posterior temporal *branch* of middle cerebral artery. SYN arteria temporalis media [TA].

muscular a., an a. with a tunica media composed principally of circularly arranged smooth muscle. SYN distributing a., medium a.

muscular a.'s (of ophthalmic artery) [TA], direct or indirect branches of the ophthalmic a. supplying the extraocular muscles. SYN arteriae musculares (arteriae ophthalmicae) [TA].

musculophrenic a. [TA], *origin*, the lateral terminal branch of internal thoracic; *distribution*, diaphragm and intercostal muscles; *anastomoses*, branches of pericardiacophrenic, inferior phrenic, and posterior intercostal arteries. SYN arteria musculophrenica [TA].

mylohyoid a., SYN mylohyoid *branch* (of inferior alveolar artery).

myometrial arcuate a.'s, branches of the uterine and ovarian a.'s.

myometrial radial a.'s, continuations of the myometrial arcuate a.'s.

Neubauer a., SYN thyroid ima a.

nutrient a. [TA], an artery of variable origin that supplies the medullary cavity of a long bone. SYN arteria nutricia [TA], nutrient vessel.

nutrient a. of femur, SYN femoral nutrient a. SYN arteria nutriciae femoris [TA], arteria nutriens femoris★.

nutrient a. of fibula, SYN fibular nutrient a.

nutrient a.'s of humerus, SYN humeral nutrient a.'s. SYN arteria nutriens humeri★.

nutrient a. of radius [TA], *origin*: radial a.; *distribution*: medullary cavity of radius. SYN arteria radii nutricia [TA], arteria nutriens radii★.

nutrient a. of the tibia, SYN tibial nutrient a.

nutrient a. of ulna [TA], *origin*: ulnar a.; *distribution*: medullary cavity of ulna. SYN arteria nutricia ulnae [TA], arteria nutriens ulnae★.

obturator a. [TA], *anastomoses*, iliolumbar, inferior epigastric, medial circumflex femoral; *origin*, anterior division of the internal iliac; *distribution*, ilium, pubis, obturator and adductor muscles; *branches*, pubic, acetabular, anterior, and posterior. SYN arteria obturatoria [TA].

occipital a. [TA], *origin*, external carotid; *branches*, sternocleidomastoid, meningeal, auricular, occipital, mastoid, and descending. SYN arteria occipitalis [TA].

omphalomesenteric a., obsolete term for vitelline a.

ophthalmic a. [TA], *origin*, internal carotid; *branches*, ciliary, central artery of retina, anterior meningeal, lacrimal, conjunctival, episcleral, supraorbital, ethmoidal, palpebral, dorsal nasal, and supratrochlear. SYN arteria ophthalmica [TA].

orbital a., SYN medial frontobasal a.

orbitofrontal a., SEE lateral frontobasal a., medial frontobasal a.

ovarian a. [TA], *origin*, aorta; *distribution*, ureter, ovary, ovarian ligament and uterine tube; *anastomoses*, uterine. SYN arteria ovarica [TA].

palmar interosseous a., SYN palmar metacarpal a.

palmar metacarpal a. [TA], one of the three arteries springing from the deep palmar arch and running in the three medial interosseous metacarpal spaces; they anastomose with the common palmar and, via perforating branches, with the dorsal metacarpal arteries. SYN arteria metacarpalis palmaris [TA], palmar interosseous a.

paracentral a., SYN paracentral *branches* (of pericallosal artery), under *branch*.

paramedian a.'s, ★official alternate term for posteromedial central a.'s.

parent a., the a. directly giving origin to a given a.; the a. of which a given a. is a branch.

parietooccipital a., SYN parieto-occipital *branches* (of anterior cerebral artery), under *branch*.

a.'s of penis, SEE dorsal a. of penis, deep a. of penis.

perforating a.'s of hand, SYN perforating *branches* of deep palmar arch.

perforating a.'s (of deep femoral artery) [TA], *origin*, a. profunda femoris; *distribution*, as three or four vessels that pass through the aponeurosis of the adductor magnus to the posterior and anterior compartments of the thigh. SYN arteriae perforantes arteriae profundae femoris [TA].

perforating a.'s (of foot), SYN perforating *branches* (of plantar metatarsal arteries), under *branch*.

perforating a.'s (of internal thoracic artery), SYN perforating *branches* of internal thoracic artery, under *branch*.

perforating a.'s of penis [TA], branches of the dorsal a. of the penis that perforate the tunica albuginea along the dorsum of the penis, especially near the glans, to supply the glans and to supplement the deep a. of the penis in supplying the cavernous spaces of the corpora cavernosa. SYN arteriae perforantes penis [TA].

perforating radiate a.'s (of kidney) [TA], continuations of the cortical radiate a.'s that perforate the capsule of the kidney and contribute to the capsular vascular plexus. SEE ALSO cortical radiate a.'s. SYN arteriae perforantes radiatae (renis) [TA].

pericallosal a. [TA], the continuation of the anterior cerebral artery after the anterior communicating artery; it supplies branches to the cerebral cortex as it passes along the corpus callosum. SYN arteria pericallosa [TA].

pericardiacophrenic a. [TA], *origin*, internal thoracic; *distribution*, pericardium, diaphragm, and pleura; *anastomoses*, musculophrenic, inferior phrenic, mediastinal and pericardial branches of the internal thoracic. SYN arteria pericardiacophrenica [TA], arteria comes nervi phrenici.

perineal a. [TA], *origin*, internal pudendal; *distribution*, superficial structures of the perineum; *anastomoses*, external pudendal arteries. SYN arteria perinealis [TA].

peroneal a., ★official alternate term for fibular a.

pipestem a.'s, a.'s hardened by calcification as seen in Mönckeberg arteriosclerosis; descriptive of the characteristic feeling to the finger of an examiner.

plantar metatarsal a. [TA], one of four branches of the plantar arterial arch that divide into plantar digital arteries to supply the toes. SYN arteria metatarsalis plantaris [TA].

polar frontal a. [TA], *origin*: as second major branch of postcommunicating part (A2 segment) of anterior cerebral a. (pericallosal a.); *distribution*: medial aspect of frontal lobe, approaching frontal pole, of cerebrum. SYN arteria polaris frontalis [TA], frontopolar a. [TA].

polar temporal a. [TA], *origin*: anterior temporal branch of middle cerebral a.; *distribution*: superomedial aspect of temporal lobe, extending to the temporal pole, of cerebrum. SYN arteria polaris temporalis [TA].

pontine a.'s, a.'s of pons [TA], branches of the basilar a. that serve the pons; divided into medial branches [TA] (rami mediales [TA]) or paramedian pontine branches [TAalt] and lateral branches [TA] (rami laterales [TA] or circumferential pontine branches [TAalt]); the circumferential pontine arteries are sometimes designated as short circumferential and long circumferential branches. SYN arteriae pontis [TA], rami ad pontem.

popliteal a. [TA], continuation of femoral a. in the popliteal space, bifurcating (at the lower border of the popliteus muscle as it passes deep to the arcus tendineus of the soleus muscle) into the anterior and posterior tibial a.'s; *branches*, lateral and medial superior genicular, middle genicular, lateral and medial inferior genicular, and sural arteries. SYN arteria poplitea [TA].

postcentral a., SYN a. of postcentral sulcus.

postcentral sulcal a., SYN a. of postcentral sulcus.

a. of postcentral sulcus [TA], a branch of the terminal part of the middle cerebral a. distributing to the cortex on either side of the postcentral sulcus. SYN arteria sulci postcentralis [TA], postcentral a., postcentral sulcal a.

posterior alveolar a., SYN posterior superior alveolar a.

posterior auricular a. [TA], *origin*: posterior aspect of external carotid just above the digastric muscle; *course*: ascends first between parotid gland and styloid process then between cartilage of auricle and the mastoid process; *branches*: muscular (digastric, stylohyoid and sternocleidomastoid), glandular (parotid), stylomastoid a., occipital and auricular; *anastomoses*: anterior tympanic a. (via the stylomastoid a.) and occipital a. SYN arteria auricularis posterior [TA].

posterior basal segmental a. of left / right lung, SYN posterior basal branch, ramus basalis posterior.

posterior cecal a. [TA], *origin*, ileocolic artery; *distribution*, posterior region of cecum. SYN arteria cecalis posterior [TA].

posterior cerebral a. [TA], formed by the bifurcation of the basilar a.; it passes around the cerebral peduncle to reach the medial aspect of the hemisphere; for descriptive purposes it is divided into three parts: 1) precommunicating part (P_1 segment of clinical terminology), which gives rise to posteromedial central a.'s [TA], short circumferential a.'s [TA], the thalamoperforating a. [TA], and the collicular a. [TA]; 2) the postcommunicating part (P_2), which gives rise to posterolateral central a.'s [TA], posterior medial choroidal branches [TA], posterior lateral choroidal branches [TA], peduncular branches [TA] the thalamogeniculate a. [TA]; and 3) the terminal or cortical part consisting of the lateral occipital a. [TA] (P_3) whose branches serve the medial aspect of the temporal lobe and the medial occipital a. [TA] (P_4), whose branches serve the medial surface of the occipital lobe; the latter includes calcarine and parietooccipital a.'s. SYN arteria cerebri posterior [TA].

posterior choroidal a., usually seen as two branches of the P_2 segment of the posterior cerebral artery [TA] that supply the choroid plexus of the third ventricle (posterior medial choroidal artery [TA]) and parts of the choroid plexus of the lateral ventricle (posterior lateral choroidal artery [TA]). SYN arteria choroidea posterior.

posterior circumflex humeral a. [TA], *origin*, axillary; *distribution*, muscles and structures of shoulder joint; *anastomoses*, anterior circumflex humeral, suprascapular, thoracoacromial, and profunda brachii. SYN arteria circumflexa humeri posterior [TA], posterior humeral circumflex a.

posterior communicating a. [TA], *origin*, internal carotid; *distribution*, optic tract, crus cerebri, interpeduncular region, and hippocampal gyrus; *anastomoses*, with posterior cerebral to form the cerebral arterial circle (circle of Willis). SYN arteria communicans posterior [TA].

posterior conjunctival a. [TA], one of a series of branches from the arterial arches of the upper and lower eyelids that supplies the conjunctiva. SYN arteria conjunctivalis posterior [TA], conjunctival a.'s.

posterior dental a., SYN posterior superior alveolar a.

posterior descending coronary a., SYN posterior interventricular branch of right coronary a.

posterior ethmoidal a. [TA], *origin*, ophthalmic; *distribution*, posterior ethmoidal cells and upper posterior part of lateral wall of nasal cavity. SYN arteria ethmoidalis posterior [TA].

posterior gastric a. [TA], *origin*: splenic a.; *distribution*: ascends retroperitoneally in posterior wall of omental bursa toward gastric fundus to reach (and supply) the gastric wall via the gastrophrenic fold. Omitted from many accounts of the blood supply of the stomach, its unexpected presence may complicate surgery involving the cardia of the stomach. SYN arteria gastrica posterior [TA].

posterior humeral circumflex a., SYN posterior circumflex humeral a.

posterior inferior cerebellar a. [TA], *origin*, intracranial part of vertebral; *distribution*, lateral medulla, choroid plexus of fourth ventricle, and cerebellum; *anastomoses*, superior cerebellar and anterior inferior cerebellar; gives rise to posterior spinal artery [TA], cerebellar tonsillar branch [TA], and choroidal branch to fourth ventricle [TA]. SYN arteria inferior posterior cerebelli [TA].

posterior intercostal a.'s 1–2, SYN first and second posterior intercostal a.'s.

posterior intercostal a.'s 3–11 [TA], one of nine pairs of a.'s arising from the thoracic aorta and distributed to the nine lower intercostal spaces, vertebral column, spinal cord, and muscles and integument of the back; they anastomose with branches of the musculophrenic, internal thoracic, superior epigastric, subcostal and lumbar. SYN arteriae intercostales posteriores III-XI [TA].

posterior interosseous a. [TA], *origin*, common interosseous artery; *distribution*, posterior compartment of forearm. SYN arteria interossea posterior [TA], dorsal interosseous a.

posterior interventricular a., SYN posterior interventricular branch of right coronary a.

posterior interventricular branch of right coronary a. [TA], continuation of right coronary a. in posterior interventricular sulcus; descends to apex to anastomose with anterior interventricular a.; supplies most of diaphragmatic aspect of ventricles and posterior third of interventricular septum. SYN ramus interventricularis posterior arteriae coronariae dextrae [TA], posterior descending coronary a., posterior interventricular a.

posterior labial a.'s, SYN posterior labial branches of internal perineal *artery*.

posterior lateral nasal a.'s [TA], branches of the sphenopalatine artery that supply the posterior parts of the conchae and lateral nasal wall. SYN arteriae nasales posteriores laterales [TA].

posterior mediastinal a.'s, SYN mediastinal *branches* of thoracic aorta, under *branch*.

posterior meningeal a. [TA], *origin*, ascending pharyngeal; *distribution*, dura mater of posterior cranial fossa; *anastomoses*, branches of middle meningeal and vertebral. SYN arteria meningea posterior [TA].

posterior pancreaticoduodenal a., SYN retroduodenal a.

posterior parietal a. [TA], the branch of the M2 segment of the middle cerebral a. distributed to the posterior part of the parietal lobe. SYN arteria parietalis posterior [TA].

posterior peroneal a.'s, SYN lateral malleolar *branch* (of fibular peroneal artery).

posterior segmental a. [TA], SEE left pulmonary a., right pulmonary a., segmental a.'s of kidney.

posterior segmental a. (of kidney) [TA], *origin*, continuation of the posterior branch of renal. SEE ALSO segmental a.'s of kidney. SYN a. of posterior segment of kidney.

a. of posterior segment of kidney, SYN posterior segmental a. (of kidney).

posterior septal a. of nose, SYN posterior septal *branch* of nose.

posterior spinal a. [TA], *origin*, intracranial part of vertebral; *distribution*, medulla, spinal cord, and pia mater; *anastomoses*, spinal branches of intercostal arteries. SYN arteria spinalis posterior [TA].

posterior superior alveolar a. [TA], *origin*, third part of maxillary a. within pterygopalatine fossa; *distribution*, molar and premolar teeth, gingiva, and mucous membrane of maxillary sinus. SYN arteria alveolaris superior posterior [TA], posterior alveolar a., posterior dental a.

posterior temporal a., SYN posterior temporal *branch* of middle cerebral artery.

posterior tibial a. [TA], the larger and more directly continuous of the two terminal branches of the popliteal; *branches*, fibular (peroneal), nutrient of fibula, lateral and medial posterior malleolar, tibial nutrient a., medial and lateral plantar. SYN arteria tibialis posterior [TA].

posterior tibial recurrent a. [TA], an inconstant branch of the posterior tibial artery (or occasionally of the anterior tibial a.), which ascends anterior to the popliteus muscle, anastomoses with branches of the popliteal artery, and sends a twig to the tibiofibular joint. SYN arteria recurrens tibialis posterior [TA].

posterior tympanic a. [TA], *origin,* stylomastoid; *distribution,* middle ear; *anastomoses,* other tympanic arteries. SYN arteria tympanica posterior [TA].

posterolateral central a.'s [TA], the circumflex mesencephalic branches, several small branches of the postcommunical part (P2 segment) of the posterior cerebral artery distributed to the lateral posterior part of the midbrain. SYN arteriae centrales posterolaterales [TA].

posteromedial central a.'s [TA], the interpeduncular perforating branches, several small branches from the precommunical part (P1 segment) of the posterior cerebral a. and the posterior communicating a. supplying the posterior medial part of the midbrain. SYN arteriae centrales posteromediales [TA], paramedian a.'s✗.

precentral a., SYN a. of precentral sulcus.

precentral sulcal a., SYN a. of precentral sulcus.

a. of precentral sulcus [TA], a branch of the terminal part of the middle cerebral a. distributed to the cortex on either side of the precentral sulcus. SYN arteria sulci precentralis [TA], pre-Rolandic a., precentral a., precentral sulcal a.

precuneal a., SYN precuneal *branches* (of anterior cerebral artery), under *branch.*

prepancreatic a. [TA], *origin:* arises from dorsal pancreatic a. as its left terminal branch; *distribution:* often double, it runs between the neck and uncinate process of the pancreas to form an arterial arch (arcade) with the anterior superior pancreaticodoudenal a. SYN arteria prepancreatica [TA].

pre-Rolandic a., SYN a. of precentral sulcus.

princeps cervicis a., SYN descending *branch* of occipital artery.

princeps pol'licis a. [TA], *origin,* radial (deep palmar (arterial) arch); *distribution,* palmar surface and sides of thumb; *anastomoses,* a.'s on dorsum of thumb. SYN arteria princeps pollicis [TA], chief a. of thumb, princeps pollicis, principal a. of thumb.

principal a. of thumb, SYN princeps pollicis a.

profunda brachii a. [TA], *origin,* brachial; *distribution,* humerus and muscles and integument of arm; *anastomoses,* posterior circumflex humeral, radial recurrent, recurrent interosseous, ulnar collateral, i.e., articular vascular *network* of elbow. SYN arteria profunda brachii [TA], ramus deltoideus arteriae profundae brachii [TA], deep a. of arm✗, deep brachial a.

profunda fem'oris a., SYN deep a. of thigh.

proper cochlear a. [TA], *origin:* common cochlear a. in modiolus; *distribution:* to cochlear duct. SYN arteria cochlearis propria [TA].

proper palmar digital a.'s [TA], terminal branches of the common palmar digital a. that pass to the side of each finger. SYN arteriae digitales palmares propriae [TA], arteria digitalis palmaris propria, collateral digital a., digital collateral a.

proper plantar digital a. [TA], one of the digital branches of the plantar metatarsal a.'s. SYN arteria digitalis plantaris propria [TA], arteriae digitales plantares propriae.

proximal medial striate a.'s [TA], *origin:* precommunicating part (A1 segment) of anterior cerebral artery; *distribution:* inferior surface of frontal lobe of cerebrum, extending into thalamus and corpus striatum. SYN arteria centralis brevis, short central a.

a. of pterygoid canal, *origin:* usually arises from the third part of the maxillary artery, but frequently from the greater palatine artery, within the pterygopalatine fossa. Passes posteriorly to run through the pterygoid canal with the corresponding nerve, supplying the contents and wall of the canal, the mucous membrane of the upper pharynx, the auditory tube, and the tympanic cavity. SYN arteria canalis pterygoidei [TA], vidian a.

pterygomeningeal a. [TA], *origin:* maxillary or middle meningeal a.; *distribution:* traverses foramen ovale to enter cranial cavity, where it supplies the trigeminal ganglion, dura mater, and bone of the floor of the middle cranial fossa; however, its main distribution is extracranially to the pterygoid and tensor tympani muscles, the sphenoid bone, and the mandibular nerves and its otic gan-

gion. SYN arteria pterygomeningealis [TA], accessory meningeal a., accessory meningeal branch, ramus meningeus accessorius.

pubic a.'s, SEE pubic *branch* of inferior epigastric vein, pubic *branch* of obturator artery.

pulmonary a., SYN pulmonary *trunk*; SEE ALSO right pulmonary a., left pulmonary a.

a. of pulp, the first section of a penicillus of the spleen.

pyloric a., SYN right gastric a.

quadrigeminal a., ✗official alternate term for collicular a.

radial a. [TA], *origin,* brachial; *branches,* radial recurrent, dorsa and palmar carpal and metacarpal, dorsal digital, princeps pollicis, radialis indicis, palmar and muscular, and perforating; usually terminates as deep palmar arch. SYN arteria radialis [TA].

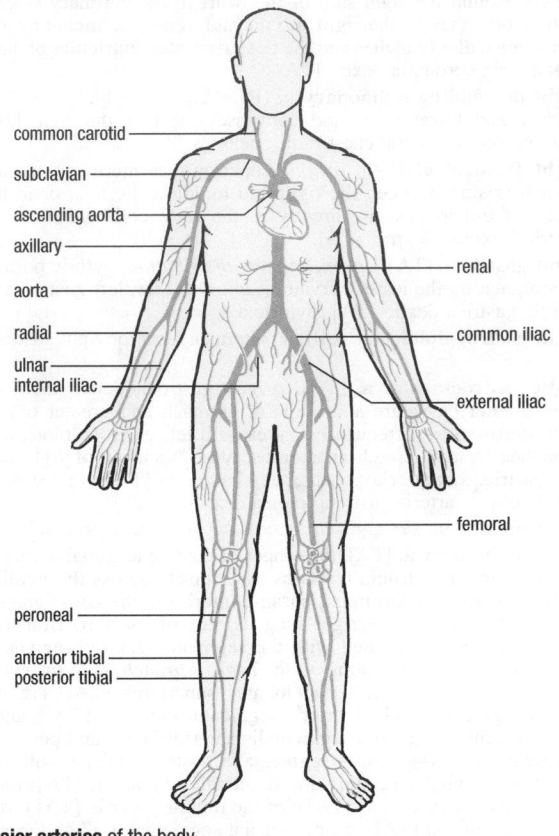

common carotid
subclavian
ascending aorta
axillary
aorta
radial
ulnar
internal iliac
renal
common iliac
external iliac
femoral
peroneal
anterior tibial
posterior tibial

major arteries of the body

radial collateral a. [TA], the anterior terminal branch of the profunda brachii, anastomosing with the radial recurrent a., forming part of the articular vascular plexus of the elbow. SYN arteria collateralis radialis [TA].

radial index a., SYN radialis indicis a.

radialis indicis a. [TA], *origin,* radial; *distribution,* radial side of index finger. SYN arteria radialis indicis [TA], arteria volaris indicis radialis, radial index a.

radial recurrent a. [TA], *origin,* radial; *distribution,* ascends around lateral side of elbow joint; *anastomoses,* radial collateral, interosseous recurrent. SYN arteria recurrens radialis [TA], recurrent radial a.

ranine a., SYN deep lingual a.

recurrent a., (1) an a. which, upon or soon after originating, reflects or turns sharply to course in the general opposite direction to that of its parent a.; (2) SYN medial striate a.

recurrent a. of Heubner, SYN medial striate a.

recurrent interosseous a. [TA], *origin,* posterior interosseous; *distribution,* elbow joint; *anastomoses,* branches of profunda brachii and inferior ulnar collateral, i.e., articular vascular *network* of elbow. SYN arteria interossea recurrens [TA].

recurrent radial a., SYN radial recurrent a.

recurrent ulnar a., SYN ulnar recurrent a.

renal a. [TA], *origin*, aorta; *branches*, segmental, ureteral, and inferior suprarenal; *distribution*, kidney. SYN arteria renalis [TA].

retroduodenal a. [TA], *origin*, one of several small branches from the gastroduodenal artery posterior to the duodenum; *distribution*, first part of duodenum. SYN arteria retroduodenalis [TA], posterior pancreaticoduodenal a.

right colic a. [TA], *origin*, superior mesenteric, sometimes by a common trunk with the ileocolic; *distribution*, ascending colon; *anastomoses*, middle colic, ileocolic. SYN arteria colica dextra [TA].

right coronary a. [TA], *origin*, right aortic sinus; *distribution*, it passes around the right side of the heart in the coronary sulcus, giving branches to the right atrium and ventricle, including the atrioventricular branches and the posterior interventricular branch. SYN arteria coronaria dextra [TA].

right descending pulmonary a. (RDPA), a. supplying the right middle and lower lobes and comprises most of the right hilar shadow on the frontal chest radiograph.

right flexural a. [TA], *origin:* superior mesenteric a.; variant branch arising between the right and middle colic a.'s, or in the place of either, passing directly to the right colic flexure. SYN arteria flexurae dextrae [TA].

right gastric a. [TA], *origin*, hepatic; *distribution*, pyloric portion of stomach on the lesser curvature; *anastomoses*, left gastric. SYN arteria gastrica dextra [TA], pyloric a.

right gastroepiploic a., ⋆official alternate term for right gastroomental a.

right gastroomental a. [TA], *origin*, gastroduodenal; *distribution*, greater curvature and walls of stomach and greater omentum; *anastomoses*, frequently unites with left gastroepiploic, and branches from this arch anastomose with branches of right and left gastric. SYN arteria gastroomentalis dextra [TA], right gastroepiploic a.⋆, arteria gastroepiploica dextra.

right hepatic a., SYN right *branch* of hepatic artery proper.

right pulmonary a. [TA], the longer of the two terminal branches of the pulmonary trunk, it passes transversely across the midline in the superior mediastinum, passing inferior to the aortic arch to enter the hilum of the right lung as part of its root. Branches divide and are distributed with the segmental and subsegmental bronchi; frequent variations occur. *Typical branches:* of the superior lobar a.'s [TA] (arteriae lobares superiores [TA]) are the apical segmental a. [TA] (arteria segmentalis apicalis [TA]), anterior segmental a. (arteria segmentalis anterior [TA]) and posterior segmental a. [TA] (arteria segmentalis posterior [TA]), with the latter two having ascending and descending branches [TA] (rami ascendens et descendens [TA]); of the middle lobar a. [TA] (arteria lobaris media [TA]) are the medial segmental a. [TA] (arteria lobaris media [TA]) and lateral segmental a. [TA] (arteria segmentalis lateralis [TA]); and of the inferior lobar a.'s [TA] (arteriae lobares inferiores [TA]) are the superior segmental a. [TA] (arteria segmentalis superior [TA]) and a basal part [TA] (pars basalis [TA]) giving rise to anterior, posterior, lateral, and medial basal segmental a.'s [TA] (arteriae segmentales basales anterior, posterior, lateralis et medialis [TA]). SYN arteria pulmonalis dextra [TA].

Rolandic sulcal a., SYN a. of central sulcus.

a. of round ligament of uterus, *origin*, inferior epigastric; *distribution*, round ligament of uterus. SYN arteria ligamenti teretis uteri.

a. to sciatic nerve [TA], *origin*, inferior gluteal; *distribution*, sciatic nerve; *anastomoses*, branches of profunda femoris. SYN arteria comitans nervi ischiadici [TA], companion a. to sciatic nerve.

screw a.'s, coiled a.'s into the uterine mucosa or in the macular region of the retina.

scrotal a.'s, SEE anterior scrotal *branch* of deep external pudendal artery, posterior scrotal *branch* of internal pudendal artery, under *branch.*

segmental a.'s of kidney [TA], the branches of the renal a. that supply the anatomical segments of kidney. Usually five in num-

ber, they are end a.'s and give off interlobar, arcuate, and interlobular a.'s in sequence. The latter send afferent arterioles to the glomeruli as well as branches to the kidney capsule. The segmental a.'s of the kidney are identified as: (1) anterior inferior (arteriae segmenti anterioris inferioris renis [NA]); (2) anterior superior (arteriae segmenti anterioris superioris renis [NA]); (3) inferior (arteriae segmenti inferioris renis [NA]); (4) posterior (arteriae segmenti posterioris renis [NA]); and (5) superior (arteriae segmenti superioris renis [NA]). SYN arteriae renis [TA], a.'s of kidney.

segmental a.'s of liver [TA], anterior and posterior segmental a.'s arising from the right branch of the hepatic a., and medial and lateral segmental a.'s arising from the left branch of the hepatic a.; the segmental a.'s serve four of the five major divisions of the liver, and then branch in turn so that each hepatic segment receives an independent blood supply. SYN arteriae segmenti hepaticae.

segmental medullary a.'s [TA], a large caliber spinal or radicular a. that courses centrally along a dorsal or ventral root, perhaps supplying it and the surrounding meninges in the fashion of any spinal/radicular a., but that continues on to reach and anastomose with the anterior or posterior (longitudinal) spinal a. Only 4–9 of the spinal a.'s are medullary spinal a.'s, found mainly in the lower cervical, lower thoracic, and upper lumbar levels, the largest of which is the segmental medullary a. SEE ALSO great segmental medullary a., spinal a.'s, (anterior and posterior) radicular a.'s. SYN arteriae medullares segmentales [TA], medullary spinal a.'s.

septal a., a branch of the superior labial a. that supplies the lower part of the nasal septum.

sheathed a., a subdivision of the penicillus of the spleen surrounded by macrophages and a reticular stroma.

short central a., SYN proximal medial striate a.'s.

short circumferential a.'s [TA], short branches of the precommunicating part (P1 segment) of the posterior cerebral a. SYN arteriae circumferentiales brevis [TA].

short gastric a.'s [TA], four or five small a.'s given off from the splenic, passing via the gastrosplenic ligament to the fundus of the stomach along the greater curvature, and anastomosing with the other arteries in that region. SYN arteriae gastricae breves [TA], vasa brevia.

short posterior ciliary a. [TA], one of approximately seven branches of the ophthalmic a. that pass around the optic nerve to supply the eyeball. Dividing into some 15–20 branches, they penetrate the sclera adjacent to the optic nerve, supplying the choroid and ciliary processes. *Anastomoses*: with central retinal a. and long and anterior ciliary arteries (at the ora serrata). SYN arteria ciliaris posterior brevis [TA].

sigmoid a.'s [TA], *origin*, inferior mesenteric; *distribution*, descending colon and sigmoid flexure; *anastomoses*, left colic, superior rectal. SYN arteriae sigmoideae [TA].

sinuatrial nodal a., SYN sinuatrial (S-A) nodal *branch* of right coronary artery.

a. to the sinoatrial (S-A) node, SYN sinuatrial (S-A) nodal *branch* of right coronary artery.

sinuatrial node a., SYN sinuatrial (S-A) nodal *branch* of right coronary artery.

sinus node a., SYN sinuatrial (S-A) nodal *branch* of right coronary artery.

small a.'s, unnamed muscular a.'s, usually with fewer than six or seven layers of muscle.

somatic a.'s, a.'s that arise in the embryo from the dorsal aorta and supply the body wall; they persist almost unchanged as the posterior intercostal, subcostal, and lumbar a.'s.

sphenopalatine a. [TA], *origin*, third part of maxillary; *distribution*, posterior portion of lateral nasal wall and septum; *anastomoses*, branches of descending palatine, superior labial, and infraorbital. SYN arteria sphenopalatina [TA].

spinal a.'s, SYN rami radiculares. SYN spinal *branches*, under *branch.*

spiral a., one of the corkscrew-like a.'s in premenstrual or progestational endometrium. SYN coiled a. of the uterus.

spiral modiolar a. [TA], a. paralleling the spiral ganglion in the root of the spiral lamina of the modiolus, serving the ganglion and the cochlear ducts and its contents; the a. forms by contributions from the common cochlear a. (serving the apical two turns of the cochlea) and the cochlear branch of the vestibulocochlear a. (serving the basal turn).

splenic a. [TA], *origin*, celiac trunk; *branches*, pancreatic, left gastroepiploic, short gastric, and (proper) splenic. SEE great segmental medullary a. SYN arteria splenica [TA], arteria lienalis*, lienal a.

stapedial a., a small a. in the embryo that passes through the ring of the stapes and is later obliterated; in most humans it is a second aortic arch derivative.

sternal a.'s, SYN sternal *branches* of internal thoracic artery, under *branch*.

sternomastoid a., SEE sternocleidomastoid *branch* of superior thyroid artery, sternocleidomastoid *branches* of occipital artery, under *branch*.

straight a.'s, *official alternate term for *vasa* recta renis, under *vas*.

stylomastoid a. [TA], *origin*, posterior auricular; *distribution*, external acoustic meatus, mastoid cells, semicircular canals, stapedius muscle, and vestibule; *anastomoses*, tympanic branches of internal carotid and ascending pharyngeal, and labyrinthine a.'s. SYN arteria stylomastoidea [TA].

subclavian a. [TA], *origin*, right from brachiocephalic, left from arch of aorta; *branches*, vertebral, thyrocervical trunk, internal thoracic; costocervical trunk, descending scapular; it continues as the axillary a. after crossing the first rib. SYN arteria subclavia [TA].

subcostal a. [TA], *origin*, thoracic aorta; *distribution*, inferior to twelfth rib in a manner similar to posterior intercostal arteries. SYN arteria subcostalis [TA].

sublingual a. [TA], *origin*, lingual; *distribution*, extrinsic muscles of tongue, sublingual gland, mucosa of region; *anastomoses*, the artery of opposite side and submental. SYN arteria sublingualis [TA].

submental a. [TA], *origin*, facial; *distribution*, mylohyoid muscle, submandibular and sublingual glands, and structures of lower lip; *anastomoses*, inferior labial, mental branch of inferior dental and sublingual. SYN arteria submentalis [TA].

subscapular a. [TA], *origin*, axillary; *branches*, circumflex scapular, thoracodorsal; *distribution*, muscles of shoulder and scapular region; *anastomoses*, branches of transverse cervical, suprascapular, lateral thoracic, and intercostals. SYN arteria subscapularis [TA].

sulcal a., a small branch of the anterior spinal a. running in the anterior median fissure of the spinal cord.

superficial brachial a. [TA], an occasional variation in which the brachial artery lies superficial to the median nerve in the arm. SYN arteria brachialis superficialis [TA].

superficial cervical a. [TA], *origin*, branch of thyrocervical trunk, running with spinal accessory nerve deep to trapezius muscle. SEE ALSO superficial *branch* of the transverse cervical artery. SYN ramus superficialis arteriae transversae cervicis [TA], arteria cervicalis superficialis.

superficial circumflex iliac a. [TA], *origin*, femoral; *distribution*, inguinal lymph nodes and integument of that region; sartorius and tensor fasciae latae muscles; *anastomoses*, deep circumflex iliac. SYN arteria circumflexa iliaca superficialis [TA].

(superficial and deep) external pudendal a.'s [TA], *origin*, from the femoral as two a.'s that pass superficial and deep to the femoral vein; *distribution*, skin over pubis, skin over penis, and skin of scrotum or labium majus via anterior scrotal (labial) arteries; *anastomoses*, dorsal artery of penis or clitoris, posterior scrotal or labial arteries. SYN arteriae pudendae externae [TA].

superficial epigastric a. [TA], *origin*, femoral; *distribution*, inguinal nodes and integument of lower abdomen; *anastomoses*, inferior epigastric, superficial circumflex iliac and external pudendal. SYN arteria epigastrica superficialis [TA].

superficial palmar a., SYN superficial palmar *branch* of radial artery.

superficial temporal a. [TA], *origin*, a terminal branch of the external carotid (with maxillary a.); *branches*, transverse facial, middle temporal, orbital, parotid, anterior auricular, frontal, and parietal. SYN arteria temporalis superficialis [TA].

superficial volar a., SYN superficial palmar *branch* of radial artery.

superior cerebellar a. [TA], *origin*, basilar; *distribution*, upper surface of cerebellum, colliculi, and most of the cerebellar nuclei; *anastomoses*, posterior inferior cerebellar; gives rise to medial branches [TA] and lateral branches [TA]. SYN arteria superior cerebelli [TA].

superior epigastric a. [TA], *origin*, the medial terminal branch of internal thoracic; *distribution*, abdominal muscles and integument, falciform ligament; *anastomoses*, inferior epigastric. SYN arteria epigastrica superior [TA].

superior gluteal a. [TA], *origin*, internal iliac; *distribution*, gluteal region; *anastomoses*, lateral sacral, inferior gluteal, internal pudendal, deep circumflex iliac, lateral circumflex femoral. SYN arteria glutea superior [TA].

superior hemorrhoidal a., SYN superior rectal a.

superior hypophysial a. [TA], a small branch of the cerebral part of the internal carotid artery supplying the hypophysis. SYN arteria hypophysialis superior [TA].

superior intercostal a., SYN supreme intercostal a.

superior internal parietal a., SYN parieto-occipital *branches* (of anterior cerebral artery), under *branch*.

superior labial a., SYN superior labial *branch* of facial artery.

superior laryngeal a. [TA], *origin*, superior thyroid; *distribution*, muscles and mucous membrane of larynx; *anastomoses*, cricothyroid branch of superior thyroid and terminal branches of inferior laryngeal. SYN arteria laryngea superior [TA].

superior lateral genicular a. [TA], *origin*, popliteal; *distribution*, knee joint; *anastomoses*, lateral circumflex femoral, third perforating, anterior tibial recurrent, lateral inferior genicular, i.e., the articular vascular network of the knee. SYN arteria superior lateralis genus [TA], lateral superior genicular a.

superior lingular a. [TA], branch (of the lingular branch) of the left pulmonary artery serving the superior lingular segment of the superior lobe of the left lung. SEE left pulmonary a. SYN arteria lingularis superior [TA], ramus lingularis superior, superior lingular branch of lingular branch of superior lobar left pulmonary artery.

superior lobar a.'s [TA], SEE left pulmonary a., right pulmonary a.

superior medial genicular a. [TA], *origin*, popliteal; *distribution*, knee joint; *anastomoses*, descending genicular, lateral superior genicular, i.e., the articular vascular network of the knee. SYN arteria superior medialis genus [TA], medial superior genicular a.

superior mesenteric a. [TA], *origin*, abdominal aorta; *branches*, inferior pancreaticoduodenal, jejunal, ileal, ileocolic, appendicular, right colic, middle colic; *anastomoses*, superior pancreaticoduodenal and left colic. SYN arteria mesenterica superior [TA].

superior phrenic a. [TA], one of a pair of small arteries given off from the thoracic aorta just superior to the diaphragm; *distribution*, diaphragm; *anastomoses*, musculophrenic, pericardiacophrenic, and inferior phrenic. SYN arteria phrenica superior [TA].

superior rectal a. [TA], *origin*, inferior mesenteric; *distribution*, upper part of rectum; *anastomoses*, middle and inferior rectal. As a tributary of the portal vein, its anastomosis with these a.'s forms a portosystemic or portocaval anastomosis. SYN arteria rectalis superior [TA], superior hemorrhoidal a.

superior segmental a. [TA], SEE left pulmonary a., right pulmonary a., segmental a.'s of kidney.

superior segmental a. of kidney [TA], *origin*, anterior branch of renal. SEE segmental a.'s of kidney. SYN a. of superior segment of kidney.

a. of superior segment of kidney, SYN superior segmental a. of kidney.

superior suprarenal a.'s [TA], *origin*, inferior phrenic artery; *distribution*, suprarenal gland. SYN arteriae suprarenales superiores [TA].

superior thoracic a. [TA], *origin*, axillary; *distribution*, muscles of superior chest; *anastomoses*, branches of suprascapular, internal thoracic, and thoracoacromial. SYN arteria thoracica superior [TA], highest thoracic a.

superior thyroid a. [TA], *origin*, external carotid; *branches*, infrahyoid, superior laryngeal, sternocleidomastoid, cricothyroid, and two terminal branches. SYN arteria thyroidea superior [TA].

superior tympanic a. [TA], *origin*, middle meningeal; *distribution*, middle ear; *anastomoses*, other tympanic arteries. SYN arteria tympanica superior [TA].

superior ulnar collateral a. [TA], *origin*, brachial; *distribution*, elbow joint; *anastomoses*, posterior ulnar recurrent and inferior ulnar collateral, as part of the articular vascular network of the elbow. SYN arteria collateralis ulnaris superior [TA].

superior vesical a. [TA], *origin*, umbilical; *distribution*, bladder, urachus, ureter; *anastomoses*, other vesical branches. SYN arteria vesicalis superior [TA].

suprachiasmatic a. [TA], *origin:* anterior communicating a.; passes superior to optic chiasm to supply region of optic recess, hypothalamic area. SYN arteria suprachiasmatica [TA].

supraduodenal a. [TA], *origin*, gastroduodenal; *distribution*, first part of duodenum. SYN arteria supraduodenalis [TA].

supraoptic a. [TA], *origin:* precommunicating part (A1 segment) of anterior cerebral a.; *distribution:* passes superior to optic nerve to orbital surface of frontal lobe of cerebrum. SYN arteria supraoptica [TA].

supraorbital a. [TA], *origin*, ophthalmic; *distribution*, frontalis muscle and scalp; *anastomoses*, branches of the superficial temporal and supratrochlear. SYN arteria supraorbitalis [TA].

suprascapular a. [TA], *origin*, thyrocervical trunk; *distribution*, clavicle, scapula, muscles of shoulder, and shoulder joint; *anastomoses*, transverse cervical circumflex scapular. SYN arteria suprascapularis [TA], transverse scapular a.

supratrochlear a. [TA], *origin*, ophthalmic; *distribution*, anterior portion of scalp; *anastomoses*, branches of supraorbital. SYN arteria supratrochlearis [TA], arteria frontalis, frontal a.

supreme intercostal a. [TA], *origin*, costocervical trunk; *distribution*, structures of first and second intercostal spaces via its terminal branches, posterior intercostal a.'s 1 and 2; *anastomoses*, anterior intercostal branches of internal thoracic. SYN arteria intercostalis suprema [TA], highest intercostal a., superior intercostal a.

sural a.'s [TA], one of four or five arteries arising (sometimes by a common trunk) from the popliteal; *distribution*, muscles and integument of the calf; *anastomoses*, posterior tibial, medial, and lateral inferior genicular. SYN arteriae surales [TA], a. of calf.

a. to tail of pancreas [TA], *origin*, splenic a. near the left gastroepiploic; *distribution*, the tail of the pancreas; *anastomoses*, with other pancreatic a.'s. SYN arteria caudae pancreatis [TA], caudal pancreatic a.

terminal a., SYN end a.

testicular a. [TA], *origin*, aorta; *branches*, ureteral, cremasteric, epididymal; *distribution*, testicle and parts designated by names of branches; *anastomoses*, branches of renal, inferior epigastric, deferential. SYN arteria testicularis [TA], arteria spermatica interna, internal spermatic a.

thoracoacromial a. [TA], *origin*, axillary; *distribution*, muscles and skin of shoulder and upper chest; *anastomoses*, branches of superior thoracic, internal thoracic, lateral thoracic, posterior and anterior circumflex humeral, and suprascapular. SYN arteria thoracoacromialis [TA], ramus deltoideus arteriae thoracoacromialis [TA], acromiothoracic a., thoracic axis (1), thoracoacromial trunk.

thoracodorsal a. [TA], *origin*, subscapular; *distribution*, muscles of upper part of back; *anastomoses*, branches of lateral thoracic. SYN arteria thoracodorsalis [TA], dorsal thoracic a.

thyroid ima a. [TA], an inconstant artery; *origin*, arch of aorta or brachiocephalic artery; *distribution*, thyroid gland. SYN arteria thyroidea ima [TA], lowest thyroid a., Neubauer a.

tibial nutrient a. [TA], a. derived from the upper part of the posterior tibial a.; it enters through the nutrient foramen on the posterior surface of the tibia. SYN arteria nutricia tibiae [TA], arteria nutriens tibiae⋆, arteria nutriens tibialis, nutrient a. of the tibia.

transverse cervical a. [TA], *origin*, thyrocervical trunk; *branch-*

es, superficial (superficial cervical) and deep (descending scapular). SYN arteria transversa colli [TA], arteria transversa cervicis⋆, transverse a. of neck.

transverse facial a. [TA], *origin*, superficial temporal; *distribution*, parotid gland, parotid duct, masseter muscle, and overlying skin; *anastomoses*, infraorbital and buccal branches of maxillary, and buccal and masseteric branches of facial. SYN arteria transversa faciei [TA].

transverse a. of neck, SYN transverse cervical a.

transverse pancreatic a., SYN inferior pancreatic a.

transverse scapular a., SYN suprascapular a.

a. of tuber cinereum [TA], small a. arising from the posterior communicating a. giving rise to lateral and medial branches supplying the tuber cinereum. SYN arteria tuberis cinerei [TA].

ulnar a. [TA], *origin*, brachial; *branches*, ulnar recurrent, common interosseous, dorsal and palmar carpal, deep palmar, and superficial palmar arch with its digital branches. SYN arteria ulnaris [TA].

ulnar recurrent a. [TA], *origin*, ulnar artery; *distribution*, two branches, anterior and posterior, pass medially in front of and behind the elbow joint; *anastomoses*, superior and inferior ulnar collateral, i.e., with articular vascular plexus of elbow. SYN arteria recurrens ulnaris [TA], recurrent ulnar a.

umbilical a. [TA], before birth this a. is a continuation of the internal iliac; after birth it is obliterated between the bladder and umbilicus, forming the medial umbilical ligament, the remaining portion, between the internal iliac artery and bladder, being reduced in size and giving off the superior vesical arteries. SYN arteria umbilicalis [TA].

uncal a. [TA], *origin:* cerebral part of internal carotid a. or occasionally from the sphenoidal part (M1 segment) of the middle cerebral a.; *distrubution:* to uncus. SYN arteria uncalis [TA].

a.'s of upper limb [TA], a.'s that supply the upper limb; all are derivatives of the axillary a. SYN arteriae membri superioris [TA].

urethral a. [TA], *origin*, perineal artery; *distribution*, membranous urethra. SYN arteria urethralis [TA].

uterine a. [TA], *origin*, internal iliac; *distribution*, uterus, upper part of vagina, round ligament, and medial part of uterine (fallopian) tube; *anastomoses*, ovarian, vaginal, inferior epigastric. Supplies maternal circulation to placenta during pregnancy. SYN arteria uterina [TA].

vaginal a. [TA], *origin*, internal iliac; *distribution*, vagina, base of bladder, rectum; *anastomoses*, uterine, internal pudendal. SYN arteria vaginalis [TA].

a. to vas deferens, ⋆official alternate term for a. to ductus deferens.

venous a., SYN pulmonary *trunk.*

ventral splanchnic a.'s, a.'s that arise in the embryo from the dorsal aorta and are distributed to the digestive tube.

ventricular a.'s, branches of the right and left coronary arteries distributed to the muscle of the ventricles. SYN arteriae ventriculares [TA].

vertebral a. [TA], the first branch of the subclavian artery; for descriptive purposes, divided into four parts: 1) prevertebral part, the portion before it enters the foramen of the transverse process of the sixth cervical vertebra; 2) cervical part, the portion in the transverse foramina of the first six cervical vertebrae; 3) atlantic (suboccipital) part, the portion running along the posterior arch of the atlas; and 4) intracranial part, the portion within the cranial cavity to its union with the artery from the other side to form the basilar artery. SYN arteria vertebralis [TA].

vestibulocochlear a. [TA], *origin:* anterior vestibular a.; *branches:* saccular, cochlear, and posterior vestibular. SYN arteria vestibulocochlearis [TA].

vidian a., SYN a. of pterygoid canal.

vitelline a., an a. carrying blood to the yolk sac from the embryo. SYN arteria vitellina.

volar interosseous a., SYN anterior interosseous a.

Zinn a., SYN central retinal a.

zygomatico-orbital a. [TA], *origin*, superficial temporal, sometimes middle temporal; *distribution*, orbicularis oculi muscle and portions of the orbit; *anastomoses,* lacrimal and palpebral branches of ophthalmic. SYN arteria zygomatico-orbitalis [TA].

⟡**arthr-.** SEE arthro-.

ar·thral (ar′thrăl). SYN articular.

ar·thral·gia (ar-thral′jē-ă). Pain in a joint, especially one not inflammatory in character. SYN arthrodynia. [G. *arthron,* joint, + *algos,* pain]

intermittent a., SYN periodic a.

periodic a. [MIM*112270], a condition in which there is pain and swelling, thought originally to involve the joints, but now known to localize to the shafts of long bones, occurring at regular intervals; there is sometimes abdominal pain, purpura, or edema. SYN intermittent a., periodic bone pain.

a. saturni′na, severe pain, chiefly on flexion of the joints of the lower extremities, in lead poisoning.

ar·thral·gic (ar-thral′jik). Relating to or affected with arthralgia. SYN arthrodynic.

ar·threc·to·my (ar-threk′tō-mē). Excision of a joint. [G. *arthron,* joint, + *ektomē,* excision]

ar·thres·the·sia (ar-thres-thē′zē-ă). SYN articular *sensibility.* [G. *arthron,* joint, + *aisthesis,* sensation]

ar·thrit·ic (ar-thrit′ik). Relating to arthritis.

ar·thrit·i·des (ar-thrit′i-dēz). Plural of arthritis.

ar·thri·tis, pl. **ar·thrit·i·des** (ar-thrī′tis, ar-thrit′i-dēz). Inflammation of a joint or a state characterized by inflammation of joints. SYN articular rheumatism. [G. fr. *arthron,* joint, + *-itis,* inflammation]

acute rheumatic a., a. due to rheumatic fever.

chronic absorptive a., SYN a. mutilans.

chylous a., a. with a high lymph content in synovial fluid, usually due to filariasis.

a. defor′mans, SYN rheumatoid a.

degenerative a., SYN osteoarthritis.

enteropathic a., a form of a. sometimes resembling rheumatoid a. which may complicate the course of ulcerative colitis, Crohn disease, or other intestinal disease.

filarial a., a. occurring in filariasis, probably due to extravasation of lipid-rich lymph resembling chyle into the joint space.

gonococcal a., joint space infection in humans caused by disseminated *Neisseria gonorrhoeae;* characteristically monarticular, but may be polyarticular. SYN gonorrheal arthritis.

gonorrheal arthritis, SYN gonococcal a.

gouty a., inflammation of the joints in gout.

hemophilic a., joint disease resulting from hemophilic bleeding into a joint.

hypertrophic a., variant of osteoarthritis characterized by afferent periarticular osteophyte formation.

Jaccoud a., a rare form of chronic a., reported to occur after attacks of acute rheumatic fever, characterized by an unusual form of bone erosion of the metacarpal heads and by ulnar deviation of the fingers; it resembles rheumatoid a., but with less overt inflammation, and rheumatoid factor is absent. SYN Jaccoud arthropathy.

juvenile a., juvenile rheumatoid a., chronic a. beginning in childhood, most cases of which are pauciarticular, i.e., affecting few joints. Several patterns of illness have been identified: in one subset, primarily affecting girls, iritis is common and antinuclear antibody is usually present; another subset, primarily affecting boys, frequently includes spinal a. resembling ankylosing spondylitis; some cases are true rheumatoid a. beginning in childhood and characterized by the presence of rheumatoid factor and destructive deforming joint changes, often undergoing remission at puberty. SEE ALSO Still *disease.* SYN juvenile chronic a.

juvenile chronic a., SYN juvenile a.

Lyme a., the arthritic manifestation of Lyme disease.

a. mu′tilans, a form of chronic rheumatoid a. in which osteolysis occurs with extensive destruction of the joint cartilages and bony surfaces with pronounced deformities, chiefly of the hands and feet; similar changes occur in some cases of psoriatic a. SYN chronic absorptive a.

neuropathic a., a. associated with an underlying neurologic disorder, e.g., syringomyelia, tabes dorsalis, diabetes mellitus.

a. nodo′sa, obsolete term for rheumatoid a.

ochronotic a., osteoarthritis occurring as a complication of ochronosis.

proliferative a., term for rheumatoid a., based on the characteristic proliferation of the synovial membrane seen in joints affected by the disease.

psoriatic a., the concurrence of psoriasis and polyarthritis, resembling rheumatoid a. but thought to be a specific disease entity, seronegative for rheumatoid factor and often involving the digits. SEE ALSO a. mutilans. SYN arthropathia psoriatica.

pyogenic a., SYN suppurative a.

reactive a., sterile, usually transient polyarthropathy following various infectious diseases.

rheumatoid a., a generalized disease, occurring more often in women, which primarily affects connective tissue; a. is the dominant clinical manifestation, involving many joints, especially those of the hands and feet, accompanied by thickening of articular soft tissue, with extension of synovial tissue over articular cartilages, which become eroded; the course is variable but often is chronic and progressive, leading to deformities and disability. SYN a. deformans, nodose rheumatism (1).

septic a., SYN suppurative a.

suppurative a., acute inflammation of synovial membranes, with purulent effusion into a joint, due to bacterial infection; the usual route of infection is hemic to the synovial tissue, causing destruction of the articular cartilage, and may become chronic, with sinus formation, osteomyelitis, deformity, and disability. SYN purulent synovitis, pyarthrosis, pyogenic a., septic a., suppurative synovitis.

⟡**arthro-, arthr-.** A joint, an articulation; corresponds to L. articul-. [G. *arthron,* a joint, fr. *ariskō,* to join, to fit together]

Arth·ro·bac·ter (ar-thrō-bak′ter). A genus of strictly aerobic, Gram-positive bacteria (family Corynebacteriaceae) whose cells undergo a change from a coccoid form to a rod shape following transfer to fresh complex growth medium. Although primarily found in soil, species identified as belonging to this genus have been found in the advancing front of lesions of dental caries. The type species is *A. globiformis.* [G. *arthron,* joint, + *baktron,* staff or rod]

ar·thro·cen·te·sis (ar′thrō-sen-tē′sis). Aspiration of fluid from a joint performed by needle puncture. [arthro- + G. *kentēsis,* puncture]

ar·thro·chon·dri·tis (ar′thrō-kon-drī′tis). Inflammation of an articular cartilage. [arthro- + G. *chondros,* cartilage, + *-itis,* inflammation]

ar·thro·cla·sia (ar-thrō-klā′zē-ă). The forcible breaking up of the adhesions in ankylosis. [arthro- + G. *klasis,* a breaking]

ar·thro·co·nid·i·um (ar′thrō-kō-nid′ē-um). A conidium released by fragmentation or separation at the septum of cells of the hypha. SYN arthrospore. [G. *arthron,* joint, + conidium]

Arth·ro·der·ma (ar′thrō-der′mă). A genus of ascomycetous fungi composed of the anamorph genera *Microsporium* and *Trichophyton* species.

ar·throd·e·sis (ar-throd′ĕ-sis, ar-thrō-dē′sis). The stiffening of a joint by operative means. SYN artificial ankylosis. [arthro- + G. *desis,* a binding together]

triple a., surgical fusion of the talonavicular, talocalcaneal, and calcaneocuboid joints.

ar·thro·dia (ar-thrō′dē-ă). SYN plane *joint.* [G. *arthrōdia,* a gliding joint, fr. *arthron,* joint, + *eidos,* form]

ar·thro·di·al (ar-thrō′dē-ăl). Relating to arthrodia.

ar·thro·dyn·ia (ar-thrō-din′ē-ă). SYN arthralgia. [arthro- + G. *odynē,* pain]

ar·thro·dyn·ic (ar-thrō-din′ik). SYN arthralgic.

ar·thro·dys·pla·sia (ar′thrō-dis-plā′zē-ă). Hereditary congenital defect of joint development. [arthro- + G. *dys,* bad, + *plasis,* a molding]

ar·thro·en·dos·co·py (ar′thrō-en-dos′kŏ-pē). SYN arthroscopy.

ar·thro·e·rei·sis (ar-thrō-ĕ-rī′sis). SYN arthrorisis.

ar·throg·e·nous (ar-throj′ĕ-nŭs). **1.** Of articular origin; starting from a joint. **2.** Forming an articulation.

ar·thro·gram (ar′thrō-gram). Imaging of a joint following the introduction of a contrast agent into the joint capsule to enhance visualization of the intraarticular structures. [arthro- + G. *gramma,* a writing]

ar·throg·ra·phy (ar-throg′ră-fē). Act of making an arthrogram. [arthro- + G. *graphō,* to describe]

ar·thro·gry·po·sis (ar′thrō-gri-pō′sis). Congenital defect of the limbs characterized by severe contractures of multiple joints. [arthro- + G. *gryphōsis,* a crooking]

a. mul′tiplex congen′ita, limitation of range of joint motion and contractures present at birth, usually involving multiple joints; a syndrome probably of diverse etiology that may result from changes in spinal cord, muscle, or connective tissue. Several forms exist, autosomal dominant [MIM*108110, 108120, 108130, 108140, 108145, 108200], recessive [MIM*208080, 208081, 208085, 208100, 208150, 208155, 208200], and X-linked [MIM*301830] SYN amyoplasia congenita.

ar·thro·ka·tad·y·sis (ar′thrō-kă-tad′i-sis). a condition of a joint with significant erosion of the concave surface, resulting in migration of the convex surface medially. SEE ALSO Otto *disease.* [arthro- + G. *katadysis,* a dipping under, a setting, fr. *dyō,* to make sink]

ar·thro·lith (ar′thrō-lith). A loose body in a joint. [arthro- + G. *lithos,* stone]

ar·thro·li·thi·a·sis (ar′thrō-li-thī′ă-sis). Rarely used term for articular *gout.*

ar·thro·lo·gia (ar-thrō-lō′jē-ă). SYN arthrology, arthrology.

ar·throl·o·gy (ar-throl′ō-jē). The branch of anatomy concerned with the joints. SYN arthrologia, syndesmologia, syndesmology, synosteology. [arthro- + G. *logos,* study]

ar·throl·y·sis (ar-throl′i-sis). Restoration of mobility in stiff and ankylosed joints through the process of disrupting intraarticular and extraarticular adhesions. [arthro- + G. *lysis,* a loosening]

ar·throm·e·ter (ar-throm′ĕ-ter). SYN goniometer (3).

ar·throm·e·try (ar-throm′ĕ-trē). Measurement of the range of movement in a joint. [arthro- + G. *metron,* measure]

ar·thro·oph·thal·mop·a·thy (ar′thrō-of′thal-mop′ă-thē). Disease affecting joints and eyes. [arthro- + ophthalmo- + G. *pathos,* suffering]

hereditary progressive a.-o. [MIM*108300], a skeletal dysplasia associated with multiple dysplasia of the epiphyses, overtubulation of long bones with metaphyseal widening, flattened vertebral bodies, pelvic bone abnormalities, hypermobility of joints, cleft palate, progressive myopia, retinal detachment, and deafness. Autosomal dominant inheritance caused by mutation in either the COL2A1 gene on 12q, COL11A1 gene on 1p or COL11A2 gene on 6p. SYN Stickler syndrome.

arthropathia psoriatica. SYN psoriatic *arthritis.*

ar·thro·pa·thol·o·gy (ar′thrō-pa-thol′ō-jē). The study of diseases of joints.

ar·throp·a·thy (ar-throp′ă-thē). Any disease affecting a joint. [arthro- + G. *pathos,* suffering]

diabetic a., a neuropathic a. occurring in diabetes.

Jaccoud a., SYN Jaccoud *arthritis.*

long-leg a., a degenerative joint disease that develops, after many years, in the hip and/or knee of the longer leg of a person with unequal leg lengths.

neuropathic a., SYN neuropathic *joint.*

static a., secondary involvement of a joint following disease in a joint of the same extremity; e.g., knee or ankle involvement in hip disease.

tabetic a., a neuropathic a. that occurs with tabes dorsalis (tabetic neurosyphilis). SEE ALSO neuropathic *joint.*

▮ar·thro·plas·ty (ar′thrō-plas-tē). **1.** Creation of an artificial joint to correct advanced degenerative arthritis, **2.** An operation to restore as far as possible the integrity and functional power of a joint. [arthro- + G. *plastos,* formed]

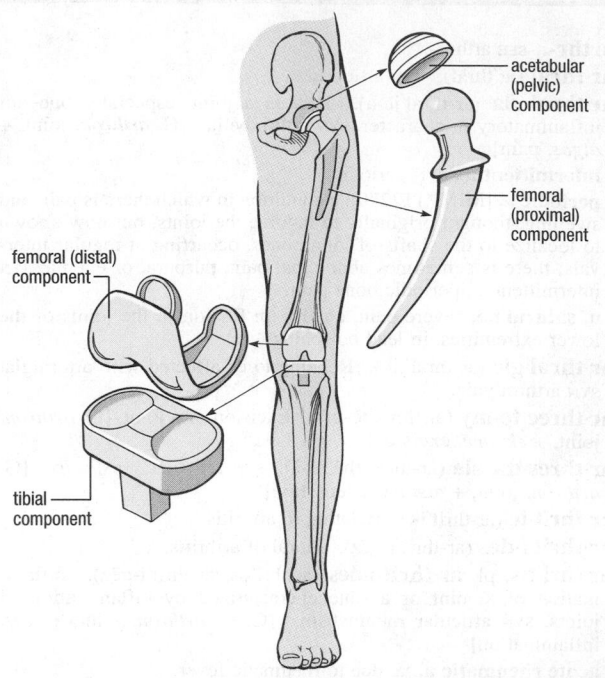

acetabular (pelvic) component

femoral (proximal) component

femoral (distal) component

tibial component

arthroplasty: showing hip and knee replacement

Charnley hip a., a form of total hip replacement consisting of the application of an acetabular cup and a femoral head prosthesis; it bears the name of John Charnley who is regarded as the pioneer in the development of this procedure.

gap a., the surgical correction of ankylosis by creating a space between the ankylosed part of a joint and the portion for which movement is desired.

interposition a., surgical correction of ankylosis by separation of the immobile part of a joint from the mobilized part and interposition of a substance (e.g., fascia, cartilage, metal, or plastic) between them.

intracapsular temporomandibular joint a., operative recontouring of the articular surface of the mandibular condyle without the removal of the articular disk.

total joint a., a. in which both joint surfaces are replaced with artificial materials, usually composed of metal and high-density plastic; currently being performed for hip, knee, shoulder, and elbow.

ar·thro·pneu·mo·ra·di·og·raph·y (ar′thrō-noo′mō-rā-dē-og′ră-fē). Radiographic examination of a joint after it has been injected with air. [arthro- + pneumo- + radiography]

ar·thro·pod (ar′thrō-pod). A member of the phylum Arthropoda. [arthro- + G. *pous,* foot]

Ar·throp·o·da (ar-throp′ŏ-dă). A phylum of the Metazoa that includes the classes Crustacea (crabs, shrimps, crayfish, lobsters), Insecta, Arachnida (spiders, scorpions, mites, ticks), Chilopoda (centipedes), Diplopoda (millipedes), Merostomata (horseshoe crabs), and various other extinct or lesser known groups. A. forms the largest assemblage of living organisms, 75% insects, of which over a million species are known. [arthro- + G. *pous,* foot]

ar·thro·po·di·a·sis (ar′thrō-pō-dī′ă-sis). Direct effects of arthropods upon vertebrates including acariasis, allergy, dermatosis, entomophobia, and actions of contact toxins.

ar·thro·po·dic, ar·throp·o·dous (ar-thrō-pō′dik, ar-throp′ŏ-dŭs). Pertaining to arthropods.

ar·thro·py·o·sis (ar′thrō-pī-ō′sis). Suppuration in a joint. [arthro- + G. *pyōsis,* suppuration]

ar·thro·ri·sis (ar'thrō-rī'sis). An operation for limiting motion in a joint in cases of undue mobility from paralysis, usually by means of a bone block. SYN arthroereisis. [arthro- + G. *ereisis*, a propping up]

ar·thro·scle·ro·sis (ar'thrō-skler-ō'sis). Stiffness of the joints, especially in the aged. [arthro- + G. *sklērōsis*, hardening]

ar·thro·scope (ar'thrō-skōp). An endoscope for examining the internal anatomy of a joint.

⑤**ar·thros·co·py** (ar-thros'kŏ-pē). Endoscopic examination of the interior of a joint. SYN arthroendoscopy. [arthro- + G. *skopeō*, to view]

⑤**ar·thro·sis** (ar-thrō'sis). **1.** SYN joint. [G. *arthrōsis*, a jointing] **2.** SYN osteoarthritis. [arthro- + G. -*osis*, condition]

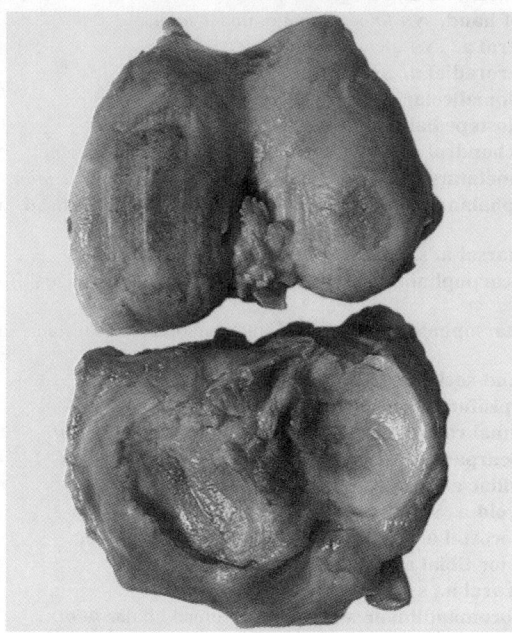

arthrosis: the cartilage of the knee is nearly destroyed

temporomandibular a., a noninfectious degenerative dysfunction of the temporomandibular joint characterized by pain, cracking, and limited mandibular opening. SEE ALSO myofascial pain-dysfunction *syndrome*.

ar·thro·spore (ar'thrō-spōr). SYN arthroconidium. [arthro- + G. *sporos*, seed]

ar·thros·to·my (ar-thros'tō-mē). Establishment of a temporary opening into a joint cavity. [arthro- + G. *stoma*, mouth]

ar·thro·sy·no·vi·tis (ar'thrō-sin-ō-vī'tis). Inflammation of the synovial membrane of a joint.

ar·thro·tome (ar'thrō-tōm). A large, strong scalpel used in cutting cartilaginous and other tough joint structures.

ar·throt·o·my (ar-throt'ō-mē). Cutting into a joint to expose its interior. [arthro- + G. *tomē*, a cutting]

ar·thro·tro·pic (ar-thrō-trop'ik). Tending to affect joints. [arthro- + G. *tropos*, a turning]

ar·thro·ty·phoid (ar-thrō-tī'foyd). Obsolete term for typhoid fever with joint involvement due to metastatic infection.

Arthus, Maurice, French bacteriologist, 1862–1945. SEE A. *phenomenon, reaction*.

ar·tic·u·lar (ar-tik'ū-lăr). Relating to a joint. SYN arthral.

ar·tic·u·la·re (ar-tik-ū-lā'rē). In cephalometrics, the point of intersection of the external dorsal contour of the mandibular condyle and the temporal bone; the midpoint is used when a profile radiograph shows double projections of the rami.

ar·tic·u·late (ar-tik'ū-lit). **1.** SYN articulated. **2.** Capable of distinct and connected meaningful speech. (ar-tik'yū-lāt). **3.** To join or connect together loosely to allow motion between the parts. **4.** To speak distinctly and connectedly. [L. *articulo*, pp. -*atus*, to articulate]

ar·tic·u·lat·ed (ar-tik'ū-lā-ted). Jointed. SYN articulate (1).

ARTICULATIO

ar·tic·u·la·tio, pl. **ar·tic·u·la·ti·o·nes** (ar-tik-ū-lā'shē-ō, -lā-shē-ō'nēz). ⭐official alternate term for synovial *joint*. [L. a forming of vines]

  a. acromioclavicula'ris [TA], SYN acromioclavicular *joint*.
  a. atlantoaxia'lis latera'lis [TA], SYN lateral atlantoaxial *joint*.
  a. atlantoaxia'lis media'na [TA], SYN median atlantoaxial *joint*.
  a. atlan'to-occipita'lis [TA], SYN atlanto-occipital *joint*.
  a. bicondyla'ris [TA], SYN bicondylar *joint*.
  a. calca'neocuboi'dea [TA], SYN calcaneocuboid *joint*.
  a. cap'itis cos'tae [TA], SYN *joint* of head of rib.
  articulationes carpi [TA], SYN carpal *joints*, under *joint*.
  a. carpi [TA], SYN carpal *joints*, under *joint*.
  articulatio'nes carpometacarpa'les [TA], SYN carpometacarpal *joints*, under *joint*.
  a. carpometacar'palis pol'licis, SYN carpometacarpal *joint* of thumb.
  a. cartilag'inis, SYN cartilaginous *joint*.
  articulatio'nes cing'uli mem'bri inferio'ris, SYN *joints* of pelvic girdle, under *joint*.
  articulationes cinguli pectoralis, ⭐official alternate term for *joints* of pectoral girdle, under *joint*.
  articulationes cinguli pelvici [TA], SYN *joints* of pelvic girdle, under *joint*.
  articulatio'nes cin'guli mem'bri superio'ris, SYN *joints* of pectoral girdle, under *joint*.
  a. complex'a, SYN complex *joint*.
  a. compos'ita [TA], SYN complex *joint*.
  a. condyla'ris, SYN condylar *joint*.
  articulationes costochondra'les [TA], SYN costochondral *joints*, under *joint*.
  a. cos'totransversa'ria, SYN costotransverse *joint*.
  articulatio'nes costovertebra'les [TA], SYN costovertebral *joints*, under *joint*.
  a. cotyl'ica, SYN ball and socket *joint*.
  a. cox'ae [TA], SYN hip *joint*.
  a. coxofemoralis, ⭐official alternate term for hip *joint*.
  articulationes cranii [TA], SYN cranial synovial *joints*, under *joint*.
  a. cricoarytenoid'ea [TA], SYN cricoarytenoid *joint*.
  a. cricothyroid'ea [TA], SYN cricothyroid *joint*.
  a. cu'biti [TA], SYN elbow *joint*.
  a. cuneonavicula'ris [TA], SYN cuneonavicular *joint*.
  a. cylindrica [TA], SYN cylindrical *joint*.
  a. dentoalveola'ris, SYN gomphosis.
  a. ellipsoi'dea [TA], SYN condylar *joint*.
  a. fibro'sa, SYN fibrous *joint*.
  a. ge'nus [TA], SYN knee *joint*.
  a. glenohumeralis, ⭐official alternate term for glenohumeral *joint*.
  a. hu'meri [TA], SYN glenohumeral *joint*.
  a. humeroradia'lis [TA], SYN humeroradial *joint*.
  a. humeroulna'ris [TA], SYN humeroulnar *joint*.
  a. incudomallea'ris [TA], SYN incudomalleolar *joint*.
  a. incudostape'dia [TA], SYN incudostapedial *joint*.
  articulatio'nes intercarpa'les, ⭐official alternate term for carpal *joints*, under *joint*.
  articulatio'nes interchondra'les [TA], SYN interchondral *joints*, under *joint*.

ar

articulationes intercuneiformes [TA], SYN intercuneiform *joints*, under *joint*.

articulatio'nes intermetacarpa'les [TA], SYN intermetacarpal *joints*, under *joint*.

articulatio'nes intermetatarsa'les [TA], SYN intermetatarsal *joints*, under *joint*.

articulatio'nes interphalan'geae ma'nus [TA], SYN interphalangeal *joints* of hand, under *joint*.

articulatio'nes interphalan'geae pe'dis [TA], SYN interphalangeal *joints* of foot, under *joint*.

articulatio'nes intertar'seae, SYN intertarsal *joints*, under *joint*.

a. lumbosacra'lis [TA], SYN lumbosacral *joint*.

a. mandibula'ris, SYN temporomandibular *joint*.

articulatio'nes ma'nus [TA], SYN *joints* of hand, under *joint*.

a. mediocarpa'lis [TA], SYN midcarpal *joint*.

articulatio'nes mem'bri inferio'ris li'beri [TA], SYN synovial *joints* of free lower limb, under *joint*.

articulatio'nes mem'bri superio'ris li'beri [TA], SYN synovial *joints* of free upper limb, under *joint*.

articulatio'nes metacarpophalan'geae [TA], SYN metacarpophalangeal *joints*, under *joint*.

articulatio'nes metatarsophalan'geae [TA], SYN metatarsophalangeal *joints*, under *joint*.

articulationes ossiculorum auditoriorum, ✩official alternate term for *joints* of auditory ossicles, under *joint*.

articulatio'nes ossiculo'rum audi'tus [TA], SYN *joints* of auditory ossicles, under *joint*.

a. os'sis pisifor'mis [TA], SYN pisiform *joint*.

a. ovoida'lis, SYN saddle *joint*.

articulatio'nes pe'dis [TA], SYN *joints* of foot, under *joint*.

a. pla'na [TA], SYN plane *joint*.

a. radiocar'palis [TA], SYN wrist *joint*.

a. radioulna'ris dista'lis [TA], SYN distal radioulnar *joint*.

a. radioulna'ris proxima'lis [TA], SYN proximal radioulnar *joint*.

a. sacrococcy'gea [TA], SYN sacrococcygeal *joint*.

a. sacroili'aca [TA], SYN sacroiliac *joint*.

a. sellar'is [TA], SYN saddle *joint*.

a. sim'plex [TA], SYN simple *joint*.

a. spheroi'dea [TA], SYN ball and socket *joint*.

a. sternoclavicula'ris [TA], SYN sternoclavicular *joint*.

articulatio'nes sternocosta'les [TA], SYN sternocostal *joints*, under *joint*.

a. subtala'ris [TA], SYN subtalar *joint*.

a. synovia'lis, SYN synovial *joint*.

a. talocalcanea, ✩official alternate term for subtalar *joint*.

a. tal'ocalca'neonavicula'ris [TA], SYN talocalcaneonavicular *joint*.

a. talocrura'lis [TA], SYN ankle *joint*.

a. tar'si transver'sa [TA], SYN transverse tarsal *joint*.

articulatio'nes tarsometatarsa'les [TA], SYN tarsometatarsal *joints*, under *joint*.

a. temporomandibula'ris [TA], SYN temporomandibular *joint*.

articulationes thoracis [TA], SYN synovial *joints* of thorax, under *joint*.

a. tibiofibula'ris [TA], SYN tibiofibular *joint*.

a. trochoid'ea [TA], SYN pivot *joint*.

articulatio'nes zygapophysia'les [TA], SYN zygapophysial *joints*, under *joint*.

---

ar·tic·u·la·tion (ar-tik-ū-lā'shŭn). **1.** SYN joint. **2.** A joining or connecting together loosely so as to allow motion between the parts. **3.** Distinct connected speech or enunciation. **4.** In dentistry, the contact relationship of the occlusal surfaces of the teeth during jaw movement. [see articulatio]

arthrodial a., SYN plane *joint*.

atlanto-occipital a., SYN atlanto-occipital *joint*.

balanced a., SYN balanced *occlusion*.

bicondylar a., SYN bicondylar *joint*.

cartilaginous a., SYN cartilaginous *joint*.

compound a., SYN complex *joint*.

condylar a., SYN condylar *joint*.

confluent a., a tendency to run the syllables together in speech.

cricoarytenoid a., SYN cricoarytenoid *joint*.

cricothyroid a., SYN cricothyroid *joint*.

cuneonavicular a., SYN cuneonavicular *joint*.

dental a., the contact relationship of the occlusal surfaces of the upper and lower teeth when moving into and away from centric occlusion. SYN gliding occlusion.

distal radioulnar a., SYN distal radioulnar *joint*.

a.'s of foot, SYN *joints* of foot, under *joint*.

glenohumeral a., SYN glenohumeral *joint*.

a.'s of hand, SYN *joints* of hand, under *joint*.

humeral a., SYN glenohumeral *joint*.

humeroradial a., SYN humeroradial *joint*.

incudomalleolar a., SYN incudomalleolar *joint*.

incudostapedial a., SYN incudostapedial *joint*.

interchondral a.'s, SYN interchondral *joints*, under *joint*.

intermetatarsal a.'s, SYN intermetatarsal *joints*, under *joint*.

interphalangeal a.'s, SYN interphalangeal *joints* of hand, under *joint*.

intertarsal a.'s, SYN intertarsal *joints*, under *joint*.

metacarpophalangeal a.'s, SYN metacarpophalangeal *joints*, under *joint*.

metatarsophalangeal a.'s, SYN metatarsophalangeal *joints*, under *joint*.

peg-and-socket a., SYN gomphosis.

a. of pisiform bone, SYN pisiform *joint*.

proximal radioulnar a., SYN proximal radioulnar *joint*.

radiocarpal a., SYN wrist *joint*.

sacroiliac a., SYN sacroiliac *joint*.

spheroid a., SYN ball and socket *joint*.

sternocostal a.'s, SYN sternocostal *joints*, under *joint*.

superior tibial a., SYN tibiofibular *joint*.

talocrural a., SYN ankle *joint*.

temporomandibular a., SYN temporomandibular *joint*.

tibiofibular a., (1) SYN tibiofibular *joint*; **(2)** SYN tibiofibular *syndesmosis*.

transverse tarsal a., SYN transverse tarsal *joint*.

trochoid a., SYN pivot *joint*.

ar·tic·u·la·tor (ar-tik'ū-lā-tŏr). A mechanical device which represents the temporomandibular joints and jaw members to which maxillary and mandibular casts may be attached. SYN occluding frame.

adjustable a., (1) an a. which may be adjusted to permit movement of the casts into recorded eccentric relationships; **(2)** an a. capable of adjustment to more than one eccentric position.

arcon a., (1) an a. with the equivalent condylar guides fixed to the upper member and the hinge axis to the lower member; **(2)** an instrument that maintains a constant relationship between the occlusal plane and the arcon guides at any position of the upper member, thereby making possible more accurate reproductions of mandibular movements.

non-arcon a., an a. with the equivalent condylar guides attached to the lower member and the hinge axis to the upper member.

ar·tic·u·la·to·ry (ar-tik'ū-lă-tō-rē). Relating to articulate speech.

ar·tic·u·lo·stat (ar-tik'ū-lō-stat). A research instrument that positions the dentition of a subject and the head of an x-ray machine in such a manner that films made at separate times may be accurately superimposed. [articulo- + G. *stasis*, a standing still]

ar·tic·u·lus (ar-tik'ū-lŭs). SYN joint. [L. joint]

ar·ti·fact (ar'ti-fakt). **1.** Anything, especially in a histologic specimen or a graphic record, that is caused by the technique used and not reflecting the original specimen or experiment. **2.** A skin lesion produced or perpetuated by self-inflicted action, as in dermatitis artefacta. [L. *ars,* art, + *facio,* pp. *factus,* to make]

chemical shift a., in magnetic resonance imaging, a dark band caused by a biochemical difference in resonant frequency of adjacent regions rather than a true anatomic separation.

thermal a., distortion of microscopic structure in a tissue specimen, because of heat generated by the instrument (e.g., loop electrocautery) used to obtain the specimen.

ar·ti·fac·ti·tious (ar′ti-fak-tish′ŭs). SYN artifactual.

ar·ti·fac·tu·al (ar-ti-fak′chū-ăl). Produced or caused by an artifact. SYN artifactitious.

Ar·ti·o·dac·ty·la (ar′ti-ō-dak′ti-lă). An order of even-toed ungulates having either two or four digits, with the axis between the third and fourth; e.g., pig and hippopotamus with four; camel, deer, giraffe, antelope, and cow with two. [G. *artios,* even in number, + *daktylos,* finger]

ar·y·ep·i·glot·tic (ar′ē-ep-i-glot′ik). Relating to the arytenoid cartilage and the epiglottis; denoting a fold of mucous membrane (aryepiglottic fold) and a muscle contained in it (aryepiglottic muscle). SYN arytenoepiglottidean.

ar·yl (ar′il). An organic radical derived from an aromatic compound by removing a hydrogen atom.

a. acylamidase, an amidohydrolase cleaving the acyl group from an anilide by hydrolysis, producing aniline and an acid anion. SYN arylamidase.

ar·yl·am·i·dase (ar-il-am′i-dās). SYN *aryl* acylamidase.

ar·yl·ar·son·ic ac·id (ar′il-ar-son′ik). An arsonic acid containing an aryl radical; e.g., arsenilic acid.

ar·yl·sul·fa·tase (ar-il-sŭl′fă-tās). An enzyme that cleaves phenol sulfates, including cerebroside sulfates (i.e., a phenol sulfate + $H_2O \rightarrow$ a phenol + sulfate anion). Some a.'s are inhibited by sulfate (type II) and some are not (type I). SYN sulfatase (2).

ar·y·te·no·ep·i·glot·tid·e·an (a-rit′ĕ-nō-ep′i-glo-tid′ē-an). SYN aryepiglottic.

ar·y·te·noid (ar-i-tē′noyd) [TA]. Denoting a cartilage (arytenoid cartilage) and muscles (oblique and transverse arytenoid muscles) of the larynx. [see arytenoideus]

ar·y·te·noi·dec·to·my (ar′ĭ-tē-noy-dek′tō-mē). Excision of an arytenoid cartilage, usually in bilateral vocal fold paralysis, to improve breathing. [arytenoid + G. *ektomē,* excision]

ar·y·te·noi·de·us (ar-ĭ-tē-noy′dē-ŭs). SYN oblique arytenoid *muscle,* transverse arytenoid (*muscle*). [G. *arytainoeides,* ladle-shaped, applied to cartilage of the larynx, fr. *arytaina,* a ladle, + *eidos,* resemblance]

ar·yt·e·noi·di·tis (ă-rit′ĕ-noy-dī′tis). Inflammation of a cricoarytenoid joint, arytenoid cartilage, or its mucosal cover.

ar·y·te·noi·do·pexy (ar′ĭ-tĕ-noy′dō-pek′sē). Fixation by surgery of an arytenoid cartilage. [arytenoid + G. *pēxis,* fixation]

A.S. Abbreviation for *auris sinistra* [L.], left ear.

As Symbol for arsenic.

as·a·fet·i·da (as-ă-fet′i-dă). A gum resin, the inspissated exudate from the root of *Ferula foetida* (family Umbelliferae); malodorous material used as a repellent against dogs, cats, and rabbits, and formerly used as an antispasmodic; in Asia, used as a condiment and flavoring agent. [Pers. *aza,* mastic, + L. *fetidus,* fetid]

Asa·rum (as′ar-ŭm). A genus of plants of the family Aristolochiaceae. [L., fr. G. *asaron,* hazelwort]

A. canaden′se, an aromatic stimulant and diaphoretic. SYN Canada snakeroot, Indian ginger, wild ginger.

A. europae′um, an emetic and cathartic. SYN European snakeroot, hazelwort.

as·bes·toid (as-bes′toyd). SYN amianthoid.

as·bes·tos (as-bes′tŏs). The commercial product, after mining and processing, obtained from a family of fibrous hydrated silicates divided mineralogically into amphiboles (amosite, anthrophyllite, and crocidolite) and serpentines (chrysotile); it is virtually insoluble and is used to provide tensile strength and moldability, thermal insulation, and resistance to fire, heat, and corrosion; inhalation of a. particles can cause asbestosis, pleural plaques, pleural fibrosis, pleural effusion, mesothelioma, and lung cancer. [G. unquenchable; so called in the erroneous belief that when heated, it could not be quenched]

as·bes·to·sis (as-bes-tō′sis). Pneumoconiosis due to inhalation of asbestos fibers suspended in the ambient air; sometimes complicated by pleural mesothelioma or bronchogenic carcinoma; ferruginous bodies are the histologic hallmark of exposure to asbestos.

as·ca·ri·a·sis (as-kă-rī′ă-sis). Disease caused by infection with *Ascaris* or related ascarid nematodes. [G. *askaris,* an intestinal worm, + *-iasis,* condition]

as·car·i·cide (as-kar′i-sīd). **1.** Causing the death of ascarid nematodes. **2.** An agent having such properties. [ascarid + L. *caedo,* to kill]

as·ca·rid (as′kă-rid). **1.** A general name for any nematode of the family Ascarididae. **2.** Pertaining to such nematodes.

As·car·i·dae (as-kar′i-dē). Former spelling for Ascarididae.

As·car·i·da·ta (as-kă-rid′ă-tă). SYN Ascaridida.

As·ca·rid·i·da (as-kă-rid′i-dă). An order of nematode worms that includes many important human, domestic animal, and fowl parasites such as *Ascaris, Ascaridia, Subuluris, Heterakis,* and *Anisakis.* SYN Ascaridata, Ascarididea, Ascaridorida.

As·ca·rid·i·dae (as-kă-rid′i-dē). A family of large intestinal roundworms that includes the important nematode of humans, *Ascaris lumbricoides,* the abundant roundworm of swine, *Ascaris suum,* and the common ascarids of dogs and cats, *Toxocara* and *Toxascaris* species. [G. *askaris,* an intestinal worm]

As·car·i·did·ea (as-kar-i-did′ē-ă). SYN Ascaridida.

As·car·i·doi·dea (as-kă-ri-doy′dē-ă). Superfamily of stout, 3-lipped intestinal roundworms that includes the family Ascarididae.

as·car·i·dole (as-kar′i-dōl). A major constituent of oil of chenopodium; an anthelmintic.

As·car·i·dor·i·da (as-kări-dōr′i-dă). SYN Ascaridida.

As·ca·ris (as′kă-ris). A genus of large, heavy-bodied roundworms parasitic in the small intestine; abundant in humans and many other vertebrates. [G. *askaris,* an intestinal worm]

A. equo′rum, SYN *Parascaris equorum.*

🔲**A. lumbricoi′des,** a large roundworm of humans, one of the commonest human parasites (8–12 inches in length); various symptoms such as restlessness, fever, and sometimes diarrhea are attributed to its presence, but usually it causes no definite symptoms; the similar species, *A. suum* (or *A. lumbricoides suum*) is very common in swine, but is not readily transmitted to humans, and vice versa; the types are morphologically and immunologically similar but apparently are host-adapted types, considered distinct species or races.

As·ca·roi·dea (as-kă-roy′dē-ă). Former spelling for Ascaridoidea.

as·ca·ron (as-kă-ron). A toxic peptone present in helminths, especially the ascaridids; symptoms of a. poisoning are similar to those of anaphylactic shock. [G. *askaris,* an intestinal worm, + *hormōn,* pres. part. of *hormaō,* to excite]

As·ca·rops stron·gy·li·na (as′kă-rops stron-ji-lī′nă). A small bloodsucking worm found in the stomach of pigs and wild boars in many parts of the world. Larvae of this species develop in coprophagous beetles; worms adhere to the gastric mucosa of the pig, and may cause inflammation and ulceration in heavy infections. [G. *askaris,* an intestinal worm; *strongylos,* round]

as·cen·dens (as-sen′denz). Ascending. Going upward, ascending, toward a higher position. [L.]

ascen·sus (ă-sen′sŭs). A moving upward; having an abnormally high position. [L. ascent]

as·cer·tain·ment (as-ser-tān′ment). In epidemiological and genetic research, the method by which a person, pedigree, or cluster is brought to the attention of an investigator; has a bearing on the interpretation of segregation ratios, concordance rates, linkage analysis, and other probability features.

complete a., method by which all families with at least one affected individual in a population are certain or have an equal chance of being identified by survey or an appropriate random sampling technique.

incomplete a., method of locating affected individuals in which probability of locating any specific patient has a known value between 0 and 1. SYN truncate a.

single a., method of a. of locating affected individuals by hospital or clinic admission or another way in which probability of encountering the same family twice approaches zero; thus, the probability that a family will be ascertained is proportional to the number of affected members.

total a., method by which all members of a population at risk of a trait are discerned or equally likely to be contained in a sample thereof.

truncate a., SYN incomplete a.

Asc·hel·min·thes (ask-hel-min'thēz). A former phylum of the Metazoa that included the class Nematoda and a disparate assortment of other pseudocelomates, each now accorded separate phylum status; they are nonsegmented, bilaterally symmetric, and cylindric or filiform, with a pseudocele body cavity and rounded or pointed ends; they vary considerably in size, and the male is usually smaller than the female.

Ascher, Karl W., U.S. ophthalmologist, 1887–1971. SEE A. aqueous influx *phenomenon, syndrome*.

Aschner, Bernhard, Austrian gynecologist, 1883–1960. SEE A. *phenomenon, reflex;* A.-Dagnini *reflex*.

Aschoff, Karl Ludwig, German pathologist, 1866–1942. SEE A. *bodies,* under *body, nodules,* under *nodule; node* of A. and Tawara; Rokitansky-A. *sinuses,* under *sinus;* A. *cell*.

as·ci·tes (ă-sī'tēz). Accumulation of serous fluid in the peritoneal cavity. SYN abdominal dropsy, hydroperitoneum, hydroperitonia. [L. fr. G. *askos,* a bag, + *-ites*]

a. adipo'sus, SYN chylous a.

chyliform a., SYN chylous a.

chylous a., a. chylo'sus, presence in the peritoneal cavity of a milky fluid containing suspended fat, ordinarily caused by an obstruction or injury of the thoracic duct or cisterna. SYN a. adiposus, chyliform a., chyloperitoneum, fatty a., milky a.

fatty a., SYN chylous a.

gelatinous a., SYN *pseudomyxoma* peritonei.

hemorrhagic a., bloody or blood-stained serous fluid, frequently resulting from metastatic carcinoma, in the peritoneal cavity.

milky a., SYN chylous a.

pseudochylous a., presence in the peritoneum of an opalescent or cloudy fluid that does not contain fat.

ascit·ic (ă-sit'ik). Of or relating to ascites.

as·ci·tog·e·nous (as-i-toj'ĕ-nŭs). Producing ascites.

as·co·carp (as'kō-karp). A fungus structure, of varying complexity, which bears asci and ascospores. [G. *askos,* bag, + *karpos,* fruit]

as·cog·e·nous (as-koj'ĕ-nŭs). Denoting ascus-bearing fungus hypha or cell.

as·co·go·ni·um (as-kō-gō'nē-ŭm). The female cell in an ascomycete that is fertilized by the male cell.

Ascoli, Alberto, Italian serologist, 1877–1957. SEE Ascoli *reaction;* Ascoli *test*.

As·co·my·ce·tes (as'kō-mī-sē'tēz). A class of fungi characterized by the presence of asci and ascospores. Such fungi have generally two distinct reproductive phases, the sexual or perfect stage and the asexual or imperfect stage. *Ajellomyces capsulatum* and *Ajellomyces dermatitidis* are pathogenic members of this class. [G. *askos,* a bag, + *mykēs,* mushroom]

as·co·my·ce·tous (as'kō-mī'sē-tus). Fungi related to the Ascomycota.

As·co·my·co·ta (as'kō-mī-kō-tă). A phylum of fungi characterized by the presence of asci and ascospores. Some mycologists have moved the class Ascomycetes to the phylum or division level.

as·cor·base (as-kōr'bās). SYN *ascorbate* oxidase.

as·cor·bate (as-kōr'bāt). A salt or ester of ascorbic acid.

a. oxidase, a copper-containing enzyme that catalyzes the oxidation of L-ascorbic acid with O_2 to L-dehydroascorbic acid. Some forms of a. use $NADP^+$ as well. Used as an antitumor enzyme. SYN ascorbase.

ascor·bic ac·id (as-kōr'bik). Used in preventing scurvy, as a strong reducing agent, and as an antioxidant. SYN antiscorbutic vitamin, cevitamic acid, vitamin C. [G. *a-* priv. + Mod.L. *scorbutus,* scurvy, fr. Germanic]

ascor·byl pal·mi·tate (as-kōr'bil pal'mi-tāt). Used as a preservative in pharmaceutical preparations.

as·co·spore (as'kō-spōr). A spore formed within an ascus; the sexual spore of Ascomycetes. [G. *askos,* bag, + *sporos,* seed]

ASCUS In the Bethesda system, acronym for atypical squamous *cells* of undetermined significance, under *cell*. SEE ALSO Bethesda *system*.

as·cus, pl. **as·ci** (as'kŭs, as'ī). The saclike cell of Ascomycetes in which ascospores develop following nuclear fusion and meiosis. [G. *askos,* bag]

-ase. A termination denoting an enzyme, suffixed to the name of the substance (substrate) upon which the enzyme acts; e.g., phosphatase, lipase, proteinase. May also indicate the reaction catalyzed, e.g., decarboxylase, oxidase. Enzymes named before the convention was established generally have an -in ending; e.g., pepsin, ptyalin, trypsin. [Fr. *(diast)ase,* an amylase that converts starch to maltose, fr. G. *diastasis,* separation, fr. *dia-,* through, apart, + *stasis,* a standing]

ase·cre·to·ry (ā-sē-krē'tō-rē). Without secretion.

Aselli (Asellius, Asellio), Gasparo, Italian anatomist at Cremona, 1581–1626. SEE A. *pancreas*.

asep·sis (ă-sep'sis, ā-). A condition in which living pathogenic organisms are absent; a state of sterility (2). [G. *a-* priv. + *sēpsis,* putrefaction]

asep·tate (ă-sep'tāt, ā-). In fungi, a term describing absence of cross walls in a hyphal filament or a spore. [G. *a-* priv. + L. *saeptum,* a partition]

asep·tic (ă-sep'tik, ā-). Marked by or relating to asepsis.

asep·ti·cism (ă-sep'ti-sizm, ā-). The practice of aseptic surgery.

ase·quence (ă-sē'kwens). Lack of normal sequence, specifically, between atrial and ventricular contractions.

asex·u·al (ā-seks'ū-ăl). **1.** Referring to reproduction without nuclear fusion in an organism. **2.** Having no sexual desire or interest. [G. *a-* priv. + sexual]

Ashby, Winifred, 20th century hematologist. SEE Ashby *method*.

Asherman, Joseph G., Czechoslovakian gynecologist, *1889. SEE A. *syndrome*.

Ashman, R., 20th century U.S. physiologist. SEE A. *phenomenon*.

asialism (ā'syal-izm). Absence of saliva. [G. *a-* priv. + *sialon* saliva + -ism]

asi·a·lo·gly·co·pro·tein (ā-sī-al'ō-glī-kō-prō-tēn). A glycoprotein without a sialic acid moiety; such proteins are recognized by a. receptors and are targeted for degradation.

asit·ia (ă-sish'ē-ă). Disgust at the sight or thought of food. [G. *a-* priv. + *sitos,* food]

Askanazy, Max, German pathologist, 1865–1940. SEE A. *cell*.

Ask-Upmark, Erik., 20th century Swedish pathologist. SEE Ask-Upmark *kidney*.

ASL Abbreviation for American Sign *Language*.

Asn (Asx) Symbol for asparagine or its mono- or diradical.

aso·cial (ā-sō'shŭl). Not social; withdrawn from society; indifferent to social rules or customs; e.g., a recluse, a regressed schizophrenic person, a schizoid personality. Cf. antisocial.

aso·ma, pl. **aso·ma·ta** (ā-sō'mă, -sō'mă-tă). A fetus with only a rudimentary body. [G. *a-* priv. + *sōma,* body]

Asp (Asx) Symbol for aspartic acid or its radical forms.

as·pal·a·so·ma (as-pal-ă-sō'mă). Obsolete term for a malformed fetus with eventration at the lower part of the abdomen, presenting separate openings for intestine, bladder, and sexual organs. [G. *aspalax,* a mole + *soma,* body]

as·par·a·gi·nase (as-par'ă-ji-nās). **1.** An enzyme catalyzing the hydrolysis of L-asparagine to L-aspartic acid and ammonia. **2.** The enzyme from *Escherichia coli,* used in the treatment of acute leukemia and other neoplastic diseases.

***Erwinia* L-a.,** L-a. from *Erwinia* bacteria, used in patients who are allergic to *Escherichia coli* L-a. SEE ALSO asparaginase.

as·par·a·gine (N, Asn) (as-par'ă-jin). NH_2COCH_2CH ($NH_3^+COO^-$; the β-amide of aspartic acid, the L-isomer is a nutritionally nonessential amino acid occurring in proteins; a diuretic.

a. ligase, an acid:ammonia ligase (amide synthetase) forming L-asparagine and L-glutamate from L-aspartate and L-glutamine, with the concomitant cleavage of ATP to AMP and pyrophosphate. Under nonphysiological conditions, the mammalian enzyme can use ammonia as the nitrogen donor. A. also displays a glutaminase-like activity. SYN a. synthetase.

a. synthetase, SYN a. ligase.

as·pa·rag·i·nyl (as-par′ă-jin-il). The aminoacyl radical of asparagine.

As·par·a·gus (as-par′ă-gŭs). A genus of plants of the family Liliaceae. *A. officinalis* is an edible vegetable, the rhizome and roots of which, together with the young edible shoots, were used as a diuretic. [L. fr. G. *asparagos*]

as·par·tame (as′par-tām). A low-calorie sweetening agent about 200 times as sweet as sucrose used by persons who must restrict sugar and caloric intake.

as·par·tase (as-par′tās). SYN *aspartate* ammonia-lyase.

as·par·tate (as-par′tāt). A salt or ester of aspartic acid.

a. aminotransferase (AST), an enzyme catalyzing the reversible transfer of an amine group from L-glutamic acid to oxaloacetic acid, forming α-ketoglutaric acid and L-aspartic acid; a diagnostic aid in viral hepatitis and in myocardial infarction. SYN a. transaminase, glutamic-aspartic transaminase, glutamic-oxaloacetic transaminase, serum glutamic-oxaloacetic transaminase.

a. ammonia-lyase, a nonmammalian enzyme catalyzing the conversion of L-aspartic acid to fumaric acid, splitting out ammonia. SYN aspartase, fumaric aminase.

a. carbamoyltransferase, an enzyme catalyzing formation of ureidosuccinate (*N*-carbamoyl-L-aspartate) and orthophosphate by the transfer of a carbamoyl moiety from carbamoylphosphate to the amino group of L-aspartate; participates in pyrimidine biosynthesis.

a. kinase, an enzyme catalyzing the phosphorylation by ATP of L-aspartate to form 4-phospho-L-aspartate (β-aspartyl phosphate) and ADP.

a. transaminase, SYN a. aminotransferase.

as·par·tate 1-de·car·box·yl·ase. SYN *glutamate* decarboxylase.

as·par·tate 4-de·car·box·yl·ase. Aspartate β-decarboxylase; a carboxy-lyase converting L-aspartate to L-alanine (releasing CO_2); it decarboxylates aminomalonate and (in bacteria) removes SO_2 from cysteinesulfinate. SEE ALSO desulfinase.

as·par·tic ac·id (Asp) (as-par′tik). $HOOC–CH_2–CH(NH_2)–COOH$; the L-isomer is one of the amino acids occurring naturally in proteins. The D-isomer is found in cell walls of many bacteria.

as·par·tyl (as-par′til). The aminoacyl radical of aspartic acid.

β-as·par·tyl(ace·tyl·glu·cos·a·mine) (as-par′til-as′e-til-gloo′kō-să-mēn). Misnomer for 1-(β-asparagino)-*N*-acetylglucosamine or 1-(β-aspartamido)-*N*-acetylglucosamine, or, formally, 1-(β-L-aspartamido)-*N*-2-acetamido-1,2-dideoxy-β-D-glucose; a compound of *N*-acetylglucosamine and asparagine, linked via the amide nitrogen of the latter and carbon-1 of the former. An important structural linkage in many glycoproteins. Elevated levels are found in certain cases of progressive mental retardation.

as·par·tyl·gly·co·sa·mine (as-par′til-glī′kō-să-mēn). Generic term for compounds of asparagine and a 2-amino sugar; e.g., β-aspartyl(acetylglucosamine).

as·par·tyl·gly·cos·a·mi·nid·ase (as-par′til-glī′kō-să-mi-ni-dās). A hydrolytic enzyme that cleaves off L-aspartate from aspartylglycosamines. A deficiency of a. can result in aspartylglycosaminuria.

as·par·tyl·gly·cos·a·mi·nu·ria (as-par′til-glī′kō-să-mi-noor′ē-ă) [MIM*208400]. A lysosomal disorder due to deficiency of aspartoglucosaminidase, resulting in accumulation of aspartlyglycosamine in the urine and spinal fluid; characterized by symptoms usually in the first few months of life, with recurrent infections and diarrhea; mental retardation, seizures, coarse facial features, and skeletal abnormalities are evident by adolescence. Autosomal recessive inheritance, caused by mutation in the aspartoglucosaminidase gene (AGA) on 4q.

as·pect (as′pekt). **1.** The manner of appearance; looks. **2.** The side

of an object that is directed in any designated direction. SYN norma (1). [L. *aspectus,* fr. *a-spicio,* pp. *-spectus,* to look at]

facial a. [TA], the outline of the skull viewed from in front. SYN norma facialis [TA], frontal a.*, norma frontalis*, norma anterior.

frontal a., *official alternate term for facial a.

lateral a. [TA], the profile of the skull; the outline of the skull viewed from either side. SYN norma lateralis [TA], norma temporalis.

occipital a. [TA], the outline of the skull viewed from behind. SYN norma occipitalis [TA], norma posterior.

superior a., the outline of the surface of the skull viewed from above. SYN norma superior [TA], norma verticalis*, vertical a.*.

vertical a., *official alternate term for superior a.

Asperger, Hans, 20th century Austrian psychiatrist. SEE A. *disorder.*

as·per·gil·lic ac·id (as-per-jil′ik). Produced by *Aspergillus flavus;* an antibiotic agent moderately active against Gram-positive and Gram-negative bacteria, but toxic to animal tissues.

as·per·gil·lin (as-per-jil′in). A black pigment obtained from various species of *Aspergillus;* improperly used to designate various antibiotics obtained from *Aspergillus.*

as·per·gil·lo·ma (as′per-ji-lō′mă). A ball-like mass of *Aspergillis* hyphae colonizing an existing cavity in the lung. [aspergillus + -oma, tumor]

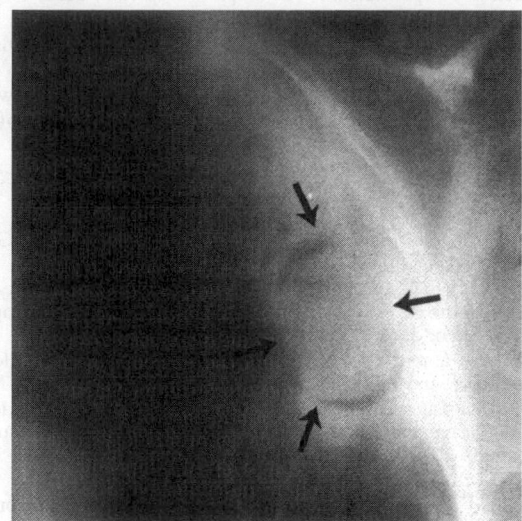

aspergilloma: tomogram showing fungal mass in a preexisting pulmonary cavity resulting from tuberculosis

as·per·gil·lo·sis (as′per-ji-lō′sis). The presence of the fungus *Aspergillus* in the tissues or invading tissue (invasive a.) or colonizing air-containing body cavities. SEE ALSO aspergilloma.

acute invasive a., an aggressive infection, particularly in severely immunocompromised people, which consists of invasion of blood vessels and tissue infarction by *Aspergillus fumigatus.* The disease often mimics the signs and symptoms of acute bacterial pneumonia.

allergic bronchopulmonary a., a disease in which the fungus grows in mucus (evoked by inflammation), which may be expectorated as yellow bronchial casts and cause intermittent bronchial obstruction, with transient infiltrates seen radiographically; asthma is often present, and bronchial wall destruction may eventually result in a proximal form of bronchiectasis.

chronic necrotizing a., an indolent but slowly progressive infection of the lungs in patients with underlying lung disease, caused by aspergillus. Most affected patients have a modest depression of the immune system, caused by diseases such as diabetes.

disseminated a., a variety of bronchopulmonary a., characterized by a generalized infection of the lung with *Aspergillus* occurring usually in subjects with defective immune response.

▪**As·per·gil·lus** (as-per-jil′ŭs). A genus of fungi (class Ascomycetes) that contains many species, a number of them with black, brown, or green spores. A few species are pathogenic for humans, avians, and other animals. There are about 300 species in this genus. [Med. L. a sprinkler, fr. L. *aspergo*, to sprinkle]

A. clava′tus, a fungal species isolated from soil and feces; it yields a carcinogenic mycotoxin known as patulin.

A. fla′vus, a fungal species with yellow-green conidia that is found growing on grains; may produce aflatoxin, which is the cause of aflatoxicosis in poultry and cattle, and is carcinogenic for rats and possibly humans; causes invasive aspergillosis in humans and animals.

A. fumiga′tus, a fungal species that yields the antibiotics fumigacin and fumigatin, and is the common cause of aspergillosis in humans and birds.

A. nid′ulans, a species that causes one form of mycetoma, and occasionally causes aspergillosis in humans and other animals.

A. ni′ger, a species with black spores, often present in the external auditory meatus but rarely pathogenic; used in the commercial manufacturing of citric and gluconic acids.

A. ter′reus, a species that produces the antibiotic citrinin; it has been isolated from otomycosis, especially in Japan and Taiwan, and occasionally causes aspergillosis in humans and animals.

asper·mat·o·gen·ic (ā-sper′mă-tō-jen′ik, ă-sper′). Failing in the production of spermatozoa. [G. *a*- priv. + *sperma*, seed, + *-gen*, production]

asper·mia (ā-sper′mē-ă, ă-sper′). Lack of secretion or expulsion of semen following ejaculation.

as·per·sion (as-per′zhŭn). A form of hydrotherapy in which water of a given temperature is sprinkled on the body. [L. *aspersio*, a sprinkling]

aspher·ic (ā-sfer′ik). Denoting a paraboloidal surface, especially of a lens or mirror, that eliminates spherical aberration. [G. *a*-priv. + *sphaira*, sphere]

as·phyg·mia (as-fig′mē-ă). Temporary absence of pulse. [G. *a*-priv. + *sphygmos*, pulse]

as·phyx·ia (as-fik′sē-ă). Impaired or absent exchange of oxygen and carbon dioxide on a ventilatory basis; combined hypercapnia and hypoxia or anoxia. [G. *a*- priv. + *sphyzō*, to throb]

cyanotic a., a. to the point of sufficient destruction of hemoglobin to produce cyanosis.

local a., stagnation of the circulation, sometimes resulting in local gangrene, especially of the fingers; one of the symptoms usually associated with Raynaud disease.

symmetric a., SYN Raynaud *syndrome*.

traumatic a., cyanotic a. due to trauma; the extravasation of blood into the skin and conjunctivae, produced by a sudden mechanical increase in venous pressure, analogous to the Rumpel-Leede test; it is common in those who have been hanged, and is seen occasionally in crush injuries. SYN pressure stasis.

as·phyx·i·al (as-fik′sē-ăl). Relating to asphyxia.

as·phyx·i·ant (as-fik′sē-ănt). **1.** Producing asphyxia. SYN asphyxiating. **2.** Anything, especially a gas, that produces asphyxia.

as·phyx·i·ate (as-fik′sē-āt). To induce asphyxia.

as·phyx·i·at·ing (as-fik′sē-āt-ing). SYN asphyxiant (1).

as·phyx·i·a·tion (as-fik-sē-ā′shŭn). The production of, or the state of, asphyxia.

As·pic·u·lu·ris tet·rap·tera (as-pik-ū-loo′ris tet-rap′ter-ă). The mouse pinworm, an abundant oxyurid nematode of the mouse cecum or large intestine, along with another common oxyurid pinworm of mice, *Syphacia obvelata;* it is also found in other rodents, including *Rattus*. [Pers. *espic*, fr. L. *spica*, ear, spike; *tetra-* + *pteron*, feather, wing]

as·pid·in (as-pid′in). A toxic active principle, $C_{25}H_{32}O_8$, contained in aspidium.

as·pid·i·nol (as-pid′i-nol). An alcohol, $C_{12}H_{16}O_4$, occurring in aspidium.

as·pid·i·um (as-pid′ē-ŭm). The rhizomes and stipes of *Dryopteris filix-mas* (European a. or male fern), or of *Dryopteris marginalis*

(American a. or marginal fern, family Polypodiaceae); used in the treatment of tapeworm infestation, usually in the form of the oleoresin or extract, but because of its potential toxicity, its use is restricted to patients who do not respond to treatment with safer drugs such as dichlorophen, niclosamide, or quinacrine. [G. *aspidion*, a little shield, dim. of *aspis*, shield]

as·pi·do·sam·ine (as′pi-dō-sam′ēn). A strong base, $C_{22}H_{28}N_2O_2$, derived from quebracho; a toxic irritant.

as·pi·do·sper·mine (as′pi-dō-sper′mēn). An alkaloid, $C_{22}H_{30}N_2O_2$, obtained from quebracho, an irritant.

as·pi·rate. 1 (as′pi-rāt′). To remove by aspiration. **2** (as′pi-rāt′). To inhale into the airways foreign particulate material, such as vomitus. **3** (as′ pi-rit). Foreign body, food, gastric contents, or fluid, including saliva that is inhaled. [L. *a-spiro*, pp. *-atus*, to breathe on, give the H sound]

as·pi·ra·tion (as-pi-rā′shŭn). **1.** Removal, by suction, of a gas, fluid, or tissue from a body cavity or organ from unusual accumulations, or from a container. **2.** The inspiratory sucking into the airways of fluid or any foreign material, especially gastric contents or food. **3.** A surgical technique for cataract, requiring a small corneal incision, severance of the lens capsule, fragmentation of the lens material, and removal with a needle. [L. *aspiratio*, fr. *aspiro*, to breathe on]

meconium a., intrauterine a. by the fetus of amniotic fluid contaminated by meconium resulting from fetal hypoxic distress.

as·pi·ra·tor (as′pi-rā-ter, -tōr). An apparatus for removing fluid, air, or tissue by aspiration from any of the body cavities; it consists usually of a hollow needle or trocar and cannula, connected by tubing with a container vacuumized by a syringe or reversed air (suction) pump.

vacuum a., an instrument for removing the products of conception by suction after cervical dilation.

water a., a jet ejector pump operated by water and commonly used as a laboratory suction pump.

as·pi·rin (as′pi-rin). A widely used analgesic, antipyretic, and anti-inflammatory agent; also used as an antiplatelet agent. SYN acetylsalicylic acid.

asple·nia (ā-splē′nē-ă). Congenital or acquired absence of the spleen (e.g., after surgical removal).

functional a., absence of splenic function due to spontaneous infarction of the spleen, as occurs in sickle cell *anemia*.

a. with cardiovascular anomalies, SYN polysplenia.

asplen·ic (ā-splen′ik). Having no spleen.

aspo·rog·e·nous (as-pō-roj′ĕ-nŭs). Not producing spores. [G. *a*-priv. + *sporos*, seed, + *-gen*, production]

aspo·rous (as-pōr′ŭs). Incapable of producing spores. [G. *a*- priv. + *sporos*, seed]

aspor·u·late (as-pōr′ū-lāt). Nonsporeforming.

as·say (as′sā, ă-sā′). **1.** The quantitative or qualitative evaluation of a substance for impurities, toxicity, etc; the results of such an evaluation. **2.** To examine; to subject to analysis. **3.** Test of purity; trial. [M.E., fr. O.Fr. *essaier*, fr. L.L. *exagium*, a weighing]

Ames a., SYN Ames *test*.

biologic a., SYN biotest.

clonogenic a., in vitro culturing of neoplastic cells to test their radiosensitivity or chemosensitivity, and probable clinical efficacy of a therapeutic agent.

competitive binding a., general term for an a. in which a substance competes for labeled versus unlabeled ligand; following separation of free and bound ligand, the concentration of unlabeled ligand is inversely proportional to the amount of labeled bound ligand. Values are compared to known standards. SEE ALSO enzyme-linked immunosorbent a., radioreceptor a., immunoassay, enzyme-multiplied *immunoassay* technique, radioimmunoassay. SYN displacement analysis, saturation analysis.

complement binding a., SYN complement *fixation*.

double antibody sandwich a., for antigen; an application of the ELISA method in which material being tested for antigen is added to wells coated with known antibody; the presence of antigen fixed to the antibody coat can be determined either directly, by adding antibody linked to the enzyme of the indicator system, or indirectly, by first adding unlabeled known antibody, the attachment of which to the antigen can be demonstrated by addition of immunoglobulin-specific antibody linked to the enzyme.

EAC rosette a. (ro-zet′ as′sā), SEE EAC *rosette.*

enzyme-linked immunosorbent a. (ELISA), an in vitro binding a. in which an enzyme and its substrate (rather than a radioactive substance) serve as the indicator system; in positive tests, the two yield a colored or other easily recognizable substance; tests are made in wells in polystyrene or other material to which immunoglobulins or antigenic preparations readily adsorb; the enzyme is linked to known immunoglobulin (or antigen) and in positive tests remains in the well as part of the antigen-antibody complex available to react with its substrate when added.

Grunstein-Hogness a., a procedure for identifying plasmid clones by colony hybridization.

hemizona a. (hem′ē-zō-nă), diagnostic test evaluating the binding capacity of sperm to the zona pellucida.

hemolytic plaque a., SYN Jerne plaque a.

immunochemical a., SYN immunoassay.

immunoradiometric a., an a. that differs from conventional radioimmunoassay in that the compound to be measured combines directly with radioactively labeled antibodies.

indirect a., for antibody; an application of the ELISA method in which serum being tested for antibody is added to wells coated with known antigen; presence of antibody bound to the antigen coat can be determined by addition of immunoglobulin-specific antibody to which is linked the enzyme of the indicator system, followed by addition of substrate to the washed aggregate.

Jerne plaque a., an a. that enumerates individual antibody-forming cells. SYN hemolytic plaque a.

Lowry-Folin a., SYN Lowry protein a.

Lowry protein a., a method for determining protein concentrations using the Folin-Ciocalteu reagent. SYN Lowry-Folin a.

radioreceptor a., a competitive binding a. in which the binder is a membrane or tissue receptor rather than an antibody.

Raji cell radioimmune a., for immune complexes; a procedure by which immune complexes adsorbed from a test serum by a standard preparation of lymphoblastoid (Raji) cells are assayed by the capacity to bind ^{125}I-labeled antibody to immunoglobulin.

assessment. Appraisal.

health risk a. (h.r.a.), method of describing an individual's chance of falling ill or dying of a specified condition, based on actuarial calculations that compare chance of acquiring condition with that of general population expressed as expected age at which death or disease will occur, and intended as a way of drawing an individual's attention to the probable health consequences of risk behavior.

Asségzat, Jules, French anthropologist, 1832–1876. SEE A. *triangle.*

as·sim·i·la·ble (ă-sim′i-lă-bl). Capable of undergoing assimilation. SEE assimilation.

as·sim·i·la·tion (ă-sim-i-lā′shŭn). **1.** Incorporation of digested materials from food into the tissues. **2.** Amalgamation and modification of newly perceived information and experiences into the existing cognitive structure. [L. *as-similo,* pp. *-atus,* to make alike]

ammonia a., the utilization of ammonia (or ammonium ions) in the net synthesis of nitrogen-containing molecules, e.g., glutamine synthetase. SYN ammonia fixation.

reproductive a., in sensorimotor theory, an active cognitive process by which past experience is applied to novel situations.

Assmann, Herbert, German internist, 1882–1950. SEE A. tuberculous *infiltrate.*

as·so·ci·ate. 1 (ă-sō′shi-ăt). Any item or individual grouped with others by some common factor. **2** (ă-sō′shē-āt). To accomplish association.

paired a.'s, words, syllables, digits, or other items learned in pairs, so that when one is given, its a. is to be recalled.

as·so·ci·a·tion (ă-sō-sē-ā′shŭn). **1.** A connection of persons, things, or ideas by some common factor. **2.** A functional connection of two ideas, events, or psychologic phenomena established through learning or experience. SEE ALSO conditioning. **3.** Statistical dependence between two or more events, characteristics, or other variables. **4.** In medical genetics, a grouping of congenital anomalies found together more frequently than otherwise expected; the use of this term implies that the cause is unknown. [L. *associo,* pp. *-sociatus,* to join to; *ad* + *socius,* companion]

CHARGE a., a particular grouping of congenital anomalies found together more frequently than otherwise expected. Affected patients have *c*oloboma of the eye, *h*eart defects (typically tetralogy of Fallot, patent ductus arteriosus, or ventricular or atrial septal defect), *a*tresia of the choanae, *r*enal anomalies and retardation of *g*rowth and/or development, *g*enital anomalies in males such as small penis or cryptorchidism, and *e*ar abnormalities or deafness. SYN CHARGE syndrome.

clang a., psychic a.'s resulting from sounds; often encountered in the manic phase of manic-depressive psychosis.

dream a.'s, the memories and emotions mentioned by a patient trying to understand a dream at the request of a psychoanalyst.

free a., an investigative psychoanalytic technique in which the patient verbalizes, without reservation or censor, the passing contents of his or her mind; the verbalized conflicts that emerge constitute resistances that are the basis of the psychoanalyst's interpretations.

genetic a., the occurrence together in a population, more often than can be readily explained by chance, of two or more traits of which at least one is known to be genetic.

independent practice a. (IPA), an a. of independent physicians or small groups of physicians formed for the purpose of contracting with one or more managed health care organizations. Member physicians provide medical services for HMO patients in their own offices and are allowed to maintain private practices. SEE ALSO managed *care,* health maintenance *organization.*

loose a.'s, a manifestation of a thought disorder whereby the patient's responses do not relate to the interviewer's questions or one paragraph, sentence, or phrase is not logically connected to those that occur before or after.

as·so·ci·a·tion·ism (ă-sō-sē-ā′shŭn-izm). In psychology, the theory that man's understanding of the world occurs through ideas associated with sensory experience rather than through innate ideas.

as·sort·ment (ă-sōrt′ment). In genetics, the relationship between nonallelic genetic traits that are transmitted from parent to child more or less independently in accordance with the degree of linkage between the respective loci.

independent a., the pattern of transmission of unlinked loci.

as·sump·tion. Belief posited at the outset of an argument as a basis for deduction and inference. Commonly confused with a hypothesis, a conclusion at the end of the argument or an inference based on empirical data.

AST Abbreviation for *aspartate* aminotransferase.

asta·sia (ă-stā′zē-ă). Inability, through muscular incoordination, to stand. [G. unsteadiness, from *a-*priv. + *stasis,* standing]

asta·sia-aba·sia (ă-stā′zē-ă-ă-bā′zē-ă). The inability to either stand or walk in a normal manner; the gait is bizarre and is not suggestive of a specific organic lesion; often the patient sways wildly and nearly falls, but recovers at the last moment; a symptom of hysteria-conversion reaction. SYN Blocq disease.

astat·ic (ā-stat′ik). Pertaining to astasia.

as·ta·tine (At) (as′tă-tēn). An artificial radioactive element of the halogen series; atomic no. 85, atomic wt. 211. [G. *astatos,* unstable]

aste·a·to·sis (ă-stē-ă-tō′sis). Diminished or arrested secretion of the sebaceous glands. [G. *a-* priv. + *stear* (steat-), fat]

a. cu′tis, dry, scaly integument with decrease in sebaceous secretion.

astem·i·zole. An H-1 type histamine-blocking drug with low sedating tendency.

as·ter (as′ter). SYN astrosphere. [Mod. L. fr. G. *astēr,* a star]

sperm a., SEE sperm-aster.

aster·e·og·no·sis (ă-stēr-og-nō′sis). SYN tactile *agnosia.* [G. *a-* priv. + *stereos,* solid + *gnōsis,* knowledge]

as·te·ri·on (ăs-tē′rē-on) [TA]. A craniometric point in the region of the posterolateral, or mastoid, fontanel, at the junction of the lambdoid, occipitomastoid and parietomastoid sutures. [G. *asterios,* starry]

as·ter·i·o·sap·on·ins (ă-stēr′ē-ō-sap′ō-ninz). SYN asteriotoxins.

as·ter·i·o·tox·ins (ă-stēr′ē-ō-tok′sinz). Toxic steroids produced by starfish (Asteroidea). SYN asteriosaponins.

aster·ix·is (as-ter-ik′sis). Involuntary jerking movements, especially in the hands, best elicited by having the patient extend the arms, dorsiflex the wrists, and spread the fingers; due to arrhythmic lapses of sustained posture; seen primarily with various metabolic and toxic encephalopathies, especially hepatic encephalopathy. SYN flapping tremor. [G. *a-* priv. + *stērixis,* fixed position]

aster·nal (ā-ster′năl). **1.** Not related to or connected with the sternum, e.g., a. rib. **2.** Without a sternum. [G. *a-* priv. + *sternon,* chest]

aster·nia (ă-ster′nē-ă). Congenital absence of the sternum.

As·ter·o·coc·cus. SYN *Mycoplasma.* [Mod. L. fr. G. *astēr,* a star, + *kokkos,* a berry]

as·ter·oid (as′tĕ-royd). Resembling a star. [G. *astēr,* star, + *eidos,* resemblance]

as·the·nia (as-thē′nē-ă). Weakness or debility. SYN adynamia (1). [G. *astheneia,* weakness, fr. *a-* priv. + *sthenos,* strength]

neurocirculatory a., an obsolete term for a type of anxiety neurosis formerly encountered often among military personnel during times of war, in which cardiorespiratory symptoms, such as palpitation, rapid pulse, and precordial pain, were prominent.

as·then·ic (as-then′ik). **1.** Relating to asthenia. **2.** Denoting a thin, delicate body habitus.

as·the·no·pia (as-thĕ-nō′pē-ă). Subjective symptoms of ocular fatigue, discomfort, lacrimation, and headaches arising from use of the eyes. SYN eyestrain. [G. *astheneia,* weakness, + *ōps,* eye]

accommodative a., a. due to errors of refraction and excessive contraction of the ciliary muscle.

muscular a., a. due to imbalance of the extrinsic ocular muscles.

nervous a., a. due to functional or organic nervous disease.

as·the·nop·ic (as-thĕ-nop′ik). Relating to or suffering from asthenopia.

as·the·no·sper·mia (as-thē-nō-sper′mē-ă). SYN asthenozoospermia. [G. *astheneia,* weakness, + *sperma,* seed, semen]

asthenozoospermia (as′thē-nō-zō-ō-sperm′ē-ă). Loss or reduction of mobility of the spermatozoa, frequently associated with infertility. SYN asthenospermia. [G. *astheneia,* weakness + *zōos,* living, + *sperma,* seed, semen, + -ia]

■ **asth·ma** (az′mă). An inflammatory disease of the lungs characterized by reversible (in most cases) airway obstruction. Originally, a term used to mean "difficult breathing"; now used to denote bronchial a. SYN reactive airway disease. [G.]

atopic a., bronchial a. due to atopy.

---

bronchial a., an acute or chronic disorder characterized by widespread and largely reversible reduction in the caliber of bronchi and bronchioles, due in varying degrees to smooth muscle spasm, mucosal edema, and excessive mucus in the lumens of airways; cardinal symptoms are dyspnea, wheezing, and cough; attacks or exacerbations may be induced by airborne allergens (e.g., molds, pollens, animal dander, dust mite and cockroach antigens), inhaled irritants (e.g., cold air, cigarette smoke, ozone), physical exercise, respiratory infection, psychological stress, or other factors; the signs and symptoms of bronchial a. are caused by the local release of spasmogens and inflammatory mediators (histamines, leukotrienes, prostaglandins) and other substances from mast cells, eosinophils, lymphocytes, neutrophils, and epithelial cells; airway caliber may be abruptly and drastically reduced during a paroxysm or after diagnostic challenge with methacholine or histamine, and may quickly return to normal after administration of a bronchodilator (inhaled β-adrenergic agonist or subcutaneous epinephrine)

Asthma is a common disease, with an incidence of about 5% in the U.S., and a leading cause of disease and disability in persons between 2 and 17 years of age. It is respon-

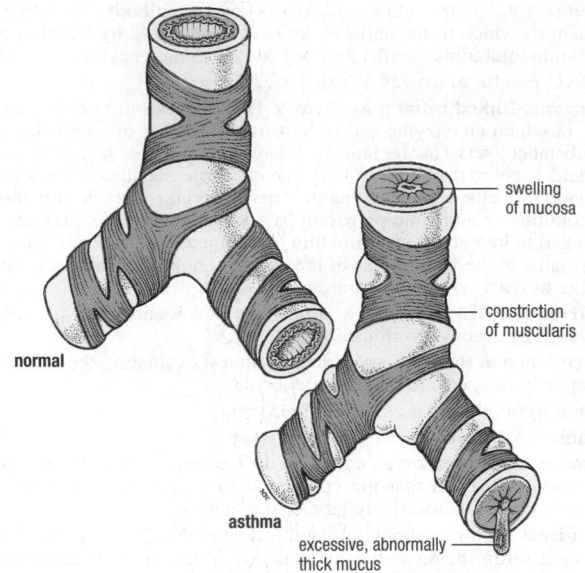

swelling of mucosa

constriction of muscularis

normal

asthma

excessive, abnormally thick mucus

asthma: showing changes in bronchiole during asthma attack

---

sible for 14.5 million outpatient visits and 5000 deaths yearly in this country. From 1980 to 1994 the prevalence of asthma increased 75%; the greatest increase (160%) occurred in children under age 5. Asthma first occurring in childhood is more likely to be allergic in origin and to show seasonal variation. Chronic sinusitis and gastroesophageal reflux disease are statistically correlated with asthma. A subset of people with allergic asthma also have nasal polyps and sensitivity to aspirin and most other nonsteroidal antiinflammatory drugs. Occupational exposure to airborne irritants or allergens is increasingly recognized as a cause of chronic asthma in adults. Current views of the pathophysiology of asthma emphasize its inflammatory component and the risk of gradual, irreversible airway remodeling due to subepithelial fibrosis in poorly controlled asthma. Current recommendations for treatment of chronic or severe asthma call for use of antiinflammatory drugs (particularly inhaled corticosteroids). Other treatments include β₂-adrenergic bronchodilators (albuterol, terbutaline, salmeterol), xanthines (theophylline, oxtriphylline, dyphylline), mast cell stabilizers (cromolyn, nedocromil), and antileukotrienes (montelukast, zafirlukast, zileuton). Self-monitoring of peak respiratory flow rate with a simple portable device helps patients adjust drug doses for optimum effect. Avoidance of allergens, irritants, and other known triggers is essential to good control.

---

bronchitic a., a. precipitated by bronchitis. SYN catarrhal a.

cardiac a., an asthmatic attack, the bronchoconstriction being secondary to the pulmonary congestion and edema of left ventricular failure.

catarrhal a., SYN bronchitic a.

cotton-dust a., SYN byssinosis.

dust a., a. aggravated by inhalation of dust, especially seen as occupational disease resulting from cotton dust.

extrinsic a., bronchial a. resulting from an allergic reaction to foreign substances, such as inhaled particles, vapors, or gases, or ingested foods, beverages, or drugs.

food a., a. caused by allergic reaction to a dietary item.

hay a., an asthmatic stage of hay fever.

intrinsic a., bronchial a. in which no extrinsic causes can be identified, and which is assumed to be due to an endogenous process, possibly allergic.

miller a., a. caused by flour or grain allergens.

miner's a., the dyspnea of anthracosis or other pneumoconioses in miners.

nervous a., a. precipitated by psychic stress.

reflex a., a. occurring as a reflex in disease of the viscera, the nose, or other parts.

spasmodic a., a. due to spasm of the bronchioles.

steam-fitter's a., a. associated with asbestosis acquired by exposure to asbestos-insulated heating and plumbing components.

stripper's a., a. associated with byssinosis.

summer a., a. associated with hay fever or allergy to summer vegetation.

triad a., syndrome comprising nasal polyps, asthma, and intolerance to aspirin.

asth·mat·ic (az-mat′ik). Relating to or suffering from asthma.

asth·ma-weed. 1. SYN lobelia. **2.** SYN *Euphorbia pilulifera.*

asth·mo·gen·ic (az′mō-jen′ik). Causing asthma.

as·tig·mat·ic (as′tig-mat′ik). Relating to or suffering from astigmatism.

astig·ma·tism (ă-stig′mă-tizm). **1.** A lens or optical system having different refractivity in different meridians. **2.** A condition of unequal curvatures along the different meridians in one or more of the refractive surfaces (cornea, anterior or posterior surface of the lens) of the eye, in consequence of which the rays from a luminous point are not focused at a single point on the retina. SYN astigmia. [G. *a-* priv. + *stigma* (*stigmat-*), a point]

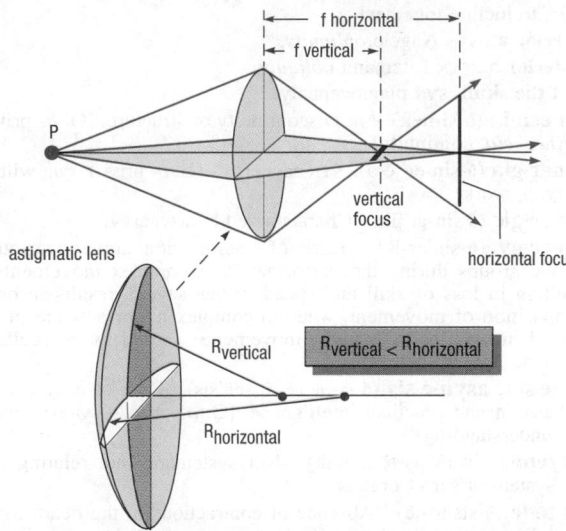

astigmatism: in an astigmatic lens, the curvatures (R) in the two meridians are unequal; thus the lens has two different focal distances and a point P appears as a line (horizontal and vertical focus); in the region between the two focal points, P appears as an ellipse

a. against the rule, a. when the greater curvature or refractive power is in the horizontal meridian.

compound hyperopic a., a. in which all meridians are hyperopic but to different degrees.

compound myopic a., a. in which all meridians are myopic but to different degrees.

corneal a., a. due to a defect in the curvature of the corneal surface.

hyperopic a., that form of a. in which one meridian is hyperopic and the one at a right angle to it is without a refractive error. SYN simple hyperopic a.

irregular a., a. in which different parts of the same meridian have different degrees of curvature.

lenticular a., a. due to defect in the curvature, position, or index of refraction of the lens.

mixed a., a. in which one meridian is hyperopic while the one at right angle to it is myopic.

myopic a., that form of a. in which one meridian is myopic and the one at right angle to it is without refractive error. SYN simple myopic a.

a. of oblique pencils, an aberration occurring when a bundle of light rays strikes a refracting medium in some other direction than parallel to the axis of the lens.

regular a., a. in which the curvature in each meridian is equal throughout its course, and the meridians of greatest and least curvature are at right angles to each other.

simple hyperopic a., SYN hyperopic a.

simple myopic a., SYN myopic a.

a. with the rule, a. when the greater curvature or refractive power is in the vertical meridian.

astig·ma·tom·e·try, as·tig·mom·e·try (ă-stig-mă-tom′ĕ-trē, as-tig-mom′ĕ-trē). Determination of the form and measurement of the degree of astigmatism.

astig·mia (ă-stig′mē-ă). SYN astigmatism.

asto·ma·tous (ă-stō′mă-tŭs). Without a mouth. SYN astomous.

asto·mia (ă-stō′mē-ă). Congenital absence of a mouth. [G. *a-* priv. + *stoma,* mouth]

asto·mous (ă-stō′mŭs). SYN astomatous.

as·trag·a·lar (as-trag′ă-lar). Relating to the astragalus or talus.

as·trag·a·lec·to·my (as-trag-ă-lek′tō-mē). Removal of the astragalus, or talus. [astragalus, + G. *ektomē,* excision]

as·trag·a·lo·cal·ca·ne·an (as-trag′ă-lō-kal-kā′nē-an). Relating to both the talus (astragalus) and the calcaneus (os calcis).

as·trag·a·lo·fib·u·lar (as-trag′ă-lō-fib′ū-lar). Relating to both the talus (astragalus) and the fibula.

as·trag·a·lo·scaph·oid (as-trag′ă-lō-scaf′oyd). SYN talonavicular.

as·trag·a·lo·tib·i·al (as-trag′ă-lō-tib′ē-ăl). Relating to both the talus (astragalus) and the tibia.

As·trag·a·lus (as-trag′ă-lŭs). A genus of plants (family Leguminosae), notably *A. mollissimus* (locoweed) on the range lands of western North America, capable of taking selenium from the soil and causing poisoning in sheep, cattle, and horses. *A. gummifer* is a source of tragacanth.

as·tral (as′trăl). Relating to an astrosphere.

as·tra·po·pho·bia (as′tră-pō-fō′bē-ă). Morbid fear of lightning. [G. *astrapē,* lightning, + *phobos,* fear]

as·tric·tion (as-trik′shŭn). **1.** Astringent action. **2.** Compression to arrest hemorrhage.

as·trin·gent (as-trin′jent). **1.** Causing contraction or shrinkage of the tissues, arrest of secretion, or control of bleeding. **2.** An agent having these effects. [L. *astringens*]

as·tro·blast (as′trō-blast). A primitive cell developing into an astrocyte. [G. *astron,* star, + *blastos,* germ]

as·tro·blas·to·ma (as′trō-blas-tō′mă). A relatively poorly differentiated glioma composed of young, immature, neoplastic cells of the astrocytic series, frequently arranged radially with short fibrils terminating on small blood vessels. [astro- + G. *blastos,* germ, + -*oma,* tumor]

as·tro·cele (as′trō-sēl). SYN centrosphere. [G. *astron,* star, + *koilia,* hollow]

as·tro·cyte (as′trō-sīt). One of the large neuroglia cells of nervous tissue. SEE ALSO neuroglia. SYN astroglia cell, astroglia, Cajal cell (2), Deiters cells (2), macroglia cell, macroglia, spider cell (1). [G. *astron,* star, + *kytos,* hollow (cell)]

Alzheimer type I a., enlarged frequently multinucleated a.'s, seen in progressive multifocal leukoencephalopathy.

Alzheimer type II a., enlarged a.'s with vesicular nuclei and one or more small basophilic nucleoli, seen in hepatocerebral disease and Wilson disease.

fibrillary a., fibrous a., stellate astrocytic cell with long processes found mainly in the white matter of the brain and spinal cord and characterized by having bundles of glial filaments in its cytoplasm; origin of most astrocytomas.

gemistocytic a., a round to oval astrocyte cell with abundant cytoplasm containing glial filaments and an eccentric nucleus;

may contain two nuclei in the cell; hypertrophy of astrocytes. SYN gemistocyte, gemistocytic cell, reactive a., reactive cell.

protoplasmic a., one form of a., found mainly in gray matter, having few fibrils and numerous branching processes.

reactive a., SYN gemistocytic a.

as·tro·cy·to·ma (as'trō-sī-tō'mă). A glioma derived from astrocytes. [G. *astron,* star, + *kytos,* cell, + *-oma,* tumor]

anaplastic a., intermediate grade a. characterized by increased cellularity, nuclear pleomorphism, mitoses, and variable vascular endothelial proliferation.

cerebellar a., a variant of a. located in the cerebellum occurring mostly in children, consists of two architectural patterns on microscopy including a loose reticular pattern and a more compact often spindled cell pattern. SYN juvenile cerebellar a.

desmoplastic cerebral a., a rare variant of a. most frequently occurring in infancy, the tumor has a spindled cell appearance.

fibrillary a., a. derived from fibrillary astrocytes.

gemistocytic a., an astrocytoma composed primarily of gemistocytic-type astrocytes. SYN gemistocytoma.

grade I a., solid or cystic a. of low grade; World Health Organization (WHO) designation including pilocytic a. and other low-grade a. variants.

grade II a., a. of low grade; World Health Organization (WHO) designation including well-differentiated fibrillary a.

grade III a., a. of intermediate grade; World Health Organization (WHO) designation. SEE ALSO anaplastic a.

grade IV a., a. of high grade; World Health Organization (WHO) designation. SEE ALSO glioblastoma multiforme.

juvenile cerebellar a., SYN cerebellar a.

low grade a., a. characterized by an increased cellularity of uneven distribution and mild nuclear pleomorphism.

pilocytic a., a slowly growing a. composed histologically of elongated astrocytes; often located in the optic chiasm region of the third ventricle, hypothalamus, or cerebellum, predominantly in younger individuals. SYN piloid astrocytoma.

piloid astrocytoma, SYN pilocytic a.

protoplasmic a., a neoplasm composed primarily of protoplasmic-type astrocytes.

subependymal giant cell a., a rare a., frequently located in the wall of the lateral ventricle, comprised of large glial cells with abundant eosinophilic cytoplasm and intermixed elongated astrocytes, associated with tuberous sclerosis.

as·tro·cy·to·sis (as'trō-sī-tō'sis). An increase in the number of astrocytes, frequently observed in an irregular, poorly or moderately well-defined zone adjacent to degenerative lesions (e.g., encephalomalacia), focal inflammations (e.g., abscesses), or certain neoplasms in the brain; in some instances, a. may be diffuse in a relatively large region; a. represents a reparative mechanism.

a. cer'ebri, SYN *gliomatosis* cerebri.

as·tro·ep·en·dy·mo·ma (as'trō-ē-pen'di-mō'mă). A glial neoplasm composed of a mixed population of astrocytic and ependymal cells.

as·trog·lia (as-trog'lē-ă). SYN astrocyte. [G. *astron,* star, + neuroglia]

as·troid (as'troyd). Star-shaped. [G. *astroeidēs,* fr. *astron,* star, + *eidos,* resemblance]

as·tro·ki·net·ic (as'trō-ki-net'ik). Relating to movement of the centrosome and astrosphere of a dividing cell. [G. *astron,* star, + *kinēsis,* movement]

as·tro·sphere (as'trō-sfēr). A set of radiating microtubules extending outward from the cytocentrum and centrosphere of a dividing cell. SYN aster, attraction sphere, Lavdovsky nucleoid, paranuclear body. [G. *astron,* star, + *sphaira,* ball]

As·tro·vi·rus (as-'rō-vī'rus). A small RNA virus and the only genus in the family Astroviridae; it is associated with diarrhea and is detected in the feces of numerous animals.

Astrup, Poul, Danish clinical chemist, *1915. SEE micro-A. *method.*

Astwood, Edwin B., U.S. endocrinologist, 1909–1976. SEE A. *test.*

as·ver·in (as'ver-in). An antitussive.

Asx Symbol meaning Asp or Asn.

asyl·la·bia (ā-si-lā'bē-ă). Form of alexia in which one recognizes individual letters, but cannot comprehend them when arranged collectively in syllables or words. [G. *a-* priv. + *syllablē,* syllable]

asy·lum (ă-sī'lŭm). Old term for an institution for the housing and care of those who by reason of age or mental or bodily infirmities are unable to care for themselves. [L. fr. G. *asylon,* a sanctuary, fr. *a-* priv. + *sylē,* right of seizure]

asym·bo·lia (ā-sim-bō'lē-ă). A form of aphasia in which the significance of signs and symbols is not appreciated. SYN sight blindness. [G. *a-* priv. + *symbolon,* an outward sign]

asym·met·ric (a) (ā-sim-et'rik). Not symmetric; denoting a lack of symmetry between two or more like parts.

asym·me·try (ā-sim'e-trē). 1. Lack of symmetry; disproportion between two normally alike parts. 2. Significant difference in amplitude or frequency of EEG activity recorded simultaneously from the two sides of the brain under identical conditions. SYN dissymmetry.

asymp·tom·at·ic (ā'simp-tō-mat'ik). Without symptoms, or producing no symptoms.

asymp·tot·ic (ā'simp-tot'ik). Pertaining to a limiting value, for example of a dependent variable, when the independent variable approaches zero or infinity.

asyn·cli·tism (ă-sin'kli-tizm). Absence of synclitism or parallelism; may be used, e.g., to refer to the axis of the presenting part of the child and the pelvic planes in childbirth, to the dental arches, or to the planes of the skull. SYN obliquity. [G. *a-* priv. + *synklinō,* to incline together]

anterior a., SYN Nägele *obliquity.*

posterior a., SYN Litzmann *obliquity.*

a. of the skull, SYN plagiocephaly.

asyn·ech·ia (ă-si-nek'ē-ă). Discontinuity of structure. [G. *a-* priv. + *synecheia,* continuity]

asy·ner·gia (ă-sin-er'jē-ă). SYN asynergy. [G. *a-* priv. + *syn,* with, + *ergon,* work]

asyn·er·gic (ā'sin-er'jik). Characterized by asynergy.

asyn·er·gy (ă-sin'er-jē). Lack of coordination among various muscle groups during the performance of complex movements, resulting in loss of skill and speed. When severe, results in decomposition of movement, wherein complex motor acts are performed in a series of isolated movements; caused by cerebellar disorders. SYN asynergia.

asy·ne·sia, asyn·e·sis (ă-si-nē'zē-ă, -nē'sis). Lack of easy comprehension and practical intelligence. [G. *a-* priv. + *synesis,* union, understanding]

asys·tem·at·ic (ā'sis-tĕ-mat'ik). Not systematic; not relating to one system or set of organs.

asys·to·le (ā-sis'tō-lē). Absence of contractions of the heart. SYN asystolia, cardiac standstill. [G. *a-* priv, + *systolē,* a contracting]

asys·to·lia (ă-sis-tō'lē-ă). SYN asystole.

asys·tol·ic (ă-sis-tol'ik). 1. Relating to asystole. 2. Not systolic.

AT Abbreviation for the adenine-thymine hydrogen-bonded base pair observed in double-stranded polynucleotides.

At Symbol for astatine.

ata Abbreviation for *atmosphere* absolute.

at·a·brine hy·dro·chlo·ride (ă'tē-brin). SYN quinacrine hydrochloride.

atac·til·ia (ā-tak-til'ē-ă). Loss of the sense of touch. [G. *a-* priv. + L. *tactilis,* relating to touch, fr. *tango,* pp. *tactus,* to touch]

at·a·rac·tic (at-ă-rak'tik). 1. Having a calming or tranquilizing effect. 2. A tranquilizer. SYN ataraxic. [G. *ataraktos,* calm]

at·a·rax·ia (at-ă-rak'sē-ă). Calmness and peace of mind; tranquility. [G. *a-* priv. + *taraktos,* disturbed, + *-ia*]

at·a·rax·ic (at-ă-rak'sik). SYN ataractic.

at·a·vism (at'ă-vizm). The appearance in an individual of characteristics presumed to have been present in some remote ancestor; reversion to an earlier biologic type, a throwback. [L. *atavus,* a remote ancestor]

at·a·vis·tic (at-ă-vis'tik). Relating to atavism.

atax·ia (ă-tak′sē-ă). An inability to coordinate muscle activity during voluntary movement; most often due to disorders of the cerebellum or the posterior columns of the spinal cord; may involve the limbs, head, or trunk. SYN ataxy, incoordination. [G. *a*-priv. + *taxis,* order]

acute a., generalized a. of abrupt onset, most often caused by drug intoxications, poisonings, or vestibular neuronitis.

Briquet a., weakening of the muscle sense and increased sensibility of the skin, in hysteria. SYN hysterical a.

Bruns a., difficulty in initiation of movement of the feet when they are in contact with the ground; a condition related to a frontal lobe lesion.

cerebellar a., loss of muscle coordination caused by disorders of the cerebellum.

chronic a., persistent a., most often caused by hereditary cerebellar or metabolic disorders.

a. cor′dis, SYN atrial *fibrillation.*

Friedreich a. [MIM*229300], a neurologic disorder characterized by a., dysarthria, scoliosis, high-arched foot or pes cavus and paralysis of the muscles, especially of the lower extremities; onset usually in childhood or youth with sclerosis of the posterior and lateral columns of the spinal cord; autosomal recessive inheritance, caused by mutation involving trinucleotide repeat expansion in Friedreich ataxia gene (FRDA) on chromosome 9q. SYN hereditary spinal a., heredotaxia.

gluten a., a. resultant from immunologic damage to cerebellulm, posterior spinal columns, and periperal nerves in gluten-senstive individuals

hereditary cerebellar a., (1) a disease of later childhood and early adult life, marked by ataxic gait, hesitating and explosive speech, nystagmus, and sometimes optic neuritis. It probably comprises several distinct conditions with diverse patterns of inheritance. (2) collective term for a number of hereditary disorders in which cerebellar signs are the most prominent finding.

hereditary spinal a. [MIM*229300], SYN Friedreich a.

hysterical a., SYN Briquet a.

kinetic a., SYN motor a.

Leyden a., SYN pseudotabes.

locomotor a., the severe gait ataxia seen with tabetic neurosyphylis. Patients walk with the feet wide apart, slapping them clumsily to the floor with each step, and depend on visual cues to maintain balance. SEE ALSO tabetic *neurosyphilis.*

Marie a., obsolete term for a variety of non-Friedreich hereditary ataxias.

motor a., a. developing upon attempting to perform coordinated muscular movements. SYN kinetic a.

optic a., an inability to guide the hand toward an object using visual information; seen in Balint *syndrome.*

respiratory a., SYN Biot *respiration.*

sensory a., an a. due to impairment of position sense caused by lesions located at some point along the central or peripheral sensory pathways.

spinal a., a. due to spinal cord disease, as in tabes dorsalis.

spinocerebellar a., the most common hereditary a., with onset in middle to late childhood, manifested as limb a., nystagmus, kyphoscoliosis, and pes cavus; the major pathologic changes are found in the posterior columns of the spinal cord; most often autosomal recessive inheritance.

static a., inability to preserve equilibrium while standing, due to loss of myesthesia; present during the resting state.

a. telangiectasia, ataxia-telangiectasia, a slowly progressive multisystem disorder with the following manifestations: a. appearing with the onset of walking; telangiectases of the conjunctiva and skin of the face, neck, and ears; athetosis and nystagmus; and recurrent infections of the respiratory system caused by immunoglobulin deficiencies. Due to an autosomal recessive trait, with major pathologic changes involving the cerebellar cortex, posterior columns, spinocerebellar tracks, anterior horn cells, dorsal roots, and peripheral nerves. A high percentage of the patients have an IgA deficiency concomitant with decreased T-helper cell function. There are numerous chromosome breaks and α-fetoprotein levels in the sera are usually elevated; caused by several

mutations in PI3′kinase gene. SYN ataxia telangiectasia syndrome, Louis-Bar syndrome.

vasomotor a., a form of autonomic a. causing irregularity in the peripheral circulation, marked by alternations of pallor and suffusion, due to spasm of the smaller blood vessels.

vestibulocerebellar a., a. due to disease of the central vestibular system or its cerebellar components, manifested clinically by an unsteady gait, nystagmus, and incoordination of arm and leg movements.

atax·i·a·dy·nam·ia (ă-tak′sē-ă-dī-nam′ē-ă). Muscular weakness combined with incoordination.

atax·i·a·gram (ă-tak′sē-ă-gram). The recording made by an ataxiagraph.

atax·i·a·graph (ă-tak′sē-ă-graf). An instrument for measuring the degree and direction of the swaying of the body and head in static ataxia, with the individual's eyes closed. SYN ataxiameter.

atax·i·a·me·ter (ă-tak′sē-ă-mē′ter). SYN ataxiagraph.

atax·i·a·pha·sia (ă-tak′sē-ă-fā′zē-ă). Inability to form connected sentences, although single words may perhaps be used intelligibly. [G. *a-* priv. + *taxis,* order, + *phasis,* an affirmation, speech]

atax·ia-tel·an·gi·ec·ta·sia. SEE *ataxia* telangiectasia.

atax·ic (ă-tak′sik). Relating to, marked by, or suffering from ataxia.

atax·i·o·pho·bia (ă-tak′sē-ō-fō′bē-ă). Morbid dread of disorder or untidiness. [G. *a-* priv. + *taxis,* order, + *phobos,* fear]

ataxy (ă-tak′sē). SYN ataxia.

-ate. Termination used as a replacement for "-ic acid" when the acid is neutralized (e.g., sodium acetate) or esterified (e.g., ethyl acetate).

at·el·ec·ta·sis (at-ĕ-lek′tă-sis). Decreased or absent air in the entire or part of a lung, with resulting loss of lung volume. Loss of lung volume itself. SEE ALSO pulmonary *collapse.* [G. *atelēs,* incomplete, + *ektasis,* extension]

adhesive a., alveolar collapse in the presence of patent airways, especially when surfactant is inactivated or absent, especially in respiratory distress syndrome of the newborn, acute radiation pneumonitis, or viral pneumonia. SYN microatelectasis, nonobstructive a.

cicatrization a., (1) the decrease in air per unit lung volume due to fibrosis, causing decreased lung compliance, and increased tissue. (2) a. due to scarring or pulmonary fibrosis.

a. of the middle ear, reduction in the volume of the middle ear because of eustachian tube obstruction followed by absorption of the oxygen in the middle ear and subsequent retraction of the tympanic membrane medially.

nonobstructive a., SYN adhesive a.

passive a., the pulmonary collapse that occurs due to a space-occupying intrathoracic process such as pneumothorax or hydrothorax. SYN relaxation a.

patchy a., decreased aeration and collapse of multiple small areas of lung.

platelike a., SYN subsegmental a.

primary a., nonexpansion of the lungs after birth, found in all stillborn infants and in liveborn infants who die before respiration is established.

relaxation a., SYN passive a.

resorption a., the slow partial collapse of a lobe that occurs when communication between alveoli and trachea is obstructed.

rounded a., an area of atelectatic lung caused by parenchymal infolding due to pleural fibrosis, most often from asbestos exposure; appears as a masslike opacity and can be mistaken for lung cancer; may be associated with a comet tail *sign*; high level of contrast enhancement on dynamic computed *tomography* aids diagnosis. SYN folded-lung syndrome.

secondary a., pulmonary collapse at any age, but particularly of infants, due to hyaline membrane disease or elastic recoil of the lungs while dying from other causes.

segmental a., partial collapse of one or more individual pulmonary segments.

subsegmental a., collapse of the portion of the lung distal to an obstructed subsegmental bronchus, manifested as a linear opacity

at

on a chest radiograph. SEE Fleischner *lines*, under *line*. SYN platelike a.

at·e·lec·tat·ic (at-ĕ-lek-tat′ik). Relating to atelectasis.

ate·lia (ă-tē′lē-ă). SYN ateliosis.

atel·i·o·sis (ă-tē′lē-ō′sis). Incomplete development of the body or any of its parts, as in infantilism and dwarfism. SYN atelia. [G. *atelēs,* incomplete, + *-osis,* condition]

atel·i·ot·ic (ă-tē-lē-ot′ik). Marked by ateliosis.

atel·op·id·tox·in (ă-tel-op′id-tok′sin). A potent poison from the skin of the golden arrow frog (*Atelopus zeteki*) of Central and South America.

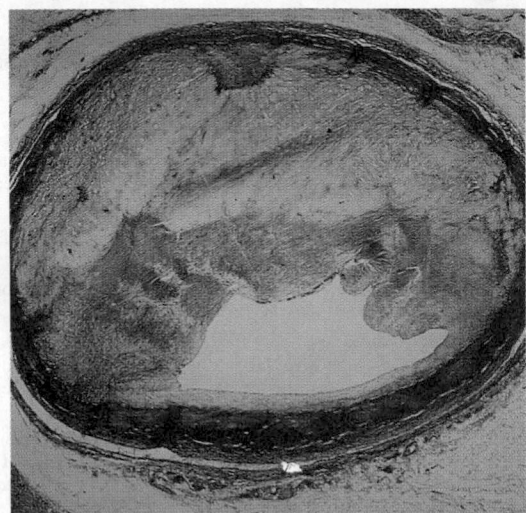

atherosclerosis: cross section of renal artery showing significant luminal narrowing by atherosclerosis; hematoxylin and eosin, ×10

aten·o·lol (ă-ten′ō-lol). A relatively cardioselective β-adrenergic blocking agent used primarily in the treatment of angina pectoris and hypertension; it possesses lower lipid solubility than other members of this class and hence apparently less central nervous system side effects.

athe·lia (ă-thē-lē-ă). Congenital absence of the nipples. [G. *a-* priv. + *thēlē,* nipple]

ath·er·ec·to·my (ath-e-rek′tō-mē). Any removal by surgery or specialized catheterization of an atheroma in the coronary or any other artery.

　coronary a., instrumental removal, via catheter, of atheromas in coronary arteries.

　directional a., removal of coronary atherometer with instrumented catheter.

ather·man·cy (ă-ther′man-sē). Impermeability to heat. [G. *athermantos,* not heated, fr. *a-* priv. + *thermaino,* to heat, fr. *thermē,* heat]

ather·ma·nous (ă-ther′mă-nŭs). Absorbing radiant heat; not permeable to heat rays.

ather·mo·sys·tal·tic (ă-ther′mō-sis-tal′tik). Not contracted or constricted by ordinary variations of temperature; said of certain tissues. [G. *a-* priv. + *thermos,* hot, + *systaltikos,* constringent]

△**athero-.** Gruel-like, soft, pasty materials; atheroma, atheromatous. [G. *athērē,* gruel, porridge]

ath·er·o·em·bo·lism (ath′er-ō-em′bō-lizm). Cholesterol embolism, with or without calcific matter, originating from an atheroma of the aorta or other diseased artery.

ath·er·o·gen·e·sis (ath′er-ō-jen′ĕ-sis). Formation of atheroma, important in the pathogenesis of arteriosclerosis.

ath·er·o·gen·ic (ath-er-ō-jen′ik). Having the capacity to initiate, increase, or accelerate the process of atherogenesis.

ath·er·o·ma (ath-er-ō′mă). The lipid deposits in the intima of arteries, producing a yellow swelling on the endothelial surface; a

characteristic of atherosclerosis. SYN atherosis. [G. *athērē,* gruel, + *-ōma,* tumor]

ath·er·om·a·tous (ath-er-ō′mă-tŭs). Relating to or affected by atheroma.

⊞ath·er·o·scle·ro·sis (ath′er-ō-skler-ō′sis). Arteriosclerosis characterized by irregularly distributed lipid deposits in the intima of large and medium-sized arteries, causing narrowing of arterial lumens and proceeding eventually to fibrosis and calcification; lesions are usually focal and progress slowly and intermittently. Limitation of blood flow accounts for most clinical manifestations, which vary with the distribution and severity of lesions. In lower animals, a. of swine and fowl closely resemble human a. SYN nodular sclerosis. [G. *athērē,* gruel, + sclerosis]

　Atherosclerosis, the most common form of arteriosclerosis, is a complex process that begins with the appearance of cholesterol-laden macrophages (foam cells) in the intima of an artery. Smooth muscle cells respond to the presence of lipid by proliferating, under the influence of platelet factors. A plaque forms at the site, consisting of smooth muscle cells, leukocytes, and further deposition of lipid; in time the plaque becomes fibrotic and may calcify. Expansion of an atherosclerotic plaque leads to gradually increasing obstruction of the artery and ischemia of tissues supplied by it. Ulceration, thrombosis, or embolization of a plaque, or intimal hemorrhage and dissection, can cause more acute and severe impairment of blood flow, with the risk of infarction. These are the principal mechanisms of coronary artery disease (arteriosclerotic heart disease with or without heart failure, angina pectoris, myocardial infarction), peripheral vascular disease (particularly occlusive disease of the lower extremity causing intermittent claudication or gangrene), and stroke (cerebral infarction due to occlusion of carotid or intracranial arteries). Independent risk factors for atherosclerosis are male sex, advancing age, the postmenopausal state, a family history of atherosclerosis, cigarette smoking, hypertension, diabetes mellitus, elevated plasma LDL cholesterol, elevated plasma homocysteine, overweight, and a sedentary lifestyle. Mounting evidence suggests that elevation of plasma levels of triglycerides, fasting insulin, fibrinogen, apolipoproteins A and B, and lipoprotein (a) are also independent risk factors. The diagnosis of atherosclerosis is usually based on history and physical examination and confirmed by angiography, Doppler ultrasonography, and other imaging techniques. Treatment is largely mechanical: balloon stretching, laser ablation, or surgical removal of plaques, and various bypass and grafting procedures. The prevention of atherosclerosis is a major objective of modern medicine. Preventive measures include regular vigorous exercise, a diet low in fat and cholesterol, maintenance of a healthful weight, avoidance of tobacco, and use of pharmacologic agents as indicated (e.g., rigorous control of hypertension and diabetes mellitus, reduction of elevated cholesterol, estrogen replacement therapy after menopause). See free radical; low-fat diet.

ath·er·o·scle·rot·ic (ath′er-ō-skler-ot′ik). Relating to or characterized by atherosclerosis.

ath·er·o·sis (ath-er-ō′sis). SYN atheroma.

ath·er·o·throm·bo·sis (ath′er-ō-throm-bō′sis). Thrombus formation in an atheromatous vessel.

ath·er·o·throm·bot·ic (ath′er-ō-throm-bot′ik). Denoting, characteristic of, or caused by atherothrombosis.

athe·toid (ath′ĕ-toyd). Resembling athetosis.

ath·e·to·sic, ath·e·tot·ic (ath-ĕ-tō′sik, -tot′ik). Pertaining to, marked by, athetosis.

ath·e·to·sis (ath-ĕ-tō′sis). A condition in which there is a constant succession of slow, writhing, involuntary movements of flexion, extension, pronation, and supination of the fingers and hands, and sometimes of the toes and feet. Usually caused by an extrapyramidal lesion. SYN extrapyramidal cerebral palsy, Hammond disease. [G. *athetos,* without position or place]

double a., a type of cerebral palsy manifested predominantly as bilateral involuntary movements, beginning at about the age of 3 years, and preceded by generalized hypotonia and delayed motor development. Due to various causes, including kernicterus and birth hypoxia. SYN congenital choreoathetosis, double congenital a., Vogt syndrome.

double congenital a., SYN double a.

posthemiplegic a., a unilateral athetosis involving hemiplegic limbs, usually seen in children. SYN posthemiplegic chorea.

aThr Abbreviation for allothreonines. SEE allothreonines.

athrep·sia, ath·rep·sy (ă-threp'sē-ă, ath'rep-sē). **1.** Obsolete term for marasmus. **2.** As used by Ehrlich, immunity to transplanted neoplastic cells due to a lack of nourishment in the sense of a deficiency of supposed substances required for the development of such cells. SYN atrepsy. [G. *a-* priv. + *threpsis,* nourishment]

ath·ro·cy·to·sis (ath'rō-sī-tō'sis). The capacity of cells to absorb and retain electronegative colloids, as shown by macrophages and at the apical surface of proximal convoluted tubule cells of the kidney. [G. *athrō,* gathered together, + *kytos,* cell, + *-osis,* condition]

athrom·bia (ă-throm'bē-ă) [MIM*209050]. A hereditary bleeding disorder characterized by prolonged bleeding time, decreased platelet adhesion and aggregation but normal plasma clotting and clot retraction, normal platelet count with platelet factor 3 availability; probably autosomal recessive inheritance. [G. *a-* priv. + thrombin]

athy·mia (ă-thī'mē-ă). **1.** Absence of affect or emotivity; morbid impassivity. **2.** Congenital absence of the thymus gland, often with associated immunodeficiency. SYN athymism. [G. *a-* priv. + *thymos,* mind, also thymus]

athy·mism (ā-thī'mizm). SYN athymia (2).

athy·rea (ă-thī'rē-ă). **1.** SYN hypothyroidism. **2.** SYN athyroidism.

athy·roid·ism (ā-thī'royd-izm). Congenital absence of the thyroid gland or suppression or absence of its hormonal secretion. SEE hypothyroidism. SYN athyrea (2), athyrosis.

athy·ro·sis (ā-thī-rō'sis). SYN athyroidism.

athy·rot·ic (ā-thī-rot'ik). Relating to athyroidism.

ATL Abbreviation for adult T-cell *leukemia* or adult T-cell *lymphoma.*

at·lan·tad (at-lan'tad). In a direction toward the atlas.

at·lan·tal (at-lan'tăl). Relating to the atlas. SYN atloid.

⚠**atlanto-, atlo-.** The atlas (the vertebra that supports the skull). [G. *Atlas, Atlantos,* Atlas, the mythical Titan who supported the dome of the sky on his shoulders]

at·lan·to·ax·i·al (at-lan'tō-ak'sē-ăl). Pertaining to the atlas and the axis; denoting the joint between the first two cervical vertebrae. SYN atlantoepistrophic, atloaxoid.

at·lan·to·did·y·mus (at-lan'tō-did'ē-mŭs). Conjoined twins with two heads on one neck and a single body. SYN atlodidymus. [atlanto- + G. *didymos,* twin]

at·lan·to·ep·i·stroph·ic (at-lan'tō-ep'i-strof'ik). SYN atlantoaxial.

at·lan·to·oc·cip·i·tal (at-lan'tō-ok-sip'i-tăl). Relating to the atlas and the occipital bone. SYN atlo-occipital.

at·lan·to·odon·toid (at-lan'tō-ō-don'toyd). Relating to the atlas and the dens of the axis.

at·las (at'las) [TA]. First cervical vertebra, articulating with the occipital bone and rotating around the dens of the axis. SYN vertebra C1✩, first cervical vertebra. [G. *Atlas,* in Greek mythology a Titan who supported the heavens on his shoulders]

⚠**atlo-.** SEE atlanto-.

at·lo·ax·oid (at-lō-ak'soyd). SYN atlantoaxial.

at·lo·did·y·mus (at-lō-did'ē-mŭs). SYN atlantodidymus.

at·loid (at'loyd). SYN atlantal.

at·lo·oc·cip·i·tal (at'lō-ok-sip'i-tăl). SYN atlanto-occipital.

atm Symbol for standard *atmosphere.*

⚠**atmo-.** Prefix denoting steam or vapor; or derived by action of steam or vapor. [G. *atmos,* steam, vapor]

at·mol·y·sis (at-mol'i-sis). Separation of mixed gases by passing them through a porous diaphragm, the lighter gases diffusing through at a faster rate. [atmo- + G. *lysis,* dissolution]

at·mom·e·ter (at-mom'ĕ-ter). An instrument for measuring the rate of evaporation. [atmo- + G. *metron,* measure]

at·mos Obsolete abbreviation for a unit of pressure; replaced by atm. [abbreviation of atmosphere]

at·mos·phere (at'mŏs-fēr). **1.** Any gas surrounding a given body; a gaseous medium. **2.** A unit of air pressure equal to 101.325 kPa. SEE ALSO standard a., torr. [atmo- + G. *sphaira,* sphere]

a. absolute (ata), a unit of absolute pressure (also known as barometric pressure) expressed in atm.

ICAO standard a., the standard a. adopted by the International Civil Aviation Organization, used for calibrating altimeters and for expressing hypobaric chamber pressures in terms of equivalent altitude; it ignores many deviations found in nature.

standard a. (atm), (1) the pressure of the a. at mean sea level at 273.15 K, equivalent to 1,013,250 dynes/cm^2 or 101,325 Pa (N/m^2 in the SI system); **(2)** a standardized expression of the relation of barometric pressure, temperature, and other atmospheric variables as a function of altitude above sea level.

at·mo·spher·i·za·tion (at'mŏ-sfēr-i-zā'shŭn). Conversion of venous into arterial blood.

At·mungs·fer·ment (aht'mungz-fer-ment). **1.** A system of cytochromes and their oxidases that participate in respiratory processes. **2.** Often, specifically, cytochrome oxidase. SYN Warburg respiratory enzyme. [Ger.]

▣**at·om** (at'ŏm). Once considered the ultimate particle of an element, believed to be as indivisible as its name indicates. Discovery of radioactivity demonstrated the existence of subatomic particles, notably protons, neutrons, and electrons, the first two comprising most of the mass of the atomic nucleus. We now know that subatomic particles are further classified into hadrons, leptons, and quarks. [G. *atomos,* indivisible, uncut]

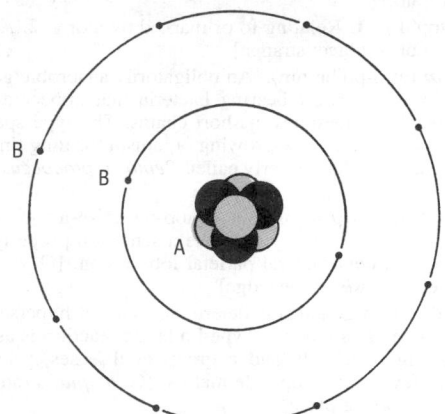

structure of an atom: (A) nucleus, containing protons (orange) and neutrons (black); (B) electrons, travelling in orbits around nucleus

activated a., an a. possessing more than normal energy as a result of input of energy. SEE ALSO excited *state.* SYN excited a.

Bohr a., a concept or model of the a. in which the negatively charged electrons move in circular or elliptical orbits around the positively charged nucleus, energy being emitted or absorbed when electrons change from one orbit to another.

excited a., SYN activated a.

ionized a., an a. that possesses an electrostatic charge as a result of loss or gain of electrons; e.g., H$^+$, Ca^{2+}, Cl$^-$, O^{2-}.

labeled a., a radioactive a., or a stable but rare one, which by its presence in a molecule helps localization or measurement of that molecule. SYN tagged a.

nuclear a., a concept or model of the a. characterized by the presence of a small, massive nucleus at its center.

quaternary carbon a., an a. of carbon to which four other carbon a.'s are attached.

radioactive a., an a. with an unstable nucleus, which emits particulate or electromagnetic radiation (radioactive emission) to achieve greater stability. SEE radionuclide, half-life, Becquerel.

recoil a., the remainder of an a. from which a nuclear particle has been emitted or ejected at high velocity; the remainder recoils with a velocity inversely proportional to its mass.

stripped a., an a. minus all its electrons; a nucleus.

tagged a., SYN labeled a.

atom·ic (ă-tom'ik). Relating to an atom.

at·om·ism (at'ŏm-izm). The approach to the study of a psychological phenomenon through analysis of the elementary parts of which it is assumed to be composed. Cf. holism.

at·om·is·tic (at-ŏm-is'tik). Pertaining to atomism or a. psychology.

at·om·i·za·tion (at-ŏm-i-zā'-shŭn). Spray production; reduction of a fluid to small droplets.

at·om·iz·er (at'ŏm-ī-zer). A device used to reduce liquid medication to fine particles in the form of a spray or aerosol; useful in delivering medication to the lungs, nose, and throat. SEE ALSO nebulizer, vaporizer. [G. *atomos*, indivisible particle]

ato·nia (ā-tō'nē-ă). SYN atony. [G. languor]

aton·ic (ă-ton'ik). Relaxed; without normal tone or tension.

at·o·nic·i·ty (at-ō-nis'i-tē). SYN atony.

at·o·ny (at'ŏ-nē). Relaxation, flaccidity, or lack of tone or tension. SYN atonia, atonicity. [G. *atonia*, languor]

postpartum a., a. of the uterine walls after childbirth. SYN metratonia.

uterine a., failure of the myometrium to contract after delivery of the placenta; associated with excessive bleeding from the placental implantation site.

at·o·pen (at'ō-pen). An old term to denote the excitant causing any form of atopy.

atop·ic (ă-top'ik). **1.** Relating to or marked by atopy. **2.** Allergic. [G. *atopos*, out of place; strange]

Ato·po·bium (at-ō-pō'bē-um). An obligatorily anaerobic genus of Gram-positive, non–spore-bearing bacteria that appear as cocci and coccobacilli, sometimes in short chains. The type species is *Atopobium parvulus,* a slow-growing organism forming tiny colonies on standard media formerly called *Peptostreptococcus parvulus* and *Streptococcus parvulus.*

atop·og·no·sia, atop·og·no·sis (ă-top-og-nō'zē-ă, -og-nō'sis). Sensory inattention; inability to locate a sensation properly. Usually caused by a contralateral parietal lobe lesion. [G. *a-* priv. + *topos,* place, + *gnōsis,* knowledge]

at·o·py (at'ō-pē). A genetically determined state of hypersensitivity to environmental allergens. Type I allergic reaction is associated with the IgE antibody and a group of diseases, principally asthma, hay fever, and atopic dermatitis. [G. *atopia,* strangeness, fr. *a-* priv. + *topos,* a place]

atox·ic (ā-tok'sik). Not toxic.

ATP Abbreviation for adenosine 5'-triphosphate.

ATPase Abbreviation for adenosine triphosphatase.

ATP cit·rate ly·ase. SEE ATP *citrate (pro-3S)*-lyase.

ATPD Symbol indicating that a gas volume has been expressed as if it had been dried at the ambient temperature and pressure.

ATP-di·phos·pha·tase. SYN apyrase.

ATPS Symbol indicating that a gas volume has been expressed as if it were saturated with water vapor at the ambient temperature and barometric pressure; the condition of an expired gas equilibrated in a spirometer.

ATP sul·fur·y·lase. SYN *sulfate* adenylyltransferase.

atrac·to·syl·id·ic ac·id (ă-trak'tō-sil-id'ik). SYN atractyligenin.

atrac·tyl·ic ac·id (ă-trak'til-ik). A highly poisonous steroid glycoside from *Atractylis gummifera L.* (*Compositae*), having a strychnine-like action that produces convulsions of a hypoglycemic nature; the aglycon, atractyliginin, is combined with glucose and isovaleric acid, and is the toxic principle. A. a. interferes with oxidative reactions, the citric acid cycle, and nerve conduction.

atrac·tyl·i·gen·in (ă-trak'til-i-jen'in). The steroid aglycon and toxic principle of atractylic acid. SYN atractosylidic acid, atractylin.

atrac·tyl·in (ă-trak'til-in). SYN atractyligenin.

atra·cu·ri·um be·syl·ate (a-tră-kūr'ē-ŭm). A nondepolarizing neuromuscular relaxant of intermediate duration of action; used as an adjunct to general anesthesia; a curare-like agent.

atrep·sy (ă-trep'sē). SYN athrepsia (2). [G. *a-* priv. + *trephō,* to nourish]

atre·sia (ă-trē'zē-ă). Congenital absence of a normal opening or normally patent lumen. SYN clausura. [G. *a-* priv. + *trēsis,* a hole]

anal a., a. a'ni, congenital absence of an anal opening due to the presence of a membranous septum (persistence of the cloacal membrane) or to complete absence of the anal canal. SYN imperforate anus, proctatresia.

aortic a., congenital absence of the valvular orifice into the aorta.

biliary a., a. of the major bile ducts, causing cholestasis and jaundice, which does not become apparent until several days after birth; periportal fibrosis develops and leads to cirrhosis, with proliferation of small bile ducts unless these are also atretic; giant cell transformation of hepatic cells also occurs. Cf. neonatal *hepatitis.*

bronchial a., severe focal narrowing or obliteration of a segmental, subsegmental, or lobar bronchus, usually associated with distal air trapping and bronchial mucoid impaction distal to the obstruction.

choanal a., a. due to congenital failure of one or both choanae to open owing to the failure of the bucconasal membrane to involute. It results in nasal obstruction and creates an emergency in newborns since they are obligatory nasal breathers.

esophageal a., congenital failure of the full esophageal lumen to develop; often associated with tracheoesophageal fistula.

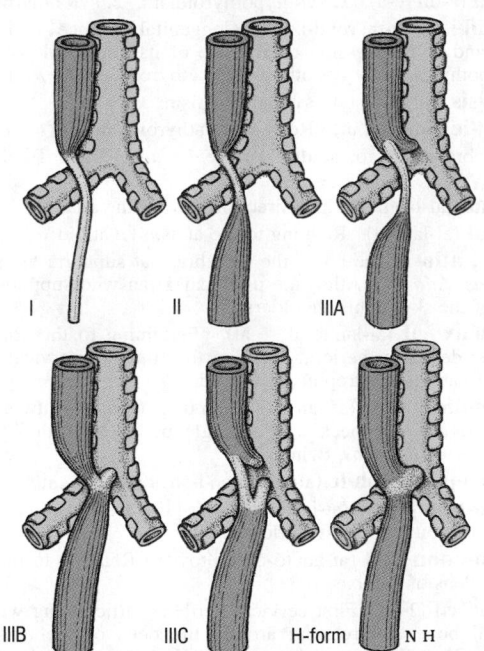

I   II   IIIA

IIIB   IIIC   H-form   N H

Vogt classification of esophageal atresia: I–IIIC and the so-called H-form type

a. follic'uli, a normal process affecting the primordial ovarian follicles in which death of the ovum results in cystic degeneration followed by cicatricial closure.

intestinal a., an obliteration of the lumen of the small intestine, with the ileum involved in 50% of cases and the jejunum and duodenum next in frequency; most frequent cause of intestinal obstruction in the newborn; etiology may be related to a failure of recanalization during early development or to some impairment of blood supply during intrauterine life.

a. i′ridis, congenital absence of the pupillary opening. SYN atretopsia.

laryngeal a., congenital failure of the laryngeal opening to develop, resulting in partial or total obstruction at or just above or below the glottis.

pulmonary a., congenital absence of the pulmonary valve orifice.

pulmonary artery a., absence of one, usually the right, pulmonary artery.

tricuspid a., congenital lack of the tricuspid orifice.

vaginal a., congenital or acquired imperforation or occlusion of the vagina, or adhesion of the walls of the vagina. SYN colpatresia.

atre·sic (ă-trē′zik). SYN atretic.

atret·ic (ă-tret′ik). Relating to atresia. SYN atresic, imperforate.

⌂**atreto-.** Lack of an opening. [G. *atrētos,* imperforate fr. *a-,* not + *trētos,* perforated, fr. *tetrainō, titrēmi,* to bore through, to pierce.]

atre·to·ble·pha·ria (ă-trē′tō-ble-fār′ē-ă). SYN symblepharon. [atreto- + G. *blepharon,* eyelid]

atre·to·cys·tia (ă-trē′tō-sis′tē-ă). Obsolete term for congenital or acquired absence of an opening of a bladder. [atreto- + G. *kystis,* bladder]

atre·to·gas·tria (ă-trē′tō-gas′trē-ă). Congenital absence of an opening of the stomach. [atreto- + G. *gastēr,* stomach]

atre·top·sia (ă-trē-top′sē-ă). SYN *atresia* iridis. [atreto- + G. *ōps,* eye]

atria (ā′trē-ă) [TA]. Plural of atrium.

atri·al (ā′trē-ăl). Relating to an atrium.

atrich·ia (ă-trik′ē-ă). Absence of hair, congenital or acquired. SYN atrichosis. [G. *a-* priv. + *thrix (trich-),* hair]

atri·cho·sis (at-ri-kō′sis). SYN atrichia.

⌂**atrio-.** The atrium; atrial. [L. *atrium,* an entrance hall]

atri·o·meg·a·ly (ā′trē-ō-meg′ă-lē). Enlargement of the atrium. [atrio- + G. *megas,* great]

atri·o·nec·tor (ā-trē-ō-nek′ter, -tōr). SYN sinuatrial *node.* [atrio- + L. *necto,* to join]

atri·o·pep·tin (ā′trē-ō-pep′tin). SYN atrial natriuretic *peptide.* [atrio- + peptide + suffix *-in,* material]

atri·o·sep·to·plas·ty (ā′trē-ō-sep′tō-plas-tē). Surgical repair of an atrial septal defect. [atrio- + L. *septum,* partition, + G. *plastos,* formed]

atri·o·sep·tos·to·my (ā′trē-ō-sep-tos′tō-mē). SYN atrial *septostomy.* [atrio- + L. *septum,* partition, + G. *stoma,* mouth]

balloon a., tearing or enlarging the foramen ovale by pulling a balloon-bearing catheter across the atrial septum for the purpose of augmenting interatrial mixing of blood in the treatment of cyanotic congenital heart disease.

atri·ot·o·my (ā-trē-ot′ō-mē). Surgical opening of an atrium. [atrio- + G. *tomē,* incision]

atri·o·ven·tric·u·lar (AV) (ā′trē-ō-ven-trik′ū-lar). Relating to both the atria and the ventricles of the heart, especially to the ordinary, orthograde transmission of conduction or blood flow.

atrip·li·cism (ă-trip′li-sizm). An intoxication caused by the ingestion of certain species of *Atriplex,* eaten as greens in China; it is marked by pain and swelling of the fingers, spreading to the forearm; bullae and ulcers form, and the fingers may become gangrenous. [L. *atriplex (-plic-),* the orach, a vegetable]

atri·um, pl. **atria** (ā′trē-ŭm, ā′trē-ă). **1** [TA]. A chamber or cavity to which are connected several chambers or passageways. **2.** SYN a. of heart. **3.** That part of the tympanic cavity that lies immediately deep to the eardrum. **4.** SYN a. of middle nasal meatus. **5.** In the lung, a subdivision of the alveolar duct from which alveolar sacs open. [L. entrance hall]

accessory a., SYN *cor* triatriatum.

a. cor′dis [TA], SYN a. of heart.

a. cordis dextrum [TA], SYN right a. of heart.

a. cordis sinistrum [TA], SYN left a. of heart.

a. dex′trum cordis, SYN right a. of heart.

a. glot′tidis, SYN *vestibule* of larynx.

a. of heart [TA], the upper chamber of each half of the heart. SYN a. cordis [TA], atrium (2).

a. of lateral ventricle [TA], portion of lateral ventricle of brain common to the frontal, occipital, and temporal horns. SYN a. ventriculi lateralis [TA], a. ventriculus lateralis [TA].

a. of lateral ventricle [TA], that portion of the lateral ventricle where the body (or central part), posterior horn, and temporal horn converge; it contains the choroid enlargement.

left a. of heart [TA], a. of the left side of the heart which receives the blood from the pulmonary veins. SYN a. cordis sinistrum [TA], a. pulmonale, a. sinistrum cordis.

a. mea′tus me′dii, SYN a. of middle nasal meatus.

a. meatus medii nasalis [TA], SYN a. of middle nasal meatus.

a. of middle nasal meatus [TA], the anterior expanded portion of the middle meatus of the nose, just above the vestibule. SYN a. meatus medii nasalis [TA], a. meatus medii, atrium (4), nasal a.

nasal a., SYN a. of middle nasal meatus.

a. pulmona′le, SYN left a. of heart.

right a. of heart [TA], right a., the a. of the right side of the heart that receives the blood from the venae cavae and coronary sinus. SYN a. cordis dextrum [TA], a. dextrum cordis.

a. sinis′trum cordis, SYN left a. of heart.

a. ventriculi lateralis [TA], SYN a. of lateral ventricle.

a. ventriculus lateralis [TA], SYN a. of lateral ventricle.

At·ro·pa (at′rō-pă). A genus of plants (family Solanaceae) of which *A. belladonna* is typical. SEE belladonna. [G. *Atropos,* one of the Fates cutting the thread of life, because of the lethal effects of the plant]

atro·phia (ă-trō′fē-ă). SYN atrophy. [G. fr. *a-* priv. + *trophē,* nourishment]

a. cu′tis, SYN atrophoderma.

a. maculo′sa variolifor′mis cu′tis, SYN anetoderma.

a. pilo′rum pro′pria, a general term that includes fragilitas crinium, trichorrhexis nodosa, monilethrix, and atrophy of the hair.

atroph·ic (ă-trof′ik). Denoting atrophy.

atro·phie blanche (ā′trō-fi blahnsh′). Small smooth ivory-white areas with hyperpigmented borders and telangiectasis, developing into atrophic stellate scars; seen especially on the legs and ankles of middle-aged women, and associated with livedo reticularis and dermal hyalinizing vasculitis. [Fr.]

at·ro·phied (at′rō-fēd). Characterized by atrophy.

at·ro·pho·der·ma (at′rō-fō-der′mă). Atrophy of the skin that may occur either in discrete localized areas or in widespread areas. SEE ALSO anetoderma. SYN atrophia cutis.

a. al′bidum, stocking-like type of atrophy affecting the extremities, probably congenital; first noted in early childhood on the lower limbs as a symmetric thinning that renders the parts sensitive.

a. diffu′sum, diffuse idiopathic cutaneous atrophy.

a. macula′tum, SYN anetoderma.

a. neurit′icum, SYN glossy *skin.*

a. of Pasini and Pierini, a form of slate-colored atrophy of the skin occurring in discrete, 2-cm or larger lesions, either singly or multiply, and occasionally confluent, increasing in number and size over a period of years and then remaining constant; thought by some to be of two types: one preceded by morphea, and the other appearing with no preceding identifiable pathology.

senile a., a. seni′lis, the loss of collagen, with thinning and decreased elasticity of the skin associated with old age.

a. stria′tum, SYN *striae* cutis distensae, under *stria.*

at·ro·pho·der·ma·to·sis (at′rō-fō-der-mă-tō′sis). Any cutaneous affection in which a prominent symptom is skin atrophy.

at·ro·phy (at′rō-fē). A wasting of tissues, organs, or the entire body, as from death and reabsorption of cells, diminished cellular proliferation, decreased cellular volume, pressure, ischemia, malnutrition, lessened function, or hormonal changes. SYN atrophia. [G. *atrophia,* fr. *a-* priv. + *trophē,* nourishment]

acute reflex bone a., SYN Sudeck a.

acute yellow a. of the liver, SYN acute massive liver *necrosis.*

alveolar a., diminution in size of the supportive tissues of the teeth due to lack of function, reduced blood supply, or unknown causes.

arthritic a., a. of muscles rendered inactive by a chronically inflamed or fixed joint.

blue a., depressed blue atrophic scars due to injections in the skin of impure substances, as seen in narcotics addicts.

brown a., a. of the heart wall, especially in the elderly, in which the muscle is dark reddish brown and reduced in volume; the muscle fibers become pigmented especially about the nuclei, by lipochrome granules.

Buchwald a., a progressive form of cutaneous a.

central areolar choroidal a., SYN areolar *choroidopathy*.

cerebellar a., a degeneration of the cerebellum, particularly the Purkinje cells, as the result of abiotrophy or of toxic agents, as in alcoholism.

choroidal vascular a., a. affecting either all choroidal vessels or only the choriocapillaris, occurring either diffusely or confined to the posterior pole of the eye.

congenital cerebellar a., familial disorder that causes degeneration of various cells in the cerebellum. Two types are recognized, one in which the granular layer cells degenerate, the other in which the Purkinje cells degenerate.

congenital microvillus a., SYN microvillus inclusion *disease*.

cyanotic a., a. due to destruction of the parenchymatous cells of an organ as a consequence of chronic venous congestion. SYN red a.

cyanotic a. of the liver, a sequela of longstanding hepatic congestion due to high pressure in the right atrium as in chronic constrictive pericarditis and severe, protracted right ventricular failure.

dentatorubral cerebellar a. with polymyoclonus, SYN *dyssynergia* cerebellaris myoclonica.

disuse a., muscle wasting caused by immobilization, such as casting.

dominant optic a., an autosomal dominant bilateral optic neuropathy characterized by insidious preschool vision loss. SYN Kjer optic a.

essential progressive a. of iris, progressive a. of the iris without inflammatory signs, characterized by patchy loss of all layers of the iris with hole formation, migration of the pupil, degeneration of the corneal endothelium, peripheral anterior synechiae, and secondary glaucoma; usually unilateral, predominantly affecting women in their middle years. SEE ALSO iridocorneal syndrome.

facioscapulohumeral a., SYN facioscapulohumeral muscular *dystrophy*.

familial spinal muscular a., SYN spinal muscular a., type I.

fatty a., fatty infiltration secondary to an a. of the essential elements of an organ or tissue.

geographic retinal a., a pattern of well-demarcated retinal pigment epithelial a. associated with choriocapillary layer and photoreceptor a. leading to vision loss.

gingival a., SYN gingival *recession*.

gyrate a. of choroid and retina [MIM*258870], a slowly progressive a. of the choriocapillaris, pigmentary epithelium, and sensory retina, with irregular confluent atrophic areas and an associated ornithinuria; autosomal recessive inheritance; due to a deficiency of ornithine δ-aminotransferase, caused by mutation in the ornithine δ-aminotransferase gene (OAT) on chromosome 10q.

Hoffmann muscular a., SYN spinal muscular a., type I.

horizontal a., a progressive loss of alveolar and supporting bone surrounding the teeth, beginning at the most coronal level of the bone. SYN horizontal resorption.

infantile muscular a., SYN spinal muscular a., type I.

infantile progressive spinal muscular a., SYN spinal muscular a., type I.

ischemic muscular a., SEE Volkmann *contracture*.

juvenile muscular a., SYN spinal muscular a., type III.

juvenile spinal muscular a., SYN spinal muscular a., type III.

Kjer optic a., SYN dominant optic a.

Leber hereditary optic a. [MIM*535000], degeneration of the optic nerve and papillomacular bundle with resulting loss of central vision and blindness, progressive for several weeks, then usually becoming stationary with permanent central scotoma; the age of onset is variable, most often in the third decade; more males than females are affected. Mitochondrial or cytoplasmic inheritance via the maternal lineage, caused by mutation in the mitochondrial gene(s) acting autonomously or in association with each other.

linear a., SYN *striae* cutis distensae, under *stria*.

macular a., SYN anetoderma.

marantic a., SYN marasmus.

multiple system a., nonhereditary, neurodegenerative disease of unknown cause, characterized clinically by the development of parkinsonism, ataxia, autonomic failure, or pyramidal track signs, in various combinations. Pathologically there are nerve cell loss, gliosis, and the accumulation of abnormal tubular structures in the cytoplasm and nucleus of oligodendrocytes and neurons in the basal ganglion, cerebellum, and intermediolateral columns of the spinal cord; can present as predominantly parkinsonism, as predominantly ataxia, or as a combination of parkinsonism, ataxia, and autonomic failure; it is a relatively rapidly progressive and fatal disorder.

muscular a., wasting of muscular tissue. Cf. myopathic a. SYN myatrophy, myoatrophy.

myopathic a., muscular a. caused by a primary disorder of muscle.

neurogenic a., SYN neurotrophic a.

neurotrophic a., abnormalities of the skin, hair, nails, subcutaneous tissues, and bone, caused by peripheral nerve lesions. SYN neurogenic a., trophoneurotic a.

nutritional type cerebellar a., a restricted type of cerebellar cortical degeneration, affecting particularly the Purkinje cells of the anterior and superior vermis; probably caused by thiamin deficiency; most frequently seen in chronic alcoholics and then called alcoholic cerebellar degeneration.

olivopontocerebellar a., a group of genetically distinct, mostly autosomal dominant progressive neurologic diseases characterized by loss of neurons in the cerebellar cortex, basis pontis, and inferior olivary nuclei; results in ataxia, tremor, involuntary movement, and dysarthria; five clinical types (four with dominant, one with recessive inheritance) have been described, each type characterized by additional findings, such as sensory loss, retinal degeneration, ophthalmoplegia, and extrapyramidal signs. Several loci are involved, autosomal dominant [MIM*164400 to *164600] and recessive [MIM*258300]. SEE ALSO spinocerebellar *ataxia*. SYN olivopontocerebellar degeneration.

periodontal a., decrease in size and/or cellular elements of the periodontium after it has reached normal maturity.

peroneal muscular a., a group of peripheral neuromuscular disorders, sharing the common feature of marked wasting of the distal parts of the extremities, particularly the peroneal muscle groups, resulting in long, thin legs; it usually involves the legs before the arms with pes cavus often the first sign. There are two forms of hereditary sensorimotor polyneuropathies, i.e., a demyelinating type and an axonal loss type. Autosomal dominant [MIM*118200 and MIM*118220], autosomal recessive [MIM*214400], and X-linked recessive [MIM*302800, MIM*302801 and MIM*302802] forms exist. SYN Charcot-Marie-Tooth disease.

Pick a., circumscribed a. of the cerebral cortex. SYN lobar sclerosis, progressive circumscribed cerebral a.

postmenopausal a., a. following menopause, as of the genital organs.

pressure a., the wasting of hard or soft tissue resulting from excessive pressure applied to tissue by a denture base.

primary idiopathic macular a., SYN anetoderma.

primary macular a. of skin, SYN anetoderma.

progressive choroidal a., SYN choroideremia.

progressive circumscribed cerebral a., SYN Pick a.

progressive infantile spinal muscular a., SYN spinal muscular a., type I.

progressive muscular a., SYN amyotrophic lateral *sclerosis*.

progressive spinal muscular a., one of the subgroups of motor neuron disease; a progressive degenerative disorder of the motor neurons of the spinal cord, manifested as progressive, often symmetrical, weakness and wasting, typically beginning in the distal portions of the limbs, particularly in the upper extremities, and spreading proximally; fasciculation potentials are often present, but evidence of corticospinal tract disease (e.g., increased deep tendon reflexes, Babinski sign) is not.

pulp a., diminution in size and/or cellular elements of the dental pulp due to interference with the blood supply.

red a., SYN cyanotic a.

scapulohumeral a., SYN Vulpian a.

senile a., wasting of tissues and organs with advancing age from decreased catabolic or anabolic processes, at times due to endocrine changes, decreased use, or ischemia. SYN geromarasmus.

spinal muscular a. (SMA), a heterogeneous group of degenerative diseases of the anterior horn cells in the spinal cord and motor nuclei of the brainstem; all are characterized by weakness. Upper motor neurons remain normal. These diseases include Werdnig-Hoffmann disease (SMA type 1), SMA type 2, and Kugelberg-Welander disease (SMA type 3). SEE ALSO Fazio-Londe *disease.*

spinal muscular a., type I [MIM*253300], the early infantile form, characterized by profound muscle weakness and wasting with onset at or shortly after birth; death occurs usually before 2 years of age. Autosomal recessive inheritance, caused by mutation in the survival motor neuron gene (SMN1) on 5q. About one-half of patients are also missing both homologs of a neighboring gene that encodes neuronal apoptosis inhibitory protein (NAIP), the loss of which is thought to influence the severity of the disease. SYN familial spinal muscular a., Hoffmann muscular a., infantile muscular a., infantile progressive spinal muscular a., progressive infantile spinal muscular a., Werdnig-Hoffmann disease, Werdnig-Hoffmann muscular a.

spinal muscular a., type II [MIM*253550], a form intermediate in severity between the infantile form (SMA type I) and the juvenile form (SMA type III); characterized by proximal muscle weakness with onset usually between 3 and 15 months and survival until adolescence; autosomal recessive inheritance, caused by mutation in the SMN1 gene on 5q.

spinal muscular a., type III [MIM*253400], the juvenile form with onset in childhood or adolescence, characterized by progressive proximal muscular weakness and wasting, primarily in the legs, followed by distal muscle involvement, caused by degeneration of motor neurons in the anterior horns of the spinal cord; autosomal recessive inheritance, caused by mutation in the SMN1 gene on 5q. SYN juvenile muscular a., juvenile spinal muscular a., Kugelberg-Welander disease, Wohlfart-Kugelberg-Welander disease.

striate a. of skin, SYN *striae* cutis distensae, under *stria.*

Sudeck a., a. of bones, commonly of the carpal or tarsal bones, following a slight injury such as a sprain. SEE ALSO causalgia, reflex sympathetic *dystrophy.* SYN acute reflex bone a., posttraumatic osteoporosis, Sudeck syndrome.

traction a., SYN *striae* cutis distensae, under *stria.*

transneuronal a., SYN transsynaptic *degeneration.*

trophoneurotic a., SYN neurotrophic a.

villous a., abnormality of the small intestinal mucosa with crypt hyperplasia, resulting in flattening of the mucosa and the appearance of a. of villi; clinically seen in malabsorption syndromes such as sprue.

Vulpian a., progressive spinal muscular a. beginning in the shoulder. SYN scapulohumeral a.

Werdnig-Hoffmann muscular a., SYN spinal muscular a., type I.

yellow a. of the liver, SEE acute yellow a. of the liver.

Zimmerlin a., a variety of hereditary progressive muscular a. in which the a. begins in the upper half of the body.

at·ro·pine (at′rō-pēn). A racemic mixture of d- and l-hyoscyamine, alkaloids obtained from the leaves and roots of *Atropa belladonna;* an anticholinergic, with diverse effects (tachycardia, mydriasis, cycloplegia, constipation, urinary retention, antisudorific) attributable to reversible competitive blockade of acetylcho-

line at muscarinic type cholinergic receptors; used in the treatment of poisoning with organophosphate insecticides or nerve gases. The (–) form is by far the more active. SYN *dl*-hyoscyamine, tropine tropate.

a. methonitrate, the methylnitrate of a., with the same actions and uses as a., but less lipid-soluble (due to the presence of a quaternary nitrogen atom that limits penetration of the blood-brain barrier) and hence with fewer central nervous system effects; a quaternary compound.

a. methylbromide, SYN methylatropine bromide.

a. sulfate, an anticholinergic; a widely used soluble salt of atropine.

atrop·in·ic (at′rō-pin-ik). Term used to indicate a sharing of pharmacologic properties with atropine. This means blocking parasympathetic neuroeffector junctions leading to a constellation of effects including tachycardia, urinary retention, dry mouth, constipation, mydriasis, cycloplegia, and other anticholinergic effects.

at·ro·pin·ism (at′rō-pin-izm). Symptoms of poisoning by atropine or belladonna.

at·ro·pin·i·za·tion (at-rō′pin-i-zā′shŭn). Administration of atropine or belladonna to the point of achieving the pharmacologic effect.

atros·cine. *dl*-Scopolamine. SEE scopolamine. [atropine + hyoscine]

at·ro·tox·in (at-rō-toks′in). A component of diamondback rattlesnake (*Crotalus atrox*) venom that specifically and reversibly increases voltage-dependent calcium ion currents in isolated myocytes.

at·tach·ment (ă-tach′ment). **1.** A connection of one part with another. **2.** In dentistry, a mechanical device for the fixation and stabilization of a dental prosthesis.

bar clip a.'s, SYN bar-sleeve a.'s.

bar-sleeve a.'s, fixed bar joints or rigid bar units used for splinting abutments with removable sleeves or clips within the partial denture for supporting and/or retaining the prosthesis. SYN bar clip a.'s.

epithelial a., SYN junctional *epithelium.*

epithelial a. of Gottlieb, SYN junctional *epithelium.*

frictional a., SYN precision a.

internal a., SYN precision a.

key a., SYN precision a.

keyway a., SYN precision a.

muscle-tendon a., the union of a muscle and tendon fiber in which sarcolemma intervenes between the two; the end of the muscle fiber may be rounded, conical, or tapered. SYN muscle-tendon junction.

parallel a., SYN precision a.

pericemental a., the tissues surrounding the cementum of the tooth, i.e., the periodontal ligament and alveolar bone.

precision a., (1) a frictional or mechanically retained unit used in fixed or removable prosthodontics, consisting of closely fitting male and female parts; (2) an a. that may be rigid in function or may incorporate a movable stress control unit to reduce the torque on the abutment. SYN frictional a., internal a., key a., keyway a., parallel a., slotted a.

slotted a., SYN precision a.

at·tack (ă-tak′). A sudden illness or an episode or exacerbation of chronic or recurrent illness.

brain a., SYN stroke (1).

drop a., an episode of sudden falling that occurs during standing or walking, without warning and without loss of consciousness, vertigo, or postictal behavior. The patients are usually elderly and have normal electroencephalograms; of unknown cause.

heart a., SYN myocardial *infarction.*

panic a., sudden onset of intense apprehension, fear, terror, or impending doom accompanied by increased autonomic nervous system activity and by various constitutional disturbances, depersonalization, and derealization.

salaam a., SYN nodding *spasm.*

transient ischemic a. (TIA), a sudden focal loss of neurological function with complete recovery usually within 24 hours; caused by a brief period of inadequate perfusion in a portion of the territory of the carotid or vertebral basilar arteries.

uncinate a., SYN uncinate *epilepsy.*

vagal a., SYN Gowers *syndrome.*

vasovagal a., SYN Gowers *syndrome.*

at·tar of rose (at′ăr). SYN *rose* oil, *oil* of rose. [Pers. *attara,* to smell sweet]

at·tend·ing (ă-tend′ing). In psychology, an aroused readiness to perceive, as in listening or looking; focusing of sense organs is sometimes involved. [L. *attendo,* to bend to, notice]

at·ten·u·ant (ă-ten′ū-ănt). 1. Denoting that which attenuates. 2. An agent, means, or method that attenuates.

at·ten·u·ate (ă-ten′ū-āt). To dilute, thin, reduce, weaken, diminish. [L. *at-tenuo,* pp. *-tenuatus,* to make thin or weak, fr. *tenuis,* thin]

at·ten·u·a·tion (ă-ten-ū-ā′shŭn). 1. The act of attenuating. 2. Diminution of virulence in a strain of an organism, obtained through selection of variants that occur naturally or through experimental means. 3. Loss of energy of a beam of radiant energy due to absorption, scattering, beam divergence, and other causes as the beam propagates through a medium. 4. Regulation of termination of transcription; involved in control of gene expression in specific tissues.

interaural a., the reduction in intensity the head provides sound presented to one ear canal before it gets to the other ear; for air conduction, the reduction approximates 35 dB, but for bone conduction, it is only about 10 dB.

at·ten·u·a·tor (ă-ten′ū-ā-tŏr, -tōr). 1. An electrical system of resistors and capacitors used to reduce the strength of electrical signals as in ultrasonography. 2. The terminator sequence in DNA at which attenuation occurs.

at·tic (at′ik). SYN epitympanic *recess.*

tympanic a., SYN epitympanic *recess.*

at·ti·co·mas·toid (at′i-kō-mas′toyd). Relating to the attic of the tympanic cavity and the mastoid antrum or cells.

at·ti·cot·o·my (at-i-kot′ō-mē). Operative opening into the tympanic attic. [attic + G. *tomē,* incision]

at·ti·tude (at′i-tood). 1. Position of the body and limbs. 2. Manner of acting. 3. In social or clinical psychology, a relatively stable and enduring predisposition or set to behave or react in a certain way toward persons, objects, institutions, or issues. [Mediev. L. *aptitudo,* fr. L. *aptus,* fit]

emotional a.'s, SYN passional a.'s.

fetal a., SYN fetal *habitus.*

passional a.'s, a.'s expressive of any of the great passions; e.g., anger, lust. SYN emotional a.'s.

at·ti·tu·di·nal (at-i-too′di-năl). Relating to a posture of the body; e.g., a. (statotonic) reflex.

△**atto- (a).** Prefix used in the SI and metric systems to signify one quintillionth (10^{-18}). [Danish *atten,* eighteen]

at·tol·lens (ă-tol′ens). Raising up; in anatomy, muscle action that lifts. [L. *at- tollo,* pres. p. *-tollens,* to lift up]

a. au′rem, a. auric′ulam, SYN auricularis superior (*muscle*).

a. oc′uli, SYN superior rectus (*muscle*).

at·trac·tin (a-trak′tin). A glycoprotein of T cell origin involved in T cell clustering and monocyte movement.

at·trac·tion (ă-trak′shŭn). The tendency of two bodies to approach each other. [L. *at-traho,* pp. *-tractus,* to draw toward]

capillary a., the force that causes fluids to rise up very fine tubes or pass through the pores of a loose material.

chemical a., the force impelling atoms of different elements or molecules to unite to form new substances or compounds.

magnetic a., the force that draws iron or steel toward a magnet.

neurotropic a., the pull of a regenerating axon toward the motor end-plate.

at·tra·hens (at′ră-henz). Drawing toward, denoting a muscle (attrahens aurem or auriculam) rudimentary in man, that tends to draw the pinna of the ear forward. SEE auricularis anterior (*muscle*). [see attraction]

at·tri·tion (ă-trish′ŭn). 1. Wearing away by friction or rubbing. 2. In dentistry, physiological loss of tooth structure caused by the abrasive character of food or from bruxism. Cf. abrasion. [L. *at-tero,* pp. *-tritus,* to rub against, rub away]

at. wt. Abbreviation for atomic *weight.*

atyp·ia (ā-tip′ē-ă). State of being not typical. SYN atypism.

atyp·i·cal (ā-tip′i-kal). Not typical; not corresponding to the normal form or type. [G. *a-* priv. + *typikos,* conformed to a type]

atyp·ism (ā-tip′izm). SYN atypia.

A.U. Abbreviation for *auris uterque* [L.], each ear or both ears.

Au Symbol for gold (aurum).

Aub, Joseph C., U.S. physician, 1890–1973. SEE A.-DuBois *table.*

Auberger blood group, Au blood group. See Blood Groups appendix.

Aubert, Hermann, German physiologist, 1826–1892. SEE A. *phenomenon.*

AUC Area under the plasma drug concentration vs. time curve; a measure of drug exposure. [abbr. *a*rea *u*nder the *c*urve]

Auch·mer·o·my·ia (awk′mer-ō-mī′yă). A genus of bloodsucking botflies (family Calliphoridae, order Diptera). [G. *auchmeros,* without rain, hence unwashed, squalid, + *myia,* a fly]

A. lute′ola, the Congo floor maggot; the bloodsucking larva of this botfly species is found in Africa south of the Sahara, usually in or near human habitations; the resistant larvae or maggots crawl to sleeping humans and suck blood for 15 to 20 minutes, detach, and hide, repeating these nightly attacks during their developmental period; no disease transmission is known from this insect.

^{198}Au col·loid. SYN radiogold colloid.

au·dile (aw′dil). 1. Relating to audition. 2. Denoting the type of mental imagery in which one recalls most readily that which has been heard rather than seen or read (i.e., having an auditory representational system). Cf. motile. 3. SYN auditive.

△**audio-.** The sense of hearing. [L. *audio,* to hear]

au·di·o·an·al·ge·sia (aw′dē-ō-an-ăl-jē′zē-ă). Use of music or sound delivered through earphones to mask pain during dental or surgical procedures.

au·di·o·gen·ic (awd′ē-ō-jen′ik). Caused by sound, especially a loud sound. [audio- + G. *genesis,* production]

▮**au·di·o·gram** (aw′dē-ō-gram). The graphic record drawn from the results of hearing tests with an audiometer, which charts the threshold of hearing at various frequencies against sound intensity in decibels. [audio- + G. *gramma,* a drawing]

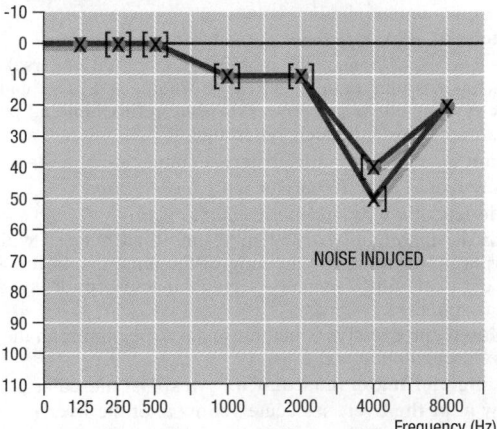

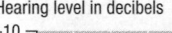

audiogram: abnormal pattern typical of noise-induced hearing loss

▮**pure tone a.,** a chart of the threshold for hearing at various frequencies usually expressed in decibels relative to normal threshold and usually covering frequencies from 250–8000 Hz.

speech a., the record of thresholds for spondaic word lists and scores for phonetically balanced word lists.

au·di·ol·o·gist (aw-dē-ol′ōjist). A specialist in evaluation and rehabilitation of those whose communication disorders stem in whole or in part from hearing impairment.

au·di·ol·o·gy (aw-dē-ol′ō-jē). The study of hearing disorders through the identification and measurement of hearing impairment as well as the rehabilitation of persons with hearing impairments.

au·di·om·e·ter (aw-dē-om′ĕ-ter). An electronic device used in measuring the threshold of hearing for pure tones of frequencies generally varying from 125–8000 Hz and speech (recorded in terms of decibels). [audio- + G. *metron,* measure]

automatic a., SYN Békésy a.

Békésy a., an automatic a. in which the tone sweeps the audiometric scale while the patient controls intensity by pressing a button when the tone is heard and releases when tone cannot be heard; may be operated either at a fixed frequency or at steadily changing frequencies. SYN automatic a.

pure-tone a., an a. that generates pure tones of selected frequencies with varying intensity. The stimuli are delivered by air conduction and bone conduction to differentiate conductive, sensorineural, or mixed hearing loss.

speech a., an a. that provides spoken material at controlled sound pressure levels to obtain speech reception thresholds, tolerance for loud speech, and discrimination ability, using either a live voice with a microphone or a recorded voice. It provides a measurement of overall performance in hearing, understanding, and responding to speech and an estimate of the degree of hearing disability.

au·di·o·met·ric (aw′dē-ō-met′rik). Related to measurement of hearing levels or to an audiometer.

au·di·om·e·trist (aw-dē-om′ĕ-trist). A person trained in the use of an audiometer in testing hearing.

au·di·om·e·try (aw-dē-om′ĕ-trē). **1.** The measurement of hearing. **2.** The use of an audiometer. **3.** Rapid measurement of the hearing of an individual or a group against a predetermined limit of normalcy; auditory responses to different frequencies presented at a constant intensity level are tested. SYN screening a.

automatic a., a. in which the subject controls increases and decreases in intensity at a fixed frequency or more usually as the frequency of the stimulus is gradually changed so that the subject traces back and forth across the threshold of hearing. SYN Békésy a.

behavioral observation a., a method of observing the motor responses of young children to test sound intensities to determine the hearing threshold.

Békésy a., SYN automatic a.

cortical a., measurement of the potentials that arise in the auditory system above the level of the brainstem.

diagnostic a., measurement of hearing threshold levels to determine the nature and degree of hearing impairment (i.e., conductive, sensorineural, or mixed).

screening a., SYN audiometry (3).

au·di·o·vi·su·al (aw′dē-ō-vizh′ū-ăl). Pertaining to a communication or teaching technique that combines both audible and visible symbols.

au·dit. An examination or review that establishes the extent to which a condition, process, or performance conforms to predetermined standards or criteria. [L. *auditus,* a hearing, fr. *audio,* to hear]

au·di·tion (aw-dish′ŭn). SYN hearing. [L. *auditio,* a hearing, fr. *audio,* to hear]

chromatic a., SYN color *hearing.*

au·di·tive (aw′di-tiv). One who recalls most readily that which has been heard. SYN audile (3).

au·di·to·ry (aw′di-tōr-ē). **1.** Pertaining to the sense of hearing or to the system serving hearing. **2.** Used to describe a person who preferentially uses verbal mental imagery. SEE ALSO internal *representation.* [L. *audio,* pp. *auditus,* to hear]

Auenbrugger, Leopold, Austrian physician, 1722–1809. SEE A. *sign.*

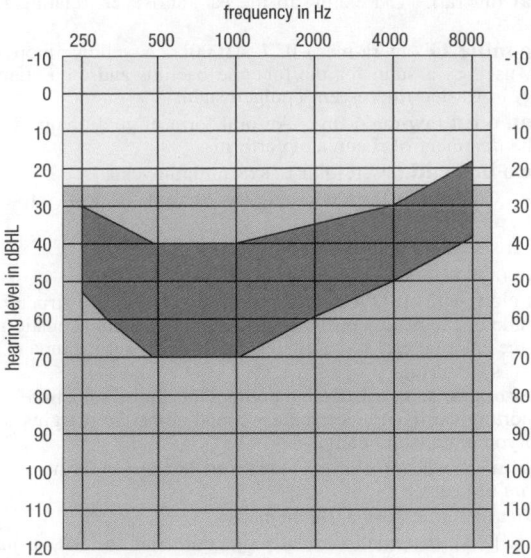

frequency in Hz

pure tone audiogram: yellow area indicates limits of normal hearing; dark green area illustrates the frequency and intensity of the English phonemes; dBHL = decibels (of) hearing loss

Auer, John, U.S. physician, 1875–1948. SEE A. *bodies,* under *body, rods,* under *rod.*

Auerbach, Leopold, German anatomist, 1828–1897. SEE A. *ganglia,* under *ganglion, plexus.*

Aufrecht, Emanuel, German physician, 1844–1933. SEE A. *sign.*

Auger (aw′ger). Pierre-Victor, French physicist, 1899–1993. SEE Auger *electron.*

aug·na·thus (awg-nā′thŭs). SYN dignathus. [G. *au,* again, + *gnathos,* jaw]

Aujeszky, Aládar, Hungarian pathologist, 1869–1933. SEE A. disease *virus.*

aur Abbreviation for auris.

au·ra, pl. **au·rae** (aw′ră, -rē). **1.** Epileptic ictal phenomenon/phenomena perceived only by the patient. **2.** Subjective symptoms at the onset of a migraine headache. [L. breeze, odor, gleam of light]

abdominal a., epileptic a. characterized by abdominal discomfort, including nausea, malaise, pain, and hunger; some phenomena reflect ictal autonomic dysfunction. SEE ALSO aura (1).

auditory a., epileptic a. characterized by illusions or hallucinations of sounds. SEE ALSO aura (1).

experiential a., epileptic a. characterized by altered perception of one's internal and/or external environment; may involve auditory, visual, olfactory, gustatory, somatosensory, or emotional altered perceptions. When one of the altered perceptions is clearly predominant, the specific a. classification should be used. SEE ALSO aura (1).

gustatory a., epileptic a. characterized by illusions or hallucinations of taste. SEE ALSO aura (1).

intellectual a., a dreamy, detached, or reminiscent a. SYN reminiscent a.

kinesthetic a., an a. consisting of a subjective feeling of movement of a part of the body.

olfactory a., epileptic a. characterized by illusions or hallucinations of smell. SEE ALSO aura (1).

reminiscent a., SYN intellectual a.

somatosensory a., epileptic a. characterized by paresthesias or abdominal somatognosia of a clearly defined regional distribution. SEE ALSO aura (1).

visual a., epileptic a. characterized by visual illusions or hallucinations, formed or unformed, including scintillations, teichopsia. SEE ALSO aura (1).

au·ral (aw′răl). **1.** Relating to the ear (auris). **2.** Relating to an aura.

au·ra·mine O (aw′ră-mēn) [C.I. 41000]. A yellow fluorescent dye, used as a stain for the tubercle bacillus and as a stain for DNA in Kasten fluorescent Feulgen stain.

au·ran·o·fin (aw-ran′ō-fin). An oral form of gold complex used in the treatment of rheumatoid arthritis.

au·re·o·lic ac·id (aw-rē-ō′lik). SYN mithramycin.

⟳**auri-.** Combining form denoting the ear. SEE ALSO ot-, oto-. [L. *auris*, an ear.]

au·ri·a·sis (aw-rī′ă-sis). SYN chrysiasis.

au·ric (aw′rik). Relating to gold (aurum).

au·ri·cle (aw′ri-kl) [TA]. **1.** The projecting shell-like structure on the side of the head, constituting, with the external acoustic meatus, the external ear. SYN auricula (1) [TA], ala auris, pinna (1). **2.** SYN a.'s (of atria).

accessory a.'s, small, fleshy nodules or folds, sometimes with supporting cartilage, occasionally found along the margins of the embryonic branchial clefts.

atrial a., SYN a.'s (of atria); SEE ALSO left *atrium* of heart, right *atrium* of heart.

cervical a., accessory a. on the neck.

left a. [TA], the small conical projection from the left atrium of the heart. SYN auricula atrii sinistra [TA], a. of left atrium, left auricular appendage.

a. of left atrium, SYN left a.

a.'s (of atria) [TA], a small conical ("ear-shaped") pouch projecting from the upper anterior portion of each atrium of the heart, increasing slightly the atrial volume. SEE left a., right a. SYN auricle (2) [TA], auricula (2) [TA], auriculae atrii [TA], atrial appendage, atrial a., atrial auricula, auricular appendix.

right a. [TA], the small conical projection from the right atrium of the heart. SYN auricula atrii dextra [TA], a. of right atrium, auricular appendage (1), right auricular appendage.

a. of right atrium, SYN right a.

au·ric·u·la, pl. **au·ric·u·lae** (aw-rik′ū-lă, -lē) [TA]. **1.** SYN auricle (1). **2.** SYN *auricles* (of atria), under *auricle*. [L. the external ear, dim. of *auris,* ear]

atrial a., SYN *auricles* (of atria), under *auricle*; SEE ALSO left *atrium* of heart, right *atrium* of heart.

auriculae atrii [TA], SYN *auricles* (of atria), under *auricle*; SEE left *atrium* of heart, right *atrium* of heart.

a. atrii dex′tra [TA], SYN right *auricle*.

a. atrii sinis′tra [TA], SYN left *auricle*.

au·ric·u·lar (aw-rik′ū-lăr). Relating to the ear, or to an auricle in any sense.

au·ric·u·la·re, pl. **au·ric·u·lar·ia** (aw-rik-ū-lā′rē, -rē-ă). A craniometric point at the center of the opening of the external acoustic meatus; or, in certain cases, the middle of the upper edge of this opening. SYN auricular point. [L. *auricularis,* pertaining to the ear]

au·ric·u·lo·cra·ni·al (aw-rik′ū-lō-krā′nē-ăl). Relating to the auricle or pinna of the ear and the cranium.

au·ric·u·lo·tem·po·ral (aw-rik′ū-lō-tem′pō-răl). Relating to the auricle or pinna of the ear and the temporal region.

au·ric·u·lo·ven·tric·u·lar (aw-rik′ū-lō-ven-trik′ū-lăr). Obsolete synonym for atrioventricular.

au·rid, pl. **au·ri·des** (aw′rid, aw′ri-dēz). A skin lesion due to injection of gold salts. [L. *aurum,* gold, + *-id* (1)]

au·ri·form (aw′ri-fōrm). Ear-shaped.

au·rin (aw′rin) [C.I. 43800]. A triphenylmethane derivative used as an indicator (changes from yellow to red at pH 6.8 to 8.2) and as a dye intermediate; also used to help differentiate tubercle bacilli from other acid-fast microorganisms. SYN corallin, *p*-rosolic acid.

au·rin·tri·car·box·yl·ic ac·id (aw′rin-trī′kar-boks-il′ik). A chelating agent that has a special affinity for beryllium and certain other materials, and may therefore be of use in combating beryllium poisoning; the ammonium salt is known as aluminon.

au·ris (a, a, aur), pl. **au·res** (aw′ris, aw′rēz) [TA]. SYN ear. [L.]

a. exte′rna, SYN external *ear.*

a. inter′na, SYN internal *ear.*

a. me′dia, SYN middle *ear.*

au·ro·chro·mo·der·ma (aw′rō-krō-mō-der′mă). SYN chrysiasis. [L. *aurum,* gold, + *chrōma,* color, + derma, skin]

au·ro·mer·cap·to·ac·et·an·i·lid (aw′rō-mer-kap′tō-as-ĕ-tan′i-lid). An organic gold compound, insoluble in water; used in the treatment of rheumatoid arthritis, and administered by intramuscular injection; more slowly absorbed than the water-soluble gold salts. SYN aurothioglycanide.

au·rone (aw′rōn). **1.** The parent compound of a series of plant pigments; they are substituted coumaranones, and may be formed from chalcones. They are often found as glycosides. **2.** A class of compounds based on a. (1). SYN benzalcoumaran-3-one.

au·ro·ther·a·py (aw-rō-thār′ă-pē). SYN chrysotherapy. [L. *aurum,* gold]

au·ro·thi·o·glu·cose (aw′rō-thī-ō-gloo′kōs). Organic gold preparation with –SAu group in place of 1-OH group of glucose; used in treatment of rheumatoid arthritis and discoid lupus erythematosus. It is thought to arrest the progression of disease. SYN gold thioglucose.

au·ro·thi·o·gly·ca·nide (aw′-rō-thī-ō-glī′kă-nīd). SYN auromercaptoacetanilid.

au·rum (aw′rŭm). SYN gold. [L.]

aus·cul·tate, aus·cult (aws′kŭl-tāt, aws-kŭlt′). To perform auscultation.

ﬧaus·cul·ta·tion (aws-kŭl-tā′shŭn). Listening to the sounds made by the various body structures as a diagnostic method. [L. *ausculto,* pp. *-atus,* to listen to]

immediate a., direct a., a. by application of the ear to the surface of the body.

ﬧmediate a., a. performed with the use of a stethoscope.

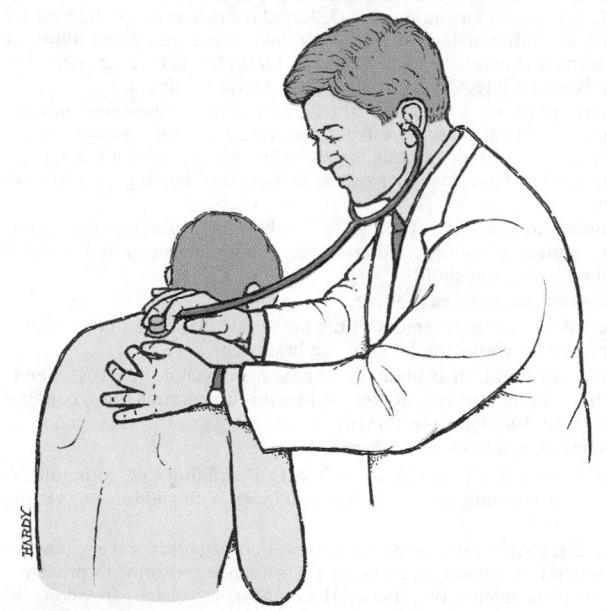

auscultation: mediate

aus·cul·ta·to·ry (aws-kŭl′tă-tō-rē). Relating to auscultation.

Auspitz, Heinrich, Austrian physician, 1835–1886. SEE Auspitz *sign.*

Austin Flint, SEE Flint.

⟳**aut-.** SEE auto-.

au·ta·coid (aw-tă′-koyd). SYN autocoid. [aut- + G. *akos,* relief, resource]

au·te·cic, au·te·cious (aw-tē′sik, aw-tē′shŭs). Denoting a parasite that infects, throughout its entire existence, the same host. [G. *autos*, same, + *oikion*, house]

au·te·me·sia (aw-tĕ-mē′zē-ă). Rarely used term for: **1.** Idiopathic or functional vomiting. **2.** Vomiting induced by provoking the gag reflex. [G. *autos*, self, + *emesis*, vomiting]

au·then·tic·i·ty (aw-then-tis′i-tē). **1.** The quality of being authentic, genuine, and valid. **2.** In psychological functioning and personality, applied to the conscious feelings, perceptions, and thoughts that one expresses and communicates honestly and genuinely. [G. *authentikos*, original, primary]

au·tism (aw′tizm). A mental disorder characterized by severely abnormal development of social interaction and verbal and nonverbal communication skills. Affected individuals may adhere to inflexible, nonfunctional rituals or routine. They may become upset with even trivial changes in their environment. They often have a limited range of interests but may become preoccupied with a narrow range of subjects or activities. They appear unable to understand others' feelings and often have poor eye contact with others. Unpredictable mood swings may occur. Many demonstrate stereotypical motor mannerisms such as hand or finger flapping, body rocking, or dipping. The disorder is probably caused by organically based central nervous system dysfunction, especially in the ability to process social or emotional information or language. [G. *autos*, self]

early infantile a., SYN infantile a.

infantile a., a severe emotional disturbance of childhood characterized by qualitative impairment in reciprocal social interaction and in communication, language, and social development. SYN childhood schizophrenia, early infantile a., Kanner syndrome.

au·tis·tic (aw-tis′tik). Pertaining to or characterized by autism.

auto-, aut-. Prefixes meaning self, same. [G. *autos*, self]

au·to·ac·ti·va·tion (aw′tō-ak-ti-vā′shŭn). SYN autocatalysis.

au·to·ag·glu·ti·na·tion (aw′to-ă-gloo-ti-nā′shŭn). **1.** Nonspecific agglutination or clumping together of cells (e.g., bacteria, erythrocytes) due to physical and/or chemical factors. **2.** The agglutination of red blood cells by specific autoantibody present in one's own serum.

au·to·ag·glu·ti·nin (aw′tō-ă-gloo′ti-nin). An agglutinating autoantibody.

anti-Pr cold a., a cold a. specific for the Pr (protease-sensitive) antigen of erythrocytes.

cold a., an antibody that agglutinates particulate antigens (i.e., bacteria) at temperatures below 37°C, often most actively at 4°C; most are the IgM class of immunoglobulins with affinity for the Ii system of erythrocyte antigens, but some are anti-Pr cold a.'s; cold a.'s may be associated with infection (e.g., primary atypical pneumonia, infectious mononucleosis and other virus infections, certain protozoan infections) and in such instances usually are not active *in vivo*.

au·to·al·ler·gic (aw′tō-ă-ler′jik). Pertaining to autoallergy.

au·to·al·ler·gi·za·tion (aw′tō-al′er-ji-zā′shŭn). Induction of autoallergy.

au·to·al·ler·gy (aw-tō-al′er-jē). An altered reactivity in which antibodies (autoantibodies) are produced against an individual's own tissues, causing a destructive rather than a protective effect. SYN autoimmunity (1).

au·to·a·nal·y·sis (aw′tō-ă-nal′i-sis). Attempted analysis, or psychoanalysis, of one's self. SYN self-analysis.

au·to·an·a·lyz·er (aw-tō-an′ă-līz-er). An instrument capable of conducting analyses automatically; commonly used in chemical analyses.

sequential multichannel a. (SMA), an automated instrument capable of performing multiple (usually chemical) analyses simultaneously by propelling samples and reagents in continuous flow fashion along tubes to the detector mechanisms.

au·to·an·a·phy·lax·is (aw′tō-an′ă-fī-lak′sis). Obsolete term for certain kinds of autoimmunity.

au·to·an·ti·body (aw-tō-an′ti-bod-ē). Antibody occurring in response to antigenic constituents of the host's tissue against self antigen, and which reacts with the inciting tissue component.

antiidiotype a., SYN idiotype a. SEE antiidiotype *antibody*.

some autoimmune diseases in humans		
disease	**self-antigen**	**immune response**
organ-specific autoimmune diseases		
Addison disease	adrenal cells	autoantibodies
autoimmune hemolytic anemia	red blood cell (RBC) membrane proteins	autoantibodies
Goodpasture syndrome	renal and lung basement membranes	autoantibodies
Graves disease	thyroid-stimulating hormone receptor	autoantibodies (stimulating)
Hashimoto thyroiditis	thyroid proteins and cells	T_{DTH} cells, autoantibodies
idiopathic thrombocytopenic purpura	platelet membrane proteins	autoantibodies
type 1 diabetes mellitus	pancreatic beta cells	T_{DTH} cells, autoantibodies
myasthenia gravis	acetylcholine receptors	autoantibody (blocking)
pernicious anemia	gastric parietal cells, intrinsic factor	autoantibody
poststreptococcal glomerulonephritis	kidney	antigen-antibody complexes
spontaneous infertility	sperm	autoantibodies
systemic autoimmune diseases		
ankylosing spondylitis	vertebrae	immune complexes
multiple sclerosis	white matter of brain and spinal cord	T_{DTH} cells and T_C cells, autoantibodies
rheumatoid arthritis	connective tissue, IgG	autoantibodies, immune complexes
scleroderma	nuclei, heart, lungs, gastrointestinal tract, kidney	autoantibodies
Sjögren syndrome	salivary gland, liver, kidney, thyroid	autoantibodies
systemic lupus erythematosus (SLE)	DNA, nuclear protein, RBC platelet membranes	autoantibodies, immune complexes

cold a., an a. that reacts at temperatures below 37°C.

Donath-Landsteiner cold a., an a. of the IgG class responsible for paroxysmal cold hemoglobinuria; it is adsorbed to red cells only at temperatures of 20°C or lower, causing the red cells to lyse in the presence of complement at higher temperatures; it has a specificity within the blood group P; it is also occasionally present for short periods of time following measles and other infections, and formerly was frequently associated with syphilis. SYN cold hemolysin.

hemagglutinating cold a., a cold autoagglutinin.

idiotype a., SYN antiidiotype a.

warm a., an a. that reacts optimally at 37°C.

au·to·an·ti·com·ple·ment (aw′tō-an-ti-com′plĕ-ment). An anticomplement that is formed in the body of an animal and inhibits or destroys the complement of the same animal.

au·to·an·ti·gen (aw-to-an′ti-jen). A "self" antigen; any tissue constituent that evokes an immune response by the host.

au·to·as·say (aw′tō-as-ā). Detection or estimation of the amount of a substance produced in an organism by means of a test object in that organism, as, for example, use of the denervated heart in situ of a cat to assay for epinephrine or sympathin liberated into its bloodstream.

au·to·aug·men·ta·tion (aw′-tō-awg′men-tā-shŭn). Augmentation of the bladder by incision and excision of detrusor muscle leaving only bladder epithelium. SYN autocystoplasty.

au·to·blast (aw′tō-blast). **1.** An independent cell. **2.** A single, independent microbe, protozoon, or single-celled (acellular) organism. [auto- + G. *blastos*, germ]

au·to·ca·tal·y·sis (aw'tō-kă-tal'i-sis). A reaction in which one or more of the products formed acts to catalyze the reaction; beginning slowly, the rate of such a reaction rapidly increases. Cf. chain *reaction*. SYN autoactivation.

au·to·cat·a·lyt·ic (aw'tō-kat-ă-lit'ik). Relating to autocatalysis.

au·to·cath·e·ter·i·za·tion, au·to·cath·e·ter·ism (aw'tō-kath-ĕ-ter-i-zā'shŭn, -kath'ĕ-ter-izm). Passage of a catheter by the patient.

au·toch·thon·ous (aw-tok'thon-ŭs). **1.** Native to the place inhabited; aboriginal. **2.** Originating in the place where found; said of a disease originating in the part of the body where found, or of a disease acquired in the place where the patient is. [auto- + G. *chthon,* land, ground, country]

au·toc·la·sis, au·to·cla·sia (aw-tok'lă-sis, aw-tō-klā'zē-ă). **1.** A breaking up or rupturing from intrinsic or internal causes. **2.** Progressive immunologically induced tissue destruction. [auto- + G. *klasis,* breaking]

au·to·clave (aw'tō-klāv). **1.** An apparatus for sterilization by steam under pressure; it consists of a strong closed boiler containing a small quantity of water and, in a wire basket, the articles to be sterilized. **2.** To sterilize in an autoclave. [auto- + L. *clavis,* a key, in the sense of self-locking]

au·to·coid (aw'tō-koyd). A chemical substance produced by one type of cell that affects the function of different types of cells in the same region, thus functioning as a local hormone or messenger. SYN autacoid substance, autacoid. [G. *autos,* self, + *eidos,* form]

au·to·crine (aw'tō-krin). Denoting self-stimulation through cellular production of a factor and a specific receptor for it. [auto- + G. *krinō,* to separate]

au·to·cys·to·plas·ty (aw-tō-sis'tō-plas-tē). SYN autoaugmentation. [auto- + G. *kystis,* bladder, + *plastos,* formed]

au·to·cy·to·ly·sin (aw'tō-sī-tol'i-sin). SYN autolysin.

au·to·cy·tol·y·sis (aw'tō-sī-tol'i-sis). SYN autolysis.

au·to·cy·to·tox·in (aw'tō-sī-tō-toks'in). A cytotoxic autoantibody.

au·to·der·mic (aw-tō-der'mik). Relating to one's own skin; denoting especially an autodermic graft or dermatoautoplasty. [auto- + G. *derma,* skin]

au·to·di·ges·tion (aw'tō-dī-jes'chŭn). SYN autolysis.

au·to·dip·loid (aw-tō-dip'loyd). SEE autoploid.

au·to·drain·age (aw-tō-drān'ij). Drainage into contiguous tissues.

au·to·ech·o·la·lia (aw'tō-ek-ō-lā'lē-ă). A morbid repetition of another person's or one's own words. [auto- + echolalia]

au·to·e·rot·ic (aw'tō-ĕ-rot'ik). Pertaining to autoerotism.

au·to·e·rot·i·cism (aw'tō-ĕ-rot'i-sizm). Sexual arousal or gratification using one's own body, as in masturbation. SYN autoerotism. [auto- + G. *erōtikos,* relating to love]

au·to·er·o·tism (aw-tō-ār'ō-tizm). SYN autoeroticism. [auto- + G. *erōtikos,* relating to love]

au·to·flu·o·ro·scope (aw-tō-flōr'ō-skōp). A type of scintillation camera consisting of a matrix of individual sodium iodide crystals, each with its separate light pipe and photomultiplier tube; used for radioisotope imaging procedures.

au·tog·a·mous (aw-tog'ă-mŭs). Relating to or characterized by autogamy.

au·tog·a·my (aw-tog'ă-mē). A form of self-fertilization in which fission of the cell nucleus occurs without division of the cell, the two pronuclei so formed reuniting to form the synkaryon; in other cases, the cell body also divides, but the two daughter cells immediately conjugate. SYN automixis. [auto- + G. *gamos,* marriage]

au·to·gen·e·sis (aw-tō-jen'ĕ-sis). **1.** The origin of living matter within the organism itself. **2.** In bacteriology, the process by which vaccine is made from bacteria obtained from the patient's own body. [auto- + G. *genesis,* production]

au·to·ge·net·ic, au·to·gen·ic (aw'tō-jĕ-net'ik, jen'ik). Relating to autogenesis. SYN autogenous (1).

au·tog·e·nous (aw-toj'ĕ-nŭs). **1.** SYN autogenetic, autologous. **2.**

Originating within the body, applied to vaccines prepared from bacteria or other cells obtained from the affected person. Cf. endogenous. [G. *autogenēs,* self-produced]

au·tog·no·sis (aw-tog-nō'sis). Recognition of one's own character, tendencies, and peculiarities. SYN self-knowledge. [auto- + G. *gnōsis,* knowledge]

au·to·graft (aw'tō-graft). Tissue or organ transferred into a new position in the body of the same individual. SYN autogeneic graft, autologous graft, autoplastic graft, autotransplant. [auto- + A.S. *graef*]

au·to·graft·ing (aw-tō-graft'ing). SYN autotransplantation.

au·to·gram (aw'tō-gram). A wheal-like lesion on the skin following pressure by a blunt instrument or by stroking. [auto- + G. *gramma,* something written]

au·tog·ra·phism (aw-tog'ră-fizm). SYN dermatographism.

au·to·hem·ag·glu·ti·na·tion (aw'tō-hē'mă-gloo-ti-nā'shŭn). Autoagglutination of autologous erythrocytes.

au·to·he·mo·ly·sin (aw'tō-hē-mol'i-sin). An autoantibody that causes lysis of erythrocytes in the presence of complement.

au·to·he·mol·y·sis (aw'tō-hē-mol'i-sis). Hemolysis occurring in certain diseases as a result of an autohemolysin.

au·to·hex·a·ploid (aw-tō-heks'ă-ployd). SEE autoploid.

au·to·hyp·no·sis (aw'tō-hip-nō'sis). Self-induced hypnosis, accomplished by concentrating on self-absorbing thought or on the idea of being hypnotized. SYN autohypnotism, idiohypnotism.

au·to·hyp·not·ic (aw'tō-hip-not'ik). Relating to autohypnosis.

au·to·hyp·no·tism (aw-tō-hip'nō-tizm). SYN autohypnosis.

au·to·im·mune (aw-tō-i-mūn'). Cells and/or antibodies arising from and directed against the individual's own tissues, as in autoimmune disease.

au·to·im·mu·ni·ty (aw'tō-i-mū'ni-tē). **1.** In immunology, the condition in which one's own tissues are subject to deleterious effects of the immune system, as in autoallergy and in autoimmune disease; specific humoral or cell-mediated immune response against the body's own tissues. SYN autoallergy. **2.** Literally, the condition in which "self" is exempt.

au·to·im·mu·ni·za·tion (aw'tō-im'ū-ni-zā'shŭn). Induction of autoimmunity.

au·to·im·mu·no·cy·to·pe·nia (aw-tō-im'oo-nō-sī-tō-pē'nē-ă). Anemia, thrombocytopenia, and leukopenia resulting from cytotoxic autoimmune reactions.

au·to·in·fec·tion (aw'tō-in-fek'shŭn). **1.** Reinfection by microbes or parasitic organisms that have already passed through an infective cycle. **2.** Self-infection by direct contagion as with pinworm (*Enterobius vermicularis*) eggs passed in the infectious state and transmitted by fingernails (anal-oral route). SYN autoreinfection, self-infection.

au·to·in·fu·sion (aw'tō-in-fū'shŭn). Forcing the blood from the extremities or other areas such as the spleen, as by the application of a bandage or pressure device, to raise the blood pressure and fill the vessels in the vital centers; resorted to after excessive loss of blood or other body fluids. Cf. autotransfusion.

au·to·in·oc·u·la·ble (aw'tō-in-ok'ū-lă-bl). Susceptible to autoinoculation.

au·to·in·oc·u·la·tion (aw'tō-in-ok-ū-lā'shŭn). A secondary infection originating from a focus of infection already present in the body.

au·to·in·tox·i·cant (aw'tō-in-toks'i-kant). An endogenous toxic agent that causes autointoxication. SYN autotoxin.

au·to·in·tox·i·ca·tion (aw'tō-in-toks-i-kā'shŭn). A disorder resulting from absorption of the waste products of metabolism, decomposed matter from the intestine, or the products of dead and infected tissue as in gangrene. SYN autotoxicosis, endogenic toxicosis, enterotoxication, enterotoxism, intestinal intoxication, self-poisoning.

au·to·i·sol·y·sin (aw'tō-ī-sol'i-sin). An antibody that in the presence of complement causes lysis of cells in the individual in whose body the lysin is formed, as well as in others of the same species.

au·to·ker·a·to·plas·ty (aw-tō-ker'ă-tō-plas-tē). Grafting of corneal tissue from one eye of a patient to the fellow eye. [auto- + G. *keras,* horn, + *plastos,* formed]

au·to·ki·ne·sia, au·to·ki·ne·sis (aw-tō-ki-ne′sē-ă, aw-tō-ki-ne′sis). Voluntary movement. [auto- + G. *kinēsis,* movement]

au·to·ki·net·ic (aw-tō-ki̇̆-net′ik). Relating to autokinesis.

au·to·le·sion (aw-tō-lē′zhŭn). A self-inflicted injury.

au·tol·o·gous (aw-tol′ŏ-gŭs). **1.** Occurring naturally and normally in a certain type of tissue or in a specific structure of the body. **2.** In transplantation, referring to a graft in which the donor and recipient areas are in the same individual, or to blood that the donor has previously donated and then receives back, usually during surgery. **3.** Sometimes used to denote a neoplasm derived from cells that occur normally at that sight, e.g., a squamous cell carcinoma in the upper esophagus. SYN autogenous (1). [auto- + G. *logos,* relation]

au·tol·y·sate (aw-tol′i-sāt). The mixture of substances resulting from autolysis.

au·to·lyse (aw′tō-līs). SYN autolyze.

au·tol·y·sin (aw-tol′i-sin). An antibody that in the presence of complement causes lysis of the cells and tissues in the body of the individual in whom the lysin is formed. SYN autocytolysin.

au·tol·y·sis (aw-tol′i-sis). **1.** Enzymatic digestion of cells (especially dead or degenerate) by enzymes present within them (autogenous). **2.** Destruction of cells as a result of a lysin formed in those cells or others in the same organism. SYN autocytolysis, autodigestion, isophagy. [auto- + G. *lysis,* dissolution]

au·to·lyt·ic (aw-tō-lit′ik). Pertaining to or causing autolysis.

au·to·lyze (aw′tō-līz). To undergo autolysis. SYN autolyse.

au·to·mal·let (aw′tō-mal-et). Obsolete term for automatic *plugger* or condenser.

au·tom·a·tism (aw-tom′ă-tizm). **1.** The state of being independent of the will or of central innervation; applicable, for example, to the heart's action. **2.** An epileptic attack consisting of stereotyped psychic, sensory, or motor phenomena carried out in a state of impaired consciousness and of which the individual usually has no knowledge. **3.** A condition in which an individual is consciously or unconsciously, but involuntarily, compelled to the performance of certain motor or verbal acts, often purposeless and sometimes foolish or harmful. SYN telergy. [G. *automatos,* self-moving, + -in]

ambulatory a., a person's automatic performance of an action or series of actions without being consciously aware of the processes involved in the performance.

immediate posttraumatic a., a posttraumatic state in which the patient performs automatically without immediate or later memory of that behavior.

au·to·mat·o·graph (aw-tō-mat′ō-graf). An instrument for recording automatic movements.

au·to·mix·is (aw-tō-miks′is). SYN autogamy. [auto- + G. *mixis,* intercourse]

au·tom·ne·sia (aw-tom-nē′zē-ă). Spontaneous revival of memories of an earlier condition of life. [auto- + G. *mnēsis,* a remembering]

au·to·my·so·pho·bia (aw′tō-mis-ō-fō′bē-ă). Morbid dread of personal uncleanliness. [auto- + G. *mysos,* dirt, + *phobos,* fear]

au·to·nom·ic (aw-tō-nom′ik). Relating to the autonomic nervous system.

au·to·nom·o·tro·pic (aw′tō-nom-ō-trop′ik). Acting on the autonomic nervous system. [autonomic + G. *trepo,* to turn]

au·ton·o·mous (aw-ton′ō-mŭs). Having independence or freedom from control by external forces or, in a narrow sense, by the cerebrospinal nerve centers.

au·ton·o·my (aw-ton′ō-mē). The condition or state of being autonomous, able to make decisions unaided by others. [auto- + G. *nomos,* law]

functional a., in social psychology, the tendency of a developed motive system (e.g., motive of acquisition) to become independent of the primary or innate drive from which it originated (e.g., need for food).

au·to·ox·i·da·tion (aw′tō-oks-i-dā′shŭn). The direct combination of a substance with molecular oxygen at ordinary temperatures. SYN autoxidation.

au·to·ox·i·diz·a·ble (aw′tō-oks-i-dīz′ă-bl). Denoting substances that react directly with oxygen (e.g., b hemochromogen in cytochrome) and do not require the action of dehydrogenases.

au·to·path·ic (aw-tō-path′ik). Rarely used synonym for idiopathic.

au·to·pen·ta·ploid (aw-tō-pen′tă-ployd). SEE autoploid.

au·to·pep·sia (aw-tō-pep′sē-ă). Rarely used term for self-digestion, said of ulceration of the gastric mucous membrane by its own secretion, or the digestion of the skin surrounding a gastrostomy or colostomy opening. [auto- + G. *pepsis,* digestion]

au·to·pha·gia (aw-tō-fā′jē-ă). **1.** Biting one's own flesh; e.g., as a symptom of Lesch-Nyhan syndrome. **2.** Maintenance of the nutrition of the whole body by metabolic consumption of some of the body tissues. **3.** SYN autophagy. [auto- + G. *phagō,* to eat]

au·to·pha·gic (aw-tō-fā′jik). Relating to or characterized by autophagia.

au·to·pha·go·ly·so·some (aw′tō-fā-gō-lī′sō-sōm). The digestive vacuole of autophagy that results from the fusion of a primary lysosome with an autophagic vacuole.

au·toph·a·gy (aw-tof′ă-jē). Segregation and disposal of damaged organelles within a cell. SYN autophagia (3). [auto- + G. *phagō,* to eat]

au·to·pho·bia (aw-tō-fō′bē-ă). Morbid fear of solitude or of self. [auto- + G. *phobos,* fear]

au·toph·o·ny (aw-tof′ŏ-nē). Increased hearing of one's own voice, breath sounds, arterial murmurs, etc., noted especially in disease of the middle ear or of the nasal fossae. SYN tympanophonia, tympanophony. [auto- + G. *phōnē,* sound]

au·to·ploid (aw′tō-ployd). Relating to an individual or cell with two or more copies of a single haploid set; depending on the number of multiples of the haploid set, a.'s are referred to as autodiploids, autotriploids, autotetraploids, autopentaploids, autohexaploids, etc. [auto- + -ploid]

au·to·ploi·dy (aw′tō-ploy-dē). The condition of being autoploid.

au·to·plug·ger (aw′tō-plŭg-er). Obsolete term for automatic *plugger.*

au·to·pod (aw′tō-pod). SYN autopodium.

au·to·po·di·um, pl. **au·to·po·dia** (aw′tō-pō′dē-ŭm, dē-ă). The distal major subdivision of a limb (hand or foot). SYN autopod. [auto- + G. *pous (pod-),* foot]

au·to·poi·son·ous (aw-tō-poy′zŭn-ŭs). SYN autotoxic.

au·to·pol·y·mer (aw-tō-pol′i-mer). SEE autopolymer *resin.*

au·to·po·lym·er·i·za·tion (aw-tō-pol′i-mer-i-zā′shŭn). Polymerization without the use of external heat, as a result of the addition of an activator and a catalyst.

au·to·pol·y·ploid (aw-tō-pol′i-ployd). An autoploid having two or more multiples of the haploid sets of chromosomes.

au·to·pol·y·ploi·dy (aw-tō-pol′i-ploy-dē). The condition of being allopolyploid.

au·top·sy (aw′top-sē). **1.** An examination of the organs of a dead body to determine the cause of death or to study the pathologic changes present. SYN necropsy. **2.** In the terminology of the ancient Greek school of empirics, the intentional reproduction of an effect, event, or circumstance that occurred in the course of a disease and observation of its influence in ameliorating or aggravating the patient's symptoms. SYN postmortem examination. [G. *autopsia,* seeing with one's own eyes]

verbal a., method of obtaining as much information as possible about a deceased person by asking questions of family and others who can describe the mode of death and circumstances preceding death; used especially in developing countries and in settings and situations in which postmortem pathological examination is not feasible.

au·to·ra·di·o·gram (aw-tō-rā′dē-ō-gram). SYN autoradiograph. [auto- + radiogram]

au·to·ra·di·o·graph (aw-tō-rā′dē-ō-graf). Image of the distribution and concentration of radioactivity in a tissue or other substance made by placing a photographic emulsion on the surface of, or in close proximity to, the substance. SYN autoradiogram.

au·to·ra·di·og·ra·phy (aw′tō-rā-dē-og′ră-fē). The process of producing an autoradiograph. SYN radioautography.

paper a., a. in which compounds are separated by paper chromatography.

autoreceptor (au′tō-rē-sep-tŏr, tōr). A site on a neuron that binds the neurotransmitter released by that neuron, which then regulates the neuron's activity. [auto- + receptor]

au·to·reg·u·la·tion (aw′tō-reg-ū-lā′shŭn). **1.** The tendency of the blood flow to an organ or part to remain at or return to the same level despite changes in the pressure in the artery which conveys blood to it. **2.** In general, any biologic system equipped with inhibitory feedback systems such that a given change tends to be largely or completely counteracted; e.g., baroreceptor reflexes form a basis for autoregulation of the systemic arterial blood pressure.

heterometric a., intrinsic regulation of the strength of cardiac contraction as a function of diastolic fiber length (volume), independent of afterload, autonomic nerves and other extrinsic influences. Heterometric a. is also known as the length-tension relationship, the relationship of end diastolic volume to end diastolic pressure, Starling law of the heart, and the Frank-Starling curve.

homeometric a., intrinsic regulation of strength of cardiac contraction in response to influences that do not depend on change in fiber length, i.e., the Frank-Starling curve, (e.g., the Anrep effect in which strength increases in response to increased afterload, and the Bowditch effect (treppe) in which strength increases in response to increased heart rate) and do not depend on extrinsic regulation (e.g., in which strength increases in response to sympathetic nerve stimulation or norepinephrine).

au·to·re·in·fec·tion (aw′tō-rē-in-fek′shŭn). SYN autoinfection.

au·to·re·pro·duc·tion (aw′tō-rē-prō-duk′shŭn). The ability of a gene or virus, or nucleoprotein molecule generally, to bring about the synthesis of another molecule like itself from smaller molecules within the cell.

au·tor·rha·phy (aw-tōr′ă-fē). Wound closure using strands of fascia from the edges of the wound. [auto- + G. *rhaphē,* sewing]

au·to·sen·si·tize (aw-tō-sen′si-tīz). To sensitize against one's own body cells. SYN isosensitize.

au·to·sep·ti·ce·mia (aw′tō-sep-ti-sē′mē-ă). Septicemia apparently originating from microorganisms existing within the individual and not introduced from without. [auto- + G. *sēpsis,* decay, + *haima,* blood]

au·to·se·ro·ther·a·py (aw′tō-sē-rō-thār′ă-pē). The treatment of certain conditions, such as dermatoses, by injection of the patient's own blood serum.

au·to·se·rum (aw-tō-sē′rŭm). Serum obtained from the patient's own blood and used in autoserotherapy.

au·to·site (aw′tō-sīt). That member of abnormal, unequal conjoined twins that is able to live independently and nourish the other member (parasite) of the pair. [auto- + G. *sitos,* food]

au·tos·mia (aw-toz′mē-ă). The smelling of one's own body odor. [auto- + G. *osmē,* smell]

au·to·so·mal (aw-tō-sō′măl). Pertaining to an autosome.

au·to·so·ma·tog·no·sis (aw-tō-sō′mă-tog-nō′sis). The sensation that an amputated portion of the body is still present. SEE phantom *limb.* [auto- + G. *sōma,* body, + *gnōsis,* recognition]

au·to·so·ma·tog·nos·tic (aw-to-sō′mă-tog-nos′tik). Pertaining to autosomatognosis.

au·to·some (aw′tō-sōm). Any chromosome other than a sex chromosome; a.'s normally occur in pairs in somatic cells and singly in gametes. SYN euchromosome. [auto- + G. *sōma,* body]

au·to·sug·gest·i·bil·i·ty (aw′tō-sŭg-jes-tĭ-bil′i-tē). A mental state in which autosuggestion (1) readily occurs.

au·to·sug·ges·tion (aw′tō-sŭg-jes′chŭn). **1.** Constant dwelling upon an idea or concept, thereby inducing some change in the mental or bodily functions. SEE ALSO autohypnosis. **2.** Reproduction in the brain of impressions previously received which become then the starting point of new acts or ideas.

au·to·syn·noia (aw′tō-sin-noy′ă). A mental disorder in which one never has a thought not connected with oneself. SYN self-centeredness. [auto- + G. *synnoia,* deep thought, fr. *syn,* with + *noeō,* to think]

au·to·syn·the·sis (aw-tō-sin′thĕ-sis). Self-reproduction or -replication.

au·to·te·lic (aw-tō-tel′ik). Denoting those traits closely associated with the central purposes of an individual. [auto- + G. *telos,* end, completeness, purpose]

au·to·tem·nous (aw-tō-tem′nŭs). Denoting a cell that propagates itself by fission without previous conjugation. [auto- + G. *temnō,* to cut]

au·to·tet·ra·ploid (aw-tō-tet′ră-ployd). SEE autoploid.

au·to·ther·a·py (aw-tō-thār′ă-pē). **1.** Self-treatment. **2.** Spontaneous cure.

au·tot·o·my (aw-tot′ŏ-mē). The act of casting off a body part as a means of escape; e.g., the limb of a crab or the tail of a lizard. [auto- + G. *tomē,* a cutting]

au·to·top·ag·no·sia (aw′tō-top′ag-nō′zē-ă). Inability to recognize or to orient any part of one's own body; caused by a parietal lobe lesion. Cf. somatotopagnosis. [auto- + G. *topos,* place, + G. *a-*priv. + *gnōsis*]

au·to·tox·e·mia (aw′tō-tok-sē′mē-ă). Autointoxicants present in the blood, usually resulting in autointoxication.

au·to·tox·ic (aw-tō-toks′ik). Relating to autointoxication. SYN autopoisonous.

au·to·tox·i·co·sis (aw′tō-tok-si-kō′sis). SYN autointoxication.

au·to·tox·in (aw-tō-tok′sin). SYN autointoxicant.

au·to·trans·fu·sion (aw′tō-tranz-fū′zhŭn). Withdrawal and reinjection/transfusion of the patient's own blood; commonly the patient's own blood is collected on several occasions over time to be reinfused during an operative procedure in which substantial blood loss is anticipated. Cf. autoinfusion.

au·to·trans·plant (aw-tō-tranz′plant). SYN autograft.

au·to·trans·plan·ta·tion (aw′tō-tranz-plan-tā′shŭn). The performance of an autograft. SYN autografting.

au·to·trip·loid (aw-tō-trip′loyd). SEE autoploid.

au·to·troph (aw′tō-trōf). A microorganism that uses only inorganic materials as its source of nutrients; carbon dioxide serves as the sole carbon source. [auto- + G. *trophē,* nourishment]

au·to·tro·phic (aw-tō-trof′ik). **1.** Self-nourishing. The ability of an organism to produce food from inorganic compounds. **2.** Pertaining to an autotroph.

au·to·tro·phy (aw′tō-trōf-ē). The state of being self-sustaining and able to produce food from inorganic compounds, with carbon dioxide serving as the sole source of carbon.

carbon a., ability to assimilate CO_2 from the air.

nitrogen a., ability to assimilate nitrate or to do nitrogen fixation.

sulfur a., ability to assimilate sulfate.

au·to·vac·ci·na·tion (aw′tō-vak-si-nā′shŭn). A second vaccination with virus from a vaccine sore or liberation of antigenic products from invading microorganisms on the same individual.

au·tox·i·da·tion (aw-tok-si-dā′shŭn). SYN auto-oxidation.

au·to·zy·gous (aw-tō-zī′gŭs). Denoting genes in a homozygote that are copies of the identical ancestral gene as a result of a consanguineous mating. [auto- + G. *zygōtos,* yoked]

auxano-, auxo-, aux-. Increase, e.g., in size, intensity, speed. [G. *auxanō,* to increase]

aux·an·o·gram (awk-san′ō-gram). A plate culture of bacteria in which variable conditions are provided in order to determine the effect of these conditions on the growth of the bacteria. [auxano- + G. *gramma,* something written]

aux·an·o·graph·ic (awk′san-ō-graf′ik). Pertaining to auxanogram or auxanography.

aux·a·nog·ra·phy (awk-să-nog′ră-fē). The study, using auxanograms, of the effects of different conditions on the growth of bacteria.

aux·an·ol·o·gy (awk-sa-nol′ō-jē). The study of growth. [auxano- + G. *logos,* study]

aux·e·sis (awk-sē′sis). Increase in size, especially as in hypertrophy. [G. increase]

aux·il·ia·ry (og-zil′yă-rē). **1.** Functioning in an augmenting capacity; supplementary. **2.** Functioning as a subordinate; secondary.

aux·il·i·o·mo·tor (awg-zil′ē-ō-mō-tŏr). Aiding motion.

aux·i·lyt·ic (awk′si-lit′ik). Increasing the destructive power of a lysin, or favoring lysis. [G. *auxō*, to increase, + *lysis*, dissolution]

△**auxo-.** SEE auxano-.

aux·o·car·dia (awk-sō-kar′dē-ă). **1.** Enlargement of the heart, either by hypertrophy or dilation. **2.** Diastole of the heart. [auxo- + G. *kardia*, heart]

aux·o·chrome (awk′sō-krōm). The chemical group within a dye molecule by which the dye is bound to reactive end groups in tissues. The a. enhances the intensity of absorption. [auxo- + G. *chrōma*, color]

aux·o·drome (awk′sō-drōm). A course of growth as plotted on a Wetzel grid. [auxo- + G. *dromos*, course]

aux·o·flore (awk′sō-flōr). An atom or group of atoms that, by its presence in a molecule, shifts the latter's fluorescent radiation in the direction of the shorter wavelength, or increases the fluorescence. Cf. bathoflore.

aux·o·gluc (awk′sō-gluk). An atomic grouping that, when present in a molecule, intensifies its sweetness. [G. *auxanō*, to increase, + *glykys*, sweet]

aux·o·ton·ic (awk-sō-ton′ik). Denoting the condition in which a contracting muscle shortens against an increasing load. Cf. isometric (2), isotonic (3).

aux·o·tox (awk′sō-toks). An atomic grouping that, when present in a molecule, intensifies its poisonous characteristics. [G. *auxanō*, to increase, + *toxikon*, poison]

aux·o·troph (awk′sō-trōf). A mutant microorganism that requires some nutrient that is not required by the organism (prototroph) from which the mutant was derived. Cf. polyauxotroph, monoauxotroph. [auxo- + G. *trophē*, nourishment]

aux·o·tro·phic (awk-sō-trof′ik, -trō′fik). Pertaining to an auxotroph.

AV Abbreviation for arteriovenous; atrioventricular.

ava Abbreviation for arteriovenous *anastomosis*.

aval·vu·lar (ā-val′vū-lăr). Nonvalvular; without valves.

avas·cu·lar (ă-vas′kū-ler, -ă). Without blood or lymphatic vessels; may be a normal state as in certain forms of cartilage, or the result of disease. SYN nonvascular.

avas·cu·lar·i·za·tion (ă-vas′kū-lar-ī-zā′shŭn, ā-). **1.** Expulsion of blood from a part, as by means of a tourniquet or other means of arterial compression. **2.** Loss of vascularity, as by scarring.

AVC Abbreviation for atrioventricular *conduction*.

AVD Abbreviation for atrioventricular *dissociation*.

Avellis, Georg, German laryngologist, 1864–1916. SEE A. *syndrome*.

ave·nin (ă-vē′nin). A prolamine, containing about 25% glutamyl residues, found in oats (*Avena*) and in various legumes; considered highly nutritious. SYN legumin, plant casein.

av·er·age. A value that represents or summarizes the relevant features of a set of values; it is usually computed by a mathematical manipulation of the individual values in a set. [M.E. *averays*, loss from damage to ship or cargo, fr. It. *avaris*, fr. Ar. '*awariya*, damaged goods, + damage]

pure-tone average, average in decibels of the thresholds for pure tones at 500, 1000, and 2000 Hz.

avermectins. A group of endectocidal drugs that includes ivermectin.

aVF, aVL, aVR Abbreviation for augmented electrocardiographic leads from the foot (left), left arm, and right arm, respectively.

Avi·ad·e·no·vi·rus (ā′vē-ad′ĕ-nō-vī′rŭs). A genus of viruses (family Adenoviridae) that includes types of viruses found in birds. [L. *avis*, bird, + G. *adēn*, gland, + virus]

avi·an (ā′vē-ăn). Pertaining to birds. [L. *avis*, bird]

av·i·din (av′i-din). A glycoprotein, obtained from egg whites, which possesses a high affinity for biotin. Labeled a. is allowed to bind to biotin-tagged antibodies in order to amplify antigen-antibody reactions that may be difficult to visualize. Ingestion of a.

can cause a biotin deficiency. SYN antibiotin. [L. *avidus*, eager fr. *aveo*, to crave + -in]

avid·i·ty (ă-vid′i-tē). The binding strength of an antibody for an antigen. [L. *avidus*, greedy, eager fr. *aveo*, to crave]

A·vi·pox·vi·rus (ā′vē-poks-vī′rŭs). The genus of viruses (family Poxviridae) that includes the poxviruses of birds, including canarypox and fowlpox viruses. [L. *avis*, bird, + pox + virus]

avir·u·lent (ā-vir′ū-lent). Not virulent.

avi·ta·min·o·sis (ā-vī′tă-min-ō′sis). Properly, hypovitaminosis.

conditioned a., a. caused by any number of pathologic states or dysfunctions in which the supply of a vitamin absorbed by the body is inadequate for the needs under particular circumstances; e.g., the reduced bacterial synthesis of the vitamins in the alimentary canal produced by antibiotic agents.

avive·ment (ah-vēv-maw′). Obsolete term for the excision of the edges of a wound to assist the healing process. [Fr. *aviver*, to quicken, revive]

AV node. Abbreviation for atrioventricular *node*.

Avogadro, Amadeo, Italian physicist, 1776–1856. SEE A. *constant, hypothesis, law, number, postulate*.

av·oir·du·pois (av′er-du-poyz′). A system of weights in which 16 ounces make a pound, equivalent to 453.59237 g. See Weights and Measures appendix. [Fr. to have weight, corrupted fr. O. Fr. *avoir*, property, + *de*, of, + *pois*, weight]

AVP Abbreviation for antiviral *protein*; arginine *vasopressin*.

A-V shunt Abbreviation for arteriovenous *shunt*.

avul·sion (ă-vŭl′shŭn). A tearing away or forcible separation. Cf. evulsion. [L. *a-vello*, pp. *-vulsus*, to tear away]

nerve a., the tearing away of a peripheral nerve at its point of origin from its parent nerve due to traction.

root a., the tearing away of the anterior and posterior primary nerve roots from the spinal cord, due to severe traction; most often the C5 through T1 roots are affected.

tooth a., the traumatic separation of a tooth from its alveolus.

AW Abbreviation for atomic *weight*.

ax Abbreviation for axis.

axen·ic (ā-zen′ik). Sterile, denoting especially a pure culture. Also used to denote "germ-free" animals born and raised in a sterile environment. SEE ALSO gnotobiote. [G. *a-* priv. + *xenos*, foreign]

ax·er·oph·thol (ak′ser-of′thōl). SYN *vitamin* A. [antixerophthalmic + -ol]

ax·es (ak′sēz). Plural of axis.

ax·i·al (ak′sē-ăl). **1** [TA]. Relating to an axis. SYN axialis [TA], axile. **2.** Relating to or situated in the central part of the body, in the head and trunk as distinguished from the limbs, e.g., axial skeleton. **3.** In dentistry, relating to or parallel with the long axis of a tooth. **4.** In radiology, an axial image is one obtained by rotating around the axis of the body, producing a transverse planar image, i.e., a section transverse to the axis.

axialis [TA]. SYN axial (1).

ax·if·u·gal (ak-sif′ū-găl). Extending away from an axis or axon. SYN axofugal. [L. *axis* + *fugio*, to flee from]

ax·il (ak′sil). SYN axilla.

ax·ile (ak′sīl). SYN axial (1).

ax·il·la, gen. and pl. **ax·il·lae** (ak′sil′ă, ak-sil′ē) [TA]. The space below the shoulder joint, bounded by the pectoralis major anteriorly, the latissimus dorsi posteriorly, the serratus anterior medially, and the humerus laterally; it has a superior opening between the clavicle, scapula, and first rib (cervicoaxillary canal), and an inferior opening or floor covered by the axillary fascia and skin; it contains the axillary artery and vein, the infraclavicular part of the brachial plexus, axillary lymph nodes and vessels, and areolar tissue. SYN armpit, axil, axillary cavity, axillary fossa, axillary space, fossa axillaris, maschale. [L.]

ax·il·lary (ak′sil-ār-ē). Relating to the axilla. SYN alar (2).

△**axio-.** An axis. SEE ALSO axo-. [L. *axis*]

ax·i·o·buc·cal (ak′sē-ō-bŭk′ăl). Referring to the junction of the axial and buccal planes of a tooth, usually a line.

ax·i·o·buc·co·gin·gi·val (ak′sē-ō-bŭk-ō-jin′ji-văl). Referring to the junction of the axial, buccal and gingival planes of teeth; usually a point.

ax·i·o·in·ci·sal (ak′sē-ō-in-sī′săl). Referring to the line angle formed by the junction of the incisal edge and axial walls of a tooth.

ax·i·o·la·bi·al (ak′sē-ō-lā′bē-ăl). Referring to the line angle of a cavity formed by the junction of the axial and the labial walls of a tooth.

ax·i·o·la·bi·o·lin·gual (ak′sē-ō-lā′bē-ō-ling′gwăl). Referring to a section from labial to lingual along the longitudinal axis of a tooth.

ax·i·o·lin·gual (ak′sē-ō-ling′gwăl). Referring to the line angle of a cavity formed by the junction of an axial and a lingual wall of a tooth.

ax·i·o·lin·guo·cer·vi·cal (ak′sē-ō-ling′gwō-ser′vi-kăl). Referring to the point angle formed by the junction of an axial, lingual, and cervical (gingival) wall of a tooth cavity.

ax·i·o·lin·guo·clu·sal (ak′sē-ō-ling′gwō-kloo′săl). Referring to the point angle formed by the junction of an axial, lingual, and occlusal wall of a tooth cavity.

ax·i·o·lin·guo·gin·gi·val (ak′sē-ō-ling′gwō-jin′ji-văl). Referring to the point angle formed by the junction of an axial, lingual, and gingival (cervical) wall of a tooth cavity.

ax·i·o·me·si·al (ak′sē-ō-mē′zē-ăl). Referring to the line angle of a tooth cavity formed by the junction of an axial and a mesial wall.

ax·i·o·me·si·o·cer·vi·cal (ak′sē-ō-mē′zē-ō-ser′vi-kăl). Referring to the point angle formed by the junction of an axial, mesial, and cervical (gingival) wall of a tooth cavity.

ax·i·o·me·si·o·dis·tal. SEE axiomesiodistal *plane.*

ax·i·o·me·si·o·gin·gi·val (ak′sē-ō-mē′zē-ō-jin′ji-văl). Referring to the point angle formed by an axial, mesial, and gingival (cervical) wall of a tooth cavity.

ax·i·o·me·si·o·in·ci·sal (ak′sē-ō-mē′zē-ō-in-sī′săl). Referring to the point angle formed by the junction of an axial, mesial, and incisal wall of a tooth cavity.

ax·i·on (ak′sē-on). The brain and spinal cord (cerebrospinal axis).

ax·io·oc·clu·sal (ak′sē-ō-ŏ-kloo′săl). Pertaining to the line angle formed by the junction of the axial and occlusal walls of a tooth.

ax·i·o·plasm (ak′sē-ō-plazm). SYN axoplasm.

ax·i·o·po·di·um, pl. **ax·i·o·po·dia** (ak′sē-ō-pō′dē-ŭm, -dē-ă). SYN axopodium.

ax·i·o·pul·pal (ak′sē-ō-pŭl′păl). Referring to the line angle formed by the junction of an axial and pulpal wall of a tooth cavity.

ax·i·o·ver·sion (ak′sē-ō-ver′zhŭn). Abnormal inclination of the long axis of a tooth.

ax·ip·e·tal (ak-sip′ĕ-tăl). SYN centripetal (2). [L. *axis* + *peto,* to seek]

ax·i·ram·if·i·cate (ak′sē-ram-if′i-kāt). Denoting a nerve cell whose axon, usually short, breaks up into many branches, e.g., Golgi type II cells. [G. *axōn,* axis + *grapho,* to write]

ax·is (ax), pl. **ax·es** (ak′sis, ak′sēz). **1** [TA]. A straight line joining two opposing poles of a spherical body, about which the body may revolve. **2** [TA]. The central line of the body or any of its parts. **3.** The vertebral column. **4.** The central nervous system. **5** [TA]. The second cervical vertebra. SYN vertebra C2*, epistropheus, odontoid vertebra, second cervical vertebra, toothed vertebra, vertebra dentata. **6.** An artery that divides, immediately upon its origin, into a number of branches, e.g., celiac axis. SEE trunk. [L. axle, axis]

basibregmatic a., a line extending from the basion to the bregma.

basicranial a., a line drawn from the basion to the midpoint of the sphenoethmoidal suture.

basifacial a., a line drawn from the subnasal point to the midpoint of the sphenoethmoidal suture. SYN facial a.

biauricular a., a straight line joining the two auricles. Cf. auriculare.

celiac a., SYN celiac (arterial) *trunk.*

cephalocaudal a., SYN long a. of body.

cerebrospinal a., the central nervous system; the brain and spinal cord. SYN encephalomyelonic a., neural a.

condylar a., a line through the two mandibular condyles around which the mandible may rotate during a part of the opening movement. SYN condyle cord.

conjugate a., SYN median *conjugate.*

craniofacial a., a straight line passing through the mesethmoid, presphenoid, basisphenoid, and basioccipital bones.

electrical a., the net direction of the electromotive forces developed in the heart during its activation, usually represented in the frontal plane. SEE triaxial reference *system.*

embryonic a., the cephalocaudal a. established in the embryo by the primitive streak.

encephalomyelonic a., SYN cerebrospinal a.

external a. of eye [TA], that part of the optic a. from the midpoint of anterior surface of the cornea to the posterior surface of the posterior pole of the external surface of the sclera. SYN a. externus bulbi oculi [TA].

a. exter′nus bul′bi oculi [TA], SYN external a. of eye.

facial a., SYN basifacial a.

axes of Fick, three axes that pass through the center of the eye vertically (Z), horizontally in the coronal plane (X), and horizontally in the sagittal plane (Y). All ocular rotations can be described by rotation along one of these axes.

hinge a., SYN transverse horizontal a.

instantaneous electrical a., the resultant a. of the electromotive forces developing in the heart at any given moment.

internal a. of eye [TA], that part of the optic a. from the midpoint of the posterior surface of the cornea to the anterior surface of the retina opposite the posterior pole. SYN a. internus bulbi oculi [TA].

a. inter′nus bul′bi oculi [TA], SYN internal a. of eye.

a. of lens, a line connecting the anterior and posterior poles of the lens of the eye. SYN a. lentis.

a. len′tis, SYN a. of lens.

long a., a line extending through the center of an object lengthwise; in dentistry, the line extending inciso- (occluso-) cervically parallel to axial surfaces of a tooth.

long a. of body, the imaginary straight line in the median plane which nearly intersects the center of all transverse planes through the body, running from the apex of the skull through the center of the perineum and continuing between the lower limbs, parallel to and equidistant from the long axes of the limbs; in theory, this is the line about which the body's mass is equally distributed. SEE ALSO embryonic a. SYN cephalocaudal a.

mandibular a., SYN transverse horizontal a.

mean electrical a., the average magnitude and direction of all the electromotive forces developed during the cardiac event under consideration; e.g., atrial or ventricular depolarization, or ventricular repolarization. SEE ALSO axis *deviation.*

neural a., SYN cerebrospinal a.

neutral a. of straight beam, the a. perpendicular to the plane of loading of a beam at stresses within the proportional limit; it lies at the gravity a. of the cross-section of the beam.

normal electrical a., a mean electrical a. of the heart situated between minus 30° and +90°. SEE hexaxial reference *system.*

opening a., an imaginary line around which the mandibular condyles may rotate during opening and closing movements. Cf. fulcrum *line.*

optic a. [TA], the a. of the eye connecting the anterior and posterior poles; it usually diverges from the visual a. by five degrees or more. SYN a. opticus [TA].

a. op′ticus [TA], SYN optic a.

orbital a., the line from the center of the optic foramen (apex of orbit) extending anteriorly, laterally, and inferiorly to the middle of the orbital opening.

pelvic a., SYN a. of pelvis.

a. pel′vis [TA], SYN a. of pelvis.

a. of pelvis [TA], a hypothetical curved line joining the center point of each of the four planes of the pelvis, marking the center of the pelvic cavity at every level. SYN a. pelvis [TA], pelvic a., plane of pelvic canal.

principal optic a., a line passing through the center of the lens of a refracting system at right angles to its surface.

pupillary a., a line perpendicular to the surface of the cornea, passing through the center of the pupil; the "direction of gaze."

rotational a., SYN fulcrum *line*.

sagittal a., in dentistry, the line in the frontal plane around which the working side condyle rotates during mandibular movement.

secondary a., any ray passing through the optical center of a lens.

a. of symmetry, an a. through a particle (e.g., a virus) on such a plane that, if the particle is rotated on the a., there are two or more positions at which the particle appears identical.

thoracic a., (1) SYN thoracoacromial *artery*; **(2)** SYN thoracoacromial *vein*.

thyroid a., SYN thyrocervical (arterial) *trunk*.

transporionic a., an imaginary line connecting the upper central points of the external auditory meatuses; used in radiographic cephalometry. SEE porion.

transverse horizontal a., an imaginary line around which the mandible may rotate through the horizontal plane. SYN hinge a., mandibular a.

vertical a., in dentistry, the line around which the working side condyle rotates in the horizontal plane during mandibular movement.

visual a., the straight line extending from the object seen, through the center of the pupil, to the macula lutea of the retina. SYN line of vision.

Y-a., a cephalometric indicator of the vertical and horizontal coordinates of mandibular growth expressed in degrees of the inferior facial angle formed by the intersection of the sella-gnathion plane with the Frankfort horizontal plane.

axo-. Axis; axion. [G. *axōn*, axis]

ax·o·ax·on·ic (ak'sō-ak-son'ik). Relating to synaptic contact between the axon of one nerve cell and that of another. SEE synapse.

ax·o·den·drit·ic (ak'sō-den-drit'ik). Pertaining to the synaptic relationship of an axon with a dendrite of another neuron. SEE synapse.

ax·of·u·gal (ak-sof'ū-găl). SYN axifugal. [axo- + L. *fugio*, to flee]

ax·o·graph (ak'sō-graf). A device for recording scales or axes of predetermined magnitude on kymographic records. [axo- + G. *graphō*, to write]

ax·o·lem·ma (ak'sō-lem'ă). The plasma membrane of the axon. SYN Mauthner sheath. [axo- + G. *lemma*, husk]

ax·ol·y·sis (ak-sol'i-sis). Destruction or dissolution of a nerve axon. [axo- + G. *lysis*, dissolution]

ax·on (ak'son). The single process of a nerve cell that under normal conditions conducts nervous impulses away from the cell body and its remaining processes (dendrites). It is a relatively even filamentous process varying in thickness from about 0.25 to more than 10 μm. In contrast to dendrites, which rarely exceed 1.5 mm in length, A.'s can extend great distances from the parent cell body (some a.'s of the pyramidal tract are 40–50 cm long). A.'s 0.5 μm thick or over are generally enveloped by a segmented myelin sheath provided by oligodendroglia cells (in brain and spinal cord) or Schwann cells (in peripheral nerves). Like dendrites and nerve cell bodies, A.'s contain a large number of neurofibrils. With some exceptions, nerve cells synaptically transmit impulses to other nerve cells or to effector cells (muscle cells, gland cells) exclusively by way of the synaptic terminals of their A. [G. *axōn*, axis]

ax·o·nal (ak'sō-năl). Pertaining to an axon.

ax·o·neme (ak'sō-nēm). **1.** The central thread running in the axis of the chromosome. **2.** SYN axial *filament*. **3.** The distinctive array of microtubules in the core of eukaryotic cilia and flagella comprising a central pair surrounded by a sheaf of nine doublet microtubules. [axo- + G. *nēma*, a thread]

ax·on·og·ra·phy (ak-sŏ-nog'ră-fē). The recording of electrical changes in axons. SYN electroaxonography.

ax·o·nop·a·thy (aks'on-op'a-thē). A disorder affecting primarily the axons of peripheral nerve fibers (although secondary demyeli-

nation occurs), in contrast to one that affects only myelin (myelinopathy).

ax·on·ot·me·sis (ak'son-ot-mē'sis). Interruption of the axons of a nerve followed by complete degeneration of the peripheral segment, without severance of the supporting structures of the nerve; such a lesion may result from pinching, crushing, or prolonged pressure. SEE ALSO neurapraxia, neurotmesis. [axon + G. *tmēsis*, a cutting]

ax·op·e·tal (ak-sop'ĕ-tăl). Extending in a direction toward an axon. [axo- + L. *peto*, to seek]

ax·o·plasm (ak'sō-plazm). Neuroplasm of the axon. SYN axioplasm.

ax·o·po·di·um, pl. **ax·o·po·dia** (ak-sō-pō'dē-ŭm, -ă). A permanent pseudopodium containing a stiff axial filament of differentiated protoplasm. SYN axiopodium. [Mod. L., fr. L. *axis* + G. *podion,* dim. of *pous* (*pod*-), foot]

ax·o·so·mat·ic (ak-sō-sō-mat'ik). Relating to the synaptic relationship of an axon with a nerve cell body. SEE synapse. [axo- + G. *sōma,* body]

ax·o·style (ak'sō-stīl). An elongate supporting rod or tubule that runs the length of certain flagellate protozoans, frequently projecting out of the posterior end. Single or multiple, filamentous or rigid, they vary with the species but serve as an endoskeletal framework and may function in locomotion as well. [axo- + G. *stylos,* pillar]

ax·ot·o·my (ak-sot'ō-mē). Incision or transection of an axon. [axo- + G. *tomē,* to cut]

ay·a·hua·sca (ī'ă-wa-skă). SYN caapi.

Ayala, G., Italian neurologist, 1878–1943. SEE A. *index, quotient*.

Ayerza, L., Argentinian physician, 1861–1918. SEE A. *disease, syndrome*.

Ayre, James Ernest, U.S. gynecologist, *1910. SEE A. *brush*.

aza·crine (ā'ză-krēn). An antimalarial; an effective schizontocide in acute falciparum infection.

aza·cy·clo·nol hy·dro·chlo·ride (ā'ză-sī'klō-nol). A structural isomer of pipradol hydrochloride partially antagonistic to its actions, used with varying results in the treatment of hallucinations and confusion.

9-aza·flu·o·rene (ā-ză-flōr'ēn). SYN carbazole.

8-aza·gua·nine (ā-ză-gwah'nēn). Guanine with N for C in position 8; a guanine antagonist that has been used in the treatment of acute leukemia. SYN guanazolo, triazologuanine.

aza·me·tho·ni·um bro·mide (ā'ză-me-thō'nē-ŭm). A ganglionic blocking agent.

aza·per·one (ā'za-per-ōn). A tranquilizing agent.

azap·e·tine phos·phate (ā-zap'ĕ-tēn). A potent adrenergic (α-receptor) blocking agent similar in action and uses to those of tolazoline; used in the treatment of peripheral vascular diseases.

aza·pir·ones (ā-za-pī'rōnz). Anxiolytics acting through agonist action at serotonin 1-A receptors.

azar·i·bine (ā-zar'i-bēn). An antipsoriatic agent no longer used because of a high incidence of severe adverse reactions.

aza·ser·ine (ā-ză-sēr'ēn). O-Diazoacetyl-Lserine; an antibiotic inhibitor of purine synthesis; a glutamine analog; mutagenic and antitumorogenic. It retards the growth of transplantable animal neoplasms.

aza·spi·ro·dec·ane·di·one (ā-ză-spī'rō-dek-ān-dī'ōn). A class of antianxiety agents not chemically or pharmacologically related to other classes of sedative and anxiolytic drugs; e.g., buspirone hydrochloride.

azat·a·dine ma·le·ate (ă-zat'ă-dēn). An antihistamine with anticholinergic and antiserotonin properties.

aza·thi·o·prine (ā-ză-thī'ō-prēn). A derivative of 6-mercaptopurine, used as a cytotoxic and immunosuppressive agent in organ transplantation and in the treatment of autoimmune diseases such as hemolytic anemias, systemic lupus erythematosus, rheumatoid arthritis and leukemias.

6-aza·thy·mine (ā-ză-thī'mēn). Thymine with N for C in position 6; an antimetabolite of thymine.

6-az·au·ri·dine (AZUR) (az-aw'ri-dēn). Uridine with N for C in position 6; a triazine analogue of uridine and an antimetabolite with selectivity for human neoplastic leukocytes; produces partial remissions in certain acute leukemias of adults.

aze·o·trope (ā-zē′ō-trōp). A mixture of two or more liquids that boils without a change in proportion of the substances either in the liquid or the vapor phase; e.g., 95% ethanol (actually 94.9% by volume, the rest being water). [G. *a-* priv. + *zeō,* to boil, + *tropos,* a turning]

halothane-ether a., an azeotropic mixture in the proportions halothane 68 to diethyl ether 32, by volume, that combines the advantages of each anesthetic yet is non-flammable.

aze·o·tro·pic (ā-zē-ō-trop′ik). Denoting or characteristic of an azeotrope.

az·ide (az′īd). A compound that contains the monovalent $-N_3$ group.

az·i·do·thy·mi·dine (AZT) (az′i-dō-thī′mi-dēn). SYN zidovudine.

az·lo·cil·lin so·di·um (az-lō-sil′in). An extended spectrum penicillin used in treatment of infections caused by *Pseudomonas aeruginosa, Escherichia coli,* and *Haemophilus influenzae.*

△**azo-.** Prefix denoting the presence in a molecule of the group ≡C–N=N–C≡. Cf. diazo-. [Fr. *azote,* name for nitrogen proposed by AL Lavoisier (1743–1794)]

az·o·bil·i·ru·bin (az′ō-bil-i-roo′bin). The red-violet pigment formed by the condensation of diazotized sulfanilic acid with bilirubin in the van den Bergh reaction.

az·o·car·mine (ā′zō-kar′min). A series of azo dyes used in preparing tissue stains.

az·o·car·mine B, az·o·car·mine G (az-ō-kar′min) [C.I. 50090, C.I. 50085]. Red acid dyes, the former more soluble in water, useful in Heidenhain azan stain.

azo·ic (ă-zō′ik, ā-). Containing no living things; without organic life. [G. *a-* priv. + *zōikos,* relating to an animal]

az·ole (az′ōl). SYN pyrrole.

az·o·lit·min (az-ō-lit′min) [old C.I. 1242]. A purplish red coloring matter obtained from natural litmus or synthesized by oxidizing orcinol in the presence of ammonia, lime, and potash; used as a broad indicator of pH (red at 4.5, blue at 8.3).

a·zo·o·sper·mia (ā-zō-ō-sper′mē-ă). Absence of living spermatozoa in the semen; failure of spermatogenesis. SEE ALSO aspermia. [G. *a-* priv. + *zōon,* animal, + *sperma,* seed]

az·o·phlox·in (az-ō-flok′sin). SYN amidonaphthol red.

az·o·pro·tein (az-ō-prō′tēn). Any of the modified proteins produced by treatment with diazonium derivatives of various aromatic amines; used to elicit antibody formation and demonstrate antibody specificity.

az·o·sul·fa·mide (az-ō-sŭl′fă-mīd). A reddish derivative, soluble in water, less toxic but less effective than sulfanilamide; it owes its antibacterial activity to the sulfanilamide released.

az·o·te·mia (az-ō-tē′mē-ă). An abnormal increase in concentration of urea and other nitrogenous substances in the blood plasma. SEE ALSO uremia. [azo- (azote) + G. *haima,* blood]

nonrenal a., prerenal a., nitrogen retention resulting from something other than primary renal disease.

az·o·tem·ic (az-ō-tēm′ik). Relating to azotemia.

az·o·ther·mia (az-ō-ther′mē-ă). Rarely used term for fever resulting from uremia. [azote + G. *thermē,* heat]

azo·tu·ria (az-ō-toor′ē-ă). An increased elimination of urea in the urine. [azo- (azote) + G. *ouron,* urine]

az·o·van blue (az′ō-van). SYN Evans blue.

AZT Abbreviation for azidothymidine.

az·tre·o·nam (az-trē′ō-nam). A synthetic bactericidal monolactam antibiotic with a wide spectrum of activity against Gram-negative aerobic pathogens.

az·ul (azh′ūl). SYN pinta. [Sp. blue]

AZUR Abbreviation for 6-azauridine.

az·ure (azh′ūr). A term for a group of metachromatic basic blue methylthionine or phenothiazine dyes; used as biologic stains, especially in blood and nuclear stains.

a. A [C.I. 52005], asymmetric dimethylthionine chloride; a blue dye used as a component of MacNeal tetrachrome blood stain and of Romanowsky-type blood stains; also used as a stain for mucins, nucleic acids, and mast cell granules; gives a metachromatic violet to red color to highly acidic substances in tissues.

a. B [C.I. 52010], trimethylthionine chloride; a blue dye used like a. A; also as a. B bromide to give metachromatic staining of RNA and DNA.

a. C [C.I. 52002], monomethylthione chloride; a blue-violet thiazin dye used in the metachromatic staining of mucins and cartilage.

a. I, a mixture of a. A and B. SYN methylene azure.

a. II, a mixture of a. I and methylene blue; the eosinate, a. II-eosin, is the principal ingredient of Giemsa stain.

az·u·res·in (azh′ū-res′in). A complex of azure A and carbacrylic resin; used as an indicator for the detection of gastric achlorhydria without intubation. SYN quinine carbacrylic resin.

az·u·ro·phil, az·u·ro·phile (azh′ū-rō-fil, -fīl). Staining readily with an azure dye, denoting especially the hyperchromatin and reddish purple granules of certain blood cells. [azure + G. *philos,* fond]

az·u·ro·phil·ia (az′ū-rō-fil′ē-ă). A condition in which the blood contains cells having azurophil granulations.

azy·go·gram (az′i-gō-gram). Radiographic demonstration of the azygos venous system after injection of contrast medium. [azygos + G. *gramma,* a writing]

azy·gog·ra·phy (az′i-gog′ră-fē). Radiography of the azygos venous system after injection of contrast medium.

az·y·gos (az′ī-gos). **1.** An unpaired (azygous) anatomical structure. **2.** SYN azygos *vein.* [G. *a-* priv. + *zygon,* a yoke]

a. continuation (of the inferior vena cava), a congenital anomaly in which the infrahepatic portion of the vena cava fails to form, and venous drainage of the lower body is maintained through a persistent right supracardinal vein, which becomes a large azygos vein.

az·y·gous (az′ī-gŭs, ă-zī′gŭs). Unpaired; single. [G. *azygos*] β **1.** Second letter of the Greek alphabet, beta. **2.** In chemistry, denotes the second in a series, the second carbon from a functional (e.g., carboxylic) group, or the direction of a chemical bond toward the viewer. For terms having this prefix, see the specific term.

β− Symbol for electron.

β⁺ Symbol for positron.

B 1. Symbol for boron; for aspartic acid or asparagine when it is unclear which of the two amino acids is present; for bromouridine; second substrate in a multisubstrate enzyme-catalyzed reaction. **2.** As a subscript, refers to barometric *pressure*.

b 1. As a subscript, refers to blood. **2.** Abbreviation for bis [L.], twice; barn.

Ba Symbol for barium.

Babbitt, Isaac, U.S. inventor, 1799–1862. SEE B. *metal*.

Babcock, Stephen M., U.S. chemist, 1843–1931. SEE B. *tube*.

Babès, Victor, Roumanian bacteriologist, 1854–1926. SEE *Babesia;* B. *nodes*, under *node*.

Ba·be·sia (bă-bē′zē-ă). The economically most important genus of the protozoan family Babesiidae; characterized by multiplication in host red blood cells to form pairs and tetrads; it causes babesiosis (piroplasmosis) in most types of domestic animals, and two species cause disease in splenectomized or normal people; vectors are ixodid or argasid ticks. [V. *Babès*]

B. diver′gens, the cause of bovine babesiosis in western and central Europe; vector tick is *Ixodes ricinus;* it has caused human babesiosis in splenectomized individuals in Europe; also found in reindeer.

B. micro′ti, a malarialike protozoan naturally parasitizing certain rodents (*Peromyscus* and *Microtus* spp.) in North America; a number of human cases have been reported in the U.S. The local tick vector is *Ixodes scapularis,* whose numbers and infection levels have greatly increased in recent years with the increase in the deer population, which serves as an abundant blood source for *I. scapularis.* SEE ALSO *Borrelia burgdorferi.*

Ba·be·si·el·la (bă-bē-zē-el′ă). SEE *Babesia.*

Ba·be·si·i·dae (ba′bē-zī′i-dē, -zē′i-dē). A family of protozoan parasites (class Sporozoea, order Piroplasmida) occurring in the red blood cells of various mammals. The organisms are piriform, round, or oval and reproduce by schizogony to form tetrads or by binary fission to form pairs in the red blood cells; transmission is effected by ticks. The family includes the genera *Babesia, Echinozoon,* and *Entopolypoides; Aegyptianella,* formerly included, is now thought to be a rickettsia. SEE ALSO Theileriidae.

ba·be·si·o·sis (bă-bē′zē-ō′sis). A disease caused by infection with a species of the protozoan *Babesia,* transmitted by ticks. In animals, the disease is characterized by fever, malaise, listlessness, severe anemia, and hemoglobulinuria; the death rate frequently is higher in adult than in young animals. SYN piroplasmosis.

human b., a rare human disease caused by infection with *Babesia* species (most frequently *B. divergens* in Europe and *B. microti* in the U.S.) that has been fatal in some splenectomized individuals.

Babinski, Joseph F., French neurologist, 1857–1932. SEE B. *phenomenon, sign, reflex, syndrome.*

ba·by (bā′bē). An infant; a newborn child.

blue b., a child born cyanotic because of a congenital cardiac or pulmonary defect causing incomplete oxygenation of the blood.

blueberry muffin b., an infant with purple skin lesions the appearance of which has been compared to that of a blueberry muffin. Lesions are caused by dermal erythropoiesis and are seen in congenital infections such as cytomegalovirus infection, toxoplasmosis, or rubella. The infection interferes with the normal production of blood cells in the bone marrow.

collodion b. [MIM*146600], a newborn child with lamellar ichthyosis; at birth, the skin is bright red, shiny, translucent, and drawn tight, giving a distorted appearance (as if having been painted with collodion) of immobilization of the face; contraction of the skin causes ectropion, a pressed down appearance of the nose, and a gaping of the mouth and the labia; autosomal dominant inheritance.

test-tube b., popular term for a b. born after uterine implantation of a maternal ovum fertilized in vitro.

bac·am·pi·cil·lin hy·dro·chlo·ride (bak′am-pi-sil′in). A semisynthetic penicillin with the same activity and uses as ampicillin, but better absorbed on oral administration.

bac·cate (bak′āt). Berrylike. [L. *bacca,* berry]

Baccelli, Guido, Italian physician, 1832–1916. SEE B. *sign.*

bac·ci·form (bak′sĭ-fōrm). Berry-shaped. [L. *bacca,* berry]

Bachman, George W., U.S. parasitologist, *1890. SEE B.-Pettit *test.*

Bachmann, Jean George, U.S. physiologist, 1877–1959. SEE B. *bundle.*

Bachmann, SEE Rivinus.

Ba·cil·la·ce·ae (bă-si-lā′sē-ē). A family of aerobic or facultatively anaerobic, sporeforming, ordinarily motile bacteria (order Eubacteriales) containing Gram-positive rods. These organisms are chemoheterotrophic. Some species are pathogenic. Ordinarily two genera, *Bacillus* and *Clostridium,* are included. The type genus is *Bacillus.*

ba·cil·lar, bac·il·la·ry (bas′i-lar, bas′i-lā-rē). Shaped like a rod; consisting of rods or rodlike elements.

ba·cil·le Calmette-Guérin (BCG) (bah-sēl′). An attenuated strain of *Mycobacterium bovis* used in the preparation of BCG vaccine that is used for immunization against tuberculosis and in cancer chemotherapy. SYN Calmette-Guérin bacillus. [Fr.]

bac·il·le·mia (bas-i-lē′mē-ă). The presence of bacilli in the circulating blood. [bacillus + G. *haima,* blood]

ba·cil·li (bă-sil′ī). Plural of bacillus.

ba·cil·li·form (ba-sil′i-fōrm). Rod-shaped. [L. *bacillus,* a rod, + *forma,* form]

ba·cil·lin (ba-sil′in). An antibiotic substance produced by *Bacillus subtilis.*

ba·cil·lo·myx·in (ba-sil-ō-mik′sin). An antibiotic active against certain pathogenic fungi obtained from cultures of *Bacillus subtilis.* [*Bacillus* + G. *mykēs,* fungus, + -in]

bac·il·lo·sis (bas-i-lō′sis). A general infection with bacilli.

bac·il·lu·ria (bas-i-loo′rē-ă). The presence of bacilli in the urine. [bacillus + G. *ouron,* urine]

Ba·cil·lus (bă-sil′ŭs). A genus of aerobic or facultatively anaerobic, sporeforming, ordinarily motile bacteria (family Bacillaceae) containing Gram-positive rods. Motile cells are peritrichous; spores are thick-walled and stain poorly with Gram stain; these organisms are chemoheterotrophic and are found primarily in soil. A few species are animal pathogens; some species evoke antibody production. The type species is *B. subtilis.* [L. dim. of *baculus,* rod, staff]

B. an′thracis, a bacterial species that causes anthrax in humans, cattle, swine, sheep, rabbits, guinea pigs, and mice; contains virulence plasmids associated with capsule and toxin production.

B. bre′vis, a bacterial species found in soil, air, dust, milk, and cheese; some strains produce the antibiotic gramicidin or tyrocidin.

B. ce′reus, a bacterial species that causes an emetic type and a diarrheal type of food poisoning in humans, and can cause infections in humans and other mammals. It can cause a highly destructive infection of the traumatized eye.

△ **Combining Forms**	☆ **Official alternate Terminologia Anatomica term**
ⓘ **Indicates term is illustrated, see Illustration Index**	
	[MIM] Mendelian Inheritance in Man
SYN Synonym	
Cf. Compare	**C.I. Colour Index**
[NA] Nomina Anatomica	
[TA] Terminologia Anatomica	**High Profile Term**

B. circulans, a bacterial species found in soil that has been incriminated in human infections including septicemia, mixed abscess infections, and wound infections.

B. hemoly'ticus, former name for *Clostridium haemolyticum.*

B. histoly'ticus, former name for *Clostridium histolyticum.*

B. megate'rium, a saprophytic bacterial species of experimental interest; strains produce bacteriocins (megacins).

B. polymyx'a, a bacterial species found in soil, water, milk, feces, and decaying vegetables; some strains produce the antibiotic polymyxin.

B. pumilis, a usually saprophytic species of bacteria that has been associated with food poisoning and rarely with abscess or bowel fistula formation.

B. sphae'ricus, a bacterial species that is an insect pathogen and that has been associated with occasional human and other mammalian infections, especially in immunocompromised hosts; human infections have included meningitis, endocarditis, and food poisoning.

B. subti'lis, a bacterial species found in soil and decomposing organic matter; some strains produce the antibiotic subtilin, subtenolin, or bacillomycin; it has been associated with human infections primarily of immunocompromised patients, and with food poisoning. It is the type species of the genus *B.* SYN grass bacillus, hay bacillus.

B. thuringien'sis, a bacterial species that is an insect pathogen used for vector control that has been implicated in human and mammalian infections. In the laboratory it may be misdiagnosed as a strain of *B. cereus.*

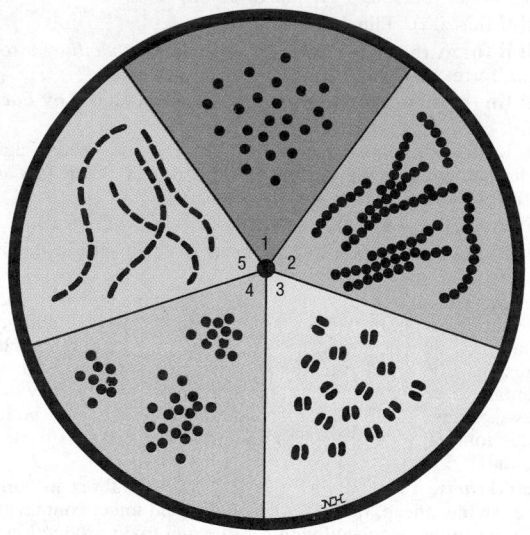

bacteria: (1) cocci, (2) streptococci, (3) diplococci, (4) staphylococci, (5) bacilli

ba·cil·lus, pl. **ba·cil·li** (ba-sil'ŭs, -ī). **1.** A vernacular term used to refer to any member of the bacterial genus *Bacillus.* **2.** Term used to refer to any rod-shaped bacterium. [L. dim. of *baculus,* a rod, staff]

abortus b., SYN *Brucella abortus.*

Battey b., SYN *Mycobacterium intracellulare.* [Battey hospital in Rome, GA]

blue pus b., SYN *Pseudomonas aeruginosa.*

Bordet-Gengou b., SYN *Bordetella pertussis.*

Calmette-Guérin b., SYN bacille Calmette-Guérin.

cholera b., SYN *Vibrio cholerae.*

coliform bacilli (kō'li-fōrm, kol'i-fōrm), common name for *Escherichia coli* that is used as an indicator of fecal contamination of water, measured in terms of coliform count; occasionally used to refer to all lactose-fermenting enteric bacteria.

colon b., SYN *Escherichia coli.*

comma b., SYN *Vibrio cholerae.*

Döderlein b., a large, Gram-positive bacterium occurring in normal vaginal secretions; although thought by some to be identical with *Lactobacillus acidophilus,* the identity of Döderlein b. is still doubtful.

Ducrey b., SYN *Haemophilus ducreyi.*

dysentery b., an organism of the genus *Shigella* which causes dysentery.

Eberth b., SYN *Salmonella typhi.*

Flexner b., SYN *Shigella flexneri.*

Friedländer b., SYN *Klebsiella pneumoniae.*

gas b., SYN *Clostridium perfringens.*

grass b., SYN *Bacillus subtilis.*

Hansen b., SYN *Mycobacterium leprae.*

hay b., SYN *Bacillus subtilis.*

Hofmann b., SYN *Corynebacterium pseudodiphtheriticum.*

influenza b., SYN *Haemophilus influenzae.*

Kitasato b., SYN *Yersinia pestis.*

Klebs-Loeffler b., SYN *Corynebacterium diphtheriae.*

Koch b., SYN *Mycobacterium tuberculosis.*

Koch-Weeks b., SYN *Haemophilus aegyptius.*

lactic acid b., a member of the genus *Lactobacillus.*

leprosy b., SYN *Mycobacterium leprae.*

Loeffler b., SYN *Corynebacterium diphtheriae.*

Moeller grass b., SYN *Mycobacterium phlei.*

Morgan b., SYN *Morganella morganii.*

Much b., an alleged non–acid-fast granular form of tubercle b.; not demonstrable by the Ziehl stain, but takes a modified Gram stain; said to be the form present in the tuberculous skin lesion.

necrosis b., SYN *Fusobacterium necrophorum.*

paracolon b., any one of a number of diverse enteric bacteria that fail to ferment lactose promptly.

paradysentery b., SYN *Shigella flexneri.*

paratyphoid b., one of the three organisms causing three forms (A, B, C) of paratyphoid fever. SEE ALSO paratyphoid *fever.*

plague b., SYN *Yersinia pestis.*

Shiga b., SYN *Shigella dysenteriae.*

Shiga-Kruse b., SYN *Shigella dysenteriae.*

tubercle b., (1) SYN *Mycobacterium tuberculosis;* **(2)** SYN *Mycobacterium bovis.*

typhoid b., SYN *Salmonella typhi.*

Vincent b., probably *Fusobacterium nucleatum.*

Weeks b., SYN *Haemophilus influenzae.*

Welch b., SYN *Clostridium perfringens.*

Whitmore b., SYN *Pseudomonas pseudomallei.*

bac·i·tra·cin (bas-i-trā'sin). An antibacterial antibiotic polypeptide of known chemical structure isolated from cultures of an aerobic, Gram-positive, spore-bearing bacillus (member of the *Bacillus subtilis* group); active against hemolytic streptococci, staphylococci, and several types of Gram-positive, aerobic, rod-shaped organisms; usually applied locally. Zinc b. is also available. [*Bacillus* + Margaret *Tracy,* source of orig. culture]

back (bak). **1.** Posterior aspect of trunk, below neck and above buttocks; **2.** Vertebral column with associated muscles (erector spinae and transversospinalis) and overlying integument. SEE dorsum.

adolescent round b., SYN Scheuermann *disease.*

hollow b., SYN lordosis.

poker b., SYN *spondylitis* deformans.

saddle b., SYN lordosis.

back·ache (bak'āk). Nonspecific term used to describe back pain; generally refers to pain below the cervical level.

back·bone (bak'bōn). SYN vertebral *column.*

back·cross (bak'kros). **1.** Mating of an individual heterozygous at one or more loci to an individual homozygous at the same loci. **2.** SYN testcross.

back·flow. The reversal of the normal flow of a fluid or current. SEE ALSO regurgitation.

pyelovenous backflow, retrograde movement of fluid (urine or injected contrast materials) from renal pelvis into the renal venous

classification of bacteria

kingdom: prokaryotes (Prokaryotae)
division I: gracilicutes (mostly Gram-negative)

Spirochetes				
order I Spirochaetales	family I	Spirochaetaceae	genera: e.g.,	*Treponema, Borrelia*
	family II	Leptospiraceae	genus:	*Leptospira*

aerobic or microaerophilic, motile, spiral or bent Gram-negative bacteria
genera: e.g., *Spirillum, Campylobacter*

Gram-negative aerobic bacilli and cocci				
	family I	Pseudomonadaceae	genera: e.g.,	*Pseudomonas, Xanthomomas*
	family VII	Legionellaceae	genus:	*Legionella*
	family VIII	Neisseriaceae	genera: e.g.	*Neisseria, Moraxella, Acinetobacter, Kingella*

other genera: e.g., *Alcaligenes, Brucella, Bordetella, Flavobacterium, Francisella*

Gram-negative facultative anaerobic bacilli				
	family I	Enterobacteriaceae	genera:	*Escherichia, Shigella, Salmonella, Citrobacter, Klebsiella, Enterobacter, Erwinia, Serratia, Hafnia, Edwardsiella, Proteus, Providencia, Morganella, Yersinia*
	family II	Vibrionaceae	genera: e.g.,	*Vibrio, Aeromonas, Plesiomonas*
	family III	Pasteurellaceae	genera:	*Pasteurella, Haemophilus, Actinobacillus*

other genera: *Zymomonas, Chromobacterium, Cardiobacterium, Calymmatobacterium, Gardnerella, Eikenella, Streptobacillus*

Anaerobic Gram-negative straight, curved, and spiral-formed bacilli				
	family	Bacteroidaceae	genera: e.g.,	*Bacteroides, Fusobacterium, Leptotrichia*

Anaerobic Gram-negative cocci				
	family	Veillonellaceae	genera: e.g.	*Veillonella, other*

Rickettsia				
order I Rickettsiales	family I	Rickettsiaceae	genera: e.g.	*Rickettsia, Coxiella*
		Ehrlichiaeae	genera: e.g.	*Ehrlichia*
	family II	Bartonellaceae	genus: e.g.,	*Bartonella*
order II Chlamydiales	family I	Chlamydiaceae	genus:	*Chlamydia*

division II: firmicutes (Gram-positive)

Gram-positive cocci				
	family	Micrococcaceae	genera:	*Micrococcus, Stomatococcus, Planococcus, Staphylococcus*
	family	Deinococcaceae	genus:	*Deinococcus*

other organisms: e.g., streptococcus, pediococcus, peptococcus, peptostreptococcus

endospore-forming Gram-positive bacilli and cocci
genera: e.g., *Bacillus, Clostridium*

regularly formed, asporogenous Gram-positive bacilli
genera: e.g., *Lactobacillus, Listeria, Erysipelothrix*

irregularly formed, asporogenous Gram-positive bacilli
genera: e.g., *Corynebacterium, Gardnerella, Brevibacterium, Propionibacterium, Eubacterium, Actinomyces, Bifidobacterium*

Mycobacteria	Family	Mycobacteriaceae	genus:	*Mycobacterium*

Nocardioforms			genus: e.g.,	*Nocardia*

division III:	Tenericutes (without cell wall)	class I:	Mollicutes	
	order I Mycoplasmatales	family I	Mycoplasmataceae	genus: *Mycoplasma, Ureaplasma*

division IV:	Mendosicutes;	
	class I: Archaeobacteria (cell wall without muramic acid)	methanogenous bacteria, extremely halophilic b., extremely thermophilic b.

system. This occurs under conditions of distal obstruction or injection of solutions into renal collecting system.

background (bak'grownd). Instrument response in the absence of a sample.

back·ing (bak'ing). In dentistry, a metal support which serves to attach a facing to a prosthesis.

back-knee (bak'nē'). SYN *genu* recurvatum.

back·pro·jec·tion (bak'prō-jek'shŭn). In computed tomography or other imaging techniques requiring reconstruction from multiple projections, an algorithm for calculating the contribution of each voxel of the structure to the measured ray data, in order to generate an image; the oldest and simplest method of image reconstruction. Cf. Fourier *analysis*. SYN apical lordotic projection. Cf. Fourier *analysis*.

back·scat·ter (bak'skat-er). Secondary radiation deflected more than 90° from the primary beam. SEE scattered *radiation*.

back·track·ing. The backwards movement of RNA polymerase along the DNA template to a state more stable than that encountered when some base pairs disrupt the attachment of the 3′ end from the active transcription site.

bac·lo·fen (bak'lō-fen). A muscle relaxant used in the symptomatic treatment of spinal cord injuries and multiple sclerosis; an agonist at $GABA_b$ receptors.

Bacon, Harry E., U.S. proctologist, *1900. SEE B. *anoscope.*

bac·te·re·mia (bak-tĕr-ē'mē-ă). The presence of viable bacteria in the circulating blood; may be transient following trauma such as dental or other iatrogenic manipulation or may be persistent or recurrent as a result of infection. SYN bacteriemia. [bacteria + G. *haima,* blood]

△**bacteri-.** SEE bacterio-.

▣**bac·te·ria** (bak-tĕr'ē-ă). Plural of bacterium.

blue-green b., SEE Cyanobacteria.

cell wall–defective b., b. with absent or damaged cell walls; morphologically, they may become spheroplasts, round structures with little or no cell wall, or they may develop filamentous forms, with or without bulbous, extruded portions.

coryneform b., common name for nondiphtheria corynebacterium, usually a nonpathogenic component of skin and oropharyngeal flora in humans and animals can cause opportunistic infections in the immunocompromised host.

bac·te·ri·al (bak-tĕr'ē-ăl). Relating to bacteria.

bac·te·ri·cho·lia (bak'tĕr-i-kō'lē-ă). Bacteria in bile.

bac·te·ri·cid·al (bak-tĕr'i-sī'dăl). Causing the death of bacteria. Cf. bacteriostatic. SYN bacteriocidal.

bac·te·ri·cide (bak-tĕr'i-sīd). An agent that destroys bacteria. Cf. bacteriostat. SYN bacteriocide. [bacteria + L. *caedo,* to kill]

specific b., a bacteriolytic substance i.e., immune serum destructive to one bacterial species or genus only.

bac·ter·id (bak'ter-id). **1.** A recurrent or persistent eruption of discrete sterile pustules of the palms and soles, thought to be an allergic response to bacterial infection at a remote site. **2.** A dissemination of a previously localized bacterial skin infection. [bacteria + -id (1)]

bac·te·ri·e·mia (bak-tĕr-ē-ē'mē-ă). SYN bacteremia.

△**bacterio-, bacteri-.** Bacteria. [see bacterium]

bac·te·ri·o·ag·glu·ti·nin (bak-tĕr'ē-ō-ă-gloo'ti-nin). An antibody that agglutinates bacteria.

bac·te·ri·o·chlo·rin (bak-tĕr'-ē-ō-klōr'in). 7,8,17,18-Tetrahydroporphyrin; the basic structure of the bacteriochlorophylls.

bac·te·ri·o·chlo·ro·phyll (bak-tĕr-ē-ō-klōr'ō-fil). Any form of chlorophyll in photosynthetic bacteria: 1) b. *a,* $-CH=CH_2$ replaced by $-CO-CH_3$ in the chlorophyll α structure, two hydrogens also being added; the photosynthetic pigments of purple bacteria; 2) b. *b,* $-CH=CH_2$ replaced by $-CO-CH_3$ and $-CH_2-CH_3$ replaced by $-C≡CH$ in the chlorophyll β structure, two hydrogens also being added.

bac·te·ri·o·cid·al (bak-tĕr'ē-ō-sī'dăl). SYN bactericidal.

bac·ter·i·o·cide (bak-tĕr'ē-ō-sīd). SYN bactericide.

bac·te·ri·o·cid·in (bak-tĕr'ē-ō-sī'din). Antibody having bactericidal activity.

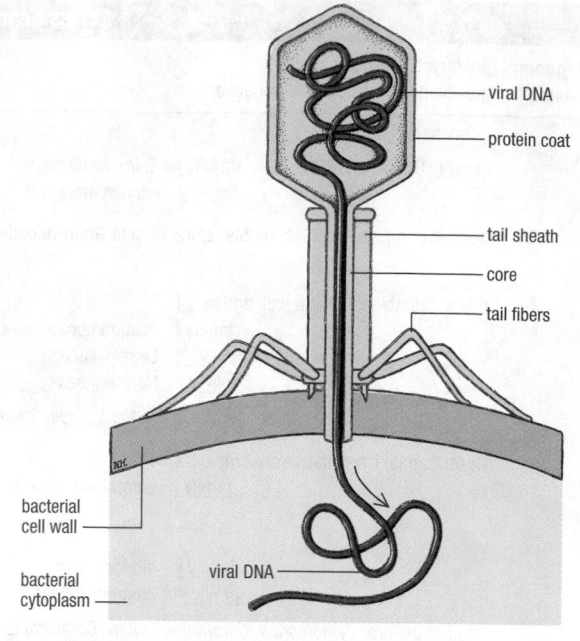

bacteriophage

bac·te·ri·o·cin·o·gens (bak-tĕr'ē-ō-sin'ō-jenz). SYN bacteriocinogenic *plasmids,* under *plasmid.*

bac·te·ri·o·cins (bak-tĕr'ē-ō-sinz). Proteins produced by certain bacteria that have bacteriocinogenic plasmids and that exert a lethal effect on closely related bacteria; in general, b. have a narrower range of activity than antibiotics and are more potent.

bac·te·ri·o·flu·o·res·cin (bak-tĕr'ē-ō-flōr-es'in). A fluorescent material produced by bacteria.

bac·te·ri·o·gen·ic (bak-tĕr'ē-ō-jen'ik). Caused by bacteria.

bac·te·ri·og·e·nous (bak-tĕr-ē-oj'e-nŭs). **1.** Producing bacteria. **2.** Of bacterial origin or causation.

bac·te·ri·oid (bak-tĕr'ē-oyd). **1.** Resembling bacteria. **2.** Intracellular forms of Rhizobium spp. in the root nodules of leguminous plants. [bacterio- + G. *eidos,* resemblance]

bac·te·ri·o·log·ic, bac·te·ri·o·log·i·cal (bak'tĕr-ē-ō-loj'ik, -i-kăl). Relating to bacteria or to bacteriology.

bac·te·ri·ol·o·gist (bak'ter-ē-ol'ŏ-jist). One who primarily studies or works with bacteria.

bac·te·ri·ol·o·gy (bak-tĕr-ē-ol'ŏ-jē). The branch of science concerned with the study of bacteria. [bacterio- + G. *logos,* study]

systematic b., that branch of b. concerned with nomenclature and classification (taxonomy).

bac·te·ri·o·ly·sin (bak-tĕr-ē-ol'i-sin). Specific antibody that combines with bacterial cells (i.e., antigen) and, in the presence of complement, causes lysis or dissolution of the cells.

bac·te·ri·ol·y·sis (bak-tĕr-ē-ol'i-sis). The dissolution of bacteria, e.g., by means of enzymes, hypotonic solutions, or specific antibody and complement. [bacterio- + G. *lysis,* dissolution]

bac·te·ri·o·lyt·ic (bak-tĕr-ē-ō-lit'ik). Pertaining to lytic destruction of bacteria; manifesting the ability to cause dissolution of bacterial cells.

bac·te·ri·o·lyze (bak-tĕr'ē-ō-līz). To cause the digestion or solution of bacterial cells.

bac·te·ri·o·pexy (bak-tĕr'ē-ō-pek-sē). Immobilization of bacteria by phagocytic cells. [bacterio- + G. *pēxis,* fixation]

▣**bac·te·ri·o·phage** (bak-tĕr'ē-ō-fāj). A virus with specific affinity for bacteria. B.'s have been found in association with essentially all groups of bacteria, including the Cyanobacteria; like other viruses they contain either (but never both) RNA or DNA and vary in structure from the seemingly simple filamentous bacterial virus to relatively complex forms with contractile "tails"; their relationships to the host bacteria are highly specific and, as in the case of temperate b., may be genetically intimate. B.'s are named after the bacterial species, group, or strain for which they are specific, e.g., corynebacteriophage, coliphage; a number of families are recognized and have been assigned provisional names: Corticoviridae, Cystoviridae, Fuselloviridae, Inoviridae, Leviviridae, Lipothrixviridae, Microviridae, Myoviridae, Plasmaviridae, Podoviridae, Styloviridae, and Tectiviridae. SEE ALSO coliphage. SYN phage. [bacterio- + G. *phagō*, to eat]

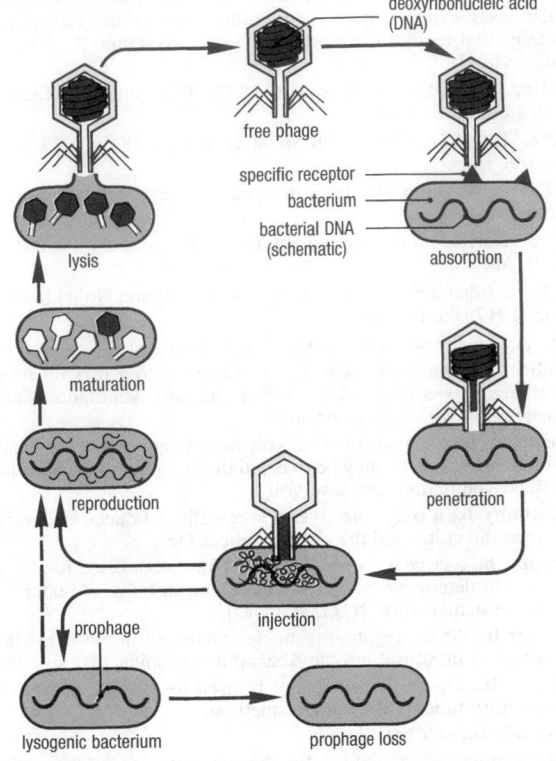

bacteriophages

defective b., a temperate b. mutant whose genome does not contain all of the normal components and cannot become a fully infectious virus, yet can replicate indefinitely in the bacterial genome as defective probacteriophage; many defective b.'s are mediators of transduction. SYN defective phage.

filamentous b., a b. that is rod-shaped and elongated lacking the head-and-tail structure characteristic of many b.'s.

mature b., the complete, infective form of b.

temperate b., b. whose genome incorporates with, and replicates with, that of the host bacterium; dissociation (and resultant development of vegetative b.) occurs at a slow rate resulting occasionally in lysis of a bacterium and release of mature b., thus rendering the bacterial culture capable of inducing general lysis if transferred to a culture of a susceptible bacterial strain.

typhoid b., b. specific for *Salmonella typhi*.

vegetative b., the form of b. in which the b. nucleic acid (lacking its coat) multiplies freely within the host bacterium, independently of bacterial multiplication.

virulent b., a b. that regularly causes lysis of the bacteria that it infects; it may exist in one or the other of only two forms, vegetative or mature; it does not have a probacteriophage form (i.e., its genome does not incorporate with that of the host bacterium), therefore it does not effect lysogenization.

bac·te·ri·o·pha·gia (bak-tēr′ē-ō-fā′jē-ă). Lysis of bacteria by a bacteriophage.

bac·te·ri·o·pha·gol·o·gy (bak-tēr′ē-ō-fă-gol′ō-jē). The study of bacteriophages. SYN protobiology.

bac·te·ri·o·phe·o·phor·bin (bak-tēr′ē-ō-fē-ō-fōr′bin). De-esterified bacteriopheophorbide, derived from bacteriochlorin.

bac·te·ri·o·phy·to·ma (bak-tēr′ē-ō-fī-tō′mă). A growth in plant tissues produced by bacteria. [bacterio- + G. *phytos*, plant, + -*oma*, growth]

bac·te·ri·o·pro·tein (bak-tēr′ē-ō-prō′tēn). One of the proteins within the cells of bacteria; these substances vary in their character and properties.

bac·te·ri·op·so·nin (bak-tēr′ē-op′sō-nin). An opsonin that may be an antibody acting upon bacteria rendering them susceptible to phagocytic cells.

bac·te·ri·o·sis (bak-tēr′ē-ō′sis). A localized or generalized bacterial infection.

bac·te·ri·o·sper·mia (bak′ter-ē-ō-sper-mē-ă). Bacteria in the semen or ejaculate.

bac·te·ri·o·sta·sis (bak-tēr-ē-os′tă-sis). An arrest or retardation of growth of bacteria. [bacterio- + G. *stasis*, a standing still]

bac·te·ri·o·stat (bak-tēr′ē-ō-stat). Any agent that inhibits or retards bacterial growth. SYN bacteriostatic agent.

bac·te·ri·o·stat·ic (bak-tēr′ē-ō-stat′ik). Inhibiting or retarding the multiplication of bacteria.

bac·te·ri·o·tox·ic (bak-tēr′ē-ō-tok′sik). Poisonous or toxic to bacteria.

bac·te·ri·o·tro·pic (bak-tēr′ē-ō-trop′ik). Turning toward or moving in the direction of bacteria; having an affinity for bacteria. [bacterio- + G. *tropē*, a turning]

bac·te·ri·ot·ro·pin (bak-tēr-ē-ot′rō-pin). A constituent of the blood, usually a specific antibody, i.e., opsonin, that combines with bacterial cells and renders them more susceptible to phagocytes.

bac·te·ri·o·tryp·sin (bak-tēr′ē-ō-trip′sin). A trypsinlike enzyme produced by bacteria, particularly *Vibrio cholerae*.

Bac·te·ri·um (bak-tēr′ē-ŭm). A bacterial generic name placed on the list of rejected names by the Judicial Commission and the International Committee on Systematic Bacteriology of the International Association of Microbiological Societies. As a consequence, *B.* is no longer used in bacteriology. Identifiable organisms formerly placed in the genus *B.* have all been transferred to other genera. Specifically, *B. anitratum* is now known as *Acinetobacter calcoaceticus; B. coli* is now called *Escherichia coli*. [Mod. L. fr. G. *baktērion*, dim. of *baktron*, a staff or club]

bac·te·ri·um (bak-tēr′ē-ŭm). A unicellular prokaryotic microorganism that usually multiplies by cell division and has a cell wall that provides a constancy of form; they may be aerobic or anaerobic, motile or nonmotile, and free-living, saprophytic, commensal, parasitic, or pathogenic. SEE ALSO Cyanobacteria. [Mod. L. fr. G. *baktērion*, dim. of *baktron*, a staff]

blue-green b., SEE Cyanobacteria.

endoteric b., a b. that forms an endotoxin.

exoteric b., a b. that secretes an exotoxin.

lysogenic b., a b. genome includes the genome (probacteriophage) of a temperate bacteriophage; in occasional instances the probacteriophage dissociates from the bacterial genome, develops into vegetative bacteriophage, and then matures, causing lysis of the respective host b. and release into the culture medium of infective temperate bacteriophage;

pyogenic b., a b. that causes a pyogenic infection usually associated with purulent exudate containing polymorphonuclear leukocytes such as the pyogenic cocci (staphylococci, streptococci, pneumococci, meningococci) and *Haemophilus influenzae*.

bac·te·ri·u·ria (bak-tēr-ē-oo′rē-ă). The presence of bacteria in the urine.

bac·te·roid (bak′ter-oyd). Resembling bacteria.

Bac·te·roi·da·ce·ae (bak′ter-oy-dā′sē-ē). A family of obligate anaerobic (microaerophilic species may occur), nonsporeforming bacteria (order Eubacteriales) containing Gram-negative rods which vary in size from minute, filterable forms to long, filamentous, branching forms; pronounced pleomorphism may occur. Motile and nonmotile species occur; motile cells are peritrichous.

Ba

Body fluids are frequently required for growth. Most species ferment carbohydrates, often with the production of acid; gas may be produced in glucose or peptone media. These organisms occur primarily in the lower intestinal tracts and mucous membranes of warm-blooded animals. They may be pathogenic. The type genus is *Bacteroides*.

Bac·te·roi·des (bak-ter-oy'dēz). A genus that includes many species of obligate anaerobic, nonsporeforming bacteria (family Bacteroidaceae) containing Gram-negative rods. Both motile and nonmotile species occur; motile cells are peritrichous. Some species ferment carbohydrates and produce combinations of succinic, lactic, acetic, formic, or propionic acids, sometimes with short-chained alcohols; butyric acid is not a major product. Those species which do not ferment carbohydrates produce from peptone either trace to moderate amounts of succinic, formic, acetic, and lactic acids or major amounts of acetic and butyric acids with moderate amounts of alcohols and isovaleric, propionic, and isobutyric acids. They are part of the normal flora of the intestinal tract and to a lesser degree, the respiratory, and urogenital cavities of humans and animals; many species formerly classified as *B.* have been reclassified as belonging to the genus *Prevotella*. Many species can be pathogenic. The type species is *B. fragilis*. [G. *bacterion + eidos*, form]

B. bivius, a species usually isolated from urogenital and abdominal infections and linked to pelvic inflammatory disease.

B. capillo'sus, a bacterial species isolated from human cysts and wounds, the mouth, and feces, and from the intestinal tracts of some animals. Its properties differ from those of most *B.* species; future reclassification is likely.

B. corro'dens, former name for *Eikenella corrodens*.

B. di'siens, SYN *Prevotella disiens*.

B. distasonis, bacterial species that is part of the normal human fecal flora; an occasional cause of intraabdominal infections.

B. frag'ilis, a bacterial species found in human and animal intestinal tracts. Although it represents only about 10–20% of B. species found in the colon, it is the primary species associated with intraabdominal abscesses and other subdiaphragmatic infections in humans, including peritonitis, rectal abscess, abdominal surgical wounds, and urogenital tract infection. Its capsule is capable of inducing abscess formation independently; characteristically, this species produces a β-lactamase that inactivates β-lactam antibiotics such as the penicillin and cephalosporin groups; it is the type species of the genus, B.

B. furco'sus, former name of *Anaerohabdus furcosis*.

B. melaninogenicus, SYN *Prevotella melaninogenica*.

B. nodo'sus, a bacterial species that causes foot rot in sheep and goats; it can be found in the human intestinal tract and has been associated with human infections; this organism has many properties different from other species of B., and its final classification is uncertain. SYN *Dichelobacter nodosus*.

B. ora'lis, former name of *Prevotella oralis*.

B. o'ris, former name of *Prevotella oris*.

B. pneumosin'tes, former name for *Dialister pneumosintes*.

B. praeacu'tus, a species isolated from the intestinal tracts of infants and adults, gangrenous lesions, lung abscesses, and blood. SYN *Tissierella praeacuta*.

B. putredi'nis, a species isolated from feces, cases of acute appendicitis, and abdominal and rectal abscesses; also from foot rot of sheep and from farm soil. Its properties are divergent from most B. species.

B. splanchnicus, a species in the indole positive group, found in normal human colonic flora, and occasionally in human specimens with unique metabolic properties that include production of large amounts of N-butyric acid; it appears to be closely related to the genus *Porphyromonas*.

B. thetaiotamicron, a bacterial species found in the intestinal tract; second only in its genus to *B. fragilis* as a cause of human subdiaphragmatic infections.

B. ureolyt'icus, a species isolated from infections of the respiratory and intestinal tracts, and from the buccal cavity, intestinal tract, urogenital tract, and blood after a dental extraction. It is closely related to *Campylobacter* species.

bac·te·roi·do·sis (bak'ter-oy-dō'sis). Rarely used term for an infection with *Bacteroides*.

bac·u·li·form (bă-kū'li-fōrm). Rod-shaped. [L. *baculum*, a rod, + *forma*, form]

Bac·u·lo·vi·ri·dae (bak-ū-lō-vir'i-dē). A family of viruses that multiply only in arthropods; virions are rod-shaped and measure 30–35 nm by 250–400 nm; genomes are of double-stranded, supercoiled DNA (90–160 kb). Baculovirus-derived vectors are frequently used to express foreign genes in insect cells. [L. *baculum*, rod]

bac·u·lo·vi·rus (bak'oo-lō-vī-rŭs). A virus that infects insect cells; used extensively in expression systems for recombinant proteins that require eucaryotic processing systems. [L. *baculum*, rod, + virus]

Baehr, George, U.S. physician, 1887–1978. SEE B.-Lohlein *lesion;* Lohlein-B. *lesion.*

Baelz, Erwin O., German physician in Tokyo, 1849–1913. SEE B. *disease.*

BAER Abbreviation for brainstem auditory evoked response. SEE evoked *response.*

Baer, Karl E. von, German-Russian embryologist, 1792–1876. SEE B. *law.*

Baeyer, Johann F.W.A. von, German chemist and Nobel laureate, 1835–1917. SEE B. *theory.*

bag. A pouch, sac, or receptacle. [A.S. *baelg*]

Ambu b., proprietary name for a self-reinflating b. with nonrebreathing valves to provide positive pressure ventilation during resuscitation with oxygen or air.

breathing b., a collapsible reservoir from which gases are inhaled and into which gases may be exhaled during general anesthesia or artificial ventilation. SYN reservoir b.

colostomy b., a bag worn over a surgically produced connection between the colon and the skin to collect feces.

Douglas b., a large b. in which expired gas is collected for several minutes to determine oxygen consumption in humans under conditions of actual work. [C.G. Douglas]

nuclear b., the aggregation of nuclei occurring in the nonstriated center of an intrafusal muscle fiber of a neuromuscular spindle.

Politzer b., a pear-shaped rubber b. used for forcing air through the auditory tube by the Politzer method.

reservoir b., SYN breathing b.

b. of waters, colloquialism for the amniotic sac and contained amniotic fluid.

bag·as·so·sis (bag-ă-sō'sis). Extrinsic allergic alveolitis following exposure to sugar-cane fiber dust (bagasse); has been attributed to inhalation of spores of soil fungi and, particularly, thermophilic actinomycetes.

Baggenstoss, Archie H., U.S. pathologist, *1908. SEE B. *change.*

Bagolini, 20th century Italian ophthalmologist. SEE B. *test.*

Baillarger, Jules G.F., French neurologist, 1809–1891. SEE B. *bands,* under *band,* *lines,* under *line.*

Bailliart, Paul, French ophthalmologist, 1877–1969. SEE B. *ophthalmodynamometer.*

Bainbridge, Francis A., English physiologist, 1874–1921. SEE B. *reflex.*

Baker, James Porter, U.S. physician, *1902. SEE Charcot-Weiss-B. *syndrome.*

Baker, John Randal, English zoologist, *1900. SEE B. *pyridine extraction,* acid *hematein.*

Baker, William M., English surgeon, 1839–1896. SEE B. *cyst.*

BAL Abbreviation for British anti-Lewisite.

BAL Abbreviation for bronchoalveolar *lavage.*

Balamuthia (bal-ă-moo'thē-ă). A genus of free-living ameba that causes granulomatous amebic encephalitis.

△**balan-.** SEE balano-.

bal·ance (bal'ans). **1.** An apparatus for weighing; e.g., scales. **2.** The normal state of action and reaction between two or more parts or organs of the body. **3.** Quantities, concentrations, and proportionate amounts of bodily constituents. **4.** The difference between intake and utilization, storage, or excretion of a substance by the body. SEE ALSO equilibrium. [L. *bi-,* twice, + *lanx,* dish, scale]

acid-base b., the normal b. between acid and base in the blood plasma, expressed in the hydrogen ion concentration or pH, resulting from the relative amounts of acidic and basic materials ingested and produced by body metabolism, compared to the relative amounts of acidic and basic materials excreted from the body and consumed by body metabolism; the normal state of acid-base b. is not one of neutrality, with equal concentrations of hydrogen and hydroxyl ions, but a more alkaline state with a certain excess of hydroxyl ions. SYN acid-base equilibrium.

nitrogen b., the difference between the total nitrogen intake by an organism and its total nitrogen loss. A zero nitrogen b. is seen in normal, healthy adults; $N_{in} > N_{out}$ is a positive nitrogen b. and $N_{in} < N_{out}$ is a negative nitrogen b.

occlusal b., a condition in which there are simultaneous contacts of the occluding units of the opposing dental arches in centric and eccentric positions within the functional range.

phonetic b., that property by which a group of words used in the measurement of hearing has the various phonemes occurring at approximately the same frequency at which they occur in ordinary conversation in that language; phonetically balanced word lists are used in determining the discrimination score.

Wilhelmy b., a device for measuring surface tension in terms of the pull exerted on a thin plate of platinum or other material suspended vertically through the surface; used in a Langmuir trough to study pulmonary surfactant.

ba·lan·ic (ba-lan′ik). Relating to the glans penis or glans clitoridis. [G. *balanos,* acorn, glans]

Ba·la·ni·tes ae·gyp·ti·a·ca (bal-ă-nī′tēz ē-jip-tī′ă-kă). A genus of trees growing in the Near East, whose berries contain an active principle that is deadly to mollusks, miracidia, cercariae, tadpoles, and fish and that is used as a prophylactic against schistosomiasis by adding it to drinking water. [L. *balanos,* acorn]

bal·a·ni·tis (bal-ă-nī′tis). Inflammation of the glans penis or clitoris. [G. *balanos,* acorn, glans, + *-itis,* inflammation]

b. circumscripta plasmacellularis, SYN plasma cell b.

b. diabet′ica, glanular inflammation in diabetics related to urinary infection or concomitant posthitis.

plasma cell b., benign circumscribed b. characterized microscopically by subepithelial plasma cell infiltration and clinically by small erythematous papular lesions. SYN b. circumscripta plasmacellularis.

b. xerot′ica oblit′erans, lichen sclerosus et atrophicus of the glans penis, which may result in meatal stenosis.

⌂**balano-, balan-.** Glans penis. [G. *balanos,* acorn, glans]

bal·a·no·plas·ty (bal′an-ō-plas-tē). Surgical reconstruction of the glans penis. [balano- + G. *plastos,* formed]

bal·a·no·pos·thi·tis (bal′an-ō-pos-thī′tis). Inflammation of the glans penis and overlying prepuce. [balano- + G. *posthē,* prepuce, + *-itis,* inflammation]

bal·an·ti·di·a·sis (bal′an-ti-dī′ă-sis). A disease caused by the presence of *Balantidium coli* in the large intestine; characterized by diarrhea, dysentery, and occasionally ulceration. SYN balantidosis.

Ba·lan·ti·di·um (bal-an-tid′ē-ŭm). A genus of ciliates (family Balantidiidae) found in the digestive tract of vertebrates and invertebrates. [G. *balantidion,* dim of *ballantion,* a bag]

B. co′li, a very large parasitic ciliate species, usually 50–80 μm in length, reaching up to 200 μm in pigs, found in the cecum or large intestine, swimming actively in the lumen; usually harmless in humans but may invade and ulcerate the intestinal wall, producing a colitis resembling amebic dysentery.

B. su′is, a species originally considered distinct from the ciliate parasite of man, *B. coli,* but now considered synonymous with it; nonpathogenic in swine.

bal·an·ti·do·sis (bal′an-ti-dō′sis). SYN balantidiasis.

bal·a·nus (bal′ă-nŭs). SYN *glans* penis. [G. *balanos,* acorn, glans penis]

bald (bawld). Having no hair, or a decrease in the amount of hair of the scalp. [M.E. *balled*]

bald·ness (bawld′nes). SYN alopecia.

common b., SYN androgenic *alopecia.*

congenital b., SYN *alopecia* congenitalis.

male pattern b., SYN male pattern *alopecia.*

Balint, Rudolph, Hungarian neurologist and psychiatrist, 1874–1930. SEE B. *syndrome.*

Ball, Sir Charles B., Irish surgeon, 1851–1916. SEE B. *operation.*

ball. 1. A round mass. SEE bezoar. 2. In veterinary medicine, a large pill or bolus.

chondrin b., one of the globular masses formed by a group of cells enclosed in a capsule, in hyaline cartilage.

food b., SYN phytobezoar.

b. of the foot, the padded portion of the sole, at the anterior extremity of the heads of the metatarsals, upon which the weight rests when the heel is raised.

fungus b., a compact mass of fungal mycelium and cellular debris, 1 to 5 cm in diameter, residing within a lung cavity, paranasal sinus, or urinary tract; aspergilloma is a type of fungus b. of the lung.

Ballance, Sir Charles A., English surgeon, 1856–1936. SEE B. *sign;* Koerte-B. *operation.*

bal·ism (bal′izm). SYN ballismus.

bal·lis·mus (bal-iz′mŭs). A type of involuntary movement affecting the proximal limb musculature, manifested as jerking, flinging movements of the extremity; caused by a lesion of or near the contralateral subthalamic nucleus. Usually only one side of the body is involved, resulting in hemiballismus. SYN ballism. [G. *ballismos,* a jumping about]

bal·lis·to·car·di·o·gram (bal-is-tō-kar′dē-ō-gram). A record of the body's recoil caused by cardiac contraction, the ejection of blood into the aorta, and ventricular filling forces; has been used as a basis for calculating the cardiac output in man, but its lack of accuracy and reproducibility has caused it to be discarded. [G. *ballō,* to throw, + *kardia,* heart, + *gramma,* something written]

bal·lis·to·car·di·o·graph (BCG) (bal-is-tō-kar′dē-ō-graf). Instrument for taking a ballistocardiogram, consisting either of a moving table suspended from the ceiling, or of an apparatus that rests upon the patient's body, usually on the shins, together with a graphic recording system.

bal·lis·to·car·di·og·ra·phy (bal-is-tō-kar-dē-og′ră-fē). 1. The graphic recording of movements of the body imparted by ballistic forces (cardiac contraction and ejection of blood, ventricular filling, acceleration, and deceleration of blood flow through the great vessels); these minute movements are amplified and recorded on moving chart paper after being translated into an electrical potential by a pickup device. 2. The study and interpretation of ballistocardiograms.

bal·lis·to·pho·bia (bal-is-tō-fō′bē-ă). Morbid fear of a projectile or missile. [G. *ballista,* catapult, fr. G. *ballistēs* fr. *ballō,* + *phobos,* fear]

bal·loon (bă-loon). 1. An inflatable spherical or ovoid device used to retain tubes or catheters in, or provide support to, various body structures. 2. A distensible device used to stretch or occlude a viscus or blood vessel. 3. To distend a body cavity with a gas or fluid to facilitate its examination, dilate a structure, or occlude its lumen. [Fr. *ballon,* fr. It. *ballone,* fr. *balla,* ball, fr. Germanic]

angioplasty b., a b. near the tip of an angiographic catheter, designed to distend narrowed vessels. SEE balloon-tip *catheter.*

detachable b., a small b., attached to the tip of a catheter, which can be released to occlude a vessel.

intraaortic b., SEE intraaortic balloon *pump.*

bal·lot·ta·ble (bal-ot′ă-bl). Capable of exhibiting the phenomenon of ballottement.

bal·lotte·ment (bal-ot-maw′). 1. Maneuver used in physical examination to estimate the size of an organ not near the surface, particularly when there is ascites, by a flicking motion of the hand or fingers similar to that involved in dribbling a basketball. 2. An obsolete method of diagnosis of pregnancy: with the tip of the forefinger in the vagina, a sharp tap is made against the lower segment of the uterus; the fetus, if present, is tossed upward and

ba

(if the finger is retained in place) will be felt to strike against the wall of the uterus as it falls back. [Fr. *balloter,* to toss up]

abdominal b., examination of the abdomen by palpation to detect excessive amounts of fluid (ascites) by causing organs to bob up and down in the fluid milieu.

renal b., a maneuver in which the kidney is moved by pressure from behind, allowing it to be felt between the hands and its size, shape, and mobility determined.

balm (bawlm). **1.** SYN balsam. **2.** An ointment, especially a fragrant one. **3.** A soothing application. [L. *balsamum,* fr. G. *balsamon,* the balsam tree]

b. of Gilead, an oleoresin from *Commiphora opobalsamum* (family Burseraceae), probably the myrrh of the Bible; used in perfumery. SYN Mecca balsam, opobalsamum.

mountain b., SYN eriodictyon.

sweet b., SYN melissa.

bal·ne·o·ther·a·peu·tics, bal·ne·o·ther·a·py (bal′nē-ō-thār-ă-pū′tiks, -thār′ă-pē). Immersion of part or all of the body in a mineral water bath as a form of therapy. [L. *balneum,* bath]

Baló, Jozsef, Hungarian physician, *1896. SEE B. *disease.*

bal·sam (bawl′sam). A fragrant, resinous or thick, oily exudate from various trees and plants. SYN balm (1), oleoresin (3). [G. *balsamon;* L. *balsamum*]

Canada b., a yellowish liquid resin from the b. fir, *Abies balsamea* (family Pinaceae); contains kinene and bornyl acetate; used for mounting histologic specimens and as a cement for lenses. SYN Canada turpentine.

b. of copaiba, SYN copaiba.

Mecca b., SYN *balm* of Gilead.

b. of Peru, a thick, dark brown liquid b. obtained from *Toluifera pereirae* (family Leguminosae), containing 60% cinnamein; used as a healing application to wounds.

Tolu b., a yellowish brown soft mass obtained from *Toluifera balsamum* (family Leguminosae), containing cinnamic and benzoic acids and esters; used as a stimulant expectorant.

bal·sam·ic (bawl-sam′ik). **1.** Relating to balsam. **2.** Fragrant.

BALT Abbreviation for bronchus-associated lymphoid *tissue.*

Bamberger, Eugen, Austrian physician, 1858–1921. SEE B.-Marie *disease, syndrome.*

Bamberger, Heinrich von, Austrian physician, 1822–1888. SEE B. *albuminuria, disease, sign.*

ba·mif·yl·line hy·dro·chlo·ride (bă-mif′i-lin). A vasodilator and smooth muscle relaxant.

bam·i·pine (bam-i-pēn). An antihistaminic.

ban·crof·ti·a·sis, ban·crof·to·sis (ban-krof-tī′ă-sis, -tō′sis). Infection with *Wuchereria bancrofti.*

band. 1. Any appliance or part of an apparatus that encircles or binds a part of the body. SEE ALSO zone. **2.** Any ribbon-shaped or cordlike anatomic structure that encircles or binds another structure or that connects two or more parts. SEE fascia, line, linea, stripe, stria, tenia. **3.** A narrow strip containing one or more macromolecules (on occasions, small molecules) detected in electrophoresis or certain types of chromatography.

A b.'s, the dark-staining anisotropic cross striations in the myofibrils of muscle fibers, comprising regions of overlapping thick (myosin) and thin (actin) filaments. SYN A disks, anisotropic disks, Q b.'s (1), Q disks.

absorption b., the range of wavelengths or frequencies in the electromagnetic spectrum where radiant energy is absorbed by passage through a gaseous, liquid, or dissolved substance; it is exploited for analytical purposes in colorimetry or spectrophotometry, and is usually described in terms of the wavelength where maximum absorbance occurs (i.e., λ_{max}).

amnionic b. [MIM*217100], strands of amnion following its rupture, which can wrap around limbs, digits, face, and internal organs, causing constriction and amputation; the genetics of which is unclear. SEE ALSO congenital *amputation.* SYN amnionic adhesions, amnionic band syndrome, anular b., constriction ring (2), Simonart b.'s (1), Simonart ligaments.

anogenital b., the first indication of the perineum in the embryo.

anular b., SYN amnionic b.

atrioventricular b., SYN atrioventricular *bundle.*

Baillarger b.'s, SYN Baillarger *lines,* under *line.*

Bechterew b., SYN b. of Kaes-Bechterew.

Broca diagonal b., a white fiber bundle descending in the precommissural septum toward the base of the forebrain, immediately rostral to the lamina terminalis; this band consists of a horizontal limb [TA] (crus horizontale [TA]), a vertical limb [TA] (crus verticale [TA]) and the cells associated with the b. form the nucleus of diagonal band [TA] (nucleus striae diagonalis [TA]); at the base, the bundle turns in the caudolateral direction; traveling through a ventral stratum of the innominate substance alongside the optic tract, it fades before reaching the amygdala. SYN diagonal b. [TA], stria diagonalis [TA].

chromosome b., a region of darker or contrasting staining across the width of a chromosome; the pattern of b.'s is characteristic for most chromosomes. SEE banding.

Clado b., SYN suspensory *ligament* of ovary.

b.'s of colon, SYN *teniae* coli, under *tenia.*

contraction b., a microscopic change in myocardial cells in which excessive contraction, associated with elevated intracellular calcium and serum norepinephrine, causes the formation of transverse amorphous b. in the fibers which are then incapable of contracting again. SYN contraction band necrosis.

diagonal b. [TA], SYN Broca diagonal b.

Essick cell b.'s, groups of cells in the developing rhombencephalon which migrate in two b.'s, one of which eventually forms the inferior olivary nucleus and the arcuate nucleus, and the other the pontine nuclei.

Gennari b., SYN *line* of Gennari.

b. of Giacomini, SYN uncus b. of Giacomini.

H b., the paler area in the center of the A b. of a striated muscle fiber, comprising the central portion of thick (myosin) filaments that are not overlapped by thin (actin) filaments. SYN H disk, Hensen disk, Hensen line.

His b., SYN atrioventricular *bundle.*

Hunter-Schreger b.'s, alternating light and dark lines seen in dental enamel that begin at the dentoenamel junction and end before they reach the enamel surface; they represent areas of enamel rods cut in cross-sections dispersed between areas of rods cut longitudinally. SYN Hunter-Schreger lines, Schreger lines.

I b., a light b. on each side of the Z line of striated muscle fibers, comprising a region of the sarcomere where thin (actin) filaments are not overlapped by thick (myosin) filaments. SYN I disk, isotropic disk.

iliotibial b., SYN iliotibial *tract.*

b. of Kaes-Bechterew, b. of horizontal myelinated fibers in the most superficial part of the third layer of the isocortex. SYN stria laminae molecularis [TA], stria of molecular layer [TA], Bechterew b., layer of Bechterew, line of Bechterew, line of Kaes.

Ladd b., a peritoneal attachment of an incompletely rotated cecum, found in malrotation of the intestine; may cause obstruction of the duodenum.

Lane b., a congenital b. on the distal ileum that may extend into the right iliac fossa causing stasis. SYN Lane kink.

longitudinal b.'s of cruciform ligament of atlas [TA], ligamentous slips forming the "upright" or vertical beam of the cruciform ligament of the atlas. SYN fasciculi longitudinales ligamenti cruciformis atlantis [TA].

M b., SYN M *line.*

Mach b., a relatively bright or dark b. perceived in a zone where the luminance increases or decreases rapidly.

Maissiat b., SYN iliotibial *tract.*

matrix b., a metal or plastic b. secured around the crown of a tooth to confine restorative material to be adapted into a prepared cavity.

Meckel b., the portion of the anterior ligament of the malleus that extends from the base of the anterior process through the petrotympanic fissure, to attach to the spine of the sphenoid. SEE anterior *ligament* of malleus. SYN Meckel ligament.

moderator b., SYN septomarginal *trabecula.*

Muehrcke b.'s, apparent leukonychia with white b.'s parallel to lanula of the nails, seen in hypoalbuminemia. SYN Muehrcke sign.

oligoclonal b., small discrete b.'s in the gamma globulin region of the spinal fluid electrophoresis, indicating local central nervous system production of IgG; b.'s are frequently seen in patients with multiple sclerosis but can also be found in other diseases of the central nervous system including syphilis, sarcoidosis, and chronic infection or inflammation.

orthodontic b., a thin strip of metal closely adapted to the crown of a tooth to which wires may be attached for tooth movement.

pecten b., a fibrous induration of the anal pecten resulting from passive congestion or a chronic form of inflammation in this region.

Q b.'s, (1) SYN A b.'s; **(2)** SEE Q-banding *stain*.

Reil b., (1) SYN septomarginal *trabecula*; **(2)** SYN medial *lemniscus*.

silastic b. (si'läs-tik), a small silastic ring placed around each fallopian tube to achieve permanent sterilization.

Simonart b.'s, (1) SYN amnionic b; **(2)** weblike band of tissue partially filling the gap between the medial and lateral portions of a cleft lip.

Soret b., the absorption b. of all porphyrins at about 400 nm.

uncus b. of Giacomini, a slender whitish b., the attenuated anterior continuation of the dentate gyrus (fascia dentata), crossing transversally the surface of the recurved part of the uncus gyri parahippocampalis. SYN b. of Giacomini, cauda fasciae dentatae, frenulum of Giacomini, tail of dentate gyrus.

ventricular b. of larynx, SYN vestibular *fold*.

Z b., SYN Z *line*.

zonular b., SYN *zona* orbicularis (articulationis coxae).

ban·dage (ban'dij). **1.** A piece of cloth or other material, of varying shape and size, applied to a body part to provide compression, protect from external contamination, prevent drying, absorb drainage, prevent motion, and retain surgical dressings. **2.** To cover a body part by application of a b.

adhesive b., a dressing of plain absorbent gauze affixed to plastic or fabric coated with a pressure-sensitive adhesive.

Barton b., a figure-of-8 b. supporting the mandible below and anteriorly; used in mandibular fracture.

capeline b., a b. covering the head or an amputation stump like a cap. [L. *capella*, a cap]

circular b., one encircling an extremity, or a portion of it, or the trunk.

cravat b., a b. made by bringing the point of a triangular b. to the middle of the base and then folding lengthwise to the desired width.

crucial b., a b. in the shape of a cross; e.g., a T-b..

demigauntlet b., a gauntlet b. that covers only the hand, leaving the fingers exposed.

Desault b., a b. for fracture of the clavicle; the elbow is bound to the side, with a pad placed in the axilla.

elastic b., a b. containing stretchable material; used to provide local compression.

Esmarch b., SYN Esmarch *tourniquet*.

figure-of-8 b., a b. applied alternately to two parts, usually two segments of a limb above and below the joint, in such a way that the turns describe the figure 8; a specific bandage used for treatment of fractures of the clavicle.

four-tailed b., a strip of cloth split in two except for a central

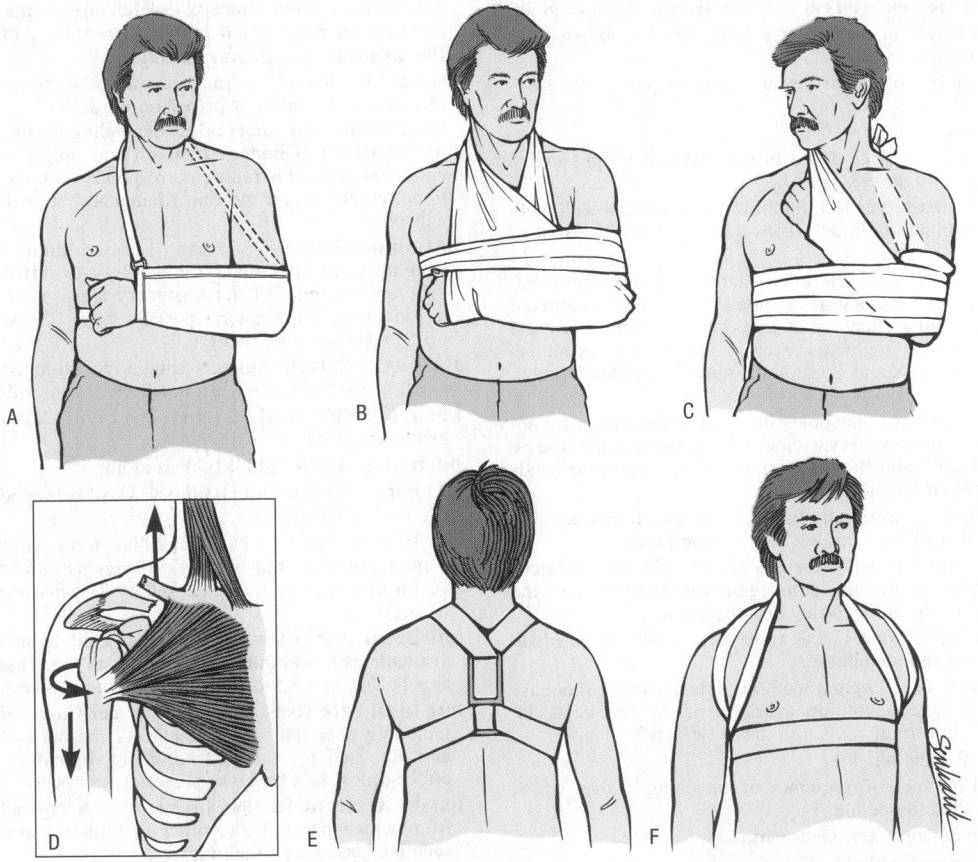

immobilization bandages: used for proximal humeral fractures, (A) commercial sling and swathe, (B) conventional sling and swathe, (C) stockinette Velpeau and swathe; (D) used for fractures of the clavicle: (E) clavicular strap, posterior view, (F) clavicular strap, anterior view

portion placed under the chin, with four tails tied over the head; used to limit motion of the mandible.

gauntlet b., a figure-of-8 b. covering the hand and fingers.

gauze b., SEE gauze.

Gibney fixation b., herring-bone strapping of the foot and leg for sprain of the ankle.

Gibson b., a b., resembling Barton b., for stabilizing a fracture of the mandible.

hammock b., a b. for retaining dressings on the head: the dressings are covered by a wide gauze strip, the ends of which are brought down over the ears and held while a narrow circular b. is passed around the head; the ends of the gauze strip are then turned up over the circular b. and other turns are made securing them firmly.

immovable b., a b. of cloth impregnated with plaster of Paris, liquid glass, or the like, which hardens soon after its application.

Martin b., a roller b. of soft rubber used to provide compression to a limb in the treatment of varicose veins or ulcers.

oblique b., a b. in which the successive turns proceed obliquely up or down the limb.

plaster b., a roller b. impregnated with plaster of Paris and applied moist; used to make a rigid dressing for a fracture or diseased joint.

roller b., a strip of material, of variable width, rolled into a compact cylinder to facilitate its application.

scarf b., SYN triangular b.

Scultetus b., a large oblong cloth, the ends of which are cut into narrow strips, which is applied to the thorax or abdomen, the strips being tied or overlapped and pinned.

spica b., successive strips of material applied to the body and the first part of a limb, or to the hand and a finger, which overlap slightly in a V to resemble an ear of grain. [L. *spica*, ear of grain]

spiral b., an oblique b. encircling a limb, the successive turns overlapping those preceding.

suspensory b., a bag of expansile fabric for supporting the scrotum and its contents.

T-b., SYN T-*binder*.

triangular b., a piece of cloth cut in the shape of a right-angled triangle, used as a sling. SYN scarf b.

Velpeau b., a b. that serves to immobilize arm to chest wall, with the forearm positioned obliquely across and upward on front of chest.

band·ing. The process of differential staining of (usually) metaphase chromosomes of cells to reveal the characteristic patterns of bands that permit identification of individual chromosomes and recognition of missing segments; each of the 22 pairs of human chromosomes and the X and Y chromosomes has an identifying b. pattern.

BrDu-b., labeling of chromosomes in proliferating tissue by adding an excess of bromodeoxyuridine, which replaces the uridine incorporated in RNA and fluoresces in ultraviolet light; the bands result from sister chromatid exchanges.

high-resolution b., b., especially in prophase, which increases the clarity and number of discernible chromosome bands.

NOR-b., a procedure which utilizes a silver stain that preferentially accumulates in the *nucleoli-organizing regions*, i.e., the satellite regions of the acrocentric chromosomes.

prometaphase b., b. done in the stage of mitosis intermediate between prophase and metaphase.

pulmonary artery b., a surgical method of decreasing pulmonary blood flow and thereby volume overload of the left ventricle, alleviating CHF in certain congenital heart defects.

reverse b., SEE R-banding *stain*.

band·width. The range of frequency or wavelengths over which a device is intended to operate.

ban·dy-leg (ban′dē-leg). SYN *genu* varum.

bane (bān). A poison or blight. [O.E. *bana*]

Bang, Bernhard L.F., Danish veterinarian and physician, 1848–1932. SEE B. *disease*.

ba·nis·te·rine (ba-nis′tĕ-rēn). SYN harmine.

Banti, Guido, Italian physician, 1852–1925. SEE B. *disease, syndrome*.

Banting, Sir Frederick G., Canadian physician, 1891–1941, co-winner of the 1923 Nobel Prize for isolating insulin from the pancreas.

bap·ti·tox·ine. SYN cytisine.

bar. 1. A unit of pressure equal to 1 megadyne (10^6 dyne) per cm^2 in the CGS system, 0.9869233 atmosphere, or 10^5 Pa (N/m^2) in the SI system. **2.** A metal segment of greater length than width that serves to connect two or more parts of a removable partial denture. SEE ALSO major *connector*. **3.** A segment of tissue or bone that unites two or more similar structures.

arch b., any one of several types of wires, b., or splints conforming to the arch of the teeth, extending from one side of the arch to the other and located labially, or lingually; used for the treatment of jaw fractures and/or stabilization of injured teeth.

b. of bladder, SYN interureteric *crest*.

clasp b., SEE clasp.

connector b., SEE major *connector*, minor *connector*.

labial b., a major connector located labial to the dental arch joining two or more bilateral parts of a mandibular removable partial denture.

lingual b., a major connector located lingual to the dental arch joining two or more bilateral parts of a mandibular removable partial denture.

median b. of Mercier, a prominent band of fibromuscular tissue involving the interureteric ridge or neck of the urinary bladder, occasionally resulting in urinary obstruction.

Mercier b., SYN interureteric *crest*.

occlusal rest b., a minor connector used to attach an occlusal rest to a major part of a removable partial denture.

palatal b., a major connector which crosses the palate and unites two or more parts of a maxillary removable partial denture.

Passavant b., SYN Passavant *ridge*.

sternal b., one of the transverse units of the developing sternum formed by the union of paired primordia.

terminal b., dark spots or b. (depending on the plane of section) in the lateral boundary between the apical ends of columnar epithelial cells; this region corresponds with the area of the junctional complex and the thin filaments that anchor on the zonula adherens.

bar·ag·no·sis (bar-ag-nō′sis). Loss of ability to appreciate the weight of objects held in the hand, or to differentiate objects of different weights. When the primary senses are intact, caused by a lesion of the contralateral parietal lobe. [G. *baros*, weight + *a*-priv., + *gnōsis*, a knowing]

Bárány, Robert, Austrian-Hungarian otologist and Nobel laureate, 1876–1936. SEE B. *sign*, caloric *test;* positional *vertigo* of B.

bar·ba (bar′bă) [TA]. **1** [NA]. The beard. **2.** A hair of the beard. SYN beard [TA]. [L.]

barb·al·o·in (bar-bal′ō-in). SYN aloin.

Barber, Glenn, 20th century U.S. orthopedic surgeon. SEE Blount-Barber *disease*.

bar·bi·e·ro (bar-bē-ā′rō). Brazilian term for the bloodsucking hemipteran triatomid bug, *Panstrongylus megistus,* an important vector of Chagas disease, caused by *Trypanosoma cruzi.* [Pg. the barber]

bar·bi·tal (bar′bi-tawl). An obsolescent hypnotic and sedative; available as b. sodium (soluble b.), with the same uses; often used as a buffer. SYN 5,5-diethylbarbituric acid, Veronal.

bar·bi·tu·rate (bar-bich′ūr-āt). A derivative of barbituric acid, including phenobarbital and others, that act as CNS depressants and are used for their tranquilizing, hypnotic, and anti-seizure effects; most b.'s have the potential for abuse.

bar·bi·tu·ric ac·id (bar-bi-chūr′ik). A crystalline dibasic acid from which barbital and other barbiturates are derived; has no sedative action. SYN malonylurea.

bar·bi·tu·rism (bar′bi-chūr-izm). Chronic poisoning by any of the derivatives of barbituric acid; symptoms, which are not very distinctive, include cutaneous eruption accompanied by chills, fever, and headache.

bar·bo·tage (bar-bō-tahzh′). A method of spinal anesthesia in which a portion of the anesthetic solution is injected into the cerebrospinal fluid, which is then aspirated back into the syringe and reinjected. [Fr. *barboter*, to dabble]

bar·bu·la hir·ci (bar′bū-lă hir′sī). The hairs growing from the tragus, antitragus, and incisura intertragica of the auricle of men after age 27 years. [L. dim. of *barba*, beard, + gen. sing. of *hircus*, goat]

Barclay, Alfred E., English physician, 1877–1949. SEE B.-Baron *disease*.

Barcroft, Sir Joseph F., English physiologist, 1872–1947. SEE B.-Warburg *apparatus, technique*.

Bard, Philip, U.S. physiologist, 1898–1945. SEE Cannon-B. *theory*.

Bardet, Georges, French physician, *1885. SEE B.-Biedl *syndrome*.

Bardinet, Barthélemy A., French physician, 1809–1874. SEE B. *ligament*.

bar·es·the·sia (bar-es-thē′zē-ă). SYN pressure *sense*. [G. *baros*, weight, + *aisthēsis*, sensation]

bar·es·the·si·om·e·ter (bar′es-thē′zē-om′ĕ-ter). An instrument for measuring the pressure sense. [G. *baros*, weight, + *aisthēsis*, sensation, + *metron*, measure]

bar·i·at·ric (bar-ē-at′rik). Relating to bariatrics.

bar·i·at·rics (bar-ē-at′riks). That branch of medicine concerned with the management (prevention or control) of obesity and allied diseases. [G. *baros*, weight, + *iatreia*, medical treatment]

ba·ric (ba′rik). Relating to barometric pressure (as in isobar) or to weight generally.

ba·ric·i·ty (ba-ris′i-tē). The weight of one substance compared to the weight of an equal volume of another substance at the same temperature. [G. *baros*, weight]

ba·ril·la (ba-ril′ă). Commercial, usually impure, sodium carbonate and sulfate.

bar·i·to·sis (bar-i-tō′sis). A form of pneumoconiosis caused by barite or barium dust.

bar·i·um (Ba) (ba′rē-ŭm, bā′rē-ŭm). A metallic, alkaline, divalent earth element; atomic no. 56, atomic wt. 137.327. Insoluble salts are often used in radiology as contrast media. [G. *barys*, heavy]

b. chloride, formerly used as a heart tonic and for varicose veins; extremely toxic.

b. hydroxide, a caustic compound combined with calcium hydroxide in a carbon dioxide absorbent; used in anesthetic circuits. SEE ALSO absorbent (3).

b. meal, oral administration of b. sulfate suspension for radiographic study of the upper gastrointestinal tract (British usage).

b. oxide, b. monoxide, it is caustic, forming the strong base, Ba(OH)$_2$, in water; used as a dehydrating agent. SYN baryta.

b. sulfate, given as a suspension orally, rectally, or through a tube, for radiographic demonstration of a part of the gastrointestinal tract. SEE enteroclysis, barium *enema*.

b. sulfide, a poisonous grayish yellow powder, used as a depilatory.

b. swallow, oral administration of b. sulfate suspension for radiographic investigation of the hypopharynx and esophagus.

bark. 1. The envelope or covering of the roots, trunk, and branches of plants. B.'s of pharmacological significance not listed below are alphabetized under specific names. **2.** SYN cinchona.

cinchona b., SYN cinchona.

cotton-root b., dried root b. of *Gossypium herbaceum* and other species of *Gossypium* (family Malvaceae). Has been used as an abortifacient and oxytocic.

Barkan, Otto, U.S. ophthalmologist, 1887–1958. SEE Barkan *membrane;* B. *operation*.

Barkman, Åke, 20th century Swedish internist. SEE B. *reflex*.

Barkow, Hans K.L., German anatomist, 1798–1873. SEE B. *ligaments*, under *ligament*.

Barlow, John B., South African cardiologist, *1924. SEE B. *syndrome*.

Barlow, Sir Thomas, British physician, 1845–1945. SEE B. *disease*.

barn (b). A unit of area for effective cross-section of atomic nuclei with respect to atomic projectiles; equal to 10^{-24} cm^2. [fr. "big as the side of a barn" by humorous comparison with much smaller areas]

Barnard, Christiaan, South African surgeon, *1922, performed the first successful heart transplant in 1967.

Barnes, Robert, British obstetrician, 1817–1907. SEE B. *curve, zone*.

Barnes, Stanley, British physician, 1875–1955.

△**baro-.** Weight, pressure. [G. *baros*, weight]

bar·o·cep·tor (bar′ō-sep-ter, -tōr). SYN baroreceptor.

bar·og·no·sis (bar′og-nō′sis). Ability to appreciate the weight of objects, or to differentiate objects of different weights. [G. *baros*, weight, + *gnōsis*, knowledge]

bar·o·graph (bar′ō-graf). A device that gives a continuous record of barometric pressure. SYN barometrograph.

bar·o·met·ro·graph (bar-ō-met′rō-graf). SYN barograph.

Baron. SEE Barclay-Baron *disease*.

bar·o·phil·ic (bar′ō-fil′ik). Thriving under high environmental pressure; applied to microorganisms. [G. *baros*, weight, + *phileō*, to love]

▣**bar·o·re·cep·tor** (bar′ō-rē-sep′ter, -tōr). **1.** In general, any sensor of pressure changes. **2.** Sensory nerve ending in the wall of the auricles of the heart, vena cava, aortic arch, and carotid sinus, sensitive to stretching of the wall resulting from increased pressure from within, and functioning as the receptor of central reflex mechanisms that tend to reduce that pressure. SYN baroceptor, pressoreceptor. [G. *baros*, weight, + receptor]

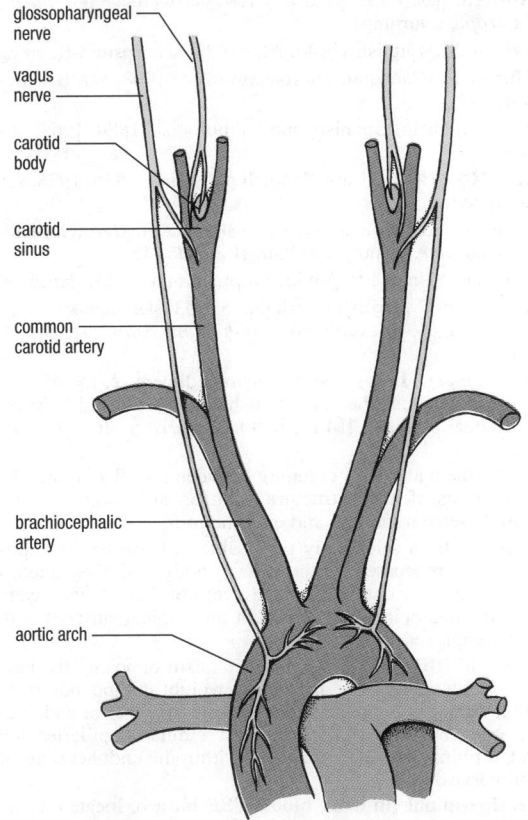

glossopharyngeal nerve

vagus nerve

carotid body

carotid sinus

common carotid artery

brachiocephalic artery

aortic arch

baroreceptors: seen in the area of the carotid sinuses and aortic arch

bar·o·re·flex (bar-ō-rē′fleks). A reflex triggered by stimulation of a baroreceptor.

bar·o·scope (bar′ō-skōp). An instrument measuring changes in atmospheric pressure.

bar·o·si·nus·i·tis (bar′ō-sī-nus-ī′tis). Inflammation of the mucous membrane of the paranasal sinuses caused by pressure difference within the sinus relative to ambient pressure, secondary to obstruction of the sinus ostium and occurring during descent in altitude. SYN aerosinusitis. [G. *baros,* weight, pressure, + sinusitis]

bar·o·stat (bar′ō-stat). A pressure-regulating device or structure, such as the baroreceptors of the carotid sinus and aortic arch, when connected to effectors providing negative feedback. [G., *baros,* weight, pressure, + *statos,* made to stand]

bar·o·tax·is (bar-ō-tak′sis). Reaction of living tissue to changes in pressure. SYN barotropism. [G. *baros,* weight, + *taxis,* order]

bar·o·ti·tis me·dia (bar-ō-tī′tis mē′dē-ă). Inflammation of the mucous membrane of the middle ear caused by pressure difference within the middle ear relative to ambient pressure, secondary to obstruction of the auditory tube or its failure to open; often occurs on descent in altitude. SYN aerotitis media.

bar·o·trau·ma (băr′ō-traw′mă). A term previously used to describe injury to the middle ear or paranasal sinuses, resulting from imbalance between ambient pressure and that within the affected cavity. Now mostly used to refer to lung injury due to pressure such as occurs when a patient is on a ventilator and is subjected to high airway pressure (pulmonary barotrauma). [G. *baros,* weight, + trauma]

otic b., injury caused to the ear by imbalance in pressure between ambient air and the air in the middle ear. SEE ALSO barotitis media.

sinus b., injury to paranasal sinuses, resulting from imbalance in pressure between ambient air and air in the paranasal sinuses. SEE ALSO barosinusitis.

bar·ot·ro·pism (bar-ot′rō-pizm). SYN barotaxis. [G. *baros,* weight, + *tropē,* a turning]

Barr, Yvonne M., English virologist, *1932. SEE Epstein-B. *virus.*

Barr, Murray L., Canadian microanatomist, *1908. SEE B. chromatin *body.*

Barraquer, Ignacio, Spanish ophthalmologist, 1884–1965. SEE B. *method.*

Barraquer Roviralta, Luis, Spanish physician, 1855–1928. SEE Barraquer *disease.*

Barré, Jean A., French neurologist, *1880. SEE B. *sign;* Guillain-B. *reflex, syndrome;* Landry-Guillain-B. *syndrome.*

bar·ren (bar′en). Unable to produce a pregnancy. [M.E. *bareyne*]

Barrett, Norman R., British physician, *1903. SEE *adenocarcinoma* in B. esophagus; B. *esophagus, epithelium, syndrome;* Barrett *metaplasia.*

bar·ri·er (bar′ē-er). **1.** An obstacle or impediment. **2.** In psychiatry, a conflictual agent that blocks behavior that could help resolve a personal struggle. [M.E., fr. O.Fr. *barriere,* fr. L.L. *barraria*]

blood-air b., the material intervening between alveolar air and the blood; it consists of a nonstructural film or surfactant, alveolar epithelium, basement lamina, and endothelium.

blood-aqueous b., a selectively permeable b. between the capillary bed in the processes of the ciliary body and the aqueous humor in the anterior chamber of the eye; consists of two layers of simple cuboidal epithelium joined at their apical surfaces with junctional complexes.

⊞ blood-brain b. (BBB), a selective mechanism opposing the passage of most ions and large–molecular weight compounds from the blood to brain tissue located in a continuous layer of endothelial cells connected by tight junctions; similar capillaries are found in the retina, iris, inner ear, and within the endoneurium of peripheral nerves.

blood-cerebrospinal fluid b., blood-CSF b., a b. located at the tight junctions which surround and connect the cuboidal epithelial cells on the surface of the choroid plexus; capillaries and connective tissue stroma of the choroid do not represent a b. to protein tracers or dyes.

blood-testis b., an occluding b. formed by Sertoli cells in the seminiferous tubules of the testis, which separates the more ma-

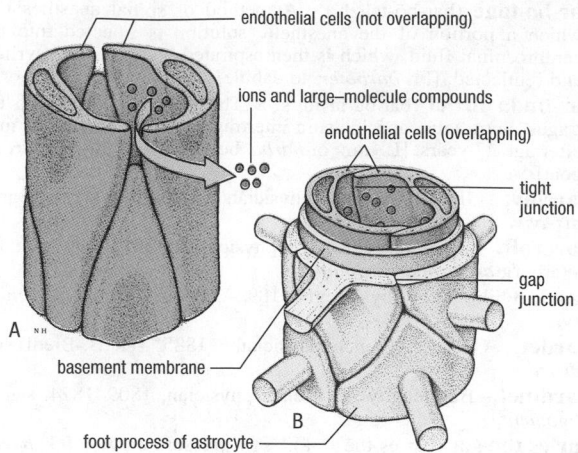

blood brain barrier: (A) in nonneural capillary, certain ions and molecules pass through gaps between endothelial cells; (B) in a neural capillary, the barrier created by "tight" junctions between endothelial cells, the basement membrane, and foot processes of astrocytes opposes the passage of these substances

ture cells of spermatogenesis in the adluminal compartment of the tubule from blood-derived products in the basal compartment.

blood-thymus b., a sheath of pericytes and epithelial reticular cells around thymic capillaries that prevents the developing T lymphocytes of the thymus from being exposed to circulating antigens.

incest b., in psychoanalysis, the learning or internalization of parental and social prohibitions against incest.

placental b., SYN placental *membrane.*

Bart, Bruce J., U.S. dermatologist, *1936. SEE B. *syndrome.*

Bartels, Peter H., German scientist in U.S., specializing in optics and computer science, *1929.

Barth, Jean B.P., Strasburg physician, 1806–1877. SEE B. *hernia.*

Bartholin, Casper, Danish anatomist, 1655–1738. SEE B. *abscess, cyst, cystectomy, duct, gland.*

Bartholin, Thomas, Danish anatomist, 1616–1680. SEE B. *anus.*

bar·tho·lin·i·tis (bar-tō-lin-ī′tis). Inflammation of a vulvovaginal (Bartholin) gland.

Bartley, Samuel H., U.S. psychologist, *1901. SEE Brücke-B. *phenomenon.*

Barton, John Rhea, U.S. surgeon, 1794–1871. SEE B. *bandage, forceps, fracture.*

Bar·ton·el·la (bar-tō-nel′ă). A genus of bacteria found in humans and in arthropod vectors; grows slowly in artificial media and may be recovered from blood cultures from infected patients; may be seen intracellularly in tissues and erythrocytes. *B.* is a minute, Gram-negative, coccobacillary organism, which may appear curved; it can cause an indolent, poorly defined, progressive disease in immunocompromised patients, including those with HIV infections. [A. L. *Barton*]

B. **bacillifor′mis,** a species found in the blood and epithelial cells of lymph nodes, spleen, and liver in Oroya fever (it is the cause of Oroya fever) and in blood and eruptive elements in verruga peruana; probably also found in sandflies (*Phlebotomus verrucarum*); known to be established only on the South American continent and perhaps in Central America; it is the type species of the genus *B.*

B. **henselae,** a bacterial species that causes catscratch *disease* in persons with normal immunity and bacillary angiomatosis in persons with AIDS. SEE ALSO catscratch *disease.*

B. **quintana,** formerly the type species of the genus *Rochalimaea,* this organism causes trench *fever* and in AIDS patients is associated with septicemia and endocarditis; arthropod vector is *Pediculus humanus,* the body louse.

Bar·ton·el·la·ceae (bar-ton-el-ā′sē-ē). A family of bacteria that currently includes the genus *Bartonella*. Based upon S16 rRNA studies, the former genera of *Rochalimaea* and *Grahamella* have been merged with the genus *Bartonella*, retaining their species names.

bar·ton·el·lo·sis (bar-tō-nel-ō′sis). A disease caused by infection with a species of bacteria belonging to the genus *Bartonella*,

Bart's. Nickname of St. Bartholomew's Hospital in London, where *hemoglobin* Bart was first isolated from a patient.

Bartter, Frederic C., U.S. physician, 1914–1983. SEE B. *syndrome*.

Baruch, Simon, U.S. physician, 1840–1921. SEE B. *law*.

bar·u·ria (bar-ū′rē-ă). Rarely used term for excretion of urine that has an unusually high specific gravity, e.g., greater than 1.025 to 1.030. [G. *barys*, heavy, + *ouron*, urine]

⌂**bary-.** Heavy. [G. *barys*]

bar·ye (ba′rē). The CGS unit of pressure, equal to 1 dyne/cm^2 or 10^{-6} bar. SEE bar (1). [G. *barys*, heavy]

ba·ry·ta (ba-rī′tă). SYN *barium* oxide. [G. *barytēs*, weight]

⌂**baryto-.** Prefix indicating the presence of barium in a mineral.

ba·sad (bā′sad). In a direction toward the base of any object or structure.

ba·sal (bā′săl) [TA]. **1.** Situated nearer the base of a pyramid-shaped organ in relation to a specific reference point; opposite of apical. SYN basalis [TA]. **2.** In dentistry, denoting the floor of a cavity in the grinding surface of a tooth. **3.** Denoting a standard or reference state of a function, as a basis for comparison. More specifically, denoting the exact conditions for measurement of basal metabolic *rate* (*q.v.*); b. conditions do not always denote a minimum value, e.g., metabolic rate in sleep is usually less than the b. rate, but is inconvenient for standard measurement.

ba·sa·lis (bā-sā′lis) [TA]. SYN basal (1). [L.]

ba·sa·loid (bā′să-loyd). Resembling that which is basal, but not necessarily basal in origin or position.

ba·sal ra·tion. Minimal diet containing only essential components.

base (bās) [TA]. **1.** The lower part or bottom; the part of a pyramidal or conical structure opposite the apex; the foundation. SYN basis [TA], basement (1). **2.** In pharmacy, the chief ingredient of a mixture. **3.** In chemistry, an electropositive element (cation) that unites with an anion to form a salt; a compound ionizing to yield hydroxyl ion. SYN alkali (2). SEE ALSO Brønsted b., Lewis b. **4.** Nitrogen-containing organic compounds (e.g., purines, pyrimidines, amines, alkaloids, ptomaines) that act as Brønsted b.'s. **5.** Cations, or substances forming cations. [L. and G. *basis*]

acrylic resin b., a form made of acrylic resin molded to conform to the tissues of the alveolar process and used to support the teeth of a prosthesis.

anterior cranial b., SYN anterior cranial *fossa*.

b. of arytenoid cartilage [TA], the part of the arytenoid cartilage that articulates with the cricoid cartilage and from which the muscular process extends laterally and the vocal process projects anteriorly. SYN basis cartilaginis arytenoideae [TA].

b. of bladder, SYN *fundus* of bladder.

b. of brain, the inferior surface of the brain, primarily the brainstem, when seen from below; commonly extended to include the inferior surface of the adjacent parts of the cerebral hemisphere. SYN basis cerebri, inferior cerebral surface.

Brønsted b., any molecule or ion that combines with a proton; e.g., OH⁻, CN⁻, NH₃; this definition replaces the older and more limited concepts of base (3).

cavity preparation b., SYN cement b.

cement b., in dentistry, a layer of dental cement, sometimes medicated, that is placed in the deep portion of a cavity preparation to protect the pulp, reduce the bulk of a metallic restoration, or eliminate undercuts. SYN cavity preparation b.

b. of cochlea [TA], the enlarged part of the cochlea that is directed posteriorly and medially and lies close to the internal acoustic meatus. SYN basis cochleae [TA].

cranial b. [TA], the sloping floor of the cranial cavity. It comprises both the external b. of skull (external view) and the internal b.

of skull (internal view). SYN basis cranii [TA], basicranium☆, b. of skull.

denture b., (1) that part of a denture which rests on the oral mucosa and to which teeth are attached; **(2)** that part of a complete or partial denture which rests upon the basal seat and to which teeth are attached. SYN saddle (2).

external b. of skull, SYN external *surface* of cranial base.

b. of heart [TA], that part of the heart that lies opposite the apex, formed mainly by the left atrium but to a small extent by the posterior part of the right atrium; it is directed backward and to the right and is separated from the vertebral column by the esophagus and aorta. SYN basis cordis [TA].

hexone b.'s, histone b.'s, the α-amino acids arginine, histidine, and lysine, which are basic by virtue of the presence in the side chains of a guanidine, imidazole, and amine group, respectively; the term "hexone" is a misnomer since histidine does not have six carbons.

b. of hyoid bone, SYN *body* of hyoid bone.

internal b. of skull, SYN internal *surface* of cranial base; SEE ALSO cranial b.

Lewis b., a b. that is an electron-pair donor.

b. of lung [TA], the lower concave part of the lung that rests upon the convexity of the diaphragm. SYN basis pulmonis [TA].

b. of mandible [TA], the rounded inferior border of the body of the mandible. SYN basis mandibulae [TA].

b. of metacarpal [TA], the expanded proximal extremity of each metacarpal that articulates with one or more of the distal row of carpal bones. SYN basis ossis metacarpalis [TA].

metal b., a metallic portion of a denture b. forming a part of the wall of the basal surface of the denture; it serves as a b. for the attachment of the plastic (resin) part of the denture and the teeth.

b. of metatarsal [TA], the expanded proximal extremity of each metatarsal bone; it articulates with one or more of the distal row of tarsal bones. SYN basis ossis metatarsalis [TA].

methamphetamine b., a form of methamphetamine that can be readily volatilized.

b. of modiolus of cochlea [TA], the part of the modiolus enclosed by the basal turn of the cochlea; it faces the lateral end of the internal acoustic meatus. SEE cochlear *area*. SYN basis modioli cochleae [TA].

nucleic acid b., a purine or pyrimidine; found in naturally occurring nucleic acids such as DNA.

ointment b., the vehicle into which active ingredients may be incorporated. Petrolatum (which may be stiffened with wax) is the most widely used greasy ointment b. and is suitable for the incorporation of oleaginous materials. Lanolin-containing b.'s will absorb water (and dissolved materials) and form water-in-oil type emulsions. Water soluble (washable) b.'s are often derived from polymers of ethylene glycol (PEGS); these will absorb water and ingredients dissolved in the water. Ointment b.'s are usually pharmacologically inert but may entrap water and serve to keep the skin from dying or to provide an emollient protective film.

b. of patella [TA], the superior border of the patella to which the tendon of the rectus femoris attaches. SYN basis patellae [TA].

b. of phalanx, the expanded proximal end of each phalanx in the hand or foot that articulates with the head of the next proximal bone in the digit. SYN basis phalangis.

b. of phalanx of foot [TA], proximal, concave, articulating end of the bones of the toes. SYN basis phalangis pedis [TA].

b. of phalanx of hand [TA], proximal, concave, articulating end of the bones of the fingers. SYN basis phalangis manus [TA].

pressor b., (1) one of several products of intestinal putrefaction believed to cause functional hypertension when absorbed; **(2)** any alkaline substance that raises blood pressure. SYN pressor amine, pressor substance.

b. of prostate [TA], the broad upper surface of the prostate contiguous with the bladder wall. SYN basis prostatae [TA].

purine b., a purine.

pyrimidine b., a pyrimidine.

record b., SYN baseplate.

b. of renal pyramid, the outer broad part of a renal pyramid that lies next to the cortex. SYN basis pyramidis renis.

b. of sacrum [TA], the upper end of the sacrum that articulates with the body of the fifth lumbar vertebra in the midline and the alae on either side. SYN basis ossis sacri [TA].

Schiff b., condensation products of aldehydes and ketones with primary amine; the compounds are stable if there is at least one aryl group on the nitrogen or carbon. Cf. ketimine. SYN aldimine.

shellac b., a resinous wafer adapted to maxillary or mandibular casts to form baseplates.

b. of skull, SYN cranial b; SEE ALSO internal *surface* of cranial base.

b. of stapes [TA], the flat portion of the stapes that fits in the oval window. SYN basis stapedis [TA], footplate (1), foot-plate★.

temporary b., SYN baseplate.

tinted denture b., a denture b. that simulates the coloring and shading of natural oral tissues.

b. of tongue, SYN *root* of tongue.

tooth-borne b., the denture b. restoring an edentulous area which has abutment teeth at each end for support; the tissue which it covers is not used for support.

trial b., SYN baseplate.

vegetable b., SYN alkaloid.

wobble b., the 3′ codon b. that is less strictly specified in the genetic code. SEE ALSO wobble, wobble *hypothesis*.

bas·e·doid (bahz′ĕ-doyd). Rarely used term denoting a condition resembling Graves disease (Basedow disease), but without toxic symptoms.

Basedow, Karl A. von, German physician, 1799–1854. SEE B. *disease, pseudoparaplegia;* Jod-B. *phenomenon;* B. *goiter.*

ba·se·dow·i·an (bahz-ĕ-dō′ē-an). Rarely used to denote terms described by or attributed to K. Basedow.

base·ment (bās′ment). **1.** SYN base (1). **2.** A cavity or space partly or completely separated from a larger space above it.

base·plate (bās′plāt). A temporary form representing the base of a denture; used for making maxillomandibular (jaw) relation records and for the arrangement of teeth. SYN record base, temporary base, trial base.

stabilized b., a b. lined with plastic material to improve its fit and stability.

base-stack·ing. An arrangement of DNA or RNA bases in which the bases lie on top of each other.

bas·fond (bah-fawn′). SYN *fundus* of bladder.

Basham mix·ture. SYN ferric and ammonium acetate *solution.*

⌂**basi-, basio-, baso-.** Base; basis. [G. and L. *basis*]

ba·si·a·lis (bā-sē-ā′lis). Relating to a basis or the basion.

ba·si·al·ve·o·lar (bā′sē-al-vē′ō-lăr). Relating to both basion and alveolar points; denoting especially the b. length, or the shortest distance between these two points.

ba·sic (bā′sik). Relating to a base.

ba·sic·i·ty (bā-sis′i-tē). **1.** The valence or combining power of an acid, or the number of replaceable atoms of hydrogen in its molecule. **2.** The characteristic(s) of being a chemical base.

ba·sic life sup·port. Emergency cardiopulmonary resuscitation, control of bleeding, treatment of shock, acidosis, and poisoning, stabilization of injuries and wounds, and basic first aid.

ba·si·cra·ni·al (bā′si-krā′nē-ăl). Relating to the base of the skull.

ba·si·cra·ni·um. ★official alternate term for cranial *base*.

Ba·sid·i·ob·o·lus (ba-sid′ē-ob′ō-lŭs). A genus of fungi belonging to the class Zygomycetes. *B. haptosporus* has been isolated from cases of zygomycosis (entomophthoramycosis basidiobolae) in humans, especially in Indonesia, tropical Africa, and Southeast Asia. [Mod. L. *basidium,* dim. of G. *basis,* base, + L. *bolus,* fr. G. *bolos,* lump or clod]

Ba·sid·i·o·my·ce·tes (ba-sid′ē-ō-mī-sēt′ez). One of the four major classes of fungi, characterized by a spore-bearing organ (basidium), usually a single clavate cell, which bears basidiospores after karyogamy and meiosis. The class comprises the smuts, rusts, mushrooms, and puffballs. Excluding mycotoxins, there is only one human pathogen, the basidiomycetous stage of *Cryptococcus neoformans.* [Mod. L. *basidium,* dim. of G. *basis,* base, + *mykēs* (*mykēt*), fungus]

Ba·sid·i·o·my·co·ta (bă-sid′ē-ō-mī-kō-tă). A phylum of fungi characterized by a spore-bearing organ, the basidium, that is usually a clavate cell that bears basidiospores after karyogamy and meiosis. Some mycologists have raised the class Basidiomycetes to the phylum or division level.

ba·sid·i·o·spore (ba-sid′ē-ō-spōr). A fungal spore borne on a basidium, characteristic of the class Basidiomycetes. [G. *basidon,* small base, + *sporos,* seed]

ba·sid·i·um, pl. **ba·sid·ia** (ba-sid′ē-ŭm, -ă). A cell or spore-bearing organ usually club-shaped that is characteristic of the Basidiomycota. It bears basidiospores externally after karyogamy and meiosis. It is composed of a swollen terminal cell situated on a slender stalk, and gives rise to slender filaments (sterigmata), usually four in number, from the ends of which the basidiospores are developed. [L., fr G. *basis,* base]

ba·si·fa·cial (bā′si-fā′shăl). Relating to the lower portion of the face.

ba·si·hy·al (bā′si-hī′ăl). SYN *body* of hyoid bone.

ba·si·hy·oid (bā-zē-hī′oyd). SYN *body* of hyoid bone.

bas·i·lar, bas·i·la·ris (bas′i-lăr, bas-i-lā′ris) [TA]. Relating to the base of a pyramidal or broad structure.

ba·si·lat·er·al (bā′si-lat′er-ăl). Relating to the base and one or more sides of any part.

ba·si·lem·ma (bā-si-lem′ă). SYN basement *membrane*. [basi- + G. *lemma,* rind]

ba·sil·i·cus (ba-sil′i-kŭs). Denoting a prominent or important part or structure. [L. fr. G. *basilikos,* royal]

ba·sin (bā′sin). A receptacle for fluids.

emesis b., kidney b., a shallow b. of curved, kidney-shaped design, used to collect body fluids or as a container for various other liquids.

pus b., a receptacle curved so as to fit closely the surface to which it is applied, used to receive the pus from a wound during drainage, cleansing, and/or redressing.

ba·si·na·sal (bā′si-nā′săl). Relating to the basion and the nasion; denoting especially the b. length, or the shortest distance between the two points.

⌂**basio-.** SEE basi-.

ba·si·oc·cip·i·tal (bā′sē-ok-sip′i-tăl). Relating to the basilar process of the occipital bone.

ba·si·oc·ci·put (bā-zē-ok′sē-put). SYN basilar *part* of occipital bone.

ba·si·o·glos·sus (bā-sē-ō-glos′ŭs). The portion of the hyoglossus muscle that originates from the body of the hyoid bone.

ba·si·on (bā′sē-on) [TA]. The middle point on the anterior margin of the foramen magnum, opposite the opisthion. [G. *basis,* a base]

ba·sip·e·tal (bă-sip′ĕ-tăl). **1.** In a direction toward the base. **2.** Pertaining to asexual conidial production in fungi, in which successive budding of the basal conidium forms in an unbranched chain with the youngest at the base. [basi- + L. *peto,* to seek]

bas·i·pho·bia (bas-i-fō′bē-ă). Morbid fear of walking. [G. *basis,* a stepping, + *phobos,* fear]

ba·sis (bā′sis) [TA]. SYN base (1). [L. and G.]

b. cartilag′inis arytenoi′deae [TA], SYN *base* of arytenoid cartilage.

b. cer′ebri, SYN *base* of brain.

b. coch′leae [TA], SYN *base* of cochlea.

b. cor′dis [TA], SYN *base* of heart.

b. cra′nii [TA], SYN cranial *base*.

b. cra′nii exter′na [TA], SYN external *surface* of cranial base.

b. cra′nii inter′na [TA], SYN internal *surface* of cranial base.

b. mandib′ulae [TA], SYN *base* of mandible.

b. modi′oli coch′leae [TA], SYN *base* of modiolus of cochlea.

b. os′sis metacarpa′lis [TA], SYN *base* of metacarpal.

b. os′sis metatarsa′lis [TA], SYN *base* of metatarsal.

b. os′sis sa′cri [TA], SYN *base* of sacrum.

b. patel′lae [TA], SYN *base* of patella.

b. pedun′culi [TA], the base of the midbrain consisting of the crus cerebri and substantia nigra. SEE ALSO cerebral *peduncle.*

b. phalan′gis, SYN *base* of phalanx.

b. phalangis manus [TA], SYN *base* of phalanx of hand.

b. phalangis pedis [TA], SYN *base* of phalanx of foot.

b. pontis, SEE basilar *part* of pons.

b. pro′statae [TA], SYN *base* of prostate.

b. pulmo′nis [TA], SYN *base* of lung.

b. pyram′idis re′nis, SYN *base* of renal pyramid.

b. stape′dis [TA], SYN *base* of stapes.

ba·si·sphe·noid (bā′si-sfē′noyd). Relating to the base or body of the sphenoid bone; denoting the independent center of ossification in the embryo that forms the posterior portion of the body of the sphenoid bone.

ba·si·tem·po·ral (bā′si-tem′pŏ-răl). Relating to the lower part of the temporal region.

ba·si·ver·te·bral (bā′si-ver′tĕ-brăl). Relating to the body of a vertebra.

bas·ket. **1.** A basketlike arborization of the axon of cells in the cerebellar cortex, surrounding the cell body of Purkinje cells. **2.** Any basketlike device or structure. [M.E., from Celtic]

fibrillar b.'s, the scleral end of neuroglia fibers of Müller that as fine, tapering, needlelike fibrillae ascend the proximal parts of rods and cones, giving them a fibrillar appearance.

Stokes b., a metal-mesh rescue stretcher.

stone b., an instrument passed through an endoscope to capture and extract urinary calculi.

Basle Nom·i·na An·a·tom·i·ca (BNA). The name adopted in 1895 in Basel, Switzerland (French spelling, Basle) by members of the German Anatomical Society that met to compile a Latin nomenclature of anatomic terms. Revisions of the resulting nomenclature were published at intervals until, in 1955 in Paris, France, the international membership of the Congress of Anatomists adopted a modification of the Basle Nomina Anatomica terminology. That modification dropped the reference to the original meeting place. SEE Nomina Anatomica, *Terminologia Anatomica.*

△**baso-.** SEE basi-.

ba·so·cyte (bā′sō-sīt). SYN basophilic *leukocyte.* [G. *basis,* base, + *kytos,* cell]

ba·so·cy·to·pe·nia (bā′sō-sī-tō-pē′nē-ă). SYN basophilic *leukopenia.*

ba·so·cy·to·sis (bā′sō-sī-to′sis). SYN basophilic *leukocytosis.*

ba·so·e·ryth·ro·cyte (bā′sō-e-rith′rō-sīt). A red blood cell that manifests changes of basophilic degeneration, such as basophilic stippling, punctate basophilia, or basophilic granules.

ba·so·e·ryth·ro·cy·to·sis (bā′sō-ĕ-rith′rō-sī-tō′sis). An increase of red blood cells with basophilic degenerative changes, frequently observed in diseases characterized by prolonged hypochromic anemia.

ba·so·lat·er·al (bā-sō-lat′er-ăl). Basal and lateral; specifically used to refer to one of the two major cytological divisions of the amygdaloid complex. SEE amygdaloid *body.*

ba·so·met·a·chro·mo·phil, ba·so·met·a·chro·mo·phile (bā′sō-met-ă-krō′mō-fil, -fīl). Staining metachromatically with a basic dye. SEE metachromasia.

ba·so·pe·nia (bā-sō-pē′nē-ă). SYN basophilic *leukopenia.* [baso- + G. *penia,* poverty]

■**ba·so·phil, ba·so·phile** (bā′sō-fil, -fīl). **1.** A cell with granules that stain specifically with basic dyes. **2.** SYN basophilic. **3.** A phagocytic leukocyte of the blood characterized by numerous basophilic granules containing heparin and histamine and leukotrines; except for its segmented nucleus, it is morphologically and physiologically similar to the mast cell though they originate from different stem cells in the bone marrow. [baso- + G. *phileō,* to love]

tissue b., SYN mast *cell.*

ba·so·phil·ia (bā-sō-fil′ē-ă). **1.** A condition in which there are more than the usual number of basophilic leukocytes in the circulating blood (basophilic leukocytosis) or an increase in the proportion of parenchymatous basophilic cells in an organ (in the bone marrow, basophilic hyperplasia). **2.** A condition in which

basophilic erythrocytes are found in circulating blood, as in certain instances of leukemia, advanced anemia, malaria, and plumbism. SYN Grawitz b. **3.** The reaction of immature erythrocytes to basic dyes whereby the cells appear blue or contain bluish granules. SYN basophilism.

Grawitz b., SYN basophilia (2).

punctate b., SYN stippling (1).

ba·so·phil·ic (bā′sō-fil′ik). Denoting tissue components having an affinity for basic dyes. SYN basophil (2), basophile.

ba·soph·i·lism (bā-sof′i-lizm). SYN basophilia.

Cushing b., SYN Cushing *syndrome.*

Cushing pituitary b., SYN Cushing *disease.*

ba·so·phil·o·cyte (bā-sō-fil′ō-sīt). SYN basophilic *leukocyte.*

ba·so·plasm (bā′sō-plazm). That part of the cytoplasm that stains readily with basic dyes.

Bassen, Frank A., U.S. physician, *1903. SEE B.-Kornzweig *syndrome.*

Bassini, Edoardo, Italian surgeon, 1844–1924. SEE B. *operation;* Bassini *herniorrhaphy.*

Bassler, Anthony, U.S. physician, 1874–1959. SEE B. *sign.*

bas·sor·in (bas′ōr-in). The insoluble portion (60 to 70%) of tragacanth that swells to form a gel; it contains complex methoxylated acids, particularly bassoric acid.

Bastedo, Walter A., U.S. physician, 1873–1952. SEE B. *sign.*

bastokinin. SYN uteroglobin.

bat. A member of the mammalian order Chiroptera. [M.E. *bakke*]

vampire b., a member of the genus *Desmodus;* an important reservoir host of rabies virus in Central and South America.

bath. **1.** Immersion of the body or any of its parts in water or any other yielding or fluid medium, or application of such medium in any form to the body or any of its parts. **2.** Apparatus used in giving a b. of any form, qualified according to the medium used, the temperature of the medium, the form in which the medium is applied, the medicament added to the medium, or according to the part bathed. **3.** Fluid used for maintenance of metabolic activities or growth of living organisms, e.g., cells derived from body tissue. [A.S. *baeth*]

colloid b., a b. prepared by adding soothing agents such as sodium bicarbonate or oatmeal to the b. water to relieve skin irritation and pruritus.

contrast b., a b. in which a part is immersed in hot water for a period of a few minutes and then in cold, the hot and cold periods alternated regularly at intervals, usually half-hours; used to increase the blood flow to the part.

douche b., the local application of water in the form of a large jet or stream.

dousing b., a luminous electric hot air b. given at a very high temperature.

electric b., electrotherapeutic b., (1) a b. in which the medium is charged with electricity; SYN hydroelectric b. **(2)** therapeutic application of static electricity, with the patient placed on an insulated platform.

Greville b., an obsolete treatment with nonluminous electric hot air given at a very high temperature.

hafussi b., a modification of the Nauheim treatment, with only the hands and feet of the patient being immersed in hot water through which carbon dioxide gas is made to pass. [Ger. *hand,* hand, + *fuss,* foot]

hydroelectric b., SYN electric b. (1).

immersion b., a therapeutic b. in which the whole person or a body part is totally immersed in the therapeutic substance.

light b., therapeutic exposure of the skin to radiant light.

Nauheim b., SYN Nauheim *treatment.*

needle b., a b. in which water is projected forcibly against the body in many very fine jets.

oil b., in chemistry, a vessel containing oil, in which a container holding a substance to be heated or evaporated can be immersed.

sand b., in chemistry, an arrangement whereby a substance to be treated is in a vessel protected from the direct action of fire by a layer of sand.

sitz b., immersion of only the perineum and buttocks, with the legs being outside the tub. [Ger. *sitzen,* to sit]

water b., in chemistry, a vessel containing water, in which a container holding a substance to be heated or evaporated can be immersed.

◊**batho-.** Depth. SEE ALSO bathy-. [G. *bathos,* depth]

bath·o·chro·mic (bath-ō-krō'mik). Denoting the shift of an absorption spectrum maximum to a longer wavelength. Opposite of hypsochromic. [batho- + G. *chrōma,* color]

bath·o·flore (bath'ō-flōr). An atom or group of atoms that, by its presence in a molecule, shifts the latter's fluorescent radiation in the direction of longer wavelength, or reduces the fluorescence. Cf. auxoflore.

bath·o·pho·bia (bath-ō-fō'bē-ă). Morbid fear of deep places or of looking into them. [G. *bathos,* depth, + *phobos,* fear]

◊**bathy-.** Depth. SEE ALSO batho-. [G. *bathys,* deep]

bath·y·an·es·the·sia (bath'ē-an-es-thē'zē-ă). Loss of deep sensibility, i.e., from muscles, ligaments, tendons, bones, and joints. [G. *bathys,* deep, + *an-* priv. + *aisthēsis,* sensation]

bath·y·car·dia (bath-ē-kar'dē-ă). A condition in which the heart occupies a lower position than normal but is fixed there, as distinguished from cardioptosia. [G. *bathys,* deep, + *kardia,* heart]

bath·y·es·the·sia (bath'ē-es-thē'zē-ă). General term for all sensation from the tissues beneath the skin, i.e., muscles, ligaments, tendons, bones and joints. SEE ALSO myesthesia. SYN deep sensibility. [G. *bathys,* deep, + *aisthēsis,* sensation]

bath·y·gas·try (bath-ē-gas'trē). SYN gastroptosis. [G. *bathys,* deep, + *gastēr,* stomach]

bath·y·hy·per·es·the·sia (bath-ē-hī'per-es-thē'zē-ă). Exaggerated sensitiveness of deep structures, e.g., muscular tissue. [G. *bathys,* deep, + *hyper,* above, + *aisthēsis,* sensation]

bath·y·hyp·es·the·sia (bath-ē-hip'es-thē'zē-ă). Impairment of sensation in the structures beneath the skin, e.g., muscle tissue. [G. *bathys,* deep, + *hypo,* under, + *aisthēsis,* sensation]

Batista, Randas, 20th century Brazilian cardiac surgeon. SEE B. *procedure.*

ba·trach·o·tox·in (ba-tra-kō-tok'sin). A neurotoxin from the Colombian arrow poison frogs (*Phyllobates* spp.). It is nontoxic when ingested. If it is injected or if there are ulcers present, it will cause an irreversible increase in permeability of sodium ions in nerve membrane, producing paralysis; used in experimental pharmacologic studies of neuromuscular transmission. [G. *batrachos,* frog, + *toxin*]

Batson, Oscar V., U.S. otolaryngologist, 1894–1979. SEE B. *plexus;* Carmody-B. *operation.*

Batten, Frederick E., British ophthalmologist, 1865–1918. SEE B.-Mayou *disease;* B. *disease.*

bat·tery (bat'er-ē). A group or series of tests administered for analytic or diagnostic purposes. [M.E. *batri,* beaten metal, fr. O.Fr. *batre,* to beat]

Halstead-Reitan b., a b. of neuropsychological tests (category test, tactual performance test, Seashore test, speech sounds perception test, finger oscillation test, trail-making test, dynamometer to measure strength of grip) used to study brain-behavior functions including determining the effects of brain damage on behavior. SYN Tactual Performance Test.

Battle, William H., English surgeon, 1855–1936. SEE B. *sign.*

Bauer, Walter, U.S. internist, *1898. SEE B. *syndrome.*

Bauer, Hans, 20th century German anatomist. SEE B. chromic acid leucofuchsin *stain.*

Bauhin, Gaspard, Swiss anatomist, 1560–1624. SEE B. *gland, valve.*

Baumé, Antoine, French chemist and pharmacist, 1728–1804. SEE B. *scale.*

Baumès symp·tom. See under symptom.

Baumgarten, Paul Clemens von, German pathologist, 1848–1928. SEE B. *veins,* under *vein;* Cruveilhier-B. *disease, murmur, sign, syndrome.*

bay (bā). **1.** In anatomy, a recess containing fluid. **2.** Especially, the lacrimal b.

celomic b., **(1)** medial and lateral recesses at either side of the urogenital mesentery of the embryo; **(2)** superior recess of the vestibule of the lesser peritoneal space; with the formation of the diaphragm, a portion of the right recess is cut off and becomes the infracardiac bursa; the portion below the diaphragm becomes the superior recess of the lesser peritoneal sac; the left recess is lost. SYN pneumatoenteric.

lacrimal b., SYN lacrimal *lake.*

bay·ber·ry bark (bā'ber-ē). SYN myrica.

Bayes, Thomas, British mathematician, 1702–1761. SEE B. *theorem.*

Bayle, Antoine L.J., French physician, 1799-1858.

Bayley, Nancy, U.S. psychologist, *1899. SEE B. *Scales* of Infant Development, under *scale.*

bay·lis·as·car·i·a·sis (bā-lē-sas'kar-ī-a-sis). The disease caused by nematode parasites of the genus *Baylisascaris;* migrating larvae of the raccoon parasite *B. procyonis* can cause a severe disease of the central nervous system in a variety of wild and domestic animal species and, rarely, in humans; human disease has been manifested as either a fatal eosinophilic meningoencephalitis or a diffuse unilateral subacute neuroretinitis.

Bay·lis·as·ca·ris (Bāy-lis-as'kă-ris). A genus of ascarid nematodes found in the intestine of mammals.

B. procyonis, a large roundworm commonly found in raccoons; has been the cause of human visceral larva migrans and ocular larva migrans, following accidental ingestion of embryonated *B. procyonis* eggs in feces of infected raccoons. SEE ALSO visceral *larva migrans.*

bay·o·net (bā-ŏ-net'). An instrument having a blade or nib that is offset and parallel to the shaft. [Fr. *bayonette,* fr. *Bayonne,* France, where first made]

Bazett, Henry C., English cardiologist, *1885. SEE Bazett *formula.*

Bazex, A., 20th century French physician. SEE Bazex *syndrome.*

Bazin, Antoine P.E., French dermatologist, 1807–1878. SEE B. *disease.*

BBB Abbreviation for blood-brain *barrier.*

BBC Abbreviation for bromobenzylcyanide.

BBOT Abbreviation for 2,5-bis(5-*t*-butylbenzoxazol-2-yl)thiophene, a liquid scintillator.

BCG Abbreviation for bacille Calmette-Guérin; ballistocardiograph.

BCL-2. An oncogene that inhibits apoptosis.

BCNU SYN carmustine.

bdel·lin (del'in). One of a group of protease inhibitors from the leech. [G. *bdella,* leech, + -in]

Bdellovibrio.

B.D.S. Abbreviation for Bachelor of Dental Surgery.

B.D.Sc. Abbreviation for Bachelor of Dental Science.

Be Symbol for beryllium.

bead·ed (bēd'ed). **1.** Marked by numerous small rounded projections, often arranged in a row like a string of beads. **2.** Applied to a series of noncontinuous bacterial colonies along the line of inoculation in a stab culture. **3.** Denoting stained bacteria in which more deeply stained granules occur at regular intervals in the organism.

bead·ing (bē'ding). **1.** Numerous small rounded projections, often in a row like a string of beads. **2.** The rounded elevation along the border of the tissue surface of the major connectors of a maxillary dental prosthesis. **3.** Protection of the formed borders of final impressions for a dental prosthesis done by placement of wax sticks or a plaster-pumice combination adjacent to the borders prior to forming the master cast.

b. of the ribs, SYN rachitic *rosary.*

beak (bēk). **1.** The nose of pliers used in dentistry for contouring and adjusting wrought or cast metal dental appliances. **2.** Sometimes used to describe a beak-shaped anatomic structure. SEE rostrum. [L. *beccus*]

beak·er (bē'ker). A thin glass vessel, with a lip (beak) for pouring, used as containers for liquids.

Beale, Lionel S., British physician, 1828–1906. SEE B. *cell.*

beam (bēm). **1.** Any bar whose curvature changes under load; in dentistry, frequently used instead of "bar." **2.** A collimated emission of light or other radiation, such as an x-ray b. [O.H.G. *Boum*]

Balkan b., SYN Balkan *frame.*

cantilever b., in dentistry, a b. that is supported by only one fixed support at only one of its ends.

continuous b., in dentistry, a b. that continues over three or more supports, those supports not at the b. ends being equally free supports.

electron b., a form of radiation used principally in superficial radiotherapy. SEE betatron.

restrained b., in dentistry, a b. that has two or more supports, at least one of which permits some freedom of rotation to the point of support but not as much as if the support were a free support.

simple b., in dentistry, a straight b. that has only two supports, one at either end.

bean (bēn). The flattened seed, contained in a pod, of various leguminous plants. B.'s of pharmacological significance are alphabetized by specific name. [O.E. *bean*]

beard [TA]. SYN barba.

bear·ing (bār'ing). A supporting point or surface.

central b., in dentistry, application of forces between the maxillae and mandible at a single point located as near as possible to the center of the supporting areas of the upper and lower jaws; used for the purpose of distributing closing forces evenly throughout the areas of the supporting structures during the recording of maxillomandibular (jaw) relations and during the correction of occlusal errors.

bear·ing down. Expulsive effort of a parturient woman in the second stage of labor.

beat (bēt). **1.** To strike; to throb or pulsate. **2.** A stroke, impulse, or pulsation, as of the heart or pulse. **3.** Activity of a cardiac chamber produced by catching a stimulus generated elsewhere in the heart. **4.** The perception of a third tone when two tones of slightly different frequencies are presented. **5.** One of a series of regularly pulsating tones created by the periodic mutual reinforcement of two simultaneously sounding tones that differ slightly in frequency. [A.S. *beatan*]

apex b., the visible and/or palpable pulsation made by the apex of the left ventricle as it strikes the chest wall in systole; normally in the fifth intercostal space, about 10 cm to the left of the median line.

atrial capture b., the cardiac cycle resulting when, after a period of A-V dissociation, the atria regain control of the ventricles; atrial depolarization due to retrograde transmission from a ventricular ectopic beat or an electronically paced ventricular impulse.

atrial fusion b., a b. that occurs when the atria are activated in part by the sinus impulse and in part by an ectopic or retrograde impulse from A-V junction or ventricle.

automatic b., in contrast to forced b., an ectopic b. that arises *de novo* and is not precipitated by the preceding b.; thus escaped and parasystolic b.'s are automatic. SYN automatic contraction.

combination b., SYN fusion b.

coupled b.'s, beats (usually premature) that recur at a fixed interval from a preceding (usually normal) beat.

dependent b., SYN forced b.

Dressler b., fusion b. interrupting a ventricular tachycardia and producing a normally narrow QRS complex as a result of the fusion of two impulses, one impulse from the ventricular tachycardia and the other from a supraventricular focus; Dressler b.'s strongly support the diagnosis of ventricular tachycardia by interruption of it.

dropped b., a heart b. that fails to appear.

echo b., extrasystole produced by the return of an impulse in the heart retrograde to a focus near its origin which then returns antegradely to produce a second depolarization.

ectopic b., a cardiac b. originating elsewhere than at the sinoatrial node.

escape b., an automatic b., usually arising from the AV junction

or ventricle, occurring after the next expected normal b. has defaulted; it is therefore always a late b., terminating a longer cycle than the normal. SYN escape contraction.

forced b., (1) an extrasystole supposedly precipitated in some way by the preceding normal b. to which it is coupled; (2) an extrasystole caused by artificial stimulation of the heart. SYN dependent b.

fusion b., a b. triggered by more than a single electrical impulse, when the wave fronts coincide to act together on a single final pathway of activity; in the electrocardiogram, the atrial or ventricular complex when either atria or ventricles are activated jointly by two simultaneous or nearly simultaneous invading impulses. SYN combination b., mixed b., summation b.

heart b., a complete cardiac cycle, including spread of the electrical impulse and the consequent mechanical contraction. SYN ictus cordis.

interference b., ventricular capture in forms of AV dissociation due to interference.

mixed b., SYN fusion b.

paired b.'s, SEE bigeminy.

parasystolic b., SYN parasystole.

premature b., SYN extrasystole.

pseudofusion b., an electrocardiographic representation of a cardiac depolarization produced by superimposition of an ineffectual electronic pacemaker spike upon a QRS-complex originating from a spontaneous focus within the heart; the pacemaker spike is ineffectual because the electronic discharge, which it represents graphically, occurred within the absolute refractory period of the spontaneous beat and is therefore not indicative of pacemaker malfunction.

reciprocal b., SEE reciprocal *rhythm.*

retrograde b., a b. occurring as an electrical activation of a portion of a heart chamber cephalad to the chamber of origin, e.g., an atrial b. triggered by an impulse originating in the ventricle.

summation b., SYN fusion b.

ventricular fusion b., a fusion b. that occurs when the ventricles are activated partly by the descending sinus or AV junctional impulse and partly by an ectopic ventricular impulse.

Beau, Joseph H.S., French physician, 1806–1865. SEE B. *lines,* under *line.*

Beau·var·ia (bō-vā'rē-ă). A genus of fungi (class Hyphomycetes). *B. bassiana* is pathogenic for insects, holds promise in the biologic control of insects, and has produced infection in humans.

be·can·thone hy·dro·chlo·ride (be-can'thōn). A schistosomicide.

Bechterew, Vladimir M. von, Russian neurologist, 1857–1927. SEE B. *band, disease; layer* of B.; B. *nucleus, sign; line* of B.; *band* of Kaes-B.; B.-Mendel *reflex;* Mendel-B. *reflex.*

Beck, Claude S., U.S. surgeon, 1894–1971. SEE B. *triad.*

Beck, E.V.V., Russian physician. SEE Bek.

Beck, Emil G., U.S. surgeon, 1866–1932. SEE B. *method.*

Becker, Samuel W., U.S. dermatologist, 1894–1964. SEE B. *nevus.*

Becker, Peter Emil, German geneticist, *1908. SEE B.-type tardive muscular *dystrophy;* B. muscular *dystrophy.*

Becker, J.P. SEE B. *disease.*

Becker stain for spi·ro·chetes. See under stain.

Beckmann, Ernst O., German chemist, 1853–1923. SEE B. *apparatus.*

Beckwith, John Bruce, U.S. pathologist, *1933. SEE B.-Wiedemann *syndrome.*

Béclard, Pierre A., French anatomist, 1785–1825. SEE ranine *anastomosis;* B. *hernia, triangle.*

be·clo·meth·a·sone di·pro·pi·o·nate (be-klō-meth'ă-sōn). A topical anti-inflammatory agent; often used by inhalation in asthma.

Becquerel, Antoine H., French physicist and Nobel laureate, 1852–1908. SEE becquerel; B. *rays,* under *ray.*

bec·que·rel (Bq) (bek-ă-rel'). The SI unit of measurement of radioactivity, equal to 1 disintegration per second; 1 Bq = 0.027 × 10^{-9} Ci. [AH *Becquerel*]

bed. 1. In anatomy, a base or structure that supports another structure. **2.** A piece of furniture used for rest, recuperation, or treatment.

b. of breast, structures against which the posterior surface of the breast lies; includes mainly the pectoralis major muscle, but also some serratus anterior and external abdominal oblique muscle; extends from second to sixth rib, and from parasternal to anterior axillary lines.

capillary b., the capillaries considered collectively and their volume capacity for blood.

fracture b., a narrow, extra-firm b. for treatment of fractures; usually incorporates an overhead frame for traction apparatus.

Gatch b., a b. with divided sections for independent elevation of a patient's head and knees.

mud b., a b. in which the mattress consists of semiliquid mud made from special clays, covered with a sheet of plastic material; used to widely distribute the pressure of the body weight over the dependent surface, for patients with burns or large anesthetic areas.

nail b., SYN nail *matrix*.

parotid b., the structures which surround and contact the parotid, forming the boundaries of the parotid space: anteriorly, the ramus of the mandible flanked by the masseter and medial pterygoid muscles; medially, the pharyngeal wall, carotid sheath and structures originating from the styloid process; posteriorly, the mastoid process, sternocleidomastoid muscle, and posterior belly of the digastric muscle; superiorly, the temporomandibular joint and the tympanic bone and cartilaginous portion of the external acoustic meatus.

b. of parotid gland, SYN parotid *space*.

b. of stomach, the structures against which the posteroinferior surface of the stomach lies, and from which it is separated, for the main part, by the omental bursa; includes diaphragm, left suprarenal gland, upper part of left kidney, splenic artery, anterior aspect of pancreatic body and tail, left colic flexure, and transverse mesocolon.

water b., a mattress in the form of a closed rubber bag filled with water; used to prevent or treat pressure sores by equalizing the distribution of the patient's weight against the support.

bed·bug. See entries under *Cimex.*

bed·lam (bed'lăm). **1.** Pejorative colloquialism for a mental hospital or institution. **2.** A place or scene of wild or riotous behavior. **3.** A disturbing uproar. [corruption or contraction of St. Mary of *Bethlehem* Hospital in London]

Bednar, Alois, Austrian physician, 1816–1888. SEE B. *aphthae,* under *aphtha.*

Bednar, Blahoslav, 20th century Czech pathologist. SEE B. *tumor.*

bed·sore (bed'sōr). SYN decubitus *ulcer.*

bed-wet·ting. SYN nocturnal *enuresis.*

bee. An insect of the genus *Apis;* the honeybee, *A. mellifica,* is the source of honey and wax. [A.S. *beó, bĭ*]

beech oil. SYN beechwood tar.

beech·wood tar (bēch'wud). A thick, oily, dark brown liquid with the odor of creosote; largely used as a source of creosote. SYN beech oil.

Beer, August, German physicist, 1825–1863. SEE B.-Lambert *law;* B. *law.*

Beer, Georg J., Austrian ophthalmologist, 1763–1821. SEE B. *knife.*

bees·wax (bēz'waks). SYN wax (1).

white b., SYN white *wax.*

bee·tu·ria (bē-too'rē-ă). Urinary excretion of betacyanin after ingestion of beets, found in most iron-deficient individuals and in some normal persons. SYN betacyaninuria.

Beevor, Charles E., English neurologist, 1854–1908. SEE B. *sign.*

Begbie, James, Scottish physician, 1798–1869.

Begg, P. Raymond, Australian orthodontist, *1898. SEE B. light wire differential force *technique.*

Béguez César, Antonio, Cuban pediatrician. SEE B.C. *disease.*

be·hav·ior (bē-hāv'yer). **1.** Any response emitted by or elicited from an organism. **2.** Any mental or motor act or activity. **3.** Specifically, parts of a total response pattern. [M.E., fr. O. Fr. *avoir,* to have]

adaptive b., any b. that enables an organism to adjust to a particular situation or environment.

appetitive b., movement of an organism toward a certain type of stimulus, such as food. Cf. aversive b.

aversive b., movement of an organism away from a certain type of stimulus, such as electric shock. Cf. appetitive b.

coronary-prone b., hostile b. that increases the risk of heart disease.

health b., combination of knowledge, practices, and attitudes that together contribute to motivate the actions we take regarding health.

hookean b., the b. of a perfectly elastic body; i.e., the strain is directly proportional to the stress. SEE ALSO Hooke *law.*

hostile b., b. that increases the risk of heart disease.

molar b., in psychology, b. described in large response units rather than smaller ones. Cf. molecular b.

molecular b., in psychology, b. described in small response units rather than larger ones; a specific response. Cf. molar b.

obsessive b., the repetitive stylized b. seen in obsessive-compulsive neurosis.

operant b., b. whose continuation and frequency is determined by its consequences on the doer; central element of behavioral conditioning theory. SEE conditioning.

passive-aggressive b., apparently compliant b., with intrinsic obstructive or stubborn qualities, to cover deeply felt aggressive feelings that cannot be more directly expressed.

respondent b., b. in response to a specific stimulus; usually associated with classical conditioning. SEE conditioning.

ritualistic b., automatic b. of psychogenic or cultural origin.

target b., (1) SYN operant; **(2)** in b. modification therapy, the prescribed b.

type A b., a b. pattern characterized by aggressiveness, ambitiousness, restlessness, and a strong sense of time urgency. New research has revealed that it is hostility, which can be commingled with other type A traits, that is associated with increased risk for coronary heart disease.

type B b., a b. pattern characterized by the absence or obverse of type A b. characteristics.

be·hav·ior·al (bē-hāv'yer-ăl). Pertaining to behavior.

be·hav·ior·al sci·enc·es. A collective term for those disciplines or branches of science, such as psychology, sociology, and anthropology, and which derive their theories, concepts, and approaches from the observation and study of the behavior of living organisms.

be·hav·ior·ism (bē-hāv'yer-izm). A branch of psychology that formulates, through systematic observation and experimentation, the laws and principles that underlie the behavior of humans and animals; its major contributions have been made in the areas of conditioning and learning. SYN behavioral psychology.

be·hav·ior·ist (bē-hāv'yer-ist). An adherent of behaviorism.

Behçet, Hulusi, Turkish dermatologist, 1889–1948. SEE B. *disease, syndrome.*

be·hen·ic ac·id (bĕ-hen'ik). $CH_3(CH_2)_{20}COOH$; a constituent of most fats and fish oils; large amounts are found in jamba, mustard seed, rapeseed oils, and cerebrosides. SYN *n*-docosanoic acid.

Behr, Carl J.P., German ophthalmologist, 1874–1943. SEE B. *disease, syndrome.*

Behring, Emil A. von, German bacteriologist and Nobel laureate, 1854–1917. SEE B. *law.*

BEI Abbreviation for butanol-extractable *iodine.*

bej·el. Nonvenereal endemic syphilis now found chiefly among Arab children; apparently due to *Treponema pallidum.* SEE ALSO nonvenereal *syphilis.* [Ar. *bajlah*]

Bek (or Beck), E.V., Russian physician. SEE Kashin-B. *disease.*

Békésy, Georg von, Hungarian biophysicist in U.S. and Nobel laureate, 1899–1972. SEE B. *audiometer, audiometry.*

bel. Unit expressing the relative intensity of a sound. The intensity in bels is the logarithm (to the base 10) of the ratio of the power of the sound to that of a reference sound. Ordinarily, the reference sound is assumed to be one with a power of 10^{-16} watts per sq cm, approximately the threshold of a normal human ear at 1000 Hz. [A.G. *Bell,* Scottish-U.S. scientist, 1847–1922]

belch·ing. SYN eructation. [A.S. *baelcian*]

bel·em·noid (be-lem′noyd). Dart-shaped. [G. *belemnon,* a dart, + *eidos,* resemblance]

Bell, John, Scottish surgeon and anatomist, 1763–1820. SEE B. *muscle.*

Bell, Sir Charles, Scottish surgeon, anatomist, and physiologist, 1774–1842. SEE B. *law;* B.-Magendie *law;* B. respiratory *nerve, palsy, spasm;* external respiratory *nerve* of B.

bel·la·don·na (bel-ă-don′ă). *Atropa belladonna* (family Solanaceae); a perennial herb with dark purple flowers and shining purplish-black berries; the leaves (0.3% b. alkaloids) and root (0.5% b. alkaloids) orginally were source of atropine and related alkaloids, which are anticholinergic. B. is used as a powder (0.3% b. alkaloids, calculated as hyoscyamine) and tincture in diarrhea, asthma, colic, and hyperacidity. SYN deadly nightshade. [It. *bella,* beautiful, + *donna,* lady]

bel·la·don·nine (bel-ă-don′ēn). An artificial alkaloid derived from atropine by warming with hydrochloric acid.

bell-crowned (bel′krownd). Denoting a tooth the crown of which has a cross-sectional diameter much greater than that of the neck.

belle in·dif·fér·ence. SEE la belle indifférence.

Bellini, Lorenzo, Italian physician and anatomist, 1643–1704. SEE B. *ducts,* under *duct, ligament.*

bel·ly (bel′ē). **1.** The abdomen. **2.** The wide swelling part of a muscle. SYN venter (2) [TA]. **3.** Popularly, the stomach or womb. [O.E. *belig,* bag]

anterior b. of digastric muscle [TA], the portion of the digastric muscle that extends anteriorly from the intermediate tendon, and attaches to the posterior aspect of the mandible. SYN venter anterior musculi digastrici [TA].

b.'s of digastric muscle, SEE anterior b. of digastric muscle, posterior b. of digastric muscle.

frontal b. of occipitofrontalis muscle [TA], the anterior b. of the occipitofrontalis muscle. SEE occipitofrontalis (*muscle*). SYN venter frontalis musculi occipitofrontalis [TA], frontalis muscle.

inferior b. of omohyoid b. [TA], the inferior b. of the omohyoid muscle, attached to the superior border of the scapula. SYN venter inferior musculi omohyoidei [TA].

occipital b. of occipitofrontalis muscle [TA], the posterior b. of the occipitofrontalis muscle. SEE occipitofrontalis (*muscle*). SYN venter occipitalis musculi occipitofrontalis [TA], occipitalis muscle.

b.'s of omohyoid muscle, SEE inferior b. of omohyoid b., superior b. of omohyoid muscle.

posterior b. of digastric muscle [TA], portion of digastric muscle posterior to the intermediate tendon, attaching to the digastric groove of the temporal bone. SYN venter posterior musculi digastrici [TA].

prune b., SYN abdominal muscle deficiency *syndrome.*

superior b. of omohyoid muscle [TA], the superior b. of the omohyoid muscle, attached to the hyoid bone. SYN venter superior musculi omohyoidei [TA].

bel·ly·ache (bel′ē-āk). Colloquialism for abdominal pain, usually colicky.

bel·ly but·ton (bel′ē bŭt′ŏn). SYN umbilicus.

bel·o·ne·pho·bia (bel′ō-nē-fō′bē-ă). Morbid fear of needles, pins, and other sharp-pointed objects. [G. *belonē,* needle, + *phobos,* fear]

Belsey, Ronald, 20th century British surgeon. SEE Belsey *fundoplication;* B. Mark *operation, procedure;* Collis-Belsey *fundoplication;* Collis-B. *procedure.*

bem·e·gride (bem′ě-grīd). A central nervous system stimulant

formerly used as an analeptic in intoxications due to barbiturates and other central nervous system depressant drugs.

ben Abbreviation for L. *bene,* well.

ben·ac·ty·zine hy·dro·chlo·ride (ben-ak′ti-zēn). An anticholinergic drug with the same actions but with approximately only one-fifth the activity of atropine; it is thought to raise the threshold of emotional reaction to external stimuli; now rarely used as a psychotherapeutic and tranquilizing agent.

Bence Jones, Henry, British physician, 1814–1873. SEE B. J. *albumin, cylinders,* under *cylinder, myeloma, proteins,* under *protein, reaction.*

ben·da·zac (ben′dă-zak). A topical anti-inflammatory agent.

Bender, Lauretta, U.S. psychiatrist, 1897–1987. SEE B. gestalt *test,* Visual Motor Gestalt *test.*

ben·dro·flu·a·zide (ben-drō-floo′ă-zīd). SYN bendroflumethiazide.

ben·dro·flu·me·thi·a·zide (ben′drō-floo′mě-thī′ă-zīd). A thiazide diuretic and antihypertensive agent. SYN bendrofluazide.

bends (bendz). Colloquialism for caisson *sickness;* decompression *sickness.* [fr. convulsive posture of those so afflicted]

ben·e·cep·tor (ben′ē-sep′ter, tōr). A nerve organ or mechanism (ceptor) for the appreciation and transmission of stimuli of a beneficial character. Cf. nociceptor. [L. *bene,* well, + *capio,* to take]

Benedek, Ladislaus (László), Austrian neurologist, 1887–1945. SEE B. *reflex.*

Benedict, Francis G., U.S. metabolist, 1870–1957. SEE B.-Roth *apparatus, calorimeter.*

Benedict, Stanley R., U.S. chemist, 1884–1936. SEE B. *solution, test* for glucose; B.-Hopkins-Cole *reagent.*

Benedikt, Moritz, Austrian physician, 1835–1920. SEE B. *syndrome.*

ben·e·fi·cence (be-nef′ĭ-sens). The ethical principle of doing good. [L. *beneficentia,* fr. *bene,* well, + *facio,* to do]

be·nign (bē-nīn′). Denoting the mild character of an illness or the nonmalignant character of a neoplasm. [through O.Fr., fr. L. *benignus,* kind]

ben·ne oil (ben′ně). SYN *sesame* oil.

Bennett, Edward H., Irish surgeon, 1837–1907. SEE B. *fracture.*

Bennett, Norman G., British dentist, 1870–1947. SEE B. *angle, movement.*

Bennhold, H., German physician, *1893. SEE B. Congo red *stain.*

ben·ox·a·pro·fen (ben-oks-ă-prō′fen). A nonsteroidal anti-inflammatory and analgesic agent, no longer clinically used.

ben·per·i·dol (ben-per′i-dol). A tranquilizer. SYN benzperidol.

ben·ser·a·zide (ben-ser′ă-zīd). An *l*-aromatic amino acid decarboxylase (dopa decarboxylase) inhibitor resembling carbidopa in action; given in combination with levodopa as an antiparkinsonian regimen. The benserazide prevents peripheral destruction of levodopa and thus reduces cardiovascular side effects of treatment.

Bensley, Robert R., U.S.-Canadian anatomist, 1867–1956. SEE B. specific *granules,* under *granule.*

ben·tir·o·mide (ben-tir′ō-mīd). A peptide used in a screening test for exocrine pancreatic insufficiency and to monitor the adequacy of supplemental pancreatic therapy.

ben·ton·ite (ben′ton-īt). Native colloidal hydrated aluminum silicate; an absorbent clay found in the western U.S.; it is sometimes used in the treatment of diarrhea and skin disorders and was used as a suspending agent in lotions. [Fort *Benton,* Montana, + -ite]

benz-. Combining form denoting association with benzene.

ben·zal·ac·e·to·phe·none (ben′zal-as-e-tō-fē′nōn). SYN chalcone.

ben·zal·cou·mar·an-3-one (ben-zal-koo′mar-an-thrē′ōn). SYN aurone.

benz·al·de·hyde (ben-zal′dě-hīd). An aldehyde produced artificially or obtained from oil of bitter almond, containing not less than 80% of b.; a flavoring agent used in orally administered medicines. SYN benzoic aldehyde.

ben·zal·ko·ni·um chlo·ride (ben-zal-kō'nē-ŭm). A mixture of alkylbenzyldimethylammonium chlorides in which the alkyls are long-chain compounds (C_8 to C_{18}); a surface-active germicide for many pathogenic nonsporulating bacteria and fungi. Aqueous solutions of this agent have a low surface tension, and possess detergent, keratolytic, and emulsifying properties that aid the penetration and wetting of tissue surfaces.

benz[a]an·thra·cene (ben-zan'thră-sēn). 1,2-Benzanthracene; a carcinogenic hydrocarbon. SYN benzanthrene.

ben·zan·threne (ben-zan'thrēn). SYN benz[a]anthracene.

ben·zene (ben'zēn). The basic structure in most aromatic compounds; a highly toxic hydrocarbon from light coal tar oil; used as a solvent. SYN benzol, coal tar naphtha. [benzoin, + -ene]
  b. bromide, a lacrimator or tear gas.

ben·zene·a·mine (ben-zēn'ă-mēn). SYN aniline.

(γ)-ben·zene hex·a·chlo·ride. SEE lindane.

ben·zes·trol (ben-zes'trol). A synthetic estrogenic substance.

benz·e·tho·ni·um chlo·ride (benz-ĕ-thō'nē-ŭm). A synthetic quaternary ammonium compound, one of the cationic class of detergents; germicidal and bacteriostatic.

ben·zi·dine (ben'zi-dēn). A colorless, crystalline compound used to detect sulfates in water analysis, for the identification of blood, and as a reagent in special stains; because it has been identified as a carcinogen, its current use is limited.

benz·im·id·az·ole (benz-im-id-ā'z-ōl). 1. A ring system comprised of a benzene ring fused with an imidazole ring; occurs in nature as part of the vitamin B_{12} molecule. 2. A class of antihelmintic, often used to treat nematodes and cestodes.

ben·zin, ben·zine (ben'zin, ben-zēn). SYN *petroleum* benzin.

ben·zin·da·mine hy·dro·chlo·ride (ben-zin'dă-mēn). SYN benzydamine hydrochloride.

ben·zi·o·da·rone (ben-zē'ō-dă-rōn). A coronary vasodilator.

ben·zo·ate (ben'zō-āt). A salt or ester of benzoic acid. The salts are often used as pharmaceutical or food preservatives.

ben·zo·at·ed (ben'zō-āt-ed). Containing benzoic acid or a benzoate, usually sodium benzoate.

ben·zo·caine (ben'zō-kān). The ethyl ester of *p*-aminobenzoic acid; a topical anesthetic agent. SYN ethyl aminobenzoate.

ben·zo·di·az·e·pine (ben'zō-dī-az'ē-pēn). 1. Parent compound for the synthesis of a number of psychoactive compounds (e.g., diazepam, chlordiazepoxide). 2. A class of compounds with antianxiety, hypnotic, anticonvulsant, and skeletal muscle relaxant properties.

ben·zo·ic (ben-zō'ik). Relating to or derived from benzoin.

ben·zo·ic ac·id. Occurs naturally in gum benzoin; it is used as a food preservative, locally as a fungistatic, and orally as an antiseptic. It is excreted rapidly as hippuric acid. SYN benzoyl hydrate, flowers of benzoin.

ben·zo·ic al·de·hyde. SYN benzaldehyde.

ben·zo·in (ben'zō-in, ben'zoyn). A balsamic resin obtained from *Styrax benzoin* (family Styracaceae), used as a stimulant expectorant, but usually by inhalation in laryngitis and bronchitis; it retards rancidification of fats and is used for this purpose in the official benzoinated lard. SYN gum benjamin, gum benzoin. [It. *benzoino*, fr. Ar. *lubān jāwīy*, Javan incense]

ben·zol (ben'zol). SYN benzene.

ben·zo·mor·phan (ben-zō-mōr'fan). The parent compound of a series of analgesics including pentazocine and phenazocine; it does not possess analgesic properties itself.

ben·zo·na·tate (ben-zō'nă-tāt). An antitussive agent related chemically to tetracaine; thought to act by depressing mechanoreceptors in the lungs.

ben·zo·pur·pu·rin 4B (ben-zō-per'pū-rin) [C.I. 23500]. A red acid dye, formerly used as a stain and as an indicator (changes from violet to red in the pH range 1.2 to 4.0).

1,4-ben·zo·qui·none (ben-zō-kwin'ōn). 1. An essential part of coenzyme Q and vitamin E, reducible to hydroquinone. SYN quinone (2). 2. One of a class of benzoquinone derivatives.

ben·zo·qui·no·ni·um chlo·ride (ben'zō-kwī-nō'nē-ŭm). A skeletal muscle relaxant.

ben·zo·res·in·ol (ben-zō-res'i-nol). A resinous constituent of benzoin.

ben·zo·sul·fi·mide (ben-zō-sŭl'fi-mīd). SYN saccharin.

ben·zo·thi·a·di·a·zides (ben'zō-thī-ă-dī'ă-zīdz). A class of diuretics that increase the excretion of sodium and chloride and an accompanying volume of water, independent of alterations in acid-base balance; most of the compounds in this group are analogues of 1,2,4-benzothiadiazine-1,1-dioxide. SEE ALSO benzthiazide.

ben·zox·i·quine (ben-zoks'i-kwin). A disinfectant. SYN benzoxyline.

ben·zox·y·line (ben-zoks'i-lēn). SYN benzoxiquine.

ben·zo·yl (ben'zō-il). The benzoic acid radical, $C_6H_5CO–$, forming benzoyl compounds.
  b. chloride, a colorless liquid of pungent odor; a reagent for acylation reactions.
  b. hydrate, SYN benzoic acid.
  b. peroxide, made by the interaction of sodium peroxide and b. chloride; used in oil as an application to ulcers and to burns and scalds, in promoting the polymerization of dental resins, and as a keratolytic in the treatment of acne.

ben·zoy·lec·gon·ine (ben'zō-il-ek'gō-nēn). A metabolite of cocaine produced by hydrolysis; it can be found in the urine. SYN ecgonine benzoate.

ben·zo·yl·pas cal·ci·um (ben-zō'il-pas). An antituberculous agent.

benz·per·i·dol (benz-per'i-dol). SYN benperidol.

benz·phet·a·mine hy·dro·chlo·ride (benz-fet'ă-mēn). A sympathomimetic agent used as an anorexiant.

benz·py·rene (benz-pī'rēn). An environmental carcinogen found in jet fuel exhaust, cigarette smoke, and charcoal broiled meats; a powerful enzyme inducer.

benz·pyr·in·i·um bro·mide (benz-pī-rin'ē-ŭm). A cholinergic drug with action and uses similar to those of neostigmine. SYN benzstigminum bromidum.

benz·quin·a·mide (benz-kwin'ă-mīd). A benzoquinoline amide used as an antiemetic agent.

benz·stig·mi·num bro·mi·dum (benz-stig'mi-nŭm). SYN benzpyrinium bromide.

benz·thi·a·zide (benz-thī'ă-zīd). A diuretic and antihypertensive agent.

benz·tro·pine mes·y·late (benz-trō'pēn). A parasympatholytic agent with atropinelike and antihistaminic actions.

ben·zyd·a·mine hy·dro·chlo·ride (ben-zid'ă-mēn). An analgesic and antipyretic. SYN benzindamine hydrochloride.

ben·zyl (ben'zil). The hydrocarbon radical, $C_6H_5CH_2–$.
  b. alcohol, $C_6H_5CH_2OH$; possesses local anesthetic and bacteriostatic properties. SYN phenmethylol, phenylcarbinol.
  b. benzoate, an agent that reduces the contractility of smooth muscular tissue, possessing marked antispasmodic properties; used now as a pediculicide and scabicide.
  b. benzoate-chlorophenothane-ethyl aminobenzoate, a mixture of three components used in emulsions or ointments.
  b. carbinol, SYN phenylethyl alcohol.
  b. cinnamate, a constituent of balsams of Peru, Tolu, and styrax. SYN cinnamein.
  b. fumarate, used for the same purposes as b. benzoate.
  b. mandelate, the b. ester of mandelic acid, having an antispasmodic action similar to that of b. benzoate.
  b. succinate, action and dosage are the same as those of b. benzoate.

ben·zyl·ic (ben-zil'ik). Relating to or containing benzyl.

ben·zyl·i·dene (ben-zil'i-dēn). The hydrocarbon radical, $C_6H_5CH=$.

ben·zyl·iso·quin·o·lines (ben'zil-ī-sō-kwin-ō-linz). A group of alkaloids found primarily in poppy plants (Papaveraceae). Curare alkaloids are bisbenzylisoquinolines.

ben·zyl·ox·y·car·bon·yl (Z, Cbz) (ben'zil-ok-sē-kar'bon-il).

Amino-protecting radical used (as the chloride) in peptide synthesis, yielding PhCH$_2$OCO–NHR. SYN carbobenzoxy-.

ben·zyl·pen·i·cil·lin (ben'zil-pen-i-sil'in). SYN *penicillin* G.

be·phen·i·um hy·drox·y·naph·tho·ate (be-fen'ē-ŭm hī-droks'ē-naf'thō-āt). A drug used against *Ancylostoma duodenale* and *Necator americanus* (hookworms of man); now largely replaced by mebendazole.

BER Abbreviation for basic electrical *rhythm*.

Beradinelli, Waldemar, Argentinian physician, 1903–1956. SEE B. *syndrome*.

Bérard, Auguste, French surgeon, 1802–1846. SEE B. *aneurysm*.

Béraud, Bruno J., French surgeon, 1825–1865. SEE B. *valve*.

ber·ber·ine (ber'ber-ēn). An alkaloid from *Hydrastis canadensis* (family Berberidaceae); has been used as an antimalarial, antipyretic, and carminative, and externally for indolent ulcers.

be·reave·ment (bĕ-rēv-ment). An acute state of intense psychological sadness and suffering experienced after the tragic loss of a loved one or some priceless possession. [M.E., *bireven*, to deprive, + -ment]

Berger, Hans, German neurologist, 1873–1941. SEE B. *rhythm*.

Berger, Jean, 20th century French nephrologist. SEE B. *disease*, focal *glomerulonephritis*.

Berger, Emil, Austrian ophthalmologist, 1855–1926. SEE B. *space*.

Berger cells. See under cell.

Bergman, Harry, U.S. urologist, 1912–1998. SEE B. *sign*.

Bergmann, Gottlieb H., German neurologist and anatomist, 1781–1861. SEE B. *cords*, under *cord*, *fibers*, under *fiber*.

Bergmeister, O., Austrian ophthalmologist, 1845–1918. SEE B. *papilla*.

Berg stain. See under stain.

ber·i·beri, beri beri (ber'ē-ber'ē). A specific nutritional deficiency syndrome occurring in endemic form in eastern and southern Asia, sporadically in other parts of the world without reference to climate, and sometimes in alcoholics, resulting mainly from a dietary deficiency of thiamine; the "dry" form is characterized by painful polyneuritis; sensory nerves are more likely to be affected than motor nerves, with symptoms beginning in the feet and working upward with the hands affected late in the course of the disease; the "wet" form is characterized by edema resulting from a high-output form of heart failure. SEE ALSO nutritional *polyneuropathy*. SYN endemic neuritis. [Singhalese, extreme weakness]

dry b., paraplegic b., affecting chiefly the peripheral nerves; its clinical pattern is predominantly that of a polyneuropathy without associated congestive failure.

infantile b., b. appearing in a breast-fed infants whose mother has b. due to thiamin deficiency. It is mainly the "wet" form of b., characterized by heart failure with marked peripheral edema (which is otherwise unusual in heart failure in infancy). An often fatal disease, acute in onset, which was formerly common in the Far Eastern countries where rice is consumed; reversible with thiamin.

ship b., a form of thiamine deficiency seen among sailors.

wet b., edematous b., in which congestive heart failure occurs in addition to polyneuropathy.

berke·li·um (Bk) (berk'lē-um). An artificial transuranium radioactive element; atomic no. 97, atomic wt. 247.07. [*Berkeley, CA,* city where first prepared]

Berlin, Rudolf, German ophthalmologist, 1833–1897. SEE B. *edema*.

Ber·lin blue [C.I. 77510]. Ferric ferrocyanide; a dye used for injection studies of blood vessels and lymphatics, and in staining of siderocytes. SYN Prussian blue.

Bernard, Jean, French physician, *1907. SEE B.-Soulier *disease,* *syndrome*.

Bernard, Claude, French physiologist, 1813–1878. SEE B. *canal, duct, puncture;* B.-Cannon *homeostasis;* B.-Horner *syndrome;* B.-Sergent *syndrome*.

Bernays, Augustus C., U.S. surgeon, 1854–1907. SEE B. *sponge*.

Bernhardt, Martin, German neurologist, 1844–1915. SEE B. *disease;* B.-Roth *syndrome*.

Bernhardt for·mu·la. See under formula.

Bernheim, P., early 20th century French physician. SEE Bernheim *syndrome*.

Bernoulli, Daniel, Swiss mathematician, 1700–1782. SEE B. *effect, law, principle, theorem*.

Bernoulli tri·al. A single random event for which there are two and only two possible outcomes that are mutually exclusive and have *a priori* fixed (and complementary) probabilities of resulting. The trial is the realization of this process. Conventionally one outcome is termed a success and is assigned the score 1, the other is a failure and has the score zero. Thus the outcome might be 0 (no heads, one tail) or 1 (1 head, no tails).

Bernstein, Lionel M., U.S. internist, *1923. SEE B. *test*.

Berry, Sir James, Canadian surgeon, 1860–1946. SEE B. *ligaments,* under *ligament*.

Berson, Solomon A., U.S. internist, 1918–1972.. SEE B. *test*.

Berthelot, Pierre Eugene Marcellin, French chemist, 1827–1907. SEE B. *reaction*.

Berthollet, Claude L., French chemist, 1748–1822. SEE B. *law*.

Bertiella studeri (ber-tē-el'ă stood-er'ē). Common tapeworm found in primates; incidental zoonotic infections in humans in the tropics have been reported.

ber·ti·el·lo·sis (ber'tē-ĕ-lō'sis). Infection of primates, including humans, with cestodes of the genus *Bertiella*.

Bertin, Exupère Joseph, French anatomist, 1712–1781. SEE B. *bones,* under *bone,* *columns,* under *column, ligament, ossicles,* under *ossicle*.

Bertrand, Ivan Georges, 20th century French neurologist. SEE Canavan-van Bogaert-Bertrand *disease*.

be·ryl·li·o·sis (be-ril-ē-ō'sis). Beryllium poisoning characterized by the occurrence of acute pneumonia or chronic interstitial granulomatous fibrosis, especially of the lungs, from inhalation of beryllium.

be·ryl·li·um (Be) (be-ril'ē-ŭm). A white metal element belonging to the alkaline earths; atomic no. 4., atomic wt. 9.012182. [G. *beryllos,* beryl]

Berzelius, J.J., Swedish chemist, 1779–1848.

Besnier, Ernest H., French dermatologist, 1831–1909. SEE B. *prurigo;* B.-Boeck-Schaumann *syndrome*.

Bes·noi·ti·i·dae (bes-noy'tē-i-dē). A family of protozoan parasites, similar to those of the family Toxoplasmatidae, to which the genus *Besnoitia* belong.

Best, Franz, German pathologist, 1878–1920. SEE B. *disease,* carmine *stain*.

bes·ti·al·i·ty (bes-tē-al'i-tē). SYN zoophilia. [L. *bestia,* beast]

be·syl·ate (bes'il-āt). USAN-approved contraction for benzenesulfonate.

be·ta (β) (bā'tă). Second letter of the Greek alphabet, β (see entry at start of letter "B's." [G.]

be·ta-block·er (bā'tă-blok'er). SYN β-adrenergic blocking *agent*.

be·ta·cism (bā'tă-sizm). A defect in speech in which the sound of *b* is given to other consonants. [G. *bēta,* the second letter of the alphabet]

be·ta·cy·a·nin (bā'tă-sī-ă-nin). One of several red plant pigments; a betalain. An example is betanin. Elevated in urine of individuals with beeturia. [L. *beta,* beet, + G. *kyanos,* dark blue substance, + -in]

be·ta·cy·a·ni·nu·ria (bā-tă-sī'ă-ni-noo'rē-ă). SYN beeturia. [beta-cyanin + G. *ouron,* urine]

Be·ta·her·pes·vir·i·nae (bā'ta-her'pez-vir'ĭ-nē). A subfamily of Herpesviridae containing Cytomegalovirus and Roseolovirus.

be·ta·his·tine hy·dro·chlo·ride (bā-tă-his'tēn). An inhibitor of diamine oxidase used as a histaminelike agent for treatment of Ménière disease.

be·ta·ine (bē'tă-ēn). **1.** An oxidation product of choline and a transmethylating intermediate in metabolism. **2.** A class of compounds related to b. (1) (i.e., $R_3N^=-CHR'-COO^-$), e.g., glycine betaine. SYN glycine betaine.

b. aldehyde, an intermediate in the interconversion of betaine and choline.

b. hydrochloride, an acidifying agent used in the treatment of achlorhydria and hypochlorhydria.

be·ta·ine-al·de·hyde de·hy·dro·gen·ase. An oxidizing enzyme that catalyzes the oxidation of betaine aldehyde with NAD^+ and water to betaine and NADH; part of the choline oxidase system and of choline metabolism.

bet·a·lains (bā'tă-lāns). A group of plant pigments found almost exclusively in the family Centrospermae, e.g., betanin. There are two groups: betacyanines (in plants with a red-violet color) and betaxanthins (in plants with a yellow color).

be·ta·meth·a·sone (bā-tă-meth'ă-sōn). A semisynthetic glucocorticoid with anti-inflammatory effects and toxicity similar to those of cortisol; not useful in the treatment of adrenal insufficiency because it causes little sodium retention. For systemic and topical therapy, its actions are similar to those of prednisone, but more potent. Also available as b. sodium phosphate, b. acetate, and b. valerate.

be·tan·i·dine sul·fate (be-tan'i-dēn). SYN bethanidine sulfate.

be·tan·in (bā'tă-nin). The red pigment in beets (*Beta vulgaris*); elevated in urine of individuals with beeturia. [fr. *betacyanin*]

be·ta sheets. A structure of proteins where the peptide is extended and stabilized by hydrogen bonding between NH and CO groups of different polypeptide chain backbones or separate regions of the same chain.

be·ta·tron (bā'tă-tron). A circular electron accelerator that is a source of either high energy electrons or x-rays.

be·tax·o·lol hy·dro·chlo·ride (be-taks'ō-lol). A β-adrenergic blocking agent used primarily in the treatment of ocular hypertension and chronic open-angle glaucoma.

be·ta·zole hy·dro·chlo·ride (bā'tă-zōl). An analogue of histamine that stimulates gastric secretion by an action on H_2 receptors with less tendency to produce the side effects seen with histamine; used, in place of histamine, to measure the gastric secretory response.

be·tel (bē'tl). The dried leaves of *Piper betle* (family Piperaceae), a climbing East Indian plant; used as a stimulant and narcotic. [Pg. *betel, betle,* fr. Malayalam or Tamil *vetila*]

be·tel nut. Areca nut, the nut of the areca palm, *Areca catechu* (family Palmae), of the East Indies, chewed by the natives; contains arecoline; produces central nervous system stimulation; stains teeth and gums red.

be·tha·ne·chol chlo·ride (be-than'ě-kol). A parasympathomimetic agent, used to relieve constipation, paralytic ileus, and urinary retention.

be·than·i·dine sul·fate (be-than'i-dēn). An adrenergic blocking agent used for palliative treatment of hypertension. SYN betanidine sulfate.

Bethesda-Ballerup Group. A group of citrate-utilizing, slow lactose-fermenting bacteria (family Enterobacteriaceae) which share a similar series of antigens with the lactose-fermenting citrobacters; these organisms are now included in the genus *Citrobacter* without a distinction between prompt and slow lactose fermentation.

Betke-Kleihauer test. See under test.

Bettendorff, Anton J., German chemist, 1839–1902. SEE B. *test.*

bet·u·la (bet'ū-lă). European white birch, bark and leaves of *Betula alba* (family Betulaceae); native to Europe, northern Asia, and North America, north of Pennsylvania. It contains betulin (betula camphor), betuloresinic acid, volatile oil, saponins, betulol (sesquiterpine alcohol), apigenin, dimethyl ether, betuloside, gaultherin, methyl salicylate, and ascorbic acid; has odor of wintergreen and is used as a pharmaceutic aid (flavor/aromatic).

Betz, Vladimir A., Russian anatomist, 1834–1894. SEE B. *cells,* under *cell.*

Beuren, Alois J., 20th century German cardiologist. SEE Beuren *syndrome.*

Bevan-Lewis, William, English physician and physiologist, 1847–1929. SEE Bevan-Lewis *cells,* under *cell.*

bev·el (bev'ěl). **1.** A surface having a sloped or slanting edge. **2.** The incline that one surface or line makes with another when not at right angles. **3.** The edge of a cutting instrument. **4.** To create a slanting edge on a body structure.

cavosurface b., the incline of the cavosurface angle of a prepared cavity wall in relation to the plane of the enamel wall.

reverse b., the sloping edge of a cutting instrument.

be·vo·ni·um meth·yl sul·fate (be-vō'nē-ŭm). An anticholinergic agent. SYN pyribenzyl methyl sulfate.

be·zoar (bē'zōr). A concretion formed in the alimentary canal of animals, and occasionally humans; formerly considered to be a useful medicine with magical properties and apparently still used for this purpose in some countries; according to the substance forming the ball, may be termed trichobezoar (hairball), trichophytobezoar (hair and vegetable fiber mixed), or phytobezoar (foodball). [Pers. *padzahr,* antidote]

Bezold, Albert von, German physiologist, 1836–1868. SEE B. *ganglion;* B.-Jarisch *reflex.*

Bezold, Friedrich, German otologist, 1842–1908. SEE B. *abscess.*

BGP Abbreviation for bone Gla *protein.*

BHA Abbreviation for butylated hydroxyanisole.

bhang (bang). Name given in the East to powdered preparation of *Cannabis sativa* that is chewed or smoked by the local residents. SEE ALSO cannabis. [Hind.]

BHN Abbreviation for Brinell hardness *number.*

BHT Abbreviation for butylated hydroxytoluene.

Bi Symbol for bismuth.

bi-. **1.** Prefix meaning twice or double, referring to double structures or dual actions. **2.** In chemistry, used to denote a partially neutralized acid (an acid salt); e.g., bisulfate. Cf. bis-, di-. [L.]

Bial, Manfred, German physician, 1869–1908. SEE B. *test.*

Bianchi, Giovanni B., Italian anatomist, 1681–1761. SEE B. *nodule.*

bi·ar·tic·u·lar (bī'ar-tik'ū-lăr). SYN diarthric.

bi·as (bī'-as). **1.** Systematic discrepancy between a measurement and the true value; may be constant or proportionate and may adversely affect test results. **2.** Any trend in the collection, analysis, interpretation, publication, or review of data that can lead to conclusions that differ systematically from the truth; deviation of results or inferences from the truth, or processes leading to deviation. [Fr. *biais,* obliquity, perh. fr. L. *bifax,* two-faced]

There is no imputation of prejudice, partisanship, or other subjective or emotional factor such as an investigator's desire to achieve a particular outcome. More than 100 varieties of bias have been described but all fall into one of a rather small number of distinct categories: 1. Systematic one-sided variation of measurements from the true value (SYN systematic error, instrumental error, or bias). 2. Variation of statistical summary measures (means, rates, measures of association, etc.) from their true values as a result of systematic variation of measurements, other flaws in data collection, or flaws in study design or analysis. 3. Deviation of inferences from the truth as a result of flaws in study design, data collection, or the analysis or interpretation of results. 4. A tendency of procedures in study design, data collection, analysis, interpretation, review or publication, to yield results or conclusions that depart from the truth. 5. Prejudice leading to the conscious or subconscious selection of study procedures that depart from the truth in a particular direction, or to one-sidedness in interpretation of results. This form of bias can arise as a result of shoddy scientific methods, or deliberately when investigators behave fraudulently in order to misrepresent the truth.

ascertainment b., systematic failure to represent equally all classes of cases or persons supposed to be represented in a sample.

cross-level b., a b. due to aggregation at the population level of causes and/or effects that are unlike at the individual level; can occur in ecologic studies.

recall b., systematic error due to differences in accuracy or completeness of recall to memory of past events or experiences.

reporting b., selective revealing or suppression of information about past medical history, e.g., details of exposure to sexually transmitted diseases.

response b., systematic error due to differences in characteristics between those who choose or volunteer to take part in a study, and those who do not.

sampling b., systematic error due to study of a nonrandom sample of a population.

bi·as·te·ri·on·ic (bī-as-ter-ē-on′ik). Relating to both asterions, especially the b. diameter, or b. width, the shortest distance from one asterion to the other.

bi·au·ric·u·lar (bī-aw-rik′ū-lăr). Relating to both auricles, in any sense.

bib. Abbreviation for L. *bibe,* drink.

bib·li·o·ma·nia (bib′lē-ō-mā′nē-ă). Morbidly intense desire to collect and possess books, especially rare books. [G. *biblion,* book, + *mania,* frenzy]

bib·u·lous (bib′ū-lŭs). SYN absorbent (1). [L. *bibulus,* drinking freely, absorbent]

bi·cam·er·al (bī-kam′er-ăl). Having two chambers; denoting especially an abscess divided by a more or less complete septum. [bi- + L. *camera,* chamber]

bi·cap·su·lar (bī-kap′soo-lăr). Having a double capsule.

bi·car·bon·ate (bī-kar′bon-āt). HCO_3^-; the ion remaining after the first dissociation of carbonic acid; a central buffering agent in blood.

standard b., the plasma b. concentration of a sample of whole blood that has been equilibrated at 37°C with a carbon dioxide pressure of 40 mm Hg and an oxygen pressure greater than 100 mm Hg; abnormally high or low values indicate metabolic alkalosis or acidosis, respectively.

bi·car·di·o·gram (bī-kar′dē-ō-gram). The composite curve of an electrocardiogram representing the combined effects of the right and left ventricles.

bi·cel·lu·lar (bī-sel′ū-lăr). Having two cells or subdivisions.

bi·ceph·a·lus (bī-sef′ă-lŭs). SYN dicephalus.

bi·ceps (bī′seps). A muscle with two origins or heads. Commonly used to refer to the biceps brachii (*muscle*). [bi- + L. *caput,* head]

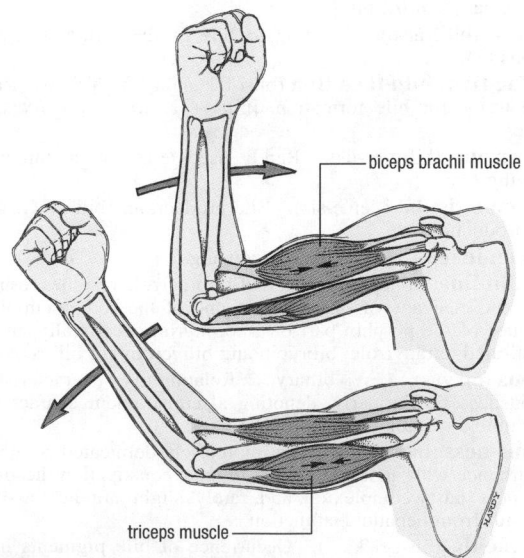

biceps brachii muscle

triceps muscle

biceps and triceps muscles: during flexion (above) and extension (below)

Bichat, Marie F.X., French anatomist, physician, and biologist, 1771–1802. SEE B. *canal, fat-pad, fissure, fossa, ligament, membrane, protuberance, tunic.*

bi·cho (bē′cho). SYN epidemic gangrenous *proctitis.*

bi·cil·i·ate (bī-sil′ē-āt). Having two cilia.

bi·cip·i·tal (bī-sip′i-tăl). **1.** Two-headed. **2.** Relating to a biceps muscle. [bi- + L. *caput,* head]

Bickel, Gustav, 19th century German physician. SEE B. *ring.*

bi·clo·nal (bī-klō′năl). Pertaining to or characterized by biclonality.

bi·clon·al·i·ty (bī-klōn-al′i-tē). A condition in which some cells have markers of one cell line and other cells have markers of another cell line, as in biclonal leukemias.

bi·con·cave (bī-kon′kāv). Concave on two sides; denoting especially a form of lens. SYN concavoconcave.

bi·con·vex (bī-kon′veks). Convex on two sides; denoting especially a form of lens. SYN convexoconvex.

bi·cor·nous, bi·cor·nu·ate, bi·cor·nate (bī-kōr′nŭs, -noo-āt, -nāt). Two-horned; having two processes or projections. [bi- + L. *cornu,* horn]

♻**bicro-.** SYN pico- (2).

bi·cron (bī′kron). SYN picometer.

bi·cu·cul·line (bī′coo-cu-lēn). An alkaloid naturally occurring in the *d*-form; found in *Dicentra cucullaria* and *Adlumia fungosa* (family Fumariaceae) and several *Corydalis* species; a powerful convulsant that acts by antagonizing γ-aminobutyric acid, an inhibitory neurotransmitter.

bi·cus·pid (bī-kŭs′pid). **1.** Having two points, prongs, or cusps. **2.** Teeth having two cusps. Humans have eight bicuspid or premolar teeth: two in front of each group of molars. SEE bicuspid *tooth.* [bi- + L. *cuspis,* point]

b. aortic valve, SEE familial aortic ectasia *syndrome.*

bi·cus·pi·di·za·tion (bī-kŭs′pi-di-zā′shŭn). Surgical change of a normally tricuspid valve into a functioning bicuspid valve; performed in correction of tricuspid valvar disease.

b.i.d. Abbreviation for L. *bis in die,* twice a day.

bi·dac·ty·ly (bī-dak′ti-lē). Abnormality in which the medial digits are lacking, with only the first and fifth represented. SEE ALSO lobster-claw *deformity,* ectrodactyly. [bi- + G. *daktylos,* finger]

bi·det (bē-dā′). A tub for a sitz bath, having also an attachment for giving vaginal or rectal infusions. [Fr. a small horse]

bi·dis·coi·dal (bī′dis-koy′dăl). Resembling, or consisting of, two disks.

BIDS [MIM*234050] Acronym for *b*rittle hair, *i*mpaired intelligence, *d*ecreased fertility, and *s*hort stature; the brittle hair may be due to an inherited deficiency of a high-sulfur protein; autosomal recessive inheritance.

bid·u·ous (bid′ū-ŭs). Rarely used term denoting of two days′ duration. [L. *biduus,* lasting two days, fr. *bi-* + *dies,* day]

Biebl, M. SEE B. *loop.*

Biebrich scar·let red [C.I. 26905]. SYN scarlet red. [*Biebrich,* Germany]

Biederman, Joseph, U.S. physician, *1907. SEE B. *sign.*

Biedl, Artur, Austrian physician, 1869–1933. SEE Bardet-B. *syndrome.*

Bielschowsky, Max, German neuropathologist, 1869–1940. SEE B. *disease, stain;* Jansky-B. *disease.*

Bielschowsky, Alfred, German ophthalmologist, 1871–1940. SEE B. *sign.*

Biemond, Avic, French neurologist, *1902. SEE B. *syndrome.*

Bier, August K.G., German surgeon, 1861–1949. SEE B. *amputation, hyperemia, method.*

Biermer, Anton, German physician, 1827–1892. SEE B. *anemia, disease;* Addison-B. *disease.*

Biesiadecki, Alfred von, Polish physician, 1839–1888. SEE B. *fossa.*

bi·fas·cic·u·lar (bī′fă-sik′ū-lăr). Involving two of the presumed three major fascicles of the ventricular conduction system of the heart.

bi·fid (bī'fid). Split or cleft; separated into two parts. [L. *bifidus,* cleft in two parts]

Bi·fi·do·bac·te·ri·um (bī'fī-dō-bak-tēr'ē-ŭm). A genus of anaerobic bacteria (family Actinomycetaceae) containing Gram-positive rods of highly variable appearance; freshly isolated strains characteristically show true and false branching, with bifurcated V and Y forms, uniform or branched, and club or spatulate forms. They frequently stain irregularly; two or more granules may stain with methylene blue, while the remainder of the cell is unstained. They are not acid fast, are nonmotile, and do not produce spores; acetic and lactic acids are produced from glucose. Pathogenicity for humans is rare, although they have been found in the feces and alimentary tract of infants, older people, and animals. The type species is *B. bifidum.* [L. *bifidus,* cleft in two parts, + bacterium]

B. bi'fidum, type species of the genus *Bifidobacterium;* it is found in the feces and alimentary tract of breast- and bottle-fed infants and of older persons, rats, turkeys, and chickens; also found in the rumen of cattle; pathogenicity for humans and other animals is rare. Associated with a growth factor belonging to a group of *N*-containing polysaccharides with a high hexosamine content and known as bifidus factor.

B. dentium, a bacterial species recovered in association with dental caries and periodontal disease. It is also an opportunistic pathogen, recovered in mixed infections associated with abscess formation.

bi·fo·cal (bī-fō'kăl). Having two foci.

bi·fo·rate (bī-fō'rāt). Having two openings. [bi- + L. *foro,* pp. *-atus,* to bore, pierce]

bi·func·tion·al (bī-fŭnc'shŭn-ăl). Referring to a molecule containing two reactive functional groups; cross-linking reagents are bifunctional compounds.

bi·fur·cate, bi·fur·cat·ed (bī-fer'kāt, -kā-ted). Forked; two-pronged; having two branches. [bi- + L. *furca,* fork]

bi·fur·ca·tio (bī'fer-kā'shē-ō) [TA]. SYN bifurcation.

b. aor'tae [TA], SYN aortic *bifurcation.*

b. tra'cheae [TA], SYN tracheal *bifurcation.*

b. trun'ci pulmona'lis [TA], SYN *bifurcation* of pulmonary trunk.

bi·fur·ca·tion (bī-fer-kā'shŭn) [TA]. A forking; a division into two branches. SYN bifurcatio [TA].

b. of aorta, SYN aortic b.

aortic b. [TA], the division of the aorta into right and left common iliac arteries; it occurs at the level of the fourth and fifth lumbar vertebral body. SYN bifurcatio aortae [TA], b. of aorta.

b. of pulmonary trunk [TA], the division of the pulmonary trunk into right and left pulmonary arteries. SYN bifurcatio trunci pulmonalis [TA].

b. of trachea, SYN tracheal b.

tracheal b. [TA], the division of the trachea into the right and left main bronchi; it occurs at the level of the fifth or sixth thoracic vertebral body and is marked internally by the presence of a carina or keellike ridge between the diverging bronchi. SYN bifurcatio tracheae [TA], b. of trachea.

Bigelow, Henry J., U.S. surgeon, 1818–1890. SEE B. *ligament, septum.*

bi·gem·i·na (bī-jem'i-nă). SYN bigeminal *pulse.*

bi·gem·i·nal (bī-jem'i-năl). Paired; double; twin.

bi·gem·i·ni (bī-jem'i-nī). SYN bigeminy.

bi·gem·i·num (bī-jem'i-nŭm). One of the corpora bigemina. [L. ntr. of *bigeminus,* doubled]

bi·gem·i·ny (bī-jem'i-nē). Pairing; especially, the occurrence of heart beats in pairs. SYN bigemini. [bi- + L. *geminus,* twin]

atrial b., pairing of atrial beats, as when an atrial extrasystole is coupled to each sinus beat.

atrioventricular junctional b., paired beats, each pair consisting of an AV nodal extrasystole coupled to a beat of the dominant, usually sinus, rhythm. SYN nodal b.

escape-capture b., paired beats, each couplet consisting of an escape beat followed by a conducted sinus beat or an escape beat followed by a conducted ectopic beat (usually atrial with retrograde P wave).

nodal b., SYN atrioventricular junctional b.

reciprocal b., paired beats, each pair consisting of an AV nodal beat followed by a reciprocal beat.

ventricular b., paired ventricular beats, the common form consisting of ventricular extrasystoles coupled to sinus beats.

bi·ger·min·al (bī-jer'min-ăl). Relating to two germs or ova.

bi·git·a·lin (bī-jit'ă-lin). SYN gitoxin.

bi·gly·can (bī'glī-kan). A small interstitial proteoglycan that contains two glycosaminoglycan chains. SYN proteoglycan I.

Bignami, Amico, Italian physician, 1862–1929. SEE Marchiafava-B. *disease.*

bi·kun·in (bik'oo-nin). A plasma glycoprotein that is found in both the free state and covalently bound to the heavy chains of certain protease inhibitors. It may participate in cell growth, oocyte cumulus expansion and stabilization.

bi·labe (bī'lāb). A forceps for seizing and removing urethral or small vesical calculi. [bi- + L. *labium,* lip]

bi·lat·er·al (bī-lat'er-ăl). Relating to, or having, two sides. [bi- + L. *latus,* side]

bi·lat·er·al·ism (bī-lat'er-ăl-izm). A condition in which the two sides are symmetrical.

bile (bīl). The yellowish brown or green fluid secreted by the liver and discharged into the duodenum where it aids in the emulsification of fats, increases peristalsis, and retards putrefaction; contains sodium glycocholate and sodium taurocholate, cholesterol, biliverdin and bilirubin, mucus, fat, lecithin, and cells and cellular debris. SYN gall (1). [L. *bilis*]

A b., b. from the common duct.

B b., b. from the gallbladder.

C b., b. from the hepatic duct.

white b., designating the relatively clear, almost colorless, clear viscid fluid that occurs in the gallbladder, intestines, or both as a result of obstruction of the b. ducts in various sites; actually the secretion of the mucous membrane, without the usual color resulting from b. pigments. SYN leukobilin.

Bilharz, Theodor M., German tropical disease specialist, 1829–1862. SEE *Bilharzia;* bilharzial *appendicitis;* bilharzial *dysentery;* bilharzial *granuloma.*

Bil·har·zia (bil-har'zē-ă). An early name for *Schistosoma.* [T. *Bilharz*]

bil·har·zi·a·sis (bil-har-zī'ă-sis). SYN schistosomiasis.

bil·har·zi·o·ma (bil-har-zē-ō'mă). A tumor-like inflammatory and fibrous swelling of the intestinal serosa, mesentery, or skin, caused by schistosomiasis.

bil·har·zi·o·sis (bil-har-zē-ō'sis). SYN schistosomiasis.

♻**bili-.** Bile. [L. *bilis,* bile]

bil·i·ary (bil'ē-ār-ē). Relating to bile or the biliary tract. SYN bilious (1).

bil·i·fac·tion, bil·i·fi·ca·tion (bil-i-fak'shŭn, -fi-kā'shŭn). Rarely used terms for bile formation. [bili- + L. *facio,* pp. *factus,* to make]

bil·if·er·ous (bil-if'er-ŭs). Rarely used term for containing or carrying bile.

bil·i·gen·e·sis (bil-i-jen'ĕ-sis). Bile production. [bili- + G. *genesis,* production]

bil·i·gen·ic (bil-i-jen'ik). Bile-producing.

bi·lin, bi·line (bī'lin). The chain of four pyrrole residues resulting from the cleavage of one bond of one of the four methylidene residues of the porphin part of a porphyrin; specifically, the unsubstituted tetrapyrrole; bilirubin and biliverdin are bilins.

bil·ious (bil'yŭs). **1.** SYN biliary. **2.** Relating to or characteristic of biliousness. **3.** Formerly, denoting a temperament characterized by a quick, irritable temper. SYN choleric.

bil·ious·ness (bil'yŭs-nes). An imprecisely delineated congestive disturbance with anorexia, coated tongue, constipation, headache, dizziness, pasty complexion, and, rarely, slight jaundice; assumed to result from hepatic dysfunction.

bil·i·ra·chia (bil-i-rā'kē-ă). Occurrence of bile pigments in the spinal fluid. [bili- + G. *rhachis,* spine]

bil·i·ru·bin (bil-i-roo'bin). A yellow bile pigment found as sodium bilirubinate (soluble), or as an insoluble calcium salt in gallstones; formed from hemoglobin during normal and abnormal destruction of erythrocytes by the reticuloendothelial system; a bilin with substituents on the 2, 3, 7, 8, 12, 13, 17, and 18 carbon atoms and with oxygens on carbons 1 and 19. Excess b. is associated with jaundice. [bili- + L. *ruber,* red]

conjugated b., SYN direct reacting b.

delta b., the fraction of b. covalently bound to albumin; in conventional methods it is measured as part of conjugated b. Because of its covalent bond during the recovery phase of hepatocellular *jaundice* it may persist in the blood for a week or more after urine clears.

direct reacting b., the fraction of serum b. which has been conjugated with glucuronic acid in the liver cell to form b. diglucuronide; so called because it reacts directly with the Ehrlich diazo reagent; increased levels are found in hepatobiliary diseases, especially of the obstructive variety. SYN conjugated b.

indirect reacting b., the fraction of serum b. which has not been conjugated with glucuronic acid in the liver cell; so called because it reacts with the Ehrlich diazo reagent only when alcohol is added; increased levels are found in hepatic disease and hemolytic conditions. SYN unconjugated b.

b. UDPglucuronyltransferase (gloo-koo′ron-il-trans′fer-ās), an enzyme that catalyzes the reaction of UDPglucuronate and bilirubin forming UDP and bilirubin-glucuronoside; a deficiency of this enzyme is associated with Crigler-Najjar syndrome.

unconjugated b., SYN indirect reacting b.

bil·i·ru·bi·ne·mia (bil′i-roo-bin-ē′mē-ă). The presence of bilirubin in the blood, where it is normally present in relatively small amounts; the term is usually used in relation to increased concentrations observed in various pathologic conditions where there is excessive destruction of erythrocytes or interference with the mechanism of excretion in the bile. Determination of the quantity of bilirubin in the blood serum reveals two fractions, namely direct reacting (conjugated) and indirect reacting (nonconjugated) bilirubin; determination of conjugated and total bilirubin in serum is an important and frequently used clinical laboratory test. [bilirubin + G. *haima,* blood]

bil·i·ru·bin·glob·u·lin (bil-i-roo′bin-glob′ū-lin). A bilirubinglobulin complex; a transport form of bilirubin to the liver where bilirubin is converted to a diglucuronic acid derivative and passes into the bile.

bil·i·ru·bin-glu·cu·ron·o·side glu·cu·ron·o·syl·trans·fer·-ase. Bilirubin monoglucuronide transglucuronidase; a transferase that transfers a glucuronoside from one molecule of bilirubin glucuronoside to another, forming bilirubin bisglucuronoside and unconjugated bilirubin (a step in heme catabolism).

bil·i·ru·bin·oids (bil-i-roo′bin-oydz). Generic term denoting intermediates in the conversion of bilirubin to stercobilin by reductive enzymes in intestinal bacteria. Included are mesobilirubin, mesobilane, mesobilene-b, urobilinogen, urobilin, reduction products of mesobilane (stercobilinogen) and mesobilene (stercobilin), and mesobiliviolin; most are found in normal urine and feces. Products related to these intermediates and found in pathological conditions (e.g., jaundice, liver disease) are the structurally indefinite probilifuscins and propentdyopents found in gallstones.

bil·i·ru·bi·nu·ria (bil′i-roo-bi-noo′rē-ă). The presence of bilirubin in the urine. [bilirubin + G. *ouron,* urine]

bil·i·ther·a·py (bil-i-thār′ă-pē). Treatment with bile or bile salts.

bil·i·u·ria (bil-ē-ū′rē-ă). The presence of various bile salts, or bile, in the urine. SYN choleuria, choluria. [bili- + G. *ouron,* urine]

bil·i·ver·din, bil·i·ver·dine (bil-i-ver′din). A green bile pigment formed from the oxidation of heme; a bilin with a structure almost identical to that of bilirubin. SYN dehydrobilirubin, verdine.

Bill, Arthur H., U.S. obstetrician, 1877–1961. SEE B. *maneuver.*

Billings, J.J., 20th century Australian gynecologist. SEE B. *method.*

Billroth, Christian A.T., Austrian surgeon, 1829–1894. SEE B. *cords,* under *cord,* operation I, operation II, *venae* cavernosae, under *vena,* I *anastomosis,* II *anastomosis.*

bi·lo·bate, bi·lobed (bī-lō′bāt, bī′lōbd). Having two lobes.

bi·lo·bec·to·my (bī′lōb-ek′tō-mē). Surgical excision of two lobes

of the right lung, either right upper and middle or right lower and middle.

bi·lob·u·lar (bī-lob′ū-lăr). Having two lobules.

bi·loc·u·lar, bi·loc·u·late (bī-lok′ū-lăr, -ū-lāt). Having two compartments or spaces. [bi- + L. *loculus,* dim. of *locus,* a place]

bi·man·u·al (bī-man′ū-ăl). Relating to, or performed by, both hands. [bi- + L. *manus,* hand]

bi·mas·toid (bī-mas′toyd). Relating to both mastoid processes.

bi·max·il·lary (bī-mak′si-lār-e). Relating to both the right and left maxillae; sometimes used when describing something affecting both halves of the upper jaw.

bi·mod·al (bī-mō′dăl). Denoting a frequency curve characterized by two peaks.

bi·mo·lec·u·lar (bī-mō-lek′ū-lăr). Involving two molecules, as in a b. reaction.

bin·an·gle (bin-ang′-ŭl). **1.** The second angle given the shank of an angled instrument to bring its working end close to the axis of the handle in order to prevent it from turning about the axis. **2.** A dental instrument possessing the above characteristics. [L. *bini,* pair, + *angulus,* angle]

bi·na·ry (bī′nār-ē). **1.** Comprising two components, elements, molecules, etc. **2.** Denoting a choice of two mutually exclusive outcomes for one event (e.g., male or female, heads or tails, affected or unaffected). [L. *binarius,* consisting of two, fr. *bini,* two at a time]

bin·au·ral (bin-aw′răl). Relating to both ears. SYN binotic. [L. *bini,* a pair, + *auris,* ear]

bind (bīnd). **1.** To confine or encircle with a band or bandage. **2.** To join together with a band or ligature. **3.** To combine or unite molecules by means of reactive groups, either in the molecules per se or in a chemical added for that purpose; frequently used in relation to chemical bonds that may be fairly easily broken (i.e., noncovalent), as in the binding of a toxin with antitoxin, or a heavy metal with a chelating agent, etc. **4.** A close interpersonal relationship in which one person feels compelled to act in a certain way to obtain the approval of the other person. [A.S. *bindan*]

double b., a type of personal interaction in which one receives two mutually conflicting verbal or nonverbal instructions or demands from the same person or different individuals, resulting in a situation in which either compliance or noncompliance with either alternative threatens one of the needed relationships.

bind·er (bīnd′er). **1.** A broad bandage, especially one encircling the abdomen. **2.** Anything that binds. SEE bind (3).

obstetrical b., a supporting garment covering the abdomen from the ribs to the trochanters, tightly pinned at the back, affording support after childbirth or, rarely, during childbirth.

T-b., two strips of cloth at right angles; used for retaining a dressing, as on the perineum. SYN T-bandage.

Binet, Alfred, French psychologist, 1857–1911. SEE B. *age, scale, test;* B.-Simon *scale;* Stanford-B. intelligence *scale.*

Bing, Richard J., U.S. physician, *1909. SEE Taussig-B. *disease, syndrome.*

Bing, Paul Robert, German neurologist, 1878–1956. SEE B. *reflex.*

Bingham, Eugene C., U.S. chemist, 1878–1945. SEE B. *flow, model, plastic.*

bin·oc·u·lar (bin-ok′ū-lăr). Adapted to the use of both eyes; said of an optical instrument. [L. *bini,* paired, + *oculus,* eye]

bi·no·mi·al (bī-nō′mē-ăl). A set of two terms or names; in the probabilistic or statistical sense it corresponds to a Bernoulli trial. SEE ALSO binary *combination.* [bi- + G. *nomos,* name]

bin·ot·ic (bin-ot′ik). SYN binaural. [L. *bini,* a pair, + G. *ous (ōt-),* ear]

Binswanger, Otto Ludwig, German neurologist, 1852–1929. SEE B. *disease, encephalopathy.*

bi·nu·cle·ar, bi·nu·cle·ate (bī-noo′klē-ăr, -klē-āt). Having two nuclei.

bi·nu·cle·o·late (bī-noo′klē-ō-lāt). Having two nucleoli.

△**bio-.** Combining form denoting life. [G. *bios,* life]

bi·o·a·cous·tics (bī′ō-ă-koos′tiks). The science dealing with the effects of sound fields or mechanical vibrations on living organisms.

bi·o·ac·tive (bī′ō-ăk′tiv). Referring to a substance that can be acted upon by a living organism or by an extract from a living organism.

bi·o·as·say (bī-ō-as′ā). Determination of the potency or concentration of a compound by its effect upon animals, isolated tissues, or microorganisms, as compared with an analysis of its chemical or physical properties.

bi·o·as·tro·nau·tics (bī′ō-as-trō-naw′tiks). The study of the effects of space travel and space habitation on living organisms.

bi·o·a·vail·a·bil·i·ty (bī′ō-ă-vāl′ă-bil′i-tē). The physiological availability of a given amount of a drug, as distinct from its chemical potency; proportion of the administered dose which is absorbed into the bloodstream.

bi·o·bur·den (bī′ō-ber′den). Degree of microbial contamination or microbial load; the number of microorganisms contaminating an object.

bi·o·cat·a·lyst (bī′ō-kat-ă-list). A substance of biologic origin that can catalyze a reaction; e.g., an enzyme.

bi·o·ce·no·sis (bī-ō-se-nō′sis). An assemblage of species living in a particular biotope. SYN biotic community. [bio- + G. *koinos*, common]

bi·o·chem·i·cal (bī-ō-kem′i-kăl). Relating to biochemistry.

bi·o·chem·is·try (bī-ō-kem′is-trē). The chemistry of living organisms and of the chemical, molecular, and physical changes occurring therein. SYN biologic chemistry, physiologic chemistry.

bi·o·chem·or·phic (bī′ō-kem-ōr′fik). Denoting the relationship between biologic action and chemical structure, as in food and drugs.

bi·o·chrome (bī′ō-krōm). SYN natural *pigment*. [bio- + G. *chrōma*, color]

bi·o·cid·al (bī-ō-sī′dăl). Destructive of life; particularly pertaining to microorganisms. [bio- + L. *caedo*, to kill]

bi·o·cli·ma·tol·o·gy (bī′ō-klī-mă-tol′ō-jē). The science of the relationship of climatic factors to the distribution, numbers, and types of living organisms; an aspect of ecology.

biocompatibility (bī′ō-kom-pat-i-bil′i-tē). The relative ability of a material to interact favorably with a biological system. [bio- + compatibility]

bi·o·cy·ber·net·ics (bī′ō-sī-ber-net′iks). The science of communication and control within a living organism, particularly on a molecular basis.

bi·o·cy·tin (bī-ō-sī′tin). ε-*N*-Biotinyl-L-lysine; biotin condensed through its carboxyl group with the ε-amino group of a lysyl residue in the apoenzymes to which biotin is the coenzyme; the predominant linkage in which biotin is found. SYN biotinyllysine.

bi·o·cy·tin·ase (bī-ō-sī′tin-ās). An enzyme in blood that catalyzes the hydrolysis of biocytin to biotin and lysine (or, lysyl residue if the lysine is in a protein).

bi·o·de·grad·a·ble (bī′ō-dē-grād′ă-bl). Denoting a substance that can be chemically degraded or decomposed by natural effectors (e.g., weather, soil bacteria, plants, animals).

bi·o·de·gra·da·tion. SYN biotransformation.

bi·o·dy·nam·ic (bī′ō-dī-nam′ik). Relating to biodynamics.

bi·o·dy·nam·ics (bī′ō-dī-nam′iks). The science dealing with the force or energy of living matter. [bio- + G. *dynamis*, force]

bi·o·e·col·o·gy (bī-ō-ē-kol′ō-jē). SYN ecology.

bi·o·el·e·ment (bī′ō-el′ĕ-ment). An element required by a living organism.

bi·o·en·er·get·ics (bī′ō-en-er-jet′iks). **1.** The study of energy changes involved in the chemical reactions within living tissue. **2.** The study of energy exchanges between living organisms and their environments.

bi·o·en·gi·neer·ing (bī′ō-en-jin-ēr′ing). SEE biomedical *engineering*.

bi·o·feed·back (bī-ō-fēd′bak). A training technique that enables an individual to gain some element of voluntary control over autonomic body functions; based on the learning principle that a desired response is learned when received information such as a recorded increase in skin temperature (feedback) indicates that a specific thought complex or action has produced the desired physiological response.

EMG b., a form of b. that uses an electromyographic measure of muscle tension as the physical symptom to be deconditioned, such as tension in the frontalis muscle in the head which can cause headaches.

bi·o·fla·vo·noids (bī-ō-flāv′on-oydz). Naturally occurring flavone or coumarin derivatives commonly found in citrus fruits having the activity of the so-called vitamin P, notably rutin and esculin.

bi·o·gen·e·sis (bī-ō-jen′ĕ-sis). **1.** Term given by Huxley to the principle that life originates from preexisting life only and never from nonliving material. SEE spontaneous *generation*, recapitulation *theory*. **2.** SYN biosynthesis. [bio- + G. *genesis*, origin]

mitochondrial b., the process by which mitochondria increase their ability to make adenosine triphosphate by synthesizing additional respiratory enzyme complexes.

bi·o·ge·net·ic (bī′ō-jĕ-net′ik). Relating to biogenesis.

bi·o·gen·ic (bī′ō-jen-ik). Produced by a living organism.

bi·o·ge·o·chem·is·try (bī′ō-jē-ō-kem′is-trē). The study of the influence of living organisms and life processes on the chemical structure and history of the earth.

bi·o·grav·ics (bī′ō-grav′iks). That field of study dealing with the effect on living organisms (particularly humans) of abnormal gravitational effects produced, e.g., by acceleration or by free fall; in the former case, heavier than normal weight is induced, and in the latter weightlessness. [bio- + L. *gravis*, weight]

bioinformatics. A scientific discipline encompassing all aspects of biologic information acquisition, processing, storage, distribution, analysis, and interpretation that combines the tools and techniques of mathematics, computer science, and biology with the aim of understanding the biologic significance of a variety of data.

bi·o·in·stru·ment (bī′ō-in′stroo-ment). A sensor or device usually attached to or embedded in the human body or other living animal to record and to transmit physiologic data to a receiving and monitoring station.

bi·o·ki·net·ics (bī′ō-ki-net′iks). The study of the growth changes and movements that developing organisms undergo. [bio- + G. *kinēsis*, motion]

bi·o·log·ic, bi·o·log·i·cal (bī′ō-loj′ik, -loj′i-kăl). Relating to biology.

bi·ol·o·gist (bī-ol′ō-jist). A specialist or expert in biology.

bi·ol·o·gy (bī-ol′ō-jē). The science concerned with the phenomena of life and living organisms. [bio- + G. *logos*, study]

cellular b., SYN cytology.

molecular b., study of phenomena in terms of b. molecular (or chemical) interactions; traditionally, the focus of molecular b. is more specific than biochemistry in that it has an emphasis on chemical interactions involved in the replication of DNA, its "transcription" into RNA, and its "translation" into or expression in protein, i.e., in the chemical reactions connecting genotype and phenotype.

oral b., that aspect of b. devoted to the study of biological phenomena associated with the oral cavity in health and disease (e.g., dental caries, mastication, periodontal disease).

pharmaceutical b., SYN pharmacognosy.

radiation b., field of science that studies the biological effects of ionizing radiation.

bi·o·lu·mi·nes·cence (bī′ō-loo-min-es′ens). **1.** Light produced by certain organisms from the oxidation of luciferins through the action of luciferases and with negligible production of heat, chemical energy being converted directly into light energy. SYN cold light (1). **2.** Any light produced by a living organism. [bio- + L. *lumen* (*-inis*), light]

bi·ol·y·sis (bī-ol′i-sis). Disintegration of organic matter through the chemical action of living organisms. [bio- + G. *lysis*, dissolution]

bi·o·lyt·ic (bī-ō-lit′ik). **1.** Relating to biolysis. **2.** Capable of destroying life.

bi·o·mac·ro·mol·e·cule (bī′ō-māk-rō-mol′ĕ-kūl). A naturally occurring substance of large molecular weight (e.g., protein, DNA).

bi·o·mass (bī′ō-mas). The total weight of all living things in a given area, biotic community, species population, or habitat; a measure of total biotic productivity.

biomaterial (bī′ō-ma-tē′rē-al). A synthetic or semisynthetic material used in a biological system to construct an implantable prosthesis and chosen for its biocompatibility. [bio- + material]

bi·ome (bī′ōm). The total complex of biotic communities occupying and characterizing a particular geographic area or zone. [bio- + -ome]

bi·o·me·chan·ics (bī-ō-me-kan′iks). The science concerned with the action of forces, internal or external, on the living body.
dental b., SYN dental *biophysics*.

bi·o·med·i·cal (bī-ō-med′i-kăl). **1.** Pertaining to those aspects of the natural sciences, especially the biologic and physiologic sciences, that relate to or underlie medicine. **2.** Biological and medical, i.e., encompassing both the science(s) and the art of medicine.

bi·o·mem·brane (bī-ō-mem′brān). A structure bounding a cell or cell organelle; it contains lipids, proteins, glycolipids, steroids, etc. SYN membrane (2).

bi·om·e·ter (bī-om′ĕ-ter). A device for measuring carbon dioxide given off by organisms and, hence, for determining the quantity of living matter present. [bio- + G. *metron*, measure]

bi·o·me·tri·cian (bī-ō-me-trish′ăn). One who specializes in the science of biometry.

bi·om·e·try (bī-om′ĕ-trē). The application of statistical methods to the study of numeric data based on biologic observations and phenomena. [bio- + G. *metron*, measure]
b. fetal, ultrasound measurement of fetal dimensions to evaluate gestational age of fetal size.

bi·o·mi·cro·scope (bī-ō-mī′krō-skōp). SYN slitlamp.

bi·o·mi·cros·co·py (bī-ō-mī-kros′kŏ-pē). **1.** Microscopic examination of living tissue in the body. **2.** Examination of the cornea, aqueous humor, lens, vitreous humor, and retina by use of a slitlamp combined with a binocular microscope.

Bi·om·pha·la·ria (bī-om-fă-lā′rē-ă). An important genus of freshwater snails (family Planorbidae, subfamily Planorbinae), several species of which serve as intermediate hosts of *Schistosoma mansoni* in Africa, Saudi Arabia and Yemen, South America, and the Caribbean. Host snails formerly were placed in the genera *Australorbis*, *Tropicorbis*, and *Taphius* but are no longer considered generically distinct.

bi·on (bī′on). A living thing. [G. pres. p. ntr. of *bioō*, to live]

Biondi, Aldolpho, Italian pathologist, 1846–1917. SEE B.-Heidenhain *stain*.

bi·o·ne·cro·sis (bī-ō-ne-krō′sis).

bi·on·ic (bī-on′ik). Relating to or developed from bionics.

bi·on·ics (bī-on′iks). **1.** The science of biologic functions and mechanisms as applied to electronic chemistry; such as computers, employing various aspects of physics, mathematics, and chemistry; e.g., improving cybernetic engineering by reference to the organization of the vertebrate nervous system. **2.** The science of applying the knowledge gained by studying the characteristics of living organisms to the formulation of nonorganic devices and techniques. [bio- + electronics]

bi·o·nom·ics (bī-ō-nom′iks). **1.** SYN bionomy. **2.** SYN ecology.

bi·on·o·my (bī-on′ō-mē). The laws of life; the science concerned with the laws regulating the vital functions. SYN bionomics (1). [bio- + G. *nomos*, law]

bi·o·phage (bī′ō-fāj). An organism that derives the nourishment for its existence from another living organism.

bi·oph·a·gism (bī-of′ă-jizm). The deriving of nourishment from living organisms. SYN biophagy. [bio- + G. *phagō*, to eat]

bi·oph·a·gous (bī-of′ă-gŭs). Feeding on living organisms; denoting certain parasites.

bi·oph·a·gy (bī-of′ă-jē). SYN biophagism.

bi·o·phar·ma·ceu·tics (bī-ō-far-mă-soo′tiks). The study of the physical and chemical properties of a drug, and its dosage form, as related to the onset, duration, and intensity of drug action, incluidng co-constituents and mode of manufacture.

bi·o·phy·lac·tic (bī-ō-fī-lak′tik). Relating to biophylaxis.

bi·o·phy·lax·is (bī-ō-fī-lak′sis). Nonspecific defense reactions of the body, e.g., phagocytosis, vascular and other reactions of inflammatory processes. [bio- + G. *phylaxis,* protection]

bi·o·phys·ics (bī-ō-phyz′iks). **1.** The study of biologic processes and materials by means of the theories and tools of physics; the application of physical methods to analyze biologic problems and processes. **2.** The study of physical processes (e.g., electricity, luminescence) occurring in organisms.
cellular b., b. concerned with cellular processes.
dental b., the relationship between the biologic behavior of oral structures and the physical influence of a dental restoration. SYN dental biomechanics.
medical b., b. related to diagnosis and therapy.
molecular b., b. concerned with membrane processes, conformational and configurational properties of macromolecules, bioelectrical phenomena, etc.
radiation b., the study of the effects of radiation on cells, tissues, biomolecules, and living organisms.

bi·o·plasm (bī′ō-plazm). Protoplasm, especially in its relation to living processes and development. [bio- + G. *plasma,* thing formed]

bi·o·plas·mic (bī-ō-plas′mik). Relating to bioplasm.

bi·o·pol·y·mer (bī′ō-pol′ĕ-mer). A naturally occurring compound that is a polymer containing identical or similar subunits.
aperiodic b., a b. consisting of nonidentical subunits present in a nonperiodic sequence.
periodic b., a b. in which there are identical, repeating subunits.

bi·op·sy (bī′op-sē). **1.** Process of removing tissue from patients for diagnostic examination. **2.** A specimen obtained by b. [bio- + G. *opsis,* vision]
aspiration b., SYN needle b.
brush b., obtained by abrading the surface of a lesion with a brush to obtain cells and tissue for microscopic examination.
chorionic villus b., transcervical or transabdominal sampling of the chorionic villi for genetic analysis.
endoscopic b., b. obtained by instruments passed through an endoscope or obtained by a needle introduced under endoscopic guidance.
excision b., excision of tissue for gross and microscopic examination in such a manner that the entire lesion is removed.
fine needle b., the aspiration and removal of tissue or suspensions of cells through a small needle.
incision b., removal of only a part of a lesion by incising into it.
needle b., any method in which the specimen for b. is removed by aspirating it through an appropriate needle or trocar that pierces the skin, or the external surface of an organ, and into the underlying tissue to be examined. SYN aspiration b.
open b., surgical incision or excision of the region from which the b. is taken.
punch b., any method that removes a small cylindrical specimen for b. by means of a special instrument that pierces the organ directly or through the skin or a small incision in the skin. SYN trephine b.
sentinal node b., b. preceded by injection of a dye or radioisotope proximal to a tumor to identify for excision the primary node draining the area; used to determine the extent of spread of a malignancy.
shave b., a b. technique performed with a surgical blade or a razor blade; used for lesions that are elevated above the skin level or confined to the epidermis and upper dermis, or to protrusions of lesions from internal sites.
sponge b., abrasion of a lesion with a suitable sponge.
trephine b., SYN punch b.
wedge b., excision of a cuneiform specimen.

bi·o·psy·chol·o·gy (bī′ō-sī-kol′ō-jē). An interdisciplinary area of study involving psychology, biology, physiology, biochemistry, the neural sciences, and related fields.

bi·o·psy·cho·so·cial (bī-ō-sī′kō-sō-shăl). Involving interplay of biologic, psychological, and social influences.

bi·op·ter·in (bī-op′ter-in). A pterin found in yeast, the fruit fly, and in normal human urine. The reduced form of b. serves as a coenzyme for a number of enzyme-catalyzed reactions.

bi·op·tome (bī-op′tōm). A biopsy instrument passed through a catheter into the heart to obtain pieces of tissue for diagnosis. [*biop*sy + G. *tomē*, a cutting]

bi·or·bit·al (bī-ōr′bī-tăl). Relating to both orbits. [bi- + G. *orbita*, orbit]

bi·o·rhe·ol·o·gy (bī′ō-rē-ol′ō-jē). The science concerned with deformation and flow in biological systems. [bio- + G. *rheō*, to flow, + *logos*, study]

bi·o·rhythm (bī′ō-rith-m). A biologically inherent cyclic variation or recurrence of an event or state, such as the sleep cycle, circadian rhythms, or periodic diseases. [bio- + G. *rhythmos*, rhythm]

bi·o·safe·ty (b-ī′ō-saf′tē). Safety measures applied to the handling of biologic materials or organisms with a known potential to cause disease in humans. Current recommendations from the Centers for Disease Control and Prevention are to follow universal precautions, that is to treat all human samples of blood and body fluid as though they were infectious.

bi·o·sis (bī-ō′sis). Life, in a general sense. [G. *biōsis*, way of living]

bi·o·so·cial (bī-ō-sō′shul). Involving the interplay of biologic and social influences.

bi·o·spec·trom·e·try (bī′ō-spek-trom′ĕ-trē). Spectroscopic determination of the types and amounts of various substances in living tissue or fluid from a living body. SYN clinical spectrometry. [bio- + L. *spectrum*, an image, + G. *metron*, measure]

bi·o·spec·tros·co·py (bī′ō-spek-tros′kō-pē). Spectroscopic examination of specimens of living tissue, including fluids removed therefrom. SYN clinical spectroscopy. [bio- + L. *spectrum*, image, + G. *skopeō*, to examine]

bi·o·spe·le·ol·o·gy (bī′ō-spē′lē-ol′ō-jē). The study of organisms whose natural habitat is wholly or partly subterranean. [bio- + G. *spēliaion*, cave]

bi·o·sphere (bī′ō-sfēr). All the regions in the world where living organisms are found. [bio- + G. *sphaira*, sphere]

bi·o·stat·ics (bī-ō-stat′iks). The science of the relation between structure and function in organisms. [bio- + G. *statikos*, causing to stand]

bi·o·sta·tis·tics (bī′ō-stă-tis′tiks). The science of statistics applied to biologic or medical data.

bi·o·syn·the·sis (bī-ō-sin′thĕ-sis). Formation of a chemical compound by enzymes, either in the organism (in vivo) or by fragments or extracts of cells (in vitro). SYN biogenesis (2).

bi·o·syn·thet·ic (bī′ō-sin-thet′ik). Relating to or produced by biosynthesis.

bi·o·sys·tem (bī′ō-sis-tem). A living organism or any complete

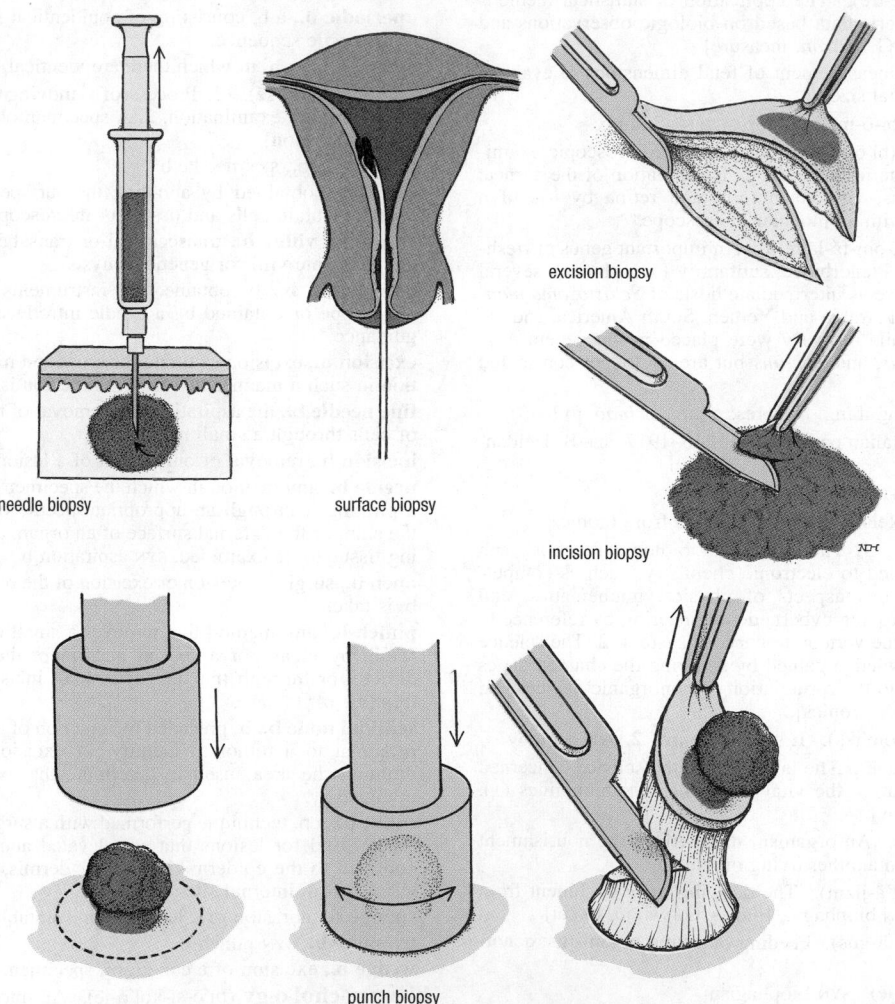

needle biopsy

surface biopsy

excision biopsy

incision biopsy

punch biopsy

biopsy

system of living things that can, directly or indirectly, interact with others.

Biot, Camille, 19th century French physician. SEE B. *breathing*, *respiration*, breathing *sign, sign.*

bi·o·ta (bī-ō′tă). The collective flora and fauna of a region. [Mod. L., fr. G. *bios,* life]

bi·o·tax·is (bī-ō-tak′sis). **1.** The classification of living beings according to their anatomic characteristics. **2.** SYN cytoclesis. [bio- + G. *taxis,* arrangement]

bi·o·tech·nol·o·gy (bī′ō-tek-nol′ō-jē). **1.** The field devoted to applying the techniques of biochemistry, cellular biology, biophysics, and molecular biology to addressing practical issues related to human beings, agriculture, and the environment. **2.** The use of recombinant DNA or hybridoma technologies for production of useful molecules, or for the alteration of biologic processes to enhance some desired property.

bi·o·te·lem·e·try (bī-ō-tel-em′ĕ-trē). The technique of monitoring vital processes and transmitting data without wires to a point remote from the subject.

bi·o·test (bī′ō-test). A method for assessing the effect of a compound, technique, or procedure on an organism. SYN biologic assay.

bi·ot·ic (bī-ot′ik). Pertaining to life.

bi·ot·ics (bī-ot′iks). The science concerned with the functions of life, or vital activity and force. [G. *biōtikos,* relating to life]

bi·o·tin (bī′ō-tin). The D-isomer component of the vitamin B_2 complex occurring in or required by most organisms and inactivated by avidin; participates in biologic carboxylations. It is a small molecule with a high affinity for avidin that can be readily coupled to a previously labeled antibody in order to allow visualization by enzymatic or histochemical means. SEE ALSO avidin. SYN coenzyme R, vitamin H, W factor.
  b. carboxylase, a subunit of a number of enzymes (e.g., acetyl-CoA carboxylase). It catalyzes the formation of carboxybiotin (on a biotin carrier protein), ADP, and P_i from ATP, CO_2 and biotin.
  b. oxidase, an enzyme (probably nonspecific) catalyzing the beta-oxidation of the b. side chain.

bi·o·tin·i·dase (bī-ō-tin′i-dās). An enzyme catalyzing the hydrolysis of biotin amide (forming biotin and ammonia), biocytin (forming biotin and lysine), and other biotinides. A deficiency of b. can lead to organic acidemia.

bi·ot·i·nides (bī-ot′i-nīdz). Compounds of biotin; e.g., biocytin.

bi·o·tin·yl·ly·sine (bī′ō-tin-il-lī′sin). SYN biocytin.

bi·o·tope (bī′ō-tōp). The smallest geographic area providing uniform conditions for life; the physical part of an ecosystem. [G. *bios,* life, + *topos,* place]

bi·o·tox·i·col·o·gy (bī′ō-tok-si-kol′ō-jē). The study of poisons produced by living organisms.

bi·o·tox·in (bī-ō-tok′sin). Any toxic substance formed in an animal body, and demonstrable in its tissues or body fluids, or both.

bi·o·trans·for·ma·tion (bī′ō-trans-fōr-mā′shŭn). The conversion of molecules from one form to another within an organism, often associated with change (increase, decrease, or little change) in pharmacologic activity; refers especially to drugs and other xenobiotics. SYN biodegradation.

bi·o·type (bī′ō-tīp). **1.** A population or group of individuals composed of the same genotype. **2.** In bacteriology, former name for biovar, referring to a variant strain of bacteria. [bio- + G. *typos,* model]

bi·o·var (bī′ō-var). A group (infrasubspecific) of bacterial strains distinguishable from other strains of the same species on the basis of physiologic characters. Formerly called biotype. [bio- + *variant*]

bi·o·vu·lar (bī′ov-ū-lar). SYN diovular.

bi·pal·a·ti·noid (bī-pal′ă-ti-noyd). A capsule with two compartments, used for making remedies in nascent form; the reaction between the two substances takes place as the capsule dissolves in the stomach, thus activating the remedy.

bi·par·a·sit·ism (bī-par′ă-sit-izm). SYN hyperparasitism.

bi·pa·ren·tal (bī-pa-ren′tăl). Having two parents, male and female.

bi·pa·ri·e·tal (bī-pa-rī′ĕ-tăl). Relating to both parietal bones of the skull. [bi- + L. *paries,* wall]

bip·a·rous (bip′ă-rŭs). Bearing two young. [bi- + L. *pario,* to give birth]

bi·par·tite (bī-par′tīt). Consisting of two parts or divisions.

bi·ped (bī′ped). **1.** Two-footed. **2.** Any animal with only two feet. [bi- + L. *pes,* foot]

bi·ped·al (bī′ped-ăl). **1.** Relating to a biped. **2.** Capable of locomotion on two feet; e.g., an iguana and some other lizards have this capability.

bi·pen·nate, bi·pen·ni·form (bī-pen′āt, pen′i-fōrm). Pertaining to a muscle with a central tendon toward which the fibers converge on either side like the barbs of a feather. [bi- + L. *penna,* feather]

bi·per·fo·rate (bī-per′fō-rāt). Having two foramina or perforations.

bi·per·i·den (bī-per′i-den). An anticholinergic agent with sedative and central effects on the basal ganglia; used in the symptomatic treatment of parkinsonism and drug-induced parkinsonism. Also available as b. hydrochloride.

bi·phen·a·mine hy·dro·chlo·ride (bī-fen′ă-mēn). An antiseborrheic agent.

bi·phe·no·typ·ic (bī′fē-nō-tip′ik). Pertaining to or characterized by biphenotypy.

bi·phe·no·ty·py (bī-fē′nō-tī′pē). The expression of markers of more than one cell type by the same cell, as in certain leukemias.

bi·phen·yl (bī-fen′il). SYN diphenyl.
  polychlorinated b. (PCB), b. in which some or all of the hydrogen atoms attached to ring carbons are replaced by chlorine atoms; a probable human carcingogen and teratogen.

bi·po·lar (bī-pō′ler). Having two poles, ends, or extremes.

Bipolaris (bī-pō-la′ris). Genus of dematiaceous fungi that are among the causes of phaeohyphomycosis; some *Drechslera* and *Helminthosporium* species are now classified as *B.* species.
  B. australiensis, species of dematiaceous fungi that is among the causes of phaeohyphomycosis.
  B. hawaiiensis, species of dematiaceous fungi that is among the causes of phaeohyphomycosis.
  B. spicifera, species of dematiaceous fungi that is among the causes of phaeohyphomycosis.

bi·po·ten·ti·al·i·ty (bī′pō-ten-shē-al′i-tē). Capability of differentiating along two developmental pathways. An example is the capacity of the gonad to develop into either an ovary or a testis.

bi·ra·mous (bī-rā′mŭs). Having two branches. [bi- + L. *ramus,* branch]

Birbeck, Michael S., contemporary British cancer researcher. SEE B. *granule.*

Birch-Hirschfeld, Felix V., German pathologist, 1842–1899. SEE Birch-Hirschfeld *stain.*

birch tar (berch). SYN birch tar oil.

birch tar oil. Pyroligneous oil obtained by the dry distillation of the wood of *Betula alba* and rectified by steam distillation; used externally in the treatment of skin diseases. SYN birch tar.

Bird, Samuel D., Australian physician, 1833–1904. SEE B. *sign.*

bi·re·frin·gence (bī-rē-frin′jens). SYN double *refraction.*

bi·re·frin·gent (bī-rē-frin′-jent). Refracting twice; splitting a ray of light in two.

Bir·na·vi·ri·dae (bir′nă-vī′rā-dā). A family of icosahedral nonenveloped viruses, 60 nm in diameter whose genome consists of two segments of linear double-stranded RNA.

Bir·navi·rus (bir′nă-vī-rŭs). A virus in the family Birnaviridae that includes infectious bursal disease virus of chickens, ducks, and turkeys and infectious pancreatic necrosis virus of fish. [bi- + RNA + virus]

bi·ro·ta·tion (bī-rō-tā′shŭn). SYN mutarotation.

birth (berth). **1.** Passage of the offspring from the uterus to the outside world; the act of being born. **2.** Specifically, in the human, complete expulsion or extraction from its mother of a fetus, irrespective of gestational age, and regardless of whether or not the umbilical cord has been cut or whether or not the placenta is attached.

average birth measurements	
length	49–52 cm
suboccipitobregmatic diameter	9.5 cm
occipitofrontal diameter	12.0 cm
occipitomental diameter	13.5 cm
suboccipitobregmatic circumference	32.0 cm
occipitofrontal circumference	34.0 cm
occipitomental circumference	35.0 cm
shoulder width	12.0 cm
shoulder girth	35.0 cm
hip width	10–11 cm
hip girth	27.0 cm

b. certificate, official, legal document recording details of a live b., usually comprising name, date, place, identity of parents, and sometimes additional information such as b. weight.

premature b., b. of an infant that has achieved a gestation of at least 20 weeks or birth weight of at least 500 g, but before 37 weeks.

birth·ing (bir'thing). Parturition; the act of giving birth.

birth·mark (berth'mark). A persistent visible lesion, usually on the skin, identified at or near birth; commonly a nevus or hemangioma. SEE nevus (1).

strawberry b., SYN strawberry *nevus*.

bis-. 1. Prefix signifying two or twice. **2.** In chemistry, used to denote the presence of two identical but separated complex groups in one molecule. Cf. bi-, di-. [L.]

bis·ac·o·dyl (bis-ak'ō-dil). A laxative used orally or rectally for constipation. Same class as phenolphthalein.

bis·a·cro·mi·al (bis'ă-krō'mē-ăl). Relating to both acromion processes.

bis·al·bu·mi·ne·mia (bis'al-bū'mi-nē'mē-ă). The concurrence of having two kinds of serum albumin that differ in mobility on electrophoresis: normal albumin (albumin A) and any one of several variant types that migrate at other speeds; individuals are heterozygous for the gene for albumin A and the gene for the variant albumin type. SEE ALSO inherited albumin *variants,* under *variant*.

bis·ax·il·lary (bis-ak'si-lār-ē). Relating to both axillae.

bis·ben·zy·liso·quinoline al·ka·loids (bis-ben'zil-ī-sō-kwin'ō-lin ăl-ka-loids). A group of alkaloids whose base structure is two fused isoquinoline rings, e.g., curare alkaloids.

2,5-bis(5-t-bu·tyl·ben·zox·a·zol-2-yl)thi·o·phene (BBOT). A scintillator used in radioactivity measurements by scintillation counting.

Bischof, W., 20th century German neurosurgeon. SEE B. *myelotomy*.

bis·cuit (bis'kit). A term associated with the firing of porcelain, and applied to the fired article before glazing. May be any stage after the fluxes have flowed enough to provide rigidity to the structure up to the stage where shrinkage is complete. Referred to as low, medium or high b., depending on the completeness of vitrification, also as hard or soft b.

bis·cuit-bake. The initial bake(s) given fusing porcelain at lower than glazing temperature to control shrinkage during the process of building up the dental restoration. SYN biscuit-firing.

bis·cuit-fir·ing. SYN biscuit-bake.

bis·de·qua·lin·i·um chlo·ride (bis'de-kwă-lin'ē-ŭm). An antiseptic.

bis in die (b.i.d.) (bis in dē'ā). Twice a day. [L.]

bi·sex·u·al (bī-seks'ū-ăl). **1.** Having gonads of both sexes. SEE ALSO hermaphroditism. **2.** Denoting an individual who engages in both heterosexual and homosexual relations.

bis·fer·i·ent (bis-fer'ē-ent). SYN bisferious.

bis·fer·i·ous (bis-fēr'ē-ŭs). Striking twice; said of the pulse. SYN bisferient. [L. *bis,* twice, + *ferio,* to strike]

Bishop, Louis F., U.S. physician, 1864–1941. SEE B. *sphygmoscope*.

bis·hy·drox·y·cou·ma·rin (bis-hī-drox'ē-koo'mă-rin). SYN dicumarol.

bis·il·i·ac (bis-il'ē-ak). Relating to any two corresponding iliac parts or structures, as the iliac bones or iliac fossae.

Bismarck brown R [C.I. 21010]. A diazo dye similar to Bismarck brown Y.

Bismarck brown Y [C.I. 21000]. A diazo dye used for staining mucin and cartilage in histologic sections, in the Papanicolaou technique for vaginal smears, and as one of Kasten Schiff-type reagents in the PAS and Feulgen stains. SYN vesuvin. [Ger. *bismarckbraun,* after Otto von *Bismarck,* Ger. chancellor]

bis·muth (Bi) (biz'mŭth). A trivalent metallic element; atomic no. 83, atomic wt. 20.98037. Several of its salts are used in medicine; some contain BiO^+, rather than Bi^{3+}, and are called subsalts. [Ger. *Wismut, weisse Masse,* white mass]

b. aluminate, a gastric antacid. SYN aluminum bismuth oxide.

b. ammonium citrate, ammoniocitrate of b.; an intestinal astringent.

b. carbonate, SYN b. subcarbonate.

b. chloride oxide, SYN b. oxychloride.

b. citrate, used in the making of b. and ammonium citrate.

b. hydroxide, used in detecting reducing sugars.

b. iodide, BiI_3; used in electron microscopy to reveal synapses. SYN b. triiodide.

b. oxide, used for the same purposes as the subnitrate.

b. oxycarbonate, SYN b. subcarbonate.

b. oxychloride, basic b. chloride, used for the same purposes as the subnitrate. SYN b. chloride oxide, bismuthyl chloride.

b. oxynitrate, SYN b. subnitrate.

b. salicylate, SEE b. subsalicylate.

b. sodium tartrate, a basic sodium b. tartrate; an antisyphilitic agent.

b. sodium triglycollamate, sodium b. complex of nitrilotriacetic acid.

b. subcarbonate, used for the same purposes as b. subnitrate, but has lower toxicity. SYN b. carbonate, b. oxycarbonate, bismuthyl carbonate.

b. subgallate, used internally in diarrhea and externally as an astringent and protective dusting powder.

b. subnitrate, a basic salt, the composition of which varies with the conditions of preparation; used internally as an intestinal astringent and externally as a mild astringent and antiseptic; the metal is used as an electron microscope stain for nucleic acids. SYN b. oxynitrate.

b. subsalicylate, used as an intestinal antiseptic.

b. tribromophenate, b. tribromophenol, used externally as an antiseptic.

b. trichloride, $BiCl_3$; addition of water results in formation of b. oxychloride. SYN butter of bismuth.

b. triiodide, SYN b. iodide.

bis·mu·tho·sis (bis-mŭ-thō'sis). Chronic bismuth poisoning.

bis·muth·yl (biz'mŭ-thil). The group, BiO^+, that behaves chemically as the ion of a univalent metal; its salts are subsalts of bismuth.

b. carbonate, SYN *bismuth* subcarbonate.

b. chloride, SYN *bismuth* oxychloride.

bis·ox·a·tin ac·e·tate (bis-ok'să-tin). A laxative.

1,4-bis(5-phen·yl·ox·a·zol-2-yl)ben·zene. A liquid scintillation agent used in radioisotope measurement.

1,3-bis·phos·pho·glyc·er·ate (1,3-P$_2$Gri) (dī-fos'fō-glis'er-āt). An intermediate in glycolysis which enzymatically reacts with ADP to generate ATP and 3-phosphoglycerate.

2,3-bis·phos·pho·glyc·er·ate (2,3-P$_2$Gri). An intermediate in the Rapoport-Luebering shunt, formed between 1,3-bisphosphoglycerate and 3-phosphoglycerate; an important regulator of the affinity of hemoglobin for oxygen; an intermediate of phosphoglycerate mutase.

2,3-b. mutase, an enzyme of the Rapoport-Luebering shunt; it catalyzes the reversible interconversion of 1,3-bisphosphoglycerate to 2,3-b.; it also has a phosphatase activity, converting 2,3-b. to orthophosphate and 3-phosphoglycerate; a deficiency of 2,3-b. mutase can result in mild erythrocytosis.

bis·phos·pho·nates (bis-fos′fō-nāts). Synthetic pyrophosphate analogs that inhibit osteoclast resorption of bone.

bi·ste·phan·ic (bī′stĕ-fan′ik). Relating to both stephanions; denoting particularly the b. width of the cranium, or b. diameter, the shortest distance from one stephanion to the other.

bi·ste·roid (bī-stēr′oyd). A molecule composed of two molecules of a given steroid joined together by a carbon-to-carbon bond.

bis·tou·ry (bis′too-rē). A long, narrow-bladed knife, with a straight or curved edge and sharp or blunt point (probe-point); used for opening or slitting cavities or hollow structures. [Fr. *bistouri,* fr. It. dialect *bistori,* perh. fr. *Pistoia,* Italy]

bi·stra·tal (bī-strā′tăl). Having two strata or layers.

bi·sul·fate (bī-sŭl′fāt). A salt containing HSO_4^-. SYN acid sulfate.

bi·sul·fide (bī-sŭl′fīd). A compound of the anion HS^-; an acid sulfide.

bi·sul·fite (bī-sŭl′fīt). A salt or ion of HSO_3^-.

bit. **1.** The smallest unit of digital information expressed in the binary system of notation (either 0 or 1). **2.** The electrical signal used in electronic computers. SYN binary digit.

bi·tar·trate (bī-tar′trāt). A salt or anion resulting from the neutralization of one of tartaric acid's two acid groups.

bitch. A female dog of breeding age. [O.E. *bicche*]

bite (bīt). **1.** To incise or seize with the teeth. **2.** The act of incision or seizure with the teeth. **3.** A morsel of food held between the teeth. **4.** Term used to denote the amount of pressure developed in closing the jaws. **5.** Undesirable jargon for terms such as interocclusal record, maxillomandibular registration, denture space, and interarch distance. **6.** A wound or puncture of the skin made by animal or insect. [A.S. *bītan*]

balanced b., SYN balanced *occlusion.*

biscuit b., SYN maxillomandibular *record.*

close b., SYN small interarch *distance.*

closed b., reduced vertical interarch distance with excessive vertical overlap of the anterior teeth.

deep b., an abnormally large vertical overlap of anterior teeth in centric occlusion.

edge-to-edge b., SYN edge-to-edge *occlusion.*

end-to-end b., SYN edge-to-edge *occlusion.*

jumping the b., an orthodontic technique for correcting a crossbite, usually anterior.

locked b., an occlusion in which the cusp arrangement restricts lateral excursions.

normal b., SYN normal *occlusion* (1).

⚑**open b.,** (1) SYN large interarch *distance*; (2) SYN apertognathia.

rest b., a misnomer for physiologic rest *position* of the mandible.

working b., SYN working *contacts,* under *contact.*

bi·tem·po·ral (bī-tem′pŏ-răl). Relating to both temples or temporal bones.

bite·plate, bite·plane (bīt′plāt, bīt′plān). A removable appliance that incorporates a plane of acrylic designed to occlude with the opposing teeth.

⚑**bite·wing** (bīt′wing). SEE bitewing *radiograph.*

bi·thi·o·nol (bī-thī′ŏ-nol). An antiparasitic agent used for treatment of the human lungworm, *Paragonimus westermani,* and the Oriental liver fluke, *Clonorchis sinensis;* also used as a bacteriostat in soaps and detergents; sodium bithionate is used as a topical bactericide and fungicide.

bi·tol·ter·ol mes·y·late (bī-tol′ter-ol). A sympathomimetic bronchodilator used in the prophylaxis and treatment of bronchial asthma and reversible bronchospasm.

Bitot, Pierre A., French physician, 1822–1888. SEE B. *spots,* under *spot.*

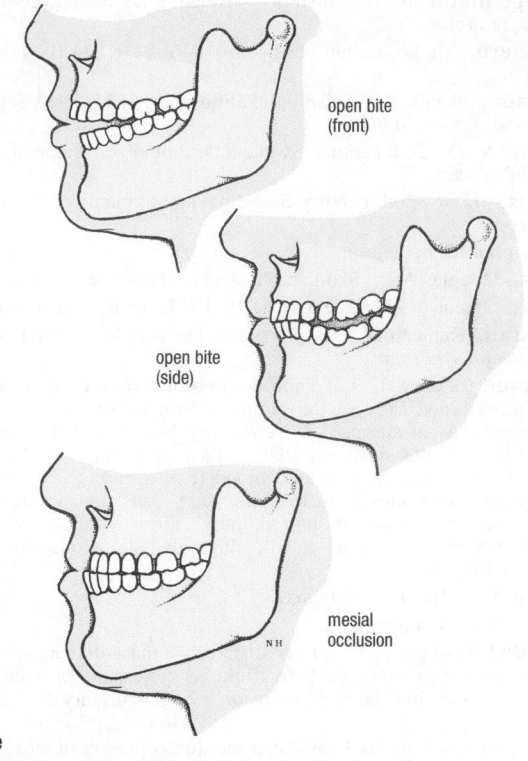

open bite (front)

open bite (side)

mesial occlusion

N H

bite

bi·tro·chan·ter·ic (bī-trō-kan-ter′ik). Relating to two trochanters, either to the two trochanters of one femur or to both greater trochanters.

bi·tro·pic (bī-trop′ik). Having a dual affinity, as in tissues or organisms. [bi- + G. *tropē,* a turning]

bit·ter ap·ple. SYN colocynth.

bit·ters. **1.** An alcoholic liquor in which bitter vegetable substances (e.g., quinine, gentian) have been steeped. **2.** Bitter vegetable drugs (e.g., quassia, gentian, cinchona), usually used as tonics. SYN amara.

aromatic b., b. with a pleasant aromatic flavor.

Bittner, John J., U.S. oncologist, 1904–1961. SEE B. *agent,* milk *factor.*

Bittorf, Alexander, German physician, 1876–1949. SEE B. *reaction.*

bi·u·ret (bī-oo-ret′). A derivative of urea obtained by heating, eliminating one NH_3 between two ureas. Used in protein determinations. SYN carbamoylurea.

bi·va·lence, bi·va·len·cy (bī-vā′lens, bī-vā′len-sē). A combining power (valence) of 2. SYN divalence, divalency.

bi·va·lent (bī-vā′lent, biv′ă-lent). **1.** Having a combining power (valence) of 2. SYN divalent. **2.** In cytology, a structure consisting of two paired homologous chromosomes, each split into two sister chromatids, as seen during the pachytene stage of prophase in meiosis. SEE ALSO tetrad.

bi·ven·ter (bī-ven′ter). Two-bellied; denoting two-bellied muscles. [bi- + L. *venter,* belly]

b. cer′vicis, SYN spinalis capitis (*muscle*).

b. mandib′ulae, SYN digastric (*muscle*) (1).

bi·ven·tral (bī-ven′tral). SYN digastric (1).

bi·ven·tric·u·lar (bī′ven-trik′oo-lar). Pertaining to both right and left ventricles.

bix·in (bik′sin). A monomethyl ester of a 24-carbon branched unsaturated dicarboxylic acid; a carotenoid (a carotene-dioic acid); the orange-red coloring matter from seeds of *Bixa orellana;* the ethyl ester is used as a food and drug colorant. SEE ALSO annotto.

bi·zy·go·mat·ic (bī′zī-gō-mat′ik). Relating to both zygomatic bones or arches.

Bizzozero, Giulio, Italian physician, 1846–1901. SEE B. *corpuscle.*

Bjerrum, Jannik P., Danish ophthalmologist, 1851–1920. SEE B. *scotoma, screen, sign.*

Björk, V. O., 20th century Swedish cardiothoracic surgeon. SEE B.-Shiley *valve.*

Björnstad, R., 20th century Scandinavian dermatologist. SEE B. *syndrome.*

Bk Symbol for berkelium.

Black, Douglas A.K., Scottish physician, *1909. SEE B. *formula.*

Black, Greene V., U.S. dentist, 1836–1915. SEE B. *classification.*

Blackfan, Kenneth D., U.S. physician, 1883–1941. SEE Diamond-B. *anemia, syndrome.*

black·out (blak′owt). **1.** Temporary loss of consciousness due to decreased blood flow to the brain. **2.** Momentary loss of consciousness, as in absence. **3.** Temporary loss of vision, without alteration of consciousness, due to positive g (gravity) forces; caused by temporary decreased blood flow in the central retinal artery, and seen mostly in aviators. **4.** A transient episode that occurs during a state of intense intoxication (alcoholic b.) for which the person has no recall, although not unconscious (as observed by others).

visual b., SEE *amaurosis* fugax.

black root. SYN leptandra.

blad·der (blad′er) [TA]. **1.** A distensible musculomembranous organ serving as a receptacle for fluid, as the urinary or gallbladder or urinary bladder. SEE detrusor. **2.** SYN urinary b. [A.S. *blaedre*]

air b., a two-chambered gas-filled sac that is present in most fish and functions as a hydrostatic organ; it is located beneath the vertebral column, and is connected with the esophagus in some fish. SYN swim b.

allantoic b., a type of b. formed as an outgrowth of the cloaca.

atonic b., a large, dilated, and nonemptying urinary b.; usually due to disturbance of innervation or to chronic obstruction.

autonomic neurogenic b., malfunctioning urinary b., secondary to low spinal cord lesions.

gall b., SYN gallbladder.

hyperreflexic b., a b. exhibiting detrusor instability.

hypertonic b., a b. with poor compliance.

ileal b., SYN ileal *conduit.*

neurogenic b., SYN neuropathic b.

neuropathic b., any defective functioning of bladder due to impaired innervation, e.g., cord b., neuropathic b. SYN neurogenic b.

nonneurogenic neurogenic b., detrusor-sphincter incoordination with urinary incontinence, constipation, UTI, upper tract changes. SYN Hinman syndrome, pseudoneurogenic b.

poorly compliant b., a b. that has high pressure at low volumes in the absence of detrusor activity.

pseudoneurogenic b., SYN nonneurogenic neurogenic b.

reflex neurogenic b., an abnormal condition of urinary b. function whereby the b. is cut off from upper motor neuron control, but the lower motor neuron arc is still intact.

swim b., SYN air b.

trabeculated b., characterized by thick wall and hypertrophied muscle bundles. Typically seen in instances of chronic obstruction.

uninhibited neurogenic b., a condition, either congenital or acquired, of abnormal urinary b. function whereby normal inhibitory control of detrusor function by the central nervous system is impaired or underdeveloped, resulting in urgency or enuresis.

unstable b., characterized by uninhibited detrusor contractions.

urinary b. [TA], a musculomembranous elastic bag serving as a storage place for the urine. SYN bladder (2) [TA], vesica urinaria [TA], vesica (1) [TA], cystis urinaria, urocyst, urocystis.

blad·der·worm (blad′er-werm). SYN *Cysticercus.*

blade·vent (blād′vent). A thin, wedge-shaped endosteal implant

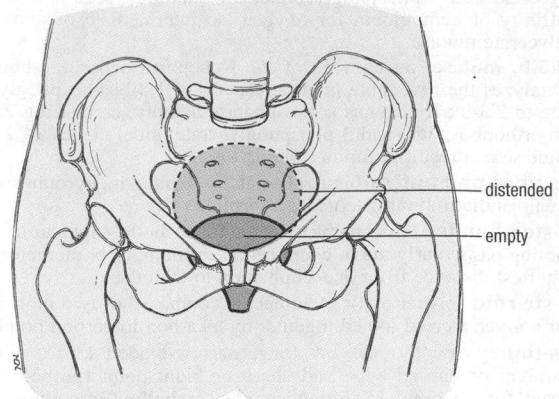

urinary bladder: shown in empty and distended states

of metal that is inserted into a surgically prepared groove in the maxilla or mandible.

Blagden, Sir Charles, British physician, 1748–1820. SEE B. *law.*

Blainville, Henri Marie Ducrotay de, French zoologist and anthropologist, 1777–1850. SEE B. *ears,* under *ear.*

Blair, Vilray P., U.S. surgeon, 1871–1955.

Blakemore, Arthur H., U.S. surgeon, 1897–1970. SEE Sengstaken-B. *tube.*

Blalock, Alfred, U.S. surgeon, 1899–1964. SEE B. *shunt;* B.-Hanlon *operation;* B.-Taussig *operation, shunt.*

Blandin, Philippe Frédéric, French anatomist and surgeon, 1798–1849. SEE B. *gland.*

blank. A solution consisting of all of the analytical components except the compound to be measured; this is used to establish a baseline of measurement intensity against which the compound of interest is compared. [M.E. white, fr. O.Fr. *blanc,* fr. Germanic]

blanket. A covering.

mucus b., the mucous covering of respiratory epithelium.

blas. Term invented by van Helmont to denote a mystical spirit or vital force which presided over and governed the various processes of the body. Each bodily function was supposed to have its own special b.; b. appears to be the counterpart of the archaeus of Paracelsus. [a Middle E. variant of *blast*]

Blaschko, Alfred, Austrian dermatologist, 1858–1922. SEE *lines* of B., under *line.*

Blasius, Gerhard (Blaes), Dutch anatomist, 1626(?)–1692. SEE B. *duct.*

blast (blăst). General term for immature or precursor cell. [G. *blastos,* germ]

-blast. An immature precursor cell of the type indicated by the preceding word. [G. *blastos,* germ]

blas·te·ma (blas-tē′mă). **1.** The primordial cellular mass (precursor) from which an organ or part is formed. **2.** A cluster of cells competent to initiate the regeneration of a damaged or ablated structure. [G. a sprout]

metanephric b., SYN metanephric *cap.*

nephric b., the extension of nephrogenic cord tissue, caudal to the mesonephros, into which the ureteric buds grow to initiate development of the definitive mammalian kidney. SYN nephroblastema.

blas·tem·ic (blas-tem′ik). Relating to the blastema.

blas·tic (blas′tik). **1.** Describing the formation of a conidium by the blowing out process of a fertile hypha before being limited by a septum. **2.** Colloquial term for osteoblastic. [G. *blastos,* germ + -ic]

blasto-. Pertaining to the process of budding (and the formation of buds) by cells or tissue. [G. *blastos,* germ]

blas·to·cele (blas′tō-sēl). The cavity in the blastula of a developing embryo. SYN blastocoele, cleavage cavity, segmentation cavity. [blasto- + G. *koilos,* hollow]

blas·to·cel·ic (blas-tō-sē′lik). Relating to the blastocele. SYN blastocoelic.

blas·to·coele (blas′tō-sēl). SYN blastocele.

blas·to·coel·ic (blas′tō-sē′lik). SYN blastocelic.

Blas·to·co·nid·i·um (blas′tō-cŏ-nid′ē-ŭm). A holoblastic conidium that is produced singly or in chains, and detached at maturity leaving a bud scar, as in the budding of a yeast cell. SYN blastospore. [blasto- + conidium]

blas·to·cyst (blas′tō-sist). The modified blastula stage of mammalian embryos, consisting of the inner cell mass and a thin trophoblast layer enclosing the blastocele. SYN blastodermic vesicle. [blasto- + G. *kystis,* bladder]

Blas·to·cys·tis (blas′tō-sis′tis). A genus of yeastlike parasites in the digestive tract of mammals; generally considered nonpathogenic. Its relationship to fungi is now being questioned owing to protozoan characteristics, such as lack of cell walls, a membrane-bound central body, pseudopod activity, protozoan type of Golgi apparatus and mitochondria, and reproduction by sporulation or binary fission rather than by budding.
B. hominis, a species of B. widespread among humans, formerly considered harmless, now recognized as a cause of diarrhea and other intestinal symptoms and eosinophilia when found in heavy infections.

blas·to·cyte (blas′tō-sīt). An undifferentiated blastomere of the morula or blastula stage of an embryo. [blasto- + G. *kytos,* cell]

blas·to·derm, blas·to·der·ma (blas′tō-derm, -tō-der′ma). The thin, disk-shaped cell mass of a young embryo and its extraembryonic extensions over the surface of the yolk; when fully formed, all three primary germ layers (ectoderm, endoderm, and mesoderm) are present. SYN germ membrane, germinal membrane, membrana germinativa. [blasto- + G. *derma,* skin]

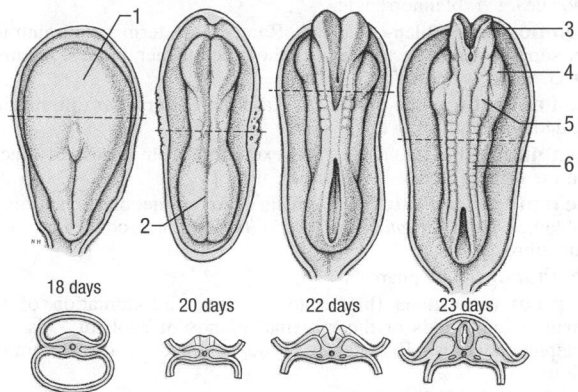

blastoderm: (above) dorsal views, (below) cross-sectional views; (1) neural plate, (2) primitive streak, (3) neural fold, (4) heart, (5) auditory placode, (6) somite

bilaminar b., the b. of a young embryo when it consists of only two of the three primary germ layers it will ultimately have.

embryonic b., that part of the b. that takes part in the formation of the embryonic body.

extraembryonic b., that part of the b. which is not incorporated in the embryo but forms membranes concerned in its nourishment and protection.

trilaminar b., the b. after all three of the primary germ layers have been established.

blas·to·der·mal, blas·to·der·mic (blas-tō-der′măl, -der′mik). Relating to the blastoderm.

blas·to·disk (blas′tō-disk). **1.** The disk of active cytoplasm at the animal pole of a telolecithal egg. **2.** The blastoderm, especially in very young stages when its extent is small.

blas·to·gen·e·sis (blas-tō-jen′ĕ-sis). **1.** Reproduction of unicellular organisms by budding. **2.** Development of an embryo during cleavage and germ layer formation. **3.** Transformation of small

lymphocytes of human peripheral blood in tissue culture into large, morphologically primitive blastlike cells capable of undergoing mitosis; can be induced by a variety of agents including phytohemagglutinin, concanavalin A, certain antigens to which the cell donor has been previously immunized, and leukocytes from an unrelated individual. [blasto- + G. *genesis,* origin]

blas·to·ge·net·ic, blas·to·gen·ic (blas′tō-je-net′ik, -tō-jen′ik). Relating to blastogenesis.

blas·tol·y·sis (blas-tol′i-sis). Dissolution or destruction of the blastocyst or blast cells and subsequent death. [blasto- + G. *lysis,* loosening]

blas·to·lyt·ic (blas-tō-lit′ik). Relating to blastolysis.

blas·to·ma (blas-tō′mă). A neoplasm composed chiefly or entirely of immature undifferentiated cells resembling those that form the blastema or primordium of the organ in which the tumor arose. [blasto- + G. *-oma,* tumor]

blas·to·mere (blas′tō-mēr). One of the cells into which the egg divides after its fertilization. SYN cleavage cell, embryonic cell. [blasto- + G. *meros,* part]

blas·to·mer·ot·o·my (blas′tō-mēr-ot′ō-mē). SYN blastotomy. [blastomere + G. *tomē,* incision]

blas·to·mo·gen·ic (blas′tō-mō-jen′ik). Causing or producing a blastoma.

Blas·to·my·ces der·ma·tit·i·dis (blas-tō-mī′sēz der-mă-tit′i-dis). A dimorphic soil fungus that causes blastomycosis. It grows in mammalian tissues as budding cells and in culture as a white to buff-colored filamentous fungus bearing spherical or ovoid conidia on terminal or lateral short, slender conidiophores. In its perfect (teleomorph) state it is known as *Ajellomyces dermatitidis.* [blasto- + G. *mykēs,* fungus]

blas·to·my·cin (blas-tō-mī′sin). An antigen for intradermal testing prepared from sterile filtrates of cultures of the filamentous form of *Blastomyces dermatitidis.*

blas·to·my·co·sis (blas-tō-mī-kō′sis). A chronic granulomatous and suppurative disease caused by *Blastomyces dermatitidis;* originates as a respiratory infection and disseminates, usually with pulmonary, osseous, and/or cutaneous involvement predominating. Formerly called North American b., the disease now has been found in African states as well as in Canada and the U.S. SYN Gilchrist disease.

Brazilian b., obsolete term for paracoccidioidomycosis.

cutaneous b., verrucous or ulcerative skin lesions seen with infection with *Blastomyces dermatitidis.*

North American b., SEE blastomycosis.

South American b., SYN paracoccidioidomycosis.

systemic b., infection with *Blastomyces dermatitidis* extending beyond the skin or the lung, the usual portals of entry; involvement of bone and genitourinary tract (esp. prostate and epididymis) are most frequent.

blas·to·neu·ro·pore (blas′tō-noo′rō-pōr). A temporary opening formed in some embryos by the union of the blastopore and neuropore. [blasto- + neuropore]

blas·to·phore (blas′tō-fōr). An early stage of division of a coccidial schizont in which spheroid or ellipsoid structures are formed with a single peripheral layer of nuclei; merozoites form at the surface of the b. over each nucleus, grow out radially, and separate from the residual body (remnant of the b.); in a first-generation schizont such as *Eimeria bovis,* about 120,000 merozoites are produced. [blasto- + G. *phorós,* bearing]

blas·to·pore (blas′tō-pōr). The opening into the archenteron formed by invagination of the blastula to form a gastrula. SYN protostoma, protostome. [blasto- + G. *poros,* opening]

Blastoschizomyces (blas′tō-skiz-ō-mī′sēz). A genus of yeastlike fungi.

B. capitatus, fungal species that causes severe disseminated infection in immunosuppressed patients; formerly classified as a species of *Geotrichum.*

blas·to·spore (blas′tō-spōr). SYN Blastoconidium. [blasto- + G. *sporos,* seed]

blas·tot·o·my (blas-tot′ō-mē). Experimental destruction of one or more blastomeres. SYN blastomerotomy. [blasto- + G. *tomē,* incision]

■**blas·tu·la** (blas'tū-lă). An early stage of an embryo formed by the rearrangement of the blastomeres of the morula to form a hollow sphere. [G. *blastos,* germ]

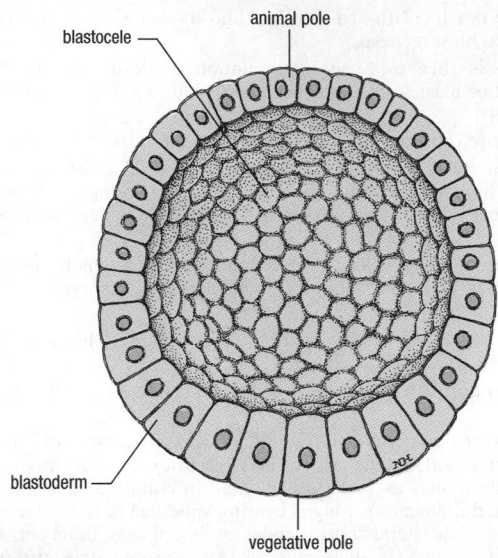

blastocele

animal pole

blastoderm

vegetative pole

blastula: hemisected

blas·tu·lar (blas'tū-lar). Pertaining to the blastula.

blas·tu·la·tion (blas-tū-lā'shŭn). Formation of the blastula or blastocyst from the morula.

Blatin, Marc, French physician, *1878. SEE B. *syndrome.*

Blat·ta (blat'ă). A genus of insects (family Blattidae) that includes the abundant oriental cockroach, *B. orientalis.* The dried insect yields antihydropin, a diuretic principle. [L. cockroach]

Blat·tel·la (bla-tel'ă). A genus of cockroaches, (family Blattidae) that includes *B. germanica,* the German cockroach or croton bug, probably the most familiar and widespread of the cockroaches. [L. *blatta,* cockroach]

Blat·ti·dae (blat'i-dē). A family of insects (order Blattaria) consisting of over 4000 species of cockroaches, largely tropical but worldwide in distribution, including a number of abundant pests of households, kitchens, and institutions or facilities, wherever food is present; noxious wherever found, yet not positively incriminated in natural transmission of pathogenic organisms to man. Common household pests include the German cockroach, *Blattella germanica,* the American cockroach, *Periplaneta americana,* and the oriental cockroach, *Blatta orientalis.* [L. *blatta,* cockroach]

bleb (blĕb). 1. A large flaccid vesicle. 2. An acquired lung cyst, usually less than 1 cm in diameter, similar to but smaller than a bulla, which is thought to be the most common cause of spontaneous pneumothorax. B.'s occur mainly in the apex of the lung.

filtering b., a blister of conjunctiva resulting from glaucoma surgery by which a flap of sclera is created in the eye wall, allowing aqueous *humor* to percolate out of the eye and underneath the conjunctiva, thus lowering intraocular *pressure.* SYN filtering cicatrix.

pulmonary b., air-filled alveolar dilation less than 1 cm in diameter on the edge of the lung at the apex of upper lobe or superior segment of lower lobe; usually occurs in young people and can rupture, producing primary pneumothorax. Cf. pulmonary *bulla.*

bleed (blēd). To lose blood as a result of rupture or severance of blood vessels.

bleed·er (blēd'er). 1. Colloquialism for a person suffering from hemophilia, Christmas disease, Osler disease, or other clotting disorder. 2. A blood vessel cut during a surgical procedure.

bleed·ing (blēd'ing). 1. Losing blood as a result of the rupture or severance of blood vessels. 2. Phlebotomy; the letting of blood.

dysfunctional uterine b., uterine b. due to a benign endocrine abnormality rather than to any organic disease.

occult b., SEE occult *blood.*

blem·ish. 1. A small circumscribed alteration of the skin considered to be unesthetic but insignificant. 2. To alter the skin, rendering an unesthetic appearance.

blen·nad·e·ni·tis (blen-ad-ĕ-nī'tis). Inflammation of the mucous glands. [G. *blennos,* mucus, + *adēn,* gland, + *-itis,* inflammation]

blen·ne·me·sis (blen-em'ĕ-sis). Rarely used term for vomiting of mucus. [G. *blennos,* mucus, + *emesis,* vomiting]

♺**blenno-, blenn-.** Mucus. [G. *blenna, blennos*]

blen·no·gen·ic (blen-ō-jen'ik). SYN muciparous. [blenno- + G. *-gen,* to produce]

blen·nog·e·nous (ble-noj'ĕ-nŭs). SYN muciparous.

blen·noid (blen'oyd). SYN muciform. [blenno- + G. *eidos,* resemblance]

blen·noph·thal·mia (blen-of-thal'mē-ă). 1. SYN conjunctivitis. 2. SYN gonorrheal *ophthalmia.*

blen·nor·rhag·ic (blen-ō-raj'ik). SYN blennorrheal.

blen·nor·rhea (blen-ō-rē'ă). 1. Rarely used term for any mucous discharge, especially from the urethra or vagina. 2. In ophthalmic usage, was synonymous with conjunctivitis, but is now obsolete. [blenno- + G. *rhoia,* a flow]

b. conjunctiva'lis, SYN gonorrheal *ophthalmia.*

inclusion b., a neonatal conjunctivitis caused by *Chlamydia trachomatis.*

b. neonato'rum, SYN *ophthalmia* neonatorum.

blen·nor·rhe·al (blen-ō-rē'ăl). Rarely used term relating to blennorrhea. SYN blennorrhagic.

blen·nos·ta·sis (blen-os'tă-sis). Rarely used term for diminution or suppression of secretion from the mucous membranes. [blenno- + G. *stasis,* standing]

blen·no·stat·ic (blen-ō-stat'ik). Rarely used term for diminishing mucous secretion.

blen·nu·ria (ble-noo'rē-ă). The excretion of an excess of mucus in the urine. [blenno- + G. *ouron,* urine]

ble·o·my·cin sul·fate (blē-ō-mī'sin). An antineoplastic antibiotic obtained from *Streptomyces verticillus.* Often produces pulmonary fibrosis.

♺**blephar-.** SEE blepharo-.

bleph·ar·ad·e·ni·tis (blef'ar-ad-ĕ-nī'tis). Inflammation of the meibomian glands or the marginal glands of Moll or Zeis. SYN blepharoadenitis. [blephar- + G. *adēn,* gland, + *-itis,* inflammation]

bleph·a·ral (blef'ă-răl). Referring to the eyelids.

bleph·a·rec·to·my (blef'a-rek'tō-mē). Excision of all or part of an eyelid. [blepharo- + G. *ektomē,* excision]

bleph·ar·e·de·ma (blef'ar-ĕ-dē'mă). Edema of the eyelids, causing swelling and often a baggy appearance.

bleph·a·ri·tis (blef'ă-rī'tis). Inflammation of the eyelids. [blepharo- + G. *-itis,* inflammation]

b. acar'ica, SYN demodectic b.

■**b. angula'ris,** inflammation of the lid margins at the angles of the commissure.

ciliary b., SYN b. marginalis.

demodectic b., inflammation of the eyelid associated with *Demodex folliculorum.* SYN b. acarica.

b. follicula'ris, a deep-seated suppurative inflammation of ciliary follicles and the glands of Zeis and Moll of the eyelid. SYN pustular b.

marginal b., SYN b. marginalis.

b. margina'lis, inflammation of the margins of the eyelids. SYN ciliary b., marginal b.

meibomian b., inflammation of the eyelid margin and the meibomian glands.

b. parasit'ica, marginal b. due to the presence of lice. SYN b. phthiriatica, pediculous b.

pediculous b., SYN b. parasitica.

b. phthiriat'ica, SYN b. parasitica.

posterior b., inflammation of eyelid margins characterized by inspissation and occlusion of tarsal glands orifices.

pustular b., SYN b. follicularis.

b. rosa'cea, inflammation of the margins of the eyelids in association with acne rosacea.

seborrheic b., a common type of chronic inflammation of the margins of the eyelids with erythema and white scales; often with an associated seborrheic dermatitis of scalp and face.

b. sic'ca, inflammation of the margins of the eyelids in which the lashes are powdered with dry scales.

staphylococcal b., inflammation of the eyelids characterized by brittle hard scales along the base of the eyelashes.

b. ulcero'sa, marginal b. with ulceration.

⌂**blepharo-, blephar-.** Eyelid. [G. *blepharon,* an eyelid]

bleph·a·ro·ad·e·ni·tis (blef'ă-rō-ad-ĕ-nī'tis). SYN blepharadenitis.

bleph·a·ro·ad·e·no·ma (blef'ă-rō-ad-ĕ-nō'mă). A tumor or adenoma of a gland of the eyelid. [blepharo- + G. *adēn,* gland, + -*oma,* tumor]

bleph·a·ro·chal·a·sis (blef'ă-rō-kal'ă-sis). A condition in which there is a redundancy of the skin of the upper eyelids so that a fold of skin hangs down, often concealing the tarsal margin when the eye is open. SYN ptosis adiposa. [blepharo- + G. *chalasis,* a slackening]

bleph·a·roc·lo·nus (blef-ar-ok'lō-nŭs). Clonic spasm of the eyelids. [blepharo- + G. *klonos,* a tumult]

bleph·a·ro·col·o·bo·ma (blef'ă-rō-kol-ō-bō'mă). SYN ankyloblepharon. [blepharo- + coloboma]

bleph·a·ro·con·junc·ti·vi·tis (blef'ă-rō-kon-jŭnk-ti-vī'tis). Inflammation of the palpebral conjunctiva.

bleph·a·ro·di·as·ta·sis (blef'ă-rō-dī-as'tă-sis). Abnormal separation or inability to completely close the eyelids. [blepharo- + G. *diastasis,* separation]

bleph·a·ro·ker·a·to·con·junc·ti·vi·tis (blef'ă-rō-ker'ă-tō-kon-jŭnk'ti-vī'tis). An inflammation involving the eyelids, cornea, and conjunctiva.

bleph·a·ron (blef'ă-ron). SYN eyelid. [G. *blepharon,* eyelid]

bleph·a·ro·phi·mo·sis (blef'ă-rō-fi-mō'sis). Decrease in the width of the palpebral aperture without fusion of lid margins. SYN blepharostenosis. [blepharo- + G. *phimōsis,* an obstruction]

bleph·a·ro·plast (blef'ă-rō-plast). SYN basal *body.* [blepharo- + G. *plastos,* formed]

bleph·a·ro·plas·tic (blef'ă-rō-plas'tik). Relating to blepharoplasty.

bleph·a·ro·plas·ty (blef'ă-ro-plast-tē). Any operation for the correction of a defect in the eyelids. [blepharo- + G. *plassō,* to form]

bleph·a·ro·ple·gia (blef'ă-rō-plē'jē-ă). Paralysis of an eyelid. [blepharo- + G. *plēgē,* stroke]

bleph·a·rop·to·sis, bleph·ar·op·to·sia (blef'ă-rop'tō-sis, -rop-tō'sē-ă). Drooping of the upper eyelid. SYN ptosis (2). [blepharo- + G. *ptōsis, a falling*]

b. adipo'sa, b. with accumulation of subcutaneous fat causing skin to hang over the free border of the eyelid.

false b., SYN pseudoptosis.

bleph·a·ro·spasm, bleph·a·ro·spas·mus (blef'ă-rō-spazm, -spaz'mŭs). Involuntary spasmodic contraction of the orbicularis oculi muscle; may occur in isolation or be associated with other dystonic contractions of facial, jaw, or neck muscles; usually initiated or aggravated by emotion, fatigue, or drugs.

bleph·a·ro·stat (blef'ă-rō-stat). SYN eye *speculum.* [blepharo- + G. *statos,* fixed]

bleph·a·ro·ste·no·sis (blef'ă-rō-ste-nō'sis). SYN blepharophimosis. [blepharo- + G. *stenōsis,* a narrowing]

bleph·a·ro·syn·ech·ia (blef'ă-rō-sin-ek'ē-ă). Adhesion of the eyelids to each other or to the eyeball. [blepharo- + G. *synecheia,* continuity, fr. *syn- echō,* to hold together]

bleph·a·rot·o·my (blef-ă-rot'ō-mē). A cutting operation on an eyelid. [blepharo- + G. *tomē,* incision]

blind (blīnd). Unable to see; without useful sight. SEE blindness.

blind·ness (blīnd'nes). **1.** Loss of the sense of sight; absolute b. connotes no light perception. SEE ALSO amblyopia, amaurosis. **2.** Loss of visual appreciation of objects although visual acuity is normal. **3.** Absence of the appreciation of sensation, e.g., taste b. SYN typhlosis.

change b., failure to observe large changes in the vision field that occur simultaneously with brief disturbances.

color b., misleading term for anomalous or deficient color vision; complete color b. is the absence of one of the primary cone pigments of the retina. SEE protanopia, deuteranopia, tritanopia.

cortical b., loss of sight due to an organic lesion in the visual cortex.

day b., SYN hemeralopia.

eclipse b., SYN solar *maculopathy.*

flash b., a temporary loss of vision produced when retinal light-sensitive pigments are bleached by light more intense than that to which the retina is physiologically adapted at that moment.

flight b., visual blackout in aviators. SEE ALSO *amaurosis* fugax.

functional b., apparent loss of vision related to suggestibility.

hysterical b., loss of vision or blurring of vision following a psychologically traumatic event such as seeing one's child being killed in an accident.

legal b., generally, visual acuity of less than 6/60 or 20/200 using Snellen test types, or visual field restriction to 20° or less in the better eye; the criteria used to define legal b. vary among different groups.

letter b., visual agnosia for letters, in which letters are seen but not identified; caused by a lesion in the occipital cortex.

mind b., visual agnosia for objects, in which objects are seen but not identified; caused by a lesion in area 18 of the occipital cortex. SYN object b., psychanopsia, psychic b.

music b., SYN musical *alexia.*

night b., SYN nyctalopia.

note b., SYN musical *alexia.*

object b., SYN mind b.

psychic b., SYN mind b.

river b., SYN ocular *onchocerciasis.*

sight b., SYN asymbolia.

sign b., visual agnosia for signs.

snow b., severe photophobia secondary to ultraviolet keratoconjunctivitis.

solar b., SYN solar *maculopathy.*

taste b., inability to appreciate gustatory stimuli.

text b., word b., SYN alexia.

blink (blink). To close and open the eyes rapidly; an involuntary act by which the tears are spread over the conjunctiva, keeping it moist. SYN wink.

blis·ter. 1. A fluid-filled thin-walled structure under the epidermis or within the epidermis (subepidermal or intradermal). **2.** To form a b. with heat or some other vesiculating agent.

blood b., a b. containing blood; resulting from a pinch or crushing injury.

fever b., colloquialism for herpes simplex of the lips.

fly b., a cantharidal b. caused by discharge of a vesicating body fluid by certain beetles, particularly members of the family Meloidae which produce cantharidin, e.g., *Lytta (Cantharis) vesicatoria,* the notorious "Spanish fly"; noncantharidin vesicating fluid is produced by other beetles, such as rove beetles (family Staphylinidae), especially the genus *Paederus,* whose fluid, on contact with the skin, produces an intensely painful b.

fracture b., superficial epidermolysis that occurs in association, most commonly, with fractures of the leg and ankle and forearm and wrist; etiology represents a combination of excessive swelling and torsional injury to the overlying soft tissues.

sucking b., superficial bullous skin lesion on neonate arm probably resultant from vigorous prenatal sucking.

blis·ter·ing. SYN vesiculation (1).

bloat, bloat·ing (blōt, blōt'ing). **1.** Abdominal distention from swallowed air or intestinal gas from fermentation. **2.** Distention of the rumen of cattle, caused by the accumulation of gases of fermentation, particularly likely to occur when the animals are pastured on rich legume grasses; if unrelieved, the condition may quickly lead to death.

Bloch, Marcel, French physician, 1885–1925. SEE B. *reaction.*

Bloch, Bruno, Swiss dermatologist, 1878–1933. SEE B.-Sulzberger *disease, syndrome.*

block (block). **1.** To obstruct; to arrest passage through. **2.** A condition in which the passage of an electrical impulse is arrested, wholly or in part, temporarily or permanently. **3.** SYN atrioventricular b. [Fr. *bloquer*]

alveolocapillary b., the presence of material that impairs the diffusion of gases between the air in the alveolar spaces and the blood in alveolar capillaries; b. can be caused by edema, cellular infiltration, fibrosis, or tumor, and results in undersaturation of peripheral arterial blood with oxygen.

antegrade b., SYN anterograde b.

anterograde b., conduction b. of an impulse traveling anywhere in its ordinary direction, for example, from the sinoatrial node toward the ventricular myocardium. SYN antegrade b.

arborization b., intraventricular b. supposedly due to widespread blockage in the Purkinje ramifications and manifested in the electrocardiogram by a pattern similar to bundle-branch b. but with complexes of low amplitude.

atrioventricular b., AV b., partial or complete b. of electric impulses originating in the atrium or sinus node preventing them from reaching the atrioventricular node and ventricles. In first degree AV b., there is prolongation of AV conduction time (PR interval); in second degree AV b., some but not all atrial impulses fail to reach the ventricles, thus some ventricular beats are dropped; in complete AV block (third degree), complete atrioventricular dissociation (2) occurs; no impulses can reach the ventricles despite even a slow ventricular rate (under 45/min); atria and ventricles beat independently. SYN block (3), heart b.

bone b., surgical procedure in which a bone graft is placed adjacent to a joint to limit motion of the joint mechanically or to improve the stability of the joint, e.g., at the ankle joint to correct foot-drop by preventing plantarflexion past 0°, but allowing dorsiflexion beyond 0°, e.g., at the glenohumeral joint to prevent posterior instability.

bundle-branch b., intraventricular b. due to interruption of conduction in one of the two main branches of the bundle of His and manifested in the electrocardiogram by marked prolongation of the QRS complex; b. of each branch has distinctive QRS morphology.

complete AV b., (1) SEE atrioventricular b; **(2)** SYN complete atrioventricular *dissociation.* SEE atrioventricular b.

conduction b., failure of impulse transmission at some point along a nerve, although conduction along the segments proximal and distal to it are unaffected; clinically, most often the result of an area of focal demyelination; when caused by focal trauma, called neurapraxia.

congenital heart b., atrioventricular b. present *in utero* or at birth and usually of advanced or complete degree.

depolarizing b., skeletal muscle paralysis associated with loss of polarity of the motor endplate, as occurs following administration of succinylcholine.

divisional b., arrest of the impulse in one of the assumed two main divisions of the left branch of the bundle of His; i.e., in either the anterior (superior) division or the posterior (inferior) division. SYN hemiblock.

entrance b., SYN protective b.

epidural b., an obstruction in the epidural space; used inaccurately to refer to epidural anesthesia.

exit b., inability of an impulse to leave its point of origin, the mechanism for which is conceived as an encircling zone of refractory tissue denying passage to the emerging impulse.

fascicular b., a condition based on the disputed concept that the left branch of the bundle of His provides two of three major fascicles of a system of conduction, of which the right bundle branch constitutes the third, for the transmission of the cardiac impulse from the atrium above to the ventricles below the AV

node; block may occur in any or all fascicles, all three together producing complete AV block. SEE ALSO hemiblock.

field b., regional anesthesia produced by infiltration of local anesthetic solution into tissues surrounding an operative field.

first degree AV b., SEE atrioventricular b.

heart b., SYN atrioventricular b.

incomplete atrioventricular b., SYN partial heart b.

interatrial b., SYN intraatrial b.

intraatrial b., impaired conduction through the atria, manifested by widened and often notched P waves in the electrocardiogram. SYN interatrial b.

intraventricular b. (IVB), IV b., delayed conduction within the ventricular conducting system or myocardium, including bundlebranch, periinfarction b.'s, fascicular b.'s, nonspecific IV b. and Wolff-Parkinson-White (preexcitation) syndrome.

Mobitz b., second degree atrioventricular b. in which there is a ratio of two or more atrial deflections (P waves) to ventricular responses.

Mobitz types of atrioventricular b., type I, the dropped beat of the Wenckebach phenomenon; type II, a dropped cardiac cycle that occurs without alteration in the conduction of the preceding intervals.

nerve b., interruption of conduction of impulses in peripheral nerves or nerve trunks by injection of local anesthetic solution.

nondepolarizing b., skeletal muscle paralysis unaccompanied by changes in polarity of the motor endplate, as occurs following administration of tubocurarine.

partial heart b., impulses penetrate the atrioventricular junction in some relation to the ventricular rate. SYN incomplete atrioventricular b.

periinfarction b., an electrocardiographic abnormality associated with a myocardial infarct and caused by delayed activation of the myocardium in the region of the infarct; characterized by an initial vector directed away from the infarcted region with the terminal vector directed toward it.

phase I b., inhibition of nerve impulse transmission across the myoneural junction associated with depolarization of the motor endplate, as in the muscle paralysis produced by succinylcholine.

phase II b., inhibition of nerve impulse transmission across the myoneural junction unaccompanied by depolarization of the motor endplate, as in the muscle paralysis produced by tubocurarine.

protective b., an incompletely understood mechanism whereby a pacemaker is protected from being discharged by the impulse from another center; the mechanism, usually conceived as an encircling zone of unidirectionally refractory tissue permitting egress of impulses from the center but preventing access to the center, is seen in operation in ventricular parasystole where the parasystolic center is protected from discharge by the sinus pacemaker and so is able to maintain its intrinsic rhythm undisturbed. SYN entrance b., protection.

pupillary b., increased resistance to flow of aqueous *humor* through the pupil from the posterior chamber to the anterior chamber, leading to anterior bowing of the peripheral iris over the trabecular *meshwork* and to angle-closure *glaucoma.*

retrograde b., impaired conduction backward from the ventricles or AV node into the atria.

reverse pupillary b., increased resistance to flow of aqueous humor through the pupil from the anterior chamber to the posterior chamber, leading to posterior bowing of the peripheral iris against the zonules; a possible mechanism for pigmentary glaucoma.

second degree AV b., SEE atrioventricular b.

sinoatrial b., S-A b., sinus b., blockade of the impulse leaving the sinus node before it can activate atrial muscle. SYN sinoauricular b.

sinoauricular b., SYN sinoatrial b.

spinal b., an obstruction to the flow of cerebrospinal fluid in the spinal subarachnoid space; used inaccurately to refer to spinal anesthesia.

stellate b., injection of local anesthetic solution in the vicinity of the stellate ganglion.

suprahisian b., atrioventricular conduction delay occurring above, or cephalad to, the bundle of His.

third degree AV b., SYN complete atrioventricular *dissociation*; SEE atrioventricular b.

unidirectional b., b. that prevents passage of an impulse when it approaches from one direction but not from the other, as when b. in the AV node prevents anterograde conduction to the ventricles while retrograde conduction to the atria remains intact.

Wenckebach b., a form of b. in any cardiac tissue (most often the atrioventricular junction) in which there is progressive lengthening of conduction (decremental conduction) until the beat is dropped.

Wolff-Chaikoff b., blocking of the organic binding of iodine and its incorporation into hormone caused by large doses of iodine; usually a transient effect, but in large doses in susceptible individuals it can be prolonged and cause iodine myxedema. SYN Wolff-Chaikoff effect.

block·ade (blok'ād). **1.** Intravenous injection of large amounts of colloidal dyes or other substances in order to block reticuloendothelial cells (e.g., phagocytosis is temporarily prevented). **2.** Receptor blockade, blocking the effect of a hormone at the cell surface. **3.** Arrest of peripheral nerve conduction or transmission at autonomic synaptic junctions, autonomic receptor sites, or myoneural junctions by a drug. **4.** The occupation of receptors by an antagonist so that usual agonists are relatively ineffective.

adrenergic b., selective inhibition by a drug of the responses of effector cells to adrenergic sympathetic nerve impulses (sympatholytic) and to epinephrine and related amines (adrenolytic).

cholinergic b., **(1)** inhibition by a drug of nerve impulse transmission at autonomic ganglionic synapses (ganglionic b.), at postganglionic parasympathetic effector cells (e.g., by atropine), and at myoneural junctions (myoneural b.); **(2)** the inhibition of a cholinergic agent.

ganglionic b., inhibition of nerve impulse transmission at autonomic ganglionic synapses by drugs such as nicotine or hexamethonium.

myoneural b., inhibition of nerve impulse transmission at myoneural junctions by a drug such as curare.

narcotic b., the use of drugs to inhibit the effects of narcotic substances, as with naloxone.

sympathetic b., interruption of transmission in sympathetic ganglia or conduction of impulses in pre- or postganglionic sympathetic nerve fibers.

virus b., the interference of one virus by another, either attenuated or unrelated.

block·er (blok'er). **1.** An instrument used to obstruct a passage. **2.** SEE blocking *agent*.

angiotensin receptor b.'s, agents, such as losartan, that bind with angiotensin receptors, thus preventing access of angiotensin II to the receptor and consequently reducing the vasoconstriction produced by this agonist; used in the treatment of hypertension.

calcium channel b., a class of drugs with the capacity to prevent calcium ions from passing through biologic membranes. These agents are used to treat hypertension, angina pectoris, and cardiac arrhythmias; examples include nifedipine, diltiazem, verapamil, amlodipine.

block·ing (blok'ing). **1.** Obstructing; arresting of passage, conduction, or transmission. **2.** In psychoanalysis, a sudden break in free association occurring when a painful subject or repressed complex is touched. **3.** Sudden cessation of thoughts and speech, which may indicate the presence of a severe thought disorder or a psychosis.

alpha b., the attenuation of the occipital alpha rhythm (8–14 Hz brain waves as seen on an electroencephalogram), produced by opening the eyes or by intense mental concentration.

block-out (blok'owt). Elimination of undercuts by filling such areas with a medium such as wax or wet pumice.

Blocq, Paul O., French physician, 1860–1896. SEE B. *disease*.

Blom, Eric D., 20th century U.S. speech-language pathologist. SEE B.-Singer *valve*.

blood (blŭd). The "circulating tissue" of the body; the fluid and its suspended formed elements that are circulated through the heart, arteries, capillaries, and veins; b. is the means by which 1) oxygen and nutritive materials are transported to the tissues, and 2) carbon dioxide and various metabolic products are removed for excretion. The b. consists of a pale yellow or gray-yellow fluid, plasma, in which are suspended red b. cells (erythrocytes), white b. cells (leukocytes), and platelets. SEE ALSO arterial b., venous b. [A.S. blōd]

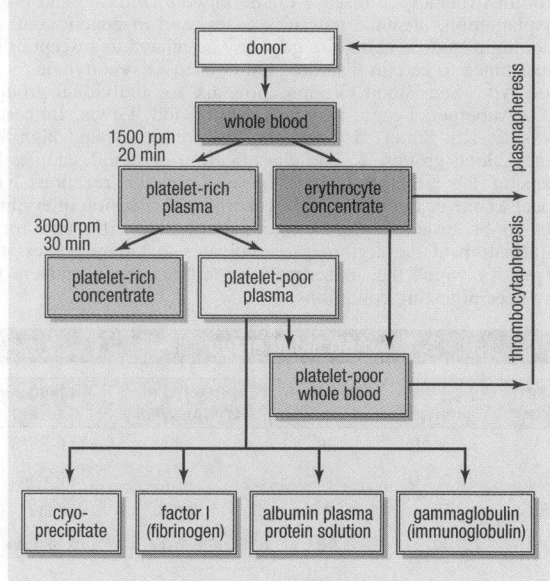

separation of blood components

arterial b., b. that is oxygenated in the lungs, found in the left chambers of the heart and in the arteries, and relatively bright red.

cord b., b. present in the umbilical vessels at the time of delivery. It is of fetal origin.

laky b., b. that is undergoing or has undergone laking. SEE lake (2), laky.

occult b., b. in the feces in amounts too small to be seen but detectable by chemical tests.

sludged b., b. in which the corpuscles, as a result of some general abnormal state, e.g., burns, traumatic shock, and similar stresses, become massed together in the capillaries, and thereby block the vessels or move slowly through them.

venous b., b. which has passed through the capillaries of various tissues, except the lungs, and is found in the veins, the right chambers of the heart, and the pulmonary arteries; it is usually dark red as a result of a lower content of oxygen.

whole b., b. drawn from a selected donor under rigid aseptic precautions; contains citrate ion or heparin as an anticoagulant; used as a b. replenisher.

blood bank. A place, usually a separate part or division of a hospital laboratory or a separtate free-standing facility, in which blood is collected from donors, typed, separated into several components, stored, and/or prepared for transfusion to recipients.

blood count. Calculation of the number of red (RBC) or white (WBC) blood cells in a cubic millimeter of blood, by means of counting the cells in an accurate volume of diluted blood.

complete b. c. (CBC), a combination of the following determinations: red blood cell count, white blood cell count, erythrocyte indices, hematocrit, differential blood count, and sometimes platelet count.

differential white b. c., an estimate of the percentage of each white blood cell type making up the total white blood cell count.

Schilling b. c., a method of counting blood in which the polymorphonuclear neutrophils are separated into four groups according to the number and arrangement of the nuclear masses in these cells. SYN Schilling index.

blood dust.   SYN hemoconia.

blood group.   **1.** A system of antigens under the control of closely linked allelic loci on the surface of the erythrocyte. Because of the antigenic differences existing between individuals, b. g.'s are significant in blood transfusions, maternal-fetal incompatibilities (hemolytic disease of the newborn), tissue and organ transplantation, disputed paternity cases, and in genetic and anthropologic studies; certain b. g.'s may be related to susceptibility or resistance to certain diseases. Often used as synonymous with blood type. See Blood Groups appendix for individual groups: ABO, Auberger, Diego, Duffy, I, Kell, Kidd, Lewis, Lutheran, MNSs, P, Rh, Sutter, Xg, and the low-frequency and high-frequency blood groups. **2.** The classification of blood samples by means of laboratory tests of their agglutination reactions with respect to one or more b. g.'s. In general, a suspension of erythrocytes to be tested is exposed to a known specific antiserum; agglutination of the erythrocytes indicates that they possess the antigen for which the antiserum is specific. Certain antisera require special testing conditions.

ABO blood group

blood group	genotype	frequency in U.S.(%)	antigens of erythrocytes	antibodies in serum
A	AA or AO	39	A	anti-B (β)
B	BB or BO	11	B	anti-A (α)
AB	AB	4	A and B	none
0	00	46	neither A nor B	α and β

private b. g., a b. g. that is known to have occurred in only one family and is traceable to one single person.

blood·less (blŭd′les).   Without blood.

blood·let·ting (blŭd′let-ing).   Removing blood, usually from a vein; formerly used as a general remedial measure, but used now in congestive heart failure and polycythemia. SEE phlebotomy.

general b., removing blood by arteriotomy or phlebotomy.

local b., removing blood from the smaller vessels, formerly by a cupping glass or by leeching.

blood rel·a·tive.   A popular term describing a relative of a person sharing a common ancestor. No special importance attaches to the blood as a vehicle of inheritance. Spouses are not ordinarily b. r.'s and when they are, the marriage is consanguineous and carries a higher risk than average of progeny homozygous by descent from ancestors in common. Such marriages are discouraged and within certain degrees of kindred may be illegal.

blood·shot (blŭd′shot).   Denoting locally congested smaller blood vessels of a part (e.g., the conjunctiva) which are dilated and visible.

blood·stream (blŭd′strēm).   The flowing blood as it is encountered in the circulatory system as distinguished from blood that has been removed from the circulatory system or sequestered in a part; thus, something added to the b. may be expected to become distributed to all parts of the body through which blood is flowing.

blood type.   The specific agglutination pattern of erythrocytes of an individual to the antisera of one blood group; e.g., the ABO blood group consists of four major b. t.'s: O, A, B, and AB. This classification depends on the presence or absence of two major antigens: A or B. Type O occurs when neither is present and type AB when both are present. The b. t. is the genetic phenotype of the individual for one blood group system and may be determined using different antisera available for testing. See Blood Groups appendix.

blood ves·sel [TA].   Any vessel conveying blood: arteries, arterioles, capillaries, venules, veins. conveying blood. SYN vas sanguineum [TA].

choroid b. v.'s [TA], the arteries and veins that, with the loose connective tissue and pigmented cells which form their matrix, comprise the vascular lamina of the choroid. SYN vasa sanguinea choroideae [TA].

intrapulmonary b. v.'s [TA], the intrasegmental branches of the pulmonary artery and vein that course within the parenchyma of the lungs. SYN vasa sanguinea intrapulmonalia [TA].

retinal b. v.'s [TA], the blood vasculature of the retina, including the branches and tributaries of the central retinal artery and vein, respectively, and the vascular circle of the optic nerve. SYN vasa sanguinea retinae [TA].

blood·worm (blŭd′werm).   **1.** The filarial parasite of sheep, *Elaeophora schneideri*. **2.** Red aquatic larvae of certain dipterous gnats and midges. **3.** Marine annelids in the family Terebellidae with soft bodies and red blood. **4.** Blood-inhabiting worms, such as the human blood flukes in the genus *Schistosoma*.

Bloom,   David, U.S. dermatologist, *1892. SEE B. *syndrome*.

blot.   SEE Northern blot *analysis*, Southern blot *analysis*, Western blot *analysis*, zoo blot *analysis*.

blotch.   Commonly used term to denote a pigmented or erythematous lesion.

Blount,   Walter P., U.S. orthopedic surgeon, *1900. SEE B. *disease*; B.-Barber *disease*.

blow·fly.   SEE *Calliphora*, *Lucilia*, *Phormia regina*.

blue (bloo).   A color between green and violet on the spectrum. For individual blue dyes, see the specific name. SYN cerulean.

blues (blooz).   State of depression or sadness. [slang, fr. *blue devils*]

postpartum b., mood disturbance (including insomnia, weepiness, depression, anxiety, and irritability) experienced by up to 50% of women the first week postpartum; apparently precipitated by progesterone withdrawal.

Blum,   Paul, French physician, 1878–1933. SEE Gougerot and B. *disease*.

Blumberg,   Jacob M., German surgeon and gynecologist, 1873–1955. SEE B. *sign*.

Blumenau,   Leonid W., Russian neurologist, 1862–1932. SEE B. *nucleus*.

Blumenbach,   Johann F., German physiologist, 1752–1840. SEE B. *clivus*.

Blumer,   George A., U.S. physician, 1858–1940. SEE B. *shelf*.

blunt-end (blunt-end).   Refers to double-stranded DNA in which there are no unpaired bases at the end of the polynucleotide.

blush (blŭsh).   **1.** A sudden and brief redness of the face and neck due to emotion. **2.** In angiography, used metaphorically to describe neovascularity or, in some cases, extravasation. [M.E., fr. O.E. *blyscan*,]

tumor b., enhancement of tumor on radiologic exams by administration of contrast agents.

BLV Abbreviation for bovine leukemia *virus*.

B-mode.   A two-dimensional diagnostic ultrasound presentation of echo-producing interfaces; the intensity of the echo is represented by modulation of the brightness of the spot, and the position of the echo is determined from the angular position of the transducer and the transit time of the acoustical pulse and its echo.

BMR Abbreviation for basal metabolic *rate*.

BNA Abbreviation for Basle Nomina Anatomica.

board.

institutional review b. (IRB), the standing committee in a hospital or other facility that is charged with responsibility for ensuring the safety and well-being of human subjects involved in research.

bob·bing (bob′ing).   An up-and-down movement.

inverse ocular b., slow downward eye movement followed by delayed quick upward return.

ocular b., sudden conjugate downward deviation of the eyes with a slow return to the normal position; seen in some comatose patients who have bilateral hemisphere lesions.

bob·i·er·rite (bōb′-ē-er-īt).   The octahydrate of magnesium phosphate; sometimes found in renal calculi. Cf. newberyite, struvite. [Pierre A. Bobierre, Fr. chemist, + -ite]

BOC, *t*-BOC Abbreviations formerly used for *t*-butoxycarbonyl; current usage is Boc.

Boc Abbreviation for *t*-butoxycarbonyl.

Bochdalek, Vincent A., Czechoslovakian anatomist, 1801–1883. SEE B. *foramen, ganglion, gap;* foramen of B. *hernia;* B. *muscle, valve;* flower basket of B.

Bock, August C., German anatomist, 1782–1833. SEE B. *ganglion.*

Bockhart, Max, German physician, 1883–1921. SEE B. *impetigo.*

BOD Abbreviation for biochemical oxygen *demand.*

Bodansky, Aaron, U.S. biochemist, 1887–1961. SEE B. *unit.*

Bödecker, Charles F., U.S. oral histologist, embryologist, and pathologist, *1880. SEE B. *index.*

Bodian, David, U.S. anatomist, *1910. SEE B. copper-PROTARGOL stain.*

Bo·do (bō′dō). A genus of free-living, ovoid or slightly pyriform protozoa with two flagella, one projecting anteriorly and the other posteriorly; may be ingested as encysted forms in food or drink, or possibly deposited in feces or urine after excretion; in either instance, cysts frequently develop into trophozoites if the specimen is permitted to remain at room temperature for a few hours prior to examination; the organisms are not pathogenic in humans.

B. cauda′tus, a species that is found in specimens of human feces (especially in tropical regions); the organisms are frequently termed coprozoic flagellates.

B. sal′tans, a species of the intestinal tract sometimes observed in ulcers.

B. urina′rius, a species found occasionally in the urine.

BODY

body (bod′ē). **1.** The head, neck, trunk, and extremities. The human body, consisting of head (caput), neck (collum), trunk (truncus), and limbs (membra). **2.** The material part of a human, as distinguished from the mind and spirit. **3.** The principal mass of any structure. **4.** A thing; a substance. SEE ALSO corpus, soma. SYN corpus (1) [TA]. [A.S. *bodig*]

acetone b., SYN ketone b.

adrenal b., SYN suprarenal *gland.*

alcoholic hyaline b.'s, SYN Mallory b.'s.

Alder b.'s, granular inclusions in polymorphonuclear leukocytes; they take on a dark color with Giemsa-Wright stain and react metachromatically with toluidine blue. SEE ALSO Alder *anomaly.*

alveolar b., SYN alveolar *process* of maxilla.

amygdaloid b. [TA], a rounded mass of gray matter in the temporal lobe internal to the cortex of the uncus and immediately anterior to the inferior horn of the lateral ventricle; its major afferents are olfactory and its efferent connections are with the hypothalamus and mediodorsal nucleus of the thalamus and it is also reciprocally associated with the cortex of the temporal lobe; it is subdivided into two major nuclear groups; basolateral and corticormedial. The individual nuclei of the amygdaloid body (or complex) are the basolateral amygdaloid nucleus [TA] (nucleus anygdalae basilis lateralis [TA]), basomedial amygdaloid nucleus [TA] (nucleus amygdalae basalis medialis [TA]), central amygdaloid nucleus [TA] (nucleus amygdalae centralis [TA]), cortical amygdaloid nucleus [TA] (nucleus amygdalae corticalis [TA]), interstitial amygdaloid nucleus [TA] (nucleus amygdalae interstitialis [TA]), lateral amygdaloid nucleus [TA] (nucleus amygdalae lateralis [TA]), medial amygdaloid nucleus [TA] (nucleus amygdalae medialis [TA]), and the nucleus of the lateral olfactory tract [TA] (nucleus tractus olfactorii lateralis [TA]). SYN amygdaloid complex [TA], corpus amygdaloideum [TA], amygdaloid nucleus, nucleus amygdalae.

amylogenic b., SYN amyloplast.

anococcygeal b., SYN anococcygeal *ligament.*

anterior quadrigeminal b., SYN superior *colliculus.*

aortic b.'s, SYN paraaortic b.'s.

Arnold b.'s, small portions or minute fragments of erythrocytes (sometimes mistaken for blood platelets), or small "ghosts" of erythrocytes.

asbestos b.'s, ferruginous b.'s with asbestos fibers as a core; a histologic hallmark of exposure to asbestos.

Aschoff b.'s, a form of granulomatous inflammation characteristically observed in acute rheumatic carditis; fully developed Aschoff b.'s consist of fibrinoid change in connective tissue, lymphocytes, occasional plasma cells, and abnormal characteristic histiocytes. SYN Aschoff nodules.

asteroid b., (1) an eosinophilic inclusion resembling a star with delicate radiating lines, occurring in a vacuolated area of cytoplasm of a multinucleated giant cell; especially frequent in sarcoidosis, but also seen in other granulomas; **(2)** a structure that is characteristic of sporotrichosis when found in the skin or secondary lesions of this mycosis; in tissue, it surrounds the 3- to 5-μm in diameter ovoid yeast of *Sporothrix schenckii.*

Auer b.'s, rod-shaped structures of uncertain nature in the cytoplasm of immature myeloid cells, especially myeloblasts, in acute myelocytic leukemia; may be an abnormal form of lysosomes; they contain peroxidase and acid phosphatase, and stain red by azure-eosin stains. SYN Auer rods.

Barr chromatin b., SYN sex *chromatin.*

basal b., an elongated centriolar structure situated at the base of each cilium at the apical margin of a cell. SYN basal corpuscle, basal granule, blepharoplast, kinetosome.

bigeminal b.'s, a bilateral single swelling of the roofplate of the embryonic midbrain that later in development becomes subdivided into a superior and an inferior colliculus. SEE quadrigeminal b.'s. SYN corpora bigemina.

b. of bladder [TA], the portion of the bladder between the apex and fundus. SYN corpus vesicae [TA].

brassy b., a dark-colored, usually shrunken erythrocyte in which there is a malarial parasite.

b. of breast [TA], the principal part of the breast, consisting of glandular tissue and its supporting fibrous tissue. It forms a conical mass converging toward the nipple and is surrounded by adipose tissue. SYN corpus mammae [TA], b. of mammary gland.

Cabot ring b.'s, ring-shaped or figure-of-eight structures that stain red with Wright stain, found in red blood cells in severe anemias, possibly a remnant of the nuclear membrane; a form of basophilic degenerative process.

Call-Exner b.'s, small fluid-filled spaces between granulosal cells in ovarian follicles and in ovarian granulosa cell tumors; they may form a rosettelike structure.

carotid b. [TA], a small epithelioid structure located just above the bifurcation of the common carotid artery on each side. It consists of granular principal cells and nongranular supporting cells, a sinusoidal vascular bed, and a rich network of sensory fibers of the glossopharyngeal nerve. It serves as a chemoreceptor organ responsive to oxygen lack, carbon dioxide excess, and increased hydrogen ion concentration. SYN glomus caroticum [TA], intercarotid b., nodulus caroticus.

b. of caudate nucleus [TA], the suprathalamic part of the caudate nucleus lying in the floor of the central part (the body) of the lateral ventricle. SYN corpus nuclei caudati [TA].

cavernous b.'s of anal canal, SYN anal *cushions,* under *cushion.*

cavernous b. of clitoris, SYN *corpus* cavernosum of clitoris.

cavernous b. of penis, SYN *corpus* cavernosum penis.

cell b., the part of the cell containing the nucleus.

central b., SYN cytocentrum.

central fibrous b., the fibrous area where the leaflets of the aortic, mitral, and tricuspid valves meet in the heart.

chromaffin b., SYN paraganglion.

chromatin b., the genetic apparatus of bacteria. SEE nucleus (2).

ciliary b. [TA], a thickened portion of the vascular tunic of the eye between the choroid and the iris; it consists of three parts or zones; orbiculus ciliaris, corona ciliaris, and ciliary muscle. SYN corpus ciliare [TA], anulus ciliaris.

Civatte b.'s, eosinophilic hyaline spherical b.'s seen in the epidermis, in lichen planus and other skin disorders; formed by apoptosis of individual basal cells. SYN colloid b.'s.

b. of clavicle, ⭐ official alternate term for *shaft* of clavicle.

b. of clitoris [TA], the shaft or pendulous portion of the clitoris, composed of two fused corpora cavernosa clitoridae, the distal end of which is the glans clitoris. SYN corpus clitoridis [TA].

coccygeal b. [TA], an arteriovenous (arteriolovenular) anastomosis supplied by the middle sacral artery and located on the pelvic surface of the coccyx. It was formerly called a gland (of Luschka) or a glomus and included with the paraganglia. SYN corpus coccygeum [TA], arteriococcygeal gland, coccygeal gland, glomus coccygeum.

colloid b.'s, SYN Civatte b.'s.

compressible cavernous b.'s, submucous venous plexuses found at the level of the pharyngoesophageal junction and anal canal, which assist in reducing or obliterating the lumen.

conchoidal b.'s, SYN Schaumann b.'s.

b. of corpus callosum, ✩official alternate term for *trunk* of corpus callosum.

Councilman b., Councilman hyaline b., an eosinophilic globule, seen in the liver in yellow fever, derived from apoptosis of a single hepatic cell.

Cowdry type A inclusion b.'s, dropletlike masses of acidophilic material surrounded by clear halos within nuclei, with margination of chromatin on the nuclear membrane as seen in human herpesvirus–infected cells.

Cowdry type B inclusion b.'s, obsolete term for dropletlike masses of acidophilic material surrounded by clear halos within nuclei, without other nuclear changes during early stages of development of the inclusion as seen in poliomyelitis.

creola b.'s, large compact clusters of ciliated columnar cells found in the sputum of some asthmatic patients.

cyanobacteriumlike b.'s, SYN *Cyclospora.*

cytoid b.'s, swollen retinal nerve fibers that on light microscopy look like cells when cut transversely; histopathologic correlative of retinal cotton-wool patches.

cytoplasmic inclusion b.'s, SEE inclusion b.'s.

Deetjen b.'s, obsolete term for platelet.

demilune b., a circular b. of extreme transparency except for a crescentic punctate substance on one edge which contains hemoglobin. The b. is much larger than a red blood cell, but is thought possibly to be a degenerated red blood cell swollen by imbibition; it has been found in malaria and in convalescence from typhoid fever; the transparent portion is called the glass b.

dense b.'s, granules in the central granulomere of blood platelets that take up and store serotonin from plasma. Electron-dense b.'s containing α-actinin in the cytoplasm of smooth muscle cells associated with the cell membrane are believed to be homologous to the Z-lines of striated muscle.

Döhle b.'s, discrete round or oval b.'s ranging in diameter from just visible to 2 μm, which stain sky blue to gray blue with Romanowsky stains, found in neutrophils of patients with infections, burns, trauma, pregnancy, or cancer. SYN Döhle inclusions, leukocyte inclusions.

Donovan b.'s, clusters of blue or black staining, bipolar chromatin condensations in large mononuclear cells in granulation tissue infected with *Calymmatobacterium granulomatis.*

Ehrlich inner b., a round oxyphil b. found in the red blood cell in case of hemocytolysis due to a specific blood poison. SYN Heinz-Ehrlich b.

elementary b.'s, (1) (E.B., EB), old term for virions, especially the largest virus particles, visible by light microscopy when stained; as in lesions of smallpox, vaccinia; **(2)** SYN platelet.

b. of epididymis [TA], the middle part that extends downward from the head to the tail of the epididymis on the posterior surface of the testis. SYN corpus epididymidis [TA].

epithelial b., SYN parathyroid *gland.*

fat b., ✩official alternate term for fat-pad.

fat b. of cheek, SYN buccal *fat-pad.*

fat b. of ischioanal fossa [TA], the fat within the ischiorectal fossa. SYN corpus adiposum fossae ischiorectalis, fat b. of ischiorectal fossa, ischiorectal fat-pad.

fat b. of ischiorectal fossa, SYN fat b. of ischioanal fossa.

fat b. of orbit, SYN retrobulbar *fat.*

b. of femur, ✩official alternate term for *shaft* of femur.

ferruginous b.'s, in the lungs, foreign inorganic or organic fibers coated by complexes of hemosiderin and glycoproteins, and believed to be formed by macrophages that have phagocytized the fibers. SEE ALSO asbestos b.'s.

b. of fibula, ✩official alternate term for *shaft* of fibula.

foreign b., anything of material substance in the tissues or cavities of the b. that has been introduced there from without, and that is not rapidly absorbable.

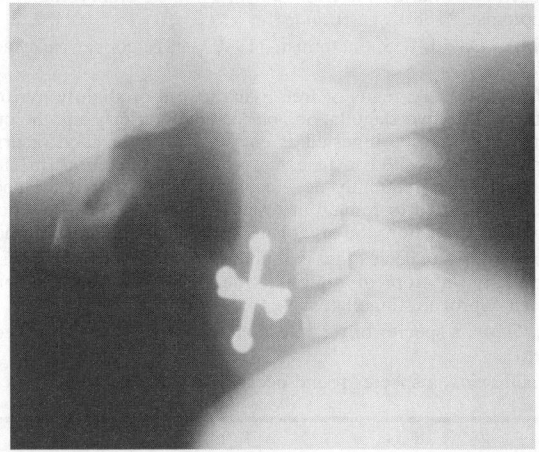

foreign body: radiograph of a 4-year-old child with a jack in cervical esophagus; lateral view of the neck shows the position of the pointed projections and the resulting tracheal compression

b. of fornix [TA], the middle part of the fornix situated ventral to the corpus callosum. SYN corpus fornicis [TA].

fruiting b., any fungal structure that bears spores.

fuchsin b.'s, (1) SYN Russell b.'s; **(2)** SYN hyaline b.'s.

b. of gallbladder [TA], the main part of the gallbladder terminating in the rounded fundus below and continuing into the neck of the gallbladder above. SYN corpus vesicae biliaris [TA], corpus vesicae felleae✩.

Gamna-Favre b.'s, characteristic, relatively large, intracytoplasmic basophilic inclusion b.'s observed in endothelial cells in lymphogranuloma venereum; probably composed of degenerated nuclear material. SEE ALSO Miyagawa b.'s.

Gamna-Gandy b.'s, small firm spheroidal or irregular foci that are yellow-brown, brown, or rusted color, occurring chiefly in the spleen in such conditions as congestive splenomegaly and sickle cell disease, and consisting of relatively dense fibrous tissue or collagenous fibers impregnated with iron pigment and calcium salts; probably result from organization and scarring of sites where small perivascular hemorrhages occurred. SYN Gamna-Gandy nodules, Gandy-Gamna b.'s, siderotic nodules.

Gandy-Gamna b.'s, SYN Gamna-Gandy b.'s.

geniculate b., SEE lateral geniculate b., medial geniculate b.

glass b., SEE demilune b.

glomus b., SYN glomus (2).

Golgi b., SYN Golgi *apparatus.*

Guarnieri b.'s, intracytoplasmic acidophilic inclusion b.'s observed in epithelial cells in variola (smallpox) and vaccinia infections, and which include aggregations of Paschen b.'s or virus particles.

Halberstaedter-Prowazek b.'s, SYN trachoma b.'s.

Hassall b.'s, SYN thymic *corpuscle.*

Hassall-Henle b.'s, hyaline b.'s on the posterior surface of Descemet membrane at the periphery of the cornea. SYN Henle warts.

Heinz b.'s, intracellular inclusions usually attached to the red cell membrane, composed of denatured hemoglobin; they occur in thalassemia, enzymopathies, hemoglobinopathies, and after splenectomy. Visualization of these usually requires examination of red cells using supravital stains or by phase microscopy.

Heinz-Ehrlich b., SYN Ehrlich inner b.

hematoxylin b.'s, hematoxyphil b.'s, poorly defined, homogeneous basophilic remnants of whole nuclei, an occasional finding in the fixed tissues of patients with systemic lupus erythematosus, but observed more frequently in the renal glomeruli and the walls of blood vessels, and probably related to the LE phenomenon; so named because of their affinity for hematoxylin stain.

Herring b.'s, accumulations of neurosecretory granules in dilated terminal endings of axons in the neurohypophysis.

Highmore b., SYN *mediastinum* of testis.

Howell-Jolly b.'s, spherical or ovoid eccentrically located granules, approximately 1 μm in diameter, occasionally observed in the stroma of circulating erythrocytes, especially in stained preparations (as compared with wet unstained films); probably represent nuclear remnants, inasmuch as they can be stained with dyes that are rather specific for chromatin; the significance of the b.'s is not exactly known; they occur most frequently after splenectomy or in megaloblastic or severe hemolytic anemia. SYN Jolly b.'s.

b. of humerus, ⁎official alternate term for *shaft* of humerus.

hyaline b.'s, homogeneous eosinophilic inclusions in the cytoplasm of epithelial cells; in renal tubules, hyaline b.'s represent droplets of protein reabsorbed from the lumen. SEE ALSO Mallory b.'s, drusen. SYN fuchsin b.'s (2).

hyaline b.'s of pituitary, accumulations of a gelatinous neurosecretory substance in the axons of the hypothalamohypophyseal tract in the posterior lobe of the hypophysis.

hyaloid b., SYN vitreous b.

b. of hyoid bone [TA], the body of the hyoid bone, from which the greater and lesser horns extend. SYN corpus ossis hyoidei [TA], base of hyoid bone, basihyal, basihyoid.

b. of ilium [TA], it forms the upper two-fifths of the acetabulum and joins the pubis and ischium in the acetabulum. It continues above into the ala or wing of the ilium. SYN corpus ossis ilii [TA].

inclusion b.'s, distinctive structures frequently formed in the nucleus or cytoplasm (occasionally in both locations) in cells infected with certain filtrable viruses; may be demonstrated by means of various stains, especially Mann eosin methylene blue or Giemsa techniques and visible by light microscopy. Nuclear inclusion b.'s are usually acidophilic and are of two morphologic types: 1) granular, hyaline, or amorphous b.'s of various sizes, i.e., Cowdry type A inclusion b.'s, occurring in such diseases as herpes simplex infection or yellow fever; 2) more circumscribed b.'s, frequently with several in the same nucleus (and no reaction in adjacent tissue), i.e., the type B b.'s, occurring in such diseases as Rift Valley fever and poliomyelitis. Cytoplasmic inclusion b.'s may be: 1) acidophilic, relatively large, spherical or ovoid, and somewhat granular, as in variola or vaccinia, rabies, and molluscum contagiosum; 2) basophilic, relatively large, complex combinations of viral and cellular material, as in trachoma, psittacosis, and lymphogranuloma venereum. In some instances, inclusion b.'s are known to be infective and probably represent aggregates of virus particles in combination with cellular material, whereas others are apparently not infective and may represent only abnormal products formed by the cell in response to injury.

b. of incus [TA], the main part of the incus that articulates with the malleus and from which the short and long limbs arise. SYN corpus incudis [TA].

infrapatellar fat b., SYN infrapatellar *fat-pad*.

intercarotid b., SYN carotid b.

intermediate b. of Flemming, SYN midbody.

b. of ischium [TA], the entire ischium with the exception of the ramus. SYN corpus ossis ischii [TA].

Jaworski b.'s, mucous shreds in the gastric contents in hyperchlorhydria.

Jolly b.'s, SYN Howell-Jolly b.'s.

juxtaglomerular b., a collection of modified smooth muscle cells around the renal glomerular arterioles that contain cytoplasmic granules, probably composed of renin. SYN periarterial pad.

juxtarestiform b. [TA], a medial (smaller) subdivision of the

inferior cerebellar peduncle composed of fibers reciprocally connecting the vestibular nuclei with the cerebellum, in particular the latter's nodulus, flocculus, and uvula vermis. It also carries primary sensory fibers from the vestibular ganglia to the cerebellum, as well as cerebellar projections to the rhombencephalic reticular formation and vestibular nuclei. SYN corpus juxtarestiforme.

ketone b., one of a group of ketones that includes acetoacetic acid, its reduction product, β-hydroxybutyric acid, and its decarboxylation product, acetone; high levels are found in tissues and body fluids in ketosis. SYN acetone b., acetone compound.

Lafora b. [MIM*254780], an autosomal recessive disorder characterized by intraneural intracytoplasmic inclusion b. composed of acid mucopolysaccharides, seen in familial myoclonic epilepsy.

Lallemand b.'s, (1) old term for small gelatinoid concretions sometimes observed in seminal fluid; (2) old term for Bence Jones *cylinders*, under *cylinder*. SYN Trousseau-Lallemand b.'s.

lateral geniculate b., the lateral of a pair of small oval masses that protrude slightly from the posteroinferior aspect of the thalamus; commonly considered a part of the metathalamus. SYN corpus geniculatum laterale [TA], corpus geniculatum externum.

b. of lateral ventricle, SYN *pars* centralis ventriculi lateralis.

L-D b., SYN Leishman-Donovan b.

LE b., the amorphous round b. in the cytoplasm of an LE cell.

Leishman-Donovan b., the intracytoplasmic, nonflagellated leishmanial form of certain intracellular parasites, such as species of *Leishmania* or the intracellular form of *Trypanosoma cruzi*; originally used for *Leishmania donovani* parasites in infected spleen or liver cells in kala azar. SYN amastigote, L-D b.

Lewy b.'s, intracytoplasmic neuronal inclusion; b.'s especially noted in pigmented brainstem neurons and seen in Parkinson disease.

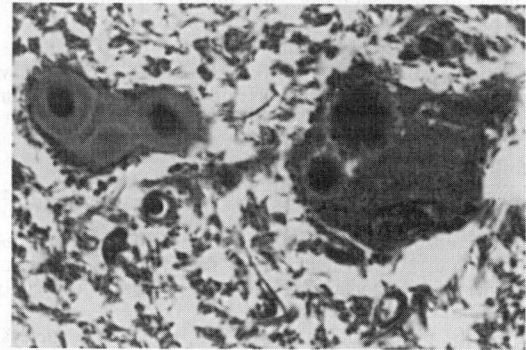

Lewy bodies: seen in two neurons with prominent central core and halo; hematoxylin and eosin, original magnification ×1000

Lieutaud b., SYN *trigone* of bladder.

Lindner b.'s, initial b.'s resembling inclusion b.'s found in scrapings of epithelial cells infected with trachoma.

loose b., a solid tissue fragment lying free in a body cavity, especially in a joint or the peritoneal cavity; e.g., joint mice, melon-seed b., rice b.

Luse b.'s, collagen fibers with abnormally long spacing (exceeding 1000 Å) between electron-dense bands.

Luys b., SYN subthalamic *nucleus*.

Mallory b.'s, large, poorly defined accumulations of eosinophilic material in the cytoplasm of damaged hepatic cells in certain forms of cirrhosis especially those due to alcoholism. SYN alcoholic hyalin, alcoholic hyaline b.'s.

malpighian b.'s, SYN splenic lymph *follicles*, under *follicle*.

b. of mammary gland, SYN b. of breast.

mammillary b. [TA], a small, round, paired cell group that protrudes into the interpeduncular fossa from the inferior aspect of the hypothalamus. It receives hippocampal fibers through the fornix and projects fibers to the anterior thalamic nuclei and into the brainstem tegmentum. SYN corpus mammillare [TA], mammillary tubercle of hypothalamus.

b. of mandible [TA], the heavy, U-shaped, horizontal portion of the mandible extending posteriorly to the angle where it is continuous with the ramus; it supports the lower teeth. SYN corpus mandibulae [TA].

b. of maxilla [TA], the central portion of the maxilla hollowed out by the maxillary sinus; it presents orbital, nasal, anterior, and infratemporal surfaces and supports four processes, frontal, zygomatic, palatine, and alveolar. SYN corpus maxillae [TA].

medial geniculate b., the medial one of a pair of small masses that protrude from the posteroinferior part of the thalamus; commonly considered a part of the metathalamus. SYN corpus geniculatum mediale [TA], corpus geniculatum internum.

melon-seed b., a small fibrous loose b. in a joint or tendon sheath.

b. of metacarpal, ✩official alternate term for *shaft* of metacarpal.

metachromatic b.'s, concentrated deposits consisting primarily of polymetaphosphate and occurring in many bacteria as well as in algae, fungi, and protozoa; m. b.'s differ in staining properties from the surrounding protoplasm. SEE metachromasia.

b. of metatarsal, ✩official alternate term for *shaft* of metatarsal.

Michaelis-Gutmann b., a rounded homogeneous or concentrically laminated b., 1 to 10 μ in diameter, containing calcium and iron; found within macrophages in malakoplakia.

Miyagawa b.'s, an obsolete term for *Chlamydia trachomatis* (*Miyagawanella lymphogranulomatosis*), the elementary b.'s that develop in the intracytoplasmic microcolonies of lymphogranuloma venereum.

molluscum b., a distinctive cytoplasmic spherical b. in the lesions of molluscum contagiosum caused by a member of the family Poxviridae; it consists of degenerated cytoplasm and the virus. SYN molluscum corpuscle.

Mooser b.'s, a term used to refer to the rickettsiae found in the exudate (and in tissue) from the tunica vaginalis in endemic typhus fever (caused by *Rickettsia typhi*).

multilamellar b., SYN cytosome (2).

multivesicular b.'s, membrane-bound b.'s, 0.5 to 1.0 μm wide, that occur in the cytoplasm of cells and contain a number of small vesicles; hydrolases (especially acid phosphatase) occur in the matrix.

myelin b., SYN myelin *figure*.

b. of nail [TA], the exposed portion of the nail distal to its root. SYN corpus unguis [TA].

Negri b.'s, eosinophilic, sharply outlined, pathognomonic inclusion b.'s (2 to 10 μm in diameter) found in the cytoplasm of certain nerve cells containing the virus of rabies, especially in Ammon horn of the hippocampus.

nerve cell b., the part of the neuron that includes the nucleus but excludes the processes.

neuroepithelial b., a corpuscular aggregate of highly innervated nonciliated cells containing neurosecretory substance found in normal intrapulmonary epithelium primarily at the bifurcations of bronchi.

Nissl b.'s, SYN Nissl *substance*.

nodular b., in fungi, a compact, roughly spherical or squarish structure formed by coiling and twisting of the end of a hypha; considered to be abortive growths toward sexual reproduction.

nu b., SYN nucleosome.

nuclear inclusion b.'s, SEE inclusion b.'s.

Odland b., SYN keratinosome.

olivary b., SYN oliva.

orbital fat b., ✩official alternate term for retrobulbar *fat*.

pacchionian b.'s, SYN arachnoid *granulations*, under *granulation*.

pampiniform b., SYN epoophoron.

b. of pancreas [TA], the part of the pancreas from the point where it crosses the portal vein to the point where it enters the lienorenal ligament. SYN corpus pancreatis [TA].

Pappenheimer b.'s, phagosomes, containing ferruginous granules, found in red blood cells in diseases such as sideroblastic anemia, hemolytic anemia, and sickle cell disease; may contribute to spurious platelet counts by electro-optical counters.

paraaortic b.'s [TA], small masses of chromaffin tissue found near the sympathetic ganglia along the aorta; they are more prom-inent during fetal life. The chromaffin cells secrete noradrenalin; chemoreceptive endings monitor levels of blood gases. SYN corpora para-aortica [TA], glomus aorticum [TA], aortic glomera✩, glomera aortica✩, aortic b.'s, corpus aorticum, organs of Zuckerkandl, Zuckerkandl b.'s.

parabasal b., a term formerly equivalent to the DNA kinetoplast, part of the giant mitochondrion of certain parasitic flagellates. The parabasal b. plus the basal b. were previously thought to comprise a kinetoplast, or locomotory apparatus, but kinetoplast is now restricted to part of the DNA giant mitochondrion and parabasal b. is a distinct structure near the nucleus, probably equivalent to the metazoan Golgi apparatus.

paranephric b., a mass of fat lying behind the renal fascia.

paranuclear b., SYN astrosphere.

paraphysial b., SYN paraphysis.

paraterminal b., SYN subcallosal *gyrus*.

Paschen b.'s, particles of virus observed in relatively large numbers in squamous cells of the skin (or the cornea of experimental animals) in variola (smallpox) or vaccinia.

b. of penis [TA], the free pendulous portion of the penis, consisting of shaft and glans penis. SYN corpus penis [TA], scapus penis.

perineal b., SYN central *tendon* of perineum.

b. of phalanx, ✩official alternate term for *shaft* of phalanx.

Pick b.'s, intracytoplasmic argentophilic neuronal inclusion b.'s seen in Pick disease.

pineal b. [TA], a small, unpaired, flattened body, shaped somewhat like a pine cone, attached at its anterior pole to the region of the posterior and habenular commissures, and lying in the depression between the two superior colliculi below the splenium of the corpus callosum; it is a glandular structure, composed of follicles containing epithelioid cells and lime concretions called brain sand; despite its attachment to the brain, it appears to receive nerve fibers exclusively from the peripheral autonomic nervous system. It produces melatonin. SYN corpus pineale [TA], glandula pinealis [TA], pineal gland [TA], conarium, epiphysis cerebri, pinus.

polar b., one of two small cells formed by the first and second meiotic division of oocytes; the first is usually released just prior to ovulation, the second not until discharge of the ovum from the ovary; in mammals, the second polar b. may fail to form unless the ovum has been penetrated by a sperm cell. SYN polar cell, polar globule, polocyte.

polyhedral b., an inclusion b. associated with replication of certain insect viruses.

pontobulbar b., a collection of nerve cells in the lower part of the medulla oblongata forming a ridge which crosses the restiform body obliquely. SYN corpus pontobulbare.

posterior quadrigeminal b., SYN inferior *colliculus*.

Prowazek b.'s, historic term for either of two types of inclusion b.'s associated with certain diseases: 1) trachoma b.'s; 2) tiny, ovoid, granular forms, frequently in pairs, observed in the cytoplasm and in Guarnieri b.'s in the cutaneous squamous cells of humans and animals infected with variola (smallpox) or vaccinia virus; probably the same as Paschen b.'s.

Prowazek-Greeff b.'s, SYN trachoma b.'s.

psammoma b.'s, (1) mineralized b.'s occurring in the meninges, choroid plexus, and in certain meningiomas; composed usually of a central capillary surrounded by concentric whorls of meningocytes in various stages of hyaline change and mineralization; can also occur in benign and malignant epithelial tumors (such as papillary ovarian or thyroid carcinoma); SYN sand b.'s. **(2)** SYN *corpora* arenacea, under *corpus*; **(3)** SYN calcospherite.

psittacosis inclusion b.'s, intracytoplasmic chlamydial microcolonies observed in bronchial epithelial cells infected with *Chlamydia psittaci*.

pubic b., b. of pubic bone, SYN b. of pubis.

b. of pubis [TA], the flattened medial portion of the pubic bone entering into the pubic symphysis. From it extend the superior and inferior rami. SYN corpus ossis pubis [TA], pubic b., b. of pubic bone.

purine b.'s, any purine.

quadrigeminal b.'s, SEE inferior *colliculus,* superior *colliculus.* SYN corpora quadrigemina.

b. of radius, ☆official alternate term for *shaft* of radius.

Renaut b., subperineurial structure comprised of loosely arranged and randomly oriented collagen fibers in a fine fibrillary material, seen in normal nerve as well as in certain pathologic states.

residual b., a cytoplasmic vacuole (lysosome) containing accumulated particulate products of metabolism, e.g., lipofuscin.

residual b. of Regaud, the excess cytoplasm that separates from the spermatozoon during spermiogenesis.

rest b., a small mass of cytoplasm remaining after the nucleus and cytoplasm of the schizont of certain sporozoan protozoa have divided into asexual spores or merozoites.

restiform b. [TA], a lateral (larger) subdivision of the inferior cerebellar peduncle located on the dorsolateral aspect of the medulla oblongata and composed of a variety of fibers including, but not limited to, olivo-, reticulo-, cuneo-, trigemino-, and dorsal spinocerebellar. SEE ALSO inferior cerebellar *peduncle.* SYN corpus restiforme [TA], eminentia restiformis, restiform eminence.

b. of rib [TA], the shaft of a rib; the portion that extends laterally, anteriorly, and then medially from the tubercle. SYN corpus costae [TA].

rice b., one of the small, loose b.'s found in hygromas, tendon sheaths, and joints; usually one of many small loose b.'s.

Rushton b., linear or curved hyaline bodies, presumably of hematogenous origin, found within the epithelial lining of odontogenic cysts.

Russell b.'s, small, discrete, variably sized, spherical, intracytoplasmic, acidophilic, hyaline b.'s that stain deeply with fuchsin; they occur in plasma cells in chronic inflammation and malignant disorders, and consist of immunoglobulin. SYN fuchsin b.'s (1).

sand b.'s, SYN psammoma b.'s (1).

Sandström b.'s, SEE parathyroid *gland.*

Savage perineal b., SYN central *tendon* of perineum.

Schaumann b.'s, concentrically laminated calcified b.'s found in granulomas, particularly in sarcoidosis. SYN conchoidal b.'s.

sclerotic b.'s, vegetative rounded muriform cells of dematiaceous fungi, characteristic of the causal agents of chromoblastomycosis in tissue. SYN copper pennies.

segmenting b., SYN schizont.

b. of sphenoid [TA], the central portion of the sphenoid bone from which the greater and lesser wings and the pterygoid processes arise. The sphenoidal sinuses lie within it. SYN corpus ossis sphenoidalis.

spongy b. of penis, SYN *corpus* spongiosum penis.

b. of sternum [TA], the middle and largest portion of the sternum, lying between the manubrium superiorly and the xiphoid process inferiorly. SYN corpus sterni [TA], gladiolus, mesosternum, midsternum.

b. of stomach [TA], the part of the stomach that lies between the fundus above and the pyloric antrum below; its boundaries are poorly defined. SYN corpus gastricum [TA].

striate b., the caudate and lentiform (lenticular) nuclei; the striate appearance on section is caused by slender fascicles of myelinated fibers. Histologically, the striate b. can be subdivided into the generally small-celled striatum, consisting of the caudate nucleus and the outer segment of the lentiform nucleus (the putamen), and a large-celled globus pallidus composed of the two segments. SYN corpus striatum [TA].

suprarenal b., SYN suprarenal *gland.*

b. of sweat gland, the coiled tubular secretory portion of a sweat gland located in the subcutaneous tissue or deep in the corium and connected to the surface of the skin by a long duct. SYN corpus glandulae sudoriferae.

Symington anococcygeal b., SYN anococcygeal *ligament.*

b. of talus [TA], the large posterior part of the talus forming the trochlea above for articulation with the tibia and fibula and articulating below with the calcaneus. SYN corpus tali [TA].

b. of thigh bone, SYN *shaft* of femur.

threshold b., SYN threshold *substance.*

thyroid b., SYN thyroid *gland.*

b. of tibia, ☆official alternate term for *shaft* of tibia.

tigroid b.'s, SYN Nissl *substance.*

b. of tongue [TA], the oral part of the tongue anterior to the terminal sulcus. SYN corpus linguae [TA].

trachoma b.'s, distinctive, complex, intracytoplasmic forms found in the conjunctival epithelial cells of persons in the acute phase of trachoma, less frequently in later stages, varying from 1) discrete acidophilic granules (approximately 250 nm in diameter), to 2) irregular clumps of such material embedded in a basophilic matrix, to 3) relatively large basophilic b.'s (approximately 700–1000 nm in diameter), to 4) large basophilic b.'s that include discrete, tiny, acidophilic granules. SYN Halberstaedter-Prowazek b.'s, Prowazek-Greeff b.'s.

trapezoid b. [TA], a plate of transverse fibers running over the dorsal (deep) border of the pontine nuclei; it is formed by ascending auditory fibers that cross to the opposite side of the brainstem. SYN corpus trapezoideum [TA], trapezoid (4) [TA].

Trousseau-Lallemand b.'s, SYN Lallemand b.'s.

tuffstone b., membrane-bound electron-dense granules, measuring about 0.5 μm in diameter, found primarily in Schwann cells of patients suffering from metachromatic leukodystrophy; the name alludes to their resemblance to volcanic limestone.

turbinated b., (1) a concha with its covering of mucous membrane and other soft parts; SYN turbinal. (2) SYN inferior nasal *concha,* middle nasal *concha,* superior nasal *concha,* supreme nasal *concha.*

tympanic b., SYN tympanic *gland.*

b. of ulna, ☆official alternate term for *shaft* of ulna.

ultimobranchial b., a diverticulum from the fourth pharyngeal pouch of an embryo, regarded by some as a rudimentary fifth pharyngeal pouch and by others as a lateral thyroid primordium; the ultimobranchial b.'s of lower vertebrates contain large amounts of calcitonin; in mammals, the ultimobranchial b.'s fuse with the thyroid gland and are thought to develop into the parafollicular cells. SEE ALSO ultimobranchial *pouch.*

b. of uterus [TA], the part of the uterus above the isthmus, comprising about two-thirds of the nonpregnant organ. SYN corpus uteri [TA].

vaccine b.'s, old term pertaining to intracellular b.'s that were erroneously thought to be forms in the life cycle of a protozoan organism, *Cytorhyctes vaccinae,* postulated to be the causal agent of vaccinia.

Verocay b.'s, hyalinized acellular areas composed of reduplicated basement membrane outlined by opposing rows of parallel nuclei; seen microscopically in neurilemomas.

b. of vertebra, SYN vertebral b.

vertebral b. [TA], the main portion of a vertebra anterior to the vertebral canal, as distinct from the arches. SYN corpus vertebrae [TA], b. of vertebra.

Virchow-Hassall b.'s, SYN thymic *corpuscle.*

vitreous b. [TA], a transparent jellylike substance filling the interior of the eyeball behind the lens of the eye; it is composed of a delicate network (vitreous stroma) enclosing in its meshes a watery fluid (vitreous humor). SYN corpus vitreum [TA], hyaloid b., vitreous (2), vitreum.

Weibel-Palade b.'s, rod-shaped bundles of microtubules seen by electron microscopy in vascular endothelial cells.

wolffian b., SYN mesonephros.

Wolf-Orton b.'s, intranuclear inclusion b.'s seen in cells of malignant neoplasms, especially those of glial cell origin.

Y b., a single fluorescent spot originating in the long arm of the Y chromosome and visible in somatic nuclei of buccal smears.

yellow b., SYN *corpus* luteum.

zebra b., metachromatically staining membrane-bound granules, measuring 0.5–1 μm in diameter and containing lamellae with a 5.8 nm spacing, reported in Schwann cells and macrophages of patients suffering from metachromatic leukodystrophy.

Zuckerkandl b.'s, SYN paraaortic b.'s.

body bur·den. Activity of a radiopharmaceutical retained by the body at a specified time following administration.

Boeck, Caesar P.M., Norwegian dermatologist, 1845–1917. SEE B. *disease, sarcoid;* Besnier-B.-Schaumann *disease, syndrome.*

Boeck, Carl W., Norwegian physician, 1808–1875. SEE Danielssen-B. *disease.*

Boehmer, F. SEE B. *hematoxylin.*

Boerhaave, Hermann, Dutch physician, 1668–1738. SEE B. *syndrome.*

bog·bean (bog′bēn). SYN buckbean.

Bogros, Antoine, 19th century French anatomist. SEE B. *serous membrane.*

Bogros, Jean-Annet, French anatomist, 1786–1823. SEE B. *space.*

Bohn, Heinrich, German physician, 1832–1888. SEE B. *nodules,* under *nodule.*

Bohr, Christian, Danish physiologist, 1855–1911. SEE B. *effect, equation.*

Bohr, Niels H.D., Danish physicist and Nobel laureate, 1885–1962. SEE B. *atom, magneton, theory.*

boil (boyl). SYN furuncle. [A.S. *byl,* a swelling]

  Aleppo b., Bagdad b., the lesion occurring in cutaneous leishmaniasis. SEE cutaneous *leishmaniasis.* SYN Biskra b.

  Biskra b., SYN Aleppo b.

  blind b., a furuncle that does not have a fluctuant central point; it appears as a dull red painful papule.

  date b., Delhi b., Jericho b., the lesion occurring in cutaneous leishmaniasis.

  Madura b., SYN mycetoma.

  Oriental b., the lesion occurring in cutaneous leishmaniasis.

  salt water b.'s, furuncles on hands and forearms of fishermen.

  tropical b., the lesion occurring in cutaneous leishmaniasis.

bol Abbreviation for bolus.

bol·din (bol′din). A glycoside from boldus; a cholagogue and diuretic. SYN boldoglucin.

bol·dine (bol′dēn). A bitter alkaloid obtained from boldus.

boldine dimethyl ether. SYN glaucine.

bol·do (bol′dō). SYN boldus.

bol·do·glu·cin (bol-dō-gloo′sin). SYN boldin.

bol·dus (bol′dŭs). The leaves of *Boldu boldus* or *Peumus boldus* (family Monimiaceae), an evergreen shrub of Chile; used in various disturbances of liver function. SYN boldo. [Chilean]

Boley gauge. See under gauge.

Boll, Franz C., German histologist and physiologist, 1849–1879. SEE B. *cells,* under *cell.*

Bollinger, Otto, German pathologist, 1843–1909. SEE B. *granules,* under *granule.*

Bollman, Jesse L., U.S. physiologist, *1896. SEE Mann-B. *fistula.*

Bolognini symp·tom. See under symptom.

bo·lom·e·ter (bō-lom′ĕ-ter). **1.** An instrument for determining minute degrees of radiant heat. **2.** An obsolete instrument for measuring the force of the heartbeat as distinguished from the blood pressure. [G. *bolē,* a throw, a sunbeam, + *metron,* measure]

bo·lus (bol) (bō′lŭs). **1.** A single, relatively large quantity of a substance, usually one intended for therapeutic use, such as a b. dose of a drug injected intravenously. **2.** A masticated morsel of food or another substance ready to be swallowed, such as a b. of barium for x-ray studies. **3.** In high-energy radiation therapy, a quantity of tissue-equivalent material placed in the radiation beam, over the surface of the irradiated region, to increase the absorbed dose in the superficial tissues. [L. fr. G. *bōlos,* lump, clod]

  intravenous b., a relatively large volume of fluid or dose of a drug or test substance given intravenously and rapidly to hasten or magnify a response; in radiology, rapid injection of a large dose of contrast medium to increase opacification of blood vessels.

bom·bard. To expose a substance to particulate or electromagnetic radiations for the purpose of making it radioactive. [Mediev. L. *bombarda,* artillery assault, fr. *bombus,* a booming sound]

bom·be·sin (bomb′ĕ-sin). Pharmacologically active tetradecapeptide found in skins of European amphibians of the family Discoglossidae, principally *Bombina bombina* and *Bombina variegata variegata.* A potent stimulant of gastric and pancreatic secretions; a bombesinlike immunoreactive peptide is found in both brain and gut. Other actions include hypertensive, antidiuretic, and hyperglycemic activity. Has a strong effect on core temperature lowering in rats. High levels of intracellular bombesin have also been found in human small-cell lung carcinoma.

bond (bond). In chemistry, the force holding two neighboring atoms in place and resisting their separation; a b. is electrovalent if it consists of the attraction between oppositely charged groups, or covalent if it results from the sharing of one, two, or three pairs of electrons by the bonded atoms.

  acylmercaptan b., –CO–S–; a "high-energy" b. formed by the condensation of a carboxyl group (–COOH) and a mercaptan (or thiol) group (–SH); widely formed in the course of intermediary metabolism, notably in the oxidation of fats, where the –SH is part of coenzyme A and the –COOH is part of the fatty acid being oxidized.

  apolar b., SEE hydrophobic *interaction.*

  conjugated double b.'s, two or more double b.'s separated by each single b.

  coordinate covalent b., SYN semipolar b.

  disulfide b., a single bond between two sulfurs; specifically, the –S–S– link binding two peptide chains (or different parts of one peptide chain); also occurs as part of the molecule of the amino acid, cystine, and is important as a structural determinant in many peptide and protein molecules, e.g., keratin, insulin, and oxytocin. A symmetric disulfide is R–S–S–R; R′–S–S–R is a mixed or asymmetric disulfide.

  double b., a covalent b. resulting from the sharing of two pairs of electrons, e.g., $H_2C=CH_2$ (ethylene).

  electrostatic b., b. between atoms or groups carrying opposite charges (or, in some cases, partial charges). SYN heteropolar b., salt bridge.

  energy-rich b., SEE high-energy *compounds,* under *compound.*

  eupeptide b., a peptide b. between the α-carboxyl group of one amino acid and the α-amino group of another amino acid. Cf. peptide b., isopeptide b.

  heteropolar b., SYN electrostatic b.

  high energy phosphate b., SEE high-energy *phosphates,* under *phosphate.*

  hydrogen b., a b. arising from the sharing of a hydrogen atom, covalently bound to a strongly electronegative element (e.g., N or O), with another strongly electronegative element (e.g., N, O, or a halogen). In substances of biologic importance, the most common hydrogen b.'s are those in which H links N to O or N; such b.'s link purines on one strand to pyrimidines on the other strand of nucleic acids, thus maintaining double-stranded structures as in the Watson-Crick helix.

  hydrophobic b., SEE hydrophobic *interaction.*

  isopeptide b., an amide linkage between a carboxyl group of one amino acid and an amino group of another amino acid in which at least one of these groups is not on the α-carbon of one of the amino acids; for example, the bond between the glutamyl residue and the cysteinyl residue of glutathione. Cf. peptide b., eupeptide b.

  noncovalent b., b. in which electrons are not shared between atoms; e.g., electrostatic b., hydrogen b.

  peptide b., the common link (–CO–NH–) between amino acids in proteins, actually a substituted amide, formed by elimination of H_2O between the –COOH of one amino acid and the $H_2N–$ of another. Cf. eupeptide b., isopeptide b.

  semipolar b., a b. in which the two electrons shared by a pair of atoms belonged originally to only one of the atoms; often represented by a small arrow pointing toward the electron receiver; e.g., nitric acid, $O(OH)N{\rightarrow}O$; phosphoric acid, $(OH)_3P{\rightarrow}O$. SYN coordinate covalent b.

  single b., a covalent b. resulting from the sharing of one pair of electrons; e.g., $H_3C–CH_3$ (ethane).

  triple b., a covalent b. resulting from the sharing of three pairs of electrons; e.g., $HC{\equiv}CH$ (acetylene).

bonding (bon′ding). Formation of a close and enduring emotional attachment, such as between parent and child, lovers, or husband and wife.

BONE

bone (bōn) [TA]. A hard connective tissue consisting of cells embedded in a matrix of mineralized ground substance and collagen fibers. The fibers are impregnated with a form of calcium phosphate similar to hydroxyapatite as well as with substantial quantities of carbonate, citrate sodium, and magnesium; by weight, b. is composed of 75% inorganic material and 25% organic material; a portion of osseous tissue of definite shape and size, forming a part of the animal skeleton; in humans there are 200 distinct b.'s in the skeleton, not including the auditory ossicles of the tympanic cavity or the sesamoid b.'s other than the two patellae. Bone consists of a dense outer layer of compact substance or cortical substance covered by the periosteum, and an inner loose, spongy substance; the central portion of a long bone is filled with marrow. SYN os [TA]. [A.S. *bān*]

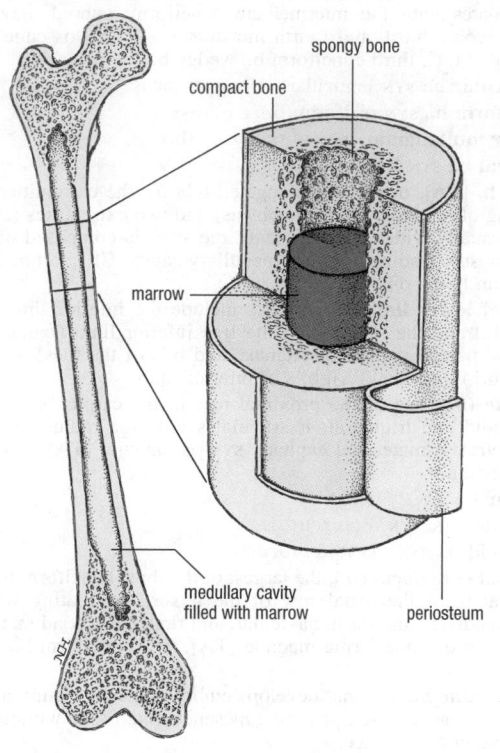

spongy bone

compact bone

marrow

medullary cavity
filled with marrow

periosteum

bone

Albrecht b., a small b. between the basioccipital and basisphenoid.

alveolar b., (1) SYN alveolar *process* of maxilla; **(2)** in dentistry, the specialized bony structure which supports the teeth; it consists of the cortical b. that comprises the tooth socket into which the roots of the tooth fit, and is supported by the trabecular b. SYN alveolar supporting b.

alveolar supporting b., SYN alveolar b. (2).

ankle b., SYN talus.

arm b., SYN humerus.

basal b., the osseus tissue of the mandible and maxillae except the alveolar processes.

basilar b., the developmental basilar process of the occipital b. that unites with the condylar portions in about the fourth or fifth

year, becoming the basilar *part* of occipital bone. SEE ALSO basilar *part* of occipital bone. SYN basioccipital b., os basilare.

basioccipital b., SYN basilar b.

basisphenoid b., in comparative anatomy, the b. in the floor of the brain case in the region of the pituitary. SEE *body* of sphenoid.

Bertin b.'s, SYN sphenoidal *conchae*, under *concha*.

blade b., SYN scapula.

breast b., SYN sternum.

Breschet b.'s, SYN suprasternal b.'s.

brittle b.'s, SYN *osteogenesis* imperfecta.

bundle b., immature b. containing thick bundles of collagen fibers arranged nearly parallel to one another with osteocytes in between; a similar type of b. is found in regions penetrated by fibers of Sharpey, as at ligament and tendon attachments.

calcaneal b., SYN calcaneus (1).

calf b., SYN fibula. [O.N. *kalfi*, fibula]

cancellous b., SYN *substantia* spongiosa.

capitate b., SYN capitate (1).

carpal b.'s [TA], eight b.'s arranged in two rows that articulate proximally with the radius and indirectly with the ulna, and distally with the five metacarpal b.'s; in domestic mammals, the b.'s of the proximal row are called radial, intermediate, ulnar, and accessory, while those of the distal row are termed first, second, third, and fourth carpal b.'s. SYN carpus (2) [TA], ossa carpi [TA].

cartilage b., SYN endochondral b.

central b., SYN *os* centrale.

central b. of ankle, SYN navicular.

cheek b., (1) SYN zygomatic b; **(2)** SYN zygomatic *arch*.

coccygeal b., SYN coccyx.

collar b., SYN clavicle.

compact b. [TA], the compact, noncancellous portion of b. that consists largely of concentric lamellar osteons and interstitial lamellae. SYN substantia compacta [TA], compact substance, substantia compacta ossium.

convoluted b., SEE inferior nasal *concha*, middle nasal *concha*, superior nasal *concha*, supreme nasal *concha*.

cortical b. [TA], the superficial thin layer of compact b. SYN substantia corticalis [TA], cortical substance.

coxal b., ☆official alternate term for hip b.

cranial b.'s, SYN b.'s of cranium.

b.'s of cranium [TA], the paired inferior nasal concha, lacrimal, maxilla, nasal, palatine, parietal, temporal, and zygomatic; and the unpaired ethmoid, frontal, occipital, sphenoid, and vomer. SYN ossa cranii [TA], b.'s of skull, cranial b.'s.

cubital b., SYN triquetrum.

cuboid (b.), the lateral b. of the distal row of the tarsus, articulating with the calcaneus, lateral cuneiform, navicular (occasionally), and fourth and fifth metatarsal b.'s. SYN os cuboideum.

cuneiform b., SEE triquetrum, intermediate cuneiform (b.), lateral cuneiform (b.), medial cuneiform (b.).

dermal b., a b. formed by ossification of the cutis.

b.'s of digits, the phalanges and sesamoid b.'s of the fingers and toes. SYN ossa digitorum ☆.

dorsal talonavicular b., an anomalous b. of the foot located near the head of the talus. SYN Pirie b.

ear b.'s, SYN auditory *ossicles*, under *ossicle*.

elbow b., SYN olecranon.

endochondral b., a b. that develops in a cartilage environment after the latter is partially or entirely destroyed by calcification and subsequent resorption. SYN cartilage b., replacement b.

epactal b.'s, SYN sutural b.'s.

epihyal b., an ossified stylomastoid ligament.

epipteric b., a sutural b. occasionally present at the pterion or junction of the parietal, frontal, greater wing of the sphenoid, and squamous portion of the temporal b.'s. SYN Flower b.

episternal b., SYN suprasternal b.'s.

ethmoid b. [TA], an irregularly shaped b. lying between the orbital plates of the frontal and anterior to the sphenoid; it consists of two lateral masses of thin plates enclosing air cells, attached above to a perforated horizontal lamina, the cribriform plate, from which descends a median vertical or perpendicular plate in the interval between the two lateral masses; the b. articulates with the sphenoid, frontal, maxillary, lacrimal, and palatine b.'s, the inferior nasal concha, and the vomer; it enters into the formation of the anterior cranial fossa, the orbits, and the nasal cavity.

exoccipital b. (eks-ok-sip′i-tăl), SYN lateral *part* of occipital bone.

facial b.'s, the b.'s surrounding the mouth and nose and contributing to the orbits; they are the paired maxillae, zygomatic, nasal, lacrimal, palatine, and inferior nasal conchae; and the unpaired ethmoid, vomer, mandible, and hyoid. SYN b.'s of visceral cranium, ossa faciei.

first cuneiform b., SYN medial cuneiform (b.).

flank b., SYN ilium.

flat b. [TA], a type of b. characterized by its thin, flattened shape, such as the scapula or certain of the cranial bones. SYN os planum [TA].

Flower b., SYN epipteric b.

b.'s of foot [TA], b.'s that collectively comprise the skeleton of the foot; includes tarsal b.'s, metatarsals (b.'s) [I–V], phalanges, and sesamoid b.'s. SYN ossa pedis [TA], foot b.'s.

foot b.'s, SYN b.'s of foot.

fourth turbinated b., SYN supreme nasal *concha.*

frontal b. [TA], the large single b. forming the forehead and the upper margin and roof of the orbit on either side; it articulates with the parietal, nasal, ethmoid, maxillary, and zygomatic b.'s, and with the lesser wings of the sphenoid. SYN os frontale [TA], coronale (1).

funny b., colloquial name for tip of olecranon.

Goethe b., SYN preinterparietal b.

greater multangular b., SYN trapezium b.

hamate (b.) [TA], the b. on the medial (ulnar) side of the distal row of the carpus; it articulates with the fourth and fifth metacarpal, triquetral, lunate, and capitate. SYN hamatum, hooked b., os hamatum, unciform b., unciforme, uncinatum.

heel b., SYN calcaneus (1).

heterotopic b.'s, b.'s that do not belong to the main skeleton but that regularly develop in certain organs, e.g., the heart, penis, clitoris, and snout of some animals.

highest turbinated b., SYN supreme nasal *concha.*

hip b. [TA], a large flat b. formed by the fusion of the ilium, ischium, and pubis (in the adult), constituting the lateral half of the pelvis; it articulates with its fellow anteriorly, with the sacrum posteriorly, and with the femur laterally. SYN os coxae [TA], coxal b.✳, pelvic b.✳, innominate b., os innominatum.

hollow b., SYN pneumatized b.

hooked b., SYN hamate (b.).

hyoid b., (1) a U-shaped bone lying between the mandible and the larynx, suspended from the styloid processes by slender stylohyoid ligaments; **(2)** SEE hyoid *apparatus.* SYN lingual b., os hyoideum, tongue b.

iliac b., SYN ilium.

incarial b., SYN interparietal b.

incisive b. [TA], the anterior and inner portion of the maxilla, which in the fetus and sometimes in the adult is a separate b.; the incisive suture runs from the incisive canal between the lateral incisor and the canine tooth; according to K. Albrecht, the incisive b. is further divided by a suture between the two incisor teeth on each side into two b.'s, the en dognathion and the mesognathion. SYN os incisivum [TA], premaxilla (1)✳, intermaxilla, intermaxillary b., os intermaxillare, os premaxillare, premaxillary b.

b.'s of inferior limb, SYN b.'s of lower limb.

inferior turbinated b., SYN inferior nasal *concha.*

innominate b., SYN hip b.

intermaxillary b., SYN incisive b.

intermediate cuneiform (b.) [TA], a b. of the distal row of the tarsus; it articulates with the medial and lateral cuneiform, navicular, and second metatarsal b.'s. SYN mesocuneiform, middle cuneiform b., os cuneiforme intermedium, second cuneiform b., wedge b.

interparietal b. [TA], the upper part of the squama of the occipi-

tal bone, developed in membrane instead of in cartilage as is the rest of the occipital, and occasionally (especially in ancient Peruvian skulls) existing as a separate bone, separated from the remainder of the occipital by the sutura mendosa. SYN os interparietale [TA], incarial b., os incae.

irregular b. [TA], one of a group of bones having peculiar or complex forms, e.g., vertebrae, many of the skull bones. SYN os irregulare [TA].

ischial b., SYN ischium.

jaw b., SYN mandible.

jugal b., SYN zygomatic b.

Krause b., small b. (secondary ossification center) in the triradiate cartilage between the ilium, the ischium, and the pubic b. in the growing acetabulum.

lacrimal b. [TA], an irregularly rectangular thin plate, forming part of the medial wall of the orbit behind the frontal process of the maxilla; it articulates with the inferior nasal concha, ethmoid, frontal, and maxillary bones. SYN os lacrimale [TA], os unguis.

lamellar b., the normal type of adult mammalian b., whether cancellous or compact, composed of parallel lamellae in the former and concentric lamellae in the latter; lamellar organization reflects a repeating pattern of collagen fibroarchitecture.

lateral cuneiform (b.) [TA], a b. of the distal row of the tarsus; it articulates with the intermediate cuneiform, cuboid, navicular, and second, third, and fourth metatarsal b.'s. SYN os cuneiforme laterale [TA], third cuneiform b., wedge b.

lenticular b., SYN lenticular *process* of incus.

lentiform b., SYN pisiform (b.).

lesser multangular b., SYN trapezoid (b.).

lingual b., SYN hyoid b.

long b. [TA], one of the elongated b.'s fof the extremities, consisting of a tubular shaft (diaphysis) and two extremities (epiphyses) usually wider than the shaft; the shaft is composed of compact b. surrounding a central medullary cavity. Cf. short b. SYN os longum [TA], pipe b.

b.'s of lower limb [TA], these include the inferior limb girdle (hip b.) and the skeleton of the free inferior limb (femur, tibia, fibula, patella, tarsus, metatarsus, and b.'s of the toes). SYN ossa membri inferioris [TA], b.'s of inferior limb.

lunate (b.), one of the proximal row in the carpus between the scaphoid and triquetral; it articulates with the radius, scaphoid, triquetral, hamate, and capitate. SYN os lunatum [TA], lunare, os intermedium.

malar b., SYN zygomatic b.

marble b.'s, SYN osteopetrosis.

mastoid b., SYN mastoid *process.*

medial cuneiform (b.), the largest of the three cuneiform b.'s, the medial b. of the distal row of the tarsus, articulating with the intermediate cuneiform, navicular, and first and second metatarsal b.'s. SYN os cuneiforme mediale [TA], first cuneiform b., wedge b.

membrane b., a b. that develops embryologically within a membrane of vascularized primitive mesenchymal tissue without prior formation of cartilage.

mesethmoid b., in comparative anatomy, the b. present in some species as the most anterior b. of the floor of the braincase.

metacarpal (b.'s) [I–V] [TA], five long b.'s (numbered I to V, beginning with the b. on the radial or thumb side) forming the skeleton of the metacarpus or palm; they articulate with the b.'s of the distal row of the carpus and with the five proximal phalanges. SYN ossa metacarpi [TA], ossa metacarpalia I–V.

metatarsal (b.'s) [I–V], the five long bones numbered I to V beginning with the bone on the medial side forming the skeleton of the anterior portion of the foot, articulating posteriorly with the three cuneiform and the cuboid bones, anteriorly with the five proximal phalanges. SYN ossa metatarsi [TA], ossa metatarsalia I–V.

middle cuneiform b., SYN intermediate cuneiform (b.).

middle turbinated b., SYN middle nasal *concha.*

multangular b., SEE trapezium, trapezoid (b.).

nasal b. [TA], an elongated rectangular b. which, with its fellow, forms the bridge of the nose; it articulates with the frontal bone superiorly, the ethmoid and the frontal process of the maxilla posteriorly, and its fellow medially. SYN os nasale [TA].

navicular (b.), SYN navicular.

navicular b. of hand, SYN scaphoid (b.).

nonlamellar b., SYN woven b.

occipital b. [TA], a bone at the lower and posterior part of the skull, consisting of three parts (basilar, condylar, and squamous), enclosing a large oval hole, the foramen magnum; it articulates with the parietal and temporal bones on either side, the sphenoid anteriorly, and the atlas below. SYN os occipitale [TA].

orbicular b., SYN lenticular *process* of incus.

palatine b. [TA], an irregularly shaped bone posterior to the maxilla, which enters into the formation of the nasal cavity, the orbit, and the hard palate; it articulates with the maxilla, inferior nasal concha, sphenoid, and ethmoid bones, the vomer and its fellow of the opposite side. SYN os palatinum [TA].

parietal b. [TA], a flat, curved bone of irregular quadrangular shape, at either side of the vault of the cranium; it articulates, with its fellow medially, with the frontal anteriorly, the occipital posteriorly, and the temporal and sphenoid inferiorly. SYN os parietale [TA].

pelvic b., ✕official alternate term for hip b.

perichondral b., in the development of a long b. a collar or cuff of osseous tissue forms in the perichondrium of the cartilage model; the connective tissue membrane of this perichondral b. then becomes periosteum. SYN periosteal b.

periosteal b., SYN perichondral b.

periotic b., SYN petrous *part* of temporal bone.

peroneal b., SYN fibula.

petrosal b., SYN petrous *part* of temporal bone.

petrous b., SYN petrous *part* of internal carotid artery.

ping-pong b., the thin shell of osseous tissue at the periphery of a giant cell tumor in a b.

pipe b., SYN long b.

Pirie b., SYN dorsal talonavicular b.

pisiform (b.), a small b. resembling a pea in size and shape, in the proximal row of the carpus, lying on the anterior surface of the triquetral, with which it articulates; it gives insertion to the tendon of the flexor carpi ulnaris muscle. SYN os pisiforme [TA], lentiform b.

pneumatic b., SYN pneumatized b.

pneumatized b. [TA], a b. that is hollow or contains many air cells, such as the mastoid process of the temporal b. SYN os pneumaticum [TA], hollow b., pneumatic b.

postsphenoid b., the posterior portion of the body of the sphenoid b.

preinterparietal b., a large sutural b. occasionally found detached from the anterior portion of the os interparietale. SYN Goethe b.

premaxillary b., SYN incisive b.

presphenoid b., in comparative anatomy, the b. in the floor of the brain case anterior to the basisphenoid b.

pubic b., SYN *mons pubis*.

pyramidal b., SYN triquetrum.

replacement b., SYN endochondral b.

reticulated b., SYN woven b.

rider's b., heterotopic bone ossification of the tendon of the adductor longus muscle from strain in horseback riding.

Riolan b.'s, several small sutural b.'s sometimes present in the petro-occipital suture.

sacred b., SYN sacrum. [so-called from belief in indestructibility of the bone as the basis for resurrection]

scaphoid (b.), the largest b. of the proximal row of the carpus on the lateral (radial) side, articulating with the radius, lunate, capitate, trapezium, and trapezoid. SYN os scaphoideum [TA], navicular b. of hand, os naviculare manus.

scroll b.'s, SEE inferior nasal *concha*, middle nasal *concha*, superior nasal *concha*, supreme nasal *concha*.

second cuneiform b., SYN intermediate cuneiform (b.).

semilunar b., obsolete term for lunate (b.).

septal b., SYN interalveolar *septum*.

sesamoid b. [TA], a bone formed after birth in a tendon where it passes over a joint, e.g., the patella. SYN os sesamoideum [TA].

shin b., SYN tibia.

short b. [TA], one whose dimensions are approximately equal; it consists of a layer of cortical substance enclosing spongy substance and marrow. Cf. long b. SYN os breve [TA].

b. sialoprotein 1, SYN osteopontin.

sieve b., SYN cribriform *plate* of ethmoid bone.

b.'s of skull, SYN b.'s of cranium.

sphenoid (b.), a b. of most irregular shape occupying the base of the skull; it is described as consisting of a central portion, or body, and six processes: two greater wings, two lesser wings and two pterygoid processes; it articulates with the occipital, frontal, ethmoid, and vomer, and with the paired temporal, parietal, zygomatic, palatine, and sphenoidal concha b.'s. SYN os sphenoidale [TA], sphenoid (2) [TA].

sphenoidal turbinated b.'s, SYN sphenoidal *conchae*, under *concha*.

spongy b. [TA], **(1)** SYN *substantia* spongiosa; **(2)** a turbinated bone.

b.'s of superior limb, SYN b.'s of upper limb.

superior turbinated b., SYN superior nasal *concha*.

suprainterparietal b., a sutural b. at the posterior portion of the sagittal suture.

suprasternal b.'s [TA], one of the small ossicles occasionally found in the ligaments of the sternoclavicular articulation. SYN ossa suprasternalia [TA], Breschet b.'s, episternal b.

supreme turbinated b., SYN supreme nasal *concha*.

sutural b.'s [TA], small irregular b.'s found along the sutures of the cranium, particularly related to the parietal b. SYN os suturarum [TA], Andernach ossicles, epactal b.'s, epactal ossicles, wormian b.'s.

tail b., SYN coccyx.

tarsal b.'s [TA], the seven b.'s of the instep: talus, calcaneus, navicular, three cuneiform (wedge), and cuboid b.'s. SYN ossa tarsi [TA], tarsale [TA], ossa tarsalia ✕.

temporal b. [TA], a large irregular b. situated in the base and side of the skull; it consists of three parts, squamous, tympanic, and petrous, which are distinct at birth; the petrous part contains the vestibulocochlear organ; the b. articulates with the sphenoid, parietal, occipital, and zygomatic b.'s, and by a synovial joint with the mandible. SYN os temporale [TA].

thigh b., ✕official alternate term for thigh.

third cuneiform b., SYN lateral cuneiform (b.).

three-cornered b., SYN triquetrum.

tongue b., SYN hyoid b.

trabecular b., ✕official alternate term for *substantia* spongiosa.

trapezium b., the lateral (radial) b. in the distal row of the carpus; it articulates with the first and second metacarpals, scaphoid, and trapezoid b.'s. SYN greater multangular b., os multangulum majus, os trapezium, trapezium (2).

trapezoid (b.), a bone in the distal row of the carpus; it articulates with the second metacarpal, trapezium, capitate, and scaphoid. SYN os trapezoideum [TA], trapezoid (3) [TA], lesser multangular b., os multangulum minus.

triangular b., SYN *os trigonum*.

triquetrum b., SYN triquetrum.

turbinated b.'s, SEE inferior nasal *concha*, middle nasal *concha*, superior nasal *concha*, supreme nasal *concha*.

tympanic b., SYN tympanic *ring*.

tympanohyal b., a small nodule of b. forming the base of the cartilaginous styloid process of the temporal b. at birth.

unciform b., SYN hamate (b.).

upper jaw b., SYN maxilla.

b.'s of upper limb [TA], these include the superior limb girdle (scapula and clavicle) and the skeleton of the free superior limb (humerus, radius, ulna, wrist bones, metacarpus, and bones of the fingers). SYN ossa membri superioris [TA], b.'s of superior limb.

Vesalius b., SYN *os* vesalianum.

b.'s of visceral cranium, SYN facial b.'s.

wedge b., SYN intermediate cuneiform (b.), lateral cuneiform (b.), medial cuneiform (b.).

wormian b.'s, SYN sutural b.'s.

woven b., bony tissue characteristic of the embryonal skeleton, in which the collagen fibers of the matrix are arranged irregularly in the form of interlacing networks. SYN nonlamellar b., reticulated b.

yoke b., SYN zygomatic b.

zygomatic b. [TA], a quadrilateral b. that forms the prominence of the cheek; it articulates with the frontal, sphenoid, temporal, and maxillary b.'s. SYN os zygomaticum [TA], cheek b. (1), jugal b., mala (2), malar b., os malare, yoke b., zygoma (1).

bone ar·chi·tec·ture. The pattern of trabeculae and associated structures. SEE ALSO Wolff *law*.

bone ash. SYN tribasic *calcium* phosphate.

bone black. SYN animal *charcoal*.

bone·let (bōn′let). SYN ossicle.

bone-salt. The main chemical compound in bone, deposited as minute amorphous crystals in a netlike matrix of collagenous fibers containing collagen; it closely resembles the naturally occurring fluorapatite $3Ca_3(PO_4)_2 \cdot CaF_2$, but is probably a hydroxyapatite in which F is replaced by OH.

Bonhoeffer, Karl, German psychiatrist, 1868–1948. SEE B. *sign*.

Bonnet, Amédée, French surgeon, 1802–1858. SEE B. *capsule*.

Bonnevie, Kristine, German physician, 1872–1950.

Bonnier, Pierre, French clinician, 1861–1918. SEE B. *syndrome*.

Bonwill, William G.A., U.S. dentist, 1833–1899. SEE B. *triangle*.

Böök, Jan A., Swedish geneticist, *1915. SEE B. *syndrome*.

BOOP Abbreviation for *bronchiolitis* obliterans with organizing pneumonia, an idiopathic form of *bronchiolitis* obliterans.

boost·er. SEE booster *dose*.

boot (boot). A boot-shaped appliance. [M.E. *bote*, fr. O.Fr.]

Gibney b., adhesive tape treatment of a sprained ankle or similar condition, applied in a basket-weave fashion under the sole of the foot and around the back of the lower leg.

bo·rac·ic ac·id (bō-ras′ik). SYN boric acid.

bo·rate (bōr′āt). A salt of boric acid.

bo·rat·ed (bōr′āt-ed). Mixed or impregnated with borax or boric acid.

bo·rax (bō′raks). SYN *sodium* borate. [Pers. *būraq*]

bor·bo·ryg·mus, pl. **bor·bo·ryg·mi** (bōr-bō-rig′mŭs, -rig′mī). Rumbling or gurgling noises produced by movement of gas, fluid, or both in the alimentary canal, and audible at a distance. [G. *borborygmos*, rumbling in the bowels]

Bordeau (Bordeu), Théophile de, French physician, 1722–1776.

bor·der (bōr′der) [TA]. The part of a surface that forms its outer boundary. SEE ALSO edge, margin, border. SYN margo [TA].

alveolar b., (1) the most occlusal edge of the alveolar bone; **(2)** SYN alveolar *process* of maxilla.

anterior b. [TA], the ventral or most forward margin of a structure. SYN margo anterior [TA], anterior margin, ventral b.

anterior b. of body of pancreas [TA], the sharp margin between the anterior and inferior surfaces of the pancreas. SYN margo anterior corporis pancreatis [TA], anterior b. of pancreas, margo anterior pancreatis.

anterior b. of eyelids, SYN anterior palpebral *margin*.

anterior b. of fibula [TA], a ridge on the shaft of the fibula to which is attached the anterior intermuscular septum of the leg. SYN margo anterior fibulae [TA].

anterior b. of lung [TA], the thin anteromedial or sternal edge of the lung that overlaps the pericardial sac anteriorly and forms the boundary between the mediastinal and costal surfaces. SYN margo anterior pulmonis [TA].

anterior b. of pancreas, SYN anterior b. of body of pancreas.

anterior b. of radius [TA], the ridge on the shaft of the radius extending from the radial tuberosity to the anterior part of the styloid process. SYN margo anterior radii [TA].

anterior b. of testis [TA], an imaginary convex line demarcating the lateral and medial surfaces. SYN margo anterior testis [TA].

anterior b. of tibia [TA], the sharp subcutaneous ridge of the tibia that extends from the tuberosity to the anterior part of the medial malleolus. SYN margo anterior tibiae [TA], anticnemion, shin, tibial crest.

anterior b. of ulna [TA], the ridge on the body of the ulna that extends from the tuberosity to the anterior part of the styloid process. SYN margo anterior ulnae [TA].

brush b., the apical epithelial surface bearing closely packed microvilli about 2 μm long, such as occur on the cells of the proximal tubule of the nephron. SYN limbus penicillatus.

ciliary b. of iris, SYN ciliary *margin* of iris.

denture b., (1) the limit or boundary or circumferential margin of a denture base; **(2)** the margin of the denture base at the junction of the polished surface with the impression (tissue) surface; **(3)** the extreme edges of a denture base at the buccolabial, lingual, and posterior limits. SYN denture edge, periphery (2).

b.'s of eyelids, SYN palpebral *margins*, under *margin*.

fibular (peroneal) b. of foot, ✗official alternate term for lateral b. of foot.

free b. [TA], unattached edge of a sturcture, often opposite the attached edge. SEE free b. of nail, free b. of ovary. SYN margo liber [TA], free margin.

free b. of nail [TA], the distal b. of the nail that overhangs the tip of the digit. SYN margo liber unguis [TA].

free b. of ovary [TA], the unattached, posterior margin of the ovary. SYN margo liber ovarii [TA].

frontal b. [TA], edge of a bone that articulates with the frontal bone. SEE frontal b. of parietal bone, frontal *margin* of sphenoid. SYN margo frontalis [TA], frontal margin.

frontal b. of parietal bone [TA], the margin of the parietal bone that articulates with the frontal bone. SYN margo frontalis ossis parietalis [TA].

frontal b. of sphenoid bone, SYN frontal *margin* of sphenoid.

hidden b. of nail [TA], the proximal b. of the nail entirely covered by the nail wall. SYN margo occultus unguis [TA], occult b. of nail, proximal b. of nail.

inferior b. [TA], the caudal or lowermost margin of a structure. SYN margo inferior [TA], inferior margin.

inferior b. of body of pancreas [TA], the b. of the pancreas separating the inferior and posterior surfaces. SYN margo inferior corporis pancreatis [TA], inferior b. of pancreas, margo inferior corporis splenis, margo inferior pancreatis.

inferior b. of liver [TA], the sharp b. of the liver that separates the diaphragmatic and visceral surfaces. SYN margo inferior hepatis [TA].

inferior b. of lung [TA], the sharp b. of the lung that separates the diaphragmatic surface from the costal and mediastinal surfaces. SYN margo inferior pulmonis [TA].

inferior b. of pancreas, SYN inferior b. of body of pancreas.

inferior b. of spleen [TA], lowermost edge of the spleen, which separates the lower visceral surface (area of renal impression) from the lower diaphragmatic surface. SYN margo inferior splenis [TA].

inner b. of iris [TA], the narrow inner zone of the iris. SYN anulus iridis minor [TA], lesser ring of iris.

interosseous b. [TA], edge of a bone to which a fibrous (interosseous) membrane is attached, by which the bone becomes attached to another bone. SEE interosseous b. of fibula, interosseous b. of radius, interosseous b. of tibia, interosseous b. of ulna. SYN margo interosseus [TA], interosseous crest, interosseous margin.

interosseous b. of fibula [TA], the ridge along the medial b. of the fibula to which is attached the interosseous membrane. SYN margo interosseus fibulae [TA].

interosseous b. of radius [TA], the ridge along the medial side of the radius to which is attached the interosseous membrane. SYN margo interosseus radii [TA].

interosseous b. of tibia [TA], the ridge along the lateral b. of the tibia to which is attached the interosseous membrane. SYN margo interosseus tibiae [TA].

interosseous b. of ulna [TA], the ridge along the lateral side of the body of the ulna to which is attached the interosseous membrane. SYN margo interosseus ulnae [TA].

b. of iris [TA], either of two zones on the anterior surface of the iris, separated by a circular line concentric with the pupillary border. SYN anulus iridis [TA], ring of iris.

lacrimal b. of maxilla, SYN lacrimal *margin* of maxilla.

lambdoid b. of occipital bone [TA], the margin of the occipital squama that articulates with the parietal bones in the lambdoid suture. SYN margo lambdoideus ossis occipitalis [TA], lambdoid margin of occipital bone, margo lambdoideus squamae occipitalis.

lateral b. [TA], the margin or edge of a structure which is farthest from the midline. SYN margo lateralis [TA], lateral margin.

lateral b. of foot [TA], the b. of the foot between the small toe and the heel. SYN margo lateralis pedis [TA], fibular (peroneal) b. of foot★, margo fibularis pedis★, peroneal b. of foot★, fibular margin of foot.

lateral b. of forearm, ★official alternate term for radial b. of forearm.

lateral b. of humerus [TA], the ridge on the humerus that extends from the greater tubercle to the lateral epicondyle. SYN margo lateralis humeri [TA].

lateral b. of kidney [TA], the convex narrow edge separating the anterior and posterior surfaces. SYN margo lateralis renis [TA].

lateral b. of nail [TA], the sides of the nail extending from the proximal to the free borders. SYN margo lateralis unguis [TA].

lateral b. of scapula [TA], the edge of the scapula extending from the glenoid fossa to the inferior angle. SYN margo lateralis scapulae [TA].

mastoid b. of occipital bone [TA], the margin of the occipital squama that articulates with the temporal bone. SYN margo mastoideus ossis occipitalis [TA], margo mastoideus squamae occipitalis, mastoid margin of occipital bone.

medial b. [TA], the b. of a structure closest to the medial plane. SYN margo medialis [TA], medial margin.

medial b. of foot [TA], the inner b. of the foot extending from heel to the great toe. SYN margo medialis pedis [TA], margo tibialis pedis★, tibial b. of foot★.

medial b. of forearm, ★official alternate term for ulnar b. of forearm.

medial b. of humerus [TA], the ridge on the humerus extending from the crest of the lesser tubercle to the medial epicondyle. SYN margo medialis humeri [TA].

medial b. of kidney [TA], the concave b. of the kidney. SYN margo medialis renis [TA].

medial b. of scapula [TA], the edge of the scapula closest to the vertebral column, extending from superior angle to inferior angle. SYN margo medialis scapulae [TA], vertebral b. of scapula.

medial b. of suprarenal gland [TA], the paravertebral edge of the suprarenal gland. SYN margo medialis glandulae suprarenalis [TA].

medial b. of tibia [TA], the rounded b. of the tibia that separates the posterior and medial surfaces. SYN margo medialis tibiae [TA].

mesovarian b. of ovary [TA], the b. of the ovary to which the mesovarium is attached. SYN margo mesovaricus ovarii, mesovarian margin of ovary.

nasal b. of frontal bone, SYN nasal *margin* of frontal bone.

occipital b. [TA], edge of a bone that articulates with the occipital bone. SEE occipital b. of parietal bone, occipital *margin* of temporal bone. SYN margo occipitalis [TA], occipital margin.

occipital b. of parietal bone [TA], the posterior margin of the parietal bone that articulates with the occipital squama. SYN margo occipitalis ossis parietalis [TA].

occipital b. of temporal bone, SYN occipital *margin* of temporal bone.

occult b. of nail, SYN hidden b. of nail.

outer b. of iris [TA], the outer, broader of the two zones of the iris. SYN anulus iridis major [TA], greater ring of iris.

parietal b. [TA], edge of a bone that articulates with the parietal bone. SEE parietal *margin* of frontal bone, parietal *margin* of greater wing of sphenoid, parietal b. of squamous part of temporal bone. SYN margo parietalis [TA], parietal margin.

parietal b. of frontal bone, SYN parietal *margin* of frontal bone.

parietal b. of sphenoid bone, SYN parietal *margin* of greater wing of sphenoid.

parietal b. of squamous part of temporal bone [TA], the b. of the squamous part of the temporal bone that articulates with the parietal bone. SYN margo parietalis partis squamosae ossis temporalis [TA], margo parietalis ossis temporalis, parietal b. of temporal bone.

parietal b. of temporal bone, SYN parietal b. of squamous part of temporal bone.

peroneal b. of foot, ★official alternate term for lateral b. of foot.

posterior b. of eyelids, SYN posterior palpebral *margin*.

posterior b. of fibula [TA], the ridge on the posterior aspect of the fibula extending from the head to the medial aspect of the peroneal groove. SYN margo posterior fibulae [TA].

posterior b. of petrous part of temporal bone [TA], the margin of the petrous part of the temporal bone that extends from the apex to the jugular notch; it articulates with the basal and jugular portions of the occipital bone. SYN margo posterior partis petrosae ossis temporalis [TA].

posterior b. of radius [TA], the ridge on the radius that extends from the tuberosity to the tubercle on the posterior aspect of the distal extremity. SYN margo posterior radii [TA].

posterior b. of testis [TA], the rounded posterior portion of the testis into which the vessels enter. SYN margo posterior testis [TA].

posterior b. of ulna [TA], the sinuous palpable subcutaneous ridge on the posterior aspect of the ulna that extends from near the olecranon to the styloid process, demarcating "anterior" (flexor) from "posterior" (extensor) compartments of forearm. SYN margo posterior ulnae [TA].

proximal b. of nail, SYN hidden b. of nail.

pupillary b. of iris, SYN pupillary *margin* of iris.

radial b. of forearm [TA], an imaginary line running along the outermost extent of the forearm separating anterior and posterior surfaces laterally. SYN margo radialis antebrachii [TA], lateral b. of forearm★, margo lateralis antebrachii★.

right b. of heart [TA], the b. between the sternocostal and diaphragmatic surfaces of the heart; it is fairly well defined in fixed hearts but is rounded and indefinite in the living heart. SYN margo dexter cordis [TA], right margin of heart.

sagittal b. of parietal bone [TA], the medial border of the parietal bone entering into the sagittal suture. SYN margo sagittalis ossis parietalis [TA].

sphenoidal b. of temporal bone, SYN sphenoidal *margin* of temporal bone.

squamosal b. [TA], edge of a bone that articulates with the squamous part of the temporal bone. SYN margo squamosus [TA], squamous b., squamous margin.

squamosal b. of parietal bone [TA], the lateral b. of the parietal bone that articulates with the squamous part of the temporal bone. SYN margo squamosus ossis parietalis [TA], squamous b. of parietal bone.

squamous b., SYN squamosal b; SEE squamosal b. of parietal bone, squamosal *margin* of greater wing of sphenoid.

squamous b. of parietal bone, SYN squamosal b. of parietal bone.

squamous b. of sphenoid bone, SYN squamosal *margin* of greater wing of sphenoid.

striated b., the free surface of the columnar absorptive cells of the intestine formed by closely packed microvilli about 1 μm long, giving the appearance of parallel striations. SYN limbus striatus.

superior b., the cranial or uppermost margin of a structure.

superior b. of body of pancreas [TA], the uppermost b. of the body of the pancreas that separates the anterior and posterior surfaces. SYN margo superior corporis pancreatis [TA], margo superior pancreatis, superior b. of pancreas.

superior b. of pancreas, SYN superior b. of body of pancreas.

superior b. of petrous part of temporal bone [TA], the margin that separates the anterior and posterior surfaces of the petrous part of the temporal bone and the lateral part of the middle cranial fossa from the posterior cranial fossa. SYN margo superior partis petrosae ossis temporalis [TA], crest of petrous part of temporal bone, crest of petrous temporal bone.

superior b. of scapula [TA], the margin of the scapula that extends from the glenoid fossa to the superior angle. SYN margo superior scapulae [TA].

superior b. of spleen [TA], the notched b. of the spleen that separates the visceral (gastric) and diaphragmatic surfaces. SYN margo superior splenis [TA].

superior b. of suprarenal gland [TA], the b. of the suprarenal gland at the superior junction of the anterior and posterior surfaces. SYN margo superior glandulae suprarenalis [TA].

tibial b. of foot, ✩official alternate term for medial b. of foot.

ulnar b. of forearm [TA], an imaginary line extrapolated from the medial epicondyle of the humerus to the styloid process of the ulna, forming a b. between the anterior and posterior surfaces. SYN margo ulnaris antebrachii [TA], margo medialis antebrachii✩, medial b. of forearm✩, ulnar margin of forearm.

b. of uterus [TA], the right or left margin of the uterus along which the broad ligament is attached. The uterine tube and round ligament attach to the uterus at the upper part of the border. SYN margo uteri [TA].

ventral b., SYN anterior b.

vermilion b., the red margin of the upper and lower lip that commences at the exterior edge of the intraoral labial mucosa ("moist line") and extends outward, terminating at the extraoral labial cutaneous junction; a thinly keratinized type of stratified squamous epithelium deeply penetrated by well-vascularized dermal papillae which show through the translucent epidermis to impart the typical red appearance of the lips. SYN vermilion zone, vermilion transitional zone.

vertebral b. of scapula, SYN medial b. of scapula.

zygomatic b. of greater wing of sphenoid bone, SYN zygomatic *margin* of greater wing of sphenoid bone.

Bordet, Jules, Belgian bacteriologist and Nobel laureate, 1870–1961. SEE *Bordetella;* B.-Gengou potato blood *agar, bacillus, phenomenon;* B. and Gengou *reaction.*

Bor·de·tel·la (bōr-dĕ-tel′ă). A genus of strictly aerobic bacteria (family Brucellaceae) containing minute, Gram-negative non-spore bearing, coccobacilli. Motile and nonmotile species occur; motile cells are peritrichous. The metabolism of these organisms is respiratory. They require nicotinic acid, cysteine, and methionine; hemin (X factor) and coenzyme I (V factor) are not required. They are parasites and pathogens of the mammalian respiratory tract; type species is *B. pertussis.* [J. *Bordet*]

B. bronchiseptica, a bacterial species found in a broad range of animal species, causing atrophic rhinitis of swine, bronchopneumonia in rodents, and a highly contagious bronchopneumonia in dogs. It is a rare cause of opportunistic respiratory tract infection in immunocomprimised patients.

B. hinzii, a newly described bacterial species isolated from a few human blood cultures and respiratory secretions, as well as from poultry respiratory secretions.

B. holmesii, a newly described bacterial species isolated from human blood cultures, primarily from mmunocompromised patients.

B. parapertus′sis, a bacterial species that causes a whooping cough-like disease, usually milder than that seen with *B. pertussis.*

B. pertus′sis, the bacterial species that is the causative agent of whooping cough, a respiratory tract infection that in infants and young children may be life-threatening; the severe cough, progressing to a paroxysmal form after 7–10 days, is associated with production of pertussis toxin, a protein consisting of 5 B subunits that bind the molecule to respiratory epithelial cells, and an A subunit, an ADP-ribosyl-transferase that interferes with proteins associated with normal signal transduction; pathology is also associated with heavy mucous secretion and hypoxia due to parox-

ysmal coughing and to blockage of air passages with mucus. SYN Bordet-Gengou bacillus.

bo·ric ac·id (bō′rik). A very weak acid, used as an antiseptic dusting powder, in saturated solution as a collyrium, and with glycerin in aphthae and stomatitis. SYN boracic acid.

bor·ism (bōr′izm). Symptoms caused by the ingestion of borax or any compound of boron.

Börjeson, Mats, Swedish physician, *1922. SEE B.-Forssman-Lehmann *syndrome.*

Born, Gustav Jacob, German embryologist, 1851–1900. SEE B. *method* of wax plate reconstruction.

bor·nane (bōr′nān). The monoterpene parent of borneols, camphene, and similar essential oils (terpenes).

bo·ro·glyc·er·in (bō-rō-glis′er-in). A soft mass obtained by heating glycerin and boric acid; an obsolete antiseptic, usually used mixed with equal parts of glycerin, constituting glycerite. SYN boroglycerol, glyceryl borate.

bo·ro·glyc·er·ol (bō-rō-glis′er-ol). SYN boroglycerin.

bo·ron (B) (bōr′on). A nonmetallic trivalent element, atomic no. 5, atomic wt. 10.811; occurs as a hard crystalline mass or as a brown powder, and forms borates and boric acid. A nutritional need has been reported for pregnant women. [Pers. *Burah*]

Borrel, Amédée, French bacteriologist, 1867–1936. SEE B. blue *stain.*

Bor·rel·ia (bō-rē′lē-ă, bo-rel′ē-ă). A genus of bacteria (family Treponemataceae) containing cells 8–16 μm in length, with coarse, shallow, irregular spirals and tapered, finely filamented ends. These organisms are parasitic on many forms of animal life, are generally hematophytic, or are found on mucous membranes; most are transmitted to animals or humans by the bites of arthropods. The type species is *B. anserina.* [A. *Borrell*]

B. afzelii, a bacterial genospecies of *Borrelia burgdorferi sensu lato* causing Lyme disease in Europe and Asia; transmitted by the tick *Ixodes ricinus* in central and western Europe and by the tick *Ixodes persulcatus* in Eurasia from the Baltic Sea to the Pacific Ocean. SEE ALSO *B. burgdorferi sensu stricto.*

B. anseri′na, a bacterial species that causes spirochetosis of fowls; found in the blood of infected geese, ducks, other fowl, and vector ticks; it is the type species of the genus *B.*

B. burgdor′feri, a bacterial species causing Lyme disease in humans and borreliosis in dogs, cattle, and possibly horses. The vector transmitting this spirochete to humans is the ixodid tick, *Ixodes dammini.*

B. burgdorferi sensu lato, a bacterial complex causing Lyme disease that is composed of several genospecies including *Borrelia burgdorferi sensu stricto, Borrelia garinii* and *Borrelia afzelii.*

B. burgdorferi sensu stricto, a bacterial genospecies of *Borrelia burgdorferi sensu lato* causing Lyme disease in North America and Europe; transmitted by the tick *Ixodes scapularis* in the eastern and central United States, by the tick *Ixodes pacificus* in the western United States, and by the tick *Ixodes ricinus* in Europe. SEE ALSO *B. garinii.*

B. cauca′sica, a bacterial species found as a cause of relapsing fever in the Caucasus; transmitted by *Ornithodoros verrucosus.*

B. crocidu′rae, a bacterial species that causes relapsing fever in North Africa, the Near East, and central Asia, and is transmitted by the small variety of the tick *Ornithodoros erraticus.*

B. dutto′nii, a bacterial species causing Central and South African relapsing fever; transmitted by a tick, *Ornithodoros moubata.*

B. garinii, a bacterial genospecies of *Borrelia burgdorferi sensu lato* causing Lyme disease in Europe and Asia; transmitted by the tick *Ixodes ricinus* in central and western Europe and by the tick *Ixodes persulcatus* in Eurasia from the Baltic Sea to the Pacific Ocean. SEE ALSO *B. burgdorferi sensu stricto.*

B. herm′sii, a bacterial species found as a cause of relapsing fever in British Columbia, California, Colorado, Idaho, Nevada, Oregon, and Washington; transmitted by a tick, *Ornithodoros hermsi.*

B. hispan′ica, a bacterial species causing relapsing fever in Spain, Portugal, and northwest Africa, transmitted by the large variety of the tick *Ornithodorus erratica.*

B. latysche′wii, a bacterial species that causes relapsing fever in

Iran and central Asia; transmitted by the tick *Ornithodoros tartakovskyi* from rodents and reptiles.

B. mazzot′tii, a bacterial species that causes relapsing fever in Mexico and Central and South America; transmitted by the tick *Ornithodoros talajé.*

B. par′keri, a bacterial species found as a cause of relapsing fever in the western United States; transmitted by a tick, *Ornithodoros parkeri.*

B. per′sica, a bacterial species that causes relapsing fever in the Middle East and central Asia; the vector is the tick *Ornithodoros tholozani.*

B. recurren′tis, a bacterial species causing relapsing fever in South America, Europe, Africa, and Asia; transmitted by the bedbug, *Cimex lectularius,* and the louse, *Pediculus humanus* subsp. *humanus.* SYN Obermeier spirillum, *Spirochaeta obermeieri.*

B. turica′tae, a bacterial species found as a cause of relapsing fever in Mexico, New Mexico, Texas, Oklahoma, and Kansas; transmitted by *Ornithodoros turicata.*

B. venezuelen′sis, a bacterial species causing spirochetal relapsing fever in Central and South America; transmitted by *Ornithodoros rudis* and *O. venezuelensis.*

bor·re·li·o·sis (bō-rē-lē-ō′sis). Disease caused by bacteria of the genus *Borrelia.*

Lyme b., SYN Lyme *disease.*

Borst, Maximilian, German pathologist, 1869–1946. SEE B.-Jadassohn type intraepidermal *epithelioma.*

Bosin dis·ease. See under disease.

boss (baws). **1.** A protuberance; a circumscribed rounded swelling. **2.** The prominence of a kyphosis. [M.E. *boce,* fr. O.Fr.]

bos·se·lat·ed (baws′ĕ-lā-ted). Marked by numerous bosses or rounded protuberances. [Fr. *bosseler,* to emboss]

bos·se·la·tion (baws-ĕ-lā′shŭn). **1.** A boss. **2.** A condition in which one or more bosses, or rounded protuberances, are present.

Boston, Leonard N., U.S. physician, 1871–1931.

Botallo (Botallus), Leonardo, Italian physician in Paris, 1530–ca.1587. SEE B. *duct, foramen, ligament.*

bot·fly (bot′flī). Robust, hairy fly of the order Diptera, often strikingly marked in black and yellow or gray, whose larvae produce a variety of myiasis conditions in humans and various domestic animals, especially herbivores.

head b.'s, flesh flies of the dipterous families Oestridae and Cuterebridae; robust, hairy, black, yellow, or gray flies that, while flying, deposit newly hatched larvae or, in some cases, eggs, on or near the nostrils of sheep, goats, deer, horses, camels, and, rarely, humans.

human b., SYN *Dermatobia hominis.*

skin b.'s, SYN *Dermatobia hominis;* SEE ALSO *Cuterebra.*

warble b., SYN *Dermatobia hominis;* SEE ALSO *Hypoderma.*

both·ria (both′rē-ă). Plural of bothrium.

both·ri·o·ceph·a·li·a·sis (both′rē-ō-sef-ă-lī′ă-sis). SYN diphyllobothriasis.

Both·ri·o·ceph·a·lus (both′rē-ō-sef′ă-lŭs). A genus of pseudophyllid tapeworms with both plerocercoid and adult stages in fishes; sometimes historically confused with *Diphyllobothrium.* [G. *bothrion,* dim. of *bothros,* pit or trench, + *kephalē,* head]

B. corda′tus, a tapeworm species common in dogs and humans in Greenland.

B. la′tus, former name for *Diphyllobothrium latum.*

B. manso′ni, former name for *Spirometra mansoni.*

B. mansonoi′des, former name for *Spirometra mansonoides.*

both·ri·um, pl. **both·ria** (both′rē-ŭm, -rē-ă). One of the slitlike sucking grooves found on the scolex of pseudophyllidean tapeworms, such as the broad fish tapeworm of man, *Diphyllobothrium latum.* [G. *bothros,* pit or trench]

bot·ry·oid (bot′rē-oyd). Having numerous rounded protuberances resembling a bunch of grapes. SYN staphyline, uviform. [G. *botryoeidēs,* like a bunch of grapes (*botrys*)]

Bot·ry·o·my·ces (bot′rē-ō-mī′sēz). A generic name applied to a supposed fungus causing botryomycosis. Since this disease is now known to be caused by several kinds of bacteria, staphylococci most commonly, the name is invalid and rarely used. The name of the disease has been retained, nevertheless, to indicate a peculiar type of tissue reaction. [G. *botrys,* a bunch of grapes, + *mykēs,* fungus]

bot·ry·o·my·co·sis (bot′rē-ō-mī-kō′sis). A chronic granulomatous condition of horses, cattle, swine, and humans, usually involving the skin but occasionally also the viscera, and characterized by granules in the pus, consisting of masses of bacteria, generally staphylococci but sometimes other types, surrounded by a hyaline capsule which sometimes exhibits clublike bodies around its periphery; the anatomic structure of the lesion resembles that of actinomycosis and mycetoma. SYN actinophytosis (2). [fr. *Botryomyces*]

bot·ry·o·my·cot·ic (bot′rē-ō-mī-kot′ik). Relating to or affected by botryomycosis.

bots. The larvae of several species of botflies. [Gael. *boiteag,* maggot]

ox b., cattle grub, the larvae of the warble flies, *Hypoderma bovis* and *H. lineatum.*

sheep b., *Oestrus ovis* larvae.

Böttcher, Arthur, Estonian anatomist, 1831–1889. SEE B. *canal, cells,* under *cell, crystals,* under *crystal, ganglion, space;* Charcot-B. *crystalloids,* under *crystalloid.*

bot·tle (bot′l). A container for liquids.

Mariotte b., a stoppered b. with bottom outlet, used as a reservoir for constant infusions; air enters only by bubbling through a tube extending down through the stopper almost to the bottom; a partial vacuum thus supports the variable height of liquid above the air inlet, providing a constant gravity head for outflow.

wash-b., **(1)** a bottle with a tube passing to the bottom, through which gases are forced into water to purify them; **(2)** a stoppered bottle with two tubes, one ending above and the other below a fluid, so that air blowing through the short tube forces liquid in a small stream from the free end of the long one; used for washing chemical apparatus.

Woulfe b., a b. with two or three necks, used in a series, connected with tubes, for working with gases (washing, drying, absorbing, etc.).

bot·u·lin (bot′ū-lin). SYN botulinus *toxin.*

bot·u·lin·o·gen·ic (bot′ū-lin-ō-jen′ik). SYN botulogenic.

bot·u·lism (bot′ū-lizm). Food poisoning usually caused by the ingestion of the neurotoxin produced by the bacterium *Clostridium botulinum* from improperly canned or preserved food; mainly affects humans, chickens, water fowl, cattle, sheep, and horses, and is characterized by paralysis in all species; can be fatal; swine, dogs, and cats are somewhat resistant. In some cases (e.g., in infants) b. may be formed in the gastrointestinal tract by ingested organisms. SEE ALSO *Clostridium botulinum.* [L. *botulus,* sausage]

wound b., b. resulting from infection of a wound.

bot·u·lis·mo·tox·in (bot′ū-liz-mō-tok′sin). SYN botulinus *toxin.*

bot·u·lo·gen·ic (bot′ū-lō-jen′ik). Botulism-producing. SYN botulinogenic.

bou·bas (boo′bahs). SYN yaws. [native Brazilian]

Bouchard, Charles Jacques, French physician, 1837–1915. SEE B. *disease.*

bouche de ta·pir (boosh-dĕ-tā′pir). SYN tapir *mouth.* [Fr.]

Bouchut, Jean A.E., French physician, 1818–1891. SEE B. *tube.*

bou·gie (boo-zhē′). A cylindrical instrument, usually somewhat flexible and yielding, used for calibrating or dilating constricted areas in tubular organs, such as the urethra or esophagus; sometimes containing a medication for local application. [Fr. candle]

b. à boule (boo-zhē′ă-bool′), a ball-tipped b.

bulbous b., a b. with a bulb-shaped tip, some of which are shaped like an acorn or an olive.

Eder-Pustow b., a metal olive-shaped b. with a flexible metal dilating system (for esophageal stricture).

elastic b., a b. made of rubber, latex, or other similarly flexible material.

elbowed b., a b. with a sharply angulated bend near its tip.

filiform b., a very slender b. usually used for gentle exploration of strictures or sinus tracts of small diameter where false passages can be encountered or created; the entering end can consist of either a straight or spiral tip, and the trailing end usually consists of a threaded cylinder into which the screw tip of a following b. can be inserted.

following b., a flexible tapered b. with a screw tip which is attached to the trailing end of a filiform b., to allow progressive dilation without danger of creating false passages.

Hurst b., a series of mercury-filled round-tipped tubes of graded diameter for dilating the cardioesophageal region.

Maloney b., a series of b.'s similar to Hurst b.'s but having cone-shaped tips.

Savary b.'s, silastic tapered-tip b.'s used over a guide wire in esophageal dilation.

tapered b., a b. with gradually increasing caliber, used to dilate strictures.

wax-tipped b., a long slender flexible b. with a wax tip, used for endoscopic passage into the ureter to confirm the presence of a calculus by scratching the surface of the tip with the sharp edges of the stone.

whip b., a b. tapered to a threadlike tip at the end.

bou·gie·nage (boo-zhē-nahzh′). Examination or treatment of the interior of any canal by the passage of a bougie or cannula.

bouil·lon (boo-yawn′). A clear beef tea. [Fr. broth, fr. *bouillir,* to boil]

Bouin, Paul, French histologist, 1870–1962. SEE B. *fixative.*

bou·lim·i·a (boo-lim′ē-ă). SYN *bulimia* nervosa.

bound (bownd). **1.** Limited, circumscribed; enclosed. **2.** Denoting a substance, such as iodine, phosphorus, calcium, morphine, or another drug, that is not in readily diffusible form but exists in combination with a high–molecular weight substance, especially protein. **3.** Fixed to a receptor, such as on a cell wall.

bou·quet (boo-ka′). A cluster or bunch of structures, especially of blood vessels, suggesting a b. [Fr.]

Riolan b., the muscles and ligaments, "les fleurs rouges et les fleurs blanches" (the red and white flowers), arising from the styloid process.

Bourgery, Marc-Jean, French anatomist and surgeon, 1797–1849. SEE B. *ligament.*

Bourneville, Désiré-Magloire, French physician, 1840–1909. SEE B. *disease;* B.-Pringle *disease.*

Bourquin, Anne, U.S. chemist, *1897. SEE Sherman-B. *unit* of vitamin B$_2$.

bou·ton (boo-ton′). A button, pustule, or knob-like swelling. [Fr. button]

axonal terminal b.'s, SYN axon *terminals,* under *terminal.*

b. de Baghdad, the lesion occurring in cutaneous leishmaniasis. SYN bouton de Biskra.

b. en chemise, small abscess of the intestinal mucosa, occurring in amebic dysentery.

b.'s en passage, consecutive synapses along the course of an axon.

synaptic b.'s, SYN axon *terminals,* under *terminal.*

terminal b.'s, b. terminaux, SYN axon *terminals,* under *terminal.*

bou·ton de Bis·kra. SYN *bouton* de Baghdad.

bou·ton·niè·re (boo-ton-nir′, -năr′). A traumatically produced slit or buttonhole-like opening. [Fr. buttonhole]

Bo·vic·o·la (bō-vik′ō-lă). A genus of biting lice that is considered by some to be a subgenus of *Damalinia;* includes the species *B. bovis* (*Trichodectes scalaris*), the common red or biting ox louse of cattle; *B. caprae* (*Trichodectes climax*), found on sheep and goats; *B. equi* (*Trichodectes parumpilosus*), the common biting louse of horses; *B. ovis* (*Trichodectes sphaerocephalus*), the common biting louse of sheep. SEE ALSO *Trichodectes.*

Bovie. An instrument used for electrosurgical dissection and hemostasis. Frequently used as a verb, i.e., to Bovie something is to dissect or cauterize it with the Bovie instrument.

bo·vine (bō′vīn, -vin). Relating to cattle. [L. *bos* (*bov*-), ox]

bow (bō). Any device bent in a simple curve or semicircle and possessing flexibility. [A.S. boga]

Cupid's b., the contour of the superior margin of the upper lip.

Logan b., heavy stainless steel wire bent in an arc and taped to both cheeks to protect a freshly repaired cleft lip.

Bowditch, Henry P., U.S. physiologist, 1840–1911. SEE B. *law, effect.*

bow·el. SYN intestine. SEE small bowel *series.* [through the Fr. from L. *botulus,* sausage]

large b., the colon.

small b., proximal portion of the intestine distal to the stomach, comprising the duodenum, jejunum, and ileum.

Bowen, John T., U.S. dermatologist, 1857–1941. SEE B. *disease,* precancerous *dermatosis;* bowenoid *papulosis;* Bowenoid *cells,* under *cell.*

Bowie, Donald James, Canadian physician, *1887. SEE Bowie *stain.*

bow·leg, bow-b. (bō′leg). SYN *genu varum.*

Bowles type steth·o·scope. See under stethoscope.

Bowman, Sir William, English ophthalmologist, anatomist, and physiologist, 1816–1892. SEE B. *capsule, disks,* under *disk, gland, membrane, muscle, probe, space.*

box (boks). Container; receptacle. [L.L. *buxis,* fr. G. *puxis,* box tree]

black b., **(1)** (Jargon) descriptive of a method of reasoning or studying a problem, in which the methods and procedures, as such, are not described, explained, or perhaps even understood: conclusions relate solely to the empirical relationships observed; **(2)** in some contexts, the term can mean a piece of apparatus or an experimental animal in which the pharmacologic or toxicologic pathway has not yet been worked out.

brain b., ✯official alternate term for neurocranium.

CAAT b., a sequence of nucleotides found in a conserved region of DNA located "upstream" (5′ direction) of the start points of eukaryotic transcription units; specific transcription factors appear to associate with it; found in many promoters at −75 bp with the consensus sequence: GG(T/C)CAATCT. It is believed to determine the efficiency of transcription.

Hogness b., SEE homeobox.

Pribnow b., SEE homeobox.

Skinner b., an experimental apparatus in which an animal presses a lever to obtain a reward or receive punishment.

TATA b., a highly conserved bacterial DNA sequence found about 25 bp upstream from the transcription start site of genes, usually flanked by GC rich sequences; binding site of transcription factors but not RNA polymerase.

view b., a light b. for display of radiographs or other photographic transparencies.

box·ing (boks′ing). In dentistry, the building up of vertical walls, usually in wax, around a dental impression after beading, to produce the desired size and form of the dental cast, and to preserve certain landmarks of the impression.

Boyce, William H., U.S. urologist, *1918. SEE Smith-B. *operation.*

Boyden, Edward A., U.S. anatomist, 1886–1976. SEE B. *meal, sphincter.*

Boyer, Baron Alexis, French surgeon, 1757–1833. SEE B. *bursa, cyst.*

Boyle, Hon. Robert, British physicist and chemist, 1627–1691. SEE B. *law.*

Bozeman, Nathan G., U.S. surgeon, 1825–1905. SEE B. *operation, position;* B.-Fritsch *catheter.*

Bozzolo, Camillo, Italian physician, 1845–1920. SEE B. *sign.*

BP Abbreviation for blood *pressure;* British Pharmacopoeia.

b.p. Abbreviation for boiling *point;* base *pair.*

Bq Abbreviation for becquerel.

Br Symbol for bromine.

Braasch, William F., U.S. urologist, 1878–1975. SEE B. *bulb, catheter.*

brace (brās). An orthosis or orthopedic appliance that supports or holds in correct position a part of the body and can allow motion at adjacent joints, in contrast to a splint, which prevents motion of the part. [M.E., fr. O.Fr., fr. L. *bracchium*, arm, fr. G. *brachion*]

Taylor back b., a steel spinal support. SYN Taylor apparatus, Taylor splint.

brac·es (brā′sez). Colloquialism for orthodontic appliances.

bra·chia (brā′kē-ă). Plural of brachium.

brach·i·al (brā′kē-ăl). Relating to the arm.

bra·chi·al·gia (brā-kē-al′jē-ă). Pain in the arm. [L. *brachium*, arm, + *algos*, pain]

b. stat′ica paresthet′ica, pain in the arm and transient paresthesia occurring only at night.

△**brachio-.** SYN arm (1). [L. *brachium*]

bra·chi·o·ce·phal·ic (brā′kē-ō-se-fal′ik). Relating to both arm and head.

bra·chi·o·cru·ral (brā′kē-ō-kroo′răl). Relating to both arm and thigh.

bra·chi·o·cu·bi·tal (brā′kē-ō-kū′bi-tăl). Relating to both arm and elbow or to both arm and forearm.

bra·chi·o·gram (brā′kē-ō-gram). Tracing of the brachial artery pulse.

bra·chi·um, pl. **bra·chia** (brā′kē-ŭm, brak′; -ă) [TA] **1.** SYN arm (1). **2.** An anatomic structure resembling an arm. [L. arm, prob. akin to G. *brachiōn*]

b. collic′uli inferio′ris [TA], SYN b. of inferior colliculus.

b. collic′uli superio′ris [TA], SYN *commissure* of superior colliculus.

b. conjuncti′vum cerebel′li, SYN superior cerebellar *peduncle*.

b. of inferior colliculus [TA], a fiber bundle passing from the inferior colliculus on either side of the brainstem along the lateral border of the superior colliculus to the posterior part of the thalamus where it enters the medial geniculate body. It forms part of the major ascending auditory pathway. SYN b. colliculi inferioris [TA], b. quadrigeminum inferius, inferior quadrigeminal b.

inferior quadrigeminal b., SYN b. of inferior colliculus.

b. pon′tis, SYN middle cerebellar *peduncle*.

b. quadrigem′inum infe′rius, SYN b. of inferior colliculus.

b. quadrigem′inum supe′rius, SYN b. of superior colliculus.

b. of superior colliculus [TA], a band of fibers of the optic tract bypassing the lateral geniculate body to terminate in the superior colliculus and pretectal region. SYN b. quadrigeminum superius, superior quadrigeminal b.

superior quadrigeminal b., SYN b. of superior colliculus.

Bracht, Erich Franz, German obstetrician and gynecologist, *1882. SEE B. *maneuver*.

Bracht, E., 20th century German pathologist. SEE B.-Wächter *lesion*.

△**brachy-.** Short. [G. *brachys*, short]

brach·y·ba·sia (brak-ē-bā′sē-ă). The shuffling gait characteristic of pyramidal tract disease. [brachy- + G. *basis*, a stepping]

brach·y·ba·so·camp·to·dac·ty·ly (brak-ē-bā′sō-kamp-tō-dak′ti-lē). Combined disproportionate shortness and crookedness of the fingers. [brachy- + G. *basis*, base, + *campylos*, curved, + *daktylos*, finger]

brach·y·ba·so·pha·lan·gia (brak-ē-bā′sō-fă-lan′jē-ă). Abnormal shortness of the proximal phalanges. [brachy- + G. *basis*, base, + phalanx]

brach·y·car·dia (brak-ē-kar′dē-ă). SYN bradycardia.

brach·y·ce·pha·lia (brak-ē-sĕ-fā′lē-ă). SYN brachycephaly.

brach·y·ce·phal·ic (brak-ē-se-fal′ik). Relating to or characterized by brachycephaly. SYN brachycephalous.

brach·y·ceph·a·lism (brak-ē-sef′ă-lizm). SYN brachycephaly. [brachy- + G. *kephalē*, head]

brach·y·ceph·a·lous (brak-ē-sef′ă-lŭs). SYN brachycephalic.

brach·y·ceph·a·ly (brak-ē-sef′ă-lē). Disproportionate shortness of head, the skull having a cephalic index of over 80; among the brachycephalic races are the Native Americans, Malays, and Bur-

mese. SYN brachycephalia, brachycephalism. [brachy- + G. *kephalē*, head]

brach·y·chei·lia, brach·y·chi·lia (brak-ē-kī′lē-ă). Abnormal shortness of the lips. [brachy- + G. *cheilos*, lip]

brach·y·cne·mic (brak-ē-nē′mik). Having short legs; specifically, relating to a tibiofemoral index of less than 82 with the leg disproportionately shorter than the thigh. [brachy- + G. *knēmē*, leg]

brach·y·cra·nic (brak-ē-krā′nik). Brachycephalic with a cephalic index of 80.0 to 84.9. [brachy- + G. *kranion*, skull]

brach·y·dac·tyl·ia (brak-ē-dak-til′ē-ă). SYN brachydactyly. [brachy- + G. *daktylos*, finger]

brach·y·dac·tyl·ic (brak-ē-dak-til′ik). Denoting brachydactyly.

brach·y·dac·ty·ly (brak-ē-dak′ti-lē). Abnormal shortness of the fingers. SYN brachydactylia. [brachy- + G. *daktylos*, finger]

brach·y·e·soph·a·gus (brak′ē-e-sof′ă-gŭs). An abnormally short esophagus. [brachy- + esophagus]

brach·y·fa·cial (brak-ē-fā′shăl). SYN brachyprosopic.

brach·y·glos·sal (brak-ē-glos′ăl). Denoting an abnormally short tongue. [brachy- + G. *glōssa*, tongue]

bra·chyg·na·thia (brak-ig-nā′thē-ă). Abnormal shortness or recession of the mandible. SEE ALSO micrognathia. SYN bird face. [brachy- + G. *gnathos*, jaw]

bra·chyg·na·thous (brak-ig′nā-thŭs). Having a receding underjaw.

brach·y·ker·kic (brak-ē-ker′kik). Relating to a radiohumeral index of less than 75, with a forearm relatively shorter than the upper arm. [brachy- + G. *kerkis*, radius]

brach·y·me·lia (brak-ē-mē′lē-ă). Disproportionate shortness of the limbs. [brachy- + G. *melos*, limb]

brach·y·me·so·pha·lan·gia (brak-ē-mes′ō-fă-lan′jē-ă). Abnormal shortness of the middle phalanges. [brachy- + G. *mesos*, middle, + phalanx]

brach·y·met·a·car·pa·lia, brach·y·met·a·car·pa·lism (brak′ē-met-ă-kar-pā′lē-ă, -met-ă-kar′pă-lizm). SYN brachymetacarpia.

brach·y·met·a·car·pia (brak′ē-met-ă-car′pē-ă). Abnormal shortness of the metacarpals, especially the fourth and fifth. SYN brachymetacarpalia, brachymetacarpalism.

brach·y·me·tap·o·dy (brak′ē-me-tap′ō-dē). Apparent shortness of toes or fingers resulting from shortness or hypoplasia of the metacarpals or metatarsals. [brachy- + G. *meta-* (tarsal) + *pous* (*pod-*), foot]

brach·y·met·a·tar·sia (brak′ē-met-ă-tar′sē-ă). Abnormal shortness of the metatarsals.

brach·y·mor·phic (brak′ē-mōr′fik). Having, or denoting, a shorter form than that of the usually accepted norm. [brachy- + G. *morphē*, form]

brach·y·o·dont (brak′ē-ō-dont). Having abnormally short teeth. [brachy- + G. *odous*, tooth]

brach·y·o·nych·ia (brak′ē-ō-nik′ē-ă). Short nails, in which the width of the nail plate and nail bed is greater than the length; may be congenital or result from nail biting, bone resorption in hyperparathyroidism, or psoriatic arthropathy. [G. *brachys*, short + *onyx, onychos*, nail, + suffix *-ia*, condition]

brach·y·pel·lic (brak-ē-pel′ik). Denoting a transverse oval pelvis. SEE brachypellic *pelvis*. SYN brachypelvic. [brachy- + pelvis]

brach·y·pel·vic (brak-ē-pel′vik). SYN brachypellic.

brach·y·pha·lan·gia (brak′ē-fă-lan′jē-ă). Abnormal shortness of the phalanges. [brachy- + phalanx]

bra·chyp·o·dous (bra-kip′ō-dŭs). Having abnormally short feet. [brachy- + G. *pous*, foot]

brach·y·pro·sop·ic (brak-ē-prō-sop′ik). Having a disproportionately short face. SYN brachyfacial. [brachy- + G. *prosōpikos*, facial]

brach·y·rhi·nia (brak-ē-rī′nē-ă). Abnormal shortness of the nose. [brachy- + G. *rhis*, nose]

brach·y·rhyn·chus (brak-ē-ring′kŭs). Abnormal shortness of the nose and maxilla, often associated with cyclopia. [brachy- + G. *rhynchos*, snout]

br

brach·y·skel·ic (brak-ē-skel′ik). Relating to abnormally short legs. [brachy- + G. *skelos*, leg]

brach·y·staph·y·line (brak-ē-staf′i-lin). Having a short palate; having a palatomaxillary index above 85. [brachy- + G. *staphylē*, uvula]

brach·y·syn·dac·ty·ly (brak′ē-sin-dak′ti-lē). Abnormal shortness of fingers or toes combined with a webbing between the adjacent digits. [brachy- + syndactyly]

brach·y·te·le·pha·lan·gia (brak-ē-tel′ĕ-fă-lan′jē-ă). Abnormal shortness of the distal phalanges. [brachy- + G. *telos*, end, + phalanx]

brach·y·ther·a·py (brak-ē-ther′ă-pē). Radiotherapy in which the source of irradiation is placed close to the surface of the body or within a body cavity; e.g., application of radium to the cervix.

high-dose-rate b., high-dose b. over time.

interstitial b., radiotherapy by implantation of radioactive needles or other sources directly into and around the tissue to be irradiated.

remote afterloading b., locally delivered radiotherapy that is loaded remotely into previously placed receptacles.

stereotactic b., radiotherapy delivered with the help of CT-guided tissue localization.

brach·y·type (brak′ē-tīp). SYN endomorph.

brac·ing (brās′ing). In dentistry, resistance to horizontal components of masticatory force. SEE *component* of force.

brack·et (brak′et). In dentistry, a small metal attachment that is soldered or welded to an orthodontic band or bonded directly to the teeth, serving to fasten the arch wire to the band or tooth.

Bradbury, Samuel, U.S. physician. SEE B.-Eggleston *syndrome.*

Bradford, Edward H., U.S. orthopedist, 1848–1926. SEE B. *frame.*

△**brady-.** Slow. [G. *bradys*, slow]

bra·dy·ar·rhyth·mia (brad′ē-ă-rith′mē-ă). Any disturbance of the heart's rhythm resulting(by convention) in a rate under 50 beats per min. [brady- + G. *a-* priv. + *rhythmos*, rhythm]

bra·dy·arth·ria (brad-ē-arth′rē-ă). A form of dysarthria characterized by an abnormal slowness or deliberation in speech. SYN bradyglossia (2), bradylalia, bradylogia. [brady- + G. *arthroō*, to utter distinctly, fr. *arthron*, a joint]

bra·dy·car·dia (brad-ē-kar′dē-ă). Slowness of the heartbeat, usually defined (by convention) as a rate under 50 beats/min. SYN brachycardia, bradyrhythmia. [brady- + G. *kardia*, heart]

central b., b. due to disease of the central nervous system, usually with increased intracranial pressure.

essential b., a slow pulse for which no cause can be discovered. SYN idiopathic b.

fetal b., a fetal heart rate of less than 120 beats/min.

idiopathic b., SYN essential b.

marked fetal b., a fetal heart rate less than 100 beats per minute.

mild fetal b., a fetal heart rate between 100-120 beats per minute.

nodal b., SYN atrioventricular junctional *rhythm.*

postinfectious b., a toxic b. occurring during convalescence from various infectious diseases, such as influenza.

sinus b., b. originating in the normal sinus pacemaker.

vagal b., any excessive cardiac slowing due to stimulation of the vagus nerves.

ventricular b., slowness of ventricular rate, usually implying the presence of atrioventricular block.

brad·y·car·di·ac (brad-ē-kar′dē-ak). Relating to or characterized by bradycardia. SYN bradycardic.

bra·dy·car·dic (brad-ē-kar′dik). SYN bradycardiac.

bra·dy·ci·ne·sia (brad-ē-si-nē′sē-ă). SYN bradykinesia.

bra·dy·crot·ic (brad-ē-krot′ik). Relating to or characterized by a slow pulse. [*brady-* + G. *krotos*, a striking]

bra·dy·di·as·to·le (brad-ē-dī-as′tō-lē). Prolongation of the diastole of the heart.

bra·dy·es·the·sia (brad-ē-es-thē′zē-ă). Slow sensory perception. [brady- + G. *aisthēsis*, sensation]

bra·dy·glos·sia (brad-ē-glos′ē-ă). 1. Slow or difficult tongue movement. 2. SYN bradyarthria. [brady- + G. *glōssa*, tongue]

bra·dy·ki·ne·sia (brad-ē-kin-ē′zē-ă). A decrease in spontaneity and movement. One of the features of extrapyramidal disorders, such as Parkinson disease. SYN bradycinesia. [brady- + G. *kinēsis*, movement]

bra·dy·ki·net·ic (brad-ē-ki-net′ik). Characterized by or pertaining to slow movement.

bra·dy·ki·nin (brad-ē-kī′nin). The nonapeptide Arg–Pro–Pro–Gly–Phe–Ser–Pro–Phe–Arg, produced from the decapeptide kallidin (bradykininogen) that is produced from α_2-globulin by kallikrein, normally present in blood in an inactive form and similar to trypsin in action; b. is one of a number of the plasma kinins, is a potent vasodilator, and is one of the physiologic mediators of anaphylaxis released from cytotropic antibody-coated mast cells following reaction with antigen (allergen) specific for the antibody. SYN kallidin 9, kallidin I, kinin 9. [brady- + G. *kineō*, to move]

bra·dy·ki·nin·o·gen (brad′ē-ki-nin′ō-jen). SYN kallidin.

bra·dy·ki·nin po·ten·ti·a·tor B. Glp–Gly–Leu–Pro–Pro–Arg–Pro–Lys–Ile–Pro–Pro; the undecapeptide precursor of bradykinin and the angiotensins.

bra·dy·la·lia (brad-ē-lā′lē-ă). SYN bradyarthria. [brady- + G. *lalia*, speech]

bra·dy·lex·ia (brad-ē-lek′sē-ă). Abnormal slowness in reading. [brady- + G. *lexis*, word]

bra·dy·lo·gia (brad-ē-lō′jē-ă). SYN bradyarthria. [brady- + G. *logos*, word]

bra·dy·pep·sia (brad-ē-pep′sē-ă). Slowness of digestion. [brady- + G. *pepsis*, digestion]

bra·dy·pha·gia (brad-ē-fā′jē-ă). Slowness in eating. [brady- + G. *phagō*, to eat]

bra·dy·pha·sia (brad-ē-fā′zē-ă). A form of aphasia characterized by abnormal slowness of speech. SYN bradyphemia. [brady- + G. *phasis*, speaking]

bra·dy·phe·mia (brad-ē-fē′mē-ă). SYN bradyphasia. [brady- + G. *phēmē*, speech]

bra·dyp·nea (brad-ip-nē′ă). Abnormal slowness of respiration, specifically a low respiratory frequency. [brady- + G. *pnoē*, breathing]

bra·dy·psy·chia (brad-ē-sī′kē-ă). Slowness of mental reactions. [brady- + G. *psychē*, soul]

bra·dy·rhyth·mia (brad-ē-rith′mē-ă). SYN bradycardia.

bra·dy·sper·ma·tism (brad-ē-sper′mă-tizm). Absence of ejaculatory force, so that the semen trickles away slowly. [brady, + G. *sperma* (*spermat*-), seed, + ism]

bra·dy·sphyg·mia (brad-ē-sfig′mē-ă). Slowness of the pulse; can occur without bradycardia, as in ventricular bigeminy when every alternate beat may fail to produce a peripheral pulse. [brady- + G. *sphygmos*, pulse]

bra·dy·stal·sis (brad-ē-stahl′sis). Slow bowel motion. [G. *bradys*, slow, + (*peri*) *stalsis*, contracting around]

bra·dy·tel·e·o·ci·ne·sia (brad′ē-tel-ē-ō-sin-ē′sē-ă). Sudden arrest of a movement just before its intended termination, then after a pause it is completed slowly or by jerks; a symptom of cerebellar disease. SYN bradyteleokinesis. [brady- + G. *teleos*, complete, + *kinēsis*, movement]

bra·dy·tel·e·o·ki·ne·sis (brad′ē-tel-ē-ō-ki-nē′sis). SYN bradyteleocinesia.

bra·dy·u·ria (brad-ē-ū′rē-ă). Slow micturition. [brady- + G. *ouron*, urine]

bra·dy·zo·ite (brad-ē-zō′īt). A slowly multiplying encysted form of sporozoan parasite typical of chronic infection with *Toxoplasma gondii.* It has also been called a merozoite or zoite; the complex of b.'s within an enclosing membrane has also been called a pseudocyst, though it is now regarded as a true cyst. [brady- + G. *zōē*, life]

braille (brāl). A system of writing and printing by means of raised dots corresponding to letters, numbers, and punctuation to enable the blind to read by touch. [Louis *Braille,* French teacher of blind, 1809–1852]

Brailsford, James Frederick, English radiologist, 1888–1961. SEE B.-Morquio *disease.*

Brain, Walter Russell, Lord, English physician, 1895–1966. SEE B. *reflex.*

brain (brān) [TA]. That part of the central nervous system contained within the cranium. SEE ALSO encephalon. Cf. cerebrum, cerebellum. [A.S. *braegen*]

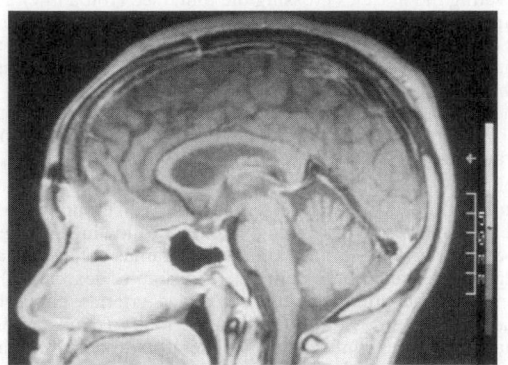

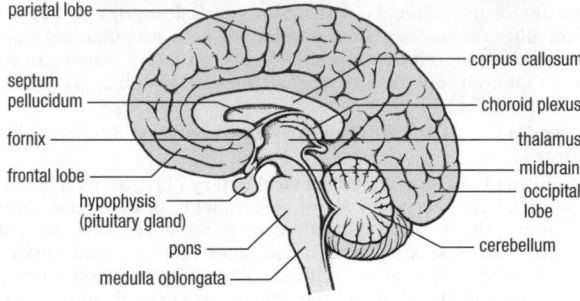

parietal lobe
septum pellucidum
fornix
frontal lobe
hypophysis (pituitary gland)
pons
medulla oblongata
corpus callosum
choroid plexus
thalamus
midbrain
occipital lobe
cerebellum

brain: (above) magnetic resonance image (MRI) of a normal brain, (below) illustration of the same midsagittal view

split b., a b. in which the corpus callosum and usually the anterior and posterior commissures have been sectioned; usually to treat certain refractory epilepsies.

visceral b., SYN limbic *system.*

brain·case (brān′kās). SYN neurocranium.

brain·stem, brain stem (brān′stem) [TA]. Originally, the entire unpaired subdivision of the brain, composed of (in anterior sequence) the rhombencephalon, mesencephalon, and diencephalon as distinguished from the brain's only paired subdivision, the telencephalon. More recently, the term's connotation has undergone several arbitrary modifications: some use it to denote no more than rhombencephalon plus mesencephalon, distinguishing that complex from the prosencephalon (diencephalon plus telencephalon); others restrict it even further to refer exclusively to the rhombencephalon. From both developmental and architectural viewpoints, the original interpretation seems preferable. SYN truncus encephali [TA].

brain·wash·ing (brān′wash′ing). Inducing a person to modify attitudes and behavior in certain directions through various forms of psychological pressure or torture.

bran. A by-product of the milling of wheat, containing approximately 20% of indigestible cellulose; a bulk cathartic, usually taken in the form of cereal or special bran products.

branch [TA]. An offshoot; in anatomy, one of the primary divisions of a nerve or blood vessel. A branch. SEE ramus, artery, nerve, vein. SYN ramus (1) [TA].

accessory meningeal b., SYN pterygomeningeal *artery.*

accessory meningeal b. of middle meningeal artery, SYN accessory b. of middle meningeal artery.

accessory b. of middle meningeal artery [TA], a b. of either the middle meningeal or maxillary artery in the infratemporal fossa and passing superiorly through the foramen ovale to supply the trigeminal ganglion, dura mater, and inner table of bone. SYN ramus accessorius arteriae meningeae mediae [TA], accessory meningeal b. of middle meningeal artery, ramus meningeus accessorius arteriae meningeae mediae.

acetabular b. [TA], an arterial b. that supplies the acetabulum; two arteries, the obturator and the medial femoral circumflex, have such b.'s. SYN ramus acetabularis [TA], acetabular artery, arteria acetabuli.

acromial b. of suprascapular artery [TA], b. of suprascapular artery that pierces the origin of the trapezius muscle to run to the acromion; *anastomoses,* acromial b. of thoracoacromial artery. SYN ramus acromialis arteriae suprascapularis [TA].

acromial b. of thoracoacromial artery [TA], a b. of the thoracoacromial artery that runs over the coracoid process and under the deltoid muscle. SYN ramus acromialis arteriae thoracoacromialis [TA], acromial artery.

anastomotic b. [TA], a blood vessel that interconnects two neighboring vessels. The term should not be used to describe internerve communication in the nervous system, because there is no analogy between a vascular anastomosing branch and a connection between nerves or their subdivisions. SYN ramus anastomoticus [TA].

anastomotic b. of middle meningeal artery with lacrimal artery [TA], a b. of the middle meningeal artery arising in the cranial cavity that runs anteriorly through the superior orbital fissure to anastomose with the lacrimal artery. SEE orbital b. of middle meningeal artery. SYN ramus anastomoticus arteriae meningeae mediae cum arteriae lacrimali [TA].

b. to angular gyrus [TA], the last b. of the terminal part of the middle cerebral artery distributed to parts of the temporal parietal and occipital lobes. SYN angular artery (2) [TA], arteria angularis [TA], arteria gyri angularis [TA], artery of angular gyrus.

anterior b. [TA], the anterior branch of the following: 1) great auricular nerve; 2) left and right superior pulmonary veins; 3) medial cutaneous nerve of the forearm; 4) obturator artery; 5) obturator nerve; 6) renal artery; 7) right branch of portal vein; 8) right hepatic duct; 9) ulnar recurrent artery. SYN ramus anterior [TA].

anterior abdominal cutaneous b. of intercostal nerve [TA], continuation of the ventral rami of spinal nerves (intercostal nerves) T7–T11 distal to the origin of the lateral cutaneous b.'s; distributed to anterior abdominal wall. SEE ALSO thoracoabdominal *nerves,* under *nerve.* SYN ramus cutaneus anterior abdominalis nervi intercostalis [TA].

anterior auricular b.'s of superficial temporal artery [TA], *distribution,* auricle, earlobe and external acoustic meatus. SYN rami auriculares anteriores arteriae temporalis superficialis [TA].

anterior basal b., SYN anterior basal segmental *artery.*

anterior basal b. of superior basal vein (of right and left inferior pulmonary veins), ⁎official alternate term for anterior basal *vein.*

anterior cutaneous b.'s of femoral nerve [TA], cutaneous b.'s of the femoral nerve distributed to the anterior and medial aspects of the thigh; convey general sensation. SYN rami cutanei anteriores nervi femoralis [TA], anterior femoral cutaneous nerves.

anterior cutaneous b. of iliohypogastric nerve [TA], *distribution,* skin on pubis. SYN ramus cutaneus anterior nervi iliohypogastrici [TA], genital b. of iliohypogastric nerve.

anterior cutaneous b.'s of intercostal nerves, medial mammary b.'s of anterior cutaneous b.'s of ventral primary rami of thoracic spinal nerves. SEE medial mammary b.'s.

anterior gastric b.'s of anterior vagal trunk [TA], anterior gastric b.'s of the vagus; b.'s of the anterior vagal trunk to the anterior surface of the stomach. SYN rami gastrici anteriores trunci vagalis anterioris [TA], gastric b.'s of anterior vagal trunk, rami gastrici anteriores nervi vagi.

anterior glandular b. of superior thyroid artery [TA], b.'s that pass deep to the sternothyroid muscle, descend along the medial side of the upper pole of the lateral lobe, and then superior margin of the isthmus, anastomosing with the contralateral artery; they mainly supply the anterior aspect of the thyroid. SYN ramus glandularis anterior arteriae thyroideae superioris [TA].

anterior intercostal b.'s of internal thoracic artery [TA], one of the arteries supplying the anterior portions of the intercostal spaces of the thoracic wall. Anterior intercostal arteries 1–6 arise as b.'s of the internal thoracic artery; 7–11 arise as b.'s of the musculophrenic artery. SYN rami intercostales anteriores arteriae thoracicae internae [TA], anterior intercostal arteries, rami intercostales anteriores.

anterior interventricular b. of left coronary artery [TA], terminal b. (with circumflex coronary artery of left coronary artery; descends in anterior interventricular groove to apex, anastomosing with posterior interventricular artery. Supplies most of sternal aspect of ventricles and anterior two-thirds of interventricular septum, including atrioventricular bundle of conducting tissue. SYN ramus interventricularis anterior arteriae coronariae sinistrae [TA], anterior interventricular artery, left anterior descending artery.

anterior labial b.'s of deep external pudendal artery [TA], b.'s to the labium majus. SYN rami labiales anteriores arteriae pudendae externae profundae [TA], anterior labial arteries, arteriae labiales anteriores.

anterior/lateral/posterior glandular b.'s of superior thyroid artery, b.'s of the b.'s of the superior thyroid artery to the thyroid gland. SYN ramus glandulares anterior/lateralis/posterior arteriae thyroideae superioris.

anterior lateral nasal b.'s of anterior ethmoidal artery [TA], b.'s of the intracranial part of the anterior ethmoidal artery that pass through the cribriform plates of the ethmoid bone, descending into the nasal cavity with the anterior ethmoidal nerves, to run in a groove on the deep surface of the nasal bone, and supply the anterosuperior aspect of the lateral wall of the cavity. SYN rami nasales anteriores laterales arteriae ethmoidalis anterioris [TA].

anterior meningeal b. (of anterior ethmoidal artery) [TA], *origin,* anterior ethmoidal; *distribution,* meninges in anterior cranial fossa; *anastomoses,* b.'s of middle meningeal and meningeal b.'s of internal carotid and lacrimal. SYN arteria meningea anterior [TA], ramus meningeus anterior arteriae ethmoidalis anterioris [TA], anterior meningeal artery.

anterior pectoral cutaneous b. of intercostal nerves [TA], continuation of the ventral rami of spinal nerves (intercostal nerves) T1–T6 distal to the origin of the lateral cutaneous b.'s; become cutaneous in the parasternal line and divide into medial (sternal) and lateral (mammary) b.'s; distributed to anterior thoracic wall. SYN ramus cutaneus anterior pectoralis nervi intercostalis [TA].

anterior b. of the renal artery [TA], SEE segmental *arteries* of kidney, under *artery.*

anterior scrotal b. of deep external pudendal artery [TA], *distribution,* skin of anterior scrotum; *anastomoses,* posterior scrotal b.'s from internal pudendal artery. SYN rami scrotales anteriores arteriae pudendae externae profundae [TA].

anterior septal b.'s of anterior ethmoidal artery [TA], b.'s of the intracranial part of the anterior ethmoidal artery that pass through the cribriform plates of the ethmoid bone, descending into the nasal cavity with the anterior ethmoidal nerves, and supply the anterosuperior aspect of the nasal septum. SYN rami septales anteriores arteriae ethmoidalis anterioris [TA].

anterior superior alveolar b.'s of infraorbital nerve, SYN anterior superior alveolar *nerves,* under *nerve.*

anterior temporal b. [TA], a b. of the insular part of the middle cerebral artery distributed to the cortex of the anterior part of the temporal lobe. SYN ramus temporalis anterior [TA], anterior temporal artery, arteria temporalis anterior.

anteromedial central b.'s, branches of the anterior communicating artery which supply part of the hypothalamus (suprachiasmatic artery [TA], median commissural artery [TA]) and a medial area of the corpus callosum (median callosal artery [TA]). SYN rami centrales anteromediales [TA].

anteromedial frontal b. of callosomarginal artery [TA], b. of initial portion of callosomarginal artery to anteroinferior portion of medial aspect of frontal lobe of cerebrum. SYN ramus frontalis anteromedialis arteriae callosomarginalis [TA].

apical b. of inferior lobar branch of right pulmonary artery,

*official alternate term for apical segmental *artery* of superior lobar artery of right lung.

apical b. of right superior pulmonary vein, *official alternate term for apical *vein.*

apicoposterior b. of left superior pulmonary vein, *official alternate term for apicoposterior *vein.*

articular b.'s [TA], b.'s distributed to joints. Almost any vessel related to a joint will supply articular rami. Most joints receive articular b.'s from the intramuscular b.'s of the motor nerves innervating the muscles crossing the joint (see Hilton *law*). At this printing, Terminologia Anatomica, however, specifically recognizes only the articular b.'s of (1) the descending genicular artery (ramus articulares arteriae descendentis genicularis) [TA]; supplying the knee joint; (2) articular b.'s of mixed spinal nerves (rami cutanei nervi mixtus); and (3) the articular b. of the posterior b. of the obturator nerves (rami articulares ramorum posteriores nervus obturatorius) supplying the hip joint. SYN rami articulares [TA], joint b.'s.

ascending b. [TA], a b. directed superiorly. Terminologia Anatomica recognizes an ascending b. of the following: 1) anterior segmental arteries of left and right lungs (ramus ascendens arteriae segmentales anteriores pulmones sinistrae et dextrae), 2) deep circumflex iliac artery (ramus ascendens arteriae circumflexae iliacae profundae), 3) inferior epigastric artery (ramus ascendens arteriae epigastricae inferiores), 4) lateral and medial circumflex femoral arteries (rami ascendens arteriae circumflexae femoris lateralis et medialis), 5) posterior segmental arteries of left and right lungs (ramus ascendens arteriae segmentales pulmones sinistrae et dextrae), and 6) superficial cervical artery (ramus ascendens ramorum superficiales arteriae transversae collie). SYN ramus ascendens [TA].

ascending b. of the inferior mesenteric artery, SYN ascending *artery* (2).

ascending b. of superficial cervical artery [TA], ascending b. of superficial cervical artery (or of superficial b. of transverse cervical artery) that passes superiorly deep to the upper (cervical) part of the trapezius, supplying it, adjacent muscles, and cervical lymph nodes; anastomoses with descending b. of occipital artery. SEE ALSO superficial b. of the transverse cervical artery. SYN ramus ascendens arteriae superficialis cervicalis [TA].

atrial b.'s [TA], b.'s of the right coronary artery and the circumflex b. of the left coronary artery distributed to the right and left atrium, respectively. SYN rami atriales [TA].

atrial anastomotic b. of circumflex branch of left coronary artery [TA], a vessel of variable origin, most commonly a b. of the circumflex artery, coursing posteriorly through the base of the interatrial septum toward the crux of the heart, anastomosing with coronary artery b.'s supplying the atrioventricular node, the atrioventricular bundle (bundle of His), and the upper posterior walls of the left ventricle. SYN ramus atrialis anastomoticus ramus circumflexus arteriae coronariae sinistrae [TA], arteria anastomotica auricularis magna, Kugel anastomotic artery.

atrioventricular nodal b. [TA], the atrioventricular b.'s or the nodal b.'s, the small arteries supplying the atrioventricular node; they usually arise from the right coronary artery where it starts to descend the posterior interventricular sulcus. SYN ramus nodi atrioventricularis [TA], artery to atrioventricular node, b. to atrioventricular node.

b. to atrioventricular node, SYN atrioventricular nodal b.

auricular b. of occipital artery [TA], *distribution,* posterior auricle; *anastomosis,* posterior auricular artery. SYN ramus auricularis arteriae occipitalis [TA].

auricular b. of posterior auricular artery [TA], arises in the groove between the auricular cartilage and the mastoid process, ascends deep to auricularis posterior muscles, and ramifies on the cranial aspect of the auricle. SYN ramus auricularis arteriae auricularis posterioris [TA].

auricular b. of vagus nerve [TA], a b. of the superior ganglion of the vagus, supplying the back of the pinna and the external acoustic meatus. SYN Arnold nerve, ramus auricularis nervi vagi.

b.'s of auriculotemporal nerve to tympanic membrane [TA], sensory b. of the auriculotemporal nerve supplying the external surface of the tympanic membrane. SYN rami membranae tympani nervi auriculotemporalis [TA], nerve of tympanic membrane.

basal tentorial b. of internal carotid artery, SYN tentorial basal b. of internal carotid artery.

bronchial b.'s of thoracic aorta [TA], the bronchial branches or arteries, vessels, or nerves distributed to the bronchi; the following have branches so named: 1) thoracic aorta; 2) internal thoracic artery; 3) vagus nerves. SYN bronchial arteries, rami bronchiales.

buccal b.'s of facial nerve, motor b.'s of the facial nerve distributed to buccina or muscle and other muscles of facial expression below orbit and above chin. SYN rami buccales nervi facialis [TA].

calcaneal b.'s [TA], the calcaneal b.'s or arteries, b.'s to the structures in the calcaneal region from 1) the posterior tibial artery and 2) the fibular artery. SYN rami calcanei [TA], calcaneal arteries.

calcarine b. of medial occipital artery [TA], b. of medial occipital artery that runs in relationship to the calcarine sulcus. SYN ramus calcarinus arteriae occipitalis medialis [TA], arteria calcarina, calcarine artery.

capsular b.'s of intrarenal arteries [TA], b.'s of arteries coursing within the renal cortex (cortical and perforate radiate arteries) that supply the fibrous capsule of the kidney. SYN rami capsulares arteriorum intrarenalium [TA].

capsular b.'s of renal artery [TA], b.'s arising from the renal artery outside the kidney that are distributed to the renal capsule. SYN rami capsulares arteriae renalis [TA].

carotid b. of glossopharyngeal nerve (CN IX), a branch of the glossopharyngeal nerve that innervates the baroreceptors in the wall of the carotid sinus and the chemoreceptors in the carotid body. SYN ramus sinus carotici nervi glossopharyngei CN IX [TA], ramus sinus carotici [TA], carotid sinus b., carotid sinus nerve, Hering sinus nerve, intercarotid nerve, nerve to carotid sinus, sinus nerve of Hering.

carotid sinus b., SYN carotid b. of glossopharyngeal nerve (CN IX).

caudate b.'s of left branch of portal vein [TA], b.'s of transverse part of left branch of portal vein distributed to the caudate lobe before the vein enters the liver. SYN rami lobi caudati rami sinistri venae portae hepatis [TA].

cavernous b. of cavernous part of internal carotid artery [TA], a number of small b.'s of the cavernous part of the internal carotid artery. SEE b.'s of internal carotid artery to trigeminal ganglion, tentorial basal b. of internal carotid artery, marginal tentorial b. of internal carotid artery. SYN ramus sinus cavernosi partis cavernosae arteriae carotidis internae [TA], cavernous arteries, cavernous sinus b. of internal carotid artery, ramus sinus cavernosi arteriae carotidis arteriae, ramus sinus cavernosi arteriae carotidis internae.

cavernous sinus b. of internal carotid artery, SYN cavernous b. of cavernous part of internal carotid artery.

celiac b.'s of posterior vagal trunk [TA], terminal b.'s of the posterior vagal trunk conveying presynaptic parasympathetic fibers to—and visceral afferent fibers from—the celiac plexus. SYN rami celiaci trunci vagi posterioris [TA], celiac b.'s of vagus nerve, rami celiaci nervi vagi.

celiac b.'s of vagus nerve, SYN celiac b.'s of posterior vagal trunk.

cervical b. of facial nerve [TA], the most inferior b. of the parotid plexus of the facial nerve, it descends to innervate the platysma muscle. SYN ramus colli nervi facialis [TA], ramus cervicalis nervi facialis*.

choroid b.'s, the choroid branches: rami choroidei posteriores laterales [TA], lateral posterior choroid branches of posterior cerebral artery distributed to the choroid plexus of the lateral ventricle; rami choroidei posteriores mediales [TA], medial posterior choroid branches of posterior cerebral artery distributed to the choroid plexus of the third ventricle; rami choroidei ventriculi lateralis [TA], lateral ventricle choroid branches of anterior choroid artery distributed to the plexus of the lateral ventricle; rami choroidei ventriculi tertii [TA], choroid branches of anterior choroid artery to the third ventricle; ramus choroideus ventriculi quarti [TA], fourth ventricle choroid branch of posterior inferior cerebellar artery. SYN rami choroidei.

cingular b. of callosomarginal artery [TA], terminal b. (with posteromedial frontal b.) of callosomarginal artery that courses in the cingulate sulcus on the medial aspect of the cerebrum. SYN ramus cingularis arteriae callosomarginalis [TA].

circumferential pontine b.'s of pontine arteries, *official alternate term for lateral b.'s of pontine arteries.

circumflex fibular b. (of posterior tibial artery) [TA], a b. of the initial (superior) part of the posterior tibial artery which winds around the neck of the fibula and joins the anastomoses around the knee joint. SYN ramus circumflexus fibularis arteriae tibialis posterioris [TA], circumflex b. of posterior tibial artery*, circumflex peroneal b. of posterior tibial artery*, ramus circumflexus peronealis arteriae tibialis posterioris*, circumflex fibular artery.

circumflex b. of left coronary artery [TA], terminal b. (with anterior interventricular artery) of left coronary artery which runs to left and then posteriorly in the coronary groove supplying atrial and ventricular b.'s. SYN ramus circumflexus arteriae coronariae sinistrae [TA].

circumflex peroneal b. of posterior tibial artery, *official alternate term for circumflex fibular b. (of posterior tibial artery).

circumflex b. of posterior tibial artery, *official alternate term for circumflex fibular b. (of posterior tibial artery).

clavicular b. of thoracoacromial artery [TA], *distribution*, subclavius muscle and sternoclavicular joint. SYN ramus clavicularis arteriae thoracoacromialis [TA].

clivus b.'s of cerebral part of internal carotid artery [TA], small b.'s arising near the ophthalmic artery that pass medially and inferiorly to the sphenoidal portion of the clivus. SYN rami clivales partis cerebralis arteriae carotidis internae [TA].

cochlear b. of labyrinthine artery, SYN cochlear b. of vestibulocochlear artery.

cochlear b. of vestibulocochlear artery [TA], terminal b. (with posterior vestibular b.) of vestibulocochlear artery; it anatomoses with a b. of the common cochlear artery forming the spiral modiolar artery; the cochlear branch specifically supplies the spiral ganglion and cochlear duct of the basal turn of the cochlea. SYN ramus cochlearis arteriae vestibulocochlearis [TA], cochlear b. of labyrinthine artery, ramus cochlearis arteriae labyrinthi.

colic b. of ileocolic artery [TA], the b. of the inferior b. of the ileocolic artery that passes superiorly up the ascending colon to communicate with a b. of the right colic artery and supplying the ascending colon. SYN arteria ascendens (1) [TA], ascending artery (1) [TA], ramus colicus arteriae ileocolicae [TA].

collateral b. of intercostal nerves [TA], inferior b. of an intercostal nerve arising medial (proximal) to the angles of the ribs and coursing in the intercostal space along the superior border of the rib below, paralleling the course of the intercostal nerve, which courses along the inferior border of the rib above. SYN ramus collateralis nervorum intercostalium [TA].

collateral b.'s of posterior intercostal arteries 3–11 [TA], b. arising near angle of rib and descending to run along superior border of rib below; *distribution:* lower half of intercostal spaces 3–11; *anastomoses:* collateral b.'s of anterior intercostal arteries. SYN ramus collateralis arteriarum intercostalium posteriorum III–XI [TA].

communicating b. [TA], a bundle of nerve fibers passing from one named nerve to join another. The term "communicating branch" is used in the nervous system to replace the inadequate "anastomosing branch" used for vascular systems. SYN ramus communicans [TA].

communicating b. of anterior interosseous nerve with ulnar nerve [TA], connection occurring occasionally between the anterior interosseous and ulnar nerves in the proximal forearm. SYN ramus communicans nervi interossei antebrachii anterioris cum nervi ulnari [TA].

communicating b.'s of auriculotemporal nerve with facial nerve [TA], b.'s conveying fibers from the auriculotemporal nerve to the facial nerve. SYN rami communicantes nervi auriculotemporalis cum nervo faciali [TA].

communicating b. of chorda tympani to lingual nerve, SYN communicating b. of chorda tympani with lingual nerve.

communicating b. of chorda tympani with lingual nerve [TA], terminal b. of chorda tympani joining the lingual nerve in the infratemporal fossa; conveys sensory fibers for taste from anterior two-thirds of tongue and presynaptic parasympathetic fibers destined for submandibular ganglion for innervation of submandibular and sublingual salivary glands. SYN ramus communicans cum chorda tympani (1) [TA], communicating b. of chorda tympani to lingual nerve, ramus communicans nervi lingualis cum chorda tympani.

communicating b. of facial nerve with glossopharyngeal nerve [TA], a small branch from the digastric branch of the facial nerve to the glossopharyngeal nerve. SYN ramus communicans nervi facialis cum nervo glossopharyngeo [TA], Haller ansa, ramus communicans cum nervo glossopharyngeo (1).

communicating b. of facial nerve with tympanic plexus, SYN communicating b. of intermediate nerve with tympanic plexus.

communicating b. of fibular artery [TA], the communicating b. of the fibular (peroneal) artery. SYN ramus communicans arteriae fibularis [TA], communicating * b. of peroneal artery*, ramus communicans arteriae peroneae*.

communicating b. of glossopharyngeal nerve with auricular branch of vagus nerve, SYN communicating b. of tympanic plexus with auricular branch of vagus nerve.

communicating b. of intermediate nerve with tympanic plexus [TA], a fine b. of facial nerve joining the tympanic b. of the glossopharyngeal nerve. SYN ramus communicans nervi intermedii cum plexu tympanico [TA], communicating b. of facial nerve with tympanic plexus, ramus communicans nervi facialis cum plexu tympanico.

communicating b. of internal laryngeal nerve with recurrent laryngeal nerve [TA], b. of internal branch of superior laryngeal nerve communicating with the recurrent laryngeal nerve in the wall of the laryngopharynx supplying sensory fibers to the latter. SYN ramus communicans nervi laryngei interni cum nervo laryngeo recurrente [TA], communicating b. of superior laryngeal nerve with recurrent laryngeal nerve, Galen anastomosis, Galen nerve, ramus communicans nervi laryngei recurrentis cum ramo laryngeo interno, ramus communicans nervi laryngei superioris cum nervo laryngeo recurrenti.

communicating b. of lacrimal nerve with zygomatic nerve [TA], nerve b. by which postsynaptic parasympathetic (secretomotor) fibers from the pterygopalatine ganglion are transferred from the zygomatic nerve to the lacrimal nerve (heretofore purely sensory) for distribution to the lacrimal gland. SYN ramus communicans nervi lacrimalis cum nervo zygomatico [TA].

communicating b.'s of lingual nerve with hypoglossal nerve [TA], communicating b.'s between the lingual nerve (from mandibular nerve) and hypoglossal nerve forming a plexus on the hyoglossus muscle. SYN rami communicantes nervi lingualis cum nervo hypoglosso [TA].

communicating b. of median nerve with ulnar nerve [TA], b. of median nerve joining the ulnar nerve in the hand; the anterior interosseous b. of the median nerve may also communicate with the ulnar nerve in the proximal forearm. SYN ramus communicans nervi mediani cum nervo ulnari.

communicating b. of nasociliary nerve with ciliary ganglion, SYN sensory *root* of ciliary ganglion.

communicating b. of otic ganglion to auriculotemporal nerve, a b. of the otic ganglion joining the roots of the auriculotemporal nerve to convey postsynaptic parasympathetic fibers to the parotid gland. SYN ramus communicans ganglii otici cum nervo auriculotemporali.

communicating b. of otic ganglion to chorda tympani, SYN communicating b. of otic ganglion with chorda tympani.

communicating b. of otic ganglion with chorda tympani, a small b. of the otic ganglion conveying sensory fibers to the chorda tympani. SYN ramus communicans cum chorda tympani (2) [TA], communicating b. of otic ganglion to chorda tympani, ramus communicans ganglii otici cum chorda tympani.

communicating b. of otic ganglion with medial pterygoid nerve, b. of otic ganglion joining the nerve to the medial pterygoid muscle. SYN ramus communicans ganglii otici cum nervo pterygoideo mediali.

communicating b. of otic ganglion with meningeal branch of mandibular nerve, a b. of otic ganglion to the meningeal branch

of mandibular nerve conveying postsynaptic parasympathetic fibers that run back to the main stem of the mandibular nerve for distribution to the parotid gland via the auriculotemporal nerve. SYN ramus communicans ganglii otici cum ramo meningeo nervi mandibularis.

communicating b. of peroneal artery, *official alternate term for communicating b. of fibular artery.

communicating b. of radial nerve with ulnar nerve [TA], connection between superficial b. of radial nerve and dorsal b. of ulnar nerve on dorsum of hand. SYN ramus communicans nervi radialis cum nervi ulnari [TA].

communicating b.'s of spinal nerves, SYN white *rami* communicantes, under *ramus*.

communicating b. of superficial radial nerve with ulnar nerve, ulnar communicating b. of superficial b. of radial nerve, joining the dorsal b. of the ulnar nerve in the hand conveying sensation from the dorsal aspect of adjacent sides of the middle and ring fingers. SYN ramus communicans ulnaris nervi radialis, ulnar communicating b. of superficial radial nerve.

communicating b. of superior laryngeal nerve with recurrent laryngeal nerve, SYN communicating b. of internal laryngeal nerve with recurrent laryngeal nerve.

communicating b.'s of sympathetic trunk, SYN gray *rami* communicantes, under *ramus*.

communicating b. of tympanic plexus with auricular branch of vagus nerve [TA], a small b. of the glossopharyngeal nerve that joins the auricular b. of the vagus, conveying tactile fibers. SYN ramus communicans plexus tympanici cum ramo auriculari nervi vagi [TA], communicating b. of glossopharyngeal nerve with auricular branch of vagus nerve, ramus communicans cum nervo glossopharyngeo (2), ramus communicans nervi glossopharyngei cum ramo auriculari nervi vagi.

cricothyroid b. of superior thyroid artery [TA], a small branch of the superior thyroid artery that supplies the cricothyroid muscle. SYN cricothyroid artery, ramus cricothyroideus (arteriae thyroideae superioris).

cutaneous b. of anterior branch of obturator nerve [TA], b. of the anterior branch of obturator nerve supplying skin of medial thigh above knee. SYN ramus cutaneus rami anterioris nervi obturatorii [TA], cutaneous b. of obturator nerve.

cutaneous b. of mixed nerve [TA], b. of a mixed spinal nerve (or its derivatives) innervating skin; such b.'s would convey mostly somatic sensory but also visceral motor fibers (postsynaptic sympathetic fibers for vasomotion and pilomotion). SYN ramus cutaneus nervi mixti [TA].

cutaneous b. of obturator nerve, SYN cutaneous b. of anterior branch of obturator nerve.

deep b. [TA], b. that passes deeply, beneath, or farther from surface; usually in contrast to a superficial b. SYN ramus profundus [TA].

deep b. of the lateral plantar nerve [TA], motor b. of lateral plantar nerve supplying lumbricals 2–4, plantar and dorsal interossei, and the adductor hallucis muscles. SYN ramus profundus nervi plantaris lateralis [TA].

deep b. of the medial circumflex femoral artery [TA], distributed to posterior aspect of femoral head and neck. SYN ramus profundus arteriae circumflexae femoris medialis [TA].

deep b. of the medial plantar artery [TA], b. running deep to abductor hallucis, supplying it and the flexor hallucis brevis muscle deep to the artery and the skin of the medial side of the distal foot. SYN ramus profundus arteriae plantaris medialis [TA].

deep palmar b. of ulnar artery [TA], b. of the ulnar artery that supplies the hypothenar muscles then passes deep into the palm to the flexor tendons and anastomoses with the deep palmar arch from the radial artery. SYN ramus palmaris profundus arteriae ulnaris [TA].

deep plantar b. of dorsalis pedis artery, SYN deep plantar *artery*. SYN arteria plantaris profundus [TA].

deep b. of radial nerve [TA], originates in cubital fossa (with superficial b.) as termination of (common) radial nerve; pierces supinator, supplying it and other extensors of forearm. Its terminal portion is the posterior interosseous nerve, which runs on the interosseous membrane in the distal third of the forearm. SEE ALSO posterior interosseous *nerve*. SYN ramus profundus nervi radialis [TA].

deep b. of the superior gluteal artery [TA], b. of superior gluteal artery that extends laterally, between the gluteus medius and minimus muscles, accompanying the superior gluteal nerve. SYN ramus profundus arteriae gluteae superioris [TA].

deep b. of the transverse cervical artery, SYN dorsal scapular *artery*.

deep b. of the ulnar nerve [TA], accompanies deep palmar b. of ulnar artery and deep palmar arch to supply wrist joint, lumbricals 3 & 4, palmar and dorsal interossei adductor pollicis and deep head of flexor pollicis brevis muscles. SYN ramus profundus nervi ulnaris [TA].

deltoid b. [TA], b.'s related to the deltoid muscle. Terminologica Anatomica lists deltoid b.'s of the following: 1) thoracoacromial artery (ramus deltoideus arteriae thoracoacromialis [TA]); 2) profunda brachii artery (ramus deltoideus arteriae profundae brachii [TA]). SYN ramus deltoideus [TA].

dental b.'s [TA], b.'s to the teeth. Terminologica Anatomica lists dental b.'s of the following: 1) anterior superior alveolar artery (rami dentales arteriarum alveolarium superiorum anteriorum [TA]); 2) inferior alveolar artery (rami dentales arteriae alveolaris inferioris [TA]); 3) posterior superior alveolar artery (rami dentales arteriae alveolaris superioris posterioris [TA]). SYN rami dentales [TA], dental rami.

descending b. [TA], b. of an artery or nerve passing inferiorly. Descending b.'s have been described for the following: (1) descending b. of hypoglossal nerve, superior root of ansa cervicalis; (2) descending branch of lateral circumflex femoral artery; (3) descending b. of the occipital artery. SYN ramus descendens [TA].

descending anterior b., SYN descending b. of anterior segmental artery of left and right lungs.

descending b. of anterior segmental artery of left and right lungs [TA], the descending anterior b. of the superior lobar b.'s of the right and left pulmonry arteries. SYN ramus descendens arteriae segmentalis anterioris pulmonis dextri et sinistri [TA], descending anterior b., ramus anterior descendens.

descending b. of hypoglossal nerve, SYN superior *root* of ansa cervicalis.

descending b. of lateral circumflex femoral artery [TA], a major b. of the lateral circumflex femoral artery accompanying the nerve to the vastus lateralis muscle along the anterior border of that muscle and deep to the rectus femoris muscle, supplying both muscles. *Anastomosis:* with lateral superior genicular artery, i.e., it contributes to the articular network of the knee. SYN ramus descendens arteriae circumflexae femoris lateralis [TA].

descending b. of medial circumflex femoral artery [TA], large artery passing deep to the rectus femoris muscle, accompanying the muscular b. of the femoral nerve to the vastus lateralis; terminates by anastomosing with the superior lateral genicular artery. SYN ramus descendens arteriae circumflexae femoris medialis [TA].

descending b. of occipital artery [TA], *origin:* occipital artery within occipital groove; *distribution:* posterior neck muscles and cervical trapezius muscle; *anastomoses:* superficial and deep cervical arteries, vertebral artery. SYN ramus descendens arteriae occipitalis [TA], princeps cervicis artery, princeps cervicis.

descending posterior b., SYN descending b. of posterior segmental artery of left and right lungs.

descending b. of posterior segmental artery of left and right lungs [TA], the descending posterior b. of the superior lobar b. of the left and right pulmonary arteries. SYN ramus descendens arteriae segmentalis posterioris pulmonis dextri et sinistri [TA], descending posterior b., ramus posterior descendens.

descending b. of superficial cervical artery [TA], descending b. of superficial cervical artery (or of superficial b. of transverse cervical artery) that passes inferiorly with the accessory nerve, deep to the middle and lower parts of the trapezius, which it supplies. SYN ramus descendens rami superficialis arteriae transversae cervicis [TA].

digastric b. of facial nerve [TA], b. of the facial nerve innervating the posterior belly of the digastric muscle. SYN ramus digastricus nervi facialis [TA].

dorsal b., (1) SYN posterior *ramus* of spinal nerve; **(2)** posteriorly-directed b.'s.

dorsal carpal b. of radial artery [TA], a b. of the radial artery that passes to the back of the wrist to join the dorsal carpal network. SYN ramus carpalis dorsalis arteriae radialis [TA], ramus carpeus dorsalis arteriae radialis.

dorsal carpal b. of ulnar artery [TA], a b. of the ulnar artery that passes to the dorsal side of the carpus to enter the dorsal carpal network. SYN ramus carpalis dorsalis arteriae ulnaris [TA], ramus carpeus dorsalis arteriae ulnaris.

dorsal b.'s of first and second posterior intercostal artery [TA], b.'s of the 1st and 2nd posterior intercostal arteries which arise as b.'s of the supreme intercostal artery. The distribtuion is the same as for the dorsal b.'s of the other posterior intercostal arteries at the T1–T2 vertebral level. SYN rami dorsales arteriarum intercostalium posteriorum primae et secundae [TA], dorsal b.'s of the superior intercostal artery, rami dorsales arteriae intercostalis supremae.

dorsal lingual b.'s of lingual artery [TA], b.'s of the lingual artery to the posterior third or root of tongue. SYN rami dorsales linguae arteriae lingualis [TA].

dorsal b. of the lumbar artery [TA], terminal b. (with ventral b.) of the 4–5 lumbar arteries, distributed to lumbar portion of back, posterior vertebral column, and spinal cord and environs. SYN ramus dorsalis arteriae lumbalis [TA].

dorsal b. of the posterior intercostal arteries 3–11 [TA], terminal b. (with ventral b.) of the 3rd through 11th posterior intercostal arteries, distributed to thoracic portion of posterior vertebral column, spinal cord and environs, and back. SYN ramus dorsalis arteriarum intercostalium posteriorum III–XI [TA].

dorsal b. of the posterior intercostal veins 4–11 [TA], major tributary of the 4th through 11th posterior intercostal veins; area drained is the same as that supplied by the dorsal b. of posterior intercostal arteries. SYN ramus dorsalis venarum intercostalium posteriorum IV–XI [TA].

dorsal b. of the subcostal artery, terminal b. (with ventral b.) of subcostal artery, distributed to posterior vertebral column, spinal cord and environs, and back at the T12–L1 vertebral level. SYN ramus dorsales arteriae subcostalis [TA], rami dorsales arteriae subcostalis.

dorsal b. of the subcostal artery [TA], b. of subcostal artery supplying muscles of the back and the overlying skin, immediately below the level of the 12th rib.

dorsal b.'s of the superior intercostal artery, SYN dorsal b.'s of first and second posterior intercostal artery.

dorsal b. of the ulnar nerve [TA], b. arising from the ulnar nerve proximal to the wrist for distribution to the medial side of the dorsum of the hand and proximal portion of the little finger and medial side of ring finger. SYN rami dorsales nervi ulnaris [TA].

duodenal b.'s of anterior superior pancreaticoduodenal artery [TA], b.'s extending to the duodenum from the arterial arcade that lies anterior to the head of the pancreas in the concavity of the duodenum. SYN rami duodenales arteriae pancreaticoduodenalis superioris anterioris [TA].

duodenal b.'s of posterior superior pancreaticoduodenal artery [TA], b.'s extending to the duodenum from the arterial arcade that lies posterior to the head of the pancreas in the concavity of the duodenum.

epiploic b.'s, SYN omental b.'s.

esophageal b.'s [TA], b.'s to the esophagus. SYN rami esophagei [TA], rami esophageales✶.

esophageal b.'s of the inferior thyroid artery [TA], *distribution:* upper one-quarter of esophagus; *anastomosis:* esophageal b.'s of thoracic aorta. SYN rami esophageales arteriae thyroideae inferioris [TA].

esophageal b.'s of the left gastric artery [TA], ascends through esophageal hiatus of diaphragm to supply lowermost (cardiac) esophagus; *anastomosis:* esophageal b.'s of thoracic aorta. SYN rami esophageales arteriae gastricae sinistrae [TA].

esophageal b.'s of the recurrent laryngeal nerve [TA], supply motor and sensory fibers to cervical esophagus on right side and

br

to cervical and upper thoracic esophagus on left. SYN rami esophagei nervi laryngei recurrentis [TA].

esophageal b.'s of the thoracic aorta [TA], b.'s arising directly from the anterior aspect of the portion of the thoracic aorta adjacent to the esophagus, by which most of the esophagus is supplied. SYN rami esophageales partis thoracicae aortae [TA], rami esophageales aortae thoracicae✕.

esophageal b.'s of thoracic ganglia [TA], cardiopulmonary splanchnic nerves conveying postsynaptic sympathetic and visceral afferent fibers from the upper thoracic paravertebral ganglia of the sympathetic trunks to the esophageal plexus of nerves. SYN rami esophageales gangliorum thoracicorum [TA].

esophageal b.'s of the vagus nerve, includes both b.'s passing directly from vagi and the b.'s from the recurrent laryngeal nerves that form the esophageal nerve plexus which surrounds esophagus, supplying it and adjacent portions of the pericardium. SEE ALSO esophageal (nervous) *plexus*. SYN rami esophagei nervi vagi.

external nasal b.'s of infraorbital nerve [TA], b.'s to external aspect of nose. The external nasal branches of 1) infraorbital nerve, rami nasales externii nervi infraorbitalis [NA], 2) nasociliary nerve, rami nasales externi nervi ethmoidalis anterioris [NA]. SYN rami nasales externi nervi infraorbitalis.

external b. of superior laryngeal nerve [TA], terminal b. of superior laryngeal nerve (with internal laryngeal nerve) supplying motor innervation to cricothyroid muscle. SYN ramus externus nervi laryngei superioris [TA].

external b. of trunk of accessory nerve [TA], portion of the accessory nerve trunk that exits independently from the jugular foramen, carrying fibers from the spinal root of the accessory nerve to the sternocleidomastoid and trapezius muscle. SYN ramus externus trunci nervi accessorii [TA].

faucial b.'s of lingual nerve, SYN b.'s of lingual nerve to isthmus of fauces.

femoral b. of genitofemoral nerve [TA], b. of genitofemoral nerve distributed to skin of uppermost part of anterior thigh. SYN ramus femoralis nervi genitofemoralis [TA].

frontal b. of middle meningeal artery [TA], the anterior and larger terminal b. (with the parietal b.) of the middle meningeal artery; runs in deep bony groove, often perforating the bone of the lateralmost part of the sphenoidal ridge, supplying the anterior portion of the lateral and superior dura and cranium. SYN ramus frontalis arteriae meningeae mediae [TA].

frontal b. of superficial temporal artery [TA], terminal b. of superficial temporal artery (with parietal b.) supplying anterolateral scalp and underlying musculature, periosteum, and outer table of cranium; *anastomosis:* across midline with contralateral partner; supratrochlear and supraorbital arteries. SYN ramus frontalis arteriae temporalis superficialis [TA].

ganglionic b. of internal carotid artery, SYN b.'s of internal carotid artery to trigeminal ganglion.

ganglionic b.'s of lingual nerve, SYN sensory *root* of submandibular ganglion.

ganglionic b.'s of lingual nerve to sublingual ganglion, ✕official alternate term for sensory *root* of sublingual ganglion.

ganglionic b.'s of lingual nerve to submandibular ganglion, ✕official alternate term for sensory *root* of sublingual ganglion.

ganglionic b.'s of maxillary nerve, SYN sensory *root* of pterygopalatine ganglion.

ganglionic b.'s of maxillary nerve to pterygopalatine ganglion, ✕official alternate term for sensory *root* of pterygopalatine ganglion.

gastric b.'s of anterior vagal trunk, SYN anterior gastric b.'s of anterior vagal trunk.

gastric b.'s of posterior vagal b., posterior gastric b.'s; b.'s of the posterior vagal trunk to the posterior surface of the stomach. SYN rami gastrici posteriores nervi vagi.

genital b. of genitofemoral nerve [TA], b. of genitofemoral nerve distributed to skin of anterior scrotum (male) or labia majora (female) and adjacent thigh and supplying a motor b. to the cremaster muscle. Usually passes through deep inguinal ring and canal. SYN ramus genitalis nervi genitofemoralis [TA], external spermatic nerve, nervus spermaticus externus.

genital b. of iliohypogastric nerve, SYN anterior cutaneous b. of iliohypogastric nerve.

glandular b.'s [TA], b.'s distributed to glands. SYN rami glandulares [TA].

glandular b.'s of facial artery [TA], b.'s of facial artery to the submandibular gland. SYN rami glandulares arteriae facialis [TA].

glandular b.'s of inferior thyroid artery [TA], b.'s of inferior thyroid artery to thyroid and parathyroid glands, anastomosing with b.'s of superior thyroid artery. SYN rami glandulares arteriae thyroideae inferioris [TA].

glandular b.'s of submandibular ganglion, b.'s of submandibular ganglion conveying postsynaptic parasympathetic fibers to the submandibular and sublingual glands. SYN rami ganglii submandibularis, rami glandulares ganglii submandibularis.

b. of glossopharyngeal nerve to stylopharyngeus muscle, SYN stylopharyngeal b. of glossopharyngeal nerve.

hepatic b.'s of anterior vagal trunk, b.'s of the anterior and posterior vagal trunks distributed to the liver. SYN rami hepatici trunci vagi anterior [TA], hepatic b.'s of vagus nerve, rami hepatici nervi vagi.

hepatic b.'s of vagus nerve, SYN hepatic b.'s of anterior vagal trunk.

iliac b. of iliolumbar artery, SYN iliacus b. of iliolumbar artery.

iliacus b. of iliolumbar artery [TA], terminal b. of iliolumbar artery (with lumbar b.) distributed to iliac fossa to supply iliac muscle, ilium, and portions of muscles having attachment to the iliac crest. SYN ramus iliacus arteriae iliolumbalis [TA], iliac b. of iliolumbar artery.

inferior b. [TA], a b. that is directed downward (caudally) or that is lowly placed, usually in contrast with another b. (superior b.), which is directed upward (rostrally) or is highly placed. SYN ramus inferior [TA].

inferior cervical cardiac b.'s of vagus nerve, the most inferior of the cervical b.'s of vagus nerve conducting presynaptic parasympathetic fibers to, and reflex afferent fibers from, the cardiac plexus; branching from the vagi at root of neck. SYN rami cardiaci cervicales inferiores nervi vagi [TA].

inferior dental b.'s of inferior dental plexus [TA], b.'s passing from the inferior dental plexus to the roots of the teeth of the lower jaw. SYN rami dentales inferiores plexus dentalis inferioris [TA], rami dentales inferiores [TA], inferior dental rami.

inferior gingival b.'s of inferior dental plexus [TA], b.'s of inferior dental plexus to the gingiva of the lower jaw. SYN rami gingivales inferiores plexus dentalis inferioris [TA].

inferior labial b. of facial artery [TA], *origin*, facial; *distribution*, structures of lower lip; *anastomoses*, the artery from the opposite side, mental and sublabial. SYN arteria labialis inferior, inferior labial artery, ramus labialis inferior arteriae facialis.

inferior labial b.'s of mental nerve, SYN labial b.'s of mental nerve.

inferior lingular b. of lingular branch of left pulmonary artery, SYN inferior lingular *artery*.

inferior b. of oculomotor nerve [TA], b. of oculomotor nerve providing motor b.'s to medial and inferior rectus and inferior oblique muscles and carrying presynaptic parasympathetic fibers that pass to the ciliary ganglion via the parasympathetic root. SYN ramus inferior nervi oculomotorii [TA].

inferior b. of pubic bone, obsolete term for inferior pubic *ramus*.

inferior b. of superior gluteal artery [TA], *distribution:* gluteus medius and minimus muscles; *anastomosis:* lateral circumflex femoral artery. SYN ramus inferior arteriae gluteae superioris [TA].

inferior b.'s of transverse cervical nerve [TA], b. of transverse cervical nerve providing cutaneous innervation in lower part of anterior triangle of neck. SYN rami inferiores nervi transversi colli✕, rami inferiores nervi transversi cervicalis [colli].

infrahyoid b. of superior thyroid artery [TA], small b. from the initial part of the superior thyroid artery coursing along the hyoid bone deep to the thyrohyoid muscle to anastomose with its contralateral partner. SYN ramus infrahyoideus arteriae thyroideae superioris [TA].

infrapatellar b. of saphenous nerve [TA], b. of saphenous nerve supplying skin over and below patella. SYN ramus infrapatellaris nervi sapheni [TA].

inguinal b.'s of deep external pudendal arteries [TA], b.'s to the inguinal region that may arise as b.'s of external pudendal arteries or as direct b.'s of the femoral artery. Supply skin and subcutaneous tissues, including inguinal lymph nodes. SYN rami inguinales arteriarum pudendarum externarum profundarum [TA].

interganglionic b.'s of sympathetic trunk [TA], the nerve strands interconnecting the ganglia of the sympathetic trunk; they consist of pre- or postganglionic fibers passing to higher or lower levels of the trunk. SYN rami interganglionares trunci sympathici [TA].

intermediate atrial b. of left coronary artery [TA], b. arising from the circumflex b. of the left coronary artery between the anterior rami (distributed to the left auricle) and the stem of the posterior atrial b.'s. SYN ramus atrialis intermedius arteriae coronariae sinistrae [TA], lateral atrial b. of left coronary artery.

intermediate atrial b. of right coronary artery [TA], arises from superior aspect of right coronary artery as or soon after it crosses the right margin on the heart; supplies posterolateral wall (sulcus/crista terminalis portion) of right atrium. SYN ramus atrialis intermedius arteriae coronariae dextrae [TA], lateral atrial b. of right coronary artery, marginal atrial b. of right coronary artery, right atrial b. of right coronary artery.

intermediate b. of hepatic artery proper [TA], smaller and central of usually three main intrahepatic branches of hepatic artery, it serves mainly the median segment (IV) of the liver. SYN ramus intermedius arteriae hepaticae propriae [TA].

intermediate temporal b.'s of lateral occipital artery [TA], the middle of three temporal b.'s of the lateral occipital artery (from posterior cerebral artery) distributed to the medial and inferior aspects of the temporal lobe of the cerebrum. SYN rami temporales intermedii arteriae occipitalis lateralis [TA], middle temporal b.'s of lateral occipital artery☆, rami temporales medii arteriae occipitalis lateralis☆.

intermediomedial frontal b. of callosomarginal artery [TA], b. of middle portion of callosomarginal artery to anterosuperior portion of medial aspect of frontal lobe of cerebrum. SYN ramus frontalis intermediomedialis arteriae callosomarginalis [TA].

b.'s of internal carotid artery to trigeminal ganglion [TA], b. to trigeminal ganglion; a small b. of the cavernous part of the internal carotid artery to the trigeminal ganglion. SYN ramus ganglionares trigeminales arteriae carotidis internae [TA], ganglionic b. of internal carotid artery, ramus ganglii trigeminalis.

internal nasal b.'s [TA], b.'s to nasal cavity. Internal nasal branches of 1) infraorbital nerve (rami nasales interni nervi infraorbitalis [NA]); 2) anterior ethmoidal nerve (rami nasales interni nervi ethmoidalis anterioris [NA]). SYN rami nasales interni [TA].

internal b. of superior laryngeal nerve [TA], terminal b. of superior laryngeal nerve (with external b.) conveying sensory fibers to the supraglottic larynx. SYN ramus internus nervi laryngei superioris [TA].

b.'s to internal capsule, genu [TA], SYN *rami* capsulae internae, under *ramus*.

b.'s to internal capsule, posterior limb [TA], SYN *rami* capsulae internae, under *ramus*.

b.'s to internal capsule, retrolentiform limb, SYN *rami* capsulae internae, under *ramus*.

internal b. of trunk of accessory nerve [TA], b. of the accessory nerve trunk that carries fibers from the cranial root and that unites with the vagus nerve in the jugular foramen. SEE ALSO accessory *nerve* [CN XI]. SYN ramus internus trunci nervi accessorii [TA], internal ramus of accessory nerve.

interventricular septal b.'s of left/right coronary artery, the interventricular septal b.'s; b.'s of the anterior and posterior interventricular arteries distributed to the muscle of the interventricular septum. SYN rami interventriculares septales arteriae coronariae sinistrae/dextrae, rami interventriculares septales, septal b.'s.

joint b.'s, SYN articular b.'s.

labial b.'s of mental nerve, b.'s of mental nerve to lower lip. SYN rami labiales nervi mentalis, inferior labial b.'s of mental nerve, rami labiales inferiores nervi mentalis.

laryngopharyngeal b.'s of superior cervical ganglion [TA], b.'s conveying postganglionic sympathetic fibers from the superior cervical ganglion to the pharyngeal plexus. SYN rami laryngopharyngei ganglii cervicalis superioris [TA].

lateral b.'s [TA], b.'s directed away from the midline, to the side. Terminologia Anatomica lists lateral b.'s (ramus lateralis/rami laterales) of the following: 1) anterior interventricular branch of left coronary artery (ramus lateralis interventricularis anterioris arteriae coronariae sinistrae [TA]); 2) anterolateral central arteries (rami laterales arteriarum centralium anterolateralium [TA]); 3) posterior primary rami of cervical/thoracic/lumbar/sacral/coccygeal spinal nerves (rami laterales ramorum posteriorum nervorum cervicalium/thoracalium/lumbalium/sacralium/coccygeum); 4) umbical part of left b. of portal vein (rami laterales partis umbilici rami sinistri venae portae hepatis [TA]); 5) left hepatic duct (ramus lateralis ductus hepatici sinistri [TA]); 6) middle lobe artery (of right lung) (ramus lateralis arteriae lobaris mediae (pulmonis dextrum) [TA]); 7) supraorbital nerve (ramus lateralis nervi supraorbitalis [TA]). SYN rami laterales [TA].

lateral abdominal/pectoral cutaneous b.'s of intercostal nerves, b.'s arising in approximately the anterior axillary line at the level of the second through sixth intercostal spaces. SYN lateral cutaneous b.'s of intercostal nerves, lateral cutaneous b.'s of ventral primary ramus of thoracic spinal nerves, ramus cutaneus lateralis abdominalis/pectoralis nervorum intercostalium.

lateral b.'s of artery of tuber cinereum [TA], b.'s arising from the lateral aspect of the artery of tuber cinereum. SEE ALSO *artery* of tuber cinereum. SYN rami laterales arteriarum tuberis cinerei [TA].

lateral atrial b. of left coronary artery, SYN intermediate atrial b. of left coronary artery.

lateral atrial b. of right coronary artery, SYN intermediate atrial b. of right coronary artery.

lateral basal b., SYN lateral basal segmental *artery.*

lateral calcaneal b.'s of sural nerve [TA], b.'s of sural nerve providing cutaneous innervation to posterior aspect of distal leg and lateral aspect of proximal portion of foot. SYN rami calcanei laterales nervi suralis [TA].

lateral costal b. of internal thoracic artery [TA], a variable b. of internal thoracic artery that runs lateral and parallel to the internal thoracic artery on the deep surface of the rib cage; *anastomosis:* posterior intercostal arteries. SYN ramus costalis lateralis arteriae thoracicae internae [TA].

lateral cutaneous b. [TA], lateral cutaneous b.'s of the following: 1) iliohypogastric nerve (ramus cutaneus lateralis nervi iliohypogastrici [TA]); 2) dorsal branch of posterior intercostal arteries (ramus cutaneos lateralis ramorum posteriorum arterieae intercostalium [TA]); 3) posterior intercostal artery (arteriae intercostales posteriores [TA]). SYN ramus cutaneus lateralis [TA].

lateral cutaneous b.'s of intercostal nerves, SYN lateral abdominal/pectoral cutaneous b.'s of intercostal nerves.

lateral cutaneous b.'s of ventral primary ramus of thoracic spinal nerves, SYN lateral abdominal/pectoral cutaneous b.'s of intercostal nerves.

lateral malleolar b. (of fibular peroneal artery) [TA], lateral malleolar branches of peroneal artery. SYN rami malleolares laterales arteriae fibularis (peronei) [TA], arteriae malleolares posteriores laterales, lateral malleolar arteries, posterior peroneal arteries.

lateral mammary b.'s, b.'s primarily distributed to the lateral portion of the breast. SYN rami mammarii laterales.

lateral mammary b.'s of lateral cutaneous branches of intercostal nerves, SYN lateral mammary b.'s of lateral cutaneous branches of thoracic spinal nerves.

lateral mammary b.'s of lateral cutaneous branches of thoracic spinal nerves, b.'s arising from the lateral cutaneous b.'s of the ventral primary rami of spinal nerves (intercostal nerves) T-3 to T-6 that run anteriorly to supply the lateral aspect of the breast. SYN lateral mammary b.'s of lateral cutaneous branches of intercostal nerves, rami mammarii laterales ramorum cutaneorum lateralis nervorum thoracicorum, rami mammarii laterales ramorum cutaneorum lateralium nervorum intercostalium.

lateral mammary b.'s of lateral thoracic artery [TA], b.'s of the lateral thoracic artery that extend around the lateral borders of the pectoral muscles to supply the lateral aspect of the breast and mammary gland. SYN rami mammarii laterales arteriae thoracicae lateralis [TA].

lateral and medial posterior choroidal b.'s of posterior cerebral artery [TA], one of two (posterior lateral and posterior medial) choroidal branches of the P_2 segment of the posterior cerebral artery that supply the choroid plexus of the body of the lateral ventricle and of the third ventricle. SYN rami choroidei posteriores arteriae cerebri posterioris laterales et mediales [TA].

lateral medullary b.'s of (intracranial part of) vertebral artery [TA], minute b.'s of the vertebral artery (or its larger b.'s) that course laterally along the ventral aspect of the medulla oblongata. SYN rami medullares laterales (partis intracranialis) arteriae vertebralis [TA].

lateral nasal b.'s of anterior ethmoidal nerve [TA], b.'s of nasociliary nerve distributed to walls of nasal cavity. SYN rami nasales laterales nervi ethmoidalis anterioris [TA].

lateral nasal b. of facial artery [TA], b. of facial artery to the side of the nose (ala and dorsum); anastomoses with its contralateral partner, as well as the septal and alar b.'s of the superior labial, the dorsal nasal b. of the ophthalmic, and the infraorbital b. of the maxillary artery. SYN ramus lateralis nasi arteriae facialis [TA], lateral nasal artery.

lateral b.'s of pontine arteries [TA], longer b.'s of the basilar artery extending across the inferior surface of the pons to reach the lateral aspects. SYN rami laterales arteriae pontis [TA], circumferential pontine b.'s of pontine arteries⋆.

lateral b. of posterior rami of spinal nerves, terminal b. (with the medial b.) of the posterior ramus of spinal nerve. In the thoracic region, the lateral b.'s of the upper thoracic spinal nerves are muscular only, not reaching the skin; the lateral b.'s of the lower thoracic spinal nerves are musculocutaneous, supplying and continuing past the muscles of the back to reach the overlying skin.

lateral sacral b.'s of median sacral artery [TA], b.'s of the sacral portion of the median sacral artery that pass laterally to anastomose with the lateral sacral arteries and send b.'s into the anterior sacral foramina. SYN rami sacrales laterales arteriae sacralis medianae [TA].

left b. [TA], of a pair of b.'s, the b. passing to the left side of the body, to the left member of a bilateral pair of structures, or to the left portion of an unpaired structure; the other member of the pair being a right b. Terminologia Anatomica lists left b.'s of 1) atrioventricular bundle, crus sinistrum fasciculus atrioventricularis; 2) hepatic artery proper, ramus sinister arteriae hepaticae proprii; 3) portal vein, ramus sinister venae portae hepatis. SYN ramus sinister [TA].

left b. of hepatic artery proper [TA], left branch of proper hepatic b.; terminal branch off proper hepatic b. supplying left lobe of the liver. SYN ramus sinister arteriae hepaticae propriae [TA], left hepatic artery.

lingual b.'s, b.'s to the tongue. Terminologia Anatomica lists lingual b.'s of 1) accessory nerv, (rami linguales nervi accessori [TA]); 2) facial nerve (inconstant) (ramus linguales nervi facialis); 3) lingual nerve (rami linguales nervi lingualis [TA]); 4) glossopharyngeal nerve (rami linguales nervi glossopharyngei [TA]). SYN rami linguales.

lingual b. of facial nerve, lingual b. (inconstant) of the stylohyoid b. of the facial nerve. SYN ramus lingualis nervi facialis.

b.'s of lingual nerve to isthmus of fauces [TA], the faucial b.'s, b.'s to the isthmus of the fauces from the lingual nerve. SYN rami isthmi faucium nervi lingualis [TA], faucial b.'s of lingual nerve, rami fauciales nervi lingualis.

lumbar b. of iliolumbar artery [TA], terminal b. of iliolumbar artery (with iliac b.) that ascends to supply psoas major and quadratus lumborum muscles; *anastomosis:* fourth lumbar artery. SYN ramus lumbalis arteriae iliolumbalis [TA].

mammary b.'s, SEE lateral mammary b.'s, medial mammary b.'s.

marginal atrial b. of right coronary artery, SYN intermediate atrial b. of right coronary artery.

marginal b. of cingulate sulcus [TA], posterior end of cingulate sulcus of cerebrum that turns superiorly to the superomedial margin of the parietal lobe. SYN ramus marginalis sulci cinguli [TA].

marginal mandibular b. of facial nerve [TA], b. of facial nerve that parallels the mandibular margin innervating risorius muscle and muscles of lower lip and chin. SYN ramus marginalis mandibulae nervi facialis [TA].

marginal b. of parietooccipital sulcus [TA], minor sulcus branching from parietooccipital sulcus as it crosses the posteromedial margin of the cerebrum. SYN ramus marginalis sulci parietooccipitalis [TA].

marginal b. [TA] of cingulate sulcus, SYN marginal *sulcus*.

marginal tentorial b. of internal carotid artery, SYN tentorial marginal b. of cavernous part of internal carotid artery.

mastoid b. of occipital artery [TA], artery passing through the mastoid foramen; *distribution*, mastoid air cells; *anastomosis*, middle meningeal b. SYN ramus mastoideus arteriae occipitalis [TA], mastoid artery.

mastoid b.'s of posterior auricular artery, SYN mastoid b.'s of posterior tympanic artery.

mastoid b.'s of posterior tympanic artery, b.'s from stylomastoid b. of posterior auricular artery arising within the facial canal, distributed to the mastoid air cells. SYN rami mastoidei arteriae tympanicae posterioris [TA], mastoid b.'s of posterior auricular artery, rami mastoidei arteriae auricularis posterioris.

medial b.'s [TA], b.'s directed toward the midline, to the middle. Terminologia Anatomica lists medial b.'s (ramus medialis/rami mediales) of the following: 1) anterolateral central arteries (rami mediales arteriarum centralium anterolateralium [TA]); 2) artery of tuber cincrum (ramus mediolis [TA]); 3) posterior primary rami of cervical/thoracic/lumbar/sacral/coccygeal spinal nerves (rami medialis ramorum posteriorum nervorum cervicalium/thoracicalium/lumbalium/sacralium/coccygeum); 4) umbilical part of left b. of portal vein (rami mediales portis umbilici rami sinistri venae portae hepatis [TA]); 5) left hepatic duct (ramus medialis ductus hepatici sinistri [TA]); 6) middle lobar artery (of right lung) (ramus medialis arteriae lobaris mediae (pulmonis dextrum) [TA]); 7) supraorbital nerve (ramus medialis nervi supraorbitalis [TA]). SYN rami mediales [TA].

medial b.'s of artery of tuber cinereum [TA], b.'s arising from the medial aspect of the artery of tuber cinereum. SEE ALSO *artery* of tuber cinereum. SYN rami mediales arteriarum tuberis cinerei [TA].

medial basal b. of pulmonary artery, SYN medial basal segmental *artery*.

medial calcaneal b.'s of tibial nerve [TA], cutaneous b.'s of tibial nerve distributed to the inferior and medial heel. SYN rami calcanei mediales nervi tibialis [TA].

medial crural cutaneous b.'s of saphenous nerve, SYN medial cutaneous *nerve* of leg.

medial cutaneous b. of dorsal branch of posterior intercostal arteries [TA], Terminologia Anatomica lists medial cutaneous b.'s of the following: 1) dorsal branch of thoracic nerves (ramus cutaneus medialis ramorum dorsalium nervorum thoracicorum [NA]); 2) dorsal branch of posterior intercostal arteries (ramus cutaneus medialis rami dorsalis arteriarum intercostalium posteriorum III–XI [NA]). SYN ramus cutaneus medialis rami dorsalis arteriarum intercostalium posteriorum III–XI.

medial malleolar b.'s (of posterior tibial artery) [TA], branches arising from the medial aspect of the posterior tibial artery at the level of the narrowest part of the leg, passing to tissues in the region of the posterior aspect of the medial malleolus; anastomose with medial malleolar branches of the anterior tibial artery. SYN rami malleolares mediales arteriae tibialis posterioris [TA], arteriae malleolares posteriores mediales, medial malleolar arteries.

medial mammary b.'s, b.'s primarily distributed to the medial portion of the breast. Terminologia Anatomica lists medial mammary b.'s (rami mammarii mediales...) of the following: 1) anterior cutaneous b.'s of intercostal nerves (...rami cutanei anterioris nervorum intercostalium); nerve b.'s accompanying the perforating b.'s of internal thoracic artery. 2) perforating b.'s of internal thoracic artery (...rami perforantes arteriae thoracicae internae [TA]). SYN rami mammarii mediales.

medial medullary b.'s of vertebral artery [TA], minute b.'s of the vertebral artery that enter the anterior median fissure of the medulla oblongata. SYN rami medullares mediales arteriae verte-bralis [TA].

medial nasal b.'s of anterior ethmoidal nerve [TA], b.'s of nasociliary nerve distributed to the nasal septum. SYN rami nasales mediales nervi ethmoidalis anterioris [TA].

medial b.'s of pontine arteries [TA], shorter b.'s of the basilar artery extending to the medial portion of the inferior surface of the pons. SYN rami mediales arteriae pontis [TA], paramedian pontine b.'s of pontine arteries⋆.

medial b. of posterior branch of spinal nerves, ⋆official alter-nate term for medial b. of posterior rami of spinal nerves.

medial b. of posterior rami of spinal nerves, terminal b. (with the lateral b.) of the posterior ramus of spinal nerves. In the thoracic region, the medial b.'s of the upper thoracic spinal nerves are musculocutaneous, supplying and continuing through the muscles of the back to reach the overlying skin; the medial b.'s of the lower thoracic spinal nerves are muscular only, terminating before reaching the skin. SYN medial b. of posterior branch of spinal nerves⋆, ramus medialis ramorum dorsalium nervorum spinalis.

mediastinal b.'s [TA], b.'s distributed to the mediastinum. SYN rami mediastinales [TA], mediastinal arteries.

mediastinal b.'s of internal thoracic artery [TA], small twigs supplying anterior mediastinal structures: mainly thymus and lymph nodes. SYN rami mediastinales arteriae thoracicae internae [TA], anterior mediastinal arteries, rami thymici.

mediastinal b.'s of thoracic aorta [TA], numerous small arteries supplying the pleura and lymph nodes of the posterior mediasti-num. SYN rami mediastinales aortae thoracicae [TA], posterior mediastinal arteries.

meningeal b.'s [TA], b.'s of vessels or nerves distributed to the coverings of the brain and spinal cord. SYN rami meningei [TA].

meningeal b. of cavernous part of internal carotid artery, a b. from the cavernous part of the internal carotid artery to the menin-ges of the anterior cranial fossa. SYN ramus meningeus partis cavernosae arteriae carotidis internae [TA], meningeal b. of inter-nal carotid artery, ramus meningeus arteriae carotidis internae.

meningeal b. of cerebral part of internal carotid artery [TA], minute artery crossing lesser wing of sphenoid to supply dura mater and bone of anterior cranial fossa and anastomose with meningeal branch of posterior ethmoidal artery. SYN ramus men-ingeus partis cerebralis arteriae carotidis internae [TA].

meningeal b. of internal carotid artery, SYN meningeal b. of cavernous part of internal carotid artery.

meningeal b. of (intracranial part of) vertebral artery [TA], one of the one or two b.'s of the intracranial part of the vertebral artery, arising near the foramen magnum, which ramify between the dura and the inner table of bone of the posterior cranial fossa, supplying dura (including falx cerebelli), inner table of bone, and diploë. SYN ramus meningeus (partis intracranialis) arteriae verte-bralis [TA].

meningeal b. of mandibular nerve [TA], a recurrent b. of the mandibular nerve that passes superiorly through foramen spino-sum to be distributed with the posterior division of the middle meningeal artery to the meninges of the posterior portion of the middle cranial fossa. SYN ramus meningeus nervi mandibularis [TA], nervus spinosus⋆.

meningeal b. of maxillary nerve, recurrent b. of maxillary nerve distributed with the anterior b. of the middle meningeal arteyr to the meninges of the anterior portion of the middle cranial fossa. SYN ramus meningeus nervi maxillaris [TA], middle meningeal b. of maxillary nerve, middle meningeal nerve, ramus meningeus medius nervi maxillaris.

meningeal b. of occipital artery [TA], one of the variable b.'s of the occipital artery that may pass through the jugular or parietal foramina or condyloid canal to reach the dura mater and bone of the posterior cranial fossa, as well as the intracranial portions of the caudal four cranial neres. SYN ramus meningeus arteriae occi-pitalis [TA].

meningeal b. of ophthalmic nerve, SEE tentorial *nerve.*

meningeal b. of spinal nerves [TA], a b. from the initial (mixed) part of each spinal nerve passing in a recurrent fashion back through the intervertebral foramen to supply spinal meninges, the posterior longitudinal ligament, posterolateral periphery of the intervertebral disk, and periosteum of the vertebrae. SYN ramus meningeus nervorum spinalium [TA], recurrent b. of spinal nerves⋆, recurrent meningeal b. of spinal nerves, sinuvertebral nerves.

meningeal b. of vagus nerve [TA], a b. of the superior ganglion of the vagus supplying the meninges of the posterior cranial fossa. SYN ramus meningeus nervi vagi [TA].

mental b.'s of mental nerve [TA], b.'s of the mental nerve providing general sensory innervation to the skin of the chin. SYN rami mentales nervi mentalis [TA].

mental b. (of inferior alveolar artery) [TA], *distribution,* chin; the terminal branch of the inferior alveolar; *anastomoses,* inferior labial artery. SYN ramus mentalis arteriae alveolaris inferioris [TA], arteria mentalis, mental artery.

middle lobe b. of right superior pulmonary vein, SYN middle lobe *vein.*

middle meningeal b. of maxillary nerve, SYN meningeal b. of maxillary nerve.

middle superior alveolar b. of infraorbital nerve [TA], the middle superior alveolar branch, a branch of the superior alveolar nerve that contributes to the superior dental plexus. SYN ramus alveolaris superior medius nervi infraorbitalis [TA].

middle temporal b. of insular part of middle cerebral artery [TA], a b. of the insular part (M2 segment) of the middle cerebral artery supplying the cortex of the temporal lobe between the anterior and posterior temporal arteries. SYN ramus temporalis medius partis insularis arteriae cerebrae mediae [TA], arteria tem-poralis intermedia, intermediate temporal artery.

middle temporal b.'s of lateral occipital artery, ⋆official alter-nate term for intermediate temporal b.'s of lateral occipital artery.

muscular b.'s [TA], b.'s of nerves or vessels that supply muscles. Most are unnamed. Terminologia Anatomica lists muscular b.'s of: 1) accessory nerve (rami musculares nervi accessorii); 2) ante-rior branch of obturator nerve (rami musculares rami anterioris nervi obturatorii); 3) anterior interosseous nerve (rami musculares nervi interossei antebrachii anterior); 4) axillary nerve (rami mus-culares nervi axillaris); 5) deep fibular nerve (rami musculares nervi fibularis profundi); 6) femoral nerve (rami musculares nervi femoralis); 7) intercostal nerves (rami musculares nervorum inter-costalium); 8) medial nerve (rami musculares nervi mediani); 9) musculocutaneous nerve (rami musculares nervi musculocutanei); 10) perineal nerves (rami musculares nervorum perinealium); 11) posterior branch of obturator nerve (rami musculares rami posteri-oris nervi obturatorii); 12) radial nerve (rami musculares nervi radialis); 13) spinal nerve (rami musculares nervorum spinalium); 14) superficial fibular nerve (rami musculares nervi fibularis su-perficialis); 15) supraclavicular part of brachial plexus (rami mus-culares partis supraclavicularis plexus brachialis); 16) of tibial nerve (rami musculares nervi tibialis); 17) ulnar nerve (rami mus-culares nervi ulnaris); 18) vertebral artery (rami musculares arteri-ae vertebralis). SYN rami musculares [TA].

mylohyoid b. (of inferior alveolar artery) [TA], branch of infe-rior alveolar artery to the mylohyoid muscle. SYN ramus mylohy-oideus arteriae alveolaris inferioris [TA], mylohyoid artery.

nasal septal b. of superior labial branch of facial artery [TA], b. of superior labial b. of facial artery that passes superiorly to ramify on the anteroinferior aspect of the nasal septum. SYN ramus septi nasi arteriae labialis superioris [TA].

obturator b. of pubic branch of inferior epigastric vein [TA], b. of the pubic b. of inferior epigastric artery that descends over the pelvic brim to anastomose with the pubic b. of the obturator artery; in 20–30% of people, this b. is larger than or replaces the obturator artery. SYN ramus obturatorius rami pubici arteriae epi-gastricae inferioris [TA].

occipital b. [TA], Terminologia Anatomica lists occipital b.'s of 1) posterior auricular artery, rami occipitalis arteriae auricularis posterior [TA]; 2) posterior auricular nerve (rami occipitalis nervi auricularis posterioris [TA]; and 3) occipital artery, rami occipita-les arteriae occipitis [TA]. SYN ramus occipitalis [TA].

b. of oculomotor nerve to ciliary ganglion, SYN parasympathetic *root* of ciliary ganglion.

omental b.'s [TA], b.'s to the greater omentum; epiploic b.'s arise from the left and right gastroomental arteries (rami omentales arteriae gastro-omentalis sinistrae et dextrae [NA]) opposite the gastric b.'s (rami gastrici [NA]) along the greater curvature of the stomach. SYN rami omentales [TA], epiploic b.'s, rami epiploicae.

orbital b.'s of maxillary nerve, b.'s of pterygopalatine ganglion traversing inferior orbital fissure, distributed in orbit to periorbita and mucosa of ethmoidal and sphenoidal sinuses. SYN rami orbitales nervi maxillaris [TA], orbital b.'s of pterygopalatine ganglion, ramus orbitalis ganglii pterygopalatini.

orbital b. of middle meningeal artery [TA], b. of middle meningeal artery traversing superior orbital fissure and running toward lacrimal gland. SEE anastomotic b. of middle meningeal artery with lacrimal artery. SYN ramus orbitalis arteriae meningeae mediae [TA].

orbital b.'s of pterygopalatine ganglion, SYN orbital b.'s of maxillary nerve.

ovarian b.'s of uterine artery [TA], terminal b. of uterine artery (with tubal b.) which runs through mesovarium supplying ovary from medial aspect and anastomosing with ovarian b. of ovarian artery. SYN rami ovarici arteriae uterinae [TA].

palmar b. of anterior interosseous nerve, b. of median nerve arising proximal to flexor retinaculum and running superficially to it to supply skin of proximal central palm and thenar eminence. Since it does not traverse carpal tunnel, it is not affected by carpal tunnel syndrome, even though it supplies skin distal to carpal tunnel. SYN ramus palmaris nervi interossei antebrachii anterioris [TA], palmar b. of median nerve, ramus palmaris nervi mediani.

palmar carpal b. of radial artery [TA], a small b. of the radial artery that passes medially across the wrist to supply the carpal joints; it anastomoses with the anterior carpal branch of the ulnar artery. SYN ramus carpalis palmaris arteriae radialis [TA], ramus carpeus palmaris arteriae radialis.

palmar carpal b. of ulnar artery [TA], a b. of the ulnar artery that supplies the carpal joints and communicates with the anterior carpal branch of the radial artery. SYN ramus carpalis palmaris arteriae ulnaris [TA], ramus carpeus palmaris arteriae ulnaris.

palmar b. of median nerve, SYN palmar b. of anterior interosseous nerve.

palmar b. of ulnar nerve [TA], b. of ulnar nerve arising in distal forearm and accompanying palmar artery into hand where it supplies skin of little finger and medial half of ring finger and adjacent parts of palm. SYN ramus palmaris nervi ulnaris [TA].

palpebral b.'s of infratrochlear nerve [TA], b.'s of infratrochlear nerve supplying skin of medial aspects of upper and lower eyelids. SYN rami palpebrales nervi infratrochlearis [TA].

pancreatic b.'s [TA], b.'s to the pancreas. Terminologia Anatomica lists pancreatic b.'s of 1) splenic artery, rami pancreatici arteriae splenicae [TA]; 2) (anterior and posterior) superior pancreaticoduodenal arteries, rami pancreatici arteriae pancreaticoduodenalis superioris (anterior et posterior) [TA]. SYN rami pancreatici [TA].

paracentral b.'s of callosomarginal artery [TA], terminal b.'s of cingulate b. of callosomarginal artery distributed to the paracentral lobule of the cerebrum. SYN rami paracentrales arteriae callosomarginalis [TA].

paracentral b.'s (of pericallosal artery), inconstant b.'s of the pericallosal artery supplying the cerebral cortex of the paracentral lobule and both sides of the medial part of the central sulcus. SYN ramus paracentrales [TA], arteria paracentralis, paracentral artery.

paramedian pontine b.'s of pontine arteries, ☆official alternate term for medial b.'s of pontine arteries.

parietal b. [TA], (**1**) b.'s coursing in relationship to and supplying the parietal bone or parietal lobe of cerebrum; (**2**) b.'s distributed to the body wall and limbs (the "parities") as opposed to visceral b.'s distributed to the body cavities. For example, the gray rami communicantes are the parietal b.'s of the sympathetic trunks (vs. the splanchnic nerves, which are visceral b.'s of the trunks). SYN rami parietales [TA].

parietal b. of medial occipital artery [TA], an anterior b. of the medial occipital artery supplying the posterior section of the parietal lobe of the cerebrum. SYN ramus parietalis arteriae occipitalis medialis [TA].

parietal b. of middle meningeal artery [TA], smaller terminal b. (with frontal b.) of middle meningeal artery supplying posterior portion of lateral and superior dura and cranium. SYN ramus parietalis arteriae meningeae mediae [TA].

parietal b. of superficial temporal artery [TA], b.'s coursing in relationship to and/or supplying the parietal lobe of the brain. SYN ramus parietalis arteriae temporalis superficialis [TA].

parieto-occipital b.'s (of anterior cerebral artery) [TA], the largest cortical b.'s of the pericallosal artery supplying the medial and superolateral surface of the parietal lobe posterior to the paracentral lobule; rarely does it extend to supply part of the occipital lobe. SYN arteriae parieto-occipitales, parietooccipital artery, superior internal parietal artery.

parieto-occipital b. (of posterior cerebral artery) [TA], a posterior b. of the medial occipital artery supplying the medial surface of the occipital lobe extending to area of the parieto-occipital sulcus of the cerebrum. SYN ramus parieto-occipitalis arteriae occipitalis medialis [TA].

parotid b.'s [TA], b.'s to parotid gland; Terminologia Anatomica lists parotid branches of 1) auriculotemporal nerve, rami parotidei nervi auriculotemporalis [TA]; 2) deep facial vein, rami parotidei venae facialis profundus [TA]; 3) posterior auricular artery, ramus parotidei arteriae auricularis posterior [TA]; 4) superficial temporal artery, ramus arteriae temporalis superficialis [TA]. SYN rami parotidei [TA].

pectoral and abdominal anterior cutaneous b. of intercostal nerves, SYN thoracoabdominal *nerves,* under *nerve.*

pectoral b.'s of thoracoacromial artery, b.'s of the thoracoacromial artery descending between and supplying the pectoralis major and minor muscles, then continuing to supply the serratus anterior muscle and, in the adult female, the upper portion of the breast. SYN rami pectorales arteriae thoracoacromialis [TA].

perforating b.'s [TA], arterial b.'s that penetrate a wall or pass from the anterior to the posterior aspect or compartment of a structure such as the hand or foot to anastomose or be distributed. SYN ramus perforans [TA].

perforating b. of anterior interosseous artery [TA], b. of anterior interosseous artery that pierces the interosseous membrane in the distal forearm to anastomose with (and actually replace distally) the posterior interosseous artery. SYN ramus perforans arteriae interossei anterioris [TA].

perforating b. of fibular artery, the b. of the peroneal artery that perforates the interosseous membrane just above the anterior tibiofibular ligament. SYN ramus perforans arteriae fibularis [TA], perforating b. of peroneal artery ☆.

perforating b.'s of internal thoracic artery [TA], small b.'s of the internal thoracic artery running between the costal cartilages to supply overlying skin and subcutaneous tissues. SYN rami perforantes arteriae thoracicae internae [TA], perforating arteries (of internal thoracic artery).

perforating b.'s (of palmar metacarpal arteries), SEE perforating *branches* of deep palmar arch.

perforating b.'s (of plantar metatarsal arteries) [TA], the perforating b.'s of the plantar metatarsal arteries, three small arteries that pass dorsally through the second, third, and fourth interosseous spaces of the foot from the plantar metatarsal arteries. SYN rami perforantes arteriarum metatarsearum plantarium [TA], perforating arteries (of foot).

perforating b. of peroneal artery, ☆official alternate term for perforating b. of fibular artery.

pericardial b. of phrenic nerve [TA], one of the b.'s of phrenic nerve distributed to the pericardium and adjacent mediastial parietal pleura. SYN ramus pericardiacus nervi phrenici [TA].

pericardial b.'s of thoracic aorta [TA], small b.'s of thoracic aorta distributed to the pericardium, in the region of the oblique pericardial sinus, and to posterior mediastinal lymph nodes. SYN rami pericardiaci aortae thoracicae [TA].

perineal b.'s of posterior cutaneous nerve of thigh, b.'s of posterior femoral cutaneous nerve that convey sensory fibers to the skin of the lateralmost perineum and adjacent portions of the upper medial thigh. SYN rami perineales nervi cutanei femoris posterioris [TA], perineal b.'s of posterior femoral cutaneous nerve ☆.

perineal b.'s of posterior femoral cutaneous nerve, ☆official alternate term for perineal b.'s of posterior cutaneous nerve of thigh.

peroneal communicating b., SYN sural communicating b. of common fibular nerve.

petrosal b. of middle meningeal artery [TA], petrous b. of middle meningeal artery; first intracranial b. of middle meningeal artery; *anastomosis:* stylomastoid artery via hiatus of facial canal. SYN ramus petrosus arteriae meningeae mediae [TA].

pharyngeal b.'s [TA], b.'s to the pharynx. SYN rami pharyngei [TA], rami pharyngeales☆, pharyngei.

pharyngeal b. of the artery of pterygoid canal [TA], distributed to uppermost nasopharynx (pharyngeal recesses). SYN ramus pharyngeus arteriae canalis pterygoidei [TA].

pharyngeal b. of the ascending pharyngeal artery [TA], *distribution:* walls of oropharynx and nasopharynx. SYN rami pharyngeales arteriae pharyngeae ascendentis [TA].

pharyngeal b. of descending palatine artery [TA], may arise as a separate b. or as a continuation of lesser palatine artery. SYN ramus pharyngeus arteriae palatinae descendentis [TA].

pharyngeal b. of glossopharyngeal nerve [TA], conveys general sensory fibers to the mucosa of the oropharynx via the pharyngeal plexus. SYN rami pharyngei nervi glossopharyngei [TA].

pharyngeal b. of inferior thyroid artery [TA], distributed to laryngopharynx. SYN rami pharyngeales arteriae thyroideae inferioris [TA].

pharyngeal b. of pterygopalatine ganglion, SYN pharyngeal *nerve.*

pharyngeal b.'s of recurrent laryngeal nerve [TA], b.'s of the recurrent laryngeal nerve that continue beyond the larynx to the inferior pharynx. SYN rami pharyngei nervi laryngei recurrentis [TA].

pharyngeal b. of vagus nerve [TA], conveys motor fibers from the cranial root of the accessory nerve to the pharyngeal constrictor muscles, the intrinsic muscles of the soft palate, and the levator palati muscle; may also bring some general sensory fibers to the pharyngeal plexus. SYN rami pharyngei nervi vagi [TA].

phrenicoabdominal b.'s of phrenic nerve, terminal b.'s of phrenic nerve providing motor innervation of diaphragm and sensory innervation to the diaphragm and the diaphragmatic pleura and peritoneum. SYN rami phrenicoabdominales nervi phrenici.

posterior b.'s [TA], b.'s directed dorsally or backward. SYN rami posteriores [TA].

posterior basal b., SYN posterior basal segmental *artery* of left / right lung.

posterior gastric b.'s of posterior vagal trunk [TA], b.'s of the posterior vagal trunk that pass posterior to the left gastric artery in the hepatogastric ligament to ramify over the posteroinferior surface of the stomach. SYN rami gastrici posteriores trunci vagalis posterioris [TA].

posterior glandular b. of superior thyroid artery, b. of superior thyroid artery that descends to supply the apical portion of the ipsilateral lobe of the thyroid, continuing along the posterior border of the gland to anastomose with the inferior thyroid artery. SYN ramus glandularis posterior arteriae thyroideae superioris [TA], posterior b. of superior thyroid artery, ramus posterior arteriae thyroideae superioris [TA].

posterior b. of great auricular nerve [TA], provides general sensory fibers to skin of posterior auricle and over mastoid process. SYN ramus posterior nervi auricularis magni [TA].

posterior inferior nasal b.'s of greater palatine nerve, SYN posterior inferior nasal *nerves,* under *nerve.*

posterior b. of inferior pancreaticoduodenal artery [TA], the more dorsal of the two b.'s into which the inferior pancreaticoduodenal artery bifurcates; supplies uncinate process and head of pancreas, as well as the third and fourth parts of the duodenum; anastomoses with the posterior branch of the superior pancreaticoduodenal artery. SYN ramus posterior arteriae pancreaticoduodenalis inferioris [TA].

posterior labial branches of internal perineal b. [TA], b.'s of the perineal artery to the posterior portion of the labium majus. SYN rami labiales posteriores arteriae perinealis [TA], posterior labial arteries, rami labiales posteriores arteriae pudendae internae.

posterior labial b.'s of perineal artery [TA], superficial b.'s of the perineal artery supplying the posterior portions of the labia majora and minora.

posterior b. of lateral cerebral sulcus, SYN posterior *ramus* of lateral cerebral sulcus.

posterior b. of medial antebrachial cutaneous nerve, SYN posterior b. of medial cutaneous nerve of forearm.

posterior b. of medial cutaneous nerve of forearm, b. of the medial antebrachial cutaneous nerve supplying the skin of the medial portion of the proximal two-thirds of the dorsal side of the forearm. SYN ramus posterior nervi cutanei antebrachii medialis [TA], posterior b. of medial antebrachial cutaneous nerve, ramus ulnaris nervi cutanei antebrachii medialis, ulnar b. of medial antebrachial cutaneous nerve.

posterior b. of obturator artery [TA], b. of obturator artery giving rise to acetabular b. and supplying muscles attached to ischium. SYN ramus posterior arteriae obturatoriae [TA].

posterior b. of obturator nerve [TA], b. supplying obturator externus muscle, then passing posterior to adductor brevis, supplying it and the adductor portion of the adductor magnus muscle. SYN ramus posterior nervi obturatorii [TA].

posterior b. of recurrent ulnar artery, SYN posterior b. of ulnar recurrent artery.

posterior b. of renal artery [TA], terminal b. of renal artery (with anterior b.) becoming the posterior segmental artery of kidney. SEE segmental *arteries* of kidney, under *artery.* SYN ramus posterior arteriae renalis [TA].

posterior b. of right branch of portal vein [TA], posterior segmental b. of portal vein; b. to posterior segments of right lobe of liver. SYN ramus posterior rami dextri venae portae hepatis [TA].

posterior b. of right hepatic duct [TA], hepatic duct b. draining bile from posterior segments of right lobe of liver. SYN ramus posterior ductus hepatici dextri [TA].

posterior b. of right superior pulmonary vein [TA], drains posterior portion of superior lobe of right lung. SYN ramus posterior venae pulmonalis dextrae superioris [TA].

posterior scrotal b.'s of internal pudendal artery, SYN posterior scrotal b.'s of perineal artery.

posterior scrotal b.'s of perineal artery, b.'s of perineal artery supplying skin of posterior scrotal sac. SYN rami scrotales posteriores arteriae perinealis [TA], posterior scrotal b.'s of internal pudendal artery, rami scrotales posteriores arteriae pudendae internae.

posterior septal b. of nose [TA], one of the b.'s of the sphenopalatine artery that supplies the nasal septum and accompanies the nasopalatine nerve. SYN ramus septi posterioris nasalis [TA], arteria nasalis posterior septi, posterior septal artery of nose, posterior septal b.'s of sphenopalatine artery.

posterior septal b.'s of sphenopalatine artery, SYN posterior septal b. of nose.

posterior b. of spinal nerves, SEE dorsal primary *ramus* of spinal nerve.

posterior superior alveolar b.'s of maxillary nerve [TA], the b.'s of the superior alveolar nerves that supply the maxillary sinus and the molar tooth. SYN rami alveolares superiores posteriores nervi maxillaris [TA].

posterior superior lateral nasal b.'s of maxillary nerve, b.'s of pterygopalatine ganglion to upper posterior part of lateral wall of nasal cavity, including superior and middle nasal concha/meatuses, and posterior ethmoidal sinuses. SYN posterior superior lateral nasal b.'s of pterygopalatine ganglion, rami nasales posteriores superiores laterales ganglii pterygopalatini, rami nasales posteriores superiores laterales nervi maxillaris.

posterior superior lateral nasal b.'s of pterygopalatine ganglion, SYN posterior superior lateral nasal b.'s of maxillary nerve.

posterior superior medial nasal b.'s of maxillary nerve [TA], usually b.'s of the nasopalatine nerve to posterior superior nasal septum. SYN rami nasales posteriores superiores mediales nervi maxillaris [TA], posterior superior medial nasal b.'s of pterygopalatine ganglion, rami nasales posteriores superiores mediales ganglii pterygopalatini.

posterior superior medial nasal b.'s of pterygopalatine ganglion, SYN posterior superior medial nasal b.'s of maxillary nerve.

posterior b. of superior thyroid artery, SYN posterior glandular b. of superior thyroid artery.

posterior temporal b. of middle cerebral artery [TA], a branch of the insular part (M2 segment) of the middle cerebral artery distributed to the cortex of the posterior part of the temporal lobe. SYN ramus temporalis posterior arteriae cerebri mediae [TA], arteria temporalis posterior, posterior temporal artery.

posterior b. of ulnar recurrent artery, contributes to blood supply of flexor carpi ulnaris and to articular network of elbow. SYN ramus posterior arteriae recurrentis ulnaris [TA], posterior b. of recurrent ulnar artery.

posterior vestibular b. of vestibulocochlear artery [TA], *origin:* terminal b., with cochlear b., of vestibulocochlear artery; *distribution:* utricle and (especially ampulla of) posterior semicircular duct. SYN ramus vestibularis posterior arteriae vestibulocochlearis [TA].

posteromedial frontal b. of callosomarginal artery [TA], terminal b. (with cingular b.) of callosomarginal artery to posterior portion of medial aspect of frontal lobe of cerebrum. SYN ramus frontalis posteromedialis arteriae callosomarginalis [TA].

precuneal b.'s (of anterior cerebral artery) [TA], the last cortical b. of the pericallosal artery; it supplies the inferior part of the precuneus. SYN rami precuneales arteriae cerebri anterioris [TA], arteria precunealis, inferior internal parietal artery, precuneal artery.

prelaminar b. of spinal branch of dorsal branch of posterior intercostal artery [TA], *origin:* spinal artery in intervertebral foramen; *distribution:* to anterior surface of laminae and ligamenta flava of thoracic vertebrae and the anterior aspects of the zygapophysial joints. SYN ramus prelaminaris rami spinalis rami dorsalis arteriae intercostalis posterioris [TA].

prostatic b.'s of inferior vesical artery [TA], b.'s of the inferior vesicle artery that descend to the prostate, comprising its major arterial supply. SYN rami prostatici arteriae vesicalis inferioris [TA].

prostatic b.'s of middle rectal artery [TA], b.'s of the middle rectal artery that anastomose with the prostatic b.'s of the inferior vesicle artery and join them in supplying the prostate. SYN rami prostatici arteriae rectalis mediae [TA].

pterygoid b.'s of maxillary artery, SYN pterygoid b. of posterior deep temporal artery.

pterygoid b. of posterior deep temporal artery, pterygoid branches of middle meningeal artery. SYN ramus pterygoideus arteriae temporalis profundae posterioris [TA], pterygoid b.'s of maxillary artery, rami pterygoidei arteriae maxillaris.

pubic b. of inferior epigastric artery [TA], b. arising from the inferior epigastric artery medial to the deep inguinal ring; runs medial to femoral ring onto posterior pubis; anastomosis, pubic b. of obturator artery. This anastomosis is frequently large, referred to as an "accessory obturator artery." In 20–30% of patients, this anastomosis replaces the obturator artery, as an "aberrant" or "replaced" obturator artery. SYN ramus pubicus arteriae epigastricae inferioris [TA].

pubic b. of inferior epigastric vein [TA], b. of inferior epigastric vein that arises medial to the deep inguinal ring and gives rise to an upper b. that anastomoses across the midline with its contralateral partner, and a lower b. that descends on the posterior aspect of the pubis; the latter gives rise to an obturator b. SEE ALSO obturator b. of pubic branch of inferior epigastric vein. SYN ramus pubicus venae epigastricae inferioris [TA].

pubic b. of obturator artery [TA], b. arising from the obturator artery just prior to its passage through the obturator canal; the b. passes superiorly on the posterior aspect of the pubis. *Anastomosis:* with contralateral partner and pubic b. of inferior epigastric artery. SEE accessory obturator *artery,* pubic b. of inferior epigastric artery. SYN ramus pubicus arteriae obturatoriae [TA].

pulmonary b.'s of autonomic nervous system, SEE pulmonary b.'s of pulmonary nerve plexus, thoracic pulmonary b.'s of thoracic ganglia. SYN rami pulmonales systematis autonomici.

pulmonary b.'s of pulmonary nerve plexus [TA], b.'s of the pulmonary nerve plexus that extend along the root of the lungs reaching the right and left lungs. SYN rami pulmonales plexi nervosi pulmonalis [TA].

pyloric b. of anterior vagal trunk [TA], b. of anterior vagal trunk that passes through the gastrohepatic ligament with the hepatic b.'s of the vagus to reach the pylorus. In selective vagotomy procedures, this b. is spared to avoid problems with gastric emptying. SYN ramus pyloricus trunci vagalis anterioris [TA].

recurrent meningeal b. of spinal nerves, SYN meningeal b. of spinal nerves.

recurrent b. of spinal nerves, ✫official alternate term for meningeal b. of spinal nerves.

renal b. of lesser splanchnic b. [TA], b. of lesser splanchnic nerve to the aorticorenal plexus/ganglion. SYN ramus renalis nervi splanchnici minoris [TA].

renal b.'s of vagus nerve [TA], b.'s of vagus nerve to kidney via the celiac plexus. SYN rami renales nervi vagi [TA].

right b. [TA], of a pair of b.'s, the b. passing to the right side of the body, to the right member of a bilateral pair of structures, or to the right portion of an unpaired structure; the other member of the pair being a left branch. SYN ramus dexter [TA].

right atrial b. of right coronary artery, SYN intermediate atrial b. of right coronary artery.

right b. of hepatic artery proper [TA], terminal b. of hepatic artery proper supplying right lobe of liver; *branch:* cystic artery. SYN ramus dexter arteriae hepaticae propriae [TA], right hepatic artery.

right marginal b. (of right coronary artery) [TA], usually the largest of the ventricular b.'s of the right coronary artery; courses along the right margin of the heart, and is of sufficient caliber and length to reach the apex. SYN ramus marginalis dexter (arteriae coronariae dextrae) [TA].

right b. of portal vein [TA], terminal b. of hepatic portal vein distributed to right lobe of liver tributary: cystic vein. SYN ramus dexter venae portae hepatis [TA].

saphenous b. of descending genicular artery [TA], b. of descending genicular artery supplying skin of the upper part of the medial aspect of the leg; *anastomosis:* medial inferior genicular artery (articular vascular *network* of knee). SYN ramus saphenus arteriae descendentis genicularis [TA].

b.'s of segmental bronchi, SYN intrasegmental *bronchi,* under *bronchus.*

septal b.'s, SYN interventricular septal b.'s of left/right coronary artery.

sinuatrial nodal b. of right coronary artery, SYN sinuatrial (S-A) nodal b. of right coronary artery.

b. to sinuatrial node, SYN sinuatrial (S-A) nodal b. of right coronary artery.

sinuatrial (S-A) nodal b. of right coronary artery [TA], ascending atrial branch, usually (55%) arising from the anterior stem of the right coronary artery (but 35–45% arising from the circumflex branch of the left coronary artery), which runs around the base of the superior vena cava to reach the sinuatrial node. SYN ramus nodi sinuatrialis arteriae coronariae dextrae [TA], artery to the sinoatrial (S-A) node, b. to sinuatrial node, sinuatrial nodal artery, sinuatrial nodal b. of right coronary artery, sinuatrial node artery, sinus node artery.

spinal b.'s [TA], b.'s of the following arteries that supply the meninges, the roots of the spinal nerves, and in some cases, the spinal cord: 1) vertebral, 2) ascending cervical, 3) dorsal b. of posterior intercostal I to XI, 4) dorsal b. of subcostal, 5) dorsal b. of lumbar arteries, 6) lumbar b. of iliolumbar, 7) lateral sacral; all spinal arteries give rise to arteries supplying dorsal and ventral roots of spinal nerves; most are exhausted in supplying the roots as radicular arteries, but some (4–9), are large enough to reach and anastomose with the anterior and posterior spinal arteries and are designated instead as segmental medullary arteries. SEE great segmental medullary *artery,* segmental medullary *arteries,* under *artery.* SYN rami spinales (1) [TA], spinal arteries.

splenic b.'s of splenic artery [TA], b.'s of proper splenic arteries; splenic artery entering spleen at hilum. SYN rami splenici arteriae splenicae [TA], rami lienales arteriae lienalis⋆.

stapedial b. of posterior tympanic artery, b. arising either directly from the posterior tympanic artery or its parent artery, the stylomastoid artery; supplies stapedius muscle. SYN ramus stapedius arteriae tympanicae posterioris [TA], ramus stapedius arteriae stylomastoideae, stapedial b. of stylomastoid artery.

stapedial b. of stylomastoid artery, SYN stapedial b. of posterior tympanic artery.

sternal b.'s of internal thoracic artery [TA], b.'s of internal thoracic artery that pass medially to supply the transversus thoracis muscle and posterior sternum. SYN rami sternales arteriae thoracicae internae [TA], sternal arteries.

sternocleidomastoid b.'s of occipital artery, b.'s of occipital artery to sternocleidomastoid muscle. One often hooks around hypoglossal nerve. It may arise as an independent b. of the external carotid, in which case it may be referred to as the sternomastoid *artery*. SYN rami sternocleidomastoidei arteriae occipitalis.

sternocleidomastoid b. of superior thyroid artery [TA], b. of superior thyroid artery to sternocleidomastoid muscle. SYN ramus sternocleidomastoideus arteriae thyroideae superioris [TA].

stylohyoid b. of facial nerve [TA], b. of facial nerve to stylohyoid muscle. SYN ramus stylohyoideus nervi facialis [TA].

stylopharyngeal b. of glossopharyngeal nerve [TA], sole motor b. of the glossopharyngeal nerve to the stylopharyngeus muscle. SYN ramus musculi stylopharyngei nervi glossopharyngei [TA], b. of glossopharyngeal nerve to stylopharyngeus muscle.

subendocardial b.'s of atrioventricular bundles, interlacing fibers formed of modified cardiac muscle cells with central granulated protoplasm containing one or two nuclei and a transversely striated peripheral portion; they are the terminal ramifications of the conducting system of the heart found beneath the endocardium of the ventricles. SEE ALSO conducting *system* of heart. SYN rami subendocardiales fasciculi atrioventricularis [TA], Purkinje fibers.

subscapular b.'s of axillary artery [TA], b.'s of axillary artery passing directly to the subscapularis muscle. SYN rami subscapulares arteriae axillaris [TA].

superficial b. [TA], b. which passes above or closer to surface; usually in contrast to a deep b. SYN ramus superficialis [TA].

superficial b. of the lateral plantar nerve [TA], mostly cutaneous b. to skin of small and lateral half of fourth toes and lateral side of sole of foot, but also supplies the flexor digiti minimi brevis muscle and the most lateral dorsal and plantar interosseous muscles. SYN ramus superficialis nervi plantaris lateralis [TA].

superficial b. of medial circumflex femoral artery [TA], small b. arising from the initial portion of the medial femoral circumflex artery that passes superficially in the superomedial thigh; after giving rise to the superficial b., the medial femoral circumflex artery continues as the deep b. SYN ramus superficialis arteriae circumflexae femoris medialis [TA].

superficial b. of the medial plantar artery [TA], gives rise to superficial digital arteries of medial three toes. SYN ramus superficialis arteriae plantaris medialis [TA].

superficial palmar b. of radial artery [TA], the superficial palmar branch of the radial artery that supplies the thenar muscles then enters the palm to communicate with the superficial palmar arch from the ulnar artery. SYN ramus palmaris superficialis arteriae radialis [TA], superficial palmar artery, superficial volar artery, superficialis volae.

superficial b. of the radial nerve [TA], cutaneous terminal b. (with deep b.) which runs under cover of brachioradialis muscle to wrist, then supplies skin of proximal portion of the dorsal aspects of thumb, index, middle and lateral half of ring fingers and the portion of the dorsum of the hand located proximally. SYN ramus superficialis nervi radialis [TA].

superficial b. of the superior gluteal artery [TA], to upper gluteus maximus muscle. SYN ramus superficialis arteriae gluteae superioris [TA].

superficial temporal b.'s of auriculotemporal nerve [TA], b.'s of auriculotemporal nerve to anterolateral scalp. SYN rami temporales superficiales nervi auriculotemporalis [TA].

superficial b. of the transverse cervical artery [TA], b. of transverse cervical artery that accompanies the spinal accessory nerve on the deep surface of the trapezius muscle. Alternatively arises as a direct b. of the thyrocervical trunk, in which case it is called the superficial cervical artery. SYN ramus superficialis arteriae transversae colli [TA].

superficial b. of the ulnar nerve [TA], b. supplying skin of palmar aspect of little and medial half of ring fingers, the portion of the palm proximal to them and the palmaris brevis muscle. SYN ramus superficialis nervi ulnaris [TA].

superior b. [TA], b. that is directed upward or cranially or which is highly placed, usually in contrast to an inferior b. SYN ramus superior [TA].

superior cervical cardiac b.'s of vagus nerve [TA], uppermost of the b.'s of vagus nerve conducting presynaptic parasympathetic fibers to, and reflex afferent fibers from, the cardiac plexus; branching from the vagi close to the base of the skull. SYN rami cardiaci cervicales superiores nervi vagi [TA].

superior dental b.'s of superior dental plexus [TA], b.'s passing from the superior dental plexus to the roots of the teeth of the upper jaw. SYN rami dentales superiores plexus dentalis superioris [TA], rami dentales superiores [TA], superior dental rami.

superior gingival b.'s of superior dental plexus [TA], b.'s of superior dental plexus to gingiva of upper jaw. SYN rami gingivales superiores plexus dentalis superioris [TA].

superior labial b. of facial artery [TA], *origin*, facial; *distribution*, structures of upper lip and, by a septal branch, the anterior and lower part of the nasal septum; *anastomoses*, the artery of the opposite side and the sphenopalatine. SYN arteria labialis superior [TA], ramus labialis superior arteriae facialis, superior labial artery.

superior labial b.'s of infraorbital nerve [TA], b.'s of infraorbital nerve to upper lip. SYN rami labiales superiores nervi infraorbitalis [TA].

superior lingular b. of lingular branch of superior lobar left pulmonary artery, SYN superior lingular *artery*.

superior b. of the oculomotor nerve [TA], b. of oculomotor nerve supplying the superior rectus and levator palpebrae superioris muscles. SYN ramus superior nervi oculomotorii [TA].

superior b. of the pubic bone, SYN superior pubic *ramus*.

superior b. of the right and left inferior pulmonary veins [TA], tributaries of the right and left inferior pulmonary veins which receive oxygenated blood from the superior [S6] bronchopulmonary segments of the inferior lobes of the right and left lungs. SYN ramus superior venae pulmonalis dextrae/sinistrae inferioris.

superior b. of the superior gluteal artery [TA], runs between gluteus medius and minimus muscles, supplying both, and continuing to reach tensor fascia lata muscle. SYN ramus superior arteriae gluteae superioris [TA].

superior b. of the transverse cervical nerve [TA], b. providing cutaneous innervation in upper part of anterior triangle of neck. SYN ramus superior nervi transversalis cervicalis (colli) [TA].

superior vermian b. (of superior cerebellar artery) [TA], *origin:* medial b. of superior cerebellar artery; *distribution:* superior vermis of cerebellum. SYN ramus vermis superior [TA].

suprahyoid b. of lingual artery [TA], b. of lingual artery that runs along hyoid bone; *anastomosis:* infrahyoid b. of superior thyroid artery and across midline with its contralateral partner. SYN ramus suprahyoideus arteriae lingualis [TA].

sural communicating b. of common fibular nerve [TA], the peroneal (fibular) communicating b. of the common peroneal (fibular) nerve; it arises from the common peroneal nerve in the popliteal space and passes over the lateral head of the gastrocnemius to the middle third of the leg, where it unites with the medial sural cutaneous nerve to form the sural nerve. SYN ramus communicans fibularis nervi fibularis communis [TA], ramus communicans nervi fibularis communis cum nervo cutaneo surae mediali⋆, ramus communicans nervi peronei communis cum nervo cutaneo surae mediali⋆, ramus communicans peroneus nervi peronei communis⋆, sural communicating b. of common peroneal nerve⋆, nervus communicans fibularis, nervus communicans peroneus, peroneal anastomotic ramus, peroneal communicating b., peroneal communicating nerve.

sural communicating b. of common peroneal nerve, ✩ official alternate term for sural communicating b. of common fibular nerve.

sympathetic b. to submandibular ganglion, SYN sympathetic *root* of submandibular ganglion.

temporal b.'s of facial nerve [TA], b.'s of facial nerve innervating the superior portion of the orbicularis oculi muscle and other muscles of facial expression above the eye. SYN rami temporales nervi facialis [TA].

tentorial basal b. of internal carotid artery [TA], a small b. from the cavernous part of the internal carotid artery to the base of the tentorium. SYN ramus basalis tentorii arteriae carotidis internae [TA], basal tentorial b. of internal carotid artery.

tentorial marginal b. of cavernous part of internal carotid artery, a small b. from the cavernous part of the internal carotid artery to the free margin of the tentorium. SYN ramus marginalis tentorii partis cavernosae arteriae carotidis internae [TA], marginal tentorial b. of internal carotid artery, ramus marginalis tentorii arteriae carotidis internae.

terminal b.'s of middle cerebral artery [TA], derivatives of the middle cerebral artery, arising distal to the M1 segment (main trunk) deep in the lateral sulcus between temporal lobe and insula; included are the superior and inferior terminal (cortical) branches (trunks) and the insular arteries. SYN rami terminales arteriae cerebri medii [TA], M2 segment of middle cerebral artery✩.

thoracic cardiac b.'s of thoracic ganglia, part of the cardiopulmonary splanchnic nerves from the second to fifth segments of the thoracic sympathetic trunk that pass medially and anteriorly to enter the cardiac plexus; they convey postsynaptic sympathetic fibers to, and visceral afferent (pain) fibers from, the heart. SYN rami cardiaci thoracici gangliorum thoracicorum [TA], nervi cardiaci thoracici, thoracic cardiac nerves, upper thoracic splanchnic nerves.

thoracic cardiac b.'s of vagus nerve [TA], b.'s of vagus nerve to the cardiac plexus that branch from the vagi at thoracic levels, conducting presynpatic parasympathetic fibers to, and reflex afferent fibers from, the cardiac plexus. SYN rami cardiaci thoracici nervi vagi [TA].

thoracic pulmonary b.'s of thoracic ganglia [TA], cardiopulmonary splanchnic nerves arising from the upper thoracic paravertebral ganglia of the sympathetic trunk conveying postsynaptic sympathetic and visceral afferent fibers to the pulmonary plexuses. SYN rami pulmonales thoracici gangliorum thoracicorum [TA].

thymic b.'s of internal thoracic artery [TA], mediastinal b.'s of the proximal (superior) portion of the internal thoracic artery which pass to the thymus. SYN rami thymici arteriae thoracicae internae [TA].

thyrohyoid b. of ansa cervicalis, derived from the cervical plexus, it contains fibers of the first and second cervical nerves that have accompanied the hypoglossal nerve to the suprahyoid region, then branch from it to reach the thyrohyoid muscle. SYN ramus thyrohyoideus ansae cervicalis [TA], nerve to thyrohyoid muscle.

tonsillar b. of the facial artery [TA], primary blood supply to palatine tonsil, with extensive anastomoses with other tonsillar arteries. SYN ramus tonsillaris arteriae facialis [TA].

tonsillar b.'s of glossopharyngeal nerve [TA], b.'s of glossopharyngeal nerve conducting sensory fibers from the palatine tonsillar fossa. SYN rami tonsillares nervi glossopharyngei.

tonsillar b.'s of lesser palatine nerves [TA], b.'s of the lesser palatine nerves that extend to the palatine tonsil and/or its bed. SYN rami tonsillares nervi palatini minores [TA].

tracheal b.'s [TA], b.'s to the trachea. Terminologia Anatomica lists tracheal branches of 1) inferior thyroid artery (rami tracheales arteriae thyroideae inferioris [TA]); 2) internal thoracic artery (rami tracheales arteria thoracicae internae [TA]); and 3) recurrent laryngeal nerve (rami tracheales nervi laryngei recurrentis [TA]). SYN rami tracheales [TA].

transverse b. of lateral femoral circumflex artery [TA], early b. of lateral femoral circumflex artery that enters the substance of the vastus lateralis and forms numerous anastomoses. SYN ramus transversus arteriae circumflexae femoris lateralis [TA].

b. to trigeminal ganglion, ganglionic b. of internal carotid artery.

tubal b. [TA], b. to a tubular structure. SYN ramus tubarius [TA].

tubal b. of ovarian artery [TA], terminal b. (with ovarian b.) of ovarian artery that passes to the distal part of the uterine tube and courses centrally to anastomose with the tubal b. of the uterine artery proper. SYN ramus tubarius arteriae ovaricae [TA].

tubal b. of the tympanic plexus [TA], sensory b. of tympanic plexus (of glossopharyngeal nerve) to pharyngotympanic (auditory) tube. SYN ramus tubarius plexus tympanici [TA].

tubal b. of the uterine artery [TA], terminal b. of uterine artery (with ovarian b.) supplying medial portion of uterine tube, anastomosing with tubal b. of ovarian artery. SYN ramus tubarius arteriae uterinae [TA].

ulnar communicating b. of superficial radial nerve, SYN communicating b. of superficial radial nerve with ulnar nerve.

ulnar b. of medial antebrachial cutaneous nerve, SYN posterior b. of medial cutaneous nerve of forearm.

ureteral b.'s, SYN ureteric b.'s.

ureteric b.'s [TA], b.'s distributed to the ureter. Although not listed in Terminologia Anatomica, ureteric b.'s also rise regularly from the 1) abdominal aorta, 2) common iliac artery, and 3) internal iliac artery. Ureteric b.'s from the inferior vesical artery are constant in occurrence and supply the terminal portion of the ureter. SYN rami ureterici [TA], ureteral b.'s.

ureteric b.'s of the inferior suprarenal artery [TA], b.'s of the right or left inferior suprarenal artery that descend to supply, with the ureteric b.'s of the renal artery, the uppermost portion of the ureter. SYN rami ureterici arteriae suprarenalis inferioris [TA].

ureteric b.'s of the ovarian artery [TA], b. of ovarian artery arising as it is crossed by the ureter in the female supplying mid portion of ureter. SYN rami ureterici arteriae ovaricae [TA].

ureteric b.'s of the patent part of umbilical artery [TA], supplies pelvic portion of ureter. SYN rami ureterici partis patentis arteriae umbilicalis [TA].

ureteric b.'s of the renal artery, supplies ureteric (renal) pelvis and superior portion of ureter. SYN rami ureterici arteriae renalis.

ureteric b.'s of the testicular artery [TA], b. of testicular artery arising as it is crossed by the ureter in the male; supplies mid portion of ureter. SYN rami ureterici arteriae testicularis [TA].

ventral b., SYN ramus ventralis. SEE ventral primary *rami* of cervical spinal nerves, under *ramus*, ventral primary *rami* of lumbar spinal nerves, under *ramus*, ventral primary *rami* of sacral spinal nerves, under *ramus*, anterior *ramus* of spinal nerve.

vestibular b.'s of labyrinthine artery, SEE posterior vestibular b. of vestibulocochlear artery, anterior vestibular *artery*.

zygomatic b.'s of facial nerve, b.'s of facial nerve crossing upper cheek to supply orbicularis oculi muscle. SYN rami zygomatici nervi facialis.

zygomaticofacial b. of zygomatic nerve [TA], penetrates zygomatic bone to supply skin of face over zygoma or cheekbone. SYN ramus zygomaticofacialis nervi zygomatici [TA].

zygomaticotemporal b. of zygomatic nerve [TA], penetrates frontal process of zygomatic bone to supply skin of face lateral to orbit. SYN ramus zygomaticotemporalis nervi zygomatici [TA].

bran·chia, pl. **bran·chi·ae** (brang′kē-ă, -ē). The gills, or organs of respiration, in water-living animals. [G. gill]

bran·chi·al (brang′kē-ăl). 1. Relating to branchiae or gills. 2. In embryology, denoting the various structures constituting the branchial *apparatus.*

branching. Dividing into parts; sending out offshoots; bifurcating. SYN ramose, ramous. [Fr. *branche,* related to L. *branchium,* arm]

false b., in bacteriology, the appearance of b. produced when a cell is pushed out of the general line of growth and develops a new line of growth while the remaining cells continue to develop along the original line of growth.

bran·chi·o·gen·ic, bran·chi·og·en·ous (brang′kē-ō-jen′ik, -kē-oj′en-ŭs). Originating from the branchial arches. [G. *branchia,* gill, *-gen,* to produce]

bran·chi·o·mere (brang′kē-ō-mēr). An embryonic segment from which a branchial arch is developed. [G. *branchia,* gill, + *meros,* part]

bran·chi·om·er·ism (brang-kē-om′er-izm). Arrangement into branchiomeres.

bran·chi·o·mo·tor (brang′kē-ō-mō′tōr). Relating to or controlling the movement of muscles associated with the branchial arches.

bran·dy. An alcoholic liquid obtained by the distillation of the fermented juice of sound ripe grapes and usually containing 48 to 54% ethyl alcohol. [Du. *brandewijn*, burnt (distilled) wine]

Branham, H.H., 19th century U.S. surgeon. SEE B. *sign*.

Branham, Sara Elizabeth, U.S. bacteriologist, 1888–1962. SEE *Branhamella*.

Bran·ha·mel·la (bran-hă-mel′ă). A subgenus of aerobic, nonmotile, nonsporeforming bacteria containing Gram-negative cocci that occur in pairs with adjacent sides flattened; these organisms are currently considered closely related to the genus *Moraxella*. They occur in the mucous membranes of the upper respiratory tract. The type species is *B. catarrhalis*. [Sara *Branham*]

B. catarrha′lis, SYN *Moraxella catarrhalis*.

bran·ny (bran′ē). Denoting desquamation of small husklike scales. [M.E. *bran*, broken coat of cereal grain]

Brasdor, Pierre, French surgeon, 1721–1798. SEE B. *method*.

Braun, Christopher Heinrich, German surgeon, 1847–1911. SEE B. *anastomosis*.

Braune, Christian W., German anatomist, 1831–1892. SEE B. *muscle, valve*.

brawny (brahw′nē). Thickened (lichenified) and dusky (a darkened hue), as of a swelling. [M.E. fleshy]

Braxton Hicks, John, British gynecologist, 1823–1897. SEE B.H. *contraction, sign*.

Bray, Charles William, U.S. otologist, *1904. SEE Wever-B. *phenomenon*.

Brazelton, T. Berry, U.S. pediatrician, *1918. SEE Brazelton Neonatal Behavioral Assessment *Scale*, under *scale*.

bra·zil·ein (bră-zil′ē-in). A red oxidation product of brazilin.

braz·i·lin (bră-zil′in) [C.I. 75280]. A red natural dye, $C_{16}H_{14}O_5$, obtained from the bark of several species of tropical trees and oxidized to the active red dye brazilein; resembles hematoxylin in origin, chemistry, and usage; used as a nuclear stain and as an indicator (red in alkalies, yellow in acids).

braz·ing (brā′zing). In dentistry, soldering.

BrDu Abbreviation for bromodeoxyuridine.

break (brāk). Separation into parts.

  double-strand b., a b. in double-stranded DNA in which both strands have been cleaved; however, the two strands have not separated from each other.

  single-strand b., a b. in double-stranded DNA in which only one of the two strands has been cleaved; both strands have not separated from each other.

breakpoint (brāk′poynt). In helminth epidemiology, the critical mean wormload in a community, below which the helminth mating frequency is too low to maintain reproduction. Below this level, helminth infection in the community will progressively decline, ultimately to zero.

break·through (brāk′throo). A sudden manifestation of new insights and more constructive attitudes following a period of resistance during psychotherapy.

breast (brest) [TA]. **1.** The pectoral surface of the thorax. **2.** The female organ of milk secretion; one of two commonly hemispheric projections anterior to the pectoral muscles including the mammary glands within a highly variable amount of fat of the subcutaneous layer and bearing the nipple superficially on either side of the chest of the mature female; it is rudimentary in the male. SYN mamma [TA], teat (2). [A.S. *breōst*]

  accessory b. [TA], a milk-secreting gland located elsewhere than at the normal place on the chest and existing in addition to the two usual mammae. SYN mamma accessoria [TA], supernumerary b., supernumerary mamma.

  chicken b., SYN *pectus* carinatum.

  funnel b., SYN *pectus* excavatum.

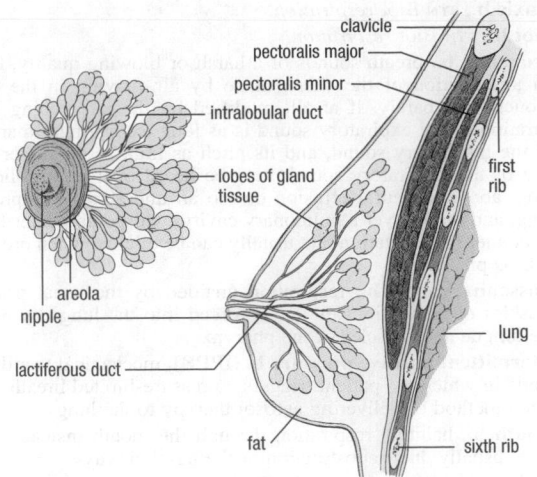

breast: glandular tissue and ducts of the mammary gland

  irritable b., swelling and induration of the b., not due to a neoplasm, and usually of comparatively brief duration.

  male b. [TA], one of the two, usually rudimentary, mammary glands and overlying nipples of the male. SYN mamma masculina [TA], mamma virilis.

  pigeon b., SYN *pectus* carinatum.

  supernumerary b., SYN accessory b.

breath (breth). **1.** The respired air. **2.** An inspiration. [A.S. *braeth*]

  liver b., SYN *fetor* hepaticus.

  uremic b., characteristic odor of the b. in patients with chronic renal failure, variously described as "fishy," "ammoniacal," and "fetid," which is indicative of the systemic accumulation of volatile metabolites, usually excreted in the urine; dimethylamine and trimethylamine have been identified and correlated with the classic fishy odor.

breath-hold·ing (breth′hōld-ing). Voluntary or involuntary cessation of breathing; often seen in young children as a response to frustration.

breath·ing (brēth′ing). Inhalation and exhalation of air or gaseous mixtures. SYN pneusis.

muscles used in breathing	
inspiration muscles	**auxiliary muscles (inspiration)**
diaphragm	sternocleidomastoid
external intercostal	scalenus anterior, medius,
internal intercostal, parasternal	and posterior
part (intercartilaginous)	pectoralis major
	pectoralis minor
	serratus posterior superior
	serratus anterior
expiration muscles	**auxiliary muscles (expiration)**
internal intercostal	rectus abdominis
transverse thoracic	transverse abdominal
subcostal	abdominal external oblique
	abdominal internal oblique
	erector spinae
	quadratus lumborum
	serratus posterior, inferior

  apneustic b., pauses in the respiratory cycle at full inspiration, caused by damage of the respiratory control centers in the more caudal pons.

ataxic b., SYN Biot *respiration*.

Biot b., SYN Biot *respiration*.

bronchial b., breath sounds of a harsh or blowing quality, heard on auscultation of the chest, made by air moving in the large bronchi and barely, if at all, modified by the intervening lung; duration of the expiratory sound is as long as or longer than that of the inspiratory sound, and its pitch as high as or higher than that of the inspiratory sound; may be heard over a consolidated lung, above a pleural effusion due to an underlying compressed lung, and rarely over a pulmonary cavity; whispered pectoriloquy is another manifestation that usually can be elicited when bronchial b. is present.

glossopharyngeal b., respiration unaided by the usual primary muscles of respiration; the air is forced into the lungs by use of the tongue and muscles of the pharynx.

intermittent positive pressure b. (IPPB), mechanical ventilating mode in which the patient triggers a pressure-limited breath. Outdated method of delivering aerosol therapy to the lungs.

mouth b., habitual respiration through the mouth instead of the nose, usually due to obstruction of the nasal airways.

positive-negative pressure b. (PNPB), inflation of the lungs with positive pressure and deflation with negative pressure by an automatic ventilator.

pursed lips b., a technique in which air is inhaled slowly through the nose and mouth and exhaled slowly through pursed lips; used by patients with chronic obstructive pulmonary disease to improve their breathing by increasing resistance to air flow, forcibly dilating small bronchi.

shallow b., a type of b. with abnormally low tidal volume.

stertorous b., SYN stertorous *respiration*.

Breda, Achille, Italian dermatologist, 1850–1933. SEE B. *disease*.

bre·douille·ment (brā-dwē-mahn′). Omission of parts of words related to extremely rapid speech. [Fr.]

breech (brēch). SYN buttocks. [A.S. *brēc*]

breed·ing (brēd′ing). Selected mating of individuals to produce a strain that is desirable or of scientific interest. SEE ALSO hybridization, linebreeding, inbreeding. [breed, fr. M.E. *breden*, fr. O.E. *brēdan*, + -ing]

breg·ma (breg′mă) [TA]. The point on the skull corresponding to the junction of the coronal and sagittal sutures. [G. the forepart of the head]

breg·mat·ic (breg-mat′ik). Relating to the bregma.

brei (brī). A fine and uniform mince or mush of tissue in which the cells are for the most part intact. Cf. homogenate. [Ger. pulp]

brems·strah·lung (bremz′strah-lŭng). Continuous spectrum radiation produced by the slowing of electrons in a beam by nuclei in their vicinity. [Ger. *Bremsstrahlung*, braking radiation]

Brenn, Lena, 20th century U.S. researcher. SEE Brown-B. *stain*.

Brenner, Fritz, German pathologist, *1877. SEE B. *tumor*.

♻**brepho-.** Prefix denoting a primitive stage of development. [G. *brephos*, embryo or newborn infant]

Breschet (Brechet), Gilbert, French anatomist, 1784–1845. SEE B. *bones*, under *bone*, *canals*, under *canal*, *hiatus*, *sinus*, *vein*.

Brescia, Michael J., U.S. nephrologist, *1933. SEE B.-Cimino *fistula*.

Breslow, Alexander, U.S. pathologist, 1928–1980. SEE B. *thickness*.

bre·tyl·i·um. **1.** An antihypertensive, which on chronic oral dosing, first releases, then diminishes the release of norepinephrine from noradrenergic nerve endings. **2.** An antiarrhythmic used to treat life-threatening ventricular arrhythmias; blocks potassium channels.

bre·tyl·i·um tos·yl·ate (bre-til′ē-ŭm). A sympatholytic agent that prevents the release of norepinephrine from the nerve ending; used in the treatment of essential hypertension. SEE ALSO bretylium.

Breuer, Josef, Austrian internist, 1842–1925. SEE Hering-B. *reflex*.

bre·ve·tox·ins (BTX) (brev′ē-tok′sins). Structurally unique neurotoxins produced by the "red tide" dinoflagellate *Ptychodiscus*

brevis Davis (*Gymnodinium breve Davis*). An algae responsible for large fish kills and mollusk and human food poisoning in the Gulf of Mexico and along the Florida coast. Unlike previously isolated dinoflagellate toxins, such as saxitoxin, which are water-soluble sodium channel blockers, the b. are lipid-soluble sodium channel activators. Used as tools in neurobiologic research.

Brev·i·bac·ter·ium (brev-ē-bak-tēr′ē-um). A bacterial genus of nonmotile, nonsporeforming, Gram-positive rods found as normal human skin flora and in raw milk and on the surface of cheeses; some species, recovered from patients with septicemia and from the peritoneum of patients undergoing peritoneal dialysis, appear to be opportunistic human pathogens.

brev·i·col·lis (brev-ē-kol′is). Abnormal shortness of the neck. [L. *brevis*, short, + *collum*, neck]

bre·vis (brev′is). Brief, short. [L. short]

Brewer, George E., U.S. surgeon, 1861–1939. SEE B. *infarcts*, under *infarct*.

Bricker, Eugene M., U.S. urologist, *1908. SEE B. *operation*.

🔲**bridge** (bridj). **1.** The upper part of the ridge of the nose formed by the nasal bones. **2.** One of the threads of protoplasm that appear to pass from one cell to another. **3.** SYN fixed partial *denture*.

arteriolovenular b., the largest capillary connecting arteriole to venule.

cantilever b., a fixed partial b. denture in which the pontic is retained only on one side by an abutment tooth. SYN extension b.

caudolenticular gray b.'s [TA], strands of neuron cell bodies that span the internal capsule, primarily its anterior limb, between the caudate nucleus and the putamen. SYN pontes grisei caudolenticulares [TA], transcapsular gray b.'s⋆.

cell b.'s, SYN intercellular b.'s.

cystine b., SYN disulfide b.

cytoplasmic b.'s, SYN intercellular b.'s.

dentin b., a deposit of reparative dentin or other calcific substances which forms across and reseals exposed tooth pulp tissue.

disulfide b., (1) a disulfide linkage between two cysteinyl residues in a poly- or oligopeptide or in a protein; (2) any disulfide linkage between any thiol-containing moieties of a larger molecule. SYN cystine b.

extension b., SYN cantilever b.

fixed b., SYN fixed partial *denture*.

Gaskell b., SYN atrioventricular *bundle*.

intercellular b.'s, slender cytoplasmic strands connecting adjacent cells; in histological sections of the epidermis and other stratified squamous epithelia, the b.'s are processes attached by a desmosome and are shrinkage artifacts of fixation; true b.'s with cytoplasmic confluence exist between incompletely divided germ cells. SYN cell b.'s, cytoplasmic b.'s.

myocardial b., a b. of cardiac muscle fibers extending over the epicardial aspect of a coronary artery; this finding, in cases of sudden unexpected death, has led to speculation that cardiac contraction during exertion could constrict the coronary artery.

removable b., SYN removable partial *denture*.

salt b., SYN electrostatic *bond*.

transcapsular gray b.'s, ⋆official alternate term for caudolenticular gray b.'s.

Wheatstone b., an apparatus for measuring electrical resistance; four resistors are connected to form the four sides or "arms" of a square; a voltage is applied to one diagonal pair of connections, while the voltage between the other diagonal pair is measured, e.g., by a galvanometer; the bridge is "balanced" when the measured voltage is zero; then, the ratios of the two pairs of adjoining resistances must be identical.

bridge·work (bridj′wŏrk). SYN partial *denture*.

bri·dle (brī′dl). **1.** SYN frenum. **2.** A band of fibrous material stretching across the surface of an ulcer or other lesion or forming adhesions between opposing serous or mucous surfaces. [M.E. *bridel*]

b. of clitoris, obsolete term for *frenulum* of clitoris.

Bright, Richard, English internist and pathologist, 1789–1858. SEE B. *disease*.

Brill, Nathan E., U.S. physician, 1860–1925. SEE B. *disease;* B.-Zinsser *disease.*

bril·liant cres·yl blue. SEE cresyl blue.

bril·liant green [C.I. 42040]. The sulfate of di-(*p*-diethylamino)-triphenyl carbinolanhydride. An indicator dye that changes from yellow to green at pH 0.0 to 2.6; also used as a topical antiseptic and as a selective bacteriostatic agent in culture media. SYN ethyl green.

bril·liant vi·tal red. SYN vital red.

bril·liant yel·low [C.I. 13085]. An indicator dye that changes from yellow to orange or red at pH 6.4 to 8.0.

brim. The upper edge or rim of a hollow structure.
pelvic b., SYN pelvic *inlet.*

brim·stone (brim'stōn). SYN sulfur. [A.S. *brinnan,* to burn]

brin·dle (brin'dl). A hair coat color in which there is a uniform mixture of gray or tawny hairs with others of white or black; a composite color. [diminutive of O.E. *brinded*]

Brinell, Johan A., Swedish metallurgist, 1849–1925. SEE B. hardness *number.*

Briquet, Paul, French physician, 1796–1881. SEE B. *ataxia, syndrome.*

brise·ment (briz-mon'fōr-sā'). Procedure infrequently used to treat frozen shoulder in which a forceful manipulation is performed to restore range of motion that usually results in torn adhesions and adjacent joint capsule. [Fr. forcible breaking]

Brissaud, Edouard, French physician, 1852–1909. SEE B. *disease, infantilism, reflex;* B.-Marie *syndrome.*

Brit·ish an·ti-Lew·is·ite (BAL) (brit'ish an-tē-loo'is-īt). SYN dimercaprol.

Brit·ish Phar·ma·co·poe·ia (BP). SEE Pharmacopeia.

broach (brōch). A dental instrument for removing the pulp of a tooth or exploring the canal.
barbed b., a root canal instrument set with barbs; used for removing a dental pulp, pulp tissue remnants, or dentinal debris.
smooth b., an exploring instrument used in endodontic practice; a root canal tine.

Broadbent, Sir William H., British physician, 1835–1907. SEE B. *law, sign.*

broad-spec·trum. SEE spectrum.

Broca, Pierre P., French surgeon, neurologist, and anthropologist, 1824–1880. SEE B. *angles,* under *angle, aphasia,* basilar *angle,* facial *angle, area,* parolfactory *area,* diagonal *band, center, field, fissure, formula,* visual *plane, pouch.*

Brock, Sir Russell C., British surgeon, *1903. SEE B. *syndrome, operation.*

Brockenbrough, E.C., U.S. surgeon, *1930. SEE B. *sign.*

bro·cre·sine (brō-krē'sēn). A histidine decarboxylase inhibitor.

Brödel, Max, German medical artist in the U.S., 1870–1941. SEE B. bloodless *line.*

Brodie, Sir Benjamin C., British surgeon, 1783–1862. SEE B. *abscess, bursa, disease, knee.*

Brodie, Charles Gordon, Scottish anatomist and surgeon, 1860–1933. SEE B. *ligament.*

Brodie, Thomas Gregor, British physiologist, 1866–1916. SEE B. *fluid.*

Brodmann, Korbinian, German neurologist, 1868–1918. SEE B. *areas,* under *area.*

Broesike, Gustav, German anatomist, *1853. SEE B. *fossa.*

△**brom-, bromo-.** 1. Foul-smelling. 2. Indicating the presence of bromine in a compound. [G. *brōmos,* a stench]

bro·mate (brō'māt). Salt or anion of bromic acid.

bro·mat·ed (brō'māt-ĕd). Combined or saturated with bromine or any of its compounds. SYN brominated.

bro·ma·ze·pam (brō-mā'zĕ-pam). An antianxiety agent of the benzodiazepine class.

bro·ma·zine hy·dro·chlo·ride (brō'mă-zēn). SYN bromodiphenhydramine hydrochloride.

brom·cre·sol green (brom-krē'sol). A substituted triphenyl-methane dye (pK_a 4.7), sparingly soluble in water but readily soluble in alcohol, diethyl ether, and ethyl acetate; used as an indicator of pH (yellow at pH 3.8, blue-green at pH 5.4).

brom·cre·sol pur·ple. A substituted triphenylmethane dye (pK_a 6.3), practically insoluble in water but soluble in alcohol and dilute alkalies; used as an indicator of pH (yellow at pH 5.2, purple at pH 6.8).

bro·me·lain, bro·me·lin (brō'mĕ-lān, -lin). One of a group of peptide hydrolases, all thiol proteinases, obtained from pineapple stem; used in tenderizing meats and in producing hydrolysates of proteins; orally administered in the treatment of inflammation and edema of soft tissues associated with traumatic injury.

Bromelius, C., Swedish botanist, 1639–1705. SEE bromelain.

brom·hex·ine hy·dro·chlo·ride (brom-hek'sēn). An expectorant with mucolytic, antitussive, and bronchodilator properties.

brom·hi·dro·sis (brom-hi-drō'sis). SYN bromidrosis.

bro·mic (brō'mik). Relating to bromine; denoting especially bromic acid, $HBrO_3$.

bro·mide (brō'mīd). The anion Br^-; salt of hydrogen bromide (HBr); several salts formerly used as sedatives, hypnotics, and anticonvulsants.

bro·mi·dro·si·pho·bia (brō'mi-drō-si-fō'bē-ă). Morbid fear of giving forth a bad odor from the body, sometimes with the belief that such an odor is present. [bromidrosis + G. *phobos,* fear]

bro·mi·dro·sis (brōm-i-drō'sis). Fetid or foul-smelling perspiration. Apocrine b. affects the axilleo after puberty, and eccrine b. is generalized, with excessive sweating. SYN bromhidrosis. [G. *brōmos,* a stench, + *hidrōs,* perspiration]

bro·min·at·ed (brō'min-āt-ĕd). SYN bromated.

bro·min·di·one (brō-min-dī'ōn). An oral anticoagulant.

bro·mine (Br) (brō'mēn, -min). A nonmetallic, reddish, volatile, liquid element; atomic no. 35, atomic wt. 79.904; valences 1–7, inclusive; it unites with hydrogen to form hydrobromic acid, and this reacts with many metals to form bromides, some of which are used in medicine. [Fr. *brome,* bromine, fr. G. *bromos,* stench]

bro·mism, bro·min·ism (brō'mizm, -min-izm). Chronic bromide intoxication, characterized by headache, drowsiness, confusion and occasionally violent delirium, muscular weakness, cardiac depression, an acneform eruption, foul breath, anorexia, and gastric distress.

△**bromo-.** SEE brom-.

bro·mo·ben·zyl·cy·an·ide (BBC) (brō'mō-benz-il-sī'a-nīd). A lacrimator used in tear gases in training and in riot control.

bro·mo·cre·sol green (brō-mō-krē'sol). Tetrabromo-m-cresolsulfonphthalein; an indicator dye changing from yellow to blue at pH 4.7; used to track DNA in agarose electrophoresis, and in a dye-binding method for analysis of serum albumin.

bro·mo·crip·tine (brō-mō-krip'tēn). A semisynthetic ergot derivative that slows dopamine turnover, inhibits prolactin secretion and release of prolactin by thyrotropin-releasing hormone, and retards tumor growth and hence is used in the treatment of hyperprolactinemia associated with various pituitary tumors; an agonist at dopamine receptors also used in Parkinson disease.

bro·mo·de·ox·y·ur·i·dine (BrDu) (brō'mō-dē-ok'sē-ūr'i-dēn). A compound that competes with uridine for incorporation in RNA and fluoresces in ultraviolet light; used in BrDu-banding.

bro·mo·der·ma (brō-mō-der'mă). An acneform or granulomatous eruption due to hypersensitivity to bromide. [bromide + G. *derma,* skin]

bro·mo·di·phen·hy·dra·mine hy·dro·chlo·ride (brō'mō-dī-fen-hī'dră-mēn). An antihistamine that may cause drowsiness and xerostomia. SYN bromazine hydrochloride.

bro·mo·hy·per·hi·dro·sis, bro·mo·hy·per·i·dro·sis (brō'mō-hī'per-hi-drō'sis, -hī'per-i-drō'sis). Excessive secretion of sweat having a fetid odor, usually eccrine and generalized or affecting the feet. [G. *brōmos,* a stench, + *hyper,* over, + *hidrōsis,* sweating]

bro·mo·phe·nol blue (brō-mō-fē'nol). SYN bromphenol blue.

bro·mo·sul·fo·phtha·lein (brō'mō-sŭl'fō-thal'ē-in). SYN sulfobromophthalein sodium.

5-bro·mo·u·ra·cil (brō-mō-ū'ră-sil). Synthetic analog (antimetabolite) of thymine, in which a bromine atom takes the place of the methyl group in thymine; a mutagen.

brom·phen·ir·a·mine ma·le·ate (brōm-fen-ir′ă-mēn). A potent antihistaminic agent.

brom·phe·nol blue (brom-fē′nol). A substituted triphenylmethane dye (MW 670, pK 4.0), used as an acid-base indicator (yellow at pH less than 3.1, blue at pH more than 4.7); also used for histochemical and electrophoretic demonstration of proteins. SYN bromophenol blue.

brom·sul·fo·phtha·lein (brom-sŭl′fō-thal′ē-in). SYN sulfobromophthalein sodium.

brom·thy·mol blue (brom-thī′mol). A substituted triphenylmethane dye (MW 624, pK 7.0), used primarily as a hydrogen ion indicator (yellow at pH 6.0, blue at pH 7.6); also a weak but toxic vital stain.

bron·ca·tar (bron′kă-tar). Camphoric acid compound (neutralized) with 2-amino-2-thiazoline (1:2); an antitussive and respiratory stimulant.

⟳**bronch-.** SEE broncho-.

bron·chi (brong′kī). Plural of bronchus.

⟳**bronchi-.** SEE broncho-.

bron·chia (brong′kē-ă). The smaller divisions of the bronchi. SEE ALSO bronchus, bronchiole. SYN bronchial tubes. [G. pl. of *bronchion,* dim. of *bronchos,* trachea]

bron·chi·al (brong′kē-ăl). Relating to the bronchi.

bron·chi·ec·ta·sia (brong′kē-ek-tā′zē-ă). SYN bronchiectasis.
　b. sicca, SYN dry *bronchiectasis.*

ℹ**bron·chi·ec·ta·sis** (brong-kē-ek′tă-sis). Chronic dilation of bronchi or bronchioles as a sequel of inflammatory disease or obstruction often associated with heavy sputum production. SYN bronchiectasia. [bronchi- + G. *ektasis,* a stretching]

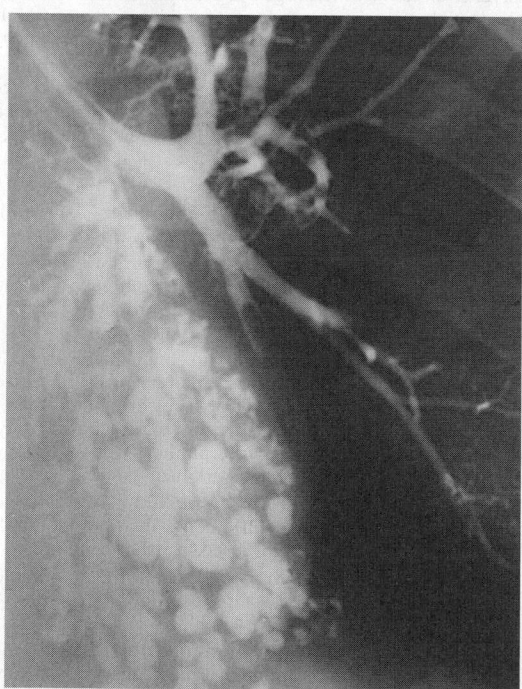

bronchiectasis: left posteroanterior bronchogram of a 10-year-old child with bronchiectasis and atelectasis of the left lower lobe subsequent to severe pneumonia

congenital b., a rare form of b. due to developmental arrest in the tracheobronchial tree; may be unilateral or bilateral.

cylindrical b., b. resulting in dilated bronchi of cylindrical shape; i.e., of uniform caliber.

ℹ**cystic b.,** b. in which the bronchi end in blind sacs greater in diameter than the draining bronchi. SEE ALSO saccular b.
　dry b., b. characterized by lack of productive cough and by occasional hemoptysis. SYN bronchiectasia sicca.
　saccular b., b. resulting in dilated bronchi of saccular or irregular shape. SEE ALSO cystic b.
　varicose b., cylindrical b. with irregular constrictions resembling varicose veins in shape.

bron·chi·ec·tat·ic (brong-kē-ek-tat′ik). Relating to bronchiectasis.

bron·chil·o·quy (brong-kil′ō-kwē). Rarely used term for bronchophony [bronchi- + L. *loquor,* to speak]

bron·chi·o·gen·ic (brong-kē-ō-jen′ik). SYN bronchogenic.

bron·chi·ole (brong′kē-ōl) [TA]. One of approximately six generations of increasingly finer subdivisions of the bronchi, all less than 1 mm in diameter, and having no cartilage in its wall, but relatively abundant smooth muscle and elastic fibers. SYN bronchiolus [TA].
　respiratory b.'s, the smallest bronchioles (0.5 mm in diameter) that connect the terminal bronchioles to alveolar ducts; alveoli rise from part of the wall. SYN bronchioli respiratorii.
　terminal b., the end of the nonrespiratory conducting airway; the lining is simple columnar or cuboidal epithelium without mucous goblet cells; most of the cells are ciliated, but a few nonciliated serous secreting cells occur. SYN bronchiolus terminalis.

bron·chi·o·lec·ta·sia (brong′kē-ō-lek-tā′zē-ă). SYN bronchiolectasis.

bron·chi·o·lec·ta·sis (brong′kē-ō-lek′tă-sis). Bronchiectasis involving the bronchioles. SYN bronchiolectasia. [bronchiole + G. *ektasis,* a stretching]

bron·chi·o·li (brong-kē′ō-lī). Plural of bronchiolus.

ℹ**bron·chi·ol·i·tis** (brong-kē-ō-lī′tis). Inflammation of the bronchioles, often associated with bronchopneumonia. [bronchiole + -*itis,* inflammation]
　constrictive b., obliteration of bronchioles by scarring following b. obliterans. Cf. proliferative b.
　exudative b., inflammation of the bronchioles, with fibrinous exudation.
　b. fibro′sa oblit′erans, obstruction of bronchioles and alveolar ducts by fibrous granulation tissue induced by mucosal ulceration; the condition may follow inhalation of irritant gases (see silofiller's *lung*) or may complicate pneumonia (see BOOP); associated with obstructive findings (see unilateral hyperlucent *lung,* Swyer-James *syndrome*). SYN b. obliterans.
　b. oblit′erans, SYN b. fibrosa obliterans.
　b. obliterans with organizing pneumonia (BOOP), b. fibrosa obliterans complicated by pneumonia with organization.
　proliferative b., b. with obliteration of bronchiolar lumen and alveoli by epithelial proliferation, which may follow influenza and giant cell pneumonia.

⟳**bronchiolo-.** Bronchiole. [L. *bronchiolus*]

bron·chi·o·lo·pul·mo·nary (brong′kē-ō-lō-pul′mō-nār-ē). Relating to the bronchioles and the lungs.

bron·chi·o·lus, pl. **bron·chi·o·li** (brong-kē′ō-lŭs, -ō-lī) [TA]. SYN bronchiole. [Mod. L. dim. of *bronchus*]
　bronchi′oli respirato′rii, SYN respiratory *bronchioles,* under *bronchiole.*
　b. termina′lis, SYN terminal *bronchiole.*

bron·chi·o·ste·no·sis (brong′kē-ō-sten-ō′sis). SYN bronchial *stenosis.*

bron·chit·ic (brong-kit′ik). Relating to bronchitis.

bron·chi·tis (brong-kī′tis). Inflammation of the mucous membrane of the bronchial tubes.
　asthmatic b., b. that causes or aggravates bronchospasm.
　Castellani b., SYN hemorrhagic b.
　chronic b., a condition of the bronchial tree characterized by cough, hypersecretion of mucus, and expectoration of sputum over a long period of time, associated with frequent bronchial infections; usually due to inhalation, over a prolonged period, of air contaminated by dust or by noxious gases of combustion.

croupous b., obsolete term for fibrinous b.

fibrinous b., inflammation of the bronchial mucous membrane, accompanied by a fibrinous exudation, which often forms a cast of the bronchial tree with severe obstruction of air flow. SYN plastic b., pseudomembranous b.

hemorrhagic b., chronic b. due to infection with spirochetes (though other bacteria are usually present and contribute to the infection) and characterized by cough and bloody sputum. SYN bronchopulmonary spirochetosis, bronchospirochetosis, Castellani b.

obliterative b., b. oblit′erans, fibrinous b. in which the exudate becomes organized, obliterating the affected portion of the bronchial tubes with consequent permanent collapse of affected portions of the lung.

plastic b., SYN fibrinous b.

pseudomembranous b., SYN fibrinous b.

putrid b., b. accompanied by an expectoration of foul-smelling sputum.

bron·chi·um (brong′kē-ŭm). SYN bronchus. [Mod. L. fr. G. *bronchion*]

⚠ **broncho-, bronch-, bronchi-.** Bronchus, and, in ancient usage, the trachea. [G. *bronchos*, windpipe]

bron·cho·al·ve·o·lar (brong′kō-al-vē′ō-lăr). SYN bronchovesicular.

bron·cho·cav·ern·ous (brong-kō-kav′er-nŭs). Relating to a bronchus or bronchial tube and a pulmonary pathologic cavity.

bron·cho·cele (brong′kō-sēl). A circumscribed dilation of a bronchus. [broncho- + G. *kēlē*, hernia]

bron·cho·con·stric·tion (brong-kō-kon-strik′shŭn). Reduction in the caliber of a bronchus or bronchi, usually referring to a dynamic process as in asthma and emphysema, rather than a fixed constriction (the latter is a bronchial stenosis). Cf. bronchospasm.

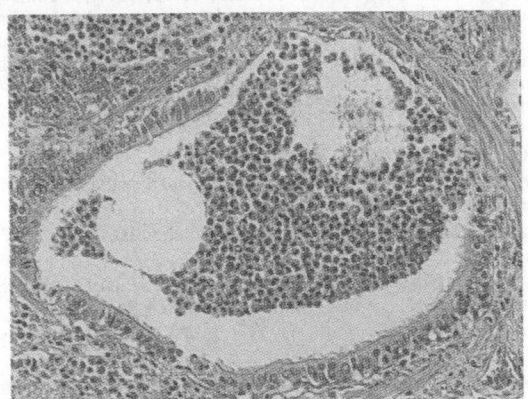

bronchiolitis: thick mass of granulocytes in a bronchiolar lumen

bron·cho·con·stric·tor (brong-kō-kon-strik′ter, -tōr). **1.** Causing a reduction in caliber of a bronchus or bronchial tube. **2.** An agent that possesses this action (e.g., histamine, acetylcholine).

bron·cho·di·la·ta·tion (brong′kō-dil-ă-tā′shŭn). SYN bronchodilation.

bron·cho·di·la·tion (brong′kō-dī-lā′shŭn). **1.** Increase in caliber of the bronchi and bronchioles in response to pharmacologically active substances or autonomic nervous activity. **2.** Rarely used term for bronchiectasis. SYN bronchodilatation.

bron·cho·di·la·tor (brong-kō-dī-lā′ter, -tōr). **1.** Causing an increase in caliber of a bronchus or bronchial tube. **2.** An agent that possesses this power (e.g., epinephrine, albuterol).

bron·cho·e·de·ma (brong′kō-ĕ-dē′mă). Swelling of the mucosa of the bronchi.

bron·cho·e·soph·a·gol·o·gy (brong′kō-ē-sof-ă-gol′ō-jē). The specialty concerned with the diagnosis and treatment of diseases of the tracheobronchial tree and esophagus by endoscopy and other means. [broncho- + G. *oisophagos*, esophagus, + *logos*, study]

bron·cho·e·soph·a·gos·co·py (brong′kō-ē-sof-ă-gos′kŏ-pē). Examination of the tracheobronchial tree and esophagus through appropriate endoscopes.

bron·cho·fi·ber·scope (brong-kō-fī′ber-skōp). SYN bronchoscope.

bron·cho·gen·ic (brong-kō-jen′ik). Of bronchial origin; emanating from the bronchi. SYN bronchiogenic.

bron·cho·gram (brong′kō-gram). A radiograph obtained by bronchography; radiographic visualization of a bronchus. [broncho- + G. *gramma*, a writing]

   air b., radiographic appearance of an air-filled bronchus surrounded by fluid-filled airspaces.

bron·chog·ra·phy (brong-kog′ră-fē). Radiographic examination of the tracheobronchial tree following introduction of a radiopaque material, usually an iodinated compound in a viscous suspension; rarely performed at this time, having been superseded by high resolution computed tomography. [broncho- + G. *graphē*, a drawing]

   tantalum b., historically, b. using insufflated metallic tantalum powder.

bron·cho·lith (brong′kō-lith). A hard concretion in a bronchus, usually resulting from the erosion of a tuberculous or other granulomatous lymph node through the bronchial wall into the lumen. SYN bronchial calculus. [broncho- + G. *lithos*, stone]

bron·cho·li·thi·a·sis (brong′kō-li-thī′ă-sis). Bronchial inflammation or obstruction caused by broncholiths.

bron·cho·ma·la·cia (brong′kō-mă-lā′shē-ă). Degeneration of elastic and connective tissue of bronchi and trachea. [broncho- + G. *malakia*, a softening]

bron·cho·mo·tor (brong-kō-mō′ter). **1.** Relating to a change in caliber, dilation, or contraction of a bronchus or bronchiole. **2.** An agent possessing this action. [broncho- + L. *motor*, mover]

bron·cho·my·co·sis (brong′kō-mī-kō′sis). Any fungus disease of the bronchial tubes or bronchi. [broncho- + G. *mykēs*, fungus]

bron·choph·o·ny (brong-kof′ō-nē). Increased intensity and clarity of voice sounds heard over a bronchus surrounded by consolidated lung tissue. SEE ALSO tracheophony. SYN bronchial voice. [broncho- + G. *phōnē*, voice]

   whispered b., SYN whispered *pectoriloquy*.

bron·cho·plas·ty (brong′kō-plas-tē). Surgical alteration of the configuration of a bronchus. [broncho- + G. *plastos*, formed]

bron·cho·pneu·mo·nia (brong′ko-nu-mo′nĭ-ă). Acute inflammation of the walls of the smaller bronchial tubes, with varying amounts of pulmonary consolidation due to spread of the inflammation into peribronchiolar alveoli and the alveolar ducts; may become confluent or may be hemorrhagic. SYN bronchial pneumonia.

   postoperative b., patchy pneumonia developing in a postoperative patient, usually following surgery to upper abdomen, with restricted diaphragmatic movement due to pain on inspiration, resulting in hypoventilation of the dependent portions of the lungs, with corresponding inadequate movement of secretions, allowing development of infection; likelihood minimized by early postoperative mobilization, deep breathing exercises.

   tuberculous b., an acute form of pulmonary tuberculosis characterized by widespread patchy consolidations.

bron·cho·pul·mo·nary (brong-kō-pul′mō-nār-ē). Relating to the bronchi and the lungs.

bron·chor·rha·phy (brong-kōr′ă-fē). Suture of a wound of the bronchus. [broncho- + G. *rhaphē*, a seam]

bron·chor·rhea (brong-kōr-rē′ă). Excessive secretions from the bronchial mucosa, resulting in copious production of thin sputum and most often due to diffuse bronchoalveolar *carcinoma* or pulmonary alveolar *proteinosis*. [broncho- + G. *rhoia*, a flow]

🔲 **bron·cho·scope** (brong′kō-skōp). An endoscope for inspecting the interior of the tracheobronchial tree, either for diagnostic purposes (including biopsy) or for the removal of foreign bodies. There are two types: flexible and rigid. SYN bronchofiberscope. [broncho- + G. *skopeō*, to view]

🔲 **bron·chos·co·py** (brong-kos′kŏ-pē). Inspection of the interior of the tracheobronchial tree through a bronchoscope.

br

bron·cho·spasm (brong′kō-spazm). Contraction of smooth muscle in the walls of the bronchi and bronchioles, causing narrowing of the lumen. Cf. bronchoconstriction.

bron·cho·spas·mo·lyt·ic (brong′kō-spazm-mō-li-tik). Relieving a bronchospasm.

bron·cho·spi·ro·che·to·sis (brong′kō-spī′rō-kē-tō′sis). SYN hemorrhagic *bronchitis*.

bron·cho·spi·rog·ra·phy (brong′kō-spī-rog′ră-fē). Use of a single-lumen endobronchial tube for measurement of ventilatory function of one lung. [broncho- + L. *spiro*, to breathe, + G. *graphō*, to write]

bron·cho·spi·rom·e·ter (brong′kō-spī-rom′ĕ-ter). A rare device for measurement of rates and volumes of air flow into each lung separately, using a double-lumen endobronchial tube. [broncho- + L. *spiro*, to breathe, + G. *metron*, measure]

bron·cho·spi·rom·e·try (brong′kō-spī-rom′ĕ-trē). Use of a bronchospirometer to measure ventilatory function of each lung separately.

bron·cho·stax·is (brong′kō-stak′sis). SYN hemoptysis. [broncho- + G. *staxis*, a dripping]

bron·cho·ste·no·sis (brong-kō-sten-ō′sis). Chronic narrowing of a bronchus.

bron·chos·to·my (brong-kos′tō-mē). Surgical formation of a new opening into a bronchus. [broncho- + G. *stoma*, mouth]

bron·chot·o·my (brong-kot′ō-mē). Incision of a bronchus.

bron·cho·tra·che·al (brong-kō-trā′kē-ăl). Relating to the trachea and bronchi.

bron·cho·ve·sic·u·lar (brong′kō-vĕ-sik′ū-lăr). Relating to the bronchi and alveoli in the lungs, especially as regards lung sound heard by auscultation. SYN bronchoalveolar.

▣ **bron·chus**, pl. **bron·chi** (brong′kŭs, brong′kī) [TA]. One of two subdivisions of the trachea serving to convey air to and from the lungs. The trachea divides into right and left main bronchi, which in turn form lobar, segmental, and intrasegmental bronchi. In structure, the intrapulmonary bronchi have a lining of pseudostratified ciliated columnar epithelium and a lamina propria with abundant longitudinal networks of elastic fibers; there are spirally arranged bundles of smooth muscle, abundant mucoserous glands, and, in the outer part of the wall, irregular plates of hyaline cartilage. SYN bronchium. [Mod. L., fr. G. *bronchos*, windpipe]

eparterial b., right superior lobar b. that passes above the right pulmonary artery.

hyparterial bronchi, those bronchi that pass below the pulmonary arteries, i.e., right middle and inferior lobar bronchi and left superior and inferior lobar bronchi.

intermediate b., the portion of the right main b. between the upper lobar b. and the origin of the middle and lower lobar bronchi. SYN b. intermedius.

b. intermedius, SYN intermediate b.

intrasegmental bronchi [TA], branches of segmental bronchi to the bronchopulmonary segments of the lungs. SYN bronchi intrasegmentales [TA], branches of segmental bronchi, rami bronchiales segmentorum.

bronchi intrasegmentales [TA], SYN intrasegmental bronchi.

left main b. [TA], it arises at the bifurcation of the trachea, passes in front of the esophagus and enters the hilum of the left lung where it divides into a superior lobe b. and an inferior lobe b. It is longer, of narrower caliber, and more nearly horizontal than the right main b., hence, aspirated objects enter it less frequently. SYN b. principalis sinister [TA].

lobar bronchi [TA], the divisions of the main bronchi that supply the lobes of the lungs; superior lobar b. (b. lobaris superior [TA]); middle lobar b. (b. lobaris medius [TA]); and inferior lobar b. (b. lobaris inferior [TA]) are the three lobar bronchi on the right; superior lobar b. (b. lobaris superior [TA]) and inferior lobar b. (b. lobaris inferior [TA]) are the two on the left. The lobar bronchi divide into segmental bronchi. SYN bronchi lobares [TA].

bronchi loba′res [TA], SYN lobar bronchi.

mucoid impaction of b., plugging of the lumen of bronchi due to thickened mucus, interfering with ventilation of corresponding lung segments and leading to characteristic clustered linear and grapelike radiologic densities and occasionally atelectasis and pneumonia; characteristically seen in cystic fibrosis but it can occur in a variety of disease states.

primary b., the main b. arising at the tracheal bifurcation and extending into the developing lung of the embryo.

b. principa′lis dex′ter [TA], SYN right main b.

b. principa′lis sinis′ter [TA], SYN left main b.

right main b. [TA], it arises at the bifurcation of the trachea and enters the hilum of the right lung, giving off the superior lobe b. and continuing downward to give off the middle and inferior lobe bronchi. It is shorter, of greater caliber, and more nearly vertical than the left main b., thus, aspirated objects more frequently lodge on the right side. SYN b. principalis dexter [TA].

▣ **segmental b.** [TA], one of the divisions of the lobar b. that supplies a bronchopulmonary segment. In the right lung there are commonly ten: *in the superior lobe*, the apical (B_1) segmental b., b. segmentalis apicalis (BI) [TA]; posterior (B_2) segmental b., b. segmentalis posterior (BII) [TA]; and anterior (B_3) segmental b., b. segmentalis anterior (BIII) [TA]; *in the middle lobe*, lateral (B_4) segmental b., b. segmentalis lateralis (BIV) [TA]; and medial (B_5) segmental b., b. segmentalis medialis (BV) [TA]; *in the inferior lobe*, superior (B_6) segmental b., b. segmentalis superior (BVI) [TA], medial basal (B_7) segmental b., b. segmentalis basalis medialis (BVII) [TA]; anterior basal (B_8) segmental b., b. segmentalis basalis anterior (BVIII) [TA]; lateral basal (B_9) segmental b., b. segmentalis basalis lateralis (BIX) [TA]; and posterior basal (B_{10}) segmental b., b. segmentalis basalis posterior (BX) [TA]. In the left lung there are commonly nine: *in the superior lobe*, the apicoposterior (B_{1+2}) segmental b., b. segmentalis apicoposterior (BI+II) [TA]; anterior (B_3) segmental b., b. segmentalis anterior (BIII) [TA]; superior lingular (B_4) segmental b., b. lingularis superior (BIV) [TA]; and inferior lingular (B_5) segmental b., b. lingularis inferior (BV) [NA]; *in the inferior lobe*, superior (B_6) segmental b., b. segmentalis superior (BVI) [TA]; medial basal (B_7) segmental b., b. segmentalis basalis medialis (cardiacus) (BVII) [TA], anterior basal (B_8) segmental b., b. segmentalis basalis anterior (BVIII) [TA]; lateral basal (B_9) segmental b., b. segmentalis basalis lateralis (BIX) [TA]; and posterior basal (B_{10}) segmental b., b. segmentalis basalis posterior (BX) [TA]. SYN b. segmentalis [TA].

b. segmenta′lis [TA], SYN segmental b.

stem b., the main b. from which the branches of the bronchial tree arise.

Brønsted, Johannes N., Danish physical chemist, 1879–1947. SEE B. *acid, base, theory.*

bron·to·pho·bia (bront-ō-fō′bē-ă). Morbid fear of thunder. SYN tonitrophobia. [G. *brontē*, thunder, + *phobos*, fear]

brood (brood). **1.** SYN litter (2). **2.** To ponder anxiously; to meditate morbidly.

Brooke, Henry A.G., English dermatologist, 1854–1919. SEE B. *tumor.*

Brooke, Bryan N., British surgeon, *1915. SEE B. *ileostomy.*

bro·tiz·o·lam (brō′tiz-ō-lam). A triazolo-benzodiazepine derivative with a sulfur and bromine atom in the molecule. Used as a sedative and hypnotic.

Broviac, J.W., 20th century U.S. surgeon. SEE B. *catheter.*

brow. 1. The eyebrow. SEE eyebrow. **2.** SYN forehead. [A.S. *brū*]

Brown, Harold W., U.S. ophthalmologist, *1898. SEE B. *syndrome.*

Brown, James, U.S. plastic surgeon, 1899–1971. SEE B.-Adson *forceps.*

Brown, James H., U.S. microbiologist, *1884. SEE B.-Brenn *stain.*

Brown, Robert, English botanist, 1773–1858. SEE brownian *motion;* brownian *movement;* brownian-Zsigmondy *movement.*

Browne, Sir Denis John, British surgeon, *1892. SEE Denis B. *pouch;* Denis B. *splint.*

brown·i·an (brown′ē-ăn). Relating to or described by Robert Brown.

Browning, William, U.S. anatomist and neurologist, 1855–1941. SEE B. *vein.*

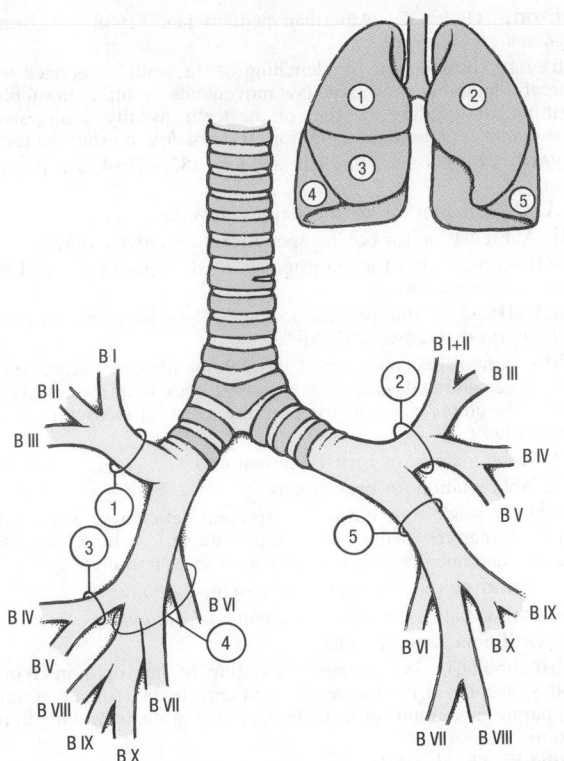

segmental bronchi: right lung: (B I) apical, (B II) posterior, (B III) anterior, (B IV) lateral, (B V) medial, (B VI) apical, (B VII) medial basal, (B VIII) anterior basal, (B IX) lateral basal, (B X) posterior basal; left lung: (BI + II) apicoposterior, (B III anterior), (B IV) superior lingular, (B V) inferior lingular, (B VI) apical, (B VII) medial basal, (B VIII) anterior basal, (B IX) lateral basal, (B X) posterior basal; lobes of lungs supplied: (1) right superior, (2) left superior, (3) right middle, (4) right inferior, (5) left inferior

---

Brown-Séquard, Charles E., French physiologist and neurologist, 1817–1894. SEE Brown-Séquard *paralysis;* Brown-Séquard *syndrome.*

Bruce, Robert A., U.S. cardiologist. SEE B. *protocol.*

Bruce, Sir David, British surgeon, 1855–1931. SEE *Brucella;* brucellosis.

Bru·cel·la (broo-sel′lă). A genus of encapsulated, nonmotile bacteria (family Brucellaceae) containing short, rod-shaped to coccoid, Gram-negative cells. These organisms do not produce gas from carbohydrates, are parasitic, invading all animal tissues and causing infection of the genital organs, the mammary gland, and the respiratory and intestinal tracts, and are pathogenic for humans and various species of domestic animals. The type species is *B. melitensis.*

B. abor′tus, a bacterial species that causes abortion in cows (bovine brucellosis), mares, and sheep, undulant fever in humans, and a wasting disease in chickens. SYN abortus bacillus.

B. ca′nis, a bacterial species causing epididymitis, brucellosis, and abortion in dogs; occasionally causes human disease.

B. meliten′sis, a bacterial species that causes brucellosis in humans, abortion in goats, and a wasting disease in chickens; it may infect cows and hogs and be excreted in their milk; it is the type species of the genus *B.*

B. su′is, a bacterial species causing abortion in swine, brucellosis in humans, and a wasting disease in chickens; may also infect horses, dogs, cows, monkeys, goats, and laboratory animals.

Bru·cel·la·ce·ae (broo-sel-ā′sē-ē). A family of bacteria (order Eubacteriales) containing small, coccoid to rod-shaped, Gram-negative cells which occur singly, in pairs, in short chains, or in groups. The cells may or may not show bipolar staining. Motile and nonmotile species occur; motile cells are peritrichous. V (phosphopyridine nucleotide) and/or X (hemin) factors are sometimes required for growth. Blood serum may be required or may enhance growth. Increased carbon dioxide tension may also favor growth, especially on primary isolation. These organisms are parasites and pathogens that affect warm-blooded animals, including humans, rarely cold-blooded animals; formerly called Parvobacteriaceae; type genus is *Brucella.*

bru·cel·ler·gin (broo-sel′er-jin). SEE brucellin.

bru·cel·lin (broo-sel′in). A preparation of antigenic material from several species of *Brucella;* used in the diagnosis of brucellosis as a skin test similar to that used for tuberculosis.

bru·cel·lo·sis (broo-sel-ō′sis). An infectious disease caused by the bacterium *Brucella,* characterized by fever, sweating, weakness, aches, and pains, and transmitted to humans by direct contact with diseased animals or through ingestion of infected meat, milk, or cheese, and particularly hazardous to veterinarians, farmers, and slaughterhouse workers; although some crossing over by species may occur, *Brucella melitensis, B. abortus, B. canis,* and *B. suis* characteristically affect goats, cattle, dogs, and swine, respectively. SYN febris undulans, Malta fever, Mediterranean fever (1), undulant fever, undulating fever.

bovine b., a disease in cattle caused by *Brucella abortus;* in pregnant cows, characterized by abortion late in pregnancy, followed by retained placenta and metritis; in bulls, orchitis and epididymitis may occur; the organism may localize in the udder and thus appear in milk from infected cows. SYN Bang disease.

Bruch, Carl W.L., German anatomist, 1819–1884. SEE B. *glands,* under *gland, membrane.*

bru·cine (broo-sēn, -in). An alkaloid from *Strychnos nux-vomica* and *S. ignatii* (family Loganiaceae), that produces paralysis of sensory nerves and peripheral motor nerves; the convulsive action which is characteristic of strychnine is almost entirely absent; formerly used as a local anodyne and tonic. [fr. *Brucea* sp., a shrub, after James Bruce, Scottish explorer, †1794]

Bruck, Alfred, German physician, *1865. SEE B. *disease.*

Brücke, Ernst W. von, Austrian physiologist, 1819–1892. SEE B. *muscle, tunic;* B.-Bartley *phenomenon.*

Brudzinski, Josef von, Polish physician, 1874–1917. SEE B. *sign.*

Bru·gi·a (broo′jē-ă). A genus of filarial worms transmitted by mosquitoes to humans, primates, felid carnivores, and a number of other mammals.

B. mala′yi, the Malayan filaria species, an important agent of human filariasis and elephantiasis in Southeast Asia and Indonesia, transmitted to humans by species of *Mansonia* and *Anopheles* mosquitoes; adult parasites cause lymphangitis and lymphadenitis, but there is less involvement of the genital region and lower extremities, and a relatively greater incidence of disease in the upper extremities than with *Wuchereria bancrofti* infection. Formerly called *Wuchereria malayi.*

bruise (brooz). An injury producing a hematoma or diffuse extravasation of blood without rupture of the skin. [M.E. *bruisen,* fr. O.Fr., fr. Germanic]

bruisse·ment (brwēs-mawhn′). A purring auscultatory sound. [Fr.]

bru·it (broo-ē′). A harsh or musical intermittent auscultatory sound, especially an abnormal one. [Fr.]

aneurysmal b., blowing murmur heard over an aneurysm.

carotid b., a systolic murmur heard in the neck but not at the aortic area; any b. produced by turbulent blood flow in a carotid artery.

b. de canon, the loud first heart sound heard intermittently in complete atrioventricular block and in interference-dissociation when the ventricles happen to contract shortly after the atria. SYN cannon sound.

b. de claquement (broo-ē′ dĕ klak-maw′), the sound of cardiac clicks. SEE click.

b. de cuir neuf (broo-ē′ dĕ kwēr nuf), the sound of new leather (also bruit de craquement); a creaking pericardial friction sound heard mainly in chronic pericarditis.

b. de diable, SYN venous *hum.* [Fr. humming-top]

b. de frolement (broo-ē′ dĕ frōl′maw), a rough, rustling sound made by a pleural or pericardial friction rub. [Fr. rustling]

b. de galop, SYN gallop. [Fr.]

b. de la roue de moulin, gurgling or splashing mill-wheel sounds heard when both fluid and air are present in the pericardial sac. [Fr. mill]

b. de lime, introduced by R. Laënnec to describe a rough rasping murmur. [Fr. file]

b. de rappel, applied by J. B. Bouillaud to describe the cadence of a split-second heart sound, or of the second sound followed by an opening snap or early third heart sound. SYN double-shock sound. [Fr. drum-beat]

b. de Roger, SYN Roger *murmur.*

b. de scie (broo-ē′ dĕ sē), a harsh heart murmur heard in systole and diastole that produces a sound resembling that of a saw. [Fr. saw]

b. de scie ou de rape, introduced by R. Laënnec to describe harsh, rasping murmurs. [Fr. saw, rasp]

b. de soufflet, introduced by R. Laënnec to describe a blowing murmur. [Fr. bellows]

b. de tabourka, a loud tambourlike or bell-like second heart sound heard at the aortic area in syphilitic aortitis. [Fr. tambour]

b. de tambour (broo-ē′ dĕ tăm-bur′), reverberating, musical tone heard as the second heart sound over the aortic area, associated with past syphilitic aortic valvular disease. SYN tambour sound. [Fr. sound of drum]

b. de triolet, introduced by L. Gallavardin to describe the triple cadence produced by a systolic click added to the first and second heart sounds. [Fr. a little trio]

Roger b. (broo-ē′), SYN Roger *murmur.*

systolic b., any abnormal sound or any murmur heard during systole.

thyroid b., vascular murmur heard over hyperactive thyroid gland, due to increased blood flow.

Traube b., SYN gallop.

Brunn, Fritz, 20th century Czechoslovakian physician. SEE B. *reaction.*

Brunn, Albert von, German anatomist, 1849–1895. SEE B. *membrane, nest.*

Brunner, Johann C., Swiss anatomist, 1653–1727. SEE B. *glands,* under *gland.*

Bruns, Ludwig von, German neurologist, 1858–1916. SEE B. *ataxia, nystagmus.*

Brunschwig, Alexander, U.S. surgeon, 1901–1969. SEE B. *operation.*

brush (brŭsh). An instrument made of some flexible material, such as bristles, attached to a handle or to the tip of a catheter. [A.S. *byrst,* bristle]

Ayre b., a device, consisting of a long flexible tube with a b. at the distal end, for collecting gastric mucosal cells in cancer detection studies; after positioning in the stomach the b. is rotated and "sweeps" cells from the mucosa.

bronchoscopic b., a small b. for insertion through a bronchoscope to wipe off cells for microscopic identification in suspected bronchial carcinoma and in obtaining microbiologic material for staining and culture.

denture b., a b. used to clean removable dentures.

Haidinger b.'s, the perception of two dark yellowish b. or sheaves radiating about 5 degrees from the point of fixation when an evenly illuminated surface, such as the blue sky, is viewed through a polarizing lens.

Kruse b., a bunch of fine platinum wires attached to a holder; used in bacteriological work to spread material over the surface of a culture medium.

polishing b., a b. usually mounted in a rotating instrument, used to polish teeth or artificial replacements.

Brushfield, Thomas, British physician, 1858–1937. SEE B. *spots,* under *spot;* B.-Wyatt *disease.*

brush·ite (brŭsh′īt). A naturally occurring acid calcium phosphate occasionally found in dental calculus and renal calculi.

Bruton, Ogden C., American pediatrician, *1908. SEE Bruton *agammaglobulinemia.*

brux·ism (brŭk′sizm). A clenching of the teeth, associated with forceful lateral or protrusive jaw movements, resulting in rubbing, gritting, or grinding together of the teeth, usually during sleep; sometimes a pathologic condition. [G. *bruchō,* to grind the teeth]

Bryant, Sir Thomas, English surgeon, 1828–1914. SEE B. *traction.*

BSA Abbreviation for bovine serum *albumin.*

BSE Abbreviation for bovine spongiform *encephalopathy.*

BSER Abbreviation for brainstem evoked *response.* SEE auditory brainstem *response.*

Bt₂cAMP $N^6,O^{2'}$-dibutyryladenosine 3′:5′-cyclic monophosphate, a dibutyryl derivative of cAMP.

BTPS Symbol indicating that a gas volume has been expressed as if it were saturated with water vapor at body temperature (37°C) and at the ambient barometric pressure; used for measurements of lung volumes.

BTU Abbreviation for British thermal *unit.*

BTX Abbreviation for brevetoxins.

bu·aki (boo-ak′ē). A nutritional (protein deficiency) disease observed in natives of the Congo and characterized by edema, skin lesions, and anemia; possibly related to kwashiorkor.

bu·ba mad·re (boo′bă mah′dre). SYN mother *yaw.*

bu·bas (boo′bahs). SYN mucocutaneous *leishmaniasis.*

b. brazilia′na, SYN espundia.

bu·bo (boo′bō). Inflammatory swelling of one or more lymph nodes, usually in the groin; the confluent mass of nodes usually suppurates and drains pus. [G. *boubōn,* the groin, a swelling in the groin]

bullet b., a hard, painless swelling of a gland in the groin, accompanying a chancre.

chancroidal b., an ulcerating b., due to *Haemophilus ducreyi.* SYN virulent b.

indolent b., an indurated enlargement of an inguinal node.

malignant b., the enlarged lymph node associated with bubonic plague.

parotid b., a swelling of the parotid gland due to secondary septic infection.

primary b., a b. occurring as the first sign of venereal infection.

tropical b., SYN venereal *lymphogranuloma.*

venereal b., an enlarged gland in the groin associated with any sexually transmitted disease, especially chancroid.

virulent b., SYN chancroidal b.

bu·bon·al·gia (boo′bon-al′jē-ă). Rarely used term for pain in the groin. [G. *boubōn,* groin, + *algos,* pain]

bu·bon·ic (boo-bon′ik). Relating in any way to a bubo.

bu·bon·u·lus (boo-bon′ū-lŭs). 1. An abscess occurring along the course of a lymphatic vessel. 2. One of a number of hard nodules, often breaking down into ulcers, which form along the course of acutely inflamed lymphatic vessels of the dorsum of the penis. [Mod. L. dim. of *bubo*]

bu·car·dia (bū-kar′dē-ă). SYN ox *heart.* [G. *bous,* ox, + *kardia,* heart]

buc·ca, gen. and pl. **buc·cae** (bŭk′ă, bŭk′sē). SYN cheek. [L.]

buc·cal (bŭk′ăl). Pertaining to, adjacent to, or in the direction of the cheek.

buc·ci·na·tor. SEE buccinator (*muscle*).

bucco-. Cheek. [L. *bucca*]

buc·co·ax·i·al (bŭk-ō-ak′sē-ăl). Referring to the line angle formed by the buccal and axial walls of a cavity.

buc·co·ax·i·o·cer·vi·cal (bŭk′ō-ak′sē-ō-ser′vi-kăl). Referring to the point angle formed by the junction of the buccal, axial, and cervical (gingival) walls of a cavity.

buc·co·ax·i·o·gin·gi·val (bŭk′ō-ak′sē-ō-jin′ji-văl). Referring to the point angle formed by the junction of a buccal, axial, and gingival (cervical) wall.

buc·co·cer·vi·cal (bŭk-ō-ser′vi-kăl). 1. Relating to the cheek and the neck. 2. In dental anatomy, referring to that portion of the buccal surface of a bicuspid or molar tooth adjacent to its cemento-enamel junction.

buc·co·clu·sal (bŭk-ō-kloo′săl).   Incorrect term referring to the line angle formed by the junction of a buccal and pulpal wall. SEE buccopulpal.

buc·co·dis·tal (buk-ō-dis′tăl).   Referring to the line angle formed by the junction of a buccal and distal wall of a cavity.

buc·co·gin·gi·val (bŭk-ō-jin′ji-văl).   Relating to the cheek and the gum.

buc·co·la·bi·al (bŭk-ō-lā′bē-ăl).   **1.** Relating to both cheek and lip. **2.** In dentistry, referring to that aspect of the dental arch or those surfaces of the teeth in contact with the mucosa of lip and cheek.

buc·co·lin·gual (bŭk-ō-ling′wăl).   **1.** Pertaining to the cheek and the tongue. **2.** In dentistry, referring to that aspect of the dental arch or those surfaces of the teeth in contact with the mucosa of the lip or cheek and the tongue.

buc·co·me·si·al (bŭk-ō-mē′zē-ăl).   Referring to the line angle formed by the junction of a buccal and mesial wall of a cavity.

buc·co·pha·ryn·ge·al (bŭk′ō-fă-rin′jē-ăl).   Relating to both cheek or mouth and pharynx.

buc·co·pul·pal (buk-ō-pŭl′păl).   Referring to the line angle formed by the junction of a buccal and pulpal wall of a cavity.

buc·co·ver·sion (bŭk′ō-ver-zhŭn).   Malposition of a posterior tooth from the normal line of occlusion toward the cheek.

buc·cu·la (bŭk′ū-lă).   A fatty puffing under the chin. SYN double chin. [L. dim. of *bucca,* cheek]

Büchner,   Hans E.A., German bacteriologist, 1850–1902. SEE B. *extract.*

Büchner,   Eduard, German chemist and Nobel laureate, 1860–1917. SEE B. *extract, funnel.*

bu·chu (boo′koo).   The dried leaves of *Barosma betulina, B. crenulata,* or *B. serratifolia* (family Rutaceae), a shrub growing in South Africa; used as a carminative, diuretic, and urinary antiseptic. SYN Hottentot tea. [native]

Buchwald,   Hermann Edmund, German physician, *1903. SEE B. *atrophy.*

Buck,   Gordon, U.S. surgeon, 1807–1877. SEE B. *extension, fascia, traction.*

buck·bean.   The leaves of *Menyanthes trifoliata* (family Gentianaceae); credited with emmenagogue, antiscorbutic, and simple bitter properties. SYN bogbean, menyanthes.

Bücklers,   Max, German ophthalmologist, 1895–1969. SEE Reis-Bücklers corneal *dystrophy.*

buck·thorn (bŭk′thōrn).   SYN Rhamnus.

Bucky,   Gustav, U.S. radiologist, 1880–1963. SEE B. *diaphragm.*

bu·cli·zine hy·dro·chlo·ride (bu′kli-zēn).   A mild sedative used for motion sickness, vertigo, and anxiety accompanying psychosomatic disorders.

buc·lo·sa·mide (buk-lō′să-mīd).   A topical antifungal agent.

bu·cry·late (bū′kri-lāt).   A tissue adhesive used in surgery.

Bucy,   Paul C., U.S. neurosurgeon, 1904–1992. SEE Klüver-B. *syndrome.*

bud (bŭd).   **1.** An outgrowth that resembles the b. of a plant, usually pluripotential, and capable of differentiating and growing into a definitive structure. **2.** To give rise to such an outgrowth. SEE ALSO gemmation. **3.** A small outgrowth from a parent cell; a form of asexual reproduction.

bronchial b., one of the outgrowths from the primordial endodermal laryngotracheal tube giving rise to the primary bronchi. SEE laryngotracheal *diverticulum.*

end b., SYN tail b.

gustatory b., SYN taste b.

limb b., an ectodermally covered mesenchymal outgrowth on the embryonic flank giving rise to either the forelimb or hindlimb.

liver b., the primordial cellular diverticulum of the embryonic foregut endoderm that gives rise to the parenchyma of the liver.

lung b., SYN tracheobronchial *diverticulum.*

median tongue b., SYN *tuberculum* impar.

metanephric b., the primordial cellular outgrowth from the mes-

onephric duct that gives rise to the epithelial lining of the ureter, of the pelvis, and calyces of the kidney, and of the straight collecting tubules. SYN ureteric b.

periosteal b., a vascular connective tissue bud from the perichondrium that invades the ossification center of the cartilaginous model of a developing long bone.

syncytial b., SYN syncytial *knot.*

tail b., the rapidly proliferating mass of cells at the caudal extremity of the embryo; remnant of the primitive node. SYN end b.

taste b., one of a number of flask-shaped cell nests located in the epithelium of vallate, fungiform, and foliate papillae of the tongue and also in the soft palate, epiglottis, and posterior wall of the pharynx; it consists of sustentacular, gustatory, and basal cells between which the intragemmal sensory nerve fibers terminate. SYN caliculus gustatorius, gustatory b., Schwalbe corpuscle, taste bulb, taste corpuscle.

tooth b., the primordial structures from which a tooth is formed; the enamel organ, the dental papilla, and the dental sac enclosing them.

ureteric b., SYN metanephric b.

vascular b., an endothelial sprout arising from a blood vessel.

Budd,   George, English physician, 1808–1882. SEE B. *syndrome;* B.-Chiari *syndrome.*

Budde,   E., Danish sanitary engineer, *1871. SEE B. *process.*

bud·ding (bŭd′ing).   SYN gemmation.

Budge,   Julius L., German physiologist, 1811–1888. SEE B. *center.*

Budin,   Pierre C., French gynecologist, 1846–1907. SEE B. obstetrical *joint.*

Buerger,   Leo, Austrian-U.S. physician, 1879–1943. SEE Winiwarter-B. *disease;* B. *disease.*

△**bufa-, bufo-.**   Combining forms denoting origin from toads; used in the systematic and trivial names of toxic substances (genins) isolated from plants and animals containing the bufanolide structure; prefixes denoting species origin are often attached. [L. *bufo,* toad]

bu·fa·di·en·o·lide (boo-fă-dī-en′ō-līd).   SEE bufanolide.

bu·fa·gen·ins (boo′fă-jen-inz).   SYN bufagins.

bu·fa·gins (boo′fă-jinz).   A group of steroids (bufanolides) in the venom of a family of toads (Bufonidae) having a digitalislike action upon the heart; cardiac glycosides having a six-membered lactone. SEE ALSO bufotoxins. SYN bufagenins, bufogenins.

bu·fan·o·lide (boo-fan′ō-līd).   The fundamental steroid lactone of several vegetable (e.g., squill) and animal (e.g., toad) venoms or toxins; also found in the form of glycosides in plants (e.g., digitalis). The steroid is essentially a 5β-androstane, with a 14β H. The lactone at C-17 is structurally related to the –CH(CH₃)-CH₂CH₂CH₃ radical attached to C-17 in the cholanes, and is in the same configuration as that of cholesterol (i.e., 20*R*); in some species, b. is formed from cholesterol. Various b. derivatives having unsaturation in the lactone ring (20, 22) or elsewhere (4) are known as **bufenolides** (one double bond), **bufadienolides** (two double bonds), **bufatrienolides** (three double bonds), etc; they have varying numbers of hydroxyl groups at positions 3, 5, 14, and 16, and these may be further substituted. For structure, see steroids.

bu·fa·tri·en·o·lide (boo-fă-trī-en′ō-līd).   SEE bufanolide.

bu·fen·o·lide (boo-fen′ō-līd).   SEE bufanolide.

buff·er (bŭf′er).   **1.** A mixture of an acid and its conjugate base (salt), such as H_2CO_3/HCO_3^-; $H_2PO_4^-/HPO_4^{2-}$, that, when present in a solution, reduces any changes in pH that would otherwise occur in the solution when acid or alkali is added to it; thus, the pH of the blood and body fluids is maintained relatively constant (pH 7.45) although acid metabolites are continually being formed in the tissues and CO_2 is lost in the lungs. SEE ALSO conjugate acid-base *pair.* **2.** To add a b. to a solution and thus give it the property of resisting a change in pH when it receives a limited amount of acid or alkali.

dipolar b., SYN zwitterionic b.

zwitterionic b., b. whose structure can include opposite charges. SYN dipolar b.

△**bufo-.**   SEE bufa-.

bu·fo·gen·ins (boo-fō-jen-inz). SYN bufagins.

Bu·fon·i·dae (boo-fon′ĭ-dē). A family of toads whose dermal glands secrete several kinds of pharmacologically active substances having a cardiac action similar to that of digitalis. [L. *bufo,* toad]

bu·for·min (boo-fōr′min). An oral hypoglycemic agent similar to metformin.

bu·fo·ten·ine (boo-fō-ten′ēn). A psychotomimetic agent isolated from the venom of certain toads (family Bufonidae) and also present in several plants and one of the active principles of cohoba; raises the blood pressure by a vasoconstrictor action and produces psychic effects including hallucinations. SYN mappine.

bu·fo·tox·ins (boo-fō-toks′inz). **1.** A group of steroid lactones (conjugates of bufagins and suberylarginine at C-3) of digitalis present in the venoms of toads (family Bufonidae); their effects are similar to but weaker than those of the bufagins. **2.** Specifically, the main toxin of the European toad (*Bufo vulgaris*).

bug. An insect belonging to the suborder Heteroptera. For organisms so called, see the specific term.

assassin b., an insect of the family Reduviidae (order Hemiptera) that inflicts irritating, painful bites in animals and humans; related to the cone-nosed bugs (triatomines), a vector of American trypanosomiasis. [Fr., fr. It. *assassino,* fr. Ar. *hashshāshin,* those addicted to hashish]

bug·gery (bŭg′ger-ē). SYN sodomy. [O.F. *bougre,* heretic, fr. Med. L. *Bulgaris,* a Bulgar (hence a heretic)]

bulb (bŭlb) [TA]. **1.** Any globular or fusiform structure. SYN bulbus [TA]. **2.** A short, vertical underground stem of plants, such as onion and garlic. [L. *bulbus,* a bulbous root]

aortic b. [TA], the dilated first part of the aorta containing the aortic semilunar valves and the aortic sinuses. SYN arterial b., bulbus aortae.

arterial b., SYN aortic b.

Braasch b., SYN Braasch *catheter.*

carotid b., SYN carotid *sinus.*

b. of corpus spongiosum, SYN b. of penis.

dental b., the papilla, derived from mesoderm, that forms the part of the primordium of a tooth that is situated within the cup-shaped enamel organ.

duodenal b., SYN duodenal *cap.*

end b., one of the oval or rounded bodies in which the sensory nerve fibers terminate in mucous membrane.

b. of eye, SYN eyeball.

hair b., SYN b. of hair.

b. of hair, hair bulb, the lower expanded extremity of the hair follicle that fits like a cap over the papilla pili. SYN bulbus pili, hair b.

jugular b., SYN b. of jugular vein.

b. of jugular vein [TA], one of two dilated parts of the internal jugular vein: (1) the superior bulb (Heister diverticulum) is a dilation at the beginning of the internal jugular vein in the jugular fossa of the temporal bone (bulbus superior venae jugularis [TA]); (2) the inferior bulb is a dilated portion of the vein just before it reaches the brachiocephalic vein (bulbus inferior venae jugularis [TA]). SYN jugular b. SYN bulbus venae jugularis [TA].

Krause end b.'s, nerve terminals in skin, mouth, conjunctiva, and other parts, consisting of a laminated capsule of connective tissue enclosing the terminal, branched, convoluted ending of an afferent nerve fiber; generally believed to be sensitive to cold. SYN bulboid corpuscles, corpuscula bulboidea.

b. of occipital horn [TA], a rounded elevation in the dorsal part of the medial wall of the posterior horn of the lateral ventricle, produced by the major forceps. SYN bulbus cornus posterioris [TA].

olfactory b. [TA], the grayish expanded rostral extremity of the olfactory tract, lying on the cribriform plate of the ethmoid and receiving the olfactory filaments. SYN bulbus olfactorius [TA].

b. of penis [TA], the expanded proximal (posterior) part of the corpus spongiosum of the penis lying in the interval between the crura of the penis and containing the somewhat dilated and angu-

lated portion of the spongy urethra. SYN bulbus penis [TA], b. of corpus spongiosum, b. of urethra, bulbus urethrae.

b. of posterior horn of lateral ventricle of brain, SYN *bulbus cornus posterioris.*

Rouget b., a venous plexus on the surface of the ovary.

speech b., a speech prosthesis used to close a cleft or other opening in the hard or soft palate, or to replace absent tissue necessary for the production of good speech.

taste b., SYN taste *bud.*

b. of urethra, SYN b. of penis.

b. of vestibule [TA], a mass of erectile tissue on either side of the vagina united anterior to the urethra by the commissura bulborum. SYN bulbus vestibuli vaginae [TA].

bul·bar (bŭl′bar). **1.** Relating to a bulb. **2.** Relating to the rhombencephalon (hindbrain). **3.** Bulb-shaped; resembling a bulb.

bul·bi (bŭl′bī). Plural of bulbus.

bul·bi·tis (bŭl-bī′tis). Inflammation of the bulbous portion of the urethra.

△**bulbo-.** Bulb; bulbus [L. *bulbus*]

bul·bo·cap·nine (bul′bō-kap′nin). Drug derived from roots of *Corydalis cava* and *C. tuberosa* (family Fumariaceae) and *Dicentra canadensis* (family Papaveraceae); blocks the effects of dopamine on peripheral dopamine receptors.

bul·bo·cav·er·no·sus (bŭl′bō-kav-er-nō′sŭs). SEE *musculus* bulbocavernosus.

bul·boid (bŭl′boyd). Bulb-shaped. [bulbo- + G. *eidos,* resemblance]

bul·bo·nu·cle·ar (bŭl-bō-noo′klē-ar). Relating to the nuclei in the medulla oblongata.

bul·bo·pon·tine (bŭl-bō-pon′tēn). Relating to the rostral part of the rhombencephalon composed of the pons and overlying tegmentum.

bul·bo·sa·cral (bŭl′bō-sā′krăl). SEE bulbosacral *system.*

bul·bo·spi·nal (bŭl-bō-spī′năl). Relating to the medulla oblongata and spinal cord, particularly to nerve fibers interconnecting the two. SYN spinobulbar.

bul·bo·u·re·thral (bŭl′bō-ū-rē′thrăl). Relating to the bulbus penis and the urethra. SYN urethrobulbar.

bul·bus, gen. and pl. **bul·bi** (bŭl′bŭs, -bī) [TA]. SYN bulb (1). [L. a plant bulb]

b. aor′tae, SYN aortic *bulb.*

b. cor′dis, a transitory dilation in the embryonic heart where the arterial trunk joins the ventral roots of the aortic arches.

b. cor′nus posterior′is [TA], SYN *bulb* of occipital horn. SYN bulb of posterior horn of lateral ventricle of brain.

b. duodeni, ✭official alternate term for *ampulla* of duodenum.

b. oc′uli [TA], SYN eyeball.

b. olfacto′rius [TA], SYN olfactory *bulb.*

b. pe′nis [TA], SYN *bulb* of penis.

b. pi′li, SYN *bulb* of hair.

b. ure′thrae, SYN *bulb* of penis.

b. ve′nae jugula′ris [TA], SYN *bulb* of jugular vein.

b. vestib′uli vaginae [TA], SYN *bulb* of vestibule.

bu·le·sis (boo-lē′sis). The will; a willing. [G. *boulēsis,* a willing]

bu·lim·ia (boo-lim′ē-ă). SYN b. nervosa. [G. *bous,* ox, + *limos,* hunger]

b. nervo′sa, a chronic morbid disorder involving repeated and secretive episodic bouts of eating characterized by uncontrolled rapid ingestion of large quantities of food over a short period of time (binge eating), followed by self-induced vomiting, use of laxatives or diuretics, fasting, or vigorous exercise in order to prevent weight gain; often accompanied by feelings of guilt, depression, or self-disgust. SYN boulimia, bulimia, hyperorexia.

bu·lim·ic (boo-lim′ik). Relating to, or suffering from, bulimia nervosa.

Bu·li·nus (bū-lī′nŭs). A genus and subgenus of freshwater snails in the family Planorbidae (subfamily Bulininae), which includes many species that are intermediate hosts of the human blood fluke, *Schistosoma haematobium,* in Africa and the Middle East; divided into two subgenera, *Physopsis* and *Bulinus,* the former being responsible for transmission of *S. haematobium* south of the Sahara, the latter responsible for transmission of this bladder blood fluke in north Africa and the Middle East. Important species include *B. truncatus* and *B. forskalii*, hosts for human and animal schistosomes and several domestic animal amphistome flukes.

bulk·age (bŭlk′ij). Anything, such as agar, that increases the bulk of material in the intestine, thereby stimulating peristalsis.

bull. Abbreviation for L. *bulliens*, *bulliat*, or *bulliant*, boiling, let boil.

bul·la, gen. and pl. **bul·lae** (bul′ă, -ē). **1.** A fluid-filled blister greater than 100 cm in diameter appearing as a circumscribed area of separation of the epidermis from the subepidermal structure (**subepidermal b.**) or as a circumscribed area of separation of epidermal cells (**intraepidermal b.**) caused by the presence of serum, or occasionally by an injected substance. **2** [NA]. A bubblelike structure. [L. bubble]

ethmoidal b. [TA], a bulging of the inner wall of the ethmoidal labyrinth in the middle meatus of the nose, just below the middle nasal concha; it is regarded as a rudimentary concha. SYN b. ethmoidalis [TA].

b. ethmoida′lis [TA], SYN ethmoidal b.

pulmonary b., air-filled emphysematous space larger than one centimeter, usually located in the lung periphery; can reach large diameter and cause symptoms by compression of normal lung tissue. Cf. pulmonary *bleb*.

bul·lec·to·my (bul-ek′tō-mē). Resection of a bulla; helpful in treating some forms of bullous emphysema, in which giant bullae compress functioning lung tissue.

bul·lous (bul′ŭs). Relating to, of the nature of, or marked by, bullae.

bu·met·a·nide (bū-met′ă-nīd). A diuretic used in the treatment of edema associated with congestive heart failure, hepatic cirrhosis, and renal disease, resembles furosemide.

Bumke, Oswald C.E., German neurologist, 1877–1950. SEE B. *pupil*.

BUN Abbreviation for blood urea *nitrogen*.

bun·am·i·dine hy·dro·chlo·ride (bŭn-am′i-dēn). An anthelmintic.

bun·dle (bŭn′dl) [TA]. A structure composed of a group of fibers, muscular or nervous; a fasciculus. SYN fasciculus (3) [TA].

aberrant b.'s, a group, or groups, of fibers from the corticobulbar or corticonuclear tract, directed to each of the motor nuclei of cranial nerves.

anterior ground b., SYN *fasciculus* proprius anterior; SEE *fasciculi* proprii, under *fasciculus*.

Arnold b., SYN temporopontine *tract*.

atrioventricular b. [TA], the bundle of modified cardiac muscle fibers that begins at the atrioventricular node as the trunk of the atrioventricular bundle and passes through the right atrioventricular fibrous ring to the membranous part of the interventricular septum where the trunk divides into two branches, the right b. (crus dextrum) of the atrioventricular b. and the left b. (crus sinistrum) of the atrioventricular b.; the two crura ramify in the subendocardium of their respective ventricles. SYN fasciculus atrioventricularis [TA], atrioventricular band, Gaskell bridge, His band, His b., Keith b., Kent b. (1), Kent-His b., truncus fascicularis atrioventricularis, trunk of atrioventricular bundle, ventriculonector.

Bachmann b., division of the theoretical anterior internodal tract that continues into the left atrium providing a specialized path for interatrial conduction. The anatomic reality of this structure has been disputed.

comma b. of Schultze, SYN semilunar *fasciculus*.

Flechsig ground b.'s [TA], fasciculus proprius anterior [TA] and fasciculus proprius lateralis [TA]. SEE *fasciculi* proprii, under *fasciculus*.

Gantzer accessory b., SEE Gantzer *muscle*.

Gierke respiratory b., SYN solitary *tract*.

ground b.'s, SYN *fasciculi* proprii, under *fasciculus*.

Held b., SYN tectospinal *tract*.

Helie b., a vertically arched b. of fibers in the superficial layer of the myometrium.

Helweg b., SYN olivospinal *tract*.

Helwig b., SYN olivospinal *fibers*, under *fiber*.

His b., SYN atrioventricular b.

Hoche b., SEE semilunar *fasciculus*.

hooked b. of Russell, SYN uncinate *fasciculus* of cerebellum.

Keith b., SYN atrioventricular b.

Kent b., (1) SYN atrioventricular b; (2) a muscle fiber b. in the mammalian heart below the atrioventricular node; may also occur in humans.

Kent-His b., SYN atrioventricular b.

Killian b., SEE inferior constrictor (*muscle*) of pharynx.

Krause respiratory b., SYN solitary *tract*.

lateral ground b., *obsolescent*. SEE *fasciculi* proprii, under *fasciculus*.

lateral proprius b., SYN *fasciculi* proprii, under *fasciculus*.

left b. of atrioventricular bundle [TA], the left limb or branch of the atrioventricular bundle that separates from the atrioventricular bundle just below the membranous portion of the interventricular septum to descend the septal wall of the left ventricle and begins to ramify subendocardially. SYN crus sinistrum fasciculi atrioventricularis, left crus of atrioventricular bundle.

Lissauer b., SYN dorsolateral *fasciculus*.

Loewenthal b., SYN tectospinal *tract*.

longitudinal pontine b.'s, SYN longitudinal pontine *fasciculi*, under *fasciculus*.

medial forebrain b. [TA], a fiber system coursing longitudinally through the lateral zone (area) of the hypothalamus, connecting the latter reciprocally with the midbrain tegmentum and with various components of the limbic system; it also carries fibers from norepinephrine-containing and serotonin-containing cell groups in the brainstem to the hypothalamus and cerebral cortex, as well as dopamine-carrying fibers from the substantia nigra to the caudate nucleus and putamen. SYN fasciculus medialis telencephali [TA].

medial longitudinal b., SYN medial longitudinal *fasciculus*.

Monakow b., SYN rubrospinal *tract*.

muscle b., a group of muscle fibers ensheathed by connective tissue (perimysium).

neurovascular b. of Walsh, the anatomic structure composed of capsular arteries and veins to the prostate and cavernous nerves that provides the macroscopic landmark used during nerve-sparing radical pelvic surgery.

oblique b. of pons, SYN oblique pontine *fasciculus*.

olfactory b., a fiber system, described by E. Zuckerkandl as "Reichbündel," descending from the transparent septum in front of the anterior commissure toward the base of the forebrain; it contains precommissural fibers of the fornix, fibers from the septum to the hypothalamus and innominate substance, as well as fibers ascending to the septum and hippocampus from the hypothalamus and midbrain; it bears no special relation to the sense of smell.

olivocochlear b., SEE olivocochlear *tract*.

Pick b., a b. of nerve fibers recurving rostralward from the pyramidal tract in the medulla oblongata, and believed to consist of corticonuclear fibers.

posterior longitudinal b., SYN medial longitudinal *fasciculus*.

precommissural b., SEE olfactory b.

predorsal b., SYN tectospinal *tract*.

b. of Rasmussen, SYN olivocochlear *tract*.

Rathke b.'s, SYN *trabeculae* carneae (of right and left ventricles), under *trabecula*.

retroflex b. of Meynert, SYN retroflex *fasciculus*.

right b. of atrioventricular bundle [TA], the right leg or branch of the atrioventricular bundle that diverges from the left crus just below the membranous portion of the interventricular septum to descend the septal wall of the right ventricle and ramify beneath the endocardium. SYN crus dextrum fasciculi atrioventricularis [TA], right crus of atrioventricular bundle.

Schütz b., SYN dorsal longitudinal *fasciculus*.

bu

solitary b., SYN solitary *tract*.

tendon b., a group of tendon fibers surrounded by a sheath of irregular connective tissue (peritendineum).

Türck b., SYN anterior corticospinal *tract*.

uncinate b. of Russell, SYN uncinate *fasciculus* of cerebellum.

Vicq d'Azyr b., SYN mammillothalamic *fasciculus*.

bun·gar·o·tox·ins (bung'gă-rō-tok'sinz). Constituent proteins of the venom of the South Asian banded krait *Bungarus multicinctus*, a snake of the Elapidae family. Used as pharmacologic tools in studying neuromuscular function.

bung·pag·ga (bŭng-păg'ă). SYN tropical *pyomyositis*.

bun·ion (bŭn'yŭn). A localized swelling at either the medial or dorsal aspect of the first metatarsophalangeal joint, caused by an inflammatory bursa; a medial b. is usually associated with hallux valgus. [O.F. *buigne,* bump on the head]

bun·ion·ec·to·my (bŭn-yŭn-ek'tō-mē). Excision of a bunion.

Keller b., excision of the proximal portion of the proximal phalanx of the first toe.

Mayo b., excision of the head of the first metatarsal.

Bunnell, Sterling, U.S. surgeon, 1882–1957. SEE B. *suture;* Paul-B. *test*.

bu·no·dont (boo'nō-dont). Having molar teeth with rounded or low conical cusps, in contrast to lophodont. [G. *bounos,* mound, + *odous* (*odont-*), tooth]

bu·no·lol hy·dro·chlo·ride (bū'nō-lol). A β-adrenergic blocking agent for treatment of cardiac arrhythmias.

bu·no·loph·o·dont (boo-nō-lof'ō-dont). Having molar teeth with transverse ridges and rounded cusps on the occlusal surface. [G. bunos, mound, + *lophos,* ridge, + *odous,* tooth]

bu·no·se·le·no·dont (boo'nō-sĕ-len'ō-dont). Having molar teeth with crescentic ridges and rounded cusps on the occlusal surface. [*bunos,* + *selēnē,* moon, + *odous,* tooth]

Bu·nos·to·mum (bū-nō-stō'mŭm). A genus of hookworms (family Ancylostomatidae, subfamily Necatorinae) found in cattle and other herbivores; similar to *Necator*. [G. *bounos,* hill, mound, + *stoma,* mouth]

B. phlebot'omum, a species that occurs in cattle, sheep, and some wild ruminants in many parts of the world.

B. trigonoceph'alum, a cosmopolitan hookworm species in the small intestines of sheep and goats.

Bunsen, Robert W., German chemist and physicist, 1811–1899. SEE B. burner, solubility *coefficient;* B.-Roscoe *law*.

Bunsen burn·er. A gas lamp supplied with lateral openings admitting sufficient air so that the carbon is completely burned, thus giving a very hot but only slightly luminous flame. [RW Bunsen, 1811–1899]

Bun·ya·vir·i·dae (bŭn-yă-vir'i-dē). A family of arboviruses composed of more than 200 virus serotypes and containing at least five genera: Bunyavirus, Hantavirus, Phlebovirus, Nairovirus, and Tospovirus. Virions in all genera except Hantavirus replicate in arthropods. Virions are 80–120 nm in diameter, sensitive to lipid solvents and detergents, and enveloped with glycopolypeptide surface projections; the nucleocapsid is of helical symmetry containing 3 molecules of single-stranded RNA (MW $5–8 \times 10^6$). [*Bunyamwere,* Uganda]

Bun·ya·vi·rus (bun'ya-vī-rus). A virus in the genus of the family Bunyaviridae that includes at least 160 types, i.e., California encephalitis virus and LaCrosse encephalitis virus.

buph·thal·mia, buph·thal·mus, buph·thal·mos (boof-thal' mē-ă, -thal'mŭs, -thal'mos). An affection of infancy, marked by an increase of intraocular pressure with enlargement of the eyeball. SYN congenital glaucoma, hydrophthalmia, hydrophthalmos, hydrophthalmus. [G. *bous,* ox, + *ophthalmos,* eye]

bu·piv·a·caine (bū-piv'ă-kān). A potent, long-acting local anesthetic used in regional anesthesia, joint and trigger point injections.

bu·pre·nor·phine hy·dro·chlo·ride (boo-pre-nōr'fēn). A semisynthetic opioid analgesic used for relief of moderate to severe pain.

bu·pro·pi·on hy·dro·chlo·ride (boo-prō'pē-on). An antidepressant. Presently widely used as an aid to smoking cessation.

bur (bŭr). **1.** A rotary cutting instrument. **2.** In ophthalmology, a device used to remove rust rings embedded in the cornea. SYN burr.

cross-cut b., a b. with blades located at right angles to its long axis.

end-cutting b., a b. with blades only on its end.

finishing b., a b. with numerous fine cutting blades placed close together; used to contour metallic restorations.

fissure b., a cylindrical or tapered rotary cutting tool intended for extending or widening fissures in a tooth, as for general surface reduction of tooth substance.

inverted cone b., a rotary cutting instrument in the shape of a truncated cone with the smaller end attached to the shaft; generally used for entering carious pits or creating undercuts in cavity preparations.

round b., a dental b. with the cutting blades spherically arranged.

Burchard, H., 19th century German chemist. SEE B.-Liebermann *reaction;* Liebermann-B. *test*.

Burdach, Karl F., German anatomist and physiologist, 1776–1847. SEE B. *column, fasciculus, nucleus, tract*.

bur·den (ber'den). SEE body burden.

clinical b., a b. that differs from genetic b. mainly in the added component of morbidity; a trait that is neither a clinical or a genetic lethal may be grossly disabling.

genetic b., the genetic debt due to harmful mutation but as yet undischarged. (In a large population of fixed size every mutation with diminished genetic fitness will eventually become extinct and depending on the details of inheritance and phenotype must be paid for by a fixed number of genetic deaths per mutation, the genetic debt.)

global b. of disease, mathematical measure of loss of healthy life years due to disabling diseases in a country's population. SEE ALSO disability-adjusted life *years,* under *year*.

bu·ret, bu·rette (boo-ret'). A graduated glass tube with a tap as its lower end; used for measuring liquids in volumetric chemical analyses. [Fr.]

Bürger, Max T.F., German physician, *1885. SEE B.-Grütz *syndrome, disease*.

Burger tri·an·gle. See under triangle.

Burk, Dean, U.S. scientist, *1904. SEE Lineweaver-B. *equation, plot*.

Burk·hol·deria (burk-hol-der'ē-ă). A genus of motile, non–spore-forming Gram-negative rods, containing significant species of human pathogens formerly classified as members of the genus *Pseudomonas*.

B. cepacia, a bacterial species found in rotted onions and in clinical specimens; commonly found in respiratory secretions in patients with cystic fibrosis, it is frequently resistant to many antibiotics. SYN *Pseudomonas cepacia*.

B. mallei, a bacterial species infectious to horses and donkeys, causing glanders and farcy. SYN *Pseudomonas mallei*.

B. pseudomallei, a species found in cases of melioidosis in humans and other animals and in soil and water in tropical regions. SYN *Pseudomonas pseudomallei*.

Burkitt, Denis P., British physician in Uganda, 1911–1993. SEE B. *lymphoma*.

Burlew disk. See under disk.

Burlew wheel. See under wheel.

Burn, Joshua Harold, 1892–1981. SEE B. and Rand *theory*.

burn (bern). **1.** To cause a lesion by heat or a similar lesion by some other agent. **2.** A sensation of pain caused by excessive heat, or similar pain from any cause. **3.** A lesion caused by heat or any cauterizing agent, including friction, caustic agents, electricity, or electromagnetic energy; types of b.'s resulting from different agents are relatively specific and diagnostic. The division of b.'s into three degrees (first degree, second degree, and third degree) reflects the severity of skin damage (erythema, blisters, charring, respectively). [A.S. *baernan*]

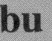

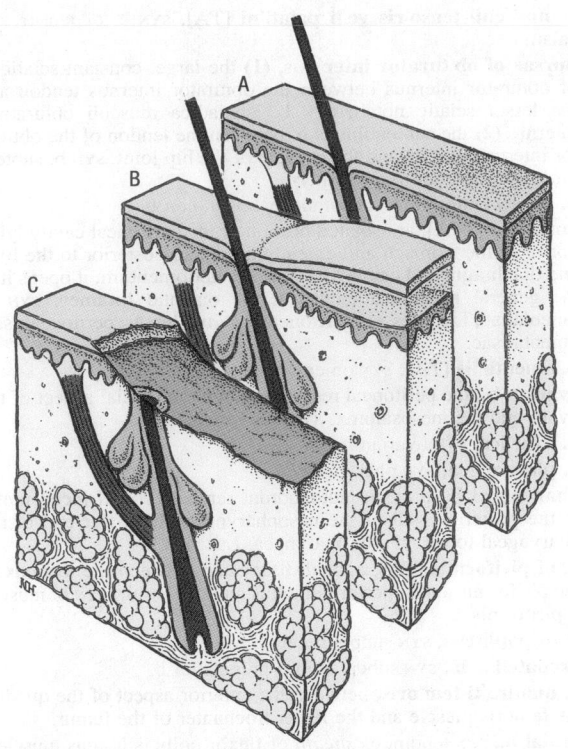

burns: (A) first degree, (B) second degree, (C) third degree

brush b., a b. caused by friction of a rapidly moving object against the skin or ground into the skin.

chemical b., a b. due to a caustic chemical.

first-degree b., a b. involving only the epidermis and causing erythema and edema without vesiculation. SYN superficial b.

flash b., a b. due to very brief exposure to intense radiant heat; the typical b. produced by atomic explosion.

full-thickness b., SYN third-degree b.

mat b., SEE brush b.

partial-thickness b., SYN second-degree b.

radiation b., a b. caused by exposure to radium, x-rays, atomic energy in any form, ultraviolet rays, etc.

rope b., SEE brush b.

☐ **second-degree b.,** a b. involving the epidermis and dermis and usually forming blisters that may be superficial, or by deep dermal necrosis, followed by epithelial regeneration extending from the skin appendages. SYN partial-thickness b.

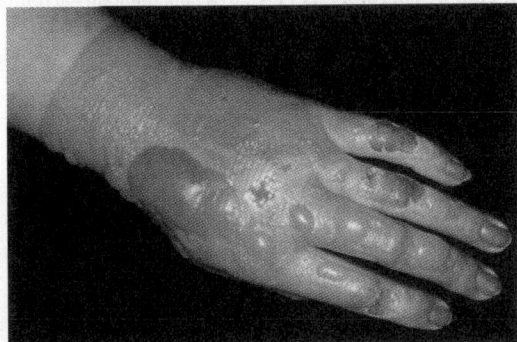

2nd degree burn: formation of blisters

superficial b., SYN first-degree b.

thermal b., a b. caused by heat.

third-degree b., a b. involving destruction of the entire skin; deep third-degree b.'s extend into subcutaneous fat, muscle, or bone and often cause much scarring. SYN full-thickness b.

burn·ers (bern'erz). Episodes of upper extremity burning pain. SEE ALSO burner *syndrome*. SYN stingers.

Burnett, Charles H., U.S. physician, 1901–1967. SEE B. *syndrome.*

bur·nish·er (bŭr'nish-er). An instrument for smoothing and polishing the surface or edge of a dental restoration. [O.F. *burnir,* to polish]

burn·out (bern'owt). **1.** In dentistry, the elimination, by heat, of an invested pattern from a set investment in order to prepare the mold to receive casting metal. **2.** A psychological state of physical and emotional exhaustion thought to be a stress reaction to a reduced ability to meet the demands of one's occupation; symptoms include fatigue, insomnia, impaired work performance, and an increased suscepibility to physical illness and substance abuse.

Burns, Allan, Scottish anatomist, 1781–1813. SEE B. *ligament,* falciform *process, space.*

Burow, Karl A. von, German surgeon, 1809–1874. SEE B. *solution, triangle, vein.*

burr (bŭr). SYN bur.

bur·row (ber'ō). **1.** A subcutaneous tunnel or tract made by a parasite, such as the scabies mite. **2.** A sinus or fistula. **3.** To undermine or create a tunnel or tract through or beneath various tissue planes.

BURSA

bur·sa, pl. **bur·sae** (ber'să, ber'sē) [TA]. A closed sac or envelope lined with synovial membrane and containing fluid, usually found or formed in areas subject to friction; e.g., over an exposed or prominent body part or where a tendon passes over a bone. [Mediev. L., a purse]

Achil′les b., SYN b. of tendo calcaneus.

b. achil′lis, SYN b. of tendo calcaneus.

b. of acromion, SYN subcutaneous acromial b.

adventitious b., a b.-like cyst formed between two parts as a result of friction.

b. anseri′na [TA], SYN anserine b.

anserine b. [TA], the b. between the tibial collateral ligament of the knee joint and the tendons of the sartorius, gracilis, and semitendinosus muscles. SYN b. anserina [TA], tibial intertendinous b.

anterior tibial b., SYN subtendinous b. of tibialis anterior.

bicipitoradial b. [TA], the b. between the tendon of the biceps brachii muscle and the anterior part of the tuberosity of the radius. SYN b. bicipitoradialis [TA].

b. bicip′itoradia′lis [TA], SYN bicipitoradial b.

Boyer b., SYN retrohyoid b.

Brodie b., (1) medial subtendinous b. of gastrocnemius muscle; (2) SYN semimembranous b.

b. of calcaneal tendon, ☆official alternate term for b. of tendo calcaneus.

Calori b., a b. between the arch of the aorta and the trachea.

coracobrachial b. [TA], a b. frequently present between the tendon of the coracobrachialis and the subscapularis muscle. SYN b. musculi coracobrachialis [TA], subcoracoid b.

b. cubita′lis interos′sea [TA], SYN interosseous cubital b.

deep infrapatellar b. [TA], the b. between the upper part of the tibia and the patellar ligament. SYN b. infrapatellaris profunda [TA].

b. of extensor carpi radialis brevis muscle, the b. between the tendon of the extensor carpi radialis brevis and the base of the third metacarpal. SYN b. musculi extensoris carpi radialis brevis.

b. fabric′ii, the b. of Fabricius in poultry, a blind saclike structure located on the posterodorsal wall of the cloaca; it performs a thymuslike function. SYN b. of Fabricius.

b. of Fabricius, SYN b. fabricii.

Fleischmann b., SYN sublingual b.

b. of gastrocnemius, SYN subtendinous bursae of gastrocnemius (muscle).

bursae of gastrocnemius, SYN subtendinous bursae of gastrocnemius (muscle).

gluteofemoral b., SYN intermuscular gluteal b.

gluteus medius bursae, SYN trochanteric bursae of gluteus medius.

gluteus minimus b., SYN trochanteric bursae of gluteus minimus.

b. of great toe, the b. between the lateral side of the base of the first metatarsal bone and the medial side of the shaft of the second metatarsal.

b. of hyoid, SYN retrohyoid b.

iliac b., SYN subtendinous b. of iliacus.

b. iliopecti′nea [TA], SYN iliopectineal b.

iliopectineal b. [TA], a large b. between the iliopsoas tendon and the iliopubic eminence. SYN b. iliopectinea [TA].

inferior subtendinous b. of biceps fem′oris [TA], the b. between the tendon of the biceps femoris and the fibular collateral ligament of the knee joint. SYN b. subtendinea musculi bicipitis femoris inferior [TA].

infracardiac b., a small serous sac sometimes present on the medial side of the base of the right lung in the embryo. SEE ALSO pneumatoenteric *recess,* celomic *bay.*

infrahyoid b. [TA], a b. sometimes found below the inferior margin of the body of the hyoid bone between the sternothyroid muscle and the median thyrohyoid membrane. SYN b. infrahyoidea [TA].

b. infrahyoi′dea [TA], SYN infrahyoid b.

b. infrapatella′ris profun′da [TA], SYN deep infrapatellar b.

infraspinatus b., SYN subtendinous b. of infraspinatus.

intermuscular gluteal b. [TA], two or three small bursae between the tendon of the gluteus maximus and the linea aspera. SYN b. intermuscularis musculorum gluteorum [TA], gluteofemoral b.

b. intermuscula′ris musculo′rum gluteor′um [TA], SYN intermuscular gluteal b.

interosseous cubital b. [TA], an inconstant b. located between the tendon of the biceps and the ulna or the oblique cord. SYN b. cubitalis interossea [TA], interosseous b. of elbow.

interosseous b. of elbow, SYN interosseous cubital b.

b. intratendin′ea olecra′ni [TA], SYN intratendinous olecranon b.

intratendinous b. of elbow, SYN intratendinous olecranon b.

intratendinous olecranon b. [TA], a b. sometimes present within the tendon of insertion of the triceps brachii. SYN b. intratendinea olecrani [TA], b. of Monro, intratendinous b. of elbow.

b. ischiad′ica mus′culi glu′tei max′imi [TA], SYN sciatic b. of gluteus maximus.

b. ischiad′ica mus′culi obturato′ris inter′ni, SYN bursae of obturator internus (1).

ischial b., SYN sciatic b. of gluteus maximus.

laryngeal b., SYN subcutaneous b. of the laryngeal prominence.

lateral malleolar subcutaneous b., SYN subcutaneous b. of lateral malleolus.

lateral malleolus b., SYN subcutaneous b. of lateral malleolus.

b. of latiss′imus dor′si, SYN subtendinous b. of latissimus dorsi.

Luschka b., SYN pharyngeal b.

medial malleolar subcutaneous b., SYN subcutaneous b. of medial malleolus.

b. of Monro, SYN intratendinous olecranon b.

b. muco′sa, SYN synovial b.

b. mus′culi bicip′itis fem′oris supe′rior [TA], SYN superior b. of biceps femoris.

b. mus′culi coracobrachia′lis [TA], SYN coracobrachial b.

b. mus′culi extenso′ris car′pi radia′lis bre′vis, SYN b. of extensor carpi radialis brevis muscle.

b. mus′culi pirifor′mis, SYN b. of piriformis.

b. mus′culi semimembrano′si, SYN semimembranous b.

b. mus′culi tenso′ris ve′li palati′ni [TA], SYN b. of tensor veli palatine.

bursae of ob′turator inter′nus, (1) the large, constant sciatic b. of obturator internus between the obturator internus tendon and the lesser sciatic notch; SYN b. ischiadica musculi obturatoris interni. **(2)** the subtendinous b. between the tendon of the obturator internus muscle and the capsule of the hip joint. SYN b. subtendinea musculi obturatoris interni.

b. of olecranon, SYN subcutaneous olecranon b.

omental b. [TA], an isolated portion of the peritoneal cavity lying dorsal to the stomach and extending craniad posterior to the liver and diaphragm and caudad into the greater omentum; it opens into the general peritoneal cavity at the omental foramen. SYN b. omentalis [TA], lesser peritoneal cavity, lesser peritoneal sac, omental sac.

b. omenta′lis [TA], SYN omental b.

ovarian b., the peritoneal recess between the medial aspect of the ovary and the mesosalpinx. SYN b. ovarica.

b. ovar′ica, SYN ovarian b.

b. pharyn′gea, SYN pharyngeal b.

pharyngeal b., a cystic notochordal remnant found inconstantly in the posterior wall of the nasopharynx at the lower end of the pharyngeal tonsil. SYN b. pharyngea, Luschka b.

b. of piriformis [TA], a small b. located between the tendons of the piriformis and superior gemellus and the femur. SYN b. musculi piriformis.

b. of popliteus, SYN subpopliteal *recess.*

prepatellar b., SYN subcutaneous prepatellar b.

b. quadra′ti fem′oris, between the anterior aspect of the quadratus femoris muscle and the lesser trochanter of the femur.

radial b., SYN tendinous *sheath* of flexor pollicis longus muscle.

retrocalcaneal b., ⋆official alternate term for b. of tendo calcaneus.

retrohyoid b. [TA], a b. between the posterior surface of the body of the hyoid bone and the thyrohyoid membrane. SYN b. retrohyoidea [TA], Boyer b., b. of hyoid, subhyoid b.

b. retrohyoi′dea [TA], SYN retrohyoid b.

rider's b., an adventitious b. on the inner side of the knee caused by horseback riding.

sartorius bursae, SYN subtendinous b. of sartorius.

sciatic b. of gluteus maximus [TA], the b. between the gluteus maximus muscle and the tuberosity of the ischium. SYN b. ischiadica musculi glutei maximi [TA], ischial b.

b. of semimembranosus muscle, SYN semimembranous b.

semimembranous b. [TA], it lies between the muscle, the head of the gastrocnemius, and the knee joint. SYN Brodie b. (2), b. musculi semimembranosi, b. of semimembranosus muscle.

subacromial b. [TA], between the acromion and the capsule of the shoulder joint. SYN b. subacromialis [TA].

b. subacromia′lis [TA], SYN subacromial b.

subcoracoid b., SYN coracobrachial b.

b. subcuta′nea acromia′lis [TA], SYN subcutaneous acromial b.

b. subcuta′nea calca′nea [TA], SYN subcutaneous calcaneal b.

b. subcuta′nea infrapatella′ris [TA], SYN subcutaneous infrapatellar b.

b. subcuta′nea malle′oli latera′lis [TA], SYN subcutaneous b. of lateral malleolus.

b. subcuta′nea malle′oli media′lis [TA], SYN subcutaneous b. of medial malleolus.

b. subcuta′nea ole′crani [TA], SYN subcutaneous olecranon b.

b. subcuta′nea prepatella′ris, SYN subcutaneous prepatellar b.

b. subcuta′nea prominen′tiae laryn′geae [TA], SYN subcutaneous b. of the laryngeal prominence.

b. subcuta′nea trochanter′ica, SYN trochanteric b. (1).

b. subcuta′nea tuberosita′tis tib′iae, SYN subcutaneous b. of tuberosity of tibia.

subcutaneous acromial b. [TA], the frequently occurring b. between the acromion and the skin. SYN b. subcutanea acromialis [TA], b. of acromion.

subcutaneous calcaneal b. [TA], a b. between the skin and the posterior surface of the calcaneus. SYN b. subcutanea calcanea [TA].

subcutaneous infrapatellar b. [TA], a b. between the patellar ligament and the skin. SYN b. subcutanea infrapatellaris [TA].

subcutaneous b. of the laryngeal prominence [TA], the b. located between the junction of the laminae of the thyroid cartilage and the skin. SYN b. subcutanea prominentiae laryngeae [TA], laryngeal b.

subcutaneous b. of lateral malleolus [TA], lateral malleolar b., the b. between the lateral malleolus and the skin. SYN b. subcutanea malleoli lateralis [TA], lateral malleolar subcutaneous b., lateral malleolus b.

subcutaneous b. of medial malleolus [TA], the b. between the medial malleolus and the skin. SYN b. subcutanea malleoli medialis [TA], medial malleolar subcutaneous b.

subcutaneous olecranon b. [TA], b. between the olecranon process of the ulna and the skin. SYN b. subcutanea olecrani [TA], b. of olecranon.

subcutaneous prepatellar b. [TA], a b. between the skin and the lower part of the patella. SYN b. subcutanea prepatellaris, prepatellar b.

subcutaneous b. of teres major [TA], b. under the tendon of the teres major near its attachment. SYN b. subtendinea musculi teretis majoris [TA], b. of teres major.

subcutaneous b. of tibial tuberosity, SYN subcutaneous b. of tuberosity of tibia.

subcutaneous b. of tuberosity of tibia [TA], the b. located superficial to the tibial tuberosity, either subcutaneous or subfascial. SYN b. subcutanea tuberositatis tibiae, subcutaneous b. of tibial tuberosity.

subdeltoid b. [TA], the b. between the deltoid muscle and the capsule of the shoulder joint. It may be combined with the subacromial b. SYN b. subdeltoidea [TA].

b. subdeltoid'ea [TA], SYN subdeltoid b.

b. subfascia'lis prepatella'ris [TA], SYN subfascial prepatellar b.

subfascial prepatellar b. [TA], a commonly occurring b. between the fascia lata and the quadriceps tendon anterior to the patella. SYN b. subfascialis prepatellaris [TA].

subhyoid b., SYN retrohyoid b.

sublingual b., an inconstant serous b. at the level of the frenulum of the tongue between the surface of the genioglossus muscle and the mucous membrane of the floor of the mouth. SYN b. sublingualis, Fleischmann b.

b. sublingua'lis, SYN sublingual b.

subscapular b., SYN subtendinous b. of subscapularis.

b. subtendin'eae mus'culi gastrocne'mii, SYN subtendinous bursae of gastrocnemius (muscle).

bursae subtendin'eae mus'culi sarto'rii [TA], SYN subtendinous b. of sartorius.

b. subtendin'ea ili'aca [TA], SYN subtendinous b. of iliacus.

b. subtendin'ea mus'culi bicip'itis fem'oris infe'rior [TA], SYN inferior subtendinous b. of biceps femoris.

b. subtendin'ea mus'culi infraspina'ti [TA], SYN subtendinous b. of infraspinatus.

b. subtendin'ea mus'culi latis'simus dor'si [TA], SYN subtendinous b. of latissimus dorsi.

b. subtendin'ea mus'culi obturatoris inter'ni, SYN bursae of obturator internus (2).

b. subtendin'ea mus'culi subscapula'ris [TA], SYN subtendinous b. of subscapularis.

b. subtendin'ea mus'culi tere'tis majo'ris [TA], SYN subcutaneous b. of teres major.

b. subtendin'ea mus'culi tibia'lis anterio'ris [TA], SYN subtendinous b. of tibialis anterior.

b. subtendin'ea mus'culi trape'zii [TA], SYN subtendinous b. of trapezius.

b. subtendin'ea mus'culi trici'pitis bra'chii [TA], SYN subtendinous b. of triceps brachii.

b. subtendin'ea prepatella'ris [TA], SYN subtendinous prepatellar b.

bursae subtendineae musculi gastrocnemii [TA], SYN subtendinous bursae of gastrocnemius (muscle).

subtendinous bursae of gastrocnemius (muscle), consist of a lateral and a medial [Brodie b. (1)] b. between the heads of the gastrocnemius and capsule of the knee joint. SYN bursae subtendineae musculi gastrocnemii [TA], b. of gastrocnemius, b. subtendineae musculi gastrocnemii, bursae of gastrocnemius.

subtendinous iliac b., SYN subtendinous b. of iliacus.

subtendinous b. of iliacus [TA], the b. at the attachment of the iliopsoas muscle into the lesser trochanter. SYN b. subtendinea iliaca [TA], iliac b., subtendinous iliac b.

subtendinous b. of infraspinatus [TA], the b. located between the tendon of the infraspinatus and the capsule of the shoulder joint. SYN b. subtendinea musculi infraspinati [TA], infraspinatus b.

subtendinous b. of latissimus dorsi [TA], a constant b. between the tendons of the teres major and the latissimus dorsi near their intersections. SYN b. subtendinea musculi latissimus dorsi [TA], b. of latissimus dorsi.

subtendinous prepatellar b. [TA], an inconstant b. between the tendon of the quadriceps and the patella. SYN b. subtendinea prepatellaris [TA].

subtendinous b. of sartorius [TA], bursae, sometimes separate from the anserine b., located between the tendons of the sartorius, semitendinosus, and gracilis muscles. SYN bursae subtendineae musculi sartorii [TA], sartorius bursae.

subtendinous b. of subscapularis [TA], b. between the tendon of the subscapularis muscle and the neck of the scapula; it communicates with the shoulder joint. SYN b. subtendinea musculi subscapularis [TA], subscapular b.

subtendinous b. of tibialis anterior, the small b. between the medial surface of the medial cuneiform bone and the tendon of the tibialis anterior. SYN b. subtendinea musculi tibialis anterioris [TA], anterior tibial b.

subtendinous b. of trapezius [TA], a b. between the tendon of the trapezius muscle and the medial end of the scapular spine. SYN b. subtendinea musculi trapezii [TA], b. of trapezius.

subtendinous b. of triceps brachii [TA], the b. located deep to the tendon of the triceps brachii near its insertion on the olecranon. SYN b. subtendinea musculi tricipitis brachii [TA], triceps b.

superior b. of biceps femoris [TA], a b. frequently found between the tendon of the long head of the biceps femoris and the ischial tuberosity and the tendon of the semimembranosus. SYN b. musculi bicipitis femoris superior [TA].

suprapatellar b. [TA], a large b. between the lower part of the femur and the tendon of the quadriceps femoris muscle. It usually communicates with the cavity of the knee joint and is pathologically distended with blood or synovial fluid in suprapatellar bursitis ("water on the knee"). SYN b. suprapatellaris [TA].

b. suprapatella'ris [TA], SYN suprapatellar b.

synovial b. [TA], a sac containing synovial fluid that occurs at sites of friction, as between a tendon and a bone over which it plays, or subcutaneously over a bony prominence. Terminologia Anatomica lists the following types: subcutaneous b., b. subcutanea [TA]; submuscular b., b. submuscularis [TA]; subfascial b., b. subfascialis [TA]; and subtendinous b., b. subtendinea [TA]. SYN b. synovialis [TA], b. mucosa.

b. synovia'lis [TA], SYN synovial b.

synovial trochlear b., SYN tendinous *sheath* of superior oblique muscle.

b. ten'dinis calca'nei, SYN b. of tendo calcaneus.

b. of tendo calca'neus [TA], b. between the tendo calcaneus and the upper part of the posterior surface of the calcaneum. SYN b. of calcaneal tendon★, retrocalcaneal b.★, Achilles b., b. achillis, b. tendinis calcanei.

b. of tensor veli palatine [TA], a small b. located where the tendon of the tensor passes around the pterygoid hamulus. SYN b. musculi tensoris veli palatini [TA].

b. of teres major, SYN subcutaneous b. of teres major.

tibial intertendinous b., SYN anserine b.

b. of trapezius, SYN subtendinous b. of trapezius.

triceps b., SYN subtendinous b. of triceps brachii.

trochanteric b. [TA], **(1)** the subcutaneous trochanteric b. between the greater trochanter of the femur and the skin; SYN b. subcutanea trochanterica. **(2)** a multilocular trochanteric b. of gluteus maximus between the gluteus maximus and the greater trochanter of the femur; SYN b. trochanterica musculi glutei maximi. **(3)** the trochanteric b. of gluteus medius between the gluteus medius and the greater trochanter; SYN bursae trochantericae musculi glutei medii [TA]. **(4)** the trochanteric b. of the gluteus minimus. SYN b. trochanterica musculi glutei minimi [TA]. SYN b. trochanterica [TA].

b. trochanterica [TA], SYN trochanteric b.

bur′sae trochanter′icae mus′culi glu′tei me′dii [TA], SYN trochanteric b. (3).

b. trochanter′ica mus′culi glu′tei max′imi, SYN trochanteric b. (2).

b. trochanter′ica mus′culi glu′tei min′imi [TA], SYN trochanteric b. (4).

trochanteric bursae of gluteus medius [TA], the b. between the tendon of the gluteus medius and the greater trochanter and the b. between the piriformis and gluteus medius. SYN gluteus medius bursae.

trochanteric bursae of gluteus minimus [TA], a fairly large b. usually located between the gluteus minimus and the greater trochanter. SYN gluteus minimus b.

trochlear synovial b., SYN tendinous *sheath* of superior oblique muscle.

ulnar b., SYN common flexor *sheath* (of hand).

---

bur·sal (ber′săl). Relating to a bursa.

bur·sec·to·my (ber-sek′tō-mē). Surgical removal of a bursa. [bursa + G. *ektomē,* excision]

bur·si·tis (ber-sī′tis). Inflammation of a bursa. SYN bursal synovitis.

anserine b., inflammation of the anserine bursa lying between the pes anserinus and the upper medial surface of the tibia.

calcific b., inflammation of a bursa that results in the deposition of calcium salts; most commonly associated with subdeltoid bursitis.

ischial b., inflammation of the bursa overlying the ischial tuberosity of the pelvis.

olecranon b., inflammation of the olecranon bursa, overlying the prominence of the elbow.

prepatellar b., SYN housemaid's *knee.*

subacromial b., inflammation of the subacromial bursa lying between the acromion above and the rotator cuff below; may be continuous with the subdeltoid *bursa.*

subdeltoid b., inflammation of the subdeltoid bursa lying between the deltoid muscle and the underlying proximal humerus and rotator cuff; may be continuous with the subacromial *bursa.*

bur·so·lith (ber′sō-lith). A calculus formed in a bursa. [bursa + G. *lithos,* stone]

bur·sop·a·thy (ber-sop′ă-thē). Any disease of a bursa.

bur·sot·o·my (ber-sot′ō-mē). Incision through the wall of a bursa. [bursa + G. *tomē,* a cutting]

burst (berst). A sudden increase in activity.

respiratory b., the marked increase in metabolic activity that occurs in phagocytes and certain other cells following binding of particles resulting in an increase in oxygen consumption, formation of superoxide anion, formation of hydrogen peroxide, and activation of the hexose monophosphate shunt.

b. size, the number of phages produced by an infected cell.

bur·su·la (ber′soo-lă). A small pouch or bag. [Mod. L. dim. of Mediev. L. *bursa,* purse]

b. tes′tium, archaic term for scrotum.

Burton, Henry, English physician, 1799–1849. SEE B. *line.*

Busacca, Archimede, Italian physician, *1893. SEE Busacca *nodules,* under *nodule.*

Buschke, Abraham, German dermatologist, 1868–1943. SEE B. *disease;* B.-Ollendorf *syndrome.*

bu·spi·rone hy·dro·chlo·ride (bū-spī′rōn). A non-benzo-

diazepine antianxiety agent used in the management of anxiety disorders or for short-term relief of the symptoms of anxiety.

Busquet, G. Paul, French physician, 1865–1930. SEE B. *disease.*

Busse, Otto, German physician, 1867–1922.

bu·sul·fan, bu·sul·phan (bū-sŭl′fan). An antineoplastic alkylating agent used in the treatment of chronic myelocytic leukemia; known to be teratogenic in humans.

bu·ta·bar·bi·tal (bū-tă-bar′bi-tawl). An obsolescent sedative and hypnotic with intermediate duration of action; available as b. sodium, with same usages.

bu·ta·caine sul·fate (bū′tă-kān). A local anesthetic.

bu·tam·ben (bū-tam′ben). SYN *butyl* aminobenzoate.

bu·tane (bū′tān). C_4H_{10}; a gaseous hydrocarbon present in natural gas; two isomers are known, both of which are anesthetically active: *n*-butane is $CH_3(CH_2)_2CH_3$ and isobutane is $CH_3CH(CH_3)$-CH_3 (or 2-methylpropane).

bu·ta·no·ic ac·id (bū-tă-nō′ik). Systematic name for normal *n*-butyric acid.

bu·ta·nol (bū′tă-nol). Preferred chemical name for *n*-butyl alcohol.

bu·tan·o·yl (bū′tan-ō-il). The radical of butanoic acid. SYN butyryl.

bu·ta·per·a·zine (bū-tă-per′ă-zēn). An antipsychotic.

bu·tav·er·ine (bū-tav′er-ēn). An antispasmodic (as hydrochloride).

bu·teth·a·mate (bū-teth′ă-māt). An intestinal antispasmodic agent.

bu·teth·a·mine hy·dro·chlo·ride (bū-teth′ă-mēn). A local anesthetic.

bu·thi·a·zide (bū-thī′ă-zīd). Has diuretic and antihypertensive actions. SYN thiabutazide.

buthionine sulfoximine (boo-thī-ō-nēn sul-fox′ĭ-mēn). A compound that decreases intracellular glutathione by inhibition of its synthesis.

bu·to·con·a·zole ni·trate (bū-tō-kō′nă-zōl). An antifungal agent used primarily in the treatment of vulvovaginal candidiasis; similar to ketoconazole and itraconazole.

bu·to·py·ro·nox·yl (bū′tō-pī-rō-nok′sil). An insect repellent, effective against the biting stable fly (*Stomoxys calcitrans*)

bu·tor·pha·nol tar·trate (bū-tōr′fă-nōl). A potent mixed agonist/antagonist narcotic analgesic agent, used by injection and in the form of a nasal spray.

bu·tox·a·mine hy·dro·chlo·ride (bū-tok′să-mēn). An antilipemic agent.

t-**bu·tox·y·car·bon·yl (BOC,** *t*-**BOC, Boc)** (bū-toks-ē-kar′bŏn-il). An amino-protecting group used in peptide synthesis. SYN *tert*-butyloxycarbonyl.

bu·trip·ty·line hy·dro·chlo·ride (bū-trip′tĭ-lēn). An antidepressant.

butt (bŭt). **1.** To bring any two square-ended surfaces in contact so as to form a joint. **2.** In dentistry, to place a restoration directly against the tissues covering the alveolar ridge.

but·ter (bŭt′er). **1.** A coherent mass of milk fat, obtained by churning or shaking cream until the separate fat globules run together, leaving a liquid residue, buttermilk. **2.** A soft solid having more or less the consistency of b. [L. *butyrum,* G. *boutyros,* prob. fr. *bous,* cow, + *tyros,* cheese]

b. of antimony, a concentrated acid solution of *antimony* trichloride.

b. of bismuth, SYN *bismuth* trichloride.

cacao b., cocoa b., SYN *theobroma* oil; SEE ALSO cacao.

b. of tin, stannic chloride pentahydrate, $SnCl_4 \cdot 5H_2O$.

b. of zinc, SYN *zinc* chloride.

but·ter·fly (bŭt′er-flī). **1.** Any structure or apparatus shaped like a butterfly with outstretched wings. **2.** A scaling erythematous lesion on each cheek, joined by a narrow band across the nose; seen in lupus erythematosus and seborrheic dermatitis. SYN butterfly eruption, butterfly patch, butterfly rash.

but·ter·milk. The fluid containing casein and lactic acid, left after the process of making butter.

but·ter yel·low [C.I. 11160]. A fat-soluble yellow dye (MW 225) that has hepatic carcinogenic action in experimental animals; used as an indicator of pH (red, at pH 2.9, yellow at pH 4.0). SYN dimethylaminoazobenzene, methyl yellow.

but·tocks (bŭt'oks) [TA]. The prominence formed by the gluteal muscles on either side. SYN nates [TA], clunes★, breech.

but·ton (bŭt'ŏn). A structure, lesion, or device of knob shape. [M.E., fr. O.Fr. *bouton*, fr. *bouter*, to thrust, fr. Germanic]

Biskra b., SYN Oriental b.

Murphy b., a device used for intestinal anastomosis; it consists of two round, hollow cylinders that insert into each end of the transected intestine; the intestine is secured to each of the components with a suture and the ends are brought into approximation and the two cylinders joined with a locking mechanism; the apparatus is degradable and within approximately 10 days dissolves and is sloughed into the lumen of the intestine. A modification of an obsolete metal device bearing the same name.

Oriental b., the lesion occurring in cutaneous leishmaniasis. SYN Biskra b.

peritoneal b., a device used to drain ascitic fluid to subcutaneous space.

but·ton·hole (bŭt'ŏn-hōl). **1.** A short straight cut made through the wall of a cavity or canal. **2.** The contraction of an orifice down to a narrow slit; i.e., the so-called mitral b. in extreme mitral stenosis. SEE buttonhole *stenosis*.

bu·tyl (bū'til). CH₃(CH₂)₃–; a radical of *n*-butane.

b. alcohol, several isomeric forms are known: **primary b. alcohol,** 1-butanol, propylcarbinol, the butyl alcohol of fermentation; **isobutyl alcohol,** isopropylcarbinol, 2-methyl-1-propanol, which is narcotic in high concentrations; **secondary b. alcohol,** ethylmethylcarbinol, 2-butanol; and **tertiary b. alcohol,** trimethylcarbinol, 2-methyl-2-propanol, a denaturant for ethanol.

b. aminobenzoate, a local anesthetic, very insoluble and only slightly absorbed. SYN butamben.

bu·tyl·at·ed hy·drox·y·an·is·ole (BHA) (boo-tĭ-lāt'ed hī'drok-sē-an'ĭ-sol). Exhibits antioxidant properties; often used with butylated hydroxytoluene propyl gallate, hydroquinone, methionine, lecithin, thiodipropionic acid, etc. Used as an antioxidant, especially in foods.

bu·tyl·at·ed hy·drox·y·tol·u·ene (BHT). Antioxidant for food, animal feed, petroleum products, synthetic rubbers, plastics, animal and vegetable oils, soap; also an antiskinning agent in paints and inks.

*tert-***bu·tyl·ox·y·car·bon·yl (tBoc)** (bū'til-oks'ē-kar'bŏn-il). SYN *t*-butoxycarbonyl.

bu·tyl·par·a·ben (bū-til-par'ă-ben). An antifungal preservative.

bu·ty·ra·ce·ous (bū-tir-ā'shĭ-us). Buttery in consistency.

bu·ty·rate (bū'ti-rāt). A salt or ester of butyric acid.

bu·ty·rate-CoA li·gase. Fatty acid thiokinase (medium chain), a ligase forming acyl-CoA's from medium-chain fatty acids and CoA with the conversion of ATP to AMP and pyrophosphate. A key step in activation of fatty acids. SYN acyl-activating enzyme (2), butyryl-CoA synthetase, octanoyl-CoA synthetase.

bu·tyr·ic (bū-tir'ik). Relating to butter.

bu·tyr·ic ac·id (bū-tir'ik). An acid of unpleasant odor occurring in butter, cod liver oil, sweat, and many other substances. It exists in two forms: **normal b. a.** (also written as *n*-butyric acid), butanoic acid, which occurs in combination with glycerol in cow's butter; and isobutyric acid, 2-methylpropanoic acid, one of the intermediates in valine catabolism, found in combination with glycerol in croton oil and elsewhere.

γ-bu·tyr·o·be·taine (bū-tir'ō-be-tān). A betaine of γ-aminobutyric acid; a precursor of carnitine by hydroxylation of the β-carbon.

bu·tyr·o·cho·lin·es·ter·ase (bū'tir-ō-kō-lin-es'ter-ās). Pseudocholinesterase or plasma cholinesterase. To be distinguished from true or tissue cholinesterase. SEE ALSO cholinesterase. SYN butyrylcholine esterase, pseudocholinesterase.

bu·ty·roid (bū'ti-royd). **1.** Buttery. **2.** Resembling butter.

bu·tyr·om·e·ter (bū-ti-rom'ĕ-ter). An instrument for determining the amount of butterfat in milk. [G. *boutyron,* butter, + *metron,* measure]

bu·ty·ro·phe·none (bū'tir-ō-fē'nōn). One of a group of derivatives of 4-phenylbutylamine that have neuroleptic activity; e.g., haloperidol.

bu·tyr·ous (bū'ti-rŭs). Denoting a tissue or bacterial growth of butterlike consistency.

bu·tyr·yl (bū'ti-ril). SYN butanoyl.

bu·tyr·yl·cho·line es·ter·ase (bū'ti-ril-kō'lēn es'ter-ās). SYN butyrocholinesterase.

bu·tyr·yl-CoA. Condensation product of coenzyme A and *n*-butanoic acid; an intermediate in fatty acid degradation and in biosynthesis.

b.-C. synthetase, SYN butyrate-CoA ligase.

Buzzard, Thomas, English physician, 1831–1919. SEE B. *maneuver.*

Buzzi, Fausto, coworker of Ernst Schweninger. SEE Schweninger-B. *anetoderma.*

Byars, Louis T., 20th century U.S. surgeon, (1906-) SEE B. *flap.*

Byler, Amish kindred in the U.S. SEE Byler *disease.*

by·pass (bī'pas). **1.** A shunt or auxiliary flow. **2.** To create new flow from one structure to another through a diversionary channel. SEE ALSO shunt.

aortocoronary b., SYN coronary artery b.

aortoiliac b., an operation in which a vascular prosthesis is united with the aorta and iliac artery to relieve obstruction of the lower abdominal aorta, its bifurcation, and the proximal iliac branches.

aortorenal b., a vascular prosthesis of synthetic material, autologous tissue, or heterologous tissue that circumvents and obstruction of the renal artery.

bowel b., SYN jejunoileal b.

cardiopulmonary b., diversion of the blood flow returning to the heart through a pump oxygenator (heart-lung machine) and then returning it to the arterial side of the circulation; used in operations upon the heart to maintain extracorporeal circulation.

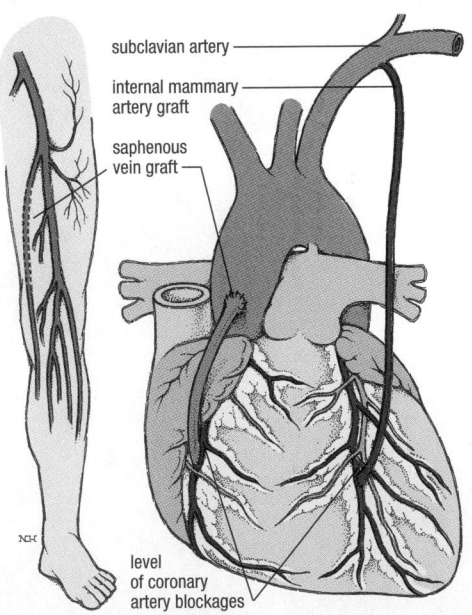

subclavian artery
internal mammary artery graft
saphenous vein graft

level of coronary artery blockages

coronary bypass: completed double bypass using the internal mammary artery and the saphenous vein

coronary artery b., conduit, usually a vein graft or internal mammary artery, surgically interposed between the aorta and a coronary artery branch to coronary shunt blood beyond an obstruction. SYN aortocoronary b.

extra-anatomic b., a vascular b. that does not conform to the preexisting anatomy.

extracranial-intracranial b., a vascular shunt created by the anastomosis of an extracranial vessel to an intracranial vessel, usually, the superficial temporal artery to a cortical branch of the middle cerebral artery.

femoropopliteal b., a vascular prosthesis of synthetic material, autologous tissue, or heterologous tissue that circumvents an obstruction in the femoral artery.

gastric b., high division of the stomach, anastomosis of the small upper pouch of the stomach to the jejunum, and closure of the distal part of the stomach that is retained; used for treatment of severe obesity.

jejunoileal b., anastomosis of the upper jejunum to the terminal ileum for treatment of severe obesity. SYN bowel b., jejunoileal shunt.

left heart b., any procedure that shunts blood returning from the pulmonary circulation to the systemic circulation without passing through the left heart. This is utilized during some cardiac surgery and experimentally during severe left heart failure or cardiogenic shock.

partial ileal b., division of the small intestine approximately 100 cm proximal to the ileocecal valve, closure of the distal end, and anastomosis of the proximal end to the cecum.

right heart b., introduction of a circuit shunting blood from the venae cavae around the right atrium and ventricle and directly into the pulmonary artery.

bys·si·no·sis (bis-i-nō'sis). Obstructive airway disease in people who work with unprocessed cotton, flax, or hemp; caused by reaction to material in the dust and thought to include endotoxin from bacterial contamination. Sometimes called "Monday morning asthma" since patients improve when away from work on the weekend. SYN cotton-dust asthma, cotton-mill fever, mill fever. [G. *byssos,* flax, + *-osis,* condition]

byte. A group of adjacent bits, commonly 4, 6, or 8, operating as a unit for the storage and manipulation of data in a computer.

C 1. Abbreviation or symbol for large *calorie*; carbon; cathodal; cathode; Celsius; cervical vertebra (C1–C7); closure (of an electrical circuit); congius (gallon); contraction; coulomb; curie; cylinder; cylindrical *lens*; cytidine; cysteine; cytosine; *component* of complement (C1–C9); third substrate in a multisubstrate enzyme-catalyzed reaction. 2. When followed by subscript letters, e.g., C_{in}, indicates renal clearance of a substance (e.g., inulin). When followed by subscript numbers, e.g., C_{19}, indicates the number of carbon atoms in a molecule, e.g., 19.

c 1. Abbreviation or symbol for centi-; small *calorie*; centum; concentration; speed of light in a vacuum; circumference. Abbreviation for curie. 2. As a subscript, refers to blood *capillary*.

c̄ Abbreviation for L. *cum*, with.

^{11}C Symbol for carbon-11.

^{12}C Symbol for carbon-12, the most common form of carbon.

^{13}C Symbol for carbon-13.

^{14}C Symbol for carbon-14.

CA Abbreviation for cancer; q; cardiac *arrest*; chronologic *age*; *cytosine* arabinoside.

CA-125. Abbreviation for cancer antigen 125 *test*.

CA125 Abbreviation for cancer antigen 125 *test*.

Ca 1. Abbreviation for cathode. 2. Symbol for calcium.

^{45}Ca Symbol for calcium-45.

^{47}Ca Symbol for calcium-47.

ca. Abbreviation for L. *circa* (about, approximately).

caa·pi (ka′pē). A hallucinogenic preparation obtained from *Banisteria caapi* (family Malpighaceae), a South American jungle vine; contains harmine and other psychotomimetic principles. SYN ayahuasca.

cab·bage tree (kab′ij trē). SYN andira.

Cabot, Richard C., U.S. physician, 1868–1939. SEE C. ring *bodies*, under *body;* C.-Locke *murmur.*

△**cac-.** SEE caco-.

ca·cao (kă-ka′ō). Prepared c., or cocoa, a powder prepared from the roasted cured kernels of the ripe seed of *Theobroma cacao* Linné (family Sterculiaceae); the tree yields a fat, theobroma oil. SYN theobroma. [native Mexican origin]

c. oil, SYN *theobroma* oil.

CaCC Abbreviation for cathodal closure *contraction.*

Cacchione, Aldo, 20th century Italian psychiatrist. SEE De Sanctis-C. *syndrome.*

ca·chec·tic (kă-kek′tik). Relating to or suffering from cachexia.

ca·chec·tin (ka-kek′tin). A polypeptide cytokine, produced by endotoxin-activated macrophages, which has the ability to modulate adipocyte metabolism, lyse tumor cells in vitro, and induce hemorrhagic necrosis of certain transplantable tumors in vivo. SYN tumor necrosis factor. [G. *kakos,* bad, + *hexis,* condition of body]

ca·chet (kă-shā′). A seal-shaped capsule or wafer made of flour for enclosing powders of disagreeable taste. The sealed dosage form is wetted and swallowed. [Fr. a seal]

ca·chex·ia (kă-kek′sē-ă). A general weight loss and wasting occurring in the course of a chronic disease or emotional disturbance. [G. *kakos,* bad, + *hexis,* condition of body]

c. aphtho′sa, SYN sprue (1).

c. aquo′sa, an edematous form of ancylostomiasis.

diabetic neuropathic c., a clinical syndrome seen almost exclusively in elderly diabetic males, consisting of the rather sudden onset of severe limb pain, marked weight loss, depression, and impotence. These patients appear to have a combination of a severe diabetic polyneuropathy, diffuse bilateral diabetic polyradiculopathy, and diabetic autonomic neuropathy.

hypophyseal c., SYN panhypopituitarism.

c. hypophys′eopri′va, a condition following total removal of the hypophysis cerebri resulting in panhypopituitarism marked by a fall of body temperature, electrolyte imbalance, and hypoglycemia, followed by coma and death.

hypophysial c., SYN panhypopituitarism.

malarial c., SYN chronic *malaria.*

pituitary c., SYN Sheehan *syndrome.*

c. strumipri′va, SYN c. thyropriva.

c. thyroid′ea, SYN c. thyropriva.

c. thyropri′va, signs and symptoms of hypothyroidism (with or without myxedema) resulting from the loss of thyroid tissue, either from surgery, radiotherapy, or disease. SYN c. strumipriva, c. thyroidea.

cach·in·na·tion (kak-i-nā′shŭn). Laughter without apparent cause, often observed in schizophrenia. [L. *cachinno,* to laugh immoderately and loudly]

△**caco-, caci-, cac-.** Bad; ill. Cf. mal-. [G. *kakos*]

cac·o·dyl (kak′ō-dil). An oil resulting from the distillation together of arsenous acid and potassium acetate. SYN dicacodyl, tetramethyldiarsine. [G. *kakōdēs,* foul-smelling]

cac·o·dyl·ate (kak′ō-dil-āt). A salt or ester of cacodylic acid. SEE cacodylic acid.

cac·o·dyl·ic (kak-ō-dil′ik). Relating to cacodyl; denoting especially c. acid.

cac·o·dyl·ic ac·id. Prepared by treating cacodyl and cacodyl oxide with mercuric oxide, and forms cacodylates with various bases that were used in skin diseases, tuberculosis, malaria, and other affections in which arsenic was considered of value. SYN dimethylarsinic acid.

cac·o·geu·sia (kak-ō-goo′sē-ă). A bad taste due to a bad-tasting substance, uncinate epilepsy, or a delusion. SEE ALSO dysgeusia. [caco- + G. *geusis,* taste]

cac·o·me·lia (kak-ō-mē′lē-ă). Congenital deformity of one or more limbs. [caco- + G. *melos,* limb]

cac·o·plas·tic (kak-ō-plas′tik). 1. Relating to or causing abnormal growth. 2. Incapable of normal or perfect formation. [caco- + G. *plastikos,* formed]

ca·cos·mia (kă-koz′mē-ă). A bad smell due to a bad smelling substance, uncinate epilepsy, or a delusion. SEE dysosmia. [G. *kakosmia,* a bad smell, fr. *kakos,* bad, + *osmē,* the sense of smell]

cac·ti·no·my·cin (kak′ti-nō-mī′sin). Produced by *Streptomyces chrysomallus.* A mixture of actinomycins C_1 (dactinomycin), C_2, and C_3 used as an antineoplastic, immunosuppressive agent. SEE ALSO actinomycin. SYN actinomycin C.

cac·u·men, pl. **cac·u·mi·na** (kak-ū′men, -mi-nă). The top or apex of a plant or an anatomic structure. [L. summit]

cac·u·mi·nal (kak-ū′mi-năl). Relating to a top or apex, particularly of a plant or anatomical structure.

ca·dav·er (kă-dav′er). A dead body. SYN corpse. [L. fr. *cado,* to fall]

ca·dav·er·ic (kă-dav′er-ik). Relating to a dead body.

ca·dav·er·ine (kă-dav′er-in). 1,5-Pentanediamine; 1,5-diaminopentane; a foul-smelling diamine formed by bacterial decarboxylation of lysine; poisonous and irritating to the skin; found in decaying meat and fish.

ca·dav·er·ous (kă-dav′er-ŭs). Having the pallor and appearance resembling a corpse.

cade oil (kād). SYN *juniper* tar.

cad·her·in (kad-hēr′-in). One of a class of integral-membrane glycoproteins that has a role in cell-cell adhesion and is important in morphogenesis and differentiation; E-c. is also known as uvomorulin and is concentrated in the belt desmosome in epithelial cells; N-c. is found in nerve, muscle, and lens cells helps maintain

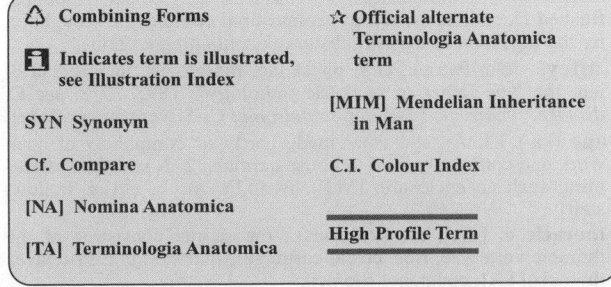

△ **Combining Forms**	☆ **Official alternate Terminologia Anatomica term**
🔲 Indicates term is illustrated, see Illustration Index	**[MIM] Mendelian Inheritance in Man**
SYN Synonym	
Cf. Compare	**C.I. Colour Index**
[NA] Nomina Anatomica	
[TA] Terminologia Anatomica	**High Profile Term**

the integrity of neuronal aggregates; P-c. is expressed in placental and epidermal cells. [cell + adhere + -in]

cad·mi·um (Cd) (kad′mē-ŭm). A metallic element, atomic no. 48, atomic wt. 112.411; its salts are poisonous and little used in medicine. Various compounds of c. are used commercially in metallurgy, photography, electrochemistry, etc.; a few have been used as ascaricides, antiseptics, and fungicides. [L. *cadmia,* fr. G. *kadmeia* or *kadmia,* an ore of zinc, calamine]

ca·du·ca (kă-doo′kă). SYN deciduous *membrane.* [L. fem. of *caducus,* fallen, falling]

🔲**ca·du·ce·us** (kă-doo′sē-ŭs). A staff with two oppositely twined serpents and surmounted by two wings; emblem of the U.S. Army Medical Corps. For veterinary medicine the double serpent was changed in 1972 to its present form with a single serpent. SEE ALSO staff of Aesculapius. [L. the staff of Mercury; G. *kēryx* herald, the staff of Hermes]

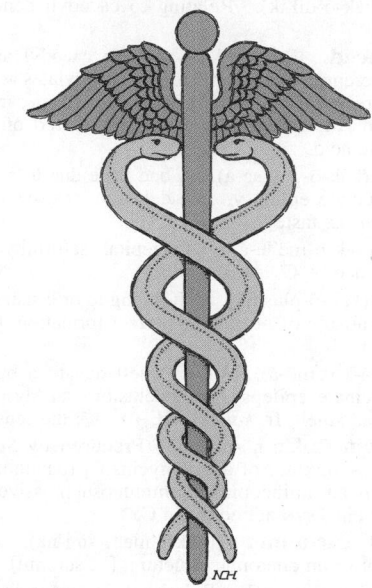

caduceus

⌒**cae-.** For words so beginning, see under ce-.

caecum. SYN cecum.

caf·fe·a·rine (kaf′ē-ă-rin). SYN trigonelline.

caf·feine (kaf′ēn). An alkaloid obtained from the dried leaves of *Thea sinensis,* tea, or the dried seeds of *Coffea arabica,* coffee; used as a central nervous system stimulant, diuretic, circulatory and respiratory stimulant, and as an adjunct in the treatment of headaches. SYN guaranine, thein.

c. citrate, citrated c., a mixture of equal parts of c. and citric acid; more water soluble than caffeine.

c. hydrate, monohydrate of c., a central nervous system stimulant.

c. and sodium salicylate, a mixture of sodium salicylate and c. formerly used for the relief of headache and neuralgia.

caf·fein·ism (kaf′ēn-izm). Caffeine intoxication characterized by restlessness, tremulousness, nervousness, excitement, insomnia, flushed face, diuresis, and gastrointestinal complaints, brought on by the ingestion of excess substances containing caffeine.

Caffey, John Patrick, U.S. physician, radiologist, and pediatrician, the "the father of pediatric radiology", 1895–1978. SEE C. *disease, syndrome;* C.-Kempe *syndrome;* C.-Silverman *syndrome.*

cage (kāj). **1.** An enclosure made partly or completely of open work and commonly used to house animals. **2.** A structure resembling such an enclosure. [M.E., fr. O.Fr., fr. L. *cavea,* hollow, stall]

thoracic c. [TA], the skeleton of the thorax consisting of the thoracic vertebrae, ribs, costal cartilages, and sternum. SYN cavea thoracis [TA], compages thoracis.

Cajal (Ramón y Cajal), Santiago, Spanish histologist and 1906 Nobel laureate, 1852–1934. SEE C. *cell;* horizontal *cell* of C.; C. astrocyte *stain;* interstitial *nucleus* of C.

caj·e·put oil, caj·u·put oil (kaj′ĕ-pŭt, -ū-pŭt). A volatile oil distilled from the fresh leaves of *Cajuputi viridiflora,* a tree of tropical Asia and Australia; a stimulant, counterirritant, and expectorant.

caj·e·put·ol, caj·u·put·ol (kaj′ĕ-pū-tol, -ŭ-pū-tol). SYN cineole.

Cal Abbreviation for large *calorie.*

cal Abbreviation for small *calorie.*

Cal·a·bar bean (kal′ă-bar bēn). SYN physostigma.

cal·a·mine (kal′ă-mīn). Zinc oxide with a small amount of ferric oxide or basic zinc carbonate suitably colored with ferric oxide; used in dusting powders, lotions, and ointments, as a mild astringent and protective agent for skin disorders. [Mediev. L. *calamina,* fr. L. *cadmia,* fr. G. *kadmia,* Theban (earth), fr. *Kadmos,* founder of Thebes]

cal·a·mus (kal′ă-mŭs). **1.** The dried, unpeeled rhizome of *Acorus calamus* (family Araceae), cultivated in Myanmar and Sri Lanka, a carminative and anthelminthic. **2.** A reed-shaped structure. [L. reed, a pen]

c. scripto′rius, inferior part of the rhomboid fossa; the narrow lower end of the fourth ventricle between the two clavae. SYN Arantius ventricle. [L. writing pen]

cal·ca·ne·al, cal·ca·ne·an (kal-kā′nē-al, kal-kā′nē-an). Relating to the calcaneus or heel bone.

⌒**calcaneo-.** The calcaneus. [L. *calcaneum,* heel]

cal·ca·ne·o·aph·y·si·tis (kal-kā′nē-ō-ă-pof-i-sī′tis). Inflammation at the posterior part of the os calcis, at the insertion of the Achilles tendon.

cal·ca·ne·o·as·trag·a·loid (kal-kā′nē-ō-as-trag′ă-loyd). Relating to the calcaneus, or os calcis, and the talus, or astragalus.

cal·ca·ne·o·cav·us (kal-ka′nē-ō-kā′vus). Combination of talipes calcaneus and talipes cavus.

cal·ca·ne·o·cu·boid (kal-kā′nē-ō-kū′boyd). Relating to the calcaneus and the cuboid bone.

cal·can·e·o·dyn·ia (kal-kā′nē-ō-din′ē-ă). SYN painful *heel.* [calcaneo- + G. *odynē,* pain]

cal·ca·ne·o·na·vic·u·lar (kal-kā′nē-ō-na-vik′ū-lăr). Relating to the calcaneus and the navicular bone. SYN calcaneoscaphoid.

cal·ca·ne·o·scaph·oid (kal-kā′nē-ō-skaf′oyd). SYN calcaneonavicular.

cal·ca·ne·o·tib·i·al (kal-kā′nē-ō-tib′ē-ăl). Relating to the calcaneus and the tibia.

cal·ca·ne·o·val·go·cav·us (kal-ka′nē-ō-val′-go-kā′vus). Combination of talipes calcaneus, valgus, and cavus.

cal·ca·ne·o·val·gus (kal-kā′nē-ō-val′gŭs). SEE *talipes* calcaneovalgus.

cal·ca·ne·o·var·us (kal-kā′nē-ō-vā′rŭs). SEE *talipes* calcaneovarus.

cal·ca·ne·um (kal-kā′nē-ŭm). SYN calcaneus (1). [L. the heel]

cal·ca·ne·us, gen. and pl. **cal·ca·nei** (kal-kā′nē-ŭs, -kā′nē-ī). **1** [TA]. The largest of the tarsal bones; it forms the heel and articulates with the cuboid anteriorly and the talus above. SYN calcaneal bone, calcaneum, heel bone, os calcis. **2.** SYN *talipes* calcaneus. [L. the heel (another form of *calcaneum*)]

cal·car (kal′kar) [TA]. **1.** A small projection from any structure; internal spurs (septa) at the level of division of arteries and confluence of veins where branches or roots form an acute angle. SEE ALSO vascular *spur.* **2.** A dull spine or projection from a bone. SYN spur [TA]. [L. spur, cock's spur]

c. a′vis [TA], SYN calcarine *spur.*

c. femora′le, a bony spur springing from the underside of the neck of the femur above and anterior to the lesser trochanter, adding to the strength of this part of the bone. SYN Bigelow septum.

c. pedis, SYN calx (2).

c. sclerae [TA], SYN scleral *spur.*

cal·car·e·ous (kal-kā′rē-ŭs). Chalky; relating to or containing lime or calcium, or calcific material. [L. *calcarius*, pertaining to lime, fr. *calx*, lime]

cal·ca·rine (kal'kă-rēn). **1.** Relating to a calcar. **2.** Spur-shaped.

cal·car·i·u·ria (kal-kar-ē-ū'rē-ă). Excretion of calcium (lime) salts in the urine. [L. *calcarius*, of lime, + G. *ouron*, urine]

cal·cer·gy (kal'ser-jē). Local calcification of soft tissue occurring at the site of injection of certain chemical compounds, such as lead acetate or cerium chloride; hydroxyapatite deposits are found in the calcified areas. [L. *calx*, chalk, calcium, + G. *ergon*, work, production]

cal·ces (kal'sēz). Plural of calx.

cal·cic (kal'sik). Relating to lime.

cal·ci·co·sis (kal-si-kō'sis). Pneumoconiosis from the inhalation of limestone dust.

cal·ci·di·ol (kal-sĭ-dī'ol). 25-Hydroxycholecalciferol (a 3,25-diol); the first step in the biologic conversion of vitamin D_3 to the more active form, calcitriol; it is more potent than vitamin D_3. SYN 25-hydroxycholecalciferol, calcifediol.

c. 1α-hydroxylase, 25-hydroxycholecalciferol 1α-hydroxylase, the monooxygenase that forms calcitriol from c. using O_2 and NADPH; a deficiency in this enzyme can result in features of a vitamin D deficiency.

cal·ci·fe·di·ol (kal-sĭ-fĕ-dī'ol). SYN calcidiol.

cal·cif·er·ol (kal-sif'er-ol). SYN ergocalciferol.

cal·cif·er·ous (kal-sif'er-ŭs). **1.** Containing lime. **2.** Producing any of the salts of calcium. SYN calcophorous.

cal·cif·ic (kal-sif'ik). Forming or depositing calcium salts.

cal·ci·fi·ca·tion (kal'si-fi-kā'shŭn). **1.** Deposition of lime or other insoluble calcium salts. **2.** A process in which tissue or noncellular material in the body becomes hardened as the result of precipitates or larger deposits of insoluble salts of calcium (and also magnesium), especially calcium carbonate and phosphate (hydroxyapatite) normally occurring only in the formation of bone and teeth. SYN calcareous infiltration. [L. *calx*, lime, + *facio*, to make]

dystrophic c., c. occurring in degenerated or necrotic tissue, as in hyalinized scars, degenerated foci in leiomyomas, and caseous nodules.

eggshell c., a thin layer of c. around an intrathoracic lymph node, usually in silicosis, seen on a chest radiograph.

metastatic c., c. occurring in nonosseous, viable tissue (i.e., tissue that is not degenerated or necrotic), as in the stomach, lungs, and kidneys (and rarely in other sites); the cells of these organs secrete acid materials and, under certain conditions in instances of hypercalcemia, the alteration in pH causes precipitation of calcium salts in these sites.

Mönckeberg c., SYN Mönckeberg *arteriosclerosis*.

Mönckeberg medial c., SYN Mönckeberg *arteriosclerosis*.

pathologic c., c. occurring in excretory or secretory passages as calculi, and in tissues other than bone and teeth.

pulp c., SYN endolith.

cal·ci·fy (kal'si-fī). To deposit or lay down calcium salts, as in the formation of bone.

cal·cig·er·ous (kal-sij'er-us). Producing or carrying calcium salts. [calcium + L. *gero*, to bear]

cal·ci·na·tion (kal-si-nā'shŭn). The process of calcining.

cal·cine (kal'sēn). To expel water and volatile matter by heat.

cal·ci·neu·rin (kal-sē-noor'in). A calcium-dependent serine-threonine phosphatase involved in T-cell signaling transcription; the reaction cascade in which it resides is referred to as the calcineurin pathway. [calcium + G. *neuron*, nerve, + -in]

cal·ci·no·sis (kal-si-nō'sis). A condition characterized by the deposition of calcium salts in nodular foci in various tissues other than the parenchymatous viscera; the two well-known forms, c. circumscripta and c. universalis, are not associated with tissue damage or demonstrable metabolic disease; other forms are the result of abnormal calcium and/or phosphorous metabolism. SEE metastatic *calcification*. [calcium + *-osis*, condition]

c. circumscrip'ta, localized deposits of calcium salts in the skin and subcutaneous tissues, usually surrounded by a zone of granu-

lomatous inflammation; clinically, the lesions resemble the tophi of gout.

c. cu'tis, a deposit of calcium in the skin; usually occurs secondary to a preexisting inflammatory, degenerative, or neoplastic dermatosis, and is frequently seen in scleroderma. SEE metastatic *calcification*. SYN dystrophic c.

dystrophic c., SYN c. cutis.

c. intervertebra'lis, calcium deposit in vertebral disk.

reversible c., a form of c. that can be reversed, as is observed in patients who constantly ingest large quantities of milk and alkaline medicines, as in the treatment of peptic ulcer. SEE ALSO milkalkali *syndrome*.

tumoral c., (1) calcification of collagen, chiefly at the site of large joints, in South African blacks; probably genetic. (2) c. that develops in association with neoplastic conditions.

c. universa'lis, diffuse deposits of calcium salts in the skin and subcutaneous tissues, connective tissue, and other sites; may be associated with dermatomyositis, occurs more frequently in young persons, and is often fatal; serum levels of calcium and phosphorus are generally within normal limits.

cal·ci·o·ki·ne·sis (kal'sē-ō-ki-nē'sis). Mobilization of stored calcium. [calcium + G. *kinēsis*, motion]

cal·ci·o·ki·net·ic (kal'sē-ō-ki-net'ik). Pertaining to or causing calciokinesis.

cal·ci·ol (kal'sē-ol). SYN cholecalciferol.

cal·ci·or·rha·chia (kal'sē-ō-ra'kē-ă). The presence of calcium in the cerebrospinal fluid. [calcium + G. *rhachis*, spine + -ia]

cal·ci·o·stat (kal'sē-ō-stat). Rarely used term denoting a postulated mechanism by which the parathyroid hormone production is increased when serum calcium is low and decreased when it is high. [calcium + G. *statos*, standing]

cal·ci·o·trau·mat·ic (kal'sē-ō-traw-mat'ik). Relating to the line of disturbed calcification that appears in the dentin of the incisor teeth of young rats placed on a rachitogenic diet: high in calcium and low in phosphorus, with no vitamin D.

cal·ci·pec·tic (kal-si-pek'tik). Pertaining to calcipexis.

cal·ci·pe·nia (kal-si-pē'nē-ă). A condition in which there is an insufficient amount of calcium in the tissues and fluids of the body. [calcium + G. *penia*, poverty]

cal·ci·pe·nic (kal-si-pē'nik). Pertaining to calcipenia.

cal·ci·pex·ic (kal-si-pek'sik). Related or pertaining to calcipexis.

cal·ci·pex·is, cal·ci·pexy (kal-si-pek'sis, kal'si-pek-sē). Fixation of calcium in the tissues, an occasional cause of tetany in infants. [calcium + G. *pēxis*, a fixing]

cal·ci·phil·ia (cal-si-fil'ē-ă). A condition in which the tissues manifest an unusual affinity for, and fixation of, calcium salts circulating in the blood. [calcium + G. *phileō*, to love]

cal·ci·phy·lax·is (kal'sī-fī-lak'sis). A condition of induced systemic hypersensitivity in which tissues respond to appropriate challenging agents with a sudden, but sometimes evanescent, local calcification.

cal·ci·priv·ia (kal-si-priv'ē-ă). Absence or deprivation of calcium in diet.

cal·ci·priv·ic (kal-si-priv'ik). Deprived of calcium.

cal·cite (kal'sīt). A naturally occurring mineral found in several forms, e.g., chalk, Iceland spar, limestone, marble. SEE ALSO *calcium* carbonate. SYN calcspar.

cal·ci·tet·rol (kal-si-tet'rol). The 1,24,25-triol (thus, a 1,3,24,24-tetrol) of cholecalciferol; the inactivation product of calcitriol.

cal·ci·to·nin (kal-si-tō'nin). A peptide hormone, of which eight forms in five species are known; composed of 32 amino acids and produced by the parathyroid, thyroid, and thymus glands; its action is opposite to that of parathyroid hormone in that c. increases deposition of calcium and phosphate in bone and lowers the level of calcium in the blood; its level in the blood is increased by glucagon and by Ca^{2+} and thus opposes postprandial hypercalcemia. SYN thyrocalcitonin. [calci- + G. *tonos*, stretching, + -in]

cal·ci·tri·ol (kal-si-trī'ol). 1α,25-Dihydroxycholecalciferol (thus, a 1,3,25-triol); formation of c. is the second step in the biological conversion of vitamin D_3 to its active form; it is more potent than calcidiol.

CALCIUM

cal·ci·um (Ca), gen. **cal·´cii** (kal′sē-ŭm, -sē-ī). A metallic bivalent element; atomic no. 20, atomic wt. 40.078, density 1.55, melting point 842°C. The oxide of c. is an alkaline earth, CaO, quicklime, which on the addition of water becomes c. hydrate, Ca(OH)$_2$, slaked lime. For some organic c. salts not listed below, see the name of the organic acid portion. Many c. salts have crucial uses in metabolism and in medicine. C. salts are responsible for the radiopacity of bone, calcified cartilage, and arteriosclerotic plaques in arteries. [Mod. L. fr. L. *calx,* lime]

c. alginate, a topical hemostatic.

c. aminosalicylate, the c. salt of *p*-aminosalicylic acid, with the same uses.

c. benzoylpas, an antituberculous agent.

c. bromide, used to meet the same indications as potassium bromide.

c. carbide, blackish crystalline lumps that when in contact with water yield acetylene gas.

c. carbimide, a fertilizer and weed seed killer that also exhibits antithyroid activity; like disulfiram, it impairs ethanol metabolism; workers in cyanamide-producing plants exhibit systemic symptoms ("Monday-morning illness") after ingestion of alcohol. SYN c. cyanamide.

c. carbonate, an astringent, antacid, and calcium dietary supplement. SEE ALSO calcite. SYN chalk, creta.

c. caseinate, the form of casein present in cow's milk; used in dietetic preparations; has been used for diarrhea in infants.

c. chloride, used to correct calcium deficiencies and in the treatment of magnesium intoxication and cardiac failure.

citrated c. carbimide, a mixture of two parts citric acid to one part c. carbimide; in the metabolism of ethanol, it slows the conversion of acetaldehyde to acetate; used in the treatment of alcoholism.

crude c. sulfide, used externally in the treatment of acne, scabies, and ringworm. SYN sulfurated lime.

c. cyanamide, SYN c. carbimide.

dibasic c. phosphate, used as a c. and phosphorus dietary supplement. SYN c. monohydrogen phosphate, secondary c. phosphate.

c. folinate, SYN *leucovorin* calcium.

c. glubionate, a calcium replenisher.

c. gluceptate, used as a nutrient. SYN c. glucoheptonate.

c. glucoheptonate, SYN c. gluceptate.

c. gluconate, a salt of c. more palatable than the chloride, sometimes used as a calcium supplement.

c. glycerophosphate, a c. and phosphorus dietary supplement.

c. hippurate, said to be a solvent of uratic gravel and calculi.

c. hydroxide, used as a carbon dioxide absorbent.

c. hypophosphite, has been used for rickets and impaired nutrition.

c. iodate, used as a dusting powder and, in lotion and ointment, as an antiseptic and deodorant.

c. iodobehenate, a c. salt, $(C_{21}H_{42}ICOO)_2Ca$, formerly used to meet the indications of the ordinary iodides.

c. ipodate, a radiopaque medium used in cholangiography and cholecystography.

c. lactate, used as a calcium replenisher.

c. lactophosphate, a mixture of c. lactate, c. acid lactate, and c. acid phosphate; used as a c. and phosphorus dietary supplement.

c. leucovorin, SEE *leucovorin* calcium.

c. levulinate, a hydrated c. salt of levulinic acid; it has the usual effects of c. administered orally or intravenously.

c. mandelate, c. salt of mandelic acid; a urinary anti-infective agent.

milk of c., densely calcified fluid, most often found radiographically in the gallbladder in association with chronic obstruction.

c. monohydrogen phosphate, SYN dibasic c. phosphate.

c. oxalate, found as sediment in the urine and in urinary calculi. Toxic end product of ethylene glycol consumption.

c. oxide, SYN lime (1).

c. pantothenate, the c. salt of pantothenic acid; a vitamin B filtrate factor.

precipitated c. carbonate, used as an antacid in the management of peptic ulcers and other conditions of gastric hyperacidity.

c. propionate, the c. salt of propionic acid; an antifungal agent.

racemic c. pantothenate, a mixture of the c. salts of the dextrorotatory and levorotatory isomers of pantothenic acid; same uses as c. pantothenate.

c. saccharate, used as an antacid in dyspepsia and flatulence, as an antidote in carbolic acid poisoning, and as a stabilizer for c. gluconate solution for parenteral administration.

secondary c. phosphate, SYN dibasic c. phosphate.

c. stearate, a soap used in the preparation of tablets as a lubricant for tablet machinery and to keep powder mixtures flowing.

c. sulfate, CaO$_4$S; used in exsiccated form to make plaster of Paris. SEE ALSO gypsum.

c. sulfite, used as an intestinal antiseptic, and locally in the treatment of parasitic skin diseases.

tertiary c. phosphate, SYN tribasic c. phosphate.

tribasic c. phosphate, used as an antacid. SYN bone ash, bone phosphate, tertiary c. phosphate, tricalcium phosphate, whitlockite.

c. trisodium pentetate, SYN pentetate trisodium calcium.

---

cal·ci·um-45 (^{45}Ca). Most easily available of the radioactive c.-45 isotopes; beta-emitter with a half-life of 162.7 days; used as a tracer.

cal·ci·um-47 (^{47}Ca). A radioisotope of calcium with a half-life of 4.54 days, used in the diagnosis of disorders of calcium metabolism.

cal·ci·um group. The metals of the alkaline earths: beryllium, magnesium, calcium, strontium, barium, and radium.

cal·ci·u·ria (kal-sē-ū′rē-ă). The urinary excretion of calcium; sometimes used as a synonym for hypercalciuria.

cal·coph·or·ous (kal-kof′er-ŭs). SYN calciferous. [L. *calx,* lime, + G. *phoros,* bearing]

cal·co·sphe·rite (kal-kō-sfēr′īt). A tiny, spheroidal, concentrically laminated body containing accretive deposits of calcium salts; found most frequently in papillary carcinoma of the thyroid and ovary, and in meningioma, probably as the result of degenerative changes in the fibrovascular stroma. SYN psammoma bodies (3). [L. *calx,* lime, + G. *sphaira,* sphere]

calc·spar (kalk′spar). SYN calcite.

cal·cu·li (kal′kū-lī). Plural of calculus.

cal·cu·lo·sis (kal-kū-lō′sis). The tendency or disposition to form calculi or stones. [L. *calculus,* small stone, + G. *-osis,* condition]

cal·cu·lus, gen. and pl. **cal·cu·li** (kal′kū-lŭs, -lī). A concretion formed in any part of the body, most commonly in the passages of the biliary and urinary tracts; usually composed of salts of inorganic or organic acids, or of other material such as cholesterol. SYN stone (1). [L. a pebble, a calculus]

apatite c., a c. in which the crystalloid component consists of calcium fluorophosphate.

arthritic c., SYN gouty *tophus.*

biliary c., SYN gallstone.

bladder c., SYN bladder *stone,* under *stone.*

blood c., an angiolith or concretion of coagulated blood. SYN hemic c.

branched c., SYN staghorn c.

bronchial c., SYN broncholith.

cerebral c., SYN encephalolith.

coral c., SYN staghorn c.

cystine c., a c. composed of cystine, soft and faintly radiopaque.

dendritic c., SYN staghorn c.

dental c., (1) calcified deposits formed around the teeth; may appear as subgingival or supragingival c.; **(2)** SYN tartar (2).

encysted c., a urinary c. enclosed in a sac developed from the wall of the bladder. SYN pocketed c.

fibrin c., a urinary c. formed largely from fibrinogen in blood.

gastric c., SYN gastrolith.

hematogenetic c., SYN serumal c. (1).

hemic c., SYN blood c.

infection c., SYN secondary renal c.

intestinal c., a concretion in the bowel, either a coprolith or an enterolith.

lacrimal c., SYN dacryolith.

mammary c., a concretion in one of the ducts of the breast.

matrix c., a yellowish-white to light tan urinary c. containing calcium salts, with the consistency of putty; composed chiefly of an organic matrix consisting of a mucoprotein and a sulfated mucopolysaccharide, and usually associated with chronic infection.

metabolic c., a stone, usually a renal stone, caused by a metabolic abnormality resulting in increased excretion of a substance of low solubility in urine, such as urate or cystine.

mulberry c., a hard nodular urinary c. composed of calcium oxalate, so-called because of its resemblance to a mulberry.

nasal c., SYN rhinolith.

oxalate c., a hard urinary c. of calcium oxalate; some are covered with minute sharp spines that can abrade the renal pelvic epithelium, whereas others are smooth.

pancreatic c., a concretion, usually multiple, in the pancreatic duct, associated with chronic pancreatitis. SYN pancreatolith, pancreolith.

pharyngeal c., SYN pharyngolith.

pleural c., SYN pleurolith.

pocketed c., SYN encysted c.

preputial c., a c. occurring beneath the foreskin. SYN postholith.

primary renal c., a c. formed in an apparently healthy urinary tract, usually composed of oxalates, urates, or cystine.

prostatic c., a concretion formed in the prostate gland, composed chiefly of calcium carbonate and phosphate (corpora amylacea). SYN prostatolith.

pulp c., SYN endolith.

renal c., a c. occurring within the kidney collecting system. SYN nephrolith.

salivary c., a c. in a salivary duct or gland.

secondary renal c., a c. associated with infection and/or obstruction, usually composed of struvite (magnesium ammonium phosphate). SYN infection c.

serumal c., (1) a greenish or dark brown calcareous deposit on the tooth, usually apical to the gingival margin; SYN hematogenetic c. **(2)** SYN subgingival c.

staghorn c., a c. occurring in the renal pelvis, with branches extending into the infundibula and calices. SYN branched c., coral c., dendritic c.

struvite c., a c. in which the crystalloid component consists of magnesium ammonium phosphate; usually associated with urinary tract infection caused by urease-producing bacteria.

subgingival c., calcareous deposit found on the tooth apical to the gingival margin. SYN serumal c. (2).

supragingival c., calcified plaques adherent to tooth surfaces coronal to the free gingival margin.

tonsillar c., SYN tonsillolith.

urethral c., a stone impacted in urethra. May have formed proximally and become stuck there or may have formed in urethra; uncommon.

urinary c., a c. in the kidney, ureter, bladder, or urethra. SYN urolith.

uterine c., a calcified myoma of the uterus. SYN uterolith.

vesical c., a urinary c. formed or retained in the bladder. SYN cystolith.

weddellite c., a c. in which the crystalloid component consists of calcium oxalate dihydrate.

whewellite c., a c. in which the crystalloid component consists of calcium oxalate monohydrate.

Cal·cu·lus Sur·face In·dex (CSI). An index that measures only dental calculus, used for evaluating new calculus formation within a large group of test subjects.

Caldani, Leopoldo M.A., Italian anatomist, 1725–1813. SEE C. *ligament.*

cal·des·mon (kal-des′mon). An F-actin cross-linking protein that, at low or absent calcium levels, binds to tropomyosin and actin and prevents myosin binding. [calcium + G. *desmos,* bond, fr. *deō,* to bind]

Caldwell, Eugene W., U.S. radiologist, 1870–1918. SEE C. *projection, view.*

Caldwell, George W., U.S. otolaryngologist, 1834–1918. SEE C.-Luc *operation.*

Caldwell, William E., U.S. obstetrician, 1880–1943. SEE C.-Moloy *classification.*

cal·e·fa·cient (kal-ĕ-fā′shent). **1.** Making warm or hot. **2.** An agent causing a sense of warmth in the part to which it is applied. [L. *calefacio,* fr. *caleo,* to be warm, + *facio,* to make]

calf, pl. **calves** (kaf, kavz). A young bovine animal, male or female. [Gael. *kalpa*]

calf-bone. 1. SYN fibula. **2.** Bone from a calf (young cow) used in orthopedic reconstruction.

cal·i·ber (kal′i-ber). The diameter of a hollow tubular structure. [Fr. *calibre,* of uncert. etym.]

cal·i·brate (kal′i-brāt). **1.** To graduate or standardize any measuring instrument. **2.** To measure the diameter of a tubular structure.

cal·i·bra·tion (kal-i-brā′shŭn). The act of standardizing or calibrating an instrument or laboratory procedure.

cal·i·bra·tor (kal′i-brā-ter, -tōr). A standard or reference material or substance used to standardize or calibrate an instrument or laboratory procedure.

cal·i·ce·al (kal′i-se′al). Relating to the calix. SYN calyceal.

cal·i·cec·ta·sis (kal-i-sek′tă-sis). SYN caliectasis. [calix + G. *ektasis,* dilation]

cal·i·cec·to·my (kal-i-sek′tō-me). SYN calicotomy. [calix, + G. *ektomē,* excision]

ca·li·ces (kal′i-sēz). Plural of calix.

cal·ic·i·form (kă-lis′i-fōrm). Shaped like a cup or goblet. SYN calyciform. [L. *calix* + *forma,* form]

cal·i·cine (kal′i-sēn). Of the nature of, or resembling a calix. SYN calycine.

Cal·i·ci·vi·ri·dae (kal′i-sē-vī′ră-dē). A family of naked icosahedral single-stranded positive sense RNA viruses 30–38 mm in diameter associated with epidemic viral gastroenteritis and certain forms of hepatitis in humans.

Ca·lic·i·vi·rus (kă-lis′i-vī′rŭs). A genus in the family Caliciviridae that is associated with gastroenteritis. SEE hepatitis E *virus,* Norwalk *agent.* [G. *kalyx,* cup, + virus]

ca·li·co·plas·ty (kā′lĭ-sō-plas-tē). SYN calioplasty. [calix, + G. *plastos,* formed]

cal·i·cot·o·my (kal-ĭ-sot′ō-me). Incision into a calix, usually for removal of a calculus. SYN calicectomy, caliotomy. [calix, + G. *tomē,* a cutting]

ca·lic·u·lus, pl. **ca·lic·u·li** (kă-lik′ū-lŭs, lī). A bud-shaped or cup-shaped structure, resembling the closed calyx of a flower. SYN calycle, calyculus. [L. dim. from G. *kalyx,* the cup of a flower]

c. gustato′rius, SYN taste *bud.*

c. ophthal′micus, SYN optic *cup.*

ca·li·ec·ta·sis (kā-lē-ek′tă-sis). Dilation of the calices, usually due to obstruction or infection. SYN calicectasis, pyelocaliectasis.

cal·i·for·ni·um (Cf) (kal-i-fōr′nē-ŭm). An artificial transuranium element, symbol Cf, atomic no. 98, atomic wt. 251.08; half-life of ^{251}Cf (the most stable known isotope) is 900 years. [*California,* state and university where first prepared]

ca·li·o·plas·ty (kā′lē-ō-plas-tē). Surgical reconstruction of a calix, usually designed to increase its lumen at the infundibulum. SYN calicoplasty.

ca·li·or·rha·phy (kā′lē-ōr-a-fē). **1.** Suturing of a calix. **2.** Plastic surgery of a dilated or obstructed calix to improve urinary drain-

ca

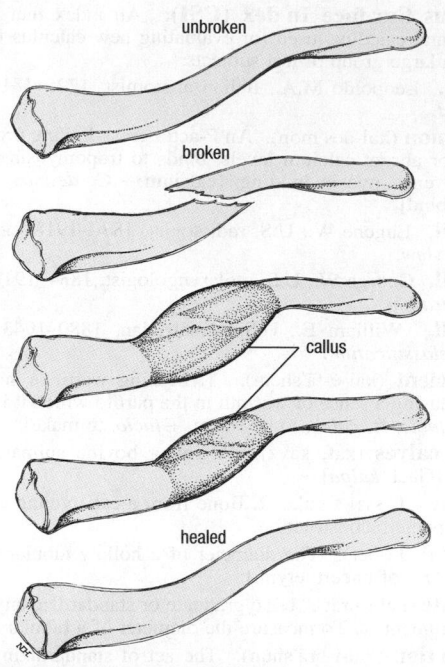

unbroken

broken

callus

healed

callus: part of the bone-fracture healing process

age, often requiring combination of two or more calices or the massive movement of renal pelvic mucosa to rebuild the caliceal drainage system. [calix, + G. *rhaphē,* suture, seam]

ca·li·ot·o·my (kā-lē-ot′ō-mē). SYN calicotomy.

cal·i·pers (kal′i-perz). An instrument used for measuring diameters. [a corruption of *caliber*]

cal·is·then·ics (kal-is-then′iks). Systematic practice of various exercises with the object of preserving health and increasing physical strength. [G. *kalos,* beautiful, + *sthenos,* strength]

ca·lix, pl. **ca·li·ces** (kā′liks, kal′i-sēz). A flower-shaped or funnel-shaped structure; specifically one of the branches or recesses of the pelvis of the kidney into which the orifices of the malpighian renal pyramids project. SYN calyx. [L. fr. G. *kalyx,* the cup of a flower]

major calices, the primary subdivisions of the renal pelvis, usually two or three in number. SYN calices renales majores.

minor calices, the subdivisions of the major calices, varying in number from 7–13, which receive the renal papillae. SYN calices renales minores.

calices rena′les majo′res, SYN major calices.

calices rena′les mino′res, SYN minor calices.

Calkins, Leroy Adelbert, U.S. obstetrician-gynecologist, 1894–1960. SEE C. *sign.*

Call, Friedrich von, Austrian physician, 1844–1917. SEE C.-Exner *bodies,* under *body.*

Callahan, John R., U.S. endodontist, 1853–1918. SEE C. *method.*

Callander, Latimer, San Francisco surgeon, 1892–1947. SEE C. *amputation.*

Calleja (Calleja y Sanchez), Camilo, Spanish anatomist, †1913. SEE *islands* of C., under *island.*

Cal·liph·o·ra (kă-lif′ō-ră). A genus of blowflies (family Calliphoridae, order Diptera), the bluebottle flies, the larvae of which feed on dead flesh. *C. vomitoria* and *C. vicina* are common species in the U.S. [G. *kalli,* beauty, + *phoros,* bearing]

Callison, James S., U.S. physician, *1873. SEE C. *fluid.*

Cal·li·tro·ga (kal-i-trō′gă). Former name for *Cochliomyia.*

cal·lo·sal (ka-lō′săl). Relating to the corpus callosum.

cal·lose (kal′ōs). A linear 1,3-β-D-glucan formed by certain enzymes from UDP-glucose, differing from cellulose (a β-1,4-glu-

can formed from GDP-glucose) and starch amylose (an α-1,4-glucan formed from ADP-glucose). Found in certain plant cell walls.

cal·los·i·ty (ka-los′i-tē). A circumscribed thickening of the keratin layer of the epidermis as a result of repeated friction or intermittent pressure. SYN callus (1), keratoma (1), poroma (1). [L. fr. *callosus,* thick-skinned]

cal·lo·so·mar·gin·al (ka-lō′sō-mar′jin-ăl). Relating to the corpus callosum and the cingulate gyrus; denoting the sulcus between them. SEE ALSO *sulcus* of corpus callosum.

cal·lous (kal′ŭs). Relating to a callus or callosity.

⊞ cal·lus (kal′ŭs). **1.** SYN callosity. **2.** A composite mass of tissue that forms at a fracture site to establish continuity between the bone ends; it is composed initially of uncallused fibrous tissue and cartilage, and ultimately of bone. [L. hard skin]

central c., the c. within the medullary cavity of a fractured bone. SYN medullary c.

definitive c., the c. which has become converted into osseous tissue. SYN permanent c.

ensheathing c., the mass of c. around the outside of the fractured bone.

medullary c., SYN central c.

permanent c., SYN definitive c.

provisional c., the c. that develops to keep the ends of the fractured bone in apposition; it is absorbed after union is complete. SYN temporary c.

temporary c., SYN provisional c.

calm·a·tive (kahl′mă-tiv). Calming, quieting; allaying excitement; denoting such an agent.

Calmette, Leon A., French bacteriologist, 1863–1933. SEE bacille C.-Guérin; bacillus C. *vaccine;* C. *test;* C.-Guérin *bacillus, vaccine.*

cal·mod·u·lin (kal-mod′ū-lin). A small, ubiquitous eukaryotic protein that binds calcium ions, thereby becoming the agent for many of the cellular effects long ascribed to calcium ions. This calcium-protein complex binds to the apoenzyme, to form the holoenzyme, of certain phosphodiesterases; through these, or other as yet unknown mechanisms, the complex regulates adenylate and guanylate cyclases, many kinases, phospholipase A_2 activity, and other basic cellular functions. [*calcium* + *modul*ate]

Calodium (ka-lō′dē-oom). One of three trichurid nematode genera, commonly referred to as *Capillaria.*

cal·o·mel (kal′ō-mel). Mild mercury chloride; mercury monochloride, protochloride, or subchloride; has been used as an intestinal antiseptic and laxative; replaced by safer agents. SYN mercurous chloride, sweet precipitate. [Mediev. L., fr. G. *kalos,* beautiful, + *melas,* black]

vegetable c., SYN podophyllum.

ca·lor (kā′lōr). Heat, as one of the four signs of inflammation (c., rubor, tumor, dolor) enunciated by Celsus. [L.]

Calori, Luigi, Italian anatomist, 1807–1896. SEE C. *bursa.*

ca·lor·ic (kă-lōr′ik). **1.** Relating to a calorie. **2.** Relating to heat. [L. *calor,* heat]

c. intake, the total number of calories in a daily diet allocation.

cal·o·rie (kal′ō-rē). A unit of heat content or energy. The amount of heat necessary to raise 1 g of water from 14.5–15.5°C (small c.). Calorie is being replaced by joule, the SI unit equal to 0.239 calorie. SEE ALSO British thermal *unit.* SYN calory. [L. *calor,* heat]

gram c., SYN small c.

kilogram c. (kcal), SYN large c.

large c. (Cal, C), the quantity of energy required to raise the temperature of 1 kg of water 1°C (more precisely from 14.5°–15.5°C); it is 1000 times the value of the small c.; used in measurements of the heat production of chemical reactions, including those involved in biology. SYN kilocalorie, kilogram c.

mean c., one hundredth of the energy required to raise the temperature of 1 g of water from 0–100°C.

small c. (cal, c), the quantity of energy required to raise the temperature of 1 g of water 1°C, or from 14.5–15.5°C in the case of normal or standard c. SYN gram c.

cal·o·rif·ic (cal-ŏ-rif′ik). Producing heat. [L. *calor,* heat]

ca·lor·i·gen·ic (kă-lōr-i-jen'ik). **1.** Capable of generating heat. **2.** Stimulating metabolic production of heat. SYN thermogenetic (2), thermogenic. [L. *calor,* heat, + G. *genesis,* production]

cal·o·rim·e·ter (kal-ō-rim'ĕ-ter). An apparatus for measuring the amount of heat liberated in a chemical reaction. [L. *calor,* heat, + G. *metron,* measure]

Benedict-Roth c., SEE Benedict-Roth *apparatus.*

bomb c., an instrument for determining the potential energy of organic substances, including those in foods. It consists of a hollow steel container, lined with platinum and filled with pure oxygen, into which a weighed quantity of substance is placed and ignited with an electric fuse; the heat produced is absorbed by water surrounding the bomb and, from the rise in temperature, the calories liberated are calculated.

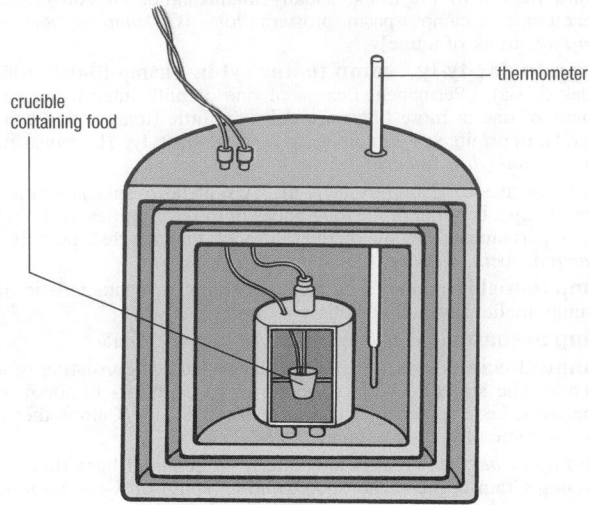

crucible containing food — thermometer

bomb calorimeter: measures heat produced by complete combustion of food sample

cal·o·ri·met·ric (kă'lōr-i-met'rik). Relating to calorimetry.

cal·o·rim·e·try (kal-ō-rim'ĕ-trē). Measurement of the amount of heat given off by a reaction or group of reactions (as by an organism).

direct c., measurement of the heat produced by a reaction, as distinguished from indirect methods, which involve measurement of something other than heat production itself.

indirect c., determination of heat production of an oxidation reaction by measuring uptake of oxygen and/or liberation of carbon dioxide and nitrogen excretion and then calculating the amount of heat produced.

ca·lor·i·tro·pic (kă-lōr'i-trop'ik). Relating to thermotropism.

cal·o·ry (kal'ō-rē). SYN calorie.

Calot, Jean-François, French surgeon, 1861–1944. SEE Calot *triangle.*

cal·pains (kal'pāns). Calcium-dependent thiol proteinases. These are cytoplasmic mammalian enzymes. [calcium + suffix *-pain,* protease, fr. *papain*]

cal·se·ques·trin (kal'sē-kwes'trin). A calcium-binding protein found in the interior of sarcoplasmic reticulum of muscles. It releases calcium ions at calcium channels. [calcium + sequester + -in]

ca·lum·ba (kă-lŭm'bă). The dried root of *Jateorrhiza palmata* (family Menispermaceae), a tall climbing vine of east Africa; used as a bitter tonic.

ca·lum·bin (kal'ŭm-bin). An amaroid from calumba that accounts for the bitterness of the crude drug.

cal·u·ster·one (kal-ū'stĕ-rōn). An antineoplastic agent.

cal·var·ia, pl. **cal·var·i·ae** (kal-vā'rē-ă, -vā'rē-ē) [TA]. The upper domelike portion of the skull. SYN roof of skull, skullcap. [L. a skull]

cal·var·i·al (kal-vār'ē-ăl). Relating to the skullcap.

cal·var·i·um (kal-vār'ē-ŭm). Incorrectly used for calvaria.

Calvé, Jacques, French orthopedic surgeon, 1875–1954. SEE C.-Perthes *disease;* Legg-C.-Perthes *disease.*

cal·vi·ti·es (kal-vish'e-ēz). SYN alopecia. [L. fr. *calvus,* bald]

calx, gen. **cal·cis,** pl. **cal·ces** (kalks, kal'sis, kal-sēs). **1.** SYN lime (1). [L. limestone] **2.** The posterior rounded extremity of the foot. SYN heel (2) [TA], calcar pedis. [L. heel]

cal·y·ce·al (kal'i-se'ăl). SYN caliceal.

ca·ly·ces (kal'i-sēz). Plural of calyx.

ca·lyc·i·form (kă-lis'i-fōrm). SYN caliciform.

ca·ly·cine (kal'i-sēn). SYN calicine.

ca·ly·cle, ca·lyc·u·lus (kal'i-kl, kă-lik'ū-lŭs). SYN caliculus.

Ca·lym·ma·to·bac·te·ri·um (kă-lim'mă-tō-bak-tēr'ē-ŭm). A genus of nonmotile bacteria (of uncertain taxonomic classification) containing Gram-negative, pleomorphic rods with single or bipolar condensations of chromatin; cells occur singly and in clusters. Outside the human body, growth occurs only in the yolk sac or amniotic fluid of a developing chick embryo or in a medium containing embryonic yolk; the organisms are pathogenic only for humans. The type species is *C. granulomatis.* [G. *kalymma,* hood, veil, + *baktērion,* rod]

C. granulo'matis, a bacterial species causing granulomatous lesions (granuloma inguinale or granuloma venereum) (donovanosis) in humans, particularly in the inguinal region; the type species of the genus *C.*

ca·lyx, pl. **ca·ly·ces** (kā'liks, kal'i-sēz). SYN calix. [G. cup of a flower]

CAM Abbreviation for cell adhesion *molecule.*

cam·ben·da·zole (kam-ben'dah-zōl). A anthelmintic.

cam·bi·um (kam'bē-ŭm). The inner layer of the periosteum in membranous ossification. [L. exchange]

cam·era, pl. **cam·er·ae, cam·er·as** (kam'er-ă, -ē) [TA]. **1.** SYN anterior *chamber* of eyeball. **2.** A closed box; especially one containing a lens, shutter, and light-sensitive film or plates for photography. [L. a vault]

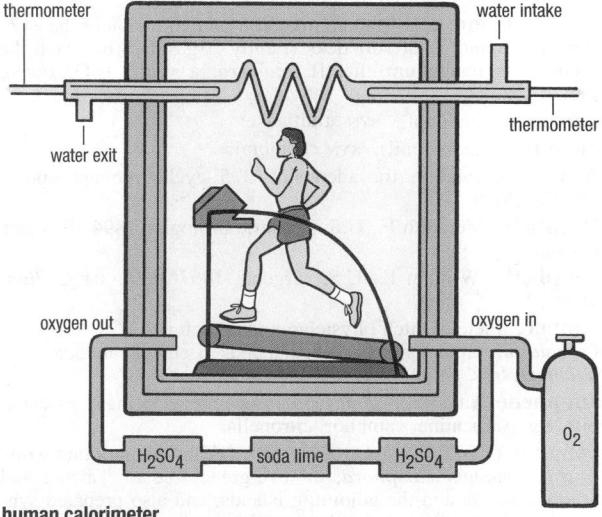

thermometer — water intake — thermometer — water exit — oxygen out — oxygen in — H_2SO_4 — soda lime — H_2SO_4 — O_2

human calorimeter

Anger c., a scintigraphic imaging system or type of gamma camera, employing a single thin crystal and multiple photodetecting circuits that views the entire field at once and is most effective in the 100- to 511-keV energy range.

c. ante'rior bul'bi [TA], SYN anterior *chamber* of eyeball.

camerae bulbi [TA], SYN *chambers* of eyeball, under *chamber.*

gamma c., any one of several scintigraphic cameras that simultaneously record counts from the entire field of view. SYN scintillation c.

multiformat c., photographic or laser printer for recording a

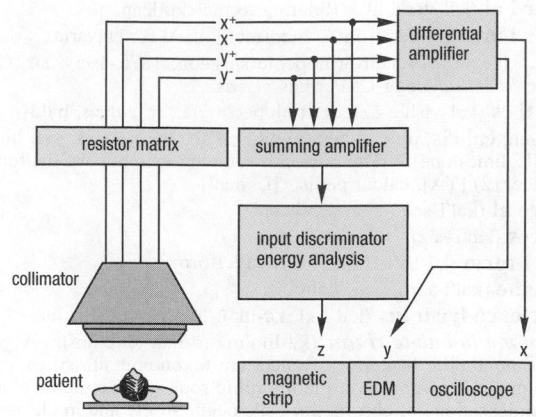

gamma camera (Anger camera) function: coordinate signals of only one photomultiplier are represented (EDM, electronic data management)

variable number of digital images on a sheet of film, as in computed tomography or ultrasound.

c. oc′uli ante′rior, SYN anterior *chamber* of eyeball.

c. oc′uli ma′jor, SYN anterior *chamber* of eyeball.

c. oc′uli mi′nor, SYN posterior *chamber* of eyeball.

c. oc′uli poste′rior, SYN posterior *chamber* of eyeball.

c. poste′rior bul′bi [TA], SYN posterior *chamber* of eyeball.

c. postrema [TA], SYN postremal *chamber* of eyeball.

retinal c., an instrument for photographing the ocular fundus.

scintillation c., SYN gamma c.

c. vitrea, ⋆official alternate term for postremal *chamber* of eyeball.

c. vi′trea bul′bi, ⋆official alternate term for postremal *chamber* of eyeball.

vitreous c., SYN postremal *chamber* of eyeball.

cam·er·o·stome (kam′er-ō-stōm). Ventral depression of the anterior cephalothorax of soft ticks (family Argasidae) in which the mouthparts (capitulum) lie. [L. *camera,* a vault, + G. *stoma,* mouth]

cam·i·sole (kam′i-sōl). SYN straitjacket.

cam·o·mile (kam′ō-mil). SYN chamomile.

cAMP Abbreviation for adenosine 3′,5′-cyclic monophosphate (cyclic AMP).

Campbell, Meredith F., U.S. pediatric urologist, 1894-1969. SEE C. *sound.*

Campbell, William F., U.S. surgeon, 1867–1926. SEE C. *ligament.*

Camper, Pieter, Dutch physician and anatomist, 1721–1789. SEE C. *chiasm;* fatty *layer* of subcutaneous tissue of abdomen; C. *ligament, line, plane.*

cam·phene (kam′fēn). A terpenoid occurring in many essential oils, e.g., turpentine, camphor, citronella.

cam·phor (kam′fōr). A ketone distilled from the bark and wood of *Cinnamonum camphora,* an evergreen tree of Taiwan and Southeast Asia and the adjoining islands, and also prepared synthetically from oil of turpentine; used in a variety of commercial products and as a topical antiinfective and antipruritic agent. [mediev. L., fr. Ar. *kāfure*]

cantharis c., SYN cantharidin.

c. liniment, a mixture of camphor and cottonseed oil, or camphor and arachis oil; a mild counterirritant. SYN camphorated oil.

monobromated c., obsolete term for an antispasmodic, soporific, and sedative.

tar c., SYN naphthalene.

thyme c., SYN thymol.

cam·pho·ra·ceous (kam-fō-rā′shŭs). Resembling camphor in appearance, consistency, or odor.

cam·phor·at·ed (kam′fō-rā-ted). Containing camphor.

cam·phor·at·ed oil. SYN *camphor* liniment.

cam·pi fo·reli (kam′pē fōr-el′ē). SYN *fields* of Forel, under *field.* [L. pl. of *campus,* field]

cam·pim·e·ter (kam-pim′ě-ter). A small tangent screen used to measure central visual field. [L. *campus,* field, + G. *metron,* measure]

camp·lo·dac·ty·ly. SYN camptodactyly.

campothecins (kam-pō-thā′sinz). Antitumor agents acting as topoisomerase inhibitors; include irinotecan and topotecan.

cAMP phos·pho·di·es·ter·ase. SYN adenosine 3′,5′-cyclic phosphate phosphodiesterase.

camp·to·cor·mia (kamp-tō-kōr′mē-ă). Static, often marked forward flexion of the trunk; usually manifestation of conversion reaction. SYN camptospasm, prosternation. [G. *kamptos,* bent, + *kormos,* trunk of a tree]

camp·to·dac·ty·ly, camp·to·dac·tyl·ia (kamp-tō-dak′ti-lē, -dak-til′ē-ă). Permanent flexion of one or both interphalangeal joints of one or more fingers, usually the little finger; often congenital in origin. SYN camplodactyly, streblodactyly. [G. *kamptos,* bent, + *daktylos,* finger]

camp·to·me·lia (kamp-tō-mē′lē-ă). A skeletal dysplasia characterized by a bending of the long bones of the extremities, resulting in a permanent bowing or curvature of the affected part. [G. *kamptos,* bent, + *melos,* limb]

camp·to·mel·ic (kamp-tō-mel′ik). Denoting or characteristic of camptomelia. SEE camptomelic *syndrome.*

camp·to·spasm (kamp′tō-spazm). SYN camptocormia.

camptothecin (kamp-tō-thek′in). Plant alkaloids consisting of a pentacyclic structure with a lactone ring; inhibitors of topoisomerase I, i.e., topotecan and irinotecan (CPT-11). [Camptotheca, genus name of botanic source]

Cam·py·lo·bac·ter (kam′pi-lō-bak′ter). A genus of bacteria containing Gram-negative, nonsporeforming, spiral or S-curved rods with a single flagellum at one or both ends of the cell; cells may also become spherical under adverse conditions; they are motile with a corkscrewlike motion and nonsacchrolytic. The type species is *C. fetus.* [G. *campylos,* curved, + *baktron,* staff or rod]

C. coli, a thermophilic bacterial species that causes first watery, then inflammatory, diarrheal disease in humans and in piglets.

C. concisus, a catalase-negative bacterial species isolated from normal human fecal flora, gingival crevices in periodontal disease, and occasionally blood.

C. fe′tus, a bacterial species that contains various subspecies which can cause human infections as well as abortion in sheep and cattle; it is the type species of the genus *C.*

C. fetus subsp. *jejuni,* former name for *C. jejuni.*

C. hyointestinalis, a bacterial species that causes an enteropathy in pigs; has been recovered from fecal specimens in humans with diarrhea and with proctitis, but its pathogenic role has not been defined.

C. jejuni, a thermophilic bacterial species that causes in humans an acute gastroenteritis of sudden onset with constitutional symptoms (malaise, myalgia, arthralgia, and headache) and cramping abdominal pain; it has been associated with a demyelinating sequela, which can present with ascending paralysis. Potential sources of human infection include poultry, cattle, sheep, pigs, and dogs. This species also causes abortion in sheep.

C. lari, a bacterial species primarily carried in birds, but associated with water-borne enteritis and occasionally septicemia in humans.

C. pylori, SYN *Helicobacter pylori.*

C. sputo′rum, a facultative, microaerophilic, catalase-negative species found in the genital tract and feces of sheep and cattle and in the human oral cavity; a cause of human bronchitis.

cam·py·lo·bac·ter·i·o·sis (kam′pi-lō-bak′ter-ē-ō′sis). Infection caused by microaerophilic bacteria of the genus *Campylobacter.*

Canada, Wilma J., U.S. radiologist. SEE Cronkhite-C. *syndrome.*

can·a·dine (kan′ă-dēn). $C_{20}H_{21}NO_4$; an alkaloid present in *Hydrastis canadensis* (family Ranunculaceae) and in *Corydalis cava* (family Fumaraceae) with sedative and muscle relaxant properties. SYN xanthopuccine.

CANAL

ca·nal (kă-nal') [TA]. A duct or channel; a tubular structure. SEE ALSO canal, duct. SYN canalis [TA]. [L. *canalis*]

abdominal c., SYN inguinal c.

accessory c., a channel leading from the root pulp laterally through the dentin to the periodontal tissue; may be found anywhere in the tooth root, but is more common in the apical third of the root. SYN lateral c.

adductor c. [TA], the space in middle third of the thigh between the vastus medialis and adductor muscles, converted into a canal by the overlying sartorius muscle. It gives passage to the femoral vessels and saphenous nerve, ending at the adductor hiatus. SYN canalis adductorius [TA], Hunter c., subsartorial c.

Alcock c., SYN pudendal c.

alimentary c., SYN digestive *tract*.

alveolar c.'s of maxilla [TA], canals in the body of the maxilla that transmit nerves and vessels from the alveolar foramina to the maxillary teeth. SYN canales alveolares corporis maxillae [TA], alveolodental c.'s, dental c.'s.

alveolodental c.'s, SYN alveolar c.'s of maxilla.

anal c. [TA], terminal portion of the alimentary canal; about 4 cm in length, beginning at the anorectal junction, where the rectal ampulla rather abruptly narrows as the alimentary canal pierces the pelvic diaphragm (levator ani), and ending at the anal verge, when the anoderm that lines the lower anal canal changes to hairy perianal skin; surrounded by the internal and external anal sphincters. SYN canalis analis [TA].

anterior condyloid c. of occipital bone, SYN hypoglossal c.

anterior semicircular c.'s, SEE semicircular c.'s of bony labyrinth.

archenteric c., invagination of the blastopore into the notochordal process to form a cavity. SEE neurenteric c. SYN notochordal c.

Arnold c., SYN *hiatus* for lesser petrosal nerve.

arterial c., SYN *ductus* arteriosus.

atrioventricular c., the c. in the embryonic heart leading from the common sinuatrial chamber to the ventricle.

auditory c., SYN external acoustic *meatus*.

basipharyngeal c., SYN vomerovaginal c.

Bernard c., SYN accessory pancreatic *duct*.

Bichat c., SYN quadrigeminal *cistern*.

birth c., cavity of the uterus and vagina through which the fetus passes. SYN parturient c.

blastoporic c., obsolete term for primitive *pit*.

bony semicircular c.'s, SYN semicircular c.'s of bony labyrinth.

Böttcher c., SYN utriculosaccular *duct*.

Breschet c.'s, SYN diploic c.'s.

carotid c. [TA], a passage through the petrous part of the temporal bone from its inferior surface upward, medially, and forward to the apex where it opens posterior and superior to the site of the foramen lacerum. It transmits the internal carotid artery and plexuses of veins and autonomic nerves. SYN canalis caroticus [TA].

carpal c., (1) SYN carpal *tunnel*; **(2)** SYN carpal *groove*.

caudal c., the space occupied by the sacral extension of the epidural space.

central c. [TA], SYN canalis centralis medullae spinalis [TA], syringocele (1), tubus medullaris. SYN central c. of spinal cord.

central c.'s of cochlea, SYN longitudinal c.'s of modiolus.

central c. of spinal cord [TA], the ependyma-lined lumen (cavity) of the neural tube, the cerebral part of which remains patent to form the ventricles of the brain, while the spinal part in the adult often is reduced to a solid strand of modified ependyma. SYN central c. [TA].

central c. of the vitreous, SYN hyaloid c.

cervical c. [TA], a fusiform canal extending from the isthmus of the uterus to the opening of the uterus into the vagina. SYN canalis cervicis uteri [TA].

cervicoaxillary c., superior opening to the axilla, bounded by clavicle anteriorly, scapula posteriorly and first rib medically. Axillary vessels and brachial plexus are transmitted.

ciliary c.'s, SYN *spaces* of iridocorneal angle, under *space*.

Civinini c., SYN anterior *canaliculus* of chorda tympani.

Cloquet c., SYN hyaloid c.

cochlear c., SYN spiral c. of cochlea.

condylar c. [TA], the inconstant opening through the occipital bone posterior to the condyle on each side that transmits the occipital emissary vein. SYN canalis condylaris [TA], condyloid c., posterior condyloid foramen.

condyloid c., SYN condylar c.

Corti c., SYN Corti *tunnel*.

Cotunnius c., SYN vestibular *aqueduct*.

craniopharyngeal c., SYN pituitary *diverticulum*.

deferent c., SYN *ductus* deferens.

dental c.'s, SYN alveolar c.'s of maxilla.

dentinal c.'s, SYN *canaliculi* dentales, under *canaliculus*.

diploic c.'s [TA], channels in the diploë that accommodate the diploic veins. SYN canales diploici [TA], Breschet c.'s.

Dorello c., a bony c. sometimes found at the tip of the temporal bone enclosing the abducens nerve and inferior petrosal sinus as these two structures enter the cavernous sinus.

Dupuytren c., SYN diploic *vein*.

ear c., SYN external acoustic *meatus*.

endodermal c., SYN primitive *gut*.

endometrial c. [TA],

facial c. [TA], the bony passage in the temporal bone through which the facial nerve passes; the facial c. commences at the internal auditory meatus with the horizontal part which passes at first anteriorly (medial crus of facial canal) then turns posteriorly at the geniculum of the facial c. to pass medial to the tympanic cavity (lateral crus of facial canal); finally, it turns downward (descending part of facial canal) to reach the stylomastoid foramen. SYN canalis nervi facialis [TA], aqueductus fallopii, fallopian aqueduct, fallopian c.

fallopian c., SYN facial c.

femoral c. [TA], the medial compartment of the femoral sheath, which is often occupied by the intermediate deep inguinal lymph node (of Cloquet), and provides both passage for lymphatics passing from lower limb to trunk and facilitates expansion of the adjacent femoral vein, as when it enlarges during a Valsalva *maneuver*. SYN canalis femoralis [TA].

Ferrein c., SYN lacrimal *pathway*.

Fontana c., SYN scleral venous *sinus*.

galactophorous c.'s, SYN lactiferous *ducts*, under *duct*.

Gartner c., SYN longitudinal *duct* of epoöphoron.

gastric c. [TA], furrow formed temporarily between longitudinal rugae of the gastric mucosa along the lesser curvature during swallowing; observed radiographically and endoscopically, it is formed because of the firm attachment of the gastric mucosa to the muscular layer, which is devoid of an oblique layer at this site; said to form a passageway favored by saliva and small quantities of masticated food and other fluids as they flow from cardia to gastroduodenal junction. SYN canalis gastricus [TA], magenstrasse.

greater palatine c. [TA], the c. formed between the maxilla and palatine bones; it transmits the descending palatine artery and the greater palatine nerve. SYN canalis palatinus major [TA], pterygopalatine c.

gubernacular c., a small c. located between the permanent tooth germ and the apex of the deciduous tooth, containing remnants of dental lamina and connective tissue.

c. of Guyon, passageway through the transverse carpal ligament by which the ulnar nerve and artery enter the palm; it is closely related to the pisiform and the hook of the hamate.

Guyon c., the superficial c. between the flexor retinaculum of the

ca

hand and flexor carpi ulnaris through which pass the ulnar nerve and vasculature between forearm and hand.

gynecophoric c., a ventral groove running the length of male schistosome flukes, into which the threadlike female worm fits.

Hannover c., the potential space between the ciliary zonule and the vitreous body.

haversian c.'s, vascular c.'s that run longitudinally in the center of haversian systems of compact osseous tissue. SYN Leeuwenhoek c.'s.

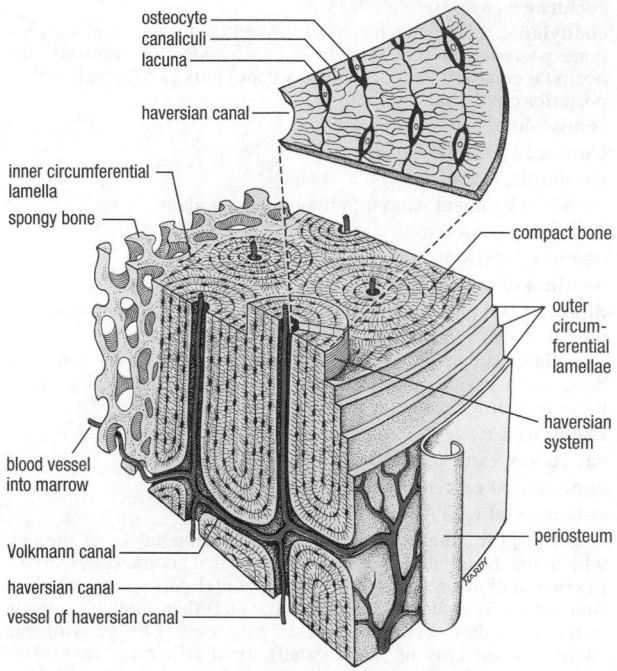

osteocyte
canaliculi
lacuna
haversian canal
inner circumferential lamella
spongy bone
compact bone
outer circumferential lamellae
haversian system
blood vessel into marrow
periosteum
Volkmann canal
haversian canal
vessel of haversian canal

haversian canals: as seen in wedge of compact bone tissue

Hensen c., SYN *ductus* reuniens.

c. of Hering, SYN cholangiole.

Hirschfeld c.'s, SYN interdental c.'s.

Holmgrén-Golgi c.'s, SYN Golgi *apparatus*.

c. of Hovius, an anastomotic circle between the anterior twigs of the venae vorticosae in the eyes of some animals, but not in normal human eyes.

Hoyer c.'s, SYN Sucquet-Hoyer c.'s.

Huguier c., SYN anterior *canaliculus* of chorda tympani.

Hunter c., SYN adductor c.

hyaloid c. [TA], a minute canal running through the vitreous from the optic disk to the lens, containing in fetal life a prolongation of the central artery of the retina, the hyaloid artery. SEE vitreous, hyaloid *artery*. SYN canalis hyaloideus [TA], central c. of the vitreous, Cloquet c., Stilling c.

hypoglossal c. [TA], the canal through which the hypoglossal nerve emerges from the skull. SYN canalis hypoglossalis [TA], anterior condyloid c. of occipital bone, anterior condyloid foramen.

incisive c.'s [TA], several bony canals leading from the floor of the nasal cavity into the incisive fossa on the palatal surface of the maxilla; they convey the nasopalatine nerves and branches of the greater palatine arteries that anastomose with the septal branch of the sphenopalatine artery. SYN canales incisivi [TA], incisor c.'s.

incisor c.'s, SYN incisive c.'s.

inferior dental c., SYN mandibular c.

infraorbital c. [TA], a canal running beneath the orbital margin of the maxilla from the infraorbital groove, in the floor of the orbit, to the infraorbital foramen; it transmits the infraorbital artery and nerve. SYN canalis infraorbitalis [TA].

inguinal c. [TA], the obliquely directed passage through the musculoaponeurotic layers of the lower abdominal wall that transmits the spermatic cord in the male and the round ligament in the female from the pelvic cavity to the scrotum or labia majora, respectively. SYN canalis inguinalis [TA], abdominal c., Velpeau c.

interdental c.'s, c.'s that extend vertically through alveolar bone between roots of mandibular and maxillary incisor and maxillary bicuspid teeth. SYN Hirschfeld c.'s.

interfacial c.'s, intercellular spaces occurring in relation to intercellular attachments by desmosomes in stratified squamous epithelium, generally resulting from shrinkage of an artifact of fixation.

Jacobson c., SYN tympanic *canaliculus.*

Kürsteiner c.'s, a fetal complex of vesicular, canalicular, and glandlike structures derived from parathyroid, thymus, or thymic cord; they are rudimentary and functionless unless persistent postnatally, when they may occur as cystic structures in the vicinity of parathyroid III and thymus III. Kürsteiner described three types, type II c.'s being associated with thyroaplasia.

lateral c., SYN accessory c.

lateral semicircular c.'s, SEE semicircular c.'s of bony labyrinth.

Laurer c., a tube originating on the surface of the ootype of trematodes, directed dorsally to or near the surface; it may have originally served as a vagina or possibly as a reservoir of excess shell material.

Lauth c., SYN scleral venous *sinus.*

Leeuwenhoek c.'s, SYN haversian c.'s.

lesser palatine c.'s [TA], c.'s located in the posterior part of the palatine bone. SYN canales palatini minores [TA], c.'s for lesser palatine nerves.

c.'s for lesser palatine nerves, SYN lesser palatine c.'s.

longitudinal c.'s of modiolus [TA], centrally placed channels that convey vessels and nerves to the apical turns of the cochlea. SYN canales longitudinales modioli [TA], central c.'s of cochlea.

Löwenberg c., SYN cochlear *duct.*

mandibular c. [TA], the canal within the mandible that transmits the inferior alveolar nerve and vessels. Its posterior opening is the mandibular foramen. SYN canalis mandibulae [TA], inferior dental c.

marrow c., SYN root c. of tooth.

mental c., SYN mental *foramen.*

musculotubal c. [TA], a canal beginning at the anterior border of the petrous portion of the temporal bone near its junction with the squamous portion, and passing to the tympanic cavity; it is divided by the cochleariform process into two semicanals: one for the pharyngotympanic (auditory) tube, the other for the tensor tympani muscle. SYN canalis musculotubarius [TA].

nasolacrimal c. [TA], the bony canal formed by the maxilla, lacrimal bone, and inferior concha that transmits the nasolacrimal duct from the orbit to the inferior meatus of the nose. SYN canalis nasolacrimalis [TA].

neural c., the c. within the embryonic neural tube; the primordium of the central c.

neurenteric c., a transitory communication between the neural tube, notochordal canal, and gut endoderm in vertebrate embryos.

notochordal c., SYN archenteric c.

c. of Nuck, SEE *processus* vaginalis of peritoneum.

nutrient c. [TA], a canal in the shaft of a long bone or in other locations in irregular bones through which the nutrient artery enters a bone. SYN canalis nutricius [TA].

obturator c. [TA], the opening in the superior part of the obturator membrane through which the obturator nerve and vessels pass from the pelvic cavity into the thigh. SYN canalis obturatorius [TA].

optic c. [TA], the short canal through the lesser wing of the sphenoid bone at the apex of the orbit that gives passage to the optic nerve and the ophthalmic artery. SYN canalis opticus [TA], foramen opticum, optic foramen.

palatovaginal c. [TA], on the undersurface of the vaginal process of the sphenoid bone, a furrow that is converted into a canal by the sphenoidal process of the palatine bone; it transmits the pharyngeal branch of the maxillary artery and the pharyngeal nerve from the pterygopalatine ganglion. SYN canalis palatovaginalis, pharyngeal c.

parturient c., SYN birth c.

pelvic c., the passage from the superior to the inferior aperture of the pelvis.

pericardioperitoneal c., the portion of the embryonic celom that joins the pericardial cavity to the peritoneal cavity, developing into the pleural cavities. SYN pleural c.

persistent atrioventricular c., a condition that is caused when the atrial and ventricular septa fail to meet, as in normal development, resulting in a low atrial and high ventricular septal defect or a common atrioventricular c. SYN endocardial cushion defect.

Petit c.'s, SYN zonular *spaces,* under *space.*

pharyngeal c., SYN palatovaginal c.

c. for pharyngotympanic (auditory) tube [TA], the inferior division of the musculotubal canal that forms the bony part of the pharyngotympanic (auditory) tube. SYN semicanalis tubae auditivae [TA], semicanal of auditory tube, semicanalis t′ubae audito′riae.

pleural c., SYN pericardioperitoneal c.

pleuropericardial c.'s, in the embryo, spaces or channels, one on each side, connecting the pericardial and pleural cavities.

pleuroperitoneal c., the communication between the embryonic pleural and peritoneal cavities.

portal c.'s, connective tissue spaces in the substance of the liver that are occupied by preterminal ramifications of the bile ducts, portal vein, and hepatic artery, as well as nerves and lymphatics.

posterior semicircular c.'s, SEE semicircular c.'s of bony labyrinth.

pterygoid c. [TA], an opening through the base of the medial pterygoid process of the sphenoid bone through which pass the artery, vein, and nerve of the pterygoid canal. SYN canalis pterygoideus [TA], vidian c.

pterygopalatine c., SYN greater palatine c.

pudendal c. [TA], the space within the obturator internus fascia lining the lateral wall of the ischioanal (ischiorectal) fossa that transmits the pudendal vessels and internal pudendal nerves. SYN canalis pudendalis [TA], Alcock c.

pulp c., SYN root c. of tooth.

pyloric c. [TA], the aboral segment (about 2–3 cm long) of the stomach; it succeeds the antrum and ends at the gastroduodenal junction. SYN canalis pyloricus [TA].

Rivinus c.'s, SEE major sublingual *duct,* minor sublingual *ducts,* under *duct.*

root c. of tooth [TA], the chamber of the dental pulp lying within the root portion of a tooth. SYN canalis radicis dentis [TA], marrow c., pulp c.

Rosenthal c., SYN spiral c. of cochlea.

sacral c. [TA], the continuation of the vertebral canal in the sacrum. SYN canalis sacralis [TA].

Santorini c., SYN accessory pancreatic *duct.*

c.'s of Scarpa, separate c.'s for the nasopalatine nerves and vessels. These c.'s normally fuse to form the incisive c.

Schlemm c., SYN scleral venous *sinus.*

semicircular c.'s, SEE semicircular c.'s of bony labyrinth.

semicircular c.'s of bony labyrinth [TA], the organ of balance; the three bony tubes in the labyrinth of the ear within which the membranous semicircular ducts are located; they lie in planes at right angles to each other and are known as anterior semicircular canal, posterior semicircular canal, and lateral semicircular canal. SYN bony semicircular c.'s, canales semicircularis ossei.

small c. of chorda tympani, SYN posterior *canaliculus* of chorda tympani.

Sondermann c., a blind outpouching of Schlemm c., extending toward, but not communicating with, the anterior chamber of the eye.

spinal c., SYN vertebral c.

spiral c. of cochlea [TA], the winding tube of the bony labyrinth that makes two and a half turns about the modiolus of the cochlea;

it is divided incompletely into two compartments by a winding shelf of bone, the bony spiral lamina. SYN canalis spiralis cochleae [TA], cochlear c., Rosenthal c.

spiral c. of modiolus [TA], the space in the modiolus in which the spiral ganglion of the cochlear nerve lies. SYN canalis spiralis modioli [TA].

Stilling c., SYN hyaloid c.

subsartorial c., SYN adductor c.

Sucquet c.'s, SYN Sucquet-Hoyer c.'s.

Sucquet-Hoyer c.'s, arteriovenular anastomoses controlling blood flow in the glomus bodies in the digits. SYN Hoyer anastomoses, Hoyer c.'s, Sucquet anastomoses, Sucquet c.'s, Sucquet-Hoyer anastomoses.

tarsal c., SYN tarsal *sinus.*

temporal c., a c. in the zygomatic bone transmitting the zygomaticofacial and zygomaticotemporal nerves and vessels.

c. for tensor tympani muscle [TA], semicanal of the tensor muscle of the tympanum; the superior division of the musculotubal canal containing the tensor tympani muscle. SYN semicanalis musculi tensoris tympani [TA], semicanal for tensor tympani muscle.

Theile c., SYN transverse pericardial *sinus.*

tubotympanic c., SEE tubotympanic *recess.*

tympanic c., SYN tympanic *canaliculus.*

uniting c., SYN *ductus* reuniens.

uterovaginal c., a median tubular structure produced in the embryo from the fusion of the caudal parts of the paramesonephric ducts.

van Horne c., SYN thoracic *duct.*

Velpeau c., SYN inguinal c.

vertebral c. [TA], the canal that contains the spinal cord, spinal meninges, and related structures. It is formed by the vertebral foramina of successive vertebrae of the articulated vertebral column. SYN canalis vertebralis [TA], spinal c., tubus vertebralis.

vesicourethral c., the cranial portion of the primitive urogenital sinus from which develop the urinary bladder and part of the urethra.

vestibular c., SYN *scala* vestibuli.

vidian c., SYN pterygoid c.

Volkmann c.'s, vascular c.'s in compact bone that, unlike those of the haversian system, are not surrounded by concentric lamellae of bone; they run for the most part transversely, perforating the lamellae of the haversian system, and communicate with the c.'s of that system.

vomerine c., SYN vomerovaginal c.

vomerobasilar c., SYN vomerorostral c.

vomerorostral c. [TA], a small canal between the superior border of the vomer and the rostrum of the sphenoidal bone. SYN canalis vomerorostralis [TA], vomerobasilar c.

vomerovaginal c. [TA], an opening between the vaginal process of the sphenoid and the ala of the vomer on either side. It conveys a branch of the sphenopalatine artery. SYN canalis vomerovaginalis [TA], basipharyngeal c., vomerine c.

Walther c.'s, SYN minor sublingual *ducts,* under *duct.*

Wirsung c., SYN pancreatic *duct.*

---

ca·na·les (kă-nā′lēz). Plural of canalis.

can·a·lic·u·lar (kan-ă-lik′ū-lăr). Relating to a canaliculus. [L. *canaliculus,* small channel, dim. fr. *canalis,* canal, + suffix *-ar,* pertaining to]

can·a·lic·u·li (kan-ă-lik′ū-lī). Plural of canaliculus.

can·a·lic·u·li·tis (kan′ă-lik-ū-lī′tis). Inflammation of the lacrimal canaliculus. [canaliculus + G. *-itis,* inflammation]

can·a·lic·u·li·za·tion (kan-ă-lik′ū-lī-zā′shŭn). The formation of canaliculi, or small canals, in any tissue.

can·a·lic·u·lus, pl. **can·a·lic·u·li** (kan-ă-lik′ū-lŭs, -lī) [TA]. A small canal or channel. SEE ALSO iter. [L. dim. fr. *canalis,* canal]

anterior c. of chorda tympani, a canal in the petrotympanic or glaserian fissure, near its posterior edge, through which the chorda tympani nerve issues from the skull. SYN Civinini canal, Huguier canal, iter chordae anterius.

auricular c., SYN mastoid c.

biliary c., one of the intercellular channels, about 1 μm or less in diameter, that occur between liver cells forming the first portion of the bile system. SYN bile capillary.

bone c., the c. interconnecting bone lacunae with one another or with a haversian canal; contains the interconnecting cytoplasmic processes of osteocytes.

caroticotympanic canaliculi [TA], small openings within the carotid canal that afford passage to the tympanic cavity of branches of the internal carotid artery and carotid sympathetic plexus. SYN canaliculi caroticotympanici [TA].

canaliculi caroticotympan'ici [TA], SYN caroticotympanic canaliculi.

c. chor'dae tym'pani [TA], SYN posterior c. of chorda tympani.

c. of chorda tympani, SYN posterior c. of chorda tympani.

c. coch'leae [TA], SYN cochlear c.

cochlear c. [TA], a minute canal in the temporal bone that passes from the cochlea inferiorly to open in front of the medial side of the jugular fossa. It contains the perilymphatic duct. SYN c. cochleae [TA].

canalic'uli denta'les, minute, wavy, branching tubes or canals in the dentin; they contain the long cytoplasmic processes of odontoblasts and extend radially from the pulp to the dentoenamel junction. SYN dental tubules, dentinal canals, dentinal tubules, tubuli dentales.

c. innomina'tus, SYN *foramen* petrosum.

intercellular c., one of the fine channels between adjoining secretory cells, such as those between serous cells in salivary glands.

intracellular c., a fine canal formed by invagination of the cell membrane into the cytoplasm of a cell, such as those of the parietal cells of the stomach.

lacrimal c. [TA], a curved canal beginning at the lacrimal punctum in the margin of each eyelid near the medial commissure and running transversely medially to empty with its fellow into the lacrimal sac. SYN c. lacrimalis [TA].

c. lacrima'lis [TA], SYN lacrimal c.

mastoid c. [TA], the canal that extends from the jugular fossa laterally through the mastoid process. It transmits the auricular branch of the vagus. SYN c. mastoideus [TA], auricular c.

c. mastoid'eus [TA], SYN mastoid c.

posterior c. of chorda tympani, a canal leading from the facial canal to the tympanic cavity through which the chorda tympani nerve enters this cavity. SYN c. chordae tympani [TA], c. of chorda tympani, iter chordae posterius, small canal of chorda tympani.

c. reu'niens, SYN *ductus* reuniens.

secretory c., SEE intercellular c., intracellular c.

Thiersch canaliculi, minute channels in newly formed reparative tissue, permitting the circulation of nutritive fluids, precursors of new vascularization.

tympanic c. [TA], a minute canal passing from the inferior surface of the petrous portion of the temporal bone between the jugular fossa and carotid canal to the floor of the tympanic cavity. Located in the wedge of bone separating the jugular canal and carotid canal, it transmits the tympanic branch of the glossopharyngeal nerve. SYN c. tympanicus [TA], Jacobson canal, tympanic canal.

c. tympan'icus [TA], SYN tympanic c.

ca·na·lis, pl. **ca·na·les** (ka-nā'lis, -lēz) [TA]. SYN canal. [L.]

c. adductor'ius [TA], SYN adductor *canal*.

cana'les alveola'res corporis maxillae [TA], SYN alveolar *canals of maxilla, under *canal*.

c. ana'lis [TA], SYN anal *canal*.

c. carot'icus [TA], SYN carotid *canal*.

c. car'pi [TA], SYN carpal *tunnel*.

c. centra'lis medul'lae spina'lis [TA], SYN central *canal*.

c. cerv'icis u'teri [TA], SYN cervical *canal*.

c. condyla'ris [TA], SYN condylar *canal*.

cana'les diplo'ici [TA], SYN diploic *canals, under *canal*.

c. femora'lis [TA], SYN femoral *canal*.

c. gastricus [TA], SYN gastric *canal*.

c. hyaloid'eus [TA], SYN hyaloid *canal*.

c. hypoglossa'lis [TA], SYN hypoglossal *canal*.

canales incisi'vi [TA], SYN incisive *canals, under *canal*.

c. infraorbita'lis [TA], SYN infraorbital *canal*.

c. inguina'lis [TA], SYN inguinal *canal*.

cana'les longitudina'les modi'oli [TA], SYN longitudinal *canals of modiolus, under *canal*.

c. mandib'ulae [TA], SYN mandibular *canal*.

c. musculotuba'rius [TA], SYN musculotubal *canal*.

c. nasolacrima'lis [TA], SYN nasolacrimal *canal*.

c. ner'vi facia'lis [TA], SYN facial *canal*.

c. ner'vi petro'si superficial'is mino'ris, SYN *hiatus* for lesser petrosal nerve.

c. nutri'cius [TA], SYN nutrient *canal*.

c. obturato'rius [TA], SYN obturator *canal*.

c. op'ticus [TA], SYN optic *canal*.

cana'les palati'ni mino'res [TA], SYN lesser palatine *canals, under *canal*.

c. palati'nus ma'jor [TA], SYN greater palatine *canal*.

c. palatovagina'lis, SYN palatovaginal *canal*.

c. pterygoi'deus [TA], SYN pterygoid *canal*.

c. pudenda'lis [TA], SYN pudendal *canal*.

c. pylor'icus [TA], SYN pyloric *canal*.

c. rad'icis den'tis [TA], SYN root *canal* of tooth.

c. reu'niens, SYN *ductus* reuniens.

c. sacra'lis [TA], SYN sacral *canal*.

canales semicircularis anterior, anterior semicurcular canal. SEE semicircular *canals* of bony labyrinth, under *canal*.

canales semicircularis lateralis, lateral semicircular canal. SEE semicircular *canals* of bony labyrinth, under *canal*.

cana'les semicircula'ris os'sei, SYN semicircular *canals* of bony labyrinth, under *canal*.

canales semicircularis posterior, posterior semicircular canal. SEE semicircular *canals* of bony labyrinth, under *canal*.

c. spira'lis coch'leae [TA], SYN spiral *canal* of cochlea.

c. spira'lis modi'oli [TA], SYN spiral *canal* of modiolus.

c. umbilica'lis, SYN umbilical *ring*.

c. vertebra'lis [TA], SYN vertebral *canal*.

c. vomerorostra'lis [TA], SYN vomerorostral *canal*.

c. vomerovagina'lis [TA], SYN vomerovaginal *canal*.

can·a·li·za·tion (kan-ăl-ī-zā'shŭn). The formation of canals or channels in a tissue.

Canavan, Myrtelle M., U.S. pathologist, 1879–1953. SEE C. *disease, sclerosis;* C.-van Bogaert-Bertrand *disease.*

can·av·a·nase (kan-av'ă-nās). SYN arginase.

can·a·van·ine (kan-ă-van'īn). 2-Amino-4-guanidinohydroxybutyric acid; an analog of arginine found in certain legumes; used in studies of arginine-dependent systems; it is also a potent growht inhibitor. [*Canavalia* + -ine]

can·cel·lat·ed (kan'sĕ-lā-ted). SYN cancellous. [L. *cancello,* to make a lattice work]

can·cel·lous (kan'sĕ-lŭs). Denoting bone that has a latticelike or spongy structure. SYN cancelled.

can·cel·lus, pl. **can·cel·li** (kan-sel'ŭs, -lī). A latticelike structure, as in spongy bone. [L. a grating, lattice]

can·cer (CA) (kan'ser). General term frequently used to indicate any of various types of malignant neoplasms, most of which invade surrounding tissues, may metastasize to several sites, and are likely to recur after attempted removal and to cause death of the patient unless adequately treated; especially, any such carcinoma or sarcoma, but, in ordinary usage, especially the former. [L. a crab, a cancer]

betel c., carcinoma of the mucous membrane of the cheek, observed in certain East Indian natives, probably as a result of irritation from chewing a preparation of betel nut and lime rolled within a betel leaf. SYN buyo cheek c.

buyo cheek c., SYN betel c. [Philippine *buyo,* betel]

chimney sweep's c., a squamous cell carcinoma of the skin of the scrotum, occurring as an occupational disease in chimney sweeps. The first reported form of occupational cancer (by Sir Percival Pott).

colloid c., SYN mucinous *carcinoma.*

conjugal c., c. à deux occurring in husband and wife.

c. à deux, carcinomas occurring at approximately the same time, or in fairly close succession, in two persons who live together. [Fr. *deux,* two]

c. en cuirasse (on-kwē-rahs′, Fr. breastplate), a carcinoma that involves a considerable portion of the skin of one or both sides of the thorax. [Fr. breastplate]

epidermoid c., SYN epidermoid *carcinoma.*

epithelial c., any malignant neoplasm originating from epithelium, i.e., a carcinoma.

familial c., c. aggregating among blood relatives; rarely the mode of inheritance is clearly mendelian, either dominant, as in retinoblastoma, basal cell nevus syndrome, neurofibromatosis, and intestinal polyposis, or recessive, as in xeroderma pigmentosum. SEE ALSO cancer *family.*

glandular c., SYN adenocarcinoma.

hereditary nonpolyposis colorectal c., an autosomal dominant predisposition to cancer of the colon and rectum.

kang c., kangri c., a carcinoma of the skin of the thigh or abdomen in certain Indian or Chinese workers; thought to result from irritation by heat from a hot brick oven (kang) or fire basket (kangri). SYN kangri burn carcinoma.

mouse c., any of various types of malignant neoplasms that occur naturally in mice, especially in certain inbred "c. strains" used for research studies.

mule-spinner's c., carcinoma of the scrotum or adjacent skin exposed to oil, observed in some workers in cotton-spinning mills.

paraffin c., carcinoma of the skin occurring as an occupational disease in paraffin workers.

pipe-smoker's c., squamous cell carcinoma of the lips occurring in pipe smokers.

pitch-worker's c., carcinoma of the skin of the face or neck, arms and hands, or the scrotum, resulting from exposure to carcinogens in pitch, which occurs naturally as asphalt, or as a residue in the distillation of tar.

scar c., SYN scar *carcinoma.*

scar c. of the lungs, a pulmonary c. intimately related to a localized area of parenchymal fibrosis.

stump c., carcinoma of the stomach developing after gastroenterostomy or gastric resection for benign disease.

telangiectatic c., a c. with numerous dilated capillaries and "lakes" of blood within relatively large endothelium-lined channels.

can·cer·o·pho·bia (kan′ser-ō-fō′bē-ă). A morbid fear of acquiring a malignant growth. SYN carcinophobia. [cancer + G. *phobos,* fear]

can·cer·ous (kan′ser-ŭs). Relating to or pertaining to a malignant neoplasm, or being afflicted with such a process.

can·cra (kang′kră). Plural of cancrum.

can·cri·form (kang′kri-fōrm). Resembling cancer. SYN cancroid (1).

can·croid (kang′kroyd). **1.** SYN cancriform. **2.** Obsolete term for a malignant neoplasm that manifests a lesser degree of malignancy than that frequently observed with carcinoma or sarcoma. [cancer + G. *eidos,* resemblance]

can·crum, pl. **can·cra** (kang′krŭm, -kră). A gangrenous, ulcerative, inflammatory lesion. [Mod. L., fr. L. *cancer,* crab]

c. na′si, gangrenous, necrotizing, and ulcerative rhinitis, especially in children.

c. o′ris, SYN noma.

can·de·la (cd) (kan′de-lă). The SI unit of luminous intensity, 1 lumen per m²; the luminous intensity, in a given direction, of a source that emits monochromatic radiation of frequency 540 × 10¹² Hz and that has a radiant intensity in that direction of 1/683 W per steradian (solid angle). SYN candle. [L.]

can·di·cans (kan′di-kanz). One of the corpora albicantia. [L. *candico,* pres. p. *-ans,* to be whitish]

can·di·ci·din (kan-di-sī′din). A fungistatic and fungicidal polyene antibiotic agent derived from a soil actinomycete similar to *Streptomyces griseus;* used in the treatment of vaginal candidiasis.

Can·di·da (kan′did-ă). A genus of yeastlike fungi commonly found in nature; a few species are isolated from the skin, feces, and vaginal and pharyngeal tissue, but the gastrointestinal tract is the source of the single most important species, *C. albicans.* [L. *candidus,* dazzling white]

C. al′bicans, a fungal species ordinarily a part of humans' normal gastrointestinal flora, but which becomes pathogenic when there is a disturbance in the balance of flora or in an impairment of the host defenses from other causes; resulting disease states may vary from limited to generalized cutaneous or mucocutaneous infections, to severe and fatal systemic disease including endocarditis, septicemia, and meningitis. SYN thrush fungus.

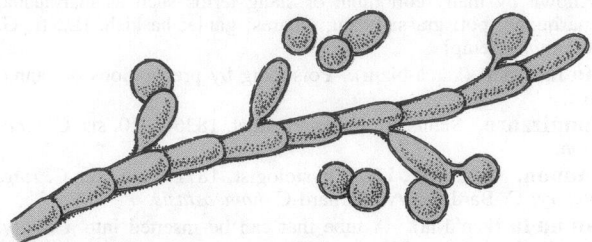

Candida albicans

C. glabrata, a fungal species that is a cause of human candidiasis; formerly classified as *Torulopsis glabrata.*

C. parapsilosis, a species of limited pathogenicity that may cause endocarditis, paronychia, and otitis externa.

C. tropicalis, a species occasionally associated with candidiasis.

can·di·de·mia (kan-di-dē′mē-ă). Presence of cells of *Candida* species in the peripheral blood. [*Candida* + G. *haima,* blood]

can·di·di·a·sis (kan-di-dī′ă-sis). Infection with, or disease caused by, *Candida,* especially *C. albicans.* This disease usually results from debilitation (as in immunosuppression and especially AIDS), physiologic change, prolonged administration of antibiotics, and iatrogenic and barrier breakage. SYN candidosis, moniliasis.

can·di·do·sis (kan-di-dō′sis). SYN candidiasis.

can·dle (kan′dl). SYN candela.

can·dle-me·ter (kan′dl-mē′ter). SYN lux.

can·dle-pow·er (kan′dl-pow′er). SYN luminous *intensity.*

Can·i·dae (kan′i-dē). A family of the *Carnivora* including the dogs, coyotes, wolves, and foxes. [L. *canis,* dog]

ca·nine (kā′nīn). **1.** Relating to a dog. **2.** Relating to the c. teeth. **3.** SYN canine *tooth.* **4.** Referring to the cuspid tooth. [L. *caninus*]

ca·ni·ni·form (kā-nī′ni-fōrm). Resembling a canine tooth.

can·is·ter (kan′is-ter). A box or container; in anesthesiology, the container for carbon dioxide absorbent.

ca·ni·ti·es (kă-nish′ē-ēz). Graying of hair. SEE ALSO poliosis. [L., fr. *canus,* hoary, gray]

canities c., SYN ectopic *eyelash.*

c. circumscrip′ta, SYN piebald *eyelash.*

rapid c., whitening of hair overnight or over a few days; in the latter case, may be seen in alopecia areata, when surviving pigmented hairs are preferentially shed from gray hair.

can·ker (kang′ker). **1.** In cats and dogs, acute inflammation of the external ear and auditory canal. SEE aphtha. **2.** In the horse, a process similar to but more advanced than thrush; the horny frog is generally underrun with a whitish, cheeselike exudate, and the entire sole and even the wall of the hoof may be undermined. [L. *cancer,* crab, malignant growth]

water c., SYN noma.

can·na·bi·di·ol (kan-ă-bi-dī′ol). A constituent of *Cannabis*, related to cannabinol.

can·nab·i·noids (ka-nab′i-noydz). Organic substances present in *Cannabis sativa*, having a variety of pharmacologic properties.

can·na·bi·nol (ka-nab′i-nol). A constituent of the resinous exudate of the pistillate flowers of *Cannabis sativa;* it has no psychotomimetic action as do the tetrahydro derivatives isolated from marijuana.

can·na·bis (kan′ă-bis). The dried flowering tops of the pistillate plants of *Cannabis sativa* (family Moraceae) containing isomeric tetrahydrocannabinols, cannabinol, and cannabidiol. Preparations of c. are smoked or ingested by members of various cultures and subcultures to induce psychotomimetic effects such as euphoria, hallucinations, drowsiness, and other mental changes. C. was formerly used as a sedative and analgesic; now available for restricted use in management of iatrogenic anorexia, especially that associated with oncologic chemotherapy and radiation therapy. Known by many colloquial or slang terms such as marihuana; marijuana; pot; grass; bhang; charas; ganja; hashish. [L., fr. G. *kannabis,* hemp]

can·na·bism (kan′ă-bizm). Poisoning by preparations of cannabis.

Cannizzaro, Stanislao, Italian chemist, 1826–1910. SEE C. *reaction.*

Cannon, Walter B., U.S. physiologist, 1871–1945. SEE C. *ring, theory;* C.-Bard *theory;* Bernard-C. *homeostasis.*

can·nu·la (kan′ū-lă). A tube that can be inserted into a cavity, usually by means of a trocar filling its lumen; after insertion of the c., the trocar is withdrawn and the c. remains as a channel for the transport of fluid. [L. dim. of *canna,* reed]

Hasson c., a laparoscopic instrument for open (rather than blind needle insufflation) placement of the initial port. The Hasson has a blunt-tipped obturator instead of a sharp trocar and a balloon on the distal portion of the sheath to hold it in place. SYN laparoscopic c.

Karman c., a flexible plastic c. used in performing early (menstrual extraction) abortion.

laparoscopic c., SYN Hasson c.

perfusion c., (1) a double-barreled c. used for irrigation of a cavity, the wash fluid passing into the cavity through one tube and out through the other. (2) c. used to perfuse an organ, i.e., used to flush a donor organ in preparation for transplantation.

washout c., a c. that can be irrigated without removal from the artery.

can·nu·la·tion, can·nu·li·za·tion (kan-ū-lā′shŭn, -ū-lī-zā′shŭn). Insertion of a cannula.

Cantelli sign. See under sign.

can·thal (kan′thăl). Relating to a canthus.

can·thar·i·dal (kan-thar′i-dăl). Relating to or containing cantharides.

can·thar·i·date (kan-thar′i-dāt). A salt of cantharidic acid.

can·thar·i·des (kan-thar′i-dēz). Plural of cantharis.

can·thar·i·dic ac·id (kan-thar′i-dik). An acid, derived from cantharis, that forms salts (cantharidates) with alkalis.

can·thar·i·din (kan-thar′i-din). The active principle of cantharis; the anhydride of cantharic acid. SYN cantharis camphor.

can·tha·ris, gen. **can·thar·i·dis,** pl. **can·thar·i·des** (kan′thar-is, kan-thar′i-dis, -dēz). A dried beetle, *Lytta (Cantharis) vesicatoria,* used as a counterirritant and vesicant. SYN Russian fly, Spanish fly. [L., fr. G. *kantharis,* a beetle]

can·thec·to·my (kan-thek′tō-mē). Excision of a palpebral canthus. [G. *kanthos,* canthus, + *ektomē,* excision]

can·thi (kan′thī). Plural of canthus.

can·thi·tis (kan-thī′tis). Inflammation of a canthus.

can·thol·y·sis (kan-thol′i-sis). SYN canthoplasty (1). [G. *kanthos,* canthus, + *lysis,* loosening]

can·tho·plas·ty (kan′thō-plas-tē). **1.** An operation for lengthening the palpebral fissure by incision through the lateral canthus. SYN cantholysis. **2.** An operation for restoration of the canthus. [G. *kanthos,* canthus, + *plassō,* to form]

can·thor·rha·phy (kan-thōr′ă-fē). Suture of the eyelids at either canthus. [G. *kanthos,* canthus, + *rhaphē,* suture]

can·thot·o·my (kan-thot′ō-mē). Slitting of the canthus. [G. *kanthos,* canthus, + *tomē,* incision]

can·thus, pl. **can·′thi** (kan′thŭs, -thī). The angle of the eye. [G. *kanthos,* corner of the eye]

external c., SYN lateral *angle* of eye.

internal c., SYN medial *angle* of eye.

lateral c., SYN lateral *angle* of eye.

medial c., SYN medial *angle* of eye.

Cantor, Meyer O., U.S. physician, *1907. SEE C. *tube.*

CaOC Abbreviation for cathodal opening *contraction.*

CAP Abbreviation for catabolite (gene) activator *protein.*

cap (kap). **1.** Any anatomic structure that resembles a c. or cover. **2.** A protective covering for an incomplete tooth. **3.** Colloquialism for restoration of the coronal part of a natural tooth by means of an artificial crown. **4.** The nucleotide structure found at the 5′-terminus of many eukaryotic messenger RNAs, consisting of a 7-methylguanosine connected, via its 5′-hydroxyl group, by a triphosphate group to the 5′-hydroxyl group of the first nucleoside encoded by the DNA; usually symbolized as $m^7G^5ppp^5N$, where N is nucleoside number 1 in the transcribed mRNA and is often itself methylated; the c. is added posttranscriptionally.

acrosomal c., a collapsed membranous vesicle that covers the anterior part of the nucleus of the spermatozoon, derived from the acrosomal granule; the carbohydrate-rich substance of the c. is associated with hydrolytic enzymes that aid in sperm penetration of the zona pellucida of the ovum. SYN head c.

apical c., a curved shadow at the apex of one or both hemithoraces on chest x-ray; caused by pleural and pulmonary fibrosis or, on the left, by blood from a traumatic rupture of the aorta.

cervical c., a contraceptive diaphragm that fits over the cervix uteri.

chin c., an extraoral appliance designed to exert an upward and backward force on the mandible by applying pressure to the chin, thereby preventing forward growth.

cradle c., colloquialism for seborrheic dermatitis of the scalp of the newborn, a red, waxy scaling seen in the third to fourth week.

dental c.'s, deciduous cheek teeth in the horse which remain attached to erupting permanent teeth.

duodenal c., the first portion of the duodenum, as seen in a radiograph or by fluoroscopy. SYN duodenal bulb.

enamel c., the enamel covering the crown of a tooth.

head c., SYN acrosomal c.

metanephric c., the concentrated mass of mesodermal cells about the metanephric bud in a young embryo; the cells of the cap form the uriniferous tubules of the permanent kidney. SYN metanephric blastema.

phrygian c., in cholecystography, an incomplete septum or a fold in the gallbladder, the shape of which suggests the liberty cap of the French Revolution.

pyloric c., obsolete term for duodenal c.

ca·pac·i·tance (kă-pas′i-tans). The quantity of electric charge that may be stored upon a body per unit electric potential; expressed in farads, abfarads, or statfarads.

ca·pac·i·ta·tion (kă-pas′i-tā′shŭn). C. is a process whereby the glycoprotein coat is modified and seminal proteins are removed from the surface of the sperm. There are no morphologic changes. C. occurs in in vitro fertilization; after c., the acrosomal reaction can occur. [L. *capacitas,* fr. *capax,* capable of]

ca·pac·i·tor (kă-pas′i-ter, -tōr). A device for holding a charge of electricity. SYN condenser (4).

ca·pac·i·ty (kă-pas′i-tē). **1.** The potential cubic contents of a cavity or receptacle. **2.** Power to do. SEE ALSO volume. [L. *capax,* able to contain; fr. *capio,* to take]

buffer c., the amount of hydrogen ion (or hydroxyl ion) required to bring about a specific pH change in a specified volume of a buffer. SEE ALSO buffer *value.*

carrying c., an estimate of the number of people that a region, a nation, or the planet can sustain.

cranial c., the cubic content of the skull obtained by determining the cubage of small shot, seeds, or beads required to fill the skull.

diffusing c. (symbol, D, followed by subscripts indicating location and chemical species), the amount of oxygen taken up by pulmonary capillary blood per minute per unit average oxygen pressure gradient between alveolar gas and pulmonary capillary blood; units are: ml/min/mm Hg; also applied to other gases such as carbon monoxide, which is used in the standard clinical measure of diffusing c.

forced vital c. (FVC), vital c. measured with the subject exhaling as rapidly as possible; data relating volume, expiratory flow, and time form the basis for other pulmonary function tests, e.g., flow-volume curve, forced expiratory volume, forced expiratory time, forced expiratory flow.

functional residual c. (FRC), the volume of gas remaining in the lungs at the end of a normal expiration; it is the sum of expiratory reserve volume and residual volume. SYN functional residual air.

heat c., the quantity of heat required to raise the temperature of a system 1°C. SYN thermal c.

inspiratory c., the volume of air that can be inspired after a normal expiration; it is the sum of the tidal volume and the inspiratory reserve volume. SYN complementary air.

iron-binding c. (IBC), the c. of iron-binding protein in serum (transferrin) to bind serum iron.

maximum breathing c. (MBC), SYN maximum voluntary *ventilation*.

oxygen c., the maximum quantity of oxygen that will combine chemically with the hemoglobin in a unit volume of blood; normally it amounts to 1.34 ml of O_2 per g of Hb or 20 ml of O_2 per 100 ml of blood.

residual c., SYN residual *volume*.

respiratory c., SYN vital c.

thermal c., SYN heat c.

total lung c. (TLC), the inspiratory c. plus the functional residual c.; i.e., the volume of air contained in the lungs at the end of a maximal inspiration; also equals vital c. plus residual volume.

vital c. (VC), the greatest volume of air that can be exhaled from the lungs after a maximum inspiration. SYN respiratory c.

cap·ac·tins (kap-ak′tinz). A class of proteins capping the ends of actin filaments.

CAPD Acronym for continuous ambulatory peritoneal *dialysis*.

Capgras, Jean Marie Joseph, French psychiatrist, 1873–1950. SEE C. *phenomenon*, *syndrome*.

cap·il·lar·ec·ta·sia (kap′i-lar-ek-tā′zē-ă). Rarely used term for dilation of the capillary blood vessels. [capillary + G. *ektasis*, extension]

Ca·pil·la·ria (kap-i-lā′rē-ă). A genus of aphasmid nematode worms, characterized by threadlike appearance; related to *Trichuris*. [L. *capillaris*, fr. *capillus*, hair]

C. hepat′ica, species of threadworm that infects the liver in rodents; occasionally reported from humans.

C. philippinen′sis, a species of threadworm that has been implicated as a cause of intestinal capillariasis among northern Philippine fishermen.

ca·pil·la·ri·a·sis (kap′i-lār-ī′ă-sis). A disease caused by infection with nematodes of the genus *Capillaria*.

intestinal c., a spruelike diarrheal disease caused by infection with *Capillaria philippinensis*, large populations of which are built up by internal autoinfection in the intestinal mucosa; characterized by abdominal pain, edema, diarrhea, cachexia, hypoproteinemia, hypotension, cardiac failure, and hyporeflexia; severe infection is often manifested as a fulminating disorder that may be fatal.

cap·il·lar·i·o·mo·tor (kap-i-lār′ē-ō-mō′tŏr). Vasomotor, with special reference to the capillaries.

cap·il·lar·i·os·co·py (kap′i-lar-ē-os′kŏ-pē). Viewing the cutaneous capillaries at the base of the fingernail through the low power of the microscope. SYN capillaroscopy, microangioscopy.

cap·il·lar·i·tis (kap′i-lar-ī′tis). Inflammation of a capillary or capillaries.

cap·il·lar·i·ty (kap-i-lar′i-tē). The rise of liquids in narrow tubes or through the pores of a loose material, as a result of capillary action.

cap·il·la·ron (kap′i-lă-ron). An anatomical module composed of parenchymal cells together with their blood capillaries and extra-capillary fluid in a compliant capsule; functions as a hydraulic unit that provides a theoretical basis for proposing that blood flow is regulated at the capillary.

cap·il·la·rop·a·thy (kap′i-lă-rop′ă-thē). Any disease of the capillaries, often applied to vascular changes in diabetes mellitus. SYN microangiopathy. [capillary + G. *pathos*, disease]

cap·il·lar·os·co·py (kap′i-lar-os′kō-pē). SYN capillarioscopy.

cap·il·lary (kap′i-lār-ē) [TA]. **1.** Resembling a hair; fine; minute. **2.** A capillary vessel; e.g., blood c., lymph c. SYN vas capillare [TA], capillary vessel. **3.** Relating to a blood or lymphatic c. vessel. [L. *capillaris*, relating to hair]

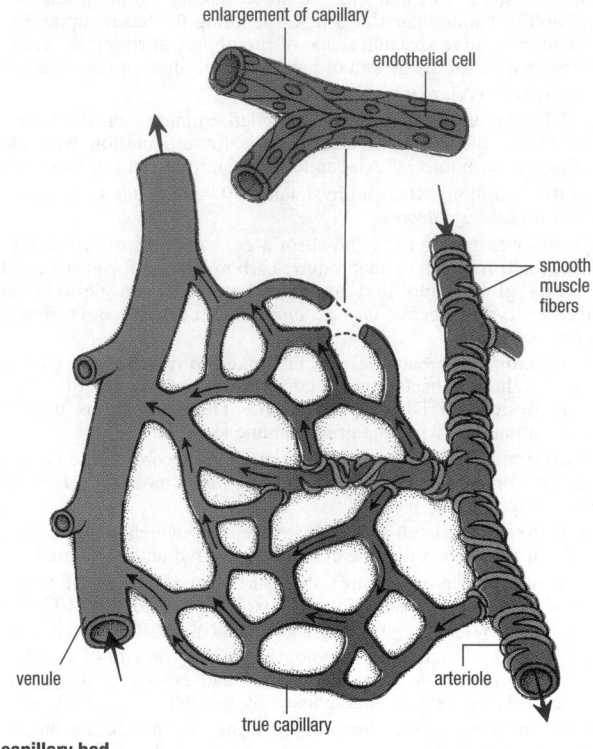

enlargement of capillary

endothelial cell

smooth muscle fibers

venule

arteriole

true capillary

capillary bed

arterial c., a c. opening from an arteriole or metarteriole.

bile c., SYN biliary *canaliculus*.

blood c. (symbol c, as a subscript), a vessel whose wall consists of endothelium and its basement membrane; its diameter, when the c. is open, is about 8 μm; with the electron microscope, fenestrated c.'s and continuous c.'s are distinguished.

continuous c., a c. in which small vesicles (caveolae) are numerous and pores are absent.

fenestrated c., a c., found in renal glomeruli, intestinal villi, and endocrine glands, in which ultramicroscopic pores of variable size occur; usually these are closed by a delicate diaphragm, although diaphragms are lacking in at least some renal glomerular c.'s.

lymph c., the beginning of the lymphatic system of vessels; it is lined with a highly attenuated endothelium with poorly developed basement membrane and a lumen of variable caliber. SEE lacteal (2).

sinusoidal c., SYN sinusoid.

venous c., a c. opening into a venule.

ca·pi·ta (kap′i-tă). Plural of caput.

cap·i·tate (kap′i-tāt) [TA]. **1.** The largest of the carpal bones; located in the distal row. SYN os capitatum [TA], capitate bone, magnum, os magnum. **2.** Head-shaped; having a rounded extremity. [L. *caput* (*capit-*), head]

capitation (kap-i-tā'shun). A system of medical reimbursement wherein the provider is paid an annual fee per covered patient by an insurer or other financial source, which aggregate fees are intended to reimburse all provided services. [L.L. *capitatio*, fr. *caput*, head]]

cap·i·tel·lum (kap-i-tel'ŭm). **1.** SYN capitulum (1). **2.** SYN *capitulum* of humerus. [L. dim. of *caput*, head]

cap·i·to·ped·al (kap-i-tō-ped'ăl). Relating to the head and the feet. [L. *caput*, head, + *pes* (*ped-*), foot]

ca·pit·u·la (kă-pit'ū-lă). Plural of capitulum.

ca·pit·u·lar (kă-pit'ū-lăr). Relating to a capitulum.

ca·pit·u·lum, pl. **ca·pit·u·la** (kă-pit'ū-lŭm, -lă) [TA]. **1** [NA]. A small head or rounded articular extremity of a bone. SYN capitellum (1). SEE ALSO caput. **2.** The bloodsucking, probing, sensing, and holdfast mouthparts of a tick, including the basal supporting structure; relative size and shape of mouthparts forming the c. are characteristic for the genera of hard ticks. [L. dim. of *caput*, head]

c. hu′meri [TA], SYN c. of humerus.

c. of humerus [TA], the small rounded eminence on the lateral half of the distal end of the humerus for articulation with the radius. SYN c. humeri [TA], capitellum (2), little head of humerus.

Caplan, Anthony, British physician, 1907–1976. SEE C. *nodules*, under *nodule*, *syndrome*.

Cap·no·cy·to·pha·ga (kap′nō-sī-tŏf′a-ga). A genus of Gram-negative, fusiform bacteria that require carbon dioxide for growth and exhibits gliding motility; associated with human periodontal disease; type species is *C. ochracea* (formerly *Bacteroides ochracea*).

C. canimor′sus, a bacterial species linked to infections from dog bites (including bacteremia, endocarditis, and meningitis. Formerly designated DF-2 by the CDC. These infections usually occur in patients with impaired immune systems.

cap·no·gram (kap′nō-gram). A continuous record of the carbon dioxide content of expired air. [G. *kapnos,* smoke, + *gramma,* something written]

cap·no·graph (kap′nō-graf). Instrument by which a continuous graph of the carbon dioxide content of expired air is obtained.

capnometry (cap′-nom-ĕ-trē). Measurement of CO_2 in the proximal airway during inspiration and expiration. End tidal CO_2 (or CO_2 at the end of exspiration) is particularly useful clinically.

cap·ping. 1. Covering. **2.** The aggregation at one end of a cell of surface antigens that have been bound and cross-linked by antibodies; this cap is then endocytosed by the cell.

direct pulp c., a procedure for covering and protecting an exposed vital pulp.

indirect pulp c., the application of a suspension of calcium hydroxide to a thin layer of dentin overlying the pulp (near exposure) in order to stimulate secondary dentin formation and protect the pulp.

Capps, Joseph A., U.S. physician, 1872–1964. SEE C. *reflex*.

cap·rate (kap′rāt). A salt or ester of capric acid.

cap·re·o·my·cin sul·fate (kap′rē-ō-mī′sin). Sulfate salt of the cyclic peptide antibiotic obtained from *Streptomyces capreolus*, used in the treatment of tuberculosis.

n-**cap·ric ac·id** (kap′rik). A fatty acid found among the hydrolysis products of fat in goat's milk, cow's milk, and other substances. Cf. *n*-caproic acid, caprylic acid. SYN *n*-decanoic acid.

ca·pril·o·quism (kă-pril′ō-kwizm). SYN egophony. [L. *caper*, goat, + *loquor*, to speak]

cap·rin (kap′rin). One of the substances found in butter upon which its flavor depends. SYN decanoin, glyceryl tricaprate.

cap·rine (kă′prīn). Relating to goats; goatlike. [L. *caprinus*, of goats]

Cap·ri·pox·vi·rus (kap′ri-poks-vī′rŭs). The genus of Poxviridae that includes the viruses of sheep-pox and goatpox. [L. *capra*, she-goat, + *virus*]

cap·ri·zant (kap′ri-zant). Bounding; leaping; denoting a form of pulse beat. [Fr., leaping, fr. L. *caper*, goat]

cap·ro·ate (kap′rō-āt). **1.** A salt or ester of *n*-caproic acid. **2.** USAN-approved contraction for hexanoate, $CH_3(CH_2)_4COO^-$.

n-**ca·pro·ic ac·id** (kap-rō′ik). A fatty acid found among the hydrolysis products of fat in butter, coconut oil, and some other substances. SYN *n*-hexanoic acid.

cap·ro·yl (kap′rō-il). The acyl radical of caproic acid. SYN hexanoyl.

cap·ro·y·late (kap′rō-i-lāt). A salt or ester of caproic acid. SYN hexanoate.

cap·ry·late (kap′ri-lāt). A salt or ester of caprylic acid. SYN octanoate.

ca·pryl·ic ac·id (kap-ril′ik). A fatty acid found among the hydrolysis products of fat in butter, coconut oil, and other substances. SYN octanoic acid.

cap·sa·i·cin (kap-sā′i-sin). Alkaloidal principle in the fruits of various species of *Capsicum*, with the same uses as capsicum. It depletes substance P from sensory nerve endings; Sometimes used for pain in postherpetic neuralgia.

cap·si·cin (kap′sī-sin). A yellowish red oleoresin containing the active principle of capsicum.

cap·si·cum (kap′si-kŭm). Cayenne, African, or red pepper, the dried ripe fruit of *Capsicum frutescens* (family Solanaceae); used as a carminative, gastrointestinal stimulant, and externally as a rubefacient.

cap·sid (kap′sid). SEE virion.

cap·so·mer, cap·so·mere (kap′sō-mēr). A subunit of the protein coat or capsid of a virus particle. SEE ALSO hexon, penton, virion.

cap·su·la, gen. and pl. **cap·su·lae** (kap′soo-lă, -lē) [TA]. **1.** SYN capsule (2). [L. dim. of *capsa,* a chest or box]

c. adiposa perirenalis [TA],

c. adipo′sa re′nis, SYN paranephric *fat*.

c. articula′ris [TA], SYN joint *capsule*.

c. articula′ris cricoarytenoi′dea [TA], SYN *capsule* of cricoarytenoid joint.

c. articula′ris cricothyroi′dea [TA], SYN *capsule* of cricothyroid joint.

c. bul′bi, SYN fascial *sheath* of eyeball.

c. cor′dis, SYN pericardium.

c. exter′na [TA], SYN external *capsule*.

c. extre′ma [TA], SYN extreme *capsule*.

c. fibro′sa, SYN fibrous *capsule*.

c. fibro′sa glan′dulae thyroi′deae [TA], SYN fibrous *capsule* of thyroid gland.

c. fibro′sa per′ivascula′ris, SYN fibrous *capsule* of liver (1).

c. fibro′sa re′nis [TA], SYN fibrous *capsule* of kidney.

c. glomer′uli, SYN glomerular *capsule*.

c. inter′na [TA], SYN internal *capsule*.

c. len′tis [TA], SYN *capsule* of lens.

c. li′enis [TA], SYN fibrous *capsule* of spleen.

c. vasculo′sa len′tis, in the embryo, the vascular mesenchymal capsule that invests the lens of the eye; the vessels of the deep part of the capsule are branches of the hyaloid artery; those of the superficial part are derived from the anterior ciliary arteries; normally all the vessels are atrophied by the end of the eighth month of intrauterine life.

cap·su·lar (kap′soo-lăr). Relating to any capsule.

cap·su·la·tion (kap-soo-lā′shŭn). Enclosure in a capsule.

cap·sule (kap′sool) [TA]. **1.** A membranous structure, usually dense collagenous connective tissue, that envelops an organ, a joint, or any other part. **2.** An anatomic structure resembling a capsule or envelope. SYN capsula (1) [TA]. **3.** A fibrous tissue layer enveloping an organ or a tumor, especially if benign. **4.** A solid dosage form in which a drug is enclosed in either a hard or soft soluble container or "shell" of a suitable form of gelatin. **5.** A hyaline polysaccharide coating around a fungal or bacterial cell. Bacteria may also have a polypeptide c. or a slime layer around the cell. [L. *capsula,* dim. of *capsa,* box]

adipose c., SYN paranephric *fat*.

adrenal c., SYN suprarenal *gland*.

articular c., ✻official alternate term for joint c.

atrabiliary c., SYN suprarenal *gland*.

auditory c., SYN otic c.

bacterial c., a layer of slime of variable composition which covers the surface of some bacteria; capsulated cells of pathogenic bacteria are usually more virulent than cells without capsules because the former are more resistant to phagocytic action.

Bonnet c., the anterior part of the vagina bulbi.

Bowman c., SYN glomerular c.

brood c.'s, small hollow projections from the lining membrane of a hydatid cyst from which the scoleces arise.

cartilage c., the more intensely basophilic and metachromatic matrix in hyaline cartilage surrounding the lacunae of chrondrocytes resulting from relatively high concentrations of chondromuco protein. SYN territorial matrix.

cricoarytenoid articular c., SYN c. of cricoarytenoid joint.

c. of cricoarytenoid joint [TA], the capsule enclosing the joint between the arytenoid and cricoid cartilages. SYN capsula articularis cricoarytenoidea [TA], cricoarytenoid articular c.

cricothyroid articular c., SYN c. of cricothyroid joint.

c. of cricothyroid joint [TA], the capsule enclosing the cricothyroid joint. SYN capsula articularis cricothyroidea [TA], cricothyroid articular c.

Crosby c., an attachment to the end of a flexible tube, used for peroral biopsy of the small intestine, by which a piece of mucosa is sucked into an opening in the c. and cut off.

crystalline c., SYN c. of lens.

external c. [TA], a thin lamina of white substance separating the claustrum from the putamen. It joins the internal c. at either extremity of the putamen, forming a c. of white matter external to the lenticular nucleus. SYN capsula externa [TA], periclaustral lamina.

extreme c. [TA], the layer of white matter separating the claustrum from the cortex of the insula, probably representing largely corticopetal and corticofugal fibers of the insular cortex. SYN capsula extrema [TA].

eye c., SYN fascial *sheath* of eyeball.

fatty renal c., SYN paranephric *fat*.

fibrous c. [TA], any fibrous envelope of a part; the fibrous capsule of an organ. SYN stratum fibrosum [TA], tunica fibrosa [TA], capsula fibrosa, stratum fibrosum capsulae articularis.

fibrous articular c., SYN fibrous *layer* of joint capsule.

fibrous c. of kidney [TA], a fibrous membrane ensheathing the kidney. SYN capsula fibrosa renis [TA], tunica fibrosa renis.

fibrous c. of liver [TA], **(1)** a layer of connective tissue ensheathing the outer surface of the liver and also the hepatic artery, portal vein, and bile ducts as these ramify within the liver; SYN capsula fibrosa perivascularis, perivascular fibrous c. **(2)** connective tissue c. surrounding the outer surface of the liver, but continuous with septae of some animals, e.g., pigs, which divide parenchyme into lobule, and with the perivascular fibrous c. at the porta hepatis. SYN tunica fibrosa hepatis [TA], Glisson c.

fibrous c. of parotid gland, SYN parotid *fascia*.

fibrous c. of spleen [TA], the fibrous capsule of the spleen, containing collagen, elastic fibers, and smooth muscle. SYN capsula lienis [TA], tunica fibrosa splenis ⭐, tunica fibrosa lienis, tunica propria lienis.

fibrous c. of thyroid gland [TA], the fibrous sheath of the thyroid gland. SYN capsula fibrosa glandulae thyroideae [TA].

Gerota c., SYN renal *fascia*.

Glisson c., SYN fibrous c. of liver (2).

glomerular c. [TA], the expanded beginning of a nephron composed of an inner and outer layer: the visceral layer consists of podocytes that surround a tuft of capillaries (glomerulus); the parietal layer is simple squamous epithelium that becomes cuboidal at the tubular pole. SYN Bowman c., capsula glomeruli, malpighian c. (1), Müller c.

internal c. [TA], a massive layer (8–10 mm thick) of white matter separating the caudate nucleus and thalamus (medial) from the more laterally situated lentiform nucleus (globus pallidus and putamen). It consists of 1) fibers ascending from the thalamus to the cerebral cortex that compose, among others, the visual, audi-

tory, and somatic sensory radiations, and 2) fibers descending from the cerebral cortex to the thalamus, subthalamic region, midbrain, hindbrain, and spinal cord. The internal c. is the major route by which the cerebral cortex is connected with the brainstem and spinal cord. Laterally and superiorly it is continuous with the corona radiata which forms a major part of the cerebral hemisphere's white matter; caudally and medially it continues, much reduced in size, as the crus cerebri which contains, among others, corticospinal fibers. On horizontal section it appears in the form of a V opening out laterally; the V's obtuse angle is called genu (knee); its anterior and posterior limbs, respectively, the crus anterior and crus posterior. The internal c. consists of an anterior limb [TA], genu of internal capsule [TA], posterior limb [TA], retrolentiform (or retrolenticular) limb [TA], and sublentiform (or sublenticular) limb [TA]. SYN capsula interna [TA].

🔢 joint c. [TA], a sac enclosing the articulating ends of the bones participating in a synovial joint, formed by an outer fibrous articular c. and an inner synovial membrane. SYN capsula articularis [TA], articular c. ⭐.

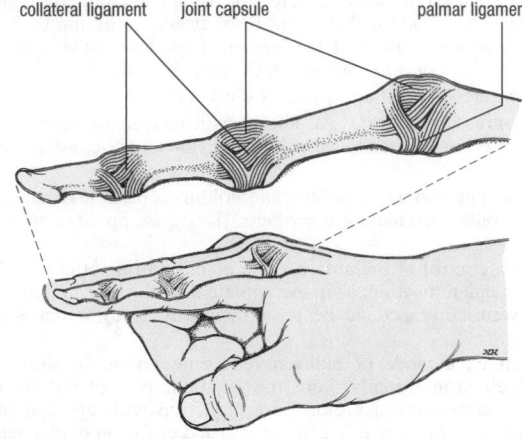

collateral ligament　joint capsule　palmar ligament

interphalangeal capsules: and associated collateral and palmar ligaments

lens c., SYN c. of lens.

c. of lens [TA], the capsule enclosing the lens of the eye. SYN capsula lentis [TA], crystalline c., lens c., lenticular c., phacocyst.

lenticular c., SYN c. of lens.

malpighian c., **(1)** SYN glomerular c; **(2)** a thin fibrous membrane enveloping the spleen and continued over the vessels entering at the hilus.

Müller c., SYN glomerular c.

nasal c., the cartilage around the developing nasal cavity of the embryo.

optic c., the concentrated zone of mesenchyme around the developing optic cup; the primordium of the sclera of the eye.

otic c., the cartilage c. surrounding the inner ear mechanism; in elasmobranchs, it remains cartilaginous in the adult; in the embryos of higher vertebrates, it is cartilaginous at first but later becomes bony (at approximately 23 weeks in humans). SYN auditory c.

perirenal fat c., SYN paranephric *fat*.

perivascular fibrous c., SYN fibrous c. of liver (1).

radiotelemetering c., an instrument that transmits measurements by radio impulses, from within the body; e.g., measurements of pressure from within the small bowel. SYN radiopill.

seminal c., SYN seminal *gland*.

suprarenal c., SYN suprarenal *gland*.

Tenon c., SYN fascial *sheath* of eyeball.

cap·sul·ec·to·my. Removal of a capsule, as around an implant or scarred tissue.

cap·su·li·tis (kap′soo-lī′tis). Inflammation of the capsule of an organ or part, as of the liver, the lens of the eye, or surrounding a joint.

adhesive c., a condition in which there is limitation of motion in a joint due to inflammatory thickening of the capsule, a common cause of stiffness in the shoulder. SYN frozen shoulder.

hepatic c., SYN perihepatitis.

cap·su·lo·len·tic·u·lar (kap′soo-lō-len-tik′ū-lăr). Referring to the lens of the eye and its capsule.

cap·su·lo·plas·ty (kap′soo-lō-plas-tē). Rearrangement of the wall of a capsule; often the capsule of a joint. [L. *capsula,* capsule, + G. *plastos,* formed]

cap·su·lor·rha·phy (kap-soo-lōr′ă-fē). Suture of a tear or surgical incision in any capsule; specifically, suture of a joint capsule to prevent recurring dislocation of the articulation. [L. *capsula,* capsule, + *rhaphē,* suture]

capsulorrhexis (kap-soo-lō-reks′sis). Technique used in cataract surgery by which a continuous circular tear is made in the anterior lens capsule. [L. *capsula,* capsule, + G. *rhēxis,* rupture]

cap·su·lo·tome (kap′soo-lō-tōm). SYN cystotome (2).

cap·su·lot·o·my (kap-soo-lot′ō-mē). **1.** Division of a capsule as around a breast implant. **2.** Creation of an opening through a capsule; e.g., of a scar that might form around a foreign body. **3.** Incision of the capsule of the lens in the extracapsular cataract operation. [L. *capsula,* capsule, + G. *tomē,* a cutting]

renal c., incision of the capsule of the kidney.

cap·to·pril (kap′tō-pril). An angiotensin converting enzyme inhibitor used in the treatment of hypertension and congestive heart failure.

cap·ture (kap′choor). Catching and holding a particle or an electrical impulse originating elsewhere. [L. *capio,* pp. *-tus,* to take, seize]

atrial c., control of the atria for one or more beats after a period of independent beating, as in incomplete AV block or in junctional or ventricular ectopic beats or tachycardias by a retrograde impulse.

electron c., a mode of radioactive disintegration, in which an orbital electron, usually from the K shell, is captured by the nucleus, converting a proton into a neutron with ejection of a neutrino and emission of a gamma ray, and emission of characteristic x-rays as the missing K-shell electron is replaced. SYN K c.

K c., SYN electron c.

ventricular c., capture of the ventricle(s) by an impulse arising in the atria or A-V junction.

Capuron, Joseph, French physician, 1767–1850. SEE C. *points,* under *point.*

ca·put, gen. **ca·pi·tis,** pl. **ca·pi·ta** (kap′ut, ka′put; kap′i-tis; kap′ĭ-tă) [TA]. [TA] SYN head. [L.]

c. angula′re quadra′ti la′bii superio′ris, SYN levator labii superioris alaeque nasi (*muscle*).

c. bre′ve [TA], SYN short *head.*

c. breve musculi bicipitis brachii [TA], SYN short *head* of biceps brachii.

c. breve musculi bicipitis fem′oris [TA], SYN short *head* of biceps femoris.

c. cos′tae [TA], SYN *head* of rib.

c. epididymid′is [TA], SYN *head* of epididymis.

c. fem′oris [TA], SYN *head* of femur.

c. fib′ulae [TA], SYN *head* of fibula.

c. gallinaginis, obsolete term for seminal *colliculus.* [Mod. L. snipe's head]

c. humera′le [TA], SYN humeral *head.*

c. humerale musculi flexoris carpi ulnaris, humeral head of flexor carpi ulnaris muscle. SEE humeral *head.*

c. humerale musculi pronatoris teretis, humeral head of pronator teres muscle. SEE humeral *head.*

c. hu′meri [TA], SYN *head* of humerus.

c. humeroulna′re musculi flexoris digitorum superificialis [TA], SYN humeroulnar *head* of flexor digitorum superficialis muscle.

c. infraorbita′le quadra′ti la′bii superio′ris, SYN levator labii superioris (*muscle*).

c. latera′le [TA], SYN lateral *head.*

c. laterale musculi gastrocnemii, lateral head of gastrocnemius muscle. SEE lateral *head.*

c. laterale musculi tricipitis brachii, lateral head of triceps brachii. SEE lateral *head.*

c. long′um [TA], SYN long *head.*

c. longum musculi bicipitis brachii, long head of biceps brachii muscle. SEE long *head.*

c. longum musculi bicipitis fem′oris, long head of biceps femoris muscle. SEE long *head.*

c. longum musculi tricipitis brachii, long head of triceps brachii muscle. SEE long *head.*

c. mal′lei [TA], SYN *head* of malleus.

c. mandib′ulae [TA], SYN *head* of mandible.

c. media′le [TA], SYN medial *head.*

c. mediale musculi gastrocnemii, medial head of gastrocnemius muscle. SEE medial *head.*

c. mediale musculi tricipitis brachii, medial head of triceps brachii muscle. SEE medial *head.*

c. medu′sae, (1) varicose veins radiating from the umbilicus, seen in the Cruveilhier-Baumgarten syndrome; **(2)** dilated ciliary arteries girdling the corneoscleral limbus in rubeosis iridis. SYN Medusa head. [*Medusa,* G. myth. char.]

c. nu′clei cauda′ti [TA], SYN *head* of caudate nucleus.

c. obli′quum [TA], SYN oblique *head.*

c. obliquum musculi adductoris hallucis, oblique head of adductor hallucis muscle. SEE oblique *head.*

c. obliquum musculi adductoris pollicis, oblique head of adductor pollicis muscle. SEE oblique *head.*

c. os′sis fem′oris, SYN *head* of femur.

c. os′sis metacarpa′lis [TA], SYN *head* of metacarpal.

c. os′sis metatarsa′lis [TA], SYN *head* of metatarsal.

c. pancrea′tis [TA], SYN *head* of pancreas.

c. phalan′gis (manus et pedis) [TA], SYN *head* of phalanx (of hand or foot).

c. profun′dum musculi flexoris pollicis brevis [TA], SYN deep *head* of flexor pollicis brevis.

c. quadra′tum, a head of large size and square shape, owing to thickened parietal and frontal eminences, seen in rachitic children.

c. ra′dii [TA], SYN *head* of radius.

c. stape′dis [TA], SYN *head* of stapes.

c. succeda′neum, an edematous swelling formed on the presenting portion of the scalp of an infant during birth; the effusion overlies the periosteum and consists of edema; contrasted with cephalhematoma, in which condition the effusion lies under the periosteum and consists of blood.

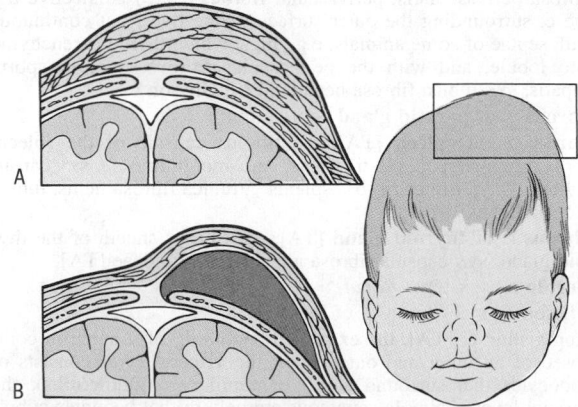

caput succedaneum (A) and **cephalhematoma** (B): in caput succedaneum, edema between skull and scalp extends across suture line; in cephalhematoma, subperiosteal hemorrhage stops at suture line

c. superficia′le musculi flexoris pollicis brevis [TA], SYN superficial *head* of flexor pollicis brevis.

c. ta′li [TA], SYN *head* of talus.

c. transver′sum [TA], SYN transverse *head*.

c. transversum musculi adductoris hallucis, transverse head of adductor hallucis muscle. SEE transverse *head*.

c. transversum musculi adductoris pollicis, transverse head of adductor pollicis muscle. SEE transverse *head*.

c. ul′nae [TA], SYN *head* of ulna.

c. ulna′re [TA], SYN ulnar *head*.

c. ulnare musculi flexoris carpi ulnaris, ulnar head of flexor carpi ulnaris muscle. SEE ulnar *head*.

c. ulnare musculi pronatoris teretis, ulnar head of pronator teres muscle. SEE ulnar *head*.

c. zygomat′icum quadra′ti la′bii superio′ris, SYN zygomaticus minor (*muscle*).

Carabelli, Georg (Edler von Lunkaszprie), Austrian dentist, 1787–1842. SEE *cusp* of C.; C. *tubercle.*

car·a·mel (kar′ă-mel). Burnt sugar; a concentrated solution of the substance obtained by heating sugar with an alkali; a thick, dark brown liquid used as a coloring and flavoring agent in pharmaceutical preparations and foods. [Sp., fr. L.L. *calamellus,* fr. L. *calamus,* reed]

ca·ram·i·phen eth·ane·di·sul·fo·nate (ka-ram′i-fen eth′ān-dī-sŭl′fō-nāt). An antitussive.

ca·ram·i·phen hy·dro·chlo·ride. A synthetic spasmolytic drug; used in the treatment of diseases of the basal ganglia, e.g., parkinsonism and hepatolenticular degeneration.

ca·ra·te (kă-rah′tē). SYN pinta.

⚖**carb-, carbo-.** Prefixes indicating carbon, especially the attachment of a group containing a carbon atom. [L. *carbo,* charcoal]

car·ba·chol (kar′bă-kol). A parasympathetic stimulant used locally in the eye for the treatment of glaucoma.

car·ba·dox (kar′bă-doks). An antibacterial agent.

car·ba·mate (kar′bă-māt). **1.** A salt or ester of carbamic acid forming the basis of urethane hypnotics. **2.** A group of cholinesterase-inhibiting insecticides resembling organophosphates; the most frequent c. is carbaril. SYN carbamoate, carbaril.

c. kinase, a phosphotransferase catalyzing the reaction of carbamoyl phosphate and ADP to form ATP, NH_3, and CO_2.

car·bam·az·e·pine (kar-bam-az′ĕ-pēn). An anticonvulsant; also useful in alleviating the pain of trigeminal neuralgia and other neurogenic pain syndromes.

car·bam·ic ac·id (kar-bam′ik). A hypothetical acid, NH_2–COOH, forming carbamates; the acyl radical is carbamoyl.

car·bam·ide (kar′bă-mīd). Obsolete term for urea.

carb·a·mi·no·he·mo·glo·bin (kar-bam′i-nō-hē-mō-glō′bin). Carbon dioxide bound to hemoglobin by means of a reactive amino group on the latter, i.e., Hb–NHCOOH; approximately 20% of the total content of carbon dioxide in blood is combined with hemoglobin in this manner. SYN carbhemoglobin, carbohemoglobin.

car·ba·moate (kar′bă-mōt). SYN carbamate.

car·bam·o·yl (kar′bă-mō-il). The acyl radical, NH_2–CO–, the transfer of which plays an important role in certain biochemical reactions; e.g., in the urea cycle, via carbamoyl phosphate.

car·bam·o·yl·as·par·tate de·hy·drase (kar′bă-mō-il-as-par′tāt). SYN dihydro-orotase.

***N*-car·bam·o·yl·as·par·tic acid** (kar′bă-mō-il-as-par′tik). SYN ureidosuccinic acid.

car·bam·o·yl·a·tion (kar-bă-mō-il-ā′shŭn). Transfer of the carbamoyl from a carbamoyl-containing molecule (e.g., carbamoyl phosphate) to an acceptor moiety such as an amino group; the second step in the urea cycle is a c.

car·bam·o·yl·car·bam·ic ac·id (kar′bă-mō-il-kar-bam′ik). SYN allophanic acid.

***N*-car·bam·o·yl·glu·tam·ic ac·id** (kar′bă-mō-il-gloo-tam′ik). An intermediate in the carbamoylation of ornithine to citrulline in the urea cycle; used in the treatment of individuals having a deficiency of the enzyme that synthesizes *N*-acetylglutamate.

car·bam·o·yl phos·phate. A reactive intermediate capable of transferring its carbamoyl group to an acceptor molecule, forming

citrulline from ornithine in the urea cycle, and ureidosuccinic acid from aspartic acid in pyrimidine ring formation.

c. p. synthetase, a phosphotransferase catalyzing the formation of c. p. There are two significant isozymes. c. p. synthetase I is a mitochondrial enzyme that catalyzes the reaction of 2ATP, NH_3, CO_2, and H_2O to c. p., 2ADP, and orthophosphate. It is activated by *N*-acetylglutamate and participates in urea biosynthesis. A deficiency of c. p. synthetase I can result in hyperammonemia. c. p. synthetase II is a cytosolic enzyme that, under physiological conditions, uses L-glutamine as the nitrogen source (producing L-glutamate) instead of NH_3, is not activated by *N*-acetylglutamate, and participates in pyrimidine biosynthesis.

car·bam·o·yl·trans·fer·as·es (kar′bă-mō-il-trans′fer-ās-ĕz) [EC 2.1.3.x]. Enzymes transferring carbamoyl groups from one compound to another (e.g., aspartate carbamoyltransferase, ornithine carbamoyltransferase). SYN transcarbamoylases.

car·bam·o·yl·u·rea (kar′bă-mō-il-ū-rē′ă). SYN biuret.

car·ba·myl (kar′bă-mil). Former spelling of carbamoyl.

car·ba·myl·a·tion (kar′bă-mil-ā′shŭn). Former spelling of carbamoylation.

carb·an·i·on (karb-an′ī-on). An organic anion in which the negative charge is on a carbon atom; the specific names are formed by adding -ide, -diide, etc., to the name of the parent compound; e.g., methanide, $(CH_3)^-$.

car·ba·pe·nems. A class of broad-spectrum bactericidal β-lactam antibiotics that bind to the penicillin-binding protein 2 and thereby interfere with cell wall structure; they are highly resistant to β-lactamases and easily penetrate bacterial walls.

car·bar·il (car-bar-il′). SYN carbamate.

car·bar·sone (kar-bar′sōn). An amebicide.

car·bar·yl (kar′bă-ril). A cholinesterase-inhibiting contact insecticide. A pediculicide and ectoparasiticide. Toxic to humans, causing nausea, vomiting, diarrhea, bronchoconstrictions, blurring vision, excessive salivation, muscle twitching, cyanosis, convulsions, coma, respiratory failure.

car·ba·zides (kar′bă-zīds). 1,3-diaminoureas. SYN carbohydrazides.

car·baz·o·chrome sa·lic·y·late (kar-baz′ō-krōm). An oxidation product of epinephrine used for the systemic control of capillary bleeding associated with increased capillary permeability.

car·ba·zole (kar′bă-zōl). Reacts with carbohydrates (including uronates and deoxypentoses) giving colors characteristic of the sugar type; used for assay and analysis of carbohydrates and formaldehyde, and as a dye intermediate; sensitive to ultraviolet light. SYN 9-azafluorene, diphenylenimine.

carb·a·zot·ic ac·id (kar-bă-zot′ik). SYN picric acid.

car·ben·i·cil·lin di·so·di·um (kar-ben-i-sil′in). A semisynthetic extended spectrum penicillin active against a wide variety of Gram-positive and Gram-negative bacteria.

car·be·ni·um (kar-ben′ē-ŭm). SEE carbonium.

car·be·ta·pen·tane cit·rate (kar′be-tă-pen′tān). It has atropine-like and local anesthetic actions and effectively suppresses acute cough due to common upper respiratory infections.

carb·he·mo·glo·bin (karb′hē-mō-glō′bin). SYN carbaminohemoglobin.

car·bide (kar′bīd). A compound of carbon with an element more electropositive than itself; e.g., CaC_2, calcium carbide.

car·bi·do·pa (kar-bi-dō′pă). A dopa decarboxylase inhibitor which does not enter the brain used in conjunction with levodopa in the treatment of Parkinson disease to reduce L-dopa doses and reduce side effects.

car·bi·ma·zole (kar-bī′mă-zōl). Used in the treatment of hyperthyroidism.

car·bi·nol (kar′bi-nol). SYN methyl *alcohol.*

car·bi·nox·a·mine ma·le·ate (kar-bi-nok′să-mēn). An antihistaminic agent.

carbo. SYN charcoal. [L. coal]

⚖**carbo-.** SEE carb-.

car·bo·ben·zoxy- (Z, Cbz) (kar′bō-ben-zok′sē). SYN benzyloxy-carbonyl.

car·bo·cat·i·on (kar-bō-kat′ĭ-on). SEE carbonium.

car·bo·gen (kar′bō-jen). A mixture of 10% carbon dioxide and 90% oxygen used for inhalation therapy to produce vasodilation. [*carbo*n dioxide + oxy*gen*]

car·bo·he·mo·glo·bin (kar′bō-hē-mō-glō′bin). SYN carbaminohemoglobin.

car·bo·hy·drates (kar-bō-hī′drāts). Class name for the aldehydic or ketonic derivatives of polyhydric alcohols, the name being derived from the fact that the most common examples of such compounds have formulas that may be written as $C_n(H_2O)_n$ (e.g., glucose, $C_6(H_2O)_6$; sucrose, $C_{12}(H_2O)_{11}$, although they are not true hydrates and the name is, in that sense, a misnomer. The group includes compounds with relatively small molecules, such as the simple sugars (monosaccharides, disaccharides, etc.), as well as macromolecular (polymeric) substances such as starch, glycogen, and cellulose. The c.'s most typical of the class contain carbon, hydrogen, and oxygen only, but carbohydrate metabolic intermediates in tissues also contain phosphorus. SEE saccharides.

car·bo·hy·drat·u·ria (kar′bō-hī-dră-too′rē-ă). General term denoting the excretion of one or more carbohydrates in the urine (e.g., glucose, galactose, lactose, pentose), thus including such conditions as glycosuria (melituria), galactosuria, lactosuria, pentosuria, etc.

car·bo·hy·dra·zides (kar-bō-hī′dră-zīdz). SYN carbazides.

car·bo·late (kar′bō-lāt). 1. SYN phenate. 2. To carbolize.

car·bo·lat·ed (kar′bō-lā-ted). SYN phenolated.

car·bol-fuch·sin (kar′bol-fuk′sin). 1. SEE Ziehl *stain*. 2. SEE carbol-fuchsin *paint*.

car·bol·ic ac·id (kar-bol′ik). SYN phenol.

car·bo·lize (kar′bō-līz). To mix with or add carbolic acid (phenol).

car·bo·lu·ria (kar-bō-loo′rē-ă). The presence of phenol (carbolic acid) in the urine. [carbolic acid + G. *ouron*, urine]

car·bo·mer (kar′bō-mer). A polymer of acrylic acid cross-linked with a polyfunctional compound, hence, a poly (acrylic acid) or polyacrylate; a suspending agent for pharmaceuticals.

car·bom·e·try (kar-bom′ĕ-trē). SYN carbonometry.

car·bo·my·cin (kar′bō-mī′sin). A macrolide antibiotic isolated from *Streptomyces halstedii;* similar to erythromycin and used as an antibacterial and antimicrobial.

car·bon (C) (kar′bŏn). A nonmetallic tetravalent element, atomic no. 6, atomic wt. 12.011; the major bioelement. It has two natural isotopes, ^{12}C and ^{13}C (the former, set at 12.00000, being the standard for all molecular weights), and two artificial, radioactive isotopes of interest, ^{11}C and ^{14}C. The element occurs in three pure forms (diamond, graphite, and in the fullerines), in amorphous form (in charcoal, coke, and soot), and in the atmosphere as CO_2. Its compounds are found in all living tissues, and the study of its vast number of compounds constitutes most of organic chemistry. [L. *carbo*, coal]

active c. dioxide, activated c. dioxide, complex of *N*-carboxybiotin (biotin + CO_2) and an enzyme; the form in which c. dioxide is added to other molecules in carboxylations; e.g., to methylcrotonyl-CoA to form β-methylglutaconyl in the catabolism of leucine, and to acetyl-CoA to form malonyl-CoA. SEE ALSO *acetyl-CoA* carboxylase.

anomeric c., the reducing c. of a sugar; C-1 of an aldose, C-2 of a 2-ketose.

c. bisulfide, SYN c. disulfide.

c. dichloride, SYN tetrachlorethylene.

c. dioxide, CO_2; the product of the combustion of c. with an excess of air; in concentrations not less than 99.0% by volume of CO_2, used as a respiratory stimulant. SYN carbonic acid gas, carbonic anhydride.

c. dioxide snow, solid c. dioxide used in the treatment of warts, lupus, nevi, and other skin affections, and as a refrigerant. SYN dry ice.

c. disulfide, an extremely flammable (flashpoint −30°C), colorless, toxic liquid with a characteristic ethereal odor (fetid when impure); it is a parasiticide. SYN c. bisulfide.

c. monoxide (CO), a colorless, practically odorless, and poisonous gas formed by the incomplete combustion of c.; its toxic action is due to its strong affinity for hemoglobin, myoglobin, and the cytochromes, reducing oxygen transport and blocking oxygen utilization.

c. tetrachloride, a colorless, mobile liquid having a characteristic ethereal odor resembling that of chloroform; it is used as a cleansing fluid and as a fire extinguisher, and has been used as an anthelmintic, especially against hookworm. SYN tetrachloromethane.

car·bon-11 (^{11}C). A cyclotron-produced, positron-emitting radioisotope of carbon with a half-life of 20.3 minutes; used in positron emission tomography (PET).

car·bon-12 (^{12}C). The standard of atomic mass, 98.90% of natural carbon.

car·bon-13 (^{13}C). A stable natural isotope, 1.1% of natural carbon.

car·bon-14 (^{14}C). A β-emitter with a half-life of 5715 years, widely used as a tracer in studying various aspects of metabolism; naturally occurring ^{14}C, arising from cosmic ray bombardment, is used to date relics containing natural carbonaceous materials.

car·bon·ate (kar′bŏn-āt). 1. A salt of carbonic acid. 2. The ion CO_3^{2-}.

c. dehydratase, SYN carbonic *anhydrase*.

c. hydro-lyase, SYN carbonic *anhydrase*.

car·bon·ic (kar-bon′ik). Relating to carbon. See also under carbonate.

car·bon·ic ac·id. H_2CO_3, formed from H_2O and CO_2.

car·bon·ic an·hy·dride. SYN carbon dioxide.

car·bo·ni·um (kar-bŏn′ē-ŭm). An organic cation in which the positive charge is on a carbon atom; e.g., $(CH_3)^+$. It is now recommended that carbocation be used as the class name and carbenium be used for specific compound names.

car·bo·nom·e·ter (kar-bō-nom′ĕ-ter). An obsolete device used in carbonometry. [L. *carbo* (*carbon*-), coal, + G. *metron*, measure]

car·bo·nom·e·try (kar-bō-nom′ĕ-trē). An obsolete method for the determination of the presence and the proportion of carbon dioxide in the air or expired breath by the precipitation of calcium carbonate from lime water. SYN carbometry.

car·bo·nu·ria (kar-bo-noo′rē-ă). Rarely used term denoting the excretion of carbon dioxide or other carbon compounds in the urine.

car·bon·yl (kar′bŏn-il). The characteristic group, –CO–, of the ketones, aldehydes, and organic acids.

car·bo·plat·in (kar′bō-plă′tin). A platinum-containing anticancer agent much like cisplatin but more toxic to the myeloid elements of bone marrow while producing less nausea and neuro-, oto-, and nephrotoxicity; used in the chemotherapy of solid tumors.

car·bo·prost tro·meth·a·mine (kar′bō-prost trō-meth′ă-mēn). A prostaglandin used as an abortifacient and in the treatment of refractory postpartum bleeding.

car·box·am·ide (kar-boks′am-īd). A molecular configuration (–CONH₂) that, together with the related carboximides (iminocarbonyls) (–CONH–), is a constituent of many hypnotics, including barbiturates, hydantoins, and thiazines. SYN aminocarbonyl.

car·box·im·ide (kar-boks′im-īd). SEE carboxamide.

carboxy-. Combining form indicating addition of CO or CO_2.

N-car·box·y·an·hy·drides (kar-bok′sē-an-hī′drīdz). Heterocyclic derivatives of amino acids from which polypeptides may be synthesized.

car·box·y·ca·thep·sin (kar-bok′sē-kă-thep′sin). SYN peptidyl dipeptidase A.

car·box·y·dis·mu·tase (kar-bok-sē-dis′moo-tās). SYN ribulose-1,5-bisphosphate carboxylase.

4-car·box·y·glu·tam·ic ac·id (Gla) (kar-bok′sē-gloo-tam′ik). A carboxylated form of glutamic acid found in certain proteins (e.g., prothrombin, factors VII, IX, and X, osteocalcin). Its synthesis is vitamin K-dependent.

car·box·y·he·mo·glo·bin (HbCO) (kar-bok′sē-hē-mō-glō′bin). A fairly stable union of carbon monoxide with hemoglobin. The formation of c. prevents the normal transfer of carbon dioxide and oxygen during the circulation of blood; thus, increasing levels of c. result in various degrees of asphyxiation, including death. SYN carbon monoxide hemoglobin, carbonmonoxy myoglobin.

car·box·y·he·mo·glo·bi·ne·mia (kar-bok′sē-hē′mō-glō-bi-nē′ mē-ă). Presence of carboxyhemoglobin in the blood, as in carbon monoxide poisoning.

car·box·yl (kar-bok′sil). The characterizing group (–COOH) of certain organic acids; e.g., HCOOH (formic acid), CH_3COOH (acetic acid), $CH_3CH(NH_2)COOH$ (alanine), etc. Cf. carboxylic acid.

car·box·yl·ase (kar-bok′sil-ās). **1.** One of several carboxy-lyases, trivially named carboxylases or decarboxylases (EC 4.1.1.x), catalyzing the addition of CO_2 to all or part of another molecule to create an additional –COOH group (e.g., ribulose-1,5-bisphosphate carboxylase). **2.** Obsolete name for *pyruvate* decarboxylase.

car·box·yl·a·tion (kar-bok-si-lā′shŭn). Addition of CO_2 to an organic acceptor, as in formation of malonyl-CoA or in photosynthesis, to yield a —COOH group; catalyzed by carboxylases.

car·box·yl·ic ac·id (kar-bok′sil-ik). An organic acid with a carboxyl group. Cf. carboxyl.

activated c. a., derivative of a carboxyl group that is more susceptible to nucleophilic attack than a free carboxyl group; e.g., acid anhydrides, thioesters.

car·box·yl·trans·fer·as·es (kar-bok-sil-trans′fer-ās-ez) [EC 2.1.3.x]. Enzymes transferring carboxyl groups from one compound to another. SYN transcarboxylases.

car·box·y·meth·yl·cel·lu·lose (kar-bok-sē-meth′il-sel′ū-lōs). A cellulose derivative which forms a colloidal dispersion in water; indigestible and nonabsorbable systemically; absorbs water and is used as a bulk laxative. Can also be used as a suspending agent.

car·box·y·pep·ti·dase (kar-bok-sē-pep′ti-dās). A hydrolase that removes the amino acid at the free carboxyl end of a polypeptide chain; an exopeptidase.

acid c., SYN serine c.

serine c., a c. of broad specificity for terminal amino acid residues of peptides; the optimum pH is 4.5 to 6.0; sensitive to diisopropyl fluorophosphate; contains a serine at the active site. SYN acid c.

car·box·y·pep·ti·dase A. A hydrolase that releases C-terminal amino acids, with the exception of C-terminal arginyl, lysyl, and prolyl residues. A zinc-containing exopeptidase.

car·box·y·pep·ti·dase B. A hydrolase that releases C-terminal lysyl or arginyl residues preferentially. A zinc-containing exopeptidase. SYN protaminase.

car·box·y·pep·ti·dase C. SEE serine *carboxypeptidase*.

car·box·y·pep·ti·dase G. SYN γ-glutamyl hydrolase.

N-**car·box·y·u·rea** (kar-bok′sē-ū-rē′ă). SYN allophanic acid.

car·bro·mal (kar′brō-mal). Obsolete hypnotic agent which is a monoureide-containing bromine.

car·bun·cle (kar′bŭng-kl). Deep-seated pyogenic infection of the skin and subcutaneous tissues, usually arising in several contiguous hair follicles, with formation of connecting sinuses. [L. *carbunculus,* dim. of *carbo,* a live coal, a carbuncle]

kidney c., renal c., formerly used term for coalescent multiple intrarenal abscesses.

car·bu·ret (kar′boo-ret). **1.** Archaic term for carbide. **2.** To combine with carbon. **3.** To enrich a gas with volatile hydrocarbons, as in a carburetor.

car·bu·ta·mide (kar-boo′tă-mīd). An oral hypoglycemic agent, e.g., tolbutamide.

car·bu·te·rol hy·dro·chlo·ride (kar-boo′tĕ-rol). A sympathomimetic drug with bronchodilatory activity.

car·cass (kar′kăs). The body of a dead animal; in reference to animals used for human food, the body after the hide, head, tail, extremities, and viscera have been removed. [F. *carcasse,* fr. It. *carcassa*]

carcino-, carcin-. Cancer; crab. [G. *karkinos,* crab, cancer]

car·ci·no·em·bry·on·ic (kar′si-nō-em-brē-on′ik). Relating to a carcinoma-associated substance present in embryonic tissue, as a c. antigen.

car·cin·o·gen (kar-sin′ō-jen, kar′si-nō-jen). Any cancer-producing substance or organism, such as polycyclic aromatic hydrocarbons, or agents such as in certain types of irradiation. [carcino- + G, -*gen,* producing]

complete c., a chemical c. that is able to induce cancer without provocation by a tumor-promoting agent introduced during therapy.

car·ci·no·gen·e·sis (kar′si-nō-jen′ĕ-sis). The origin or production, or development of cancer, including carcinomas and other malignant neoplasms. [carcino- + G. *genesis,* generation]

field c., increased susceptibility of an entire area to c.; the upper aerodigestive tract and colon, e.g., tend to develop synchronous as well as metachronous cancers.

car·ci·no·gen·ic (kar′si-nō-jen′ik). Causing cancer.

carcinogenicity (kar′-sin-ō-jen-is′ĭ-tē). Ability to cause cancer.

car·ci·noid (kar′si-noyd). SEE carcinoid *tumor*, carcinoid *syndrome*.

car·ci·no·lyt·ic (kar′si-nō-lit′ik). Destructive to the cells of carcinoma. [carcino- + G. *lytikos,* causing a solution]

CARCINOMA

car·ci·no·ma (CA), pl. **car·ci·no·mas, carcinomata** (kar-si-nō′mă, -măz). Any of various types of malignant neoplasm derived from epithelial cells, chiefly glandular (adenocarcinoma) or squamous (squamous cell c.); the most commonly occurring kind of cancer. [G. *karkinōma,* fr. *karkinos,* cancer, + -*oma,* tumor]

Like other malignant neoplasms, carcinomas display uncontrolled cellular proliferation, anaplasia (regression of cells and tissues to a more primitive or undifferentiated state), and a tendency to invade adjacent tissues and to spread to distant sites by metastasis. A carcinoma arises from a single cell whose genome either contains an inherited aberration (oncogene) or has acquired one as a consequence of spontaneous mutation or damage by chemical toxins (carcinogens), radiation, viral infection, chronic inflammation, or other external assault. Probably a complex sequence of biochemical and genetic injuries must take place for a carcinoma to develop. Some carcinomas (e.g., prostate, breast) depend partly on the presence of hormones (androgen, estrogen) for their proliferation. Carcinomas are graded histologically according to evidence of invasiveness and changes that indicate anaplasia, i.e., loss of polarity of nuclei, loss of orderly maturation of cells (especially in squamous cell types), variation in the size and shape of cells, hyperchromatism of nuclei with clumping of chromatin, and increase in the nuclear-cytoplasmic ratio. Carcinomas may be undifferentiated, or the neoplastic tissue may resemble to varying degrees one of the types of normal epithelium. Carcinomas can secrete a variety of hormonelike factors capable of inducing systemic (paraneoplastic) effects (e.g., hypercalcemia, thrombophlebitis). The most common site of origin of carcinoma in both sexes is the skin; the second most common site in men is the prostate and in women the breast. However, the most frequently lethal carcinoma in both sexes is bronchogenic carcinoma.

acinar c., SYN acinic cell *adenocarcinoma.*

acinic cell c., SYN acinic cell *adenocarcinoma.*

adenoid cystic c., a histologic type of c. characterized by large epithelial masses containing round, glandlike spaces or cysts that frequently contain mucus or collagen and are bordered by a few or many layers of epithelial cells without intervening stroma, forming a cribriform pattern like a slice of Swiss cheese; perineural invasion and hematogenous metastasis are common; occurs most commonly in salivary glands and skin. SYN cylindromatous c.

adenosquamous c., a type of lung tumor exhibiting areas of clear cut glandular and squamous cell differentiation.

adnexal c., a c. arising from sweat or sebaceous glands.

adrenal cortical carcinoma, a c. arising in the adrenal cortex that may cause virilism or Cushing syndrome.

alveolar cell c., a c., subtype of adenocarcinoma, thought to be derived from epithelium of terminal bronchioles, in which the neoplastic tissue extends along the alveolar walls and grows in small masses within the alveoli; involvement may be uniformly diffuse and massive, or nodular, or lobular; microscopically, the neoplastic cells are cuboidal or columnar and form papillary structures; mucin may be demonstrated in some of the cells and in the material in the alveoli, which also includes denuded cells; metastases in regional lymph nodes, and even in more distant sites, are known to occur, but are infrequent. SYN bronchiolar adenocarcinoma, bronchiolar c., bronchiolo-alveolar c., bronchioloalveolar adenocarcinoma, bronchoalveolar c.

anaplastic c., c. with absence of epithelial structural differentiation.

apocrine c., (1) a c. composed predominantly of cells with abundant eosinophilic granular cytoplasm, occurring in the breast or other sites; **(2)** a c. of the apocrine glands.

basal cell c., a slow-growing, invasive, but usually non-metastasizing neoplasm recapitulating normal basal cells of the epidermis or hair follicles, most commonly arising in sun-damaged skin of the elderly and fair-skinned. SYN basal cell epithelioma.

basaloid c., SYN cloacogenic c.

basal squamous cell c., SYN basosquamous c.

basosquamous c., basisquamous c., a c. of the skin which in structure and behavior is considered transitional between basal cell and squamous cell c. The term should not be used for the much more common keratotic variety of basal cell c., in which the tumor cells are of basal type but which contains small foci of abrupt keratinization. SYN basal squamous cell c.

bronchiolar c., SYN alveolar cell c.

bronchiolo-alveolar c., SYN alveolar cell c.

bronchoalveolar c., SYN alveolar cell c.

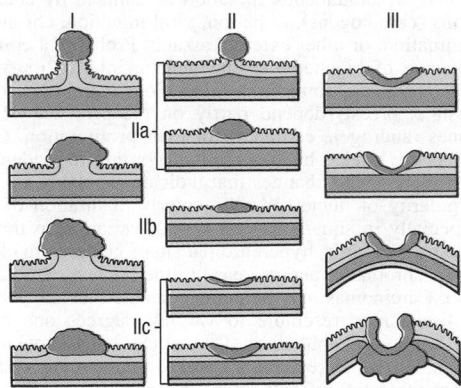

carcinoma: patterns of development in carcinomas of the stomach; I, polypoid or fungating; II, superficial extension (a, elevated; b, plaquelike; c, depressed); III, ulcerating

bronchogenic c., originally described only c. arising in a bronchus, usually squamous or small cell, but now generally agreed to refer to any lung cancer. Includes squamous or epidermoid, small cell or large cell c., and adenocarcinoma. Observed radiologically as an enlarging lung mass; malignant tumor cells can be detected in the sputum. They metastasize early to the thoracic lymph nodes and to the brain, adrenal glands, and other organs through the bloodstream.

canine c. 1, one of the few transplantable tumors of animals.

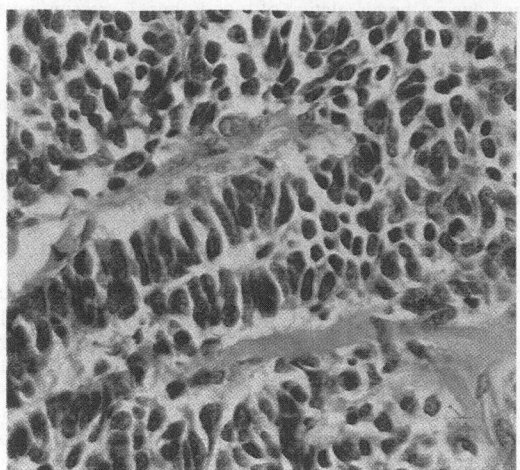

bronchogenic carcinoma: small cell

c. of the breast, a malignant tumor arising from epithelial cells of the female (and occasionally the male) breast, usually adenocarcinoma arising from ductal epithelium.

The impact of breast cancer on Western society is enormous. Breast cancer is the most common noncutaneous malignancy in women. A woman's lifetime risk of developing breast cancer is 8%, and approximately 182,000 cases are newly diagnosed each year in the United States. With 46,000 deaths yearly, it ranks second only to lung cancer as a cause of cancer deaths in women. Most breast cancers are estrogen-dependent adenocarcinomas. Many factors, including age, race, family history, and reproductive history, influence a woman's risk of developing breast cancer. The risk rises with advancing age: it is less than 0.1% at age 30, about 2% at age 50, and 10% at age 80. African-American women have the highest mortality and lowest survival rates for breast cancer. Asian women living in the U.S. have the lowest rates, but some studies suggest that their cancer risk increases as they become acculturated. The risk of breast cancer is slightly increased by nulliparity or first pregnancy after age 35 and by early menarche or late menopause. About 10% of breast cancers are induced by inherited genetic mutations (particularly BRCA1 and BRCA2 mutations, which together account for about one-third of familial breast cancers), the rest by spontaneous, non-inherited mutations. The HER-2/neu oncogene, which encodes a 185-kDa transmembrane oncoprotein, is amplified, overexpressed, or both in 10–30% of invasive breast cancers and in 40–60% of intraductal breast carcinomas. Detection of this gene in cancer tissue by fluorescent in-situ hybridization is associated with poor prognosis (30% greater likelihood of recurrence and cancer death). Women with a strong family history of breast cancer tend to develop it at an earlier age and may also be at risk for ovarian and other malignancies. Other risk factors are cigarette smoking, daily alcohol use, exposure to environmental radon, therapeutic and diagnostic radiation including that from mammograms, and possibly estrogen replacement therapy (with or without a progestogen). Preventive, diagnostic, and therapeutic options continue to be vigorously explored. The possibility of identifying inherited oncogenes has generated controversy as to the appropriateness of prophylactic mastectomy for women at risk for early mammary carcinoma. Tamoxifen, an estrogen antagonist used in the treatment of estrogen-dependent breast cancer, has been found effective in reducing the risk for those with strong family history of breast cancer. Authorities recommend annual mammography for all women over 40, and for high-risk women (those with a strong family history of breast cancer and those who have received irradiation treatment for Hodgkin disease) over 25. Because some 10% of breast cancers that can be felt on examination are missed by mammography, annual examination of the breasts by a physician is also recommended. Recent studies have shown no survival advantage for women practicing breast self examination. Treatments for breast cancer include surgical excision, limited or extensive, with or without radical dissection and removal of axillary lymph nodes; irradiation; and chemotherapy, depending on the type and stage of the disease. Limited resection of small invasive tumors, with preservation of the breast, affords survival rates similar to those after modified radical mastectomy. Chemotherapeutic agents in standard use include doxorubicin, epirubicin, cyclophosphamide, and paclitaxel. Trastuzumab, a monoclonal antibody to the HER-2/neu oncogene, shrinks tumors that contain this gene, but its use is associated with a high incidence of cardiac dysfunction. Known or suspected metastases from an estrogen-responsive tumor are treated with tamoxifen or oophorectomy. See Also BRCA1 gene, BRCA2 gene, mammography, tamoxifen.

c. of the prostate, a malignant neoplasm arising from glandular epithelial cells of the prostate gland.

Prostatic adenocarcinoma (PA) is the most commonly occurring cancer in men, and it ranks second only to lung cancer as a cause of cancer deaths in men. Each year 200,000 new cases are diagnosed in the U.S., and more than 38,000 men die of the disease. Foci of PA are found at autopsy in 40% of men dying after age 50. The neoplasm is androgen-dependent and does not occur in eunuchs. It is both more common and more aggressive in African-American men. A family history of PA, and possibly vasectomy, are other risk factors. PA must be differentiated diagnostically from benign prostatic hyperplasia, which is not a premalignant lesion. PA usually arises in the periphery of the gland and may extend through the capsule into the periprostatic tissues, to seminal vesicles, and regional lymph nodes. At the time of diagnosis, more than 40% of patients have disease that has spread beyond the gland. Bones of the axial skeleton are the usual sites of distant metastasis; the liver, lungs, and brain are other common sites. Early disease is asymptomatic; the diagnosis is most often made by screening of apparently healthy men with digital rectal examination, assay of prostate-specific antigen (PSA), or both. Advanced disease may present as urinary obstruction or bone pain due to metastasis. Men with nodular asymmetry or induration in the prostate gland on digital examination, or elevation of PSA, are evaluated by transrectal ultrasonography of the prostate with ultrasonically directed needle biopsy. Testing for osseous metastases includes measurement of serum alkaline phosphatase, radionuclide bone scan, computed tomography, and magnetic resonance imaging. PA is graded by the Gleason scoring method, which reflects the degree of histologic differentiation in the two most prominent malignant foci. Anatomic staging is based on extension of the tumor beyond the prostatic capsule, not on tumor size. A low or undetectable level of p27 protein in prostatic tissue is a marker of more aggressive malignancy. Treatment depends on the grade and stage of disease and the age and general condition of the patient. In elderly men and those with concurrent life-threatening illness, benign neglect may be the treatment of choice. Radical prostatectomy (removal of the entire gland along with the seminal vesicles) is generally reserved for patients with early or limited disease and a life expectancy of at least 10 years. This treatment is associated with a substantial risk of urinary incontinence and impotence. Radiotherapy with external beam radiation or transperineal implantation of radioactive isotopes may be employed in addition to or instead of surgery. Androgen blockade by orchidectomy or by administration of estrogen, an androgen antagonist, or a gonadotropin-releasing hormone is palliative in advanced disease. Between 1984 and 1992, the number of cases of AP diagnosed nearly doubled, apparently because of extensive PSA screening. Since 1992 the number of new cases has regressed nearly to its former level. The mortality of PA has declined substantially since 1990. Many observers attribute this decline to the ability of PSA screening to detect cancer at a curable stage. In addition, one large case-control study showed that men dying of PA were one-half as likely as population-based controls to have had a digital rectal examination during the preceding 10 years. Some authorities oppose digital rectal examination and PSA screening of asymptomatic men with life expectancies of less than 10 years, on the grounds that the risks of false-negative results and of adverse consequences of aggressive treatment outweigh any possible benefit in survival or quality of life.

clear cell c., SYN mesonephroma.

clear cell c. of kidney, SYN renal *adenocarcinoma.*

clear cell c. of salivary glands, a malignant tumor, comprising several subtypes such as clear cell oncocytoma, hyalinizing clear cell carcinoma, epithelial-myoepithelial (intercalated duct) c.

cloacogenic c., (1) a type of squamous cell c. of the anus originating in tissues arising from, or in remnants of, the cloaca. (2) in oncology, anal cancer arising proximal to the pectinate line. SYN basaloid c., cuboidal c. [cloaca + -genic]

colloid c., SYN mucinous c.

cuboidal c., SYN cloacogenic c.

cylindromatous c., SYN adenoid cystic c.

cystic c., a c. in which true epithelium-lined cysts are formed, or degenerative changes may result in cystlike spaces.

duct c., ductal c., a c. derived from epithelium of ducts, e.g., in the breast or pancreas.

embryonal c., a malignant neoplasm of the testis or ovary, composed of anaplastic cells with indistinct cellular borders, amphophilic cytoplasm, and ovoid, round, or bean-shaped nuclei that may have large nucleoli; in some instances, the neoplastic cells may form tubular or papillary structures.

endometrioid c., adenocarcinoma of the ovary or prostate resembling endometrial adenocarcinoma.

epidermoid c., squamous cell c. of the skin or lung. SYN epidermoid cancer.

epithelial myoepithelial c. (mī′yō-ep-i-thē′lē-al), a salivary gland malignancy composed of an inner layer of ductal cells surrounded by a layer of clear myoepithelial cells.

fibrolamellar liver cell c., primary hepatic c. in which malignant hepatocytes are intersected by fibrous lamellated bands. SYN oncocytic hepatocellular tumor.

follicular carcinoma, c. of the thyroid composed of well or poorly differentiated epithelial follicles without papillary formation, which is difficult to distinguish from adenoma; the criteria include blood vessel invasion and the finding of metastases of follicular thyroid tissue in other structures such as cervical lymph nodes and bone; follicular c. may take up radioactive iodine.

giant cell c., a malignant epithelial neoplasm characterized by unusually large anaplastic cells.

giant cell c. of thyroid gland, a rapidly progressive undifferentiated c. observed in the thyroid gland, characterized by numerous, unusually large, anaplastic cells derived from glandular epithelium of the thyroid gland.

glandular c., SYN adenocarcinoma.

hepatocellular c., a malignant tumor composed of neoplastic liver cells; may be well, moderately, or poorly differentiated; secretes α-fetoprotein, which serves as a useful serologic marker. SYN hepatocarcinoma, liver cell c., malignant hepatoma.

Hürthle cell c., a salivary or thyroid c. composed of cells that have eosinophilic cytoplasm. SEE ALSO Hürthle cell *adenoma.* SYN oncocytic c., oxyphilic c.

inflammatory c., c. of the breast presenting with edema, hyperemia, tenderness, and rapid enlargment of the breast; microscopically, there is extensive invasion of dermal lymphatics by the c.

intraductal c., a form of c. derived from the epithelial lining of ducts, especially in the breast, where most carcinomas arise from ductal epithelium; the neoplastic cells proliferate in irregular papillary projections or masses, filling the lumens, that are solid, cribriform, or centrally necrotic; intraductal c. is a form of c. in situ as it is contained by the ductal basement membrane; when it invades surrounding stroma or metastasizes it is referred to as ductal c.

intraepidermal c., c. in situ of the skin; e.g., Bowen disease.

intraepithelial c., SYN c. in situ.

invasive c., a neoplasm in which collections of epithelial cells infiltrate or destroy the surrounding tissue.

juvenile c., SYN secretory c.

kangri burn c., SYN kang *cancer*.

large cell c., an anaplastic c., particularly bronchogenic, composed of cells which are much larger than those in oat cell c. of the lung.

latent c., an epithelial neoplasm showing microscopic features of malignancy believed to have remained localized and asymptomatic for a long period; e.g., small c. of the prostate in old men, often found incidentally at autopsy.

lateral aberrant thyroid c., obsolete term for a cervical nodule of thyroid c. situated outside the thyroid gland, formerly thought to arise from ectopic thyroid tissue but now believed to be metastatic from an occult c. within the gland.

leptomeningeal c., SYN meningeal c.

liver cell c., SYN hepatocellular c.

lobular c., a form of adenocarcinoma, especially of the breast, where lobular c. is less common than ductal c. and usually is composed of small cells.

lobular c. in situ, SYN noninfiltrating lobular c.

medullary c., a malignant neoplasm, comparatively soft and brainlike in consistency, that consists chiefly of neoplastic epithelial cells, with only a scant amount of fibrous stroma.

medullary c. of breast, a subtype of breast c. composed of sheets of large epithelial cells surrounded by scant fibrous stroma; it is soft and well circumscribed and has a better prognosis than invasive ductal c.

medullary c. of thyroid, a malignant thyroid neoplasm composed of calcitonin producing C-cells and amyloid rich stroma; it may be sporadic or familial; the familial form may be part of the multiple endocrine neoplasia syndrome, type 2A and 2B.

meningeal c., an infiltration of c. cells in the arachnoid and subarachnoid space; may be primary or secondary. SYN leptomeningeal c., leptomeningeal carcinomatosis, meningeal carcinomatosis.

metaplastic c., a c. in which some of the tumor cells are spindle shaped, suggesting a sarcoma, or in which the stroma shows foci of bone or cartilage; such carcinomas occur in the upper respiratory or alimentary tract or in the breast.

metastatic c., a c. that has appeared in a region remote from its site of origin, as in metastasis (2). SYN secondary c.

microinvasive c., a variety of c. seen most frequently in the uterine cervix, in which c. in situ of squamous epithelium, on the surface or replacing the lining of glands, is accompanied by small collections of abnormal epithelial cells that infiltrate a very short distance into the stroma; this represents the earliest stage of invasion.

mucinous c., a variety of adenocarcinoma in which the neoplastic cells secrete conspicuous quantities of mucin, and, as a result, the neoplasm is likely to be glistening, sticky, and gelatinoid in consistency. SYN colloid cancer, colloid c.

mucoepidermoid c., most commonly a salivary gland c. of low grade malignancy composed of mucous, epidermoid, and intermediate cells, with mucous cells abundant only in low-grade c.; recurrence is frequent, and high-grade c. metastasize to cervical nodes. SYN mucoepidermoid tumor.

nasopharyngeal c., a squamous cell c. arising from the surface epithelium of the nasopharynx; three histologic variants are recognized: keratinizing, nonkeratinizing, and undifferentiated c.

noninfiltrating lobular c., c. of the breast in which small tumor cells fill preexisting acini within lobules, without invading the surrounding stroma. SYN lobular c. in situ, lobular neoplasia.

oat cell c., SYN small cell c.

occult c., a small c., either asymptomatic or giving rise to metastases without symptoms due to the primary c.

oncocytic c., SYN Hürthle cell c.

oxyphilic c., SYN Hürthle cell c.

papillary c., a malignant neoplasm characterized by the formation of numerous, irregular, fingerlike projections of fibrous stroma that is covered with a surface layer of neoplastic epithelial cells.

polymorphous low-grade c. of salivary glands, a low-grade malignant tumor of salivary glands showing several histologic patterns, such as cribriform, ductal, and papillary growth. SYN terminal duct c.

primary c., c. at the site of origin, with local invasion in that organ.

primary neuroendocrine c. of the skin, SYN Merkel cell *tumor*.

renal cell c., SYN renal *adenocarcinoma*.

sarcomatoid c., SYN spindle cell c.

scar c., c. of the lung, usually adenocarcinoma, arising from a peripheral lung scar or associated with interstitial fibrosis in a honeycomb lung. SYN scar cancer.

scirrhous c., a hard c., fibrous in nature, resulting from a desmoplastic reaction by the stromal tissue to the presence of the neoplastic epithelium.

secondary c., SYN metastatic c.

secretory c., c. of the breast with pale-staining cells showing prominent secretory activity, as seen in pregnancy and lactation, but found mostly in children. SYN juvenile c.

signet-ring cell c., a poorly differentiated adenocarcinoma composed of cells with a cytoplasmic droplet of mucus that compresses the nucleus to one side along the cell membrane; arises most frequently in the stomach, occasionally in the large bowel or elsewhere.

c. in si′tu (CIS), a lesion characterized by cytologic changes of the type associated with invasive c., but with the pathologic process limited to the lining epithelium and without histologic evidence of extension to adjacent structures; the distinctive changes are usually more apparent in the nucleus, i.e., variation in size and shape, increase in chromatin, and numerous mitoses (including some that are atypical) in all layers of the epithelium, with loss of orderly maturation. The lesion is presumed to be the histologically recognizable precursor of invasive c., i.e., a localized and curable phase of c. SYN intraepithelial c.

small cell c., (1) an anaplastic c. composed of small cells; **(2)** an anaplastic, highly malignant, and usually bronchogenic c. composed of small ovoid cells with very scanty cytoplasm. SYN oat cell c.

spindle cell c., a c. composed of elongated cells, frequently a poorly differentiated squamous cell c. which may be difficult to distinguish from a sarcoma. SYN sarcomatoid c.

squamous cell c., a malignant neoplasm derived from stratified squamous epithelium, but which may also occur in sites such as bronchial mucosa where glandular or columnar epithelium is normally present; variable amounts of keratin are formed, in relation to the degree of differentiation, and, if the keratin is not on the surface, it may accumulate in the neoplasm as a keratin pearl; in instances in which the cells are well differentiated, intercellular bridges may be observed between adjacent cells.

sweat gland c., usually a solitary tumor, nodular and fixed to the skin and underlying structure, having slow growth for long periods followed by rapid growth and dissemination.

terminal duct c., SYN polymorphous low-grade c. of salivary glands.

trabecular c., SYN Merkel cell *tumor*.

transitional cell c., SYN urothelial c.

tubular c., a well-differentiated form of ductal breast c. with invasion of the stroma by small epithelial tubules.

urothelial c., a malignant neoplasm derived from transitional epithelium, occurring chiefly in the urinary bladder, ureters, or renal pelves (especially if well differentiated); frequently papillary; these carcinomas are graded according to the degree of anaplasia. So-called transitional cell c. of the upper respiratory tract is more properly classified as squamous cell c. Transitional cell c. is also a rare tumor of the ovary. SYN transitional cell c.

V-2 c., a transplantable, highly malignant c. of experimental animals that developed as a result of malignant change in a virus-induced papilloma of a domestic rabbit.

verrucous c., a well-differentiated papillary squamous cell c., especially of the oral cavity or penis, that may invade locally but rarely metastasizes; the usual cytologic features of malignancy are absent. Genital verrucous c. may be associated with pre-existing condyloma acuminatum.

villous c., a form of c. in which there are numerous, closely packed, papillary projections of neoplastic epithelial tissue.

wolffian duct c., SYN mesonephroma.

yolk sac c., SYN endocervical sinus *tumor*.

car·ci·no·ma ex ple·o·mor·phic ad·e·no·ma. Carcinoma arising in a benign mixed tumor of a salivary gland, characterized by rapid enlargement and pain.

car·ci·no·ma·ta (kar-si-nō′mă-tă). Alternative plural of carcinoma.

car·ci·no·ma·to·sis (kar′si-nō-mă-tō′sis). A condition resulting from widespread dissemination of carcinoma in multiple sites in various organs or tissues of the body; sometimes also used in relation to involvement of a relatively large region of the body.

leptomeningeal c., SYN meningeal *carcinoma*.

lymphangitic c., a condition in which lymph vessels are filled with tumor cells or blocked by tumor cells.

meningeal c., SYN meningeal *carcinoma*.

car·ci·nom·a·tous (kar-si-nom′ă-tŭs). Pertaining to or manifesting the characteristic properties of carcinoma.

car·ci·no·pho·bia (kar′sin-ō-fō′bē-ă). SYN cancerophobia.

car·ci·no·sar·co·ma (kar′si-nō-sar-kō′mă). A malignant neoplasm that contains elements of carcinoma and sarcoma so extensively intermixed as to indicate neoplasia of epithelial and mesenchymal tissue. SEE ALSO collision *tumor*.

car·ci·no·stat·ic (kar′si-nō-stat′ik). 1. Pertaining to an arresting or inhibitory effect on the development or progression of a carcinoma. 2. An agent that manifests such an effect.

car·co·ma (kar-kō′mă). Dark red-brown or mahogany-colored granular material that occurs in human feces in tropical regions; it yields a chemical reaction similar to that of urobilinogen and is composed of calcium oxide, iron, phosphoric and carbonic acids, urobilinogen, cholerythrogen, and other organic matter in varying proportions. [Sp. wood dust under the bark of a tree, caused by the wood louse]

car·da·mom (kar′dă-mom). Grains of paradise. Dried ripe seeds of *Elettaria cardamomum;* used for flavoring baked goods, confectionery, curry powder, and in the manufacture of *oil* of cardamom which is used for flavoring liqueurs. Pharmaceutical aid (flavor); adjuvant and carminative.

Carden, Henry D., British surgeon, †1872. SEE C. *amputation*.

car·den·o·lide (kar-den′ō-līd). A class of cardiac glycosides containing a five-membered lactone ring (e.g., the *Digitalis* glycosides).

△**cardi-.** SEE cardio-.

car·dia (kar′dē-ă) [TA]. The area of the stomach close to the esophageal opening (cardiac orifice or cardia) that contains the cardiac glands. SYN pars cardiaca gastricae [TA], cardiac part of stomach, cardial part of stomach, gastric cardia, pars cardiaca ventriculi. [G. *kardia*, heart]

car·di·ac (kar′dē-ak). 1. Pertaining to the heart. 2. Pertaining to the esophageal opening of the stomach. 3. (Obsolete). A remedy for heart disease. [L. *cardiacus*]

car·di·ac bal·let (kar′dē-ak bal-ā′). Short runs of cardiac dysrhythmia consisting of uniform sequences of repetitive multiform extrasystoles; so called from its undulating appearance, originally described by Bellet. SEE ALSO torsade de pointes.

car·di·al·gia (kar-dē-al′jē-ă). 1. Obsolete term for pyrosis. 2. SYN cardiodynia. [cardi- + G. *algos*, pain]

car·di·a·tax·ia (kar′dē-ă-tak′sē-ă). Extreme irregularity in the action of the heart. [cardi- + G. *ataxia*, disorder]

car·di·a·te·lia (kar′dē-ă-tē′lē-ă). Incomplete development of the heart. [cardi- + G. *atelēs*, incomplete]

car·di·ec·ta·sia (kar′dē-ek-tā′zē-ă). Dilation of the heart. [cardi- + G. *ektasis*, a stretching]

car·di·ec·to·my (kar-dē-ek′tō-mē). Excision of the cardiac part of the stomach. [cardi-(2) + G. *ektomē*, excision]

car·di·ec·to·pia (kar-dē-ek-tō′pē-ă). Abnormal placement of the heart. SEE *ectopia* cordis. [cardi- + G. *ektopos*, out of place]

car·di·nal (kar′di-năl). Chief or principal; in embryology, relating to the main venous drainage. [L. *cardinalis*, principal]

card·ing. The procedure of placing individual sets of anterior or posterior teeth in trays lined with a wax strip.

△**cardio-, cardi-.** 1. The heart. 2. The cardia (ostium cardiacum). [G. *kardia*, heart]

car·di·o·ac·cel·er·a·tor (kar′dē-ō-ak-sel′er-ā-ter). Accelerator of the heart beat.

car·di·o·ac·tive (kar′dē-ō-ak′tiv). Influencing the heart.

car·di·o·an·gi·og·ra·phy (kar′dē-ō-an-jē-og′ră-fē). SYN angiocardiography.

car·di·o·a·or·tic (kar′dē-ō-ā-ōr′tik). Relating to the heart and the aorta.

car·di·o·ar·te·ri·al (kar′dē-ō-ar-tēr′ē-ăl). Relating to the heart and the arteries.

Car·di·o·bac·te·ri·um (kar′dē-ō-bak-tē′rē-ŭm). A genus of nonmotile, pleomorphic, Gram-negative, facultatively anaerobic, rod-shaped bacteria found in the nasal flora and associated with endocarditis in humans. The type species is *C. hominis.*

C. hom′inis, a bacterial species that causes endocarditis in humans. The type species of *Cardiobacterium.* SEE HACEK *group.*

C. violaceum, a motile, Gram-negative, non–spore-bearing rod, found in soil in tropical and subtropical environments; a cause of human infections including septicemia, pneumonia, wound infections, and abscesses; it can be rapidly fatal, and may relapse after cessation of antibiotic therapy.

car·di·o·cele (kar′dē-ō-sēl). A herniation or protrusion of the heart through an opening in the diaphragm, or through a wound. [cardio- + G. *kēlē*, hernia]

car·di·o·cha·la·sia (kar′dē-ō-kă-lā′zē-ă). Achalasia of the cardia.

car·di·o·di·o·sis (kar′dē-ō-dē-ō′sis). Rarely used term for maneuver to dilate the gastric cardia. [cardio- (2) + G. *diōsis*, a spreading open]

car·di·o·dy·nam·ics (kar′dē-ō-dī-nam′iks). The mechanics of the heart's action, including its movement and the forces generated thereby.

car·di·o·dyn·ia (kar′dē-ō-din′ē-ă). Pain in the heart. SYN cardialgia (2). [cardio- + G. *odynē*, pain]

car·di·o·e·soph·a·ge·al (kar′dē-ō-ē-sof-ă-jē′ăl). Denoting the area at the junction of the esophagus and cardiac part of the stomach.

car·di·o·gen·e·sis (kar-dē-ō-gen′ĕ-sis). Formation of the heart in the embryo. [cardio + G. *genesis*, origin]

car·di·o·gen·ic (kar′dē-ō-jen′ik). Of cardiac origin.

car·di·o·gram (kar′dē-ō-gram). 1. The graphic tracing made by the stylet of a cardiograph. 2. Generally used for any recording derived from the heart, with such prefixes as apex-, echo-, electro-, phono-, or vector- being understood. [cardio- + G. *gramma*, a diagram]

esophageal c., tracing of left atrial contractions made by recording displacements of the column of air in a sensor-equipped esophageal transducer tube or wire.

car·di·o·graph (kar′dē-ō-graf). An instrument for recording graphically the movements of the heart, constructed on the principle of the sphygmograph. [cardio- + G. *graphō*, to write]

car·di·og·ra·phy (kar-dē-og′ră-fē). Use of the cardiograph. SEE ALSO electrocardiography.

ultrasonic c., SYN echocardiography.

ultrasound c., SYN echocardiography.

car·di·o·he·mo·throm·bus (kar′dē-ō-hē-mō-throm′bŭs). SYN cardiothrombus.

car·di·o·he·pat·ic (kar′dē-ō-hĕ-pat′ik). Relating to the heart and the liver.

car·di·o·he·pa·to·meg·a·ly (kar′dē-ō-hep′ă-tō-meg′ă-lē). Enlargement of both heart and liver.

car·di·oid (kar′dē-oyd). Resembling a heart. [cardi- + G. *eidos,* resemblance]

car·di·o·in·hib·i·to·ry (kar′dē-ō-in-hib′ĭ-tō-rē). Arresting or slowing the action of the heart.

car·di·o·ky·mo·gram (kar′dē-ō-kī′mō-gram). Record made by a cardiokymograph.

car·di·o·ky·mo·graph (kar′dē-ō-kī′mō-graf). Noninvasive device, placed on the chest, capable of recording anterior left ventricle segmental wall motion; consists of a 5-cm diameter capacitive plate transducer as part of a high frequency, low-power oscillator with recording probe; changes in wall motion affect the magnetic field and thus the oscillatory frequency, which is then recorded on a multichannel analog waveform polygraph.

car·di·o·ky·mog·ra·phy (kar′dē-ō-kī-mog′ră-fē). Use of a cardiokymograph.

car·di·o·lip·in (kar′dē-ō-lip′in). A 1,3-bis(phosphatidyl)glycerol found in many biomembranes with immunologic properties; used in serologic diagnosis of syphilis. When mixed with lecithin and cholesterol c. will combine with the Wassermann antibody but not with the treponema-immobilizing antibody. SYN acetone-insoluble antigen, heart antigen.

car·di·ol·o·gist (kar-dē-ol′ō-jist). Physician specializing in cardiology.

car·di·ol·o·gy (kar-dē-ol′ō-jē). The medical specialty concerned with the diagnosis and treatment of heart disease. [cardio- + G. *logos,* study]

car·di·ol·y·sis (kar-dē-ol′i-sis). An obsolete operation for breaking up the adhesions in chronic mediastinopericarditis; access is gained by resection of a portion of the sternum and the corresponding costal cartilages. [cardio- + G. *lysis,* loosening]

car·di·o·ma·la·cia (kar′dē-ō-mă-lā′shē-ă). Softening of the walls of the heart. [cardio- + G. *malakia,* softness]

car·di·o·meg·a·ly (kar′dē-ō-meg′ă-lē). Enlargement of the heart. SYN macrocardia, megacardia, megalocardia. [cardio- + G. *megas,* large]

glycogen c., a form of glycogenosis due to abnormal storage of glycogen within the heart muscle cells.

glycogenic c., enlargement of the heart due to glycogen storage disease; most often occurs in type II (lysosomal acid glucosidase deficiency), especially in infancy and childhood.

car·di·om·e·try (kar-dē-om′ĕ-trē). Measurement of the dimensions of the heart or the force of its action. [cardio- + G. *metron,* measure]

car·di·o·mo·til·i·ty (kar′dē-ō-mō-til′ĭ-tē). Movements of the heart.

car·di·o·mus·cu·lar (kar′dē-ō-mŭs′kū-lăr). Pertaining to the cardiac musculature.

▓**car·di·o·my·op·a·thy** (kar′dē-ō-mī-op′ă-thē). Disease of the myocardium. As a disease classification, the term is used in several different senses, but is limited by the World Health Organization to: "Primary disease process of heart muscle in absence of a known underlying etiology" when referring to idiopathic cardiomyopathy. SYN myocardiopathy. [cardio- + G. *mys,* muscle, + *pathos,* disease]

alcoholic c., myocardial disease occurring in some chronic alcoholics; may result from alcohol toxicity, thiamin deficiency, or be of unknown pathogenesis. SYN alcoholic myocardiopathy, beer heart.

congestive c., SYN dilated c.

dilated c., decreased function of the left ventricle associated with its dilation; most patients have global hypokinesia, although discrete regional wall movement abnormalities may occur; usually manifested by signs of overall cardiac failure, with congestive

etiologic classification of cardiomyopathies

primary myocardial involvement

idiopathic (D, R, H)	familial (D, H)
eosinophilic endomyocardial disease (R)	endomyocardial fibrosis (R)

secondary myocardial involvement

infective myocarditis (D)	
viral	bacterial
fungal	protozoal
metazoal	spirochetal
rickettsial	
metabolic (D)	
familial storage disease (D, R)	
glycogen storage disease	mucopolysaccharidoses
hemochromatosis	Fabry disease
deficiency (D)	
electrolyte	nutritional
connective tissue disorders (D)	
systemic lupus erythematosus	polyarteritis nodosa
rheumatoid arthritis	progressive systemic sclerosis
dermatomyositis	
infiltration and granulomas (R, D)	
amyloidosis	sarcoidosis
malignancy	
neuromuscular (D)	
muscular dystrophy	myotonic dystrophy
Friedreich ataxia (H, D)	
sensitivity and toxic reactions (D)	
alcohol	radiation
drugs	
peripartum heart disease (D)	

NOTE: The principal clinical manifestation(s) of each etiologic grouping is denoted by D (dilated), R (restrictive), or H (hypertrophic) cardiomyopathy.

SOURCE: Adapted from the WHO/ISFC task force report on the definition and classification of cardiomyopathies, 1980.

findings, as well as by fatigue indicative of a low output state. SYN congestive c.

familial hypertrophic c., familial occurrence of hypertrophic c. exhibiting an autosomal dominant pattern of inheritance. Familial c. of various kinds occurs with autosomal dominant inheritance [MIM*115200]. There is also an asymmetrical form affecting the ventricles and the interventricular septum [MIM*192600].

hypertrophic c., thickening of the ventricular septum and walls of the left ventricle with marked myofibril disarray; often associated with greater thickening of the septum than of the free wall resulting in narrowing of the left ventricular outflow tract and dynamic outflow gradient; diastolic compliance is greatly impaired.

idiopathic c., SYN primary c. (1).

peripartum c., cardiac failure due to heart muscle disease in the period before, during, or after delivery.

postpartum c., cardiomegaly and congestive heart failure developing in the puerperium in the absence of any of the known causes of heart disease.

primary c., (1) c. of unknown or obscure cause; SYN idiopathic c. **(2)** a disease that affects mainly the heart muscle, sparing other cardiac structures and usually resulting in fibrosis, hypertrophy, or both.

restrictive c., a diverse group of conditions characterized by restriction of diastolic filling; often confused with constrictive pericarditis and the infiltrative cardiomyopathies; left ventricular size and systolic function may be preserved but dyspnea results primarily from increase in left ventricular diastolic pressure; signs of right ventricular failure may be prominent.

secondary c., disease that affects the myocardium secondarily to systemic disease, infection, or metabolic disease.

car·di·o·my·o·plas·ty. An operation that uses stimulated latissimus dorsi muscle to assist cardiac function. The latissimus dorsi muscle is mobilized from the chest wall and moved into the thorax through the bed of the resected 2nd or 3rd rib. The muscle is then wrapped around the left and right ventricles and stimulated to contract during cardiac systole by means of an implanted burst-stimulator. SYN cardiac muscle wrap.

car·di·o·my·ot·o·my (kar′dē-ō-mī-ot′ō-mē). SYN esophagomyotomy. [cardio- (2) + G. *mys*, muscle, + *tomē*, cutting]

car·di·o·nat·rin. SYN atrial natriuretic *peptide*. [cardio- + Mod. L. *natrium*, sodium, + suffix -in, material]

car·di·o·ne·cro·sis (kar′dē-ō-nĕ-krō′sis). Necrosis of the myocardium.

car·di·o·nec·tor (kar′dē-ō-nek′tŏr, -tōr). Archaic term sometimes used for conducting *system* of heart. [cardio- + L. *necto*, to join]

car·di·o·neph·ric (kar′dē-ō-nef′rik). SYN cardiorenal.

car·di·o·neu·ral (kar′dē-ō-noor′ăl). Relating to the nervous control of the heart. [cardio- + G. *neuron*, nerve]

car·di·o·neu·ro·sis (kar′dē-ō-noo-rō′sis). SYN cardiac *neurosis.*

car·di·o·o·men·to·pexy (kar′dē-ō-ō-men′tō-pek-sē). Operation for the attachment of omentum to the heart with the object of improving its blood supply. [cardio- + omentum, + G. *pēxis*, fixation]

car·di·o·pal·u·dism (kar′dē-ō-pal′oo-dizm). Irregularity in the heart's action due to malaria. [cardio- + paludism, malaria, fr. L. *palus*, marsh]

car·di·o·path (kar′dē-ō-path). A sufferer from heart disease.

car·di·o·path·ia nig·ra (kar-dē-ō-path′ē-ă nī′gra). SYN Ayerza *syndrome.*

car·di·op·a·thy (kar-dē-op′ă-thē). Any disease of the heart. [cardio- + G. *pathos*, disease]

car·di·o·pho·bia (kar′dē-ō-fō′bē-ă). Morbid fear of heart disease.

car·di·o·phone (kar′dē-ō-fōn). A stethoscope specially modified to aid in listening to the sounds of the heart. [cardio- + G. *phōnē*, sound]

car·di·oph·o·ny (kar′dē-of′ō-nē). A rarely used term for phonocardiography (1).

car·di·o·phre·nia (kar′dē-ō-frē′nē-ă). SYN phrenocardia.

car·di·o·plas·ty (kar′dē-ō-plas-tē). An operation on the cardia of the stomach. SYN esophagogastroplasty. [cardio- (2) + G. *plastos*, formed]

car·di·o·ple·gia (kar′dē-ō-plē′jē-ă). **1.** Paralysis of the heart. **2.** An elective stopping of cardiac activity temporarily by injection of chemicals, selective hypothermia, or electrical stimuli. [cardio- + G. *plēgē*, stroke]

antegrade c., c. effected by delivery of solutions through the coronary arteries.

retrograde c., c. effected by delivery of solutions via the coronary veins.

car·di·o·ple·gic (kar-dē-ō-plē′jik). Relating to cardioplegia.

car·di·op·to·sia (kar′dē-op-tō′sē-ă). A condition in which the heart is unduly movable and displaced downward, as distinguished from bathycardia. SEE ALSO *cor* mobile, *cor* pendulum. SYN drop heart. [cardio- + G. *ptōsis*, a falling]

car·di·o·pul·mo·nary (kar′dē-ō-pŭl′mo-nār-ē). Relating to the heart and lungs. SYN pneumocardial.

car·di·o·py·lo·ric (kar′dē-ō-pī-lōr′ik, -pi-lōr′ik). Relating to the cardiac and pyloric extremities of the stomach.

car·di·o·re·nal (kar′dē-ō-rē′năl). Relating to the heart and the kidney. SYN cardionephric, nephrocardiac, renicardiac.

car·di·or·rha·phy (kar-dē-ōr′ă-fē). Suture of the heart wall. [cardio- + G. *rhaphē*, suture]

car·di·or·rhex·is (kar-dē-ō-rek′sis). Rupture of the heart wall. [cardio- + G. *rhēxis*, rupture]

car·di·o·scope (kar′dē-ō-skōp). An instrument for inspecting the interior of the living heart. [cardio- + G. *skopeō*, to view]

car·di·o·se·lec·tive (kar′dē-ō-sĕ-lek′tiv). Denoting or having the properties of cardioselectivity.

car·di·o·se·lec·tiv·i·ty (kar′dē-ō-sĕ-lek-tiv′i-tē). The relatively predominant cardiovascular pharmacologic effect of a drug with multipharmacologic effects; used especially when describing beta-blocking agents.

car·di·o·spasm (kar′dē-ō-spazm). SYN esophageal *achalasia.*

car·di·o·sphyg·mo·graph (kar′dē-ō-sfig′mō-graf). An instrument for recording graphically the movements of the heart and the radial pulse. [cardio- + G. *sphygmos*, pulse, + *graphō*, to write]

car·di·o·ta·chom·e·ter (kar′dē-ō-tă-kom′ĕ-ter). An instrument for measuring the heart rate. [cardio- + G. *tachos*, rapidity, + *metron*, measure]

car·di·o·throm·bus (kar′dē-ō-throm′bŭs). A clot of blood within one of the heart's chambers. SYN cardiohemothrombus.

car·di·o·thy·ro·tox·i·co·sis (kar′dē-ō-thī-rō-tok-si-kō′sis). Hyperthyroidism with cardiac complications.

car·di·ot·o·my (kar-dē-ot′ō-mē). **1.** Incision of a heart wall. **2.** Incision of the cardiac part of the stomach. [cardio- + G. *tomē*, incision]

car·di·o·ton·ic (kar′dē-ō-ton′ik). Exerting a favorable, so-called tonic effect upon the action of the heart; usually intended to indicate increased force of contraction. [cardio- + G. *tonos*, tension]

car·di·o·tox·ic (kar′dē-ō-tok′sik). Having a deleterious effect upon the action of the heart, due to poisoning of the cardiac muscle or of its conducting system. [cardio- + G. *toxikon*, poison]

car·di·o·tox·in (kar′dē-ō-tok′sin). **1.** A poisonous glycoside with specific cardiac effects. For example, causes irreversible depolarization of cell membranes. **2.** Specifically, one of the toxic principles from cobra venom. **3.** Any substance that can cause heart damage with toxic doses.

car·di·o·val·vu·li·tis (kar′dē-ō-val-vū-lī′tis). Inflammation of the heart valves.

car·di·o·vas·cu·lar (CV) (kar′dē-ō-vas′kū-lăr) [TA]. Relating to the heart and the blood vessels or the circulation. SYN cardiovasculare [TA], vasculocardiac. [cardio- + L. *vasculum*, vessel]

cardiovasculare [TA]. SYN cardiovascular.

car·di·o·vas·cu·lo·re·nal (kar′dē-ō-vas′kū-lō-rē′năl). Relating to the heart, arteries, and kidneys, especially as to function or disease.

car·di·o·ver·sion (kar′dē-ō-ver′zhŭn). Restoration of the heart's rhythm to normal by electrical countershock or by medications (chemical cardioversion). [cardio- + con*version*]

car·di·o·vert (car′dē-ō-vert). The act of cardioversion.

car·di·o·ver·ter (kar′dē-ō-ver′ter). A machine used to perform cardioversion.

Car·di·o·vi·rus (kar′dē-ō-vī-rŭs). A genus of RNA viruses in the family Picornaviridae that are rarely associated with human disease and are recovered frequently from rodents, i.e., Columbia S.K. virus, mengo virus.

car·di·tis (kar-dī′tis). Inflammation of the heart.

rheumatic c., pancarditis occurring in rheumatic fever, characterized by formation of Aschoff bodies in the cardiac interstitial tissue; may be associated with acute cardiac failure, endocarditis with small fibrin vegetations on the margins of closure of valve cusps (especially the mitral), and fibrinous pericarditis; it is frequently followed by scarring of the valves.

care (kār). In medicine and public health, a general term for the application of knowledge to the benefit of a community or individual.

comprehensive medical c., a concept that includes not only the traditional c. of the acutely or chronically ill patient, but also the prevention and early detection of disease and the rehabilitation of the disabled.

end-of-life c., multidimensional and multidisciplinary physical, emotional, and spiritual c. of the patient with terminal illness, including support of family and caregivers.

End-of-life care has received increasing attention in recent years. The pioneer studies of Elisabeth Kübler-Ross on death and dying, begun in the 1960s, have afforded valuable insights into the evolving emotions, experiences, and needs of the dying person. Health professionals have formally recognized the importance of rendering humane and competent care at the end of life in ways that preserve the dignity and autonomy of the patient. Physicians, particularly oncologists, who treat patients with terminal illness have focused on the need to distinguish clearly between aggressive and palliative forms of treatment and to establish guidelines for the care of patients for whom further cure-oriented treatment will be of no benefit. In particular, they have recognized the importance of providing adequate pain relief to persons with advanced cancer. Increased attention has also been given to the control of nausea and dyspnea, which often occur in terminal illness. Studies have shown that pain relief in terminal patients is often inadequate because physicians fear to induce narcotic addiction or to be accused of hastening death. Wider use of opioid analgesics and development of patient-controlled analgesia and anesthesia systems have improved control of pain in terminal cancer and AIDS. Professional nurses have embraced the obligation to provide relief of suffering, comfort, companionship, and, when possible, a death that is congruent with the dying person's wishes. The hospice movement has established programs and facilities within the organized health care system that focus on the special needs of dying persons for comfort and care rather than efforts at cure. These programs include support of caregivers and family members during and after the patient's final illness. End-of-life care emphasizes the importance of frank, timely, supportive discussion of such matters as preferences for life-extending care, including cardiopulmonary resuscitation, before such measures become necessary. Legislatures have sought to preserve the dignity and independence of persons nearing the end of life by allowing them to enact advance directives for their care in the event that they become incompetent or comatose. The integrity of the relationship between patients and health professionals has been threatened by growing social and legal toleration of physician-assisted suicide. The American Medical Association and the American Nurses Association have issued official position statements opposing assisted suicide. See Also advance directive; physician-assisted suicide.

health c., services provided to individuals or communities by agents of the health services or professions for the purpose of promoting, maintaining, monitoring, or restoring health.

intensive c., management and c. of critically ill patients. SEE ALSO intensive care *unit*.

managed c., a contractual arrangement whereby a third-party payer (e.g., insurance company, government agency, or corporation) mediates between physicians and patients, negotiating fees for service and overseeing the types of treatment given. SEE ALSO health maintenance *organization*.

Managed care has largely replaced traditional medical indemnity insurance plans, under which payment is automatic and oversight procedures are minimal. Under managed care, the third-party payer controls specialty referrals, chiefly by appointing primary care physicians as "gatekeepers"; restricts the scope of covered services (particularly diagnostic procedures, choice of drugs prescribed, and length of hospital stay) for each diagnosis; and requires precertification review before hospital admission and a second opinion before elective surgery. Standards of care are regulated by practice guidelines, which may be set forth in oversimplified algorithms featuring binary (yes/no) choices. Prescribing alternatives are typically restricted to drugs listed in the plan's formulary. Practice guidelines, formulary choices, and other policies affecting patient care incorporate contemporary medical knowledge and professional standards but also strongly reflect strategies for loss control and for the even distribution of actuarial risk over all beneficiaries. The plan may bargain with physicians, hospitals, diagnostic laboratories, and pharmacies for wholesale prices, or may compensate providers by capitation rather than by fees for services. Managed care organizations typically employ cost-containment measures such as emphasis on preventive medicine, audits of medical records, intensive review of claims, and punitive action against noncompliant providers.

medical c., the portion of c. under a physician's direction.

primary medical c., c. of a patient by a member of the health c. system who has initial contact with the patient.

secondary medical c., medical c. by a physician who acts as a consultant at the request of the primary physician.

tertiary medical c., specialized consultative c., usually on referral from primary or secondary medical c. personnel, by specialists working in a center that has personnel and facilities for special investigation and treatment.

ca·ri·bi (kă-rē′bē). SYN epidemic gangrenous *proctitis*.

car·i·ca (kar′i-kă). SYN papaya.

car·ies (kār′ēz). **1.** Microbial destruction or necrosis of teeth. **2.** Obsolete term for tuberculosis of bones or joints. [L. dry rot]

active c., microbial-induced lesions of teeth that are increasing in size.

arrested dental c., carious lesions that have become inactive and stopped progressing; they may exhibit changes in color and/or consistency.

buccal c., c. beginning with decay on the buccal surface of a tooth.

cemental c., c. of the cementum of a tooth.

compound c., (1) c. involving more than one surface of a tooth; (2) two or more carious lesions joined to form one cavity.

dental c., a localized, progressively destructive disease of the teeth which starts at the external surface (usually the enamel) with the apparent dissolution of the inorganic components by organic acids that are produced in immediate proximity to the tooth by the enzymatic action of masses of microorganisms (in the bacterial plaque) on carbohydrates; the initial demineralization is followed by an enzymatic destruction of the protein matrix with subsequent cavitation and direct bacterial invasion; in the dentin, demineralization of the walls of the tubules is followed by bacterial invasion and destruction of the organic matrix. SYN saprodontia.

distal c., loss of structure on the tooth surface that is directed away from the median plane of the dental arch.

fissure c., c. beginning in a fissure on the occlusal surfaces of posterior teeth.

incipient c., beginning c. or decay.

interdental c., c. between the teeth.

mesial c., c. on the tooth surface that is directed toward the median plane of the dental arch.

nursing bottle c., c. and tooth enamel erosion that result from permitting infants and children to go to sleep while sucking intermittently from a bottle of formula, whole milk, or fruit juice. SYN baby bottle syndrome.

occlusal c., c. starting from the occlusal surface of a tooth.

pit c., a carious lesion, usually small, beginning in a pit on the labial, buccal, lingual, or occlusal surface of a tooth.

pit and fissure c., c. initiated in the areas where developmental pits and fissures are located on the tooth surface.

primary c., initial lesions produced by direct extension from an external surface.

proximal c., c. occurring in the proximal surface, either distal or mesial, of a tooth.

radiation c., c. of the cervical regions of the teeth, incisal edges, and cusp tips secondary to xerostomia induced by radiation therapy to the head and neck.

recurrent c., c. recurring in an area due to inadequate removal of the initial decay, usually beneath a restoration or new decay at a site where caries has previously occurred.

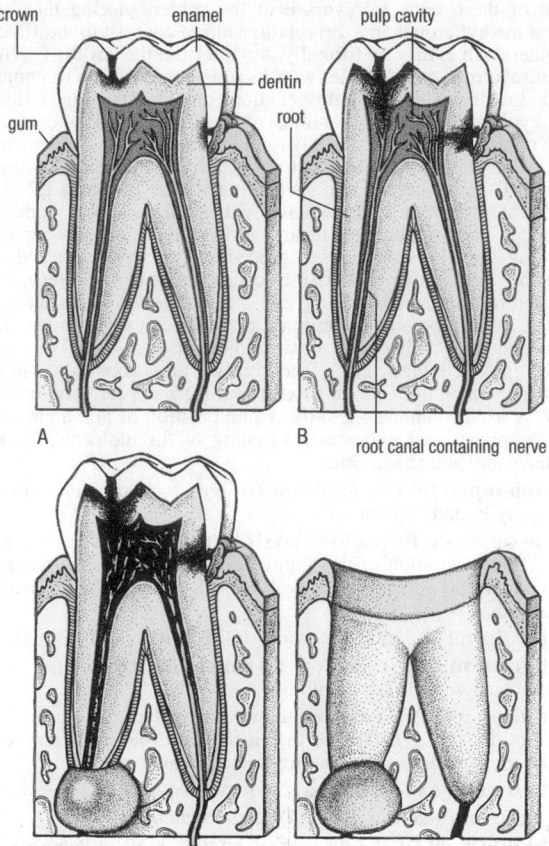

crown | enamel | pulp cavity

gum | dentin | root

root canal containing nerve

A | B

C | D

caries: (A) acid, enzymes, or both produced by oral bacteria break down enamel to form cavities; (B) bacteria penetrate dentin to invade pulp cavity; (C) infection destroys pulp and extends through left root canal to cause peri-apical disease; (D) tooth has been lost, leaving periapical cyst on the left

root c., c. of the root surface of a tooth, usually appearing as a broad shallow defect in the area of the cemento-enamel junction.

secondary c., c. of enamel beginning at the dento-enamel junction due to a rapid lateral spread of decay from the original decay.

senile dental c., c. occurring in old age, usually interproximally and in the cementum.

smooth surface c., c. initiated on the smooth surfaces of teeth.

ca·ri·na, pl. **ca·ri·nae** (kă-rī′nă, -rī′nē). **1.** In humans, a term applied or applicable to several anatomic structures forming a projecting central ridge. **2.** That portion of the sternum in a bird, bat, or mole that serves as the origin of the pectoral muscles; it is not found in flightless birds and most mammals. [L. the keel of a boat]

c. for′nicis, a ridge running along the undersurface of the fornix of the brain.

▮**c. of trachea** [TA], the ridge separating the openings of the right and left main bronchi at their junction with the trachea. SYN c. tracheae [TA], tracheal c.

c. tra′cheae [TA], SYN c. of trachea.

tracheal c., SYN c. of trachea.

c. urethra′lis vagi′nae, SYN urethral c. of vagina.

urethral c. of vagina, the ridge formed by the lower part of the anterior column of the vaginal rugae in relation with the urethra, which parallels the vagina indenting the wall here. SYN c. urethralis vaginae, c. vaginae.

c. vagi′nae, SYN urethral c. of vagina.

car·i·nate (kar′i-nāt). Shaped like a keel; relating to or resembling a carina.

△**cario-.** Caries. [L. *caries*]

car·i·o·gen·e·sis (ka′rē-ō-jen′ĕ-sis). The process of producing caries; the mechanism of caries production.

car·i·o·gen·ic (ka′rē-ō-jen′ik). Producing caries; usually said of diets.

car·i·o·ge·nic·i·ty (ka′rē-ō-jĕ-nis′i-tē). Potential for caries production.

car·i·ol·o·gy (ka-rē-ol′ō-jē). The study of dental caries and cariogenesis.

car·i·o·stat·ic (kār-ē-ō-stat′ik). Exerting an inhibitory action upon the progress of dental caries.

car·i·ous (kār′ē-oos). Relating to or affected with caries.

car·i·so·pro·date (kar′i-sō-prō′dāt). SYN carisoprodol.

car·i·so·pro·dol (kar′i-sō-prō′dol). A skeletal muscle relaxant, chemically related to meprobamate and having abuse potential. SYN carisoprodate.

ca·ris·sin (ka-ris′sin). A glucoside obtained from *Carissa ovata stolonifera* of Australia; a powerful cardiac poison.

Carlen, Eric, 20th century Swedish otolaryngologist. SEE Carlen *tube.*

carm·al·um (kar-mal′ŭm). A 1% solution of carmine in 10% alum water, used as a stain in histology.

Carman. Russell D., U.S. radiologist, 1875–1926. SEE Carman *sign.*

car·mi·nate (kar′mi-nāt). A red salt of carminic acid.

car·min·a·tive (kar-min′ă-tiv). **1.** Preventing the formation or causing the expulsion of flatus. **2.** An agent that relieves flatulence. [L. *carmino,* pp. *-atus,* to card wool; special Mod. L. usage, to expel wind]

car·mine (kar′min, kar′mēn) [C.I. 75470]. Red coloring matter used as a histology stain produced from coccinellin derived from cochineal; treatment of coccinellin with alum forms an aluminum lake of carminic acid, the essential constituent of c. [Mediev. L. *carminus,* contr. fr. *carmisinus,* fr. Ar. *qirmizē,* the cochineal insect]

lithium c., a vital stain for marophages.

Schneider c., a stain consisting of a 10% solution of c. in 45% acetic acid, used for fresh chromosome preparations.

car·min·ic ac·id (kar-min′ik). A glucoside of an anthracenequinone carboxylic acid; the essential constituent of carmine.

car·min·o·phil, car·min·o·phile, car·mi·noph·i·lous (kar-min′ō-fil, -fīl, kar-mi-nof′i-lŭs). Staining readily with carmine dyes. [G. *phileō,* to love]

Carmody, Thomas Edward, U.S. oral surgeon, *1875. SEE C.-Batson *operation.*

car·mus·tine (kar-mŭs′tēn). An antineoplastic agent. SYN BCNU.

car·nas·si·al (kar-nas′ē-ăl). Adapted for shearing flesh; denoting those teeth designed to cut flesh. [Fr. *carnassier,* carnivorous, fr. L. *caro,* flesh]

car·ne·ous (kar′nē-ŭs). Fleshy. [L. *carneus*]

car·nes (kar′nēz). Plural of caro. [L.]

Carnett, J. B., 20th century U.S. physician. SEE Carnett *sign.*

Carney, J.A., contemporary American physician. SEE Carney *complex.*

Carney, J. Aldan, U.S. pathologist, *1934. SEE C. *complex.*

car·ni·fi·ca·tion (kar′ni-fi-kā′shŭn). A change in tissues, whereby they become fleshy, resembling muscular tissue. [L. *caro* (carn-), flesh, + *facio,* to make]

car·ni·tine (kar′ni-tēn). A trimethylammonium (betaine) derivative of γ-amino-β-hydroxybutyric acid, formed from $N^{\epsilon},N^{\epsilon},N^{\epsilon}$-trimethyllysine and from γ-butyrobetaine; the L-isomer is a thyroid inhibitor found in muscle, liver, and meat extracts; L-c. is an acyl carrier with respect to the mitochondrial membrane; it thus stimulates fatty acid oxidation. SYN B_T factor, vitamin B_T. [L. *caro carn-,* flesh + ine]

c. acetyltransferase, an enzyme found in mitochondria that catalyzes the reversible transfer of an acetyl group from acetyl-CoA to c., forming *O*-acetylcarnitine and coenzyme A. Acetylcarnitine is an important fuel source in sperm.

ca

c. **acylcarnitine translocase,** a transport protein found in the inner mitochondrial membrane. Transports acylcarnitine derivatives into the mitochondria and transports c. out of the mitochondria. An important step in fatty acid oxidation.

c. **palmitoyltransferase, (1)** an enzyme that reversibly forms acylcarnitines and coenzyme A from carnitine and acylcoenzyme A (often, palmitoyl-CoA); important in fatty acid oxidation. Deficiency of isozyme I results in ketogenesis with hypoglycemia; deficiency of isozyme II affects primarily skeletal muscle.

Car·niv·o·ra (kar-niv′ŏ-ră). An order of chiefly flesh-eating mammals that includes the cats, dogs, bears, civets, minks, and hyenas, as well as the raccoon and panda; some species are omnivorous or herbivorous. [L. *carnivorus,* fr. *caro* (*carn-*), flesh, + *voro,* to devour]

car·ni·vore (kar′ni-vōr). One of the Carnivora.

car·niv·o·rous (kar-niv′ŏ-rŭs). Flesh-eating; subsisting on animals as food. SYN zoophagous.

car·nos·in·ase (kar′nō-si-nās). Mammalian enzyme that catalyzes the hydrolysis of carnosine, producing histidine and β-alanine; a deficiency of the serum enzyme leads to elevated carnosine levels.

car·no·sine (kar′nō-sēn). *N*-β-Alanyl-L-histidine; the dominant nonprotein nitrogenous component of brain tissue, first found in relatively high amounts in muscle; chelates copper and activates myosin ATPase. SYN ignotine, inhibitine. [L. *carnosus,* fleshy, fr. *caro,* flesh, + -ia]

car·nos·ine·mia (kar′nō-si-nē′mē-ă). An autosomal recessive congenital disease, characterized by the presence of excess amounts of carnosine in the blood and urine and caused by a genetic deficiency of the enzyme carnosinase. Clinically characterized by progressive neurologic damage, severe mental retardation, and myoclonic seizures. [carnosine + G. *haima,* blood + -ia]

car·nos·i·ty (kar-nos′i-tē). **1.** Fleshiness. **2.** A fleshy protuberance.

Carnoy, Jean Baptiste, French biologist, 1836–1899. SEE C. *fixative.*

ca·ro, gen. **car·nis,** pl. **car·nes** (kā′rō, kar′nis, -nes). The fleshy parts of the body; muscular and fatty tissues. [L.]

c. **quadra′ta syl′vii,** SYN quadratus plantae (*muscle*).

car·ob flour (kar′ob). SYN algaroba.

Caroli, J., 20th century French physician. SEE C. *disease.*

car·o·ten·ase (kar′-ō-ten-ās). SYN β-carotene 15,15′-dioxygenase.

car·o·tene (kar′ō-tēn). A class of carotenoids, yellow-red pigments (lipochromes) widely distributed in plants and animals, notably in carrots, and closely related in structure to the xanthophylls and lycopenes and to the open-chain squalene; of particular interest in that they include precursors of the vitamins A (provitamin A carotenoids). Chemically, they consist of 8 isoprene units in a symmetrical chain with the two isoprenes at each end cyclized, forming either α-carotene or β-carotene (γ-carotene has only one end cyclized). The cyclic ends of β-carotene are identical β-ionine-like structures; thus, on oxidative fission, β-carotene yields 2 molecules of vitamin A. The cyclic ends of α-carotene differ: one is an α-ionone, the other a β-ionone; on fission, α-carotene, like γ-carotene, yields 1 molecule of vitamin A (a β-ionone derivative).

c. **oxidase,** SYN lipoxygenase.

β-car·o·tene 15,15′-di·ox·y·gen·ase. An enzyme catalyzing the reaction of β-carotene plus O_2, producing two retinals. SYN β-carotene-cleavage enzyme, carotenase.

car·o·ten·e·mia (kar′ō-te-nē′mē-ă). Carotene in the blood, especially pertaining to increased quantities, which sometimes cause a pale yellow-red pigmentation of the skin that may resemble icterus. SYN carotinemia, xanthemia.

car·o·ten·o·der·ma (ka-rot′en-ō-der-mă). SYN carotenosis cutis. [carotene + G. *derma,* skin]

ca·rot·e·noid (ka-rot′e-noyd). **1.** Resembling carotene; having a yellow color. **2.** One of the carotenoids.

ca·rot·e·noids (ka-rot′e-noydz). Generic term for a class of carotenes and their oxygenated derivatives (xanthophylls) consisting of 8 isoprenoid units (thus, tetraterpenes) joined so that the orien-

tation of these units is reversed at the center, placing the two central methyl groups in a 1,6 relationship in contrast to the 1,5 of the others. All c. may be formally derived from the acyclic $C_{40}H_{56}$ structure known as lycopene, with its long central chain of conjugated double bonds by hydrogenation, dehydrogenation, oxidation, cyclization, or combinations of these. Included as c.'s are some compounds arising from certain rearrangements or degradations of the carbon skeleton, but not retinol and related C_{20} compounds. The nine-carbon end groups may be acyclic with 1,2 and 5,6 double bonds or cyclohexanes with a single double bond at 5,6 or 5,4 or cyclopentanes or aryl groups; these are now designated by Greek letter prefixes preceding "carotene" (α and δ, which are used in the trivial names α-carotene and δ-carotene, are not used for that reason). Suffixes (-oic acid, -oate, -al, -one, -ol) indicate certain oxygen-containing groups (acid, ester, aldehyde, ketone, alcohol); all other substitutions appear as prefixes (alkoxy-, epoxy-, hydro-, etc.). The configuration about all double bonds is *trans* unless *cis* and locant numbers appear. The prefix *retro-* is used to indicate a shift of one position of all single and double bonds; *apo-* indicates shortening of the molecule. Many c.'s have anticancer activities.

car·o·ten·o·pro·tein (ka-rot′en-ō-prō-tēn). A protein with a covalently-bound carotenoid.

car·o·te·no·sis cu·tis (kar-ō-te-nō′sis kū′tis). A harmless, reversible yellow coloration of the skin caused by an increase in carotene content; the sclera is not involved. SYN carotenoderma, carotinosis cutis.

ca·rot·ic (kă-rot′ik). SYN stuporous. [G. *karōtikos,* stupefying]

ca·rot·i·co·tym·pan·ic (ka-rot′i-kō-tim-pan′ik). Relating to the carotid canal and the tympanum.

ca·rot·id (ka-rot′id). Pertaining to any c. structure. [G. *karōtides,* the carotid arteries, fr. *karoō,* to put to sleep (because compression of the c. artery results in unconsciousness)]

car·o·ti·dyn·ia (kă-rot′i-din′ē-ă). SYN carotodynia.

car·o·tin·e·mia (kar′ō-ti-nē′mē-ă). SYN carotenemia.

ca·rot·i·no·sis cu·tis (ka-rot-i-nō′sis kū′tis). SYN carotenosis cutis.

ca·rot·o·dyn·ia (kă-rot′ō-din′ē-ă). Pain caused by pressure on the carotid artery. SYN carotidynia. [G. *odynē,* pain]

car·pal (kar′păl). Relating to the carpus.

car·pec·to·my (kar-pek′tō-mē). Excision of a portion or all of the carpus. [G. *karpos,* wrist, + *ektomē,* excision]

Carpenter, George Alfred, British physician, 1859–1910. SEE C. *syndrome.*

Carpentier, Alain, 20th century French cardiothoracic surgeon. SEE Carpentier-Edwards *valve.*

car·phen·a·zine ma·le·ate (kar-fen′ă-zēn). A phenothiazine tranquilizer of the piperazine group. Functionally classified as an antipsychotic agent, it is used in the treatment of chronic and acute schizophrenia; also possesses antiemetic, adrenolytic, anticholinergic, and dopamine-blocking actions.

car·po·car·pal (kar-pō-kar′păl). SYN midcarpal (2).

Car·po·gly·phus (kar-pō-glif′us). A genus of mites including C. *passularum,* the fruit mite, which causes a dermatitis among handlers of dried fruit. [G. *karpos,* fruit, + *glyphō,* , to carve]

car·po·met·a·car·pal (kar′pō-met-ă-kar′păl). Relating to both carpus and metacarpus.

car·po·ped·al (kar′pō-ped′ăl). Relating to the wrist and the foot, or the hands and feet; denoting especially c. spasm. [G. *karpos,* wrist, + L. *pes* (*ped-*), foot]

car·pop·to·sis, car·pop·to·sia (kar-pop-tō′sis, -tō′zē-ă). SYN *wrist*-drop. [G. *karpos,* wrist, + *ptōsis,* a falling]

Carpue, Joseph C., British surgeon, 1764–1846.

car·pus, gen. and pl. **car·pi** (kar′pŭs, kar′pī) [TA]. **1.** SYN wrist. **2.** SYN carpal *bones,* under *bone.* [Mod. L. fr. Gr. *karpos*]

c. **cur′vus,** SYN Madelung *deformity.*

Carr, Francis H., British chemist, *1874. SEE C.-Price *reaction.*

car·ra·geen, car·ra·gheen (kar′ă-jēn, -gēn). **1.** SYN chondrus (2). **2.** SYN carrageenan.

car·ra·gee·nan, car·ra·gee·nin (kar-ă-gē′nan, -nin). A polysaccharide vegetable gum obtained from Irish moss; a galactosan sulfate resembling agar in molecular structure. SYN carrageen (2), carragheen. [*Carragheen*, Irish village]

car·re·four sen·si·tif (kar-foor′son-sē-tēf′). A term given by Charcot to the posterior portion of the caudal limb of the internal capsule. [Fr. sensory crossroads]

Carrel, Alexis, French-U.S. surgeon and Nobel laureate, 1873–1944. SEE C. *treatment;* C.-Lindbergh *pump;* Dakin-C. *treatment.*

car·ri·er (ka′rē-er). **1.** A person or animal that harbors a specific infectious agent in the absence of discernible clinical disease and serves as a potential source of infection. **2.** Any chemical capable of accepting an atom, radical, or subatomic particle from one compound, then passing it to another; e.g., cytochromes are electron c.'s; homocysteine is a methyl c. **3.** A substance that, by having chemical properties closely related to or indistinguishable from those of a radioactive tracer, is thus able to carry the tracer through a precipitation or similar chemical procedure; the best c.'s are the nonradioactive isotopes of the tracer in question. SEE ALSO label, tracer. **4.** A large immunogen that, when coupled to a hapten, will facilitate an immune response to the hapten. **5.** A component of a membrane that causes the transfer of a substance from one side of the membrane to the other. **6.** The mobile phase in chromatography.

amalgam c., an instrument used to transport triturated amalgam to a cavity preparation and to deposit it therein.

convalescent c., an individual who is clinically recovered from an infectious disease but is still capable of transmitting the infectious agent to others.

genetic c., a person heterozygous for a mutant allele that, in homozygous form, causes a recessive condition.

hydrogen c., a molecule that, in conjunction with a tissue enzyme system, carries hydrogen from one metabolite (oxidant) to another (reductant) or to molecular oxygen to form H_2O. SYN hydrogen acceptor.

incubatory c., an individual capable of transmitting an infectious agent to others during the incubation period of the disease.

latent c., typically a prospective parent, bearing the appropriate genotype of a trait (homozygous for recessive, homozygous or heterozygous for dominant, hemizygous or homozygous for X-linked) that manifests the trait only under certain conditions, e.g., age, an environmental insult, etc.

manifesting c., SYN manifesting *heterozygote.*

translocation c., a person with balanced translocation.

car·ri·er-free. Said of a substance in which a radioactive or other tagged atom is found in every molecule; the highest possible specific activity.

Carrión, Daniel A., Peruvian medical student, 1859–1885, who inoculated himself with a disease later designated as Carrión *disease,* and died thereof. SEE C. *disease.*

carry-over (kar′ē-ō′ver). The phenomenon by which part of the analyte present in a sample appears to be present in the next or following samples in the same analytic process. This is most noticeable when a sample of low analyte concentration follows one of very high concentration.

Carteaud, Alexandre, French physician, *1897. SEE Gougerot-C. *syndrome.*

car·te·sian (kar-tē′zhŭn). Relating to Cartesius, Latinized form of Descartes.

car·tha·mus (kar′tha-mŭs). The dried florets of *Carthamus tinctorius* (family Compositae). SEE ALSO safflower oil. SYN safflower. [Ar. *qurtum,* fr. *qartama,* paint; the plant yields a dye]

CARTILAGE

car·ti·lage (kar′ti-lij) [TA]. A connective tissue characterized by its nonvascularity and firm consistency; consists of cells (chondrocytes), an interstitial matrix of fibers (collagen), and a ground substance (proteoglycans). There are three kinds of c.: hyaline c.,

elastic c., and fibrocartilage. Nonvascular, resilient, flexible connective tissue found primarily in joints, the walls of the thorax, and tubular structures such as the larynx, air passages, and ears; comprises most of the skeleton in early fetal life, but is slowly replaced by bone. For gross anatomic description, see cartilago and its subentries. SYN cartilago [TA], chondrus (1), gristle. [L. *cartilago (cartilagin-),* gristle]

accessory c., a sesamoid c.

accessory nasal c.'s [TA], variable small plates of cartilage located in the interval between the greater alar and lateral nasal cartilages. SYN cartilagines nasales accessoriae [TA], sesamoid c.'s of nose.

accessory quadrate c., SYN minor alar c.

c. of acoustic meatus [TA], the cartilage that forms the wall of the lateral part of the external acoustic meatus. It is incomplete above and is firmly attached to the margins of the bony part of the external meatus. SYN cartilago meatus acustici [TA], meatal c.

alisphenoid c., the c. in the embryo from which the greater wing of the sphenoid bone is developed.

anular c., SYN cricoid c.

arthrodial c., SYN articular c.

articular c., the cartilage covering the articular surfaces of the bones participating in a synovial joint. SYN arthrodial c., cartilago articularis, diarthrodial c., investing c.

arytenoid c. [TA], one of a pair of small triangular pyramidal laryngeal cartilages that articulate with the lamina of the cricoid cartilage. It gives attachment at its anteriorly directed vocal process to the posterior part of the corresponding vocal ligament and to several muscles at its laterally directed muscular process. The base of the cartilage is hyaline but the apex is elastic. SYN cartilago arytenoidea [TA], triquetrous c. (2).

c. of auditory tube, SYN c. of pharyngotympanic tube.

auricular c. [TA], the cartilage of the auricle. SYN cartilago auriculae [TA], c. of ear, conchal c.

basilar c., the c. filling the foramen lacerum. SYN basilar fibrocartilage, fibrocartilago basalis.

branchial c.'s, c.'s developing within the embryonic branchial arches; they form the cartilaginous viscerocranium. SYN pharyngeal c.'s.

calcified c., c. in which calcium salts are deposited in the matrix; it occurs prior to replacement by osseous tissue and sometimes in aging c.

cellular c., an embryonic or immature stage of c. in which it consists chiefly of cells with very little matrix. SYN parenchymatous c.

ciliary c., incorrect term sometimes applied to the inferior and superior tarsi. SEE tarsus (2).

circumferential c., (1) SYN acetabular *labrum;* **(2)** SYN glenoid *labrum* of scapula.

conchal c., SYN auricular c.

connecting c., the c. in a cartilaginous joint such as the symphysis pubis. SYN interosseous c., uniting c.

corniculate c. [TA], a conical nodule of elastic cartilage surmounting the apex of each arytenoid cartilage. SYN cartilago corniculata [TA], corniculum laryngis, Santorini c., supra-arytenoid c.

costal c. [TA], the cartilage forming the anterior continuation of a rib, providing the means by which it reaches and articulates with the sternum. SYN cartilago costalis [TA], costicartilage.

cricoid c. [TA], the lowermost of the laryngeal cartilages; it is shaped like a signet ring, being expanded into a nearly quadrilateral plate (lamina) posteriorly; the anterior portion is called the arch (arcus). SYN cartilago cricoidea [TA], anular c.

cuneiform c. [TA], a small nonarticulating rod of elastic cartilage in the aryepiglottic fold anterolateral and somewhat superior to the corniculate cartilage. SYN cartilago cuneiformis [TA], Morgagni c., Morgagni tubercle, Wrisberg c.

diarthrodial c., SYN articular c.

c. of ear, SYN auricular c.

elastic c., a c. in which the cells are surrounded by a territorial capsular matrix outside of which is an interterritorial matrix con-

ca

taining elastic fiber networks in addition to type II collagen fibers and ground substance. SYN yellow c.

ensiform c., ensisternum c., obsolete term for xiphoid *process*.

epiglottic c. [TA], a thin lamina of elastic cartilage forming the central portion of the epiglottis. SYN cartilago epiglottica [TA].

epiphysial c. [TA], particular type of new c. produced by the epiphysis of a growing long bone; located on the epiphysial (distal) side of the zone of growth c., it is a zone of relatively quiescent chondrocytes (the resting zone) of the epiphyseal (growth) plate that unites the epiphysis with the shaft. SEE ALSO epiphysial *plate*. SYN cartilago epiphysialis [TA].

falciform c., SYN medial *meniscus*.

floating c., a loose piece of c. within a joint cavity, detached from the articular c. or from a meniscus. SYN loose c.

greater alar c., SYN major alar c.

Huschke c.'s, two horizontal cartilaginous rods at the edge of the cartilaginous septum of the nose.

hyaline c., c. having a frosted glass appearance, with interstitial substance containing fine type II collagen fibers obscured by the ground substance; in adult c., the cells are present in isogenous groups.

hypsiloid c., SYN Y c.

interosseous c., SYN connecting c.

intervertebral c., SYN intervertebral *disk*.

intraarticular c., (1) SYN articular *disk*; (2) SYN meniscus *lens*.

intrathyroid c., a narrow slip of c. sometimes found joining the laminae of the thyroid c. of the larynx in infancy.

investing c., SYN articular c.

Jacobson c., SYN vomeronasal c.

c.'s of larynx, SEE thyroid c., cricoid c., arytenoid c., cuneiform c., triticeal c., corniculate c., sesamoid c. of cricopharyngeal ligament, epiglottic c. SYN cartilagines laryngis.

lateral c. of nose, SYN lateral *process* of septal nasal cartilage.

lesser alar c.'s, SYN minor alar c.

loose c., SYN floating c.

Luschka c., a small cartilaginous nodule sometimes found in the anterior portion of the vocal cord.

major alar c. [TA], one of a pair of cartilages that form the tip of the nose. It consists of a medial crus that extends into the nasal septum with its fellow of the opposite side, and a lateral crus that forms the anterior part of the wing of the nose. SYN cartilago alaris major, greater alar c.

mandibular c., a c. bar in the mandibular arch that forms a temporary supporting structure in the embryonic mandible; the cartilagenous primordia of the malleus and incus develop from its proximal end, and it also gives rise to the sphenomandibular and anterior malleolar ligaments. SYN Meckel c.

meatal c., SYN c. of acoustic meatus.

Meckel c., SYN mandibular c.

Meyer c.'s, the anterior sesamoid c.'s at the anterior attachments of the vocal ligaments.

minor alar c. [TA], the 2–4 cartilaginous plates of the wing of the nose posterior to the greater alar cartilage. SYN accessory quadrate c., cartilagines alares minores, lesser alar c.'s.

Morgagni c., SYN cuneiform c.

nasal septal c., SYN septal nasal c.

c. of nasal septum, SYN septal nasal c.

c.'s of nose, SEE lateral *process* of septal nasal cartilage, major alar c., septal nasal c., vomeronasal c., minor alar c., accessory nasal c.'s. SYN cartilagines nasi.

ossifying c., SYN temporary c.

parachordal c., c. primordia adjacent on either side to the cephalic portion of the notochord in young embryos; they represent an initial step in the formation of the chondrocranium.

paraseptal c., SYN vomeronasal c.

parenchymatous c., SYN cellular c.

periotic c., a cartilaginous mass on either side of the chondrocranium surrounding the developing auditory vesicle in the fetus; the otic capsule in its early cartilaginous stage.

permanent c., c. that is not replaced by bone.

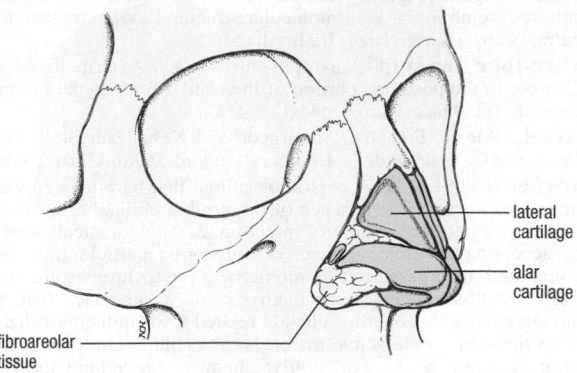

cartilage of the nose

pharyngeal c.'s, SYN branchial c.'s.

c. of pharyngotympanic tube [TA], the trough-shaped cartilage that forms the medial wall, roof, and part of the lateral wall of the pharyngotympanic tube. SYN cartilago tubae auditivae [TA], c. of auditory tube, tubal c.

precursory c., SYN temporary c.

primordial c., c. in an early stage in its development.

quadrangular c., SYN septal nasal c.

Reichert c., a c. in the mesenchyme of the second branchial arch in the embryo, from which develop the stapes, the styloid processes, the stylohyoid ligaments, and the lesser cornua of the hyoid bone.

reticular c., retiform c., rarely used terms for fibrocartilage.

Santorini c., SYN corniculate c.

Seiler c., a small rod of c. attached to the vocal process of the arytenoid c.

semilunar c., one of the articular menisci of the knee joint. SEE lateral *meniscus*, medial *meniscus*.

septal c., SYN septal nasal c.

septal nasal c. [TA], a thin cartilaginous plate located between vomer, perpendicular plate of the ethmoid, and nasal bones, and completing the nasal septum anteriorly. SYN cartilago septi nasi [TA], c. of nasal septum, cartilaginous septum, nasal septal c., pars cartilaginea septi nasi, quadrangular c., septal c.

sesamoid c. of cricopharyngeal ligament [TA], a small nodule of elastic cartilage sometimes present on the lateral border of the arytenoid cartilage. SYN cartilago sesamoidea ligamentum cricopharyngeum [TA], cartilago sesamoidea laryngis, sesamoid c. of larynx.

sesamoid c. of larynx, SYN sesamoid c. of cricopharyngeal ligament.

sesamoid c.'s of nose, SYN accessory nasal c.'s.

slipping rib c., subluxation of rib c., at the costo-chondral junction, causing pain and audible click.

sternal c., a costal c. of one of the true ribs.

supra-arytenoid c., SYN corniculate c.

tarsal c., incorrect term sometimes applied to the inferior tarsus and superior tarsus. SEE tarsus (2).

temporary c., a c. that is normally replaced by bone, to form a part of the skeleton. SYN ossifying c., precursory c.

thyroid c. [TA], the largest of the cartilages of the larynx; it is formed of two approximately quadrilateral plates (*laminae*) joined anteriorly at an angle of from 90–20°, the prominence so formed constituting the laryngeal prominence (Adam's apple). SYN cartilago thyroidea [TA].

tracheal c.'s [TA], the 16–20 incomplete rings of hyaline cartilage forming the skeleton of the trachea; the rings are deficient posteriorly for from one-fifth to one-third of their circumference. SYN cartilagines tracheales [TA], tracheal ring.

triangular c., SYN articular *disk* of distal radioulnar joint.

triquetrous c., (1) SYN articular *disk* of distal radioulnar joint; **(2)** SYN arytenoid c.

triticeal c. [TA], a rounded nodule of cartilage, the size of a grain of wheat, occasionally present in the posterior margin of the lateral thyrohyoid ligament. SYN cartilago triticea [TA], corpus triticeum, triticeum.

tubal c., SYN c. of pharyngotympanic tube.

uniting c., SYN connecting c.

vomerine c., SYN vomeronasal c.

vomeronasal c. [TA], a narrow strip of c. located between the lower edge of the c. of the nasal septum and the vomer. SYN cartilago vomeronasalis [TA], Jacobson c., paraseptal c., vomer cartilagineus, vomerine c.

Weitbrecht c., SYN articular *disk* of acromioclavicular joint.

Wrisberg c., SYN cuneiform c.

xiphoid c., SYN xiphoid *process.*

Y c., Y-shaped c., the connecting c. for the ilium, ischium, and pubis; it extends through the acetabulum. SYN hypsiloid c.

yellow c., SYN elastic c.

---

car·ti·la·gi·nes (kar-ti-laj′i-nĕz). Plural of cartilago.

car·ti·lag·i·noid (kar-ti-laj′i-noyd). SYN chondroid (1).

car·ti·lag·i·nous (kar-ti-laj′i-nŭs). Relating to or consisting of cartilage. SYN chondral.

car·ti·la·go, pl. **car·ti·la·gi·nes** (kar-ti-lā′gō, -laj′i-nēs) [TA]. SYN cartilage. For histologic description, see cartilage. [L. gristle]

cartila′gines ala′res mino′res, SYN minor alar *cartilage.*

c. ala′ris ma′jor, SYN major alar *cartilage.*

c. articula′ris, SYN articular *cartilage.*

c. arytenoi′dea [TA], SYN arytenoid *cartilage.*

c. auric′ulae [TA], SYN auricular *cartilage.*

c. cornicula′ta [TA], SYN corniculate *cartilage.*

c. costa′lis [TA], SYN costal *cartilage.*

c. cricoi′dea [TA], SYN cricoid *cartilage.*

c. cuneifor′mis [TA], SYN cuneiform *cartilage.*

c. epiglot′tica [TA], SYN epiglottic *cartilage.*

c. epiphysialis [TA], SYN epiphysial *cartilage.*

cartila′gines laryn′gis, SYN *cartilages* of larynx, under *cartilage.*

c. mea′tus acus′tici [TA], SYN *cartilage* of acoustic meatus.

cartila′gines nasa′les accessor′iae [TA], SYN accessory nasal *cartilages,* under *cartilage.*

cartila′gines na′si, SYN *cartilages* of nose, under *cartilage.*

c. na′si latera′lis, SYN lateral *process* of septal nasal cartilage.

c. sep′ti na′si [TA], SYN septal nasal *cartilage.*

c. sesamoi′dea laryn′gis, SYN sesamoid *cartilage* of cricopharyngeal ligament.

c. sesamoidea ligamentum cricopharyngeum [TA], SYN sesamoid *cartilage* of cricopharyngeal ligament.

c. thyroid′ea [TA], SYN thyroid *cartilage.*

cartila′gines trachea′les [TA], SYN tracheal *cartilages,* under *cartilage.*

c. tritic′ea [TA], SYN triticeal *cartilage.* [L. *triticum,* wheat]

c. tu′bae auditi′vae [TA], SYN *cartilage* of pharyngotympanic tube.

c. vomeronasa′lis [TA], SYN vomeronasal *cartilage.*

ca·run·cle (kar′ŭng-kl) [TA]. A small, fleshy protuberance, or any structure suggesting such a shape. SYN caruncula (1) [TA].

lacrimal c. [TA], a small reddish body at the medial angle of the eye, containing modified sebaceous and sweat glands. SYN caruncula lacrimalis [TA].

Morgagni c., SYN middle *lobe* of prostate.

Santorini major c., SYN major duodenal *papilla.*

Santorini minor c., SYN minor duodenal *papilla.*

urethral c., a small, fleshy, sometimes painful protrusion of the mucous membrane at the meatus of the female urethra; it may be telangiectatic, papillomatous, or composed of granulation tissue.

ca·run·cu·la, pl. **ca·run·cu·lae** (kă-rŭng′kū-lă, -lē) [TA]. **1**

[TA]. SYN caruncle. **2.** In ungulates, one of about 200 specific disklike areas of the uterine endometrium that, in conjunction with the fetal cotyledon, forms a placentome of the placenta; as a site of fetal-maternal contact, the c. remains constant in position but enlarges greatly during pregnancy. [L. a small fleshy mass, fr. *caro,* flesh]

hymenal c. [TA], one of the numerous tabs or projections surrounding the orifice of the vagina. SYN c. hymenalis [TA], c. myrtiformis.

c. hymena′lis, pl. **carun′culae hymena′les** [TA], SYN hymenal c.

c. lacrima′lis [TA], SYN lacrimal *caruncle.*

c. myrtifor′mis, pl. **carun′culae myrtifor′mes,** SYN hymenal c.

c. saliva′ris, SYN sublingual c.

sublingual c. [TA], a papilla on each side of the frenulum of the tongue marking the opening of the submandibular duct. SYN c. sublingualis [TA], c. salivaris.

c. sublingua′lis [TA], SYN sublingual c.

Carus, Karl G., German anatomist and zoologist, 1789–1869. SEE C. *circle, curve.*

car·va·crol (kar′vă-krol). An isomer of thymol that occurs in several volatile oils (marjoram, origanum, savory, and thyme), with properties and activity that closely resemble those of thymol; has antiseptic properties, but is used chiefly as a perfume.

Carvallo, SEE Rivero-Carvallo.

car·ve·di·lol (kar′vē-dil-ol). An agent used as an antihypertensive and antianginal, and in congestive heart failure.

carv·er (kar′ver). A dental hand instrument, available in a wide variety of end shapes, used for forming and contouring wax, filling materials, etc.

△**caryo-.** Nucleus. SEE karyo-. [G. *karyon,* nut, kernel]

car·y·o·phyl·lus, car·y·o·phyl·lum (kar′ē-ō-fī′lŭs, -ŭm). Clove. [G. *karyophyllon,* clove tree, fr. *karyon,* nut, + *phyllon,* leaf]

car·y·o·the·ca (kar′ē-ō-thē′kă). SYN nuclear *envelope.* [caryo- + G. *thēkē,* sheath, box]

Casal, Gasper, Spanish physician, 1691–1759. SEE C. *necklace.*

cas·a·mi·no ac·ids (kās′ă-mē′nō). Trivial term for the mixture of amino acids derived by hydrolysis of casein; used in bacterial and similar growth media.

cas·cade (kas-kād′). **1.** A series of sequential interactions, as of a physiological process, which once initiated continues to the final one; each interaction is activated by the preceding one, sometimes with cumulative effect. **2.** To spill over, especially rapidly. [Fr., fr. It. *cascare,* to fall]

cas·cara (kas-kar′ă). SYN c. sagrada.

c. amara, the dried bark of a species of *Picramnia* (family Simarubaceae); used as a bitter tonic. SYN Honduras bark.

c. sagrada, the dried bark of *Rhamnus purshiana* (family Rhamnaceae); used as a laxative. SYN cascara.

case (kās). **1.** An instance of disease with its attendant circumstances. Cf. patient. **2.** A box or container. [L. *casus,* an occurrence]

borderline c., a patient, whose clinical findings are suggestive, but not fully convincing, of a specific diagnosis.

index c., SYN proband.

trial c., in refraction, a box containing lenses for testing.

ca·se·a·tion (kā-sē-ā′shŭn). A form of coagulation necrosis in which the necrotic tissue resembles cheese and contains a mixture of protein and fat that is absorbed very slowly; occurs particularly in tuberculosis. SEE ALSO caseous *necrosis.* SYN tyrosis (2). [L. *caseus,* cheese]

ca·sein (cā′sē-in, kā′sēn). The principal protein of cow's milk and the chief constituent of cheese. It is insoluble in water, soluble in dilute alkaline and salt solutions, forms a hard insoluble plastic with formaldehyde, and is used as a constituent of some glues; various components are designated α-, β-, and κ-caseins. β-C. is converted to γ-c. by milk proteases. There are several isoforms of α-c. κ-C. is not precipitated by calcium ions.

c. iodine, iodinated c., a compound of c. with iodine formed by incubating the protein with the element, which becomes attached to tyrosine groups in the protein. SYN caseo-iodine.

ca

plant c., SYN avenin.

ca·sein·ate (kā′sē-in-āt). A salt of casein.

ca·sein·o·gen (kā-sē-in′ō-jen). "Soluble" or κ-casein which, when acted upon by rennin, is converted into paracasein.

ca·seo·io·dine (kā′sē-ō-i′ō-dīn). SYN *casein* iodine.

ca·se·ose (kā′sē-ōs). Nondescript term for product resulting from the hydrolysis or digestion of casein.

ca·se·ous (kā′sē-ŭs). Pertaining to or manifesting the gross and microscopic features of tissue affected by caseation.

Casoni, Tommaro, Italian physician, 1880–1933. SEE Casoni *antigen;* C. intradermal *test,* skin *test.*

cas·sa·va starch (kă-sah′vah). SYN tapioca.

Casselberry, William E., U.S. laryngologist, 1858–1916. SEE C. *position.*

Casser (Casserio), Giulio, Italian anatomist, 1556–1616. SEE C. *fontanelle,* perforated *muscle.*

cas·se·ri·an (ka-sē′rē-an). Relating to or described by Casser.

cas·sette (kă-set′). **1.** A plate, film, or tape holder for use in photography or radiography. A radiographic c. contains two intensifying screens and a sheet of x-ray film. **2.** A perforated holder in which tissue blocks are placed for paraffin embedding. [Fr., dim. of *casse,* box]

susceptibility c., a common sequence of amino acids in residues 70–74 in the HLA-DRB1 chains, found in alleles associated with rheumatoid arthritis. It is one of two variations: glutamine[Q]-lysine[K]-arginine[R]-alanine[A]-alanine[A] or QRRAA. These susceptibility cassettes are found in many different DRB1 alleles. The alpha and beta chains that form these antigen-presenting molecules have a configuration not unlike a trough or rain gutter; antigens are bound by sequences of amino acids in a pocket along the bottom and sides of the trough or cavity, and this complex forms a heterotrimer with the T-cell receptor on CD4+ cells. SYN rheumatoid pocket, shared epitope.

cas·sia bark (kash′yă). SYN cinnamon.

cas·sia fis·tu·la. The dried ripe fruit of *Cassia fistula,* used as a laxative. SYN purging cassia.

cas·sia oil. SYN cinnamon oil.

cast (kast). **1.** An object formed by the solidification of a liquid poured into a mold. **2.** Rigid encasement of a part, as with plaster, plastic, or fiberglass, for purposes of immobilization. **3.** An elongated or cylindrical mold formed in a tubular structure (e.g., renal tubule, bronchiole) that may be observed in histologic sections or in material such as urine or sputum; results from inspissation of fluid material secreted or excreted in the tubular structures. **4.** Restraint of a large animal, usually a horse, with ropes and harnesses in a recumbent position. **5.** In dentistry, a positive reproduction of the form of the tissues of the upper or lower jaw, which is made by the solidification of plaster, metal, etc., poured into an impression, and over which denture bases or other dental restorations may be fabricated. [M.E. *kasten,* fr. O.Norse *kasta*]

bacterial c., a c. in the urine composed of bacteria.

blood c., a c. usually formed in renal tubules, but may occur in bronchioles; consists of inspissated material that includes various elements of blood (i.e., erythrocytes, leukocytes, fibrin, and so on), resulting from bleeding into the glomerulus or tubule, or into the alveolus or bronchiole.

coma c., a renal c. of strongly refracting granules said to be indicative of imminent coma in diabetes. SYN Külz cylinder.

decidual c., a mold of the interior of the uterus formed of the exfoliated mucous membrane in cases of extrauterine gestation.

dental c., a positive likeness of a part or parts of the oral cavity.

diagnostic c., a positive replica of the form of the teeth and tissues made from an impression.

epithelial c., a c. that contains epithelial cells and their remnants; occurs most frequently in renal tubules and urine as a marker for renal tubular necrosis.

false c., an elongated, ribbonlike mucous thread with poorly defined edges and pointed or split ends, often confused with a true urinary c. SYN cylindroid, mucous c., pseudocast, spurious c.

fatty c., a renal or urinary c. consisting largely of fat globules;

those containing doubly refractile bodies (composed of cholesterol) are found in the nephrotic syndrome.

fibrinous c., a yellow c. that somewhat resembles a waxy c.; more likely to occur in the urine of certain patients with acute nephritis.

granular c., a relatively dark, dense urinary c. of coarsely or finely particulate cellular debris and other proteinaceous material, frequently seen in chronic renal disease but also in the recovery phase of acute renal failure. SEE ALSO waxy c.

hair c., a c. composed of parakeratotic scales attached to scalp hair but freely movable up and down the hair shaft; found in scaling dermatitis of the scalp, including dandruff, psoriasis, and seborrheic dermatitis. SYN pseudonit.

halo c., a c. applied to the shoulders in which metal bars are set that extend over the head to a halo, from which traction may be applied to the head by means of tongs or a halter.

hyaline c., a relatively transparent renal c. seen in the urine and composed of proteinaceous material derived from disintegration of cells; seen in patients with renal disease or transiently with exercise, fever, congestive heart failure, and diuretic therapy.

investment c., SYN refractory c.

master c., a replica of the prepared tooth surfaces, residual ridge areas, and/or other parts of the dental arch as reproduced from an impression.

mucous c., SYN false c.

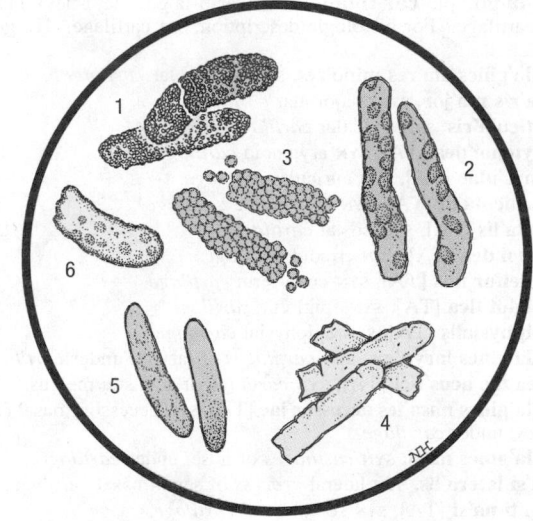

urinary casts: (1) coarse granular casts; (2) epithelial cell casts; (3) red blood cell casts; (4) waxy casts; (5) hyaline casts; (6) casts with pyocytes

red blood cell c., a urinary c. composed of a matrix containing red cells in various stages of degeneration and visibility, characteristic of glomerular disease or renal parenchymal bleeding. SYN red cell c.

red cell c., SYN red blood cell c.

refractory c., a c. made of material that will withstand the high temperatures of metal casting or soldering without disintegrating. SYN investment c.

renal c., any type of c. formed in a renal tubule, and found in the urine consisting of various materials, e.g., albumin, cells, blood. SYN tube c.

spica c., a c. of layers overlapping in a V pattern, covering two body parts greatly different in size, as the hip and waist, thumb and wrist, etc.

spurious c., SYN false c.

tube c., SYN renal c.

urinary c.'s, c.'s discharged in the urine.

waxy c., a form of urinary c. consisting of homogeneous proteinaceous material that has a high refractive index, in contrast to the low refractive index of hyaline c.'s; waxy c.'s probably represent an advanced stage of the disintegrative process that results in coarsely and finely granular c.'s, and are usually indicative of advanced renal disease.

white blood cell c., a urinary c. composed of polymorphonuclear leukocytes, characteristic of tubulointerstitial disease, especially pyelonephritis.

white cell c., a c. in the urine composed of white blood cells.

cast brace (kast brās). A specially designed plaster or plastic cast incorporating hinges and other brace components; used in the treatment of fractures to provide immobilization and to promote early activity and early joint motion.

Castellani, Sir Aldo, Italian physician, 1877–1971. SEE C. *bronchitis, paint.*

cast·ing (kas'ting). **1.** A metallic object formed in a mold. **2.** The act of forming a c. in a mold.

centrifugal c., c. molten metal into a mold by spinning the metal from a crucible at the end of a revolving arm.

ceramo-metal c., a c. made of alloys containing or excluding precious metals, to which dental porcelain can be fused.

gold c., a c. made of gold, usually formed to represent and replace lost tooth structure.

vacuum c., the c. of a metal in the presence of a vacuum.

Castle, William B., U.S. physician, 1897–1991. SEE C. intrinsic *factor.*

Castleman, Benjamin, U.S. pathologist, 1906–1982. SEE C. *disease.*

cas·tor bean (kas'ter bēn). SYN Ricinus.

cas·tor oil. A fixed oil expressed from the seeds of *Ricinus communis* (family Euphorbiaceae); a purgative.

aromatic c. o., contains cinnamon oil 3, clove oil 1, vanillin 1, saccharin 0.5, alcohol 30, in c. o. to make 1000; a cathartic.

cas·trate (kas'trāt). To remove the testicles or the ovaries. [L. *castro,* pp. *-atus,* to deprive of generative power (male or female)]

cas·tra·tion (kas-trā'shŭn). **1.** Removal of the testicles or ovaries. **2.** SEE castration *complex, castrate.*

functional c., gonadal atrophy produced by prolonged treatment with sex hormones.

ca·su·al·ty (kazh'oo-ăl-tē). An injury, or the victim of an accident.

CAT Abbreviation for *chloramphenicol* acetyl transferase; obsolete abbreviation for computerized axial *tomography* (CT).

△**cata-.** Down; opposite of ana-. SEE ALSO kata-. Cf. de-. [G. *kata,* down]

cat·a·ba·si·al (kat-ă-bā'sē-ăl). Denoting a skull in which the basion is lower than the opisthion. [cata- + Mod. L. *basion*]

cat·a·bi·ot·ic (kat'ă-bī-ot'ik). Used up in the carrying on of the vital processes other than growth, or in the performance of function, referring to the energy derived from food. [cata- + G. *biōtikos,* relating to life]

cat·a·bol·ic (kat-ă-bol'ik). Relating to or promoting catabolism.

ca·tab·o·lism (kă-tab'ō-lizm). **1.** The breaking down in the body of complex chemical compounds into simpler ones (e.g., glycogen to CO_2 and H_2O), often accompanied by the liberation of energy. **2.** The sum of all degradative processes. SYN dissimilation (2). Cf. anabolism, metabolism. [G. *katabolē,* a casting down]

ca·tab·o·lite (kă-tab'ō-līt). Any product of catabolism.

cat·a·chron·o·bi·ol·o·gy (kat'ă-kron'ō-bī-ol'ō-jē). The study of the deleterious effects of time on a living system. [cata- + G. *chronos,* time, + biology]

cat·a·crot·ic (kat-ă-krot'ik). Denoting a pulse tracing in which the downstroke is interrupted by one or more upward waves.

ca·tac·ro·tism (kă-tak'rō-tizm). A condition of the pulse in which there are one or more secondary expansions of the artery following the main beat, producing secondary upward waves on the downstroke of the pulse tracing. [cata- + G. *krotos,* beat]

cat·a·di·crot·ic (kat'ă-dī-krot'ik). Denoting a pulse tracing in which there are two minor elevations interrupting the downstroke.

cat·a·di·cro·tism (kat-ă-dī'krō-tizm). A condition of the pulse marked by two minor expansions of the artery following the main

beat, producing two secondary upward waves on the downstroke of the pulse tracing. [cata + G. *di-,* two, + *krotos,* beat]

cat·a·did·y·mus (kat-ă-did'i-mŭs). SYN *duplicitas* anterior. [cata- + G. *didymus,* twin]

cat·a·di·op·tric (kat-ă-dī-op'trik). Employing both reflecting and refractive optical systems.

cat·a·dro·mous (kat-a-drō'mus). Migrating from fresh water to the ocean to spawn. SEE ALSO anadromous.

cat·a·gen (kat'ă-jen). A regressing phase of the hair growth cycle during which cell proliferation ceases, the hair follicle shortens, and an anchored club hair is produced.

cat·a·gen·e·sis (kat-ă-jen'ě-sis). SYN involution. [cata- + G. *genesis,* origin]

cat·a·lase (kat'ă-lās). A hemoprotein catalyzing the decomposition of hydrogen peroxide to water and oxygen ($2H_2O_2 \rightarrow O_2 + 2H_2O$); a deficiency of c. is associated with acatalasemia.

cat·a·lep·sy (kat'ă-lep-sē). A condition characterized by waxy rigidity of the limbs, which may be placed in various positions that are maintained for a time, lack of response to stimuli, mutism and inactivity; occurs with some psychoses, especially catatonic schizophrenia. [G. *katalēpsis,* a seizing, catalepsy, fr. *kata,* down, + *lēpsis,* a seizure]

cat·a·lep·tic (kat-ă-lep'tik). Relating to, or suffering from, catalepsy.

cat·a·lep·toid (kat-ă-lep'toyd). Simulating or resembling catalepsy.

ca·tal·y·sis (kă-tal'i-sis). The effect that a catalyst exerts upon a chemical reaction. [G. *katalysis,* dissolution]

contact c., a process wherein the catalyst is a solid and the catalyzed reaction is produced after the reactants (usually gases) have made contact with the solid.

surface c., c. at the surface of a solid particle or interface, or of a macromolecule.

cat·a·lyst (kat'ă-list). A substance that accelerates a chemical reaction but is not consumed or changed permanently thereby. SYN catalyzer.

inorganic c., a c. such as a finely divided metal (Pt, Rh), carbon, etc.

negative c., a c. that retards a reaction.

organic c., (1) SYN enzyme, ribozyme; **(2)** a c. that is an organic molecule.

Raney c., SYN Raney Nickel.

cat·a·lyt·ic (kat-ă-lit'ik). Relating to or effecting catalysis.

cat·a·lyze (kat'ă-līz). To act as a catalyst.

cat·a·lyz·er (kat'ă-līz-er). SYN catalyst.

cat·am·ne·sis (kat-am-nē'sis). The medical history of a patient after an illness; the follow-up history. [cata- + G *mnēmē,* memory]

cat·am·nes·tic (kat-am-nes'tik). Related to catamnesis.

cat·a·pasm (kat'ă-pazm). A dusting powder applied to raw surfaces or ulcers. [G. *katapasma,* a powder; *katapassō,* to sprinkle over]

cat·a·pho·re·sis (kat'ă-fō-rē'sis). Movement of positively charged particles (cations) in a solution or suspension toward the cathode in electrophoresis. Cf. anaphoresis. [cata- + G. *phorēsis,* a being carried]

cat·a·pho·ret·ic (kat'ă-fō-ret'ik). Relating to cataphoresis.

cat·a·pla·sia, cat·a·pla·sis (kat-ă-plā'sē-ă, -plā'sis). A degenerative change in cells or tissues that is the reverse of the constructive or developmental change; a return to an earlier or embryonic stage. SYN retrograde metamorphosis (1), retrogression, retromorphosis. [cata- + G. *plasis,* a molding]

cat·a·plasm (kat'ă-plazm). SYN poultice. [G. *kataplasma,* poultice, fr. *kataplassō,* to spread over]

cat·a·plec·tic (kat-ă-plek'tik). **1.** Developing suddenly. **2.** Pertaining to cataplexy.

cat·a·plexy (kat'ă-plek-sē). A transient attack of extreme generalized weakness, often precipitated by an emotional response, such as surprise, fear, or anger; one component of the narcolepsy quadrad. [cata- + G. *plēxis,* a blow, stroke]

ca

CATARACT

cat·a·ract (kat'ă-rakt). Complete or partial opacity of the ocular lens. SYN cataracta. [L. *cataracta,* fr. G. *katarrhaktēs,* a downrushing, a waterfall, fr. *katarrhēgnymi,* to break down, rush down]

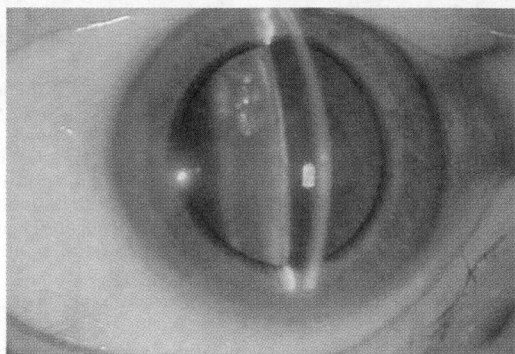

cataract

anular c., congenital c. in which a central white membrane replaces the nucleus. SYN disk-shaped c., life-belt c., umbilicated c.

atopic c., a c. associated with atopic dermatitis.

axial c., a lenticular opacity in the visual axis of the lens.

black c., a c. in which the lens is hardened and a dark brown. In the 19th century, German black c. meant gutta serena (q.v.). SYN cataracta brunescens, cataracta nigra.

blue c., coronary c. of bluish color. SYN cataracta cerulea.

capsular c., a c. in which the opacity affects the capsule only.

capsulolenticular c., a c. in which both the lens and its capsule are involved. SEE ALSO membranous c.

central c., congenital c. limited to the embryonic nucleus.

cerulean c. [MIM*115660], a congenetal c. with bluish coloring and radial lesions; autosomal dominant inheritance in some cases.

complete c., SYN mature c.

complicated c., SYN secondary c. (1).

concussion c., traumatic c. occurring with or without a hole in the lens capsule.

congenital c., c., usually bilateral, present at birth. It occurs as an autosomal recessive condition in calves of the Jersey breed. In humans approximately 25% of bilateral congenital c.'s are autosomal dominant [MIM*116200, *116700]; X-linked forms also exist [MIM*302200, *302300]. Most congenital c.'s are sporadic, some the result of prematurity, intrauterine infection, drug-related toxicity, injury, or chromosomal or metabolic disorders.

copper c., SYN *chalcosis* lentis.

coralliform c., congenital c. with round or elongated processes radiating from the center of the lens.

coronary c., peripheral cortical developmental c. occurring just after puberty; transmitted as a hereditary dominant characteristic.

cortical c., a c. in which the opacity affects the cortex of the lens. SYN peripheral c.

crystalline c., a hereditary c. with a coralliform or needle-shaped accumulation of crystals in the axial region of an otherwise clear lens.

cuneiform c., cortical c. in which the opacities radiate from the periphery like spokes of a wheel.

cupuliform c., a common form of senile c. often confined to a region just within the posterior capsule. SYN saucer-shaped c.

dendritic c., a congenital sutural c. with complicated branching.

diabetic c., c. occurring in insulin-dependent diabetes mellitus.

disk-shaped c., SYN anular c.

electric c., a c. caused by contact with a high-power electric current, or a lightning bolt. SYN cataracta electrica.

embryonic c. [MIM*115650], a congenital c. situated near the anterior Y suture of the fetal lens nucleus. Inheritance heterogeneous.

embryopathic c., congenital c. as a result of intrauterine infection, e.g., rubella.

fibroid c., fibrinous c., a sclerotic hardening of the capsule of the lens, following exudative iridocyclitis.

floriform c., a congenital c. with opacities arranged like the petals of a flower.

furnacemen's c., SYN infrared c.

fusiform c., SYN spindle c.

galactose c., a neonatal c. associated with intralenticular accumulation of galactose alcohol. SEE galactosemia.

glassworker's c., SYN infrared c.

glaucomatous c., a nuclear opacity usually seen in absolute glaucoma.

gray c., a c. of gray color, usually seen in senile, mature, or cortical c.

hard c., SYN nuclear c.

hook-shaped c., congenital c. with hooklike figures between the fetal and embryonic nuclei.

hypermature c., a c. in which the lens cortex becomes liquid, with the nucleus gravitating within the capsule (Morgagni c.). SYN overripe c.

hypocalcemic c., a c. occurring with low serum calcium.

immature c., a stage of partial lens opacification.

infantile c., a c. affecting a very young child.

infrared c., a c. secondary to absorption of heat by the lens, or by transmission from the adjacent iris. SYN furnacemen's c., glassworker's c.

intumescent c., a c. swollen because of fluid absorption.

juvenile c., a soft c. occurring in a child or young adult.

lamellar c., a c. in which the opacity is limited to the cortex. SYN zonular c.

life-belt c., SYN anular c.

mature c., a c. in which both the nucleus and cortex are opaque. SYN complete c., ripe c.

membranous c., a secondary c. composed of the remains of the thickened capsule and degenerated lens fibers.

Morgagni c., a hypermature c. in which the nucleus gravitates within the capsule. SYN sedimentary c.

myotonic c., c. occurring in myotonic dystrophy.

nuclear c., a c. involving the nucleus. SYN hard c.

overripe c., SYN hypermature c.

perinuclear c., a lamellar c. in which the nucleus is clear but is surrounded by a ring of opacity.

peripheral c., SYN cortical c.

pisciform c., a hereditary c. with bilateral fish-shaped opacities in the axial region of the fetal nucleus.

polar c., a capsular c. limited to an area of the anterior or posterior pole of the lens.

posterior subcapsular c., a c. involving the cortex at the posterior pole of the lens.

progressive c., a c. in which the opacification process progresses to involve the entire lens.

punctate c., an incomplete c. in which there are opaque dots scattered through the lens.

pyramidal c., a cone-shaped, anterior polar c.

radiation c., a c. caused by excessive or prolonged exposure to ultraviolet rays, x-rays, radium, gamma rays, heat, or radioactive isotopes.

reduplicated c., a type of congenital c. with opacities situated at various levels in the lens.

ripe c., SYN mature c.

rubella c., embryopathic c. secondary to intrauterine rubella infection.

saucer-shaped c., SYN cupuliform c.

secondary c., (1) a c. that accompanies or follows some other eye disease such as uveitis; SYN complicated c. (2) a c. occurring in the retained lens or capsule after a c. extraction.

sedimentary c., SYN Morgagni c.

senile c., a c. occurring spontaneously in the elderly; mainly a cuneiform c., nuclear c., or posterior subcapsular c., alone or in combination.

siderotic c., a c. resulting from deposition of iron from an iron-containing intraocular foreign body.

soft c., an advanced or mature c. in which the nucleus is not well developed.

spindle c., a c. in which the opacity is fusiform, extending from one pole to the other. SYN fusiform c.

stationary c., a c. that does not progress.

stellate c., congenital c. with lens opacities radiating toward the periphery, with subcapsular and cortical changes.

subcapsular c., a c. in which the opacities are concentrated beneath the capsule.

sugar c., any c. associated with intralenticular accumulation of pentose or hexose alcohols.

sunflower c., SYN *chalcosis* lentis.

sutural c., a congenital type of c. with opacities along the Y sutures of the fetal lens nucleus; usually does not affect vision.

tetany c., a c. that develops in hypocalcemia.

total c., a c. involving the entire lens.

toxic c., a c. caused by drugs or chemicals.

traumatic c., a c. caused by contusion, rupture, or a foreign body.

umbilicated c., SYN anular c.

vascular c., congenital c. in which the degenerated lens is replaced with mesodermal tissue. SYN cataracta adiposa, cataracta fibrosa.

zonular c., SYN lamellar c.

---

cat·a·rac·ta (kat-ă-rak′tă). SYN cataract. [L.]

c. adipo′sa, SYN vascular *cataract.*

c. brunes′cens, SYN black *cataract.*

c. ceru′lea, SYN blue *cataract.*

c. elec′trica, SYN electric *cataract.*

c. fibro′sa, SYN vascular *cataract.*

c. ni′gra, SYN black *cataract.*

cat·a·rac·to·gen·e·sis (kat′ă-rak-tō-jen′ĕ-sis). The process of cataract formation. [cataract + G. *genesis,* production]

cat·a·rac·to·gen·ic (kat′ă-rak-tō-jen′ik). Cataract-producing.

cat·a·rac·tous (kat-ă-rak′tŭs). Relating to a cataract.

ca·tar·ia (ka-tā′rē-ă). The dried flowering tops of *Nepeta cataria* (family Labiatae); an emmenagogue and antispasmodic; also reported to produce psychic effects. SYN catnep, catnip. [L. *cattus,* male cat (post-class)]

ca·tarrh (kă-tahr′). Inflammation of a mucous membrane with increased flow of mucus or exudate. [G. *katarrheō,* to flow down]

nasal c., SYN rhinitis.

vernal c., SYN vernal *conjunctivitis.*

ca·tarrh·al (kă-tah′răl). Relating to or affected with catarrh.

cat·a·stal·sis (kat-ă-stal′sis). A contraction wave resembling ordinary peristalsis but not preceded by a zone of inhibition. [G. *katastellō,* to put in order, check]

cat·a·stal·tic (kat-ă-stal′tik). Inhibitory, restricting, or restraining. [cata- + G. *staltos,* contracted, fr. *stellō,* to contract]

ca·tas·ta·sis (kă-tas′tă-sis). 1. A condition or state. 2. Restoration to a normal condition or a normal place. [G.]

cat·a·to·nia (kat-ă-tō′nē-ă). A syndrome of psychomotor disturbances characterized by periods of physical rigidity, negativism, or stupor; may occur in schizophrenia, mood disorders, or organic mental disorders. [G. *katatonos,* stretching down, depressed, fr. *kata,* down, + *tonos,* tone]

excited c., c. in which the patient is excited, impulsive, hyperactive, and combative.

periodic c., regularly reappearing phases of catatonic excitement.

stuporous c., c. in which the patient is subdued, mute, and nega-

tivistic, accompanied by varying combinations of staring, rigidity, and cataplexy.

cat·a·ton·ic, cat·a·to·ni·ac (kat-ă-ton′ik, -tō′nē-ak). Relating to, or characterized by, catatonia.

cat·a·tri·chy (kat′ă-tri-kē) [MIM*116850]. Presence of a forelock of hair that is separate or different in appearance; may be inherited as an autosomal dominant. SEE Waardenburg *syndrome.* [cata- + G. *thrix,* hair]

cat·a·tri·crot·ic (kat′ă-trī-krot′ik). Denoting a pulse tracing with three minor elevations interrupting the downstroke.

cat·a·tri·cro·tism (kat-ă-trī′krō-tizm). A condition of the pulse marked by three minor expansions of the artery following the main beat, producing three secondary upward waves on the downstroke of the pulse tracing. [cata- + G. *tri-,* three, + *krotos,* beat]

cat·e·chase (kat′ĕ-kās). SYN catechol 1,2-dioxygenase.

cat·e·chin (kat′ĕ-kin). Derived from catechu, and used as an astringent in diarrhea and as a stain. SYN catechinic acid, catechuic acid, cyanidol.

cat·e·chin·ic ac·id (kat-ĕ-kin′ik). SYN catechin.

cat·e·chol (kat′ĕ-kol). 1. SYN pyrocatechol. 2. Term loosely used for catechin, which contains an *o*-c. moiety, and as the root of catecholamines, which are pyrocatechol derivatives.

c.-*O*-methyltransferase, a transferase that catalyzes the methylation of the hydroxyl group at the 3 position of the aromatic ring of c.'s, including the catecholamines norepinephrine and epinephrine (thus, converting to normetanephrine and metanephrine, respectively), the methyl group coming from *S*-adenosyl-L-methionine. An important step in the catabolism of the catecholamines.

c. oxidase, an enzyme oxidizing c.'s to 1,2-benzoquinones, with O_2. SEE ALSO monophenol monooxygenase. SYN diphenol oxidase, *o*-diphenolase.

c. oxidase (dimerizing), an enzyme oxidizing a c., with O_2, to a diphenylenedioxide quinone (e.g., 4 c. + $3O_2$ → 2 dibenzo[1,4]-2,3-dione + $6H_2O$).

cat·e·chol·a·mines (kat-ĕ-kol′ă-mēnz). Pyrocatechols with an alkylamine side chain; examples of biochemical interest are epinephrine, norepinephrine, and L-dopa. C.'s are major elements in responses to stress.

cat·e·chol 1,2-di·ox·y·gen·ase. An oxidoreductase catalyzing oxidation of pyrocatechol, with O_2, to *cis-cis*-muconate. SYN catechase, pyrocatechase.

cat·e·chol 2,3-di·ox·y·gen·ase. An oxidoreductase oxidizing catechol, with O_2, to 2-hydroxymuconate semialdehyde. SYN metapyrocatechase.

cat·e·chu·ic ac·id (kat-ĕ-choo′ik, -koo′ik). SYN catechin.

cat·e·chu ni·grum. Black c. n., an extract of the heart wood of *Acacia catechu* (family Leguminosae), used as an astringent in diarrhea. SYN cutch.

cat·e·lec·trot·o·nus (kat′ē-lek-trot′ō-nŭs). The changes in excitability and conductivity in a nerve or muscle in the neighborhood of the cathode during the passage of a constant electric current. [cathode + electrotonus]

cat·e·nate (kat′en-āt). To connect in a series of links like a chain; for example, two rings of mitochondrial DNA are often catenated. [L. *catenatus,* chained together, fr. *catena,* chain]

cat·e·nat·ing (kat′en-āt-ing). Occurring in a chain or series. [L. *catenatus,* chained]

cat·e·nin (ka-tēn′in). Cytoplasmic molecule that serves as a link between cadherins and the cytoskeleton of cells, allowing the formation of adherent junctions. There are two types: β-c., which is linked to the cadherin itself and α-c., which associates with actin microfilaments. [L. *catena,* chain, + -in]

cat·e·noid (kat′ĕ-noyd). 1. Like a chain, such as a chain of fungus spores or a colony of protozoa in which the individuals are joined end to end. SYN catenulate. 2. Surface of net zero curvature generated by the rotation of a catenary (curve of repose of a suspended chain); the interventricular septum of the heart in idiopathic hypertrophic subaortic stenosis resembles a c., which makes it ineffective in increasing intracavity pressure or in reducing its volume as defined in Laplace law. [L. *catena,* chain, + G. *eidos,* resemblance]

ca·ten·u·late (ka-ten′ū-lāt). SYN catenoid (1).

cat·er·pil·lar (kat′er-pil′er). The wormlike larval stage of a butterfly or a moth. [M.E. *catirpeller*, fr. O.Fr. *cate*, cat, + *pelose*, hairy]

dermatitis-causing c., one of several species whose hairs can cause an allergic dermatitis; the saddleback c. (*Sabine stimulea*) and the brown-tail moth (*Euproctis chrysorrhoea*) are common examples.

saddleback c., *Sabine stimulea,* a cause of caterpillar dermatitis.

stinging c., caterpillar with urticarious hairs or spines that cause allergic dermatitis, e.g., the Io moth and the puss c.

cat·gut (kat′gŭt). An absorbable surgical suture material made from the collagenous fibers of the submucosa of certain animals (usally from sheep or cows); misnamed catgut. [probably from *kit,* a small violin, through confusion with *kit,* a small cat]

chromic c., c. impregnated with chromium salts to prolong its tensile strength and retard its absorption.

silverized c., c. prepared by immersion in a 2% solution of colloidal silver for 1 week and then in 95% alcohol for 15 to 30 minutes.

Catha ed·u·lis (kath′ă ed′ū-lis). A plant of Ethiopia and Arabia (family Celastraceae), cultivated for use as a stimulant; khat (the fresh leaves and twigs) is chewed or used in the preparation of a beverage; the active principle is pharmacologically related to the amphetamines, probably *d*-norisoephedrine. [Ar. *khat*]

Cath·ar·an·thus al·ka·loids (kath-ăr-ran′thus). SYN Vinca *alkaloids,* under *alkaloid.*

ca·thar·sis (kă-thar′sis). 1. SYN purgation. 2. The release or discharge of emotional tension or anxiety by psychoanalytically guided emotional reliving of past, especially repressed, events. SYN psychocatharsis. [G. *katharsis,* purification, fr. *katharos,* pure]

ca·thar·tic (kă-thar′tik). 1. Relating to catharsis. 2. An agent having purgative action.

ca·thec·tic (kă-thek′tik). Pertaining to cathexis.

ca·them·o·glo·bin (ka-thēm-ō-glō′bin). An artificial derivative of hemoglobin in which the globin is denatured and the iron oxidized.

ca·thep·sin (kă-thep′sin). One of a number of intracellular proteinases and peptidases (all endopeptidases) of animal tissues of varying specificities.

cath·e·ter (kath′ĕ-ter). 1. A tubular instrument to allow passage of fluid from or into a body cavity or blood vessel. SEE ALSO line (4). 2. Especially a c. designed to be passed through the urethra into the bladder to drain it of retained urine. [G. *kathetēr,* fr. *kathiēmi,* to send down]

acorn-tipped c., a c. used in ureteropyelography to occlude the ureteral orifice and prevent backflow from the ureter during and following the injection of an opaque medium.

angiography c., a thin-walled tube suitable for percutaneous insertion and power injection of contrast media for radiography; c. diameter is measured on the French scale. SEE Seldinger *technique.*

balloon c., a c. used in arterial embolectomy or to float into the pulmonary artery.

balloon-tip c., a single- or double-lumen tube with a balloon at its tip that can be inflated or deflated without removal after installation; the balloon may be inflated to facilitate passage of the tube through a blood vessel (propelled by the bloodstream) or to occlude the vessel in which the tube alone would allow free flow; such c.'s are used to enter the pulmonary artery to facilitate hemodynamic measurements. SEE ALSO Swan-Ganz c.

bicoudate c., c. bicoudé (bī-koo-dā′), an elbowed c. with a double bend. [bi + Fr. *coudé,* bent]

Bozeman-Fritsch c., a slightly curved double-channel uterine c. with several openings at the tip.

Braasch c., a bulb-tipped c. used for dilation and calibration. SYN Braasch bulb.

Broviac c., a type of long-term central venous c. with an external port for administration of medication.

brush c., a ureteral c. with a finely bristled brush tip that is endoscopically passed into the ureter or renal pelvis and by gentle to-and-fro movement brushes cells from the surface of suspected tumors.

cardiac c., SYN intracardiac c.

central venous c., a c. passed through a peripheral or central vein, ending in the superior vena cava or right atrium, for measurement of central venous pressure or for infusion of hyperosmolar solutions.

conical c., a c. with a cone-shaped tip designed to dilate the ureter.

c. coudé (koo-da′), a c. with an angular bend near the beak; used to rise over prostatic obstruction. SYN elbowed c., prostatic c. [Fr. *coudé,* bent]

c. à demeure (ă-dem-ër′), an obsolete term for a c. that is retained for a considerable period in the urethra. [Fr. *demeurer,* to dwell]

de Pezzer c., a self-retaining c. with a bulbous extremity.

double-channel c., a c. with two lumens, allowing irrigation and aspiration or injection and pressure measurement. SYN two-way c.

elbowed c., SYN c. coudé.

eustachian c., a c. for the middle ear through the eustachian tube.

female c., a short, nearly straight c. for passage into the female urethra.

Fogarty embolectomy c., a c. with an inflatable balloon near its tip; used to remove emboli and thrombi from blood vessels or to remove stones from the biliary ducts.

Foley c., urethral c. with a retaining balloon.

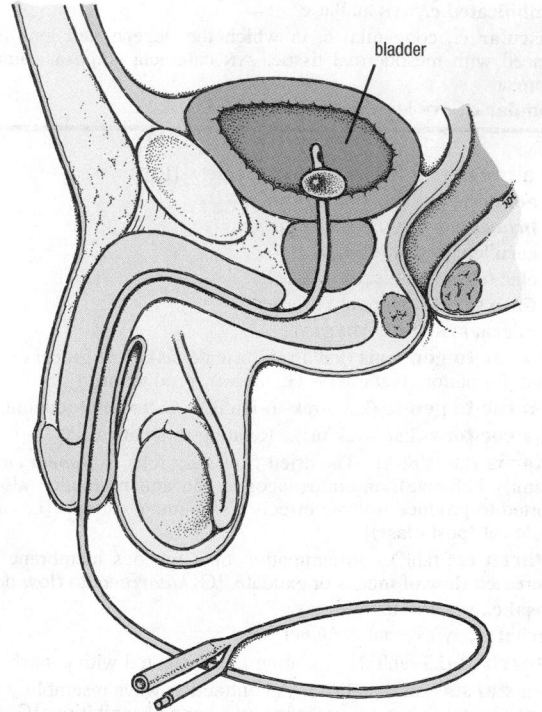

bladder

Foley catheter

Gouley c., a solid curved steel instrument grooved on its inferior surface so that it can be passed over a guide through a urethral stricture.

Hickman c., long-term, central venous indwelling c. with external port(s).

indwelling c., a c. left in place in the bladder, usually a balloon c.

intracardiac c., a c. that can be passed into the heart through a vein or artery, to withdraw samples of blood, measure pressures within the heart's chambers or great vessels, and inject contrast media; used mainly in the diagnosis and evaluation of congenital, rheumatic, and coronary artery lesions and to evaluate systolic and diastolic cardiac function. SYN cardiac c.

Malecot c., a two- or four-winged c.

Nélaton c., a flexible c. of red rubber.

olive-tipped c., a ureteral c. with an olive-shaped tip, used to dilate a constricted ureteral orifice; larger sizes are also used for dilating or calibrating urethral strictures.

pacing c., a cardiac c. with one or more electrodes at its tip which can be used to artificially pace the heart.

Pezzer c., SEE de Pezzer c.

Phillips c., a c. with a filiform guide for the urethra.

pigtail c., a c. with a tightly curled end and multiple side holes to reduce the impact of the injectant on the vessel wall or to remain in a chamber or space for drainage.

prostatic c., SYN c. coudé.

pulmonary artery c., SYN Swan-Ganz c.

Robinson c., a straight urethral c. with two to six holes to facilitate drainage, especially in the presence of blood clots which may occlude one or more openings.

self-retaining c., a c. so constructed that it remains in urethra and bladder until removed, e.g., indwelling c.; Foley c.

spiral tip c., a c. with a helical filiform tip.

Swan-Ganz c., a balloon-tipped flexible c. commonly used in the treatment of critically ill patients; introduced via a major peripheral vein, usually jugular or subclavian, and floated under pressure *waveform* guidance, with or without fluoroscopy, sequentially through the right atrium, right ventricle, and pulmonary artery, ultimately to wedge, when the balloon is inflated, in a small arterial branch where the tip measures pressure-transmitted retrograde from the left side of the heart, which is assumed to represent left ventricular end-diastolic pressure; side holes allow measurement of central venous pressure; with the balloon deflated, c. measures pulmonary artery systolic, diastolic, and mean pressures; also allows infusion via c.; some c.'s are fitted with pacing electrodes. SYN pulmonary artery c.

two-way c., SYN double-channel c.

vertebrated c., a c. made of several segments moving on each other like the links of a chain.

whistle-tip c., a c. with an opening at the end and side.

winged c., a soft rubber c. with little flaps at each side of the beak to retain it in the bladder.

cath·e·ter·i·za·tion (kath′ĕ-ter-ī-zā′shŭn). Passage of a catheter.

clean intermittent bladder c. (CIC), a common way for patients with neurogenic bladders that do not empty normally to empty their bladders on a routine schedule.

cath·e·ter·ize (kath′ĕ-ter-īz). To pass a catheter.

cath·e·ter·o·stat (kath′ĕ-ter-ō-stat). A stand for holding catheters. [catheter + G. *statos,* standing]

ca·thex·is (kă-thek′sis). A conscious or unconscious attachment of psychic energy to an idea, object, or person. [G. *kathexis,* a holding in, retention]

cath·o·dal (C) (kath′ō-dăl). Of, pertaining to, or emanating from a cathode. SYN cathodic.

cath·ode (Ca, C) (kath′ōd). The negative pole of a galvanic battery or the electrode connected with it; the electrode toward which positively charged ions (cations) migrate and are reduced, and into which electrons are fed from their source (anode or generator). Cf. anode. SYN negative electrode. [G. *kathodos,* a way down, fr. *kata,* down, + *hodos,* a way]

ca·thod·ic (kă-thod′ik). SYN cathodal.

cath·ol·y·sis (kath-ol′ē-sis). Electrolysis with a cathode needle.

cat·i·on (kat′ī-on). An ion carrying a charge of positive electricity, therefore going to the negatively charged cathode. [G. *katiōn,* going down]

cat·i·on ex·change. The process by which a cation in a liquid phase exchanges with another cation present as the counter ion of a negatively charged solid polymer (cation exchanger). A cation-exchange reaction in removal of the Na^+ of a sodium chloride solution is $RSO_3^-H^+ + Na^+ \rightarrow RSO_3^-Na^+ + H^+$ (R is the polymer, RSO_3^- is the cation exchanger); if this is combined with the anion-exchange reaction, NaCl is removed from the solution (desalting). Cation exchange may also be used chromatographically, to separate cations, and medicinally, to remove a cation; e.g., H^+,

from gastric contents, or Na^+ and K^+ in the intestine. SEE anion exchange.

cat·i·on ex·chang·er. An insoluble solid (usually a polystyrene or a polysaccharide) that has negatively charged radicals attached to it (e.g., $-COO^-$, $-SO_3^-$), which can attract and hold cations that pass by in a moving solution if these are more attracted to the acid groups than the counter ion present.

cat·i·on·ic (kat-ī-on′ik). Referring to positively charged ions and their properties.

cat·i·on·o·gen (kat-ī-on′ō-jen). A substance that gives rise to positively charged ions.

cat·lin, cat·ling (kat′lin, -ling). A long, sharp-pointed, double-edged knife used in amputations.

cat·nep, cat·nip (kat′nep, kat′nip). SYN cataria.

cat·o·chus (kat′ō-kŭs). The trancelike phase of catalepsy in which the patient is conscious but cannot move or speak. [G. *katochē,* epilepsy (Galen), fr. *katechō,* to hold fast]

ca·top·tric (ka-top′trik). Relating to reflected light. [G. *katoptron,* mirror]

cau·da, pl. **cau·dae** (kaw′dă, kaw′dē) [TA]. SYN tail (1). [L. a tail]

c. epididym′idis [TA], SYN *tail* of epididymis.

c. equi′na [TA], the bundle of spinal nerve roots arising from the lumbosacral enlargement and medullary cone and running through the lumbar cistern (subarachnoid space) within the vertebral canal below the first lumbar vertebra; it comprises the roots of all the spinal nerves below the first lumbar. [L. horse tail]

c. fas′ciae denta′tae, SYN uncus *band* of Giacomini.

c. hel′icis [TA], SYN *tail* of helix.

c. nu′clei cauda′ti [TA], SYN *tail* of caudate nucleus.

c. pancrea′tis [TA], SYN *tail* of pancreas.

c. stria′ti, SYN *tail* of caudate nucleus.

cau·dad (kaw′dad). **1.** In a direction toward the tail. **2.** Situated nearer the tail in relation to a specific reference point; opposite of craniad. SEE ALSO inferior.

cau·dal (kaw′dăl) [TA]. Pertaining to the tail. SYN caudalis [TA]. [Mod. L. *caudalis*]

cau·da·lis (kaw-dā′lis) [TA]. SYN caudal.

cau·date (kaw′dāt). **1.** Tailed; possessing a tail. **2.** SYN caudate *nucleus.*

cau·da·to·len·tic·u·lar (kaw-dā′tō-len-tik′ū-lăr). Relating to the caudate nucleus and lenticularis. SYN caudolenticular.

cau·da·tum (kaw-dā′tŭm). SYN caudate *nucleus.*

cau·do·ceph·a·lad (kaw-dō-sef′ăl-ad). In a direction from the tail toward the head.

cau·do·len·tic·u·lar (kaw′dō-len-tik′ū-lăr). SYN caudatolenticular.

caul, cowl (kawl). **1.** The amnion, either as a piece of membrane capping the baby's head at birth or the whole membrane when delivered unruptured with the baby. SYN galea (4), veil (2), velum (2). **2.** SYN greater *omentum.* [Gaelic, *call,* a veil]

cau·sal·gia (kaw-zal′jē-ă). Persistent severe burning pain, usually following injury of a peripheral nerve (especially median and tibial) or the brachial plexus, accompanied by trophic changes. [G. *kausis,* burning, + *algos,* pain]

cau·sal·i·ty (kawz′al-i-tē). The relating of causes to the effects they produce; the pathogenesis of disease, and epidemiology, are largely concerned with causality.

cause (kawz). That which produces an effect or condition; that by which a morbid change or disease is brought about. [L. *causa*]

constitutional c., a c. acting from within or through some systemic process or inborn error.

exciting c., the direct provoking c. of a condition. SYN procatarxis (1).

necessary c., an etiologic factor without which a result in question will not occur; the occurrence of the result is proof that the factor is operating.

precipitating c., a factor that brings on the onset of manifestations of a disease process.

ca

predisposing c., anything that produces a susceptibility or disposition to a condition without actually causing it.

proximate c., the immediate c. that precipitates a condition.

specific c., a c. the action of which can definitely produce the condition in question.

sufficient c., an etiologic factor that guarantees that a result in question will occur; non-occurrence of the result is proof that the factor is not operating.

caus·tic (kaws'tik). **1.** Chemically exerting an effect resembling a burn. **2.** An agent producing this effect. **3.** Denoting a solution of a strong alkali; e.g., caustic soda, NaOH. SYN pyrotic (2). [G. *kaustikos,* fr. *kaiō,* to burn]

cau·ter·ant (kaw'ter-ant). **1.** Cauterizing. **2.** A cauterizing agent.

cau·ter·i·za·tion (kaw-ter-ī-zā'shŭn). The act of cauterizing. SEE ALSO cautery.

cau·ter·ize (kaw'ter-īz). To apply a cautery; to burn with a cautery.

cau·tery (kaw'ter-ē). **1.** An agent or device used for scarring, burning, or cutting the skin or other tissues by means of heat, cold, electric current, ultrasound, or caustic chemicals. **2.** Use of a cautery. [G. *kautērion,* a branding iron]

actual c., a c., such as electrocautery, acting directly through heat and not by chemical means. SYN technocausis.

BICAP c., a form of bipolar electrocoagulation frequently used to arrest gastrointestinal bleeding.

bipolar c., electrocautery by high frequency electrical current passed through tissue from an active to a passive electrode; used for hemostasis.

chemical c., SYN chemocautery.

cold c., SYN cryocautery.

electric c., SYN electrocautery.

gas c., c. by means of a measured amount of a lighted gas jet.

monopolar c., electrocautery by high frequency electrical current passed from a single electrode, where the cauterization occurs, the patient's body serving as a ground.

ca·va (kā'vă). SEE inferior *vena* cava, superior *vena* cava.

ca·va·gram (kā'vă-gram). SYN cavogram.

ca·val (kā'văl). Relating to a vena cava.

cave (kāv) [TA]. A hollow or enclosed space or cavity. SEE cavity, cavitas, cavernous *space.* SYN cavea.

trigeminal c. [TA], the cleft in the meningeal layer of dura of the middle cranial fossa near the tip of the petrous part of the temporal bone; it encloses the roots of the trigeminal nerve and the trigeminal ganglion. SYN cavum trigeminale [TA], trigeminal cavity ⚹, Meckel cavity, Meckel space.

cavea. SYN cave.

cavea thoracis [TA], SYN thoracic *cage.*

cav·e·o·la, pl. **cav·e·o·lae** (kav-ē-ō'lă, -lē). A small pocket, vesicle, cave, or recess communicating with the outside of a cell and extending inward, indenting the cytoplasm and the cell membrane. Such caveolae may be pinched off to form free vesicles within the cytoplasm. They are considered to be sites of uptake of materials into the cell, expulsion of materials from the cell, or sites of addition or removal of cell (unit) membrane to or from the cell surface. [L.]

cav·ern (kav'ern). SYN cavernous *space.*

c.'s of corpora cavernosa, SYN cavernous *spaces* of corpora cavernosa, under *space.*

c.'s of corpus spongiosum, SYN cavernous *spaces* of corporus spongiosum, under *space.*

ca·ver·na, pl. **ca·ver·nae** (kă-ver'nă, -nē). SYN cavernous *space.* [L. a grotto, fr. *cavus,* hollow]

cavernae cor'poris spongio'si [TA], SYN cavernous *spaces* of corporus spongiosum, under *space.*

cavernae cor'porum cavernoso'rum [TA], SYN cavernous *spaces* of corpora cavernosa, under *space.*

cav·er·nil·o·quy (kav-er-nil'ō-kwē). Low-pitched resonant pectoriloquy heard over a lung cavity. [L. *caverna,* cavern, + *loquor,* to talk]

cav·er·ni·tis (kav-er-nī'tis). Inflammation of the corpus cavernosum penis. SYN cavernositis.

fibrous c., c. occasionally associated with Peyronie disease.

cav·er·no·si·tis (kav'er-nō-sī'tis). SYN cavernitis.

cav·ern·ous (kav'er-nŭs). Relating to a cavern or a cavity; containing many cavities.

Ca·via (kā'vē-ă). A genus of the family Caviidae that includes the guinea pigs. [Mod. L., fr. native Indian]

C. porcel'lus, a rodent with a very short tail that is not visible externally; native to South America, where it is raised for food; used widely as a laboratory animal in medical research. SYN guinea pig.

cav·i·tary (kav'i-tā-rē). **1.** Relating to a cavity or having a cavity or cavities. **2.** Denoting any animal parasite that has an enteric canal or body cavity and that lives within the host's body.

cav·i·tas, pl. **cav·i·ta·tes** (kav'i-tas, -tā'tēs). SYN cavity. [Mod. L.]

c. abdomina'lis [TA], SYN abdominal *cavity.*

c. abdominis et pelvis [TA], SYN abdominopelvic *cavity.*

c. articula'ris [TA], SYN articular *cavity.*

c. conchae [TA], SYN *cavity* of concha.

c. coronae [TA], SYN crown *cavity.*

c. corona'lis, SYN pulp *cavity* of crown.

c. cranii [TA], SYN cranial *cavity.*

c. den'tis [TA], SYN pulp *cavity.*

c. glenoida'lis, SYN mandibular *fossa.*

c. glenoidalis scapulae [TA], SYN glenoid *cavity* of scapula.

c. infraglottica [TA], SYN infraglottic *cavity.*

c. infraglot'ticum, SYN infraglottic *cavity.*

c. laryn'gis [TA], SYN laryngeal *cavity.*

c. medulla'ris [TA], SYN medullary *cavity.*

c. na'si [TA], SYN nasal *cavity.*

c. o'ris [TA], SYN oral *cavity.*

c. o'ris pro'pria [TA], SYN oral *cavity* proper.

c. pelvina, ⚹official alternate term for pelvic *cavity.*

c. pel'vis [TA], SYN pelvic *cavity.*

c. pericardiaca [TA], SYN pericardial *cavity.*

c. peritonea'lis [TA], SYN peritoneal *cavity.*

c. pharyn'gis [TA], SYN *cavity* of pharynx.

c. pleura'lis [TA], SYN pleural *cavity.*

c. pulparis, ⚹official alternate term for pulp *cavity.*

c. thora'cis [TA], SYN thoracic *cavity.*

c. tympan'ica [TA], SYN tympanic *cavity.*

c. u'teri [TA], SYN uterine *cavity.*

cav·i·ta·tion (kav-i-tā'shŭn). **1.** Formation of a cavity, as in the lung in tuberculosis or with development of a bacterial lung abscess. **2.** The production of small vapor-containing bubbles or cavities in a liquid or tissue by ultrasound.

ca·vi·tis (kā-vī'tis). SYN celophlebitis.

cav·i·ty (kav'i-tē). **1.** A hollow space; hole. SEE cave, cavity, cavitas, cavernous *space.* **2.** Lay term for the loss of tooth structure due to dental caries. SYN cavum [TA], cavitas. [L. *cavus,* hollow]

abdominal c. [TA], the space bounded by the abdominal walls, the diaphragm, and the pelvis; it usually is arbitrarily separated from the pelvic cavity by a plane across the superior aperture of the pelvis; however, it may include the pelvis with the abdomen (see abdominopelvic c.); within the c. lie the greater part of the organs of digestion, the spleen, the kidneys, and the suprarenal glands. SYN cavitas abdominalis [TA], cavum abdominis, enterocele (2).

abdominopelvic c. [TA], the combined and continuous abdominal and pelvic c.'s. SEE ALSO abdominal c. SYN cavitas abdominis et pelvis [TA].

amnionic c., the fluid-filled c. inside the amnion that contains the developing embryo.

articular c. [TA], a joint cavity, the potential space bounded by the synovial membrane and articular cartilages of all synovial joints. Normally, the articular c. contains only sufficient synovial fluid to lubricate the internal surfaces. SYN cavitas articularis [TA], cavum articulare.

axillary c., SYN axilla.

body c., the collective visceral c. of the trunk (thoracic c. plus abdominopelvic c.), bounded by the superior thoracic aperture above, the pelvic floor below, and the body walls (parietes) in between. SYN celom (2), celoma, coelom.

buccal c., SYN oral *vestibule.*

cleavage c., SYN blastocele.

c. of concha [TA], the space within the lower, larger portion of the concha below the crus helicis; it forms the vestibule leading into the external acoustic meatus. SYN cavitas conchae [TA], cavum conchae⁎.

c.'s of corpora cavernosa, SYN cavernous *spaces* of corpora cavernosa, under *space.*

c.'s of corpus spongiosum, SYN cavernous *spaces* of corporus spongiosum, under *space.*

cotyloid c., SYN acetabulum.

cranial c. [TA], the space within the skull occupied by the brain, its coverings, and cerebrospinal fluid. SYN cavitas cranii [TA], intracranial c.

crown c., SYN pulp c. of crown. SYN cavitas coronae [TA].

ectoplacental c., SYN epamniotic c.

ectotrophoblastic c., a developmental c. appearing between the trophoblast and the embryonic disk ectoderm in some mammals.

epamniotic c., a developmental c. that exists in some mammals and is derived by division of the proamniotic space; it is further removed from the embryo than the amniotic c. in some mammals. SYN ectoplacental c.

epidural c., SYN epidural *space.*

glenoid c., SYN mandibular *fossa.*

glenoid c. of scapula [TA], the hollow in the head of the scapula that receives the head of the humerus to make the shoulder joint; SYN cavitas glenoidalis scapulae [TA], glenoid fossa (1).

greater peritoneal c., SYN peritoneal c.

head c., the cephalic region in the embryos of vertebrates containing the modified somites that give rise to the extrinsic eye muscles.

idiopathic bone c., SYN solitary bone *cyst.*

inferior laryngeal c., SYN infraglottic c.

infraglottic c. [TA], the part of the cavity of the larynx immediately below the glottis. SYN cavitas infraglottica [TA], aditus glottidis inferior, cavitas infraglotticum, cavum infraglotticum, inferior laryngeal c., infraglottic space.

intermediate laryngeal c., portion of the c. of the larynx between the vestibular and vocal folds, with which the ventricles communicate. SYN aditus glottidis superior.

intracranial c., SYN cranial c.

laryngeal c. [TA], a cavity that is continuous above with the pharynx at the level of the aryepiglottic folds and extends downward through the rima glottidis to the infraglottic space. SYN cavitas laryngis [TA], c. of larynx, cavum laryngis.

c. of larynx, SYN laryngeal c.

lesser peritoneal c., SYN omental *bursa.*

Meckel c., SYN trigeminal *cave.*

medullary c. [TA], the marrow cavity in the shaft of a long bone. SYN cavitas medullaris [TA], cavum medullare.

c. of middle ear, SYN tympanic c.

nasal c. [TA], the cavity on either side of the nasal septum, lined with ciliated respiratory mucosa, extending from the naris anteriorly to the choana posteriorly, and communicating with the paranasal sinuses through their orifices in the lateral wall, from which also project the three conchae; the cribriform plate, through which the olfactory nerves are transmitted, forms the roof; the floor is formed by the hard palate. SYN cavitas nasi [TA], cavum nasi.

nephrotomic c., SYN nephrocele (2).

oral c. [TA], the region consisting of the vestibulum oris, the narrow cleft between the lips and cheeks, and the teeth and gums, and the cavitas oris propria. SYN cavitas oris [TA], cavum oris, mouth (1).

oral c. proper [TA], the space between the dental arches, limited posteriorly by the isthmus of the fauces (palatoglossal arch). SYN cavitas oris propria [TA].

orbital c., SYN orbit.

pelvic c. [TA], the space bounded at the sides by the bones of the pelvis, above by the superior aperture of the pelvis, and below by the pelvic diaphragm; it contains the pelvic viscera. SYN cavitas pelvis [TA], cavitas pelvina⁎, cavum pelvis.

pericardial c. [TA], (1) the potential space between the parietal and the visceral layers of the serous pericardium; (2) in the embryo, that part of the primary celom containing the heart; originally it is in open communication with the pericardioperitoneal c.'s and indirectly, through them, with the peritoneal part of the celom. SYN cavitas pericardiaca [TA], cavum pericardii.

peritoneal c. [TA], the interior of the peritoneal sac, normally only a potential space between the parietal and visceral layers of the peritoneum. SYN cavitas peritonealis [TA], cavum peritonei, greater peritoneal c.

perivisceral c., the space between the ectoderm and endoderm in the gastrula. SYN primitive perivisceral c.

pharyngonasal c., SYN nasopharynx.

c. of pharynx [TA], it consists of a nasal part (nasopharynx) continuous anteriorly with the nasal cavity and receiving the openings of the auditory tubes, an oral part (oropharynx) opening through the fauces into the oral cavity, and a laryngeal part (laryngopharynx) leading into the vestibule of the larynx and to the esophagus. SYN cavitas pharyngis [TA], cavum pharyngis.

pleural c. [TA], the potential space between the parietal and visceral layers of the pleura. SYN cavitas pleuralis [TA], cavum pleurae, pleural space.

pleuroperitoneal c., that part of the embryonic celom later partitioned to give rise to the pleural and peritoneal c.'s.

primitive perivisceral c., SYN perivisceral c.

pulmonary c., one of the bilateral subdivisions of the thoracic c. lying on either side of the mediastinum, lined with parietal pleura and occupied by a lung; the space existing when a lung is removed. The term is not synonymous with pleural c., which is a space between the parietal and visceral pleura that is normally empty except for a fine layer of pleural fluid and that surrounds (but does not contain) the lung.

pulp c. [TA], the central hollow of a tooth consisting of the crown cavity and the root canal; it contains the fibrovascular dental pulp and is lined throughout by odontoblasts. SYN cavitas dentis [TA], cavitas pulparis⁎, c. of tooth, cavum dentis.

pulp c. of crown [TA], the space within the crown of a tooth continuous with the root canal. SYN cavitas coronalis, cavum coronale, crown c.

Retzius c., SYN retropubic *space.*

segmentation c., SYN blastocele.

c. of septum pellucidum, a slitlike, fluid-filled space of variable width between the left and right transparent septum, which occurs in fewer than 10% of human brains and may communicate with the third ventricle. SYN cavum septum pellucidum [TA], Duncan ventricle, fifth ventricle, pseudocele, pseudoventricle, sylvian ventricle, ventricle of Sylvius, ventriculus quintus, Vieussens ventricle, Wenzel ventricle.

somite c., SYN myocele (2).

splanchnic c., the celom or one of the body c.'s derived from it. SYN visceral c.

subarachnoid c., SYN subarachnoid *space.*

subdural c., SYN subdural *space.*

subgerminal c., SYN primitive *gut.*

superior laryngeal c., SYN *vestibule* of larynx.

thoracic c. [TA], the space within the thoracic walls, bounded below by the diaphragm and above by the neck. SYN cavitas thoracis [TA], cavum thoracis.

c. of tooth, SYN pulp c.

trigeminal c., ⁎official alternate term for trigeminal *cave.*

tympanic c. [TA], an air chamber in the temporal bone containing the ossicles; it is lined with mucous membrane and is continuous with the auditory tube anteriorly and the tympanic antrum and mastoid air cells posteriorly. SYN cavitas tympanica [TA], c. of middle ear, cavum tympani.

ca

uterine c., c. of uterus [TA], the space within the uterus extending from the cervical canal to the openings of the uterine tubes. SYN cavitas uteri [TA], cavum uteri.

visceral c., SYN splanchnic c.

ca·vo·gram (kā'vō-gram). An angiogram of a vena cava. SYN cavagram. [(vena) cava + G. *gramma,* a writing]

ca·vog·ra·phy (kā-vog'ră-fē). SYN venacavography.

ca·vo·sur·face (kā-vō-sŭr'făs). Relating to a cavity and the surface of a tooth.

ca·vum, pl. **ca·va** (ka'vŭm, -vă) [TA]. SYN cavity. [L. ntr. of adj. *cavus,* hollow]

c. abdom'inis, SYN abdominal *cavity.*

c. articula're, SYN articular *cavity.*

c. con'chae, ✶official alternate term for *cavity* of concha.

c. corona'le, SYN pulp *cavity* of crown.

c. den'tis, SYN pulp *cavity.*

c. doug'lasi, SYN rectouterine *pouch.*

c. epidura'le, SYN epidural *space.*

c. infraglot'ticum, SYN infraglottic *cavity.*

c. laryn'gis, SYN laryngeal *cavity.*

c. mediastina'le, an inappropriate name sometimes applied to the mediastinum.

c. medulla're, SYN medullary *cavity.*

c. na'si, SYN nasal *cavity.*

c. o'ris, SYN oral *cavity.*

c. pel'vis, SYN pelvic *cavity.*

c. pericar'dii, SYN pericardial *cavity.*

c. peritone'i, SYN peritoneal *cavity.*

c. pharyn'gis, SYN *cavity* of pharynx.

c. pleu'rae, SYN pleural *cavity.*

c. psalte'rii, SYN Verga *ventricle.*

c. ret'zii, SYN retropubic *space.* [A.A. Retzius]

c. sep'tum pellu'cidum [TA], SYN *cavity* of septum pellucidum.

c. subarachnoid'eum, SYN subarachnoid *space.*

c. subdura'le, SYN subdural *space.*

c. thora'cis, SYN thoracic *cavity.*

c. trigemina'le [TA], SYN trigeminal *cave.*

c. tym'pani, SYN tympanic *cavity.*

c. u'teri, SYN uterine *cavity.*

c. ver'gae, SYN Verga *ventricle.*

c. vesicouteri'num, SYN vesicouterine *pouch.*

Cb Symbol for columbium.

C-band·ing. SEE C-banding *stain.*

CBC Abbreviation for complete *blood count.*

CBF Abbreviation for cerebral or coronary blood flow.

CBG Abbreviation for corticosteroid-binding *globulin.*

Cbl Abbreviation for cobalamin.

Cbz Abbreviation for carbobenzoxy- (benzyloxycarbonyl).

C.C. Abbreviation for chief complaint, as recorded on a patient's medical history.

cc, c.c. Abbreviation for cubic *centimeter.*

CCA Abbreviation for chimpanzee coryza *agent.*

CCC Abbreviation for cathodal closure *contraction.*

CCDM Abbreviation for *Control of Communicable Diseases Manual.*

CCK Abbreviation for cholecystokinin.

CCNU SYN lomustine.

CCU Abbreviation for coronary care *unit;* critical care *unit.*

CD Abbreviation for curative *dose;* circular *dichroism;* cluster of differentiation.

CD 54. SEE intercellular adhesion *molecule*-1.

CD^{50} 1. Abbreviation for curative *dose.* **2.** In a study of a therapeutic agent, the dose that cures 50% of the test subjects.

Cd Symbol for cadmium.

cd Symbol for candela.

CDC Abbreviation for Centers for Disease Control and Prevention; previously known as the Communicable Disease Center.

CDE blood group. See Rh blood group, Blood Groups appendix.

cDNA Abbreviation for complementary DNA, sometimes used as copy DNA.

CDP Abbreviation for cytidine 5'-diphosphate.

CDP-cho·line Abbreviation for cytidine diphosphocholine.

CDP-glyc·er·ide Abbreviation for cytidine diphosphoglyceride.

CDP-sug·ar Abbreviation for cytidine diphosphosugar.

Ce Symbol for cerium.

CEA Abbreviation for carcinoembryonic *antigen.*

ce·bo·ceph·a·ly (sē-bō-sef'ă-lē). Malformation of the head in which the features are suggestive of a monkey, with defective or absent nose and closely set eyes; part of the holoprosencephaly spectrum. [G. *kēbos,* monkey, + *kephalē,* head]

♻**cec-.** SEE ceco-.

ce·ca (sē'kă). Plural of cecum.

ce·cal (sē'kăl). **1.** Relating to the cecum. **2.** Ending blindly or in a cul-de-sac.

ce·cec·to·my (sē-sek'tō-mē). Excision of the cecum. SYN typhlectomy. [ceco- + G. *ektomē,* excision]

Cecil, Arthur Bond, U.S. urologist, 1885–1967. SEE Cecil *urethroplasty.*

ce·ci·tis (sē-sī'tis). Inflammation of the cecum. SYN typhlenteritis, typhlitis, typhloenteritis.

♻**ceco-, cec-.** The cecum. SEE ALSO typhlo- (1). Cf. typhlo-. [L. *caecum,* cecum, blind]

ce·co·co·los·to·my (sē'kō-kō-los'tō-mē). Formation of an anastomosis between cecum and colon.

ce·co·fix·a·tion (sē'kō-fik-sā'shŭn). SYN cecopexy.

ce·co·il·e·os·to·my (sē'kō-il-ē-os'tō-mē). SYN ileocecostomy.

ce·co·pexy (sē'kō-pek-sē). Operative anchoring of a movable cecum. SYN cecofixation, typhlopexy, typhlopexia. [ceco- + G. *pexis,* fixation]

ce·co·pli·ca·tion (sē'kō-pli-kā'shŭn). Operative reduction in size of a dilated cecum by the formation of folds or tucks in its wall. [ceco- + L. *plico,* pp. *-atus,* to fold]

ce·cor·rha·phy (sē-kōr'ă-fē). Suture of the cecum. SYN typhlorrhaphy. [ceco- + G. *rhaphē,* suture]

ce·co·sig·moid·os·to·my (sē'kō-sig-moy-dos'tō-mē). Formation of a communication between the cecum and the sigmoid colon.

ce·cos·to·my (sē-kos'tō-mē). Operative formation of a cecal fistula. SYN typhlostomy. [ceco- + G. *stoma,* mouth]

ce·cot·o·my (sē-kot'ō-mē). Incision into the cecum. SYN typhlotomy. [ceco- + G. *tome,* incision]

ce·co·u·re·ter·o·cele (sē'cō-ū-rē'ter-ō-sēl). A ureterocele that extends far along the urethra, sometimes even out the urethral meatus.

ce·cro·pins (sē-krō-pinz). Antibacterial peptides consisting of two amphipathic α-helix components.

ce·cum, pl. **ce·ca** (sē'kŭm, sē'kă) [TA]. **1.** The cul-de-sac, about 6 cm in depth, lying below the terminal ileum forming the first part of the large intestine. SYN blind gut, intestinum cecum, typhlon. **2.** Any similar structure ending in a cul-de-sac. SYN caecum. [L. ntr. of *caecus,* blind]

cupular c. of the cochlear duct [TA], the upper blind extremity of the cochlear duct. SYN c. cupulare [TA], cupular blind sac, lagena (1).

c. cupula're [TA], SYN cupular c. of the cochlear duct.

intestinal c.,

vestibular c. of the cochlear duct [TA], the lower extremity of the cochlear duct, occupying the cochlear recess in the vestibule. SYN c. vestibulare [TA], vestibular blind sac.

c. vestibula're [TA], SYN vestibular c. of the cochlear duct.

ce·dar leaf oil (sē'der). Oil obtained by steam distillation from the fresh leaves of *Thuja occidentalis;* used as an insect repellent and counterirritant, and in perfumery. SYN thuja oil.

ce·dar wood oil. Volatile oil obtained from the wood of *Juniperus virginiana* (family Pinaceae); used as an insect repellent, in perfumery, and as a clearing agent in microscopy.

Ced·e·cea (sed-e′sē-ă). A genus in the Enterobacteriaceae group that includes the species *C. davisae,* (the type strain), *C. lapagei,* and *C. neteri;* they have been recovered from the human respiratory tract, but their role in disease has not yet been delineated.

Ceelen, Wilhelm, 1884–1964. SEE C.-Gellerstedt *syndrome.*

cef·a·clor (sef′ă-klōr). A semisynthetic broad spectrum antibiotic derived from cephalosporin C; used orally.

cef·a·drox·il (sef-ă-drok′sil). A semisynthetic broad spectrum antibiotic derived from cephalosporin C; used orally.

cef·a·man·dole nafate (sef-ă-man′dōl naf′āt). A semisynthetic broad spectrum antibiotic derived from cephalosporin C; used by injection.

ce·faz·o·lin (se-faz′ō-lin). A broad spectrum cephalosporin antibiotic used to treat a wide variety of serious infections; available as the sodium salt for intramuscular or intravenous administration.

ce·fon·i·cid di·so·di·um (se-fon′ĭ-sid). A broad-spectrum long acting cephalosporin antibiotic structurally related to cefamandole.

ce·fo·per·a·zone so·di·um (se-fō-per′ă-zōn). A semisynthetic piperazine-cephalosporin antibiotic.

ce·for·a·nide (se-fōr′ă-nīd). A broad-spectrum long-acting cephalosporin antibiotic.

ce·fo·tax·ime so·di·um (se-fō-taks′ēm). A broad-spectrum cephalosporin antibiotic.

cef·o·te·tan di·so·di·um (sef′ō-te-tan). A broad-spectrum cephalosporin antibiotic.

ce·fox·i·tin so·di·um (se-fok′si-tin). A semisynthetic antibiotic derived from cephamycin C, but structurally and pharmacologically similar to the cephalosporins; used by injection.

cef·taz·i·dime so·di·um (sef-taz′i-dēm). A cephalosporin antibiotic especially effective against enterobacteria and species of *Pseudomonas.*

cef·ti·zox·ime so·di·um (sef-ti-zoks′ēm). A broad spectrum cephalosporin antibiotic similar to cefotaxime sodium.

cef·tri·ax·one di·so·di·um (sef-trī-aks′ōn). A semisynthetic parenteral cephalosporin antibiotic.

cel (sel). A unit of velocity; 1 cm per second. [L. *celer,* swift]

-cele. Swelling; hernia. [G. *kēlē,* tumor]

ce·len·ter·on (sē-len′ter-on). SYN primitive *gut.* [G. *koilos,* hollow, + *enteron,* intestine]

cel·ery seed (sel′er-ē). The dried ripe fruit of *Apium graveolens* (family Umbelliferae); has been used in dysmenorrhea and as a sedative.

Celestin, Felix, French physician, *1900. SEE C. *tube.*

ce·les·tine blue B (sĕ-les′tēn) [C.I. 51050]. A dye recommended as a substitute for hematoxylin when it is unavailable.

ce·li·ac (sē′lē-ak). Relating to the abdominal cavity. [G. *koilia,* belly]

ce·li·ag·ra (sē-lē-ag′ră). Rarely used term for sudden painful affection of the stomach or other abdominal organs. [G. *koilia,* belly, + *agra,* seizure]

celio-. The abdomen. SEE ALSO celo- (3). [G. *koilia,* belly]

ce·li·o·cen·te·sis (sē′lē-ō-sen-tē′sis). Rarely used term for paracentesis of the abdomen. [celio- + G. *kentēsis,* puncture]

ce·li·o·my·al·gia (sē′lē-ō-mī-al′jē-ă). Rarely used term for pain in the abdominal muscles. [celio- + G. *mys,* muscle, + *algos,* pain]

ce·li·o·my·o·si·tis (sē′lē-ō-mī-ō-sī′tis). Inflammation of the abdominal muscles. [celio- + G. *mys,* muscle, + *-itis,* inflammation]

ce·li·o·par·a·cen·te·sis (sē′lē-ō-par-ă-sen-tē′sis). Rarely used term for paracentesis of the abdomen. [celio- + G. *parakentēsis,* a puncture for dropsy]

ce·li·op·a·thy (sē-lē-op′ă-thē). Rarely used term for any abdominal disease. [celio- + G. *pathos,* disease]

ce·li·or·rha·phy (sē-lē-ōr′ă-fē). Suture of a wound in the abdominal wall. SYN laparorrhaphy. [celio- + G. *rhaphē,* seam]

ce·li·os·co·py (sē-lē-os′kŏ-pē). SYN peritoneoscopy. [celio- + G. *skopeō,* to view]

ce·li·ot·o·my (sē-lē-ot′ō-mē). Transabdominal incision into the peritoneal cavity. SYN abdominal section, laparotomy (2), ventrotomy. [celio- + G. *tomē,* incision]

vaginal c., opening the peritoneal cavity through the vagina. SYN culdotomy (2).

ce·li·tis (sē-lī′tis). Any inflammation of the abdomen. [G. *koilia,* belly, + *-itis,* inflammation]

CELL

---

cell (sel). **1.** The smallest unit of living structure capable of independent existence, composed of a membrane-enclosed mass of protoplasm and containing a nucleus or nucleoid. C.'s are highly variable and specialized in both structure and function, though all must at some stage replicate proteins and nucleic acids, utilize energy, and reproduce themselves. **2.** A small closed or partly closed cavity; a compartment or hollow receptacle. **3.** A container of glass, ceramic, or other solid material within which chemical reactions generating electricity take place or solutions are placed for photometric assays. [L. *cella,* a storeroom, a chamber]

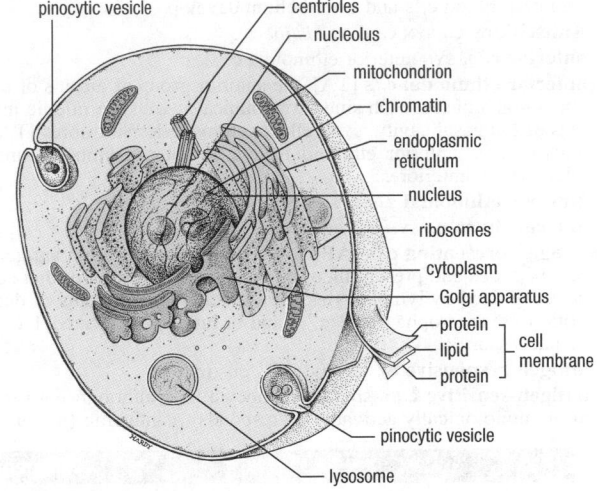

cell with typical organelles

A c.'s, alpha c.'s of pancreas or of anterior lobe of hypophysis.

absorption c., a small glass chamber with parallel sides, in which absorption spectra of solutions can be obtained.

absorptive c.'s of intestine, c.'s on the surface of villi of the small intestine and the luminal surface of the large intestine that are characterized by having microvilli on their free surface.

accessory c., SYN antigen-presenting c.'s.

acid c., SYN parietal c.

acidophil c., a c. whose cytoplasm or granules stain with acid dyes.

acinar c., any secreting c. lining an acinus, especially applied to the c.'s of the pancreas that furnish pancreatic juice and enzymes to distinguish them from the c.'s of ducts and the islets of Langerhans. SYN acinous c.

acinous c., SYN acinar c.

acoustic c., a hair c. of the organ of Corti.

adipose c., SYN fat c.

adventitial c., SYN pericyte.

air c.'s, (1) SYN pulmonary *alveolus;* **(2)** air-containing spaces in the skull.

air c.'s of auditory tube, SYN tubal air c.'s (of pharyngotympanic tube).

albuminous c., (1) SYN serous c; **(2)** SYN zymogenic c.

algoid c., a c. appearing like c.'s of algae, sometimes found in chronic diarrhea.

alpha c.'s of anterior lobe of hypophysis, acidophil c.'s that constitute about 35% of the c.'s of the anterior lobe. There are two varieties: one that elaborates somatotropin, another that elaborates prolactin.

alpha c.'s of pancreas, c.'s of the islets of Langerhans that secrete glucagon.

alveolar c., any of the c.'s lining the alveoli of the lung, including the squamous alveolar c.'s, the great alveolar c.'s, and the alveolar macrophages. SYN pneumocyte.

amacrine c., a nerve c. with short branching dendrites but believed to lack an axon; Cajal described and named such cells in the retina.

ameboid c., a c. such as a leukocyte, having ameboid movements, with a power of locomotion. SYN wandering c. SYN migratory c.

amniogenic c.'s, c.'s from which the amnion develops.

anabiotic c., c. that is capable of resuscitation after apparent death; the existence of anabiotic tumor c.'s is postulated to explain the recurrence of a cancer after a very long symptomless period following operation.

anaplastic c., (1) a c. that has reverted to an embryonal state; **(2)** an undifferentiated c., characteristic of malignant neoplasms.

angioblastic c.'s, those c.'s in the early embryo from which primitive blood c.'s and endothelium develop.

Anitschkow c., SYN cardiac *histiocyte*.

anterior c.'s, SYN anterior ethmoidal c.'s.

anterior ethmoidal c.'s [TA], the anterior group of air c.'s of the ethmoidal sinuses; each sinus communicates with the middle meatus of the nasal cavity. SYN cellulae ethmoidales anteriores [TA], anterior c.'s, anterior ethmoidal air c.'s, anterior sinuses, sinus ethmoidales anteriores.

anterior ethmoidal air c.'s, SYN anterior ethmoidal c.'s.

anterior horn c., SYN motor *neuron*.

ⓘ **antigen-presenting c.'s (APC),** c.'s that process protein antigens into peptides and present them on their surface in a form that can be recognized by lymphocytes. APCs include Langerhans c., dendritic c.'s, macrophages, B c.'s, and in humans, activated T c.'s. SYN accessory c.

antigen-responsive c., SYN antigen-sensitive c.

antigen-sensitive c., a small lymphocyte that, although not itself an immunologically activated c., responds to antigenic (immuno-genic) stimulus by a process of division and differentiation that results in the production of immunologically activated cells. SYN antigen-responsive c.

apolar c., a neuron without processes.

APUD c.'s, SEE APUD.

argentaffin c.'s, c.'s that contain granules which precipitate silver from an ammoniacal silver nitrate solution. SEE ALSO enteroendocrine c.'s.

argyrophilic c.'s, c.'s that bind silver salts but that precipitate silver only in the presence of a reducing agent. SEE ALSO enteroendocrine c.'s.

Aschoff c., a large cell component of rheumatic nodules in the myocardium with a characteristic nucleus and relatively little cytoplasm.

Askanazy c., SYN Hürthle c.

astroglia c., SYN astrocyte.

atypical glandular c.'s of undetermined significance, the term in the Bethesda system for reporting cervical and/or vaginal cytologic diagnosis describing c.'s that show either endometrial or endocervical differentiation and display nuclear atypia that exceed reactive or reparative changes but lack definite features of invasive adenocarcinoma. SEE ALSO Bethesda *system*.

atypical squamous c.'s of undetermined significance (AS-CUS), the term in the Bethesda system for reporting cervical/vaginal cytologic diagnosis describing cellular abnormalities that are more marked than those attributable to reactive changes but that quantitatively or qualitatively fall short of a definitive diagnosis of squamous intraepithelial lesion (LSIL); may reflect a benign or a potentially serious lesion. SEE ALSO Bethesda *system*, reactive *changes*, under *change*.

auditory receptor c.'s, columnar c.'s in the epithelium of the organ of Corti, having hairs (stereocilia) on their apical ends. SEE Corti c.'s.

B c., (1) β c. of pancreas or of anterior lobe of hypophysis; **(2)** SYN B *lymphocyte*.

balloon c., (1) an unusually large degenerated c. with pale-staining vacuolated or reticulated cytoplasm, as in viral hepatitis or in degenerated epidermal c.'s in herpes zoster; **(2)** a large form of nevus c. with abundant nonstaining cytoplasm, formed by vacular degeneration of melanosomes.

ⓘ **band c.,** any c. of the granulocytic (leukocytic) series that has a nucleus that could be described as a curved or coiled band, no matter how marked the indentation, if it does not completely

antigen presenting cells

	dendrite cell	macrophage		B lymphocyte	
		resting	activated	resting	activated
antigen uptake	endocytosis phagocytes (by Langerhans cells)	phagocytosis	phagocytosis	receptor-mediated endocytosis	receptor-mediated endocytosis
class II MHC expression	constitutive (+++)	inducible (−)	inducible (++)	constitutive (++)	constitutive (+++)
costimulatory activity	constitutive B7 (+++)	inducible B7 (−)	inducible B7 (++)	inducible B7 (−)	inducible B7 (++)
T-cell activation	naive T cells effector T cells memory T cells	(−)	effector T cells memory T cells	effector T cells memory T cells	naive T cells effector T cells memory T cells

MHC, major histocompatibility complex; LPS, lipopolysaccharide; IFN-γ, interferon gamma

segment the nucleus into lobes connected by a filament. SYN band neutrophil, rod nuclear c., Schilling band c., stab c., stab neutrophil, staff c.

basal c., a c. of the deepest layer of stratified epithelium. SYN basilar c.

basaloid c., a c., usually of the epidermis, resembling a basal c.

basilar c., SYN basal c.

basket c., (1) a neuron enmeshing the cell body of another neuron with its terminal axon ramifications; (2) SYN smudge c.'s; (3) a myoepithelial c. with branching processes that occurs basal to the secretory c.'s of certain salivary gland and lacrimal gland alveoli.

basophil c. of anterior lobe of hypophysis, SYN beta c. of anterior lobe of hypophysis.

beaker c., SYN goblet c.

Beale c., a bipolar ganglion c. of the heart with one spiral and one straight prolongation.

Berger c.'s, SYN hilus c.'s.

berry c., a crenated red blood c. with surface spicules.

beta c. of anterior lobe of hypophysis, one of a population of functionally diverse c.'s that contain basophilic granules and secrete hormones such as ACTH, lipotropin, thyrotropin, and the gonadotropins. SYN basophil c. of anterior lobe of hypophysis.

beta c. of pancreas, the predominant c. of the islets of Langerhans that secretes insulin.

Betz c.'s, large pyramidal c.'s in the motor area of the precentral gyrus of the cerebral cortex. SYN Bevan-Lewis c.'s.

Bevan-Lewis c.'s, SYN Betz c.'s.

bipolar c., a neuron having two processes, such as those of the retina or the spiral and vestibular ganglia of the eighth nerve.

Bizzozero red c.'s, nucleated red blood c.'s in human blood.

blast c., an immature precursor c.; e.g., erythroblast, lymphoblast, neuroblast. SEE ALSO -blast.

blood c., one of the cells of the blood, a leukocyte or erythrocyte. SYN blood corpuscle.

Boll c.'s, basal c.'s in the lacrimal gland.

bone c., SYN osteocyte.

border c.'s, c.'s forming the inner boundary of the organ of Corti.

Böttcher c.'s, c.'s of the basilar membrane of the cochlea.

Bowenoid c.'s, c.'s characteristic of Bowen disease; scattered large, round intraepidermal keratinocytes with a hyperchromatic nucleus and pale cytoplasm.

bristle c., hair c. of the inner ear.

bronchic c.'s, SYN pulmonary *alveolus*.

bronchiolar exocrine c., SYN Clara c.

brood c., SYN mother c.

burr c., a crenated red blood c.

C c., (1) a c. of the pancreatic islets of the guinea pig; SYN gamma c. of pancreas. SEE ALSO medullary *carcinoma* of thyroid; (2) calcitonin-secreting round or spindle shaped follicular thyroid c.; ultrastructurally contains numerous 60–550 nm neuroendocrine granules; best identified immunohistochemically with antibodies to calcitonin. SYN light c.'s of thyroid, parafollicular c.'s.

Cajal c., (1) SYN horizontal c. of Cajal; (2) SYN astrocyte.

caliciform c., SYN goblet c.

capsule c., SYN amphicyte.

carrier c., SYN phagocyte.

cartilage c., SYN chondrocyte.

castration c.'s, altered basophilic c.'s of the anterior lobe of the pituitary that develop following castration; the body of the c. is occupied by a large vacuole that displaces the nucleus to the periphery, giving the c. a resemblance to a signet ring. SYN signet ring c.'s.

caterpillar c., SYN cardiac *histiocyte*.

centroacinar c., a c. of the pancreatic ductule that occupies the lumen of an acinus; it secretes bicarbonate and water, providing an alkaline pH necessary for enzyme activity in the intestine.

chalice c., SYN goblet c.

chief c., the predominant cell type of a gland.

chief c. of corpus pineale, SYN pinealocyte.

chief c. of parathyroid gland, a round clear c. with a centrally located nucleus; secretes parathyroid hormone.

chief c. of stomach, SYN zymogenic c.

chromaffin c., a c. that stains with chromic salts, in adrenal medulla and paraganglia of the sympathetic nervous system.

chromophobe c.'s of anterior lobe of hypophysis, c.'s of the adenohypophysis that are devoid of specific acidophilic or basophilic granules when stained with common differential stains.

Clara c., a rounded, club-shaped, nonciliated c. protruding between ciliated c.'s in bronchiolar epithelium; believed to be secretory in function. SYN bronchiolar exocrine c.

Clarke c.'s, large multipolar c.'s characteristic of the thoracic nucleus (Clarke nucleus in lamina VII) of the spinal cord.

Claudius c.'s, columnar c.'s on the floor of the ductus cochlearis external to the organ of Corti.

clear c., (1) a c. in which the cytoplasm appears empty with the light microscope, as occurs in certain secretory c.'s of eccrine sweat glands and in the parathyroid glands when the glycogen is unstained; (2) any c., particularly a neoplastic one, containing abundant glycogen or other material that is not stained by hematoxylin or eosin, so that the c. cytoplasm is very pale in routinely stained sections.

cleavage c., SYN blastomere.

cleaved c., a c. with single or multiple clefts in the nuclear membrane.

clonogenic c., a c. that has the potential to proliferate and give rise to a colony of c.'s; some daughter c.'s from each generation retain this potential to proliferate.

clue c., a type of vaginal epithelial c. that appears granular and is coated with coccobacillary organisms; seen in bacterial vaginosis.

cochlear hair c.'s, sensory c.'s in the organ of Corti in synaptic contact with sensory as well as efferent fibers of the cochlear (auditory) nerve; from the apical end of each c. about 100 stereocilia extend from the surface and make contact with the tectorial membrane. SYN Corti c.'s.

column c.'s, neurons in the gray matter of the spinal cord whose axons are confined within the central nervous system.

commissural c., a neuron whose axon passes to the opposite side of the neuraxis. SYN heteromeric c.

compound granule c., SYN gitter c.

cone c. of retina, SYN cone (2).

connective tissue c., any of the c.'s of varied form occurring in connective tissue.

contrasuppressor c.'s, a subpopulation of T c.'s, distinct from T helper c.'s, which allegedly inhibit T suppressor c. function.

Corti c.'s, SYN cochlear hair c.'s.

crescent c., SYN sickle c.

cytomegalic c.'s, c.'s containing large intranuclear and intracytoplasmic cytomegalic inclusion bodies caused by cytomegalovirus; a member of the family Herpesviridae.

cytotoxic c., (1) a subset of CD8 T lymphocytes that bind to other c.'s via class I MHC and are involved in their destruction. SYN T cytotoxic c. (2) other c.'s of the immune system capable of killing pathogens or abberant c.'s, i.e., macrophages, NK cells, K cells.

cytotrophoblastic c.'s, stem c.'s that fuse to form the overlying syncytiotrophoblast of placental villi. SYN Langhans c.'s (2).

D c., SYN delta c. of pancreas.

dark c.'s, c.'s in eccrine sweat glands having many ribosomes and mucoid secretory granules.

daughter c., one of the two or more c.'s formed in the division of a parent c.

Davidoff c.'s, SYN Paneth granular c.'s.

decidual c., an enlarged, ovoid connective tissue c. appearing in the endometrium of pregnancy.

decoy c., benign exfoliated epithelial c. with pyknotic nucleus seen in urinary infections; may be mistaken for malignant c.

deep c., SYN mesangial c.

Deiters c.'s, (1) SYN phalangeal c; (2) SYN astrocyte.

delta c. of anterior lobe of hypophysis, a variety of c. having basophilic granules.

delta c. of pancreas, a c. of the islets having fine granules and containing somatostatin. SYN D c.

dendritic c., c. of neural crest origin with extensive processes; they develop melanin early.

Dogiel c.'s, the different cell types in cerebrospinal ganglia.

dome c., one of the rounded surface c.'s of the periderm layer of the fetal epidermis.

Downey c., the atypical lymphocyte of infectious mononucleosis.

dust c., SYN alveolar *macrophage.*

effector c., a terminally differentiated leukocyte that performs one or more specific functions. SEE ALSO effector.

egg c., the unfertilized ovum.

embryonic c., SYN blastomere.

enamel c., SYN ameloblast.

end c., a fully differentiated c., the mature c. of a lineage.

endodermal c., embryonic c.'s forming the yolk sac and giving rise to the epithelium of the alimentary and respiratory tracts and to the parenchyma of associated glands. SYN entodermal c.

endothelial c., one of the squamous c.'s forming the lining of blood and lymph vessels and the inner layer of the endocardium. SYN endotheliocyte.

enterochromaffin c.'s, SYN enteroendocrine c.'s.

enteroendocrine c.'s, c.'s, scattered throughout the digestive tract that are of several varieties and are believed to produce at least 20 different gastrointestinal hormones and neurotransmitters; they contain granules that may be either argentaffinic or argyrophilic. SYN enterochromaffin c.'s, Kulchitsky c.'s.

entodermal c., SYN endodermal c.

ependymal c., a c. lining the central canal of the spinal cord (those of pyramidal shape) or one of the brain ventricles (those of cuboidal shape).

epidermic c., one of the c.'s of the epidermis.

epithelial c., one of the many varieties of c.'s that form epithelium.

epithelial reticular c., one of the many-branched epithelial c.'s that collectively form the supporting stroma for lymphocytes in the thymus; believed to produce thymosin and other factors that control thymic function.

epithelioid c., (1) a nonepithelial c. having certain characteristics of epithelium; (2) large mononuclear histiocytes having certain epithelial characteristics, particularly in areas of granulomatous inflammation where they are polygonal and have eosinophilic cytoplasm.

erythroid c., a c. of the erythrocytic series.

ethmoid c.'s, ethmoidal air cells; evaginations of the mucous membrane of the middle and superior meatuses of the nasal cavity into the ethmoidal labyrinth forming multiple small paranasal sinuses; they are subdivided into anterior, middle and posterior ethmoidal sinuses. SEE anterior ethmoidal c.'s, middle ethmoidal c.'s, posterior ethmoidal c.'s. SYN cellulae ethmoidales [TA], ethmoid air c.'s [TA], ethmoid c.'s [TA], antra ethmoidalia, ethmoidal sinuses, sinus ethmoidales.

ethmoid air c.'s [TA], SYN ethmoid c.'s.

ethmoidal c.'s [TA], SYN ethmoid c.'s.

external pillar c.'s, SEE pillar c.'s.

exudation c., SYN exudation *corpuscle.*

Fañanás c., a specialized astrocyte found in the cerebellar cortex.

fasciculata c., a c. of the zona fasciculata of the adrenal cortex that contains numerous lipid droplets due to the presence of corticosteroids.

fat c., a connective tissue c. distended with one or more fat globules, the cytoplasm usually being compressed into a thin envelope, with the nucleus at one point in the periphery. SYN adipocyte, adipose c.

fat-storing c., a multilocular fat-filled c. present in the perisinusoidal space in the liver. SYN lipocyte.

Ferrata c., SYN hemohistioblast.

flame c., primitive, ciliated excretory c. in trematodes; the movement of the cilia on this c. within the miracidium larva within a schistosome egg indicates egg viability.

foam c.'s, c.'s with abundant, pale-staining, finely vacuolated cytoplasm, usually histiocytes that have ingested or accumulated material that dissolves during tissue preparation, especially lipids. SEE ALSO lipophage.

follicular epithelial c., a c. lining a follicle such as that of the thyroid gland.

follicular ovarian c.'s, c.'s of an ovarian follicle that surround the developing ovum; they form the stratum granulosum ovarii and cumulus oophorus.

foreign body giant c., a multinucleate "cell" or syncytium formed around particulate matter in chronic inflammatory reactions, formed by a fusion of macrophages.

formative c., inner cell mass c. of the blastocyst; collectively, these c.'s give rise to the embryo.

foveolar c.'s of stomach, theca c.'s of the foveolae of the stomach.

fuchsinophil c., a c. with a special affinity for fuchsin.

fusiform c.'s of cerebral cortex, spindle-shaped c.'s in the sixth layer of the cerebral cortex.

G c.'s, enteroendocrine c.'s that secrete gastrin, found primarily in the mucosa of the pyloric antrum of the stomach.

gamma c. of pancreas, SYN C c. (1).

ganglion c., originally, any nerve c. (neuron); in current usage, a neuron the c. body of which is located outside the limits of the brain and spinal cord, hence forming part of the peripheral nervous system; ganglion c.'s are either 1) the pseudounipolar c.'s of the sensory spinal and cranial nerves (sensory ganglia), or 2) the peripheral multipolar motor neurons innervating the viscera (visceral or autonomic ganglia). SYN gangliocyte.

ganglion c.'s of dorsal spinal root, pseudounipolar nerve c. bodies in the ganglia of the dorsal spinal nerve roots; the sensory spinal nerves are composed of the peripheral axon branches of these sensory ganglion c.'s, whereas the central axon branch of each such c. enters the spinal cord as a component of the dorsal root.

ganglion c.'s of retina, the nerve c.'s of the retina whose central processes (axons) form the optic nerve; their peripheral processes synapse with the bipolar c.'s and through them with the rod and cone c.'s; these c. bodies are round or flask-shaped and vary considerably in size. SEE ALSO ganglionic *layer.*

Gaucher c.'s, large, finely and uniformly vacuolated c.'s derived from the reticuloendothelial system, and found especially in the spleen, lymph nodes, liver, and bone marrow of patients with Gaucher disease; Gaucher c.'s contain kerasin (a cerebroside), which accumulates as a result of a genetically determined absence of the enzyme glucosylceramidase.

gemistocytic c., SYN gemistocytic *astrocyte.*

germ c., SYN sex c.

germinal c., a c. from which other c.'s proliferate.

ghost c., (1) a dead c. in which the outline remains visible, but without other cytoplasmic structures or stainable nucleus; (2) an erythrocyte after loss of its hemoglobin.

giant c., a c. of large size, often with many nuclei.

Gierke c.'s, small c.'s characteristic of the substantia gelatinosa (lamina II) of the dorsal horn of the spinal cord.

gitter c., a lipid-laden microglial phagocyte commonly seen at the edge of healing brain infarcts, a result of cellular phagocytosis of lipid from necrotic or degenerating brain c.'s. SYN compound granule c., gitterzelle. [Ger. *Gitterzelle,* fr. *Gitter,* lattice, wire-net]

glia c.'s, SEE neuroglia.

glitter c.'s, polymorphonuclear leukocytes that stain pale blue with gentian violet and contain cytoplasmic granules that exhibit brownian movement; observed in urine sediment and characteristic of pyelonephritis.

globoid c., a large c. of mesodermal origin that is found clustered in the intracranial tissues in globoid cell leukodystrophy.

glomerulosa c., a c. of the zona glomerulosa of the adrenal cortex that is the source of aldosterone; the c.'s are arranged in spherical or oval groups.

goblet c., an epithelial c. that becomes distended with a large accumulation of mucous secretory granules at its apical end, giving it the appearance of a goblet. SYN beaker c., caliciform c., chalice c.

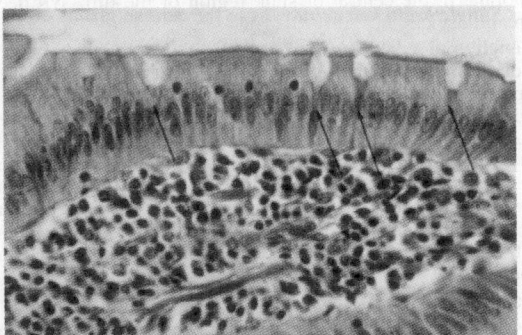

goblet cells: photomicrograph of intestinal epithelium showing single goblet cells (arrows) dispersed among absorptive cells

Golgi c.'s, SEE Golgi type I *neuron*, Golgi type II *neuron*.

Golgi epithelial c., a glial cell found in the cerebellar cortex. SEE Bergmann *fibers*, under *fiber*.

Goormaghtigh c.'s, SYN juxtaglomerular c.'s.

granule c.'s, (1) small nerve cell bodies in the external and internal granular layers of the cerebral cortex; **(2)** small nerve cell bodies in the granular layer of the cerebellar cortex.

granule c. of connective tissue, SYN mast c.

granulosa c., a c. of the membrana granulosa lining the vesicular ovarian follicle that becomes a luteal c. of the corpus luteum after ovulation.

granulosa lutein c.'s, c.'s derived from the membrana granulosa of a mature ovarian follicle that secrete both estrogen and progesterone, and form the major component of the corpus luteum.

great alveolar c.'s, cuboidal c.'s connected with the squamous pulmonary alveolar c.'s and having in their cytoplasm lamellated bodies (cytosomes) that represent the source of the surfactant that coats the alveoli. SYN granular pneumonocytes, type II c.'s.

guanine c., a c. whose cytoplasm contains glistening crystals of guanine.

gustatory c.'s, SYN taste c.'s.

gyrochrome c., SEE gyrochrome.

hair c.'s, sensory epithelial c.'s present in the organ of Corti, in the maculae and cristae of the membranous labyrinth of the ear, and in taste buds; they are characterized by having long stereocilia or kinocilia (or both) which, with the light microscope, appear as fine hairs. SEE ALSO vestibular hair c.'s, cochlear hair c.'s, taste c.'s.

hairy c.'s, medium-sized leukocytes that have features of reticuloendothelial c.'s and multiple cytoplasmic projections (hairs) on the c. surface, but which may be a variety of B lymphocyte; they are found in hairy cell leukemia.

Haller c., a variant of ethmoidal air cell developing into the floor of the orbit adjacent to the natural ostium of the maxillary sinus. A diseased Haller c. is capable of obstructing that ostium and producing a maxillary sinusitis.

heart failure c., macrophage in the lung during left heart failure that often carries large amounts of hemosiderin. SEE ALSO siderophore.

HeLa c.'s, the first continuously cultured human malignant c.'s, derived from a cervical carcinoma of a patient, Henrietta Lacks; used in the cultivation of viruses.

helmet c., a schistocyte shaped like a military helmet, seen in hemolytic anemia.

helper c.'s, SYN T helper c.'s.

HEMPAS c.'s, the abnormal erythrocytes of type II congenital dyserythropoietic anemia. SEE HEMPAS.

Hensen c., one of the supporting c.'s in the organ of Corti, immediately to the outer side of the c.'s of Deiters.

heteromeric c., SYN commissural c.

hilus c.'s, c.'s in the hilus of the ovary that produce androgens; they are thought to be the ovarian counterpart of the interstitial c.'s of the testis. SYN Berger c.'s.

hobnail c., c. characteristic of a clear cell adenocarcinoma; a round expansion of clear cytoplasm projects into the lumen of neoplastic tubules, but the basal part of the c. containing the nucleus is narrow.

Hofbauer c., a large c. in the connective tissue of the chorionic villi; it appears to be a type of phagocyte.

horizontal c. of Cajal, a small fusiform c. found in the superficial layer of the cerebral cortex with its long axis placed horizontally. SYN Cajal c. (1).

horizontal c.'s of retina, c.'s in the outer part of the inner nuclear layer of the retina that lie with their axes more or less parallel with the surface. They are thought to connect the rods of one part of the retina with cones of another part.

horny c., SYN corneocyte.

Hortega c.'s, SYN microglia.

host c., a c. (e.g., a bacterium) in which a vector can be propagated.

Hürthle c., a large, granular eosinophilic c. derived from thyroid follicular epithelium by accumulation of mitochondria, e.g., in Hashimoto disease. SYN Askanazy c.

I c., a cultured skin fibroblast containing membrane-bound inclusions; characteristic of mucolipidosis II. SYN inclusion c.

immunologically activated c., an immunocyte that is in an elevated state of reactivity capable of carrying out an immune response.

immunologically competent c., a small lymphocyte capable of being immunologically activated by exposure to a substance that is antigenic (immunogenic) for the respective c.; activation involves either the capacity to produce antibody or the capacity to participate in cell-mediated immunity.

inclusion c., SYN I c.

indifferent c., an undifferentiated, nonspecialized c.

inducer c., an old term for T helper 1 subset.

innocent bystander c., the destruction of a c. by an immune process even though that c. was not directly targeted.

intercapillary c., SYN mesangial c.

interdigitating reticulum c., an antigen-presenting c. in the paracortex of lymph nodes, interacting with T lymphocytes.

internal pillar c.'s, SEE pillar c.'s.

interstitial c.'s, (1) c.'s between the seminiferous tubules of the testis that secrete testosterone; SYN Leydig c.'s. **(2)** c.'s derived from the theca interna of atretic follicles of the ovary; they resemble luteal c.'s and are an important source of estrogens; **(3)** pineal c.'s similar to glial c.'s with long processes.

irritation c., SYN Türk c.

islet c., one of the c.'s of the pancreatic islets.

Ito c.'s, fat-containing c.'s lining hepatic sinusoids.

Jurkat c.'s, a line of T c.'s often employed in immunologic research, originally derived from a Burkitt lymphoma.

juvenile c., SYN metamyelocyte.

juxtaglomerular c.'s, c.'s located at the vascular pole of the renal corpuscle that secrete renin and form a component of the juxtaglomerular complex; they are modified smooth muscle c.'s primarily of the afferent arteriole of the renal glomerulus. SYN Goormaghtigh c.'s.

K c.'s, SYN killer c.'s.

karyochrome c., SEE karyochrome.

keratinized c., SYN corneocyte.

killer c.'s, cytotoxic c.'s involved in antibody-dependent c.-mediated immune responses; they may be T lymphocytes with receptors for the Fc portion of IgG molecules, and lyse or damage IgG coated target c.'s without mediation of complement. SEE antibody-dependent cell-mediated *cytotoxicity*. SYN K c.'s, null c.'s (1).

Kulchitsky c., SYN enteroendocrine c.

Kupffer c.'s, phagocytic c.'s of the mononuclear phagocyte series found on the luminal surface of the hepatic sinusoids. SYN stellate c.'s of liver.

lacis c. (lah-sē′), one of the c.'s of the juxtaglomerular apparatus found at the vascular pole of the renal corpuscle. [Fr. *lacis*, meshwork]

Langerhans c.'s, (1) dendritic clear c.'s in the epidermis, containing distinctive granules that appear rod- or racket-shaped in section, but lacking tonofilaments, melanosomes, and desmosomes; they carry surface receptors for immunoglobulin (Fc) and complement (C3), and are believed to be antigen fixing and processing c.'s of monocytic origin; active participants in cutaneous delayed hypersensitivity. **(2)** c.'s seen in eosinophilic granuloma and lymphoma of the lungs.

Langhans c.'s, (1) multinucleated giant c.'s seen in tuberculosis and other granulomatous diseases; the nuclei are arranged in an arciform manner at the periphery of the c.'s; SYN Langhans-type giant c.'s. **(2)** SYN cytotrophoblastic c.'s.

Langhans-type giant c.'s, SYN Langhans c.'s (1).

LE c., a polymorphonuclear leukocyte containing an amorphous round body that is a phagocytosed nucleus from another cell plus serum antinuclear globulin (IgG) and complement; formed in vitro in the blood of patients with systemic lupus erythematosus. SYN lupus erythematosus c.

Leishman chrome c.'s, basophilic granular leukocytes (basophils) observed in the circulating blood of some persons with blackwater fever.

lepra c.'s, distinctive, large, mononuclear phagocytes (macrophages) with a foamlike cytoplasm, and also poorly staining saclike structures resulting from degeneration of such c.'s, observed characteristically in leprous inflammatory reactions; indistinct staining results from numerous, fairly closely packed leprosy bacilli, which are acid-fast and resistant to staining by ordinary methods.

Leydig c.'s, SYN interstitial c.'s (1).

light c.'s of thyroid, SYN C c. (2).

lining c., SYN littoral c.

Lipschütz c., SYN centrocyte (1).

littoral c., the c.'s lining the lymphatic sinuses of lymph nodes and the blood sinuses of bone marrow. SYN lining c. [L. *littoralis*, the seashore]

Loevit c., obsolete term for erythroblast.

lupus erythematosus c., SYN LE c.

luteal c., lutein c., a c. of the corpus luteum of the ovary that is derived from the granulosa cells of the preovulatory follicle; it secretes progesterone and estrogen.

lymph c., SYN lymphocyte.

lymphoid c., white blood c.'s of the immune system.

M c., SYN microfold c.

macroglia c., SYN astrocyte.

malpighian c., a c. of the stratum spinosum of the epidermis.

Marchand wandering c., a c. of the mononuclear phagocyte system.

marrow c., any c. of bone marrow, especially hemopoietic c.'s.

Martinotti c., a small multipolar nerve c. with short branching dendrites scattered through various layers of the cerebral cortex; its axon ascends toward the surface of the cortex.

mast c., a connective tissue c. that contains coarse, basophilic, metachromatic secretory granules; the granules contain heparin, histamine and eosinophilic chemotactic factor. These c.'s are involved in immediate hypersensitivity reactions and play a role in the regulation of the composition of ground substance. SYN granule c. of connective tissue, labrocyte, mastocyte, tissue basophil.

mastoid c.'s [TA], numerous small intercommunicating cavities in the mastoid process of the temporal bone that empty into the mastoid or tympanic antrum. SYN cellulae mastoideae [TA], mastoid air c.'s, mastoid sinuses.

mastoid air c.'s, SYN mastoid c.'s.

memory B c.'s, b lymphocytes that mediate immunologic memory; these allow for enhanced immunologic reaction when an immunologically competent organism is reexposed to an antigen.

memory T c.'s, t lymphoctyes that mediate immunologic memory; these allow for enhanced immunologic reaction when an immunologically competent organism is reexposed to an antigen.

Merkel tactile c., SYN tactile *meniscus*.

mesangial c., a phagocytic c. in the capillary tuft of the renal glomerulus, interposed between endothelial c.'s and the basement membrane in the central or stalk region of the tuft. SYN deep c., intercapillary c.

mesenchymal c.'s, fusiform or stellate c.'s found between the ectoderm and endoderm of young embryos; the shape of the c.'s in fixed material is indicative of the fact that in life they were moving from their place of origin to areas where they would become reaggregated and specialized; most mesenchymal c.'s are derived from mesoderm, but in the cephalic region they also develop from neural crest or surface ectoderm; they are the most strikingly pluripotential c.'s in the embryonic body, developing at different locations into any of the types of connective or supporting tissues, to smooth muscle, to vascular endothelium, and to blood cells.

mesoglial c.'s, SYN mesoglia.

mesothelial c., one of the flat c.'s of mesodermal origin that form the superficial layer of the serosal membranes lining the body cavities of the abdomen and thorax.

Mexican hat c., SYN target c. (1).

Meynert c.'s, solitary pyramidal c.'s found in the cortex in the region of the calcarine fissure.

microfold c., specialized intestinal epithelial c.'s found in association with the lymphoid follicles in Peyer patches of the ileum; characterized by elaborate invaginations of their apical c. surface that harbor numerous lymphocytes and macrophages; believed to phagocytose antigens and present them to underlying lymphoid c.'s. SYN M c.

microglia c.'s, microglial c.'s, SYN microglia.

middle c.'s, SYN middle ethmoidal c.'s.

middle ethmoidal c.'s [TA], the middle group of air c.'s of the ethmoidal sinuses; each sinus communicates with the middle meatus of the nasal cavity. SYN cellulae ethmoidales mediae [TA], middle c.'s, middle ethmoidal air c.'s, middle ethmoidal sinuses, sinus ethmoidales mediae.

middle ethmoidal air c.'s, SYN middle ethmoidal c.'s.

midget bipolar c.'s, bipolar c.'s in the inner nuclear layer of the retina that synapse with individual cone c.'s in the outer plexiform layer; other larger bipolar c.'s in the inner nuclear layer synapse with both rod and cone c.'s; the axons of both types synapse in the inner plexiform layer with the dendrites of the ganglion c.'s.

migratory c., SYN ameboid c.

Mikulicz c.'s, foamy macrophages containing *Klebsiella rhinoscleromatis;* found in the mucosal nodules in rhinoscleroma.

mirror-image c., (1) a c. whose nuclei have identical features and are placed in the cytoplasm in similar fashion; **(2)** a binucleate form of Reed-Sternberg c. often found in Hodgkin disease; the twin nuclei are disposed in relation to an imaginary plane between them like a single nucleus together with its image in a mirror.

mitral c.'s, large nerve c.'s in the olfactory lobe of the brain whose dendrites synapse (in glomeruli) with axons of the olfactory receptor c.'s of the nasal mucous membrane, and whose axons pass centrally in the olfactory tract to the olfactory cortex.

monocytoid c., a c. having morphologic characteristics of a monocyte but which is nonphagocytic.

mossy c., one of the two types of neuroglia c.'s, consisting of a rather large body with numerous short branching processes.

mother c., a c. which, by division, gives rise to two or more daughter c.'s. SYN brood c., metrocyte, parent c.

motor c., a neuron whose axon innervates peripheral effector c.'s such as muscle fibers or gland c.'s.

mucoalbuminous c.'s, SYN mucoserous c.'s.

mucoserous c.'s, glandular c.'s intermediate in histologic characteristics between serous and mucous c.'s. SYN mucoalbuminous c.'s, seromucous c.'s.

mucous c., a c. secreting mucus; e.g., a goblet c.

mucous neck c., one of the acidic mucin-secreting c.'s in the neck of a gastric gland.

Müller radial c.'s, SYN Müller *fibers* (2), under *fiber*.

multipolar c., a nerve c. with a number of dendrites arising from the c. body.

mural c., a nonendothelial c. enclosed within the basement membrane of retinal capillaries.

myeloid c., specifically, any young c. that develops into a mature granulocyte of blood, but frequently used as a synonym for marrow c.

myoepithelial c., a smooth muscle-like c. of ectodermal origin, found between the epithelium and basement membrane in a number of organs such as mammary, sweat, and lacrimal glands.

myoid c.'s, flattened smooth muscle-like c.'s of mesodermal origin that lie just outside the basal lamina of the seminiferous tubule. SYN peritubular contractile c.'s.

Nageotte c.'s, c.'s found in the cerebrospinal fluid, one or two per cubic millimeter in health, but in greater numbers in various diseases.

natural killer c.'s, large granular lymphocytes which do not express markers of either T or B c. lineage. These c.'s do possess Fc receptors for IgG and can kill target c.'s using antibody-dependent cell-mediated cytotoxicity. NK c.'s can also use perforin to kill c.'s in the absence of antibody. Killing occurs without previous sensitization. SYN NK c.'s.

nerve c., SYN neuron.

neurilemma c.'s, SYN Schwann c.'s.

neuroendocrine c., (1) SEE neuroendocrine (2); (2) SYN paraneurone.

neuroendocrine transducer c., an endocrine c. that releases its hormonal product into the bloodstream only upon receipt of a nervous impulse.

neuroepithelial c.'s, SYN neuroepithelium.

neuroglia c.'s, SEE neuroglia.

neurolemma c.'s, SYN Schwann c.'s.

neurosecretory c.'s, nerve c.'s, such as those of the hypothalamus, that elaborate a chemical substance (such as a releasing factor, neuropeptide, or, more rarely, a true hormone) that influences the activity of another structure (e.g., anterior lobe of the hypophysis). See also neurosecretion.

nevus c., the c. of a pigmented cutaneous nevus that differs from a normal melanocyte in that it lacks dendrites. SYN nevocyte.

nevus c., A-type, melanocytes in the epidermis in pigmented nevi, resembling epithelial c.'s and frequently containing melanin.

nevus c., B-type, small, usually non-pigmented melanocytes in the mid-dermis in pigmented nevi.

nevus c., C-type, non-pigmented spindle-shaped melanocytes in the lower dermis in pigmented nevi.

Niemann-Pick c., SYN Pick c.

NK c.'s, SYN natural killer c.'s.

nonclonogenic c., a c. that does not give rise to a colony of c.'s (large numbers of c.'s that are genetically identical); may undergo two or more c. divisions, but all daughter c.'s are destined to die or differentiate (losing all potential to divide).

null c.'s, (1) SYN killer c.'s; **(2)** large granular lymphocytes that lack surface markers or membrane-associated proteins of either B or T lymphocytes.

nurse c.'s, SYN Sertoli c.'s.

oat c., SYN small c.

OKT c.'s, old term for c.'s recognized by monoclonal antibodies to T lymphocyte antigens; OKT-3 c.'s are T lymphocytes as a class, because all share a common leukocyte differentiation antigen; OKT-4 c.'s are helper c.'s; OKT-8 c.'s are suppressor c.'s. OKT-4/OKT-8 expresses the ratio of helper to suppressor c.'s, sometimes used as a measure of the functional status of the immune system and thus a basis for clinical diagnosis and prognosis. Current usage favors using CD designations. [*Ortho-Kung T cell*]

olfactory c.'s, SYN olfactory receptor c.'s.

olfactory receptor c.'s, very slender nerve c.'s, with large nuclei and surmounted by six to eight long, sensitive cilia in the olfactory epithelium at the roof of the nose; they are the receptors for smell. SYN olfactory c.'s, Schultze c.'s.

oligodendroglia c.'s, SEE oligodendroglia.

Onodi c., a variant of a posterior ethmoidal air c. in intimate relationship with the optic nerve just distal to the optic chiasm.

Opalski c., a characteristic altered glial c. in the basal ganglia and thalamus in hepatocerebral degeneration and Wilson disease.

osseous c., SYN osteocyte.

osteochondrogenic c., one of the undifferentiated c.'s in the inner layer of the periosteum of an endochondrally developing bone capable of developing into an osteoblast or a chondroblast.

osteogenic c., one of the c.'s in the inner layer of the periosteum that forms osseous tissue.

osteoprogenitor c., a mesenchymal c. that differentiates into an osteoblast. SYN preosteoblast.

oxyntic c., SYN parietal c.

oxyphil c., c. of the parathyroid gland that increase in number with age; the cytoplasm contains numerous mitochondria and stains with eosin. Similar c.'s, and tumors composed of them, are found in salivary glands and the thyroid; in the latter, also called Hürthle c.

P c., a characteristic specialized c., with probable pacemaker function, found in the S-A node and A-V junction.

packed human blood c.'s, whole blood from which plasma has been removed; may be prepared any time during the dating period of the whole blood from which it is derived, but not later than 6 days after the blood has been drawn if separation of plasma and c.'s is achieved by centrifugation.

Paget c.'s, relatively large, neoplastic epithelial c.'s (carcinoma c.'s) with hyperchromatic nuclei and abundant palely staining cytoplasm; in Paget disease of the breast, such c.'s occur in neoplastic epithelium in the ducts and in the epidermis of the nipple, areola, and adjacent skin.

pagetoid c.'s, atypical melanocytes resembling Paget c.'s, q.v., found in some cutaneous melanomas of the superficial spreading type.

Paneth granular c.'s, c.'s, located at the base of intestinal glands of the small intestine, which contain large acidophilic refractile granules and may produce lysozyme. SYN Davidoff c.'s.

parafollicular c.'s, SYN C c. (2).

paraganglionic c.'s, c.'s of the embryonic sympathetic nervous system that become chromaffin c.'s.

paraluteal c., SYN theca lutein c.

paralutein c., SYN theca lutein c.

parenchymal c., SEE parenchyma.

parenchymatous c. of corpus pineale, SYN pinealocyte.

parent c., SYN mother c.

parietal c., one of the c.'s of the gastric glands; it lies upon the basement membrane, covered by the chief c.'s, and secretes hydrochloric acid that reaches the lumen of the gland through fine intracellular and intercellular canals (canaliculi). SYN acid c., oxyntic c.

peptic c., SYN zymogenic c.

pericapillary c., SYN pericyte.

peripolar c., a granular c. located where the parietal and visceral capsules of the renal corpuscle meet; part of the c. faces the filtration space of Bowman.

perithelial c., SYN pericyte.

peritubular contractile c.'s, SYN myoid c.'s.

permissive c., a c. in which the late phase of viral infection follows the early phase and cell death is coupled with massive synthesis of virus; e.g., monkey c.'s are permissive for SV40.

pessary c., a red blood c. in which the hemoglobin has disappeared from the center, leaving only the periphery visible.

phalangeal c., the supporting c.'s of the organ of Corti, attached to the basement membrane and receiving the hair c.'s between their free extremities. SEE ALSO phalanx (2). SYN Deiters c.'s (1).

photo c., a light-detecting electronic device used to measure x-ray transmission through a patient for automatic termination of the exposure or to calculate a digital image.

photoreceptor c.'s, rod and cone c.'s of the retina.

physaliphorous c., c.'s containing a bubbly or vacuolated cytoplasm, e.g., as characteristically seen in chordoma.

Pick c., a relatively large, rounded or polygonal, mononuclear c., with indistinctly or palely staining, foamlike cytoplasm that contains numerous droplets of a phosphatide, sphingomyelin; such c.'s are widely distributed in the spleen and other tissues, especially those rich in reticuloendothelial components, in patients with Niemann-Pick disease. SYN Niemann-Pick c.

pigment c., a c. containing pigment granules.

pigment c.'s of iris, c.'s of the stromal layer of the iris; in dark eyes (but not in blue) they contain granules of pigment.

pigment c.'s of retina, c.'s in the outermost layer of the retina that contain pigment granules.

pigment c. of skin, SYN melanocyte.

pillar c.'s, c.'s forming the outer and inner walls of the tunnel in the organ of Corti. SYN Corti pillars, Corti rods, pillar c.'s of Corti, tunnel c.'s.

pillar c.'s of Corti, SYN pillar c.'s.

pineal c.'s, c.'s of the corpus pineale or pinealocyte.

plasma c., an ovoid c. with an eccentric nucleus; the cytoplasm is strongly basophilic because of the abundant RNA in its endoplasmic reticulum; plasma c.'s are derived from B lymphocytes and are active in the formation and secretion of antibodies. SYN plasmacyte.

pluripotent c.'s, primordial c.'s that may still differentiate into various specialized types of tissue elements; e.g., mesenchymal c.'s.

polar c., SYN polar body.

polychromatic c., a primitive erythrocyte in bone marrow, with basophilic material as well as hemoglobin (acidophilic) in the cytoplasm. SYN polychromatophil c.

polychromatophil c., SYN polychromatic c.

posterior c.'s, SYN posterior ethmoidal c.'s.

posterior ethmoidal c.'s [TA], the posterior group of air c.'s of the ethmoidal sinuses; each sinus communicates with the superior meatus of the nasal cavity. SYN cellulae ethmoidales posteriores [TA], posterior c.'s, posterior ethmoidal air c.'s, sinus ethmoidales posteriores.

posterior ethmoidal air c.'s, SYN posterior ethmoidal c.'s.

pregnancy c.'s, hypophysial chromophobe c.'s that increase in number and accumulate eosinophil granules during pregnancy.

pregranulosa c.'s, capsular c.'s surrounding the primordial ova in the embryonic ovary; they are derived from celomic epithelium.

prickle c., one of the c.'s of the stratum spinosum of the epidermis; so called because of typical shrinkage artifacts that occur in histologic preparations, resulting in intercellular bridges at points of desmosomal adhesion. SYN spine c.

primary embryonic c., in a very young embryo, a c. still capable of differentiation.

primitive reticular c., SYN reticular c.

primordial c., a c. from a group that constitutes the primordium of an organ or part of the embryo.

primordial germ c., the most primitive undifferentiated sex cell, found initially outside the gonad. SYN gonocyte.

prolactin c., SYN mammotroph.

pseudo-Gaucher c., a plasma c., microscopically resembling a Gaucher c., found in the bone marrow in some cases of multiple myeloma.

pseudounipolar c., SYN unipolar neuron.

pseudoxanthoma c., relatively large phagocytic c.'s (macrophages) that contain numerous small lipid vacuoles or hemosiderin (or both), in organizing hemorrhagic or inflammatory lesions.

pulpar c., the specific macrophagic c. of the spleen substance.

Purkinje c.'s, SYN Purkinje cell layer.

pus c., SYN pus corpuscle.

pyramidal c.'s, neurons of the cerebral cortex which, in sections perpendicular to the cortical surface, exhibit a triangular shape with a long apical dendrite directed toward the surface of the cortex; there are also lateral dendrites, and a basal axon that descends to deeper layers.

pyrrol c., pyrrhol c., a c. of the mononuclear macrophage system that has a special affinity for pyrrol blue, taking up the dye by a process of pinocytosis.

Raji c., a c. of a cultured line of lymphoblastoid c.'s derived from a Burkitt lymphoma; it possesses numerous receptors for certain complement components and is thus suitable for use in detection

of immune complexes. It expresses certain complement receptors as well as Fc receptors for immunoglobulin G.

reactive c., SYN gemistocytic astrocyte.

red blood c. (rbc, RBC), SYN erythrocyte.

Reed c., SYN Reed-Sternberg c.

Reed-Sternberg c., large transformed lymphocytes, probably B cell in origin, generally regarded as pathognomonic of Hodgkin lymphoma; a typical c. has a pale-staining acidophilic cytoplasm and one or two large nuclei showing marginal clumping of chromatin and unusually conspicuous deeply acidophilic nucleoli; binucleate Reed-Sternberg c. frequently shows a mirror-image form (mirror-image c.). SYN Reed c., Sternberg c., Sternberg-Reed c.

Renshaw c.'s, inhibitory interneurons that are innervated by collaterals from motoneurons and in turn form synapses with the same and adjacent motoneurons to exert inhibition; identified physiologically and by intracellular injection technic.

resting c., a quiescent c.; one not undergoing mitosis.

resting wandering c., SYN fixed macrophage.

restructured c., the viable c. produced by fusion of a karyoplast with a cytoplast.

reticular c., c. with processes making contact with those of other similar c.'s to form a cellular network ensheathing a network of reticular fibers, which constitutes the stroma of all lymphoid organs except the thymus. SYN primitive reticular c.

reticularis c., a c. of the zona reticularis of the innermost part of the adrenal cortex.

reticuloendothelial c., a c. of the reticuloendothelial system.

rhagiocrine c., SYN macrophage.

Rieder c.'s, abnormal myeloblasts (12 to 20 μm in diameter) in which the nucleus may be widely and deeply indented (i.e., suggestive of lobulation), or may actually be a bi- or multilobate structure; such c.'s are frequently observed in acute leukemia, and probably represent a more rapid maturation of the nucleus than that of the cytoplasm.

rod nuclear c., SYN band c.

rod c. of retina, SYN rod (2).

Rolando c.'s, the nerve c.'s in Rolando gelatinous substance of the spinal cord.

rosette-forming c.'s, term usually used for T lymphocytes with an affinity for sheep erythrocytes and which, when suspended in serum, bind the uncoated, nonsensitized erythrocytes in a rosette formation.

sarcogenic c., SYN myoblast.

satellite c.'s, neuroglial c.'s surrounding the c. body of a ganglion c. in the spinal, cranial, and autonomic ganglia.

satellite c. of skeletal muscle, an elongated spindle-shaped c. occupying depressions in the sarcolemma and between it and the basal lamina; believed to play a role in muscle repair and regeneration by fusing with adjacent myofiber. SYN sarcoplast.

scavenger c., SYN phagocyte.

Schilling band c., SYN band c.

Schultze c.'s, SYN olfactory receptor c.'s.

Schwann c.'s, c.'s of ectodermal (neural crest) origin that compose a continuous envelope around each nerve fiber of peripheral nerves; such c.'s are comparable to the oligodendroglia c.'s of brain and spinal cord; like the latter, they may form membranous expansions that wind around axons and thus form the axon's myelin sheath. SYN neurilemma c.'s, neurolemma c.'s.

segmented c., a polymorphonuclear leukocyte matured beyond the band c. so that two or more lobes of the nucleus occur.

sensitized c., (1) a c. that has been either exposed to antigen or opsonized with antibodies and/or complement. (2) a small, "committed," c. derived, by division and differentiation, from a resting lymphocyte; (3) a c., including a bacterial c., that has combined with specific antibody to form a complex capable of reacting with complement components;

sensory c., a c. in the peripheral nervous system that receives afferent (sensory) input; sensory receptor c.'s.

septal c., a round pale c. of the lungs in the septa between the pulmonary alveoli.

seromucous c.'s, SYN mucoserous c.'s.

serous c., a c., especially of the salivary gland, that secretes a watery or thin albuminous fluid, as opposed to a mucous c. SYN albuminous c. (1).

Sertoli c.'s, elongated c.'s in the seminiferous tubules that ensheathe spermatids, providing a microenvironment that supports spermiogenesis; they secrete androgen-binding protein and establish the blood-testis barrier by forming tight junctions with adjacent Sertoli c.'s. SYN nurse c.'s.

sex c., a spermatozoon or an ovum. SYN germ c.

Sézary c., an atypical T lymphocyte seen in the peripheral blood in the Sézary syndrome; it has a large convoluted nucleus and scanty cytoplasm containing PAS-positive vacuoles.

shadow c.'s, SYN smudge c.'s.

sickle c., an abnormal, crescentic erythrocyte that is characteristic of sickle c. anemia, resulting from an inherited abnormality of hemoglobin (hemoglobin S) causing decreased solubility at low oxygen tension. SYN crescent c., drepanocyte, meniscocyte.

signet ring c.'s, SYN castration c.'s.

silver c., one of a number of c.'s seen in plaques of multiple sclerosis, having round or oval nuclei, the body of the c. containing many yellow or light brown particles; the c.'s are characteristic of multiple sclerosis, but are found in other conditions, including syphilis.

skein c., SYN reticulocyte.

small c., a short, blunty spindle-shaped c. that contains a relatively large, hyperchromatic nucleus, frequently observed in some forms of undifferentiated bronchogenic carcinoma. SYN oat c.

small cleaved c., a lymphoid c. of follicular center c. origin that has an irregularly shaped nucleus with clumped chromatin, absent nucleoli, and one or more clefts in the nuclear membrane.

smudge c.'s, immature leukocytes of any type that have undergone partial breakdown during preparation of a stained smear or tissue section, because of their greater fragility; smudge c.'s are seen in largest numbers in chronic lymphocytic leukemia. SYN basket c. (2), Gumprecht shadows, shadow c.'s.

somatic c.'s, the c.'s of an organism, other than the germ c.'s.

sperm c., SYN spermatozoon.

spider c., (1) SYN astrocyte; (2) a c. in a rhabdomyoma of the heart, with central nucleus and cytoplasmic mass connected to the cell wall by strands of cytoplasm separated by clear glycogen-filled areas.

spindle c., a fusiform c., such as those in the deeper layers of the cerebral cortex.

spine c., SYN prickle c.

splenic c.'s, large round ameboid c.'s (macrophages) in the splenic pulp.

spur c., a spiculated red c. with 5–10 spiny projections of varying length distributed irregularly over the c. surface; seen in patients with liver disease and abetalipoproteinemia.

squamous c., a flat scalelike epithelial c.

squamous alveolar c.'s, highly attentuated squamous c.'s that form the gas-permeable epithelium lining the alveoli of the lungs. SYN type I c.'s.

stab c., SYN band c.

staff c., SYN band c.

standard c., an electrical c. having a definite known voltage; used to calibrate other electric c.'s.

stellate c.'s of cerebral cortex, small star-shaped c.'s in the second and fourth layers of the cortex, and large stellate c.'s in the deeper part of the third layer in the visual cortex.

stellate c.'s of liver, SYN Kupffer c.'s.

stem c., (1) any precursor cell; (2) a c. whose daughter c.'s may differentiate into other c. types.

Sternberg c., SYN Reed-Sternberg c.

Sternberg-Reed c., SYN Reed-Sternberg c.

stichochrome c., SEE stichochrome.

strap c., an elongated tumor c. of uniform width that may show cross-striations; found in rhabdomyosarcoma.

supporting c., SYN sustentacular c.

suppressor c.'s, cells of the immune system that inhibit or help to terminate an immune response, e.g., suppressor macrophages and suppressor T cells.

surface mucous c.'s of stomach, c.'s lining the gastric surface and foveolae; an acid-resistant mucous product at the apical end of each c. that apparently diffuses out to lubricate and protect the mucosal surface. SYN theca c.'s of stomach.

sustentacular c., one of the ordinary elongated c.'s resting on the basement membrane that surround and serve as a support to the shorter specialized c.'s in certain organs, such as the labyrinth of the inner ear or olfactory epithelium. SYN supporting c.

sympathetic formative c., a neuroblast of the embryonic autonomic nervous system.

sympathicotropic c.'s, large epithelioid c.'s in the hilum of the ovary associated with unmyelinated nerve fibers.

sympathochromaffin c., the c. type in the embryonic suprarenal gland from which both sympathetic ganglion c.'s and chromaffin c.'s are developed.

synovial c., fibrotoplastlike c.'s that form 1–6 epithelioid layers in the synovial membrane of joints; believed to contribute proteoglycans and hyaluronate to the synovial fluid.

T c., SYN T lymphocyte.

Tγ c.'s, a subset of T c.'s that have an Fc receptor for immunoglobulin G molecules.

Tμ c.'s, t helper c.'s that have an Fc receptor for immunoglobulin M molecules.

tactile c., one of the epithelioid c.'s of a corpusculum tactus. SYN touch c.

tanned red c.'s, erythrocytes subjected to mild treatment with chemicals such as tannic acid so that they adsorb onto their surface soluble antigens; used in hemagglutination tests.

target c., (1) an erythrocyte with a dark center surrounded by a light band that again is encircled by a darker ring; it thus resembles a shooting target; such c.'s appear in target-cell anemias or after splenectomy; SYN Mexican hat c. (2) a c. lysed by cytotoxic T lymphocytes, as in graft rejection.

tart c., a monocyte with an engulfed nucleus in which the structure is still well preserved.

taste c.'s, darkly staining c.'s in a taste bud that appear to have extending into the gustatory pore long hairlike microvilli containing a number of closely packed microtubules; the taste c.'s stand in synaptic contact with sensory nerve fibers of the facial, glossopharyngeal, or vagus nerves. SYN gustatory c.'s.

T cytotoxic c.'s (Tc), SYN cytotoxic c. (1).

TDTH c.'s, a functional subset of T helper c.'s that are involved in delayed-type hypersensitivity reactions.

tendon c.'s, elongated fibroblastic c.'s arranged in rows between the collagenous tendon fibers.

theca lutein c., a steroid secretory c. of the corpus luteum that comes from the theca interna of the ovarian follicle at the time of ovulation and secretes progesterone under the control of prolactin. SYN paraluteal c., paralutein c.

theca c.'s of stomach, SYN surface mucous c.'s of stomach.

T helper c.'s (Th), a subset of lymphocytes that secrete various cytokines that regulate the immune response: *subset 1,* which synthesize gamma interferon and interleukin 2 and are involved in cell-mediated immunity; *subset 2,* which synthesize interleukins 4, 5, 10, and are involved in immunoglobulin synthesis. SYN helper c.'s.

T helper subset 1 c.'s, a subset of CD4⁺ T c.'s that can secrete interferon gamma and IL-2 and are responsible for cellular immunity.

T helper subset 2 c.'s, a subset of CD4⁺ T c.'s that synthesize IL-4, IL-5, and IL-10 and facilitate immunoglobulin synthesis.

Tiselius electrophoresis c., the special container in a Tiselius apparatus containing the solution to be analyzed electrophoretically.

Toker c., an epithelial c. with clear cytoplasm found in 10% of normal nipples; contains keratin 7, like Paget carcinoma c.'s, from which it must be distinguished cytologically.

totipotent c., an undifferentiated c. capable of developing into any type of body c.

touch c., SYN tactile c.

T-helper subsets		
TH subtype	cytokines secreted	major immunologic effects[1]
T_H1	IFN-γ	activate macrophages
		promote B-cell proliferation and class switching to IgG1
	IL-2	promotion, activation of antigen-specific T_H and T_C cells
	TNFβ	activate macrophages and neutrophils
		promote B-cell growth and immunoglobulin production
T_H2	IL-4	chemoattract lymphocytes, mast cells, and basophils
		enhance growth of mast cells and eosinophils
		promote B-cell proliferation and class switching to IgE and IgG4
		inhibit T_H1-cell differentiation
		inhibit cytokine production by macrophages
	IL-5	enhance growth and development of eosinophils
	IL-6	promote B-cell growth and immunoglobulin production
	IL-10	inhibit production of cytokines (including IFN-γ) by T_H1 cells, macrophages, and other APCs
		inhibit T_H1-cell differentiation
		promote B-cell growth and immunoglobulin production
	IL-13	same as IL-4

Abbreviations: IFN-γ = interferon gamma, IL = interleukin, TNFβ = tumor necrosis factor beta, APC = antigen-presenting cell.

[1] Only a few pertinent effects of these cytokines are listed here. Each of the processes listed is enhanced by the cytokine unless otherwise stated.

Touton giant c., a xanthoma c. in which the multiple nuclei are grouped around a small island of nonfoamy cytoplasm.

transducer c., any c. responding to a mechanical, thermal, photic, or chemical stimulus by generating an electrical impulse synaptically transmitted to a sensory neuron in contact with the c.

transitional c., any c. thought to represent a phase of development from one form to another.

tubal air c.'s (of pharyngotympanic tube) [TA], occasional small air cells in the inferior wall of the pharyngotympanic tube, near the tympanic orifice, communicating with the tympanic cavity. SYN cellulae pneumaticae tubae auditivae [TA], air c.'s of auditory tube.

tufted c., a particular type of c. in the olfactory bulb comparable to the bulb's mitral c. with respect to afferent and efferent relationships, but smaller and more superficially located.

tunnel c.'s, SYN pillar c.'s.

Türk c., a relatively large, immature c. with certain morphologic features resembling those of a plasma c., although the nuclear pattern is similar to that of a myeloblast; found in circulating blood only in pathologic conditions. SYN irritation c., Türk leukocyte.

tympanic c.'s [TA], numerous groovelike depressions in the walls of the tympanic cavity, communicating with the tubal air cells. SYN cellulae tympanicae [TA], tympanic air c.'s.

tympanic air c.'s, SYN tympanic c.'s.

type I c.'s, SYN squamous alveolar c.'s.

type II c.'s, SYN great alveolar c.'s.

Tzanck c.'s, acantholytic epithelial c.'s seen in the Tzanck test.

undifferentiated c., a primitive c. that has not assumed the morphologic and functional characteristics it will later acquire.

unipolar c., SYN unipolar *neuron.*

vasoformative c., SYN angioblast (1).

veil c., an antigen-presenting c. that has veil-like cytoplasmic processes and circulates in the blood and lymph. SYN veiled c.'s (1).

veiled c.'s, (1) SYN veil c; **(2)** SEE Langerhans c.'s.

vestibular hair c.'s, c.'s in the sensory epithelium of the maculae and cristae of the membranous labyrinth of the inner ear; afferent and efferent nerve fibers of the vestibular nerve end synaptically upon them; from the apical end of each c. a bundle of stereocilia and a kinocilium extend into the statoconial membrane of the maculae and the cupula of the cristae.

Virchow c.'s, (1) the lacunae in osseous tissue containing the osteocytes; **(2)** an obsolete term for the osteocytes themselves; **(3)** SYN corneal *corpuscles,* under *corpuscle.*

virus-transformed c., a c. that has been genetically changed to a tumor c., the change being subsequently transmitted to all descendent c.'s; c.'s transformed by oncogenic RNA viruses continue to produce virus in high concentration without being killed; DNA tumor virus-transformed c.'s develop (along with other changes) tumor-associated antigens and rarely produce virus.

visual receptor c.'s, the rod and cone c.'s of the retina.

vitreous c., a c. occurring in the peripheral part of the vitreous body that may be responsible for production of hyaluronic acid and possibly of collagen. SYN hyalocyte.

wandering c., SYN ameboid c.

Warthin-Finkeldey c.'s, giant c.'s with multiple overlapping nuclei, found in lymphoid tissue in measles, especially during the prodromal stage.

wasserhelle c., SYN water-clear c. of parathyroid.

water-clear c. of parathyroid, a variety of chief c., so called because the cytoplasm contains much glycogen that is not preserved or stained in the usual preparation. SYN wasserhelle c.

white blood c. (WBC), SYN leukocyte.

WI-38 c.'s, the first normal human cells, derived from fetal lung tissue, continuously cultivated. [*Wistar Institute*]

wing c., one of the polyhedral c.'s in the corneal epithelium beneath the surface layer.

yolk c.'s, primitive embryonic c.'s lying between the endoderm and mesoderm; they probably give rise to the endothelium of vitelline vessels.

zymogenic c., a c. that secretes an enzyme; specifically a chief c. of a gastric gland or an acinar c. of the pancreas. SYN albuminous c. (2), chief c. of stomach, peptic c.

---

cel·la, gen. and pl. **cel·lae** (sel′ă, sel′ē). A room or cell. [L. storeroom, or compartment]

c. me′dia, SYN *pars* centralis ventriculi lateralis.

cel·lic·o·lous (se-lik′ō-lŭs). Living within cells. [L. *cella,* cells, + *colo,* to abide in]

cel·lo·bi·ase (sel-ō-bī′ās). SYN β-D-glucosidase.

cel·lo·bi·ose (sel-ō-bī′ōs). A disaccharide obtained from cellulose and lichenin; a glucose-β(1→4)-glucoside, differing only from maltose in the nature of the glycosidic bond.

cel·lo·hex·ose (sel-ō-heks′ōs). SYN D-glucose.

cel·loi·din (se-loy′din). A solution of pyroxylin in ether and alcohol, used for embedding histologic specimens.

cel·lon (sel′on). SYN tetrachloroethane.

cel·lo·na (sel-ō′nă). A cellulose bandage impregnated with plaster of Paris.

cel·lu·la, gen. and pl. **cel·lu·lae** (sel′ū-lă, -lē). **1** [NA]. In gross anatomy, a small but macroscopic compartment. SYN cellule. **2.** In histology, a cell. [L. a small chamber, dim. of *cella*]

cel′lulae co′li, SYN *haustra* of colon, under *haustrum.*

cel′lulae ethmoida′les [TA], SYN ethmoid *cells,* under *cell;* SEE ALSO anterior ethmoidal *cells,* under *cell,* middle ethmoidal *cells,* under *cell,* posterior ethmoidal *cells,* under *cell.*

cel′lulae ethmoidales anterio′res [TA], SYN anterior ethmoidal *cells,* under *cell.*

cel'lulae ethmoidales me'diae [TA], SYN middle ethmoidal *cells*, under *cell*.

cel'lulae ethmoidales posterio'res [TA], SYN posterior ethmoidal *cells*, under *cell*.

cel'lulae mastoid'eae [TA], SYN mastoid *cells*, under *cell*.

cel'lulae pneumat'icae tu'bae auditi'vae [TA], SYN tubal air *cells* (of pharyngotympanic tube), under *cell*.

cel'lulae tympan'icae [TA], SYN tympanic *cells*, under *cell*.

cel·lu·lar (sel'ū-lăr). **1.** Relating to, derived from, or composed of cells. **2.** Having numerous compartments or interstices. [L. *cellula*, dim. of *cella*, storeroom]

cel·lu·lar·i·ty (sel-ū-lar'i-tē). The degree, quality, or condition of cells that are present.

cel·lu·lase (sel'ū-lās). Endo-1,4-β-glucase; an enzyme catalyzing the hydrolysis of 1,4-β-glucoside links in cellulose, lichenin, and other β-D-glucans; found in a variety of microorganisms in soil and in the digestive tracts of herbivores. Used to produce digestive tablets and in the removal of cellulose from foods for special diets.

cel·lule (sel'ūl). SYN cellula (1).

cel·lu·li·ci·dal (sel-ū-li-sī'dăl). Destructive to cells. [cellula + L. *caedo*, to kill]

cel·lu·lif·u·gal (sel-ū-lif'ū-găl). Moving from, or extending in a direction away from, a cell or cell body; denoting certain cells repelled by other cells, or processes extending from the body of a cell. [cellula + L. *fugio*, to flee]

cel·lu·lin (sel'ū-lin). SYN cellulose.

cel·lu·lip·e·tal (sel-ū-lip'ĕ-tăl). Moving toward, or extending in a direction toward, a cell or cell body. [cellula + L. *peto*, to seek]

cel·lu·lite (sel'ū-līt). **1.** Colloquial term for deposits of fat and fibrous tissue causing dimpling of the overlying skin. **2.** SYN lipoedema.

cel·lu·li·tis (sel-ū-lī'tis). Inflammation of subcutaneous, loose connective tissue (formerly called cellular tissue).

acute scalp c., deep inflammation of the scalp without suppuration.

anaerobic c., infection with subcutaneous soft tissues with any of a variety of anaerobic bacteria, usually a mixed culture including Bacteroides species, anaerobic cocci, and clostridia.

dissecting c., SYN *perifolliculitis* abscedens et suffodiens.

eosinophilic c., recurrent cellulitis followed by brawny edematous skin lesions or sometimes urticarial papular, annular, or gyrate lesions; affected skin and subcutis are heavily infiltrated by eosinophils and histiocytes, with scattered small necrotic foci (flame figures); of varied etiology; sometimes follows an arthropod bite. SYN Wells syndrome.

gangrenous c., infection of soft tissue with organisms that produce extensive tissue necrosis and local vascular occlusions; streptococci, clostridia, and anaerobes are known causes, but most cases recently have been polymicrobial. SYN necrotizing c.

necrotizing c., SYN gangrenous c.

orbital c., c. that involves the tissue layers posterior to the orbital septum.

pelvic c., SYN parametritis.

periorbital c., SYN preseptal c.

preseptal c., infection involving the superficial tissue layers anterior to the orbital septum. SYN periorbital c.

cel·lu·los·an (sel'ū-lō-san). SYN hemicellulose.

cel·lu·lose (sel'ū-lōs). A linear B1→4 glucan, composed of cellobiose residues, differing in this respect from starch, which is comprised of maltose residues; it forms the basis of vegetable and wood fiber and is the most abundant organic compound; useful in providing bulk in the diet. SYN cellulin. [L. *cellula*, cell, + -ose]

c. acetate, a polymer commonly used as a support medium for electrophoresis.

c. acetate phthalate, a reaction product of phthalic anhydride and a partial acetate ester of c.; used as a tablet-coating agent.

carboxymethyl c., c. in which some of the OH groups are modified to contain –CH$_2$–COOH groups; used in column chromatography. SYN CM-cellulose.

O-**diethylaminoethyl c.,** c. to which diethylaminoethyl groups have been attached; used in anion-exchange chromatography. SYN DEAE-cellulose.

microcrystalline c., purified, partially depolymerized c., prepared by treating α-cellulose, obtained as a pulp from fibrous plant material, with mineral acids; used as a tablet diluent.

oxidized c., (1) cellulosic acid in the form of an absorbable gauze; used as a hemostatic in operations where ligation is not feasible (capillary or venous bleeding from small vessels) because cellulosic acid has a pronounced affinity for hemoglobin and produces an artificial clot; (2) a sterile absorbable substance prepared by the oxidation of cotton containing not less than 16% and not more than 22% of carboxyl. SEE ALSO oxycellulose.

TEAE-c., c. to which triethylaminoethyl groups have been attached; used in ion-exchange chromatography. SYN *O*-(triethylaminoethyl) c.

O-**(triethylaminoethyl) c.,** SYN TEAE-c.

cel·lu·los·ic ac·id (sel-ū-los'ik). SEE oxidized *cellulose*.

⌂**celo-.** **1.** The celom. [G. *koilōma*, hollow (celom)] **2.** Hernia. [G. *kēlē*, hernia] **3.** The abdomen. SEE ALSO celio-. [G. *koilia*, belly]

ce·lom, ce·lo·ma (sē'lom, sē-lō'mă). **1.** The cavity between the splanchnic and somatic mesoderm in the embryo. **2.** SYN body cavity. [G. *koilōma*, a hollow]

extraembryonic c., that portion of the c. that extends beyond the confines of the embryonic body.

ce·lom·ic (sē-lom'ik). Relating to the body *cavity*.

ce·lo·phle·bi·tis (sē-lō-flĕ-bī'tis). Inflammation of a vena cava. SYN cavitis. [G. *koilos*, hollow, + phlebitis]

ce·lo·scope (sē'lō-skōp). Rarely used term for an optic device for examining the interior of a body cavity. [G. *koilos*, hollow, + *skopeō*, to view]

ce·los·co·py (sē-los'kŏ-pē). Rarely used term for examination of any body cavity with an optical instrument.

ce·lo·so·mia (sē-lō-sō'mē-ă). Congenital protrusion of the abdominal or thoracic viscera, usually with a defect of the sternum and ribs as well as of the abdominal walls. SYN kelosomia. [G. *kēlē*, hernia, + *sōma*, body]

Ce·lo·vi·rus (sel'ō-vī-rŭs). An adenovirus found in chickens.

ce·lo·zo·ic (sē-lō-zō'ik). Inhabiting any of the cavities of the body; applied to certain parasitic protozoa, chiefly gregarines. [G. *koilos*, hollow, + *zoikos*, pertaining to animals]

Celsius, Anders, Swedish astronomer, 1701–1744. SEE Celsius *scale*.

Cel·si·us (C). SEE Celsius *scale*.

ce·ment (se-ment') [TA]. **1.** A layer of bonelike mineralized tissue covering the dentin of the root and neck of a tooth that serves to anchor the fibers of the periodontal ligament. SYN cementum [TA], substantia ossea dentis, tooth c. **2.** In dentistry, a nonmetallic material used for luting, filling, or permanent or temporary restorative purposes, made by mixing components into a plastic mass that sets, or as an adherent sealer in attaching various dental restorations in or on the tooth. [see cementum]

composite dental c., an organic dental c. modified by the inclusion of inorganic materials treated with a coupling agent to bond them to the polymers.

copper phosphate c., a dental preparation, the combination of a solution of orthophosphoric acid with a c. powder (usually zinc oxide) modified with varying proportions of copper oxide.

dental c., SEE cement (2).

glass ionomer c., a dental c. produced by mixing a powder prepared from a calcium aluminosilicate glass with an aqueous solution of polyacrylic acid. [ion + -mer (1)]

inorganic dental c., a dental c. consisting usually of metallic salts or oxides which, when mixed with a specific liquid, form a plastic mass that sets.

intercellular c., a hypothetical adhesive substance formerly believed to occur between some epithelial cells.

modified zinc oxide-eugenol c., dental c. obtained by mixing zinc oxide and eugenol with one or more additives.

organic dental c., a dental c. consisting mainly of synthetic polymers.

polycarboxylate c., a powder containing primarily zinc oxide mixed with a liquid containing polyacrylic acid which reacts to form a hard crystalline mass upon standing; when used to lute metal castings to teeth, it has the potential of bonding to the calcium contained in tooth structure as well as to any base metals contained in the casting.

resin c., a monomer or monomer/polymer system used as a dental luting agent; used in cementation of restorations or orthodontic brackets to the teeth.

silicate c., a dental filling material prepared by mixing a modified phosphoric acid solution with a powdered silica alumina fluoride glass.

tooth c., SYN cement (1). SEE cement (2).

unmodified zinc oxide-eugenol c., a dental c. obtained by mixing zinc oxide and eugenol without modifiers.

zinc phosphate c., a powder, containing primarily zinc oxide mixed with a liquid containing orthophosphoric acid to form a hard crystalline mass on standing, used in dentistry as a luting agent for cast metal restorations and orthodontic bands, and as a temporary restorative material, or a base under restorations, particularly in deep cavities.

ce·men·ta·tion (sē-men-tā′shŭn). **1.** The process of attaching parts by means of a cement. **2.** In dentistry, attaching a restoration to natural teeth by means of a cement.

ce·ment·i·cle (se-men′ti-kl). A calcified spherical body, composed of cementum lying free within the periodontal membrane, attached to the cementum or imbedded within it.

ce·ment·i·fi·ca·tion (se-men′ti-fi-kā′shŭn). Metaplastic production of cementum or cementoid within a less differentiated connective tissue, e.g., c. of a fibroma.

ce·ment·o·blast (se-men′tō-blast). A cell of mesenchymal origin concerned with the formation of the layer of cementum on the roots of teeth. [L. *cementum*, cement, + G. *blastos*, germ]

ce·ment·o·blas·to·ma (se-men′tō-blas-tō′mă). A benign odontogenic tumor of functional cementoblasts; it appears as a mixed radiolucent-radiopaque lesion attached to a tooth root and may cause expansion of the bone cortex or be associated with pain. SYN benign c., true cementoma.

benign c., SYN cementoblastoma.

ce·ment·o·cla·sia (se-men-tō-klā′zē-ă). Destruction of cementum by cementoclasts. [L. *cementum*, cement, + G. *klasis*, fracture]

ce·ment·o·clast (se-men′tō-klast). One of the multinucleated giant cells, identical with osteoclasts, that are associated with the resorption of cementum. [L. *cementum*, cement, + G. *klastos*, broken]

ce·ment·o·cyte (se-men′tō-sīt). An osteocyte-like cell with numerous processes, trapped in a lacuna in the cementum of the tooth. [L. *cementum*, cement, + G. *kytos*, cell]

ce·ment·o·den·tin·al (se-men′tō-den′ti-năl). SYN dentinocemental.

ce·men·to·gen·e·sis (se-men′to-jen′ĕ-sis). The development of the cementum over the root dentin of a tooth. [cementum + G. *genesis*, production]

ce·men·to·ma (se-men-tō′mă). Nonspecific term referring to any benign cementum-producing tumor; four types are recognized: 1) periapical cemental dysplasia, 2) central ossifying fibroma, 3) cementoblastoma, 4) sclerotic cemental mass. When the type is not specified, c. usually refers to periapical cemental *dysplasia*. [L. *cementum*, cement, + G. *-ōma*, tumor]

gigantiform c., the familial occurrence of cemental masses in the jaws; inherited as an autosomal dominant characteristic. SEE ALSO sclerotic cemental *mass*.

true c., SYN cementoblastoma.

ce·men·tum (se-men′tŭm) [TA]. SYN cement (1). [L. *caementum*, rough quarry stone, fr. *caedo*, to cut]

afibrillar c., c. which, with the electron microscope, appears as laminated, electron-dense reticular material that sometimes overlies the enamel of the tooth.

primary c., c. that has no cementocytes; may cover the entire root of the tooth, but often is missing on the apical third of the root.

secondary c., c. that forms on the root surface after eruption; it contains cementocytes.

ce·nes·the·sia (sē-nes-thē′zē-ă). The general sense of bodily existence; the sensation caused by the functioning of the internal organs. SYN coenesthesia. [G. *koinos*, common, + *aisthēsis*, sensation]

ce·nes·the·sic, ce·nes·thet·ic (sē-nes-thē′zik, -sik; -thet′ik). Relating to cenesthesia.

△**ceno-. 1.** Shared in common. [G. *koinos*, common] **2.** New, fresh. [G. *kainos*, new] **3.** Emptiness (rare). SEE ALSO coeno-. [G. *kenos*, empty]

ce·no·cyte (sē′nō-sīt). A multinucleate cell or hypha without cross walls, characteristic of the hyphae of zygomycetes. SEE ALSO nonseptate *mycelium*. SYN coenocyte. [G. *koinos*, common, + *kytos*, cell]

ce·no·cyt·ic (sē-nō-sit′ik). Pertaining to or having characteristics of a cenocyte. SYN coenocytic.

cen·o·site (sē′nō-sīt). A facultative commensal organism; one that can sustain itself apart from its usual host. [G. *koinos*, common, + *sitos*, food]

ce·no·trope (sē′nō-trōp). A scientifically more accurate term than the earlier "instinct", denoting the behavior pattern shown by all members of a large group having the same biologic equipment and same experience. [G. *koinos*, common, + *tropē*, a turning]

cen·sor (sen′sōr). In psychoanalytic theory, the psychic barrier that prevents certain unconscious thoughts and wishes from coming to consciousness unless they are so cloaked or disguised as to be unrecognizable. [L. a judge, critic, fr. *censeo*, to value, judge]

censoring (sen′sōr-ing). In epidemiology, (1) Loss of subjects from a follow-up study for unknown reasons. (2) Observations with unknown values from one end of a frequency distribution, beyond a measurement threshold.

cen·sus. An enumeration of a population, originally for taxation and military purposes, now with many other purposes; basic facts about all persons—age, sex, occupation, nature of residence, etc.— are recorded in the census, which often also includes some information about health status. [L., fr. *censeo*, to count]

cen·ter (sen′ter) [TA]. **1.** The middle point of a body; loosely, the interior of a body. A center of any kind, especially an anatomical center. **2.** A group of nerve cells governing a specific function. SYN centrum [TA]. [L. *centrum*; G. *kentron*]

active c., the part of a macromolecule at which a substrate or ligand, upon binding, produces biologic activity; for an enzyme, this is the catalytic c., the site on an enzyme that catalyzes the reaction.

anospinal c., the c. in the spinal cord that controls the contraction of the anal sphincter.

birthing c., a facility, usually in a hospital, that provides labor and delivery services in a comfortable, homelike setting.

Broca c., the posterior part of the inferior frontal gyrus of the left or dominant hemisphere, corresponding approximately to Brodmann area 44; Broca identified this region as an essential component of the motor mechanisms governing articulated speech. SYN Broca area, Broca field, motor speech c.

Budge c., SYN ciliospinal c.

catalytic c., SEE active c.

cell c., SYN cytocentrum.

chondrification c., a site of earliest cartilage formation in the body.

ciliospinal c., the preganglionic motor neurons in the first thoracic segment of the spinal cord which give rise to the sympathetic innervation that eventually influences the dilator muscle of the eye's pupil. SYN Budge c.

dentary c., a specific ossification c. of the mandible that gives rise to the lower border of its outer plate.

diaphysial c., primary c. of ossification in the shaft of a long bone.

epiotic c., the c. of ossification of the petrous part of the temporal bone that appears posterior to the posterior semicircular canal.

expiratory c., the region of the medulla oblongata that is electrically active during expiration and where electrical stimulation produces sustained expiration.

feeding c., a region of the lateral zone of the hypothalamus, electrical stimulation of which in the rat elicits uninterrupted eating; destruction of the region causes long-lasting anorexia.

germinal c. of Flemming, the lightly staining c. in a lymphatic nodule in which the predominant cells are large lymphocytes and macrophages. SYN reaction c.

inspiratory c., the region of the medulla oblongata that is electrically active during inspiration and where electrical stimulation produces sustained inspiration.

Kerckring c., an occasional independent ossification c. in the occipital bone; it appears in the posterior margin of the foramen magnum at about the sixteenth week of gestation. SYN Kerckring ossicle.

medullary c., SYN *centrum* semiovale.

microtubule-organizing c., a locus in interphase and mitotic cells from which most microtubules radiate; in the center of this c. is the centriole; this c. determines the polarity of cellular microtubules.

motor speech c., SYN Broca c.

ossific c., SYN ossification c.

c. of ossification, SYN ossification c. SYN centrum ossificationis [TA].

ossification c. [TA], the site of earliest bone formation via accumulation of osteoblasts within connective tissue (membranous ossification) or of earliest destruction of cartilage prior to onset of ossification (endochondral ossification). SYN c. of ossification, ossific c., point of ossification, punctum ossificationis.

primary c. of ossification, SYN primary ossification c. SYN centrum ossificationis primarium [TA].

primary ossification c. [TA], this is the first site where bone begins to form in the shaft of a long bone or in the body of an irregular bone. SYN primary c. of ossification, primary point of ossification, punctum ossificationis primarium.

reaction c., SYN germinal c. of Flemming.

respiratory c., the region in the medulla oblongata concerned with integrating afferent information to determine the signals to the respiratory muscles; the inspiratory and expiratory c.'s considered together.

c. of ridge, the buccolingual midline of the residual ridge.

c. of rotation, a point or line around which all other points in a body move. SEE axis.

satiety c., a term referring to the region of the ventromedial nucleus in the hypothalamus; destruction of this small region in the rat leads to continuous eating and extreme obesity.

secondary c. of ossification, SYN secondary ossification c. SYN centrum ossificationis secundarium [TA].

secondary ossification c. [TA], this is the center of bone formation appearing later than the punctum ossificationis primarium, usually in epiphysis. SYN punctum ossificationis secundarium, secondary c. of ossification, secondary point of ossification.

semioval c., SYN *centrum* semiovale.

sensory speech c., SYN Wernicke c.

speech c.'s, areas of the cerebral cortex centrally involved in speech function; one is in the left inferior frontal gyrus, a second one in the supramarginal, angular, and first and second temporal gyri. SEE ALSO Broca c., Wernicke c.

sphenotic c., one of the paired c.'s of ossification of the sphenoid bone.

vasomotor c., diffuse area of the reticular formation in the lateral medulla containing neurons that control vascular tone; consists of separate vasodepressor and vasopressor areas.

vital c., c. essential to life; usually refers to the centers located in the medulla oblongata which are necessary for the maintenance of respiration and circulation.

Wernicke c., the region of the cerebral cortex thought to be essential for understanding and formulating coherent, propositional speech; it encompasses a large region of the parietal and temporal lobes near the lateral sulcus of the left cerebral hemisphere; corresponding approximately to Brodmann areas 40, 39,

and 22. SYN sensory speech c., Wernicke area, Wernicke field, Wernicke region, Wernicke zone.

Cen·ters for Dis·ease Con·trol and Pre·ven·tion (CDC). The federal facility for disease eradication, epidemiology, and education headquartered in Atlanta, Georgia, which encompasses the Center for Infectious Diseases, Center for Environmental Health, Center for Health Promotion and Education, Center for Prevention Services, Center for Professional Development and Training, and Center for Occupational Safety and Health. Formerly named Center for Disease Control (1970), Communicable Disease Center (1946).

cen·te·sis (sen-tē′sis). Puncture, especially when used as a suffix, as in paracentesis. [G. *kentēsis,* puncture, fr. *kenteō,* to prick, pierce]

centi- (c). Prefix used in the SI and metric systems to signify one hundredth (10^{-2}). [L. *centum,* one hundred]

cen·ti·bar (sen′ti-bar). One hundredth of a bar.

cen·ti·grade (C) (sen′ti-grād). 1. Basis of the former temperature scale in which 100 degrees separated the melting and boiling points of water. SEE Celsius *scale.* 2. One hundredth of a circle, equal to 3.6° of the astronomical circle. [L. *centum,* one hundred, + *gradus,* step, degree]

cen·ti·gram (sen′ti-gram). One hundredth of a gram; 0.15432358 grain.

cen·tile (sen′til). One-hundredth. SEE quantile. [L. *centum,* one hundred, + *-ilis,* adj. suffix]

cen·ti·li·ter (sen′ti-lē-ter). 10 mL; one hundredth of a liter; 162.3073 minims (U.S.).

cen·ti·me·ter (cm) (sen′ti-mē-ter). One hundredth of a meter; 0.3937008 inch.

cubic c. (cc, c.c.), one thousandth of a liter; 1 mL.

cen·ti·mor·gan (cM) (sen′ti-mōr-găn). SEE morgan.

cen·ti·nor·mal (sen-ti-nōr′măl). One-hundredth normal; denoting the concentration of a solution.

cen·ti·pede (sen′ti-pēd). A venomous predatory arthropod of the order Chilopoda, characterized by one pair of legs per leg-bearing segment. The venom is injected through the first pair of leglike appendages, modified into piercing claws; the bites may be painful and locally necrotic, but seldom are dangerous, except to very young children. Genera found in the U.S. include *Scutigera, Lithobius, Scolopendra,* and *Geophilus.* [L. *centum,* hundred, + *pes (ped-),* foot]

cen·ti·poise (sen′ti-poyz). One hundredth of a poise.

cen·tra (sen′trǎ). Plural of centrum.

cen·trad (sen′trad). 1. Toward the center. 2. A unit of measurement of the refracting strength of a prism; it corresponds to the deviation of a ray of light, the arc of which is $^1/_{100}$ of the radius of the circle, or 0.57°.

cen·trage (sen′trāj). The condition in which the optical centers of all the reflecting and refracting surfaces of an optical system are on the same axis.

cen·tra·lis (sen-trā′lis). Central; in the center. [L.]

cen·tre mé·di·an de Luys (sen′tr mā-dē-an). SYN centromedian *nucleus.* [Fr.]

cen·tren·ce·phal·ic (sen′tren-se-fal′ik). Relating to the center of the encephalon.

cen·tri- (sen′tri). Combining form denoting center.

centric (sen′trik). Having a center (of a specific kind or number) or having a specific thing as its center (of interest, focus, etc.). [G. *kentron,* center]

cen·tric·i·put (sen-tris′i-put). The central portion of the upper surface of the skull, between the occiput and the sinciput. [L. *centrum,* center, + *caput,* head]

cen·trif·u·gal (sen-trif′ū-găl). 1. Denoting the direction of the force pulling an object outward (away) from an axis of rotation. 2. Sometimes, by analogy, extended to describe any movement away from a center. Cf. eccentric (2). [L. *centrum,* center, + *fugio,* to flee]

cen·trif·u·gal·i·za·tion (sen-trif′ū-găl-i-zā′shŭn). SYN centrifugation.

cen·trif·u·gal·ize (sen-trif′ū-găl-īz). SYN centrifuge (2).

cen·trif·u·ga·tion (sen-trif-ū-gā′shŭn). Subjection to sedimentation, by means of a centrifuge, of solids suspended in a fluid. SYN centrifugalization.

band c., SYN density gradient c.

density gradient c., ultracentrifugation of substances in concentrated solutions of cesium salts or of sucrose; at equilibrium, the medium exhibits a concentration (hence density) gradient increasing in the direction of centrifugal force and the substances of interest collect in layers at the levels of their densities. SEE isopycnic *zone.* SYN band c., zone c.

zone c., SYN density gradient c.

cen·tri·fuge (sen′tri-fooj). **1.** An apparatus by means of which particles in suspension in a fluid are separated by spinning the fluid, the centrifugal force throwing the particles to the periphery of the rotated vessel. **2.** To submit to rapid rotary action, as in a c. SYN centrifugalize.

cen·tri·lob·u·lar (sen-tri-lob′ū-lăr). At or near the center of a lobule, e.g., of the liver.

cen·tri·ole (sen′trē-ōl). Tubular structures, 150 nm by 300 to 500 nm, with a wall having 9 triple microtubules, usually seen as paired organelles lying in the cytocentrum; c.'s may be multiple and numerous in some cells, such as the giant cells of bone marrow. [G. *kentron,* a point, center]

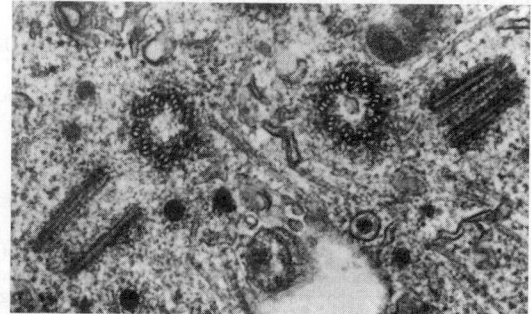

centriole: electron micrograph showing both parent and daughter centrioles in a fibroblast × 90,000

anterior c., SYN proximal c.

distal c., the c. in the developing spermatozoon from which the flagellum develops. SYN posterior c.

posterior c., SYN distal c.

proximal c., the c. that lies in a depression in the wall of the posterior portion of the nucleus of the developing spermatozoon. SYN anterior c.

cen·trip·e·tal (sen-trip′ĕ-tăl). **1.** SYN afferent. **2.** Denoting the direction of the force pulling an object toward an axis of rotation. SYN axipetal. [L. *centrum,* center, + *peto,* to seek]

centro-. Combining form denoting center. [G. *kentron*]

cen·tro·blast (sen′trō-blast). A lymphocyte with a large noncleaved nucleus. [centro- + G. *blastos,* germ]

Cen·tro·ces·tus (sen-trō-ses′tŭs). A genus of extremely small fish-borne flukes (family Heterophyidae) that may produce intestinal lesions similar to those caused by *Heterophyes heterophyes. C. formosana* has been reported in humans in Taiwan. [G. *kentron,* point, center, + *kestos,* belt, both words fr. *kenteō,* to pierce]

cen·tro·cyte (sen′trō-sīt). **1.** A cell whose protoplasm contains single and double granules of varying size stainable with hematoxylin; seen in lesions of lichen planus. SYN Lipschütz cell. **2.** A lymphocyte with a cleaved nucleus. **3.** A nondividing, activated B cell that expresses membrane immunoglobulin. [centro- + G. *kytos,* cell]

cen·tro·ki·ne·sia (sen′trō-ki-nē′sē-ă). Movement excited by a stimulus of central origin. [centro- + G. *kinēsis,* movement]

cen·tro·ki·net·ic (sen′trō-ki-net′ik). **1.** Relating to centrokinesia. **2.** SYN excitomotor.

cen·tro·lec·i·thal (sen-trō-les′i-thăl). Denoting an ovum in which

the deutoplasm accumulates centrally. [centro- + G. *lekithos,* yolk]

cen·tro·mere (sen′trō-mēr). **1.** The nonstaining primary constriction of a chromosome which is the point of attachment of the spindle fiber; provides the mechanism of chromosome movement during cell division; the c. divides the chromosome into two arms, and its position is constant for a specific chromosome: near one end (acrocentric), near the center (metacentric), or between (submetacentric). [centro- + G. *meros,* part]

cen·tro·plasm (sen′trō-plazm). The substance of the cytocentrum. [centro- + G. *plasma,* thing formed]

cen·tro·some (sen′trō-sōm). SYN cytocentrum. [centro- + G. *sōma,* body]

cen·tro·sphere (sen′trō-sfēr). The specialized, often gelated cytoplasm of the cytocentrum. Contains the centrioles from which the astral fibers (microtubules) extend during mitosis. SYN astrocele, statosphere. [centro- + G. *sphaira,* a ball, sphere]

cen·tro·stal·tic (sen-trō-stal′tik). Relating to the center of motion. [centro- + G. *stallein,* set forth, fetch]

cen·trum, pl. **cen·tra** (sen′trŭm, sen′tră) [TA]. SYN center. [L. fr. G. *kentron*]

c. media′num, SYN centromedian *nucleus.*

c. medulla′re, SYN c. semiovale.

c. ossificationis [TA], SYN *center* of ossification.

c. ossificationis primarium [TA], SYN primary *center* of ossification.

c. ossificationis secundarium [TA], SYN secondary *center* of ossification.

c. ova′le, SYN c. semiovale.

c. semiova′le, the great mass of white matter composing the interior of the cerebral hemisphere; the name refers to the general shape of this white core in horizontal sections of the hemisphere. SYN c. medullare, c. ovale, medullary center, semioval center, Vicq d'Azyr c. semiovale, Vieussens c.

c. tendin′eum diaphrag′matis [TA], SYN central *tendon* of diaphragm.

c. tendin′eum perine′i [TA], SYN central *tendon* of perineum.

c. of a vertebra, (1) the ossification center of the central mass of the body of a vertebra; **(2)** *body* of vertebra (as distinct from the arches).

Vicq d'Azyr c. semiova′le, SYN c. semiovale.

Vieussens c., SYN c. semiovale.

Willis c. nervo′sum, SYN celiac *ganglia,* under *ganglion.*

Cen·tru·roi·des (sen-tru-roy′dēz). A genus of North American scorpions, the commonest species of which are *C. gracilis,* the margarite scorpion; *C. vittatus,* the stripe-back scorpion; and *C. sculpturatus,* the deadly sculptured scorpion. SEE ALSO Scorpionida.

cen·tum (c) (sen′tum). One hundred. [L. one hundred]

cen·u·ris, coe·nu·ris (se-nū′ris). A tapeworm bladderworm with multiple inverted scoleces attached to the inner germinative layer; produced by taeniid cestodes of the genus *Multiceps,* typically found in the brain or tissues of herbivores and the adult worm in the intestine of wolves, dogs, or other canids; rare cases of c. infections in humans have been reported. [G. *kenos,* empty, + G. *uris,* tail]

cen·u·ro·sis, ce·nu·ri·a·sis (sen-ū-rō′sis, sen-ū-rī′ă-sis). Disease produced by the presence of a cenuris cyst that, in sheep, causes a brain infection known as "gid" for the giddy gait induced in the infected animal; human c. has been reported but is extremely unusual, in contrast with hydatid disease. SYN coenurosis.

ce·pha·e·line (sef-a′ĕ-lēn). An alkaloid of ipecac; an emetic and amebicide.

Ceph·a·e·lis (sef-ă-ē′lis). SYN *Uragoga.* [G. *kephalē,* head, + *eilō,* to roll up, pack close]

cephal-. SEE cephalo-.

ceph·a·lad (sef′ă-lad). In a direction toward the head. SEE ALSO cranial (1).

ceph·a·lal·gia (sef′al-al′jē-ă). SYN headache. [cephal- + G. *algos,* pain]

benign coital c., SYN coital *headache.*

histaminic c., SYN cluster *headache.*

Horton c., SYN cluster *headache.*

ceph·al·e·de·ma (sef′al-ĕ-dē′mǎ). Edema of the head.

ceph·a·le·mia (sef-ă-lē′-mē-ă). Congestion, active or passive, of the brain. [cephal- + G. *haima,* blood]

ceph·a·lex·in (sef-ă-lek′sin). A broad-spectrum antibiotic derived from cephalosporin C.

ceph·al·he·ma·to·cele (sef′ăl-hē-mat′ō-sēl). A cephalhematoma under the pericranium communicating with the dural sinuses. SYN cephalohematocele. [cephal- + G. *haima,* blood, + *kēlē,* tumor]

ceph·al·he·ma·to·ma (sef′ăl-hē-mă-tō′mǎ). A collection of blood due to an effusion of blood beneath the periosteum frequently in a newborn as a result of birth trauma; contrasted with caput succedaneum, in which the effusion overlies the periosteum and consists of serum. SYN cephalohematoma. [cephal- + G. *haima,* blood, + *-ōma,* tumor]

ceph·al·hy·dro·cele (sef-ăl-hī′drō-sēl). An accumulation of serous or watery fluid under the pericranium. [cephal- + G. *hydōr,* water, + *kēlē,* tumor]

ce·phal·ic (se-fal′ik). SYN cranial (1).

ceph·a·lin (sef′ă-lin). A term formerly applied to a group of phosphatidic esters resembling lecithin but containing either 2-ethanolamine or L-serine in the place of choline; these are now known as phosphatidylethanolamine and phosphatidylserine. They are widely distributed in the body, especially in the brain and spinal cord, and are used as local hemostatics and as reagents in liver function test. SYN kephalin.

ceph·a·line (sef′ă-līn). Denoting members of the protozoan suborder Cephalina (order Eugregarinida), characterized by bodies divided into chambers (anterior protomerite and posterior deutomerite, or anterior epimerite, protomerite, and terminal deutomerite); all are parasites of invertebrates.

ceph·a·li·tis (sef-ă-lī′tis). Obsolete term for encephalitis.

ceph·a·li·za·tion (sef′ăl-ĭ-zā′shŭn). **1.** Evolutionary tendency for important functions of the nervous system to move forward in the brain. **2.** Initiation and concentration of the growth tendency at the anterior end of the embryo.

⌂**cephalo-, cephal-.** The head. [G. *kephalē*]

ceph·a·lo·cau·dal (sef′ă-lō-kaw′dăl). Relating to both head and tail, i.e., to the long axis of the body. [cephalo- + L. *cauda,* tail]

ceph·a·lo·cele (sef′ă-lō-sēl). Protrusion of part of the cranial contents, e.g., meningocele, encephalocele. SEE ALSO encephalocele.

ceph·a·lo·cen·te·sis (sef′ă-lō-sen-tē′sis). Passage of a hollow needle or trocar and cannula into the brain to drain or aspirate an abscess or the fluid of a hydrocephalus. [cephalo- + G. *kentēsis,* puncture]

ceph·a·lo·chord (sef′ă-lō-kōrd). Intracranial portion of the notochord in the embryo.

ceph·a·lo·did·y·mus (sef′ă-lō-did′i-mŭs). Conjoined twins fused except in the cephalic region; a variety of duplicitas posterior. SEE conjoined *twins,* under *twin.* [cephalo- + G. *didymos,* twin]

ceph·a·lo·di·pros·o·pus (sef′ă-lō-dī-pros′ō-pŭs). Asymmetrical conjoined twins with the head of the autosite carrying a reduced parasitic head. SEE conjoined *twins,* under *twin,* diprosopus. [cephalo- + G. *di-,* two, + *prosōpon,* face]

ceph·a·lo·dyn·ia (sef′ă-lō-din′ē-ă). Headache. [cephalo- + G. *odynē,* pain]

ceph·a·lo·gen·e·sis (sef′ă-lō-jen′ĕ-sis). Formation of the head in the embryonic period. [cephalo- + G. *genesis,* production]

ceph·a·lo·gly·cin (sef′ă-lō-glī′sin). A semisynthetic broad-spectrum antibiotic produced from cephalosporin C.

ceph·a·lo·gram (sef′ă-lō-gram). SYN cephalometric *radiograph.*

ceph·a·lo·gy·ric (sef′ă-lō-jī′rik). Relating to rotation of the head. [cephalo- + G. *gyros,* a circle]

ceph·a·lo·he·ma·to·cele (sef′ă-lō-hē-mat′ō-sēl). SYN cephalhematocele.

ceph·a·lo·he·ma·to·ma (sef′ă-lō-hē-mă-tō′mǎ). SYN cephalhematoma.

ceph·a·lo·he·mom·e·ter (sef′ă-lō-hē-mom′ĕ-ter). An instrument showing the degree of intracranial blood pressure. [cephalo- + G. *haima,* blood, + *metron,* measure]

ceph·a·lo·meg·a·ly (sef′ă-lō-meg′ă-lē). Enlargement of the head. [cephalo- + G. *megas,* great]

ceph·a·lom·e·lus (sef-ă-lom′ĕ-lŭs). Malformed individual with an accessory limb, resembling a leg or arm, growing from the head. [cephalo- + G. *melos,* a limb]

ceph·a·lo·men·in·gi·tis (sef′ă-lō-men-in-jī′tis). Obsolete term for meningitis. [cephalo- + G. *mēninx* (*mēning-*), membrane]

ceph·a·lom·e·ter (sef-ă-lom′ĕ-ter). An instrument used to position the head to produce oriented, reproducible lateral and posterior-anterior head films. SYN cephalostat. [cephalo- + G. *metron,* measure]

ceph·a·lo·met·rics (sef-ă-lō-met′riks). In oral surgery and orthodontics: **1.** The scientific measurement of the bones of the cranium and face, utilizing a fixed, reproducible position for lateral radiographic exposure of skull and facial bones. SEE ALSO cephalometry. **2.** A scientific study of the measurements of the head with relation to specific reference points; used for evaluation of facial growth and development, including soft tissue profile. [cephalo- + G. *metron,* measure]

ceph·a·lom·e·try (sef-ă-lom′ĕ-trē). Scientific measurements, often taken by means of radiographic imaging, of the head in the living, or of the cadaver head with soft tissues in place, utilizing specific reference points and sufficient standardization to allow reproducible results. Commonly used to document age based on cephalic growth (as in obstetric ultrasonography) or to plan or measure progress in cephalic remodeling (as in orthodontics). SEE ALSO craniometry, cephalometrics. [cephalo- + G. *metron,* measure]

ultrasonic c., measurement of the fetal head by ultrasound.

ceph·a·lo·mo·tor (sef′ă-lō-mō′ter). Relating to movements of the head.

Ceph·a·lo·my·ia (sef′ă-lō-mī′yă). Former name for *Oestrus.* [cephalo- + G. *myia,* fly]

ceph·a·lont (sef′ă-lont). Adult stage of a cephaline gregarine, a sporozoan parasite commonly found in arthropods and other invertebrate hosts. The body is usually divided by a septum into an anterior epimerite and protomerite and a posterior deutomerite; acephaline gregarines lack a dividing septum. [cephalo- + G. *ōn* (*ont-*), being]

ceph·a·lop·a·gus (sef-ă-lop′ă-gŭs). Conjoined twins with heads fused but the remainder of the bodies separate. SEE conjoined *twins,* under *twin.* SEE ALSO craniopagus, *duplicitas* posterior. [cephalo- + G. *pagos,* something fixed]

ceph·a·lo·pel·vic (sef-ă-lō-pel′vik). Pertaining to the size of the fetal head in relation to the maternal pelvis.

ceph·a·lo·pel·vim·e·try (sef′ă-lō-pel-vim′ĕ-trē). Radiographic measurement of the dimensions of the pelvis and the fetal head; the technique has been largely abandoned. SYN pelvicephalography, pelvocephalography. [cephalo- + pelvimetry]

ceph·a·lo·pha·ryn·ge·us (sef′ă-lō-fă-rin′jē-ŭs). SEE superior pharyngeal constrictor (*muscle*).

ceph·a·lor·i·dine (sef-ă-lōr′i-dēn). A broad-spectrum antimicrobial derived from cephalosporin C.

ceph·a·lor·rha·chid·i·an (sef-ă-lō-ra-kid′ē-an). Relating to the head and the spine. [cephalo- + G. *rhachis,* spine]

ceph·a·lo·spor·an·ic ac·id (sef′ă-lō-spōr-an′ik). The basic chemical nucleus upon which cephalosporin antibiotic derivatives are based.

ceph·a·lo·spo·rin (sef′ă-lō-spōr′in). This is an antibiotic produced by a *Cephalosporium,* but since the antibiotic was discovered the name Cephalosporium has been removed and the new name is Acremonium.

c. C, an antibiotic whose activity is due to the 7-aminocephalosporanic acid portion of the cephalosporanic acid molecule; it is effective against Gram-positive and Gram-negative bacteria, but is less potent than c. N. Addition of side chains produced semisynthetic broad spectrum antibiotics with greater antibacterial activity than that of c. C; the antibiotic activity is due to interference with bacterial cell-wall synthesis.

c. N, an antibiotic active against Gram-positive and Gram-negative bacteria, but inactivated by penicillinase; on hydrolysis it yields penicillamine. SYN penicillin N, synnematin B.

c. P, a steroid antibiotic produced by *Cephalosporium*, chemically related to fusidic and helvolic acids, that is active only against Gram-positive bacteria.

ceph·a·lo·spor·i·nase (sef′ă-lō-spōr′i-nās). SYN β-lactamase.

Ceph·a·lo·spo·ri·um (sef′ă-lō-spō′rē-ŭm). Former name of *Acremonium*.

ceph·a·lo·stat (sef′ă-lō-stat). SYN cephalometer. [cephalo- + G. *statos,* stationary]

ceph·a·lo·thin (sef-ă-lō′thin). Chemically modified cephalosporin C, a broad-spectrum antibiotic.

ceph·a·lo·tho·rac·ic (sef′ă-lō-thō-ras′ik). Relating to the head and the chest.

ceph·a·lo·tho·ra·cop·a·gus (sef′ă-lō-thōr-ă-kop′ă-gŭs). Conjoined twins with the bodies fused in the cephalic and thoracic regions. SEE conjoined *twins,* under *twin.* [cephalo- + G. *thorax,* chest, + *pagos,* something fixed]

c. asym′metros, SYN c. monosymmetros.

c. disym′metros, a form of c. with the fused head showing equally developed faces directed laterally.

c. monosym′metros, a form of c. in which only one of the faces is well developed. SYN c. asymmetros.

ceph·a·lo·tome (sef′ă-lō-tōm). Instrument formerly used for cutting into the fetal head to permit its compression in cases of dystocia. [cephalo- + G. *tomē,* a cutting]

ceph·a·lot·o·my (sef-ă-lot′ō-mē). Formerly used operation of cutting into the head of the fetus.

ceph·a·lo·tox·in (sef′ă-lō-tok′sin). A poison, believed to be a protein, found in the salivary glands of cephalopods (octopus). SEE ALSO eledoisin.

ceph·a·lo·tribe (sef′ă-lō-trīb). Forcepslike instrument, with strong blades and a screw handle, formerly used to crush the fetal head in cases of dystocia. [G. *tribō,* to rub, bruise]

ceph·a·my·cins (sef′ă-mī′sin). A family of β-lactam antibiotics (similar to penicillin and cephalosporins) produced by various *Streptomyces* species.

ceph·a·pi·rin so·di·um (sef-ă-pī′rin). A semisynthetic broad spectrum antibiotic derived from cephalosporin C; it is used by injection.

ceph·ra·dine (sef′ră-dēn). A semisynthetic broad-spectrum antibiotic derived from cephalosporin C; used orally and by injection.

cep·tor (sep′ter, tōr). SYN receptor (2). [L. *capio,* pp. *captus,* to take]

chemical c., c. that initiates chemical reactions in response to the appropriate stimuli.

contact c., a nerve c. in the surface layer of skin or mucous membrane by means of which impulses contributed by direct physical impact are received.

distance c., a nerve mechanism of one of the organs of special sense whereby the subject is brought into relation with the distant environment.

△**-ceptor.** Combining form denoting taker, receiver. [L. *capio,* pp. *captus,* to take]

ce·ra (sē′ră). SYN wax (1). [L.]

ce·ra·ceous (se-rā′shŭs). Waxen. [L. *cera,* wax]

cer·am·i·dase (ser-am′i-dās). An enzyme that hydrolyzes ceramides into sphingosine and a fatty acid; acylsphirgosine deacylase. A deficiency of this enzyme is associated with Farber disease.

cer·a·mide (ser′ă-mīd). Generic term for a class of sphingolipid, *N*-acyl (fatty acid) derivatives of a long chain base or sphingoid such as sphinganine or sphingosine; e.g., $CH_3(CH_2)_{12}CH=CH-CHOH-CH(CH_2OH)-NH-CO-R$, where R is the fatty-acyl residue, attached in this example to 4-sphingenine (sphingosine) in amide linkage. C.'s accumulate in individuals with Farber disease.

c. dihexoside, the accumulated glycolipid noted in glycolipid lipidosis.

c. lactosidase, a hydrolytic enzyme (a β-galactosidase) that acts on c. lactoside, producing glucosylceramide and galactose. A deficiency of this enzyme can result in c. lactoside liposis. Cf. cytolipin.

c. lactoside, a lactosylceramide that accumulates in individuals with c. lactoside liposis. Cf. cytolipin.

c. 1-phosphorylcholine, SYN sphingomyelins.

c. saccharide, SYN glycosphingolipid.

cer·a·sin (ser′ă-sin). SYN kerasin.

△**cerat-.** SEE kerat-.

ce·rate (sē′rāt). A rarely used unctuous solid preparation, harder than an ointment, containing sufficient wax to prevent it from melting when applied to the skin. [L. *cera,* wax]

cer·a·tin (ser′a-tin). SYN keratin.

△**cerato-.** SEE kerato-.

cer·a·to·cri·coid (ser′ă-tō-krī′koyd). Relating to the inferior cornua of the thyroid cartilage and to the cricoid cartilage, or the cricothyroid articulation. SYN keratocricoid.

cer·a·to·hy·al (ser′ă-tō-hī′ăl). Relating to one of the cornua of the hyoid bone. SYN keratohyal.

Cer·a·to·phyl·li·dae (ser′ă-tō-fil′i-dē). A family of mammal and bird fleas, many of which have a wide host range and serve as important vectors of plague, sustaining the infection among wild and domestic rodent hosts. Important genera include *Nosopsyllus* and *Ceratophyllus.* [G. *keras,* horn, + *phyllōdēs,* like leaves]

Cer·a·to·phyl·lus (ser-ă-tof′-ă-lŭs). A genus of fleas (family Ceratophyllidae) found in temperate climates; includes important fleas of poultry such as *C. niger,* the western chicken flea, and *C. gallinae,* the European chicken flea, although these fleas have a wide range of hosts, including humans. [cerat- (kerat-) + G. *phyllon,* leaf]

C. punjaten′sis, a species of flea abundant on wild and domestic rodents in India; may serve as a liaison agent between wild rodents and humans in the transmission of plague.

cer·car·ia, pl. **cer·car·i·ae** (ser-kā′rē-ă, -rē-ē). The free-swimming trematode larva that emerges from its host snail; it may penetrate the skin of a final host (as in *Schistosoma* of humans), encyst on vegetation (as in *Fasciola*), in or on fish (as in *Clonorchis*), or penetrate and encyst in various arthropod hosts. Body and tail are greatly varied in form, and specialized function is adapted to the particular life cycle demands of each species. SEE ALSO sporocyst (1), redia. [G. *kerkos,* tail]

cer·ci (ser′sī). Plural of cercus.

cer·clage (sair-klazh′). **1.** Bringing into close opposition and binding together the ends of an obliquely fractured bone by a ring or by an encircling, tightly drawn wire loop. **2.** Operation for retinal detachment in which the choroid and retinal pigment epithelium are brought in contact with the detached sensory retina by a band encircling the sclera posterior to the insertion of the ocular rectus muscles. **3.** The placing of a nonabsorbable suture around an incompetent cervical os. [Fr. an encircling, hooping, banding]

cer·co·cys·tis (ser-kō-sis′tis). A specialized form of tapeworm cysticercoid larva that develops within the vertebrate host villus rather than in an invertebrate host; e.g., the c. of *Hymenolepis nana* in its direct or egg-borne cycle in man. SEE ALSO cysticercus, cysticercoid. [G. *kerkos,* tail, + *kystis,* bladder]

cer·co·mer (ser′kō-mer). The caudal appendage of a larval cestode, the procercoid stage of pseudophyllid cestodes; it may also be found on the cysticercoid larvae of taenioid cestodes, as well as in many of the hymenolepidids (e.g., *Hymenolepis nana*). This appendage frequently bears the hooks originally used by the hexacanth in clawing its way into the intermediate host in which the procercoid or other larval stage develops. [G. *kerkos,* tail + *meros,* part]

cer·co·mo·nad (ser-kō-mō′nad). Common name for members of the genus *Cercomonas.*

Cer·co·mo·nas (ser-kō-mō′nas). A genus of freshwater and coprophilic protozoan flagellates in which members have one anterior and one posterior flagellum. Species have been described from the intestine or feces of humans and several types of domestic livestock, but have usually proved to be other genera such as *Trichomonas* or *Chilomastix*. [G. *kerkos*, tail + *monas (monad-)*, unit, monad]

Cer·co·pi·the·coi·dea (ser′kō-pith-ĕ-koy′dē-ă). One of the three superfamilies of the suborder Anthropoidea; includes apes, Old World monkeys, and humans. [G. *kerkos*, tail, + *pithēkos*, monkey]

Cer·co·pi·the·cus (ser-kō-pith-ē′kŭs). A genus of the family Cercopithecidae, represented by guenons and common African monkeys.

cer·cus, gen. and pl. **cer·ci** (ser′kŭs, ker′kŭs; -sē, -kē). **1.** A stiff hairlike structure. **2.** A pair of specialized sensory appendages on the 11th abdominal segment of most insects. [Mod. L., fr. G. *kerkos*, tail]

ce·rea flex·i·bil·i·tas (sē′rē-ă flek-si-bil′i-tas). "Waxy flexibility," in which the limb remains where placed; often seen in catatonia. [L.]

cer·e·bel·lar (ser-e-bel′ar). Relating to the cerebellum.

cer·e·bel·lin (ser-ĕ-bel′in). A cerebellum-specific hexadecapeptide localized in the perikarya and dendrites of cerebellar Purkinje cells; used as a marker for Purkinje cell maturation studies of neural development.

cer·e·bel·li·tis (ser-ĕ-bel-ī′tis). Obsolete term for inflammation of the cerebellum.

△**cerebello-.** The cerebellum. [L. *cerebrum*, brain, + *-ellum*, dim. suff.]

cer·e·bel·lo·len·tal (ser-e-bel′ō-len′tăl). Relating to the cerebellum and the lens of the eye.

cer·e·bel·lo·med·ul·lary (ser-e-bel′ō-med′ū-lār-ē). Relating to the cerebellum and the medulla oblongata.

cer·e·bel·lo·ol·i·vary (ser-e-bel′ō-ol′i-vār-ē). Relating to the connections of the cerebellum with the inferior olive.

cer·e·bel·lo·pon·tine (ser-e-bel′ō-pon′tēn). Relating to the cerebellum and the pons; denoting especially the c. recess or angle between these two structures.

cer·e·bel·lo·ru·bral (ser-e-bel′ō-roo′brăl). Relating to the connections of the cerebellum with the red nucleus. [cerebello- + L. *ruber*, red]

cer·e·bel·lum, pl. **ce·re·bel·la** (ser-e-bel′ŭm, -bel′ă) [TA]. The large posterior brain mass lying dorsal to the pons and medulla and ventral to the tentorium cerebelli and posterior portion of the cerebrum; it consists of two lateral hemispheres united by a narrow middle portion, the vermis. [L. dim. of *cerebrum*, brain]

△**cerebr-.** SEE cerebro-.

ce·re·bral (ser′ĕ-brăl, sĕ-rē′brăl). Relating to the cerebrum.

cer·e·bra·tion (ser-ĕ-brā′shŭn). Activity of the mental processes; thinking. SEE ALSO mentation, cognition.

△**cerebri-.** SEE cerebro-.

cer·e·bri·form (se-rē′bri-fōrm). Resembling the external fissures and convolutions of the brain. [cerebri- + L. *forma*, shape, appearance, nature]

cer·e·bri·tis (ser-ĕ-brī′tis). Focal inflammatory infiltrates in the brain parenchyma.

suppurative c., inflammation (phlegmon) of the brain with suppuration.

△**cerebro-, cerebr-, cerebri-.** The cerebrum. SEE ALSO encephalo-. [L. *cerebrum*, brain]

cer·e·bro·cu·pre·in (ser′ĕ-brō-koo′prē-in). SYN cytocuprein.

cer·e·bro·ma. SYN encephaloma.

cer·e·bro·ma·la·cia (ser′ĕ-brō-mă-lā′shē-ă). SYN encephalomalacia.

cer·e·bro·men·in·gi·tis (ser′ĕ-brō-men-in-jī′tis). SYN meningoencephalitis.

cer·e·bron (ser′ĕ-bron). SYN phrenosin.

cer·e·bron·ic ac·id (ser-ĕ-bron′ik). A constituent of brain cerebrosides and other glycolipids. SYN phrenosinic acid.

cer·e·bro·path·ia (ser′ĕ-brō-path′ē-ă). SYN encephalopathy.

cer·e·brop·a·thy (ser-ĕ-brop′ă-thē). SYN encephalopathy.

cer·e·bro·phys·i·ol·o·gy (ser′ĕ-brō-fiz-ē-ol′ō-jē). The physiology of the cerebrum.

cer·e·bro·scle·ro·sis (ser′ĕ-brō-sklēr-ō′sis). Encephalosclerosis, hardening of the cerebral hemispheres. [cerebro- + G. *sklērōsis*, hardening]

cer·e·bro·side (ser′ĕ-brō-sīd). A class of glycosphingolipid; specifically, a monoglycosylceramide (ceramide monosaccharide), the sugar being attached to the –CHOH– moiety of the sphingoid. C.'s are found in the myelin sheath of nerve tissue; e.g., kerasin, nervon, oxynervon, phrenosin, these names also being used for the fatty acid involved. C. is sometimes prefixed by gluco-, galacto-, etc., in place of the correct glucosylceramide, etc. The sulfate esters of c.'s are among the sulfatidates.

c.-sulfatase, c. sulfatidase, an enzyme that cleaves sulfate from a sulfated glycosphingolipid (such as a cerebroside 3-sulfate).

cer·e·bro·si·do·sis (ser′ĕ-brō-sī-dō′sis). A lipidosis as in Gaucher *disease*.

cer·e·bro·spi·nal (ser′ĕ-brō-spī′năl, sĕ-rē′brō-). Relating to the brain and the spinal cord. SYN encephalorrhachidian, encephalospinal.

cer·e·bro·ste·rol (ser′ĕ-brō-stēr′ol). A hydroxylated cholesterol found in the brain and spinal cord.

cer·e·brot·o·my (ser-ĕ-brot′ō-mē). Incision of the brain. [cerebro- + G. *tomē*, incision]

cer·e·bro·vas·cu·lar (ser′ĕ-brō-vas′kū-lăr). Relating to the blood supply to the brain, particularly with reference to pathologic changes.

cer·e·brum, pl. **ce·re·bra**, **cer·e·brums** (ser′ĕ-brŭm, sĕ-rē′brŭm; -brä; -brŭmz) [TA]. Originally referred to the largest portion of the brain, including practically all parts within the skull except the medulla, pons, and cerebellum; it now usually refers only to the parts derived from the telencephalon and includes mainly the cerebral hemispheres (cerebral cortex and basal ganglia). [L., brain]

cere·cloth (sēr′kloth). Gauze or cheese cloth impregnated with wax containing an antiseptic; used in surgical dressings. [L. *cera*, wax]

Cerenkov, (Cherenkov) Pavel A., Russian physicist and Nobel laureate, *1904. SEE C. *radiation*.

cer·e·sin (ser′ĕ-sin). A natural mixture of hydrocarbons of high molecular weight; a substitute for beeswax, also used in dentistry for impressions. SYN cerin, cerosin, earth wax, mineral wax (2), purified ozokerite.

ce·rin (se′rin). SYN ceresin.

Cer·i·thid·ea (ser-i-thid′ē-ă). A genus of marine and brackish water operculate (prosobranch) snails that serve as first intermediate hosts of a number of trematodes. *C. cingulata* serves as host for *Heterophyes heterophyes* in Japan and Southeast Asia; *C. scalariformis* for cercariae that induce swimmer's itch in the southeastern U.S. from Florida to Texas.

ce·ri·um (Ce) (sēr′ē-ŭm). A metallic element, atomic no. 58, atomic wt. 140.115. [fr. *Ceres*, the planetoid]

c. oxalate, a mixture of the oxalates of c., lanthanum, and other rare earths; has been used in the treatment of vomiting.

△**cero-.** Wax. [L. *cera*, wax]

ce·roid (sē′royd). A waxlike, golden or yellow-brown pigment first found in fibrotic livers of choline-deficient rats, and also known to be present in some of the cirrhotic livers (and certain other tissues) of human beings. C. is acid fast, insoluble in fat solvents, and probably a type of lipofuscin, although differing from true lipofuscins by failing to stain with Schmorl ferric-ferricyanide reduction stain; it also exhibits autofluorescence. Accumulates in Hermansky-Pudlak syndrome. [L. *cera*, wax, + G. *eidos*, appearance]

ce·ro·plas·ty (sē′rō-plas-tē). The manufacture of wax models of anatomic and pathologic specimens or of skin lesions. [G. *kēros*, wax, + *plassō*, to mold]

cer·o·sin (ser′ō-sin). SYN ceresin.

ce·ro·tin·ic ac·id (ser-ō-tin′ik). A long-chain fatty acid found in natural waxes, wool fat, and certain lipids.

cer·ti·fi·a·ble (ser-ti-fī′ă-bl). Denoting a person showing disordered behavior of sufficient gravity to justify involuntary mental hospitalization.

cer·ti·fi·ca·tion (ser'ti-fi-kā'shŭn). **1.** Acknowledgment by a medical specialty board of successful completion of requirements for recognition as a specialist. **2.** The court procedure by which a patient is committed to a mental institution. **3.** Involuntary mental hospitalization.

cer·ti·fied nurse-mid·wife (C.N.M.). A registered nurse with at least a master's degree in nursing and advanced education in the management of the entire maternity cycle. Achieved through an organized program of study and national testing by the American College of Nurse-Midwives.

cer·ti·fy (ser'ti-fī). To commit a patient to a mental hospital in accordance with the laws of the state. [L. *certus,* certain, + *facio,* to make]

ce·ru·le·an (se-roo'lē-ăn). SYN blue. [L. *caeruleus,* blue, fr. *caelum,* sky]

ce·ru·le·in (se-roo'lē-in). A decapeptide with hypotensive activity; stimulates smooth muscle and increases digestive secretions; it is similar in structure to cholecystokinin and the gastrins, but much more potent as a stimulant to gallbladder contraction; also stimulates release of insulin. It inhibits fatty acid biosynthesis. [fr. *Cephalosporium caerulea,* from which isolated]

ce·ru·lo·plas·min (sĕ-roo'lō-plaz-min). A blue, copper-containing α-globulin of blood plasma, with a molecular weight of about 122,000 and 6 or 7 atoms of copper per molecule; involved in copper transport and regulation, and can reduce O_2 directly without known intermediates; has ferroxidase and polyamine oxidase activities. C. is absent in congenital Wilson disease. [L. *caeruleus,* dark blue]

ce·ru·men (sĕ-roo'men). The soft, brownish yellow, waxy secretion (a modified sebum) of the ceruminous glands of the external auditory meatus. SYN ear wax, earwax. [L. *cera,* wax]

c. inspissa'tum, inspissated c., dried earwax plugging the external auditory canal.

ce·ru·mi·nal (se-roo'mi-năl). Relating to cerumen.

ce·ru·mi·no·lyt·ic (sĕ-roo'mi-nō-lit'ik). One of several substances instilled into the external auditory canal to soften wax. [cerumen, + G. *lysis,* a loosening]

ce·ru·mi·no·ma (sĕ-roo-mi-nō'mă). A usually benign adenomatous tumor of ceruminous glands of the external auditory canal.

ce·ru·mi·no·sis (se-roo-mi-nō'sis). Excessive formation of cerumen.

ce·ru·mi·nous (sĕ-roo'mi-nŭs). Relating to cerumen.

ce·ruse (sē'roos). SYN lead carbonate. [L. *cerussa*]

cer·veau iso·lé (ser-vō' ē-so-lā'). An animal with its mesencephalon transected; it breathes spontaneously but is unresponsive, with abnormal pupils (usually dilated) and a continuous sleep pattern in the electroencephalogram. Cf. encéphale isolé. [Fr. detached brain]

cer·vi·cal (ser'vĭ-kal). Relating to a neck, or cervix, in any sense. SYN cervicalis. [L. *cervix (cervic-),* neck]

cer·vi·ca·lis (ser-vi-kā'lis). SYN cervical.

c. ascen'dens, (1) SYN iliocostalis cervicis *(muscle);* **(2)** SYN ascending cervical *artery.*

cer·vi·cec·to·my (ser-vi-sek'tō-mē). Excision of the cervix uteri. SYN trachelectomy. [cervix + G. *ektomē,* excision]

cer·vi·ces (ser'vi-sēz). Plural of cervix.

cer·vi·ci·tis (ser-vi-sī'tis). Inflammation of the mucous membrane, frequently involving also the deeper structures, of the cervix uteri. SYN trachelitis.

♻**cervico-.** A cervix, or neck, in any sense. [L. *cervix,* neck]

cer·vi·co·brach·i·al (ser'vi-kō-brā'kē-ăl). Relating to the neck and the arm.

cer·vi·co·buc·cal (ser'vi-kō-bŭk'ăl). Relating to the buccal region of the neck of a premolar or molar tooth.

cer·vi·co·dyn·ia (ser'vi-kō-din'ē-ă). Neck pain. [cervico- + G. *odynē,* pain]

cer·vi·co·fa·cial (ser'vi-kō-fā'shăl). Relating to the neck and the face.

cer·vi·cog·ra·phy (ser-vi-kog'ră-fē). Technique, equivalent to colposcopy, for photographing part or all of the uterine cervix. [cervix + G. *graphō,* to write]

cer·vi·co·la·bi·al (ser'vi-kō-lā'bē-ăl). Relating to the labial region of the neck of an incisor or canine tooth.

cer·vi·co·lin·gual (ser'vi-kō-ling'gwăl). Relating to the lingual region of the cervix of a tooth.

cer·vi·co·lin·guo·ax·i·al (ser'vi-kō-ling'gwō-ak'sē-ăl). Referring to the point angle formed by the junction of the cervical (gingival), lingual, and axial walls of a cavity.

cer·vi·co·oc·cip·i·tal (ser'vi-kō-ok-sip'i-tăl). Relating to the neck and the occiput.

cer·vi·co·plas·ty (ser'vi-kō-plas-tē). Rearrangement of tissue of the cervix uteri or the neck.

cervicoscopy. SYN visual inspection with acetic acid.

cer·vi·co·tho·rac·ic (ser'vi-kō-thōr-as'ik). Relating to: **1.** The neck and thorax; **2.** The transition between the neck and thorax; **3.** The fusion of these vertebrae.

cer·vi·cot·o·my (ser-vi-kot'ō-mē). Incision into the cervix uteri. SYN trachelotomy. [cervico- + G. *tomē,* incision]

cer·vi·co·ves·i·cal (ser'vi-kō-ves'i-kăl). Relating to the cervix of the uterus and the bladder.

cer·vi·lax·in. SYN relaxin.

cer·vix, gen. **cer·vi·cis,** pl. **cer·vi·ces** (ser'viks, ser-vī'sis, -sēz) [TA]. **1.** SYN neck. **2.** Any necklike structure. **3.** SYN c. of uterus. [L. neck]

c. of the axon, the constricted portion of the axon just before the myelin sheath begins.

c. colum'nae posterio'ris, a slight constriction of the posterior gray column of the spinal cord, seen on cross-section just behind the gray commissure.

c. den'tis [TA], SYN *neck* of tooth.

strawberry c., macular erythema of the uterine cervix, characteristic of vaginitis due to *Trichomonas vaginalis.*

c. of tooth, ✶official alternate term for *neck* of tooth.

c. u'teri [TA], SYN c. of uterus.

c. of uterus [TA], the lower part of the uterus extending from the isthmus of the uterus into the vagina. It is divided into supravaginal and vaginal parts by its passage through the vaginal wall. SYN c. uteri [TA], cervix (3) [TA], neck of uterus, neck of womb.

c. vesi'cae urina'riae [TA], SYN *neck* of (urinary) bladder.

ce·ryl (sēr'il). The hydrocarbon radical $C_{26}H_{53}-$ of ceryl alcohol (hexacosanol). SYN hexacosyl.

ce·sar·e·an (se-zā'rē-ăn). Denoting a c. section, which was included under *lex cesarea,* Roman law (715 B.C.); not because performed at the birth of Julius Caesar (100 B.C.).

ce·si·um (Cs) (sē'zē-ŭm). A metallic element, atomic no. 55, atomic wt. 132.90543; a member of the alkali metal group. ^{137}Cs (half-life equal to 30.1 years) is used in the treatment of certain malignancies. [L. *caesius,* bluish gray]

Cestan, Raymond, French neurologist, 1872–1934. SEE C.-Chenais *syndrome.*

Ces·to·da (ses-tō'dă). A subclass of tapeworms (class Cestoidea), containing the typical members of this group, including the segmented tapeworms that parasitize humans and domestic animals. SYN Eucestoda. [G. *kestos,* girdle]

Ces·to·dar·ia (ses-tō-dā'rē-ă). A subclass of the class Cestoidea, containing tapeworms that lack a scolex and are unsegmented (monozoic), in contrast to the typical tapeworms in the subclass Cestoda; larvae of c. (called lycophora) characteristically have 10 hooklets rather than six. C. are believed to be primitive tapeworms, parasitizing the intestine and celomic cavities of certain fish and a few reptiles.

ces·tode, ces·toid (ses'tōd, -toyd). Common name for tapeworms of the class Cestoidea or its subclasses, Cestoda and Cestodaria.

ces·to·di·a·sis (ses-tō-dī'ă-sis). Disease caused by infection with a cestode.

Ces·toi·dea (ses-toy'dē-ă). The tapeworms, a class of platyhelminth flatworms characterized by lack of an alimentary canal and, in typical forms (subclass Cestoda), by a segmented body with a scolex or holdfast organ at one end; adult worms are vertebrate parasites, usually found in the small intestine. [G. *kestos,* girdle, + *eidos,* form]

ce·ta·ce·um (sĕ-tā′shē-ŭm). SYN spermaceti. [G. *kētos,* a whale]

cet·al·ko·ni·um chlo·ride (set′al-kō′nē-ŭm). An antibacterial agent.

cet·hex·o·ni·um bro·mide (set-heks-ō′nē-ŭm). An antiseptic.

ce·to·ste·a·ryl al·co·hol (se-tō-stē′ă-ril). A component of the hydrophilic ointment ingredient known as emulsifying wax; a mixture of solid aliphatic alcohols consisting chiefly of stearyl and cetyl alcohols.

ce·trar·ia (se-trā′rē-ă). The dried plant, *Cetraria islandica* (family Parmeliaceae), a lichen, not a moss, used as a demulcent and as a folk remedy for bronchitis. SYN Iceland moss. [L. *caetra,* a short Spanish shield (from shape of the apothecia)]

ce·tri·mo·ni·um bro·mide (se-trī-mō′nē-ŭm). An antiseptic.

ce·tyl (sē′til). The univalent radical $C_{16}H_{33}-$ of cetyl alcohol.

c. alcohol, the 16-carbon alcohol corresponding to palmitic acid, so called because it is isolated from among the hydrolysis products of spermaceti; it is used as an emulsifying aid and in the preparation of "washable" (oil in water emulsions) ointment bases. SYN 1-hexadecanol, palmityl alcohol.

c. palmitate, a wax; the chief constituent of spermaceti.

ce·tyl·pyr·i·din·i·um chlo·ride (sē′til-pī-ri-din′ē-ŭm). The monohydrate of the quaternary salt of pyridine and cetyl chloride; a cationic detergent with antiseptic action against nonsporulating bacteria.

ce·tyl·tri·meth·yl·am·mo·ni·um bro·mide (sē′til-trī-me′thil-ă-mō′nē-ŭm). A mixture of dodecyl-, tetradecyl-, and hexadecyl-trimethylammonium bromides; an odorless surface-active agent, readily soluble in water; a disinfectant with a strong bacteriostatic action, used for the sterilization of instruments and utensils.

cev·a·dil·la (se-vă-dil′ă). SYN sabadilla. [Sp. dim. of *cebada,* barley]

cev·a·dine (sev′ă-dēn). An alkaloid occurring in the seeds of *Schoenocaulon officinale* (*Sabadilla officinarum*), family Liliaceae; highly irritating to skin and mucous membranes. SEE ALSO veratrine.

ce·vi·tam·ic ac·id (sev-i-tam′ik). SYN ascorbic acid.

CF Abbreviation for citrovorum *factor;* coupling factor.

Cf Symbol for californium.

CFF Abbreviation for critical fusion frequency. SEE critical flicker fusion *frequency.*

CG Abbreviation for chorionic *gonadotropin;* phosgene.

CGA Abbreviation for catabolite gene *activator.*

cGMP Abbreviation for cyclic *guanosine* 3′,5′-monophosphate.

CGP Abbreviation for chorionic "growth *hormone*-prolactin".

CGRP Abbreviation for calcitonin gene-related *peptide.*

CGS, cgs Abbreviation for centimeter-gram-second. SEE centimeter-gram-second *system,* centimeter-gram-second *unit.*

CH Abbreviation for crown-heel *length.*

Chaddock, Charles G., U.S. neurologist, 1861–1936. SEE C. *reflex, sign.*

Chadwick, James R., U.S. gynecologist, 1844–1905. SEE C. *sign.*

chae·ta (kē′tă). SYN seta. [Mod. L. fr. G. *chaitē,* stiff hair]

chafe (chāf). To cause irritation of the skin by friction. [Fr. *chauffer,* to heat, fr. L. *calefacio,* to make warm]

Chagas, Carlos, Brazilian physician, 1879–1934. SEE C. *disease;* C.-Cruz *disease.*

cha·go·ma (sha-gō′mă). Small granuloma in the skin caused by early multiplication of *Trypanosoma cruzi* (Chagas disease).

chain (chān). **1.** In chemistry, a series of atoms held together by one or more covalent bonds. **2.** In bacteriology, a linear arrangement of living cells that have divided in one plane and remain attached to each other. **3.** A series of reactions. **4.** In anatomy, a linked series of structures, e.g., ossicular c., chain *ganglia,* under *ganglion.* SEE ALSO sympathetic *trunk.* [L. *catena*]

A c., (1) the shorter polypeptide component of insulin containing 21 amino acyl residues, beginning with a glycyl residue (NH$_2$-

terminus); insulin is formed by the linkage of an A c. to a B c. by two disulfide bonds; the amino-acid composition of the A c. is a function of species; (2) in general, one of the polypeptides in a multiprotein complex.

B c., (1) the longer polypeptide component of insulin containing 30 amino acyl residues, beginning with a phenylalanyl residue (NH$_2$-terminus); insulin is formed by the linkage of a B c. to an A c. by two disulfide bonds; the amino acid composition of the B c. is a function of species; (2) the light chain of an immunoglobulin.

behavior c., related behaviors in a series in which each response serves as a stimulus for the next response.

C c., SYN C-peptide.

cold c., a system of protection against high environmental temperatures for heat-labile vaccines, sera, and other biological preparations.

electron-transport c., SYN respiratory c.

ganglionic c., SYN sympathetic *trunk.*

heavy c., a polypeptide c. of high molecular weight (about 400–500 amino acyl residues), as the γ, α, μ, δ, or ε c.'s in immunoglobulin, determining the immunoglobulin class and subclass. This chain also determines if complement can be bound and if the chain can pass through the placenta. There are two identical chains in each immunoglobulin. SYN H chain.

J c., a glycopeptide, cysteine-rich polypeptide that is bonded to polymeric IgA and IgM; its function is to ensure correct polymerization of the subunits of IgA and IgM and to be secreted externally. [*joining* chain]

L c., SYN light c.

light c., a polypeptide c. of low molecular weight (about 200 amino acyl residues), as the κ or λ c.'s in immunoglobulin. There are two identical light c.'s in each immunoglobulin monomer. SYN L c.

long c., in bacteriology, a continuous line of more than eight cells.

ossicular c., SYN auditory *ossicles,* under *ossicle.*

respiratory c., a sequence of energy-liberating oxidation-reduction reactions whereby electrons are accepted from reduced compounds and eventually transferred to oxygen with the formation of water. SYN cytochrome system, electron-transport c., electron-transport system.

short c., in bacteriology, a string of two to eight cells.

side c., (1) a c. of noncyclic atoms linked to a benzene ring, or to any cyclic c. compound; (2) the atoms of an α-amino acid other than the α-carboxyl group, the α-amino group, the α-carbon, and the hydrogen attached to the α-carbon.

chain·ing (chān′ing). Learning related behaviors in a series in which each response serves as a stimulus for the next response.

cha·la·sia, cha·la·sis (kă-lā′zē-ă, -lā′sis). Inhibition and relaxation of any previously sustained contraction of muscle, usually of a synergic group of muscles. [G. *chalaō,* to loosen]

cha·la·za (kă-lā′ză). **1.** SYN chalazion. **2.** Suspensory ligament of the yolk in a bird's egg. [G. hail; a small tubercle, a sty (Galen)]

cha·la·zi·on, pl. **cha·la·zia** (ka-lā′zē-on, -zē-ă). A chronic inflammatory granuloma of a meibomian gland. SYN chalaza (1), meibomian cyst, tarsal cyst. [G. dim. of *chalaza,* a sty]

acute c., SYN hordeolum internum.

collar-stud c., a c. that extends through the tarsal plate anteriorly (c. externum) and toward the conjunctiva.

chal·cone (kal′kōn). The parent compound of a series of plant pigments. All are flavonoids and typically are yellow to orange in color. SYN benzalacetophenone.

chal·co·sis (kal-kō′sis). Chronic copper poisoning. SYN chalkitis. [G. *chalkos,* copper, brass]

c. len·tis, a cataract caused by excessive intraocular copper. SYN copper cataract, sunflower cataract.

chal·i·co·sis (kal-i-kō′sis). Pneumoconiosis caused by the inhalation of dust incident to the occupation of stone cutting. SYN flint disease. [G. *chalix,* gravel]

chalk (chawk). SYN *calcium* carbonate. [L. *calx*]

French c., SYN talc.

prepared c., purified native calcium carbonate, usually molded into cones; used as a mild astringent and antacid.

chal·ki·tis (kal-kī′tis). SYN chalcosis. [G. *chalkos,* copper, brass]

cha·lone (kā′lōn). Originally, a hormone (e.g., enterogastrone) that inhibits rather than stimulates; now, any one of a number of mitotic inhibitors (often glycoproteins) elaborated by a tissue and active only on that type of tissue, regardless of species; thus, a reversible tissue-specific mitotic inhibitor. [G. + *chalaō,* to relax, + -one]

cha·ly·be·ate (kal-ib′ē-āt). Obsolete term for impregnated with or containing iron salts and for a therapeutic agent containing iron. [G. *chalyps* (*chalyb-*), steel]

cham·ber (chām′ber) [TA]. A compartment or enclosed space. SEE ALSO camera. [L. *camera*]

altitude c., a decompression c. for simulating a high altitude environment, particularly its low barometric pressure. SYN high altitude c.

anechoic c., a room designed to absorb all sound so as to eliminate all echoes; used for research on hearing and sensory deprivation.

anterior c. of eyeball [TA], the space between the cornea anteriorly and the iris/pupil posteriorly, filled with a watery fluid (aqueous humor) and communicating through the pupil with the posterior chamber. SYN camera anterior bulbi [TA], camera (1) [TA], camera oculi anterior, camera oculi major.

aqueous c.'s, the combined anterior and posterior c.'s of the eye containing the aqueous humor. SEE anterior c. of eyeball, posterior c. of eyeball; SEE ALSO anterior *segment*.

▣ **counting c.,** a device for counting microscopic objects suspended in fluid, as cells and platelets in dilute whole blood or bacteria in broth culture. It consists of a microscope slide containing a shallow cavity of uniform depth whose floor is ruled with a grid and which, when closed with a cover glass, holds a precise volume of fluid. A calculation based on the number of objects counted within the grid lines, the dilution of the fluid, and the volume of the counting c. yields an estimate of the concentration of objects in the fluid before dilution. SEE ALSO hemocytometer.

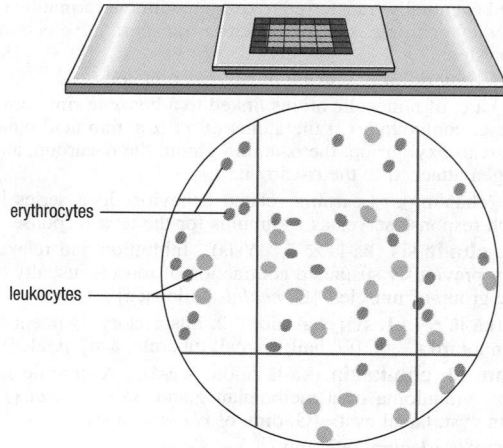

erythrocytes

leukocytes

Zappert counting chamber: (top) slide containing chamber, (bottom) view as seen through microscope

decompression c., a c. for exposing organisms to pressures below that of the atmosphere.

c.'s of eyeball [TA], the cavities within the eyeball: anterior and posterior c.'s, filled with aqueous, and the postremal (vitreous) chamber, occupied by the vitreous. SEE ALSO anterior c. of eyeball, posterior c. of eyeball, postremal c. of eyeball. SYN camerae bulbi [TA].

high altitude c., SYN altitude c.

hyperbaric c., a c. providing pressures greater than atmospheric, commonly used to treat decompression sickness and to provide hyperbaric oxygenation.

ionization c., a c. for detecting ionization of the enclosed gas;

used for determining intensity of ionizing radiation. SEE ALSO Geiger-Müller *counter.*

posterior c. of eyeball, the ringlike space, filled with aqueous humor, between the iris/pupil anteriorly and the lens and ciliary body posteriorly. SYN camera posterior bulbi [TA], camera oculi minor, camera oculi posterior.

postremal c. of eyeball [TA], the large space between the lens and the retina; it is filled with the vitreous body. SYN camera postrema [TA], camera vitrea bulbi✶, camera vitrea✶, vitreous c.✶, posterior segment of eyeball, vitreous camera, vitreous c. of eye.

pulp c., that portion of the pulp cavity which is contained in the crown or body of the tooth.

relief c., a recess in the impression surface of a denture to reduce or eliminate pressure from that specific area of the mouth.

Sandison-Clark c., a c. that can be fitted over a hole punched in a rabbit's ear, so that tissue will grow to fill the defect between two transparent plates; if the distance between the plates is small, the living tissue can be studied microscopically.

sinuatrial c., the common c. formed by the single embryonic atrium and the right and left horns of the sinus venosus.

vitreous c., ✶official alternate term for postremal c. of eyeball.

vitreous c. of eye, SYN postremal c. of eyeball.

Zappert counting c., a special, standardized glass slide used for counting cells (especially erythrocytes and leukocytes) and other particulate material in a measured volume of fluid; the central portion is precisely ground in such a manner that the uniformly flat surface is exactly 0.1 mm lower than that of two parallel ridges on which a special, uniformly flat coverslip may be placed; accurately etched lines on the flat central portion form the boundaries of groups of squares of known areas, thereby providing the basis for determining the volume of fluid in which the cells are counted. Glass slides of this type are frequently known as hemocytometers.

Chamberlain, W. Edward, U.S. radiologist, 1891–1947. SEE C. *line.*

Chamberlen, Peter, English obstetrician, 1560–1631. SEE C. *forceps.*

cham·e·ce·phal·ic (kam-ĕ-se-fal′ik). Having a flat head; denoting a skull with a vertical index of 70 or less; similar to tapinocephalic. SYN chamecephalous. [G. *chamai,* on the ground (low, stunted), + *kephalē,* head]

cham·e·ceph·a·lous (kam-ĕ-sef′ă-lus). SYN chamecephalic.

cham·e·pro·sop·ic (kam′ĕ-prō-sop′ik). Having a broad face. [G. *chamai* (adv.), on the ground (low, spread out), + *prosōpikos,* facial]

cham·fer (sham′fer). A marginal finish on an extracoronal cavity preparation of a tooth which describes a curve from an axial wall to the cavosurface. [fr. O.Fr. *chanfrein*(t), beveled edge]

cham·o·mile (kam′ō-mīl). The flowering heads of *Anthemis nobilis* (family Compositae); a stomachic. SYN camomile. [G. *chamaimēlon,* chamomile, fr. *chamai,* on the ground, + *mēlon,* apple]

Champy, Christian, French physician, *1885. SEE C. *fixative.*

Chanarin, I., 20th century British hematologist. SEE Dorfman-C. *syndrome.*

Chance, G.Q., 20th century British radiologist. SEE C. *fracture.*

chan·cre (shan′ker). The primary lesion of syphilis, which begins at the site of cutaneous or mucosal infection after an interval of 10–30 days as a papule or area of infiltration, of dull red color, hard, and insensitive; the center usually becomes eroded or breaks down into an ulcer that heals slowly after 4–6 weeks. Finding *Treponema pallidum* on dark-field examination is diagnostic, except in oral ulcers, in which *T. microdentium* is normally present. SYN hard c., hard sore, hard ulcer, syphilitic ulcer (1). [Fr. indirectly from L. *cancer*]

hard c., SYN chancre.

mixed c., a sore resulting from simultaneous inoculation of a site with syphilis and chancroid.

monorecidive c., a c. that recurs at the site of a previously healed lesion.

c. re′dux, a second c. occurring in a syphilitic subject, possibly an allergic reaction without the presence of the specific spirochete.

soft c., SYN chancroid.

sporotrichositic c., the initial lesion at the site of skin infection in sporotrichosis.

tularemic c., the primary lesion, usually of finger, thumb, or hand, in tularemia.

chan·cri·form (shang′kri-fōrm). Resembling chancre.

chan·croid (shang′kroyd). An infectious, painful, ragged venereal ulcer at the site of infection by *Haemophilus ducreyi,* beginning after an incubation period of 3–7 days; seen more commonly in men; Gram-negative streptobacilli may be identified by staining material from the ulcer. SYN soft chancre, soft sore, soft ulcer, venereal sore, venereal ulcer. [chancre + G. *eidos,* resemblance]

chan·croi·dal (shang-kroy′dăl). Relating to or of the nature of chancroid.

chan·crous (shang′krŭs). Characterized by having a chancre.

Chandler, Paul A., U.S. ophthalmologist, *1896. SEE C. *syndrome.*

change (chānj). An alteration; in pathology, structural alteration of which the cause and significance is uncertain. SYN shift.

Armanni-Ebstein c., SYN Armanni-Ebstein *kidney.*

Baggenstoss c., distention of pancreatic acini by proteinaceous secretion, seen in dehydration.

Crooke hyaline c., replacement of cytoplasmic granules of basophil cells of the anterior pituitary by homogeneous hyaline material; a characteristic finding in Cushing syndrome, but usually not present in the cells of a basophil adenoma. SYN Crooke hyaline degeneration.

fatty c., SYN fatty *metamorphosis.*

c. of life, colloquialism for (1) menopause; (2) climacteric.

reactive c.'s, term in the Bethesda classification system for reporting cervical/vaginal cytologic diagnosis that refers to c.'s benign in nature, associated with inflammation (including typical repair), atrophy with inflammation, radiation, an intrauterine device, and other nonspecific causes. SEE ALSO Bethesda *system,* AGUS, LSIL, HSIL.

trophic c.'s, changes resulting from interruption of nerve supply. SEE ALSO neurotrophic *atrophy.*

Changeux, Jean-Pierre, French 20th century biochemist. SEE Monod-Wyman-Changeux *model.*

chan·nel (chan′ĕl). A furrow, gutter, or groovelike passageway. SEE ALSO canal. [L. *canalis*]

ion c., a specific macromolecular protein pathway, with an aqueous "pore," that traverses the lipid bilayer of a cell's plasma membrane and maintains or modulates the electrical potential across this barrier by allowing controlled influx or exit of small inorganic ions such as Na^+, K^+, Cl^-, and Ca^{2+}. It plays an important role in propagation of the action potential in neurons, but also may control transduction of extracellular signals and contraction in muscle cells. In general, ion c.'s are characterized by their selectivity for certain ions, their specific regulation or gating of these ions, and their specific sensitivity to toxins.

ligand-gated c., a class of ion c.'s whose ionic permeability is regulated by cell membrane receptors that respond to specific extracellular chemical signals.

transnexus c., a hexagonal 15–20Å hydrophilic c. capable of transporting small ions between cardiac muscle cells.

voltage-gated c., a class of ion c.'s that open and close in response to change in the electrical potential across the plasma membrane of the cell; voltage-gated Na^+ c.'s are important for conducting action potential along nerve cell processes.

channelopathies (chan-el-op′ath-ēz). SYN ion channel *disorders,* under *disorder.* [channel + G. *pathos,* disease]

Chantemesse, André, French bacteriologist, 1851–1919. SEE C. *reaction.*

cha·os (kā′ŏs). 1. State of such total disorganization that it has no constructive predicates. 2. A state in which no causal relationships are operating. [G., primeval formless void]

mathematical c., a dynamic system so sensitive to its precise current state (which in practice will never be known exactly) that

its behavior, though deterministic, is indistinguishable from random.

cha·o·tro·pic (kā-ō-trōp′ik). Pertaining to chaotropism.

cha·o·tro·pism (kā-ō-trōp′izm). The property of certain substances, usually ions (e.g., SCN^-, ClO_4^-, guanidinium), to disrupt the structure of water and thereby promote the solubility of nonpolar substances in polar solvents (e.g., water), the unfolding of proteins, the elution from or movement through a chromatographic medium of an otherwise tightly bound substance, etc. [G. *chaos,* disorder, confusion, + *tropē,* a turning]

CHAP Acronym for cyclophosphamide, hexamethylmelamine, doxorubicin (Adriamycin), and cisplatin, a chemotherapy regimen used in the treatment of ovarian cancer.

cha·pe·rone (shap-ĕ-rōn). 1. A protein required for the proper folding and/or assembly of another protein or protein complex. 2. One who accompanies a physician during examination of a patient of the opposite sex (from the physician). [Eng. escort, protector, fr. Fr. *chaperon,* hood, fr. *chape,* cape, fr. L.L. *cappa,* fr. L. *caput,* head]

chap·pa (chap′pǎ). A disease marked by subcutaneous nodules, the size of a pigeon's egg, which break down, release a fatty looking material, and form ulcers; the eruption is preceded by severe muscular and articular pains. [W. Af.]

chapped (chapt). Having or pertaining to skin, especially of the hands, that is dry, scaly, and fissured, owing to the action of cold or to the excess rate of evaporation of moisture from the skin surface. SEE hand *eczema.* [M.E. *chap,* to chop, split]

char·ac·ter (kar′ak-ter). An attribute in individuals that is amenable to formal and logical analysis and may be used as the basis of generalizations about classes and other statements that transcend individuality. SYN characteristic (1). [G. *charakter,* stamp, mark, fr. *charassō,* to engrave]

acquired c., a c. developed in a plant or animal as a result of environmental influences during the individual's life.

classifiable c., a c. that allows individuals to be sorted into distinct but not quantitative classes, e.g., blood types.

compound c., an inherited c. dependent upon two or more distinct genes.

denumerable c., classifiable c. that is also countable (e.g., number of progeny, number of teeth). SYN discrete c.

discrete c., SYN denumerable c.

dominant c., an inherited c. determined by one kind of allele. SEE phenotype.

inherited c., a discrete attribute of an animal or plant that is transmitted at one genetic locus from generation to generation in accordance with Mendel law. SEE gene. SYN unit c.

mendelian c., an inherited c. under the control of a single locus (although perhaps modified by genes at other loci).

primary sex c.'s, the sex glands, testes or ovaries, and the accessory sex organs.

recessive c., an inherited c. determined by an allele in homozygous state only. SEE *dominance* of traits.

secondary sex c.'s, those c.'s peculiar to the male or female that develop at puberty, e.g., men's beards and women's breasts.

sex-linked c., an inherited c. determined by a gene on a gonosome. SEE gene.

unit c., SYN inherited c.

char·ac·ter ar·mor. A habitual pattern of organized defenses against anxiety.

char·ac·ter·is·tic (kar′ak-ter-is′tik). 1. SYN character. 2. Typical or distinctive of a particular disorder.

receiver operating c. (ROC), a plot of the sensitivity of a diagnostic test as a function of nonspecificity (one minus the specificity). The ROC curve indicates the intrinsic properties of a test's diagnostic performance and can be used to compare the relative merits of competing procedures.

char·ac·ter·i·za·tion (kar′ak-ter-i-zā′shŭn). The discernment, description, or attributing of distinguishing traits.

denture c., modification of the form and color of the denture base and/or teeth to produce a more lifelike appearance.

cha·ras (char′as). A resin obtained from mature leaves of selected varieties of *Cannabis sativa;* used for smoking.

char·bon (shar-bawn′). SYN anthrax (2). [Fr. coal]

char·coal (char′kōl). Carbon obtained by heating or burning wood with restricted access of air. SYN carbo.

activated c., the residue from the destructive distillation of various organic materials, treated to increase its adsorptive power; used in diarrhea, as an antidote in various forms of poisoning, and in purification processes in industry and research. SYN medicinal c.

animal c., c. produced by incomplete combustion of animal tissues, especially bone. SYN animal black, bone black, bone c.

bone c., SYN animal c.

medicinal c., SYN activated c.

vegetable c., c. obtained by charring vegetable tissues, especially the wood of willow, beech, birch, or oak. SYN wood c.

wood c., SYN vegetable c.

Charcot, Jean M., French neurologist, 1825–1893. SEE C. *arteries, disease,* intermittent *fever, gait, joint, syndrome, triad, vertigo;* C.-Leyden *crystals,* under *crystal;* C.-Neumann *crystals,* under *crystal;* C.-Robin *crystals,* under *crystal;* C.-Böttcher *crystalloids,* under *crystalloid;* C.-Marie-Tooth *disease;* C.-Weiss-Baker *syndrome;* Erb-C. *disease.*

Chargaff, Erwin, Austrian-U.S. biochemist, *1905. SEE C. *rule.*

charge trans·fer. SEE charge transfer *complex.*

char·la·tan (shar′lă-tan). A medical fraud claiming to cure disease by useless procedures, secret remedies, and worthless diagnostic and therapeutic machines. SYN quack. [Fr., fr. It. *ciarlare,* to prattle]

char·la·tan·ism (shar′lă-tan-izm). A fraudulent claim to medical knowledge; treating the sick without knowledge of medicine or authority to practice medicine. SYN quackery.

Charles, Jacques, French physicist, 1746–1823. SEE C. *law.*

char·ley horse (char′lē hōrs). Localized pain or muscle stiffness following a contusion of a muscle. [slang]

Charlton, Willy, German physician, *1889. SEE Schultz-C. *phenomenon, reaction.*

Charnley, Sir John, English orthopedic surgeon, 1911–1982. SEE C. hip *arthroplasty.*

Charrière, Joseph F.B., French instrument maker, 1803–1876. SEE C. *scale.*

🔲**chart. 1.** A recording of clinical data relating to a patient's case. **2.** SYN curve (2). **3.** In optics, symbols of graduated size for measuring visual acuity, or test types for determining far or near vision. SEE Snellen *test types.* [L. *charta,* sheet of papyrus]

Amsler c., a 10-cm square divided into 5-mm squares upon which an individual may project a defect in the central visual field. SYN Amsler grid.

isometric c., a c. or graph that displays three dimensions on a plane surface.

Levey-Jennings c., SYN quality control c.

Pickles c., day-by-day plots of new cases of infectious disease used to demonstrate the progress of an epidemic in a small, relatively isolated population.

quality control c., a c. illustrating the allowable limits of error in laboratory test performance, the limits being a defined deviation from the mean of a control serum, most commonly ±2 SD. SEE ALSO quality *control.* SYN Levey-Jennings c.

Tanner growth c., a series of c.'s showing distribution of parameters of physical development, such as stature, growth curves, and skinfold thickness, for children by sex, age, and stages of puberty.

Walker c., a system of plotting the relative fetal and placental sizes.

Charters, W.J., U.S. dentist. SEE C. *method.*

chart·ing. Making a record in tabular or graph form of the progress of a patient's condition. SYN clinical recording.

Chassaignac, Edouard P.M., French surgeon, 1804–1879. SEE C. *space, tubercle.*

Chaudhry, Anand P. SEE Gorlin-C.-Moss *syndrome.*

Chauffard, Anatole M.E., French physician, 1855–1932. SEE C. *syndrome;* Still-C. *syndrome.*

chaul·moo·gra oil (chawl-moo′grä). The fixed oil expressed from seeds of *Taraktogenos kurzii* and *Hydnocarpus wightiana* (family Flacourtiaceae); formerly used in the treatment of leprosy. SYN gynocardia oil, hydnocarpus oil.

Chaussier, François, French physician, 1746–1828. SEE C. *line, sign.*

Chayes, Herman E.S., U.S. prosthodontist, 1880–1933. SEE C. *method.*

Ch.B. Abbreviation for *Chirurgiae Baccalaureus,* Bachelor of Surgery.

Ch.D. Abbreviation for *Chirurgiae Doctor,* Doctor of Surgery.

Cheadle, Walter B., English pediatrician, 1835–1910. SEE C. *disease.*

Cheatle, Sir George L., British surgeon, 1865–1951. SEE C. *slit.*

Δ **check.** SYN *delta* check.

check·bite (chek′bīt). SYN interocclusal *record.*

check·er·ber·ry oil (chek′er-bār′ē). SYN methyl salicylate.

Chédiak, Moisés, 20th century Cuban physician. SEE C.-Higashi *disease;* C.-Steinbrinck-Higashi *anomaly, syndrome.*

cheek (chēk). The side of the face forming the lateral wall of the mouth. SYN bucca, gena, mala (1). [A. S. *ceáce*]

△**cheil-.** SEE cheilo-.

chei·lal·gia, chi·lal·gia (kī-lal′jē-ă). Pain in the lip. [cheil- + G. *algos,* pain]

chei·lec·to·my, chi·lec·to·my (kī-lek′tō-mē). **1.** Excision of a portion of the lip. **2.** Chiseling away bony irregularities at osteochondral margin of a joint cavity that interfere with movements of the joint. [cheil- + G. *ektomē,* excision]

cheil·ec·tro·pi·on, chil·ec·tro·pi·on (kī-lek-trō′pē-on). Eversion of the lips or a lip. [cheil- + G. *ektropos,* a turning out]

chei·li·on (kī′lē-on). A cephalometric point located at the angle (corner) of the mouth. [G. *cheilos,* lips]

chei·li·tis, chi·li·tis (kī-lī′tis). Inflammation of the lips or of a lip. SEE ALSO cheilosis. [cheil- + G. *-itis,* inflammation]

actinic c., SYN solar c.

angular c., inflammation and fissuring radiating from the commissures of the mouth secondary to predisposing factors such as lost vertical dimension in denture wearers, nutritional deficiencies, atopic dermatitis, or *Candida albicans* infection. SYN angular stomatitis, commissural c., perlèche.

commissural c., SYN angular c.

contact c., inflammation of the lips resulting from contact with a primary irritant or specific allergen, including ingredients of lipsticks. SYN c. venenata.

🔲**c. exfoliati′va,** an exfoliative dermatitis; it may be related to atopic dermatitis or to contact sensitivity.

c. glandula′ris, an acquired disorder, of unknown etiology, of the lower lip characterized by swelling, ulceration, crusting, mucous gland hyperplasia, abscesses, and sinus tracts. SYN Baelz disease, myxadenitis labialis, Volkmann c.

c. granulomato′sa, chronic, diffuse, soft swelling of the lips, of unknown etiology, microscopically characterized by noncaseating granulomatous inflammation. SEE ALSO Melkersson-Rosenthal *syndrome.* SYN Meischer syndrome.

impetiginous c., pyoderma of the lips with yellow crusts due to *Staphylococcus aureus* or streptococcal infection.

solar c., mucosal atrophy with drying, crusting, and fissuring of the vermilion border of the lower lip in older fair-skinned individuals, resulting from chronic exposure to sunlight; dysplastic (premalignant) changes are noted microscopically, analogous to solar keratosis. SYN actinic c.

c. venena′ta, SYN contact c.

Volkmann c., SYN c. glandularis.

△**cheilo-, cheil-.** Lips. SEE ALSO chilo-, labio-. [G. *cheilos,* lip]

chei·lo·gnath·o·glos·sos·chi·sis (kī′lō-nath′ō-glos-os′ki-sis). Associated condition of cleft mandible and lower lip, and bifid tongue. [cheilo- + G. *gnathos,* jaw, + *glōssa,* tongue, + *schisis,* cleft]

chei·lo·gnath·o·pal·a·tos·chi·sis (kī′lō-nath′ō-pal-ă-tos′ki-sis). SYN cheilognathouranoschisis.

chei·lo·gnath·o·u·ra·nos·chi·sis (kī-lō-nath′ō-ū-ră-nos′ki-sis). Cleft lip with cleft upper jaw and palate. SYN cheilognathopalatoschisis. [cheilo- + G. *gnathos,* jaw, + *ouranos,* sky (roof of mouth), + *schisis,* cleft]

chei·lo·pha·gia, chi·lo·pha·gia (kī-lō-fā′jē-ă). Biting of the lips. [cheilo- + G. *phagō,* to eat]

chei·lo·plas·ty (kī′lō-plas-tē). Old term for plastic surgery of the lips. [cheilo- + G. *plastos,* formed]

chei·lor·rha·phy (kī-lōr′ă-fē). Suturing of the lip. [cheilo- + G. *rhaphē,* suture]

chei·lo·sis, chi·lo·sis (kī-lō′sis). A condition characterized by dry scaling and fissuring of the lips, attributed by some to riboflavin and other nutritional deficiencies. SEE ALSO cheilitis. [cheil- + G. *-osis,* condition]

chei·lot·o·my (kī-lot′ō-mē). Incision into the lip. [cheilo- + G. *tomē,* incision]

♻**cheir-.** SEE cheiro-.

cheiralgia (kīr-al′jē-ă, -jya). Obsolete term for pain and paresthesia in the hand.

   c. paresthetica, compression neuropathy of the superficial branch of the radial nerve, marked by pain and paresthesia over the course of the nerve.

chei·rar·thri·tis (kī′rar-thrī′tis). Obsolete term for inflammation of the joints of the hand. SYN chirarthritis. [cheir- + arthritis]

♻**cheiro-, cheir-.** Hand. SEE ALSO chiro-. [G. *cheir,* a hand]

chei·rog·nos·tic (kī′rog-nos′tik). Able to distinguish between right and left, as of the hands or of which side of the body is touched. SYN chirognostic. [cheiro- + G. *gnostikos,* perceptive]

chei·ro·kin·es·the·sia (kī′rō-kin-es-thē′zē-ă). The subjective sensation of movement of the hands. SYN chirokinesthesia. [cheiro- + G. *kinēsis,* movement, + *aisthēsis,* sensation]

chei·ro·kin·es·thet·ic (kī′rō-kin-es-thet′ik). Relating to cheirokinesthesia.

chei·rol·o·gy, chi·rol·o·gy (kī-rol′ō-jē). SYN dactylology. [cheiro- + G. *logos,* word]

chei·ro·meg·a·ly, chi·ro·meg·a·ly (kī′rō-meg′ă-lē). SYN macrocheiria. [cheiro- + G. *megas,* large]

chei·ro·po·dal·gia (kī′rō-pō-dal′jē-ă). Rarely used term for pain in the hands and in the feet. SYN chiropodalgia. [cheiro- + G. *pous,* foot, + *algos,* pain]

chei·ro·pom·pho·lyx (kī-rō-pom′fō-liks). SYN dyshidrosis. [cheiro- + G. *pompholyx,* a bubble, fr. *pomphos,* a blister]

chei·ro·spasm (kī′rō-spazm). Rarely used term for spasm of the muscles of the hand, as in writers' cramp. SYN chirospasm. [cheiro- + G. *spasmos,* spasm]

che·late (kē′lāt). 1. To effect chelation. 2. Pertaining to chelation. 3. A complex formed through chelation.

che·la·tion (kē-lā′shŭn). Complex formation involving a metal ion and two or more polar groupings of a single molecule; thus, in heme, the Fe^{2+} ion is chelated by the porphyrin ring. C. can be used to remove an ion from participation in biological reactions, as in the c. of Ca^{2+} of blood by EDTA, which thus acts as an anticoagulant. [G. *chēlē,* claw]

che·lic·era, pl. **che·lic·er·ae** (ke-lis′ĭ-ră, -ĭ-rē). One of the two anterior appendages of arachnids; in ticks and parasitic mites, the chelicerae are piercing and cutting structures, and constitute important feeding organs. [G. *chēlē,* claw, + *keras,* horn]

chel·i·don (kel′ĕ-don). SYN cubital *fossa.* [G. *chelidōn,* a swallow, because of fancied resemblance to the shape of a swallow's tail]

che·loid (kē′loyd). SYN keloid.

♻**chem-.** SEE chemo-.

chem·ex·fo·li·a·tion (kem′eks-fō-lē-ā′shŭn). A chemosurgical technique designed to remove acne scars or treat chronic skin changes caused by exposure to sunlight. SYN chemical peeling.

chem·i·a·try (kem′i-ă-trē). Obsolete term for iatrochemistry.

chem·i·cal (kem′i-kăl). Relating to chemistry.

chem·i·co·cau·tery (kem′i-kō-kaw′ter-ē). SYN chemocautery.

chem·i·lu·mi·nes·cence (kem′ē-loo-min-es′ens). Light produced by chemical action usually at, or below, room temperature. SYN chemoluminescence.

chem·i·o·tax·is (kem′ē-ō-taks′is). SYN chemotaxis.

che·mise (shem-ēz′). A square of gauze fastened to a catheter passed through its center; used to retain a tampon packed around the catheter inserted into a wound, such as that resulting from a perineal resection. [Fr. shirt]

chem·ist (kem′ist). 1. A specialist or expert in chemistry. 2. Pharmacist (British).

chem·is·try (kem′is-trē). 1. The science concerned with the atomic composition of substances, the elements, and their interreactions, as well as the formation, decomposition, and properties of molecules. 2. The chemical properties of a substance. 3. Chemical processes. [G. *chēmeia,* alchemy]

   analytic c., the application of c. to the determination and detection of composition and identification of specific substances.

   applied c., the application of the theories and principles of chemistry to practical purposes.

   biologic c., SYN biochemistry.

   clinical c., (1) the c. of human health and disease; (2) c. in connection with the management of patients, as in a hospital laboratory.

   ecologic c., (1) c. that concentrates on the effects of human-made chemicals on the environment as well as the development of agents that are not harmful to the environment; (2) the study of the molecular interactions between species and between species and the environment.

   epithermal c., so-called "hot atom" c.; the science concerned with the chemical reactions of recoil atoms and free radicals produced in low energy nuclear processes.

   inorganic c., the science concerned with compounds not involving carbon-containing molecules.

   macromolecular c., the c. of macromolecules (e.g., proteins, nucleic acids) and polymers (nylon, polyethylene, etc).

   medicinal c., SYN pharmaceutical c.

   nuclear c., the science concerned with the c. of nuclear reactions and processes.

   organic c., that branch of c. concerned with covalently linked atoms, centering around carbon compounds of this type; originally, and still including, the c. of natural products.

   pharmaceutical c., medicinal c. in its application to the analysis, development, preparation, and the manufacture of drugs. SYN medicinal c., pharmacochemistry.

   physiologic c., SYN biochemistry.

   radiopharmaceutical c., the science concerned with the labeling of pharmaceuticals with radionuclides.

   synthetic c., the formation or building up of complex compounds by uniting the more simple ones.

♻**chemo-, chem-.** Chemistry. [G. *chēmeia,* alchemy]

chemo·at·tract·ants (kem′ă-trak′tinz). Chemical substances that influence the migration of cells. [chem- + attract + -i]

che·mo·au·to·troph (kem′ō-aw′tō-trōf, kē′mō). An organism that depends on chemicals for its energy and principally on carbon dioxide for its carbon. SYN chemolithotroph. [chemo- + G. *autos,* self, + *trophikos,* nourishing]

che·mo·au·to·tro·phic (kem′ō-aw-tō-trof′ik, kē′mo-). Pertaining to a chemoautotroph. SYN chemolithotrophic.

che·mo·bi·o·dy·nam·ics (kem′ō-bī-ō-dī-nam′iks, kē′mo-). Study devoted to elucidation of correlations between the chemical constitution of various materials and their ability to modify the function and morphology of biological systems. [chemo- + G. *bios,* life, + *dynamis,* power]

che·mo·cau·tery (kem′ō-kaw-ter-ē, kē′mō-). Any substance that destroys tissue upon application. SYN chemical cautery, chemicocautery.

che·mo·cep·tor (kē′mō-sep-tŏr). SYN chemoreceptor.

che·mo·dec·to·ma (kem′ō-dek-tō′mă, kē′mō-). Aortic body, carotid body, chemoreceptor, or glomus jugulare tumor; nonchro-

ch

maffin paraganglioma; receptoma; a relatively rare, usually benign neoplasm originating in the chemoreceptor tissue of the carotid body, glomus jugulare, and aortic bodies; consisting histologically of rounded or ovoid hyperchromatic cells that tend to be grouped in an alveoluslike pattern within a scant to moderate amount of fibrous stroma and a few large thin-walled vascular channels. Cf. paraganglioma. SYN aortic body tumor, carotid body tumor, nonchromaffin paraganglioma. [chemo- + G. *dektēs*, receiver, fr. *dechomai*, to receive, + *-oma*, tumor]

che·mo·dec·to·ma·to·sis (kem'ō-dek-tō-mă-to'sis, kē'mō-). Multiple tumors of perivascular tissue of carotid body or presumed chemoreceptor type, which have been reported in the lungs as minute neoplasms.

che·mo·dif·fer·en·ti·a·tion (kem'ō-dif-er-en-shē-ā'shŭn, kē'mō-). Differentiation of the cellular chemical constituents in the embryo prior to cytodifferentiation; sometimes recognizable histochemically. SYN invisible differentiation.

che·mo·het·er·o·troph (kem'ō-het'er-ō-trōf, kē'mō-). SYN chemoorganotroph. [chem- + G. *heteros*, other, + *trophē*, nourishment]

che·mo·het·er·o·troph·ic (kem'ō-het-er-ō-trof'ik, kē'mō-). SYN chemoorganotrophic.

che·mo·im·mu·nol·o·gy (kem'ō-im-ū-nol'ō-jē, kē'mō-). An obsolete term for immunochemistry.

che·mo·kines (kē'mō-kinz). Several groups composed of usually 8–10 kD polypeptide cytokines that are chemokinetic and chemotactic stimulating leukocyte movement and attraction. SYN intercrines. [chemo- + G. *kineō*, to set in motion]

che·mo·ki·ne·sis (kem'ō-ki-nē'sis, kē'mō-). Stimulation of an organism by a chemical. [chemo- + G. *kinēsis*, movement]

che·mo·ki·net·ic (kem'-ō-ki-net'ik, kē'mo-). Referring to chemokinesis.

che·mo·lith·o·troph (kem'ō-lith'ō-trōf, kē'mō-). SYN chemoautotroph.

che·mo·lith·o·tro·phic (kem'ō-lith-ō-trof'ik, kē'mō-). SYN chemoautotrophic.

che·mo·lith·o·tro·phy (kem'ō-lith'ō-trōf-ē). The utilization of inorganic compounds or ions to obtain reducing equivalents and energy. [chemo- + G. *lithos*, stone, mineral, + *trophe*, nourishment]

che·mo·lu·mi·nes·cence (kem'ō-loo-min-es'ens, kē'mō-). SYN chemiluminescence.

chem·ol·y·sis (kem-ol'i-sis). Chemical decomposition. [chemo- + G. *lysis*, dissolution]

che·mo·nu·cle·ol·y·sis (kem'ō-noo-klē-ol'i-sis, kē'mō-). Injection of chymopapain into the nucleus pulposus of an intervertebral disk. A therapeutic option for the treatment of a herniated nucleus pulposis, e.g., "slipped disk."

che·mo·or·ga·no·troph (kem'ō-ōr'gă-nō-trōf, kē'mō-). An organism that depends on organic chemicals for its energy and carbon. SYN chemoheterotroph. [chemo- + G. *organon*, organ, + *trophē*, nourishment]

che·mo·or·ga·no·tro·phic (kem'ō-ōr-gă-nō-trof'ik, kē'mō-). Pertaining to a chemoorganotroph. SYN chemoheterotrophic.

che·mo·pal·li·dec·to·my (kem'ō-pal-i-dek'tō-mē, kē'mō-). Destruction of the globus pallidus by injection of a chemical agent. SYN chemopallidotomy. [chemo- + globus pallidus + G. *ektomē*, excision]

che·mo·pal·li·do·thal·a·mec·to·my (kem'ō-pal'i-dō-thal-ă-mek'tō-mē, kē'mō-). Destruction of portions of the globus pallidus and thalamus by injection of a chemical substance. [chemo- + globus pallidus + thalamus + G. *ektomē*, excision]

che·mo·pal·li·dot·o·my (kēm'ō-pal-i-dot'ō-mē, kē'mō-). SYN chemopallidectomy. [chemo- + globus pallidus + G. *tomē*, incision]

chem·o·pre·ven·tion. The use of drugs or other agents to inhibit the development or progression of malignant changes in cells.

che·mo·pro·phy·lax·is (kem'ō-pro'fi-lak'sis, kē'mō-). Prevention of disease by the use of chemicals or drugs.

che·mo·re·cep·tion (kēm-ō-rē-sep'shun). The ability to perceive

chemicals in the environment that are odorants or tastants. SYN chemosensation.

che·mo·re·cep·tive (kē-mō-rē-sep'tiv). Relating to chemoreception.

che·mo·re·cep·tor (kē'mō-rē-sep'tor). Any cell that is activated by a change in its chemical milieu and results in a nerve impulse. Such cells can be either 1) "transducer" cells innervated by sensory nerve fibers (e.g., the gustatory receptor cells of the taste buds; cells in the carotid body sensitive to changes in the oxygen and carbon dioxide content of the blood); or 2) nerve cells proper, such as the olfactory receptor cells of the olfactory mucosa, and certain cells in the brainstem that are sensitive to changes in the composition of the blood or cerebrospinal fluid. SYN chemoceptor.

medullary c., the c.'s in or near the ventrolateral surface of the medulla that are stimulated by local acidity.

peripheral c., the c.'s in the carotid and aortic bodies that are stimulated by chemical changes in the composition of the blood such as hypoxia.

che·mo·re·flex (kem-ō-rē'fleks, kē-mō-). A reflex initiated by the stimulation of chemoreceptors, e.g., of a carotid body.

che·mo·re·sis·tance (kem'ō-rē-zis'tans, kē'mō-). The resistance of bacteria or malignant cells to the inhibiting action of certain chemical substances used in treatment.

che·mo·re·sponse (kē-mō-rē-sponz'). A reaction to chemical stimulation.

che·mo·sen·sa·tion (kē-mō-sen-sā'shun). SYN chemoreception.

che·mo·sen·si·tive (kem-ō-sen'si-tiv, kē-mō-). Capable of perceiving changes in the chemical composition of the environment, e.g., changes in the oxygen and carbon dioxide content of the blood.

che·mo·se·ro·ther·a·py (kem'ō-sē-r'ō-thār-ă-pē, kē'mō-). An obsolete treatment of disease with a combination of drugs and serum.

che·mo·sis (kē-mō'sis). Edema of the bulbar conjunctiva, forming a swelling around the cornea. [G. *chēmē*, a yawning, the cockle (from its gaping shell)]

chem·os·mo·sis (kem-os-mō'sis). Chemical reaction between substances initially separated by a membrane. [chem- + G. *ōsmos*, a thrusting, an impulsion]

che·mo·stat (kem'ō-stat). A fermenter for microbial growth in which the ratio of growth to synthesis of secondary products is controlled by the rate at which new medium is added to the culture.

che·mo·sur·gery (kem'ō-ser-jer-ē, kē'mō-). Excision of diseased tissue after it has been fixed in situ by chemical means.

Mohs c., a technique for removal of skin tumors with a minimum of normal tissue, by prior necrosis with zinc chloride paste, mapping of the tumor site, and excision and microscopic examination of frozen section of thin horizontal layers of tissue, until all of the tumor is removed. More recently, the preliminary step of chemical necrosis has been omitted. SYN microscopically controlled surgery, Mohs micrographic surgery, Mohs surgery.

che·mo·syn·the·sis (ke-m'ō-sin'thĕ-sis). 1. Chemical synthesis. 2. Chemolithotrophy.

che·mo·tac·tic (kē-mō-tak'tik). Relating to chemotaxis.

che·mo·tax·is (kē-mo-tak'sis). 1. Movement of cells or organisms in response to chemicals, whereby the cells are attracted (**positive c.**) or repelled (**negative c.**) by substances exhibiting chemical properties. 2. The migration of polymorphonuclear leukocytes and macrophages toward higher concentrations of certain fragments of complement. SYN chemiotaxis, chemotropism. [chemo- + G. *taxis*, orderly arrangement]

che·mo·thal·a·mec·to·my (kem'ō-thal-ă-mek'tō-mē, kē'mō-). Chemical destruction of a part of the thalamus, usually for relief of pain or dyskinesia. SYN chemothalamotomy. [chemo- + thalamus, + G. *ektomē*, excision]

che·mo·thal·a·mot·o·my (kem'ō-thal-ă-mot'ō-mē, kē'mō-). SYN chemothalamectomy.

che·mo·ther·a·peu·tic (kem'ō-thār-ă-pū'tik, kē'mō-). Relating to chemotherapy.

che·mo·ther·a·peu·tics (kem′ō-thār-ă-pū′tiks, kē′mō-). The branch of therapeutics concerned with chemotherapy.

che·mo·ther·a·py (kem′ō-thār-ă-pē, kē′mō-). Treatment of disease by means of chemical substances or drugs; usually used in reference to neoplastic disease. SEE ALSO pharmacotherapy.

adjuvant c., c. given in addition to surgical therapy, in order to reduce the risk of local or systemic relapse.

combination c., c. with more than one drug, to benefit from their dissimilar toxicities.

consolidation c., repetitive cycles of treatment during the immediate post-remission period, used especially for leukemia. SYN intensification c.

cytostatic c., c. that does not allow tumor cell proliferation, but may not kill cells.

cytotoxic c., c. designed to kill tumor cells.

induction c., use of c. as initial treatment before surgery or radiotherapy of a malignancy.

intensification c., SYN consolidation c.

salvage c., use of c. in a patient with recurrence of a malignancy following initial treatment, in hope of a cure or prolongation of life. SYN salvage therapy.

che·mot·ic (kē-mot′ic). Relating to chemosis.

che·mo·trans·mit·ter (kem-ō-trans′mit-er, kē-mō-). A chemical substance produced to diffuse across the space between cells (synapse) and cause responses of neurons or effector cells.

che·mo·troph (ke-mō-trōf). An organism that obtains its energy by the oxidation of inorganic or organic nutrients (i.e., exogenous chemical sources).

che·mo·tro·pism (kĕ-mot′rŏ-pi-zŭm). SYN chemotaxis. [chemo- + G. *tropos,* direction, turn]

Chenais, Louis J., French physician, 1872–1950. SEE Cestan-C. *syndrome.*

Cheney, William D., U.S. radiologist, *1918. SEE C. *syndrome.*

che·no·de·ox·y·cho·lic ac·id (kē′nō-dē-oks-ē-kō′lik). A major bile acid in many vertebrates, usually conjugated with glycine or taurine, which facilitates cholesterol excretion and fat absorption; administered to dissolve cholesterol gallstones. SYN chenodiol.

che·no·di·ol (kē-nō-dī′ol). SYN chenodeoxycholic acid.

che·no·po·di·um (kē-nō-pō′dē-ŭm). The dried ripe fruit of *Chenopodium ambrosoides* (family Chenopodiaceae), American wormwood, from which a volatile oil is distilled and used as an anthelmintic. SYN Jesuit tea, Mexican tea, wormseed (2). [G. *chēn,* goose, + *pous (pod-),* foot]

Cherenkov, SEE Cerenkov.

cher·ry juice (chār′ē). The juice expressed from the fresh ripe fruit of *Prunus cerasus,* containing not less than 1.0% of malic acid; used as a flavoring agent, and as a vehicle for cough syrups and other preparations for oral administrations.

che·rub·ism (che-r′ŭb-izm) [MIM*118400]. Hereditary giant cell lesions of the jaws beginning in early childhood; multilocular radiolucencies and progressive symmetric painless swelling of the jaws; bilateral; occurs with no associated systemic manifestations. SYN fibrous dysplasia of jaws. [Hebr. *kerubh,* cherub]

chest. The anterior wall of the thorax. SEE ALSO thorax. SYN pectus. [A.S. *cest,* a box]

alar c., SYN flat c.

barrel c., a c. permanently resembling the shape of a barrel, i.e., with increased anteroposterior diameter, roughly equaling the lateral diameter; usually with some degree of kyphosis; seen in cases of emphysema.

flail c., loss of stability of thoracic cage following fracture of sternum, ribs, or both; can cause respiratory failure.

flat c., a c. in which the anteroposterior diameter is shorter than the average. SYN alar c., pterygoid c.

foveated c., funnel c., SYN *pectus* excavatum.

keeled c., SYN *pectus* carinatum.

phthinoid c., a long narrow c., the lower ribs being more oblique than usual and sometimes reaching almost to the crest of the ilium, with the scapulae projecting backward, the manubrium

sterni depressed, and Louis angle sharper than normal; such a c. was once considered indicative of pulmonary tuberculosis.

pigeon c., SYN *pectus* carinatum.

pterygoid c., SYN flat c.

Cheyne, John, Scottish physician, 1777–1836. SEE C.-Stokes *psychosis, respiration.*

chi (kī). 1. The 22nd letter of the Greek alphabet, χ. 2. In chemistry, denotes the 22nd in a series. 3. Symbol for the dihedral angle between the α-carbon and the side chains of amino acids in peptides and proteins.

Chiari, Johann B., German obstetrician, 1817–1854. SEE C.-Frommel *syndrome.*

Chiari, Hans, German pathologist, 1851–1916. SEE Arnold-C. *deformity, malformation, syndrome;* C. *disease, net, syndrome,* II *syndrome;* C.-Budd *syndrome;* Budd-C. *syndrome.*

chi·asm (kī′azm). 1. An intersection or crossing of two lines. 2 [TA]. In anatomy, a decussation or crossing of two fibrous bundles, such as tendins, nerves, or tracts. 3. In cytogenetics, the site at which two homologous chromosomes make contact (thus appearing to be crossed), enabling the exchange of genetic material during the prophase stage of meiosis. SYN chiasma [TA]. [G. *chiasma*]

Camper c., SYN tendinous c. of the digital tendons.

optic c. [TA], a flattened quadrangular body in front of the tuber cinereum and infundibulum, the point of crossing or decussation of the axons of the optic nerves; axons from the nasal retina cross to the opposite side while axons from the temporal retina run directly caudal without crossing, some pass transversely on the posterior surface between the two optic tracts and others pass transversely on the anterior surface between the two optic nerves. SYN chiasma opticum [TA], optic decussation.

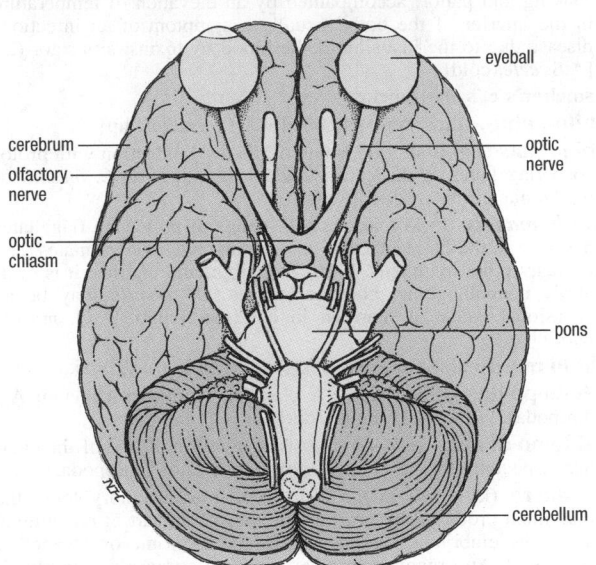

optic chiasm

tendinous c. of the digital tendons [TA], crossing of the tendons, the passage of the tendons of the flexor digitorum profundus (flexor digitorum longus in the foot) through the interval left by the decussation of the fibers of the tendons of the flexor digitorum superficialis (flexor digitorum brevis in the foot). SYN chiasma tendinum [TA], Camper c.

chi·as·ma, pl. **chi·as·ma·ta** (kī-az′mă, kī-az′mă-tă) [TA]. SYN chiasm. [G. *chiasma,* two crossing lines, fr. the letter *chi,* 3]

c. op′ticum [TA], SYN optic *chiasm.*

c. ten′dinum [TA], SYN tendinous *chiasm* of the digital tendons.

chi·as·ma·pexy (kī-as′mă-pek-sē). Surgical fixation of the optic chiasma. [G. *chiasma,* decussation, + *pēxis,* fixation]

chi·as·mat·ic (kī-az-mat′ik). Relating to a chiasm.

chick·en·pox (chik′en-poks). SYN varicella.

Chick-Martin test. See under test.

chi·cle (chik′el). 1. The partially evaporated viscous, milky juice from *Manilkara zapotilla* (sapotaceae), which is native to the West Indies, Mexico, and Central America. 2. A mixture of gutta with triterpene alcohols. Used in the manufacture of chewing gum. [Sp., from Nahuatl *chictli*]

Chievitz, Johan H., Danish anatomist, 1850–1901. SEE C. *layer*, *organ*.

chig·ger (chig′er). The six-legged larva of *Trombicula* species and other members of the family Trombiculidae; a bloodsucking stage of mites that includes the vectors of scrub typhus.

chig·oe (chig′ō). Common name for *Tunga penetrans*.

⌂**chil-.** SEE chilo-.

Chilaiditi, Demetrius, Austrian radiologist, *1883. SEE C. *syndrome*.

chil·blain (chil′blān). Erythema, itching, and burning, especially of the dorsa of the fingers and toes, and of the heels, nose, and ears caused by vascular constriction on exposure to extreme cold (usually associated with high humidity); lesions can be single or multiple, and can become blistered and ulcerated. SYN erythema pernio, perniosis. [chill + A.S. *blegen*, a blain]

CHILD SEE CHILD *syndrome*.

child·bear·ing (chīld′bār-ing). Pregnancy and parturition.

child·birth (chīld′berth). The process of labor and delivery in the birth of a child. SEE ALSO birth, accouchement. SYN parturition.

child·hood (chīld′hud). The period of life between infancy and puberty.

chill. 1. A sensation of cold. 2. A feeling of cold with shivering or shaking and pallor, accompanied by an elevation of temperature in the interior of the body; usually a symptom of an infectious disease due to the invasion of the blood by toxins. SYN rigor (2). [A.S. *cele*, cold]

smelter's c.'s, SYN smelter's *fever*.

⌂**chilo-, chil-.** Lips. SEE ALSO cheilo-. [G. *cheilos*, lip]

chi·lo·mas·ti·gi·a·sis (kī′lō-mas-ti-gī′ă-sis). Infection with protozoan flagellates of the genus *Chilomastix*, such as *C. mesnili* of the human cecum. SYN chilomastosis.

Chi·lo·mas·tix (kī-lō-mas′tiks). A genus of protozoan flagellates parasitic in the large intestine of humans and other primates, and in many other mammals, birds, amphibia, and reptiles; it is ordinarily nonpathogenic, but one species, *C. mesnili*, may be an occasional cause of diarrhea in children. [chilo- + G. *mastix*, whip]

chi·lo·mas·to·sis (kī′lō-mas-tō′sis). SYN chilomastigiasis.

Chi·lo·po·da (kī-lop′ŏ-dă). A class of centipedes (phylum Arthropoda). [chilo- + G. *pous*, foot]

chi·lo·po·di·a·sis (kī′lō-pō-dī′ă-sis). Invasion of one of the cavities, especially the nasal cavity, by a species of Chilopoda.

chi·me·ra (kī-mēr′ă, kī-). 1. In experimental embryology, the individual produced by grafting an embryonic part of one animal on to the embryo of another, either of the same or of another species. 2. An organism that has received a transplant of genetically and immunologically different tissue, such as bone marrow. 3. Dizygotic twins that retain each other as immunologically distinct types of erythrocytes. 4. A protein fusion in which two different proteins are linked via peptide bonds; usually genetically engineered. Chimeric antibodies may have the Fab fragment from one species fused with the Fc fragment from another. 5. Any macromolecule fusion formed by two or more macromolecules from different species or from different genes. [L. *Chimaera*, G. *Chimaira*, mythic monster (lit. a she-goat)]

radiation c., an individual that has been subjected to whole body irradiation in order to lower immune response to foreign donor cells and therefore has the immunologic characteristics of both host and donor after a bone marrow graft from the antigenically different donor.

chi·mer·ic (kī-mēr′ik). 1. Relating to a chimera. Cf. mosaicism. 2. Composed of parts that are of different origin and are seemingly incompatible.

chi·me·rism (kī-mē-r′izm). The state of being a chimera.

chim·pan·zee (chim-pan′zē, chim′pan-zē′). Generic name for the apes *Pan panisus* and *P. troglodytes*. [African dial.]

chin [TA]. The prominence formed by the anterior projection of the mandible, or lower jaw. SYN mentum [TA]. [A.S. *cin*]

double c., SYN buccula.

chi·ni·o·fon (ki-nī′ē-ō-fon). A mixture of 7-iodo-8-hydroxyquinoline-5-sulfonic acid and sodium bicarbonate, used in the treatment of amebic dysentery.

chin·o·le·ine (chin′ō-lē-in). SYN quinoline (1).

chip. A small fragment resulting from breakage, cutting, or avulsion.

bone c.'s, small pieces of cancellous bone generally used to fill in bony defects and to promote reossification.

chip-blow·er. An instrument for blowing the debris out of, or drying, a tooth cavity that is being excavated for a filling; it consists of a rubber bulb with a metal nozzle.

chi·ral (kī′răl). Denoting an object, such as a molecule in a given configuration or conformation, that possesses chirality. A c. molecule has no plane, axis, or center of symmetry.

chi·ral·i·ty (kī-ral′i-tē). The property of nonidentity of an object with its mirror image; used in chemistry with respect to stereochemical isomers. [G. *cheir*, hand]

chi·rar·thri·tis (kī-rar-thrī′tis). SYN cheirarthritis.

⌂**chiro-, chir-.** The hand. SEE ALSO cheiro-. [G. *cheir*, hand]

chi·rog·nos·tic (kī-rog-nos′tik). SYN cheirognostic.

chi·ro·kin·es·the·sia (kī-rō-kin-es-thē′zē-ă). SYN cheirokinesthesia.

chi·ro·po·dal·gia (kī′rō-pō-dal′jē-ă). SYN cheiropodalgia.

chi·rop·o·dist (kī-rop′ō-dist). SYN podiatrist. [chiro- + G. *pous*, foot]

chi·rop·o·dy (kī-rop′ō-dē). SYN podiatry.

chi·ro·pom·pho·lyx (kī-rō-pom′fō-liks). SYN dyshidrosis.

chi·ro·prac·tic (kī-rō-prak′tik). A system that, in theory, uses the recuperative powers of the body and the relationship between the musculoskeletal structures and functions of the body, particularly of the spinal column and the nervous system, in the restoration and maintenance of health. [chiro- + G. *praktikos*, efficient]

chi·ro·prac·tor (kī-rō-prak′tŏr). One who is licensed and certified to practice chiropractic.

Chiropsalmus. A genus of the invertebrate phylum Cnidaria that includes the sea wasp.

C. quadrumanus, the sea wasp, the most venomous jellyfish inhabiting the waters surrounding the United States. SEE ALSO jellyfish. SYN box jelly, sea wasp.

Chi·rop·te·ra (kī-rop′ter-ă). The bats, an order of placental mammals of worldwide distribution, characterized by a modification of the forelimbs that enables them to fly. They are capable of emitting ultrasonic sounds that enable them to echolocate, find flying insect prey, and avoid objects in the dark. Though mostly insectivorous, some species feed on nectar, fruit, fish, and blood; the blood-feeding and insectivorous species are important reservoir hosts of rabies. [chiro- + G. *pteron*, wing]

chi·ro·scope (kī′rō-skōp). A haploscopic instrument used for coordinating hand and eye as the patient draws while looking through it. [chiro- + G. *skopeō*, to view]

chi·ro·spasm (kī′rō-spazm). SYN cheirospasm.

chirurg. Abbreviation for L. *chirurgicalis*, surgical.

chi·rur·geon (kī-rer′jon). Obsolete term for surgeon. [G. *cheirourgos*, fr. *cheir*, hand, + *ergon*, work]

chi·rur·gery (kī-rer′jer-ē). Obsolete term for surgery. [G. *cheirourgia*]

chi·rur·gi·cal (kī-rer′ji-kăl). Obsolete term for surgical. [L. surgical, fr. *chirurgia*, surgery, fr. G. *cheirourgia*, handicraft, fr. *cheir*, hand + *ergon*, work]

chis·el (chiz′l). A single beveled end-cutting blade with a straight or angled shank used with a thrust along the axis of the handle for cutting or splitting dentin and enamel.

binangle c., a c. with an angled shank to which a second angle is added in order to bring the cutting edge nearly in line with the axis of the handle so as to restore balance and to prevent it from turning about the axis; used when a c. must be angled for access.

chi-square (kī′ skwăr). A statistical technique whereby variables are categorized to determine whether a distribution of scores is due to chance or experimental factors.

chi·tin (kī′tin). A linear polymer of *N*-acetyl-D-glucosamine, linked β(1→4), similar in structure to cellulose and the second most abundant polysaccharide in nature, comprising the horny substance in the exoskeleton of beetles, crabs, certain microorganisms, etc., as well as in some plants and fungi.

chi·ti·nase (kī′ti-nās). An enzyme catalyzing the random hydrolysis of β(1→4) linkages in chitin (ultimately releasing *N*-acetyl-D-glucosamine); some enzymes of this type display lysozyme activity. SYN poly-β-glucosaminidase.

chi·tin·ous (kī′tin-ŭs). Of or relating to chitin.

chi·to·bi·ose (kī-tō-bī′ōs). The disaccharide repeating unit in chitin; differs from cellobiose only in the presence of an *N*-acetylamino group on carbon-2 in place of the hydroxyl group. However, the nonacetylated form is also referred to as c.

chi·to·sa·mine (kī-tō′să-mēn). D-Glucosamine. SEE glucosamine.

chi·u·fa (chē-oo′fä). An acute gangrenous proctitis and colitis with high fever, seen in southern Africa and South America at high altitudes; in women, the vulva and vagina may be affected. SYN kanyemba.

CHL Abbreviation for crown-heel *length*.

Chla·myd·i·a (kla-mid′ē-ă). The only genus of the family Chlamydiaceae, including all the agents of the psittacosis-lymphogranuloma-trachoma disease groups; chlamydia are obligatory intracellular spherical or ovoid bacteria with a complex intracellular life cycle; the infective form is the elementary body, which penetrates the host cell, replicating as the rediculate body by binary fission; replication occurs in a vacuole called the inclusion body; chlamydia lack peptidoglycan in their cell walls; the type species is *C. trachomitis*. Formerly called *Betsonia*. SYN *Chlamydozoon*. [G. *chlamys,* cloak]

C. pneumo′niae, a bacterial species first isolated in 1986 and currently recognized as a common cause of pneumonia, bronchitis, rhinosinusitis, and pharyngitis in both adults and children. SYN TWAR.

> *Chlamydia pneumoniae* is responsible for about 25% of cases of acute bronchitis and 10% of community-acquired pneumonia. Recent studies have suggested that it may also play a role in the genesis of cardiovascular disease and late-onset Alzheimer dementia. Like *C. trachomatis* and *C. psittaci*, this organism is an occasional cause of myocarditis and endocarditis. Elevated levels of antibody to *C. pneumoniae* are found in persons with acute myocardial infarction (MI), and in persons showing significant atheroma formation at autopsy, significantly more often than in control groups. The organism has been detected by immunocytochemistry, polymerase chain reaction, and electron microscopy in macrophages and smooth muscle cells of atheromatous plaques of the aorta, coronary arteries, and carotid arteries (surgical and autopsy specimens), but not in normal arteries. The incidence of acute infection in MI patients, as detected by throat culture, is higher than in the general public. A retrospective review of medical records of persons with acute MI showed that they were less likely than matched controls to have been treated during the preceding 3 years with tetracycline or quinolone antibiotics, which are active against *C. pneumoniae*. To date, however, prospective studies have not shown an association between the presence of IgG antibody to *C. pneumoniae* and an increased risk of atherothrombotic disease. Researchers have speculated that infection with *C. pneumoniae* may be one of several factors capable of initiating changes that culminate in atherosclerosis, or that reinfection may trigger coronary atherothrombosis. Antibody to *C. pneumoniae* is also found in persons with severe hypertension at about twice the incidence rate for the general public. In addition, the organism has been detected in

microglia and astroglia of the hippocampus and temporal cortex in persons with late-onset Alzheimer disease with much greater frequency than in normal brains.

C. psi′ttaci, bacterial organisms that resemble *C. trachomatis,* but that form loosely bound intracytoplasmic microcolonies up to 12 μm in diameter, do not produce glycogen in sufficient quantity to be detected by iodine stains, and are not susceptible to sulfadiazine. Various strains of this species cause psittacosis in humans and ornithosis in nonpsittacine birds; pneumonitis in cattle, sheep, swine, cats, goats, and horses; enzootic abortion of ewes; bovine sporadic encephalomyelitis; enteritis of calves; epizootic chlamydiosis of muskrats and hares; encephalitis of opossum; and conjunctivitis of cattle, sheep, and guinea pigs.

C. tracho′matis, spherical nonmotile bacteria that are obligatory intracellular organisms; they form compact intracytoplasmic microcolonies up to 10 μm in diameter which (by division) give rise to infectious spherules 0.3 μm or more in diameter, accumulate glycogen for a limited period in sufficient quantity to be detected by iodine stain, and are usually susceptible to sulfadiazine, tetracycline, and quinalones; various strains of this species cause trachoma, inclusion and neonatal conjunctivitis, lymphogranuloma venereum, mouse pneumonitis, nonspecific urethritis, epididymitis, cervicitis, salpingitis, proctitis, and pneumonia; chief agent of bacterial sexually transmitted diseases in the U.S.; the type species of the genus *C.*

chla·myd·ia, pl. **chla·myd·i·ae** (kla-mid′ē-ă, -mid′ē-ē). A vernacular term used to refer to any member of the genus *Chlamydia.*

Chlam·y·di·a·ce·ae (kla-mid′ē-ā′sē-ē). A family of the order Chlamydiales (formerly included in the order Rickettsiales) that includes the agents of the psittacosis-lymphogranuloma-trachoma group. The family contains small, coccoid, Gram-negative bacteria that resemble rickettsiae but that differ from them significantly by possessing a unique, obligately intracellular developmental cycle; intracytoplasmic microcolonies give rise to infectious forms by division. The classification of these organisms previously was in a state of flux, but they are now placed in a single genus, *Chlamydia,* the type genus of the family.

chla·myd·i·al (kla-mid′ē-ăl). Relating to or caused by any bacterium of the genus *Chlamydia.*

chla·myd·i·o·sis (klă-mid-ē-ō′sis). General term for diseases caused by *Chlamydia* species. SEE ALSO ornithosis, psittacosis.

chlam·y·do·co·nid·i·um (klam′i-dō-kŏ-nid′ē-um). A thallic conidium that is thick-walled and may be terminal or intercalary. Seen in a form of asexual reproduction. [G. *chlamys,* cloak, + conidium]

Chlam·y·do·phrys (kla-mid′ō-fris). A genus of shelled amebas, commonly found as fecal protozoans. [G. *chlamys,* cloak, + *ophrys,* brow]

Chlam·y·do·zo·on (klam′i-dō-zō′on). SYN *Chlamydia.*

chlo·as·ma (klō-az′mă). Melanoderma or melasma characterized by the occurrence of extensive brown patches of irregular shape and size on the skin of the face and elsewhere; the pigmented facial patches if confluent are also called the mask of pregnancy, and are associated most commonly with pregnancy and use of oral contraceptives. SEE ALSO melasma. [G. *chloazō,* to become green]

c. bronzi′num, a bronze-colored pigmentation, probably produced by hormone imbalance, occurring in gradually increasing areas on the face, neck, and chest in persons exposed continuously to the tropical sun; similar to c. of the temperate zone, but intensified because of strong sunlight. SYN tropical mask.

chlo·phe·di·a·nol hy·dro·chlo·ride (klō-fē-dī′ă-nol). An antitussive agent related chemically to the antihistamines.

chlor-, chloro-. 1. Combining form denoting green. 2. Combining form denoting association with chlorine. [G. *chloros,* green]

chlor·a·ce·tic ac·id (klōr-ă-sē′tik). SYN chloroacetic acid.

chlor·ac·ne (klōr-ak′nē). An acnelike eruption due to occupational contact, by inhalation or ingestion or through the skin, with certain chlorinated compounds (naphthalenes and diphenyls) used as insulators, insecticides, fungicides, and herbicides, including Agent Orange; keratinous plugs (comedones) form in the pilose-

ch

baceous orifices, and variously sized small papules (2 to 4 mm) develop. SYN tar acne.

chlo·ral (klōr′ăl). A thin oily liquid with a pungent odor, formed by the action of chlorine gas on alcohol. SYN anhydrous c.

anhydrous c., SYN chloral.

c. betaine, the adduct formed by chloral hydrate and betaine; it is slowly hydrolyzed in the alimentary tract to chloral hydrate; used as a hypnotic and sedative.

c. hydrate, a hypnotic, sedative, and anticonvulsant; it is also used externally as a rubefacient, anesthetic, and antiseptic.

_m_-chlo·ral. A polymer of chloral obtained by prolonged contact with sulfuric acid; it has properties similar to those of chloral hydrate. SYN metachloral, _p_-chloral, trichloral.

_p_-chlo·ral. SYN _m_-chloral.

chlo·ral al·co·hol·ate. A complex of chloral and ethanol. Prepared by refluxing trichloroacetaldehyde (chloral) or chloral hydrate with alcohol. Alleged to be an active constituent of a "Mickey Finn."

chlo·ral·ism (klōr′ăl-izm). Habitual use of chloral compounds as an intoxicant, or the symptoms caused thereby.

α-chlor·a·lose (klōr′ă-lōs). A conjugate of chloral and glucose used as an anesthetic in laboratory animals; it does not depress cardiovascular reflexes as much as most other anesthetic agents.

chlor·am·bu·cil (klōr-am′bū-sil). A nitrogen mustard derivative that depresses lymphocytic proliferation and maturation. SYN chloraminophene, chloroambucil.

chlo·ra·mine B (klōr′ă-mēn). A nontoxic antiseptic substance used in wound irrigation as a substitute for chloramine T.

chlo·ra·mine T. A nontoxic but strong antiseptic used in the irrigation of wounds and infected cavities. SYN chlorazene.

chlor·am·i·no·phene (klōr-am′i-nō-fēn). SYN chlorambucil.

chlor·am·i·phene (klōr-am′i-fēn). SYN clomiphene citrate.

chlor·am·phen·i·col (klōr-am-fen′i-kol). An antibiotic originally obtained from _Streptomyces venezuelae_. It is effective against a number of pathogenic microorganisms including _Staphylococcus aureus_, _Brucella abortus_, Friedländer bacillus, and the organisms of typhoid, typhus, and Rocky Mountain spotted fever; active by mouth. A serious reaction resulting in marrow damage with agranulocytosis or aplastic anemia may occur. Gray baby syndrome may occur in newborns due to a lack of glucoronyltransferase needed to metabolize the drug.

c. acetyl transferase (CAT), a bacterial enzyme often used as a marker for examining the control of eucaryotic gene expression.

c. palmitate, same action and use as c.; was widely used in suspension for pediatric injections.

c. sodium succinate, the water-soluble sodium succinate derivative of c., suitable for parenteral administration; antibacterial activity, uses, and side effects are similar to those of the parent compound.

chlo·rate (klōr′āt). A salt of chloric acid.

chlo·raz·a·nil (klō-raz′ă-nil). A diuretic.

chlor·a·zene (klōr′ă-zēn). SYN chloramine T.

chlo·ra·zol black E (klor′ă-zol) [C.I. 30235]. An acid dye, used as a fat and general tissue stain, and to stain protozoa in fecal smears or in tissues.

chlor·ben·zox·a·mine (klōr-ben-zok′să-mēn). An anticholinergic agent. SYN chlorbenzoxyethamine.

chlor·ben·zox·y·eth·a·mine (klōr′ben-zok-sē-eth′ă-mēn). SYN chlorbenzoxamine.

chlor·bet·a·mide (klōr-bet′ă-mīd). An amebicide.

chlor·bu·tol (klōr-bū′tol). SYN chlorobutanol.

chlor·cy·cli·zine hy·dro·chlo·ride (klōr-sik′li-zēn). An H₁ antihistaminic agent.

chlor·dane (klōr′dān). A chlorinated hydrocarbon used as an insecticide; it may be absorbed through the skin with resultant severe toxic effects: hyperexcitability of central nervous system, tremors, lack of muscular coordination, convulsions, and death; also causes damage to the liver, kidneys, and spleen. It is only mildly toxic to animals.

chlor·dan·to·in (klōr-dan′tō-in). A topical antifungal agent.

chlor·di·az·e·pox·ide hy·dro·chlo·ride (klōr′dī-az-ē-pok′sīd). The hydrochloride of 7-chloro-2-methylamino-5-phenyl-3_H_-1,4-benzodiazepine-4-oxide; an antianxiety agent. An early benzodiazepine.

chlor·e·mia (klōr-ē′-mē-ă). 1. SYN chlorosis. 2. SYN hyperchloremia.

chlor·eth·ene ho·mo·pol·y·mer (klōr′eth-ēn). SYN polyvinyl chloride.

chlor·gua·nide hy·dro·chlo·ride (klōr-gwah′nīd). SYN chloroguanide hydrochloride.

chlor·hex·i·dine hy·dro·chlo·ride (klōr-hek′si-dēn). A topical antiseptic.

chlor·hy·dria (klōr-hī′drē-ă). SYN hyperchlorhydria.

chlo·ric ac·id (klōr′ik). An acid of pentavalent chlorine, HClO₃, existing only in solution and as chlorates.

chlo·ride (klōr′īd). A compound containing chlorine, at a valence of −1, as in the salts of hydrochloric acid.

carbamylcholine c., a cholinomimetic drug that reacts with and activates both muscarinic and nicotinic receptors. It is slowly hydrolyzed and thus its effects far outlast those of acetylcholine. Used medically to stimulate smooth muscle, as in paralytic ileus following surgery.

chlor·i·dim·e·try (klōr-ĭ-dim′ē-trē). The process of determining the amount of chlorides in the blood or urine, or in other fluids.

chlor·i·dom·e·ter (klōr-i-dom′ē-ter). An apparatus for determining the amount of chlorides in blood or urine, or other fluids.

chlor·i·du·ria (klōr-i-doo′rē-ă). SYN chloruresis.

chlo·rin (klōr′in). 2,3-Dihydroporphin(e); 2,3-dihydroporphyrin; one of the root structures of the chlorophylls (for structure, see porphyrin). Addition of the two-carbon bridge (see structure of chlorophyll) to c. yields phorbin(e); addition of side chains yields the phorbides, distinguished by a number of arbitrary prefixes (those found in the chlorophylls are pheo- and bacteriopheophorbide); esterification of the propionic group by phytyl yields the respective phytins, and the addition of magnesium yields the chlorophylls (magnesium phytinates). SEE porphyrins.

chlo·ri·nat·ed (klōr′in-āt-ĕd). Having been treated with chlorine.

chlor·in·da·nol (klōr-in′dă-nol). A spermicide.

chlo·rine (Cl) (klōr′ēn). 1. A greenish, toxic, gaseous element; atomic no. 17, atomic wt. 35.4527; a halogen used as a disinfectant and bleaching agent in the form of hypochlorite or of c. water, because of its oxidizing power. One of the bioelements. 2. The molecular form of c. (1), Cl₂ (dichloride). [G. _chloros_, greenish yellow]

chlo·rine group. The halogens.

chlor·i·o·dized (klōr-ī′ō-dīzd). Containing both chlorine and iodine.

chlor·i·o·dized oil. Chlorinated and iodized peanut oil formed by the chemical addition of iodine monochloride; formerly used for radiography of sinuses and bronchi. SYN iodochlorol.

chlor·i·o·do·quin (klōr′ē-ō-dō′kwin). SYN iodochlorhydroxyquin.

chlor·i·son·da·mine chlo·ride (klōr-i-son′dă-mēn). A quaternary ammonium compound with ganglionic blocking action similar to, but more potent than, hexamethonium and pentolinium; was used in the management of severe hypertension, including the malignant phase.

chlo·rite (klōr′īt). A salt of chlorous acid; the radical ClO₂⁻.

chlor·mad·i·none ac·e·tate (klōr-mad′i-nōn). A progesterone derivative used in conjunction with estrogen as an oral contraceptive.

chlor·mer·od·rin (klōr-mer′od-rin). A mercurial diuretic chemically related to meralluride.

chlor·mez·a·none (klōr-mez′ă-nōn). A muscle relaxant and tranquilizing agent with pharmacologic actions and uses similar to those of meprobamate.

⌂chloro-. SEE chlor-.

chlo·ro·a·ce·tic ac·id (klōr′ō-ă-sē′tik). An acetic acid in which one or more of the hydrogen atoms are replaced by chlorine. According to the number of atoms so displaced the acid is called monochloroacetic (chloroacetic), dichloroacetic, or trichloroacetic. SYN chloracetic acid.

chlo·ro·ac·e·to·phe·none (klōr′ō-as′ĕ-tō-fē′nōn). A lacrimatory gas; used in training and in riot control.

chlo·ro·am·bu·cil (klōr-ō-am′bū-sil). SYN chlorambucil.

chlo·ro·a·ne·mia (klōr′ō-ă-nē′mē-ă). SYN chlorosis.

chlo·ro·az·o·din (klōr-ō-az′ō-din). A bactericidal agent used as a surgical antiseptic.

o-chlo·ro·benz·al·mal·o·no·ni·trile (ōr′thō-klōr′ō-ben-zal-ma-lon′ō-nī-trīl). A strong lacrimator used in riot control.

chlo·ro·bu·ta·nol (klōr-ō-bū′tă-nol). A hypnotic sedative and local anesthetic; used chiefly in dermatologic preparations and as a preservative in multiple-dose vials for parenteral use. SYN acetone chloroform, chlorbutol.

chlo·ro·cre·sol (klōr-ō-krē′sol). Used as an antiseptic and disinfectant; it is more active in acid than in alkaline solutions.

chlo·ro·cru·o·rin (klōr-ō-kroo′ōr-in). A greenish hemoglobin-like pigment found in certain worms; contains a porphyrin differing from protoporphyrin by a formyl group in place of the 2-vinyl group.

chlo·ro·eth·ane (klōr-ō-eth′ān). SYN *ethyl* chloride.

chlo·ro·eth·yl·ene (klōr-ō-eth′i-lēn). SYN *vinyl* chloride.

chlo·ro·form (klōr′ō-fōrm). Formerly used by inhalation to produce general anesthesia; also used as a solvent. SYN trichloromethane. [chlor(ine) + form(yl)]
acetone c., SYN chlorobutanol.

chlo·ro·form·ism (klōr′ō-fōrm-izm). Habitual chloroform inhalation, or the symptoms caused thereby.

chlo·ro·gua·nide hy·dro·chlo·ride (klōr-ō-gwah′nīd). An antimalarial drug. SYN chlorguanide hydrochloride, proguanil hydrochloride.

chlo·ro·he·min (klōr-ō-hē′min). SYN hemin.

chlo·ro·ma (klō-rō′mă). A condition characterized by the development of multiple localized green masses of abnormal cells (in most instances, myeloblasts), especially in relation to the periosteum of the skull, spine, and ribs; the clinical course is similar to that of acute myeloid leukemia, although the tumors may precede the findings in blood and bone marrow; observed more frequently in children and young adults. SEE ALSO granulocytic *sarcoma*. [chloro- + G. -ōma, tumor]

p-chlo·ro·mer·cu·ri·ben·zo·ate (PCMB, *p*CMB, *p*-CMB) (klōr′ō-mer′cūr-ē-ben′zō-āt). Organic mercury compound that reacts with –SH groups of proteins; an inhibitor of action of those proteins (enzymes) that depend on –SH reactivity. SEE ALSO *p*-mercuribenzoate.

chlo·ro·meth·ane (klōr-ō-meth′ān). A refrigerant with anesthetic properties when inhaled; it hydrolyzes to methanol. SYN methyl chloride.

chlo·rom·e·try (klo-rom′ĕ-trē). The measurement of chlorine content, or the use of analytical techniques involving the release or titration of chlorine.

chlo·ro·pe·nia (klōr-ō-pē′nē-ă). A deficiency in chloride. [chloro- + G. *penia,* poverty]

chlo·ro·per·cha (klōr-ō-per′chă). A solution of gutta-percha in chloroform, used in dentistry as an agent to lute gutta-percha filling material to the wall of a prepared root canal.

chlo·ro·phe·nol (klōr-ō-fē′nol). One of several substitution products obtained by the action of chlorine on phenol; used as antiseptics.

o-chlo·ro·phe·nol. An antiseptic liquid, used in the treatment of lupus.

p-chlo·ro·phe·nol. SYN parachlorophenol.

chlo·ro·phen·o·thane (klōr-ō-fen′ō-thān). SYN dichlorodiphenyl-trichloroethane.

chlo·ro·phyll (klōr′ō-fil). The magnesium complex of the phorbin derivative found in photosynthetic organisms; light-absorbing green plant pigments that, in living plants, convert light energy into oxidizing and reducing power, thus fixing CO_2 and evolving O_2; the naturally occurring forms are c. *a*, *b*, *c*, and *d*. SEE ALSO phorbin.

c. *a*, magnesium(II) pheophytinate *a* [(pheophytinato *a*)-magnesium(II)]; the major pigment found in all oxygen-evolving photosynthetic organisms (higher plants, and red and green algae).

c. *b*, (CH_3 at 7 replaced by CHO in the c. structure), magnesium-(II) pheophytinate *b* [(pheophytinato *b*) magnesium(II)]; the c. generally characteristic of higher plants (including the *Chlorophyta, Euglenaphyta,* and green algae). Absent in other types of algae.

c. *c*, the c. present in brown algae, diatoms, and flagellates. Two variants are known: c_1, in which two hydrogens are lost from C-17 and C-18, thus resembling phytoporphyrin, and the side chain at C-17 becomes an acrylic residue, $–CH=CH_2COOH$; c_2, in which the same changes are noted, but two more hydrogens are lost from the ethyl group at C-8, making this a vinyl residue like that at C-3. The two compounds can thus be named in terms of phytoporphyrin: magnesium $3^1,3^2,17^1,17^2$-tetradehydro-13^2-(methoxycarbonyl)phytoporphyrinate and magnesium $3^1,3^2,8^1,8^2,17^1,17^2$-hexadehydro-$13^2$-(methoxycarbonyl)-phytoporphyrinate.

c. *d*, ($–CH=CH_2$ replaced by $–CO–CH_3$ in the c. structure), the c. found in red algae (*Rhodophyceae*), together with c. *a*.

c. esterase, SYN chlorophyllase.

water-soluble c. derivatives, the copper complex of sodium and/or potassium salts of saponified c., used topically for deodorization of chronic lesions and to promote wound repair.

chlo·ro·phyl·lase (klōr-ō-fil′-ās). A reversible hydrolyzing enzyme catalyzing the removal of the phytyl group from a chlorophyll, leaving a chlorophyllide. SYN chlorophyll esterase.

chlo·ro·phyl·lide, chlo·ro·phyl·lid (klōr-ō-fil-id). That which remains of a chlorophyll molecule when the phytyl group is removed.

chlo·ro·pic·rin (klōr-ō-pik′rin). A toxic lung irritant and lacrimatory gas; it also causes vomiting, colic, and diarrhea, and therefore is called vomiting gas. SYN nitrochloroform.

chlo·ro·plast (klōr′ō-plast). A plant cell inclusion body containing chlorophyll; occurs in cells of leaves and young stems. Site of photosynthesis in higher plants. [chloro- + G. *plastos,* formed]

chlo·ro·pred·ni·sone (klōr-ō-pred′ni-sōn). A topical anti-inflammatory agent.

chlo·ro·pro·caine hy·dro·chlo·ride (klōr-ō-prō′kān). A local anesthetic similar in action and use to procaine hydrochloride.

chlo·rop·sia (klo-rop′sē-ă). A condition in which objects appear to be colored green, as may occur in digitalis intoxication. SYN green vision. [chloro- + G. *opsis,* eyesight]

chlo·ro·pyr·a·mine (klōr-ō-pir′ă-mēn). An H_1 antihistaminic agent.

chlo·ro·quine (klōr′ō-kwīn). An antimalarial agent used for the treatment and suppression of *Plasmodium vivax, P. malariae,* and *P. falciparum;* available as the phosphate and sulfate. It does not produce a radical cure because it has no effect on the exoerythrocytic stages; c.-resistant strains of *P. falciparum* have developed in Southeast Asia, Africa, and South America. It is also used for hepatic amebiasis and for certain skin diseases, e.g., lupus erythematosus and lichen planus.

chlo·ro·sis (klōr-ō′sis). Rarely used term for a form of chronic hypochromic microcytic (iron deficiency) anemia, characterized by a great reduction in hemoglobin out of proportion to the decreased number of red blood cells; observed chiefly in females from puberty to the third decade and usually associated with diets deficient in iron and protein. SYN asiderotic anemia, chloremia (1), chloroanemia, chlorotic anemia, green sickness. [chloro- + G. -*osis,* condition]

chlo·ro·then cit·rate (klōr′ō-then). An antihistaminic agent.

chlo·ro·thi·a·zide (klōr-ō-thī′ă-zīd). An orally effective diuretic inhibiting renal tubular reabsorption of sodium; used in the treatment of edema due to congestive heart failure, liver disease, pregnancy, premenstrual tension, and drugs; also used as an adjunct in the management of hypertension.

c. sodium, c. suitable for parenteral administration.

chlo·ro·thy·mol (klōr-ō-thī′mol). An antibacterial for topical use. SYN chlorthymol.

ch

chlo·rot·ic (klō-rot′ik). Pertaining to or having the characteristic features of chlorosis.

chlo·ro·tri·an·i·sene (klōr′ō-trī-an′i-sēn). A synthetic estrogen derived from stilbene, active by mouth.

chlo·rous (klōr′ŭs). 1. Relating to chlorine. 2. Denoting compounds of chlorine in which its valence is +3; e.g., c. acid.

chlo·rous ac·id. HClO₂; an acid forming chlorites with bases.

β-chlo·ro·vi·nyl·di·chlo·ro·ar·sine (klōr′ō-vī′nil-dī-klōr′ō-ar′sēn). SYN lewisite.

chlo·ro·zo·to·cin (klōr′ō-zō-tō-sin). A nitrogen mustard compound that is a chloroethylnitrosourea compound used in cancer chemotherapy; an antineoplastic.

chlor·phen·e·sin (klōr-fen′ĕ-sin). A topical antifungal agent.

c. carbamate, a skeletal muscle relaxant in which actions are exerted in the central nervous system.

chlor·phen·in·di·one (klōr-fen-in-dī′ōn). An anticoagulant related chemically to phenindione.

chlor·phen·ir·a·mine ma·le·ate (klōr-fen-ir′ă-mēn). An H₁ antihistamine.

chlor·phe·nol red (klōr-fē′nol). An acid-base indicator (MW 423, pK 6.0): yellow at pH values below 5.1, red above 6.7.

chlor·phen·ox·a·mine (klōr-fen-ok′să-mēn). Used in the management of idiopathic, arteriosclerotic, and postencephalitic parkinsonism, usually with concomitant administration of other antiparkinsonian agents.

chlor·phen·ter·mine hy·dro·chlo·ride (klōr-fen′ter-mēn). A sympathomimetic amine used as an anorexiant; resembles amphetamine.

chlor·pro·guan·il hy·dro·chlo·ride (klōr-prō′gwah-nil). The 3,4-dichloro homologue of chloroguanide; used for causal prophylaxis and suppression of falciparum malaria.

chlor·prom·a·zine (klōr-prō′mă-zēn). A phenothiazine antipsychotic agent with antiemetic, antiadrenergic, and anticholinergic actions.

c. hydrochloride, c. suitable for oral, intramuscular, and intravenous administration.

chlor·prop·a·mide (klōr-prō′pă-mīd). An orally effective hypoglycemic agent related chemically and pharmacologically to tolbutamide; used in controlling hyperglycemia in selected patients with adult onset (type II) diabetes mellitus.

chlor·pro·thix·ene (klōr-prō-thik′sēn). An antipsychotic of the thioxanthene group; it also possesses antiemetic, adrenolytic, spasmolytic, and antihistaminic actions.

chlor·quin·al·dol (klōr-kwin′al-dol). A keratoplastic, antibacterial, and antifungal agent used in the treatment of cutaneous bacterial and mycotic infections.

chlor·tet·ra·cy·cline (klōr′tet-ră-sī′klēn). Active against a wide range of pathogenic microorganisms including hemolytic streptococci, staphylococci, typhoid bacilli, and brucellae, as well as against certain viruses. Also available as c. hydrochloride.

chlor·thal·i·done (klōr-thal′i-dōn). An orally effective diuretic and antihypertensive agent, used in the treatment of edema associated with congestive heart failure, renal disease, hepatic cirrhosis, pregnancy, and premenstrual tension; it produces an increase in the excretion of sodium, chloride, potassium, and water.

chlor·then·ox·a·zin (klōr-then-ok′să-zin). An antipyretic and analgesic.

chlor·thy·mol (klōr-thī′mol). SYN chlorothymol.

chlor·u·re·sis (klōr-ū-rē′sis). The excretion of chloride in the urine. SYN chloriduria, chloruria.

chlor·u·ret·ic (klōr-ū-ret′ik). Relating to an agent that increases the excretion of chloride in the urine, or to such an effect.

chlor·u·ria (klōr-ū′rē-ă). SYN chloruresis.

chlor·zox·a·zone (klōr-zok′să-zōn). A centrally acting skeletal muscle relaxant used in the treatment of painful muscle spasm due to musculoskeletal disorder.

cho·a·nae (kō′an-ă) [TA]. The opening into the nasopharynx of the nasal cavity on either side. SYN posterior nasal apertures☆, isthmus pharyngonasalis, posterior nares, postnaris. [Mod. L. fr. G. *choanē,* a funnel]

primary c., primitive c., initial opening of the nasal pits and olfactory sac of the embryo into the rostral part of the primordial oronasal cavity, before the formation of the secondary palate.

secondary c., the definitive c. opening into the nasopharynx, after the nasal chambers have been lengthened by the formation of the secondary palate. SYN internal nostril.

cho·a·nal (kō′ă-năl). Pertaining to a choana.

cho·a·nate (kō′an-āt). Having a funnel, i.e., with a ring or collar.

cho·a·no·flag·el·late (kō′an-ō-flaj′ĕ-lāt). SYN choanomastigote.

cho·a·noid (kō′ă-noyd). Funnel-shaped. SYN infundibuliform. [G. *choanē,* funnel, + *eidos,* resemblance]

cho·a·no·mas·ti·gote (kō′an-ō-mas′tī-gōt). A term, in the series used to describe developmental stages of the parasitic flagellates, denoting the "barleycorn" form of the flagellate in the genus *Crithidia* characterized by a collarlike extension surrounding the anterior and through which the single flagellum emerges. SEE ALSO amastigote, epimastigote, promastigote, trypomastigote. SYN choanoflagellate, collared flagellate. [G. *choanē,* a funnel, + *mastix,* whip]

Cho·a·no·tae·nia in·fun·dib·u·lum (kō-ā-nō-tē′nē-ă). An important species of cosmopolitan tapeworm of fowls, occurring in the small intestine and transmitted by houseflies and stableflies; related to *Dipylidium,* the double-pored dog tapeworm. [G. *choanē,* a funnel, + L., fr. G. *tainia,* tapeworm]

Chodzko re·flex. See under reflex.

choke (chōk). 1. To prevent respiration by compression or obstruction of the larynx or trachea; common expression for laryngospasm. 2. Any obstruction of the esophagus in herbivorous animals by a partly swallowed foreign body. [M.E. *choken,* fr. O.E. *ăceócian*]

chokes (chōks). A manifestation of decompression sickness or altitude sickness characterized by dyspnea, coughing, and choking.

△**chol-.** SEE chole-.

cho·la·gog·ic (kō-lă-goj′ik). SYN cholagogue (2).

cho·la·gogue (kō′lă-gog). 1. An agent that promotes the flow of bile into the intestine, especially as a result of contraction of the gallbladder. 2. Relating to such an agent or effect. SYN cholagogic. [chol- + G. *agōgos,* drawing forth]

cho·la·ic ac·id (kō-lā′ik). SYN taurocholic acid.

cho·lal·ic ac·id (kō-lal′ik). SYN cholic acid.

cho·lane, 5β-cho·lane (kō′lān). Parent hydrocarbon of the cholanic acids (cholic acids); androstane with a –CH(CH₃)- CH₂CH₂CH₃ group in the 17 position. 5α-Cholane is sometimes called allocholane. For structures, see steroids.

chol·a·ner·e·sis (kō-lă-ner′ĕ-sis). Increase in output of cholic acid or its conjugates. [cholane + G. *hairesis,* a taking]

cho·lan·ge·i·tis (kō′lan-jē-ī′tis). SYN cholangitis.

chol·an·gi·ec·ta·sis (kō-lan-jē-ek′tă-sis). Dilation of the bile ducts, usually as a sequel to obstruction or from a congenital lack of a portion of the ductal wall. [chol- + G. *angeion,* vessel, + *ektasis,* a stretching]

chol·an·gi·o·car·ci·no·ma (kō-lan′jē-ō-kar-si-nō′mă). An adenocarcinoma, primarily in intrahepatic bile ducts, composed of ducts lined by cuboidal or columnar cells that do not contain bile, with abundant fibrous stroma; cirrhosis is usually absent.

chol·an·gi·o·en·ter·os·to·my (kō-lan′jē-ō-en-ter-os′tō-mē). Surgical anastomosis of bile duct to intestine.

chol·an·gi·o·fi·bro·sis (kō-lan′jē-ō-fī-brō′sis). Fibrosis of the bile ducts. [chol- + G. *angeion,* vessel, + fibrosis]

chol·an·gi·o·gas·tros·to·my (kō-lan′jē-ō-gas-tros′tō-mē). Formation of a communication between a bile duct and the stomach. [chol- + G. *angeion,* vessel, + *gastēr,* belly, + *stoma,* mouth]

chol·an·gi·o·gram (kō-lan′jē-ō-gram). The radiographic record of the bile ducts obtained by cholangiography.

▪**chol·an·gi·og·ra·phy** (kō-lan-jē-og′ră-fē). Radiographic examination of the bile ducts with contrast medium. [chol- + G. *angeion,* vessel, + *graphō,* to write]

cystic duct c., radiography of the biliary system after introduction of contrast medium through the cystic duct.

intravenous c., c. of bile ducts opacified by hepatic secretion of an intravenously injected contrast medium.

percutaneous c., radiography of the biliary system after introduction of contrast medium by inserting a needle through the skin, inferior to the right costal margin, into the substance of the liver or into the gallbladder.

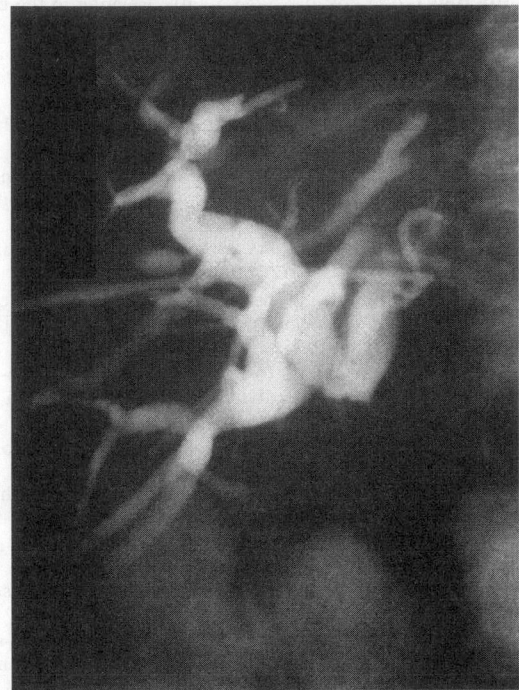

percutaneous transhepatic cholangiography: showing obstruction of common bile duct by tumor (dark area below center of image)

🔲**percutaneous transhepatic c. (PTHC),** contrast radiographic examination of biliary system performed by injection of radiopaque dye through a percutaneously placed needle inserted into an intrahepatic bile duct.

chol·an·gi·ole (kō-lan′jē-ōl). A ductule occurring between a bile canaliculus and an interlobular bile duct. SYN canal of Hering. [chol- + G. *angeion*, vessel, + *-ole*, small]

chol·an·gi·o·li·tis (kō-lan′jē-ō-lī′tis). Inflammation of the small bile radicles or cholangioles.

chol·an·gi·o·ma (kō-lan′jē-ō′mă). A neoplasm of bile duct origin, especially within the liver; may be either benign or malignant (cholangiocarcinoma). [chol- + G. *angeion*, vessel, + *-oma*, tumor]

chol·an·gi·o·pan·cre·a·tog·ra·phy (kō-lan′jē-ō-pan-krē-ă-tog′ră-fē). Contrast radiographic examination of the bile and pancreatic ducts after the injection of radiopaque dye.

endoscopic retrograde c. (ERCP), a method of c. using an endoscope to inspect and cannulate the ampulla of Vater, with injection of contrast medium for radiographic examination of the pancreatic, hepatic, and common bile ducts.

chol·an·gi·os·co·py (kō-lan-jē-os′kŏ-pē). Visual examination of bile ducts utilizing a fiberoptic endoscope. [chol- + G. *angeion*, vessel, + *skopeō*, to examine]

chol·an·gi·os·to·my (kō-lan-jē-os′tō-mē). Formation of a fistula into a bile duct. [chol- + G. *angeion*, vessel, + *stoma*, mouth]

chol·an·gi·ot·o·my (ko-lan-jĭ-ot′o-mĭ). Incision into a bile duct. [chol- + G. *angeion*, vessel, + *tome*, incision]

chol·an·gi·tis (kō-lan-jī′tis). Inflammation of a bile duct or the entire biliary tree. SYN angiocholitis, cholangeitis. [chol- + G. *angeion*, vessel, + *-itis,* inflammation]

ascending c., SYN c. lenta.

c. lenta (len-tă′), low-grade bacterial infection of the biliary tract; sometimes a cause of fever of unknown origin. SYN ascending c.

primary sclerosing c., recurrent or persistent obstructive jaundice, frequently with ulcerative colitis, due to extensive obliterative fibrosis of the extrahepatic or intrahepatic bile ducts; generally progresses to cirrhosis, portal hypertension, and liver failure; seen most commonly in young men.

recurrent pyogenic c., repeated attacks of c., most commonly noted among Asians living in Asia, associated with the presence of multiple intrahepatic and extrahepatic bile duct strictures and stones.

cho·lan·ic ac·id (kō-lan′ik). SYN cholic acid.

cho·lan·o·poi·e·sis (kō′lan-ō-poy-ē′sis). Synthesis by the liver of cholic acid or its conjugates, or of natural bile salts. [chol- + G. *anō,* upward, + *poiēsis,* making]

cho·lan·o·poi·et·ic (kō′lan-ō-poy-et′ik). Pertaining to or promoting cholanopoiesis.

chol·an·threne (kō-lan′thrēn). A polycyclic, somewhat carcinogenic hydrocarbon, structural parent of the highly carcinogenic 3 (or 20)-methylcholanthrene.

cho·las·cos (kō-las′kos). Rarely used term for escape of bile into the free peritoneal cavity. [chol- + G. *askos,* bag]

cho·late (kō′lāt). A salt or ester of a cholic acid.

c. ligase, an enzyme that converts c., coenzyme A, and ATP, to choloyl-coenzyme A, AMP, and pyrophosphate. SYN choloyl-coenzyme A synthetase.

c. synthetase, c. thiokinase, cholate-CoA ligase.

♻**chole-, chol-, cholo-.** Bile. Cf. bili-. [G. *cholē*]

cho·le·cal·cif·er·ol (kō′lē-kal-sif′er-ol). (5Z,7E)-(3S)-9,10-Secocholesta-5,7,10(19)-trien-3-ol; formed by breakage of the 9,10 bond in 7-dehydrocholesterol by ultraviolet irradiation, yielding a double bond between C-10 and C-19; probably the vitamin D of animal origin found in the skin, fur, and feathers of animals and birds exposed to sunlight, and also in butter, brain, fish oils, and egg yolk. SYN vitamin D_3. SYN calciol.

cho·le·chro·mo·poi·e·sis (kō′lē-krō-mō-poy-ē′sis). Synthesis of bile pigments by the liver. [chole- + G. *chrōma,* color, + *poiesis,* making]

cho·le·cyst (kō′le-sist). SYN gallbladder.

cho·le·cys·ta·gog·ic (kō′lē-sis-tă-goj′ik). Stimulating activity of the gallbladder.

cho·le·cys·ta·gogue (kō-lē-sis′tă-gog). A substance that stimulates activity of the gallbladder. [chole- + G. *kystis,* bladder, + *agōgos,* leader]

cho·le·cys·tat·o·ny (kō′lē-sis-tat′ō-nē). Atonia, weakness, or failure of function of the gallbladder. [chole- + G. *kystis,* bladder, + *atonia,* atony]

cho·le·cys·tec·ta·sia (kō′lē-sis-tek-tā′zē-ă). Rarely used term for dilation of the gallbladder. [chole- + G. *kystis,* bladder, + *ektasis,* extension]

🔲**cho·le·cys·tec·to·my** (kō′lē-sis-tek′tō-mē). Surgical removal of the gallbladder. [chole- + G. *kystis,* bladder, + *ektomē,* excision]

cho·le·cyst·en·ter·os·to·my (kō′lē-sist-en-ter-os′tō-mē). Formation of a direct communication between the gallbladder and the intestine. SYN enterocholecystostomy. [chole- + G. *kystis,* bladder, + *enteron,* intestine, + *stoma,* mouth]

cho·le·cyst·en·ter·ot·o·my (kō′lē-sist-en-ter-ot′ō-mē). Incision of both intestine and gallbladder. SYN enterocholecystotomy. [chole- + G. *kystis,* bladder, + *enteron,* intestine, + *tome,* a cutting]

cho·le·cys·tic (kō-lē-sis′tik). Relating to the cholecyst, or gallbladder.

cho·le·cys·tis (kō-lē-sis′tis). SYN gallbladder. [chole- + G. *kystis,* bladder]

cho·le·cys·ti·tis (kō′lē-sis-tī′tis). Inflammation of the gallbladder. [chole- + G. *kystis,* bladder, + *-itis,* inflammation]

acute c., inflammation and/or hemorrhagic necrosis, with variable infection, ulceration, and neutrophilic infiltration of the gallbladder wall; usually due to impaction of a stone in the cystic duct.

chronic c., chronic inflammation of the gallbladder, usually secondary to lithiasis, with lymphocytic infiltration and fibrosis that may produce marked thickening of the wall.

emphysematous c., c. due to infection with gas-producing bacteria, giving rise to gas in the gallbladder.

xanthogranulomatous c., chronic c. with conspicuous nodular infiltration by lipid macrophages; may be associated with biliary obstruction by calculi.

cho·le·cys·to·du·o·de·nos·to·my (kō-lē-sis′tō-doo-ō-dē-nos′tō-mē). Establishment of a direct communication between the gallbladder and the duodenum. SYN duodenocholecystostomy, duodenocystostomy (1). [chole- + G. *kystis*, bladder, + L. *duodenum* + G. *stoma*, mouth]

cho·le·cys·to·gas·tros·to·my (kō-lē-sis′tō-gas-tros′tō-mē). Establishment of a communication between the gallbladder and the stomach. [chole- + G. *kystis*, bladder, + *gastēr*, stomach, + *stoma*, mouth]

cho·le·cys·to·gram (kō-lē-sis′tō-gram). The radiographic record of gallbladder structure and function obtained by cholecystography.

cho·le·cys·tog·ra·phy (kō-lē-sis-tog′ră-fē). Radiographic study of the gallbladder after oral administration of a cholecystopaque; or scintigraphic imaging of the gallbladder and central bile ducts after administration of a radiopharmaceutical secreted by the liver. SYN Graham-Cole test. [chole- + G. *kystis*, bladder, + *grapho*, to write]

cho·le·cys·to·il·e·os·to·my (kō-lē-sis′tō-il-ē-os′tō-mē). Establishment of a communication between the gallbladder and the ileum. [chole- + G. *kystis*, bladder, + ileum + G. *stoma*, mouth]

cho·le·cys·to·je·ju·nos·to·my (kō-lē-sis′tō-jē-joo-nos′tō-mē). Establishment of a communication between the gallbladder and the jejunum. [chole- + G. *kystis*, bladder, + jejunum, + G. *stoma*, mouth]

cho·le·cys·to·ki·nase (kō-lē-sis-tō-kī′nās). An enzyme catalyzing the hydrolysis of cholecystokinin.

cho·le·cys·to·ki·net·ic (kō′lē-sis′tō-ki-net′ik). Promoting emptying of the gallbladder.

cho·le·cys·to·ki·nin (CCK) (kō′lē-sis-tō-kī′nin). A polypeptide hormone (the human peptide has 33 residues) liberated by the upper intestinal mucosa on contact with gastric contents; stimulates contraction of the gallbladder and secretion of pancreatic juice. SEE ALSO sincalide. SYN pancreozymin.

cho·le·cys·to·li·thi·a·sis (kō-lē-sis′tō-li-thī′ă-sis). Presence of one or more gallstones in the gallbladder. [chole- + G. *kystis*, bladder, + *lithos*, stone]

cho·le·cys·to·lith·o·trip·sy (kō-lē-sis′tō-lith′ō-trip-sē). Fragmentation of a gallstone most commonly by the application of transcutaneously applied sonic energy focused on the stone. [chole- + G. *kystis*, bladder, + *lithos*, stone, + *tripsis*, a rubbing]

cho·le·cys·to·my (kō-lē-sis′tō-mē). SYN cholecystotomy.

cho·le·cys·to·paque (kō-lē-sis′tō-pāk). A radiographic contrast medium that opacifies the gallbladder following oral administration, by virtue of hepatic secretion and gallbladder concentration; used in cholecystography.

cho·le·cys·top·a·thy (kō′lē-sis-top′ă-thē). Disease of the gallbladder.

cho·le·cys·to·pexy (kō-lē-sis′tō-pek-sē). Suture of the gallbladder to the abdominal wall. [chole- + G. *kystis*, bladder, + *pēxis*, fixation]

cho·le·cys·tor·rha·phy (kō′lē-sis-tōr′ă-fē). Suture of an incised or ruptured gallbladder. [chole- + G. *kystis*, bladder, + *rhaphē*, sewing]

cho·le·cys·to·so·nog·ra·phy (kō-lē-sis′tō-sō-nog′ră-fē). Ultrasonic examination of the gallbladder. [cholecysto- + sonography]

cho·le·cys·tos·to·my (kō′lē-sis-tos′tō-mē). Establishment of a fistula into the gallbladder. [chole- + G. *kystis*, bladder, + *stoma*, mouth]

cho·le·cys·tot·o·my (kō′lē-sis-tot′ō-mē). Incision into the gallbladder. SYN cholecystomy. [chole- + G. *kystis*, bladder, + *tomē*, incision]

laparoscopic c., minimally invasive surgical technique for removal of the gallbladder whereby four or five small (less than 10

mm) incisions are used for the insertion of a laparoscope and various instruments into the abdominal cavity, therefore avoiding the traditional incision.

cho·le·doch (kō′lē-dok). SYN bile *duct* (1). [G. *cholēdochos*, containing bile, fr. *cholē*, bile, + *dechomai*, to receive]

♻**choledoch-.** SEE choledocho-.

cho·le·doch·al (kō-lē-dok′ăl, kō-led′ō-kal). Relating to the common bile duct.

cho·led·o·chec·to·my (kō-led-ō-kek′tō-mē). Surgical removal of a portion of the common bile duct. [choledoch- + G. *ektomē*, excision]

cho·led·o·chen·dy·sis (kō′led-ō-ken′dī-sis). SYN choledochotomy. [choledoch- + G. *endysis*, an entering in]

cho·led·o·chi·arc·tia (kō′led-ō-ki-ark′tē-ă). Obsolete term for stenosis of the gall duct. [choledoch- + L. *artus* (improperly *arctus*), narrow]

cho·led·o·chi·tis (kō-led-ō-kī′tis). Inflammation of the common bile duct. [choledoch- + G. *-itis*, inflammation]

♻**choledocho-, choledoch-.** The ductus choledochus (the common bile duct). [G. *cholēdochos*, containing bile, fr. *cholē*, bile, + *dechomai*, to receive]

cho·led·o·cho·cho·led·o·chos·to·my (kō-led′ō-kō-kō-led′ō-kos′tō-mē). Operative joining of divided portions of common bile duct. [choledocho- + choledocho- + G. *stoma*, mouth]

cho·led·o·cho·du·o·de·nos·to·my (kō-led′ō-kō-doo′ō-dē-nos′tō-mē). Formation of a communication, other than the natural one, between the common bile duct and the duodenum. [choledocho- + duodenum + G. *stoma*, mouth]

cho·led·o·cho·en·ter·os·tomy (kō-led′ō-kō-en-ter-os′tō-mē). Establishment of a communication, other than the natural one, between the common bile duct and any part of the intestine. [choledocho- + G. *enteron*, intestine, + *stoma*, mouth]

cho·led·o·cho·je·ju·nos·to·my (kō-led′ō-kō-jě-joo-nos′tō-mē). Anastomosis between the common bile duct and the jejunum. [choledocho- + jejuno- + G. *stoma*, mouth]

cho·led·o·cho·lith (kō-led′ō-kō-lith). Stone in the common bile duct. [choledocho- + G. *lithos*, stone]

cho·led·o·cho·li·thi·a·sis (kō-led′ō-kō-lith-ī′ă-sis). Presence of a stone in the common bile duct.

cho·led·o·cho·li·thot·o·my (kō-led′ō-kō-li-thot′ō-mē). Incision of the common bile duct for the extraction of a stone. [choledocho- + G. *lithos*, stone, + *tomē*, incision]

cho·led·o·cho·lith·o·trip·sy (kō-led′ō-kō-lith′ō-trip-sē). Fragmentation of a gallstone in the common bile duct either by transcutaneous sonic energy or endoscopically directed laser. SYN choledocholithotrity. [choledocho- + G. *lithos*, stone, + *tripsis*, rubbing]

cho·led·o·cho·li·thot·ri·ty (kō-led′ō-kō-li-thot′ri-tē). SYN choledocholithotripsy.

cho·led·o·cho·plas·ty (kō-led′ō-kō-plas-tē). Rearrangement of tissues of the common bile duct. [choledocho- + G. *plastos*, formed]

cho·led·o·chor·rha·phy (kō-led-ō-kōr′ă-fē). Suturing together the divided ends of the common bile duct. [choledocho- + G. *rhaphē*, suture]

cho·led·o·chos·to·my (kō-led-ō-kos′tō-mē). Establishment of a fistula into the common bile duct. [choledocho- + G. *stoma*, mouth]

cho·led·o·chot·o·my (kō-led-ō-kot′ō-mē). Incision into the common bile duct. SYN choledochendysis. [choledocho- + G. *tomē*, incision]

cho·led·o·chous (kō-led′ō-kŭs). Containing or conveying bile.

cho·led·o·chus (kō-led′ō-kŭs). SYN bile *duct* (1). [see choledoch]

cho·le·glo·bin (kō-lē-glō′bin). A pigmented compound of globin and iron porphyrin (with an open ring due to cleavage of the α-methene bridge by α-methyl oxygenase); the first intermediate in the degradation of hemoglobin, further degraded successively to verdohemochrome, biliverdin, and bilirubin. SYN bile pigment hemoglobin, green hemoglobin, verdohemoglobin.

cho·le·he·ma·tin (kō-lē-hē′mă-tin). A red pigment in the bile of herbivorous animals; derived from chlorophyll and a product of hematin oxidation.

cho·le·he·mia (kō-lē-hē'mē-ă). SYN cholemia. [chole- + G. *haima,* blood]

cho·le·ic (kō-lē'ik). SYN cholic.

cho·le·ic ac·ids. Compounds of bile acids and sterols.

cho·le·lith (kō'lē-lith). SYN gallstone. [chole- + G. *lithos,* stone]

▣**cho·le·li·thi·a·sis** (kō'lē-li-thī'ă-sis). Presence of concretions in the gallbladder or bile ducts. SYN chololithiasis.

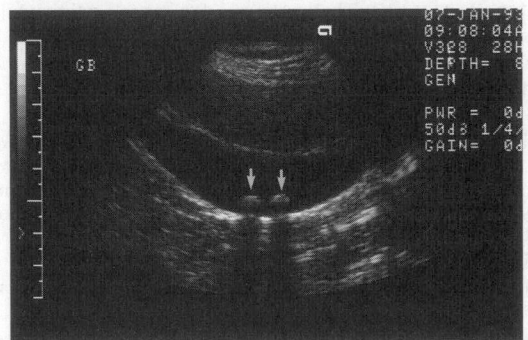

cholelithiasis: sonogram of two stones present in the gallbladder

cho·le·li·thot·o·my (kō'lē-li-thot'ō-mē). Operative removal of a gallstone. [chole- + G. *lithos,* stone, + *tomē,* incision]

cho·le·lith·o·trip·sy (kō-lē-lith'ō-trip-sē). Rarely used term for the crushing of a gallstone. [chole- + G. *lithos,* stone, + *tripsis,* a rubbing]

cho·le·li·thot·ri·ty (kō-lē-li-thot'ri-tē). Rarely used term for the crushing of a gallstone. [chole- + G. *lithos,* stone, + L. *tero,* pp. *tritus,* to rub]

cho·lem·e·sis (kō-lem'ě-sis). Vomiting of bile. [chole- + G. *emesis,* vomiting]

cho·le·mia (kō-lē'mē-ă). The presence of bile salts in the circulating blood. SYN cholehemia. [chole- + G. *haima,* blood]

cho·lem·ic (kō-lē'mik). Relating to cholemia.

cho·le·path·ia (kō-lē-path'ē-ă). **1.** Disease of bile ducts. **2.** Irregularity in contractions of the bile ducts.

c. spas'tica, spastic contraction of the bile ducts.

cho·le·per·i·to·ni·tis (kō'le-per-i-tō-nī'tis). SYN bile *peritonitis.*

cho·le·poi·e·sis (kō'lē-poy-ē'sis). Formation of bile. SYN cholopoiesis. [chole- + G. *poiēsis,* making]

cho·le·poi·et·ic (kō'lē-poy-et'ik). Relating to the formation of bile.

chol·era (kol'er-ă). An acute epidemic infectious disease caused by the bacterium *Vibrio cholerae.* A soluble toxin elaborated in the intestinal tract by the bacterium activates the adenylate cylase of the mucosa, causing active secretion of an isotonic fluid resulting in profuse watery diarrhea, extreme loss of fluid and electrolytes, and dehydration and collapse, but no gross morphologic change in the intestinal mucosa. SYN Asiatic c. [L. a bilious disease, fr. G. *cholē,* bile]

Asiatic c., SYN cholera.

c. infan'tum, old term for a disease of infants, characterized by vomiting, profuse watery diarrhea, fever, prostration, and collapse.

c. mor'bus, old term for acute severe gastroenteritis of unknown etiology, marked by severe colic, vomiting, and diarrhea with watery stools; formerly common during hot weather.

pancreatic c., SYN *diarrhea* pancreatica.

c. sic'ca, an old term for a malignant form of disease seen during epidemics of Asiatic c. in which death occurs without diarrhea.

typhoid c., old term for c. (2) with predominantly cerebral manifestations such as confusion or dementia.

chol·er·a·gen (kol'er-ă-jen). A term suggested for a factor(s)

produced during growth in vitro of the cholera vibrio and causes diarrhea. [cholera + G. *-gen,* producing]

chol·er·a·ic (kol'er-ā'ik). Relating to cholera.

chol·er·a·phage (kol'er-ă-fāj). Bacteriophage of *Vibrio cholerae.* [cholera + G. *phagō,* to eat]

cho·le·re·sis (kō-ler-ē'sis). The secretion of bile, as opposed to the expulsion of bile, by the gallbladder. [chole- + G. *hairesis,* a taking]

cho·le·ret·ic (kol-er-et'ik). **1.** Relating to choleresis. **2.** An agent, usually a drug, that stimulates the liver to increase output of bile.

chol·er·rhe·ic (kol-ě-rē'ik). Denoting diarrhea produced secondary to unabsorbed bile salts. [chole- + G. *hairesis,* a taking]

chol·er·ic (kol'er-ik). SYN bilious (3).

chol·er·i·form (kol'er-i-fōrm). Resembling cholera. SYN choleroid.

chol·er·i·gen·ic, chol·er·ig·en·ous (kol'er-i-jen'ik, -ij'en-ŭs). Causing or engendering cholera.

chol·er·ine (kol'er-ēn). A mild form of diarrhea seen during epidemics of Asiatic cholera.

chol·er·oid (kol'er-oyd). SYN choleriform.

cho·ler·rha·gia (kō-lē-rā'jē-ă). Extensive flow of bile. [chole- + G. *rhegnymi,* to burst forth]

cho·ler·rha·gic (kō-lē-raj'ik). Referring to the flow of bile.

chol·e·scin·tig·ra·phy (kō-lē-sin-tig'ră-fē). Examination of the gall bladder and bile ducts by nuclear medicine scanning; radionuclide cholecystography. [chole- + scintigraphy]

cho·les·tane (kō'les-tān). The parent hydrocarbon of cholesterol. For structure, see steroids.

cho·les·ta·nol (kō-les'tan-ol). Differing from cholesterol in the absence of the double bond.

cho·les·tan·one (kō-les'tan-ōn). An oxidation product of cholestanol, differing from it in the presence of a ketone oxygen in place of the 3-hydroxyl group; an isomer of coprostanone.

cho·le·sta·sia, cho·le·sta·sis (kō-les-tā'sē-ă, -les'tă-sis). An arrest in the flow of bile; c. due to obstruction of bile ducts is accompanied by formation of plugs of inspissated bile in the small ducts, canaliculi in the liver, and elevation of serum direct bilirubin and some enzymes. [chole- + G. *stasis,* a standing still]

cho·le·sta·sis (-les'tă-sis). SEE cholestasia.

intrahepatic cholestasis of pregnancy, intrahepatic cholestasis with centrilobular bile staining without inflammatory cells or proliferation of mesenchymal cells; clinically characterized by pruritus and/or icterus; of unknown cause but associated with high estrogen levels. SYN cholestasis of pregnancy, cholestatic hepatosis icterus gravidarum, recurrent jaundice of pregnancy.

cholestasis of pregnancy, SYN intrahepatic cholestasis of pregnancy.

cho·le·stat·ic (kō-les-tat'ik). Tending to diminish or stop the flow of bile.

▣**cho·les·te·a·to·ma** (kō-les-tē-ă-tō'mă). **1.** A mass of keratinized squamous cell epithelium and cholesterol in the middle ear, usually resulting from chronic otitis media, with squamous metaplasia or extension of squamous epithelium inward to line an expanding cystic cavity that may involve the mastoid and erode surrounding bone. **2.** An epidermoid cyst arising in the central nervous system in humans or animals. [cholesterol + G. *stear (steat-),* tallow, + *-ōma,* tumor]

cho·les·te·at·om·a·tous (kō-les-tē-ă-tō'mă-tŭs). Of or pertaining to cholesteatoma.

cho·les·ten·one (kō-les'ten-ōn). A dehydrocholestanone, differing from cholestanone by the presence of a double bond between carbons 4 and 5.

cho·les·ter·e·mia (kō-les-ter-ē'mē-ă). The presence of enhanced quantities of cholesterol in the blood. SYN cholesterinemia, cholesterolemia. [cholesterol + G. *haima,* blood]

cho·les·ter·in·e·mia (kō-les'ter-in-ē'mē-ă). SYN cholesteremia.

cho·les·ter·in·o·sis (kō-les'ter-in-ō'sis). SYN cholesterolosis.

cho·les·ter·i·nu·ria (kō-les'ter-i-noo'rē-ă). SYN cholesteroluria. [cholesterin + G. *ouron,* urine]

cho·les·ter·ol (kō-les'ter-ol). 5-Cholesten-3β-ol (cholestane with a 5,6 double bond and a 3β-hydroxyl group); the most abundant steroid in animal tissues, especially in bile and gallstones, and present in food, especially food rich in animal fats; circulates in the plasma complexed to proteins of various densities and plays an important role in the pathogenesis of atheroma formation in arteries. SEE ALSO lipoprotein.

cho·les·ter·ol·e·mia (kō-les′ter-ol-ē′mē-ă). SYN cholesteremia. [cholesterol + G. *haima,* blood]

cho·les·ter·ol·o·gen·e·sis (kō-les′ter-ol-ō-jen′ĕ-sis). The biosynthesis of cholesterol.

cho·les·ter·ol·o·sis (kō-les′ter-ol-ō′sis). **1.** A condition resulting from a disturbance in metabolism of lipids, characterized by deposits of cholesterol in tissue, as in Tangier disease. **2.** Cholesterol crystals in the anterior chamber of the eye, as in aphakia with associated retinal separation. SYN cholesterinosis.

cho·les·ter·ol·u·ria (kō-les′ter-ol-oo′rē-ă). The excretion of cholesterol in the urine. SYN cholesterinuria.

cho·le·styr·a·mine (kō-les′tēr-ă-mēn). An anion exchange resin used to bind dietary cholesterol and hence prevent its systemic absorption. Used to treat hypercholesteremia. Can bind many acidic drugs in the gastrointestinal tract and prevent their absorption.

cho·le·u·ria (kō-lē-ū′rē-ă). SYN biliuria.

cho·lic (kō′lik). Relating to the bile. SYN choleic.

cho·lic ac·id. A family of steroids comprising the bile acids (or salts), generally in conjugated form (e.g., glycocholic and taurocholic acids). Chemically, c. a.'s are cholan-24-oic (cholanic) acids (the terminal C_{24} of cholane becoming a –COOH group); biologically, c. a.'s are derived from cholesterol (a cholestane derivative) and display varying degrees of oxidation (OH groups) and orientation at positions 3, 7, and 12. It is these oxidations and orientations that distinguish the several c. a.'s; e.g., c. a. is 3α,7α,12α-trihydroxy-5β-cholan-24-oic acid, deoxycholic acid is 3α,12α-dihydroxy-5β-cholanic acid. C. a. is a naturally occurring detergent that aids in the digestion of fats. SYN cholalic acid, cholanic acid.

cho·li·cele (kō′li-sēl). Enlargement of the gallbladder due to retained fluids. [G. *cholē,* bile, + *kēlē,* tumor]

cho·line (kō′lēn). (2-Hydroxyethyl)trimethylammonium ion; found in most animal tissues either free or in combination as lecithin (phosphatidylcholine), acetate (acetylcholine), or cytidine diphosphate (cytidine diphosphocholine). It is included in the vitamin B complex; as acetylcholine (choline esterified with acetic acid), it is essential for synaptic transmission. Several salts of choline are used in medicine. SYN lipotropic factor, transmethylation factor.

c. acetylase, SYN c. acetyltransferase.

c. acetyltransferase, an enzyme catalyzing the condensation of choline and acetyl-coenzyme A, forming *O*-acetylcholine and coenzyme A. SYN c. acetylase.

activated c., SYN cytidine diphosphocholine.

c. chloride, a lipotropic agent.

c. dihydrogen citrate, a lipotropic agent.

c. esterase I, SYN acetylcholinesterase.

c. esterase II, SYN cholinesterase.

c. kinase, an enzyme that catalyzes the formation of *O*-phosphocholine and ADP from choline and ATP. SYN c. phosphokinase.

c. phosphatase, SYN *phospholipase* D.

c. phosphate cytidylyltransferase, an enzyme that catalyzes a key step in lecithin biosynthesis: CTP + phosphocholine ↔ pyrophosphate + CDP-choline.

c. phosphokinase, SYN c. kinase.

c. salicylate, c. salt of salicyclic acid, an analgesic and antipyretic (because of the salicylate moiety).

c. theophyllinate, SYN oxtriphylline.

cho·line·phos·pho·trans·fer·ase (kō′lēn-fos-fō-trans′fer-ās). An enzyme catalyzing the reaction between CDP-choline and 1,2-diacylglycerol to form a phosphatidylcholine and CMP. The last step in lecithin biosynthesis.

cho·lin·er·gic (kol-in-er′jik). Relating to nerve cells or fibers that employ acetylcholine as their neurotransmitter. Cf. adrenergic. [choline + G. *ergon,* work]

cho·lin·es·ter (kō′lin-es-ter). An ester of choline; e.g., acetylcholine.

cho·lin·es·ter·ase (kō-lin-es′ter-ās). One of a family of enzymes capable of catalyzing the hydrolysis of acylcholines and a few other compounds. In mammals, found in white matter of brain, liver, heart, pancreas, and serum. It is also found in cobra venom. SEE ALSO acetylcholinesterase. SYN choline esterase II, nonspecific c., "s"-type c.

"e"-type c., SYN acetylcholinesterase. ["e" as in erythrocyte]

nonspecific c., SYN cholinesterase.

specific c., SYN acetylcholinesterase.

"s"-type c., SYN cholinesterase. ["s" as in serum]

true c., SYN acetylcholinesterase.

cho·lin·es·ter·ase re·ac·ti·va·tor. A drug that reacts directly with the alkylphosphorylated enzyme to free the active unit; the drugs used therapeutically to reactivate phosphorylated forms of acetylcholinesterase are oximes, e.g., diacetylmonoxime, monoisonitrosoacetone, 2-pralidoxime.

cho·lin·o·cep·tive (kō′lin-ō-sep′tiv). Referring to chemical sites in effector cells with which acetylcholine unites to exert its actions. Cf. adrenoceptive. [acetylcholine + L. *capio,* to take]

cho·li·no·lyt·ic (kō′lin-ō-lit′ik). Preventing the action of acetylcholine. [acetylcholine + G. *lysis,* loosening]

chol·i·no·mi·met·ic (kol′i-nō-mi-met′ik). Having an action similar to that of acetylcholine, the substance liberated by cholinergic nerves; term proposed to replace the less accurate term, parasympathomimetic. Cf. adrenomimetic. [acetylcholine + G. *mimētikos,* imitating]

cho·lin·o·re·ac·tive (kō′lin-ō-rē-ak′tiv). Responding to acetylcholine and related compounds.

chol·i·no·re·cep·tors (kol′i-nō-rē-sep′terz, -tōrz). SEE cholinergic *receptors,* under *receptor.*

cho·lis·tine sul·pho·meth·ate so·di·um (kō-lis′tēn sul-fō-meth′āt). SYN colistimethate sodium.

△**cholo-.** SEE chole-.

chol·o·li·thi·a·sis (kol-ō-li-thī′ă-sis). SYN cholelithiasis.

chol·o·pla·nia (kol-ō-plā′nē-ă). The presence of bile salts in the blood or tissues. [cholo- + G. *planē,* a wandering]

chol·o·poi·e·sis (kō-lō-poy-ē′sis). SYN cholepoiesis.

chol·or·rhea (kol-ō-rē′ă). Obsolete term for an excessive secretion of bile. [cholo- + G. *rhoia,* a flow]

cho·los·co·py (kō-los′kŏ-pē). Rarely used term for cholangioscopy. [cholo- + G. *skopeō,* to view]

chol·o·tho·rax (kō-lō-thōr′aks). Bile in the pleural cavity.

cho·lo·yl (kō′lō-il). The radical of cholic acid or cholate.

chol·ur·ia (kō-loo′rē-ă). SYN biliuria. [G. *cholē,* bile, + *ouron,* urine]

cho·lyl-co·en·zyme A (kō′lil-kō-en′zīm). A condensation product of cholic acid and coenzyme A; an intermediate in the formation of bile salts from bile acids, such as taurocholic acid from cholic acid.

c.-c. A synthetase, SYN *cholate* ligase.

chon·dral (kon′drăl). SYN cartilaginous. [G. *chondros,* cartilage]

chon·dral·lo·pla·sia (kon′dral-ō-plā′zē-ă). Occurrence of cartilage in abnormal situations in the bony skeleton. [G. *chondros,* cartilage, + *allos,* other, + *plasia,* formed]

chon·drec·to·my (kon-drek′tō-mē). Excision of cartilage. [G. *chondros,* cartilage, + *ektomē,* excision]

chon·dri·fi·ca·tion (kon′dri-fi-kā′shŭn). Conversion into cartilage. [G. *chondros,* cartilage, + L. *facio,* to make]

chon·dri·fy (kon′dri-fī). To become cartilaginous.

△**chondrio-.** SEE chondro-.

chon·dri·tis (kon-drī′tis). Inflammation of cartilage. [G. *chondros,* cartilage, + *-itis,* inflammation]

costal c., SYN costochondritis.

△**chondro-, chondrio-.** **1.** Cartilage or cartilaginous. **2.** Granular or gritty substance. [G. *chondrion,* dim. of *chondros,* groats (coarsely ground grain), grit, gristle, cartilage]

chon·dro·blast (kon′drō-blast). A dividing cell of growing cartilage tissue. SYN chondroplast. [chondro- + G. *blastos,* germ]

chon·dro·blas·to·ma (kon′drō-blas-tō′mă). A benign tumor arising in the epiphyses of long bones, consisting of highly cellular tissue resembling fetal cartilage.

chon·dro·cal·cin (kon′drō-kal-sin). A 69,000 molecular weight protein believed to play a role in mineralization in hard tissue.

chon·dro·cal·ci·no·sis (kon′drō-kal-si-nō′sis). Calcification of cartilage. [chondro- + calcium + G. *-osis,* condition]

articular c. [MIM*118600], a disease characterized by deposits of calcium pyrophosphate crystals free of urate in synovial fluid, articular cartilage, and adjacent soft tissue; causes various forms of arthritis commonly characterized by goutlike attacks of pain, swelling of joints, and radiologic evidence of calcification in articular cartilage (pseudogout); inherited as an autosomal dominant trait in some cases, and associated with certain diseases in others.

chon·dro·clast (kon′drō-klast). A multinucleated cell (giant cell) involved in the resorption of calcified cartilage; morphologically identical to osteoblasts. [chondro- + G. *klastos,* broken in pieces]

chon·dro·cos·tal (kon-drō-kos′tăl). SYN costochondral. [chondro- + L. *costa,* rib]

chon·dro·cra·ni·um (kon-drō-krā′nē-ŭm). A cartilaginous skull; the cartilaginous parts of the developing skull. [chondro- + G. *kranion,* skull]

chon·dro·cyte (kon′drō-sīt). A nondividing cartilage cell; occupies a lacuna within the cartilage matrix. SYN cartilage cell. [chondro- + G. *kytos,* a hollow (cell)]

isogenous c.'s, a clone of cartilage cells derived from one cell by division; occur in a cluster called an isogenous nest.

chon·dro·der·ma·ti·tis no·du·la·ris chron·i·ca he·li·cis (kon-drō-der-ma-tī′tis nod-ū-lar′is kron′i-kă hel′i-sis). A benign, chronic, small, painful nodule or (nodules) on the helix of the ear in the elderly, which may occasionally become ulcerated and results from habitually sleeping on the affected side.

chon·dro·dys·pla·sia (kon′drō-dis-plā′zē-ă) [MIM*118650]. SYN chondrodystrophy. [chondro- + G. *dys,* bad, + *plasis,* a molding]

c. calcif′icans congen′ita [MIM*118650], autosomal dominant inheritance characterized by asymmetric calcifications and dysplastic skeletal changes, less frequent occurrence of congenital cataracts and ichthyosis compared to other forms, and relatively good prognosis. SYN Conradi disease, Conradi-Hünermann disease.

Nance-Sweeney c., SYN *chondrodystrophy* with sensorineural deafness.

c. puncta′ta, a developmental disorder characterized by epiphyseal stippling, coronal clefting of the vertebrae, dwarfism with rhizomelic shortening of the limbs, joint contractures, congenital cataracts, ichthyosis, and mental retardation. Autosomal dominant and recessive and X-linked forms exist. SYN dysplasia epiphysialis punctata, hypoplastic fetal chondrodystrophy, stippled epiphysis.

rhizomelic c. punctata [MIM*215100], autosomal recessively inherited lethal c. caused by mutation in the PEX 7 gene encoding the peroxisomal type 2 targeting signal (PTS2) receptor on chromosomal 6q.

chon·dro·dys·tro·phy (kon-drō-dis′trō-fē). A disturbance in the development of the cartilage primordia of the long bones, especially the region of the epiphysial plates, resulting in arrested growth of the long bones and dwarfism in which the extremities are abnormally short, but the head and trunk are essentially normal; autosomal recessive inheritance. SYN chondrodysplasia. [chondro- + G. *dys,* bad, + *trophē* nourishment]

asphyxiating thoracic c., SYN asphyxiating thoracic *dystrophy.*

asymmetric c., SYN enchondromatosis.

hereditary deforming c., (1) SYN hereditary multiple *exostoses,* under *exostosis;* **(2)** SYN enchondromatosis.

hypoplastic fetal c., SYN *chondrodysplasia* punctata.

myotonic c., a rare congenital disease that causes myotonia, mus-

cular hypertrophy, joint and long bone abnormalities, and weakness. SYN Schwartz-Jampel disease.

c. with sensorineural deafness [MIM*215150], a skeletal dysplasia characterized by dwarfism, flat nasal bridge, cleft palate, sensorineural deafness, large epiphyses, and flattening of the vertebral bodies; autosomal recessive inheritance, caused by mutation in the type XI collagen gene (COL11A2) on chromosome 6p; dominant forms exist. SYN Nance-Insley syndrome, Nance-Sweeney chondrodysplasia, OSMED, otospondylomegaepiphyseal dysplasia.

chon·dro·ec·to·der·mal (kon′drō-ek-tō-der′măl). Relating to ectodermally derived cartilage; e.g., branchial cartilages that have developed from the neural crest.

chon·dro·fi·bro·ma (kon′drō-fī-brō′mă). SYN chondromyxoid *fibroma.*

chon·dro·gen·e·sis (kon-drō-jen′ĕ-sis). Formation of cartilage. [chondro- + G. *genesis,* origin]

chon·dro·glos·sus (kon-drō-glos′ŭs). SEE chondroglossus *muscle.* [chondro- + G. *glossa,* tongue]

chon·droid (kon′droyd). **1.** Resembling cartilage. SYN cartilaginoid. **2.** Uncharacteristically developed cartilage, primarily cellular with a basophilic matrix and thin or nonexistent capsules. [chondro- + G. *eidos,* resemblance]

chon·dro·i·tin (kon-drō′i-tin). A (muco)polysaccharide (proteoglycan) composed of alternating residues of β-D-glucuronic acid and *N*-acetyl-D-galactosamine sulfate in alternating β(1-3) and β(1-4) linkages; present among the ground substance materials in the extracellular matrix of connective tissue.

c. sulfate A, c. with sulfuric residues esterifying the 4-hydroxyl groups of the galactosamine residues; found in connective tissue.

c. sulfate B, SYN dermatan *sulfate.*

c. sulfate C, c. with sulfuric residues esterifying the 6-hydroxyl groups of the galactosamine residues.

chon·drol·o·gy (kon-drol′ō-jē). The study of cartilage. [chondro- + G. *logos,* treatise]

chon·drol·y·sis (kon-drol′i-sis). Disappearance of articular cartilage as the result of disintegration or dissolution of the cartilage matrix and cells.

chon·dro·ma (kon-drō′mă). A benign neoplasm derived from mesodermal cells that form cartilage. [chondro- + G. *-ōma,* tumor]

extraskeletal c., a c. located in soft tissues, usually of the fingers, hands, and feet, not connected to underlying bone or periosteum.

juxtacortical c., SYN periosteal c.

periosteal c., a c. that develops from periosteum or periosteal connective tissue. SYN juxtacortical c.

chon·dro·ma·la·cia (kon′drō-mă-lā′shē-ă). Softening of any cartilage. [chondro- + G. *malakia,* softness]

c. feta′lis, an intrauterine form of c. in which the fetus is born dead with soft pliable limbs.

generalized c., SYN relapsing *polychondritis.*

c. of larynx, the presence of soft laryngeal cartilage, most often seen in epiglottis of young children. SYN laryngomalacia.

c. patel′lae, a softening of the articular cartilage of the patella; may cause patellalgia.

systemic c., SYN relapsing *polychondritis.*

chon·dro·ma·to·sis (kon′drō-mă-tō′sis). Presence of multiple tumor-like foci of cartilage.

synovial c., c. or osteocartilaginous nodules occurring in the synovial membrane of a joint. SYN synovial osteochondromatosis.

chon·dro·ma·tous (kon-drō′mă-tŭs). Pertaining to or manifesting the features of a chondroma.

chon·drome (kon′drōm). The genetic information contained in all of the mitochondria of a cell. [mitochondria + -ome]

chon·dro·mere (kon′drō-mēr). A cartilage unit of the fetal axial skeleton developing within a single metamere of the body; a primordial cartilaginous vertebra together with its costal component. [chondro- + G. *meros,* part]

chon·dro·myx·o·ma (kon′drō-mik-sō′mă). SYN chondromyxoid *fibroma.*

chon·dro·nec·tin (kon-drō-nek'tin). A glycoprotein of cartilage matrix that mediates the adhesion of chondrocytes to type II collagen. [chondro- + L. *necto,* to bind, + -in]

chon·dro·os·se·ous (kon-drō-os'ē-ŭs). Relating to cartilage and bone, either as a mixture of the two tissues or as a junction between the two, such as the union of a rib and its costal cartilage.

chon·dro·os·te·o·dys·tro·phy (kon'drō-os'tē-ō-dis'trō-fē). Term used for a group of disorders of bone and cartilage which includes Morquio syndrome and similar conditions. SYN osteochondrodystrophia deformans, osteochondrodystrophy.

chon·drop·a·thy (kon-drop'ă-thē). Any disease of cartilage. [chondro- + G. *pathos,* suffering]

chon·dro·pha·ryn·ge·us (kon'drō-făr-in-jē'ŭs). SEE middle constrictor (*muscle*) of pharynx.

chon·dro·phyte (kon'drō-fīt). An abnormal cartilaginous mass that develops at the articular surface of a bone. [chondro- + G. *phytos,* a growth]

chon·dro·plast (kon'drō-plast). SYN chondroblast. [chondro- + G. *plastos,* formed]

chon·dro·plas·ty (kon'drō-plas-tē). Reparative or plastic surgery of cartilage. [chondro- + G. *plastos,* formed]

chon·dro·po·ro·sis (kon'drō-pōr-ō'sis). Condition of cartilage in which spaces appear, either normal (in the process of ossification) or pathologic. [chondro- + L. *porosus,* porous]

chon·dro·sar·co·ma (kon'drō-sar-kō'mă). A malignant neoplasm derived from cartilage cells, occurring most frequently in pelvic bones or near the ends of long bones, in middle-aged and older people; most c.'s arise *de novo,* but some may develop in a preexisting benign cartilaginous lesion.

chon·dro·sin, chon·dro·sine (kon'drō-sin). A disaccharide composed of one molecule of D-glucuronic acid and one of D-galactosamine (chondrosamine); a component of the chondroitins.

chon·dro·skel·e·ton (kon'drō-skel'ĕ-tŏn). A skeleton formed of hyaline cartilage; e.g., that of the human embryo or of certain adult fishes such as the shark or ray.

chon·dro·ster·nal (kon-drō-ster'năl). **1.** Relating to a sternal cartilage. **2.** Relating to the costal cartilages and the sternum.

chon·dro·ster·no·plas·ty (kon-drō-ster'nō-plas-tē). Surgical correction of malformations of the sternum.

chon·dro·tome (kon'drō-tōm). A very stiff scalpel-shaped knife used in cutting cartilage. SYN cartilage knife. [chondro- + G. *tomē,* cutting]

chon·drot·o·my (kon-drot'ō-mē). Division of cartilage. [chondro- + G. *tomē,* a cutting]

chon·dro·tro·phic (kon-drō-trof'ik). Influencing the nutrition and thereby the development and growth of cartilage. [chondro- + G. *trophē,* nourishment]

chon·dro·xi·phoid (kon-drō-zif'oyd). Relating to the xiphoid or ensiform cartilage. [chondro- + G. *xiphos,* sword, + *eidos,* appearance]

chon·drus (kon'drŭs). **1.** SYN cartilage. **2.** The plant *Chondrus crispus, Fucus crispus,* or *Gigartina mamillosa* (family Gigartinaceae); a demulcent in chronic and intestinal disorders. SYN carrageen (1), carragheen, Irish moss, pearl moss. [G. *chondros,* gristle]

CHOP Acronym for cyclophosphamide, doxorubicin, vincristine, and prednisone, a chemotherapy regimen for treatment of lymphomas.

Chopart, François, French surgeon, 1743–1795. SEE C. *amputation, joint.*

△**chord-.** Cord. SEE ALSO cord-. [G. *chordē*]

chor·da, pl. **chor·dae** (kōr'dă, -dē) [TA]. A tendinous or a cord-like structure. SEE ALSO cord. [L., cord]

  c. arteriae umbilicalis [TA], SYN cord of umbilical artery.

  c. chirurgica'lis, surgical catgut. [L.]

  c. dorsa'lis, SYN notochord (2).

  false chordae tendineae [TA], tendinous cords that, unlike the true chordae tendineae, do not attach to the leaflets of the atrioventricular valves. Instead they connect papillary muscles to each other or to the ventricular wall (including the interventricular septum), or merely pass between two points on the ventricular wall (including the septum). SYN chordae tendineae falsae [TA], chordae tendineae spuriae✩, false tendinous cords✩.

  c. mag'na, SYN calcaneal *tendon.*

  c. obli'qua membranae interosseae antebrachii [TA], SYN oblique *cord* of interosseous membrane of forearm.

  c. spermat'ica, SYN spermatic *cord.*

  c. spina'lis, SYN spinal *cord.*

  chordae tendineae cordis [TA], SYN chordae tendineae of heart.

  chordae tendineae falsae [TA], SYN false chordae tendineae.

  chor'dae tendin'eae of heart [TA], the tendinous strands running from the papillary muscles to the leaflets of the atrioventricular valves (mitral and tricuspid). Based on their shape, position, or specific area of attachment to the leaflets, several varieties have been described: fan-shaped chordae, rough zone chordae, free-edge chordae, deep chordae, and basal chordae. SYN chordae tendineae cordis [TA], tendinous cords✩.

  chordae tendineae spuriae, ✩official alternate term for false chordae tendineae.

  c. tym'pani [TA], a nerve given off from the facial nerve in the facial canal which passes through the posterior canaliculus of the c. tympani into the tympanic cavity, crosses over the tympanic membrane and handle of the malleus, and passes out through the anterior canaliculus of the c. tympani in the petrotympanic fissure to join the lingual branch of the mandibular nerve in the infratemporal fossa; it conveys taste sensation from the anterior two-thirds of the tongue and carries parasympathetic preganglionic fibers to the submandibular ganglion, for innervation of the submandibular and sublingual salivary glands. SYN cord of tympanum, parasympathetic root of submandibular ganglion, radix parasympathica ganglii submandibularis, tympanichord.

  c. umbilica'lis, SYN umbilical *cord.*

  c. vertebra'lis, obsolete term for notochord (2).

  c. voca'lis, pl. **chor'dae voca'les,** SYN vocal *fold.*

  chor'dae willis'ii, SYN Willis *cords,* under *cord.*

chord·al (kōr'dăl). Relating to any chorda or cord, especially to the notochord.

chor·da·me·so·derm (kōr-dă-mes'ō-derm). That part of the epiblast of a young embryo that has the potentiality of forming notochord and mesoderm.

Chor·da·ta (kor-dā'tă). The phylum that includes the vertebrates, defined by possession of: 1) a single dorsal nerve cord (the brain and spinal cord of mammals); 2) a cartilaginous rod, the notochord, which forms dorsal to the primitive gut in the early embryo, and is surrounded and replaced by the vertebral column in the subphylum vertebrata; 3) by presence at some stage in development of gill slits in the pharynx or throat. [L. *chorda,* fr. G. *chordē,* a string]

chor·date (kōr'dāt). An animal of the phylum *Chordata.*

chor·dee (kōr-dē'). **1.** Painful erection of the penis in gonorrhea or Peyronie disease, with curvature resulting from lack of distensibility of the corpus cavernosum urethrae. SYN gryposis penis. **2.** Ventral curvature of the penis, most apparent on erection, as seen in hypospadias. [Fr. corded]

chor·di·tis (kōr-dī'tis). Inflammation of a cord; usually a vocal cord. [G. *chordē,* cord, + *-itis,* inflammation]

  c. voca'lis infe'rior, an inflammation limited mainly to the undersurface of the vocal cords and adjacent parts. SYN chronic subglottic laryngitis.

chor·do·ma (kōr-dō'mă). A rare neoplasm of skeletal tissue in adults, derived from persistent portions of the notochord; composed of cells arranged in lobules, with abundant myxoid stroma; some cells contain vacuoles that resemble soap bubbles (physaliphorous cells); most frequently in region clivus or lumbar-sacral cord. [(noto)chord + G. *-oma,* tumor]

chor·do·skel·e·ton (kōr-dō-skel'ĕ-tŏn). The part of the embryonic skeleton that develops in conjunction with the notochord.

cho·rea (kōr-ē'ă). Irregular, spasmodic, involuntary movements of the limbs or facial muscles, often accompanied by hypotonia. The location of the responsible cerebral lesion is not known. [L. fr. G. *choreia,* a choral dance, fr. *choros,* a dance]

c.-acanthocytosis, a slowly progressive familial chorea with associated mental deterioration, diminished deep tendon reflexes, bilateral atrophy of the putamen and caudate nuclei and acanthocytosis (thorny appearance of blood erythrocytes); the disorder typically begins around late adolescence; inheritance is usually autosomal recessive. SYN acanthocytosis with c.

acanthocytosis with c., SYN c.-acanthocytosis.

acute c., SYN Sydenham c.

benign familial c., a rare, nonprogressive movement disorder characterized by c. and athetosis appearing in early childhood, most commonly manifested as gait ataxia and upper limb coordination. Intellect is unaffected. Probably autosomal-dominance inheritance with incomplete penetrance.

chronic progressive c., SYN Huntington c.

dancing c., SYN procursive c.

degenerative c., SYN Huntington c.

electric c., (1) progressively fatal spasmodic disorder, possibly of malarial origin, occurring chiefly in Italy; (2) a severe form of Sydenham c., in which the spasms are rapid and of a specially jerky character.

fibrillary c., SYN myokymia.

c. gravida′rum, sydenham chorea occurring in pregnancy.

habit c., SYN tic.

hemilateral c., SYN hemichorea.

Henoch c., SYN spasmodic *tic*.

hereditary c., SYN Huntington c.

Huntington c. [MIM*143100], a neurodegenerative disorder, with onset usually in the third or fourth decade, characterized by chorea and dementia; pathologically, there is bilateral marked atrophy of the putamen and the head of the caudate nucleus. Autosomal dominant inheritance with complete penetrance, caused by mutation associated with trinucleotide repeat expansion in the Huntington gene (HD) on chromosome 4p. SYN chronic progressive c., degenerative c., hereditary c., Huntington disease.

hysterical c., conversion hysteria in which involuntary, quick, and purposeless (choreiform) movements constitute the chief feature.

juvenile c., SYN Sydenham c.

laryngeal c., a spasmodic tic involving the muscles, resulting in a halting manner of speaking, as in spasmotic dysphonia.

c. mi′nor, SYN Sydenham c.

Morvan c., SYN myokymia.

posthemiplegic c., SYN posthemiplegic *athetosis*.

procursive c., a form in which the patient whirls around, runs forward, or exercises a sort of rhythmic dancing movement. SYN dancing c.

rheumatic c., SYN Sydenham c.

rhythmic c., patterned movement in conversion hysteria.

saltatory c., rhythmic dancing movements, as in procursive c.

senile c., a disorder resembling Sydenham c., not associated with cardiac disease or dementia, occurring in the aged.

Sydenham c., a postinfectious c. appearing several months after a streptococcal infection with subsequent rheumatic fever. The c. typically involves the distal limbs and is associated with hypotonia and emotional lability. Improvement occurs over weeks or months and exacerbations occur without associated infection recurrence. SYN acute c., c. minor, juvenile c., rheumatic c., Sydenham disease.

cho·re·al (kōr-ē′ăl). Relating to chorea.

cho·re·ic (kōr-ē′ik). Relating to or of the nature of chorea.

cho·re·i·form (kōr-ē′i-fōrm). SYN choreoid.

△**choreo-.** Chorea.

cho·re·o·ath·e·toid (kōr′ē-ō-ath′ĕ-toyd). Pertaining to or characterized by choreoathetosis.

cho·re·o·ath·e·to·sis (kōr′ē-ō-ath-ĕ-tō′sis). Abnormal movements of body of combined choreic and athetoid pattern. [choreo- + G. *athētos*, unfixed, + *-ōsis*, condition]

congenital c., SYN double *athetosis*.

cho·re·oid (kōr′ē-oyd). Resembling chorea. SYN choreiform.

△**chorio-.** Any membrane, especially that which encloses the fetus. [G. *chorion*, membrane]

cho·ri·o·ad·e·no·ma (kō′rē-ō-ad-ĕ-nō′mă). A benign neoplasm of chorion, especially with hydatidiform mole formation.

c. des′truens, hydatidiform mole in which there is an unusual degree of invasion of the myometrium or its blood vessels, causing hemorrhage, necrosis, and occasionally rupture of the uterus or embolism of molar tissue to the lungs; there is marked proliferation of the trophoblast, but avascular villi may also be found. SYN invasive mole.

cho·ri·o·al·lan·to·ic (kō′rē-ō-al-an-tō′ik). Pertaining to the chorioallantois.

cho·ri·o·al·lan·to·is (kō′rē-ō-ă-lan′tō-is). Extraembryonic membrane formed by the fusion of the allantois with the serosa or false chorion. In mammals it forms the fetal portion of the placenta; in avian embryos it is fused with the shell.

cho·ri·o·am·ni·o·ni·tis (kō′rē-ō-am′nē-ō-nī′tis). Infection involving the chorion, amnion, and amniotic fluid; usually the placental villi and decidua are also involved.

cho·ri·o·an·gi·o·ma (kō′rē-ō-an-jē-ō′mă). Benign tumor of placental blood vessels (hemangioma), usually of no clinical significance; large tumors may be associated with placental insufficiency and fetal hydrops; in some instances, the stroma is edematous and may resemble myxomatous tissue. SEE ALSO chorioangiosis. [chorion + angioma]

cho·ri·o·an·gi·o·ma·to·sis (kō′rē-ō-an′jē-ō-mă-tō′sis). SYN chorioangiosis.

cho·ri·o·an·gi·o·sis (kō′rē-ō-an-jē-ō′sis). An abnormal increase in the number of vascular channels in placental villi; severe c. is associated with a high incidence of neonatal death and major congenital malformations. SYN chorioangiomatosis. [chorio- + G. *angeion*, vessel, + *-osis*, condition]

cho·ri·o·cap·il·la·ris (kō′rē-ō-kap-i-lā′ris). SYN capillary *lamina* of choroid.

cho·ri·o·car·ci·no·ma (kō′rē-ō-kar-si-nō′mă). A highly malignant neoplasm derived from placental syncytial trophoblasts and cytotrophoblasts which forms irregular sheets and cords, which are surrounded by irregular "lakes" of blood; villi are not formed; neoplastic cells invade blood vessels. Hemorrhagic metastases develop relatively early in the course of the illness, and are frequently found in the lungs, liver, brain, and vagina, and various other pelvic organs; c. may follow any type of pregnancy, especially hydatidiform mole, and occasionally originates in teratoid neoplasms of the ovaries or testes. SYN chorioepithelioma.

cho·ri·o·cele (kō′rē-ō-sēl). A hernia of the choroid coat of the eye through a defect in the sclera. [chorio- + G. *kēlē*, hernia]

cho·ri·o·ep·i·the·li·o·ma (kō′rē-ō-ep-i-thē-lē-ō′mă). SYN choriocarcinoma.

cho·ri·o·go·nad·o·tro·pin (kō′rē-ō-gon′ă-dō-trō-pin). SYN chorionic *gonadotropin*.

△**chorioid-, chorioido-.** For words beginning thus and not found here, see choroid-, choroido-.

cho·ri·o·mam·mo·tro·pin (kō′rē-ō-mam′ō-trō-pin). SYN human placental *lactogen*.

cho·ri·o·men·in·gi·tis (kō-rē-ō-men-in-jī′tis). A cerebral meningitis in which there is a more or less marked cellular infiltration of the meninges, often with a lymphocytic infiltration of the choroid plexuses, particularly of the third and fourth ventricles.

lymphocytic c., a form of viral meningitis that usually occurs in young adults during the fall and winter months. Caused by a virus carried by the common house mouse. SEE ALSO lymphocytic choriomeningitis *virus*.

cho·ri·on (kō′rē-on). The multilayered, outermost fetal membrane consisting of extraembryonic somatic mesoderm, trophoblast, and, on the maternal surface, villi bathed by maternal blood; as pregnancy progresses, part of the c. becomes the definitive fetal placenta. SYN chorionic sac, membrana serosa (1). [G. *chorion*, membrane enclosing the fetus]

c. frondo′sum, the part of the c. where the villi persist, forming the fetal part of the placenta. SYN shaggy c.

c. lae′ve, the portion of the c. from which the villi disappear in the later stages of pregnancy. SYN smooth c.

previllous c., SYN primitive c.

primitive c., the c. before its villi are well formed. SYN previllous c.

shaggy c., SYN c. frondosum.

smooth c., SYN c. laeve.

cho·ri·on·ic (kō-rē-on′ik). Relating to the chorion.

cho·ri·o·ret·i·nal (kō-rē-ō-ret′i-năl). Relating to the choroid coat of the eye and the retina. SYN retinochoroid.

cho·ri·o·ret·i·ni·tis (kō′rē-ō-ret-i-nī′tis). SYN retinochoroiditis.

c. sclopeta′ria, proliferation of fibrous tissue in the choroid and retina as the result of contusion of the sclera by a high velocity missile. [L. *sclopetum,* 14th century Italian handgun]

cho·ri·o·ret·i·nop·a·thy (kō′rē-ō-ret-i-nop′ă-thē). A primary abnormality of the choroid with extension to the retina. SEE ALSO choroidopathy.

cho·ris·ta (kō-ris′tă). A focus of tissue that is histologically normal per se, but is not normally found in the organ or structure in which it is located; e.g., tissue displaced, during development, from its normal site. Cf. choristoma. [G. *chōristos,* separated]

cho·ris·to·blas·to·ma (kō-ris′tō-blas-tō′mă). An autonomous neoplasm composed of relatively undifferentiated cells of a choristoma. [choristoma + blastoma]

cho·ris·to·ma (kō-ris-tō′mă). A mass formed by maldevelopment of tissue of a type not normally found at that site. [G. *chōristos,* separated, + *-ōma*]

cho·roid (ko′royd) [TA]. The middle vascular tunic of the eye lying between the pigment epithelium and the sclera. SYN choroidea [TA]. [G. *choroeidēs,* a false reading for *chorioeidēs,* like a membrane]

cho·roi·dal (kō-roy′dăl). Relating to the choroid (choroidea).

cho·roi·dea (kō-royd′ē-ă) [TA]. SYN choroid. [see choroid]

cho·roi·der·e·mia (kō-roy-der-ē′mē-ă) [MIM*303100]. Progressive degeneration of the choroid in males, occasionally in females, beginning with peripheral pigmentary retinopathy, followed by atrophy of the retinal pigment epithelium and of the choriocapillaris, night blindness, progressive constriction of visual fields, and finally complete blindness; X-linked inheritance caused by mutation in the Rab escort protein-1 (REP1) gene on Xq; heterozygous females show a pigmentary retinopathy but without visual defect or peripheral progression. SYN progressive choroidal atrophy, progressive tapetochoroidal dystrophy. [choroid + G. *erēmia,* absence]

cho·roid·i·tis (kō-roy-dī′tis). Inflammation of the choroid. Cf. choroidopathy, chorioretinopathy. SYN posterior uveitis.

anterior c., disseminated c. restricted to peripheral choroid.

areolar c., inflammation of the choroid, with prominent pigment proliferation occurring first in the macular region and then more peripherally.

diffuse c., a widespread exudative inflammation of the choroid, with progressive resolution of older lesions as new ones occur.

disseminated c., chronic inflammation of the choroid, with multiple isolated foci.

exudative c., a circumscribed inflammation of the choroid, often with multiple lesions.

juxtapupillary c., c. adjacent to the optic disk.

metastatic c., inflammation of the choroid arising from microbial emboli.

multifocal c., macular, peripapillary, and peripheral c., often designated presumed ocular histoplasmosis.

posterior c., disseminated c. restricted to the central choroid.

proliferative c., the dense scar tissue produced by severe choroiditis.

suppurative c., purulent inflammation of the choroid.

vitiliginous c., SYN bird shot *retinochoroiditis.*

△**choroido-.** The choroid.

cho·roid·o·cy·cli·tis (kō-roy′dō-sī-klī′tis). Inflammation of the choroid coat and the ciliary body. [choroido- + G. *kyklos,* circle]

cho·roi·dop·a·thy (kō-roy-dop′ă-thē). Noninflammatory degeneration of the choroid.

areolar c., a slowly progressive pigmentary degeneration in young persons; characterized by black foci closely set together and coalescent at the posterior pole and macular region. SYN central areolar choroidal atrophy, central areolar choroidal sclerosis.

central serous c., an idiopathic sensory retinal detachment in the macula; more common in males. SYN central angiospastic retinopathy, central serous retinopathy.

Doyne honeycomb c., obsolete term for macular *drusen.*

geographic c., SYN serpiginous c.

helicoid c., SYN serpiginous c.

myopic c., chronic degeneration of the sclera and choroid with posterior staphyloma, accompanying high myopia.

serpiginous c., bilateral acquired abnormality of retinal pigment epithelium and choroid in which irregular multiple progressive swelling is followed by atrophic scars in linear patterns. SYN geographic c., helicoid c.

cho·roi·do·sis (ko′-roy-dō′sis). Obsolete term for choroidopathy.

Chotzen, F., 20th century German physician. SEE C. *syndrome.*

Christensen, Erna, Danish neuropathologist, 1906–1967. SEE C.-Krabbe *disease.*

Christian, Henry A., U.S. internist, 1876–1951. SEE C. *disease, syndrome;* Hand-Schüller-C. *disease;* Weber-C. *disease.*

Christison, Sir Robert, Scottish physician, 1797–1882. SEE C. *formula.*

Christmas. Surname of a child (Stephen Christmas) with the disease subsequently called Christmas *disease;* first case studied in detail. SEE Christmas *disease,* Christmas *factor.* SEE ALSO Christmas *factor, hemophilia* B.

△**chrom-, chromat-, chromato-, chromo-.** Color. [G. *chrōma*]

chro·maf·fin (krō′maf-in). Giving a brownish yellow reaction with chromic salts; denoting certain cells in the medulla of the adrenal glands and in paraganglia. SYN chromaphil, chromatophil (3), chromophil (3), chromophile, pheochrome (1). [chrom- + L. *affinis,* affinity]

chro·maf·fin·o·ma (krō-maf-in-ō′mă). A neoplasm composed of chromaffin cells occurring in the medullae of adrenal glands, the organs of Zuckerkandl, or the paraganglia of the thoracolumbar sympathetic chain; may secrete catecholamines. SEE ALSO pheochromocytoma. SYN chromaffin tumor.

chro·maf·fin·op·a·thy (krō′maf-in-op′ă-thē). Obsolete term for any pathologic condition of chromaffin tissue, as in the medullae of adrenal glands or the organs of Zuckerkandl. [chromaffin + G. *pathos,* suffering]

chro·man, chro·mane (krō′man, -mān). Fundamental unit of the tocopherols (vitamin E). SEE ALSO chromanol, chromene, chromenol.

chro·man·ol (krō′man-ol). 6-Hydroxychroman (6-chromanol) is the fundamental unit of the tocopherols (vitamin E), tocols, and tocotrienols, as well as of ubi-, toco-, and phyllochromanol. SEE ALSO chroman, chromene, chromenol. SYN hydroxychroman.

chro·ma·phil (krō′mă-fil). SYN chromaffin.

△**chromat-.** SEE chrom-.

chro·mate (krō′māt). A salt of chromic acid.

sodium c. Cr 51, anionic hexavalent radioactive chromium in the form of sodium c. ($Na_2{}^{51}CrO_4$) with a half-life of 27.8 days; used for the determination of circulating red cell volume and red cell survival time.

chro·mat·ic (krō-mat′ik). Of or pertaining to color or colors; produced by, or made in, a color or colors.

chro·ma·tid (krō′mă-tid). Each of the two strands formed by longitudinal duplication of a chromosome that becomes visible during prophase of mitosis or meiosis; the two c.'s are joined by the still undivided centromere; after the centromere has divided at metaphase and the two c.'s have separated, each c. becomes a chromosome. [G. *chrōma,* color, + *-id* (2),]

chro·ma·tin (krō′ma-tin). The genetic material of the nucleus, consisting of deoxyribonucleoprotein, which occurs in two forms during the phase between mitotic divisions: 1) as heterochromatin, seen as condensed, readily stainable clumps; 2) as euchromatin, dispersed lightly staining or nonstaining material. During mitotic division the c. condenses into chromosomes. [G. *chroma*, color]

heteropyknotic c., SYN heterochromatin.

oxyphil c., SYN oxychromatin.

sex c., a small condensed mass of the inactivated X-chromosome usually located just inside the nuclear membrane of the interphase nucleus; the number of sex c. bodies per nucleus is one less than the number of X-chromosomes, hence normal males and females with Turner syndrome (XO) have none (sex c. negative), normal females and males with Klinefelter syndrome (XXY) have one, and XXX-females have two c. masses. For technical reasons only about half the cells in a preparation show typical masses. SEE ALSO Lyon *hypothesis*. SYN Barr chromatin body.

chro·ma·ti·nol·y·sis (krō′mă-ti-nol′i-sis). SYN chromatolysis.

chro·mat·i·nor·rhex·is (krō-mat′i-nō-rek′sis). Fragmentation of the chromatin. [chromatin + G. *rhēxis*, rupture]

chro·ma·tism (krō′mă-tizm). **1.** Abnormal pigmentation. **2.** SYN chromatic *aberration*. [G. *chrōma*, color]

△**chromato-.** SEE chrom-.

chro·ma·tog·e·nous (krō-mă-toj′ĕ-nŭs). Producing color; causing pigmentation. [chromato- + *-gen,* producing]

chro·mat·o·gram (krō-mat′ō-gram). The graphic record produced by chromatography.

chro·mat·o·graph (krō-mat′ō-graf). To perform chromatography.

chro·mat·o·graph·ic (krō′mat-ō-graf′ik). Pertaining to chromatography.

chro·ma·tog·ra·phy (krō-mă-tog′ră-fē). The separation of chemical substances and particles (originally plant pigments and other highly colored compounds) by differential movement through a two-phase system. The mixture of materials to be separated is percolated through a column or sheet of some suitable chosen absorbent (e.g., an ion-exchange material); the substances least absorbed are least retarded and emerge the earliest; those more strongly absorbed emerge later. SYN absorption c. [chromato- + G. *graphō,* to write]

absorption c., SYN chromatography.

adsorption c., c. in which separation of substances is achieved by the difference in degree of adsorption of the compounds to a stationary phase.

affinity c., c. where the absorbent has a unique chemical affinity for a particular component of the passing solution. SYN affinity column.

column c., a form of partition, adsorption, ion exchange, or affinity c. in which one phase is liquid (aqueous) flowing down a column packed with the second phase, a solid; the dissolved substances form a partition between the solid and liquid phases depending on the chemical and physical conditions of each phase; the more strongly adsorbed solutes reach the bottom of the column later than the less strongly adsorbed ones.

gas c., a chromatographic procedure in which the mobile phase is a mixture of gases or vapors, which are separated in the process by their differential adsorption on a stationary phase.

gas-liquid c. (GLC), gas c., with the stationary phase being liquid rather than solid.

gel filtration c., SEE gel *filtration*.

high-performance liquid c. (HPLC), a chromatographic technology used to separate and quantitate mixtures of substances in solution. A sample is injected into a moving stream of solvent that flows through a column and detector. Separation during passage through the column occurs by absorption, partition, ion exchange, or size exclusion. The technique is commonly used in laboratories to measure organic compounds including steroid hormones, pesticides and poisons, toxic and carcinogenic compounds, and drugs. SYN high-pressure liquid chromatography.

high-pressure liquid chromatography (HPLC), SYN high-performance liquid c.

ion exchange c., c. in which cations or anions in the mobile phase

are separated by electrostatic interactions with the stationary phase. SEE ALSO anion exchange, cation exchange.

liquid-liquid c., c. in which both the moving phase and the stationary (or reverse-moving) phase are liquids, as in countercurrent distribution.

paper c., partition c. in which the moving phase is a liquid and the stationary phase is paper.

partition c., the separation of similar substances by repeated divisions between two immiscible liquids, so that the substances, in effect, cross the partition between the liquids in opposite directions; where one of the liquids is bound as a film on filter paper, the process is termed paper partition c. or paper c.

reversed phase c., a form of partitionary c. in which the stationary phase is less polar than the mobile phase.

thin-layer c. (TLC), c. through a thin layer of cellulose or similar inert material supported on a glass or plastic plate.

two-dimensional c., paper c. in which a spot, located originally in one corner of a sheet, is developed in one direction along one side of the sheet, after which the sheet is rotated 90° and developed, with another solvent, in the new direction; the resultant spots are thus spread over the entire paper, giving a "map" or "fingerprint." Also generalized to include c. followed by electrophoresis (or vice versa), column c. followed by paper c., etc.

chro·ma·toid (krō′mă-toyd). A refractile substance composed of chromatin, thought to be a nonglycogen food reserve contained within the cytoplasm of certain protozoa; seen in cysts of *Entamoeba histolytica* as rounded bars or chromatoidal bodies in contrast to the splintery form of c. bodies in cysts of *Entamoeba coli.* [chromato- + G. *eidos,* form]

chro·mat·o·ki·ne·sis (krō′mă-tō-ki-nē′sis). Rearrangement of the chromatin into various forms. [chromato- + G. *kinēsis,* movement]

chro·ma·tol·y·sis (krō-mă-tol′i-sis). The disintegration of the granules of chromophil substance (Nissl bodies) in a nerve cell body that may occur after exhaustion of the cell or damage to its peripheral process; other changes considered part of c. include swelling of the perikaryon and shifting of the nucleus from its central position to the periphery. SYN chromatinolysis, chromolysis, tigrolysis. [chromato- + G. *lysis,* dissolution]

central c., c. associated with significant axonal injury. SYN retrograde c.

retrograde c., SYN central c.

transsynaptic c., SYN transsynaptic *degeneration*.

chro·mat·o·lyt·ic (krō-mă-tō-lit′ik). Relating to chromatolysis.

chro·ma·tom·e·ter (krō-mă-tom′ĕ-ter). SYN colorimeter. [chromato- + G. *metron,* measure]

chro·mat·o·pec·tic (krō′mă-tō-pek′tik). Relating to or causing chromatopexis. SYN chromopectic.

chro·mat·o·pex·is (krō′mă-tō-pek′sis). The fixation of color or staining fluid, i.e., as the liver functions in forming bilirubin. SYN chromopexis. [chromato- + G. *pēxis,* fixation]

chro·mat·o·phil (krō-mat′ō-fil). **1.** SYN chromophilic. **2.** SYN chromophil (2). **3.** SYN chromaffin.

chro·mat·o·phil·ia (krō′mă-tō-fil′ē-ă). SYN chromophilia.

chro·mat·o·phil·ic, chro·ma·toph·i·lous (krō′mă-tō-fil′ik, -tof′i-lŭs). SYN chromophilic.

chro·mat·o·pho·bia (krō′mă-tō-fō′bē-ă). SYN chromophobia.

chro·mat·o·phore (krō-mat′ō-fōr). **1.** A colored plastid, due to the presence of chlorophyll or other pigments, found in certain forms of protozoa. **2.** Melanophage; a pigment-bearing phagocyte found chiefly in the skin, mucous membrane, and choroid coat of the eye, and also in melanomas. **3.** SYN chromophore. **4.** A colored plastid in plants; e.g., chloroplasts, leukoplasts, etc. [chromato- + G. *phoros,* bearing]

chro·mat·o·pho·ro·tro·pic (krō′mă-tō-fōr′ō-trop′ik). Denoting the attraction of chromatophores to the skin or other organs. [chromatophore + G. *tropos,* a turning]

chro·mat·o·plasm (krō′mă-tō-plazm). The part of the cytoplasm containing pigment.

chro·ma·top·si·a (krō-mă-top′sē-ă). A condition in which objects appear to be abnormally colored or tinged with color; designated

ch

according to the color seen: xanthopsia, yellow vision; erythropsia, red vision; chloropsia, green vision; cyanopsia, blue vision. SYN chromatic vision, colored vision, tinted vision. Cf. dyschromatopsia. [chromato- + G. *opsis,* vision]

chro·mat·o·some (krō-ma′tō-sōm). A nucleosome with one bound histone-1 protein.

chro·ma·to·tro·pism (krō-mat′rō-pizm). 1. A change of color. 2. The phenomenon of orientation in response to color. [chromato- + G. *trope,* turn]

chro·ma·tu·ria (krō-mă-too′rē-ă). Abnormal coloration of the urine. [chromato- + G. *ouron,* urine]

chrome (krōm). Chromium, especially as a source of pigment. [G. *chroma,* color]

♻**-chrome.** A word termination indicating relationship to color. [G. *chroma* color]

chro·mene (krō′mēn). 2*H*-1-Benzopyran; fundamental unit of the tocopherolquinones. SEE ALSO chroman, chromanol, chromenol.

chro·men·ol (krō′men-ol). 6-Hydroxychromene (6-chromenol) is the fundamental unit of the tocopherolquinones (oxidized tocopherol) and plastochromenol-8. SEE ALSO chroman, chromanol, chromene. SYN hydroxychromene.

chrome red. Basic lead chromate.

chro·mes·the·sia (krō-mes-thē′zē-ă). 1. The color sense. 2. A condition in which nonvisual stimuli, such as taste or smell, cause the perception of color. [G. *chroma,* color, + *aisthesis,* sensation]

chrome yel·low [C.I. 77600]. A fine yellow powder used in paints and dyes. SYN lead chromate, Leipzig yellow, lemon yellow, Paris yellow.

chrom·hi·dro·sis (krōm-hī-drō′sis). A rare condition characterized by the excretion of sweat containing pigment. SYN chromidrosis. [chrom- + G. *hidros,* sweat]

apocrine c., excretion of colored sweat, usually black, from apocrine glands.

chro·mic ac·id (krō′mik). H_2CrO_4 or $H_2Cr_2O_7$; a strong oxidizing agent formed by dissolving chromium trioxide (CrO_3) in water. Has been used in solution as a topical antiseptic.

chro·mid·ia (krō-mid′ē-ă). Plural of chromidium.

chro·mid·i·a·tion (krō-mid-ē-ā′shŭn). SYN chromidiosis.

chro·mid·i·o·sis (krō-mid-ē-ō′sis). An outpouring of nuclear substance and chromatin into the cell protoplasm. SYN chromidiation.

chro·mid·i·um, pl. **chro·mid·ia** (krō-mid′ē-ŭm, -ē-ă). A basophilic particle or structure in the cell cytoplasm, rich in RNA, often found in specialized cells. [G. *chroma,* color, + *-idion,* a diminutive termination]

chro·mi·dro·sis (krō-mi-drō′sis). SYN chromhidrosis.

chro·mi·um (Cr) (krō′mē-ŭm). A metallic element, atomic no. 24, atomic wt. 51.9961. A dietary essential bioelement. ^{51}Cr (half-life of 27.70 days) is used as a diagnostic aid in many disorders (e.g., gastrointestinal protein loss). [G. *chroma,* color]

c. trioxide, CrO_3; chromic acid, a strong oxidizing agent used as a caustic in the removal of warts and other small growths from the skin and genitals; the hydrated acid, H_2CrO_4, forms variously colored salts with potassium, lead, and other bases.

♻**chromo-.** SEE chrom-.

Chro·mo·bac·te·ri·um (krō-mō-bak-tēr′ē-ŭm). A genus of bacteria containing Gram-negative, motile rods. These microorganisms produce a violet pigment (violacein) and are occasionally pathogenic to humans and other animals. The type species is *C. violaceum.*

C. viola′ceum, type species of the genus *C.;* it is found in soil and water.

chro·mo·blast (krō′mō-blast). An embryonic cell with the potentiality of developing into a pigment cell. [chromo- + G. *blastos,* germ]

chro·mo·blas·to·my·co·sis (krō′mō-blas′tō-mī-kō′sis). A localized chronic mycosis of the skin and subcutaneous tissues characterized by skin lesions so rough and irregular as to present a cauliflowerlike appearance; caused by dematiaceous fungi such as *Phialophora verrucosa, Exophiala (wangiella) dermatitidis, Fonsecaea pedrosoi, F. compacta,* and *Cladosporium carrionii;*

fungal cells resembling copper pennies form rounded sclerotic bodies in tissue, with epidermal hyperplasia and intraepidermal microabscesses. SYN chromomycosis. [chromo- + G. *blastos,* germ, + *myke,* fungus, + *-osis,* condition]

chro·mo·cen·ter (krō′mō-sen-ter). SYN karyosome.

chro·mo·cyte (krō′mō-sīt). Any pigmented cell, such as a red blood corpuscle. [chromo- + G. *kytos,* cell]

chro·mo·gen (krō′mō-jen). 1. A substance, itself without definite color, that may be transformed into a pigment; denoting especially benzene and its homologs toluene, xylene, quinone, naphthalene, and anthracene, from which the aniline dyes are manufactured. 2. A microorganism that produces pigment. 3. A compound, containing a chromophore, that is colorless if that chromophore is removed.

Porter-Silber c.'s, yellow phenylhydrazones formed by the reaction of 17,21-dihydroxy-20-oxosteroids with a phenylhydrazine-ethanol-sulfuric acid reagent; used chiefly to determine plasma cortisol concentrations and the urinary output of 17-hydroxycorticoids.

chro·mo·gen·e·sis (krō-mō-jen′ĕ-sis). Production of coloring matter or pigment, often via an enzyme-catalyzed reaction. [chromo- + G. *genesis,* production]

chro·mo·gen·ic (krō-mō-jen′ik). 1. Denoting a chromogen. 2. Relating to chromogenesis.

chro·mo·gran·ins (krō′mō-gran-inz). Soluble proteins of chromaffin granules; c. A, an acidic glycoprotein, accounts for approximately half of the total protein of the granule matrix.

chro·mo·i·som·er·ism (krō′mō-ī-som′er-izm). Isomerism in which the isomers display different colors.

chro·mo·lip·id (krō-mō-lip′id). SYN lipochrome (1).

chro·mol·y·sis (krō-mol′i-sis). SYN chromatolysis.

chro·mo·mere (krō′mō-mēr). 1. A condensed segment of a chromonema; densely staining bands visible in chromosomes under certain conditions. 2. SYN granulomere. [chromo- + G. *meros,* a part]

chro·mom·e·ter (krō-mom′ĕ-ter). SYN colorimeter.

chro·mo·my·co·sis (krō′mō-mī-kō′sis). SYN chromoblastomycosis. [chromo- + G. *mykes,* fungus, + *-osis,* condition]

chro·mone (krō′mōn). 4*H*-1-Benzopyran-4-one; fundamental unit of various plant pigments and other substances. SEE ALSO flavone, chromene, chroman.

chro·mo·ne·ma, pl. **chro·mo·ne·ma·ta** (krō-mō-nē′mă, -ma-tă). The coiled filament in which the genes are located, which extends the entire length of a chromosome and exhibits an intensely positive Feulgen test for DNA. SYN chromatic fiber. [chromo- + G. *nema,* thread]

chro·mo·nych·ia (krō-mō-nik′ē-ă). Abnormality in the color of the nails. [chromo- + G. *onyx (onych-),* nail]

chro·mo·pec·tic (krō-mō-pek′tik). SYN chromatopectic.

chro·mo·pex·is (krō-mō-pek′sis). SYN chromatopexis.

chro·mo·phil, chro·mo·phile (krō′mō-fil, krō′mō-fīl). 1. SYN chromophilic. 2. A cell or any histologic element that stains readily. SYN chromatophil (2). 3. SYN chromaffin. [chromo- + G. *phileo,* to love]

chro·mo·phil·ia (krō-mō-fil′ē-ă). The property possessed by most cells of staining readily with appropriate dyes. SYN chromatophilia. [chromo- + G. *phileo,* to love]

chro·mo·phil·ic, chro·moph·i·lous (krō-mō-fil′ik, -mof′i-lŭs). Staining readily; denoting certain cells and histologic structures. SYN chromatophil (1), chromatophilic, chromatophilous, chromophil (1), chromophile.

chro·mo·phobe (krō′mō-fōb). Resistant to stains, staining with difficulty or not at all; denoting certain degranulated cells in the anterior lobe of the pituitary gland. SYN chromophobic. [chromo- + G. *phobos,* fear]

chro·mo·pho·bia (krō-mō-fō′bē-ă). 1. Resistance to stains on the part of cells and tissues. 2. A morbid dislike of colors. SYN chromatophobia. [chromo- + G. *phobos,* fear]

chro·mo·pho·bic (krō-mō-fō′bik). SYN chromophobe. [chromo- + *phobos,* fear]

chro·mo·phore (krō′mō-fōr). The atomic grouping upon which the color of a substance depends. SYN chromatophore (3), color radical. [chromo- + G. *phoros,* bearing]

chro·mo·phor·ic, chro·moph·o·rous (krō-mō-fōr′ik, -mof′ŏr-ŭs). **1.** Relating to a chromophore. **2.** Producing or carrying color; denoting certain microorganisms.

chro·mo·pho·to·ther·a·py (krō′mō-phō′tō-thār′ă-pē). SYN chromotherapy. [chromo- + photo- + G. *therapeia,* medical treatment]

chro·mo·plast (krō′mō-plast). A plastid filled with carotenoid pigments.

chro·mo·plas·tid (krō-mō-plas′tid). A pigmented plastid, containing chlorophyll, formed in certain protozoans. [chromo- + G. *plastos,* formed, + *-id* (2)]

chro·mo·pro·tein (krō-mō-prō′tēn). One of a group of conjugated proteins, consisting of a combination of pigment (i.e., a colored prosthetic group) with a protein; e.g., hemoglobin.

chro·mo·som·al (krō′mō-sō′măl). Pertaining to chromosomes.

chro·mo·some (krō′mō-sōm). One of the bodies (normally 46 in somatic cells in humans) in the cell nucleus that is the bearer of genes, has the form of a delicate chromatin filament during interphase, contracts to form a compact cylinder segmented into two arms by the centromere during metaphase and anaphase stages of cell divison, and is capable of reproducing its physical and chemical structure through successive cell divisons. In bacteria and other prokaryotes, the c. is not enclosed within a nuclear membrane and not subject to a mitotic mechanism. Prokaryotes may have more than one c. [chromo- + G. *sōma,* body]

chromosome (set)					
n = haploid					
2n = diploid					
3n = triploid					
4n = tetraploid		anorthoploid	euploid or polyploid		
5n = pentaploid		orthoploid			
6n = hexaploid					heteroploid
n + 1	= simple disomal		aneuploid or polysomic		
2n + 1	= simple trisomal				
2n + 2 (same)	= simple tetrasomal				
2n + 2 (diff.)	= double trisomal				

accessory c., a supernumerary c. that is not an exact replica of any of the c.'s in the normal cellular complement. SYN monosome (1), odd c., unpaired allosome, unpaired c.

acentric c., a fragment of a c. lacking a centromere and unable to attach to the mitotic spindle, therefore unable to take part in the division of a nucleus and randomly distributed in daughter cells. SYN acentric fragment.

acrocentric c., a c. with the centromere placed very close to one end so that the short arm is very small, often with a satellite.

bivalent c., a pair of c.'s temporarily united.

Christchurch c., an obsolete term describing an abnormal small acrocentric c. (no. 21 or 22) with complete or almost complete deletion of the short arm; found in cultured leukocytes in some cases of chronic lymphocytic leukemia, also in some normal relatives of patients.

derivative c., an anomalous c. generated by translocation. SYN translocation c.

dicentric c., a c. with two centromeres that may result from reciprocal translocation.

double minute c.'s, paired, extrachromosomal elements lacking centromeres, often associated with a drug resistance gene.

fragile X c., an X c. with a fragile site near the end of the long arm, resulting in the appearance of an almost detached fragment; demonstrated only under special culture conditions; frequently associated with X-linked mental retardation. SEE Renpenning *syndrome*.

giant c., (1) SYN polytene c; **(2)** SYN lambrush c.

heterotypical c., c. that pairs with an unequal partner, e.g., the X and Y c.'s.

homologous c.'s, members of a single pair of c.'s.

lampbrush c., lamp-brush c., (1) a large c. found in oocytes of certain animals characterized by many fine lateral projections giving the appearance of a test tube brush or lampbrush. **(2)** multiply looped chromosomal area of the chromatin of some species. SYN giant c. (2).

late replicating c., a c. (often anomalous) that is shown, e.g., by incorporation of a labeled nucleotide, to undergo delayed duplication preliminary to mitosis; formerly used as a means of distinguishing members of a group of c.'s.

marker c., a c. with cytologically distinctive characteristics.

metacentric c., a c. with a centrally placed centromere that divides the c. into two arms of approximately equal length.

mitochondrial c., the DNA component of mitochondria, the chief function of which is synthesis of adenosine triphosphate and the management of cellular energy; the c. contains some 16,000 base pairs arranged in a circle. The inheritance is matrilineal, and the mutation rate is unusually high; since each cell contains thousands of copies,s a mutant form may assume an almost continuous gradation as in a galtonian process. Most of the mutations known have their impact on the respiratory chain.

nonhomologous c.'s, c.'s that are not members of the same pair.

nucleolar c., a c. regularly associated with a nucleolus.

odd c., SYN accessory c.

Philadelphia c. (Ph1), an abnormally shortened chromosome 22, formed by translocation of a portion of the long arm of c. 22 to c. 9; found in cultured leukocytes of many patients with chronic granulocytic leukemia.

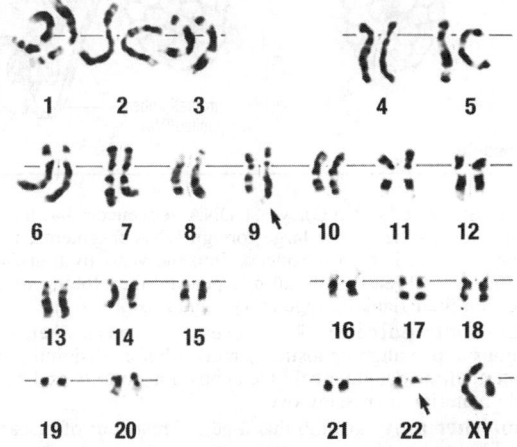

Philadelphia chromosome translocation: karyotype from a patient with chronic granulocytic leukemia showing the Philadelphia chromosome translocation, t(9:22)(q34;q11); the Philadelphia chromosome is chromosome number 22

polytene c., a stage of c. division that forms the giant c. found in the salivary gland of dipterous insects; the great width is the result of repeated divisions of the chromonema without subsequent lengthwise separation of the filaments. SYN giant c. (1).

c. puffs, expansions of particular c. regions; sites of RNA syntheses.

ring c., a c. with ends joined to form a circular structure. The ring form is abnormal in humans but the normal form of the c. in certain bacteria.

sex c.'s, the pair of c.'s responsible for sex determination. In humans and most animals, the sex c.'s are designated X and Y; females have two X c.'s, males have one X and one Y c. In certain birds, insects, and fishes the sex c.'s are designated Z and W; males have two Z c.'s, females may have one Z and one W c., or one Z and no W c. SYN gonosome.

ch

submetacentric c., a c. with the centromere so placed that it divides the c. into two arms of strikingly unequal length.

telocentric c., a c. with a terminal centromere; such c.'s in humans are unstable and arise by misdivision or breakage near the centromere and are usually eliminated within a few cell divisions.

translocation c., SYN derivative c.

unpaired c., SYN accessory c.

W c., X c., Y c., Z c., SEE sex c.'s.

c. walking, sequential isolation of overlapping sequences of DNA (i.e., clones); with this procedure large regions of the chromosome can be spanned. SYN overlap hybridization.

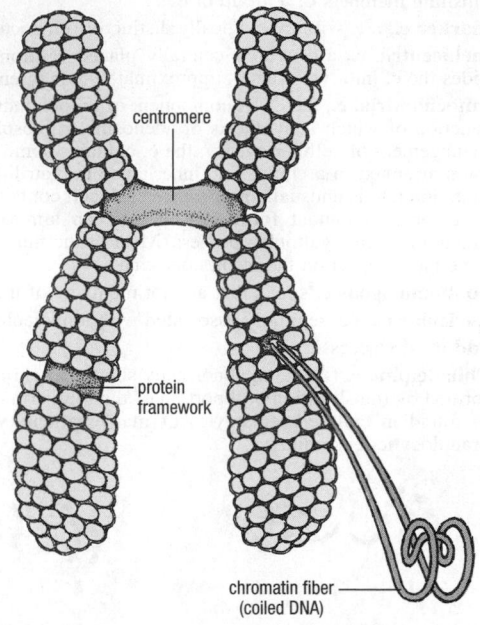

centromere

protein
framework

chromatin fiber
(coiled DNA)

chromosome

---

yeast artificial c.'s (YAC), yeast DNA sequences that have incorporated into them very large foreign DNA fragments; the recombinant DNA is then introduced into the yeast by transformation; the use of yeast artificial c.'s permits the cloning of large genes with their flanking regulatory sequences.

chro·mo·some pair·ing. The process in synapsis whereby homologous c. p.'s align opposite each other before disjoining in the formation of the daughter cell; the apposition permits exchange of genetic material in crossing-over.

chro·mo·ther·a·py (krō-mō-thār′ă-pē). Treatment of disease by colored light. SYN chromophototherapy.

chro·mo·tox·ic (krō-mō-tok′sik). Caused by a toxic action on the hemoglobin, as in chromotoxic hyperchromemia, or resulting from the destruction of hemoglobin.

chro·mo·trich·ia (krō-mō-trik′ē-ă). Colored or pigmented hair. [chromo- + G. *thrix* (*trich-*), hair]

chro·mo·trich·i·al (krō-mō-trik′ē-ăl). Pertaining to the coloring of hair.

chro·mo·trope (krō′mō-trōp). Any of several dyes containing chromotropic acid and which have the property of changing from red to blue on afterchroming.

chro·mo·trope 2R [C.I. 16570]. A red acid dye used as a counterstain and for staining red blood cells in sections.

chro·mo·tro·pic ac·id (krō′mō-trōp-ik). Used as a reagent and in chromotropes.

chro·nax·ia (krō-nak′sē-ă). SYN chronaxie.

chro·nax·ie (krō′nak-sē). A measurement of excitability of nervous or muscular tissue; the shortest duration of an effective electrical stimulus having a strength equal to twice the minimum strength required for excitation. SYN chronaxia, chronaxis, chronaxy. [G. *chronos,* time, + *axia,* value]

chro·nax·im·e·ter (krō-nak-sim′ĕ-ter). An instrument for measuring chronaxie.

chro·nax·im·e·try (krō-nak-sim′ĕ-trē). The measurement of chronaxie. [G. *chronos,* time, + *axia,* value, + *metrein,* to measure]

chro·nax·is (krō-nak′sis). SYN chronaxie.

chro·naxy (krō′nak-sē). SYN chronaxie.

chron·ic (krŏn′ik). **1.** Referring to a health-related state, lasting a long time. **2.** Referring to exposure, prolonged or long-term, sometimes meaning also low intensity. **3.** The U.S. National Center for Health Statistics defines a chronic condition as one of 3 months' duration or longer. [G. *chronos,* time]

chro·nic·i·ty (kron-is′i-tē). The state of being chronic.

△**chrono-.** Time. [G. *chronos*]

chro·no·bi·ol·o·gy (kron′ō-bī-ol′ō-jē). That aspect of biology concerned with the timing of biological events, especially repetitive or cyclic phenomena in individual organisms. [chrono- + G. *bios,* life, + *logos,* study]

chron·og·no·sis (kron-og-nō′sis). Perception of the passage of time. [chrono- + G. *gnōsis,* knowledge]

chro·no·graph (kron′ō-graf). An instrument for graphic measurement and recording brief periods of time. [chrono- + G. *graphō,* to record]

chro·nom·e·try (krō-nom′ĕ-tre). Measurement of intervals of time. [chrono- + G. *metron,* measure]

mental c., study of the duration of mental and behavorial processes.

chron·o·on·col·o·gy (kron′ō-on-kol′ō-jē). The study of the influence of biological rhythms on neoplastic growth; also used to describe anti-cancer treatment based on the timing of drug administration. [G. *chronos,* time, + oncology]

chro·no·phar·ma·col·o·gy (kron′ō-far-mă-kol′ō-jē). A branch of chronobiology concerned with the effects of drugs upon the timing of biological events and rhythms, and the relation of biological timing to the effects of drugs.

chro·no·pho·bia (kron′ō-fō′bē-ă). Morbid fear of the duration or immensity of time.

chro·no·pho·to·graph (kron-ō-fō′tō-graf). A photograph taken as one of a series for the purpose of showing successive phases of a motion.

chro·no·ta·rax·is (kron′ō-tă-rak′sis). Distortion or confusion of the sense of time. [chrono- + G. *taraxis,* confusion]

chronotherapy (krō′nō-ther′ă- pē). The practice of administering chemotherapy at certain times of the day that are thought to be optimal for enhanced activity or lessened toxicity. SEE ALSO chrono-oncology. [chrono- + therapy]

chro·no·tro·pic (kron′ō-trop′ik). Affecting the rate of rhythmic movements such as the heartbeat.

chro·not·ro·pism (kron-ot′rō-pizm). Modification of the rate of a periodic movement, e.g., the heartbeat, through some external influence. [chrono- + G. *tropē,* turn, change]

negative c., retardation of movement, especially of the heart rate.

positive c., acceleration of movement, especially of the heart rate.

chro·o·coc·cals (krō-ō-kok-alz). A class of cyanobacteria in which the cells are solitary or colonial. [*Chroococcus* fr. G. *chrōs, chroos,* color, + coccus]

△**chrys-, chryso-.** Gold; corresponds to L. auro-. [G. *chrysos*]

chry·san·the·mum-car·box·yl·ic ac·ids (kri-san′thĕ-mŭm-kar-bok′si-lik). Cyclopropane carboxylic acids substituted in one position by two methyl groups, the other by 2-methyl-1-propenyl (chrysanthemum monocarboxylic acid) or by 3-methoxy-2-methyl-3-oxo-1-propenyl (chrysanthemum dicarboxylic acid methyl ester); these acids, esterified with allethrolone or pyrethrolone, are the allethrins and pyrethrins, respectively.

Chrys·a·or·a (kris′-a-ōr-a). A genus of the invertebrate phylum Cnidaria that includes the sea nettle.

C. quinquecirrha, the sea nettle, a jellyfish that can inflict moderate to severe stings. SEE ALSO jellyfish. SYN sea nettle.

chrys·a·ro·bin (kris-ă-rō′bin). An extract of Goa powder; a complex mixture of reduction products of chrysophanic acid, emodin, and emodin monomethyl ether; used locally in ringworm, psoriasis, and eczema. [G. *chrysos,* gold, + Brazil Ind. *araroba,* bark]

chrys·a·zine (kris′ă-zin). SYN danthron.

chry·si·a·sis (kri-sī′ă-sis). A permanent slate-gray discoloration of the skin and sclera resulting from deposition of gold in macrophages. SYN auriasis, aurochromoderma. [G. *chrysos,* gold]

chrys·o·cy·a·no·sis (kris′ō-sī-ă-nō′sis). Pigmentation of skin due to reaction to therapeutic use of gold salts.

chrys·oi·din (kris′oy-din) [C.I. 11270]. A dye (MW 249) made from aniline, used in histology and as an indicator (changing from orange to yellow at pH 4.0 to 7.0); also employed as a substitute for Bismarck brown. C. citrate and c. thiocyanate are used as antiseptics.

Chrys·o·my·ia (kris-ō-mī′yă). A genus of myiasis-producing fleshflies (family Calliphoridae) with medium-sized metallic-colored adults; includes the Old World screw worm, *C. bezziana* (sometimes called *Cochliomyia bezziana*), which is a primary invader, comparable to *Cochliomyia hominivorax,* the New World screw worm fly, whereas *C. megacephala* is an Old World equivalent to *Cochliomyia macellaria,* both being secondary or saprophytic invaders. [G. *chrysos,* gold, + *myia,* fly]

Chrys·ops (kris′ops). The deerfly, a genus of biting flies with about 80 North American species, characterized by a splotched wing pattern; *C. discalis* is a vector of *Francisella tularensis* in the U.S.; *C. dimidiatus* and *C. silaceus* are the principal vectors of *Loa loa* in west Africa. [G. *chrysos,* gold, + *ōps,* eye]

Chrys·o·spo·ri·um par·vum (kris-ō-spōr′ē-ŭm par′vŭm). Former name for *Emmonsia parva.*

chrys·o·ther·a·py (kris-ō-thār′ă-pē). Treatment of disease by the administration of gold salts. SYN aurotherapy. [G. *chrysos,* gold]

chunk·ing (chŭnk′ing). The process within short-term memory of combining disparate items of information so that they take up as little as possible of the limited space in short-term memory; e.g., combining into one percept the three individual letters making up the word "cat".

Churg, Jacob, U.S. pathologist, *1910. SEE C.-Strauss *syndrome.*

chut·ta (chŭt′ă). Cancer of the roof of the mouth developing in Asians who smoke cigars with the lighted end inside the mouth. A similar association has been reported from South America and Sardinia.

Chvostek, Franz, Austrian surgeon, 1834–1884. SEE C. *sign.*

⌂chyl-. SEE chylo-.

chy·lan·gi·o·ma (kī-lan-jē-ō′mă). A mass of prominent, dilated lacteals and larger intestinal lymphatic vessels. [chyl- + G. *angeion,* vessel, + *-ōma,* tumor]

chy·la·que·ous (kī-lā′kwē-ŭs). Referring to watery chyle. [chyl- + L. *aqua,* water]

chyle (kīl). A turbid white or pale yellow fluid taken up by the lacteals from the intestine during digestion and carried by the lymphatic system via the thoracic duct into the circulation. The milky appearance is due to chylomicrons in the lymph. [G. *chylos,* juice]

chy·le·mia (kī-lē′mē-ă). The presence of chyle in the circulating blood. [chyl- + G. *haima,* blood]

chy·li·dro·sis (kī-li-drō′sis). Sweating of a milky fluid resembling chyle. [chyl- + G. *hidrōs,* sweat]

chy·li·fac·tion (kī-li-fak′shŭn). SYN chylopoiesis. [chyl- + L. *facio,* to make]

chy·li·fac·tive (kī-li-fak′tiv). SYN chylopoietic.

chy·lif·er·ous (kī-lif′er-ŭs). Conveying chyle. SYN chylophoric. [chyl- + L. *fero,* to carry]

chy·li·fi·ca·tion (kī′li-fi-kā′shŭn). SYN chylopoiesis.

chy·li·form (kī′li-fōrm). Resembling chyle.

⌂chylo-, chyl-. Chyle. [G. *chylos,* juice.]

chy·lo·cele (kī′lō-sēl). An effusion of chyle into the tunica vaginalis propria and space of the tunica vaginalis testis. [chylo- + G. *kēlē,* tumor]

parasitic c., SYN *elephantiasis* scroti.

chy·lo·cyst (kī′lō-sist). SYN *cisterna* chyli. [chylo- + G. *kystis,* bladder]

chy·lo·me·di·as·ti·num (kī′lō-mē-dē-as-tī′nŭm). Abnormal presence of chyle in the mediastinum.

chy·lo·mi·cron, pl. **chy·lo·mi·cra, chy·lo·mi·crons** (kī-lō-mi′kron, -mī′krä, -mi′kronz). A large lipid droplet (between 0.8 and 5 nm in diameter) of reprocessed lipid synthesized in epithelial cells of the small intestine and containing triacylglycerols, cholesterol esters, and several apolipoproteins (e.g., A-I, B-48, C-I, C-II, C-III, E); the least dense (less than 1.006 g/mL) of the plasma lipoproteins that functions as a transport vehicle. [chylo- + G. *micros,* small]

chy·lo·mi·cro·ne·mia (kī′lō-mī-krō-nē′mē-ă). The presence of chylomicrons, especially an increased number, in the circulating blood, as in type I familial hyperlipoproteinemia. SEE ALSO familial chylomicronemia *syndrome.*

chy·lo·per·i·car·di·um (kī′lō-pār-i-kar′dē-ŭm). A milky pericardial effusion resulting from obstruction of the thoracic duct, from trauma, or of idiopathic origin.

chy·lo·per·i·to·ne·um (kī′lō-pār-i-tō-nē′ŭm). SYN chylous *ascites.*

chy·lo·phor·ic (kī-lō-fōr′ik). SYN chyliferous. [chylo- + G. *phoros,* bearing]

chy·lo·pleu·ra (kī-lō-ploor′ă). SYN chylothorax.

chy·lo·pneu·mo·tho·rax (kī′lō-noo-mō-thōr′aks). Free chyle and air in the pleural space.

chy·lo·poi·e·sis (kī′lō-poy-ē′sis). Formation of chyle in the intestine. SYN chylifaction, chylification. [chylo- + G. *poiesis,* a making]

chy·lo·poi·et·ic (kī′lō-poy-et′ik). Relating to chylopoiesis. SYN chylifactive.

chy·lor·rhea (kī-lō-rē′ă). The flow or discharge of chyle. [chylo- + G. *rhoia,* flow]

chy·lo·sis (kī-lō′sis). The formation of chyle from the food in the intestine, its digestion and absorption by the intestinal mucosa, and its mixture with the blood and conveyance to the tissues.

chy·lo·tho·rax (kī-lō-thōr′aks). An accumulation of chylous fluid in the pleural space. SYN chylopleura, chylous hydrothorax.

chy·lous (kī′lŭs). Relating to chyle.

chy·lu·ria (kī-loo′rē-ă). The passage of chyle in the urine; a form of albiduria. [chyl- + G. *ouron,* urine]

chy·mase (kī′mās). SYN chymosin.

chyme (kīm). The semifluid mass of partly digested food passed from the stomach into the duodenum. SYN pulp (3) [TA], chymus. [G. *chymos,* juice]

chy·mi·fi·ca·tion (kī-mi-fi-kā′shŭn). SYN chymopoiesis. [G. *chymos,* juice, + L. *facio,* to make]

chy·mo·pa·pa·in (kī′mō-pap-ā′in). A cysteine proteinase similar to papain in specificity; on rare occasions, it is used to shrink slipped disks as an alternative to surgery; used as a meat tenderizer. It is the major endopeptidase of papaya.

chy·mo·poi·e·sis (kī′mō-poy-ē′sis). The production of chyme; the physical state of food (semifluid) brought about by digestion in the stomach. SYN chymification. [G. *chymos,* juice, chyme, + *poiesis,* a making]

chy·mor·rhea (kī-mō-rē′ă). The flow of chyme. [G. *chymos,* juice, + *rhoia,* flow]

chy·mo·sin (kī′mō-sin). An aspartic proteinase structurally homologous with pepsin, formed from prochymosin; the milk-curdling enzyme obtained from the glandular layer of the stomach of the calf. Acts on a single peptide bond (–Phe–Met–) in κ-casein. SYN chymase, pexin, rennase, rennet, rennin.

chy·mo·sin·o·gen (kī-mō-sin′ō-jen). SYN prochymosin.

chy·mo·sta·tin (kī′mō-sta-tin). An oligopeptide that is known to inhibit chymotrypsin-like proteases (e.g., cathepsin A, B, and D, and papain).

chy·mo·tryp·sin (kī-mō-trip′sin). C. A or B; a serine proteinase of the gastrointestinal tract that preferentially cleaves carboxyl links of hydrophobic amino acids, particularly at tyrosyl, tryptophanyl, phenylalanyl, and leucyl residues; synthesized in the pancreas as chymotrypsinogen, and subsequently converted to π-, δ-, and finally α-c. by successive trypsin-dependent cleavages;

proposed for use in the treatment of inflammation and edema associated with trauma and to facilitate intracapsular cataract extraction; c. A has the specificity above, c. B is homologous to c. A, and c. C has a broader specificity (e.g., additionally acting on carboxyl links of methionyl, glutaminyl, and asparaginyl residues).

chy·mo·tryp·sin·o·gen (kī′mō-trip-sin′ō-jen). The precursor of chymotrypsin. Converted to π-chymotrypsin by the action of trypsin.

chy·mous (kī′mŭs). Relating to chyme.

chy·mus (kī′mŭs). SYN chyme.

chytide. A skin wrinkle.

Ci Abbreviation for curie.

Ciaccio, Carmelo, Italian pathologist, 1877–1956. SEE Ciaccio *stain*.

Ciaccio, Giuseppe V., Italian anatomist, 1824–1901. SEE Ciaccio *glands*, under *gland*.

cib. Abbreviation for L. *cibus*, food.

ci·bo·pho·bia (sī-bō-fō′bē-ă). Fear of eating, or loathing for, food. [L. *cibus*, food, + G. *phobos*, fear]

CIC Abbreviation for completely in the canal *hearing aid*.

CIC Abbreviation for clean intermittent bladder *catheterization*.

cic·a·trec·to·my (sik-ă-trek′tō-mē). Excision of a scar. [L. *cicatrix*, scar, + G. *ektomē*, excision]

cic·a·tri·ces (si-kā′tri-sēz). Plural of cicatrix.

cic·a·tri·cial (sik-ă-trish′ăl). Relating to a scar.

cic·a·tri·cot·o·my, cic·a·tri·sot·o·my (sik′ă-trī-kot′ō-mē, -sot′ō-mē). Cutting a scar. [L. *cicatrix*, scar, + G. *tomē*, cutting]

cic·a·trix, pl. **cic·a·tri·ces** (sik′ă-triks, si-kā′triks; sik-ă-trī′sēz). A scar. [L.]

　brain c., a scarring of the brain resulting from injury (reactive gliosis), characterized by proliferation of mesodermal (vascular) and ectodermal (glial) elements. SEE ALSO isomorphous *gliosis*.

　filtering c., SYN filtering *bleb*.

　meningocerebral c., scarring and adhesions involving contiguous brain and meninges; typically caused by head injury.

　vicious c., a c. that by its contraction causes a deformity.

cic·a·tri·zant (sik-at′ri-zant). **1.** Causing or favoring cicatrization. **2.** An agent with such action.

cic·a·tri·za·tion (sik′ă-tri-zā′shŭn). **1.** The process of scar formation. **2.** The healing of a wound otherwise than by first intention.

ci·clo·pir·ox·ol·a·mine (sī-klō-pir′oks ōl′ă-mēn). A broad-spectrum antifungal agent used to treat a variety of fungus and yeast skin infections.

cic·u·tox·in (sik-ū-tok′sin). A toxic principle present in water hemlock, *Cicuta virosa* (family Umbelliferae); pharmacologic action is similar to that of picrotoxin.

△**-cide.** A word ending denoting an agent that kills (e.g., insecticide), or the act of killing (e.g., suicide). [L. *-cida, -cidium*, fr. *caedo*, to kill]

CIDP Abbreviation for chronic inflammatory demyelinating *polyneuropathy*.

ci·gua·te·ra (sē′gwah-tār′ă). An acute toxic syndrome with predominantly gastrointestinal and neuromuscular features induced by ingestion of the flesh or viscera of various marine fish of the Caribbean and tropical Pacific reefs that contain ciguatoxin. [Sp. fr. *cigua*, sea snail]

　Sporadic cases of ciguatera occur along the east coast of the United States from Vermont to southern Florida and in the U.S. Virgin Islands, Puerto Rico, and Hawaii. Occasional outbreaks result from group consumption of large catches of contaminated fish. The condition is probably underreported, many cases being dismissed as viral syndromes or seasickness. The lipid-soluble, heat-stable toxin is produced by the dinoflagellate *Gambierdiscus toxicus*, which is epiphytic on red and brown algae. Herbivorous fish foraging on reef algae consume the flagellates and are in turn consumed by carnivorous fish; the toxin becomes increasingly concentrated as it passes up the food chain.

The heads and viscera of affected fish contain higher concentrations than other parts. Some 400 species of fish have been associated with human intoxication, including particularly predators such as amberjack, barracuda, grouper, moray eels, red snapper, sea bass, Spanish mackerel, and surgeon fish. Contaminated fish look, smell, and taste normal, and ciguatoxin is not destroyed by cooking, drying, salting, or freezing. Symptoms come on 3–12 hours after exposure (occasionally within minutes) and include vomiting and diarrhea, myalgia, dysesthesia and paresthesia of the extremities and perioral region, pruritus, headache, weakness, and diaphoresis. Bradycardia and hypotension may occur. A few deaths due to respiratory paralysis have been reported. Toxic effects usually resolve spontaneously in about 1 week but residual symptoms may persist for months. Repeated exposure can increase the sensitivity of an individual to the toxin. Diagnosis is confirmed by identification of toxin in uneaten portions of seafood or in the patient's serum. Treatment is purely supportive.

ci·gua·tox·in (sēg-wă-tok′sin). A marine saponin of unknown structure but with the empirical formula $C_{35}H_{65}NO_8$; the toxic substance causing ciguatera.

ci·la·stat·in so·di·um (sī-lă-stat′in). An inhibitor of the renal dipeptidase, dehydropeptidase 1, used, in conjunction with antibiotics subject to metabolism in the kidneys, to increase therapeutic response to the antibiotic.

△**cili-.** SEE cilio-.

cil·ia (sil′ē-ă). Plural of cilium.

cil·i·ary (sil′ē-ar-ē). **1.** Relating to any cilia or hairlike processes, specifically, the eyelashes. **2.** Relating to certain of the structures of the eyeball. [Mod. L. *ciliaris*, relating to or resembling an eyelid, or eyelash, fr. L. *cilium*, eyelid]

cil·i·a·stat·ic (sil-ē-ă-stat′ik). Denoting a drug or condition that slows or stops the beating of cilia (generally used with reference to respiratory mucous membrane cilia).

Ci·li·a·ta (sil-ē-ā′tă). Formerly considered a class of Protozoa whose members bear cilia or structures derived from them, such as cirri or membranelles, but now placed within the phylum Ciliophora. Typical members, such as *Paramecium* or *Balantidium coli* (a parasite of humans) possess two distinctive nuclei, a macronucleus and a micronucleus; only the latter bears the hereditary material exchanged in conjugation, a form of sexual reproduction found only in the C. [L. *cilium*, eyelid]

cil·i·at·ed (sil′ē-ā-ted). Having cilia.

cil·i·ates (sil′ē-āts). Common name for members of the Ciliata.

cil·i·ec·to·my (sil-ē-ek′tō-mē). SYN cyclectomy.

△**cilio-, cili-.** Cilia or meaning ciliary, in any sense; eyelashes. [L. *cilium*, eyelid (eyelash)]

cil·i·o·cy·toph·thor·ia (sil′ē-ō-sī-tō- thōr′ē-a). Detached ciliary tufts (remnants of ciliated epithelium) that can be seen in a variety of body fluids, especially peritoneal, amnionic, and respiratory specimens; they are motile and can be confused with ciliated or flagellated protozoa. [Pl. of ciliocytophthorium, fr. cilio- + cyto- + G. *phthora* corruption, decay, + *-ium*, noun suffix]

cil·i·o·gen·e·sis (sil′ē-ō-jen′ĕ-sis). The formation of cilia.

Ci·li·oph·o·ra (sil′ē-of′ō-ră). A phylum of protozoa that includes the abundant free-living ciliates and the sessile suctorians; formerly classified as a subphylum of the phylum Protozoa. [cilio- + G. *phoros*, bearing]

cil·i·o·ret·i·nal (sil′ē-ō-ret′i-năl). Pertaining to the ciliary body and the retina.

cil·i·o·scle·ral (sil′ē-ō-sklē′răl). Relating to the ciliary body and the sclera.

cil·i·o·spi·nal (sil′ē-ō-spī′nal). Relating to the ciliary body and the spinal cord; denoting in particular the ciliospinal *center*.

cil·i·o·tox·ic·i·ty (sil′ē-ō-tok-sis′i-tē). The characteristic of a drug or other substance that impairs ciliary activity (generally refers to respiratory mucous membrane cilia) (e.g., tobacco smoke).

▣**cil·i·um,** pl. **cil·ia** (sil′ē-ŭm, -ă). **1** [NA]. SYN eyelash. **2.** A motile extension of a cell surface, e.g., of certain epithelial cells, containing nine longitudinal double microtubules arranged in a peripheral ring, together with a central pair. [L. an eyelid]

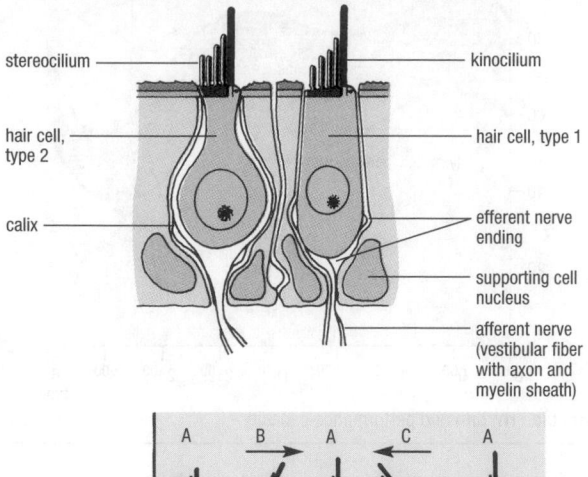

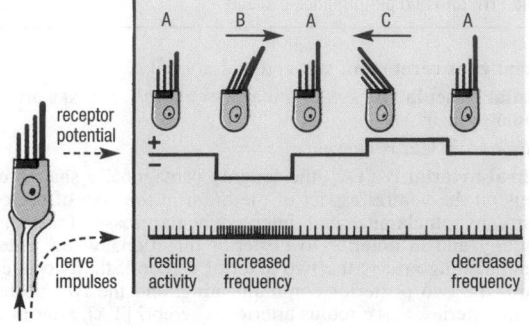

cilia: excitatory and inhibitory responses of stereocilia and kinocilia on hair cells (types I and II) of the vestibular apparatus to stimulation by movement in opposite direction; (A) resting state, (B) stimulation, (C) inhibition

---

Cil·lo·bac·te·ri·um (sil'ō-bak-tēr'ē-ŭm). An obsolete genus of motile, anaerobic bacteria containing Gram-positive, straight or curved rods.

ci·met·i·dine (si-met'i-dēn). A histamine analogue and antagonist used to treat peptic ulcer and hypersecretory conditions by blocking histamine H₂ receptor sites, thus inhibiting gastric acid secretion.

Ci·mex (sī'meks). A genus of bedbugs of the family Cimicidae in the order Hemiptera, with flat, reddish-brown, wingless bodies, prominent lateral eyes, a three-jointed beak, and a characteristic odor from thoracic stink glands; an abundant pest in human abodes. Although its bite produces characteristic linear groups of pruritic wheals with a central hemorrhagic punctum, the bedbug is not a proven vecter of human disease, with the possible exception of hepatitis B. [L. *cimex,* bug, L. *lectulus,* a bed]
   C. hemipterus, a bedbug frequently found in the tropics.
   C. lectularius, the common bedbug.

Cimino, James E., U.S. nephrologist, *1928. SEE Brescia-C. *fistula.*

cIMP Abbreviation for cyclic inosine 3,5-monophosphate.

△**cin-.** SEE cine-.

cin·an·es·the·sia (sin'an-es-thē'zē-ă). SYN kinanesthesia.

ci·nan·ser·in hy·dro·chlo·ride (si-nan'ser-in). A serotonin inhibitor.

cin·chol (sin'kol). SYN β-sitosterol.

cin·cho·na (sin-kō'nă). The dried bark of the root and stem of various species of *Cinchona,* a genus of evergreen trees (family Rubiaceae), native of South America but cultivated in various tropical regions. The cultivated bark contains 7 to 10% of total alkaloids; about 70% is quinine. C. contains more than 20 alkaloids, of which two pairs of isomers are most important: quinine

and quinidine, and cinchonidine and cinchonine. SYN bark (2), cinchona bark, Jesuits bark, Peruvian bark, quina, quinaquina, quinquina. [*Cinchona,* fr. Countess of *Chinch'on*]

cin·chon·ic (sin-kon'ik). Relating to cinchona.

cin·cho·nine (sin'kō-nēn). A quinoline alkaloid prepared from the bark of several species of *Cinchona;* a tonic and antimalarial agent. Several c. salts are available.

cin·cho·nism (sin'kō-nizm). Poisoning by cinchona, quinine, or quinidine; characterized by tinnitus, headache, deafness, and occasionally, anaphylactoid shock. SYN quininism.

cin·cho·phen (sin'kō-fen). An analgesic, antipyretic, and uricosuric agent that may produce liver damage and gastric lesions; used in experimental animals to produce gastric ulcer.

cin·cli·sis (sing'kli-sis). Rapid repetition of a movement, e.g., rapidly repeated winking. [G. *kingklizō,* to wag the tail, change constantly]

△**cine-, cin-.** Movement, usually relating to motion pictures. SEE ALSO kin-. [G. *kineō,* to move]

cin·e·an·gi·o·car·di·og·ra·phy (sin'ē-an'jē-ō-kar-dē-og'ră-fē). Motion pictures of the passage of a contrast medium through chambers of the heart and great vessels.

cin·e·flu·o·rog·ra·phy (sin'ē-flōr-og'ră-fē). SYN cineradiography.

cin·e·flu·o·ros·co·py (sin'ē-flōr-os'kŏ-pē). SYN cineradiography.

cin·e·gas·tros·co·py (sin'ē-gas-tros'kō-pē). Motion pictures of gastroscopic observations.

cin·e·mat·ics (sin-ē-mat'iks). SYN kinematics.

cin·e·ole, cin·e·ol (sin'ē-ōl, -ol). A stimulant expectorant obtained from the volatile oil of *Eucalyptus globulus* and other species of *Eucalyptus.* SYN cajeputol, cajuputol, eucalyptol.

cin·e·pho·to·mi·crog·ra·phy (sin'ē-fō'tō-mī-krog'ră-fē). The making of a motion picture of microscopic objects; time lapse photography is often used.

cin·e·plas·tics (sin-ē-plas'tiks). SYN cineplastic *amputation.*

cin·e·ra·di·og·ra·phy (sin'ē-rā-dē-og'ră-fē). Radiography of an organ in motion, e.g., the heart, the gastrointestinal tract. SYN cinefluorography, cinefluoroscopy, cineroentgenography.

ci·ne·rea (si-nē'rē-ă). **1.** The gray matter of the brain and other parts of the nervous system. **2.** Obsolete term for mantle *layer.* [L. fem. of *cinereus,* ashy, fr. *cinis,* ashes]

ci·ne·re·al (si-nē'rē-ăl). Relating to the gray matter of the nervous system.

ci·ner·i·tious (si-ner-ish'ŭs). Ashen; denoting the gray matter of the brain, spinal cord, and ganglia.

cin·e·roent·gen·og·ra·phy (sin'ē-rent-gen-og'ră-fē). SYN cineradiography.

ci·ne·seis·mog·ra·phy (sin'ē-sīz-mog'ră-fē). A technique for measuring movements of the body by continuous photographic recording of shaking or vibration.

ci·ne·to·plasm, ci·ne·to·plas·ma (sin-et'ō-plazm, sin-et-ō-plaz'mă). SYN kinetoplasm.

cin·gu·late (sin'gū-lāt). Relating to a cingulum.

cin·gu·lec·to·my (sin-gū-lek'tō-mē). SYN cingulotomy. [cingulum + G. *ektomē,* excision]

cin·gu·lot·o·my (sin-gū-lot'ō-mē). Formerly, a unilateral or bilateral surgical excision of the anterior half of the cingulate gyrus, but now accomplished by electrolytic destruction of the anterior cingulate gyrus and callosum. SYN cingulectomy. [cingulum + G. *tomē,* a cutting]

cin·gu·lum, gen. **cin·gu·li,** pl. **cin·gu·la** (sin'gū-lŭm, -lē, -lă) [TA]. **1.** SYN girdle. **2.** A well-marked fiber bundle passing longitudinally in the white matter of the cingulate gyrus; the bundle extends from the region of the anterior perforated substance back over the dorsal surface of the corpus callosum; behind the latter's splenium it curves down and then forward in the white matter of the parahippocampal gyrus; composed largely of fibers from the anterior thalamic nucleus to the cingulate and parahippocampal gyri, it also contains association fibers connecting these gyri with the frontal cortex, and their various subdivisions with each other. [L. girdle, fr. *cingo,* to surround]
   c. den'tis [TA], SYN c. of tooth.

c. mem′bri inferior′is, ✭official alternate term for pelvic *girdle*.

c. mem′bri superior′is, ✭official alternate term for pectoral *girdle*.

c. pectorale [TA], SYN pectoral *girdle*.

c. pelvici [TA], SYN pelvic *girdle*.

c. of tooth [TA], a U- or W-shaped ridge at the base of the lingual surface of the crown of the upper incisors and cuspid teeth, the lateral limbs running for a short distance along the linguoproximal line angles, the central portion just above the gingiva. SYN c. dentis [TA], basal ridge (2), lingual lobe.

cin·na·mal·de·hyde (sin-ă-mal′de-hīd). Chief constituent of cinnamon oil. SYN cinnamic aldehyde.

cin·na·mate (sin′ă-māt). A salt or ester of cinnamic acid.

cin·nam·e·in (sin′am-ē-in). SYN *benzyl* cinnamate.

cin·na·mene (sin′ă-mēn). SYN styrene.

cin·nam·ic (si-nam′ik). Relating to cinnamon.

cin·nam·ic ac·id. Obtained from cinnamon oil, Peruvian and tolu balsams, or storax. It has been used in lupus as paint and in infectious diseases to promote leukocytosis. SYN cinnamylic acid, phenylacrylic acid.

cin·nam·ic al·co·hol. SYN styrone.

cin·nam·ic al·de·hyde. SYN cinnamaldehyde.

cin·na·mon (sin′ă-mon). **1.** The dried bark of *Cinnamomum loureirii* Nees (family Lauraceae), an aromatic bark used as a spice and, in medicine, as an adjuvant, carminative, and aromatic stomachic. SYN Saigon c. **2.** The dried inner bark of the shoots of *Cinnamomum zeylanicum.* SYN Ceylon c. SYN cassia bark. [L. fr. G. *kinnamōmon,* cinnamon]

cassia c., *Cinnamomum cassia* Nees (family Lauraceae); the unofficial source of most of the cinnamon in the shops; the source of c. oil. SYN Chinese c.

Ceylon c., SYN cinnamon (2).

Chinese c., SYN cassia c.

Saigon c., SYN cinnamon (1).

cin·na·mon oil. The volatile oil distilled with steam from the leaves and twigs of *Cinnamomum cassia;* it contains not less than 80% by volume of the total aldehydes of cinnamon oil. SYN cassia oil.

cin·na·myl·ic ac·id (sin-ă-mil′ik). SYN cinnamic acid.

cin·nar·i·zine (si-nar′i-zēn). An H_1 antihistaminic. SYN cinnipirine.

cin·nip·i·rine (si-nip′i-rēn). SYN cinnarizine.

cin·o·cen·trum (sin-ō-sen′trŭm). SYN cytocentrum.

ci·nox·a·cin (si-noks′ă-sin). A synthetic organic acid, chemically related to nalidixic acid, used as an antibacterial to treat urinary tract infections.

ci·nox·ate (si-nok′sāt). An ultraviolet screen for topical application on the skin.

ci·on (sī′on). Archaic term for uvula. [G. *kiōn,* pillar, the uvula]

cip·ro·flox·a·cin hy·dro·chlo·ride (sip-rō-floks′ă-sin). A synthetic fluoroquinolone broad-spectrum antibacterial with activity against a wide range of Gram-negative and Gram-positive organisms.

cir·an·tin (sir-an′tin). SYN hesperidin.

🔲 **cir·ca·di·an** (ser-kā′dē-ăn). Relating to biologic variations or rhythms with a cycle of about 24 hours. Cf. infradian, ultradian. [L. *circa,* about, + *dies,* day]

cir·cel·lus (sir-sel′ŭs). A small circle. [L.]

c. veno′sus hypoglos′si, SYN venous *plexus* of canal of hypoglossal nerve.

cir·cho·ral (ser-kō′răl). Occurring cyclically about once an hour.

cir·ci·nate (ser′si-nāt). Circular; ring-shaped. [L. *circinatus,* made round, pp. of *circino,* to make round, fr. *circinus,* a pair of compasses]

cir·cle (ser′kl). **1** [TA]. In anatomy, a ring-shaped structure or group of structures, as formed by anastomosing arteries or veins, or by connected (communicating) nerves, **2.** A line or process with every point approximately equidistant from the center. SYN circulus [TA]. [L. *circulus*]

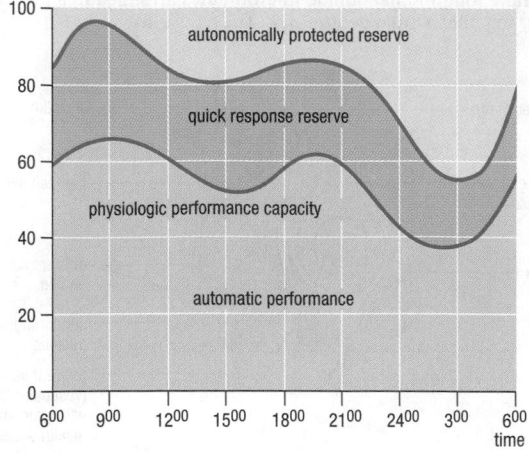

performance/time for performance in %

autonomically protected reserve

quick response reserve

physiologic performance capacity

automatic performance

time

circadian rhythm and performance capacity

arterial c. of cerebrum, SYN cerebral arterial c.

articular vascular c., SYN articular vascular *plexus*; SEE articular vascular *network*.

Carus c., SYN Carus *curve.*

cerebral arterial c. [TA], the roughly pentagonally shaped c. of vessels on the ventral aspect of the brain in the area of the optic chiasm, hypothalamus, and interpeduncular fossa; formed, sequentially and in anterior to posterior direction, by the anterior communicating artery, the two anterior cerebral, the two internal carotid, the two posterior communicating, and the two posterior cerebral arteries. SYN circulus arteriosus cerebri [TA], arterial c. of cerebrum, c. of Willis.

closed c., a circuit for administration of an inhalation anesthetic in which there is complete rebreathing with carbon dioxide absorption.

defensive c., obsolete term for the addition of a secondary affection that limits or arrests the progress of the primary affection, as thought to occur when pneumothorax supervenes on pulmonary tuberculosis, the former having a therapeutic effect on the latter.

greater arterial c. of iris, SYN major arterial c. of iris.

Haller c., (1) SYN vascular c. of optic nerve; **(2)** SYN areolar venous *plexus.*

Huguier c., anastomosis around the isthmus of the uterus (junction of the cervix with the body) between the right and left uterine arteries.

least confusion c., in the configuration of rays emerging from a spherocylindrical lens system, the place where diverging rays of the lens first forming a line image are balanced by converging rays of the second lens.

lesser arterial c. of iris, SYN minor arterial c. of iris.

major arterial c. of iris, an arterial circle at the ciliary border of the iris. SYN circulus arteriosus iridis major [TA], major circulus arteriosus of iris [TA], greater arterial c. of iris.

minor arterial c. of iris, an arterial circle near the pupillary margin of the iris. SYN circulus arteriosus iridis minor [TA], minor circulus arteriosus of iris [TA], lesser arterial c. of iris.

Pagenstecher c., in the case of a freely movable abdominal tumor, the mass is moved throughout its entire range, its position at intervals being marked on the abdominal wall; when these points are joined, a c. is formed, the center of which marks the point of attachment of the tumor.

Ridley c., SYN circular *sinus* (1).

rolling c., a mechanism for the replication of circular DNA.

semi-closed c., a circuit for administration of an inhalation anesthetic in which partial rebreathing with carbon dioxide absorption is combined with loss from the circuit of a portion of respired gases through valves.

vascular c., (1) the c. around the mouth formed by the inferior and superior labial arteries; (2) SYN areolar venous *plexus*.

vascular c. of optic nerve [TA], a network of branches of the short ciliary arteries on the sclera around the point of entrance of the optic nerve. SYN circulus vasculosus nervi optici [TA], circulus arteriosus halleri, circulus zinnii, Haller c. (1), Zinn corona, Zinn vascular c.

venous c. of mammary gland, SYN areolar venous *plexus*.

vicious c., the mutually augmenting action of two independent diseases or phenomena, or of a primary and secondary affection;

Vieth-Müller c., a geometric c. passing through the optical centers of two eyes by which points adjacent to the point of fixation, both lying on the circle, theoretically fall on corresponding retinal points.

c. of Willis, SYN cerebral arterial c.

Zinn vascular c., SYN vascular c. of optic nerve.

cir·cuit (ser′kit). The path or course of flow of cases or electric or other currents. [L. *circuitus,* a going round, fr. *circum,* around, + *eo,* pp. *itus,* to go]

anesthetic c., equipment used during inhalation anesthesia to regulate concentrations of inhaled gases; includes a reservoir bag and usually directional valves, breathing tubes, and a carbon dioxide absorber.

Papez c., a long circuitous conduction chain in the mammalian forebrain, leading from the hippocampus by way of the fornix to the mammillary body and thence returning to the hippocampus by way of, sequentially, the anterior thalamic nuclei, cingulate gyrus, and parahippocampal gyrus.

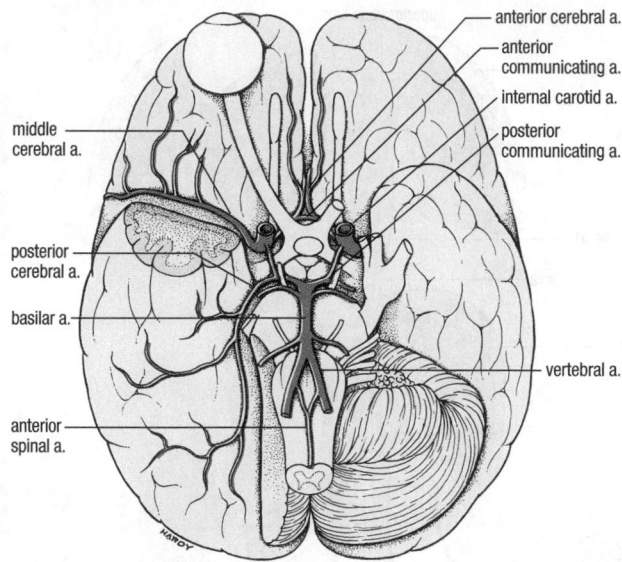

middle cerebral a.
posterior cerebral a.
basilar a.
anterior spinal a.
anterior cerebral a.
anterior communicating a.
internal carotid a.
posterior communicating a.
vertebral a.

HARDY

circle of Willis: view of arteries at the base of the brain

reverberating c., a theory of periodic conduction through the cerebral cortex of trains of impulses traveling in c.'s of neurons.

signal-processing c.'s, the electronic hardware of hearing aids that allows alteration in the amplification of various bands of frequencies of the acoustic signal.

cir·cu·la·tion (ser-kū-lā′shŭn). Movements in a circle, or through a circular course, or through a course that leads back to the same point; usually referring to blood c. unless otherwise specified. [L. *circulatio*]

assisted c., application of external devices to improve pressure, flow, or both in the heart or arteries.

blood c., the course of the blood from the heart through the arteries, capillaries, and veins back again to the heart.

capillary c., the course of the blood through the capillaries.

collateral c., c. maintained in small anastomosing vessels when the main vessel is obstructed.

compensatory c., c. established in dilated collateral vessels when the main vessel of the part is obstructed.

cross c., c. to an animal or one of its parts from the c. of another animal.

embryonic c., the basic plan of the c. of a young mammalian embryo, at first similar to that in aquatic forms, with an unpartitioned heart and conspicuous aortic arches in the branchial region; as gestation progresses, the arrangement of the major blood vessels gradually approaches that of an adult, but the routing of blood through the heart, characteristic of an adult, cannot be attained until lung breathing begins at birth.

enterohepatic c., c. of substances such as bile salts which are absorbed from the intestine and carried to the liver, where they are secreted into the bile and again enter the intestine.

extracorporeal c., the c. of blood outside of the body through a machine that temporarily assumes an organ's functions, e.g., through a heart-lung machine or artificial kidney.

fetal c., the c. which serves the fetus in utero, with the placental circuit responsible for supplying oxygen and nutritive material and for eliminating CO_2 and nitrogenous wastes. SEE ALSO embryonic c.

greater c., SYN systemic c.

hypophysial portal c., SYN portal hypophysial c.

hypothalamohypophysial portal c., SYN portal hypophysial c.

lesser c., SYN pulmonary c.

lymph c., the slow passage of lymph through the lymphatic vessels and glands.

placental c., the c. of blood through the placenta during intrauterine life, serving the needs of the fetus for aeration, absorption, and excretion; also, maternal circulation through the intervillous space of the placenta.

portal c., (1) c. of blood to the liver from the small intestine, the right half of the colon, and the spleen via the portal vein; sometimes specified as the hepatic portal c.; (2) more generally, any part of the systemic circulation in which blood draining from the capillary bed of one structure flows through a larger vessel(s) to supply the capillary bed of another structure before returning to the heart; e.g., the hypothalamohypophysial portal system.

portal hypophysial c., a capillary network that carries hypophyseotropic hormones from the hypothalamus, where they are secreted into blood, to their sites of action in the anterior hypophysis. SEE portal c., pituitary *gland,* hypothalamus. SYN hypophyseoportal system, hypophysial portal c., hypophysial portal system, hypophysioportal system, hypothalamohypophysial portal c., hypothalamohypophysial portal system (1).

pulmonary c., the passage of blood from the right ventricle through the pulmonary artery to the lungs and back through the pulmonary veins to the left atrium. SYN lesser c.

Servetus c., obsolete eponym for the pulmonary c.

systemic c., the c. of blood through the arteries, capillaries, and veins of the general system, from the left ventricle to the right atrium. SYN greater c.

thebesian c. (thē-bē′sē-an), the system of smaller veins in the myocardium.

cir·cu·la·to·ry (ser′kū-lă-tō-rē). **1.** Relating to the circulation. **2.** SYN sanguiferous.

cir·cu·lus, gen. and pl. **cir·cu·li** (ser′kū-lŭs, -lī) [TA]. SYN circle. **2.** A circle formed by connecting arteries, veins, or nerves. [L. dim. of *circus,* circle]

c. arterio′sus cer′ebri [TA], SYN cerebral arterial *circle*.

c. arterio′sus hal′leri, SYN vascular *circle* of optic nerve.

c. arterio′sus ir′idis ma′jor [TA], SYN major arterial *circle* of iris.

c. arterio′sus ir′idis mi′nor [TA], SYN minor arterial *circle* of iris.

c. articula′ris vasculo′sus, SYN articular vascular *plexus*.

major c. arteriosus of iris [TA], SYN major arterial *circle* of iris.

minor c. arteriosus of iris [TA], SYN minor arterial *circle* of iris.

c. vasculo′sus ner′vi op′tici [TA], SYN vascular *circle* of optic nerve.

c. veno′sus hal′leri, SYN areolar venous *plexus*.

c. veno′sus rid′leyi, SYN circular *sinus* (1).

ci

c. zin'nii, SYN vascular *circle* of optic nerve.

△**circum-.** A circular movement, or a position surrounding the part indicated by the word to which it is joined. SEE ALSO peri-. [L. around]

cir·cum·a·nal (ser-kŭm-ā'năl). Surrounding the anus. SYN perianal, periproctic.

cir·cum·ar·tic·u·lar (ser'kŭm-ar-tik'ū-lăr). Surrounding a joint. SYN periarthric, periarticular. [circum- + L. *articulus*, joint]

cir·cum·ax·il·lary (ser-kŭm-ak'si-lār-ē). Around the axilla. SYN periaxillary.

cir·cum·bul·bar (ser-kŭm-bŭl'bar). SYN peribulbar.

cir·cum·cise (ser'kŭm-sīz). To remove the prepuce or other tissue by circumferential incision (circumcision).

cir·cum·ci·sion (ser-kŭm-sizh'ŭn). **1.** Operation to remove part or all of the prepuce. **2.** Cutting around an anatomic part (e.g., the areola of the breast). SYN peritectomy (2). [L. *circumcido*, to cut around, fr. *circum*, around, + *caedo*, to cut]

female c., a broad term referring to many forms of female genital cutting, ranging from removal of the clitoral prepuce to the removal of the q.v., clitoris, labia minora and parts of the labia majora, and infibulation; done for cultural, not medical, reasons.

cir·cum·cor·ne·al (ser-kŭm-kōr'nē-ăl). SYN pericorneal.

circumductio [TA]. SYN circumduction.

cir·cum·duc·tion (ser-kŭm-dŭk'shŭn) [TA]. **1.** Movement of a part, e.g., an extremity, in a circular direction. **2.** SYN cycloduction. SYN circumductio [TA]. [circum- + L. *duco*, pp. *ductus*, to draw]

cir·cum·fer·ence (c) (ser-kŭm'fer-ens) [TA]. The outer boundary, especially of a circular area. SYN circumferentia [TA]. [L. *circumferentia, a bearing around*]

articular c. of head of radius [TA], the portion of the head of the radius that articulates with the radial notch of the ulna. SYN circumferentia articularis capitis radii [TA].

articular c. of head of ulna [TA], the portion of the head of the ulna that articulates with the ulnar notch of the radius. SYN circumferentia articularis capitis ulnae [TA].

cir·cum·fer·en·tia (ser-kŭm-fer-en'shē-ă) [TA]. SYN circumference. [L. a bearing around]

c. articula'ris capitis ra'dii [TA], SYN articular *circumference* of head of radius.

c. articula'ris capitis ul'nae [TA], SYN articular *circumference* of head of ulna.

cir·cum·flex (ser'kŭm-fleks). Describing an arc of a circle or that which winds around something; denotes several anatomic structures: arteries, veins, nerves, and muscles. [circum- + L. *flexus*, to bend]

cir·cum·gem·mal (ser-kŭm-jem'ăl). Surrounding a budlike or bulblike body; denoting a mode of nerve termination by fibrils surrounding an end bulb. SYN perigemmal. [circum- + L. *gemma*, a bud]

cir·cum·in·tes·ti·nal (ser'kŭm-in-tes'ti-năl). SYN perienteric.

cir·cum·len·tal (ser-kŭm-len'tăl). SYN perilenticular.

cir·cum·man·dib·u·lar (ser'kŭm-man-dib'ū-lăr). Around or about the mandible.

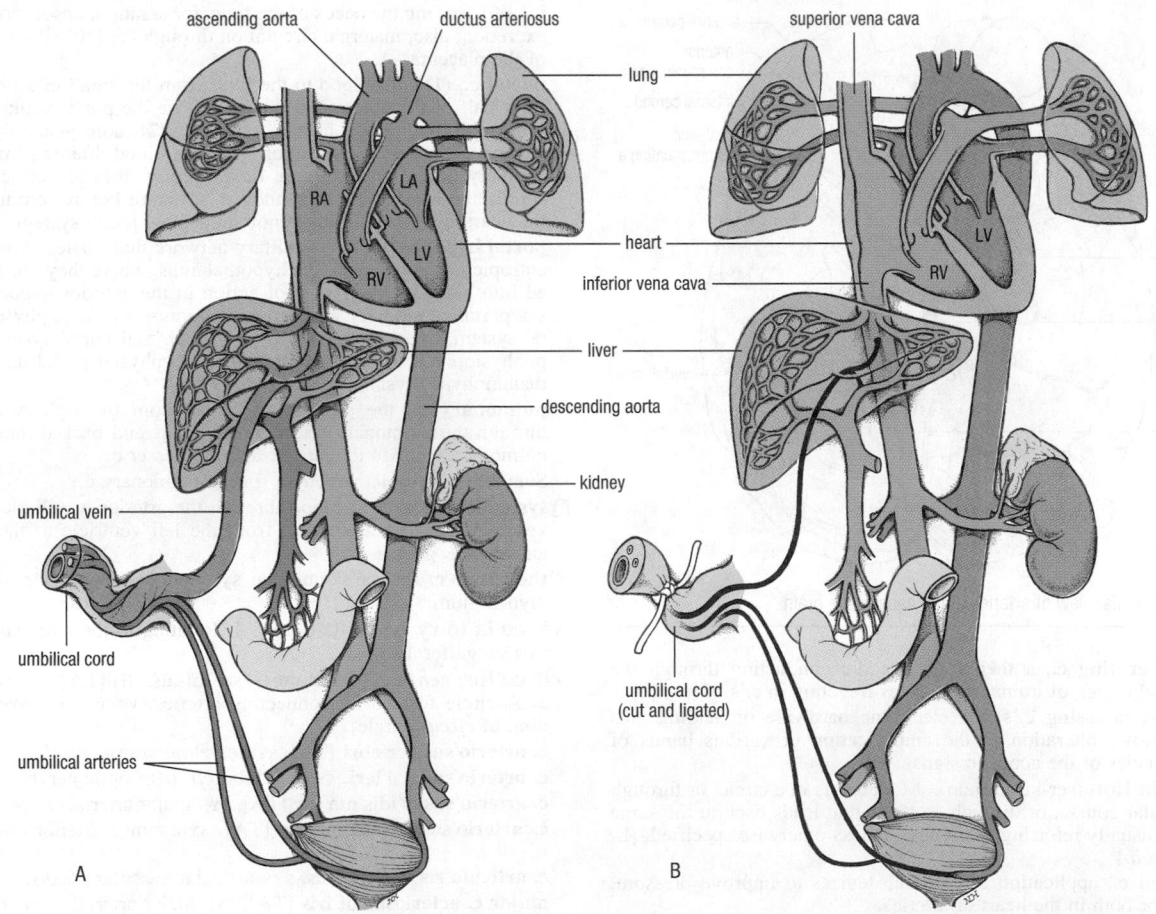

fetal circulation: (A) during pregnancy, oxygen diffuses from the maternal circulation to the fetal circulation in the placenta; oxygenated blood (red) returns to fetus through umbilical vein; (B) after birth, umbilical cord is cut and blood is oxygenated as it passes through the lungs; (RA) right atrium, (LA) left atrium, (LV) left ventricle, (RV) right ventricle

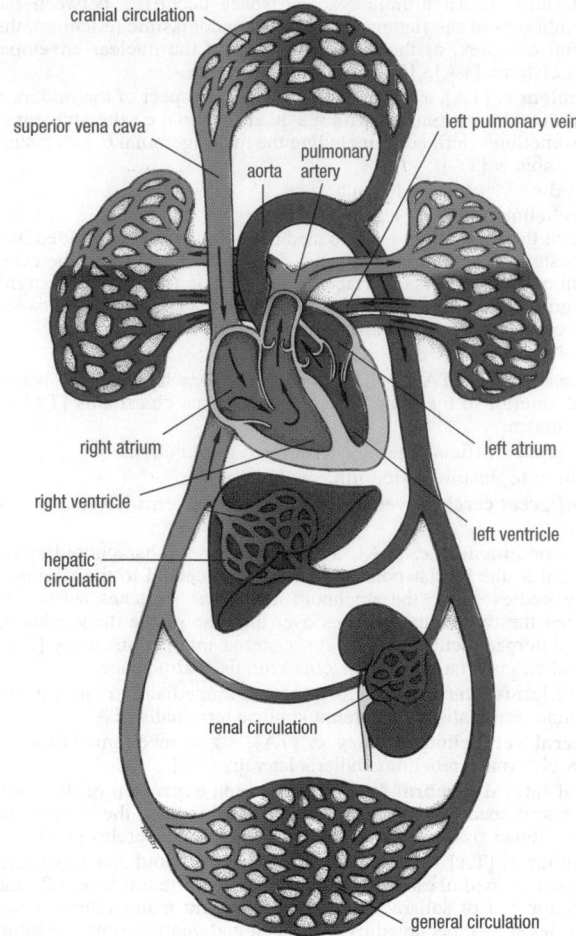

cranial circulation

superior vena cava

aorta

pulmonary artery

left pulmonary veins

right atrium

left atrium

right ventricle

left ventricle

hepatic circulation

renal circulation

general circulation

pulmonary circulation: through the lungs, from the right ventricle to the left atrium

systemic circulation: through the body, from the left ventricle to the right atrium

---

cir·cum·nu·cle·ar (ser-kŭm-noo′klē-ăr). SYN perinuclear.

cir·cum·oc·u·lar (ser-kŭm-ok′ū-lăr). Around the eye. SYN periocular, periophthalmic. [circum- + L. *oculus,* eye]

cir·cum·o·ral (ser-kŭm-ōr′ăl). SYN perioral. [circum- + L. *os* (*oris*), mouth]

cir·cum·or·bit·al (ser-kŭm-ōr′bi-tăl). Around the orbit. SYN periorbital (2).

cir·cum·re·nal (ser-kŭm-rē′năl). SYN perinephric. [circum- + L. *ren,* kidney]

cir·cum·scribed (ser′kŭm-skrībd). Bounded by a line; limited or confined. SYN circumscriptus. [circum- + L. *scribo,* to write]

cir·cum·scrip·tus (ser-kŭm-skrip′tŭs). SYN circumscribed. [L.]

cir·cum·stan·ti·al·i·ty (ser′kŭm-stan-shē-al′i-tē). A disturbance in the thought process, either voluntary or involuntary, in which one gives an excessive amount of detail (circumstances) that is often tangential, elaborate, and irrelevant, to avoid making a direct statement or answer to a question; observed in schizophrenia and in obsessional disorders. Cf. tangentiality. [L. *circum-sto,* pr. p. *-stans,* to stand around]

cir·cum·val·late (ser-kŭm-val′āt). Denoting a structure surrounded by a wall, as the c. (vallate) papillae of the tongue. [circum- + L. *vallum,* wall]

cir·cum·vas·cu·lar (ser-kŭm-vas′kū-lăr). SYN perivascular. [circum- + L. *vasculum,* vessel]

cir·cum·ven·tric·u·lar (ser′kŭm-ven-trik′ū-lăr). Around or in the area of a ventricle, as are the c. organs.

cir·cum·vo·lute (ser-kŭm-vol′oot). Twisted around; rolled about. [L. *circum-volvo,* pp. *-volutus,* to roll around]

cir·rhog·e·nous, cir·rho·gen·ic (sir-roj′ĕ-nŭs, -rō-jen′ik). Rarely used term for tending to the development of cirrhosis. [G. *kirrhos,* yellow (liver), + *-gen,* producing]

cir·rhon·o·sus (sir-ron′ō-sŭs). A disease of the fetus marked anatomically by a yellow staining of the peritoneum and pleura. [G. *kirrhos,* yellow (liver), + *nosos,* disease]

cir·rho·sis (sir-rō′sis). Endstage liver disease characterized by diffuse damage to hepatic parenchymal cells, with nodular regeneration, fibrosis, and disturbance of normal architecture; associated with failure in the function of hepatic cells and interference with blood flow in the liver, frequently resulting in jaundice, portal hypertension, ascites, and ultimately biochemical and functional signs of hepatic failure. [G. *kirrhos,* yellow (liver), + *-osis,* condition]

alcoholic c., c. that frequently develops in chronic alcoholism, characterized in an early stage by enlargement of the liver due to fatty change with mild fibrosis, and later by Laënnec c. with contraction of the liver.

biliary c., c. due to biliary obstruction, which may be a primary intrahepatic disease or secondary to obstruction of extrahepatic bile ducts; the latter may lead to cholestasis and proliferation in small bile ducts with fibrosis, but marked disturbance of the lobular pattern is infrequent. SEE ALSO primary biliary c.

capsular c. of liver, SYN Glisson c.

cardiac c., an extensive fibrotic reaction within the liver as a result of chronic constrictive pericarditis or prolonged congestive heart failure; true c. with fibrous bridging of lobules is unusual. SYN cardiac liver, congestive c., pseudocirrhosis, stasis c.

congestive c., SYN cardiac c.

cryptogenic c., c. of unknown etiology, with no history of alcoholism or previous acute hepatitis.

fatty c., early nutritional c., especially in alcoholics, in which the liver is enlarged by fatty change, with mild fibrosis.

Glisson c., chronic perihepatitis with thickening and subsequent contraction, resulting in atrophy and deformity of the liver. SYN capsular c. of liver.

Hanot c., SYN primary biliary c.

juvenile c., SYN chronic active *hepatitis.*

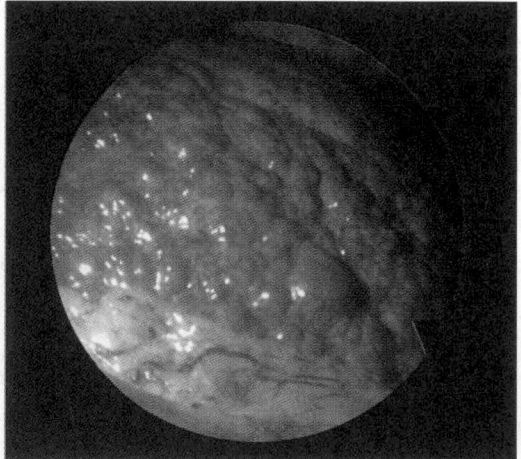

cirrhosis of the liver: small-node type (laparoscopic view)

Laënnec c., c. in which normal liver lobules are replaced by small regeneration nodules, sometimes containing fat, separated by a fairly regular framework of fine fibrous tissue strands (hob-nail liver); usually due to chronic alcoholism. Can cause severe impairment of liver function, portal hypertension with ascites and esophageal varices, and life-threatening complications. SYN portal c.

necrotic c., SYN postnecrotic c.

nutritional c., c. occurring in persons or animals with general or specific dietary deficiencies; methionine and cystine deficiency may produce changes of c. in animals, but it is uncertain whether malnutrition in humans leads to c. or only to reversible fatty infiltration of the liver.

periportal c., c. of the liver with wide bands of fibrosis surrounding large segments of liver, with regenerative nodules.

pigment c., c. of the liver associated with dark brown discoloration seen in hemochromatosis.

pigmentary c., c. resulting from excessive deposits of iron in the liver, usually seen in hemochromatosis.

pipe stem c., c. of the liver with fingerlike fibrosis predominantly around portal tracts, seen in schistosomiasis. Leads to portal hypertension but rarely to functional failure of the liver.

portal c., SYN Laënnec c.

posthepatitic c., SYN chronic active *hepatitis*.

postnecrotic c., c. characterized by necrosis involving whole hepatic lobules, with collapse of the reticular framework to form large scars; regeneration nodules are also large; may follow viral or toxic necrosis, or develop as a result of ischemic necrosis. SYN necrotic c.

primary biliary c., a condition occurring mainly in middle-aged women, characterized by obstructive jaundice with hyperlipemia, pruritis, and hyperpigmentation of the skin; no obstruction of large bile ducts or proliferation of small bile ducts is found; the liver shows c. with marked portal infiltration by lymphocytes and plasma cells, and frequently by epithelioid cell granulomas; serum antimitochondrial antibodies are present in 85–90% of patients. SYN Hanot c.

pulmonary c., fibrosis of the lungs; usually interstitial pulmonary fibrosis.

stasis c., SYN cardiac c.

syphilitic c., c. of the liver occurring as a result of tertiary or congenital syphilis.

toxic c., c. of the liver resulting from chronic poisoning, as by lead or carbon tetrachloride.

cir·rhot·ic (sir-rot′ik). Relating to or affected with cirrhosis or advanced fibrosis.

cir·ri (sir′ī). Plural of cirrus.

cir·rose, cir·rous (sir′ōs, sir′ŭs). Relating to or having cirri.

cir·rus, pl. **cir·ri** (sir′rŭs, -rī). A structure formed from a cluster or tuft of fused cilia, constituting one of the sensory or locomotor organs of certain ciliate protozoa. [L. a curl]

cir·soid (ser′soyd). SYN variciform. [G. *kirsos,* varix, + *eidos,* appearance]

cir·som·pha·los (ser-som′fă-los). Rarely used term for *caput* medusae [G. *kirsos,* varix, + *omphalos,* umbilicus]

cir·soph·thal·mia (ser-sof-thal′mē-ă). Varicose dilation of the conjunctival blood vessels. [G. *kirsos,* varix, + *ophthalmos,* eye]

CIS Abbreviation for *carcinoma in situ.*

⌂**cis-.** **1.** Prefix (in italics) meaning on this side, on the near side; opposite of *trans-.* **2.** In genetics, a prefix denoting the location of two or more genes on the same chromosome of a homologous pair, in coupling. **3.** In organic chemistry (in italics), a form of geometric isomerism in which similar functional groups are attached on the same side of the plane that includes two adjacent, fixed carbon atoms (e.g., the 2- and 3-OH groups of ribofuranose) in a ring structure. SEE entgegen. **4.** In organic chemistry, a form of geometric isomerism with regard to carbon-carbon double bonds. Identical functional groups on the same side of the double bond are *cis-.* When the four moieties attached to the carbons of the double bond are all different, then the *E/Z* nomenclature has to be followed. SYN zusammen (1). SEE entgegen, zusammen. [L.]

cis·plat·in (sis′pla-tin). A chemotherapeutic agent with antitumor activity; c. binds DNA and interferes with DNA synthesis; strongly emetogenic.

cis·tern (sis′tern) [TA]. **1** [TA]. Any cavity or enclosed space serving as a reservoir, especially for chyle, lymph, or cerebrospi-

nal fluid. **2.** An ultramicroscopic space occurring between the membranes of the flattened sacs of the endoplasmic reticulum, the Golgi complex, or the two membranes of the nuclear envelope. SYN cisterna [TA]. [L. *cisterna*]

ambient c. [TA], a c. located on the lateral aspect of the midbrain and dorsally continuous with the quadrigeminal c.; the ambient c. is sometimes defined as including the quadrigeminal c. SYN cisterna ambiens [TA].

basal c., SYN interpeduncular c.

cerebellomedullary c., the largest of the subarachnoid c.'s between the cerebellum and the medulla oblongata; it is divided into a posterior cerebellomedullary c. [TA] located between the cerebellum and the dorsal surface of the medulla (also called cisterna magna), and a lateral cerebellomedullary c. [TA] located between the cerebellum and the lateral aspect of the medulla.

c. of chiasm, SYN chiasmatic c.

chiasmatic c. [TA], a dilation of the subarachnoid space below and anterior to the optic chiasm. SYN cisterna chiasmatis [TA], c. of chiasm.

chyle c., ☆official alternate term for *cisterna* chyli.

c. of cytoplasmic reticulum, SEE cisterna.

c. of great cerebral vein, ☆official alternate term for quadrigeminal c.

interpeduncular c. [TA], a dilation of the subarachnoid space rostral to the basilar pons and ventral and caudal to the mammillary bodies where the arachnoid membrane stretches across between the two temporal lobes over the base of the diencephalon. SEE interpeduncular *fossa.* SYN cisterna interpeduncularis [TA], basal c., cisterna basalis, cisterna cruralis, Tarin space.

c. of lamina terminalis [TA], located immediately rostral to the lamina terminalis. SYN cisterna laminae terminalis [TA].

lateral cerebellomedullary c. [TA], SEE cerebellomedullary c. SYN cisterna cerebellomedullaris lateralis [TA].

c. of lateral cerebral fossa, an elongated expansion of the subarachnoid space where the arachnoid bridges over the opening of the Sylvian fissure. SYN cisterna fossae lateralis cerebri [TA].

lumbar c. [TA], enlargement of the subarachnoid space between the conus medullaris of spinal cord (about vertebral level L2) and inferior end of subarachnoid space and dura mater (about vertebral level S2); occupied by the dorsal and ventral roots constituting the cauda equina, the terminal filum, and cerebrospinal fluid. Site for lumbar puncture and spinal anesthesia.

c. of nuclear envelope, SYN *cisterna* caryothecae.

Pecquet c., SYN *cisterna* chyli.

pericallosal c. [TA], located immediately adjacent to the full length of the corpus callosum, contains portions of pericallosal artery, a branch of the anterior cerebral artery. SYN cisterna pericallosa [TA].

pontine c., SYN pontocerebellar c.

pontocerebellar c. [TA], located on lateral aspects of the pons at its junction with the cerebellum, may be divided into superior and inferior portions. SYN cisterna pontocerebellaris [TA], cisterna pontis, pontine c., prepontine c.

posterior cerebellomedullary c. [TA], SEE cerebellomedullary c. SYN cisterna cerebellomedullaris posterior [TA], cisterna magna☆.

prepontine c., SYN pontocerebellar c.

quadrigeminal c. [TA], an expansion of the subarachnoid space extending forward between the corpus callosum and the thalamus; it encloses the internal cerebral veins which caudally join to form the vena magna cerebri (Galen vein). SYN cisterna quadrigeminalis [TA], c. of great cerebral vein☆, cisterna venae magnae cerebri☆, Bichat canal, superior c.

quadrigeminal c. [TA], slightly enlarged portion of the subarachnoid space located immediately dorsal to the tectum of the mesencephalon; contains parts of the great cerebral vein and of the medial posterior choroidal arteries.

subarachnoid c.'s [TA], widening portions of the subarachnoid space within the cranium where the arachnoid bridges over a depression on the surface of the brain. SYN cisternae subarachnoideae [TA].

superior c., SYN quadrigeminal c.

Sylvian c., the subarachnoid space associated with the lateral cerebral sulcus (Sylvian fissure); contains the M1 segment of the middle cerebral artery and the origin of lenticulostriate arteries, and proximal parts of the middle cerebral artery.

cis·ter·na, gen. and pl. **cis·ter·nae** (sis-ter′nă, -ter′nē) [TA]. SYN cistern. [L. an underground cistern for water, fr. *cista,* a box]

c. am′biens [TA], SYN ambient *cistern.*

c. basa′lis, SYN interpeduncular *cistern.*

c. caryothe′cae, the space between the internal and external membranes of the nuclear envelope; may be continuous in places with cisterns of the endoplasmic reticulum. SYN cistern of nuclear envelope, perinuclear space.

c. cerebellomedullaris lateralis [TA], SYN lateral cerebellomedullary *cistern.*

c. cerebellomedulla′ris posterior [TA], SYN posterior cerebellomedullary *cistern;* SEE cerebellomedullary *cistern.*

c. chiasmatica [TA],

c. chias′matis [TA], SYN chiasmatic *cistern.*

c. chy′li [TA], a dilated sac at the lower end of the thoracic duct into which the intestinal trunk and two lumbar lymphatic trunks open; it occurs inconsistently and when present is located posterior to the aorta on the anterior aspect of the bodies of the first and second lumbar vertebrae. SYN chyle cistern✩, ampulla chyli, chylocyst, Pecquet cistern, Pecquet reservoir, receptaculum chyli, receptaculum pecqueti.

c. crura′lis, SYN interpeduncular *cistern.*

c. fos′sae latera′lis cer′ebri [TA], SYN *cistern* of lateral cerebral fossa.

c. interpeduncula′ris [TA], SYN interpeduncular *cistern.*

c. laminae terminalis [TA], SYN *cistern* of lamina terminalis.

c. lumbalis [TA], SYN lumbar *cistern.*

c. mag′na, ✩official alternate term for posterior cerebellomedullary *cistern.*

c. pericallosa [TA], SYN pericallosal *cistern.*

c. perilymphat′ica, SYN perilymphatic *space.*

c. pon′tis, SYN pontocerebellar *cistern.*

c. pontocerebellaris [TA], SYN pontocerebellar *cistern.*

c. quadrigeminalis [TA], SYN quadrigeminal *cistern;* SEE *cistern* of great cerebral vein.

cisternae subarachnoideae [TA], SYN subarachnoid *cisterns,* under *cistern.*

subsurface c., a cistern of the endoplasmic reticulum that lies close to the plasma membrane; such cisternae occur especially in the cell bodies of neurons.

terminal cisternae, pairs of transversely oriented tubules of the sarcoplasmic reticulum occurring at regular intervals in skeletal muscle fibers; together with an intermediate T tubule they make up a triad.

c. ve′nae mag′nae cer′ebri, ✩official alternate term for quadrigeminal *cistern.*

cis·ter·nal (sis-ter′năl). Relating to a cisterna.

cis·tern·og·ra·phy (sis′tern-og′ră-fē). The radiographic study of the basal cisterns of the brain after the subarachnoid introduction of an opaque or other contrast medium, or a radiopharmaceutical with a suitable detector. [cisterna + G. *graphō,* to write]

cerebellopontine c., the radiographic study of the cerebellopontine angle and contiguous structures after the introduction of a radiopaque contrast medium into the subarachnoid space.

radionuclide c., scintigraphic imaging of the cisterns at the base of the brain following subarachnoid injection of a gamma-emitting radiopharmaceutical.

cis·tron (sis′tron). **1.** The smallest functional unit of heritability; a length of chromosomal DNA associated with a single biochemical function. Under classical concepts, a gene might consist of more than one c.; in modern molecular biology, the c. is essentially equivalent to the structural gene. **2.** The genetic unit defined by the *cis/trans* test. [*cis tr*-ans + -on]

cis·ves·tism, cis·ves·ti·tism (sis-ves′tizm, -ves′ti-tizm). The practice of dressing in clothes inappropriate to one's position or status. Cf. transvestism. [L. *cis,* on the near side of, + *vestio,* to dress]

Ci·tel·lus (si-tel′ŭs). Former name for genus *Spermophilus.* [Mod. L.]

cito disp. Abbreviation for L. *cito dispensetur,* let it be dispensed quickly.

cit·ral (sit′răl). A monoterpene aldehyde consisting of both geometric isomers found in oils from lemon, orange, verbena, and lemon grass; c.-A is the trans-isomer and c.-B is the cis-isomer (neral).

cit·rase, cit·ra·tase (sit′rās, -ră-tās). SYN *citrate* lyase.

cit·rate (sit′rāt, sī′trāt). A salt or ester of citric acid; used as anticoagulants because they bind calcium ions.

c. aldolase, SYN c. lyase.

ATP c. (*pro-3S*)-lyase, an enzyme that catalyzes the reaction of ATP, citrate, and coenzyme A to form ADP, orthophosphate, oxaloacetate, and acetyl-CoA. An important step in fatty acid biosynthesis. SYN citrate-cleavage enzyme.

c. lyase, c. (*pro-3S*)-lyase; an enzyme that catalyzes the cleavage of citrate to oxaloacetate and acetate, in the absence of coenzyme A. SYN citrase, citratase, c. aldolase.

c. synthase, c. (*si*)-synthase; an enzyme catalyzing the condensation of oxaloacetate, water, and acetyl-CoA, forming citrate and coenzyme A; an important step in the tricarboxylic acid cycle. SYN condensing enzyme, oxaloacetate transacetase.

cit·rat·ed (sit′rā-ted). Containing a citrate; specifically denoting blood serum or milk to which has been added a solution of potassium or sodium citrate, or both.

cit·ric ac·id (sit′rik). 2-Hydroxypropane-1,2,3-tricarboxylic acid; the acid of citrus fruits, widely distributed in nature and a key intermediate in intermediary metabolism.

cit·rin (sit′rin). SYN *vitamin* P.

Cit·ro·bac·ter (sit′rō-bak-ter). A genus of motile bacteria (family Enterobacteriaceae) containing Gram-negative rods which use citrate as a source of carbon; the motile cells are peritrichous. Fermentation of lactose by these organisms is delayed or absent; they produce trimethylene glycol from glycerol. The type species is *C. freundii.*

C. amalona′tica, a bacterial species found in feces, soil, water, and sewage; isolated from clinical specimens as an opportunistic pathogen. SYN *Levinea amalonatica.*

C. diver′sus, a bacterial species found in feces, soil, water, sewage, and food; isolated from urine, throat, nose, sputum, and wounds; reported in cases of neonatal meningitis where it frequently is severe, resulting in brain abscess formation. SYN *C. koseri, Levinea diversus, Levinea malonatica.*

C. freun′dii, a bacterial species found in water, feces, and urine; it is an inhabitant of the normal intestine, but it may occur in alimentary infections and in infections of the urinary tract, gallbladder, middle ear, and meninges; it is the type species of the genus *C.*

C. ko′seri, SYN *C. diversus.*

cit·ro·nel·la (sit-rō-nel′ă). *Cymbopogon (Andropogon) nardus* (family Gramineae); a fragrant grass of Ceylon, from which is distilled a volatile oil (c. oil) used as a perfume and insect repellent.

cit·ro·nel·lal (sit′-rō-nel′ăl). Principal volatile ingredient of lemon grass and citronella oil. Used in soap perfumes and as an insect repellent.

ci·trul·line (sit′rul-ēn). N^5-(Aminocarbonyl)-L-ornithine; α-amino-δ-ureidovaleric; 5-ureidonorvaline; an amino acid formed from L-ornithine in the course of the urea cycle as well as a product in nitric oxide biosynthesis; also found in watermelon (*Citrullus vulgaris*) and in casein. Elevated in individuals with a deficiency of argininosuccinate synthetase or argininosuccinate lyase.

cit·rul·li·ne·mia (sit′rul-i-nē′mē-ă) [MIM*215700]. Urea cycle disorder in which citrulline concentrations in the blood, urine, and cerebrospinal fluid are elevated, because of deficiency of argininosuccinate synthetase (ASS); manifested clinically by lethargy, vomiting, ammonia intoxication, and mental retardation with onset usually in infancy; autosomal recessive inheritance, caused by mutation in the ASS gene on chromosome 9 in some patients.

ci

cit·rul·li·nu·ria (sit′rŭl-i-noo′rē-ă). Enhanced urinary excretion of citrulline; a manifestation of citrullinemia.

Civatte, Achille, French dermatologist, 1877-1956. SEE C. *bodies,* under *body; poikiloderma* of C.

Civinini, Filippo, Italian anatomist, 1805–1844. SEE C. *canal, ligament, process.*

CJD Abbreviation for Creutzfeldt-Jakob *disease.*

CK Abbreviation for *creatine* kinase.

Cl Symbol for chlorine.

clad·i·o·sis (klad-ē-ō′sis). A dermatophytosis resembling sporotrichosis, characterized by verrucous lesions and ascending lymphangitis; caused by *Scopulariopsis blochii.* SEE *Scopulariopsis.* [G. *klados,* branch or root, + *-osis,* condition]

Clado, Spiro, French gynecologist, 1856–1905. SEE C. *anastomosis, band, ligament, point.*

Cla·dor·chis wat·soni (kla-dōr′kis wat-sō′nī). Incorrect term for *Watsonius watsoni.*

clad·o·spo·ri·o·sis (klad′ō-spō-rē-ō′sis). Infection with a fungus of the genus *Cladosporium.*

  cerebral c., cerebral phaeohyphomycosis, a mycotic brain infection usually due to *Cladosporium trichoides* (*Xylohypha bantianum*).

Clad·o·spo·ri·um (klad-ō-spōr′i-ŭm). A genus of fungi having dematiaceous or dark-colored conidiophores with oval or round spores, commonly isolated in soil or plant residues. [G. *klados,* a branch, + *sporos,* seed]

  C. carrion′ii, a species of fungi that is a cause of chromoblastomycosis in humans.

  C. cladosporioides, a species reported to cause local infection at the site of a skin test in an HIV-infected patient.

  C. wernec′kii, SYN *Exophiala werneckii.*

  C. (Xylohypha) bantia′num, a species of fungi that causes cerebral cladosporiosis; probably synonymous with *C. trichoides.*

clair·voy·ance (klār-voy′ans). Perception of objective events (past, present, or future) not ordinarily discernible by the senses; a type of extrasensory perception. [Fr.]

clam·ox·y·quin hy·dro·chlo·ride (klam-ok′si-kwin). An amebicide.

■**clamp** (klamp). An instrument for compression or holding a structure. Cf. forceps. [M.E., fr. Middle Dutch *klampe*]

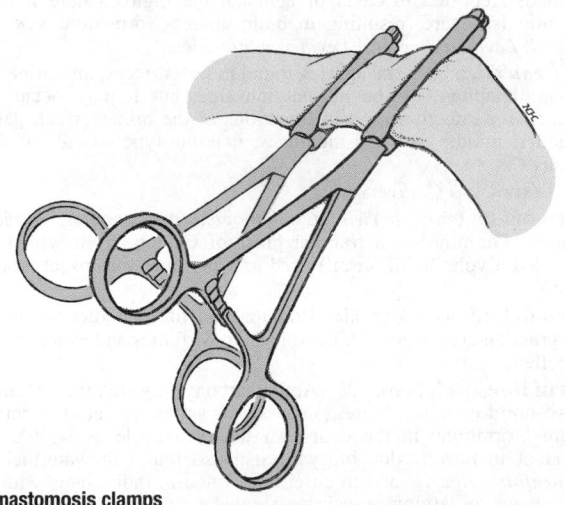

anastomosis clamps

Cope c., a c. used in excision of colon and rectum.

Crafoord c., a c. used in heart, lung, and vascular operations.

Crile c., a c. for temporary stoppage of blood flow.

Fogarty c., a c. with rubber-shod blades having serrated surfaces, to provide an atraumatic grip on tissues.

Gant c., a right-angled c. used in hemorrhoidectomy.

Gaskell c., an instrument for crushing the atrioventricular bundle in experimental animals and thus producing heart block.

gingival c., a springlike metal piece encircling or grasping the cervix of a tooth and shaped so as to retract the gingival tissue.

Kelly c., a curved hemostat without teeth, introduced for gynecological surgery.

Kocher c., a heavy, straight hemostat with interlocking teeth on the tip.

liver-shod c., a c. with jaws covered by cloth to minimize injury to structures such as bowel when c. is closed.

Mikulicz c., a c. used to crush walls between proximal and distal colon in two-stage colectomy.

Mixter c., a right angle c.

Mogen c., a circumcision instrument. [Hebrew star]

mosquito c., a small hemostat, straight or curved, with or without teeth; used to hold delicate tissue or for hemostasis. SYN mosquito forceps.

Ochsner c., a straight hemostat with teeth.

patch c., SYN *patch* clamping.

Payr c., a large, slightly curved c. used in gastrectomy or enterectomy.

Potts c., a fine-toothed, multiple-point, vascular fixation c. that imparts limited trauma to the vessel while securely holding it.

Rankin c., a three-bladed c. used in resection of colon.

right angle c., a c. with a short 90° bend to its tip frequently used for dissection or passage of ligatures around vessels.

rubber dam c., a springlike metal piece encircling or grasping the cervix of a tooth and so shaped as to prevent a rubber dam from coming off the tooth.

rubber-shod c., a small rubber-tipped c. that holds sutures in place during surgery.

clamp con·nec·tion. In fungi, a short hypha which bypasses a hyphal septum and is attached to the two cells adjacent to the septum; characteristic of most members of the phylum Basidiomycetes.

cla·po·tage, cla·pote·ment (kla-pō-tahz′, kla-pōt-mawn′). The splashing sound heard on succussion of a dilated stomach. [Fr.]

Clapton, Edward, English physician, 1830–1909. SEE C. *line.*

Clara, Max, Austrian anatomist, 1899–1966. SEE C. *cell.*

cla·rif·i·cant (kla-rif′i-kant). An agent that makes a turbid liquid clear. [L. *clarus,* clear, + *facio,* to make]

clar·i·fi·ca·tion (klar′i-fi-kā′shŭn). The process of making a turbid liquid clear. SYN lucidification.

Clark, Alonzo, U.S pharmacologist, 1807–1887. SEE C. *weight rule.*

Clark, Eliot R., U.S. anatomist, 1881–1963. SEE Sandison-C. *chamber.*

Clark, Wallace H., Jr., U.S. dermatopathologist, *1924. SEE C. *level.*

Clark, Leland, Jr., U.S. biochemist, *1918. SEE C. *electrode.*

Clarke, Jacob A.L., English anatomist, 1817–1880. SEE C. *column, nucleus.*

Clarke, Cecil. SEE C.-Hadfield *syndrome.*

clas·mat·o·cyte (klaz-mat′ō-sīt). Obsolete term for macrophage. [G. *klasma,* a fragment, + *kytos,* a hollow (cell)]

clas·ma·to·sis (klaz-mă-tō′sis). The extension of pseudopodia-like processes in unicellular organisms and blood cells by plasmolysis rather than by a true formation of pseudopodia. [G. *klasma,* a fragment, + *-osis,* condition]

clasp. 1. A part of a removable partial denture that acts as a direct retainer and/or stabilizer for the denture by partially surrounding or contacting an abutment tooth. 2. A direct retainer of a removable partial denture, usually consisting of two arms joined by a body which connects with an occlusal rest; at least one arm of a clasp usually terminates in the infrabulge (gingival convergence) area of the tooth enclosed.

  bar c., (1) a c. whose arms are bar-type extensions from major connectors or from within the denture base; the arms pass adjacent to the soft tissues and approach the point of contact on the tooth in a gingivo-occlusal direction; (2) a c. consisting of two or more separate arms located opposite to each other on the tooth; the bar arms arise from the framework or from a connector and may traverse the soft tissue; one arm (bar), the retentive arm, usually terminates in the infrabulge (gingival convergence) area of the tooth; the other, the reciprocal arm, usually terminates on the suprabulge (occlusal convergence) area. SYN Roach c.

circumferential c., (1) a c. that encircles more than 180° of a tooth, including opposite angles, and which usually contacts the tooth throughout the extent of the c., at least one terminal being in the infrabulge (gingival convergence) area; **(2)** a c. consisting of two circumferential c. arms, both of which originate from the same minor connector and are located on opposite surfaces of the abutment tooth.

continuous c., SYN continuous bar *retainer.*

extended c., a c. that extends from its minor connector along the lingual and/or facial surface of two or more teeth.

Roach c., SYN bar c.

class (klas). In biologic classification, the next division below the phylum (or subphylum) and above the order. [L. *classis,* a class, division]

clas·si·fi·ca·tion (klas′i-fi-kā′shŭn). A systematic arrangement into classes or groups based on perceived common characteristics; a means of giving order to a group of disconnected facts.

adansonian c., the c. of organisms based on giving equal weight to every character of the organism; this principle has its greatest application in numerical taxonomy. [M. *Adanson*]

▣ Angle c. of malocclusion, a c. of different types of malocclusion, based on the mesiodistal relationship of the permanent molars upon their eruption and locking, and comprised of three classes; *Class I:* normal relationship of the jaws, wherein the mesiobuccal cusp of the maxillary first molar occludes in the buccal groove of the mandibular first permanent molar; *Class II:* distal relationship of the mandible, wherein the distobuccal cusp of the maxillary first permanent molar occludes in the buccal groove of the mandibular first molar, and further classified as Division 1, labioversion of maxillary incisor teeth, and Division 2, linguoversion of maxillary central incisors, both of which may be unilateral conditions; *Class III:* mesial relationship of the mandible, wherein the mesiobuccal cusp of the maxillary first molar occludes in the embrasure between the mandibular first and second permanent molars, further classified as a unilateral condition.

Angle classification of malocclusion	
classes	**anomalies**
I	normal relationship of the jaws; neutroclusion
II	distal relationship of mandible; distoclusion
II div. 1	labioversion of maxillary incisors
div. 2	linguoversion of maxillary incisors
	– "pure class II": distoclusion without anomalies of teeth
	– class II "right" or "left": anomalies of teeth on right or left sides
III	mesial relationship of the mandible; mesioclusion

Arneth c., a c. of the polymorphonuclear neutrophils according to the number of their nuclear lobes. SEE Arneth *stages,* under *stage.*

Astler-Coller c., a staging system that is a modification of Dukes c. for colon cancer.

Bethesda c., SYN Bethesda *system.*

Black c., a c. of cavities of the teeth based upon the tooth surface(s) involved.

Caldwell-Moloy c., a c. of the variations in the female pelvis; namely gynecoid, android, anthropoid, and platypelloid pelvis, based on the type of the posterior and anterior segments of the inlet.

Cummer c., a listing of several types of removable partial dentures in accordance with the distribution of direct retainers.

DeBakey c., consists of three types: Type I extends into the transverse arch and distal aorta and type II is confined to the ascending aorta; type III dissections begin in the descending aor-

ta, with type IIIA extending toward the diaphragm and type IIIB extending below it.

Denver c., a system of nomenclature for human mitotic chromosomes, based on length and position of the centromere. [*Denver,* Colorado, where agreed upon]

Dukes c., a c. of the extent of invasion of a resected adenocarcinoma of the colon or rectum commonly modified as follows: A (Dukes A), confined to the mucosa; B_1, into the muscularis mucosae; B_2, through the muscularis mucosae; C_1, limited to the bowel wall, with nodal metastases; C_2, through the bowel wall, with nodal metastases.

FAB c., French-American-British c. of acute leukemias based on the study of microscopic features and cytochemistry of blast cells; it subdivides acute myelogenous leukemias into 8 groups (M_0–M_7) and acute lymphoblastic leukemias into 3 groups (L_1–L_3); widely used in clinical practice. SYN French-American-British c.

French-American-British c., SYN FAB c.

Gell and Coombs C. (gel koomz), a c. system that differentiates the 4 types of hypersensitivity reactions: Type I: anaphylactic reactions, Type II: cytotoxic reactions, Type III: immune complex reactions, and Type IV: cell-mediated/delayed hypersensitivity reactions.

International Labour Organization C., ILO 1980 International Classification of Radiographs of the Pneumoconioses; a system for qualitative and semiquantitative description of the chest radiographic findings caused by pneumoconiosis, designed for epidemiologic studies; supersedes classifications of 1950, 1958, 1968, and 1971.

Jansky c., the c. of human blood groups now designated O, A, B, and AB.

Kennedy c., a listing of several forms of partially edentulous jaws in accordance with the distribution of the missing teeth.

Kiel c., c. of non-Hodgkin lymphoma into low-grade malignancy (lymphocytic, lymphoplasmacytoid, centrocytic, and centroblastic-centrocytic types) and high-grade malignancy (centroblastic, lymphoblastic of Burkitt or convoluted cell, and immunoblastic types). SYN Lennert c.

Lancefield c., a serologic c. dividing hemolytic streptococci into groups (A to O) which bear a definite relationship to their sources, based upon precipitation tests depending upon group-specific substances that are carbohydrate in nature; e.g., *Group A* contains strains most pathogenic for humans; *B,* strains from mastitis in cows and from normal milk, including strains from the human throat and vagina; *C,* strains from various lower animals, including a number from cattle and the human throat; *D,* strains from cheese and humans; *E,* strains from certified milk; *F,* strains mainly from the human throat, associated with tonsillitis; *G,* strains from humans, a few from monkeys and dogs; and *H, K,* and *O,* nonpathogenic strains occasionally from normal human respiratory tracts.

Lennert c., SYN Kiel c.

Lukes-Collins c., a c. of lymphomas according to the immunologic nature of the cell of origin, based on histologic and clinical data.

multiaxial c., a procedure used in DSM-III-R for diagnosing patients on five axes: 1) psychiatric syndrome present; 2) patient's history of personality and developmental disorders; 3) possible nonmental medical disorders; 4) severity of psychosocial stressors; 5) highest level of adaptive functioning in the past year.

New York Heart Association c., a functional c. to assess cardiovascular disability. Class I: patients with cardiac disease without limitation of physical activity. Ordinary activity does not cause symptoms. Class II: patients with cardiac disease with slight limitation of activity; comfortable at rest. Ordinary physical activity results in fatigue, palpitation, dyspnea or angina. Class III: patients with cardiac disease producing marked limitation of activity: comfortable at rest. Less than ordinary physical activity causes symptoms. Class IV: patients with cardiac disease resulting in inability to carry on any physical activity without discomfort. Symptoms may be present even at rest.

Rappaport c., a histologic c. of lymphomas in use before the availability of recent methods for identification of B- and T-type lymphocytes.

cl

REAL c., a c. of lymphoma first published in 1994 and based on the correlation of clinical features of lymphomas with their histopathology and immunophenotype and genotype of neoplastic cells; groups lymphoproliferative diseases into chronic leukemia/lymphoma, nodal or extranodal lymphoma, acute leukemia lymphoma, plasma cell disorders, and Hodgkin disease. [*R*evised *E*uropean-*A*merican *l*lymphoma classification]

Runyon c., a classification scheme for mycobacteria other than *Mycobacterium tuberculosis* that divides species into four categories: 1) photochromogens, species that produce a yellow to brown carotene pigment when grown in the presence of light; 2) scotochromogens, which produce pigment in presence or absence of light; 3) nonpigmented, which do not produce pigment; and 4) rapid growers, which grow on solid media in 5–10 days rather than 4–8 weeks. This classification has no clinical or genetic significance but remains of limited value in identification of some clinical isolates.

Rye c., c. of Hodgkin disease according to lymphocyte predominance, nodular sclerosing, mixed cellularity, and lymphocyte depletion types. [*Rye*, NY, 1965]

Salter-Harris c. of epiphysial plate injuries, the c. of epiphysial plate injuries into five groups (I to V), according to the pattern of damage to epiphysis, physis, and/or metaphysis; the c. correlates with different prognoses regarding the effects of the injury on subsequent growth and subsequent deformity of the epiphysis.

Tessier c., an anatomical c. of facial, craniofacial, and laterofacial clefts that utilizes the orbit as the primary structure for reference. Fifteen locations for clefts are differentiated.

class switch. Change in the isotype of antibody produced after a B cell has encountered an antigen.

clas·tic (klas′tik). Breaking up into pieces, or exhibiting a tendency so to break or divide. [G. *klastos*, broken]

clas·to·gen (klas′tō-jen). An agent (e.g., certain chemicals, x-rays, ultraviolet light) that causes breaks in chromosomes. [G. *klastos*, broken, + *genos*, birth]

clas·to·gen·ic (klas-tō-jen′ik). Relating to the action of a clastogen.

clath·rate (klath′rāt). A type of inclusion compound in which small molecules are trapped in the cagelike lattice of macromolecules. [L. *clathrare*, pp. *-atus*, to furnish with a lattice]

clath·rin (klath′rin). The principal constituent of a polyhedral protein lattice that coats eukaryotic cell membranes (vesicles) and coated pits and appears to be involved in protein secretion. This protein also occurs in synaptic vesicles. [L. *clathri*, lattice]

Clauberg, Karl W., German bacteriologist, *1893. SEE C. *test, unit.*

Claude, Henri, French psychiatrist, 1869–1945. SEE C. *syndrome.*

clau·di·ca·tion (klaw-di-kā′shŭn). Limping, usually referring to intermittent c. [L. *claudicatio*, fr. *claudico*, to limp]

intermittent c., a condition caused by ischemia of the muscles; characterized by attacks of lameness and pain, brought on by walking, chiefly in the calf muscles; however, the condition may occur in other muscle groups. SYN Charcot syndrome, myasthenia angiosclerotica.

neurogenic c., c. with neurologic injury, usually in association with lumbar spinal stenosis.

clau·di·ca·tory (klaw′di-kă-tōr-ē). Relating to claudication, especially intermittent claudication.

Claudius, Friedrich M., German anatomist, 1822–1869. SEE C. *cells*, under *cell, fossa.*

Clausen. J., Danish physician. SEE Dyggve-Melchior-Clausen *syndrome.*

claus·tra (klaws′tră). Plural of claustrum.

claus·tral (klaws′trăl). Relating to the claustrum.

claus·tro·pho·bia (klaw-strō-fō′bē-ă). A morbid fear of being in a confined place. [L. *claustrum*, an enclosed space, + G. *phobos*, fear]

claus·tro·pho·bic (klaw-strō-fō′bik). Relating to or suffering from claustrophobia.

claus·trum, pl. **claus·tra** (klaws′trŭm, klaws′tră). **1.** One of several anatomic structures bearing a resemblance to a barrier. **2**

[TA]. A thin, vertically placed lamina of gray matter lying close to the putamen, from which it is separated by the external capsule. C. consists of two parts: 1) an insular part and 2) a temporal part between putamen and the temporal lobe. Cells of the c. have reciprocal connections with sensory areas of the cerebral cortex. [L. barrier]

c. gut′turis, c. o′ris, obsolete term for soft *palate.*

c. virgina′le, an obsolete term for hymen.

clau·su·ra (klaw-soo′ră). SYN atresia. [L. a lock, bolt, fr. *claudo*, to close]

cla·va (klā′vă). SYN gracile *tubercle*. [L. a club]

cla·val (klā′văl). Relating to the clava.

cla·vate (klā′vāt). Club-shaped. [L. *clava*, a club]

Clav·i·ceps pur·pu·rea (klav′i-seps poor-poo′rē-ă). SEE ergot. [L. *clava*, club, + *caput*, head]

clav·i·cle (klav′i-kl) [TA]. A doubly curved long bone that forms part of the shoulder girdle. Its medial end articulates with the manubrium sterni at the sternoclavicular joint, its lateral end with the acromion of the scapula at the acromioclavicular joint. SYN clavicula [TA], collar bone.

cla·vic·u·la, pl. **cla·vic·′u·lae** (klă-vik′oo-lă, -lī) [TA]. SYN clavicle. [L. *clavicula*, a small key, fr. *clavis*, key]

cla·vic·u·lar (kla-vik′ū-lăr). Relating to the clavicle.

cla·vic·u·lus, pl. **cla·vic·u·li** (kla-vik′ū-lŭs, -lī). One of the perforating collagen fibers of bone. [Mod. L. dim. of L. *clavus*, nail]

clav·u·lan·ic ac·id (klav-ū-lan′ik). A beta-lactam structurally related to the penicillins that inactivate β-lactamase enzymes in penicillin-resistant organisms; usually used in combination with penicillins to enhance and broaden the spectrum of the penicillins.

cla·vus, pl. **cla·vi** (klā′vŭs, -vī). **1.** A small conical callosity caused by pressure over a bony prominence, usually on a toe. SYN corn. [L. a nail, wart, corn]

claw (klaw). A sharp, slender, usually curved nail on the paw of an animal. [L. *clavus*, a nail]

claw·foot (klaw′fut). A condition of the foot characterized by hyperextension at the metatarsophalangeal joint and flexion at the interphalangeal joints, as a fixed contracture.

claw·hand (klaw′hand). Atrophy of the interosseous muscles of the hand with hyperextension of the metacarpophalangeal joints and flexion of the interphalangeal joints; develops as a result of nerve injury either at the spinal cord or peripheral nerve level.

Claybrook, Edwin B., U.S. surgeon, 1871–1931. SEE C. *sign.*

CLB Abbreviation for cyanobacterialike, coccidialike or *Cryptosporidium*-like organisms that have now been identified as coccidia in the genus *Cyclospora* (C. *cayetanensis*).

clean·ing (klēn′ing). In dentistry, a procedure whereby accretions are removed from the teeth or from a dental prosthesis. SEE ALSO dental *prophylaxis.*

ultrasonic c., in dentistry, the use of a high-frequency vibrating point to remove deposits from tooth structure; also the process of cleaning dentures by placing them in a special liquid in a container that generates high-frequency vibrations.

clear·ance (klēr′ans). **1** (*C* with a subscript indicating the substance removed). Removal of a substance from the blood, e.g., by renal excretion, expressed in terms of the volume flow of arterial blood or plasma that would contain the amount of substance removed per unit of time; measured in mL/min. Renal c. of any substance except urea or free water is calculated as the urine flow in mL/min multiplied by the urinary concentration of the substance divided by the arterial plasma concentration of the substance; normal human values are commonly expressed per 1.73 m^2 body surface area. **2.** A condition in which bodies may pass each other without hindrance, or the distance between bodies. **3.** Removal of something from some place; e.g., "esophageal acid c." refers to removal from the esophagus of some acid that has refluxed into it from the stomach, evaluated by the time taken for restoration of a normal pH in the esophagus.

p-aminohippurate c., a good measure of renal plasma flow, which it slightly underestimates; when a low plasma concentration of *p*-aminohippurate (PAH) is maintained by intravenous infusion, the kidney extracts and excretes almost all of the PAH from the plasma before it reaches the renal vein.

creatinine c., measurement of the clearance of endogenous creatinine, used for evaluating the glomerular filtration rate (GFR).

endogenous creatinine c., a term distinguishing measurements based on the creatinine normally present in plasma; since no infusion is necessary, an average value may be obtained by collecting urine for a long period, e.g., 24 hours.

exogenous creatinine c., a term distinguishing measurements based on infusing creatinine intravenously to raise its plasma concentration and facilitate its accurate chemical determination.

free water c., the amount of water excreted in the urine beyond that which would accompany the excreted solutes if the urine were isosmotic with plasma; it represents the loss of body water in excess of solute tending to raise body osmolality and making urine hyposmotic. Unlike other c.'s, it is calculated by subtracting the osmolal c. from the actual volume of urine excreted per minute. A negative value for free water c. represents the amount of water that the body has reclaimed from isosmotic tubule fluid to make the urine hyperosmotic and to lower body osmolality.

interocclusal c., SYN freeway *space.*

inulin c., an accurate measure of the rate of filtration through the renal glomeruli, because inulin filters freely with water and is neither excreted nor reabsorbed through tubule walls. Inulin is not a normal constituent of plasma and must be infused continuously to maintain a steady plasma concentration and a steady rate of urinary excretion during the measurement. Inulin c. in a normal adult person is about 120 mL/min (range 100–150) per 1.73 m^2 body surface area.

isotope c., the rate at which an isotope is removed (usually by blood flow) from a tissue or organ such as the brain.

maximum urea c., the urea c. when the urine flow exceeds 2 ml/min; normal value is about 75 mL blood/min per 1.73 m^2 body surface area.

mucociliary c., the movement of the mucous covering of the respiratory epithelium by the beating of cilia: rapid, forward (effective) stroke and slow, return (recovery) stroke.

occlusal c., a condition in which the opposing occlusal surfaces may glide over one another without any interfering projection.

osmolal c., the volume of urine that would be excreted per minute if the urinary solutes were accompanied by just enough water to make the urine isosmotic with plasma, i.e., so that the solute excretion did not change the osmolality of body fluids. To calculate it, the volume of urine excreted per minute is multiplied by the urinary osmolality (usually measured by freezing point depression) and divided by the plasma osmolality. Osmolal c. is less than actual urine flow when urine is hyposmotic and exceeds it when urine is hyperosmotic.

standard urea c., the value obtained when the square root of the urine flow (when below 2 mL/min) is multiplied by the urine urea concentration and divided by the whole blood urea concentration; represents an old empirical adjustment for the effect of low urine flow on urea excretion; sometimes corrected for body size by dividing by some function of body weight or surface area. Later, plasma concentration was substituted for blood concentration in the calculation. The normal value is about 54 mL/min per 1.73 m^2 in an adult person. SYN Van Slyke formula.

urea c., the volume of plasma (or blood) that would be completely cleared of urea by one minute's excretion of urine; originally calculated as urine flow multiplied by urine urea concentration divided by concentration of urea in whole blood rather than plasma, representing blood urea c. rather than plasma urea c.

clear·er (klēr'er). An agent, used in histological preparations, which is miscible in both the dehydrating or fixing fluid and the embedding substance.

cleav·age (klēv'ij). **1.** Series of mitotic cell divisions occurring in the ovum immediately following its fertilization. SYN segmentation (2). SEE ALSO cleavage *division.* **2.** Splitting of a complex molecule into two or more simpler molecules. SYN scission (2). **3.** Linear clefts in the skin indicating the direction of the fibers in the dermis. SEE ALSO tension *lines,* under *line.* **4.** Midline depression or furrow between mature female breasts (common).

abnormal c. of cardiac valve, congenital malformation of a valve leaflet with a defect extending from the free margin.

adequal c., c. resulting in the formation of blastomeres of approximately equal size.

complete c., SYN holoblastic c.

determinate c., c. resulting in blastomeres each capable of developing only into a particular embryonic structure.

discoidal c., meroblastic c. limited to the small cap (animal pole) of protoplasm of large-yolked eggs, such as the telolecithal eggs of birds.

enamel c., the splitting of enamel in a plane parallel to the direction of the enamel rods.

equal c., c. producing blastomeres of like size.

equatorial c., c. in which the plane of cytoplasmic division is at right angles to the axis of the ovum.

holoblastic c., c. in which the blastomeres are completely separated; the entire egg participates in cell division. SYN complete c., total c.

hydrolytic c., SYN hydrolysis.

incomplete c., SYN meroblastic c.

indeterminate c., c. resulting in blastomeres of similar developmental potencies, each capable, when isolated, of producing an entire embryonic body.

meridional c., c. in a plane through the axis of the zygote.

meroblastic c., incomplete separation of the blastomeres, with the divisions being limited to the nonyolked portion of the egg. SYN incomplete c.

phosphoroclastic c., SYN phosphorolysis.

progressive c., in fungi, a type of sporulation in which c. planes in the cytoplasm first produce protospores and then sporangiospores in a sporangium.

pudendal c., SYN pudendal *cleft.*

subdural c., SYN subdural *space.*

superficial c., meroblastic c. with the divisions limited to the peripheral (surface) cytoplasm of a centrolecithal egg.

thioclastic c., the splitting of a bond in fashion analogous to hydrolysis or phosphorolysis except that the elements of a substituted hydrogen sulfide (usually coenzyme A) are added across the break.

total c., SYN holoblastic c.

unequal c., c. producing blastomeres of different sizes at the two poles.

yolk c., segmentation of the vitellus.

cleav·er (klē'ver). A heavy knife for cutting or chopping.

enamel c., an instrument with a heavy shank and a very short blade at about 90° to the axis of the handle; used with a hoeing motion to strip enamel from the axial surfaces of a tooth in preparation for a crown.

cleft (kleft) [TA]. A fissure.

anal c., SYN intergluteal c.

branchial c.'s, a bilateral series of slitlike openings into the pharynx through which water is drawn by aquatic animals; in the walls of the c.'s are the vascular gill filaments that take up oxygen from the water passing through the c.'s; sometimes loosely applied to the branchial ectodermal grooves of mammalian embryos, which are imperforate, rudimentary homologues of complete gill c.'s. SYN gill c.'s.

cholesterol c., a space caused by the dissolving out of cholesterol crystals in sections of tissue embedded in paraffin.

complete posterior laryngeal c., SEE laryngotracheoesophageal c.

facial c., a c. resulting from incomplete merging or fusion of embryonic processes normally uniting in the formation of the face, e.g., c. lip or c. palate. SYN prosopoanoschisis.

first visceral c., SYN hyomandibular c.

gill c.'s, SYN branchial c.'s.

gingival c., a fissure associated with pocket formation and lined by mixed gingival and pocket epithelium.

gluteal c., SYN intergluteal c.

hyobranchial c., the c. caudal to the hyoid arch of the embryo.

hyomandibular c., the c. between the hyoid and mandibular arches of the embryo; the external auditory meatus is developed from its dorsal portion. SYN first visceral c.

intergluteal c. [TA], the sulcus between the buttocks (nates). SYN crena analis [TA], crena ani⋆, crena interglutealis⋆, natal c.⋆, anal c., crena clunium, gluteal c.

interneuromeric c.'s, c.'s between the neuromeric or segmental elevations in the primitive rhombencephalon.

Larrey c., SYN *trigonum* sternocostale.

laryngotracheoesophageal c., absence of fusion of the musculature or cricoid cartilaginous laminae of varying severity: type 1, submucous c. of the interarytenoid muscles (known also as occult posterior laryngeal c. or submucous laryngeal c.); type 2, partial cricoid c. (known also as partial posterior laryngeal c.); type 3, total cricoid c. (known also as laryngotracheoesophageal c. or total cricoid c.); and type 4, extension of the c. into the esophagus.

Maurer c.'s, SYN Maurer *dots*, under *dot*.

median maxillary anterior alveolar c., an asymptomatic midline defect of the maxillary anterior ridge; the result of a failure of fusion or development of the lateral halves of the palate.

natal c., ⋆official alternate term for intergluteal c.

oblique facial c., SYN prosoposchisis.

occult posterior laryngeal c., SEE laryngotracheoesophageal c.

partial cricoid c., SEE laryngotracheoesophageal c.

partial posterior laryngeal c., SEE laryngotracheoesophageal c.

posterior laryngeal c., laryngotracheoesophageal cleft (type 2 or 3).

pudendal c. [TA], the cleft between the labia majora. SYN rima pudendi [TA], fissura pudendi, pudendal cleavage, pudendal slit, rima vulvae, urogenital c., vulvar slit.

residual c., the remnants of the pituitary diverticulum that occur between the pars distalis and pars intermedia; a distinct lumen is present in some animals, but, in humans, is present only during prenatal development and sometimes in young children. SYN residual lumen.

Schmidt-Lanterman c.'s, SYN Schmidt-Lanterman *incisures*, under *incisure*.

subdural c., SYN subdural *space*.

submucous laryngeal c., SEE laryngotracheoesophageal c.

synaptic c., the space about 20 nm wide between the axolemma and the postsynaptic surface. SEE ALSO synapse.

total cricoid c., SEE laryngotracheoesophageal c.

urogenital c., SYN pudendal c.

visceral c., any c. between two branchial (visceral) arches in the embryo.

⌂**cleid-.** SEE cleido-.

clei·dag·ra, cli·dag·ra (klī-dag′ră). Rarely used term for a sudden severe pain in the clavicle, resembling gout. [cleid- + G. *agra*, seizure]

clei·dal (klī′dăl). Relating to the clavicle. SYN clidal.

⌂**cleido-, cleid-.** The clavicle; also spelled clido-, clid-. [G. *kleis*, bar, bolt]

clei·do·cos·tal (klī-dō-kos′tăl). Relating to the clavicle and a rib. SYN clidocostal. [cleido- + L. *costa*, rib]

clei·do·cra·ni·al (klī′dō-krā′nē-ăl). Relating to the clavicle and the cranium. SYN clidocranial. [G. *kleis*, clavicle, + *kranion*, cranium]

clei·dot·o·my (klī-dot′ō-mē). Cutting the clavicle of a dead fetus to effect a vaginal delivery. [cleido- + -tomy]

⌂**-cleisis.** Closure. [G. *kleisis*, a closing]

cleis·to·the·ci·um (klīs-tō-thē′sē-ŭm). In fungi, an ascocarp that is closed, with randomly dispersed asci. [G. *kleistos*, enclosed, + *thēkē*, box]

Cleland, W. Wallace, U.S. biochemist, *1930. SEE C. *reagent*.

clem·as·tine (klem′as-tēn). An H₁ antihistaminic. SYN meclastine.

cle·oid (klē′oyd). A dental instrument with a pointed elliptical cutting end, used in excavating cavities or carving fillings and waxes. [A. S. *cle*, claw + G. *eidos*, resemblance]

clep·to·par·a·site (klep-tō-par′ă-sīt). A parasite that develops on the prey of the parasite's host. [G. *kleptō*, to steal, + parasite]

Cléret, M. Francois, French physician, 1876–1968. SEE Launois-C. *syndrome*.

Clevenger, Shobal V., U.S. neurologist, 1843–1920. SEE C. *fissure*.

CLIA Abbreviation for Clinical Laboratory Improvement Amendments.

click (klik). A slight, sharp sound.

ejection c., a clicking ejection sound. SEE sound.

mitral c., the opening snap of the mitral valve.

systolic c., a sharp, clicking sound heard during cardiac systole; when heard in early systole it is usually an ejection sound; in late systole the c. usually signifies mitral insufficiency, as in the dysfunction of the mitral valvular apparatus when it prolapses into the left atrium during systole (see Barlow syndrome); rarely may also be due to pleuropericardial adhesions or other extracardiac mechanisms.

click·ing (klik′ing). A snapping, crepitant noise noted on excursions of the temporomandibular articulation, due to an asynchronous movement of the disk and condyle.

⌂**clid-.** SEE clido-.

cli·dal (klī′dăl). SYN cleidal.

cli·din·i·um bro·mide (klī-din′ē-ŭm). An anticholinergic.

⌂**clido-, clid-.** The clavicle. SEE ALSO cleido-. [G. *kleis*, bar, bolt]

cli·do·cos·tal (klī-dō-kos′tăl). SYN cleidocostal.

cli·do·cra·ni·al (klī-dō-krā′nē-ăl). SYN cleidocranial.

cli·ma·co·pho·bia (klī′mă-kō-fō′bē-ă). Morbid fear of stairs or of climbing. [G. *klimax*, ladder, + *phobos*, fear]

cli·mac·ter·ic (klī-mak′ter-ik, klī-mak-ter′ik). **1.** The period of endocrinal, somatic, and transitory psychologic changes occurring in the transition to menopause. **2.** A critical period of life. SYN climacterium. [G. *klimaktēr*, the rung of a ladder]

cli·mac·ter·i·um (klī-mak-tēr′ē-ŭm). SYN climacteric.

cli·ma·tol·o·gy (klī-mă-tol′ō-jē). The study of climate and its relation to disease.

cli·ma·to·ther·a·py (klī′mă-tō-thār′ă-pē). Treatment of disease by removal of the patient to a region having a climate more favorable for recovery.

cli·max (klī′maks). **1.** The height or acme of a disease; its stage of greatest severity. **2.** SYN orgasm. [G. *klimax*, staircase]

cli·mo·graph (klī′mō-graf). A diagram showing the effect of climate on health. [G. *klima*, climate, + *graphō*, to record]

clin·da·my·cin (klin-dă-mī′sin). An antibacterial and antibiotic.

cline (klīn). A systematic relation between location and the frequencies of alleles; lines connecting points of equal frequency are termed isoclines, and the direction of the c. at any point is at right angles to an isocline. [G. *klinō*, to slope]

clin·ic (klin′ik). **1.** An institution, building, or part of a building where ambulatory patients are cared for. **2.** An institution, building, or part of a building in which medical instruction is given to students by means of demonstrations in the presence of the sick. **3.** A lecture or symposium on a subject relating to disease. [G. *klinē*, bed]

clin·i·cal (klin′i-kl). **1.** Relating to the bedside of a patient or to the course of the disease. **2.** Denoting the symptoms and course of a disease, as distinguished from the laboratory findings of anatomical changes. **3.** Relating to a clinic. [G. *klinē*, bed, + -al]

Clin·i·cal Lab·o·ra·tory Im·prove·ment A·mend·ments (CLIA). Federal legislation, and the personnel and procedures established by it under the aegis of the Health Care Financing Administration (HCFA), for the surveillance and regulation of all clinical laboratory procedures in the U.S.

The Clinical Laboratory Improvement Amendments of 1988 (CLIA '88) were passed by Congress in response to public concerns about the quality of laboratory testing, particularly in physician office laboratories and in Pap smear interpretation. This legislation brought all 150,000 U.S. clinical laboratories, including physician office laboratories, under uniform regulations. A clinical laboratory is defined as any facility where materials derived from the human body are examined for the purpose of providing information for the diagnosis, prevention, or treatment of disease or the assessment of health. Standards applied to laboratory personnel and procedures are based on test complexity and potential harm to the patient. The regulations establish application procedures and fees for CLIA registration, enforcement and surveillance methods, and sanctions applicable when laboratories fail to meet standards. CLIA regulations define three categories of testing complexity: waived, moderate, and high. A subcategory for physician-performed microscopy exists at the moderate complexity level. For tests of moderate or high complexity, the laboratory must participate in a continuing program of proficiency testing whereby an independent laboratory periodically submits specimens of known composition for testing. The imposition and enforcement of CLIA regulations have elicited opposition, particularly from private physicians performing office testing. Opponents of the legislation claim that, while there is little, if any, demonstrable evidence that the CLIA rules have resulted in an improvement in patient care, regulation of office laboratories impedes the ability of physicians to serve their patients' needs. Patients and third-party payers have had to absorb increases in the cost of laboratory testing due to compliance with CLIA regulations. In addition, about one-third of physicians have discontinued some or all office testing as a result of CLIA. This has led to added inconvenience and expense for both patients and physicians. Particularly for children, the poor, and the elderly, the difficulty of arranging repeated visits and of complying with monitoring schedules decreases the quality of overall patient care. Delayed receipt by physicians of laboratory test results diminishes patient compliance, leads to delays or errors in diagnosis, and requires the use of anticipatory treatment, which leads to unnecessary expense and in some cases avoidable hospitalization.

cli·ni·cian (klin-ish′ŭn). A health professional engaged in the care of patients, as distinguished from one working in other areas.

clin·i·co·path·o·log·ic (klin′i-kō-path-ō-loj′ik). Pertaining to the signs and symptoms manifested by a patient, and also the results of laboratory studies, as they relate to the findings in the gross and histologic examination of tissue by means of biopsy or autopsy, or both.

△**clino-.** A slope (inclination or declination) or bend. [G. *klinō*, to slope, incline, or bend]

cli·no·ce·phal·ic, cli·no·ceph·a·lous (klī-nō-se-fal′ik, -sef′ă-lŭs). Relating to clinocephaly.

cli·no·ceph·a·ly (klī′nō-sef′ă-lē). Craniosynostosis in which the upper surface of the skull is concave, presenting a saddle-shaped appearance in profile. SYN saddle head. [clino- + G. *kephalē*, head]

cli·no·dac·ty·ly (klī′nō-dak′ti-lē). Permanent deflection of one or more fingers. [clino- + G. *daktylos*, finger]

cli·nog·ra·phy (klin-og′ră-fē). Graphic representation of the signs and symptoms exhibited by a patient. [G. *klinē*, bed, + *graphō*, to write]

cli·noid (klī′noyd). **1.** Resembling a four-poster bed. **2.** SYN clinoid *process*. [G. *klinē*, bed, + *eidos*, resemblance]

cli·o·quin·ol (klī-ō-kwin′ol). SYN iodochlorhydroxyquin.

cli·ox·a·nide (klī-ok′să-nīd). An anthelmintic.

clip (klip′). **1.** A fastener used to hold a part or thing together with another. **2.** A fastener used to close off a small vessel.

wound c., a metal clasp or device for surgical approximation of skin incisions.

clith·ro·pho·bia (klīth-rō-fō′bē-ă). Morbid fear of being locked in. [G. *kleithron*, a bolt, + *phobos*, fear]

clit·i·on (klit′ē-on). A craniometric point in the middle of the highest part of the clivus on the sphenoid bone. [G. *klitos*, a declivity]

clit·o·rid·e·an (klit′ō-ri-dē′an). Relating to the clitoris.

clit·o·ri·dec·to·my (klit′ō-ri-dek′tō-mē). Removal of the clitoris. [clitoris + G. *ektomē*, excision]

clit·o·ri·di·tis (klit′ō-ri-dī′tis). Inflammation of the clitoris. SYN clitoritis. [clitoris + G. *-itis*, inflammation]

clit·o·ris, pl. **cli·to·ri·des** (klit′ō-ris, -tōr′i-dēz; klī′tō-ris) [TA]. A cylindric, erectile body, rarely exceeding 2 cm in length, situated at the most anterior portion of the vulva and projecting between the branched limbs or laminae of the labia minora, which form its prepuce and frenulum. It consists of a glans, a corpus, and two crura, and is the homolog of the penis in the male, except that it is not perforated by the urethra and does not possess a corpus spongiosum. [G. *kleitoris*]

clit·o·rism (klit′ō-rizm). Prolonged and usually painful erection of the clitoris; the analogue of priapism.

clit·o·ri·tis (klit-ō-rī′tis). SYN clitoriditis.

clit·or·o·meg·a·ly (klit′ōr-ō-meg′ă-lē). An enlarged clitoris. [clitoris + G. *megas*, great]

clit·or·o·plas·ty (klit′ō-rō-plas′tē). Any plastic surgery procedure on the clitoris. [clitoris + G. *plastos*, formed]

cli·val (klī′văl). Pertaining to the clivus.

cli·vus, pl. **cli·vi** (klī′vŭs, -vē) [TA]. **1.** A downward sloping surface. **2** [TA]. The sloping surface from the dorsum sellae to the foramen magnum composed of part of the body of the sphenoid and part of the basal part of the occipital bone. SYN Blumenbach c. [L. slope]

Blumenbach c., SYN clivus (2).

c. ocula′ris, the sloping walls of the fovea leading to the foveola.

clo·a·ca (klō-ā′kă). **1.** In early embryos, the endodermally lined chamber into which the hindgut and allantois empty. **2.** In birds and monotremes, the common chamber into which open the hindgut, bladder, and genital ducts. [L. sewer]

ectodermal c., the proctodeum of the embryo.

endodermal c., terminal portion of the hindgut internal to the cloacal membrane of the embryo.

persistent c., a condition in which the urorectal fold has failed to divide the c. of the embryo into rectal and urogenital portions. SYN sinus urogenitalis, urogenital sinus (2).

clo·a·cal (klō-ā′kăl). Pertaining to the cloaca.

clo·ba·zam (klō-bă-zam). A novel benzodiazepine psychotherapeutic agent in which the nitrogens in the heterocyclic ring are in the 1,5- rather than in the more usual 1,4- positions; an anxiolytic.

clo·be·ta·sol pro·pi·o·nate (klō-bā′tă-sōl). An anti-inflammatory corticosteroid usually used in topical preparations.

clo·cor·to·lone (klō-kōr′tō-lōn). An anti-inflammatory corticosteroid usually used in topical preparations; available as the acetate and the pivalate.

clo·faz·i·mine (klō-faz′ĭ-mēn). A tuberculostatic and leprostatic agent.

clo·fen·a·mide (klō-fen′ă-mid). A diuretic. SYN monochlorphenamide.

clo·fi·brate (klō′fi-brāt). An antilipemic agent that reduces plasma levels of cholesterol, triglycerides, and uric acid; used in the treatment of hypercholesterolemia and atherosclerosis.

clo·ges·tone ac·e·tate (klō-jes′tōn). A progestational agent.

clo·ma·cran phos·phate (klō′mă-kran). A tranquilizer.

clo·me·ges·tone ac·e·tate (klō-me-jes′tōn). A progestational drug.

clo·mi·phene cit·rate (klō′mi-fēn). An analog of the nonsteroid estrogen, chlorotrianisene; a pituitary gonadotropin stimulant used therapeutically to induce ovulation; it competes with estrogen at the hypothalamic level, interrupting the negative feedback system and resulting in increased gonadotropin secretion; use often results in multiple births. SYN chloramiphene.

clo·mip·ra·mine hy·dro·chlo·ride (klō-mip′ră-mēn). An antidepressant.

clo·nal (klō′năl). Pertaining to a clone.

clo·na·ze·pam (klō-nā′zē-pam). An anticonvulsant drug in the benzodiazepine class.

clone (klōn). **1.** A colony or group of organisms (or an individual organism), or a colony of cells derived from a single organism or cell by asexual reproduction, all having identical genetic constitutions. **2.** To produce such a colony or individual. **3.** A short section of DNA that has been copied by means of gene cloning. SEE cloning. **4.** A homogeneous population of DNA molecules. [G. *klōn*, slip, cutting used for propagation]

cDNA c., a duplex DNA, representing an mRNA, carried in a cloning vector.

genomic c., a cell with a vector containing a fragment of DNA from a different organism.

clo·nic (klon'ik). Relating to or characterized by clonus.

clon·ic·i·ty (klon-is'i-tē). The state of being clonic.

clon·i·co·ton·ic (klon'i-kō-ton'ik). Both clonic and tonic; said of certain forms of muscular spasm.

clo·ni·dine hy·dro·chlo·ride (klō'ni-dēn). An antihypertensive agent with central and peripheral actions; it stimulates adrenergic receptors in the brain leading to reduced sympathetic nervous system output; used as an adjunct to lessen drug withdrawal symptoms.

clon·ing (klōn'ing). **1.** Growing a colony of genetically identical cells or organisms in vitro. **2.** Transplantation of a nucleus from a somatic cell to an ovum, which then develops into an embryo; many identical embryos can thus be generated by asexual reproduction. **3.** With blastocysts, dividing a cluster of cells through microsurgery and transferring one-half of the cells to a zona pellucida that has been emptied of its contents. The resulting embryos, genetically identical, may be implanted in an animal for gestation. **4.** A recombinant DNA technique used to produce millions of copies of a DNA fragment. The fragment is spliced into a cloning vehicle (i.e., plasmid, bacteriophage, or animal virus). The cloning vehicle penetrates a bacterial cell or yeast (the host), which is then grown in vitro or in an animal host. In some cases, as in the production of genetically engineered drugs, the inserted DNA becomes activated and alters the chemical functioning of the host cell.

The successful cloning of an apparently normal and fertile sheep has shown the possibilities of the technique, but announcement of a proposal to clone a human being has generated controversy and threats of legal prohibition. Opponents of human cloning object to the experimental creation of human embryos that would never have the opportunity for implantation and whose eventual destruction would be tantamount to abortion. Many bioethics authorities object even to implantation of an artificially created human embryo into a human uterus. Supporters of cloning research fear that legal prohibition will impede needed investigations into human reproduction and infertility. In 1997 the National Bioethics Advisory Commission, after considering the scientific and ethical dimensions of cloning, recommended a 5-year ban on all human cloning research. Nineteen European nations have signed an agreement prohibiting the artificial genetic replication of human beings.

A/T c., cloning of fragments where the only overhanging (or uncomplemented) ends are the A or T bases; occurs often in use of specific enzymes to cut or make DNA fragments.

positional c., SYN reverse *genetics*.

clo·nism (klon'izm). A long continued state of clonic spasms.

clo·no·gen·ic (klō-nō-jen'ik). Arising from or consisting of a clone.

clon·o·graph (klon'ō-graf). An instrument for registering the movements in clonic spasm. [G. *klonos*, tumult, + *graphō*, to write]

clo·nor·chi·a·sis (klō-nōr-kī'ă-sis). A disease caused by the fluke *Clonorchis sinensis*, affecting the distal bile ducts of humans and other fish-eating animals after ingestion of raw, smoked, or undercooked fish or raw crayfish; initial infection may be benign, but repeated or chronic infection induces an intense proliferative and granulomatous condition. SYN clonorchiosis.

clo·nor·chi·o·sis (klō-nōr-kē-ō'sis). SYN clonorchiasis.

Clo·nor·chis si·nen·sis (klō-nōr'kis sī-nen'sis). The Asiatic liver fluke, a species of trematodes (family Opisthorchiidae) that in the Far East infects the bile passages of humans and other fish-eating animals; cyprinoid fish serve as chief second intermediate hosts, and various operculate snails serve as the first intermediate hosts. SYN *Opisthorchis sinensis*.

clo·nus (klō'nŭs). A form of movement marked by contractions and relaxations of a muscle, occurring in rapid succession seen with, among other conditions, spasticity and some seizure disorders. SEE ALSO contraction. [G. *klonos*, a tumult]

ankle c., a rhythmic contraction of the calf muscles following a sudden passive dorsiflexion of the foot, the leg being semiflexed.

toe c., alternating movements of flexion and extension of the great toe following forcible extension at the metatarsophalangeal joint.

wrist c., rhythmical contractions and relaxations of the muscles of the forearm excited by a forcible passive extension of the hand.

clo·pam·ide (klō-pam'īd). A diuretic and antihypertensive agent.

Cloquet, Hippolyte, French anatomist, 1787–1840. SEE C. *space*.

Cloquet, Jules G., French anatomist, 1790–1883. SEE C. *canal*, *hernia*, *septum;* proximal deep inguinal *lymph node*.

clor·az·e·pate (klōr-az'ĕ-pāt). The mono- or dipotassium salt is used as an anti-anxiety agent; a benzodiazepine prodrug for nordiazepam.

clor·pren·a·line hy·dro·chlo·ride (klōr-pren'ă-lēn). A bronchodilator. SYN isoprophenamine hydrochloride.

clos·trid·ia (klos-trid'ē-ă). Plural of clostridium.

clos·trid·i·al (klos-trid'ē-ăl). Relating to any bacterium of the genus *Clostridium*.

clos·trid·i·o·pep·ti·dase A (klos-trid'ē-ō-pep'ti-dās). SYN *Clostridium histolyticum* collagenase.

clos·trid·i·o·pep·ti·dase B. SYN clostripain.

CLOSTRIDIUM

Clos·trid·i·um (klos-trid'ē-ŭm). A genus of anaerobic (or anaerobic, aerotolerant), spore-forming, motile (occasionally nonmotile) bacteria (family Bacillaceae) containing Gram-positive rods; motile cells are peritrichous. Many of the species are saccharolytic and fermentative, producing various acids and gases and variable amounts of neutral products; other species are proteolytic, some attacking proteins with putrefaction or more complete proteolysis. Some species fix free nitrogen. These organisms sometimes produce exotoxins; they are generally found in soil and in the mammalian intestinal tract, where they may cause disease. The type species is *C. butyricum*. [G. *klōstēr*, a spindle]

C. bifermen'tans, a bacterial species found in putrid meat and gaseous gangrene; also commonly found in soil, feces, and sewage. Its pathogenicity (largely due to an edema-producing toxin) varies from strain to strain.

C. botuli'num, a bacterial species that occurs widely in nature and is a frequent cause of food poisoning (botulism) from preserved meats, fruits, or vegetables that have not been properly sterilized before canning. The main types, A to F, are characterized by antigenically distinct, but pharmacologically similar, very potent neurotoxins, each of which can be neutralized only by the specific antitoxin; group C toxin contains at least two components; the recorded cases of human botulism have been due mainly to types A, B, E, and F; infant botulism occurs when colonization of the gastrointestinal tract with *C. botulinum* results in absorption of the toxin through the gastrointestinal wall; type Cα causes botulism in domestic and wild water fowl; Cβ and D are associated with intoxications in cattle. Type E is usually associated with improperly processed fish products.

C. butyr'icum, a bacterial species that occurs in naturally soured milk, in naturally fermented starchy plant substances, and in soil; formerly considered nonpathogenic, it is now known to include neurotoxin-producing strains; the type species of the genus *C*.

C. cadav'eris, a bacterial species found in a human feces and in the pleural fluid of a sheep; it is not pathogenic for guinea pigs or rabbits, but has been a rare cause of gas gangrene in humans.

C. car'nis, a bacterial species found in a rabbit inoculated with soil; it is pathogenic for laboratory animals, in which an exotoxin produces edema, necrosis, and death.

C. chauvoe'i, a bacterial species that causes blackleg, black quarter, or symptomatic anthrax in cattle and other animals and that produces an exotoxin.

C. cochlear'ium, a bacterial species found in human war wounds and septic infections; it is not pathogenic for guinea pigs.

C. difficile (di-fi'-sēl), a bacterial species found in feces of humans and animals. It colonizes newborn infants, who are spared from toxin induced diarrheal disease. Pathogenic for human beings, guinea pigs, and rabbits; frequent cause of colitis and diarrhea following antibiotic use. Found to be a cause of pseudomembranous colitis and associated with a number of intestinal diseases that are linked to antibiotic therapy; also the chief cause of nosocomial diarrhea. [L. difficult]

C. fal'lax, a bacterial species found in war wounds, appendicitis, and black leg of sheep; it produces a weak exotoxin.

C. haemoly'ticum, a bacterial species found in cattle dying of icterohemoglobinuria; it is pathogenic and toxic for guinea pigs and rabbits and produces an unstable, hemolytic toxin.

C. histoly'ticum, a bacterial species found in war wounds, where it induces necrosis of tissue; it produces cytolytic exotoxins that cause local necrosis and sloughing on injection; it is not toxic on feeding; it is pathogenic for small laboratory animals.

C. innomina'tum, a bacterial species found in septic and gangrenous war wounds.

C. nigri'ficans, former name for *Desulfotomaculum nigrificans.*

C. no'vyi, a bacterial species consisting of three types, A, B, and C; type A, from a case of gaseous gangrene and from human necrotic hepatitis, produces γ-toxin (a hemolytic lecithinase); B, from black disease (infectious necrotic hepatitis) of sheep, produces β-toxin (a hemolytic lecithinase); and C, found in bacillary osteomyelitis of water buffaloes, does not produce toxin. SYN *C. oedematiens.*

C. oedema'tiens, SYN *C. novyi.*

C. parabotuli'num, a bacterial species containing formerly referred to as *C. botulinum* types A and B; the types are identified by protection tests with known type antitoxin; it produces a powerful exotoxin and is pathogenic for humans and other animals.

C. paraputri'ficum, a bacterial species found in feces (especially of infants), gaseous gangrene, and postmortem fluid and tissue cultures; it is not pathogenic for rabbits or guinea pigs.

C. perfrin'gens, a bacterial species that is the chief causative agent of gas gangrene in humans and a cause of gas gangrene in other animals, especially sheep; it may also be involved in causing enteritis, appendicitis, and puerperal fever; it is one of the most common causes of food poisoning in the U. S. This organism is found in soil, water, milk, dust, sewage, and the intestinal tract of humans and other animals. SYN *C. welchii,* gas bacillus, Welch bacillus.

C. ramo'sum, a bacterial species found in the natural cavities of humans and other animals as well as in seawater and in feces; it is also found in association with mastoiditis, otitis, pulmonary gangrene, putrid pleurisy, appendicitis, intestinal infections, balanitis, liver abscess, osteomyelitis, septicemia, and urinary infections. It was formerly the type species of the obsolete genus *Ramibacterium.*

C. sep'ticum, a bacterial species found in malignant edema of animals, in human war wounds, and in cases of appendicitis; it is pathogenic for guinea pigs, rabbits, mice, and pigeons and produces an exotoxin that is lethal and hemolytic. SYN *Vibrion septique.*

C. sordellii, a bacterial strain that produces multiple toxins including a lecithinase, hemolysin, and a fibrinolysin, which result in edema and potentially fatal hypotension, and necrotic infections in humans. It is especially associated with abdominal and gynecologic posttraumatic and postoperative wound infection; also causes big head in rams.

C. sphenoi'des, a bacterial species found in gangrenous war wounds; it is not pathogenic for guinea pigs or rabbits.

C. sporo'genes, a bacterial species found in intestinal contents, gaseous gangrene, and soil; it is not pathogenic for guinea pigs or rabbits, but does produce a slight, temporary, local tumefaction.

C. ter'tium, a bacterial species found in wounds, but that is nonpathogenic for laboratory animals.

C. tet'ani, the bacterial species that causes tetanus; it produces a potent exotoxin (neurotoxin) that is intensely toxic for humans and other animals when formed in tissues or injected, but not when ingested.

C. thermosaccharoly'ticum, a bacterial species of thermophilic bacteria found in "hard swell" of canned goods; it is not pathogenic to laboratory animals.

C. welch'ii, SYN *C. perfringens.*

clos·trid·i·um, pl. **clos·trid·ia** (klos-trid'ē-ŭm, -ă). A vernacular term used to refer to any member of the genus *Clostridium.*

Clos·trid·i·um his·to·lyt·i·cum **col·la·gen·ase.** An enzyme that catalyzes the hydrolysis of collagen, preferentially at peptide bonds on the amino side of a glycylprolyl sequence. SYN clostridiopeptidase A, collagenase A, collagenase I, microbial collagenase.

Clos·trid·i·um his·to·lyt·i·cum **pro·tein·ase B.** SYN clostripain.

clos·tri·pain (klos'tri-pān). A cysteine proteinase cleaving preferentially at the carboxyl side of arginyl and lysyl residues. It also has an esterase activity. SYN clostridiopeptidase B, *Clostridium histolyticum* proteinase B.

clo·sure (klō'zhŭr). **1.** The completion of a reflex pathway. **2.** The place of coupling between stimuli in the establishment of conditioned learning. **3.** To achieve or experience a sense of completion in a mental task.

flask c., in dentistry, the procedure of bringing the two halves or parts of a flask together; trial flask c.'s are preliminary c.'s made to eliminate excess denture-base material and to ensure that the mold is completely filled; the final flask c. is the last c. of a flask before curing, following trial packing of the mold with denture-base material.

velopharyngeal c., the apposition of the velum (soft palate) and the upper pharyngeal walls as in deglutition and in some speech sounds.

clo·sy·late (klō'si-lāt). USAN-approved contraction for *p*-chlorobenzenesulfonate.

clot (klot). **1.** To coagulate, said especially of blood. **2.** A soft, nonrigid, insoluble mass formed when a liquid (e.g., blood or lymph) gels. [O.E. *klott,* lump]

agonal c., intravascular thrombosis ascribed to the process of dying.

antemortem c., a blood c., found at autopsy, formed in any of the heart cavities or the great vessels before death.

blood c., the coagulated phase of blood; the soft, coherent, jelly-like red mass resulting from the conversion of fibrinogen to fibrin, thereby entrapping the red blood cells (and other formed elements) within the coagulated plasma.

chicken fat c., c. formed in vitro or postmortem from leukocytes and plasma of sedimented blood.

currant jelly c., a jellylike mass of red blood cells and fibrin formed by the in vitro or postmortem clotting of whole or sedimented blood.

laminated c., a c. formed in a succession of layers such as occurs in the natural course of an aneurysm.

passive c., a c. formed in an aneurysmal sac consequent to the cessation or slowing of circulation through the aneurysm.

postmortem c., a c. formed in the heart or great vessels after death.

clo·trim·a·zole (klō-trim'ă-zōl). An antifungal agent used topically to treat a variety of fungal and yeast infections.

clot·tage (klot'ij). Obsolete term for blocking of any canal or duct by a blood clot.

Cloudman, Arthur M., U.S. zoologist and pathologist, *1901. SEE *C. melanoma.*

clove oil (klōv). SYN *oil of clove.*

clox·a·cil·lin so·di·um (klok-să-sil'in). A penicillinase-resistant penicillin.

clo·za·pine (klō'ză-pēn). A sedative and antipsychotic tricyclic dibenzodiazepine regarded as atypical because of low central antidopaminergic activity.

CLQ Abbreviation for cognitive laterality *quotient*.

club·bing (klŭb'ing). A condition affecting the fingers and toes in which proliferation of distal soft tissues, especially the nail beds, results in thickening and widening of the extremities of the digits; the nails are abnormally curved nail beds excessively compressible, and skin over them red and shiny. SEE Hippocratic *nails*, under *nail*.

   hereditary c. [MIM*119900], simple hereditary c. of the digits without associated pulmonary or other progressive disease, often more severe in males; most common in black patients; autosomal dominant inheritance. SYN acropachy.

club·foot (klŭb'fut). SYN *talipes* equinovarus.

club·hand (klŭb'hand). Congenital or acquired angulation deformity of the hand associated with partial or complete absence of radius or ulna; usually with intrinsic deformities in the hand in congenital variants.

   radial c., c. with angular deviation toward radial side of limb associated with partial or complete absence of the radius.

   ulnar c., c. with angular deviation toward ulnar side of limb associated with partial or complete absence of the ulna.

clump (klŭmp). To form into clusters, small aggregations, or groups. [A.S. *clympre,* a lump]

clump·ing (klŭmp-ing). The massing together of bacteria or other cells suspended in a fluid.

clu·ne·al (kloo'nē-ăl). Pertaining to the clunes.

clu·nes (kloo'nēz). ⋆official alternate term for buttocks. [pl. of L. *clunis,* buttock]

clu·pan·o·don·ic ac·id (kloo-pan'ō-don'ik). An ω-3 fatty acid with 22 carbons and five double bonds; found in fish oils and phospholipids in brain.

CLUSTER OF DIFFERENTIATION

---

cluster of differentiation. Cell membrane molecules that are used to classify leukocytes into subsets. CD molecules are classified by monoclonal antibodies. There are four general types: type I transmembrane proteins have their COOH-termini in the cytoplasm and their NH2-termini outside the cell; type II transmem-

brane proteins have their NH2-termini in the cytoplasm and their COOH-termini outside the cell; type III transmembrane proteins cross the plasma membrane more than once and hence may form transmembrane channels; and glycosylphosphatidylinositol-anchored proteins (type IV), which are tethered to the lipid bilayer via a glycosylphosphatidylinositol anchor.

CD1a, a type I transmembrane protein found on thymocytes, Langerhans cell, brain astrocytes, and dermal cells that is involved in nonclassical antigen presentation or is a receptor for an undefined ligand or hormone; expressed in patients with T-cell acute lymphoblastic leukemia, histiocytosis X, and thymomas.

CD1b, a type I transmembrane protein found on cortical thymocytes, dermal cells, and brain astrocytes that is involved in nonclassical antigen presentation or is a receptor for an undefined ligand or hormone; expressed in patients with T-cell acute lymphoblastic leukemia, T-cell lymphoma, and thymomas.

CD1c, a type I transmembrane protein found on cortical thymocytes, dermal cells, and brain astrocytes that is involved in nonclassical antigen presentation or is a receptor for an undefined ligand or hormone; expressed in patients with T-cell acute lymphoblastic leukemia, B-cell chronic lymphocytic leukemias, and B cells in severe combined immunodeficiency disease.

CD2, a type I transmembrane protein found on thymocytes, T cells, and some natural killer cells that acts as a ligand for CD58 and CD59 and is involved in signal transduction and cell adhesion; expressed in T-cell acute lymphoblastic leukemia and T-cell lymphoma.

CD2r, a type I transmembrane protein found on T cells and some natural killer cells that is unrelated to binding sites for CD58 and CD59; expressed on activated T cells in autoimmune diseases.

CD3, a type I transmembrane protein found on T cells that forms the signal transduction unit for the T cell; expressed in patients with T-cell lymphomas.

CD4, a type I transmembrane protein found on helper/inducer T cells, monocytes, macrophages, and dendritic cells that is involved in T-cell recognition of antigens; expressed in mycosis fungoides, Sézary syndrome, and T-cell lymphomas.

CD5, a type I transmembrane protein found on T cells, thymocytes, and some B cells that is a ligand for CD72 and is involved in cellular activation or adhesion; expressed in B-cell chronic lymphocytic leukemia and T-cell lymphoma.

CD6, a type I transmembrane protein found on T cells, medullary thymocytes, some cortical thymocytes, a few B cells, and in brain. CD6 is phosphorylated on cellular activation and possibly plays a role in signal transduction; expressed in some B-cell chronic lymphocytic leukemias.

CD7, a type I transmembrane protein found on thymocytes, some T cells, monocytes, natural killer cells, and hemopoietic stem cells; expressed in patients with mycosis fungoides, some patients

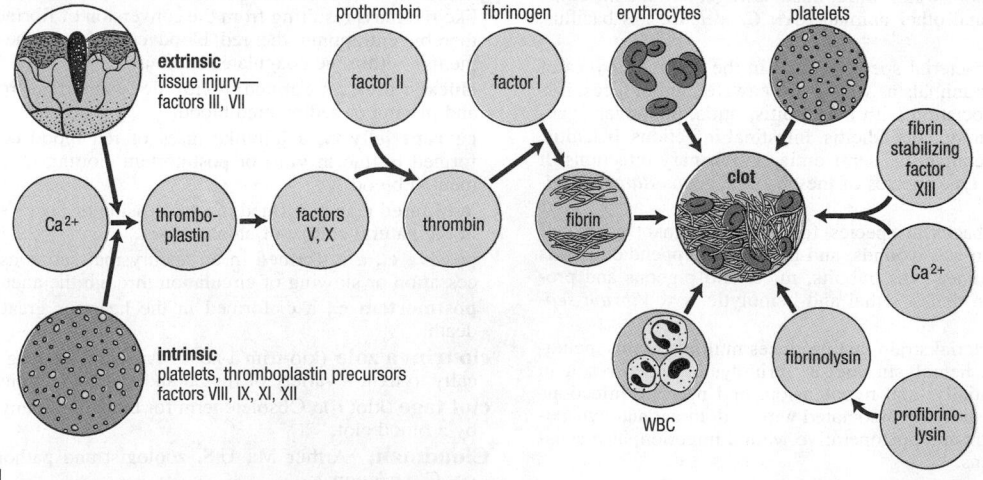

blood clotting

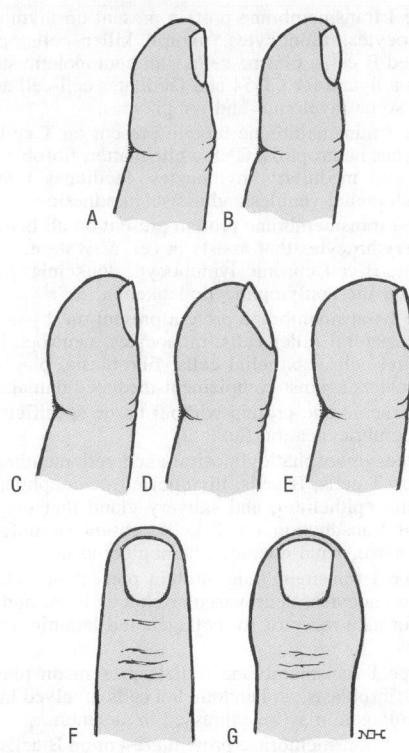

varieties of digital clubbing: (A) normal, (B) increased curvature of nail, (C) mild clubbing, (D) parrot's beak type, (E) watch glass type, (F) normal, (G) drumstick type

with T-cell acute lymphoblastic lymphoma, and a few patients with acute nonlymphocytic lymphoma.

CD8, a type I transmembrane protein found on suppressor (cytotoxic) T cells, some natural killer cells, and most thymocytes that is involved in T-cell antigen recognition; expressed in some T-cell lymphomas and large granular lymphocyte leukemias.

CD9, a type III transmembrane protein found on platelets, megakaryocytes, monocytes, pre-B cells, eosinophils, basophils, and activated T cells; plays a role in signal transduction leading to platelet activation and aggregation; expressed in some T-cell acute lymphocytic leukemias and some acute nonlymphocytic leukemias.

CD10, a type II transmembrane protein found on pre-B cells, germinal-center B cells, some neutrophils, kidney cells, T-cell precursors, and epithelial cells that acts as a zinc metalloprotease cleaving peptide bonds on the amino side of hydrophobic amino acids; expressed in acute lymphocytic leukemia and follicular-center–cell lymphomas.

CD11a, a type I transmembrane protein found on lymphocytes, neutrophils, monocytes, and macrophages that facilitates cell adhesion and cell activation; expressed in lymphomas.

CD11b, a type I transmembrane protein found on monocytes, macrophages, granulocytes, some B cells, dendritic cells, and natural killer cells that facilitates cell adhesion, phagocytosis, and/or chemotaxis; expressed in some B-cell chronic lymphocytic leukemias, most acute nonlymphocytic leukemias, and some hairy cell leukemias.

CD11c, a type I transmembrane protein found on monocytes, macrophages, neutrophils, and some B cells that induces cellular activation and helps trigger neutrophil respiratory burst; expressed in hairy cell leukemias, acute nonlymphocytic leukemias, and some B-cell chronic lymphocytic leukemias.

CDw12, a membrane protein found on monocytes, neutrophils, and platelets; the function of this moiety is unknown.

CD13, a type II transmembrane protein found on myeloid cells that acts as a zinc-binding metalloprotease catalyzing removal of NH2-terminal amino acids from peptides; expressed in some types of acute nonlymphocytic leukemia.

CD14, a transmembrane protein found on monocytes, macrophages, neutrophils, some B cells, and dendritic cells that is involved in signal transduction leading to oxidative burst and/or synthesis of tumor necrosis factor-α; expressed in some patients with acute nonlymphocytic leukemia and in B-cell chronic lymphocytic leukemia.

CD15, a phosphatidylinositol-anchored transmembrane protein found on neutrophils and which may be involved in phagocytosis; expressed in patients with Hodgkin disease, some B-cell chronic lymphocytic leukemias, acute lymphoblastic leukemias, and most acute nonlymphocytic leukemias.

CD15s, a transmembrane protein found on neutrophils, monocytes, myeloid cells, and some T cells that serves as the major ligand for CD62E; expressed on squamous cell carcinomas.

CD16, a type I transmembrane protein found on natural killer cells and macrophages that is involved in directing NK cell activation.

CD16b, a glycosylphosphatidylinositol-anchored protein present on neutrophils; deficient in patients with paroxysmal nocturnal hemoglobinemia and expressed in large granular lymphocytic leukemias and natural killer cell leukemias.

CDw17, a type I transmembrane protein found on monocytes, neutrophils, and platelets that may play a role in granule content packaging or exocytosis.

CD18, a type I transmembrane protein found on lymphocytes, neutrophils, monocytes, macrophages, some B cells, dendritic cells, and natural killer cells that appears active in signal transduction; expressed in some patients with B-cell chronic lymphocytic leukemia, most acute nonlymphocytic leukemia, and some hairy cell leukemia.

CD19, a type I transmembrane protein found on all B cells and B-cell precursors and some follicular dendritic cells that acts as an accessory molecule for B cell signal transduction; expressed in all B-cell neoplasms.

CD20, a type III transmembrane protein found on B cells that forms a calcium channel in the cell wall allowing for the influx of calcium required for cell activation; expressed in B-cell lymphomas, hairy cell leukemia, and B-cell chronic lymphocytic leukemia.

CD21, a type I transmembrane protein found on B cells, follicular dendritic cells, pharyngeal and cervical epithelial cells, some thymocytes, and some T cells that plays a role in signal transduction; expressed in hairy cell leukemia, B-cell lymphoma, and some T-cell acute lymphocytic leukemias.

CD22, a type I transmembrane protein found in the cytoplasm of pre-B cells and on the surface of mature B cells that facilitates signal transduction; expressed in patients with hairy cell leukemias and in some with B-cell lymphomas.

CD22α, a type I transmembrane protein found on mature B cells that facilitates adhesion of B cells to monocytes and red blood cells.

CD22β, a type I transmembrane protein found on mature B cells that facilitates adhesion of B cells to CD4-positive T cells.

CD23, a type II transmembrane protein found on mature B cells, monocytes, activated macrophages, eosinophils, platelets, and dendritic cells that enhances capture and processing of antigen complexed with IgE.

CD24, a glycosylphosphatidylinositol-anchored protein present on B cells, pre-B cells, neutrophils, and a few thymocytes that may play a role in inducing B-cell proliferation and differentiation; expressed in patients with B-cell lymphomas and some with B-cell chronic lymphocytic leukemias.

CD25, a type I transmembrane protein present on activated T cells, activated B cells, some thymocytes, myeloid precursors, and oligodendrocytes that associates with CD122 to form a heterodimer that can act as a high-affinity receptor for IL-2; expressed in most B-cell neoplasms, some acute nonlymphocytic leukemias, and neuroblastomas.

CD26, a type II transmembrane protein present on mature T cells, some B cells, apical membranes of epithelial and endothelial cells, kidney, intestinal brush borders, and liver bile canaliculi that combines with collagen and associates with adenosine deaminase.

CD27, a type I transmembrane protein present on mature T cells, medullary thymocytes, and some B cells that is a ligand for CD70 and serves as a member of the nerve growth factor family; expressed in chronic lymphocytic leukemia.

CD28, a type I transmembrane protein present on most CD4 T cells, many CD8 T cells, and most plasma cells that enhances the transcription and stability of IL-2 messenger RNA.

CD29, a type I transmembrane protein present on some CD4 helper T cells, platelets, and dendritic cells that is involved in cell-cell or cell-matrix adhesion.

CD30, a type I transmembrane protein present on activated T and B cells that may play a role in cell activation and/or differentiation; expressed in Hodgkin disease, some T-cell lymphomas, and anaplastic large cell lymphomas.

CD30l, a type III transmembrane protein present on activated T cells and monocytes that can induce differential responses in CD30-expressing cells ranging from growth to cell death.

CD31, a type I transmembrane protein present on myeloid cells, platelets, endothelial cells, natural killer cells, monocytes, and subsets of CD4-positive T cells that acts as a cosignal transducer for macrophages, inducing respiratory burst; plays a key role in the transmigration of leukocytes through intercellular junctions of vascular endothelium and mediates calcium-dependent heterophilic aggregation; expressed in neoplastic endothelial cells.

CD32, a type I transmembrane protein present on monocytes, B cells, neutrophils, placental trophoblasts, and endothelium; acts as a signal transducer for IgG-mediated phagocytosis and neutrophil and monocyte oxidative burst; transduces an inhibitory signal on B cells and may play a role in placental IgG transport.

CD33, a type I transmembrane protein present on myeloid cells and myeloid precursors; expressed in many acute nonlymphoblastic leukemias and some B-cell chronic lymphocytic leukemias.

CD34, a type I transmembrane protein present on myeloid cells and myeloid precursors that plays a role in signal transduction; expressed in some acute nonlymphocytic leukemias and some acute lymphocytic leukemias.

CD35, a type I transmembrane protein present on monocytes, granulocytes, dendritic cells, red blood cells, some T cells, and glomerular podocytes that facilitates phagocytosis and/or binding of immune complexes; expressed in Wilms tumor.

CD36, a transmembrane protein present on monocytes, platelets, megakaryocytes, umbilical vein, small-vessel endothelium, reticulocytes, and mammary epithelium that may be involved in signal transduction; expressed in myeloproliferative disorders.

CD37, a type III transmembrane protein present on mature B cells, some T cells, and monocytes that may play a role in ion transport; expressed on B-cell lymphomas, B-cell chronic lymphocytic leukemia, and hairy cell leukemia.

CD38, a transmembrane protein present on macrophages, dendritic cells, and activated cells of the natural killer, B- and T-cell lines that can facilitate B-cell adhesion.

CD39, a transmembrane protein present on macrophages, dendritic cells, and activated lymphoid cells that facilitates B-cell adhesion.

CD40, a type I transmembrane protein present on mature B cells, monocytes, dendritic cells, and epithelial cells involved in signal transduction leading to cell activation, proliferation, adhesion, and/or differentiation; expressed in B-cell chronic lymphocytic leukemias, lymphomas, and some carcinomas.

CD40l, a type II transmembrane protein present on activated CD4-positive T cells, a few activated CD8-activated T cells, and blood basophils; a ligand for CD40 that induces activation, proliferation, and/or differentiation of CD40-expressing cells.

CD41, a type I transmembrane protein present on platelets and megakaryocytes that serves as a receptor for fibrinogen, fibronectin, vitronectin, von Willebrand factor, and other factors and facilitates platelet adhesion and aggregation.

CD42, a type I transmembrane protein present on platelets and megakaryocytes that mediates platelet binding to damaged blood vessels.

CD43, a type I transmembrane protein present on thymocytes, T cells, granulocytes, monocytes, natural killer cells, platelets, brain, activated B cells, plasma cells, and hemopoietic stem cells that serves as a ligand for CD54 and facilitates cell-cell adhesion; expressed on some myelomas and lymphomas.

CD44, a type I transmembrane protein present on T cells, pre-B cells, monocytes, neutrophils, CNS white matter, fibroblasts, skeletal muscle, and medullary thymocytes; facilitates lymphocyte binding to endothelial venules and assists in adhesion.

CD45, a type I transmembrane protein present on all hemopoietic cells except erythrocytes that assists in cell activation; expressed in lymphomas, B-cell chronic lymphocytic leukemia, hairy cell leukemia, and acute nonlymphocytic leukemia.

CD46, a type I transmembrane protein present on thymocytes, T cells, B cells, natural killer cells, monocytes, neutrophils, platelets, endothelial cells, epithelial cells, fibroblasts, placenta, and sperm that protects against complement-mediated damage.

CD47, a transmembrane protein without tissue specificity that is involved in membrane cation flux.

CD48, a glycosylphosphatidylinositol-anchored membrane protein present on T cells, B cells, thymocytes, eosinophils, neutrophils, bronchial epithelium, and salivary gland that may play a role in signal transduction on T cells; absent or defective in patients with paroxysmal nocturnal hemoglobinuria.

CD49a, a type I transmembrane protein present on activated T and B cells, monocytes, neurovascular endothelium, and smooth muscle that forms a receptor for collagen and laminin; expressed on melanomas.

CD49b, a type I transmembrane protein present on platelets, T cells, B cells, fibroblasts, and endothelial cells involved in platelet adhesion of collagen; may be expressed in melanomas.

CD49c, a type I transmembrane protein present on B cells, kidney glomerulus, thyroid, and some basement membranes that may play a role in cell-cell adhesion; expressed in most cultured cell lines.

CD49d, a type I transmembrane protein present on B and T cells, natural killer cells, eosinophils, monocytes, erythroblasts, thymocytes, and myoblasts that facilitates cell-cell adhesion and leukocyte migration and aids in lymphocyte activation; expressed in melanomas.

CD49e, a type I transmembrane protein present on monocytes, neutrophils, leukocytes, fibroblasts, platelets, and myoblasts that helps form a receptor for fibronectin and activates the sodium-hydrogen antiporter; may serve an accessory role to T-cell activation.

CD49f, a type I transmembrane protein present on platelets, macrophages, monocytes, thymocytes, T cells, and adherent cell lines that forms a receptor for invasion and laminin; expressed in some acute lymphocytic leukemias.

CD50, a type I transmembrane protein present on thymocytes, B cells, monocytes, and neutrophils; involved in intracellular adhesion.

CD51, a type I transmembrane protein present on endothelial cells, monocytes, macrophages, platelets, some B cells, osteoclasts, and uterine cells; plays a role in platelet aggregation and/or endothelial cell adhesion and in monocyte migration.

CD52, a glycosylphosphatidylinositol-anchored membrane protein present on thymocytes, T cells, B cells, some granulocytes, seminal vesicles, epididymis, and spermatozoa; plays a role in signal transduction.

CD53, a type III transmembrane protein present on leukocytes, platelets, osteoblasts, and osteoclasts; contributes to the transduction of CD2-generated signals in T cells and natural killer cells; facilitates cytoplasmic calcium flux in B cells, monocytes, and granulocytes; and plays a role in activation of the monocyte oxidative burst; expressed in hemopoietic neoplasms and myelomas.

CD54, a type I transmembrane protein present on leukocytes and endothelial cells and inducible on lymphocytes, dendritic cells, keratinocytes, chondrocytes, fibroblasts, and epithelial cells; acts as a ligand for CD11 and CD18 and aids in intercellular adhesion.

CD55, a glycosylphosphatidylinositol-anchored membrane protein present on all hemopoietic cells and spermatozoa that neutralizes complement activation; absent or defective in paroxysmal nocturnal hemoglobinuria.

CD57, a membrane protein present on natural killer cells, some T cells, a few B cells, and monocytes of unknown function; expressed in large granular lymphocyte leukemias.

CD58, a membrane protein present on many hemopoietic cells and fibroblasts that acts as a ligand for CD2 and may be involved in T-cell function.

CD59, a glycosylphosphatidylinositol-anchored membrane protein present on many hemopoietic cells, vascular endothelium, epithelial cells, and placenta that inhibits membrane complement attack and may be involved in T-cell signal transduction; absent or defective in paroxysmal nocturnal hemoglobinuria.

CDw60, a membrane protein present on T-cell subsets, some monocytes, and platelets that may play a role in signal transduction leading to cell activation; present on cutaneous T-cell lymphomas.

CD61, a membrane protein present on platelets, megakaryocytes, endothelial cells, osteoclasts, and uterine cells that facilitates platelet aggregation and adhesion.

CD62e, a type I transmembrane protein present on endothelium that facilitates adhesion of neutrophils, monocytes, and some T cells to vascular endothelium; enhanced expression occurs at sites of chronic inflammation.

CD62l, a type I transmembrane protein present on B cells, T cells, neutrophils, thymocytes, monocytes, eosinophils, erythroid and myeloid progenitor cells, and natural killer cells that functions as a peripheral lymph node homing receptor and facilitates binding to endothelium at inflammatory sites; found on many malignant leukocytes.

CD62p, a type I transmembrane protein present on activated platelets, endothelial cells, and megakaryocytes that facilitates adhesion of monocytes and neutrophils to activated platelets and to endothelial cells.

CD63, a type III transmembrane protein present on activated platelets, monocytes, macrophages, and in secretory granules of vascular endothelial cells and platelet-dense granules; facilitates adhesion to activated endothelium.

CD64, a type I transmembrane protein present on monocytes, megakaryocytes, and activated neutrophils that acts as a high-affinity receptor for IgG; present in some cases of acute nonlymphocytic leukemia.

CDw65, a membrane protein present on myeloid cells and some monocytic cells that is involved in signal transduction leading to formation of the respiratory burst; present in some acute nonlymphocyte leukemias.

CD66a, a type I transmembrane protein, present on neutrophils, histiocytes, some myeloid progenitor cells, and the brush border of colonic epithelial cells, that facilitates adhesion and neutrophilic activation; expressed in chronic myelocytic leukemia and some cases of acute lymphocytic leukemia.

CD66b, a glycosylphosphatidylinositol-anchored membrane protein present on neutrophils that induces aggregation and activation; expressed in chronic myelocytic leukemia.

CD66c, a glycosylphosphatidylinositol-anchored membrane protein present on neutrophils that induces aggregation and activation; expressed in chronic myelocytic leukemia.

CD66d, a type I transmembrane protein present on neutrophils that facilitates adhesion and neutrophil activation; expressed in chronic myelocytic leukemia.

CD66e, a glycosylphosphatidylinositol-anchored membrane protein present in tissues derived from all three germ layers during embryogenesis and adult colon epithelial cells that facilitates calcium-independent adhesion during embryogenesis; expressed in most colon carcinomas and other carcinomas.

CD68, a type I transmembrane protein present on monocytes, macrophages, osteoclasts, mast cells, cytoplasmic granules, activated platelets, and large lymphocytes; expressed in neuroma Schwann cells, in nerves undergoing wallerian degeneration, in myeloid cell tumors, and in anaplastic lymphomas and epithelial tumors.

CD69, a type II transmembrane protein present on platelets, CD4-positive or CD8-positive thymocytes, activated lymphocytes, and activated T or natural killer cells that functions as a signal transducer, enhancing cell activation and/or platelet aggregation.

CD70, a type II transmembrane protein present on activated B cells and some activated T cells that enhances activation of T cells; expressed in Reed-Sternberg cells, some lymphomas, and monocyte lineage–derived tumors.

CD71, a type II transmembrane protein present on activated or proliferating cells that facilitates cellular iron uptake; expressed in many acute leukemias and some lymphomas.

CD72, a type II transmembrane protein present on all B cells and macrophages that plays a role in signal transduction or adhesion; expressed in B-cell acute lymphoblastic leukemia, B-cell lymphomas, and B-cell chronic lymphocytic leukemia.

CD73, a glycosylphosphatidylinositol-anchored membrane protein present on some B cells, some T cells, thymocytes, some epithelial and endothelial cells, and dendritic cells; expressed on most B-cell acute lymphoblastic leukemias, breast carcinomas, and large granular leukocyte leukemias.

CD74, a type II transmembrane protein present on B cells, monocytes, dendritic cells, and activated T cells that prevents binding of endogenous peptides; expressed in B-cell chronic lymphocytic leukemia, hairy cell leukemia, and large granular leukocyte lymphomas.

CDw75, a type II transmembrane protein present on mature B cells and some T cells that may facilitate B-cell adhesion; expressed in B-cell lymphomas of follicular cell origin.

CDw76, a membrane protein present on mature B cells, some T cells, melanocytes, endothelial cells, hepatocytes, and kidney tubular cells; expressed in mature B-cell lymphomas and B-cell chronic lymphocytic leukemias.

CD77, a membrane protein present on germinal center B cells, follicular dendritic cells, endothelium, and some epithelial cells which may act as a receptor for toxins of *Escherichia coli* or *Shigella dysenteriae;* expressed in Burkitt lymphomas and B-cell lymphomas of follicular center cell origin.

CDw78, a membrane protein present on B-cells and tissue macrophages that may be involved in signal transduction; expressed in some acute lymphoblastic leukemias, B-cell lymphomas, and some acute nonlymphocytic leukemias.

CD79a, a type I transmembrane protein present on B cells that mediates signal transduction; expressed in mature B-cell neoplasms.

CD79b, a type I transmembrane protein on B cells that mediates signal transduction; expressed in B-cell tumors and B-cell acute leukoblastic leukemias.

CD80, a type I transmembrane protein on activated B cells, activated monocytes, activated follicular dendritic cells, and some activated T cells that provide a costimulatory signal to T cells during antigen presentation; expressed in B lymphoblastoid cells.

CD81, a type III transmembrane protein present on many cell types, including lymphocytes, that facilitates signal transduction; expressed on lymphomas, leukemias, melanomas, and neuroblastomas.

CD82, a type III transmembrane protein present on epithelial cells, endothelium, and activated lymphocytes that may play a role in calcium flux.

CD83, a type I transmembrane protein, present on dendritic cells, Langerhans cells, B cells, and interdigitating reticular cells, that may play a role in antigen presentation or the cellular interactions that follow lymphocyte activation.

CDw84, a membrane protein present on monocytes, early B cells, platelets, germinal-center B cells, mantle-zone B cells, and circulating lymphocytes.

CD85, a membrane protein present on plasma cells, B cells, and monocytes.

CD86, a membrane protein present on some germinal-center B cells, mitogen-activated B cells, and monocytes that serves as a B-cell activator; expressed in anaplastic large cell lymphomas, on Reed-Sternberg cells, and on Epstein Barr virus–transformed B cells.

CD87, a glycosylphosphatidylinositol-anchored membrane protein present on activated T cells, monocytes, and activated neutrophils that plays a role in cell-surface plasminogen activation; expressed on macrophages at sites of inflammation.

CD88, a type III transmembrane protein present on neutrophils, macrophages, eosinophils, mast cells, and smooth muscle cells that helps trigger chemotaxis and aids in cellular activation, respiratory burst, and degranulation; expressed in monocytoid tumors.

CD89, a type I transmembrane protein present on neutrophils, monocytes, macrophages, and some T and B cells that assists in triggering granulocyte respiratory burst; expressed in monocytoid tumors.

CDw90, a glycosylphosphatidylinositol-anchored membrane protein of unknown function present on prothymocytes and in brain and other nonlymphoid tissues.

CD91, a membrane protein on monocytes and macrophages that may facilitate endocytosis.

CDw92, a membrane protein present on neutrophils, platelets, and monocytes; of unknown function.

CD93, a membrane protein present on neutrophils, monocytes, and endothelial cells; of unknown function.

CD94, a membrane protein expressed on natural killer cells and a few T cells that stimulates natural killer cell cytolysis and release of tumor necrosis factor.

CD95, a type I transmembrane protein present on T cells and myeloid cells that may induce apoptosis.

CD96, a type I transmembrane protein present on T cells, natural killer cells, and activated B cells that is expressed primarily upon cellular activation, suggesting ligand-binding activity.

CD97, a membrane protein of unknown function present on monocytes and mature granulocytes.

CD98, a type II transmembrane protein present on monocytes, cardiac muscle cells, endothelial cells, T cells, B cells, and natural killer cells; probably involved in regulating calcium fluxes; increased on T cells in some autoimmune disease or in chronic hepatitis.

CD99, a type I transmembrane protein present on thymocytes, lymphocytes, and myeloid cells involved in rosette formations with sheep erythrocytes.

CD99r, a type I transmembrane protein similar to CD99 but present on myeloid cells.

CD100, a membrane protein present on hemopoietic cells that can induce proliferative responses.

CDw101, a membrane protein of unknown function present on neutrophils, monocytes, and some T cells.

CD102, a type I transmembrane protein present on endothelial cells, platelets, monocytes, dendritic cells, subsets of lymphocytes, and in splenic sinusoids that may facilitate recirculation of memory T cells.

CD103, a type I transmembrane protein present on intestinal intraepithelial lymphocytes, some circulating leukocytes, and some T cells that facilitates adhesion to epithelia; expressed in hairy cell leukemia and some B-cell chronic lymphocytic leukemias.

CD104, a type I transmembrane protein present on epithelia and thymocytes that facilitates adhesion of cells to the extracellular matrix; expressed in squamous cell carcinoma.

CD105, a type II transmembrane protein present on endothelium, proerythroblasts, activated monocytes and macrophages, and follicular dendritic cells that may play a role in adhesion; expressed in leukemic cells of B-lymphoid and myeloid origin.

CD106, a type I transmembrane protein present on activated endothelial cells, macrophages, dendritic cells, marrow stroma, myoblasts, and myotubules that facilitates recruitment of leukocytes to sites of inflammation.

CD107a, a type I transmembrane protein present on activated platelets; increased expression noted on transformation of cells with metastatic potential and on embryonic cells.

CD107b, a type I transmembrane protein present on activated platelets; increased expression noted on transformation of cells with metastatic potential and on embryonic cells.

CDw108, a glycosylphosphatidylinositol-anchored protein of unknown function present on activated T cells.

CDw109, a glycosylphosphatidylinositol-anchored membrane protein of unknown function present on activated T cells, activated platelets, and endothelial cells.

CD115, a type I transmembrane protein present on placenta, macrophages, monocytes, and monocyte-precursors that is involved in proliferation and differentiation of monocytes and their progenitors; expressed in choriocarcinomas.

CDw116, a type I transmembrane protein present on monocytes, granulocytes, endothelial cells, dendritic cells, and fibroblasts that stimulates cell proliferation and differentiation; expressed in osteogenic sarcoma and breast and lung carcinomas.

CD117, a type I transmembrane protein present on hemopoietic progenitors, mast cells, melanocytes, spermatogonia, oocytes, and some natural killer cells that assists in signal transduction to transfected cell lines; expressed in colon carcinomas.

CD120a, a type I transmembrane protein present on many cell types that has a high affinity for tumor necrosis factors.

CD120b, a type I transmembrane protein present on many cell types that has a high affinity for tumor necrosis factors.

CDw121a, a type I transmembrane protein present on T cells, thymocytes, chondrocytes, synovial cells, endothelial cells, fibroblasts, keratinocytes, and hepatocytes that aids in stimulation of cellular proliferation and/or activation.

CDw121b, a type I transmembrane protein present on B cells, monocytes, and macrophages that is involved in interaction with interleukins.

CDw122, a type I transmembrane protein present on activated T cells, B cells, monocytes, and natural killer cells that may complex with CD25.

CD123, a type I transmembrane protein present on pluripotent stem cells and committed hemopoietic progenitor cells that is involved in cell proliferation and/or differentiation.

CDw124, a type I transmembrane protein present on mature B cells, T cells, epithelium, hemopoietic precursors, and fibroblasts that induces cell proliferation and/or activation; expressed in lymphomas and pancreatic, hepatic, and bladder tumors.

CD125, a type I transmembrane protein present on eosinophils and basophils that stimulates cellular proliferation and/or differentiation.

CD126, a type I transmembrane protein present on plasma cells, leukocytes, epithelial cells, fibroblasts, neural cells, and hepatocytes that stimulates cell growth and/or differentiation; possible growth factor for myelomas.

CDw127, a type I transmembrane protein present on B-cell precursors, thymocytes, mature T cells, and monocytes that induces cell growth and/or differentiation.

CDw128, a type III transmembrane protein present on neutrophils, basophils, monocytes, keratinocytes, and some T cells that induces chemotaxis and/or cell activation; expressed on melanoma cells.

CD129, a type I transmembrane protein present on some T cells, myeloid and erythroid precursors, and mast cells that induces cell growth and/or differentiation; expressed in Hodgkin disease, large cell lymphomas, and megakaryoblastic leukemia.

CDw130, a type I transmembrane protein present on most leukocytes, epithelial cells, fibroblasts, hepatocytes, and neural cells; interacts with leukemia inhibitor factors, interleukins, and other cell-proliferative factors.

---

clut·ter·ing (klŭt′er-ing). A speech disorder usually occurring in childhood characterized by abnormally rapid rate, disturbed fluency, erratic rhythm, and poor articulation that makes it difficult to understand the speaker.

Clutton, Henry H., British surgeon, 1850–1909. SEE C. *joints,* under *joint.*

cly·sis (klī′sis). **1.** An infusion of fluid, usually subcutaneously, for therapeutic purposes. **2.** Formerly, a fluid enema; later, the washing out of material from any body space or cavity by fluids. [G. *klysis,* a drenching by a clyster]

△**-clysis.** Combining form referring to injection or enema. [G. *klysis,* a drenching by a clyster]

clys·ter (klis′ter). An old term for enema. [G. *klystēr*, fr. *klyzō*, fut. *klysō*, to wash out]

C.M. Abbreviation for *Chirurgiae Magister*, Master in Surgery.

△**CM-** Symbol for carboxymethyl radical.

Cm Symbol for curium.

cM Abbreviation for centimorgan.

cm Abbreviation for centimeter; cm² for square centimeter; cm³ for cubic *centimeter*.

CMA Abbreviation for Certified Medical Assistant.

p-**CMB** Abbreviation for *p*-chloromercuribenzoate.

cmc Abbreviation for critical micelle *concentration*.

CM-cel·lu·lose. SYN carboxymethyl *cellulose*.

CMG Abbreviation for cystometrogram.

CMI Abbreviation for cell-mediated *immunity*.

CML 1. Abbreviation for cell-mediated lymphocytotoxicity. **2.** Acronym for chronic myelogenous *leukemia*.

CMO Abbreviation for calculated mean *organism*.

CMP Symbol for cytidine 5′-monophosphate (secondarily, for any cytidine monophosphate).

c-mp1. A cell-surface receptor on megakaryocytes, platelets, and CD34-positive hematopoietic precursor cells; appears to be the receptor for regulation of megakaryocytopoiesis and platelet production.

CMT Abbreviation for Certified Medical Transcriptionist. SEE medical transcriptionist.

CMV 1. Abbreviation for controlled mechanical *ventilation*; Cytomegalovirus. **2.** A cancer drug combination treatment consisting of cisplatin, methotrexate, and vinblastine, used in the treatment of bladder and other malignancies.

cne·mi·al (ne′mē-ăl). Relating to the leg, especially to the shin. [G. *knēmē*, leg]

cne·mis (nē′mis). The shin. [G. *knēmis* (*knēmid*-), a legging]

cni·da, pl. **cni·dae** (nī′dă, nī′dē). SYN nematocyst. [G. *knidē*, nettle]

cni·do·cyst (nī′dō-sist). SYN nematocyst.

Cnid·o·spora (nī-dō-spōr′ă). SYN Microspora. [G. *knidē*, nettle, sea nettle, + *sporos*, seed]

Cni·do·spo·rid·ia (nī′dō-spō-rid′ēă). SYN Microsporida. [G. *knidē*, nettle, sea nettle, + Mod. L., fr. G. *sporos*, seed]

C.N.M. Abbreviation for certified nurse-midwife.

CNS 1. Abbreviation for central nervous *system*. **2.** Symbol for the thiocyanate radical, CNS⁻ or –CNS.

CO Symbol for *carbon* monoxide.

Co Symbol for cobalt; coccygeal.

⁵⁷Co Symbol for cobalt-57.

⁶⁰Co Symbol for cobalt-60.

⁵⁸Co Symbol for cobalt-58.

△**co-.** SEE con-.

CoA Abbreviation for coenzyme A.

co·ac·er·vate (kō-as′er-vāt). An aggregate of colloidal particles separated out of an emulsion (coacervation) by the addition of some third component (coacervating agent). [L. *coacervare*, pp. *-atus*, to collect in a mass]

co·ac·er·va·tion (kō-as-er-vā′shŭn). Formation of a coacervate.

co·ad·ap·ta·tion (kō′ad-ap-tā′shŭn). The operation of selection jointly on two or more loci.

co·ag·glu·ti·nation (kō-ă-gloo′tin-a′shun). Aggregation of particulate antigens bound with agglutinins of more than one specificity.

co·ag·u·la (kō-ag′ū-lă). Plural of coagulum.

co·ag·u·la·ble (kō-ag′ū-lă-bl). Capable of being coagulated or clotted.

co·ag·u·lant (kō-ag′ū-lant). **1.** An agent that causes, stimulates, or accelerates coagulation, especially with reference to blood. **2.** SYN coagulative.

co·ag·u·late (kō-ag′ū-lāt). **1.** To convert a fluid or a substance in

solution into a solid or gel. **2.** To clot; to curdle; to change from a liquid to a solid or gel. [L. *coagulo*, pp. *-atus*, to curdle]

co·ag·u·la·tion (kō-ag-ū-lā′shŭn). **1.** Clotting; the process of changing from a liquid to a solid, said especially of blood (i.e., blood c.). In vertebrates, blood c. is a result of cascade regulation from fibrin. **2.** A clot or coagulum. **3.** Transformation of a sol into a gel or semisolid mass; e.g., the c. of the white of an egg by means of boiling. In any colloidal suspension, the dispersion of the disperse phase from the continuous phase is greatly reduced, thereby leading to a complete or partial separation of the latter; usually an irreversible phenomenon unless the basic nature of the substance is chemically altered.

disseminated intravascular c. (DIC), a hemorrhagic syndrome that occurs following the uncontrolled activation of clotting factors and fibrinolytic enzymes throughout small blood vessels; fibrin is deposited, platelets and clotting factors are consumed, and fibrin degradation products inhibit fibrin polymerization, resulting in tissue necrosis and bleeding. SEE ALSO consumption *coagulopathy*.

co·ag·u·la·tive (kō-ag′ū-lă-tiv). Causing coagulation. SYN coagulant (2).

▣**co·ag·u·lop·a·thy** (kō-ag-ū-lop′ă-thē). A disease affecting the coagulability of the blood.

coagulopathy	
some of the most important causes of consumption coagulopathy (often used as a synonym for disseminated intravascular coagulation)	
acute	**subacute/chronic**
abruptio placentae	septic abortion
amniotic fluid embolism	toxemia of pregnancy
hemolytic transfusion reaction	carcinoma (lung, prostate)
Waterhouse-Friderichsen syndrome	Kasabach-Merritt syndrome
Gram-negative sepsis	dead fetus syndrome
heat stroke	acute hemorrhagic pancreatitis
snake bite	acute leukemia
acute promyelocytic leukemia	decompensated cirrhosis of liver
shock	
purpura fulminans	

consumption c., a disorder in which marked reductions develop in blood concentrations of platelets with exhaustion of the coagulation factors in the peripheral blood; often used as a synonym for disseminated intravascular coagulation.

co·ag·u·lum, pl. **co·ag·u·la** (kō-ag′ū-lŭm, -lă). A clot or a curd; a soft, nonrigid, insoluble mass formed when a sol. undergoes coagulation. [L. a means of coagulating, rennet]

co-alcoholic (kō-al-kō-hol′ik). **1.** The person(s) who enables an alcoholic by assuming responsibilities on the alcoholic's behalf, minimizing or denying the problem drinking, or making amends for the alcoholic's behavior. **2.** Pertaining to the co-alcoholic or to co-alcoholism. SEE ALSO splinting.

co-alcoholism (kō-al′kō-hol-izm). The constellation of attitudes, attributes, and behaviors of the person who enables the alcoholic, which are necessary for the attainment of a symbiotic balance between alcoholic and co-alcoholic. SEE ALSO symbiosis.

co·a·les·cence (kō-ă-les′ens). Fusion of originally separate parts. SYN concrescence (1).

coal oil (kōl). SYN petroleum.

coal tar. A by-product obtained during the destructive distillation of bituminous coal; a very dark semisolid of characteristic naphthalenelike odor and a sharp, burning taste; used in the treatment of skin diseases.

co·apt (kō′apt). To join or fit together.

co·ap·ta·tion (kō-ap-tā′shŭn). Joining or fitting together of two surfaces; e.g., the lips of a wound or the ends of a broken bone. [L. *co-apto*, pp. *-aptatus*, to fit together]

co·arct (kō-arkt′). To restrict or press together. SYN coarctate (1). [L. *co-arcto*, pp. *-arctatus*, to press together]

co·arc·tate (kō-ark′tāt). **1.** SYN coarct. **2.** Pressed together.

co·arc·ta·tion (kō-ark-tā′shŭn). A constriction, stricture, or stenosis.

aortic c., congenital narrowing of the aorta, usually located just distal to the left subclavian *artery*, causing upper-extremity hypertension, excess left ventricular workload, and diminished blood flow to the lower extremities and abdominal viscera.

reversed c., aortic arch syndrome in which blood pressure in the arms is lower than in the legs.

co·arc·tec·to·my (kō′ark-tek′tō-mē). Excision of a coarctation (of the aorta).

co·arc·tot·o·my (kō-ark-tot′ō-mē). Division of a stricture. [coarct + G. *tomē*, cutting]

CoAS–, CoASH Symbols for the coenzyme A radical and reduced coenzyme A, respectively.

coat (kōt). **1.** The outer covering or envelope of an organ or part. **2.** One of the layers of membranous or other tissues forming the wall of a canal or hollow organ. SEE tunic.

buffy c., the upper, lighter portion of the blood clot (coagulated plasma and white blood cells), occurring when coagulation is delayed so that the red blood cells have had time to settle; the portion of centrifuged, anticoagulated blood which contains leukocytes and platelets. SYN crusta inflammatoria, crusta phlogistica, leukocyte cream.

muscular c., ☆official alternate term for muscular *layer*.

muscular c. of bronchi, ☆official alternate term for muscular *layer* of bronchi.

muscular c. of colon, ☆official alternate term for muscular *layer* of colon.

muscular c. of ductus deferens, ☆official alternate term for muscular *layer* of ductus deferens.

muscular c. of esophagus, ☆official alternate term for muscular *layer* of esophagus.

muscular c. of female urethra, ☆official alternate term for muscular *layer* of female urethra.

muscular c. of gallbladder, ☆official alternate term for muscular *layer* of gallbladder.

muscular c. of intermediate part of male urethra, ☆official alternate term for muscular *layer* of intermediate part of (male) urethra.

muscular c. of intermediate part of male urethra, ☆official alternate term for muscular *layer* of prostatic urethra.

muscular c. of large intestine, ☆official alternate term for muscular *layer* of large intestine.

muscular c. of male urethra, SYN muscular *layer* of male urethra.

muscular c. of pharynx, ☆official alternate term for muscular *layer* of pharynx.

muscular c. of prostatic urethra, SYN muscular *layer* of prostatic urethra.

muscular c. of rectum, ☆official alternate term for muscular *layer* of rectum.

muscular c. of small intestine, ☆official alternate term for muscular *layer* of small intestine.

muscular c. of spongy part of male urethra, ☆official alternate term for muscular *layer* of spongy (male) urethra.

muscular c. of stomach, ☆official alternate term for muscular *layer* of stomach; SEE ALSO oblique *fibers* of muscular layer of stomach, under *fiber*.

muscular c. of trachea, ☆official alternate term for muscular *layer* of trachea.

muscular c. of ureter, ☆official alternate term for muscular *layer* of ureter.

muscular c. of urinary bladder, ☆official alternate term for muscular *layer* of urinary bladder.

muscular c. of uterine tube, ☆official alternate term for muscular *layer* of uterine tube.

muscular c. of uterus, SYN myometrium.

muscular c. of vagina, ☆official alternate term for muscular *layer* of vagina.

sclerotic c., SYN sclera.

serous c., ☆official alternate term for serosa.

serous c. of peritoneum, ☆official alternate term for *serosa* of peritoneum.

coat·ing (kōt′ing). A covering; a layer of some substance spread over a surface.

antireflection c., a film of magnesium fluoride spread on a lens to minimize reflections.

CoA trans·fer·as·es [EC 2.8.3.x]. Thiaphorases; enzymes transferring CoA from acetyl-CoA or succinyl-CoA to other acyl radicals.

Coats, George, British ophthalmologist, 1876–1915. SEE C. *disease*.

co·bal·a·min (Cbl) (kō-bal′ă-min). General term for compounds containing the dimethylbenzimidazolylcobamide nucleus of vitamin B_{12}.

ATP c. adenoxyltransferase, an enzyme that catalyzes the reaction of ATP, water, and cobalamin to form orthophosphate, pyrophosphate, and adenoxylcobalamin. Adenosylcobalamin is required by methylmalonyl-CoA mutase. A deficiency of ATP c. adenosyltransferase will lead to methylmalonic acidemia.

c. concentrate, the dried, partially purified product resulting from the growth of selected *Streptomyces* cultures or other cobalamin-producing microorganisms; contains at least 500 μg of c. in each gram.

co·balt (Co) (kō′bawlt). A steel-gray metallic element, atomic no. 27, atomic wt. 58.93320; a bioelement and a constituent of vitamin B_{12}; certain of its compounds are pigments, e.g., c. blue. [Ger. *kobalt*, goblin or evil spirit]

co·balt-57 (^{57}Co). Half-life, 271.8 days; decays by electron capture with emission of a medium energy (122.06 keV) gamma ray. Used as a diagnostic aid with some metabolic disorders.

co·balt-58 (^{58}Co). Positron emitter with half-life of 70.88 days.

co·balt-60 (^{60}Co). Half-life, 5.271 years; emits beta particles and energetic gamma rays, for which reason it is used in radiation teletherapy and diagnostics in place of radium (radon) or x-rays. It is also used as a diagnostic aid in vitamin B_{12}-related problems.

co·bal·tous chlo·ride (kō-bawl′tŭs). Used in the treatment of various types of refractory anemia to improve the hematocrit, hemoglobin, and erythrocyte count.

Cobb, Stanley, U.S. neuropathologist, 1887–1968. SEE C. *syndrome*.

co·bra (kō′bră). Most cobras are members of the highly venomous snake genus, *Naja* (family Elapidae); six species are recognized, all African except for the Asiatic c.; typical behavior includes spreading of the neck (hood), rearing one-third of the body off of the ground, and, in some species, the spitting of venom, which is primarily neurotoxic. There are also cobras that belong to the genera *Pseudohaje, Hemachatus,* and *Ophiophagus*. [Port. snake, from L. *coluber,* snake]

co·bro·tox·in (kō′brō-tok-sin). A polypeptide of 62 residues; action on cells is similar to that of melittin in that it promotes disruption of membranes; used as an investigational antirheumatic agent. SYN cobra toxin, direct lytic factor of cobra venom.

co·byr·ic ac·id (kō-bir′ik). The hexa-amide of cobyrinic acid; a part of the vitamin B_{12} structure. SYN cobyrinamide, factor V_{1a}.

co·byr·in·a·mide (kō-bir-in′ă-mīd). SYN cobyric acid.

co·byr·in·ic ac·id (kō-bir-in′ik). Corrin with 8 methyl groups at positions 1, 2, 5, 7, 12 (2), 15, and 17; $-CH_2COOH$ groups at positions 2, 7, and 18; $-CH_2CH_2COOH$ groups at positions 3, 8, 13, and 17; and divalent cobalt centered among the four nitrogens. The acid side chains are designated, in numeric order, *a, b, c, d, e, f,* and *g*. It is a part of the vitamin B_{12} structure.

COC Abbreviation for cathodal opening *contraction*.

co·ca (kō′kă). The dried leaves of *Erythroxylon coca*, yielding not less than 0.5% of ether-soluble alkaloids; the source of cocaine and several other alkaloids. [S. Am.]

co·caine (kō-kān′). $C_{17}H_{21}NO_4$; Benzoylmethylecgonine; a crystalline alkaloid obtained from the leaves of *Erythroxylon coca* (family Erythroxylaceae) and other species of *Erythroxylon*, or by synthesis from ecgonine or its derivatives; a potent central nervous system stimulant, vasoconstrictor, and topical anesthetic, widely abused as a euphoriant and associated with the risk of severe adverse physical and mental effects.

The coca bush is indigenous to Bolivia and Peru, where for centuries natives have chewed its leaves along with limestone pellets or plant ashes in order to withstand hunger, thirst, and fatigue. During the 19th century cocaine was widely used in medicine as a stimulant, antidepressant, and topical anesthetic, but because of its strong potential for inducing dependency it is no longer administered systemically. Its popularity as a recreational drug waned slightly after amphetamines became available in the 1920s but returned in the 1960s. Cocaine is generally sold on the street as the hydrochloride salt, a fine white powder known as "coke," "C," "snow," "flake," or "blow." Street dealers cut or adulterate it with inert substances such as cornstarch, talcum powder, and sugar, or with active drugs such as procaine and benzocaine. In powder form it is usually "snorted" into the nostrils, although it may also be absorbed through the buccal, vaginal, or rectal mucosa or injected. A smokable form of cocaine can be prepared from the hydrochloride by a process called "free-basing." Production of pure free-base cocaine is hazardous because it employs highly flammable solvents. The drug commonly called "crack" is a crude form of free base prepared from cocaine hydrochloride with ammonia or sodium bicarbonate and water. The hardened product of this process is cracked into irregular fragments called "rock," "ready rock," "french fries," or "teeth." Street use of crack exploded upon its introduction in the 1980s, causing increases in emergency department admissions for cocaine overdose, drug-related deaths, and births of cocaine-dependent babies.

Administration of cocaine quickly produces intense euphoria, accompanied by a sense of increased energy, alertness, and self-confidence and diminished need for food and sleep. Pulse, blood pressure, and respiratory rate are increased. Higher doses can lead to bizarre or violent behavior, paranoia, chest pain, tremors, seizures, coma, and death due to coronary artery spasm or respiratory arrest. Smoked crack cocaine reaches the brain more quickly than snorted cocaine. The effects of either form wear off in less than 30 minutes, to be succeeded by profound depression, irritability, and fatigue ("coke crash"). Prolonged use of cocaine leads to chronic symptoms including restlessness, irritability, depression, insomnia, and a reversible psychosis characterized by paranoia, hallucinations, and delusions. Repeated snorting of cocaine causes rhinitis, which can culminate in perforation of the nasal septum. Cocaine is not truly addictive because tolerance does not develop; in fact, some regular users note increasing sensitivity to its physical and psychologic effects. But psychological dependency can develop in less than 2 weeks. Withdrawal is associated with intense craving for another dose; sustained abstinence may lead to anxiety, depression, and disorders of appetite and sleep.

----

crack c., a derivative of cocaine, usually smoked, resulting in a brief, intense high. C. is relatively inexpensive and extremely addictive. SEE street *drug.*

c. hydrochloride, a water-soluble salt used for local anesthesia of the eye or mucous membranes.

co·cain·i·za·tion (kō′kăn-i-zā′shŭn). Production of topical anesthesia of mucous membranes by the application of cocaine.

co·car·box·yl·ase (kō-kar-boks′i-lās). SYN *thiamin* pyrophosphate.

co·car·cin·o·gen (kō-kar′si-nō-jen). A substance that works symbiotically with a carcinogen in the production of cancer.

Coc·ca·ce·ae (kok-kā′sē-ē). An obsolete term for a family of Eubacteriales which included all the spherical cells dividing in one (*Streptococcus*), two (*Micrococcus*), or three (*Sarcina*) planes, then forming cells, pairs, tetrads, cubes or larger packets, or chains. [G. *kokkos,* a berry]

coc·cal (kok′ăl). Relating to cocci.

coc·ci (kok′sī). Plural of coccus.

Coc·cid·i·a (kok-sid′ē-ă). A subclass of important protozoa (class Sporozoea, phylum Apicomplexa) in which the mature trophozoites are small and typically intracellular; schizogony and sporogony can occur in the same host, in contrast to the gregarines (subclass Gregarinia of class Sporozoea), which have large extracellular trophozoites in various invertebrates and do not reproduce by schizogony. SYN Coccidiasina. [Mod. L., fr. G. *kokkos,* berry]

coc·cid·ia (kok-sid′ē-ă). Plural of coccidium.

coc·cid·i·al (kok-sid′ē-ăl). Relating to coccidia.

Coc·ci·di·as·i·na (kok-sid′ē-ā-sī′nă). SYN Coccidia.

coc·cid·i·oi·dal (kok-sid-ē-oy′dăl). Referring to the disease or to the infecting organism of coccidioidomycosis.

Coc·cid·i·oi·des (kok-sid-ē-oy′dēz). A genus of fungi found in the soil of the semi-arid areas of the Southwestern U.S. and smaller areas throughout Central and South America, but has not been found elsewhere. The only pathogenic species, *C. immitis,* causes coccidioidomycosis. [coccidium + G. *eidos,* resemblance]

coc·cid·i·oi·din (kok-sid-ē-oy′din). A sterile solution containing the by-products of growth of *Coccidioides immitis;* used as an intracutaneous skin test, diagnostically more valuable in nonendemic areas.

coc·cid·i·oi·do·ma (kok-sid′ē-oy-dō′mă). A benign localized residual granulomatous lesion or scar in a lung following primary coccidioidomycosis.

coc·cid·i·oi·do·my·co·sis (kok-sid-ē-oy′dō-mī-kō′sis). A variable, benign, severe, or sometimes fatal systemic mycosis due to inhalation of arthroconidia of *Coccidioides immitis.* In benign forms of the infection, the lesions are limited to the upper respiratory tract, lungs, and near lymph nodes; in a low percentage of cases, the disease disseminates to other visceral organs, meninges, bones, joints, and skin and subcutaneous tissues. SYN Posadas disease. [coccidioides + G. *mykēs,* fungus, + *-osis,* condition]

disseminated c., a severe, chronic, and progressive form of c. with spread from the lung to other organs. Patients with this disease are usually significantly immunocompromised.

primary c., a disease common in the San Joaquin Valley of California and certain additional areas in the southwestern U.S. as well as the Chaco region of Argentina, caused by inhalation of the arthroconidia of *Coccidioides immitis;* acute onset of respiratory symptoms accompanied by fever, aches, malaise, arthralgia, headache, and occasionally an early erythematous or papular eruption; erythema multiforme or erythema nodosum may appear. SYN desert fever, San Joaquin fever, San Joaquin Valley disease, San Joaquin Valley fever, valley fever.

primary extrapulmonary c., a rare form of c. presenting near the site of local trauma with painless firm nodules occurring at one to two weeks, accompanied by regional adenopathy, with spontaneous healing in a few weeks.

secondary c., progressive or disseminated extrapulmonary granulomatous lesions following primary c. SYN coccidioidal granuloma.

subclinical c., a form of c. that does not come to medical attention because respiratory symptoms are mild and self-limited.

coc·cid·i·o·sis (kok-sid-ē-ō′sis). Group name for diseases due to any species of coccidia; a common and serious protozoan disease of many species of domestic animals and birds and many wild animals kept in captivity; both intestinal and pulmonary c. have been reported in humans with AIDS.

coc·cid·i·o·stat (kok-sid′ē-ō-stat). A chemical agent generally added to animal feed to partially inhibit or delay the development of coccidiosis.

coc·cid·i·um, pl. **coc·cid·i·a** (kok-sid′ē-ŭm, -ē-ă). Common name given to protozoan parasites (order Eucoccidiida) in which schizogony occurs within epithelial cells, generally in the intestine, but in some species in the bile ducts and kidney; the final product of sexual fusion and differentiation that occurs within the host, the oocyst, generally passes to the soil in the feces, undergoes sporulation, and then acts as the infective form for another host. Coccidia are parasitic in most domestic and wild birds and mammals, occasionally in humans, and are highly host-specific; the majority are nonpathogenic, but certain species rank among the most serious and economically important pathogens, causing coccidiosis in birds and mammals. SEE *Isospora, Cryptosporidium.* [Mod. L. dim. of G. *kokkos,* berry]

coc·ci·nel·la (kok-sin-el′ă). SYN cochineal.

coc·ci·nel·lin (kok-si-nel′in). The coloring principle derived from cochineal.

coc·co·bac·il·lary (kok′ō-bas′i-lār-ē). **1.** Relating to a coccobacillus. **2.** Of organisms exhibiting coccal, bacillary, and intermediate forms.

coc·co·ba·cil·lus (kok′ō-bă-sil′ŭs). A short, thick bacterial rod of the shape of an oval or slightly elongated coccus. [G. *kokkos,* berry]

coc·coid (kok′oyd). Resembling a coccus. [G. *kokkos,* berry, + *eidos,* resemblance]

coc·cu·lin (kok′ū-lin). SYN picrotoxin.

coc·cus, pl. **coc·ci** (kok′ŭs, kok′sī). **1.** A bacterium of round, spheroidal, or ovoid form. **2.** SYN cochineal. [G. *kokkos,* berry]

Neisser c., SYN *Neisseria gonorrhoeae.*

Weichselbaum c., SYN *Neisseria meningitidis.*

coc·cy·ceph·a·ly (kok′si-sef′ă-lē). A malformation in which the cephalic profile suggests a beak. [G. *kokkyx,* cuckoo, + *kephalē,* head]

coc·cy·dyn·ia (kok-sē-din′ē-ă). Pain in the coccygeal region. SYN coccygodynia, coccyodynia. [coccyx + G. *ōdyne, pain*]

coc·cyg·eal (Co) (kok-sij′ē-ăl). Relating to the coccyx.

coc·cy·gec·to·my (kok-sē-jek′tō-mē). Removal of the coccyx. [coccyx + G. *ektomē,* excision]

coc·cyg·e·us *muscle.* SEE coccygeus.

coc·cy·go·dyn·ia (kok′si-gō-din′ē-ă). SYN coccydynia. [coccyx + G. *odynē,* pain]

coc·cy·got·o·my (kok-sē-got′ō-mē). Operation for freeing the coccyx from its attachments. [coccyx + G. *tomē,* a cutting]

coc·cy·o·dyn·ia (kok′sē-ō-din′ē-ă). SYN coccydynia.

coc·cyx, gen. **coc·cy·gis,** pl. **coc·cy·ges** (kok′siks, -si-jis, -si-jēs) [TA]. The small bone at the end of the vertebral column in humans, formed by the fusion of four rudimentary vertebrae; it articulates above with the sacrum. SYN os coccygis [TA], coccygeal bone, tail bone. [G. *kokkyx,* a cuckoo, the coccyx]

coch·i·neal (kotch′i-nēl) [C.I. 75470]. The dried female insects, *Coccus cacti,* enclosing the young larvae, or the dried female insect, *Dactylopius coccus,* containing eggs and larvae, from which coccinellin is obtained; used as a red coloring agent and a stain. SEE carmine. SYN coccinella, coccus (2). [O.Sp. *cochinilla,* wood louse, fr. G. *kokkinos,* berry]

🔲**co·chlea,** pl. **co·chle·ae** (kok′lē-ă, lē-ē) [TA]. A conical cavity in the petrous portion of the temporal bone, forming one of the divisions of the labyrinth or internal ear. It consists of a spiral canal making two and a half turns around a central core of spongy bone, the modiolus; this spiral canal of the cochlea contains the membranous cochlea, or cochlear duct, in which is the spiral organ (Corti). [L. snail shell]

membranous c., SYN cochlear *duct.*

co·chle·ar (kok′lē-ăr). Relating to the cochlea.

cochlear microphonic (kok′lē-ar mī-krō-fon′ik), bioelectric potentials produced by the hair cells of the organ of Corti in response to sound that faithfully represent the frequency and intensity of the acoustic stimulation. SYN cochlear potential, Wever-Bray phenomenon.

co·chle·a·re (kō-klē′ă, kok-lē-ā′rē). A spoon. [L.]

c. am′plum, a tablespoonful. [L.]

c. mag′num, a tablespoonful. [L.]

c. me′dium, a dessertspoonful. [L.]

c. mod′icum, a dessertspoonful. [L.]

c. par′vum, a teaspoonful. [L.]

co·chle·ar·i·form (kok-lē-ar′i-fōrm). Spoon-shaped. [L. *cochleare,* spoon, + *forma,* form]

co·chle·ate (kok′lē-āt). **1.** Resembling a snail shell. **2.** Denoting the appearance of a form of plate culture. [L. *cochlea,* a snail shell]

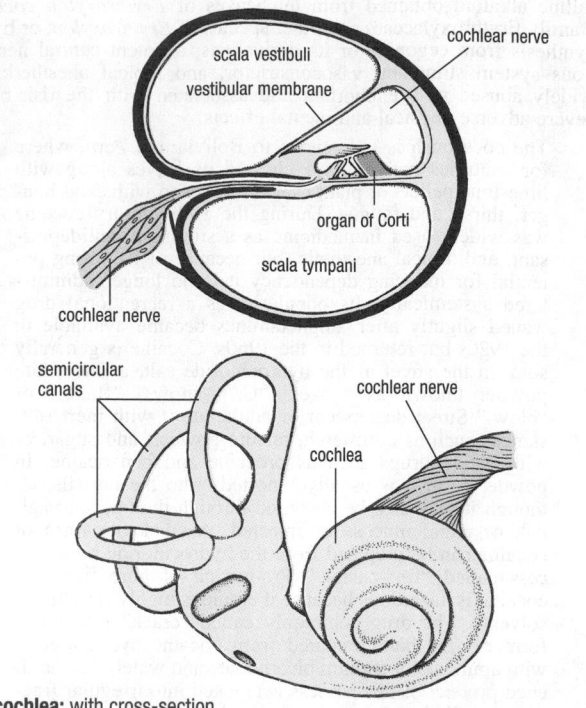

cochlea: with cross-section

coch·le·i·tis (kō-klē-ī′tis). Inflammation of the cochlea. [cochlea + G. *-itis,* inflammatio]

co·chle·o·sac·cu·lot·o·my (kok′lē-ō-sac-ū-lot′ō-mē). An operation for Ménière disease performed through the round window to create a shunt between the cochlear duct and the saccule.

coch·le·o·topic (kō-klē-ō-top′ik). Referring to the frequency-responsive organization of the central auditory pathways in the brain. [cochlea + G. *topos,* place, + -ic]

co·chle·o·ves·tib·u·lar (kok′lē-ō-ves-tib′ū-lăr). Relating to the cochlea and the vestibule of the ear.

Co·chli·o·my·ia (kok′lē-ō-mī′yă). A genus of fleshflies (family Calliphoridae) whose larvae develop in decaying flesh or carrion or in wounds or sores.

C. american′a, incorrect name for *C. hominivorax.*

C. homini′vorax, the screw-worm fly, a species that is a serious pest of livestock from Mexico to Argentina and is the primary cause of myiasis in the western hemisphere; attracted by fresh blood, it deposits eggs on wounds, tick bites, or intact moist areas of the body, and the larvae invade living tissues, causing severe myiasis and often death; it is known to attack humans, especially in the nose, although wounds, eyes, and other body openings have also been attacked.

Cochrane, A.L., British epidemiologist, 1909–1988. SEE C. *collaboration.*

co·cil·la·na (ko′sĕ-lah′nă). The dried bark of *Guarea rusbyi,* a Bolivia tree, used as an expectorant in bronchitis.

Cockayne, Edward A., British physician, 1880–1956. SEE C. *disease, syndrome;* Weber-C. *syndrome.*

cock·tail (kok′tāl). A mixture that includes several ingredients or drugs.

Brompton c., a c. of morphine and cocaine usually used for analgesia in terminal cancer patients; the formulations vary, but typically it contains 15 mg of morphine hydrochoride and 10 mg of cocaine hydrochloride per 10 ml of the c. [*Brompton* Chest Hospital, London, England, where developed]

Philadelphia c., SYN Rivers c.

Rivers c., an intravenous slow injection of from 1000 to 2000 ml of 10% dextrose in isotonic saline to which thiamine hydrochloride and 25 units of insulin are added; used in acute alcoholism. SYN Philadelphia c.

co·coa (kō′kō). A powder prepared from the roasted kernels of the ripe seed of *Theobroma cacao* (family Sterculiaceae); used in the preparation of c. syrup, a flavoring agent. SEE ALSO cacao.

co·con·scious·ness (kō-kon′shŭs-nes). **1.** A splitting of consciousness into two streams. **2.** Awareness by one personality of the thoughts of another personality in dissociative disorder.

co·con·ver·sion (kō′kon-ver′shŭn). The simultaneous correction of two sites on DNA during gene conversion.

cocto-. Prefix indicating boiled or modified by heat. [L. *coctus*, cooked]

coc·to·la·bile (kok-tō-lā′bil, -bīl). Subject to alteration or destruction when exposed to the temperature of boiling water.

coc·to·sta·bile, coc·to·sta·ble (kok-tō-stā′bil, -bīl; -stā′bl). Resisting the temperature of boiling water without alteration or destruction.

code (kōd). **1.** A set of rules, principles, or ethics. **2.** Any system devised to convey information or facilitate communication. **3.** Term used in hospitals to describe an emergency requiring situation trained members of the staff, such as a cardiopulmonary resuscitation team, or the signal to summon such a team. **4.** A numeric system for ordering and classifying information, e.g., about diagnostic categories. [L. *codex*, book]

genetic c., the genetic information carried by the specific DNA molecules of the chromosomes; specifically, the system whereby particular combinations of three consecutive nucleotides in a DNA molecule control the insertion of one particular amino acid in equivalent places in a protein molecule. The genetic c. is almost universal throughout the prokaryotic, plant, and animal kingdoms. There are two known exceptions. In ciliated protozoans, the triplets AGA and AGG are read as termination signals instead of as L-arginine. This is also true of the human mitochondrial c., which, in addition, uses AUA as a code for L-methionine (instead of isoleucine) and UGA for L-tryptophan (instead of a termination signal).

soundex c., a sequence of letters used for recording names phonetically, especially in record linkage.

co·deine (kō′dēn). Obtained from opium, which contains 0.7 to 2.5%, but usually made from morphine. Used as an analgesic and antitussive; drug dependence (physical and psychic) may develop, but c. is less liable to produce addiction than is morphine; c. is biotransformed to morphine, which accounts for most of c. effects. SYN methylmorphine. [G. *kōdeia*, head, poppy head]

Co·dex med·i·ca·men·tar·i·us (kō′deks med′i-kă-men-tār′ē-ŭs). The official title of the French Pharmacopeia. [L. a book pertaining to drugs]

cod·ing. Translation of information, e.g., diagnoses, questionnaire responses, into numbered categories for entry into a data processing system.

place coding, frequency coding as determined by the activation of the organ of Corti from the base to the apex of the cochlea in a gradation with higher frequencies transmitted from near the base and lower frequencies from near the apex.

cod liv·er oil. The partially desteariated fixed oil extracted from the fresh livers of the codfish (*Gadus morrhuae*) and other species of the family Gadidae, containing vitamins A and D; used as a supplementary source of vitamins A and D.

Codman, Ernest Amory, U.S. surgeon, 1869–1940. SEE C. *triangle, tumor.*

co·do·gen·ic (kō-dō-jen-ik). Formed by a code; specifically, the genetic code.

co·dom·i·nant (kō-dom′i-nant). In genetics, denoting an equal degree of dominance of two genes, both being expressed in the phenotype of the individual; e.g., genes A and B of the ABO blood group are codominant; individuals with both are type AB.

co·don (kō′don). A set of three consecutive nucleotides in a strand of DNA or RNA that provides the genetic information to code for a specific amino acid which will be incorporated into a protein chain or serve as a termination signal. SYN triplet (3). [code + -on]

amber c., the termination codon UAG.

genetic code					
1. Position	**2. Position**				**3. Position**
	U(A)	C(G)	A(T)	G(C)	
U(A)	Phe	Ser	Tyr	Cys	U(A)
	Phe	Ser	Tyr	Cys	C(G)
	Leu	Ser	End	End	A(T)
	Leu	Ser	End	Trp	G(C)
C(G)	Leu	Pro	His	Arg	U(A)
	Leu	Pro	His	Arg	C(G)
	Leu	Pro	Gln	Arg	A(T)
	Leu	Pro	Gln	Arg	G(C)
A(T)	Ile	Thr	Asn	Ser	U(A)
	Ile	Thr	Asn	Ser	C(G)
	Ile	Thr	Lys	Arg	A(T)
	Met	Thr	Lys	Arg	G(C)
G(C)	Val	Ala	Asp	Gly	U(A)
	Val	Ala	Asp	Gly	C(G)
	Val	Ala	Glu	Gly	A(T)
	Val	Ala	Glu	Gly	G(C)

The so-called "code lexicon": it shows the relationship of mRNA codons (in parentheses) to the coded amino acids. The triplets are arranged according to nucleic acid bases (A=adenine; C=cytosine; G=guanine; T=thymine; U=uracil; "End" (white) indicates chain termination codons). The three colors indicate whether the amino acids are hydrophobic (yellow), hydrophilic (blue), or ambiphilic (pink).

initiating c., the trinucleotide AUG (or sometimes GUG) that codes for the first amino acid in protein sequences, formylmethionine; the latter is often removed post-transcriptionally. SYN start c.

initiation c., a specific mRNA sequence (usually AUG, but sometimes GUG) that is the signal for the addition of fMet-tRNA and the beginning of translation.

nonsense c., SYN termination c.

ochre c., the termination c. UAA.

opal c., SYN umber c.

punctuation c., SYN termination c.

start c., SYN initiating c.

stop c., SYN termination c.

termination c., trinucleotide sequence (UAA, UGA, or UAG) that specifies the end of translation or transcription. Cf. amber c., ochre c., umber c. SYN nonsense c., punctuation c., stop c., termination sequence, termination signal.

umber c., the termination c. UGA. SYN opal c.

coe-. For words so beginning, and not found here, see ce-.

co·ef·fi·cient (kō-ĕ-fish′ĕnt). **1.** The expression of the amount or degree of any quality possessed by a substance, or of the degree of physical or chemical change normally occurring in that substance under stated conditions. **2.** The ratio or factor that relates a quantity observed under one set of conditions to that observed under standard conditions, usually when all variables are either 1 or a simple power of 10. [L. *co-* + *efficio* (*exfacio*), to accomplish]

absorption c., (**1**) the milliliters of a gas at standard temperature and pressure that will saturate 100 mL of liquid; (**2**) the amount of light absorbed in passing through 1 cm of a 1 molar solution of a given substance, expressed as a constant in Beer-Lambert law; Cf. specific absorption c; (**3**) a measure of the rate of decrease of intensity of an x-ray beam in its passage through a substance, resulting from a combination of scattering and conversion to other forms of energy.

activity c. (γ), SEE activity (2).

biological c., rarely used term denoting the energy expended by the body at rest.

Bunsen solubility c. (α), the milliliters of gas STPD dissolved per milliliter of liquid and per atmosphere (760 mm Hg) partial pressure of the gas at any given temperature.

c. of consanguinity, SYN c. of inbreeding.

CO

correlation c., a measure of association that indicates the degree to which two variables have a linear relationship; this c., represented by the letter r, can vary between +1 and −1; when r = +1, there is a perfect positive linear relationship in which one variable relates directly with the other; when r = −1, there is a perfect negative linear relationship between the variables.

creatinine c., the number of milligrams of creatinine excreted daily per kilogram of body weight.

diffusion c., the mass of material diffusing across a unit area in unit time under a concentration gradient of unity. SYN diffusion constant.

distribution c., the ratio of concentrations of a substance in two immiscible phases at equilibrium; the basis of many chromatographic separation procedures. SYN partition c.

economic c., in growth and cultivation of microorganisms, the ratio of the mass produced to the substrate consumed.

extinction c. (ε), SYN specific absorption c.

extraction c., the percentage of a substance removed from the blood or plasma in a single passage through a tissue; e.g., the extraction c. for *p*-aminohippuric acid (PAH) in the kidney is the difference between arterial and renal venous plasma PAH concentrations, divided by the arterial plasma PAH concentration.

filtration c., a measure of a membrane's permeability to water; specifically, the volume of fluid filtered in unit time through a unit area of membrane per unit pressure difference, taking into account both hydraulic and osmotic pressures.

Hill c., the slope of the line in a Hill plot; a measure of the degree of cooperativity. SYN Hill constant.

hygienic laboratory c., SYN Rideal-Walker c.

c. of inbreeding, the probability that the progeny of a consanguineous marriage will be homozygous for a specific autosomal allele derived from a common ancestor. SYN c. of consanguinity.

isotonic c., the amount of salts in the blood plasma, or the amount that should be added to distilled water in order to prepare an isotonic solution.

c. of kinship, the probability that two genes at the same locus, picked at random from each of two individuals, are identical by descent.

lethal c., that concentration of disinfectant that kills bacteria at 20–25°C in the shortest period of time.

linear absorption c., that fraction of ionizing radiation absorbed in a unit thickness of a substance or tissue. SEE ALSO absorption c. (3); Cf. attenuation.

Long c., SYN Long *formula.*

molar absorption c. (ε), absorbance (of light) per unit path length (usually the centimeter) and per unit of concentration (moles per liter); a fundamental unit in spectrophotometry. SYN absorbancy index (2), absorptivity (2), molar absorbancy index, molar absorptivity, molar extinction c.

molar extinction c., SYN molar absorption c.

Ostwald solubility c. (Λ), the milliliters of gas dissolved per milliliter of liquid and per atmosphere (760 mm Hg) partial pressure of the gas at any given temperature. This differs from Bunsen solubility c. (α) in that the amount of dissolved gas is expressed in terms of its volume at the temperature of the experiment, instead of STPD. Thus, $\lambda = \alpha (1 + 0.00367t)$, where t = temperature in degrees Celsius.

oxygen utilization c., the extraction c. for oxygen in any given tissue.

partition c., SYN distribution c.

permeability c., a c. associated with simple diffusion through a membrane that is proportional to the partition coefficient and the diffusion coefficient and inversely proportional to membrane thickness.

phenol c., SYN Rideal-Walker c.

Poiseuille viscosity c., an expression of the viscosity as determined by the capillary tube method; the coefficient $\eta = (\pi P r^4 t / 8 v l)$, where P is the pressure difference between the inlet and outlet of the tube, r the radius of the tube, l its length, and v the volume of liquid delivered in the time t. If volume is in cubic centimeters, time is in seconds, and l and r are in centimeters, then η will be in poise.

reflection c. (σ), a measure of the relative permeability of a particular membrane to a particular solute; calculated as the ratio of observed osmotic pressure to that calculated from van't Hoff law; also equal to 1 minus the ratio of the effective pore areas available to solute and to solvent.

c. of relationship, the probability that a gene present in one mate is also present in the other and is derived from the same source.

reliability c., an index of the consistency of measurement often based on the correlation between scores obtained on the initial test and a retest (test-retest reliability) or between scores on two similar forms of the same test (equivalent-form reliability).

respiratory c., SYN respiratory *quotient.*

Rideal-Walker c., a figure expressing the disinfecting power of any substance; it is obtained by dividing the figure indicating the degree of dilution of the disinfectant that kills a microorganism in a given time by that indicating the degree of dilution of phenol that kills the organism in the same space of time under similar conditions. SYN hygienic laboratory c., phenol c.

sedimentation c. (s), SYN sedimentation *constant.*

selection c. (s), the proportion of progeny or potential progeny not surviving to sexual maturity; usually defined artificially by expressing the fitness of a phenotype as a fraction of the mean or optimal fitness to give the relative fitness, and subtracting this fraction from unity. If the mean size of family in the population is 3.2 and that for a particular genotype is 2.4 then the fitness of the phenotype is 2.4/3.2 = 0.75 and the selection coefficient = 1 − 0.75 = .25.

specific absorption c. (*a*), absorbance (of light) per unit path length (usually the centimeter) and per unit of mass concentration. Cf. molar absorption c. SYN absorbancy index (1), absorptivity (1), extinction c., specific extinction.

temperature c., the fractional change in any physical property per degree rise in temperature.

ultrafiltration c., the filtration c. of a semipermeable membrane.

c. of variation (CV), the ratio of the standard deviation to the mean.

velocity c., the rate of transformation of a unit mass of substance in a chemical reaction.

c. of viscosity, the value of the force per unit area required to maintain a unit relative velocity between two parallel planes a unit distance apart.

Coe·len·ter·a·ta (sē-len-tĕ-rā′tă). One of the major phyla of invertebrates, to which such forms as jellyfish belong.

coe·len·ter·ate (sē-len′ter-at). Common name for members of the Coelenterata.

coe·lom (sē′lom). SYN body *cavity.*

co·en·es·the·sia (kō-en-es-thē′zē-ă). SYN cenesthesia.

coeno-. Shared in common. SEE ALSO ceno-. [G. *koinos,* common]

coe·no·cyte (sē′nō-sīt). SYN cenocyte.

coe·no·cyt·ic (sē-nō-sit′ik). SYN cenocytic.

coe·nu·ro·sis (sē-noo-rō′sis). SYN cenurosis.

Coe·nu·rus (sē-noo′rŭs). Former generic name, now used to designate larval forms of taenioid cestodes in which a bladder is formed with a number of invaginated scoleces developing within; distinguished from a hydatid cyst by the absence of free-floating daughter cyst colonies budded off within the bladder; C. larvae are found in members of the genus *Multiceps.* [G. *koinos,* common, + *oura,* tail]

C. cerebra′lis, the coenurus larvae of the tapeworm *Multiceps multiceps,* found in the brain and spinal cord of sheep, goats, and other ruminants (a few have been recorded in humans); adults are found in the intestine of dogs, foxes, coyotes, and jackals.

C. seria′lis, the coenurus larvae of the tapeworm *Multiceps serialis,* found in subcutaneous and intramuscular tissues of rabbits and hares (a few have been recorded in humans); adult worms are found in the intestine of dogs, foxes, and jackals.

co·en·zyme (kō-en′zīm). A substance (excluding solo metal ions) that enhances or is necessary for the action of enzymes; c.'s are of smaller molecular size than the enzymes themselves, are dialyzable and relatively heat-stable, and are usually easily dissociable from the protein portion of the enzyme; several vitamins are c. precursors. SYN cofactor (1).

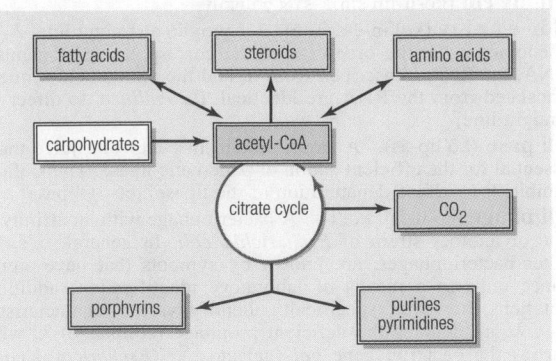

coenzyme: central position of acetylcoenzyme A in the interchange of intermediate substances

co·en·zyme A (CoA). A coenzyme containing pantothenic acid, adenosine 3'-phosphate 5'-pyrophosphate, and cysteamine; involved in the transfer of acyl groups, notably in transacetylations.

co·en·zyme F (kō-en'zīm). SYN tetrahydrofolic acid.

co·en·zyme Q (CoQ, Q). Quinones with isoprenoid side chains (specifically, ubiquinones) that mediate electron transfer between cytochrome *b* and cytochrome *c;* chemically similar to vitamins E and K, and to other tocopherols, quinones, and tocols.

co·en·zyme R. SYN biotin.

coeur (koor). SYN heart. [Fr.]

c. en sabot (awn sah-bo'), the radiographic configuration of the heart in the tetralogy of Fallot; the elevated apex gives a silhouette like that of a wooden shoe. SYN sabot heart, wooden-shoe heart.

co·ev·o·lu·tion (kō-ev-ō-loo'shŭn). The process whereby genes or gene fragments are changing together and not diverging.

co·fac·tor (kō'fak'ter, tōr). **1.** SYN coenzyme. **2.** An atom or molecule essential for the action of a large molecule; e.g., heme in hemoglobin, magnesium in chlorophyll. Solo metal ions are regarded as c.'s for proteins, but not as coenzymes.

cobra venom c., equivalent in action to C3B, which means that it can activate the alternative complement pathway.

molybdenum c. (mō-lib'dĕ-nŭm), a complex of molybdenum and molybdopterin required for a number of enzymes. A deficiency of this c. will result in lower activities of sulfite oxidase, xanthine dehydrogenase, and aldehyde oxidase causing elevated levels of sulfite, thiosulfite, xanthine, etc.

platelet c. I, SYN *factor* VIII.

platelet c. II, SYN *factor* IX.

Coffey, Robert, U.S. surgeon, 1869–1933. SEE C. *suspension.*

Coffin, Grange S., U.S. pediatrician, *1923. SEE C.-Lowry *syndrome;* C.-Siris *syndrome.*

Cogan, David G., U.S. ophthalmologist, 1908–1993. SEE C. *syndrome;* C.-Reese *syndrome.*

cog·ni·tion (kog-ni'shŭn). **1.** Generic term embracing the mental activities associated with thinking, learning, and memory. **2.** Any process whereby one acquires knowledge. [L. *cognitio*]

cog·ni·tive (kog'ni-tiv). Pertaining to cognition.

co·he·sion (kō-hē'zhŭn). The attraction between molecules or masses that holds them together. [L. *co-haereo,* pp. *-haesus,* to stick together]

Cohnheim, Julius F., German histologist, pathologist, and physiologist, 1839–1884. SEE C. *area, field.*

co·ho·ba (kō-hō'bă). A psychotomimetic hallucinogenic substance obtained from *Acacia niopo* (family Leguminosae), a Central American plant, *Piptadenia peregrina,* and other plants; among its constituents are bufotenine and dimethyltryptamine; used in native localities as snuff or enema.

co·hort (kō'hōrt). **1.** Component of the population born during a particular period and identified by period of birth so that its characteristics can be ascertained as it enters successive time and age periods. **2.** Any designated group followed or traced over a period, as in an epidemiological cohort study. [L. *cohors,* retinue, military unit]

coil (kōil). **1.** A spiral or series of loops. **2.** An object made of wire wound in a spiral configuration, used in electronic applications, or a loop of wire used as an antenna. **3.** A spiral loop of wire used to embolize an artery to obstruct it.

detector c., a c. used in magnetic resonance imaging as an antenna to record radiofrequency emissions of stimulated nuclei, e.g., body coil, head coil.

random c., a structure of a macromolecule (typically, a biopolymer) which changes with time.

surface c., a detector c. applied directly to a body part for high resolution magnetic resonance imaging; often a single loop of metal.

coin-count·ing (koyn'kownt'ing). A sliding movement of the tips of the thumb and index finger, occurring in paralysis agitans.

co·in·te·grate. A structure resulting from replicative transposition where the transposon is duplicated.

co·i·tal (kō'i-tăl). Pertaining to coitus.

Coiter (Koyter), Volcher, Dutch surgeon and anatomist, 1534–1576. SEE C. *muscle.*

co·i·tion (kō-ish'ŭn). SYN coitus. [L. *co-eo,* pp. *-itus,* to come together]

co·i·to·pho·bia (kō'i-tō-fō'bē-ă). Morbid fear of sexual intercourse. [L. *coitus,* sexual intercourse, + G. *phobos,* fear]

co·i·tus (kō'i-tŭs). Sexual union between male and female. SYN coition, copulation (1), pareunia, sexual intercourse. [L.]

c. interrup'tus, sexual intercourse that is interrupted before the male ejaculates.

c. reserva'tus, c. in which ejaculation is postponed or suppressed.

Co·ker·o·my·ces (kō'ker-ō-mī'sēz). A fungal genus in the order Mucorales; a rare cause of disease in humans.

col (kol). A craterlike area of the interproximal oral mucosa joining the lingual and buccal interdental papillae.

△**col-.** SEE con-.

co·la (kō'lă). **1.** SYN kola. **2.** [L.] strain (imperative form).

col·chi·cine (kol'chi-sin) [USP]. An alkaloid obtained from *Colchicum autumnale* (family Liliaceae); used in the chronic treatment of gout. Inhibits microtuble formation.

Col·chi·cum corm (kōl'chĭ-kum). Dried corm of *Colchicum autumnale,* the botanical source for colchicine, an alkaloidal drug used for the treatment of gout.

cold (kōld). **1.** A low temperature; the sensation produced by a temperature notably below an accustomed norm or a comfortable level. **2.** Popular term for a virus infection involving the upper respiratory tract and characterized by congestion of the mucous membrane, watery nasal discharge, and general malaise, with a duration of 3–5 days. SEE ALSO rhinitis, coryza. SYN frigid (1).

head c., SYN acute *rhinitis.*

rose c., allergic rhinitis occurring in the spring and early summer.

cold-blood·ed (kōld-blŭd'ed). SYN poikilothermic.

Coldman, Andrew James, 20th century Canadian epidemiologist (1952-). SEE Goldie-C. *hypothesis.*

Cole, Laurent, French pathologist, *1903. SEE Benedict-Hopkins-C. *reagent.*

Cole, Rufus Ivory, U.S. physician, 1872–1966.

Cole, Warren Henry, surgeon, *1898. Co-developer with E. A. Graham of cholecystography, first described in 1924. SEE Graham-Cole *test.*

Cole-Cecil mur·mur. See under murmur.

co·lec·ta·sia (kō-lek-tā'zē-ă). Distention of the colon. [G. *kolon,* colon, + *ektasis,* a stretching]

col·ec·to·my (kō-lek'tō-mē). Excision of a segment or all of the colon. [G. *kolon,* colon, + *ektomē,* excision]

△**coleo-.** Sheath, specifically, the vagina. [G. *koleos,* sheath]

Co·le·op·te·ra (kō-lē-op'ter-ă). An order of insects, the beetles, characterized by the possession of a pair of hard, horny wing covers overlying a pair of delicate membranous flying wings; it is the largest of the insect orders with the largest number of species of any animal or plant order. [G. *koleos,* sheath + *pteron,* wing]

co·le·op·to·sis (kō-lē-op'tō-sis). SYN coloptosis.

co·le·ot·o·my (kol-ē-ot'ō-mē). SYN colpotomy. [G. *koleos,* sheath, + *tomē,* incision]

co·les·ti·pol (kō-les'ti-pol). An antilipemic drug resembling cholestyramine.

colet. Abbreviation for L. *coletur,* let it be strained.

co·li·bac·il·lo·sis (kō'li-bas-i-lō'sis). Diarrheal disease caused by the bacterium *Escherichia coli.* Often called enteric c.

co·li·ba·cil·lus, pl. **co·li·ba·cil·li** (kō'li-bă-sil'ŭs). SYN *Escherichia coli.*

col·ic (kol'ik). **1.** Relating to the colon. **2.** Spasmodic pains in the abdomen. **3.** In young infants, paroxysms of gastrointestinal pain, with crying and irritability, due to a variety of causes, such as swallowing of air, emotional upset, or overfeeding. [G. *kōlikos,* relating to the colon]

appendicular c., colicky pain occurring early in acute appendicitis. SYN vermicular c.

biliary c., intense spasmodic pain felt in the right upper quadrant of the abdomen from impaction of a gallstone in the cystic duct. SYN gallstone c., hepatic c.

copper c., an affection similar to lead c. occurring in chronic poisoning by copper.

Devonshire c., SYN lead c.

gallstone c., SYN biliary c.

gastric c., colicky pain associated with gastritis or peptic ulcer.

hepatic c., SYN biliary c.

infantile c., episodes of abdominal pain due to abnormal muscular contraction of the intestine in infants.

lead c., severe colicky abdominal pain, with constipation, symptomatic of lead poisoning. SYN Devonshire c., painter's c., Poitou c., saturnine c.

meconial c., abdominal pain of newborn infants.

menstrual c., intermittent cramplike lower abdominal pains associated with menstruation.

ovarian c., lower abdominal pain due to torsion or twisting of an ovary, as with an ovarian cyst.

painter's c., SYN lead c.

pancreatic c., severe colicky abdominal pain, resembling that of biliary c., caused by the passage of a pancreatic calculus.

Poitou c., SYN lead c.

renal c., severe colicky pain caused by the impaction or passage of a calculus in the ureter or renal pelvis.

salivary c., periodic attacks of pain in the region of a salivary duct or gland, accompanied by an acute swelling of the gland, occurring in cases of salivary calculus.

saturnine c., SYN lead c.

tubal c., lower abdominal pain due to spasmodic contraction of the oviduct excited by a blood clot, other irritant, or the injection of gas or oil.

ureteral c., paroxysm of pain due to abrupt obstruction of ureter from a calculus or blood clot in most instances.

uterine c., painful cramps of the uterine muscle sometimes occurring at the menstrual period, or in association with uterine disease.

vermicular c., SYN appendicular c.

zinc c., c. resulting from chronic zinc poisoning.

col·i·ca (kol'i-kă). A colic artery. SEE artery.

col·i·cin (kol'i-sin). Bacteriocin produced by strains of *Escherichia coli* and by other enterobacteria (*Shigella* and *Salmonella*) that carry the necessary plasmids. Many are toxic to related bacterial strains and bind to specific cellular receptors interfering with normal function. [(*Escherichia*) *coli* + bacteriocin]

col·i·ci·nog·e·ny (kol'i-si-noj'ĕ-nē). The bacterial property of producing a colicin.

col·icky (kol'i-kē). Denoting or resembling the pain of colic.

col·i·co·ple·gia (kol'i-kō-plē'jē-ă). Lead poisoning marked by both colic and palsy. [G. *kolikos,* suffering from colic, + *plēgē,* stroke]

co·li·my·cin (kō-li-mī'sin). SYN colistin.

col·in·e·ar·i·ty (kol'in-ē-ar'i-tē). **1.** Lying in a straight line. **2.** The phenomona that the orderings of the corresponding elements of DNA, the RNA transcribed from it, and the amino acid sequence translated from the RNA are identical. [L. *collineo,* to direct in a straight line]

co·li·pase (kō'lip-ās). A small protein in pancreatic juice that is essential for the efficient action of pancreatic lipase. This cofactor inhibits the surface denaturation of the lipase. [co- + lipase]

co·li·phage (kō'li-fāj, kol'i-). A bacteriophage with an affinity for one or another strain of *Escherichia coli.* In general, c.'s, like other bacteriophages, are known by symbols that have significance only as a means of laboratory identification; additional notations, however, specifically identify variant characteristics, e.g., λdgal denotes the deficient prophage (coliphage) λ, which carries the bacterial gene *gal* (galactose). [(*Escherichia*) *coli* + bacteriophage]

co·li·pli·ca·tion (kō'li-pli-kā'shŭn). SYN coloplication.

co·li·punc·ture (kō'li-pŭnk-choor). SYN colocentesis.

co·lis·ti·meth·ate so·di·um (kō-lis-ti-meth'āte). Contains the pentasodium salt of the penta(methanesulfonic acid) derivative of colistin A as the major component, with a small proportion of the pentasodium salt of the same derivative of colistin B; an effective antibiotic against most Gram-negative bacilli (except *Proteus*), given intramuscularly. SEE ALSO *colistin* sulfate, polymyxin. SYN cholistine sulphomethate sodium, colistin sulfomethate sodium.

co·lis·tin (kō-lis'tin). A mixture of cyclic polypeptide antibiotics from a strain of *Bacillus polymyxa;* separable into polymyxins. SYN colimycin.

c. sulfate, the sulfate salt of an antibacterial substance produced by the growth of a strain of *Bacillus polymyxa,* consisting primarily of colistin A with small amounts of colistin B; it is effective against most Gram-negative bacteria (except *Proteus*); given orally for intestinal antibacterial action. SEE ALSO colistimethate sodium, polymyxin.

c. sulfomethate sodium, SYN colistimethate sodium.

co·li·tis (kō-lī'tis). Inflammation of the colon. [G. *kōlon,* colon, + *-itis,* inflammation]

amebic c., inflammation of the colon in amebiasis.

collagenous c., c. occurring mostly in middle-aged women and characterized by persistent watery diarrhea and a deposit of a band of collagen beneath the basement membrane of colon surface epithelium.

c. cys'tica profun'da, intramural mucus-containing cysts of the large bowel; the condition may be mistaken for mucinous carcinoma but is not neoplastic.

c. cys'tica superficia'lis, a form of c. in which there is superficial cyst formation in the colon.

granulomatous c., changes, identical to those of regional enteritis, involving the colon.

hemorrhagic c., abdominal cramps and bloody diarrhea, without fever, attributed to a self-limited infection by a strain of *Escherichia coli.*

mucous c., an affection of the mucous membrane of the colon characterized by colicky pain, constipation or diarrhea (sometimes alternating), and passage of mucous or slimy pseudomembranous shreds and patches. SYN mucocolitis, myxomembranous c.

myxomembranous c., SYN mucous c.

pseudomembranous c., SYN pseudomembranous *enterocolitis.*

ulcerative c., a chronic disease of unknown cause characterized by ulceration of the colon and rectum, with rectal bleeding, mucosal crypt abscesses, inflammatory pseudopolyps, abdominal pain, and diarrhea; frequently causes anemia, hypoproteinemia, and electrolyte imbalance, and is less frequently complicated by peritonitis, toxic megacolon, or carcinoma of the colon.

uremic c., c. characterized by hemorrhages in the mucosa, occurring in renal failure, possibly owing to the irritant effect of ammonia formed by breakdown of increased urea in the intestinal secretions.

col·i·tose (kol'ĭ-tōs). A polysaccharide somatic antigen of *Salmonella* species.

col·la (kol'ă). Plural of collum.

collaboration.

Cochrane c., a worldwide network of clinical epidemiologists who review and publish results of randomized controlled trials. The aim is to provide improved data for use in evidence-based medicine and for setting clinical practice guidelines. SEE ALSO evidence-based *medicine,* clinical practice *guidelines,* under *guideline.*

col·la·cin (kol'ă-sin). Degenerated collagen. SYN collastin.

col·la·gen (kol'lă-jen). The major protein (comprising over half of that in mammals) of the white fibers of connective tissue, cartilage, and bone, that is insoluble in water but can be altered to easily digestible, soluble gelatins by boiling in water, dilute acids, or alkalis. It is high in glycyl, L-alanyl, L-prolyl, and L-4-hydroxyprolyl residues, but is low in sulfur and has no L-tryptophanyl residues. It comprises a family of genetically distinct molecules all of which have a unique triple helix configuration of three polypeptide subunits known as α-chains; at least 13 types of c. have been identified, each with a different polypeptide chain. SEE ALSO collagen *fiber.* SYN ossein, osseine, ostein, osteine. [G. *koila,* glue, + *-gen,* producing]

type I c., the most abundant c., which forms large well-organized fibrils having high tensile strength.

type II c., c. unique to cartilage, nucleus pulposis, notochord, and vitreous body; it forms as thin highly glycosylated fibrils.

type III c., c. characteristic of reticular fibers.

type IV c., a less distinctly fibrillar form of c. characteristic of basement membranes.

col·la·gen·ase (kol-ă'jĕ-nās). A proteolytic enzyme that acts on one or more of the collagens.

microbial c., SYN *Clostridium histolyticum* collagenase.

col·la·gen·ase A, col·la·gen·ase I. SYN *Clostridium histolyticum* collagenase.

col·la·ge·na·tion (kol'ă-jĕ-nā'shŭn). SYN collagenization.

col·la·gen·ic (kol-ă-jen'ik). SYN collagenous.

col·lag·e·ni·za·tion (ko-laj'ĕ-ni-zā'shŭn). **1.** Replacement of tissues or fibrin by collagen. **2.** Synthesis of collagen by fibroblasts. SYN collagenation.

col·lag·e·no·lyt·ic (ko-laj'ĕ-nō-lit'ik). Causing the lysis of collagen, gelatin, and other proteins containing proline. [collagen + G. *lysis,* dissolving]

col·lag·e·no·sis (ko-laj-i-nō'sis). SEE collagen *disease.*

reactive perforating c., a rare skin disorder characterized by extrusion of collagen fibers through the epidermis; usually begins in infancy or childhood and appears clinically as recurrent umbilicated papules that resolve spontaneously. The condition may be inherited or acquired; the latter is associated with diabetes and renal insufficiency and differs from Kyrle disease in that follicular involvement is absent.

col·lag·e·nous (ko-laj'ĕ-nŭs). Producing or containing collagen. SYN collagenic.

col·lapse (kō-laps'). **1.** A condition of extreme prostration, similar or identical to hypovolemic shock and due to the same causes. **2.** A state of profound physical depression. **3.** A falling together of the walls of a structure. **4.** The failure of a physiologic system. **5.** The falling away of an organ from its surround structure e.g., collapse of the lung. [L. *col-labor,* pp. *-lapsus,* to fall together]

absorption c., pulmonary c. due to rapid complete obstruction of a large bronchus.

circulatory c., failure of the circulation, either cardiac or peripheral.

c. of dental arch, movement of teeth to fill a space which would normally be filled by another, missing tooth, creating a malpositioning of adjacent and opposing teeth.

massive c., relatively sudden atelectasis of an entire lung or of a lobe.

pressure c., pulmonary c. due to external compression of the lung, as by a pleural effusion or pneumothorax.

pulmonary c., secondary atelectasis due to bronchial obstruction, pleural effusion or pneumothorax, cardiac hypertrophy, or enlargement of other structures adjacent to the lungs.

col·lar (kol'ăr). A band, usually denoting one encircling the neck.

renal c., in the embryo, a ring of veins around the aorta below the origin of the superior mesenteric artery.

col·lar·ette (kol'er-et'). **1.** The sinuous, scalloped line in the iris that divides the central pupillary zone from the peripheral ciliary zone and marks the embryonic site of the atrophied minor vascular circle of the iris. **2.** Brittle scales encircling eyelashes in staphylococcal blepharitis. SYN iris frill.

col·las·tin (kol-as'tin). SYN collacin.

col·lat·er·al (ko-lat'er-ăl). **1.** Indirect, subsidiary, or accessory to the main thing; side by side. **2.** A side branch of a nerve axon or blood vessel.

col·lec·tins. A family of molecules that recognize and opsonize microbes during the preimmune response of a host and may activate the complement pathway.

Colles, Abraham, Irish surgeon, 1773–1843. SEE C. *fascia, fracture, ligament, space.*

Collet, Frédéric-Justin, French otolaryngologist, 1870–1965.

col·lic·u·lec·to·my (ko-lik-ū-lek'tō-mē). Excision of the colliculus seminalis.

col·lic·u·lus, pl. **col·lic·u·li** (ko-lik'ū-lŭs, -lī) [TA]. A small elevation above the surrounding parts. [L. mound, dim. of *collis,* hill]

c. of arytenoid cartilage [TA], the elevation on the anterolateral surface of the arytenoid cartilage above the triangular fovea. SYN c. cartilaginis arytenoideae [TA].

c. cartila´ginis arytenoi´deae [TA], SYN c. of arytenoid cartilage.

facial c. [TA], prominent portion of the medial eminence, just rostral to the medullary striae in the rhomboidal fossa; it is formed by the internal genu of the facial nerve and the abducens nucleus around which the facial fibers curve. SYN c. facialis [TA], abducens eminence, eminentia abducentis, eminentia facialis, facial eminence, facial hillock.

c. facia´lis [TA], SYN facial c.

c. infe´rior [TA], SYN inferior c.

inferior c. [TA], the ovoid, paired, inferior eminence of the laminae of mesencephalic tectum; it receives the lateral lemniscus and projects by way of the brachium of inferior colliculus to the medial geniculate body of the thalamus, and is thus an essential way-station in the central auditory pathway. SYN c. inferior [TA], corpus quadrigeminum posterius, inferior nasal c., posterior quadrigeminal body.

inferior nasal c., SYN inferior c.

seminal c. [TA], an elevated portion of the urethral crest upon which open the two ejaculatory ducts and the prostatic utricle. SYN c. seminalis [TA], c. urethralis, seminal hillock, verumontanum.

c. semina´lis [TA], SYN seminal c.

superior c. [TA], the paired, larger, rounded anterior eminence of the laminae of mesencephalic tectum; major afferent connections of the superficial layers are the retina and striate cortex; input to deep layers of the c. are polymodal. Its efferent connections are with the lower brainstem and spinal cord (tectobulbar tract and tectospinal tract) and with the pulvinar and other cell groups in the caudal part of the thalamus; participates in extrageniculate visual pathway. The layers of the superior colliculus from superficial to deep are: zonal layer (stratum zonale), superficial gray layer (stratum griseum superficial), optic layer (stratum opticum), intermediate gray layer (stratum griseum intermedium), intermediate white layer (stratum medullare intermedium), deep gray layer (stratum griseum profundum), deep white layer (stratum medullare profundum). SYN c. superior [TA], anterior quadrigeminal body, corpus quadrigeminum anterius.

c. supe´rior [TA], SYN superior c.

c. urethra´lis, SYN seminal c.

Collier, James S., English physician, 1870–1935. SEE C. *tract, sign.*

col·li·ga·tion (kol-i-gā'shŭn). **1.** A combination in which the components are distinguishable from one another. **2.** The bringing of isolated events into a unified experience. **3.** The formation of a covalent bond by means of two combining groups. [L. *cum*, together, + *ligo*, to bind]

col·li·ga·tive (ko-lig'ă-tiv). **1.** Depending on numbers of particles. **2.** Referring to properties of solutions that depend only on the concentration of dissolved substances and not on their nature (e.g., osmotic pressure, elevation of boiling point, vapor pressure lowering, freezing point depression).

col·li·ma·tion (kol-i-mā'shŭn). The method, in radiology, of restricting and confining the x-ray beam to a given area and, in nuclear medicine, of restricting the detection of emitted radiations from a given area of interest. [L. *collineo*, to direct in a straight line]

col·li·ma·tor (kol'i-mā-ter). A device of high absorption coefficient material used in collimation.

Col·lins. SEE Lukes-Collins *classification*, Treacher Collins *syndrome*.

col·li·ot·o·my (kol-ē-ot'ō-mē). Obsolete term for adhesiotomy. [G. *kolla*, glue, + G. *tomē*, incision]

Collip, James B., Canadian endocrinologist, 1892–1965. SEE Noble-C. *procedure;* Anderson-C. *test*.

col·li·qua·tion (kol-i-kwā'shŭn). **1.** Excessive discharge of fluid. **2.** Liquefaction in the process of necrosis. [L. *col-*, together, + *liquo*, pp. *liquatus*, to cause to melt]

col·liq·ua·tive (ko-lik'wă-tiv). Denoting or characteristic of colliquation.

Collis, John Leighton, British thoracic surgeon, *1911. SEE C. *gastroplasty;* Collis-Nissen *fundoplication;* Collis-Belsey *fundoplication;* C.-Belsey *procedure*.

col·lo·di·on (ko-lō'dē-on). A liquid made by dissolving pyroxylin or gun cotton in ether and alcohol; on evaporation it leaves a glossy contractile film; used as a protective for cuts or as a vehicle for the local application of medicinal substances. SYN collodium. [Mod. L. *collodium*, fr. G. *kolla*, glue]

blistering c., SYN cantharidal c.

cantharidal c., a powdered chloroform extract of cantharides in flexible c.; a vesicant. SYN blistering c., c. vesicans.

flexible c., a mixture of camphor, castor oil, and c., or a mixture of castor oil, Canada turpentine, and c., used for the same purposes as c., but its film possesses the advantage, for certain conditions, of not contracting.

hemostatic c., SYN styptic c.

iodized c., a 5% solution of iodine in flexible c.; a counterirritant.

salicylic acid c., a keratolytic agent used in the treatment of corns and verrucae.

styptic c., tannic acid in flexible c.; an astringent and local hemostatic. SYN hemostatic c., styptic colloid, xylostyptic ether.

c. vesicans, SYN cantharidal c.

col·lo·di·um (ko-lō'dē-ŭm). SYN collodion. [G. *kolla*, glue, + *eidos*, appearance]

col·loid (kol'oyd). **1.** Aggregates of atoms or molecules in a finely divided state (submicroscopic), dispersed in a gaseous, liquid, or solid medium, and resisting sedimentation, diffusion, and filtration, thus differing from precipitates. SEE ALSO hydrocolloid. **2.** Gluelike. **3.** A translucent, yellowish, homogeneous material of the consistency of glue, less fluid than mucoid or mucinoid, found in the cells and tissues in a state of c. degeneration. SYN colloidin. **4.** The stored secretion within follicles of the thyroid gland. For individual c.'s not listed below, see the specific name. [G. *kolla*, glue, + *eidos*, appearance]

bovine c., SYN conglutinin.

dispersion c., SYN dispersoid.

emulsion c., SYN emulsoid.

hydrophil c., hydrophilic c., SYN emulsoid.

hydrophobic c., SYN suspensoid.

irreversible c., a c. that is not again soluble in water after having been dried at ordinary temperature. SYN unstable c.

lyophilic c., SYN emulsoid.

lyophobic c., SYN suspensoid.

protective c., a c. that has the power of preventing the precipitation of suspensoids under the influence of an electrolyte.

c. pseudomilium, SYN colloid milium.

reversible c., a c. that is again soluble in water after having been dried at ordinary temperature. SYN stable c.

stable c., SYN reversible c.

styptic c., SYN styptic *collodion*.

suspension c., SYN suspensoid.

thyroid c., the semifluid material that occupies the lumen of thyroid follicles; it mainly contains thyroglobulin.

unstable c., SYN irreversible c.

col·loi·dal (ko-loyd'ăl). Denoting or characteristic of a colloid.

col·loi·din (ko-loy'din). SYN colloid (3).

col·loid mil·i·um (kol'loyd mil'ē-ŭm). Yellow papules developing in sun-damaged skin of the head and backs of the hands, composed of colloid material in the dermis resembling amyloid but with a different ultrastructure. Filaments less than 2.0 nm in diameter are present that may be a form of elastic tissue produced by actinically damaged fibroblasts. SYN colloid pseudomilium, elastosis colloidalis conglomerata. [L. *milium*, millet]

col·loi·do·cla·sia, col·loi·do·cla·sis (ko-loy-dō-klā'sē-ă, -sis). Obsolete term for a rupture of the colloid equilibrium in the body. [colloid + G. *klasis*, fracture]

col·loi·do·clas·tic (ko-loy-dō-klas'tik). Obsolete term denoting colloidoclasia.

col·loi·do·gen (ko-loy'dō-jen). A substance capable of giving rise to a colloidal solution or suspension.

col·lox·y·lin (ko-lok'si-lin). SYN pyroxylin. [G. *kolla*, glue, + *xylinos*, woody, fr. *xylon*, wood]

col·lum, pl. **col·la** (kol'ŭm, kol'ă). ⋆official alternate term for neck. [L.]

c. anatom'icum hu'meri [TA], SYN anatomical *neck* of humerus.

c. chirur'gicum hu'meri [TA], SYN surgical *neck* of humerus.

c. cos'tae [TA], SYN *neck* of rib.

c. den'tis, SYN *neck* of tooth.

c. fem'oris [TA], SYN *neck* of femur.

c. fib'ulae [TA], SYN *neck* of fibula.

c. folli'culi pi'li, SYN *neck* of hair follicle.

c. glan'dis [TA], SYN *neck* of glans.

c. hu'meri, SEE anatomical *neck* of humerus, surgical *neck* of humerus.

c. mal'lei [TA], SYN *neck* of malleus.

c. mandib'ulae [TA], SYN *neck* of mandible.

c. os'sis fem'oris, SYN *neck* of femur.

c. ra'dii [TA], SYN *neck* of radius.

c. scap'ulae [TA], SYN *neck* of scapula.

c. ta'li [TA], SYN *neck* of talus.

c. vesicae, ⋆official alternate term for *neck* of (urinary) bladder.

c. vesi'cae biliar'is [TA], SYN *neck* of gallbladder.

c. vesi'cae fel'leae, ⋆official alternate term for *neck* of gallbladder.

col·lu·to·ri·um (kol-ū-tō'rē-ŭm). SYN mouthwash. [Mod. L. fr. *col-luo*, pp. -*lutus*, to wash thoroughly]

col·lu·tory (kol'ū-tor-ē). SYN mouthwash. [L. *colluere*, to rinse]

col·lyr·i·um (ko-lir'ē-ŭm). Originally, any preparation for the eye; now, an eyewash. [G. *kollyrion*, poultice, eye salve]

colo-. The colon. [G. *kolon*]

col·o·bo·ma (kol-ō-bō'mă). Any defect, congenital, pathologic, or artificial, especially of the eye due to incomplete closure of the optic fissure. [G. *kolobōma*, lit., the part taken away in mutilation, fr. *koloboō*, to dock, mutilate]

c. of choroid, a congenital defect of the choroid and retinal pigment epithelium exposing the sclera; the defect is usually situated below the optic disk in the region of the fetal (choroid) fissure.

Fuchs c., a congenital inferior crescent on the choroid at the edge of the optic disk; not associated with myopia. SYN congenital conus.

c. i'ridis, (1) retention of the choroid fissure causing a congenital cleft of the iris, often associated with c. of the choroid; **(2)**

obsolete term for the iris defect resulting from a large surgical iridectomy.

c. len'tis, a segment of the lens equator devoid of zonular fibers, giving the appearance of a notch.

c. lo'buli, congenital fissure of the lobule of the ear.

macular c., a defect of the central retina as a result of arrested development or intrauterine retinal inflammation.

c. of optic nerve, a congenital notch in the formation of the optic nerve, appearing as a craterlike excavation at the optic disk. SEE optic *pit*.

c. palpebra'le, a congenital notch in the eyelid margin.

c. of vitreous, a congenital indentation of the vitreous body by mesenchyme; associated with severe myopia.

co·lo·cen·te·sis (kō'lō-sen-tē'sis). Puncture of the colon with a trochar or scalpel to relieve distention. SYN colipuncture, colopuncture. [colo- + G. *kentēsis,* a puncture]

co·lo·col·ic (kō-lō-kol'ik). From colon to colon; said of a spontaneous or induced anastomosis between two parts of the colon.

co·lo·co·los·to·my (kō'lō-kō-los'tō-mē). Establishment of a communication between two noncontinuous segments of the colon. [colo- + colo- + G. *stoma,* mouth]

col·o·cynth (kol'ō-sinth). The peeled dried fruit of *Citrullus colcynthis* (family Cucurbitaceae), an herb of the sandy shores of the Mediterranean, resembling somewhat the watermelon plant; formerly widely used as a cathartic and laxative. SYN bitter apple. [G. *kolokynthē,* the round gourd or pumpkin]

co·lo·cys·to·plas·ty (kō-lō-sis'tō-plas-tē). Enlargement of the urinary bladder by attaching a segment of colon to it.

co·lo·en·ter·i·tis (kō'lō-en-ter-ī'tis). SYN enterocolitis.

co·lo·hep·a·to·pexy (kō-lō-hep'ă-tō-pek'sē). Attachment of the colon to the liver by adhesions. [colo- + G. *hēpar (hēpat-),* liver, + *pēxis,* fixation]

co·lol·y·sis (kō-lol'i-sis). Procedure of freeing the colon from adhesions. [colo- + G. *lysis,* loosening]

col·o·min·ic ac·id (kol-ō-min'ik). Polymer of α(1,5)-*N*-acetylneuraminic acid; found in *Escherichia coli.*

co·lon (kō'lon) [TA]. The division of the large intestine extending from the cecum to the rectum. [G. *kolon*]

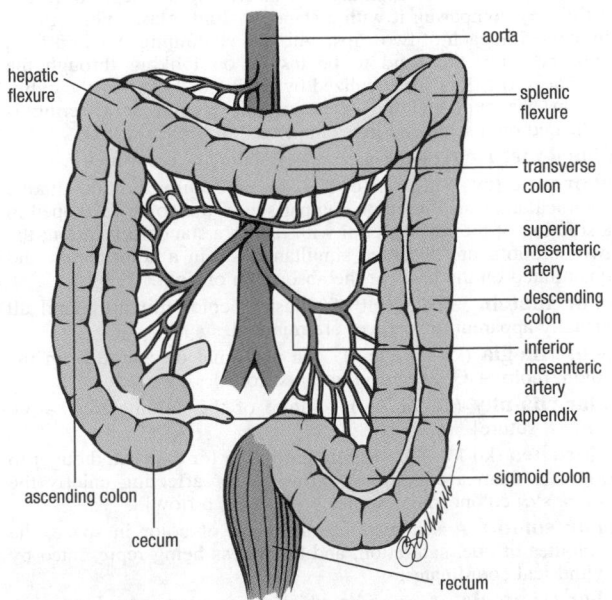

colon: anatomy and blood supply

hepatic flexure

aorta

splenic flexure

transverse colon

superior mesenteric artery

descending colon

inferior mesenteric artery

appendix

sigmoid colon

ascending colon

cecum

rectum

c. ascen'dens [TA], SYN ascending c.

ascending c. [TA], the portion of the c. between the ileocecal orifice and the right colic flexure. SYN c. ascendens [TA].

c. descen'dens [TA], SYN descending c.

descending c. [TA], the part of the c. extending from the left colic flexure to the pelvic brim. SYN c. descendens [TA].

giant c., SYN megacolon.

iliac c., that portion of the descending c. which occupies the left iliac fossa, between the crest of the left ilium and the pelvic brim.

irritable c., tendency to colonic hyperperistalsis, sometimes with colicky pains and diarrhea.

lead-pipe c., the scarred rigid c. of advanced ulcerative colitis. SYN stove-pipe c.

c. pelvi'num, SYN sigmoid c.

sigmoid c. [TA], the part of the c. describing an S-shaped curve between the pelvic brim and the third sacral segment; it is continuous with the rectum. SYN c. sigmoideum [TA], c. pelvinum, flexura sigmoidea, sigmoid flexure.

c. sigmoi'deum [TA], SYN sigmoid c.

spastic c., nonspecific term used to describe symptoms such as abdominal pain, flatulence, and alternating diarrhea with constipation thought to reflect increased muscular function of the colon.

stove-pipe c., SYN lead-pipe c.

transverse c. [TA], the part of the c. between the right and left colic flexures. It may extend somewhat transversely across the abdomen, but more often sags centrally, frequently to subumbilical levels. SYN c. transversum [TA].

c. transver'sum [TA], SYN transverse c.

co·lon·al·gia (ko-lon-al'jē-ă). Rarely used term for pain in the colon. [colon + G. *algos,* pain]

co·lon·ic (ko-lon'ik). Relating to the colon.

col·o·ni·za·tion (kol'on-i-zā'shŭn). **1.** SYN innidiation. **2.** The formation of compact population groups of the same type of microorganism, as the colonies that develop when a bacterial cell begins reproducing. **3.** The care of certain persons, e.g., lepers, mental patients, in community groups.

genetic c., propagation of a gene by a host into which the gene has been introduced, naturally or artificially.

co·lon·o·gram (ko-lon'ō-gram). Graphic recording of movements of the colon.

co·lo·nom·e·ter (kō'lō-nom'ĕ-ter). A device for counting bacterial colonies.

co·lon·op·a·thy (kō-lŏ-nop'ă-thē). Rarely used term for any disordered condition of the colon. SYN colopathy.

fibrosing c., colonic fibrosis seen in cystic fibrosis patients, thought to be due to pancreatins.

co·lon·or·rha·gia (kō-lon-ō-rā'jē-ă). Rarely used term for colorrhagia.

co·lon·or·rhea (kō'lon-ō-rē'ă). SYN colorrhea.

co·lon·o·scope (kō-lon'ō-skōp). A long, flexible fiberoptic endoscope.

co·lon·os·co·py (kō-lon-os'kŏ-pē). Visual examination of the inner surface of the colon by means of a colonoscope. SYN coloscopy. [colon + G. *skopeō,* to view]

col·o·ny (kol'ŏ-nē). **1.** A group of cells growing on a solid nutrient surface, each arising from the multiplication of an individual cell; a clone. **2.** A group of people with similar interests, living in a particular location or area. [L. *colonia,* a colony]

daughter c., a secondary c. growing on the surface of an older c.; it is smaller and may have characteristics different from those of the mother c.

filamentous c., in bacteriology, a c. composed of long, interwoven, irregularly disposed threads.

H c., a c. of motile organisms forming a thin film of growth. Cf. O c. [Ger. *Hauch,* breath]

lenticular c., a bacterial c. shaped like a lentil or a double-convex lens.

mother c., a c. which gives rise to a secondary c. (a daughter c.), the latter growing on the surface of the former; the mother c. is larger than the daughter c., and the characteristics of the c.'s may differ.

mucoid c., a c. showing viscous or sticky growth typical of an organism producing large quantities of a carbohydrate capsule.

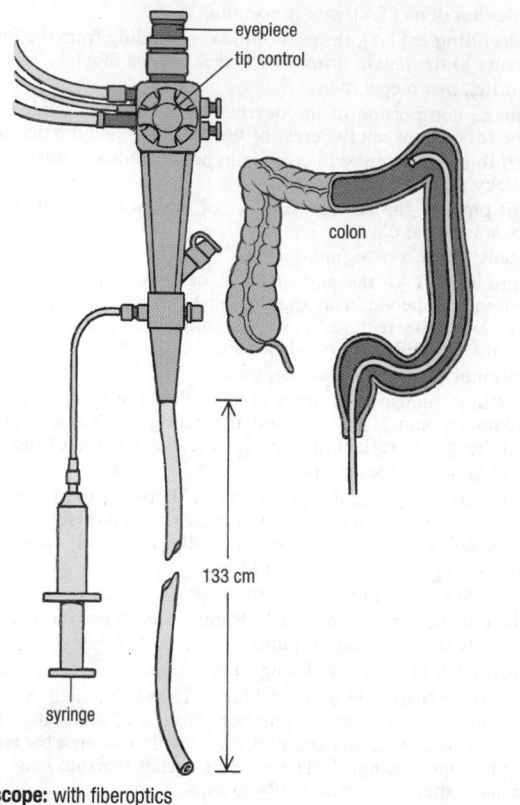

eyepiece
tip control
colon
133 cm
syringe

colonoscope: with fiberoptics

O c., growth of a nonmotile bacterium in discrete, compact c.'s in contrast to a film of growth produced by some motile bacteria. Cf. H c. [Ger. *ohne Hauch*, without breath]

rough c., a bacterial c. with a granular, flattened surface; this type of c. is usually associated with loss of virulence with respect to that of smooth c.'s.

smooth c., a bacterial c. with a glistening, rounded surface; this type of c. is usually associated with increased virulence with respect to that of rough c.'s.

spheroid c., a c. of protozoa in which the individual cells are held together in a coherent spherical mass by a gelatinoid material.

co·lop·a·thy (kō-lop′ă-thē). SYN colonopathy.

co·lo·pex·os·to·my (kō′lō-peks-os′tō-mē). Rarely used term for establishment of connection between the lumen of the colon and the skin after the colon's fixation to the abdominal wall. [colo- + G. *pēxis*, fixation, + *stoma*, mouth]

co·lo·pex·ot·o·my (kō′lō-pek-sot′ō-mē). Rarely used term for incision into the colon after its fixation to the abdominal wall. [colo- + G. *pēxis*, fixation, + *tomē*, incision]

col·o·pexy (kol′ō-pek-sē). Attachment of a portion of the colon to the abdominal wall. [colo- + G. *pēxis*, fixation]

co·lo·pho·ny (kō-lof′ō-nē). SYN rosin. [*Colophon*, Summit, a town in Ionia]

co·lo·pli·ca·tion (kō′lō-pli-kā′shŭn). Reduction of the lumen of a dilated colon by making folds or tucks in its walls. SYN coliplication. [colo- + Mod. L. *plica*, fold]

co·lo·proc·ti·tis (kō′lō-prok-tī′tis). Inflammation of both colon and rectum. SYN colorectitis, proctocolitis, rectocolitis. [colo- + G. *prōktos*, anus (rectum), + *-itis*, inflammation]

co·lo·proc·tos·to·my (kō′lō-prok-tos′tō-mē). Establishment of a communication between the rectum and a discontinuous segment of the colon. SYN colorectostomy. [colo- + G. *prōktos*, anus (rectum), + *stoma*, mouth]

co·lop·to·sis, co·lop·to·sia (kō-lop-tō′sis, -tō′sē-ă). Downward displacement, or prolapse, of the colon, especially of the transverse portion. SYN coleoptosis. [colo- + G. *ptōsis*, a falling]

co·lo·punc·ture (kō-lō-pŭnk′choor). SYN colocentesis.

col·or (kŭl′ŏr). **1.** That aspect of the appearance of objects and light sources that may be specified as to hue, lightness (brightness), and saturation. **2.** That portion of the visible (370–760 nm) electromagnetic spectrum specified as to wavelength, luminosity, and purity. [L.]

complementary c.'s, pairs of different colors of light that produce white light when combined.

confusion c.'s, a set of c.'s (usually of colored wools), cream, buff, pale blue, gray, brown, green, violet, etc., used in tests for c. blindness.

extrinsic c., c. applied to the external surface of a dental prosthesis.

intrinsic c., the addition of c. pigment within the material of a dental prosthesis.

opponent c., pairs of c. that share c. channels in the retina (red-green, blue-yellow, black-white).

primary c., the three c.'s of the retinal cone pigments (red, green, blue) that may be combined to match any hue. SYN simple c.

pure c., a visual sensation produced by light of a specific wavelength.

reflected c.'s, those c.'s seen in light falling upon a pigmented surface.

saturated c., a c. containing a minimum amount of whiteness.

simple c., SYN primary c.

structural c., a c. created by an optical effect (e.g., via interference, refraction, or diffraction). Many naturally occurring blues fall in this class. Cf. natural *pigment*. SYN schemochromes.

tone c., SYN timbre.

co·lo·rec·tal (kol′ō-rek′tăl). Relating to the colon and rectum, or to the entire large bowel.

co·lo·rec·ti·tis (kō′lō-rek-tī′tis). SYN coloproctitis.

co·lo·rec·tos·to·my (kō′lō-rek-tos′tō-mē). SYN coloproctostomy.

col·or·im·e·ter (kŏl-er-im′ĕ-ter). An optic device for determining the color and/or intensity of the color of a liquid. SYN chromatometer, chromometer.

Duboscq c., an early apparatus for measuring the depth of tint in a fluid by comparing it with a standard fluid; glass cylinders are immersed in each of two cups, with one containing standard fluid and the other the fluid to be tested; on looking through the cylinders, the tints are equalized by raising or lowering the cylinder in one cup, and the extent of this raising or lowering is indicated on a scale and gives the exact difference in tint.

col·or·i·met·ric (kŏl-er-i-met′rik). Relating to colorimetry.

col·or·im·e·try (kol-er-im′ĕ-trē). A procedure for quantitative chemical analysis, based on comparison of the color developed in a solution of the test material with that in a standard solution; the two solutions are observed simultaneously in a colorimeter, and quantitated on the basis of the absorption of light.

col·or match. The result of adjusting color mixtures until all visually apparent differences are minimal.

col·or·rha·gia (kō-lō-rā′jē-ă). An abnormal discharge from the colon. [colo- + G. *rhēgnymi*, to burst forth]

col·or·rha·phy (kō-lŏr′ă-fē). Suture of the colon. [colo- + G. *rhaphē*, suture]

col·or·rhea (kō-lō-rē′ă). Rarely used term for diarrhea thought to originate from a condition confined to or affecting chiefly the colon. SYN colonorrhea. [colo- + G. *rhoia*, a flow]

col·or sol·id. A schematic arrangement of color in space, the attributes of hue, saturation, and brightness being represented by cylindrical coordinates.

col·or tri·an·gle. A graph on which chromaticity coordinates are plotted.

co·los·co·py (kō-los′kŏ-pē). SYN colonoscopy. [colo- + G. *skopeō*, to view]

co·lo·sig·moi·dos·to·my (kō′lō-sig-moy-dos′tŏ-mē). Establishment of an anastomosis between any other part of the colon and the sigmoid colon.

co·los·to·my (kō-los'tō-mē). Establishment of an artificial connection between the lumen of the colon and the skin. [colo- + G. *stoma*, mouth]

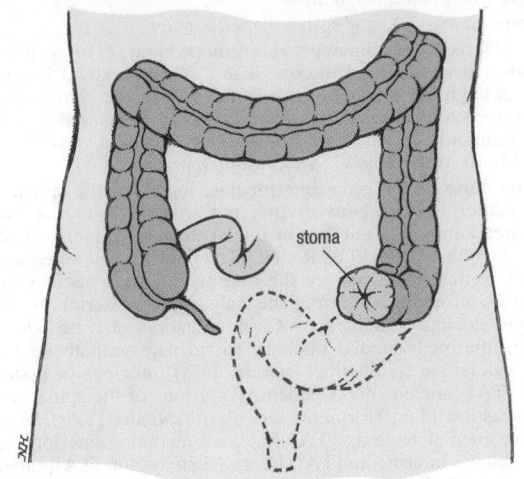

colostomy

co·los·tror·rhea (kō-los-trōr-rē'ă). Abnormally profuse secretion of colostrum. [colostrum, + G. *rhoia*, flow]

co·los·trous (kō-los'trŭs). Containing colostrum.

co·los·trum (kō-los'trŭm). A thin white opalescent fluid, the first milk secreted at the termination of pregnancy; it differs from the milk secreted later by containing more lactalbumin and lactoprotein; c. is also rich in antibodies which confer passive immunity to the newborn. SYN foremilk. [L.]

co·lot·o·my (kō-lot'ō-mē). Incision into the colon. [colo- + G. *tomē*, incision]

Col·our In·dex. A publication concerned with the chemistry of dyes, with each listed dye identified by a five-digit C.I. number, e.g., methylene blue is C.I. 52015.

△**colp-.** SEE colpo-.

col·pa·tre·sia (kol-pa-trē'zē-ă). SYN vaginal *atresia*. [colp- + G. *atrētos*, imperforate]

col·pec·ta·sis, col·pec·ta·sia (kol-pek'tă-sis, -pek-tā'si-ă). Distention of the vagina. [colp- + G. *aktasis*, stretching]

col·pec·to·my (kol-pek'tō-mē). SYN vaginectomy. [colp- + G. *ektomē*, excision]

△**colpo-, colp-.** The vagina. SEE ALSO vagino-. [G. *kolpos*, fold or hollow]

col·po·cele (kol'pō-sēl). 1. A hernia projecting into the vagina. SYN vaginocele. 2. SYN colpoptosis. [colpo- + G. *kēlē*, hernia]

col·po·clei·sis (kol-pō-klī'sis). Operation for obliterating the lumen of the vagina. [colpo- + G. *kleisis*, closure]

col·po·cys·to·plas·ty (kol-pō-sis'tō-plas-tē). Plastic surgery to repair the vesicovaginal wall. [colpo- + G. *kystis*, bladder, + *plastos*, formed]

col·po·cys·tot·o·my (kol'pō-sis-tot'ō-mē). Incision into the bladder through the vagina. [colpo- + G. *kystis*, bladder, + *tomē*, incision]

col·po·cys·to·u·re·ter·ot·o·my (kol'pō-sis'tō-ū-rē-ter-ot'ō-mē). Incision into the ureter by way of the vagina and the bladder. [colpo- + G. *kystis*, bladder, + *ourēter*, ureter, + *tomē*, incision]

col·po·dyn·ia (kol-pō-din'ē-ă). SYN vaginodynia. [colpo- + G. *odynē*, pain]

col·po·hys·ter·ec·to·my (kol'pō-his-ter-ek'tō-mē). SYN vaginal *hysterectomy*. [colpo- + G. *hystera*, uterus, + *ektomē*, excision]

col·po·hys·ter·o·pexy (kol-pō-his'ter-ō-pek-sē). Operation for fixation of uterus performed through the vagina. [colpo- + G. *hystera*, uterus, + *pēxis*, fixation]

col·po·hys·ter·ot·o·my (kol'pō-his-ter-ot'ō-mē). SYN vaginal *hysterotomy*. [colpo- + G. *hystera*, uterus, + *tomē*, incision]

col·po·mi·cro·scope (kol-pō-mī'krō-skōp). Special microscope for direct visual examination of the cervical tissue.

col·po·mi·cros·co·py (kol'pō-mī-kros'kŏ-pē). Direct observation and study of cells in the vagina and cervix magnified in vivo, in the undisturbed tissue, by means of a colpomicroscope.

col·po·my·co·sis (kol'pō-mī-kō'sis). SYN vaginomycosis.

col·po·my·o·mec·to·my (kol'pō-mī-ō-mek'tō-mē). SYN vaginal *myomectomy*. [colpo- + myoma + G. *ektomē*, excision]

col·po·per·i·ne·o·plas·ty (kol'pō-pār-i-nē'ō-plas-tē). SYN vagino-perineoplasty. [colpo- + perineum, + G. *plastos*, formed]

col·po·per·i·ne·or·rha·phy (kol'pō-pār-i-nē-ōr'ă-fē). SYN vagi-noperineorrhaphy. [colpo- + perineum, + G. *rhaphē*, sewing]

col·po·pexy (kol'pō-pek-sē). SYN vaginofixation. [colpo- + G. *pēxis*, fixation]

col·po·plas·ty (kol'pō-plas-tē). SYN vaginoplasty. [colpo- + G. *plastos*, formed]

col·po·poi·e·sis (kol'pō-poy-ē'sis). Surgical construction of a vagina. [colpo- + G. *poiēsis*, a making]

col·po·pto·sis, col·po·pto·sia (kol'pō-tō'sis, -tō'sē-ă; kol-pop-tō'sis). Prolapse of the vaginal walls. SYN colpocele (2). [colpo- + G. *ptōsis*, a falling]

col·po·rec·to·pexy (kol-pō-rek'tō-pek-sē). Repair of a prolapsed rectum by suturing it to the wall of the vagina. [colpo- + rectum + G. *pēxis*, fixation]

col·por·rha·phy (kol-pōr'ă-fē). Repair of a rupture of the vagina by excision and suturing of the edges of the tear. [colpo- + G. *rhaphē*, suture]

col·por·rhex·is (kol-pō-rek'sis). SYN vaginal *laceration*. [colpo- + G. *rhēxis*, rupture]

col·po·scope (kol'pō-skōp). Endoscopic instrument that magnifies cells of the vagina and cervix in vivo to allow direct observation and study of these tissues.

col·pos·co·py (kol-pos'kŏ-pē). Examination of vagina and cervix by means of an endoscope. [colpo- + G. *skopeō*, to view]

Colposcopy is used chiefly to identify areas of cervical dysplasia in women with abnormal Pap smears and as an aid in biopsy or excision procedures including cautery, cryotherapy, laser vaporization, and loop electrosurgical excision. The colposcope is a stationary instrument with self-contained lighting and magnification adjustable from 2× to 20× or higher. It is used in conjunction with a standard vaginal speculum to view the cervix, particularly the transformation zone, and the vaginal mucosa. A green filter enhances visualization of blood vessels and identification of abnormal (punctate, mosaic, or atypical) vascular patterns. Application of 5% acetic acid solution accentuates areas of increased cellular protein and increased nuclear density, which are likely to represent zones of squamous cell change. Lugol solution (iodine-potassium iodide), which stains only squamous epithelial cells that have a normal glycogen content, may also be applied to delineate abnormal squamous epithelium. Colposcopically directed cervical biopsy is the procedure of choice following a Pap smear showing atypical squamous cells of uncertain significance, low-grade or high-grade squamous intraepithelial lesions, koilocytosis, carcinoma in situ, or higher grade carcinomas.

col·po·spasm (kol'pō-spazm). Spasmodic contraction of the vagina.

col·po·stat (kol'pō-stat). Appliance for use in the vagina, such as a radium applicator, for treatment of cancer of the cervix. [colpo- + G. *statos*, standing]

col·po·ste·no·sis (kol'pō-sten-ō'sis). Narrowing of the lumen of the vagina. [colpo- + G. *stenōsis*, narrowing]

col·po·ste·not·o·my (kol'pō-sten-ot'ō-mē). Surgical correction of a colpostenosis. [colpo- + G. *stenōsis*, narrowing, + *tomē*, incision]

col·po·sus·pen·sion (kol′pō-sus-pen′shun). Suture fixation of the lateral vaginal fornix to Cooper ligament on each side, as a modification and enhancement of the standard Marshall-Marchetti-Kranz urethrovesical suspension for stress urinary incontinence due to cystocele. [colpo- + suspension]

col·pot·o·my (kol-pot′ō-mē). A cutting operation in the vagina. SYN coleotomy, vaginotomy. [colpo- + G. *tomē*, incision]

col·po·u·re·ter·ot·o·my (kol′pō-ū-rē-ter-ot′ō-mē). Incision into a ureter through the vagina. [colpo- + G. *tomē*, incision]

col·po·xe·ro·sis (kol-pō-zē-rō′sis). Abnormal dryness of the vaginal mucous membrane. [colpo- + G. *xērōsis*, dryness]

Col·ti·vi·rus (kol′tē-vī-rus). A genus in the family Reoviridae that causes Colorado tick fever. [*Colo*rado *ti*ck fever + virus]

Co·lu·bri·dae (kol-ū′bri-dē). A family of largely nonpoisonous or mildly poisonous snakes comprising over 1000 species, found in North and South America, Asia, and Africa. [L. *coluber*, serpent]

co·lum·bi·um (Cb) (kol-ŭm′bē-ŭm). Former name for niobium. [*Columbia*, name for America]

col·u·mel·la, pl. **col·u·mel·lae** (kol-oo-mel′ă, -mel′ē). **1.** A column, or a small column. SYN columnella. **2.** In fungi, a sterile invagination of a sporangium, as in Zygomycetes. [L. dim. of *columna*, column]

c. coch′leae, SYN *modiolus* of angle of mouth.

c. na′si, the fleshy lower margin (termination) of the nasal septum.

col·umn (kol′ŭm) [TA]. **1.** An anatomic part or structure in the form of a pillar or cylindric funiculus. SEE ALSO fascicle. **2.** A vertical object (usually cylindrical), mass, or formation. SYN columna [TA]. [L. *columna*]

affinity c., SYN affinity *chromatography*.

anal c.'s [TA], a number of vertical ridges in the mucous membrane of the upper half of the anal canal formed as the caliber of the canal is sharply reduced from that of the rectal ampulla. SYN columnae anales [TA], Morgagni c.'s, rectal c.'s.

anterior c. [TA], the pronounced, ventrally oriented ridge of gray matter in each half of the spinal cord; it corresponds to the anterior or ventral horn appearing in transverse sections of the cord, and contains the motor neurons innervating the skeletal musculature of the trunk, neck, and extremities. SEE ALSO gray c.'s. SYN columna anterior [TA].

anterior gray c., SYN central and lateral intermediate *substances*, under *substance*.

anterior c. of medulla oblongata, SYN *pyramid* of medulla oblongata.

anterolateral c. of spinal cord, SYN lateral *funiculus*.

Bertin c.'s, SYN renal c.'s.

branchial efferent c., SYN special visceral efferent c.

Burdach c., SYN cuneate *fasciculus*.

Clarke c., SYN posterior thoracic *nucleus*.

dorsal c. of spinal cord, SYN posterior c.

c. of fornix [TA], that part of the fornix that curves down rostral to the dorsal thalamus and adjacent to the interventricular foramen of Monro, then continues through the hypothalamus to the mamillary body; consisting primarily of fibers originating in the hippocampus and subiculum, the c. of fornix is the direct continuation of the body of the fornix. SYN columna fornicis [TA], anterior pillar of fornix.

general somatic afferent c., in the embryo, a c. of gray matter in the hindbrain and spinal cord, represented in the adult by the sensory nuclei of the trigeminal nerve and relay cells in the dorsal horn.

general somatic efferent c., a c. of gray matter in the embryo, represented in the adult by the nuclei of the oculomotor, trochlear, abducens, and hypoglossal nerves and by motor neurons of the ventral horn of the spinal cord.

general visceral afferent c., a c. of gray matter in the hindbrain and spinal cord of the embryo, developing into the nucleus of the solitary tract and relay cells of the spinal cord.

general visceral efferent c., a c. of gray matter in the hindbrain and spinal cord of the embryo, represented in the adult by the

dorsal nucleus of the vagus, the superior and inferior salivatory and Edinger-Westphal nuclei and the visceral motor neurons of the spinal cord.

Goll c., SYN gracile *fasciculus*.

Gowers c., SYN anterior spinocerebellar *tract*.

gray c.'s, the three somewhat ridge-shaped masses of gray matter (anterior, posterior, and intermediate c.'s) that extend longitudinally through the center of each lateral half of the spinal cord; in transverse sections these c.'s appear as gray horns and are therefore commonly called ventral or anterior, dorsal or posterior, and lateral respectively. SYN columnae griseae [TA].

intermediate c. [TA], the intermediate region of the spinal cord gray matter located between the posterior and anterior horns. This area contains a number of nuclei that collectively comprise spinal lamina VIII [TA] of Rexed. The nuclei of the intermediate c., or intermediate zone, are the intermediolateral nucleus in the lateral horn, central intermediate substance, posterior or dorsal thoracic nucleus (nucleus of Clarke), lateral intermediate substance, intermediomedial nucleus, sacral parasympathetic nuclei [TA] (nuclei parasympathici sacrales [TA]), nucleus of pudendal nerve [TA] (nucleus nervi pudendi), portions of the spinal reticular formation [TA] (formatio reticularis spinalis [TA]), and the anterior medial nucleus [TA] (nucleus medialis anterior [TA]). SYN columna intermedia [TA], intermediate region [TA], intermediate zone [TA].

intermediolateral cell c. of spinal cord, SYN intermediolateral *nucleus*.

lateral c., a slight protrusion of the gray matter of the spinal cord into the lateral funiculus of either side, especially marked in the thoracic region where it encloses preganglionic motor neurons of the sympathetic division of the autonomic nervous system; it corresponds to the lateral horn appearing in transverse sections of the spinal cord. SEE ALSO gray c.'s. SYN columna lateralis, lateral c. of spinal cord.

lateral c. of spinal cord, SYN lateral c.

Lissauer c., SYN dorsolateral *fasciculus*.

Morgagni c.'s, SYN anal c.'s.

posterior c. [TA], the pronounced, dorsolaterally oriented ridge of gray matter in each lateral half of the spinal cord, corresponding to the posterior or dorsal horn appearing in transverse sections of the cord. SYN columna posterior [TA], dorsal c. of spinal cord, posterior c. of spinal cord [TA].

posterior c. of spinal cord, (1) SYN posterior c; (2) in clinical parlance, the term often refers to the posterior funiculus of the spinal cord.

rectal c.'s, SYN anal c.'s.

renal c.'s [TA], the prolongations of cortical substance separating the pyramids of the kidney. SYN columnae renales [TA], Bertin c.'s.

Rolando c., a slight ridge on either side of the medulla oblongata related to the descending trigeminal tract and nucleus.

rugal c.'s of vagina, SYN vaginal c.'s.

Sertoli c.'s, SEE Sertoli *cells*, under *cell*.

special somatic afferent c., a c. of gray matter in the hindbrain of the embryo, represented in the adult by the nuclei of the auditory and vestibular nerves.

special visceral efferent c., a c. of gray matter in the hindbrain of the embryo, represented in the adult by the trigeminal and facial nuclei and the nucleus ambiguus. SYN branchial efferent c.

spinal c., SYN vertebral c.

c. of Spitzka-Lissauer, SEE dorsolateral *fasciculus*.

Stilling c., SYN posterior thoracic *nucleus*.

Türck c., SYN anterior corticospinal *tract*.

vaginal c.'s, two slight longitudinal ridges, anterior and posterior, in the vaginal mucous membrane, each marked by a number of transverse mucosal folds. SYN columnae rugarum, rugal c.'s of vagina.

ventral white c. [TA], SYN white *commissure*.

vertebral c. [TA], the series of vertebrae that extend from the cranium to the coccyx, providing support and forming a flexible bony case for the spinal cord. SYN columna vertebralis [TA], spine

(2) [TA], backbone, dorsal spine, rachis, spina dorsalis, spinal c., vertebrarium.

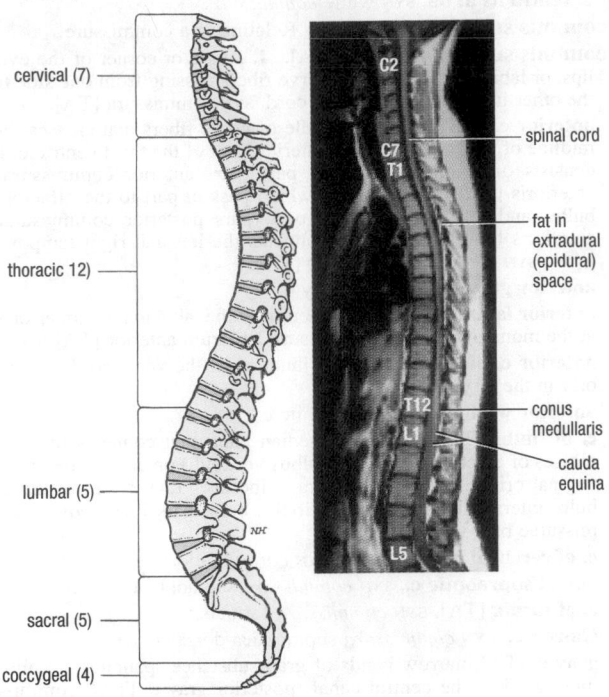

vertebral column: (left) lateral view of complete column, (right) sagittal magnetic resonance image from atlas to fifth lumbar vertebra

Labels: cervical (7), thoracic 12), lumbar (5), sacral (5), coccygeal (4); C2, C7, T1, spinal cord, fat in extradural (epidural) space, T12, L1, conus medullaris, cauda equina, L5

co·lum·na, gen. and pl. **co·lum·nae** (ko-lŭm′nă, -nē) [TA]. SYN column. [L.]

colum′nae ana′les [TA], SYN anal *columns*, under *column*.

c. ante′rior [TA], SYN anterior *column*.

colum′nae car′neae, SYN *trabeculae* carneae (of right and left ventricles), under *trabecula*.

c. for′nicis [TA], SYN *column* of fornix.

colum′nae gris′eae [TA], SYN gray *columns*, under *column*.

c. intermedia [TA], SYN intermediate *column*.

c. latera′lis, SYN lateral *column*.

c. poste′rior [TA], SYN posterior *column*.

colum′nae rena′les [TA], SYN renal *columns*, under *column*.

colum′nae ruga′rum, SYN vaginal *columns*, under *column*.

c. vertebra′lis [TA], SYN vertebral *column*.

co·lum·nel·la, pl. **col·um·nel·lae** (ko-lŭm-nel′ă, -nel′ē). SYN columella (1). [L. dim. of *columna*, a column; another form of *columella*]

co·ly·pep·tic (kō-lē-pep′tik). Rarely used term for retarding digestion. [G. *kōlyō*, to hinder, + *pepsis*, digestion]

△**com-**. SEE con-.

co·ma (kō′mă). **1.** A state of profound unconsciousness from which one cannot be roused; may be due to the action of an ingested toxic substance or of one formed in the body, to trauma, or to disease. [G. *kōma*, deep sleep, trance] **2.** An aberration of spherical lenses; occurring in cases of oblique incidence (e.g., the image of a point becomes comet-shaped). [G. *kome*, hair] **3.** SYN coma *aberration*.

delayed c. after hypoxia, c. that develops a few days to 3 weeks after an acute hypoxic insult; the latter was usually severe enough to cause an initial bout of coma, which cleared, and was followed by a transient interval of apparent normality. SYN severe postanoxic encephalopathy.

diabetic c., c. that develops in severe and inadequately treated cases of diabetes mellitus and is commonly fatal, unless appropri-

ate therapy is instituted promptly; results from reduced oxidative metabolism of the central nervous system that, in turn, stems from severe ketoacidosis and possibly also from the histotoxic action of the ketone bodies and disturbances in water and electrolyte balance. SYN Kussmaul c.

hepatic c., c. that occurs with advanced hepatic insufficiency and portal-systemic shunts, caused by elevated blood ammonia levels; characteristic findings include asterixis in the precoma stage and paroxysms of bilaterally synchronous triphasic waves on EEG examination.

hyperosmolar (hyperglycemic) nonketotic c. (hī′per-os-mō-lăr), a complication seen in *diabetes* mellitus in which very marked hyperglycemia occurs (such as levels over 800 mg/dL) causing osmotic shifts in water in brain cells and resulting in coma. It can be fatal or lead to permanent neurologic damage. Ketoacidosis does not occur in these cases. SYN nonketotic hyperglycemia.

hypoglycemic c., a metabolic encephalopathy caused by hypoglycemia; usually seen in diabetics, and due to exogenous insulin excess.

hypoventilation c., coma seen with advanced lung failure and resultant hypoventilation. SYN CO_2 narcosis, hypoxic-hypercarbic encephalopathy, pulmonary encephalopathy.

Kussmaul c., SYN diabetic c.

metabolic c., coma resulting from diffuse failure of neuronal metabolism, caused by such abnormalities as intrinsic disorders of neuron or glial cell metabolism, or extracerebral disorders that produce intoxication or electrolyte imbalances.

thyrotoxic c., c. preceding death in severe hyperthyroidism, as in thyroid storm or thyrotoxic crisis.

trance c., SYN lethargic *hypnosis*.

uremic c., a metabolic encephalopathy caused by renal failure.

co·ma·tose (kō′mă-tōs). In a state of coma.

com·bi·na·tion (kom-bi-nā′shŭn). **1.** The act of combining (i.e., by joining, uniting, or otherwise bringing into close association) separate entities. **2.** The state of being so combined.

binary c., the name of a species of bacteria consisting of two parts: a generic name and a specific epithet.

new c., the new name that results from the transfer of a microorganism from one genus to another; the generic name changes but, in most cases, the specific epithet remains the same.

com·bi·na·to·ri·al (kom′bin-ă-tor′ē-ăl). Any system using a random assortment of components at any positions in the linear arrangement of atoms, i.e., a combinatorial library of mutations could contain positions where all four bases have been randomly inserted.

com·bus·ti·ble (kom-bus′ti-bl). Capable of combustion.

com·bus·tion (kom-bŭs′chŭn). Burning, the rapid oxidation of any substance accompanied by the production of heat and light. [L. *comburo*, pp. -*bustus*, to burn up]

slow c., SEE decay.

spontaneous c., the ignition of a mass of material by heat developed within it by the oxidation of the substances composing it without external ignition.

Comby, Jules, French pediatrician, 1853–1947. SEE C. *sign*.

com·e·do, pl. **com·e·dos**, **com·e·do·nes** (kom′ē-dō, kō-mē′dō; kom′ē-dōz; kom-ē-dō′nēz). A dilated hair follicle infundibulum filled with keratin squamae, bacteria, particularly *Propionibacterium acnes*, and sebum; the primary lesion of acne vulgaris. [L. a glutton, fr. *com-edo*, to eat up]

closed c., a c. with a narrow or obstructed opening on the skin surface; closed comedos may rupture, producing a low-grade dermal inflammatory reaction. SYN whitehead (2).

open c., a c. with a wide opening on the skin surface capped with a melanin-containing blackened mass of epithelial debris.

solar c., SYN Favre-Racouchot *disease*.

com·e·do·car·ci·no·ma (kō-mē′dō-kar-si-nō′mă). Form of carcinoma of the breast or other organ in which plugs of necrotic malignant cells may be expressed from the ducts.

com·e·do·gen·ic (kom′ē-dō-jen′ik). Tending to promote the formation of comedones. [comedo + G. *genesis*, production]

com·e·do·ne·cro·sis (kom′ē-dō-nek-rō′sis). A type of necrosis occurring with glands in which there is central luminal inflammation with devitalized cells, usually occurring in the breast in intraductal carcinoma. [comedo + necrosis]

co·mes, pl. **com·i·tes** (kō'mēz, kom'i-tēz). A blood vessel accompanying another vessel or a nerve; the veins accompanying an artery, often two in number, are called venae comitantes or venae comites. [L. a companion, fr. *com-*, together, + *eo*, pp. *itus*, to go]

com·i·tance (kom'ē-tans). A characteristic of strabismus in which the misalignment of the eyes is maintained in all directions of gaze.

com·i·tant (komitant). Having comitance; in a c. strabismus the same angle of misalignment of the eyes is maintained in all directions of gaze. SYN concomitant.

com·men·sal (kŏ-men'săl). **1.** Pertaining to or characterized by commensalism. **2.** An organism participating in commensalism.

com·men·sal·ism (kŏ-men'săl-izm). A symbiotic relationship in which one species derives benefit and the other is unharmed; e.g., *Entamoeba coli* in the human large intestine. Cf. metabiosis, mutualism, parasitism. [L. *con-*, with, together, + *mensa*, table]
  epizoic c., SYN phoresis (2).

com·mi·nut·ed (kom'i-noo-ted). Broken into several pieces; denoting especially a fractured bone. [L. *com-minuo*, pp. *-minutus*, to make smaller, break into pieces, fr. *minor*, less]

com·mi·nu·tion (kom-i-noo'shŭn). A breaking into several pieces.

com·mis·su·ra, gen. and pl. **com·mis·su·rae** (kom-i-sūr'ă, -sūr'ē) [TA]. SYN commissure. [L. a joining together, seam, fr. *committo*, to send together, combine]
  c. alba anterior [TA], SYN white *commissure.*
  c. al'ba posterior [TA], SYN white *commissure.*
  c. ante'rior [TA], SYN anterior *commissure.*
  c. ante'rior gris'ea, SEE *substantia* intermedia centralis.
  c. bulbor'um [TA], SYN *commissure* of bulbs.
  c. cine'rea, SYN interthalamic *adhesion.*
  c. colliculo'rum inferi'orum [TA], SEE *commissure* of inferior colliculus.
  c. colliculo'rum superio'rum [TA], SEE *commissure* of superior colliculus.
  c. epithalamica, SYN c. posterior.
  c. for'nicis [TA], the triangular subcallosal plate of commissural fibers resulting from the converging of the right and left fornix bundles which exchange numerous fibers and which curve back in the contralateral fornix to end in the hippocampus of the opposite side. SYN commissure of fornix [TA], c. hippocampi, delta fornicis, hippocampal commissure, psalterium, transverse fornix.
  c. grisea posterior [TA], SEE gray *commissure.*
  c. gris'ea, (1) SYN interthalamic *adhesion*; **(2)** SEE *substantia* intermedia centralis.
  c. grisea anterior, SEE gray *commissure.*
  c. habenula'rum [TA], the connection between the right and left habenular nuclei; the decussation of fibers of the two striae medullares, forming the dorsal portion of the peduncle of the pineal body. SYN habenular commissure [TA], commissure of habenulae.
  c. hippocam'pi, SYN c. fornicis.
  c. labio'rum [TA], SYN *commissure* of lips.
  c. labio'rum ante'rior [TA], SYN anterior labial *commissure.*
  c. labio'rum poste'rior [TA], SYN posterior labial *commissure.*
  c. lateralis palpebrum [TA], SYN lateral palpebral *commissure.*
  c. medialis palpebrum [TA], SYN medial palpebral *commissure.*
  c. palpebra'rum latera'lis, SYN lateral palpebral *commissure.*
  c. palpebra'rum media'lis, SYN medial palpebral *commissure.*
  c. poste'rior [TA], a thin band of white matter, crossing from side to side beneath the habenula of the pineal body and over the aditus ad aqueductum cerebri; it is largely composed of fibers interconnecting the left and right pretectal region and related cell groups of the midbrain; dorsally, it marks the junction of the diencephalon and mesencephalon. SYN c. epithalamica, posterior commissure.
  c. supraop'tica dorsalis [TA], the commissural fibers that lie above and behind the optic chiasm. SYN dorsal supraoptic com-

missure, Ganser commissure, Gudden commissure, Meynert commissure.
  c. ventra'lis al'ba, SYN white *commissure.*

com·mis·sur·al (kom-i-sūr'ăl). Relating to a commissure.

com·mis·sure (kom'i-shŭr) [TA]. **1.** Angle or corner of the eye, lips, or labia. **2.** A bundle of nerve fibers passing from one side to the other in the brain or spinal cord. SYN commissura [TA].
  anterior c. [TA], a round bundle of nerve fibers that crosses the midline of the brain near the anterior limit of the third ventricle. It consists of a smaller anterior part (pars anterior commissurae anterioris [TA]), the fibers of which pass in part to the olfactory bulbs, and a larger posterior part (pars posterior commissurae anterioris [TA]), which interconnects the left and right temporal lobes. SYN commissura anterior [TA].
  anterior gray c. [TA], SEE gray c.
  anterior labial c. [TA], the junction of the labia majora anteriorly at the mons pubis. SYN commissura labiorum anterior [TA].
  anterior c. of the larynx, the junction of the vocal cords anteriorly in the larynx.
  anterior white c. [TA], SYN white c.
  c. of bulbs [TA], a narrow median band that connects the two masses of erectile tissue (the bulbus vestibuli) on either side of the vaginal orifice. SYN commissura bulborum [TA], c. of vestibular bulb, intermediate part of vestibular bulb, pars intermedia commissurae bulborum.
  c. of cerebral hemispheres, SYN *corpus* callosum.
  dorsal supraoptic c., SYN *commissura* supraoptica dorsalis.
  c. of fornix [TA], SYN *commissura* fornicis.
  Ganser c., SYN *commissura* supraoptica dorsalis.
  gray c. [TA], narrow bands of gray substance spanning the midline dorsal to the central canal (posterior gray c. [TA], commissura griesa posterior [TA]) and ventral to the central canal (anterior gray c. [TA], *commissura* grisea anterior [TA])
  Gudden c., SYN *commissura* supraoptica dorsalis.
  c. of habenulae, SYN *commissura* habenularum.
  habenular c., SYN *commissura* habenularum.
  hippocampal c., SYN *commissura* fornicis.
  c. of inferior colliculus [TA], nerve fibers on the midline between the two inferior colliculi connecting the colliculi and containing some fibers originating from nontectal nuclei.
  labial c. [TA], junction of upper and lower lip which occurs at corner of mouth. SEE ALSO *angle* of mouth.
  lateral palpebral c. [TA], the union of the upper and lower eyelids adjacent to the lateral angle. SYN commissura lateralis palpebrum [TA], commissura palpebrarum lateralis.
  c. of lips, the junction of the lips lateral to the angle of the mouth. SYN commissura labiorum [TA], junction of lips.
  medial palpebral c. [TA], the union of the upper and lower eyelids adjacent to the medial angle. SYN commissura medialis palpebrum [TA], commissura palpebrarum medialis.
  Meynert c., SYN *commissura* supraoptica dorsalis.
  posterior c., SYN *commissura* posterior.
  posterior gray c. [TA], SEE gray c.
  posterior labial c. [TA], a slight fold uniting the labia majora posteriorly in front of the anus. SYN commissura labiorum posterior [TA].
  posterior c. of the larynx, SYN interarytenoid *fold.*
  c. of superior colliculus [TA], nerve fibers interconnecting corresponding and noncorresponding portions of the two superior colliculi across the midline; may contain fibers originating outside the tectum. SYN brachium colliculi superioris [TA].
  ventral white c. [TA], SYN white c.
  c. of vestibular bulb, SYN c. of bulbs.
  Wernekinck c., the decussation of the brachia conjunctiva before their entrance into the red nucleus of the tegmentum.
  white c., a narrow band of white matter that crosses the midline of the spinal cord dorsal to the central canal and posterior gray commissure (posterior white commissure [TA]) and ventral to the central canal and the anterior gray commissure (anterior white commissure [TA]). SYN anterior white c. [TA], commissura alba

anterior [TA], commissura alba posterior [TA], ventral white column [TA], ventral white c. [TA], commissura ventralis alba.

com·mis·sur·ot·o·my (kom′i-sŭr-ot′ō-mē). **1.** Surgical division of any commissure, fibrous band, or ring via an incision or disruption e.g., balloon inflation. **2.** SYN midline *myelotomy*.

mitral c., opening the narrowed mitral orifice for the relief of mitral stenosis.

com·mit·ment (kŏ-mit′ment). Legal consignment, by certification, or voluntarily, of an individual to a mental hospital or institution. [L. *com-mitto*, to deliver, consign]

com·mon ve·hi·cle spread. Spread of disease agent from a source that is common to those who acquire the disease, e.g., water, milk, air, syringe contaminated by infectious or noxious agents.

com·mo·tio (kō-mō′shē-ō). SYN concussion (2). [L. a moving, commotion, fr. *commoveo*, pp. *-motus*, to set in motion, agitate]

c. cer′ebri, SYN brain *concussion*.

c. re′tinae, concussion of the retina that may produce a milky edema in the posterior pole that clears up after a few days.

com·mu·ni·ca·ble (kŏ-mūn′i-kă-bl). Capable of being communicated or transmitted; said especially of disease.

com·mu·ni·cans, pl. **com·mu·ni·can·tes** (kŏ-mū′ni-kans, kŏ-mū-ni-kan′tēz). Communicating; connecting or joining. [L. pres. p. of *communico*, pp. *-atus*, to share with someone, make common]

com·mu·ni·ca·tion (kŏ-mū-ni-kā′shŭn). **1.** An opening or connecting passage between two structures. **2.** In anatomy, a joining or connecting, said of fibrous, solid structures, e.g., tendons and nerves. Anastomosis is incorrectly used as a synonym. **3.** Information or ideas transmitted from one party to another. [L. *com-municatio*]

human c., the production and reception of oral, written, signed, or gestured information among human beings; involves the use of symbols known as language received through the auditory, tactile, proprioceptive, and visual systems and generated through voice and speech, writing, manual signs, and gestures; c. among humans may at times involve the vestibular, olfactory, and gustatory senses.

simultaneous c., SYN total c.

total c., an approach to the education of deaf children that uses a combination of sign language, finger spelling, and oral communication. SEE ALSO oral auditory *method*, manual visual *method*, combined *methods*, under *method*. SYN simultaneous c.

com·mu·ni·ty (kŏ-mū′ni-tē). A given segment of a society or a population.

biotic c., SYN biocenosis.

therapeutic c., a specially structured mental hospital or community health center milieu that provides an effective environment for behavioral changes in patients through resocialization and rehabilitation.

com·mu·ni·ty men·tal health cen·ter. A mental health treatment center located in a neighborhood catchment area close to the homes of patients, introduced in the 1960s via new federal legislation designed to replace the large state hospitals, which usually were located in remote rural areas; features include offering a series of comprehensive services by one or more members of the four mental health professions, provision of continuity of care, participation of consumers in the centers, community location to provide accessibility, a combination of indirect or preventive and direct services, the use of program-centered as well as case-centered consultation, a requirement for program evaluation, and various linkages to a variety of health and human services.

co·mor·bid·i·ty (kō-mōr-bid′i-tē). A concomitant but unrelated pathologic or disease process; usually used in epidemiology to indicate the coexistence of two or more disease processes. [co- + L. *morbidus*, diseased]

com·pac·ta (kom-pak′tă). SYN *stratum* compactum.

com·pa·ges tho·ra·cis (kom-pā′jēz thō-rā′sis). SYN thoracic *cage.*

com·par·a·scope (kom-par′ă-skōp). A microscope accessory by means of which an observer may directly compare simultaneously

the findings in two microscopic preparations. [L. *comparo,* to compare, + G. *skopeō,* to view]

com·par·ti·men·tum. SYN compartment.

c. antebrachii anterius [TA], SYN anterior *compartment* of forearm.

c. antebrachii extensorum, ☆official alternate term for posterior *compartment* of forearm.

c. antebrachii flexorum, ☆official alternate term for anterior *compartment* of forearm.

c. antebrachii posterius [TA], SYN posterior *compartment* of forearm.

c. brachii anterius [TA], SYN anterior *compartment* of arm.

c. brachii extensorum, ☆official alternate term for posterior *compartment* of arm.

c. brachii flexorum [TA], SYN anterior *compartment* of arm.

c. brachii posterius [TA], SYN posterior *compartment* of arm.

c. cruris, SYN lateral *compartment* of leg.

c. cruris anterius [TA], SYN anterior *compartment* of leg.

c. cruris extensorum, ☆official alternate term for anterior *compartment* of leg.

c. cruris fibularium, ☆official alternate term for lateral *compartment* of leg.

c. cruris flexorum, ☆official alternate term for posterior *compartment* of leg.

c. cruris laterale peroneorum [TA], SYN lateral *compartment* of leg.

c. cruris posterius [TA], SYN posterior *compartment* of leg.

c. femoris adductorum, ☆official alternate term for medial *compartment* of thigh.

c. femoris anterius [TA], SYN anterior *compartment* of thigh.

c. femoris extensorum [TA], SYN anterior *compartment* of thigh.

c. femoris flexorum, ☆official alternate term for posterior *compartment* of thigh.

c. femoris mediale [TA], SYN medial *compartment* of thigh.

c. femoris posterius [TA], SYN posterior *compartment* of thigh.

compartment. **1.** Partitioned off portion of a larger bound space; a separate section or chamber; the compartments of the limbs are bound deeply by bones and intermuscular septa and superficially by deep fascia and generally are not in communication with the other compartments, and thus infection or increased pathologic pressure may be limited to a compartment; muscles contained within the compartments of the limbs share similar functions and innervation. **2.** A separate division; specifically, a structural or biochemical portion of a cell that is separated from the rest of the cell. SYN compartimentum.

adductor c. of thigh, ☆official alternate term for medial c. of thigh.

anterior c. of arm [TA], anterior portion of the space enclosed by the brachial fascia, separated from the posterior c. by the humerus and the lateral and medial intermuscular septa that extend from it; contains muscles that produce flexion, all innervated by the musculocutaneous nerve. SYN compartimentum brachii anterius [TA], compartimentum brachii flexorum [TA], flexor c. of arm☆.

anterior c. of forearm [TA], anterior portion of the space enclosed by the antebrachial fascia, separated from the posterior c. by the radius and ulna and by the intervening interosseous membrane; the spaces are demarcated superficially by the subcutaneous border of the ulna and the (pulse of the) radial artery; contains the pronators of the forearm, flexors of the wrist, and long flexors of the digits, innervated by the median (mostly) and ulnar nerves; is unusual among limb c.'s since it communicates via the carpal tunnel with the midpalmar space. SYN compartimentum antebrachii anterius [TA], compartimentum antebrachii flexorum☆, flexor c. of forearm☆.

anterior c. of leg [TA], anterior portion of space enclosed by the deep fascia of the leg, separated from the posterior c. by the tibia and fibula by the intervening interosseous membrane, and from the lateral c. by the anterior intermuscular septum; contains the dorsiflexors of the foot and long extensors of the toes, all innervated by the deep fibular (peroneal) nerve. SYN compartimentum cruris anterius [TA], compartimentum cruris extensorum★, extensor c. of leg★, dorsiflexor c. of leg.

anterior c. of thigh [TA], anterior portion of the space enclosed by the fascia lata, separated from the medial and lateral c.'s by the medial and lateral intermuscular septa, respectively; contains the shaft of the femur and the muscles that produce flexion at hip and/or extension at the knee, innervated by the femoral nerve. SYN compartimentum femoris anterius [TA], compartimentum femoris extensorum [TA], extensor c. of thigh★, c. of thigh for extensors of knee, c. of thigh for flexors of hip.

dorsiflexor c. of leg, SYN anterior c. of leg.

extensor c. of arm, ★official alternate term for posterior c. of arm.

extensor c. of forearm, ★official alternate term for posterior c. of forearm.

extensor c. of leg, ★official alternate term for anterior c. of leg.

extensor c. of thigh, ★official alternate term for anterior c. of thigh.

fibular c. of leg, ★official alternate term for lateral c. of leg.

flexor c. of arm, ★official alternate term for anterior c. of arm.

flexor c. of forearm, ★official alternate term for anterior c. of forearm.

flexor c. of leg, ★official alternate term for posterior c. of leg.

flexor c. of thigh, ★official alternate term for posterior c. of thigh.

lateral c. of leg [TA], lateral portion of space enclosed by the deep fascia of the leg, separated from the anterior and posterior c.'s by the anterior and posterior intermuscular septa of leg, respectively; contains evertors of the foot, innervated by the superficial fibular (peroneal) nerve. SYN compartimentum cruris laterale peroneorum [TA], compartimentum cruris fibularium★, fibular c. of leg★, peroneal c. of leg★, compartimentum cruris.

medial c. of thigh [TA], medial portion of the space enclosed by the fascia lata, separated from the anterior and posterior c.'s by the medial and posterior femoral intermuscular septa, respectively; contains muscles that adduct the thigh at the hip joint, all of which are innervated by the obturator nerve. SYN compartimentum femoris mediale [TA], adductor c. of thigh★, compartimentum femoris adductorum★.

nonplasmatic c., c. surrounded by a single biomembrane (e.g., vacuoles, lysosomes).

peroneal c. of leg, ★official alternate term for lateral c. of leg.

plantarflexor c. of leg, SYN posterior c. of leg.

plasmatic c., c. surrounded by a double biomembrane and containing polynucleotides (e.g., mitochondria).

posterior c. of arm [TA], posterior portion of the space enclosed by the brachial fascia, separated from the anterior c. by the humerus and the lateral and medial intermuscular septa that extend from it; contains the triceps muscles that extend the forearm at the elbow joint and are innervated by the radial nerve. SYN compartimentum brachii posterius [TA], compartimentum brachii extensorum★, extensor c. of arm★.

posterior c. of forearm [TA], posterior portion of the space enclosed by the antebrachial fascia, separated from the anterior c. by the radius and ulna and by the intervening interosseous membrane; the spaces are demarcated superficially by the subcutaneous border of the ulna and the (pulse of the) radial artery; contains a supinator of the forearm, extensors of the hand at the wrist, and long extensors of the digits, all innervated by the radial nerve. SYN compartimentum antebrachii posterius [TA], compartimentum antebrachii extensorum★, extensor c. of forearm★.

posterior c. of leg [TA], posterior portion of space enclosed by the deep fascia of the leg, separated from the anterior c. by the tibia and fibula by the intervening interosseous membrane, and from the lateral compartment by the posterior intermuscular septum of the leg; contains the plantarflexors of the foot and long flexors of the toes, all innervated by the tibial nerve. SYN compartimentum cruris posterius [TA], compartimentum cruris flexorum★, flexor c. of leg★, plantarflexor c. of leg.

posterior c. of thigh [TA], posterior portion of the space enclosed by the fascia lata, separated from the medial and anterior c.'s by the posterior and lateral intermuscular septa, respectively;

contains the hamstring muscles (extensor of the thigh at the hip joint and flexors of the leg at the knee joint) and the short head of the biceps; all innervated by the sciatic nerve (the former by the tibial nerve portion, the latter by the fibular nerve portion). SYN compartimentum femoris posterius [TA], compartimentum femoris flexorum★, flexor c. of thigh★, c. of thigh for extensors of hip joint, c. of thigh for flexors of knee.

c. of thigh for extensors of hip joint, SYN posterior c. of thigh.

c. of thigh for extensors of knee, SYN anterior c. of thigh.

c. of thigh for flexors of hip, SYN anterior c. of thigh.

c. of thigh for flexors of knee, SYN posterior c. of thigh.

com·part·men·ta·tion (kom-part′ment-ā′shŭn). The division of a cell into different regions, either structurally or biochemically.

com·pat·i·bil·i·ty (kom-pat-ĭ-bil′i-tē). The condition of being compatible.

com·pat·i·ble (kom-pat′ĭ-bl). 1. Capable of being mixed without undergoing destructive chemical change or exhibiting mutual antagonism; said of the elements in a properly constructed pharmaceutical mixture. 2. Denoting the ability of two biologic entities to exist together without nullification of, or deleterious effects on, the function of either; e.g., blood, tissues, or organs that cause no reaction when transfused or no rejection when transplanted. 3. Denoting satisfactory relationships between two or more people as in work or in marriage or in sexual activities. [L. con-, with, + patior, to suffer]

com·pen·sa·tion (kom-pen-sā′shŭn). 1. A process in which a tendency for a change in a given direction is counteracted by another change so that the original change is not evident. 2. An unconscious mechanism by which one tries to make up for fancied or real deficiencies. [L. com-penso, pp. -atus, to weigh together, counterbalance]

attenuation c., SYN time-gain c.

depth c., SYN time-gain c.

gene dosage c., the putative mechanism that adjusts the X-linked phenotypes of males and females to compensate for the haploid state in males and the diploid state in females. It is now largely ascribed to lyonization which compensates the mean of the dose but not its variance, which is greater in females.

time-gain c. (TGC), in ultrasonography, an increase in receiver gain with time to compensate for loss in echo amplitude with depth, usually due to attenuation. SYN attenuation c., depth c., time compensation gain, time-compensated gain, time-varied gain control, time-varied gain.

com·pen·sa·to·ry (kom-pen′să-tōr-ē). Providing compensation; making up for a deficiency or loss.

com·pe·tence (kom′pĕ-tens). 1. The quality of being competent or capable of performing an allotted function. 2. The normal tight closure of a cardiac valve. 3. The ability of a group of embryonic cells to respond to an inducer. 4. The ability of a (bacterial) cell to take up free DNA, which may lead to transformation. 5. In psychiatry, the mental ability to distinguish right from wrong and to manage one's own affairs, or to assist one's counsel in a legal proceeding. 6. The state of reactivity of a cell, tissue, or organism that allows it to respond to certain stimuli. [Fr. competence, fr. L.L. competentia, congruity]

cardiac c., ability of the ventricles to pump the blood returning to the atria, so that atrial pressure does not rise abnormally.

immunologic c., capability of mounting an immunologic response.

com·pe·ti·tion (kom-pĕ-tish′ŭn). The process by which the activity or presence of one substance interferes with, or suppresses, the activity of another substance with similar affinities.

antigenic c., c. that occurs when two different antigens, each of which can evoke an immunologic response when inoculated alone, are mixed and inoculated together; the response may be to only one, that to the other being largely or entirely suppressed.

com·plaint (kom-plānt′). A disorder, disease, or symptom, or the description of it. [O.Fr. complainte, fr. L. complango, to lament]

chief c., the primary symptom that a patient states as the reason for seeking medical care.

com·ple·ment (kom′plĕ-ment). Ehrlich term for the thermolabile substance, normally present in serum, that is destructive to certain bacteria and other cells sensitized by a specific complement-fixing antibody. C. is a group of at least 20 distinct serum proteins, the activity of which is affected by a series of interactions resulting in enzymatic cleavages and which can follow one or the other of at least two pathways. In the case of immune hemolysis (classical pathway), the complex comprises nine components (designated C1 through C9) that react in a definite sequence and the activation of which is usually effected by the antigen-antibody complex; only the first seven components are involved in chemotaxis, and only the first four are involved in immune adherence or phagocytosis or are fixed by conglutinins. An alternative pathway (see properdin *system*) may be activated by factors other than antigen-antibody complexes and involves components other than C1, C4, and C2 in the activation of C3. SEE ALSO *component* of complement. [L. *complementum,* that which completes, fr. *com-pleo,* to fill up]

heparin c., the protein component of heparin in blood.

c. pathways, (1) the classical c. pathway (initiated usually by binding of C1 to IgG or IgM antibody to C1)is a complex of three subunits: C1q, C1r, and C1s. After C1q is bound, $\overline{C1r}$ (an overbar indicates enzymatic activity) cleaves C1s to $\overline{C1s}$. $\overline{C1s}$ cleaves both C4 into C4a and C4b as well as C2 into C2a and C2b. C2b combines with C4b to form C4b2b, which is a C3 convertase. C3 convertase cleaves C3 into C3a and C3b. C3b joins C4bC2b to form a C5 convertase (also known as C4b2b3b), which cleaves C5 into C5a and C5b. Once C5b is bound to the cell surface the remainder of the c. components (C6–C9) as well as C5b form the membrane attack complex (MAC). MAC causes a hole in the cell membrane. **(2)** in the alternative c. pathway, surface-bound C3b binds Factor B, which is cleaved by Factor D into Ba and Bb. C3bBb is an unstable C3 convertase unless properdin (P) binds to it to form C3bBbP. The stable C3 convertase generates more C3b. When a complex of C3bBbC3b is formed, this is the alternative pathway C5 convertase. From C5b through C9, the classical and alternative pathways are the same. **(3)** In the lectin-binding pathway, mannose-binding protein (MBP) initiates the pathway, which then uses components of the classical c. pathway. Some of the "a" components of both pathways have various biologic activities, i.e., C3a is an anaphylatoxin.

com·ple·men·tar·i·ty (kom-plĕ-men-tār′i-tē). **1.** The degree of base-pairing (A opposite U or T, G opposite C) between two sequences of DNA and/or RNA molecules. **2.** The degree of affinity, or fit, of antigen- and antibody-combining sites.

com·ple·men·ta·tion (kom′plĕ-men-tā′shŭn). **1.** Functional interaction between two defective viruses permitting replication under conditions inhibitory to the single virus. **2.** Interaction between two genetic units, one or both of which are defective, permitting the organism containing these units to function normally, whereas it could not do so if either unit were absent.

intergenic c., c. between pieces of genetic material that regulate the same function, such as a multienzyme pathway, but have defects in regions of separate genetic function; such c. permits synthesis of a normal end-product.

intragenic c., c. between pieces of genetic material, each of which has a different defect within the same locus; the resultant product of each is defective and nonfunctional, but the defective products may associate to produce a product which has some activity.

com·plex (kom′pleks). **1.** An organized constellation of feelings, thoughts, perceptions, and memories that may be in part unconscious and may strongly influence associations and attitudes. **2.** In chemistry, the relatively stable combination of two or more compounds into a larger molecule without covalent binding. **3.** A composite of chemical or immunologic structures. **4.** A structural anatomic entity made up of three or more interrelated parts. **5.** An informal term used to denote a group of individual structures known or believed to be anatomically, embryologically, or physiologically related. [L. *complexus,* woven together]

aberrant c., an anomalous electrocardiographic c., more specifically an abnormal ventricular c. caused by abnormal intraventricular conduction of a supraventricular impulse.

AIDS dementia c. (ADC), a subacute or chronic HIV-1 encephalitis, the most common neurologic complication in the later stages of HIV infection; manifested clinically as a progressive dementia, accompanied by motor abnormalities. SYN AIDS dementia, HIV encephalopathy.

AIDS-related c. (ARC), manifestations of AIDS in persons who have not yet developed major deficient immune function, characterized by fever with generalized lymphadenopathy, diarrhea, weight loss, minor opportunistic infections, cytopenias.

amygdaloid c. [TA], SYN amygdaloid *body.*

anomalous c., a c. in the electrocardiogram differing significantly from the physiologic type in the same lead.

antigen-antibody c., SEE immune c.

antigenic c., a composite of different antigenic structures, such as a cell or a bacterium, or, by extension, a molecule containing two or more determinant groups of different antigenic specificities.

apical c., a set of anterior structures that characterize one or several developmental stages of members of the protozoan phylum Apicomplexa; includes the following structures, visible by electron microscopy: polar ring, conoid, rhoptries, micronemes, and subpellicular tubules.

atrial c., p wave in the electrocardiogram. SYN auricular c.

auricular c., SYN atrial c.

binary c., a noncovalent c. of two molecules; often referring to the enzyme-substrate c. in an enzyme-catalyzed reaction. Cf. central c., Michaelis c. SYN enzyme-substrate c.

brain wave c., a specific combination of fast and slow electroencephalographic activity that recurs frequently enough to be identified as a discrete phenomenon.

brother c., SYN Cain c.

Cain c., a rarely used term for extreme envy or jealousy of a brother, leading to hatred. SYN brother c. [*Cain,* biblical personage]

Carney c., an autosomal dominant condition of Cushing syndrome due to immunoglobulin-mediated ACTH receptor inhibition, cardiac and cutaneous myxomas, lentigines, melanotic schwannomas, and pituitary and testicular tumors.

castration c., (1) a child's fear of injury to the genitals by the parent of the same sex as punishment for unconcious guilt over oedipal feelings; **(2)** fantasied loss of the penis by a female or fear of its actual loss by a male; **(3)** unconscious fear of injury from those in authority. SYN castration anxiety.

caudal pharyngeal c., the ultimobranchial body associated with the embryonic fourth and transitory fifth pharyngeal pouches.

central c., in an enzyme-catalyzed reaction, the structural complex of the enzyme and all of the enzyme's substrates (or the enzyme with all of the enzyme's products) equivalent to the binary c. for a one-substrate enzyme. Cf. binary c., Michaelis c.

charge transfer c., (1) a c. between two organic molecules in which an electron from one (the donor) is transferred to the other (the acceptor), becoming generally distributed throughout the latter; subsequent transfer of a hydrogen atom completes the reduction of the acceptor; such c.'s are generally highly colored and may be so observed; **(2)** a network of hydrogen bridges at the catalytic center of certain proteases. SYN charge transfer system.

Diana c., a rarely used term for ideas leading to the adoption of masculine traits and behavior in a female. [*Diana,* L. myth. char.]

diphasic c., a c. consisting of both positive and negative deflections.

EAHF c., a combination of allergies consisting of *e*czema, *a*sthma and *h*ay *f*ever.

Eisenmenger c., the combination of ventricular septal defect with pulmonary hypertension and consequent right-to-left shunt through the defect, with or without an associated overriding aorta. SYN Eisenmenger defect, Eisenmenger disease, Eisenmenger tetralogy.

Electra c., female counterpart of the Oedipus c. in the male; a term used to describe unresolved conflicts during childhood development toward the father which subsequently influence a woman's relationships with men. SYN father c. [*Electra,* daughter of Agamemnon]

electrocardiographic c., a deflection or group of deflections in the electrocardiogram.

enzyme-substrate c., SYN binary c.

CO

equiphasic c., SYN isodiphasic c.

father c., SYN Electra c.

femininity c., in psychoanalysis, the unconscious fear, in boys and men, of castration at the hands of the mother with resultant identification with the aggressor and envious desire for breasts and vagina.

Ghon c., SYN Ghon *tubercle.*

Golgi c., SYN Golgi *apparatus.*

H-2 c., term that denotes genes of the major histocompatibility c. in the mouse.

histocompatibility c., a family of fifty or more genes on the sixth human chromosome that code for cell surface proteins and play a role in the immune response.

> Histocompatibility genes control the production of proteins on the outer membranes of tissue and blood cells, especially lymphocytes, and are essential elements in cell-cell recognition and interaction. Surface proteins also determine the level and type of immune response, are involved in the presentation of antigens to the immune system, and may serve other biochemical and immunologic functions. In the case of allografts, the greater the histocompatibility (i.e., the closer the match between donor and recipient cell surface antigens), the less the likelihood of rejection. The major histocompatibility determinants are the human leukocyte antigens (HLA). HLA typing of a potential marrow donor and a potential transplant recipient is used to predict graft rejection and graft-versus-host disease.

HLA c., the major histocompatibility c. in humans. SEE ALSO human leukocyte *antigens,* under *antigen.*

immune c., antigen combined with specific antibody, to which complement may also be fixed, and which may precipitate or remain in solution. Frequently associated with autoimmune disease.

inferiority c., a sense of inadequacy which is expressed in extreme shyness, diffidence, or timidity, or as a compensatory reaction in exhibitionism or aggressiveness.

inferior olivary c. [TA], the three nuclei that collectively form what is commonly called the inferior olivary nucleus. These are the principal olivary nucleus (with its dorsal, ventral, and lateral lamellae) and the medial accessory and posterior (dorsal) accessory olivary nuclei. SEE ALSO principal olivary *nucleus.* SYN complexus olivaris inferior [TA].

iron-dextran c., a colloidal solution of ferric hydroxide in c. with partially hydrolyzed dextran; used in the treatment of iron deficiency anemias by intramuscular injection.

isodiphasic c., a diphasic c. whose positive and negative deflections are approximately equal. SYN equiphasic c.

j-g c., SYN juxtaglomerular c.

Jocasta c., a rarely used term for a mother's libidinous fixation on a son. [*Jocasta,* mother and wife of Oedipus]

junctional c., the attachment zone between epithelial cells, typically consisting of the zonula occludens, the zonula adherens, and the macula adherens (desmosome).

juxtaglomerular c., a c. consisting of the juxtaglomerular cells, which are modified smooth muscle cells in the wall of the afferent glomerular arteriole and sometimes also the efferent arteriole; extraglomerular mesangium lacis cells, which are located in the angle between the afferent and efferent glomerular arterioles; the macula densa of the distal convoluted tubule; and granular epithelial peripolar cells located at the angle of reflection of the parietal to the visceral capsule of the renal corpuscle; believed to provide some feedback control of extracellular fluid volume and glomerular filtration rate. SYN j-g c., juxtaglomerular apparatus.

K c., high amplitude, diphasic frontocental slow waves in the electroencephalogram related to arousal from sleep by a sound; characteristic of sleep stages 2, 3, and 4.

α-keto acid dehydrogenase c., SEE α-*keto acid* dehydrogenase.

α-ketoglutarate dehydrogenase c., SYN α-*ketoglutarate* dehydrogenase.

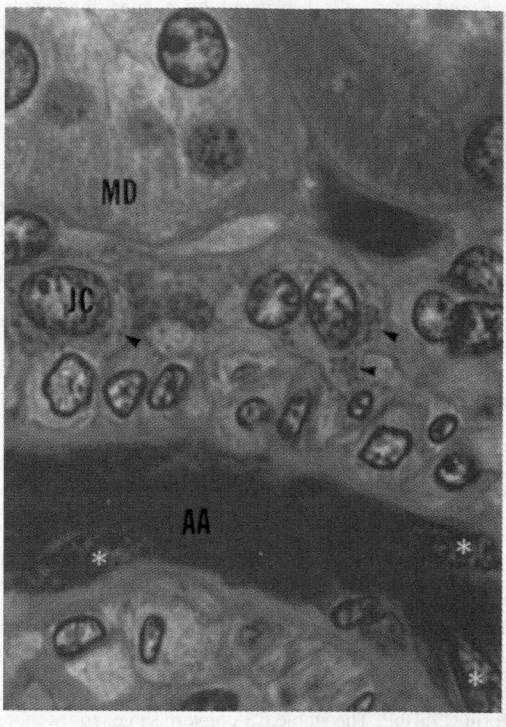

juxtaglomerular apparatus: kidney of monkey; plastic section, composed of the macula densa (MD) region of the distal tubule and juxtaglomerular cells (JC), modified smooth muscle cells of the afferent glomerular arteriole (AA); observe the granules (arrowheads) in the juxtaglomerular cells and the nuclei (asterisks) of the endothelial cells lining the afferent glomerular arteriole; ×1325

Lear c., a rarely used term for a father's libidinous fixation on a daughter. [*Lear,* Shakespearean character]

MAC c., SYN membrane attack c.

major histocompatibility c. (MHC), a group of linked loci, collectively termed H-2 c. in the mouse and HLA c. in humans, that codes for cell-surface histocompatibility antigens and is the principal determinant of tissue type and transplant compatibility. SEE ALSO human leukocyte *antigens,* under *antigen.*

mediator c., co-activation proteins involved in RNA polymerase transcription of DNA segments.

membrane attack c. (MAC), a c. of complement components (C5–C9) that, when activated, bind to the membrane of a target cell, penetrating it with a hydrophobic residue exteriorly and a hydrophilic residue in the interior of the cell; this allows passage of ions and water, swelling of the cell and subsequent lysis. SYN MAC c.

Meyenburg c., clusters of small bile ducts occurring in polycystic livers, separate from the portal areas.

Michaelis c., binary c. of an enzyme.

minor histocompatibility c. (MHC), genes outside of MHC that are present on various chromosomes that encode antigens contributing to graft rejection.

monophasic c., a c. in the electrocardiogram that is entirely negative or entirely positive.

multienzyme c., a structurally distinct and ordered collection of enzymes, often catalyzing successive steps in a metabolic pathway (e.g., pyruvate dehydrogenase c.).

Oedipus c., a developmentally distinct group of associated ideas, aims, instinctual drives, and fears generally observed in male children 3 to 6 years old: coinciding with the peak of the phallic phase of psychosexual development, the child's sexual interest is attached primarily to the parent of the opposite sex and is accompanied by aggressive feelings toward the parent of the same sex;

in psychoanalytic theory, it is replaced by the castration c. [*Oedipus*, G. myth. char.]

ostiomeatal c., point where the frontal and maxillary sinuses normally drain into the nasal cavity; obstruction produces inflammation of affected sinus cavities. SYN ostiomeatal unit.

persecution c., a feeling that others have evil designs against one's well-being.

primary c., SYN Ranke c.

pyruvate dehydrogenase c., SEE *pyruvate* dehydrogenase.

QRS c., portion of electrocardiogram corresponding to the depolarization of ventricular cardiac cells.

Ranke c., the typical lesions of primary pulmonary tuberculosis, consisting of a small peripheral focus of infection (Ghon focus), with hilar or paratracheal lymph node involement. SYN primary c.

ribosome-lamella c., a cylindric cytoplasmic inclusion composed of concentrically arranged sheets of membranes alternating with rows of ribosomes; characteristic of the hairy cell in leukemic reticuloendotheliosis.

Shone c., an obstructive lesion of the mitral valve c. with left ventricular outflow obstruction and coarctation of the aorta.

sicca c., dryness of the mucous membranes, as of the eyes and mouth, in the absence of a connective tissue disease such as rheumatoid arthritis.

spike and wave c., a generalized, synchronous pattern seen on the electroencephalogram, consisting of a sharply contoured fast wave followed by a slow wave; particularly found in patients with generalized epilepsies. Spike and wave complexes are often characterized by their frequency, e.g., slow spike and wave, fast spike and wave.

superiority c., term sometimes given to the compensatory behavior, e.g., aggressiveness, self-assertion, associated with inferiority c.

superior olivary c., ☆official alternate term for superior olivary *nucleus.*

symptom c., (1) SEE syndrome; (2) SEE complex (1).

synaptinemal c., a submicroscopic structure interposed between the homologous chromosome pairs during synapsis. SYN synaptonemal c.

synaptonemal c., SYN synaptinemal c.

Tacaribe c. of viruses, a group of arenaviruses (New World) that includes the antigenically related arboviruses Amapari, Junin, Latino, Machupo, Parana, Pichinde, Tacaribe, and Tamiami.

ternary c., term used to describe the tripartite combination of, for example, enzyme-cofactor-substrate or enzyme-substrate$_1$-substrate$_2$ for a multisubstrate enzyme, the active form involved in many enzyme-catalyzed reactions.

triple symptom c., SYN Behçet *syndrome.*

VATER c., a constellation of *v*ertebral defects, *a*nal atresia, *tr*acheoesophageal fistula with *e*sophageal atresia, and *r*enal and *r*adial anomalies; associated with Fanconi anemia.

ventricular c., the continuous QRST waves of each beat in the electrocardiogram.

ventrobasal c. [TA], the large posterior part of the ventral nucleus of the thalamus receiving the somatic sensory lemnisci (medial lemniscus, spinothalamic tract, trigeminal lemniscus) and the ascending gustatory (taste) lemniscus and projecting in turn by way of the internal capsule to the cortex of the postcentral gyrus. This complex of nuclei is somatotopically organized and subdivided into a ventral posterolateral nucleus [TA] (nucleus ventralis posterolateralis [TA]) representing the leg, a ventral posterior intermediate nucleus representing the arm, and a ventral posteromedial nucleus [TA] (nucleus ventralis posteromedialis [TA]) representing the face and an arcuate nucleus of thalamus receiving the gustatory lemniscus. SYN nuclei ventrobasales [TA], ventrobasal nuclei (complex) [TA], nucleus ventralis posterior thalami.

com·plex·ion (kom-plek′shŭn). The color, texture, and general appearance of the skin of the face. [L. *complexio,* a combination, (later) physical condition]

com·plex·i·ty (kom-pleks′i-tē). The state of consisting of many interrelated parts.

chemical c., the number of different sequences in DNA as defined by hybridization kinetics.

com·plex·us (kom-plek′sŭs). Obsolete term for semispinalis capitis (*muscle*). [L. an embracing, encircling]

c. olivaris inferior [TA], SYN inferior olivary *complex.*

c. stimulans cordis [TA], SYN conducting *system* of heart.

com·pli·ance (kom-plī′ans). **1.** A measure of the distensibility of a chamber expressed as a change in volume per unit change in pressure. **2.** The consistency and accuracy with which a patient follows the regimen prescribed by a physician or other health professional. Cf. adherence (2), maintenance. **3.** A measure of the ease with which a structure or substance may be deformed. In medicine and physiology, usually a measure of the ease with which a hollow viscus (e.g., lung, urinary bladder, gallbladder) may be distended, *i.e.,* the volume change resulting from the application of a unit pressure differential between the inside and outside of the viscus; the reciprocal of elastance. [M.E. fr. O.Fr., fr. L. *compleo,* to fulfill]

bladder c., change in volume of bladder for a given change in pressure; can be calculated from a cytometrogram's pressure volume curve. SYN c. of bladder, detrusor c.

c. of bladder, SYN bladder c.

detrusor c., SYN bladder c.

dynamic c. of lung, the value obtained when lung c. is estimated during breathing by dividing the tidal volume by the difference in instantaneous transpulmonary pressures at the ends of the respiratory excursions, when flow in the airway is momentarily zero; this value deviates markedly from static c. in patients in whom resistances and compliances are not uniform throughout the lung (i.e., uneven time constants).

c. of heart, the reciprocal of passive or diastolic stiffness of the ventricle of the heart, most commonly of the left ventricle; one may distinguish between c. of the muscle and c. of the supportive structures, although ordinarily both are considered together (chamber c.); a hypertrophied or scarred heart will manifest a stiff wall, i.e., decreased c.

specific c., (1) the c. of a structure divided by its initial volume; (2) more specifically for the lungs, the c. divided by the functional residual capacity.

static c., the value obtained when c. is measured at true equilibrium, i.e., in the absence of any motion.

thoracic c., that portion of total ventilatory c. ascribable to c. of the thoracic cage.

ventilatory c., the sum of dynamic c. of the lung and thoracic c.

com·pli·cat·ed (kom′pli-kā-ted). Made complex; denoting a disease upon which a morbid process or event has been superimposed, altering symptoms and modifying its course for the worse. [L. *com-plico,* pp. *-atus,* to fold together]

com·pli·ca·tion (kom-pli-kā′shŭn). A morbid process or event occurring during a disease that is not an essential part of the disease, although it may result from it or from independent causes.

com·po·nent (kom-pō′nent). An element forming a part of the whole. [L. *com-pono,* pp. *-positus,* to place together]

anterior c. of force, a force operating to move teeth anteriorly.

▣ **c. of complement (C),** any one of the nine distinct protein units designated C1 through C9. SEE complement; SEE ALSO *complement* pathways.

c. of force, (1) one of the factors from which a resultant force may be compounded or into which it may be resolved; (2) one of the vectors into which a force may be resolved.

c.'s of mastication, the various jaw movements that are made during the act of mastication, as determined by the neuromuscular system, the temporomandibular articulations, the teeth, and the food being chewed; divided, for purposes of analysis or description, into opening, closing, left lateral, right lateral, and anteroposterior c.'s.

c.'s of occlusion, the various factors involved in occlusion, such as the temporomandibular joint, the associated neuromusculature, the teeth, and the denture-supporting structures.

plasma thromboplastin c. (PTC), SYN *factor* IX.

secretory c., a polypeptide chain found in external secretions (e.g., tears, saliva, colostrum) associated with the immunoglobulins IgA and IgM. It also may occur in free form. The secretory

CO

com-ponent	mol. wt. (kD)	serum conc. (μg/ml)	no. of poly-peptides	function
C1q	410	150	18	form a Ca^{++} linked complex – C1q
C1r	83	50	1	$C1r_2$ $C1s_2$; C1q binds to complexed Ig
C1s	83	50	1	to activate the classical pathway
C4	210	550	3	classical pathway molecules, activated by C1s to form a C3
C2	115	25	1	convertase, C4b.2a
C3	180	1200	2	active C3 (C3b) opsonizes anything to which it binds and activates the lytic pathway. C3a causes mast cell degranulation and smooth muscle contraction. iC3b, C3d, C3e, and C3g are breakdown products of C3b
C5	180	70	2	C5b on membranes initiates the lytic pathway. C5a is chemotactic for macrophages and neutrophils, causes smooth muscle contraction, mast cell degranulation, and increased capillary permeability
C6	130	60	1	lytic pathway components that assemble in the presence of C5b to form the membrane attack complex and so may cause cell lysis
C7	120	50	1	
C8	155	55	3	
C9	75	60	1	
B	95	200	1	B binds to C3b in the presence of alternative pathway activators, then is cleaved by D, an active serum enzyme to form a C3 convertase C3b, Bb
D	25	10	1	
P (properdin)	185	25	4	stabilizes C3b, Bb to potentiate amplification loop activity
MBL	540	1	18	binds bacterial carbohydrate activates C4 and C2
MASP	94	?	1	
C4bp	550	250	7	C4bp binds C4b, and H binds C3b to act as cofactors for I, which cleaves and inactivates C3b and C4b
H(β_1H)	150	500	1	
I(C3bina)	100	30	2	
C1inh	100	185	1	binds and inactivates $\overline{C1r_2}$ and $\overline{C1s_2}$
S-protein (vitronectin)	83	505	1	binds C5b-7, prevents attachment to membranes

complement components

piece is derived by proteolytic cleavage of the immunoglobulin receptor on epithelial cells.

com·pos·ite (kom-poz′-it). A colloquial term for resin materials used in restorative dentistry. [L. *compositus*, put together, fr. *compono*, to put together]

com·po·si·tion (kom-pō-zish′ŭn). In chemistry, the kinds and numbers of atoms constituting a molecule. [L. *compono*, to arrange]

base c., the proportions of the four bases (adenine, cytosine, guanine, and thymine or uracil) present in DNA or RNA; usually expressed as the percentage (mol %) of G plus C.

modeling c., SYN modeling *plastic.*

com·pos men·tis (kom′pos men′tis). Of sound mind; usually used in its opposite form, *non compos mentis.* [L. possessed of one's mind; *compos,* having control, + *mens* (*ment-*), mind]

com·pound (kom′pownd). **1.** In chemistry, a substance formed by the covalent or electrostatic union of two or more elements, generally differing entirely in physical characteristics from any of its components. **2.** In pharmacy, denoting a preparation containing several ingredients. For c.'s not listed here, see the specific chemical or pharmaceutical names. [through O.Fr., fr. L. *compono*]

acetone c., SYN ketone *body.*

acyclic c., an organic c. in which the chain does not form a ring. SYN aliphatic c., open chain c.

addition c., (1) strictly, a complex of two or more complete molecules in which each preserves its fundamental structure and no covalent bonds are made or broken (e.g., hydrates of salts, adducts); **(2)** loosely, association of acids with basic organic c.'s (e.g., amines with HCl); **(3)** more loosely, addition of two molecules without loss of any atom, but forming new covalent bonds (e.g., $CH_2=CH_2 + Br_2 \rightarrow BrCH_2–CH_2Br$).

alicyclic c.'s, SEE cyclic c.

aliphatic c., SYN acyclic c.

APC c., an analgesic tablet drug combination containing aspirin, phenacetin, and caffeine. Very widely used in the 1940s through 1960s; original constituents of popular over-the-counter pain remedies. Use currently much diminished due to concerns about potential renal injury due to the phenacetin.

aromatic c., SEE cyclic c.

carbamino c., any carbamic acid derivative formed by the combination of carbon dioxide with a free amino group to form an *N*-carboxy group, –NH–COOH, as in hemoglobin forming carbaminohemoglobin.

closed chain c., SYN cyclic c.

condensation c., a c. resulting from the combination of two or more simple substances, with the splitting off of some other substance, such as alcohol or water; e.g., a peptide. Cf. conjugated c.

conjugated c., a c. formed by the union of two c.'s (as by the elimination of water between an alcohol and an organic acid to form an ester) and easily converted to the original c.'s (hydrolysis). SEE ALSO conjugation (4); Cf. condensation c.

cyclic c., any c. in which the constituent atoms, or any part of them, form a ring. Used mainly in organic chemistry where: 1) numerous c.'s contain rings of carbon atoms (carbocyclic c.'s) or carbon atoms plus one or more atoms of other types (heterocyclic c.'s), usually nitrogen, oxygen, or sulfur; 2) where the atoms in the ring are all of the same element (homocyclic or isocyclic c.'s); 3) where the ring is saturated or contains nonconjugated double bonds (alicyclic c.), the c. is similar in properties to the corresponding acyclic c. (e.g., cyclohexane resembles hexane); 4) where the ring contains conjugated double bonds in a closed loop in which there are $4n + 2$ (where n is an integer) delocalized π electrons (Hückel rule) (aromatic c.; e.g., benzene, pyridine), it is more stable than the corresponding saturated ring and exhibits unusual chemical properties characteristic of itself and not of other types of rings or of acyclic c.'s. These aromatic c.'s have the ability to sustain an induced ring current. SYN closed chain c., ring c.

genetic c., SYN compound *heterozygote.*

glycosyl c., the c. formed between a sugar and another organic substance in which the OH of the reducing (hemiacetal) group of the former is removed; e.g., the natural nucleosides, in which a heterocyclic N becomes linked directly to the C-1 of ribose (or deoxyribose) to yield ribosyl compounds. Cf. glycoside.

heterocyclic c., SEE cyclic c.

high-energy c.'s, classically, a group of phosphoric esters whose hydrolysis takes place with a standard free energy change of −5 to −15 kcal/mol (or −20 to −63 kJ/mol) (in contrast to −1 to −4 kcal/mol, or −4 to −17 kJ/mol) for simple phosphoric esters like glucose 6-phosphate or α-glycerophosphates, thus being capable of driving energy-consuming reactions in living cells or reconstituted cell-free systems; adenosine 5′-triphosphate, with respect to the β- and γ-phosphates, is the best known and is regarded as the immediate energy source for most metabolic syntheses. Other examples include acid anhydrides, phosphoric esters of enols, phosphamic acid ($R–NH–PO_3H_2$) derivatives, acyl thioesters (e.g., of coenzyme A), sulfonium c.'s ($R_3–S^+$), and aminoacyl esters of ribosyl moieties. SEE ALSO high-energy *phosphates,* under *phosphate.*

homocyclic c., SEE cyclic c.

impression c., SYN modeling *plastic.*

inclusion c., the mechanical trapping of small molecules within spaces between other molecules; e.g., the inclusion of iodine molecules by starch molecules to form the well-known red-to-black "addition c."

inorganic c., a c. in which the atoms or radicals consist of elements other than carbon and are typically held together by electrostatic forces rather than by covalent bonds; often are capable of dissociation into ions in polar solvents (e.g., H_2O). Cf. organic c.

isocyclic c., SEE cyclic c.

Kendall c.'s, a group of corticosteroids. Kendall's compound A (11-dehydrocorticosterone, Kendall compound B (corticosterone), Kendall compound E (cortisone), Kendall compound F (cortisol). SYN Kendall substance.

***meso* c.'s,** c.'s containing more than one asymmetric carbon atom, with configurations about them so balanced that the molecule as a whole possesses a plane of symmetry, although the individual carbon atoms do not; such compounds are not optically active; e.g., ribitol, mucic acid, *meso*-inositol, *meso*-cystine.

methonium c.'s, agents that either block impulses in ganglia (e.g., hexamethonium) and are used in arterial hypertension or block at neuromuscular junctions and are used for neuromusclar paralysis in surgery (e.g., decamethonium).

modeling c., SYN modeling *plastic*.

nonpolar c., a c. composed of molecules that possess a symmetrical distribution of charge, so that no positive or negative poles exist, and that are not ionizable in solution; e.g., hydrocarbons. SEE ALSO organic c.

open chain c., SYN acyclic c.

organic c., a c. composed of atoms (some of which are carbon) held together by covalent (shared electron) bonds. Cf. inorganic c.

polar c., a c. in which the electric charge is not symmetrically distributed, so that there is a separation of charge or partial charge and formation of definite positive and negative poles; e.g., H_2O. See also inorganic c.

Reichstein c., SYN Reichstein *substance*.

ring c., SYN cyclic c.

Wintersteiner c. F, SYN cortisone.

com·pre·hen·sion (kom-prē-hen′shŭn).   Knowledge or understanding of an object, situation, event, or verbal statement.

com·press (kom′pres).   A pad of gauze or other material applied for local pressure. [L. *com-primo,* pp. *-pressus,* to press together]

graduated c., layers of cloth thickest in the center, becoming thinner toward the periphery.

wet c., gauze moistened with saline or antiseptic solution.

com·pres·sion (kom-presh′ŭn).   A squeezing together; the exertion of pressure on a body in such a way as to tend to increase its density; the decrease in a dimension of a body under the action of two external forces directed toward one another in the same straight line.

c. of brain, SYN cerebral c.

cerebral c., pressure upon the intracranial tissues by an effusion of blood or cerebrospinal fluid, an abscess, a neoplasm, a depressed fracture of the skull, or an edema of the brain. SYN c. of brain.

c. limiting, a hearing aid circuit in which amplification is reduced at high input levels.

c. of tissue, SYN tissue *displaceability.*

wide dynamic range c., a hearing aid circuit in which amplification is increased across the frequency range at low input levels.

com·pres·sor (kom-pres′er, -ōr).   **1.** A muscle, contraction of which causes compression of any structure. **2.** An instrument for making pressure on a part, especially on an artery to prevent loss of blood. SYN compressorium.

c. urethrae [TA], part of female external urethral sphincter arising from the ischiopubic rami, posterior to the plane of the urethra, passing anteriorly and medially to fuse with the contralateral muscle anterior to the urethra and blending with the other parts of the external urethral sphincter (sphincter urethrovaginalis inferiorly and sphincter urethrae superiorly). SEE ALSO external urethral *sphincter.*

c. ve′nae dorsa′lis pe′nis, a variation of the bulbospongiosus

muscle in which some fibers pass dorsal to the dorsal vein of the penis; thought at one time to be an important component in the mechanism of erection. SYN Houston muscle.

com·pres·sor·i·um (kom-pres-ōr′ē-ŭm).   SYN compressor (2).

Compton, Arthur H., U.S. physicist and Nobel laureate, 1892–1962. SEE C. *effect,* scattering.

Compton scat·ter·ing. SYN Compton *effect.*

com·pul·sion (kom-pŭl′shŭn).   Uncontrollable thoughts or impulses to perform an act, often repetitively, as an unconscious mechanism to avoid unacceptable ideas and desires which, by themselves, arouse anxiety; the anxiety becomes fully manifest if performance of the compulsive act is prevented; may be associated with obsessive thoughts. [L. *com-pello* pp. *-pulsus,* to drive together, compel]

com·pul·sive (kom-pŭl′siv).   Influenced by compulsion; of a compelling and irresistible nature.

com·put·er. A programmable electronic device that can be used to store and manipulate data in order to carry out designated functions; the two fundamental components are hardware, i.e., the actual electronic device, and software, i.e., the instructions or program used to carry out the function.

△**con-.** With, together, in association; appears as com- before p, b, or m, as col- before l, and as co- before a vowel; corresponds to G. syn-. [L. *cum,* with, together]

conA, con A Abbreviation for concanavalin A.

con·al·bu·min (kon-al-bū′min).   A glycoprotein containing D-mannose and D-galactose, constituting about 12% of total solids of egg white. It will bind iron ions. SYN ovotransferrin.

con·a·nine (kon′ă-nēn).   A steroid alkaloid; pregnane with a methylimino group bridging C-18 and C-20 (in α-configuration). SEE ALSO conessine.

co·nar·i·um (kō-nā′rē-ŭm).   SYN pineal *body.* [G. *kōnarion* (dim. of *kōnos,* cone), the pineal body]

co·na·tion (kō-nā′shŭn).   The conscious tendency to act, usually an aspect of mental process; historically aligned with cognition and affection, but more recently used in the wider sense of impulse, desire, purposeful striving. [L. *conātio,* an undertaking, effort]

co·na·tive (kon′ă-tiv).   Pertaining to, or characterized by, conation.

co·na·tus (kō-nah′tŭs, -nā′tŭs).   A striving toward self-preservation and self-affirmation. [L. attempt]

con·cam·er·a·tion (kon-kam-er-ā′shŭn).   A system of interconnecting cavities. [L. *concameratio,* a vault; fr. *concamero,* pp. *-atus,* to vault over, fr. *camera,* a vault]

con·ca·nav·a·lin A (conA, con A) (kon-kă-nav′ă-lin).   A phytomitogen, extracted from the jack bean (*Canavalia ensiformis*) that agglutinates the blood of mammals and reacts with glucosans; like other phytohemagglutinins, conA stimulates T lymphocytes more vigorously than it does B lymphocytes.

con·ca·ta·mer (kon-kāt-ă-mer).   A linear repeat of restriction fragments. [*concat*enate + -mer]

con·cat·e·nate (kon-kat′ĕ-nāt).   Denoting the arrangement of a number of structures, e.g., enlarged lymph glands, in a row like the links of a chain. [L. *concateno,* pp. *-atus,* to link together, fr. *catena,* a chain]

Concato, Luigi M., Italian physician, 1825–1882. SEE C. *disease.*

con·cave (kon′kāv).   Having a depressed or hollowed surface. [L. *concavus,* arched or vaulted]

con·cav·i·ty (kon-kav′i-tē).   A hollow or depression, with more or less evenly curved sides, on any surface.

con·ca·vo·con·cave (kon-kā′vō-kon′kāv).   SYN biconcave.

con·ca·vo·con·vex (kon-kā′vō-kon′veks).   Concave on one surface and convex on the opposite surface.

con·cen·tra·tion (c) (kon-sen-trā′shŭn).   **1.** A preparation made by extracting a crude drug, precipitating from the solution, and drying. **2.** Increasing the amount of solute in a given volume of solution by evaporation of the solvent. **3.** The quantity of a substance per unit volume or weight. In renal physiology, symbol U for urinary c., P for plasma c.; in respiratory physiology, symbol

C for amount per unit volume in blood, F for fractional c. (mole fraction or volume per volume) in dried gas; subscripts indicate location and chemical species. [L. *con-*, together, + *centrum*, center]

Baermann c., preparation that relies on the principle that active nematode larvae will migrate from a fresh fecal specimen through several layers of gauze into tap water, from which the larvae can be recovered by centrifugation.

buffy coat c., centrifugation of whole blood containing anticoagulant to obtain a buffy coat layer containing white blood cells; blood films for staining can be prepared from this layer of cells and examined for the presence of parasites (trypanosomes and intracellular leishmaniae).

critical micelle c. (cmc), the c. at which an amphipathic molecule (e.g., a phospholipid) will form a micelle.

fecal c., preparation using centrifugation and either flotation or sedimentation methods to separate parasitic elements from fecal debris.

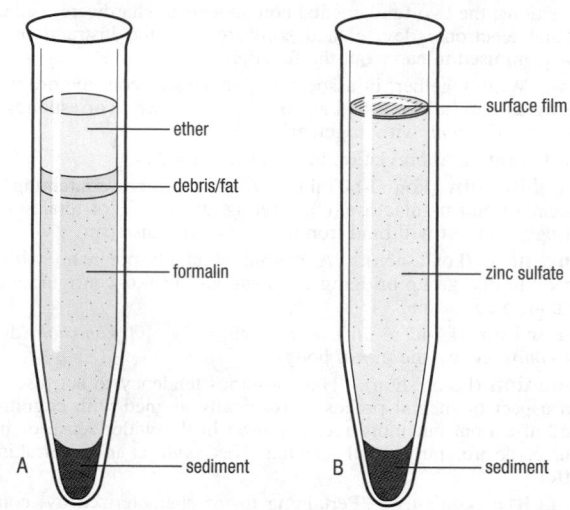

fecal concentration procedures: various layers seen in tubes after centrifugation; (A) formalin-ether (or ethyl acetate) ; (B) zinc sulfate (the surface film should be within 2 to 3 mm of the tube rim)

formalin-ether sedimentation c., a sedimentation method to separate parasitic elements from fecal debris through centrifugation and the use of ether to trap debris in a separate layer from the parasites.

formalin-ethyl acetate sedimentation c., a sedimentation method to separate parasitic elements from fecal debris through centrifugation and the use of ethyl acetate (substitute for ether) to trap debris in a separate layer from the parasites.

gravity c., a method of separating parasites from debris through gravity sedimentation of fecal suspensions.

M c., the maximum number of bacterial cells which can be produced in a unit volume of growth medium.

mean corpuscular hemoglobin c. (MCHC), Hgb/Hct; the average hemoglobin c. in a given volume of packed red cells, calculated from the hemoglobin therein and the hematocrit, in erythrocyte indices.

microhematocrit c., the centrifugation of whole, anticoagulated blood, using microhematocrit tubes, to obtain a buffy coat layer containing white blood cells; blood films for staining can be prepared from this layer of cells and examined for the presence of parasites (trypanosomes and intracellular leishmaniae).

minimal alveolar c., the end-alveolar c. of an inhalation anesthetic that prevents somatic response to a painful stimulus in 50% of individuals; an index of relative potency of inhalation anesthetics. SYN minimal anesthetic c.

minimal anesthetic c. (MAC), SYN minimal alveolar c.

minimal alveolar concentration (MAC) values of inhalation anesthetics, in order of increasing effectiveness		
	MAC values (% atm)	
	100% O_2	with 70% N_2O
halothane	0.75	0.29
isoflurane	1.15	0.50
sevoflurone	1.4–3.2	0.7–2.0
desflurone	6.0	3.0
N_2O	110	–

minimal inhibitory c. (MIC), the lowest concentration of antibiotic sufficient to inhibit bacterial growth when tested in vitro.

molar c., SEE molar (4).

normal c. (N), SEE normal (3).

zinc sulfate flotation c., a method using saturated zinc sulfate to separate parasitic elements from fecal debris through differences in specific gravity; most parasite cysts, oocysts, spores, eggs, and larvae can be found in the surface film after centrifugation.

con·cen·tric (kon-sen′trik). Having a common center, such that two or more spheres, circles, or segments of circles are within one another.

con·cept (kon′sept). **1.** An abstract idea or notion. **2.** An explanatory variable or principle in a scientific system. SYN conception (1). [L. *conceptum,* something understood, pp. ntr. of *concipio,* to receive, apprehend]

no-threshold c., that the biologic effect of radiation is proportional to dose, even for minutely small doses.

self-c., an individual's sense of self, including self-definition in the various social roles one enacts, including assessment of one's own status with respect to a single trait or to many human dimensions, using societal or personal norms as criteria.

con·cep·ti (kon-sep′tī). Plural of conceptus.

con·cep·tion (kon-sep′shŭn). **1.** SYN concept. **2.** Act of forming a general idea or notion. **3.** Act of conceiving; the implantation of the blastocyte in the endometrium. [L. *conceptio;* see concept]

imperative c., a concept that does not arise from association but appears spontaneously and refuses to be banished.

retained products of c., fragments of fetal, placental, or membrane tissue remaining in utero following delivery or abortion, posing an increased risk of bleeding or infection.

con·cep·tu·al (kon-sep′chŭ-ăl). Relating to the formation of ideas, usually higher order abstractions, to mental conceptions.

con·cep·tus, pl. **con·cep·ti** (kon-sep′tŭs, -sep′tī). The product of conception, i.e., embryo or fetus and membranes.

con·cha, pl. **con·chae** (kon′kă, kon′kē) [TA]. In anatomy, a structure comparable to a shell in shape, as the auricle or pinna of the ear or a turbinate bone in the nose. [L. a shell]

c. of auricle [TA], the large hollow, or floor of the auricle, between the anterior portion of the helix and the antihelix; it is divided by the crus of the helix into the cymba above and the cavum below. SYN c. auriculae [TA], c. of ear.

c. auric′ulae [TA], SYN c. of auricle.

c. bullosa, abnormal pneumatization of the middle turbinate that may interfere with normal ventilation of sinus ostia and can result in recurrent sinusitis.

c. of ear, SYN c. of auricle.

highest c., SYN supreme nasal c.

inferior nasal c. [TA], **(1)** a thin, spongy, bony plate with curved margins, on the lateral wall of the nasal cavity, separating the middle from the inferior meatus; it articulates with the ethmoid, lacrimal, maxilla, and palate bones; **(2)** the above bony plate and its thick mucoperiosteum containing an extensive cavernous vascular bed for heat exchange. SYN c. nasalis inferior [TA], inferior turbinated bone, turbinated body (2).

middle nasal c. [TA], **(1)** the middle thin, spongy, bony plate with curved margins, part of the ethmoidal labyrinth, projecting from the lateral wall of the nasal cavity and separating the superior or meatus from the middle meatus; (2) the above bony plate and its thick mucoperiosteum containing a cavernous vascular bed for heat exchange. SYN c. nasalis media [TA], middle turbinated bone, turbinated body (2).

Morgagni c., SYN superior nasal c.

c. nasa′lis infe′rior [TA], SYN inferior nasal c.

c. nasa′lis me′dia [TA], SYN middle nasal c.

c. nasa′lis supe′rior [TA], SYN superior nasal c.

c. nasa′lis supre′ma [TA], SYN supreme nasal c.

Santorini c., c. santori′ni, SYN supreme nasal c.

sphenoidal conchae [TA], pyramidal paired ossicles, the spines of which are in contact with the medial pterygoid lamina, the bases forming the roof of the nasal cavity. SYN conchae sphenoidales [TA], Bertin bones, Bertin ossicles, sphenoidal turbinated bones.

con′chae sphenoida′les [TA], SYN sphenoidal conchae.

superior nasal c. [TA], (1) the upper thin, spongy, bony plate with curved margins, part of the ethmoidal labyrinth, projecting from the lateral wall of the nasal cavity and separating the superior or meatus from the sphenoethmoidal recess; (2) the above bony plate and its thick mucoperiosteum, which is less vascular than that of the middle and inferior conchae. SYN c. nasalis superior [TA], Morgagni c., superior turbinated bone, turbinated body (2).

supreme c., SYN supreme nasal c.

supreme nasal c. [TA], a small c. frequently present on the posterosuperior part of the lateral nasal wall; it overlies the supreme nasal meatus. SYN c. nasalis suprema [TA], fourth turbinated bone, highest c., highest turbinated bone, Santorini c., c. santorini, supraturbinal, supreme c., supreme turbinated bone, turbinated body (2).

con·choi·dal (kon-koy′dăl). Shaped like a shell; having alternate convexities and concavities on the surface. [concha + G. *eidos,* appearance]

con·com·i·tance (kon-kom′i-tăns). In esotropia, one eye accompanying the other in all excursions, as in concomitant strabismus. [con- + L. *comito-,* pp. *-atus,* to accompany]

con·com·i·tant. SYN comitant.

con·cor·dance (kon-kōr′dans). 1. Agreement in the types of data that occur in natural pairs. For example, in a trait like schizophrenia, a pair of identical twins is concordant if both are affected or both are unaffected; it is discordant if one of them only is affected. Likewise, the pairs might be non-identical twins, or sibs, or husband and wife, etc. 2. A negotiated, shared agreement between clinician and patient concerning treatment regimen(s), outcomes, and behaviors; a more cooperative relationship than those based on issues of compliance and noncompliance. [L. *concordia,* agreeing, harmony]

con·cor·dant (kon-kōr′dant). Denoting or exhibiting concordance.

con·cre·ment (kon′krē-ment). A concretion; a deposit of calcareous material in a part. [L. *con- cresco,* to grow together]

con·cres·cence (kon-kres′ens). 1. SYN coalescence. 2. In dentistry, the union of the roots of two adjacent teeth by cementum. [see concrement]

con·cre·tio cor·dis (kon-krē′shē-ō kōr′dis). Extensive adhesion between parietal and visceral layers of the pericardium with partial or complete obliteration of the pericardial cavity. SYN internal adhesive pericarditis.

con·cre·tion (kon-krē′shŭn). The formation of solid material by aggregation of discrete units or particles. [L. *cum,* together, + *crescere,* to grow]

con·cret·i·za·tion (kon′krēt-i-zā′shŭn). Inability to abstract with an overemphasis on specific details; seen in mental disorders, such as dementia and schizophrenia, and also normally in children. [L. *con-cresco,* pp. *-cretus,* to grow together, harden]

con·cus·sion (kon-kŭsh′ŭn). 1. A violent shaking or jarring. 2. An injury of a soft structure, as the brain, resulting from a blow or violent shaking. SYN commotio. [L. *concussio,* fr. *con- cutio,* pp. *-cussus,* to shake violently]

brain c., a clinical syndrome due to mechanical, usually traumat-

ic, forces; characterized by immediate and transient impairment of neural function, such as alteration of consciousness, disturbance of vision and equilibrium, etc. SYN commotio cerebri.

spinal c., SYN spinal cord c.

spinal cord c., injury to the spinal cord due to a blow to the vertebral column with transient or prolonged dysfunction below the level of the lesion. SYN spinal c.

con·den·sa·tion (kon-den-sā′shŭn). 1. Making more solid or dense. 2. The change of a gas to a liquid, or of a liquid to a solid. 3. In psychoanalysis, an unconscious mental process in which one symbol stands for a number of others. 4. In dentistry, the process of packing a filling material into a cavity, using such force and direction that no voids result. [L. *con-denso,* pp. *-atus,* to make thick, condense]

aldol c., formation of an aldol (a β-hydroxy carbonyl compound) from two carbonyl compounds; the reverse reaction is an aldol cleavage; fructose 1,6-bisphosphate aldolase catalyzes such a reaction.

Claisen c., the formation of a β-keto ester from two esters, one of which has an α-hydrogen atom; malate synthase, citrate synthase, and ATP citrate lyase all catalyze such reactions.

con·dense (kon-dens′). To pack; to increase the density of; applied particularly to insertion of gold foil or silver amalgam in a cavity prepared in a tooth.

con·dens·er (kon-den′ser). 1. An apparatus for cooling a gas to a liquid, or a liquid to a solid. 2. In dentistry, a manual or powered instrument used for packing a plastic or unset material into a cavity of a tooth; variation in sizes and shapes allows conformation of the mass to the cavity outline. 3. The simple or compound lens on a microscope that is used to supply the illumination necessary for visibility of the specimen under observation. 4. SYN capacitor.

Abbé c., a system of two or three wide-angle, achromatic, convex and planoconvex lenses that may be moved upward or downward beneath the stage of a microscope, thereby regulating the concentration of light (directly from a bulb or reflected from a mirror) that passes through the material to be examined on the stage.

automatic c., SYN automatic *plugger.*

cardioid c., a type of dark-field c.

dark-field c., an apparatus for throwing reflected light through the microscope field, so that only the object to be examined is illuminated, the field itself being dark.

paraboloid c., a type of dark-field c.

con·di·tion (kon-dish′ŭn). 1. To train; to undergo conditioning. 2. A certain response elicited by a specifiable stimulus or emitted in the presence of certain stimuli with reward of the response during prior occurrence. 3. Referring to several classes of learning in the behavioristic branch of psychology. [L. *conditio,* fr. *condico,* to agree]

fibrocystic c. of the breast, a benign c. common in women of the third, fourth, and fifth decades characterized by formation, in one or both breasts, of small cysts containing fluid which may appear as blue dome cysts; associated with stromal fibrosis and with variable degrees of intraductal epithelial hyperplasia and sclerosing adenosis. SYN cystic hyperplasia of the breast.

con·di·tion·ing (kon-dish′ŭn-ing). The process of acquiring, developing, educating, establishing, learning, or training new responses in an individual. Used to describe both respondent and operant behavior; in both usages, refers to a change in the frequency or form of behavior as a result of the influence of the environment.

assertive c., SYN assertive *training.*

aversive c., SYN aversive *training.*

avoidance c., the technique whereby an organism learns to avoid unpleasant or punishing stimuli by learning the appropriate anticipatory response to protect it from further such stimuli. Cf. escape c. SYN avoidance training.

classical c., a form of learning, as in Pavlov experiments, in which a previously neutral stimulus becomes a conditioned stimulus when presented together with an unconditioned stimulus. Also called stimulus substitution because the new stimulus evokes the response in question. SEE ALSO respondent c. SYN stimulus substitution.

escape c., the technique whereby an organism learns to terminate unpleasant or punishing stimuli by making the appropriate new response which stops the delivery of such stimuli. Cf. avoidance c. SYN escape training.

higher order c., the use of a previously conditioned stimulus to condition further responses, in much the same way unconditioned stimuli are used.

instrumental c., c. in which the response is a prerequisite to achieving some goal; often used as a synonym for operant c., but some psychologists make distinctions in the usages of these two terms.

operant c., a type of c. developed by Skinner in which an experimenter waits for the target response (head scratching) to be conditioned to occur (emitted) spontaneously, immediately after which the organism is given a reinforcer reward; after this procedure is repeated many times, the frequency of emission of the targeted response will have significantly increased over its pre-experiment base rate. SEE ALSO *schedules* of reinforcement, under *schedule.* SYN skinnerian c.

pavlovian c., SYN respondent c.

respondent c., a type of c., first studied by I. P. Pavlov, in which a previously neutral stimulus (bell sound) elicits a response (salivation) as a result of pairing it (associating it contiguously in time) a number of times with an unconditioned or natural stimulus for that response (food shown to a hungry dog). SYN pavlovian c.

second-order c., the use of a previously successfully conditioned stimulus as the unconditioned stimulus for further c.

skinnerian c., SYN operant c.

trace c., c. when there is no temporal overlap between the c. stimulus and the unconditioned stimulus.

con·dom (kon′dom). Sheath or cover for the penis or vagina for use in the prevention of conception or infection during coitus.

con·duc·tance (kon-dŭk′tans). **1.** A measure of conductivity; the ratio of the current flowing through a conductor to the difference in potential between the ends of the conductor; the c. of a circuit is the reciprocal of its resistance. **2.** The ease with which a fluid or gas enters and flows through a conduit, air passage, or respiratory tract; the flow per unit pressure difference.

con·duc·tion (kon-dŭk′shŭn). **1.** The act of transmitting or conveying certain forms of energy, such as heat, sound, or electricity, from one point to another, without evident movement in the conducting body. **2.** The transmission of stimuli of various sorts by living protoplasm. [L. *con-* *duco,* pp. *ductus,* to lead, conduct]

aberrant ventricular c., abnormal intraventricular c. of a supraventricular beat, especially where surrounding beats are normally conducted. SYN ventricular aberration.

accelerated c., any pathologically increased speed of c.; usually occurs between the atrium and ventricles as in the Wolff-Parkinson-White and Lown-Ganong-Levine syndromes; such accelerated pathways provide the bases for particular forms of reentry tachycardia.

air c., in relation to hearing, the transmission of sound to the inner ear through the external auditory canal and the structures of the middle ear.

anomalous c., c. of cardiac electrical impulses through any abnormal pathway.

antegrade c., SYN anterograde c.

anterograde c., c. in the expected normal direction between any cardiac structures. SYN antegrade c., forward c., orthograde c.

atrioventricular c. (AVC), AV c., forward c. of the cardiac impulse from atria to ventricles via the AV node or any bypass tract, represented in the electrocardiogram by the PR interval. PH c. time is from the onset of the P wave to the first high-frequency component of the His bundle electrogram (normally 119 ± 38 msec); A-H c. time is from the onset of the first high-frequency component of the atrial electrogram to the first high-frequency component of the His bundle electrogram (normally 92 ± 38 msec); P-A conduction time is from the onset of the P wave to the onset of the atrial electrogram (normally 27 ± 18 msec).

avalanche c., the discharge of an impulse from a neuron into a large number of neurons of the same physiologic system, thus producing the liberation of a very large amount of nervous energy by a given stimulus.

bone c., in relation to hearing, the transmission of sound to the inner ear through vibrations applied to the bones of the skull. SYN osteophony.

concealed c., c. of an impulse through a part of the heart without direct evidence of its presence in the electrocardiogram; c. is inferred only because of its influence on the subsequent cardiac cycle.

decremental c., impaired c. in a portion of a fiber because of progressively lessening response of the unexcited portion of the fiber to the action potential coming toward it; it is manifested by decreasing speed of c., amplitude of action potential, and extent of spread of the impulse.

delayed c., first-degree AV block. SEE atrioventricular *block,* intraventricular *block,* bundle-branch *block.*

forward c., SYN anterograde c.

intraatrial c., c. of the cardiac impulse through the atrial myocardium, represented by the P wave in the electrocardiogram.

intraventricular c., c. of the cardiac impulse through the ventricular myocardium, represented by the QRS complex in the electrocardiogram. HR c. time is from the onset of the first high frequency component of the His bundle electrogram to the onset of the QRS complex of the surface electrocardiogram (normally 43 ± 12 msec); HV c. time is from the onset of the first high-frequency component of the His bundle electrogram to the onset of the ventricular electrogram (normally approximates the HR interval but may be a little shorter). SYN ventricular c.

nerve c., the transmission of an impulse along a nerve fiber.

orthograde c., SYN anterograde c.

Purkinje c., c. of the cardiac impulse through the Purkinje system.

retrograde VA c., c. backward from the ventricles or from the AV node into and through the atria. SYN retroconduction, ventriculoatrial c., VA c.

saltatory c., c. in which the nerve impulse jumps from one node of Ranvier to the next.

sinoventricular c., a rare form of c. of the sinus impulse during paralysis of the atrial muscle by hyperkalemia. The impulse leaves the sinus node and enters the internodal tracts rapidly achieving the junctional tissues but without inscribing a P wave due to the inactivation of the atrial muscle cells.

supernormal c., SYN supranormal c.

supranormal c., transmission of an impulse during the brief period of the cardiac cycle when it would be expected to fail if it occurred outside this time interval; considered to be better than expected rather than better than normal. Cf. supranormal *excitability.* SYN supernormal c.

synaptic c., the c. of a nerve impulse across a synapse.

ventricular c., SYN intraventricular c.

ventriculoatrial c. (VAC), VA c., SYN retrograde VA c.

con·duc·tiv·i·ty (kon-dŭk-tiv′i-tē). **1.** The power of transmission or conveyance of certain forms of energy, as heat, sound, and electricity, without perceptible motion in the conducting body. **2.** The property, inherent in living protoplasm, of transmitting a state of excitation; e.g., in muscle or nerve.

hydraulic c., ease of pressure filtration of a liquid through a membrane; specifically, $Kf = \eta(\dot{Q}/A)\,(\delta x/\delta P)$, where Kf = hydraulic c., η = viscosity of the liquid being filtered, $\dot{Q}/A$ = volume of liquid filtered per unit time and unit area, and $\delta x/\delta P$ = reciprocal of the pressure gradient through the membrane; solute concentrations should be identical on both sides of the membrane. Also applied more loosely to measurements on a total membrane of unknown area and thickness with unmeasured fluid viscosity ($K = \dot{Q}/\delta P$).

con·duc·tor (kon-dŭk′ter, -tōr). **1.** A probe or sound with a groove along which a knife is passed in slitting open a sinus or fistula; a grooved director. **2.** Any substance possessing conductivity.

con·duit (kon′doo-it). A channel.

apical-aortic c., a valved c. between the LV apex and aorta, used to treat severe otherwise unapproachable LV outflow tract obstruction.

ileal c., an isolated segment of ileum serving as a cutaneous replacement for the urinary bladder, into which ureters can be implanted, the lumen of which is connected to the skin; used following total cystectomy or other loss of normal bladder function requiring supravesical diversion. SYN ileal bladder.

con·du·pli·cate (kon-doo'pli-kāt). Folded upon itself lengthwise. [L. *con-*, with, + *duplico*, pp. *-atus*]

con·du·pli·ca·to cor·pore (kon-doo-pli-kā'tō kōr'pōr-ē). Condition in which the fetus is doubled up on itself in shoulder presentation.

con·du·ran·go (kon-doo-rang'gō). The bark of *Gonolobus condurango, Marsdenia condurango* (family Asclepiadaceae), a shrub of Ecuador and Peru; an aromatic bitter and astringent. [Peruv.]

con·dy·lar (kon'di-lăr). Relating to a condyle.

con·dy·lar·thro·sis (kon'di-lar-thrō'sis). A joint, like that of the knee, formed by condylar surfaces. [G. *kondylos*, condyle, + *arthrōsis*, a jointing]

con·dyle (kon'dīl) [TA]. A rounded articular surface at the extremity of a bone. SYN condylus [TA].

balancing side c., in dentistry, the mandibular c. on the side away from which the mandible moves in a lateral excursion.

c. of humerus [TA], the distal end of the humerus, including the trochlea, capitulum and the olecranon, coronoid and radial fossae. SYN condylus humeri [TA].

lateral c. [TA], c. farthest from the midline. SYN condylus lateralis [TA].

lateral c. of femur [TA], the lateral c. is longer than the medial c. SYN condylus lateralis femoris [TA].

lateral c. of tibia [TA], the lateral c. is longer than the medial c. SYN condylus lateralis tibiae [TA].

mandibular c., SYN condylar *process* of mandible.

medial c. [TA], c. closest to midline. SYN condylus medialis [TA].

medial c. of femur [TA], the shorter c. closest to the midline. SYN condylus medialis femoris [TA].

medial c. of tibia [TA], the shorter c. closest to the midline. SYN condylus medialis tibiae [TA].

occipital c. [TA], one of two elongated oval facets on the undersurface of the occipital bone, one on each side of the foramen magnum, which articulate with the atlas. SYN condylus occipitalis [TA].

working side c., in dentistry, the mandibular c. on the side toward which the mandible moves in a lateral excursion.

con·dy·lec·to·my (kon-di-lek'tō-mē). Excision of a condyle. [G. *kondylos*, condyle, + *ektomē*, excision]

con·dyl·i·on (kon-dil'ē-on). A point on the lateral outer or medial inner surface of the condyle of the mandible. [G. *kondylion*, dim. of *kondylos*, condyle]

con·dy·loid (kon'di-loyd). Relating to or resembling a condyle. [G. *kondylōdēs*, like a knuckle, fr. *kondylos*, condyle, + *eidos*, resemblance]

con·dy·lo·ma, pl. **con·dy·lo·ma·ta** (kon-di-lō'mă, -mah'tă). A wartlike excrescence at the anus or vulva, or on the glans penis. [G. *kondylōma*, a knob]

🔳**c. acumina′tum,** a contagious projecting warty growth on the external genitals or at the anus, consisting of fibrous overgrowths covered by thickened epithelium showing koilocytosis, due to sexual contact with infection by human papilloma virus; it is usually benign, although malignant change has been reported, associated with particular types of the virus. SYN genital wart, venereal wart.

flat c., (1) SYN c. latum; **(2)** a c. of the uterine cervix or other site caused by human papilloma virus infection and characterized histologically by koilocytosis without papillomatosis.

giant c., a large type of c. acuminatum found in the anus, vulva, or preputial sac of the penis of middle-aged, uncircumcised men; it tends to extend deeply and recur. SEE ALSO verrucous *carcinoma*.

c. la′tum, a secondary syphilitic eruption of flat-topped papules,

occurring in groups covered by a necrotic layer of epithelial detritus, and secreting a seropurulent fluid; they are found at the anus and wherever contiguous folds of skin produce heat and moisture. SYN flat c. (1), moist papule, mucous papule.

con·dy·lom·a·tous (kon-di-lō'mă-tŭs). Relating to a condyloma.

con·dy·lot·o·my (kon-di-lot'ō-mē). Division, without removal of a condyle. [G. *kondylos*, condyle, + *tomē*, incision]

con·dy·lus (kon'di-lŭs) [TA]. SYN condyle. [L. fr. G. *kondylos*, knuckle, the knuckle of any joint]

c. hu′meri [TA], SYN condyle of humerus.

c. latera′lis [TA], SYN lateral *condyle*.

c. latera′lis fem′oris [TA], SYN lateral *condyle* of femur.

c. latera′lis tib′iae [TA], SYN lateral *condyle* of tibia.

c. media′lis [TA], SYN medial *condyle*.

c. media′lis fem′oris [TA], SYN medial *condyle* of femur.

c. media′lis tibiae [TA], SYN medial *condyle* of tibia.

c. occipita′lis [TA], SYN occipital *condyle*.

cone (kōn). **1.** A surface joining a circle to a point above the plane (containing the circle). **2.** The photosensitive, outward-directed, conical process of a c. cell essential for sharp vision and color vision; c.'s are the only photoreceptor in the fovea centralis and become interspersed with increasing numbers of rods toward the periphery of the retina. SYN cone cell of retina. **3.** Metallic cylinder or truncated c., either circular or square in cross-section, used to confine a beam of x-rays to. SYN conus (1). [G. *kōnos*, cone]

antipodal c., the set of astral rays of a dividing cell extending from the centriole in a direction opposite to the equatorial plate.

arterial c., SYN *conus* arteriosus.

c. down, to confine a beam of x-rays to a region of interest using a collimator or c. (3); colloq., to focus one's attention or activities.

elastic c., SYN *conus* elasticus.

gutta-percha c., a c.-shaped, semirigid root canal filling material composed of gutta-percha and zinc oxide.

Haller c.'s, SYN *lobules* of epididymis, under *lobule*.

implantation c., SYN axon *hillock*.

c. of light, SYN light *reflex* (3).

medullary c. [TA], SYN *conus* medullaris.

nerve growth c., a highly motile structure at the leading edge of an elongating axon.

ocular c., the c. of light in the interior of the eyeball with the base formed by the rays entering through the pupil and the apex focused on the retina.

Politzer luminous c., SYN light *reflex* (3).

pulmonary c., SYN *conus* arteriosus.

retinal c.'s, SEE cone (2).

silver c., pure silver c. with standard conical shape, used with cement to obturate dental root canals.

theca interna c., the conical thickening of thecal cells of an ovarian follicle with its apex pointed toward the surface.

twin c., two retinal c.'s fused together.

vascular c.'s, SYN *lobules* of epididymis, under *lobule*.

♻**-cone.** The cusp of a tooth in the upper jaw.

co·nes·si (ko-nes'e). The bark of *Holarrhena antidysenterica* (family Apocynaceae), an Indian tree; used as an astringent and in the treatment of dysentery and amebiasis. SYN kurchi bark. [E. Ind.]

co·nes·sine (kon'ĕ-sēn). A steroid alkaloid derived from *Holarrhena antidysenterica* (conessi); a yellow astringent, used in the treatment of amebic dysentery and vaginal trichomoniasis. SYN neriine, wrightine.

co·nex·us, pl. **co·nex·us** (ko-nek'sŭs). SYN connection. [L.]

c. intertendin′eus, SYN intertendinous *connections* of extensor digitorum, under *connection*.

con·fab·u·la·tion (kon'fab-ū-lā'shŭn). The making of bizarre and incorrect responses, and a readiness to give a fluent but tangential answer, with no regard whatever to facts, to any question put; seen in amnesia and Wernicke-Korsakoff syndrome. [L. *con-fabulor*, pp. *-fabulatus,* to talk together, fr. *fabula*, narrative]

con·fec·tio, gen. **con·fec·ti·o·nis,** pl. **con·fec·ti·o·nes** (kon-fek′

shē-ō, -ō′nis, -ō′nēz). SYN confection. [L. fr. *conficio,* pp. *-fectus,* to make ready, prepare]

con·fec·tion (kon-fek′shŭn). A pharmaceutical preparation consisting of a drug mixed with honey or syrup; a soft solid, sometimes used as an excipient for pill masses. SYN confectio, conserve, electuary. [L. *confectio*]

con·fer·tus (kon-fer′tŭs). Arranged closely together; coalescing. [L. *confercio,* pp. *-fertus,* to cram together, fr. *farcio,* to fill full, cram]

con·fi·den·ti·al·i·ty (kon′fi-den-shē-al′i-tē). The statutorily protected right afforded to (and duty required of) specifically designated health professionals not to disclose information discerned during consultation with a patient. [L. *con-fido,* to trust, be assured]

con·fig·u·ra·tion (kon-fig-ū-rā′shŭn). **1.** The general form of a body and its parts. **2.** In chemistry, the spatial arrangement of atoms in a molecule. The c. of a compound (e.g., a sugar) is the unique spatial arrangement of its atoms such that no other arrangement of these atoms is superimposable thereon with complete correspondence, regardless of changes in conformation (*i.e.,* twisting or rotation about single bonds); change of c. requires breaking and rejoining of bonds, as in going from D to L c.'s of sugars. Cf. conformation.
cis c., (1) SEE cis- (4); **(2)** the property of two or more sites on the same molecule of DNA.

con·fine·ment (kon-fīn′ment). Lying-in; giving birth to a child. [L. *confine* (ntr.), a boundary, confine, fr. *con-* + *finis,* boundary]

con·flict (kon′flikt). Tension or stress experienced by an organism when satisfaction of a need, drive, motive, or wish is thwarted by the presence of other attractive or unattractive needs, drives, or motives.
approach-approach c., a situation of indecision and vacillation when an individual is confronted with two equally attractive alternatives.
approach-avoidance c., a situation of indecision and vacillation when the individual is confronted with a single object or event which has both attractive and unattractive qualities.
avoidance-avoidance c., a situation of indecision and vacillation when the individual is confronted with two equally unattractive alternatives.
c. of interest, a c. between the professional or personal interests and needs of a health provider and his or her professional responsibilities toward a patient or other consumer.
interpersonal c., relating to a conflict in the relations and social exchanges between persons. Cf. intrapersonal c.
intrapersonal c., a conflict that occurs solely in the psychological dynamics of the individual's own mind. SEE intrapsychic.
role c., the dilemma an individual experiences when required to play two different parts (e.g., spouse and aggressive business competitor) that cannot be easily harmonized.

con·flu·ence (kon′floo-ĕns) [TA]. A flowing together; a joining of two or more streams. SYN confluens [TA]. [L. *confluens*]
c. of sinuses [TA], a meeting place, at the internal occipital protuberance, of the superior sagittal, straight, occipital, drained by the two transverse sinuses of the dura mater. SYN confluens sinuum [TA].

con·flu·ens (kon-floo′enz) [TA]. SYN confluence, confluence. [L.]
c. si′nuum [TA], SYN *confluence* of sinuses.

con·flu·ent (kon′floo-ent). **1.** Joining; running together; denoting certain skin lesions which become merged, forming a patch; denoting a disease characterized by lesions which are not discrete, or distinct one from the other. **2.** Denoting a bone formed by the blending together of two originally distinct bones. [L. *con-fluo,* to flow together]

con·fo·cal (kon-fō′kal). SEE confocal *microscope.*

con·for·ma·tion (kon-fōr-mā′shŭn). The spatial arrangement of a molecule achieved by rotation of groups about single covalent bonds, without breaking any covalent bonds; the latter restriction differentiates c. from configuration (as in anomers and related stereoisomers) where a bond or bonds must be broken in going from one form (configuration) to another. C. is one of the most

important aspects of sugar chemistry and is basic to an understanding of the chemical properties of sugars. Cf. configuration.
boat c., SEE Haworth conformational formulas of cyclic *sugars.*
envelope c., SEE Haworth conformational formulas of cyclic *sugars.*

con·form·er (kon-fōr′mer). A mold, usually of plastic material, used in surgical repair to maintain space in a cavity or to prevent closing by healing of an artificial or natural opening. [L. *conformo,* to fashion]

con·found·ing. 1. A situation in which the effects of two or more processes are not separated; the distortion of the apparent effect of an exposure on risk, brought about by the association with other factors that can influence the outcome. **2.** A relationship between the effects of two or more causal factors observed in a set of data, such that it is not logically possible to separate the contribution of any single causal factor to the observed effects.

con·fron·ta·tion (kon-frŏn-tā′shŭn). The act by the therapist, or another patient in a therapy group, of openly interpreting a patient's resistances, attitudes, feelings, or effects upon either the therapist, the group, or its member(s).

con·fu·sion (kon-fū′zhŭn). A mental state in which reactions to environmental stimuli are inappropriate because the person is bewildered, perplexed, or unable to orientate himself. [L. *con-fusio,* a confounding]

con·fu·sion·al (kon-fū′zhŭn-ăl). Characterized by, or pertaining to, confusion.

con·ge·ner (kon′jē-ner). **1.** One of two or more things of the same kind, as of animal or plant with respect to classification. **2.** One of two or more muscles with the same function. [L. *con-,* with, + *genus,* race]

con·ge·ner·ous (kon-jen′er-ŭs). **1.** Having the same function; denoting certain muscles that are synergistic. **2.** Derived from the same source, or of a similar nature. [see congener]

con·gen·ic (kon-jen′ik). Relating to an inbred strain of animals produced by repeated crossing of one gene line onto another inbred (isogenic) line. [con- + G. *genos,* birth, + -ic]

con·gen·i·tal (kon-jen′i-tăl). Existing at birth, referring to certain mental or physical traits, anomalies, malformations, diseases, etc. which may be either hereditary or due to an influence occurring during gestation up to the moment of birth. SYN congenitus. [L. *congenitus,* born with]

con·gen·i·tus (kon-jen′i-tŭs). SYN congenital. [L.]

con·gest·ed (kon-jes′ted). Containing an abnormal amount of blood; in a state of congestion.

con·ges·tion (kon-jes′chŭn). Presence of an abnormal amount of fluid in the vessels or passages of a part or organ; especially, of blood due either to increased influx or to an obstruction to outflow. SEE ALSO hyperemia. [L. *congestio,* a bringing together, a heap, fr. *con-gero,* pp. *-gestus,* to bring together]
active c., c. due to an increased flow of arterial blood to a part.
brain c., increased volume of the intravascular compartment of the brain; often associated with brain swelling. SYN encephalemia.
functional c., hyperemia occurring during functional activity of an organ. SYN physiologic c.
hypostatic c., c. due to pooling of venous blood in a dependent part. SYN hypostasis (2).
passive c., c. caused by obstruction or slowing of the venous drainage, resulting in partial stagnation of blood in the capillaries and venules.
physiologic c., SYN functional c.
venous c., overfilling and distention of the veins with blood as a result of mechanical obstruction or right ventricular failure.

con·ges·tive (kon-jes′tiv). Relating to congestion.

con·glo·bate (kon-glō′bāt). Formed in a single rounded mass. [L. *con-globo,* pp. *-atus,* to gather into a *globus,* ball]

con·glo·ba·tion (kon-glō-bā′shŭn). An aggregation of numerous particles into one rounded mass.

con·glom·er·ate (kon-glom′ĕ-rāt). Composed of several parts aggregated into one mass. [L. *conglomero,* pp. *-atus,* to roll together, fr. *glomus,* a ball]

con·glu·ti·nant (kon-gloo′ti-nant). Adhesive, promoting the union of a wound. [L. *con-glutino,* pp. *-atus,* to glue together, fr. *gluten,* glue]

con·glu·ti·na·tion (kon-gloo-ti-nā′shŭn). **1.** SYN adhesion (1). **2.** Agglutination of antigen(erythrocyte)-antibody-complement complex by normal bovine serum (and certain other colloidal materials); the procedure provides a means of detecting the presence of nonagglutinating antibody.

con·glu·ti·nin (kon-gloo′ti-nin). Bovine serum protein that, when absorbed by erythrocyte-antibody-complement complexes, causes them to agglutinate; it is comparatively thermostable and apparently dissociates when diluted with physiologic saline solution. SYN bovine colloid.

con·go·phil·ic (kon-gō-fil′ik). Denoting any substance that takes a Congo red stain.

Con·go red (kong′gō) [C.I. 22120]. An acid direct cotton dye, it is absorbed by amyloid and induces green fluorescence to amyloid in polarized light; used as a laboratory aid in the diagnosis of amyloidosis, as a histologic stain, and as an indicator (pH 3.0, blue-violet, to pH 5.0, red) in testing for free hydrochloric acid in gastric contents. SEE Bennhold Congo red *stain.*

co·ni (kō′nī). Plural of conus.

con·ic, con·i·cal (kon′ik, kon′i-kăl). Resembling a cone.

△**-conid.** The cusp of a tooth in the lower jaw.

co·nid·ia (ko-nid′ē-ă). Plural of conidium.

co·nid·i·al (ko-nid′ē-ăl). Relating to a conidium.

Co·nid·i·o·bo·lus (ko-nid′ē-ō-bō′lŭs). A genus of fungi containing two species, *C. coronatus* and *C. incongruus,* both of which cause zygomycosis (entomophthoramycosis).

co·nid·i·og·e·nous (ko-nid-ē-oj′ĕ-nŭs). Denoting a cell that gives rise to a conidium, e.g., a phialide.

co·nid·i·o·phore (ko-nid′ē-ō-fōr). A specialized hypha which bears conidia in fungi. [conidium + G. *phoros,* bearing]

Phialophore-type c., a type of spore formation, characteristic of the genus *Phialophora,* in which conidia are formed endogenously in flasklike c.'s called phialids.

co·nid·i·um, pl. **co·nid·ia** (ko-nid′ē-ŭm, -ē-ă). An asexual spore of fungi borne externally in various ways. [Mod. L. dim. fr. G. *konis,* dust]

co·ni·ine (kō′nē-ēn). The toxic active alkaloid of conium (hemlock); hydrobromide and hydrochloride salts have been used as an antispasmodic; principal toxin of poison hemlock (*Conium maculatum*).

co·ni·o·fi·bro·sis (kō′nē-ō-fī-brō′sis). Fibrosis produced by dust, especially of the lungs by inhaled dust. [G. *konis,* dust, + fibrosis]

co·ni·o·lymph·sta·sis (kō′nē-ō-limf′stă-sis). Stasis of lymph caused by dust, presumably through the intervention of fibrosis. [G. *konis,* dust, + lymph + G. *stasis,* a standing]

co·ni·om·e·ter (kō-nē-om′ĕ-ter). A device for estimating the amount of dust in the air. [G. *konis,* dust, + *metron,* measure]

co·ni·o·phage (kō′nē-ō-fāj). SYN alveolar *macrophage.* [G. *konis,* dust, + *phagō* to eat]

co·ni·o·sis (kō-nē-ō′sis). Any disease or morbid condition caused by dust. [G. *konis,* dust]

co·ni·ot·o·my (kō-nē-ot′ō-mē). Incision of the laryngeal conus elasticus. SEE ALSO cricothyrotomy.

co·ni·um (kō-nē′ŭm). The dried unripe fruit of *Conium maculatum* (family Umbelliferae), also known as spotted cowbane or spotted parsley; it has been used as a sedative, antispasmodic, and anodyne. SYN hemlock. [L. fr. G. *kōneion,* hemlock]

con·i·za·tion (kō-nī-zā′shŭn). Excision of a cone of tissue, e.g., mucosa of the cervix uteri.

cautery c., removal of a cone shape of endocervical tissue with electrocautery.

cold knife c., obtaining a cone of endocervical tissue with a cold knife blade so as to preserve histological characteristics and avoid desiccating tissue.

con·ju·gant (kon′joo-gant). A member of a mating pair of organisms or gametes undergoing conjugation. SEE ALSO exconjugant. [L. *con-jugo,* to join]

con·ju·ga·ta (kon-joo-gā′tă) [TA]. Conjugate diameters of the

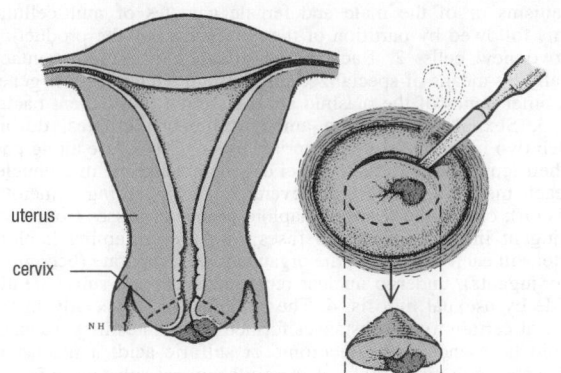

conization: malignancy shown in red, dashed line shows extent of resection

pelvis. SEE conjugate. [L. fem. of *conjugatus,* pp. of *con-jugo,* to join together]

c. anatomica [TA], SYN anatomical *conjugate.*

c. diagonal′is [TA], SYN diagonal *conjugate.*

c. externa [TA], SYN external *conjugate.*

c. recta [TA], SYN straight *conjugate.*

c. vera [TA], SYN true *conjugate.*

con·ju·gate (kon′joo-gāt) [TA]. **1.** Joined or paired. SYN conjugated. **2.** Conjugate diameters of the pelvis. The distance between any two specified points on the periphery of the pelvic canal. [L. *conjugatus,* joined together. See conjugata]

anatomical c. [TA], measure of pelvic dimension describing the distance between the sacral promontory and the inferior border of the pubic symphysis, measured manually per vagina or by ultrasonography. It is used to extrapolate the true c. SYN conjugata anatomica [TA].

diagonal c. [TA], the anteroposterior dimension of the inlet that measures the clinical distance from the promontory of the sacrum to the lower margin of the symphysis pubica. SYN conjugata diagonalis [TA], diagonal conjugate diameter, false c. (1).

effective c., the internal c. measured from the nearest lumbar vertebra to the symphysis, in spondylolisthesis. SYN false c. (2).

external c. [TA], the distance in a straight line between the depression under the last spinous process of the lumbar vertebrae and the upper edge of the pubic symphysis. SYN conjugata externa [TA], external conjugate diameter.

false c., (1) SYN diagonal c; (2) SYN effective c.

folic acid c., a folate with three molecules of glutamic acid (pteropterin) instead of one, or with seven (pteroylheptaglutamic acid or vitamin B_c conjugate).

internal c., SYN median c.

median c. [TA], distance from the promontory of the sacrum to the upper posterior edge of the pubic symphysis. SYN anteroposterior diameter of the pelvic inlet, conjugate axis, conjugate diameter of pelvic inlet, c. of pelvic inlet, internal c.

obstetric c., SYN true c.

obstetric c. of pelvic outlet, the c. of the pelvic outlet lengthened by the posterior displacement of the coccyx.

c. of pelvic inlet, SYN median c.

c. of pelvic outlet, SYN straight c; SEE ALSO obstetric c. of pelvic outlet.

straight c. [TA], the distance from the tip of the coccyx to the lower edge of the pubic symphysis. SYN conjugata recta [TA], conjugate diameter of pelvic outlet, c. of pelvic outlet.

true c. [TA], the diameter that represents the shortest diameter through which the head must pass in descending into the superior strait and measures, by means of x-ray, the distance from the promontory of the sacrum to a point on the inner surface of the symphysis a few millimeters below its upper margin. SYN conjugata vera [TA], obstetric conjugate diameter, obstetric c.

con·ju·gat·ed (kon′joo-gāt-ed). SYN conjugate (1).

con·ju·ga·tion (kon-jŭ-gā′shŭn). **1.** The union of two unicellular

co

organisms or of the male and female gametes of multicellular forms followed by partition of the chromatin and the production of two new cells. **2.** Bacterial c., effected by simple contact, usually by means of specialized pili through which transfer genes and other genes of the plasmid are transferred to recipient bacteria. **3.** Sexual reproduction among protozoan ciliates, during which two individuals of appropriate mating types fuse along part of their lengths; their macronuclei degenerate and the micronuclei in each macronucleus divide several times (including a meiotic division); one of the resulting haploid pronuclei passes from each conjugant into the other and fuses with the remaining haploid nucleus in each conjugant; the organisms then separate (becoming exconjugants), undergo nuclear reorganization, and subsequently divide by asexual mitosis. **4.** The combination, especially in the liver, of certain toxic substances formed in the intestine, drugs, or steroid hormones with glucuronic or sulfuric acid; a means by which the biologic activity of certain chemical substances is terminated and the substances made ready for excretion. **5.** The formation of glycyl or tauryl derivatives of the bile acids. **6.** An alternating sequence of multiple and single chemical bonds in a chemical compound in which there is some delocalization of π-electrons. **7.** The joining together of two compounds. [L. *conjugo*, pp. *-jugatus*, to join together]

con·junc·ti·va, pl. **con·junc·ti·vae** (kon-jŭnk-tī′vă, -vē) [TA]. The mucous membrane investing the anterior surface of the eyeball and the posterior surface of the lids. SYN tunica conjunctiva [TA]. [L. fem. of *conjunctivus*, from *conjungo*, pp. *-junctus*, to bind together]

bulbar c. [TA], the part of the conjunctiva covering the anterior surface of the sclera and the surface epithelium of the cornea. SYN tunica conjunctiva bulbi [TA], conjunctival layer of bulb.

palpebral c. [TA], the part of the conjunctiva lining the posterior surface of the eyelids and continuous with the bulbar conjunctiva at the conjunctival fornices. SYN tunica conjunctiva palpebrarum [TA], conjunctival layer of eyelids.

con·junc·ti·val (kon-jŭnk-tī′văl). Relating to the conjunctiva.

con·junc·tive (kon-jŭnk′tiv). Joining; connecting; connective.

con·junc·ti·vi·plas·ty (kon-jŭnk-tī′vi-plas-tē). SYN conjunctivo-plasty.

con·junc·ti·vi·tis (kon-jŭnk-ti-vī′tis). Inflammation of the conjunctiva. SYN blennophthalmia (1).

actinic c., SYN ultraviolet *keratoconjunctivitis*.

acute contagious c., an obsolete term for an acute c. marked by intense hyperemia and profuse mucopurulent discharge. SYN acute epidemic c., pinkeye.

acute epidemic c., SYN acute contagious c.

acute hemorrhagic c., specific acute endemic c. with eyelid swelling, tearing, conjunctival hemorrhages, and follicles; usually caused by Enterovirus type 70.

acute viral c., an epidemic inflammation of the conjunctiva marked by follicles, especially in the lower fornix; may be caused by adenoviruses, herpesvirus, and Newcastle disease virus.

allergic c., an immunologic reaction mediated by immunoglobulin E associated with itching, redness, and tearing; it is typically seasonal and may affect up to 10% of the population.

angular c., a subacute bilateral conjunctival inflammation sometimes caused by the *Moraxella* bacillus, marked by redness of the lateral canthi and scanty, stringy discharge that adheres to the lashes. SYN *Moraxella* c.

arc-flash c., SYN ultraviolet *keratoconjunctivitis*.

c. ar′ida, SYN xerophthalmia.

chemical c., conjunctival inflammation due to chemical irritants.

chronic c., a persistent, bilateral, conjunctival hyperemia with scanty exudation; there is a tendency toward remission and exacerbation.

chronic follicular c., indolent inflammation of the conjunctiva, with discrete follicles in fornices that may be infective, toxic, or irritant in nature.

cicatricial c., a chronic progressive ocular affection that produces scarring of the conjunctiva primarily and of the cornea sequentially.

diphtheritic c., a severe conjunctival inflammation caused by

Corynebacterium diphtheriae and characterized by an infiltrating membrane which on removal leaves a raw surface. SYN membranous c.

follicular c., c. associated with hypertrophic lymphoid tissue in the conjunctival fornices.

giant papillary c., conjunctival inflammation characterized by large papillae and associated with sensitization to antigenic material present on the surface of a contact lens.

gonococcal c., a type of hyperacute, purulent c.

gonorrheal c., SYN gonorrheal *ophthalmia*.

granular c., SYN trachomatous c.

hyperacute purulent c., c. caused by *Neisseria gonorrhea* and marked by swollen congested conjunctiva, edematous eyelids, and a purulent discharge.

inclusion c., a follicular c. caused by *Chlamydia trachomatis*.

infantile purulent c., SYN *ophthalmia* neonatorum.

larval c., c. due to imbedding of larvae in the eye. SEE ophthalmo-myiasis.

ligneous c., c. characterized typically by woody induration of the upper tarsal conjunctiva, whitish pseudomembrane, and, in severe cases, corneal opacity; usually bilateral.

c. medicamento′sa, a c. caused by medicine or toxin instilled into the conjunctival sac. SYN toxicogenic c.

membranous c., SYN diphtheritic c.

molluscum c., c. associated with lesions of molluscum contagiosum of the eyelid.

***Moraxella* c.,** SYN angular c.

necrotic infectious c., a unilateral, suppurative, necrotic inflammation of the conjunctiva characterized by scattered, elevated white spots in the fornices and palpebral conjunctiva, and ipsilateral swelling of preauricular, parotid, and submaxillary lymph glands. SYN Pascheff c.

neonatal c., SYN *ophthalmia* neonatorum.

Parinaud c., a chronic necrotic inflammation of the conjunctiva characterized by large, irregular, reddish follicles and regional lymphadenopathy.

Pascheff c., SYN necrotic infectious c.

phlyctenular c., a circumscribed c. accompanied by the formation of small red nodules of lymphoid tissue (phlyctenulae) on the conjunctiva. SYN phlyctenular ophthalmia.

pseudomembranous c., a nonspecific inflammatory reaction characterized by the appearance on the conjunctiva of a coagulated fibrinous plaque that may be peeled off from intact epithelium.

purulent c., a violently acute inflammation of the conjunctiva, with copious pus and a marked tendency for corneal involvement.

simple c., acute viral c., self-limited and of short duration.

snow c., SYN ultraviolet *keratoconjunctivitis*.

spring c., SYN vernal c.

squirrel plague c., one of the causes of Parinaud c. SYN tularemic c., c. tularensis.

swimming pool c., a nonspecific red eye that can be caused by pool chlorination, adenovirus, and rarely, *Chlamydia*.

toxicogenic c., SYN c. medicamentosa.

trachomatous c., a chronic infection of the conjunctiva due to *Chlamydia trachomatis*, characterized by conjunctival follicles and subsequent cicatrization. SEE ALSO trachoma. SYN granular c.

tularemic c., c. tularen′sis, SYN squirrel plague c.

vernal c., a chronic, bilateral conjunctival inflammation with photophobia and intense itching that recurs seasonally during warm weather; characterized in the palpebral form by cobblestone papillae in the upper palpebral conjunctiva and in the bulbar form by gelatinous nodules adjacent to the corneoscleral limbus. SYN spring c., spring ophthalmia, vernal catarrh, vernal keratoconjunctivitis.

welder's c., SYN ultraviolet *keratoconjunctivitis*.

con·junc·ti·vo·chal·a·sis (kon-junk′-ti-vō-kal′ă-sis). Condition in which redundant bulbar *conjunctiva* billows over the eyelid margin or covers the lower punctum. [conjunctiva + G. *chalasis*, loosening]

con·junc·ti·vo·dac·ry·o·cys·to·rhi·nos·to·my (kon-jŭnk′ti-vō-dak′rē-ō-sis′tō-rī-nos′tō-mē). A procedure for providing lacrimal drainage when the canaliculi are closed; plastic tubes are inserted that extend from the conjunctival sac through the lacrimal sac to the nose; the opening so produced. [conjunctiva + G. *dakryon*, tear, + *kystis*, cyst, + *ris* (*rhin*-), nose, + *stoma*, mouth]

con·junc·ti·vo·dac·ry·o·cys·tos·to·my (kon-jŭnk'ti-vō-dak'rē-ō-sis-tos'tō-mē). **1.** A surgical procedure through the conjunctiva, which provides an opening into the lacrimal sac. **2.** The opening so produced. [conjunctiva + G. *dakryon*, tear, + *kystis*, sac, + *stoma*, mouth]

con·junc·ti·vo·plas·ty (kon-jŭnk-tī'vō-plas-tē, kon-jŭnk'ti-vō-). Plastic surgery on the conjunctiva. SYN conjunctiviplasty.

con·junc·ti·vo·rhi·nos·to·my (kon-jŭnk'ti-vō-rī-nos'tō-mē). **1.** A surgical procedure to construct a passageway through the conjunctiva into the nasal cavity. **2.** The opening so produced. [conjunctiva + G. *ris* (*rhin*), nose, + *stoma*, mouth]

Conn, Harold J., U.S. microbiologist, 1886–1975. SEE Hucker-C. *stain.*

Conn, Jerome, U.S. physician, *1907. SEE C. *syndrome.*

con·nec·tins (kon-nek'tinz). Collective term for the protein components of the cytoskeleton (connective tissue); originally described in muscle, but later observed in erythrocyte and other cell membranes.

con·nec·tion (kŏ-nek'shŭn). A union of elements or things; a connecting structure. SYN conexus, connexus.

  ambiguous atrioventricular c.'s, c.'s in which half the atrioventricular junction is connected concordantly and the other half is discordantly connected.

  anomalous pulmonary venous c.'s, total or partial, c.'s in which some or all of the pulmonary veins connect to the right atrium or one of its tributaries.

  atrioventricular c.'s, the five distinct and discrete ways in which the atrial chambers may be connected to the ventricles are concordant, discordant, ambiguous, double inlet, and univentricular.

  concordant atrioventricular c.'s, c.'s in which the atrial chambers connect to the morphologically appropriate ventricles.

  discordant atrioventricular c.'s, c.'s in which each atrium is connected with a morphologically inappropriate ventricle.

  double inlet atrioventricular c.'s, c.'s in which both atrial chambers connect to the same ventricle.

  intertendinous c.'s of extensor digitorum [TA], fibrous bands passing obliquely between the diverging tendons of the extensor digitorum on the dorsum of the hand. SYN connexus intertendinei musculi extensoris digitorum [TA], conexus intertendineus, juncturae tendinum.

  marrow-mesenchyme c.'s, uninterrupted continuations between bone marrow and mesenchyme of fetal and newborn middle ears.

  partial anomalous pulmonary venous c.'s, SEE anomalous pulmonary venous c.'s, total or partial.

  univentricular c.'s, c.'s in which one of the atrial chambers is connected to a ventricle, but the other has no connection with the ventricular mass at all.

con·nec·tor (kŏ-nek'tŏr, -tōr). In dentistry, a part of a partial denture which unites its components.

  major c., a plate or bar (lingual bar, palatal bar) used for the purpose of uniting partial denture bases.

  minor c., the connecting link (tang) between the major c. or base of a partial denture and other units of the prosthesis, such as clasps, indirect retainers, and occlusal rests.

  nonrigid c., a c. or joint that is not rigid or solid. SYN stress-broken c., stress-broken joint.

  rigid c., a c. that is solid or rigid, as a soldered joint.

  stress-broken c., SYN nonrigid c.

Connell, F. Gregory, U.S. surgeon, 1875–1968. SEE C. *suture.*

con·nex·in 26 (kon-eks'in). The gap junction protein, the gene for which (Cx26) when mutated, accounts for a major portion of recessive nonsyndromic hearing impairment.

con·nex·ins, con·nex·ons (kon-neks'inz, -onz). Complex protein assemblies that traverse the lipid bilayer of the plasma membrane and forms a continuous channel with a pore diameter of approximately 1.5 nm; a pair of c.'s from two adjacent cells join to form a gap junction that bridges the 2–4-nm gap between the

cells, resulting in both electrical and metabolic couplings; one type of c.'s makes up the gap junction in heart and may coordinate the beating of all muscle cells in one section of the heart.

con·nex·us (ko-nek'sŭs). SYN connection. [L.]

  c. intertendin'ei musculi extensoris digitorum [TA], SYN intertendinous *connections* of extensor digitorum, under *connection.*

co·noid (kō'noyd). **1.** A cone-shaped structure. **2.** Part of the apical complex characteristic of the protozoan subphylum, Apicomplexa; seen in sporozoites, merozoites, or other developmental stages of sporozoans, less well developed in the piroplasms (families Babesiidae and Theileriidae). The function of the c. is unknown, but it is thought to be an organelle of penetration into the host cell, possibly aided by a protrusible form of the c. [G. *kōnoeidēs,* cone-shaped]

  Sturm c., in optics, the pattern of rays formed after passage through a spherocylindrical combination.

co·no·my·oi·din (kō-nō-mī'oy-din). Contractile protoplasm at the inner end of the inner segment of retinal cones; motility is most evident in fishes and amphibians, and slight or absent in mammals. [G. *kōnos,* cone, + *mys,* muscle, + *eidos,* resemblance]

con·qui·nine (kon'kwi-nēn). SYN quinidine.

Conradi, Andrew, Norwegian physician, 1809–1869. SEE C. *line.*

Conradi, Erich, 20th century German physician. SEE C. *disease.*

con·san·guin·e·ous (kon-sang-gwin'ē-ŭs). Denoting consanguinity. [L. *cum,* with, + *sanguis,* blood: *consanguineus*]

con·san·guin·i·ty (kon-sang-gwin'i-tē). Kinship because of common ancestry. SEE ALSO relationship. [L. *consanguinitas,* blood relationship]

con·scious (con'shŭs). **1.** Aware; having present knowledge or perception of oneself, one's acts and surroundings. **2.** Denoting something occurring with the perceptive attention of the individual, as a c. act or idea, distinguished from automatic or instinctive. [L. *conscius,* knowing]

con·scious·ness (con'shŭs-nes). The state of being aware, or perceiving physical facts or mental concepts; a state of general wakefulness and responsiveness to environment; a functioning sensorium. [L. *con-scio,* to know, to be aware of]

  clouding of c., a state in which the patient's mental state is clouded and thus not fully in contact with the environment.

  double c., a condition in which one lives in two seemingly unrelated mental states, being, while in one, unaware of the other or of the acts performed in the other. SEE ALSO dual *personality.*

  field of c., the content of awareness at any given moment.

con·sen·su·al (kon-sen'shoo-ăl). **1.** With consent; by mutual agreement of all parties. **2.** Pertaining to a reflex elicited by indirect stimulation of a receptor, as pupillary constriction in 1 eye when the other is stimulated by light. [L. *con-sentio,* pp. *consensus,* to agree, to feel at the same time + -al]

con·ser·va·tion (kon-ser-vā'shŭn). **1.** Preservation from loss, injury, or decay. **2.** In sensorimotor theory, the mental operation by which an individual retains the idea of an object after its removal in time or space. [L. *conservatio,* a preserving, keeping]

  c. of energy, the principle that the total amount of energy in a closed system remains always the same, none being lost or created in any chemical or physical process or in the conversion of one kind of energy into another, within that system.

con·ser·va·tive (kon-ser'vă-tiv). Denoting treatment by gradual, limited, or well-established procedures, as opposed to radical.

con·serve (kon'serv). SYN confection.

con·sol·i·dant (kon-sol'i-dant). A substance that promotes healing or union.

con·sol·i·da·tion (kon-sol-i-dā'shŭn). Solidification into a firm dense mass; applied especially to inflammatory induration of a normally aerated lung due to the presence of cellular exudate in the pulmonary alveoli as commonly seen in pneumonia. [L. *consolido,* to make thick, condense, fr. *solidus,* solid]

con·spe·cif·ic (kon-spe-sif'ik). Of the same species. [L. *con-,* with, + specific]

con·spi·cu·i·ty (kon-spi-kū'i-tē). The visibility of a structure of interest on a radiograph, a function of the inherent contrast of the structure and the complexity (noise) of the surrounding image.

CO

con·stan·cy (kon'stan-sē). The quality of being unchanging [L. *constantia*, fr. *consto*, to stand still]

color c., unchanging perception of the color of an object despite changes in lighting or viewing conditions.

object c., (1) the tendency for objects to be perceived as unchanging despite variations in the positions in and conditions under which the objects are observed; e.g., a book's shape is always perceived as a rectangle regardless of the visual angle from which it is viewed. **(2)** in psychoanalysis, the relatively enduring emotional investment in another person.

con·stant (kon'stănt). A quantity that, under stated conditions, does not vary with changes in the environment.

association c., (1) in experimental immunology, a mathematical expression of hapten-antibody interaction: average association c., K = [hapten-bound antibody]/[free antibody][free hapten]; **(2)** (K_a), the equilibrium c. involved in the association of two or more compounds or ions into a new compound; the reciprocal of the dissociation c. SYN binding c.

Avogadro c., SYN Avogadro *number*.

binding c., SYN association c.

decay c., the fractional change in the number of atoms of a radionuclide that occurs in unit time; the constant λ in the equation for the fraction (dN/N) of the number of atoms (N) of a radionuclide disintegrating in time dt, $dN/N = -\lambda dt$. SYN disintegration c., radioactive c., transformation c.

diffusion c., SYN diffusion *coefficient*.

disintegration c., SYN decay c.

dissociation c. (K_d, K), the equilibrium c. involved in the dissociation of a compound into two or more compounds or ions. The reciprocal of the association c. (2).

dissociation c. of an acid (K_d, K_a), expressed by the general equation [H^+][A^-]/[HA] = K_a, where HA is the undissociated acid.

dissociation c. of a base (K_b), expressed by the general equation [B^+][OH^-]/[BOH] = K_b, where BOH is the undissociated base.

dissociation c. of water, expressed by the equation [H^+][OH^-] = $K_w = 10^{-14}$ at 25°C.

equilibrium c. (K_{eq}), in the reaction A + B $\leftrightarrow$ C + D at equilibrium (i.e., no net change in concentrations of A, B, C, or D), the concentrations of the four components are related by the equation K_{eq} = [C][D]/[A][B]; K_{eq} is the equilibrium c. If any component in the reaction has a multiplier (e.g., $H_2 \leftrightarrow 2H$), that multiplier appears as an exponent in the calculation of K (e.g., $K_{eq} = [H]^2/[H_2]$). When this equation is applied to the ionization of a substance in solution, K_{eq} is called the dissociation c. (K_d) and its negative logarithm (base 10) is the pK_d. SEE ALSO Henderson-Hasselbalch *equation*, mass-action *ratio*.

Faraday c. (F), SEE faraday.

flotation c. (S_f), characteristic sedimentation behavior of a lipoprotein fraction of plasma in a centrifugal field in a medium of appropriate density, achieved by adding a salt or D_2O to the plasma. SYN negative S, Svedberg of flotation.

gas c. (R), $R = 8.314 \times 10^7$ ergs K^{-1} mol^{-1} = 8.314 J K^{-1} mol^{-1}.

Hill c., SYN Hill *coefficient*.

Michaelis c., (1) the true dissociation constant for the enzyme-substrate binary complex in a single-substrate rapid equilibrium enzyme-catalyzed reaction (usually symbolized by K_s); **(2)** the concentration of the substrate at which half the true maximum velocity of an enzyme-catalyzed reaction is achieved (when velocities are measured under initial rate and steady state conditions); the ratio of rate constants ($k_2 + k_3$)/k_1 in the single-substrate enzyme-catalyzed reaction: E + S $\leftrightarrow$ ES $\leftrightarrow$ E + products where E represents the free enzyme, S is the substrate, and ES is the central binary complex. The expression for the Michaelis c. will be more complex for multisubstrate reactions. An apparent Michaelis c. is a c. determined either under conditions that are not strictly steady state and initial rate or one that varies with the concentration of one or more cosubstrates. SEE Michaelis-Menten *equation*. SYN Michaelis-Menten c.

Michaelis-Menten c. (K_m), SYN Michaelis c.

Newtonian c. of gravitation (G), a universal c. relating the gravitational force, F, attracting two masses, m_1 and m_2, toward each other when they are separated by a distance, r, in the equation: F = G($m_1 m_2/r^2$); it has the value of 6.67259×10^{-8} dyne cm^2 g^{-2} = 6.67259×10^{-11} m^3 kg^{-1} s^{-2} in SI units.

permeability c., a measure of the ease with which an ion can cross a unit area of membrane driven by a 1.0 mol/L difference in concentration; usually expressed in centimeters per second. Cf. permeability *coefficient*.

Planck c. (*h*), a c., $6.6260755 \times 10^{-34}$ J · s or $6.6260755 \times 10^{-27}$ erg-seconds = $6.6260755 \times 10^{-34}$ J Hz^{-1}.

radioactive c. (Λ), SYN decay c.

rate c.'s (*k*), proportionality c.'s equal to the initial rate of a reaction divided by the concentration of the reactant(s); e.g., in the reaction A $\rightarrow$ B + C, the rate of the reaction equals $-d[A]/dt = k_1[A]$. The rate c. k_1 is a unimolecular rate c. since there is only one molecular species reacting and has units of reciprocal time (e.g., s^{-1}). For the reverse reaction, B + C $\rightarrow$ A, the rate equals $-d[B]/dt = d[A]/dt = k_2[B][C]$. The rate c. k_2 is a bimolecular rate c. and has units of reciprocal concentration-time (e.g., M^{-1} s^{-1}). SYN velocity c.'s.

sedimentation c., the c. s in Svedberg equation for estimating the molecular weight of a protein from the rate of movement in a centrifugal field:

$$M = s\frac{RT}{D(1 - \bar{V}\rho)}$$

where M is the molecular weight, R the gas constant, T the absolute temperature, D the diffusion constant (in square centimeters per second), $\bar{V}$ the partial specific volume of the protein, ρ the density of the solvent. The constant s, with dimensions of time per unit of field force ($s = {}^{dr/dt}/_{\omega^2 r_o}$ where r_b is the position at time t, r_0 is the position at time 0, and ω is the angular velocity) is usually between 1×10^{-13} and 200×10^{-13} s. The Svedberg unit (S) is arbitrarily set at 1×10^{-13} s and is very often used to describe the sedimentation rate of macromolecules; e.g., 4S RNA. SYN sedimentation coefficient.

specificity c., ratio of the maximum velocity (V_{max}) or k_{cat} to the true K_m value for a specific substrate in an enzyme-catalyzed reaction.

time c., that part of a circuit that determines the time interval over which the rate of electrical events will be averaged; in pulmonary physiology, the factors determining rate of flow in the airways.

transformation c., SYN decay c.

velocity c.'s (*k*), SYN rate c.'s.

con·stel·la·tion (kon-stel-ā'shŭn). In psychiatry, all the factors that determine a particular action. [L.L. *constellatio*, fr. *cum*, together, + *stella*, star]

con·sti·pate (kon'sti-pāt). To cause constipation.

con·sti·pat·ed (kon'sti-pāt-ed). Suffering from constipation.

con·sti·pa·tion (kon-sti-pā'shŭn). A condition in which bowel movements are infrequent or incomplete. SYN costiveness. [L. *con-stipo*, pp. *-atus*, to press together]

con·sti·tu·tion (kon-sti-too'shŭn). **1.** The physical makeup of a body, including the mode of performance of its functions, the activity of its metabolic processes, the manner and degree of its reactions to stimuli, and its power of resistance to the attack of pathogenic organisms or other disease processes. **2.** In chemistry, the number and kind of atoms in the molecule and the relation they bear to each other. [L. *constitutio*, constitution, disposition, fr. *constituo*, pp. *-stitutus*, to establish, fr. *statuo*, to set up]

con·sti·tu·tion·al (kon-sti-too'shŭn-ăl). **1.** Relating to a body's constitution. **2.** General; relating to the system as a whole; not local.

con·sti·tu·tive (kon-sti'too-tiv). **1.** SEE constitutive *enzyme*. **2.** In genetics, descriptive of a gene that is controlled by constantly active promoter.

constric'tio [TA]. SYN constriction (1).

c. bronchoaortica esophagea, [★]official alternate term for thoracic *constriction* of esophagus.

c. diaphragmatica esophagea, [★]official alternate term for diaphragmatic *constriction* of esophagus.

c. partis thoracicae esophagea [TA], SYN thoracic *constriction* of esophagus.

c. pharyngoesophagealis [TA], SYN pharyngoesophageal *constriction*.

c. phrenica esophagea [TA], SYN diaphragmatic *constriction* of esophagus.

con·stric·tion (kon-strik'shŭn). **1** [TA]. A normally or pathologically constricted or narrowed portion of a structure. SYN constrictio [TA]. SEE ALSO stricture, stenosis. **2.** The act or process of binding or contracting, becoming narrowed; the condition of being constricted. squeezed. **3.** A subjective sensation of pressure or tightness, as if the body or any part were tightly bound or squeezed. [L. *con-stringo,* pp. *-strictus,* to draw together]

broncho-aortic c., ☆official alternate term for thoracic c. of esophagus.

diaphragmatic c. of esophagus [TA], normal narrowing of the esophagus, demonstrated radiographically following a barium swallow, caused by the passage of the esophagus through the esophageal hiatus of the diaphragm. SYN constrictio phrenica esophagea [TA], constrictio diaphragmatica esophagea☆, inferior esophageal c.

esophageal c.'s, three narrowings of the esophagus normally demonstrated radiographically following a barium swallow. SEE ALSO pharyngoesophageal c., thoracic c. of esophagus, diaphragmatic c. of esophagus. SYN impressions of esophagus.

inferior esophageal c., SYN diaphragmatic c. of esophagus.

middle esophageal c., SYN thoracic c. of esophagus.

pharyngoesophageal c. [TA], normal narrowing of the alimentary tract, demonstrated radiographically following a barium swallow, at the junction of the pharynx with the esophagus (C5 vertebral level) caused by the tonic or active contraction of the cricopharyngeal part of the inferior constrictor of the pharynx (upper esophageal sphincter). SEE ALSO cricopharyngeal *part* of inferior constrictor (muscle) of pharynx. SYN constrictio pharyngoesophagealis [TA], upper esophageal c.

primary c., the narrowing between the two arms of the chromosome represented by the centromere.

pyloric c., circular groove on the external aspect of the gut at the gastroduodenal junction overlying the pyloric sphincter, thus demarcating the pyloric orifice.

secondary c., a subsidiary narrowing of the chromosome associated in some cases with satellites, e.g., the short arms of acrocentric autosomes.

thoracic c. of esophagus [TA], normal left-sided narrowing of the esophagus, demonstrated radiographically following a barium swallow, at the T4–T5 vertebral level, where the esophagus is impressed by the left main bronchus and the arch of the aorta. SYN constrictio partis thoracicae esophagea [TA], broncho-aortic c.☆, constrictio bronchoaortica esophagea☆, middle esophageal c.

upper esophageal c., SYN pharyngoesophageal c.

c.'s of ureter, normal physiological narrowings of the ureter observable in a pyelogram; the uppermost occurs at the origin of the ureter from the renal pelvis; a second occurs as the ureter crosses the iliac vessels and pelvic brim; the inferiormost occurs as the ureter penetrates the wall of the urinary bladder.

con·stric·tor (kon-strik'ter, -tōr). **1.** Anything that binds or squeezes a part. SEE ALSO inferior constrictor (*muscle*) of pharynx, middle constrictor (*muscle*) of pharynx, superior pharyngeal constrictor (*muscle*). **2.** A muscle, the action of which is to narrow a canal; a sphincter. [L. fr. *constringo,* to draw together]

con·struct (kon'strukt). The combination of a bone graft, metal instrumentation, prosthetic devices and/or bone cement applied to a specific level of the spinal column in the setting of segmental spinal instability.

con·sul·tand (kon-sŭl'tand). A person about whose future offspring the genetic counselor is to make predictions; not to be confused with proband. [consult (for counsel) + L. *-andus,* gerundive suffix]

dummy c., a person in the line of descent from the leading ancestor to the c. proper; for logical simplicity, the dummy c. is analyzed as if the c. proper.

con·sul·tant (kon-sŭl'tant). **1.** A physician or surgeon who does not take full responsibility for a patient, but acts in an advisory capacity, deliberating with and counseling the attending physician or surgeon. **2.** A member of a hospital staff who has no active service but stands ready to advise in any case, at the request of the attending physician or surgeon. [L. *consulto,* pp. *-atus,* to deliberate, ask advice]

con·sul·ta·tion (kon-sŭl-tā'shŭn). Meeting of two or more physicians or surgeons to evaluate the nature and progress of disease in a particular patient and to establish diagnosis, prognosis, and/or therapy.

con·sump·tion (kon-sŭmp'shŭn). **1.** The using up of something, especially the rate at which it is used. **2.** Obsolete term for a wasting of the tissues of the body, usually tuberculous. [L. *con-sumo,* pp. *-sumptus,* to take up wholly, use up, waste]

oxygen c. ($\dot{V}_{O_2}$), (1) (Qo or Qo_2), the rate at which oxygen is used by a tissue; units: microliters of oxygen STPD used per milligram of tissue per hour; **(2)** ($\dot{V}_{O_2}$), the rate at which oxygen enters the blood from alveolar gas, equal in the steady state to the consumption of oxygen by tissue metabolism throughout the body; units: milliliters of oxygen STPD used per minute or mmol/min.

con·sump·tive (kon-sŭmp'tiv). Relating to, or suffering from, consumption.

con·tact (kon'takt). **1.** The touching or apposition of two bodies. **2.** A person who has been exposed to a contagious disease. [L. *con- tingo,* pp. *-tactus,* to touch, seize, fr. *tango,* to touch]

balancing c., (1) the c.'s between upper and lower dentures on the balancing or mediotrusive side for the purpose of stabilizing the dentures; **(2)** the c.'s between upper and lower dentures at the opposite side from the working or laterotrusive side (anteroposteriorly or laterally) for the purpose of stabilizing the dentures; **(3)** the c.'s between upper and lower natural or artificial teeth at the opposite side from the working or laterotrusive side. SYN balancing occlusal surface.

centric c., SYN centric *occlusion.*

deflective occlusal c., a condition of tooth c.'s which diverts the mandible from a normal path of closure to centric jaw relation. SYN cuspal interference, interceptive occlusal c., premature c.

initial c., (1) the first meeting of opposing teeth upon elevation of the mandible toward the maxillae; **(2)** the initial occlusal c. of opposing teeth when the jaw is closed.

interceptive occlusal c., SYN deflective occlusal c.

premature c., SYN deflective occlusal c.

proximal c., proximate c., the area where the surfaces of two adjacent teeth in the same arch touch.

c. with reality, correctly interpreting external phenomena in relation to the norms of one's social or cultural milieu.

working c.'s, working or occlusion; c.'s of teeth made on the side of the occlusion toward which the mandible has been moved. SYN working bite, working occlusion.

con·tac·tant (kon-tak'tănt). Any of a heterogeneous group of allergens that elicit manifestations of delayed hypersensitivity by direct contact with skin or mucosa.

con·ta·gion (kon-tā'jŭn). **1.** SYN contagium. **2.** Transmission of infection by direct contact, droplet spread, or contaminated fomites. The term originated long before development of modern ideas of infectious disease and has since lost much of its significance, being included under the more inclusive term "communicable disease." **3.** Production via suggestion or imitation of a neurosis or psychosis in several or more members of a group. [L. *contagio;* fr. *contingo,* to touch closely]

psychic c., communication of a nervous disorder or lesser psychological symtoms by imitation, as in mass hysteria.

con·ta·gious (kon-tā'jŭs). Relating to contagion; communicable or transmissible by contact with the sick or their fresh secretions or excretions.

con·ta·gious·ness (kon-tā'jŭs-nes). The quality of being contagious.

con·ta·gium (kon-tā'jē-ŭm). The agent of an infectious disease. SYN contagion (1). [L. a touching]

con·tain·ment. The concept of regional or global eradication of communicable disease, proposed by Fred Lowe Soper (1893-1977) in 1949 for the eradication of smallpox.

con·tam·i·nant (kon-tam'i-nant). An impurity; any material of an extraneous nature associated with a chemical, a pharmaceutical preparation, a physiologic principle, or an infectious agent.

con·tam·i·nate (kon-tam′i-nāt). To cause or result in contamination. [L. *con-tamino,* to mingle, corrupt]

con·tam·i·na·tion (kon-tam-i-nā′shŭn). **1.** The presence of an infectious agent on a body surface; also on or in clothes, bedding, toys, surgical instruments or dressings, or other inanimate articles or substances including water, milk, and food or that infectious agent itself. **2.** In epidemiology, the situation that exists when a population being studied for one condition or factor also possesses other conditions or factors that modify results of the study. **3.** Freudian term for a fusion and condensation of meanings of words, percepts, or motivations for behavior. **4.** The presence of foreign material that adulterates or renders impure a material whose composition is degraded. [L. *contamino,* pp. *-atus,* to stain, defile]

con·tent (kon′tent). **1.** That which is contained within something else, usually in this sense in the plural form, contents. **2.** In psychology, the form of a dream as presented to consciousness. **3.** Ambiguous usage for concentration (3); e.g., blood hemoglobin c. could mean either its concentration or the product of its concentration and the blood volume. [L. *contentus,* fr. *con- tineo,* pp. *-tentus,* to hold together, contain]

carbon dioxide c., the total carbon dioxide available from serum or plasma following addition of acid; measured routinely in hospital laboratories as a component of electrolyte profiles.

GC c., the amount of guanine and cytosine in a polynucleic acid usually expressed in mole fraction (or percentage) of total bases; the melting temperature of such biopolymers varies with the GC c.

latent c., the hidden, unconscious meaning of thoughts or actions, especially in dreams or fantasies.

manifest c., those elements of fantasy and dreams which are consciously available and reportable.

con·tig. SEE contig *map.*

con·ti·gu·i·ty (kon-ti-gū′i-tē). **1.** Contact without actual continuity, e.g., the contact of the bones entering into the formation of a cranial suture. Cf. continuity. **2.** Occurrence of two or more objects, events, or mental impressions together in space (**spatial c.**) or time (**temporal c.**). [L. *contiguus,* touching, fr. *contingo,* to touch]

con·tig·u·ous (kon-tig′oo-ŭs). Adjacent or in actual contact.

con·ti·nence (kon′ti-nens). **1.** The ability to retain urine and/or feces until a proper time for their discharge. **2.** Moderation, temperance, or self-restraint in respect to the appetites, especially to sexual intercourse. [L. *continentia,* fr. *con- tineo,* to hold back]

con·ti·nent (kon′ti-nent). Denoting continence.

con·tin·ued (kon-tin′ūd). Continuous; without intermission; said especially of protracted fever without apyretic intervals, such as typhoid fever, compared with the paroxysms of fever in malaria. [L. *continuo,* to join together, make continuous]

con·ti·nu·i·ty (kon-ti-nu′i-tē). Absence of interruption, a succession of parts intimately united, e.g., the unbroken conjunction of cells and structures that make up a single bone of the skull. Cf. contiguity. [L. *continuus,* continued]

con·tour (kon′toor). **1.** The outline of a part; the surface configuration. **2.** In dentistry, to restore the normal outlines of a broken or otherwise misshapen tooth, or to create the external shape or form of a prosthesis. [L. *con-* (intens.), + *torno,* to turn (in a lathe), fr. *tornus,* a lathe]

flange c., the design of the flange of a denture.

gingival c., the shape or form of the gingiva, either natural or artificial, around the necks of the teeth. SYN gum c.

gum c., SYN gingival c.

height of c., SEE *height* of contour.

△**contra-.** Opposed, against. SEE ALSO counter-. Cf. anti-. [L.]

con·tra·an·gle (kon′tră-ang′gl). **1.** One of the double or triple angles in the shank of an instrument by means of which the cutting edge or point is brought into the axis of the handle. **2.** An extension piece added to the end of a dental handpiece which, through a set of bevel gears, changes the angle of the axis of rotation of the bur in relation to the axis of the handpiece.

con·tra·ap·er·ture (kon′tră-ap′er-choor). SYN counteropening.

con·tra·bev·el (kon′tră-bev′ĕl). A bevel located on the side opposite the customary side.

con·tra·cep·tion (kon-tră-sep′shŭn). Prevention of conception or impregnation.

emergency hormonal c., SYN morning after *pill.* SYN postcoital c.

postcoital c., SYN emergency hormonal c.

con·tra·cep·tive (kon-tră-sep′tiv). **1.** An agent for the prevention of conception. **2.** Relating to any measure or agent designed to prevent conception. [L. *contra,* against, + conceptive]

barrier c., a mechanical device designed to prevent spermatozoa from penetrating the cervical os; usually used in combination with a spermicidal agent, i.e., vaginal diaphragm.

combination oral c., a mixture of a steroid having progestational activity and an estrogen.

intrauterine c. device, SEE intrauterine contraceptive *devices,* under *device.*

oral c., any orally effective preparation designed to prevent conception.

con·tract. **1** (kon-trakt′). To shorten; to become reduced in size; in the case of muscle, either to shorten or to undergo an increase in tension. **2** (kon-trakt′). To acquire by contagion or infection. **3** (kon′trakt). An explicit bilateral commitment by psychotherapist and patient to a defined course of action to attain the goal of the psychotherapy. [L. *con-traho,* pp. *-tractus,* to draw together]

con·trac·tile (kon-trak′tīl). Having the property of contracting.

con·trac·til·i·ty (kon-trak-til′i-tē). The ability or property of a substance, especially of muscle, of shortening, or becoming reduced in size, or developing increased tension.

cardiac c., a measure of cardiac pump performance, the degree to which muscle fibers can shorten when activated by a stimulus independent of preload and afterload.

con·trac·tion (C) (kon-trak′shŭn). **1.** A shortening or increase in tension; denoting the normal function of muscle. **2.** A shrinkage or reduction in size. **3.** Heart beat, as in premature c. See also entries under beat. [L. *contractus,* drawn together]

after-c., SEE aftercontraction.

anodal closure c. (ACC, AnCC), obsolete term for the momentary c. of a muscle under the influence of the positive pole when the electrical circuit is established.

anodal opening c. (AnOC, AOC), obsolete term for the momentary c. of a muscle under the influence of the positive pole when the circuit is broken.

automatic c., SYN automatic *beat.*

Braxton Hicks c., rhythmic myometrial activity occurring during the course of a pregnancy that usually causes no pain for the patient.

cathodal closure c. (CaCC, CCC), obsolete term for the momentary c. of a muscle under the influence of the negative pole when an electrical circuit is established.

cathodal opening c. (CaOC, COC), obsolete term for the momentary c. of a muscle under the influence of the negative pole when the circuit is broken.

closing c., c. produced at the time of closing of the circuit when using direct current to stimulate the muscle.

escape c., SYN escape *beat.*

escape ventricular c., an escape beat arising in the ventricle.

fibrillary c.'s, c.'s occurring spontaneously in individual muscle fibers; they are seen commonly a few days after damage to the motor nerves supplying the muscle, and this type of activity is distinguished from fasciculation, which is related to activation of motor units.

front-tap c., c. of the calf muscles when the anterior surface of the leg is struck. SYN Gowers c.

Gowers c., SYN front-tap c.

hourglass c., constriction of the middle portion of a hollow organ, such as the stomach or the gravid uterus.

hunger c.'s, strong c.'s of the stomach associated with hunger pains.

idiomuscular c., SYN myoedema.

isometric c., force development at constant length. Cf. isotonic c.

isotonic c., shortening at constant force development. Cf. isometric c. SYN isotonic exercise.

myotatic c., a reflex c. of a skeletal muscle that occurs as a result of stimulation of the stretch receptors in the muscle, i.e., as part of a myotatic reflex.

opening c., a c. produced at the time of opening the circuit when using direct current to stimulate the muscle or a motor nerve.

paradoxical c., a tonic c. of the anterior tibial muscles when a sudden passive dorsal flexion of the foot is made.

postural c., maintenance of muscular tension (usually isometric) sufficient to maintain posture.

premature c., SEE extrasystole.

reflex detrusor c., normal coordinated function of the bladder with sustained contractions of the bladder matched by simultaneous relaxation of the sphincteric outlet mechanisms to empty the bladder.

tetanic c., SEE tetanus (2).

tonic c., sustained contraction of a muscle, as employed in the maintenance of posture.

uterine c., rhythmic activity of the myometrium associated with menstruation, pregnancy, or labor.

con·trac·ture (kon-trak′choor). Static muscle shortening due to tonic spasm or fibrosis, to loss of muscular balance, the antagonists being paralyzed or to a loss of motion of the adjacent joint. [L. *contractura,* fr. *con-traho,* to draw together]

Dupuytren c., a disease of the palmar fascia resulting in thickening and shortening of fibrous bands on the palmar surface of the hand and fingers resulting in a characteristic flexion deformity of the fourth and fifth digits.

fixed c., SYN organic c.

functional c., muscular shortening that ceases during sleep or general anesthesia, caused by prolonged active muscle contraction.

ischemic c. of the left ventricle, irreversible contraction of the left ventricle of the heart, seen as a complication in the early period of cardiopulmonary bypass and now avoided by appropriate cardioplegic solutions. SYN myocardial rigor mortis, stone heart.

organic c., c., usually due to fibrosis within the muscle that persists whether the subject is conscious or unconscious. SYN fixed c.

Volkmann c., ischemic c. resulting from irreversible necrosis of muscle tissue, produced by a compartment syndrome; classically involves the forearm flexor muscles.

con·tra·fis·sura (kon′tră-fi-shoor′ă). Fracture of a bone, as in the skull, at a point opposite that where the blow was received. [L. *contra,* against, counter, + *fissura,* fissure]

con·tra·in·di·cant (kon-tră-in′di-kant). Indicating the contrary, i.e., showing that a method of treatment that would otherwise be proper is inadvisable by special circumstances in the individual case.

con·tra·in·di·ca·tion (kon-tră-in-di-kā′shŭn). Any special symptom or circumstance that renders the use of a remedy or the carrying out of a procedure inadvisable, usually because of risk.

con·tra·lat·er·al (kon-tră-lat′er-ăl). Relating to the opposite side, as when pain is felt or paralysis occurs on the side opposite to that of the lesion. SYN heterolateral. [L. *contra,* opposite, + *latus,* side]

c. partner, the corresponding structure on the opposite side.

con·trast (kon′trast). **1.** A comparison in which differences are demonstrated or enhanced. **2.** In radiology, the difference between the image densities of two areas is the c. between them; this is a function of the number of x-ray photons transmitted or the strength of the signals emitted by the two regions and the response of the recording medium. [L. *contra,* against, + *sto,* pp. *status,* to stand]

simultaneous c., the enhancement of the visual sensation of white when a white object is viewed adjacent to a black object; the black object also appears blacker as a result of the contiguity of white. Adjacent complementary colors also appear brighter; e.g., green appears a brighter green and red a brighter red if these two colors are viewed side by side.

successive c., the visual effect caused by viewing a brightly colored object and then a gray surface; the latter appears tinged with the complementary color of the object. Viewing a surface colored in the complementary color of the object rather than in gray enhances the color intensity of the surface.

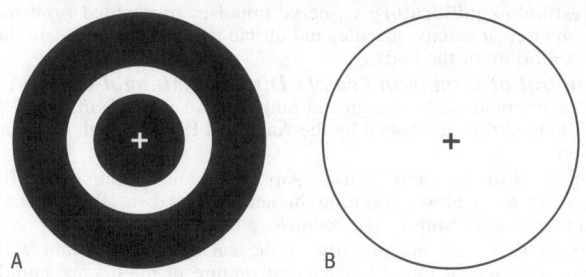

successive contrast: stare at white cross in (A) for about 30 seconds and then look at black cross in (B); the image of (A) reappearing in the white field of (B) is a successive contrast

con·tre·coup (kawn-tr-koo′). Denoting the manner of a contrafissura, as in the skull, at a point opposite that at which the blow was received. SEE ALSO contrecoup *injury* of brain. [Fr. counter-blow]

cont. rem. Abbreviation for L. *continuenter remedia,* continue the medicines.

con·trol (kon-trōl′). **1.** (v.) To regulate, restrain, correct, restore to normal. **2.** (n.) Ongoing operations or programs aimed at reducing a disease. **3.** (n.) Members of a comparison group who differ in disease experience or allocation to a regimen from the subjects of a study. **4.** (v.) In statistics, to adjust or take into account extraneous influences. [Mediev. L. *contrarotulum,* a counterroll for checking accounts, fr. L. *rotula,* dim. of *rota,* a wheel]

autogenous c., regulation by the action of a gene product on the gene that codes for that product.

automatic gain c. (AGC), a feature of some hearing aids that reduces amplification at high-input intensity levels.

aversive c., control of the behavior of another individual by use of psychologically noxious means; e.g., attempting to force better study habits by withholding a child's allowance, or withholding sexual contact unless the partner complies with a request.

biologic c., c. of living organisms, including vectors and reservoirs of disease, by using their natural enemies (predators, parasites, competitors).

birth c., (1) restriction of the number of offspring by means of contraceptive measures; (2) projects, programs, or methods to control reproduction, by either improving or diminishing fertility.

idiodynamic c., nervous impulses from the medulla that preserve the normal trophic condition of the muscles.

negative c., regulation of an enzyme activity by an inhibitor of that enzyme or regulation of a protein by repression of transcription.

own c.'s, a method of experimental c. in which the same subjects are used in both experimental and c. conditions.

positive c., regulation of an enzyme activity by an activator of that enzyme. Also, regulation via induction of a specific protein's biosynthesis or activation of a protein's processing.

quality c., the c. of laboratory analytical error by monitoring analytical performance with control sera and maintaining error within established limits around the mean control values, most commonly ±2 SD.

reflex c., nerve impulses transmitted to the muscles to maintain normal reflex action.

social c., the influence on the behavior of a person exerted by other persons or by society as a whole; e.g., through appropriate social norms, ostracism, or the criminal law.

stimulus c., the use of conditioning techniques to bring the target behavior of an individual under environmental c. SEE classical *conditioning.*

synergic c., impulses transmitted from the cerebellum regulating the muscular activity of the synergic units of the body.

time-varied gain c. (TGC), SYN time-gain *compensation.*

tonic c., nerve impulses that maintain a normal tonus or level of activity in muscle or other effector organs.

vestibulo-equilibratory c., nerve impulses transmitted from the semicircular canals, saccule, and utricle that serve to maintain the equilibrium of the body.

Con·trol of Com·mun·i·ca·ble Dis·eases Manual (CCDM). The internationally recognized authoritative manual, in the 17th (2000) edition, published by the American Public Health Association.

con·tu·sion (kon-too′shŭn). Any mechanical injury (usually caused by a blow) resulting in hemorrhage beneath unbroken skin. SEE ALSO bruise. [L. *contusio,* a bruising]

brain c., a bruising, usually of the surface, of the brain with extravasation of blood but without rupture of the pia-arachnoid; healing results in a superficial depressed sclerotic area, possibly with incorporated meninges. SEE ALSO brain *cicatrix.*

scalp c., intracutaneous or subcutaneous extravasation of blood without gross disruption of skin.

con·u·lar (kon′ū-lăr). Cone-shaped.

Co·nus (kō′nŭs). A genus of shellfish that inhabits the shores of some South Pacific islands. Several species, *C. geographus, C. textilis, C. aulicus, C. tulipa,* and *C. marmoreus* are poisonous, their sting or spine causing acute pain, edema, numbness, spreading paralysis, and sometimes coma and death.

co·nus, pl. **co·ni** (kō′nŭs, -nī). **1** [TA]. SYN cone. **2.** Posterior staphyloma in myopic choroidopathy. [L. fr. G. *kōnos,* cone]

c. arterio′sus [TA], the left or anterosuperior, smooth-walled portion of the cavity of the right ventricle of the heart, which begins at the supraventricular crest and terminates in the pulmonary trunk. SYN arterial cone, infundibulum (4), pulmonary cone, pulmonary c.

congenital c., SYN Fuchs *coloboma.*

distraction c., a c. in which the optic nerve passes through the scleral canal in a markedly oblique direction.

c. elas′ticus [TA], thicker lower portion of the elastic membrane of the larynx, extending between the cricoid cartilage and the vocal ligaments, the latter actually being a thickening of the free, superior margin of the c. elasticus; SYN cricovocal membrane*,* elastic cone.

co′ni epididym′idis, *official alternate term for *lobules* of epididymis, under *lobule.*

c. medulla′ris [TA], the tapering lower extremity of the spinal cord. SYN medullary cone [TA].

myopic c., SYN myopic *crescent.*

pulmonary c., SYN c. arteriosus.

supertraction c., a reddish yellow c. or ring at the nasal margin of the optic disk, produced by displacement of the retinal pigment epithelium and lamina vitrea of the choroid; occurs in high myopia.

co′ni vasculo′si, SYN *lobules* of epididymis, under *lobule.*

con·va·les·cence (kon-vă-les′ens). A period between the end of a disease and the patient's restoration to complete health. [L. *con-valesco,* to grow strong, fr. *valeo,* to be strong]

con·va·les·cent (kon-vă-les′ent). **1.** Getting well or one who is getting well. **2.** Denoting the period of convalescence.

con·val·lar·ia (kon-va-lār′ē-ă). The flower, rhizome, and roots of *Convallaria majalis* (family Liliaceae), lily of the valley; they contain glycosides with digitalis-like action (e.g., convallatoxin). [L. *convallis,* an enclosed valley]

con·vec·tion (kon-vek′shŭn). Conveyance of heat in liquids or gases by movement of the heated particles, as when the layer of water at the bottom of a heated pot rises or the warm air of a room ascends to the ceiling. [L. *con-veho,* pp. *-vectus,* to carry or bring together]

con·ver·gence (kon-ver′jens). **1.** The tending of two or more objects toward a common point. **2.** The direction of the visual lines to a near point. [L. *con-vergere,* to incline together]

accommodative c., the meter angle of c. expressed in diopters;

equal to the product of the meter angles of c. times the interpupillary distance measured in centimeters.

amplitude of c., the distance between the near point and far point of c. SYN range of c.

angle of c., the angle that the visual axis makes with the median line when a near object is viewed.

far point of c., the point to which the visual lines are directed when c. is at rest.

near point of c., the point to which the visual lines are directed when c. is at its maximum.

negative c., the slight divergence of the visual axes when c. is at rest, as when observing the far point or during sleep.

positive c., inward deviation of the visual axes even when c. is at rest, as in cases of convergent squint.

range of c., SYN amplitude of c.

unit of c., SEE meter *angle.*

con·ver·gent (kon-ver′jent). Tending toward a common point.

con·ver·sion (kon-ver′zhŭn). **1.** SYN transmutation. **2.** An unconscious defense mechanism by which the anxiety which stems from an unconscious conflict is converted and expressed symbolically as a physical symptom; transformation of an emotion into a physical manifestation, as in c. hysteria. SEE conversion *hysteria.* **3.** In virology, the acquisition by bacteria of a new property associated with presence of a prophage. SEE ALSO lysogeny. [L. *con-verto,* pp. *-versus,* to turn around, to change]

con·ver·tase (kon′ver-tās). Proteases of complement that convert one component into another. SEE *component* of complement.

con·ver·tin (kon-ver′tin). Active form of factor VII designated VIIa.

con·vex (kon′veks, kŏn-veks′). Applied to a surface that is evenly curved outward, the segment of a sphere. [L. *convexus,* vaulted, arched, convex, fr. *con-veho,* to bring together]

high c., the segment of a sphere of short radius.

low c., the segment of a sphere of long radius.

con·vex·i·ty (kon-veks′i-tē). **1.** The state of being convex. **2.** A convex structure.

cortical c., SYN superolateral *surface* of cerebrum.

con·vex·o·ba·sia (kon-vek-sō-bā′sē-ă). Forward bending of the occipital bone. [L. *convexus,* outwardly curved, + *basis,* foundation]

con·vex·o·con·cave (kon-vek′sō-kon′kāv). Convex on one surface and concave on the opposite surface.

con·vex·o·con·vex (kon-vek′sō-kon′veks). SYN biconvex.

con·vo·lute (kon′vō-loot). Rolled together with one part over the other; in the shape of a roll or scroll. SYN convoluted. [L. *con-volvo,* pp. *-volutus,* to roll together]

con·vo·lut·ed (kon′vō-loo-ted). SYN convolute.

con·vo·lu·tion (kon-vō-loo′shŭn). **1.** A coiling or rolling of an organ. **2.** Specifically, a gyrus of the cerebral or cerebellar cortex. [L. *convolutio*]

angular c., SYN angular *gyrus.*

anterior central c., SYN precentral *gyrus.*

ascending frontal c., SYN precentral *gyrus.*

ascending parietal c., SYN postcentral *gyrus.*

callosal c., SYN cingulate *gyrus.*

cingulate c., SYN cingulate *gyrus.*

first temporal c., SYN superior temporal *gyrus.*

hippocampal c., SYN parahippocampal *gyrus.*

inferior frontal c., SYN inferior frontal *gyrus.*

inferior temporal c., SYN inferior temporal *gyrus.*

middle frontal c., SYN middle frontal *gyrus.*

middle temporal c., SYN middle temporal *gyrus.*

posterior central c., SYN postcentral *gyrus.*

second temporal c., SYN middle temporal *gyrus.*

superior frontal c., SYN superior frontal *gyrus.*

superior temporal c., SYN superior temporal *gyrus.*

supramarginal c., SYN supramarginal *gyrus.*

third temporal c., SYN inferior temporal *gyrus.*

transitional c., SYN transitional *gyrus.*

transverse temporal c.'s, SYN transverse temporal *gyri*, under *gyrus*.

Zuckerkandl c., SYN subcallosal *gyrus*.

con·vul·sant (kon-vŭl′sant). A substance that produces convulsions. SEE ALSO eclamptogenic, epileptogenic.

con·vul·sion (kon-vŭl′shŭn). **1.** A violent spasm or series of jerkings of the face, trunk, or extremities. **2.** SYN seizure (2). [L. *convulsio,* fr. *convello,* pp. *-vulsus,* to tear up]

benign neonatal c.'s, a familial, self-limited epilepsy, beginning at 2, 3, or 6 days of age and resolving spontaneously by six months of age; autosomal dominant inheritance.

clonic c., a c. in which the contractions are intermittent, the muscles alternately contracting and relaxing.

complex febrile c., a febrile c. that is prolonged (greater than 15 minutes' duration) or is associated with focal neurologic deficits.

febrile c., a brief seizure, lasting less than 15 minutes, seen in a neurologically normal infant or young child, associated with fever. SYN febrile seizure.

hysterical c., hysteroid c., SEE hysteria.

immediate posttraumatic c., a c. beginning very soon after injury.

infantile c., any c. occurring in infancy (0–2 years of age).

salaam c.'s, SYN infantile *spasm.*

tetanic c., SYN tonic c.

tonic c., a c. in which muscle contraction is sustained. SYN tetanic c.

con·vul·sive (kon-vŭl′siv). Relating to convulsions; marked by or producing convulsions.

Cooke, A. Bennett, U.S. physician, *1869. SEE C. *speculum.*

Cooley, Denton, U.S. cardiothoracic surgeon, *1920, noted for inventing many surgical instruments.

Cooley, Thomas B., U.S. pediatrician, 1871–1945. SEE C. *anemia.*

Coolidge, William D., U.S. physicist, 1873–1975. SEE C. *tube.*

Coomassie bril·liant blue R-250 [C.I. 42660]. A general protein stain used in electrophoresis because of its unusual sensitivity. [originally, a proprietary name of Imperial Chemical; Coomassie (Kumasi), Ghana]

Coombs, Carey F., English physician, 1879–1932. SEE Carey C. *murmur;* C. *murmur.*

Coombs, Robin R.A., English veterinarian and immunologist, *1921. SEE Gell and C. *reactions,* under *reaction;* C. *serum, test;* direct C. *test;* indirect C. *test.*

Cooper, Sir Astley Paston, English anatomist and surgeon, 1768–1841. SEE C. *fascia, hernia, herniotome, ligaments,* under *ligament;* suspensory *ligaments* of C., under *ligament.*

co·op·er·a·tiv·i·ty. A property of certain proteins (often enzymes) in which the binding curves or saturation curves or, in the case of enzymes, a plot of initial rates as a function of initial substrate concentration, are nonhyperbolic; suggests that the binding of a ligand has a different affinity at different ligand concentrations. Both allosterism and hysteresis are models that will display c. Cf. allosterism, hysteresis.

negative c., c. in which successive ligand molecules appear to bind with decreasing affinity.

positive c., c. in which successive ligand molecules appear to bind with increasing affinity.

Coo·pe·ria (koo-pē′rē-ă). A genus of small, slender nematodes (family Trichostrongylidae) inhabiting the small intestine, rarely the abomasum, of ruminants; when fresh they are a bright pink color; they produce serious effects only when present in large numbers. In partly immune animals, these worms become enclosed in nodules in the wall of the intestine; they are less pathogenic in sheep and goats than the trichostrongyles *Haemonchus, Ostertagia,* and *Trichostrongylus.*

C. biso′nis, species that occurs in cattle, sheep, bison, and pronghorn antelopes.

C. curti′cei, species that occurs in sheep, goats, and wild deer in Europe, although cosmopolitan in distribution.

C. fiel′dingi, SYN *C. punctata.*

C. oncoph′ora, species that occurs in cattle and domestic and wild sheep, but rarely in the horse; although worldwide in distribution, it is most common in the northern U.S. and Canada. SYN *Strongylus radiatus, Strongylus ventricosus.*

C. pectina′ta, species that occurs in cattle, sheep, water buffalo, dromedary camels, and various wild ruminants; it is common in the southern U.S.

C. puncta′ta, species that occurs mainly in cattle, less commonly in sheep, water buffalo, and several wild ruminants; although worldwide in distribution, it is especially widespread in North America and common in Hawaii. SYN *C. fieldingi.*

C. spatula′ta, a species that occurs in cattle and sheep in the southern U.S., Kenya, Australia, and Malaysia.

co·or·di·nate. **1** (kō-ōr′di-nit). Any of the scales or magnitudes that serve to define the position of a point. **2** (kō-ōr′di-nāt). To perform the act of coordination. [see coordination]

co·or·di·na·tion (kō-ōr′di-nā′shun). The harmonious working together, especially of several muscles or muscle groups in the execution of complicated movements. [L. *co-,* together, + *ordino,* pp. *-atus,* to arrange, fr. *ordo* (*ordin-*), arrangement, order]

co·os·si·fi·ca·tion (kō-os′i-fi-kā′shŭn). State of being joined by bone formation.

co·os·si·fy (kō-os′i-fī). To unite into one bone. [L. *co-,* together, + *os,* bone, + *facio,* to make]

co·pai·ba (kō-pī′bă). The oleoresin of *Copaifera officinalis* and other species of *Copaifera* (family Leguminosae), a South American plant; c. oil is used as an expectorant, diuretic, and stimulant. SYN balsam of copaiba. [Sp.]

COPD Abbreviation for chronic obstructive pulmonary *disease.*

Cope, Sir Vincent Z., English surgeon, 1881–1974. SEE C. *clamp.*

cope (kōp). **1.** The upper half of a flask in the casting art; hence applicable to the upper or cavity side of a denture flask. **2.** An act that enables one to adjust to the environmental circumstances.

co·pe·pod (kō′pē-pod). Any member of the order Copepoda.

Co·pep·o·da (kō-pep′ō-dă). An order of abundant, free-living, freshwater and marine crustaceans of basic importance in the aquatic food chain in both the marine and freshwater environments; some species are commonly called water fleas. Some are ectoparasites of both cold-blooded and warm-blooded aquatic vertebrates; the parasitic copepods of fish and whales are often highly modified for deep penetration of the skin or for adherence by suckers and hooks (e.g., the fish lice, *Argulus*). Certain copepods (*Cyclops, Diaptomus*) are important as intermediate hosts of the tapeworm *Diphyllobothrium latum* and of the nematode *Dracunculus medinensis.* [G. *kōpē,* an oar, + *pous* (*pod-*), a foot]

cop·ing (kōp′ing). **1.** A thin metal covering or cap. **2.** An adaptive or otherwise successful method of dealing with individual or environmental situations that involve psychologic or physiologic stress or threat.

transfer c., in dentistry, a metallic, acrylic resin or other covering or cap used to position a die in an impression.

co·pol·y·mer (kō′pol-i-mer). A polymer in which two or more monomers or base units are combined.

c.-1, acetate salt of a mixture of synthetic polypeptides composed of four amino acids; used to reduce the relapse rate with relapsing-remitting multiple sclerosis.

cop·per (Cu) (kop′er). A metallic element, atomic no. 29, atomic wt. 63.546; several of its salts are used in medicine. A bioelement found in a number of proteins. [L. *cuprum,* orig. *Cyprium,* fr. Cyprus, where it was mined]

c. arsenite, SYN cupric arsenite.

c. bichloride, SYN cupric chloride.

c. chloride, SYN cupric chloride.

c. citrate, SYN cupric citrate.

c. dichloride, SYN cupric chloride.

c. sulfate, c. sulphate, SYN cupric sulfate.

cop·per-64 (^{64}Cu). Beta and positron emitter with a half-life of 12.82 hr. Used in the study of Wilson disease and in brain scans for tumors.

cop·per-67 (^{67}Cu). Beta and gamma emitter with a half-life of 2.580 days.

CO

cop·per·as (kop′er-as). The impure commercial variety of ferrous sulfate.

cop·per·head (kop′er-hed). A poisonous snake of the genus *Agkistrodon* in the U.S.

cop·per pen·nies. SYN sclerotic *bodies*, under *body*.

Coppet, Louis de, French physicist, 1841–1911. SEE C. *law.*

co·pre·cip·i·ta·tion (kō′prē-sip-i-tā′shŭn). Precipitation of unbound antigen along with an antigen-antibody complex; may occur particularly when a soluble complex is precipitated by a second antibody specific for the Fc fragment of the immunoglobulin of the complex.

cop·rem·e·sis (kop-rem′ĕ-sis). SYN fecal *vomiting.* [G. *kopros,* dung, + emesis]

△**copro-.** Filth, dung, usually used in referring to feces. SEE ALSO scato-, sterco-. [G. *kopros,* dung]

cop·ro·an·ti·bod·ies (kop′rō-an′ti-bod-ēz). Antibodies found in the intestine and in feces; they probably are formed by plasma cells in the intestinal mucosa and consist chiefly of the IgA class.

cop·ro·la·lia (kop-rō-lā′lē-ă). Involuntary utterances of vulgar or obscene words; seen in Gilles de la Tourette syndrome. SYN coprophrasia. [copro- + G. *lalia,* talk]

cop·ro·lith (kop′rō-lith). SYN fecalith. [copro- + G. *lithos,* stone]

co·prol·o·gy (kop-rol′ō-jē). SYN scatology (1). [copro- + G. *logos,* study]

cop·ro·ma (kop-rō′mă). SYN fecaloma. [copro- + G. *-ōma,* tumor]

cop·ro·pha·gia (kop′rō-fā′jyă). The eating of excrement. SYN coprophagy, scatophagy.

co·proph·a·gous (kō-prof′ă-gŭs). Feeding on excrement.

co·proph·a·gy (kŏ-prof′ă-jē). SYN coprophagia. [copro- + G. *phagō,* to eat]

cop·ro·phil, cop·ro·phil·ic (kop′rō-fil, -fil′ik). 1. Denoting microorganisms occurring in fecal matter. 2. Relating to coprophilia. [see coprophilia]

cop·ro·phile (kop′rō-fīl). An organism that ingests fecal material from other organisms.

cop·ro·phil·ia (kop-rō-fil′ē-ă). 1. Attraction of microorganisms to fecal matter. 2. In psychiatry, a morbid attraction to, and interest in (with a sexual element), fecal matter. SYN mysophilia. [copro- + G. *philos,* fond]

cop·ro·pho·bia (kop-rō-fō′bē-ă). Morbid fear of defecation and feces. [copro- + G. *phobos,* fear]

cop·ro·phra·sia (kop-rō-frā′zē-ă). SYN coprolalia.

cop·ro·plan·e·sia (kop-rō-plan-ē′zē-ă). Rarely used term for passage of feces through a fistula or artificial anus. [copro- + G. *planēsis,* a wandering]

cop·ro·por·phyr·ia (kop′rō-pōr-fir′ē-ă). Presence of coproporphyrins in the urine, as in variegate porphyria.

  hereditary c., an inherited (autosomal dominant) disorder of a deficiency of coproporphyrinogen oxidase, resulting in overproduction of porphyrin precursors leading to neurological disturbances and photosensitivity.

cop·ro·por·phy·rin (kop-rō-pōr′fi-rin). One of two porphyrin compounds found normally in feces as a decomposition product of bilirubin (hence, from hemoglobin); certain c.'s are elevated in certain porphyrias. SEE ALSO porphyrinogens.

cop·ro·por·phy·rin·o·gen (kop′rō-pōr-fi-rin′ō-jen). SEE porphyrinogens.

  c. oxidase, an enzyme that catalyzes a step in porphyrin biosynthesis, reacting coproporphyrinogen III and O_2 to form protoporphyrinogen IX and $2CO_2$. A deficiency of this enzyme will result in hereditary coproporphyria.

cop·ro·stane (kop-ros′tān). The parent hydrocarbon of coprosterol.

3β-co·pros·ta·nol (kop-ros′tan-ol). SYN coprosterol.

epi-**co·pros·ta·nol.** 5β-Cholestan-3α-ol. For the structure of cholestane, see steroids. SYN *epi*-coprosterol.

cop·ros·tan·one (kop-ros′tan-ōn). 5β-Cholestan-3-one, an oxidation product of coprosterol.

cop·ro·sta·sis (kop-rō-stā′sis). Rarely used term for fecal impaction. [copro- + G. *stasis,* a standing]

cop·ros·ten·ol (kop-ros′ten-ol). SYN allocholesterol.

co·pros·ter·ol (kop-ros′ter-ol). 5β-Cholestan-3β-ol; the main sterol of the feces produced by the reduction of cholesterol by intestinal bacteria. For structure of coprostane and cholestane, see steroids. SYN 3β-coprostanol, stercorin.

epi-**co·pros·ter·ol.** SYN *epi*-coprostanol.

cop·ro·stig·mas·tane (kop-rō-stig-mas′tān). The 5β isomer of stigmastane.

cop·ro·zoa (kop-rō-zō′ă). Protozoa that can be cultivated in fecal matter, although not necessarily living in feces within the intestine. [copro- + G. *zōon,* animal]

cop·ro·zo·ic (kop-rō-zō′ik). Relating to coprozoa.

cop·to·sis (kop-tō′sis). A state of perpetual fatigue. [G. *kopto,* to tire, + *osis,* condition]

cop·u·la (kop′ū-lă). 1. In anatomy, a narrow part connecting two structures, e.g., the body of the hyoid bone. 2. A swelling that is formed during the early development of the tongue by the medial portion of the second branchial arch; it is overgrown by the hypobranchial eminence and is not present in the adult tongue. 3. Obsolete term for zygote. [L. a bond, tie]

  His c., SYN hypobranchial *eminence.*

  c. lin′guae, SYN hypobranchial *eminence.*

cop·u·la·tion (kop-ū-lā′shŭn). 1. SYN coitus. 2. In protozoology, conjugation between two cells that do not fuse but separate after mutual fertilization; observed in the ciliophora, as in *Paramecium.* [L. *copulatio,* a joining]

copulines. Substances that occur in vaginal secretions; men who were exposed to copulines rated women as more attractive, especially those women considered less attractive by controls tested with water. Copulines from ovulatory (but not menstrual or premenstrual) women caused a rise in salivary testosterone in men.

CoQ Abbreviation for coenzyme Q.

co·quille (kō-kēl′). A spherical curved lens of uniform thickness. [Fr.]

cor, gen. **cor·dis** (kōr, kōr′dis) [TA]. SYN heart. [L.]

  c. adipo′sum, SYN fatty *heart* (2).

  c. bilocula′re, a heart in which the interatrial and interventricular septa are absent or incomplete.

  c. bovi′num (kōr bō′vī-nŭm), SYN ox *heart.*

  c. mo′bile, a heart that moves unduly on change of bodily position; associated with large defects or absence (congenital or surgical) of the pericardium. SYN movable heart.

  c. pen′dulum, an extreme form of c. mobile in which the heart appears to be suspended by the great vessels. SYN pendulous heart.

  c. pulmona′le, chronic c. p. is characterized by hypertrophy of the right ventricle resulting from disease of the lungs, except for lung changes in diseases that primarily affect the left side of the heart and pulmonary artery and excluding congenital heart disease; acute c. p. is characterized by dilation and failure of the right side of the heart due to pulmonary embolism. In both types, characteristic electrocardiogram changes occur, and in later stages there is usually right-sided cardiac failure.

  c. triatria′tum, a heart with three atrial chambers, the left atrium being subdivided by a transverse septum with a single small opening which separates the openings of the pulmonary veins from the mitral valve. SYN accessory atrium.

  c. trilocula′re, three-chambered heart due to absence of the interatrial or the interventricular septum.

  c. trilocula′re biatria′tum, absence of the interventricular septum.

  c. trilocula′re biventricula′re, absence of the interatrial septum.

cor·a·cid·i·um (kō-ră-sid′ē-ŭm). The ciliated first-stage aquatic embryo of pseudophyllid and other cestodes with aquatic cycles; within the ciliated embryophore is a hooked larva, the hexacanth, that develops in the intermediate host, usually an aquatic crustacean, into the next larval stage, the procercoid.

cor·a·co·a·cro·mi·al (kōr′ă-kō-ă-krō′mē-ăl). Relating to the coracoid and acromial processes. SYN acromiocoracoid.

cor·a·co·bra·chi·a·lis (kōr′ă-kō-brā-kē-ā′lis). Relating to the coracoid process of the scapula and the arm. SEE ALSO coracobrachialis *muscle,* coracobrachial *bursa.*

cor·a·co·cla·vic·u·lar (kōr′ă-kō-kla-vik′ū-lăr). Relating to the coracoid process and the clavicle. SYN scapuloclavicular (2).

cor·a·co·hu·mer·al (kōr′ă-kō-hū′mer-ăl). Relating to the coracoid process and the humerus.

cor·a·coid (kōr′ă-koyd). Shaped like a crow's beak; denoting a process of the scapula. [G. *korakōdēs,* like a crow's beak, fr. *korax,* raven, + *eidos,* appearance]

cor·al·lin (kōr′ă-lin). SYN aurin.

yellow c., a sodium salt of aurin.

cord (kōrd) [TA]. **1.** In anatomy, any long ropelike structure. A small, cordlike structure composed of several to many longitudinally oriented fibers, vessels, ducts, or combinations thereof. SEE ALSO chorda. **2.** In histopathology, a line of tumor cells only one cell in width. SYN fasciculus (2) [TA], funiculus [TA], funicle. [L. *chorda,* a string]

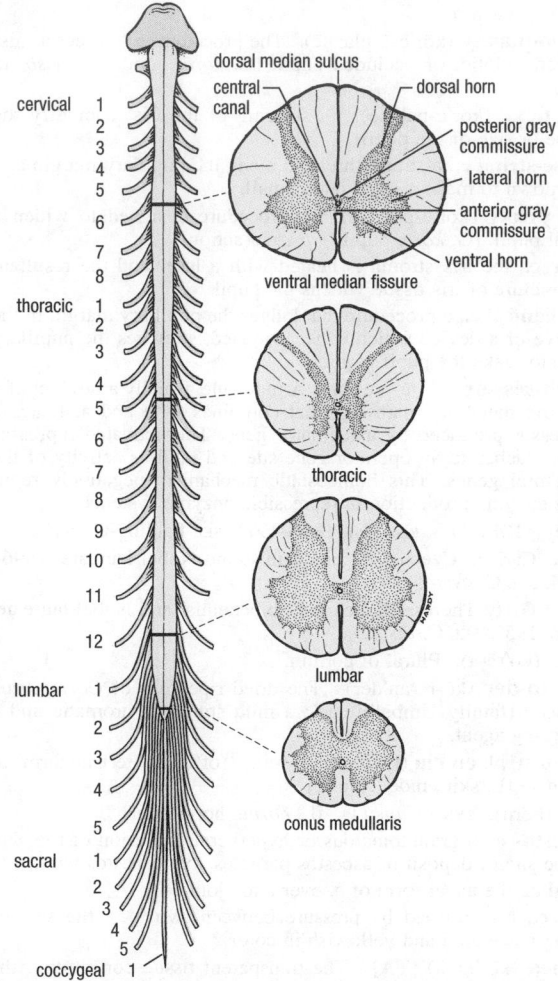

spinal cord: including cross-sectional views showing regional variations in the gray matter

Labels (left figure, top to bottom): cervical 1 2 3 4 5 6 7 8; thoracic 1 2 3 4 5 6 7 8 9 10 11 12; lumbar 1 2 3 4 5; sacral 1 2 3 4 5; coccygeal 1

Labels (cross sections): dorsal median sulcus; central canal; dorsal horn; posterior gray commissure; lateral horn; anterior gray commissure; ventral horn; ventral median fissure; thoracic; lumbar; conus medullaris

Bergmann c.'s, SYN medullary *striae* of fourth ventricle, under *stria.*

Billroth c.'s, SYN splenic c.'s.

condyle c., SYN condylar *axis.*

dental c., an aggregation of epithelial cells forming the rudimentary enamel organ.

false tendinous c.'s, ✰official alternate term for false *chordae tendineae,* under *chorda.*

false vocal c., SYN vestibular *fold.*

Ferrein c.'s, SYN vocal *fold.* SEE vocal *fold.*

ganglated c., SYN sympathetic *trunk.*

genital c., one of a pair of mesenchymal ridges bulging into the caudal part of the celom of a young embryo and containing the mesonephric and paramesonephric duct.

germinal c.'s, the gonadal c.'s of the embryonic ovary or testis. SYN sex c.'s.

gonadal c.'s, columns of germinal and follicle cells penetrating centripetally into the embryonic ovarian or testicular cortex.

gubernacular c., the content of the gubernacular canal, usually composed of remnants of dental lamina and connective tissue.

hepatic c.'s, liver laminae as seen in sections.

lateral c. of brachial plexus [TA], in the brachial plexus, the bundle of nerve fibers formed by the anterior divisions of the superior and middle trunks which is located lateral to the axillary artery. This cord gives off the lateral pectoral nerve and terminates by dividing into the musculocutaneous nerve and the lateral root of the median nerve. SYN fasciculus lateralis plexus brachialis [TA].

lymph c.'s, SYN medullary c.'s (1).

medial c. of brachial plexus [TA], in the brachial plexus, the bundle of nerve fibers formed by the anterior division of the inferior trunk which lies medial to the axillary artery; it gives off the medial pectoral nerve, the medial brachial cutaneous, and medial antebrachial cutaneous nerves and end by dividing into the medial root of the median nerves and the ulnar nerve. SYN fasciculus medialis plexus brachialis [TA].

medullary c.'s, **(1)** c.'s of dense lymphoid tissue between the sinuses in the medulla of a lymph node; SYN lymph c.'s. **(2)** SYN rete c.'s.

nephrogenic c., a longitudinal dorsolateral tract of intermediate mesoderm; the primordium for both mesonephric and metanephric tubules.

nuchal c., loop(s) of umbilical c. around the fetal neck, posing risk of intrauterine hypoxia, fetal distress, or death.

oblique c. of interosseous membrane of forearm [TA], a slender band extending from the lateral part of the coronoid process of the ulna distad and laterad to the radius immediately distal to the bicipital tuberosity. SYN chorda obliqua membranae interosseae antebrachii [TA], oblique ligament of elbow joint, round ligament of elbow joint, Weitbrecht c., Weitbrecht ligament.

omphalomesenteric c., SYN vitelline c.

posterior c. of brachial plexus [TA], in the brachial plexus, the bundle of nerve fibers formed by the posterior divisions of the upper, middle and lower trunks which lies posterior to the axillary artery; it gives rise to the upper and lower subscapular and thoracodorsal nerves, terminates by dividing into the axillary, and radial nerves. SYN fasciculus posterior plexus brachialis [TA].

psalterial c., SYN *stria* vascularis of cochlear duct.

red pulp c.'s, SYN splenic c.'s.

rete c.'s, primordial cell c.'s (medullary c.'s and sex c.'s) in the embryonic gonads that connect with some of the mesonephric tubules and from which the rete testis of the male and the rete ovarii of the female develop. SYN medullary c.'s (2).

sex c.'s, SYN germinal c.'s.

spermatic c. [TA], the cord formed by the ductus deferens and its associated structures extending from the deep inguinal ring through the inguinal canal into the scrotum. SEE ALSO *coverings* of spermatic cord, under *covering.* SYN funiculus spermaticus [TA], chorda spermatica, testicular c.

spinal c. [TA], the elongated cylindrical portion of the cerebrospinal axis, or central nervous system, which is contained in the spinal or vertebral canal. SYN medulla spinalis [TA], chorda spinalis, spinal marrow.

splenic c.'s, the tissue occurring between the venous sinuses in the red pulp of the spleen. SYN Billroth c.'s, red pulp c.'s.

tendinous c.'s, ✰official alternate term for *chordae* tendineae of heart, under *chorda.*

testicular c., SYN spermatic c.

testis c.'s, the germinal c.'s of the embryonic testis.

true vocal c., SYN vocal *fold*.

c. of tympanum, SYN *chorda* tympani.

umbilical c., the definitive connecting stalk between the embryo or fetus and the placenta; at birth it is primarily composed of Wharton jelly in which the umbilical vessels are embedded. SYN chorda umbilicalis, funiculus umbilicalis, funis (1).

c. of umbilical artery [TA], the obliterated umbilical artery that persists as a fibrous cord passing upward alongside the bladder to the umbilicus. SYN chorda arteriae umbilicalis [TA], ligamentum umbilicale mediale, medial umbilical ligament.

vitelline c., a persistent yolk stalk in the form of a solid cord of tissue connecting ileum to umbilicus. SYN omphalomesenteric c.

vocal c., SYN vocal *fold*.

Weitbrecht c., SYN oblique c. of interosseous membrane of forearm.

Wilde c.'s, transverse markings on the corpus callosum.

Willis c.'s, several fibrous c.'s crossing the superior sagittal sinus. SYN chordae willisii.

⌂**cord-.** SEE chord-.

cor·date (kōr′dāt). Heart-shaped.

cor·dec·to·my (kōr-dek′tō-mē). Excision of a part or whole of a vocal cord. [G. *chordē*, cord, + *ektomē*, excision]

cor·dial (kōr′jŭl). A sweet aromatic liquor. [Mediev. L. *cordialis*, fr. *cor (cord-)*, heart]

cor·di·a·nine (kor-dī′ă-nēn). SYN allantoin.

cor·di·form (kōr′di-fōrm). Heart-shaped. [L. *cor (cord-)*, heart, + *forma*, shape]

cor·dis (kōr′dis). Of the heart. [gen. of L. *cor*, heart]

diastasis c. (dī-as′tă-sis), any period of mechanical inactivity of the heart and particularly of the ventricles, usually appearing normally during slow heart rates when the ventricles complete their filling early and appear to be inactive.

cor·do·cen·te·sis (cor-dō-cen-tē′sis). Transabdominal blood sampling of the fetal umbilical cord, performed under ultrasound guidance. SYN funipuncture. [cord + G. *kentēsis*, puncture]

cor·don san·i·taire (kor-don′ san-i-tayr′). The barrier erected around a focus of infection. [Fr., sanitary barrier]

cor·do·pexy (kōr′dō-pek-sē). **1.** Operative fixation of any displaced anatomic cord. **2.** Lateral fixation of one or both vocal cords to correct glottic stenosis. [G. *chordē*, cord, + *pēxis*, fixation]

cor·dot·o·my (kōr-dot′ō-mē). **1.** Any operation on the spinal cord. **2.** Division of tracts of the spinal cord, which may be performed percutaneously (stereotactic c.) or after laminectomy (open c.) by various techniques such as incision or radio frequency coagulation. **3.** Incision through the membranous portion of the vocal fold to widen the posterior glottis in bilateral vocal paralysis. [G. *chordē*, cord, + *tomē*, a cutting]

anterolateral c., division of the anterolateral quadrant of the spinal cord to section the spinothalamic tract. SYN anterolateral tractotomy, spinal tractotomy, spinothalamic c.

open c., SEE cordotomy (2).

posterior column c., division of the posterior column of the spinal cord.

spinothalamic c., SYN anterolateral c.

stereotactic c., SEE cordotomy (2).

Cor·dy·lo·bia (kor-di-lō′bē-ă). A genus of calliphorid fleshflies. [G. *kordylē*, a cudgel, swelling, or tumor]

C. anthropoph′aga, tumbu fly of Africa south of the Sahara; a species that causes a boil-like furuncular myiasis; many animals besides humans are attacked, especially domestic dogs, though rats are probably the chief reservoir of human infection.

cor·dy·lo·bi·a·sis (kōr′di-lō-bī′ă-sis). Infection of humans and animals with larvae of flies of the genus *Cordylobia*. SYN African furuncular myiasis, tumbu dermal myiasis.

core (kōr). **1.** The central mass of necrotic tissue in a boil. **2.** A metal casting, usually with a post in the canal of a tooth root, designed to retain an artificial crown. **3.** A sectional record, usu-

ally of plaster of Paris or one of its derivatives, of the relationships of parts, such as teeth, metallic restorations, or copings. [L. *cor*, heart]

atomic c., the nucleus plus the nonvalence electrons.

central transactional c., the reticular activating system of the brain.

⌂**core-, coreo-, coro-.** The pupil (of the eye). [G. *korē*, pupil]

co-receptor. A cell surface protein that increases the sensitivity of the antigen receptor to antigen by binding to other ligands.

B cell co-receptor, a complex of three proteins associated with the B-cell receptor (CR2, CD19, and TAPA-1).

cor·ec·to·pia (kōr-ek-tō′pē-ă). Eccentric location of the pupil so that it is not in the center of the iris. [G. *korē*, pupil, + *ektopos*, out of place]

co·rel·y·sis (kō-rē-lī′sis). A rarely used term for freeing of adhesions between lens capsule and the iris. [G. *korē*, pupil, + *lysis*, loosening]

co·re·mi·um (kō-rē′mē-ŭm). A sheaflike tuft of conidiophores. [G. *korēma*, filth, refuse]

⌂**coreo-.** SEE core-.

cor·e·o·plas·ty (kōr′ē-ō-plas-tē). The procedure to correct a misshapen, miotic, or occluded pupil. [G. *korē*, pupil, + *plassō*, to form]

cor·e·pexy (kōr′ē-pek-sē). A suturing of the iris to modify the shape or size of the pupil.

purse-string c., a suture threaded along the pupillary margin and tied down to make a large pupil small.

cor·e·praxy (kōr′ē-prak′sē). A procedure designed to widen a small pupil. [G. *korē*, pupil, + *praxis*, action]

laser c., the iris stroma is heated with a laser and the resultant contracture of iris tissue widens the pupil.

mechanical c., a procedure that lodges the pupillary margin in the groove of a device which, when widened, stretches the pupillary edge to make the pupil larger.

co·re·pres·sor (kō-rē-pres′ŏr). A molecule, usually a product of a specific metabolic pathway, that combines with and activates a repressor produced by a regulator gene. The activated repressor then attaches to an operator gene site and inhibits activity of the structural genes. This homeostatic mechanism negatively regulates enzyme production in repressible enzyme systems.

Corey, R.B., U.S. chemist, 1897–1971. SEE Pauling-C. helix.

Cori, Carl F., Czech-U.S. biochemist and Nobel laureate, 1896–1984. SEE C. cycle, ester.

Cori, Gerty Theresa, Czech-U.S. biochemist and Nobel laureate, 1896–1957. SEE C. disease.

co·ria (kō′rē-ă). Plural of corium.

co·ri·an·der (kō-rē-an′der). The dried ripe fruit of *Coriandrum sativum* (family Umbelliferae); a mild stimulant aromatic and a flavoring agent.

co·ri·um, pl. **co·ria** (kō′rē-ŭm, -rē-ă). ✶official alternate term for dermis. [L. skin, hide, leather]

corn (kōrn). SYN clavus (1). [L. *cornu*, horn, hoof]

asbestos c., a granulomatous or hyperkeratotic lesion of the skin at the site of deposit of asbestos particles. SYN asbestos wart.

hard c., the usual form of c. over a toe joint.

soft c., a c. formed by pressure between two toes, the surface being macerated and yellowish in color.

cor·nea (kōr′nē-ă) [TA]. The transparent tissue constituting the anterior sixth of the outer wall of the eye, with a 7.7-mm radius of curvature as contrasted with the 13.5 mm of the sclera; it consists of stratified squamous epithelium continuous with that of the conjunctiva, a substantia propria, substantially regularly arranged collagen imbedded in mucopolysaccharide, and an inner layer of endothelium. It is the chief refractory structure of the eye. [L. fem. of *corneus*, horny]

conical c., SYN keratoconus.

c. farina′ta, bilateral speckling of the posterior part of the corneal stroma. SYN floury c.

floury c., SYN c. farinata.

c. plana, a congenital disorder in which the arc curvature of the cornea is flatter than normal, leaving the eye hyperopic.

c. uri′ca, bilateral deposition of crystalline deposits of urea and sodium urate within corneal stroma.

c. verticilla′ta, congenital whorl-like opacities in the c. SYN Fleischer vortex.

cor·ne·al (kŏr′nē-ăl). Relating to the cornea.

cor·ne·o·bleph·a·ron (kŏr′nē-ō-blef′ă-ron). Adhesion of the eyelid margin to the cornea. [cornea + G. *blepharon,* eyelid]

cor·ne·o·cyte (kŏr′nē-ō-sīt). The dead keratin-filled squamous cell of the stratum corneum. SYN horny cell, keratinized cell. [*cornea,* L. fem. of *corneus,* horny, + G. *kytos,* cell]

cor·ne·o·sclera (kŏr′nē-ō-sklēr′ă). The combined cornea and sclera when considered as forming the external coat of the eyeball.

cor·ne·o·scler·al (kŏr′nē-ō-sklēr′ăl). Pertaining to the cornea and sclera.

Corner, Edred M., English surgeon, 1873–1950. SEE C. *tampon.*

Corner, George W., U.S. anatomist, 1889–1981. SEE C.-Allen *test, unit.*

cor·ne·um (kŏr′nē-ŭm). SEE *stratum* corneum epidermidis, *stratum* corneum unguis. [L., ntr. of *corneus,* horny, fr. *cornu,* horn]

cor·nic·u·late (kŏr-nik′ū-lāt). **1.** Resembling a horn. **2.** Having horns or horn-shaped appendages. [L. *corniculatus,* horned]

cor·nic·u·lum (kŏr-nik′ū-lŭm). A small cornu. [L. dim. of *cornu,* horn]

c. laryn′gis, SYN corniculate *cartilage.*

cor·ni·fi·ca·tion (kŏr-ni-fi-kā′shŭn). SYN keratinization. [L. *cornu,* horn, + *facio,* to make]

cor·ni·fied (kŏr′ni-fīd). SYN keratinized.

corn oil. The refined fixed oil expressed from the embryo of *Zea mays* (family Gramineae); a solvent. SYN maise oil.

corn·silk (kŏrn′silk). SYN zea.

corn smut (kŏrn′smŭt). SYN *Ustilago maydis.*

cor·nu, gen. **cor·nus,** pl. **cor·nua** (kŏr′noo, -nŭs, -noo-ă). **1** [TA]. SYN horn. **2.** Any structure composed of horny substance. **3.** One of the coronal extensions of the dental pulp underlying a cusp or lobe. **4.** The major subdivisions of the lateral ventricle in the cerebral hemisphere (the frontal horn, occipital horn, and temporal horn). SEE ALSO lateral *ventricle.* **5.** The major divisions of the gray columns of the spinal cord (anterior horn, lateral horn, posterior horn). [L. horn]

c. ammo′nis, SYN Ammon *horn.*

c. ante′rius [TA], SYN anterior *horn.*

coccygeal c., two processes that project upward from the dorsum of the base of the coccyx to articulate with the sacral c. SYN c. coccygeum [TA], coccygeal horn, cornua coccygealia.

cornua coccygea′lia, SYN coccygeal c.

c. coccygeum [TA], SYN coccygeal c.

c. cuta′neum, SYN cutaneous *horn.*

cornua of falciform margin of saphenous opening, SEE inferior *horn* of falciform margin of saphenous opening, superior *horn* of falciform margin of saphenous opening.

c. frontale ventriculi lateralis [TA], SYN cornua of lateral ventricle.

cornua of hyoid bone, SEE greater *horn* of hyoid bone, lesser *horn* of hyoid.

c. infe′rius [TA], SYN inferior *horn.*

c. infe′rius cartila′ginis thyroi′deae [TA], SYN inferior *horn* of thyroid cartilage.

c. infe′rius mar′ginis falcifor′mis hia′tus saphe′ni [TA], SYN inferior *horn* of falciform margin of saphenous opening.

c. infe′rius ventric′uli latera′lis [TA], SYN inferior *horn* of lateral ventricle.

c. latera′le [TA], SYN lateral *horn.*

cornua of lateral ventricle, SYN c. frontale ventriculi lateralis [TA], c. occipitale ventriculi lateralis [TA], c. temporale ventriculi lateralis [TA]. SEE anterior *horn* (1), inferior *horn,* posterior *horn.*

c. ma′jus os′sis hyoi′dei [TA], SYN greater *horn* of hyoid bone.

c. mi′nus os′sis hyoi′dei [TA], SYN lesser *horn* of hyoid.

c. occipitale ventriculi lateralis [TA], SYN cornua of lateral ventricle.

c. posterius [TA], SYN posterior *horn.*

c. poste′rius ventric′uli latera′lis [TA], SYN posterior *horn.*

sacral c. [TA], the most caudal parts of the intermediate sacral crest. On each side they form the lateral margin of the sacral hiatus and articulate with the coccygeal cornua. SYN c. sacrale [TA], sacral horn☆.

c. sacra′le [TA], SYN sacral c.

c. of spinal cord, SYN posterior *horn.* SEE anterior *horn* (2), lateral *horn.*

styloid c., SYN lesser *horn* of hyoid.

c. supe′rius cartila′ginis thyroi′deae [TA], SYN superior *horn* of thyroid cartilage.

c. supe′rius margin′alis falcifor′mis [TA], SYN superior *horn* of falciform margin of saphenous opening.

c. temporale ventriculi lateralis [TA], SYN inferior *horn* of lateral ventricle.

c. temporale ventriculi lateralis [TA], SYN cornua of lateral ventricle.

cornua of thyroid cartilage, SEE inferior *horn* of thyroid cartilage, superior *horn* of thyroid cartilage.

c. u′teri [TA], SYN uterine *horn.*

cor·nua (kŏr′noo-ă). Plural of cornu.

cor·nu·al (kŏr′noo-ăl). Relating to a cornu.

♲coro-. SEE core-.

co·ro·na, pl. **co·ro·nae** (kō-rō′nă, -nē) [TA]. SYN crown. [L. garland, crown, fr. G. *korōnē*]

c. cap′itis, the topmost part of the head. SYN crown of head.

c. cilia′ris [TA], the circular figure on the inner surface of the ciliary body, formed by the processes and folds (plicae) taken together. SYN ciliary crown, ciliary wreath.

c. clin′ica, SYN clinical *crown.*

c. den′tis, SYN *crown* of tooth.

c. glan′dis penis [TA], SYN c. of glans penis.

c. of glans penis [TA], the prominent posterior border of the glans penis. SYN c. glandis penis [TA].

c. radia′ta, **(1)** [TA], a fan-shaped fiber mass on the white matter of the cerebral cortex, composed of the widely radiating fibers of the internal capsule; **(2)** a single layer of columnar cells derived from the cumulus oophorus, which anchor on the pellucid zone of the oocyte in a secondary follicle. SYN radiate crown.

c. seborrhe′ica, a red band at the hair line along the upper border of the forehead and temples occasionally observed in seborrheic dermatitis of the scalp.

c. vene′ris, papular syphilitic lesions (secondary eruption) along the anterior margin of the scalp or on the back of the neck. SEE ALSO *crown* of Venus.

Zinn c., SYN vascular *circle* of optic nerve.

cor·o·nad (kŏr′ŏ-nad). In a direction toward any corona.

cor·o·nal (kŏr′ŏ-năl) [TA]. Relating to a corona or the coronal plane. SYN coronalis [TA].

cor·o·na·le (kŏr-ō-nā′lē). **1.** SYN frontal *bone.* **2.** One of the two most widely separated points on the coronal suture at the poles of the greatest frontal diameter. [L. neuter of *coronalis,* pertaining to a *corona,* crown]

cor·o·na·lis (kŏr-ō-nā′lis) [TA]. SYN coronal.

cor·o·na·ria (kŏr-ō-nā′rē-ă). A coronary artery, of the heart.

cor·o·nar·ism (kŏr′ō-nār-izm). **1.** SYN coronary *insufficiency.* **2.** SYN *angina* pectoris. [coronary (artery) + *-ism*]

cor·o·na·ri·tis (kŏr′ō-nă-rī′tis). Inflammation of coronary artery or arteries.

cor·o·nary (kŏr′o-nār-ē). **1.** Relating to or resembling a crown. **2.** Encircling; denoting various anatomical structures, e.g., nerves, blood vessels, ligaments. **3.** Specifically, denoting the c. blood vessels of the heart and, colloquially, c. thrombosis. [L. *coronarius;* fr. *corona,* a crown]

CO

cafe c., sudden collapse while eating that results from food impaction closing the glottis; often erroneously thought to stem from coronary artery disease.

Co·ro·na·vir·i·dae (kō-rō′nă-vir′i-dē). A family of single-stranded RNA-containing viruses with 3 or 4 major antigens corresponding to each of the major viral proteins; some of which cause upper respiratory tract infections in humans similar to the "common cold"; others cause animal infections (infectious avian bronchitis, swine encephalitis, mouse hepatitis, neonatal calf diarrhea, and others). The viruses resemble myxoviruses except for the petal-shaped projections that give an impression of the solar corona. Virions are 120–160 nm in diameter, enveloped, and ether-sensitive. Nucleocapsids are thought to be of helical symmetry; they develop in cytoplasm and are enveloped by budding into cytoplasmic vesicles. Coronavirus and Torovirus are the only recognized genera. [L. *corona,* garland, crown]

Co·ro·na·vi·rus (kō-rō′nă-vī′rŭs). A genus in the family Coronaviridae that is associated with upper respiratory tract infections and possibly gastroenteritis in man.

co·ro·na·vi·rus (kō-rō′nă-vī′rŭs). Any virus of the family Coronaviridae.

cor·o·ner (kŏr′on-er). An official whose duty it is to investigate sudden, suspicious, or violent death to determine the cause; in some communities, the office has been replaced by that of medical examiner. [L. *corona,* a crown]

co·ro·ni·on (kŏ-rō′nē-on). The tip of the coronoid process of the mandible; a craniometric point. SYN koronion. [G. *korōnē,* crow]

cor·o·noid (kŏr′ŏ-noyd). Shaped like a crow's beak; denoting certain processes and other parts of bones. [G. *korōnē,* a crow, + *eidos,* resembling]

cor·o·noi·dec·to·my (kŏr′ŏ-noy-dek′tō-mē). Surgical removal of the coronoid process of the mandible. [coronoid + G. *ektomē,* excision]

cor·po·ra (kŏr′pōr-ă). Plural of corpus.

cor·po·re·al (kŏr-pō′rē-ăl). Pertaining to the body, or to a corpus.

cor·po·rin (kŏr′pŏ-rin). Obsolete term for corpus luteum hormone.

corpse (kōrps). SYN cadaver. [L. *corpus,* body]

corps ronds (kōr-ron′). Dyskeratotic round cells occurring in the epidermis, with a central round basophilic mass surrounded by a clear halo; characteristically found in keratosis follicularis. [Fr. round bodies]

cor·pu·lence, cor·pu·len·cy (kŏr′pū-lens, -len-sē). SYN obesity. [L. *corpulentia,* magnification of *corpus,* body]

cor·pu·lent (kŏr′pū-lent). SYN obese.

CORPUS

cor·pus, gen. **cor·po·ris,** pl. **cor·po·ra** (kōr′pŭs, -pōr-is, -pōr-ă) [TA]. **1.** SYN body. **2.** Any body or mass. **3.** The main part of an organ or other anatomic structure, as distinguished from the head or tail. SEE ALSO body, diaphysis, soma. [L. body]

c. adipo′sum [TA], SYN fat-pad.

c. adipo′sum buc′cae [TA], SYN buccal *fat-pad.*

c. adiposum fossae ischioanalis [TA],

c. adipo′sum fos′sae ischiorecta′lis, SYN fat *body* of ischioanal fossa.

c. adipo′sum infrapatella′re [TA], SYN infrapatellar *fat-pad.*

c. adipo′sum or′bitae [TA], SYN retrobulbar *fat.*

c. al′bicans, a retrogressed c. luteum characterized by increasing cicatrization and shrinkage of the cicatricial core with an amorphous, convoluted, completely hyalinized lutein zone surrounding the central plug of scar tissue. SYN albicans (2), atretic c. luteum, c. candicans.

c. amygdaloi′deum [TA], SYN amygdaloid *body.*

c. amyla′ceum, pl. **cor′pora amyla′cea,** one of a number of small ovoid or rounded, sometimes laminated, bodies resembling a

grain of starch and found in nervous tissue, in the prostate, and in pulmonary alveoli; of little pathological significance, and apparently derived from degenerated cells or proteinaceous secretions. SYN amnionic corpuscle, amylaceous corpuscle, amyloid corpuscle, colloid corpuscle.

c. aor′ticum, SYN paraaortic *bodies,* under *body.*

c. aran′tii, SYN *nodules* of semilunar cusps, under *nodule.*

cor′pora arena′cea, small calcareous concretions in the stroma of the pineal and other central nervous system tissues. SYN acervulus, brain sand, psammoma bodies (2).

atretic c. luteum, SYN c. albicans.

c. atret′icum, SYN atretic ovarian *follicle.*

cor′pora bigem′ina, SYN bigeminal *bodies,* under *body.*

c. callo′sum [TA], the great commissural plate of nerve fibers interconnecting the cortical hemispheres (with the exception of most of the temporal lobes which are interconnected by the anterior commissure). Lying at the floor of the longitudinal fissure, and covered on each side by the cingulate gyrus, it is arched from behind forward and is thick at each extremity (splenium [TA] and genu [TA]) but thinner in its long central portion (truncus [TA]); it curves back underneath itself at the genu to form the rostrum [TA] of the c. callosum. SYN commissure of cerebral hemispheres.

c. can′dicans, SYN c. albicans.

corpora cavernosa recti, SYN anal *cushions,* under *cushion.*

c. caverno′sum clitor′idis [TA], SYN c. cavernosum of clitoris.

c. cavernosum of clitoris [TA], one of the two parallel columns of erectile tissue forming the body of the clitoris; they diverge at the root to form the crura of the clitoris. SYN c. cavernosum clitoridis [TA], cavernous body of clitoris.

c. caverno′sum con′chae, SYN cavernous (vascular) *plexus* of conchae.

c. caverno′sum pe′nis [TA], one of two parallel columns of erectile tissue forming the dorsal part of the body of the penis; they are separated posteriorly, forming the crura of the penis. SYN cavernous body of penis.

c. caverno′sum ure′thrae, SYN c. spongiosum penis.

c. cilia′re [TA], SYN ciliary *body.*

c. clavic′ulae [TA], SYN shaft of clavicle.

c. clitor′idis [TA], SYN *body* of clitoris.

c. coccy′geum [TA], SYN coccygeal *body.*

c. cos′tae [TA], SYN *body* of rib.

c. denta′tum, SYN dentate *nucleus* of cerebellum.

c. epididym′idis [TA], SYN *body* of epididymis.

c. fem′oris, SYN shaft of femur.

c. fibro′sum, the small fibrous cicatricial mass in the ovary formed following the atresia of an ovarian follicle; similar to a corpus albicans but smaller.

c. fib′ulae [TA], SYN shaft of fibula.

c. fimbria′tum, (1) SYN *fimbria* hippocampi; **(2)** the outer, ovarian extremity of the oviduct.

c. for′nicis [TA], SYN *body* of fornix.

c. gas′tricum [TA], SYN *body* of stomach.

c. genicula′tum exter′num, SYN lateral geniculate *body.*

c. genicula′tum inter′num, SYN medial geniculate *body.*

c. genicula′tum latera′le [TA], SYN lateral geniculate *body.*

c. genicula′tum media′le [TA], SYN medial geniculate *body.*

c. glan′dulae sudorif′erae, SYN *body* of sweat gland.

c. hemorrhag′icum, a hematoma with a lining formed by the thinned-out bright yellow lutein zone; gradual resorption of the blood elements leaves a cavity filled with a clear fluid, i.e., a c. luteum cyst. SYN corpus luteum hematoma.

c. high′mori, c. highmoria′num, SYN *mediastinum* of testis.

c. hu′meri [TA], SYN shaft of humerus.

c. incu′dis [TA], SYN *body* of incus.

c. juxtarestiforme, SYN juxtarestiform *body.*

c. lin′guae [TA], SYN *body* of tongue.

c. lu′teum, the yellow endocrine body, 1–1.5 cm in diameter, formed in the ovary at the site of a ruptured ovarian follicle immediately after ovulation; there is an early stage of proliferation and vascularization before full maturity; later, there is a festooned and bright yellowish lutein zone traversed by trabeculae of theca interna containing numerous blood vessels; the c. luteum secretes estrogen, as did the follicle, and also secretes progesterone. If pregnancy does not occur, it is called a **c. luteum spurium**, which undergoes progressive retrogression to a c. albicans. If pregnancy does occur, it is called a **c. luteum verum**, which increases in size, persisting to the fifth or sixth month of pregnancy before retrogression. SYN yellow body.

c. luy′si, SYN subthalamic *nucleus.*

c. mam′mae [TA], SYN *body* of breast.

c. mammilla′re [TA], SYN mammillary *body.*

c. mandib′ulae [TA], SYN *body* of mandible.

c. maxil′lae [TA], SYN *body* of maxilla.

c. medulla′re cerebel′li [TA], the interior white substance of the cerebellum.

c. metacarpale [TA], SYN *shaft* of metacarpal.

c. metatarsale [TA], SYN *shaft* of metatarsal.

c. nu′clei cauda′ti [TA], SYN *body* of caudate nucleus.

c. oliva′re, SYN oliva.

c. os′sis fem′oris [TA], SYN *shaft* of femur.

c. os′sis hyoi′dei [TA], SYN *body* of hyoid bone.

c. os′sis il′ii [TA], SYN *body* of ilium.

c. os′sis isch′ii [TA], SYN *body* of ischium.

c. os′sis metacarpa′lis, the shaft of one of the metacarpal bones.

c. os′sis pu′bis [TA], SYN *body* of pubis.

c. os′sis sphenoida′lis, SYN *body* of sphenoid.

c. pampinifor′me, SYN epoophoron.

c. pancrea′tis [TA], SYN *body* of pancreas.

c. papilla′re, SYN *stratum* papillare corii.

cor′pora para-aor′tica [TA], SYN paraaortic *bodies,* under *body.*

c. paratermina′le, SYN subcallosal *gyrus.*

c. pe′nis [TA], SYN *body* of penis.

c. phalan′gis [TA], SYN *shaft* of phalanx.

c. pinea′le [TA], SYN pineal *body.*

c. pon′tobulba′re, SYN pontobulbar *body.*

cor′pora quadrigem′ina, SYN quadrigeminal *bodies,* under *body;* SEE inferior *colliculus,* superior *colliculus.*

c. quadrigem′inum ante′rius, SYN superior *colliculus.*

c. quadrigem′inum poste′rius, SYN inferior *colliculus.*

c. ra′dii [TA], SYN *shaft* of radius.

c. restifor′me [TA], SYN restiform *body.*

c. spongio′sum pe′nis [TA], the median column of erectile tissue located between and ventral to the two corpora cavernosa penis; posteriorly it expands into the bulbus penis and anteriorly it terminates as the enlarged glans penis; it is traversed by the urethra. SYN c. cavernosum urethrae, spongy body of penis.

c. spongio′sum ure′thrae mulie′bris, the submucous coat of the female urethra, containing a venous network that insinuates itself between the muscular layers, giving to them an erectile nature.

c. ster′ni [TA], SYN *body* of sternum.

c. stria′tum [TA], SYN striate *body.*

c. ta′li [TA], SYN *body* of talus.

c. tib′iae [TA], SYN *shaft* of tibia.

c. trapezoid′eum [TA], SYN trapezoid *body.*

c. triti′ceum, SYN triticeal *cartilage.*

c. ul′nae [TA], SYN *shaft* of ulna.

c. un′guis [TA], SYN *body* of nail.

c. u′teri [TA], SYN *body* of uterus.

c. ver′tebrae [TA], SYN vertebral *body.*

c. vesi′cae [TA], SYN *body* of bladder.

c. vesi′cae bilia′ris [TA], SYN *body* of gallbladder.

c. vesi′cae fell′eae, ☆ official alternate term for *body* of gallbladder.

c. vit′reum [TA], SYN vitreous *body;* SEE ALSO vitreous.

---

①cor·pus·cle (kōr′pŭs-l). **1.** A small mass or body. **2.** A blood cell. SYN corpusculum. [L. *corpusculum,* dim. of *corpus,* body]

amnionic c., SYN *corpus* amylaceum.

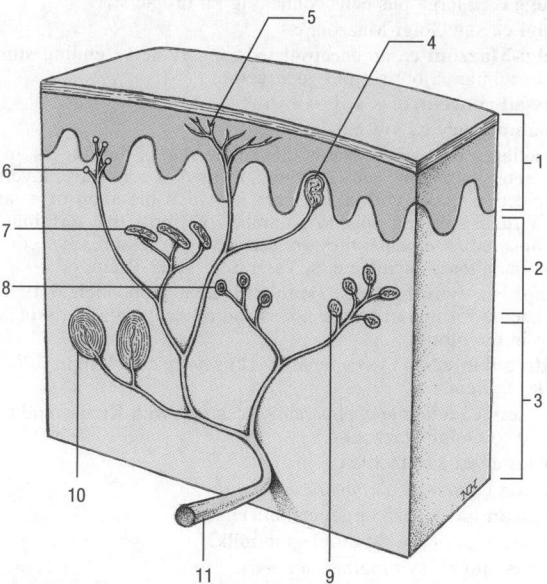

sensory corpuscles: (4) Meissner c. (touch), (5) free nerve ending (pain), (6) Merkel disk (light touch), (7) c. of Ruffini (heat), (8) Golgi c. (light pressure), (9) c. of Krause (cold), (10) pacinian c. (heavy pressure), (11) nerve fiber; and skin layers (1) epidermis (touch), (2) dermis (temperature), (3) subcutaneous tissue (pressure)

---

amylaceous c., amyloid c., SYN *corpus* amylaceum.

articular c.'s, encapsulated nerve terminations within joint capsules. SYN corpuscula articularia.

axis c., axile c., the central portion of a tactile c.

basal c., SYN basal *body.*

Bizzozero c., SYN platelet.

blood c., SYN blood *cell.*

bone c., SYN osteocyte.

bridge c., SYN desmosome.

bulboid c.'s, SYN Krause end *bulbs,* under *bulb.*

calcareous c.'s, rounded masses composed of concentric layers of calcium carbonate, characteristic of tapeworm tissue.

cement c., a cementocyte contained within a lacuna or crypt of the cementum of a tooth; an entrapped cementoblast.

chyle c., a cell of the same appearance as a leukocyte, present in chyle.

colloid c., SYN *corpus* amylaceum.

colostrum c., one of numerous bodies present in the colostrum, supposed to be modified leukocytes containing fat droplets. SYN Donné c., galactoblast.

concentrated human red blood c., c. prepared from one or more preparations of whole human blood that are not more than 14 days old and each of which has already been directly matched with the blood of the intended recipient.

corneal c.'s, connective tissue cells found between the laminae of fibrous tissue in the cornea. SYN Toynbee c.'s, Virchow cells (3), Virchow c.'s.

Dogiel c., an encapsulated sensory nerve ending.

Donné c., SYN colostrum c.

dust c.'s, SYN hemoconia.

Eichhorst c.'s, the globular forms sometimes occurring in the poikilocytosis of pernicious anemia.

exudation c., a cell present in an exudate that assists in the organization of new tissue. SYN exudation cell, inflammatory c., plastic c.

genital c.'s, special encapsulated nerve endings found in the skin of the genitalia and nipple. SYN corpuscula genitalia.

ghost c., SYN achromocyte.

Gluge c.'s, large pus cells containing fat droplets.

Golgi c., SEE Golgi-Mazzoni c.

Golgi-Mazzoni c., an encapsulated sensory nerve ending similar to a pacinian c. but simpler in structure.

Hassall concentric c.'s, SYN thymic c.

inflammatory c., SYN exudation c.

lamellated c.'s, small oval bodies in the skin of the fingers, in the mesentery, tendons, and elsewhere, formed of concentric layers of connective tissue with a soft core in which the axon of a nerve fiber runs, splitting up into a number of fibrils that terminate in bulbous enlargements; they are sensitive to pressure. SYN corpuscula lamellosa, pacinian c.'s, Vater c.'s, Vater-Pacini c.'s.

lymph c., lymphatic c., lymphoid c., a mononuclear type of leukocyte formed in lymph nodes and other lymphoid tissue, and also in the blood.

malpighian c.'s, (1) SYN renal c; **(2)** SYN splenic lymph *follicles,* under *follicle.*

Mazzoni c., a tactile c. apparently identical with Krause end bulb. SEE ALSO Golgi-Mazzoni c.

Meissner c., SYN tactile c.

Merkel c., SYN tactile *meniscus.*

Mexican hat c., SEE target cell *anemia.*

milk c., one of the fat droplets in milk.

molluscum c., SYN molluscum *body.*

Negri c.'s, obsolete term for Negri *bodies,* under *body.*

Norris c.'s, decolorized red blood cells that are invisible or almost invisible in the blood plasma, unless they are appropriately stained.

oval c., SYN tactile c.

pacchionian c.'s, SYN arachnoid *granulations,* under *granulation.*

pacinian c.'s, SYN lamellated c.'s.

pessary c., an elongated red blood cell with hemoglobin concentrated in the peripheral portion.

phantom c., SYN achromocyte.

plastic c., SYN exudation c.

Purkinje c.'s, SYN Purkinje cell *layer.*

pus c., one of the polymorphonuclear leukocytes that comprise the chief portion of the formed elements in pus. SYN pus cell, pyocyte.

Rainey c.'s, rounded, ovoidal, or sickle-shaped spores or bradyzoites, 12–16 by 4–9 μm, found within the elongated cysts (Miescher tubes) of the protozoan *Sarcocystis.*

red c., SYN erythrocyte.

renal c., the tuft of glomerular capillaries and the capsula glomeruli that encloses it. SYN corpusculum renis, malpighian c.'s (1).

reticulated c., SYN reticulocyte.

Ruffini c.'s, sensory end-structures in the subcutaneous connective tissues of the fingers, consisting of an ovoid capsule within which the sensory fiber ends with numerous collateral knobs.

salivary c., one of the leukocytes present in saliva.

Schwalbe c., SYN taste *bud.*

shadow c., SYN achromocyte.

splenic c.'s, SYN splenic lymph *follicles,* under *follicle.*

tactile c., one of numerous oval bodies found in the dermal papillae of thick skin, especially those of the fingers and toes; they consist of a connective tissue capsule in which the axon fibrils terminate around and between a pile of wedge-shaped epithelioid cells; believed to be mechanoreceptors for tactile sensation. SYN corpusculum tactus, Meissner c., oval c., touch c.

taste c., SYN taste *bud.*

terminal nerve c.'s, generic term denoting specialized encapsulated nerve endings such as the articular, bulboid, genital, lamellated, and tactile c.'s, and the tactile meniscus. SYN corpuscula nervosa terminalia.

third c., SYN platelet.

thymic c., small spherical bodies of keratinized and usually squamous epithelial cells arranged in a concentric pattern around clusters of degenerating lymphocytes, eosinophils, and macrophages; found in the medulla of the lobules of the thymus. SYN Hassall bodies, Hassall concentric c.'s, Virchow-Hassall bodies.

touch c., SYN tactile c.

Toynbee c.'s, SYN corneal c.'s.

Traube c., SYN achromocyte.

Tröltsch c.'s, minute spaces, resembling c.'s, between the radial fibers of the drum membrane of the ear.

Valentin c.'s, small bodies, probably amyloid, found occasionally in nerve tissue.

Vater c.'s, SYN lamellated c.'s.

Vater-Pacini c.'s, SYN lamellated c.'s.

Virchow c.'s, SYN corneal c.'s.

white c., any type of leukocyte.

Zimmermann c., SYN platelet.

cor·pus·cu·la (kōr-pŭs'kū-lă). Plural of corpusculum.

cor·pus·cu·lar (kōr-pŭs'kū-lăr). Relating to a corpuscle.

cor·pus·cu·lum, pl. **cor·pus·cu·la** (kōr-pŭs'kū-lŭm, -kū-lă). SYN corpuscle.

corpus'cula articula'ria, SYN articular *corpuscles,* under *corpuscle.*

corpus'cula bulboi'dea, SYN Krause end *bulbs,* under *bulb.*

corpus'cula genita'lia, SYN genital *corpuscles,* under *corpuscle.*

corpus'cula lamello'sa, SYN lamellated *corpuscles,* under *corpuscle.*

corpus'cula nervo'sa termina'lia, SYN terminal nerve *corpuscles,* under *corpuscle.*

c. re'nis, pl. **corpus'cula re'nis,** SYN renal *corpuscle.*

c. tac'tus, pl. **corpus'cula tac'tus,** SYN tactile *corpuscle.*

cor·rec·tion (kō-rek'shŭn). The act of reducing a fault; the elimination of an unfavorable quality.

occlusal c., (1) the c. of malocclusion, by whatever means is employed; **(2)** elimination of disharmony of occlusal contacts.

spontaneous c. of placenta previa, the upward "migration" of the placenta away from the internal os by the differential growth rates of upper and lower uterine segments.

cor·rec·tive (kō-rek'tiv). **1.** Counteracting, modifying, or changing what is injurious. **2.** A drug that modifies or corrects an undesirable or injurious effect of another drug. SYN corrigent. [L. *cor-rigo (conr-),* pp. *-rectus,* to set right, fr. *rego,* to keep straight]

cor·re·la·tion (kōr-ĕ-lā'shŭn). **1.** The mutual or reciprocal relation of two or more items or parts. **2.** The act of bringing into such a relation. **3.** The degree to which variables change together.

product-moment c., a statistical procedure which yields the correlation coefficient referred to as *r* (−1.00 to +1.00) and involves the actual values, rather than the ranks (rank order) of the measurements.

rank-difference c., the relationship between paired series of measurements, each ranked according to magnitude, which yields a coefficient known as *rho;* the value of *rho* varies from zero (no relationship) to +1.00 (perfect relationship).

Correra line. See under line.

cor·re·spon·dence (kōr-ĕ-spon'dens). In optics, those points on each retina that have the same visual direction.

abnormal c., SYN anomalous retinal c.

anomalous retinal c., abnormal c., a condition, frequent in strabismus, in which corresponding retinal points do not have the same visual direction; the fovea of one eye corresponds to an extrafoveal area of the fellow eye. SYN abnormal c.

dysharmonious retinal c., a type of anomalous retinal c. in which the angle of the visual direction of the two retinas is different from the objective angle of the strabismus.

harmonious retinal c., a type of anomalous retinal c. in which the angle of the visual direction of the two retinas is equal to the objective angle of strabismus.

Corrigan, Sir Dominic J., Irish pathologist and clinician, 1802–1880. SEE C. *disease, pulse, sign.*

cor·ri·gent (kōr'i-jent). SYN corrective.

cor·rin (kōr'in). The cyclic system of four pyrrole rings forming corrinoids, which are the central structure of the vitamins B_{12} and related compounds, differing from porphin (porphyrin) in that two of the pyrrole rings are directly linked (C-19 to C-1). [fr. *core* (of vitamin B_{12} molecule)]

cor·rin·oid (kōr′rin-oid). A compound containing a corrin ring.

cor·rode (kŏ-rōd′). To cause, or to be affected by, corrosion.

cor·ro·sion (kŏ-rō′shŭn). **1.** Gradual deterioration or consummation of a substance by another, especially by biochemical or chemical reaction. Cf. erosion. **2.** The product of corroding, such as rust. [L. *cor-rodo* (*conr-*), pp. *-rosus,* to gnaw]

cor·ro·sive (kŏ-rō′siv). **1.** Causing corrosion. **2.** An agent that produces corrosion; e.g., a strong acid or alkali.

cor·ru·ga·tor (kōr′ŭ-gā-ter, -tōr). A muscle that draws together the skin, causing it to wrinkle. [L. *cor-rugo* (*conr-*), pp. *-atus,* to wrinkle, fr. *ruga,* a wrinkle]

CORTEX

cor·tex, gen. **cor·ti·cis**, pl. **cor·ti·ces** (kōr′teks, -ti-sis, -ti-sēz) [TA]. The outer portion of an organ, such as the kidney, as distinguished from the inner, or medullary, portion. [L. bark]

adrenal c., SYN c. of suprarenal gland.

agranular c., SEE cerebral c.

association c., generic term denoting the large expanses of the cerebral c. that are not sensory or motor in the customary sense, but are involved in advanced stages of sensory information processing, multisensory integration, or sensorimotor integration. SEE ALSO cerebral c. SYN association areas.

auditory c., the region of the cerebral c. that receives the auditory radiation from the medial geniculate body, a thalamic cell group receiving auditory input from the cochlear nuclei in the rhombencephalon; it corresponds approximately to Brodmann areas 41 and 42 and is tonotopically organized. SYN auditory area.

cerebellar c., the thin gray surface layer of the cerebellum, consisting of an outer molecular layer or stratum moleculare, a single layer of Purkinje cells (the Purkinje cell layer), and an inner granular layer or stratum granulosum. SYN c. cerebelli [TA].

c. cerebel′li [TA], SYN cerebellar c.

⬛**cerebral c.** [TA], the gray cellular mantle (1–4 mm thick) covering the entire surface of the cerebral hemisphere of mammals; characterized by a laminar organization of cellular and fibrous components such that its nerve cells are stacked in defined layers varying in number from one, as in the archicortex of the hippocampus, to five or six in the larger neocortex; the outermost (molecular or plexiform) layer contains very few cell bodies and is composed largely of the distal ramifications of the long apical dendrites issued perpendicularly to the surface by pyramidal and fusiform cells in deeper layers. From the surface inward, the layers as classified in K. Brodmann's parcellation are: 1) molecular layer [TA]; 2) external granular layer [TA]; 3) external pyramidal layer [TA]; 4) internal granular layer [TA]; 5) internal pyramidal layer [TA]; and 6) multiform layer [TA], many of which are fusiform. This multilaminate organization is typical of the neocortex (homotypic c.; isocortex [TA] in O. Vogt terminology), which in humans covers the largest part by far of the cerebral hemisphere. The more primordial heterotypic c. or allocortex (Vogt) has fewer cell layers. A form of c. intermediate between isocortex and allocortex, called juxtallocortex (Vogt) covers the ventral part of the cingulate gyrus and the entorhinal area of the parahippocampal gyrus.

On the basis of local differences in the arrangement of nerve cells (cytoarchitecture), Brodmann outlined 47 areas in the cerebral c. which, in functional terms, can be classified into three categories: motor c. (areas 4 and 6), characterized by a poorly developed internal granular layer (agranular c.) and prominent pyramidal cell layers; sensory c., characterized by a prominent internal granular layer (granular c. or koniocortex) and comprising the somatic sensory c. (areas 1 to 3), the auditory c. (areas 41 and 42), and the visual c. (areas 17 to 19); and association c., the vast remaining expanses of the cerebral c. SYN c. cerebri [TA], pallium [TA], brain mantle, mantle (2).

c. cer′ebri [TA], SYN cerebral c.

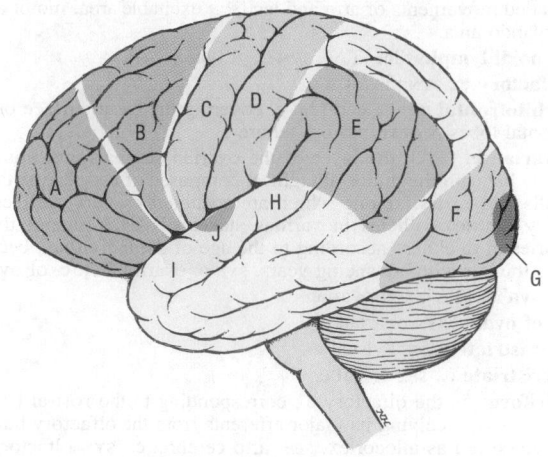

cerebral cortex: major functional areas: (A) biologic intelligence, (B) premotor, (C) somatomotor, (D) somatosensory, (E) bodily awareness, (F) visual psychic, (G) visual sensory, (H) speech understanding, (I) auditory psychic, (J) auditory sensory

deep c., SYN paracortex.

dysgranular c., the region of the cerebral c. that is transitional between the agranular c. of the precentral gyrus and the granular frontal cortex (Brodmann area 8).

fetal adrenal c., an extensive area of the adrenal gland present in primates during fetal life and for a short period after birth; located between the definitive cortex and the medulla, it contains large steroid-secreting cells arranged in a reticular pattern; involution of this zone in humans is largely completed by three months after birth. SYN androgenic zone (2), fetal reticularis (1), fetal zone, provisional c.

frontal c., c. of the frontal lobe of the cerebral hemisphere; **(1)** originally, the entire cortical expanse anterior to the central sulcus, including the agranular motor and premotor c. (Brodmann areas 4 and 6), the dysgranular c. (area 8), and the granular frontal (prefrontal) c. anterior to the latter; **(2)** now more often refers to the granular frontal (prefrontal) c. SYN frontal area.

c. glan′dulae suprarena′lis [TA], SYN c. of suprarenal gland.

granular c., SEE cerebral c.

c. of hair shaft, the principal structural component of the hair shaft, composed of closely packed fusiform keratinized cells and invested by the cuticula pili.

heterotypic c., SYN allocortex.

homotypic c., SYN isocortex.

insular c., SYN insula (1).

laminated c., neocortex [TA] and allocortex [TA].

c. of lens [TA], the softer, more superficial part of the lens of the eye that encloses the central part or nucleus; its refractive power is less than that of the nucleus. SYN c. lentis [TA].

c. len′tis [TA], SYN c. of lens.

c. of lymph node [TA], the outer portion of the lymph node underneath its capsule, consisting of fibrous trabeculae separating densely packed masses of lymphocytes arranged in nodules and separated from the trabeculae and capsule by lymph sinuses. SYN c. nodi lymphatici [TA].

mastoid c., the plate of bone on the lateral surface of the mastoid process of the temporal bone.

motor c., the region of the cerebral c. most nearly immediately influencing movements of the face, neck and trunk, and arm and leg; it corresponds approximately to Brodmann areas 4 and 6 of the precentral gyrus and immediately adjacent portions of the superior and middle frontal gyri; its effects upon the motor neurons innervating the skeletal musculature are mediated by corticospinal fibers (pyramidal tract) and corticonuclear fibers and are particularly essential for the human capacity to perform finely graded movements of arm and leg. SYN excitable area, motor area, Rolando area.

c. no'di lymphat'ici [TA], SYN c. of lymph node.

olfactory c., SYN piriform c.

orbitofrontal c., the cerebral c. covering the basal surface of the frontal lobes. SYN fronto-orbital area.

ovarian c. [TA], the layer of the ovarian stroma lying immediately beneath the tunica albuginea, composed of connective tissue cells and fibers, among which are scattered primary and secondary (antral) follicles in various stages of development; the c. varies in thickness according to the age of the individual, becoming thinner with advancing years. SYN c. ovarii [TA], c. of ovary.

c. ova'rii [TA], SYN ovarian c.

c. of ovary, SYN ovarian c.

parastriate c., SEE visual c.

peristriate c., SEE visual c.

piriform c., the olfactory c., corresponding to the rostral half of the uncus; receiving its major afferents from the olfactory bulb, it is classified as allocortex. SEE ALSO cerebral c. SYN olfactory c., piriform area.

prefrontal c., SEE frontal c.

premotor c., a somewhat ill-defined term usually referring to the agranular cortex of Brodmann area 6. SYN premotor area.

primary visual c., SEE visual c.

provisional c., SYN fetal adrenal c.

renal c. [TA], the part of the kidney consisting of renal lobules in the outer zone beneath the capsule and also the lobules of the renal columns that are extensions inward between the pyramids; contains the renal corpuscles and the proximal and distal convoluted tubules. SYN c. renalis [TA].

c. rena'lis [TA], SYN renal c.

secondary sensory c., a cortical region occupying the parietal operculum (upper lip of the lateral sulcus) closely posterior to the foot of the postcentral gyrus; like the primary somatic-sensory c. of the postcentral gyrus, this region receives sensory impulses originating in face, trunk, and limbs; projections to the s.s.c. are from the ventral basal complex (ventral posteromedial and posterolateral thalamic nuclei) and from the primary somesthetic cortex.

secondary visual c., SEE visual c.

sensory c., formerly denoting specifically the somatic sensory c., but now used to refer collectively to the somatic sensory, auditory, visual, and olfactory regions of the cerebral c.

somatic sensory c., somatosensory c., the region of the cerebral c. receiving the somatic sensory radiation from the ventrobasal nucleus of the thalamus; it represents the primary cortical processing mechanism for sensory information originating at the body surfaces (touch) and in deeper tissues such as muscle, tendons, and joint capsules (position sense); it corresponds approximately to Brodmann areas 1, 2, 3 on the postcentral gyrus. SYN somesthetic area.

striate c., SEE visual c.

supplementary motor c., a region from which, by electrical stimulation, the musculature of all bodily parts can be activated, as it also can by stimulation of the motor c. of the precentral gyrus; the region corresponds approximately to the expansion of Brodmann area 6 over the medial surface of the cerebral hemisphere; this area has largely a bilateral representation and is concerned primarily with tonic and postural motor activities.

suprarenal c., SYN c. of suprarenal gland.

c. of suprarenal gland [TA], the outer part of the adrenal gland, consisting of three zones from without inward: zona glomerulosa, zona fasciculata, and zona reticularis; this part of the adrenal c. yields steroid hormones such as corticosterone, deoxycorticosterone, and estrone. SYN c. glandulae suprarenalis [TA], adrenal c., suprarenal c.

temporal c., SYN temporal *lobe*.

tertiary c., SYN paracortex.

c. thymi [TA], SYN c. of thymus.

c. of thymus [TA], the outer part of a lobule of the thymus; it surrounds the medulla and is composed of masses of closely packed lymphocytes. SYN c. thymi [TA].

visual c., the region of the cerebral c. occupying the entire surface of the occipital lobe, and composed of Brodmann areas 17–19. Area 17 (which is also called striate c. or area because the line of Gennari is grossly visible on its surface) is the primary visual c., receiving the visual radiation from the lateral geniculate body of the thalamus. The surrounding areas 18 (parastriate c. or area) and 19 (peristriate c. or area) are probably involved in subsequent steps of visual information processing; area 18 is referred to as the secondary visual c. SYN visual area.

cor·tex·o·lone (kōr-teks'ō-lōn). A mineralocorticoid hormone from the adrenal cortex.

cor·tex·one (kōr-teks'ōn). SYN deoxycorticosterone.

Corti, Marquis Alfonso, Italian anatomist, 1822–1876. SEE C. arch, canal, cells, under *cell, ganglion, membrane, organ, pillars,* under *pillar, rods,* under *rod,* auditory *teeth,* under *tooth, tunnel;* pillar *cells* of C., under *cell.*

cor·ti·cal (kōr'ti-kăl). Relating to a cortex.

cor·ti·cal·i·za·tion (kōr'ti-kăl-i-zā'shŭn). In phylogenesis, the migration of function from subcortical centers to the cortex. SYN encephalization, telencephalization.

cor·ti·cal·os·te·ot·o·my (kōr'ti-kăl-os-tē-ot'ō-mē). An osteotomy through the cortex at the base of the dentoalveolar segment, which serves to weaken the resistance of the bone to the application of orthodontic forces.

cor·ti·cec·to·my (kōr-ti-sek'tō-mē). Removal of a specific portion of the cerebral cortex. [cortic- + G. *ektomē,* excision]

cor·ti·ces (kōr'ti-sēz). Plural of cortex.

cor·ti·cif·u·gal (kōr-ti-sif'ū-găl). SYN corticofugal.

cor·ti·cip·e·tal (kōr-ti-sip'e-tăl). Passing in a direction toward the outer surface; denoting nerve fibers conveying impulses toward the cerebral cortex. SYN corticoafferent. [L. *cortex,* rind, bark, + *peto,* to seek]

cor·ti·co·af·fer·ent (kōr'ti-kō-af'er-ent). SYN corticipetal.

cor·ti·co·bul·bar (kōr'ti-kō-bŭl'bar). SEE corticobulbar *fibers,* under *fiber,* corticonuclear *fibers,* under *fiber.*

cor·ti·co·cer·e·bel·lum (kor'ti-kō-ser-ĕ-bel'ŭm). SYN neocerebellum.

cor·ti·co·ef·fer·ent (kōr'ti-kō-ef'er-ent). SYN corticofugal.

cor·ti·cof·u·gal (kōr'ti-kō-fū'găl). Passing in a direction away from the outer surface; denoting especially nerve fibers conveying impulses away from the cerebral cortex. SYN corticifugal, cortico-efferent. [L. *cortex,* rind, bark, + *fugio,* to flee]

cor·ti·coid (kōr'ti-koyd). **1.** Having an action similar to that of a hormone of the adrenal cortex. **2.** Any substance exhibiting this action. **3.** SYN corticosteroid.

cor·ti·co·me·di·al (kōr'ti-kō-mē'dē-ăl). Cortical and medial; specifically used to refer to one of the two major cytological divisions of the amygdaloid complex. SEE *corpus* amygdaloideum.

cor·ti·co·ste·roid (kōr'ti-kō-stēr'oyd). A steroid produced by the adrenal cortex (i.e., adrenal corticoid); a corticoid containing a steroid. SYN adrenocorticoid, corticoid (3), cortin.

cor·ti·cos·ter·one (kōr-ti-kos'ter-ōn). A corticosteroid that induces some deposition of glycogen in the liver, sodium conservation, and potassium excretion; the principal glucocortoid in the rat.

cor·ti·co·tha·lam·ic (kōr'ti-kō-thal'ă-mik). Pertaining to cortex and thalamus; the term is applied to fibers projecting from the cerebral cortex to the thalamus, the corticothalamic fibers [TA].

cor·ti·co·troph (kōr'ti-kō-trof). A cell of the adenohypophysis that produces adrenocorticotropic hormone (ACTH).

cor·ti·co·tro·pin (kōr'ti-kō-trō'pin). **1.** SYN adrenocorticotropic *hormone.* **2.** SYN β-corticotropin. [G. *tropē,* a turning]

c.-zinc hydroxide, purified c. absorbed on zinc hydroxide; same uses as c. but with a prolonged duration of action.

β-cor·ti·co·tro·pin. Acid- or pepsin-degraded β-corticotropin. SYN corticotropin (2).

Cor·ti·co·vir·i·dae (kōr'ti-kō-vir'i-dē). Name for a family of nonenveloped, ether-sensitive bacterial viruses of medium size, with a lipid-containing capsid and genome of circular, double-stranded DNA (MW 5×10^6), which accounts for about 12% of virion weight.

corticovirus. Only genus in family of Corticoviridae.

cor·ti·lymph (kōr′tē-limf). The fluid in Corti tunnel.

cor·tin (kōr′tin). SYN corticosteroid.

cor·ti·sol (kōr′ti-sol). SYN hydrocortisone.

c. acetate, SYN *hydrocortisone* acetate.

cor·ti·sone (kōr′ti-sōn). A glucocorticoid not normally secreted in significant quantities by the human adrenal cortex. Endogenously, it is probably a metabolite of hydrocortisone but exhibits no biological activity until converted to hydrocortisone (cortisol); it acts upon carbohydrate metabolism and influences the nutrition and growth of connective (collagenous) tissues. It was the first glucocorticoid available for therapy. SYN Wintersteiner compound F.

α-cor·tol (kōr′tol). The 5β enantiomer of α-allocortol; a reduction product of cortisone, present in the urine, differing from cortisone in that the three keto groups are reduced to hydroxyls.

β-cor·tol. α-Cortol with a 20β-OH group; the 5β enantiomer of β-allocortol, found in urine.

α-cor·to·lone (kōr′tŏ-lōn). The 5β enantiomer of α-allocortolone; a reduction product of cortisone, present in the urine, differing from cortisone in that two of the keto groups (at positions 3 and 20) are reduced to hydroxyls.

β-cor·to·lone. α-Cortolone with a 20β-OH group; the 5β enantiomer of β-allocortolone, found in urine.

co·run·dum (ko-rŭn′dŭm). Native crystalline aluminum oxide. [Hind. *kurand*]

Corvisart des Marets, Baron Jean N., French clinician, 1755–1821. SEE Corvisart *facies*.

co·rym·bi·form (kŏ-rim′bi-fōrm). Denoting the flowerlike clustering configuration of skin lesions in granulomatous diseases (e.g., syphilis, tuberculosis). [L. *corymbus,* cluster, garland]

cor·y·ne·bac·te·ria (kŏ-rī′nē-bak-tēr′ē-ă). Plural of corynebacterium.

cor·y·ne·bac·te·ri·o·phage (kŏ-rī′nē-bak-tēr′ē-ō-fāj). Any one of the bacteriophages specific for corynebacteria.

β c., a DNA-containing bacteriophage that induces toxigenicity in strains of *Corynebacterium diphtheriae* that are lysogenic for its prophage. SYN β phage.

Cor·y·ne·bac·te·ri·um (kŏ-rī′nē-bak-tēr′ē-ŭm). A genus of nonmotile (except for some plant pathogens), aerobic to anaerobic bacteria (family Corynebacteriaceae) containing irregularly staining, Gram-positive, straight to slightly curved, often club-shaped rods which, as a result of snapping division, may show a picket fence arrangement. These organisms are widely distributed in nature. The best known species are parasites and pathogens of humans and domestic animals. The type species is *C. diphtheriae.* [G. *coryne,* a club, + *bacterium,* a small rod]

C. ac′nes, former name for *Propionibacterium acnes.*

C. amycolatum, a species found as normal skin flora, it causes septicemia, frequently associated with venous access devices, and has also been recovered from urinary tract infections and mixed flora abscesses.

C. diphthe′riae, a bacterial species that causes diphtheria and produces a powerful exotoxin causing degeneration of various tissues, notably myocardium, in humans and experimental animals and catalyzes the ADP-ribosylation of elongation factor II; virulent strains of this organism are lysogenic; it is commonly found in membranes in the pharynx, larynx, trachea, and nose in cases of diphtheria; it is also found in apparently healthy pharynx and nose in carriers, and is occasionally found in the conjunctiva and in superficial wounds; it occasionally infects the nasal passages and wounds of horses; it is the type species of the genus C. SYN Klebs-Loeffler bacillus, Loeffler bacillus.

C. e′qui, SYN *Rhodococcus equi.*

C. glucuronolyticum, a species isolated from patients with urinary tract infections.

C. haemoly′ticum, former name for *Arcanobacterium haemolyticum.*

C. hofman′nii, former name for *C. pseudodiphtheriticum.*

C. jeikeium, species associated with septicemia and skin lesions in immunocompromised patients, especially associated with venous access devices.

C. matruchotii, a species recovered in mixed infections from human eye specimens.

C. minutis′simum, a bacterial species that is a component of normal skin flora, causes erythrasma in humans.

C. par′vum, former name for *Propionibacterium acnes.*

C. pseudodiphtherit′icum, a rarely pathogenic species found in normal throats. SYN Hofmann bacillus.

C. stria′tum, a bacterial species found in nasal mucus and in the throat; also found in udders of cows with mastitis; pathogenic to laboratory animals; a rare cause of infection to immnocompromised patients.

C. xero′sis, a bacterial species found in normal and diseased conjunctiva; there is no evidence that this organism is pathogenic.

cor·y·ne·bac·te·ri·um, pl. **cor·y·ne·bac·te·ria** (kŏ-rī′nē-bak-tēr′ē-ŭm, -ă). A vernacular term used to refer to any member of the genus *Corynebacterium.*

co·ry·za (kŏ-rī′ză). SYN acute *rhinitis.* [G.]

allergic c., SYN hay *fever.*

Co·ry·za·vi·rus (kŏ-rī′ză-vī′rŭs). Obsolete name for Rhinovirus.

cos·me·sis (koz-mē′sis). A concern in therapeutics for the appearance of the patient; i.e., an operation that improves appearance. [G. *kosmēsis,* an adorning, fr. *kosmeō,* to order, arrange, adorn, fr. *kosmos,* order]

cos·met·ic (koz-met′ik). **1.** Relating to cosmesis. **2.** Relating to the use of cosmetics.

cos·met·ics (koz-met′iks). Composite term for a variety of camouflages applied to the skin, lips, hair, and nails for purposes of beautifying in accordance with cultural dictates.

cos·mid (koz′mid). A recombinantly engineered plasmid, a circular DNA containing, in order: a plasmid origin of replication and a drug-resistance marker, the *cos* (cohesive end) site from bacteriophage λ, and a fragment of eukaryotic DNA to be cloned; c.'s are constructed to permit cloning of fragments of up to about 40,000 base pairs in length, with one or more unique restriction sites being necessary to facilitate cloning.

cos·mo·pol·i·tan (koz-mō-pol′i-tan). In the biologic sciences, a term denoting worldwide distribution. [G. *kosmos,* universe, + *polis,* city-state]

cos·ta, gen. and pl. **cos·tae** (kos′tă, -tē). **1** [TA]. [I–XII]. SYN rib [I–XII]. **2.** A rodlike internal supporting organelle that runs along the base of the undulating membrane of certain flagellate parasites such as *Trichomonas.* SYN basal rod. [L.]

c. cervica′lis [TA], SYN cervical *rib.*

cos′tae fluctuan′tes [XI–XII], SYN floating *ribs* [XI–XII], under *rib [I–XII].*

cos′tae fluitan′tes, SYN floating *ribs* [XI–XII], under *rib [I–XII].*

c. lumbalis [TA],

c. prima [I] [TA], SYN first *rib* [I].

cos′tae spu′riae [VII–XII] [TA], SYN false *ribs,* under *rib [I–XII].*

cos′tae ve′rae [I–VII] [TA], SYN true *ribs* [I–VII], under *rib [I–XII].*

cos·tal (kos′tăl). Relating to a rib.

cos·tal·gia (kos-tal′jē-ă). SYN pleurodynia. [L. *costa,* rib, + G. *algos,* pain]

cos·tec·to·my (kos-tek′tō-mē). Excision of a rib. [L. *costa,* rib, + G. *ektomē,* excision]

Costen, James B., U.S. otolaryngologist, 1895–1962. SEE C. *syndrome.*

cos·ti·car·ti·lage (kos-ti-kar′ti-lij). SYN costal *cartilage.*

cos·ti·form (kos′ti-fōrm). Rib-shaped. [L. *costa,* rib, + *forma,* form]

cos·tive (kos′tiv). Pertaining to or causing constipation. [contraction from L. *constipo,* to press together]

cos·tive·ness (kos′tiv-ness). SYN constipation.

△**costo-.** The ribs. [L. *costa,* rib]

cos·to·cen·tral (kos-tō-sen′trăl). SYN costovertebral.

CO

cos·to·chon·dral (kos-tō-kon′drăl). Relating to the costal cartilages. SYN chondrocostal.

cos·to·chon·dri·tis (kos′tō-kon-drī′tis). Inflammation of one or more costal cartilages, characterized by local tenderness and pain of the anterior chest wall that may radiate, but without the local swelling typical of Tietze syndrome. SYN costal chondritis. [costo- + G. *chondros,* cartilage, + *-itis,* inflammation]

cos·to·cla·vic·u·lar (kos-tō-klă-vik′ū-lăr). Relating to the ribs and the clavicle.

cos·to·cor·a·coid (kos-tō-kōr′ă-koyd). Relating to the ribs and the coracoid process of the scapula.

cos·to·gen·ic (kos-tō-jen′ik). Arising from a rib.

cos·to·in·fe·ri·or (kos-tō-in-fēr′ē-ōr). Relating to the lower ribs.

cos·to·scap·u·lar (kos-tō-skap′ū-lăr). Relating to the ribs and the scapula.

cos·to·sca·pu·la·ris (kos-tō-skap-ū-lā′ris). SYN serratus anterior (*muscle*).

cos·to·ster·nal (kos-tō-ster′năl). Pertaining to the ribs and the sternum.

cos·to·ster·no·plas·ty (kos-tō-ster′nō-plas-tē). Operation to correct a malformation of the anterior chest wall. [costo- + G. *sternon,* chest, + *plastos,* formed]

cos·to·su·pe·ri·or (kos-tō-soo-pēr′ē-ōr). Relating to the upper ribs.

cos·to·tome (kos′tō-tōm). An instrument, knife or shears, designed for cutting through a rib.

cos·tot·o·my (kos-tot′ō-mē). Division of a rib. [costo- + G. *tomē,* a cutting]

cos·to·trans·verse (kos-tō-trans-vers′). Relating to the ribs and the transverse processes of the vertebrae articulating with them. SYN transversocostal.

cos·to·trans·ver·sec·to·my (kos′tō-tranz-ver-sek′tō-mē). Excision of a proximal portion of a rib and the articulating transverse process.

cos·to·ver·te·bral (kos-tō-ver′tĕ-brăl). Relating to the ribs and the bodies of the thoracic vertebrae with which they articulate. SYN costocentral, vertebrocostal (1).

cos·to·xi·phoid (kos-tō-zī′foyd). Relating to the ribs and the xiphoid cartilage of the sternum.

co·sub·strate (kō-sŭb′strāt). The second or other substrate of a multisubstrate enzyme; often, specifically refers to the coenzyme.

co·syn·tro·pin (kō-sin-trō′pin). α^{1-24}- or β^{1-24}-Corticotropin; a synthetic corticotrophic agent, comprising the first 24 amino acyl residues of human ACTH, which sequence is found in several other species and which retains the full biologic activity of the complete ACTH; the remaining 15 residues differ among species and confer specific immunologic properties. SYN tetracosactide, tetracosactin.

Cotard, Jules, French neurologist, 1840–1887. SEE C. *syndrome.*

co·tar·nine (kō-tar′nēn). An alkaloidal principle, $C_{12}H_{15}NO_4$, derived from narcotine by oxidation; an astringent. [anagram of *narcotine*]

COTe Abbreviation of cathodal opening tetanus.

co·ti·nine (kō′ti-nēn). One of the major detoxication products of nicotine; eliminated rapidly and completely by the kidneys. [anagram of *nicotine*]

co·trans·la·tion·al (kō′tranz-lā′shun-ăl). Any process involving the maturation or delivery of a protein that occurs during the process of translation.

co·trans·port (kō-trans′pōrt). The transport of one substance across a membrane, coupled with the simultaneous transport of another substance across the same membrane in the same direction.

Cotte, Gaston, French surgeon, 1879–1951. SEE C. *operation.*

Cotton, Frank A., U.S. chemist, *1930. SEE C. *effect.*

cot·ton (kot′ŭn). The white, fluffy, fibrous covering of the seeds of a plant of the genus *Gossypium* (family Malvaceae); used extensively in surgical dressings. [Ar. *qútun*]

absorbent c., c. from which all fatty matter has been extracted, so that it readily takes up fluids.

purified c., absorbent c. in which the hairs of the seed of varieties of *Gossypium* and other allied species are freed from adhering impurities, deprived of fatty matter, bleached, and sterilized; used for tampons, etc.

soluble gun c., SYN pyroxylin.

styptic c., absorbent c. wet with a dilute solution of ferric chloride, and then dried; applied locally as a hemostatic.

cot·ton·pox (kot′ŭn-poks). Obsolete name for *variola* minor.

cot·ton·seed oil (kot′ŭn-sēd). The refined fixed oil obtained from the seed of cultivated plants of various varieties of *Gossypium hirsutum* or of other species of *Gossypium* (family Malvaceae); a solvent.

Cotunnius (Cotugno), Domenico, Italian anatomist, 1736–1822. SEE C. *aqueduct, canal, liquid, space; aqueductus* cotunnii; *liquor* cotunnii.

cot·y·le (kot′i-lē). **1.** Any cup-shaped structure. **2.** SYN acetabulum. [G. *kotylē,* anything hollow, the cup or socket of a joint]

cot·y·le·don (kot-i-lē′don). **1.** SEE maternal c., fetal c. **2.** In plants, a seed leaf, the first leaf to grow from a seed. **3.** A placental unit. SEE maternal c. [G. *kotylēdon,* any cup-shaped hollow]

fetal c., a unit of the fetal placenta supplied by the vessels of a stem villus; several such c.'s may occur between two placental septa; traditionally called embryologists' c.

maternal c., a unit of the placenta made up of trophoblastic cells, fibrous tissue, and abundant blood vessels, which is visible grossly on the maternal surface as an irregularly shaped lobe circumscribed by a deep cleft and made up of a stem villus with numerous branching free villi and anchoring villi; placental vessels in the chorionic plate supply the stem villus and its branches, allowing gas and metabolite exchange across the trophoblastic layer with maternal blood in the intervillous space; traditionally called clinicians' c.

Cot·y·lo·gon·i·mus (kot-i-lō-gon′i-mŭs). A group of heterophyid flukes, now properly included in the genus *Heterophyes.* [G. *kotylē,* cup, + *gonimos,* productive]

cot·y·loid (kot′i-loyd). **1.** Cup-shaped; cuplike. **2.** Relating to the cotyloid cavity or acetabulum. [G. *kotylē,* a small cup, + *eidos,* appearance]

cough (kawf). **1.** A sudden explosive forcing of air through the glottis, occurring immediately on opening the previously closed glottis, excited by mechanical or chemical irritation of the trachea or bronchi or by pressure from adjacent structures. **2.** To force air through the glottis by a series of expiratory efforts. [echoic]

aneurysmal c., c. due to impingement of an aortic aneurysm on the recurrent laryngeal nerve or other nearby structures.

brassy c., loud metallic barking c. associated with subglottic edema.

habit c., a persistent c. due to a tic or to psychological causes.

privet c., an allergic c., occurring in China during May and June, supposed to be caused by inhalation of the pollen of a species of privet (*Lingustrum*); it is analogous to the laurel fever seen in New England.

reflex c., a c. excited reflexly by irritation in some distant part, as the ear or the stomach.

weaver's c., term for c., dyspnea, and sense of constriction of the chest, caused in persons working with mildewed yarns.

whooping c., SYN pertussis.

cou·lomb (C, Q) (koo-lom′). The unit of electrical charge, equal to 3×10^9 electrostatic units; the quantity of electricity delivered by a current of 1 A in 1 s equal to 1/96,485 faraday. [CA de *Coulomb,* Fr. physicist, 1736–1806]

cou·mar·a·none (koo-mar′ă-nōn). 3(2*H*)-Benzofuranone; the basis of many plant products; e.g., aurone.

cou·ma·ric an·hy·dride (koo-mā′rik). SYN coumarin.

cou·ma·rin (koo′mă-rin). **1.** A general descriptive term applied to anticoagulants and other drugs derived from dicumarol, a component of the Tonka bean. **2.** A fragrant neutral principle obtained from the Tonka bean, *Dypterix odorata,* and made synthetically from salicylic aldehyde; it is used to disguise unpleasant odors.

SYN coumaric anhydride, cumarin. [*coumarou,* native name of Tonka bean]

cou·met·a·rol (koo-met′ă-rol). An oral anticoagulant. SYN cumetharol, cumethoxaethane.

Councilman, William T., U.S. pathologist, 1854–1933. SEE C. *body.*

Coun·cil·ma·nia (kown-sil-man′ē-ă). Obsolete generic term for a group of amebae now recognized as *Entamoeba.* [W. Councilman]

coun·sel·ing (kown′sel-ing). A professional relationship and activity in which one person endeavors to help another to understand and to solve his or her adjustment problems; the giving of advice, opinion, and instruction to direct the judgment or conduct of another. SEE psychotherapy. [L. *consilium,* deliberation]

genetic c., the process whereby an expert in genetic disorders provides information about risk and clinical burden of a disorder or disorders to patients or relatives in families with genetic disorders as an aid to making informed and responsible decisions about marriage, children, early diagnosis, and prognosis.

marital c., the process whereby a trained counselor assists married couples to resolve problems that arise and trouble them in their relationship; husband and wife are seen by the same counselor in separate and joint c. sessions focusing on immediate family problems.

pastoral c., the use of psychotherapeutic methods by members of the clergy, members of a religious community, and/or lay therapists for parishioners seeking help with personal problems.

count (kownt). 1. A reckoning, enumeration, or accounting. 2. To enumerate or score.

Addis c., a quantitative enumeration of the red blood c., white blood c., and casts in a 12-hr urine specimen; used to follow the progress of known renal disease.

Arneth c., the percentage distribution of polymorphonuclear neutrophils, based on the number of lobes in the nuclei (from 1 to 5). SEE ALSO Arneth *index.*

blood c., SEE blood count.

CD4/CD8 c., The ratio of helper-inducer T lymphocytes to cytotoxic-suppressor T lymphocytes in peripheral blood. T-cell subset analysis is performed by flow cytometry of lymphocytes after incubation with fluorescently tagged monoclonal antibodies to the CD4 surface antigen found on helper-inducer T cells and the CD8 surface antigen found on cytotoxic-suppressor T cells. In healthy persons, the CD4/CD8 ratio ranges between 1.6 and 2.2.

epidermal ridge c., an index of the frequency of sweat pores on the fingertips by enumeration along a set of arbitrarily defined lines; a classic example of a galtonian trait determined almost exclusively by genetic factors.

filament-nonfilament c., a differential c. of the number of neutrophils showing nuclear division and those showing no such division.

total cell c., number of cells in a given area or volume.

viable cell c., number of cells in a given area or volume that are thriving.

count·er (kown′ter). A device that counts, usually scintillations.

automated differential leukocyte c., an instrument using digital imaging or cytochemical techniques to differentiate leukocytes.

electronic cell c., an automatic blood cell c. in which cells passing through an aperture alter resistance and are counted as voltage pulses, or in which cells passing through a flow cell deflect light; some types of c. are capable of multiple simultaneous measurements on each blood sample; e.g., leukocyte count, red cell count, hemoglobin, hematocrit, and red cell indices.

Geiger-Müller c., an instrument for measuring radioactivity by counting the emission of radioactive particles; it consists of a metallic cylinder, negatively charged, in a tube containing a fine, positively charged wire at its center; radiations produce ionization of the gas molecules between the cylinder and the wire and result in an electrical discharge independent of the energy of the impinging particle or ray.

proportional c., a Geiger-Müller c. operating in the voltage range and under conditions in which pulse height is proportional to the energy of the particles or rays being counted, thus making dis-

crimination between particles or rays of different energies possible.

scintillation c., an instrument used for the detection of radioactivity; the radiation is absorbed by a scintillator (a crystal or a compound, such as POPOP, in solution) which results in minute flashes of light that are detected by a photocathode. The resultant electron emission is amplified by a photomultiplier and an amplifier. SYN scintillometer, spinthariscope.

well c., a scintillation crystal shaped with a central hole to receive a small sample, plus associated detector and electronics.

whole-body c., shielding and instrumentation, usually involving more than one detector, designed to evaluate the total-body burden of various gamma-emitting nuclides.

△**counter-.** Opposite, opposed, against. SEE ALSO contra-. [L. *contra,* against]

count·er·bal·anc·ing (kown-ter-bal′ăn-sing). A procedure in behavorial research for distributing unwanted but unavoidable influences equally among the different experimental conditions or subjects.

count·er·con·di·tion·ing (kown′ter-kon-dish′ŭn-ing). Any of a group of specific behavior therapy techniques in which a second conditioned response (e.g., approaching or even touching a snake) is introduced for the express purpose of counteracting or nullifying a previously conditioned or learned response (fear and avoidance of snakes).

count·er·cur·rent (kown′ter-ker′ent). 1. Flowing in an opposite direction. 2. A current flowing in a direction opposite to another current.

count·er·cur·rent ex·chang·er. A system in which heat or chemicals passively diffuse across a membrane separating two c. e. streams so that at each end the fluid leaving along one side of the membrane nearly resembles, in temperature or composition, the fluid entering the other; e.g., the venae comites in the arms serve as a c. e. exchanger, the arterial blood serving to rewarm the cooler venous blood.

count·er·cur·rent mul·ti·pli·er. A system in which energy is used to transport material across a membrane separating two c. m. tubes connected at one end to form a hairpin shape; by this means a concentration can be achieved in the fluid in the hairpin bend, relative to the inflow and outflow fluids, that is much greater than the transport mechanism could produce between the two sides of the membrane at any point; e.g., the nephronic loops in the renal medulla act as c. m.'s.

count·er·die (kown′ter-dī). The reverse image of a die, usually made of a softer and lower fusing metal than the die.

count·er·ex·ten·sion (kown′ter-eks-ten′shŭn). SYN countertraction.

count·er·im·mu·no·e·lec·tro·pho·re·sis (kown′ter-im′ū-nō-ē-lek′trō-fōr-ē′-sis). A modification of immunoelectrophoresis in which antigen (e.g., serum containing hepatitis B virus) is placed in wells cut in the sheet of agar gel toward the cathode, and antiserum is placed in wells toward the anode; antigen and antibody, moving in opposite directions, form precipitates in the area between the cells where they meet in concentrations of optimal proportions.

count·er·in·ci·sion (kown′ter-in-sizh′ŭn). A second incision in the region of a primary incision designed to take tension off the primary closure.

count·er·in·vest·ment (kown′ter-in-vest′ment). SYN anticathexis.

count·er·ir·ri·tant (kown-ter-ir′i-tant). 1. An agent that causes irritation or a mild inflammation of the skin in order to relieve symptoms of a deep-seated inflammatory process. 2. Relating to or producing counterirritation. Enhances blood flow to affected area.

count·er·ir·ri·ta·tion (kown′ter-ir-i-tā′shŭn). Irritation or mild inflammation (redness, vesication, or pustulation) of the skin excited for the purpose of relieving symptoms of an inflammation of the deeper structures.

count·er·o·pen·ing (kown′ter-ō-pen-ing). A second opening made at the dependent part of an abscess or other cavity containing fluid, which is not draining satisfactorily through a previous opening. SYN contraaperture, counterpuncture.

count·er·pho·bic (kown-ter-fō′bik). **1.** Denoting a state of actual preference, on the part of a phobic person, for the very situation of which that person is afraid. **2.** Opposed to the phobic impulse, as in c. mastery of a feared action by repeated engagement in the action.

count·er·pul·sa·tion (kown′ter-pŭl-sā′shŭn). A means of assisting the failing heart by automatically removing arterial blood just before and during ventricular ejection and returning it to the circulation during diastole; a balloon catheter is inserted into the aorta and activated by an automatic mechanism triggered by the ECG.

intra-aortic balloon c., rhythmic inflation and deflation of a catheter-borne balloon placed in the aorta distal to the aortic valve to facilitate ejection during systole and to limit regurgitation during diastole by the appropriate application of pressures. Usually an emergency treatment for cardiogenic shock or for intractable angina.

count·er·punc·ture (kown′ter-pŭnk-choor). SYN counteropening.

count·er·shock (kown′ter-shok). An electric shock applied to the heart to terminate a disturbance of its rhythm.

count·er·stain (kown′ter-stān). A second stain of different color, having affinity for tissues, cells, or parts of cells other than those taking the primary stain, used to render more distinct the parts taking the first stain.

count·er·trac·tion (kown-ter-trak′shŭn). The resistance, or back-pull, made to traction or pulling on a limb; e.g., in the case of traction made on the leg, c. may be effected by raising the foot of the bed so that the weight of the body pulls against the weight attached to the limb. SYN counterextension.

count·er·trans·fer·ence (kown′ter-trans-fer′ens). In psychoanalysis, the analyst's transference (often unconscious) to the patient of emotional needs and conflicts from the analyst's past experiences or the analyst's current emotional responses to the manifestation of the patient's transference.

count·er·trans·port (kown-ter-tranz′pōrt). The transport of one substance across a membrane, coupled with the simultaneous transport of another substance across the same membrane in the opposite direction.

coup de sa·bre (koo-dĕ-sahb′). Linear scleroderma found over the scalp with scarring alopecia, face, or forehead. [Fr. stroke of a sword]

cou·ple (kŭ′pl). To copulate; to perform coitus; said especially of the lower animals.

cou·pling (kŭp′ling). **1.** Usually the result of the repeated pairing of a normal sinus beat with a ventricular extrasystole. **2.** SEE coupling *phase.* **3.** A condition in which one or more products of a reaction are the subsequent reactants (or substrates) of a second reaction.

constant c., SYN fixed c.

fixed c., where several premature beats are seen, the interval between each of them and the preceding normal beat is constant. SYN constant c.

variable c., where several extrasystoles are seen, the interval between each of them and the preceding sinus beat varies.

Courvoisier, Ludwig G., French surgeon, 1843–1918. SEE C. *law, sign, gallbladder.*

cou·vade (koo-vahd′). A primitive custom in certain cultures in which a man develops labor pains while his wife is in labor and then submits to the same postpartum purification rites and taboos. [Fr. *couver,* to hatch]

Couvelaire, Alexandre, French obstetrician, 1873–1948. SEE C. *uterus.*

cou·ver·cle (koo-ver′kl). Rarely used term for an external coagulum, especially a blood clot formed extravascularly. [Fr. cover, lid]

co·va·lent (kō-vāl′ent). Denoting an interatomic bond characterized by the sharing of 2, 4, or 6 electrons.

cov·er·age. A measure of the extent to which the services rendered cover the potential need for these services in a community;

applied specifically to such services as immunization in developing countries.

cov·er·ing (kov′er-ing). A surrounding layer; something that covers or encloses, forming an outer layer. SEE ALSO tunica.

c.'s of spermatic cord, c.'s of the spermatic cord, including external and internal spermatic fasciae, and cremasteric muscle and fascia. SYN tunicae funiculi spermatici.

cov·er·slip (kŭv′er-slip). SYN cover *glass.*

cow (kow). **1.** A generator for short-lived isotopes based upon successively eluting or otherwise separating ("milking") a short-lived radioactive daughter from a longer-lived parent; e.g., ^{99m}Tc from ^{99}Mo, ^{113m}In from ^{113}Sn. **2.** The mature female of domestic cattle (genus *Bos*); also the mature female of certain other animals such as buffalo, elephant, and whale.

Cowden. Surname of the family from which the condition subsequently known as Cowden *disease* was first reported.

Cowdry, Edmund Vincent, U.S. cytologist, 1888–1975. SEE C. type A inclusion *bodies,* under *body,* type B inclusion *bodies,* under *body.*

cowl. SEE caul.

Cowling rule. See under rule.

Cowper, William, English anatomist, 1666–1709. SEE C. *cyst, gland, ligament.*

cow·per·i·an (kow-pēr′ē-an). Relating to or described by Cowper.

Cox, H.R., U.S. bacteriologist, *1907.

coxa, gen. and pl. **cox·ae** (kok′să, -sē) [TA]. **1.** SYN hip (1). **2.** SYN hip *joint.* [L]

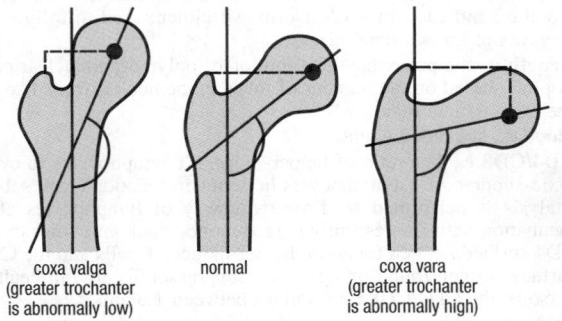

coxa valga
(greater trochanter
is abnormally low)

normal

coxa vara
(greater trochanter
is abnormally high)

coxa valga, coxa vara: varying configurations of the angle of the hip-joint

c. adduc′ta, SYN c. vara.

false c. va′ra, approximation of the head of the femur to the shaft, due not to deformity of the neck of the femur, but to curvature of the shaft.

c. mag′na, enlargement and often deformation of the femoral head; usually refers to a sequela of Legg-Calvé-Perthes disease or osteoarthritis.

c. pla′na, SYN Legg-Calvé-Perthes *disease.*

c. val′ga, alteration of the angle made by the axis of the femoral neck to the axis of the femoral shaft, so that the angle exceeds 135°; the femoral neck is in more of a straight-line relationship to the shaft of the femur.

c. va′ra, alteration of the angle made by the axis of the femoral neck to the axis of the femoral shaft so that the angle is less than 135°; the femoral neck becomes more horizontal. SYN c. adducta.

c. va′ra lux′ans, c. vara with dislocation of the femoral head.

cox·al·gia (koks-al′jē-ă). SYN coxodynia. [L. *coxa,* hip, + G. *algos,* pain]

Cox·i·el·la (kok-sē-el′ă). A genus of filterable bacteria (order Rickettsiales) containing small, pleomorphic, rod-shaped or coccoid, Gram-negative cells that occur intracellularly in the cytoplasm of infected cells and possibly extracellularly in infected ticks. These organisms have not been cultivated in cell-free media; they are parasitic on humans and other animals; type species is *C. burnetii.*

C. burnet′ii, a bacterial species that causes Q fever in humans; it is more resistant than other rickettsiae and may be passed via aerosols as well as living vectors. Acute pneumonia and chronic endocarditis are also associated with this species. The type species of the genus *Coxiella*.

cox·i·tis (koks-ī′tis). Inflammation of the hip.

cox·o·dyn·ia (koks-ō-din′ē-ă). Pain in the hip joint. SYN coxalgia. [L. *coxa*, hip, + G. *odynē*, pain]

cox·o·fem·o·ral (kok-sō-fem′ŏ-răl). Relating to the hip bone and the femur.

cox·o·tu·ber·cu·lo·sis (koks′ō-too-ber-kū-lō′sis). Tuberculous hip-joint disease.

cox·sack·ie·vi·rus (kok-sak′ē-vī′rŭs). A group of picornaviruses, included in the genus Enterovirus, of icosahedral shape, stable at acid pH, and about 28 nm in diameter, causing myositis, paralysis, and death in young mice, and responsible for a variety of diseases in man, although inapparent infections are common. They are divided antigenically into two groups, A and B, each of which includes a number of serological types, e.g., Enterovirus coxsackie A1 to 24 and Enterovirus coxsackie B1 to 6. Type A viruses cause human herpangina and hand-foot-and-mouth disease; type B viruses cause epidemic pleurodynia; both type viruses may cause aseptic meningitis, myocarditis and pericarditis, and acute onset juvenile diabetes. [*Coxsackie*, N.Y., where first isolated]

c.p. Abbreviation for chemically pure.

CPAP Abbreviation for continuous positive airway *pressure*.

CPEO Acronym for chronic progressive external *ophthalmoplegia*.

C-pep·tide. The 30-amino-acid chain that connects the A and B chains of insulin in proinsulin; removed in the conversion of proinsulin to insulin. SYN C chain.

CPK Abbreviation for *creatine* phosphokinase.

CPM Abbreviation for continuous passive *motion*.

cpm Abbreviation for counts per minute.

CPPD Abbreviation for calcium pyrophosphate deposition *disease*.

CPPV Abbreviation for continuous positive pressure *ventilation*.

CPR Abbreviation for cardiopulmonary *resuscitation*.

cps Abbreviation for cycles per second.

CR Abbreviation for conditioned *reflex*; crown-rump *length*; computed *radiography*.

Cr 1. Symbol for chromium. **2.** Abbreviation for creatinine.

crab (krab). **1.** A crustacean, many varieties of which are edible. **2.** An insect, the crab louse, *Pthirus pubis*.

Crabtree, Herbert G., 20th century English physician and biochemist. SEE C. *effect*.

crack (krăk). **1.** A fissure. **2.** SEE crack *cocaine*. [slang]

    lacquer c.'s, breaks in Bruch *membrane* seen in pathologic myopia.

crac·kle (krak′l). SYN rale. [echoic]

cra·dle (krā′dl). A frame used to keep bedclothes from coming in contact with a patient. [M.E. *cradel*]

Crafoord, Clarence, Swedish thoracic surgeon, 1899–1984. SEE C. *clamp*.

Craig·ia (krā′gē-ă). Obsolete generic term for a group of amebae now recognized as *Entamoeba*. [C. *Craig*]

Cramer, Friedrich, German surgeon, 1847–1903. SEE C. wire *splint*.

cramp (kramp). **1.** A painful muscle spasm caused by prolonged tetanic contraction. **2.** A localized muscle spasm related to occupational use, qualified according to the occupation of the sufferer; e.g., seamstress's c., writer's c. [M.E. *crampe*, fr. O.Fr., fr. Germanic]

    heat c.'s, muscle spasms induced by severe exertion in intense heat, accompanied by considerable pain; sometimes related to salt deficiency, hyperventilation, or overindulgence in alcohol. SYN myalgia thermica.

    intermittent c., SYN tetany.

miner's c.'s, c.'s caused by excessive salt loss through perspiration. SYN stoker's c.'s.

musician's c., an occupational dystonia, affecting those who play on musical instruments, and named usually according to the instrument played upon.

pianist's c., piano-player's c., an occupational dystonia affecting the muscles of the fingers and forearms in piano players.

seamstress's c., an occupational dystonia occurring in the fingers of women who sew.

shaving c., an occupational dystonia affecting the hands and fingers of barbers.

stoker's c.'s, SYN miner's c.'s.

tailor's c., an occupational dystonia affecting the forearms and hands of tailors.

typist's c., an occupational dystonia affecting chiefly the long flexor muscles of the hands of typists.

violinist's c., a occupational dystonia affecting the digits of the fingering hand, or sometimes the bowing arm, in violin players.

waiter's c., an occupational dystonia characterized by spasm of the muscles of the back and dominant arm in persons who wait tables.

watchmaker's c., an occupational dystonia characterized by spasm of the orbicularis palpebrarum muscle from holding the lens to the eye and spasm of the muscles of the hand from performing the delicate movements of watch repairing.

writer's c., an occupation dystonia affecting chiefly the muscles of the thumb and two adjoining fingers of the writing hand, induced by excessive use of a writing instrument. SYN dysgraphia (2), graphospasm, scrivener's palsy.

Crampton, Sir Philip, Irish surgeon, 1777–1858. SEE C. *line*, *muscle*.

Crampton, Charles Ward, U.S. physician, *1877. SEE C. *test*.

Crandall, Barbara F., U.S. physician. SEE Crandall *syndrome*.

△**crani-.** SEE cranio-.

cra·nia (krā′nē-ă). Plural of cranium.

cra·ni·ad (krā′nē-ad). Situated nearer the head in relation to a specific reference point; opposite of caudad. SEE ALSO superior.

cra·ni·al (krā′nē-ăl). **1** [TA]. Relating to the cranium or head. SYN cranialis [TA], cephalic. SEE ALSO cephalad. **2.** SYN superior (2).

cra·ni·a·lis (krā-nē-ā′lis) [TA]. SYN cranial (1).

cra·ni·am·phit·o·my (krā-nē-am-fit′ō-mē). A decompression operation in which the entire circumference of the calvarium is divided. [G. *kranion*, skull, + *amphi*, around, + *tomē*, cutting]

Cra·ni·a·ta (krā-nē-ā′tă). SYN Vertebrata. [Mediev. L. *cranium*, fr. G. *kranion*, skull]

cra·ni·ec·to·my (krā′nē-ek′tō-mē). Excision of a portion of the skull, without replacement of the bone, e.g., subtemporal or suboccipital. [G. *kranion*, skull, + *ektomē*, excision]

    linear c., excision of a strip of cranium containing a prematurely fused suture.

△**cranio-, crani-.** The cranium. Cf. cerebro-. [G. *kranion*, skull]

cra·ni·o·au·ral (krā′nē-ō-aw′răl). Relating to the skull and the ear.

cra·ni·o·cele (krā′nē-ō-sēl). SYN encephalocele. [cranio- + G. *kēlē*, hernia]

cra·ni·o·ce·re·bral (krā′nē-ō-ser′ē-brăl). Relating to the skull and the brain.

cra·ni·o·cla·sia, cra·ni·o·cla·sis (krā-nē-ō-klā′sē-ă, krā-nē-ok′lă-sis). Formerly used operation for crushing of the fetal skull in cases of dystocia. [cranio- + G. *klasis*, a breaking]

cra·ni·o·clast (krā′nē-ō-klast). Instrument like a strong forceps formerly used for crushing and extracting the fetal head after perforation. [cranio- + G. *klaō*, to break in pieces]

cra·ni·o·clei·do·dys·os·to·sis (krā′nē-ō-klī′dō-dis-os-tō′sis). SYN cleidocranial *dysostosis*. [cranio- + G. *kleis*, clavicle, + dysostosis]

cra·ni·o·did·y·mus (krā′nē-ō-did′i-mŭs). Conjoined twins with fused bodies but with two heads. SEE conjoined *twins*, under *twin*. [cranio- + G. *didymos*, twin]

cr

cra·ni·o·fa·cial (krā′nē-ō-fā′shăl). Relating to both the face and the cranium.

cra·ni·o·fe·nes·tria (krā′nē-ō-fe-nes′trē-ă). SYN craniolacunia. [cranio- + L. *fenestra*, window]

cra·ni·og·no·my (krā-nē-og′nō-mē). SYN phrenology. [cranio- + G. *gnōme*, judgment]

cra·ni·o·graph (krā′nē-ō-graf). An instrument for making drawings to scale of the diameters and general configuration of the skull.

cra·ni·og·ra·phy (krā-nē-og′ră-fē). The art of representing, by drawings made from measurements, the configuration of the skull and the relations of its angles and craniometric points. [cranio- + G. *graphō*, to write]

cra·ni·o·la·cu·nia (krā′nē-ō-lă-koo′nē-ă). Incomplete formation of the bones of the vault of the fetal skull so that there are nonossified areas in the calvaria. SYN craniofenestria. [cranio- + L. *lacuna*, cleft]

cra·ni·ol·o·gy (krā-nē-ol′ō-jē). The science concerned with variations in size, shape, and proportion of the cranium, especially with the variations characterizing the different races of humans. [cranio- + G. *logos*, study]

cra·ni·o·ma·la·cia (krā′nē-ō-mă-lā′shē-ă). Softening of the bones of the skull. [cranio- + G. *malakia*, softness]

circumscribed c., SYN craniotabes.

cra·ni·o·me·nin·go·cele (krā′nē-ō-mĕ-ning′gō-sēl). Protrusion of the meninges through a defect in the skull. [cranio- + G. *mēninx*, membrane, + *kēlē*, hernia]

cra·ni·om·e·ter (krā-nē-om′ĕ-ter). An instrument for measuring the diameters of the skull.

cra·ni·o·met·ric (krā-nē-ō-met′rik). Relating to craniometry.

cra·ni·om·e·try (krā-nē-om′ĕ-trē). Measurement of the dry skull after removal of the soft parts, and study of its topography. [cranio- + G. *metron*, measure]

cra·ni·op·a·gus (krā-nē-op′ă-gŭs). Conjoined twins with fused skulls. SEE conjoined *twins*, under *twin*. SEE ALSO janiceps, syncephalus. [cranio- + G. *pagos*, something fixed]

c. occipita′lis, conjoined twins united at the occipital region of the skull. SYN iniopagus.

c. parasit′icus, a variety of c. in which one fetus is rudimentary in form and parasitic on the other. SEE ALSO epicomus.

cra·ni·op·a·thy (krā-nē-op′ă-thē). Any pathologic condition of the cranial bones. [cranio- + G. *pathos*, suffering]

metabolic c., SYN Morgagni *syndrome*.

cra·ni·o·pha·ryn·ge·al (krā′nē-ō-fă-rin′jē-ăl). Relating to the skull and to the pharynx.

cra·ni·o·pha·ryn·gi·o·ma (krā′nē-ō-fă-rin-jē-ō′mă). A suprasellar neoplasm, which may be cystic, that develops from the nests of epithelium derived from Rathke pouch; the histologic pattern, similar to that observed in adamantinomas, consists of nesting of squamous epithelium bordered by radially arranged cells; frequently accompanied by calcium deposition; may occassionally have a papillary architecture microscopically. SYN Erdheim tumor, pituitary adamantinoma, pituitary ameloblastoma, Rathke pouch tumor, suprasellar cyst. [cranio- + pharyngio- + -oma]

ameloblastomatous c., a form of c. resembling an ameloblastoma.

cystic papillomatous c., a form of c. characterized by large cysts within which are fungating, irregular outgrowths of stratified squamous epithelium.

cra·ni·o·phore (krā′nē-ō-fōr). An apparatus for holding a skull while its angles and diameters are measured. [cranio- + G. *phoros*, bearing]

cra·ni·o·plas·ty (krā′nē-ō-plas-tē). An operation to correct a cranial defect, such as burring or onlay bone grafting or application of alloplastic material. [cranio- + G. *plastos*, formed]

cra·ni·o·punc·ture (krā′nē-ō-pŭnk′choor). Puncture of the brain for exploratory purposes.

cra·ni·or·rha·chid·i·an (krā′nē-ō-ră-kid′ē-an). SYN craniospinal. [cranio- + G. *rhachis*, spine]

cra·ni·or·rha·chis·chi·sis (krā′nē-ō-ră-kis′ki-sis). Severe congenital malformation in which there is incomplete closure of the skull and spinal column. [cranio- + G. *rhachis*, spine, + *schisis*, a cleaving]

cra·ni·o·sa·cral (krā′nē-ō-sā′krăl). Denoting the cranial and sacral origins of the parasympathetic division of the autonomic nervous system.

cra·ni·os·chi·sis (krā-nē-os′ki-sis). Congenital malformation in which there is incomplete closure of the skull. Usually accompanied by grossly defective development of the brain. [cranio- + G. *schisis*, a cleavage]

cra·ni·o·scle·ro·sis (krā′nē-ō-skler-ō′sis). Thickening of the skull. [cranio- + G. *sklēros*, hard, + *-osis*, condition]

cra·ni·os·co·py (krā-nē-os′kŏ-pē). Examination of the skull in the living subject for craniometric or diagnostic purposes. [cranio- + G. *skopeō*, to view]

cra·ni·o·spi·nal (krā′nē-ō-spī′năl). Relating to the cranium and spinal column. SYN craniorrhachidian.

cra·ni·o·ste·no·sis (krā′nē-ō-sten-ō′sis). Premature closure of cranial sutures resulting in malformation of the skull. [cranio- + G. *stenōsis*, a narrowing]

cra·ni·os·to·sis (krā′nē-os-tō′sis). SYN craniosynostosis. [cranio- + G. *osteon*, a bone, + *-osis*, condition]

cra·ni·o·syn·os·to·sis (krā′nē-ō-sin′os-tō′sis). Premature ossification of the skull and obliteration of the sutures. The particular sutures involved determine the resultant shape of the malformed head. SYN craniostosis.

cra·ni·o·tabes (krā′nē-ō-tā′bēz). A disease marked by the presence of areas of thinning and softening in the bones of the skull and widening of the sutures and fontanelles. Usually of syphilitic or rachitic origin. SYN circumscribed craniomalacia. [cranio- + L. *tabes*, a wasting]

cra·ni·o·tome (krā′nē-ō-tōm). Instrument formerly used for perforation and crushing of the fetal skull.

cra·ni·ot·o·my (krā-nē-ot′ō-mē). **1.** Opening into the skull. **2.** Formerly used operation for perforation of the head of the fetus, removal of the contents, and compression of the empty skull, when delivery by natural means is impossible. [cranio- + G. *tomē*, incision]

attached c., c. with a segment of the calvaria and attached soft tissues turned as a flap to expose the cranial cavity. SYN attached cranial section, osteoplastic c.

detached c., c. with section of cranium separated from its soft tissue attachments. SYN detached cranial section.

osteoplastic c., SYN attached c.

cra·ni·o·to·nos·co·py (krā′nē-ō-tō-nos′kŏ-pē). Auscultatory percussion of the cranium. [cranio- + G. *tonos*, tone, + *skopeō*, to examine]

cra·ni·o·try·pe·sis (krā′nē-ō-tri-pē′sis). Trephining of the skull. [cranio- + G. *trypēsis*, a boring]

cra·ni·o·tym·pan·ic (krā′nē-ō-tim-pan′ik). Relating to the skull and the middle ear.

cra·ni·um, pl. **cra·nia** (krā′nē-ŭm, -ă) [TA]. The bones of the head collectively. In a more limited sense, the neurocranium, the bony brain case containing the brain, excluding the bones of the face (viscerocranium). SYN skull. [Mediev. L. fr. G. *kranion*]

c. bif′idum, bifid c., SYN encephalocele.

c. cerebra′le, cerebral c., SYN neurocranium.

c. viscera′le, visceral c., SYN viscerocranium.

crap·u·lent, crap·u·lous (krap′ū-lent, -lŭs). Rarely used term for drunken; due to alcoholic intoxication. [L. *crapula*, drunkenness]

crash cart. A movable collection of emergency equipment and supplies meant to be readily available for resuscitative effort. It includes medication as well as the equipment for defibrillation, intubation, intravenous medication, and passage of central lines.

cras·sa·men·tum (kras-ă-men′tŭm). **1.** Old term for blood *clot*. **2.** Old term for coagulum. [L. thickness, fr. *crassus*, thick]

cra·ter (krā′ter). The most depressed, usually central portion of an ulcer.

cra·ter·i·form (krā-ter′i-fōrm). Hollowed like a bowl or a saucer. [L. *crater,* bowl, + *forma,* shape]

cra·ter·i·za·tion (krā-ter-ī-zā′shŭn). SYN saucerization.

craw-craw (kraw′kraw). A term applied in west Africa to a pruritic papular skin eruption, which may lead to ulceration; some cases are caused by *Onchocerca.*

Crawford, Brian H., British physicist, *1906. SEE Stiles-C. *effect.*

craz·ing (krā′zing). In dentistry, the appearance of minute cracks on the surface of plastic restorations such as filling materials, denture teeth, or denture bases.

cream (krēm). **1.** The upper fatty layer that forms in milk on standing or which is separated from it by centrifugalization; it contains about the same amount of sugar and protein as milk, but from 12 to 40% more fat. **2.** Any whitish viscid fluid resembling c. **3.** A semisolid emulsion of either the oil-in-water or the water-in-oil type, ordinarily intended for topical use. [L. *cremor,* thick juice, broth]

cleansing c., a form of cold c. used to remove grime and cosmetics from the skin.

cold c., a water-in-oil emulsion of various oils, waxes, and water; the standard formula, rose water ointment, contains expressed almond oil, rose water, spermaceti, white paraffin wax, and sodium borate; used as a cleansing or lubricating c.

greaseless c., SYN vanishing c.

leukocyte c., SYN buffy *coat.*

lubricating c., a form of cold c. used as a massage c. or night c.; it contains lanolin or its derivatives.

vanishing c., an oil-in-water emulsion containing potassium, ammonium, or sodium stearate with water and holding in emulsified form more or less free stearic acid; it also contains a hygroscopic ingredient such as glycerol, and a small amount of a fatty ingredient; it leaves a protective, invisible film of stearic acid on the skin. SYN greaseless c.

crease (krēs). A line or linear depression as produced by a fold. SEE ALSO fold, groove, line.

digital c., one of the grooves on the palmar surface of a finger, at the level of an interphalangeal joint. SYN digital flexion c., digital furrow.

digital flexion c., SYN digital c.

ear lobe c., a diagonal c. found on one or both earlobes with a possible connection to coronary heart disease in males.

flexion c., a permanent c. in the skin on the flexor aspect of a movable joint.

palmar c., any of the several flexion c.'s normally found on the palm of the hand, occurring proximal to, but as a consequence of flexion at, the metacarpophalangeal joints.

simian c., a single transverse palmar c. formed by fusion of the proximal and distal palmar c.'s, so called because of its similarity to the transverse flexion crease seen in some monkeys; a common but not pathognomonic feature of Down syndrome; also found in 1% of the normal population.

Sydney c., a variation of the proximal transverse palmar flexion c. that reaches the ulnar side of the palm; associated with acute lymphocytic anemia in early childhood, rubella embryopathy, and Down syndrome. SYN Sydney line.

cre·a·ti·nase (krē′ă-tĭ-nās). An enzyme catalyzing the hydrolysis of creatine to sarcosine and urea.

cre·a·tine (krē′ă-tēn, -tin). *N*-(Aminoiminomethyl)-*N*-methylglycine; occurs in urine, sometimes as such, but generally as creatinine, and in muscle, generally as phosphocreatine. Elevated in urine in individuals with muscular dystrophy.

c. kinase (CK), an enzyme catalyzing the reversible transfer of phosphate from phosphocreatine to ADP, forming creatine and ATP; of importance in muscle contraction. Certain isozymes are elevated in plasma following myocardial infarctions. SYN c. phosphokinase.

c. phosphate, SYN phosphocreatine.

c. phosphokinase (CPK), SYN c. kinase.

cre·a·ti·ne·mia (krē′ă-ti-nē′mē-ă). The presence of abnormal concentrations of creatine in peripheral blood. [creatine + G. *haima,* blood]

cre·at·i·nin·ase (krē-at′i-nin-ās). An amidohydrolase catalyzing the conversion of creatine to creatinine.

cre·at·i·nine (Cr) (krē-at′i-nēn, -nin). A component of urine and the final product of creatine catabolism; formed by the nonenzymatic dephosphorylative cyclization of phosphocreatine to form the internal anhydride of creatine.

cre·a·tin·u·ria (krē′ă-ti-noo′rē-ă). The urinary excretion of increased amounts of creatine. [creatine + G. *ouron,* urine]

Credé, Karl S.F., German obstetrician and gynecologist, 1819–1892. SEE C. *methods,* under *method.*

credentialing (krĭ-den′shal-ing). A formal review of the qualifications of a provider who has applied to participate in a health care system or plan. [*credential,* proof of authenticity, fr. Med. L. *credentialis,* fr. *credo,* to believe, + -ing]

creep (krēp). Any time-dependent strain developing in a material or an object in response to the application of a force or stress.

cre·mas·ter (krē-mas′ter). SEE cremasteric *fascia,* cremaster *muscle.* [G. *kremastēr,* a suspender, in pl. the muscles by which the testicles are retracted, fr. *kremannymi,* to hang]

crem·as·ter·ic (krēm-as-ter′ik). Relating to the cremaster.

crem·no·cele (krem′nō-sēl). A protrusion of intestine into the labium majus. [G. *krēmnos,* overhanging cliff, labium pudendi, + *kēlē,* hernia]

crem·no·pho·bia (krem-nō-fō′bē-ă). Morbid fear of precipices or steep places. [G. *krēmnos,* precipice, + *phobos,* fear]

cre·na, pl. **cre·nae** (krē′nă, krē′nē). A V-shaped cut or the space created by such a cut; one of the notches into which the opposing projections fit in the cranial sutures. [L. a notch]

c. analis [TA], SYN intergluteal *cleft.*

c. a′ni, ✱ official alternate term for intergluteal *cleft.*

c. clu′nium, SYN intergluteal *cleft.*

c. cor′dis, (1) SYN anterior interventricular *sulcus;* **(2)** SYN posterior interventricular *sulcus.*

c. interglutealis, ✱ official alternate term for intergluteal *cleft.*

cre·nate, cre·nat·ed (krē′nāt, -nā-ted). Indented; denoting the outline of a shriveled red blood cell, as observed in a hypertonic solution. [L. *crena,* a notch]

cre·na·tion (krē-nā′shŭn). The process of becoming, or state of being, crenated.

cre·no·cyte (krē′nō-sīt). A red blood cell with serrated, notched edges. [L. *crena,* a notch, + G. *kytos,* a hollow (cell)]

cre·no·cy·to·sis (krē′nō-sī-tō′sis). The presence of crenocytes in the blood. [crenocyte + G. *-osis,* condition]

Cren·o·so·ma vul·pis (krē′nō-sō-mă vŭl′pis). A metastrongyle lungworm species of the fox, wolf, dog, raccoon, and other small carnivores in Europe, Asia, and North America; it occurs in the bronchi, causing bronchitis. [G. *krēnē,* a (mineral) spring, + *sōma,* body; L. *vulpes,* fox]

cre·oph·a·gy, cre·oph·a·gism (krē-of′ă-jē, krē-of′ă-jizm). Carnivorousness; flesh-eating. [G. *kreas,* flesh, + *phagō,* to eat]

cre·o·sol (krē′ō-sol). A slightly yellowish aromatic liquid distilled from guaiac or from beechwood tar; a constituent of creosote. Cf. cresol.

cre·o·sote (krē′ō-sōt). A mixture of phenols (chiefly methyl guaiacol, guaiacol, and creosol) obtained during the distillation of wood-tar, preferably that derived from beechwood; used as a disinfectant and wood preservative. [G. *kreas,* flesh, + *sōtēr,* preserver]

crep·i·tant (krep′i-tant). **1.** Relating to or characterized by crepitation. **2.** Denoting a fine bubbling noise (rale) produced by air entering fluid in lung tissue; heard in pneumonia and in certain other conditions. **3.** The sensation imparted to the palpating finger by gas or air in the subcutaneous tissues.

crep·i·ta·tion (krep-i-tā′shŭn). **1.** Crackling; the quality of a fine bubbling sound (rale) that resembles noise heard on rubbing hair between the fingers. **2.** The sensation felt on placing the hand over the seat of a fracture when the broken ends of the bone are moved, or over tissue, in which gas gangrene is present. SYN bony crepitus. **3.** Noise or vibration produced by rubbing bone or irregular degenerated cartilage surfaces together as in arthritis and other conditions. SYN crepitus (1). [see crepitus]

crep·i·tus (krep′i-tŭs). **1.** SYN crepitation. **2.** A noisy discharge of gas from the intestine. [L. fr. *crepo*, to rattle]

articular c., the grating of a joint, often in association with osteoarthritis.

bony c., SYN crepitation (2).

cres·cent (kres′ent). **1.** Any figure of the shape of the moon in its first quarter. **2.** The figure made by the gray columns or cornua on cross-section of the spinal cord. **3.** SYN malarial c. [L. *cresco*, pp. *cretus*, to grow]

articular c., SYN meniscus *lens*.

Giannuzzi c.'s, SYN serous *demilunes*, under *demilune*.

glomerular c., proliferated epithelial cells partly encircling a renal glomerulus; it occurs in glomerulonephritis.

Heidenhain c.'s, SYN serous *demilunes*, under *demilune*.

malarial c., the male or female gametocyte(s) of *Plasmodium falciparum*, whose presence in human red blood cells is diagnostic of falciparum malaria. SYN crescent (3), sickle form.

myopic c., a white or grayish white crescentic area in the fundus of the eye located on the temporal side of the optic disk; caused by atrophy of the choroid, permitting the sclera to become visible. SYN myopic conus.

sublingual c., the crescent-shaped area on the floor of the mouth formed by the lingual wall of the mandible and the adjacent part of the floor of the mouth.

cres·cen·tic (kres-sen′tik). Shaped like a crescent.

cres·co·graph (kres′kō-graf). A device for recording the degree and rate of growth. [L. *cresco*, to grow, + G. *graphō*, to draw or write]

cre·sol (krē′sol). A mixture of the three isomeric cresols, *o*-, *m*-, and *p*-cresol, obtained from coal tar. Its properties are similar to those of phenol, but it is less poisonous; used as an antiseptic and disinfectant. SYN tricresol.

m-cre·sol. A local antiseptic with a higher germicidal power than phenol and less toxicity to tissues; used in disinfectants and fumigants; its acetate derivative is used as a topical antiseptic and fungicide. SYN metacresol.

cre·so·lase (krē′sō-lās). SYN monophenol monooxygenase (1).

cre·sol red. An acid-base indicator with a pK value of 8.3; yellow at pH values below 7.4, red above 9.0.

CREST Acronym for *c*alcinosis, *R*aynaud phenomenon, *e*sophageal motility disorders, *s*clerodactyly, and *t*elangiectasia. SEE CREST *syndrome*.

CREST

---

crest (krest) [TA]. **1.** A ridge, especially a bony ridge. SEE ALSO crista. **2.** The ridge of the neck of a male animal, especially of a stallion or bull. **3.** Feathers on the top of a bird's head, or fin rays on the top of a fish's head. SYN crista [TA]. [L. *crista*]

acoustic c., SYN ampullary c.

alveolar c., **(1)** the portion of the alveolar bone extending beyond the periphery of the socket, lying interproximally; **(2)** the top of the residual alveolar bone.

c. of alveolar ridge, the top of the alveolar ridge or residual ridge; the highest continuous surface of the ridge, but not necessarily the center of the ridge.

ampullary c. [TA], an elevation on the inner surface of the ampulla of each semicircular duct; filaments of the vestibular nerve pass through the c. to reach hair cells on its surface; the hair cells are capped by the cupula, a gelatinous protein-polysaccharide mass. SEE ALSO *neuroepithelium* of ampullary crest. SYN crista ampullaris [TA], acoustic c., transverse septum (1).

ampullary c. (of semicircular ducts) [TA], crescentic ridge invaginating the lumen of the ampullae of the semicircular ducts

bearing sensory epithelium on a base of nerve fibers and connective tissue. SYN crista ampullaris (ductuum semicircularium) [TA].

anterior lacrimal c. [TA], a vertical ridge on the lateral surface of the frontal process of the maxilla that forms part of the medial rim of the orbit. SYN crista lacrimalis anterior [TA].

arched c., SYN arcuate c. of arytenoid cartilage.

arcuate c., SYN arcuate c. of arytenoid cartilage.

arcuate c. of arytenoid cartilage [TA], the ridge on the anterior surface of the arytenoid cartilage that separates the triangular from the oblong fovea. SYN crista arcuata cartilaginis arytenoideae [TA], arched c., arcuate c.

articular c., SYN intermediate sacral c.

basal c. of cochlear duct [TA], sharp extension of the central portion of the spiral ligament that continues as the basilar membrane. SYN crista basalaris ductus cochlearis [TA], crista spiralis ductus cochlearis☆, spiral c. of cochlear duct☆.

basilar c. of cochlear duct, an inward projection of the spiral ligament of the cochlea to which is attached the basilar membrane forming the floor of the cochlear duct. SYN crista basilaris ductus cochlearis [TA].

c. of body of rib [TA], the sharp inferior margin of the shaft of a rib. SYN crista corporis costae [TA].

buccinator c., a ridge passing from the base of the coronoid process of the mandible to the region of the last molar tooth; it gives attachment to the mandibular part of the buccinator muscle. SYN crista buccinatoria.

c. of cochlear opening, SYN c. of round window.

conchal c. [TA], bony ridge that articulates with, or provides attachment for, the inferior nasal concha. SEE conchal c. of body of maxilla, conchal c. of palatine bone. SYN crista conchalis [TA], turbinated c.

conchal c. of body of maxilla [TA], ridge of the nasal surface of the body of the maxilla that articulates with the inferior nasal concha. SYN crista conchalis corporis maxillae [TA].

conchal c. of palatine bone [TA], the ridge on the nasal surface of the perpendicular part of the palatine bone to which the inferior nasal concha attaches. SYN crista conchalis ossis palatini [TA].

deltoid c., SYN deltoid *tuberosity* (of humerus).

dental c., the maxillary ridge on the aleveolar processes of the maxillary bones in the fetus. SYN crista dentalis.

ethmoidal c. [TA], bony ridge which articulates with, or provides attachment for, any part of the ethmoid bone, especially the middle nasal concha. SEE ethmoidal c. of maxilla, ethmoidal c. of palatine bone. SYN crista ethmoidalis [TA].

ethmoidal c. of maxilla [TA], a ridge on the upper part of the nasal surface of the frontal process of the maxilla that gives attachment to the anterior portion of the middle nasal concha. SYN crista ethmoidalis maxillae [TA].

ethmoidal c. of palatine bone [TA], a ridge on the medial surface of the perpendicular part of the palatine bone to which the middle nasal concha attaches posteriorly. SYN crista ethmoidalis ossis palatini [TA].

external occipital c. [TA], a ridge extending from the external occipital protuberance to the border of the foramen magnum. SYN crista occipitalis externa [TA], linea nuchae mediana.

falciform c., SYN transverse c. of internal acoustic meatus.

c. of fenestrae cochleae, SYN c. of round window.

frontal c. [TA], a ridge arising at the termination of the sagittal sulcus on the cerebral surface of the frontal bone and ending at the foramen caecum. SYN crista frontalis [TA].

ganglionic c., SYN neural c.

gingival c., SYN gingival *margin*.

gluteal c., SYN gluteal *tuberosity*.

c. of greater tubercle [TA], the ridge below the greater tubercle of the humerus into which the pectoralis major muscle inserts. SYN crista tuberculi majoris [TA], bicipital ridges, pectoral ridge.

c. of head of rib [TA], the ridge that separates the superior and inferior articular surfaces of the head of a rib. SYN crista capitis costae [TA].

iliac c. [TA], the long, curved upper border of the wing of the ilium. SYN crista iliaca [TA].

incisor c., the front part of the nasal c. of the palatine process of the maxilla.

infratemporal c. of greater wing of sphenoid [TA], a rough ridge marking the angle of union of the temporal and infratemporal surfaces of the greater wing of the sphenoid bone. SYN crista infratemporalis alaris majoris ossis sphenoidalis [TA], pterygoid ridge of sphenoid bone.

inguinal c., an elevation in the body wall of the embryo at the internal opening of the inguinal canal; part of the gubernaculum testis develops within it.

intermediate sacral c. [TA], c.'s formed by the fusion of articular processes of all the sacral vertebrae. SYN crista sacralis medialis [TA], articular c., crista sacralis intermedia.

internal occipital c. [TA], a ridge running from the internal occipital protuberance to the posterior margin of the foramen magnum, giving attachment to the falx cerebelli. SYN crista occipitalis interna [TA].

interosseous c., SYN interosseous *border.*

intertrochanteric c. [TA], the rounded ridge that connects the greater and lesser trochanters of the femur posteriorly and marks the junction of the neck and shaft of the bone. SYN crista intertrochanterica [TA], trochanteric c.

interureteric c. [TA], a fold of mucous membrane extending from the orifice of the ureter of one side to that of the other side. SYN plica interureterica [TA], bar of bladder, interureteric fold, Mercier bar, plica ureterica, torus uretericus, ureteric fold.

lateral epicondylar c., SYN lateral supraepicondylar *ridge.*

lateral sacral c. [TA], c.'s which are rough ridges lying lateral to the sacral foramina; they represent the fused transverse processes of sacral vertebrae. SYN crista sacralis lateralis [TA].

lateral supracondylar c., SYN lateral supraepicondylar *ridge.*

c. of lesser tubercle [TA], the ridge below the lesser tubercle of the humerus into which the teres major muscle inserts. SYN crista tuberculi minoris [TA], bicipital ridges.

marginal c. of tooth [TA], the rounded borders that form the mesial and distal margins of the occlusal surface of a tooth. SYN crista marginalis dentis [TA], marginal ridge.

medial epicondylar c., SYN medial supraepicondylar *ridge.*

medial c. of fibula [TA], a ridge of bone, on the posterior surface of the fibula, separating the attachment of the posterior tibial muscle from that of the flexor hallucis longus and soleus muscles. SYN crista medialis fibulae [TA].

medial supracondylar c., SYN medial supraepicondylar *ridge.*

median sacral c. [TA], an unpaired c. formed by the fused spinous processes of the upper four sacral vertebrae. SYN crista sacralis mediana [TA].

c.'s of nail bed,

c.'s of nail matrix [TA], the numerous longitudinal ridges of the nail bed distal to the lunula. SYN cristae matricis unguis.

nasal c. [TA], the midline ridge in the floor of the nasal cavity, formed by the union of the paired maxillae and palatine bones; the vomer attaches to the crest. SYN crista nasalis [TA], semicrista incisiva.

nasal c. of horizontal plate of palatine bone [TA], superiorly (nasally) directed bony c., formed at the meeting of the horizontal processes of the right and left palatine bones, for attachment of the nasal septum. SYN crista nasalis laminae horizontalis ossis palatini [TA].

nasal c. of palatine process of maxilla [TA], superiorly (nasally) directed bony c., formed at the meeting of the palatine processes of the right and left maxillae, for attachment of the nasal septum. SYN crista nasalis processus palatini maxillae [TA].

c. of neck of rib [TA], the sharp upper margin of the neck of a rib. SYN crista colli costae [TA].

neural c., neuroectodermal cells that originate in the dorsal aspect of the neural folds or neural tube; these cells leave the neural tube or folds and differentiate into various cell types including dorsal-root ganglion cells, autonomic ganglion cells, the chromaffin cells of the adrenal medulla, Schwann cells, sensory ganglia cells of cranial nerves, 5, 9, and 10, part of the meninges, or integumentary pigment cells. SYN ganglion ridge, ganglionic c.

obturator c. [TA], a ridge that extends from the pubic tubercle to

the acetabular notch, giving attachment to the pubofemoral ligament of the hip joint. SYN crista obturatoria [TA].

c. of palatine bone, palatine c., SYN palatine c. of horizontal process of palatine bone.

palatine c. of horizontal process of palatine bone [TA], a transverse ridge near the posterior border of the bony palate, located on the inferior surface of the horizontal plate of the palatine bone. SYN crista palatina laminae horizontalis ossis palatini [TA], c. of palatine bone, palatine c., crista palatina.

c. of petrous part of temporal bone, SYN superior *border* of petrous part of temporal bone.

c. of petrous temporal bone, SYN superior *border* of petrous part of temporal bone.

posterior lacrimal c. [TA], a vertical ridge on the orbital surface of the lacrimal bone that, together with the anterior lacrimal crest, bounds the fossa for the lacrimal sac. SYN crista lacrimalis posterior [TA].

pubic c. [TA], the rough anterior border of the body of the pubis, continuous laterally with the pubic tubercle. SYN crista pubica [TA].

c. of round window [TA], the edge of the opening of the cochlear window to which the secondary tympanic membrane is attached. SYN crista fenestrae cochleae [TA], c. of cochlear opening, c. of fenestrae cochleae.

sacral c. [TA], one of three rough irregular ridges on the posterior surface of the sacrum; median sacral c.; lateral sacral c.'s. SYN crista sacralis [TA].

sagittal c., a prominent ridge along the sagittal suture of the skull, present in some animals as a result of temporal muscle development.

c. of scapular spine, the posterior subcutaneous border of the spine of the scapula that expands in its medial part into a smooth triangular area.

sphenoidal c. [TA], a vertical ridge in the midline of the anterior surface of the sphenoid bone that articulates with the perpendicular plate of the ethmoid bone. SYN crista sphenoidalis [TA].

spiral c., SYN spiral *ligament* of cochlear duct.

spiral c. of cochlear duct, ✩official alternate term for basal c. of cochlear duct.

c. of supinator muscle, SYN supinator c. (of ulna).

supinator c. (of ulna) [TA], the proximal part of the interosseous border of the ulna from which a portion of the supinator muscle takes origin. SYN crista musculi supinatoris ulnae [TA], c. of supinator muscle.

supramastoid c. [TA], the ridge that forms the posterior root of the zygomatic process of the temporal bone. SYN crista supramastoidea [TA].

suprastyloid c. of radius [TA], lateral border of the distal radius leading to the styloid process; site of insertion of the brachioradialis muscle. SYN crista suprastyloidea radii [TA].

supraventricular c. [TA], the internal muscular ridge that separates the conus arteriosus from the remaining part of the cavity of the right ventricle of the heart. SYN crista supraventricularis [TA].

temporal c. of mandible [TA], ridge along anteromedial aspect of the coronoid process and upper ramus of the mandible into which the temporalis muscle inserts. SYN crista temporalis mandibulae [TA].

terminal c., SYN *crista* terminalis of right atrium.

tibial c., SYN anterior *border* of tibia.

transverse c., (1) SYN transverse c. of internal acoustic meatus; (2) SYN *crista* transversalis.

transverse c. of internal acoustic meatus [TA], a horizontal ridge that divides the fundus of the internal acoustic meatus into a superior and an inferior area. In the former are the introitus of the facial canal and openings for the branches of the vestibular nerve to the utricle and to the ampullae of the anterior and lateral semicircular canals. In the latter are openings for the cochlear nerve, and for branches of the vestibular nerve to the saccule and to the ampulla of the posterior semicircular canal. SYN crista transversa meatus acustici interni [TA], falciform c., transverse c. (1).

triangular c., SYN *crista* triangularis.

trigeminal c., that part of the cranial neural c. from which part of the ganglion of the fifth cranial nerve develops.

trochanteric c., SYN intertrochanteric c.

turbinated c., SYN conchal c.

urethral c. [TA], longitudinal mucosal fold in the dorsal wall of the urethra. SEE urethral c. of female, urethral c. of male. SYN crista urethralis [TA].

urethral c. of female [TA], a conspicuous longitudinal fold of mucosa on the posterior wall of the urethra. SYN crista urethralis femininae [TA].

urethral c. of male [TA], a longitudinal fold on the posterior wall of the urethra extending from the uvula of the bladder through the prostatic urethra; prominent in its midportion is the seminal colliculus. SYN crista urethralis masculinae [TA], crista phallica.

vertical c. of internal acoustic meatus [TA], bony ridge of the fundus of the internal acoustic meatus separating the superior vestibular area from the facial area above the more prominent transverse c., and the inferior vestibular area from the cochlear area below the transverse c. SYN crista verticalis meatus acustici interni [TA].

vestibular c. [TA], an oblique ridge on the inner wall of the vestibule of the labyrinth, bounding the spherical recess above and posteriorly. SYN crista vestibuli [TA], c. of vestibule.

c. of vestibule, SYN vestibular c.

vomerine c. of choana [TA], the concave posterior border of the vomer and overlying respiratory epithelium that forms the medial boundary of and separates the right and left choanae. SYN crista choanalis vomeris [TA].

---

cres·ta (kres'tă). A small membranous organelle characteristic of certain flagellate protozoa, located near the pelta and seen in the living organism as an independently moving structure. [L. *crispus*, trembling]

cres·yl·ate (kres'i-lāt). A salt of cresylic acid, or cresol.

cres·yl blue, cres·yl blue bril·liant (kres'il) [C.I. 51010]. A basic oxazin dye used for staining the reticulum in young erythrocytes (reticulocytes); also used in vital staining and as a selective stain for gastric surface epithelial mucin and other acid mucopolysaccharides.

cres·yl echt, cres·yl fast vi·o·let. A metachromatic basic oxazin dye, closely related to cresyl violet acetate and used for the same purposes.

cres·yl vi·o·let ac·e·tate. A metachromatic basic oxazin dye, used as a stain for nuclei and Nissl substance; related to German derived dye known as cresyl echt violet or cresyl fast violet.

cre·ta (krē'tă). SYN *calcium* carbonate. [L. orig. adj. fr. *Creta*, Crete, *i.e.* Cretan earth, chalk]

cre·tin (krē'tin). An individual exhibiting cretinism. [Fr. *crétin*]

cre·tin·ism (krē'tin-izm). Obsolete term for congenital *hypothyroidism.* SEE infantile *hypothyroidism.*

cre·tin·is·tic (krē'tin-is-tik). SYN cretinous.

cre·tin·oid (krē'tin-oyd). Resembling a cretin; presenting symptoms similar to those of cretinism.

cre·tin·ous (krē'tin-ŭs). Relating to cretinism or a cretin; affected with cretinism. SYN cretinistic.

Creutzfeldt, Hans Gerhard, German neuropsychiatrist, 1885–1964. SEE Creutzfeldt-Jakob *disease.*

crev·ice (krev'is). A crack or small fissure, especially in a solid substance. [Fr. *crevasse*]

    gingival c., SYN gingival *sulcus.*

cre·vic·u·lar (krĕ-vik'ū-lăr). 1. Relating to any crevice. 2. In dentistry, relating especially to the gingival crevice or sulcus.

CRF Abbreviation for corticotropin-releasing *factor.*

CRH Abbreviation for corticotropin-releasing *hormone.*

cri·bra (krī'bră, krib'ră). Plural of cribrum.

crib·rate (krib'rāt). SYN cribriform.

cri·bra·tion (kri-brā'shŭn). 1. Sifting; passing through a sieve. 2. The condition of being cribrate or numerously pitted or punctured.

crib·ri·form (krib'ri-fōrm) [TA]. Sievelike; containing many perforations. SYN cribrate, polyporous. [L. *cribrum*, a sieve, + *forma*, form]

cri·brum, pl. **cri·bra** (krī'brŭm, krib'rŭm; -bră, -ra). SYN cribriform *plate* of ethmoid bone. [L. a sieve]

Cri·cet·i·nae (krī-sē'ti-nē). A subfamily of rodents (family Muridae) that includes hamsters and native American rats.

Cri·ce·tu·lus (kri-sē'tū-lŭs). One of four genera of hamsters; *C. griseus*, the striped hamster native to Europe and Asia, is a reservoir for visceral leishmaniasis.

Cri·ce·tus (kri-sē'tŭs). One of four genera of hamsters; *C. cricetus* is used extensively as a research animal.

Crick, Francis H.C., British biochemist and Nobel laureate, *1916. SEE Watson-C. *helix.*

cri·co·ar·y·te·noid (krī'kō-ar-i-tē'noyd). Relating to the cricoid and arytenoid cartilages.

cri·co·ar·y·te·noi·de·us (krī'kō-ar-i-te-noy'dē-ŭs). SEE lateral cricoarytenoid (*muscle*), posterior cricoarytenoid (*muscle*).

cri·coid (krī'koyd). Ring-shaped; denoting the cricoid cartilage. [L. *cricoideus*, fr. G. *krikos*, a ring, + *eidos*, form]

cri·coi·dyn·ia (krī'koy-din'ē-ă). Pain in the cricoid. [cricoid + G. *odynē*, pain]

cri·co·pha·ryn·ge·al (krī'kō-fă-rin'jē-ăl). Relating to the cricoid cartilage and the pharynx; a part of the inferior constrictor muscle of the pharynx. SEE inferior constrictor (*muscle*) of pharynx.

cri·co·thy·roid (krī-kō-thī'royd). Relating to the cricoid and thyroid cartilages.

cri·co·thy·roi·de·us (krī'kō-thī-roy'dē-ŭs). SEE cricothyroid *muscle.*

cri·co·thy·roi·dot·o·my (krī'kō-thī-roy-dot'ō-mē). SYN cricothyrotomy.

cri·co·thy·rot·o·my (krī'kō-thī-rot'ō-mē). Incision through the skin and cricothyroid membrane for relief of respiratory obstruction; used prior to or in place of tracheotomy in certain emergency respiratory obstructions. SEE ALSO coniotomy. SYN cricothyroidotomy, inferior laryngotomy, intercricothyrotomy. [cricoid + thyroid + G. *tomē*, incision]

cri·cot·o·my (krī-kot'ō-mē). Division of the cricoid cartilage, as in cricoid split, to enlarge the subglottic airway. [cricoid + G. *tomē*, incision]

Crigler, John F., U.S. physician, *1919. SEE C.-Najjar *disease*, *syndrome.*

Crile, George W., U.S. surgeon, 1864–1943. SEE C. *clamp.*

crim·i·nol·o·gy (krim-i-nol'ō-jē). The branch of science concerned with the physical and mental characteristics and behavior of criminals. [L. *crimen*, crime, + G. *logos*, study]

crin·in (krin'in). Old term for a substance that will stimulate the production of secretions by specific glands. [G. *krinō*, to secrete, + -in]

crin·o·gen·ic (krin-ō-jen'ik). Causing secretion; stimulating a gland to increased function. [G. *krinō*, to separate, + -gen, to produce]

crin·oph·a·gy (krin-of'ă-jē). Disposal of excess secretory granules by lysosomes.

crip·pled (krip'ld). Denoting a person who, owing to a physical defect or injury, is partially or completely disabled. [A.S. *creopan*, to creep]

cri·sis, pl. **cri·ses** (krī'sis, -sēz). 1. A sudden change, usually for the better, in the course of an acute disease, in contrast to the gradual improvement by lysis. 2. A paroxysmal pain in an organ or circumscribed region of the body occurring in the course of tabetic neurosyphilis. SYN tabetic c. 3. A convulsive attack. [G. *krisis*, a separation, crisis]

    addisonian c., SYN acute adrenocortical *insufficiency.*

    adolescent c., the emotional turmoil often accompanying adolescence.

    adrenal c., SYN acute adrenocortical *insufficiency.*

    anaphylactoid c., (1) SYN anaphylactoid *shock*; (2) SYN pseudoanaphylaxis.

    blast c., a sudden alteration in the status of a patient with leukemia in which the peripheral blood cells are almost exclusively blast cells of the type characteristic of leukemia; usually accompanied by a decrease in numbers of other formed elements of the blood, fever, and rapid clinical deterioration.

blood c., **(1)** the appearance of a large number of nucleated red blood cells in the peripheral blood, accompanied by reticulocytosis and occurring in "exhausted" bone marrow in pernicious anemia and in hemolytic icterus; **(2)** a suddenly appearing leukocytosis, indicating a change for the better in the course of a grave blood disease.

Dietl c., intermittent pain, sometimes with nausea and emesis, caused by intermittent proximal obstruction of ureter. Originally believed due to a mobile kidney that caused ureter to kink with positional changes. SYN incarceration symptom.

febrile c., the stage in a febrile disease when spontaneous defervescence occurs.

gastric c., an attack, usually lasting several days, with severe pain in the abdomen or around the waist, accompanied by nausea and vomiting and occasionally diarrhea; occurs in tabetic neurosyphilis.

glaucomatocyclitic c., a form of monocular secondary open-angle glaucoma due to recurrent mild cyclitis.

hemolytic c., massive hemolysis with severe anemia associated with hemolytic disease such as sickle cell disease.

identity c., a disorientation concerning one's sense of self, values, and role in society, often of acute onset and related to a particular and significant event in one's life.

laryngeal c., an attack of paralysis of the abductor, or spasm of the adductor, muscles of the larynx with dyspnea and noisy respiration, occurring in tabetic neurosyphilis.

midlife c., a point in a sequence of events during the middle years of life at which certain trends of prior and subsequent events in one's life are pondered, generally involving an aggregate of personal, career, or sexual dissatisfactions.

myasthenic c., severe, life-threatening exacerbation of the manifestations of *myasthenia* gravis requiring intensive treatment.

myelocytic c., a temporary but conspicuous and sudden increase in cells of the myelocytic series in the circulating blood.

ocular c., sudden and severe pain in the eyes.

oculogyric crises, incapacitating attacks of upward eye rolling seen in encephalitis lethargica and with phenothiazine drugs.

otolithic c., a sudden drop attack without loss of consciousness, vertigo, auditory disturbances, or autonomic manifestations.

salt-depletion c., severe illness resulting from loss of sodium chloride, usually in urine (i.e., salt-losing nephritis), in sweat following severe exercise in hot weather, or in intestinal secretions, as in cholera. Can occur as result of Addison disease or Addisonian crisis; characterized by hypovolemia, hypotension.

sickle cell c., SEE sickle cell *anemia.*

tabetic c., SYN crisis (2).

therapeutic c., a turning point leading to positive or negative change in psychiatric treatment.

thyrotoxic c., thyroid c., the exacerbation of symptoms of hyperthyroidism; severe thyrotoxicosis; can follow shock or injury or thyroidectomy; marked by rapid pulse (140–170/minute), nausea, diarrhea, fever, loss of weight, extreme nervousness, and a sudden rise in the metabolic rate; coma and death may occur; occasionally the entire clinical picture is that of profound prostration, weakness, and collapse, without the phase of muscular overactivity and tachycardia. SYN thyroid storm.

vasoocclusive c., SYN sickle cell *anemia.*

visceral crises, attacks of severe, spreading epigastric pain that occur in patients with tabetic neurosyphilis.

cris·pa·tion (kris-pā'shŭn). **1.** A "creepy" sensation due to slight, fibrillary muscular contractions. **2.** Retraction of a divided artery or of muscular fibers or other tissues when cut across. [L. *crispo,* pp. -*atus,* to curl]

CRISTA

cris·ta, pl. **cris·tae** (kris'tă, -tē) [TA]. SYN crest. [L. crest]
c. ampulla′ris [TA], SYN ampullary *crest.*
c. ampullaris (ductuum semicircularium) [TA], SYN ampullary *crest* (of semicircular ducts).
c. arcua′ta cartila′ginis arytenoi′deae [TA], SYN arcuate *crest* of arytenoid cartilage.
c. basalaris ductus cochlearis [TA], SYN basal *crest* of cochlear duct.
c. basila′ris duc′tus cochlea′ris [TA], SYN basilar *crest* of cochlear duct.
c. buccinator′ia, SYN buccinator *crest.*
c. cap′itis cos′tae [TA], SYN *crest* of head of rib.
c. choanalis vomeris [TA], SYN vomerine *crest* of choana.
c. col′li cos′tae [TA], SYN *crest* of neck of rib.
c. concha′lis [TA], SYN conchal *crest.*
c. concha′lis corporis maxil′lae [TA], SYN conchal *crest* of body of maxilla.
c. concha′lis os′sis palati′ni [TA], SYN conchal *crest* of palatine bone.
c. corporis costae [TA], SYN *crest* of body of rib.
cris′tae cu′tis [TA], SYN dermal *ridges,* under *ridge.*
c. denta′lis, SYN dental *crest.*
c. div′idens, the lower free edge of the septum secundum, forming the upper margin of the fetal foramen ovale; the limbus of the foramen ovale.
c. ethmoida′lis [TA], SYN ethmoidal *crest.*
c. ethmoida′lis maxil′lae [TA], SYN ethmoidal *crest* of maxilla.
c. ethmoida′lis os′sis palati′ni [TA], SYN ethmoidal *crest* of palatine bone.
c. fenes′trae coch′leae [TA], SYN *crest* of round window.
c. fronta′lis [TA], SYN frontal *crest.*
c. gal′li [TA], the triangular midline process of the ethmoid bone extending superiorly from the cribriform plate; it gives anterior attachment to the falx cerebri.
c. glu′tea, SYN gluteal *tuberosity.*
c. hel′icis, SYN *crus* of helix.
c. ili′aca [TA], SYN iliac *crest.*
c. infratempora′lis alaris majoris ossis sphenoidalis [TA], SYN infratemporal *crest* of greater wing of sphenoid.
c. intertrochanter′ica [TA], SYN intertrochanteric *crest.*
c. lacrima′lis ante′rior [TA], SYN anterior lacrimal *crest.*
c. lacrima′lis poste′rior [TA], SYN posterior lacrimal *crest.*
c. margina′lis dentis [TA], SYN marginal *crest* of tooth.
cris′tae ma′tricis un′guis, SYN *crests* of nail matrix, under *crest.*
c. media′lis fi′bulae [TA], SYN medial *crest* of fibula.
cristae of mitochondria, cris′tae mitochondria′les, shelflike infoldings of the inner membrane of a mitochondrion.
c. mus′culi supinato′ris ulnae [TA], SYN supinator *crest* (of ulna).
c. nasa′lis [TA], SYN nasal *crest.*
c. nasalis laminae horizontalis ossis palatini [TA], SYN nasal *crest* of horizontal plate of palatine bone.
c. nasalis processus palatini maxillae [TA], SYN nasal *crest* of palatine process of maxilla.
c. obturato′ria [TA], SYN obturator *crest.*
c. occipita′lis exter′na [TA], SYN external occipital *crest.*
c. occipita′lis inter′na [TA], SYN internal occipital *crest.*
c. palati′na, SYN palatine *crest* of horizontal process of palatine bone.
c. palatina laminae horizontalis ossis palatini [TA], SYN palatine *crest* of horizontal process of palatine bone.
c. phal′lica, SYN urethral *crest* of male.
c. pu′bica [TA], SYN pubic *crest.*

cr

c. quar'ta, a ridge that projects into the posterior end of the lateral semicircular duct of the labyrinth.

c. sacra'lis [TA], SYN sacral *crest*.

c. sacra'lis interme'dia, SYN intermediate sacral *crest*.

c. sacra'lis latera'lis [TA], SYN lateral sacral *crest*.

c. sacralis medialis [TA], SYN intermediate sacral *crest*.

c. sacra'lis median'a [TA], SYN median sacral *crest*.

c. sphenoida'lis [TA], SYN sphenoidal *crest*.

c. spira'lis, SYN spiral *ligament* of cochlear duct.

c. spiralis ductus cochlearis, ☆official alternate term for basal *crest* of cochlear duct.

c. supracondyla'ris latera'lis, ☆official alternate term for lateral supraepicondylar *ridge*.

c. supracondyla'ris media'lis, ☆official alternate term for medial supraepicondylar *ridge*.

c. supraepicondylaris lateralis [TA], SYN lateral supraepicondylar *ridge*.

c. supraepicondylaris medialis [TA], SYN medial supraepicondylar *ridge*.

c. supramastoi'dea [TA], SYN supramastoid *crest*.

c. suprastyloidea radii [TA], SYN suprastyloid *crest* of radius.

c. supraventricula'ris [TA], SYN supraventricular *crest*.

c. temporalis mandibulae [TA], SYN temporal *crest* of mandible.

c. termina'lis, SYN c. terminalis of right atrium.

c. terminalis atrii dextri [TA], SYN c. terminalis of right atrium.

c. terminalis of right atrium [TA], a vertical crest on the interior wall of the right atrium that lies to the right of the sinus of the vena cava and separates this from the remainder of the right atrium. SYN c. terminalis atrii dextri [TA], c. terminalis, tenia terminalis, terminal crest.

c. transversa'lis [TA], a crest or ridge on the occlusal surface of a tooth formed by the union of two triangular crests. SYN transverse ridge [TA], transverse crest (2).

c. transver'sa meatus acustici interni [TA], SYN transverse *crest* of internal acoustic meatus.

c. triangula'ris [TA], a crest or ridge which extends from the apex of a cusp of a premolar or molar tooth toward the central part of the occlusal surface. SYN triangular ridge [TA], triangular crest.

c. tuber'culi majo'ris [TA], SYN *crest* of greater tubercle.

c. tuber'culi mino'ris [TA], SYN *crest* of lesser tubercle.

c. urethra'lis [TA], SYN urethral *crest*.

c. urethra'lis femini'nae [TA], SYN urethral *crest* of female.

c. urethra'lis masculi'nae [TA], SYN urethral *crest* of male.

c. verticalis meatus acustici interni [TA], SYN vertical *crest* of internal acoustic meatus.

c. vestib'uli [TA], SYN vestibular *crest*.

---

cri·te·ri·on, pl. **cri·te·ria** (krī-tēr'ē-on, -ē-ă). **1.** A standard or rule for judging; usually plural (criteria) denoting a set of standards or rules. **2.** In psychology, a standard such as school grades against which test scores on intelligence tests or other measured behaviors are validated. **3.** A list of manifestations of a disease or disorder, a certain number of which must be present to warrant diagnosis in a given patient. [G. *kritērion,* a standard]

Amsel criteria, c. for clinical diagnosis of bacterial vaginosis; the diagnosis is made if three of the following four c. are positive: homogeneous discharge, pH $\geq$ 4.8, presence of clue cells, and amine odor with the application of KOH to the discharge.

Hill's criteria of evidence, a set of epidemiologic criteria that help to indicate whether a statistically significant relationship obtained in epidemiologic and other studies is a causal relationship. The criteria are consistency, specificity, strength, dose-response relationship, temporality, biologic plausibility, coherence, and capability of experimental confirmation. Temporality is the only absolute c.: the putative cause must precede the effect in time.

Jones criteria, criteria (proposed by T.D. Jones in 1944 and modified in 1965) used to make the diagnosis of rheumatic fever. There are five major criteria: carditis, polyarthritis, chorea, ery-

thema marginatum, and subcutaneous nodules; minor criteria include fever, arthralgia, elevated erythrocyte sedimentation rate or C reactive protein, and prolonged PR interval on ECG. Diagnosis requires evidence of recent group A β-hemolytic streptococcal infection, plus two major and one minor criteria, or one major and two minor criteria; revised Jones criteria allow the diagnosis when indolent carditis or chorea exists with no other cause, or in patients with a previous history of rheumatic fever who have one major or two minor criteria in association with a recent streptococcal infection.

Spiegelberg criteria (for diagnosis of ovarian pregnancy), 1) the oviduct on the affected side must be intact; 2) the amnionic sac must occupy the position of the ovary; 3) the amnionic sac must be connected to the uterus by the ovarian ligament; and 4) ovarian tissue must be present in the wall of the amnionic sac.

Cri·thid·i·a (kri-thid'ē-ă). A genus of asexual, monogenetic, insect-parasitizing flagellates in the family Trypanosomatidae. [Mod. L., fr. G. *krithidion,* dim. of *krithē,* barley]

cri·thid·i·a (kri-thid'ē-ă). Former term for epimastigote. [Mod. L. fr. G. *krithidion,* dim. of *krithē,* barley]

crit·i·cal (krit-i-kăl). **1.** Denoting or of the nature of a crisis. **2.** Denoting a morbid condition in which death is possible. **3.** In sufficient quantity as to constitute a turning point.

CRL Abbreviation for crown-rump *length*.

CRM Abbreviation for certified reference *material*.

CRM Abbreviation for cross-reacting *material*.

C.R.N.A. Abbreviation for certified registered *nurse* anesthetist.

cRNA Abbreviation for complementary ribonucleic acid.

CRO Abbreviation for cathode ray *oscilloscope*.

Crocq, Jean, Belgian physician, 1868–1925. SEE C. *disease*.

cro·cus (krō'kŭs). The dried stigmas of *Crocus sativus* (*C. officinalis*) (family Iridaceae), formerly used occasionally in flatulent dyspepsia; also formerly used as an antispasmodic in asthma and dysmenorrhea and as a coloring and flavoring agent. SYN saffron. [L. fr. G. *krokos,* the crocus, saffron (made from its stigmas)]

Crohn, Burrill B., U.S. gastroenterologist, 1884–1983. SEE C. *disease*.

cro·mo·lyn so·di·um (krō'mō-lin). Used for the prevention of asthmatic attack. Stabilizes mast cell membranes to prevent the release of leukotrienes and other bronchospasm-inducing substances. SYN sodium cromoglycate.

Cronkhite, Leonard W., Jr., U.S. physician, *1919. SEE C.-Canada *syndrome*.

Crooke, Arthur, English pathologist, *1905. SEE C. *granules*, under *granule*, hyaline *change*, hyaline *degeneration*.

Crookes, Sir William, British physicist and chemist, 1832–1919; winner of the Nobel Prize in chemistry in 1907. SEE C. *glass*; C.-Hittorf *tube*.

Crosby, William Holmes, Jr., U.S. physician, *1914. SEE C. *capsule*.

cross (kros). **1.** Any figure in the shape of a c. formed by two intersecting lines. SYN crux. **2.** SYN *crux* of heart. **3.** A method of hybridization or the hybrid so produced. [F. *croix,* L. *crux*]

back c., the mating between an animal that is homozygous at a locus of interest and an animal that is heterozygous, commonly from the same ancestral stock.

double back c., a mating that is a back c. at each of two loci of interest; of special value and importance in linkage analysis.

hair c.'s [TA], crosslike figures formed by hairs growing from two directions that meet and then separate in a direction perpendicular to the original orientation. SYN cruces pilorum [TA].

maltese c., a tetrad formation of the early ringlike parasites within the red blood cell seen in babesiosis.

Ranvier c.'s, black or brown figures in the shape of a c., marking Ranvier nodes in the longitudinal section of a nerve stained with silver nitrate.

test c., in experimental genetics, a deliberate mating designed to test claims about the pattern of inheritance of one or more traits.

cross·bite (kros'bīt). An abnormal relation of one or more teeth of one arch to the opposing tooth or teeth of the other arch due to labial, buccal, or lingual deviation of tooth position, or to abnormal jaw position.

cross·breed (kros′brēd). **1.** SYN hybrid. **2.** To breed a hybrid.

cross·breed·ing (kros′brēd-ing). SYN hybridization.

cross-dress·ing. Clothing oneself in the clothes of the opposite sex. SEE transvestism.

cross-eye (kros′ī). Alternative spelling for crossed *eyes*, under *eye*.

cross·ing-over, cross·over (kros-ing-ō′ver, kros′ō-ver). Reciprocal exchange of material between two paired chromosomes during meiosis, resulting in the transfer of a block of genes from each chromosome to its homologue. In contrast to genetic recombination (2), which is a phenotypic phenomenon, c.-o. is genotypic. Any even number of c.-o. between two loci will cancel out phenotypically and no recombination will occur.

somatic c.-o., c.-o. that occurs during the mitosis of somatic cells, in contrast to that which occurs in meiosis.

uneven c.-o., unequal c.-o., c.-o. that happens when the breaks do not occur at precisely homologous points in two chromatid strands, and hence results in localized duplication of genetic material in one chromatid and complementary deletion in the other.

cross-link (kros-lingk). A covalent linkage between two polymers or between two different regions of the same polymer.

cross-match·ing (kros′match-ing). **1.** A test for incompatibility between donor and recipient blood, carried out prior to transfusion to avoid potentially lethal hemolytic reactions between the donor's red blood cells and antibodies in the recipient's plasma, or the reverse; performed by mixing a sample of red blood cells of the donor with plasma of the recipient (*major crossmatch*) and the red blood cells of the recipient with the plasma of the donor (*minor crossmatch*). Incompatibility is indicated by clumping of red blood cells and contraindicates use of the donor's blood. **2.** In allotransplantation of solid organs (e.g., kidney), a test for identification of antibody in the serum of potential allograft recipients which reacts directly with the lymphocytes or other cells of a potential allograft donor; presence of these antibodies usually, if not always, contraindicates the performance of the transplantation because virtually all such grafts will be subject to a hyperacute type of rejection.

cross·over. Refers to the phenomenon of sound presented to one ear may be perceived in the other ear by passing around the head by air conduction or through the head by bone conduction.

cross-sec·tion. 1. A transverse section through a structure. **2.** The probability of an activation (5) by a nuclear reaction when a material is bombarded by neutrons, as in the production of radionuclides in a pile; unit: barn (10^{-24} cm^2/atom).

cross-sec·tion·al. SEE synchronic.

cross-taper (kros tā′per). A practice in pharmacotherapy of lowering the dose of one medication while simultaneously increasing the dose of another medication.

cross·way (kros′wā). The crossing of two nerve paths.

sensory c., the postlenticular portion of the posterior limb of the internal capsule of the brain.

Crosti, A., 20th century Italian dermatologist. SEE Gianotti-C. *syndrome.*

cro·ta·lid (krō′tă-lid). Any member of the snake family Crotalidae.

Cro·tal·i·dae (krō-tal′i-dē). A family of New World vipers characterized by the presence of a heat-sensitive loreal pit between each eye and nostril, and folding, caniculated, long anterior fangs.

cro·ta·lin (krot′ă-lin). A protein in rattlesnake venom. [*Crotalus,* a genus of rattlesnakes]

cro·tal·ism (krō′tal-izm). SYN crotalaria *poisoning.*

Cro·ta·lus (krot′ă-lŭs). A genus of rattlesnakes (family Crotalidae) native to North America, having large fangs that are replaced periodically throughout life and a venom that is both neurotoxic and hemolytic. The largest species are the diamondbacks of the southern states (*C. adamanteus*) and western states (*C. atrox*); the smallest are the pigmy rattlers. [G. *krotalon,* a rattle, fr. *krotos,* a rattling noise]

cro·tam·i·ton (krō-tam′i-ton). A sarcopticide for topical use in scabies.

cro·taph·i·on (krō-taf′ē-on). The tip of the greater wing of the sphenoid bone; a point in craniometry. [G. *krotaphos,* the temple of the head]

cro·ton·ase (krō′ton-ās). SYN enoyl-CoA hydratase.

cro·ton oil (krō′ton). A fixed oil expressed from the seeds of *Croton tiglium* (family Euphorbiaceae), an East Indian shrub; used as an irritant purgative, and externally as a counterirritant and vesicant.

cro·to·nyl-ACP re·duc·tase (krō′to-nil). SYN enoyl-ACP reductase.

cro·tox·in (krō-tok′sin). The toxin from the venom of the North American rattlesnake. [*Crotalus* + toxin]

crot·tle (krot′el). SYN cudbear.

croup (kroop). **1.** Acute obstruction of upper airway in infants and children characterized by a barking cough with difficult and noisy respiration. **2.** Laryngotracheobronchitis in infants and young children caused by parainfluenza viruses 1 and 2. [Scots, probably from A.S. *kropan,* to cry aloud]

croup·ous (kroo′p-ŭs). Relating to croup; marked by a fibrinous exudation.

croupy (kroo′pē). Having the characteristics of croup, as a c. cough.

Crouzon, Octave, French physician, 1874–1938. SEE C. *disease, syndrome.*

Crow, R.S., British physician. SEE C.-Fukase *syndrome.*

crowd·ing (krowd′ing). A condition in which the teeth are crowded, assuming altered positions such as bunching, overlapping, displacement in various directions, torsiversion, etc.

Crowe, Samuel J., U.S. physician, 1883–1955. SEE C.-Davis mouth *gag.*

◨ **crown** (krown) [TA]. **1.** Any structure, normal or pathologic, resembling or suggesting a crown or a wreath. **2.** In dentistry, that part of a tooth that is covered with enamel, or an artificial substitute for that part. SYN corona [TA]. [L. *corona*]

anatomical c., SYN c. of tooth.

artificial c., a fixed restoration of the major part of the entire coronal part of a natural tooth; usually of gold, porcelain, or acrylic resin.

bell-shaped c., the c. of a tooth that has an exaggerated occlusogingival contour; human deciduous molars typify the bell-shaped c.

ciliary c., SYN *corona* ciliaris.

clinical c., that part of the crown of a tooth visible in the oral cavity. SYN corona clinica.

c. of head, SYN *corona* capitis.

jacket c., a hollow c. of acrylic resin, fused porcelain or cast gold, combinations of gold and acrylic or gold and porcelain; it fits over the prepared stump of the natural c.

radiate c., SYN *corona* radiata.

c. of tooth, the portion of a tooth covered with enamel. SYN anatomical c., corona dentis.

c. of Venus, papular lesions of secondary syphilis on the forehead near the hair margin.

crown·ing (krown′ing). **1.** Preparation of the natural crown of a tooth and covering the prepared crown with a veneer of suitable dental material (gold or non-precious metal casting, porcelain, plastic, or combinations). **2.** That stage of childbirth when the fetal head has negotiated the pelvic outlet and the largest diameter of the head is encircled by the vulvar ring.

CRP Abbreviation for cAMP receptor *protein*; C-reactive *protein.*

CRT Abbreviation for cathode ray *tube.*

cru·ces (kroo′sēz). Plural of crux.

cru·ci·ate (kroo′shē-āt). Shaped like, or resembling, a cross. [L. *cruciatus*]

cru·ci·ble (kroo′si-bl). A vessel used as a container for reactions or meltings at high temperature. [Mediev. L. *crucibulum,* a night lamp, later, a melting pot]

cru·fo·mate (kroo′fō-māt). A veterinary anthelmintic.

crunch (krunch). Sound heard on auscultation of the chest synchronous with cardiac contraction, indicating presence of air in the mediastinum. [onomatopoetic]

cruor (kroo′ōr). Coagulated blood. [L. blood (that flows from a wound)]

cru·ra (kroo′ră). Plural of crus.

cru·ral (kroo′răl). Relating to the leg or thigh, or to any crus.

cru·re·us (kroo-rē′ŭs). SYN vastus intermedius (*muscle*). [Mod. L.]

crus, gen. **cru·ris**, pl. **cru·ra** (kroos, kroo′ris, -ră) [TA]. **1.** SYN leg. **2.** Any anatomical structure resembling a leg; usually (in the plural) a pair of diverging bands or elongated masses. SEE ALSO limb. [L.]

    ampullary crura of semicircular ducts, SYN ampullary membranous *limbs* of semicircular ducts, under *limb*.

    anterior c. of stapes, SYN anterior *limb* of stapes.

    c. ante′rius cap′sulae inter′nae [TA], SYN anterior *limb* of internal capsule.

    c. ante′rius stape′dis [TA], SYN anterior *limb* of stapes.

    crura anthel′icis, SYN crura of antihelix.

    crura antihelicis [TA], SYN crura of antihelix.

    crura of antihelix [TA], two ridges, inferior and superior, bounding the fossa triangularis, by which the antihelix begins at the upper part of the auricle. SYN crura antihelicis [TA], crura anthelicis, leg of antihelix.

    crura of bony semicircular canals, SYN bony *limbs* of semicircular canals, under *limb*.

    c. bre′ve incu′dis [TA], SYN short *limb* of incus.

    c. cer′ebri [TA], specifically, the massive bundle of corticofugal nerve fibers passing longitudinally on the ventral surface of the midbrain on each side of the midline; it consists of fibers descending from the cortex to the tegmentum of the brainstem, pontine gray matter, and spinal cord. SEE ALSO cerebral *peduncle*, *basis* pedunculi.

    c. clitor′idis [TA], SYN c. of clitoris.

    c. of clitoris [TA], the continuation on each side of the corpus cavernosum of the clitoris that diverges from the body posteriorly and is attached to the pubic arch. SYN c. clitoridis [TA].

    common c. of semicircular ducts, SYN common membranous *limb* of semicircular ducts.

    c. cor′poris caverno′si pe′nis, SYN c. of penis.

    c. dex′trum diaphrag′matis [TA], SYN right c. of diaphragm.

    c. dex′trum fasci′culi atrioventricula′ris [TA], SYN right *bundle* of atrioventricular bundle; SEE ALSO atrioventricular *bundle*.

    c. for′nicis [TA], that part of the fornix that rises in a forward curve behind the thalamus to continue forward as the body for fornix ventral to the corpus callosum. SYN c. of fornix [TA], posterior pillar of fornix.

    c. of fornix [TA], SYN c. fornicis.

    c. hel′icis [TA], SYN c. of helix.

    c. of helix [TA], a transverse ridge continuing backward from the helix of the auricle, dividing the concha into an upper portion (cymba) and a lower portion (cavity of concha). SYN c. helicis [TA], crista helicis, limb of helix.

    c. inferius marginis falciformis hiatus sapheni, ✮official alternate term for inferior *horn* of falciform margin of saphenous opening.

    lateral c., limb or leglike portion of a structure, farthest from midline. SYN c. laterale, lateral limb.

    c. latera′le, SYN lateral c.

    c. latera′le an′uli inguina′lis superficia′lis [TA], SYN lateral c. of the superficial inguinal ring.

    c. latera′le cartila′ginis ala′ris major′is [TA], SYN lateral c. of the major alar cartilage of the nose.

    lateral c. of facial canal, laterally placed, posteriorly directed second portion of the horizontal part of the facial canal. SEE horizontal *part* of facial canal. SYN lateral c. of horizontal part of the facial canal.

    lateral c. of horizontal part of the facial canal, SYN lateral c. of facial canal; SEE horizontal *part* of facial canal.

    lateral c. of the major alar cartilage of the nose [TA], portion of cartilage extending laterally and posteriorly in a winglike fashion, supporting the wing of the nose and keeping the nostril patent. SYN c. laterale cartilaginis alaris majoris [TA].

    lateral c. of the superficial inguinal ring [TA], portion of the external oblique aponeurosis that passes lateral to the superficial inguinal ring blending into the inguinal ligament and forming the lateral boundary of the ring. SYN c. laterale anuli inguinalis superficialis [TA].

    left c. of atrioventricular bundle, SYN left *bundle* of atrioventricular bundle.

    🔲 **left c. of diaphragm** [TA], the muscular origin of the diaphragm from the upper two or three lumbar vertebrae that ascends to the left of the aorta to reach the central tendon. SYN c. sinistrum diaphragmatis [TA].

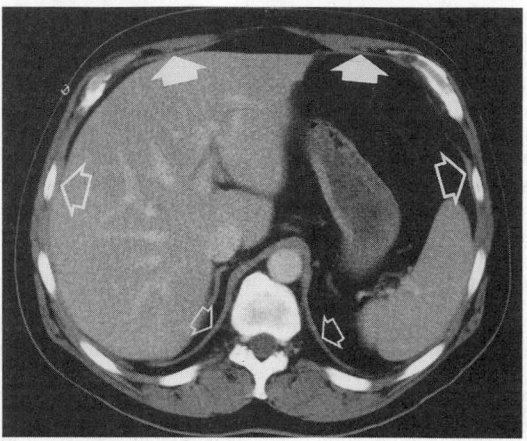

crura of diaphragm: normal anatomy on CT; scan through upper abdomen demonstrates crura of the diaphragm posteriorly (small open arrows), the costal origins of the diaphragm laterally (large open arrows), and costal cartilaginous origins anterolaterally (solid arrows)

    long c. of incus, SYN long *limb* of incus.

    c. lon′gum incu′dis [TA], SYN long *limb* of incus.

    medial c. [TA], limb or leglike portion of a structure closest to the midline. SYN c. mediale [TA], medial limb.

    c. media′le [TA], SYN medial c.

    c. media′le an′uli inguina′lis superficia′lis [TA], SYN medial c. of the superficial inguinal ring.

    c. media′le cartila′ginis ala′ris major′is [TA], SYN medial c. of major alar cartilage of nose.

    medial c. of facial canal, medially placed, anteriorly directed first portion of the horizontal part of the facial canal. SEE horizontal *part* of facial canal. SYN medial c. of the horizontal part of the facial canal.

    medial c. of the horizontal part of the facial canal, SYN medial c. of facial canal; SEE horizontal *part* of facial canal.

    medial c. of major alar cartilage of nose [TA], portion of cartilage that forms the anterioinferior portion of the cartilaginous septum between nostrils. SYN c. mediale cartilaginis alaris majoris [TA].

    medial c. of the superficial inguinal ring [TA], portion of the external oblique aponeurosis which passes medial to the superficial inguinal ring forming the medial boundary of the ring. SYN c. mediale anuli inguinalis superficialis [TA].

    cru′ra membrana′cea ampulla′ria duc′tuum semicircula′rium [TA], SYN ampullary membranous *limbs* of semicircular ducts, under *limb*.

    c. membrana′ceum commu′ne duc′tuum semicircula′rium [TA], SYN common membranous *limb* of semicircular ducts.

    c. membrana′ceum sim′plex duc′tus semicircula′ris [TA], SYN simple membranous *limb* of semicircular duct.

    cru′ra os′sea cana′lium semicircula′rium, SYN bony *limbs* of semicircular canals, under *limb*.

c. pe′nis [TA], SYN c. of penis.

c. of penis [TA], the posterior, tapering portion of the corpus cavernosum penis which diverges from its contralateral partner to be attached to the ischiopubic ramus. SYN c. penis [TA], c. corporis cavernosi penis.

posterior c. of stapes, SYN posterior *limb* of stapes.

c. poste′rius cap′sulae inter′nae [TA], SYN posterior *limb* of internal capsule.

c. poste′rius stape′dis [TA], SYN posterior *limb* of stapes.

right c. of atrioventricular bundle, SYN right *bundle* of atrioventricular bundle.

right c. of diaphragm [TA], the muscular origin of the diaphragm from the bodies of the upper three or four lumbar vertebrae that passes upward to the right of the aorta toward the central tendon; the esophageal hiatus is a parting of the fibers of the right c. to allow passage of the esophagus. SYN c. dextrum diaphragmatis [TA].

short c. of incus, SYN short *limb* of incus.

simple c. of semicircular duct, SYN simple membranous *limb* of semicircular duct.

c. sinis′trum diaphrag′matis [TA], SYN left c. of diaphragm.

c. sinis′trum fasci′culi atrioventricula′ris, SYN left *bundle* of atrioventricular bundle; SEE ALSO atrioventricular *bundle*.

c. superius marginis falciformis hiatus sapheni, SYN superior *horn* of falciform margin of saphenous opening.

crus I (kroos). SYN superior semilunar *lobule*.

crus II (kroos). SYN inferior semilunar *lobule*.

crush (krŭsh). **1.** To squeeze injuriously between two hard bodies. **2.** A bruise or contusion from pressure between two solid bodies. [O.Fr. *cruisir*]

crus·ot·o·my (kroos-ot′ō-mē). A mesencephalic pyramidal tractotomy. [L. *crus*, leg, + G. *tomē*, incision]

■**crust** (krŭst). **1.** A hard outer layer or covering; cutaneous crusts are often formed by dried serum or pus on the surface of a ruptured blister or pustule. **2.** A scab. SYN crusta. [L. *crusta*]
milk c., SYN *crusta lactea*.

crus·ta, pl. **crus·tae** (krŭs′tă, -tē). SYN crust. [L.]
c. inflammato′ria, SYN buffy *coat*.
c. lac′tea, seborrhea of the scalp in an infant. SYN milk crust.
c. phlogis′tica, SYN buffy *coat*.

Crus·ta·cea (krŭs-tā′shē-ă). A very large class of aquatic animals (phylum Arthropoda) with a chitinous exoskeleton and jointed appendages; e.g., the crab, lobster, crayfish, shrimp, isopods, ostracods, and amphipods. Some, such as certain copepods, are parasitic; others serve as intermediate hosts for parasitic worms which cause disease in humans and various other vertebrates. SEE ALSO Copepoda. [L. *crusta*, a crust]

crutch (krŭtch). A device used singly or in pairs to assist in walking when the act is impaired by a lower extremity (or trunk) disability; it transfers all or part of weight-bearing to the upper extremity. [A. S. *cryce*]

Cruveilhier, Jean, French pathologist and anatomist, 1791–1874. SEE C. *fascia, fossa; fossa* navicularis Cruveilhier; C. *joint, ligaments,* under *ligament, plexus;* C.-Baumgarten *disease, murmur, sign, syndrome*.

crux, pl. **cru·ces** (krŭks, kroo′sēz). A junction or crossing. SYN cross (1). [L.]
c. of heart, the zone of junction of the septa and walls of the four chambers of the heart. SYN cross (2).
cru′ces pilo′rum [TA], SYN hair *crosses,* under *cross*.

Cruz, Oswaldo, Brazilian physician, 1872–1917. SEE Chagas-C. *disease;* C. *trypanosomiasis*.

△**cry-.** SEE cryo-.

cry·al·ge·sia (krī-al-jē′zē-ă). Pain caused by cold. [G. *kryos,* cold, + *algos,* pain]

cry·an·es·the·sia (krī′an-es-thē′zē-ă). Inability to perceive cold. [G. *kryos,* cold, + *an-* priv. + *aisthēsis,* sensation]

cry·es·the·sia (krī-es-thē′zē-ă). **1.** A subjective sensation of cold. **2.** Sensitiveness to cold. [G. *kryos,* cold, + *aisthēsis,* sensation]

cry for help. Telephone calls, notes left in conspicuous places,

and other behaviors that communicate extreme distress and possible consideration of suicide.

△**crymo-.** Cold. SEE ALSO cryo-, psychro-. [G. *krymos,* cold]

cry·mo·phil·ic (krī-mō-fil′ik). Preferring cold; denoting microorganisms which thrive best at low temperatures. SYN cryophilic. [crymo- + G. *philos,* fond]

cry·mo·phy·lac·tic (krī′mō-fi-lak′tik). Resistant to cold, said of certain microorganisms that are not destroyed even by freezing temperatures. SYN cryophylactic. [crymo- + G. *phylaxis,* a guarding against]

△**cryo-, cry-.** Cold. SEE ALSO crymo-, psychro-. [G. *kryos,* cold]

cry·o·an·es·the·sia (krī′ō-an-es-thē′zē-ă). Localized application of cold as a means of producing regional anesthesia. SYN refrigeration anesthesia.

cry·o·bi·ol·o·gy (krī′ō-bī-ol′ō-jē). The study of the effects of low temperatures on living organisms.

cry·o·cau·tery (krī′ō-kaw′ter-ē). Any substance, such as liquid nitrogen or carbon dioxide snow, or a low temperature instrument, the application of which causes destruction of tissue by freezing. SYN cold cautery.

cry·o·con·i·za·tion (krī′ō-kon-ī-zā′shŭn). Freezing of a cone of endocervical tissue *in vivo* with a cryoprobe.

cry·o·ex·trac·tion (krī′ō-ek-strak′shŭn). Removal of cataracts by the adhesion of a freezing probe to the lens; now rarely done.

cry·o·ex·trac·tor (krī′ō-ek-strak′tŏr, -tōr). An instrument, artificially cooled, for extraction of the lens by freezing contact.

cry·o·fi·brin·o·gen (krī′ō-fī-brin′ō-jen). An abnormal type of fibrinogen very rarely found in human plasma; it is precipitated upon cooling, but redissolves when warmed to room temperature.

cry·o·fi·brin·o·gen·e·mia (krī′ō-fī-brin′ō-je-nē′mē-breve;a). The presence in the blood of cryofibrinogens.

cry·o·flu·o·rane (krī-ō-flōr′ān). Used as a refrigerant and aerosol propellant; may be irritating to the respiratory tract and mildly narcotic.

cry·o·frac·ture (kri′ō-frak′choor). SYN freeze *fracture*. [cryo- + fracture]

cry·o·gen (krī′ō-jen). A freezing substance used to produce very low temperatures.

cry·o·gen·ic (krī-ō-jen′ik). **1.** Denoting or characteristic of a cryogen. **2.** Relating to cryogenics.

cry·o·gen·ics (krī-ō-jen′iks). The science concerned with the production and effects of very low temperatures, particularly temperatures in the range of liquid helium (<4.25 K). [cryo- + G. *-gen,* producing]

cry·o·glob·u·lin·e·mia (krī′ō-glob′ū-li-nē′mē-ă). The presence of abnormal quantities of cryoglobulin in the blood plasma.

cry·o·glob·u·lins (krī-ō-glob′ū-linz). **1.** Abnormal plasma proteins (paraproteins), now grouped with gamma globulins, characterized by precipitating, gelling, or crystallizing when serum or solutions of them are cooled; distinguished from Bence Jones proteins by their larger molecular weight (approximately 200,000 compared with 35,000–50,000); they may appear in patients with multiple myeloma. **2.** Any globulin that forms a gel or flocculent precipitate on cooling.

cry·o·hy·drate (krī-ō-hī′drāt). A eutectic system of a salt and water.

cry·o·hy·poph·y·sec·to·my (krī′ō-hī-pof′i-sek′tō-mē). Destruction of hypophysis by the application of extreme cold. [cryo- + hypophysis + G. *ektomē,* excision]

cry·ol·y·sis (krī-ol′i-sis). Destruction by cold. [cryo- + G. *lysis,* dissolution]

cry·om·e·ter (krī-om′ĕ-ter). A device for measuring very low temperatures. [cryo- + G. *metron,* measure]

cry·o·pal·li·dec·to·my (krī′ō-pal-i-dek′tō-mē). Destruction of the globus pallidus by the application of extreme cold. [cryo- + globus pallidus + G. *ektomē,* excision]

cry·op·a·thy (krī-op′ă-thē). A morbid condition in which exposure to cold is an important factor. SYN frigorism. [cryo- + G. *pathos,* suffering]

cry·o·pexy (krī′ō-pek-sē). In retinal detachment surgery, sealing the sensory retina to the pigment epithelium and choroid by a freezing probe applied to the sclera. [cryo- + G. *pēxis,* a fixing in place]

cry·o·phil·ic (krī-ō-fil'ik). SYN crymophilic. [cryo- + G. *philos,* fond]

cry·o·phy·lac·tic (krī'ō-fī-lak'tik). SYN crymophylactic.

cry·o·pre·cip·i·tate (krī'ō-prē-sip'i-tāt). Precipitate that forms when soluble material is cooled, especially with reference to the precipitate that forms in normal blood plasma which has been subjected to cold precipitation and which is rich in factor VIII.

cry·o·pre·cip·i·ta·tion (krī'ō-prē-sip-i-tā'shŭn). The process of forming a cryoprecipitate from solution.

cry·o·pres·er·va·tion (krī'ō-pres-er-vā'shŭn). Maintenance of the viability of excised tissues or organs at extremely low temperatures.

cry·o·probe (krī'ō-prōb). An instrument used in cryosurgery to apply extreme cold to a selected area. [cryo- + L. *probo,* to test]

cry·o·pros·ta·tec·to·my (krī'ō-pros-tă-tek'tō-mē). Destruction of the prostate gland by freezing, utilizing a specially designed cryoprobe. [cryo- + L. *prostata,* prostate, + G. *ektomē,* excision]

cry·o·pro·tein (krī-ō-prō'tēn). A protein that precipitates from solution when cooled and redissolves upon warming.

cry·o·pul·vi·nec·to·my (krī'ō-pŭl-vi-nek'tō-mē). Destruction of the pulvinar by the application of extreme cold. [cryo- + pulvinar + G. *ektomē,* excision]

cry·o·scope (krī'ō-skōp). An instrument for measuring the freezing point.

cry·os·co·py (krī-os'kŏ-pē). The determination of the freezing point of a fluid, usually blood or urine, compared with that of distilled water. SYN algoscopy. [cryo- + G. *skopeō,* to examine]

cry·o·spasm (krī'ō-spazm). Spasm produced by cold. [cryo- + G. *spasmos,* convulsion]

cry·o·stat (krī'ō-stat). A freezing chamber. [cryo- + G. *statos,* standing]

cry·o·sur·gery (krī-ō-ser'jer-ē). An operation using freezing temperature (achieved by liquid nitrogen or carbon dioxide) as an independent agent or in an instrument to destroy tissue.

cry·o·thal·a·mec·to·my (krī'ō-thal-ă-mek'tō-mē). Destruction of the thalamus by the application of extreme cold. [cryo- + thalamus + G. *ektomē,* excision]

cry·o·ther·a·py (krī'ō-thār'ă-pē). The use of cold in the treatment of disease.

cry·o·tol·er·ant (krī-ō-tol'er-ant). Tolerant of very low temperatures.

crypt (kript) [TA]. A pitlike depression or tubular recess. SYN crypta [TA].

anal c.'s, SYN anal *sinuses,* under *sinus.*

dental c., the space filled by the dental follicle.

enamel c., the narrow, mesenchyme-filled space between the dental ledge and an enamel organ. SYN enamel niche.

c.'s of Henle, infoldings of conjunctiva.

c.'s of iris, (1) pits near the pupillary margin of the anterior surface of the iris. **(2)** spaces in the anterior iris stroma through which the aqueous washes with every pupillary movement.

c.'s of Lieberkühn, SYN intestinal *glands,* under *gland.*

c.'s of Lieberkühn of large intestine, SYN *glands* of large intestine, under *gland.*

c.'s of Lieberkühn of small intestine, SYN *glands* of small intestine, under *gland.*

lingual c., a pit lined with epithelium in the lingual tonsil.

Morgagni c.'s, SYN anal *sinuses,* under *sinus.*

synovial c., a diverticulum of the synovial membrane of a joint.

tonsillar c. [TA], one of the variable number of deep recesses that extend into the lingual, palatine, pharyngeal, and tubal tonsils from the free surface where they open at the tonsillar fossa. SYN crypta tonsillaris [TA].

△**crypt-.** SEE crypto-.

cryp·ta, pl. **cryp·tae** (krip'tă, -tē) [TA]. SYN crypt. [L. fr. G. *kryptos,* hidden]

c. tonsilla′ris, pl. **cryp′tae tonsilla′res** [TA], SYN tonsillar *crypt.*

cryp·tec·to·my (krip-tek'tō-mē). Excision of a tonsillar or other crypt. [crypt + G. *ektomē,* excision]

cryp·ten·a·mine ac·e·tates, cryp·ten·a·mine tan·nates (kripten'ă-mēn). Acetate or tannate salts of alkaloids from a nonaqueous extract of *Veratrum viride,* containing the hypotensive alkaloids protoveratrines A and B, germitrine, neogermetrine, germerine, germidine, jervine, rubijervine, isorubijervine, and germubide; used as antihypertensive agents. SEE ALSO protoveratrine A and B.

cryp·tic (krip'tik). Hidden; occult; larvate. [G. *kryptikos*]

cryp·ti·tis (krip-tī'tis). Inflammation of a follicle or glandular tubule, particularly in the colon.

△**crypto-, crypt-.** Hidden, obscure; without apparent cause. [G. *kryptos,* hidden, concealed]

cryptochrome (krip'tō-krōm). Flavoprotein ultraviolet-A receptor involved in circadian rhythm entrainment in plants, insects, and mammals.

cryp·to·coc·co·ma (krip'tō-kok-ō'mă). An infectious granuloma, typically in the brain, but also found in the lung and elsewhere, caused by *Cryptococcus neoformans.* [*Cryptococcus* (genus name) + -oma]

cryp·to·coc·co·sis (krip'tō-kok-ō'sis). An acute, subacute, or chronic infection by *Cryptococcus neoformans,* causing a pulmonary, disseminated, or meningeal mycosis. The pulmonary form may resolve spontaneously in previously normal persons but dissemination to other organs is fatal if untreated; the most common clinical manifestation is meningitis.

🔟 *Cryp·to·coc·cus* (krip-tō-kok'ŭs). A genus of yeastlike fungi that reproduce by budding. [crypto- + G. *kokkos,* berry]

C. neofor′mans, a species that causes cryptococcosis in humans and other mammals, particularly the cat family. Cells are spherical and reproduce by budding; a prominent feature is a polysaccharide capsule. *C. neoformans var. neoformans* has a worldwide distribution and can often be isolated from weathered pigeon droppings. *C. neoformans var. gattii* causes cryptococcosis in subtropical and tropical climates. This variety has been isolated from foliage and litter of species of eucalyptus.

cryp·to·crys·tal·line (krip-tō-kris'tă-lēn). Having very minute crystals.

Cryp·to·cys·tis trich·o·dec·tis (krip-tō-sis'tis trī-kō-dek'tis). Name formerly applied to the larval form of the dog tapeworm, *Dipylidium caninum,* named for the cysticercoids found in the dog louse, *Trichodectes.* [crypto- + G. *kystis,* bladder; tricho- + G. *dektēs,* a beggar]

cryp·to·did·y·mus (krip'tō-did'i-mŭs). Conjoined twins, with the poorly developed parasitic twin concealed within the larger autosite. SEE conjoined *twins,* under *twin.* [crypto- + G. *didymos,* twin]

Cryp·to·gam·ia (krip-tō-gam'ē-ă). A montaxonomic division of the plant kingdom containing all forms of plant life that do not reproduce by means of seeds; included are the algae, bacteria, fungi, lichens, mosses, liverworts, ferns, horsetails, and club mosses. [crypto- + G. *gamos,* marriage]

cryp·to·gen·ic (krip-tō-jen'ik). Of obscure, indeterminate etiology or origin, in contrast to phanerogenic. [crypto- + G. *genesis,* origin]

cryp·to·lith (krip'tō-lith). A concretion in a gland follicle. [crypto- + G. *lithos,* stone]

cryp·to·men·or·rhea (krip'tō-men-ō-rē'ă). Occurrence each month of the general symptoms of the menses without any flow of blood, as in cases of imperforate hymen. [crypto- + G. *mēn,* month, + *rhoia,* flow]

cryp·toph·thal·mus, cryp·toph·thal·mia (krip-tof-thal'mŭs, -thal'mē-ă). Congenital absence of eyelids, with the skin passing continuously from the forehead onto the cheek over a rudimentary eye. [crypto- + G. *ophthalmos,* eye]

cryp·to·po·dia (krip-tō-pō'dē-ă). A swelling of the lower part of the leg and the foot, in such a manner that there is great distortion and the sole seems to be a flattened pad. [crypto- + G. *pous,* foot]

cryp·to·pyr·role (krip-tō-pir'ōl). 3-Ethyl-2,4-dimethylpyrrole;

one of the pyrrole derivatives obtained by the drastic reduction of heme.

cryp·tor·chid (krip-tōr′kid). Relating to or characterized by cryptorchism. [crypto- + G. *orchis,* testis]

cryp·tor·chi·dism (krip-tōr′ki-dizm). SYN cryptorchism.

cryp·tor·chism (krip-tōr′kizm). Failure of one or both of the testes to descend. SYN cryptorchidism.

cryp·to·scope (krip′tō-skōp). Obsolete term for a simple x-ray fluoroscope. [G. *kryptos,* something hidden, + *skopeō,* to examine]

cryp·to·spo·rid·i·o·sis (krip′tō-spō-rid-ē-ō′sis). An enteric disease caused by waterborne protozoan parasites of the genus *Cryptosporidium;* characterized pathologically by villous atrophy and fusion and clinically by diarrhea in humans, calves, lambs, and other animals; disease in immunocompetent persons is manifest as a self-limiting diarrhea, whereas in immunocompromised persons it is manifest as a prolonged severe diarrhea that can be fatal.

Cryp·to·spo·rid·i·um (krip′tō-spō-rid′ē-ŭm). A genus of coccidian sporozoans (family Cryptosporiidae, suborder Eimeriina) that are important pathogens of calves and other domestic animals, and common opportunistic parasites of humans that flourish under conditions of compromised immune function; can cause self-limiting diarrhea in immunocompetent persons.

C. parvum, sporozoan species that is an important cause of neonatal diarrhea in calves and lambs; causes mild, self-limiting to severe, chronic diarrhea in humans.

Cryp·to·stro·ma cor·ti·ca·le (krip-tō-strō′mă kōr-ti-kā′lē). A species of fungus that is a common allergen, growing profusely under the bark of stacked maple logs; handlers who inhale the massive number of spores may develop pneumonitic as well as allergic reactions, including maple bark disease. [crypto- + G. *stroma,* bed]

cryp·to·tia (krip-tō′shē-ă). A rare abnormality in which the superior portion of the auricle is hidden under the scalp. [crypto- + G. *ōtos,* ear]

cryp·to·xan·thin (krip-tō-zan′thin). (3*R*)-β,β-Caroten-3-ol; β-caroten-3-ol; carotenoid (specifically, a xanthophyll) yielding 1 mol of vitamin A per mole. Found in many fruits and berries.

cryp·to·zo·ite (krip′tō-zō′īt). The exoerythrocyte stage of the malarial organism that develops directly from the sporozoite inoculated by the infected mosquito; development of the first generation of merozoites in vertebrate host tissues occurs in the liver parenchyma. [crypto- + G. *zōē,* life]

cryp·to·zy·gous (krip-toz′i-gŭs, -tō-zī′gŭs). Having a narrow face compared with the width of the cranium, so that, when the skull is viewed from above, the zygomatic arches are not visible. [crypto- + G. *zygon,* yoke]

crys·tal (kris′tăl). A solid of regular shape and, for a given compound, characteristic angles, formed when an element or compound solidifies slowly enough, as a result either of freezing from the liquid form or of precipitating out of solution, to allow the individual molecules to take up regular positions with respect to one another. [G. *krystallos,* clear ice, crystal]

asthma c.'s, SYN Charcot-Leyden c.'s.

blood c.'s, SYN hematoidin.

Böttcher c.'s, small c.'s observed microscopically in prostatic fluid that is treated with a drop or two of 1% solution of ammonium phosphate.

Charcot-Leyden c.'s, c.'s in the shape of elongated double pyramids, formed from eosinophils, found in the sputum in bronchial asthma and in other exudates or transudates containing eosinophils. SYN asthma c.'s, Charcot-Neumann c.'s, Charcot-Robin c.'s, Leyden c.'s.

Charcot-Neumann c.'s, SYN Charcot-Leyden c.'s.

Charcot-Robin c.'s, SYN Charcot-Leyden c.'s.

chiral c., an enantiomorphic, dysymmetric, optically active c.

chlorohemin c.'s, SYN Teichmann c.'s.

clathrate c., latticelike arrangement of molecules of one substance surrounding molecules of another substance.

ear c.'s, SYN otoliths.

Florence c.'s, brown rhombic c.'s formed at the interface between a drop of Lugol solution and a drop of fluid that contains semen; not a specific test for the latter.

hematoidin c.'s, SYN hematoidin.

hydrate c., one of several possible microstructural arrangements of water molecules based on intermolecular forces; suggested as being involved in the mode of action of inhalation anesthetics.

knife-rest c., a c. of ammoniomagnesium phosphate found in alkaline urine.

Leyden c.'s, SYN Charcot-Leyden c.'s.

Lubarsch c.'s, intracellular c.'s in the testis resembling sperm c.'s.

sperm c., spermin c., a c. of spermin phosphate found in the semen; possibly identical to Böttcher c.'s.

Teichmann c.'s, rhombic c.'s of hemin; used in microscopic detection of blood. SEE hemin. SYN chlorohemin c.'s.

thorn apple c.'s, ammonium urate c.'s in the shape of rounded bodies with many projecting points.

twin c., two c.'s that have grown together along a common face.

Virchow c.'s, yellow-brown, amber, or burnt orange c.'s of hematoidin, frequently observed in extravasated blood in tissues.

whetstone c.'s, xanthine c.'s occasionally observed in urine.

crys·tal·lin (kris′tă-lin). One of several water-soluble proteins found in the lens of the eye; alpha (an embryonic single protein), beta, and gamma varieties (based on precipitibility) are known. Reptiles and birds have a δ-c. as well. ε-C. is identical with lactate dehydrogenase.

gamma c., the least rapidly mobile form of c. on electrophoresis.

crys·tal·line (kris′tă-lēn). 1. Clear; transparent. 2. Relating to a crystal or crystals.

crys·tal·li·za·tion (kris′tăl-i-zā′shŭn). Assumption of a crystalline form when a vapor or liquid becomes solidified, or a solute precipitates from solution.

crys·tal·lo·gram (kris′tă-lō-gram). A photograph produced when x-rays are diffracted by a crystal. [G. *krystallos,* crystal, + *gramma,* something written]

crys·tal·log·ra·phy (kris-tăl-log′ră-fē). The study of the shape and atomic structure of crystals.

crys·tal·loid (kris′tăl-oyd). 1. Resembling a crystal, or being such. 2. A body that in solution can pass through a semipermeable membrane, as distinguished from a colloid, which cannot do so.

Charcot-Böttcher c.'s, spindle-shaped c.'s 10–25 μm long, found in human Sertoli cells.

Reinke c.'s, rod-shaped crystal-like structures with pointed or rounded ends present in the interstitial cells of the testis (Leydig cells) and ovary.

crys·tal·lo·pho·bia (kris′tăl-ō-fō′bē-ă). SYN hyalophobia. [G. *krystallon,* crystal, + *phobos,* fear]

crys·tal·lu·ria (kris-tă-loo′rē-ă). The excretion of crystalline materials in the urine.

crys·tal vi·o·let (kris′tăl) [C.I. 42555]. A compound that has been used in the external treatment of burns, wounds, and fungal infections of skin and mucous membranes, and internally for pinworm and certain fluke infections; used also as a stain for chromatin, amyloid, platelets in blood, fibrin, and neuroglia, and to differentiate among bacteria. SYN methylrosaniline chloride.

Cs Symbol for cesium.

CSD Abbreviation for catscratch *disease.*

C-sec·tion. SEE cesarean *section.*

CSF Abbreviation for cerebrospinal *fluid*; colony-stimulating *factors,* under *factor.*

CSI. Abbreviation for Calculus Surface Index.

CT Abbreviation for computed *tomography.*

dynamic CT, SYN dynamic computed *tomography.*

helical CT, SYN spiral computed *tomography.*

spiral CT, SYN spiral computed *tomography.*

CTD Abbreviation for cumulative trauma *disorders,* under *disorder.*

Cte·no·ce·phal·i·des (tē-nō-se-fal′i-dēz). A genus of fleas. *C. canis* (dog flea) and *C. felis* (cat flea) are nearly universal ectopar-

CT

asites of household pets; will attack humans when starving owing to absence of pets. [G. *ktenōdēs*, like a cockle, + *kephalē*, head]

CTL Abbreviation for cytotoxic T lymphocytes.

CTP Abbreviation for cytidine 5′-triphosphate.

Cu Symbol for copper.

⁶⁷Cu Symbol for copper-67.

⁶⁴Cu Symbol for copper-64.

cu·beb (kū′beb). The dried unripe, nearly full-grown fruit of *Piper cubeba* (family Piperaceae), a climbing plant of the West Indies, used as stimulant, carminative, and local irritant; c. oil has been used as a mild urinary antiseptic. [Ar. and Hindu, *kababa*]

cu·bi·tal (kū′bi-tăl). Relating to the elbow or to the ulna.

cu·bi·tus, gen. and pl. **cu·bi·ti** (kū′bi-tŭs, -tī) [TA]. **1.** SYN elbow (2). **2.** SYN ulna. [L. elbow]

c. val′gus, deviation of the extended forearm to the outer (radial) side of the axis of the limb.

c. va′rus, deviation of the extended forearm to the inward (ulnar) side of the axis of the limb.

cu·boid, cu·boi·dal (kū′boyd, kū-boy′dăl) [TA]. **1.** Resembling a cube in shape. **2.** Relating to the os cuboideum. [G. *kybos*, cube, + *eidos*, resemblance]

cud·bear (kŭd′bār). Purple-red coloring agent derived from the lichen *Ochrolechia tartarea* (family Lecanoraceae) and for the coloring principles from Roccellaceae used for coloring liquid pharmaceutical preparations. SYN crottle.

cue (kū). In conditioning and learning theory, a pattern of stimuli to which an individual has learned or is learning to respond.

response-produced c.'s, successive stimulus c.'s in a behavior chain, each response serving as a reinforcer for the previous response and as a stimulus, or c., for the next response. SEE higher order *conditioning*, behavior *chain*.

cuff (kŭf). Any structure shaped like a c.

musculotendinous c., SYN rotator c. of shoulder.

perivascular c.'s, SEE cuffing.

rotator c. of shoulder, the anterior, superior, and posterior aspects of the capsule of the shoulder joint reinforced by the tendons of insertion of the *supraspinatus, infraspinatus, teres* minor, and *subscapularis* (SITS) muscles. SYN musculotendinous c.

vaginal c., the portion of the vaginal vault remaining open to the peritoneum following hysterectomy.

cuff·ing (kŭf′ing). **1.** A perivascular accumulation of various leukocytes seen in infectious, inflammatory, or autoimmune diseases. **2.** To surround a structure with fluid or cells, as with a cuff; in chest radiography, thickening of bronchial walls on the image. [M.E. *cuffe*, mitten]

cui·rass (kwē-ras′). The anterior surface of the thorax in relation to symptoms or disease changes. [Fr. *cuirasse*, a breastplate]

analgesic c., SYN tabetic c.

tabetic c., an analgesic or hypalgesic zone in the proximal thoracic region, found in tabetic neurosyphilis. SYN analgesic c., Hitzig girdle.

cul-de-sac, pl. **culs-de-sac** (kool-de-sak′). **1.** A blind pouch or tubular cavity closed at one end; e.g., diverticulum; cecum. **2.** SYN rectouterine *pouch.* [Fr. bottom of a sack]

conjunctival cul-de-sac, SYN conjunctival *fornix.*

Douglas cul-de-sac, SYN rectouterine *pouch.*

greater cul-de-sac, SYN *fundus* of stomach.

Gruber cul-de-sac, a lateral diverticulum in the suprasternal space beside the medial extremity of the clavicle behind the sternal attachment of the sternocleidomastoid muscle.

lesser cul-de-sac, SYN pyloric *antrum.*

cul·do·cen·te·sis (kŭl′dō-sen-tē′sis). Aspiration of fluid from the cul-de-sac (rectouterine excavation) by puncture of the vaginal vault near the midline between the uterosacral ligaments. [cul-de-sac + G. *kentēsis*, puncture]

cul·do·plas·ty (kŭl′dō-plas-tē). Plastic surgery to remedy relaxation of the posterior fornix of the vagina. [cul-de-sac + G. *plastos*, formed]

cul·do·scope (kŭl′dō-skōp). Endoscopic instrument used in culdoscopy.

cul·dos·co·py (kŭl-dos′kŏ-pē). Introduction of an endoscope through the posterior vaginal wall for viewing the rectovaginal pouch and pelvic viscera. [cul-de-sac + G. *skopeō*, to view]

cul·dot·o·my (kŭl-dot′ō-mē). **1.** Cutting through the posterior vaginal wall into the cul-de-sac of Douglas. **2.** SYN vaginal *celiotomy.* [cul-de-sac + G. *tomē*, incision]

Cu·lex (kū′leks). A genus of mosquitoes (family Culicidae) including over 2000 species. Largely tropical but worldwide in distribution; they are vectors for a number of diseases of humans and of domestic and wild animals and birds. [L. gnat]

C. nigripalpus, mosquito species that is a vector of St. Louis encephalitis within the United States.

C. pi′piens, a subspecies complex of the abundant polytypic species, the brown house mosquito or rainbarrel mosquito of temperate climates, which breeds commonly in standing water, especially in artificial containers, and has a 5- to 6-day cycle under optimal conditions; closely related forms are found in tropical areas.

C. quinquefasciatus, mosquito species that could serve as a vector of *Wuchereria bancrofti*, if this filarial infection were introduced into the United States.

C. restuans, mosquito species that is a secondary or suspected vector of Eastern equine encephalitis and Western equine encephalitis within the United States.

C. salinarius, mosquito species that is a secondary or suspected vector of Eastern equine encephalitis within the United States.

C. tarsa′lis, a mosquito species that is an important vector of St. Louis and Western equine encephalomyelitis viruses in horses, birds, and humans.

Cu·lic·i·dae (kū-lis′i-dē). A family of insects (order Diptera) that includes the true mosquitoes, which are all included in the subfamily Culicinae.

cu·li·ci·dal (kū-li-sī′dăl). Destructive to mosquitoes. [L. *culex*, gnat, + *caedo*, to kill]

cu·li·cide (kū′li-sīd). An agent that destroys mosquitoes.

cu·lic·i·fuge (kū-lis′i-fooj). **1.** Driving away gnats and mosquitoes. **2.** An agent that keeps mosquitoes from biting. [L. *culex*, gnat + *fugo*, to drive away]

Cu·li·coi·des (kū-li-koy′dēz). A genus of minute biting gnats or midges, vectors of several nonpathogenic human filariae (*Mansonella, Dipetalonema*), of *Onchocerca* in horses and cattle, and of several viral agents of domestic sheep and fowl. [L. *culex*, gnat]

C. aus′teni, species that is an intermediate host of the filarial worm, *Mansonella perstans*, chiefly in equatorial Africa.

C. fu′rens, species that is a vector of *Mansonella ozzardi*, in the West Indies.

C. mil′nei, a species that is one of the vectors of *Mansonella perstans* in West Africa.

Culiseta (kū-lis′ē-ta). A genus of mosquitoes (family Culicidae). They are vectors for a number of diseases of humans and of domestic and wild animals and birds.

C. inornata, mosquito species that is a secondary or suspected vector of Western equine encephalitis and California group encephalitis within the United States.

C. melanura, a species of mosquito that is the principal endemic vector of Eastern equine encephalomyelitis virus; since this species feeds primarily on birds, other mosquitoes (*Aedes* spp.) transmit the virus from birds to humans and horses.

Cullen, Thomas S., U.S. gynecologist, 1868–1953. SEE C. *sign.*

cul·men, pl. **cul·′mi·na** (kul′men) [TA]. The anterior prominent portion of the monticulus of the vermis of the cerebellum; vermal lobule rostral to the primary fissure; divided into an anterior part [TA] (lobule IV of Larsell) and a posterior part [TA] (lobule V of Larsell). SYN lobulus culminis. [L. summit]

Culp, Ormond S., U.S. urologist, 1910–1977. SEE C. *pyeloplasty.*

cult (kŭlt). A system of beliefs and rituals based on dogma or religious teachings and characterized by devoted adherents who display a readiness to obey, an unrealistic idealization of the leader, an abandonment of personal ambition and goals, and an eschewing of traditional societal values. [L. *cultus,* an honoring, adoration]

cul·ti·va·tion (kŭl-ti-vā'shŭn). SYN culture. [Mediev. L. *cultivo,* pp. -*atus,* fr. L. *colo,* pp. *cultus,* to till]

cul·tur·al di·ver·si·ty. The inevitable variety in customs, attitudes, practices, and behavior that exists among groups of individuals from different ethnic, racial, or national backgrounds who come into contact.

cul·ture (kŭl'chŭr). **1.** The propagation of microorganisms on or in media of various kinds. **2.** A mass of microorganisms on or in a medium. **3.** The propagation of mammalian cells, i.e., cell culture. SEE cell c. **4.** Set of beliefs, values, artistic, historical, religious characteristics, customs, etc. common to a community or nation. SYN cultivation. [L. *cultura,* tillage, fr. *colo,* pp. *cultus,* to till]

batch c., a technique for large-scale production of microbes or microbial products in which, at a given point in time, the fermenter is stopped and the c. is worked up.

cell c., the maintenance or growth of dispersed cells after removal from the body, commonly on a glass surface immersed in nutrient fluid.

continuous c., a technique for production of microbes or microbial products in which nutrients are continuously supplied to the fermenter.

discontinuous c., a technique for production of microbes or microbial products in which the organisms are grown in a closed system until one nutrient factor becomes rate-limiting.

elective c., a method of isolating microorganisms capable of utilizing a specific substrate by incubating an inoculum in a medium containing the substrate; the medium usually contains substances or has characteristics that inhibit the growth of unwanted microorganisms. SYN enrichment c.

enrichment c., SYN elective c.

hanging-block c., the propagation of microorganisms on a cube of solidified agar medium which is inoculated, attached to a cover glass, and inverted over a moist chamber or hollowed slide.

Harada-Mori filter paper strip c., a combination of filter paper, fecal specimen, and tap water placed in a centrifuge tube; provides an environment for nematode eggs to hatch and larvae to develop.

mixed lymphocyte c., SEE mixed lymphocyte culture *test.*

monoxenic c., c. of parasites grown in association with a single known bacterium.

needle c., SYN stab c.

neotype c., SYN neotype *strain.*

organ c., the maintenance or growth of tissues, organ primordia, or the parts or whole of an organ in vitro in such a way as to allow differentiation or preservation of the architecture or function.

Petri dish c., a combination of filter paper, fecal specimen, and tap water placed in a Petri dish; provides an environment for nematode eggs to hatch and larvae to develop.

plastic envelope c., simplified method for transport and culture of specimens for the diagnosis of infection with *Trichomonas vaginalis;* liquid culture medium is examined microscopically through the envelope, so pipette sampling of the medium is not required.

pouch c., plastic c. systems used for transport of specimens, culture, and examination chambers for the isolation, growth, and detection of *Trichomonas vaginalis.*

pure c., in the ordinary bacteriologic sense, a c. consisting of a single species and strain of a bacterium.

roll-tube c., a c. in a tube of medium which has been melted and allowed to solidify while the tube is being spun; the inside of the tube is thereby coated with a thin layer of solidified medium.

sensitized c., a live c. of an organism to which a specific antiserum is added; after the mixture is incubated for several minutes (during which the antibody in the serum combines with the organisms), the excess serum is removed by means of centrifugation, washing in physiologic saline solution, and recentrifugation; the sensitized organisms may then be resuspended in physiologic saline solution.

shake c., a c. made by inoculating a liquefied gelatin or agar medium, distributing the inoculum thoroughly by agitation, and

then allowing the medium to solidify in the tube in an upright position.

slant c., a c. made on the slanting surface of a medium which has been solidified in a test tube inclined from the perpendicular so as to give a greater area than that of the lumen of the tube. SYN slope c.

slope c., SYN slant c.

smear c., a c. obtained by spreading material presumed to be infected on the surface of a solidified medium.

stab c., a c. produced by inserting an inoculating needle with inoculum down the center of a solid medium contained in a test tube. SYN needle c.

stock c., a c. of a microorganism maintained solely for the purpose of keeping the microorganism in a viable condition by subculture, as necessary, into fresh medium.

streak c., a c. produced by lightly stroking an inoculating needle or loop with inoculum over the surface of a solid medium.

tissue c., the maintenance of live tissue after removal from the body, by placing in a vessel with a sterile nutritive medium.

type c., a type strain of microorganism preserved in a c. collection as the standard.

xenic c., c.'s of parasites grown in association with an unknown microbiota. [G. *xenikos,* alien, foreign, fr. *xenos,* guest, stranger]

cum (kum). With [L.]

cu·ma·rin (kū'mă-rin). SYN coumarin.

cu·meth·a·rol (kū-meth'ă-rol). SYN coumetarol.

cu·me·thox·a·eth·ane (kū-me-thoks'ă-eth-ān). SYN coumetarol.

Cummer, William E., Canadian dentist, 1879–1942. SEE C. *classification, guideline.*

cUMP Abbreviation for cyclic *uridine* 3',5'-monophosphate.

cu·mu·la·tive (kū'mū-lă-tiv). Tending to accumulate or pile up, as with certain drugs that may have a c. effect.

cu·mu·lus, pl. **cu·mu·li** (kū'mū-lŭs, -lī). A collection or heap of cells. [L. a heap]

c. oöph′orus, a mass of epithelial granulosa cells surrounding the ovum in the ovarian follicle. SYN ovigerus, proligerous disk, proligerous membrane. [NA]

c. ova′ricus, rarely used term for c. oöphorus.

cu·ne·ate (kū'nē-āt). Wedge-shaped. [L. *cuneus,* wedge]

cu·ne·i·form (kū'nē-i-fōrm). Wedge-shaped. SEE intermediate cuneiform (*bone*), lateral cuneiform (*bone*), medial cuneiform (*bone*).

cu·ne·o·cu·boid (kū'nē-ō-kū'boyd). Relating to the lateral cuneiform and the cuboid bones.

cu·ne·o·na·vic·u·lar (kū-nē-ō-na-vik'ū-lăr). Relating to the cuneiform and the navicular bones. SYN cuneoscaphoid.

cu·ne·o·scaph·oid (kū-nē-ō-skaf'oyd). SYN cuneonavicular.

cu·ne·us, pl. **cu·nei** (kū'nē-ŭs, koo'nē-ī) [TA]. That region of the medial aspect of the occipital lobe of each cerebral hemisphere bounded by the parietooccipital fissure and the calcarine fissure. [L. wedge]

cu·nic·u·lus, pl. **cu·nic·u·li** (kū-nik'ū-lŭs, -lī). The burrow of the scabies mite in the epidermis. [L. a rabbit; an underground passage]

cun·ni·lin·gus (kŭn-i-ling'gŭs). Oral stimulation of the vulva or clitoris; a type of oral-genital sexual activity; contrasted with fellatio, which is the oral stimulation of the penis. [L. *cunnus,* pudendum, + *lingo,* to lick]

Cun·ning·ham·el·la el·e·gans (kŭn-ing-ha-mel'ă el'ě-ganz). One of several species of fungi that can cause mucormycosis in humans.

cun·nus (kŭn'ŭs). SYN vulva. [L.]

cup (kŭp). **1.** An excavated or hallowed structure, either anatomic or pathologic. SYN poculum. **2.** SYN cupping *glass.* [A.S. *cuppe*]

Diogenes c., SYN c. of palm.

dry c., a cupping glass formerly applied to the unbroken skin to draw blood to the area but without removing it.

eye c., a small oval receptacle used to apply a liquid to the external eye.

glaucomatous c., a bean-pot-like depression of the optic disk caused by glaucoma. SYN glaucomatous excavation.

ocular c., SYN optic c.

optic c., the double-walled c. formed by the invagination of the embryonic optic vesicle; its inner component becomes the sensory layer of the retina, its outer layer, the pigment layer. SYN caliculus ophthalmicus, ocular c.

c. of palm, the palm of the hand when contracted and deepened by the action of the muscles on either side. SYN Diogenes c., poculum diogenis.

perilimbal suction c., a device for increasing intraocular pressure by impeding circulation and aqueous humor flow from the eye.

physiologic c., SYN *depression* of optic disk.

suction c., one of the cupping glasses of various shapes, formerly used to produce local hyperemia according to Bier method.

wet c., a cupping glass formerly applied to a part previously scarified or incised to draw and remove blood.

cu·po·la (koo′pŏ-lă, kū′). SYN cupula.

cupped (kŭpt). Hollowed; made cup-shaped.

cup·ping (kŭp′ing). 1. Formation of a hollow, or cup-shaped excavation. 2. Application of a c. glass. SEE ALSO cup.

cu·pric (koo′prik, kū-). Pertaining to copper, particularly to copper in the form of a doubly charged positive ion.

cu·pric ac·e·tate, cu·pric ac·e·tate nor·mal. A stimulating local caustic to ulcers.

cu·pric ar·se·nite. A poisonous green crystalline powder, obsolete as a medicinal agent; now used as an insecticide and pigment. SYN copper arsenite, Scheele green.

cu·pric chlo·ride. Has been used as an antiseptic in the treatment of water supplies, ponds, and pools. SYN copper bichloride, copper chloride, copper dichloride.

cu·pric cit·rate. A salt of copper used as an astringent and antiseptic. SYN copper citrate.

cu·pric sul·fate. A blue salt highly poisonous to algae, it is a prompt and active emetic, and is used as an irritant, astringent, and fungicide. SYN copper sulfate, copper sulphate.

cu·pri·u·re·sis (koo′pri-ū-rē′sis, kū′-). The urinary excretion of copper. [L. *cuprum,* copper, + G. *ourēsis,* a urinating]

cu·pu·la, pl. **cu·pu·lae** (koo′poo-lă, -lē; kū′pū-lă) [TA]. A cup-shaped or domelike structure. SYN cupola. [L. dim. of *cupa,* a tub]

ampullary c., SYN c. ampullaris.

c. ampulla′ris [TA], a gelatinous mass that overlies the hair cells of the ampullary crests of the semicircular ducts; movement of endolymphatic fluid causes the c. to move across the hair cells of the ampullary crest. SYN ampullary c.

c. of cochlea, SYN cochlear c.

c. coch′leae [TA], SYN cochlear c.

cochlear c. [TA], the domelike apex of the cochlea. SYN c. cochleae [TA], c. of cochlea.

c. pleu′rae [TA], SYN cervical *pleura.*

pleural c., ☆official alternate term for cervical *pleura.*

cu·pu·lar (koo′poo-lăr, kū′pū-lăr). 1. Relating to a cupula. 2. Dome-shaped. SYN cupulate, cupuliform.

cu·pu·late (koo′poo-lāt, kū′pū-). SYN cupular (2).

cu·pu·li·form (koo′pŭ-lĭ-fōrm, kū′pū-). SYN cupular (2).

cu·pu·lo·gram (koo′poo-lō-gram). A graphic representation of vestibular function relative to normal performance.

cu·pu·lo·lith·i·a·sis (koo′poo-lō-li-thī′a-sis). SYN benign paroxysmal positional *vertigo.*

cu·rage (kū′rij, koo-rahzh′). Curettage by means of the finger rather than the curet. [Fr. a cleansing]

cu·ra·re (koo-rah′rē). An extract of various plants, especially *Strychnos toxifera, S. castelnaei, S. crevauxii,* and *Chondodendron tomentosum,* that produces nondepolarizing paralysis of skeletal muscle after intravenous injection by blocking transmission at the myoneuronal junction; used clinically (e.g., as *d*-tubocurarine chloride, metocurine iodide) to provide muscle relaxation during surgical operations. Often classified by the vessels with which Amazon and Orinoco Indians stored c. SYN arrow poison (1). [S. Am.]

calabash c., (packed by Indians in hollow gourds), c. from *Strychnos* sp.; contains yohimbine, indole, and strychnine-type alkaloids.

pot c., (c. stored in clay pots), c. from *Chondodendron* sp.

tube c., (c. stored in bamboo tubes), c. from *Chondodendron* sp.; contains the alkaloid tubocurarine.

cu·ra·ri·form (koo-rar′i-fōrm). Denoting a drug having an action like curare.

cu·rar·i·mi·met·ic (koo-rar′i-mī-met′ik). Having a curarelike action.

cu·ra·rine (kū′ră-rēn). The alkaloid principle of calabash curare.

cu·ra·ri·za·tion (kū-rah-ri-zā′shŭn). Induction of muscular relaxation or paralysis by the administration of curare or related compounds that have the ability to block nerve impulse transmission at the myoneural junction.

cur·a·tive (kūr′ă-tiv). 1. That which heals or cures. 2. Tending to heal or cure.

cur·cum·in (kur′koo-min) A yellow pigment from roots and pods of *Curcuma longa;* used in liver and bile ailments; found in curry powder; used as an indicator; it inhibits 5-lipoxygenase. SYN tumeric yellow.

curd (kerd). The coagulum of milk.

cure (kūr). 1. To heal; to make well. 2. A restoration to health. 3. A special method or course of treatment. SEE dental *curing.* [L. *curo,* to care for]

cu·ret. SEE curette.

cu·ret·tage (kū-rĕ-tahzh′, koo-). A scraping, usually of the interior of a cavity or tract, for the removal of new growths or other abnormal tissues, or to obtain material for tissue diagnosis. SYN curettement.

periapical c., (1) removal of a cyst or granuloma from its pathologic bony crypt, utilizing a curette; (2) the removal of tooth fragments and debris from sockets at the time of extraction or subsequent removal of bone sequestra.

subgingival c., removal of subgingival calculus, ulcerated epithelial and granulation tissues found in periodontal pockets. SYN apoxesis.

suction c., a form of abortion in which the cervix is dilated if necessary and the products of conception removed by use of a canula attached to a suction source; technique used to complete a spontaneous incomplete abortion or as a form of induced abortion. SYN dilation and suction.

cu·rette, cu·ret (kū-ret′, koo-). Instrument in the form of a loop, ring, or scoop with sharpened edges attached to a rod-shaped handle, used for curettage. [Fr.]

Hartmann c., a c., cutting on the side, for the removal of adenoids.

cu·rette·ment (kū-ret′ment, koo-). SYN curettage.

cu·rie (C, c, Ci) (kū′rē). A unit of measurement of radioactivity, 3.70×10^{10} disintegrations per second; formerly defined as the radioactivity of the amount of radon in equilibrium with 1 gm. of radium; superseded by the S.I. unit, the becquerel (1 disintegration per second). [Marie (1867–1934) and Pierre (1859–1906) *Curie,* French chemists and physicists and Nobel laureates]

cur·ing (kūr′ing). 1. The act of accomplishing a cure. 2. A process by which something is prepared for use, as by heating, aging, etc.

dental c., the process by which plastic materials become rigid to form a denture base, filling, impression tray, or other appliance.

cu·ri·um (Cm) (kū′rē-ŭm). An element, atomic no. 96, atomic wt. 247.07, not occurring naturally on earth, but first formed artificially in 1944 by bombarding ^{239}Pu with alpha particles; the most stable of the c. isotopes is ^{247}Cm, with a half-life of 15.6 million years. [see curie]

Curling, Thomas B., English surgeon, 1811–1888. SEE stress *ulcer.*

cur·rent (ker′rĕnt). A stream or flow of fluid, air, or electricity. [L. *currens,* pres. p. of *curro,* to run]

action c., an electrical c. induced in muscle fibers when they are effectively stimulated; normally it is followed by contraction.

after-c., SEE aftercurrent.

alternating c. (AC), a c. that flows first in one direction then in the other; e.g., 60-cycle c.

anodal c., a c. produced in tissues under the anode when the circuit is closed.

ascending c., the direction of c. flow in a nerve when the anode is placed peripheral to the cathode, in contrast to descending c.; the convention used is that c. flows from positive to negative. SYN centripetal c.

axial c., the central rapidly moving portion of the bloodstream in an artery.

centrifugal c., SYN descending c.

centripetal c., SYN ascending c.

d'Arsonval c., SYN high-frequency c.

demarcation c., SYN c. of injury.

descending c., the direction of c. flow in a nerve when the cathode is placed peripheral to the anode, in contrast to ascending c. SYN centrifugal c.

direct c. (DC), a c. that flows only in one direction; e.g., that derived from a battery; sometimes referred to as galvanic c. SEE ALSO galvanism.

electrotonic c., SEE electrotonus.

galvanic c., SEE direct c., galvanism (1).

high-frequency c., an alternating electric c. having a frequency of 10,000 or more cycles per second; it produces no muscular contractions and does not affect the sensory nerves. SYN d'Arsonval c., Tesla c.

c. of injury, the c. generated when an injured part of a nerve, muscle, or other excitable tissue is connected through a conductor with the uninjured region; the injured tissue is negative to the uninjured. SYN demarcation c.

labile c., an electrical c. applied to the body by means of electrodes that are constantly shifted about.

Tesla c., SYN high-frequency c.

Curschmann, Heinrich, German physician, 1846–1910. SEE C. *spirals*, under *spiral*.

curse (kers). An affliction thought to be invoked by a malevolent spirit.

Ondine c., idiopathic central alveolar hypoventilation in which involuntary control of respiration is depressed, but voluntary control of ventilation is not impaired. [*Ondine,* char. in play by J. Giraudoux, based on Undine, Ger. myth. char.]

Curtis, Arthur H., U.S. gynecologist, 1881–1955. SEE Fitz-Hugh and C. *syndrome.*

cur·va·tu·ra, pl. **cur·va·tu·rae** (ker′vă-too′ră, -too′rē). SYN curvature. [L.]

c. primaria columnae vertebralis [TA], SYN primary *curvature* of vertebral column.

curvaturae secondariae columnae vertebralis [TA], SYN secondary *curvatures* of vertebral column, under *curvature.*

c. ventric′uli ma′jor [TA], SYN greater *curvature* of stomach.

c. ventric′uli mi′nor [TA], SYN lesser *curvature* of stomach.

cur·va·ture (ker′vă-choor). A bending or flexure. SEE angulation. SYN curvatura. [L. *curvatura,* fr. *curvo,* pp. *-atus,* to bend, curve]

angular c., a gibbous deformity, i.e., a sharp angulation of the spine, occurring in Pott disease. SYN Pott c.

anterior c., c. in which a more distal or cephalad part is deviated anteriorly with respect to the coronal anatomic plane.

backward c., c. in which a more distal or cephalad part is deviated posteriorly with respect to the coronal anatomic plane. SYN posterior c.

gingival c., the rounding of the gum along its line of attachment to the neck of a tooth.

greater c. of stomach [TA], the border of the stomach to which the greater omentum is attached. SYN curvatura ventriculi major [TA].

lateral c., c. in which a more distal part is deviated away from the anatomic sagittal plane, producing valgus alignment.

lesser c. of stomach [TA], the right border of the stomach to which the lesser omentum is attached. SYN curvatura ventriculi minor [TA].

occlusal c., SYN *curve* of occlusion.

posterior c., SYN backward c.

Pott c., SYN angular c.

primary c. of vertebral column [TA], the ventrally concave curve of the fetal vertebral column, retained in the thoracic and sacral regions as the thoracic and sacral kyphoses. SEE ALSO kyphosis. SYN curvatura primaria columnae vertebralis [TA].

secondary c.'s of vertebral column [TA], ventrally convex curves of the vertebral column that develop postnatally in the cervical and lumbar regions: the cervical and lumbar lordoses. SEE

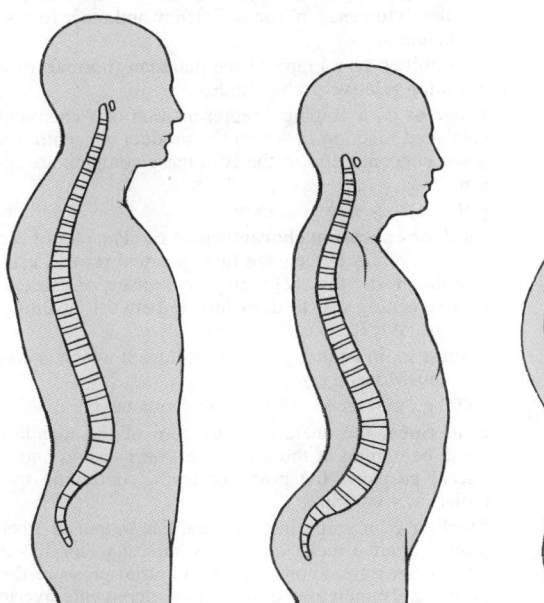
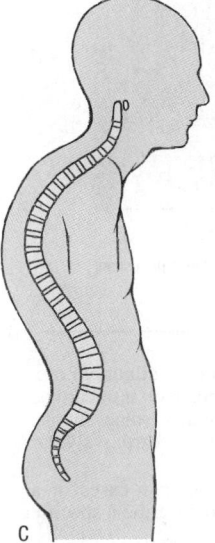
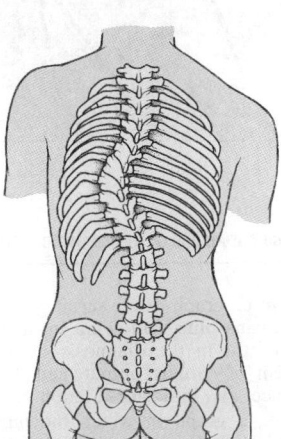

spinal curvatures: (A) normal, (B) lordosis, (C) kyphosis, (D) scoliosis

ALSO lordosis. SYN curvaturae secondariae columnae vertebralis [TA].

spinal c., SEE kyphosis, lordosis, scoliosis.

curve (kerv). **1.** A nonangular continuous bend or line. **2.** A chart or graphic representation, by means of a continuous line connecting individual observations, of the course of a physiologic activity, of the number of cases of a disease in a given period, or of any entity that might be otherwise presented by a table of figures. SYN chart (2). [L. *curvo,* to bend]

active length-tension c., the relationship between active isometric tension and preload (rest length) for a contracting muscle.

alignment c., the line passing through the center of the teeth laterally in the direction of the c. of the dental arch.

anti-Monson c., SYN reverse c.

Barnes c., a c. corresponding in general with Carus c., being the segment of a circle whose center is the promontory of the sacrum.

buccal c., the line of the dental arch from the canine, or cuspid tooth to the third molar.

calibration c., the graphic or mathematic relationship between the readings obtained in an analytic process and the quantity of analyte in a calibration. The relationship is often a straight line rather than a c.

Carus c., an imaginary curved line obtained from a mathematical formula, supposed to indicate the outlet of the pelvic canal. SYN Carus circle.

cephalic c., c. conforming to that of the fetal head, used in reference to the shape of obstetrical forceps.

characteristic c., sensitometric c. of radiographic film, a plot of the film density versus the logarithm of the relative exposure. SYN H and D c., Hunter and Driffield c.

compensating c., the anteroposterior and lateral curvature in the alignment of the occluding surfaces and incisal edges of artificial teeth; used to develop balanced occlusion.

distribution c., a systematic grouping of data into classes or categories according to the frequency of occurrence of each successive value or ranges of such values, resulting in a graph of a frequency distribution. SYN frequency c.

dose-response c., a graph showing the relationship between the dose of a drug, infectious agent, etc. and the biological response.

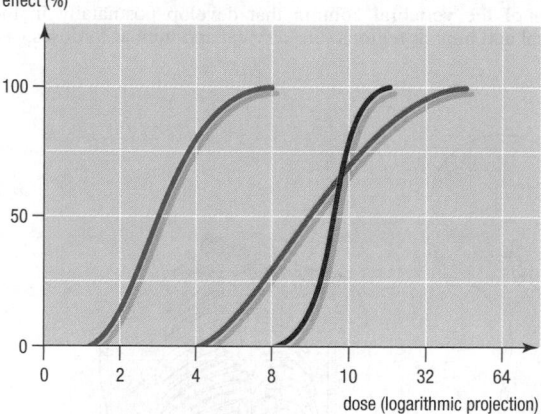

effect (%)

dose response curve: one of several expressions

dye-dilution c., graph of the serial concentrations (dilutions) of a dye, e.g., Evans blue, following its intravascular or intracardiac injection; useful in the diagnosis of congenital cardiac shunts, measurement of cardiac output, and detection of cardiovalvular incompetence. SYN indicator-dilution c.

epidemic c., a graph in which the number of new cases of a disease is plotted against an interval of time to describe a specific epidemic or outbreak.

flow-volume c., the graph produced by plotting the instantaneous flow of respiratory gas against the simultaneous lung volume, usually during maximal forced expiration.

force-velocity c., the relationship between isotonic velocity of shortening and afterload for a contracting muscle.

Frank-Starling c., SYN Starling c.

frequency c., SYN distribution c.

Friedman c., SYN partogram.

gaussian c., SYN normal *distribution.*

growth c., a graphic representation of the change in size of an individual or a population over a period of time.

H and D c., SYN characteristic c.

Heidelberger c., SYN precipitation c.

Hunter and Driffield c., SYN characteristic c.

indicator-dilution c., SYN dye-dilution c.

intracardiac pressure c., c. of pressure recorded within the atrium or ventricle (intra-atrial and intraventricular pressure c.'s).

isovolume pressure-flow c., the relationship between transpulmonary pressure and respiratory air flow, expressed as a function of lung volume.

labor c., SYN partogram.

logistic c., an S-shaped c. which depicts the growth of a population in an area of fixed limits.

milled-in c.'s, SYN milled-in *paths,* under *path.*

Monson c., the c. of occlusion in which each cusp and incisal edge touches or conforms to a segment of the surface of a sphere 8 inches in diameter with its center in the region of the glabella.

muscle c., SYN myogram.

c. of occlusion, (1) a curved surface which makes simultaneous contact with the major portion of the incisal and occlusal prominences of the existing teeth; **(2)** the c. of a dentition on which the occlusal surfaces lie. SYN occlusal curvature.

passive length-tension c., the relationship between passive tension and preload (rest length) for a muscle at rest.

Pleasure c., a c. of occlusion which when viewed in sagittal section conforms to a line that is convex upward except for the last molars.

precipitation c., a graph of the quantity of precipitate formed as a function of the quantity of antigen added during the titration of an antibody with an antigen. SYN Heidelberger c.

Price-Jones c., a distribution c. of the measured diameters of red blood cells; it is to the right of the normal c. (i.e., indicating larger diameters) in instances of pernicious anemia and other forms in which macrocytes are present, and to the left (i.e., indicating smaller diameters) in iron deficiency and other forms of microcytic anemia.

probability c., a graph of the gaussian (normal) distribution representing relative probabilities.

progress c., a graphical representation of a chemical or enzyme-catalyzed reaction in which the product concentration or the substrate concentration or the ES binary complex are plotted against time.

pulse c., SYN sphygmogram.

receiver operating characteristic c., (1) a plot of percentage true positive versus percentage false positive results, usually in a trial of a diagnostic test. **(2)** a graphical means of assessing the ability of a screening test to discriminate between healthy and diseased persons. SYN ROC c.

reverse c., in dentistry, a c. of occlusion which is convex upward. SYN anti-Monson c.

ROC c., SYN receiver operating characteristic c.

c. of Spee, the anatomic curvature of the mandibular occlusal plane beginning at the tip of the lower cuspid and following the buccal cusps of the posterior teeth, continuing to the terminal molar. SYN von Spee c.

Starling c., a graph in which cardiac output or stroke volume is plotted against mean atrial or ventricular end-diastolic pressure; with increasing venous return and atrial pressure the output proportionately increases until further increments overload the heart and the output falls. SYN Frank-Starling c.

strength-duration c., a graph relating the intensity of an electrical stimulus to the length of time it must flow to be effective. SEE chronaxie, rheobase.

stress-strain c., a c. showing the ratio of deformation to load during the testing of a material in tension.

tension c., the direction of the trabeculae in cancellous bone tissue that forms as an adaptation to resist stress.

Traube-Hering c.'s, slow oscillations in blood pressure usually extending over several respiratory cycles; related to variations in vasomotor tone; rhythmical variations in blood pressure. SYN Traube-Hering waves.

tuning c., a graph of acoustic threshold intensity at various frequencies for a single neuron.

volume-time c., volume of an expelled breath plotted against time. This is the basic c. generated by so-called "simple spirometry."

von Spee c., SYN c. of Spee.

whole-body titration c., a graphic representation of the in vivo changes in hydrogen ion, Pa_{CO_2}, and bicarbonate which occur in arterial blood in response to primary acid-base disturbances.

Cur·vu·la·ria (ker-vū-lā′rē-ă). A genus of dark-colored fungi that grow rapidly on culture media. Generally regarded as contaminants, two species, *C. lunata* and *C. geniculata*, are among the species capable of producing mycetoma in humans, keratomycosis, sinusitis, and phaeohyphomycosis.

Cushing, Hayward W., U.S. surgeon, 1854–1934. SEE C. *suture.*

Cushing, Harvey W., U.S. neurosurgeon, 1869–1939. SEE C. *basophilism, disease, syndrome, syndrome medicamentosus, effect, phenomenon, response,* pituitary *basophilism.*

cush·ing·oid (kush′ing-oyd). Resembling the signs and symptoms of Cushing disease or syndrome: moon facies, buffalo hump obesity, striations, adiposity, hypertension, diabetes, and osteoporosis, usually due to exogenous corticosteroids.

cush·ion (kush′ŭn). In anatomy, any structure resembling a pad or c.

anal c.'s, vascular prominences formed by clusters of normally sacculated veins of the superior rectal venous plexus, fed by arteriovenous anastomoses that cause their engorgement, and which are usually found to lie laterally on the left and antero- and posterolaterally on the right side of the anal canal. SYN cavernous bodies of anal canal, corpora cavernosa recti, hemorrhoidal c.'s, threshold pads of anal canal.

atrioventricular canal c.'s, a pair of mounds of embryonic connective tissue covered by endothelium, bulging into the embryonic atrioventricular canal; located one dorsally and one ventrally, they grow together and fuse with each other and with the lower edge of the septum primum, dividing the originally single canal into right and left atrioventricular orifices. SYN endocardial c.'s.

endocardial c.'s, SYN atrioventricular canal c.'s.

c. of epiglottis, SYN epiglottic *tubercle.*

eustachian c., SYN *torus* tubarius.

hemorrhoidal c.'s, SYN anal c.'s.

levator c., SYN *torus* levatorius.

Passavant c., SYN Passavant *ridge.*

pharyngoesophageal c.'s, venous plexuses on the anterior and posterior walls of the pharyngoesophageal junction. SYN pharyngoesophageal pads.

sucking c., SYN buccal *fat-pad.*

cusp (kŭsp) [TA]. **1.** In dentistry, a conical elevation arising on the surface of a tooth from an independent calcification center. SEE ALSO dental *tubercle.* **2.** A leaflet of one of the heart's valves. SYN cuspis [TA]. [L. *cuspis,* point]

anterior c. of left atrioventricular valve, ☆official alternate term for anterior c. of mitral valve.

anterior c. of mitral valve [TA], the ventrally placed and larger of the two leaflets that come together during ventricular systole to close the left atrioventricular orifice; it attaches to the septal aspect of the orifice. SYN cuspis anterior valvae atrioventricularis sinistrae [TA], anterior c. of left atrioventricular valve☆, cuspis anterior valvae mitralis☆.

anterior c. of right atrioventricular valve, ☆official alternate term for anterior c. of tricuspid valve.

anterior c. of tricuspid valve [TA], the largest and most ventrally placed of the three leaflets that come together during ven-

tricular systole to close the right atrioventricular orifice. SYN cuspis anterior valvae atrioventricularis dextrae [TA], anterior c. of right atrioventricular valve☆, cuspis anterior valvae tricuspidalis☆.

c. of Carabelli, a fifth c. found on the maxillary first molars, usually located lingual to the mesiolingual c.

posterior c. of left atrioventricular valve, ☆official alternate term for posterior c. of mitral valve.

posterior c. of mitral valve [TA], the dorsally placed and smaller of the two leaflets that come together during ventricular systole to close the left atrioventricular orifice; it attaches to the mural aspect of the orifice. SYN cuspis posterior valvae atrioventricularis sinistrae [TA], cuspis posterior valvae mitralis☆, posterior c. of left atrioventricular valve☆.

posterior c. of right atrioventricular valve, ☆official alternate term for posterior c. of tricuspid valve.

posterior c. of tricuspid valve [TA], the medium-sized and most dorsally placed of the three leaflets that come together during ventricular systole to close the right atrioventricular orifice. SYN cuspis posterior valvae atrioventricularis dextrae [TA], cuspis posterior valvae tricuspidalis☆, posterior c. of right atrioventricular valve☆.

semilunar c., one of the three semilunar segments serving as the three c.'s of a valve preventing regurgitation at the beginning of the aorta; a similar valve guards the entrance of the pulmonary trunk; the segments are named, respectively, anterior, right, and left in the pulmonary valve, and posterior, right, and left in the aortic valve.

septal c. of right atrioventricular valve, ☆official alternate term for septal c. of tricuspid valve.

septal c. of tricuspid valve [TA], the leaflet of the tricuspid valve located adjacent to the interventricular septum. SYN cuspis septalis valvae atrioventricularis dextrae [TA], cuspis septalis valvae tricuspidalis☆, septal c. of right atrioventricular valve☆.

talon c., an anomalous c. that projects lingually from the cingulum of permanent incisors. [Eng. claw, heel, fr. O.Fr., fr. L. *talus,* ankle]

c. of tooth [TA], an elevation or mound on the crown of a tooth making up a part of the occlusal surface. SYN cuspis dentis [TA], cuspis coronae.

cus·pad (kŭs′păd). In a direction toward the cusp of a tooth. [L. *ad,* to]

cus·pal (kŭs′păl). Pertaining to a cusp.

cus·pid (kŭs′pid). **1.** Having but one cusp. SYN cuspidate. **2.** SYN canine *tooth.* [L. *cuspis,* point]

cus·pi·date (kŭs′pi-dāt). SYN cuspid (1).

cus·pis, pl. **cus·pi·des** (kŭs′pis, kŭs′pi-dēz) [TA]. SYN cusp. [L. a point]

c. anterior valvae atrioventricularis dextrae [TA], SYN anterior *cusp* of tricuspid valve.

c. anterior valvae atrioventricularis sinistrae [TA], SYN anterior *cusp* of mitral valve.

c. anterior valvae mitralis, ☆official alternate term for anterior *cusp* of mitral valve.

c. anterior valvae tricuspidalis, ☆official alternate term for anterior *cusp* of tricuspid valve.

c. coro′nae, SYN *cusp* of tooth, *cusp* of tooth.

c. den′tis [TA], SYN *cusp* of tooth.

c. posterior valvae atrioventricularis dextrae [TA], SYN posterior *cusp* of tricuspid valve.

c. posterior valvae atrioventricularis sinistrae [TA], SYN posterior *cusp* of mitral valve.

c. posterior valvae mitralis, ☆official alternate term for posterior *cusp* of mitral valve.

c. posterior valvae tricuspidalis, ☆official alternate term for posterior *cusp* of tricuspid valve.

c. septa′lis val′vae atrioventricula′ris dex′trae [TA], SYN septal *cusp* of tricuspid valve.

c. septalis valvae tricuspidalis, ☆official alternate term for septal *cusp* of tricuspid valve.

cu

cu·sum (koo′sum). Acronym for cumulative sum of a series of measurements; used primarily in Great Britain.

cut (kŭt). **1.** In molecular biology, a hydrolytic cleavage of two opposing phosphodiester bonds in a double-stranded nucleic acid. Cf. nick. **2.** To sever or divide. **3.** To separate into fractions. **4.** An informal term for a fraction.

cu·ta·ne·o·mu·co·sal (kū-tā′nē-ō-mū-kō′săl). SYN mucocutaneous.

cu·ta·ne·ous (kū-tā′nē-ŭs). Relating to the skin. [L. *cutis,* skin]

cutch (kŭtch). SYN catechu nigrum.

cut·down (kŭt′down). Dissection of a vein or artery for insertion of a cannula or needle for the administration of intravenous fluids or medication or for measurement of pressure. SYN venostomy.

Cu·te·reb·ra (kū-te-rē′bră). A genus of botflies with large blue or black bumble-bee-like adults, whose larvae most commonly infest rodents and lagomorphs (hares and rabbits); the larvae develop into large spiny grubs, usually in the subcutaneous connective tissue of the neck. Similar grubs, probably of other species, are not uncommon in cats and are sometimes found in dogs and in humans. [L. *cutis,* skin, + *terebro,* to bore, fr. *terebra,* an auger]

cu·ti·cle (kū′ti-kl). **1.** An outer thin layer, usually horny in nature. SYN cuticula (1). **2.** The layer, chitinous in some invertebrates, which occurs on the surface of epithelial cells. **3.** SYN epidermis. [L. *cuticula,* dim. of *cutis,* skin]

acquired c., acquired enamel c., SYN acquired *pellicle.*

dental c., SYN enamel c.

enamel c., the primary enamel cuticle, consisting of two extremely thin layers (the inner one clear and structureless, the outer one cellular), covering the entire crown of newly erupted teeth and subsequently abraded by mastication; it is evident microscopically as an amorphous material between the attachment epithelium and the tooth. SYN adamantine membrane, cuticula dentis, dental c., membrana adamantina, Nasmyth c., Nasmyth membrane, skin of teeth.

c. of hair, SYN *cuticula* pili.

c. of nail, the exposed distal prolongation of the corneal layer of the deep surface of the proximal nail fold (eponychium (2)), seen as a thin "skin" overlapping and adherent to the body of the nail at its proximal portion (the area of the lunula). It is formed as a remnant of the eponychium (1) which otherwise degenerates by the eighth month of pregnancy.

Nasmyth c., SYN enamel c.

posteruption c., SYN acquired *pellicle.*

c. of root sheath, SYN *cuticula* vaginae folliculi pili.

cu·tic·u·la, pl. **cu·tic·u·lae** (kū-tik′ū-lă, -lē). **1** [NA]. SYN cuticle (1). **2.** SYN epidermis. [L. cuticle]

c. 2,

c. den′tis, SYN enamel *cuticle.*

c. pi′li, a layer of overlapping shinglelike cells that invest the hair cortex and serve to enclose the cortical cells of the hair and lock the hair shaft in its follicle. SYN cuticle of hair.

c. vagi′nae follic′uli pi′li, cuticle of overlapping shinglelike cells lining the follicle of the hair. SYN cuticle of root sheath.

cu·tin (kū′tin). A specially prepared, thin, animal membrane used as a protective covering for wounded surfaces. [L. *cutis,* skin]

cu·tis (kū′tis) [TA]. SYN skin. [L.]

c. anseri′na, contraction of the arrectores pilorum produced by cold, fear, or other stimulus, causing the follicular orifices to become prominent. SYN goose flesh, gooseflesh.

c. lax′a [MIM*123700], SYN dermatochalasis.

c. marmora′ta, a normal, physiologic, pink, marblelike mottling of the skin in infants, persisting abnormally in some children on exposure to cold.

c. marmorata telangiectatica congenita, capillary-venous cutaneous malformation with "marbled" appearance. SYN Van Lohuizen syndrome.

c. rhomboida′lis nu′chae, geometric furrowed configurations of the skin of the back of the neck as a result of prolonged exposure to sunlight with solar elastosis.

c. ve′ra, SYN dermis.

c. ver′ticis gyra′ta, a congenital condition in which the skin of the scalp is hypertrophied and thrown into folds forming anterior to posterior furrows; it may be a component of pachydermoperiostosis.

cu·ti·za·tion (kū-ti-zā′shŭn). The transition from mucous membrane to skin at the mucocutaneous margins.

cutpoint (kut′poynt). Arbitrary value on an ordinal scale such as blood pressure, beyond which values are regarded as clinically abnormal.

cu·vet, cu·vette (koo-vet′). A small container or cup in which solutions are placed for photometric analysis.

Cuvier, Baron Georges L.C.F.D. de la, French scientist, 1769–1832. SEE C. *ducts,* under *duct, veins,* under *vein.*

CV Abbreviation for *coefficient* of variation; cardiovascular; closing *volume.*

CVA Abbreviation for cerebrovascular *accident.*

CVP Abbreviation for central venous *pressure.*

CX Abbreviation for *phosgene* oxime.

CxT Abbreviation for concentration × time. SEE AUC.

△**cyan-.** SEE cyano-.

cy·an·al·co·hols (sī-an-al′kō-holz). SYN cyanohydrins.

cy·an·a·mide (sī-an′i-mīd). An irritating and caustic water-soluble substance, H_2NCN or $HN=C=NH$; often used in referring to calcium cyanamide.

cy·a·nate (sī′an-āt). The radical $-O-C≡N$ or ion $(CNO)^-$.

cy·a·ne·mia (sī-a-ne′mē-ă). Obsolete term for cyanosis. [cyan- + G. *haima,* blood]

cy·a·nide (sī′an-īd). **1.** The radical $-CN$ or ion $(CN)^-$. The ion is extremely poisonous, forming hydrocyanic acid in water, it has the odor of almond oil; inhibits respiratory proteins (cytochromes) at the cellular level. **2.** A salt of HCN or a cyano-containing molecule.

c. methemoglobin, SYN cyanmethemoglobin.

cy·a·nid·e·non (sī-ă-nid′ĕ-non). SYN luteolin.

cy·an·i·dol (sī′an-i-dol). SYN catechin.

cy·an·met·he·mo·glo·bin (sī′an-met-hē′mō-glō-bin). A relatively nontoxic compound of cyanide with methemoglobin, which is formed when methylene blue is administered in cases of cyanide poisoning. SYN cyanide methemoglobin.

△**cyano-, cyan-.** **1.** Combining form meaning blue. **2.** Chemical prefix frequently used in naming compounds that contain the cyanide group, CN. [G. *kyanos,* a dark blue substance]

Cy·a·no·bac·te·ria (sī′ă-nō-bak-tēr′ē-ă). A division of the kingdom Prokaryotae consisting of unicellular or filamentous bacteria that are either nonmotile or possess a gliding motility, reproduce by binary fission, and perform photosynthesis with the production of oxygen. These blue-green bacteria were formerly referred to as blue-green algae. SYN Cyanophyceae.

cy·a·no·chro·ic, cy·an·och·rous (sī-an-ō-krō′ik, sī-an-ok′rŭs). SYN cyanotic. [cyano- + G. *chroia,* color]

cy·a·no·co·bal·a·min (sī′an-ō-kō-bal′ă-min). A complex of cyanide and cobalamin, as in vitamin B_{12}, in which a cyanide group has filled the sixth coordinate position of the cobalt atom.

radioactive c., cyano[^{57}Co]cobalamin, cyano[^{58}Co]cobalamin, or cyano[^{60}Co]cobalamin produced by the growth of certain microorganisms on a medium containing cobalt-57, cobalt-58, or cobalt-60; used in the investigation of the absorption and metabolism of cyanocobalamin (vitamin B_{12}).

cy·an·o·gen (sī-an′ō-jen). **1.** A compound of two cyano radicals, NC–CN. **2.** Highly toxic compounds (general formula X–CN, where X is a halogen) that are used in chemical syntheses and as tissue preservatives. An example is c. bromide.

c. chloride, CNCl; a highly volatile liquid; a systemic poison used as a warning agent in fumigation with hydrogen cyanide.

cy·a·no·gen·ic (sī′an-ō-jen′ik). Capable of producing hydrocyanic acid; said of plants such as sorghum, Johnson grass, arrowgrass, and wild cherry which may cause cyanide poisoning in herbivorous animals.

cy·a·no·hy·drins (sī′an-ō-hī′drinz). R–CHOH–CN; addition compounds of HCN and aldehydes. SYN cyanalcohols.

cy·an·o·phil, cy·an·o·phile (sī'an-ō-fil, -fil). A cell or element that is differentially colored blue by a staining procedure. [cyano- + G. *philos,* fond]

cy·a·noph·i·lous (sī-ă-nof'i-lŭs). Readily stainable with a blue dye.

Cy·a·no·phy·ce·ae (sī'ă-nō-fī'sē-ē). SYN Cyanobacteria. [cyano- + G. *phykos,* seaweed]

cy·a·no·pia (sī-ă-nō'pē-ă). SYN cyanopsia.

cy·a·nop·sia (sī-ă-nop'sē-ă). A condition in which all objects appear blue; may temporarily follow cataract extraction. SYN blue vision, cyanopia. [cyano- + G. *opsis,* vision]

cy·a·nosed (sī'ă-nōst). SYN cyanotic.

cy·a·no·sis (sī-ă-nō'sis). A dark bluish or purplish discoloration of the skin and mucous membrane due to deficient oxygenation of the blood, evident when reduced hemoglobin in the blood exceeds 5 g/100 ml. [G. dark blue color, fr. *kyanos,* blue substance]

compression c., c. accompanied by edema and petechial hemorrhages over the head, neck, and upper part of the chest, as a venous reflex resulting from severe compression of the thorax or abdomen; the conjunctiva and retinas are similarly affected.

enterogenous c., apparent c. caused by the absorption of nitrites or other toxic materials from the intestine with the formation of methemoglobin or sulfhemoglobin; the skin color change is due to the chocolate color of methemoglobin.

false c., c. due to the presence of an abnormal pigment, such as methemoglobin, in the blood, and not resulting from a deficiency of oxygen.

hereditary methemoglobinemic c., SYN congenital *methemoglobinemia.*

late c., c. due to right to left shunt in congenital heart disease appearing only after cardiac failure. SYN cyanose tardive, tardive c.

c. ret'inae, venous congestion of the retina.

shunt c., any blue color of the entire skin or a region of the skin or mucous membrane due to a right to left shunt permitting unoxygenated blood to reach the left side of the circulation.

tardive c., SYN late c.

toxic c., c. due to methemoglobin formation resulting from the action of certain drugs, e.g., nitrites.

cy·a·not·ic (sī-ă-not'ik). Relating to or marked by cyanosis. SYN cyanochroic, cyanochrous, cyanosed.

cy·a·nu·ria (sī-ă-noo'rē-ă). The presence of blue urine. [cyano- + G. *ouron,* urine]

cy·a·nu·ric ac·id (sī-ă-noor'ik). A cyclic product formed by heating urea; used industrially and as an herbicide.

Cy·a·tho·sto·ma (sī-ă-thos'tō-mă). A genus of gapeworms of poultry in the nematode family Syngamidae, so called because of the gaping habit of fowl infected by these worms in their upper respiratory tract. [G. *kyathos,* cup, cup-shaped, + *stoma,* mouth]

C. bronchia'lis, a species found in wild geese and domestic ducks, geese, and swans; occurs in the larynx, trachea, and bronchi and causes distress and symptoms similar to those produced by the chicken gapeworm, *Syngamus trachea;* its life cycle is thought to be similar to that of *Syngamus trachea.*

Cy·a·tho·sto·mum (sī-ă-thos'tō-mŭm). A genus of strongyle nematodes (family Cyasthostomidae, formerly part of the family Strongylidae); it includes many of the small strongyles of horses formerly placed in the genus *Trichonema,* which have been variously divided into a number of genera and subgenera. [see *Cyathostoma*]

cy·ber·net·ics (sī-ber-net'iks). **1.** The comparative study of computers and the human nervous system, with intent to explain the functioning of the brain. **2.** The science of control and communication in both living and nonliving systems; characteristically, control is governed by feedback, that is, by communication within the system concerning the difference between the actual and the desired result, action then being modified so as to minimize this

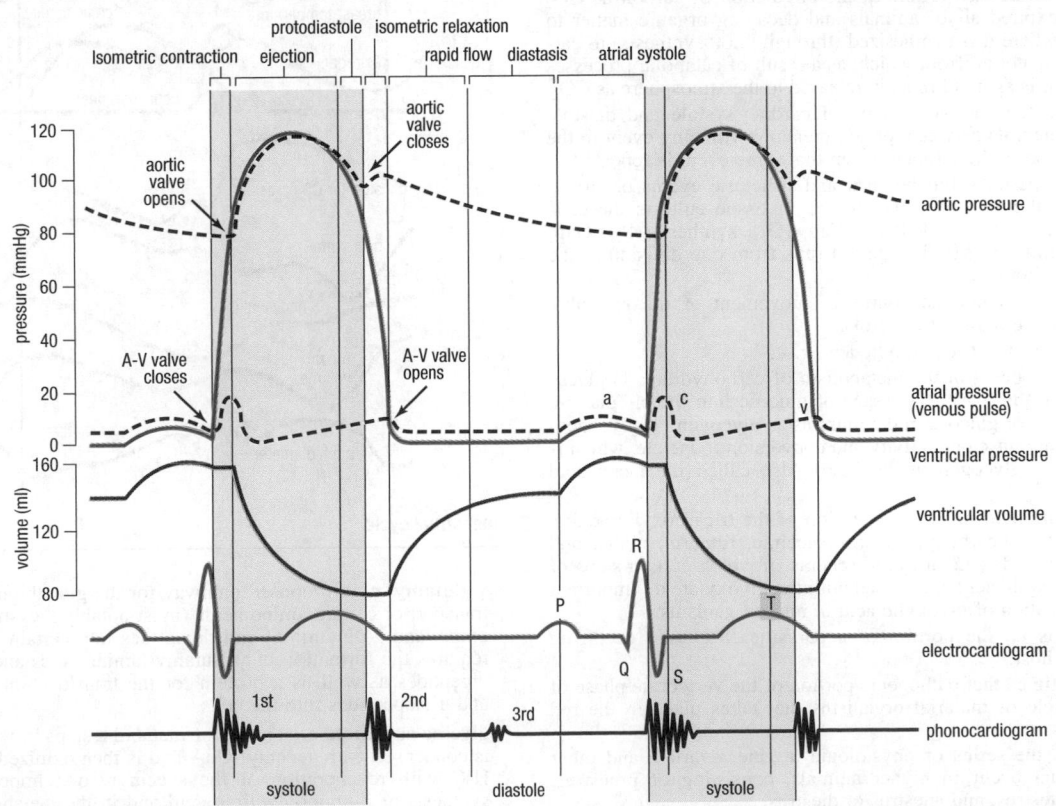

cardiac cycle: showing changes in heart pressures and volumes, electrocardiogram, and phonocardiogram; A–V, atrioventricular difference. SEE ALSO feedback. [G. *kybernētica,* things pertaining to control or piloting]

cy·brid (sī′brid). A cell with cytoplasm from two different cells as a result of cell hybridization. [cell + hybrid]

△**cycl-.** SEE cyclo-.

cy·cla·mate (sī′klă-māt). A salt or ester of cyclamic acid; the calcium and sodium are noncaloric artificial sweetening agents.

cy·clam·ic ac·id (sī-klam′ik). A sweetening agent, usually used as sodium or calcium cyclamate. SYN cyclohexanesulfamic acid, cyclohexylsulfamic acid.

cy·cla·mide (sī′klă-mīd). SYN glycyclamide.

cy·clan·de·late (sī-klan′de-lāt). An antispasmodic similar in action to papaverine; used for obliterative vascular diseases and vasospastic conditions.

cy·clar·thro·di·al (sī-klar-thrō′dē-ăl). Relating to a cyclarthrosis.

cy·clar·thro·sis (sī-klar-thrō′sis). A joint capable of rotation. [cyclo- + G. *arthrōsis,* articulation]

cy·clase (sī′klās). Descriptive name applied to an enzyme that forms a cyclic compound; e.g., adenylate cyclase.

CYCLE

cy·cle (sī′kl). **1.** A recurrent series of events. **2.** A recurring period of time. **3.** One successive compression and rarefaction of a wave, as of a sound wave. [G. *kyklos,* circle]

anovulatory c., a sexual c. in which no ovum is discharged.

brain wave c., the complete upward and downward excursion of a single wave, complex, or impulse as seen on an electroencephalogram.

carbon dioxide c., carbon c., the circulation of carbon as CO_2 from the expired air of animals and decaying organic matter to plant life where it is synthesized (through photosynthesis) to carbohydrate material, from which, as a result of catabolic processes in all life, it is again ultimately released to the atmosphere as CO_2.

cardiac c., the complete round of cardiac systole and diastole with the intervals between, or commencing with, any event in the heart's action to the moment when that same event is repeated.

cell c., the periodic biochemical and structural events occurring during proliferation of cells such as in tissue culture; the c. is divided into phases called: G_0, Gap_1 (G_1), synthesis (S_1), Gap_2 (G_2), and mitosis (M). The period runs from one division to the next. SYN mitotic c.

chewing c., a complete course of movement of the mandible during a single masticatory stroke.

citric acid c., SYN tricarboxylic acid c.

Cori c., the phases in the metabolism of carbohydrate: 1) glycogenolysis in the liver; 2) passage of glucose into the circulation; 3) deposition of glucose in the muscles as glycogen; 4) glycogenolysis during muscular activity and conversion to lactate, which is converted to glycogen in the liver. Also called the lactic acid cycle.

dicarboxylic acid c., (1) that portion of the tricarboxylic acid c. involving the dicarboxylic acids (succinic, fumaric, malic, and oxaloacetic acids); **(2)** a cyclic scheme in which certain steps of the tricarboxylic acid c. are used with the glyoxylate c.; important in the utilization of glyoxylic acid in microorganisms.

endogenous c., the portion of a parasitic life cycle occurring within the host.

erythrocytic c., that pathogenic portion of the vertebrate phase of the life cycle of malarial organisms that takes place in the red blood cells.

estrous c., the series of physiologic uterine, ovarian, and other changes that occur in higher animals, consisting of proestrus, estrus, postestrus, and anestrus or diestrus.

exoerythrocytic c., that nonpathogenic portion of the vertebrate phase of the life cycle of malarial organisms that takes place in liver cells, outside of the blood cells.

exogenous c., the portion of a parasitic life cycle occurring outside the host.

fatty acid oxidation c., a series of reactions involving acyl-coenzyme A compounds, whereby these undergo beta oxidation and thioclastic cleavage, with the formation of acetyl-coenzyme A; the major pathway of fatty acid catabolism in living tissue.

forced c., a cardiac c. (atrial or ventricular) that is cut short by a forced beat.

futile c., a c. of phosphorylation and dephosphorylation catalyzed by two enzymes which normally function in two different metabolic pathways; the net effect is the hydrolysis of ATP and the generation of heat; e.g., the futile c. from the unregulated action of 6-phosphofructokinase and fructose-1,6-bisphosphatase in muscle; such c.'s may have important roles in heat production, in the fine tuning of the regulation of certain pathways and may be a factor in malignant hyperthermia. SYN substrate c.

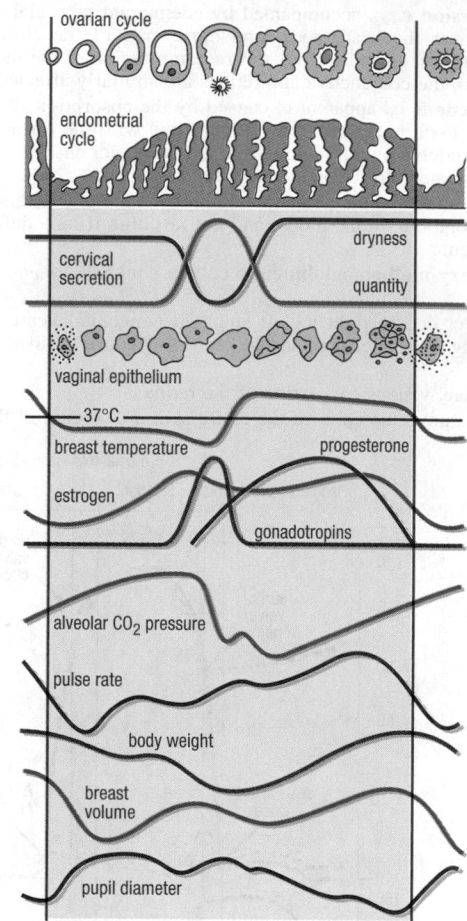

menstrual cycle

γ-glutamyl c., a proposed pathway for the glutathione-dependent transport of certain amino acids (most notably L-cystine, L-methionine, and L-glutamine) and dipeptides into certain cells; this c. requires the formation of γ-glutamyl amino acids and γ-glutamyl dipeptides as well as a protein for the translocation of these di- and triisopeptides into the cells.

glycine-succinate c., a series of metabolic steps in which glycine is condensed with succinyl-CoA and is then oxidized to CO_2 and H_2O with regeneration of the succinyl-CoA; important in the synthesis of δ-aminolevulinic acid and in the metabolism of red blood cells. SYN Shemin c.

glyoxylic acid c., a catabolic c. in plants and microorganisms like that of the tricarboxylic acid c. in animals; its key reaction is the condensation of acetyl-CoA with glyoxylic acid to malic acid (analogous to the condensation of acetyl-CoA and oxaloacetic acid to form citric acid in the tricarboxylic acid c.). SYN Krebs-Kornberg c.

gonadotrophic c. (gō'nad-ō-trōf'ik), one complete round of ovarian development in the insect vector from the time when the blood meal is taken to the time when the fully developed eggs are laid.

hair c., the cyclical phases of growth (anagen), regression (catagen), and quiescence (telogen) in the life of a hair.

heterogonic life c., free-living stage of life c. of an organism (e.g., *Strongyloides stercoralis*) that also has a parasitic stage.

homogonic life c., parasitic stage of life cycle of an organism (e.g., *Strongyloides stercoralis*) that also has a free-living stage.

Krebs c., SYN tricarboxylic acid c.

Krebs-Henseleit c., Krebs ornithine c., Krebs urea c., SYN urea c.

Krebs-Kornberg c., SYN glyoxylic acid c.

life c., the entire life history of a living organism.

masticating c.'s, the patterns of mandibular movements formed during the chewing of food.

menstrual c., the period in which an ovum matures, is ovulated, and enters the uterine lumen via the fallopian tubes; ovarian hormonal secretions effect endometrial changes such that, if fertilization occurs, nidation will be possible; in the absence of fertilization, ovarian secretions wane, the endometrium sloughs, and menstruation begins; this c. lasts an average of 28 days, with day 1 of the c. designated as that day on which menstrual flow begins.

mitotic c., SYN cell c.

nitrogen c., the series of events in which the nitrogen of the atmosphere is fixed, thus made available for plant and animal life, and is then returned to the atmosphere: nitrifying bacteria convert N_2 and O_2 to NO_2^- and NO_3^-, the latter being absorbed by plants and converted to protein; if plants decay, the nitrogen is in part given up to the atmosphere and the remainder is converted by microorganisms to ammonia, nitrites, and nitrates; if the plants are eaten, the animals' excreta or bacterial decay return the nitrogen to the soil and air.

ornithine c., SYN urea c.

ovarian c., the normal sex c. which includes development of an ovarian (graafian) follicle, rupture of the follicle with discharge of the ovum, and formation and regression of a corpus luteum.

pentose phosphate c., SYN pentose phosphate *pathway*.

reproductive c., the c. which begins with conception and extends through gestation and parturition.

restored c., an atrial or ventricular cardiac c. that follows the returning c. and resumes the normal rhythm.

returning c., an atrial or ventricular cardiac c. that begins with an extrasystole or a forced beat.

Ross c., the life c. of the malaria parasite.

Shemin c., SYN glycine-succinate c.

substrate c., SYN futile c.

succinic acid c., a series of oxidation reduction reactions in which succinic acid and other acids containing four-carbon atoms (fumaric, malic, oxaloacetic) take part in the oxidation of pyruvic acid as part of the tricarboxylic acid c. SEE ALSO dicarboxylic acid c.

tricarboxylic acid c., together with oxidative phosphorylation, the main source of energy in the mammalian body and the end toward which carbohydrate, fat, and protein metabolism are directed; a series of reactions, beginning and ending with oxaloacetic acid, during the course of which a two-carbon fragment is completely oxidized to carbon dioxide and water with the production of 12 high-energy phosphate bonds. So called because the first four substances involved (citric acid, *cis*-aconitic acid, isocitric acid, and oxalosuccinic acid) are all tricarboxylic acids; from oxalosuccinate, the others are, in order, α-ketoglutarate, succinate, fumarate, L-malate, and oxaloacetate, which condenses with acetyl-CoA (from fatty acid degradation) to form citrate (citric acid) again. SYN citric acid c., Krebs c.

urea c., the sequence of chemical reactions, occurring primarily in the liver, that results in the production of urea; the key reaction is the hydrolysis of L-arginine by arginase to L-ornithine and urea;

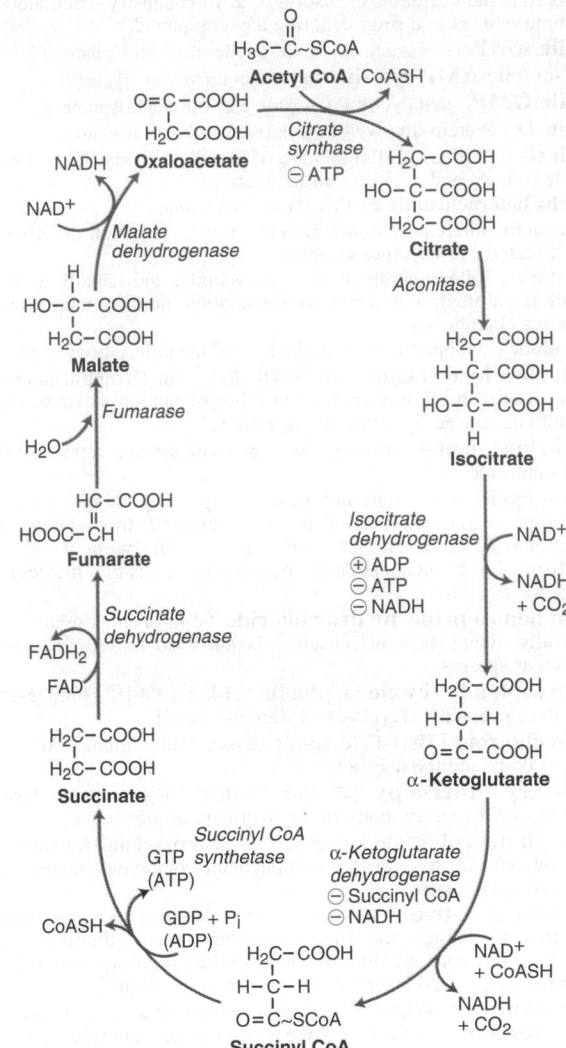

tricarboxylic acid cycle (citric acid cycle, Krebs cycle): + = activator, − = inhibitor, *italicized terms* = enzyme names, ~ = high-energy bonds

L-ornithine is then converted to L-citrulline by a carbamoylation reaction, then to L-argininosuccinate by an amination reaction involving L-aspartic acid, and finally there is a lyase-dependent step that generates arginine and fumarate. SYN Krebs-Henseleit c., Krebs ornithine c., Krebs urea c., ornithine c.

visual c., the transformation of carotenoids involved in the bleaching and regeneration of the visual pigment.

cy·clec·to·my (sī-klek'tō-mē, sik-lek'tō-mē). Excision of a portion of the ciliary body. SYN ciliectomy. [cyclo- + G. *ektomē*, excision]

cy·clen·ceph·a·ly, cy·clen·ce·pha·lia (sī-klen-sef'ă-lē, -se-fā'lē-ă). Condition in a malformed fetus characterized by poor development and a varying degree of fusion of the two cerebral hemispheres. SYN cyclocephaly, cyclocephalia. [cyclo- + G. *enkephalos*, brain]

cy·cles per sec·ond (cps). The number of successive compressions and rarefactions per second of a sound wave. The preferred designation for this unit of frequency is hertz.

cy·clic (sī'klik, sik'lik). 1. Pertaining to, or characteristic of, a cycle; occurring periodically, denoting the course of the symptoms in certain diseases or disorders. **2.** In chemistry, continuous, without end, as in a ring; denoting a c. compound.

cy·clic AMP. SYN adenosine 3′,5′-cyclic monophosphate.

3′,5′-cy·clic AMP syn·the·tase. SYN *adenylate* cyclase.

cy·clic GMP. SYN cyclic *guanosine* 3′,5′-monophosphate.

cyclin D. Protein involved in progression to cell division.

cy·cli·tis (sī-klī′tis). Inflammation of the ciliary body. [G. *kyklos,* circle (ciliary body), + *-itis,* inflammation]

Fuchs heterochromic c., SYN Fuchs *syndrome.*

heterochromic c., a chronic inflammatory c. in which the iris of the affected eye becomes atrophic.

plastic c., inflammation of the ciliary body, and usually of the entire uveal tract, with a fibrinous exudation into the anterior and vitreous chambers.

purulent c., suppurative inflammation of the ciliary body.

cy·cli·zine hy·dro·chlo·ride (sī′kli-zēn). An H₁ antihistamine agent useful in the prevention and relief of motion sickness and symptoms caused by vestibular disorders.

cy·cli·zine lac·tate. An agent with the same use and action as the hydrochloride.

⚘**cyclo-, cycl-. 1.** Combining forms relating to a circle or cycle; or denoting an association with the ciliary body. **2.** In chemistry, a combining form indicating a continuous molecule, without end, or the formation of such a structure between two parts of a molecule. [G. *kyklos,* circle]

cy·clo·ben·za·prine hy·dro·chlo·ride (sī-klō-ben′ză-prēn). A centrally acting skeletal muscle relaxant used to relieve acute muscular spasms.

cy·clo·ceph·a·ly, cy·clo·ce·pha·lia (sī-klō-sef′ă-lē, -sĕ-fā′lē-ă). SYN cyclencephaly. [cyclo- + G. *kephalē,* head]

cy·clo·cho·roid·i·tis (sī′klō-kō-roy-dī′tis). Inflammation of the ciliary body and the choroid.

cy·clo·cry·o·ther·a·py (sī′klō-krī′ō-thār′ă-pē). Transscleral freezing of the ciliary body in the treatment of glaucoma.

cy·clo·cu·ma·rol (sī-klō-kū′mă-rol). 4-Hydroxycoumarin anticoagulant No. 63; a synthetic anticoagulant compound, related to bishydroxycoumarin.

cy·clo·des·truc·tive (sī′klō-dis-truk′tiv). Relating to a procedure designed to damage the ciliary body in order to diminish the production of aqueous fluid in patients with glaucoma. SEE cyclocryotherapy, cyclodiathermy, cyclophotocoagulation.

cy·clo·di·al·y·sis (sī′klō-dī-al′i-sis). Establishment of a communication between the anterior chamber and the suprachoroidal space in order to reduce intraocular pressure in glaucoma. [cyclo- + G. *dialysis,* separation]

cy·clo·di·a·ther·my (sī′klō-dī-ă-ther′mē). Diathermy applied to the sclera adjacent to the ciliary body in the treatment of glaucoma.

cy·clo·duc·tion (sī-klō-dŭk′shŭn). Rotation of the eye around its visual axis. SYN circumduction (2) [TA], cyclotorsion. [cyclo- + L. *duco,* pp. *ductus,* to draw]

cy·clo·guan·il pam·o·ate (sī-klō-gwahn′il). A long-acting antimalarial agent that prevents the growth or survival of the pre-erythrocytic and erythrocytic parasites.

cy·clo·hex·ane·sul·fam·ic ac·id (sī-klō-heks′an-sŭl-fam′ik). SYN cyclamic acid.

cy·clo·hex·i·mide (sī-klō-heks′i-mīd). An antibiotic obtained from certain strains of *Streptomyces griseus;* used in biochemical research to inhibit in vitro protein synthesis; also a fungicide and rat repellent.

cy·clo·hex·yl·sul·fam·ic ac·id (sī-klō-hek′sil-sŭl-fam′ik). SYN cyclamic acid.

cy·cloid (sī′kloyd). Suggesting cyclothymia; a term applied to a person who tends to have periods of marked swings of mood, but within normal limits. [cyclo- + G. *eidos,* resembling]

cy·clol (sī′klol). A cyclic dipeptide postulated as occurring in proteins; it does occur in some of the ergot alkaloids.

cy·clo·na·mine (sī-klō-nā′mēn). SYN ethamsylate.

cy·clo·ox·y·gen·ase (sī′klō-oks′ē-jen-ās). SYN *prostaglandin* endoperoxide synthase.

cy·clo·pea (sī-klō′pē-ă). SYN cyclopia.

cy·clo·pe·an (sī-klō′pē-an). SYN cyclopian.

cy·clo·pent·a·mine hy·dro·chlo·ride (sī-klō-pent′ă-mēn). A sympathomimetic amine, similar in action to ephedrine.

cy·clo·pen·tane (sī-klō-pen′tān). A closed ring hydrocarbon containing five carbon atoms, isomeric with pentene.

cy·clo·pen·ta[*a*]phen·an·threne (sī-klō-pen-ta[ā]fen′ă-thrēn). Phenanthrene, to the *a* side of which a three-carbon fragment is fused; as the perhydro (saturated) derivative, it is the basic structure of the steroids.

cy·clo·pen·thi·a·zide (sī′klō-pen-thī′ă-zīd). A benzothiadiazide diuretic.

cy·clo·pen·to·late hy·dro·chlo·ride (sī-klō-pen′tō-lāt). An anticholinergic, spasmolytic drug, used in refraction determinations; causes cycloplegia and mydriasis; an atropinelike agent with brief duration of action.

cy·clo·pep·tide (sī-klō-pep′tīd). A polypeptide lacking terminal –NH₂ and –COOH groups by virtue of their combination to form another peptide link, forming a ring.

cy·clo·phen·a·zine hy·dro·chlo·ride (sī-klō-fen′ă-zēn). A tranquilizing drug.

cy·clo·pho·ras·es (sī-klō-fōr′ās-ez). The group of enzymes in mitochondria that catalyze the complete oxidation of pyruvic acid to carbon dioxide and water; essentially, those enzymes and coenzymes involved in the tricarboxylic acid cycle.

cy·clo·pho·ria (sī-klō-fō′rē-ă). Abnormal tendency for each eye to rotate around its anteroposterior axis, the rotation being prevented by visual fusional impulses. [cyclo- + G. *phora,* movement]

cy·clo·phos·pha·mide (sī-klō-fos′fă-mīd). An alkylating agent with antitumor activity and uses similar to those of its parent compound, nitrogen mustard (mechlorethamine hydrochloride); also a suppressor of B-cell activity and antibody formation, used to treat autoimmune diseases.

cy·clo·pho·to·co·ag·u·la·tion (sī′klō-fō′tō-kō-ag-ū-lā′shŭn). Photocoagulation of the ciliary processes to reduce the secretion of aqueous humor in glaucoma. [cyclo- + photocoagulation]

Cy·clo·phyl·li·dae (sī-klō-fil′i-dē). An order of tapeworms that includes most of the common parasites of humans and domestic animals. [cyclo- + G. *phyllon,* leaf]

cy·clo·pia (sī-klō′pē-ă). A congenital defect in which the two orbits are united to form a single cavity containing one eye, which typically results from union of the right and left optic primordia, usually combined with holoprosencephaly or cyclencephaly. SYN cyclopea, synophthalmia, synophthalmus. [G. *Kyklōps,* fr. *kyklos,* circle, + *ōps,* eye]

cy·clo·pi·an (sī-klō′pē-an). Denoting or relating to cyclopia. SYN cyclopean.

cy·clo·ple·gia (sī-klō-plē′jē-ă). Loss of power in the ciliary muscle of the eye; may be by denervation or by pharmacologic action. [cyclo- + G. *plēgē,* stroke]

cy·clo·ple·gic (sī-klō-plē′jik). **1.** Relating to cycloplegia. **2.** A drug that paralyzes the ciliary muscle and thus the power of accommodation.

cy·clo·pro·pane (sī-klō-prō′pān). An explosive gas of characteristic odor; in the past, widely used for producing general anesthesia. SYN trimethylene.

cy·clops (sī′klops). An individual with cyclopia. SYN monoculus (1), monophthalmus, monops. [see cyclopia]

cy·clo·ser·ine (sī-klō-ser′ēn). An antibiotic produced by strains of *Streptomyces orchidaceus* or *S. garyphalus* with a wide spectrum of antibacterial activity. SYN orientomycin.

cy·clo·sis (sī-klō′sis). The movement of the protoplasm and contained plastids within the protozoan cell. [G., fr. *kykloō,* to move around]

Cy·clo·spo·ra (sī-klō-spōr′ah). A *Cryptosporidium*-like genus of coccidian parasites reported from millipedes, reptiles, insectivores, and a rodent species. C. is characterized by acid-fast oocysts with two sporocysts, each with two sporozoites. C. is implicated as the cause of a widespread, prolonged but self-limited human diarrhea in patients in the Americas, Caribbean countries,

Southeast Asia, and eastern Europe previously reported as caused by cyanobacteriumlike bodies. SYN cyanobacteriumlike bodies.

C. cayetanensis, a species causing enteritis with persistent diarrhea; usually acquired by ingestion of contaminated water or food.

cy·clo·spor·in A (sī-klō-spōr'in). SYN cyclosporine.

cy·clo·spor·ine (sī-klō-spōr'ēn). A cyclic oligopeptide immunosuppressant produced by the fungus *Tolypocladium inflatum Gams;* used to inhibit organ transplant rejection. SYN cyclosporin A.

cy·clo·thi·a·zide (sī-klō-thī'ă-zīd). A diuretic and antihypertensive.

cy·clo·thy·mia (sī-klō-thī'mē-ă). A mental disorder characterized by marked swings of mood from depression to hypomania but not to the degree that occurs in bipolar disorder. SYN cyclothymic disorder. [cyclo- + G. *thymos,* rage]

cy·clo·thy·mi·ac, cy·clo·thy·mic (sī-klō-thī'mē-ăk, -thī'mik). Relating to cyclothymia.

cy·clot·o·my (sī-klot'ō-mē). Operation of cutting the ciliary muscle. [cyclo- + G. *tomē,* incision]

cy·clo·tor·sion (sī'klō-tōr'shun). SYN cycloduction.

cy·clo·tron (sī'klō-tron). An accelerator that produces high-speed ions (e.g., protons and deuterons) under the influence of an alternating magnetic field, for bombardment and disruption of atomic nuclei. Used to produce clinically useful positron-emitting radionuclides. [cyclo- + G. *-tron,* instrumental suffix]

cy·clo·tro·pia (sī-klō-trō'pē-a). A disparity of ocular position in which one eye is rotated around its visual axis, with respect to the other eye. [cyclo- + G. *tropē,* a turn, turning]

cy·clo·zo·o·no·sis (sī'klō-zō-ō-nō'sis). A zoonosis that requires more than one vertebrate host (but no invertebrate) for completion of the life cycle; e.g., various taenioid cestodes such as *Taenia saginata* and *T. solium* in which humans are an obligatory host; hydatid disease, a c. in which humans are not obligatory host. [cyclo- + G. *zōon,* animal, + *nosos,* disease]

Cyd Symbol for cytidine.

cy·e·sis (sī-ē'sis). Obsolete term for pregnancy. [G. *kyēsis*]

cyl. Abbreviation for cylinder, or cylindrical *lens.*

cyl·in·der (cyl., C) (sil'in-der). **1.** A cylindrical *lens.* **2.** A cylindrical or rodlike renal cast. **3.** A cylindrical metal container for gases stored under high pressure. [G. *kylindros,* a roll]

Bence Jones c.'s, slightly irregular, relatively smooth, rod-shaped or cylindroid bodies of fairly tenacious, viscid proteinaceous material in the fluid of the seminal vesicles.

crossed c.'s, a lens used in refraction to determine the strength and axis of a cylindrical lens to correct astigmatism; a combination of concave and convex cylinders of like power whose axes are at right angles to each other.

Külz c., SYN coma *cast.*

cyl·in·drax·is (sil-in-drak'sis). Historical precursor of the term axon, based on an interpretation of the myelinated nerve fiber as a cylinder of which the axon formed the axis.

cy·lin·dri·cal (si-lin'dri-kăl). Shaped like a cylinder; referring to a cylinder.

cyl·in·dro·ad·e·no·ma (sil'in-drō-ad-ĕ-nō'mă). SYN cylindroma.

cyl·in·droid (sil'in-droyd). SYN false *cast.* [G. *kylindrōdēs,* fr. *kylindros,* roll, cylinder, + *eidos,* appearance]

cyl·in·dro·ma (sil-in-drō'mă). A histologic type of epithelial neoplasm, frequently malignant, characterized by islands of neoplastic cells embedded in a hyalinized stroma which may represent a thickened basement membrane; may form from ducts of glands, especially in salivary glands, skin, and bronchi; in the salivary glands, also termed adenoid cystic carcinoma. SYN cylindroadenoma. [G. *kylindros,* cylinder, *-oma,* tumor]

cyl·in·dru·ria (sil-in-droo'rē-ă). The presence of renal cylinders or casts in the urine.

cyl·lo·so·ma (sil-ō-sō'mă). One-sided congenital defect of the lower abdominal wall (eventration) with defective development of the corresponding lower limb. [G. *kyllos,* deformed, esp. clubfooted or bandylegged, + *sōma,* body]

cy·ma·rin (sī'mă-rin). K-Strophanthin-α, a glycoside of cymarose present in the seeds of *Strophanthus kombé;* the aglycone is strophanthin; a cardiotonic.

cym·ba con·chae (sim'bă kong'kē) [TA]. The upper, smaller part of the external ear lying above the crus helicis. [G. *kymbē,* the hollow of a vessel, a cup, bowl, a boat]

cym·bo·ce·phal·ic, cym·bo·ceph·a·lous (sim-bō-se-fal'ik, -sef'ă-lŭs). Relating to cymbocephaly.

cym·bo·ceph·a·ly (sim-bō-sef'ă-lē). SYN scaphocephaly. [G. *kymbē,* the hollow of a vessel, a boat-shaped structure, + *kephalē,* head]

cy·nan·thro·py (sī-nan'thrō-pē). A delusion in which one barks and growls, imagining oneself to be a dog. [G. *kyōn,* dog, + *anthrōpos,* man]

cy·no·ceph·a·ly (sī-nō-sef'ă-lē). Craniostenosis in which the skull slopes back from the orbits, producing a resemblance to the head of a dog. [G. *kyōn,* dog, + *kephalē,* head]

cyn·o·dont (sī'nō-dont). **1.** A canine tooth. **2.** A tooth having one cusp or point. [G. *kyōn,* dog, + *odous (odont-),* tooth]

cy·no·pho·bia (sī-nō-fō'bē-ă). Morbid fear of dogs. [G. *kyōn,* dog, + *phobos,* fear]

Cyon, Elie de, Russian physiologist, 1843–1912. SEE C. *nerve.*

CYP. Abbreviation for cytochrome P450 enzymes; usually followed by an arabic numeral, a letter, and another arabic numeral (e.g., CYP 2D6). These enzymes are found in and on the smooth endoplasmic reticulum of liver and other cells and are responsible for a large number of drug biotransformation reactions.

CYP 1A2, microsomal enzyme, the substrates of which include theophylline, antidepressants, and tacrine. It is inhibited by grapefruit juice and quinolones, and induced by smoking, phenobarbital, phenytoin, rifampin, and omeprazole.

CYP 2C9, microsomal enzyme responsible for the oxidation of S-warfarin, phenytoin, and numerous NSAIDs. Inhibitors include azole antifungals (e.g., ketoconazole, itraconazole, metronidazole); induced by rifampin.

CYP 2C19, microsomal enzyme partially responsible for the oxidation of clomipramine, diazepam, propranolol, imipramine, and omeprazole. Inhibited by fluoxetine, sertraline, omeprazole, and ritinovir.

CYP 2D6, the isoenzyme that metabolizes many antidepressants, antipsychotic agents, beta adrenergic blockers, and codeine. It is inhibited by cimetidine and several antidepressants and antipsychotics.

CYP 2E1, microsomal enzyme that participates in the oxidation of ethanol and acetaminophen. Inhibited by disulfiram and induced by ethanol and isoniazid (INH). Believed to be responsible for the hepatotoxic metabolite of acetaminophen.

CYP 3A, a cytochrome P450 isoform found in the gastrointestinal tract as well as hepatic and other cells; substrates include benzodiazepines, calcium channel blockers, antihistamines, steroid hormones, and protease inhibitors. Inhibited by antidepressants, azole antifungals, cimetidine, and erythromycin. Induced by phenobarbital, phenytoin, rifampin, and carbamazepine.

cy·pri·do·pho·bia (sī'pri-dō-fō'bē-ă). Morbid fear of venereal disease or of sexual intercourse. [G. *Kypris,* Aphrodite, + *phobos,* fear]

cy·pro·hep·ta·dine hy·dro·chlo·ride (sī-prō-hep'tă-dēn). A potent antagonist of histamine and serotonin, with H₁ antihistaminic and antipruritic actions.

cy·pro·ter·one ac·e·tate (sī-prō'ter-ōn). A synthetic steroid capable of inhibiting the biological effects exerted by endogenous or exogenous androgenic hormones; an antiandrogen.

Cys Symbol for cysteine (half-cystine) or its mono- or diradical.

CYST

cyst (sist). **1.** A bladder. **2.** An abnormal sac containing gas, fluid, or a semisolid material, with a membranous lining. SEE ALSO pseudocyst. [G. *kystis*, bladder]

adventitious c., SYN pseudocyst (1).

allantoic c., SYN urachal c.

alveolar hydatid c., a hydatid c. of a multiloculate type, usually in the liver, caused by *Echinococcus multilocularis*, adults of which are in foxes; larvae (alveolar hydatid) are found chiefly in microtine rodents, but also among humans such as trappers and others handling pelts of infected foxes and other carnivores; growth is by exogenous budding and is not limited by an outer laminated membrane as in the hydatid c. from *E. granulosus*; necrosis, cavitation, contiguous spread, and death usually ensue. SYN multilocular hydatid c., multiloculate hydatid c.

aneurysmal bone c., a solitary benign osteolytic lesion expanding a long bone or within a vertebra, consisting of blood-filled spaces, and separated by fibrous tissue containing multinucleated giant cells; may cause swelling, pain, and tenderness and compromise the structural integrity of the involved bone.

angioblastic c., mesenchymal tissue capable of forming blood in the embryo.

apical periodontal c., an inflammatory odontogenic c. derived histogenetically from Malassez epithelial rests surrounding the root apex of a nonvital tooth. SYN periapical c., radicular c., root end c.

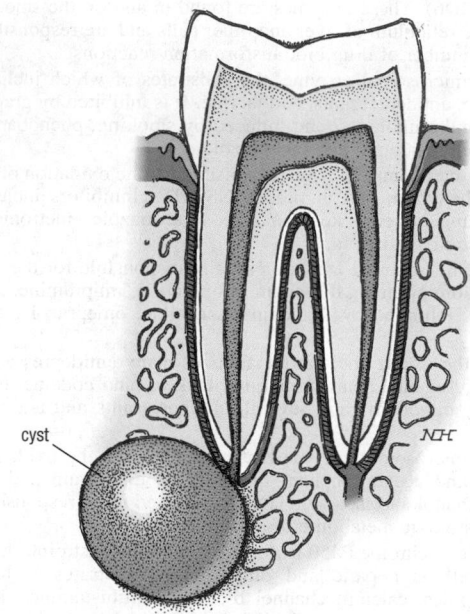

cyst

apical periodontal cyst

apoplectic c., a pseudocyst formed of extravasated blood as in a stroke.

arachnoid c., a fluid-filled c. lined with arachnoid membrane, frequently situated near the lateral aspect of the fissure of Sylvius; usually congenital in origin. SYN leptomeningeal c.

Baker c., a collection of synovial fluid which has escaped from the knee joint or a bursa and formed a new synovial-fluid lined sac in the popliteal space; seen in degenerative or other joint diseases that produce increased amounts of synovial fluid.

Bartholin c., a c. arising from the major vestibular gland or its ducts.

bile c., SYN gallbladder.

blood c., SYN hemorrhagic c.

blue dome c., (1) one of a number of small dark blue nodules or c.'s in the vaginal fornix due to retained menstrual blood in endometriosis affecting this region; **(2)** a benign retention c. of the mammary gland in fibrocystic disease, containing a pale slightly yellow fluid which gives a blue color to the c. when seen through the surrounding fibrous tissue.

bone c., SEE solitary bone c.

botryoid odontogenic c., a type of lateral periodontal c. that shows a multilocular growth pattern.

Boyer c., a subhyoid c.

branchial c., a cervical c. arising from developmental persistence of ectodermal branchial grooves or endodermal pharyngeal pouches. SYN branchial cleft c.

branchial cleft c., SYN branchial c.

bronchogenic c., a c. lined by ciliated columnar epithelium believed to represent bronchial differentiation; smooth muscle and mucous glands may be present.

bursal c., a retention c. in a bursa.

calcifying and keratinizing odontogenic c., SYN calcifying odontogenic c.

calcifying odontogenic c., a mixed radiolucent-radiopaque lesion of the jaws with features of both a c. and a solid neoplasm; characterized microscopically by an epithelial lining showing a palisaded layer of columnar basal cells, presence of ghost cell keratinization, dentinoid, and calcification. SYN calcifying and keratinizing odontogenic c., Gorlin c.

cerebellar c., a c. usually occurring in the lateral cerebellar white matter; often a part of cerebellar astrocytoma.

chocolate c., c. of the ovary with intracavitary hemorrhage and formation of a hematoma containing old brown blood; often seen with endometriosis of the ovary but occasionally with other types of c.'s.

choledochal c., c. originating from common bile duct; usually becomes apparent early in life as a right upper abdominal mass in association with jaundice.

chyle c., a circumscribed dilation of a lymphatic channel of the mesentery, containing chyle.

colloid c., a c. with gelatinous contents.

compound c., SYN multilocular c.

corpora lutea c., persistent corpora lutea with c. formation.

Cowper c., a retention c. of a bulbourethral gland.

daughter c., a secondary c., usually multiple, derived from a mother c.

dentigerous c., an odontogenic c. derived from the reduced enamel epithelium surrounding the crown of an impacted or embedded tooth. SYN follicular c. (2).

dermoid c., a tumor consisting of displaced ectodermal structures along lines of embryonic fusion, the wall being formed of epithelium-lined connective tissue, including skin appendages and containing keratin, sebum, and hair. SYN dermoid tumor, dermoid (2).

dermoid c. of ovary, a common benign cystic teratoma of the ovary, lined for the most part by skin, and containing hair and sebum, but also usually containing a variety of other well differentiated structures within a small inwardly projecting mass of solid tissue.

distention c., SYN retention c.

duplication c., a congenital cystic malformation attached to or originating from any part of the alimentary canal, from the base of the tongue to the anus, which reproduces the structure of the adjacent alimentary tract.

echinococcus c., SYN hydatid c.

endodermal c., c. lined by columnar epithelium; presumed dermal in origin.

endometrial c., a c. resulting from endometrial implantation outside the uterus, as in endometriosis.

endothelial c., a serous c. whose sac is lined with endothelium.

enterogenous c., mediastinal c. derived from cells sequestered from the primitive foregut; may be classified histologically as bronchogenic, esophageal, or gastric.

ependymal c., a circumscribed distention of some portion of the central canal of the spinal cord or of the cerebral ventricles. SYN neural c.

epidermal c., a c. formed of a mass of epidermal cells which, as a result of trauma, has been pushed beneath the epidermis; the c. is lined with stratified squamous epithelium and contains concentric layers of keratin. SYN implantation c., inclusion c. (1), inclusion dermoid.

epidermoid c., a spherical, unilocular c. of the dermis, comprised of encysted keratin and sebum; the c. is lined by a keratinizing epithelium resembling the epidermis derived from the follicular infundibulum.

epithelial c., a c. lined with epithelium.

eruption c., a form of dentigerous c. in the soft tissues in conjunction with an erupting tooth; seen on the alveolar ridge of children.

extravasation c., obsolete term for hemorrhagic c.

exudation c., a c. resulting from distention of a closed cavity, such as a bursa, by an excessive secretion of its normal fluid contents.

false c., SYN pseudocyst (1).

fissural c., a c. derived from epithelial remnants entrapped along the fusion line of embryonal processes. SYN inclusion c. (2).

follicular c., (1) a cystic graafian follicle; (2) SYN dentigerous c.

Gartner c., a c. of the principal duct in the vestigial structures of the paroöphoron in the cervix or anterolateral vaginal wall, corresponding to the sexual portion of mesonephros in the male.

gas c., a c. with gaseous instead of the ordinary liquid or pultaceous contents.

gingival c., a c. derived from remnants of the dental lamina situated in the attached gingiva, occasionally producing superficial erosion of the cortical plate of bone; most are located in the cuspid-premolar region.

globulomaxillary c. (glō′boo-lō-maks′il-lar-ē) a c. of odontogenic origin found between the roots of the maxillary lateral incisor and canine teeth.

glomerular c., c. formed by dilation of Bowman capsule, found in rare cases of congenital polycystic kidneys.

Gorlin c., SYN calcifying odontogenic c.

granddaughter c., a tertiary c. sometimes developed within a daughter c., as in the hydatid cyst of *Echinococcus.*

hemorrhagic c., a c. containing blood or resulting from the encapsulation of a hematoma. SYN blood c., hematocele (1), hematocyst, sanguineous c.

hepatic c., congenital c. thought to originate from an obstruction of biliary ductules; may be solitary and range in size from small to enormous; polycystic disease may also occur.

heterotrophic oral gastrointestinal c., a c. of the oral cavity lined by gastric or intestinal mucosa from misplaced embryonic rests.

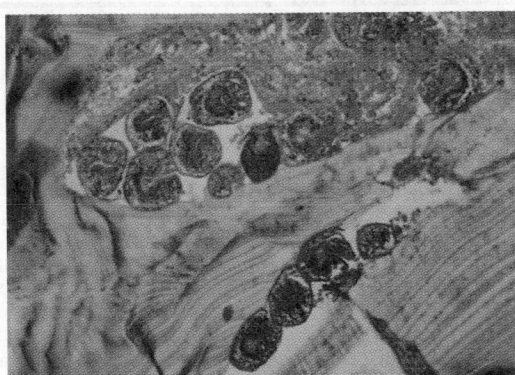

hydatid cyst: section containing numerous protoscolices between the laminated layers; hematoxylin and eosin, × 32

🔲**hydatid c.,** a c. formed in the liver, or, less frequently, elsewhere, by the larval stage of *Echinococcus,* chiefly in ruminants; two morphologic forms caused by *Echinococcus granulosus* are found in humans: the unilocular hydatid c. and the osseous hydatid c.; a third form in humans is the alveolar hydatid c., caused by *Echinococcus multilocularis.* SYN echinococcus c., hydatid (1).

implantation c., SYN epidermal c.

incisive canal c., a c. in or near the incisive canal, arising from proliferation of epithelial remnants of the nasopalatine duct; the most common maxillary development c. SYN median anterior maxillary c., nasopalatine duct c.

inclusion c., (1) SYN epidermal c; (2) SYN fissural c.

junctional c., a c. of the testis arising from the structures connecting the rete testis with the epididymis.

keratinous c., an epithelial c. containing keratin.

Klestadt c., SYN nasoalveolar c.

lacteal c., a retention c. in the mammary gland resulting from closure of a lactiferous duct. SYN milk c.

lateral periodontal c., an intraosseous c., usually encountered in the cuspid-premolar region of the mandible, derived from the remnants of the dental lamina and representing the intraosseous counterpart of the gingival c.

leptomeningeal c., SYN arachnoid c.

lymphoepithelial c., a cervical c. arising from salivary gland epithelium entrapped in lymph nodes during embryogenesis. Also seen within the oral cavity.

median anterior maxillary c., SYN incisive canal c.

median palatal c., a developmental c. located in the midline of the hard palate.

median raphe c. of the penis, a c. of the raphe penis resulting from incomplete closure of the urethral groove, becoming clinically evident in childhood or later.

meibomian c., SYN chalazion.

milk c., SYN lacteal c.

morgagnian c., SYN vesicular *appendages* of epoophoron, under *appendage.*

mother c., a hydatid c. from the inner, or germinal, layer, from which secondary c.'s containing scoleces (daughter c.'s) are developed; sometimes tertiary c.'s (granddaughter c.'s) are developed within the daughter c.'s; occurs most frequently in the liver, but may be found in other organs and tissues; symptoms are those of a tumor of the part affected. SYN parent c.

mucous c., a retention c. resulting from obstruction in the duct of a mucous gland. SYN mucocele (1).

multilocular c., a c. containing several compartments formed by membranous septa. SYN compound c.

multilocular hydatid c., multiloculate hydatid c., SYN alveolar hydatid c.

myxoid c., SYN ganglion (2).

nabothian c., a retention c. that develops when a mucous gland of the cervix uteri is obstructed; of no pathologic significance. SYN nabothian follicle.

nasoalveolar c., a soft tissue c. located near the attachment of the ala over the maxilla; probably derived from the lower anterior part of the nasolacrimal duct. SYN Klestadt c., nasolabial c.

nasolabial c., SYN nasoalveolar c.

nasopalatine duct c., SYN incisive canal c.

necrotic c., a c. due to a circumscribed encapsulated area of necrosis with subsequent liquefaction of the dead tissue.

neural c., SYN ependymal c.

neurenteric c.'s, paravertebral c.'s commonly connected to the meninges or a portion of the gastrointestinal tract that develop due to incomplete separation of endoderm from the notochord during early fetal life; often symptomatic.

odontogenic c., a c. derived from odontogenic epithelium. [odont- + G. *genos*, birth, origin, + suffix -*ic*, pertaining to]

oil c., a c. resulting from loss of the epithelial lining of a sebaceous, dermoid, or lacteal c., or from the subcutaneous injection of oil or fat material.

omphalomesenteric c., cystic lesion found within the umbilical cord, presumed to develop from remnants of the omphalomesenteric duct early in gestation. May be found on antenatal ultrasound. SYN omphalomesenteric duct c.

omphalomesenteric duct c., SYN omphalomesenteric c.

oophoritic c., SYN ovarian c.

osseous hydatid c., a morphologic form of hydatid c. caused by *Echinococcus granulosus,* and found in the long bones or the pelvic arch of humans if the embryo is filtered out in bony tissue;

in this site no limiting membrane forms and the c. grows in an uncontrolled fashion, producing cancellous structures and inducing fracture, followed by spread to new sites.

ovarian c., a cystic tumor of the ovary, either non-neoplastic (follicle, lutein, germinal inclusion, or endometrial) or neoplastic; usually restricted to benign c.'s, i.e., mucinous serous cystadenoma, or dermoid c.'s. SYN oophoritic c.

paraphysial c.'s, c.'s arising from vestigial remnants of the paraphysis; they are the possible origin of some third ventricular colloid c.'s.

parasitic c., a c. formed by the larva of a metazoan parasite, such as a hydatid or trichinal c.

parent c., SYN mother c.

paroophoritic c., a c. arising from the paroöpheron.

parvilocular c., a tumor composed of multiple small c.'s.

pearl c., a mass of epithelial cells introduced into the interior of the eye by a perforating injury.

periapical c., SYN apical periodontal c.

phaeomycotic c., a subcutaneous cystic granuloma caused by pigmented fungi, usually solitary and located on the extremities.

pilar c., a common c. of the skin, especially the scalp, which contains sebum and keratin, and is lined by pale-staining stratified epithelial cells derived from follicular trichilemma. SYN sebaceous c., trichilemmal c.

piliferous c., a dermoid c. containing hair.

pilonidal c., SEE pilonidal *sinus.*

pineal c., a c. of the pineal gland; rarely of clinical importance.

posttraumatic leptomeningeal c., a persistent cystic accumulation of cerebrospinal fluid with progressive loss of bone and dura, occurring at the site of a previous fracture.

primordial c., a c. that develops in place of a tooth through cystic degeneration of the enamel organ before formation of calcified odontogenic tissue.

proliferating tricholemmal c., SYN pilar *tumor* of scalp.

proliferation c., proliferative c., proliferous c., a mother c. containing daughter c.'s; a c. with tumorous formation at one portion of the sac.

protozoan c., infectious form of many protozoan parasites such as *Entamoeba histolytica, Giardia lamblia, Balantidium coli,* usually passed in the feces and provided with a highly condensed cytoplasm and resistant cell wall.

pseudomucinous c., a c. containing a gelatinous fluid, formerly thought to differ significantly from mucin, occurring especially in the ovary.

radicular c., SYN apical periodontal c.

Rathke cleft c., an intrasellar or suprasellar c. lined by cuboidal epithelium derived from remnants of Rathke pouch.

residual c., the persistence of an apical periodontal c. that remains after tooth extraction.

retention c., a c. resulting from some obstruction to the excretory duct of a gland. SYN distention c., secretory c.

rete c. of ovary, a c. derived from the germinal cords in the hilum of the ovary.

root end c., SYN apical periodontal c.

sanguineous c., SYN hemorrhagic c.

sebaceous c., SYN pilar c.

secretory c., SYN retention c.

seminal vesical c., a c., usually congenital, of the seminal vesicle.

sequestration c.,

serous c., a c. containing clear serous fluid, such as a hygroma.

simple bone c., SYN solitary bone c.

solitary bone c., a unilocular c. containing serous fluid and lined with a thin layer of connective tissue, occurring usually in the shaft of a long bone in a child. SYN idiopathic bone cavity, osteocystoma, simple bone c., traumatic bone c., unicameral bone c.

Stafne bone c., SYN lingual salivary gland *depression.*

static bone c., SYN lingual salivary gland *depression.*

sterile c., a hydatid c. without brood capsules or viable scoleces.

sublingual c., SYN ranula (2).

sudoriferous c., a c. caused by a blocked excretory duct of Moll *glands,* under *gland.* SYN apocrine hidrocystoma.

suprasellar c., SYN craniopharyngioma.

surgical ciliated c., a c. that arises from maxillary sinus epithelium implanted along a line of surgical entry.

synovial c., SYN ganglion (2).

Tarlov c., a perineural c. found in the proximal radicles of the lower spinal cord; it is usually productive of symptoms.

tarry c., a c. or collection of old blood having a tarry or black, sticky appearance; usually due to endometriosis.

tarsal c., SYN chalazion.

teratomatous c., a c. containing structures derived from all three of the primary germ layers of the embryo.

thyroglossal duct c., thyrolingual c., a c. in the midline of the neck resulting from nonclosure of a segment of the ductus thyroglossus.

Tornwaldt c., inflammation or obstruction of the pharyngeal bursa or an adenoid cleft with the formation of a cyst containing pus. SYN Tornwaldt disease.

traumatic bone c., SYN solitary bone c.

trichilemmal c., SYN pilar c.

tubular c., SYN tubulocyst.

umbilical c., SYN vitellointestinal c.

unicameral c., SYN unilocular c.

unicameral bone c., SYN solitary bone c.

unilocular c., a c. having a single sac. SYN unicameral c.

unilocular hydatid c., the commonest form of hydatid c. in man, caused by *Echinococcus granulosus* and found in the liver, lungs, or any other site where the hexacanth embryo may settle if it passes the hepatic or pulmonary capillary filters; characterized by large balloonlike forms lined internally with a germinative membrane, enclosed externally in a laminated membrane within a host-parasite capsule, and filled with fluid (hydatid fluid) and infectious scoleces of the young tapeworms (hydatid sand).

urachal c., a c. of the urachus which may communicate with the umbilicus or bladder, or give rise to a midline swelling. SYN allantoic c.

urinary c., SYN urinoma.

utricular c., dilation of the utricular lumen; usually unilocular.

vitellointestinal c., a small red sessile or pedunculated tumor at the umbilicus in an infant; it is due to the persistence of a segment of the vitellointestinal duct. SYN umbilical c.

wolffian c., a c. lying in the broad ligaments of the uterus and arising from any mesonephric structures.

---

cyst-. SEE cysto-.

cys·ta·canth (sis′tă-kanth). The fully developed larva of Acanthocephala, infective to the final host and with an inverted fully formed proboscis characteristic of the adult worm. [cyst- + G. *akantha,* thorn or spine]

cyst·ad·e·no·car·ci·no·ma (sist-ad′en-ō-kar-si-nō′mă). A malignant neoplasm derived from glandular epithelium, in which cystic accumulations of retained secretions are formed; the neoplastic cells manifest varying degrees of anaplasia and invasiveness, and local extension and metastases occur; c.'s develop frequently in the ovaries, where pseudomucinous and serous types are recognized.

cyst·ad·e·no·ma (sist′ad-ĕ-nō′mă). A histologically benign neoplasm derived from glandular epithelium, in which cystic accumulations of retained secretions are formed; in some instances, considerable portions of the neoplasm, or even the entire mass, may be cystic. SYN cystoadenoma.

papillary c. lymphomato′sum, SYN adenolymphoma.

cyst·al·gia (sist-al′jē-ă). Pain in a bladder, especially the urinary bladder. [cyst- + G. *algos,* pain]

cys·ta·mine (sis′tă-mēn). Decarboxycystine; forms when cystine is distilled. The disulfide of cysteamine.

cys·ta·thi·o·nase (sis-tă-thī′ō-nās). SYN cystathionine γ-lyase.

β-cys·ta·thi·o·nase. SYN cystathionine β-lyase.

γ-cys·ta·thi·o·nase. SYN cystathionine γ-lyase.

cys·ta·thi·o·nine (sis-tă-thī′ō-nēn). The L-isomer is an intermediate in the conversion of L-methionine to L-cysteine; cleaved by cystathionases.

cys·ta·thi·o·nine β-ly·ase. An enzyme catalyzing the hydrolysis of L-cystathionine to pyruvate, L-homocysteine, and NH₃. SEE ALSO cystathionine γ-lyase. SYN β-cystathionase, cystine lyase.

cys·ta·thi·o·nine γ-ly·ase. A liver enzyme, requiring pyridoxal phosphate as coenzyme, that catalyzes the hydrolysis of L-cystathionine to L-cysteine and 2-ketobutyrate, releasing NH₃; also catalyzes formation of 2-ketobutyrate from L-homoserine, of pyruvate (and NH₃ and H₂S) from L-cysteine, and of thiocysteine, pyruvate, and NH₃ from cystine. A deficiency of this enzyme results in cystathioninuria. It catalyzes a step in methionine catabolism and in cysteine biosynthesis. SEE ALSO cystathionine β-lyase. SYN cystathionase, cysteine desulfhydrase, cystine desulfhydrase, γ-cystathionase, homoserine deaminase, homoserine dehydratase.

cys·ta·thi·o·nine β-syn·thase. An enzyme catalyzing the reversible hydrolysis of L-cystathionine to L-serine and L-homocysteine. A step in cysteine biosynthesis and in methionine catabolism. A deficiency of this enzyme leads to vascular thrombosis, dislocation of ocular lens, and abnormal development. SEE ALSO cystathionine γ-synthase. SYN β-thionase, cysteine synthase, serine sulfhydrase.

cys·ta·thi·o·nine γ-syn·thase. SYN *O*-succinylhomoserine (thiol)-lyase.

cys·ta·thi·o·nin·u·ria (sis-tă-thī′ō-nin-oo′rē-ă) [MIM*219500]. A disorder characterized by inability to metabolize cystathionine, normally due to deficiency of cystathionase, with high concentration of the amino acid in blood, tissue, and urine; mental retardation is an associated condition; autosomal recessive inheritance.

cys·te·a·mine (sis-tā′a-mēn). Sulfhydryl compound used experimentally to produce ulcers in rats and as a radioprotective agent; antidote to acetaminophen.

cys·tec·to·my (sis-tek′tō-mē). **1.** Excision of the the urinary bladder. **2.** Excision of the gallbladder (cholecystectomy). **3.** Removal of a cyst. [cyst- + G. *ektomē*, excision]

    Bartholin c., removal of a cyst of a major vestibular gland. SYN vulvovaginal c.

    partial c., removal of a part or segment of the bladder.

    radical c., removal of the entire bladder, surrounding fatty tissues, and regional lymph nodes.

    salvage c., removal of the bladder, after failed chemotherapy and radiation for malignancy.

    total c., removal of the entire bladder.

    vulvovaginal c., SYN Bartholin c.

cys·te·ic ac·id (sis-tā′ik). An oxidation product of cysteine, and a precursor of taurine and isethionic acid. SYN 3-sulfoalanine.

cys·te·ine (C, Cys) (sis′ta-ēn). Amino-3-mercaptopropionic acid; the L-isomer is found in most proteins; especially abundant in keratin.

    c. desulfhydrase, SYN cystathionine γ-lyase.

    c. synthase, SYN cystathionine β-synthase.

cys·te·ine sul·fin·ic ac·id (sis′tē-ēn-sul-fin′ik). A natural oxidation product of cysteine; an intermediate in the formation of taurine (via cysteic acid).

cys·tein·yl (sis′tēn-il). Aminoacyl radical of cysteine.

⚠️**cysti-.** SEE cysto-.

cys·tic (sis′tik). **1.** Relating to the urinary bladder or gallbladder. **2.** Relating to a cyst. **3.** Containing cysts.

cys·ti·cer·coid (sis-ti-ser′koyd). A larval tapeworm resembling a cysticercus but having a smaller bladder, containing little or no fluid, in which scolex of the future adult tapeworm is found; the larval form is typically found in insect intermediate hosts. [cysti- + G. *kerkos*, tail, + *eidos*, resemblance]

cys·ti·cer·co·sis (sis′ti-ser-kō′sis). **1.** Disease caused by encystment of cysticercus larvae of some tapeworms (e.g., *Taenia solium* or *T. saginata*) in subcutaneous, muscle, or central nervous system tissues; c. is typically developed in swine and cattle, producing measly pork and beef. In humans, it results from the hatching of the eggs of *Taenia solium* in the intestines or by

accidental ingestion of eggs from human feces; encystment in the brain may cause serious nervous damage, and encystment in the eye (usually the rear chamber) may cause ophthalmic damage. **2.** Larval infections in animals with other taeniid tapeworm larvae. SYN cysticercus disease.

Cys·ti·cer·cus (sis-ti-ser′kŭs). Originally described as a genus of bladderworms, now known to be the encysted larvae of various taenioid tapeworms; the generic name is, however, retained as a convenience in referring to the larval encysted forms. SEE cysticercus. SYN bladderworm. [G. *kystis*, bladder, + *kerkos*, tail]

    C. bo′vis, the cysticercus larva of *Taenia saginata* in cattle; the cause of measly beef.

    C. cellulo′sae, the cysticercus larva of *Taenia solium* in pigs; also the cause of human cysticercosis.

cys·ti·cer·cus, pl. **cys·ti·cer·ci** (sis-ti-ser′kŭs, -ser′sī). The larval form of certain *Taenia* species, typically found in muscles of mammalian intermediate hosts that serve as a prey of various predators; it consists of a fluid-filled bladder in which the invaginated cestode scolex develops. SEE ALSO *Taenia saginata*, *Taenia solium*. [G. *kystis*, bladder, + *kerkos*, tail]

cys·ti·form (sis′ti-fōrm). SYN cystoid (1).

⬛**cys·tine** (sis′tīn). 3,3′-Dithiobis(2-aminopropionic acid); the disulfide product of two cysteines in which two –SH groups become one –S–S– group; if two cysteinyl residues in polypeptide chains form a disulfide linkage, then the two polymers are cross-linked; sometimes occurs as a deposit in the urine, or forming a vesical calculus. Cf. *meso*-cystine. SYN dicysteine.

    c. desulfhydrase, SYN cystathionine γ-lyase.

    half c., refers to one-half of a cystine molecule or of a cystinyl residue in a protein or peptide.

    c. lyase, SYN cystathionine β-lyase.

***meso*-cys·tine.** An isomer of cystine in which the configuration about one of the α-carbons is D, about the other, L, so that the molecule as a whole possesses a plane of symmetry and is optically inactive. Note that *meso*-cystine is not DL-cystine. DL-cystine is a racemic mixture of DD-cystine and LL-cystine.

cys·ti·ne·mia (sis-ti-nē′mē-ă). The presence of cystine in the blood. [cystine + G. *haima*, blood]

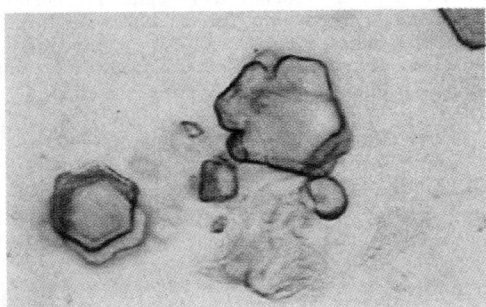

cystinosis: microscopic view of cystine crystals in the urine

⬛**cys·ti·no·sis** (sis-ti-nō′sis) [MIM*219800]. A lysosomal storage disorder with various forms, all with autosomal recessive inheritance. The nephropathic form of early childhood is characterized by widespread deposits of cystine crystals throughout the body, including the bone marrow, cornea, and other tissues, with mild elevation of plasma cystine and cystinuria; associated with a marked generalized aminoaciduria, glycosuria, polyuria, chronic acidosis, hypophosphatemia with vitamin D-resistant rickets, and often with hypokalemia; other extrarenal manifestations include photophobia and hypothyroidism; due to a defect in the transport of cystine across lysosomal membranes caused by mutation in the CTNS gene on 17p. There is a milder form with onset in adolescence [MIM*219900] and one with onset in adulthood without kidney damage [MIM*219750]; the latter two forms are thought to be allelic to the nephropathic form of early childhood. SYN cystine storage disease. [cystine + G. *-osis*, condition]

cys·ti·nu·ria (sis-ti-noo′rē-ă) [MIM*220100, *104614, *600918].

Excessive urinary excretion of cystine, along with lysine, arginine, and ornithine, arising from defective transport systems for these acids in the kidney and intestine; renal function is sometimes compromised by cystine crystalluria and nephrolithiasis. There are at least three forms of c., which are distinguished by the severity of urinary excretion of cystine in obligate carriers; all with autosomal recessive inheritance. Types I and II c. are allelic disorders caused by mutation in the solute carrier family 3 gene (SLC3A1), which is an amino acid transporter gene on chromosome 2q. Type III is caused by mutation at a separate locus. [cystine + G. *ouron*, urine]

cys·tin·yl (sis′tin-il). Aminoacyl radical of cystine.

cys·tis, pl. **cys·ti·des** (sis′tis, sis′ti-dēz). SEE cyst, pouch, sac. [G. *kystis*]

　c. fel′lea, SYN gallbladder.

　c. urina′ria, SYN urinary *bladder.*

cys·ti·stax·is (sis-ti-stak′sis). Obsolete term for oozing of blood from the epithelial lining of the bladder. [cysti- + G. *staxis*, trickling]

cys·ti·tis (sis-tī′tis). Inflammation of the urinary bladder. [cyst- + G. -*itis*, inflammation]

　bacterial c., bladder inflammation caused by bacteria.

　c. col′li, inflammation of the neck of the bladder.

　c. cys′tica, c. glandularis with the formation of cysts.

　emphysematous c., inflammation of the bladder wall caused by gas-forming bacteria, usually secondary to diabetes mellitus.

　eosinophilic c., bladder inflammation with many eosinophils in urinary sediment as well as bladder wall.

　follicular c., chronic c. characterized by small mucosal nodules due to lymphocytic infiltration.

　c. glandula′ris, chronic c. with glandlike metaplasia of urothelium.

　hemorrhagic c., bladder inflammation with macroscopic hematuria. Generally the result of a chemical or other traumatic insult to the bladder (chemotherapy, radiation therapy).

　incrusted c., bladder inflammation with deposition of inorganic minerals on luminal wall. There generally is evidence of chronic inflammation.

　interstitial c., a chronic inflammatory condition of unknown etiology involving the epithelium and muscularis of the bladder, resulting in reduced bladder capacity, pain relieved by voiding, and severe bladder irritative symptoms. SEE ALSO Hunner *ulcer.*

　viral c., bladder inflammation due to a viral infection.

△**cysto-, cysti-, cyst-.** Combining forms relating to: **1.** The bladder. **2.** The cystic duct. **3.** A cyst. Cf. vesico-. [G. *kystis*, bladder, pouch]

cys·to·ad·e·no·ma (sis′tō-ad-ĕ-nō′mǎ). SYN cystadenoma.

cys·to·car·ci·no·ma (sis′tō-kar-si-nō′mǎ). A carcinoma in which cystic degeneration has occurred; sometimes used incorrectly as a term for cystadenocarcinoma.

cys·to·cele (sis′tō-sēl). Hernia of the bladder usually into the vagina and introitus. SYN vesicocele. [cysto- + G. *kēlē*, hernia]

cys·to·chro·mos·co·py (sis′tō-krō-mos′kǒ-pē). Examination of the interior of the bladder after administration of a colored dye to aid in the identification or study of the function of the ureteral orifices. [cysto- + G. *chrōma*, color + *skopeō*, to view]

cys·to·du·o·de·nos·to·my (sis′tō-doo′ō-dē-nos′tō-mē). Drainage of a cyst, usually pancreatic pseudocyst, into duodenum. SYN duodenocystostomy (2). [cysto- + duodenum, + G. *stoma*, mouth]

　pancreatic c., surgical or endoscopic drainage of pancreatic pseudocyst into duodenum. SYN duodenocystostomy (3).

cys·to·en·ter·o·cele (sis-tō-en′ter-ō-sēl). Hernial protrusion of portions of the bladder and of the intestine, usually into the vagina and introitus. [cysto- + G. *enteron*, intestine, + *kēlē*, hernia]

cys·to·en·ter·os·to·my (sis′tō-en-ter-os′tō-mē). Internal drainage of pancreatic pseudocysts into some portion of the intestinal tract preferably stomach, duodenum, or small intestine. [cysto- + G. *enteron*, intestine, + *stoma*, mouth]

cys·to·e·pip·lo·cele (sis-tō-e-pip′lō-sēl). Hernial protrusion of portions of the bladder and of the omentum. [cysto- + G. *epiploon*, omentum, + *kēlē*, tumor]

cys·to·fi·bro·ma (sis′tō-fī-brō′mǎ). A fibroma in which cysts or cystlike foci have formed.

cys·to·gas·tros·to·my (sis′tō-gas-tros′tō-mē). Drainage of a pancreatic pseudocyst, into the stomach. [cysto- + G. *gastēr*, stomach, + *stoma*, mouth]

cys·to·gram (sis′tō-gram). Radiographic demonstration of the bladder filled with contrast medium.

　voiding c., SYN voiding *cystourethrogram.*

cys·tog·ra·phy (sis-tog′rǎ-fē). Radiography of the bladder following injection of a radiopaque substance. [cysto- + G. *graphō*, to write]

　antegrade c., c. in which the contrast medium enters the urinary bladder via ureters or cystotomy.

cys·toid (sis′toyd). **1.** Bladderlike, resembling a cyst. SYN cystiform, cystomorphous. **2.** A tumor resembling a cyst, with fluid, granular, or pulpy contents, but without a capsule. [cysto- + G. *eidos*, appearance]

cys·to·je·ju·nos·to·my (sis′tō-je-joo-nos′tō-mē). Drainage of a pancreatic pseudocyst, into the jejunum. [cysto- + jejunum, + G. *stoma*, mouth]

cys·to·lith (sis′tō-lith). SYN vesical *calculus.* [cysto- + G. *lithos*, stone]

cys·to·li·thi·a·sis (sis′tō-li-thī′ǎ-sis). The presence of a vesical calculus. SYN vesicolithiasis. [cysto- + G. *lithos*, stone, + -*iasis*, condition]

cys·to·lith·ic (sis-tō-lith′ik). Relating to a vesical calculus.

cy·sto·lith·o·la·paxy (sis′tō-lith-ō-lā-paks-ē). Removal of bladder calculi by intravesical crushing and then irrigating to remove fragments. [cysto- + G. *lithos*, stone, + *lapaxis*, and emptying out]

cys·to·li·thot·o·my (sis′tō-li-thot′ō-mē). Removal of a stone from the bladder through an incision in its wall. SYN vesical lithotomy. [cysto- + G. *lithos*, stone, + *tomē*, incision]

cys·to·ma (sis-tō′mǎ). A cystic tumor; a new growth containing cysts. [cyst- + G. -*oma*, tumor]

cys·tom·e·ter (sis-tom′ě-ter). A device for studying bladder function by measuring capacity, sensation, intravesical pressure, and residual urine. [cysto- + G. *metron*, measure]

cys·to·met·ro·gram (CMG) (sis-tō-met′rō-gram). A graphic recording of urinary bladder pressure at various volumes. [cysto- + G. *metron*, measure, + *gramma*, a writing]

cys·to·me·trog·ra·phy (sis′tō-mě-trog′rǎ-fē). SYN cystometry.

cys·tom·e·try (sis-tom′ě-trē). Measurement of the pressure/volume relationship of the bladder. SYN cystometrography. [see cystometer]

cys·to·mor·phous (sis-tō-mōr′fǔs). SYN cystoid (1). [cysto- + G. *morphē*, form]

cys·to·my·o·ma (sis′tō-mī-ō′mǎ). A myoma in which cysts or cystlike foci have developed.

cys·to·myx·o·ad·e·no·ma (sis-tō-mik′sō-ad-ě-nō′mǎ). An adenoma in which there are cysts or cystlike foci in association with myxomatous change in the stroma.

cys·to·myx·o·ma (sis′tō-mik-sō′mǎ). A myxoma in which cysts or cystlike foci have formed.

cys·to·pan·en·dos·co·py (sis′tō-pan-en-dos′kǒ-pē). Inspection of the interior of the bladder and urethra by means of specially designed endoscopes introduced in retrograde fashion through the urethra and into the bladder. [cysto- + panendoscope]

cys·to·pa·ral·y·sis (sis-tō-pǎ-ral′i-sis). SYN cystoplegia.

cys·to·pexy (sis′tō-pek-sē). Surgical attachment of the gallbladder or of the urinary bladder to the abdominal wall or to other supporting structures. SYN ventrocystorrhaphy. [cysto- + G. *pēxis*, fixation]

cys·to·pho·tog·ra·phy (sis′tō-fō-tog′rǎ-fē). Photographing the interior of the bladder.

cys·to·plas·ty (sis′tō-plas-tē). Any reconstructive operation on the urinary bladder. Cf. ileocystoplasty, colocystoplasty. [cysto- + G. *plastos*, formed]

cys·to·ple·gia (sis-tō-plē′jē-ǎ). Paralysis of the bladder. SYN cystoparalysis. [cysto- + G. *plēgē*, a stroke]

cysto·pros·ta·tec·to·my (sis′tō-pros-tă-tek′tō-mē). Surgical removal of bladder, prostate, and seminal vesicles simultaneously.

cys·to·py·e·li·tis (sis′tō-pī-el-ī′tis). Inflammation of both the bladder and the pelvis of the kidney. [cysto- + G. *pyelos*, trough (pelvis), + *-itis*, inflammation]

cys·to·py·e·lo·ne·phri·tis (sis-tō-pī′el-ō-nef-rī′tis). Inflammation of the bladder, the pelvis of the kidney, and the kidney parenchyma. [cysto- + G. *pyelos*, trough (pelvis), + *nephros*, kidney, + *-itis*, inflammation]

cys·tor·rha·phy (sis-tōr′ă-fē). Suture of a wound or defect in the urinary bladder. [cysto- + G. *rhaphē*, a sewing]

cys·tor·rhea (sis′tō-rē-ă). A mucous discharge from the bladder. [cysto- + G. *rhoia*, a flow]

cys·to·sar·co·ma (sis′tō-sar-kō′mă). A sarcoma in which the formation of cysts or cystlike foci has occurred.
　c. phyllo′des, a circumscribed or infiltrating fibroadenomatous tumor that may be partly cystic, of the breast, prostate, or other organs and either benign or malignant; the stroma is cellular and resembles a fibrosarcoma.

cys·to·scope (sis′tō-skōp). A lighted tubular endoscope for examining the interior of the bladder. [cysto- + G. *skopeō*, to examine]

█ cys·tos·co·py (sis-tos′kŏ-pē). The inspection of the interior of the bladder by means of a cystoscope.

cys·to·spasm (sis′tō-spazm). Bladder spasm; unintentional, painful contraction of the bladder, often without micturition.

cys·tos·to·my (sis-tos′tō-mē). Creation of an opening into the urinary bladder. SYN vesicostomy. [cysto- + G. *stoma*, mouth]

cys·to·tome (sis′tō-tōm). **1.** An instrument for incising the urinary bladder or gallbladder. **2.** A surgical instrument used for incising the capsule of a lens. SYN capsulotome.

cys·tot·o·my (sis-tot′ō-mē). Incision or puncture into urinary bladder or gallbladder. SYN vesicotomy. [cysto- + G. *tomē*, incision]
　suprapubic c., opening into the bladder through an incision or puncture above the symphysis pubis.

cys·to·u·re·ter·i·tis (sis′tō-ū-rē-ter-ī′tis). Inflammation of the bladder and of one or both ureters.

cys·to·u·re·ter·o·gram (sis′tō-ū-rē′ter-ō-gram). Radiographic demonstration of the bladder and ureters.

cys·to·u·re·ter·og·ra·phy (sis′tō-oo-rē′ter-og′ră-fē). Radiography of the bladder and ureters.

cys·to·u·re·thri·tis (sis′tō-ū-rē-thrī′tis). Inflammation of the bladder and of the urethra.

cys·to·u·re·thro·cele (sis′tō-ū-rē′thrō-sēl). Hernia of the urinary bladder and urethra. [cysto- + urethra + G. *kēlē*, hernia]

cys·to·u·re·thro·gram (sis-tō-ū-rēth′rō-gram). SYN voiding c.
　micturating c., SYN voiding c.
　retrograde c., a c. performed by injection of contrast via urethral meatus or distal urethra.
　voiding c. (VCUG), an x-ray image made during voiding and with the bladder and urethra filled with contrast medium to demonstrate the urethra. SYN cystourethrogram, micturating c., voiding cystogram.

cys·to·u·re·throg·ra·phy (sis′tō-ū′rē-throg′ră-fē). Radiography of the bladder and urethra during voiding, following filling of the bladder with a radiopaque contrast medium either by intravenous injection or retrograde catheterization.

cys·to·u·re·thro·scope (sis-tō-ū-rē′thrō-skōp). An instrument combining the uses of a cystoscope and a urethroscope, whereby both the bladder and urethra can be visually inspected.

Cys·to·vir·i·dae (sis′tō-vir′i-dē). Provisional name for a family of monotypic bacterial viruses, the type species of which is phage Φ6. Virions are 86 nm in diameter, isometric, have lipid envelopes, and adsorb to the sides of pili of *Pseudomonas* species. Capsids are of cubic symmetry, and the genomes are of double-stranded RNA in three pieces (MW 13×10^6). [G. *kystis*, bladder]

cys·tyl·a·mi·no·pep·ti·dase (sis′til-a-mi-nō-pep′ti-dās). Oxytocinase; an enzyme that degrades cystine-containing peptides, such as oxytocin.

Cyt Symbol for cytosine.

△**cyt-.** SEE cyto-.

cy·ta·pher·e·sis (sī′tă-fĕ-rē′sis). A procedure in which various cells can be separated from the withdrawn blood and retained, with the plasma and other formed elements retransfused into the donor. [cyt- + G. *aphairesis*, a withdrawal]

cy·tar·a·bine (sī′tar-ă-bēn). SYN arabinosylcytosine.

cy·tase (sī′tās). An obsolete term, coined by Metchnikoff, for alexin or complement, which he held to be a digestive secretion of the leukocyte.

△**-cyte.** Suffix meaning cell. [G. *kytos*, a hollow (cell)]

cyt·i·dine (C, Cyd) (sī′ti-dēn). A major component of ribonucleic acids. SYN 1-β-D-ribofuranosylcytosine, cytosine ribonucleoside.
　c. diphosphate choline, SYN cytidine diphosphocholine.
　c. phosphate, SEE cytidylic acid.

cyt·i·dine 5′-di·phos·phate (CDP). An ester, at the 5′ position, between cytidine and diphosphoric acid.

cyt·i·dine di·phos·pho·cho·line (CDP-cho·line) (sī′ti-dēn-dī′fos-fō-kō′lēn). An intermediate in the formation of phosphatidylcholine (lecithin) and sphingomyelins; formed by the action of cytidine 5′-triphosphate on phosphocholine, linking the choline phosphate group to the α-phosphate of the cytidine 5′-triphosphate to give a pyrophosphate. SYN activated choline, cytidine diphosphate choline.

cyt·i·dine di·phos·pho·glyc·er·ide (CDP-glyc·er·ide) (sī′ti-dēn dī′fos-fō-gli′cer-īd). An intermediate in the formation of phospholipids (e.g., cardiolipin) formed by the action on CTP and 1,2-diacylglycerols by a cytidyl transferase, releasing CDP-glyceride and pyrophosphate.

cyt·i·dine di·phos·pho·sug·ar (CDP-sug·ar). An activated form of a sugar.

cyt·i·dine 5′-tri·phos·phate (CTP). An ester, at the 5′ position, between cytidine and triphosphoric acid.

cyt·i·dyl·ic ac·id (sī-ti-dil′ik). Cytidine monophosphate (five are possible, depending on the site of attachment of the phosphate to the ribosyl OH's); a constituent of ribonucleic acids.

cy·ti·sine (sit′i-sin). A toxic selective nicotinic cholinergic agonist; an alkaloid from the seed of *Laburnum anagyroides* and other Leguminosae. Used in pharmacological studies of nicotinic cholinergic receptors in the brain. SYN baptitoxine.

△**cyto-, cyt-.** A cell. [G. *kytos*, a hollow (cell)]

cy·to·an·a·lyz·er (sī-tō-an′ă-lī-zer). An electronic optical machine that screens smears containing cells suspected of malignancy. [cyto- + analyzer]

cy·to·ar·chi·tec·ton·ics (sī′tō-ar-ki-tek-ton′iks). SYN cytoarchitecture. [cyto- + G. *architektonikē*, architectural]

cy·to·ar·chi·tec·tur·al (sī-tō-ar-ki-tek′chŭr-ăl). Pertaining to cytoarchitecture.

cy·to·ar·chi·tec·ture (sī′tō-ar′ki-tek-chŭr). The arrangement of cells in a tissue; e.g., the arrangement of nerve-cell bodies in the brain, especially the cerebral cortex. SYN architectonics, cytoarchitectonics.

cy·to·bi·ol·o·gy (sī′tō-bī-ol′ō-jē). SYN cytology.

cy·to·bi·o·tax·is (sī′tō-bī-ō-tak′sis). SYN cytoclesis. [cyto- + G. *bios*, life, + *taxis*, arrangement]

cy·to·cen·trum (sī-tō-sen′trŭm). A zone of cytoplasm containing one or two centrioles but devoid of other organelles; usually located near the nucleus of a cell. SYN cell center, central body, centrosome, cinocentrum, kinocentrum, microcentrum. [cyto- + G. *kentron*, center]

cy·to·chal·a·sins (sī-tō-kal′ă-zinz). A group of substances derived from molds that disaggregate the microfilaments of the cell and interfere with the division of cytoplasm, inhibit cell movement, and cause extrusion of the nucleus; used for investigations in cell biology. [cyto- + G. *chalasis*, a relaxing]

cy·to·chem·is·try (sī′tō-kem′is-trē). The study of intracellular distribution of chemicals, reaction sites, enzymes, etc., often by means of staining reactions, radioactive isotope uptake, selective metal distribution in electron microscopy, or other methods. SYN histochemistry.

cy

cy·to·chrome (sī'tō-krōm). A class of hemoprotein whose principal biologic function is electron and/or hydrogen transport by virtue of a reversible valency change of the heme iron. C.'s are classified in four groups (*a*, *b*, *c*, and *d*) according to spectrochemical characteristics; many variants exist, particularly among bacteria and in green plants and algae, one being a variant of the *c* type cytochrome called cytochrome *f*. The mitochondrial system of c.'s provides electron transport through cytochrome *c* oxidase to molecular oxygen as the terminal electron acceptor (respiration). [cyto- + G. *chrōma*, color]

cy·to·chrome aa_3. SYN cytochrome *c* oxidase.

cy·to·chrome *b*. A cytochrome of the respiratory chain. A deficiency of this cytochrome leads to chronic granulomatous disease.

cy·to·chrome b_5. A cytochrome in the endoplasmic reticulum that acts with a number of oxygenases; a deficiency of this cytochrome results in a form of hereditary methemoglobinemia.

cy·to·chrome b_5 re·duc·tase. A flavoenzyme catalyzing the reduction of 2ferricytochrome b_5 to 2ferrocytochrome b_5 at the expense of NADH; has a role in fatty acid desaturation; a deficiency can lead to hereditary methemoglobinemia (type I, only observed in erythrocyte cytosol; type II, deficiency in all tissues; type III, deficiency in all hematopoetic cells).

cy·to·chrome *c*. The mobile cytochrome that transports electrons from Complex III to Complex IV of the respiratory chain.

cy·to·chrome *cd*. SYN cytochrome oxidase (*Pseudomonas*).

cy·to·chrome c_3 hy·dro·gen·ase. A hydrogenase enzyme catalyzing reduction of 2ferricytochrome c_3 by H_2 to 2ferrocytochrome c_3 and $2H^+$.

cy·to·chrome *c* ox·i·dase. A cytochrome of the *a* type, containing copper, that catalyzes the oxidation of 4ferrocytochrome *c* by molecular oxygen to 4ferricytochrome *c* and $2H_2O$. A part of Complex IV of the respiratory chain. A deficiency of one or more of the polypeptides of this complex results in neuronal loss in brain leading to psychomotor retardation and neurodegenerative disease. SYN cytochrome aa_3, indophenol oxidase, indophenolase.

cy·to·chrome *c* re·duc·tase. SYN *NADH* dehydrogenase.

cy·to·chrome c_2 re·duc·tase. SYN *NADPH*-cytochrome c_2 reductase.

cy·to·chrome ox·i·dase (*Pseu·do·mo·nas*). An enzyme with action identical to that of cytochrome *c* oxidase, but acting on ferrocytochrome c_2. SYN cytochrome *cd*.

cy·to·chrome P-450$_{SCC}$. Cholesterol monooxygenase (side chain cleaving). [*450 nm*, the absorption maximum that the reduced cytochrome complexed with carbon monoxide exhibits]

cy·to·chrome per·ox·i·dase. A hemoprotein enzyme catalyzing the reaction between H_2O_2 and 2ferrocytochrome *c* to yield 2ferricytochrome *c* and $2H_2O$.

cy·to·chrome re·duc·tase. SYN *NADPH*-ferrihemoprotein reductase.

cy·to·chy·le·ma (sī'tō-kī-lē'mă). The more fluid portion of the cytoplasm. [cyto- + G. *chylos*, juice]

cy·toc·i·dal (sī-tō-sī'dăl). Causing the death of cells. [cyto- + L. *caedo*, to kill]

cy·to·cide (sī'tō-sīd). An agent that is destructive to cells. [cyto- + L. *caedo*, to kill]

cy·toc·la·sis (sī-tok'lă-sis). Fragmentation of cells. [cyto- + G. *klasis*, a breaking]

cy·to·clas·tic (sī-tō-klas'tik). Relating to cytoclasis.

cy·to·cle·sis (sī-tō-klē'sis). The influence of one cell on another. SYN biotaxis (2), cytobiotaxis. [cyto- + G. *klēsis*, a call]

cy·to·cu·prein (sī-tō-koo'prē-in). Former terms for copper-containing proteins found in human erythrocytes and other tissues. SEE *superoxide* dismutase, ceruloplasmin. SYN cerebrocuprein, erythrocuprein, hemocuprein, hepatocuprein.

cy·to·cyst (sī'tō-sist). Rarely used term for the bladderlike remains of the red blood cell or tissue cell that encloses a mature schizont. [cyto- + G. *kystis*, bladder]

cy·to·di·ag·no·sis (sī'tō-dī-ag-nō'sis). Diagnosis of the type and, when feasible, the cause of a pathologic process by means of microscopic study of cells in an exudate or other form of body fluid.

cy·to·di·er·e·sis (sī'tō-dī-er'ē-sis). SYN cytokinesis. [cyto- + G. *diairesis*, division]

cy·to·gene (sī'tō-jēn). SYN plasmagene.

cy·to·gen·e·sis (sī-tō-jen'ě-sis). The origin and development of cells. [cyto- + G. *genesis*, origin]

cy·to·ge·net·i·cist (sī'tō-jě-net'i-sist). A specialist in cytogenetics.

cy·to·ge·net·ics (sī'tō-jě-net'iks). The branch of genetics concerned with the structure and function of the cell, especially the chromosomes.

> Cytogenetics arose as a fusion of 19th century cytology and 20th century genetics, which came into being in 1903 with the articulation of the chromosome theory of inheritance. The developing field concerned itself with detailing the behavior of chromosomes and their functional subunits, the genes, during reproduction, and with relating that behavior statistically to characteristics of the resulting cells or animals. Modern molecular cytogenetics involves the microscopic study of chromosomes that have been fixed in mitosis and stained with various agents to delineate characteristic bands. DNA probes can be applied to locate specific gene sequences. Karyotyping is the arrangement of photographs of stained chromosomes in a standard format. Cytogenetic techniques are used to test for inborn errors of metabolism and genomic aberrations such as Down syndrome and to determine sex in cases where anatomy is inconclusive.

cy·to·gen·ic (sī-tō-jen'ik). Relating to cytogenesis.

cy·tog·e·nous (sī-toj'ě-nŭs). Cell-forming.

cy·to·glu·co·pe·nia (sī'tō-gloo-kō-pē'nē-ă). An intracellular deficiency of glucose. [cyto- + glucose + G. *penia*, poverty]

cy·toid (sī'toyd). Resembling a cell. [cyto- + G. *eidos*, resemblance]

cy·to·ker·a·tin (sī-tō-ker-a-tinz). SYN keratin.

cy·to·kine (sī'tō-kīn). Any of numerous hormonelike, low-molecular-weight proteins, secreted by various cell types, that regulate the intensity and duration of immune response and mediate cell-cell communication. SEE interferon, interleukin, lymphokine, chemokines. See entries under various growth factors. SEE ALSO interferon, interleukin, lymphokine. [cyto- + G. *kinēsis*, movement]

> Cytokines are produced by macrophages, B and T lymphocytes, mast cells, endothelial cells, fibroblasts, and stromal cells of the spleen, thymus, and bone marrow. They are involved in mediating immunity and allergy and in regulating the maturation, growth, and responsiveness of particular cell populations, sometimes including the cells that produce them (autocrine activity). A given cytokine may be produced by more than one type of cell. Some cytokines enhance or inhibit the action of other cytokines. The first cytokines to be identified were named according to their functions (e.g., T cell growth factor), but this nomenclature became awkward because several cytokines can have the same function, and the function of a cytokine can vary with the circumstances of its elaboration. Later, as the chemical structure of each cytokine was determined, it was designated an interleukin and assigned a number (e.g., interleukin-2 [IL-2], formerly T cell growth factor). Cytokines have been implicated in the generation and recall of long-term memory and the focusing of attention. Some of the degenerative effects of aging may be due to a progressive loss of regulatory capacity by cytokines. Because cytokines derived from the immune system (immunokines) are cytotoxic, they have been used against certain types of cancer.

c. network, a group of c.'s which together modulate and regulate key cellular functions.

cy·to·ki·ne·sis (sī′tō-ki-nē′sis). Changes occurring in the cytoplasm of the cell outside the nucleus during cell division. SYN cytodieresis. [cyto- + G. *kinēsis,* movement]

cy·to·lem·ma (sī-tō-lem′mă). SYN cell *membrane.* [cyto- + G. *lemma,* husk]

cy·to·lip·in (sī-tō-lip′in). A glycosphingolipid, specifically a ceramide oligosaccharide; **c. H,** a lactosylceramide, may display immunological properties under certain conditions; **c. K** is probably identical with globoside. Cf. *ceramide* lactosidase.

cy·to·log·ic (sī-tō-loj′ik). Relating to cytology.

cy·tol·o·gist (sī-tol′ō-jist). One who specializes in cytology.

cy·tol·o·gy (sī-tol′ō-jē). The study of the anatomy, physiology, pathology, and chemistry of the cell. SYN cellular biology, cytobiology. [cyto- + G. *logos,* study]

exfoliative c., the examination, for diagnostic purposes, of cells denuded from a neoplasm (or other type of lesion) and recovered from the sediment of the exudate, secretions, or washings from the tissue (e.g., sputum, vaginal secretion, gastric washings, urine). SYN cytopathology (2).

cy·tol·y·sin (sī-tol′i-sin). A substance i.e., an antibody that effects

cy

cytokines and chemokines: molecular weight, source, and function

human cytokines	MW (kDa)	cellular source	major functions
IL–1α	17.5	monocytes, MØ, B cells, T cells, NK cells, dendritic cells	↑ fever and acute phase protein synthesis; ↑ thymocyte and T-cell activation and B-cell growth, differentiation, and immunoglobulin secretion
IL–1β	17.5	monocytes, MØ, B cells, T cells, NK cells, dendritic cells	↑ fever and acute phase protein synthesis; ↑ thymocyte and T-cell activation and B-cell growth, differentiation, and immunoglobulin secretion
IL–2	15–20	T cells	↑ growth and differentiation of T cells, B cells, and NK cells
IL–3	14–30	T cells, mast cells, and eosinophils	↑ growth of hematopoietic stem cells and mast cells
IL–4	15–19	T cells, mast cells, and basophils	↑ differentiation of B cells and Th2 cells; ↑ IgG$_4$ and IgE synthesis; ↓ proinflammatory Th1 cell and MØ function
IL–5	45 homodimer	T cells, mast cells, and eosinophils	↑ growth and differentiation of eosinophils and B cells (IgA synthesis)
IL–6	26	monocytes, MØ, B cells, T cells, vascular endothelial cells	↑ acute phase protein synthesis; ↑ thymocyte and T cell activation; B cell growth, differentiation and Ig production
IL–7	20–28	fibroblasts, endothelial cells and T cells, BMC and thymic stromal cells	growth of pre-B; ↑ growth and differentiation of pre-T cells and mature T cells
IL–9	32–39	T cells	↑ T cell and mast-cell activation; ↑ IL-4 -induced IgE and IgC expression
IL–10	35–40	T cells, B1 B cells, and MØ	↓ Th1, NK cell, and MØ function including cytokine synthesis/release; ↑B-cell and mast cell proliferation
IL–11	23	fibroblasts and BMC stromal cells	↑ megakaryocyte (platelet progenitor) growth
IL–12	35,40 subunits heterodimer	B cells and MØ	↑ NK cells, CTL and Th1 generation, ↑ IFN-γ production by NK cells and T cells; ↑ NK and ADCC activity; costimulates T cell proliferation
IL–13	9–17	T cells	growth factor for B cells; ↑ IgM, IgE, and IgG4 synthesis; ↑B cell membrane CD23 and MHC class II Ag expression; ↓ monocyte/M Ø functions including proinflammatory cytokine synthesis
IL–14	60	follicular dendritic cells, T cells	↑ B cell proliferation and memory B cell generation; ↓ immunoglobulin synthesis
IL–15	14–15	monocytes, epithelial cells, muscle	↑ the growth and differentiation of T cells
IL–16	17	T cells, brain, thymus, spleen and pancreas	chemotactic for CD4 cells induces proliferation of T cell lines
IL–17	30–38 homodimer	CD4 T cells	↑ epithelial, endothelial, and fibroblastic cells to secrete IL-6, IL-8, GM-CSF
IL–18	18	monocytes/MØ	↑ IFN-γ production by T cells; ↑ NK activity
G–CSF	18–22	BMC stromal cells and monocytes/MØ	↑ growth, differentiation, and activation of precursor and mature granulocytes
M–CSF	45–90	T cells and monocytes/MØ	↑ growth, differentiation, and activation pf precursor and mature MØs
GM–CSF	22	T cells and monocytes/MØ	↑ growth, differentiation, and activation of precursor and mature granulocytes and MØs
TGF–β	25 homodimer	many cell types including T cells and monocytes/MØ	↑ IgA production and activation of naive T cells; ↓ activation of monocytes and memory T cells; active in fibroblast growth/wound healing
IFN–γ	40–70 homodimer	T cells and NK cells	antiviral; ↑ MØ and NK cell function; ↑ MHC class I and II cell surface antigen expression
TNF–a	17 homotrimer	many cell types including monocytes/MØ, B cells, T cells	expressed as cell surface homotrimer, also shed in soluble form by enzymatic cleavage; ↑ fever and septic shock; cytotoxic for many tumor cell types
LT–α (TNF–β)	20–25 subunits homotrimer or heterotrimer	T cells	(*aka* lymphotoxin) secreted as homotrimer or complexed with LT-β and expressed as cell surface heterotrimer; involved in 2° lymphoid tissue organogenesis
LIF	46	T cells, myelomonocytic lineages	↑ acute phase protein synth; ↑ MØ differentiation and hematopoietic stem cell proliferation

cytokines and chemokines: molecular weight, source, and function (cont.)			
human chemokines	Mw (kDa)	cellular source	major functions
IL–8	6–8	many cell types including monocytes, lymphocytes, and granulocytes	chemotactic and activating for neutrophils promotes angiogenesis
GROα	7–11	monocytes, epithelial and endothelial cells, and tumor cells *eg* melanoma	chemotactic and activating for neutrophils promotes angiogenesis and growth of certain tumors
IP–10	10–11	endothelial cells, monocytes and fibroblasts, thymic and splenic stromal cells	chemotactic for activated T cells inhibits endothelial cell proliferation
SDF–1	10	stromal cells, liver, muscle	stimulates growth of pre-B cells chemotactic for monocytes and T cells
MIG	14–15	IFN-γ treated monocytes and macrophages	chemotactic for tumor infiltrating lymphocytes
MCP–1	11–17	many cell types including monocyte/macrophages, fibroblasts and certain tumors	chemotactic for T cells, and induces chemotaxis and activation of monocytes
MCP–2	7.5–11	many cell types including monocyte/macrophages, fibroblasts and certain tumors	chemotactic for T cells, and induces chemotaxis and activation of monocytes
MCP–3	11	many cell types including monocyte/macrophages, fibroblasts, and certain tumors	chemotactic for eosinophils and T cells, induces chemotaxis and activation of monocytes
MIP–1α	10	many cell types including monocytes, lymphocytes, and stromal cells	chemotactic for monocytes and T cells; inhibits proliferation of hemopoietic stem cells
MIP–1β	10	many cell types including monocytes, lymphocytes, and tumor cells	chemotactic for monocytes and T cells; inhibits proliferation of hemopoietic stem cells
RANTES	10	many cell types including T cells, monocytes, fibroblasts, and certain tumor cell lines	chemotaxis of T cells, monocytes, and eosinophils
eotaxin	8–9	endothelial cells, alveolar macrophages, lung, intestine, heart, thymus, spleen, liver, kidney	eosinophil chemotaxis
lymphotactin	10	thymocytes, activated T cells	T-cell chemotaxis
I–309	10–16	T cells, mast cells	chemotaxis of neutrophils

abbreviations

↑	= increases (stimulates)	IL	= interleukin	NK cells	= natural killer cells
↓	= decreases (suppresses)	LIF	= leukocyte inhibitory factor	Th1	= type 1 T helper cell
BMC	= bone marrow cell	LT	= long terminal	Th2	= type 2 T helper cell
CTL	= cytototoxic T-lymphocytes	MØ	= macrophage	TNF	= tumor necrosis factor
GM-CSF	= granulocyte macrophage–colony stimulating factor	MHC	= major histocompatibilty complex		
IFN	= interferon	MIP	= macrophage inhibitory protein		

partial or complete destruction of an animal cell; may require complement. SEE ALSO perforin.

cy·tol·y·sis (sī-tol′i-sis). The dissolution of a cell. [cyto- + G. *lysis,* loosening]

cy·to·ly·so·some (sī-tō-lī′sō-sōm). A variety of secondary lysosome that contains the remnants of mitochondria, ribosomes, or other organelles. SYN autophagic vacuole.

cy·to·lyt·ic (sī-tō-lit′ik). Pertaining to cytolysis; possessing a solvent or destructive action on cells.

cy·to·ma·trix (sī-tō-mā′triks). SYN cytoplasmic *matrix.*

cy·to·me·ga·lic (sī-tō-meg′ă-lik). Denoting or characterized by markedly enlarged cells. [cyto- + G. *megas,* big]

⊞Cy·to·meg·a·lo·vi·rus (CMV) (sī-tō-meg′ă-lō-vī′rŭs). A group of viruses in the family Herpesviridae infecting humans and other animals, many of the viruses having special affinity for salivary glands, and causing enlargement of cells of various organs and development of characteristic inclusions (owl eye) in the cytoplasm or nucleus. Infection of embryo in utero may result in malformation and fetal death. They are all species-specific and include salivary virus, inclusion body rhinitis virus of pigs, and others. SYN visceral disease virus. [cyto- + G. *megas,* big]

cy·to·mem·brane (sī-tō-mem′brān). SYN cell *membrane.*

cy·to·mere (sī′tō-mēr). The structure separating the portions of the contents of a large schizont in the course of schizogony, as in some of the sporozoans undergoing exoerythrocytic asexual division. C.'s are caused by complex invaginations of the surface of the schizont, which isolates them; ultimately, c.'s complete the budding process in the formation of large numbers of merozoites. [cyto- + G. *meros,* part]

cy·tom·e·ter (sī-tom′ĕ-ter). A standardized, usually ruled glass slide or small glass chamber of known volume, used in counting and measuring cells, especially blood cells. [cyto- + G. *metron,* measure]

image c., apparatus for measuring various qualitative tests, such as antibody density.

cy·tom·e·try (sī-tom′ĕ-trē). The counting of cells, especially blood cells, using a cytometer or hemocytometer.

Feulgen c., a form of cytometry using Feulgen-stained nuclei to characterize the chromatin pattern and nuclear distribution of DNA of cells.

flow c., a method of measuring fluorescence from stained cells that are in suspension and flowing through a narrow orifice, usually in combination with one or two lasers to activate the dyes; used to measure cell size, number, viability, and nucleic acid content with the aid of acridine orange, Kasten fluorescent Feulgen stain, ethidium bromide, trypan blue, and other selected staining reagents. SYN flow cytophotometry.

cy·to·mi·cro·some (sī-tō-mī′krō-sōm). SEE microsome. [cyto- + G. *mikros,* small, + *sōma,* body]

cy·to·mor·phol·o·gy (sī′tō-mōr-fol′ō-jē). The study of the structure of cells.

cy·to·mor·pho·sis (sī′tō-mōr-fō′sis). Changes that the cell undergoes during the various stages of its existence. SEE ALSO prosoplasia. [cyto- + G. *morphōsis,* a shaping]

diagnosis of cytomegalovirus (CMV)	
histology	liver, kidney, lung, salivary glands, and other organs
cytology	urine; inclusion bodies in epithelial cells,especially in children up to 3 mos.; saliva
immuno-fluorescence	specific intranuclear and intracytoplasmic inclusions in tissue sections
virus culture	tissue cultures from urine, throat cultures,lymphocytes, cervical secretion, biopsy and necropsy materials (sperm, breast milk)
hybridization treatment	separation of cellular from viral DNA
serologic antibody evidence	complement binding reaction (CBR), passive hemoagglutination, immunofluorescence, neutralization test in tissue cultures,determination of IgM antibodies if active infection is suspected

cy·to·path·ic (sī-tō-path′ik). Pertaining to or exhibiting cytopathy.

cy·to·path·o·gen·ic (sī′tō-path-ō-jen′ik). Pertaining to an agent or substance that causes a diseased condition in cells, in contrast to histologic changes; used especially with reference to effects observed in cells in tissue cultures.

cy·to·path·o·log·ic, cy·to·path·o·log·i·cal (sī′tō-pa-thō-loj′ik, -loj′i-kăl). **1.** Denoting cellular changes in disease. **2.** Relating to cytopathology.

cy·to·pa·thol·o·gist (sī′tō-pa-thol′ō-jist). A physician, usually skilled in anatomical pathology, who is specially trained and experienced in cytopathology.

cy·to·pa·thol·o·gy (sī′tō-pa-thol′ō-jē). **1.** The study of disease changes within individual cells or cell types. **2.** SYN exfoliative *cytology.*

cy·top·a·thy (sī-top′ă-thē). Any disorder of a cell or anomaly of any of its constituents. [cyto- + G. *pathos,* disease]

cy·to·pemp·sis (sī-tō-pemp′sis). SYN transcytosis. [cyto- + G. *pempis,* sending through]

cy·to·pe·nia (sī-tō-pē′nē-ă). A reduction, i.e., hypocytosis, or a lack of cellular elements in the circulating blood. [cyto- + G. *penia,* poverty]

cy·toph·a·gy (sī-tof′ă-jē). Devouring of other cells by phagocytes. [cyto- + G. *phagō,* to devour]

cy·to·phan·ere (sī′tō-fă-nēr). A radial spine seen in certain cysts of *Sarcocystis,* as in rabbit and sheep tissue cysts. [cyto- + G. *phaneros,* visible, evident, open]

cy·to·phar·ynx (sī′tō-far′inks). An organelle in certain flagellates and ciliates that serves as a gullet through which food material passes from the cytostome to the cell interior; food passed is collected in food vacuoles, into which digestive enzymes are secreted.

cy·to·phil·ic (sī-tō-fil′ik). SYN cytotropic. [cyto- + G. *philos,* fond]

cy·to·pho·tom·e·try (sī′tō-fō-tom′ĕ-trē). A method of measuring the absorption of monochromatic light by stained microscopic structures (e.g., chromosomes, nuclei, whole cells) with the aid of a photoelectric cell; also used to measure emitted light from such objects by fluorescence in combination with selected fluorochrome dyes. [cyto- + G. *phōs,* light + *metron,* measure]

flow c., SYN flow *cytometry.*

cy·to·phy·lac·tic (sī′tō-fī-lak′tik). Relating to cytophylaxis.

cy·to·phy·lax·is (sī′tō-fī-lak′sis). Protection of cells against lytic agents. [cyto- + G. *phylaxis,* a guarding]

cy·to·phy·let·ic (sī′tō-fī-let′ik). Relating to the genealogy of a cell. [cyto- + G. *phylē,* a tribe]

cy·to·pi·pette (sī′tō-pi-pet′). A slightly curved, blunt end pipette usually made of glass and fitted with a rubber bulb to provide gentle negative pressure for the collection of vaginal secretions for cytological examination.

cy·to·plasm (sī′tō-plazm). The substance of a cell, exclusive of the nucleus, which contains various organelles and inclusions within a colloidal protoplasm. SEE ALSO protoplasm, hyaloplasm, cytosol. [cyto- + G. *plasma,* thing formed]

ground-glass c., uniform finely granular eosinophilic c. seen in hepatocytes in carriers of hepatitis B virus, and also in epidermal cells in keratoacanthoma.

cy·to·plas·mic (sī-tō-plaz′mik). Relating to the cytoplasm.

cy·to·plas·mon (sī-tō-plaz′mon). The total extranuclear genetic information of a eukaryotic cell excluding that of mitochondria and plastids.

cy·to·plast (sī′tō-plast). The living intact cytoplasm that remains following cell enucleation. [cyto- + G. *plastos,* formed]

cy·to·poi·e·sis (sī-tō-poy-ē′sis). Formation of cells. [cyto- + G. *poiēsis,* a making]

cy·to·prep·a·ra·tion (sī′tō-prep-ă-rā′shŭn). Laboratory preparation of a cellular specimen for cytologic examination.

cy·to·py·ge (sī-tō-pī′jē). The anal orifice (cell "anus") found in certain structurally complex protozoa, such as the rumen-dwelling ciliates of herbivores, through which waste matter is ejected. [cyto- + G. *pygē,* buttocks]

cy·to·ryc·tes, cy·tor·rhyc·tes (sī-tō-rik′tēz). Obsolete term for inclusion *bodies,* under *body.* [cyto- + G. *oryktēs,* a digger]

cytoscreener (sī′tō-skrēn′er). SYN cytotechnologist.

cy·to·sides (sī′tō-sīdz). Ceramide disaccharides. SEE glycosphingolipid.

cy·to·sine (Cyt) (sī′tō-sēn). a pyrimidine found in nucleic acids.

c. arabinoside (CA, AraC), (1) a synthetic nucleoside used as an antimetabolite in the treatment of neoplasms; **(2)** incorrect term for arabinosylcytosine.

c. ribonucleoside, SYN cytidine.

cy·to·sis (sī-tō′sis). **1.** A condition in which there is more than the usual number of cells, as in the c. of spinal fluid in acute leptomeningitis. **2.** Frequently used with a prefixed combining form as a means of describing certain features pertaining to cells; e.g., isocytosis, equality in size; polycytosis, abnormal increase in number. [cyto- + G. *-osis,* condition]

cy·to·skel·e·ton (sī-tō-skel′ĕ-ton). The tonofilaments, keratin, desmin, neurofilaments, or other intermediate filaments serving to act as supportive cytoplasmic elements to stiffen cells or to organize intracellular organelles.

cy·to·smear (sī′tō-smēr). SYN cytologic *smear.*

cy·to·sol (sī′tō-sol). Cytoplasm exclusive of the mitochondria, endoplasmic reticulum, and other membranous components. [cyto- + "sol," abbrev. of soluble]

cy·to·sol·ic (sī-tō-sol′ik). Relating to or contained in the cytosol.

cy·to·some (sī′tō-sōm). **1.** The cell body exclusive of the nucleus. **2.** Distinctive granule found in great alveolar (type II) cells of the lung that releases pulmonary surfactant on the alveolar surfaces. SYN multilamellar body. [cyto- + G. *sōma,* body]

cy·tos·ta·sis (sī-tos′tă-sis). The slowing of movement and accumulation of blood cells, especially polymorphonuclear leukocytes, in the capillaries, as in a region of inflammation; obstruction of a capillary as the result of accumulated leukocytes. [cyto- + G. *stasis,* standing]

cy·to·stat·ic (sī-tō-stat′ik). Characterized by cytostasis.

cy·to·stome (sī′tō-stōm). The cell "mouth" of certain complex protozoa, usually with a short gullet or cytopharynx leading food into the organism, where it is collected into food vacuoles, then circulated inside the body, eventually to be excreted through the cytopyge. [cyto- + G. *stoma,* mouth]

cy·to·tac·tic (sī-tō-tak′tik). Relating to cytotaxis.

cy·to·tax·is, cy·to·tax·ia (sī-tō-tak′sis, -tak′sē-ă). The attraction (**positive c.**) or repulsion (**negative c.**) of cells for one another. [cyto- + G. *taxis,* arrangement]

cytotechnologist (sī′tō-tek-nol′ŏ-jist). A person with special training in cytopathology who is responsible for screening Pap smears and determining which are negative and which require further review by a pathologist. SEE ALSO Pap *smear*, Pap *test*. SYN cytoscreener.

cy·toth·e·sis (sī-toth′ĕ-sis). The repair of injury in a cell; the restoration of cells. [cyto- + G. *thesis,* a placing]

cy·to·tox·ic (sī-tō-tok′sik). Detrimental or destructive to cells.

cy·to·tox·ic·i·ty (sī′tō-tok-sis′i-tē). The quality or state of being cytotoxic.

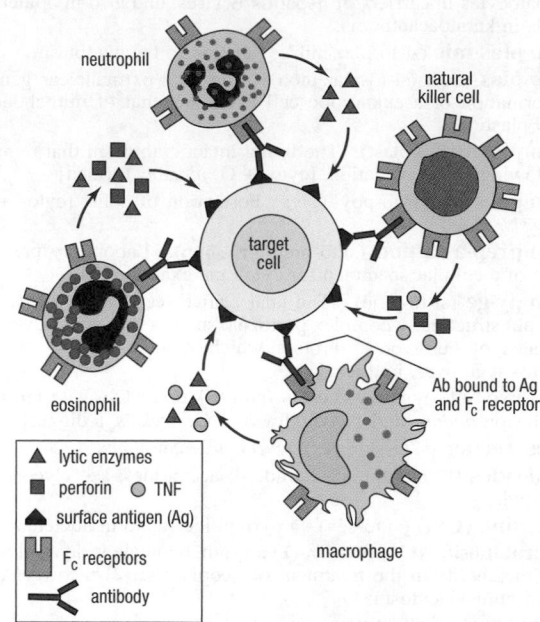

antibody-dependent cell-mediated cytotoxicity (ADCC): nonspecific cytotoxic cells are directed to specific target cells by binding to Fc region of antibody bound to surface antigens on target cells; various substances (e.g., lytic enzymes, tumor necrosis factor (TNF), perforin) secreted by nonspecific cytotoxic cells then mediate target-cell destruction

antibody-dependent cell-mediated c. (ADCC), a form of cell-mediated cytotoxicity that functions by binding of the FC region of IgG antibodies to Fc receptors on leukocytes. The FAB region of the antibody binds to the target cell. Killing of the target cell may be through various modalities, e.g., perforin, reactive oxygen intermediates, cytokines.

lymphocyte-mediated c., the toxic or lytic activity of lymphocytes, which may or may not be mediated by antibodies. Cytotoxic T lymphocytes may cause lysis of cells by production of cytolytic proteins such as perforin. B cells may cause lysis of cells by antibody-complement binding to a target cell. Natural killer cells are cytotoxic without prior sensitization. SEE ALSO antibody-dependent cell-mediated c.

cy·to·tox·in (sī′tō-tok′sin). A specific substance, which may or may not be antibody, that inhibits or prevents the functions of cells, causes destruction of cells, or both. SEE ALSO perforin. [cyto- + G. *toxikon,* poison]

vero c., a cell c. produced by enterohemorrhagic *Escherichia coli* that appears to contribute to the occurrence of hemorrhagic colitis and hemolytic uremic syndrome. SYN Shigalike toxin.

cy·to·tro·pho·blast (sī-tō-trof′ō-blast). The inner layer of the trophoblast. SYN Langhans layer.

cy·to·tro·pic (sī-tō-trop′ik). Having an affinity for cells. SYN cytophilic.

cy·tot·ro·pism (sī-tot′rō-pizm). **1.** Affinity for cells. **2.** Affinity for specific cells, especially the ability of viruses to localize in and damage specific cells. [cyto- + G. *tropos,* a turning]

cy·to·zo·ic (sī-tō-zō′ik). Living in a cell; denoting certain parasitic protozoa.

cy·to·zo·on (sī-tō-zō′on). A protozoan cell or organism. [cyto- + G. *zōon,* animal]

cy·tu·ria (sī-too′rē-ă). The passage of cells in unusual numbers in the urine. [G. *kytos,* cell, + *ouron,* urine]

Czapek, Friedrich J.F., Czechoslovakian botanist, 1868–1921. SEE C. solution *agar;* C.-Dox *medium.*

CZE Abbreviation for capillary zone *electrophoresis.*

Czerny, Vincenz, German surgeon, 1842–1916. SEE C. *suture;* C.-Lembert *suture.*

Δ, δ **1.** Fourth letter of the Greek alphabet, delta. **2.** In chemistry, denotes a double bond, usually with a superscript to indicate position in a chain (Δ^5); application of heat in a reaction (A $\xrightarrow{\Delta}$ B); absence of heat treatment ($\not\Delta$); distance between two atoms in a molecule; or position of a substituent located on the fourth atom from the carboxyl or other primary functional group (δ); change (Δ); thickness (δ); chemical shift in NMR (δ).

D 1. Symbol for the vitamin D potency of cod liver oil, multiples of which (5D, 100D, etc.) are used to designate the vitamin D potency of irradiated ergosterol (viosterol) or other substances; for deuterium; for dihydrouridine in nucleic acids; for diffusing capacity; for aspartic acid; dihydrouridine; diffusion *coefficient* (in italics). **2.** In optics, abbreviation for diopter; for dexter (right). **3.** In electrodiagnosis, abbreviation for duration, the current flowing and the circuit being closed. **4.** In dental formulas, abbreviation for deciduous (2). **5.** As a subscript, refers to dead *space*. SEE physiologic dead *space*. **6.** D line in Na emission spectra.

2,4-D Abbreviation for (2,4-dichlorophenoxy) acetic acid.

d Symbol for deci-; abbreviation for *dexter* [L], right; diameter; day.

△**D-.** Prefix indicating that a chemical compound is sterically related to D-glyceraldehyde, the basis of stereochemical nomenclature. Cf. L-.

△**d-.** Prefix indicating a chemical compound to be dextrorotatory; should be avoided when (+) or (−) could be used. Cf. *l-*.

△**-d.** Suffix indicating the presence of deuterium in a compound in concentrations above normal, thus labeling the compound; subscripts (d_2, d_3, etc.) indicate the number of such atoms so fortified.

DA Abbreviation for developmental *age* (2).

Da Symbol for dalton.

dA, dAdo Abbreviation for deoxyadenosine.

da Symbol for deca-.

Daae, Anders, Norwegian physician, 1838–1910. SEE D. *disease.*

DAB Abbreviation for 3'3-diaminobenzidine HCl; in the immunoperoxidase technique, used to produce a colored complex at the site of peroxidase activity.

da·car·ba·zine (DTIC) (dă-kar′bă-zēn). An antineoplastic agent used in the treatment of malignant melanoma and sarcoma.

△**dacry-.** SEE dacryo-.

dac·ry·ad·e·ni·tis (dak′rē-ad-ĕ-nī′tis). SYN dacryoadenitis.

△**dacryo-, dacry-.** Tears; lacrimal sac or duct. [G. *dakryon*, tear]

dac·ry·o·ad·e·ni·tis (dak-rē-ō-ad-ĕ-nī′tis). Inflammation of the lacrimal gland. SYN dacryadenitis. [dacryo- + G. *adēn*, gland, + -*itis*, inflammation]

dac·ry·o·blen·nor·rhea (dak-rē-ō-blen-ō-rē′ă). A chronic discharge of mucus from a lacrimal sac. [dacryo- + G. *blenna*, mucus, + *rhoia*, flow]

dac·ry·o·cele (dak′rē-ō-sēl). SYN dacryocystocele.

dac·ry·o·cyst (dak′rē-ō-sist). SYN lacrimal *sac.* [dacryo- + G. *kystis*, sac]

dac·ry·o·cys·tal·gia (dak′rē-ō-sis-tal′jē-ă). Pain in the lacrimal sac. [dacryocyst + G. *algos*, pain]

dac·ry·o·cys·tec·to·my (dak′rē-ō-sis-tek′tō-mē). Surgical removal of the lacrimal sac. [dacryocyst + G. *ektomē*, excision]

🔲**dac·ry·o·cys·ti·tis** (dak′rē-ō-sis-tī′tis). Inflammation of the lacrimal sac. [dacryocyst + G. -*itis*, inflammation]

dac·ry·o·cys·to·cele (dak′rē-ō-sis′tō-sēl). Enlargement of the lacrimal sac with fluid. SYN dacryocele. [dacryocyst + G. *kēlē*, hernia]

dac·ry·o·cys·to·gram (dak′rē-ō-sis′tō-gram). A radiograph of the lacrimal apparatus obtained after injection of contrast material for the purpose of determining the presence of and localizing a site of obstruction; this procedure has been largely replaced by the CT and MRI. [dacryocyst + G. *gramma*, a writing]

dac·ry·o·cys·to·rhi·nos·to·my (dak′rē-ō-sis′tō-rī-nos′tō-mē). An operation providing an anastomosis between the lacrimal sac and the nasal mucosa through an opening in the lacrimal bone. [dacryocyst + G. *rhis* (rhin-), nose, + *stoma*, mouth]

dac·ry·o·cys·tot·o·my (dak′rē-ō-sis-tot′ō-mē). Incision of the lacrimal sac. [dacryocyst + G. *tomē*, incision]

dac·ry·o·hem·or·rhea (dak′rē-ō-hem-ō-rē′ă). Bloody tears. [dacryo- + G. *haima*, blood, + *rhoia*, flow]

dac·ry·o·lith (dak′rē-ō-lith). A concretion in the lacrimal apparatus. SYN lacrimal calculus, ophthalmolith, tear stone. [dacryo- + G. *lithos*, stone]

Desmarres d.'s, SYN Nocardia d.'s.

Nocardia d.'s, white pseudoconcretions, composed of masses of *Nocardia* species found in the lacrimal canaliculi. SYN Desmarres d.'s.

dac·ry·o·li·thi·a·sis (dak′rē-ō-li-thī′ă-sis). The formation and presence of dacryoliths.

dac·ry·on (dak′rē-on). The point of junction of the frontomaxillary and lacrimomaxillary sutures on the medial wall of the orbit. See figure under craniometric *points*, under *point*. [G. a tear]

dac·ry·ops (dak′rē-ops). **1.** Excess of tears in the eye. **2.** A cyst of a duct of the lacrimal gland. [dacryo- + G. *ōps*, eye]

dac·ry·o·py·or·rhea (dak′rē-ō-pī-ō-rē′ă). The discharge of tears containing leukocytes. [dacryo- + G. *pyon*, pus, + *rhoia*, flow]

dac·ry·or·rhea (dak′rē-ō-rē′ă). An excessive secretion of tears. [dacryo- + G. *rhoia*, flow]

dac·ry·o·ste·no·sis (dak′rē-ō-ste-nō′sis). Stricture of the lacrimal duct. [dacryo- + G. *stenōsis*, narrowing]

dac·ti·no·my·cin (dak′ti-nō-mī′sin). Produced by several species of *Streptomyces* (e.g., *S. parvulus*); an antineoplastic antibiotic used especially for Ewing sarcoma, rhabdomyosarcoma, and Wilms tumor in children and for trophoblastic disease in women. SEE ALSO actinomycin. SYN actinomycin D.

dac·tyl (dak′til). SYN digit. [G. *daktylos*]

△**dactyl-.** SEE dactylo-.

dac·ty·lal·gia (dak-ti-lal′jē-ă). Pain in the fingers. SYN dactylodynia. [dactyl- + G. *algos*, pain]

Dac·ty·la·ria (dak-ti-lā′rē-ă). A genus of dematiaceous soildwelling fungi. *D. gallopava* is a causative agent of phaeohyphomycosis in chickens and turkeys. [G. *daktylos*, finger]

dac·ty·li·tis (dak-ti-lī′tis). Inflammation of one or more fingers. **blistering distal d.,** infection of the volar fat pad of the distal phalanx of the finger by group A β-hemolytic streptococci. **sickle cell d.,** SYN hand-and-foot *syndrome.*

△**dactylo-, dactyl-.** The fingers and (less often) toes. See entries under digit. [G. *daktylos*, finger]

dac·ty·lo·camp·sis (dak′ti-lō-kamp′sis). Permanent flexion of the fingers. [dactylo- + G. *kampsis*, bending]

dac·ty·lo·camp·so·dyn·ia (dak′ti-lō-kamp′sō-din′ē-ă). Painful contraction of one or more fingers. [dactylo- + G. *kampsis*, a bending, + *odynē*, pain]

dac·ty·lo·dyn·ia (dak′tĭ-lō-din′ē-ă). SYN dactylalgia.

dac·ty·lo·gry·po·sis (dak′ti-lō-gri-pō′sis). Contraction of the fingers. [dactylo- + G. *grypōsis*, a crooking]

dac·ty·lol·o·gy (dak′ti-lol′ō-jē). The use of the finger alphabet in communicating. SYN cheirology, chirology. [dactylo- + G. *logos*, word]

dac·tyl·o·meg·a·ly (dak′til-ō-meg′ă-lē). SYN megadactyly. [dactylo- + G. *megas*, large]

<table>
<tr><td>△ Combining Forms</td><td>☆ Official alternate
Terminologia Anatomica
term</td></tr>
<tr><td>🔲 Indicates term is illustrated,
see Illustration Index</td><td></td></tr>
<tr><td>SYN Synonym</td><td>[MIM] Mendelian Inheritance
in Man</td></tr>
<tr><td>Cf. Compare</td><td>C.I. Colour Index</td></tr>
<tr><td>[NA] Nomina Anatomica</td><td>High Profile Term</td></tr>
<tr><td>[TA] Terminologia Anatomica</td><td></td></tr>
</table>

dac·ty·los·co·py (dak-ti-los′kŏ-pē). An examination of the markings in prints made from the fingertips; employed as a method of personal identification. SEE Galton system of classification of *fingerprints*, under *fingerprint*. [dactylo- + G. *skopeō*, to examine]

dac·ty·lo·spasm (dak′ti-lō-spazm). Spasmodic contraction of the fingers or toes.

dac·ty·lus, pl. **dac·ty·li** (dak′ti-lŭs, -lī). SYN digit. [G. *daktylos*]

dac·u·ro·ni·um (dak-ū-rō′nē-ŭm). A nondepolarizing steroid neuromuscular blocking agent with more rapid onset and shorter duration of action than pancuronium.

Da Fano, Corrado D., Italian-American anatomist, 1879–1927. SEE Da F. *stain*.

DAG Abbreviation for diacylglycerol.

dag·ga (dag′ă). Leaves of *Leonotis leonurus*, a plant found in South Africa, where it is smoked like tobacco with mild sedative effect; a term mistakenly applied to Indian hemp, *Cannabis sativa*. [aborigines′ term]

Dagnini, Giuseppe, Italian physician, 1866–1928. SEE Aschner-D. *reflex*.

DAH Abbreviation for disordered action of heart.

dah·lia (dal′yah). A violet dye, methyl-triethyl-amino-triphenyl-carbinol chloride. Also called Hoffman violet.

dah·lin. SYN inulin. [fr. *dahlia*, after A. *Dahl*, Swedish botanist, 1751–1789]

dahll·ite (dah′līt). A naturally occurring calcium phosphate, similar in structure to the mineral portions of bones and teeth. SYN podolite.

dai·sy (dā′zē). Colloquial term descriptive of the segmented forms (merozoites) of the mature schizont of *Plasmodium malariae*.

Dakin, Henry, U.S. chemist, 1880–1952. SEE D. *fluid, solution;* D.-Carrel *treatment*.

Dale, Sir Henry Hallett, English physiologist and Nobel laureate, 1875–1968. SEE D. *reaction;* D.-Feldberg *law;* Schultz-D. *reaction*.

Dalen, Johan A., Swedish ophthalmologist, 1866–1940. SEE D.-Fuchs *nodules*, under *nodule*.

Dalgarno, Lynn, contemporary Australian molecular biologist.

Dalrymple, John, English oculist, 1803–1852. SEE D. *sign*.

Dalton, John, English chemist, mathematician, and natural philosopher, 1766–1844. SEE D. *law;* D.-Henry *law;* daltonian; daltonism.

dal·ton (Da) (dawl′tŏn). Term unofficially used to indicate a unit of mass equal to $^{1}/_{12}$ the mass of a carbon-12 atom, 1.0000 in the atomic mass scale; numerically, but not dimensionally, equal to molecular or particle weight (atomic mass units). [J *Dalton*]

dal·to·ni·an (dawl-tō′nē-ăn). **1.** Attributed to or described by John Dalton. **2.** Pertaining to daltonism.

dal·ton·ism (dawl′tŏn-izm). A color vision deficiency, especially deuteranomaly or deuteranopia. [J. *Dalton*]

DALYs Abbreviation for disability-adjusted life *years*, under *year*.

DAM Abbreviation for diacetylmonoxime.

Dam, C.P. Henrik, Danish biochemist and Nobel laureate, 1895–1976. SEE D. *unit*.

dam. **1.** Any barrier to the flow of fluid. **2.** In surgery and dentistry, a sheet of thin rubber arranged so as to shut off the part operated upon from the access of fluid. [A.S. *fordemman*, to stop up]

post d., SYN posterior palatal *seal*.

rubber d., (1) in surgery, thin strips of rubber used as a surgical drain or barrier; **(2)** a thin sheet of rubber with holes that is placed over teeth to isolate them from the oral cavity.

damage.

diffuse alveolar damage, SYN adult respiratory distress *syndrome*.

Dam·a·lin·ia (dam-ă-lin′ē-ă). A genus of biting lice containing a number of species found on domestic and wild animals; they are all highly host-specific, one species being confined to each species of mammal. SEE ALSO *Bovicola, Trichodectes.*

dam·mar. A resin resembling copal, obtained from various species of *Shorea* (family Dipterocarpaceae) in the East Indies; used, dissolved in chloroform, for mounting microscopic specimens. [Hind. *dāmar*, resin]

dam meth·yl·ase. An enzyme responsible for the methylation of adenine residues in specific sequences. SYN deoxyadenosine methylase.

dAMP Abbreviation for deoxyadenylic acid.

damp. **1.** Humid; moist. **2.** Atmospheric moisture. **3.** Foul air in a mine; air charged with carbon oxides (black or choke d.) or with various explosive hydrocarbon vapors (firedamp).

damp·ing. Bringing a mechanism to rest with minimal oscillation; e.g., in echocardiography, electrical or mechanical loading to reduce duration of echo, transmitter pulse, and transmitter complex. [M.E. *damp*, poisonous vapor]

Damus-Kaye-Stancel pro·ce·dure. See under procedure.

Dana, Charles L., U.S. neurologist, 1852–1935. SEE D. *operation;* Putnam-D. *syndrome*.

da·na·zol (dā′nă-zol). An anterior pituitary suppressant used in the treatment of endometriosis, fibrocystic breast disease, and angioedema.

Dance, Jean B.H., French physician, 1797–1832. SEE D. *sign*.

dance (dans). Involuntary movements related to brain damage.

hilar d., vigorous pulmonary arterial pulsations due to increased blood flow, often seen fluoroscopically in patients with congenital left-to-right shunts, especially atrial septal defects.

Saint Anthony d., Saint Vitus d., Saint John d., obsolete eponyms for Sydenham *chorea*.

dan·der. **1.** A fine scaling of the skin and scalp. SEE ALSO dandruff. **2.** A normal effluvium of animal hair or coat capable of causing allergic responses in atopic persons.

dan·druff (dan′drŭf). The presence, in varying amounts, of white or gray scales in the hair of the scalp, due to excessive or normal branny exfoliation of the epidermis. SEE ALSO seborrheic *dermatitis*. SYN pityriasis capitis, scurf, seborrhea sicca (2).

Dandy, Walter E., U.S. neurosurgeon, 1886–1946. SEE D. *operation;* D.-Walker *syndrome*.

Dane, D.S., 20th century British virologist. SEE D. *particles,* under *particle*.

Dane stain. See under stain.

Danforth, William Clark, U.S. obstetrician-gynecologist, 1878–1949. SEE D. *sign*.

Danielssen, Daniel C., Norwegian physician, 1815–1894. SEE D. *disease;* D.-Boeck *disease*.

Danlos, Henri A., French dermatologist, 1844–1912. SEE Ehlers-D. *syndrome*.

DANS Abbreviation for 1-dimethylaminonaphthalene-5-sulfonic acid; a green fluorescing compound used in immunohistochemistry to detect antigens.

dan·syl (Dns, DNS) (dan′sil). The 5-dimethylaminonaphthalene-1-sulfonyl radical; a blocking agent for NH_2 groups, used in peptide synthesis.

dan·thron. An anthraquinone laxative. SYN chrysazine.

dan·tro·lene so·di·um (dan′trō-lēn). A synthetic skeletal muscle relaxant that acts directly on muscle by uncoupling electrical from mechanical events; also, the specific agent for prevention and treatment of malignant hyperthermia.

Danysz, Jan, Polish pathologist in France, 1860–1928. SEE D. *phenomenon*.

DAPI Abbreviation for 4′6-diamidino-2-phenylindole·2HCl, a fluorescent probe for DNA. SEE DAPI *stain*.

dap·sone (dap′sōn). An antibiotic used in the treatment of leprosy and certain cutaneous diseases such as dermatitis herpetiformis, is active against the tubercle bacillus, is used in the treatment of bovine coccidiosis and streptococcal mastitis, and is used as a second-line agent in *Pneumocystis carinii* pneumonia, a disease common in AIDS patients.

d′Arcet, Jean, French chemist, 1725–1801. SEE d′A. *metal*.

Darier, Jean F., French dermatologist, 1856–1938. SEE D. *disease, sign*.

Darkschewitsch (Darkshevich), Liverij O., Russian neurologist, 1858–1925. SEE *nucleus* of D.

Darling, Samuel Taylor, U.S. physician in Panama, 1872–1925. SEE D. *disease.*

Darrow red. A basic oxazin dye used as a substitute for cresyl violet acetate in the staining of Nissl substance. [Mary A. *Darrow,* U.S. stain technologist, 1894–1973]

d'Arsonval, Jacques Arsène, French biophysicist, 1851–1940. SEE d'A. *current, galvanometer.*

dar·to·ic, dar·toid (dar-tō′ik, dar′toyd). Resembling tunica dartos in its slow involuntary contractions. [G. *dartos,* flayed]

dar·tos (dar′tōs). SEE dartos *fascia.* [G. skinned or flayed, fr. *derō,* to skin]

d. mulieb′ris, a very thin layer of smooth muscle in the integument of the labia majora; less well-developed than the tunica dartos of the scrotum.

Darwin, Charles R., English biologist and evolutionist, 1809–1882. SEE darwinian *ear;* darwinian *evolution;* darwinian *reflex;* darwinian *theory;* darwinian *tubercle.*

dar·win·i·an (dar-win′ē-an). Relating to or ascribed to Darwin.

Das·y·proc·ta (das′ē-prok′tă). A genus of rodents of the guinea pig family, a reservoir host of *Trypanosoma cruzi.* SYN *agouti.* [G. *dasyprōktos,* having hairy buttocks]

da·ta. Multiple facts (usually but not necessarily empirical) used as a basis for inference, testing, models, etc. The word is plural and takes a plural verb.

da·ta pro·cess·ing. Conversion of crude information into usable or storable form; statistical analysis of data by a computer program.

da·tum (dā′tŭm). An individual piece of information used in a scholarly field. [L., *given,* fr. *do,* pp. *datum,* to give]

Da·tu·ra (da-too′ră). A genus of solanaceous plants. Several species (*D. arborea, D. fastuosa, D. ferox,* and *D. sanguinea*) are used in Brazil, India, and Peru to produce unconsciousness. The seeds contain hyoscine (scopolamine), an alkaloid with an anticholinergic action similar to that of atropine. [Hind.]

D. me′tel, *D. fastuosa* L. var. *alba;* a species that contains scopolamine as its chief alkaloid and traces of hyoscyamine and atropine.

D. stramo′nium, a species that is the main source of stramonium. SYN Jamestown weed, jimson weed, stink weed, thorn apple.

da·tu·rine (da-too′rin, -rēn). SYN hyoscyamine.

Daubenton (D'Aubenton), Louis J.M., French physician, 1716–1799. SEE D. *angle, line, plane.*

daugh·ter (daw′ter). In nuclear medicine, an isotope that is the disintegration product of a radionuclide. SEE daughter *isotope,* radionuclide *generator.* [O.E. *dohtor*]

DES (diethylstilbestrol) daughter, the daughter of a woman who received diethylstilbestrol during pregnancy; DES daughters are at risk of deformity, adenosis, and other epithelial changes of the vagina and cervix, including clear cell adenocarcinoma.

dau·no·my·cin (daw-nō-mī′sin). SYN daunorubicin.

dau·no·ru·bi·cin (daw-nō-roo′bi-sin). An antibiotic of the rhodomycin group, obtained from *Streptomyces peucetius;* used in the treatment of acute leukemia; also used in cytogenetics to produce Q-type chromosome bands. SYN daunomycin.

Davidoff, M. von, German histologist, †1904. SEE D. *cells,* under *cell.*

Davidson, Edward C., U.S. surgeon, 1894–1933. SEE D. *syringe.*

Daviel, Jacques, French oculist, 1693–1762. SEE D. *operation, spoon.*

Davies, J.N.P., U.S. pathologist, *1915. SEE D. *disease.*

Davis, Hallowell, U.S. physiologist, 1896–1992. SEE D. battery model of *transduction.*

Davis, John Staige, U.S. surgeon, 1872–1946. SEE D. *graft;* Crowe-D. mouth gag.

Davis, David M., U.S. urologist, *1886.

Davis in·ter·lock·ing sound. See under sound.

Dawson, James R., U.S. pathologist, *1908. SEE D. *encephalitis.*

Day, Richard H., U.S. physician, 1813–1892. SEE D. *test.*

Day, Richard L., U.S. pediatrician, *1905. SEE Riley-D. *syndrome.*

daz·zling. The consequence of illumination too intense for adaptation by the eye; in contrast to glare, d. is alleviated by appropriate tinted glasses.

dB, db Abbreviation for decibel.

DBP Abbreviation for vitamin D–binding *protein.*

DC Abbreviation for direct *current.*

D & C Abbreviation for dilation and curettage.

D.C. Abbreviation for Doctor of Chiropractic.

dCMP Abbreviation for deoxycytidylic acid.

DDA Abbreviation for dideoxyadenosine.

DDI Abbreviation for dideoxyinosine.

d-dimer (dī′mer). A covalently cross-linked degradation product released from the cross-linked fibrin polymer during plasmin-mediated fibrinolysis; laboratory measurements of this product made using latex bead or ELISA assays can be used to identify the presence of fibrinolysis.

D.D.S. Abbreviation for Doctor of Dental Surgery.

DDT Abbreviation for dichlorodiphenyltrichloroethane.

D & E Abbreviation for dilation and evacuation. **2.** Abbreviation for *dilation* and extraction

de-. **1.** Away from, cessation, without; sometimes has an intensive force. **2.** For names with this prefix not found here, see under the principal part of the name. [L. *de,* from, away]

de·a·cid·i·fi·ca·tion (dē-a-sid′i-fi-kā′shŭn). The removal or neutralization of acid.

de·ac·ti·va·tion (dē-ak-ti-vā′shŭn). The process of rendering or of becoming inactive.

de·ac·yl·ase (dē-as′il-ās). **1.** A member of the subclass of hydrolases (EC class 3), especially of that subclass of esterases, lipases, lactonases, and hydrolases (EC subclass 3.1). **2.** Any enzyme catalyzing the hydrolytic cleavage of an acyl group (R–CO–) in an ester linkage; also includes enzymes cleaving amide linkages (EC subclass 3.5) and similar acyl compounds.

dead (ded). **1.** Without life. SEE ALSO death. **2.** Numb.

DEAE-cel·lu·lose. SYN *O*-diethylaminoethyl *cellulose.*

deaf (def). Unable to hear. [A.S. *deáf*]

de·af·fer·en·ta·tion (dē-af′er-en-tā′shŭn). A loss of the sensory input from a portion of the body, usually caused by interruption of the peripheral sensory fibers. [L. *de,* from, + afferent]

deaf·ness (def′nes). General term for inability to hear.

deafness due to developmental dysplasias of the cochlea		
type of inner-ear defect	**principal characteristics**	**morphologic changes**
Michel type (1863)	complete aplasia	aplasia of petrosal portion of temporal bone or osseous labyrinth
Mondini type (1791)	severe hypoplasia of osseous and membranous labyrinth	absence of spiral lamina in proximal part of cochlea; widening of endolymphatic sac and duct; defect of Corti's organ
Sceibe type (1892)	aplasia of membranous labyrinth (cochlea and sacculus)	sacculus is widened or collapsed; cochlear duct is widened; Corti's organ is aplastic or hypoplastic, with defective supporting or hair cells

central d., d. due to disorder of the auditory system of the brainstem or cerebral cortex.

cortical d., d. resulting from bilateral lesions of the primary receptive area of the temporal lobe.

hereditary d., SEE hereditary *hearing impairment.*

nerve d., neural d., former terms for sensorineural hearing loss.

postlingual d., hearing impairment occurring after speech and language skills have been developed.

prelingual d., hearing impairment occurring before development of speech and language skills.

sudden d., a profound sensory hearing loss that develops in 24 hrs or less; generally thought to be due to a viral infection in the inner ear.

word d., SYN auditory *aphasia.*

de·al·ba·tion (dē-al-bā′shŭn). The act of whitening, bleaching, or blanching. [L. *de-albo,* pp. *-atus,* to whiten]

de·al·co·hol·i·za·tion (dē-al′kō-hol-i-zā′shŭn). The removal of alcohol from a fluid; in histologic technique, the removal of alcohol from a specimen that has been previously immersed in this fluid.

de·al·ler·gize (dē-al′er-jīz). Obsolete term for desensitize.

de·am·i·das·es (dē-am′i-dā-sez). SYN amidohydrolases.

de·am·i·da·tion, de·am·i·di·za·tion (dē-am-i-dā′shŭn, dē-am′i-di-zā′shŭn). The hydrolytic removal of an amide group.

de·am·i·dize (dē-am′i-dīz). To perform deamidation. SYN desamidize.

de·am·i·nas·es (dē-am′i-nā-sez) [EC 3.5.4.x]. Enzymes catalyzing simple hydrolysis of C–NH_2 bonds of purines, pyrimidines, and pterins, thus producing ammonia (usually named in terms of the substrate, e.g., guanine d., adenosine d., AMP d., pterin d.); not generally used for deamination of noncyclic amides. D. are distinguished from ammonia-lyases (EC 4.3.1.x) in that the latter produce an unsaturation at the point of NH_3 removal. SYN deaminating enzymes.

de·am·i·na·tion, de·am·i·ni·za·tion (dē-am-i-nā′shŭn, dē-am′i-ni-zā′shŭn). Removal, usually by hydrolysis, of the NH_2 group from an amino compound.

oxidative d., d. by enzymes that uses flavin or pyridine nucleotides (such as FAD or NAD^+).

de·am·in·ize (dē-am′i-nīz). To perform deamination.

Dean, Henry Trendley, U.S. dentist and epidemiologist, 1893–1962. SEE D. fluorosis *index.*

de·a·nol ac·et·a·mi·do·ben·zo·ate (dē′ă-nol as-ĕ-tam′i-dō-ben′zō-āt). The *p*-acetamidobenzoic acid salt of 2-dimethylaminoethanol; a central nervous system stimulant.

death (dĕth). The cessation of life. In lower multicellular organisms, d. is a gradual process at the cellular level, because tissues vary in their ability to withstand deprivation of oxygen; in higher organisms, a cessation of integrated tissue and organ functions; in humans, manifested by the loss of heartbeat, by the absence of spontaneous breathing, and by cerebral d. SYN mors. [A.S. *dēath*]

black d., term applied to the worldwide epidemic of the 14th century, of which some 60 million persons are said to have died; the descriptions indicate that it was pneumonic plague.

brain d., SYN cerebral d.

cerebral d., a clinical syndrome characterized by the permanent loss of cerebral and brainstem function, manifested by absence of responsiveness to external stimuli, absence of cephalic reflexes, and apnea. An isoelectric electroencephalogram for at least 30 minutes in the absence of hypothermia and poisoning by central nervous system depressants supports the diagnosis. SYN brain d.

d. certificate, official, legal document and vital record, signed by a licensed physician or other designated authority, that includes cause of d., decedent's name, sex, place of residence, date of d.; other information, e.g., birth date, birth place, occupation may be included; the immediate cause of d. is recorded on the first line of the certificate, followed by the condition(s) giving rise to this, with the underlying cause on the last line; the underlying cause is coded and tabulated in official publications of mortality.

cot d., SYN sudden infant death *syndrome.*

crib d., SYN sudden infant death *syndrome.*

crude d. rate, SYN death *rate.*

fetal d., d. prior to the complete expulsion or extraction from the mother of a product of conception, irrespective of the duration of pregnancy. Fetal death is considered *early* if it takes place in the first 20 weeks of gestation; *middle* (intermediate) if it takes place

from 21–28 weeks of gestation, and *late* if it takes place after 28 weeks.

genetic d., d. of the bearer of a gene at any age before generating living offspring. May be compatible with good health and long life. SEE ALSO genetic *lethal.*

infant d., d. of a liveborn infant within the first year.

local d., d. of a part of the body or of a tissue by necrosis.

maternal d., d. of a woman while pregnant or within 42 days after the termination of gestation, irrespective of the duration and site of pregnancy and the cause of d.; two periods are recognized in the 42-day interval: period one includes day 1 to day 7; period two includes day 8 to day 42. Maternal d.'s are further classified as: **direct maternal d.,** d. resulting from obstetric complications of the gestation, labor, or puerperium, and from interventions, omissions, incorrect treatment, or a chain of events caused by any of the above; **indirect maternal d.,** an obstetric d. resulting from previously existing disease or from disease developing during pregnancy, labor, or the puerperium; it is not directly due to obstetric causes, but to conditions aggravated by the physiologic effects of pregnancy.

neonatal d., d. of a young, liveborn infant; classified as: **early neonatal d.,** d. of a liveborn infant occurring fewer than 7 completed days (168 hours) from the time of birth; **late neonatal d.,** d. of a liveborn infant occurring after 7 completed days of age but before 28 completed days.

perinatal d., an inclusive term referring to both stillborn infants and neonatal d.'s.

programmed cell d., SYN apoptosis.

somatic d., systemic d., d. of the entire body, as distinguished from local d.

sudden d., d. occurring rapidly and generally unexpectedly; usually from a cardiac dysrhythmia or myocardial infarction, but also from any cause of rapid d., e.g., pulmonary embolus, stroke, ruptured aortic aneurysm, aortic dissection.

death-rat·tle (deth′rat′l). A respiratory gurgling or rattling in the pharynx or trachea of a dying person, caused by the loss of the cough reflex and accumulation of mucus.

Deaver, John Blair, U.S. surgeon, 1855–1931. SEE D. incision.

Deaver, George G., U.S. physiatrist, 1890–1973. SEE D. *method.*

DeBakey, Michael Ellis, U.S. heart surgeon, *1908. SEE DeBakey *classification,* DeBakey *forceps.*

de·band·ing (dē-band′ing). The removal of fixed orthodontic appliances.

de·bil·i·tant (dē-bil′i-tant). **1.** Weakening; causing debility. **2.** Obsolete term for a quieting agent or one that subdues excitement. [L. *debilito,* to weaken, fr. *de,* neg., + *habilis,* able]

de·bil·i·tat·ing (dĕ-bil′i-tāt-ing). Denoting or characteristic of a morbid process that causes weakness.

de·bil·i·ty (dĕ-bil′i-tē). Weakness. [L. *debilitas,* fr. *debilis,* weak, fr. *de-* priv. + *habilis,* able]

debond (dē-bond′). To separate a dental appliance such as an orthodontic band from the tooth to which it has been attached or bonded by a resin cement. [de- + bond]

de·bouch (dĕ-boosh′). To open or empty into another part. [Fr. *bouche,* mouth]

dé·bouche·ment (dā-boosh-mon′). Opening or emptying into another part. [Fr.]

Debré, Robert, French pediatrician and infectious disease specialist, 1882–1978. SEE D. *phenomenon;* D.-Sémélaigne *syndrome;* Kocher-D.-Sémélaigne *syndrome.*

dé·bride·ment (dā-brēd-mon′). Excision of devitalized tissue and foreign matter from a wound. [Fr. unbridle]

debris (de-brē′). A useless accumulation of miscellaneous particles; waste in the form of fragments. [Fr. *débris,* fr. O.Fr. *desbrisier,* to break apart, (fr. *des-* down, away + *brisier* to break) rubble, rubbish]

particulate wear d., microscopic particles produced by friction between articulating surfaces in a total joint replacement; d. can include particles of metal, polyethylene, and polymethylmethacrylate cement, and can induce osteolysis.

de·bris·o·quine sul·fate (dĕ-bris′ō-kwin). An antihypertensive agent resembling guanethidine; also used in drug metabolism studies.

debt (det). A deficit; a liability. [L. *debitum*, debt]

alactic oxygen d., that part of the oxygen d. that is not lactacid oxygen d.; during recovery, stores of ATP and creatine phosphate must be replenished by oxidative metabolism, and a small amount of oxygen is also needed to restore the normal oxyhemoglobin levels throughout the circulating blood.

lactacid oxygen d., that part of an oxygen d. represented by the production of lactic acid by anaerobic glycolysis during exercise and, therefore, by the need to eliminate it by oxidative metabolism during recovery.

oxygen d., the extra oxygen, taken in by the body during recovery from exercise, beyond the resting needs of the body; sometimes used as if synonymous with oxygen deficit.

deca- (da). Prefix used in the SI and metric system to signify multiples of 10. Also spelled deka-. [G. *deka*, ten]

dec·a·gram (dek′ă-gram). Ten grams.

de·cal·ci·fi·ca·tion (dē′kal-si-fi-kā′shŭn). **1.** Removal of lime or calcium salts, chiefly tricalcium phosphate, from bones and teeth, either in vitro or in vivo as a result of a pathologic process. **2.** Precipitation of calcium from blood as by oxalate or fluoride, or the conversion of blood calcium to an un-ionized form as by citrate, thus preventing or delaying coagulation. [L. *de-*, away, + *calx* (calc-), lime, + *facio*, to make]

de·cal·ci·fy (dē-kal′si-fī). To remove lime or calcium salts, especially from bones or teeth.

de·cal·ci·fy·ing (dē-kal′si-fī-ing). Denoting an agent, measure, or process that causes decalcification.

dec·a·li·ter (dek′ă-lē-ter). Ten liters.

de·cal·vant (dē-kal′vant). Removing the hair; making bald. [L. *decalvare*, to make bald]

dec·a·me·ter (dek′ă-mē-ter). Ten meters.

dec·a·me·tho·ni·um bro·mide (dek-ă-me-thō′nē-ŭm). A synthetic nondepolarizing neuromuscular blocking agent used to produce muscular relaxation during general anesthesia.

dec·a·mine (dek′ă-mēn). SYN dequalinium acetate.

***n*-dec·ane** (dek′ān). A paraffin hydrocarbon, CH_3–$(CH_2)_8$–CH_3.

de·can·nul·a·tion (dē-kan-ū-lā′shun). Planned or accidental removal of a tracheostomy tube.

***n*-dec·a·no·ic ac·id** (dek-ă-nō′ik). SYN *n*-capric acid.

dec·a·no·in (dek-ă-nō′in). SYN caprin.

dec·a·nor·mal (dek-ă-nōr′măl). Rarely used term denoting the concentration of a solution 10 times that of normal.

de·cant (dē-kant′). To pour off gently the upper clear portion of a fluid, leaving the sediment in the vessel. [Mediev. L. *decantho*, fr. *de-* + *canthus*, the beak of a jug, fr. G. *kanthos*, corner of the eye]

de·can·ta·tion (dē-kan-tā′shŭn). Pouring off the clear upper portion of a fluid, leaving a sediment or precipitate.

de·ca·pac·i·ta·tion (dē′kă-pas-i-tā′shŭn). Prevention of spermatozoa from undergoing capacitation and thus from becoming able to fertilize ova. SEE ALSO decapacitation *factor*.

dec·a·pep·tide (dek′ă-pep′tīd). An oligopeptide containing 10 amino acids.

de·cap·i·tate (dē-kap′i-tāt). **1.** To cut off the head; specifically, to remove the head of a fetus to facilitate delivery in cases of irremediable dystocia; to cut off the head of an animal in preparation for certain physiologic experiments; obsolete term. **2.** Relating to an experimental animal with the head removed. [L. *de-*, away, + *caput*, head]

de·cap·i·ta·tion (dē-kap-i-tā′shŭn). Removal of a head. SEE decapitate.

de·cap·su·la·tion (dē-kap-soo-lā′shŭn). Incision and removal of a capsule or enveloping membrane.

d. of kidney, removing or stripping off the capsule of the kidney.

de·car·bo·ni·za·tion (dē-kar′bon-i-zā′shŭn). Rarely used term denoting the process of arterialization of the blood by oxygenation and the removal of carbon dioxide in the lungs.

de·car·box·yl·ase (dē-kar-boks′ē-lās). Any enzyme (EC 4.1.1.x)

that removes a molecule of carbon dioxide from a carboxylic group (e.g., from an α-amino acid, converting it into an amine).

de·car·box·yl·a·tion (dē′kar-boks-ē-lā′shŭn). A reaction involving the removal of a molecule of carbon dioxide from a carboxylic acid.

oxidative d., d. requiring the participation of coenzymes such as NAD^+, $NADP^+$, FAD, or FMN.

de·cay (dē-kā′). **1.** Destruction of an organic substance by slow combustion or gradual oxidation. **2.** SYN putrefaction. **3.** To deteriorate; to undergo slow combustion or putrefaction. **4.** In dentistry, caries. **5.** In psychology, loss of information registered by the senses and processed into short-term memory. SEE ALSO memory. **6.** Loss of radioactivity with time; spontaneous emission of radiation or charged particles or both from an unstable nucleus. [L. *de*, down, + *cado*, to fall]

free induction d. (FID), in magnetic resonance imaging, the d. curve that is detected by the receiver coil after the application of an excitation pulse, without additional pulses.

de·cel·er·a·tion (dē-sel-er-ā′shŭn). **1.** The act of decelerating. **2.** The rate of decrease in velocity per unit of time.

early d., slowing of the fetal heart rate early in the uterine contraction phase, denoting compression of the fetal head.

late d., any transient fetal bradycardia, the nadir of which occurs after the peak of the uterine contraction. This may represent uteroplacental insufficiency.

variable d., transient fetal bradycardia usually denoting compression of the umbilical cord, which may occur at any time in relation to a uterine contraction.

de·cen·tra·tion (dē-sen-trā′shŭn). Removal from the center.

de·cer·e·brate (dē-ser′ĕ-brāt). **1.** To cause decerebration. **2.** Denoting an animal so prepared, or a patient whose brain has suffered an injury which renders the patient, in neurologic behavior, comparable to a decerebrate animal.

de·cer·e·bra·tion (dē-ser′ĕ-brā′shŭn). Removal of the brain above the lower border of the corpora quadrigemina, or a complete section of the brain at this level or somewhat below.

bloodless d., destroying the function of the cerebrum by tying the basilar artery at about the middle of the pons and the common carotid arteries in the neck.

de·cer·e·brize (dē-ser′ĕ-brīz). To remove the brain.

de·chlo·ri·da·tion (dē′klōr-i-dā′shŭn). Reduction of sodium chloride in the tissues and fluids of the body by reducing its intake or increasing its excretion. SYN dechlorination, dechloruration.

de·chlo·ri·na·tion (dē′klōr-i-nā′shŭn). SYN dechloridation.

de·chlo·ru·ra·tion (dē′klōr-oo-rā′shŭn). SYN dechloridation.

de·cho·les·ter·ol·i·za·tion (dē′kō-les′ter-ol-i-zā′shŭn). Therapeutic reduction of the cholesterol concentration of the blood.

deci- (d). Prefix used in the SI and metric system to signify one-tenth (10^{-1}). [L. *decimus*, tenth]

dec·i·bel (dB, db) (des′i-bel). One-tenth of a bel; unit for expressing the relative intensity of sound on a logarithmic scale. [L. *decimus*, tenth, + bel]

de·cid·ua (dē-sid′ū-ă). SYN deciduous *membrane*. [L. *deciduus*, falling off (qualifying *membrana*, membrane, understood)]

d. basa′lis, the area of endometrium between the implanted chorionic vesicle and the myometrium, which develops into the maternal part of the placenta. SYN d. serotina.

d. capsula′ris, the layer of endometrium overlying the implanted chorionic vesicle; it becomes progressively attenuated as the chorionic vesicle enlarges and, by the fourth month, is squeezed against the d. parietalis and thereafter undergoes rapid regression. SYN d. reflexa, membrana adventitia (2).

ectopic d., decidual cells which may be found in the cervix, appendix, or areas other than the endometrium.

d. menstrua′lis, the succulent mucous membrane of the nonpregnant uterus at the menstrual period.

d. parieta′lis, the altered mucous membrane lining the main cavity of the pregnant uterus other than at the site of attachment of the chorionic vesicle. SYN d. vera.

d. polypo'sa, d. parietalis showing polypoid projections of the endometrial surface.

d. reflex'a, SYN d. capsularis.

d. seroti'na, SYN d. basalis.

d. spongio'sa, the portion of the d. basalis attached to the myometrium.

d. ve'ra, SYN d. parietalis.

de·cid·u·al (dē-sid'ū-ăl). Relating to the decidua.

de·cid·u·ate (dē-sid'ū-āt). Relating to those mammals (e.g., humans, dogs, rodents) that shed maternal uterine tissue when expelling the placenta at birth, in contrast to indeciduate mammals (horse, pig). [see deciduation]

de·cid·u·a·tion (dē-sid-ū-ā'shŭn). Shedding of endometrial tissue during menstruation. [L. *deciduus,* falling off]

de·cid·u·i·tis (dē-sid-ū-ī'tis). Inflammation of the decidua.

de·cid·u·o·ma (dē-sid-ū-ō'mă). An intrauterine mass of decidual tissue, probably the result of hyperplasia of decidual cells retained in the uterus. SYN placentoma.

Loeb d., mass of decidual tissue produced in the uterus, in the absence of a fertilized ovum, by means of mechanical or hormonal stimulation.

de·cid·u·ous (dē-sid'ū-ŭs). **1.** Not permanent; denoting that which eventually falls off. **2 (D)** (in dental formulas). In dentistry, often used to designate the first or primary dentition. SEE deciduous *tooth.* [L. *deciduus,* falling off]

dec·i·gram (des'i-gram). One-tenth of a gram.

dec·i·li·ter (des'i-lē-ter). One-tenth of a liter.

dec·i·me·ter (des'i-mē-ter). One-tenth of a meter.

dec·i·mor·gan (des'i-mōr-găn). SEE morgan.

dec·i·nor·mal (des-i-nōr'măl). One-tenth of normal, denoting the concentration of a solution.

decision.

limiting d., an understanding of self achieved as a result of response to a significant or traumatic event. SEE ALSO Time-Line *therapy.*

de·ci·sion tree. Alternative choices available at each stage of deciding how to manage a clinical problem, displayed graphically; at each branch or decision node, the probabilities of each outcome that can be predicted are shown; the relative worth of each outcome is described in terms of its utility or quality of life, e.g., as measured by probability of death, life expectancy, or freedom from disability.

de Clerambault, G., French psychiatrist, 1872–1934. SEE de C. *syndrome.*

dec·lin·a·tor (dek'lin-ā-ter, -tōr). A retractor that holds certain structures out of the way during an operation.

de·clive (dē-klīv') [TA]. The posterior sloping portion of the monticulus of the vermis of the cerebellum; vermal lobule immediately caudal to the primary fissure; lobule VI. SYN declivis, lobulus clivi. [L. *declivis,* sloping downward, fr. *clivus,* a slope]

de·cli·vis (dē-klī'vis). SYN declive.

de·coc·tion (dē-kok'shŭn). **1.** The process of boiling. **2.** The pharmacopeial name for preparations made by boiling crude vegetable drugs, and then straining, in the proportion of 50 g of the drug to 1000 mL of water. SYN apozem, apozema. [L. *decoctio,* fr. *de-coquo,* pp. *-coctus,* to boil down]

dé·colle·ment (dā-kŭl-mon'). Rarely used term for surgical separation of tissues or organs which are adherent, either normally or pathologically. [Fr. ungluing]

de·com·pen·sa·tion (de'kom-pen-sā'shŭn). **1.** A failure of compensation in heart disease. **2.** The appearance or exacerbation of a mental disorder due to failure of defense mechanisms.

corneal d., corneal edema resulting from failure of the corneal endothelium to maintain deturgescence.

de·com·pose (dē'kom-pōz). **1.** To resolve a compound into its component parts; to disintegrate. **2.** To decay; to putrefy. [L. *de,* from, down, + *com-pono,* pp. *-positus,* to put together]

de·com·po·si·tion (dē'kom-pō-zish'ŭn). SYN putrefaction.

de·com·pres·sion (dē'kom-presh-ŭn). Removal of pressure. [L. *de-,* from, down, + *com-primo,* pp. *-pressus,* to press together]

cardiac d., incision into the pericardium or aspiration of fluid from the pericardium to relieve pressure due to blood or other fluid in the pericardial sac. SYN pericardial d.

cerebral d., removal of a piece of the cranium, with incision of the dura, to relieve intracranial pressure.

explosive d., SYN rapid d.

internal d., removal of intracranial tissue, usually tumor, hematoma, or brain tissue; to relieve pressure.

nerve d., release of pressure on a nerve trunk by the surgical excision of constricting bands or widening of a bony canal.

optic nerve sheath d., a venting of the optic nerve sheath into the retrobulbar space, by slitting or by fenestrating the sheath. SEE optic nerve sheath *fenestration.*

orbital d., removal of a portion of the bony orbit, usually superior (Naffziger operation), lateral (Krönlein operation), or inferior (Ogura operation).

pericardial d., SYN cardiac d.

rapid d., sudden severe expansion of gases due to a reduction in ambient pressure. SYN explosive d.

spinal d., the removal of pressure upon the spinal cord as created by a tumor, cyst, hematoma, herniated nucleus pulposus, abscess, or bone.

suboccipital d., d. of the posterior fossa by occipital craniectomy and opening of the dura.

subtemporal d., d. of the brain by temporal craniectomy and opening of the dura over the inferolateral surface of the temporal lobe.

trigeminal d., d. of the trigeminal nerve root.

de·con·ges·tant (dē-kon-jes'tant). **1.** SYN decongestive. **2.** An agent that possesses this action.

de·con·ges·tive (dē-kon-jes'tiv). Having the property of reducing tissue swelling. SYN decongestant (1).

de·con·tam·i·na·tion (dē'kon-tam-i-nā'shŭn). Removal or neutralization of poisonous gas or other injurious agents from the environment.

de·con·vo·lu·tion (dē-con-vō-loo'shŭn). A mathematic technique for solution of functions whose input includes their output; used to solve for the image elements in computed tomography or magnetic resonance imaging. [de- + L. *convulutio,* a rolling up, fr. *convolvo,* to roll up]

de·cor·ti·ca·tion (dē-kōr-ti-kā'shŭn). **1.** Removal of the cortex, or external layer, beneath the capsule from any organ or structure. **2.** An operation for removal of the residual clot and/or newly organized scar tissue that form after a hemothorax or neglected empyema. [L. *decortico,* pp. *-atus,* to deprive of bark, fr. *de,* from, + *cortex,* rind, bark]

cerebral d., destruction of the cerebral cortex, usually due to anoxia.

reversible d., a temporary loss of function of the cerebral cortex.

dec·re·ment (dek'rĕ-ment). **1.** Decrease. **2.** Decrease in conduction velocity at a particular point; a result of altered properties at that point. SEE ALSO decremental *conduction.* [L. *decrementum,* fr. *decresco,* to decrease]

de·crep·i·ta·tion (dē-krep-i-tā'shŭn). Crackling; the snapping of certain salts when heated. [L. *de,* from, + *crepo,* pp. *crepitus,* to crackle]

de·cru·des·cence (dē-kroo-des'ens). Abatement of the symptoms of disease. [L. *de,* from, + *crudesco,* to become worse, fr. *crudus,* crude]

de·cu·bi·tal (dē-kū'bi-tăl). Relating to a decubitus ulcer.

de·cu·bi·tus (dē-kū'bi-tŭs). **1.** The position of the patient in bed; e.g., dorsal d., lateral d. SEE decubitus *film.* **2.** Sometimes used in referring to a decubitus *ulcer.* [L. *decumbo,* to lie down]

Andral d., position assumed by the patient who lies on the sound side in cases of beginning pleurisy.

ventral d., pressure sores (decubitus ulceration) occurring in ventral locations, such as the abdominal wall or the anterior surface of an extremity.

de·cur·rent (dē-kŭr'ent). Extending downward. [L. *de-curro,* pp. *-cursus,* to run down]

de·cus·sate (dē'kŭ-sāt, dē-kŭs'āt). **1.** To cross. **2.** Crossed like the arms of an X. [L. *decusso,* pp. *-atus,* to make in the form of an X, fr. *decussis,* a large, bronze Roman (2nd c. BC), 10-unit coin marked with an X to indicate its denomination]

de·cus·sa·tio, pl. **de·cus·sa·ti·o·nes** (dē-kŭ-sā′shē-ō, -ō′nēz) [TA]. **1.** In general, any crossing over or intersection of parts. **2.** The intercrossing of two homonymous fiber bundles as each crosses over to the opposite side of the brain in the course of its ascent or descent through the brainstem or spinal cord. SYN decussation. [L. (see decussate)]

d. bra′chii conjuncti′vi, SYN *decussation* of superior cerebellar peduncles.

d. fibrarum nervo′rum trochlear′ium [TA], SYN *decussation* of trochlear nerve fibers.

d. fontina′lis, SEE decussationes tegmentales.

d. lemnisci mediales [TA], SYN *decussation* of medial lemniscus.

d. moto′ria, SYN *decussation* of pyramids.

d. pedunculo′rum cerebella′rium superio′rum [TA], SYN *decussation* of superior cerebellar peduncles.

d. pyram′idum [TA], SYN *decussation* of pyramids.

d. senso′ria, SYN *decussation* of medial lemniscus.

decussatio′nes tegmen′tales [TA], SYN tegmental *decussations,* under *decussation.*

d. tegmentalis anterior [TA], SEE tegmental *decussations,* under *decussation.*

d. tegmentalis posterior [TA], SEE tegmental *decussations,* under *decussation.*

de·cus·sa·tion (dē-kŭ-sā′shŭn). SYN decussatio. [L. *decussatio*]

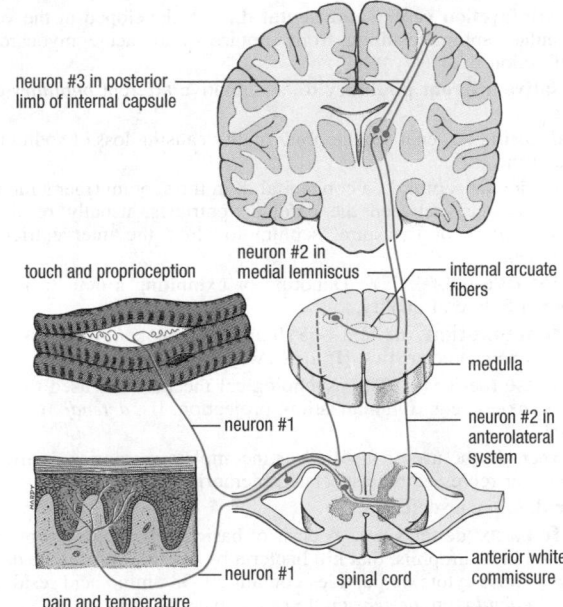

diagrammatic representation of the decussations of some ascending tracts; first order neurons for touch and proprioception ascend in the posterior columns to synapse on second order neurons in the medulla; the axons of these second order neurons cross the midline and ascend to the thalamus via the medial lemniscus; first order neurons for pain and temperature enter the posterior horn to synapse on second order neurons located therein; the axons of these second order neurons cross the midline in the anterior white commissure and ascend to the thalamus within the anterolateral system; third order neurons connect the thalamus to the cerebral cortex

anterior tegmental d. [TA], SEE tegmental d.'s (2).

d. of brachia conjunctiva, SYN d. of superior cerebellar peduncles.

dorsal tegmental d. [TA], SEE tegmental d.'s.

d. of the fillet, SYN d. of medial lemniscus.

Forel d., SEE tegmental d.'s (2).

fountain d., SEE tegmental d.'s (1).

Held d., the crossing of some of the fibers arising from the cochlear nuclei to form the lateral lemniscus.

d. of medial lemniscus, the intercrossing of the fibers of the left and right medial lemniscus ascending from the gracile and cuneate nuclei, immediately rostral to the level of the decussation of the pyramidal tracts in the medulla oblongata. SYN decussatio lemnisci mediales [TA], decussatio sensoria, d. of the fillet, sensory d. of medulla oblongata.

Meynert d., SEE tegmental d.'s (1).

motor d., SYN d. of pyramids.

optic d., SYN optic *chiasm.*

posterior tegmental d. [TA], SEE tegmental d.'s (1).

d. of pyramids [TA], the intercrossing of the bundles of corticospinal fibers at the lower border region of the medulla oblongata. SYN decussatio pyramidum [TA], decussatio motoria, motor d.

rubrospinal d., SEE tegmental d.'s (2).

sensory d. of medulla oblongata, SYN d. of medial lemniscus.

d. of superior cerebellar peduncles [TA], the decussation of the left and right superior cerebellar peduncles in the tegmentum of the caudal mesencephalon. SYN decussatio pedunculorum cerebellarium superiorum [TA], decussatio brachii conjunctivi, d. of brachia conjunctiva, Wernekinck d.

tectospinal d., SEE tegmental d.'s (1).

tegmental d.'s, (1) the posterior tegmental decussation [TA] (dorsal tegmental decussation [TA], fountain d., Meynert's d.) is formed by the crossing of the left and right tectospinal and tectobulbar tracts; **(2)** the anterior tegmental decussation [TA] (ventral tegmental decussation [TA], Forel's decussation) is formed by the crossing of the left and right rubrospinal and rubrobulbar tracts; both d.'s are located in the mesencephalon. SYN decussationes tegmentales [TA].

d. of trochlear nerve fibers [TA], the crossing of the two trochlear nerves at their exit through the velum medullare anterius. SYN decussatio fibrarum nervorum trochlearium [TA].

ventral tegmental d., SEE tegmental d.'s (2).

Wernekinck d., SYN d. of superior cerebellar peduncles.

de·cus·sa·ti·o·nes (dē-kŭs-ā-shē-ō′nēz). Plural of decussatio.

de·den·ti·tion (dē-den-tish′ŭn). Obsolete term denoting loss of teeth.

de·dif·fer·en·ti·a·tion (dē-dif′er-en-shē-ā′shŭn). **1.** The return of parts to a more homogeneous state. **2.** SYN anaplasia.

de·do·la·tion (dē-dō-lā′shŭn). A slicing wound made by a sharp instrument grazing the surface. [L. *de-dolo,* pp. *-atus,* to hew away]

de·duc·tion (dē-duk′shun). The logical derivation of a conclusion from certain premises. The conclusion will be true if the premises are true and the deductive argument is valid. Cf. induction (9).

de·ef·fer·en·ta·tion (dē-ef-er-en-tā′shŭn). A loss of the motor nerve fibers to an area of the body. [L. *de,* from, + efferent]

deep (dēp) [TA]. Situated at a deeper level in relation to a specific reference point. Cf. superficialis. SYN profundus [TA].

de·ep·i·car·di·al·i·za·tion (dē-ep-i-kar′dē-al-i-zā′shŭn). Obsolete surgical destruction of the epicardium, usually by the application of phenol, designed (unsuccessfully) to promote collateral circulation to the myocardium.

Deetjen, Hermann, German physician, 1867–1915. SEE D. *bodies,* under *body.*

def, DEF Abbreviation for decayed, extracted, and filled tooth. SEE def caries *index.*

de·fat·i·ga·tion (dē-fat-i-gā′shŭn). Weariness, exhaustion, or extreme fatigue. [L. *de-fatigo,* pp. *-atus,* to tire out]

def·e·cate (def′ĕ-kāt). To perform defecation.

def·e·ca·tion (def-ĕ-kā′shŭn). The discharge of feces from the rectum. SYN motion (2), movement (3). [L. *defaeco,* pp. *-atus,* to remove the dregs, purify]

de·fec·og·ra·phy (de-fĕ-kog′ră-fē). Radiographic examination of the act of defecation of a radiopaque stool. [defecation + G. *graphō,* to write]

de·fect (dē′fekt). An imperfection, malformation, dysfunction, or absence; an attribute of quality, in contrast with deficiency, which is an attribute of quantity. [L. *deficio*, pp. *-fectus*, to fail, to lack]

aortic septal d., aorticopulmonary septal d., a small congenital opening between the aorta and pulmonary artery about 1 cm above the semilunar valves, e.g., aorticopulmonary window. SYN aorticopulmonary window.

atrial septal d., a congenital d. in the septum between the atria of the heart, due to failure of the foramen primum or secundum to close normally; may involve atrioventricular canal cushions; occasionally there is strong evidence of autosomal dominant inheritance [MIM*108800]. In varying degree, it is also a common feature of the autosomal recessive Ellis-van Creveld *syndrome* [MIM*225500] and the autosomal dominant Holt-Oram *syndrome* [MIM*142900].

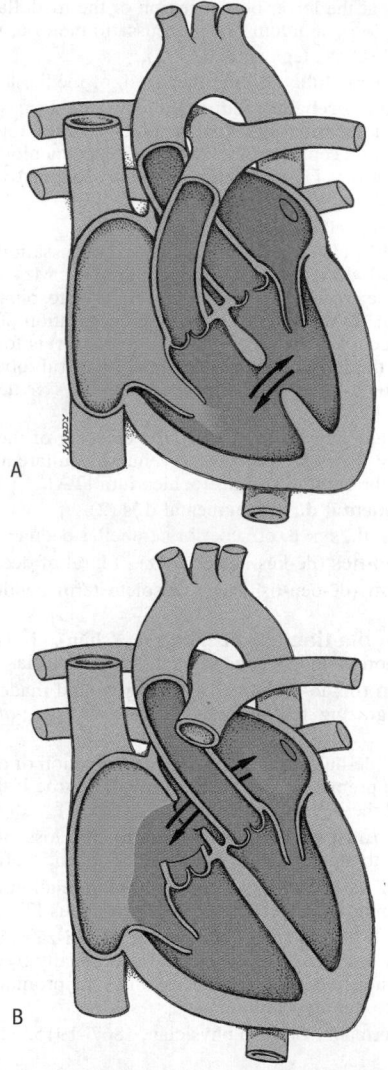

A

B

septal defects: (A) interventricular defect, (B) interatrial defect

atrial ventricular canal d., a d. caused by deficient or absent septal tissue immediately above and below the normal level of the atrioventricular valves, including the region normally occupied by the A-V septum in hearts with two ventricles. The A-V valves are abnormal to a varying degree.

birth d., d. present at birth; sometimes referred to as congenital d.

congenital ectodermal d., SYN congenital ectodermal *dysplasia*.

coupling d., SEE familial *goiter*.

Eisenmenger d., SYN Eisenmenger *complex*.

endocardial cushion d., SYN persistent atrioventricular *canal*.

fibrous cortical d., a common 1 to 3 cm d. in the cortex of a bone, most commonly the lower femoral shaft of a child, filled with fibrous tissue. Nonosteogenic or nonossifying *fibroma* by convention refers to lesions greater than 3 cm in diameter. SEE ALSO nonossifying *fibroma*. SYN nonosteogenic fibroma.

filling d., displacement of contrast medium by a space-occupying lesion in a radiographic study of a contrast-filled hollow viscus, such as a polyp on a barium enema; also applied to defects in the otherwise uniform distribution of radionuclide in an organ, such as a metastasis in the liver on a ^{99m}Tc-sulfur colloid scan.

Gerbode d., a defect in the interventricular portion of the membranous septum, associated with a communication between the right ventricle and the right atrium through an abnormality in the tricuspid valve.

iodide transport d., SEE familial *goiter*.

iodotyrosine deiodinase d., SEE familial *goiter*.

luteal phase d., a condition characterized by inadequate secretion of progesterone during the luteal phase of the menstrual cycle, with resultant infertility; subnormal luteal function commonly attributed to abnormal pituitary gonadotropin secretion. SYN luteal phase deficiency.

metaphyseal fibrous cortical d., a small fibrous cortical d. located in the metaphysis of a long bone.

organification d., SEE familial *goiter*.

osteoporotic marrow d. (ŏs'tē-ō-pō-rŏ'tik), focal osteoporotic bone marrow d. of the jaw; a focal radiolucent d. composed of normal marrow.

postinfarction ventricular septal d., a d. developed in the ventricular septum resulting from rupture of an acute myocardial infarction.

relative afferent pupillary d., SEE relative afferent *pupillary* defect.

salt-losing d., renal tubular abnormality causing loss of sodium in the urine.

ventricular septal d., a congenital d. in the septum (membranous or muscular) between the cardiac ventricles, usually resulting from failure of the spiral septum to close the interventricular foramen.

de·fec·tive (dē-fek'tiv). Denoting or exhibiting a defect; imperfect; a failure of quality.

de·fem·i·na·tion (dē-fem-i-nā'shŭn). A weakening or loss of feminine characteristics. [L. *de-*, away, + *femina*, woman]

de·fense (dē-fens'). The psychological mechanisms used to control anxiety, e.g., rationalization, projection. [L. *defendo*, to ward off]

screen d., the use of falsified or incomplete memories or affects to cover repressed but associated memories and affects.

ur-d.'s, SEE ur-defenses.

de·fen·sins (dē-fen'sinz). A class of basic antibiotic polypeptides, found in neutrophils, that kill bacteria by causing membrane damage. These cytotoxic peptides contain 29–38 amino acid residues. [L. *de-fendo*, pp. *de-fensum*, to repel, avert, + -in]

def·er·ent (def'er-ent). Carrying away. [L. *deferens*, pres. p. of *defero*, to carry away]

def·er·en·tial (def-er-en'shăl). Relating to the ductus deferens.

def·er·en·ti·tis (def'er-en-tī'tis). Inflammation of the ductus deferens. SYN vasitis.

de·fer·ox·a·mine mes·y·late (de-fer-ok'să-mēn). Chelate used in the treatment of iron poisoning. SYN desferrioxamine mesylate.

de·fer·ves·cence (def-er-ves'ens). Falling of an elevated temperature; abatement of fever. [L. *de-fervesco*, to cease boiling, fr. *de-* neg. + *fervesco*, to begin to boil]

de·fi·bril·la·tion (dē-fib-ri-lā'shŭn). The arrest of fibrillation of the cardiac muscle (atrial or ventricular) with restoration of the normal rhythm, if successful.

de·fi·bril·la·tor (dē-fib'ri-lā-ter). **1.** Any agent or measure, e.g., an electric shock, that arrests fibrillation of the ventricular muscle and restores the normal beat. **2.** The machine designed to administer a defibrillating electric shock.

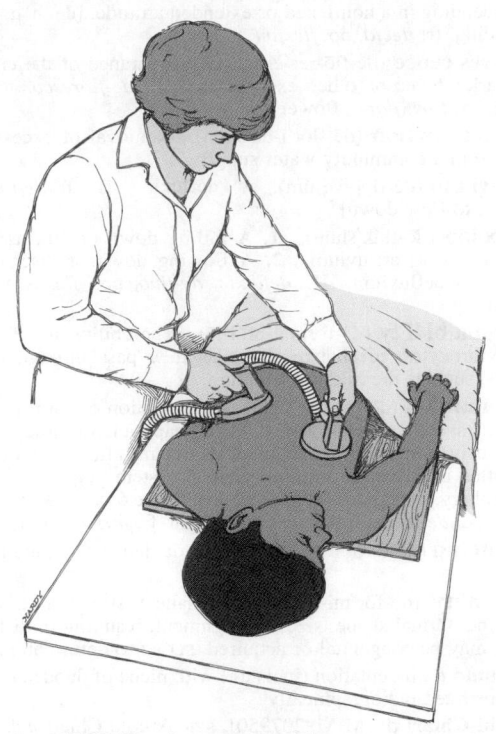

ventricular defibrillation: placement of paddles

external d., a d. that delivers its defibrillating shock through the unopened chest wall.

de·fi·bri·na·tion (dē-fī-bri-nā'shŭn). Removal of fibrin from the blood, usually by means of constant agitation while the blood is collected in a container with glass beads or chips.

de·fi·cien·cy (dē-fish'en-sē). An insufficient quantity of some substance (as in dietary d. or hemoglobin d. in marrow aplasia); organization (as in mental d.); activity (as in enzyme d. or reduced oxygen-carrying capacity of the blood), etc., of which the amount present is of normal quality. SEE ALSO deficiency *disease*. [L. *deficio*, to fail, fr. *facio*, to do]

adult lactase d., onset of lactase d., with resulting milk intolerance and malabsorption, in adulthood. Inherited forms may not be manifested until adulthood; any process that damages the intestinal lining cells can cause lactase d. in adults.

antitrypsin d., d. of α_1-antitrypsin, a serum protease inhibitor (PI), is associated with emphysema and/or liver cirrhosis. By isoelectric focusing, numerous variants have been identified, with different levels of normal activity; autosomal recessive inheritance, caused by mutation in the P1 gene on chromosomal 14q.

α_1-antitrypsin d., absence of a serum proteinase inhibitor that may cause relapsing nodular nonsuppurative panniculitis.

arch length d., the difference between the available circumference of the dental arch and that required to accommodate the succedaneous teeth in proper alignment.

arginosuccinate lyase d., SYN argininosuccinic *aciduria*.

arylsulfatase A d., SYN metachromatic *leukodystrophy*.

arylsulfatase B d., SYN Maroteaux-Lamy *syndrome*.

biotinidase d., a rare, autosomal recessive disease causing loss of excessive biotin; clinical manifestations may be absent, but extreme manifestations include seizures, alopecia, dermatitis, hypotonia, optic atrophy, ataxia, developmental delay, hearing deficits, and occasionally immunodeficiency; trait has a prevalence of 1 in 60,000.

carnitine d., a condition associated with many disorders of fatty acid oxidation. Fatty acids are linked to carnitine as they are transported across the inner mitochondrial membrane; errors in this process lead to problems with energy production; patients may experience episodes of hypoglycemia or metabolic acidosis and may have cardiomyopathy or skeletal muscle weakness.

debrancher d., SYN brancher glycogen storage *disease*.

familial high density lipoprotein d., SYN analphalipoproteinemia.

fructokinase d., SYN essential *fructosuria*.

galactokinase d. [MIM*230200], an inborn error of metabolism due to congenital d. of galactokinase (GALK), resulting in increased blood galactose concentration (galactosemia), cataracts, hepatomegaly, and mental deficiency; autosomal recessive inheritance, caused by mutation in the GALK gene on 17q. Galactose epimerase d. [MIM*230350] and galactose-1-phosphate uridyl transferase d. [MIM*230400] produce much the same clinical picture.

glucose-6-phosphate dehydrogenase d., a d. of glucose-6-phosphate dehydrogenase, an enzyme important for maintaining cellular concentrations of reduced nucleotides. An X-linked disorder with various polymorphic forms, it can cause a variety of anemias including favism, primaquine sensitivity and other drug sensitivity anemias, anemia of the newborn, and chronic nonspherocytic hemolytic anemia.

glucosephosphate isomerase d. [MIM*172400], an enzyme d. characterized by chronic nonspherocytic hemolytic anemia; autosomal recessive inheritance. SYN phosphohexose isomerase d.

β-*d*-glucuronidase d., a rare d. of β-*d*-glucuronidase; an autosomal recessive disorder with several allelic forms, characterized by abnormal mucopolysaccharide metabolism leading to progressive mental deterioration, splenic and hepatic enlargement, and dysostosis multiplex. SYN mucopolysaccharidase.

glutathione synthetase d., an inborn error of metabolism associated with massive urinary excretion of 5-oxyproline, elevated levels of 5-oxyproline in the blood and cerebrospinal fluid, severe metabolic acidosis, tendency toward hemolysis, and defective central nervous systems function. Glutathione synthetase d. has been reported as a generalized condition or with a d. restricted to erythrocytes.

11-hydroxylase d., a type of congenital adrenal hyperplasia, with multiple manifestations, including hypertensive types and salt-wasting varieties.

21-hydroxylase d., one form of congenital adrenal hyperplasia, with variable presentations, including simple virilizing, salt-wasting, or nonclassic types.

hypoxanthine guanine phosphoribosyltransferase d., a sex-linked inherited metabolic disorder; complete d. results in Lesch-Nyhan syndrome; incomplete d. is associated with acute gouty arthritis and renal stones.

immune d., SYN immunodeficiency.

immunity d., SYN immunodeficiency.

immunologic d., SYN immunodeficiency.

LCAT d., a rare condition characterized by corneal opacities, hemolytic anemia, proteinuria, renal insufficiency, and premature atherosclerosis, and very low levels of lecithin cholesterol acyltransferase (LCAT) activity; results in accumulation of unesterfied cholesterol in plasma and tissues.

leukocyte adhesion d. (LAD), an inherited disorder (autosomal recessive) in which there is a defective CD18 adherence complex that disturbs chemotaxis. It is characterized by recurrent bacterial pyogenic infections and impaired wound healing.

long-chain 3-hydroxyacyl-CoA dehydrogenase d., a fatty acid oxidation disorder; patients may experience episodes of acute hypoketotic hypoglycemia (similar to that found in MCAD deficiency), cardiomyopathy, muscle weakness, and liver abnormalities.

long-chain/very long-chain acyl-CoA dehydrogenase d., a disorder of fatty acid oxidation in patients who lack the enzyme very long chain acyl-CoA dehydrogenase; sometimes manifested as weakness, hypotonia, cardiomyopathy, rhabdomyolysis, and episodes of hypoglycemia during fasting.

luteal phase d., SYN luteal phase *defect*.

medium-chain acyl-CoA dehydrogenase d., the most common fatty acid oxidation disorder, presenting as acute episodes triggered by prolonged fasting for more than 12–16 hours, with

de

hypoglycemia, vomiting, and lethargy, which may progress to seizures, coma, or cardiopulmonary collapse, usually presenting before age 3.

mental d., SYN mental *retardation*.

muscle phosphorylase d., type V glycogen storage disease, affecting muscle, caused by d. of muscle phosphorylase.

phosphohexose isomerase d., SYN glucosephosphate isomerase d.

placental sulfatase d., an enzyme defect in the placenta which results in failure of conversion of 16α-hydroxydehydroepiandrosterone to estriol; women with this condition rarely enter into spontaneous labor.

primary carnitine d., a rare defect in carnitine metabolism due to a defect in carnitine transport; patients may present with hypoketotic hypoglycemia and develop cardiomyopathy or skeletal muscle weakness.

proximal femoral focal d. (PFFD), a congenital defect in which variable portions of the upper end of the femur are reduced or absent.

pseudocholinesterase d. [MIM*177400], an autosomal dominant disorder manifested by exaggerated responses to drugs ordinarily hydrolyzed by serum pseudocholinesterase (e.g., succinylcholine); believed to entail production of a variant enzyme that is less active than the normal enzyme in hydrolyzing appropriate substrates, but also abnormally resistant to the effects of anticholinesterases, caused by mutation in the pseudocholinesterase E1 gene (CHE1) on 3q.

pyruvate kinase d. [MIM*266200], a disorder in which there is a d. of pyruvate kinase in red blood cells; characterized by hemolytic anemia varying in degree from one patient to another; autosomal recessive inheritance, caused by mutation in the pyruvate kinase liver and red blood cell gene (PKLR) on chromosome 1q.

riboflavin d., SEE ariboflavinosis.

secondary antibody d., SYN secondary *immunodeficiency*.

short-chain acyl-CoA dehydrogenase d., a disorder of fatty acid oxidation; patients may have chronic acidosis, failure to thrive, muscle weakness, and developmental delay.

taste d. [MIM*171200], reduced or absent ability to detect a bitter taste in a group of compounds of which phenylthiocarbamide is the prototype, due to the homozygous state of a common allele. SEE ALSO phenylthiourea.

def·i·cit (def′i-sit). The result of consuming or using something faster than it is being replenished or replaced. [L. *deficio,* to fail]

base d., a decrease in the total concentration of blood buffer base, indicative of metabolic acidosis or compensated respiratory alkalosis.

oxygen d., the difference between oxygen uptake of the body during early stages of exercise and during a similar duration in a steady state of exercise; sometimes considered as the formation of the oxygen debt.

pulse d., (1) the absence of palpable pulse waves in a peripheral artery for one or more heart beats, as is often seen in atrial fibrillation; **(2)** the number of such missing pulse waves (usually expressed as heart rate minus pulse rate per minute).

sleep d., a lack of sleep time or a relative lack of one of the stages of sleep as determined by a sleep study.

def·i·ni·tion (def′i-nish′ŭn). In optics, the power of a lens to give a distinct image. SEE ALSO resolving *power*. [L. *de-finio,* pp. *-finitus,* to bound, fr. *finis,* limit]

de·flec·tion (dē-flek′shŭn). **1.** A moving to one side. **2.** In the electrocardiogram, a deviation of the curve from the isoelectric base line; any wave or complex of the electrocardiogram. [L. *de-flecto,* pp. *-flexus,* to bend aside]

intrinsic d., with the electrode in direct contact with the muscle fiber, a rapid downward d. from the peak of latest positivity, signifying that the activation front has reached the subjacent muscle.

intrinsicoid d., the abrupt downstroke from latest positivity when the electrode is placed not directly on the muscle but at a distance, as in the unipolar chest leads in clinical electrocardiography.

de·flex·ion (dē′fleks-shŭn). Term used to describe the position of the fetal head in relation to the maternal pelvis in which the head

is descending in a nonflexed or extended attitude. [de- + L. *flexio,* a bending, fr. *flecto,* pp. *flexum,* to bend]

def·lo·res·cence (dē-flō-res′ens). Disappearance of the eruption in scarlet fever or other exanthemas. [L. *de-floresco,* to fade, wither, fr. *flos* (*flor-*), flower]

de·flu·o·ri·da·tion (dē-flōr′i-dā′shŭn). Removal of excess fluorides from a community water supply.

de·flu·vi·um (dē-floo′vē-ŭm). SYN defluxion. [L., fr. *de-fluo,* pp. *-fluxus,* to flow down]

de·flux·ion (dē-flŭk′shŭn). **1.** A falling down or out, as of the hair. SEE ALSO effluvium. **2.** A flowing down or discharge of fluid. SYN defluvium. [L. *defluxio, de-fluo,* pp. *-fluxus,* to flow down]

de·for·ma·bi·li·ty (dē-form′ă-bil′i-tē). The ability of cells, such as erythrocytes, to change shape as they pass through narrow spaces, such as the microvasculature.

de·for·ma·tion (dē-fōr-mā′shŭn). **1.** Deviation of form from the normal; specifically, an alteration in shape and/or structure of a previously normally formed part. It occurs after organogenesis and often involves the musculoskeletal system (e.g., clubfoot). **2.** In rheology, the change in the physical shape of a mass by applied stress. [L. *de-formo,* pp. *-atus,* to deform, fr. *forma,* form]

de·form·ing (dē-fōrm′ing). Causing a deviation from the normal form.

de·for·mi·ty (dē-fōr′mi-tē). A permanent structural deviation from the normal shape, size, or alignment, resulting in disfigurement; may be congenital or acquired. SEE ALSO deformation (1).

Åkerlund d., indentation (incisura) with niche of duodenal cap as demonstrated radiographically.

Arnold-Chiari d. [MIM*207950], SYN Arnold-Chiari *malformation*.

bell clapper d., a testis and epididymis free of the usual posterior attachment of the tunica vaginalis such that the tunic inserts high on the spermatic cord leaving the gonad more likely to undergo torsion.

boutonnière d., flexion of the proximal interphalangeal joint with hyperextension of the distal interphalangeal joint of the finger, caused by separation of the extensor hood and protrusion of the head of the proximal phalanx through the resulting "buttonhole"; can result from degeneration (rheumatoid arthritis) or trauma.

contracture d., d. of a limb without discernable primary changes of bone.

Erlenmeyer flask d., a d. at the distal end of the femur caused by a failure of the shaft of the bone to develop to its normal tubular shape, with the result that the bone is wide for a much longer distance up the shaft than normal; encountered in Gaucher disease. [resemblance to an E. flask]

gunstock d., a form of cubitus varus resulting from supracondylar or condylar fracture at the elbow in which the axis of the extended forearm is not continuous with that of the arm but is displaced toward midline.

Haglund d., SYN Haglund *disease.*

J-sella d., pear-shaped or J-shaped d. of sella turcica caused by increased pressure on growing sphenoid bone; noted in the mucopolysaccharide storage diseases.

keyhole d., mucosal ectropion at the posterior edge of the anus following sphincterotomy at that location.

lobster-claw d., SEE ectrodactyly.

Madelung d., a distal radioulnar subluxation due to a relative deficiency of axial growth of the medial side of the distal radius, which, as a consequence, is abnormally inclined proximally and ulnarwards. SYN carpus curvus.

mermaid d., SYN sirenomelia.

parachute d., SYN parachute mitral *valve.*

reduction d., congenital absence or attenuation of one or more body parts; usually of the limbs or limb components.

silver-fork d., the d. resembling the curve of the back of a fork seen in Colles (distal radius) fracture.

Sprengel d., congenital elevation of the scapula. SYN scapula elevata.

swan-neck d., hyperextension of the proximal interphalangeal joint with flexion of the distal interphalangeal joint of the finger.

torsional d., in orthopedics, a d. caused by an abnormal rotation of a portion of an extremity with relationship to the long axis of the entire extremity.

whistling d., d. caused by insufficient tissue in the lower border of a repaired cleft lip, giving the appearance of whistling.

Whitehead d., circumferential mucosal ectropion at the anus following Whitehead operation.

de·fur·fur·a·tion (dē-fer-fer-ā′shŭn). The shedding of the epidermis in the form of fine scales. SYN branny desquamation. [L. *de,* away from, + *furfur,* bran]

de·gan·gli·on·ate (dē-gang′glē-on-āt). To deprive of ganglia.

de·gen·er·a·cy (dē-jen′er-ă-sē). 1. A condition marked by deterioration of mental, physical, or moral processes. 2. The fact that several different triplet codons encode the same amino acid. [L. *de,* from, + *genus,* (*gener-*), race]

de·gen·er·ate. 1 (dē-jen′er-āt). To pass to a lower level of mental, physical, or moral state; to fall below the normal or acceptable type or state. 2 (dē-jen′ĕ-răt). Below the normal or acceptable; that which has passed to a lower level.

de·gen·er·a·tio (dē-jen-er-ā′shē-ō). SYN degeneration. [L. *degenero,* pp. *-atus,* fr. *de,* from, + *genus,* race]

DEGENERATION

---

de·gen·er·a·tion (dē-jen-er-ā′shŭn). 1. Deterioration; passing from a higher to a lower level or type. 2. A worsening of mental, physical, or moral qualities. 3. A retrogressive pathologic change in cells or tissues, in consequence of which their functions are often impaired or destroyed; sometimes reversible; in the early stages, necrosis results. SYN retrograde metamorphosis. SYN degeneratio. [L. *degeneratio*]

adipose d., SYN fatty d.

adiposogenital d., SYN adiposogenital *dystrophy.*

age-related macular d., a common macular d. beginning with drusen of the macula and pigment disruption and sometimes leading to severe loss of central vision.

amyloid d., infiltration of amyloid between cells and fibers of tissues and organs. SYN waxy d. (1).

angiolithic d., calcareous d. of the walls of the blood vessels.

ascending d., (1) retrograde d. of an injured nerve fiber; i.e., toward the nerve cell of the fiber; (2) spinal cord d. that begins in one region and then progresses cephalad.

atheromatous d., focal accumulation of lipid material (atheroma) in the intima and subintimal portion of arteries, eventually resulting in fibrous thickening or calcification.

axon d., SYN axonal d.

axonal d., a type of peripheral nerve fiber response to insult, wherein axon death and subsequent breakdown occurs, with secondary breakdown of the myelin sheath associated; caused by focal injury to peripheral nerve fibers; often referred to as wallerian d. SYN axon d.

ballooning d., an obsolete term for cells that are infected with certain viruses, resulting in conspicuous swelling of the cell and cytoplasmic vacuolation.

basophilic d., blue staining of connective tissues when hematoxylin-eosin stain is used; found in such conditions as solar elastosis.

calcareous d., in a precise sense, not a degenerative process *per se,* but the deposition of insoluble calcium salts in tissue that has degenerated and become necrotic, as in dystrophic calcification.

carneous d., SYN red d.

caseous d., SYN caseous *necrosis.*

colloid d., a d. similar to mucoid d., in which the material is inspissated.

cone d., SYN cone *dystrophy.*

corticobasal d., a rare, progressive disease involving both cerebral cortex and extrapyramidal structures; clinically manifest as disturbances of voluntary movements and rigidity; pathologic characteristics include degeneration of the cerebral cortex with balloon neurons and degeneration of the substantia nigra.

Crooke hyaline d., SYN Crooke hyaline *change.*

descending d., (1) wallerian d. of an injured nerve fiber; i.e., d. distal to the lesion; (2) d. caudal to the level of a spinal cord lesion.

disciform d., foveal or parafoveal subretinal neovascularization with retinal separation and hemorrhage leading finally to a circular mass of fibrous tissue with marked loss of visual acuity. SYN disciform macular d.

disciform macular d., SYN disciform d.

ectatic marginal d. of cornea, SYN pellucid marginal corneal d.

elastoid d., (1) SYN elastosis (2); (2) hyaline d. of the elastic tissue of the arterial wall, seen during involution of the uterus.

elastotic d., SYN elastosis (2).

familial pseudoinflammatory macular d. [MIM*136900], macular d. that occurs during the fifth decade of life, with sudden development of a central scotoma in one eye followed rapidly by a similar lesion in the opposite eye; autosomal dominant inheritance. SYN Sorsby macular d.

fascicular d., d. restricted to certain fascicles of nerves or muscles.

fatty d., abnormal formation of microscopically visible droplets of fat in the cytoplasm of cells, as a result of injury. SYN adipose d., steatosis (2).

fibrinoid d., fibrinous d., a process resulting in poorly defined, deeply acidophilic, homogeneous refractile deposits with some staining reactions that resemble fibrin, occurring in connective tissue, blood vessel walls, and other sites.

fibrous d., not a d. *per se,* but rather a reparative process; cells and foci of tissue previously affected with degenerative processes, and necrosis, are replaced by cellular fibrous tissue.

granular d., SYN cloudy *swelling.*

granulovacuolar d., d. of hippocampal brain cells in elderly persons, characterized by basophilic granules surrounded by a clear zone in hippocampal neurons; occurs more frequently in Alzheimer disease.

gray d., d. of the white substance of the spinal cord, the fibers of which lose their myelin sheaths and become darker in color.

hepatolenticular d., SYN Wilson *disease* (1).

hyaline d., a group of several degenerative processes that affect various cells and tissues, resulting in the formation of rounded masses ("droplets") or relatively broad bands of substances that are homogeneous, translucent, refractile, and moderately to deeply acidophilic; may occur in the collagen of old fibrous tissue, smooth muscle of arterioles or the uterus, and as droplets in parenchymal cells.

hyaloideoretinal d. [MIM*143200], progressive liquefaction and destruction of the vitreous humor with grayish-white preretinal membranes, myopia, cataract, retinal detachment, and hyper- and hypopigmentation; autosomal dominant inheritance. SYN Wagner disease, Wagner syndrome.

hydropic d., SYN cloudy *swelling.*

infantile neuronal d., degenerative disorder of infants with widespread neuronal loss in thalamus, cerebellum, pons, and spinal cord, resembling infantile muscular atrophy.

liquefaction d., (1) necrosis with softening, as in ischemic brain tissue; (2) dissolution of the basal epidermal layer by necrosis of scattered cells with vacuolization, observed in lichen planus, lupus erythematosus, and other dermatologic conditions.

macular d., any ocular d. affecting predominantly the posterior fundus, but most commonly age-related macular d.

Mönckeberg d., SYN Mönckeberg *arteriosclerosis.*

mucinoid d., a term including both mucoid and colloid d., the essential cellular changes in both being similar, the only difference being that, in colloid d., the substance is firmer and more inspissated than in mucoid d., in which it is thin and jellylike.

mucoid d., a conversion of any of the connective tissues into a gelatinous or mucoid substance. SYN myxoid d., myxomatous d., myxomatosis (1).

mucoid medial d., SYN cystic medial *necrosis.*

myelinic d., formation of myelin figures in the cytoplasm of cells, possibly by degradation or hydration of lipoprotein of self-digested organelles.

myopic d., association of crescent of the optic disk, atrophy of the choroid and macular pigment, subretinal neovascularization, hemorrhage, and pigment proliferation in pathologic myopia.

myxoid d., myxomatous d., SYN mucoid d.

neurofibrillary d., formation of coarse, argentophilic, intracytoplasmic fibers, often in complex tangles within intracranial nerve cells. SEE ALSO Alzheimer *disease.*

Nissl d., d. of the cell body occurring after transection of the axon; characterized by dispersion of the granular endoplasmic reticulum, swelling of the soma, and an eccentric position of the nucleus of the cell.

olivopontocerebellar d., SYN olivopontocerebellar *atrophy.*

parenchymatous d., SYN cloudy *swelling.*

pellucid marginal corneal d., bilateral opacification and vascularization of the periphery of the cornea, progressing to formation of a gutter and ectasia. SYN ectatic marginal d. of cornea.

primary neuronal d., SYN Alzheimer *disease.*

primary pigmentary d. of retina, SYN tapetoretinal d.

primary progressive cerebellar d., a familial ataxic condition related to cerebellar d.

pseudotubular d., obsolete term for a form of d. observed in adrenal glands, especially those of patients with febrile infectious disease; the shrunken, lipid-depleted cells of the zona fasciculata (and sometimes the zona glomerulosa) are arranged in a circular pattern about spaces that may be empty or partly filled with fibrin, necrotic cells, or amorphous material.

red d., obsolete term for necrosis, with staining by hemoglobin, which may occur in uterine myomas, especially during pregnancy; marked by softening and a red color resembling partly cooked meat. SYN carneous d.

reticular d., severe epidermal edema resulting in multilocular bullae.

retrograde d., retrograde cell d. with chromatolysis of Nissl bodies and peripheral displacement of the nucleus of the cell of origin of a nerve fiber injured or sectioned.

Salzmann nodular corneal d., large and prominent nodules of a solid, opaque material that stands out from the surface of the cornea; occurs occasionally in persons previously affected by phlyctenular keratitis.

senile d., the process of involution occurring in old age.

snail track d., circumferential line of fine white dots in the peripheral retina associated with atrophic retinal holes.

Sorsby macular d., SYN familial pseudoinflammatory macular d.

spheroidal d., SYN climatic *keratopathy.*

spongy d. of infancy, SYN Canavan *disease.*

subacute combined d. of the spinal cord, a subacute or chronic disorder of the spinal cord, such as that occurring in certain patients with vitamin B_{12} deficiency, characterized by a slight to moderate degree of gliosis in association with spongiform degeneration of the posterior and lateral columns. SYN combined sclerosis, combined system disease, funicular myelitis (2), Putnam-Dana syndrome, vitamin B_{12} neuropathy.

tapetoretinal d. [MIM*272600], a hereditary disorder of the retina mainly affecting photoreceptors and retinal pigment epithelium; this may be a manifestation of Friedreich *ataxia,* Refsum *disease,* and abetalipoproteinemia. SYN primary pigmentary d. of retina.

Terrien marginal d., a form of pellucid marginal corneal d.

transsynaptic d., an atrophy of nerve cells following damage to the axons that make synaptic connection with them; noted especially in the lateral geniculate body. SYN transneuronal atrophy, transsynaptic chromatolysis.

Türck d., d. of a nerve fiber and its sheath distal to the point of injury or section of the axon; usually applied to d. within the central nervous system.

vacuolar d., formation of nonlipid vacuoles in cytoplasm, most frequently due to accumulation of water by cloudy swelling.

vitelliform d. [MIM*153700], SYN Best *disease.* SYN vitelliruptive d.

vitelliruptive d., SYN vitelliform d.

wallerian d., the degenerative changes the distal segment of a peripheral nerve fiber (axon and myelin) undergoes when its continuity with its cell body is interrupted by a focal lesion.

waxy d., (1) SYN amyloid d; (2) SYN Zenker d.

xerotic d., scarring of the conjunctiva associated with keratinized epithelium.

Zenker d., obsolete term for a form of severe hyaline d. or necrosis in skeletal muscle, occurring in severe infections. SYN waxy d. (2).

---

de·gen·er·a·tive (dē-jen′er-ă-tiv). Relating to degeneration.

de·glov·ing (dē-glov′ing). **1.** Intraoral surgical exposure of the anterior mandible used in various orthognathic surgical operations such as genioplasty or mandibular alveolar surgery. **2.** Intraoral exposure of the midfacial skeleton used in various operations on the nose and paranasal sinuses particularly for excision of neoplasms. **3.** SEE degloving *injury.*

deglut. Abbreviation for L. *deglutiatur,* swallow.

de·glu·ti·tion (dē-gloo-tish′ŭn). The act of swallowing. [L. *de-glutio,* to swallow]

de·glu·ti·tive (dē-gloo′ti-tiv). Relating to deglutition.

Degos, Robert, French dermatologist, *1904. SEE D. *disease, syndrome;* Kohlmeier-D. *syndrome.*

deg·ra·da·tion (deg-ră-dā′shŭn). The change of a chemical compound into a less complex compound. [L. *degradatus,* degrade]

de·gran·u·la·tion (dē-gran-ū-lā′shŭn). Disappearance or loss of cytoplasmic granules (lysosomes) from a cell.

de·gree (dĕ-grē′). **1.** One of the divisions on the scale of a measuring instrument such as a thermometer, barometer, etc. See Comparative Temperature Scales appendix. SEE scale. **2.** The 360th part of the circumference of a circle. **3.** A position or rank within a graded series. **4.** A measure of damage to tissue. [Fr. *degré;* L. *gradus,* a step]

d.'s of freedom, in statistics, the number of independent comparisons that can be made between the members of a sample (e.g., subjects, test items and scores, trials, conditions); in a contingency table it is one less than the number of row categories multiplied by one less than the number of column categories.

de·gus·ta·tion (dē-gŭs-tā′shŭn). **1.** The act of tasting. **2.** The sense of taste. [L. *degustatio,* fr. *de-gusto,* pp. *-atus,* to taste]

de·hal·o·gen·ase (dē-hal′ō-jen-ās). Any enzyme (EC subclass 3.8) removing halogen atoms from organic halides.

Dehio, Karl K., Russian physician, 1851–1927. SEE D. *test.*

de·his·cence (dē-his′ens). A bursting open, splitting, or gaping along natural or sutured lines. [L. *dehisco,* to split apart or open]

iris d., a defect of the eye characterized by multiple holes in the iris.

root d., a loss of the buccal or lingual bone overlaying the root portion of a tooth, leaving that area covered by soft tissue only.

wound d., disruption of apposed surfaces of a wound.

de·hu·man·i·za·tion (dē-hū′măn-i-zā′shŭn). Loss of human characteristics; brutalization by either mental or physical means; stripping one of self-esteem. [*de-* + *humanus,* human, fr. *homo,* man]

de·hy·drase (dē-hī′drās). Former name for dehydratase.

de·hy·dra·tase (dē-hī′drā-tās). A subclass (EC 4.2.1.x) of lyases (hydro-lyases) that remove H and OH as H_2O from a substrate, leaving a double bond, or add a group to a double bond by the elimination of water from two substances to form a third; synthase is sometimes used when the synthetic aspect of the reaction is emphasized. Some trivial names of enzymes in this subclass bear the generic term hydratase, emphasizing the reverse reaction.

de·hy·drate (dē-hī′drāt). **1.** To extract water from. **2.** To lose water. [L. *de,* from + G. *hydōr* (*hydr-*), water]

de·hy·dra·tion (dē-hī-drā′shŭn). **1.** Deprivation of water. SYN anhydration. **2.** Reduction of water content. **3.** SYN exsiccation (2). **4.** SYN desiccation.

absolute d., actual water deficit as measured by a difference from the normal or from a given water content.

relative d., water deficit relative to content of solutes contributing effective osmotic pressure; a state of increased effective osmotic pressure of body fluids.

voluntary d., that physiologic lag or deficit that results when sensations of thirst are not strong enough to bring about complete replacement of water loss, as in rapid sweating.

○**dehydro-.** Prefix used in the names of those chemical compounds that differ from other and more familiar compounds in the absence of two hydrogen atoms; e.g., dehydroascorbic acid, which resembles ascorbic acid in all structural features except for its lack of two hydrogen atoms that are present in the ascorbic acid molecule. In systematic nomenclature, didehydro- is preferred as being more exact.

de·hy·dro·a·ce·tic ac·id (dē-hī′drō-ă-sē′tik). An antimicrobial agent used as a preservative in cosmetics.

L-de·hy·dro·a·scor·bic ac·id (dē-hī′drō-as-kōr′bik). The reversibly oxidized form of ascorbic acid; it is antiscorbutic, but is converted in the body to 2,3-diketo-L-gulonic acid, which has no vitamin C activity.

de·hy·dro·bil·i·ru·bin (dē-hī′drō-bil-ē-roo′bin). SYN biliverdin.

de·hy·dro·cho·late (dē-hī-drō-kō′lāt). A salt or ester of dehydrocholic acid.

7-de·hy·dro·cho·les·ter·ol (dē-hī′drō-kō-les′ter-ol). A zoosterol in skin and other animal tissues that upon activation by ultraviolet light becomes antirachitic and is then referred to as cholecalciferol (vitamin D$_3$). SYN provitamin D$_3$.

24-de·hy·dro·cho·les·ter·ol. SYN desmosterol.

de·hy·dro·cho·lic ac·id (dē-hī-drō-kol′ik). Has a stimulating effect upon the secretion of bile by the liver (choleretic), and improves the absorption of essential food materials in states associated with deficient bile formation.

11-de·hy·dro·cor·ti·co·ster·one (dē-hī′drō-kōr-ti-ko-s′ter-ōn). Principally, a metabolite of corticosterone, found in the adrenal cortex.

de·hy·dro·em·e·tine (dē-hī-drō-em′ĕ-tēn). A synthetic derivative of emetine; used in the treatment of intestinal amebiasis.

d. resinate, a derivative of emetine.

dehydroepiandrosterone. Steroid agent related to male hormones that have been advocated as able to prevent physiologic consequences of aging, without studies that show benefit or safety.

de·hy·dro-3-ep·i·an·dros·ter·one (DHEA) (dē-hī′drō-ep-ē-an-dros′ter-ōn). a steroid secreted chiefly by the adrenal cortex, but also by the testis; it is the principal precursor of urinary 17-ketosteroids. Weakly androgenic itself, it is metabolized to delta-5 androstenediol, a hormone with both androgenic and estrogenic effects, and is one of the precursors of testosterone. Serum levels are elevated in adrenal virilism. It may function as a neurotransmitter. SYN androstenolone, dehydroisoandrosterone.

> DHEA secretion begins during fetal life, reaches a peak in the 3rd decade, and declines steadily thereafter; the level at age 80 is only 10–20% of the peak level. This decline has been speculatively associated with the changes of aging. Commercial formulations of DHEA are marketed as dietary supplements, although this substance is neither a nutrient nor a component of the human food chain. Available from health food stores in 10-, 25-, and 50-mg capsules, DHEA has been promoted for the prevention of degenerative diseases including atherosclerosis, Alzheimer dementia, and parkinsonism, and other effects of aging. None of the alleged benefits have been demonstrated in large, randomized clinical trials. Long-term administration to postmenopausal women has been associated with insulin resistance, hypertension, and reduction of LDL cholesterol. An analysis of 16 preparations of DHEA by high-performance liquid chromatography showed a variation in content from 0–150% of the labeled strength; only 7 products fell between the expected 90–110% of labeled strength.

de·hy·dro·gen·ase (dē-hī′drō-jen-ās). Class name for those enzymes that oxidize substrates by catalyzing removal of hydrogen from metabolites (hydrogen donors) and transferring it to other substances (hydrogen acceptors), which are thus reduced; most of the oxidative enzymes (oxidoreductases, EC class 1) perform their oxidations in this manner.

aerobic d., an enzyme (usually a metalloflavoenzyme) catalyzing the transfer of hydrogen from some metabolite to oxygen, forming hydrogen peroxide in the process; e.g., xanthine oxidase and others in several sub-subclasses (e.g., EC 1.1.3, 1.2.3, 1.7.3, 1.8.3, 1.10.3).

anaerobic d., an enzyme (usually a pyridinoenzyme) catalyzing the transfer of hydrogen from some metabolite to some acceptor molecule (e.g., NAD$^+$, cytochrome) other than oxygen; e.g., lactate d.'s, isocitrate d.'s, and others in EC class 1, excluding those listed under aerobic d.

α-keto acid d., SEE α-*keto acid* dehydrogenase.

Robison ester d., SYN glucose-6-phosphate dehydrogenase.

de·hy·dro·gen·ate (dē-hī′drō-jen-āt). To subject to dehydrogenation.

de·hy·dro·gen·a·tion (dē-hī′drō-jen-ā′shŭn). Removal of a pair of hydrogen atoms from a compound by the action of enzymes (dehydrogenases) or other catalysts.

de·hy·dro·i·so·an·dros·ter·one (dē-hī′drō-ī-sō-an-dros′ter-ōn). SYN dehydro-3-epiandrosterone.

de·hy·dro·ret·i·nal·de·hyde (dē-hī′drō-ret-i-nal′dĕ-hīd). Dehydroretinol with –CHO instead of –CH$_2$OH at the terminal carbon of the side chain. SYN retinene-2, vitamin A$_2$ aldehyde.

de·hy·dro·ret·i·no·ic ac·id (dē-hī′drō-ret-i-nō′ik). Dehydroretinol with –COOH in place of –CH$_2$OH at the terminal carbon of the side chain.

de·hy·dro·ret·i·nol (dē-hī-drō-ret′i-nol). Retinol with an additional double bond in the 3-4 position of the cyclohexane ring. SYN vitamin A$_2$.

de·hy·dro·sug·ars (dē-hī′drō-shug-erz). SYN anhydrosugars.

de·hyp·no·tize (dē-hip′nō-tīz). To bring out of the hypnotic state.

de·im·i·nas·es (dē-im′i-nās-ez). SYN iminohydrolases.

de·in·sti·tu·tion·al·i·za·tion (dē′in-sti-too′shŭn-ăl-i-zā-shŭn). The discharge of institutionalized patients from a mental hospital into treatment programs in half-way houses and other community-based programs.

de·i·on·i·za·tion (dē-ī′-on-ī-zā′shŭn). The production of a mineral-free state by the removal of ions.

Deiters, Otto F.K., German anatomist, 1834–1863. SEE D. *cells,* under *cell,* terminal *frames,* under *frame, nucleus.*

dé·jà vou·lu (dā-zhă′ voo-loo′). A term for a type of disturbance of memory in which the individual believes that his or her present desires are exactly the same as the desires the individual had some time before.

dé·jà vu (dā-zhah-voo′). Feeling of having been in a place before. SEE déjà vu *phenomenon.* SEE phenomenon. [Fr. already seen]

de·jec·ta (dē-jek′tă). SYN dejection (3). [L. neut, pl. of *de-jectus,* fr. *de-jicio,* to cast down]

de·jec·tion (dē-jek′shŭn). **1.** SYN depression (4). **2.** The discharge of excrementitious matter. **3.** The matter so discharged. SYN dejecta. [L. *dejectio,* fr. de- *jicio,* pp. *-jectus,* to cast down]

Dejerine, Joseph J., Paris neurologist, 1849–1917. SEE D. *disease,* hand *phenomenon, reflex, sign;* D.-Roussy *syndrome;* D.-Sottas *disease;* D.-Klumpke *syndrome;* Landouzy-D. *dystrophy.*

Dejerine-Klumpke, Augusta, French neurologist (born in the U.S.), 1859–1927. SEE Klumpke *palsy;* Klumpke *paralysis;* Dejerine-Klumpke *palsy;* Dejerine-Klumpke *syndrome.*

○**deka-.** SEE deca-.

Delafield, Francis, U.S. physician and pathologist, 1841–1915. SEE D. *hematoxylin.*

de·lam·i·na·tion (dē-lam-i-nā′shŭn). Division into separate layers. [L. *de,* from, + *lamina,* a thin plate]

de

Delaney clause. A clause of the Food Additive Amendment of the U.S. Federal law specifying that no substance that has been found to induce cancer in any animal may be incorporated into food. [James F. *Delaney*, U.S. Congressman]

de Lange, Cornelia, Dutch pediatrician, 1871–1950. SEE de L. *syndrome.*

Delbet, Pierre L.E., French surgeon, 1861–1925. SEE D. *sign.*

Del Castillo, E.B., 20th century Argentinian physician. SEE Del C. *syndrome.*

de·lead (dē-lēd'). To cause the mobilization and excretion of lead deposited in the bones and other tissues, as by the administration of a chelating agent.

del·e·te·ri·ous (del-ĕ-tēr'ē-ŭs). Injurious; noxious; harmful. [G. *dēlētērios,* fr. *dēleomai,* to injure]

de·le·tion (dĕ-lē'shŭn). In genetics, any spontaneous elimination of part of the normal genetic complement, whether cytogenetically visible (chromosomal d.) or found by molecular techniques. [L. *deletio,* destruction]

    chromosomal d., a microscopically evident loss of part of a chromosome. SEE ALSO monosomy.

    gene d., d. of a segment of a chromosome too small to be detected cytogenetically, inferred from the phenotype at one particular locus.

    interstitial d., d. that does not involve the terminal parts of a chromosome.

    nucleotide d., d. of a single nucleotide, which in a transcribed gene will lead to a frame-shift mutation. SYN point d. (2).

    point d., (1) d. involving a submicroscopic loss of genetic material too small to be resolved by linkage analysis; **(2)** SYN nucleotide d.

    terminal d., d. involving the terminal part of a chromosome and leading to a adhesive terminus.

del·i·cate (del'ĭ-kăt). Of feeble resisting power. [L. *delicatus,* soft, luxurious, fr. *de,* from, + *lacio,* to entice]

de·lim·i·ta·tion (dē-lim-i-tā'shŭn). Marking off; putting bounds or limits; preventing the spread of a morbid process in the body or of a disease in the community. [L. *de-limito,* pp. *-atus,* to bound, fr. *limes,* boundary]

del·i·quesce (del-i-kwes'). To undergo deliquescence.

del·i·ques·cence (del-i-kwes'ens). Becoming damp or liquid by absorption of water from the atmosphere and then dissolving in the water taken up; a property found in certain salts, such as $CaCl_2$. [L. *de-liquesco,* to melt or become liquid]

del·i·ques·cent (del-i-kwes'ent). Denoting a solid capable of deliquescence.

de·li·ria (dē-lir'ē-ă). Plural of delirium. SEE delirium.

de·lir·i·ous (dē-lir'ē-ŭs). In a state of delirium.

de·lir·i·um, pl. **de·li·ria** (dē-lir'ē-ŭm, dē-lir'ē-ă). An altered state of consciousness, consisting of confusion, distractibility, disorientation, disordered thinking and memory, defective perception (illusions and hallucinations), prominent hyperactivity, agitation and autonomic nervous system overactivity; caused by a number of toxic, structural, and metabolic disorders. [L. fr. *deliro,* to be crazy, fr. *de-* + *lira,* a furrow (*i.e.,* go out of the furrow)]

    acute d., d. of recent, rapid onset.

    alcohol withdrawal d., the d. experienced by an alcohol-habituated individual caused by the abrupt cessation of alcohol intake.

    anxious d., d. in which the predominating symptom is an incoherent apprehension or anxiety.

    d. cor'dis, obsolete term for atrial *fibrillation.*

    posttraumatic d., d. caused by a structural traumatic brain injury.

    senile d., d. associated with senile dementia.

    toxic d., d. caused by the action of a poison.

    d. tre'mens (DT), a severe, sometimes fatal, form of d. due to alcoholic withdrawal following a period of sustained intoxication. [L. pres. p. of *tremo,* to tremble]

del·i·tes·cence (del-i-tes'ens). Rarely used term for: **1.** Sudden subsidence of symptoms; disappearance of a tumor or a cutaneous lesion. **2.** Period of incubation of an infectious disease. [L. *delitesco,* to lie hidden away]

de·liv·er (dē-liv'er). **1.** To assist a woman in childbirth. **2.** To extract from an enclosed place, as the fetus from the womb, an object or foreign body, e.g., a tumor from its capsule or surroundings, or the lens of the eye in cases of cataract. [fr. O. Fr. fr. L. *de-* + *liber,* free]

de·liv·ery (dē-liv'er-ē). Passage of the fetus and the placenta from the genital canal into the external world.

    assisted cephalic d., extraction of a fetus that presents by the head.

    breech d., extraction or expulsion of a fetus that presents by the buttocks or feet.

    forceps d., assisted birth of the child by an instrument designed to grasp the fetal head.

    high forceps d., d. by forceps applied to the fetal head before engagement has taken place.

    low forceps d., d. by forceps applied to the fetal head at station $\geq$ +2 cm and not on the pelvic floor. This classification of forceps delivery may be with or without rotation of the fetal head.

    midforceps d., d. by forceps applied to the fetal head at above +2 station, but after engagement has taken place.

    outlet forceps d., d. by forceps applied to the fetal head when it has reached the perineal floor and is visible between contractions.

    perimortem d., SYN postmortem d.

    postmortem d., extraction of the fetus after the death of its mother. SYN perimortem d.

    premature d., birth of a fetus between 20 and 37 weeks' gestation. SEE ALSO premature *birth.*

    spontaneous cephalic d., unassisted expulsion of a fetus that presents by the head.

del·le (del'eh). The central lighter-colored portion of the erythrocyte, as observed in a stained film of blood. [Ger. *Delle,* low ground, pit]

del·len. Shallow, saucerlike, clearly defined excavations at the margin of the cornea, about 1.5 by 2 mm, due to localized dehydration; also called Fuchs dellen. [Ger. pl. of *Delle,* low ground, pit]

del·o·mor·phous (del-ō-mōr'fŭs). Of definite form and shape; a term applied in the past to the parietal cells of the gastric glands. [G. *dēlos,* manifest, + *morphē,* form]

de·louse (dē-lows'). To remove lice from; to free from infestation with lice; used especially of prophylaxis of louse-borne diseases.

del·phi·nine (del'fin-ēn). A toxic alkaloid, an aconine derivative, from *Delphinium staphisagria;* it resembles aconitine in its action and chemical structure.

Del·phin·i·um aja·cis (del-fin'ē-ŭm ă-jā'sis). A species of plant (family Ranunculaceae) containing the alkaloids ajacine and ajaconine; the dried ripe seeds have been used externally as a parasiticide in pediculosis; rarely used now because of its toxicity. SYN larkspur. [G. *delphinion,* larkspur]

del·ta (Δ) (del'tă). **1.** Fourth letter of the Greek alphabet, Δ (capital), δ (lower case). **2.** In anatomy, a triangular surface.

    d. check, a comparison of consecutive values for a given test in a patient's laboratory file used to detect abrupt changes, usually generated as a part of computer-based quality control programs. SYN Δ check.

    d. for'nicis, SYN *commissura* fornicis.

    Galton d., (1) a more or less well-marked triangle, in a fingerprint, on either side where the straight ridges near the joint of the distal phalanx are succeeded by arches, loops, or whorls; SEE ALSO Galton system of classification of *fingerprints,* under *fingerprint;* **(2)** SYN triradius.

    d. mesoscap'ulae, the flat triangular surface at the vertebral extremity of the spine of the scapula over which glides the tendon for the lower fibers of the trapezius muscle.

del·toid (del'toyd). Resembling the Greek letter delta (Δ); triangular. [G. *deltoeidēs,* shaped like the letter *delta*]

de·lu·sion (dē-loo'zhŭn). A false belief or wrong judgment held with conviction despite incontrovertible evidence to the contrary. [L. *de-ludo,* pp. *-lusus,* to play false, deceive, fr. *ludo,* to play]

    d. of control, d. of being controlled, a d. in which one experiences one's feelings, impulses, thoughts, or actions as not one's own, but as being imposed on by some external force. SYN d. of passivity.

encapsulated d., a d. that usually relates to one specific topic or belief but does not pervade an individual's life or level of functioning.

expansive d., SYN d. of grandeur.

d. of grandeur, a d. in which one believes oneself possessed of great wealth, intellect, importance, power, etc. SYN expansive d., grandiose d.

grandiose d., SYN d. of grandeur.

d. of negation, a d. in which one imagines that the world and all that relates to it have ceased to exist. SYN nihilistic d.

nihilistic d., SYN d. of negation.

organic d.'s, false beliefs experienced in the delirium associated with dementia in conjunction with traumatic injury to the brain, or an organic change in the brain such as in Alzheimer syndrome, or in cocaine or other drug intoxication.

d. of passivity, SYN d. of control.

d. of persecution, persecutory d., a false notion that one is being persecuted; characteristic symptom of paranoid schizophrenia.

d. of reference, a delusional idea that external events, etc., refer to the self.

somatic d., a d. having reference to a nonexistent lesion or alteration of some organ or part of the body; sometimes indistinguishable from hypochondriasis.

systematized d., a d. that is logically constructed from a false premise and embraces a specific sector of the patient's life.

unsystematized d., one of a group of apparently discrete, disconnected d.'s.

de·lu·sion·al (dē-loo′zhŭn-ăl). Relating to a delusion.

de·mand (dē-mand′). A quantity of a substance, commodity, or service wanted or required.

biochemical oxygen d. (BOD), the rate at which dissolved oxygen is consumed by an organism (often, a microorganism) or a culture of cells.

de·mar·ca·tion (dē-mar-kā′shŭn). A setting of limits; a boundary. [Fr. fr. L. *de,* from, + Mediev. L. *marco,* to mark]

Demarquay, Jean N., French surgeon, 1814–1875. SEE D. *sign.*

de·mas·cu·lin·iz·ing (dē-mas′kū-lin-īz′ing). Depriving of male characteristics or inhibiting development of such characteristics.

De·mat·i·a·ce·ae (dē-mat-ē-ā′sē-ē). A family of soil-inhabiting, brown or black melanin-producing fungi found in decaying vegetables, rotting wood, and forest carpets, and including several of the dark-colored genera that cause chromoblastomycosis in humans, such as *Exophiala, Phialophora, Fonsecaea,* and *Cladosporium.*

de·mat·i·a·ceous (dē-mat-ē-ā′shŭs). Denoting dark conidia and/or hyphae, usually brown or black; used frequently to denote dark-colored fungi.

deme (dēm). A local, small, highly inbred group or kinship. Cf. isolate. [G. *dēmos,* people]

dem·e·car·i·um bro·mide (dem-ĕ-kar′ē-ŭm). A potent cholinesterase inhibitor used in the treatment of glaucoma and accommodative esotropia; it is stable in aqueous solution.

dem·e·clo·cy·cline (dem′ĕ-klō-sī′klēn). A broad-spectrum antibiotic that is more slowly excreted and more stable in acid and alkali than are other forms of the tetracyclines; available as the hydrochloride.

dem·e·col·cine (dem-ĕ-kol′sēn). An alkaloid from *Colchicum autumnale* (family Liliaceae) similar chemically to colchicine except that the acetyl group is replaced by a methyl group; used for gout and leukemia, is said to be less toxic than colchicine, and has an action upon mitosis similar to that of colchicine.

de·ment·ed (dē-ment′ed). Suffering from dementia.

de·men·tia (dē-men′shē-ă). The loss, usually progressive, of cognitive and intellectual functions, without impairment of perception or consciousness; caused by a variety of disorders including severe infections and toxins, but most commonly associated with structural brain disease. Characterized by disorientation, impaired memory, judgment, and intellect, and a shallow labile affect. SYN amentia (2). [L. fr. *de-* priv. + *mens,* mind]

AIDS d., SYN AIDS dementia *complex.*

Alzheimer d., SYN Alzheimer *disease.*

catatonic d., d. with catatonic symptoms.

dialysis d., SYN dialysis encephalopathy *syndrome.*

epileptic d., d. occurring in an individual afflicted with epilepsy, and thought to be a result of prolonged seizures, the epileptogenic brain lesion, or antiepileptic drugs.

hebephrenic d., d. with hebephrenic symptoms.

Lewy body d., SYN diffuse Lewy body *disease.*

multi-infarct d., SYN vascular d.

paralytic d., d. and paralysis resulting from a chronic syphilitic meningoencephalitis. SYN d. paralytica.

d. paralytica, SYN paralytic d.

posttraumatic d., d. caused by traumatic brain injury.

d. prae′cox, any one of the group of psychotic disorders known as the schizophrenias; formerly used to describe schizophrenia as a single entity. [L. precocious]

presenile d., d. preseni′lis, (1) d. of Alzheimer disease developing before age 65; **(2)** SYN Alzheimer *disease.*

primary d., d. occurring independently as a mental disorder.

primary senile d., SYN Alzheimer *disease.*

secondary d., chronic d. following and due to a psychosis or some other underlying disease process.

senile d., d. of Alzheimer disease developing after age 65.

toxic d., d. caused by an exogenous agent.

vascular d., a steplike deterioration in intellectual functions with focal neurologic signs, as the result of multiple infarctions of the cerebral hemispheres. SYN multi-infarct d.

de·meth·yl·ase (dē-meth′i-lās). SYN methyltransferase.

de·meth·yl·a·tion. The enzymatic removal of methyl groups.

⚬demi-. Half, lesser. SEE ALSO hemi-, semi-. [Fr. fr. L. *dimidius,* half]

dem·i·gaunt·let (dem-ē-gawnt′let). A glovelike bandage for the fingers and hand. [demi- + *gauntlet,* armored glove, fr. M.E., fr. O.Fr., fr. Germanic]

dem·i·lune (dem′ē-loon). **1.** A small body with a form similar to that of a half-moon or a crescent. **2.** Term frequently used for the gametocyte of *Plasmodium falciparum.* [Fr. half-moon]

Giannuzzi d.'s, SYN serous d.'s.

Heidenhain d.'s, SYN serous d.'s.

serous d.'s, the serous cells at the distal end of a mucous, tubulo-alveolar secretory unit of certain salivary glands. SYN Giannuzzi crescents, Giannuzzi d.'s, Heidenhain crescents, Heidenhain d.'s.

de·min·er·al·i·za·tion (dē-min′er-ăl-ī-zā′shŭn). A loss or decrease of the mineral constituents of the body or individual tissues, especially of bone.

dem·i·pen·ni·form (dem′ē-pen′i-fōrm). SYN semipennate.

Dem·o·dex (dem′ō-deks). A genus of very minute (0.1–0.4 mm) follicular mites (family Demodicidae) that inhabit the skin and are usually found in the sebaceous glands and hair follicles of mammals, including humans. Some cases of blepharitis in humans have been attributed to *Demodex* infection; use of facial creams promotes D. infection in older women, resulting in facial erythema with follicular scaling. [G. *dēmos,* tallow, + *dēx,* a woodworm]

D. folliculo′rum, a very common, universally distributed, and usually nonpathogenic species of mite that inhabits the hair follicles and sebaceous glands of humans, commonly of the face around the nose and scalp margins. SYN *Acarus folliculorum.*

de·mog·ra·phy (dĕ-mog′ra-fē). The study of populations, especially with reference to size, density, fertility, mortality, growth rate, age distribution, migration, and vital statistics. [G. *demos,* people, + *graphō,* to write]

dynamic d., a study of the functioning of a community, including statistical records.

Demoivre, Abraham, English mathematician, 1667–1754. SEE D. *formula.*

de·mo·ni·ac (dē-mō′nē-ak). Frenzied, fiendish, as if possessed by evil spirits. [G. *daimōn,* a spirit]

dem·on·stra·tor (dem′on-strā-ter, -tōr). An assistant to a professor of anatomy, surgery, etc., who prepares for the lecture by dissections or collection of patients, or who instructs small classes supplementary to the regular lectures; a d. corresponds in a general way to the Dozent of a German university. [L. *de-monstro,* pp. *-atus,* to point out]

De Morgan, Campbell, English physician, 1811–1876. SEE De M. *spots,* under *spot.*

de·mor·phin·i·za·tion (dē-mōr′fin-i-zā′shŭn). **1.** Removal of morphine from an opiate. **2.** Gradual withdrawal of morphine as a method of overcoming morphine dependence.

de Morsier, Georges, 20th century Swiss neurologist. SEE de M. *syndrome.*

de·mu·co·sa·tion (dē-mū-kō-sā′shŭn). Rarely used term for excision or stripping of the mucosa of any part.

de·mul·cent (de-mŭl′sent). **1.** Soothing; relieving irritation. **2.** An agent, such as a mucilage or oil, that soothes and relieves irritation, especially of the mucous surfaces. [L. *de-mulceo,* pp. *-mulctus,* to stroke lightly, to soften]

de Musset, Alfred. SEE Musset.

de·my·e·li·na·tion, de·my·e·lin·i·za·tion (dē-mī′ĕ-li-nā′shŭn, dē-mī′ĕ-lin-i-za′shŭn). Loss of myelin with preservation of the axons or fiber tracts. Central demyelination occurs within the central nervous system (e.g., the demyelination seen with multiple sclerosis); peripheral demyelination affects the peripheral nervous system (e.g., the demyelination seen with Guillain-Barré syndrome).

de·nar·co·tize (dē-nar′kō-tīz). To remove narcotic properties from an opiate; to deprive of narcotic properties.

de·na·to·ni·um ben·zo·ate (dē-nă-tō′nē-ŭm). An alcohol denaturant.

de·na·tur·a·tion (dē-na-tū-rā′shŭn). The process of becoming denatured.

de·na·tured (dē-nā′tūrd). **1.** Made unnatural or changed from the normal in any of its characteristics; often applied to proteins or nucleic acids heated or otherwise treated to the point where tertiary structural characteristics are altered. **2.** Adulterated, as by addition of methanol to ethanol.

den·dri·form (den′dri-fōrm). Tree-shaped, or branching. SYN arborescent, dendritic (1), dendroid. [G. *dendron,* tree, + L. *forma,* form]

den·drite (den′drīt). **1.** One of the two types of branching protoplasmic processes of the nerve cell (the other being the axon). SYN dendritic process, dendron, neurodendrite, neurodendron. **2.** A crystalline treelike structure formed during the freezing of an alloy. [G. *dendritēs,* relating to a tree]
   apical d., SYN apical *process.*

den·drit·ic (den-drit′ik). **1.** SYN dendriform. **2.** Relating to the dendrites of nerve cells.

den·dro·gram (den′drō-gram). A treelike figure used to represent graphically a hierarchy. [*dendron,* tree, + *gramma,* a drawing]

den·droid (den′droyd). SYN dendriform. [G. *dendron,* tree, + *eidos,* appearance]

den·dron. SYN dendrite (1). [G. a tree]

de·ner·vate (dē-ner′vāt). To cause denervation.

de·ner·va·tion (dē-ner-vā′shŭn). Loss of nerve supply.

den·gue (den′gā). A disease of tropical and subtropical regions that occurs epidemically, is caused by dengue virus, a member of the family Flaviviridae. There are 4 antigenic types, and they are transmitted by a mosquito of the genus *Aedes* (usually *A. aegypti,* but frequently *A. albopictus*). Four grades of severity are recognized: grade I, fever and constitutional symptoms; grade II, grade I plus spontaneous bleeding (of skin, gums, or gastrointestinal tract); grade III, grade II plus agitation and circulatory failure; grade IV, profound shock. SYN Aden fever, bouquet fever, breakbone fever, dandy fever, date fever, dengue fever, dengue hemorrhagic fever, exanthesis arthrosia, polka fever, scarlatina rheumatica, solar fever (1). [Sp. corruption of "dandy" fever]
   hemorrhagic d., a more severe form of d. characterized by hemorrhagic skin lesions, which has erupted in a number of epidemic outbreaks in the Pacific basin.

de·ni·al (dē-nī′ăl). An unconscious defense mechanism used to allay anxiety by denying the existence of important conflicts, troublesome impulses, events, actions, or illness. SYN negation. [M.E., fr O.Fr., fr. L. *denegare,* to say no]

den·i·da·tion (den-i-dā′shŭn). Exfoliation of the superficial portion of the mucous membrane of the uterus; stripping off of the menstrual decidua. [L. *de,* from, + *nidus,* nest]

de·ni·tra·tion (dē-nī-trā′shŭn). SYN denitrification.

de·ni·tri·fi·ca·tion (dē-nī′tri-fi-kā′shŭn). **1.** Removal of nitrogen from any material or chemical compound; especially from the soil, as by certain (denitrifying) bacteria that render the nitrogen unavailable for plant growth. **2.** Withdrawal of nitrogen from soil by plant growth. SYN denitration.

de·ni·tri·fy (dē-nī′tri-fī). To remove nitrogen from any material or chemical compound.

de·ni·tro·gen·a·tion (dē-nī′trō-jĕ-nā′shŭn). Elimination of nitrogen from lungs and body tissues by breathing gases devoid of nitrogen.

Dennie, Charles Clayton, U.S. dermatologist, 1883–1971. SEE D.-Morgan *fold;* D. *line.*

de·nom·in·a·tor (dē-nōm′i-nā-tor). The lower portion of a fraction used to calculate a rate or ratio; the population at risk in the calculation of a rate or ratio.

Denonvilliers, Charles P., French surgeon, 1808–1872. SEE D. *aponeurosis, ligament.*

de novo (di-nō′vō). Anew; often applied to particular biochemical pathways in which metabolites are newly biosynthesized (e.g., de novo purine biosynthesis). [L.]

dens, pl. **den·tes** (denz, den′tēz) [TA]. **1.** SYN tooth. **2.** A strong toothlike process projecting upward from the body of the axis, or epistropheus, around which the atlas rotates. SYN d. axis [TA], odontoid process of epistropheus, odontoid process. [L.]
   den′tes acus′tici [TA], SYN acoustic *teeth.*
   d. angula′ris, SYN canine *tooth.*
   d. axis [TA], SYN dens (2).
   d. bicus′pidus, pl. **den′tes bicus′pidi,** SYN premolar *tooth.*
   d. cani′nus, pl. **den′tes cani′ni** [TA], SYN canine *tooth.*
   d. cuspida′tus, pl. **den′tes cuspida′ti,** SYN canine *tooth.*
   d. decid′uus, pl. **den′tes deci′dui** [TA], SYN deciduous *tooth.*
   d. in den′te, a developmental disturbance in tooth formation resulting from invagination of the epithelium associated with crown development into the area destined to become pulp space; after calcification there is an invagination of enamel and dentin into the pulp space, giving the radiographic appearance of a "tooth within a tooth." SYN d. invaginatus.
   d. incisi′vus, pl. **den′tes incisi′vi** [TA], SYN incisor *tooth.*
   d. invaginatus (denz in′vă-gē-nā′-tus), SYN d. in dente. [Mediev. L. folded inward, fr. L. *vagina,* sheath]
   d. lac′teus, SYN deciduous *tooth.*
   d. molaris, pl. **den′tes mola′res** [TA], SYN molar *tooth;* SEE ALSO molar.
   d. molaris tertius [TA], SYN third-year molar *tooth.*
   d. per′manens, pl. **den′tes permanen′tes** [TA], SYN permanent *tooth.*
   d. premola′ris, pl. **den′tes premola′res** [TA], SYN premolar *tooth.*
   d. sapien′tiae, SYN third-year molar *tooth.* [L. *sapientia,* wisdom]
   d. seroti′nus, ✱official alternate term for third-year molar *tooth.*
   d. succeda′neus, SYN permanent *tooth.*

den·sim·e·ter (den-sim′ĕ-ter). SYN densitometer (1). [L. *densitas,* density, + G. *metron,* measure]

den·si·tom·e·ter (den-si-tom′ĕ-ter). **1.** An instrument for measuring the density of a fluid. SYN densimeter. **2.** An instrument for measuring, by virtue of relative turbidity, the growth of bacteria in broth; useful in microbiologic assay of nutrients and antibiotics, phage studies, etc. **3.** An instrument for measuring the density of components (e.g., protein fractions) separated by electrophoresis or chromatography, utilizing light absorption or reflection. **4.** An electronic instrument for measuring the blackening of radiographic film by x-ray exposure; used for film sensitometry, bone densitometry, measurement of line spread function (microdensitometer). **5.** An instrument for measuring the extent to which a material absorbs or reflects light. [L. *densitas,* density, + G. *metron,* measure]

den·si·tom·e·try (den-si-tom′ĕ-trē). A procedure utilizing a densitometer.

den·si·ty (ρ) (den′si-tē). **1.** The compactness of a substance; the ratio of mass to unit volume, usually expressed as g/cm³ (kg/m³ in the SI system). **2.** The quantity of electricity on a given surface or in a given time per unit of volume. **3.** In radiological physics, the opacity to light of an exposed radiographic or photographic film; the darker the film, the greater the measured d. **4.** In clinical radiology, a less exposed area on a film, corresponding to a region of greater x-ray attenuation (radiopacity) in the subject; the more light transmitted by the film, the greater the d. of the subject; this is not actually the opposite of the prior definition, since one concerns film d. and the other subject d. [L. *densitas,* fr. *densus,* thick]

bone d., quantitative measurement of the mineral content of bone, used as an indicator of the structural strength of the bone and as a screen for osteoporosis

buoyant d., the d. that allows a substance to float in some standard fluid.

count d., SYN photon d.

flux d., (1) SYN flux (4); **(2)** either particle flux d., the particle fluence rate, or energy flux d., the energy fluence rate of intensity. Cf. fluence.

incidence d., the person-time incidence rate.

optic d. (OD), SYN absorbance.

photon d., the number of counted events recorded in scintigraphy per square centimeter or per square inch of imaged area. SYN count d.

spin d., the number of nuclear dipoles per unit volume.

vapor d., the mass per unit volume of a vapor; since the vapor d. changes with temperature and pressure, it is commonly expressed as a specific gravity, i.e., the weight of the vapor divided by the weight of an equal volume of a reference gas (e.g., oxygen or hydrogen) at the same temperature and pressure.

♻**dent-, denti-, dento-.** Teeth; dental. SEE ALSO odonto-. [L. *dens,* tooth]

den·tal (den′tăl). Relating to the teeth. [L. *dens,* tooth]

den·tal en·gine. The motive power of a dental handpiece that causes it to rotate.

den·tal·gia (den-tal′jē-ă). SYN toothache. [L. *dens,* tooth, + G. *algos,* pain]

den·tate (den′tāt). Notched; toothed; cogged. [L. *dentatus,* toothed]

den·ta·tec·to·my (den-tă-tek′tō-mē). Surgical destruction of the dentate nucleus of the cerebellum. [dentate (nucleus) + G. *ectomē,* excision]

den·ta·tum (den-tā′tŭm, den-tah′tŭm). SYN dentate *nucleus* of cerebellum. [L. neut. of *dentatus,* toothed]

den·tes (den′tēz). Plural of dens. [L.]

♻**denti-.** SEE dent-.

den·tia (den-tē′a). The process of tooth development or eruption. Also serves to denote a relationship to the teeth. [dent- + suffix -ia, condition, process]

d. praecox (den-tē′a prē-coks), premature tooth eruption. [L. premature]

d. tarda (den-tēa′ tar′dă), delayed tooth eruption. [L. delayed]

den·ti·cle (den′ti-kl). **1.** SYN endolith. **2.** A toothlike projection from a hard surface. [L. *denticulus,* a small tooth]

den·tic·u·late, den·tic·u·lat·ed (den-tik′ū-lāt, -lāt-ed). **1.** Finely dentated, notched, or serrated. **2.** Having small teeth.

den·ti·form (den′ti-fōrm). Tooth-shaped; pegged. SEE ALSO odontoid (1). [denti- + L. *forma,* form]

den·ti·frice (den′ti-fris). Any preparation used in the cleansing of the teeth, e.g., a tooth powder, toothpaste, or tooth wash. [L. *dentifricium,* fr. *dens,* tooth, + *frico,* pp. *frictus,* to rub]

den·tig·er·ous (den-tij′er-ŭs). Arising from or associated with teeth, as a d. cyst. [denti- + L. *gero,* to bear]

den·ti·la·bi·al (den′ti-lā′bē-ăl). Relating to the teeth and lips. [denti- + L. *labium,* lip]

den·ti·lin·gual (den-ti-ling′gwăl). Relating to the teeth and tongue. [denti- + L. *lingua,* tongue]

den·tin (den′tin). SYN dentine. [L. *dens,* tooth]

hereditary opalescent d., (1) SYN *dentinogenesis* imperfecta; **(2)** SYN opalescent d.

hypersensitive d., exposed d., usually at the cervical portion of a tooth, painful to touch, sweetness, or temperature changes.

interglobular d., imperfectly calcified matrix of d. situated between the calcified globules near the dentinal periphery.

irregular d., irritation d., SYN tertiary d.

opalescent d., d. usually associated with dentinogenesis imperfecta. It gives an unusual opalescent or translucent appearance to the teeth. SYN hereditary opalescent d. (2).

peritubular d., an electron-dense layer of d. observed adjacent to the odontoblastic process.

primary d., d. which forms until the root is completed.

reparative d., SYN tertiary d.

sclerotic d., d. characterized by calcification of the dentinal tubules as a result of injury or normal aging. SYN transparent d.

secondary d., d. formed by normal pulp function after root end formation is complete.

tertiary d., morphologically irregular d. formed in response to an irritant. SYN irregular d., irritation d., reparative d.

transparent d., SYN sclerotic d.

vascular d., SYN vasodentin.

den·ti·nal (den′ti-năl). Relating to dentin.

den·ti·nal·gia (den-ti-nal′jē-ă). Dentinal sensitivity or pain. [dentin + G. *algos,* pain]

den·tine (den′tēn) [TA]. The ivory forming the mass of the tooth. About 20% is organic matrix, mostly collagen, with some elastin and a small amount of mucopolysaccharide; the inorganic fraction (70%) is mainly hydroxyapatite, with some carbonate, magnesium, and fluoride. The d. is traversed by a large number of fine tubules running from the pulp cavity outward; within the tubules are processes from the odontoblasts. SYN dentinum [TA], dentin, ebur dentis, substantia eburnea.

den·tin·o·ce·ment·al (den′ti-nō-se-men′tăl). Relating to the dentin and cementum of teeth. SYN cementodentinal.

den·tin·o·e·nam·el (den′ti-nō-ē-nam′ĕl). Relating to the dentin and enamel of teeth. SYN amelodentinal.

den·tin·o·gen·e·sis (den′ti-nō-jen′ĕ-sis). The process of dentin formation in the development of teeth. [dentin + G. *genesis,* production]

d. imperfec′ta [MIM*125490 & MIM*125500], an autosomal dominant disorder of the teeth characterized clinically by translucent gray to yellow-brown teeth involving both primary and permanent dentition; the enamel fractures easily, leaving exposed dentin, which undergoes rapid attrition; radiographically, the pulp chambers and canals appear obliterated and the roots are short and blunted; sometimes occurs in association with osteogenesis imperfecta; autosomal dominant inheritance. SYN hereditary opalescent dentin (1).

den·ti·noid (den′ti-noyd). **1.** Resembling dentin. **2.** SYN dentinoma. [dentin + G. *eidos,* resembling]

den·ti·no·ma (den′ti-nō′mă). A rare benign odontogenic tumor consisting microscopically of dysplastic dentin and strands of epithelium within a fibrous stroma. SYN dentinoid (2). [dentin + G. *-oma,* tumor]

den·ti·num (den′ti-nŭm) [TA]. SYN dentine. [L. *dens,* tooth]

den·tip·a·rous (den-tip′ă-rŭs). Tooth-bearing. [denti- + L. *pario,* to bear]

den·tist. A legally qualified practitioner of dentistry.

▫**den·tis·try** (den′tis-trē). The healing science and art concerned with the structure and function of the oral-facial complex, and with the prevention, diagnosis, and treatment of deformities, pa-

de

thoses, and traumatic injuries thereof. SYN odontology, odontonosology.

community d., public health d., with an academic base, emphasizing the professional obligation to foster the delivery of prevention, education, and care to populations.

ℹ️ **esthetic d.,** a field of d. concerned especially with the appearance of the dentition as achieved through its arrangement, form, and color.

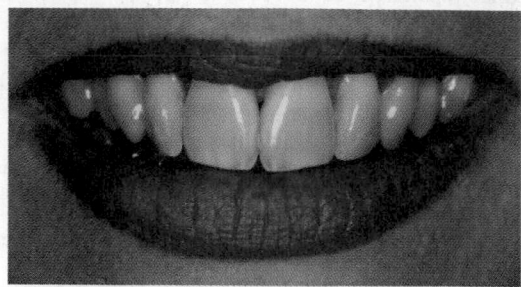

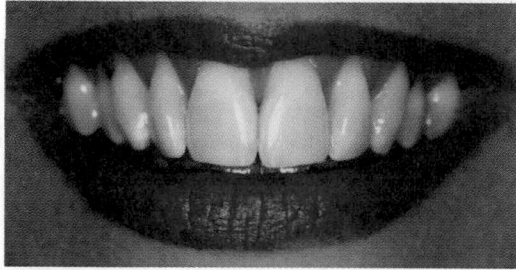

vital bleaching: of natural teeth for esthetic reasons; (top) before; (bottom) after

forensic d., (1) the relation and application of dental facts to legal problems, as in using the teeth for identifying the dead; (2) the law in its bearing on the practice of dentistry. SYN dental jurisprudence, forensic odontology, legal d.

legal d., SYN forensic d.

operative d., usually, the individual restoration of teeth by means of metallic or nonmetallic materials. SYN restorative d.

pediatric d., SYN pedodontics.

preventive d., a philosophy and method of dental practice that seeks to prevent the initiation, progression, and recurrence of dental disease.

prosthetic d., SYN prosthodontics.

public health d., that specialty of d. concerned with the prevention and control of dental diseases and promotion of oral health through organized community efforts.

restorative d., SYN operative d.

ℹ️ **den·ti·tion** (den-tish'ŭn). The natural teeth, as considered collectively, in the dental arch; may be deciduous, permanent, or mixed. [L. *dentitio,* teething]

artificial d., SYN denture (1).

deciduous d., SYN deciduous *tooth.*

delayed d., delayed eruption of the teeth.

first d., SYN deciduous *tooth.*

mandibular d., SYN mandibular dental *arcade.*

maxillary d., SYN maxillary dental *arcade.*

natural d., SEE dentition.

primary d., SYN deciduous *tooth.*

retarded d., d. in which growth phenomena such as calcification, elongation, and eruption occur later than in the average range of normal variation as a result of some systemic metabolic dysfunction (e.g., hypothyroidism).

secondary d., SYN permanent *tooth.*

succedaneous d., SYN permanent *tooth.*

🔺**dento-.** SEE dent-.

den·to·al·ve·o·lar (den'to-al-vē'ō-lăr). Usually, denoting that portion of the alveolar bone immediately about the teeth; used also to denote the functional unity of teeth and alveolar bone.

den·tode (den'tōd). An exact reproduction of a tooth on a gnathographically mounted cast.

den·toid (den'toyd). SYN odontoid (1). SEE ALSO dentiform. [dent- + G. *eidos,* resemblance]

den·to·le·gal (den-tō-lē'găl). Relating to both dentistry and the law. SEE forensic *dentistry.*

den·to·li·va (den-tō-lī'vă). Rarely used term for oliva. [L. *dens,* tooth, + *oliva,* olive]

den·tu·lous (den'tū-lŭs). Having natural teeth present in the mouth.

den·ture (den'tūr). **1.** An artificial substitute for missing natural teeth and adjacent tissues. SYN artificial dentition. **2.** Sometimes used to denote the dentition of animals.

bar joint d., SYN overlay d.

complete d., a dental prosthesis which is a substitute for the lost natural dentition and associated structures of the maxillae or mandible. SYN full d.

design d., a planned visualization of the form and extent of a dental prosthesis, made after a study of all factors involved.

fixed partial d., a restoration of one or more missing teeth which cannot be readily removed by the patient or dentist; it is permanently attached to natural teeth or roots which furnish the primary support to the appliance. SYN bridge (3), fixed bridge.

full d., SYN complete d.

immediate d., a complete or partial d. constructed for insertion immediately following the removal of natural teeth. SYN immediate insertion d.

immediate insertion d., SYN immediate d.

implant d., a d. that receives its stability and retention from a substructure which is partially or wholly implanted under the soft tissues of the d. basal seat. SEE ALSO implant denture *substructure,* implant denture *superstructure,* subperiosteal *implant.*

interim d., a dental prosthesis to be used for a short interval of time for reasons of esthetics, mastication, occlusal support, or convenience, or to condition the patient to accept an artificial substitute for missing natural teeth until more definite prosthetic dental treatment can be provided. SYN provisional d., temporary d.

overlay d., a complete d. that is supported by both soft tissue and natural teeth that have been altered so as to permit the d. to fit over them. The altered teeth may have been fitted with short or long copings, locking devices, or connecting bars. SYN bar joint d., hybrid prosthesis, overdenture, telescopic d.

partial d., a dental prosthesis which restores one or more, but less than all, of the natural teeth and/or associated parts and which is supported by the teeth and/or the mucosa; it may be removable or fixed. SYN bridgework.

partial d., distal extension, a removable partial d. that is retained by natural teeth at one end of the d. base segments only, and in which a portion of the functional load is carried by the residual ridge.

provisional d., SYN interim d.

removable partial d., a partial d. which supplies teeth and associated structures on a partially edentulous jaw, and which can be readily removed from the mouth. SYN removable bridge.

telescopic d., SYN overlay d.

temporary d., SYN interim d.

transitional d., a partial d. which is to serve as a temporary prosthesis to which teeth will be added as more teeth are lost, and which will be replaced after postextraction tissue changes have occurred; a transitional d. may become an interim d. when all of the teeth have been removed from the dental arch.

treatment d., a dental prosthesis used for the purpose of treating or conditioning the tissues which are called upon to support and retain a denture base.

trial d., a setup of artificial teeth so fabricated that it may be placed in the patient's mouth to verify esthetics, for the making of records, or for any other operation deemed necessary before final completion of the d. SYN wax model d.

wax model d., SYN trial d.

den·ture ser·vice. Those procedures performed in the diagnosis, construction, and maintenance of artificial substitutes for missing natural teeth.

den·tur·ist (den'tūr-ist). A dental technician who fabricates and fits dentures without supervision of a dentist.

Denucé, Jean L.P., French surgeon, 1824–1889. SEE D. *ligament.*

de·nu·cle·at·ed (dē-noo'klē-ā-ted). Deprived of a nucleus.

de·nu·da·tion (den-ū-dā'shŭn). Depriving of a covering or protecting layer; the act of laying bare, as in the removal of the epithelium from a surface. [L. *de-nudo,* to lay bare, fr. *de,* from, + *nudus,* naked]

de·nude (dē'nood). To perform denudation.

Denys, Joseph, Belgian bacteriologist, 1857–1932. SEE D.-Leclef *phenomenon.*

de·o·dor·ant (dē-ō'der-ant). **1.** Eliminating or masking a smell, especially an unpleasant one. **2.** An agent having such an action; especially a cosmetic combined with an antiperspirant. SYN deodorizer. [L. *de-* priv. + *odoro,* pp. *-atus,* to give an odor to, fr. *odor,* a smell]

de·o·dor·ize (dē-ō'der-īz). To use a deodorant.

de·o·dor·iz·er (dē-ō'der-īz-er). SYN deodorant (2).

de·on·tol·o·gy (dē-on-tol'ō-jē). The study of professional ethics and duties. [G. *deon* (*deont-*), that which is binding, pr. part. ntr. of *dei,* (impers.) it behooves, fr. *deō,* to bind, + *logos,* study]

de·or·sum·duc·tion (dē-ōr'sŭm-dŭk'shŭn). Rotation of one eye downward. SYN infraduction. [L. *deorsum,* downward, + *duco,* to lead]

de·os·si·fi·ca·tion (dē-os'i-fi-kā'shŭn). Removal of the mineral constituents of bone. SEE demineralization. [L. *de,* from, + *os,* bone, + *facio,* to make]

de·ox·i·da·tion (dē'oks-i-dā'shŭn). Depriving a chemical compound of its oxygen.

de·ox·i·dize (dē-oks'i-dīz). To remove oxygen from its chemical combination.

△**deoxy-.** Prefix to chemical names of substances to indicate replacement of an –OH by an H. The older desoxy- has been retained in some instances.

de·ox·y·a·den·o·sine (dA, dAdo) (dē-oks'ē-ă-den'ō-sēn). 2'-Deoxyribosyladenine, one of the four major nucleosides of DNA (the others being deoxycytidine, deoxyguanosine, and thymidine). The 5' derivative is also an important component of one form of vitamin B_{12}. D. accumulates in individuals with severe combined immunodeficiency disease.

de·ox·y·a·den·o·sine meth·yl·ase. SYN dam *methylase.*

5'-de·ox·y·ad·e·no·syl·co·bal·a·min (dē-oks'ē-ă-den-ō-sil-kō-bal'ă-min). An active coenzyme form of vitamin B_{12}; required in the conversion of methylmalonyl-CoA to succinyl-CoA. A deficiency of 5'-d. will result in methylmalonic acidemia.

de·ox·y·ad·e·nyl·ic ac·id (dAMP) (dē-oks'ē-ad-en-il'ik). Deoxyadenosine monophosphate, a hydrolysis product of DNA, differing from adenylic acid in containing deoxyribose in place of ribose. SYN adenine deoxyribonucleotide.

de·ox·y·bar·bi·tu·rate (dē-oks-ē-bar-bit'ŭr-āt). A barbiturate compound lacking the oxygen atom at the #2 position in the ring; example of a deoxybarbiturate is the antiepileptic drug, primidone. SEE ALSO barbiturate.

de·ox·y·cho·late (DOC) (dē-oks-ē-kō'lāt). A salt or ester of deoxycholic acid.

de·ox·y·cho·lic ac·id (dē-oks-ē-kō'lik). 7-Deoxycholic acid; 3α,12α-dihydroxy-5β-cholanic acid; a bile acid and choleretic; used in biochemical preparations as a detergent.

de·ox·y·co·for·my·cin (dē'oks-ē-cō-fōr-mī'sin). A purine analog which acts as an antimetabolite; potent inhibitor of adenosine deaminase. Used as an antineoplastic agent. SEE ALSO pentostatin.

2-de·ox·y·co·for·my·cin. SYN pentostatin.

de·ox·y·cor·ti·cos·ter·one (DOC) (dē-oks'ē-kōr-ti-kos'ter-ōn). An adrenocortical steroid, principally a biosynthetic precursor of corticosterone, that occasionally appears in adrenocortical secretions; a potent mineralocorticoid with no appreciable glucocorticoid activity. SYN 21-hydroxyprogesterone, cortexone, deoxycortone, desoxycortone.

d. acetate, acetate salt used for intramuscular injection for replacement therapy of the adrenocortical steroid.

d. pivalate, pivalate salt of the steroid.

de·ox·y·cor·tone (dē-oks-ē-kōr'tōn). SYN deoxycorticosterone.

de·ox·y·cyt·i·dine (dē-oks-ē-sī'ti-dēn). 2'-Deoxyribosylcytosine,

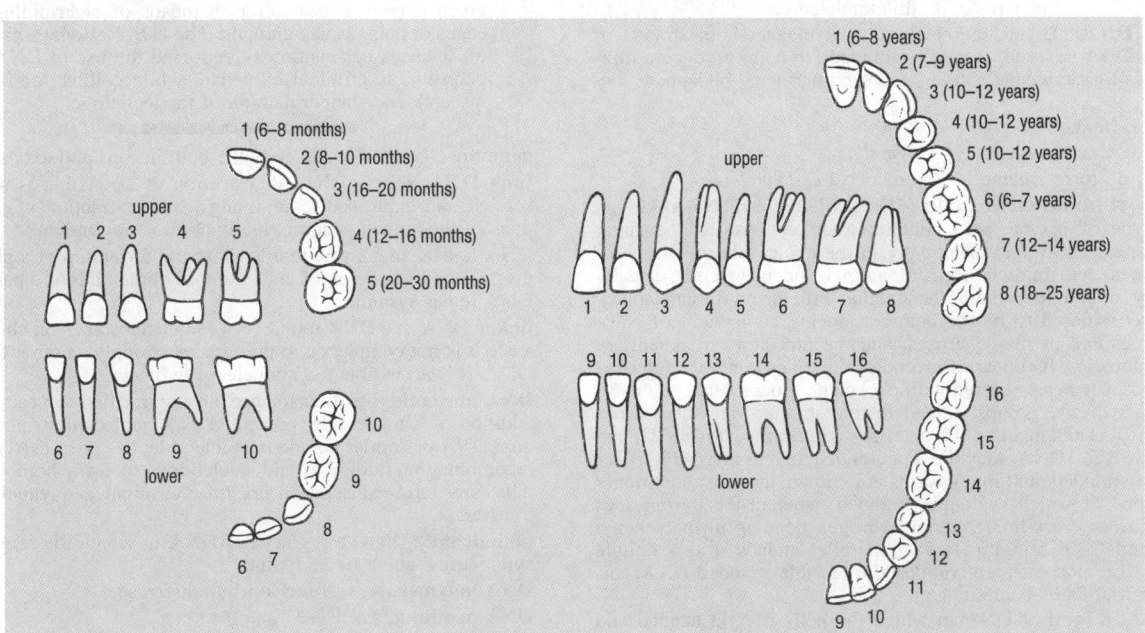

deciduous dentition: left; (1, 6) central incisor; (2, 7) lateral incisor; (3, 8) canine; (4, 9) first molar; (5, 10) second molar

permanent dentition: right; (1, 9) central incisor; (2, 10) lateral incisor; (3, 11) canine; (4, 12) first bicuspid; (5, 13) second bicuspid; (6, 14) first molar; (7, 15) second molar; (8, 16) third molar

de

one of the four major nucleosides of DNA (the others being deoxyadenosine, deoxyguanosine, and thymidine).

de·ox·y·cyt·i·dyl·ic ac·id (dCMP) (dē-oks'ē-sī-ti-dil'ik). Deoxycytidine monophosphate, a hydrolysis product of DNA.

de·ox·y·ep·i·neph·rine (dē-oks'ē-ep-i-nef'rēn). A sympathomimetic amine used as a vasoconstrictor.

de·ox·y·gua·no·sine (dē-oks-ē-gwan'ō-sēn). 2'-Deoxyribosylguanine, one of the four major nucleosides of DNA (the others being deoxyadenosine, deoxycytidine, and thymidine). Found to accumulate in individuals with purine nucleoside phosphorylase deficiency.

de·ox·y·gua·nyl·ic ac·id (dGMP) (dē-oks-ē-gwan-il'ik). Deoxyguanosine monophosphate, a hydrolysis product of DNA. SYN guanine deoxyribonucleotide.

de·ox·y·hex·ose (dē-oks-ē-heks'ōs). A 6-carbon deoxy-sugar in which one OH is replaced by H.

de·ox·y·nu·cle·o·side (dē-oks'ē-noo'klē-ō-sīd). SEE deoxyribonucleoside.

de·ox·y·nu·cle·o·tide (dē-oks'ē-noo'klē-ō-tīd). SEE deoxyribonucleoside.

de·ox·y·pen·tose (dē-oks-ē-pen'tōs). A 5-carbon deoxy-sugar in which one OH is replaced by H.

de·ox·y·ri·bo·al·dol·ase (dē-oks'ē-rī-bō-al'dō-lās). SYN deoxyribosephosphate aldolase.

de·ox·y·ri·bo·di·py·rim·i·dine pho·to·ly·ase (dē-oks'ē-rī'bō-dī-pī-rim'i-dēn). An enzyme in yeast that is activated by light, whereupon it can reverse a previous photochemical reaction by cleaving the cyclobutane ring of the thymine dimer. SYN dipyrimidine photolyase, photoreactivating enzyme.

de·ox·y·ri·bo·nu·cle·ase (DNASe, DNAase, DNase) (de-oks' ē-rī-bō-noo'klē-ās). Any enzyme (phosphodiesterase) hydrolyzing phosphodiester bonds in DNA. SEE ALSO endonuclease, nuclease.

acid d., SYN d. II.

d. I, DNase I, an endonuclease that cleaves primarily double-stranded DNA to a mixture of oligodeoxyribonucleotides, each ending in a 5'-phosphate; streptodornase is a similar enzyme. Under appropriate conditions, it can produce single-strand nicks in DNA; used in nick translation and in the mapping of hypersensitive sites. SYN pancreatic d., thymonuclease.

d. II, DNase II, an endonuclease that cleaves both strands of native DNA (as well as single-stranded DNA) to produce a mixture of oligodeoxynucleotides, each ending in a 3'-phosphate. SYN acid d.

pancreatic d., SYN d. I.

d. S₁, SYN endonuclease S₁ *Aspergillus.*

spleen d., former name for micrococcal *endonuclease.*

de·ox·y·ri·bo·nu·cle·ic ac·id (DNA) (dē-oks'ē-rī'bō-noo-klē'ic). The type of nucleic acid containing deoxyribose as the sugar component and found principally in the nuclei (chromatin, chromosomes) and mitochondria of animal and plant cells, usually loosely bound to protein (hence the term deoxyribonucleoprotein); considered to be the autoreproducing component of chromosomes and of many viruses, and the repository of hereditary characteristics. Its linear macromolecular chain consists of deoxyribose molecules esterified with phosphate groups between the 3'- and 5'-hydroxyl groups; linked to this structure are the purines adenine (A) and guanine (G) and the pyrimidines cytosine (C) and thymine (T). DNA may be open-ended or circular, single- or double-stranded, and many forms are known, the most commonly described of which is double-stranded, wherein the pyrimidines and purines cross-link through hydrogen bonding in the schema A-T and C-G, bringing two antiparallel strands into a double helix. Chromosomes are composed of double-stranded DNA; mitochondrial DNA is circular.

A-DNA, a form of DNA in which the helix is right-handed and the overall appearance is short and broad.

antisense DNA, the strand of DNA complementary to the one bearing the genetic message and from which it may be reconstructed. A DNA sequence complementary to a portion of mRNA. Used as potential therapeutic to stop transcription or translation of pathogens or inappropriately expressed host gene.

B-DNA, a form of DNA in which the helix is right-handed and the overall appearance is long and thin.

blunt-ended DNA, double-stranded DNA in which at least one of the ends has no unpaired bases.

competitor DNA, dNA from a test organism that is denatured and then used in in vitro hybridization experiments in which it competes with DNA (homologous) from a reference organism; used to determine the relationship of the test organism to the reference organism.

complementary DNA (cDNA), (1) single-stranded DNA that is complementary to messenger RNA; **(2)** dNA that has been synthesized from mRNA by the action of reverse transcriptase.

extrachromosomal DNA, dNA that occurs naturally outside of the nucleus (e.g., mitochondrial DNA).

DNA fingerprinting, a technique used to compare individuals by molecular genotyping. DNA isolated from a biological specimen is digested and fractionated. Southern hybridization with a radiolabeled repetitive DNA provides an autoradiographic pattern unique to the individual. SYN DNA profiling, DNA typing.

A technique developed in 1985 for comparing sets of DNA by locating identical sequences of nucleotides. Forensic applications of DNA fingerprinting are based on the premise that no 2 persons have exactly the same genetic makeup. The most distinctive features of an individual's genome are not the genes themselves but the variable number of tandem repeats (VNTRs) that occur between genes. While these do not transmit genetic information, they are highly consistent within the cells of an individual and highly variable from one individual to another. In DNA fingerprinting, the specimen is split into nucleotide fragments by treatment with restriction enzymes and then subjected to gel electrophoresis so as to yield a characteristic pattern of banding. Radioactive probes, composed of short nucleotide sequences (10–15 base pairs), then identify sites of tandem repeats and hybridize with them. Comparing the results from 2 or more DNA sources reveals their degree of relatedness. DNA fingerprinting offers a statistical basis for evaluating the probability that samples of blood, hair, semen, or tissue have originated from a given person. It also offers a means of determining lineages of humans and animals. The U.S. National Academy of Sciences has cautiously endorsed the use of DNA fingerprints as criminal evidence, while calling for further research and standardization of the technique.

genomic DNA, dNA that contains both introns and exons.

junk DNA, selfish DNA; that portion of DNA that is not transcribed and expressed, comprising a major fraction of the base pairs of the human genome; its function is not known.

DNA ligase, an enzyme that leads to the formation of a phosphodiester bond at a break of one strand in duplex DNA; a part of the DNA repair system.

linker DNA, the DNA found between nucleosomes on chromatin; since it is not complexed to proteins as strongly as other forms of DNA, it is accessible to exonuclease hydrolysis.

DNA nucleotidylexotransferase, an enzyme that can catalyze the addition of a nucleotide, presented as a nucleoside triphosphate, on a DNA or similar polydeoxynucleotide; has been used in DNA recombination studies to add nucleotides to form homopolymer tails. SYN terminal addition enzyme, terminal deoxynucleotidyltransferase.

palindromic DNA, a segment of DNA in which the sequence is symmetrical about its midpoint.

DNA polymerase, SEE nucleotidyltransferases.

DNA profiling, SYN DNA fingerprinting.

recombinant DNA, altered DNA resulting from the insertion into the chain, by chemical, enzymatic, or biologic means, of a sequence (a whole or partial chain of DNA) not originally (biologically) present in that chain.

repetitive DNA, a segment of DNA that consists of a linear array of multiple copies of the same sequence of nucleotides.

satellite DNA, dNA in the satellite regions of acrocentric chromosomes.

sticky-ended DNA, double-stranded DNA in which one of the strands protrudes from the other strand (i.e., has a number of unpaired bases) at one end or more.

DNA typing, SYN DNA fingerprinting.

Z-DNA, a form of DNA in which the helix is left-handed, and the overall appearance is elongated and slim.

zero time-binding DNA, DNA that has become the duplex form at the start of a reassociation process.

de·ox·y·ri·bo·nu·cle·o·pro·tein (DNP, Dnp) (dē-oks′ē-rī-bō-noo′klē-ō-prō′tēn). The complex of DNA and protein in which DNA is usually found upon cell disruption and isolation.

de·ox·y·ri·bo·nu·cle·o·side (dē-oks′ē-rī-bō-noo′klē-ō-sīd). A nucleoside component of DNA containing 2-deoxy-D-ribose; the condensation product of deoxy-D-ribose with purines or pyrimidines.

de·ox·y·ri·bo·nu·cle·o·tide (dē-oks′ē-rī-bō-noo′klē-ō-tīd). A nucleotide component of DNA containing 2-deoxy-D-ribose; the phosphoric ester of deoxyribonucleoside; formed in nucleotide biosynthesis.

de·ox·y·ri·bose (dē-oks-ē-rī′bōs). A deoxypentose, 2-deoxy-D-ribose being the most common example, occurring in DNA and responsible for its name.

d. phosphate, SEE deoxyribonucleotide.

de·ox·y·ri·bose·phos·phate al·dol·ase (dē-oks′ē-rī-bōs-fos′fāt). An enzyme catalyzing cleavage of 2-deoxy-D-ribose 5-phosphate to D-glyceraldehyde 3-phosphate and acetaldehyde. SYN deoxyriboaldolase.

de·ox·y·ri·bo·side (dē-oks-ē-rī′bō-sīd). Deoxyribose combined via its 1-O atom with a radical derived from an alcohol; not to be confused with deoxyribosyl compounds such as deoxyribonucleosides. Cf. deoxyribosyl.

de·ox·y·ri·bo·syl (dē-oks-ē-rī′bō-sil). The radical formed from deoxyribose by removal of the OH from the C-1 carbon; e.g., deoxyadenosine. Cf. deoxyriboside.

de·ox·y·ri·bo·syl·trans·fer·as·es (dē-oks′ē-rī′bō-sil-trans′fer-ās-es). Enzymes that catalyze the transfer of 2-deoxy-D-ribose from deoxyribosides to free bases.

de·ox·y·ri·bo·tide (dē-oks-ē-rī′bō-tīd). Misnomer for deoxyribonucleotide or deoxynucleotide derived, by analogy with nucleoside-nucleotide, from incorrect usage of deoxyriboside.

de·ox·y·ribo·vi·rus (dē-ok′sē-vī′rŭs). SYN DNA virus.

de·ox·y·thy·mi·dine (dT) (dē-oks′ē-thi′mi-dēn). SYN thymidine.

de·ox·y·thy·mi·dyl·ic ac·id (dTMP) (dē-oks′ē-thī-mi-dil′ik). A component of DNA; originally and properly called thymidylic acid, but use of deoxy- is less ambiguous, as ribothymidylic acid is now known to exist. SYN thymine deoxyribonucleotide.

de·ox·y·ur·i·dine (dē-oks′ē-ūr′i-dēn). A derivative of uridine in which one or more of the hydroxyl groups on the ribose moiety has been replaced by a hydrogen; e.g., 2′-deoxyuridine is a rare naturally occurring deoxynucleoside.

de·o·zon·ize (dē-ō′zō-nīz). To deprive of ozone.

de·pen·dence (dē-pen′dens). The quality or condition of relying upon, being influenced by, or being subservient to a person or object reflecting a particular need. [L. *dependeo,* to hang from]

anchorage d., the need of normal cells to have an appropriate surface to attach to in order for them to grow in culture.

substance d., a pattern of behavioral, physiologic, and cognitive symptoms that develop due to substance use or abuse; usually indicated by tolerance to the effects of the substance and withdrawal symptoms that develop when use of the substance is terminated.

de·pen·den·cy (dē-pen′dens-ē). The state of being dependent.

pyridoxine d. with seizure, an inherited disorder (autosomal recessive) apparently associated with deficient brain type I glutamate decarboxylase; seizures can be controlled with vitamin B₆.

De·pen·do·vi·rus (dē-pen′dō-vī-rŭs). A genus of small defective single-stranded DNA viruses in the family Parvoviridae that depend on adenoviruses for replication. SYN adeno-associated virus, adenosatellite virus. [L. *dependeo,* to be dependent upon, + virus]

de·per·son·al·i·za·tion (dē-per′sŏn-ăl-i-zā′shŭn). A state in which one loses the feeling of one's own identity in relation to others in one's family or peer group, or loses the feeling of one's own reality. SYN depersonalization syndrome.

de Pezzer, O., 19th century French physician. SEE de P. *catheter.*

de·phas·ing. In magnetic resonance imaging, following alignment by a radiofrequency pulse, the gradual loss of orientation of the magnetic atomic nuclei due to random molecular energy transfer or relaxation.

de·phos·pho·ryl·a·tion (dē-fos′fōr-i-lā′shŭn). Removal of a phosphoric group, usually hydrolytically and by enzyme action, from a compound.

de·pig·men·ta·tion (dē-pig-men-tā′shŭn). Loss of pigment which may be partial or complete. SEE ALSO achromia (1).

dep·i·late (dep′i-lāt). To remove hair by any means. Cf. epilate. [L. *de-pilo,* pp. *-atus,* to deprive of hair, fr. *de-* neg. + *pilo,* to grow hair]

dep·i·la·tion (dep-i-lā′shŭn). SYN epilation.

de·pil·a·to·ry (dē-pil′ă-tō-rē). 1. SYN epilatory (1). 2. An agent that causes the falling out of hair. SYN epilatory (2).

chemical d., a topically applied d. substance.

de·ple·tion (dē-plē′shŭn). 1. The removal of accumulated fluids or solids. 2. A reduced state of strength from too many free discharges. 3. Excessive loss of a constituent, usually essential, of the body, e.g., salt, water, etc.

salt d., excessive loss of sodium chloride from the body in urine, sweat, etc.; a cause of secondary dehydration.

water d., reduction in the total volume of body water; dehydration.

de·po·lar·i·za·tion (dē-pō′lăr-i-zā′shŭn). 1. A relative reduction in magnitude of polarization; in nerve cells, depolarization may result from an increase in the permeability of the cell membrane to sodium ions. 2. The destruction, neutralization, or change in direction of polarity.

dendritic d., the loss of a negative charge in the dendrites of a nerve cell.

de·po·lar·ize (dē-pō′lăr-īz). To deprive of polarity.

de·pol·y·mer·ase (dē-pol′i-mer-ās). Name used originally, before hydrolytic action was understood, for an enzyme catalyzing the hydrolysis of a macromolecule to simpler components. SEE nuclease.

de·pos·it (dē-poz′it). 1. A sediment or precipitate. 2. A pathological accumulation of inorganic material in a tissue. [L. *de-pono,* pp. *-positus,* to lay down]

brickdust d., a sediment of urates in the urine. SYN sedimentum lateritium.

dep·ra·va·tion (dep′ră-vā′shŭn). SYN depravity. [L. *depravatio,* fr. *depravo,* pp. *-atus,* to corrupt]

de·praved (dē-prāvd′). Deteriorated or degenerate; corrupt. [L. *depravo,* to corrupt]

de·prav·i·ty (dē-prav′i-tē). A depraved act or the condition of being depraved. SYN depravation.

de·pre·nyl (dē′pren-il). An inhibitor of monoamine oxidase selective for the type B isozyme. The drug is used as an antiparkinsonian agent. It does not give rise to the hypertensive crisis that can occur when nonselective monoamine oxidase inhibitors are taken in the presence of dietary sources of tyramine. SYN selegiline.

de·pres·sant (dē-pres′ănt). 1. Diminishing functional tone or activity. 2. An agent that reduces nervous or functional activity, such as a sedative or anesthetic. [L. *de-primo,* pp. *-pressus,* to press down]

de·pressed (dē-prest′). 1. Flattened from above downward. 2. Below the normal level or the level of the surrounding parts. 3. Below the normal functional level. 4. Dejected; lowered in spirits.

de·pres·sion (dē-presh′ŭn) [TA]. 1. Reduction of the level of functioning. 2. SYN excavation (1). 3. Displacement of a part downward or inward. 4. A temporary mental state or chronic mental disorder characterized by feelings of sadness, loneliness, despair, low self-esteem, and self-reproach; accompanying signs include psychomotor retardation or less frequently agitation, withdrawal from social contact, and vegetative states such as loss of

de

appetite and insomnia. SYN dejection (1), depressive reaction, depressive syndrome. [L. *depressio*, fr. *deprimo*, to press down]

agitated d., d. with excitement and restlessness.

anaclitic d., impairment of an infant's physical, social, and intellectual development following separation from its mother or from a mothering surrogate; characterized by listlessness, withdrawal, and anorexia.

clinical d., SYN major d.

endogenous d., any depressive disorder occurring in the absence of external precipitants and believed to have a biologic origin. SYN endogenomorphic depression, nonreactive d.

exogenous d., similar signs and symptoms as endogenous d. but the precipitating factors are social or environmental and outside the individual.

involutional d., depression or psychosis first occurring in the involutional years (40 to 55 for women, 50 to 65 for men).

lingual salivary gland d., an indentation on the lingual surface of the mandible within which a portion of the submandibular gland lies; it appears radiographically as a sharply circumscribed ovoid radiolucency between the mandibular canal and the inferior border of the posterior mandible. SYN Stafne bone cyst, static bone cyst.

---

major d., a mental disorder characterized by sustained depression of mood, anhedonia, sleep and appetite disturbances, and feelings of worthlessness, guilt, and hopelessness. Diagnostic criteria (*DSM-IV*) for a major depressive episode include a depressed mood, a marked reduction of interest or pleasure in virtually all activities, or both, lasting for at least 2 weeks. In addition, 3 or more of the following must be present: gain or loss of weight, increased or decreased sleep, increased or decreased level of psychomotor activity, fatigue, feelings of guilt or worthlessness, diminished ability to concentrate, and recurring thoughts of death or suicide. SEE endogenous d., exogenous d., bipolar *disorder*. SYN clinical d., major depressive disorder.

Approximately 20 million persons a year suffer depressive illness in the U.S. About 10% of men and 25% of women experience major depression at some time in their lives, and 15–30% of these commit suicide. The negative impact of this disease on the economy of the U.S. is estimated at $16 billion annually. Risk factors for depression are drug or alcohol abuse, chronic physical illness, stressful life events, social isolation, a history of physical or sexual abuse, and a family history of depressive illness. Depression can be masked by substance abuse. In elderly persons it may be mistaken for senile dementia, and vice versa; the two may coexist. The disorder is believed to represent an electrochemical malfunction of the limbic system involving disturbances in the metabolism of the neurotransmitters dopamine and serotonin. In persons with familial depression, the number of glial cells in the subgenual prefrontal cortex is significantly smaller than in mentally healthy persons. Treatment with psychopharmaceutical agents, including tricyclic antidepressants, selective serotonin reuptake inhibitors (SSRIs), monoamine oxidase (MAO) inhibitors, and others, effectively controls most cases of clinical depression. Cognitive psychotherapy has demonstrated some success in reversing depression. Refined methods of electroconvulsive shock therapy (ECT) have been used with increasing frequency since the 1980s, generally for cases that do not respond to other treatment. Even in severe depression the response rate with ECT is 80% or higher. This mode of therapy has a faster onset of action, causes fewer side effects than drug therapy, and is particularly useful in elderly patients.

---

nonreactive d., SYN endogenous d.

d. of optic disk [TA], the normally occurring d. or pit in the center of the optic disk. SYN excavatio disci [TA], excavatio papillae, excavation of optic disk, physiologic cup, physiologic excavation.

pacchionian d.'s, SYN granular *foveolae*, under *foveola*.

postdrive d., slowing of the heart, often with a rate-dependent blockade of AV and/or VA conduction following rapid atrial stimulation.

pterygoid d., SYN pterygoid *fovea*.

reactive d., a psychological state occasioned directly by an intensely sad external situation (frequently loss of a loved person), relieved by the removal of the external situation (e.g., reunion with a loved person).

spreading d., a decrease of activity evoked by local stimulation of the cerebral cortex and spreading slowly over the whole cortex.

de·pres·sive (dē-pres′iv). **1.** Pushing down. **2.** Pertaining to or causing depression.

de·pres·sor (dē-pres′ŏr). **1.** A muscle that flattens or lowers a part. **2.** Anything that depresses or retards functional activity. **3.** An instrument or device used to push certain structures out of the way during an operation or examination. **4.** An agent that decreases blood pressure. SYN hypotensor, vasodepressor (2). [L. *de-primo*, pp. *-pressus*, to press down]

tongue d., an instrument with a broad flat extremity used for pressing down the tongue to facilitate examination of the oral cavity and pharynx.

dep·ri·va·tion (dep′ri-vā′shŭn). Absence, loss, or withholding of something needed.

emotional d., lack of adequate and appropriate interpersonal or environmental experiences, or both, usually in the early developmental years.

sensory d., diminution or absence of usual external stimuli or perceptual experiences, commonly resulting in psychological distress and aberrant functioning if continued too long.

dep·si·pep·tide (dep′sē-pep′tīd). An oligo- or polypeptide containing one or more ester bonds as well as peptide bonds. SEE ALSO peptolide. [G. *deseō*, to knead, blend, + peptide]

depth (depth). Distance from the surface downward.

anesthetic d., the degree of central nervous system depression produced by a general anesthetic agent; a function of potency of the anesthetic and the concentration in which it is administered.

focal d., d. of focus, the greatest distance through which an object point can be moved while maintaining a clear image. SYN penetration (3).

dep·tro·pine cit·rate (dep′trō-pēn). An antihistaminic agent with anticholinergic properties. SYN dibenzheptropine citrate.

de·pu·li·za·tion (dē-pū′li-zā′shŭn). Destruction of fleas which convey the plague bacillus from animals to humans. [L. *de*, from, + *pulex* (*pulic-*), flea]

dep·u·rant (dep′ū-rant). **1.** An agent or means used to effect purification. **2.** An agent that promotes the excretion and removal of waste material. [L. *de-* intens. + *puro*, pp. *-atus*, to make pure]

dep·u·ra·tion (dep-ū-rā′shŭn). Purification; removal of waste products or foul excretions.

dep·u·ra·tive (dep′ū-ră-tiv). Tending to depurate; depurant.

de·qua·lin·i·um ac·e·tate (dē-kwah-lin′ē-ŭm). An antimicrobial agent. SYN decamine.

de·qua·lin·i·um chlo·ride. Dequalinium acetate, with chloride replacing acetate, used as an antimicrobial agent primarily in lozenges for the treatment of mouth and throat infections.

de Quervain, Friedrich Joseph, Swiss surgeon, 1868–1940. SEE de Q. *disease;* de Quervain *tenosynovitis;* de Q. *thyroiditis*.

der·a·del·phus (dār-ă-del′fŭs). Conjoined twins with a single head and neck and separate bodies below the thoracic level. SEE conjoined *twins*, under *twin*. [G. *derē*, neck, + *adelphos*, brother]

de·rail·ment (dē-rāl′ment). A symptom of a thought disorder in which one constantly gets "off the track" in one's thoughts and speech; similar to loosening of association.

der·an·en·ceph·a·ly, der·an·en·ce·pha·lia (dār-an′en-sef′ă-lē, -se-fā′lē-ă). **1.** Congenital malformation in which the head is absent, although there is a rudimentary neck. **2.** Defect of the brain and upper part of the spinal cord. [G. *derē*, neck, + *an-*, priv., + *kephalē*, head]

de·range·ment (dē-rānj′ment). **1.** A disturbance of the regular order or arrangement. **2.** Rarely used term for a mental disturbance or disorder. [Fr.]

Dercum, Francis X., U.S. neurologist, 1856–1931. SEE D. *disease*.

de·re·al·i·za·tion (dē-rē′ă-li-zā′shŭn). An alteration in one's perception of the environment such that things that are ordinarily familiar seem strange, unreal, or two-dimensional.

de·re·ism (dē′rē-izm). Mental activity in fantasy in contrast to reality. [L. *de*, away, + *res*, thing]

de·re·is·tic (dē-rē-is′tik). Living in imagination or fantasy with thoughts that are incongruent with logic or experience.

der·en·ce·pha·lia (dār-en-se-fā′lē-ă). SYN derencephaly.

der·en·ceph·a·lo·cele (dār-en-sef′ă-lō-sēl). In derencephaly, protrusion of the rudimentary brain through a defect in the upper cervical spinal canal. [G. *derē*, neck, + *enkephalos*, brain, + *kēlē*, hernia]

der·en·ceph·a·ly (dār-en-sef′ă-lē). Cervical rachischisis and anencephaly, a malformation involving an open cranial vault with a rudimentary brain usually crowded back toward bifid cervical vertebrae. SYN derencephalia. [G. *derē*, neck, + *enkephalos*, brain]

de·re·pres·sion (dē-rē-presh′ŭn). A homeostatic mechanism for regulating enzyme production in an inducible enzyme system: an inducer, usually a substrate of a specific enzyme pathway, by combining with an active repressor (produced by a regulator gene) deactivates it; the release of the previously repressed operator is followed by enzyme production.

der·i·va·tion (dār-i-vā′shŭn). **1.** The source or process of an evolution. SYN revulsion. **2.** The drawing of blood or the body fluids to one part to relieve congestion in another. [L. *derivatio*, fr. *derivo*, pp. -*atus*, to draw off, fr. *rivus*, a stream]

de·riv·a·tive (dĕ-riv′ă-tiv). **1.** Relating to or producing derivation. **2.** Something produced by modification of something preexisting. **3.** Specifically, a chemical compound that may be produced from another compound of similar structure in one or more steps, as in replacement of H by an alkyl, acyl, or amino group.

⬠**derm-, derma-.** The skin; corresponds to L. cut-. See entries under cut. [G. *derma*]

der·ma·brad·er (derm′ă-brād-er). A motor-driven device used in dermabrasion.

der·ma·bra·sion (der-mă-brā′zhŭn). Operative procedure to efface acne scars or pits performed with sandpaper, rotating wire brushes, or other abrasive materials.

Der·ma·cen·tor (der-mă-sen′ter). An ornate, characteristically marked genus of hard ticks (family Ixodidae) that possess eyes and 11 festoons; it consists of some 20 species whose members commonly attack dogs, humans, and other mammals. [derm- + G. *kentōr*, a goader]

D. albopic′tus, the winter tick, a species found principally on horses, cattle, elk, moose, and deer in Canada and the northern and western United States; it is a one-host tick, but humans are sometimes attacked when skinning or dressing deer.

D. anderso′ni, the wood tick; the vector of Rocky Mountain spotted fever; also transmits tularemia and causes tick paralysis; there are characteristic black and white markings on the large scutum of the male.

D. marginatus, a tick species found across Europe and the vector of a human rickettsiosis caused by *Rickettsia slovaca*.

D. occidenta′lis, the Pacific Coast tick, a species found on all domestic herbivores, deer, dogs, humans, and other animals in California and Oregon.

D. reticula′tus, a common species attacking sheep, oxen, goats, and deer, and sometimes troublesome to humans; it is found in Europe, Asia, and America.

D. varia′bilis, the American dog tick, a species that is a common pest of dogs along the eastern seaboard of the U.S., a vector of tularemia, and a principal vector of *Rickettsia rickettsii* which causes Rocky Mountain spotted fever in the central and eastern U.S.; may also cause tick paralysis.

Der·ma·coc·cus (der-ma-kok′ŭs). A genus of Gram-positive, aerobic cocci found on human skin.

der·mad (der′mad). In the direction of the outer integument. [derm- + L. *ad*, to]

der·mal (der′măl). Relating to the skin. SYN dermatoid (2).

Der·ma·nys·sus gal·li·nae (der-mă-nis′ŭs ga-lē′-nē). The red hen-mite, a parasite of chickens, pigeons, and other birds; it sometimes attacks humans and causes an itching eruption, especially in sensitized individuals. SYN *Acarus gallinae*. [derm- + G. *nyssō*, to prick; L. *gallina*, hen]

⬠**dermat-.** The skin. SEE ALSO derm-, dermato-, dermo-. [G. *derma*]

der·ma·tal·gia (der-mă-tăl′jē-ă). Localized pain, usually confined to the skin. SYN dermatodynia. [dermat- + G. *algos*, pain]

▣**der·ma·ti·tis,** pl. **der·ma·tit·i·des** (der-mă-tī′tis, -tit′i-dēz). Inflammation of the skin. [derm- + G. -*itis*, inflammation]

dermatitis – division into types	
endogenous	**contact (or exogenous) dermatitis**
atopic	direct irritation
seborrheic	not photosensitive
nummular	phototoxic
chronic hand and foot dermatitis	allergic
exfoliative	not photosensitive
stasis dermatitis	photoallergic
circumscribed neurodermatitis	
pruritus ani/vulvae	
drug eruption	

actinic d., SYN photodermatitis.

d. aestiva′lis, eczema recurring during the summer.

allergic contact d., a delayed type IV allergic reaction of the skin with varying degrees of erythema, edema, and vesiculation resulting from cutaneous contact with a specific allergen. SYN contact allergy.

ancylostoma d., SYN cutaneous *larva migrans*.

d. artefac′ta, self-induced skin lesions resulting from habitual rubbing, scratching or hair-pulling, malingering, or mental disturbance. SYN factitial d., feigned eruption.

atopic d., d. characterized by the distinctive phenomena of atopy, including infantile and flexural eczema. SYN atopic eczema.

berloque d., berlock d., a type of photosensitization resulting in deep brown pigmentation on exposure to sunlight after application of bergamot oil and other essential oils in perfumes and colognes.

blastomycetic d., d. blastomycot′ica, cutaneous blastomycosis.

bubble gum d., allergic contact d. developing about the lips in children who chew bubble gum; caused by plastics in the gum substance.

d. calor′ica, SYN *erythema* ab igne.

caterpillar d., allergic contact d. caused by the larva of the brown-tail moth, puss caterpillar, gypsy moths, and other caterpillars. SYN caterpillar rash.

chemical d., allergic contact d. or primary irritation d. due to application of chemicals; usually characterized by erythema, edema, and vesiculation of the exposed or contacted site, and in some cases acne or pigmentary disturbances.

d. combustio′nis, inflammation of the skin following a burn.

▣**contact d.,** a T lymphocyte–mediated d. (type IV hypersensitivity) resulting from cutaneous contact with a specific allergen (allergic contact d.) or irritant (nonallergic contact d.). SYN contact hypersensitivity (1).

contagious pustular d., SYN orf *virus*.

cosmetic d., a cutaneous eruption that results from the application of a cosmetic; due to allergic sensitization or primary irritation.

diaper d., colloquially referred to as diaper rash; d. of thighs and buttocks resulting from exposure to urine and feces in infants' diapers. Formerly attributed to ammonia formation; moisture, bacterial growth, and alkalinity may all induce lesions. SEE ALSO intertrigo. SYN diaper rash.

de

d. exfoliati′va infan′tum, d. exfoliati′va neonato′rum, a generalized pyoderma accompanied by exfoliative d., with constitutional symptoms, affecting young infants, which may result from atopic d., Leiner disease, or staphylococcal scalded skin syndrome. SYN impetigo neonatorum (1).

exfoliative d., rapidly extending erythema followed in a few days by generalized exfoliation with scaling of the skin and associated in some cases with lymphadenopathy or loss of water and electrolytes; may be a drug reaction or associated with various benign dermatoses, lupus erythematosus, or lymphoma, or be of undetermined cause. SYN Wilson disease (2).

exudative discoid and lichenoid d., d. resembling an exudative form of nummular eczema, occurs especially in Jewish males, with oval lesions on the penis, trunk, and face. SYN Sulzberger-Garbe disease, Sulzberger-Garbe syndrome.

factitial d., SYN d. artefacta.

d. gangreno′sa infan′tum, a bullous or pustular eruption, of uncertain origin, followed by necrotic ulcers or extensive gangrene in children under 2 years of age; if untreated, death may result from hematogenous infection, such as liver abscess. SYN disseminated cutaneous gangrene, ecthyma gangrenosum, pemphigus gangrenosus (1).

d. herpetifor′mis, a chronic disease of the skin marked by a symmetric itching eruption of vesicles and papules that occur in groups; relapses are common; associated with gluten-sensitive enteropathy and IgA together with neutrophils beneath the epidermis of lesional and perilesional skin. SYN Duhring disease.

d. hiema′lis, SYN winter itch.

infectious eczematoid d., an inflammatory reaction of skin adjacent to the site of a pyogenic infection; e.g., purulent otitis, the area around a colostomy, or intranasal infection; thought to spread by autoinoculation.

irritant contact d., skin reactions ranging from erythema and scaling to necrotic burns resulting from nonimmunologic damage by chemicals in contact with the skin immediately or repeatedly.

mango d., a perioral contact d. resulting from sensitization to the resinous coating on the peel of the mango fruit.

meadow d., meadow grass d., a photoallergic reaction to contact with a plant containing furocoumarin in which the bizarre configuration of the eruption is that of the streaky pattern of the plant contact; often occurs after sunbathing.

d. medicamento′sa, SYN drug eruption.

nickel d., allergic d. due to contact with, or in some cases ingestion of, nickel or other metals containing nickel (e.g., stainless steel).

d. nodo′sa, a papular eruption on the legs, related to onchocerciasis (q.v.).

d. nodula′ris necrot′ica, a recurrent eruption of vesicles, papules, and papulonecrotic lesions on the buttocks and extensor surfaces of the extremities, accompanied by fever, sore throat, diarrhea, and eosinophilia; probably a variant of vasculitis, it can be of varying and increasing severity and duration and can occasionally involve the heart, kidneys, and gastrointestinal tract. SYN Werther disease.

nummular d., SYN nummular eczema.

papular d. of pregnancy, intensely pruritic papular eruption of torso and extremities occurring throughout pregnancy, with no systemic toxicity; may be similar to pruritic urticarial papules and plaques of pregnancy.

d. pediculoi′des ventrico′sus, SYN straw itch.

primary irritant d., a frequently cumulative reaction of irritation on exposure of the skin to substances which are toxic to epidermal or connective tissue cells; lesions are usually erythematous and papular, but can be purulent or necrotic, depending on the nature of the toxic material applied.

proliferative d., SYN dermatophilosis.

rat mite d., an eruption of wheals, papules, or vesicles caused by the rat mite.

d. re′pens, SYN pustulosis palmaris et plantaris. [L. creeping]

rhus d., contact d. caused by cutaneous exposure to urushiol from species of Toxicodendron (Rhus), such as poison ivy, oak, or sumac.

sandal strap d., allergic contact on the dorsal surfaces of the feet, caused by synthetic rubber sandal straps or additives to natural rubber.

schistosomal d., a sensitization response to repeated cutaneous invasion by cercariae of bird, mammal, or human schistosomes. SYN swimmer's itch, water itch (2).

seborrheic d., d. seborrhe′ica, a common scaly macular eruption that occurs primarily on the face, scalp (dandruff), and other areas of increased sebaceous gland secretion, especially during infancy and after puberty; the lesions are covered with a slightly adherent oily scale. Effectiveness of treatment with betaconazole supports an etiologic role for Pityrosporum ovale infection. SYN seborrheic eczema, Unna disease.

solar d., a d. in photosensitive persons caused by exposure to the sun's rays.

stasis d., erythema and scaling of the lower extremities due to impaired venous circulation, seen commonly in older women or secondary to deep vein thrombosis, the latter with rapid onset and swelling.

subcorneal pustular d., SYN subcorneal pustular dermatosis.

traumatic d., any d. caused by an irritant substance or by a physical agent.

d. veg′etans, a benign fungating granulomatous mass caused by chronic pyogenic infection. SYN pyoderma vegetans.

dermato-. SEE derm-. [G. derma, skin]

der·mat·o·ar·thri·tis (der′mă-tō-ar-thrī′tis). Associated skin disease and arthritis.

lipoid d., a multicentric reticulohistiocytosis.

Der·ma·to·bia (der-mă-tō′bē-ă). A genus of flies (family Oestridae) found in tropical America. [dermato- + G. bios, way of living]

D. cyaniven′tris, SYN D. hominis.

D. hom′inis, a large, blue, brown-winged species whose larvae develop in open boillike lesions in the skin of humans, many domestic animals, and some fowl. It is a very serious and damaging cattle parasite and frequently attacks small children in Central and South America. Its eggs are laid on the legs or abdomen of another insect, such as the mosquito; the eggs later hatch, when stimulated by warmth or other factors, to release the botfly larvae on the skin of the mosquito's bloodmeal host, and the larvae quickly invade the skin to initiate myiasis. SYN D. cyaniventris, human botfly, skin botflies, warble botfly.

der·ma·to·bi·a·sis (der′mă-tō-bī′ă-sis). Infection of humans and animals with larvae of the fly Dermatobia hominis. SYN human botfly myiasis.

der·mat·o·cel·lu·li·tis (der′mă-tō-sel-ū-lī′tis). Inflammation of the skin and subcutaneous connective tissue.

der·mat·o·cha·la·sis (der′mă-tō-kă-lā′sis). A congenital or acquired condition characterized by deficient elastic fibers of the skin, which may hang in folds; vascular anomalies may be present; inheritance is either autosomal dominant or recessive, the latter sometimes in association with pulmonary emphysema and diverticula of the alimentary tract or bladder. The dominant form is caused by mutation in the elastin gene (ELN) on 7q. There is also an X-linked form that is due to mutation in the Menkes gene (MNK), encoding copper-transporting ATPase on Xq. SYN cutis laxa, generalized elastolysis, loose skin. [conjunctiva + G. chalasis, a loosening]

der·mat·o·co·ni·o·sis (der′mă-tō-kō-nī-o′sis). An occupational dermatitis caused by local irritation from dust. [dermato- + G. konis, dust, + -osis, condition]

der·mat·o·cyst (der′mă-tō-sist). A cyst of the skin.

der·mat·o·dyn·ia (der′mă-tō-din′ē-ă). SYN dermatalgia. [dermato- + G. odynē, pain]

der·mat·o·fi·bro·ma (der′mă-tō-fī-brō′mă). A slowly growing benign skin nodule consisting of poorly demarcated cellular fibrous tissue enclosing collapsed capillaries, with scattered hemosiderin-pigmented and lipid macrophages. The following terms are considered by some to be synonymous with, and by others to be varieties of, d.: sclerosing hemangioma (2), fibrous histiocytoma, nodular subepidermal fibrosis. SYN fibrous histiocytoma, sclerosing hemangioma (2).

der·mat·o·fi·bro·sar·co·ma pro·tu·ber·ans (der′mă-tō-fī′brō-sar-kō′mă prō-too′ber-ans). A relatively slowly growing dermal neoplasm consisting of one or several firm nodules that are usually covered by dark red-blue skin, which tends to be fixed to the palpable masses; histologically, the neoplasm resembles a cellular dermatofibroma with a pronounced storiform pattern; metastases are unusual, but the incidence of recurrence is fairly high.

pigmented d. p., an uncommon variant of d. p. containing heavily pigmented dendritic melanocytes scattered between spindle cells of the tumor. SYN Bednar tumor, storiform neurofibroma.

der·ma·to·fi·bro·sis len·tic·u·lar·is dis·sem·i·na·ta (der′mă-tō-fī-brō′sis len-tik-ū-lā′ris di-sem-i-nā′tă) [MIM*166700]. Small papules or discs of increased dermal elastic tissue appearing in early life; when osteopoikilosis is also present, the condition is called osteodermatopoikilosis or Buschke-Ollendorf syndrome; autosomal dominant inheritance.

der·mat·o·glyph·ics (der′mă-tō-glif′iks). **1.** The configurations of the characteristic ridge patterns of the volar surfaces of the skin; in the human hand, the distal segment of each digit has three types of configurations: whorl, loop, and arch. SEE ALSO fingerprint. **2.** The science or study of these configurations or patterns. [dermato- + *glyphē,* carved work]

der·mat·o·graph (der-mat′ō-graf). The linear wheal made in the skin in dermatographism.

der·ma·tog·ra·phism (der-mă-tog′ră-fizm). A form of urticaria in which whealing occurs in the site and in the configuration of application of stroking (pressure, friction) of the skin. The resulting white line response appears early in flares of atopic dermatitis. SYN autographism, factitious urticaria, skin writing. [dermato- + G. *graphō,* to write]

der·ma·toid (der′mă-toyd). **1.** Resembling skin. SYN dermoid (1). **2.** SYN dermal.

der·ma·tol·o·gist (der-mă-tol′ō-jist). A physician who specializes in the diagnosis and treatment of cutaneous diseases and related systemic diseases.

der·ma·tol·o·gy (der-mă-tol′ō-jē). The branch of medicine concerned with the study of the skin, diseases of the skin, and the relationship of cutaneous lesions to systemic disease. [dermato- + G. *logos,* study]

der·ma·tol·y·sis (der-mă-tol′i-sis). Loosening of the skin or atrophy of the skin by disease; erroneously used as a synonym for cutis laxa. SYN dermolysis. [dermato- + G. *lysis,* a loosening]

der·ma·to·ma (der-mă-tō′mă). A circumscribed thickening or hypertrophy of the skin. [dermato- + G. *-oma,* tumor]

der·ma·tome (der′mă-tōm). **1.** An instrument for cutting thin sections of epidermis/dermis for grafting, or excising small lesions. **2.** The dorsolateral part of an embryonic somite. SYN cutis plate. **3.** The area of skin supplied by cutaneous branches from a single spinal nerve; neighboring d.'s can overlap. SYN dermatomal distribution, dermatomic area. [dermato- + G. *tomē,* a cutting]

der·mat·o·meg·a·ly (der′mă-tō-meg′ă-lē). Congenital or acquired defect in which the skin hangs in folds; may be part of a syndrome or may occur in isolation as cutis laxa, dermatochalasis, or dermatolysis. [dermato- + G. *megas,* large]

der·mat·o·mere (der′mă-tō-mēr). A metameric area of the embryonic integument. [dermato- + G. *meros,* part]

der·mat·o·my·co·sis (der′mă-tō-mī-kō′sis). Fungus infection of the skin caused by dermatophytes, yeasts, and other fungi. Cf. dermatophytosis.

d. ped′is, SYN *tinea* pedis.

der·mat·o·my·o·ma (der′mă-tō-mī-ō′mă). SYN *leiomyoma* cutis. [dermato- + G. *mys,* muscle, + *-oma,* tumor]

der·mat·o·my·o·si·tis (der′mă-tō-mī-ō-sī′tis). A progressive condition characterized by symmetric proximal muscular weakness with elevated serum levels of muscle enzymes and a skin rash, typically a purplish-red erythema on the face, and edema of the eyelids and periorbital tissue; affected muscle tissue shows degeneration of fibers with a chronic inflammatory reaction; occurs in children and adults, and in the latter may be associated with visceral cancer or other disorders of connective tissue. [dermato- + G. *mys,* muscle, + *-itis,* inflammation]

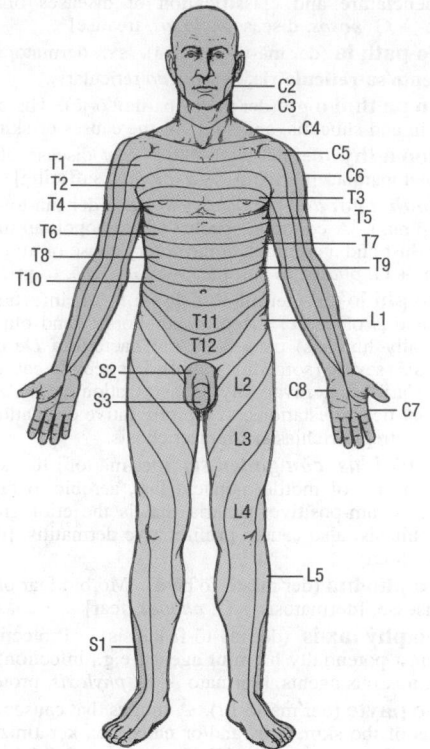

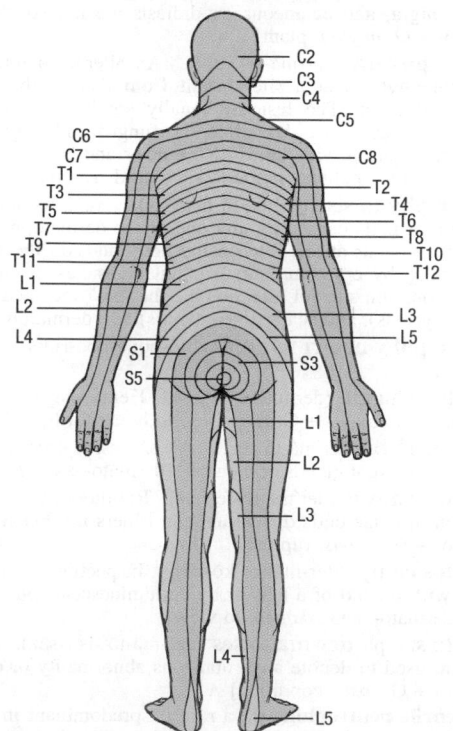

dermatomes

der·mat·o·neu·ro·sis (der′mă-tō-noo-ro′sis). Any cutaneous eruption due to emotional stimuli.

der·mat·o·no·sol·o·gy (der′mă-tō-nō-sol′ō-jē). The science of

de

the nomenclature and classification of diseases of the skin. [dermato- + G. *nosos,* disease, + *logos,* treatise]

der·mat·o·path·ia (der'mă-tō-path'ē-ă). SYN dermatopathy.

d. pigmento'sa reticula'ris, SYN *livedo* reticularis.

der·mat·o·pa·thol·o·gy (der'mă-tō-pa-thol'ō-jē). Histopathology of the skin and subcutis, and study of the causes of skin disease.

der·ma·top·a·thy (der'mă-top'ă-thē). Any disease of the skin. SYN dermatopathia. [dermato- + G. *pathos,* suffering]

Der·ma·toph·a·goi·des pter·o·nys·si·nus (der-mă-tof-ă-goy'dēz ter-ō-ni-si'nŭs). A common species of cosmopolitan mites found in house dust and a common contributory cause of atopic asthma. [dermato- + G. *phagō,* to eat; ptero- + G. *nyssō,* to prick, stab]

der·ma·to·phi·lo·sis (der'mă-tō-fi-lō'sis). An infectious exudative dermatitis of cattle, sheep, goats, horses, and other animals (occasionally humans) caused by the bacterium *Dermatophilus congolensis;* severe (sometimes fatal) d. is seen in cattle in Africa and the Caribbean, invariably in association with *Amblyomma variegatum* tick infestations. SYN proliferative dermatitis, streptothrichosis, streptotrichiasis, streptotrichosis.

Der·ma·toph·i·lus con·go·len·sis (der-mă-tof'i-lŭs kon-gō-len' sis). A species of motile, nonacid fast, aerobic to facultatively anaerobic, Gram-positive bacteria that is the etiologic agent of dermatophilosis; also causes proliferative dermatitis. [dermato- + G. *philos,* fond]

der·mat·o·pho·bia (der'mă-tō-fō'bē-ă). Morbid fear of acquiring a skin disease. [dermatosis + G. *phobos,* fear]

der·mat·o·phy·lax·is (der'mă-tō-fī-lak'sis). Protection of the skin against potentially harmful agents; e.g., infection, excessive sunlight, noxious agents. [dermato- + G. *phylaxis,* protection]

der·mat·o·phyte (der'mă-tō-fīt). A fungus that causes superficial infections of the skin, hair, and/or nails, i.e., keratinized tissues. Species of *Epidermophyton, Microsporum,* and *Trichophyton* are regarded as dermatophytes, but causative agents of tinea versicolor, tinea nigra, and cutaneous candidiasis are not so classified. [dermato- + G. *phyton,* plant]

der·mat·o·phy·tid (der'mă-tof'i-tid). An allergic manifestation of dermatophytosis at a site distant from that of the primary fungous infection. The lesions, usually small vesicles on the hands and/or arms, are devoid of the fungus and may become extensive, covering wide areas of the body and causing extreme discomfort to the patient. SEE ALSO -id (1), id *reaction.*

der·mat·o·phy·to·sis (der'mă-tō-fī-tō'sis). An infection of the hair, skin, or nails caused by any one of the dermatophytes. The lesions may occur at any site on the body and, on the skin, are characterized by erythema, small papular vesicles, fissures, and scaling. Common sites of infection are the feet (tinea pedis), nails (onychomycosis), and scalp (tinea capitis). Cf. dermatomycosis.

der·mat·o·pol·y·neu·ri·tis (der'mă-tō-pol'ē-noo-rī'tis). SYN acrodynia (2).

der·ma·tor·rha·gia (der'mă-tō-rā'jē-ă). Hemorrhage from or into the skin. [dermato- + G. *rhēgnymi,* to break forth]

der·ma·tor·rhea (der'mă-tō-rē'ă). An excessive secretion of the sebaceous or sweat glands of the skin. [dermato- + G. *rhoia,* flow]

der·ma·tor·rhex·is (der'mă-tō-rek'sis). Rupture of the skin; e.g., as is seen in striae cutis distensae or in Ehlers-Danlos syndrome. [dermato- + G. *rhēxis,* rupture]

der·ma·tos·co·py (der-mă-tos'kŏ-pē). Inspection of the skin, usually with the aid of a lens or by epiluminescence *microscopy,* (q.v.). [dermato- + G. *skopeō,* to view]

der·ma·to·sis, pl. **der·ma·to·ses** (der-mă-tō'sis, -sēz). Nonspecific term used to denote any cutaneous abnormality or eruption. [dermato- + G. *-osis,* condition]

acute febrile neutrophilic d., a rare d., predominant in women, of rapid onset and characterized by plaquelike lesions, usually multiple, on the face, neck, and upper extremities, accompanied by conjunctivitis, mucosal lesions, fever, malaise, arthralgia, and peripheral blood neutrophilia in many cases; biopsy reveals polymorphonuclear infiltrate of the dermis; rapid remission occurs with systemic steroid therapy. SYN Sweet disease.

ashy d., SYN *erythema* dyschromicum perstans.

Bowen precancerous d., SYN Bowen *disease.*

chronic bullous d. of childhood, a rare, self-limiting bullous disease, chiefly of the trunk, perioral, and pelvic areas, with onset in the first decade, successively less severe recurrences, and total remission at adolescence; linear epidermal basement membrane zone deposit of IgA is found in involved and in normal skin. SYN linear IgA bullous disease in children.

dermolytic bullous d., SYN *epidermolysis* bullosa dystrophica.

digitate d., SEE *parapsoriasis* en plaque. SYN small plaque parapsoriasis.

juvenile plantar d., a painful dermatitis, occurring primarily in children, that causes the plantar skin to appear glazed and fissured; may be associated with hyperhidrosis.

lichenoid d., any chronic skin eruption, characterized clinically by induration and thickening of the skin with accentuation of skin markings, and microscopically by a bandlike lymphocytic infiltration of the papillary dermis.

d. medicamento'sa, SYN drug *eruption.*

d. papulo'sa ni'gra, dark brown papular lesions, observed in blacks, on the face and upper trunk; histologically and clinically, they resemble seborrheic keratoses.

pigmented purpuric lichenoid d., an eruption comprised of lichenoid papules variously pigmented from the hemosiderin of the associated purpura; found on the legs, usually in men over 40 years of age. SYN Gougerot and Blum disease.

progressive pigmentary d., chronic purpura, especially of the legs in men, spreading to form red-brown patches and puncta described as cayenne pepper spots; associated microscopically with perivascular lymphocytic infiltration, diapedesis, and hemosiderosis. SYN Schamberg fever.

radiation d., skin changes at the site of ionizing radiation, particularly erythema in the acute stage, temporary or permanent epilation, and chronic changes in the epidermis and dermis resembling actinic keratosis, from which squamous cell carcinoma may develop.

subcorneal pustular d., a pruritic chronic annular eruption of sterile vesicles and pustules beneath the stratum corneum. SYN Sneddon-Wilkinson disease, subcorneal pustular dermatitis.

transient acantholytic d., a pruritic papular eruption, with histologic suprabasal acantholysis, of the chest, with scattered lesions of the back and lateral aspects of the extremities, lasting from a few weeks to several months; seen predominantly in males over 40. SYN Grover disease.

der·mat·o·ther·a·py (der'mă-tō-thār'ă-pē). Treatment of skin diseases.

der·mat·o·thla·si·a (der'mă-tō-thlā'zē-ă). An uncontrollable impulse to pinch and bruise the skin. [dermato- + G. *thlasis,* a bruising]

der·mat·o·tro·pic (der'mă-tō-trop'ik). Having an affinity for the skin. SYN dermotropic. [dermato- + G. *trōpe,* a turning]

der·mat·o·zo·on (der'mă-tō-zō'on). An animal parasite of the skin. [dermato- + G. *zōon,* animal]

der·mat·o·zo·o·no·sis (der'mă-tō-zō-ō-nō'sis, -zō-on'ō-sis). Infestation of the skin by an animal parasite. [dermato- + G. *zōon,* animal, + *nosos,* disease]

der·ma·tro·phia, der·mat·ro·phy (der-mă-trō'fē-ă, der-mat'rō-fē). Atrophy or thinning of the skin.

der·men·chy·sis (der-men'ki-sis). Rarely used term for subcutaneous administration of remedies. [derm- + G. *enchysis,* a pouring in]

der·mis [TA]. A layer of skin composed of a superficial thin layer that interdigitates with the epidermis, the stratum papillare, and the stratum reticulare; it contains blood and lymphatic vessels, nerves and nerve endings, glands, and, except for glabrous skin, hair follicles. SYN corium✲, cutis vera. [G. *derma,* skin]

△**dermo-.** SEE derm-. [G. *derma,* skin]

Der·mo·bac·ter (der-mō-bak'ter). A bacterial genus of nonmotile, non–spore-bearing Gram-positive rods, recovered on human skin. *Dermobacter hominis* has been associated with positive blood cultures.

der·mo·blast (der'mō-blast). One of the mesodermal cells from which the dermis is developed. [dermo- + G. *blastos,* germ]

der·mo·cy·ma (der′mō-sī′mă). Unequal conjoined twins in which the smaller parasite is buried in the integument of the autosite. [dermo- + G. *kyma,* fetus]

der·moid (der′moyd). **1.** SYN dermatoid (1). **2.** SYN dermoid *cyst.* [dermo- + G. *eidos,* resemblance]

inclusion d., SYN epidermal *cyst.*

der·moi·dec·to·my (der-moy-dek′tō-mē). Rarely used term for operative removal of a dermoid cyst. [dermoid + G. *ektomē,* excision]

der·mol·y·sis (der-mol′i-sis). SYN dermatolysis.

der·mo·ne·crot·ic (der′mō-nĕ-krot′ik). Pertaining to any application or illness which may cause necrosis of the skin.

der·mop·a·thy (der-mop′ă-thē). SYN dermatopathy.

diabetic d., small macules and papules of the extensor surfaces of the extremities, most commonly the shins of diabetics, which become atrophic, hyperpigmented, and occasionally undergo ulceration with scarring; may be a manifestation of microangiopathy.

der·mo·phle·bi·tis (der′mō-flĕ-bī′tis). Inflammation of the superficial veins and the surrounding skin. [dermo- + G. *phleps,* vein, + *-itis,* inflammation]

der·mo·skel·e·ton (der-mō-skel′ĕ-tŏn). SYN exoskeleton (1).

der·mo·ste·no·sis (der′mō-stĕ-nō′sis). Pathologic contraction of the skin. [dermo- + G. *stenōsis,* a narrowing]

der·mo·tox·in (der-mō-tok′sin). A substance elaborated by a living agent, especially an exotoxin formed by bacteria, and characterized by its ability to cause pathologic changes in skin, e.g., erythema, degenerative changes, necrosis.

der·mo·tro·p·ic (der-mō-trop′ik). SYN dermatotropic.

der·mo·vas·cu·lar (der-mō-vas′kū-lăr). Pertaining to the blood vessels of the skin. [dermo- + L. *vasculum,* small vessel]

der·o·did·y·mus (dār′ō-did′i-mŭs). SYN *dicephalus* diauchenos. [G. *derē,* neck, + *didymos,* twin]

de·ro·ta·tion (dē-rō-tā′shŭn). **1.** A turning back. **2.** In orthopedics, the correction of a rotation deformity by turning or rotating the deformed structure toward a normal position. [L. *de,* away, + *rotatio,* turning]

DES Abbreviation for diethylstilbestrol.

⌂**des-.** In chemistry, a prefix indicating absence of some component of the principal part of the name; largely replaced by "de-" (e.g., deoxyribonucleic acid, dehydro-) but retained where "de-" could be taken for D- or *d-,* as part of "desmo-" (e.g., desmosterol), and in such terms as desoxycortone.

des·am·i·dize (dē-sam′i-dīz). SYN deamidize.

De Sanctis, Carlo, Italian psychiatrist, *1888. SEE De S.-Cacchione *syndrome.*

de·sat·u·rate (dē-sat′ū-rāt). To produce desaturation.

de·sat·u·ra·tion (dē′sat-ū-rā′shŭn). **1.** The act, or the result of the act, of making something less completely saturated; more specifically, the percentage of total binding sites remaining unfilled, e.g., when hemoglobin is 70% saturated with oxygen and nothing else, its d. is 30%. Cf. saturation (5). **2.** The process or reaction of removal of two hydrogen atoms from a molecule, resulting in the formation of a double bond.

Desault, Pierre-Joseph, French surgeon, 1744–1795. SEE D. *bandage.*

Descartes (Cartesius), René, French philosopher, mathematician, physiologist, 1596–1650. The founder of modern philosophy and proponent of the mechanistic *school* or iatromathematical *school.* SEE D. *law.*

Descemet, Jean, French physician, 1732–1810. SEE D. *membrane.*

des·ce·me·ti·tis (des′ĕ-mĕ-tī′tis). Inflammation of Descemet membrane.

des·ce·met·o·cele (des-ĕ-met′ō-sēl). A bulging forward of Descemet membrane caused by the destruction of the substance of the cornea by infection.

de·scen·dens (dē-sen′denz). SYN descending. [L.]

d. cervica′lis, SYN inferior *root* of ansa cervicalis.

d. hypoglos′si, SYN superior *root* of ansa cervicalis.

de·scend·ing (dē-send′ing). Running downward or toward the periphery. SYN descendens. [L. *de-scendo,* pp. *-scensus,* to come down, fr. *scando,* to climb]

de·scen·sus (dē-sen′sŭs). A falling away from a higher position. SEE ALSO ptosis, procidentia. SYN descent (1). [L.]

d. tes′tis, descent of the testis from the abdomen into the scrotum during the seventh and eighth months of intrauterine life.

d. u′teri, SYN *prolapse* of the uterus.

d. ventric′uli, SYN gastroptosis.

de·scent (dē-sent′). **1.** SYN descensus. **2.** In obstetrics, the passage of the presenting part of the fetus into and through the birth canal. [L. descensus]

Deschamps, Joseph F.L., French surgeon, 1740–1824. SEE D. *needle.*

de·sen·si·tiz·a·tion (dē-sen′si-ti-zā′shŭn). **1.** The reduction or abolition of allergic sensitivity or reactions to the specific antigen (allergen). SYN antianaphylaxis. **2.** The act of removing an emotional complex. SYN hyposensitization.

heterologous d., stimulation by one agonist which leads to a broad pattern of unresponsiveness to further stimulation by a variety of other agonists.

homologous d., loss of sensitivity only to the class of agonist used to desensitize the tissue.

systematic d., a type of behavior therapy for eliminating phobias or anxieties: the patient and therapist construct a list of imagined scenes eliciting the phobia, ranked from least to most anxiety producing; the patient then is trained in deep muscle relaxation, and is repeatedly asked to imagine him or herself in the presence of the least anxiety-producing scene on the list until the patient feels fully relaxed while doing so; the procedure is repeated for each scene on the list until the patient develops the capacity to feel relaxed with any of the anxiety-producing scenes; real life scenes are then substituted for the imagined scenes. SYN reciprocal inhibition (2).

de·sen·si·tize (dē-sen′si-tīz). **1.** To reduce or remove any form of sensitivity. **2.** To effect desensitization (1). **3.** In dentistry, to eliminate or subdue the painful response of exposed, vital dentin to irritative agents or thermal changes.

de·ser·pi·dine (dē-ser′pi-dēn). Ester alkaloid isolated from *Rauwolfia canescens* (family Apocynaceae) with the same actions and uses as reserpine.

des·e·tope (dē′se-tōp). That part of the Class II major histocompatibility molecule that interacts with the antigen. The term desetope is derived from determinant selection. [*de*terminant *se*lection + -*tope*]

des·fer·ri·ox·a·mine mes·y·late (des′făr-ē-ok′să-mēn). SYN deferoxamine mesylate.

des·flu·rane (dés′floor′ān). An inhalation anesthetic with physical characteristics that provide rapid induction of and recovery from anesthesia.

des·hy·dre·mia (des′hī-drē′mē-ă). Hemoconcentration due to the loss of water from blood plasma. [L. *de-,* away from, + G. *hydor,* water, + *haima,* blood + -ia]

des·ic·cant (des′i-kant). **1.** Drying; causing or promoting dryness. SYN desiccative. **2.** An agent that absorbs moisture; a drying agent. SYN exsiccant. [L. *de-sicco,* pp. *-siccatus,* to dry up]

des·ic·cate (des′i-kāt). To dry thoroughly; to render free from moisture. SYN exsiccate.

des·ic·ca·tion (des-i-kā′shŭn). The process of being desiccated. SYN dehydration (4), exsiccation (1).

des·ic·ca·tive (des-i-kā′tiv). SYN desiccant (1).

des·ic·ca·tor (des′i-kā-ter, tōr). **1.** SYN desiccant (2). **2.** An apparatus, such as a glass chamber containing calcium chloride, sulfuric acid, or other drying agent, in which a material is placed for drying.

vacuum d., a d. that can be evacuated.

de·si·pra·mine hy·dro·chlo·ride (des-ip′ră-mēn). A dibenzazepine derivative; an antidepressant similar to imipramine hydrochloride. Selectively blocks reuptake of norepinephrine back into central aminergic neurons.

de

des·lan·o·side (des-lan'ō-sīd). A rapidly acting steroid glycoside obtained from lanatoside C (*Digitalis lanata*) by alkaline hydrolysis; a cardiotonic.

△**desm-.** SEE desmo-.

Desmarres, Louis A., French ophthalmologist, 1810–1882. SEE D. *dacryoliths,* under *dacryolith;* Desmarres *retractor.*

des·min (dez'minz). Proteins found in intermediate filaments that copolymerizes with vimentin to form constituents of connective tissue, cell walls, filaments, etc. Found in Z disk of skeletal and cardiac muscle cells.

des·mi·tis (dez-mī'tis). Inflammation of a ligament. [desm- + G. -*itis,* inflammation]

△**desmo-, desm-.** Fibrous connection; ligament. [G. *desmos,* a band]

des·mo·cra·ni·um (dez-mō-krā'nē-ŭm) [TA]. The mesenchymal primordium of the cranium.

des·mo·den·ti·um [TA]. The collagen fibers, running from the cementum to the alveolar bone, that suspend a tooth in its socket; they include apical, oblique, horizontal, and alveolar crest fibers, indicating that the orientation of the fibers varies at different levels. SYN desmodontium [TA], periodontal fiber✩, periodontal ligament fibers.

des·mo·don·ti·um [TA]. SYN desmodentium.

Des·mo·dus (dez'mō-dŭs). A blood-feeding genus of Chiroptera, known generally as vampire bats, found in Trinidad, Mexico, and Central and South America; *D. artibaeus, D. rotundus,* and *D. rufus,* three species present in Trinidad and South America, are reservoir hosts of rabies virus. [desmo- + G. *odous,* tooth]

des·mog·e·nous (dez-moj'ĕ-nŭs). Of connective tissue or ligamentous origin or causation; e.g., denoting a deformity due to contraction of ligaments, fascia, or a scar. [desmo- + G. -*gen,* producing]

des·mog·ra·phy (dez-mog'ră-fē). A description of, or treatise on, the ligaments. [desmo- + G. *graphō,* to describe]

des·moid (dez'moyd). **1.** Fibrous or ligamentous. **2.** A nodule or relatively large mass of unusually firm scarlike connective tissue resulting from active proliferation of fibroblasts, occurring most frequently in the abdominal muscles of women who have borne children; the fibroblasts infiltrate surrounding muscle and fascia. SYN abdominal fibromatosis, desmoid tumor. [desmo- + G. *eidos,* appearance, form]

  extra-abdominal d., a deep-seated firm tumor, most frequently occurring on the shoulders, chest, or back of young men or women, consisting of collagenous fibrous tissue that infiltrates surrounding muscle; frequently recurs but does not metastasize.

des·mo·las·es (dez'mō-lā'sez). Old and nonspecific term for enzymes catalyzing reactions other than those involving hydrolysis; e.g., those involving oxidation and reduction, isomerization, the breaking of carbon-carbon bonds.

des·mol·o·gy (dez-mol'ō-jē). The branch of anatomy concerned with the ligaments. [desmo- + G. *logos,* study]

des·mop·a·thy (dez-mop'ă-thē). Any disease of the ligaments. [desmo- + G. *pathos,* suffering]

des·mo·pla·sia (dez-mō-plā'zē-ă). Hyperplasia of fibroblasts and disproportionate formation of fibrous connective tissue, especially in the stroma of a carcinoma. [desmo- + G. *plasis,* a molding]

des·mo·plas·tic (dez-mō-plas'tik). **1.** Causing or forming adhesions. **2.** Causing fibrosis in the vascular stroma of a neoplasm.

des·mo·pres·sin (des-mō-pres'in). An analog of vasopressin (antidiuretic hormone, ADH) possessing powerful antidiuretic activity.

  d. acetate, a synthetic analog of vasopressin and an antidiuretic hormone.

des·mo·sine (dez'mō-sēn). A cross-linking amino acid formed from lysyl residues found in elastin. [G. *desmos,* bond, fr. *deō,* to bind, + -ine]

des·mo·some (dez'mō-sōm). A site of adhesion between two epithelial cells, consisting of a dense attachment plaque separated from a similar structure in the other cell by a thin layer of extracellular material. SYN bridge corpuscle, macula adherens. [desmo- + G. *sōma,* body]

des·mos·te·rol (dez-mos'ter-ol). 5α-Cholesta-5,24-diene-3β-ol; postulated intermediate in cholesterol biosynthesis from lanosterol via zymosterol; accumulates after prolonged administration of substances interfering with cholesterol biosynthesis. SYN 24-dehydrocholesterol.

des·o·nide (des'ō-nīd). An anti-inflammatory corticosteroid used in topical preparations.

des·ox·i·met·a·sone (des-ok-si-met'ă-sōn). An anti-inflammatory corticosteroid used in topical preparations.

△**desoxy-.** SEE deoxy-.

des·ox·y·cor·ti·cos·ter·one (dēs-oks-ē-kōr'tĭ-kōs-ter-ōn). A steroid derived from the adrenal cortex with strong mineralocorticoid activity.

des·ox·y·cor·tone (des-oks-ē-kōr'tōn). SYN deoxycorticosterone.

de·spe·ci·a·tion (dē-spē'shē-ā'shŭn). **1.** Alteration of, or loss of species characteristics. **2.** Removal of species-specific antigenic properties from a foreign protein.

D'Éspine, Jean H.A., French physician, 1846–1930. SEE D. *sign.*

des·pu·ma·tion (des-pū-mā'shŭn). **1.** The rising of impurities to the surface of a liquid. **2.** The skimming off of impurities on the surface of a liquid. [L. *de-spumo,* pp. -*atus,* to skim, fr. *spumo,* to foam, fr. *spuma,* foam]

des·qua·mate (des'kwă-māt). To shred, peel, or scale off, as the casting off of the epidermis in scales or shreds, or the shedding of the outer layer of any surface. [L. *desquamo,* pp. -*atus,* to scale off, fr. *squama,* a scale]

des·qua·ma·tion (des-kwă-mā'shŭn). The shedding of the cuticle in scales or of the outer layer of any surface.

  branny d., SYN defurfuration.

des·qua·ma·tive (des-kwam'ă-tiv). Relating to or marked by desquamation.

des·thi·o·bi·o·tin (des'thī-ō-bī'ō-tin). A compound derived from biotin by the removal of the sulfur atom; a precursor of biotin in bacteria and molds; it can substitute for biotin in some microorganisms, but is without effect on or is inhibitory to the growth of others.

de·stru·do (dē-stroo'dō). Energy associated with the death or destructive instinct. [coinage on the analogy of *libido* fr. L. *destruo,* to destroy]

de·sulf·hy·dras·es (dē'sulf-hī'drā-sez). Enzymes or groups of enzymes catalyzing the removal of a molecule of H_2S or substituted H_2S from a compound, as in the conversion of cysteine to pyruvic acid by cysteine desulfhydrase (cystathionine γ-lyase). SYN desulfurases.

de·sul·fi·nase (dē-sŭl'fi-nās). Term sometimes applied to the enzyme (aspartate-4-decarboxylase) removing sulfite: 1) from cysteinesulfinate, an intermediate in cysteine degradation, yielding alanine; 2) from sulfinylpyruvate, previously postulated to be formed by deamination of cysteinesulfinate, yielding pyruvate; degradation of sulfinylpyruvate is now considered to be spontaneous, not requiring an enzyme.

De·sul·fo·to·ma·cu·lum (dē-sul-fō-tō-mak'ū-lŭm). A genus of rod-shaped (straight or curved), anaerobic, chemoorganotrophic motile bacteria that stain Gram-negative but have Gram-positive cell walls. Found in soil, the rumen and elsewhere. The type species is *D. nigrificans.*

  D. nigri'ficans, a species found in spoiled foods showing "sulfur stinker " spoilage as a result of hydrogen sulfide production. It is not pathogenic.

de·sul·fu·ras·es (dē-sŭl'fūr-ās-ez). SYN desulfhydrases.

de·syn·chro·nous (de-sin'kron-ŭs). Lack of synchrony, as in brain waves. [de- + G. *syn,* with, + *chronos,* time]

DET Abbreviation for diethyltryptamine.

det. Abbreviation for L. *detur,* give. [let it be given]

de·tach·ment (dē-tach'ment). **1.** A voluntary or involuntary feeling or emotion that accompanies a sense of separation from normal associations or environment. **2.** Separation of a structure from its support.

  exudative retinal d., d. of the retina without retinal breaks, arising from inflammatory disease of choroid, retinal tumors, and retinal angiomatosis.

retinal d., d. of retina, loss of apposition between the sensory retina and the retinal pigment epithelium. SYN detached retina, separation of retina.

rhegmatogenous retinal d., retinal separation associated with a break, a hole, or a tear in the sensory retina.

vitreous d., separation of the peripheral vitreous humor from the retina.

de·tec·tion (dē-tek′shun). 1. The act of discovery. 2. In chromatography, visualization of the separated material.

de·tec·tor (dē-tek′ter, -tōr). The component of a laboratory instrument which detects the chemical or physical signal indicating the presence or quantity of the substance of interest.

solid-state d., a d. that uses a crystalline scintillating material rather than an ionization chamber to detect or measure radiation.

de·ter·gent (dē-ter′jent). 1. Cleansing. 2. A cleansing or purging agent, usually salts of long-chain aliphatic bases or acids (e.g., quaternary ammonium or sulfonic acid compounds) which, through a surface action that depends on their possessing both hydrophilic and hydrophobic properties, exert cleansing (oil-dissolving) and antibacterial effects; acridine derivatives (e.g., acriflavine, proflavine) as well as other dyes (e.g., brilliant green, crystal violet) have d. properties for the same reasons. SYN detersive. [L. *de-tergeo,* pp. *-tersus,* to wipe off]

anionic d.'s, d.'s, such as soaps (alkali metal salts of long-chain fatty acids), that carry a negative electric charge on a lipidlike molecule and exert a limited antibacterial effect.

cationic d.'s, d.'s, such as the amine salts or quaternary ammonium or pyridinium compounds of long-chain fatty acids, that have positively charged groups attached to the larger hydrophobic portions.

zwitterionic d., SYN zwittergents.

de·te·ri·o·ra·tion (dē-tēr′i-ō-rā′shŭn). The process or condition of becoming worse. [L. *deterior,* worse]

alcoholic d., dementia occurring in persons chronically addicted to alcohol. SEE chronic *alcoholism.*

senile d., a slowly progressing decline in physical and mental health, apparently due to natural causes attendant upon the processes of aging. SEE Alzheimer *disease.*

de·ter·mi·nant (dē-ter′mi-nănt). The factor that contributes to the generation of a trait. [L. *determans,* determining, limiting]

allotypic d.'s, antigenic d.'s of allotypes.

antigenic d., the particular chemical group of a molecule that determines immunological specificity. SYN determinant group.

disease d.'s, any variables that directly or indirectly influence the frequency of occurrence and/or the distribution of any given disease; they include specific disease agents, host characteristics, and environmental factors.

genetic d., any antigenic d. or identifying characteristic, particularly those of allotypes. SYN genetic marker.

idiotypic antigenic d., SYN idiotope.

isoallotypic d.'s, genetic d.'s that are both isotypic and allotypic in that they appear on heavy chains of all members of at least one subclass of immunoglobulin but also on heavy chains of another subclass of the same species.

mathematical d., a formal algebraic operation on the terms of a square matrix of quantities, fundamental in solving multiple simultaneous equations and widely used in regression analysis, notably in epidemiology and quantitative genetics. If d. is zero, the equations have no unambiguous solution.

de·ter·mi·na·tion (dē-ter-mi-nā′shŭn). 1. A change, for the better or for the worse, in the course of a disease. 2. A general move toward a given point. 3. The measurement or estimation of any quantity or quality in scientific or laboratory investigation. 4. Discernment of a state or category (e.g., in diagnosis). 5. A process, both necessary and sufficient, whereby an effect is caused. [L. *de-termino,* pp. *-atus,* to limit, determine, fr. *terminus,* a boundary]

cell d., the process by which embryonic cells, previously undifferentiated, take on a specific developmental character. SEE morphogenesis, induction, evocator.

sex d., d. of the sex of a fetus *in utero* by identification of fetal chromosomes.

de·ter·mi·nism (dē-ter′mi-nizm). The proposition that all behavior is caused exclusively by genetic and environmental influences with no random components, and independent of free will. [L. *determino,* to limit, fr. *terminus,* boundary + -ism]

psychic d., in psychoanalysis, the concept that all psychological and behavioral phenomena result from antecedent, unconsciously operating causes.

de·ter·sive (dē-ter′siv). SYN detergent.

de·tox·i·cate (dē-tok′si-kāt). To diminish or remove the poisonous quality of any substance; to lessen the virulence of any pathogenic organism. SYN detoxify. [L. *de,* from, + *toxicum,* poison]

de·tox·i·ca·tion (dē-tok-si-kā′shŭn). SYN detoxification.

ammonia d., the d. of ammonia and ammonium ion by the formation of ammonium salts, specific nitrogen-excretion products, or L-glutamine.

de·tox·i·fi·ca·tion (dē-tok′si-fi-kā′shŭn). 1. Recovery from the toxic effects of a drug. 2. Removal of the toxic properties from a poison. 3. Metabolic conversion of pharmacologically active principles to pharmacologically less active principles. SYN detoxication.

de·tox·i·fy (dē-tok′si-fī). SYN detoxicate.

de·tri·tion (dē-trish′ŭn). A wearing away by use or friction. [L. *de-tero,* pp. *-tritus,* to rub off]

de·tri·tus (dē-trī′tŭs). Any broken-down material, carious or gangrenous matter, gravel, etc. [L. (see detrition)]

de·tru·sor (dē-troo′ser, -sōr). 1. A muscle that has the action of expelling a substance. 2. SEE detrusor (*muscle*). [L. *detrudo,* to drive away]

de·tru·sor·rha·phy (dē-troo′-sor-a-fē). A procedure in which bladder muscle (detrusor) is reconstructed around the ureterovesical junction to form a competent one-way valve. SEE ALSO ureteroneocystostomy. SYN extravesical reimplantation. [detrusor + G. *rhaphē,* a seam]

de·tu·mes·cence (dē-too-mes′ens). Subsidence of a swelling. [L. *de,* from, + *tumesco,* to swell up, fr. *tumeo,* to swell]

de·tur·ges·cence (dē-toor-ges′ens). The mechanism by which the stroma of the cornea remains relatively dehydrated. [L. *de,* from, + *turgesco,* to begin to swell]

deut-. SEE deutero-.

deu·ten·ceph·a·lon (doo′ten-sef′ă-lon). Rarely used term for diencephalon. [G. *deuteros,* second, + *enkephalos,* brain]

deu·ter·a·nom·a·ly (doo′ter-ă-nom′ă-lē). A form of anomalous trichromatism due to a defect of the green-sensitive retinal cones. [G. *deuteros,* second, + *anōmalia,* anomaly]

deu·ter·an·ope (doo′ter-ă-nōp). A person affected with deuteranopia.

deu·ter·an·o·pia (doo′ter-ă-nō′pē-ă). A congenital abnormality of the retina in which there are two rather than three retinal cone pigments (dichromatism) and complete insensitivity to middle wavelengths (green). [G. *deuteros,* second, + anopia]

deuterio-. Prefix indicating "containing deuterium."

deu·te·ri·um (D) (doo-tē-r′ē-ŭm). SYN hydrogen-2. [G. *deuteros,* second]

d. oxide, SYN heavy *water.*

deutero-, deut-, deuto-. Combining forms meaning two, or second (in a series); secondary. [G. *deuteros,* second]

deu·ter·o·my·ce·tes (du′ter-ō-mī-sē′tēz). Members of the class Deuteromycetes or the phylum Deuteromycota.

Deu·ter·o·my·co·ta (doo′ter-ō-mī-kō-tă). A phylum in which the sexual (teleomorph or perfect) part of the life cycle has not been discovered; only the asexual (anamorph or imperfect) part of the life cycle has been found. SEE ALSO Fungi Imperfecti.

deu·ter·on (doo′ter-on). The nucleus of hydrogen-2, composed of one neutron and one proton; it thus has the one positive charge characteristic of a hydrogen nucleus. SYN deuton, diplon.

deu·ter·o·path·ic (doo′ter-ō-path′ik). Relating to a deuteropathy.

deu·ter·op·a·thy (doo-ter-op′ă-thē). A secondary disease or symptom. [deutero- + G. *pathos,* suffering]

de

deu·ter·o·plasm (doo′ter-ō-plazm). SYN deutoplasm. [deutero- + G. *plasma*, thing formed]

deu·ter·o·por·phy·rin (doo′ter-ō-pōr′fi-rin). A porphyrin derivative resembling the protoporphyrins except that the two vinyl side chains are replaced by hydrogen.

deu·ter·o·some (doo′ter-ō-sōm). Dense spherical fibrous granules that occur in the centrosphere and act in the development of centrioles or basal bodies. SYN procentriole organizer.

deu·ter·o·to·cia (doo′ter-ō-tō′sē-ă). A form of parthenogenesis in which the female has offspring of both sexes. SYN deuterotoky. [deutero- + G. *tokos*, childbirth]

deu·ter·ot·o·ky (doo-ter-ot′ō-kē). SYN deuterotocia.

deuto-. SEE deutero-.

deu·to·gen·ic (doo-tō-jen′ik). Of secondary origin following an inductive influence. [deuto- + G. -*gen*, production]

deu·tom·er·ite (doo-tom′er-īt). The posterior nucleated portion of an attached cephalont in a gregarine protozoan, separated by an ectoplasmic septum from the anterior portion, or protomerite. [deuto- + L. *meros*, part]

deu·ton (doo′ton). SYN deuteron.

deu·to·nymph (doo′to-nimt). The third stage of a mite.

deu·to·plasm (doo′tō-plazm). The yolk of a meroblastic egg; the nonliving material in the cytoplasm, especially that stored in the ovum as food for the developing embryo, the commonest types being lipoid droplets and yolk granules. SYN deuteroplasm. [deuto- + G. *plasma*, thing formed]

deu·to·plas·mic (doo-tō-plaz′mik). Relating to the deutoplasm.

deu·to·plas·mi·gen·on (doo′tō-plaz-mi-jen′on). That which produces or gives rise to deutoplasm. [deutoplasm + G. *genos*, birth]

deu·to·plas·mol·y·sis (doo′tō-plaz-mol′i-sis). The disintegration of deutoplasm. [deutoplasm + G. *lysis*, dissolution]

Deutschländer, Carl E. W., German surgeon, 1872–1942. SEE D. *disease*.

DEV Abbreviation for duck embryo origin *vaccine*.

de·vas·cu·lar·i·za·tion (dē-vas′kū-lăr-i-zā′shŭn). Occlusion of all or most of the blood vessels to any part or organ. [L. *de*, away, + *vasculum*, small vessel, + G. *izo*, to cause]

de·vel·op (dē-vel′ŏp). To process an exposed photographic or radiographic film in order to turn the latent image into a permanent one. [O.Fr. *desveloper*, to unwrap, fr. *voloper*, to wrap]

de·vel·op·er (dē-vel′ŏp-er). **1.** An individual or procedure that develops. **2.** SYN eluent. **3.** The chemicals used to develop film by reducing the light-activated silver halide molecules to atomic silver. **4.** The factor(s) causing a cell, organ, or organism to undergo a series of orderly changes.

de·vel·op·ment (dē-vel′ŏp-ment). **1.** The act or process of natural progression in physical and psychological maturation from a previous, lower, or embryonic stage to a later, more complex, or adult stage. **2.** The process of chromatography.

cognitive d., the evolving d. of the infant's and child's intellectual functions.

life-span d., development and mastery (or loss) of differing biologic, intellectual, behavioral, and social skills in different epochs of the life-span from the prenatal through the gerontological periods of growth.

psychosexual d., maturation and development of the psychic and behavioral phases of sexuality from birth to adult life through the oral, anal, phallic, latency, and genital phases.

Deventer, Hendrik van, Dutch obstetrician, 1651–1724. SEE D. *pelvis*.

de·vi·ance (dē′vē-ans). SYN deviation (3).

de·vi·ant (dē′vē-ant). **1.** Denoting or indicative of deviation. **2.** An individual exhibiting deviation, especially sexual.

de·vi·a·tion (dē-vē-ā′shŭn). **1.** A turning away or aside from the normal point or course. **2.** An abnormality. **3.** In psychiatry and the behavioral sciences, a departure from an accepted norm, role, or rule. SYN deviance. **4.** A statistical measure representing the difference between an individual value in a set of values and the mean value in that set. [L. *devio*, to turn from the straight path, fr. *de*, from, + *via*, way]

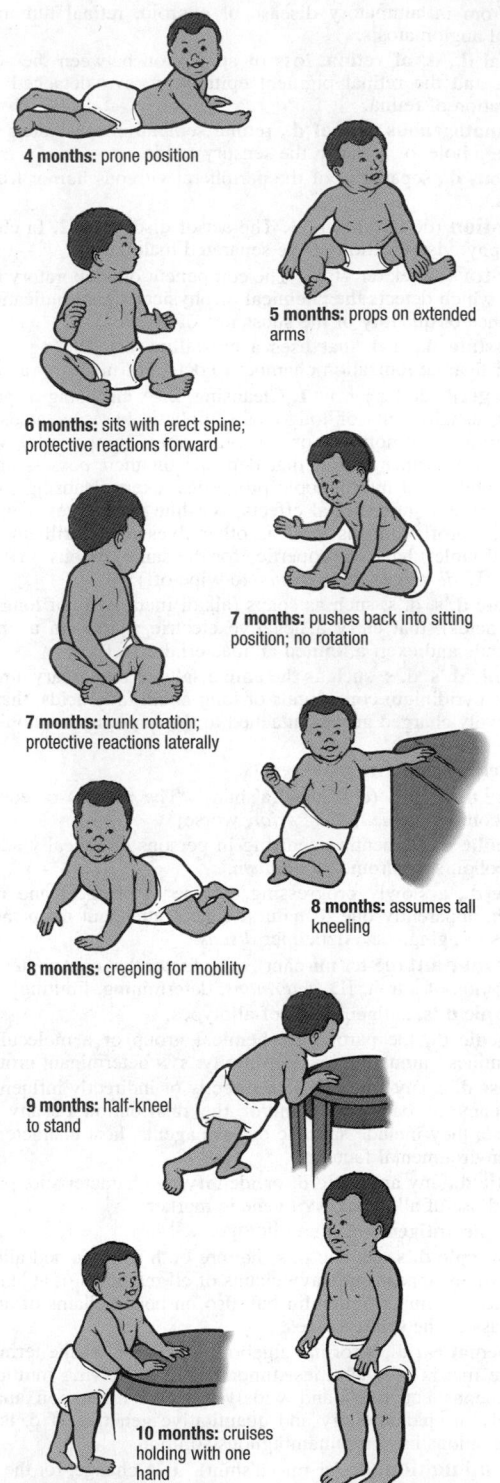

4 months: prone position

5 months: props on extended arms

6 months: sits with erect spine; protective reactions forward

7 months: pushes back into sitting position; no rotation

7 months: trunk rotation; protective reactions laterally

8 months: assumes tall kneeling

8 months: creeping for mobility

9 months: half-kneel to stand

10 months: cruises holding with one hand

11 months: stands alone

developmental milestones

axis d., deflection of the electrical axis of the heart to the right or left of the normal. SEE ALSO left axis d., right axis d., axis. SYN axis shift.

conjugate d. of the eyes, (1) rotation of the eyes equally and simultaneously in the same direction, as occurs normally; (2) a condition in which both eyes are turned to the same side as a result of either paralysis or muscular spasm.

dissociated horizontal d., a tendency often associated with re-paired congenital esotropia in which an eye abducts when it is covered, in violation of Herring *law*.

dissociated vertical d., a tendency often associated with congenital esotropia, in which an eye elevates, abducts, and extorts when covered, in violation of Herring *law*.

immune d., SYN split *tolerance*.

d. to the left, SYN *shift* to the left (1).

left axis d., a mean electrical axis of the heart pointing to −30° or more negative. SEE hexaxial reference *system*.

primary d., the ocular deviation seen in paralysis of an ocular muscle when the nonparalyzed eye is used for fixation.

d. to the right, SYN *shift* to the right (1).

right axis d., a mean electrical axis of the heart pointing to the right of +90°. SEE hexaxial reference *system*.

secondary d., ocular deviation seen in paralysis of an ocular muscle when the paralyzed eye is used for fixation.

sexual d., a sexual practice that is biologically atypical, considered morally wrong, or legally prohibited. SEE bestiality, pedophilia. SYN sexual perversion.

skew d., a hypertropia in which the eyes move in opposite directions equally; an acquired hypertropia, often fairly comitant, not fitting the characteristic pattern of trochlear nerve damage or of ocular muscle abnormality; often due to a brainstem or cerebellar lesion.

standard d. (SD, σ), (1) statistical index of the degree of d. from central tendency, namely, of the variability within a distribution; the square root of the average of the squared d.'s from the mean. **(2)** a measure of dispersion or variation used to describe a characteristic of a frequency distribution.

Devic, Eugène, French physician, 1869–1930. SEE D. *disease*.

de·vice (dē-vīs'). An appliance, usually mechanical, designed to perform a specific function, such as prosthesis or orthesis. [M.E., fr. O.Fr. *devis*, fr. L. *divisum*, divided]

central-bearing d., in dentistry, a d. which provides a central point of bearing, or support, between upper and lower record bases; it consists of a contacting point which is attached to one base and a plate attached to the other which provides the surface on which the bearing point rests or moves.

central-bearing tracing d., in dentistry, a central-bearing d. used for making a tracing and/or for support between upper and lower bases.

contraceptive d., a d. used to prevent pregnancy; e.g., occlusive diaphragm, condom, intrauterine d.

intrauterine d.'s (IUD), pieces of plastic or metal of various shapes (e.g., coil, loop, bow "T") inserted into the uterus to exert a contraceptive effect. SYN intrauterine contraceptive d.'s.

intrauterine contraceptive d.'s (IUCD), SYN intrauterine d.'s.

left-ventricular assist d., mechanical pump inserted at some point in the circulation to parallel the activity of the left ventricle and thereby reduce its load.

ventricular assist d., any of a variety of mechanical d.'s that

motor, social, and verbal and cognitive development of the normal child			
age	**motor**	**skill area social**	**verbal and cognitive**
2–3 months	lifts head when lying on stomach	smiles in response to a human face ("social smile")	coos, gurgles
5–6 months	turns over, sits unassisted	forms an attachment to primary caregiver, recognizes parents	babbles (repeats a single sound over and over)
7–11 months	pulls up to standing position	shows fear in response to unfamiliar people ("stranger anxiety")	imitates sounds, uses gestures
12–15 months	walks unassisted	fears separation from primary caregiver ("separation anxiety")	says first word
16 months–2½ years	climbs stairs, makes marks with a crayon on paper	plays independently, shows negativity (e.g., favorite word is "no")	speaks in two-word sentences (e.g., "Me do."), names body parts and objects
2½–4 years	rides a tricycle, undresses and partially dresses without help; copies a circle, line, or cross; identifies color	plays alongside, but not with, another child ("parallel play"), can spend much of the day with adults other than parents (e.g., preschool), develops core gender identity by age 3	speaks in complete sentences (e.g., "I can do it myself.")
4–6 years	draws a person in detail (e.g., with arms, legs, body, eyes, hair), dresses independently, skips using alternate feet, ties shoelaces by 6 years of age, copies a square or triangle	plays cooperatively with other children; may have imaginary companions; has curiosity about the body, plays "doctor"; has romantic feeling about the opposite-sex parent ("the oedipal phase")	good verbal self-expression (e.g., tells detailed stories)
6–11 years	engages in complex motor tasks (e.g., plays ball, rides a bicycle, skips rope)	prefers to play with children of the same sex, is hardworking and industrious, develops a moral sense of right and wrong, learns to follow rules, identifies with the parent of the same sex, has relationships with adults other than parents (e.g., teachers, group leaders)	develops the capacity for logical thought; understands that objects have more than one property (e.g., can be both wood and blue); learns to read, write, and calculate (Piaget's "concrete operations" stage)
11–14 years	has greater body strength, participates in individual and team sports	shows preoccupation with gender roles, body image, and popularity; continues to separate from family; forms stronger relationships with peers	develops abstract reasoning (beginning of Piaget's "formal operations" stage) and creativity
14–17 years	shows motor skills that approach those of the adult	has feelings of omnipotence that lead to risk-taking behavior (e.g., failing to use birth control devices, driving fast)	continues development as intellectual capacity nears its peak
17–20 years	reaches adult level of motor skills	shows concern about humanitarian issues, morality, and self-control; may have an identity crisis that causes role confusion (manifested by criminal behavior or joining a cult)	shows further development of abstract mathematic reasoning (e.g., calculus)

de

support or replace the pumping function of the left (LVAD) or right ventricle (RVAD). The inflow end of the pump is connected to the ventricle and the outflow end to the aorta (LVAD) or pulmonary artery (RVAD). Most or all of the cardiac output is directed through the d. to allow time for recovery of the patient's damaged heart muscle after myocardial infraction or heart surgery. Also used as "a bridge to transplantation," i.e., to maintain the patient whose heart will not recover until a donor heart becomes available.

de·vi·om·e·ter (dē-vē-om′ĕ-ter). A form of strabismometer.

de·vi·tal·i·za·tion (dē-vi′tăl-i-zā′shŭn). **1.** Deprivation of vitality or of vital properties. **2.** In dentistry, the process by which tooth pulp is destroyed; e.g., by chemical means, by infection, or by extirpation.

de·vi·tal·ize (dē-vī′tăl-īz). To deprive of vitality or of vital properties.

de·vi·tal·ized (dē-vī′tăl-īzd). Devoid of life; dead.

dev·o·lu·tion (dev-ō-loo′shŭn). A continuing process of degeneration or breaking down, in contrast to evolution. SEE ALSO involution, catabolism. [L. *de-volvo*, pp. *-volutus*, to roll down]

Dewar, Sir James, English chemist, 1842–1923. SEE D. *flask.*

de Wecker, Louis H., French physician, 1832–1906. SEE de W. *scissors.*

dex·a·meth·a·sone (dek-să-meth′ă-sōn). A potent synthetic analogue of cortisol, with similar biological action; used as an anti-inflammatory agent and as a test material for adrenal cortical function.

dex·am·phet·a·mine (deks-am-fet′ă-mēn). SYN dextroamphetamine sulfate.

d. sodium phosphate, the water-soluble ester of d., with the same actions and uses.

dex·brom·phen·ir·a·mine ma·le·ate (deks′brom-fen-ir′ă-mēn). The dextrorotatory isomer of brompheniramine; an antihistamine.

dex·chlor·phen·ir·a·mine ma·le·ate (deks′klōr-fen-ir′ă-mēn). The dextrorotatory isomer of chlorpheniramine; an antihistamine.

dex·i·o·car·dia (deks-ē-ō-kar′dē-ă). SYN dextrocardia.

dex·pan·the·nol (deks-pan′thĕ-nol). Pantothenic acid with –CH₂OH replacing the terminal –COOH; a cholinergic agent and a dietary source of pantothenic acid. SYN panthenol, pantothenyl alcohol.

dex·ter (D) (deks′ter). Located on or relating to the right side. [L. fr. *dextra,* neut. *dextrum*]

♻ **dextr-.** SEE dextro-.

dex·trad (deks′trad). Toward the right side. [L. *dexter,* right, + *ad,* to]

dex·tral (deks′trăl). SYN right-handed.

dex·tral·i·ty (deks-tral′i-tē). Right-handedness; preference for the right hand in performing manual tasks.

dex·tran (deks′tran). **1.** Any of several water-soluble high molecular weight glucose polymers (average MW 75,000; ranging between 1,000 and 40,000,000) produced by the action of members of the family Lactobacillaceae and certain other microorganisms on sucrose; used in isotonic sodium chloride solution for the treatment of shock, and in distilled water for the relief of the edema of nephrosis; lower molecular weight d. (e.g., MW 40,000) improves blood flow in areas of stasis by reducing cellular aggregation. **2.** Poly(α-1,6-glucose); α-1,6-glucan with branch points (1,2; 1,3; 1,4) and spacing of these characteristic of the species; used as plasma substitutes or expanders. SEE dextransucrase.

d. 110, d. (average MW 110,000) available as 5% solution in water or saline solution; used as a plasma volume expander.

d. 40, d. (average MW 40,000) used as a plasma volume expander and blood flow adjuvant.

d. 70, d. (average MW 70,000) used as a plasma volume expander.

d. 75, d. (average MW 75,000) used as a plasma volume expander.

acid d., the product of acid and heat treatment of d.

animal d., SYN glycogen.

blue d., high molecular weight d. containing a blue chlorotriazine dye, Cibacron Blue; used to measure the void volumes in gel filtration columns, as well as checking column packing.

d. sulfate, the sodium salt of sulfuric acid esters of the polysaccharide d.; it contains not less than 10 units per mg and not less than 14% of sulfate; an anticoagulant.

dex·tran·ase (deks′tran-ās). An enzyme hydrolyzing α-1,6-D-glucosidic linkages in dextran; used in the prevention of caries.

dex·tran·su·crase (deks-tran-su′krās). A glucosyltransferase that builds poly(α-1,6-D-glucosyl), i.e., polyglucoses, dextrans, or α-glucans, from sucrose, releasing D-fructose residues.

dex·trase (deks′trās). Nonspecific term for the complex of enzymes that converts dextrose (D-glucose) into lactic acid.

dex·tri·fer·ron (deks-tri-fer′on). A colloidal solution of ferric hydroxide in complex with partially hydrolyzed dextrin, used in the treatment of iron-deficiency anemia; it is suitable for intravenous administration and contains 20 mg of iron per ml.

dex·trin (deks′trin). A mixture of oligo(α-1,4-D-glucose) molecules formed during the enzymic or acid hydrolysis of starch, amylopectin, or glycogen; on further hydrolysis they are converted into D-glucose. D.'s are of much lower molecular weight than dextrans, hence are not suitable as plasma expanders; d. (usually white d.) is used in pharmaceutical preparations. SYN starch gum.

acid d., the product of acid and heat treatment of d.

limit d., the polysaccharide fragments remaining at the end (limit) of exhaustive hydrolysis of amylopectin or glycogen by α-1,4-glucan maltohydrolase or β-amylase, which cannot hydrolyze the α-1,6 bonds at branch points; accumulates in individuals with type III glycogen storage disease. SYN dextrin limit.

Schardinger d.'s, cyclic rings of glucose monomer (usually 6 to 8) linked α-1,4; the result of action of *Bacillus macerans* on starch.

dex·tri·nase (deks′tri-nās). Any of the enzymes catalyzing the hydrolysis of dextrins; e.g., amylo-1,6-glucosidase, dextrin dextranase.

limit d., (1) SYN α-dextrin endo-1,6-α-glucosidase; **(2)** SYN oligo-α-1,6-glucosidase.

dex·trin dex·tran·ase. A glucosyltransferase transferring 1,4-α-D-glucosyl residues, thus catalyzing the synthesis of dextrans (with 1,6 links between monosaccharide units) from dextrins (with 1,4 links) by glucose transfer. SYN dextrin → dextran transglucosidase, dextrin 6-glucosyltransferase.

dex·trin → dex·tran trans·glu·co·si·dase. SYN dextrin dextranase.

α-dex·trin en·do-1,6-α-glu·co·si·dase. An enzyme with action similar to that of isoamylase; it cleaves 1,6-α-glucosidic linkages in pullalan, amylopectin, and glycogen, and in α- and β-amylase limit-dextrins of amylopectin and glycogen. Cf. isoamylase. SYN limit dextrinase (1), pullulanase, R enzyme.

dex·trin 6-α-D-glu·co·si·dase. SYN amylo-1,6-glucosidase.

dex·trin 6-glu·co·syl·trans·fer·ase. SYN dextrin dextranase.

dex·trin gly·co·syl·trans·fer·ase. SYN 4-α-D-glucanotransferase.

dex·trin lim·it. SYN limit *dextrin.*

dex·trin·o·gen·ic (deks′trin-ō-jen′ik). Capable of producing dextrin.

dex·tri·no·sis (deks-trin-ō′sis). SYN glycogenosis.

debranching deficiency limit d., limit d., SYN type 3 *glycogenosis.*

dex·trin trans·gly·co·syl·ase. SYN 4-α-D-glucanotransferase.

dex·tri·nu·ria (deks-tri-noo′rē-ă). The passage of dextrin in the urine.

♻ **dextro-, dextr-. 1.** Prefixes meaning right, toward, or on the right side. **2.** Chemical prefixes meaning dextrorotatory. [L. *dexter,* on the right-hand side]

dex·tro·am·phet·a·mine phos·phate (deks′trō-am-fet′ă-mēn). Same actions and uses as dextroamphetamine sulfate. SYN *d*-amphetamine phosphate.

dex·tro·am·phet·a·mine sul·fate. Similar in action to racemic amphetamine sulfate, but is more stimulating to the central nervous system; sympathomimetic and appetite depressant. SYN *d*-amphetamine sulfate, dexamphetamine.

dex·tro·car·dia (deks′trō-kar′dē-ă). Displacement of the heart to the right, either as dextroposition, with simple displacement to the right, or as cardiac heterotaxia, with complete transposition of the right and left chambers, resulting in a heart that is the mirror image of a normal heart. SYN dexiocardia. [dextro- + G. *kardia,* heart]

corrected d., displacement and rotation of the heart into the right side of the chest but without mirror transposition of the cardiac chambers. SYN dextroversion of the heart, false d., type 3 d.

false d., SYN corrected d.

isolated d., d. with mirror-image transposition of the cardiac chambers but without displacement of the abdominal viscera. SYN type 2 d.

mirror image d., perfect right to left congenital reversal of the heart sometimes with other congenital abnormalities, sometimes normal except for position.

secondary d., dextroposition of the heart by some disease of the lungs, pleura, or diaphragm. SYN type 4 d.

type 1 d., SYN d. with situs inversus.

type 2 d., SYN isolated d.

type 3 d., SYN corrected d.

type 4 d., SYN secondary d.

d. with si′tus inver′sus, displacement of the heart to the right side of the chest with mirror-image transposition of the cardiac chambers together with transposition of the abdominal viscera. SYN type 1 d.

dex·tro·car·di·o·gram (deks′trō-kar′dē-ō-gram). That part of the electrocardiogram that is derived from the right ventricle.

dex·tro·ce·re·bral (deks′trō-ser′ĕ-brăl). Having a dominant right cerebral hemisphere.

dex·troc·u·lar (deks-trok′ū-lăr). Rarely used term for indicating right ocular dominance; denoting one who prefers the right eye in monocular work, such as microscopy. SYN right-eyed. [dextro- + L. *oculus,* eye]

dex·tro·cy·clo·duc·tion (deks′trō-sī-klō-dŭk′shŭn). Rotation of the upper pole of the cornea to the right. SEE excycloduction. [dextro- + cyclo- + L. *duco,* pp. *ductus,* to lead]

dex·tro·duc·tion (deks-trō-dŭk′shŭn). Rarely used term for rotation of one eye to the right. [dextro- + L. *duco,* pp. *ductus,* to lead]

dex′tro·gas′tria (deks-trō-gas′trē-ă). Condition in which the stomach is displaced to the right; may represent either simple displacement or situs inversus. Usually associated with dextrocardia. [dextro- + G. *gastēr,* stomach]

dex·tro·glu·cose (deks-trō-gloo′kōs). SEE D-glucose.

dex·tro·gram (deks′trō-gram). Electrocardiographic record in an experimental animal representing spread of impulse through the right ventricle alone.

dex·tro·gy·ra·tion (deks′trō-jī-rā′shŭn). A twisting to the right. [dextro- + L. *gyro,* pp. *-atus,* to turn in a circle, fr. *gyrus,* circle]

dex·tro·man·u·al (deks-trō-man′ū-ăl). SYN right-handed. [dextro- + L. *manus,* hand]

dex·tro·meth·or·phan hy·dro·bro·mide (deks′trō-meth-ōr′fan hī-drō-brō′mīd). A synthetic morphine derivative used as an antitussive agent. Inferior to codeine but seemingly lacking in dependence production. It has weak central depressant action.

dex·tro·mor·a·mide tar·trate (deks-trō-mōr′ă-mīd). A narcotic analgesic related chemically and pharmacologically to methadone.

dex·trop·e·dal (deks-trop′ĕ-dăl). Denoting one who uses the right leg in preference to the left. SYN right-footed. [dextro- + L. *pes (ped-),* foot]

dex·tro·po·si·tion (deks′trō-pō-zi′shŭn). Abnormal right-sided location or origin of a normally left-sided structure, e.g., origin of the aorta from the right ventricle.

d. of the heart, SEE dextrocardia.

dex·tro·pro·pox·y·phene hy·dro·chlo·ride (deks′trō-prō-pok′sē-fēn). SYN propoxyphene hydrochloride.

dex·tro·pro·pox·y·phene nap·syl·ate. SYN propoxyphene napsylate.

dex·tro·ro·ta·tion (deks′trō-rō-tā′shŭn). A turning or twisting to the right; especially, the clockwise twist given the plane of plane-polarized light by solutions of certain optically active substances. Cf. levorotation.

dex·tro·ro·ta·to·ry (deks-trō-rō′tă-tōr-ē). Denoting dextrorotation, or certain crystals or solutions capable of such action; as a chemical prefix, usually abbreviated *d*-. Cf. levorotatory.

dex·trose (deks′trōs). SEE D-glucose.

dex·tro·si·nis·tral (deks′trō-si-nis′trăl). In a direction from right to left. [dextro- + L. *sinister,* left]

dex·tro·thy·rox·ine so·di·um (deks-trō-thī-roks′ēn). An antihypercholesterolemic agent.

dex·tro·tor·sion (deks-trō-tōr′shŭn). **1.** A twisting to the right. **2.** In ophthalmology, a seldom-used term for a conjugate rotation of the upper pole of both corneas to the right. [dextro- + L. *torsio,* a twisting]

dex·tro·tro·p·ic (dek-trō-trop′ik). Turning to the right. [dextro- + G. *tropos,* a turn]

dex·tro·ver·sion (deks′trō-ver′zhŭn). **1.** Version toward the right. **2.** In ophthalmology, a conjugate rotation of both eyes to the right. [dextro- + L. *verto,* pp. *versus,* to turn]

d. of the heart, SYN corrected *dextrocardia.*

d.f.. Abbreviation for *degrees* of freedom, under *degree.*

df, DF Abbreviation for decayed and filled teeth. SYN df caries *index.*

DFP Abbreviation for diisopropyl fluorophosphate.

dGlc Abbreviation for 2-deoxyglucose.

dGMP Abbreviation for deoxyguanylic acid.

DHAP Abbreviation for *dihydroxyacetone* phosphate.

Dharmendra an·ti·gen. See under antigen.

DHEA Abbreviation for dehydroepiandrosterone.

DHEA Abbreviation for dehydro-3-epiandrosterone.

DHEAS Abbreviation for the sulfate salt of dehydroepiandrosterone.

d'Herelle, Felix H., Canadian physician and bacteriologist, 1873–1949. SEE d'H. *phenomenon;* Twort-d'H. *phenomenon.*

DHF Abbreviation for dihydrofolic acid.

DHFR Abbreviation for dihydrofolate reductase.

D. Hy. Abbreviation for Doctor of Hygiene.

DI Abbreviation for dental *index.*

di-. **1.** Two, twice. **2.** In chemistry, often used in place of bis-when not likely to be confusing; e.g., dichloro- compounds. Cf. bi-, bis-. [G. *dis,* two]

dia-. Through, throughout, completely. [G. *dia,* through]

di·a·be·tes (dī-ă-bē′tēz). Either d. insipidus or d. mellitus, diseases having in common the symptom polyuria; when used without qualification, refers to d. mellitus. [G. *diabētēs,* a compass, a siphon, diabetes]

adult-onset d., non-insulin-dependent d. mellitus.

alimentary d., SYN alimentary *glycosuria.*

alloxan d., experimental d. mellitus produced in animals by the administration of alloxan, which damages the insulin-producing islet cells of the pancreas.

brittle d., d. mellitus in which there are marked fluctuations in blood glucose concentrations that are difficult to control.

bronze d., d. mellitus associated with hemochromatosis, with iron deposits in the skin, liver, pancreas, and other viscera, often with severe liver damage and glycosuria. SEE ALSO hemochromatosis. SYN bronzed d., bronzed disease.

bronzed d., SYN bronze d.

calcinuric d., SYN hypercalciuria.

chemical d., SYN latent d.

galactose d., SYN galactosemia.

gestational d., carbohydrate intolerance of variable severity with onset or first recognition during pregnancy.

di

Gestational diabetes occurs in 3–6% of all pregnancies, and although it typically resolves after delivery, as many as 60% of women with this disorder eventually develop type 2 diabetes. Diabetes occurring during pregnancy increases the risk of maternal pyelonephritis and of certain congenital anomalies, and is often associated with polyhydramnios and fetal macrosomia, with resultant dystocia. It is recommended that all pregnant women be screened for gestational diabetes between the 24th and 28th week of pregnancy by determination of the plasma glucose level 1 hour after a 50 g oral glucose load. A level above 140 mg/dL (7.8 mmol/L) is an indication for a 3-hour glucose tolerance test. Gestational diabetes can usually be managed by diet alone, but insulin is sometimes required.

growth-onset d., SYN insulin-dependent d. mellitus.

d. in′nocens, obsolete term for renal *glycosuria.*

d. insip′idus, chronic excretion of very large amounts of pale urine of low specific gravity, causing dehydration and extreme thirst; ordinarily results from inadequate output of pituitary antidiuretic hormone; the urine abnormalities may be mimicked as a result of excessive fluid intake, as in psychogenic polydipsia. Several types exist: central, neurohypophyseal, and nephrogenic. Autosomal dominant [MIM*125700, *125800, *192340], X-linked [MIM*304800 and *304900], and even autosomal recessive forms [MIM*222000] have been described. SEE ALSO nephrogenic d. insipidus.

insulin-dependent d. mellitus (IDDM), severe d. mellitus, often brittle, usually of abrupt onset during the first two decades of life but can develop at any age; characterized by polydipsia, polyuria, increased appetite, weight loss, low plasma insulin levels, and susceptibility to ketoacidosis; immune-mediated destruction of pancreatic B cells; insulin therapy and dietary regulation are necessary. Term declared obsolete by American Diabetes Association. SYN growth-onset d., juvenile-onset d., type I d.

insulinopenic d., any form of d. mellitus resulting from inadequate secretion of insulin.

d. intermit′tens, d. mellitus in which there are periods of relatively normal carbohydrate metabolism followed by relapses to the previous diabetic state.

juvenile d., d. mellitus appearing in a child or adolescent; often fatal before the discovery of insulin, usually of abrupt onset during first or second decades of life; characterized by polyuria, polydipsia, weight loss; usually severe, insulin dependent, and prone to periods of ketoacidosis; can be familial, follow a viral infection such as mumps; thought to be due to virus-induced or immune destruction of pancreatic islets. SYN type I d. mellitus.

juvenile-onset d., SYN insulin-dependent d. mellitus.

ketosis-prone d., type I or juvenile d. mellitus, in which inadequate treatment leads to development of ketoacidosis.

ketosis-resistant d., type II or adult onset d. mellitus, in which episodes of ketoacidosis rarely occur.

latent d., a mild form of d. mellitus in which the patient displays no overt symptoms, but displays certain abnormal responses to diagnostic procedures, such as an elevated fasting blood glucose concentration or reduced glucose tolerance. Term declared obsolete by American Diabetes Association. SYN chemical d.

lipoatrophic d., SYN lipoatrophy.

lipogenous d., d. and obesity combined.

maturity-onset d., non-insulin-dependent d. mellitus.

maturity onset d. of youth, a relatively mild, non-insulin requiring form of d. mellitus beginning at a younger age than usual.

d. melli′tus (DM), a chronic metabolic disorder in which utilization of carbohydrate is impaired and that of lipid and protein enhanced; it is caused by an absolute or relative deficiency of insulin and is characterized, in more severe cases, by chronic hyperglycemia, glycosuria, water and electrolyte loss, ketoacidosis, and coma; long-term complications include neuropathy, retinopathy, nephropathy, generalized degenerative changes in large and small blood vessels, and increased susceptibility to infection. [L. sweetened with honey]

---

diabetes mellitus (DM): etiologic classification

I. Primary diabetes mellitus (types 1 and 2)

II. Secondary diabetes

  A. pancreatic diabetes:
    – after total or partial pancreatectomy
    – with extensive destruction of pancreas
    – through tumor or wound
    – pancreatitis; hemochromatosis

  B. extrapancreatic/endocrine diabetes
    – with hypersomatotropism (acromegaly)
    – with hyperadrenalism (Cushing syndrome; Conn syndrome, pheochromocytoma)
    – with hyperthyroidism
    – with glucagonoma

  C. drug-induced diabetes
    – (somatotropin; ACTH; adrenocorticoid [steroid diabetes]; thyroid hormone)
    – thiazides

III. Rare, exceptional forms of diabetes
  e.g., lipoatrophic diabetes
  (Lawrence); myatonic diabetes (Prader-Labhart-Willi); disturbance of insulin receptors; DM with certain genetic syndromes

---

Diabetes mellitus affects at least 16 million Americans, ranks seventh as a cause of death in the United States, and costs the national economy over $100 billion yearly. About 95% of persons with DM have type 2, in which the pancreatic beta cells retain some insulin-producing potential, and the rest have type 1, in which exogenous insulin is required for long-term survival. In type 1 DM, which typically causes symptoms before age 25, an autoimmune process is responsible for beta cell destruction. Type 2 DM is characterized by insulin resistance in peripheral tissues as well as a defect in insulin secretion by beta cells. Insulin regulates carbohydrate metabolism by mediating the rapid transport of glucose and amino acids from the circulation into muscle and other tissue cells, by promoting the storage of glucose in liver cells as glycogen, and by inhibiting gluconeogenesis. The normal stimulus for the release of insulin from the pancreas is a rise in the concentration of glucose in circulating blood, which typically occurs within a few minutes after a meal. When such a rise elicits an appropriate insulin response, so that the blood level of glucose falls again as it is taken into cells, glucose tolerance is said to be normal. The central fact in diabetes mellitus is an impairment of glucose tolerance of such a degree as to threaten or impair health. Revised diagnostic criteria for DM were published by the American Diabetes Association in June 1997. All criteria depend on the glucose concentration of venous plasma. The diagnosis is confirmed when any 2 tests performed on different days yield levels at or above established thresholds: in the fasting state, 126 mg/dL (7.0 mmol/L); 2 hours postprandially (after a 75-g glucose load), or at random, 200 mg/dL (11.1 mmol/L).

Long recognized as an independent risk factor for cardiovascular disease, DM is often associated with other risk factors, including disorders of lipid metabolism, obesity, hypertension, and impairment of renal function. Current recommendations for the management of DM emphasize education and individualization of therapy. Controlled studies have shown that rigorous maintenance of plasma glucose levels as near to normal as possible at all times substantially reduces the incidence and severity of long-term complications, particularly microvascular complications (retinopathy, neuropathy, and nephropathy). Such control involves limitation of dietary carbohydrate and saturated fat; monitoring of blood glucose, including self-testing by the patient and periodic determination of glycosylated hemoglobin; and administration of insulin (particularly in type 1 DM), drugs that stimulate endogenous insulin production (in type 2 DM), or both. Some studies suggest that the risk of cardiovascular disease may be increased in some patients by intensive treatment of DM because of elevation of body weight, blood pressure, triglycerides, and total and low-density cholesterol. Pharmaceutical agents developed during the 1990s have improved control of DM by enhancing responsiveness of cells to insulin, counteracting insulin resistance, and reducing postprandial carbohydrate absorption. See Also insulin resistance; alpha-reductase inhibitor.

metahypophysial d., (1) d. mellitus caused by large quantities of endogenous or exogenous pituitary growth hormone; **(2)** term used to designate the irreversible phase of d. mellitus in acromegaly.

Mosler d., inosituria with excretion of large quantities of water.

nephrogenic d. insipidus [MIM*304800], d. insipidus due to inability of the kidney tubules to respond to antidiuretic hormone; X-linked inheritance, caused by mutation in the vasopressin V2 receptor gene (AVPR2) on Xq. There is also an autosomal dominant form [MIM*125800], caused by mutation in the aquaphorin 2 gene (AQP2) on 12q. SYN vasopressin-resistant d.

non-insulin-dependent d. mellitus (NIDDM), an often mild form of d. mellitus of gradual onset, usually in obese individuals over age 35; absolute plasma insulin levels are normal to high, but relatively low in relation to plasma glucose levels; ketoacidosis is rare, but hyperosmolar coma can occur; responds well to dietary regulation and/or oral hypoglycemic agents, but diabetic complications and degenerative changes can develop. Term declared obsolete by American Diabetes Association.

pancreatic d., (1) d. mellitus demonstrably dependent upon a pancreatic lesion; **(2)** d. following removal of the pancreas in an animal.

phlorizin d. (flō-rid′zin), SYN phlorizin *glycosuria.*

phosphate d., excessive secretion of phosphate in the urine due to a defect in tubular reabsorption; usually part of a more generalized abnormality, such as Fanconi syndrome.

piqûre d., SYN puncture d. [Fr.]

pregnancy d., SEE subclinical d.

puncture d., experimental d. produced in animals by puncture of the floor of the fourth ventricle of the brain. SYN piqûre d.

renal d., SYN renal *glycosuria.*

starvation d., after prolonged fasting, glycosuria following the ingestion of carbohydrate or glucose because of reduced output of insulin and/or reduced rate of glucose metabolism with a reduced ability to form glycogen.

steroid d., d. mellitus produced by pharmacological doses of steroid hormones, particularly glucocorticoids or estrogens; characterized by one or more of the typical manifestations of d. mellitus.

steroidogenic d., abnormal glucose tolerance, often frank d. mellitus, induced by the metabolic effects of adrenocortical steroid hormones such as cortisone or therapeutic analogues such as prednisone. The effect may be temporary, resolving when the steroid therapy is discontinued, or d. mellitus may persist.

subclinical d., a form of d. mellitus that is clinically evident only under certain circumstances, such as pregnancy or extreme stress; persons so afflicted may, in time, manifest more severe forms of the disease. Term declared obsolete by American Diabetes Association.

thiazide d., impaired carbohydrate metabolism associated with the use of thiazide diuretic drugs; severe manifestations are seen in persons having d. mellitus, but impairment is mild or absent in nondiabetic individuals.

type I d., SYN insulin-dependent d. mellitus.

type II d., non-insulin-dependent d. mellitus.

type I d. mellitus, SYN juvenile d.

vasopressin-resistant d., SYN nephrogenic d. insipidus.

di·a·bet·ic (dī-ă-bet′ik). **1.** Relating to or suffering from diabetes. **2.** One who suffers from diabetes.

di·a·be·to·gen·ic (dī′ă-bet-ō-jen′ik, -bē-tō-jen′ik). Causing diabetes.

di·a·be·tog·en·ous (dī′ă-bĕ-toj′en-ŭs). Caused by diabetes.

di·a·be·tol·o·gy (dī′ă-be-tol′ō-jē). The field of medicine concerned with diabetes.

di·a·cele (dī′ă-sēl). Rarely used term for third *ventricle.* [G. *dia-,* through, + *koilia,* a hollow]

di·ac·e·tal (dī-as′ē-tal). SEE diacetyl.

di·ac·e·tate (dī-as′ĕ-tāt). **1.** SYN acetoacetate. **2.** A compound containing two acetate residues.

di·ac·e·te·mia (dī-as-ĕ-tē′mē-ă). A form of acidosis resulting from the presence of acetoacetic (diacetic) acid in the blood.

di·ac·e·ton·u·ria (dī-as′ĕ-tō-noo′rē-ă). SYN diaceturia.

di·ac·e·tu·ria (dī-as-ĕ-too′rē-ă). The urinary excretion of acetoacetic (diacetic) acid. SYN diacetonuria.

di·a·ce·tyl, di·ac·e·tal (dī-as′ē-til, dī-as′ē-tal). A yellow liquid, $(CH_3CO)_2$, having the pungent odor of quinone and carrying the aromas of coffee, vinegar, butter, and other foods; a byproduct of carbohydrate degradation.

di·a·ce·tyl·cho·line (dī-as′ĕ-til-kō′lēn). SYN succinylcholine.

di·a·ce·tyl·mon·ox·ime (DAM) (dī-as′ĕ-til-mon-ok′sīm). A 2-oxo-oxime that can reactivate phosphorylated acetylcholinesterase in vitro and in vivo; it penetrates the blood-brain barrier. SImilar to 2-PAM.

di·a·ce·tyl·mor·phine (dī-as′ĕ-til-mōr′fēn). SYN heroin.

di·a·ce·tyl·tan·nic ac·id (dī-as′ĕ-til-tan′ik). SYN acetyltannic acid.

di·a·chron·ic (dī-ă-kron′ik). Systematically observed over time in the same subjects throughout as opposed to synchronic or cross-sectional; the inferences are equivalent only where there is strict stability of all elements. [dia- + G. *chronos,* time]

di·ac·id (dī-as′id). Denoting a substance containing two ionizable hydrogen atoms per molecule; more generally, a base capable of combining with two hydrogen ions per molecule.

di·ac·la·sis, di·a·cla·sia (dī-ak′lă-sis, dī-ă-klā′zē-ă). SYN osteoclasis. [G. *diaklasis,* a breaking up, fr. *dia,* through, + *klasis,* a breaking]

di·ac·ri·nous (dī-ak′ri-nŭs). Excreting by simple passage through a gland cell. [G. *diakrinō,* to separate one from another]

di·ac·ri·sis (dī-ak′ri-sis). SYN diagnosis. [G. *dia-,* through, + *krisis,* a judgment]

di·a·crit·ic, di·a·crit·i·cal (dī-ă-krit′ik, -krit′i-kăl). Distinguishing; diagnostic; allowing of distinction. [G. *diakritikos,* able to distinguish]

di·ac·tin·ic (dī′ak-tin′ik). Having the property of transmitting light capable of bringing about chemical reactions. [G. *dia,* through, + *aktis,* ray]

di·ac·yl·glyc·er·ol (DAG) (dī′as-il-glis′er-ol). Diglyceride; glycerol with two esterified acyl moieties, either 1,3-d. or 1,2-d.; if the two acyl groups are nonidentical, there are four possible stereoisomers; 1,2-d. is an intermediate in the synthesis of triacylglycerols and of lecithin; also serves as a second messenger in stimulating the activity of protein kinase C.

d. acyltransferase, an enzyme, in fat biosynthesis, that catalyzes the transfer of an acyl moiety from acyl-CoA to 1,2-d. thus forming free coenzyme A and triacylglycerol.

d. lipase, SYN lipoprotein lipase.

di·ad (dī′ad). **1.** The transverse tubule and a cisterna in cardiac muscle fibers. **2.** SYN dyad (1).

di·ad·o·cho·ci·ne·sia (dī-ad′ō-kō-si-nē′zē-ă). SYN diadochokinesia.

di·ad·o·cho·ki·ne·sia, di·ad·o·cho·ki·ne·sis (dī-ad′ō-kō-ki-nē′zē-ă, -ki-nē′sis). The normal power of alternately bringing a limb into opposite positions, as of flexion and extention or of pronation and supination. SYN diadochocinesia. [G. *diadochos,* working in turn, + *kinēsis,* movement]

di·ad·o·cho·ki·net·ic (dī-ad′ō-kō-ki-net′ik). Relating to diadochokinesia.

di·ag·nose (dī-ag-nōs′). To make a diagnosis.

di·ag·no·sis (dī-ag-nō′sis). The determination of the nature of a disease, injury, or congenital defect. SYN diacrisis. [G. *diagnōsis,* a deciding]

di

antenatal d., SYN prenatal d.

clinical d., a d. made from a study of the signs and symptoms of a disease.

differential d., the determination of which of two or more diseases with similar symptoms is the one from which the patient is suffering, by a systematic comparison and contrasting of the clinical findings. SYN differentiation (2).

d. by exclusion, a d. made by excluding those diseases to which only some of the patient's symptoms might belong, leaving one disease as the most likely d., although no definitive tests or findings establish that d.

laboratory d., a d. made by a chemical, microscopic, microbiologic, immunologic, or pathologic study of secretions, discharges, blood, or tissue.

neonatal d., systematic evaluation of the newborn for evidence of disease or malformations, and the conclusion reached.

pathologic d., a d., sometimes postmortem, made from an anatomic and/or histologic study of the lesions present.

physical d., (1) a d. made by means of physical examination of the patient. **(2)** the process of a physical examination.

prenatal d., d. utilizing procedures available for the recognition of diseases and malformations *in utero*, and the conclusion reached. SYN antenatal d.

di·ag·nos·tic (dī-ag-nos′tik). **1.** Relating to or aiding in diagnosis. **2.** Establishing or confirming a diagnosis.

di·ag·nos·ti·cian (dī′ag-nos-tish′ăn). One who is skilled in making diagnoses; formerly, a name for specialists in internal medicine.

Diagnostic and Statistical Manual of Mental Disorders (DSM). A system of classification, published by the American Psychiatric Association, that divides recognized mental disorders into clearly defined categories based on sets of objective criteria. Representing a majority view (rather than a consensus) of hundreds of contributors and consultants, DSM is widely recognized as a diagnostic standard and widely used for reporting, coding, and statistical purposes.

The first edition (1952), based on the sixth revision of the *International Classification of Diseases (ICD-6)*, was intended to promote uniformity in the naming and reporting of psychiatric disorders. It contained definitions of all named disorders, but no sets of diagnostic criteria. While its classification of mental disorders showed the influence of Freudian psychoanalysis, its nomenclature (e.g., depressive reaction, anxiety reaction, schizophrenic reaction) reflected the theories of Adolf Meyer (1866–1950). The second edition (*DSM-II*, 1968) preserved the psychoanalytic orientation but dropped the "reaction" terminology. The third edition (*DSM-III*, 1980) abandoned much of the rigidly psychodynamic thinking of the earlier editions and, for the first time, provided explicit diagnostic criteria and introduced a multiaxial system whereby different aspects of a patient's condition could be separately assessed. Briefly stated, the axes are I, clinical disorders; II, personality disorders and mental retardation; III, general medical disorders; IV, psychosocial and environmental stressors; and V, overall level of functioning. A revised version of the third edition (*DSM-IIIR*, 1987) incorporated a number of improvements and clarifications. The fourth edition (*DSM-IV*) appeared in May, 1994. It follows its two predecessors closely in general outline, and like them is coordinated with and partly derived from *ICD-9*. For many observers, the most significant change in *DSM-IV* is the renaming of the category formerly called "Organic Mental Syndromes and Disorders" as "Delirium, Dementia, and Amnestic and Other Cognitive Disorders," a shift in terminology intended to avoid the implication that mental disorders in other categories are not organic.

---

di·a·gram. A simple, graphic depiction of an idea or object.

Dieuaide d., SYN triaxial reference *system*.

flow d., a d. composed of blocks connected by arrows representing steps in a process such as decision analysis.

Venn d., pictorial representation of the extent to which two or more quantities or concepts are mutually inclusive and exclusive.

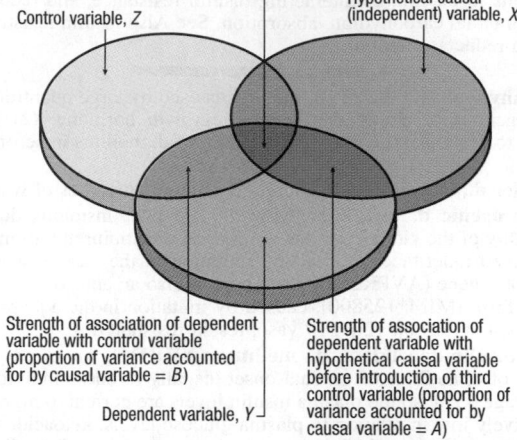

Overlap, in associations with dependent variable, of hypothetical causal variable and control variable (≈C)

Control variable, Z

Hypothetical causal (independent) variable, X

Strength of association of dependent variable with control variable (proportion of variance accounted for by causal variable = B)

Strength of association of dependent variable with hypothetical causal variable before introduction of third control variable (proportion of variance accounted for by causal variable = A)

Dependent variable, Y

Venn diagram

---

di·a·ki·ne·sis (dī′ă-ki-nē′sis). Final stage of prophase in meiosis I, in which the chiasmata present during the diplotene stage disappear, the chromosomes continue to shorten, and the nucleolus and nuclear membrane disappear. [G. *dia,* through, + *kinēsis,* movement]

dial (dī′ăl, dīl). A clock face or instrument resembling a clock face. [L. *dies,* day]

astigmatic d., a diagram of radiating lines, used to test for astigmatism.

Di·a·lis·ter (dī-ăl-is′ter). An obsolete name for a genus of bacteria, the type species of which, *D. pneumosintes,* is now placed in the genus *Bacteroides.*

di·al·lyl (dī-al′il). A compound containing two allyl groups.

di·al·y·sance (dī-al′i-sans). The number of milliliters of blood completely cleared of any substance by an artificial kidney or by peritoneal dialysis in a unit of time; conventional clearance formulas are expressed as mm/min. [fr. dialysis]

di·al·y·sate (dī-al′i-sāt). That part of a mixture that passes through a dialyzing membrane; the material that does not pass through is referred to as the retentate. SYN diffusate.

di·al·y·sis (dī-al′i-sis). **1.** A form of filtration to separate crystalloid from colloid substances (or smaller molecules from larger ones) in a solution by interposing a semipermeable membrane between the solution and dialyzing fluid; the crystalloid (smaller) substances pass through the membrane into the dialyzing fluid on the other side, the colloids do not. **2.** The separation of substances across a semipermeable membrane on the basis of particle size and/or concentration gradients. **3.** A method of artificial kidney function. [G. a separation, fr. *dialyo,* to separate]

continuous ambulatory peritoneal d. (CAPD), method of peritoneal d. performed in ambulatory patients with influx and efflux of dialysate during normal activities.

equilibrium d., in immunology, a method for determination of association constants for hapten-antibody reactions in a system in which the hapten (dialyzable) and antibody (nondialyzable) solutions are separated by semipermeable membranes. Since at equilibrium the quantity of free hapten will be the same in the two compartments, quantitative determinations can be made of hapten-bound antibody, free antibody, and free hapten.

extracorporeal d., hemodialysis performed through an apparatus outside the body.

peritoneal d., removal from the body of soluble substances and water by transfer across the peritoneum, utilizing a d. solution which is intermittently introduced into and removed from the peritoneal cavity; transfer of diffusable solutes and water between the blood and the peritoneal cavity depends on the concentration gradient between the two fluid compartments.

d. ret′i·nae, congenital or traumatic separation of the peripheral sensory retina from the retinal pigment epithelium at the ora serrata, often causing a retinal detachment. SYN retinodialysis.

di·a·lyze (dī′ă-līz). To perform dialysis; to separate a substance from a solution by means of dialysis.

di·a·lyz·er (dī′ă-lī-zer). The apparatus for performing dialysis; a membrane used in dialysis.

di·a·mag·net·ic (dī′ă-mag-net′ik). Having the property of diamagnetism.

di·a·mag·net·ism (dī-ă-mag′nĕ-tizm). The property displayed by substances that have a very small negative magnetic susceptibility, given by molecules in which all electrons are paired; an unpaired electron yields a magnetic movement, hence the molecule containing such exhibits paramagnetism.

di·a·me·lia (dī-ă-mē′lē-ă). Absence of two limbs.

di·am·e·ter (dī-am′ĕ-ter). **1.** A straight line connecting two opposite points on the surface of a more or less spherical or cylindrical body, or at the boundary of an opening or foramen, passing through the center of such body or opening. **2.** The distance measured along such a line. [G. *diametros,* fr. *dia,* through, + *metron,* measure]

anteroposterior d. of the pelvic inlet, SYN median *conjugate.*

biparietal d., the d. of the fetal head between the two parietal eminences.

buccolingual d., the d. of the crown of a tooth measured from the buccal to the lingual surfaces.

conjugate d. of pelvic inlet, SYN median *conjugate.*

conjugate d. of pelvic outlet, SYN straight *conjugate.*

diagonal conjugate d., SYN diagonal *conjugate.*

external conjugate d., SYN external *conjugate.*

d. obli′qua [TA], SYN oblique d.

oblique d. [TA], a measurement across the pelvic inlet from the sacroiliac joint of one side to the opposite iliopectineal eminence. SYN d. obliqua [TA].

obstetric conjugate d., SYN true *conjugate.*

occipitofrontal d., the d. of the fetal head from the external occipital protuberance to the most prominent point of the frontal bone in the midline.

occipitomental d., the d. of the fetal head from the external occipital protuberance to the midpoint of the chin.

posterior sagittal d., distance from the sacrococcygeal junction to the middle of an imaginary line running between the left and right ischial tuberosities.

suboccipitobregmatic d., the d. of the fetal head from the lowest posterior point of the occipital bone to the center of the anterior fontanelle.

total end-diastolic d. (TEDD), cross sectional d. of the left ventricle including the septum and posterior wall thicknesses in diastole.

total end-systolic d. (TESD), cross sectional d. of the left ventricle including the septum and posterior wall thicknesses in systole.

trachelobregmatic d., the d. of the fetal head from the middle of the anterior fontanelle to the neck.

d. transver′sa [TA], SYN transverse d.

transverse d. [TA], the transverse d. of the pelvic inlet, measured between the terminal lines. SYN d. transversa [TA].

zygomatic d., the extreme breadth of the skull at the zygomatic arches.

di·am·ide (dī′am-id, -īd). A compound containing two amide groups.

di·am·i·dines (dī-am′i-dēnz). A group of compounds containing two amidine groups; e.g., stilbamidine, propamidine.

di·a·mine (dī′ă-mēn, -min). An organic compound containing two amine groups per molecule; e.g., ethylenediamine, $NH_2CH_2CH_2NH_2$.

d. oxidase, SYN *amine* oxidase (copper-containing), *amine* oxidase (flavin-containing).

di·am·ni·ot·ic (dī-am-nē-ot′ik). Exhibiting two amniotic sacs.

Diamond, Louis K., U.S. physician, 1902–1995. SEE D.-Blackfan *anemia, syndrome;* Gardner-D. *syndrome;* Shwachman-Diamond *syndrome.*

di·am·tha·zole di·hy·dro·chlo·ride (dī-am′thă-zōl). An antifungal agent for topical use. SYN dimazole dihydrochloride.

di·an·dry, di·an·dria (dī′an-drē, dī-an′drē-ă). The phenomenon in which a single ovum is fertilized by a diploid sperm and hence produces a triploid fetus. Cf. digyny. [di- + G. *andros,* male]

di·a·no·et·ic (dī′ă-nō-et′ik). Of or pertaining to reason or other intellectual functions. [G. *dia,* through, + *noeō,* to think]

di·a·pause (dī′ă-pawz). A period of biological quiescence or dormancy with decreased metabolism; an interval in which development is arrested or greatly slowed. [dia- + G. *pausis,* pause]

embryonic d., a d. in the course of embryogenesis; postulated to occur in instances of double parturition and possibly of delayed implantation.

di·a·pe·de·sis (dī′ă-pĕ-dē′sis). The passage of blood, or any of its formed elements, through the intact walls of blood vessels. SYN migration (2). [G. *dia,* through, + *pēdēsis,* a leaping]

di·a·phan·og·ra·phy (dī-ă-fă-nog′ră-fē). Examination of a body part by transillumination, especially for the detection of breast cancer. [G. *diaphanēs,* transparent, + *graphō,* to write]

di·aph·a·nos·cope (dī-af′ă-nō-skōp). An instrument for illuminating the interior of a cavity to determine the translucency of its walls. SYN polyscope. [G. *diaphanēs,* transparent, + *skopeō,* to examine]

di·aph·a·nos·co·py (dī-af-ă-nos′kŏ-pē). Examination of a cavity with a diaphanoscope.

di·a·phe·met·ric (dī′ă-fĕ-met′rik). Relating to the determination of the degree of tactile sensibility. [G. *dia,* through, + *haphē,* touch, + *metron,* measure]

di·a·phen hy·dro·chlo·ride (dī′ă-fen). An antihistaminic agent with anticholinergic properties.

di·aph·o·rase (dī-af′ōr-ās). Originally, a series of flavoproteins with reductase activity in mitochondria; now dihydrolipoamide dehydrogenase.

di·a·pho·re·sis (dī′ă-fō-rē′sis). SYN perspiration (1). [G. *diaphorēsis,* fr. *dia,* through, + *phoreō,* to carry]

di·a·pho·ret·ic (dī-ă-fō-ret′ik). **1.** Relating to, or causing, perspiration. **2.** An agent that increases perspiration.

di·a·phragm (dī′ă-fram). **1.** The musculomembranous partition between the abdominal and thoracic cavities. SYN diaphragma (2) [TA], interseptum, midriff, phren (1). **2.** A thin disk pierced with an opening, used in a microscope, camera, or other optical instrument in order to shut out the marginal rays of light, thus giving a more direct illumination. **3.** A flexible ring covered with a dome-shaped sheet of elastic material used in the vagina to prevent pregnancy. **4.** In radiography, a grid (2) or a lead sheet with an aperture. SEE collimator. [G. *diaphragma*]

aperture d., a metal device that limits the area of the beam emerging from an x-ray tube.

Bucky d., in radiography, a d. with a moving grid that avoids grid shadows. SYN Potter-Bucky d.

d. of mouth, SYN mylohyoid (*muscle*).

pelvic d., the paired levator ani and coccygeus muscles together with the fascia above and below them. SYN d. of pelvis, diaphragma pelvis.

d. of pelvis, SYN pelvic d.

Potter-Bucky d., SYN Bucky d.

d. sellae, SYN *diaphragma* sellae.

sellar d., ✶official alternate term for *diaphragma* sellae.

d. of sella turcica, SYN *diaphragma* sellae.

urogenital d., an obsolete concept of a trilaminar, triangular sheet of muscle and fascia spanning the ischiopubic rami; composed of the sphincter urethrae and the deep transverse perineal muscles (which were said to be flat muscles forming a continuous sheet), plus the perineal membrane below and a superior fascia of the

di

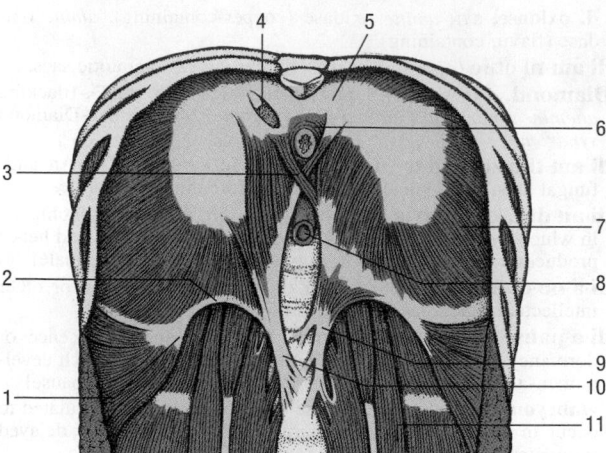

diaphragm (abdominal surface): (1) lateral arcuate ligament, (2) medial arcuate ligament, (3) median arcuate ligament, (4) caval opening, (5) central tendon, (6) esophageal hiatus with esophagus, (7) costal part of diaphragm, (8) aortic hiatus with aorta, (9) left crus, (10) right crus, (11) muscles of posterior abdominal wall

diaphragm above. Evidence of the latter is lacking. The muscle-containing space between the fascial structures was formerly referred to as the deep perineal space. The terms urogenital d. and deep perineal *space* are not recognized by Terminologia Anatomica due to more accurate understanding of the morphology, especially of the sphincter urethrae. SYN diaphragma urogenitale.

di·a·phrag·ma, pl. **di·a·phrag·ma·ta** (dī-ă-frag′mă, -frag′mă-tă) [TA]. **1.** A thin partition separating adjacent regions. **2.** SYN diaphragm (1). [G. *diaphragma,* a partition wall, midriff]

d. oris, SYN mylohyoid (*muscle*).

d. pel′vis, SYN pelvic *diaphragm.*

d. sel′lae [TA], a fold of dura mater extending transversely across the sella turcica and roofing over the hypophyseal fossa; it is perforated in its center for the passage of the infundibulum. SYN sellar diaphragm✩, diaphragm of sella turcica, diaphragm sellae, tentorium of hypophysis.

d. urogenita′le, SYN urogenital *diaphragm.*

di·a·phrag·mal·gia (dī′ă-frag-mal′jē-ă). Rarely used term for a pain in the diaphragm. SYN diaphragmodynia. [diaphragm + G. *algos,* pain]

di·a·phrag·mat·ic (dī′ă-frag-mat′ik). Relating to a diaphragm. SYN phrenic (1).

di·a·phrag·mat·o·cele (dī′ă-frag-mat′ō-sēl). Rarely used term for diaphragmatic *hernia.* [diaphragm + G. *kēlē,* hernia]

di·a·phrag·mo·dyn·ia (dī′ă-frag-mō-din′ē-ă). SYN diaphragmalgia. [diaphragm + G. *odynē,* pain]

di·aph·y·se·al (dī-ă-fiz′ē-ăl). SYN diaphysial.

di·a·phy·sec·to·my (dī′ă-fi-sek′tō-mē). Partial or complete removal of the shaft of a long bone. [diaphysis + G. *ektomē,* excision]

di·a·phys·i·al (dī-ă-fiz′ē-ăl). Relating to a diaphysis. SYN diaphyseal.

di·aph·y·sis, pl. **di·aph·y·ses** (dī-af′i-sis, -sēz) [TA]. An elongated rodlike structure, as the part of a long bone between the epiphysial extremities. The shaft of a long bone, as distinguished from the epiphyses, or extremities, and apophyses, or outgrowths. SYN shaft [TA]. [G. a growing between]

di·aph·y·si·tis (dī-af-i-sī′tis). Inflammation of the shaft of a long bone.

di·a·pi·re·sis (dī′ă-pī-rē′sis). Passage of colloidal or other small particles of suspended matter through the unruptured walls of the blood vessels. SEE ALSO diapedesis. [G. *diapeirō,* to drive through, fr. *peirō,* to pierce]

di·a·pla·cen·tal (dī′ă-pla-sen′tăl). Passing through or "across" the placenta.

di·a·plex·us (dī-ă-plek′sŭs). Rarely used term for choroid *plexus* of third ventricle. [G. *dia,* through, + L. *plexus,* a plaiting]

di·ap·no·ic, di·ap·not·ic (dī-ap-nō′ik, -not′ik). **1.** Relating to, or causing perspiration, especially insensible perspiration. **2.** A mild sudorific.

diapophysis. SYN superior articular *process.*

Di·ap·to·mus (dī-ap′tō-mŭs). A genus of copepod crustacea, the principal intermediate host for *Diphyllobothrium latum* in North America.

▌**di·ar·rhea** (dī-ă-rē′ă). An abnormally frequent discharge of semi-solid or fluid fecal matter from the bowel. [G. *diarrhoia,* fr. *dia,* through, + *rhoia,* a flow, a flux]

cachectic d., d. occurring in patients with severe wasting. Usually due to underlying gastrointestinal disease.

choleraic d., SYN summer d.

chronic bacillary d., prolonged diarrhea occurring in association with bacterial infection, usually occurring in patients with gastrointestinal stasis, allowing bacterial proliferation in the intestine with secondary malabsorption. Occurs in blind-loop syndrome after intestinal surgery, following vagotomy, and occasionally in scleroderma or diabetes.

Cochin China d., obsolete term for tropical *sprue.*

colliquative d., d. associated with excessive discharge of fluid.

dientamoeba d., d. thought to be due to infection with the flagellate, *Dientamoeba fragilis.*

dysenteric d., d. in bacillary or amebic dysentery.

fatty d., d. seen in malabsorption syndromes including chronic pancreatic disease, characterized by foul smelling stools with increased fat content that usually float in water. SYN pimelorrhea.

flagellate d., d. due to infection with flagellate *Giardia lamblia.*

gastrogenous d., a d. that may occur in achylia gastrica, or that is caused by excess secretion of gastric and other intestinal juices.

lienteric d., d. in which undigested food appears in the stools.

morning d., a form in which there are several loose stools in the early morning and during the forenoon, the bowels being quiet during the remainder of the day and night.

mucous d., d. with the presence of considerable mucus in the stools.

nocturnal d., d. that occurs chiefly at night, usually in association with diabetic autonomic neuropathy.

pancreatic d., SYN d. pancreatica.

d. pancreatica (pan-krē-a′ti-kă), d. characterized by severe, watery, secretory d. and hyperkalemia; most patients have hypercalcemia, many have hyperglycemia; results from excessive secretion of VIP (vasoactive intestinal peptide) by an islet cell tumor of the pancreas. Sometimes called WDHA *syndrome.* SEE Verner-Morrison *syndrome,* WDHA *syndrome.* SYN pancreatic cholera, pancreatic d.

pancreatogenous d., d. in which the stools are bulky, pale, foul, greasy, and oily, as a result of malabsorption of fat due to deficient secretion of pancreatic enzymes in chronic pancreatitis.

serous d., d. characterized by watery stools.

summer d., d. of infants in hot weather, usually an acute gastroenteritis due to the presence of *Shigella* or *Salmonella.* SYN choleraic d.

toddler's d., recurrent loose stools usually seen in otherwise healthy, normally growing children between the ages of 1 and 3 years, and occurring in daytime; often due to excessive fluid intake.

traveler's d., d. of sudden onset, often accompanied by abdominal cramps, vomiting, and fever, occurring sporadically in travelers usually during the first week of a trip; most commonly caused by unfamiliar strains of enterotoxigenic *Escherichia coli.*

tropical d., SYN tropical *sprue.*

di·ar·rhe·al, di·ar·rhe·ic (dī-ă-rē′ăl, -rē′ik). Relating to diarrhea. SYN diarrhetic.

di·ar·rhe·tic. SYN diarrheal.

di·ar·thric (dī-ar′thrik). Relating to two joints. SYN biarticular, diarticular. [G. *di-*, two, + *arthron*, joint]

di·ar·thro·sis, pl. **di·ar·thro·ses** (dī-ar-thrō′sis, -sēz). ⁕official alternate term for synovial *joint*. [G. articulation]

di·ar·tic·u·lar (dī-ar-tik′ū-lăr). SYN diarthric.

di·as·chi·sis (dī-as′ki-sis). A sudden inhibition of function produced by an acute focal disturbance in a portion of the brain at a distance from the original site of injury, but anatomically connected with it through fiber tracts. [G. a splitting]

di·a·scope (dī′ă-skōp). A flat glass plate through which one can examine superficial skin lesions by means of pressure. [G. *dia*, through, + *skopeō*, to view]

di·as·co·py (dī-as′kŏ-pē). Examination of superficial skin lesions with a diascope. [G. *dia*, through, + *skopeō*, to see]

di·a·stal·sis (dī-ă-stal′sis). The type of peristalsis in which a region of inhibition precedes the wave of contraction, as seen in the intestinal tract. [G. an arrangement]

di·a·stal·tic (dī-ă-stal′tik). Pertaining to diastalsis.

di·a·stase (dī′as-tās). A mixture, obtained from malt and containing amylolytic enzymes (principally α- and β-amylases), that converts starch into dextrin and maltose; used to make soluble starches, to aid in digestion of starches in certain types of dyspepsia, and to digest glycogen in histologic sections. [Fr., fr. G. *diastasis*, separation, fr. *dia*, apart + *histēmi*, to make to stand]

di·as·ta·sis (dī-as′tă-sis). **1.** Any simple separation of normally joined parts. SYN divarication. **2.** The mid-portion of diastole when the blood enters the ventricle slowly or ceases to enter prior to atrial systole. Diastasis duration is in inverse proportion to heart rate and is absent at very high heart rates. [G. a separation]
    d. rec′ti, separation of rectus abdominis muscles away from the midline, sometimes seen during or following pregnancy.

di·as·tas·u·ria (dī-as-tās-ū′rē-ă). SYN amylasuria.

di·a·stat·ic (dī-ă-stat′ik). Relating to a diastasis.

di·a·ste·ma, pl. **di·a·ste·ma·ta** (dī′ă-stē′mă, -stē′mă-tă) [TA]. **1.** Fissure or abnormal opening in any part, especially if congenital. **2** [NA]. Space between two adjacent teeth in the same dental arch. **3.** Cleft or space between the maxillary lateral incisor and canine teeth, into which the lower canine is received when the jaws are closed; abnormal in humans but normal in dogs and many other animals. [G. *diastēma*, an interval]

di·a·ste·ma·to·cra·nia (dī-ă-stē′mă-tō-krā′nē-ă). Congenital sagittal fissure of the skull. [G. *diastēma*, an interval, + *kranion*, skull]

di·a·ste·ma·to·my·e·lia (dī-ă-stē′mă-tō-mī-e′lē-ă). Complete or incomplete sagittal division of the spinal cord by an osseous or fibrocartilaginous septum. [G. *diastēma*, interval, + *myelon*, marrow]

di·a·ster (dī′as-ter). SYN amphiaster. [G. *di-*, two, + *astēr*, star]

di·a·ste·re·o·i·so·mers (dī′ă-stār-ē-ō-ī′sō-merz). Optically active isomers that are not enantiomorphs (mirror images); e.g., D-glucose and D-galactose.

di·as·to·le (dī-as′tō-lē). Normal postsystolic dilation of the heart cavities, during which they fill with blood; d. of the atria precedes that of the ventricles; d. of either chamber alternates rhythmically with systole or contraction of that chamber. [G. *diastolē*, dilation]
    atrial d., period of relaxation and repolarization of the atrial muscle.
    electrical d., period from end of T wave to beginning of next Q wave.
    gastric d., a phase of relaxation of stomach peristalsis seen fluoroscopically or with the gastroscope.
    late d., SYN presystole.
    ventricular d., period of relaxation and repolarization of the ventricular muscle.

di·a·stol·ic (dī-ă-stol′ik). Relating to diastole.

di·as·tol·ogy (dī-as-tol′ō-jē). The study or science of cardiac diastole and its components.

di·as·tro·phism (dī-as′trof-izm). Distortion that occurs in objects as a result of bending. [G. *diastrophē*, fr. *diastrephein*, distortion]

di·a·tax·ia (dī′ă-tak′sē-ă). Ataxia affecting both sides of the body.
    cerebral d., the ataxic type of cerebral birth palsy.

di·a·te·la (dī-ă-tē′lă). Rarely used term for *tela* choroidea of third ventricle. [G. *dia*, through, between, + L. *tela*, web]

di·a·ther·mal (dī-ă-ther′mal). SYN diathermic. [G. *dia*, through, + *thermē*, heat]

di·a·ther·man·cy (dī-ă-ther′man-sē). The condition of being diathermic.

di·a·ther·ma·nous (dī-ă-ther′man-ŭs). Permeable by heat rays. SYN transcalent. [G. *dia-thermaino*, to heat through, fr. *thermos*, hot]

di·a·ther·mic (dī-ă-ther′mik). Relating to, characterized by, or affected by diathermy. SYN diathermal.

di·a·ther·mo·co·ag·u·la·tion (dī-ă-ther′mō-kō-ag-ū-lā′shŭn). SYN surgical *diathermy*.

di·a·ther·my (dī′ă-ther-mē). Local elevation of temperature within the tissues, produced by high frequency current, ultrasonic waves, or microwave radiation. SYN transthermia. [G. *dia*, through, + *thermē*, heat]
    medical d., d. of mild degree causing no destruction of tissue. SYN thermopenetration.
    short wave d., therapeutic elevation of temperature in the tissues by means of an oscillating electric current of extremely high frequency (10–100 million Hz) and short wavelength of 3–30 meters.
    surgical d., electrocoagulation with a high frequency electrocautery, resulting in local tissue destruction; usually used to seal blood vessels and arrest bleeding. SYN diathermocoagulation.
    ultrashortwave d., shortwave d. in which the wavelength is under 10 meters.

di·ath·e·sis (dī-ath′ĕ-sis). The constitutional or inborn state disposing to a disease, group of diseases, or metabolic or structural anomaly. [G. arrangement, condition]
    contractural d., an older term denoting a tendency to have contractures in hysteria.
    cystic d., a condition in which multiple cysts form in the liver, kidneys, and other organs.
    gouty d., a state of susceptibility to attacks of gout or development of tophi, usually associated with hyperuricemia or hyperexcretion of urate in urine.
    spasmophilic d., a condition in which there is an abnormal excitability of the motor nerves, shown by a tendency to tetany, laryngeal spasm, or general convulsions.

di·a·thet·ic (dī-ă-thet′ik). Relating to a diathesis.

di·a·tom (dī′ă-tom). An individual of microscopic unicellular algae, the shells of which compose a sedimentary infusorial earth. [G. *diatomos*, cut in two]

di·a·to·ma·ceous (dī′ă-tō-mā′shŭs). Pertaining to diatoms or their fossil remains.

di·a·tom·ic (dī-ă-tom′ik). **1.** Denoting a compound with a molecule made up of two atoms. **2.** Denoting any ion or atomic grouping composed of two atoms only.

di·a·tor·ic (dī′ă-tōr′ik). **1.** The vertical cylindric aperture formed in the base of artificial porcelain teeth and extending into the body of the tooth, serving as a mechanical means of attaching the tooth to the denture base. **2.** Denoting teeth that contain a d. [G. *diatoros*, pierced]

di·a·tri·zo·ate. Salt of 3,5-diacetamido-2,4,6-triiodobenzoic acid. SEE *sodium* diatrizoate.

di·az·e·pam (dī-az′ĕ-pam). A skeletal muscle relaxant, sedative, and antianxiety agent; also used as an anticonvulsant, particularly in the treatment of status epilepticus by the parenteral route.

di·a·zines (dī′ă-zēnz). A group of synthetic tuberculostatic drugs, such as pyrazine carboxamide and pyridazine-3-carboxamide.

di·az·in·on (dī-az′in-on). A sulfur-containing organophosphate compound used as an insecticide and cholinesterase inhibitor.

△**diazo-.** Prefix denoting a compound containing the R—N=N—X or R=N_2 grouping, where X is not carbon (except for CN). An example is diazomethane, CH_2N_2. Cf. azo-. [G. *di-*, two, + Fr. *azote*, nitrogen]

di·az·o·tize (dī-az′ō-tīz). To introduce the diazo group into a chemical compound, usually through the treatment of an amine with nitrous acid.

di·az·ox·ide (dī-ă-zok′sīd). An antihypertensive agent.

di·ba·sic (dī-bā′sik). Having two replaceable hydrogen atoms, denoting an acid with two ionizable hydrogen atoms.

di·ben·a·mine (dī-ben′ă-mēn). A nonspecific and irreversible antagonist at alpha-adrenergic receptors. Prevents vasoconstriction produced by epinephrine and norepinephrine and similar agents causing vasoconstriction by an action on alpha adrenergic receptors.

di·benz·e·pin hy·dro·chlo·ride (dī-benz′ĕ-pin). An antidepressant.

di·benz·hep·tro·pine cit·rate (dī-benz-hep′trō-pēn). SYN deptropine citrate.

di·ben·zo·pyr·i·dine (dī-ben′zō-pir′i-dēn). SYN acridine.

di·ben·zo·thi·a·zine (dī-ben′zō-thī′ă-zēn). SYN phenothiazine.

di·benz·thi·one (dī-benz-thī′ōn). An antifungal antiseptic. SYN sulbentine.

Di·both·ri·o·ceph·a·lus (dī-both′rē-ō-sef′ă-lŭs). Former name for *Diphyllobothrium.* [G. *di-,* two, + *bothrion,* dim. of *bothros,* a pit, + *kephalē,* head]

D. la′tus, SYN *Diphyllobothrium latum.*

di·bro·mo·pro·pam·i·dine is·e·thi·o·nate (dī-brō′mō-prō-pam′i-dēn). An antiseptic.

di·brom·sa·lan (dī-brom′să-lan). A disinfectant.

di·bu·caine (dī′boo-kān). A potent local anesthetic with a long duration of action used by injection or topically on skin or mucous membranes.

di·bu·caine hy·dro·chlo·ride (dī-bū′kān). A potent local anesthetic (surface and spinal anesthesia).

di·bu·caine num·ber (DN). A test for differentiation of one of several forms of atypical pseudocholinesterases that are unable to inactivate succinylcholine at normal rates; based upon percent inhibition of the enzymes by dibucaine, normal enzyme has a DN of 75 and above, heterozygous atypical enzyme has a DN of 40-70, and homozygous atypical enzyme has a DN of less than 20. SEE ALSO fluoride number.

di·bu·to·line sul·fate (dī-bū′tō-lēn). An anticholinergic agent used as a mydriatic, a cycloplegic, and a gastrointestinal antispasmodic.

di·bu·tyl phthal·ate (dī-bū′til thal′āt). An insect repellent.

DIC Abbreviation for disseminated intravascular *coagulation.*

di·cac·o·dyl (dī-kak′ō-dil). SYN cacodyl.

di·ce·lous (dī-sē′lŭs). Having two cavities or excavations on opposite surfaces. [G. *di-,* two, + *koilos,* hollow]

di·cen·tric (dī-sen′trik). Referring to a structural chromosome having two centromeres, an abnormal state.

di·ceph·a·lous (dī-sef′ă-lŭs). Having two heads.

di·ceph·a·lus (dī-sef′ă-lŭs). Symmetrical conjoined twins with two separate heads. SEE conjoined *twins,* under *twin.* SYN bicephalus, diplocephalus. [G. *di-,* two, + *kephalē,* head]

d. di′auchenos, a d. with separate necks. SYN derodidymus.

d. di′pus dibra′chius, a d. in which there are only two arms and two legs for a body with two axes.

d. di′pus tetrabra′chius, a d. with two legs and four separate arms.

d. di′pus tribra′chius, a d. with two legs and three arms.

d. dip′ygus, SYN anakatadidymus; SEE conjoined *twins,* under *twin.*

d. mon′auchenos, a d. in which union involves the cervical region so that the two heads are on a single neck.

di·chei·lia, di·chi·lia (dī-kī′lē-ă). A lip appearing to be double because of the presence of an abnormal fold of mucosa. [G. *di-,* two, + *cheilos,* lip]

di·chei·ria, di·chi·ria (dī-kī′rē-ă). Complete or incomplete duplication of the hand. SEE ALSO polydactyly. SYN diplocheiria, diplochiria. [G. *di-,* two, + *cheir,* hand]

Di·chel·o·bac·ter no·do·sus. SYN *Bacteroides nodosus.*

di·chlo·ra·mine-T (dī-klōr′ă-mēn). Used as an antiseptic in surgical dressings.

di·chlo·ride (dī-klōr′īd). A compound with a molecule containing two atoms of chlorine to one of another element.

di·chlo·ri·sone (dī-klōr′i-sōn). A topical antipruritic agent.

di·chlo·ro·ben·zene (dī-klōr′ō-ben′zēn). An insecticide used chiefly as a moth repellent.

di·chlo·ro·di·flu·o·ro·meth·ane (dī-klōr′ō-dī-floo-rō-meth′ān). An easily liquefiable gas used as a refrigerant and aerosol propellant.

***p,p′*-di·chlo·ro·di·phen·yl meth·yl car·bi·nol (DMC)** (dī-chlōr′ō-dī-fen′il). A synthetic compound found effective as a miticide.

di·chlo·ro·di·phen·yl·tri·chlo·ro·eth·ane (DDT) (dī-chlōr′ō-dī-fen′il-trī-klōr-ō-eth′ān). An insecticide that came into prominence during and after World War II. For a time it proved very effective, but insect populations rapidly developed tolerance for it, hence much of its original effectiveness has been lost; general usage is now widely discouraged because of the toxicity that results from the environmental persistence of this agent. SYN chlorophenothane, dicophane.

di·(2-chlo·ro·eth·yl)sul·fide. SYN mustard *gas.*

di·chlo·ro·for·mox·ime. SYN *phosgene* oxime.

di·chlo·ro·hy·drin (dī-klōr′ō-hī′drin). A colorless, odorless fluid prepared by heating anhydrous glycerin with sulfur monochloride; a solvent of resins. SYN dichloroisopropyl alcohol.

2,6-di·chlo·ro·in·do·phe·nol (dī-klōr′ō-in-dō-fē′nol). A reagent for the chemical assay of ascorbic acid that depends upon the reducing properties of the latter. It is red in acid solution; in the presence of the vitamin C it undergoes reduction and becomes colorless, the vitamin being oxidized to dehydroascorbic acid. Often misnamed dichlorophenol-indophenol.

di·chlo·ro·i·so·pro·pyl al·co·hol (dī-klōr′ō-is-ō-prō′pil). SYN dichlorohydrin.

di·chlo·ro·phen (dī-klōr′ō-fen). Used topically as a fungicide and bactericide, and internally in the treatment of infections by tapeworms of humans and domestic animals.

di·chlo·ro·phen·ar·sine hy·dro·chlo·ride (dī-klōr′ō-fen-ar′sēn). (3-Amino-4-Hydroxyphenyl)dichloroarisine hydrochloride, formerly used as an arsenical antisyphilitic.

2,6-di·chlo·ro·phe·nol-in·do·phe·nol (dī′klōr-ō-fē′nol-in-dō-fē′nol). Misnomer for 2,6-dichloroindophenol.

(2,4-di·chlo·ro·phen·oxy) ace·tic ac·id (2,4-D). An herbicide, more toxic to broad-leaved dicotyledonous plants (weeds) than to monocotyledonous ones (grains and grass), used with (2,4,5-trichlorophenoxy)acetic acid as a constituent of Agent Orange.

di·chlo·ro·vos (dī-klōr′ō-vos). SYN dichlorvos.

di·chlor·phen·a·mide (dī-klōr-fen′ă-mīd). A carbonic anhydrase inhibitor with actions similar to those of acetazolamide.

di·chlor·vos (dī-klōr′vos). An anthelmintic in veterinary and human medicine. SYN dichlorovos.

di·cho·ri·al, di·cho·ri·on·ic (dī-kō′rē-ăl, dī-kō-rē-on′ik). Showing evidence of two chorions. [G. *di-,* two, + chorion]

di·chot·ic (dī-kot′ik). **1.** SYN dichotomous. **2.** Simultaneous presentation of a different sound to each ear.

di·chot·o·mous (dī-kot′ō-mŭs). Denoting or characterized by dichotomy. SYN dichotic (1).

di·chot·o·my (dī-kot′ō-mē). Division into two parts. [G. *dichotomia,* a cutting in two, fr. *dicha,* in two, + *tomē,* a cutting]

di·chro·ic (dī-krō′ik). Relating to dichroism.

di·chro·ism (dī′krō-izm). The property of seeming to be differently colored when viewed from emitted light and from transmitted light. [G. *di-,* two, + *chrōa,* color]

circular d. (CD), the change from circular polarization to elliptical polarization of monochromatic, circularly polarized light in the immediate vicinity of the absorption band of the substance through which the light passes. SEE ALSO Cotton *effect.*

di·chro·mat (dī′krō-mat). An individual with dichromatism.

di·chro·mate (dī-krō′māt). A compound containing the radical $Cr_2O_7^=$.

di·chro·mat·ic (dī-krō-mat′ik). **1.** Having or exhibiting two colors. **2.** Relating to dichromatism (2).

di·chro·ma·tism (dī-krō′mă-tizm). **1.** The state of being dichromatic (1). **2.** The abnormality of color vision in which only two of the three retinal cone pigments are present, as in protanopia, deuteranopia, and tritanopia. SYN dichromatopsia. [G. *di-*, two, + *chrōma*, color]

di·chro·ma·top·sia (dī-krō-mă-top′sē-ă). SYN dichromatism (2). [G. *di-*, two, + *chrōma*, color, + *opsis*, vision]

di·chro·mic (dī-krō′mik). Having, or relating to, two colors.

di·chro·mo·phil, di·chro·mo·phile (dī-krō′mō-fil, dī-krō′mō-fīl). Taking a double stain; denoting a tissue or cell taking both acid and basic dyes in different parts. [G. *di-*, two, + *chrōma*, color, + *philos*, fond]

Dick, George Frederick, U.S. internist, 1881–1967. SEE D. *method*, *test*, test *toxin*.

Dick, Gladys R.H., U.S. internist, 1881–1963. SEE D. *method*, *test*, test *toxin*.

Dickens, Frank, British biochemist, *1899. SEE D. *shunt;* Warburg-Lipmann-D.-Horecker *shunt*.

di·clo·fen·ac (dī-klō′fén-ák). One of several nonsteroidal antiinflammatory drugs used in the treatment of rheumatic disorders such as rheumatoid arthritis; also used in osteoarthritis and other conditions. Acts by preventing prostaglandin synthesis.

di·clox·a·cil·lin so·di·um (dī-klok-să-sil′in). A semisynthetic penicillin resistant to penicillinase.

DICOM Abbreviation for Digital Imaging and Communications in Medicine, a joint standard of the American College of Radiology and National Equipment Manufacturers Association; specifies entities (or objects) and functions (or services) to allow communication between various image sources and other computer devices, such as archives or workstations.

di·co·phane (dī′kō-fān). SYN dichlorodiphenyltrichloroethane.

di·co·ria (dī-kō′rē-ă). SYN diplocoria. [G. *di-*, two, + *korē*, pupil]

di·cot·yl·ed·on. Plant (shrub, herb, or tree) whose seeds consist of two cotyledons, i.e., the primary or rudimentary leaf of the embryo of seed plants.

di·cro·coe·li·o·sis (dī′krō-sē-li-ō′sis). Infection of animals and, rarely, humans with trematodes of the genus *Dicrocoelium*.

Di·cro·coe·li·um (dīk-rō-sē′lē-ŭm). A genus of digenetic trematodes inhabiting the bile ducts and gallbladder of herbivores. The species D. *dentriticum* (lancet fluke) is rarely found in humans, but is an important parasite of sheep in some localities. [G. *dikroos*, forked, + *koilia*, belly]

di·crot·ic (dī-krot′ik). Relating to dicrotism. [G. *dikrotos*, double-beating]

di·cro·tism (dī′krō-tizm). That form of the pulse in which a double beat can be appreciated at any arterial pulse for each beat of the heart; due to accentuation of the dicrotic wave. [G. *di-*, two, + *krotos*, a beat]

dicta- (dik′ta). Prefix used to signify two hundred. [G.]

dic·ty·o·ma (dik-tē-ō′mă). A benign tumor of the ciliary epithelium with a netlike structure resembling embryonic retina. [G. *dikyton*, net (retina), + *-oma*, tumor]

dic·ty·o·some (dik′tē-ō-sōm). SYN Golgi *apparatus*. [G. *diktyon*, net, + *-some*]

dic·ty·o·tene (dik′tē-ō-tēn). The state of meiosis at which the oocyte is arrested during the several years between late fetal life and menarche. [G. *diktyon*, net, + *tainia*, band]

di·cu·ma·rol (dī-koo′mă-rol). An anticoagulant that inhibits the formation of prothrombin in the liver. Acts as an antagonist of vitamin K; discovered as the causative agent in spoiled hay, which produced bleeding in cattle (sweet clover disease). SYN bishydroxycoumarin.

di·cy·clo·mine hy·dro·chlo·ride (dī-sī′klō-mēn). An anticholinergic agent.

di·cys·te·ine (dī-sis′tēn). SYN cystine.

di·dac·tic (dī-dak′tik). Instructive; denoting medical teaching by lectures or textbooks, as distinguished from clinical demonstrations with patients or laboratory exercises. [G. *didaktikos*, fr. *didaskō*, to teach]

di·dac·ty·lism (dī-dak′ti-lizm). Congenital condition of having only two fingers on a hand or two toes on a foot. [G. *di-*, two, + *daktylos*, finger or toe]

di·del·phic (dī-del′fik). Having or relating to a double uterus. [G. *di-*, two, + *delphys*, womb]

Di·del·phis (dī-del′fis). A genus of marsupials, commonly called opossums, that serve as reservoir hosts of *Trypanosoma cruzi*. D. *marsupialis* is the common North American variety; D. *paraguayensis* is a South American form. [G. *di-*, two, + *delphys*, womb]

di·de·ox·y·aden·o·sine (DDA) (dī′dē-oks′ē-ă-den′ō-sēn). An antiviral agent used in the treatment of AIDS, similar to DDC.

di·de·ox·y·cy·ti·dine (dī′-dē-ok′-sē-sī′-ti-dēn). Pyrimidine nucleoside analog with antiviral activity; used in the treatment of AIDS.

di·de·ox·y·in·o·sine (DDI) (dī′-dē-oks-ē-ī′-nō-sēn). Antiviral agent; has been used in treatment of AIDS.

DIDMOD An acronym for Wolfram *syndrome*, which comprises *d*iabetes *i*nsipidus, *d*iabetes *m*ellitus, *o*ptic atrophy, and *d*eafness.

⚠️**didym-, didymo-.** The didymus, testis. [G. *didymos*, twin]

did·y·mus (did′ē-mŭs). SYN testis. [G. *didymos*, a twin, pl. *didymoi*, testes]

⚠️**-didymus.** A conjoined twin, with the first element of the complete word designating fused parts. SEE ALSO -dymus, -pagus. [G. *didymos*, twin]

die (dī). In dentistry, the positive reproduction of the form of a prepared tooth in any suitable hard substance, usually in metal or specially prepared artificial stone. SEE ALSO counterdie.

dieb. alt. Abbreviation for L. *diebus alternis*, every other day.

di·e·cious (dī-ē′shŭs). Denoting animals or plants that are sexually distinct, the individuals being of one or the other sex. [G. *di-*, two, + *oikia*, house]

Dieffenbach, Johann F., German surgeon, 1792–1847.

Diego blood group, Di blood group. See Blood Groups appendix.

di·el (dī′el). Term frequently used synonymously with diurnal (2) or circadian. [irreg., fr. L. *dies,* day]

di·el·drin (dī-el′drin). A chlorinated hydrocarbon used as an insecticide; may cause toxic effects in persons and animals exposed to its action through skin contact, inhalation, or food contamination.

di·e·lec·trog·ra·phy (dī-ē-lek-trog′ră-fē). SYN impedance *plethysmography*.

di·e·lec·trol·y·sis (dī′ē-lek-trol′i-sis). SYN electrophoresis.

Diels, Otto, German chemist and Nobel laureate, 1876–1954. SEE D. *hydrocarbon*.

di·en·ceph·a·lo·hy·po·phy·si·al (dī-en-sef′ă-lō-hī-pō-fiz′ē-ăl). Relating to the diencephalon and hypophysis.

di·en·ceph·a·lon, pl. **di·en·ceph·a·la** (dī-en-sef′ă-lon, -sef′ă-lă) [TA]. The caudal part of the prosencephalon composed of the epithalamus, thalamus, and hypothalamus. [G. *dia*, through, + *enkephalos*, brain]

die·ner (dē′ner). A laboratory worker who assists in cleaning; most commonly applied to laboratory workers who assist in the performance of autopsies and maintenance of morgues. [Ger. *Diener,* servant]

di·en·es·trol (dī-en-es′trol). An estrogenic agent. SYN estrodienol.

Di·ent·a·moe·ba frag·i·lis (dī-ent-ă-mē′bă fraj′i-lis). A species of small amebalike flagellates, formerly considered a true ameba, now recognized as an ameboflagellate related to *Trichomonas*, parasitic in the large intestine of humans and certain monkeys; may be nonpathogenic, but believed to be capable of sometimes causing low-grade inflammation with mucous diarrhea and gastrointestinal disturbance in humans.

di·er·e·sis (dī-er′ĕ-sis). SYN *solution* of continuity. [G. *diairesis,* a division]

di

di·e·ret·ic (dī-er-et′ik). **1.** Relating to dieresis. **2.** Dividing; ulcerating; corroding.

di·es·ter·ase (dī-es′ter-ās). SEE phosphodiesterases.

di·es·trous (dī-es′trŭs). Pertaining to diestrus.

di·es·trus (dī-es′trŭs). A period of sexual quiescence intervening between two periods of estrus. [G. *dia,* between, + *oistros,* desire]

di·et (dī′et). **1.** Food and drink in general. **2.** A prescribed course of eating and drinking in which the amount and kind of food, as well as the times at which it is to be taken, are regulated for therapeutic purposes. **3.** Reduction of caloric intake so as to lose weight. **4.** To follow any prescribed or specific d. [G. *diaita,* a way of life; a diet]

acid-ash d., SYN alkaline-ash d.

alkaline-ash d., a d. consisting mainly of fruits, vegetables, and milk (with minimal amounts of meat, fish, eggs, cheese, and cereals), which, when catabolized, leave an alkaline residue to be excreted in the urine. SYN acid-ash d., basic d.

balanced d., a d. containing the essential nutrients with a reasonable ration of all the major food groups.

basal d., (1) a d. having a caloric value equal to the basal heat production and sufficient quanties of essential nutrients to meet basic needs; **(2)** in experiments in nutrition, a d. complete and adequate except for a single constituent (e.g., a vitamin, mineral, or amino acid), the nutritional value of which is to be determined, is omitted for a period and the effects observed; the subject is observed for a second period during which the ingredient being studied is added to the d.

basic d., SYN alkaline-ash d.

bland d., a regular d. omitting foods that mechanically or chemically irritate the gastrointestinal tract.

BRAT d., a limited diet often used in regimens for acute gastroenteritides; acronym for *b*ananas, *r*ice, *a*pples (juice or sauce), and *t*oast.

challenge d., a d. in which one or more specific substances are included for the purpose of determining whether an abnormal reaction occurs.

clear liquid d., a d., often used postoperatively, consisting usually of water, tea, coffee, gelatin preparations, and clear soups or broth.

diabetic d., a dietary adjustment for patients with *diabetes* mellitus intended to decrease the need for insulin or oral diabetic agents and control weight by adjusting caloric and carbohydrate intake.

elimination d., a d. designed to detect what ingredient of the food causes allergic manifestations in the patient; food items to which the patient may be sensitive are withdrawn separately and successively from the d. until that which causes the symptoms is discovered.

full liquid d., a d. consisting only of liquids but including cream soups, ice cream, and milk.

Giordano-Giovannetti d., a d. designed for patients with renal failure; it provides small amounts of protein, primarily as essential amino acids, along with alpha-keto derivatives of amino acids; breakdown of protein in skeletal muscle is retarded and, because transaminase reactions are reversible, a small proportion of the ammonia released by urea breakdown is used for synthesis of nonessential amino acids. SYN Giovannetti d.

Giovannetti d., SYN Giordano-Giovannetti d.

gluten-free d., elimination of all wheat, rye, barley, and oat gluten from the d.; treatment for gluten-sensitive enteropathy (celiac disease). SEE celiac *disease.*

gout d., a d. containing a minimal quantity of purine bases (meats); liver, kidney, and sweetbread especially are excluded and replaced by dairy products, fruits, and cereals; alcoholic beverages also are excluded. SYN purine-free d.

high-calorie d., a d. containing upward of 4,000 calories per day.

high-fat d., a d. containing large amounts of fat.

high-fiber d., a d. high in the nondigestible part of plants, which is fiber. Fiber is found in fruits, vegetables, whole grains, and legumes. Insoluble fiber increases stool bulk, decreases transit time of food in the bowel, and decreases constipation and the risk of colon cancer. Soluble fiber delays absorption of glucose, which

helps to control blood sugar in diabetes mellitus, and delays absorption of lipids, which helps to control hyperlipidemia. Recommended in treatment of diverticular disease of the colon.

Kempner d., SYN rice d.

ketogenic d., a high-fat, low-carbohydrate, and normal protein d. causing ketosis.

low-calorie d., a d. of 1,200 calories or less per day.

low-fat d., a d. containing a minimal proportion of fat.

Diets containing low amounts of fat and cholesterol are designed to reduce the risk of cardiovascular disease, specifically atherosclerosis. The National Cholesterol Education Program recommends maintaining a total cholesterol level of no more than 200 mg/dL, with LDL cholesterol less than 130 mg/dL and HDL cholesterol at least 60 mg/dL. (According to the National Institutes of Health, LDL cholesterol in patients with atherosclerotic heart disease should not exceed 100 mg/dL.) About one-half of adult Americans exceed these total cholesterol and LDL cholesterol limits; for many, the reason is an inborn metabolic disorder of lipid metabolism not correctable by dietary restrictions alone. A low-fat diet should derive less than 10% of its calories from saturated fat (meats, dairy products) and should be low in cholesterol (<300 mg/d) and trans fatty acids (e.g., hydrogenated oils as in stick margarine and shortening) and rich in whole grains, fresh fruits and vegetables, and legumes. People who follow an extremely low-fat diet experience some reversal in atherosclerosis despite a concomitant decrease in HDL cholesterol. A low-fat diet may also help decrease body weight or prevent weight gain, because fats and oils yield more than twice as many calories per gram as carbohydrate and protein foods. See atherosclerosis; free radical.

low purine d., a d. low in precursors of purines (such as tissues rich in cells with abundant nuclei, as in liver, glandular meats, etc.) to minimize formation of uric acid. Useful in treatment of patients with gout or urate-containing renal calculi.

low residue d., a d. that leaves minimal unabsorbed components in the intestine, to minimize functional stress on the colon.

low salt d., a d. with restricted amounts of sodium chloride, useful in the treatment of some cases of hypertension, heart failure, and other syndromes characterized by fluid retention and/or edema formation.

macrobiotic d., a d. claimed to promote longevity, often by promoting an emphasis on natural foods and restrictions on noncereal foods, as well as liquids.

Meulengracht d., a feeding program for patients with peptic ulcer disease, containing a relatively full diet free of acidic or highly seasoned food.

Minot-Murphy d., the use of large amounts of raw liver in the treatment of pernicious *anemia.* First successes in the treatment of this disease occurred with this diet and led to development of liver extract for treatment.

Ornish prevention d.'s, relaxed versions of the Ornish reversal d., which is designed to prevent coronary artery disease. These d.'s reduce dietary fat in proportion to blood cholesterol level.

Ornish reversal d., a d. designed by Dean Ornish, who has evidence that it will reverse coronary artery disease. It consists of 10% of calories from fat (mostly polyunsaturated or monounsaturated, with 5 mg cholesterol per day), 70–75% from carbohydrate, and 15–20% from protein.

purine-free d., SYN gout d.

purine-restricted d., SEE gout d.

rachitic d., a d. that will induce rickets in susceptible experimental animals.

reducing d., a d. in which caloric expenditure is greater than caloric intake.

rice d., a d. of rice, fruit, and sugar, plus vitamin and iron supplements, devised by Kempner to treat hypertension. In 2,000 calories, the d. contains 5 gm or less of fat, about 20 gm of protein, and not more than 150 mg of sodium. SYN Kempner d.

Schmidt d., SYN Schmidt-Strassburger d.

Schmidt-Strassburger d., an obsolete d. designed to facilitate examination of the stools in patients with diarrhea, consisting of milk, zwieback, oatmeal gruel, eggs, butter, small amounts of beef and potato. SYN Schmidt d.

Sippy d., a d. formerly used in the initial stages of treatment of peptic ulcer, beginning with milk and cream every hour or two to keep gastric acid neutralized, gradually increasing to include cereal, eggs and crackers after three days, pureed vegetables later.

smooth d., a d. containing little roughage; used primarily in diseases of the colon.

soft d., a normal d. limited to soft foods for those who have difficulty chewing or swallowing; there are no restrictions on seasoning or method of food preparation.

subsistence d., a meager d. providing barely enough for sustenance.

Wilder d., obsolete d., low in potassium, for treating Addison *disease.*

di·e·tary (dī′ĕ-tār-ē). Relating to the diet.

Dieterle stain. See under stain.

di·e·tet·ic (dī′ĕ-tet′ik). **1.** Relating to the diet. **2.** Descriptive of food that, naturally or through processing, has a low caloric content.

di·e·tet·ics (dī-ĕ-tet′iks). The practical application of diet in the prophylaxis and treatment of disease.

di·eth·a·di·one (dī-eth-ă-dī′ōn). An analeptic.

di·eth·a·nol·a·mine (dī-eth-ă-nol′ă-mēn). Used as an emulsifier and as a dispersing agent in cosmetics and pharmaceuticals. SYN diethylolamine.

di·eth·a·zine (dī-eth′ă-zēn). An anticholinergic agent.

di·eth·yl (dī-eth′il). A compound containing two ethyl radicals.

5,5-di·eth·yl·bar·bi·tu·ric ac·id (dī-eth′il-bar-bi-tū′rik). SYN barbital.

di·eth·yl·car·bam·a·zine cit·rate (dī-eth′il-kar-bam′ă-zēn). An effective microfilaricide, although relatively ineffective against the adult filariae.

di·eth·yl·ene·di·a·mine (dī-eth′il-ēn-dī′ă-mēn). SYN piperazine.

1,4-di·eth·yl·ene di·ox·ide (dī-eth′il-ēn). SYN dioxane.

di·eth·yl·ene gly·col (dī-eth′il-ēn). An organic solvent chemically related to ethylene glycol. Upon metabolic conversion it becomes oxalic acid, which is toxic to the kidney. A sweet, viscous liquid that was used to make the infamous elixir of sulfanilamide that proved fatal to over 100 children in 1937, leading to the mandate to the FDA to monitor drug safety.

di·eth·yl·ene·tri·a·mine pen·ta·a·ce·tic ac·id (DTPA) (dī-eth′il-ēn-trī′ă-mēn pen-ta-ă-sē′tik as′id). An important chelating agent used in therapy (e.g., in therapy for lead poisoning), and in metal-containing diagnostic agents for magnetic resonance imaging and nuclear scanning.

di·eth·yl ether. A flammable, volatile organic solvent formerly widely used in surgical procedures; was used as an inhalation anesthetic; shortcomings include: irritating vapor, slow onset and prolonged recovery phase, explosion hazard. SYN ethyl ether, ethyl oxide, sulfuric ether.

di·eth·y·lol·a·mine (dī-eth-i-lol′ă-mēn). SYN diethanolamine.

di·eth·yl·pro·pi·on hy·dro·chlo·ride (dī-eth-il-prō′pē-on). A sympathomimetic drug resembling amphetamine in its actions and used as an appetite suppressant. Increases blood pressure, heart rate.

di·eth·yl·stil·bes·trol (DES) (dī-eth′il-stil-bes′trol). A synthetic nonsteroidal estrogenic compound. Sometimes used as a postcoital antipregnancy agent to prevent implantation of the fertilized ovum. The first demonstrated transplacental carcinogen responsible for a delayed clear cell vaginal carcinoma in female offspring of mothers who took the drug during pregnancy when the drug was erroneously thought to prevent threatened abortion. SYN stilbestrol.

di·eth·yl·tol·u·am·ide (dī-eth′il-tō-loo′ă-mīd). An insect repellent.

di·eth·yl·tryp·ta·mine (DET) (dī-eth-il-trip′tă-mēn). A hallucinogenic agent similar to dimethyltryptamine.

di·e·ti·tian (dī-ĕ-tish′ŭn). An expert in dietetics.

Dietl, Józef, Polish physician, 1804–1878. SEE D. *crisis.*

Dieuaide di·a·gram. See under diagram.

Dieulafoy, Georges, French physician, 1839–1911. SEE D. *erosion.*

di·far·ne·syl group (di-far′nĕ-sil). A 30-carbon open chain hexaisoprenoid hydrocarbon radical; occurs as a side chain in vitamin K_2.

di·fen·ox·in (dī-fen-ok′sin). An antidiarrheal agent with actions similar to those of difenoxylic acid. SYN difenoxylic acid.

di·fen·ox·y·lic ac·id (dī-fen-ok′si-lik). SYN difenoxin.

dif·fer·ence (dif′er-ens). The magnitude or degree by which one quality or quantity differs from another of the same kind.

alveolar-arterial oxygen d., the d. or gradient between the partial pressure of oxygen in the alveolar spaces and the arterial blood: $P_{(A-a)}O_2$. Normally in young adults this value is less than 20 mm Hg. SEE ALSO alveolar gas *equation.*

arteriovenous carbon dioxide d., the d. in carbon dioxide content (in mL per 100 mL blood) between arterial and venous blood.

arteriovenous oxygen d., the d. in the oxygen content (in mL per 100 mL blood) between arterial and venous blood.

AV d., abbreviation for arteriovenous difference of concentration of a substance.

cation-anion d., SYN anion *gap.*

individual d.'s, in clinical psychology, deviations of individuals from the group average or from each other.

light d., **(1)** the d. in light sensitivity of the two eyes; **(2)** SYN brightness difference *threshold.*

masking level d., a technique of comparing threshold responses with masking noise presented in phase and out of phase with the test signal; release from masking is normal and indicates an intact brainstem auditory pathway.

standard error of d., a statistical index of the probability that a d. between two sample means is greater than zero.

dif·fer·en·tial (dif-er-en′shăl). Relating to, or characterized by, a difference; distinguishing. [L. *dif-fero,* to carry apart, differ, fr. *dis,* apart]

threshold d., SYN differential *threshold.*

dif·fer·en·ti·at·ed (dif-er-en′shē-ā-ted). Having a different character or function from the surrounding structures or from the original type; said of tissues, cells, or portions of the cytoplasm.

dif·fer·en·ti·a·tion (dif′er-en-shē-ā′shŭn). **1.** The acquisition or possession of one or more characteristics or functions different from that of the original type. SYN specialization (2). **2.** SYN differential *diagnosis.* **3.** Partial removal of a stain from a histologic section to accentuate the staining differences of tissue components.

correlative d., d. due to the interaction of different parts of an organism.

echocardiographic d., the processing of a signal so that the output depends upon the rate of change of the input; e.g., it will display changes in amplitude but will reduce the duration of the waveform.

invisible d., SYN chemodifferentiation.

pressure pulse d., the processing of a pressure pulse signal so that the output depends upon the rate of change of the input, yielding dP/dt (pressure) or, for noninvasively recorded pulses, dD/dt (rate of change of displacement).

dif·flu·ence (dif′loo-ens). The process of becoming fluid. [L. *diffluo,* to flow in different directions, dissolve]

dif·frac·tion (di-frak′shŭn). Deflection of the rays of light from a straight line in passing by the edge of an opaque body or in passing an obstacle of about the size of the wavelength of the light. [L. *dif- fringo,* pp. *-fractus,* to break in pieces]

dif·frac·tion grat·ing. A variety of filter composed of lined grooves in a thin layer of aluminum-copper alloy on a glass surface; used in spectrophotometers to disperse light into a spectrum. SEE monochromator.

di

dif·fu·sate (di-fū′zāt). SYN dialysate. [L. *dif-fundo*, pp. *-fusus*, to pour in different directions]

dif·fuse (di-fūs). **1** (di-fūz′). To disseminate; to spread about. **2** (di-fūs′). Disseminated; spread about; not restricted. [L. *dif-fundo*, pp. *-fusus*, to pour in different directions]

dif·fus·i·ble (di-fūz′i-bl). Capable of diffusing.

dif·fu·sion (di-fū′zhŭn). **1.** The random movement of molecules or ions or small particles in solution or suspension under the influence of brownian (thermal) motion toward a uniform distribution throughout the available volume; the rate is relatively rapid among liquids and gases, but takes place very slowly among solids. **2.** Light scattering.

facilitated d., SEE facilitated *transport*.

gel d., d. in a gel, as in the case of gel d. precipitin tests in which the immune reactants diffuse in agar. SEE ALSO immunodiffusion.

passive d., SEE facilitated *transport*.

di·flor·a·sone di·ac·e·tate (dī-flōr′ă-sōn). An anti-inflammatory corticosteroid used in topical preparations.

di·flu·cor·to·lone (dī-floo-kōr′ti-lōn). A synthetic glucocorticoid steroid analog.

di·flu·ni·sal (dī-floo′ni-saul). A salicyclic acid derivative with anti-inflammatory, analgesic, and antipyretic actions used in chronic disorders such as rheumatoid arthritis and osteoarthritis.

di·ga·met·ic (dī-gă-met′ik). SYN heterogametic.

di·gas·tric (dī-gas′trik). **1.** Having two bellies; denoting especially a muscle with two fleshy parts separated by an intervening tendinous part. SYN biventral. SEE digastric (*muscle*). **2.** Relating to the d. muscle; denoting a fossa or groove with which it is in relation and a nerve supplying its posterior belly. SYN digastricus (1). [G. *di-*, two, + *gastēr*, belly]

di·gas·tri·cus (dī-gas′tri-kŭs). **1.** SYN digastric. **2.** Denoting the *musculus* digastricus. [L.]

Di·ge·nea (dī-jē′nē-ă). Subclass of parasitic flatworms (class Trematoda) characterized by a complex life cycle involving developmental multiplying stages in a mollusk intermediate host, an adult stage in a vertebrate, and often involving an additional transport host or an additional intermediate host; includes all of the common flukes of humans and other mammals. [G. *di-*, two, + *genesis*, generation]

di·gen·e·sis (dī-jen′ĕ-sis). Reproduction in distinctive patterns in alternate generations, as seen in the nonsexual (invertebrate) and the sexual (vertebrate) cycles of digenetic trematode parasites. [G. *di-*, two, + G. *genesis*, generation]

di·ge·net·ic (dī-jĕ-net′ik). **1.** Pertaining to or characterized by digenesis. SYN heteroxenous. **2.** Pertaining to the digenetic fluke.

DiGeorge, Angelo M., U.S. pediatrician, *1921. SEE DiG. *syndrome.*

di·gest. 1 (di-jest′, dī-). To soften by moisture and heat. **2** (di-jest′, dī-). To hydrolyze or break up into simpler chemical compounds by means of hydrolyzing enzymes or chemical action, as in the action of the secretions of the alimentary tract upon food. **3** (dī′jest). The materials resulting from digestion or hydrolysis. [L. *digero*, pp. *-gestus*, to force apart, divide, dissolve]

di·ges·tant (di-jes′tănt, dī-). **1.** Aiding digestion. **2.** An agent that favors or assists the process of digestion. SYN digestive (2).

di·ges·tion (di-jes′chŭn, dī-). **1.** The process of making a digest. **2.** The mechanical, chemical, and enzymatic process whereby ingested food is converted into material suitable for assimilation for synthesis of tissues or liberation of energy. [L. *digestio*. See digest]

buccal d., that part of d. carried on in the mouth; e.g., the action of salivary amylases.

duodenal d., that part of d. carried on in the duodenum.

gastric d., that part of d., chiefly of the proteins, carried on in the stomach by the enzymes of the gastric juice. SYN peptic d.

intercellular d., d. in a cavity by means of secretions from the surrounding cells, such as occurs in the metazoa.

intestinal d., that part of d. carried on in the intestine; it affects all the foodstuffs: starches, fats, and proteins.

intracellular d., d. within the boundaries of a cell, such as occurs in the protozoa and in phagocytes.

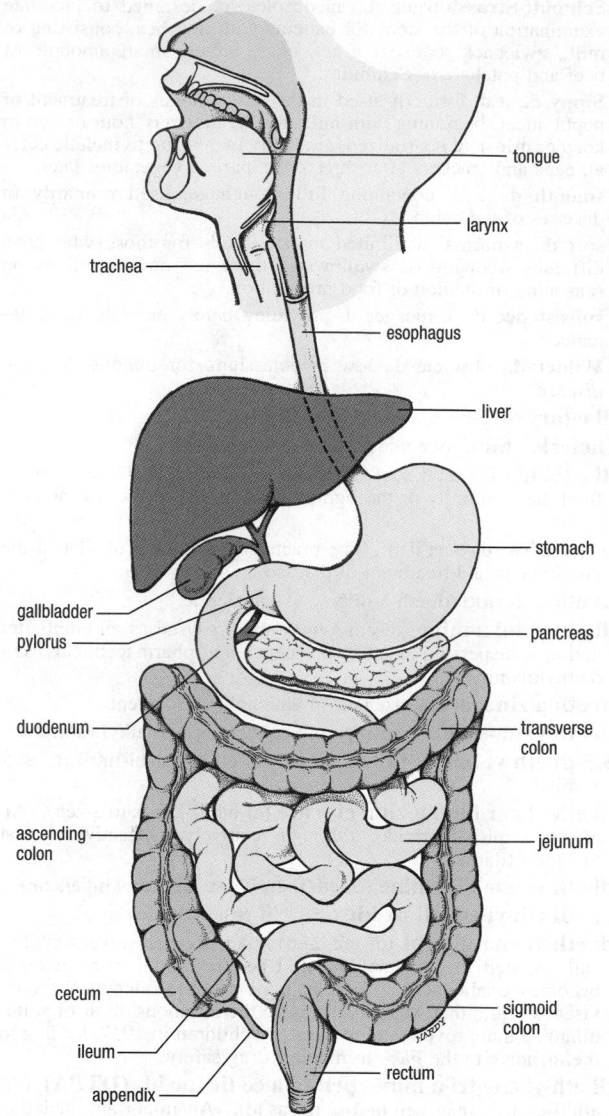

digestive organs and associated structures

pancreatic d., d. in the intestine by the enzymes of the pancreatic juice.

peptic d., SYN gastric d.

primary d., d. in the alimentary tract.

salivary d., the conversion of starch into sugar by the action of salivary amylase.

secondary d., the change in the chyle effected by the action of the cells of the body, whereby the final products of d. are assimilated in the process of metabolism.

di·ges·tive (di-jes′tiv, dī-). **1.** Relating to digestion. **2.** SYN digestant (2).

dig·it (dij′it) [TA]. A finger or toe. SEE ALSO finger, toe. SYN digitus [TA], dactyl, dactylus. [L. *digitus*]

binary d., SYN bit.

clubbed d., SEE clubbing.

d.'s of foot, ✕ official alternate term for toe.

primary d. of foot, SYN great *toe* I.

dig·i·tal (dij′i-tăl). Relating to or resembling a digit or digits or an impression made by them; based on numeric methodology.

dig·i·tal·in (dij-i-tal′in). A standardized mixture of digitalis glycosides used as a cardiotonic in the treatment of congestive heart failure.
    crystalline d., SYN digitoxin.

Dig·i·tal·is (dij-i-tal′is, -ta′lis). A genus of perennial flowering plants of the family Schrophulariaceae. *D. lanata,* a European species, and *D. purpurea,* purple foxglove, are the main sources of cardioactive steroid glycosides used in the treatment of certain heart diseases, especially congestive heart failure; also used to treat tachyarrhythmias of atrial origin. SYN foxglove. [L. *digitalis,* relating to the fingers; in allusion to the fingerlike flowers]

dig·i·tal·ism (dij′i-tal-izm). The symptoms caused by digitalis poisoning or overdosage.

dig·i·tal·i·za·tion (dij′i-tal-i-zā′shŭn). Administration of digitalis by any one of a number of schedules until sufficient amounts are present in the body to produce the desired therapeutic effects.

dig·i·tate (dij′i-tāt). Marked by a number of fingerlike processes or impressions. [L. *digitatus,* having fingers, fr. *digitus,* finger]

dig·i·ta·tion (dij-i-tā′shŭn). A process resembling a finger. [Mod. L. *digitatio*]

dig·i·ta·ti·o·nes hip·po·cam·pi (dij-i-tā-shē-ō′nēz hip-ō-kam′pē). SYN *foot* of hippocampus. [Mod. L. pl. of *digitatio*]

di·gi·ti (dij′i-tī). Plural of digitus. [L.]

dig·i·tin (dij′i-tin). SYN digitonin.

dig·i·to·nin (dij-i-tō′nin). **1.** A steroid glycoside obtained from *Digitalis purpurea* that has no cardiac action; used as a reagent in the determination of plasma cholesterol and steroids having a 3-hydroxyl group in beta configuration. **2.** A mixture of four different steroids found in the seeds of *Digitalis purpurea;* a strong hemolytic poison. They can act as nonionic detergents in the solubilization of membrane proteins. SYN digitin.

dig·i·tox·i·gen·in (dij′i-toks′ĭ-jen-in). The aglycon derived from digitoxin; can be prepared by refluxing digitoxin in a mixture of water, alcohol, and hydrochloric acid.

dig·i·tox·in (dij-i-tok′sin). A cardioactive glycoside obtained from the leaves of *Digitalis purpurea;* it is more completely absorbed from the gastrointestinal tract than is digitalis. Largely eliminated by hepatic metabolism. SYN crystalline digitalin.

dig·i·tox·ose (dij′ĭ-toks′ōs). The sugar moiety obtained by mild acid hydrolysis of the glycosides digitoxin, gitoxin, and digoxin. The hydrolysis yields 3 moles of d. for each mole of the respective aglycon.

D-dig·i·tox·ose (dij′i-toks′ōs). The carbohydrate moiety found in digitalis glycosides; 2,6-dideoxy-D-*ribo*-hexose.

dig·i·tus, pl. **di·gi·ti** (dij′i-tŭs, -tī) [TA]. SYN digit. [L.]
    d. anula′ris [TA], SYN ring *finger.*
    d. auricula′ris, SYN little *finger.*
    dig′iti hippocrat′ici, obsolete term for clubbed digits or fingers. SEE clubbing.
    d. ma′nus [TA], SYN finger.
    d. (manus) me′dius [TA], SYN middle *finger.*
    d. (manus) min′imus [TA], SYN little *finger.*
    d. (manus) pri′mus, ✕official alternate term for thumb.
    d. (manus) quartus IV, ✕official alternate term for ring *finger.*
    d. (manus) quin′tus [V], SYN little *finger.*
    d. (manus) secun′dus [II], ✕official alternate term for index *finger.*
    d. (manus) ter′tius [III], ✕official alternate term for middle *finger.*
    d. ped′is [TA], SYN toe.
    d. (pedis) minimus [V] [TA], SYN little *toe* [V].
    d. pedis primus I, ✕official alternate term for great *toe* I.
    d. (pedis) quartus [IV] [TA], SYN fourth *toe* [IV].
    d. (pedis) quintus [V], ✕official alternate term for little *toe* [V].
    d. (pedis) secundus [II] [TA], SYN second *toe* [II].
    d. (pedis) tertius [III] [TA], SYN third *toe* [III].
    d. val′gus, permanent deviation of one or more fingers to the radial side.
    d. va′rus, permanent deviation of one or more fingers to the ulnar side.

di·glos·sia (dī-glos′ē-ă). A developmental condition that results in a longitudinal split in the tongue. SEE bifid *tongue.* [G. *di-,* two, + *glōssa,* tongue]

di·glyc·er·ide li·pase (dī-glis′er-īd). SYN lipoprotein lipase.

di·gly·co·coll hy·dro·i·o·dide-io·dine (dī-glī′kō-kol hī-drō-ī′ō-dīd-ī′ō-dīn). Two moles of diglycocoll hydroiodide combined with two atomic weights of iodine; an antibacterial agent used in tablet form to disinfect drinking water.

di·gna·thus (dī-nath′ŭs). A malformed fetus with a double mandible. SYN augnathus. [G. *di-,* two, + *gnathos,* jaw]

di·gox·i·gen·in (dī-joks′ĭ-jen-in). The aglycon of digoxin that is joined by 3 moles of digitoxose to form the glycoside, digoxin.

di·gox·in (dī-jok′sin). A cardioactive steroid glycoside obtained from *Digitalis lanata.* Largely eliminated by the kidneys.

Di Guglielmo, Giovanni, Italian physician, 1886–1961. SEE Di G.'s *disease, syndrome.*

di·gy·ny, di·gyn·ia (dī′ji-nē, dī-jin′ē-ă). Fertilization of a diploid ovum by a sperm, which results in a triploid zygote. Cf. diandry. [di- + G. *gynē,* woman]

di·het·er·o·zy·gote (dī-het′er-ō-zī′gōt). An individual heterozygous at two loci of interest, especially in genetic linkage analysis.

di·hy·brid (dī-hī′brid). The offspring of parents differing in two characters. [G. *di-,* two, + L. *hybrida,* offspring of a tame sow and a wild boar]

di·hy·dral·a·zine (dī-hī-drăl′ă-zēn). An antihypertensive agent.

di·hy·drate (dī-hī′drāt). A compound with two molecules of water of crystallization.

di·hy·dra·zone (dī-hī′dră-zōn). SYN osazone.

△**dihydro-.** Prefix indicating the addition of two hydrogen atoms. [G. *di,* two + *hydor,* water]

di·hy·dro·a·scor·bic ac·id (dī-hī′drō-as-kōr′bik). SYN L-gulonolactone.

di·hy·dro·bi·op·ter·in (dī-hī′drō-bī-op′ter-in). Precursor to tetrahydrobiopterin, a required cofactor for a number of enzymes, including the biosynthesis of L-tyrosine; the inability to synthesize d. can result in a form of malignant hyperphenylalaninemia.
    d. reductase, SYN dihydropteridine reductase.

di·hy·dro·co·deine tar·trate (dī-hī-drō-kō′dēn). An analgesic derivative of codeine, about one-sixth as potent as morphine; a narcotic antitussive.

di·hy·dro·co·de·i·none (dī-hī-drō-kō′dēn-ōn). SYN hydrocodone.

4,5α-di·hy·dro·cor·ti·sol (dī-hī-drō-kōr′ti-sol). SYN hydrallostane.

di·hy·dro·cor·ti·sone (dī-hī-drō-kōr′ti-sōn). A metabolite of cortisone, reduced at the 4,5 double bond.

di·hy·dro·er·go·cor·nine (dī-hī′drō-er-gō-kōr′nīn). An ergot alkaloid derivative prepared by the hydrogenation of ergocornine and less toxic than the latter. SEE dihydroergotoxine mesylate.

di·hy·dro·er·go·cris·tine (dī-hī′drō-er-gō-kris′tēn). An ergot alkaloid derivative prepared by the hydrogenation of ergocristine and less toxic than the latter. SEE dihydroergotoxine mesylate.

di·hy·dro·er·go·cryp·tine (dī-hī′drō-er-gō-krip′tēn). An ergot alkaloid derivative prepared by the hydrogenation of ergocryptine and less toxic than the latter. SEE dihydroergotoxine mesylate.

di·hy·dro·er·got·a·mine (dī-hī′drō-er-got′ă-mēn). An ergot alkaloid derivative prepared by the hydrogenation of ergotamine; used in the treatment of migraine; less toxic and less oxytocic than ergotamine.

di·hy·dro·er·go·tox·ine mes·y·late (dī-hī′drō-er-gō-tok′sēn). A mixture of dihydroergocornine methanesulfate, dihydroergocristine methanesulfate, and dihydroergocryptine methane sulfate; used as an α-adrenergic blocking agent for relief of cardiovascular insufficiency.

di·hy·dro·fo·late re·duc·tase (DHFR) (dī-hī-drō-fō′lāt). An enzyme reversibly oxidizing tetrahydrofolate to 7,8-dihydrofolate with NADP⁺. A crucial enzyme in one-carbon metabolism; used as a marker of drug resistance to methotrexate. SYN 5,6,7,8-tetrahydrofolate dehydrogenase.

7,8-di·hy·dro·fo·lic ac·id (dī-hī-drō-fō′lik). Intermediate between folic acid and 5,6,7,8-tetrahydrofolic acid, oxidation of the latter requiring NADP$^+$ and dehydrofolate reductase.

dihydrogen. SYN hydrogen (2).

di·hy·dro·lip·o·am·ide S-ace·tyl·trans·fer·ase (dī-hī′drō-lip-ō-am′id ă-sē-til-trans′fer-āz). An enzyme catalyzing the transfer of an acetyl grout from S^6-acetyldihydrolipoamide to coenzyme A. A part of many enzyme complexes (e.g., pyruvate dehydrogenase complex). SYN lipoate acetyltransferase, thioltransacetylase A.

di·hy·dro·lip·o·am·ide de·hy·dro·gen·ase (dī-hī′drō-lip-ō-am′id dī-hī-dro′jen-āz). A flavoenzyme oxidizing dihydrolipoamide at the expense of NAD$^+$; completes the oxidative decarboxylation of pyruvate; a part of several enzyme complexes (e.g., α-ketoglutarate dehydrogenase complex). Decreased activity leads to neuronal loss in brain resulting in psychomotor retardation. SYN coenzyme factor, lipoamide dehydrogenase, lipoamide reductase (NADH), lipoyl dehydrogenase.

di·hy·dro·li·po·ic ac·id (dī-hī′drō-lip-ō′ik). Reduced lipoic acid, formed by cleavage of the –S–S– bond as a result of the acceptance of two hydrogens. Cf. lipoic acid.

di·hy·dro·mor·phi·none hy·dro·chlo·ride (dī-hī-drō-mōr′fi-nōn). SYN hydromorphone hydrochloride.

di·hy·dro·or·o·tase (dī-hī′drō-ōr-ō′tās). An enzyme catalyzing ring closure of N-carbamoyl-L-aspartate to form L-5,6-dihydroorotate and water; an enzyme in pyrimidine biosynthesis. SYN carbamoylaspartate dehydrase.

di·hy·dro·or·o·tate (dī-hī′drō-ōr-ō′tāt). L-5,6-Dihydroorotate; an intermediate in the biosynthesis of pyrimidines.

di·hy·dro·pter·i·dine re·duc·tase. An enzyme that catalyzes the reversible formation of tetrahydrobiopterin from dihydrobiopterine using NADPH; a deficiency of this enzyme can result in malignant hyperphenylalaninemia. SYN dihydrobiopterin reductase.

di·hy·dro·pte·ro·ic ac·id (dī-hī′drō-te-rō′ik). An intermediate in the formation of folic acid; a compound of 6-hydroxymethylpterin and p-aminobenzoic acid, the combining of which is inhibited by sulfonamides.

di·hy·dro·py·rim·i·dine de·hy·dro·gen·ase (dī-hī-drō′pī-rim′i-dēn dē-hī-dro′jen-ās). An enzyme in pyrimidine biosynthesis that reacts 5,6-dihydrouracil with NADP$^+$ to form uracil and NADPH; it also acts on dihydrothymine; a deficiency of this enzyme can result in hyperuracil thyminuria. SYN dihydrouracil dehydrogenase.

di·hy·dro·strep·to·my·cin (dī-hī′drō-strep-tō-mī′sin). An aminoglycoside antibiotic similar in action to streptomycin but with a higher risk of ototoxicity.

di·hy·dro·ta·chys·ter·ol (dī-hī′drō-tă-kis′ter-ōl). SEE tachysterol.

di·hy·dro·tes·tos·ter·one (dī-hī′drō-tes-tos′ter-ōn). SYN stanolone.

di·hy·dro·ur·a·cil (dī-hī-drō-ūr′ă-sil). 5,6-Dihydrouracil; a reduction product of uracil and one of the intermediates of uracil catabolism.

di·hy·dro·ur·a·cil de·hy·dro·gen·ase. SYN dihydropyrimidine dehydrogenase.

di·hy·dro·ur·i·dine (hU, hu, D) (dī-hī-drō-ūr′i-dēn). Uridine in which the 5,6-double bond has been saturated by addition of two hydrogen atoms; a rare constituent of transfer ribonucleic acids.

⌂**dihydroxy-.** Prefix denoting addition of two hydroxyl groups; as a suffix, becomes -diol.

di·hy·drox·y·ac·e·tone (dī′hī-drok-sē-as′e-tōn). HOCH$_2$-CO-CH$_2$OH; 1,3-dihydroxy-2-propanone; glycerone; the simplest ketose. SYN glycerulose.

d. phosphate (DHAP), one of the intermediates in the glycolytic pathway and in fat biosynthesis; glycerone phosphate.

d. phosphate acyltransferase, an enzyme that catalyzes an important step in plasmalogen biosynthesis; an acyl group from acyl-CoA is transferred to d. phosphate producing free coenzyme A and 1-acyldihydroxyacetone phosphate.

2,8-di·hy·drox·y·ad·en·ine (di-hī-drok′sē-ad′ĕ-nēn). An insoluble minor product of adenine catabolism that is elevated in individuals with an absence of adenine phosphoribosyltransferase.

di·hy·drox·y·a·lu·mi·num ami·no·ac·e·tate (dī-hī-drok′sē-ă-loo′mi-nŭm am′i-nō-as′ĕ-tāt). Basic aluminum glycinate, a basic aluminum salt of aminoacetic acid containing small amounts of aluminum hydroxide and aminoacetic acid; used as an antacid in hyperchlorhydria and peptic ulcer.

di·hy·drox·y·a·lu·mi·num so·di·um car·bon·ate. A gastric antacid.

1α,25-di·hy·drox·y·cho·le·cal·cif·er·ol (dī-hī-drok′sē-ko′lē-kal-si′fer-ol). An active form of vitamin D formed in the proximal convoluted tubules of the kidney. A deficiency of the receptor for 1α,25-dihydroxycholecalciferol results in all of the features of a vitamin D$_3$ deficiency.

1,25-di·hy·drox·y·er·go·cal·cif·er·ol (dī-hī-drok′sē-er′gō-kal-sif′er-ol). A biologically active metabolite of vitamin D$_2$. SYN ercalcitriol.

3,4-di·hy·drox·y·phen·yl·al·a·nine (dī-hī-droks′e-fen-il-al′ă-nēn). SYN dopa.

di·i·o·dide (dī-ī′ō-dīd). A compound containing two atoms of iodine per molecule.

⌂**diiodo-.** Prefix indicating two atoms of iodine. [G. di, + ioeidēs, violet flower color]

di·i·o·do·hy·drox·y·quin (dī-ī-ō′dō-hī-drok′si-kwin). C$_9$H$_5$I$_2$NO; an antiprotozoal agent, used in the treatment of intestinal amebiasis. SYN diodoquin.

di·i·o·do·ty·ro·sine (DIT) (dī′ī-ō-dō-tī′rō-sēn). An intermediate in the biosynthesis of thyroid hormone.

di·i·so·pro·mine (dī-ī-sō-prō′mēn). A cholagogue. SYN disopromine.

di·i·so·pro·pyl flu·o·ro·phos·phate (DFP) (dī-ī-sō-prō′pil flōr-ō-fos′fāt). SYN isofluorphate.

di·i·so·pro·pyl im·in·o·di·ace·tic ac·id (DISIDA) (dī-ē-sō-prō′pil im′i- nō-dī-ă-sē-tik). A radiopharmaceutical labeled with ^{99m}Tc, used for cholescintigraphy. SYN disofenin.

2,6-di·i·so·pro·pyl phe·nol. SYN propofol.

2,3-di·ke·to·L·gul·on·ate. A product of catabolism of vitamin C; formed from L-dehydroascorbate; it has no vitamin C activity.

di·ke·to·hy·drin·dyl·i·dene-di·ke·to·hy·drin·da·mine (dī-kē′tō-hī-drin-dil′i-dēn dī-kē′tō-hī-drind′ă-mēn). The colored product formed in the reaction of an α-amino acid and ninhydrin (triketohydrindene hydrate); a reaction used in the quantitative assay of α-amino acids.

di·ke·tone (dī-kē′tōn). A molecule containing two carbonyl groups; e.g., acetylacetone (CH$_3$COCH$_2$COCH$_3$).

di·ke·to·pi·per·a·zines (dī-kē′tō-pī-per′ă-zēnz). A class of organic compounds with a closed ring structure formed from two α-amino acids by the joining of the α-amino group of each to the carboxyl group of the other, with the loss of two molecules of water.

dil. Abbreviation for L. dilue, dilute, or L. dilutus, diluted.

di·lac·er·a·tion (dī-las-er-ā′shŭn). Displacement of some portion of a developing tooth which is then further developed in its new relation, resulting in a tooth with sharply angulated root(s). [L. di-lacero, pp. laceratus, to tear in pieces, fr. lacer, mangled]

di·la·tan·cy (dī-lā′tan-sē). An increasing viscosity with increasing rate of shear accompanied by volumetric expansion. [L. dilato, to dilate]

dil·a·ta·tion (dil-ă-tā′shŭn). SYN dilation.

digital d., use of the finger or finger-tip to enlarge an orifice or opening, such as enlarging the orifice of a sclerosed mitral valve surgically.

dil·a·ta·tor (dil′ă-tā-tĕr, -tōr). SYN dilator.

di·late (dī′lāt). To perform or undergo dilation.

di·la·tion (dī-lā′shŭn). **1.** Physiologic or artificial enlargement of a hollow structure or opening. **2.** The act of stretching or enlarging an opening or the lumen of a hollow structure. SYN dilatation. [L. dilato, pp. dilatatus, to spread out, dilate]

d. and extraction, a form of abortion in which the cervix is dilated and the fetus extracted in pieces using surgical forceps; technique used to complete a second trimester spontaneous abortion or as a form of induced abortion.

di *(margin tab)*

post-stenotic d., d. of an artery, most commonly the pulmonary artery or the aorta, distal to an area of narrowing.

d. and suction, SYN suction *curettage.*

urethral d., increasing the caliber of the urethra by passage of a dilator.

di·la·tion and cu·ret·tage (D & C). Dilation of the cervix and curettement of the endometrium.

di·la·tion and evac·u·a·tion (D & E). Dilation of the cervix and removal of the products of conception.

di·la·tor (dī′lă-tĕr). **1.** An instrument designed for enlarging a hollow structure or opening. **2.** A muscle that pulls open an orifice. **3.** A substance that causes dilation or enlargement of an opening or the lumen of a hollow structure. SEE ALSO bougie. SYN dilatator.

Chevalier-Jackson d., an esophageal dilator that passes through a rigid endoscope.

Hanks d., uterine d.'s of solid metal construction.

Hegar d.'s, a series of cylindrical bougies of graduated sizes used to dilate the cervical canal.

hydrostatic d., an instrument for dilating esophageal strictures; fluid pressure is delivered into a flexible area of the instrument placed in the stricture to establish a uniform dilating pressure.

d. ir′idis, SYN dilator pupillae *muscle.*

Kollmann d., a metallic expandable instrument used to dilate urethral strictures.

pneumatic d., any of a variety of catheters fitted with distal balloons that can be inflated to desired pressures for overcoming obstructions in hollow viscera; most often used to rupture the lower esophageal sphincter to treat achalasia.

Pratt d.'s, cylindrical metal rods of graduated sizes used to dilate the cervical canal.

d. of pupil, SYN dilator pupillae *muscle.*

Walther d., a gently curved instrument that tapers to an increased diameter, used to dilate the female urethra.

dil·do, dil·doe (dil′dō). An artificial penis; an object having the approximate shape and size of an erect penis, and commonly made of wood, plastic, or rubber; utilized for sexual pleasure.

di·lem·ma.

masking dilemma, a problem encountered in establishing the bone conduction thresholds in severe bilateral conductive hearing loss, in which the amount of masking of the nontest ear exceeds the interaural attenuation so that enough masking is too much masking.

dill oil. A volatile oil distilled from the fruit of *Anethum graveolens* (family Umbelliferae); a carminative.

di·lox·a·nide fu·ro·ate (dī-lok′să-nīd fū′rō-āt). An amebicide used in the treatment of dysentery.

dil·ti·a·zem hy·dro·chlo·ride (dil-tī′ă-zem). A calcium channel blocking agent used as a coronary vasodilator, an antiarrhythmic, and antihypertensive.

dil·u·ent. 1. Ingredient in a medicinal preparation that lacks pharmacologic activity but is pharmaceutically necessary or desirable. In tablet or capsule dosage forms, this may be lactose or starch; it is particularly useful in increasing the bulk of potent drug substances whose mass is too small for dosage form manufacture or administration. May be a liquid for the dissolution of drug(s) to be injected, ingested, or inhaled. **2.** Denoting that which dilutes; the diluting agent.

di·lute (dil.) (dī-loot′). **1.** To reduce a solution or mixture in concentration, strength, quality, or purity. **2.** Diluted; denoting a solution or mixture so effected. [L. *di-luo,* to wash away, dilute]

di·lu·tion (dī-loo′shŭn). **1.** The act of being diluted. **2.** A diluted solution or mixture. **3.** In microbiologic techniques, a method for counting the number of viable cells in a suspension; a sample is diluted to the point where an aliquot, when plated, yields a countable number of separate colonies.

dim. Abbreviation for L. *dimidius,* one-half.

di·ma·zole di·hy·dro·chlo·ride (dī′mā-zōl). SYN diamthazole dihydrochloride.

di·ma·zon (dī-mā′zon). An azo compound occurring in red crystals; used with petrolatum as an ointment to stimulate epithelial cell proliferation and thus promote the healing of superficial wounds.

di·me·lia (dī-mē′lē-ă). Congenital duplication of the whole or a part of a limb. [G. *di-,* two, + *melos,* limb]

di·men·hy·dri·nate (dī-men-hī′dri-nāt). The 8-chlorotheophylline salt of the antihistamine, diphenhydramine; used for the prevention of motion sickness, as an antihistamine and mild sedative. Also used in the treatment of Parkinson disease, as it has appreciable anticholinergic properties.

di·men·sion (di-men′shŭn). Scope, size, magnitude; denoting, in the plural, linear measurements of length, width, and height.

buccolingual d., the diameter or d. of a premolar or molar tooth from buccal to lingual surface.

occlusal vertical d. of the face when the teeth or occlusion rims are in contact in centric occlusion; *decrease* in occlusal vertical d. may result from modification of tooth form by attrition or grinding, drifting of teeth, or, in edentulous patients, by resorption of residual ridges; *increase* may result from modifications of tooth form, tooth position, height of occlusion rims, rebasing or relining, or occlusal splints.

rest vertical d., the vertical d. of the face with the jaws in rest relation; *decrease* in rest vertical d. may or may not accompany a decrease in occlusal vertical d.; it may occur without a decrease in occlusal vertical d. in patients with a preponderant activity of the jaw-closing musculature, as in patients with muscular hypertenseness or in chronic gum chewers; *increase* in rest vertical d. may or may not accompany an increase in occlusal vertical d.; it sometimes occurs after the removal of remaining occlusal contacts, perhaps as a result of the removal of noxious reflex stimuli.

vertical d., a vertical measurement of the face between any two arbitrarily selected points which are conveniently located, one above and one below the mouth, usually in the midline. SYN vertical opening.

di·mer (dī′mer). A compound or unit produced by the combination of two like molecules; in the strictest sense, without loss of atoms (thus nitrogen tetroxide, N_2O_4, is the d. of nitrogen dioxide, NO_2), but usually by elimination of H_2O or a similar small molecule between the two (e.g., a disaccharide), or by simple noncovalent association (as of two identical protein molecules); higher orders of complexity are called trimers, tetramers, oligomers, and polymers. [G. *di-,* two, + -mer]

pyrimidine d., a product of ultraviolet radiation of pyrimidines in nucleic acids; most frequently thymidine d.'s.

thymine d., a product of ultraviolet irradiation of thymine (free in ice or bound in nucleic acids) in which two thymine residues become linked by formation of a cyclobutane ring involving both C-5's and both C-6's at the expense of the two double bonds; several stereoisomeric forms are possible.

di·mer·cap·rol (dī-mer-kap′rol). A chelating agent, developed as an antidote for lewisite and other arsenical poisons. It acts by competing for the metal with the essential —SH groups in the pyruvate oxidase system of the cells and forms, with arsenic, a stable, relatively nontoxic cyclic compound, the metal having a greater affinity for it than for the —SH groups of the cell proteins; also used as an antidote for antimony, bismuth, chromium, mercury, gold, and nickel. SYN antilewisite, British anti-Lewisite.

di·mer·cur·i·on (dī-mer′kŭr-ī′on). The mercuric ion, Hg^{2+}.

di·mer·ic (dī′mer-ik). Having the characteristics of a dimer.

dim·er·ous (dim′er-ŭs). Consisting of two parts. [G. *di-,* two, + *meros,* part]

di·met·a·crine tar·trate (dī-met′ă-krēn). An antidepressant.

di·meth·a·di·one (dī-meth-ă-dī′ōn). The active metabolite formed by the N-demethylation of trimethadione, an oxazolidinedione type antiepileptic agent. Can be used for *in vivo* measurement of intracellular pH.

di·meth·i·cone (dī-meth′i-kōn). A silicone oil consisting of dimethylsiloxane polymers, usually incorporated into a petrolatum base or a nongreasy preparation and used for the protection of normal skin against various, chiefly industrial, skin irritants; may also be used to prevent diaper dermatitis.

di·meth·in·dene ma·le·ate (dī-meth′in-dēn). An antihistamine also used as an antipruritic.

di·me·this·ter·one (dī-me-this′ter-ōn). A modified testosterone or ethisterone; an orally effective synthetic progestin used alone or in combination with ethynyl estradiol as a contraceptive agent.

di·meth·o·thi·a·zine mes·y·late (dī-meth-ō-thī′ă-zēn). SYN fonazine mesylate.

di·me·thox·a·nate hy·dro·chlo·ride (dī′me-thok′să-nāt). A non-narcotic antitussive agent, less effective than codeine.

di·me·thox·y·am·phet·a·mine (DMA). A hallucinogen with properties resembling *lysergic acid* diethylamide (LSD).

2,5-di·me·thox·y-4-meth·yl·am·phet·a·mine (DOM). An hallucinogenic agent chemically related to amphetamine and mescaline, a drug of abuse.

di·meth·yl·al·lyl·py·ro·phos·phate (di-meth′il-ăl′lil-pī′rō -fos′ fāt). An intermediate in steroid and terpene biosynthesis.

di·meth·yl·a·mi·no·az·o·ben·zene (dī-meth′il-ă-mē-nō-az-ō-ben′zēn) [C.I. 11160]. SYN butter yellow.

di·meth·yl·ar·sin·ic ac·id (dī-meth′il-ar-sin′ik). SYN cacodylic acid.

di·meth·yl·ben·zene (dī-meth-il-ben′zēn). SYN xylol.

5,6-di·meth·yl·benz·im·id·a·zole (dī-meth′il-benz-ē-mid-a-zōl). A structural moiety found in one of the cobalamins.

di·meth·yl·car·bi·nol (dī-meth-il-kar′bi-nol). SYN isopropyl alcohol.

di·meth·yl-1-car·bo·me·thox·y-1-pro·pen-2-yl phos·phate. An organic phosphorus compound used as a systemic poison for the extermination of such pests as mites, aphids, and houseflies.

β,β-di·meth·yl·cys·teine (dī-meth-il-sis′tē-ēn). SYN penicillamine.

di·meth·yl im·in·o·di·ace·tic ac·id (HIDA) (dī-meth′il im′i-nō-dī-ă-sē-tik). A radiopharmaceutical labeled with ^{99m}Tc, an early agent used for cholescintigraphy.

di·meth·yl ke·tone (dī-meth′il kē′tōn). SYN acetone.

di·meth·yl·mer·cu·ry (dī-meth-il-mer′kū-rē). A contaminant of seafood products synthesized in sediments from mercury and mercury-containing chemicals dumped in waters supporting marine life. The methylmercury is concentrated in aquatic life forms and can thus be deposited in fishes intended for human consumption. Probable cause of Minimata disease, a teratogenic condition characterized by multiple birth defects. An inorganic reagent. SEE ALSO Minamata *disease*. SYN methylmercury.

di·meth·yl·phe·nol (dī-meth-il-fē′nol). SYN xylenol.

di·meth·yl·phen·yl·pi·per·a·zin·i·um (DMPP) (dī-meth′il-fe-n′il-pi-pār-ă-zin′ē-ŭm). A highly selective stimulant of autonomic ganglionic cells; used experimentally.

di·meth·yl phthal·ate (dī-meth′il thal′āt). An insect repellent.

di·meth·yl·pi·per·a·zine tar·trate (dī-meth′il-pi-pār′ă-zēn). A diuretic, also used as a uric acid solvent.

di·meth·yl sul·fate. An industrial chemical (sulfuric acid dimethyl ester $(CH_3)_2SO_4$), used in synthesis as an alkylating agent; it causes nystagmus, convulsions, and death from pulmonary complications.

di·meth·yl sulf·ox·ide (DMSO) (dī-meth′il). Me_2SO; a penetrating solvent, enhancing absorption of therapeutic agents from the skin; an industrial solvent that has been proposed as an effective analgesic and anti-inflammatory agent in arthritis and bursitis.

***N,N*-di·meth·yl·tryp·ta·mine (DMT)** (dī-meth′il-trip′tă-mēn). A psychotomimetic agent present in several South American snuffs (e.g., cohoba snuff) and in the leaves of *Prestonia amazonica* (family Apocynaceae). Effects are similar to those of LSD, but with more rapid onset, greater likelihood of a panic reaction, and a shorter duration (1 to 2 hours, "businessman's trip"); it produces pronounced autonomic effects, including a marked increase in blood pressure.

di·meth·yl *d*-tu·bo·cu·ra·rine. SYN metocurine iodide.

di·meth·yl tu·bo·cu·ra·rine chlo·ride. Dimethyl ether of *d*-tubocurarine chloride; a skeletal muscle relaxant. SEE tubocurarine chloride.

di·meth·yl tu·bo·cu·ra·rine io·dide. SYN metocurine iodide.

di·me·tria (dī-mē′trē-ă). Obsolete term for *uterus* didelphys. [G. *di-*, two, + *mētra*, womb]

Dimmer, Friedrich, Austrian ophthalmologist, 1855–1926. SEE D. *keratitis.*

di·mor·phic (dī-mōr′fik). **1.** In fungi, a term referring to growth and reproduction in two forms: mold and yeast. SYN dimorphous (2). **2.** SYN dimorphous (1).

di·mor·phism (dī-mōr′fizm). **1.** Existence in two shapes or forms; denoting a difference of crystalline form exhibited by the same substance, or a difference in form or outward appearance between individuals of the same species (e.g., sexual dimorphism). **2.** The occurrence in plants of two distinct forms of leaves or other parts in the same individual plant. [G. *di-*, two, + *morphē*, shape]

sexual d., the somatic differences within species between male and female individuals that arise as a consequence of sexual maturation; inclusive of, but not restricted to, the secondary sexual characters.

di·mor·phous (dī-mōr′fŭs). **1.** Having the property of dimorphism. SYN dimorphic (2). **2.** SYN dimorphic (1).

dim·ple (dim′pl). **1.** A natural indentation, usually circular and of small area, in the chin, cheek, or sacral region. **2.** A depression of similar appearance to a d., resulting from trauma or the contraction of scar tissue. **3.** To cause d.'s.

coccygeal d., SYN coccygeal *foveola.*

postanal d., SYN coccygeal *foveola.*

dimp·ling. 1. Causing dimples. **2.** A condition marked by the formation of dimples, natural or artificial.

di·ner·ic (dī-ner′ik). Denoting the interface between two mutually immiscible liquids (e.g., oil and water) in the same container. [di- + G. *nerōn*, water]

di·ni·tro·cel·lu·lose (dī-nī-trō-sel′ū-lōs). SYN pyroxylin.

4,6-di·ni·tro-*o*-cre·sol. An insecticide used against mites in the form of a spray or dust; also used as a weed killer.

di·ni·tro·gen mon·ox·ide (dī-nī′trō-jen). SYN nitrous oxide.

2,4-di·ni·tro·phe·nol (DNP, Dnp) (dī-nī-trō-fē′nol). N_2pH-OH; a toxic dye, chemically related to trinitrophenol (picric acid), used in biochemical studies of oxidative processes where it uncouples oxidative phosphorylation; it is also a metabolic stimulant.

di·no·flag·el·late (dī′nō-flaj′ĕ-lāt). A plantlike flagellate of the subclass Phytomastigophorea, some species of which (e.g., *Gonyaulax cantanella*) produce a potent neurotoxin that may cause severe food intoxication following ingestion of parasitized shellfish. [G. *dinos*, whirling, + L. *flagellum*, a whip]

Dinoflagellida. An order in the phylum Sareomastigophorea characterized by the presence of two flagella so placed as to cause the organism to have a whirling motility. Its outer surface is composed of cellulose-containing plates whose size and number vary with genus and species.

di·no·prost (dī′nō-prost). An oxytocic agent. SYN prostaglandin $F_{2\alpha}$.

d. tromethamine, an oxytocic agent. SYN prostaglandin $F_{2\alpha}$ tromethamine.

di·no·pros·tone (dī-nō-pros′tōn). An oxytocic agent used as an abortifacient. SYN prostaglandin E_2.

di·nu·cle·o·tide (dī-noo′klē-ō-tīd). A compound containing two nucleotides; e.g., NAD^+, ApGp.

Di·oc·to·phy·ma (dī-ok-tō-fī′mă). A genus of very large nematode worms infecting the kidney. [L. fr. G. *dionkoō*, to distend, + *phyma*, growth]

D. rena′le, a large blood-red nematode found in the pelvis of the kidney and the peritoneal cavity of the dog; fairly common in wild carnivores like the mink, but rarely found in humans; the life cycle is via leeches ectoparasitic on crayfish, which are then eaten by various fishes and finally by humans or any of a number of other mammalian fish-eating hosts.

di·oc·to·phy·mi·a·sis (dī-ok′tō-fi-mī′ă-sis). Infection of animals and rarely humans with the giant kidney worm, *Dioctophyma renale.*

di·oc·tyl cal·ci·um sul·fo·suc·ci·nate (dī-ok′til kal′sē-ŭm sŭl-fō-sŭk′si-nāt). SYN docusate calcium.

di·oc·tyl so·di·um sul·fo·suc·ci·nate. SYN docusate sodium.

Di·o·don (dī′ō-don). A genus of porcupine fishes related to balloon fish, globefish, and puffers. Although the common puffer is widely eaten as "sea squab" in the United States, many puffers, especially in the Pacific, are poisonous because of the presence of a neurotoxin, tetrodotoxin, in the liver and ovary. [G. *di-*, two, + *odous* (*odont-*), tooth]

di·o·done (dī′ō-dōn). SYN iodopyracet.

di·o·do·quin (dī-ō′dō-kwin). SYN diiodohydroxyquin.

Diogenes, Of Sinope, Greek philosopher, 412–323 B.C. SEE D. *cup; poculum* diogenis.

-diol (dī′ol). **1.** Suffix form of the prefix dihydroxy. **2.** A member of a class of compounds containing two hydroxyl groups.

gym-diol, *gym-diol,* a compound in which both hydroxyl groups are attached to the same carbon atom; an intermediate in many reactions.

di·ol·a·mine (dī-ōl′ă-mēn). USAN-approved contraction for diethanolamine.

di·op·ter (D) (dī-op′ter). The unit of refracting power of lenses, denoting the reciprocal of the focal length expressed in meters. [G. *dioptra,* a leveling instrument]

prism d. (p.d.), the unit of measurement of the deviation of light in passing through a prism, being a deflection of 1 cm at a distance of 1 m.

di·op·trics (dī-op′triks). The branch of optics concerned with the refraction of light.

di·os·cin (dī-ōs-in). A steroid saponin found in yams (Dioscorea) and trilliums.

di·ose (dī′ōs). SYN glycolaldehyde.

di·os·gen·in (dī′os-jen′in). The aglycon of dioscing a sapogenin derived from the saponins dioscin and trillin found in the roots of plants such as the yam; its steroid portion serves as a source from which pregnenolone and progesterone can be prepared.

di·otic (dī-ot′ik). Simultaneous presentation of the same sound to each ear. [di- + otic]

di·ov·u·lar (dī′ov-ū-lar). Relating to two ova. SYN biovular. [di- + Mod. L. *ovulum,* dim. of L. *ovum,* egg]

di·ov·u·la·to·ry (dī-ō′vū-lă-tō′rē). Releasing two ova in one ovarian cycle.

di·ox·ane (dī-oks′ān). 1,4-Dioxane; a colorless liquid used as a solvent for cellulose esters and in histology as a drying agent. SYN 1,4-diethylene dioxide.

di·ox·ide (dī-oks′īd). A molecule containing two atoms of oxygen; e.g., carbon dioxide, CO_2.

di·ox·in (dī-oks′in) **1.** A ring consisting of two oxygen atoms, four CH groups, and two double bonds; the positions of the oxygen atoms are specified by prefixes, as in 1,4-dioxin. **2.** Abbreviation for dibenzo[*b,e*][1,4]dioxin which may be visualized as an anhydride of two molecules of 1,2-benzenediol (pyrocatechol), thus forming two oxygen bridges between two benzene moieties, or as a 1,4-dioxin with a benzene ring fused to catch each of the two CH=CH groups. **3.** A contaminant in the herbicide, 2,4,5-T; it is potentially toxic, teratogenic, and carcinogenic.

di·ox·y·ben·zone (dī-ok-sē-ben′zōn). An ultraviolet screen for topical application to the skin.

di·ox·y·gen·ase (dī-oks′ē-jen-ās). An oxidoreductase that incorporates two atoms of oxygen (from one molecule of O_2) into the (reduced) substrate.

D.I.P. Abbreviation for desquamative interstitial *pneumonia.*

dip. **1.** A downward inclination or slope. **2.** A preparation for coating a surface by submersion, as for the destruction of skin parasites. [M.E. *dippen*]

Cournand d., in constrictive pericarditis, rapid early diastolic fall and reascent of the ventricular pressure curve to an elevated plateau (square root configuration).

di·pep·ti·dase (dī-pep′ti-dās). A hydrolase catalyzing the hydrolysis of a dipeptide to its constituent amino acids.

methionyl d., a hydrolase catalyzing the hydrolysis of an L-methionyl-amino acid to L-methionine and an amino acid.

di·pep·tide (dī-pep′tīd). A combination of two amino acids by means of a peptide (–CO–NH–) link.

di·pep·ti·dyl car·box·y·pep·ti·dase (dī-pep′ti-dil). SYN peptidyl dipeptidase A.

di·pep·ti·dyl pep·ti·dase. A hydrolase occurring in a number of forms: d. p. I, dipeptidyl transferase, cleaving dipeptides from the amino end of polypeptides; d. p. II, with properties similar to those of I, has a different specificity and acts preferably on tripeptides; d. p. III acts on longer peptides.

di·pep·ti·dyl trans·fer·ase. Cleaving dipeptides from the amino end of polypeptides. SEE dipeptidyl peptidase.

Di·pet·a·lo·ne·ma (dī-pet′ă-lō-nē′mă). A genus of nematode filariae with species in humans and many other mammals; as with other filarial worms, it produces microfilariae in blood or tissue fluids, with adults found in deep connective tissue, membranes, or visceral surfaces. [G. *di-*, two, + *petalon,* leaf, + *nēma,* thread]

D. recondi'tum, a filarial species found in dogs, transmitted by fleas and lice, in contrast to the canine heartworm, *Dirofilaria immitis,* which is transmitted by mosquitoes.

D. streptocer'ca, former name for *Mansonella streptocerca.*

di·phal·lus (dī-fal′ŭs). A rare congenital anomaly in which the penis is partly or completely duplicated; may be symmetrical, or placed one above the other; often there are associated urogenital or other anomalies; occurs when two genital tubercles develop. May also be associated with exstrophy of the urinary bladder and splitting of the genital tubercle. SYN bifid penis. [G. *di-*, two, + *phallos,* penis]

di·pha·sic (dī-fā′zik). Occurring in or characterized by two phases or stages.

di·phe·ma·nil meth·yl·sul·fate (dī-fē′mă-nil). An anticholinergic agent.

di·phem·e·thox·i·dine (dī-fem-ĕ-thok′si-dēn). An anorexigenic drug.

di·phen·a·di·one (dī-fen-ă-dī′ōn). An orally effective anticoagulant with actions and uses similar to those of bishydroxycoumarin.

di·phen·an (dī′fen-ān, dī-fen′an). Used as a vermicide in oxyuriasis.

di·phen·hy·dra·mine hy·dro·chlo·ride (dī-fen-hī′dră-mēn). An H_2 antihistaminic with anticholinergic and sedative properties.

di·phen·i·dol (dī-fen′i-dol). An antiemetic.

o-di·phe·no·lase (dī-fen′ō-lās). SYN *catechol* oxidase.

di·phe·nol ox·i·dase (dī-fen′ol). SYN *catechol* oxidase.

di·phe·nox·y·late hy·dro·chlo·ride (dī-fen-ok′si-lāt). An antidiarrheal agent, chemically related to meperidine, that inhibits rhythmic contraction of smooth muscle; it has modest addiction liability. Similar to loperamide.

di·phen·yl (dī-fen′il). Colorless liquid; used as heat transfer agent, frequently as polychlorinated biphenyls (PCBs); as fungistat for oranges (applied to inside of shipping container or wrappers); and in organic syntheses. Produces convulsions and central nervous system depression. SYN biphenyl, phenylbenzene.

diphenyl-. Prefix denoting two independent phenyl groups attached to a third atom or radical, as in diphenylamine.

di·phen·yl·chlor·ar·sine (dī-fen′il-klōr-ar′sēn). A sternutator, inhalation of which causes violent sneezing, cough, salivation, headache, and retrosternal pain; a common vomiting agent used in mob and riot control.

di·phen·yl·cy·an·o·ar·sine (dī-fen′il-sī-an-ō-ar-sēn). A common vomiting agent used for mob and riot control.

di·phen·yl·en·i·mine (dī′fen-il-ēn′i-mēn). SYN carbazole.

di·phen·yl·hy·dan·to·in (dī′fen-il-hī-dan′tō-in). SEE phenytoin.

5,5-di·phen·yl·hy·dan·to·in (dī-fen′il-hī-dan′tō-in). SYN phenytoin.

2,5-di·phen·yl·ox·a·zole (PPO) (dī′fen-il-oks′ă-zōl). A scintillator used in radioactivity measurements by liquid scintillation counting.

di·phen·yl·pyr·a·line hy·dro·chlo·ride (dī-fen-il-pir′ă-lēn).

di

An H$_1$ antihistaminic similar in action and use to diphenhydramine.

di·phos·gene (dī-fos′jēn). A poison gas used in World War I; it is also slightly lacrimatoric.

di·phos·pha·tase (dī-fos′fa-tāz). SYN pyrophosphatase.
   inorganic diphosphatase, SYN inorganic *pyrophosphatase*.

di·phos·phate. SYN pyrophosphate.

di·phos·pho·thi·a·min (dī′fos-fō-thī′ă-min). SYN *thiamin* pyrophosphate.

diph·the·ria (dif-thē-r′ĕă). A specific infectious disease due to the bacterium *Corynebacterium diphtheriae* and its highly potent toxin; marked by severe inflammation that can form a membranous coating, with formation of a thick fibrinous exudate, of the mucous membrane of the pharynx, the nose, and sometimes the tracheobronchial tree; the toxin produces degeneration in peripheral nerves, heart muscle, and other tissues, d. had a high fatality rate, especially in children, but now rare because of an effective vaccine. [G. *diphthera,* leather]
   cutaneous d., a "punched-out" shallow ulcer sometimes bordered or followed by a bulla, resulting from infection of the skin by *Corynebacterium diphtheriae;* systemic manifestations are the same as those of pharyngeal d.
   false d., SYN diphtheroid (1).
   faucial d., severe pharyngitis affecting the fauces, the usual site affected by infection with *Corynebacterium diphtheriae.*
   laryngeal d., d. affecting the larynx, usually with asphyxiation due to obstruction of the airway by the membrane that forms, with fatal outcome. SYN laryngotracheal d.
   laryngotracheal d., SYN laryngeal d.

diph·the·ri·al, diph·the·rit·ic (dif-thē-r′ē-ăl, dif-thĕ-rit′ik). Relating to diphtheria, or the membranous exudate characteristic of this disease. SYN diphtheric.

diph·ther·ic. SYN diphtherial.

diph·the·roid (dif′thĕ-royd). **1.** One of a group of local infections suggesting diphtheria, but caused by microorganisms other than *Corynebacterium diphtheriae.* SYN Epstein disease, false diphtheria, pseudodiphtheria. **2.** Any microorganism resembling *Corynebacterium diphtheriae.* [diphtheria + G. *eidos,* resemblance]

diph·the·ro·tox·in (dif′thĕr-ō-tok′sin). The toxin of diphtheria.

di·phyl·lo·both·ri·a·sis (dī-fil′ō-both-rī′ă-sis). Infection with the cestode *Diphyllobothrium latum;* human infection is caused by ingestion of raw or inadequately cooked fish infected with the plerocercoid larva. Leukocytosis and eosinophilia may occur; if the worm is high enough in the alimentary canal, it may preempt the supply of vitamin B$_{12}$ or alter its absorption, leading to hyperchromic macrocytic anemia resembling pernicious anemia, although the condition is rare, even in hyperendemic areas. SYN bothriocephaliasis.

Di·phyl·lo·both·ri·um (dī-fil-lō-both′rē-ŭm). A large genus of tapeworms (order Pseudophyllidea) characterized by a spatulate scolex with dorsal and ventral sucking grooves or bothria. Several species are found in humans, although only one, *D. latum,* is of widespread importance. [G. *di-,* two, + *phyllon,* leaf, + *bothrion,* little ditch]
   D. corda′tum, a species found in dogs, sea mammals, and occasionally humans, in Greenland.
   D. dendriticum, adult form of the tapeworm found in the intestine of fish-eating birds; infective for humans.
   D. hians, tapeworm species found in humans in Japan.
   D. houghtoni, canine and feline tapeworm; found in humans in China.
   D. la′tum, the broad or broad fish tapeworm, a species that causes diphyllobothriasis, found in humans and fish-eating mammals in many parts of northern Europe, Japan and elsewhere in Asia, and in Scandinavian populations of the American north central states; it often has 3 or 4 thousand segments, broader than long; the head has typical bothria characteristic of the genus. SYN *Dibothriocephalus latus.*
   D. linguloi′des, SYN *Spirometra mansoni.*
   D. man′soni, SYN *Spirometra mansoni.*
   D. mansonoi′des, SYN *Spirometra mansonoides.*

D. nihonkaiense, tapeworm species closely related to *Diphyllobothrium latum;* found in Japan with increasing numbers of human infections.

D. orcini, tapeworm species found in humans in Japan.

D. pacificum, tapeworm species found in sea lions; has been described as a human tapeworm acquired from marine fishes; found in Japan, Peru, and Ecuador.

D. scoticum, tapeworm species found in humans in Japan.

di·phy·o·dont (dī-f′ē-ō-dont). Possessing two sets of teeth, as occurs in humans and most other mammals. [G. *di-,* two, + *phyō,* to produce, + *odous* (odont-), tooth]

di·pi·pro·ver·ine (dī-pī-prō′ver-ēn). An intestinal antispasmodic.

di·piv·e·frin hy·dro·chlo·ride (dī-piv′ĕ-frin). An adrenergic epinephrine prodrug used in drop form in initial therapy for control of intraocular pressure in chronic open-angle glaucoma.

dip·la·cu·sis (dip-lă-koo′sis). Abnormal perception of sound, either in time or in pitch, so that one sound is heard as two. [G. *diplous,* double, + *akousis,* a hearing]
   d. binaura′lis, a condition in which the same sound is heard differently by the two ears.
   d. dysharmon′ica, a condition in which the same sound is heard as a different pitch in each ear.
   d. echo′ica, a condition in which sound heard in the affected ear is repeated.
   d. monaura′lis, a condition in which one sound is perceived as two in the same ear.

di·ple·gia (dī-plē′jē-ă). Paralysis of corresponding parts on both sides of the body. SYN double hemiplegia. [G. *di-,* two, + *plēgē,* a stroke]
   congenital facial d., SYN Möbius *syndrome.*
   facial d., paralysis of both sides of the face.
   infantile d., SYN spastic d.
   masticatory d., paralysis of all the muscles of mastication.
   spastic d., a type of cerebral palsy in which there is bilateral spasticity, with the lower extremities more severely affected. Cf. flaccid *paralysis.* SYN Erb-Charcot disease (1), infantile d., Little disease, spastic spinal paralysis.

⟐**diplo-.** Double, twofold. SEE haplo-. [G. *diploos,* double]

dip·lo·al·bu·mi·nu·ria (dip′lō-al-bū-mi-noo′rē-ă). The coexistence of nephritic, or pathologic, and nonnephritic, or physiologic, albuminuria.

dip·lo·ba·cil·lus (dip′lō-bă-sil′ŭs). Two rod-shaped bacterial cells linked end to end. [diplo- + bacillus]

dip·lo·blas·tic (dip-lō-blas′tik). Formed of two germ layers. [diplo- + G. *blastos,* germ]

dip·lo·car·dia (dip-lō-kar′dē-ă). An anomaly in which the left and right halves of the heart are separated to varying degrees by a central fissure. [diplo- + G. *kardia,* heart]

dip·lo·ceph·a·lus (dip-lō-sef′ă-lŭs). SYN dicephalus.

dip·lo·chei·ria, dip·lo·chi·ria (dip′lō-kī′rē-ă). SYN dicheiria. [diplo- + G. *cheir,* hand]

dip·lo·coc·ce·mia (dip-lō-kok-sē′mē-ă). The presence of diplococci in the blood; used especially in referring to *Neisseria meningitidis* (meningococci) in circulating blood.

dip·lo·coc·ci (dip′lō-kok′sī). Plural of diplococcus.

dip·lo·coc·cin (dip-lō-kok′sin). An antibiotic crystalline substance isolated from cultures of lactic acid-producing cocci present in milk active against lactobacilli and certain Gram-positive cocci, but inactive against Gram-negative bacteria.

Dip·lo·coc·cus (dip′lō-kok′ŭs). Species of this former genus of bacteria are now assigned to other genera. *Diplococcus pneumoniae,* the type species of *D.,* is a member of the genus *Streptococcus.* SEE *Neisseria, Peptococcus, Streptococcus.* [diplo- + G. *kokkos,* berry]

dip·lo·coc·cus, pl. **dip·lo·coc·ci** (dip′lō-kok′ŭs, -kok′sī). **1.** Spherical or ovoid bacterial cells joined together in pairs. **2.** Common name of any organism belonging to the former bacterial genus *Diplococcus.* [diplo- + G. *kokkos,* berry]

dip·lo·co·ri·a (dip-lō-kō′rē-ă). The occurrence of two pupils in the eye. SYN dicoria. [diplo- + G. *korē,* pupil]

dip·lo·ë (dip′lō-ē) [TA]. The central layer of spongy bone between the two layers of compact bone, outer and inner plates, or tables, of the flat cranial bones. [G. *diploë*, fem. of *diplous*, double]

dip·lo·gen·e·sis (dip-lō-jen′ĕ-sis). Production of a double fetus or of one with some parts doubled. [diplo- + G. *genesis*, production]

Dip·lo·go·nop·o·rus (dip′lō-gō-nop′ŏ-rŭs). A genus of tapeworms found in Japan (*D. grandis*) and probably also in Rumania (*D. brauni*) [diplo- + G. *gonos*, seed, + *poros*, pore]

di·plo·ic (dip-lō′ik). Relating to the diploë.

dip·loid (dip′loyd). Denoting the state of a cell containing two haploid sets derived from the father and from the mother respectively; the normal chromosome complement of somatic cells (in humans, 46 chromosomes). [diplo- + G. *eidos* resemblance]

dip·lo·kar·y·on (dip′lō-kar′ē-on). A cell nucleus containing four haploid sets; i.e., a tetraploid nucleus. SEE ALSO polyploidy. [diplo- + G. *karyon*, nut (nucleus)]

dip·lo·mel·i·tu·ria (dip′lō-mel-i-too′rē-ă). The occurrence of diabetic and nondiabetic glycosuria in the same individual. [diplo- + G. *meli*, honey, + *ouron*, urine]

dip·lo·my·e·lia (dip-lō-mī-ē′lē-ă). Complete or incomplete doubling of the spinal cord; may be accompanied by a bony septum of the vertebral canal. [diplo- + G. *myelon*, marrow]

dip·lon (dip′lon). SYN deuteron.

dip·lo·ne·ma (dip-lō-nē′mă). The doubled form of the chromosome strand visible at the diplotene stage of meiosis. [diplo- + G. *nēma*, thread]

dip·lo·neu·ral (dip-lō-noo′răl). Supplied by two nerves from different sources, said of certain muscles. [diplo- + G. *neuron*, nerve]

dip·lop·a·gus (dip-lop′ă-gŭs). General term for conjoined twins, each with fairly complete bodies, although one or more internal organs may be in common. SEE conjoined *twins*, under *twin*. [diplo- + G. *pagos*, something fixed]

dip·lo·pia (di-plō′pē-ă). The condition in which a single object is perceived as two objects. SYN double vision. [diplo- + G. *ōps*, eye]

crossed d., d. in which the image seen by the right eye is to the left of the image seen by the left eye. SYN heteronymous d.

heteronymous d., SYN crossed d.

homonymous d., SYN homonymous *images*, under *image*.

monocular d., a double image or an extra ghost image produced in one eye, almost always by an aberration of the ocular media; for example, a corneal or lenticular irregularity, an uncorrected astigmatism or an irregularity of the vitreous or the retina. If a similar process occurs in both eyes (bilateral monocular diplopia), that is, the doubling is still present with either eye covered, the patient may still only see two images; seeing multiple images (polyopia) is rare.

simple d., SYN homonymous *images*, under *image*.

uncrossed d., SYN homonymous *images*, under *image*.

dip·lo·po·dia (dip-lō-pō′dē-ă). Duplication of digits of the foot. [diplo- + G. *pous*, foot]

dip·lo·some (dip′lō-sōm). Paired allosomes; the pair of centrioles of mammalian cells. SYN paired allosome. [diplo- + G. *sōma*, body]

dip·lo·so·mia (dip-lō-sō′mē-ă). Condition in which twins who seem functionally independent are joined at one or more points. SEE conjoined *twins*, under *twin*. [diplo- + G. *sōma*, body]

dip·lo·tene (dip′lō-tēn). The late stage of prophase in meiosis in which the paired homologous chromosomes begin to repel each other and move apart, but are usually held together by chiasmata. The chiasmata are associated with breakage of two chromatids at corresponding points followed by refusion of the broken ends with exchange of segments between the chromatids; this is considered to be the cytologic basis for the crossing-over of genes. [diplo- + G. *tainia*, band]

di·po·dia (dī-pō′dē-ă). **1.** A developmental anomaly involving complete or incomplete duplication of a foot. **2.** In conjoined twins and sirenomelia, a degree of union leaving two feet evident. [G. *di-*, two, + *pous* (*pod-*), foot]

di·pole (dī′pōl). A pair of separated electrical charges, one or more positive and one or more negative; or a pair of separated partial charges. SYN doublet (2).

di·po·tas·si·um phos·phate (dī-pō-tas′ē-ŭm). SYN *potassium phosphate*.

di·pre·nor·phine (dī-pren′ōr-fēn). A narcotic antagonist resembling naloxone but more potent.

di·pro·pyl·tryp·ta·mine (dī-prō-pil-trip′tă-mēn). A hallucinogenic agent similar to dimethyltryptamine.

di·pro·so·pus (dī-pros′ō-pŭs, dī-prō-sō′pus). Conjoined twins with almost complete fusion of the bodies and with normal limbs. Part or all of the face may be duplicated. SEE conjoined *twins*, under *twin*. [G. *di-*, two + *prosopon*, face]

dip·se·sis (dip-sē′sis). An abnormal or excessive thirst, or a craving for unusual forms of drink. SYN dipsosis, morbid thirst. [G. *dipseō*, to thirst]

dip·so·gen (dip′sō-jen). A thirst-provoking agent. [G. *dipsa*, thirst, + *-gen*, producing]

dip·so·ma·nia (dip-sō-mā′nē-ă). A recurring compulsion to drink alcoholic beverages to excess. SEE alcoholism. [G. *dipsa*, thirst, + *mania*, madness]

dip·so·sis (dip-sō′sis). SYN dipsesis. [G. *dipsa*, thirst, + *-osis*, condition]

dip·so·ther·a·py (dip′sō-thār′ă-pē). Treatment of certain diseases by abstention, as far as possible, from liquids.

Dip·tera (dip′ter-ă). An important order of insects (the two-wing flies and gnats), including many significant disease vectors such as the mosquito, tsetse fly, sandfly, and biting midge. [G. *di-*, two, + *pteron*, wing]

dip·ter·an (dip′ter-an). Denoting insects of the order Diptera.

dip·ter·ous (dip′ter-ŭs). Relating to or characteristic of the order Diptera.

Di·pus sa·git·ta (dī′pŭs saj′i-tă). A small rodent of southern Russia that serves as a vector, through fleas, of *Yersinia pestis* (plague bacillus). [G. *dipous*, jerboa, two-footed; L. *sagitta*, arrow]

di·py·gus (dī-pī′gŭs, dip′ē-gŭs). Conjoined twins with a single head and thorax and the pelvis and lower extremities duplicated; when the duplications of the lower parts are symmetric, usually called duplicitas posterior. SEE conjoined *twins*, under *twin*. [G. *di-*, two, + *pyge*, buttocks]

dip·y·lid·i·a·sis (dip′i-li-dī′ă-sis). Infection of carnivores and humans with the cestode *Dipylidium caninum*.

Dip·y·lid·i·um ca·ni·num (dip-ĭ-lid′ē-ŭm kā-nī′nŭm). The commonest species of dog tapeworm, the double-pored tapeworm, the larvae of which are harbored by dog fleas or lice; the worm occasionally infects humans, especially children licked by dogs that have recently nipped infected fleas. [G. *dipylos*, with two entrances; L. ntr. of *caninus*, pertaining to *canis*, dog]

di·py·rid·am·ole (dī-pir-id′ă-mōl). A coronary vasodilator that also has a weak action to reduce platelet aggregation; commonly used in place of exercise for studies of myocardial contractility.

di·py·rim·i·dine pho·to·ly·ase (dī-pi-rim′i-dēn). SYN deoxyribodipyrimidine photolyase.

di·py·rine (dī-pī′rēn). SYN aminopyrine.

di·py·rone (dī-pī′rōn). An analgesic, anti-inflammatory, and antipyretic agent rarely used because of a high incidence of agranulocytosis. SYN methampyrone.

directive.

advance d., a legal document giving instructions as to the type and degree of medical care to be administered in the event that the person signing the document becomes mentally incompetent during the course of a terminal illness, or becomes permanently comatose (persistent vegetative state).

State legislatures have enacted so-called Death with Dignity laws to protect the rights of patients to refuse medical care, including life-prolonging and palliative care in terminal illness, as well as to clarify the role of physicians and indemnify them against the accusation of euthanasia or physician-assisted suicide when they withhold such care in compliance with patients' wishes. These laws spell out

di

strict procedural requirements, including the need for the signing of an advance directive to be duly witnessed, and make it easier to revoke an advance directive than to establish one. When an advance directive provides instructions for the types of care the patient does or does not want to receive, it is known as a living will. When it names another person to make such decisions, it is known as a durable power-of-attorney for health care decisions. An advance directive can contain both types of instruction. An agent making end-of-life decisions on behalf of a patient is required to follow the patient's instructions, interpreting them when necessary in the light of the patient's personal philosophy, religious beliefs, and ethical values, and with due consideration for the likelihood that the patient will regain competency or will recover.

di·rec·tor (di-rek′ter, -tōr, dī-). **1.** A smoothly grooved instrument used with a knife to limit the incision of tissues. SYN staff (2). **2.** The head of a service or specialty division. [L. *dirigo*, pp. *-rectus*, to arrange, set in order]

Di·ro·fil·a·ria (dī-rō-fi-lā′rē-ă). A genus of filaria (family Onchocercidae, superfamily Filarioidea); *D.* species are usually found in mammals other than man, but rare examples of human infection are known, as by *D. immitis*. [L. *dirus*, dread, + *filum*, thread]
D. conjuncti′vae, name assigned to filarial worms removed from tumors and abscesses in various sites in human cases, especially palpebral conjunctivae and other eye tissues, but also subcutaneous tissues from other sites; probably caused by a number of species of animal origin.
D. im′mitis, a species of filarial worms of dogs and other canids in tropical and subtropical areas, found chiefly in the right ventricle and pulmonary arteries of dogs; sometimes a serious pathogen of racing and show dogs, especially in the southern U.S. where mosquito vectors are common; *D. immitis* and its canine host have been used to test chemotherapeutic agents, and an extract of *D. immitis* may be used as a nonspecific intradermal antigen in the diagnosis of human filariasis and in complement-fixation tests. SEE ALSO *Dipetalonema reconditum*. SYN heartworm.

di·ro·fil·a·ri·a·sis (dir′ō-fil-ă-rī′ă-sis). Infection of animals and, rarely, humans with nematodes of the genus *Dirofilaria*.

dirt-eat·ing. SYN geophagia.

△**dis-.** In two, apart; un-, not; very. Cf. dys-. [L. separation]

dis·a·bil·i·ty (dis-ă-bil′i-tē). **1.** According to the "International Classification of Impairments, Disabilities and Handicaps" (World Health Organization), any restriction or lack of ability to perform an activity in a manner or within the range considered normal for a human being. The term disability reflects the consequences of impairment in terms of functional performance and activity by the individual; disabilities thus represent disturbances at the level of the person. **2.** An impairment or defect of one or more organs or members.
developmental d., loss of function brought on by prenatal and postnatal events in which the predominant disturbance is in the acquisition of cognitive, language, motor, or social skills; e.g., mental retardation, autistic disorder, learning disorder, and attention-deficit hyperactivity disorder.
learning d., a disorder in one or more of the basic cognitive and psychological processes involved in understanding or using written or spoken language; may be manifested in age-related impairment in the ability to read, write, spell, speak, or perform mathematical calculations.

di·sac·cha·rid·as·es (dī-sak′ă-rid-ăs-ez). A group of enzymes that catalyze the hydrolysis of disaccharides, producing two monosaccharides.

di·sac·cha·ride (dī-sak′ă-rīd). A condensation product of two monosaccharides by elimination of water (usually between an alcoholic OH and a hemiacetal OH); e.g., sucrose, lactose, maltose.

dis·ag·gre·ga·tion (dis′ag-grĕ-gā′shŭn). **1.** A breaking up into component parts. **2.** An inability to coordinate various sensations and failure to comprehend their mutual relations. [L. *dis-*, separating, + *ag- grego* (*adg-*), pp. *-gregatus*, to add to something]

dis·ar·tic·u·la·tion (dis-ar-tik-ū-lā′shŭn). Amputation of a limb through a joint, without cutting of bone. [L. *dis-*, apart, + *articulus*, joint]

dis·as·sim·i·la·tion (dis′ă-sim-i-lā′shŭn). Destructive or retrograde metabolism. SYN dissimilation (1).

dis·as·so·ci·a·tion (dis′ă-sō-sē-ā′shŭn). SYN dissociation (1).

disc (disk). SEE disk.

△**disc-.** SEE disco-.

disc·ec·to·my (disk-ek′tō-mē). Excision, in part or whole, of an intervertebral disk. SYN discotomy. [disco- + G. *ektomē*, excision]

dis·charge (dis′charj). **1.** That which is emitted or evacuated, as an excretion or a secretion. **2.** The activation or firing of a neuron.
after-d., SEE afterdischarge.
early d., d. of a woman and the newborn from the hospital within 24 hours of a vaginal delivery.

Dische, Zacharias, 20th century Austrian-U.S. biochemist, 1895–1988. SEE D. *reaction, reagent*; D.-Schwarz *reagent*.

dis·chro·na·tion (dis-krō-nā′shŭn). A disturbance in the consciousness of time. [L. *dis-*, apart, + G. *chronos*, time]

dis·ci (dis′kī). Plural of discus.

dis·ci·form (dis′i-fōrm). Disk-shaped.

dis·cis·sion (di-sish′ŭn). **1.** Incision or cutting through a part. **2.** In ophthalmology, opening of the capsule and breaking up of the cortex of the lens with a needle knife or laser. [L. *di- scindo*, pp. *-scissus*, to tear asunder]

dis·ci·tis (dis-kī′tis). Inflammation of an intervertebral disk or disk space often related to infections. SYN diskitis.

△**disco-, disc-.** A disk; disk-shaped. [G. *diskos*]

dis·co·blas·tic (dis-kō-blas′tik). Denoting a discoblastula.

dis·co·blas·tu·la (dis′kō-blas′tū-lă). A blastula of the type produced by the meroblastic discoidal cleavage of a large-yolked ovum.

dis·co·gas·tru·la (dis′kō-gas′troo-lă). A gastrula of the type formed after the discoidal cleavage of a large-yolked ovum.

dis·co·gen·ic (dis′kō-gen′ik). Denoting a disorder originating in or from an intervertebral disk. [disco- + G. *genesis*, origin]

dis·coid (dis′koyd). **1.** Resembling a disk. **2.** In dentistry, an excavating or carving instrument having a circular blade with a cutting edge around the periphery. [disco- + G. *eidos*, appearance]

dis·con·ju·gate (dis-cŏn′joo-gāt). Not paired in action or joined together; the opposite of conjugate. SEE disconjugate *movement* of eyes. [L. *dis-*, apart, + *jugatus*, yoked]

dis·cop·a·thy (dis-kop′ă-thē). Disease of a disk, particularly of an invertebral disk. [disco- + G. *pathos*, disease]
traumatic cervical d., an injury characterized by fissuration, laceration and/or fragmentation of a cervical disk or surrounding ligaments, with or without displacement of fragments against spinal cord, nerve roots, or ligaments.

dis·co·pla·cen·ta (dis-kō-pla-sen′tă). A placenta of discoid shape.

dis·cor·dance (dis-kōr′dans). **1.** Dissociation of two characteristics in the members of a sample from a population; used as a measure of dependence. **2.** In genetics, the presence of a given trait in only one member of a twin pair. Cf. concordance.

dis·cot·o·my (dis-kot′ō-mē). SYN discectomy. [disco- + G. *tome*, incision]

dis·crete (dis-krēt′). Separate; distinct; not joined to or incorporated with another; denoting especially certain lesions of the skin. [L. *dis- cerno*, pp. *-cretus*, to separate]

dis·crim·i·na·tion (dis′krim-i-nā′shŭn). In conditioning, responding differentially, as when an organism makes one response to a reinforced stimulus and a different response to an unreinforced stimulus. [L. *discrimino*, pp. *-atus*, to separate]

dis·cus, pl. **dis·ci** (dis′kŭs, -kī) [TA]. SYN lamella (2). [L. fr. G. *diskos*, a quoit, disk]
d. articula′ris [TA], SYN articular *disk*.
d. articula′ris acromioclavicula′ris [TA], SYN articular *disk* of acromioclavicular joint.

d. articula′ris radioulna′ris distalis [TA], SYN articular *disk* of distal radioulnar joint.

d. articula′ris sternoclavicula′ris [TA], SYN articular *disk* of sternoclavicular joint.

d. articularis temporomandibularis [TA], SYN articular *disk* of temporomandibular joint.

d. interpu′bicus [TA], SYN interpubic *disk.*

d. intervertebra′lis [TA], SYN intervertebral *disk.*

d. lentifor′mis, rarely used term for subthalamic *nucleus.*

d. ner′vi op′tici [TA], SYN optic *disk.*

d. prolig′erus, the attachment point of the cumulus oöph′orus to the most peripheral granulosa cells of an antral follicle.

dis·di·a·clast (dis-dī′ă-klast). A doubly refractive element in striated muscular tissue. [G. *dis,* twice, + *dia,* through, + *klastos,* broken]

DISEASE

dis·ease (di-zēz′). **1.** An interruption, cessation, or disorder of body function, system, or organ. SYN illness, morbus, sickness. **2.** A morbid entity characterized usually by at least two of these criteria: recognized etiologic agent(s), identifiable group of signs and symptoms, or consistent anatomic alterations. SEE ALSO syndrome. **3.** Literally, dis-ease, the opposite of ease, when something is wrong with a bodily function. [Eng. *dis-* priv. + ease]

aaa d., endemic anemia of ancient Egypt, ascribed in the Papyrus Ebers to intestinal infestation with ancylostoma; now called ancylostomiasis.

ABO hemolytic d. of the newborn, erythroblastosis fetalis due to maternal-fetal incompatibility with respect to an antigen of the ABO blood group; the fetus possesses A or B antigen which is lacking in the mother, and the mother produces immune antibody which causes hemolysis of fetal erythrocytes.

accumulation d., a disease characterized by abnormal accumulation of a metabolic product in certain cells and tissues; examples include the mucopolysaccharidoses, lipoidoses.

Acosta d., SYN altitude *sickness.*

Adams-Stokes d., SYN Adams-Stokes *syndrome.*

adaptation d.'s, d.'s falling theoretically into Selye concept of the general-adaptation syndrome.

Addison d., SYN chronic adrenocortical *insufficiency.*

Addison-Biermer d., SYN pernicious *anemia.*

akamushi d., SYN tsutsugamushi d.

Albers-Schönberg d., SYN osteopetrosis.

Albright d., SYN McCune-Albright *syndrome.*

Alexander d., a rare, fatal central nervous system degenerative disease of infants, characterized by psychomotor retardation, seizures, and paralysis; megaloencephaly is associated with widespread leukodystrophic changes, especially in the frontal lobes.

Almeida d., SYN paracoccidioidomycosis.

Alpers d., SYN *poliodystrophia* cerebri progressiva infantilis.

altitude d., SYN altitude *sickness.*

Alzheimer d., a progressive degenerative d. of the brain that causes impairment of memory and dementia manifested by confusion, visual-spatial disorientation, inability to calculate, and deterioration of judgment; delusions and hallucinations may occur. The most common degenerative brain disorder, Alzheimer d. makes up 70% of all cases of dementia. Onset is usually in late middle life, and death typically ensues in 5–10 years. SYN Alzheimer dementia, presenile dementia (2), dementia presenilis, primary neuronal degeneration, primary senile dementia.

> Alzheimer disease (AD) ranks 4th as a cause of death in the U.S., and its annual cost to the nation is nearly $100 billion. Onset is typically insidious, with a progressive deterioration in the ability to learn and retain information. In recalling and repeating new material, the patient makes

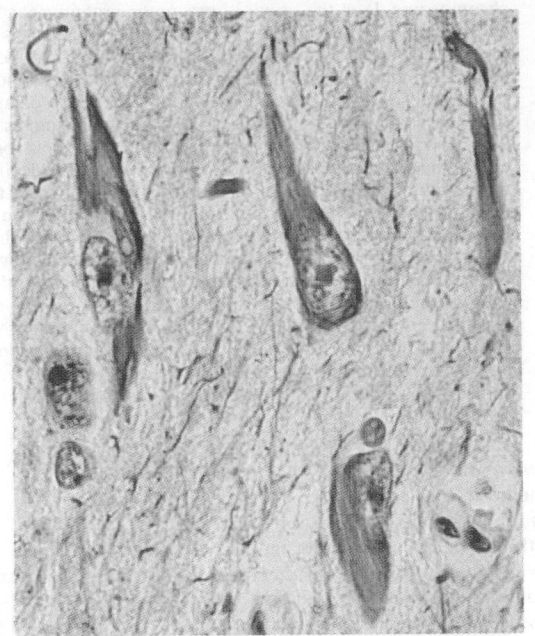

Alzheimer disease: neurofibrillary tangles in the distended cytoplasm of pyramidal neurons impregnated with silver

intrusion errors (insertion of irrelevant words or ideas) and resorts to confabulation. Orientation and judgment decline; 50% of patients experience depression, 20% delusions. Agitation occurs in 70%. Numerous drugs, including many not considered psychoactive, can aggravate the symptoms of AD; clinical depression can mask dementia, and vice versa. Behavioral disturbances are the major indications for the use of psychotropic drugs and physical restraints, and substantially influence the quality of life of demented elderly patients. Neurologic findings may be essentially normal, but myoclonus, bradykinesia, rigidity, and seizures can occur late in the disease. Death is usually due to sepsis associated with urinary or pulmonary infection. Atrophy of the cerebral cortex, with consequent enlargement of sulci and ventricles, may be grossly evident on imaging studies. Histologically the cortex, hippocampus, and amygdala show atrophy of neurons, with cytoplasmic vacuoles and argentophilic granules; distortion of intracellular neurofibrils (neurofibrillary tangles) due to excessive phosphorylation of microtubular tau proteins; and plaques composed of granular or filamentous argentophilic masses with a core of the 42-aminoacid form of β-amyloid (Aβ42). The concentration of tau protein in the cerebrospinal fluid is increased while that of Aβ42 is decreased. Lewy bodies (eosinophilic inclusions in the cytoplasm of CNS neurons, believed to be products of altered neurofilament metabolism and recognized as a hallmark of idiopathic parkinsonism) occur in cortical neurons of some persons with dementia, including AD. Dementia associated with Lewy bodies tends to appear before age 60, to progress rapidly, and to display parkinsonian features (tremor, rigidity). Nearly all persons with Down syndrome who live past the age of 40 develop cognitive decline associated with histologic findings typical of AD. Advancing age and a history of head injury are also risk factors for AD. Although most cases are sporadic, about 10% of patients have a family history of AD. Familial disease, which is often characterized by early onset and rapid course, has been traced to mutations of several genes. At least half of all patients with early-onset familial AD show mutations in the presenilin-1 gene on chromosome 14. Mutations in the presenilin-2 gene on chromosome 1 or the amyloid precursor protein gene on chromosome 21 have been found in smaller kindreds with familial disease. Late-onset familial disease has been traced to mutations in an apolipoprotein E (APOE) locus on chromosome 19. All of these mutations are associated with increased production of Aβ42. It has been suggested that incorporation of presenilin proteins into neurons programs them for death through apoptosis. Cognitive decline in AD has been attributed in part to a deficiency of the neurotransmitter acetylcholine, and therapy with reversible cholinesterase inhibitors (donezepil, galanthamine, metrifonate, tacrine) has improved cognition and slowed progression of dementia in some patients. Numerous other agents (including nicotine, ginkgo extract, vitamin E, selegiline, ergoloid mesylates, and ibuprofen) have shown slight efficacy in some studies. Experimental evidence suggests that administration of estrogen to postmenopausal women retards onset and progression of nonfamilial AD.

---

anarthritic rheumatoid d., rheumatoid d. without arthritis.

Anders d., SYN *adiposis* dolorosa.

Andersen d., SYN type 4 *glycogenosis*.

antibody deficiency d., SYN antibody deficiency *syndrome*.

aortoiliac occlusive d., obstruction of the abdominal aorta and its main branches by atherosclerosis.

Aran-Duchenne d., SYN amyotrophic lateral *sclerosis*.

Australian X d., SYN Murray Valley *encephalitis*.

autoimmune d., any disorder in which loss of function or destruction of normal tissue arises from humoral or cellular immune responses to the body's own tissue constituents; may be systemic, as systemic lupus erythematosus, or organ specific, as thyroiditis.

aviator's d., syndrome resembling decompression sickness occurring in occupants of airplanes that reach very high altitudes without adequate pressurization of the cabin. SEE ALSO decompression *sickness*.

Ayerza d., SYN Ayerza *syndrome*.

Azorean d., SYN Machado-Joseph d.

Baelz d., SYN *cheilitis* glandularis.

Baló d., SYN *encephalitis* periaxialis concentrica.

Baltic myoclonus d., one of the familial light sensitive myoclonic epilepsies. Unlike Lafora body polymyoclonus, where inclusion bodies are seen in the brain cells, the prognosis is often favorable. Probably an autosomal recessive disorder.

Bamberger d., (1) SYN saltatory *spasm*; (2) SYN polyserositis.

Bamberger-Marie d., SYN hypertrophic pulmonary *osteoarthropathy*.

Bang d., SYN bovine *brucellosis*.

Banti d., SYN Banti *syndrome*.

Barclay-Baron d., SYN vallecular *dysphagia*.

Barlow d., SYN infantile *scurvy*.

Barraquer d., SYN progressive *lipodystrophy*.

Basedow d., SYN Graves d.

Batten d., cerebral *sphingolipidosis*, late juvenile type. SYN ceroid lipofuscinosis.

Batten-Mayou d., cerebral *sphingolipidosis*, late infantile and juvenile types.

Bazin d., SYN *erythema* induratum.

Bechterew d., SYN *spondylitis* deformans.

Becker d., an obscure South African cardiomyopathy leading to rapidly fatal congestive heart failure and idiopathic mural endomyocardial d.

Béguez César d., SYN Chédiak-Higashi *syndrome*.

Behçet d., SYN Behçet *syndrome*.

Behr d., SYN Behr *syndrome*.

Berger d., SYN focal *glomerulonephritis*.

Bernard-Soulier d. (ber-nar′-sool-ya), an autosomal recessive disorder of absent or decreased platelet membrane glycoproteins Ib, IX, and V (the receptor for factor VIII R). This deficiency can lead to a failure to bind von Willebrand factor, causing moderate bleeding.

Bernhardt d., SYN *meralgia* paresthetica.

Besnier-Boeck-Schaumann d., SYN sarcoidosis.

Best d. [MIM*153700], autosomal dominant macular degeneration beginning during the first years of life. SYN vitelliform degeneration, vitelliform retinal dystrophy.

Bielschowsky d., early childhood type of lipofuscinosis.

Biermer d., SYN pernicious *anemia*.

Binswanger d., one of the causes of multi-infarct dementia, in which there are many infarcts and lacunae in the white matter, with relative sparing of the cortex and basal ganglia. SYN Binswanger encephalopathy, encephalitis subcorticalis chronica, subcortical arteriosclerotic encephalopathy.

bird-breeder's d., SYN bird-breeder's *lung*.

blinding d., SYN onchocerciasis.

Bloch-Sulzberger d., SYN *incontinentia* pigmenti.

Blocq d., SYN astasia-abasia.

Blount d., tibia vara; nonrachitic bowlegs in children. SYN Blount-Barber d.

Blount-Barber d., SYN Blount d.

blue d., SYN Rocky Mountain spotted *fever*.

Boeck d., SYN sarcoidosis.

Bornholm d., SYN epidemic *pleurodynia*. [*Bornholm,* Danish island in the Baltic where the d. was first described]

Bosin d., SYN subacute sclerosing *panencephalitis*.

Bouchard d., myopathic dilation of the stomach.

Bourneville d., SYN tuberous *sclerosis*.

Bourneville-Pringle d., facial lesions with tuberous sclerosis, first reported as adenoma sebaceum, but now recognized as angiofibromas.

Bowen d., a form of intraepidermal carcinoma characterized by the development of slowly enlarging pinkish or brownish papules or eroded plaques covered with a thickened horny layer; microscopically, there is dyskeratosis with large round epidermal cells with large nuclei and pale-staining cytoplasm which are scattered through all levels of the epidermis. SYN Bowen precancerous dermatosis.

Brailsford-Morquio d., SYN Morquio *syndrome*.

brancher glycogen storage d., type of glycogen storage d., due to deficiency of amylo-1,4-1,6-transglucosidase (brancher enzyme). SYN brancher deficiency glycogenosis, debrancher deficiency.

Breda d., SYN espundia.

Bright d., nonsuppurative nephritis with albuminuria and edema, associated in fatal cases with large white kidneys; or with hematuria and red kidneys; or with contracted granular kidneys, corresponding to the stages of glomerulonephritis now termed subacute or membranous, acute, and chronic, respectively.

Brill d., SYN Brill-Zinsser d.

Brill-Zinsser d., an endogenous reinfection associated with the "carrier state" in persons who previously had epidemic typhus fever; it is a rather mild d. and may be mistaken for endemic (murine) typhus; first described by Brill in New York City but not recognized as a recrudescent form of epidemic typhus until after the work of Zinsser. SYN Brill d., recrudescent typhus fever, recrudescent typhus.

Briquet d., hysterical neurosis, conversion type.

Brissaud d., SYN tic.

broad beta d., type III familial hyperlipoproteinemia.

Brodie d., (1) SYN Brodie *knee*; (2) hysterical spinal neuralgia, simulating Pott disease, following a trauma.

bronzed d., SYN bronze *diabetes*; SEE hemochromatosis.

Bruck d., a d. marked by osteogenesis imperfecta, ankylosis of the joints, and muscular atrophy.

Brushfield-Wyatt d., a familial disorder characterized by unilateral nevus, contralateral hemiplegia, hemianopia, cerebral angioma, and mental retardation; possibly a variant of Sturge-Weber syndrome. SYN nevoid amentia.

Buerger d., SYN *thromboangiitis* obliterans.

bulging eye d., SYN gedoelstiosis.

bulky d., term used for large tumors or lymph nodes; usually more resistant to conventional therapy. SYN bulky lymphadenopathy.

Bürger-Grütz d., obsolete term for idiopathic *hyperlipemia*.

Buschke d., SYN *scleredema* adultorum.

Busquet d., an osteoperiostitis of the metatarsal bones, leading to exostoses on the dorsum of the foot.

Byler d. [MIM*211600], progressive intrahepatic cholestasis, with early onset of loose, foul-smelling stools, jaundice, hepatosplenomegaly, dwarfism, and occasionally death; due to an error in conjugated bile salt metabolism; autosomal recessive inheritance, caused by mutation in the familial intrahepatic cholestasis 1 gene (FIC1) on chromosome 18q. [*Byler,* an Amish kindred]

Caffey d., SYN infantile cortical *hyperostosis*.

caisson d. (kā′son), SYN decompression *sickness*. [Fr. *caisson* (fr. *caisse,* a chest) a water-tight box or cylinder containing air under high pressure used in sinking structural pilings underwater]

calcium pyrophosphate deposition d. (CPPD), a crystal deposition arthritis that may simulate gout.

Calvé-Perthes d., SYN Legg-Calvé-Perthes d.

Canavan d. [MIM*271900], progressive degenerative d. of infancy; mostly affecting Ashkenazi Jewish babies; onset typically within the first 3–4 months of birth; characterized by megalencephaly, optic atrophy, blindness, psychomotor regression, hypotonia, and spasticity; there is increased urinary excretion of *N*-acetylaspartic acid. MRI shows enlarged brain, decreased attenuation of cerebral and cerebellar white matter, and normal ventricles; pathologically, there is increased brain volume and weight and spongy degeneration in the subcortical white matter. Autosomal recessive inheritance, caused by mutation in the aspartoacylase A gene (ASPA) on chromosome 17p in Jewish and non-Jewish affected individuals. SEE ALSO leukodystrophy. SYN Canavan sclerosis, Canavan-van Bogaert-Bertrand d., spongy degeneration of infancy.

Canavan-van Bogaert-Bertrand d., SYN Canavan d.

Caroli d. [MIM*263200], congenital cystic dilation of the intrahepatic bile ducts, sometimes associated with intrahepatic stones and biliary obstruction; may be a part of the phenotype of infantile polycystic kidney d.

Carrington d., SYN chronic eosinophilic *pneumonia*.

Carrión d., SYN Oroya *fever*.

Castleman d., SYN benign giant lymph node *hyperplasia*.

cat-bite d., rat-bite fever, presumably spread from rats to cats and thus to humans. SYN cat-bite fever.

_____

catscratch d. (CSD), an infection that causes chronic benign adenopathy in most cases, especially in children and young adults, usually associated with a cat scratch or bite. In most cases it is caused by the bacterium *Bartonella henselae.* The lymphadenopathy usually resolves spontaneously within a period of several months. The infection may cause other clinical symptoms such as fever of unknown origin, encephalitis, microabscess in the liver and spleen, and osteomyelitis. SYN benign inoculation lymphoreticulosis, benign inoculation reticulosis, catscratch fever, regional granulomatous lymphadenitis.

A primary lesion (typically a solitary papule 2–5 mm in diameter) develops at the site of inoculation in 50–95% of cases, usually within 1–2 weeks of inoculation. Regional lymphadenopathy commonly follows, in 75% of patients involving only a single lymph node. The node is usually tender and approximately 10% suppurate. Histopathologic study of an infected node shows lymphoid hyperplasia and granuloma formation with central areas of stellate necrosis containing neutrophils. About one-third of patients experience transitory systemic symptoms such as fever, headache, malaise, or rash. Spontaneous resolution of lymphadenopathy generally occurs in 6–12 weeks. Recovery from CSD confers immunity to further attacks. The Centers for Disease Control estimates the incidence of CSD in the U.S. at 2.5 cases per 100,000 population per year. Most patients are under 21 years of age, and males are affected more often than females. In 1988, a bacterium named *Afipia felis* was cultured from the lymph nodes of patients with CSD, and for a time was believed to be the cause of the disease. More recently, serologic studies have shown that *Bartonella hensalae,* a Gram-negative bacterium, is probably the cause of most typical cases of CSD. The organism can sometimes be visualized with Warthin-Starry silver stain in infected lymph nodes. A serum immunofluorescent antibody test is available. Cats are the principal reservoir for *Bartonella henselae;* 25–40% of clinically healthy cats in the U.S. have antibody to the organism. Fleas have been shown to transmit infection from one cat to another. The majority of infected cats do not become ill. Although CSD is generally benign and self-limited, infection with *Bartonella henselae* is occasionally associated with severe or systemic involvement, including Parinaud's oculoglandular syndrome (granulomatous conjunctivitis with preauricular lymphadenitis), encephalopathy, myelitis, osteolytic lesions, erythema nodosum, etythema marginatum, thrombocytopenic purpura, nonimmune hemolytic anemia, arthritis, and pneumonia. In immunocompromised persons, particularly those with AIDS, infection with *Bartonella henselae* (perhaps not always associated with cats) takes the form of bacillary angiomatosis (BA), in which nodular tumors made up of densely proliferating blood vessels appear in the skin, bone, brain, liver, spleen, and other tissues. Antibiotic treatment is not recommended in uncomplicated catscratch disease. Doxycycline, ciprofloxacin, and gentamicin may be used in encephalitis or disseminated disease. Whereas these agents consistently lead to rapid improvement in bacillary angiomatosis, the response of glandular inflammation and other symptoms of catscratch disease is unpredictable.

_____

celiac d., a disease occurring in children and adults characterized by sensitivity to gluten, with chronic inflammation and atrophy of the mucosa of the upper small intestine; manifestations include diarrhea, malabsorption, steatorrhea, and nutritional and vitamin deficiencies. SYN celiac sprue, celiac syndrome, gluten enteropathy.

cement d., the osteolysis that frequently occurs in association with loosening of cemented total hip replacements; the microscopic particles of polymethylmethacrylate cement induce a biologic reaction by osteoclasts leading to bone resorption and progressive bone loss.

central core d. [MIM*117000], a congenital myopathy characterized by hypotonia, delay of motor development in infancy, and nonprogressive or slowly progressive muscle weakness; on biopsy the central core of muscle fibers stains abnormally, myofibrils are abnormally compact, and there is virtual absence of mitochondria and sarcoplasmic reticulum; histochemically, the cores are devoid of oxidative enzyme, phosphorylase, and ATPase activity; autosomal dominant inheritance, often subclinical, caused by mutation in the ryanodine receptor-1 gene (RYR1) on 19q.

cerebrovascular d., general term for a brain dysfunction caused by an abnormality of the cerebral blood supply.

Chagas d., SYN South American *trypanosomiasis*.

Chagas-Cruz d., SYN South American *trypanosomiasis*.

α chain d., a vague or indefinite term; could be used for α-heavy-chain d. (a lymphoplasma cell proliferative d. usually seen in Mediterranean men, characterized by intestinal involvement with steatorrhea, often progressive with fatal outcome) or α *thalassemia* (a genetic abnormality in the alpha globin chain of hemoglobin).

Charcot d., SYN amyotrophic lateral *sclerosis*.

Charcot-Marie-Tooth d., SYN peroneal muscular *atrophy*.

Cheadle d., SYN infantile *scurvy*.

Chédiak-Higashi d., SYN Chédiak-Higashi *syndrome*.

Chiari d., SYN Chiari *syndrome*.

Chicago d., obsolete term for North American *blastomycosis*.

cholesterol ester storage d. [MIM*278000], a lipidosis caused by a deficiency of lysosomal acid lipase activity resulting in widespread accumulation of cholesterol esters and triglycerides in viscera with xanthomatosis, adrenal calcification, hepatosplenomegaly, foam cells in bone marrow and other tissues, and vacuo-

di

lated lymphocytes in peripheral blood; autosomal recessive inheritance, caused by mutation in the lysosomal acid lipase gene (LIPA) on chromosome 10q. SYN cholesteryl ester storage d., Wolman d., Wolman xanthomatosis.

cholesteryl ester storage d., SYN cholesterol ester storage d.

Christensen-Krabbe d., SYN *poliodystrophia* cerebri progressiva infantilis.

Christian d., (1) SYN Hand-Schüller-Christian d; (2) SYN relapsing febrile nodular nonsuppurative *panniculitis*.

Christmas d., SYN *hemophilia* B.

chronic active liver d., SYN chronic *hepatitis*.

chronic granulomatous d., a congenital defect in the killing of phagocytosed bacteria by polymorphonuclear leukocytes, which cannot increase their oxygen metabolism either because of defective cytochrome [MIM*233710 and MIM*233690] or other specific factor deficiencies [MIM*233700 and MIM*306400]. As a result there is an increased susceptibility to severe infection by catalase-positive microorganisms; inheritance is usually autosomal recessive or X-linked. SYN congenital dysphagocytosis, granulomatous d.

chronic hypertensive d., the chronic accumulative effects of long-standing high blood pressure on such vital organs as the heart, kidney, and brain.

chronic obstructive pulmonary d. (COPD), general term used for those diseases with permanent or temporary narrowing of small bronchi, in which forced expiratory flow is slowed, especially when no etiologic or other more specific term can be applied.

chylomicron retention d., an inherited disorder in which apolipoprotein B-48 is retained in intestine and absent in plasma; results in fat malabsorption.

Coats d., SYN exudative *retinitis*.

Cockayne d., SYN Cockayne *syndrome*.

cold hemagglutinin d., a condition associated with the presence of hemagglutinating autoantibody active in vivo but in vitro particularly or solely active in the cold; when the concentration of IgM antibody is high there may be increased serum viscosity, but clinical manifestations (due to hemagglutination) usually appear following exposure to cold; hemolysis usually is mild but may be severe, resulting in autoimmune hemolytic anemia, cold antibody type. SYN cold agglutinin syndrome.

collagen d., collagen-vascular d., a group of generalized d.'s affecting connective tissue and frequently characterized by fibrinoid necrosis or vasculitis; in some collagen d.'s, auto-immunization, particularly antinuclear antibodies, has been shown and circulating immune complexes are found. The term is not entirely acceptable because there is no evidence that collagen is primarily involved; "collagen" was once synonymous with "connective tissue" rather than describing a specific fibrinous protein in that tissue. SEE ALSO connective-tissue d.

combined system d., SYN subacute combined *degeneration* of the spinal cord.

communicable d., any d. that is transmissible by infection or contagion directly or through the agency of a vector.

Concato d., SYN polyserositis.

connective-tissue d., a group of generalized d.'s affecting connective tissue, especially those not inherited as mendelian characteristics; rheumatic fever and rheumatoid arthritis were first proposed as such d.'s, and other so-called collagen d.'s have been added.

Conradi d. [MIM*215100 & MIM*302950], SYN *chondrodysplasia* calcificans congenita.

Conradi-Hünermann d., SYN *chondrodysplasia* calcificans congenita.

contagious d., an infectious d. transmissible by direct or indirect contact; now used synonymously with communicable d.

Cori d., SYN type 3 *glycogenosis*.

Corrigan d., SYN aortic *regurgitation*.

Cowden d. [MIM*158350], hypertrichosis and gingival fibromatosis from infancy, accompanied by postpubertal fibroadenomatous breast enlargement; papules of the face are characteristic of multiple trichilemmomas. SYN multiple hamartoma syndrome.

Creutzfeldt-Jakob d. (CJD), a progressive neurologic disorder, one of the subacute spongiform encephalopathies caused by prions. Clinical features of CJD include a progressive cerebellar syndrome, including ataxia, abnormalities of gait and speech, and dementia. In most patients, these symptoms are followed by involuntary movements (myoclonus) and the appearance of a typical diagnostic electroencephalogram tracing (burst suppression, consisting of intermittent sharp and slow wave complexes on a flat background). The average survival is less than 1 year after onset of symptoms. Changes in the CSF are absent or nonspecific. Mild cortical atrophy and ventricular dilation may be grossly evident. On microscopic examination the distinctive finding is spongiform encephalopathy in gray matter throughout the brain and spinal cord. Severe neuronal loss and gliosis are also present and mild demyelination may occur. Ultrastructural changes include formation of intracytoplasmic vacuoles, the basis for the spongy appearance. CJD occurs worldwide at a rate of about 1–2 cases per million population per year; most cases are sporadic, but 10–12% are inherited. The peak incidence is between 55 and 65 years of age; the d. is rare before age 30. Cases of iatrogenic Creutzfeldt-Jakob d. have been associated with corneal transplants, electrode implants, dura mater grafts, and administration of human growth hormone. CJD is caused by a prion protein (an abnormal isoform of amyloid protein) that serves as a nucleating factor, inducing abnormalities in other proteins. This protein is detectable by Western blot early in the course of clinical d. Prion d.'s besides CJD include Gerstmann-Sträussler-Scheinker syndrome, fatal familial insomnia, and kuru in humans; scrapie in sheep and goats; bovine spongiform encephalopathy (mad cow d.) in cattle; and similar encephalopathies and wasting syndromes in other species. All these d.'s have been shown to be transmissible in laboratory animals. SEE ALSO bovine spongiform *encephalopathy*.

> An unusual number of cases of Creutzfeldt-Jakob disease were reported in young persons in Great Britain during the 1990s. These patients displayed ataxia, memory impairment, dementia, and myoclonus. Besides the characteristic spongiform changes of CJD, autopsy specimens from these patients showed unusual amyloid plaques with dense eosinophilic centers extensively distributed throughout the cerebrum and cerebellum. These plaques, visible with routine staining methods, had not previously been noted in Creutzfeldt-Jakob disease, but did resemble plaques seen in kuru. In addition, these patients did not display the EEG changes characteristic of classical CJD. An association is suspected between this regional cluster of variant Creutzfeldt-Jakob disease and an epizootic of bovine spongiform encephalopathy that affected more than 150,000 cattle in Britain between 1986 and 1996. However, review of mortality statistics shows no increase in deaths due to CJD among butchers, farmers, and veterinarians in England and Wales between 1979 and 1996. See Also bovine spongiform *encephalopathy*.

Crigler-Najjar d., SYN Crigler-Najjar *syndrome*.

Crocq d., SYN acrocyanosis.

Crohn d., SYN regional *enteritis*.

Crouzon d., SYN Crouzon *syndrome*.

Cruveilhier-Baumgarten d., SYN Cruveilhier-Baumgarten *syndrome*.

Cushing d., adrenal hyperplasia (Cushing syndrome) caused by an ACTH-secreting basophil adenoma of the pituitary. SYN Cushing pituitary basophilism.

Cushing d. of the omentum, central obesity in association with glucocorticoid excess, in which adipose stromal cells of the omental fat, but not subcutaneous tissue; can generate active cortisol from inactive cortisone. Patients have increased cortisol production and urinary cortisol excretion but no abnormality in the hypothalamico-pituitary-adrenal axis.

cystic d. of the breast, fibrocystic condition of the breasts.

cysticercus d., SYN cysticercosis.

cystic d. of renal medulla [MIM*256100], presence of small cysts in the renal medulla associated with anemia, sodium depletion, and chronic renal failure. It is of two types: 1) fatal autosomal recessive or juvenile type (also called familial juvenile nephrophthisis), beginning at about age 10 with an average duration of 6–8 years; 2) autosomal dominant or adult type. SYN microcystic d. of renal medulla.

cystine storage d., SYN cystinosis.

cytomegalic inclusion d., caused by Cytomegalovirus, a member of the Herpesviridae family; the presence of inclusion bodies within the cytoplasm and nuclei of enlarged cells of various organs of newborn infants dying with jaundice, hepatomegaly, splenomegaly, purpura, thrombocytopenia, and fever; the condition also occurs, at all ages, as a complication of other d.'s in which immune mechanisms are severely depressed, and has been found incidentally in salivary gland epithelium, apparently as a localized or mild infection (salivary gland virus d.). SYN cytomegalovirus d., inclusion body d.

cytomegalovirus d., SYN cytomegalic inclusion d.

Daae d., SYN epidemic *pleurodynia.*

Danielssen d., SYN anesthetic *leprosy.*

Danielssen-Boeck d., SYN anesthetic *leprosy.*

Darier d., SYN *keratosis* follicularis.

Darling d., SYN histoplasmosis.

Davies d., SYN endomyocardial *fibrosis.*

decompression d., SYN decompression *sickness.*

deer-fly d., SYN tularemia.

deficiency d., any d. resulting from undernutrition or an inadequacy of calories, proteins, essential amino acids, fatty acids, vitamins, or trace minerals.

degenerative joint d., SYN osteoarthritis.

Degos d., SYN malignant atrophic *papulosis.*

Dejerine d., SYN Dejerine-Sottas d.

Dejerine-Sottas d., a familial type of demyelinating sensorimotor polyneuropathy that begins in early childhood and is slowly progressive; clinically characterized by foot pain and paresthesias, followed by symmetrical weakness and wasting of the distal limbs; one of the causes of stork legs; patients are wheelchairbound at an early age; peripheral nerves are palpably enlarged and non-tender; pathologically, onion bulb formation is seen in the nerves: whorls of overlapping, intertwined Schwann cell processes that encircle bare axons; usually autosomal recessive inheritance; an autosomal dominant form also exists; both forms can be caused by mutations in the peripheral myelin protein gene 22 (PMP22) on 17q or in the myelin protein zero gene (MPZ) on 1q. SYN Dejerine d., hereditary hypertrophic neuropathy, progressive hypertrophic polyneuropathy.

demyelinating d., generic term for a group of d.'s, of unknown cause, in which there is extensive loss of the myelin in the central nervous system, as in multiple sclerosis and Schilder disease.

dense-deposit d., SEE membranoproliferative *glomerulonephritis.*

de Quervain d., fibrosis of the sheath of a tendon of the thumb. SYN radial styloid tendovaginitis.

Dercum d., SYN *adiposis* dolorosa.

Deutschländer d., tumor of one of the metatarsal bones;

Devic d., SYN *neuromyelitis* optica.

diffuse Lewy body d., a degenerative cerebral disorder of the elderly, characterized initially by progressive dementia or psychosis, and subsequently by parkinsonian findings, usually with severe rigidity; other manifestations include involuntary movements, myoclonus, dysphagia, and orthostatic hypotension. Pathologically, Lewy bodies are present diffusely in the nuclei of the hypothalamus, basal forebrain, and brainstem. SYN Lewy body dementia.

Di Guglielmo d., the acute form of erythremic myelosis. SYN Di Guglielmo syndrome.

disappearing bone d., extensive decalcification of a single bone; of unknown cause, sometimes associated with angioma. SYN Gorham d., Gorham syndrome.

diverticular d., symptomatic congenital or acquired diverticula of any portion of the gastrointestinal tract. Such diverticula occur in about 15% of the population but rarely cause symptoms.

dog d., SYN phlebotomus *fever.*

dominantly inherited Lévi d., SYN snub-nose *dwarfism.*

Donohue d., SYN leprechaunism.

drug-induced d., a toxic reaction to or morbid condition resulting from the administration of a drug.

Dubois d., SYN Dubois *abscesses,* under *abscess.*

Duchenne d., SYN Duchenne *dystrophy.*

Duchenne-Aran d., SYN amyotrophic lateral *sclerosis.*

Duhring d., SYN *dermatitis* herpetiformis.

Dukes d., SYN *exanthema* subitum.

Duncan d. [MIM*308240], SYN X-linked lymphoproliferative *syndrome.* SYN lymphoproliferative syndrome.

Dupuytren d. of the foot, SYN plantar *fibromatosis.*

Duroziez d., congenital stenosis of the mitral valve.

Dutton d., african tick-borne relapsing fever caused by *Borrelia duttonii* and spread by the soft tick, *Ornithodoros moubata.* SYN Dutton relapsing fever.

Eales d., peripheral retinal periphlebitis causing recurrent retinal or intravitreous hemorrhages in young adults.

Ebstein d., SYN Ebstein *anomaly.*

echinococcus d., SYN echinococcosis.

Eisenmenger d., SYN Eisenmenger *complex.*

elephant man's d., (1) SYN Proteus *syndrome;* **(2)** SYN neurofibromatosis.

elevator d., respiratory distress arising in persons who work in grain elevators resulting from inhalation of dusts or insects.

emotional d., SEE mental *illness.*

endemic d., continued prevalence of a d. in a specific population or area. SEE ALSO endemic, enzootic.

Engelmann d., SYN diaphysial *dysplasia.*

English sweating d., a d. of unknown nature that appeared in England and spread over Europe in 1485, 1508 and 1528–30 and was characterized by heavy sweats, prostration, and a high fatality rate. SYN sudor anglicus.

eosinophilic endomyocardial d., a restrictive cardiomyopathy associated with hyperproduction of eosinophiles and their cardiac infiltration, clinically characterized by diastolic and later systolic ventricular failure. Sometimes associated with Churg-Strauss syndrome or eosinophilic pericarditis.

epidemic d., marked increase in prevalence of a d. in a specific population or area, usually with an environmental cause, such as an infectious or toxic agent.

Epstein d., SYN diphtheroid (1).

Erb d., SYN progressive bulbar *paralysis.*

Erb-Charcot d., (1) SYN spastic *diplegia;* **(2)** SYN spastic *paraplegia.*

Erdheim d., SYN cystic medial *necrosis.*

ergot alkaloid-associated heart d., heart d. caused by endomyocardial fibrosis which extends into valve structures, producing stenosis and/or regurgitation, associated with ergot alkaloid use.

Eulenburg d., SYN congenital *paramyotonia.*

exanthematous d., SEE exanthema.

extramammary Paget d., an intraepidermal form of mucinous adenocarcinoma, most commonly in the anogenital region, presenting as erythematous plaques in the elderly, which may be associated with sweat gland or regional visceral carcinoma. SYN Paget d. (3).

extrapyramidal d., a general term for a number of disorders caused by abnormalities of the basal ganglia or certain brainstem or thalamic nuclei; characterized by motor deficits, loss of postural reflexes, bradykinesia, tremor, rigidity, and various involuntary movements. SYN extrapyramidal motor system d.

extrapyramidal motor system d., SYN extrapyramidal d.

Fabry d. [MIM*301500], due to deficiency of α-galactosidase and characterized by abnormal accumulations of neutral glycolipids (e.g., globotriaosylceramide) in endothelial cells in blood vessel walls; clinical findings include angiokeratomas on the thighs, buttocks, and genitalia, hypohidrosis, paresthesia in extremities, cornea verticillata, and spokelike posterior subcapsular cataracts; death results from renal, cardiac, or cerebrovascular complica-

di

tions; X-linked recessive inheritance caused by mutation the α-galactosidase gene (GLA) on Xq. SYN diffuse angiokeratoma, glycolipid lipidosis.

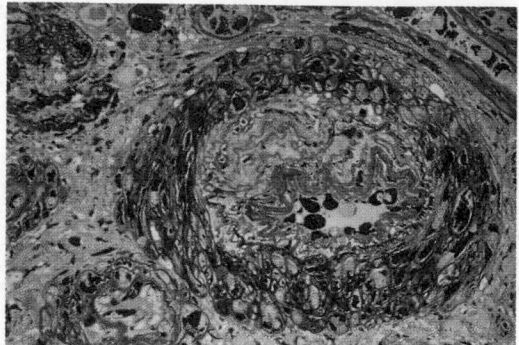

Fabry disease: artery showing accumulation of periodic acid–Schiff (PAS)-positive droplets in muscle cells of the media; intima shows considerable thickening; osmium fixation, periodic acid-Schiff stain, ×250

Fahr d., progressive calcific deposition in the walls of blood vessels of the basal ganglia, in young to middle-aged persons; occasionally associated with mental retardation and extrapyramidal symptoms.

Farber d., SYN disseminated *lipogranulomatosis*.

Favre-Durand-Nicholas d., SYN venereal *lymphogranuloma*.

Favre-Racouchot d., comedones developing on sun-damaged skin due to obstruction of pilosebaceous follicles by solar elastosis. SYN Favre-Racouchot syndrome, solar comedo.

Fazio-Londe d. [MIM*211500], a progressive bulbar palsy affecting the brainstem; due to motor neuron degeneration; a variant of spinal muscular atrophy (q.v.).

Feer d., SYN acrodynia (2).

femoropopliteal occlusive d., obstruction of the femoral and popliteal arteries by atherosclerosis.

fibrocystic d. of the pancreas, SYN cystic *fibrosis*.

fifth d., SYN *erythema* infectiosum. [after scarlatina, morbilli, rubella, and fourth d.]

Filatov d., SYN Filatov-Dukes d.

Filatov-Dukes d., an exanthem-producing infectious disease of childhood of unknown etiology. SYN Filatov d., parascarlatina, scarlatinella, scarlatinoid (2).

fish eye d., an inherited disorder resulting in low HDL cholesterol and corneal opacities; also, low LCAT activity.

flax-dresser's d., chronic obstructive pulmonary d. caused by inhalation of particles of unprocessed flax; a form of byssinosis. SEE ALSO byssinosis.

Flegel d., SYN *hyperkeratosis* lenticularis perstans.

flint d., SYN chalicosis.

focal metastatic d., presence of a single area of metastasis of a malignant tumor or infection distant from the primary lesion.

Folling d., SYN phenylketonuria.

foot-and-mouth d. (FMD), a highly infectious disease of wide distribution and great economic importance, occurring in cattle, swine, sheep, goats and all wild and domestic cloven-footed animals caused by a picornavirus (genus Aphthovirus) and characterized by vesicular eruptions in the mouth, tongue, hoofs, and udder; humans are rarely affected. SYN aftosa.

Forbes d., SYN type 3 *glycogenosis*.

Fordyce d., SYN Fordyce *spots*, under *spot*.

Forestier d., SYN diffuse idiopathic skeletal *hyperostosis*.

Fothergill d., **(1)** SYN trigeminal *neuralgia*; **(2)** SYN anginose *scarlatina*.

Fournier d., infective gangrene involving the scrotum. SYN Fournier gangrene, syphiloma of Fournier.

fourth d., SYN *exanthema* subitum.

Fox-Fordyce d., a chronic pruritic eruption of dry papules and distended ruptured apocrine glands, seen mostly in women, with follicular hyperkeratosis of the nipples, axillae, and pubic and sternal regions. SYN apocrine miliaria.

Franklin d., SYN γ-heavy-chain d.

Freiberg d., osteonecrosis of second metatarsal head. SYN Freiberg infarction.

Friend d., mouse leukemia caused by the Friend leukemia virus, a member of the family Retroviridae.

functional d., SYN functional *disorder*.

functional cardiovascular d., a euphemism for cardiovascular symptoms deemed to be psychogenic. More generally, sometimes used for abnormal cardiac function.

fusospirochetal d., infection of the mouth and/or pharynx associated with fusiform bacilli and spirochetes, commonly part of the normal flora of the mouth. SEE ALSO necrotizing ulcerative *gingivitis*.

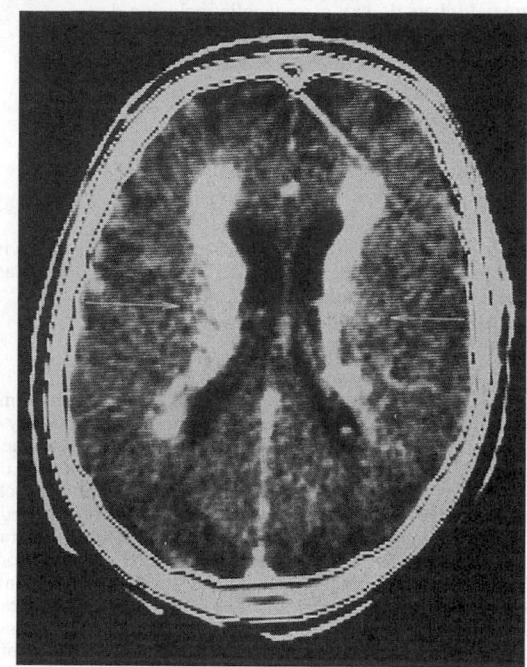

Fahr disease: arteriosclerotic calcification of the basal ganglia, on both sides (computed tomogram)

Gairdner d., attacks of cardiac distress accompanied by apprehension. SYN angina pectoris sine dolore, angor pectoris (1).

Gamna d., a form of chronic splenomegaly characterized by conspicuous thickening of the capsule and the presence of multiple, small, rustlike, brown foci (Gamna-Gandy bodies), which contain iron; this condition may be observed in fibrocongestive splenomegaly, sickle cell d., and some examples of hemochromatosis.

Gandy-Nanta d., siderotic splenomegaly, probably the same as Gamna d.

garapata d., tick fever occurring in Spain.

Garré d., SYN sclerosing *osteitis*.

gastroesophageal reflux d. (GERD), a syndrome due to structural or functional incompetence of the lower esophageal sphincter, which permits retrograde flow of acidic gastric juice into the esophagus.

Although the underlying abnormality in GERD is apparently inborn and irreversible, the incidence increases with age. In addition to reflux, most cases involve disordered gastric motility and prolonged gastric emptying time. Symptoms include recurring epigastric and retrosternal distress, usually described as heartburn, along with varying degrees of belching, nausea, gagging, cough, or hoarseness. GERD is increasingly recognized as a cause of throat irritation and chronic cough. The incidence of GERD among adults with asthma may be as high as 80%. The disorder is more common in men. The likelihood of symptomatic reflux is increased by obesity, pregnancy, cigarette smoking, diabetes mellitus, scleroderma, and other connective tissue diseases. Symptoms can be induced by recumbency, strenuous exercise, heavy lifting, smoking, eating large meals, or consuming alcohol, chocolate, fatty foods, and drugs such as theophylline, calcium channel blockers, and anticholinergic agents. Acid reflux can cause peptic esophagitis, ulcer formation, or esophageal stricture. Metaplastic changes in esophageal squamous epithelium, called Barrett's esophagus, can progress to carcinoma. Diagnosis is by history, esophageal pH monitoring, radiologic study showing reflux of swallowed barium, and endoscopy to identify ulceration or stricture and permit biopsy to rule out malignancy. Treatment includes avoidance of known causes and administration of antacids, H_2 antagonists, prokinetic agents, and proton pump inhibitors.

Gaucher d., a lysosomal storage disorder due to a deficiency of glucocerebrosidase resulting in accumulation of glucocerebroside; high incidence among persons of Ashkenazi Jewish descent; occurs most severely in infants, characterized by hepatosplenomegaly, hematologic abnormalities, bone lesions, neurological manifestations with ataxia, spastic paraplegia, seizures, and dementia, and presence of characteristic histiocytes (Gaucher cells) in the viscera; autosomal recessive inheritance, caused by mutation in the glucocerebrosidase A gene (GBA) on chromosome 1q. There are three main forms: type I, noncerebral juvenile [MIM*230800]; type II, cerebral juvenile [MIM*230900]; and type III, adult cerebral [MIM*231000]; the juvenile forms are most severe. SYN cerebroside lipidosis.

Gerhardt-Mitchell d., SYN erythromelalgia.

Gerlier d., SYN vestibular *neuronitis.*

gestational trophoblastic d., SYN hydatidiform *mole.*

Gierke d., SYN type 1 *glycogenosis.*

Gilbert d., SYN familial nonhemolytic *jaundice.*

Gilchrist d., SYN blastomycosis.

Gilles de la Tourette d., SYN Tourette *syndrome.*

Glanzmann d., SYN Glanzmann *thrombasthenia.*

glycogen-storage d., SYN glycogenosis.

Goldflam d., SYN *myasthenia* gravis.

Gorham d., SYN disappearing bone d.

Gougerot and Blum d., SYN pigmented purpuric lichenoid *dermatosis.*

Gougerot-Sjögren d., SYN Sjögren *syndrome.* [Sjögren, Henrik S.C.]

Gowers d., (1) SYN saltatory *spasm*; **(2)** a distal type of progressive muscular dystrophy.

graft versus host d., an incompatibility reaction (that may be fatal) in a subject (host) of low immunologic competence who has been the recipient of immunologically competent lymphoid tissue from a donor who is immunologically different from the recipient; the reaction, or disease, is the result of action of the transplanted cells against those host tissues that possess an antigen not found in the donor. Seen most commonly following bone marrow transplantation, acute d. is seen after 7–30 days and chronic d. weeks to months after transplantation, affecting, principally, the gastrointestinal tract, liver, and skin. SYN GVH d.

granulomatous d., SYN chronic granulomatous d.

Graves d., (1) toxic goiter characterized by diffuse hyperplasia of the thyroid gland, a form of hyperthyroidism; exophthalmos is a common, but not invariable, concomitant; **(2)** thyroid dysfunction and all or any of its clinical associations; **(3)** an organ-specific autoimmune disease of the thyroid gland. SEE thyrotoxicosis, Hashimoto *thyroiditis*, goiter, myxedema. SYN Basedow d., ophthalmic hyperthyroidism, Parry d.

Griesinger d., bilious typhoid of Griesinger, a severe form of louse-borne relapsing fever caused by *Borrelia recurrentis* and

causing high fever, epistaxis, dyspnea, intense jaundice, purpura, and splenomegaly.

Grover d., SYN transient acantholytic *dermatosis.*

GVH d., SYN graft versus host d.

Haff d., rhabdomyolysis resultant from an unidentified toxin contained in some fishes, including turbot and biffalo fish. [*Haff*, an arm of the Baltic Sea in East Prussia]

Haglund d., an abnormal prominence of the posterior superior lateral aspect of the os calcis. SYN Haglund deformity.

Hailey-Hailey d., SYN benign familial chronic *pemphigus.*

Hallervorden-Spatz d., SYN Hallervorden-Spatz *syndrome.*

Hallopeau d., SYN *pemphigus* vegetans (2).

Hamman d., SYN Hamman *syndrome.*

Hammond d., SYN athetosis.

hand-foot-and-mouth d., an exanthematous eruption in small children usually consisting of small, pearl-gray vesicles of the fingers, toes, palms, and soles, accompanied by often painful vesicles and ulceration of the buccal mucous membrane and the tongue and by slight fever; the d. lasts 4–7 days, and is usually caused by coxsackie virus type A-16, but other types have been identified.

Hand-Schüller-Christian d., the chronic disseminated form of Langerhans cell histiocytosis. The classic triad of signs consists of diabetes insipidus, exophthalmos, and bony lesions composed of histiocytes. SYN Christian d. (1), Christian syndrome, normal cholesteremic xanthomatosis, Schüller d., Schüller syndrome.

Hansen d., SYN leprosy.

Harada d., SYN Harada *syndrome.*

Hartnup d. [MIM*234500], an autosomal recessively inherited metabolic disorder characterized by aminoaciduria which is due to defective renal tubular transport of neutral α-amino acids; there is increased urinary excretion of tryptophan derivatives caused by defective intestinal absorption and bacterial degradation of unabsorbed tryptophan in the gut; manifestations include pellagralike, light-sensitive skin rash with temporary cerebellar ataxia. SYN Hartnup syndrome.

Hashimoto d., SYN Hashimoto *thyroiditis.*

heavy chain d., a term used for a group of d.'s, the paraproteinemias, characterized by production of homogeneous immunoglobulins or fragments, and associated with malignant disorders of the plasmacytic and lymphoid cell series. Three types have been recognized: γ-heavy-chain d., α-heavy-chain d., and μ-heavy-chain d.; each is diagnosed by the finding of the appropriate heavy-chain fragment in the serum, urine, or both.

α-heavy-chain d., the most common form of heavy-chain d., characterized by a finding in the serum of a protein reactive with antisera to α-chains but not light chains; clinical features include diarrhea, steatorrhea, and severe malabsorption.

γ-heavy-chain d., heavy-chain d. characterized by a finding in the serum and urine of a broad protein peak that is reactive with antisera to γ-chains and unreactive with antisera to light chains; common features include anemia, lymphocytosis, eosinophilia, thrombocytopenia, hyperuricemia, lymphadenopathy, and hepatosplenomegaly. SYN Franklin d.

μ-heavy-chain d., the rarest form of heavy-chain d., primarily seen in patients with long-standing chronic lymphatic leukemia; diagnosis is made on immunoelectrophoresis by finding a component reactive with antisera to μ-chains but not to light chains.

Heck d., SYN focal epithelial *hyperplasia.*

Heerfordt d., SYN uveoparotid *fever.*

hemoglobin C d., the homozygous state of hemoglobin C.

hemoglobin H d., SEE *hemoglobin* H.

hemolytic d. of newborn, SYN *erythroblastosis* fetalis.

hemorrhagic d. of the newborn, a syndrome characterized by spontaneous internal or external bleeding accompanied by hypoprothrombinemia, slightly decreased platelets, and markedly elevated bleeding and clotting times, usually occurring between the third and sixth days of life and effectively treated with vitamin K.

herring-worm d., SYN anisakiasis.

Hers d., SYN type 6 *glycogenosis.*

Hirschsprung d., SYN congenital *megacolon.*

di

Hodgkin d., a d. marked by chronic enlargement of the lymph nodes, often local at the onset and later generalized, together with enlargement of the spleen and often of the liver, no pronounced leukocytosis, and commonly anemia and continuous or remittent (Pel-Ebstein) fever; considered to be a malignant neoplasm of lymphoid cells of uncertain origin (Reed-Sternberg cells), associated with inflammatory infiltration of lymphocytes and eosinophilic leukocytes and fibrosis; can be classified into lymphocytic predominant, nodular sclerosing, mixed cellularity, and lymphocytic depletion type; a similar disease occurs in domestic cats. SYN Hodgkin lymphoma, lymphadenoma (2).

Hodgson d., dilation of the arch of the aorta associated with insufficiency of the aortic valve.

holoendemic d. (hol′ō-en-dem′ik), a d. for which a high prevalent level of infection begins early in life and affects most or all of the child population, leading to a state of equilibrium, such that the adult population shows evidence of the disease much less frequently than do the children.

hookworm d., SEE ancylostomiasis, necatoriasis.

Huntington d. [MIM*143100], SYN Huntington *chorea*.

Hurler d., SYN Hurler *syndrome*.

Hurst d., SYN acute necrotizing hemorrhagic *encephalomyelitis*.

Hutchinson-Gilford d., SYN progeria.

hyaline membrane d. of the newborn, a d. seen especially in premature neonates with respiratory distress; characterized postmortem by atelectasis and alveolar ducts lined by an eosinophilic membrane; also associated with reduced amounts of lung surfactant. SYN hyaline membrane syndrome, respiratory distress syndrome of the newborn.

hydatid d., infection of humans, sheep, and most other herbivorous and omnivorous mammals with larvae of the tapeworm *Echinococcus*.

hyperendemic d., a d. that is constantly present at a high incidence and/or prevalence rate and affects all age groups equally.

Iceland d., SYN epidemic *neuromyasthenia*.

I-cell d., SYN *mucolipidosis* II.

idiopathic d., a d. of unknown cause or mechanism.

immune complex d., an immunologic category of d.'s evoked by the deposition of antigen-antibody in the microvasculature. Complement is frequently involved and the breakdown products of complement attract polymorphonuclear leukocytes to the site of deposition. Damage to tissue is frequently caused by the process of "frustrated" phagocytosis by polymorphonuclear cells. Vasculitis or nephritis is common. Arthus phenomenon and serum sickness are classic examples, but many other disorders, including most of the connective tissue d.'s, may belong in this immunologic category; immune complex d.'s can also occur during a variety of d.'s of known etiology, such as subacute bacterial endocarditis. SEE ALSO autoimmune d. SYN immune complex disorder, type III hypersensitivity reaction.

immunoproliferative small intestinal d., diffuse lymphoplasmacytic infiltration of the proximal small bowel mucosa and mesenteric lymph nodes resulting in diarrhea, weight loss, abdominal pain, and clubbing of fingers and toes; seen in poor people in developing countries. SYN Mediterranean lymphoma.

inborn lysosomal d., inherited disorder of one or more degradative enzymes normally located in lysosomes leading to accumulation (storage) of abnormal quantities of a substance, such as a glycosaminoglycan as in Hurler *syndrome* or a lipopolysaccharide as in Gaucher d.

inclusion body d., SYN cytomegalic inclusion d.

inclusion cell d., SYN *mucolipidosis* II.

industrial d., a morbid condition resulting from exposure to an agent discharged by a commercial enterprise into the environment. Cf. occupational d.

infantile celiac d., gluten-sensitive enteropathy appearing in infancy, often before the age of 9 months and characterized by acute onset, diarrhea, abdominal pain, and "failure to thrive."

infectious d., infective d., a d. resulting from the presence and activity of a microbial agent.

intercurrent d., a new d. occurring during the course of another d., not related to the primary disease process.

⊟interstitial d., a d. occurring chiefly in the connective-tissue framework of an organ, the parenchyma suffering secondarily.

iron-storage d., the storage of excess iron in the parenchyma of many organs, as in idiopathic hemochromatosis or transfusion hemosiderosis.

island d., SYN tsutsugamushi d.

Itai-Itai d., a form of cadmium poisoning described in Japanese people, characterized by renal tubular dysfunction, osteomalacia, pseudofractures, and anemia, caused by ingestion of contaminated shellfish or other sources containing cadmium.

Jaffe-Lichtenstein d., obsolete term for fibrous *dysplasia* of bone.

Jansky-Bielschowsky d., cerebral *sphingolipidosis*, early juvenile type.

Jensen d., SYN *retinochoroiditis* juxtapapillaris.

jumping d., jumper d., one of the pathologic startle syndromes found in isolated parts of the world, characterized by greatly exaggerated responses, such as jumping, flinging the arms and yelling, to minimal stimuli. SYN jumping Frenchmen of Maine d., jumper d. of Maine.

jumping Frenchmen of Maine d., jumper d. of Maine, SYN jumping d.

Jüngling d., SYN *osteitis* tuberculosa multiplex cystica.

Kashin-Bek d., a form of generalized osteoarthrosis limited to areas of Asia, including the Urov river; believed to result from ingestion of wheat infected with the fungus *Fusarium sporotrichiella*.

Katayama d., acute early egg-laying phase of schistosomiasis, a toxemic syndrome in heavy primary infections, rarely seen in chronic cases. It is considered a form of immune complex d. or serum sickness–like condition. Described for *schistosomiasis japonica*, but observed with other forms as well. SYN Katayama fever. [town in Japan where the d. is common]

Kawasaki d., a systemic vasculitis of unknown origin that occurs primarily in children under 8 years of age. Symptoms include a fever lasting more than 5 days, polymorphic rash, erythematous, dry, cracking lips; conjunctival injection, swelling of the hands and feet, irritability, adenopathy, and a perineal desquamative rash. Approximately 20% of untreated patients may develop coronary artery aneurysms. As the child recovers from the illness, thrombocytosis and peeling of the fingertips occurs. SYN Kawasaki syndrome, mucocutaneous lymph node syndrome.

Kennedy d., an X-linked recessive disorder characterized by progressive spinal and bulbar muscular atrophy; associated features include distal degeneration of sensory axons, and signs of endocrine dysfunction, including diabetes mellitus, gynecomastia, and testicular atrophy. SYN X-linked recessive bulbospinal neuronopathy.

Kienböck d., osteonecrosis of the lunate bone resulting from unknown etiology, although can occur after trauma. SYN lunatomalacia.

Kikuchi d., necrotizing lymphadenitis of unknown etiology, most often encountered in young women in Japan but also in other parts of the world; lymph node enlargement, associated with fever, subsides spontaneously.

Kimmelstiel-Wilson d., SYN Kimmelstiel-Wilson *syndrome*.

Kimura d., SYN angiolymphoid *hyperplasia* with eosinophilia.

kinky-hair d., kinky hair d. [MIM*309400], an inborn error of copper metabolism with onset within a few weeks of birth; manifested by short, sparse, poorly pigmented kinky hair; failure to thrive; development of seizures; spasticity; and progressive mental deterioration leading to death. X-linked recessive inheritance due to a defect of copper transport, caused by mutation in the Menkes gene (MNK), which encodes a copper-transporting ATPase on Xq. SYN Menkes syndrome, trichopoliodystrophy.

Köhler d., osteonecrosis of the tarsal navicular bone or of the patella.

kok d., SYN hyperekplexia.

Krabbe d., SYN globoid cell *leukodystrophy*.

Kufs d., cerebral *sphingolipidosis*, adult type.

Kugelberg-Welander d., SYN spinal muscular *atrophy*, type III.

Kussmaul d., SYN *polyarteritis* nodosa.

Kyasanur Forest d., a d. occurring among forest workers in the Kyasanur Forest and in Mysore, India, caused by a Flavivirus in the family Flaviviridae transmitted chiefly by *Haemaphysalis spinigera*, although other ticks have been implicated as well; symptoms include fever, headache, back and limb pains, diarrhea, and intestinal bleeding; central nervous system symptoms do not occur.

Kyrle d., SYN *hyperkeratosis* follicularis et parafollicularis.

Lafora d., SYN Lafora body d.

Lafora body d. [MIM*254780], a form of progressive myoclonus epilepsy beginning from age 6–19; characterized by generalized tonic-clonic seizures, resting and action myoclonus, ataxia, dementia, and classic EEG findings, including polyspike and wave discharges; basophilic cytoplasmic inclusion bodies present in portions of the brain, the liver, and skin, as well as the duct cells of the sweat glands. Death usually occurs within 10 years of onset; autosomal recessive inheritance, caused by mutation in the progressive myoclonic epilepsy 2 gene (EPM2A) on chromosome 6q. SYN Lafora d.

Lane d., SYN *erythema* palmare hereditarium.

L-chain d., SYN Bence Jones *myeloma*.

Legg-Calvé-Perthes d., Legg-Perthes d., Legg d., epiphysial osteonecrosis of the upper end of the femur. SYN Calvé-Perthes d., coxa plana, osteochondritis deformans juvenilis, Perthes d., pseudocoxalgia, quiet hip d.

Legionnaires d., an acute infectious d., caused by *Legionella pneumophila*, with prodromal influenzalike symptoms and a rapidly rising high fever, followed by severe pneumonia and production of usually nonpurulent sputum, and sometimes mental confusion, hepatic fatty changes, and renal tubular degeneration. It has a high case-fatality rate; acquired from contaminated water, usually by aerosolization rather than being transmitted from person-to-person. SYN legionellosis. [American *Legion* convention, 1976, at which many delegates were so affected]

Leigh d. [MIM*256000], subacute encephalomyelopathy affecting infants, causing seizures, spasticity, optic atrophy, and dementia; the genetic causation is heterogeneous; may be associated with deficiency of cytochrome c oxidase or NADH-ubiquinone oxidoreductase or other enzymes involved in energy metabolism. Autosomal recessive, X-linked recessive and mitochondrial inheritance have been described; mutations have been identified in the surfeit-1 gene (SURF) [MIM*185620] on chromosome 9, in a mtDNA-encoded subunit of ATP synthase [MIM*516060], in the X-linked E1-alpha subunit of pyruvate dehydrogenase [MIM*312170], and in several subunits of mitochondrial complex I [MIM*161015 and MIM*620141]. SYN necrotizing encephalomyelopathy, necrotizing encephalopathy.

Leiner d., SYN *erythroderma* desquamativum.

Lenègre d., SYN Lenègre *syndrome*.

lenticular progressive d., SYN wilson *disease*.

Leri-Weill d., SYN dyschondrosteosis.

Letterer-Siwe d., the acute disseminated form of Langerhans cell histiocytosis. SYN nonlipid histiocytosis.

Lev d., SYN Lev *syndrome*.

Lindau d., SYN von Hippel-Lindau *syndrome*.

linear IgA bullous d. in children, SYN chronic bullous *dermatosis* of childhood.

Little d., SYN spastic *diplegia*.

Lobo d., SYN lobomycosis.

Löffler d., SYN Löffler *endocarditis*.

Lorain d., SYN idiopathic *infantilism*.

Lou Gehrig d., SYN amyotrophic lateral *sclerosis*.

Luft d. [MIM*238800], a metabolic d. due to relative uncoupling of phosphorylation in skeletal muscle causing myopathy and general hypermetabolism; a mitochondial myopathy.

lung fluke d., infection with the lung fluke, *Clonorchis sinensis*.

Lutz-Splendore-Almeida d., SYN paracoccidioidomycosis.

Lyell d., SYN staphylococcal scalded skin *syndrome*.

Lyme d., a subacute inflammatory disorder caused by infection with *Borrelia burgdorferi*, a nonpyogenic spirochete transmitted by *Ixodes scapularis*, the deer tick, in the eastern U.S. and *I. pacificus*, the western black-legged tick, in the western U.S.; the characteristic skin lesion, erythema chronicum migrans, is usually preceded or accompanied by fever, malaise, fatigue, headache, and stiff neck; neurologic, cardiac, or articular manifestations may occur weeks to months later. Tick nymphs are thought to be responsible for about 90% of transmission to human beings. Nymphs and larvae feed especially on the white-footed mouse, *Peromyscus leucopus*, while the preferred host of adults is the deer. Infected reservoir animals and ticks do not become ill. Residual articular or neurologic symptoms, which may persist for months or years after the initial infection, probably represent an immune response to the organism. Variations in clinical features or severity from one patient to another may be due to inborn variations in immune response, perhaps linked to the human lymphocytic antigen system. SYN Lyme borreliosis. [Lyme, CT, where first observed]

Because of media coverage, Lyme disease has a higher profile than its occurrence warrants. Fewer than 18,000 cases are confirmed annually in the U.S. It is generally a benign, self-limited disease, even when untreated. Antibody studies in endemic areas suggest that as many as 50% of persons who contract the infection never show symptoms. The case fatality rate is virtually zero. The diagnosis is essentially clinical. Serologic tests for antibody to *B. burgdorferi* are notoriously poor in both sensitivity and specificity. In nonendemic areas, false-positive test results statistically outnumber true positives. IgM antibody appears and peaks relatively late, so that one-half of patients are seronegative during the first month following appearance of the rash. Antibiotic treatment administered early can alter or prevent the expected acute immune response. IgG antibody persists for months or years after infection and hence affords no help in diagnosing acute disease. Given the nonspecific and variable clinical picture and the unreliability of laboratory diagnostic measures, it is inevitable that many cases of Lyme disease are missed, and that, conversely, the diagnosis is often wrongly made. A study assessing the costs of misdiagnosis of Lyme disease found that 60% of patients referred to a Lyme disease clinic had never had the disease and another 19% had a history of infection but no current disease. The drug of choice is doxycycline administered orally for several weeks. Amoxicillin is the standard alternative for children and pregnant patients. Recovery does not confer immunity to future attacks; in fact, in highly endemic areas, the reinfection rate may be as high as 20%. Infectious disease authorities do not recommend antibiotic prophylaxis after a tick bite, even in highly endemic areas, nor do they countenance treatment of asymptomatic persons who have serologic evidence of past infection. A vaccine consisting of outer surface protein A (OspA) of *B. burgdorferi* synthesized by a nonvirulent strain of recombinant *Escherichia coli* was released in 1998. Antibody induced by the vaccine enters a feeding tick and binds any spirochetes present, preventing their mobilization. Three doses of the vaccine administered over a 12-month period confer about 80% protection against Lyme disease. The vaccine is not approved for persons under age 15 and is recommended only for those living or working in highly endemic areas.

lysosomal d., a d. due to inadequate functioning of a lysosomal enzyme; most such d.'s are associated with a storage d.

Machado-Joseph d. [MIM*109150], a rare form of hereditary ataxia, characterized by onset in early adult life of progressive, spinocerebellar and extrapyramidal disease with external ophthalmoplegia, rigidity dystonia symptoms, and, often, peripheral amyotrophy; found predominantly in people of Azorean ancestry; autosomal dominant inheritance, caused by a trinucleotide repeat expansion mutation in the Machado-Joseph gene (MJD1) on 14q. SYN Azorean d., Portuguese-Azorean d. [Surnames of two families studied in major descriptions of the disease.]

mad cow d., SYN bovine spongiform *encephalopathy*.

Madelung d., SYN multiple symmetric *lipomatosis*.

di

Manson d., SYN *schistosomiasis* mansoni.

maple bark d., hypersensitivity pneumonitis caused by spores of *Cryptostroma corticale* growing under the bark of stacked maple logs.

maple syrup urine d. [MIM*248600], an inborn error of metabolism caused by defective oxidative decarboxylation of α-keto acids of leucine, isoleucine, and valine; these branched-chain amino acids are present in the blood and urine in high concentrations; manifestations of d. include feeding difficulties, physical and mental retardation, and a urine odor similar to that of maple syrup; neonatal death is common. Autosomal recessive inheritance, caused by mutation in the E1, E2 or E3 subunit of the branched-chain α-keto acid dehydrogenase gene (BCKDH) on 19q. There are various forms differentiated by the subunit of BCKDH mutated. SYN branched chain ketoaciduria, branched chain ketonuria, ketoacidemia.

marble bone d., SYN osteopetrosis.

Marburg d., infection with an unusual rhabdovirus composed of RNA and lipid, tentatively assigned to the family of Filoviridae. Virus is "pantropic" and affects most organ systems.The disease is characterized by a prominent rash and hemorrhages in many organs and is often fatal. First seen among laboratory workers in Marburg, Germany, exposed to African green monkeys. Some person-to-person spread has been observed. Attempts to isolate virus should be done only in high-security laboratories. SYN Marburg virus d.

Marburg virus d., SYN Marburg d.

Marchiafava-Bignami d., a disorder recognized primarily by its pathological features, consisting of demyelination of the corpus callosum and cortical laminar necrosis involving the frontal and temporal lobes. Occurs predominantly in chronic alcoholics, particularly wine drinkers.

Marfan d., SYN Marfan *syndrome*.

margarine d., erythema multiforme caused by an emulsifying agent used in the manufacture of margarine.

Marie-Strümpell d., SYN ankylosing *spondylitis*.

Marion d., a congenital obstruction of the posterior urethra.

Martin d., a periosteoarthritis of the foot from excessive walking.

McArdle d., SYN type 5 *glycogenosis*.

McArdle-Schmid-Pearson d., SYN type 5 *glycogenosis*.

mechanobullous d., SYN *epidermolysis* bullosa. [G. *mechanē*, machine, + bullous]

Meige d. [MIM*153200], autosomal dominant lymphedema with onset at about the age of puberty.

Ménétrier d., gastric mucosal hyperplasia, either mucoid or glandular; the latter type may be associated with the Zollinger-Ellison syndrome. SYN giant hypertrophy of gastric mucosa, hypertrophic gastritis, Ménétrier syndrome.

Ménière d., an affection characterized clinically by vertigo, nausea, vomiting, tinnitus, and progressive hearing loss due to hydrops of the endolymphatic duct. SYN endolymphatic hydrops, Ménière syndrome.

mental d., SEE mental *illness*.

Merzbacher-Pelizaeus d., SYN Pelizaeus-Merzbacher d.

metabolic d., generic term for disease caused by an abnormal metabolic process. It can be congenital, due to inherited enzyme abnormality, or acquired, due to disease of an endocrine organ or failure of function of a metabolic important organ such as the liver.

Meyenburg d., SYN relapsing *polychondritis*.

Meyer-Betz d., SYN myoglobinuria.

Mibelli d., SYN porokeratosis.

microcystic d. of renal medulla, SYN cystic d. of renal medulla.

micrometastatic d., the condition of a patient who has had all clinically evident cancer removed, but who may be expected to have a recurrence from metastases that are too small to be apparent.

microvillus inclusion d., a condition that begins at birth with persistent watery diarrhea and life-threatening malabsorption associated with villus atrophy and crypt hypoplasia in the small bowel; electron microscopy reveals microvillus inclusions in enterocytes. SYN congenital microvillus atrophy.

Mikulicz d., benign swelling of the lacrimal, and usually also of the salivary glands in consequence of an infiltration of and replacement of the normal gland structure by lymphoid tissue. SEE ALSO Mikulicz *syndrome*, Sjögren *syndrome*.

Milroy d. [MIM*153100], the congenital type of autosomal dominant lymphedema.

Minamata d., a neurologic disorder caused by methyl mercury intoxication; first described in the inhabitants of Minamata Bay, Japan, resulting from their eating fish contaminated with mercury industrial waste. Characterized by peripheral sensory loss, tremors, dysarthria, ataxia, and both hearing and visual loss.

miner's d., (1) SYN ancylostomiasis, miner's *nystagmus*.

minimal-change d., SYN lipoid *nephrosis*.

mixed connective-tissue d., d. with overlapping features of various systemic connective-tissue d.'s and with serum antibodies to nuclear ribonucleoprotein.

molecular d., a d. in which the manifestations are due to alterations in molecular structure and function.

Mondor d., thrombophlebitis of the thoracoepigastric vein of the breast and chest wall.

Monge d., SYN chronic mountain *sickness*.

Morgagni d., SYN Adams-Stokes *syndrome*.

Morquio d., SYN Morquio *syndrome*.

Morquio-Ullrich d., SYN Morquio *syndrome*.

Morvan d., SYN syringomyelia.

motor neuron d. (MND), a general term including progressive spinal muscular atrophy (infantile, juvenile, and adult), amyotrophic lateral sclerosis, progressive bulbar paralysis, and primary lateral sclerosis; frequently a familial d. SYN motor system d.

motor system d., SYN motor neuron d.

mountain d., a term that can mean acute altitude sickness; also used for chronic disease characterized by low oxygen saturation of hemoglobin, due to low partial pressure of oxygen in inspired air plus alveolar hypoventilation that develops in some individuals, especially older people. Polycythemia leads to florid skin color but cyanosis appears on mild exertion, along with dyspnea, fatigue, headache, and mental torpor. A person so afflicted returns to normal shortly after return to lower altitude.

moyamoya d., a cerebrovascular disorder occurring predominantly in the Japanese, in which the vessels of the base of the brain become occluded and revascularized with a fine network of vessels; it occurs commonly in young children and is manifested by convulsions, hemiplegia, mental retardation, and subarachnoid hemorrhage; the diagnosis is made by the angiographic picture. [Jap. addlebrained]

Mucha-Habermann d., SYN *pityriasis* lichenoides et varioliformis acuta.

multicore d., nonprogressive congenital myopathy characterized by weakness of proximal muscles, multifocal degeneration of the muscle fibers, and eccentric areas of decreased or absent oxidative enzyme activity in muscles.

Neumann d., SYN *pemphigus* vegetans (1).

neutral lipid storage d., SYN Dorfman-Chanarin *syndrome*.

Newcastle d., an acute febrile, and contagious d. of fowls resembling fowl plague, caused by a Paramyxovirus (Newcastle d. virus) and characterized by high infectivity and respiratory and nervous symptoms; it is readily transmissible to humans, in whom it causes a severe but transient conjunctivitis. SYN Ranikhet d. [*Newcastle*–upon–Tyne, England, where first reported]

Nicolas-Favre d., SYN venereal *lymphogranuloma*.

Niemann d., SYN Niemann-Pick d.

Niemann-Pick d. [MIM*257200], lipidosis with accumulation of sphingomyelin in histiocytes in the liver, spleen, lymph nodes, and bone marrow due to a deficiency of sphingomyelinase; associated with hepatosplenomegaly, physical, and mental retardation and neurologic manifestations; macular cherry-red spots may occur at a later stage; occurs most commonly in Ashkenazi Jewish infants and leads to early death; a more benign form may occur in adults. There are several variants: Type A, the classic infantile form; Type B, the visceral form; Type C, the juvenile form; Type

D, the Nova Scotia variant; and Type E, the adult form; all are of autosomal recessive inheritance with Types A and B caused by mutation in the acid sphingomyelinase gene (SMPD) on chromosome 11p. SYN Niemann d., sphingomyelin lipidosis.

Niemann-Pick C1 d. [MIM*257220], a rare inherited lipid storage disorder, affecting viscera and central nervous system, inherited as an autosomal recessive. There are two types of disease, with same clinical manifestations and biochemical abnormalities, resulting from abnormalities in two separate genes, NPC-1, the major locus, and NPC-2, the minor locus; then two types have identical clinical and biochemical phenotypes. Cells from NPC patients are defective in the esterification and release of cholesterol from lysosomes; lysosomal sequestration of LDL-derived cholesterol, including delayed down-regulation of LDL uptake and de novo synthesis occur.

nil d., SYN lipoid *nephrosis.*

nodular d., esophagostomiasis in herbivores and primates, characterized by nodules in the wall of the large intestine, cecum, and occasionally, the ileum; the nodules are filled with caseous material and result from host response to encystment of the larvae of *Oesophagostomum* species.

Norrie d. [MIM*310600], congenital bilateral masses of tissue arising from the retina or vitreous and resembling glioma (pseudoglioma), usually with atrophy of iris and development of cataract; associated mental retardation and deafness; X-linked recessive inheritance, caused by mutation in the Norrie disease gene (NDP) on Xp.

notifiable d., a d. that, by statutory requirements, must be reported to the public health or veterinary authorities when the diagnosis is made because of its importance to human or animal health. SYN reportable d.

oasthouse urine d. [MIM*250900], an autosomal recessively inherited metabolic defect in the absorption of methionine which is converted by intestinal bacteria to α-hydroxybutyric acid; characterized by diarrhea, tachypnea, and marked urinary excretion of α-hydroxybutyric acid (causing an odor like that of an oasthouse). [*oast,* kiln for drying hops, malt, or tobacco]

occupational d., a morbid condition resulting from exposure to an agent during the usual performance of one's occupation. Cf. industrial d.

Ofuji d., SYN eosinophilic pustular *folliculitis.*

Oguchi d. [MIM*258100], a rare congenital nonprogressive night blindness with diffuse yellow or gray coloration of fundus; after 2 or 3 hours in total darkness, fundus resumes normal color; autosomal recessive inheritance, caused by mutation in either the arrestin gene (SAG) on 2q or the rhodopsin kinase gene (RHOK) on 13q.

Ollier d., SYN enchondromatosis.

Oppenheim d., SYN *amyotonia* congenita.

organic d., a d. in which there are anatomic or pathophysiologic changes in some bodily tissue or organ, in contrast to a functional disorder; particularly one of psychogenic origin.

Ormond d., SYN retroperitoneal *fibrosis.*

orphan d., a d. for which no treatment has been developed because of its rarity (affecting no more than 200,000 persons in the U.S.). SEE ALSO orphan *products,* under *product.*

Osgood-Schlatter d., inflammation of the growth center (apophysis) that forms the tibial tubercle. SYN apophysitis tibialis adolescentium, Schlatter d., Schlatter-Osgood d.

Osler d., SYN *polycythemia* vera.

Osler-Vaquez d., SYN *polycythemia* vera.

Otto d., a d. characterized by an inward bulging of the acetabulum into the pelvic cavity, resulting in protrusion of the femoral head; found in association with arthritis of the hip joints, usually rheumatoid arthritis. SYN Otto pelvis, protrusio acetabuli.

Owren d. [MIM*227400], a congenital deficiency of factor V, resulting in prolongation of prothrombin time; bleeding and clotting times are consistently prolonged; autosomal recessive inheritance caused by mutation in the F5 gene on chromosome 1q.

Paas d., a familial skeletal deformation marked by coxa valga, double patella, shortening of the middle and terminal phalanges of fingers and toes, deformities of the elbows, scoliosis, and spondy-

litis deformans of the lumbar vertebrae; all these manifestations may be unilateral or bilateral.

Paget d., (1) a generalized skeletal disease, frequently familial, of older persons in which bone resorption and formation are both increased, leading to thickening and softening of bones (e.g., the skull), and bending of weight-bearing bones; SYN osteitis deformans. **(2)** a d. of elderly women, characterized by an infiltrated, somewhat eczematous lesion surrounding and involving the nipple and areola, and associated with subjacent intraductal cancer of the breast and infiltration of the lower epidermis by malignant cells; **(3)** SYN extramammary Paget d.

Panner d., epiphysial osteonecrosis of the capitellum of the humerus. SYN little league elbow.

paper mill worker's d., extrinsic allergic alveolitis caused by moldy wood pulp containing spores of *Alternaria* fungi.

parasitic d., a d. due to the presence and vital activity of a parasite, or as a reaction to a parasite.

Parkinson d., SYN parkinsonism (1).

Parrot d., (1) pseudoparalysis in infants, due to syphilitic osteochondritis; **(2)** SYN marasmus; **(3)** SYN psittacosis.

Parry d., SYN Graves d.

Pavy d., cyclic or recurrent physiologic albuminuria.

pearl-worker's d., inflammatory hypertrophy of the bones affecting grinders of mother-of-pearl.

Pel-Ebstein d., SYN Pel-Ebstein *fever.*

Pelizaeus-Merzbacher d. [MIM*311601, *312080, *260600], a sudanophilic leukodystrophy with a tigroid appearance of the myelin resulting from patchy demyelination. Type 1, classic, nystagmus and tremor appearing in the first few months of life, followed by slow motor development sometimes with choreoathetosis, spasticity, optic atrophy and seizures, with death in early adulthood, X-linked recessive inheritance caused by mutation in the proteolipid protein gene (PLP) on Xq; there is an autosomal recessive form as well; type 2, contralateral form with death in months to years after birth, X-linked recessive inheritance; type 3, transitional, with death in the first decade; type 4, adult form associated with involuntary movements, ataxia and hyperreflexia, but without nystagmus; autosomal dominant inheritance [MIM*169500]; type 5, variant forms. Cockayne is sometimes included as a sixth form. SYN Merzbacher-Pelizaeus d.

Pellegrini d., a calcific density in the medial collateral ligament and/or bony growth on the medial aspect of the medial condyle of the femur. SYN Pellegrini-Stieda d.

Pellegrini-Stieda d., SYN Pellegrini d.

pelvic inflammatory d. (PID), acute or chronic suppurative inflammation of female pelvic structures (endometrium, uterine tubes, pelvic peritoneum) due to infection by *Neisseria gonorrhoeae*, *Chlamydia trachomatis*, or other organisms, typically a complication of sexually transmitted infection of the lower genital tract, may be precipitated by menstruation, parturition, or surgical procedures including abortion; complications include tubo-ovarian abscess, tubal stenosis with resulting infertility or sterility and heightened risk of ectopic pregnancy, and peritoneal adhesions.

periodic d., any condition or d. in which episodes tend to recur at regular intervals; many such cases are manifestations of familial Mediterranean fever; the cause of the periodicity is usually unknown.

Perthes d., SYN Legg-Calvé-Perthes d.

Pette-Döring d., SYN nodular *panencephalitis.*

Peyronie d., a d. in which plaques or strands of dense fibrous tissue surrounding the corpus cavernosum of the penis cause penile bending and pain on erection; sometimes associated with Dupuytren contracture. SYN penile fibromatosis, van Buren d.

Pick d., progressive circumscribed cerebral atrophy; a rare type of cerebrodegenerative disorder manifested primarily as dementia, in which there is striking atrophy of portions of the frontal and temporal lobes. SYN Pick syndrome. [F. Pick]

pink d., SYN acrodynia (2).

Plummer d., eponym sometimes applied to hyperthyroidism resulting from a nodular toxic goiter, usually not accompanied by exophthalmos.

polycystic d. of kidneys, SYN polycystic *kidney.*

di

polycystic liver d., SYN polycystic *liver*.

Pompe d., SYN type 2 *glycogenosis*.

Portuguese-Azorean d., SYN Machado-Joseph d.

Posadas d., SYN coccidioidomycosis.

posttransplant lymphoproliferative d., a complication of organ transplantation in children; characterized by a mononucleosislike syndrome, tonsillar enlargement, and Epstein-Barr virus seroconversion.

Pott d., SYN tuberculous *spondylitis*.

Potter d., SYN Potter *facies*.

poultry handler's d., extrinsic allergic alveolitis similar to birdbreeder's lung, caused by inhalation of particulate emanations from domesticated fowl such as chickens and turkeys.

primary d., a d. that arises spontaneously and is not associated with or caused by a previous disease, injury, or event, but which may lead to a secondary d.

Pringle d., SYN *adenoma* sebaceum.

pseudo-Hurler d., SYN infantile, generalized G_{M1} *gangliosidosis*.

pulseless d., SYN Takayasu *arteritis*.

Purtscher d., SYN Purtscher *retinopathy*.

quiet hip d., SYN Legg-Calvé-Perthes d.

ragpicker's d., SYN pulmonary *anthrax*.

ragsorter's d., SYN pulmonary *anthrax*.

Ranikhet d., SYN Newcastle d. [Ranikhet, town in northern India]

rat-bite d., SYN rat-bite *fever*.

Rayer d., SYN biliary *xanthomatosis*.

Raynaud d., SYN Raynaud *syndrome*.

reactive airway d., SYN asthma.

Recklinghausen d. of bone, SYN *osteitis* fibrosa cystica.

Refsum d. [MIM*266500], a rare degenerative disorder due to a deficiency of phytanic acid α-hydroxylase; clinically characterized by retinitis pigmentosa, ichthyosis, demyelinating polyneuropathy, deafness, and cerebellar signs; autosomal recessive inheritance caused by mutation in the gene encoding phytanoyl-CoA hydroxylase (PAHX or PAYH) on chromosome 10p. Infantile Refsum d. [MIM*266510] is an impaired peroxisomal function with accumulation of phytanic acid, pipecolic acid; autosomal recessive inheritance, caused by mutation in the PEX 1 gene on 7q. SYN heredopathia atactica polyneuritiformis, Refsum syndrome.

Reiter d., SYN Reiter *syndrome*.

reportable d., SYN notifiable d.

rhesus d., sensitization of the mother during pregnancy to Rh factor in fetal blood, leading to erythroblastosis fetalis.

rheumatic d., SEE rheumatism.

rheumatic heart d., d. of the heart resulting from rheumatic fever, chiefly manifested by abnormalities of the valves.

rheumatoid d., rheumatoid *arthritis*, referring particularly to nonarticular lesions such as subcutaneous nodules.

Ribas-Torres d., a mild form of smallpox. SEE ALSO *variola* minor.

rice d., beriberi, the original outbreaks of which were caused by feeding people rice from which the husks had been removed (polished rice), decreasing the vitamin B_1 content of the rice.

Riedel d., SYN Riedel *thyroiditis*.

Riga-Fede d., ulceration of the lingual frenum in teething infants, related to abrasion of the tissue against the new central incisors.

Roger d., a congenital cardiac anomaly consisting of a small, isolated, asymptomatic defect of the interventricular septum, often with a loud murmur and definite thrill. SYN maladie de Roger.

Rokitansky d., (1) SYN acute massive liver *necrosis*; (2) SYN Chiari *syndrome*.

Romberg d., SYN facial *hemiatrophy*.

Rosai-Dorfman d., SYN sinus *histiocytosis* with massive lymphadenopathy.

Rougnon-Heberden d., SYN *angina* pectoris.

Roussy-Lévy d. [MIM*180800], dominantly inherited disorder consisting of a motor-sensory demyelinating polyneuropathy and a coexisting essential tremor. SYN Roussy-Lévy syndrome.

runt d., a graft versus host reaction in mice first observed following intravenous injection of allogeneic spleen cells into newborn animals. SYN wasting d.

salivary gland d., disorder of salivary glands; i.e., Sjögren *syndrome*.

salivary gland virus d., SEE cytomegalic inclusion d.

Salla d. (sal'ya), an autosomal recessive disorder in which there is a defect in the transport of free sialic acid across lysosomal membranes.

Sandhoff d. [MIM*268800], an infantile form of G_{M2} gangliosidosis characterized by a defect in the production of hexosaminidases A and B; it resembles Tay-Sachs disease, but occurs predominantly (if not entirely) in non-Jewish children; accumulation of glucoside and ganglioside G_{m2}, caused by mutation in hexoaminidase B gene (HEX B) on chromosome 5q.

sandworm d., an inflammatory eruption on the inner side of the sole, observed in certain parts of Australia, marked by a patch of erythema spreading in spirals, and disappearing spontaneously; probably a form of creeping eruption similar to larva migrans.

San Joaquin Valley d., SYN primary *coccidioidomycosis*.

Schenck d., SYN sporotrichosis.

Scheuermann d., epiphysial osteonecrosis of adjacent vertebral bodies in the thoracic spine. SYN adolescent round back, juvenile kyphosis, osteochondritis deformans juvenilis dorsi.

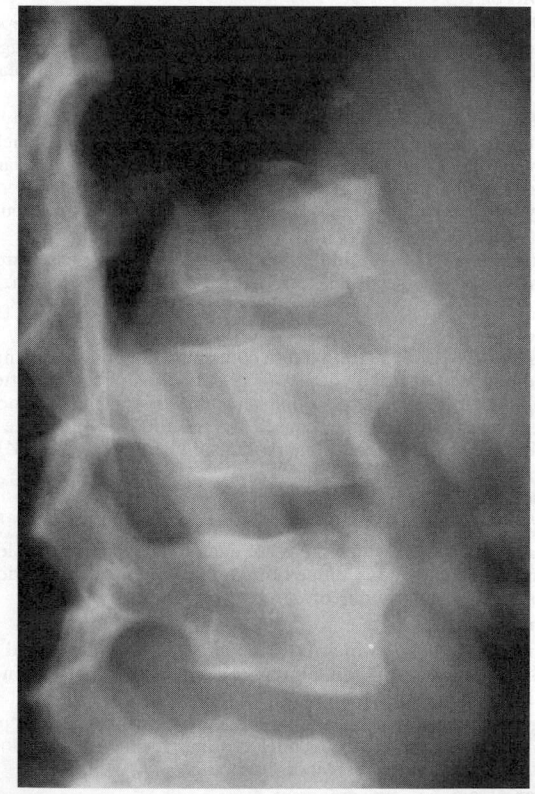

Scheuermann disease: avascular necrosis of apophyseal rings of vertebral bodies is called Scheuermann disease; it is most commonly seen without kyphosis or pain and with few vertebral bodies involved

Schilder d., term used to describe at least two separate disorders described by Schilder: 1) Diffuse sclerosis or encephalitis periaxialis diffusa; a nonfamilial disorder affecting primarily children and young adults and characterized by progressive dementia, visual disturbances, deafness, pseudobulbar palsy, and hemiplegia or quadriplegia. Most patients die within a few years of onset; pathologically, there is a large, asymmetric area of myelin destruction, sometimes involving an entire cerebral hemisphere, and typically with extension across the corpus callosum. 2) The leukodystrophies. SYN encephalitis periaxialis diffusa.

Schindler d. (shind′ler), an autosomal recessive disorder with deficient activity of α-*N*-acetylgalactosaminidase resulting in accumulation of glycoproteins and other substrates that are deposited in terminal axons, primarily in gray matter.

Schlatter d., Schlatter-Osgood d., SYN Osgood-Schlatter d.

Scholz d., former eponym for the juvenile form of metachromatic leukodystrophy.

Schüller d., SYN Hand-Schüller-Christian d.

Schwartz-Jampel d., SYN myotonic *chondrodystrophy*.

sclerocystic d. of the ovary, SYN polycystic ovary *syndrome*.

sea-blue histiocyte d. [MIM*269600], splenomegaly and mild thrombocytopenia, with histiocytes in the bone marrow which contain cytoplasmic granules that stain bright blue; sometimes familial; perhaps a lipidosis; autosomal recessive inheritance.

secondary d., (1) a d. that follows and results from an earlier disease, injury, or event; **(2)** a wasting disorder that follows successful transplantation of bone marrow into a lethally irradiated host; frequently severe and usually associated with fever, anorexia, diarrhea, dermatitis, and desquamation. SEE ALSO graft versus host d.

self-limited d., a d. process that resolves spontaneously with or without specific treatment.

Senear-Usher d., SYN *pemphigus* erythematosus.

serum d., SYN serum *sickness*.

Sever d., an osteochondrosis of the heel, probably secondary to microfractures in the bone where the Achilles tendon attaches to the posterior calcaneus; an overuse injury and a common cause of heel pain in older children. SYN calcaneal apophysitis.

sexually transmitted d. (STD), SEE venereal disease.

Shaver d., SYN bauxite *pneumoconiosis*.

shimamushi d., SYN tsutsugamushi d.

sickle cell d., SYN sickle cell *anemia*.

sickle cell C d. [MIM*141900], a d. resulting from abnormal sickle-shaped erythrocytes (containing hemoglobins C and S) which appear in response to a lowering of the partial pressure of oxygen; characterized by anemia, crises due to hemolysis or vascular occlusion, chronic leg ulcers and bone deformities, and infarcts of bone or of the spleen.

sickle cell-thalassemia d., d. clinically resembling sickle cell d., in which individuals are compound heterozygous for the sickle cell gene and a thalassemia gene; about 60–80% of hemoglobin is Hb S, up to 20% Hb F, and the remainder Hb A. SYN microdrepanocytic anemia.

silo-filler′s d., a pulmonary lesion produced by oxides of nitrogen due to fresh silage; in its acute form it may lead to death from pulmonary edema or may go on to a subacute or chronic proliferative pulmonary disease sometimes leading to chronic pulmonary invalidism.

Simmonds d., SYN Sheehan *syndrome*.

Simons d., SYN progressive *lipodystrophy*.

sixth d., SYN *exanthema* subitum.

Sjögren d., SYN Sjögren *syndrome*.

skinbound d., scleroderma (usually applied to extensive involvement).

slow virus d., a d. that follows a slow, progressive course spanning months to years, frequently involving the central nervous system and ultimately leading to death; examples are visna and maedi of sheep, caused by viruses of the genus Lentivirus (family Retroviridae), and subacute sclerosing panencephalitis, apparently caused by the measles virus. Spongiform encephalopathies, including kuru of humans, scrapie of sheep, and transmissible encephalopathy of mink may also be classified under slow virus d. but are now considered to be prion diseases.

Sneddon-Wilkinson d., SYN subcorneal pustular *dermatosis*.

specific d., a d. produced by the action of a special pathogenic microorganism.

Spielmeyer-Sjögren d., cerebral *sphingolipidosis*, late juvenile type.

Spielmeyer-Stock d., retinal atrophy in amaurotic familial idiocy.

Spielmeyer-Vogt d., cerebral *sphingolipidosis*, late juvenile type. SYN Vogt-Spielmeyer d.

stable d., in oncology, less than 25% increase or less than 50% decrease in the size of all tumors.

Stargardt d. [MIM*248200], fundus flavimaculatus initiated with atrophic macular lesions, caused by mutationin the ATP-binding cassette transporter, retina-specific gene (ABCR) on 1p.

startle d., SYN hyperekplexia.

Steele-Richardson-Olszewski d., SYN progressive supranuclear *palsy*.

Steinert d., SYN myotonic *dystrophy*.

Still d., a form of juvenile chronic arthritis (formerly called juvenile rheumatoid arthritis) characterized by high fever and signs of systemic illness that can exist for weeks or months before the onset of arthritis.

Stokes-Adams d., SYN Adams-Stokes *syndrome*.

stone-mason′s d., SYN silicosis.

storage d., a generic term that includes any accumulation of a specific substance within tissues, generally because of congenital deficiency of an enzyme necessary for further metabolism of the substance; e.g., glycogen-storage d.'s.

Strümpell d., (1) SYN *spondylitis* deformans; **(2)** SYN acute epidemic *leukoencephalitis*.

Strümpell-Marie d., SYN ankylosing *spondylitis*.

Sturge-Weber d., SYN Sturge-Weber *syndrome*.

Sulzberger-Garbe d., SYN exudative discoid and lichenoid *dermatitis*.

Sutton d., SYN *aphthae* major, under *aphtha*; [R. L. Sutton, Jr.]

Sweet d., SYN acute febrile neutrophilic *dermatosis*.

swineherd′s d., a leptospirosis caused by a leptospira occurring in those who attend swine or who are occupied in the slaughtering or processing of pork, and characterized by aches and pains throughout the body, fever, headache, dizziness, and nausea.

swine vesicular d., a contagious disease of swine caused by a porcine enterovirus of the family Picornaviridae, closely related to the human enterovirus Coxsackie B-5, and characterized by vesicular lesions and erosions of the epithelium of the mouth, nares, snout, and feet; human infections have been reported in laboratory workers.

swollen belly d., a fatal d. of infants infected with *Strongyloides fuelleborni* subsp. *kellyi*; appears in localized areas of New Guinea. SYN swollen belly syndrome.

Sydenham d., SYN Sydenham *chorea*.

Sylvest d., SYN epidemic *pleurodynia*.

systemic autoimmune d.'s, a group of connective tissue d.'s characterized by the presence of autoantibodies responsible for immunopathologically mediated tissue lesions; systemic lupus erythematosus is the prototype.

systemic febrile d.'s, generic term for diseases characterized by fever.

Takahara d., SYN acatalasia.

Takayasu d., SYN Takayasu *arteritis*.

Tangier d., SYN analphalipoproteinemia. [an island in the Chesapeake Bay, home of the family of first cases described]

Taussig-Bing d., SYN Taussig-Bing *syndrome*.

Taylor d., diffuse idiopathic cutaneous atrophy.

Tay-Sachs d., a lysosomal storage disease, resulting from hexosaminidase A deficiency. The monosialoganglioside is stored in central and peripheral neuronal cells. Infants present with hyperacusis and irritability, hypotonia, and failure to develop motor skills. Blindness with macular cherry red spots and seizures are evident in the first year. Death occurs within a few years. Autosomal-recessive transmission; found primarily in Jewish populations. SYN infantile G_{M2} gangliosidosis.

Thiemann d., SYN Thiemann *syndrome*.

third d., SYN rubella.

Thomsen d., SYN *myotonia* congenita.

Thygeson d., SYN superficial punctate *keratitis*.

thyrocardiac d., heart d. resulting from hyperthyroidism.

thyrotoxic heart d., cardiac symptoms, signs, and physiologic

di

impairment due to overactivity of the thyroid gland usually due to excessive sympathetic stimulation.

Tommaselli d., hemoglobinuria and pyrexia due to quinine intoxication.

Tornwaldt d., SYN Tornwaldt *cyst.*

torsion d. of childhood, SYN *dystonia* musculorum deformans.

Tourette d., SYN Tourette *syndrome.*

Trevor d., SYN tarsoepiphyseal *aclasis.*

tropical d.'s, infectious and parasitic d.'s endemic in tropical and subtropical zones, including Chagas disease, leishmaniasis, leprosy, malaria, onchocerciasis, schistosomiasis, sleeping sickness, yellow fever, and others; often water- or insect-borne. SEE ALSO emerging *viruses,* under *virus.*

tsutsugamushi d., an acute infectious disease, caused by *Rickettsia tsutsugamushi* and transmitted by *Trombicula akamushi* and *T. deliensis,* that occurs in harvesters of hemp in some parts of Japan; characterized by fever, painful swelling of the lymphatic glands, a small blackish scab on the genitals, neck, or axilla, and an eruption of large dark red papules. SYN akamushi d., flood fever, inundation fever, island d., island fever, Japanese river fever, kedani fever, mite typhus, scrub typhus, shimamushi d., tropical typhus, tsutsugamushi fever.

tunnel d., SYN ancylostomiasis.

Unna d., SYN seborrheic *dermatitis.*

Unverricht d. [MIM*254800], a progressive myoclonic epilepsy; one of the degenerative gray matter disorders characterized by myoclonus and generalized seizures, with progressive neurologic and intellectual decline; age of onset between 8–13 years of age; autosomal recessive inheritance, caused by mutation in the cystatin B gene (CSTB) on 21q22.

Urbach-Wiethe d., SYN lipoid *proteinosis.*

vagabond's d., SYN parasitic *melanoderma.*

vagrant's d., SYN parasitic *melanoderma.*

van Buren d., SYN Peyronie d.

Vaquez d., SYN *polycythemia* vera.

venereal d., any contagious d. acquired during sexual contact; e.g., syphilis, gonorrhea, chancroid.

venoocclusive d. of the liver, obliterating endophlebitis of small hepatic vein radicles, described in Jamaican children, associated with ingestion of toxic plant substances in bush tea; causes ascites, which may progress to cirrhosis.

Vincent d., SYN necrotizing ulcerative *gingivitis.*

Virchow d., SYN megacephaly.

virus X d., an old term applied to a number of virus d.'s of obscure etiology, e.g., Australian X d. (Murray Valley encephalitis).

Vogt-Spielmeyer d., SYN Spielmeyer-Vogt d.

Voltolini d., infectious d. of the labyrinth, leading to meningitis in young children.

von Economo d., a unique encephalitis, presumably viral in origin, which followed the influenza pandemic of 1914–1918. Symptoms included ophthalmoplegia and marked somnolence, and in many survivors, the delayed development of Parkinson disease; the basis for postencephalitic Parkinsonism. SYN encephalitis lethargica, polioencephalitis infectiva.

von Gierke d., SYN type 1 *glycogenosis.*

von Recklinghausen d., type 1 neurofibromatosis. SEE neurofibromatosis.

von Willebrand d. [MIM*193400], a hemorrhagic diathesis characterized by tendency to bleed primarily from mucous membranes, prolonged bleeding time, normal platelet count, normal clot retraction, partial and variable deficiency of factor VIIIR, and possibly a morphologic defect of platelets; autosomal dominant inheritance with reduced penetrance and variable expressivity, caused by mutation in the von Willebrand factor gene (VWF) on 12p. Type III von Willebrand d. is a more severe disorder with markedly reduced factor VIIIR levels. There is a recessive version of this disease [MIM*277480] which has the remarkable property that it represents a mutation at the same locus as the dominant form.

Voorhoeve d., SYN *osteopathia* striata.

Wagner d., SYN hyaloideoretinal *degeneration.*

wasting d., SYN runt d.

Weber-Christian d., term used for cases of relapsing febrile nodular nonsuppurative *panniculitis* (q.v.) of undetermined cause. SYN relapsing febrile nodular nonsuppurative *panniculitis.*

Wegner d., SYN syphilitic *osteochondritis.*

Weil d., a form of leptospirosis generally caused by *Leptospira interrogans* serogroup *icterohaemorrhagiae,* believed to be acquired by contact with the urine of infected rats; characterized clinically by fever, jaundice, muscular pains, conjunctival congestion, and albuminuria; agglutinins regularly appear in the serum. SYN infectious icterus, infectious jaundice (1).

Werdnig-Hoffmann d., SYN spinal muscular *atrophy,* type I.

Werlhof d., formerly used term for idiopathic thrombocytopenic *purpura.*

Wernicke d., SYN Wernicke *syndrome.*

Werther d., SYN *dermatitis* nodularis necrotica.

Wesselsbron d., SYN Wesselsbron *fever.*

Whipple d., a rare d. characterized by steatorrhea, frequently generalized lymphadenopathy, arthritis, fever, and cough; many "foamy" macrophages are found in the jejunal lamina propria; caused by *Tropheryma whippleii.*

white spot d., SYN *morphea* guttata.

Whitmore d., SYN melioidosis.

Wilkie d., SYN superior mesenteric artery *syndrome.*

Wilson d. [MIM*277900], **(1)** a disorder of copper metabolism, characterized by liver cirrhosis, basal ganglia degeneration, neurological manifestations, and deposition of green or golden brown pigment in the periphery of the cornea; the plasma levels of copper and ceruloplasmin are decreased, urinary excretion of copper is increased, and the amounts of copper in the liver, brain, kidneys, and lenticular nucleus are unusually high while cytochrome oxidase is reduced; autosomal recessive inheritance caused by mutation in the copper-transporting ATPase gene (ATP7B) on chromosome 13q. SYN hepatolenticular degeneration. SEE ALSO Kayser-Fleischer *ring;* [S.A.K. Wilson] **(2)** SYN exfoliative *dermatitis.*

Winiwarter-Buerger d., SYN *thromboangiitis* obliterans.

Wohlfart-Kugelberg-Welander d., SYN spinal muscular *atrophy,* type III.

Wolman d., SYN cholesterol ester storage d.

woolsorter's d., SYN pulmonary *anthrax.*

Woringer-Kolopp d., SYN pagetoid *reticulosis.*

X d., one of several viral d.'s of obscure etiology.

X-linked lymphoproliferative d., SYN X-linked lymphoproliferative *syndrome.*

yellow d., SYN xanthochromia.

Ziehen-Oppenheim d., SYN *dystonia* musculorum deformans.

---

dis·en·gage·ment (dis-en-gāj′ment). **1.** The act of setting free or extricating; in childbirth, the emergence of the head from the vulva. **2.** Ascent of the presenting part from the pelvis after the inlet has been negotiated. [Fr.]

dis·e·qui·lib·ri·um (dis-ē′kwi-lib′rē-ŭm). A disturbance or absence of equilibrium.

genetic d., a state in the genetic composition of a population which under selection may be expected to change toward an equilibrium or absorbing state.

linkage d., a state involving two loci in which the probability of a joint gamete is not equal to the product of the probabilities of the constituent genes. The difference between these quantities is the increase of the d.; there are many causes of the d.

dis·flu·en·cy (dis-floo′en-sē). Inability to produce a smooth flow of speech sounds in connected discourse; the flow of speech is characterized by frequent interruptions and repetitions. [dis- + fluency]

dis·flu·ent (dis-floo′ent). Relating to disfluency.

dis·ger·mi·no·ma (dis-jer-mi-nō′mă). SYN dysgerminoma.

DISH Abbreviation for diffuse idiopathic skeletal *hyperostosis.*

dish. A shallow container, usually concave.

Petri d., a small, shallow, circular d. made of thin glass or clear plastic with a loosely fitting, overlapping cover used especially in microbiology for the cultivation of microorganisms on solid media; it is frequently referred to as a plate.

Stender d., a flat shallow vessel used in staining sections.

dis·har·mo·ny (dis-har′mŏ-nē). **1.** The state of being deranged or lacking in orderliness. **2.** In a complex sound, the absence of a mathematical relationship among the frequencies of the fundamental tone and its overtones so that the frequencies of the overtones are not whole-number multiples or partials of the frequency of the fundamental tone. The auditory effect has a noisy or unpleasant quality, as opposed to music.

occlusal d., (1) contacts of opposing occlusal surfaces of teeth which are not in harmony with other tooth contacts and with the anatomic and physiologic control of the mandible; (2) occlusions which do not coincide with their respective jaw relations. SEE ALSO deflective occlusal *contact.*

DISIDA Abbreviation for diisopropyl iminodiacetic acid or disofenin.

dis·im·pac·tion (dis′im-pak′shŭn). **1.** Separation of impaction in a fractured bone. **2.** Removal of feces, usually manually, in fecal impaction.

dis·in·fect (dis-in-fekt′). To destroy pathogenic microorganisms in or on any substance or to inhibit their growth and vital activity.

dis·in·fec·tant (dis-in-fek′tănt). **1.** Capable of destroying pathogenic microorganisms or inhibiting their growth activity. **2.** An agent that possesses this property.

complete d., a d. that kills both vegetative forms and spores.

incomplete d., a d. that kills only the vegetative forms, leaving the spores uninjured.

dis·in·fec·tion (dis-in-fek′shŭn). Destruction of pathogenic microorganisms or their toxins or vectors by direct exposure to chemical or physical agents.

concurrent d., application of disinfective measures as soon as possible after discharge of infectious material from the body of an infected person, or after soiling of articles with such infectious discharges.

terminal d., application of disinfective measures after the patient has been removed, e.g., by death, or has ceased to be a source of infection.

dis·in·fes·ta·tion. Physical or chemical process to destroy or remove small undesirable animal forms, particularly arthropods or rodents, present upon the person, clothing, or environment of an individual or domestic animals.

dis·in·hi·bi·tion (dis′in-hi-bish′ŭn). **1.** Removal of an inhibition, such as by a toxic or organic process. **2.** Removal of an inhibitory effect by a stimulus, as when a conditioned reflex has undergone extinction but is restored by some extraneous stimulus.

dis·in·sec·tion, dis·in·sec·ti·za·tion (dis-in-sek′shŭn, dis′in-sek-ti-zā′shŭn). Freeing an area from insects. [L. *dis-,* apart, + insect]

dis·in·te·gra·tion (dis-in-tĕ-grā′shŭn). **1.** Loss or separation of the component parts of a substance, as in catabolism or decay. **2.** Disorganization of psychic and behavioral processes. [dis- + L. *integer,* whole, intact]

dis·in·vag·i·na·tion (dis′in-vaj-i-nā′shŭn). Relieving an invagination.

dis·junc·tion (dis-jŭnk′shŭn). The normal separation of pairs of chromosomes at the anaphase stage of meiosis I or II. [dis- + L. *junctio,* a joining, fr. *jungo,* pp. *junctum,* to join]

disk [TA]. **1.** A round, flat plate; any approximately flat circular structure. **2.** SYN lamella (2). **3.** In dentistry, a circular piece of thin paper or other material, coated with an abrasive substance, used for cutting and polishing teeth and fillings. [L. *discus;* G. *diskos,* a quoit, disk]

A d.'s, SYN A *bands,* under *band.*

acromioclavicular d., SYN articular d. of acromioclavicular joint.

Airy d., the image of a circular blur formed by a distant point source of light on the retina because of diffraction by the edge of the pupillary aperture where the diameter of the image decreases as the aperture increases.

anisotropic d.'s, SYN A *bands,* under *band.*

articular d. [TA], a plate or ring of fibrocartilage attached to the joint capsule and separating the articular surfaces of the bones for a varying distance, sometimes completely; it serves to adapt two articular surfaces that are not entirely congruent. SYN discus articularis [TA], fibrocartilago interarticularis, fibroplate, interarticular fibrocartilage, intraarticular cartilage (1).

articular d. of acromioclavicular joint [TA], the articular disk of fibrocartilage usually found between the acromial end of the clavicle and the medial border of the acromion. SYN discus articularis acromioclavicularis [TA], acromioclavicular d., Weitbrecht cartilage.

articular d. of distal radioulnar joint [TA], the disk that holds together the distal ends of the radius and ulna; it is attached by its apex to a depression between the styloid process and distal surface of the head of the ulna, and by its base to the ridge separating the ulnar notch from the carpal surface of the radius. SYN discus articularis radioulnaris distalis [TA], radioulnar d., radioulnar articular d., triangular cartilage, triangular d. of wrist, triquetrous cartilage (1).

articular d. of sternoclavicular joint [TA], the fibrocartilaginous disk that subdivides the sternoclavicular joint into two cavities. SYN discus articularis sternoclavicularis [TA], sternoclavicular d., sternoclavicular articular d.

articular d. of temporomandibular joint [TA], the fibrocartilaginous plate that separates the joint into upper and lower cavities. SYN discus articularis temporomandibularis [TA], mandibular d., temporomandibular articular d.

blastodermic d., the aggregation of blastomeres of a telolecithal ovum after cleavage has occurred.

blood d., SYN platelet.

Bowman d.'s, d.'s resulting from transverse segmentation of striated muscular fiber treated with weak acids, certain alkaline solutions, or freezing.

Burlew d., an abrasive-impregnated rubber wheel used in dentistry for polishing. SYN Burlew wheel.

choked d., SYN papilledema.

ciliary d., SYN orbiculus ciliaris.

cone d.'s, membranous d.'s of flattened sacs about 14 nm thick that occur in the outer segment of cones of the retina.

cuttlefish d., a circle of paper or thin plastic coated with ground cuttlefish bone; used, when attached to a mandrel and rotated by a dental handpiece, for fine smoothing and finishing of dental materials and tooth.

diamond d., a steel d. with the cutting surface(s) covered with fine diamond chips, for use in a dental handpiece.

embryonic d., SYN germinal d.

emery d.'s, d.'s of paper or other materials coated with emery powder used to abrade or smooth the surface of teeth or fillings.

germinal d., germ d., the point in a telolecithal ovum where the embryo begins to be formed. SYN embryonic d., germinal area, area germinativa.

H d., SYN H *band.*

hair d., a richly innervated area of skin around a hair follicle, consisting of a thickened layer of epithelial cells in which ramify unmyelinated terminals of a single axon.

Hensen d., SYN H *band.*

herniated d., protrusion of a degenerated or fragmented intervertebral d. into the intervertebral foramen with potential compression of a nerve root or into the spinal canal with potential compression of the cauda equina in the lumbar region or the spinal cord at higher levels. SYN protruded d., ruptured d.

I d., SYN I *band.*

intercalated d., a specialized intercellular attachment of cardiac muscle comprising gap junctions, fascia adherens, and occasionally desmosomes.

intermediate d., SYN Z line.

interpubic d., SYN interpubic *disk.*

intervertebral d., a disk interposed between the bodies of adjacent vertebrae. It is composed of an outer fibrous part (annulus fibrosus) that surrounds a central gelatinous mass (nucleus pulposus). SYN discus intervertebralis [TA], fibrocartilago intervertebralis, intervertebral cartilage.

di

isotropic d., SYN I *band*.

mandibular d., SYN articular d. of temporomandibular joint.

Merkel tactile d., SYN tactile *meniscus*.

Newton d., a d. on which are seven colored sectors, each occupying proportionally the same space as the corresponding primary color in the spectrum; when the disk is rapidly rotated it appears white.

optic d. [TA], an oval area of the ocular fundus devoid of light receptors where the axons of the retinal ganglion cell converge to form the optic nerve head; SYN discus nervi optici [TA], blind spot (3), Mariotte blind spot, optic nerve head, optic papilla, papilla nervi optici, porus opticus.

Placido da Costa d., SYN keratoscope.

proligerous d., SYN *cumulus* oöphorus.

protruded d., SYN herniated d.

Q d.'s, SYN A *bands*, under *band*.

radioulnar d., radioulnar articular d., SYN articular d. of distal radioulnar joint.

Ranvier d.'s, tactile nerve endings, of cupped disklike form, in the skin.

rod d.'s, membranous d.'s of flattened sacs about 14 nm thick that occur in the outer segment of rods of the retina.

ruptured d., SYN herniated d.

sacrococcygeal d., a thin plate of fibrocartilage interposed between the sacrum and coccyx.

sandpaper d.'s, d.'s of paper coated with various grits of silica; used to abrade or smooth the surface of teeth or dental materials.

stenopeic d., stenopaic d., a metallic or other opaque d. with a narrow slit through which one looks; used as a test for astigmatism.

sternoclavicular d., sternoclavicular articular d., SYN articular d. of sternoclavicular joint.

stroboscopic d., a revolving d. that gives successive views of a moving object.

tactile d., SYN tactile *meniscus*.

temporomandibular articular d., SYN articular d. of temporomandibular joint.

transverse d., one of the dark transverse bands seen on examining a striated muscular fiber under the microscope.

triangular d. of wrist, SYN articular d. of distal radioulnar joint.

Z d., SYN Z *line*.

dis·ki·tis (dis-kī'tis). SYN discitis.

disko-. SEE disco-.

dis·ko·gram (dis'kō-gram). The graphic record, usually radiographic, of diskography.

dis·kog·ra·phy (dis-kog'ră-fē). Historically, radiographic demonstration of intervertebral disk by injection of contrast media into the nucleus pulposus. [disco- + G. *graphō*, to write]

dis·lo·cate (dis'lō-kāt). To luxate; to put out of joint.

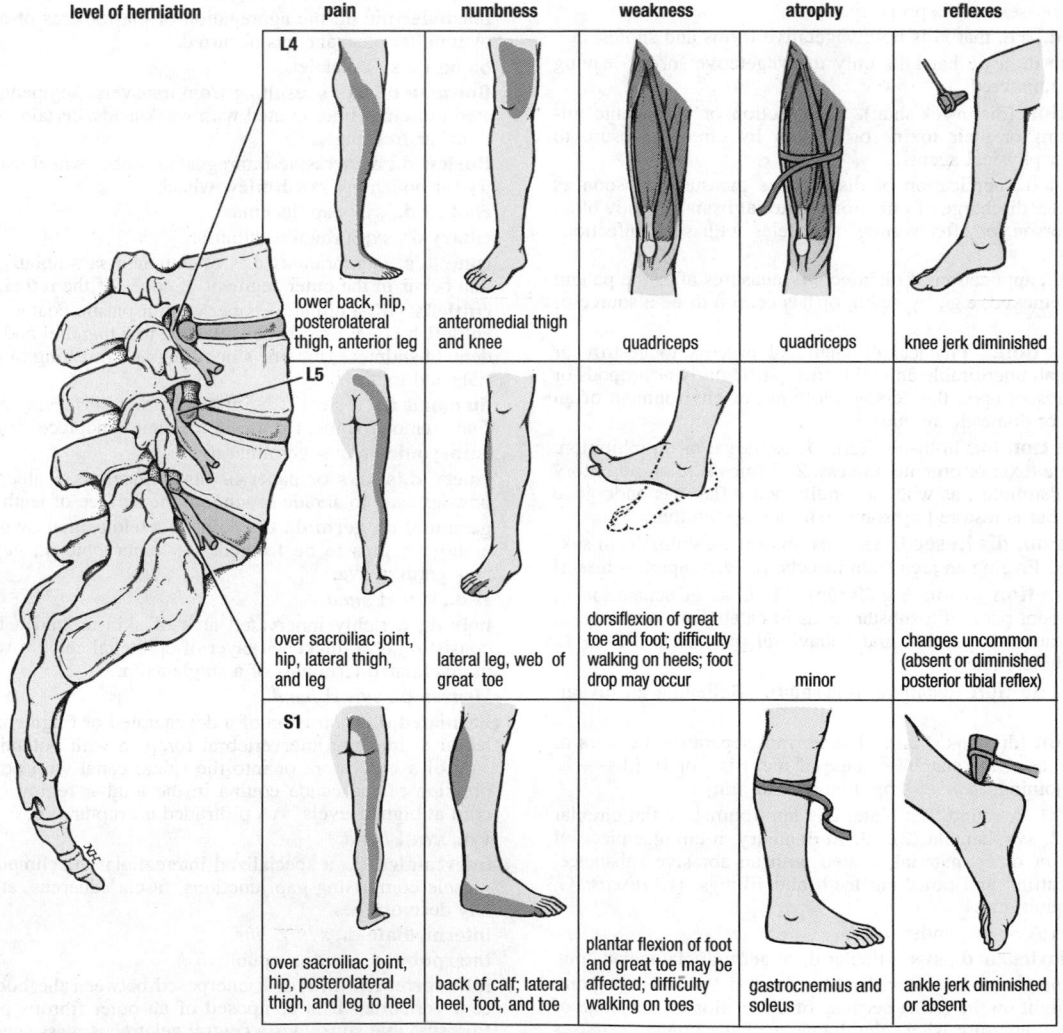

level of herniation	pain	numbness	weakness	atrophy	reflexes
L4	lower back, hip, posterolateral thigh, anterior leg	anteromedial thigh and knee	quadriceps	quadriceps	knee jerk diminished
L5	over sacroiliac joint, hip, lateral thigh, and leg	lateral leg, web of great toe	dorsiflexion of great toe and foot; difficulty walking on heels; foot drop may occur	minor	changes uncommon (absent or diminished posterior tibial reflex)
S1	over sacroiliac joint, hip, posterolateral thigh, and leg to heel	back of calf; lateral heel, foot, and toe	plantar flexion of foot and great toe may be affected; difficulty walking on toes	gastrocnemius and soleus	ankle jerk diminished or absent

intervertebral disk herniation

dis·lo·ca·tio (dis-lō-kā′shē-ō). SYN dislocation. [L.]
d. erec′ta, a subglenoid dislocation of the shoulder in which the humerus is in an abducted postion with the head of the humerus displaced inferiorly.

dis·lo·ca·tion (dis-lō-kā′shŭn). Displacement of an organ or any part; specifically a disturbance or disarrangement of the normal relation of the bones at a joint. The direction of the dislocation is determined by the position of the distal part of the articulation. SYN dislocatio, luxation (1). [L. *dislocatio,* fr. *dis-,* apart, + *locatio,* a placing]

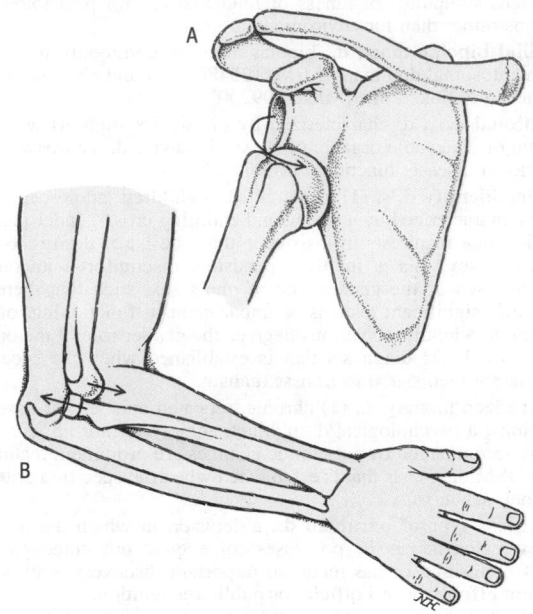

dislocation: (A) subglenoid dislocation of shoulder, (B) dislocation of elbow

d. of articular processes, complete d. of one or both articular processes, usually with overriding of the inferior articular process of the vertebra above into a position anterior to the superior articular process of the vertebra below. SYN locked facets.
arytenoid d., separation of the cricoarytenoid joint with subluxation of the arytenoid cartilage. SYN arytenoid subluxation.
closed d., a d. not complicated by an external wound. SYN simple d.
compound d., SYN open d.
fracture d., dislocation associated with or accompanied by a fracture of one of the bones forming the articulation.
Kienböck d., d. of semilunar bone.
open d., a d. complicated by a wound opening from the surface down to the affected joint. SYN compound d.
perilunar d., d. of carpal bones around the lunate, which remains in its normal anatomic position in relation to the radius; distinguish from d. of lunate, Kienböck d.
simple d., SYN closed d.

dis·mem·ber (dis-mem′ber). **1.** To amputate an arm or leg. **2.** To divide the body (corpus) in parts.

dis·mu·tase (dis′mū-tās). Generic name for enzymes catalyzing the reaction of two identical molecules to produce two molecules in differing states of oxidation (e.g., superoxide dismutase) or of phosphorylation (e.g., glucose-1-phosphate phosphodismutase).

dis·mu·ta·tion (dis′mū-tā′shŭn). A reaction involving a single substance but producing two products; e.g., two molecules of acetaldehyde may react, producing an oxidation product (acetic acid) and a reduction product (ethyl alcohol).

dis·o·bli·ter·a·tion (dis′ob-lit-er-ā′shŭn). Opening of a pathologically closed channel.

di·so·fen·in (dī′sō-fen-in). SYN diisopropyl iminodiacetic acid.

di·so·mic (dī-sō′mik). Relating to disomy.

di·so·my (dī′sō-mē). **1.** The state of an individual or cell having two members of a pair of homologous chromosomes; the normal state in humans, in contrast to monosomy and trisomy. **2.** An abnormal chromosome represented twice in a single cell. [G. *dis,* two, + *sōma,* body]

di·so·pro·mine (di-sō-prō′mēn). SYN diisopromine.

di·so·pyr·a·mide (dī-sō-pir′ă-mīd). An antiarrhythmic drug resembling quinidine with substantial anticholinergic properties.

dis·or·der (dis-ōr′der). A disturbance of function, structure, or both, resulting from a genetic or embryonic failure in development or from exogenous factors such as poison, trauma, or disease.

adjustment d.'s, (1) a group of mental and behavioral d.'s in which the development of symptoms is related to the presence of some environmental stressor or life event and is expected to remit when the stress ceases; **(2)** a d. whose essential feature is a maladaptive reaction to an identifiable psychological stress, or stressors, that occurs within weeks of the onset of the stressors and persists for up to six months; the maladaptive nature of the reaction is indicated by impairment in occupational (including school) functioning, or in usual social activities or relationships with others, or with symptoms that are in excess of a normal or expectable reaction to the stressor.

affective d.'s, a group of mental d.'s characterized by a disturbance in mood.

antisocial personality d., (1) an enduring and pervasive pattern characterized by continuous and chronic antisocial behavior with disregard for and violation of the rights and safety of others, beginning before the age of 15; early childhood signs include chronic lying, stealing, fighting, and truancy; in adolescence there may be unusually early or aggressive sexual behavior, excessive drinking, and use of illicit drugs, such behavior continuing in adulthood. **(2)** a DSM diagnosis that is established when the specified criteria are met.

anxiety d.'s, a group of interrelated mental illnesses involving anxiety reactions in response to stress. The types include: 1) generalized anxiety, by far the most prevalent condition, which strikes slightly more females than males, mostly in the 20–35 age group; 2) panic d., in which a person suffers repeated panic attacks. Some 2–5% of Americans are subject to this ailment, about twice as many women as men; 3) obsessive-compulsive d., afflicting 2–3% of the U.S. population; 4) posttraumatic stress disorder, most frequent among combat veterans or survivors of major physical trauma; and 5) the phobias (e.g., fear of snakes, crowds, confinement, heights, etc.), which on a minor scale affect about one in eight people in the U.S. SEE neurosis.

articulation d.'s, errors in pronunciation including phoneme omissions, substitutions, distortions, and additions.

Asperger d., (1) a pervasive developmental d. characterized by severe and enduring impairment in social skills and restrictive and repetitive behaviors and interests, leading to impaired social and occupational functioning but without significant delays in language development. **(2)** a DSM diagnosis that is established when the specified criteria are met.

asthenic personality d., SYN asthenic *personality.*

attention deficit d., a d. of attention, organization and impulse control appearing in childhood and sometimes persisting to adulthood. Hyperactivity may be a feature, but is not necessary for the diagnosis.

attention deficit hyperactivity d., (1) a disorder of childhood and adolescence manifested at home, in school, and in social situations by developmentally inappropriate degrees of inattention, impulsiveness, and hyperactivity. **(2)** a DSM diagnosis that is established when the specified criteria are met. SYN hyperactive child syndrome.

autistic d., (1) a severe form of pervasive developmental disorder. SEE ALSO autism, infantile *autism*; **(2)** a DSM diagnosis that is established when the specified criteria are met. SEE autism, infantile *autism.*

avoidant d. of adolescence, SEE avoidant d. of childhood.

avoidant d. of childhood, a mental d. occurring in childhood or adolescence characterized by an excessive shrinking away from contact with people who are unfamiliar.

avoidant personality d., (1) an enduring and pervasive pattern in adulthood characterized by hypersensitivity to rejection, humiliation, shame, feelings of inadequacy resulting in social inhibition, and an unwillingness to enter into relationships without unusually strong guarantees of uncritical acceptance. (2) a DSM diagnosis that is established when the specified criteria are met. SYN avoidant personality.

behavior d., general term used to denote mental illness or psychological dysfunction, specifically those mental, emotional, or behavioral subclasses for which organic correlates do not exist. SEE antisocial personality d.

bipolar d., an affective d. characterized by the occurrence of alternating periods of euphoria (mania) and depression. SYN manic-depressive psychosis.

body dysmorphic d., (1) a psychosomatic (somatoform) d. characterized by preoccupation with some imagined defect in appearance in a normal-appearing person. (2) a DSM diagnosis that is established when the specified criteria are met. SYN dysmorphophobia.

borderline personality d., (1) an enduring and pervasive pattern that begins by early adulthood and is characterized by impulsivity and unpredictability, unstable interpersonal relationships, inappropriate or uncontrolled affect, especially anger, identity disturbances, rapid shifts of mood, suicidal acts, self-mutilations, job and marital instability, chronic feelings of emptiness or boredom, and intolerance of being alone. (2) a DSM diagnosis that is established when the specific criteria are met.

character d., an older term referring to a group of behavioral d.'s, now replaced by a more general term, personality d.

conduct d., (1) a mental d. of childhood or adolescence characterized by a persistent pattern of violating societal norms and the rights of others; children with the d. may exhibit physical aggression, cruelty to animals, vandalism and robbery, along with truancy, cheating, and lying. (2) a DSM diagnosis that is established when the specified criteria are met. SEE antisocial personality d.

conversion d., (1) a mental d. in which an unconscious emotional conflict is expressed as an alteration or loss of physical functioning, usually controlled by the voluntary nervous system. (2) a DSM diagnosis that is established when the specified criteria are met.

cumulative trauma d.'s (CTD), chronic d.'s involving connective tissue (muscles, tendons) and nerve, often resulting from work-related physical activities. SYN repetitive strain d.'s, repetitive stress d.'s.

cyclothymic d., SYN cyclothymia.

cyclothymic personality d., SYN cyclothymic *personality*.

delusional d., a severe mental d. characterized by the presence of delusions. The delusions may be related to paranoid, grandiose, somatic, or erotic themes.

dependent personality d., (1) an enduring and pervasive pattern in adulthood characterized by submissive and clinging behavior and excessive reliance on others to meet one's emotional, social, or economic needs. (2) a DSM diagnosis that is established when the specified criteria are met. SYN dependent personality.

depersonalization d., (1) a d. characterized by persistent or recurrent experiences of detachment from one's mental processes or body, as if one is an automaton, an outside observer, or in a dream; reality testing remains intact and there is clinically significant distress impairment. (2) a DSM diagnosis is established when the specified criteria are met.

dissociative d.'s, a group of mental d.'s characterized by disturbances in the functions of identity, memory, consciousness, or perception of the environment; this group includes dissociative (older term, psychogenic) amnesia, dissociative fugue, dissociative identity (older term, multiple personality) disorder, and depersonalization d.

dissociative identity d., (1) a d. in which two or more distinct conscious personalities alternately prevail in the same person, sometimes without any one personality being aware of the other(s). (2) a DSM diagnosis that is established when the specified criteria are met. SYN multiple personality.

dysthymic d., (1) a chronic disturbance of mood characterized by mild depression or loss of interest in usual activities. SEE depression; (2) a DSM diagnosis is established when the specified criteria are met.

eating d.'s, a group of mental d.'s including anorexia nervosa, bulimia nervosa, pica, and rumination d. of infancy.

emotional d., SEE mental *illness*, behavior d.

erotomanic d., the false belief that one is loved by another such as a movie star or a casual acquaintance.

factitious d., a mental d. in which the individual intentionally produces symptoms of illness or feigns illness for psychological reasons rather than for environmental goals.

familial bipolar mood d., bipolar mood d. commonly inherited as an autosomal dominant [MIM*125480] trait and also occasionally as an X-linked one [MIM*309200].

functional d., a d. characterized by physical symptoms with no known or detectable organic basis. SEE behavior d., neurosis. SYN functional disease, functional illness.

gender identity d.'s, (1) a mental d. in children, adolescents, or adults characterized by a strong and enduring cross-gender identification that manifests in insistence that one is, or desires to be, the other sex; this d. involves persistent discomfort with one's assigned sex or the gender role of one's sex, such that there is clinically significant distress or impairment in functioning, often leading to adopting to various degrees the gender role of the other sex. (2) a DSM diagnosis that is established when the specific criteria are met. SEE ALSO transsexualism.

generalized anxiety d., (1) chronic, repeated episodes of anxiety reactions; a psychological d. in which anxiety or morbid fear and dread accompanied by autonomic changes are prominent features. (2) a DSM diagnosis that is established when the specified criteria are met. SEE anxiety.

grandiose type of paranoid d., a delusion in which the person believes that he or she possesses some great but unrecognized talent or insight, or has made an important discovery, with subsequent efforts toward official or public recognition.

histrionic personality d., (1) an enduring and pervasive pattern of behavior in adulthood characterized by excessive, dramatic, and shallow emotionality; attention-seeking; and demands for approval and reassurance, beginning in early childhood and present in a variety of contexts. (2) a DSM diagnosis that is established when the specified criteria are met. SYN hysterical personality d., hysterical personality.

hysterical personality d., SYN histrionic personality d.

identity d., a mental d. in which one suffers severe distress regarding one's ability to reconcile aspects of the self into a coherent acceptable sense of self.

immune complex d., SYN immune complex *disease*.

immunoproliferative d.'s, d.'s in which there is a continuing proliferation of cells of the immune system that can result in γ-globulin abnormalities such as in chronic lymphocytic leukemia, "macroglobulinemias," and multiple myeloma.

impulse control d., a group of mental d.'s characterized by a person's failure to resist an impulse to perform some act harmful to self or to others; includes pathologic gambling, pedophilia, kleptomania, pyromania, trichotillomania, intermittent and isolated explosive d.'s.

induced psychotic d., a severe mental disorder brought about by a toxic agent such as a drug or hallucinogen. SEE psychosis.

intermittent explosive d., (1) a disorder that may begin in early childhood, or following head injury at any age, characterized by repeated acts of violent, aggressive behavior in otherwise normal persons that is markedly out of proportion to the event that provokes it. (2) a DSM diagnosis that is established when the specified criteria are met. SYN dyscontrol, episodic dyscontrol syndrome.

internet addiction d., a posited clinical syndrome involving excessive time spent "surfing the net"; without clearly established criteria or etiology.

ion channel d.'s, a number of diseases, mostly inherited and episodic in nature, caused by dysfunction of the calcium, chloride, potassium, or sodium channels of nerve or muscle; the inherited myotonias and periodic paralyses are included in this category; there is usually dominant inheritance, with the primary defect due to mutations of gene encoding on locus 7q32, 17q, or 1q31-32. SYN channelopathies.

isolated explosive d., a d. of impulse control characterized by a single episode of failure to resist a violent, externally directed act which had serious impact on others.

jealous type of paranoid d., the false belief that one's spouse or lover is unfaithful, leading to repeated confrontation, or the taking of extraordinary steps to intervene in the imagined infidelity.

late luteal phase dysphoric d., SYN premenstrual *syndrome.*

LDL receptor d., abnormality in clearance of LDL from the plasma due to abnormality in LDL receptor activity; causes hypercholesterolemia.

lymphoplasmacellular d.'s, term used to refer to a group of disorders including plasmacytoma, multiple myeloma, lymphoplasmacytic lymphoma, MALT lymphoma, and amyloidosis.

major depressive d., SYN major *depression.*

major mood d., SEE bipolar d., affective *psychosis,* endogenous *depression,* dysthymia, manic-depressive d.

manic-depressive d., obsolete term for bipolar disorder.

mental d., a psychological syndrome or behavioral pattern that is associated with subjective distress and/or objective impairment. SEE ALSO mental *illness,* behavior d.

mitochondrial d.'s, a group of diverse hereditary d.'s caused by genetic mutation of mitochrondrial DNA; includes ragged red fiber myopathy; progressive external ophthalmoplegia; Leigh syndrome; myoclonic epilepsy with ragged red fiber myopathy (MERRF); mitochondrial myopathy, encephalopathy, lacta cidosis, and stroke (MELAS); and Lieber optic neuropathy.

mood d.'s, a group of mental disorders involving a disturbance of mood, accompanied by either a full or partial manic or depressive syndrome that is not due to any other mental disorder. Mood refers to a prolonged emotion that colors the whole psychic life; it generally involves either depression or elation; e.g., manic episode, major depressive episode, bipolar disorders, and depressive disorder (see separate entries for each).

multiple personality d., older term for dissociative identity disorder.

narcissistic personality d., (1) a pervasive pattern in adulthood of self-centeredness, self-importance, lack of empathy for others, sense of entitlement, and viewing others largely as objects to meet one's needs, manifested in a variety of contexts. (2) a DSM diagnosis that is established when the specified criteria are met.

neuropsychologic d., cerebral dysfunction from any physical cause manifested by changes in mood, behavior, perception, memory, cognition, or judgment and/or psychophysiology.

neurotic d., SYN neurosis.

obsessive-compulsive d., (1) a type of anxiety d. whose essential feature is recurrent obsessions, persistent, intrusive ideas, thoughts, impulses or images, or compulsions (repetitive, purposeful, and intentional behaviors performed in response to an obsession) sufficiently severe to cause marked distress, be time-consuming, or significantly interfere with the individual's normal routine, occupational functioning, or usual social activities or relationships with others. (2) a DSM diagnosis that is established when the specified criteria are met. SEE ALSO obsessive-compulsive personality d.

obsessive-compulsive personality d., (1) a pervasive pattern in adulthood characterized by unattainable perfectionism; preoccupation with rules, details, and orderliness; unreasonable attempts to control others; excessive devotion to work; and rumination to the point of indecisiveness, all at the expense of flexiblity, openness, and efficiency. (2) a DSM diagnosis that is established when the specified criteria are met. SYN compulsive personality, obsessive personality, obsessive-compulsive personality.

oppositional d., SYN oppositional defiant d.

oppositional defiant d., (1) a d. of childhood or adolescence characterized by a recurrent pattern of negativistic, hostile, and disobedient behavior toward authority figures. (2) a DSM diagno-

sis that is established when the specified criteria are met. SYN oppositional d.

organic mental d., a psychological, cognitive, or behavioral abnormality associated with transient or permanent dysfunction of the brain, usually characterized by the presence of an organic brain syndrome.

overanxious d., a mental d. of childhood or adolescence marked by excessive worrying and fearful behavior not related specifically to separation or due to recent stress, now included within generalized anxiety d.

panic d., recurrent panic attacks that occur unpredictably. SEE generalized anxiety d.

paranoid d., SYN persecutory type of paranoid d.

paranoid personality d., (1) a personality d. that is less debilitating than is the paranoid or delusional paranoid d.; the essential feature is a pervasive and unwarranted tendency, beginning in early adulthood and present in a variety of contexts, to misinterpret the actions of others as deliberately exploitive, harmful, demeaning, or threatening. (2) a DSM diagnosis that is established when the specified criteria are met. SYN paranoid personality.

persecutory type of paranoid d., one of the most common of the types of paranoid disorders, it involves a single theme or series of connected themes, such as being conspired against, cheated, spied on, followed, poisoned or drugged, maligned, harassed, or obstructed in the pursuit of long-term goals; small slights may be exaggerated and become the focus of a delusional system. SEE paranoia; Cf. paranoid personality d. SYN paranoid d.

personality d., general term for a group of behavioral d.'s characterized by usually lifelong ingrained maladaptive patterns of subjective internal experience and deviant behavior, lifestyle, and social adjustment, which patterns may manifest in impaired judgement, affect, impulse control and interpersonal functioning.

pervasive developmental d., a group of mental d.'s of infancy, childhood, or adolescence characterized by distortions in the acquisition of the multiple basic psychologic funtions necessary for the elaboration of social skills, language skills, and imagination; also characterized by restricted or stereotypical activities and interests. SEE ALSO Rett *syndrome,* Asperger d.

plasma iodoprotein d., SEE familial *goiter.*

posttraumatic stress d., (1) development of characteristic symptoms following a psychologically traumatic event that is generally outside the range of usual human experience; symptoms include numbed responsiveness to environmental stimuli, a variety of autonomic and cognitive dysfunctions, and dysphoria. (2) a DSM diagnosis that is established when the specified criteria are met.

premenstrual dysphoric d., (1) a pervasive pattern occurring during the last week of the luteal phase in most menstrual cycles for at least a year and remitting within a few days of the onset of the follicular phase, with some combination of depressed mood, mood lability, marked anxiety, or irritability; various specific physical symptoms; and significant functional impairment; the symptoms are comparable in severity to those seen in a major depressive episode, distinguishing this d. from the far more common premenstrual syndrome. SEE ALSO premenstrual *syndrome;* (2) a specified set of criteria in the DSM, proposed for the purpose of futher research.

psychogenic pain d., a d. in which the principal complaint is pain that is out of proportion to objective findings and that is related to psychological factors.

psychosomatic d., psychophysiologic d., a d. characterized by physical symptoms of psychic origin, usually involving a single organ system innervated by the autonomic nervous system; physiological and organic changes stem from a sustained disturbance.

psychotic d., SYN psychosis.

reactive attachment d., (1) a mental d. of infancy or early childhood characterized by disturbed social relatedness; thought to be caused by grossly pathologic care. (2) a DSM diagnosis that is established when the specified criteria are met.

REM behavior d., a d. characterized by lack of the atonia of voluntary muscles that normally occurs in REM sleep.

repetitive strain d.'s, SYN cumulative trauma d.'s.

repetitive stress d.'s, SYN cumulative trauma d.'s.

di

rumination d., (1) a mental d. occurring in infancy characterized by repeated regurgitation of food, usually accompanied by weight loss or failure to gain weight. **(2)** a DSM diagnosis that is established when the specified criteria are met.

schizoid personality d., (1) an enduring and pervasive pattern of behavior in adulthood characterized by social withdrawal, emotional coldness or aloofness or restriction, and indifference to others. **(2)** a DSM diagnosis that is established when the specific criteria are met. SYN schizoid personality.

schizophreniform d. (skiz'ō-fren'ĭ-fōrm), **(1)** a d. whose essential features are identical with those of schizophrenia, with the exception that the duration including prodromal, active, and residual phases is less than six months. **(2)** a DSM diagnosis that is established when the specified criteria are met.

schizotypal personality d., (1) an enduring and pervasive pattern of behavior in adulthood characterized by discomfort with and reduced capacity for close relationships, cognitive or perceptual distortions, and eccentric behavior. **(2)** a DSM diagnosis that is established when the specific criteria are met. SYN schizotypal personality.

seasonal affective d. (SAD), a depressive mood disorder that occurs at approximately the same time year after year and spontaneously remits at the same time each year. The most common type is winter depression and it is characterized by morning hypersomnia, low energy, increased appetite, weight gain, and carbohydrate craving, all of which remit in the spring.

separation anxiety d., (1) a mental d. occurring in childhood characterized by excessive anxiety when the child is separated from someone to whom the child is attached, usually a parent. **(2)** a DSM diagnosis that is established when the specified criteria are met.

sexual d.'s, a group of behavioral and psychophysiologic d.'s in which there is symptomatic variability in sexual functioning, including either the eroticized behavior associated with sexual activity (the paraphilias) or with disturbances of desire, arousal, and orgasm.

shared psychotic d., SYN *folie* à deux.

sleep terror d., SEE night terrors.

somatization d., (1) a mental d. characterized by presentation of a complicated medical history and of physical symptoms referring to a variety of organ systems, but without a detectable or known organic basis. SEE conversion, hysteria, Briquet *syndrome*; **(2)** a DSM diagnosis that is established when the specified criteria are met.

somatoform d., a group of d.'s in which physical symptoms suggesting physical d.'s for which there are no demonstrable organic findings or known physiologic mechanisms, and for which there is positive evidence, or a strong presumption that the symptoms are linked to psychological factors; e.g., hysteria, conversion disorder, hypochondriasis, pain disorder, somatization disorder, body dysmorphic disorder, and Briquet syndrome.

substance abuse d.'s, a group of mental d.'s in which maladaptive behavioral and biologic changes are associated with regular use of alcohol, drugs, and related substances that affect the central nervous system and result in failure to meet significant obligations in personal and social functioning.

substance dependence d., a maladaptive pattern of use of alcohol, drugs, or other substances, with tolerance and/or withdrawal symptoms, drug-seeking behavior, and lack of success in discontinuation of use, to the detriment of social, interpersonal, and occupational activities.

substance-induced organic mental d.'s, mental d.'s caused by use of drugs, e.g., cocaine, alcohol, etc.

thought d., SYN thought process d.

thought process d., an intellectual function symptom of schizophrenia, manifested by irrelevance and incoherence of verbal productions ranging from simple blocking and mild circumstantiality to total loosening of associations. SYN thought d.

triple repeat d.'s, a group of hereditary d.'s in which a gene mutation on a specific chromosome produces an abnormal form of protein terminated by a long chain of amino acid glutamate repeats; includes Huntington disease, Kennedy disease, Machado-

Joseph disease, myotonic dystrophy, fragile X syndrome, and some spinal cerebellar d.'s.

visceral d., an obsolete term used in reference to psychosomatic d.

dis·or·ga·ni·za·tion (dis-ōr'gan-i-zā'shŭn). Destruction of an organ or tissue with consequent loss of function.

dis·o·ri·en·ta·tion (dis'ōr-ē-en-tā'shŭn). Loss of the sense of familiarity with one's surroundings (time, place, and person); loss of one's bearings.

dis·par·ate (dis'pa-răt). Unequal; not alike. [L. *disparo*, pp. *-atus*, to separate, fr. *paro*, to prepare]

dis·par·i·ty (dis-par'i-tē). The condition of being disparate. [L. *dispar*, dissimilar]

fixation d., the amount of heterophoria possible with fusion present.

retinal d., the slight difference in retinal images that arises because of the lateral separation of the two eyes that stimulates stereoscopic vision.

dis·pen·sa·ry (dis-pen'ser-ē). **1.** A physician's office, especially the office of one who dispenses medicines. **2.** The office of a hospital pharmacist, where medicines are given out on physicians' orders. **3.** An outpatient department of a hospital. [L. *dis-penso*, pp. *-atus*, to distribute by weight, fr. *penso*, to weigh]

Dis·pen·sa·to·ry (dis-pen'să-tō-rē). A work originally intended as a commentary on the Pharmacopeia, but now more of a supplement to that work, which contains an account of the sources, mode of preparation, physiologic action, and therapeutic uses of most of the agents, official and nonofficial; used in the treatment of disease. [L. *dispensator*, a manager, steward; see dispensary]

dis·pense (dis-pens'). To give out medicine and other necessities to the sick; to fill a medical prescription.

di·sper·my, di·sperm·ia (dī'sper-mē, dī-sperm'ē-ă). Entrance of two spermatozoa into one ovum.

dis·per·sal (dis-per'săl). SYN dispersion (1).

flash d., the property of rapid disintegration of a tablet when placed on the tongue.

dis·perse (dis-pers'). To dissipate, to cause disappearance of, to scatter, to dilute.

dis·per·sion (dis-per'zhŭn). **1.** The act of dispersing or of being dispersed. SYN dispersal. **2.** Incorporation of the particles of one substance into the mass of another, including solutions, suspensions, and colloidal dispersions (solutions). **3.** Specifically, what is usually called a colloidal *solution*. **4.** The extent or degree in which values of a statistical frequency distribution are scattered about a mean or median value. [L. *dispersio*]

coarse d., SYN suspension (4).

colloidal d., SYN colloidal *solution*.

molecular d., d. in which the dispersed phase consists of individual molecules; if the molecules are of less than colloidal size, the result is a true solution.

optic rotatory d. (ORD), the change in optic rotation with the wavelength of the incident monochromatic polarized light; the displacement of the former from zero within the absorption band is known as the Cotton *effect.*

temporal d., asynchronous repolarization of myocardial fibers that predisposes to abnormal current flow and ectopic rhythms (especially with bradyarrhythmias or ventricular tachyarrhythmias).

dis·per·si·ty (dis-per'si-tē). The extent to which the dimensions of particles have been reduced in colloid formation.

dis·per·soid (dis-per'soyd). A colloidal solution in which the dispersed phase can be concentrated by centrifugation. SYN dispersion colloid, molecular dispersed solution.

di·spi·reme (dī-spī'rēm). The double chromatin skein in the telophase of mitosis. [G. *di-*, twice, + *speirēma,* coil, convolution]

dis·place·a·bil·i·ty (dis-plās-ă-bil'i-tē). The capability of, or susceptibility to, displacement.

tissue d., the property of tissue that permits it to be moved from an initial or relaxed position or form. SYN compression of tissue.

dis·place·ment (dis-plās'ment). **1.** Removal from the normal location or position. **2.** The adding to a fluid (particularly a gas) in an open vessel one of greater density whereby the first is expelled. **3.** In chemistry, a change in which one element, radical, or molecule is replaced by another, or in which one element exchanges electric charges with another by reduction or oxidation. **4.** In psychiatry, the transfer of impulses from one expression to another, as from fighting to talking.

affect d., a shift of feeling from the object originally arousing it to some associated object.

mesial d., SYN mesioversion.

tissue d., the change in the form or position of tissues as a result of pressure.

display.

differential d., the use of RT-PCR-based technologies to amplify mRNA from specific cells or tissues and then to compare them directly with amplified mRNA from another cell or tissue.

dis·pro·por·tion (dis-prō-pōr'shun). Lack of proportion or symmetry.

cephalopelvic d., a condition in which the fetal head is too large to traverse the maternal pelvis.

Disse, Josef, German anatomist, 1852–1912. SEE D. *space.*

dis·sect (di-sekt', dī-). **1.** To cut apart or separate the tissues of the body for study. **2.** In an operation, to separate the different structures along natural lines by dividing the connective tissue framework. [L. *dis-seco,* pp. -*sectus,* to cut asunder]

dis·sec·tion (di-sek'shŭn, dī-). The act of dissecting. SYN anatomy (3) [TA], necrotomy (1).

aortic d., a pathologic process, characterized by splitting of the media layer of the aorta, which leads to formation of a dissecting aneurysm. Classified according to location as follows: type I involves the ascending aorta, transverse arch, and distal aorta; type II is confined to the ascending aorta; type III extends distally in the descending aorta usually from a starting point just distal to the left subclaviar artery.

functional neck d., operation to remove metastases to the lymph nodes of the neck; differs from a radical neck dissection by preserving any of the following structures: the sternocleidomastoid muscle, the spinal accessory nerve, and the internal jugular vein. SYN limited neck d.

limited neck d., SYN functional neck d.

radical neck d., an operation for the removal of metastases to the lymph nodes of the neck in which all of the tissue is removed between the superficial and the deep cervical fascia from the mandible to the clavicle. SEE ALSO functional neck d.

dis·sec·tor (dis-ek'ter). **1.** One who dissects. **2.** A written guide for dissection. **3.** Instrument for dissecting.

dis·sem·i·nat·ed (di-sem'i-nā-ted). Widely scattered throughout an organ, tissue, or the body. [L. *dissemino,* pp. -*atus,* to scatter seed, fr. *semen* (-*min*-), seed]

dis·sep·i·ment (di-sep'i-ment). A separating tissue, partition, or septum. [L. *dis- sepio,* pp. -*septus,* to divide by a fence]

dis·sim·i·la·tion (di-sim-i-lā'shŭn). **1.** SYN disassimilation. **2.** SYN catabolism.

dis·sim·u·la·tion (di-sim-ū-lā'shŭn). Concealment of the truth about a situation, especially about a state of health or during a mental status examination, as by a malingerer or someone with a factitious disorder. [L. *dissimulatio,* fr. *dissimulo,* to feign, fr. *dis,* apart, + *simillis,* same]

dis·so·ci·a·tion (di-sō-sē-ā'shŭn, -shē-ā'shŭn). **1.** Separation, or a dissolution of relations. SYN disassociation. **2.** The change of a complex chemical compound into a simpler one by any lytic reaction, by ionization, by heterolysis, or by homolysis. **3.** An unconscious separation of a group of mental processes from the rest, resulting in an independent functioning of these processes and a loss of the usual associations; for example, a separation of affect from cognition. SEE multiple *personality.* **4.** A state used as an essential part of a technique for healing in psychology and psychotherapy, for instance in hypnotherapy or the neurolinguistic programming technique of time-line therapy. SEE ALSO Time-Line *therapy.* **5.** The translocation between a large chromosome and a small supernumerary one. **6.** Separation of the nuclear components of a heterokaryotic dikaryon. [L. *dis-socio,* pp. -*atus,* to disjoin, separate, fr. *socius,* partner, ally]

albuminocytologic d., increased protein in the cerebrospinal fluid without increase in cell count, characteristic of the Guillain-Barré syndrome; it is also associated with spinal block and with intracranial neoplasia, and is seen in the last phases of poliomyelitis.

atrial d., mutually independent beating of the two atria or of parts of the atria.

atrioventricular d. (AVD), AV d., (1) any situation in which atria and ventricles are activated and contract independently, as in complete AV block; **(2)** more specifically, the d. between atria and ventricles that results from slowing of the atrial pacemaker or acceleration of the ventricular pacemaker at nearly equal (rarely equal) rates, each depolarizing its own chamber, thus interfering with depolarization by the other (interference-dissociation).

complete atrioventricular d., complete AV d., AV d. not interrupted by ventricular captures. SYN complete AV block (2), third degree AV block.

electromechanical d., persistence of electrical activity in the heart without associated mechanical contraction; often a sign of cardiac rupture. SYN pulseless electrical activity.

incomplete atrioventricular d., incomplete AV d., AV d. interrupted by ventricular captures.

interference d., the simultaneous operation of two separate cardiac pacemaking foci that are unassociated because of interference (a normal physiologic phenomenon) due to rendering their respective territories refractory to each other. Usually atrioventricular d. is indicated, the rates being quite close to each other with the atrial rate slightly slower than that of the pacemaker in control of the ventricles. Capture is in either direction, usually the ventricle by the atrium, in incomplete d. h SYN d. by interference.

d. by interference, SYN interference d.

isorhythmic d., AV d. characterized by equal or closely similar atrial and ventricular rates.

light-near d., SYN *pupillary* light-near dissociation.

longitudinal d., d. between parallel chambers of the heart, as between one atrium and the other or between one ventricle and the other, in contrast to d. between atria and ventricles.

pupillary light-near d., SEE *pupillary* light-near dissociation.

sleep d., SYN sleep *paralysis.*

syringomyelic d., loss of pain and temperature sensation with relative retention of tactile sensation, related to a cavity in the central portion of the cord interrupting the decussation of nerve fibers.

tabetic d., loss of proprioceptive sensation with retained pain and temperature sensation due to involvement of the posterior columns of the spinal cord.

visual-kinetic d., the neurolinguistic programming process of removing a synesthesia from a person's internal experience. SEE ALSO neurolinguistic *programming.*

dis·solve (di-zolv'). To change or cause to change from a solid to a dispersed form by immersion in a fluid of suitable properties. [L. *dis-solvo,* pp. -*solutus,* to loose asunder, to dissolve]

dis·so·nance (di'sō-nans). In social psychology and attitude theory, an aversive state which arises when an individual is minimally aware of inconsistency or conflict within himself. SEE cognitive dissonance *theory.* [L. *dissonus,* discordant, confused]

cognitive d., a motivational state studied by social and clinical psychologists which exists when a person's attitudes, perceptions, and related d. state are inconsistent with each other, e.g., hating blacks but admiring Martin Luther King.

dis·sym·me·try (di-sim'ĕ-trē). SYN asymmetry. [dis- + symmetry]

dis·tad (dis'tad). Toward the periphery; in a distal direction.

dis·tal (dis'tăl) [TA]. **1.** Situated away from the center of the body, or from the point of origin; specifically applied to the extremity or distant part of a limb or organ. **2.** In dentistry, away from the median sagittal plane of the face, following the curvature of the dental arch. SYN distalis [TA]. [L. *distalis*]

dis·ta·lis (dis-tā'lis) [TA]. SYN distal.

dis·tance (dis'tans). The measure of space between two objects. [L. *distantia,* fr. *di-sto,* to stand apart, be distant]

focal d., the d. from the center of a lens to its focus.

infinite d., the limit of distant vision, the rays entering the eyes from an object at that point being practically parallel. SYN infinity.

interarch d., (1) the vertical d. between the maxillary and mandibular arches under conditions of vertical dimensions which must be specified; **(2)** the vertical d. between maxillary and mandibular ridges. SYN interalveolar space, interridge d.

interocclusal d., (1) the vertical d. between the opposing occlusal surfaces, assuming rest relation unless otherwise designated; SYN interocclusal rest space (1). **(2)** SYN freeway *space.*

interridge d., SYN interarch d.

large interarch d., a large d. between the maxillary and mandibular arches; may also imply an excessive vertical dimension. SYN open bite (1).

pupillary d., the d. between the center of each pupil; the major reference points in measuring for fitting of spectacle frames and lenses.

reduced interarch d., an occluding vertical dimension which results in an excessive interocclusal d. when the mandible is in rest position, and in a reduced interridge d. when the teeth are in contact.

small interarch d., a small d. between the maxillary and mandibular arches. SYN close bite.

sociometric d., some measurable degree of mutual or social perception, acceptance, and understanding; hypothetically, greater sociometric d. is associated with more inaccuracy in evaluating a relationship (e.g., it is easier to understand and deal with a native than a foreigner).

dis·ten·si·bil·i·ty (dis-ten-si-bil′i-tē). The capability of being distended or stretched. [L. *dis- tendo,* to stretch apart]

dis·ten·tion, dis·ten·sion (dis-ten′shŭn). The act or state of being distended or stretched. SEE ALSO dilation. [L. *dis-tendo,* to stretch apart]

dis·ti·chi·a·sis (dis′tĭ-kī′ă-sis). A congenital, abnormal, accessory row of eyelashes. [G. *di-* double, + *stichos,* row]

dis·till (dis-til′). To extract a substance by distillation.

dis·til·late (dis′ti-lāt). The product of distillation.

dis·til·la·tion (dis-ti-lā′shŭn). Volatilization of a liquid by heat and subsequent condensation of the vapor; a means of separating the volatile from the nonvolatile, or the more volatile from the less volatile, part of a liquid mixture. [L. *de-(di-)stillo,* pp. *-atus,* to drop down]

destructive d., SYN dry d.

dry d., submission of an organic substance to heat in a closed vessel so that oxygen is absent and combustion prevented, with the objective of effecting its decomposition with release of volatile constituents and the formation of new substances. SYN destructive d.

fractional d., d. of a compound liquid at varying degrees of heat whereby the components of different boiling points are collected separately.

molecular d., d. in high vacuum, intended to make possible use of low temperatures to minimize damage to thermally labile molecules that would be decomposed by boiling at higher temperatures.

dis·to·buc·cal (dis-tō-bŭk′kăl). Relating to the distal and buccal surfaces of a tooth; denoting the angle formed by their junction.

dis·to·buc·co·oc·clu·sal (dis′tō-bŭk′ŏ-ō-kloo′săl). Relating to the distal, buccal, and occlusal surfaces of a bicuspid or molar tooth; denoting especially the angle formed by the junction of these surfaces.

dis·to·buc·co·pul·pal (dis′tō-bŭk′ō-pŭl′păl). Relating to the point (trihedral) angle formed by the junction of a distal, buccal, and pulpal wall of a cavity.

dis·to·cer·vi·cal (dis-tō-ser′vi-kăl). Relating to the line angle formed by the junction of the distal and cervical (gingival) walls of a class V cavity.

dis·to·clu·sal (dis-tō-kloo′săl). **1.** Relating to or characterized by distoclusion. **2.** Denoting a compound cavity or restoration involving the distal and occlusal surfaces of a tooth. **3.** Denoting the line angle formed by the distal and occlusal walls of a class V cavity. SYN disto-occlusal.

dis·to·clu·sion (dis-tō-kloo′zhŭn). A malocclusion in which the mandibular arch articulates with the maxillary arch in a position distal to normal; in Angle classification, a Class II malocclusion. SYN distal occlusion (2).

dis·to·gin·gi·val (dis-tō-jin′ji-văl). Relating to the junction of the distal surface with the gingival line of a tooth.

dis·to·in·ci·sal (dis′tō-in-sī′zăl). Relating to the line (dihedral) angle formed by the junction of the distal and incisal walls of a class V cavity in an anterior tooth.

dis·to·la·bi·al (dis-tō-lā′bē-ăl). Relating to the distal and labial surfaces of a tooth; denoting the angle formed by their junction.

dis·to·la·bi·o·pul·pal (dis′tō-lā′bē-ō-pŭl′păl). Relating to the point (trihedral) angle formed by the junction of distal, labial and pulpal walls of the incisal part of a class IV (mesioincisal) cavity.

dis·to·lin·gual (dis-tō-ling′gwăl). Relating to the distal and lingual surfaces of a tooth; denoting the angle formed by their junction.

dis·to·lin·guo·oc·clu·sal (dis′tō-ling′gwō-ŏ-kloo′zăl). Relating to the distal, lingual, and occlusal surfaces of a bicuspid or molar tooth; denoting especially the angle formed by the junction of these surfaces.

Dis·to·ma (dis′tō-mă). Obsolete term for various digenetic flukes, now referred to other genera; e.g., *Fasciola, Fasciolopsis, Paragonimus, Opisthorchis, Clonorchis, Dicrocoelium, Heterophyes,* and *Schistosoma.* SYN *Distomum.* [G. *di-,* two, + *stoma,* mouth]

dis·to·mi·a·sis, dis·to·ma·to·sis (dis′tō-mī′ă-sis, -mă-tō′sis). Presence in any of the organs or tissues of digenetic flukes formerly classified as Distoma or Distomum; in general, infection by any parasitic trematode or fluke.

hemic d., SYN schistosomiasis.

pulmonary d., SYN paragonimiasis.

dis·to·mo·lar (dis-tō-mō′lăr). A supernumerary tooth located in the region posterior to the third molar tooth.

Dis·to·mum (dis′tō-mŭm). SYN *Distoma.*

dis·to·oc·clu·sal (dis′tō-ŏ-kloo′săl). SYN distoclusal.

dis·to·oc·clu·sion (dis′tō-ŏ-kloo′zhŭn). SYN distal *occlusion* (1).

dis·to·place·ment (dis′tō-plās-ment). SYN distoversion.

dis·to·pul·pal (dis-tō-pŭl′păl). Relating to the line (dihedral) angle formed by the junction of the distal and pulpal walls of a cavity.

dis·tor·tion (dis-tōr′shŭn). **1.** In psychiatry, a defense mechanism that helps to repress or disguise unacceptable thoughts. **2.** In dental impressions, the permanent deformation of the impression material after the registration of an imprint. **3.** A twisting out of normal shape or form. **4.** In ophthalmology, unequal magnification over a field of view. [L. *distortio,* fr. *dis-torqueo,* to wrench apart]

barrel d., irregular image produced when peripheral magnification is greater than axial magnification. SEE Petzval *surface.*

parataxic d., an attitude toward another person based on a distorted evaluation, usually because of too close an identification of that person with emotionally significant figures in the patient's past life.

pincushion d., irregular image produced when axial magnification is greater than peripheral magnification. SEE Petzval *surface.*

dis·to·ver·sion (dis′tō-ver-zhŭn). Malposition of a tooth distal to normal, in a posterior direction following the curvature of the dental arch. SYN distoplacement.

dis·tract·i·bil·i·ty (dis-trak-tĭ-bil′i-tē). A disorder of attention in which the mind is easily diverted by inconsequential occurrences; seen in mania and attention deficit disorder.

dis·trac·tion (dis-trak′shŭn). **1.** Difficulty or impossibility of concentration or fixation of the mind. **2.** A force applied to a body part to separate bony fragments or joint surfaces. [L. *dis-traho,* pp. *-tractus,* to pull in different directions]

dis·tress (dis-tres′). Mental or physical suffering or anguish. [L. *distringo,* to draw asunder]

fetal d., SYN nonreassuring fetal *status.*

dis·tri·bu·tion (dis-tri-bū′shŭn). **1.** The passage of the branches of arteries or nerves to the tissues and organs. **2.** The area in which the branches of an artery or a nerve terminate, or the area supplied by such an artery or nerve. **3.** The relative numbers of individuals in each of various categories or populations such as in different age, sex, or occupational samples. SEE frequency d. **4.** Partition. **5.** The pattern of occurrence of a substance within or between cells, tissues, organisms, or taxa. [L. *distribuo,* pp. *-tributus,* to distribute, fr. *tribus,* a tribe]

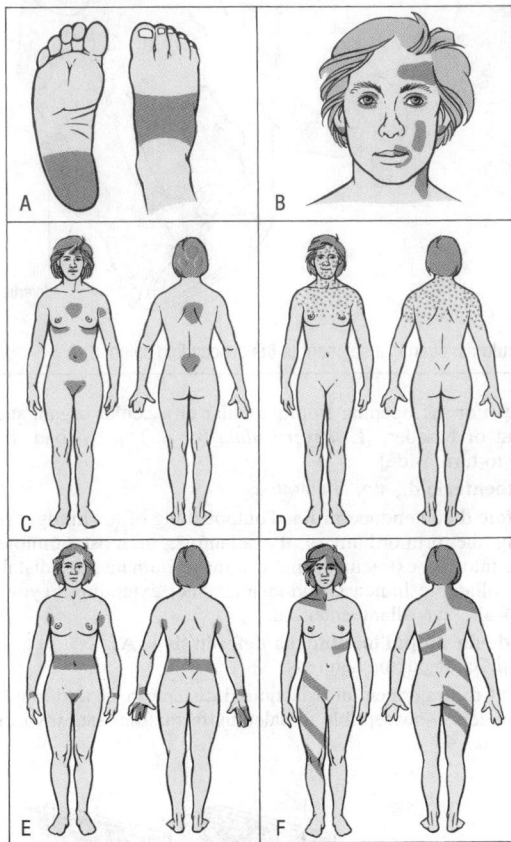

anatomic distribution of common skin disorders: (A) contact dermatitis (shoes); (B) contact dermatitis (cosmetics, perfumes, earrings); (C) seborrheic dermatitis; (D) acne; (E) scabies; (F) herpes zoster (shingles)

Bernoulli d., the probability d. associated with two mutually exclusive and exhaustive outcomes, e.g., death or survival.

binomial d., (1) a probability d. associated with two mutually exclusive outcomes, e.g., presence or absence of a clinical sign. **(2)** the possible array of the number of successes in the outcomes from a fixed number, n, of independent Bernoulli trials; the probabilities associated with each constitute a binomial process of order n.

chi-square d. (kī), a variable is said to have a chi-square d. with K degrees of freedom if it is distributed like the sum of the squares of K independent random variables, each of which has a normal (gaussian) d. with mean zero and variance one. The chi square d. is the basis for many variations of the chi-square(d) test, perhaps the most widely used test for statistical significance in biology and medicine.

countercurrent d., a method of separation of two or more substances by repeated distribution between two immiscible liquid phases that move past each other in opposite directions; a form of liquid-liquid chromatography.

dermatomal d., SYN dermatome (3).

epidemiological d., SEE histogram.

exponential d., the time until failure of a process at constant hazard.

f d., the d. of the ratio of two independent quantities each of which is distributed like a variance in normally distributed samples. So named in honor of the English statistician and geneticist R.A. Fisher.

frequency d., a statistical description of raw data in terms of the number or frequency of items characterized by each of a series or range of values of a continuous variable.

gaussian d., SYN normal d.

lognormal d., if a variable y is such that x = log y, it is said to have a lognormal d.; this is a skew d.

multinomial d., probability distribution associated with the classification of each of a sample of individuals into one of several mutually exclusive and exhaustive categories.

normal d., a specific bell-shaped frequency d. commonly assumed by statisticians to represent the infinite population of measurements from which a sample has been drawn; characterized by two parameters, the mean (x) and the standard deviation (σ), in the equation: SYN gaussian curve, gaussian d.

Poisson d., (1) a discontinuous d. important in statistical work and defined by the equation $p(x) = e^{-\mu}\mu^x / x!$, where e is the base of natural logarithms, x is the sequence of integers, μ is the mean, and $x!$ represents the factorial of x. **(2)** a d. function used to describe the occurrence of rare events, or the sampling d. of isolated counts in a continuum of time or space.

skew d., an asymmetrical frequency d.; in biology and medicine it is usually a lognormal d.

t d., the d. of the quotient of independent random variables, the numerator of which is a standardized normal variate and the denominator the positive square root of the quotient of a chi-square distributed variate and its number of degrees of freedom.

dis·tri·chi·a·sis (dis-tri-kī′ă-sis). Growth of two hairs in a single follicle. [G. *dis,* double, + *thrix* (*trich-*), hair]

dis·trix (dis′triks). Splitting of the hairs at their ends. [G. *dis,* twice, + *thrix,* hair]

dis·tro·pin. SYN dystrophin.

dis·tur·bance (dis-ter′bans). Deviation from, interruption of, or interference with a normal state.

emotional d., mental d., SEE mental *illness,* behavior *disorder.*

di·sulf·am·ide (dī-sul′fă-mīd). A diuretic.

di·sul·fate (dī-sŭl′fāt). A molecule containing two sulfates.

di·sul·fide (dī-sŭl′fīd). **1.** A molecule containing two atoms of sulfur to one of the reference element, e.g., CS_2, carbon disulfide. **2.** A compound containing the –S–S– group, e.g., cystine.

asymmetric d., SYN mixed d.

mixed d., d. which is not symmetric on both sides of the –S–S– linkage; e.g., the d. formed between coenzyme A and glutathione or between cysteine and coenzyme A or glutathione. SYN asymmetric d.

symmetric d., d. that is symmetric on both sides of the –S–S– linkage; i.e., d. formed from identical thiol-containing compounds; e.g., cystine, glutathione disulfide.

di·sul·fi·ram (dī-sŭl′fi-ram). An antioxidant that interferes with the normal metabolic degradation of alcohol in the body, resulting in increased acetaldehyde concentrations in blood and tissues. Used in the treatment of chronic alcoholism; when a small quantity of alcohol is consumed an unpleasant reaction results. Also used as a chelator in copper and nickel poisoning. SYN tetraethylthiuram disulfide.

DIT Abbreviation for diiodotyrosine.

di·ter·penes (dī-ter′pēnz). Hydrocarbons or their derivatives containing four isoprene units, hence containing 20 carbon atoms and four branched methyl groups; e.g., vitamin A, retinene, aconitine.

di·thi·az·a·nine io·dide (dī-thī-az′ă-nēn). A broad spectrum anthelmintic, effective against *Strongyloides.*

di·thi·o·thre·i·tol (dī-thē′ō-thrē-tol). A donor of thiol groups used in biochemical and pharmacological studies. SYN Cleland reagent.

di·thra·nol (dith′ră-nol). SYN anthralin.

Dittrich, Franz, German pathologist, 1815–1859. SEE D. *plugs,* under *plug, stenosis.*

Di

di·u·re·sis (dī-ū-rē'sis). Excretion of urine; commonly denotes production of unusually large volumes of urine. [G. *dia,* throughout, completely, + *ourēsis,* urination]

alcohol d., d. following the ingestion of alcoholic beverages; due, in part, to inhibition of the output of antidiuretic hormone by the neurohypophysis.

osmotic d., d. due to a high concentration of osmotically active substances in the renal tubules (e.g., urea, sodium sulfate), which limit the reabsorption of water.

water d., d. following the drinking of water; due to reduced secretion of the antidiuretic hormone of the neurohypophysis in response to the lowered osmotic pressure of the blood.

di·u·ret·ic (dī-ū-ret'ik). **1.** Promoting the excretion of urine. **2.** An agent that increases the amount of urine excreted.

cardiac d., a d. that acts by increasing function of the heart, and thereby improves renal perfusion.

direct d., a d. whose primary effect is on renal tubular function.

indirect d., a d. that acts by increasing cardiac function or by increasing the state of hydration.

loop d., a class of d. agents (e.g., furosemide, ethacrynic acid) that act by inhibiting reabsorption of sodium and chloride, not only in the proximal and distal tubules but also in Henle loop.

mercurial d.'s, d. drugs containing organic mercury (e.g., Mercuhydrin) that promote substantial salt and water loss through the kidney. Among the first potent d. agents used in congestive heart failure, but now obsolescent.

osmotic d.'s, drugs, such as mannitol, which by their osmotic effects retain water during urine formation and thus dilute electrolytes in the urine, making resorption less efficient; they promote the elimination of water and electrolytes in the urine.

potassium sparing d.'s, d. agents that, unlike most d.'s, retain potassium; examples are triamterene and amiloride. Often used together with d.'s that promote the loss of both sodium and potassium. Used in hypertension and in congestive heart failure.

di·ur·nal (dī-er'năl). **1.** Pertaining to the daylight hours; opposite of nocturnal. **2.** Repeating once each 24 hours, e.g., a d. variation or a d. rhythm. Cf. circadian. [L. *diurnus,* of the day]

di·va·lence, di·va·len·cy (dī-vā'lens, dī-vā'len-sē). SYN bivalence.

di·va·lent (dī-vā'lent, div'ă-). SYN bivalent (1).

di·val·pro·ex so·di·um (dī-val'prō-eks). Pentanoic acid, 2-propyl-, sodium salt (2:1); an anticonvulsant used in absence seizures and related seizure disorders. Derived from valproic acid.

di·var·i·ca·tion (dī'var-i-kā'shŭn). SYN diastasis (1). [L. *divaricare,* to spread asunder]

di·ver·gence (dī-ver'jens). **1.** A moving or spreading apart or in different directions. **2.** The spreading of branches of the neuron to form synapses with several other neurons. [L. *di-,* apart, + *vergo,* to incline]

di·ver·gent (dī-ver'jent). Moving in different directions; radiating.

di·ver·tic·u·la (dī-ver-tik'ū-lă). Plural of diverticulum.

di·ver·tic·u·lar (dī-ver-tik'ū-lăr). Relating to a diverticulum.

di·ver·tic·u·lec·to·my (dī'ver-tik-ū-lek'tō-mē). Excision of a diverticulum.

di·ver·tic·u·li·tis (dī'ver-tik-ū-lī'tis). Inflammation of a diverticulum, especially of the small pockets in the wall of the colon which fill with stagnant fecal material and become inflamed; rarely, they may cause obstruction, perforation, or bleeding.

di·ver·tic·u·lo·ma (dī'ver-tik-ū-lō'mă). Development of a granulomatous mass in the wall of the colon. [diverticulum + G. *-oma,* tumor]

di·ver·tic·u·lo·pexy (dī-ver-tik'ū-lō-pek-sē). An operation to obliterate a diverticulum without resecting it, usually by securing the tip to a nearby structure so the diverticulum no longer fills. [diverticulum + G. *pēxis,* fixation]

di·ver·tic·u·lo·sis (dī'ver-tik-ū-lō'sis). Presence of a number of diverticula of the intestine, common in middle age; the lesions are acquired pulsion diverticula.

di·ver·tic·u·lum, pl. **di·ver·tic·u·la** (dī-ver-tik'ū-lŭm, ū-lă) [tA].

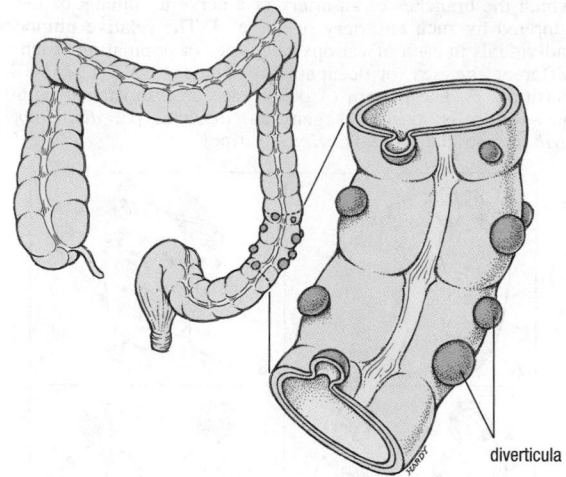

diverticula

diverticulosis: seen in a segment of the descending colon

A pouch or sac opening from a tubular or saccular organ, such as the gut or bladder. [L. *diverticulum* (or *di-*), a by-road, fr. *deverto,* to turn aside]

allantoenteric d., SYN allantoic d.

allantoic d., an endoderm-lined outpouching of the hindgut representing the primordium of the allantois; in most amniotes, it grows into the extraembryonic celom; in humans, the distal part of the allantoic lumen is rudimentary, not extending beyond the body stalk. SYN allantoenteric d.

diverticula ampul'lae duc'tus deferen'tis [TA], SYN diverticula of ampulla of ductus deferens.

caliceal d., a congenital or acquired distention of a kidney calix that renders it susceptible to calculus formation. SEE ALSO Fraley *syndrome.*

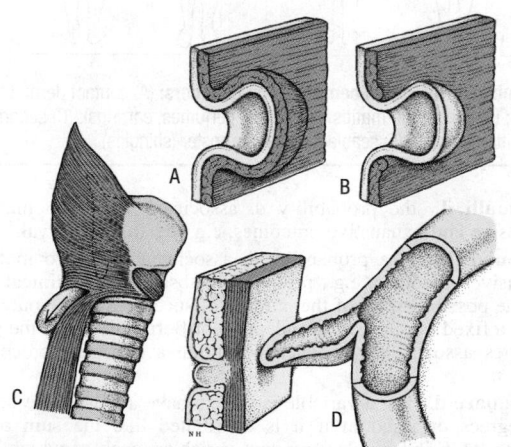

diverticulum: (A) true diverticulum (includes all layers of wall), (B) false diverticulum of ileum (includes only mucosa); (C) Zenker diverticulum of esophagus, (D) Meckel diverticulum of ileum

cervical d., a d. in the neck derived from retention of part of one of the pharyngeal pouches (endodermal) or branchial grooves (ectodermal) of the embryo.

diverticula of colon, diverticula, which are herniations of mucosa and submucosa through or between fibers of the major muscle layer (muscularis propria) of the colon. Usually multiple, it occurs in 50% of western populations above the age of 70, but is much less common in other populations. Can cause bleeding and episodes of severe inflammation. SYN colonic diverticula.

colonic diverticula, SYN diverticula of colon.

diverticula of ampulla of ductus deferens [TA], the irregular sacculations of the ampullary part of the ductus deferens near its termination in the ejaculatory duct. SYN diverticula ampullae ductus deferentis [TA].

duodenal d., a d. of the duodenum, often of large size, that is occasionally found projecting from the duodenum near the duodenal papilla.

epiphrenic d., a d. which originates just above the cardioesophageal junction and usually protrudes to the right side of the lower mediastinum.

false d., a d. of the intestine that passes through a defect in the muscular wall of the gut and thus does not include a layer of muscle in its wall.

Heister d., SEE *bulb* of jugular vein.

hypopharyngeal d., SYN pharyngoesophageal d.

Kommerell d., not a true d., but a bulblike swelling at the origin of the left subclavian artery due to a remnant of the left fourth aortic arch; associated vascular ring compression syndromes involve persistent right aortic arch; the left subclavian artery may pass behind the esophagus; the d. may be large enough to compress the trachea and esophagus even after the vascular ring has been divided and may need to be resected or affixed to the chest wall or vertebral fascia.

laryngotracheal d., a d. from the floor of the caudal end of the pharynx which gives rise to the epithelium and glands of the larynx, trachea, bronchi, and lungs. Once this d. separates from the foregut, it is referred to as a tube.

Meckel d., the remains of the yolk stalk of the embryo, which, when persisting abnormally as a blind sac or pouch in the adult, is located on the ileum a short distance above the cecum; it may be attached to the umbilicus and, if the lining includes gastric mucosa, peptic ulceration and bleeding may result.

metanephric d., an outgrowth from the caudal portion of the mesonephric duct on either side, which grows cephalodorsally to make contact with the masses of metanephrogenous tissue (nephric blastemas) and give rise to the epithelial lining of the ureter and of the pelvis and the collecting ducts of the kidney.

Nuck d., SYN *processus* vaginalis of peritoneum.

pancreatic diverticula, the ventral and dorsal endodermal buds from the embryonic foregut that constitute the primordia of the parenchyma of the pancreas.

Pertik d., an abnormally deep recessus pharyngeus.

pharyngoesophageal d., most common d. of the esophagus; a pulsion d. developing between the inferior pharyngeal constrictor and the cricopharyngeus muscle. SYN hypopharyngeal d., Zenker d.

pituitary d., a tubular outgrowth of ectoderm from the stomodeum of the embryo; it grows dorsad toward the infundibular process of the diencephalon, around which it forms a cuplike mass, giving rise to the pars distalis and pars juxtaneuralis of the hypophysis. SYN craniopharyngeal canal, hypophyseal pouch, Rathke d., Rathke pocket, Rathke pouch.

pulsion d., a d. formed by pressure from within, frequently causing herniation of mucosa through the muscularis.

Rathke d., SYN pituitary d.

thyroid d., thyroglossal d., the endodermal bud from the floor of the embryonic pharynx; the primordium of the parenchyma of the thyroid gland.

tracheobronchial d., the endodermal lung primordium which will give rise to the epithelial lining of the respiratory tract. SYN lung bud.

traction d., a d. formed by the pulling force of contracting bands of adhesion, occurring mainly in the distal esophagus, from tuberculous hilar or mediastinal lymphadenitis.

true d., a term denoting a d. that includes all the layers of the wall from which it protrudes.

urethral d., a saclike outpouching of the urethral wall, either from a congenital defect or, more commonly, as a result of chronic penetrating inflammation.

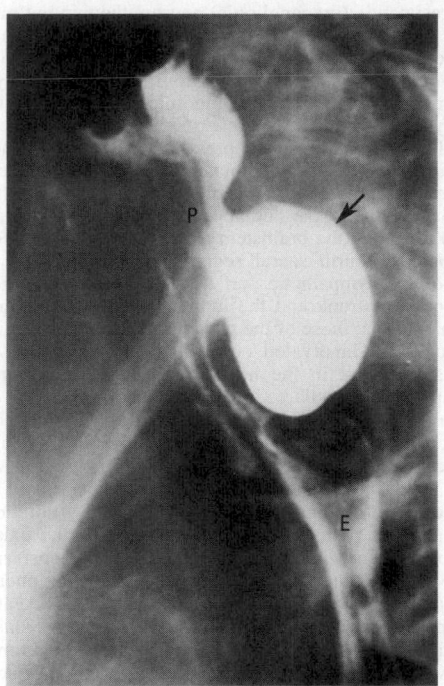

pharyngoesophageal diverticulum (arrow): contrast radiography, lateral view; note aspiration of contrast material; P=pharynx, E=esophagus

ventricular d., a congenital outpouching of the right or left ventricle.

vesical d., a d. of the bladder wall; may be either true or false type.

Zenker d., SYN pharyngoesophageal d.

di·vic·ine (dī′vis-ēn). A base with alkaloidal properties present in *Lathyrus sativus* that is responsible, in part at least, for the latter's poisonous action. SEE lathyrism.

divisio. SYN division.

d.'s anteriores plexus brachialis [TA], SYN anterior *divisions* of (trunks of) brachial plexus, under *division*.

d. autonomica systematis nervosi peripherici [TA], SYN autonomic *division* of nervous system.

d. lateralis dextra hepatis [TA], SYN right lateral *division* of liver.

d. lateralis sinistra, ✫official alternate term for left *lobe* of liver.

d. lateralis sinistra hepatis [TA], SYN left lateral *division* of liver.

d. medialis dextra hepatis [TA], SYN right medial *division* of liver.

d. medialis sinistra hepatis [TA], SYN left medial *division* of liver.

d.'s posteriores plexus brachialis [TA], SYN posterior *divisions* of (trunks of) brachial plexus, under *division*.

di·vi·sion (di-vizh′ŭn). A separating into two or more parts. SEE ALSO ramus. SYN divisio.

anterior primary d., SYN anterior *ramus* of spinal nerve.

anterior d.'s of (trunks of) brachial plexus [TA], portion of the superior, middle, and inferior trunks of the brachial plexus that are destined to serve the anterior or flexor compartments of the upper limb. SYN divisiones anteriores plexus brachialis [TA].

autonomic d. of nervous system [TA], that part of the nervous system which represents the motor innervation of smooth muscle, cardiac muscle, and gland cells. It consists of two physiologically and anatomically distinct, mutually antagonistic components: the sympathetic and parasympathetic parts. In both of these parts the pathway of innervation consists of a synaptic sequence of two motor neurons, one of which lies in the spinal cord or brainstem as the presynaptic (preganglionic) neuron, the thin but myelinated axon of which (presynaptic (preganglionic) or B fiber) emerges with an outgoing spinal or cranial nerve and synapses with one or more of the postsynaptic (postganglionic or, more strictly, ganglionic) neurons composing the autonomic ganglia; the unmyelinated postsynaptic fibers in turn innervate the smooth muscle, cardiac muscle, or gland cells. The presynaptic neurons of the sympathetic part lie in the intermediolateral cell column of the thoracic and upper two lumbar segments of the spinal gray matter; those of the parasympathetic part compose the visceral motor (visceral efferent) nuclei of the brainstem as well as the lateral column of the second to fourth sacral segments of the spinal cord. The ganglia of the sympathetic part are the paravertebral ganglia of the sympathetic trunk and the lumbar and sacral prevertebral or collateral ganglia; those of the parasympathetic part lie either near the organ to be innervated or as intramural ganglia within the organ itself except in the head, where there are four discrete parasympathetic ganglia (ciliary, otic, pterygopalatine, and submandibular). Impulse transmission from presynaptic to postsynaptic neuron is mediated by acetylcholine in both the sympathetic and parasympathetic parts; transmission from the postsynaptic fiber to the visceral effector tissues is classically said to be by acetylcholine in the parasympathetic part and by noradrenalin in the sympathetic part; recent evidence suggests the existence of further noncholinergic, nonadrenergic classes of postsynaptic fibers. SYN divisio autonomica systematis nervosi peripherici [TA], pars autonomica systematis nervosi peripherici [TA], autonomic part of peripheral nervous system ⋆, autonomic nervous system, involuntary nervous system, systema nervosum autonomicum, vegetative nervous system, visceral motor system, visceral nervous system.

cleavage d., the rapid mitotic d. of the zygote with decrease in size of individual cells or blastomeres and the formation of a morula. SEE ALSO cleavage (1).

conjugate d., simultaneous d. of haploid nuclei, as in Basidiomycota.

craniosacral d. of autonomic nervous system, SYN parasympathetic *part* of autonomic division of peripheral nervous system.

direct nuclear d., SYN amitosis.

equatorial d., nuclear d. in which each chromosome divides equally.

indirect nuclear d., SYN mitosis.

lateral d. of left liver, ⋆official alternate term for left *lobe* of liver.

left lateral d. of liver [TA], in the surgical schema for subdividing the liver, the portion that lies to the left of the approximately vertical plane of the left hepatic vein and includes the left posterior and anterior lateral segments (hepatic segments II and III); it corresponds with the left anatomic lobe of the liver, and so is demarcated externally by the falciform ligament on the diaphragmatic surface and by the fissures for the ligamentum venosum and ligamentum teres on the viscera surface. SYN divisio lateralis sinistra hepatis [TA].

left medial d. of liver [TA], in the surgical schema for subdividing the liver, the portion that lies between the approximately vertical planes of the left and middle hepatic veins and includes the left medial segment (hepatic segment IV); on the diaphragmatic surface, it is approximately the left third of the anatomic right lobe of the liver; on the visceral surface, its inferior portion corresponds to the quadrate lobe. SYN divisio medialis sinistra hepatis [TA].

meiotic d., SYN meiosis.

mitotic d., SYN mitosis.

multiplicative d., reproduction by simultaneous d. of a mother cell into a number of daughter cells. If the process occurs without fertilization of the mother cell, or encystment, the daughter cells are called merozoites; if they develop within a cyst, and usually after fertilization, they are called sporozoites.

posterior primary d., SYN posterior *ramus* of spinal nerve.

posterior d.'s of (trunks of) brachial plexus [TA], portion of the superior, middle, and inferior trunks of the brachial plexus that are destined to serve the posterior or extensor compartments of the upper limb. SYN divisiones posteriores plexus brachialis [TA].

reduction d., SEE *reduction* of chromosomes.

Remak nuclear d., SYN amitosis.

right lateral d. of liver [TA], in the surgical schema for subdividing the liver, the portion that lies to the right of the approximately vertical plane of the right hepatic vein and includes the right anterior and posterior lateral segments (hepatic segments VI and VII); it is approximately the right third of the right anatomic lobe of the liver. SYN divisio lateralis dextra hepatis [TA].

right medial d. of liver [TA], in the surgical schema for subdividing the liver, the portion that lies between the approximately vertical planes of the right and middle hepatic veins and includes the right anterior and posterior medial segments (hepatic segments V and VIII); it is approximately the middle third of the anatomic right lobe of the liver. SYN divisio medialis dextra hepatis [TA].

div. in p. aeg. Abbreviation for L. *divide in partes aequales,* divide into equal parts.

di·vulse (di-vŭls′). To tear away or apart. [L. *divello,* pp. *di-vulsus,* to pull apart]

di·vul·sion (di-vŭl′shŭn). **1.** Removal of a part by tearing. **2.** Forcible dilation of the walls of a cavity or canal.

di·vul·sor (di-vŭl′sĕr, -sōr). An instrument for forcible dilation of the urethra or other canal or cavity.

Dix. M.R., 20th century British otologist. SEE Dix-Hallpike *maneuver.*

di·xyr·a·zine (dī-zir′ă-zēn). A phenothiazine compound used as an antipsychotic.

di·zy·got·ic, di·zy·gous (dī′zī-got′ik, dī-zī′gŭs). Relating to twins derived from two separate zygotes, i.e., bearing the same genetic relationship as full sibs but sharing a common intrauterine environment. [G. *di-,* two, + *zygotos,* yoked together]

diz·zi·ness (diz′i-nes). Imprecise term commonly used to describe various symptoms such as faintness, giddiness, imbalance, lightheadedness, unsteadiness, or vertigo. SEE ALSO vertigo. [A. S. *dyzig,* foolish]

djen·kol·ic ac·id (jeng-kol′ik). *S,S′*-Methylenebiscysteine; a sulfur-containing amino acid, resembling cystine but with a methylene bridge between the two sulfur atoms; very insoluble. [*djenkol* bean, bean in which first isolated]

△**DL-.** Prefix (in small capital letters) denoting a substance consisting of equal quantities of the two enantiomorphs, D and L; replaces the older *dl-* as a more exact definition of structure.

*dl***-nar·co·tine** (nar′kō-tēn). SYN gnoscopine.

DM Abbreviation for adamsite; *diabetes* mellitus; diastolic *murmur;* dopamine.

DMA Abbreviation for dimethoxyamphetamine.

DMARD Acronym for disease modifying antirheumatic *drugs,* under *drug.*

DMC Abbreviation for *p,p,′*-dichlorodiphenyl methyl carbinol.

D.M.D. Abbreviation for Doctor of Dental Medicine.

dmf, DMF Abbreviation for decayed, missing, and filled teeth. SEE ALSO dmfs caries *index.*

dmfs, DMFS Abbreviation for decayed, missing, and filled surfaces. SEE ALSO dmfs caries *index.*

DMPP Abbreviation for dimethylphenylpiperazinium.

DMSA. SEE ^{99m}Tc-dimercaptosuccinic acid.

DMSO Abbreviation for dimethyl sulfoxide.

DMT Abbreviation for *N,N*-dimethyltryptamine.

DN Abbreviation for dibucaine number.

▮**DNA** Abbreviation for deoxyribonucleic acid. For terms bearing this abbreviation, see subentries under deoxyribonucleic acid.

DNA diagnostics. SYN genetic *testing.* SEE DNA markers, familial *screening,* prenatal *screening.*

dnaG SYN primase.

DNA markers. Segments of chromosomal DNA known to be linked with heritable traits or diseases. Although the markers themselves do not produce the conditions, they exist in concert with the genes responsible and are passed on with them. Certain markers, restriction fragment length polymorphisms, consist of

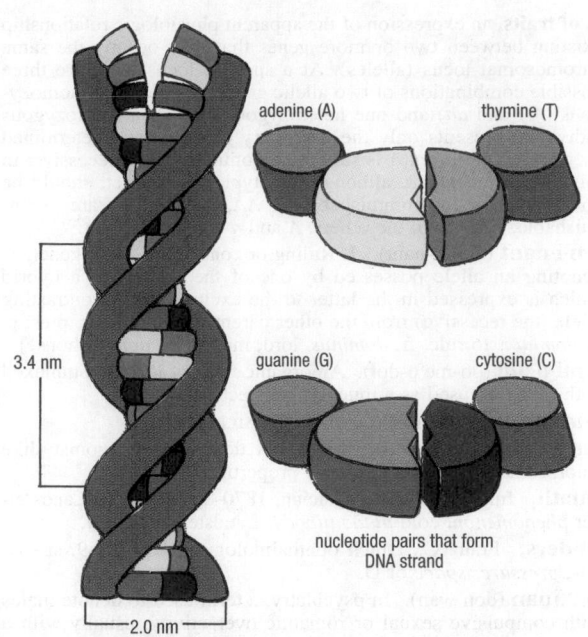

adenine (A)

thymine (T)

3.4 nm

guanine (G)

cytosine (C)

nucleotide pairs that form
DNA strand

2.0 nm

DNA (deoxyribonucleic acid)

segments of DNA that can be identified on autoradiographs (produced after digestion of the DNA by restriction enzymes and segregation of the resulting fragments through gel electrophoresis).

DNAse, DNAase, DNase Abbreviations for deoxyribonuclease.

DNP, Dnp 1. Abbreviation for 2,4-dinitrophenol. **2.** Abbreviation for deoxyribonucleoprotein.

DNR Abbreviation for "do not resuscitate."

Dns, DNS Abbreviations for dansyl.

D.O. Abbreviation for Doctor of Osteopathy.

DOA Abbreviation for dead on arrival.

do·bu·ta·mine (dō-bū′tă-mēn). A synthetic derivative of dopamine characterized by prominent inotropic but weak chronotropic and arrhythmogenic properties; a cardiotonic agent.

DOC Abbreviation for deoxycorticosterone; deoxycholate.

d'Ocagne, Philbert M., French mathematician, 1862–1938. SEE d'O. *nomogram.*

***n*-doc·o·sa·no·ic ac·id** (dō′kō-san-ō′ik). SYN behenic acid.

doc·tor (dok′ter). **1.** A title conferred by a university on one who has followed a prescribed course of study, or given as a title of distinction; as d. of medicine, laws, philosophy, etc. **2.** A physician, especially one upon whom has been conferred the degree of M.D. by a university or medical school. [L. a teacher, fr. *doceo,* pp. *doctus,* to teach]

doc·trine (dok′trin). A particular system of principles taught or advocated. [L. *doceo,* to teach]

Arrhenius d., the theory of electrolytic dissociation (1887) that became the basis of our modern understanding of electrolytes: in an electrically conductive solution (e.g., acid, base, or salt), free ions are present before electrolysis, and the proportion of molecules dissociated into ions can be calculated from measurements of electrical conductivity as well as of osmotic pressure. SYN Arrhenius law.

humoral d., the ancient Greek theory of the four body humors (blood, yellow and black bile, and phlegm) that determined health and disease. The humors were associated with the four elements (air, fire, earth, and water), which in turn were paired with one of the qualities (hot, cold, dry, and moist). A proper and evenly balanced mixture of the humors characterized health of body and mind; an imperfect balance resulted in disease. Temperament of body or mind also was supposed to be determined, e.g., sanguine

(blood), choleric (yellow bile), melancholic (black bile), or phlegmatic (phlegm). SYN fluidism, humoralism, humorism.

Monro d., a d. that states that the cranial cavity is a closed rigid box and that therefore a change in the quantity of intracranial blood can occur only through the displacement of or replacement by cerebrospinal fluid. SYN Monro-Kellie d.

Monro-Kellie d., SYN Monro d.

doc·u·sate cal·ci·um (dok′ū-sāt). A surface-active agent used in the treatment of constipation as a nonlaxative fecal softener. SYN dioctyl calcium sulfosuccinate.

doc·u·sate so·di·um. A surface-active agent used as a dispersing agent in topically applied preparations. After oral administration it lowers the surface tension of the gastrointestinal tract and is used in the treatment of constipation as a wetting agent and stool softener. SYN dioctyl sodium sulfosuccinate.

do·de·cane (dō′dĕ-kān). n-$C_{12}H_{26}$; a straight, unbranched, saturated hydrocarbon containing 12 carbon atoms; the 12th member of the alkane series that begins with methane.

***n*-do·dec·a·no·ic ac·id** (dō-dek′ă-nō-ik). SYN lauric acid.

do·dec·an·o·yl-CoA syn·the·tase (dō-dek′ăn-ō-il-kō-āsin′the-tās). SYN long-chain fatty acid-CoA ligase.

do·de·car·bo·ni·um chlo·ride (dō-dē-kar-bō′nē-ŭm). An antiseptic.

do·de·cyl (dō′dĕ-sil). The radical of dodecane.

d. gallate, an antioxidant.

d. sulfate, SEE *sodium* dodecyl sulfate.

Döderlein, Albert, S.G., German obstetrician, 1860–1941. SEE D. *bacillus.*

Doerfler, Leo G., U.S. audiologist, *1919. SEE D.-Stewart *test.*

Dogiel, Alexander S., Russian histologist, 1852–1922. SEE D. *corpuscle.*

Dogiel, Jan von, Russian anatomist and physiologist, 1830–1905. SEE D. *cells,* under *cell.*

dog·ma. A theory or belief that is formally stated, defined, and thought to be true.

central d., the proposition that while genetic information is transferred from parent to offspring via DNA duplication, within the cell, genetic information is transferred from DNA to mRNA (transcription) and then to protein (translation); proposed by Francis Crick.

dog·mat·ic (dog-mat′ik). SEE dogmatic *school.* [G. *dogmatikos,* concerning opinions; *d. iatroi,* physicians who go by general principles; fr. *dogma,* an opinion]

dog·ma·tist (dog′mă-tist). A follower of the dogmatic *school.*

Döhle, Karl G.P., German histologist and pathologist, 1855–1928. SEE D. *bodies,* under *body, inclusions,* under *inclusion.*

Doisy, Edward A., U.S. biochemist and Nobel laureate, 1893–1986. SEE Allen-D. *test, unit.*

dol (dōl). A unit measure of pain. [L. *dolor,* pain]

⚠**dolicho-.** Long. [G. *dolichos*]

dol·i·cho·ce·phal·ic, dol·i·cho·ceph·a·lous (dol-i-kō-sĕ-fal′ik, -sef′ă-lŭs). Having a disproportionately long head; denoting a skull with a cephalic index below 75. SYN dolichocranial. [dolicho- + G. *kephalē,* head]

dol·i·cho·ceph·a·ly, dol·i·cho·ceph·a·lism (dol-i-kō-sef′ă-lē, sef′ă-lizm). The condition of being dolichocephalic.

dol·i·cho·co·lon (dol-i-kō-kō′lŏn). A colon of abnormal length. [dolicho- + G. *kōlon,* colon]

dol·i·cho·cra·ni·al (dol-i-kō-krā′nē-ăl). SYN dolichocephalic.

dol·i·cho·fa·cial (dol-i-kō-fā′shăl). SYN dolichoprosopic.

dol·i·chol (dol′i-kol). Polyisoprenes in which the terminal member is saturated and oxidized to an alcohol, usually phosphorylated and often glycosylated; found in endoplasmic reticulum, but not in mitochondrial or plasma membranes; urinary levels are elevated in disorders exhibiting abnormal skin, rectal, or brain profiles in electron microscopy of biopsies.

d. phosphate, an intermediate in the glycosylation of proteins and lipids; contains 11–24 isoprene units; a product of the isoprenylation pathway; participates in the formation of glycosylphosphatidylinositol anchors of proteins in biomembranes.

do

dol·i·cho·pel·lic, dol·i·cho·pel·vic (dol-i-kō-pel'ik, -pel'vik). Having a disproportionately long pelvis; denoting a pelvis with a pelvic index above 95. [dolicho- + G. *pellis,* bowl (pelvis)]

dol·i·cho·pro·sop·ic, dol·i·cho·pro·so·pous (dol-i-kō-pros-ō' pik, -kō-pros'ō-pŭs). Having a disproportionately long face. SYN dolichofacial. [dolicho- + G. *prosōpikos,* facial]

dol·i·cho·sten·o·me·lia (dol'i-kō-sten'ō-mē'lē-ă). Narrow body habitus which, like arachnodactyly, is a common feature of several kinds of hereditary disorders of connective tissue. [dolicho- + G. *stenos,* narrow, + *melos,* limb]

dol·i·cho·u·ran·ic, dol·i·chu·ran·ic (dol'i-kō-ū-ran'ik, dol-ik-ū-). Having a long palate, with a palatal index below 110. [dolicho- + G. *ouranos,* vault of the palate]

Doll, Richard, British epidemiologist, *1912. SEE Armitage-D. model.

do·lor (dō'lōr). Pain, as one of the four signs of inflammation (d., calor, rubor, tumor) enunciated by Celsus. [L.]

d. cap'itis, headache, especially due to changes in the scalp or bones rather than in the intracranial structures.

do·lo·rif·ic (dō-lōr-if'ik). Pain-producing.

do·lo·rim·e·try (dō-lō-rim'ĕ-trē). The measurement of pain. [L. *dolor,* pain, + G. *metron,* measure]

do·lor·ol·o·gy (dō-lōr-ol'ō-jē). The study and treatment of pain. [L. *dolor,* pain, + G. *logos,* study]

DOM Abbreviation for 2,5-dimethoxy-4-methylamphetamine.

do·main (dō-mān'). **1.** Homologous unit of approximately 110–120 amino acids, groups of which make up the light and heavy chains of the immunoglobulin molecule; each serves a specific function. The light chain has two d.'s, one in the variable region and one in the constant region of the chain; the heavy chain has four to five d.'s, depending upon the class of immunoglobulin, one in the variable region and the remaining ones in the constant region. **2.** A region of a protein having some distinctive physical feature or role. **3.** An independently folded, globular structure composed of one section of a polypeptide chain. A d. may interact with another d.; it may be associated with a particular function. D.'s can vary in size. [Fr. *domaine,* fr. L. *dominium,* property, dominion]

dinucleotide d., SYN dinucleotide *fold.*

Dombrock blood group. See Blood Groups appendix.

dome.

d. of pleura, ✕ official alternate term for cervical *pleura.*

do·mes·tic vi·o·lence. Intentionally inflicted injury perpetrated by and on family member(s); varieties include spouse abuse, child abuse, and sexual abuse, including incest. Various kinds of abuse, such as sexual abuse, also happen outside the family unit. The American Medical Association, like similar organizations in other countries, has issued advisory notices to physicians on the detection and treatment of d. v.

dom·i·cil·i·at·ed (dō-mi-sil'ē-āt-ed). A state of close association of an organism within human abodes or activities, such that partial domestication results, leading to the organism's dependence on continued association with the human environment; this frequently results in the d. organism becoming a noxious pest, a vector, or an intermediate host of human disease. [L. *domicilium,* a dwelling]

dom·i·nance (dom'i-nans). The state of being dominant.

cerebral d., the fact that one hemisphere is dominant over the other and will exercise greater influence over certain functions; the left cerebral hemisphere is usually dominant in the control of speech, language and analytical processing, and mathematics, while the right hemisphere (usually nondominant) processes spatial concepts and language as related to certain types of visual images; handedness (right-handed people have left cerebral d.) is considered a general example of cerebral d.

false d., SYN quasidominance.

genetic d., denoting a pattern of inheritance of an autosomal mendelian trait due to a gene that always manifests itself phenotypically; generally, the phenotype in the homozygote is more severe than in the heterozygote, but details depend on what criterion of phenotyping is used.

d. of traits, an expression of the apparent physiologic relationship existing between two or more genes that may occupy the same chromosomal locus (alleles). At a specific locus there are three possible combinations of two allelic genes, A and a: two homozygous (AA and aa) and one heterozygous (Aa). If a heterozygous individual presents only the hereditary characteristic determined by gene A, but not a, A is said to be dominant and a recessive; in this case, AA and Aa, although genotypically distinct, should be phenotypically indistinguishable. If AA, Aa, and aa are distinguishable, each from the others, A and a are codominant.

dom·i·nant (dom'i-nant). **1.** Ruling or controlling. **2.** In genetics, denoting an allele possessed by one of the parents of a hybrid which is expressed in the latter to the exclusion of a contrasting allele (the recessive) from the other parent. [L. *dominans,* pres. p. of *dominor,* to rule, fr. *dominus,* lord, master, fr. *domus,* house]

do·mi·o·dol (do-mē'ō-dol). An organic form of iodine complexed with glycerol; used as a mucolytic/expectorant.

do·mi·phen bro·mide (dō'mi-fen). An antiseptic.

dom·per·i·done (dom-per'ĭ-dōn). A dopamine antagonist (like chlorpromazine) with antiemetic properties.

Donath, Julius, German physician, 1870–1950. SEE D.-Landsteiner *phenomenon,* cold *autoantibody;* Landsteiner-D. *test.*

Donders, Franz C., Dutch ophthalmologist, 1818–1889. SEE D. *law, pressure; space* of D.

Don Juan (don wan). In psychiatry, a term used to denote males with compulsive sexual or romantic overactivity, usually with a succession of female partners. [legendary Spanish nobleman]

Don Juan·ism (don wăn'izm). SEE Don Juan.

Donnan, Frederick G., English physical chemist, 1870–1956. SEE D. *equilibrium;* Gibbs-D. *equilibrium.*

Donné, Alfred, French physician, 1801–1878. SEE D. *corpuscle.*

Donohue, William L., Canadian pediatric pathologist, 1906–1984. SEE D. *disease.*

do·nor (dō'ner). **1.** An individual from whom blood, tissue, or an organ is taken for transplantation. **2.** A compound that will transfer an atom or a radical to an acceptor; e.g., methionine is a methyl d.; glutathione is a glutamyl d. **3.** An atom that readily yields electrons to an acceptor; e.g., nitrogen, which will donate both electrons to a shared pool in forming a coordinate bond. [L. *dono,* pp. *donatus,* to donate, to give]

hydrogen d., a metabolite from which hydrogen is removed (by a dehydrogenase system) and transferred by a hydrogen carrier to another metabolite, which is thus reduced.

universal d., in blood grouping, a person belonging to group O; i.e., one whose erythrocytes do not contain either agglutinogen A or B and are, therefore, not agglutinated by plasma containing either of the ordinary isoagglutinins.

Donovan, Charles, Irish surgeon, 1863–1951. SEE D. *bodies,* under *body;* Leishman-D. *body.*

Doose, H., 20th century German pediatrician and epileptologist. SEE D. *syndrome.*

do·pa, DO·PA, Do·pa (dō'pă). An intermediate in the catabolism of L-phenylalanine and L-tyrosine, and in the biosynthesis of norepinephrine, epinephrine, and melanin; the L form, levodopa, is biologically active. SEE dopa *reaction.* SYN 3,4-dihydroxyphenylalanine.

alpha methyl d., SYN methyldopa.

d. decarboxylase, SYN aromatic D-amino acid decarboxylase.

decarboxylated d., SYN dopamine.

d. oxidase, provisional name given the enzyme(s) catalyzing the formation of melanins from d.; it now appears that the copper-containing monophenol monooxygenases and/or catechol oxidases are responsible for the oxidation of L-tyrosine to d. and d. quinone.

d. quinone, an oxidation product of d. and an intermediate in the formation of melanin from tyrosine.

L-dopa. SYN levodopa.

do·pa·mine (DM) (dō'pă-mēn). An intermediate in tyrosine metabolism and precursor of norepinephrine and epinephrine; it accounts for 90% of the catecholamines; its presence in the central nervous system and localization in the basal ganglia (caudate and lentiform nuclei) suggest that d. may have other functions. Depletion of d. produces Parkinson *disease*. SYN 3-hydroxytyramine, decarboxylated dopa.

d. hydrochloride, a biogenic amine and neural transmitter substance, used as a vasopressor agent for treatment of shock.

do·pa·mine β-hy·drox·y·lase. SYN dopamine β-monooxygenase.

do·pa·mine β-mon·o·ox·y·gen·ase. A copper-containing enzyme catalyzing oxidation of ascorbate and 3,4-dihydroxyphenylethylamine simultaneously by O_2 to yield norepinephrine, dehydroascorbate, and water; a crucial step in catecholamine metabolism. The enzyme is stimulated by fumarate. SYN dopamine β-hydroxylase.

do·pa·min·er·gic (dō′pă-min-er′jik). Relating to nerve cells or fibers that employ dopamine as their neurotransmitter. [dopamine + G. *ergon,* work]

dope (dōp). **1.** Any drug, either stimulating or depressing, administered for its temporary effect, or taken habitually or addictively. **2.** To administer or take such a drug. [Dutch, *doop,* sauce]

dop·ing (dōp′ing). The administration of foreign substances to an individual; often used in reference to athletes who try to stimulate physical and psychological strength.

Doppler, Johann Christian, Austrian mathematician and physicist, 1803–1853. SEE D. *echocardiography, effect, phenomenon, shift, ultrasonography.*

Dop·pler. A diagnostic instrument that emits an ultrasonic beam into the body; the ultrasound reflected from moving structures changes its frequency (Doppler effect). Of diagnostic value in peripheral vascular and cardiac disease.

do·ra·pho·bia (dō-ră-fō′bē-ă). Morbid fear of touching the skin or fur of animals. [G. *dora,* hide, skin, + *phobos,* fear]

Dorello, P., Italian anatomist, *1872. SEE D. *canal.*

Dorendorf, H., German physician, *1866. SEE D. *sign.*

Dorfman, Maurice L., 20th century Israeli dermatologist. SEE D.-Chanarin *syndrome.*

Döring, G., 20th century German neurologist. SEE Pette-D. *disease.*

dor·nase (dōr′nās). Obsolete contraction of deoxyribonuclease. SEE ALSO streptodornase.

pancreatic d., a stabilized deoxyribonuclease preparation from beef pancreas; used by inhalation in the form of aerosols to reduce thick mucopurulent secretions in certain bronchopulmonary infections.

Dorno, Carl, Swiss climatologist, 1865–1942.

do·ro·ma·ni·a (dō-rō-mā′nē-ă). An abnormal desire to give presents. [G. *dōron,* gift, + *mania,* insanity]

dor·sa (dōr′să). Plural of dorsum.

dor·sab·dom·i·nal (dōr-sab-dom′i-nal). Relating to the back and the abdomen.

dor·sad (dor′sad). Toward or in the direction of the back. [L. *dorsum,* back, + *ad,* to]

dor·sal (dōr′săl) [TA]. **1.** Pertaining to the back or any dorsum. SYN tergal. **2.** SYN posterior (2). **3.** In veterinary anatomy, pertaining to the back or upper surface of an animal. Often used to indicate the position of one structure relative to another; i.e., nearer the back surface of the body. **4.** Old term meaning thoracic, in a limited sense; e.g., d. vertebrae. [Mediev. L. *dorsalis,* fr. *dorsum,* back]

dor·sa·lis (dōr-sā′lis) [TA]. SYN posterior (2). [L.]

Dorset, Marion, U.S. bacteriologist, 1872–1935. SEE D. culture egg *medium.*

dor·si·duct (dōr′si-dŭkt). To draw backward or toward the back. [L. *dorsum,* back, + *duco,* pp. *ductus,* to draw]

dor·si·flex·ion (dōr-si-flek′shŭn). Upward movement (extension) of the foot or toes or of the hand or fingers.

dor·si·scap·u·lar (dōr′si-skap′ū-lăr). Relating to the dorsal surface of the scapula.

dor·si·spi·nal (dōr′si-spī′năl). Relating to the vertebral column, especially to its dorsal aspect.

dor·so·ceph·a·lad (dōr′sō-sef′ă-lad). Toward the occiput, or

back of the head. [L. *dorsum,* back, + G. *kephalē,* head, + L. *ad,* to]

dor·so·lat·er·al (dōr-sō-lat′er-ăl). Relating to the back and the side.

dor·so·lum·bar (dōr-sō-lŭm′bar). Referring to the back in the region of the lower thoracic and upper lumbar vertebrae.

dor·so·ven·trad (dōr-sō-ven′trad). In a direction from the dorsal to the ventral aspect.

dor·sum, gen. **dor·si,** pl. **dor·sa** (dōr′sŭm, -sī, -să) [TA]. **1.** The back of the body. **2.** The upper or posterior surface, or the back, of any part. SYN tergum. [L. back]

d. ephip′pii, SYN d. sellae.

d. of foot [TA], the back, or upper surface, of the foot. SYN d. pedis [TA].

d. of hand [TA], the back of the hand; surface of hand opposite the palm.

d. lin′guae [TA], SYN d. of tongue.

d. ma′nus [TA], SYN dorsum of *hand.*

d. na′si [TA], SYN d. of nose.

d. of nose [TA], the external ridge of the nose, looking forward and upward. SYN d. nasi [TA].

d. pe′dis [TA], SYN d. of foot.

d. of penis [TA], the aspect of the penis opposite to that of the urethra. SYN d. penis [TA].

d. pe′nis [TA], SYN d. of penis.

d. scap′ulae, the posterior surface of the scapula.

d. sel′lae [TA], a square portion of bone on the body of the sphenoid posterior to the sella turcica or hypophysial fossa. SYN d. ephippii.

d. of tongue [TA], the back of the tongue; the upper surface of the tongue divided by the sulcus terminalis into an anterior two-thirds, the pars presulcalis (presulcal part), and a posterior one-third, the pars postsulcalis (postsulcal part). SYN d. linguae [TA].

dos·age (dō′sij). **1.** The giving of medicine or other therapeutic agent in prescribed amounts. **2.** The determination of the proper dose of a remedy. Cf. dose. **3.** In nuclear medicine, quantity of radiopharmaceutical given.

dose (dōs). **1.** The quantity of a drug or other remedy to be taken or applied all at one time or in fractional amounts within a given period. Cf. dosage (2). **2.** In nuclear medicine, amount of energy absorbed per unit mass of irradiated material (absorbed d.). SEE ALSO dosage (3). [G. *dosis,* a giving]

absorbed d., the amount of energy absorbed per unit mass of irradiated material at the target site; in radiation therapy, the former unit for absorbed d. is the rad (100 ergs/g); the current (SI) unit is the gray (1 J/kg or 100 rad).

air d., SYN exposure d.

bone marrow d., the cumulative d. to the blood-forming organ from therapeutic or nuclear fallout irradiation; the presumed leukemogenic d.

booster d., a d. given at some time after an initial d. to enhance the effect, said usually of antigens for the production of antibodies.

cumulative d., the total d. resulting from repeated exposures to radiation or chemotherapy of the same part of the body or of the whole body.

curative d. (CD, CD^{50}), (1) the quantity of any substance required to effect the cure of a disease or that will correct the manifestations of a deficiency of a particular factor in the diet; **(2)** effective d. used with therapeutically applied compounds. SEE ALSO CD^{50}. SYN therapeutic d.

daily d., the total amount of a remedy that is to be taken within 24 hours.

depth d., the d. of radiation at a distance beneath the surface, including secondary radiation or scatter, in proportion to the d. at the surface.

divided d., a definite fraction of a full d.; given repeatedly at short intervals so that the full d. is taken within a specified period, usually one day. SYN fractional d.

effective d. (ED), (1) the d. that produces a specific effect; when followed by a subscript (generally "ED_{50}"), it denotes the d.

do

having such an effect on a certain percentage (e.g., 50%) of the test animals; ED_{50} is the median effective dose; **(2)** in radiation protection, the sum of the equivalent d.'s in all tissues and organs of the body weighted for tissue effects of radiation. The SI unit of effective d. is the sievert (Sv) (=100 rem). **(3)** in diagnostic radiology, if a patient weighing W absorbs A joules of energy, and the experimentally derived ratio of effective dose to energy absorbed in an anthropomorphic phantom with mass M is R, then the effective d. is $A \cdot R \cdot M/W$. This formula results in a larger value for children despite their lesser absorption of radiation.

epilation d., the minimum amount of radiation sufficient to produce hair loss, usually in 10 to 14 days.

equianalgesic d., the qualitative ratio between actual milligram potency of comparable analgesics required to achieve the equivalent therapeutic effect.

equivalent d., in radiation protection, the absorbed d. averaged over a tissue or organ and weighted for the quality of the type of radiation. The unit of equivalent d. is the sievert.

erythema d., the minimum amount of x-rays or other form of radiation sufficient to produce erythema; historically, this d. was indicated by the Sabouraud meter as the B tint, the Holzknecht as 5(5H), the Hampson as 4, and the Kienbock as 10.

exit d., the exposure dose of radiation leaving a body opposite the portal of entry.

exposure d., the radiation d., expressed in roentgens, delivered at a point in free air. SYN air d.

fractional d., SYN divided d.

gonad d., the exposure d. to the male or female gonad, usually from incidental secondary radiation in diagnostic or therapeutic irradiation, or from whole-body irradiation. SYN gonadal d.

gonadal d., SYN gonad d.

initial d., SYN loading d.

integral d., the total energy absorbed by the body, the product of the mass of tissue irradiated and the absorbed d.; unit, the gram rad.

L d.'s, a group of terms that indicate the relative activity or potency of diphtheria toxin; the L d.'s are distinctly different from the minimal lethal d. and minimal reacting d., inasmuch as the latter two represent the direct effects of toxin, whereas the L d.'s pertain to the combining power of toxin with specific antitoxin. ["L" for L. *limes,* limit, boundary]

L^+ d., L_+ d., alternatives for L†, the limes tod d. of diphtheria toxin, i.e., the smallest amount of toxin that, when mixed with one unit of antitoxin and injected subcutaneously into a 250-g guinea pig, results in death of the animal within 96 hours (based on the average in a series); on theoretical grounds, one might expect that the difference between the L_+ and L_0 d.'s would be identical to 1 MLD, but this is not so in actual practice; with various toxic filtrates, the difference may range from several to more than 100 MLDs, indicating that the toxin-antitoxin combination is *not* a firm chemical union that occurs in constant proportions.

lethal d. (LD), the d. of a chemical or biologic preparation (e.g., a bacterial exotoxin or a suspension of bacteria) that is likely to cause death; it varies in relation to the type of animal and the route of administration; when followed by a subscript (generally "LD_{50}" or median lethal d.), it denotes the d. likely to cause death in a certain percentage (e.g., 50%) of the test animals; median lethal d. is LD_{50}, absolute lethal d. is LD_{100}, and minimal lethal d. is LD_{05}.

Lf d., L_f d., the limes flocculation d. of diphtheria toxin, i.e., the smallest amount of toxin that, when mixed with one unit of antitoxin, yields the most rapid flocculation in the Ramon test (in vitro); in general, the L_f d. is slightly less than the L_r d.

Lo d., L_0 d., the limes nul d. of diphtheria toxin, i.e., the largest amount of toxin that, when mixed with one unit of antitoxin and injected subcutaneously into a 250-g guinea pig, yields no recognizable reaction in the average of a series; actually, the L_0d. is usually recorded as the one that causes a barely perceptible local edema at the site of inoculation.

loading d., a comparatively large d. given at the beginning of treatment to start getting the effect of a drug, especially one with slow clearance thus requiring a long period to achieve stable blood levels without a high initial dose. SYN initial d.

Lr d., L_r d., the limes reacting d. of diphtheria toxin, i.e., the smallest amount of toxin that, when mixed with one unit of antitoxin and injected intracutaneously in the shaved skin of a susceptible guinea pig, yields a minimal, positive reaction and inflammation localized to the region of the injection; the L_rd. closely approximates the L_0d., as would be expected, inasmuch as a slight excess of unneutralized toxin results in a reaction.

maintenance d., SEE maintenance drug *therapy.*

maximal d., the largest amount of a drug or physical procedure that an adult can take with safety.

maximal permissible d., SEE maximum permissible d.

maximum permissible d. (MPD), defined by the International Commission on Radiological Protection as the greatest d. of radiation which, in the light of present knowledge, is not expected to cause detectable bodily injury to persons at any time during their lifetime. This d. has been reduced with each Commission report. The MPD is given in terms of acute or chronic exposure of the whole body or of organs, systems, or regions of the body and differs for persons who are occupationally exposed versus the public at large.

maximum tolerated d., d. that produces grade 3 (severe) or grade 4 (life-threatening) toxicity in 30% or fewer of the patients tested.

median effective dose (ED_{50}), SEE effective d.

minimal d., the smallest amount of a drug or physical procedure that will produce a desired physiologic effect in an adult.

minimal infecting d. (MID), the smallest quantity of infectious material regularly producing infection; usually expressed as $I.D._{-50}$, the quantity causing infection in 50% of a suitable series of animals or cells (cell cultures).

minimal lethal d. (MLD, mld), (1) the minimal d. of a toxic substance or infectious agent that is lethal, as assayed in various experimental animals (e.g., the least amount of diphtheria toxin that, on an average, kills a 250-g guinea pig within 96 h after subcutaneous inoculation); when followed by a subscript (generally "MLD_{50}"), denotes the minimal dose that is lethal to a certain percentage (e.g., 50%) of animals so assayed; **(2)** ld_{05}. SEE lethal d.

minimal reacting d. (MRD, mrd), the minimal d. of a toxic substance causing a reaction, as manifested in the skin of a series of susceptible test animals; the assay is based on the development of a characteristic, minimal but definite, "standard," focal inflammation (congestion and edema, induration, degenerative changes, and desquamation of epidermal cells).

optimum d., the d. of a drug or radiation that will produce the desired effect with minimum likelihood of undesirable symptoms.

preventive d., the smallest amount of any substance that will prevent occurrence of symptoms of a disease or the consequences of a lack of a particular factor in the diet.

sensitizing d., in experimental anaphylaxis, the antigenic inoculum that renders an animal susceptible (sensitive) to anaphylactic shock following a subsequent inoculum (shocking d.) of the same antigen (anaphylactogen).

shocking d., in experimental anaphylaxis, the inoculum of antigen that causes anaphylactic shock in an animal sensitized by a previous inoculum (sensitizing d.) of the same antigen.

skin d., the absorbed dose of radiation delivered to the skin surface.

therapeutic d., SYN curative d.

tissue culture infectious d. (TCID$_{50}$, TCD$_{50}$), the quantity of a cytopathogenic agent, such as a virus, that will produce a cytopathic effect in 50% of the cultures inoculated.

tolerance d., the largest d. of a remedy that can be accepted without the production of injurious symptoms.

dos·im·e·ter (dō-sim′ĕ-ter). A device for measuring radiation, especially x-rays. [G. *dosis,* dose, + *metron,* measure]

do·sim·e·try (dō-sim′ĕ-trē). Measurement of radiation exposure, especially x-rays or gamma rays; calculation of radiation dose from internally administered radionuclides.

thermoluminescence d., the calculation of a radiation dose by measuring the light output after heating a special absorbent material (e.g., lithium fluoride) placed in the radiation beam; the light output is proportional to the amount of radiation exposure.

x-ray d., SYN roentgenometry.

dot (dŏt). A small spot.

Gunn d.'s, minute, highly glistening, white or yellowish specks usually seen in the posterior part of the fundus; nonpathologic.

Horner-Trantas d.'s, evanescent white cellular infiltrates occurring in the bulbar form of vernal keratoconjunctivitis.

Maurer d.'s, finely granular precipitates or irregular cytoplasmic particles that usually occur diffusely in red blood cells infected with the trophozoites of *Plasmodium falciparum,* occasionally those of *P. malariae;* rarely observed in *P. falciparum* blood smears because its trophozoites seldom are seen in peripheral blood. SYN Maurer clefts.

Mittendorf d., a small d. visible on the posterior aspect of the lens capsule on ophthalmologic examination that represents a remnant of the primitive hyaloid vascular system.

Schüffner d.'s, fine, round, uniform red or red-yellow d.'s (as colored with Romanovsky stains) characteristically observed in erythrocytes infected with *Plasmodium vivax* and *P. ovale,* but not ordinarily found in *P. malariae* and *P. falciparum* infections. SYN Schüffner granules.

Trantas d.'s, pale, grayish red, uneven nodules of gelatinous aspect at the limbal conjunctiva in vernal conjunctivitis.

Ziemann d.'s, fine d.'s seen in erythrocytes in malariae malaria. SYN Ziemann stippling.

dot·age (dō'tij). The deterioration of previously intact mental powers, common in old age.

dou·blet (dŭb'let). **1.** A combination of two lenses designed to correct the chromatic and spherical aberration. **2.** SYN dipole. **3.** Any sequence of two nucleotides in a polynucleotide strand. **4.** A closely spaced pair of peaks or lines in a spectrum.

Wollaston d., a combination of two planoconvex lenses in the eyepiece of a microscope designed to correct the chromatic aberration.

douche (doosh). **1.** A current of water, gas, or vapor directed against a surface or projected into a cavity. **2.** An instrument for giving a d. **3.** To apply a d. [Fr. fr. *doucher,* to pour]

Douglas, Claude G., English physiologist, 1882–1963. SEE D. *bag.*

Douglas, John C., Irish obstetrician, 1777–1850. SEE D. *mechanism.*

Douglas, James, Scottish anatomist in London, 1675–1742. SEE D. *abscess, cul-de-sac, fold, line, pouch; cavum* douglasi.

Douglas, Beverly, U.S. surgeon, 1891–1975.

dove·tail (dŭv'tāl). A widened portion of a cavity preparation usually established to increase the retention and resistance form.

dow·el (dow'l). **1.** A cast gold or preformed metal pin placed into a root canal for the purpose of providing retention for a crown. **2.** A preformed metal pin placed in a copper-plated die to provide a die stem. **3.** A pin or rod that aligns or joins two structures by fitting into holes in both of them; d.'s of various materials are used in orthopaedic surgery and dentistry. **4.** SYN dowel *graft.*

Down, John Langdon H., English physician, 1828–1896. SEE D. *syndrome.*

Downey, Hal, U.S. hematologist, 1877–1959. SEE D. *cell.*

down·growth (doun-grōth). Something that grows downward; the process of growing in a downward direction.

epithelial d., the invasion of surface epithelium into the interior of the eye as a consequence of a penetrating ocular wound.

down-reg·u·la·tion. Development of a refractory or tolerant state consequent upon repeated administration of a pharmacologically or physiologically active substance; often accompanied by an initial decrease in affinity of receptors for the agent and a subsequent diminution in the number of receptors.

Downs, William B., U.S. orthodontist, 1899–1966. SEE D. *analysis.*

Dox, Arthur W., U.S. chemist, *1882. SEE Czapek-D. *medium.*

dox·a·cu·ri·um chlo·ride (doks'a-koo'rē-um). A nondepolarizing neuromuscular blocking drug similar to pancuronium but without cardiovascular side effects.

dox·a·pram hy·dro·chlo·ride (doks'ă-pram). A central nervous system stimulant, advocated but infrequently used as a respiratory stimulant in anesthesia.

dox·a·zo·cin (doks'ă-zō-sin). An antihypertensive agent that selectively blocks the α_1 (postjunctional) subtype of α-adrenergic receptors; resembles prazocin in pharmacologic actions. Prevents the blood pressure elevating effects of norepinephrine, phenylephrine, and other agonists at vascular α_1-receptors.

dox·e·pin hy·dro·chlo·ride (dok'sĕ-pin). An antidepressant agent.

dox·o·phyl·line (doks'ō-fil'in). A theophyllinelike drug used, though rarely in the U.S., as a bronchodilator in asthma and chronic obstructive pulmonary disease.

dox·o·ru·bi·cin (dok'sō-roo'bi-sin). An antineoplastic antibiotic isolated from *Streptomyces peucetius;* also used in cytogenetics to produce Q-type chromosome bands. SYN adriamycin.

dox·y·cy·cline (dok-sē-sī'klēn). A broad-spectrum antibiotic.

dox·yl·a·mine suc·ci·nate (dok-sil'ă-mēn). An antihistaminic. SYN mereprine.

Doyère, Louis, French physiologist, 1811–1863. SEE D. *eminence.*

Doyle, J.B., U.S. gynecologist, *1907. SEE D. *operation.*

Doyne, Robert Walter, English ophthalmologist, 1857–1916. SEE D. honeycomb *choroidopathy.*

D.P. Abbreviation for Doctor of Podiatry.

D.P.H. Abbreviation for Department of Public Health; Doctor of Public Health; Diploma of Public Health.

D.P.M. Abbreviation for Doctor of Podiatric Medicine.

DPT. Abbreviation for diphtheria-pertussis-tetanus (vaccine). SEE diphtheria toxoid, tetanus toxoid, and pertussis *vaccine.*

DR Abbreviation for digital *radiography.*

Dr. Abbreviation for doctor.

dr Abbreviation for dram.

drachm (dram). SYN dram. [G. *drachmē,* an ancient Greek weight, equivalent to about 60 gr]

dra·cun·cu·li·a·sis, dra·cun·cu·lo·sis (dra-kŭng-kū-lī'ă-sis, -kū-lō'sis). Infection with *Dracunculus medinensis.*

ⓘ*Dra·cun·cu·lus* (dra-kŭng'kū-lŭs). A genus of nematodes (superfamily Dracunculoidea) that have some resemblances to true filarial worms; however, adults are larger (females being as long as 1 m), and the intermediate host is a freshwater crustacean rather than an insect. [L. dim. of *draco,* serpent]

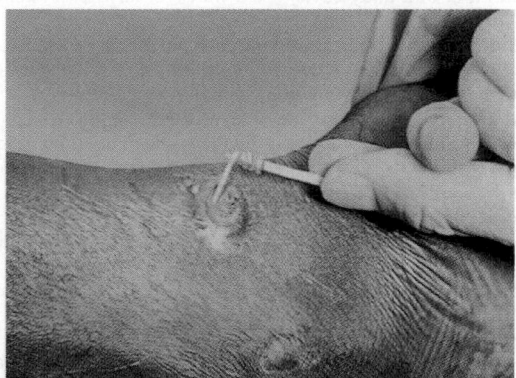

Dracunculus medinensis: an adult worm being removed by being wound on a stick

D. lova, old incorrect term for *Loa loa.*

D. medinen'sis, a species of skin-infecting, yard-long nematodes, formerly incorrectly classed as *Filaria;* adult worms live anywhere in the body of humans and various semi-aquatic mammals; the females migrate along fascial planes to subcutaneous tissues, where troublesome chronic ulcers are formed in the skin; when the host enters water, larvae are discharged from the ulcers, from which the head of the female worm protrudes; these larvae, if

dr

ingested by *Cyclops* species, develop in the intermediate host to the infective stage; humans and various animals contract the infection from accidental ingestion of infected *Cyclops* in drinking water. Popularly known as guinea, Medina, serpent, or dragon worm, and frequently thought to be the "fiery serpent" that plagued the Israelites. [L. of Medina]

D. oc′uli, old incorrect term for *Loa loa.*

D. persa′rum, old term for *D. medinensis.* [L. of the Persians]

draft. 1. A current of air in a confined space. **2.** A quantity of liquid medicine ordered as a single dose. SYN draught.

drag. 1. The lower or cast side of a denture flask. **2.** Any tendency for one moving thing to pull something else along with it.

solvent d., the influence exerted by a flow of solvent through a membrane on the simultaneous movement of a solute through the membrane.

dra·gée (dra-zhā′). A sugar-coated pill or capsule. [Fr.]

Dragendorff, Georg J.N., German physician and pharmaceutical chemist, 1836–1898. SEE D. *test.*

Drager, Glenn A., U.S. neurologist, *1917. SEE Shy-D. *syndrome.*

Dräger, Heinrich, German manufacturer of industrial and diving respiratory apparatus and anesthesia machines, 1847–1917. SEE D. *respirometer.*

drain (drān). **1.** To remove fluid from a cavity as it forms, e.g., to drain an abscess. **2.** A device, usually in the shape of a tube or wick, for removing fluid as it collects in a cavity, especially a wound cavity. [A. S. *drehnian,* to draw off]

cigarette d., a wick of gauze wrapped in a thin, soft rubberlike material, providing capillary drainage.

Mikulicz d., a d. made of several strings of gauze held together by a single layer of gauze.

Penrose d., a soft, tubular, rubberlike drain.

stab d., a d. passed into a cavity through a puncture made at a dependent part away from the wound of operation, designed to prevent infection of the wound.

sump d., a d. consisting of an outer tube vented to the outside with a smaller tube within it which is attached to a suction pump; both have multiple perforations that allow fluid and air to be carried away through the suction tube.

drain·age (drān′ij). Continuous withdrawal of fluids from a wound or other cavity.

capillary d., d. by means of a wick of gauze or other material.

closed d., d. of a body cavity via a water- or air-tight system. Cf. sump *drain.*

dependent d., d. from the lowest part and into a receptacle at a level lower than the structure being drained. SYN downward d.

downward d., SYN dependent d.

infusion-aspiration d., a type of d. in which antibiotics are continuously infused into a cavity at the same time fluid is being drained (aspirated) from the cavity.

open d., d. allowing air to enter.

🛈**postural d.,** d. used in bronchiectasis and lung abscess. The patient's body is positioned so that the trachea is inclined downward and below the affected chest area.

suction d., closed drainage of a cavity, with a suction apparatus attached to the drainage tube.

through d., d. obtained by the passage of a perforated tube, open at both extremities, through a cavity; in addition, the cavity can be washed out by a solution passed through the tube.

tidal d., d. of the urinary bladder by means of an intermittent filling and emptying apparatus.

Wangensteen d., continuous d. by suction through an indwelling gastric or duodenal tube.

dram (dr). A unit of weight: ¹/₈ oz.; 60 gr, apothecaries' weight; ¹/₁₆ oz., avoirdupois weight. SYN drachm. [see drachm]

drape (drāp). **1.** To cover parts of the body other than those to be examined or operated upon. **2.** The cloth or materials used for such cover. [M.E., fr. L.L. *drappus,* cloth]

Draper, John William, English chemist, 1811–1882. SEE D. *law.*

draught (draft). SYN draft.

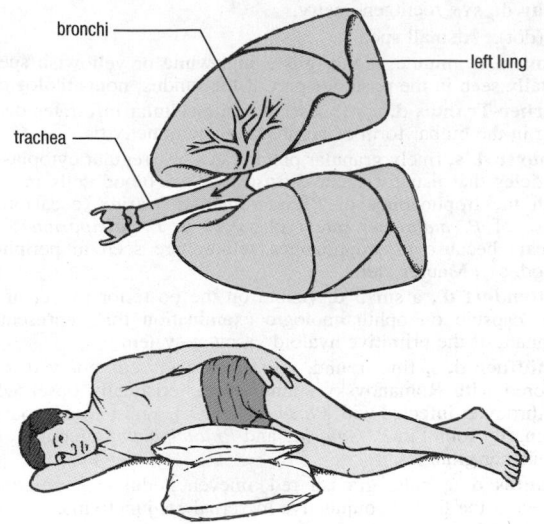

postural drainage of left lung

draw-sheet (draw′shēt). A narrow sheet placed crosswise on the bed under the patient to assist in moving the patient or in changing soiled bed coverings.

dream (drēm). Mental activity during sleep in which events, thought, emotions, and images are experienced as real.

anxiety d., a d. (or nightmare) in which morbid fear and anxiety form an important part.

wet d., a true physiologic orgasm during sleep including, in males, a nocturnal seminal emission usually accompanying a d. with sexual content.

dream-work. In psychoanalysis, the process by which the change from latent to manifest content of a dream is effected.

Drechs·lera (dresh′ler-ă). A saprobic genus of fungi, frequently recovered in the clinical laboratory, characterized by conidia attached to a zigzagged conidiophore. Most species in this genus that cause phaeohyphomycosis in humans, cats, and horses have been transferred to the genera *Bipolaris* or *Exserohilum.*

Dreifuss, Fritz E., *1926. SEE Emery-D. muscular *dystrophy.*

drep·a·nid·i·um (drep-ă-nid′ē-ŭm). A young sickle-shaped or crescentic form of a gregarine. [G. *drepanē,* a sickle]

drep·a·no·cyte (drep′ă-nō-sīt). SYN sickle *cell.* [G. *drepanē,* sickle, + *kytos,* a hollow (cell)]

drep·a·no·cyt·ic (drep′ă-nō-sit′ik). Relating to or resembling a sickle cell.

dress·er (dres′ĕr). In Great Britain, a surgical assistant whose primary duty is bandaging and dressing wounds.

dress·ing (dres′ing). The material applied, or the application itself of material, to a wound for protection, absorbance, drainage, etc.

adhesive absorbent d., a sterile individual d. consisting of a plain absorbent compress affixed to a film of fabric coated with a pressure-sensitive adhesive.

antiseptic d., a sterile d. of gauze impregnated with an antiseptic.

bolus d., SYN tie-over d.

dry d., dry gauze or other material applied to a wound.

fixed d., a d. stiffened with a substance that produces immobilization when it dries.

Lister d., the first type of antiseptic d., one of gauze impregnated with carbolic acid.

occlusive d., a d. that hermetically seals a wound.

pressure d., a d. by which pressure is exerted on the area covered to prevent the collection of fluids in the underlying tissues; most commonly used after skin grafting and in the treatment of burns.

tie-over d., a d. placed over a skin graft or other sutured wound and tied on by the sutures which have been left of sufficient length for that purpose. SYN bolus d.

water d., an application of gauze or other material that is kept wet with sterilized water or saline solution.

wet-to-dry d., a d. that is applied moist with saline and allowed to dry before it is removed.

Dressler, William, U.S. physician, 1890–1969. SEE D. *beat, syndrome.*

Dreyer, Georges, English pathologist, 1873–1934. SEE D. *formula.*

DRG Abbreviation for diagnosis-related *group.*

drib·ble (dri′bl). **1.** To drool, slaver, drivel. **2.** To fall in drops, as the urine from a distended bladder.

drift. 1. A gradual movement, as from an original position. **2.** A gradual change in the value of a random variable over time as a result of various factors, some random and some systematic effects of trend, manipulation, etc.

antigenic d., the process of "evolutionary" changes in molecular structure of DNA/RNA in microorganisms during their passage from one host to another; it may be due to recombination, deletion, or insertion of genes, point mutations or combinations of these events; it leads to alteration (usually slow and progressive) in the antigenic composition, and therefore in the immunologic responses of individuals and populations to exposure to the microorganism concerned; common with influenzavirus.

genetic d., a change in the frequencies of genetic traits or allele frequencies over generations.

pure random d., that which has random components only with an average value of zero and no systematic effects. Brownian movement in a still container shows pure random d. but in the Mississippi shows a steady downstream tendency.

drift·ing. Random movement of a tooth to a position of greater stability.

drifts (drifts). Slow ocular movements of greater amplitude than flicks, occurring during ocular fixation. SYN drift movements.

drill. 1. To make a hole in bone or other hard substance. **2.** An instrument for making or enlarging a hole in bone or in a tooth. [Middle Dutch *drillen,* to bore]

bur d., SEE bur.

dental d., a rotary power-driven instrument into which cutting points may be inserted. SEE ALSO handpiece.

drill-out. A drilling away; scooping out.

cochlear d.-o., implantation of electrodes in a cochlea in which the lumen of the scala tympani has been obliterated by the deposition of new bone due to the inflammatory process in labyrinthitis; the cochlear wall and new bone are drilled away so that the electrodes can be placed close to the remaining neurons of the auditory division of the 8th cranial nerve.

Drinker, Philip, U.S. industrial hygienist, 1893–1972. SEE D. *respirator.*

drip. 1. To flow a drop at a time. **2.** A flowing in drops.

alkaline milk d., a variable mixture of sodium bicarbonate in whole milk dripped into the stomach through a small oral or nasal tube to produce constant achlorhydria; a now obsolete therapy for certain ulcers.

intravenous d., the slow but continuous introduction of solutions intravenously, a drop at a time.

Murphy d., SYN proctoclysis.

postnasal d., term sometimes used to describe sensation of mucoid or mucopurulent discharge from the posterior nares.

drive. 1. In psychoanalysis, a basic compelling urge. **2.** In psychology, classified as either innate (e.g., hunger) or learned (e.g., hoarding) and appetitive (e.g., hunger, thirst, sex) or aversive (e.g., fear, pain, grief). SEE ALSO motive, motivation.

acquired d.'s, SYN secondary d.'s.

exploratory d., the d. typical of toddlers and some animals to investigate the unfamiliar or unknown.

learned d., SYN motive (1).

meiotic d., differential fitness in males and females.

physiological d.'s, those d.'s such as hunger and thirst which stem from the biological needs of an organism. SYN primary d.'s.

primary d.'s, SYN physiological d.'s.

secondary d.'s, those d.'s not directly related to biological needs; a secondary d. can be learned as an offshoot of a primary d., in which case it is often referred to as a motive. SYN acquired d.'s.

driv·ing (drīv′ing). The induction of a frequency in the electroencephalogram by sensory stimulation at this frequency.

photic d., a normal EEG phenomenon whereby the frequency of the activity recorded over the parieto-occipital regions is time-locked to the flash frequency during photic stimulation.

drom·o·ma·nia (drom-ō-mā′nē-ă). An uncontrollable impulse to wander or travel. [G. *dromos,* a running, + *mania,* insanity]

dro·mo·stan·o·lone pro·pi·o·nate (drō-mos′tan-ō-lōn, drō-mō-stan′ō-lōn). An antineoplastic agent.

dro·nab·i·nol (drō-nab′i-nol). The principal psychoactive substance present in *Cannabis sativa,* used therapeutically as an antinauseant to control the nausea and vomiting associated with cancer chemotherapy. SEE ALSO tetrahydrocannabinol.

drop. 1. To fall, or to be dispensed or poured in globules. **2.** A liquid globule. **3.** A volume of liquid regarded as a unit of dosage, equivalent in the case of water to about 1 minim. SEE ALSO drops. **4.** A solid confection in globular form, usually intended to be allowed to dissolve in the mouth. [A.S. *droppan*]

enamel d., SYN enameloma.

hanging d., a d. of liquid on the undersurface of the object glass for examination under the microscope.

dro·per·i·dol (drō-per′i-dol). A butyrophenone drug used in neuroleptanalgesia and preanesthetic medication; the pharmacology is similar to that of haloperidol; a dopamine receptor blocker. Exhibits antiemetic effects.

dropfoot. SEE footdrop.

drop·let (drop′let). A diminutive drop, such as a particle of moisture discharged from the mouth during coughing, sneezing, or speaking; these may transmit infections to others by their airborne passage. [drop + -*let,* dim. suffix]

drop·per. SYN instillator.

drops. A popular term for a medicine taken in doses measured by d.'s, usually a tincture, or applied by dropping, as an eyewash.

eye d., SEE eyewash, ophthalmic *solutions,* under *solution.*

knock-out d., a popular name for chloral alcoholate given with criminal intent to produce unconsciousness rapidly; it is formed by adding chloral hydrate to beer or some stronger alcoholic liquor.

nose d., a liquid preparation intended for intranasal administration with a medicine dropper. Most frequently used for decongestion of the nasal passages but can be used for any other appropriate indication.

stomach d., a stomachic tonic, usually tincture of gentian, alone or with other stomachics.

drop·si·cal (drop′si-kăl). SYN hydropic.

drop·sy (drop′sē). Old term for generalized edema, most often associated with cardiac failure. [G. *hydrōps*]

abdominal d., SYN ascites.

cardiac d., edema due to heart failure.

epidemic d., a disease causing occasional epidemics in India and Mauritius; marked by edema, anemia, eruptive angiomatosis, and mild fever; may be associated with nutritional deficiency.

famine d., edema occurring with the hypoproteinemia of low protein intake occurring as starvation of a large population group.

nutritional d., edema due to hypoproteinemia secondary to malnutrition.

d. of pericardium, SYN pericardial *effusion.*

drown·ing. Death within 24 hours of immersion in liquid, either due to anoxia or cardiac arrest caused by sudden extreme lowering of temperature (immersion syndrome). SEE ALSO near d.

dry d., d. by asphyxiation in an individual whose laryngeal reflexes are brisk, resulting in spasm that prevents inhalation of water; may be associated with the highest recovery rate.

near d., initial survival following immersion in liquid; the victim may die more than 24 hours later, e.g., from ARDS.

secondary d., pulmonary edema and resulting asphyxia, resulting from hypoxia and increased permeability of pulmonary capillaries

dr

occurring in a patient who has been immersed in and aspirated some water.

drows·i·ness (drow′zē-nes). A state of impaired awareness associated with a desire or inclination to sleep.

Dr.P.H. Abbreviation of Doctor of Public Health.

drug (drŭg). **1.** Therapeutic agent; any substance, other than food, used in the prevention, diagnosis, alleviation, treatment, or cure of disease. For types or classifications of d.'s, see the specific name. SEE ALSO agent. **2.** To administer or take a d., usually implying an overly large quantity or a narcotic. **3.** General term for any substance, stimulating or depressing, that can be habituating or addictive, especially a narcotic. [M.E. *drogge*]

addictive d., any d. that creates a certain degree of euphoria and has a strong potential for addiction.

crude d., an unrefined preparation, usually of plant origin, that occurs either in the entire, nearly entire, broken, cut, or powdered state.

disease modifying antirheumatic d.'s, agents that apparently alter the course and progression of rheumatoid arthritis, as opposed to more rapidly acting substances that suppress inflammation and decrease pain, but do not prevent cartilage or bone erosion or progressive disability.

d. holiday, interval when a chronically medicated patient temporarily stops taking the medication; used to allow some recuperation of normal functions, to maintain sensitivity to the drug, and to reduce the likelihood of side-effects.

nonsteroidal anti-inflammatory d.'s (NSAID), a large number of d.'s exerting anti-inflammatory (and also usually analgesic and antipyretic) actions; examples include aspirin, acetaminophen, diclofenac, indomethacine, ketorolac, ibuprofen, and naproxen. A contrast is made with steroidal compounds (such as hydrocortisone or prednisone) exerting anti-inflammatory activity.

orphan d.'s, SYN orphan *products,* under *product.*

psychedelic d., SYN hallucinogen.

psychodysleptic d., SYN hallucinogen.

psycholytic d., SYN hallucinogen.

psychotomimetic d., SYN hallucinogen.

psychotropic d., any d. that affects the mind.

recreational d., SYN street d.

scheduled d., a d. assigned to any of the five schedules in the Controlled Substances Act (1970). SEE ALSO controlled *substance.*

street d., a controlled substance taken for non-medical purposes. Street d.'s comprise various amphetamines, anesthetics, barbiturates, opiates, and psychoactive drugs, and many are derived from natural sources (e.g., the plants *Papaver somniferum, Cannibis sativa, Amanita pantherina, Lophophora williamsii*). Slang names include acid (lysergic acid diethylamide), angel dust (phencyclidine), coke (cocaine), downers (barbiturates), grass (marijuana), hash (concentrated tetrahydrocannibinol), magic mushrooms (psilocybin), and speed (amphetamines). During the 1980s, a new class of "designer drugs" arose, mostly analogs of psychoactive substances intended to escape regulation under the Controlled Substances Act. Also, crack cocaine, a potent, smokable form of cocaine, emerged as a major public health problem. In the U.S. illicit use of drugs such as cocaine, marijuana, and heroin historically has occurred in cycles. SYN recreational d.

drug-fast. Pertaining to microorganisms that resist or become tolerant to an antibacterial agent.

drug·gist (drŭg′ist). Old common term for pharmacist.

drug in·ter·ac·tions. The pharmacological result, either desirable or undesirable, of drugs interacting with other drugs, with endogenous physiologic chemical agents (e.g., MAOI with epinephrine), with components of the diet, and with chemicals used in diagnostic tests or the results of such tests.

drum, drum·head (drŭm, drŭm′hed). SYN tympanic *membrane.*

Drummond, Sir David, English physician, 1852–1932. SEE *artery* of D.; D. *sign.*

drunk·en·ness (drŭnk′en-nes). Intoxication, usually alcoholic. SEE ALSO acute *alcoholism.*

sleep d., a half-waking condition in which the faculty of orientation is in abeyance, and under the influence of nightmarelike ideas

the person may become actively excited and violent. SYN somnolentia (2).

dru·sen (droo′sen). Small bright structures seen in the retina and in the optic disk. [Ger. pl. of *Druse,* stony nodule, geode]

basal laminar d., small, round, translucent lesions measuring 25–75 μm in diameter, which represent nodular thickening of the basement membrane of the retinal pigment *epithelium,* often with an overlying focal detachment of the retinal pigment epithelium from Bruch *membrane.* SYN cuticular d.

basal linear d., deposits of long-spaced collagen located between the plasma *membrane* and basement *membrane* of the retinal pigment *epithelium.*

cuticular d., SYN basal laminar d.

exudative d., accumulations of an amorphous and granular material, cytoplasmic processes, and bent fibers between the basement membrane of the retinal pigment epithelium and the inner collagenous zone of Bruch *membrane;* types of exudative d. include hard d. and soft d. SYN typical d.

hard d., type of exudative or typical d. that appear ophthalmoscopically as discrete, yellow nodules characterized histopathologically by well-defined accumulations of hyaline material in the inner and outer collagenous zones of Bruch *membrane.*

intrapapillary d., SYN d. of the optic nerve head.

d. of the macula, excrescences of Bruch membrane that produce a window in the retinal pigment epithelium and are a feature of age-related macular retinal degeneration. SYN macular d.

macular d., SYN d. of the macula.

d. of the optic nerve head, basophilic, laminated, calcareous acellular masses that resemble crystals within the nerve head, anterior to the lamina cribrosa, that may simulate papilledema and/or cause visual field defects. SYN intrapapillary d.

soft d., type of exudative d. that appear ophthalmoscopically as placoid, yellow lesions characterized histopathologically by localized serous detachments of the retinal pigment *epithelium* from the Bruch *membrane.*

typical d., SYN exudative d.

dry ice (drī īs). SYN *carbon* dioxide snow.

ds Abbreviation for double-stranded.

DSA Abbreviation for digital subtraction *angiography.*

DSM Abbreviation for the *Diagnostic and Statistical Manual of Mental Disorders.*

DT Abbreviation for *delirium* tremens.

dT Abbreviation for deoxythymidine.

DTaP Abbreviation for diphtheria, tetanus, and acellular pertussis vaccine.

DT-di·aph·o·rase. SYN *NADPH* dehydrogenase (quinone).

dTDP Abbreviation for thymidine 5′-diphosphate.

dTDP-sug·ars. Sugars or sugar derivatives bonded to dTDP.

DTH Abbreviation for delayed-type hypersensitivity.

dThd Abbreviation for thymidine.

DTIC Abbreviation for dacarbazine.

dTMP Abbreviation for deoxythymidylic acid; thymidine 5′-monophosphate.

DTP Abbreviation for distal *tingling* on percussion; diphtheria toxoid, tetanus toxoid, and pertussis *vaccine;* and Demerol, Thorazine, and Phenergan, sometimes used as a sedative.

DTPA Abbreviation for diethylenetriamine pentaacetic acid.

DTPA Abbreviation for diethylenetriamine pentaacetic acid.

DTR Abbreviation for deep tendon *reflex.*

dTTP Abbreviation for thymidine 5′-triphosphate.

du·al·ism (doo′ăl-izm). **1.** In chemistry, a theory advanced by Berzelius that every compound, no matter how many elements enter into it, is composed of two parts, one electrically negative, the other positive; still applicable, with modification, to polar compounds, but inapplicable to nonpolar compounds. **2.** In hematology, the concept that blood cells have two origins, i.e., lymphogenous and myelogenous. **3.** The theory that the mind and body are two distinct systems, independent and different in nature. [L. *dualis,* relating to two, fr. *duo,* two]

Duane, Alexander, U.S. ophthalmologist, 1858–1926. SEE D. *syndrome.*

Dubin, I. Nathan, U.S. pathologist, 1913–1980. SEE D.-Johnson *syndrome.*

DuBois, Eugene F., U.S. physiologist, 1882–1959. SEE DuB. *formula;* Aub-DuB. *table.*

Dubois, Paul A., French obstetrician, 1795–1871. SEE D. *abscesses,* under *abscess, disease.*

du·boi·sine (doo-boy′sēn). An alkaloid obtained from the leaves of *Duboisia myoporoides* (family Solanaceae). SEE hyoscyamine.

Du Bois-Reymond, Emil H., German physiologist, 1818–1896. SEE Du Bois-Reymond *law.*

Duboscq, Jules, French optician, 1817–1886. SEE D. *colorimeter.*

Dubowitz, Victor, South African-English pediatrician, *1931. SEE D. *score.*

Dubreuil-Chambardel, Louis, French dentist, 1879–1927. SEE Dubreuil-Chambardel *syndrome.*

Duchenne, Guillaume B.A., French neurologist, 1806–1875. SEE D. *disease, sign;* D.-Aran *disease;* Aran-D. *disease;* D.-Erb *paralysis;* D. *dystrophy.*

Duckworth, Sir Dyce, English physician, 1840–1928. SEE D. *phenomenon.*

Ducrey, Augusto, Italian dermatologist, 1860–1940. SEE D. *bacillus, test.*

DUCT

duct (dŭkt) [TA]. A tubular structure giving exit to the secretion of a gland or organ, capable of conducting fluid. SEE ALSO canal. SYN ductus [TA]. [L. *duco,* pp. *ductus,* to lead]

aberrant d.'s, SYN aberrant *ductules,* under *ductule.*

aberrant bile d.'s, small d.'s occasionally present in the ligaments of the liver or originating from the surface of the liver.

accessory pancreatic d. [TA], the excretory duct of the head of the pancreas, one branch of which joins the pancreatic duct, the other opening independently into the duodenum at the lesser duodenal papilla. SYN ductus pancreaticus accessorius [TA], Bernard canal, Bernard d., ductus dorsopancreaticus, Santorini canal, Santorini d.

alveolar d., (1) the part of the respiratory passages distal to the respiratory bronchiole; from it arise alveolar sacs and alveoli; (2) the smallest of the intralobular d.'s in the mammary gland, into which the secretory alveoli open. SYN ductulus alveolaris.

amnionic d., the transitory opening between the seroamnionic folds in birds just before they fuse to form the seroamnionic raphe.

anal d.'s, short d.'s lined with simple columnar to stratified columnar epithelium that extend from the valvulae anales to the sinus anales.

arterial d., SYN *ductus* arteriosus.

Bartholin d., SYN major sublingual d.

Bellini d.'s, SYN papillary d.'s.

Bernard d., SYN accessory pancreatic d.

bile d., (1) a d. formed by the union of the hepatic and cystic d.'s; it discharges at the duodenal papilla. SYN ductus choledochus [TA], choledoch d., choledoch, choledochus, common bile d. (2) any of the d.'s conveying bile between the liver and the intestine, including hepatic, cystic, and common bile d. a duct formed by the union of the hepatic and cystic ducts; it discharges at the duodenal papilla. SYN ductus biliaris [TA], biliary d.

biliary d., SYN bile d. (2).

Blasius d., SYN parotid d.

Botallo d., SYN *ductus* arteriosus.

bucconeural d., SYN craniopharyngeal d.

d. of bulbourethral gland [TA], the long slender duct on each side passing down through the inferior fascia of the urogenital diaphragm to enter the bulb of the penis and course forward 2 or 3 cm before terminating in the urethra. SYN ductus glandulae bulbourethralis [TA].

canalicular d.'s, (1) SYN lactiferous d.'s; **(2)** SYN biliary *ductules,* under *ductule.*

carotid d., SYN *ductus* caroticus.

cervical d., SEE cervical *diverticulum.*

choledoch d., SYN bile d. (1).

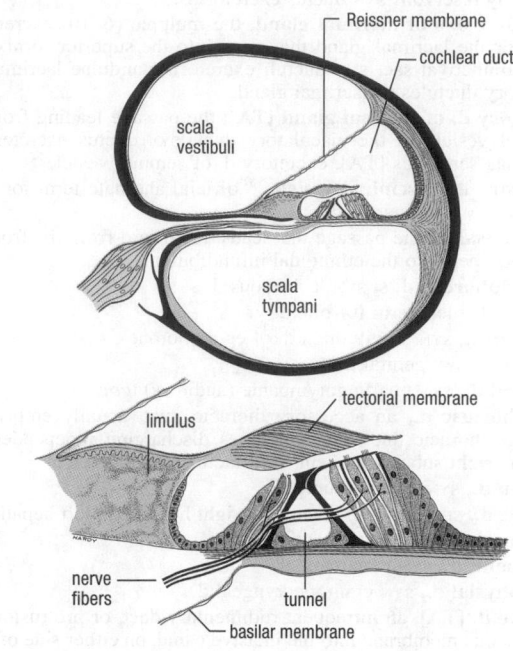

cochlear duct and spiral organ: cross-section showing nerve fibers and cells (yellow), substentacular cells (purple), cells of Hensen (red), stria vascularis (green), outer hair cells (dark blue), inner hair cells (black)

cochlear d. [TA], a spirally arranged membranous tube suspended within the cochlea, lying between and separating the scala vestibuli and scala tympani; it begins by a blind extremity, the vestibular cecum, in the cochlear recess of the vestibule, terminating in another blind extremity, the cecum cupulare or lagena, at the cupola of the cochlea; it contains endolymph and communicates with the sacculus by the ductus reuniens; the spiral organ (of Corti), the neuroepithelial receptor organ for hearing, occupies the floor of the duct. SYN ductus cochlearis [TA], Löwenberg canal, Löwenberg scala, membranous cochlea, scala media.

common bile d., SYN bile d. (1).

common hepatic d. [TA], the part of the biliary duct system that is formed by the confluence of right and left hepatic ducts. At the porta hepatis it is joined by the cystic duct to become the common bile duct. SYN ductus hepaticus communis [TA], hepatocystic d.

craniopharyngeal d., the slender tubular part of the hypophysial diverticulum; the stalk of Rathke pocket. SYN bucconeural d., hypophysial d.

Cuvier d.'s, obsolete term for the common cardinal veins.

cystic d. [TA], the d. leading from the gallbladder; it joins the hepatic duct to form the common bile duct. SYN ductus cysticus [TA], cystic gall d.

cystic gall d., SYN cystic d.

deferent d., SYN *ductus* deferens.

efferent d., SYN efferent *ductules* of testis, under *ductule.*

ejaculatory d. [TA], the duct formed by the union of the deferent duct and the excretory duct of the seminal vesicle, which opens into the prostatic urethra. SYN ductus ejaculatorius [TA], spermiduct (2).

endolymphatic d. [TA], a small membranous canal, connecting with both saccule and utricle of the membranous labyrinth, passing through the aqueduct of vestibule, and terminating in a dilated blind extremity, the endolymphatic sac, on the posterior surface of the petrous portion of the temporal bone beneath the dura mater. SYN ductus endolymphaticus [TA].

d. of epididymis [TA], a convoluted tube into which the efferent ductules open and which itself terminates in the ductus deferens. SYN ductus epididymidis [TA].

excretory d., a d. carrying the secretion from a gland or a fluid from any reservoir. SYN ductus excretorius.

excretory d.'s of lacrimal gland, the multiple (6–10) excretory ducts of the lacrimal gland that open into the superior fornix of the conjunctival sac. SYN ductuli excretorii glandulae lacrimalis, excretory ductules of lacrimal gland.

excretory d. of seminal gland [TA], the passage leading from a seminal vesicle to the ejaculatory duct. SYN ductus excretorius vesiculae seminalis [TA], excretory d. of seminal vesicle ☆.

excretory d. of seminal vesicle, ☆ official alternate term for excretory d. of seminal gland.

frontonasal d., the passage that leads downward from the frontal sinus to open into the ethmoidal infundibulum.

galactophorous d.'s, SYN lactiferous d.'s.

gall d., obsolete term for bile d.

Gartner d., SYN longitudinal d. of epoöphoron.

genital d., SYN genital *tract*.

guttural d., SYN pharyngotympanic (auditory) *tube*.

hemithoracic d., an accessory thoracic duct, usually emptying into the thoracic duct but sometimes discharging independently into the right subclavian vein. SYN ductus hemithoracicus.

Hensen d., SYN *ductus* reuniens.

hepatic d., SEE common hepatic d., right hepatic d., left hepatic d.

hepatocystic d., SYN common hepatic d.

Hoffmann d., SYN pancreatic d.

hypophysial d., SYN craniopharyngeal d.

incisive d. [TA], an infrequent rudimentary duct, or protrusion of the mucous membrane into the incisive canal, on either side of the anterior extremity of the nasal crest. SYN ductus incisivus [TA].

intercalated d.'s, the minute d.'s of glands, such as the salivary and the pancreas, that lead from the acini; they are lined by low cuboidal cells.

interlobar d., a d. draining the secretion of the lobe of a gland and formed by the junction of a number of interlobular d.'s.

interlobular d., any d. leading from a lobule of a gland and formed by the junction of the intralobular d.'s.

intralobular d., a d. that lies within a lobule of a gland.

jugular d., SYN jugular lymphatic *trunk*.

lactiferous d.'s [TA], one of the d.'s, numbering 15–20, which drain the lobes of the mammary gland; they open at the nipple. SYN ductus lactiferi [TA], canalicular d.'s (1), galactophore, galactophorous canals, galactophorous d.'s, mammillary d.'s, mammary d.'s, milk d.'s, tubuli galactophori, tubuli lactiferi.

left d. of caudate lobe of liver [TA], a tributary to the left hepatic duct draining bile from the left half of the caudate lobe. SYN ductus lobi caudati sinister hepatis [TA].

left hepatic d. [TA], the duct that drains bile from the left half of the liver, including the quadrate lobe and the left part of the caudate lobe. SYN ductus hepaticus sinister [TA].

longitudinal d. of epoöphoron [TA], a rudimentary vestige of the mesonephric duct in the female into which the tubules of the epoöphoron open; it is located in the broad ligament of the uterus, parallel with the lateral part of the uterine tube, and in the lateral walls of the cervix and vagina. SYN ductus longitudinalis epoöphori [TA], ductus deferens vestigialis, Gartner canal, Gartner d.

Luschka d.'s, glandlike tubular structures in the wall of the gallbladder, especially in the part covered with peritoneum.

lymphatic d., one of the two large lymph channels, right lymphatic d. or thoracic d.

major sublingual d. [TA], the duct that drains the anterior portion of the sublingual gland; it opens at the sublingual papilla. SYN ductus sublingualis major [TA], Bartholin d.

mamillary d.'s, SYN lactiferous d.'s.

mammary d.'s, SYN lactiferous d.'s.

mesonephric d., a duct in the embryo draining the mesonephric tubules; in the male it becomes the ductus deferens; in the female it becomes vestigial. SEE ALSO longitudinal d. of epoöphoron. SYN ductus mesonephricus, wolffian d.

metanephric d., the slender tubular portion of the metanephric diverticulum; the primordium of the epithelial lining of the ureter. SEE epoophoron, longitudinal d. of epoöphoron.

milk d.'s, SYN lactiferous d.'s.

minor sublingual d.'s [TA], from 8–20 small ducts of the sublingual salivary gland that open into the mouth on the surface of the sublingual fold; a few join the submandibular ducts. SYN ductus sublinguales minores [TA], Rivinus d.'s, Walther canals, Walther d.'s.

Müller d., müllerian d., SYN paramesonephric d.

nasal d., SYN nasolacrimal d.

🔲**nasolacrimal d.** [TA], the passage leading downward from the lacrimal sac on each side to the anterior portion of the inferior meatus of the nose, through which tears are conducted into the nasal cavity. SYN ductus nasolacrimalis [TA], nasal d.

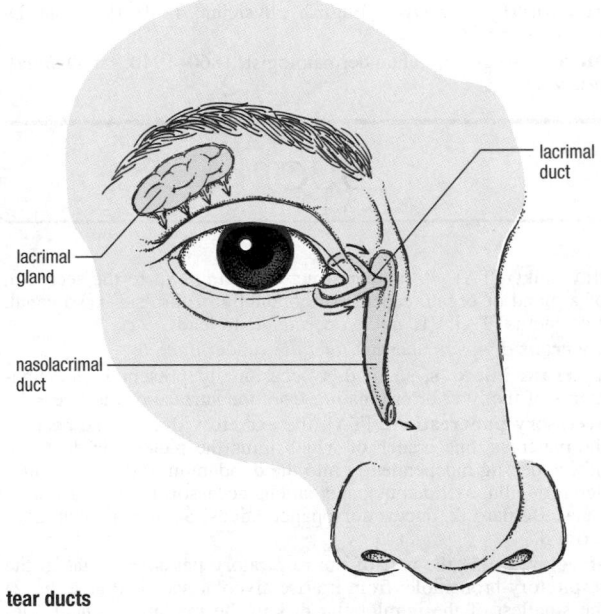

lacrimal duct

lacrimal gland

nasolacrimal duct

tear ducts

nephric d., SYN pronephric d.

omphalomesenteric d., obsolete term for yolk *stalk*.

pancreatic d. [TA], the excretory duct of the pancreas that extends through the gland from tail to head where it empties into the duodenum at the greater duodenal papilla. SYN ductus pancreaticus [TA], Hoffmann d., Wirsung canal, Wirsung d.

papillary d.'s, the largest straight excretory d.'s in the kidney medulla and papillae whose openings form the area cribrosa that open into a minor calyx; they are a continuation of the collecting tubules. SYN Bellini d.'s.

paramesonephric d., either of the two paired embryonic tubes extending along the mesonephros roughly parallel to the mesonephric duct and emptying into the cloaca; in the female, the upper parts of the ducts form the uterine tubes, while the lower fuse to form the uterus and part of the vagina; in the male, vestiges of the ducts form the vagina masculina and the appendix testis. SYN ductus paramesonephricus, Müller d., müllerian d.

paraurethral d.'s [TA], inconstant ducts along the side of the female urethra that convey the mucoid secretion of Skene glands to the vestibule. SYN ductus paraurethrales [TA], d.'s of Skene glands, Schüller d.'s.

parotid d. [TA], the duct of the parotid gland opening from the cheek into the vestibule of the mouth opposite the neck of the superior second molar tooth. SYN ductus parotideus [TA], Blasius d., Stensen d., Steno d.

Pecquet d., SYN thoracic d.

perilymphatic d., SYN cochlear *aqueduct.*

pharyngobranchial d.'s, SEE *ductus* pharyngobranchialis III, *ductus* pharyngobranchialis IV.

pronephric d., the d. of the pronephros. SYN nephric d.

prostatic d.'s, SYN prostatic *ductules,* under *ductule.*

right d. of caudate lobe of liver [TA], the bile duct from the right half of the caudate lobe, a tributary to the right hepatic duct. SYN ductus lobi caudati dexter hepatis [TA].

right hepatic d. [TA], the duct that transmits bile to the common hepatic duct from the right half of the liver and the right part of the caudate lobe. SYN ductus hepaticus dexter [TA].

right lymphatic d. [TA], one of the two terminal lymph vessels, a short trunk, about 2 cm in length, formed by the union of the right jugular lymphatic vessel and vessels from the lymph nodes of the right superior limb, thoracic wall, and both lungs; it lies on the right side of the root of the neck and empties into the right brachiocephalic vein. Frequently, no right lymphatic d. is formed, with the vessels that normally contribute to its formation entering the venous system independently. SYN ductus lymphaticus dexter [TA], ductus thoracicus dexter ☆.

Rivinus d.'s, SYN minor sublingual d.'s.

saccular d. [TA], saccular portion of the utriculosaccular duct; extends between the sacculus and the endolymphatic d. SEE ALSO utriculosaccular d. SYN ductus saccularis [TA].

salivary d., SYN striated d.

Santorini d., SYN accessory pancreatic d.

Schüller d.'s, SYN paraurethral d.'s.

secretory d., SYN striated d.

semicircular d.'s [TA], three small membranous tubes in the bony semicircular canals that lie within the bony labyrinth and form loops of about two-thirds of a circle. The three semicircular ducts: anterior semicircular d. [TA] (ductus semicircularis anterior [TA]), lateral semicircular d. [TA] (ductus semicircularis lateralis [TA]), and posterior semicircular d. [TA] (ductus semicircularis posterior [TA]), lie in planes at right angles to each other and open into the vestibule by five openings of which one is common to the anterior and lateral ducts. Each duct has an ampulla at one end within which filaments of the vestibular nerve terminate. SYN ductus semicirculares [TA].

seminal d., any one of the d.'s conveying semen from the epididymis to the urethra, ductus deferens, or ejaculatory d. SYN gonaduct (1).

d.'s of Skene glands, SYN paraurethral d.'s.

spermatic d., SYN *ductus* deferens.

Stensen d., Steno d., SYN parotid d.

striated d., a type of intralobular d. found in some salivary glands that modifies the secretory product; it derives its name from extensive infolding of the basal membrane. SYN salivary d., secretory d.

subclavian d., SYN subclavian lymphatic *trunk.*

submandibular d., [TA], the duct of the submandibular salivary gland; it opens at the sublingual papilla near the frenulum of the tongue. SYN ductus submandibularis [TA], ductus submaxilaris, submaxillary d., Wharton d.

submaxillary d., SYN submandibular d.

sudoriferous d., SYN d. of sweat glands.

sweat d., SYN d. of sweat glands.

d. of sweat glands, the superficial portion of the sweat gland that passes through the corium and epidermis, opening on the surface by the porus sudoriferus or sweat pore. SYN ductus sudoriferus, sudoriferous d., sweat d.

testicular d., SYN *ductus* deferens.

▣thoracic d. [TA], the largest lymph vessel in the body, beginning at the cisterna chyli at about the level of the second lumbar vertebra; the abdominal part extends superiorly to pass through the aortic opening of the diaphragm, where it becomes the thoracic part and crosses the posterior mediastinum to form the arch of the thoracic duct and discharge into the left venous angle (origin

of the brachiocephalic vein). SYN ductus thoracicus [TA], Pecquet d., van Horne canal.

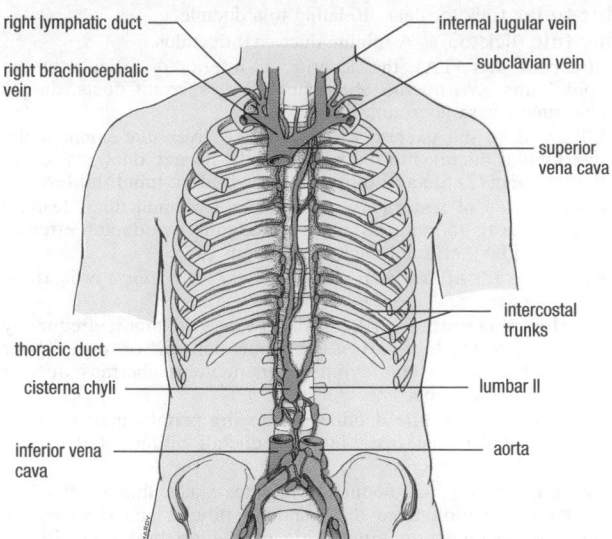

right lymphatic duct — internal jugular vein
right brachiocephalic vein — subclavian vein
superior vena cava
intercostal trunks
thoracic duct —
cisterna chyli — lumbar II
inferior vena cava — aorta

thoracic and right lymphatic ducts: deep lymphatic vessels and nodes are also shown

thyroglossal d. [TA], a transitory endodermal tube in the embryo, carrying thyroid-forming tissue at its caudal end; normally, the duct disappears after the thyroid has moved to its definitive location in the neck; its point of origin is regularly marked on the root of the adult tongue by the foramen cecum; occasionally, its incomplete regression results in the formation of cysts along its embryonic course. SEE ALSO pyramidal *lobe* of thyroid gland. SYN ductus thyroglossus [TA], thyrolingual d.

thyrolingual d., SYN thyroglossal d.

umbilical d., SYN yolk *stalk.*

uniting d., SYN *ductus* reuniens.

utricular d. [TA], utricular portion of the utriculosaccular d.; extends between the utriculus and the endolymphatic duct. SEE ALSO utriculosaccular d. SYN ductus utricularis [TA].

utriculosaccular d. [TA], a duct that connects the inner aspect of the utricle with the endolymphatic duct a short distance from its origin from the saccule. SYN ductus utriculosaccularis [TA], Böttcher canal.

vitelline d., vitellointestinal d., SYN yolk *stalk.*

Walther d.'s, SYN minor sublingual d.'s.

Wharton d., SYN submandibular d.

Wirsung d., SYN pancreatic d.

wolffian d., SYN mesonephric d.

duc·tal (dŭk′tăl). Relating to a duct.

duc·tile (dŭk′tĭl). Denoting the property of a material that allows it to be bent, drawn out (as a wire), or otherwise deformed without breaking. [L. *ductilis,* capable of being led or drawn]

duc·tion (dŭk′shŭn). **1.** The act of leading, bringing, conducting. **2.** In ophthalmology, ocular rotations with reference to one eye; usually additionally designating direction of movement of the eye; e.g., rotation toward the nose, adduction; toward the temple, abduction; upward, supra- or sursumduction; downward, deorsumduction; of the upper pole of one cornea, cycloduction; of the upper pole of one cornea outward, excycloduction; of the upper pole of one cornea inward, incycloduction. [L. *duco,* to lead]

forced d., a maneuver to determine whether a mechanical obstruction is present in the eye; with forceps grasping an eye muscle, an attempt is made to passively move the eyeball in the direction of restricted rotation. SYN passive d.

passive d., SYN forced d.

duct·less (dŭkt′les). Having no duct; denoting certain glands having only an internal secretion.

duc·tu·lar (dŭk′too-lăr). Relating to a ductule.

duc·tule (dŭk′tool). A minute duct. SYN ductulus.

aberrant d.'s [TA], the superior or inferior diverticula of the epididymis. SYN ductuli aberrantes [TA], aberrant ducts, ductus aberrantes, vasa aberrantia.

biliary d.'s, the excretory ducts of the liver that connect the interlobular ductules to the right (or left) hepatic duct. SYN canalicular ducts (2), ductuli biliferi, ductus biliferi, tubuli biliferi.

efferent d.'s of testis [TA], 12–14 small seminal ducts leading from the testis to the head of the epididymis. SYN ductuli efferentes testis [TA], efferent duct, vas efferens (3).

excretory d.'s of lacrimal gland, SYN excretory *ducts* of lacrimal gland, under *duct*.

inferior aberrant d. [TA], a narrow, coiled tubule frequently connected to the first part of the ductus deferens or to the lower part of the ductus epididymitis. SYN ductulus aberrans inferior [TA], Haller vas aberrans.

interlobular d.'s, bile ductules occupying portal canals between hepatic lobules that open into the ductuli biliferi. SYN ductuli interlobulares.

prostatic d.'s [TA], about 20 minute canals that receive the prostatic secretion from the glandular tubules and discharge it through openings on either side of the urethral crest in the posterior wall of the urethra. SYN ductuli prostatici [TA], ductus prostatici, prostatic ducts.

superior aberrant d. [TA], a diverticulum from the head of the epididymis. SYN ductulus aberrans superior [TA].

transverse d.'s of epoöphoron [TA], a series of 10–15 short tubules that open into the longitudinal duct of the epoöphoron and represent vestiges of the mesonephric duct. SYN ductuli transversi epoöphori [TA], tubuli epoöphori.

duc·tu·lus, pl. **duc·tu·li** (dŭk′too-lŭs, -too-lī). SYN ductule. [Mod. L. dim. of L. *ductus,* duct]

d. aberrans infe′rior [TA], SYN inferior aberrant *ductule*.

d. aberrans supe′rior [TA], SYN superior aberrant *ductule*.

ductuli aberran′tes [TA], SYN aberrant *ductules*, under *ductule*.

d. alveola′ris, pl. **duc′tuli alveola′res,** SYN alveolar *duct*.

duc′tuli bilif′eri, SYN biliary *ductules*, under *ductule*.

ductuli efferen′tes tes′tis [TA], SYN efferent *ductules* of testis, under *ductule*.

duc′tuli excreto′rii glan′dulae lacrima′lis, SYN excretory *ducts* of lacrimal gland, under *duct*.

duc′tuli interlobula′res, SYN interlobular *ductules*, under *ductule*.

duc′tuli paroöph′ori, tubular remnants of the embryonic mesonephros forming the paroöphoron. SYN tubuli paroöphori.

duc′tuli prostat′ici [TA], SYN prostatic *ductules*, under *ductule*.

duc′tuli transver′si epoöph′ori [TA], SYN transverse *ductules* of epoöphoron, under *ductule*; SEE ALSO epoophoron.

DUCTUS

duc·tus, gen. and pl. **duc·tus** (dŭk′tŭs) [TA]. SYN duct. [L. a leading, fr. *duco,* pp. *ductus,* to lead]

d. aber′rantes, SYN aberrant *ductules*, under *ductule*.

d. arterio′sus, a fetal vessel connecting the left pulmonary artery with the descending aorta; in the first two months after birth, it normally changes into a fibrous cord, the ligamentum arteriosum; persistent postnatal patentcy is a correctable cardiovascular handicap. SYN arterial canal, arterial duct, Botallo duct.

d. biliaris [TA], SYN bile *duct* (2).

d. bilif′eri, SYN biliary *ductules*, under *ductule*.

d. carot′icus, a portion of the embryonic dorsal aorta between points of juncture with the third and fourth arch arteries; it disappears early in development. SYN carotid duct.

d. choled′ochus [TA], SYN bile *duct* (1).

d. cochlea′ris [TA], SYN cochlear *duct*.

d. cys′ticus [TA], SYN cystic *duct*.

d. def′erens [TA], the secretory duct of the testicle, running from the epididymis, of which it is the continuation, to the prostatic urethra where it terminates as the ejaculatory duct. SYN deferent canal, deferent duct, spermatic duct, spermiduct (1), testicular duct, vas deferens.

d. def′erens vestigia′lis, SYN longitudinal *duct* of epoöphoron.

d. diverticulum, SYN ductal *aneurysm*.

d. dorsopancreat′icus, SYN accessory pancreatic *duct*.

d. ejaculato′rius [TA], SYN ejaculatory *duct*.

d. endolymphat′icus [TA], SYN endolymphatic *duct*.

d. epididym′idis [TA], SYN *duct* of epididymis.

d. excreto′rius, SYN excretory *duct*.

d. excretorius glandulae vesiculosae [TA],

d. excreto′rius vesic′ulae semina′lis [TA], SYN excretory *duct* of seminal gland.

d. glan′dulae bulbourethra′lis [TA], SYN *duct* of bulbourethral gland.

d. hemithorac′icus, SYN hemithoracic *duct*.

d. hepat′icus commu′nis [TA], SYN common hepatic *duct*.

d. hepat′icus dex′ter [TA], SYN right hepatic *duct*.

d. hepat′icus sinis′ter [TA], SYN left hepatic *duct*.

d. incisi′vus [TA], SYN incisive *duct*.

d. lactif′eri [TA], SYN lactiferous *ducts*, under *duct*.

d. lingua′lis, a pit on the upper surface of the tongue at the apex of the sulcus terminalis; it marks the point of origin of the d. thyroglossus of the embryo; known more commonly as the foramen cecum.

d. lo′bi cauda′ti dex′ter hepatis [TA], SYN right *duct* of caudate lobe of liver.

d. lo′bi cauda′ti sinis′ter hepatis [TA], SYN left *duct* of caudate lobe of liver.

d. longitudina′lis epoöph′ori [TA], SYN longitudinal *duct* of epoöphoron; SEE ALSO epoophoron.

d. lymphat′icus dex′ter [TA], SYN right lymphatic *duct*.

d. mesoneph′ricus, SYN mesonephric *duct*; SEE ALSO longitudinal *duct* of epoöphoron.

d. nasolacrima′lis [TA], SYN nasolacrimal *duct*.

d. pancreat′icus [TA], SYN pancreatic *duct*.

d. pancreat′icus accesso′rius [TA], SYN accessory pancreatic *duct*.

d. paramesoneph′ricus, SYN paramesonephric *duct*.

d. paraurethra′les [TA], SYN paraurethral *ducts*, under *duct*.

d. parotid′eus [TA], SYN parotid *duct*.

patent d. arterio′sus, SEE d. arteriosus.

d. perilymphat′icus, SYN cochlear *aqueduct*.

d. pharyngobranchia′lis III, a narrow communication between the third branchial pouch and the pharynx in the embryo.

d. pharyngobranchia′lis IV, a narrow communication between the fourth branchial pouch and the pharynx in the embryo.

d. prostat′ici, SYN prostatic *ductules*, under *ductule*.

d. reun′iens [TA], a short membranous tube passing from the lower end of the saccule to the cochlear duct of the membranous labyrinth. SYN canaliculus reuniens, canalis reuniens, Hensen canal, Hensen duct, uniting canal, uniting duct.

d. saccularis [TA], SYN saccular *duct*.

d. semicircula′res [TA], SYN semicircular *ducts*, under *duct*.

d. sublingua′les mino′res [TA], SYN minor sublingual *ducts*, under *duct*.

d. sublingua′lis ma′jor [TA], SYN major sublingual *duct*.

d. submandibula′ris [TA], SYN submandibular *duct*.

d. submaxilla′ris, SYN submandibular *duct*.

d. sudorif′erus, SYN *duct* of sweat glands.

d. thorac′icus [TA], SYN thoracic *duct*.

d. thorac′icus dex′ter, ☆official alternate term for right lymphatic *duct*.

d. thyroglos′sus [TA], SYN thyroglossal *duct*.

d. utricularis [TA], SYN utricular *duct*.

d. utric´ulosaccula´ris [TA], SYN utriculosaccular *duct.*

d. veno´sus, in the fetus, continuation of the left umbilical vein through the liver to the vena cava inferior; after birth, its lumen becomes obliterated, forming the ligamentum venosum.

d. veno´sus aran´tii, rarely used term for d. venosus.

Duddell, Benedict, 18th century British oculist. SEE D. *membrane.*

Duffy blood group. See Blood Groups appendix.

Dugas, Louis A., U.S. physician, 1806–1884.

Duhring, Louis A., U.S. dermatologist, 1845–1913. SEE D. *disease.*

Dührssen, Alfred, German obstetrician-gynecologist, 1862–1933. SEE D. *incisions,* under *incision.*

Duke, William Waddell Duke, U.S. pathologist, 1883–1945. SEE D. bleeding time *test.*

Dukes, Cuthbert E., British pathologist, 1890–1977. SEE D. *classification.*

Dukes, Clement, English physician, 1845–1925. SEE D. *disease;* Filatov-D. *disease.*

dul·cin (dŭl´sin). Has been used as a substitute for sugar, being 200 times as sweet as cane sugar. Because of hydrolysis to aminophenol, it may produce an injurious effect when used over long periods of time.

dul·cite, dul·ci·tol, dul·cose (dŭl´sīt, -si´tol, -kōs). Galactitol.

dull (dŭl). Not sharp or acute, in any sense; qualifying a surgical instrument, the action of the mind, pain, a sound (especially the percussion note), etc. [M.E. *dul*]

dull·ness, dul·ness (dŭl´nes). The character of the sound obtained by percussing over a solid part incapable of resonating; usually applied to an area containing less air than those which can resonate.

shifting d., a sign of free peritoneal fluid wherein the d. of percussion shifts, generally from one side to the other, as the patient is turned from side to side.

Dulong, Pierre L., French chemist, 1785–1838. SEE D.-Petit *law.*

dum·my (dŭm´ē). SYN pontic.

Dumontpallier, Alphonse, French physician, 1827–1899. SEE D. *pessary.*

dump·ing (dŭmp´ing). SEE dumping *syndrome.*

Duncan, James M., Scottish gynecologist, 1826–1890. SEE Duncan *folds,* under *fold,* Duncan *mechanism,* Duncan *placenta,* Duncan *ventricle.*

Duncan. Surname of first studied patients afflicted with what is now known as Duncan *disease.*

Dunn, Richard L. SEE Lison-D. *stain.*

du·o·crin·in (doo-ō-krin´in). A postulated gastrointestinal hormone that is liberated by the contact of gastric contents with the intestine and that stimulates the secretory activity of the duodenal glands (Brunner glands). [duodenum + G. *krinō,* to secrete, + -in]

du·o·de·nal (doo´ō-dē´năl, doo-od´ĕ-năl). Relating to the duodenum.

du·o·de·nec·to·my (doo-ō-dĕ-nek´tō-mē). Excision of the duodenum. [duodenum + G. *ektomē,* excision]

du·o·de·ni·tis (doo-od-ĕ-nī´tis). Inflammation of the duodenum.

duodeno-. Combining form relating to the duodenum. [L. *duodenum, scil., digitorum* breadth of 12 fingers]

du·o·de·no·cho·lan·gi·tis (doo-ō-dē´nō-kō-lan-jī´tis). Inflammation of the duodenum and common bile duct. [duodeno- + G. *cholē,* bile, + *angeion,* vessel, + -*itis,* inflammation]

du·o·de·no·cho·le·cys·tos·to·my (doo-ō-dē´nō-kō-lē-sis-tos´tō-mē). SYN cholecystoduodenostomy. [duodeno- + G. *cholē,* bile, + *kystis,* bladder, + *stoma,* mouth]

du·o·de·no·cho·led·o·chot·o·my (doo-ō-dē´nō-kō-led-ō-kot´ō-mē). Incision into the common bile duct and the adjacent portion of the duodenum. [duodeno- + G. *cholèdochus,* bile duct, + *tomē,* incision]

du·o·de·no·cys·tos·to·my (doo-ō-dē´nō-sis-tos´tō-mē). **1.** SYN cholecystoduodenostomy. **2.** SYN cystoduodenostomy. **3.** SYN pancreatic *cystoduodenostomy.*

du·o·de·no·en·ter·os·to·my (doo-ō-dē´nō-en-ter-os´tō-mē). Establishment of communication between the duodenum and another part of the intestinal tract. [duodeno- + G. *enteron,* intestine, + *stoma,* mouth]

du·o·de·no·je·ju·nos·to·my (doo-ō-dē´nō-jĕ-joo-nos´tō-mē). Operative formation of an artificial communication between the duodenum and the jejunum. [duodeno- + jejunum, + G. *stoma,* mouth]

du·o·de·nol·y·sis (doo-ō-dĕ-nol´i-sis). Incision of adhesions to the duodenum. [duodeno- + G. *lysis,* a freeing]

du·o·de·nor·rha·phy (doo-ō-dĕ-nōr´ă-fē). Suture of a tear or incision in the duodenum. [duodeno- + G. *rhaphē,* a seam]

du·o·de·nos·co·py (doo-ō-dĕ-nos´kŏ-pē). Inspection of the interior of the duodenum through an endoscope. [duodeno- + G. *skopeō,* to examine]

du·o·de·nos·to·my (doo-ō-dĕ-nos´tō-mē). Establishment of a fistula into the duodenum. [duodeno- + G. *stoma,* mouth]

du·o·de·not·o·my (doo-ō-dĕ-not´ō-mē). Incision of the duodenum. [duodeno- + G. *tomē,* incision]

du·o·de·num, gen. **du·o·de·ni,** pl. **du·o·de·na** (doo-ō-dē´nŭm, doo-od´ĕ-nŭm; -od´ĕ-nă, -dē´nă) [TA]. The first division of the small intestine, about 25 cm or 12 fingerbreadths (hence the name) in length, extending from the pylorus to the junction with the jejunum at the level of the first or second lumbar vertebra on the left side. It is divided into the superior part, the first part of which is the duodenal cap, the descending part, into which the bile and pancreatic ducts open, the horizontal (inferior) part and the ascending part, terminating at the duodenojejunal junction. [Mediev. L. fr. L. *duodeni,* twelve]

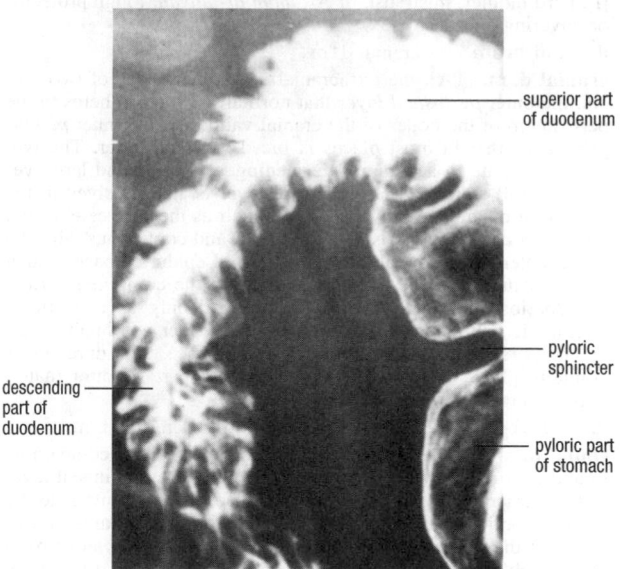

descending part of duodenum

superior part of duodenum

pyloric sphincter

pyloric part of stomach

duodenum: radiograph after barium swallow

du·o·vi·rus (doo´ō-vī´rŭs). SYN rotavirus.

du·plex (doo´pleks). Providing two functions. SEE duplex *ultrasonography.*

du·pli·ca·tion (doo-pli-kā´shŭn). **1.** A doubling. SEE ALSO reduplication. **2.** Inclusion of two copies of the same genetic material in a genome; an important step in diversification of genomes, as in the evolution of the (nonallelic) hemoglobin chains from a common ancestor. SYN gene d. [L. *duplicatio,* a doubling, fr. *duplico,* to double]

d. of chromosomes, a chromosome aberration resulting from unequal crossing over or exchange of segments between two homologous chromosomes; one chromosome of the pair loses a small segment, while the other gains this segment; the chromosome gaining the segment has undergone d. while its homologue has undergone deletion. SEE *hemoglobin* Lepore.

gene d., SYN duplication (2).

du·plic·i·tas (doo-plis′i-tahs). Doubling of a part. [L. a doubling, fr. *duplex (duplic-),* two-fold]

d. ante′rior, conjoined twins in which there are two thoraces and two heads and a single pelvis with one pair of lower extremities. SEE conjoined *twins,* under *twin;* SEE ALSO cephalodidymus, ileadelphus, iliadelphus. SYN catadidymus.

d. poste′rior, conjoined twins in which there is a single head and upper body and duplicated buttocks and legs. SEE conjoined *twins,* under *twin;* SEE ALSO dipygus. SYN anadidymus, ileadelphus, iliadelphus.

Dupré, 17th Century Paris surgeon and anatomist. SEE D. *muscle.*

Dupuytren, Baron Guillaume, French surgeon and surgical pathologist, 1777–1835. SEE D. *amputation, canal, contracture, disease* of the foot, *fascia, fracture, hydrocele, sign, suture, tourniquet.*

du·ra (doo′ră) [TA]. SYN dura mater. [L. fem. of *durus,* hard]

d. mater cranialis [TA], SYN cranial *dura mater.*

dur·a·en·ceph·a·lo·syn·an·gi·o·sis (door′a-en-sef′a-lō-sin-anj-ē-ō′sis). Surgical transposition of the superficial temporal artery with attached galea to the underlying dura with hope for cerebral revascularization; most commonly used in moyamoya syndrome. SYN encephaloduroarteriosynangiosis.

du·ral (doo′răl). Relating to the dura mater. SYN duramatral.

du·ra mat·er (doo′ră mā′ter) [TA]. Pachymeninx (as distinguished from leptomeninx, the combined pia mater and arachnoid); a tough, fibrous membrane forming the outer covering of the central nervous system. SYN dura [TA], pachymeninx [TA]. [L. hard mother, mistransl. of Ar. *umm al-jāfīyah,* tough protector or covering]

ⅰ d. m. of brain, SYN cranial d. m.

cranial d. m. [TA], the intracranial d. m., consisting of two layers: the outer *periosteal layer* that normally always adheres to the periosteum of the bones of the cranial vault; and the inner *meningeal layer* that in most places is fused with the outer. The two layers separate to accommodate meningeal vessels and large venous (dural) sinuses. The meningeal layer is also involved in the formation of the various dural folds, such as the falx cerebri and tentorium cerebelli and is comparable to and continuous with the dural mater of the spinal cord. The cranial epidural space is then an artifactual space between the bone and the combined periosteum/periosteal layer of the d. m. realized only as a result of pathologic or traumatic processes and is neither continuous with or comparable to the vertebral epidural space. SYN dura mater cranialis [TA], d. m. encephali☆, cerebral part of dura mater, d. m. of brain.

d. m. enceph′ali, ☆ official alternate term for cranial d. m.

spinal d. m. [TA], single-layered strong membrane, comparable to and continuous with (at foramen magnum) the meningeal layer of the intracranial d. m. of the brain. It does not (in contrast to the d. m. of brain) adhere to the enveloping bony structures (vertebrae) or their periosteum, being separated from the latter by a considerable space, the vertebral epidural space—a true space containing the internal vertebral venous plexus embedded in a matrix of epidural fat. SYN d. m. spinalis [TA], d. m. of spinal cord, endorrhachis, theca vertebralis.

d. m. of spinal cord, SYN spinal d. m.

d. m. spina′lis [TA], SYN spinal d. m.

du·ra·ma·tral (doo-ră-mā′trăl). SYN dural.

Duran-Reynals, Francisco, U.S. bacteriologist, 1899–1958. SEE Duran-Reynals permeability *factor.*

du·ra·plas·ty (doo′ră-plas-tē). A reconstructive operation on the open dura mater that involves a primary closure or secondary closure with another soft tissue material (e.g., muscle, fascia, allograft dura). [dura (mater) + G. *plastos,* formed]

du·ra·tion (D) (doo-ră′shŭn). A continuous period of time.

half amplitude pulse d., the time, in milliseconds, required for a wave form to reach half of its full magnitude.

pulse wave d., the interval between onset of the leading edge and the end of the trailing edge of a pulse wave.

Dürck, Hermann, German pathologist, 1869–1941. SEE D. *nodes,* under *node.*

dur. dolor. Abbreviation for L. *duarte dolare,* while pain lasts.

Duret, Henri, French neurosurgeon, 1849–1921. SEE D. *lesion, hemorrhage.*

Durham, Arthur E., English surgeon, 1834–1895. SEE D. *tube.*

Duroziez, Paul L., French physician, 1826–1897. SEE D. *disease, murmur, sign.*

DUSN Acronym for diffuse unilateral subacute *neuroretinitis.*

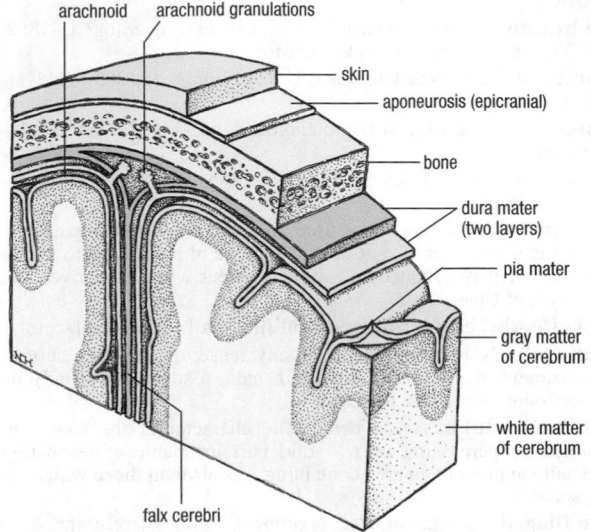

dura mater: and associated structures of the scalp, skull, and meninges (coronal view)

dUTP Abbreviation for deoxyuridine 5-triphosphate.

Dutton, Joseph Everett, English physician, 1877–1905. SEE D. *disease,* relapsing *fever.*

Duverney, Guichaud Joseph, French anatomist, 1648–1730. SEE D. *fissures,* under *fissure, gland, muscle.*

dwarf (dwōrf). An abnormally undersized person with disproportion among the bodily parts. SEE dwarfism. [A.S. *dweorh*]

hypophysial d., dwarfism as result of failure of growth hormone production because of hypothalamic or pituitary abnormality. SYN pituitary d.

hypothyroid d., dwarfism associated with lack of thyroid function.

pituitary d., SYN hypophysial d.

dwarf·ism (dwōrf′izm). A condition or a group of conditions in which the standing height of the person is below the 3rd percentile.

achondroplastic d., SEE achondroplasia.

acromelic d., SYN acromesomelic d.

acromesomelic d., a form of short-limb d. characterized by pugnose and shortening particularly striking in the distal segment of the limbs, i.e., the forearms and lower legs, fingers and toes; autosomal recessive inheritance. SYN acromelic d., acromesomelia.

aortic d., underdevelopment of physical stature associated with severe aortic stenosis.

asexual d., d. in which adult sexual development is deficient.

ateliotic d., SYN panhypopituitarism.

camptomelic d., d. with shortening of the lower limbs due to anterior bending of the femur and tibia.

chondrodystrophic d., SEE chondrodystrophy.

deprivation d., short stature due to emotional deprivation. SYN psychosocial d.

diastrophic d. [MIM*222600], SYN diastrophic *dysplasia*.

disproportionate d., d. characterized by more significant shortening of the limbs or the trunk; when the limbs are primarily involved, the shortening may predominate in the proximal segments (rhizomelia), middle segments (mesomelia), or distal segments (acromelia); usually results from hereditary intrinsic skeletal dysplasias.

Fröhlich d., d. with Fröhlich syndrome.

Hunter-Thompson d. [MIM*201250], a severe form of acromesomelic d., characterized by shortening of the distal segments of the limbs; lower extremities are more severely affected than the upper limbs; often associated with dislocations of elbows, knees, and hips. Autosomal recessive inheritance, caused by mutations in the cartilage-derived morphogenetic protein 1 (CDMP1) gene on chromosome 20q.

hypothyroid d., SYN infantile *hypothyroidism*.

infantile d., SYN infantilism (1).

Laron type d., d. associated with an absent or very low levels of somatomedin C (insulinlike growth factor I) or abnormalities in receptor activity.

lethal d., d. leading to intrauterine or neonatal death.

Lorain-Lévi d., SYN pituitary d.

mesomelic d., d. with shortness of the forearms and lower legs.

metatropic d. [MIM*250600], a skeletal dysplasia characterized by disproportionate d. in which the trunk is long relative to the limbs at birth but undergoes reversal of this proportion with subsequent development with severe and progressive kyphoscoliosis; there is metaphyseal flare of long bones, the pelvis is halberd-shaped, and the coccyx is long, resulting in a sacral appendage; autosomal recessive inheritance.

micromelic d., d. with abnormally short or small limbs.

panhypopituitary d., type I is an autosomal recessive disorder with deficient human growth hormone, ACTH, FSH, etc., having delayed sexual development, hypothyroidism, and adrenal insufficiency; type II is similar but is an X-linked disorder.

phocomelic d., d. in which the diaphyses of the long bones are abnormally short or the intermediate parts of the limbs are absent.

physiologic d., d. characterized by normal development that is at a strikingly lesser rate than that for members of the same family, race, or other races. SYN primordial d., true d.

pituitary d., a rare form of d. caused by the absence of a functional anterior pituitary gland; may be present at birth or develop during early childhood. SYN Lorain-Lévi d., Lorain-Lévi infantilism, Lorain-Lévi syndrome, pituitary infantilism.

primordial d., SYN physiologic d.

proportionate d., d. characterized by a symmetric shortening of the limbs and trunk; generally results from chemical, endocrine, nutritional, or nonosseous abnormalities.

psychosocial d., SYN deprivation d.

rhizomelic d., one of the syndromes of chondrodysplasia punctata (q.v.), autosomal recessive, with variable skin keratinization disorders and variable facial, cardiac, optic, and central nervous system abnormalities; epiphyseal stippling is also present. There are multiple enzymatic defects, including peroxisomal ones, and affected infants fail to thrive and usually die in infancy.

Robinow d., SYN Robinow *syndrome*.

Seckel d., SYN Seckel *syndrome*.

senile d., d. characterized by craniofacial anomalies with progeroid appearance.

sexual d., d. with normal sexual development.

Silver-Russell d., SYN Silver-Russell *syndrome*.

snub-nose d. [MIM*127100], d. characterized by low birth weight, snub nose, and stocky build; autosomal dominant inheritance. There is a similar autosomal recessive phenotype [MIM*223600]. SYN dominantly inherited Lévi disease.

thanatophoric d., a lethal d. characterized by micromelia, bowed long bones, enlarged head, flattened vertebral bodies, and muscular hypotonia; lack of pulmonary ventilation causes respiratory difficulties with cyanosis leading to death within the first few hours or days after birth.

true d., SYN physiologic d.

Dwyer, Frederick, English orthopaedic surgeon, 1920–1975. SEE D. *osteotomy*.

Dy Symbol for dysprosium.

dy·ad (dī′ad). **1.** A pair. SYN diad (2). **2.** In chemistry, a bivalent element. **3.** A pair of persons in an interactional situation, e.g., patient and therapist, husband and wife. **4.** The double chromosome resulting from the splitting of a tetrad during meiosis. **5.** Two units treated as one. **6.** A pair of cells resulting from the first meiotic division. [G. *dyas,* the number two, duality]

dy·clo·nine hy·dro·chlo·ride (dī′klō-nēn). A topical local anesthetic.

dy·dro·ges·ter·one (dī-drō-jes′ter-ōn). A synthetic steroid, derived from retroprogesterone, with progestational effects.

dye (dī). A stain or coloring matter; a compound consisting of chromophore and auxochrome groups attached to one or more benzene rings, its color being due to the chromophore and its dyeing affinities to the auxochrome. D.'s are used for intravital coloration of living cells, staining tissues and microorganisms, as antiseptics and germicides, and some as stimulants of epithelial growth. For individual d.'s, see the specific names. Commonly but improperly used for radiographic contrast medium. [A.S. *deah, deag*]

acidic d.'s, d.'s that ionize in solution to produce negatively charged ions or anions; they consist of sodium salts of phenols and carboxylic acid dyes; their solutions tend to be neutral or slightly alkaline; examples are eosin and aniline blue.

acridine d.'s, derivatives of the compound acridine that is closely related to xanthene; important as fluorochromes in histology, cytochemistry, and chemotherapy; examples include acriflavine, acridine orange, and quinacrine mustard.

azin d.'s, d. derivatives of phenazine that include important histologic stains, such as neutral red, azocarmine G., and safranin O.

azo d.'s, d.'s in which the azo group is the chromophore and joins benzene or naphthalene rings; they include a large number of biologic stains, such as Congo red and oil red O; also used clinically to promote epithelial growth in the treatment of ulcers, burns, and other wounds; many have anticoagulant action.

azocarmine d.'s, d.'s giving a dark purplish red color as histologic stains.

basic d.'s, d.'s which ionize in solution to give positively charged ions or cations; the auxochrome group is an amine which can form a salt with an acid like HCl; solutions are usually slightly acidic; examples include basic fuchsin and toluidine blue O.

chlorotriazine d.'s, d.'s containing one or more chlorotriazine moieties that react with polysaccharides.

diphenylmethane d.'s, d.'s in which the central carbon connecting two phenyl groups lacks an amino or imino group; the chromophore is the quinoid ring; an alternative formulation is as a ketonimide; the most common example is auramine O.

ketonimine d.'s, d.'s in which the chromophore is $=C=NH$ connected to two benzene rings; alkylamino groups are added para to the methane carbon on both rings. The most important member for biological purposes is auramine O; an alternative formulation is as a diphenylmethane dye.

natural d.'s, d.'s obtained from animals or plants; examples include carmine, obtained from cochineal in the dried female insect *Dactylopius coccus* of Central America, and hematoxylin, extracted from the bark of the logwood tree *Haematoxylon campechianum* in the Caribbean area.

nitro d.'s, d.'s in which the chromophore is $-NO_2$, which is so acidic that all dyes in this group are of the acid type; important examples in cytoplasmic staining are picric acid and naphthol yellow S.

oxazin d.'s, similar to azin d.'s except that one of the connecting N atoms is replaced by O; most important representatives are brilliant cresyl blue, orcein, litmus, and cresyl violet.

rosanilin d.'s, several triaminotriphenylmethane d.'s or mixtures of them often sold under the name of basic fuchsin; rosanilin d.'s differ from other triphenylmethane d.'s in that the amino groups

dy

are unsubstituted, and they may have methyl groups introduced directly onto the benzene rings; the four possible such dyes are pararosanilin, rosanilin, new fuchsin, and magenta II.

salt d., SYN neutral *stain*.

synthetic d.'s, organic d. compounds originally derived from coal-tar derivatives; presently produced by synthesis from benzene and its derivatives; examples include eosin, methylene blue, and fluorescein.

thiazin d.'s, similar to azin d.'s except that one of the connecting N atoms is replaced by S; includes many important biologic stains, especially in hematology, e.g., azure A, azure B, and methylene blue.

triphenylmethane d.'s, a group of d.'s that includes pararosanilin, as well as many others used in histology and cytology; employed as nuclear, cytoplasmic, and connective tissue stains; important in histochemistry as in the preparation of Schiff reagent.

xanthene d.'s, derivatives of the compound xanthene; include the pyronins, rhodamines, and fluoresceins.

Dyggve, Holger, Danish pediatrician, 1913–1984. SEE D.-Melchior-Clausen *syndrome*.

○**-dymus.** **1.** Suffix to be combined with number roots; e.g., didymus, tridymus, tetradymus. **2.** Occasionally used shortened form -didymus. [G. *-dymos,* fold]

dy·nam·ics (dī-nam′iks). **1.** The science of motion in response to forces. **2.** In psychiatry, used as a contraction of psychodynamics. **3.** In the behavioral sciences, any of the numerous intrapersonal and interpersonal influences or phenomena associated with personality development and interpersonal processes. [G. *dynamis,* force]

group d., a term used to represent the study of underlying features of group behavior, e.g., motives, attitudes; it is concerned with group change rather than with static characteristics.

○**dynamo-.** Combining form denoting force, energy. [G. *dynamis,* power]

dy·na·mo·gen·e·sis (dī′nă-mō-jen′ĕ-sis). The production of force, especially of muscular or nervous energy. SYN dynamogeny. [dynamo- + G. *genesis,* production]

dy·na·mo·gen·ic (dī′nă-mō-jen′ik). Producing power or force, especially nervous or muscular power or activity.

dy·na·mog·e·ny (dī-nă-moj′ĕ-nē). SYN dynamogenesis.

dy·nam·o·graph (dī-nam′ō-graf). An instrument for recording the degree of muscular power. [dynamo- + G. *graphō,* to write]

dy·na·mom·e·ter (dī-nă-mom′ĕ-ter). An instrument for measuring the degree of muscular power. SYN ergometer. [dynamo- + G. *metron,* measure]

dy·nam·o·scope (dī-nam′ō-skōp). A modified stethoscope for auscultation of the muscles. [dynamo- + G. *skopeō,* to examine]

dy·na·mos·co·py (dī-nă-mos′kŏ-pē). Auscultation of a contracting muscle.

dy·na·therm (dī′nă-therm). An apparatus for inducing diathermy. [G. *dynamis,* force, + *thermē,* heat]

dyne (dīn). The unit of force in the CGS system, replaced in the SI system by the newton ($1 N = 10^5$ dynes), that gives a body of 1 g mass an acceleration of 1 cm/sec^2; expressed as F (dynes) $= m$ (grams) $\times a$ (cm/sec^2). [G. *dynamis,* force]

dyn·ein (dīn′ēn). A protein associated with motile structures, exhibiting adenosine triphosphatase activity; it forms "arms" on the outer tubules of cilia and flagella. It functions as a molecular motor. SEE ALSO tubulin, dynein *arm.* [dyne + protein]

dy·nor·phin (dī′nōr-fin). An endogenous opioid ligand that acts as an agonist at opiate receptors. Extremely potent, widely distributed neuropeptide that has 17 amino acid residues and contains leu^5-enkephalin as its NH$_2$-terminal sequence.

dy·phyl·line (dī-fil′in). Exhibits characteristic peripheral vasodilator and bronchodilator actions of other theophylline compounds.

○**dys-.** Bad, difficult, un-, mis-; opposite of eu-. Cf. dis-. [G.]

dys·a·cou·sia, dys·a·cu·sia (dis-ă-kū′sē-ă). SYN dysacusis.

dys·a·cu·sis (dis-ă-kū′sis). **1.** Any impairment of hearing involving difficulty in processing details of sound as opposed to any loss of sensitivity to sound. **2.** Pain or discomfort in the ear from exposure to sound. SYN dysacousia, dysacusia. [dys- + G. *akousis,* hearing]

dys·ad·ap·ta·tion (dis′ad-ap-tā′shŭn). Inability of the retina and iris to accommodate well to varying intensities of light.

dys·an·ti·graph·ia (dis′an-tē-graf′ē-ă). A form of agraphia in which the subject is unable to copy written or printed matter. [dys- + G. *antigraphō,* to write back]

dys·a·phia (dis-ā′fē-ă, dis-af′ē-ă). Impairment of the sense of touch. [dys- + G. *haphē,* touch]

dys·a·phic (dis-ā′fik). Relating to impaired tactile sensibility.

dys·ar·te·ri·ot·o·ny (dis-ar-tēr-ē-ot′ō-nē). Abnormal blood pressure, either too high or too low. [dys- + G. *artēria,* artery, + *tonos,* tension]

dys·ar·thria (dis-ar′thrē-ă). A disturbance of speech due to emotional stress, to brain injury, or to paralysis, incoordination, or spasticity of the muscles used for speaking. SYN dysarthrosis (1). [dys- + G. *arthroō,* to articulate]

ataxic d., d. caused by cerebellar lesions.

hyperkinetic d., d. caused by chorea and myoclonus.

hypokinetic d., d. caused by the rigid types of extrapyramidal *disease*.

lower motor neuron d., d. caused by dysfunction of the motor nuclei and the lower pons or medulla, or other neural connections, central and peripheral to the muscles of articulation.

rigid d., SYN spastic d.

spastic d., d. caused by lesions along the corticobulbar tracts. SYN rigid d.

dys·ar·thric (dis-ar′thrik). Relating to dysarthria.

dys·ar·thro·sis (dis-ar-thrō′sis). **1.** SYN dysarthria. **2.** Malformation of a joint. **3.** A false joint. [dys- + G. *arthrōsis,* joint]

dys·au·to·no·mia (dis′aw-tō-nō′mē-ă). Abnormal functioning of the autonomic nervous system. [dys- + G. *autonomia,* self-government]

familial d. [MIM*223900], a congenital syndrome with specific disturbances of the nervous system and aberrations in autonomic nervous system function such as indifference to pain, diminished lacrimation, poor vasomotor homeostasis, motor incoordination, labile cardiovascular reactions, hyporeflexia, frequent attacks of bronchial pneumonia, hypersalivation with aspiration and difficulty in swallowing, hyperemesis, emotional instability, and an intolerance for anesthetics; autosomal recessive inheritance. Mapped to human chromosome 9q31–q33. SYN Riley-Day syndrome.

dys·ba·rism (dis′bar-izm). General term for the symptom complex resulting from exposure to decreased or changing barometric pressure, including all physiologic effects resulting from such changes with the exception of hypoxia, and including the effects of rapid decompression. [dys- + G. *baros,* weight]

dys·ba·sia (dis-bā′zē-ă). **1.** Difficulty in walking. **2.** The difficult or distorted walking that occurs in persons with certain mental disorders. [dys- + G. *basis,* a step]

d. angiosclerot′ica, d. angiospas′tica, obsolete terms meaning intermittent difficulty in walking due to peripheral vascular causes.

d. lordot′ica progressi′va, an affection characterized by lordoscoliosis of the lower portion of the vertebral column, occurring when the patient stands or walks and usually disappearing when the patient lies down. SYN torsion neurosis.

dys·be·ta·lip·o·pro·tei·ne·mia (dis-bā′tă-lip-ō-prō′tēn-ē′mē-ă). SYN type III familial *hyperlipoproteinemia*.

dys·bo·lism (dis′bō-lizm). Abnormal, but not necessarily morbid, metabolism, as in alkaptonuria. [dys- + G. *bolē (metabolē),* + *-ismos,* metabolism]

dys·bu·lia (dis-boo′lē-ă). Weakness and uncertainty of volition. [dys- + G. *boulē,* will]

dys·bu·lic (dis-boo′lik). Relating to, or characterized by, dysbulia.

dys·cal·cu·lia (dis-kal-kū′lē-ă). Difficulty in performing simple mathematical problems; commonly seen in parietal lobe lesions. [dys- + L. *calculo,* to compute, fr. *calculus,* pebble, counter]

dys·ce·pha·lia (dis-sĕ-fā′lē-ă). Malformation of the head and face. SYN dyscephaly. [dys- + G. *kephalē*, head]

d. mandib′ulo-oculofacia′lis [MIM*234100], a syndrome of bony anomalies of the calvaria, face, and jaw, with brachygnathia, narrow curved nose, and multiple ocular defects including microphthalmia, microcornea, and cataract, often with alopecia overlying skull sutures, or alopecia areata, or absence of eyebrows. The pattern of inheritance is undecided. SYN Hallermann-Streiff syndrome, Hallermann-Streiff-François syndrome, mandibulo-oculofacial syndrome, oculomandibulodyscephaly, oculomandibulofacial syndrome, progeria with cataract, progeria with microphthalmia.

dys·ceph·a·ly (dis-sef′ă-lē). SYN dyscephalia.

dys·chei·ral, dys·chi·ral (dis-kī′răl). Relating to dyscheiria.

dys·chei·ria, dys·chi·ria (dis-kī′rē-ă). A disorder of sensibility in which, although there is no apparent loss of sensation, the patient is unable to tell which side of the body has been touched (acheiria), or refers it to the wrong side (allocheiria), or to both sides (syncheiria). [dys- + G. *cheir*, hand]

dys·che·zia (dis-kē′zē-ă). Difficulty in defecation. [dys- + G. *chezō*, to defecate]

dys·chon·dro·gen·e·sis (dis-kon-drō-jen′ĕ-sis). Abnormal development of cartilage. [dys- + G. *chondros*, cartilage, + *genesis*, production]

dys·chon·dro·pla·sia (dis-kon-drō-plā′zē-ă). SYN enchondromatosis. [dys- + G. *chondros*, cartilage, + *plasis*, a forming]

d. with hemangiomas, SYN Maffucci *syndrome.*

dys·chon·dros·te·o·sis (dis′kon-dros-tē-ō′sis) [MIM*127300]. A skeletal dysplasia, more severe in females and with a female preponderance, characterized by bowing of radius, dorsal dislocation of the distal ulna with limited movement of the elbow and wrist (wrist deformity is called Madelung deformity), and mesomelic dwarfism; dominant inheritance, caused by mutation in the short stature homeobox gene (SHOX) on the pseudoautosomal region of Xp. Langer mesomelic dysplasia, the homozygous form of d., is also caused by homozygous mutations in the SHOX gene. SYN Leri pleonosteosis, Leri-Weill disease, Leri-Weill syndrome. [dys- + G. *chondros*, cartilage, + *osteon*, bone, + *-osis*, condition]

dys·chroia, dys·chroa (dis-kroy′ă, -krō′ă). A bad complexion; discoloration of the skin. [dys- + G. *chroia, chroa*, color]

dys·chro·ma·top·sia (dis′krō-mă-top′sē-ă). A condition in which the ability to perceive colors is not fully normal. Cf. anomalous *trichromatism*, dichromatism, monochromatism, chromatopsia. [dys- + G. *chrōma*, color, + *opsis*, vision]

dys·chro·ma·to·sis (dis-krō-mă-tō′sis). An asymptomatic anomaly of pigmentation occurring among the Japanese; may be localized or diffuse. [dys- + G. *chrōma*, color, + *-osis*, condition]

dys·chro·mia (dis-krō′mē-ă). Any abnormality in the color of the skin.

dys·ci·ne·sia (dis′si-nē′zē-ă). SYN dyskinesia.

dys·con·trol (dis-kon-trōl′). SYN intermittent explosive *disorder.*

dys·co·ria (dis-kō′rē-ă). Abnormality in the shape of the pupil. [dys- + G. *korē*, pupil of eye]

dys·cra·sia (dis-krā′zē-ă). **1.** A morbid general state resulting from the presence of abnormal material in the blood, usually applied to diseases affecting blood cells or platelets. **2.** Old term indicating disease. [G. bad temperament, fr. dys- + *krasis*, a mixing]

blood d., a diseased state of the blood; usually refers to abnormal cellular elements of a permanent character.

dys·cra·sic, dys·crat·ic (dis-krā′sik, krat′ik). Pertaining to or affected with dyscrasia.

dys·di·ad·o·cho·ki·ne·sia, dys·di·ad·o·cho·ci·ne·sia (dis-dī-ad′ō-kō-ki-nē′zē-ă). Impairment of the ability to perform rapidly alternating movements. [dys- + G. *diadochos*, working in turn, + *kinēsis*, movement]

dys·di·a·do·cho·ki·ne·sis (dis′dī-ad-ō-kō-ki-nē′sis). SYN adiadochokinesis.

dys·e·mia (dis-ē′mē-ă). Any abnormal condition or disease of the blood. [dys- + G. *haima*, blood]

dys·en·ce·pha·lia splanch·no·cys·ti·ca (dis′en-se-fā′lē-ă

splangk-nō-sis′ti-kă) [MIM*249000]. A malformation syndrome, lethal in the perinatal period, and characterized by intrauterine growth retardation, sloping forehead, occipital encephalocele, ocular anomalies, cleft palate, polydactyly, polycystic kidneys, and other malformations; autosomal recessive inheritance. Mapped to human chromosome 17q21–q24. SYN Meckel syndrome, Meckel-Gruber syndrome.

dys·en·ter·ic (dis-en-tār′ik). Relating to or suffering from dysentery.

dys·en·tery (dis-en-tār-ē). A disease marked by frequent watery stools, often with blood and mucus, and characterized clinically by pain, tenesmus, fever, and dehydration. [G. *dysenteria,* fr. *dys-,* bad, + *entera,* bowels]

amebic d., diarrhea resulting from ulcerative inflammation of the colon, caused chiefly by infection with *Entamoeba histolytica;* may be mild or severe and also may be associated with amebic infection of other organs.

bacillary d., infection with *Shigella dysenteriae, S. flexneri,* or other organisms.

balantidial d., a type of colitis resembling in many respects amebic d.; caused by the parasitic ciliate, *Balantidium coli.*

bilharzial d., d. due to infection with *Schistosoma mansoni, S. haematobium,* or *S. japonicum.*

fulminating d., SYN malignant d.

helminthic d., d. caused by infection with parasitic worms.

malignant d., d. in which the symptoms are intensely acute, leading to prostration, collapse, and often death. SYN fulminating d.

viral d., profuse watery diarrhea thought to be caused by infection with a virus.

dys·er·e·thism (dis-er′ĕ-thizm). A condition of slow response to stimuli. [dys- + G. *erethismos,* irritation]

dys·er·gia (dis-er′jē-ă). Lack of harmonious action between the muscles concerned in executing any definite voluntary movement. [dys- + G. *ergon,* work]

dys·es·the·sia (dis-es-thē′zē-ă). **1.** Impairment of sensation short of anesthesia. **2.** A condition in which a disagreeable sensation is produced by ordinary stimuli; caused by lesions of the sensory pathways, peripheral or central. **3.** Abnormal sensations experienced in the absence of stimulation. [G. *dysaisthēsia,* fr. *dys-,* hard, difficult, + *aisthēsis,* sensation]

dys·fi·brin·o·ge·ne·mia (dis′fī-brin′ō-jĕ-nē′mē-ă) [MIM*134820]. An autosomal dominant disorder of qualitatively abnormal fibrinogens of various types; each type is named for the city in which the abnormal fibrinogen was discovered. Examples include: 1) Amsterdam, Bethesda II, Cleveland, Los Angeles, Saint Louis, Zurich I and II: major defect, aggregation of fibrin monomers; thrombin time prolonged; inhibitory effect on normal clotting; asymptomatic; 2) Bethesda I and Detroit: major defect, fibrinopeptide release; thrombin time prolonged; inhibitory effect on normal clotting; abnormal bleeding; 3) Baltimore: major defect, fibrinopeptide release; thrombin time prolonged; no inhibitory effect on normal clotting; bleeding and thrombosis; 4) Leuven: major defect, questionable aggregation of fibrin monomers; thrombin time prolonged; slight inhibitory effect on normal clotting; abnormal bleeding; 5) Metz: major defect unreported; thrombin time infinite; effect on normal clotting unreported; abnormal bleeding; 6) Nancy: major defect, aggregation of fibrin monomers; thrombin time prolonged; slight inhibitory effect on normal clotting; asymptomatic; 7) Oklahoma: major defect unreported; thrombin time infinite; no effect on normal clotting; abnormal bleeding; 8) Oslo: major defect unreported; thrombin time shortened; effect on normal clotting unreported; abnormal thrombosis; 9) Parma: major defect unreported; thrombin time infinite; no inhibitory effect on normal clotting; abnormal bleeding; 10) Paris I: major defect unreported; thrombin time infinite; inhibitory effect on normal clotting; asymptomatic; 11) Paris II: major defect unreported; thrombin time prolonged; inhibitory effect on normal clotting; asymptomatic; 12) Troyes: major defect unreported; thrombin time prolonged; effect on normal clotting unreported; asymptomatic; 13) Vancouver: major defect unreported; thrombin time prolonged; no effect on normal clotting; abnormal bleeding; 14) Wiesbaden: major defect, aggregation of fibrin

dy

monomers; thrombin time prolonged; inhibitory effect on normal clotting; bleeding and thrombosis.

dys·func·tion (dis-fŭnk′shŭn). Abnormal or difficult function.

constitutional hepatic d., SYN familial nonhemolytic *jaundice.*

dental d., abnormal functioning of dental structures.

minimal brain d., SEE attention deficit *disorder.*

papillary muscle d., impaired function of a papillary muscle, usually due to ischemia or infarction, with resulting incompetence of the mitral (rarely tricuspid) valve. SYN papillary muscle syndrome.

phagocyte d. (fã′gō-sīt), disorder of phagocytic function.

placental d., SYN dysmature (3).

psychosexual d., sexual d., a disturbance of sexual functioning, e.g., impotence, premature ejaculation, anorgasmia, presumed to be of psychological rather than physical etiology.

sphincter of Oddi d., structural or functional abnormality of the sphincter of Oddi that interferes with bile or pancreatic duct drainage. SYN biliary dyskinesia.

temporomandibular joint d. (TMD, TMJ), chronic or impaired function of the temporomandibular articulation. SEE temporomandibular *arthrosis,* myofascial pain-dysfunction *syndrome.*

dys·gam·ma·glob·u·lin·e·mia (dis-gam′ă-glob′ū-li-nē′mē-ă). An immunoglobulin abnormality, a disturbance of the percentage distribution of γ-globulins or selective deficiency of one or more immunoglobulins.

dys·gen·e·sis (dis-jen′ĕ-sis). Defective development. [dys- + G. *genesis,* generation]

cortical d., SYN cortical *dysplasia.*

gonadal d., defective gonadal development, varying types and degrees of which have been identified, including gonadal aplasia or agenesis, rudimentary gonads, congenitally defective gonads, and true hermaphroditism; the character of the external genitalia, genital ducts, and secondary sexual development are only sometimes uniquely related to a given type of gonadal d. **XO gonadal d.** consists of monosomy X with a gonadal streak rather than a true ovary, notably seen in Turner syndrome; **XX gonadal d.** is an autosomal recessive disorder with a female karyotype, streaked gonads, and primary amenorrhea, but with no body features of Turner syndrome; **XY gonadal d.** is an X-linked disorder associated with a male karyotype and a female habitus, streaked gonads, and absence of secondary sexual characteristics.

iridocorneal mesenchymal d., d. of cornea and iris, producing pupillary anomalies, posterior embryotoxon, and secondary glaucoma, resulting in part from anomalous development of the ocular mesenchyme.

seminiferous tubule d., rarely used term for a disorder in which the seminiferous tubules exhibit an abnormal cytoarchitecture and extensive hyalinization; the testes are small, and few spermatozoa are formed; the body habitus may be eunuchoid, and gynecomastia may be present; urinary gonadotropin output is usually high, and the incidence of mental deficiency and illness increased; sex chromatin may be male or female, and androgen secretion ranges from subnormal to normal. It is a constant feature of (and the term may be used synonymously with) Klinefelter *syndrome.* SYN germinal aplasia.

testicular d. [MIM*305700], a congenital derangement of seminiferous tubular structure and function, resulting in male infertility; the defect in spermatogenesis may be incomplete, as in maturational arrest or premature sloughing, or spermatogenesis may be completely absent, as in the Sertoli-cell-only syndrome.

dys·gen·ic (dis-jen′ik). Applying to factors that have a detrimental effect upon hereditary qualities, physical or mental.

dys·ger·mi·no·ma (dis-jer-mi-nō′mă). A malignant neoplasm of the ovary (counterpart of seminoma of the testis), composed of undifferentiated gonadal germinal cells and occurring more frequently in patients less than 20 years of age. The neoplasms are gray-yellow and firm, contain foci of necrosis and hemorrhage, and tend to be encapsulated; characteristically, they spread by way of lymphatic vessels, but widespread metastases also occur. SYN disgerminoma. [dys- + L. *germen,* a bud or sprout, + G. *-ōma,* tumor]

dys·geu·sia (dis-goo′sē-ă). Distortion or perversion in the percep-

tion of a tastant. An unpleasant perception may occur when a normally pleasant taste is present, or the perception may occur when no tastant is present (gustatory hallucination). SYN parageusia. [dys- + G. *geusis,* taste]

dys·gna·thia (dis-nath′ē-ă). Any abnormality that extends beyond the teeth and includes the maxilla or mandible, or both. [dys- + G. *gnathos,* jaw]

dys·gnath·ic (dis-nath′ik). Pertaining to or characterized by abnormality of the maxilla and mandible.

dys·gno·sia (dis-nō′sē-ă). Any cognitive disorder, i.e., any mental illness. [G. *dysgnōsia,* difficulty of knowing]

dys·gon·ic (dis-gon′ik). A term used to indicate that the growth of a bacterial culture is slow and relatively poor; used especially in reference to the growth of cultures of the bovine tubercle bacillus (*Mycobacterium bovis*) SEE ALSO eugonic. [dys- + G. *gonikos,* relating to the seed or offspring]

dys·graph·ia (dis-graf′ē-ă). **1.** Difficulty in writing. **2.** SYN writer's *cramp.* [dys- + G. *graphē,* writing]

dys·hem·a·to·poi·e·sis (dis-hē′mă-tō-poy-ē′sis). Defective formation of the blood. SYN dyshemopoiesis. [dys- + G. *haima* (*haimat-*), blood, + *poiēsis,* making]

dys·hem·a·to·poi·et·ic (dis-hē′mă-tō-poy-et′ik). Pertaining to or characterized by dyshematopoiesis. SYN dyshemopoietic.

dys·he·mo·poi·e·sis (dis-hē′mō-poy-ē′sis). SYN dyshematopoiesis.

dys·he·mo·poi·et·ic (dis-hē′mō-poy-et′ik). SYN dyshematopoietic.

dys·hid·ria (dis-hid′rē-ă). SYN dyshidrosis.

▣**dys·hi·dro·sis** (dis-i-drō′sis). A vesicular or vesicopustular eruption of multiple causes that occurs primarily on the volar surfaces of the hands and feet; the lesions spread peripherally but have a tendency to central clearing. SYN cheiropompholyx, chiropompholyx, dyshidria, dyshidrotic eczema, pompholyx. [dys- + G. *hidrōs,* sweat]

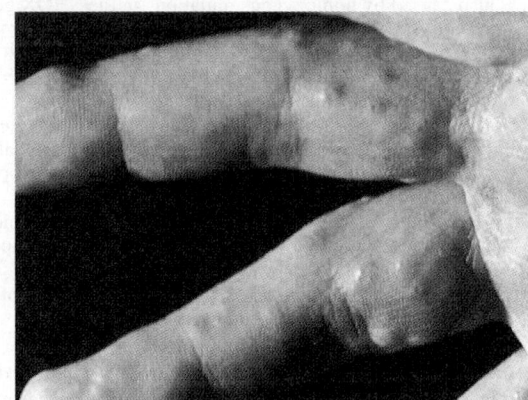

dyshidrosis: note deep-seated vesicles on the sides and flexural aspects of the fingers

dysjunction. A separation of parts or structures normally joined; cleavage.

Le Fort III craniofacial d., SYN craniofacial dysjunction *fracture.*

dys·kar·y·o·sis (dis-kar-ē-ō′sis). Abnormal maturation seen in exfoliated cells that have normal cytoplasm but hyperchromatic nuclei, or irregular chromatin distribution; may be followed by the development of a malignant neoplasm. [dys- + G. *karyon,* nucleus, + *-ōsis,* condition]

dys·kar·y·ot·ic (dis-kar-ē-ot′ik). Pertaining to or characterized by dyskaryosis.

dys·ker·a·to·ma (dis-ker-ă-tō′mă). A skin tumor exhibiting dyskeratosis. [dys- + G. *keras,* horn, + *-oma,* tumor]

warty d., a benign solitary tumor of the skin, usually of the scalp, face, or neck, with a central keratotic plug; it appears to arise from a hair follicle, and microscopically resembles a lesion of keratosis follicularis but is larger, with more extensive epithelial downgrowth. SYN isolated dyskeratosis follicularis.

dys·ker·a·to·sis (dis′ker-ă-tō′sis). **1.** Premature keratinization in individual epithelial cells that have not reached the keratinizing surface layer; dyskeratotic cells generally become rounded and they may break away from adjacent cells and fall off. **2.** Epidermalization of the conjunctival and corneal epithelium. **3.** A disorder of keratinization. [dys- + G. *keras,* horn, + *-osis,* condition]

benign d., d. that may occur in congenital and bullous diseases of the skin.

d. congen′ita [MIM*305000], nail dystrophy, oral leukoplakia, and reticular pigmentation of the skin, testicular atrophy with anemia progressing most commonly to pancytopenia; X-linked recessive inheritance, caused by mutation in the DKC1 gene encoding dyskenin on Xq.

intraepithelial d. [MIM*127600], an autosomal dominant condition consisting of white spongy lesions of the buccal mucosa, floor of the mouth, ventral lateral tongue, gingiva and palate. Transient gelatinous plaques form over the cornea, which may produce temporary blindness;

isolated d. follicula′ris, SYN warty *dyskeratoma.*

dys·ker·a·tot·ic (dis′ker-a-tot′ik). Relating to or characterized by dyskeratosis.

dys·ki·ne·sia (dis-ki-nē′zē-ă) [MIM*242650]. Difficulty in performing voluntary movements. Term usually used in relation to various extrapyramidal disorders. SYN dyscinesia. [dys- + G. *kinēsis,* movement]

biliary d., SYN sphincter of Oddi *dysfunction.*

extrapyramidal d.'s, abnormal involuntary movements attributed to pathologic states of one or more parts of the striate body and characterized by insuppressible, stereotyped, automatic movements that cease only during sleep; e.g., Parkinson disease; chorea; athetosis; hemiballism.

lingual-facial-buccal d., SYN tardive d.

tardive d., involuntary movements of the facial muscles and tongue, often persistent, that develop as a late complication of some neuroleptic therapy, more likely with typical antipsychotics. SYN lingual-facial-buccal d.

tracheobronchial d., degeneration of elastic and connective tissue of bronchi and trachea.

dys·ki·ne·sis. SYN dyskinesia.

ciliary dyskinesis, (1) absent or impaired motion of the cilia, occurring as a primary or secondary disorder; SEE ALSO Kartagener *syndrome;* (2) associated with recurrent infections in the respiratory tract.

dys·ki·net·ic (dis-ki-net′ik). Denoting or characteristic of dyskinesia.

dys·lex·ia (dis-lek′sē-ă). Impaired reading ability with a competence level below that expected on the basis of the individual's level of intelligence, and in the presence of normal vision and letter recognition and normal recognition of the meaning of pictures and objects. SYN incomplete alexia. [dys- + G. *lexis,* word, phrase]

dys·lex·ic (dis-lek′sik). Relating to, or characterized by, dyslexia.

dys·lo·gia (dis-lō′jē-ă). Impairment of speech and reasoning as the result of a mental disorder. [dys- + G. *logos,* speaking, reason]

dys·ma·se·sis (dis-mă-sē′sis). Difficulty in mastication. [dys- + G. *masēsis,* chewing]

dys·ma·ture (dis′mă-tūr). **1.** Denoting faulty development or ripening; often connoting structural and/or functional abnormalities. **2.** In obstetrics, denoting an infant whose birth weight is inappropriately low for its gestational age. **3.** Immature development of the placenta so that normal function does not occur. SYN placental dysfunction.

dys·ma·tu·ri·ty (dis′mă-choor-i-tē). Syndrome of an infant born with relative absence of subcutaneous fat, wrinkling of the skin, prominent finger and toe nails, and meconium staining of the infant's skin and of the placental membranes; often associated with postmaturity or placental insufficiency.

dys·me·lia (dis-mē′lē-ă). Congenital abnormality characterized by missing or foreshortened limbs. SEE amelia, phocomelia. [dys- + G. *melos,* limb]

dys·men·or·rhea (dis-men-ōr-ē′ă). Difficult and painful menstruation. SYN menorrhalgia. [dys- + G. *mēn,* month, + *rhoia,* a flow]

functional d., SYN primary d.

mechanical d., d. due to obstruction of discharge of menstrual blood, as in cervical stenosis. SYN obstructive d.

membranous d., d. accompanied by an exfoliation of the menstrual decidua.

obstructive d., SYN mechanical d.

ovarian d., a form of secondary d. due to disease of an ovary.

primary d., d. due to a functional disturbance and not due to inflammation, new growths, or anatomic factors. SYN functional d.

secondary d., d. due to inflammation, infection, tumor, or anatomical factors.

spasmodic d., d. accompanied by painful contractions of the uterus.

tubal d., a form of secondary d. due to stenosis or other abnormal condition of the fallopian tubes.

ureteric d., a form of secondary d. characterized by pain due to spasm of the ureter occurring at the time of the menses.

uterine d., a form of secondary d. resulting from disease of the uterus.

vaginal d., a form of secondary d. due to obstruction or other abnormal condition in the vagina.

dys·met·ria (dis-mē′trē-ă, -met′rē-ă). An aspect of ataxia, in which the ability to control the distance, power, and speed of an act is impaired. Usually used to describe abnormalities of movement caused by cerebellar disorders. SEE ALSO hypermetria, hypometria. [dys- + G. *metron,* measure]

ocular d., abnormality of ocular movements in which the eyes overshoot on attempting to fixate an object.

dys·mor·phia (dis-mōr′fē-ă). SYN dysmorphism.

dys·mor·phism (dis-mōr′fizm). Abnormality of shape. SYN dysmorphia. [G. *dysmorphia,* badness of form]

dys·mor·pho·gen·e·sis (dis′mōr-fō-jen′ĕ-sis). The process of abnormal tissue formation. [dys- + G. *morphē,* form, + *genesis,* production]

dys·mor·phol·o·gy (dis-mōr-fol′ŏ-jē). General term for the study of, or the subject of, abnormal development of tissue form. A branch of clinical genetics. [dys- + G. *morphē,* form, + *logos,* study]

dys·mor·pho·pho·bia (dis′mōr-fō-fō′bē-ă). SYN body dysmorphic *disorder.* [dys- + G. *morphē,* form, + *phobos,* fear]

dys·my·e·li·na·tion (dis-mī-ĕ-li-nā′shŭn). Improper laying down or breakdown of a myelin sheath of a nerve fiber, caused by abnormal myelin metabolism.

dys·my·o·to·nia (dis-mī-ō-tō′nē-ă). Abnormal muscular tonicity (either hyper- or hypo-). SEE dystonia. [dys- + G. *mys,* muscle, + *tonos,* tension, tone]

dys·nys·tax·is (dis-nis-tak′sis). A condition of half sleep. SYN light sleep. [dys- + G. *nystaxis,* drowsiness]

dys·o·don·ti·a·sis (dis′ō-don-tī′ă-sis). Difficulty or irregularity in the eruption of the teeth. [dys- + G. *odous,* tooth, + *-iasis,* condition]

dys·on·to·gen·e·sis (dis′on-tō-jen′ĕ-sis). Defective embryonic development. [dys- + G. *ōn,* being, + *genesis,* origin]

dys·on·to·ge·net·ic (dis′on-tō-jĕ-net′ik). Characterized by dysontogenesis.

dys·o·rex·ia (dis-ō-rek′sē-ă). Diminished or perverted appetite. [dys- + G. *orexis,* appetite]

dys·os·mia (dis-oz′mē-ă). Distortion or perversion in the perception of an odorant; an unpleasant perception may occur when a normally pleasant odor is present, or the perception may occur when no odorant is present (olfactory hallucination). SYN parosmia, parosphresia. [dys- + G. *osmē,* smell]

dys·os·te·o·gen·e·sis (dis′os-tē-ō-jen′ĕ-sis). Defective bone formation. SYN dysostosis. [dys- + G. *osteon,* bone, + *genesis,* production]

dys·os·to·sis (dis-os-tō'sis). SYN dysosteogenesis. [dys- + G. *osteon,* bone, + *-osis,* condition]

acrofacial d., mandibulofacial d. associated with malformations of the extremities such as defective radius and thumbs, and radio-ulnar synostosis. SEE ALSO Treacher Collins *syndrome.* SYN acrofacial syndrome.

cleidocranial d., clidocranial d. [MIM*119600], a developmental disorder characterized by absence or hypoplasia of clavicles, box-shaped skull with open sutures, frontal bossing, womian bones, ability to oppose shoulders, and missing teeth; autosomal dominant inheritance, caused by mutation in the transcription factor gene (CBFA1) encoding core-binding factor, runt domain, alpha-subunit 1 on 6p. There is an autosomal recessive form [MIM*216330]. SYN cleidocranial dysplasia, clidocranial dysplasia, craniocleidodysostosis.

craniofacial d. [MIM*123500], SYN Crouzon *syndrome.*

mandibuloacral d. [MIM*248370], an autosomal recessive disorder characterized by hypoplastic mandible, dental crowding, acro-osteolysis, stiff joints, and atrophy of the skin of the hands and feet; clavicles are hypoplastic, cranial sutures are wide, and multiple wormian bones are present.

mandibulofacial d., a variable syndrome of malformations primarily of derivatives of the first branchial arch; characterized by palpebral fissures sloping outward and downward with notches or colobomas in the outer third of the lower lids, bony defects or hypoplasia of malar bones and zygoma, hypoplasia of the mandible, macrostomia with high or cleft palate and malposition and malocclusion of teeth, low-set malformed external ears, atypical hair growth, and occasional pits or clefts between mouth and ear. SEE ALSO Treacher Collins *syndrome.* SYN mandibulofacial dysotosis syndrome, mandibulofacial dysplasia.

metaphysial d., a rare developmental abnormality of the skeleton in which metaphyses of tubular bones are expanded by deposits of cartilage.

d. mul'tiplex, specific pattern of radiographic changes observed in many lysosomal storage disorders.

orodigitofacial d., SYN orofaciodigital *syndrome.*

otomandibular d., hypoplasia of the mandible, often with malformation of the temporomandibular joint, associated with malformations of the ear but not eye malformations or malar defects. SYN otomandibular syndrome.

peripheral d. [MIM*170700], d. of the metacarpals and metatarsals, accompanied by variable facial features; possibly autosomal dominant inheritance.

dys·pal·lia (dis-pal'ē-ă). Developmental distortion of the brain mantle. [dys- + L. *pallium,* cloak]

dys·pa·reu·nia (dis-pa-roo'nē-ă). Occurrence of pain during sexual intercourse. [dys- + G. *pareunos,* lying beside, fr. *para,* beside, + *eunē,* a bed]

dys·pep·sia (dis-pep'sē-ă). Impaired gastric function or "upset stomach" due to some disorder of the stomach; characterized by epigastric pain, sometimes burning, nausea, and gaseous eructation. SYN gastric indigestion. [dys- + G. *pepsis,* digestion]

acid d., d. associated with excess gastric acidity.

adhesion d., pain, d., and other symptoms alleged to result from perigastric adhesions.

atonic d., d. with impaired tone in the muscular walls of the stomach. SYN functional d. (1).

fermentative d., d. accompanied by fermentation of the contents of the stomach, usually occurring in gastric dilation.

flatulent d., d. with frequent eructations of swallowed air, sometimes without underlying organic disease.

functional d., (1) SYN atonic d; (2) SYN nervous d.

nervous d., d. associated with nervousness, tension, or anxiety. SYN functional d. (2).

reflex d., functional d. excited by reflex irritation from disease elsewhere than in the stomach or intestines.

dys·pep·tic (dis-pep'tik). Relating to or suffering from dyspepsia.

dys·pha·gia, dys·pha·gy (dis-fā'jē-ă, dis'fă-jē). Difficulty in swallowing. SEE ALSO aglutition. [dys- + G. *phagō,* to eat]

d. luso'ria, d. said to be due to compression by the right subclavi-

an artery arising abnormally from the descending aorta and passing behind the esophagus. [coinage from L. *lusus naturae,* a sport of nature]

d. nervo'sa, nervous d., SYN esophagism.

sideropenic d., SYN Plummer-Vinson *syndrome.*

vallecular d., d. caused by food becoming lodged in a vallecula above the epiglottis. SYN Barclay-Baron disease.

dys·pha·go·cy·to·sis (dis-fag'ō-sī-tō'sis). Disordered phagocytosis, especially failure of cells to ingest and digest bacteria.

congenital d., SYN chronic granulomatous *disease.*

dys·pha·sia (dis-fā'zē-ă). Impairment in the production of speech and failure to arrange words in an understandable way; caused by an acquired lesion of the brain. SYN dysphrasia. [dys- + G. *phasis,* speaking]

dys·phe·mia (dis-fē'mē-ă). Disordered phonation, articulation, or hearing due to emotional or mental deficits. [dys- + G. *phēmē,* speech]

dys·pho·nia (dis-fō'nē-ă). Altered voice production. [dys- + G. *phōnē,* voice]

abductor spasmodic d., a breathy form of spasmodic d. caused by excessive and long vocal cord opening for voiceless phonemes extending into vowels.

adductor spasmodic d., a form of spasmodic d. in which excessive closure of the vocal cords affects the initiation and maintenance of phonation.

d. pli'cae ventricula'ris, phonation with the ventricular bands rather than with the vocal cords.

spasmodic d., a spasmodic contradiction of the intrinsic muscles of the larynx excited bt attempted phonation, producing either adductor or abductor subtypes caused by a central nervous system disorder. A localized form of movement disorder. SYN d. spastica, spastic d.

spastic d., SYN spasmodic d.

d. spas'tica, SYN spasmodic d.

dys·pho·ria (dis-fōr'ē-ă). A mood of general dissatisfaction, restlessness, depression, and anxiety; a feeling of unpleasantness or discomfort. [dys- + G. *phora,* a bearing]

late luteal phase d., SYN premenstrual *syndrome.*

dys·phra·sia (dis-frā'zē-ă). SYN dysphasia. [dys- + G. *phrasis,* speaking]

dys·pig·men·ta·tion (dis'pig-men-tā'shŭn). Any abnormality in the formation or distribution of pigment, especially in the skin; usually applied to an abnormal reduction in pigmentation (depigmentation). SEE ALSO albinism.

dys·pin·e·al·ism (dis-pin'ē-ăl-izm). Obsolete term for the syndrome supposed to result from the deficiency of pineal gland secretion.

dys·pi·tu·i·tar·ism (dis-pi-too'i-ter-izm). The complex of phenomena due to excessive or deficient secretion by the pituitary gland.

dys·pla·sia (dis-plā'zē-ă). Abnormal tissue development. SEE ALSO heteroplasia. [dys- + G. *plasis,* a molding]

anhidrotic ectodermal d. [MIM*305100], a disorder characterized by absent or defective sweat glands, saddle-shaped nose, hyperpigmentation around the eyes, malformed or missing teeth, sparse hair, dysplastic nails, smooth, finely wrinkled skin, syndactyly, absent breast tissue, and occasionally mental retardation; X-linked recessive inheritance, caused by mutation in the ED1 gene on chromosome Xq. There is also an autosomal recessive form [MIM*224900]. SYN hypohidrotic ectodermal d.

anterofacial d., anteroposterior facial d., anteroposterior d., abnormal growth of the face or cranium in an anteroposterior direction as seen and measured with a cephalogram.

asphyxiating thoracic d. [MIM*208500], SYN asphyxiating thoracic *dystrophy.*

branchiootorenal d., an autosomal dominant disorder manifested by branchial cysts, preauricular skin tags or sinuses, ear anomalies, and kidney malformations. SYN BOR syndrome.

bronchopulmonary d., chronic pulmonary insufficiency seen primarily in infants born prematurely; defined clinically as a persistent supplemental oxygen requirement at 1 month of age and typically seen in infants who required positive pressure ventilation.

cerebral d., abnormal development of the telencephalon.

cervical d., d. of the uterine cervix, epithelial atypia involving part or all of the thickness of cervical squamous epithelium, occurring most often in young women; appears to regress frequently, but may progress over a long period to carcinoma; severe d. may be microscopically indistinguishable from carcinoma in situ.

chondroectodermal d. [MIM*225500], triad of chondrodysplasia, ectodermal d., and polydactyly, with congenital heart defects in over half of patients; autosomal recessive inheritance. Maps to human chromosome 4p16. SYN Ellis-van Creveld syndrome.

cleidocranial d., clidocranial d., SYN cleidocranial *dysostosis.*

cochlear d., failure of the bony cochlea to develop completely.

congenital ectodermal d., incomplete development of the epidermis and skin appendages; the skin is smooth and hairless, the facies abnormal, and the teeth and nails may be affected; sweating may be deficient. SYN congenital ectodermal defect.

congenital hip d., SYN developmental hip d.

cortical d., a malformative disorganization of the cytoarchitecture of the cortex relative to neurons. SYN cortical dysgenesis, neuronal migration abnormality.

craniocarpotarsal d., SYN craniocarpotarsal *dystrophy.*

craniodiaphysial d. [MIM*218300], small stature, thickening of the cranial bones with sclerosis and diaphysial widening of tubular bones; autosomal recessive inheritance. There may also be an autosomal dominant form [MIM 122860].

craniometaphysial d., syndrome of metaphysial d. associated with severe sclerosis and overgrowth of bones of the skull (leontiasis ossea) and with hypertelorism.

dentin d., a hereditary disorder of the teeth, involving both primary and permanent dentition, in which the clinical morphology and color of the teeth are normal, but the teeth radiographically exhibit short roots [MIM125400], obliteration of the pulp chambers and canals, and mobility and premature exfoliation; autosomal dominant inheritance. In another type of d. the teeth are opalescent [MIM 125420].

developmental hip d., a developmental abnormality in which a neonate's hips easily become dislocated; etiology is complex, with mechanical, familial, hormonal, and birthing presentation all contributing; female predominance is 9:1. SYN congenital hip d.

diaphysial d., progressive, symmetrical fusiform enlargement of the shafts of long bones characterized by the formation of excessive new periosteal and endosteal bone and irregular conversion of this cortical bone into cancellous bone; anemia does not occur as a rule, as in osteopetrosis. SYN Engelmann disease.

diastrophic d. [MIM*222600], a skeletal d. characterized by scoliosis, hitchhiker thumb due to shortening of the first metacarpal bone, cleft palate, malformed ear with calcification, chondritis, shortening of the Achilles tendon, clubbed foot, and characteristic radiologic findings; autosomal recessive inheritance, caused by mutation in the diastrophic dysplasia sulfate transporter gene (DTDST) on chromosome 5q. SYN diastrophic dwarfism.

ectodermal d., a congenital defect of the ectodermal tissues, including the skin and its appendages; associated with dysplasia of the teeth and hyperthermia. SEE anhidrotic ectodermal d., hidrotic ectodermal d.

enamel d., SYN *amelogenesis* imperfecta.

d. epiphysea'lis mul'tiplex, SYN multiple epiphyseal d.

d. epiphysia'lis hemime'lia, SYN tarsomegaly.

d. epiphysia'lis puncta'ta, SYN *chondrodysplasia* punctata.

epithelial d., a disorder of differentiation of epithelial cells which may regress, remain stable, or progress to invasive carcinoma.

faciodigitogenital d., a syndrome of ocular hypertelorism, anteverted nostrils, broad upper lip, saddle-bag or shawl scrotum, protruding umbilicus, and laxity of ligaments resulting in genu recurvatum, flat feet, and hyperextensible fingers; the X-linked form [MIM*305400] is caused by mutation in the FGD1 gene on Xp; autosomal dominant [MIM*100050] and recessive [MIM*227300] forms also exist. SYN Aarskog-Scott syndrome.

familial white folded d., SYN white sponge *nevus.*

fibromuscular d., idiopathic nonatherosclerotic disease leading to stenosis of arteries, usually the renal arteries, and hypertension; two varieties are fibromuscular hyperplasia and perimuscular fibrosis.

fibrous d. of bone, a disturbance of medullary bone maintenance in which bone undergoing physiologic lysis is replaced by abnormal proliferation of fibrous tissue, resulting in asymmetric distortion and expansion of bone; may be confined to a single bone (monostotic fibrous d.) or involve multiple bones (polyostotic fibrous d.).

fibrous d. of jaws, SYN cherubism.

florid osseous d., cemental d., SYN sclerotic cemental *mass.*

hidrotic ectodermal d. [MIM*129500], congenital dystrophy of the nails and hair with thickened nails and sparse or absent scalp hair; often associated with keratoderma of the palms and soles; teeth and sweat gland function are normal; autosomal dominant inheritance.

hypohidrotic ectodermal d., SYN anhidrotic ectodermal d.

mandibulofacial d., SYN mandibulofacial *dysostosis.*

McKusick metaphyseal d., SYN cartilage-hair *hypoplasia.*

metaphysial d., an abnormality that occurs when new bone at the metaphyses of long bones fails to undergo remodeling to the normal tubular structure; the ends of long bones appear to be expanded and porotic, with thin cortex; there may be an associated overgrowth of cranial bones (craniometaphysial d.).

Mondini d., congenital anomaly of osseus and membranous otic labyrinth characterized by aplastic cochlea, and deformity of the vestibule and semicircular canals with partial or complete loss of auditory and vestibular function; may be associated with spontaneous cerebrospinal fluid otorrhoea resulting in meningitis. SEE ALSO Mondini *hearing impairment.*

monostotic fibrous d., fibrous d. of a single bone. SYN localized osteitis fibrosa, osteitis fibrosa circumscripta.

mucoepithelial d. [MIM*158310], an epithelial cell dishesive disease characterized by red, periorificial mucosal lesions of oral, nasal, vaginal, urethral, anal, bladder, and conjunctival mucosa, with cataracts, follicular keratosis, nonscarring alopecia, frequent pulmonary infections, pneumothorax, and sometimes cor pulmonale; autosomal dominant inheritance.

multiple epiphyseal d. (EDM), a disorder of epiphyses characterized by difficulty in walking, pain and stiffness of joints, stubby fingers, and often short stature; on X-ray examination, the epiphyses are irregular and mottled, the ossification centers are late in appearance and may be multiple, but the vertebrae are normal. There are at least 3 forms of autosomal dominant inheritance: EDM1 [MIM*132400] due to mutation in the cartilage oligomeric matrix protein gene (COMP) on chromosome 19p; EDM2 [MIM*600304], due to mutation in the type IX collagen gene (COL9A2) on 1p; and EDM3 [MIM*600969], which is linked to an unknown locus. There is also an autosomal recessive form [MIM*226900]. SYN d. epiphysealis multiplex.

neuronal intestinal d., SYN neuronal *hyperplasia.*

oculoauriculovertebral d., OAV d. [MIM*257700], a syndrome characterized by epibulbar dermoids, preauricular appendages, micrognathia, and vertebral and other anomalies. SYN Goldenhar syndrome, OAV syndrome.

oculodentodigital d. [MIM*164200], microphthalmia, coloboma, or anomalies of the iris associated with malformed and malpositioned teeth and with anomalies of the fingers including syndactyly, campylodactyly, or absent phalanges; autosomal dominant inheritance. There is also a recessive form in which the ocular manifestation is more severe [MIM*257850].

oculovertebral d., microphthalmia, colobomas, or anophthalmia with small orbit, twisted face due to unilateral d. of maxilla, macrostomia with malformed teeth and malocclusion, vertebral malformations, and branched and hypoplastic ribs. SYN oculovertebral syndrome, Weyers-Thier syndrome.

odontogenic d., SYN odontodysplasia.

ophthalmomandibulomelic d. [MIM*164900], an autosomal dominant disorder with corneal clouding and multiple abnormalities of the mandible and limbs.

dy

otospondylomegaepiphyseal d., SYN *chondrodystrophy* with sensorineural deafness.

periapical cemental d., a benign, painless, non-neoplastic condition of the jaws which occurs almost exclusively in middle-aged black females; lesions are usually multiple, most frequently involve vital mandibular anterior teeth, surround the root apices, and are initially radiolucent (becoming more opaque as they mature). SYN periapical osteofibrosis.

polyostotic fibrous d., the occurrence of lesions of fibrous d. in multiple bones, commonly on one side of the body; may occur with areas of pigmentation and endocrine dysfunction (McCune-Albright syndrome). SYN multifocal osteitis fibrosa, osteitis fibrosa disseminata.

pseudoachondroplastic spondyloepiphysial d., SYN pseudoachondroplasia.

retinal d., an overgrowth of glial tissue compensating for aplasia of sensory elements.

septooptic d., congenital optic nerve hypoplasia associated with midline cerebral anomalies. SYN de Morsier syndrome.

skeletal d.'s, a heterogeneous group of disorders (over 120 types), each of which results in numerous disturbances of the skeletal system and most of which include dwarfism. SEE ALSO chondrodystrophy.

spondyloepiphyseal d., a group of conditions characterized by growth deficiency of the vertebral column with flattening of the vertebrae or platyspondyly, lack of ossification of the epiphyses, short-trunk dwarfism with limb shortening, and sometimes with other malformations; autosomal dominant [MIM*183900 and MIM*184100], autosomal recessive [MIM*208230 and MIM*271600], and X-linked recessive [MIM*313400] inheritance have been described.

spondyloepiphyseal d. congenita (SEDC) [MIM*183900], a skeletal d. characterized by short-trunk dwarfism with short limbs, delayed ossification of the pubic rami and femoral and tibial epiphyses, flattening of the vertebral bodies, myopia, retinal detachment, and cleft palate; autosomal dominant inheritance caused by mutation in the type II collagen gene (COL2A1) on 12q.

spondyloepiphyseal d. tarda, a skeletal d. of later onset, usually in the second decade, characterized by short stature, flattening of the vertebrae, epiphyseal involvement with bony fusion of the hip joint, premature osteoarthritis, and distinctive radiographic findings. Autosomal dominant [MIM*184100] and X-linked recessive [MIM*313400] forms exist.

ventriculoradial d., a congenital syndrome consisting of a ventricular septal defect with associated absence of thumb or radius.

dys·plas·tic (dis-plas'tik). Pertaining to or marked by dysplasia.

dysp·nea (disp-nē'ă). Shortness of breath, a subjective difficulty or distress in breathing, usually associated with disease of the heart or lungs; occurs normally during intense physical exertion or at high altitude. [G. *dyspnoia,* fr. *dys-,* bad, + *pnoē,* breathing]

cardiac d., shortness of breath of cardiac origin.

exertional d., excessive shortness of breath after exercise.

expiratory d., difficulty with the expiratory phase of breathing, often due to obstruction in the larynx or large bronchi, such as by a foreign body.

functional d., shortness of breath without apparent underlying disease.

nocturnal d., d. occurring at night, several hours after assuming recumbent position. Occurs in heart failure and results from reabsorption of water from dependent areas after removal of effect of gravity, causing hypervolemia, aggravating left-ventricular failure.

paroxysmal nocturnal d., acute d. appearing suddenly at night, usually waking the patient from sleep; caused by pulmonary congestion with or without pulmonary edema that results from left-sided heart failure following mobilization of fluid from dependent areas after lying down.

Traube d., obsolete eponym for inspiratory d. with maximal expansion of the chest and a slow respiratory rhythm.

dysp·ne·ic (disp-nē'ik). Out of breath; relating to or suffering from dyspnea.

dys·prax·ia (dis-prak'sē-ă). Impaired or painful functioning in any organ. [dys- + G. *praxis,* a doing]

dys·pro·si·um (Dy) (dis-prō'sē-ŭm). A metallic element of the lanthanide (rare earth) series, atomic no. 66, atomic wt. 162.50. [G. *dysprositos,* hard to get at]

dys·pro·tein·e·mia (dis-prō'tēn-ē'mē-ă). An abnormality in plasma proteins, usually in immunoglobulins.

dys·pro·tein·e·mic (dis-prō-tēn-ē'mik). Relating to dysproteinemia.

dys·ra·phism, dys·raph·ia (dis'ră-fizm, dis-raf'ē-ă). Defective fusion, especially of the neural folds, resulting in status dysraphicus or neural tube defect. [dys- + G. *rhaphē,* suture]

spinal d., a general term used to describe a collection of congenital abnormalities that include defects in the vertebrae and underlying spine or nerve roots.

dys·rhyth·mia (dis-rith'mē-ă). Defective rhythm. See also entries under rhythm. Cf. arrhythmia. [dys- + G. *rhythmos,* rhythm]

cardiac d., any abnormality in the rate, regularity, or sequence of cardiac activation.

electroencephalographic d., a diffusely irregular brain wave tracing.

esophageal d., abnormal motility of the muscular layers of the esophageal wall, such as occurs in esophageal spasm.

paroxysmal cerebral d., a diffusely abnormal electroencephalogram often seen with epilepsy.

dys·som·nia (dis-som'nē-ă). Disturbance of normal sleep or rhythm pattern.

dys·spon·dy·lism (dis-spon'di-lizm). An abnormality of development of the spine or vertebral column. [dys- + G. *spondylos,* vertebra]

dys·sta·sia (dis-stā'sē-ă). Difficulty in standing. SYN dystasia. [dys- + G. *stasis,* standing]

dys·stat·ic (dis-tat'ik). Marked by difficulty in standing.

dys·syl·la·bia (dis-il-lā'bē-ă). SYN syllable-stumbling. [dys- + G. *syllabē,* syllable]

dys·syn·er·gia (dis-in-er'jē-ă). An aspect of ataxia, in which an act is not performed smoothly or accurately because of lack of harmonious association of its various components; usually used to describe abnormalities of movement caused by cerebellar disorders. [dys- + G. *syn,* with, + *ergon,* work]

d. cerebellaris myoclonica, a familial disorder beginning in late childhood, characterized by progressive cerebellar ataxia, action myoclonus and preserved intellect. Probably due to multiple causes, mitochondrial abnormalities being one. SYN dentatorubral cerebellar atrophy with polymyoclonus.

detrusor sphincter d., a disturbance of the normal relationship between bladder (detrusor) contraction and sphincter relaxation during voluntary or involuntary voiding efforts.

dys·tas·ia. SYN dysstasia.

dys·tel·e·pha·lan·gy (dis-tel'ē-fă-lan'jē). Bowing of the distal phalanx of the little finger. [dys- + G. *telos,* end, + phalanx]

dys·thy·mia (dis-thī'mē-ă). A chronic mood disorder manifested as depression for most of the day, more days than not, accompanied by some of the following symptoms: poor appetite or overeating, insomnia or hypersomnia, low energy or fatigue, low self-esteem, poor concentration, difficulty making decisions, and feelings of hopelessness. SEE mood *disorders,* under *disorder,* endogenous *depression,* exogenous *depression.* [dys- + G. *thymos,* mind, emotion]

dys·thy·mic (dis-thī'mik). Relating to dysthymia.

dys·to·cia (dis-tō'sē-ă). Difficult childbirth. [G. *dystokia,* fr. *dys-,* difficult, + *tokos,* childbirth]

arrest of active phase d., stoppage of further cervical dilation for longer than 2 hours after labor has entered active phase (generally defined as active contraction with at least 4 cm of cervical dilatation); causes include inadequate uterine contractions and cephalopelvic disproportion.

arrest of descent d., failure of fetus to descend after an hour in second stage despite maternal effort; typically due to inadequate maternal effort, fetal malposition, or fetal size.

fetal d., d. due to an abnormality of the fetus.

maternal d., d. caused by an abnormality or physical problem in the mother.

placental d., retention or difficult delivery of the placenta.

shoulder d., arrest of normal labor after delivery of the head by impaction of the anterior shoulder against the symphysis pubis.

dys·to·nia (dis-tō′nē-ă). A state of abnormal (either hypo- or hyper-) tonicity in any of the tissues resulting in impairment of voluntary movement. [dys- + G. *tonos,* tension]

d. lenticula′ris, d. resulting from a lesion of the lenticulate nucleus.

d. musculo′rum defor′mans, a genetic, environmental, or idiopathic disorder, usually beginning in childhood or adolescence, marked by muscular contractions that distort the spine, limbs, hips, and sometimes the cranial-innervated muscles. The abnormal movements are increased by excitement and, at least initially, abolished by sleep. The musculature is hypertonic when in action, hypotonic when at rest. Hereditary forms usually begin with involuntary posturing of the foot or hand (autosomal recessive form [MIM*224500]) or of the neck or trunk (autosomal dominant form [MIM*128100]); both forms may progress to produce contortions of the entire body. SYN torsion disease of childhood, torsion d., Ziehen-Oppenheim disease.

torsion d., SYN d. musculorum deformans.

dys·ton·ic (dis-ton′ik). Pertaining to dystonia.

dys·to·pia (dis-tō′pē-ă). Faulty or abnormal position of a part or organ. SYN allotopia, malposition. [dys- + G. *topos,* place]

pituitary d., failure of union of neurohypophysis and adenohypophysis.

dys·top·ic (dis-top′ik). Pertaining to, or characterized by, dystopia. SEE ALSO ectopic.

dys·tro·phia (dis-trō′fē-ă). SYN dystrophy. [L. fr. G. *dys-,* bad, + *trophē,* nourishment]

d. adipo′sogenita′lis, SYN adiposogenital *dystrophy.*

d. brevicol′lis, a condition marked by symptoms of d. adiposogenitalis together with a deforming shortness of the neck, but without synostosis of the cervical vertebrae seen in Klippel-Feil syndrome.

d. myoton′ica, SYN myotonic *dystrophy.*

d. un′guium, dystrophy of the nails.

dys·tro·phic (dis-trof′ik). Relating to dystrophy.

dys·tro·phin (dis-trō′fin). A protein found in the sarcolemma of normal muscle; it is missing in individuals with pseudohypertrophic muscular dystrophy and in other forms of muscular dystrophy; its role may be in the linkage of the cytoskeleton of the muscle cell to extracellular protein. SYN distrophin, dystropin.

dys·tro·phy (dis′trō-fē). Progressive changes that may result from defective nutrition of a tissue or organ. SYN dystrophia. [dys- + G. *trophē,* nourishment]

adiposogenital d., a disorder characterized primarily by obesity and hypogonadotrophic hypogonadism in adolescent boys; dwarfism is rare, and when present is thought to reflect hypothyroidism. Visual loss, behavioral abnormalities, and diabetes insipidus may occur. Fröhlich syndrome often is used synonymously for this disorder. Although the original case involved a pituitary tumor, most cases are thought to result from hypothalamic dysfunction in areas regulating appetite and gonadal development. The most common causes are pituitary and hypothalamic neoplasms. SYN adiposis orchica, adiposogenital degeneration, adiposogenital syndrome, dystrophia adiposogenitalis, Fröhlich syndrome, hypophysial syndrome, hypothalamic obesity with hypogonadism, Launois-Cléret syndrome.

adult foveomacular retinal d., an autosomal dominant disorder presenting in the fifth decade with a mild decrease in vision and subfoveal, round yellow lesion with a central hyperpigmented spot.

adult pseudohypertrophic muscular d. [MIM*310200.0002], SYN Becker muscular d.

anterior corneal d., corneal opacification with involvement of the epithelium, basement *membrane,* or Bowman *membrane* of the cornea.

asphyxiating thoracic d. [MIM*208500], hereditary hypoplasia of the thorax, associated with pelvic skeletal abnormality. SYN asphyxiating thoracic chondrodystrophy, asphyxiating thoracic dysplasia, Jeune syndrome, thoracic-pelvic-phalangeal d.

Becker muscular d., a hereditary muscle disorder of late onset, usually in the second or third decade, affecting the proximal muscles with characteristic pseudohypertrophy of the calves; clinical features similar to Duchenne muscular d. but much milder and not a genetic lethal; X-linked recessive inheritance, with both Becker and Duchenne d.'s caused by mutation in the dystrophin gene on Xp. Cf. Duchenne d. SYN adult pseudohypertrophic muscular d., Becker-type tardive muscular d.

Becker-type tardive muscular d., SYN Becker muscular d.

central areolar choroidal d., an autosomal dominant progressive disorder of vision loss with well-demarcated areas of atrophy of retinal pigment *epithelium* and choriocapillaris.

central cloudy corneal d. of François, an autosomal dominant opacification of the central corneal stroma consisting of cloudy polygonal areas.

central crystalline corneal d. of Snyder, an autosomal dominant opacification of the central corneal stroma by needle-shaped polychromatic crystals.

childhood muscular d., SYN Duchenne d.

Cogan d., SYN map-dot-fingerprint d.

cone d., a retinal abnormality in which color perception is severely deficient and typical changes occur in electroretinogram. SEE achromatopsia. SYN cone degeneration.

cone-rod retinal d., a disorder affecting the retinal cones more than the rods, characterized by diminished central vision and color vision.

congenital hereditary endothelial d., a dominantly or recessively inherited condition characterized by a cloudy, thickened cornea at birth or in the neonatal period.

corneal d. [MIM*217600], central corneal opacification, usually bilateral, symmetrical, involving predominantly epithelial, stromal, or endothelial layers, often in a typical pattern; autosomal recessive inheritance.

craniocarpotarsal d. [MIM*193700], a syndrome characterized by specific facial features with sunken eyes, hypertelorism, long philtrum, small nose, and small mouth with pursing of lips as in whistling, and skeletal malformations with ulnar deviation of hands, camptodactyly, talipes equinovarus, and frontal bone defects; autosomal dominant inheritance. SYN craniocarpotarsal dysplasia, Freeman-Sheldon syndrome, whistling face syndrome.

Duchenne d., the most common childhood muscular d., with onset usually before age 6. Characterized by symmetric weakness and wasting of first the pelvic and crural muscles and then the pectoral and proximal upper extremity muscles; pseudohypertrophy of some muscles, especially the calf; heart involvement; sometimes mild mental retardation; progressive course and early death, usually in adolescence. X-linked inheritance (affects males and transmitted by females). SYN childhood muscular d., Duchenne disease, pseudohypertrophic muscular d.

Emery-Dreifuss muscular d., a generally benign type of muscular d., with onset in childhood or early adulthood. Weakness begins with the pectoral girdle and proximal upper extremity muscles and spreads to the pelvic girdle and distal lower extremity muscles. Contractures of the elbow, flexors, neck flexors, and calf muscles often occur; muscle pseudohypertrophy and mental retardation do not occur. A cardiomyopathy is common. An X-linked inherited disorder, nonallelic to Duchenne muscular d.

facioscapulohumeral muscular d. [MIM*158900], a highly variable hereditary disorder with onset in childhood or adolescence, characterized by weakness and wasting, sometimes asymmetrical, mainly of the muscles of the face, shoulder girdle, arms, and later, pelvic girdle and legs; autosomal dominant inheritance. SYN facioscapulohumeral atrophy, Landouzy-Dejerine d.

Favre d., SYN vitreotapetoretinal d.

fingerprint d., a condition wherein fine parallel lines in a fingerprint configuration area are seen in the basal epithelial layer and basement membrane of the corneal epithelium. SEE ALSO map-dot-fingerprint d.

dy

fleck d. of cornea [MIM*121850], a bilateral occurrence of subtle spots in the corneal stroma; the spots vary in size and shape, and have sharp margins and clear centers; photophobia may occur; autosomal dominant inheritance.

Fuchs endothelial d., common corneal d. with autosomal dominant inheritance, characterized by keratopathia guttata with loss of endothelium and progressive corneal edema.

gelatinous droplike corneal d., a bilateral, autosomal recessive condition characterized by mulberrylike elevated amyloid deposits involving the epithelium and anterior corneal stroma.

granular corneal d., an autosomal dominant disorder characterized by hyaline deposits in the corneal stroma.

Groenouw corneal d., (1) a granular type of corneal d., with autosomal dominant inheritance [MIM*121900], caused by mutation in the transforming growth factor, beta-induced, gene (TGFB1) encoding keratoepithelin on chromosome 5q; **(2)** a progressive macular type of corneal d., characterized by punctate opacities and episodes of photophobia, corneal erosion, and foreign body sensation; autosomal recessive inheritance.

gutter d. of cornea, a marginal furrow usually inferiorly about 1 mm from the limbus; and sometimes bilateral. SYN keratoleptynsis (1).

hereditary epithelial d., SYN Meesman d.

hypertrophic d., SYN squamous cell *hyperplasia*.

infantile neuroaxonal d., a rare, familial disorder of early childhood manifested as progressive psychomotor deterioration, increased reflexes, Babinski sign, hypotonia and progressive blindness. Pathologically, eosinophilic spheroids of swollen axoplasm are found in various central nervous system nuclei.

Landouzy-Dejerine d., SYN facioscapulohumeral muscular d.

lattice corneal d. [MIM*122200], a corneal d. due to localized accumulation of amyloid in a reticular pattern; manifest at puberty and progressing slowly until eventually useful vision is lost; autosomal dominant inheritance, caused by mutation in the transforming growth factor, beta-induced, gene (TGFB1) encoding keratoepithelin on 5q.

Leyden-Möbius muscular d., SYN limb-girdle muscular d.

limb-girdle muscular d. [MIM*253600], a group of muscular d.'s, probably heterogeneous in nature. Onset usually in childhood or early adulthood and both sexes affected. Characterized by weakness and wasting, usually symmetrical, of the pelvic girdle muscles, the shoulder girdle muscles, or both, but not the facial muscles. Muscle pseudohypertrophy, heart involvement, and mental retardation are absent. Autosomal dominant and recessive inheritance have been described. SYN Leyden-Möbius muscular d., pelvofemoral muscular d., scapulohumeral muscular d.

macular corneal d., an autosomal recessive disorder characterized by glycosaminoglycan deposits in the corneal stroma.

macular retinal d., a group of disorders involving predominantly the posterior portion of the ocular fundus, due to degeneration in the sensory layer of the retina, retinal pigment epithelium, Bruch membrane, choroid, or a combination of these tissues. SEE Stargardt *disease*, Best *disease*.

map-dot-fingerprint d., fingerprint d. accompanied by maplike patterns and microcystic epithelial inclusions. SYN Cogan d.

Meesman d. [MIM*122100], epithelial d. characterized by progressive cysts and opacities of the corneal epithelium, with onset in infancy; autosomal dominant inheritance with incomplete penetrance. SYN hereditary epithelial d.

microcystic epithelial d., bilateral, symmetrical intraepithelial cysts in the central area of the cornea of healthy women, without hereditary predisposition.

mucopolysaccharide keratin d., a histologic finding seen in the surface epithelium of oral inflammatory fibrous hyperplasia, consisting of homogeneous eosinophilic pools of material in the superficial spinous layer.

muscular d., a general term for a number of hereditary, progressive degenerative disorders affecting skeletal muscles, and often other organ systems as well. SYN myodystrophy, myodystrophia.

myotonic d. [MIM*160900], the most common adult muscular d., characterized by progressive muscle weakness and wasting of

some of the cranial innervated muscles, as well as the distal limb muscles; other clinical features include myotonia, cataracts, hypogonadism, cardiac abnormalities, and frontal balding; onset usually in the third decade; autosomal dominant inheritance caused by abnormal trinucleotide repeat expansion in the dystrophia myotonica protein kinase gene (DMPK) on chromosome 19q. This disorder demonstrates anticipation (increase in severity in successive generations because of successive amplification of the trinucleotide repeats); the severe congenital form is almost always confined to the offspring of affected women. SYN dystrophia myotonica, myotonia atrophica, myotonia dystrophica, Steinert disease.

neuroaxonal d., a rare disorder that begins in the second year of life and is relentlessly progressive; clinically characterized initially by walking difficulties, weakness, and areflexia, later followed by corticospinal and pseudobulbar findings, blindness, loss of pain appreciation, and mental deterioration; pathologically, eosinophilic spheroids of swollen axoplasm are found in various central nuclei; autosomal recessive inheritance.

oculopharyngeal d., a dominantly inherited form of chronic progressive external *ophthalmoplegia* usually presenting in middle life or old age with chronic ptosis and/or difficulty swallowing. Many sufferers have French-Canadian ancestry.

pattern retinal d., a spectrum of autosomal dominant diseases affecting the retinal pigment *epithelium*, leading to mild to moderate vision loss.

pelvofemoral muscular d., SYN limb-girdle muscular d.

posterior corneal d., opacification with primary involvement of the endothelium of the cornea.

posterior polymorphous corneal d., an autosomal dominant condition characterized by vesicular and linear abnormalities of the corneal endothelium; occasionally leads to corneal edema.

pre-Descemet corneal d., opacification with primary involvement of the posterior stroma of the cornea.

progressive tapetochoroidal d., SYN choroideremia.

pseudohypertrophic muscular d., SYN Duchenne d.

reflex sympathetic d. (RSD), diffuse persistent pain usually in an extremity often associated with vasomotor disturbances, trophic changes, and limitation or immobility of joints; frequently follows some local injury. SEE ALSO causalgia. SYN shoulder-hand syndrome, sympathetic reflex d.

Reis-Bücklers corneal d., an autosomal dominant disorder of Bowman *membrane* of the cornea, characterized by a reticular haze and associated with recurrent corneal erosions.

ringlike corneal d. [MIM*121900], threadlike opacities of the anterior corneal stroma, with acute, painful onset followed by decreased vision; autosomal dominant inheritance, caused by mutationin the transforming growth factor, beta-induced, gene (TGFB1) encoding keratoepithelium on chromosome 5q.

scapulohumeral muscular d., SYN limb-girdle muscular d.

stromal corneal d., opacification with involvement of the middle layer of the cornea.

sympathetic reflex d., SYN reflex sympathetic d.

thoracic-pelvic-phalangeal d., SYN asphyxiating thoracic d.

twenty-nail d., longitudinal ridging of all of the nails; seen in alopecia areata and lichen planus.

vitelliform retinal d., SYN Best *disease*.

vitreotapetoretinal d. [MIM*268100], autosomal recessive bilateral peripheral and central retinoschisis with pigmentary degeneration of the retina, chorioretinal atrophy, vitreous degeneration, and night blindness. SYN Favre d.

vortex corneal d., a swirling pattern of abnormally pigmented corneal epithelial cells, seen in Fabry *disease* and in response to certain medications (including chloroquine, chlorpromazine, and amiodarone).

vulvar d., a spectrum of vulvar eruptions consisting of white atrophic papules, including lichen sclerosus et atrophicus, squamous cell hyperplasia (hypertrophic dystrophy), or a combination of these (mixed dystrophy). SEE ALSO *lichen* sclerosus et atrophicus.

dystropin. SYN dystrophin.

dys·tro·py (dis′trō-pē). Abnormal or eccentric behavior. [dys- + G. *tropos,* a turning]

dys·u·ria (dis-ū′rē-ă). Difficulty or pain in urination. SYN dysury. [dys- + G. *ouron,* urine]

dys·u·ric (dis-ū′rik). Relating to or suffering from dysuria.

dys·u·ry (dis′ū-rē). SYN dysuria.

dys·ver·sion (dis-ver′zhŭn). A turning in any direction, less than inversion; particularly d. of the optic nerve head (situs inversus of the optic disk). [dys- + L. *verto,* to turn]

E

ε **1.** Fifth letter of the Greek alphabet, epsilon. **2.** Symbol for molar absorption *coefficient* or extinction *coefficient*. For terms beginning with this prefix, see the specific term. **3.** In chemistry, denotes a position of a substituent located on the fifth atom from the carboxyl or other primary functional group. For terms beginning with this prefix, see the specific term.

E 1. Symbol for exa-; extraction *ratio*; glutamic acid; energy; electromotive *force*; glutamyl; internal *energy*. **2.** As a subscript, refers to expired *gas*; obsolete symbol for einsteinium.

E_0^+, E^0, E_h Symbols for oxidation-reduction potential.

E_2 Symbol for estradiol.

E_1 Symbol for estrone.

E Abbreviation for entgegen.

E_a Abbreviation for *energy* of activation.

e Symbol for elementary charge; base of natural, or Napierian, logarithms (2.71828...). It is the limit of 1 + (1/n!).

EAE Abbreviation for experimental allergic *encephalitis*.

Eagle, Harry, U.S. physician and cell biologist, 1905–1992. SEE E. basal *medium*, minimum essential *medium*.

Eagle, Watt W., 20th century U.S. otolaryngologist.

Eales, Henry, English ophthalmologist, 1852–1913. SEE E. *disease*.

ear (ēr) [TA]. The organ of hearing: composed of the **external e.**, which includes the auricle and the external acoustic, or auditory, meatus; the **middle e.**, or the tympanic cavity with its ossicles; and the **internal e.** or **inner e.**, or labyrinth, which includes the semicircular canals, vestibule, and cochlea. SEE ALSO auricle. SYN auris [TA]. [A.S. *eáre*]

Aztec e., an auricle with the lobule absent.

bat e., SYN lop-ear.

bladder e., protrusion of a portion of the bladder into proximal inguinal canal; often seen in pediatric VCUGs and rarely of clinical significance.

Blainville e.'s, asymmetry in size or shape of the auricles.

boxer's e., SYN cauliflower e.

Cagot e. (kă-gō′), an auricle having no lobulus. [a people in the Pyrenees among whom physical stigmata are common]

cauliflower e., thickening and induration of the e. with distortion of contours following extravasation of blood within its tissues. SYN boxer's e.

darwinian e., an auricle in which the upper border is not rolled over to form the helix, but projects upward as a flat, sharp edge.

dog e., redundant corner of skin, usually the result of mismatch of skin edges in a wound closure, leaving an excessive hump or triangular bit of tissue.

external e., SYN auris externa. SEE ALSO auricle, external acoustic *meatus*, pinna.

glue e., middle e. inflammation with thick mucoid effusion caused by long-standing eustachian tube obstruction.

internal e., SYN auris interna. SEE ALSO labyrinth.

lop e., SYN outstanding e. SEE lop-ear.

middle e., SYN auris media. SEE ALSO tympanic *cavity*.

Morel e., a large, misshapen, outstanding auricle, with obliterated grooves and thinned edges.

Mozart e., a deformity of the pinna where the two crura of the

⌂ **Combining Forms**	☆ **Official alternate Terminologia Anatomica term**
Indicates term is illustrated, see Illustration Index	**[MIM] Mendelian Inheritance in Man**
SYN Synonym	**C.I. Colour Index**
Cf. Compare	
[NA] Nomina Anatomica	
[TA] Terminologia Anatomica	**High Profile Term**

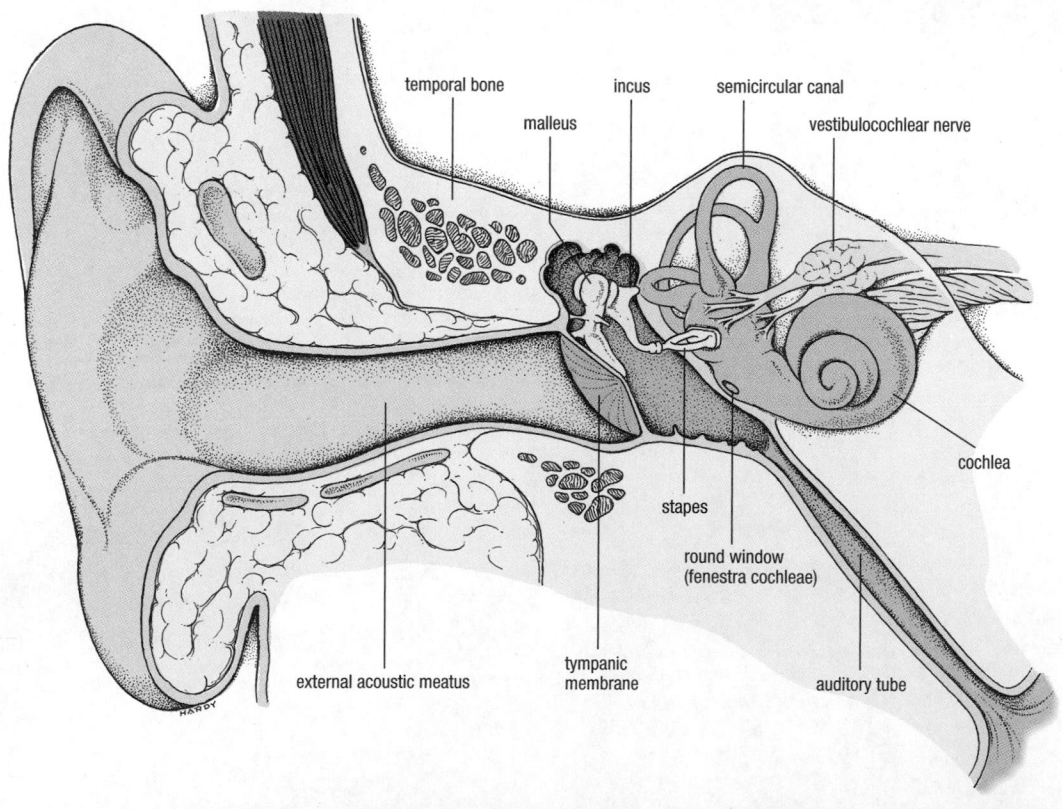

temporal bone · incus · semicircular canal · malleus · vestibulocochlear nerve · stapes · round window (fenestra cochleae) · cochlea · external acoustic meatus · tympanic membrane · auditory tube

ear

antihelix and the crus of the helix are fused, giving a bulging appearance of the superior part of the pinna. [Wolfgang Amadeus Mozart, 1756–1791, composer, said to have had this deformity]

outstanding e., excessive protrusion of the ear from the head, usually due to failure of the antihelical fold to develop. SYN lop e., protruding e.

protruding e., SYN outstanding e.

scroll e., a deformity of the external e. in which the pinna is rolled forward.

Stahl e., a deformed external e., in which the fossa ovalis and upper portion of the scaphoid fossa are covered by the helix; once regarded as a stigma of degenerate constitution.

swimmer's e., SYN otitis externa.

telephone e., noise-induced hearing loss due to exposure to static over telephones.

Wildermuth e., an e. in which the helix is turned backward and the anthelix is prominent.

ear·ache (ēr'āk). Pain in the ear. SYN otalgia, otodynia.

ear·drum (ēr'drŭm). The middle ear. Cf. tympanic *membrane.* SYN tympanum.

Earle, Wilton R., U.S. pathologist, 1902–1964. SEE E. L *fibrosarcoma, solution.*

ear·piece (ēr-pēs). A part of a device inserted into the external auditory canal to deliver sound to the ear.

ear·plug (ēr'plug). Generic term for occlusive devices for the external auditory canal for protection of hearing against noise-induced hearing loss or to prevent water from getting into the ear. SEE ALSO hearing *protectors,* under *protector.*

earth (erth). **1.** Soil; the soft material of the land, as opposed to rock and sand. **2.** An easily pulverized mineral. **3.** An insoluble oxide of aluminum or of certain other elements characterized by a high melting point. [A.S. *eorthe*]

alkaline e.'s, SEE alkaline earth *elements,* under *element.*

diatomaceous e., a powder made of desiccated diatom material; used as a filtering agent, adsorbent, and abrasive in many chemical operations.

fuller's e., (1) an amorphous variety of kaolin of varying composition, containing an aluminum magnesium silicate. The name is derived from an ancient process of cleansing or "fulling" wool to remove the oil and dirt particles with a water slurry of e. or clay. (2) a refined clay sometimes used as a dusting powder or applied moistened with water as a form of poultice. Currently refers to any clay that can be used for the purpose of decolorizing in oil refining. Used as decolorizer for oils and other liquids, filtering medium, filler for rubber, and in agricultural formulations. [fr. *fulling,* an old process of cleaning wool, with earth or clay]

rare e.'s, SEE lanthanides.

ear·wax (ēr'waks). SYN cerumen.

eat (ēt). **1.** To take solid food. **2.** To chew and swallow any substance as one would food. **3.** To corrode. [A.S. *etan*]

Eaton, Lee M., U.S. neurologist, 1905–1958. SEE E.-Lambert *syndrome.*

Eaton, Monroe A., U.S. microbiologist, *1904. SEE E. *agent.*

E.B., EB Abbreviation for elementary *bodies* (1), under *body.*

Ebbinghaus, Hermann, German, 1850–1909. SEE E. *test.*

Eberth, Karl J., German physician, 1835–1926. SEE E. *bacillus, lines,* under *line, perithelium.*

Ebner, Victor von. SEE von Ebner.

e·bo·na·tion (ē-bō-nā'shŭn). Removal of loose fragments of bone from a wound. [L.]

ébran·le·ment (ā-brahn-la-mon'). Twisting a polyp on its stalk to cause atrophy. [Fr.]

Ebstein, Wilhelm, German physician, 1836–1912. SEE E. *anomaly, disease, sign;* Armanni-E. *change, kidney;* Pel-E. *disease, fever.*

EBT Abbreviation for electron beam *tomography.*

eb·ul·lism (eb'ū-lizm). Formation of water vapor bubbles in the tissues brought on by an extreme reduction in barometric pressure; occurs if the body is exposed to pressures above an altitude of 63,000 feet, or if a diver rises rapidly from a great depth to the surface. [L. *ebullire,* to boil out]

ebur (ē'bŭr). A tissue resembling ivory in outward appearance or structure. [L. ivory]

e. den'tis, SYN dentine.

eb·ur·na·tion (ē-bŭr-nā'shŭn). A change in exposed subchondral bone in degenerative joint disease in which it is converted into a dense substance with a smooth surface like ivory. SYN bone sclerosis. [L. *eburneus,* of ivory]

e. of dentin, a condition observed in arrested dental caries wherein decalcified dentin is burnished and takes on a polished, often brown-stained appearance.

ebur·ne·ous (ē-bŭr'nē-ŭs). Resembling ivory, especially in color.

ebur·ni·tis (ē-bŭr-nī'tis). Increased density and hardness of dentin, which may occur after the dentin is exposed. [L. *eburneus,* of ivory, + G. -itis, inflammation]

EBV Abbreviation for Epstein-Barr *virus.*

EC Abbreviation for Enzyme Commission of the International Union of Biochemistry, used in conjunction with a unique number to define a specific enzyme in the Enzyme Commission's list [*Enzyme Nomenclature*] (1984); e.g., EC 1.1.1.1 defines an alcohol dehydrogenase and EC 2.6.1.1 defines aspartate aminotransferase, also known as glutamic-oxalacetic transaminase (GOT).

ec-. Out of, away from. [G.]

E-cad·her·in (ē-căd-hěr'in). SYN uvomorulin.

écar·teur (ā-kar-ter'). A type of retractor. [Fr. *écarter,* to separate]

ecau·date (ē-kaw'dāt). Tailless. [L. e- priv. + *cauda,* tail]

ec·bo·line (ek'bŏ-lēn). SYN ergotoxine.

ec·cen·tric (ek-sen'trik). **1.** Abnormal or peculiar in ideas or behavior. SYN erratic (1). **2.** Proceeding from a center. Cf. centrifugal (2). **3.** SYN peripheral. [G. *ek,* out, + *kentron,* center]

ec·cen·tro·chon·dro·pla·sia (ek-sen'trō-kon-drō-plā'zē-ă). Abnormal epiphysial development from eccentric centers of ossification. [G. *ek,* out + *kentron,* center, + *chondros,* cartilage, + *plasis,* a molding]

ec·cen·tro·pi·e·sis (ek-sen'trō-pī-ē'sis). Pressure exerted from within outward. [G. *ek,* out, + *kentron,* center, + *piesis,* pressure]

ec·chon·dro·ma (ek-kon-drō'mă). **1.** A cartilaginous neoplasm arising as an overgrowth from normally situated cartilage, as a mass protruding from the articular surface of a bone, in contrast to enchondroma. **2.** An enchondroma which has burst through the shaft of a bone and become pedunculated. SYN ecchondrosis. [G. *ek,* from, + *chondros,* cartilage, + *-oma,* tumor]

ec·chon·dro·sis (ek-kon-drō'sis). SYN ecchondroma.

ec·chor·do·sis phy·sa·li·phor·'a (ek-kor-dō'sis fiz-ăl-ē-for'-mē-a). A notochordal rest of the cranial clivus that may form a small tumor.

ec·chy·mo·ma (ek-i-mō'mă). A slight hematoma following a bruise. [G. *ek,* out, + *chymos,* juice, + *-oma,* tumor]

ec·chy·mo·sis (ek-i-mō'sis). A purplish patch caused by extravasation of blood into the skin, differing from petechiae only in size (larger than 3 mm diameter). [G. *ekchymōsis,* ecchymosis, fr. *ek,* out, + *chymos,* juice]

bilateral medial orbital e.'s, SYN raccoon *eyes,* under *eye.*

Tardieu e.'s, subpleural and subpericardial petechiae or ecchymoses (or both), as observed in the tissues of persons who have been strangled, or otherwise asphyxiated. SYN Tardieu petechiae, Tardieu spots.

ec·chy·mot·ic (ek-i-mot'ik). Relating to an ecchymosis.

Eccleston. SEE Paget-Eccleston *stain.*

ec·crine (ek'rin). **1.** SYN exocrine (1). **2.** Denoting the flow of sweat from skin glands unconnected to hair follicles. [G. *ek-krino,* to secrete]

ec·cri·nol·o·gy (ek-ri-nol'ō-jē). The branch of physiology and of anatomy concerned with the secretions and the secreting (exocrine) glands. [G. *ekdrino,* to secrete, + *logos,* study]

ec·cri·sis (ek'ri-sis). **1.** The removal of waste products. **2.** Any waste product; excrement. [G. separation]

ec

ec·crit·ic (e-krit′ik). **1.** Promoting the expulsion of waste matters. **2.** An agent that promotes excretion.

ec·cy·e·sis (ek-sī-ē′sis). SYN ectopic *pregnancy*. [G. *ek*, out, + *kyēsis*, pregnancy]

ec·dem·ic (ek-dem′ik). Denoting a disease brought into a region from without. [G. *ekdēmos*, foreign, from home, fr. *dēmos*, people]

ec·dys·i·asm (ek-diz′ē-azm). A morbid tendency to undress to produce sexual desire in others. [fr. G. *ekdyō*, to remove one's clothes]

ec·dy·sis (ek′di-sis). Desquamation, sloughing, or molting as a necessary phenomenon to permit growth in arthropods and skin renewal in amphibians and reptiles. [G. *ekdysis*, shedding]

ec·dys·ist (ek-dis-ist). A person who engages in ecdysiasm.

ECF Abbreviation for extracellular *fluid*.

ECF-A Abbreviation for eosinophil chemotactic *factor* of anaphylaxis.

ECFV Abbreviation for extracellular fluid *volume*.

ECG Abbreviation for electrocardiogram.

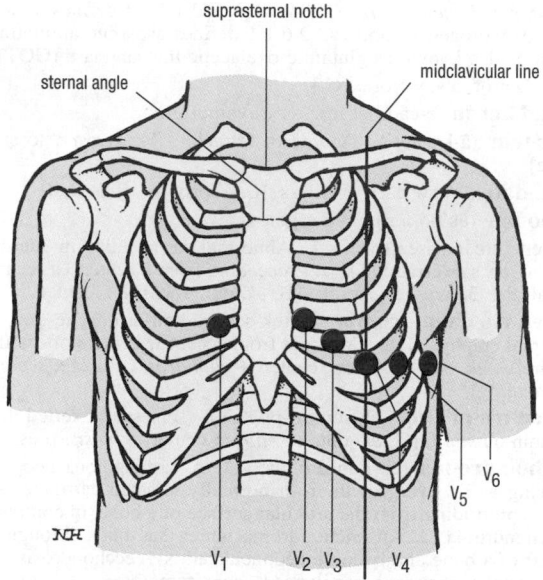

sternal angle · suprasternal notch · midclavicular line · V_6 · V_5 · V_1 · V_2 · V_3 · V_4

ECG lead placement: landmarks for chest lead placement

ec·go·nine (ek′gō-nēn, -nin). The important part of the cocaine molecule; a topical anesthetic; basis of many coca alkaloids.
    ecgonine e., SYN benzoylecgonine.

Echid·noph·a·ga gal·li·na·cea (ek-id-nof′ă-gă gal-i-nā′sē-ă). The sticktight flea, a serious pest of poultry in subtropical America; also frequently attacks domestic mammals and humans.

echin-. SEE echino-.

echi·nate (ek′i-nāt). SYN echinulate.

echino-, echin-. Prickly, spiny. [G. *echinos*, hedgehog, sea urchin]

Echi·no·chas·mus (ĕ-kī-nō-kaz′mŭs). A genus of digenetic flukes (family Echinostomatidae), particularly common in wading and fish-eating birds; the species *E. perfoliatus* var. *japonicus* is reported as a rare intestinal parasite of humans in Japan. [echino- + G. *chasma*, open mouth]

echi·no·coc·ci·a·sis (ĕ-kī′nō-kok-sē′ā-sis). SYN echinococcosis.

echi·no·coc·co·sis (ĕ-kī′nō-kok-kō′sis). Infection with *Echinococcus;* larval infection is called hydatid *disease.* SYN echinococciasis, echinococcus disease.

Echi·no·coc·cus (ĕ-kī′nō-kok′ŭs). A genus of very small taeniid tapeworms, two to five segments in adult worms; adults are found in various carnivores but not in humans; larvae, in the form of hydatid cysts, are found in the liver and other organs of rumi-

nants, pigs, horses, rodents, and, under certain epidemiologic circumstances, humans (e.g., sheep herders living closely with their infected dogs). [echino- + G. *kokkos*, a berry]

E. granulo'sus, hydatid tapeworm, a species in which adults infect canids and the larval form (osseous and unilocular hydatid cysts) infects sheep and other ruminants, pigs, and horses; may also occur in humans, giving rise to a large cyst in the liver or other organs and tissues.

E. multilocula'ris, a north temperate and Arctic species of tapeworm that occurs, in the adult form, in foxes; the larva (alveolar hydatid cyst) is found in the liver of microtine rodents and in humans; it produces a proliferative, often slow-growing cyst in the liver that, in humans, is usually fatal.

E. voge'li, a species reported from humid tropical forests of Panama and northern South America causing a polycystic form of human hydatid disease intermediate between cystic and alveolar hydatid disease; the typical cycle involves domestic dogs and wild canids as host of the adult tapeworm, and rodents such as the paca (*Cuniculus paca*) as the intermediate host for the cystic form.

echi·no·cyte (ek′i-nō-sīt). A crenated red blood cell. [echino- + G. *kytos,* cell]

echi·no·derm (e-kī′nō-derm). A member of the phylum Echinodermata.

Echi·no·der·ma·ta (e-kī-nō-der′mă-tă). A phylum of Metazoa that includes starfish, sea urchins, sea lilies, and other classes. All but the sea cucumbers (Holothuroidea) are basically radially symmetrical and most possess a calcareous endoskeleton with external spines. They inhabit the sea bottom, some near shore, others in deep water. [echino- + G. *derma,* skin]

Echi·no·rhyn·chus (e-kī-nō-ring′kŭs). A genus of acanthocephalid (thorny-headed) worms which originally included species now contained in *Macracanthorhynchus, Gigantorhynchus,* and other genera. [echino- + G. *rhynchos,* snout]

ech·i·no·sis (ek-i-nō′sis). A condition in which the red blood cells have lost their smooth outlines, resembling an echinus or sea urchin. [echino- + G. *-osis,* condition]

Echi·no·sto·ma (ĕ-kī-nō-stō′mă, ek-i-nos′tō-mă). A genus of digenetic flukes (family Echinostomatidae) with characteristic oral spines; widely distributed and parasitic in a broad range of bird and mammal hosts; several species have been reported in humans from Southeast Asia. [echino- + G. *stoma,* mouth]

E. iloca'num, a species reported from humans in the Philippines.

E. malay'anum, a species typically found in the pig, but reported occasionally from humans in Malaysia; infection results from ingestion of snails with infective cysts (metacercariae).

echi·no·sto·mi·a·sis (ĕ-kī′nō-stō-mī′ă-sis). Infection of birds and mammals, including humans, with trematodes of the genus *Echinostoma.*

echin·u·late (e-kin′ū-lāt). Prickly or spinous. Covered with small spines. SYN echinate. [Mod. L. *echinulus,* dim. of L. *echinus,* hedgehog]

Ech·is (ek′is, ē′kis). The saw-scaled or carpet viper, a genus of small (under 1 m), irritable, and alert snakes with a highly toxic venom; they are responsible for numerous snakebite cases with many fatalities. [G. *echis,* a viper]

ech·o (ek′ō). **1.** A reverberating sound sometimes heard during auscultation of the chest. **2.** In ultrasonography, the acoustic signal received from scattering or reflecting structures or the corresponding pattern of light on a CRT or ultrasonogram. **3.** In magnetic resonance imaging, the signal detected following an inverting pulse. [G.]

atrial e., electrical reactivation of the atrium by a retrograde impulse returning from the A-V node while the antegrade impulse continues to the ventricle; characterized electrocardiographically, by a pair of P waves enclosing a QRS complex, the second P wave being opposite in polarity (usually inverted in lead II), indicating that it is the reverse (the retrograde pathway) of the pathway of the first P wave (the antegrade pathway).

navigator e., a method of respiratory *gating* q.v., used in magnetic resonance *imaging* to limit respiratory motion artifact; a signal is derived from the top of the diaphragm, and image data are collected only when it is in a selected range.

nodus sinuatrialis e., NS e., a postectopic sinus beat occurring earlier than would be expected from the preceding sinus node discharge interval; i.e., the interval following a premature beat of supraventricular origin is less than the ordinary cycle length between sinus beats, whereas ordinarily the interval would be expected to exceed cycle length.

e. planar, a method of magnetic resonance imaging that allows rapid image acquisition during free induction decay, using technically demanding rapidly oscillating radiofrequency gradients.

spin e., a commonly used technique to recover T1 and T2 relaxation signals in magnetic resonance imaging, by using a 180° inverting pulse in the pulse sequence to compensate for loss of transverse magnetization caused by magnetic field inhomogeneities.

ech·o·a·cou·sia (ek′ō-ă-koo′zē-ă). A subjective disturbance of hearing in which a sound appears to be repeated. [echo + G. *akouō*, to hear]

ech·o·a·or·tog·ra·phy (ek′ō-ā-ōr-tog′ră-fē). Application of ultrasound techniques to the diagnosis and study of the aorta. [echo + aortography]

ech·o·car·di·o·gram (ek-ō-kar′dē-ō-gram). The record obtained by echocardiography. SEE ultrasonography.

ech·o·car·di·og·ra·phy (ek′ō-kar-dē-og′ră-fē). The use of ultrasound in the investigation of the heart and great vessels and diagnosis of cardiovascular lesions. SYN ultrasonic cardiography, ultrasound cardiography. [echo + cardiography]

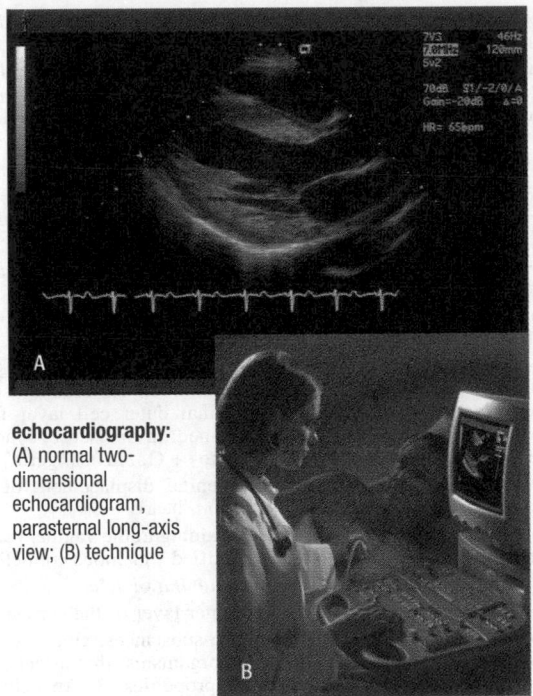

echocardiography:
(A) normal two-dimensional echocardiogram, parasternal long-axis view; (B) technique

contrast e., the injection of contrast media of high echo reflectants (e.g., bubbles) to outline a chamber or delineate a shunt within the heart.

cross-sectional e., SYN two-dimensional e.

Doppler e., use of Doppler ultrasonography techniques to augment two-dimensional e. by allowing velocities to be registered within the echocardiographic image. SEE duplex *ultrasonography*, Doppler *ultrasonography*.

M-mode e., SEE M-mode.

real-time e., SYN two-dimensional e.

sector e., two-dimensional e. with a stationary transducer.

stress e., echocardiographic monitoring of a circulatory challenge, usually exercise.

transesophageal e., recording of the echocardiogram from a transducer swallowed by the patient to predetermined distances in the esophagus and stomach.

transthoracic e., the standard e. recorded from echocardiographic "windows" on the chest wall, jugular notch, or epigastrium.

two-dimensional e., e. in which an image is reconstructed from the echoes stimulated and detected by a linear array or moving transducers. SYN cross-sectional e., real-time e.

ech·o·en·ceph·a·log·ra·phy (ek′ō-en-sef-ă-log′ră-fē). The use of reflected ultrasound in the diagnosis of intracranial processes. [echo + encephalography]

echo-free (ek′ō-frē). SYN anechoic.

ech·o·gen·ic (ek-ō-jen′ik). Pertaining to a structure or medium (e.g., tissue) that has internal echoes. Cf. hypoechoic, hyperechoic, and anechoic, which refer, respectively, to paucity, abundance, and absence of echoes displayed in the image of a structure.

ech·o·gram (ek′ō-gram). A record obtained using acoustic reflection techniques in any one of the various display modes, especially an echocardiogram. SEE ALSO ultrasonogram. [echo + G. *gramma*, a diagram]

echog·ra·pher (e-kog′ră-fer). SYN ultrasonographer.

ech·o·graph·ia (ek-ō-graf′ē-ă). A form of agraphia in which one cannot write spontaneously, but can write from dictation or copy. [echo + G. *graphō*, to write]

echog·ra·phy (e-kog′ră-fē). SYN ultrasonography. [echo + G. *graphō*, to write]

ech·o·la·lia (ek-ō-lā′lē-ă). Involuntary parrotlike repetition of a word or sentence just spoken by another person. Usually seen with schizophrenia. SYN echo reaction, echo speech, echophrasia. [echo + G. *lalia*, a form of speech]

ech·o·lo·ca·tion (ek′ō-lō-kā′shŭn). Term applied to the method by which bats direct their flight and avoid solid objects. The creatures emit high-pitched cries that, though inaudible to human ears, are heard by the bats themselves as reflected sounds (echoes) from objects in their path.

ech·o·mo·tism (ek′ō-mō′tizm). SYN echopraxia. [echo + L. *motio*, motion]

e·chop·a·thy (ĕ-kop′ă-thē). A form of psychopathology, usually associated with schizophrenia, in which the words (echolalia) or actions (echopraxia) of another are imitated and repeated. [echo + G. *pathos*, suffering]

e·choph·o·ny, ech·o·pho·nia (ĕ-kof′ō-nē, ek-ō-fō′nē-ă). A duplication of the voice sound occasionally heard during auscultation of the chest. [echo + G. *phōnē*, voice]

ech·o·phra·sia (ek-ō-frā′zē-ă). SYN echolalia. [echo + *phrasis*, speech]

ech·o·prax·ia (ek′ō-prak′sē-ă). Involuntary imitation of movements made by another. SEE echopathy. SYN echomotism. [echo + G. *praxis*, action]

ech·o·scope (ek′ō-skōp). Instrument for displaying echoes by means of ultrasonic pulses on an oscilloscope to demonstrate structures lying at depths within the body. [echo + G. *skopeō*, to view]

ech·o·thi·o·phate io·dide (ek-ō-thī′ō-fāt). A potent organophosphorus compound and cholinesterase inhibitor, used in the eye in the treatment of glaucoma.

Ec·ho·vi·rus 28 (ek′ō-vī′rŭs). Reclassified as Rhinovirus type 1.

ech·o·vi·rus (ek′ō-vī-rŭs). SYN ECHO *virus*.

Eck, Nikolai V., Russian physiologist, 1849–1917. SEE E. *fistula;* reverse E. *fistula*.

Ecker, Enrique Eduardo, U.S. bacteriologist, 1887–1966. SEE Rees-E. *fluid*.

Ecker, Alexander, German anatomist, 1816–1887. SEE E. *fissure*.

ec·la·bi·um (ek-lā′bē-ŭm). Eversion of a lip. [G. *ek*, out, + L. *labium*, lip]

ec·lamp·sia (ek-lamp′sē-ă). Occurrence of one or more convulsions, not attributable to other cerebral conditions such as epilepsy or cerebral hemorrhage, in a patient with preeclampsia. [G. *eklampsis*, a shining forth]

puerperal e., convulsions and coma associated with hypertension, edema, or proteinuria occurring in a woman following delivery.

superimposed e., convulsions occuring in a woman with superimposed preeclampsia.

ec·lamp·tic (ek-lamp'tik). Relating to eclampsia.

ec·lamp·to·gen·ic, ec·lamp·tog·e·nous (ek-lamp-tō-jen'ik, -tog'ĕ-nŭs). Causing eclampsia.

ec·lec·tic (ek-lek'tik). Picking out from different sources what appears to be the best or most desirable. [G. *eklektikos*, selecting, fr. *ek*, out, + *lego*, to select]

ec·lec·ti·cism (ek-lek'ti-sizm). **1.** A now defunct system of medicine that advocated use of indigenous plants to effect specific cures of certain signs and symptoms. **2.** A system of medicine practiced by ancient Greek and Roman physicians who were not affiliated with a medical sect but who adopted the practice and teachings that they considered best from other systems.

⌂**eco-.** The environment. [G. *oikos*, house, household, habitation]

eco·en·do·cri·nol·o·gy (ē′kō-en′dō-kri-nol′ō-jē). The study of the interactions of endocrine systems with the environment.

ECoG Abbreviation for electrocorticography.

eco·log·i·cal fal·la·cy. The bias that may occur because an association observed between variables at an aggregate level does not necessarily represent an association that exists at an individual level; an error of inference due to failure to distinguish between different levels of organization.

e·col·o·gy (ē-kol′ō-jē). The branch of biology concerned with the total complex of interrelationships among living organisms, encompassing the relations of organisms to each other, to the environment, and to the entire energy balance within a given ecosystem. SYN bioecology, bionomics (2). [eco- + G. *logos*, study]

human e., the relations of persons to their total (biologic and social) environment.

landscape e., the study of the reciprocal effects of spatial pattern on ecologic processes.

econ·a·zole (e-kōn′ă-zōl). A broad spectrum antifungal agent used in the treatment of tinea pedis and related fungal infections.

Economo. SEE von Economo.

econ·o·my (ē-kon′ō-mē). System; the body regarded as an aggregate of functioning organs. [G. *oikonomia*, management of the house, fr. *oikos*, house, + *nomos*, usage, law]

ec·o·spe·cies (ē-kō-spē′shēz). Two or more populations of a species isolated by ecologic barriers, theoretically able to exchange genes and interbreed, but partially separated from one another by differences in habitat or behavior.

ec·o·sys·tem (ē′kō-sis-tem). **1.** The fundamental unit in ecology, comprising the living organisms and the nonliving elements that interact in a defined region. **2.** A biocenosis (biotic community) and its biotope. SYN ecological system.

parasite-host e., SYN parasitocenose.

ec·o·tax·is (ē-kō-tak′sis). Migration of lymphocytes "homing" from the thymus and bone marrow into tissues possessing an appropriate microenvironment. [eco- + G. *taxis*, order, arrangement]

écou·vil·lon (ā-koo-vē-yōhn′). A brush with firm bristles for freshening sores or abrading the interior of a cavity. [Fr., cleaning brush]

ECP Abbreviation for eosinophil cationic *protein*.

ec·phy·ma (ek-fī′mă). A warty growth or protuberance. [G. a pimply eruption]

ECS Abbreviation for electrocerebral silence.

ec·sta·sy (ek′stă-sē). Mental exaltation, and/or a rapturous experience. [G. *ekstasis*, astonishment]

ec·stat·ic (ek-stat′ik). Relating to or marked by ecstasy.

ec·stro·phe (ek′strō-fē). SYN exstrophy.

ECT Abbreviation for electroconvulsive *therapy*, electroshock *therapy*.

⌂**ect-.** SEE ecto-.

ec·tad (ek′tad). Outward. [G. *ektos*, outside, + L. *ad*, to]

ec·tal (ek′tăl). Outer; external. [G. *ektos*, outside]

ec·ta·sia, ec·ta·sis (ek-tā′zē-ă, ek′tă-sis). Dilation of a tubular structure. [G. *ektasis*, a stretching]

annuloaortic e., supravalvular dilation of the aorta involving both its wall and the valve ring, which, however, remains of smaller diameter than the more distal ectatic wall; many cases are related to Marfan syndrome. SYN aortoannular e.

aortoannular e., SYN annuloaortic e.

e. cor′dis, dilation of the heart.

corneal e., SYN keratoectasia.

diffuse arterial e., spontaneous enlargement with dilation of the vessels.

familial aortic e. (ek′tā-zē-ă), SYN familial aortic ectasia *syndrome*.

hypostatic e., dilation of a blood vessel, usually a vein, in a dependent portion of the body, as in varicose veins of the leg.

mammary duct e., dilation of mammary ducts by lipid and cellular debris in older women; rupture of ducts may result in granulomatous inflammation and infiltration by plasma cells. SEE ALSO plasma cell *mastitis*.

scleral e., SYN sclerectasia.

e. ventric′uli paradox′a, SYN hourglass *stomach*.

⌂**-ectasia, -ectasis.** Dilation, expansion. [G. *ektasis*, a stretching]

ec·tat·ic (ek-tat′ik). Relating to, or marked by, ectasis.

ec·ten·tal (ek-ten′tăl). Relating to both ectoderm and endoderm; denoting the line where these two layers join. SYN ectoental. [G. *ektos*, outside, + *entos*, within]

ect·eth·moid (ekt-eth′moyd). SYN ethmoidal *labyrinth*. [G. *ektos*, outside, + ethmoid]

ec·thy·ma (ek-thī′mă). A pyogenic infection of the skin initiated by β-hemolytic streptococci and characterized by adherent crusts beneath which ulceration occurs; the ulcers may be single or multiple, and heal with scar formation. [G. a pustule]

contagious e., SYN orf.

e. gangreno′sum, SYN *dermatitis* gangrenosa infantum.

ec·ti·ris (ek-tī′ris). The outer layer of the iris. [G. *ektos*, outside, + iris]

⌂**ecto-, ect-.** Outer, on the outside. SEE ALSO exo-. [G. *ektos*, outside]

ec·to·an·ti·gen (ek-tō-an′ti-jen). Any toxin or other excitor of antibody formation, separate or separable from its source. SYN exoantigen.

ec·to·blast (ek′tō-blast). **1.** SYN ectoderm. **2.** As used by some experimental embryologists, the original outer cell layer from which the primary germ layers are formed; in this sense, synonymous with epiblast. **3.** A cell wall. [ecto- + G. *blastos*, germ]

ec·to·car·dia (ek-tō-kar′dē-ă). Congenital displacement of the heart. SYN exocardia. [ecto- + G. *kardia*, heart]

ec·to·cer·vi·cal (ek′tō-ser′vi-kăl). Pertaining to the vaginal part of the cervix of the uterus lined with stratified squamous epithelium.

ec·to·chor·oi·dea. SYN suprachoroid *lamina* of sclera.

ec·to·cor·nea (ek-tō-kōr′nē-ă). The outer layer of the cornea.

ec·to·crine (ek′tō-krin). **1.** Relating to substances, either synthesized or arising by decomposition of organisms, that affect plant life. **2.** A compound with ectocrine properties. **3.** An ectohormone. Cf. endocrine, exocrine. [ecto- + G. *krinō*, to separate]

ecological e., a chemical substance that undergoes biosynthesis in one species and that exerts an effect on the function of another species through mechanisms of the external environment; e.g., the biosynthesis of vitamins by ruminants and their subsequent ingestion by other animals. SEE ALSO ectohormone.

ec·to·cyst (ek′tō-sist). The outer layer of a hydatid cyst. [ecto- + G. *kystis*, bladder]

ec·to·derm (ek′tō-derm). The outer layer of cells in the embryo, after establishment of the three primary germ layers (ectoderm, mesoderm, endoderm), the germ layer in contact with the amnionic cavity. SYN ectoblast (1). [ecto- + G. *derma*, skin]

amnionic e., inner layer of the amnion continuous with body ectoderm.

chorionic e., SYN trophoblast.

epithelial e., that part of the e. separating from the neuroectoderm at about the fourth week of embryonic life; the epidermis and its specialized derivatives develop from it. SYN superficial e.

extraembryonic e., derivative of epiblast outside the embryo's body.

superficial e., SYN epithelial e.

ec·to·der·mal (ek-tō-der′măl). Relating to the ectoderm. SYN ectodermic.

ec·to·der·ma·to·sis (ek′tō-der-mă-tō′sis). SYN ectodermosis.

ec·to·der·mic (ek-tō-der′mik). SYN ectodermal.

ec·to·der·mo·sis (ek′tō-der-mō′sis). A disorder of any organ or tissue developed from the ectoderm. SYN ectodermatosis.

ec·to·en·tad (ek-tō-en′tad). From without inward.

ec·to·en·tal (ek-tō-en′tăl). SYN ectental.

ec·to·en·zyme (ek-tō-en′zīm). **1.** An enzyme that is excreted externally and that acts outside the organism. **2.** An enzyme that is attached to the external surface of the plasma membrane of a cell.

ec·to·eth·moid (ek-tō-eth′moyd). SYN ethmoidal *labyrinth*.

ec·tog·e·nous (ek-toj′e-nŭs). SYN exogenous. [ecto- + G. *-gen,* producing]

ec·to·hor·mone (ek′tō-hōr-mōn). A parahormonal chemical mediator of ecologic significance which is secreted, largely by an organism (usually an invertebrate) into its immediate environment (air or water); it can alter the behavior or functional activity of a second organism, often of the same species as that secreting the e. SEE ALSO ecological *ectocrine*.

ec·to·mere (ek′tō-mēr). One of the blastomeres involved in formation of ectoderm. [ecto- + G. *meros,* part]

ec·to·me·rog·o·ny (ek′tō-mĕ-rog′ō-nē). The production of merozoites in the asexual reproduction of sporozoan parasites at the surface of schizonts and of blastophores, or by infolding into the schizont, as contrasted with endomerogony; e. has been observed in various species of *Eimeria.* [ecto- + G. *meros,* part, + *gonē,* generation]

ec·to·mes·en·chyme (ek-tō-mes′en-kīm). SYN mesectoderm (2). [ecto- + G. *mesos,* middle, + *enkyma,* infusion]

ec·to·morph (ek′tō-mōrf). A constitutional body type or build (biotype or somatotype) in which tissues originating from the ectoderm predominate; from a morphological standpoint, the limbs predominate over the trunk. SYN longitype. [ecto- + G. *morphē,* form]

ec·to·mor·phic (ek-tō-mōrf′ik). Relating to, or having the characteristics of, an ectomorph.

△**-ectomy.** Removal of an anatomical structure. SEE ALSO -tomy. [G. *ektomē,* a cutting out]

ec·top·a·gus (ek-top′ă-gŭs). Conjoined twins in which the bodies are joined laterally. SEE conjoined *twins,* under *twin.* [ecto- + G. *pagos,* something fixed]

ec·to·par·a·site (ek-tō-par′ă-sīt). A parasite that lives on the surface of the host body.

ec·to·par·a·sit·i·cide (ek′tō-par-ă-sit′i-sīd). An agent that is applied directly to the host to kill ectoparasites. [ectoparasite + L. *caedo,* to kill]

ec·to·par·a·sit·ism (ek′tō-par′ă-sī-tizm). SYN infestation.

ec·to·per·i·to·ni·tis (ek′tō-pār-i-tō-nī′tis). Inflammation beginning in the deeper layer of the peritoneum which is next to the viscera or the abdominal wall.

ec·to·phyte (ek′tō-fīt). A plant parasite of the skin. [ecto- + G. *phyton,* plant]

ec·to·pia (ek-tō′pē-ă). Congenital displacement or malposition of any organ or part of the body. SYN ectopy, heterotopia (1). [G. *ektopos,* out of place, fr. *ektos,* outside, + *topos,* place]

e. cloa′cae, SYN cloacal *exstrophy.*

e. cor′dis, congenital condition in which the heart is exposed on the chest wall because of maldevelopment of the sternum and pericardium.

crossed renal e., ectopic kidney located on opposite (contralateral) side of midline from its ureteral insertion into bladder. In most instances, the two renal moieties are fused (crossed fused ectopia).

crossed testicular e., testis that has crossed the midline to join its contralateral mate in the contralateral inguinal canal or hemiscrotum.

e. len′tis, displacement of the lens of the eye. SYN dislocation of lens.

e. lentis et pupillae, disorder characterized by corectopia and a subluxed or dislocated lens.

e. mac′ulae, a condition in which one macula is displaced so that the two foveas are not at corresponding retinal points. SYN heterotopia maculae.

e. pupil′lae congen′ita, displacement of the pupil present at birth.

e. re′nis, displacement of the kidney.

e. tes′tis, SYN testis e.

testis e., testis that is malpositioned other than along the normal path of descent. SYN e. testis, parorchidium.

thoracoabdominal e. cordis, SYN *pentalogy* of Cantrell.

ureteral e., abnormal termination of ureter within the bladder, the urethra, or outside the urinary tract.

e. vesi′cae, SYN *exstrophy* of the bladder.

ec·top·ic (ek-top′ik). **1.** Out of place; said of an organ not in its proper position, or of a pregnancy occurring elsewhere than in the cavity of the uterus. SYN aberrant (3), heterotopic (1). **2.** In cardiography, denoting a heartbeat that has its origin in some abnormal focus; developing from a focus other than the sinoatrial node. [see ectopia]

ec·to·pla·cen·tal (ek′tō-pla-sen′tăl). **1.** Outside, beyond, or surrounding the placenta; in primates, referring especially to the parts of the trophoblast not directly involved in the formation of the placenta. **2.** In rodents, referring to the actively growing part of the trophoblast involved in the formation of the placenta.

ec·to·plasm (ek′tō-plazm). The peripheral, more viscous cytoplasm of a cell; it contains microfilaments but is lacking in other organelles. SYN exoplasm. [ecto- + G. *plasma,* something formed]

ec·to·plas·mat·ic, ec·to·plas·mic, ec·to·plas·tic (ek-tō-plas-mat′ik, -plas′mik, -plas′tik). Relating to the ectoplasm.

ec·to·py (ek′tō-pē). SYN ectopia.

ec·to·ret·i·na (ek′tō-ret′i-nă). SYN pigmented *layer* of retina.

ec·to·sarc (ek′tō-sark). The outer membrane, or ectoplasm, of a protozoon. [ecto- + G. *sarx,* flesh]

ec·tos·co·py (ek-tos′kŏ-pē). An obsolete method of diagnosis of disease of any of the internal organs by a study of movements of the abdominal wall or thorax caused by phonation. [ecto- + G. *skopeō,* to examine]

ec·tos·te·al (ek-tos′tē-ăl). Relating to the external surface of a bone. [ecto- + G. *osteon,* bone]

ec·tos·to·sis (ek-tos-tō′sis). Ossification in cartilage beneath the perichondrium, or formation of bone beneath the periosteum. [ecto- + G. *osteon,* bone, + *-osis,* condition]

ec·to·thrix (ek′tō-thriks). A sheath of spores (conidia) on the outside of a hair. [ecto- + G. *thrix,* hair]

ec·to·tox·in (ek-tō-tok′sin). SYN exotoxin.

ec·to·zo·on (ek-tō-zō′on). An animal parasite living on the surface of the body. [ecto- + G. *zōon,* animal]

△**ectro-.** Congenital absence of a part. [G. *ektrōsis,* miscarriage]

ec·tro·chei·ry, ec·tro·chi·ry (ek-trō-kī′rē). Total or partial absence of a hand. [ectro- + G. *cheir,* hand]

ec·tro·dac·ty·ly, ec·tro·dac·tyl·ia, ec·tro·dac·tyl·ism (ek-trō-dak′ti-lē, -dak-til′i-ă, -dak′ti-lizm). Congenital absence of all or part of one or more fingers or toes. There are several varieties and the pattern of inheritance may be autosomal dominant with reduced penetrance [MIM*183600 and MIM*183802], autosomal recessive [MIM*225290 and MIM*225300], or X-linked [MIM*313350]. [ectro- + G. *daktylos,* finger]

ec·tro·gen·ic (ek-trō-jen′ik). Relating to ectrogeny.

ec·trog·e·ny (ek-troj′ĕ-nē). Congenital absence or defect of any bodily part. [ectro- + G. *-gen,* producing]

ec·tro·me·lia (ek-trō-mē′lē-ă). **1.** Congenital hypoplasia or aplasia of one or more limbs. **2.** A disease of mice caused by the ectromelia virus, a member of the family *Poxviridae;* characterized by gangrenous loss of feet and necrotic areas in the internal organs; in laboratory mouse colonies, it usually results in high mortality rates. [ectro- + G. *melos,* limb]

ec·tro·mel·ic (ek-trō-mel'ik). Pertaining to, or characterized by, ectromelia.

ec·tro·pi·on, ec·tro·pi·um (ek-trō'pē-on, -pē-ŭm). A rolling outward of the margin of a part, e.g., of an eyelid. [G. *ek,* out, + *tropē,* a turning]

atonic e., e. of the lower eyelid following paralysis of the orbicularis oculi muscle. SYN flaccid e., paralytic e.

cicatricial e., e. of the eyelids after burns, lacerations, or skin infection.

flaccid e., SYN atonic e.

paralytic e., SYN atonic e.

spastic e., e. of the lower eyelid as a result of ocular irritation and/or orbicularis oculi muscle contraction.

e. u'veae, eversion of the pigmented posterior epithelium of the iris at the pupillary margin.

ec·trop·o·dy (ek-trop'ō-dē). Total or partial absence of a foot. [ectro- + G. *pous,* foot]

ec·tro·syn·dac·ty·ly (ek'trō-sin-dak'ti-lē). Congenital abnormality marked by the absence of one or more digits and the fusion of others. [ectro- + G. *syn,* together, + *daktylos,* finger]

ec·tyl·u·rea (ek'til-ū-rē'ă). A mild obsolete sedative used in the treatment of nervous tension and anxiety.

ec·type (ek'tīp). Extreme somatotype, such as ectomorph (longitype) or endomorph (brachytype). [G. *ek,* out, + *typos,* stamp, model]

ec·u·re·sis (ek-ū-rē'sis). A condition in which urinary excretion and intake of water act to produce an absolute dehydration of the body. SEE ALSO emuresis. [G. *ek,* out, + *ourēsis,* urination]

ec·ze·ma (ek'ze-mă, eg'ze-mă, eg-ze'mă). Generic term for inflammatory conditions of the skin, particularly with vesiculation in the acute stage, typically erythematous, edematous, papular, and crusting; followed often by lichenification and scaling and occasionally by duskiness of the erythema and, infrequently, hyperpigmentation; often accompanied by sensations of itching and burning; the vesicles form by intraepidermal spongiosis; often hereditary and associated with allergic rhinitis and asthma. [G. fr. *ekzeō,* to boil over]

allergic e., macular, papular, or vesicular eruption due to an allergic reaction, e.g., contact dermatitis.

atopic e., SYN atopic *dermatitis.*

baker e., allergic e. due to contact with flour, yeast, or other ingredients handled by bakers.

chronic e., SYN lichenoid e.

dyshidrotic e., SYN dyshidrosis.

e. erythemato'sum, a dry form of e. marked by extensive areas of redness with scaly desquamation.

flexural e., e. of skin at the flexures of elbow, knees, wrists, etc., associated with atopy persisting through childhood.

hand e., e. that predominantly and persistently affects the hands; of multiple causation, including allergic, industrial, irritant, dyshidrotic, bacterial, and atopic mechanisms; distinguished from chapped hands by the presenc of vesiculation or spongiosis.

e. herpet'icum, a febrile condition caused by cutaneous dissemination of herpesvirus type 1, occurring most commonly in children, consisting of a widespread eruption of vesicles rapidly becoming umbilicated pustules; clinically indistinguishable from a generalized vaccinia. The two may be distinguished by electron microscopy or demonstration of inclusion bodies in smears, which are intranuclear in e. herpeticum and intracytoplasmic in e. vaccinatum. SYN pustulosis vacciniformis acuta.

infantile e., e. in infants; the clinical appearance varies according to the dominant causative mechanism, e.g., contact-type hypersensitivity, candidiasis, atopy, seborrhea, or a combination including intertrigo and diaper dermatitis.

e. intertri'go, SEE intertrigo.

lichenoid e., thickening of skin with accentuated skin lines in e. SYN chronic e.

nummular e., discrete, coin-shaped patches of e. SYN nummular dermatitis.

e. papulo'sum, a dermatitis marked by an eruption of discrete or aggregated reddish excoriated papules.

e. parasit'icum, eczematous eruption precipitated by parasite infestation.

e. pustulo'sum, a later stage of vesicular e., in which the vesicles have become secondarily infected; the lesions become covered with purulent crusts.

seborrheic e., SYN seborrheic *dermatitis.*

stasis e., eczematous eruption on legs due to or aggravated by vascular stasis.

tropical e., e. occurring in plaques on extensors of the extremities; of common occurrence and unknown etiology.

e. tylot'icum, hyperkeratotic dyshidrosis.

varicose e., e. occurring over areas in which the skin has been compromised by varicosities.

e. verruco'sum, e. with hyperkeratosis; chronic lichenified e.

e. vesiculo'sum, dermatitis marked by an eruption of vesicles upon erythematous patches that rupture and exude serum.

weeping e., a moist, eczematous dermatitis.

winter e., e. resulting from accelerated evaporation of moisture (including insensitive sweat) from the cutaneous surface; occurs as dry crackled plaques, usually on the extremities, but not infrequently also on the trunk in any season under circumstances (occupational, environmental) of excessively rapid drying out of the skin.

ec·zem·a·ti·za·tion (ek-zem'ă-ti-zā'shŭn). **1.** Formation of an eruption resembling eczema. **2.** Occurrence of eczema secondary to a preexisting dermatosis.

ec·ze·ma·toid (ek-zem'ă-toyd). Resembling eczema in appearance.

ec·ze·ma·tous (ek-zem'ă-tŭs). Marked by or resembling eczema.

ED Abbreviation for effective *dose;* ethyldichloroarsine.

ED₅₀ Abbreviation for median effective dose.

edath·a·mil (ĕ-dath'ă-mil). SYN ethylenediaminetetraacetic acid.

EDC Abbreviation for estimated date of confinement. SEE Nägele *rule.*

e·de·a (e-dē'ă). The external genitals. [G. *aidoia,* genitals]

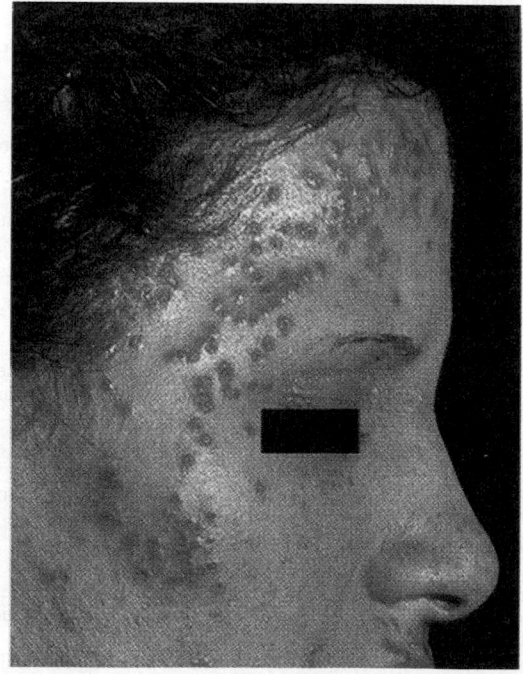

eczema herpeticum

ede·ma (e-dē'mă). An accumulation of an excessive amount of watery fluid in cells or intercellular tissues. [G. *oidēma,* a swelling]

ambulant e., e. forming during periods of walking with the legs dependent.

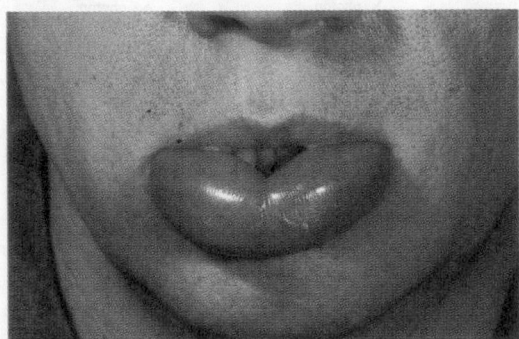**angioneurotic e.,** SYN angioedema.

angioneurotic edema: seen in the lower lip

Berlin e., retinal e. after blunt trauma to the globe.

blue e., the swelling and cyanosis of an extremity in hysterical paralysis.

brain e., SYN cerebral e.

brawny e., SYN nonpitting e.

brown e., e. of the lungs associated with chronic passive congestion.

bullous e., a reddened, swollen appearance of the ureteral orifice in the bladder wall, frequently observed with distal ureteral calculi or in tuberculosis of the ureter.

bullous e. vesi′cae, a prominent area of focal e. involving the bladder epithelium, consisting of elevated masses of edematous tissue or clusters of clear fluid-filled vesicles; often associated with chronic inflammation or irritation secondary to tubes, foreign bodies, or perivesical inflammation.

cachectic e., e. occurring in diseases characterized by wasting and hypoproteinemia; due to low plasma oncotic pressure. SYN marantic e.

cardiac e., e. resulting from congestive heart failure.

cerebral e., brain swelling due to increased volume of the extravascular compartment from the uptake of water in the neuropile and white matter. SEE ALSO brain *swelling.* SYN brain e.

cystoid macular e., e. of the posterior pole of the eye secondary to abnormal permeability of capillaries of the central sensory retina.

dependent e., a clinically detectable increase in extracellular fluid volume localized in a dependent area, as of a limb, characterized by swelling or pitting.

gestational e., occurrence of a generalized and excessive accumulation of fluid in the tissues of greater than 1+ pitting after 12 hours' bed rest, or of a weight gain of 5 pounds or more in 1 week due to the influence of pregnancy.

e. glot′tidis, e. of the larynx.

heat e., e. caused by excessively high external temperature.

hereditary angioneurotic e. (HANE) [MIM*106100], a relatively rare form of e. characterized by onset, usually in adolescence, of erythema followed by e., involving the upper respiratory or gastrointestinal tracts, associated with either a deficiency of C1 esterase inhibitor or a functionally inactive form of the inhibitor. There are two clinically indistinguishable forms: type I, in which the serum level of C1 esterase inhibitor is low (up to 30% of normal) and type II, in which the level is normal or elevated. There is uncontrolled activation of early complement components and production of a kininlike factor that induces the angioedema; death may occur from upper respiratory tract e. and asphyxia. Inheritance is autosomal dominant, caused by mutation in the C1-esterase inhibitor gene (C1NH) on chromosome 11q.

hydremic e., obsolete term for e. occurring in states marked by pronounced hydremia.

infantile acute hemorrhagic e. of the skin, a generally benign form of cutaneous vasculitis, characterized by ecchymotic purpura, often in a cockade pattern, and inflammatory e. in infants.

inflammatory e., a swelling due to effusion of fluid in the soft parts surrounding a focus of inflammation.

lymphatic e., e. due to stasis in the lymph channels.

marantic e., SYN cachectic e.

menstrual e., retention of water and increase in weight, which occurs during or preceding menstruation.

e. neonato′rum, a diffuse, firm, and commonly fatal e. occurring in the newborn, usually beginning in the legs and spreading upward.

nephrotic e., e. resulting from renal dysfunction.

noninflammatory e., e. due to mechanical or other causes, not marked by inflammation or congestion.

nonpitting e., swelling of subcutaneous tissues which cannot be indented easily by compression. Usually due to metabolic abnormality, such as increased glycosaminoglycan content, like that which occurs in Graves *disease* (pretibial myxedema) or in early phase of scleroderma. SYN brawny e.

nutritional e., a form of swelling caused by insufficient protein intake resulting in hypoproteinemia and low plasma oncotic pressure.

periodic e., SYN angioedema.

pitting e., e. that retains for a time the indentation produced by pressure.

premenstrual e., SEE menstrual e.

pulmonary e., e. of lungs usually resulting from mitral stenosis or left ventricular failure.

salt e., e. from excessive intake or retention of sodium chloride.

solid e., infiltration of the subcutaneous tissues by mucoid material, as in myxedema.

Yangtze e., SYN gnathostomiasis.

edem·a·ti·za·tion (e-dem′ă-ti-zā′shŭn). Making edematous.

edem·a·tous (e-dem′ă-tŭs). Marked by edema.

eden·tate (ē-den′tāt). SYN edentulous. [L. *edentatus*]

eden·tu·lous (ē-den′tū-lŭs). Toothless, having lost the natural teeth. SYN edentate. [L. *edentulus,* toothless]

edes·tin (ĕ-des′tin). A hexameric globulin derived from the castor oil bean, hemp seed, and other seeds. It will support the growth of animals in the absence of other dietary proteins.

ed·e·tate (ed′ĕ-tāt). USAN-approved contraction for ethylenediaminetetraacetate, the anion of ethylenediaminetetraacetic acid; various ed.e.'s are used as chelating agents to carry cations in (e.g., ferric sodium e. as an iron ion carrier) or out (e.g., sodium e. for calcium or heavy metal ion removal).

ed·e·tate cal·ci·um di·so·di·um. Contracted name for a salt of ethylenediaminetetraacetate, an agent used as a chelator of lead and some other heavy metals. Available in several forms: disodium, sodium, and trisodium.

edet·ic ac·id (ĕ-det′ik). SYN ethylenediaminetetraacetic acid.

edge (ej). A line at which a surface terminates. SEE ALSO border, margin.

cutting e., (1) the beveled, knifelike, sharpened working angle of a dental hand instrument; **(2)** SYN incisal *margin.*

denture e., SYN denture *border.*

incisal e., SYN incisal *margin.*

leading e., the initial part of a waveform.

shearing e., SYN incisal *margin.*

Edinger, Ludwig, German anatomist, 1855–1918. SEE E.-Westphal *nucleus.*

edis·y·late (e-dis′i-lāt). USAN-approved contraction for 1,2-ethanedisulfonate, $^-O_3S(CH_2)_2SO_3^-$.

Edlefsen, Gustav J.F., German physician, 1842–1910. SEE E. *reagent.*

EDM Abbreviation for multiple epiphyseal *dysplasia.*

Edman, Pehr, Australian scientist, 1916–1977. SEE E. *method, reagent.*

EDRF Acronym for endothelium-derived relaxing *factor*, now known to be nitric oxide.

Edridge-Green, Frederick W., English ophthalmologist, 1863–1953. SEE Edridge-Green *lamp*.

ed·ro·pho·ni·um chlo·ride (ed-rō-fō′nē-ŭm). A short-duration competitive antagonist of skeletal muscle relaxants (curare derivatives and gallamine triethiodide) and an anticholinesterase, used as an antidote for curariform drugs, as a diagnostic agent in myasthenia gravis, and in myasthenic crisis.

EDS Abbreviation for Ehlers-Danlos *syndrome*.

EDSS Abbreviation for expanded disability status *scale*.

EDTA Abbreviation for ethylenediaminetetraacetic acid.

educt (ē′dŭkt). An extract.

edul·co·rant (e-dŭl′kō-rant). Sweetening.

edul·co·rate (e-dŭl′kō-rāt). To sweeten or render less acrid. [L. *e*-intensive, + *dulcoro*, to sweeten, fr. *dulcor*, sweetness, fr. *dulcis*, sweet]

Edwards, James Hilton, English physician and medical geneticist, *1928. SEE E. *syndrome*.

Edwards, M.L., U.S. physician, *1906. SEE Carpentier-Edwards *valve*; Starr-Edwards *valve*.

Ed·ward·si·el·la (ed′ward-sē-el′lă). A genus of Gram-negative, facultatively anaerobic bacteria (family Enterobacteriaceae) containing motile, peritrichous, nonencapsulated rods. The type species is *E. tarda*, which is occasionally isolated from the stools of both healthy humans and those with diarrhea, from the blood of humans and other animals, and from human urine. *E. tarda* is an etiologic agent of gastroenteritis in humans. The two other species in this genus are *E. hoshinae* and *E. ictaluri*.

EEE Abbreviation for eastern equine *encephalomyelitis*.

EEG Abbreviation for electroencephalogram; electroencephalography.

eel (ēl). Any of a number of scaleless, snakelike fish. [M.E. *ele*, fr. O.E. *ael*]

    vinegar e., SYN *Turbatrix aceti*.

EENT Abbreviation for eye, ear, nose, and throat. See also ENT.

ef·face·ment (ē-fās′ment). The thinning out of the cervix just before or during labor.

ef·fect (e-fekt′). The result or consequence of an action. [L. *efficio*, pp. *effectus*, to accomplish, fr. *facio*, to do]

    abscopal e., a reaction produced following irradiation but occurring outside the zone of actual radiation absorption.

    additive e., an e. wherein two or more substances or actions used in combination produce a total e., the same as the arithmetic sum of the individual e.'s.

    after-e., SEE aftereffect.

    Anrep e., a small transient positive inotropic e. of abrupt increases of systolic aortic and left ventricular pressures related to recovery from transient subendocardial ischemia (e.g., cold pressor test).

    Arias-Stella e., SYN Arias-Stella *phenomenon*.

    autokinetic e., in psychology, the apparent drifting about of a small, fixed, spot of light which is being observed in a dark room.

    Bernoulli e., the decrease in fluid pressure that occurs in converting potential to kinetic energy when motion of the fluid is accelerated, in accordance with Bernoulli law; applied in water aspirators, atomizers, and humidifiers in which a gas is accelerated across the end of a narrow, fluid-filled orifice.

    Bohr e., the influence exerted by carbon dioxide on the oxygen dissociation curve of blood, i.e., the curve is shifted to the right, which means an apparent reduction in the affinity of hemoglobin for oxygen. Cf. Haldane e.

    Bowditch e., homeometric autoregulation of cardiac function induced by changing heart rate.

    Circe e., an e. observed in enzyme catalysis in which accelerated diffusion of the substrate occurs through attractive forces of the enzyme's active site.

    clasp-knife e., SYN clasp-knife *spasticity*.

    Compton e., in the absorption of electromagnetic radiation of medium energy, a decrease in energy of the bombarding photon

with the dislodgement of an orbital electron, usually from an outer shell. SYN Compton scattering.

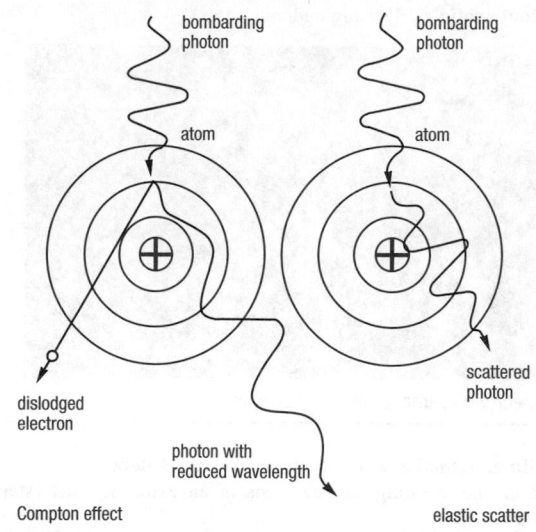

bombarding photon

bombarding photon

atom

atom

dislodged electron

scattered photon

photon with reduced wavelength

Compton effect

elastic scatter

Compton effect and elastic scatter

    Cotton e., the positive and negative displacement from zero of the rotation of plane polarized monochromatic light and the change of monochromatic circularly polarized light into elliptically polarized light in the immediate vicinity of the absorption band of the substance through which the light passes. SEE ALSO optic rotatory *dispersion*, circular *dichroism*.

    Crabtree e., inhibition of cellular respiration of isolated systems by high concentrations of glucose; a "reciprocal" of Pasteur e.; due, in part, to the inhibition of hexokinase by elevated glucose 6-phosphate. Cf. Pasteur e.

    cumulative e., the condition in which repeated administration of a drug may produce e.'s that are more pronounced than those produced by the first dose. SYN cumulative action.

    Cushing e., SYN Cushing *phenomenon*.

    cytopathic e., degenerative changes in cells (especially in tissue culture) associated with the multiplication of certain viruses; when, in tissue culture, spread of virus is restricted by an overlay of agar (or other suitable substance) the cytopathic e. may lead to formation of plaque.

    Doppler e., a change in frequency observed when the sound source and observer are in relative motion away from or toward each other. SEE ALSO Doppler *shift*. SYN Doppler phenomenon.

    electrophonic e., the sensation of hearing produced when an alternating current of suitable frequency and magnitude is passed from an external source through the head of a person.

    experimenter e.'s, the influence of the experimenter's behavior, personality traits, or expectancies on the results of that person's own research. SEE double blind *study*.

    Fahraeus-Lindqvist e., the decrease in apparent viscosity that occurs when a suspension, such as blood, is made to flow through a tube of smaller diameter; observed in tubes less than about 0.3 mm in diameter. SYN sigma e.

    Fenn e., the increased liberation of heat in a stimulated muscle when it is allowed to do mechanical work; the amount of heat liberated is increased in proportion to the distance the muscle is allowed to shorten and in proportion to the tension it must develop (e.g., the weight it lifts) during shortening; thus increased chemical energy is consumed both to liberate increased heat and to do increased mechanical work.

    first-pass e., SYN first-pass *metabolism*.

flash-lag e., the apparent lagging behind a moving object of a portion of it that flashes briefly.

founder e., an unusually high frequency of a gene in a particular population derived from a small set of unrepresentative ancestors.

gene dosage e., in codominant alleles, the more or less linear relationship between the phenotypic value and the number of genes of one type substituted by another type.

generation e., variation in health status arising from the different causal factors of disease to which each successive generation born is exposed as it passes through life.

Haldane e., the promotion of carbon dioxide dissociation in blood by an increase in the oxygenation of hemoglobin.

halo e., (1) the e. (usually beneficial) that the manner, attention, and caring of a provider have on a patient during a medical encounter, regardless of what medical procedure or services the encounter involves; (2) the influence upon an observation of the observer's perception of the characteristics of the individual observed (other than the characteristics under study) or the influence of the observer's recollection or knowledge of findings on a previous occasion.

Hawthorne e., the e. (usually positive or beneficial) of being under study, upon the persons being studied; their knowledge of the study often influences their behavior. [city in Illinois; site of the Western Electric plant]

healthy worker e., phenomenon observed initially in studies of occupational diseases; workers usually exhibit lower overall death rates than the general population because severely ill and disabled people are excluded from employment.

hyperchromic e., an increase in absorptivity (or extinction) at a particular wavelength of light by a solution or substance due to structural changes in a molecule.

hypochromic e., a phenomenon in which an individual molecule, containing several chromophores, has a certain absorptivity (or optical density) at a given wavelength that is less than the sum of the optical densities of the individual chromophores (at that same wavelength).

Mach e., the appearance of a light or dark line on a radiograph where there is a concave or convex interface in the subject, a physiologic optical form of edge enhancement. SEE ALSO Mach *band.*

e. modifier, a factor that modifies the e. of a putative causal factor under study; e.g., age is an e. modifier for many conditions.

nuclear Overhauser e. (NOE), an e. seen in nuclear magnetic resonance in which there is a through-space nearest-neighbor interaction.

Orbeli e., the fatigue of a muscle stimulated by its nerve (i.e., indirectly) is reduced by concurrent stimulation of sympathetic fibers to the muscle; thought to be caused by norepinephrine diffusing from adrenergic fibers which innervate blood vessels in the muscle.

oxygen e., enhancement of radiosensitivity of cells by a high concentration of oxygen, and, conversely, decreased radiosensitivity in a hypoxic environment.

Pasteur e., the inhibition of fermentation by oxygen, first observed by Pasteur; either not observed, or only slightly observed, in malignant tumors. Cf. Crabtree e.

photechic e., the ability of an agent, other than light, to make a developable latent image in a photographic film emulsion. SYN Russell e.

photoelectric e., (1) the loss of electrons from the surface of a metal upon exposure to light; (2) a mode of interaction of radiation with matter in which all of the energy of the incident photon is absorbed, with ejection of a photoelectron and characteristic radiation from filling the vacancy from another shell; since the energy absorption per gram of tissue is proportional to the cube of the atomic number, this mode is important in diagnostic radiography.

piezoelectric e., the property of certain crystalline or ceramic materials to emit electricity when deformed and to deform when an electric current is passed across them, a mechanism of interconverting electrical and acoustic energy; an ultrasound transducer sends and receives acoustic energy using this e.

position e., a change in the phenotypic expression of one or more genes due to a change in its physical location with respect to other genes; may result from change in chromosome structure or from crossing-over.

Purkinje e., SYN Purkinje *phenomenon.*

quantal e., an e. that can be expressed only in binary terms, as occurring or not occurring.

Raman e., a change in frequency undergone by monochromatic light scattered in passage through a transparent substance whose characteristics determine the amount of change, yielding a spectrum in which the incident wavelength band is flanked by small satellite bands of greater and lesser wavelengths.

Rivero-Carvallo e., inspiratory increase in the systolic murmur of tricuspid insufficiency; the characteristic distinguishing tricuspid insufficiency from mitral insufficiency.

Russell e., SYN photechic e.

second gas e., when a constant concentration of an anesthetic like halothane is inspired, the increase in alveolar concentration is accelerated by concomitant administration of nitrous oxide, because alveolar uptake of the latter creates a potential subatmospheric intrapulmonary pressure that leads to increased tracheal inflow.

sigma e., SYN Fahraeus-Lindqvist e.

Somogyi e., in diabetes, a rebound phenomenon of reactive hyperglycemia in response to a preceding period of relative hypoglycemia that has increased secretion of hyperglycemic agents (epinephrine, norepinephrine, glucagon, cortisol, and growth hormone); described in diabetic patients given too much insulin who developed unrecognized nocturnal hypoglycemia that made them hyperglycemic (suggesting insufficient insulin) when tested the next morning.

Staub-Traugott e., in normal persons, a drop in blood glucose which follows a second oral dose of glucose given 30 minutes or so after the first.

Stiles-Crawford e., light that enters through the center of the pupil produces a greater visual effect than light that enters obliquely.

synergistic e., SYN synergism.

Tyndall e., SYN Tyndall *phenomenon.*

Venturi e., term applied to the operation of a Venturi tube and similar systems.

Wedensky e., a relatively long enhancing e. following application of a maximal shock or stimulus to a neuromuscular preparation during which a subthreshold stimulation, otherwise too small to evoke a response, will produce a response; a relatively prolonged lowered threshold of excitability following a maximal shock.

Wolff-Chaikoff e., SYN Wolff-Chaikoff *block.*

Zeeman e., the splitting of spectral lines into three or more symmetrically placed lines when the light source is subjected to a magnetic field.

ef·fec·tive·ness. **1.** A measure of the accuracy or success of a diagnostic or therapeutic technique when carried out in an average clinical environment. Cf. efficacy. **2.** The extent to which a treatment achieves its intended purpose.

relative biologic e. (RBE), a factor used to compare the biologic effect of absorbed doses of different types and energies of ionizing radiation. It is determined by the ratio of an absorbed dose of the particular radiation in question to the absorbed dose of a reference radiation required to produce an identical biologic effect in a specific organism, organ, or tissue.

ef·fec·tor (ē-fek′tŏr, -tōr). **1.** C. Sherrington term for a peripheral tissue that receives nerve impulses and reacts by contraction (muscle), secretion (gland), or a discharge of electricity (electric organ of certain bony fishes). **2.** A small metabolic molecule that by combining with a repressor gene depresses the activity of an operon. **3.** A small molecule that binds to a protein and, in so doing, alters the activity of that protein. **4.** A substance, technique, procedure, or individual that causes an effect. [L. *producer*]

ef·fem·i·na·tion (e-fem-i-nā′shŭn). Acquisition of feminine characteristics, either physiologically as part of female maturation, or pathologically by individuals of either sex. [L. *ef-femino,* pp. *-atus,* to make feminine, fr. *ex,* out, + *femina,* woman]

ef

ef·fer·ent (ef'er-ent). Conducting (fluid or a nerve impulse) outward from a given organ or part thereof; e.g., the efferent connections of a group of nerve cells, efferent blood vessels, or the excretory duct of an organ. [L. *efferens*, fr. *effero*, to bring out]

gamma e., the thin axon of a gamma motor neuron innervating the intrafusal muscle fibers of a muscle spindle.

ef·fer·vesce (ef-er-ves'). To boil up or form bubbles rising to the surface of a fluid in large numbers, as in the evolution of CO_2 from aqueous solution when the pressure is reduced. [L. *ef-ferves-co*, to boil up, from *ferveo*, to boil]

ef·fer·ves·cent (ef-er-ves'ent). 1. Boiling; bubbling; effervescing. 2. Causing to effervesce, as an e. powder. 3. Tending to effervesce when freed from pressure, as an e. solution.

ef·fi·ca·cy (ef'ĭ-ka-sē). The extent to which a specific intervention, procedure, regimen, or service produces a beneficial result under ideal conditions. Cf. effectiveness. [L. *efficacia*, fr, *ef-ficio*, to perform, accomplish]

ef·fi·cien·cy (ĕ-fish'en-sē). 1. The production of the desired effects or results with minimum waste of time, money, effort, or skill. 2. A measure of effectiveness; specifically, the useful work output divided by the energy input.

quantum e., SYN quantum *yield*.

visual e., a rating used in computing compensation for industrial ocular injuries, incorporating measurements of central acuity, visual field, and ocular motility.

ef·fleu·rage (e-fler-ahz'). A stroking movement in massage. [Fr. *effleurer*, to touch lightly]

ef·flo·resce (e-flōr-es'). To become powdery by losing the water of crystallization on exposure to a dry atmosphere. [L. *ef-floresco* (*exf-*), to blossom, fr. *flos* (*flor-*), flower]

ef·flo·res·cent (e-flōr-es'ent). Denoting a crystalline body that gradually changes to a powder by losing its water of crystallization on exposure to a dry atmosphere.

ef·flu·vi·um, pl. **ef·flu·via** (e-floo'vē-ŭm, -ē-ă). Shedding of hair. SEE ALSO defluxion (1). [L. a flowing out, fr. *ef-fluo*, to flow out]

anagen e., sudden diffuse hair shedding with cancer chemotherapy or radiation, usually reversible when treatment ends.

telogen e., increased transient shedding of normal club hairs by premature development of telogen in anagen follicles, resulting from various kinds of stress, e.g., childbirth, shock, drug intake or cessation of an oral contraceptive, fever, and dieting with marked weight loss.

ef·fort (ef'ert). Deliberate exertion of physical or mental power.

distributed e., in psychology, learning that involves small units of work and interpolated rest periods, as contrasted with massed learning, in which the individual works continually until the skill is mastered.

ef·fuse (ef-ūz'). Thin and widely spread; denoting the surface character of a bacterial culture. [L. *ef-fundo*, pp. *-fusus;* to pour out]

ef·fu·sion (e-fū'zhŭn). 1. The escape of fluid from the blood vessels or lymphatics into the tissues or a cavity. 2. A collection of the fluid effused. [L. *effusio*, a pouring out]

complex pleural e., a pleural e. without actual infection but with signs of a high degree of inflammation (e.g., low pH, low glucose, high lactate dehydrogenase, many white cells).

joint e., increased fluid in synovial cavity of a joint.

loculated pleural e., pleural e. that is confined to one or more fixed pockets in the pleural space.

middle-ear e., a condition in which the air in the middle ear has been replaced with serous or mucoid fluid as a consequence of otitis media. SYN secretory otitis media, serous otitis media.

parapneumonic e., pleural e. associated with pneumonia

pericardial e., increased fluid within the pericardial sac; can cause circulatory compromise by compression of the heart; most often caused by inflammation, infection, malignancy, and uremia. SYN dropsy of pericardium.

pleural e., increased fluid in the pleural space; can cause shortness of breath by compression of the lung and/or increased intrathoracic pressure resulting in mediastinal shift and increased work

of breathing; a transudative e. has low protein content and is usually due to heart failure, uremia, or hypoalbuminemia; an exudative e. has high protein and cell count and is due most often to inflammation, malignancy, or infection; an infected pleural e. is an empyema; a pleural e. associated with pneumonia is a parapneumonic e.; a pleural e. without actual infection but with signs of a high degree of inflammation (e.g., low pH, low glucose, high lactate dehydrogenase, many white cells) is a complex pleural e. and is frequently associated with pneumonia; a loculated pleural e. is not free-flowing in the pleural space but rather confined to one or more fixed pockets. SYN hydrothorax.

subpulmonic e., a collection of fluid in the pleural space mostly located radiographically between the diaphragm and the basal surface of the lung.

eflor·ni·thine hy·dro·chlo·ride (ē-flōr'ni-thēn). An antineoplastic and antiprotozoal orphan drug used in the treatment of *Pneumocystis carinii* pneumonia in AIDS and of *Trypanosoma brucei gambiense* sleeping sickness.

EGD Abbreviation for esophagogastroduodenoscopy.

eges·ta (ē-jes'tă). Unabsorbed food residues that are discharged from the digestive tract. [L. *e-gero*, pp. *-gestus*, to carry out, discharge]

EGF Abbreviation for epidermal growth *factor*.

EGFR Abbreviation for epidermal growth factor *receptor* .

egg (eg). The female sexual cell, or gamete; after fertilization and fusion of the pronuclei it is a zygote and no longer an egg. In reptiles and birds, the egg is provided with a protective shell, membranes, albumin, and yolk for the nourishment of the embryo. SEE ALSO oocyte, ovum. [A.S. *aeg*]

centrolecithal e., an e. in which the yolk is concentrated near the center of the e. cell, as is the case in many of the insects.

homolecithal e., an e. in which the total amount of yolk is small and fairly uniformly distributed throughout the cytoplasm. SYN isolecithal e.

isolecithal e., SYN homolecithal e.

microlecithal e., an e. containing a small amount of deutoplasm.

telolecithal e., an e. containing a relatively large quantity of deutoplasm concentrated at the abapical pole; e.g., e.'s of reptiles and birds.

egg clus·ter. One of the clumps of cells resulting from the breaking up of the gonadal cords in the ovarian cortex; these clumps later develop into primary ovarian follicles.

Egger, Fritz, Swiss internist, 1863–1938. SEE E. *line*.

Eggleston, Cary, U.S. physician, 1884–1966. SEE E. *method;* Bradbury-Eggleston *syndrome*.

egg·shell. The calcareous envelope of a bird's egg.

eglan·du·lous (ē-glan'doo-lŭs). Without glands. [L. *e*, without, + gland or glandula]

Eglis glands. See under gland.

e·go (ē'gō). In psychoanalysis, one of the three components of the psychic apparatus in the freudian structural framework, the other two being the id and superego. Although the e. has some conscious components, many of its functions are learned and automatic. It occupies a position between the primal instincts (pleasure principle) and the demands of the outer world (reality principle), and therefore mediates between the person and external reality by performing the important functions of perceiving the needs of the self, both physical and psychological, and the qualities and attitudes of the environment. It evaluates, coordinates, and integrates these perceptions so that internal demands can be adjusted to external requirements, and is also responsible for certain defensive functions to protect the person against the demands of the id and superego. [L. I]

ego-al·ien (ē'gō-ā'lē-en). SYN ego-dystonic.

ego·bron·choph·o·ny (ē'gō-brong-kof'ō-nē). Egophony with bronchophony. [G. *aix* (*aig-*), goat, + *bronchos*, bronchus, + *phōnē*, voice]

ego·cen·tric (ē-gō-sen'trik). Marked by extreme concentration of attention upon oneself, i.e., self-centered. Cf. allocentric. SYN egotropic. [ego + G. *kentron*, center]

ego·cen·tric·i·ty (ē′gō-sen-tris′i-tē). The condition of being egocentric.

ego-dys·ton·ic (ē′gō-dis-ton′ik). Repugnant to or at variance with the aims of the ego and related psychological needs of the individual (e.g., an obsessive thought or compulsive behavior); the opposite of ego-syntonic. SYN ego-alien. [ego + G. *dys,* bad, + *tonos,* tension]

ego-ideal. In psychoanalysis, a more or less conscious ideal of personal excellence toward which an individual strives, and that is derived from a composite image of the personal characteristics of a parent, public figure, or one or more other individuals the person admires.

ego·ma·nia (ē-gō-mā′nē-ă). Extreme self-centeredness, self-appreciation, or self-content. [ego + G. *mania,* frenzy]

ego·phon·ic (ē-gō-fon′ik). Relating to egophony.

egoph·o·ny (ē-gof′ō-nē). A peculiar broken quality of the voice sounds, like the bleating of a goat, heard about the upper level of the fluid in cases of pleurisy with effusion. SYN capriloquism, tragophonia, tragophony. [G. *aix* (*aig*-), goat, + *phōnē,* voice]

ego-syn·ton·ic (ē′gō-sin-ton′ik). Acceptable to the aims of the ego and the related psychological needs of the individual (e.g., a delusion); the opposite of ego-dystonic. [ego + G. *syn,* together, + *tonos,* tension]

ego·tro·pic (ē-gō-trop′ik). SYN egocentric. [ego + G. *tropē,* a turning]

EGTA Abbreviation for ethyleneglycotetraacetic acid.

EHEC Abbreviation for enterohemorrhagic *Escherichia coli.*

Ehlers, Edward L., Danish dermatologist, 1863–1937. SEE E.-Danlos *syndrome.*

Ehrenritter, Johann, Austrian anatomist, †1790. SEE E. *ganglion.*

Ehret, Heinrich, German physician, *1870. SEE E. *phenomenon.*

Ehrlich, Paul, German bacteriologist, immunologist, and Nobel laureate, 1854–1915. SEE *Ehrlichia;* E. *anemia,* inner *body, phenomenon, postulate,* diazo *reagent, theory;* E.-Türk *line.* See entries under stain; reaction.

Ehr·lich·ia (er-lik′ē-ă). A genus of small, often pleomorphic, coccoid to ellipsoidal, nonmotile, Gram-negative bacteria (order Rickettsiales) that occur either singly or in compact inclusions in circulating mammalian leukocytes; species are the etiologic agents of ehrlichiosis and are transmitted by ticks. The type species is E. *canis.* [P. *Ehrlich*]

E. *ca′nis,* the bacterial species causing the tick-borne disease canine ehrlichiosis in dogs (transmitted by the tick *Rhipicephalus sanguineus*); it is the type species of the genus E. Occasionally causes tick-borne infection in humans.

E. *chaffee′nsis,* a recently described bacterial species associated with human ehrlichiosis; infects human monocytes and is carried by the tick vector, *Amblyomma americanum,* the Lone Star tick.

E. *equi,* a bacterial species that causes human granulocytic ehrlichiosis; occurs in the Midatlantic, southern New England, and southern Midwest and is spread by ticks (*Ixodes*).

E. *phagocytophila,* a bacterial species that causes human granulocytic ehrlichiosis; also causes tick-borne fever in cattle; occurs in the Midatlantic, southern New England, and southern Midwest and is spread by ticks (*Ixodes*).

E. *ristic′ii,* the bacterial species causing equine monocytic ehrlichiosis.

E. *sennet′su,* the bacterial species causing Sennetsu fever in humans. SYN *Rickettsia sennetsu.*

Ehr·lic·hi·eae. Members of the Rickettsiaceae family; obligate intracellular parasites of peripheral blood leukocytes.

ehr·lich·i·o·sis (er-lik-ē-ō′sis). Infection with leukocytic rickettsiae of the genus *Ehrlichia;* in humans, especially by E. *sennetsu* that produces manifestations similar to those of Rocky Mountain spotted fever.

Species of *Ehrlichia* have long been recognized as causes of febrile hemorrhagic disease of variable severity in animals, including dogs and horses. Human infection with E. *sennetsu,* limited to the Far East, is a mononucleosislike illness. The first human case of ehrlichiosis in the western hemisphere was reported in 1986. Since then 2 distinct forms of the disease, each associated with a different species of *Ehrlichia* and a different group of tick vectors, have been recognized in human beings. More than 90% of patients give a history of having been bitten by several ticks. An animal reservoir has not yet been identified, but rodents and deer are suspected. After an incubation period of 1–4 weeks, infection begins as a nonspecific febrile illness with chills, sweating, headache, and joint and muscle pains. One-fourth of patients have a transitory nonspecific rash not related to the site of tick bite. Systemic complications may involve the respiratory tract (sore throat, cough, pulmonary infiltrates, acute respiratory distress syndrome), the digestive system (nausea, vomiting, abdominal pain, gastrointestinal bleeding), or the liver (80% have hepatitis). Other possible complications include meningitis, pericarditis, renal failure, and disseminated intravascular coagulation. Early studies of these infections, based on populations with more conspicuous and readily identifiable disease, overestimated case fatality rates. With treatment, the case fatality rate in the 2 forms of ehrlichiosis probably does not exceed 1%. Human granulocytic ehrlichiosis is clinically indistinguishable from human monocytic ehrlichiosis, but in the former, morulae are found in neutrophils rather than in monocytes, and the disease is somewhat more severe. For both forms of ehrlichiosis, polymerase chain reaction technology has yielded the most sensitive and specific serologic testing. Tetracycline and doxycycline are highly effective in arresting progression of either form of human ehrlichiosis. Because other agents, including chloramphenicol, have not been found to be effective, tetracyclines are used even in children, in whom they are generally contraindicated because of the risk of dental mottling and suppression of bone growth. Treatment is often begun on suspicion, pending confirmation of the clinical diagnosis by serologic test. Drug therapy is continued for 14 days.

human e., a form of e. that presents clinically as a undifferentiated acute febrile illness characterized by fever, chills, diarrhea, and headache, following tick bite(s), probably by the Lone Star tick, *Amblyomma americanum.* Usually caused by *Ehrlichia chaffeensis.* First described in 1987. (Thought to be predominantly a monocytic form of ehrlichiosis.)

human granulocytic e. (HGE), an acute infectious disease characterized by fever, chills, headache, joint and muscle pains, and sometimes respiratory, gastrointestinal, hepatic, or other systemic involvement; first described in 1994 in northeastern and northern midwestern states and California; the causative agent can be distinguished only by molecular studies from *Ehrlichia equi,* the cause of equine e. The deer tick, *Ixodes scapularis,* is the principal vector, and the peak incidence is in July. Hematologic studies show depression of RBC, WBC, and platelets. Clusters of developing organisms called morulae may be seen in neutrophils on stained blood smears, but serologic testing is more sensitive.

human monocytic e. (HME), an acute infectious disease characterized by fever, chills, headache, muscle and joint pain, and variable respiratory, gastrointestinal, and systemic involvement; hematologic studies show depression of RBC, WBC, and platelets. The finding of clumps of developing organisms, called morulae, in the cytoplasm of monocytes in a stained smear of peripheral blood establishes the diagnosis, but their detection is often difficult. Serologic testing shows antibody to *Ehrlichia chaffeensis,* an organism closely resembling the agent of canine e., E. *canis.* This disease has been largely confined to the southeastern and south central United States. The Lone Star tick (*Amblyomma americanum*) and the American dog tick (*Dermacentor variabilis*) are the principal vectors, and the incidence is highest from April to September, during the peak activity of these ticks.

Eichhorst, Hermann L., Swiss physician, 1849–1921. SEE E. *corpuscles,* under *corpuscle, neuritis.*

Eicken, Karl von, German laryngologist, 1873–1960. SEE E. *method.*

Ei

***n*·ei·co·sa·no·ic ac·id** (ī'kō-să-nō'ik). SYN arachidic acid.

ei·co·sa·noids (ī'kō-să-noydz). The physiologically active substances derived from arachidonic acid, i.e., the prostaglandins, leukotrienes, and thromboxanes; synthesized via a cascade pathway. [G. *eicosa-*, twenty, + *eidos*, form]

9-ei·co·se·no·ic ac·id (ī'kō-sĕ-nō'ik). SYN gadoleic acid.

ei·det·ic (ī-det'ik). **1.** Relating to the power of visualization of and memory for objects previously seen which reaches its height in children aged 8 to 10. **2.** A person possessing this power to a high degree. [G. *eidon*, saw (aorist of verb)]

EIEC Abbreviation for enteroinvasive *Escherichia coli.*

Ei·ken·el·la cor·ro·dens (ī-kĕ-nel'ă kōr-rō'denz). A species of nonmotile, rod-shaped, Gram-negative, facultatively anaerobic bacteria that characteristically pits the agar under its colonies; it is part of the normal flora of the adult human oral cavity but may be an opportunistic pathogen, in pure or mixed culture especially in immunocompromised hosts. [M. *Eiken*, 1958]

ei·ko·nom·e·ter (ī-kō-nom'ĕ-ter). **1.** An instrument for determining the magnifying power of a microscope, or the size of a microscopic object. **2.** An instrument for determining the degree of aniseikonia. [G. *eikon*, image, + *metron*, measure]

ei·loid (ī'loyd). Resembling a coil or roll. [G. *eilō*, to roll up, + *eidos*, appearance]

Eimer, Gustav Heinrich Theodor, German zoologist, 1843–1898.

Ei·me·ri·i·dae (ī-mēr-ī'i-dē). A family of sporozoan coccidia; important genera are *Eimeria* and *Isospora*, infections by *Eimeria* being by far the most common and most serious in domesticated animals. [see *Eimeria*]

Einarson gal·lo·cy·a·nin-chrome al·um stain. See under stain.

ein·stein (īn'stīn). A unit of energy equal to 1 mol quantum, hence to 6.0221367×10^{23} quanta. The value of e., in kJ, is dependent upon the wavelength. [A. *Einstein*, German-born U.S. theoretical physicist and Nobel laureate, 1879–1955]

ein·stein·i·um (Es) (īn-stīn'ē-ŭm). An artificially prepared transuranium element, atomic no. 99, atomic wt. 252.0; it has many isotopes, all of which are radioactive (^{252}Es has the longest known half-life, 1.29 years).

Einthoven, Willem, Dutch physiologist and Nobel laureate, 1860–1927. SEE E. *equation, law*, string *galvanometer, triangle.*

Eisenlohr, Carl, German physician, 1847–1896.

Eisenmenger, Victor, German physician, 1864–1932. SEE E. *complex, defect, disease, syndrome, tetralogy.*

ei·sod·ic (ī-sod'ik). Rarely used term for afferent. [G. *eis*, into, + *hodos*, a way]

ejac·u·late (ē-jak'ū-lāt). **1.** To expel suddenly. **2.** Semen expelled in ejaculation. [see ejaculation]

ejac·u·la·tion (ē-jak-ū-lā'shŭn). The process that results in propulsion of semen from the genital ducts and urethra to the exterior; caused by the rhythmic contractions of the muscles surrounding the internal genital organs and the ischiocavernous and bulbocavernous muscles, resulting in an increase in pressure on the semen in the internal genital glands and the internal urethra. [L. *e-iaculo*, pp. *-atus*, to shoot out]

premature e., during sexual intercourse, too rapid achievement of climax and e. in the male relative to his own or his partner's wishes.

retrograde e., delivery of semen ejaculate into the bladder; seen in neurologic disease, diabetes, and occasionally after prostate surgery.

ejac·u·la·to·ry (ē-jak'ū-lă-tōr-ē). Relating to an ejaculation.

ejec·ta (ē-jek'tă). SYN ejection (2). [L. ntr. pl. of *ejectus*, pp. of *ejicio*, to throw out]

ejec·tion (ē-jek'shŭn). **1.** The act of driving or throwing out by physical force from within. **2.** That which is ejected. SYN ejecta. [L. *ejectio*, from *ejicio*, to cast out]

ejec·tor (ē-jek'tŏr, -tōr). A device used for forcibly expelling (ejecting) a substance.

saliva e., a hollow, perforated suction tube used in the evacuation

of saliva or liquid debris from the oral cavity. SYN dental pump, saliva pump.

EJP Abbreviation for excitatory junction *potential.*

Ejrup, Erick, 20th century Swedish internist. SEE E. *maneuver.*

⌂eka-. Prefix used to denote an undiscovered or just discovered element in the periodic system before a proper and official name is assigned by authorities; e.g., eka-osmium, now plutonium. [Sanskrit *eka*, one]

Ekbom, Karl A., Swedish neurologist, *1907. SEE E. *syndrome.*

EKG Abbreviation for electrocardiogram.

eki·ri (ē-kī'rī). An acute, toxic form of dysentery of infants seen in Japan and due to *Shigella sonnei*. [Jap.]

EKY Abbreviation for electrokymogram.

elab·o·ra·tion (ē-lab'ōr-ā'shŭn). The process of working out in detail by labor and study. [L. *e-laborō*, pp. *-atus*, to labor, endeavor, fr. *labor*, toil, to work out]

secondary e., the mental process occurring partly during dreaming and partly during the recalling or telling of a dream by means of which the latent (relatively disorganized and psychologically painful) content of the dream is brought into increasingly more coherent and logical order, resulting in the manifest content of the dream; an aspect of dream work.

Elae·oph·o·ra schnei·deri (ē-lē-of'ō-ră schnī'der-ī). The bloodworm of sheep; a species of nematodes causing filarial dermatosis. [Mod. L. *elaea*, fr. G. *elaia*, olive, + *agnos*, sheep, + *phoros*, to bear]

el·a·id·ic ac·id (el-ā-id'ik). An unsaturated monobasic *trans*-isomer of oleic acid; found in ruminant fats. Cf. oleic acid.

elai·o·path·ia (el'ā-ō-path'ē-ă). SYN eleopathy. [G. *elaion*, oil, + *pathos*, suffering]

E-LAM Abbreviation for endothelial-leukocyte adhesion *molecule.*

el·a·pid (el'ă-pid). Any member of the snake family Elapidae.

Elap·i·dae (ē-lap'i-dē). A family of highly venomous snakes characterized by a pair of comparatively short, permanently erect deeply grooved fangs at the front of the mouth. There are over 150 species, including the cobra, krait, mamba, and coral snakes. [G. *elops*, a serpent]

elas·tance (ē-las'tans). A measure of the tendency of a structure to return to its original form after removal of a deforming force. In medicine and physiology, usually a measure of the tendency of a hollow viscus (e.g., lung, urinary bladder, gallbladder) to recoil toward its original dimensions upon removal of a distending or compressing force, the recoil pressure resulting from a unit distention or compression of the viscus; the reciprocal of compliance. The relationship between elasticity and e. is of the same nature as that between the specific inductive capacity of an insulator material and the capacitance of a particular condenser made from that material.

elas·tase (ĕ-las'tās). A serine proteinase hydrolyzing elastin; other e.-like enzymes have been identified (e.g., pancreatic e. [pancreatopeptidase E] and leukocyte e. [lysosomal or neutrophil e.]) with different sequences and kinetic parameters; all have fairly broad specificities.

elas·tic (ĕ-las'tik). **1.** Having the property of returning to the original shape after being stretched, compressed, bent, or otherwise distorted. **2.** A rubber or plastic band used in orthodontics as either a primary or adjunctive source of force to move teeth. The term is generally modified by an adjective to describe the direction of the force or the location of the terminal connecting points. [G. *elastreō*, epic form of *elaunō*, drive, push]

intermaxillary e., material used to provide e. traction between the upper and lower teeth.

vertical e., e. material used in a direction perpendicular to the occlusal plane, connecting one arch wire to the other, and usually used to improve intercuspation.

elas·ti·ca (ĕ-las'ti-kă). **1.** The elastic layer in the wall of an artery. **2.** SYN elastic *tissue.*

elas·ti·cin (ĕ-las'ti-sin). SYN elastin.

elas·tic·i·ty (ĕ-las-tis'i-tē). The quality or condition of being elastic.

physical e. of muscle, the quality of muscle that enables it to yield to passive physical stretch.

physiologic e. of muscle, the biologic quality, unique for muscle, of being able to change and resume size under neuromuscular control.

total e. of muscle, the combined effect of physical and physiologic e. of muscle.

elas·tin (ĕ-las'tin). A yellow elastic fibrous mucoprotein that is the major connective tissue protein of elastic structures (e.g., large blood vessels, tendons, ligaments, etc.); e.'s precursor is proelastin. SYN elasticin.

elas·to·fi·bro·ma (ĕ-las'tō-fī-brō'mă). A nonencapsulated slow-growing mass of poorly cellular, collagenous, fibrous tissue and elastic tissue; occurs usually in subscapular adipose tissue of old persons. [G. *elastos,* beaten, + L. *fibra, -oma* tumor]

elas·toi·din (ĕ-las'toy-din). A complex collagen.

elas·tol·y·sis. Dissolution of elastic fibers. [elasto- + G. *lysis,* loosening, fr. *luō,* to loosen]

generalized e., SYN dermatochalasis.

elas·to·ma (ĕ-las-tō'mă). A tumorlike deposit of elastic tissue.

juvenile e., a connective tissue nevus characterized by an increase in the number and size of the elastic fibers. SEE ALSO osteodermatopoikilosis.

Miescher e., circinate groups of hyperkeratotic papules that become dislodged, leaving a small bloody depression; associated with pseudoxanthoma elasticum.

elas·tom·e·ter (ĕ-las-tom'ĕ-ter). A device for measuring the elasticity of any body or of the animal tissues.

elas·to·mu·cin (ĕ-las-tō-mū'kin). The mucoprotein of connective tissue; e.g., elastin.

elas·tor·rhex·is (ĕ-las-tō-rek'sis). Fragmentation of elastic tissue in which the normal wavy strands appear shredded and clumped, and take a basophilic stain. [G. *rhēxis,* rupture]

elas·to·sis (ĕ-las-tō'sis). **1.** Degenerative change in elastic tissue. **2.** Degeneration of collagen fibers, with altered staining properties resembling elastic tissue. SYN elastoid degeneration (1), elastotic degeneration.

e. colloida'lis conglomera'ta, SYN colloid milium.

e. dystroph'ica, SYN angioid *streaks,* under *streak.*

e. per'forans serpigino'sa, circinate groups of asymptomatic keratotic papules; the epidermis is thickened around a central plug of dermal elastic tissue which is extruded through the epidermis.

solar e., e. seen histologically in the sun-exposed skin of the elderly or in those who have chronic actinic damage.

ela·tion (ē-lā'shŭn). The feeling or expression of excitement or gaiety; if prolonged and inappropriate, a characteristic of mania. [L. *elatio,* fr. *ef-fero,* pp. *e-latus,* to lift up]

e·laun·in (ē-law'nin). A component of elastic fibers formed from a deposition of elastin between oxytalan fibers; found in the connective tissue of the dermis, particularly in association with sweat glands. [G. *elaunō,* to drive]

Elaut, Leon J.S., 20th century Belgian pathologist. SEE E. *triangle.*

el·bow (el'bō). **1.** The region of the upper limb between arm and forearm surrounding the elbow joint, especially posteriorly. **2.** The joint between the arm and the forearm. SYN cubitus (1) [TA], ancon. **3.** An angular body resembling a flexed e. [A.S. *elnboga*]

little league e., SYN Panner *disease.*

Little Leaguer's e., an epicondylitis of the medial epicondyle at the origin of the flexor muscles of the forearm; related to throwing and usually seen in children or adolescents.

miner's e., inflammation with fluid distention of the olecranon bursa.

nursemaid's e., subluxation of the radial head from the annular ligament. SYN Malgaigne luxation.

tennis e., chronic inflammation at the origin of the extensor muscles of the forearm from the lateral epicondyle of the humerus, as a result of unusual or repetitive strain (not necessarily from playing tennis). SYN epicondylalgia externa, lateral humeral epicondylitis.

el·bowed (el'bōd). Angular; kneed.

el·der, el·'der flow·ers. SYN sambucus.

electro-. Electric, electricity. [G. *ēlektron,* amber (on which static electricity can be generated by friction)]

elec·tro·an·al·ge·sia (ē-lek'trō-an-ăl-jē'zē-ă). Analgesia induced by the passage of an electric current.

elec·tro·a·nal·y·sis (ē-lek'trō-ă-nal'i-sis). Quantitative analysis of metals by electrolysis.

elec·tro·an·es·the·sia (ē-lek'trō-an-es-thē'zē-ă). Anesthesia produced by an electric current.

elec·tro·ax·on·og·ra·phy (ē-lek'trō-ak-son-og'ră-fē). SYN axonography.

elec·tro·bi·os·co·py (ē-lek'trō-bī-os'kŏ-pē). Rare term for use of electricity as a means of determining whether life is present or not. [electro- + G. *bios,* life, + *skopeō,* to examine]

elec·tro·car·di·o·gram (**ECG, EKG**) (ē-lek-trō-kar'dē-ō-gram). Graphic record of the heart's integrated action currents obtained with the electrocardiograph displayed as voltage changes over time. [electro- + G. *kardia,* heart, + *gramma,* a drawing]

concordant changes e., the presence of more than one waveform change, each in the same direction (polarity).

discordant changes e., the presence of more than one waveform change, each in a different direction (polarity).

scalar e. (skāl'ar), electrocardiographic lead output that can be displayed on one plane of the body in contradistinction to vector electrocardiogram in which the display is on two or more planes.

unipolar e., an e. taken with the exploring electrode placed on the chest overlying the heart or upon a single limb, the indifferent ("zero" potential) electrode being the central terminal.

elec·tro·car·di·o·graph (ē-lek-trō-kar'dē-ō-graf). An instrument for recording the potential of the electrical currents that traverse the heart.

elec·tro·car·di·og·ra·phy (ē-lek'trō-kar-dē-og'ră-fē). **1.** A method of recording electrical currents traversing the heart muscle. **2.** The study and interpretation of electrocardiograms.

fetal e., recording the electrocardiogram of the fetus *in utero.*

precordial e., recording of electrocardiographic signals from the anterior left chest; conventionally six electrode positions are used but any number may be applied.

elec·tro·car·di·o·pho·no·gram (ē-lek'trō-kar-dē-ō-fōn'ō-gram). The record obtained by electrocardiophonography.

elec·tro·car·di·o·pho·nog·ra·phy (ē-lek'trō-kar-dē-ō-fō-nog'ră-fē). Method of electrically recording the heart sounds. [electro- + G. *kardia,* heart, + *phōnē,* sound, + *graphō,* to write]

elec·tro·cau·ter·i·za·tion (ē-lek'trō-caw'ter-i-zā'shŭn). Cauterization by passage of high-frequency current through tissue or by a metal device that has been electrically heated.

elec·tro·cau·tery (ē-lek'trō-caw'ter-ē). **1.** An instrument for directing a high frequency current through a local area of tissue. **2.** A metal cauterizing instrument heated by an electric current. SYN electric cautery.

elec·tro·ce·re·bral in·ac·tiv·i·ty. SYN electrocerebral silence.

elec·tro·ce·re·bral si·lence (**ECS**) (ē-lek'trō-ser-ē'brăl sī'lens). Flat or isoelectric encephalogram; an electroencephalogram with absence of cerebral activity over 2 μv from symmetrically placed electrode pairs 10 or more centimeters apart, and with interelectrode resistance between 100 and 10,000 ohms; if such a record is present for 30 minutes in a clinically brain dead adult and if drug intoxication, hypothermia, and recent hypotension have been excluded, the diagnosis of cerebral death is supported. SYN electrocerebral inactivity, flat electroencephalogram, isoelectric electroencephalogram.

elec·tro·chem·i·cal (ē-lek'trō-kem'i-kăl). Denoting chemical reactions involving electricity, and the mechanisms involved.

elec·tro·co·ag·u·la·tion (ē-lek'trō-kō-ag-ū-lā'shŭn). Coagulation produced by an electrocautery.

elec·tro·co·chle·o·gram (ē-lek'trō-kok'lē-ō-gram). The record obtained by electrocochleography.

elec·tro·co·chle·og·ra·phy (ē-lek'trō-kok-lē-og'ră-fē). A measurement of the electrical potentials generated in the inner ear as a result of sound stimulation. [electro- + L. *cochlea,* snail shell, + G. *graphō,* to write]

elec·tro·con·trac·til·i·ty (ē-lek′trō-kon-trak-til′i-tē). The power of contraction of muscular tissue in response to an electrical stimulus.

elec·tro·con·vul·sive (ē-lek′trō-kon-vŭl′siv). Denoting a convulsive response to an electrical stimulus. SEE electroshock *therapy.*

elec·tro·cor·ti·co·gram (ē-lek-trō-kōr′ti-kō-gram). A record of electrical activity derived directly from the cerebral cortex.

elec·tro·cor·ti·cog·ra·phy (ECoG) (ē-lek′trō-kōr-ti-kog′ră-fē). The technique of recording the electrical activity of the cerebral cortex by means of electrodes placed directly on it.

elec·tro·cute (ē-lek′trō-kūt). To cause death by the passage of an electric current through the body. [electro- + execute]

elec·tro·cu·tion (ē-lek-trō-kū′shŭn). Death caused by electricity. SEE electrocute. SYN electrothanasia.

elec·tro·cys·tog·ra·phy (ē-lek′trō-sis-tog′ră-fē). Recording of electric currents or changes in electric potential from the urinary bladder.

elec·trode (ē-lek′trōd). **1.** Device to record one of the two extremities of an electric circuit; one of the two poles of an electric battery or of the end of the conductors connected thereto. **2.** An electrical terminal specialized for a particular electrochemical reaction. [electro- + G. *hodos,* way]

active e., a small e. whose exciting effect is used to stimulate or record potentials from a localized area. SYN exciting e., localizing e., therapeutic e.

calomel e., an e. in which the wire is connected through a pool of mercury to a paste of mercurous chloride (Hg_2Cl_2, calomel) in a potassium chloride solution covered by more potassium chloride solution; commonly used as a reference e.

carbon dioxide e., a glass e. in a film of bicarbonate solution covered by a thin plastic membrane permeable to carbon dioxide but impermeable to water and electrolytes; the carbon dioxide pressure of a gas or liquid sample quickly equilibrates through the membrane and is measured in terms of the resulting pH of the bicarbonate solution, as sensed by the glass e.; commonly used to analyze arterial blood samples for CO_2. SYN Severinghaus e.

central terminal e., in electrocardiography, an e. in which connections from the three limbs (right arm, left arm, and left leg) are joined and led to the electrocardiograph to form the indifferent e., theoretically at zero potential for the system.

Clark e., an oxygen e. consisting of the tip of a platinum wire exposed to a thin film of electrolyte covered by a plastic membrane permeable to oxygen but not to water or the electrolyte. When a certain voltage is applied, oxygen is destroyed at the platinum surface; the flow of current is then proportional to the rate at which oxygen can diffuse to the platinum surface from the gas or liquid sample outside the membrane and is thus a measure of the oxygen pressure in the sample; commonly used to measure oxygen pressure in arterial blood samples.

dispersing e., SYN indifferent e.

exciting e., SYN active e.

exploring e., an e. placed on or near an excitable tissue; in unipolar electrocardiography, the e. is placed on the chest in the region of the heart and paired with an indifferent electrode.

glass e., a thin-walled glass bulb containing a standard buffer solution, quinhydrone, and a platinum wire; when immersed in an unknown solution, a potential difference develops that varies with the pH of the unknown solution; this difference can be made to give the pH; used in pH meters.

hydrogen e., the ultimate standard of reference in all pH determinations, limited and technically difficult to use, consisting of a piece of spongy platinum black partly immersed in a solution in a small glass tube; the tube above the solution is filled with hydrogen gas that is bubbled through the solution and absorbed by the platinum; the electrode thus measures the potential between H_2 and H^+, the "standard" potential of which (1 atmosphere, 1 molar) is taken as zero; hence, the hydrogen e. potential measures $[H^+]$ or pH.

indifferent e., in unipolar electrocardiography, a remote e. placed either upon a single limb or connected with the central terminal and paired with an exploring e.; the indifferent e. is supposed to

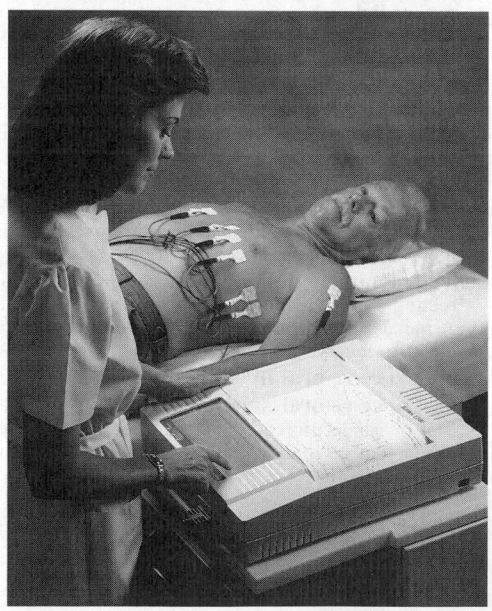

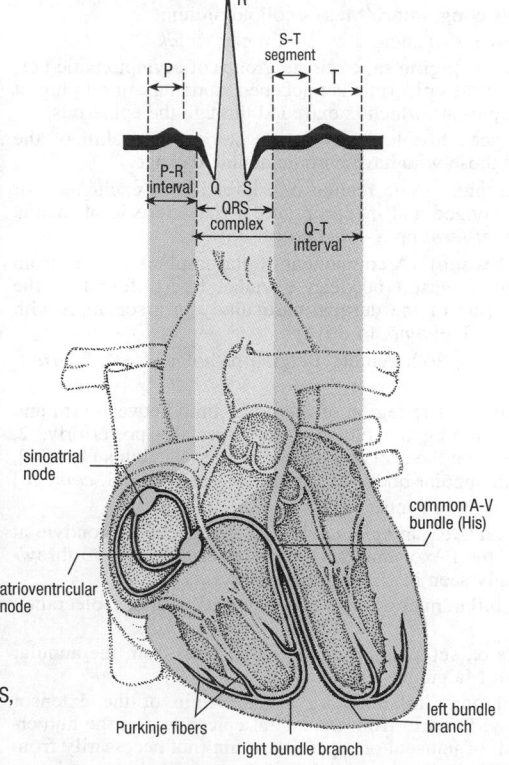

electrocardiography (ECG): (left) resting electrocardiogram; (right) an electrical picture of the heart is represented by positive and negative deflections on a graph labeled with the letters P, Q, R, S, and T, corresponding to the events of the cardiac cycle

R

P

S-T segment

T

P-R interval

Q S

QRS complex

Q-T interval

sinoatrial node

common A-V bundle (His)

atrioventricular node

left bundle branch

Purkinje fibers

right bundle branch

contribute little or nothing to the resulting record. SYN dispersing e., silent e.

ion-selective e.'s, glass, liquid ion-exchange, or solid state e.'s used to measure electrolyte and calcium ion activity in biological fluids.

localizing e., SYN active e.

negative e., SYN cathode.

oxidation-reduction e., an e. capable of measuring oxidation-reduction potential. SEE quinhydrone e. SYN redox e.

oxygen e., an e., usually consisting of a platinum wire or dropping mercury, used to measure the dioxygen concentration in a solution.

positive e., SYN anode.

quinhydrone e., one of several oxidation-reduction e.'s in which the ratio of the two forms (quinone-quinhydrone), determined by the hydrogen ion concentration, sets up a potential that can be measured and converted to a pH value (fails above pH 8).

redox e., SYN oxidation-reduction e.

reference e., an e. expected to have a constant potential, such as a calomel e., and used with another e. to complete an electrical circuit through a solution; e.g., when a reference e. is used with a glass e. for pH measurement, changes in voltage between the two e.'s can be attributed to the effects of pH on the glass e. alone.

resectoscope e., a wire loop e. that allows removal of tissue as well as cautery of the raw surface; used in endometrial ablation.

rollerball e., a ball e. that rolls like a paint roller over surface tissue, cauterizing it; used in endometrial ablation.

Severinghaus e., SYN carbon dioxide e.

silent e., SYN indifferent e.

therapeutic e., SYN active e.

elec·tro·der·mal (ē-lek′trō-der′măl). Pertaining to electric properties of the skin, usually referring to altered resistance. [electro- + G. *derma,* skin]

elec·tro·des·ic·ca·tion (ē-lek′trō-des-i-kā′shŭn). Destruction of lesions or sealing off of blood vessels (usually of the skin, but also of available surfaces of mucous membrane) by monopolar high-frequency electric current. [electro- + L. *desicco,* to dry up]

elec·tro·di·ag·no·sis (ē-lek′trō-dī-ag-nō′sis). **1.** The use of electronic devices for diagnostic purposes. **2.** By convention, the studies performed in the EMG laboratory, i.e., nerve conduction studies and needle electrode examination (EMG proper). SYN electroneurography. **3.** Determination of the nature of a disease through observation of changes in electrical activity. SYN evoked electromyography.

elec·tro·di·al·y·sis (ē-lek′trō-dī-al′i-sis). In an electric field, the removal of ions from larger molecules and particles. Cf. electro-osmosis.

elec·tro·en·ceph·a·lo·gram (EEG) (ē-lek′trō-en-sef′ă-lō-gram). The record obtained by means of the electroencephalograph.

flat e., SYN electrocerebral silence.

isoelectric e., SYN electrocerebral silence.

elec·tro·en·ceph·a·lo·graph (ē-lek′trō-en-sef′ă-lō-graf). A system for recording the electric potentials of the brain derived from electrodes attached to the scalp. [electro- + G. *encephalon,* brain, + *graphō,* to write]

elec·tro·en·ceph·a·log·ra·phy (EEG) (ēlek′trō-en-sef′ă-log′ră-fē). Registration of the electrical potentials recorded by an electroencephalograph.

elec·tro·en·dos·mo·sis (ē-lek′trō-en-dos-mō′sis). Endosmosis produced by means of an electric field.

elec·tro·focus·ing (ē-lek′trō-fō-kus-ing). The process of separating macromolecules or small molecules via electrophoresis in a pH gradient.

elec·tro·gas·tro·gram (ē-lek′trō-gas′trō-gram). The record obtained with the electrogastrograph.

elec·tro·gas·tro·graph (ē-lek′trō-gas′trō-graf). An instrument used in electrogastrography. [electro- + G. *gastēr,* stomach, + *graphō,* to write]

elec·tro·gas·trog·ra·phy (ē-lek′trō-gas-trog′ră-fē). The recording of the electrical phenomena associated with gastric secretion and motility.

elec·tro·gram (ē-lek′trō-gram). **1.** Any record on paper or film made by an electrical event. **2.** In electrophysiology, a recording taken directly from the surface by unipolar or bipolar leads.

His bundle e. (HBE), an e. recorded from the His bundle, either in the experimental animal or in humans during electrophysiologic cardiac catheterization.

elec·tro·he·mo·sta·sis (ē-lek′trō-hē-mos′tă-sis, -hē-mō-stā′sis). Arrest of hemorrhage by means of an electrocautery. [electro- + G. *haima,* blood, + *stasis,* halt]

elec·tro·hys·ter·o·graph (ē-lek′trō-his′ter-ō-graf). Instrument that records uterine electrical activity. [electro- + G. *hystera,* womb, + *graphō,* to write]

elec·tro·im·mu·no·dif·fu·sion (ē-lek′trō-im′ū-nō-di-fū′zhŭn). An immunochemical method that combines electrophoretic separation with immunodiffusion by incorporating antibody into the support medium.

elec·tro·ky·mo·gram (EKY) (ē-lek-trō-kī′mō-gram). An obsolete technique for making a graphic record of the heart's movements produced by the electrokymograph.

elec·tro·ky·mo·graph (ē-lek-trō-kī′mō-graf). An obsolete apparatus for recording, from changes in the x-ray silhouette, the movements of the heart and great vessels; consists of a fluoroscope, x-ray tube, and a photomultiplier tube together with an electrocardiograph.

elec·trol·y·sis (ē-lek-trol′i-sis). **1.** Decomposition of a salt or other chemical compound by means of an electric current. **2.** Destruction of hair follicles by means of galvanic electricity. [electro- + G. *lysis,* dissolution]

elec·tro·lyte (ē-lek′trō-līt). **1.** Any compound that, in solution or in molten form, conducts electricity and is decomposed (electro-

el

				physiologic variations of potential		
type of wave	shape	frequency per sec.	amplitude in μV	in waking EEG		in sleeping EEG
				adult	child	all ages
beta		14–30	5–50	frontal and precentral prominent, in clusters	seldom prominent	beta-activity ("spindles") sign of light sleep
alpha		8–13	20–120	predominant activity	predominant activity, age 5 and above	not a sign of sleep
theta		4–7	20–100	constant, not prominent	predominant activity, from 18 mos. to 5 yrs.	normal sign of sleep
delta		0.5–3	5–250	not prominent	predominant activity until 18 mos.	concomitant sign of deep sleep
gamma	—	31–60	–10	laws governing predominance and localization not fully known		

electroencephalogram

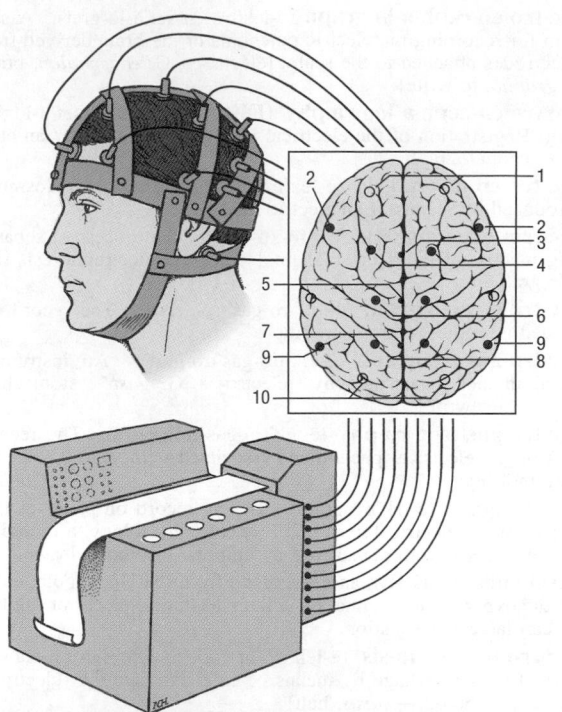

electroencephalography: insert shows leads used, (1) frontal, (2) temporal (front), (3) bregma, (4) precentral, (5) vertex, (6) central, (7) lambda, (8) parietal, (9) temporal (rear), (10) occipital

lyzed) by it. **2.** An ionizable substance in solution. [electro- + G. *lytos,* soluble]

amphoteric e., an e. that can either give up or take on a hydrogen ion and can thus behave as either an acid or a base. SYN ampholyte.

elec·tro·lyt·ic (ē-lek-trō-lit′ik). Referring to or caused by electrolysis.

elec·tro·lyze (ē-lek′trō-līz). To decompose chemically by means of an electric current.

elec·tro·lyz·er (ē-lek′trō-līz-er). An obsolete apparatus for the treatment of strictures, fibromas, etc., by electrolysis.

elec·tro·mag·net (ē-lek-trō-mag′net). A bar of soft iron rendered magnetic by an electric current encircling it.

elec·tro·mas·sage (ē-lek′trō-mas-sazh′). Massage combined with the application of electricity.

elec·tro·mic·tu·ra·tion (ē-lek′trō-mik-too-rā′shŭn). Electrical stimulation of the conus medullaris to empty the urinary bladder of paraplegics. [electro- + L. *micturio,* to desire to make water]

e·lec·tro·morph (ē-lek′trō-mōrf). A mutant form of a protein, phenotypically distinguished by its electrophoretic mobility. [electro- + G. *morphē,* form, shape]

elec·tro·mo·til·ity (ē-lek′trō-mō-til′ĭ-tē). The motility of the auditory outer hair cells in response to electrical stimulation.

elec·tro·my·o·gram (EMG) (ē-lek-trō-mī′ō-gram). A graphic representation of the electric currents associated with muscular action.

elec·tro·my·o·graph (ē-lek-trō-mī′ō-graf). An instrument for recording electrical currents generated in an active muscle.

elec·tro·my·og·ra·phy (ē-lek′trō-mī-og′ră-fē). **1.** The recording of electrical activity generated in muscle for diagnostic purposes; both surface and needle recording electrodes can be used, although characteristically the latter is employed, so that the procedure is also called needle electrode examination. **2.** Umbrella term for the entire electrodiagnostic study performed in the EMG laboratory, including not only the needle electrode examination, but

also the nerve conduction studies. [electro- + G. *mys,* muscle, + *graphō,* to write]

evoked e., SYN electrodiagnosis.

elec·tron (β−) (ē-lek′tron). One of the negatively charged subatomic particles that orbit the positive nucleus, in one of several energy levels called shells; in mass they are estimated to be 1/1836.15 of a proton; when emitted from inside the nucleus of a radioactive substance, e.'s are called β particles. A nucleus and its e.'s constitute an atom. SEE ALSO shell. [electro- + -on]

Auger e., an e. ejected from an orbital by photoelectric interaction with a photon emitted when another electron, in a higher energy orbital, passed from a higher to a lower energy level; the Auger e. recoils with energy equal to the characteristic radiation less the difference in shell binding energies. SEE photoelectric *effect,* transition e.

conversion e., an internal conversion e.

emission e., a beta particle resulting from radioactive decay.

internal conversion e., an e., similar to an Auger e., released from one of the e. orbits of the atom upon activation by a gamma ray from that atom's nucleus; the e. has kinetic energy equal to the net energy transition of the disintegration.

positive e., SYN positron.

transition e., an e. that moves from one energy level to another to fill a vacancy in a shell, with the emission of characteristic radiation.

valence e., one of the e.'s that take part in chemical reactions of an atom.

elec·tro·nar·co·sis (ē-lek′trō-nar-kō′sis). Production of insensibility to pain by the use of electrical current.

elec·tro·neg·a·tive (ē-lek-trō-neg′ă-tiv). **1.** Relating to or charged with negative electricity. **2.** Referring to an element whose uncharged atoms have a tendency to ionize by adding electrons, thus becoming anions (e.g., oxygen, fluorine, chlorine).

elec·tro·neu·rog·ra·phy (ē-lek′trō-noo-rog′ră-fē). SYN electrodiagnosis (2).

elec·tro·neu·rol·y·sis (ē-lek′trō-noo-rol′i-sis). Destruction of nerve tissue by electricity.

elec·tro·neu·ro·my·og·ra·phy (ē-lek′trō-noor′ō-mī-og′ră-fē). SEE electrodiagnosis (2).

elec·tron·ic (ē-lek-tron′ik). **1.** Pertaining to electrons. **2.** Denoting devices or systems utilizing the flow of electrons in a vacuum, gas, or semiconductor.

elec·tron-volt (eV, ev). The energy imparted to an electron by a potential of 1 V; equal to 1.60218×10^{-12} erg in the CGS system, or 1.60218×10^{-19} J in the SI system.

elec·tro·nys·tag·mog·ra·phy (ENG) (ē-lek′trō-nis′tag-mog′ră-fē). A method of nystagmography based on electrooculography; skin electrodes are placed at outer canthi to register horizontal nystagmus or above and below each eye for vertical nystagmus. [electro- + nystagmus + G. *graphō,* to write]

elec·tro·oc·u·lo·gram (ē-lek′trō-ok′ū-lō-gram). A record of electric currents in electro-oculography.

elec·tro·oc·u·log·ra·phy (EOG) (ē-lek′trō-ok′ū-log′ră-fē). Oculography in which electrodes placed on the skin adjacent to the eyes measure changes in standing potential between the front and back of the eyeball as the eyes move; a sensitive electrical test for detection of retinal pigment epithelium dysfunction.

elec·tro·ol·fac·to·gram (EOG) (ē-lek′trō-ol-fak′tō-gram). An electronegative wave of potential occurring on the surface of the olfactory epithelium in response to stimulation by an odor. SYN osmogram, Ottoson potential.

elec·tro·os·mo·sis (ē-lek′trō-os-mō′sis). The diffusion of a substance through a membrane in an electric field. Cf. electrodialysis.

elec·tro·para·cen·te·sis (ē-lek′tro-par′ă-sen-tē′sis). Removal of fluid, as from the eye, with an electrically activated instrument.

elec·tro·pher·o·gram (ē-lek-trō-fer′ō-gram). The densitometric or colorimetric pattern obtained from filter paper or similar porous strips on which substances have been separated by electrophoresis; may also refer to the strips themselves. SYN electropheretogram, ionogram, ionopherogram.

elec·tro·phil, elec·tro·phile (ē-lek′trō-fil, -fīl). **1.** The electron-

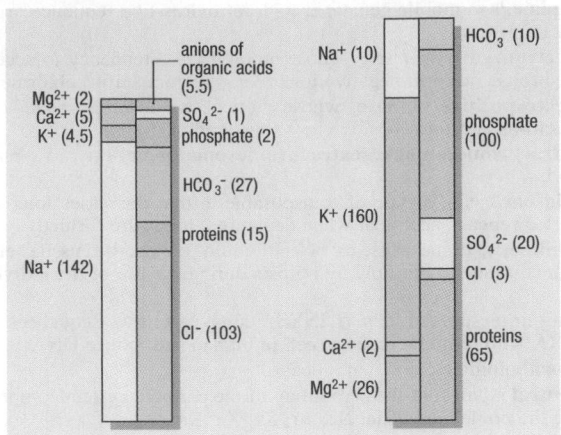

electropherogram: of blood plasma (left) and of intracellular fluid (right); concentration levels of ions are given in parentheses (in mmol/l)

attracting atom or agent in an organic reaction. Cf. nucleophil. **2.** Relating to an electrophil. SYN electrophilic. [electro- + G. *philos,* fond]

elec·tro·phil·ic (ē-lek-trō-fil′ik). SYN electrophil (2).

elec·tro·pho·bia (ē-lek-trō-fō′bē-ă). Morbid fear of electricity. [electro- + G. *phobos,* fear]

elec·tro·pho·re·sis (ē-lek-trō-fōr′e-sis). The movement of particles in an electric field toward an electric pole (anode or cathode); used to separate and purify biomolecules. SEE ALSO electropherogram. SYN dielectrolysis, ionophoresis, phoresis (1). [electro- + G. *phorēsis,* a carrying]

capillary zone e. (CZE), a method for separating molecules extremely rapidly based on their electrophoretic mobility.

carrier e., e. done on a carrier (such as paper, polyacrylamide gel, etc.).

disk e., a modification of gel e. in which a discontinuity (pH, gel pore size) is introduced near the origin to produce a lamina (disk) of the materials being separated; the separating bands retain their discoid shape as they move through the gel.

free e., e. of substances placed in a solution in a U-shaped tube.

gel e., e. through a gel, usually a cylindrical tube or on a slab consisting of a gel of uniform composition.

isoenzyme e., electrophoretic separation of serum enzymes; separation of lactate dehydrogenase and creatine phosphokinase is commonly used for diagnosis of acute myocardial infarction.

lipoprotein e., electrophoretic separation of plasma lipoproteins.

lipoprotein electrophoresis

S_f	D	ultracentrifuge (S_f) specific gravity (D)		electrophoresis
− 4 - 10^4	− 0.94			
		① chylomicrons		
− 400	− 0.98	VLDL (very low density lipoproteins)	②	pre-β lipoproteins
− 20	− 1.006	LDL (low density lipoproteins)	③	
− 0	− 1.063			β-lipoproteins
		HDL (high density lipoproteins)	④	α-lipoproteins
	− 1.210			

lipoprotein groups in normal blood; beta and pre-beta lipoproteins are reversed in electrophoretic separation (S_f = Svedberg unit = flotation unit)

polyacrylamide gel e. (PAGE), a gel formed by cross-linking of acrylamide that is used for the separation of proteins or nucleic acids. These substances are separated on the basis of both size and charge.

pulsed-field gel e., SYN pulse-field gel e.

pulse-field gel e., gel e. in which, after electrophoretic migration has begun, the current is briefly stopped and reapplied in a different orientation; allows for the purification of long DNA molecules. SYN pulsed-field gel e.

thin-layer e. (TLE), electrophoretic migrations (separations) through a thin layer of inert material, such as cellulose, supported on a glass or plastic plate.

elec·tro·pho·ret·ic (ē-lek′trō-phōr-et′ik). Relating to electrophoresis, as an e. separation. SYN ionophoretic.

elec·tro·pho·ret·o·gram (ē-lek′trō-fōr-et′ō-gram). SYN electropherogram.

elec·tro·phren·ic (ē-lek′trō-fren′ik). Denoting electrical stimulation of the phrenic nerve usually at its motor point in the neck. SEE ALSO electrophrenic *respiration.*

elec·tro·phys·i·ol·o·gy (ē-lek′trō-fiz-ē-ol′ō-jē). The branch of science concerned with electrical phenomena that are associated with physiologic processes. Electrical phenomena are prominent in neurons and effectors.

elec·tro·por·a·tion (ē-lek′trō-pōr-ā-shŭn). A technique in which a brief electric shock is applied to cells; momentary holes open briefly in the plasma membrane, allowing the entry of macromolecules (e.g., a way of introducing new DNA into a cell).

elec·tro·pos·i·tive (ē-lek′trō-pos′i-tiv). **1.** Relating to or charged with positive electricity. **2.** Referring to an element whose atoms tend to lose electrons; e.g., sodium, potassium, calcium.

elec·tro·punc·ture (ē-lek′trō-pŭnk′choor). Passage of an electrical current through needle electrodes piercing the tissues.

elec·tro·ra·di·ol·o·gy (ē-lek′trō-rā-dē-ol′ō-jē). Obsolete term for the use of electricity and x-ray in treatment.

elec·tro·ra·di·om·e·ter (ē-lek′trō-rā-dē-om′ĕ-ter). A modified electroscope designed for the differentiation of radiant energy. [electro- + L. *radius,* ray, + G. *metron,* measure]

elec·tro·ret·i·no·gram (ERG) (ē-lek′trō-ret′i-nō-gram). A record of the retinal action currents produced in the retina by an adequate light stimulus. [electro- + retina + G. *gramma,* something written]

elec·tro·ret·i·nog·ra·phy (ē-lek′trō-ret′i-nog′ră-fē). The recording and study of the retinal action currents.

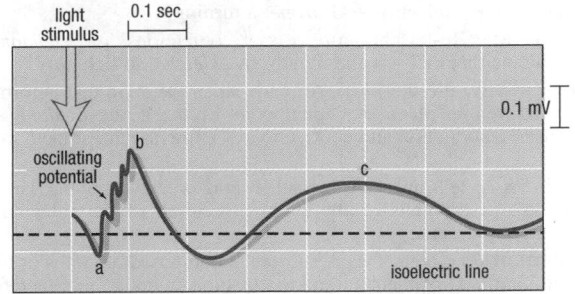

electroretinography: electroretinogram with a, b, and c waves

elec·tro·scis·sion (ē-lek′trō-si-shŭn). Division of tissues by means of an electrocautery knife. [electro- + L. *scissio,* a splitting, fr. *scindo,* to split]

elec·tro·scope (ē-lek′trō-skōp). An instrument for the detection of electrical charges or ionization of gas by beta or x-rays; consists of two strips of gold leaf suspended from an insulated conductor and enclosed in an airtight container viewed with a low-power microscope. [electro- + G. *skopeō,* to examine]

elec·tro·shock (ē-lek′trō-shok). SEE electroshock *therapy.*

elec·tro·sol (ē-lek′trō-sol). SYN colloidal *metal.*

elec·tro·spec·trog·ra·phy (ē-lek′trō-spek-trog′ră-fē). The recording, study, and interpretation of electroencephalographic wave patterns.

elec·tro·spi·no·gram (ē-lek-trō-spī′nō-gram). The record obtained by electrospinography.

elec·tro·spi·nog·ra·phy (ē-lek′trō-spī-nog′ră-fē). The recording of spontaneous electrical activity of the spinal cord.

elec·tro·ste·nol·y·sis (ē-lek′trō-stĕ-nol′ĭ-sis). The precipitation of metals in membrane pores in the course of electrolysis.

elec·tro·steth·o·graph (ē-lek′trō-steth′ō-graf). Electrical instrument that amplifies or records the respiratory and cardiac sounds of the chest. [electro- + G. *stēthos,* chest, + *graphō,* to record]

elec·tro·stric·tion (ē-lek-trō-strik′shŭn). **1.** The contraction in volume in a protein solution during proteolysis due to the formation of new charged groups. **2.** The reversible change in dimensions of a substance or material when an electric field is applied to it.

elec·tro·sur·gery (ē-lek-trō-ser′jer-ē). Division of tissues by high frequency current applied locally with a metal instrument or needle. SEE ALSO electrocautery. SYN electrotomy.

elec·tro·tax·is (ē-lek-trō-tak′sis). Reaction of plant or animal protoplasm to either an anode or a cathode. SEE ALSO tropism. SYN electrotropism, galvanotaxis, galvanotropism. [electro- + G. *taxis,* orderly arrangement]

negative e., e. by which an organism is attracted toward an anode or repelled from a cathode.

positive e., e. by which an organism is attracted toward a cathode or repelled from an anode.

elec·tro·tha·na·sia (ē-lek′trō-thă-nā′zē-ă). SYN electrocution. [electro- + G. *thanatos,* death]

elec·tro·ther·a·peu·tics, elec·tro·ther·a·py (ē-lek′trō-thār-ă-pū′tiks, -thār′ă-pē). Use of electricity in the treatment of disease.

elec·tro·therm (ē-lek′trō-therm). A flexible sheet of resistance coils used for applying heat to the surface of the body. [electro- + G. *thermē,* heat]

elec·tro·tome (ē-lek′trō-tōm). An electric scalpel.

elec·trot·o·my (ē-lek-trot′ō-mē). SYN electrosurgery. [electro- + G. *tomē,* incision]

elec·tro·ton·ic (ē-lek-trō-ton′ik). Relating to electrotonus.

elec·trot·o·nus (ē-lek-trot′ō-nŭs). Changes in excitability and conductivity in a nerve or muscle cell caused by the passage of a constant electric current. SEE ALSO catelectrotonus, anelectrotonus. SYN galvanotonus (1). [electro- + G. *tonos,* tension]

elec·trot·ro·pism (ē-lek-trot′rō-pizm, ē-lek-trō-trō′pizm). SYN electrotaxis. [electro- + G. *tropē,* a turning]

elec·tu·ar·y (ē-lek′choo-ā-rē). SYN confection. [G. *eleikton,* a medicine that melts in the mouth, fr. *ekleichō,* to lick up]

el·e·doi·sin (el-ĕ-doy′sin). An undecapeptide toxin that is formed in the venom gland of cephalopods of the genus *Eledone* and causes vasodilation and contraction of extravascular smooth muscle.

ele·i·din (ē-lē′ĭ-din). A refractile and weakly staining keratin present in the cells of the stratum lucidum of the palmar and plantar epidermis.

el·e·ment (el′ĕ-ment). **1.** A substance composed of atoms of only one kind, i.e., of identical atomic (proton) number, that therefore cannot be decomposed into two or more e.'s and that can lose its chemical properties only by union with some other e. or by a nuclear reaction changing the proton number. **2.** An indivisible structure or entity. **3.** A functional entity, frequently exogenous, within a bacterium, such as an extrachromosomal e. [L. *elementum,* a rudiment, beginning]

actinide e.'s, SYN actinides.

alkaline earth e.'s, those e.'s in the family Be, Mg, Ca, Sr, Ba, and Ra, the hydroxides of which are highly ionized and hence alkaline in water solution.

amphoteric e., an e., one or more of whose oxides unite with water to form hydroxides that may act as acids or as bases (e.g., aluminum).

anatomical e., any anatomical unit, such as a cell. SYN morphologic e.

copia e.'s, a mobile genetic e. with retrovirus-like sequence organization.

electronegative e., an e. whose atoms have a tendency to accept electrons and form negative ions (e.g., oxygen, sulfur, chlorine).

electropositive e., an e. whose atoms have a tendency to lose electrons and form positive ions (e.g., sodium).

extrachromosomal e., extrachromosomal genetic e., SYN plasmid.

fold-back e.'s, a type of transposable e. that possesses long inverted repeats, such that when denatured, loops are formed.

labile e.'s, tissue cells, as of epithelium, connective tissue, etc., that continue to multiply by mitosis during the life of the individual.

long interspersed e.'s (LINES), long repetitive sequences in DNA with terminal repeats seen in human and mouse DNA.

morphologic e., SYN anatomical e.

neutral e., an e. of the zero group of the periodic system comprising the noble gases, He, Ne, Ar, Kr, Xe, Rn.

noble e., SYN noble *metal.*

P e.'s, a class of transposable e.'s in Drosophila responsible for hybrid dysgenesis; utilized as tools for introducing genes into new locations in the genome.

picture e., SEE pixel.

rare earth e.'s, SYN lanthanides.

short interspersed e.'s (SINES), highly repetitive sequences of DNA of about 300 base pairs in length that occur about every 3000–5000 bp in the genome.

trace e.'s, e.'s present in minute amounts in the body, many of which are essential in metabolism or for the manufacture of essential compounds; e.g., Zn, Se, V, Ni, Mg, Mn. SYN microelements, microminerals.

transposable e., a DNA sequence that can move from one location in the genome to another; the transposition event can involve both recombination and replication, producing two copies of the moving piece of DNA; the insertion of these DNA fragments can disrupt the integrity of the target gene, possibly causing activation of dormant genes, deletions, inversions, and a variety of chromosomal aberrations. SEE ALSO transposon.

volume e., SEE voxel.

eleo-. Oil. SEE ALSO oleo-. [G. *elaion,* olive oil]

el·e·o·ma (el-ē-ō′mă). SYN lipogranuloma. [G. *elaion,* oil, + *-oma,* tumor]

el·e·om·e·ter (el-ē-om′ĕ-ter). SYN oleometer. [G. *elaion,* oil, + *metron,* measure]

el·e·op·a·thy (el-ē-op′ă-thē). A rare condition in which there is boggy swelling of the joints, said to be due to a fatty deposit following contusion; or possibly a condition resulting from the injection of paraffin oil as a form of malingering. SYN elaiopathia.

el·e·o·stear·ic ac·id (el-ē-ō-stē′ă-rik, -stēr′ik). An 18-carbon fatty acid with three double bonds (at carbons 9, 11, and 13); isomeric with linolenic acid; found in plant fats.

el·e·o·ther·a·py (el-ē-ō-thār′ă-pē). SYN oleotherapy. [G. *elaion,* oil]

el·e·phan·ti·a·sis (el-ĕ-fan-tī′ă-sis). Hypertrophy, edema, and fibrosis of the skin and subcutaneous tissue, especially of the lower extremities and genitalia with hydrocele, or enlargement of a limb, usually caused by long-standing obstructed lymphatic vessels, most commonly the result of years of infection by the filarial worm *Wuchereria bancrofti* or *Brugia malayi.* SEE ALSO filariasis. SYN elephant leg. [G. fr. *elephas,* elephant]

congenital e., congenital enlargement of one or more of the limbs or other parts, due to dilation of the lymphatics. See also entries under hereditary *lymphedema,* congenital type.

gingival e., a fibrous hyperplasia of the gingiva.

e. neuromato′sa, enlargement of a limb due to diffuse neurofibromatosis of the skin and subcutaneous tissue.

e. scro′ti, brawny swelling of the scrotum as a result of chronic lymphatic obstruction. SYN lymph scrotum, parasitic chylocele.

e. telangiecto′des, hypertrophy of the skin and subcutaneous tissues accompanied by and dependent upon dilation of the blood vessels.

e. vul′vae, SYN chronic hypertrophic *vulvitis.*

el·e·va·tion (el-ĕ-vā′shŭn) [TA]. SYN torus (1).

e. of levator palati, SYN *torus* levatorius.

tactile e.'s [TA], small areas in the skin of the palms and soles especially rich in sensory nerve endings. SYN toruli tactiles [TA].

el·e·va·tor (el′ĕ-vā-tĕr). **1.** An instrument for prying up a sunken part, as the depressed fragment of bone in fracture of the skull, or for elevating tissues from their attachment to bone. **2.** A surgical instrument used to luxate and remove teeth and roots that cannot be engaged by the beaks of forceps, or to loosen teeth and roots prior to forceps application. SYN dental lever. [L. fr. *e-levo,* pp. *-atus,* to lift up]

periosteal e., an instrument used for separating the periosteum from the bone. SYN rugine (1).

screw e., a dental instrument with a threaded extremity used for extracting the root of a broken tooth.

elim·i·nant (ē-lim′i-nant). **1.** An evacuant that promotes excretion or the removal of waste. **2.** An agent that increases excretion.

elim·i·na·tion (ē-lim-i-nā′shŭn). Expulsion; removal of waste material from the body; the getting rid of anything. [L. *elimino,* pp. *-atus,* to turn out of doors, fr. *limen,* threshold]

carbon dioxide e. ($\dot{V}_{CO2}$) ($\dot{V}_{CO_2}$), the rate at which carbon dioxide enters the alveolar gas from the blood, equal in the steady state to the metabolic production of carbon dioxide by tissue metabolism throughout the body; units: ml/min STPD or mmol/min.

elin·gua·tion (ē-ling-gwā′shŭn). SYN glossectomy. [L. *e,* out, + *lingua,* tongue]

el·i·nin (el′i-nin). A lipoprotein fraction of red blood cells that contains the Rh and A and B factors.

ELISA Abbreviation for enzyme-linked immunosorbent *assay.*

elix·ir (ē-lik′ser). A clear, sweetened, hydroalcoholic liquid intended for oral use; e.'s contain flavoring substances and are used either as vehicles or for the therapeutic effect of the active medicinal agents. [Mediev. L., fr. Ar. *al- iksir,* the philosopher's stone]

phenobarbital e., a palatable, colored hydroalcoholic (12–15% alcohol) mixture containing 20 mg of phenobarbital per 5 ml (teaspoonful); useful in administering the drug to children or persons who have difficulty swallowing tablets; used as an anticonvulsant and sedative.

Ellik, Milo, U.S. urologist, *1905. SEE E. *evacuator.*

Elliot, John W., U.S. surgeon, 1852–1925. SEE E. *position.*

Elliot, Robert Henry, British ophthalmologist, 1864–1936. SEE E. *operation.*

Elliott, Thomas R., British physician, 1877–1961. SEE E. *law.*

el·lip·sis (ē-lip′sis). Omission of words or ideas, leaving the whole to be completed by the reader or listener. [G. *ek-,* out, + *leipsis,* leaving]

el·lip·soid (ē-lip′soyd). **1.** A spherical or spindle-shaped condensation of phagocytic macrophages in a reticular stroma investing the wall of the splenic arterial capillaries shortly before they release their blood in the cords of red pulp. **2.** The outer end of the inner segment of the retinal rods and cones. **3.** Having the shape of an ellipse or oval. SYN sheath of Schweigger-Seidel. [G. *ellips,* oval, + *eidos,* form]

el·lip·to·cy·to·sis (ē-lip′tō-sī-tō′sis). A hematologic disorder in which 50–90% of the red blood cells consist of rod forms and elliptocytes; often associated with a hemolytic anemia. There are several autosomal dominant forms [MIM*130500, MIM*130600, and MIM*179650], with one form linked to the Rh blood group, caused by mutation in the gene encoding erythrocyte membrane protein band 4.1 (EPB41) on chromosome 1p, while the unlinked form is due to mutation either in the alpha-spectrin gene on 1q, or in the beta-spectrin gene on 14q or the band 3 gene on 17q. There is one autosomal recessive form [MIM*225450] known. SYN ovalocytosis.

Ellis, Richard W.B., English physician, 1902–1966. SEE E.-van Creveld *syndrome.*

Ellison, Edwin H., U.S. physician, 1918–1970. SEE Zollinger-E. *syndrome, tumor.*

Ellsworth, Read McLane, U.S. physician, 1899–1970. SEE E.-Howard *test.*

Eloesser, Leo, U.S. thoracic surgeon, 1881–1976. SEE Eloesser *flap;* E. *procedure.*

elon·ga·tion (ē-lon-gā′shŭn). **1.** The increase in the gauge length measured after fracture in tension within the gauge length, expressed in percentage of original gauge length. **2.** The lengthening of a macromolecule; e.g., in the synthesis of long-chain fatty acids or in the synthesis of a protein.

Elschnig, Anton, German ophthalmologist, 1863–1939. SEE E. *pearls,* under *pearl,* *spots,* under *spot;* Koerber-Salus-E. *syndrome.*

el·u·ant (el′ū-ant). The material that has been eluted.

el·u·ate (el′ū-āt). The solution emerging from a column or paper in chromatography. SEE ALSO elution.

el·u·ent (el′ū-ent). The mobile phase in chromatography. SEE ALSO elution. SYN developer (2), elutant.

elu·tant (ē-loo′tant). SYN eluent.

elute (ē-loot′). To perform or accomplish an elution. SYN elutriate.

elu·tion (ē-loo′shŭn). **1.** The separation, by washing, of one solid from another. **2.** The removal, by means of a suitable solvent, of one material from another that is insoluble in that solvent, as in column chromatography. **3.** The removal of antibodies absorbed onto the erythrocyte surface. SYN elutriation. [L. *e-luo,* pp. *lutus,* to wash out]

gradient e., e. in column chromatography in which a changing pH or ionic strength is used to separate substances.

elu·tri·ate (ē-loo′trē-āt). SYN elute.

elu·tri·a·tion (ē-loo-trē-ā′shŭn). SYN elution. [L. *elutrio,* pp. *-atus,* to wash out, decant, fr. *e-luo,* to wash out]

elytro-. The vagina. SEE ALSO colpo-, vagino-. [G. *elytron,* sheath (vagina)]

em-. SEE en-.

EMA Abbreviation for epithelial membrane *antigen.*

ema·ci·a·tion (ē-mā-sē-ā′shŭn). Becoming abnormally thin from extreme loss of flesh. SYN wasting (1). [L. *e-macio,* pp. *-atus,* to make thin]

emac·u·la·tion (ē-mak-ū-lā′shŭn). Removal of spots or other blemishes from the skin. [L. *emaculo,* pp. *-atus,* to clear from spots, fr. *e-,* out, + *macula,* spot]

em·a·na·tion (em-ă-nā′shŭn). **1.** Any substance that flows out or is emitted from a source or origin. **2.** The radiation from a radioactive element. [L. *e- mano,* pp. *-atus,* to flow out]

actinium e., radon-219. SEE emanon.

radium e., radon-222. SEE emanon.

thorium e., radon-220. SEE emanon.

em·a·na·tor·i·um (em′ă-nā-tōr′ē-ŭm). An institution where, formerly, radiation treatment now considered dangerous (using radioactive waters and the inhalation of radium emanations) was administered.

eman·ci·pa·tion (ē-man-si-pā′shŭn). In embryology, delimitation of a specific area in an organ-forming field, giving definite shape and limits to the organ primordium.

em·a·non (em′ă-non). Obsolete term once used to denote all radon isotopes collectively, when the term radon was restricted to the isotope radon-222, the naturally occurring intermediate of the uranium-238 radioactive series; so called because original names for radon-219, radon-220, and radon-222 were, respectively, "actinium emanation," "thorium emanation," and "radium emanation." [L. *emano,* to flow out + *-on*]

em·a·no·ther·a·py (em′ă-nō-thār′ă-pē). An obsolete treatment of various diseases by means of radium emanation (radon), or other emanation.

emar·gi·nate (ē-mar′ji-nāt). Nicked; with broken margin. SYN notched. [L. *emargino,* to deprive of its edge, fr. *e-* priv. + *margo* (*margin-*), edge]

emar·gi·na·tion (ē-mar′ji-nā′shŭn). SYN notch.

emas·cu·la·tion (ē-mas-kū-lā′shŭn). Castration of the male by removal of the testes and/or penis. SYN eviration (1). [L. *emasculo,* pp. *-atus,* to castrate, fr. *e-* priv. + *masculus,* masculine]

EMB Abbreviation for eosin-methylene blue. SEE eosin-methylene blue *agar.*

EM

Em·ba·dom·o·nas (em-bă-dom′ō-nas, em′bă-dō-mō′nas). Old name for *Retortamonas*. [G. *embadon*, surface, + *monas*, unit, monad]

em·balm (em-bahlm′). To treat a dead body with balsams or other chemicals to preserve it from decay. [L. *in*, in, + *balsamum*, balsam]

Embden, Gustav G., German biochemist, 1874–1933. SEE E. *ester;* Robison-E. *ester;* E.-Meyerhof *pathway;* E.-Meyerhof-Parnas *pathway*.

em·bed (em-bed′). To surround a pathological or histological specimen with a firm and sometimes hard medium such as paraffin, wax, celloidin, or a resin, in order to make possible the cutting of thin sections for microscopic examination. SYN imbed.

em·be·lin (em′bě-lin). The active principle from the dried fruit of *Embelia ribes* and *E. robusta* (family Myrsinaceae); has been used as a teniacide.

em·boite·ment (awm-bwaht-mawn′). SYN preformation *theory*. [Fr., encasement]

em·bo·le (em′bō-lē). **1.** Reduction of a limb dislocation. SYN embolia. **2.** Formation of the gastrula by invagination. SYN emboly. [G. *embolē*, insertion]

em·bo·lec·to·my (em-bō-lek′tō-mē). Removal of an embolus. [G. *embolos*, a plug (embolus), + *ektomē*, excision]

em·bo·le·mia (em-bō-lē′mē-ă). The presence of emboli in the circulating blood. [G. *embolos*, a plug (embolus), + *haima*, blood]

em·bo·li (em′bō-lī). Plural of embolus.

em·bo·lia (em-bō′lē-ă). SYN embole (1).

em·bol·ic (em-bol′ik). Relating to an embolus or to embolism.

em·bol·i·form (em-bol′i-fōrm). Shaped like an embolus. [G. *embolos*, plug (embolus), + L. *forma*, form]

⬛ **em·bo·lism** (em′bō-lizm). Obstruction or occlusion of a vessel by an embolus. [G. *embolisma*, a piece or patch; lit. something thrust in]

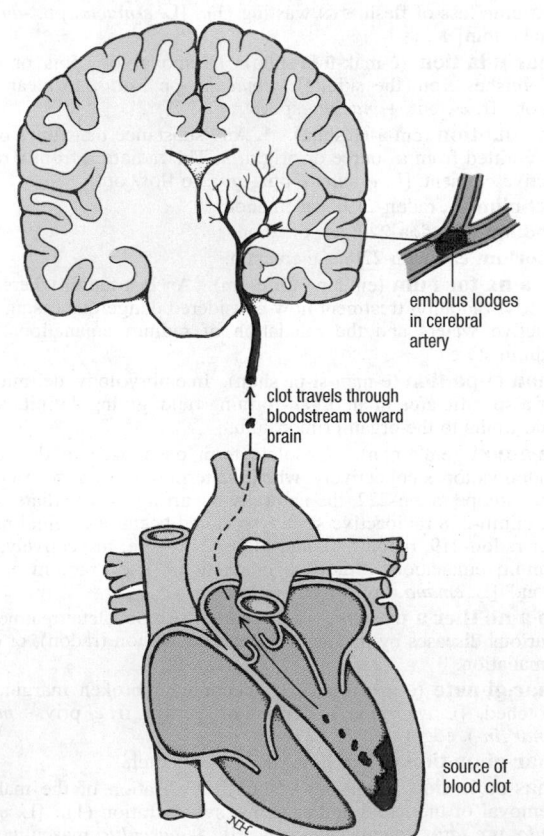

embolus lodges in cerebral artery

clot travels through bloodstream toward brain

source of blood clot

embolism

air e., an e. caused by air bubbles in the vascular system; venous air e. can result from air introduced via intravenous lines, especially central lines, and generally must be substantial to block pulmonary blood flow and cause symptoms; arterial air e. is also usually iatrogenic, caused by cardiopulmonary *bypass* or other intravascular interventions, rarely after penetrating lung injury; small amounts of arterial air can cause death by blockage of coronary and/or cerebral arteries; small bubbles introduced into the venous system may similarly cause symptoms if they reach the arterial side. Cf. paradoxical e. SYN gas e.

amnionic fluid e., obstruction and constriction of pulmonary blood vessels by amniotic fluid entering the maternal circulation, causing obstetric shock. SEE ALSO amnionic fluid *syndrome*.

atheromatous e., SYN cholesterol e.

bland e., e. by simple nonseptic material.

bone marrow e., obstruction of a vessel by bone marrow, usually following fracture of a bone.

cellular e., e. due to a mass of cells transported from disintegrating tissue.

cholesterol e., e. of lipid debris from an ulcerated atheromatous deposit, generally from a large artery to small arterial branches; it is usually small and rarely causes infarction. SYN atheromatous e.

cotton-fiber e., e. by cotton fibers from sterile gauze used in intravenous medication or transfusion; may form as foreign body granulomas in small pulmonary arteries.

crossed e., SYN paradoxical e.

direct e., e. occurring in the direction of the blood current.

fat e., the occurrence of fat globules in the circulation following fractures of a long bone, in burns, in parturition, and in association with fatty degeneration of the liver; the emboli most commonly block pulmonary or cerebral vessels when symptoms referable to either or both of these regions appear. SYN oil e.

gas e., SYN air e.

hematogenous e., e. occurring via a blood vessel.

infective e., SYN pyemic e.

lymph e., lymphogenous e., e. occurring in a lymphatic vessel.

miliary e., e. occurring simultaneously in a number of capillaries. SYN multiple e. (1).

multiple e., (1) SYN miliary e; **(2)** e. caused by the arrest of a number of small emboli.

obturating e., complete closing of the lumen of a vessel by an embolism.

oil e., SYN fat e.

paradoxical e., (1) obstruction of a systemic artery by an embolus originating in the venous system which passes through a septal defect, patent foramen ovale, or other shunt to the arterial system; **(2)** obstruction by a minute embolism that passes through the pulmonary capillaries from the venous to the arterial system. SYN crossed e.

pulmonary e., e. of pulmonary arteries, most frequently by detached fragments of thrombus from a leg or pelvic vein, commonly when thrombosis has followed an operation or confinement to bed.

pyemic e., plugging of an artery by an embolus detached from a suppurating source. SYN infective e.

retinal e., e. of an artery of the retina.

retrograde e., e. of a vein by an embolus carried in a direction opposite to that of the normal blood current, after being diverted into a smaller vein. SYN venous e.

riding e., SYN straddling e.

saddle e., a straddling e. at any vascular bifurcation, e.g., of the aorta which occludes both common iliac arteries.

straddling e., e. occurring at the bifurcation of an artery and blocking more or less completely both branches. SYN riding e.

tumor e., e. by neoplastic tissue transported from a tumor site and which may grow as a metastasis.

venous e., SYN retrograde e.

em·bo·li·za·tion (em′bol-i-zā′shŭn). **1.** The formation and release of an embolus into the circulation. **2.** Therapeutic introduction of various substances into the circulation to occlude vessels, either to arrest or prevent hemorrhaging, to devitalize a structure, tumor, or organ by occluding its blood supply, or to reduce blood flow to an arteriovenous malformation.

em·bo·lo·my·cot·ic (em′bō-lō-mī-kot′ik). Relating to or caused by an infective embolus. [G. *embolos,* a plug (embolus), + *mykēs,* fungus]

em·bo·lo·ther·a·py (em-bō-lō-thăr′ă-pē). Occlusion of arteries by insertion of blood clots, Gelfoam, coils, balloons, etc., with an angiographic catheter; used for control of inoperable hemorrhage or preoperative management of highly vascular neoplasms. [G. *embolos,* plug, + *therapeia,* medical treatment]

em·bo·lus, pl. **em·bo·li** (em′bō-lŭs, -lī). **1.** A plug, composed of a detached thrombus or vegetation, mass of bacteria, or other foreign body, occluding a vessel. **2.** SYN emboliform *nucleus.* [G. *embolos,* a plug, wedge or stopper]

catheter e., coiled worm-shaped platelet and fibrin aggregates produced during vascular catheterization, originating on the catheter or its guide wire; embolization of the catheter itself.

em·bo·ly (em′bō-lē). SYN embole (2).

em·bouche·ment (ahm-boosh-mon′). The opening of one blood vessel into another. [Fr.]

em·bra·sure (em-brā′shoor). In dentistry, an opening that widens outwardly or inwardly; specifically, that space adjacent to the interproximal contact area that spreads toward the facial, gingival, lingual, occlusal, or incisal aspect. [Fr. an opening in a wall for cannon]

buccal e., a space existing on the facial aspect of the interproximal contact area between adjacent posterior teeth.

gingival e., a space existing cervical to the interproximal contact area between adjacent teeth.

incisal e., a space existing on the incisal aspect of the interproximal contact area between adjacent anterior teeth.

labial e., a space existing on the facial aspect of the interproximal contact area between adjacent anterior teeth.

lingual e., a space existing on the lingual aspect of the interproximal contact area between adjacent teeth.

occlusal e., a space existing on the occlusal aspect of the interproximal contact areas between adjacent posterior teeth.

em·bro·ca·tion (em-brō-kā′shŭn). Rarely used term for liniment or for the application of a liniment. [G. *embrochē,* a fomentation]

♻**embry-.** SEE embryo-.

🔲**em·bryo** (em′brē-ō). **1.** An organism in the early stages of development. **2.** In humans, the developing organism from conception until approximately the end of the second month; developmental stages from this time to birth are commonly designated as fetal. **3.** A primordial plant within a seed. [G. *embryon,* fr. *en,* in, + *bryō,* to be full, swell]

heterogametic e., a male e. with XY karyotype.

hexacanth e., the e. of tapeworms of the subclass Cestoda, such as *Taenia saginata,* characterized by three pairs of hooks used for penetration through the gut of an intermediate host. SYN oncosphere e.

homogametic e., a female e. with XX karyotype.

oncosphere e., SYN hexacanth e.

presomite e., an e. before the appearance of the first pair of somites, which are notable about 20–21 days after fertilization in humans.

previllous e., the e. of a placental mammal prior to the formation of chorionic villi.

♻**embryo-, embry-.** The embryo. [G. *embryon,* a young one]

em·bry·o·blast (em′brē-ō-blast). SYN inner cell *mass.* [embryo- + G. *blastos,* germ]

em·bry·o·car·dia (em′brē-ō-kar′dē-ă). A condition in which the cadence of the heart sounds resembles that of the fetus, the first and second sounds becoming alike and evenly spaced; a sign of serious myocardial disease. SYN pendulum rhythm, tic-tac rhythm, tic-tac sounds. [embryo- + G. *kardia,* heart]

em·bry·o·gen·e·sis (em′brē-ō-jen′ĕ-sis). That phase of prenatal development involved in establishment of the characteristic configuration of the embryonic body; in humans, e. is usually regarded as extending from the end of the second week, when the embryonic disk is formed, to the end of the eighth week, after

which the conceptus is usually spoken of as a fetus. [embryo- + G. *genesis,* origin]

em·bry·o·gen·ic, em·bry·o·ge·ne·tic (em-brē-ō-jen′ik, -jĕ-net′ik). Producing an embryo; relating to the formation of an embryo.

em·bry·og·e·ny (em-brē-oj′ĕ-nē). The origin and growth of the embryo.

em·bry·oid (em′brē-oyd). SYN embryonoid.

em·bry·ol·o·gist (em-brē-ol′ō-jist). One who specializes in embryology.

em·bry·ol·o·gy (em-brē-ol′ōjē). Science of the origin and development of the organism from fertilization of the ovum to the end of the eighth week. Sometimes used to include all stages of prenatal life. [embryo- + G. *logos,* study]

em·bry·o·ma (em-brē-ō′mă). SYN embryonal *tumor.*

em·bry·o·mor·phous (em′brē-ō-mōr′fŭs). **1.** Relating to the formation and structure of the embryo. **2.** Applied to structures or tissues in the body similar to those in the embryo, or embryonal rests. [embryo- + G. *morphē,* shape]

em·bry·o·nal (em′brē-ō′năl). Relating to an embryo. SYN embryonate (1).

em·bry·o·nate (em′brē-ō-nāt). **1.** SYN embryonal. **2.** Containing an embryo. **3.** Impregnated.

em·bry·on·ic (em-brē-on′ik). Of, pertaining to, or in the condition of an embryo.

em·bry·on·i·form (em-brē-on′i-fōrm). SYN embryonoid.

em·bry·on·i·za·tion (em′brē-on-i-zā′shŭn). Reversion of a cell or tissue to an embryonic form.

em·bry·o·noid (em′brē-ō-noyd). Resembling an embryo or a fetus. SYN embryoid, embryoniform. [embryo- + G. *eidos,* appearance]

em·bry·o·ny (em′brē-ō-nē). The forming of an embryo.

em·bry·op·a·thy (em-brē-op′ă-thē). A morbid condition in the embryo or fetus. SYN fetopathy. [embryo- + G. *pathos,* disease]

em·bry·o·phore (em′brē-ō-fōr). A membrane or wall around the hexacanth embryo of tapeworms, forming the inner portion of the eggshell. In the genus *Taenia,* the e. is exceptionally thick, with radial striations that form a highly protective structure; in the genus *Diphyllobothrium,* the e. is ciliated and enhances the aquatic life cycle of this and other pseudophyllid cestodes. SEE ALSO coracidium. [embryo- + G. *phoros,* bearing]

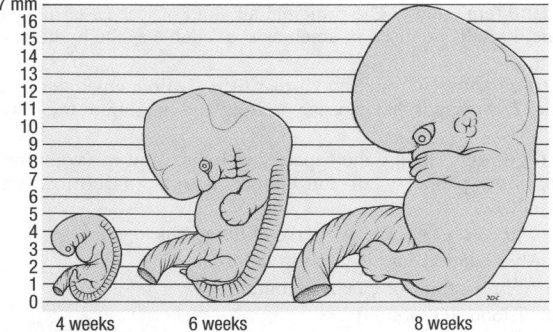

human embryos

em·bry·o·plas·tic (em-brē-ō-plas′tik). **1.** Producing an embryo. **2.** Relating to the formation of an embryo. [embryo- + G. *plassō,* to form]

em·bry·ot·o·my (em-brē-ot′ō-mē). Any mutilating operation on the fetus to make possible its removal when delivery is impossible by natural means. [embryo- + G. *tomē,* cutting]

em·bry·o·tox·ic·i·ty (em′brē-ō-tok-sis′i-tē). Injury to the embryo, which may result in death, growth retardation, or abnormal development of a part that may affect either its structure or function.

em·bry·o·tox·on (em′brē-ō-tok′son). Congenital opacity of the periphery of the cornea, a feature of osteogenesis imperfecta. [embryo- + G. *toxon,* bow]

anterior e., SYN *arcus* senilis.

posterior e., a common developmental abnormality marked by a prominent white ring of Schwalbe.

em·bry·o·troph (em′brē-ō-trōf). **1.** Nutritive material supplied to the embryo during development. Cf. hemotroph, histotroph. **2.** In the implantation stages of deciduate placental mammals, fluid adjacent to the blastodermic vesicle; a mixture of the secretion of the uterine glands, cellular debris resulting from the trophoblastic invasion of the endometrium, and exudated plasma. [embryo- + G. *trophē,* nourishment]

em·bry·o·tro·phic (em′brē-ō-trof′ik). Relating to any process or agency involved in the nourishment of the embryo.

em·bry·ot·ro·phy (em′brē-ot′rō-fē). The nutrition of the embryo. [embryo- + G. *trophē,* nourishment]

emed·ul·late (ē-med′ū-lāt). To extract any marrow. [L. *e-,* from, + *medulla,* marrow]

emei·o·cy·to·sis (ē′mē-ō-sī-tō′sis). SYN exocytosis (2). [L. *emitto,* to send forth, + G. *kytos,* cell, + *-osis,* condition]

emer·gence (ē-mer′jens). **1.** Recovery of normal function following a period of unconsciousness, especially that associated with a general anesthetic. **2.** SEE property e.

property e., properties in a complex system that are not present in the component parts, e.g., symmetry; i.e., in an ecologic hierarchy, populations have properties not expressed by an individual or a community.

emer·gen·cy (ē-mer′jen-sē). A patient's condition requiring immediate treatment. [L. *e-mergo,* pp. *-mersus,* to rise up, emerge, fr. *mergo,* to plunge into, dip]

emer·gent (ē-mer′jent). **1.** Arising suddenly and unexpectedly, calling for quick judgment and prompt action. **2.** Coming out; leaving a cavity or other part.

Emery, Alan E. H., Contemporary British physician. SEE E.-Dreifuss muscular *dystrophy.*

em·ery (em′er-ē). An abrasive containing aluminum oxide and iron. [O.Fr. *emeri,* fr. L.L. *smericulum,* fr. G. *smiris*]

em·e·sis (em′ĕ-sis). **1.** SYN vomiting. **2.** Combining form, used in the suffix position, for vomiting. [G. fr. *emeō,* to vomit]

emet·ic (ĕ-met′ik). **1.** Relating to or causing vomiting. **2.** An agent that causes vomiting, e.g., ipecac syrup. [G. *emetikos,* producing vomiting, fr. *emeō,* to vomit]

em·e·tine (em′ĕ-tēn). The principal alkaloid of ipecac, used as an emetic; its salts are used in amebiasis; available as the hydrochloride.

em·e·to·ca·thar·tic (em′ĕ-tō-kă-thar′tik). **1.** Both emetic and cathartic. **2.** An agent that causes vomiting and purging of the lower intestines.

eme·to·gen·ic. Having the capacity to induce emesis (vomiting), a common property of anticancer agents, narcotics, and amorphine.

e·me·to·ge·nic·i·ty. The property of being emetogenic.

EMF Abbreviation for electromotive *force.*

EMG Abbreviation for electromyogram.

△**-emia.** Blood. [G. *haima*]

emic·tion (ē-mik′shŭn). Rarely used term for urination.

em·i·gra·tion (em-i-grā′shŭn). The passage of white blood cells through the endothelium and wall of small blood vessels. [L. *e-migro,* pp. *-atus,* to emigrate]

EMINENCE

em·i·nence (em′i-nens) [TA]. A circumscribed area raised above the general level of the surrounding surface, particularly on a bone surface. SYN eminentia [TA]. [L. *eminentia*]

abducens e., SYN facial *colliculus.*

arcuate e. [TA], a prominence on the anterior surface of the petrous portion of the temporal bone indicating the position of the superior semicircular canal. SYN eminentia arcuata [TA].

articular e. of temporal bone, SYN articular *tubercle* of temporal bone.

canine e., an elevation on the maxilla corresponding to the socket of the canine tooth. SYN canine prominence.

collateral e. [TA], a longitudinal elevation of the floor of the collateral trigone of the lateral ventricle of the brain, between the hippocampus and the calcar avis, caused by the proximity of the floor of the collateral fissure. SYN eminentia collateralis [TA].

e. of concha [TA], the prominence on the cranial surface of the auricle corresponding to the concha. SYN eminentia conchae [TA], apophysis conchae.

cruciate e., SYN cruciform e.

cruciform e. [TA], bony cross-like elevation on the internal aspect of the squamous portion of the occipital bone formed by the intersection of the groove for the transverse sinuses and the internal occipital crest, with the internal occipital protuberance at the center of the "cross." SYN eminentia cruciformis [TA], cruciate e.

deltoid e., SYN deltoid *tuberosity* (of humerus).

Doyère e., the slightly elevated area of the striated muscle fiber's surface that corresponds to the site of the motor *endplate.*

facial e., SYN facial *colliculus.*

forebrain e., SYN frontonasal *prominence.*

frontal e., ✭official alternate term for frontal *tuber.*

genital e., in very young embryos, the vaguely outlined median elevation immediately cephalic to the proctodeum; its central part develops into the genital tubercle.

hypobranchial e., a median elevation in the floor of the embryonic pharynx caudal to the tuberculum impar; it merges laterally with the ventral part of the second and third branchial arches, and in later development is incorporated in the root of the tongue. SYN copula linguae, His copula.

hypoglossal e., SYN hypoglossal *trigone.*

hypothenar e. [TA], the fleshy mass at the medial side of the palm. SYN hypothenar (1) [TA], eminentia hypothena′ris✭, antithenar, hypothenar prominence.

ileocecal e., SYN ileal *papilla.*

iliopectineal e., SYN iliopubic e.

iliopubic e. [TA], a rounded elevation on the superior surface of the hip bone at the junction of the ilium and the superior ramus of the pubis. SYN eminentia iliopubica [TA], iliopectineal e.

intercondylar e. [TA], an elevation on the proximal extremity of the tibia between the two articular surfaces. SYN eminentia intercondylaris [TA], eminentia intercondyloidea, intercondyloid e., spinous process of tibia.

intercondyloid e., SYN intercondylar e.

maxillary e., SYN maxillary *tuberosity.*

medial e., term originally used to describe a longitudinal elevation of the rhomboid fossa extending throughout the length of the rhombencephalon and made up of named elevations such as the facial colliculus and the hypoglossal and vagal trigones; now used to describe only the medial elevation in the floor of fourth ventricle immediately rostral to the facial colliculus, the other elevations being separately named. SYN eminentia medialis, eminentia teres, funiculus teres, round e.

median e. [TA], the slightly prominent lower segment of the infundibulum of the hypothalamus, immediately proximal to the hypophysial stalk; the region is characterized by the capillary tufts of the infundibular arteries, from which the hypothalamohypophysial portal system of veins arises. SYN eminentia mediana.

olivary e., SYN oliva.

omental e. of pancreas [TA], a bulge on the anterior surface of the body of the pancreas to the left of the superior mesenteric vessels. SYN tuber omentale pancreatis [TA], omental tuber.

orbital e. of zygomatic bone, SYN orbital *tubercle* (of zygomatic bone).

parietal e., ✭official alternate term for parietal *tuber.*

pyramidal e., SYN *eminentia* pyramidalis.

radial e. of wrist, a rather large flat e. on the radial side of the palmar aspect of the wrist, due to the tuberosity of scaphoid and the ridge on the trapezium. SYN eminentia carpi radialis.

restiform e., SYN restiform *body.*

round e., SYN medial e.

e. of scapha [TA], the prominence on the cranial surface of the auricle corresponding to the scapha. SYN eminentia scaphae [TA].

thenar e. [TA], the fleshy mass on the lateral side of the palm; the radial palm; the ball of the thumb. SYN eminentia thena'ris✩, thenar prominence.

thyroid e., SYN laryngeal *prominence.*

e. of triangular fossa of auricle [TA], the prominence on the cranial surface of the auricle corresponding to the triangular fossa. SYN eminentia fossae triangularis auricularis [TA], agger perpendicularis, eminentia triangularis.

ulnar e. of wrist, an e. smaller than the radial, on the ulnar side of the palmar aspect of the wrist, due to presence of the pisiform bone. SYN eminentia carpi ulnaris.

---

em·i·nen·tia, pl. **em·i·nen·ti·ae** (em-i-nen'shē-ă, -shē-ē) [TA]. SYN eminence. [L. prominence, fr. *e-mineo,* to stand out, project]

e. abducen'tis, SYN facial *colliculus.*

e. arcua'ta [TA], SYN arcuate *eminence.*

e. articula'ris os'sis tempora'lis, SYN articular *tubercle* of temporal bone.

e. car'pi radia'lis, SYN radial *eminence* of wrist.

e. car'pi ulna'ris, SYN ulnar *eminence* of wrist.

e. collatera'lis [TA], SYN collateral *eminence.*

e. con'chae [TA], SYN *eminence* of concha.

e. crucifor'mis [TA], SYN cruciform *eminence.*

e. facia'lis, SYN facial *colliculus.*

e. fos'sae triangula'ris auricula'ris [TA], SYN *eminence* of triangular fossa of auricle.

e. fronta'lis, ✩official alternate term for frontal *tuber,* frontal *tuber.*

e. hypoglos'si, SYN hypoglossal *trigone.*

e. hypothena'ris, ✩official alternate term for hypothenar *eminence.*

e. iliopu'bica [TA], SYN iliopubic *eminence.*

e. intercondyla'ris [TA], SYN intercondylar *eminence.*

e. intercondyloid'ea, SYN intercondylar *eminence.*

e. maxil'lae, SYN maxillary *tuberosity,* maxillary *tuberosity.*

e. media'lis, SYN medial *eminence.*

e. media'na, SYN median *eminence.*

e. orbita'lis (os'sis zygoma'tici), SYN orbital *tubercle* (of zygomatic bone).

e. parieta'lis, ✩official alternate term for parietal *tuber.*

e. pyramida'lis [TA], a conical projection posterior to the vestibular window in the middle ear; it is hollow and contains the stapedius muscle. SYN pyramid of tympanum, pyramidal eminence, pyramis tympani.

e. restifor'mis, SYN restiform *body.*

e. sca'phae [TA], SYN *eminence* of scapha.

e. sym'physis, SYN mental *tubercle* (of mandible).

e. te'res, SYN medial *eminence.*

e. thena'ris, ✩official alternate term for thenar *eminence.*

e. triangula'ris, SYN *eminence* of triangular fossa of auricle.

va'gi e., SYN vagal (nerve) *trigone.*

em·i·o·cy·to·sis (ē'mē-ō-sī-tō'sis). SYN exocytosis (2). [L. *emitto,* to send forth, + G. *kytos,* cell, + *-osis,* condition]

em·is·sar·i·um (em-i-sā'rē-ŭm). SYN emissary *vein.* [L. an outlet, fr. *e-mitto,* pp. *-missus,* to send out]

e. condyloid'eum, SYN condylar emissary *vein.*

e. mastoid'eum, SYN mastoid emissary *vein.*

e. occipita'le, SYN occipital emissary *vein.*

e. parieta'le, SYN parietal emissary *vein.*

em·is·sary (em'i-sār-ē). **1.** Relating to, or providing an outlet or drain. **2.** SYN emissary *vein.* [see emissarium]

emis·sion (ē-mish'ŭn). A discharge; referring usually to a dis-

charge of the male internal genital organs into the internal urethra; the contents of the organs, including sperm cells, prostatic fluid, and seminal vesicle fluid, mix in the internal urethra with mucus from the bulbourethral glands to form semen. [L. *emissio,* fr. *e-mitto,* to send out]

characteristic e., SYN characteristic *radiation.*

continuous otoacoustic e., a form of evoked otoacoustic e. in which the e. is of the same frequency as the stimulus and persists as long as the stimulus.

distortion-product otoacoustic e., a form of evoked otoacoustic e. in which a third frequency is produced when two pure tones are used as the stimulus.

evoked otoacoustic e., a form resulting from acoustic stimulation, as opposed to spontaneous otoacoustic e.

otoacoustic e., sound emanating from the ear that can be recorded from minute microphones placed in the external auditory canal and is thought to be produced by the outer hair cells in the cochlea. Otoacoustic e.'s occur spontaneously and can be evoked by acoustic stimuli; they are more prominent in women than in men and are particularly robust in infants. Indicative of the integrity of the auditory hair cells, they are measured to screen newborns for hearing impairment.

transient evoked otoacoustic e., a form in which the response is limited in time.

emis·siv·i·ty (ē-mi-siv'i-tē). The giving off of heat rays; a perfect "black body" has an e. of 1, a highly polished metallic surface may have an e. as low as 0.02.

EMIT Abbreviation for enzyme-multiplied *immunoassay* technique.

Emmet, Thomas A., U.S. gynecologist, 1828–1919. SEE E. *needle, operation.*

em·me·tro·pia (em-ĕ-trō'pē-ă). The state of refraction of the eye in which parallel rays, when the eye is at rest, are focused exactly on the retina. [G. *emmetros,* according to measure, + *ōps,* eye]

em·me·tro·pic (em-ĕ-trop'ik). Pertaining to or characterized by emmetropia.

em·me·trop·i·za·tion (em'ĕ-trōp-i-zā'shŭn). The process by which the refraction of the anterior ocular segment and the axial length of the eye tend to balance each other to produce emmetropia.

Emmonsia.

E. parva var. *crescens,* the main fungal species causing adiaspiromycosis in animals and the only agent of human adiaspiromycosis; infection is acquired by inhaling conidia from the fungus growing in soil.

E. parva var. *parva,* a fungal species causing adiaspiromycosis in animals.

Em·mon·si·el·la cap·su·la·ta (e-mon-sī-el'ă kap-soo-lā'tă). SYN Ajellomyces capsulatum.

em·o·din (em'ō-din). A crystalline substance (cathartic) found in rhubarb, senna, cascara sagrada, and other purgative drugs. SYN archin, frangulic acid.

emol·lient (ē-mol'ē-ent). **1.** Soothing to the skin or mucous membrane. **2.** An agent that softens the skin or soothes irritation in the skin or mucous membrane. SYN malactic. [L. *emolliens,* pres. p. of *e- mollio, emollire,* to soften]

emo·tion (ē-mō'shŭn). A strong feeling, aroused mental state, or intense state of drive or unrest, which may be directed toward a definite object and is evidenced in both behavior and in psychologic changes, with accompanying autonomic nervous system manifestations. [L. *e-moveo,* pp. *-motus,* to move out, agitate]

emo·tion·al (ē-mō'shŭn-ăl). Relating to or marked by an emotion.

emo·ti·o·vas·cu·lar (ē-mō'shē-ō-vas'kū-ler). Relating to the vascular changes, such as pallor and blushing, caused by emotions of various kinds.

em·pasm, em·pas·ma (em'pazm, em-paz'mă). A dusting powder. [G. *empasma,* fr. *em-passo,* to sprinkle on]

em·path·ic (em-path'ik). Relating to or marked by empathy.

em·pa·thize (em'pă-thīz). To feel empathy in relation to another person; to put oneself in another's place.

em·pa·thy (em'pă-thē). **1.** The ability to intellectually and emo-

types of emphysema	
1. centrilobular/centriacinar emphysema	beginning near terminal bronchiole in center of lobule (also called proximal acinar emphysema)
2. panlobular/panacinar emphysema	affecting the entire lung from the periphery inward (also called generalized emphysema)
3. localized emphysema	one, or a very few, sites of alveolar destruction, surrounded by normal pulmonary architecture (also called bullous, distal acinar, or paraseptal emphysema)
4. perifocal emphysema	occurring in the vicinity of focal lesions or scarring (also called paracicatricial or irregular emphysema)

tionally sense the emotions, feelings, and reactions that another person is experiencing and to effectively communicate that understanding to the individual. Cf. sympathy (3). **2.** The anthropomorphization or humanizing of objects and the feeling of oneself as being in and part of them. [G. *en (em)*, in, + *pathos*, feeling]

generative e., the inner experience of sharing in and comprehending the momentary psychologic state of another person.

em·per·i·po·le·sis (em-pār′i-pō-lē′sis). Active penetration of one cell by another, which remains intact; observed in tissue cultures in which leukocytes have entered macrophages and subsequently left. [G. *en (em)*, inside, + *peri*, around, + *poleomai*, to wander about]

em·phrax·is (em-frak′sis). **1.** A clogging or obstruction of the mouth of the sweat gland. **2.** An impaction. [G. a stoppage]

em·phy·se·ma (em-fizē′mă). **1.** Presence of air in the interstices of the connective tissue of a part. **2.** A condition of the lung characterized by increase beyond the normal in the size of air spaces distal to the terminal bronchiole (those parts containing alveoli), with destructive changes in their walls and reduction in their number. Clinical manifestation is breathlessness on exertion, due to the combined effect (in varying degrees) of reduction of alveolar surface for gas exchange and collapse of smaller airways with trapping of alveolar gas in expiration; this causes the chest to be held in the position of inspiration ("barrel chest"), with prolonged expiration and increased residual volume. Symptoms of chronic bronchitis often, but not necessarily, coexist. Two structural varieties are panlobular (panacina) e. and centrilobular (centriacinar) e.; paracicatricial, paraseptal, and bullous e. are also common. SYN pulmonary e. [G. inflation of stomach, etc. fr. *en*, in, + *physēma*, a blowing, fr. *physa*, bellows]

alveolar duct e., e. in which the primary involvement is in the alveolar ducts and respiratory bronchioles, as opposed to panacinar e.

bullous e., e. in which the enlarged airspaces are 1 to several cm in diameter, often visible on chest radiographs. Thin-walled air sacs, under tension, compress pulmonary tissue, either single or multiple; sometimes amenable to surgical resection with improvement in pulmonary function.

centriacinar e., SYN centrilobular e.

centrilobular e., e. affecting the central portion of secondary pulmonary lobules, around the central bronchiole, typically involving the superior part of the lungs or lobes; may be related to inflammation of the bronchioles and to the effects of inhaled dust, which aggregates next to respiratory bronchioles; seen in coalworker's pneumoconiosis and (in mild form) asymptomatic city dwellers. SYN centriacinar e.

compensating e., compensatory e., increase in the air capacity of a portion of the lung when another portion is consolidated, shrunken, or unable to perform its respiratory function; the alveoli are distended, but there is no destruction of alveolar walls, and hence, no true e., as this term is now defined.

congenital lobar e., common cause of neonatal respiratory distress which usually involves the left upper lobe.

cutaneous e., SYN subcutaneous e.

diffuse obstructive e., the major component of chronic obstructive lung disease.

ectatic e., obstructive airway disease with areas of dilation of alveoli acini. Seen primarily in association with inherited deficiency of α-1-antitrypsin. SEE panlobular e.

familial e., e. inherited in association with severe α-1 antitrypsin deficiency. It may occur as an isolated feature [MIM*130700, 130710] or with *cutis* laxa and hemolytic *anemia* [MIM*235360].

gangrenous e., SYN gas *gangrene*.

generalized e., SYN panlobular e.

increased markings e., a term applied to mixed obstructive lung disease in which radiographic findings of emphysema coexist with nonvascular shadows, probably related to bronchial inflammation.

interlobular e., interstitial e. in the connective tissue septa between the pulmonary lobules.

interstitial e., (1) presence of air in the pulmonary tissues consequent upon rupture of the air cells; (2) presence of air or gas in the connective tissue.

intestinal e., SYN *pneumatosis* cystoides intestinalis.

irregular e., e. that shows no consistent relationship to any portion of the acinus; always associated with fibrosis.

mediastinal e., SYN pneumomediastinum.

panacinar e., SYN panlobular e.

panlobular e., e. affecting all parts of the secondary pulmonary lobule, typically involving the inferior part of the lung and often asociated with a α₁-antitrypsin deficiency. SYN generalized e., panacinar e.

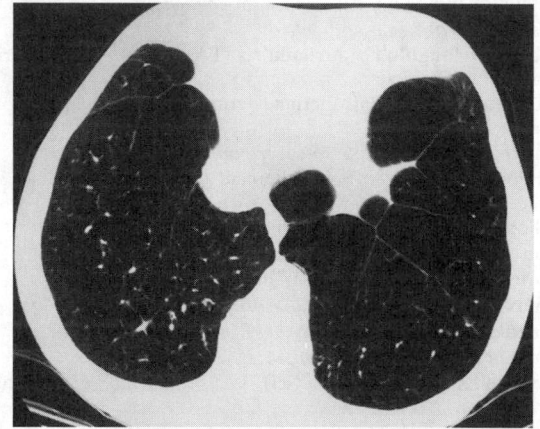

panlobular emphysema: high-resolution CT through lower lobes shows uniform destruction of secondary pulmonary lobules

paracicatricial e., dilated terminal air spaces adjacent to a scar in the lung. SEE ALSO paraseptal e.

paraseptal e., e. involving the periphery of the pulmonary lobules. SYN scar e.

pulmonary e., SYN emphysema (2).

scar e., SYN paraseptal e.

senile e., e. consequent upon the physiologic atrophy of old age.

subcutaneous e., the presence of air or gas in the subcutaneous tissues. SYN aerodermectasia, cutaneous e., pneumoderma, pneumohypoderma.

subgaleal e., collection of air or gas between the inner layer of the scalp and the cranium.

surgical e., subcutaneous e. from gas trapped in the tissues by an operation or injury, frequently seen after carbon dioxide insufflation during laproscopic procedures.

unilateral lobar e., radiographically hyperlucent lobe (or lung) secondary to bronchiolitis obliterans, with air trapping. SYN Macleod syndrome, Swyer-James syndrome (1), Swyer-James-MacLeod syndrome.

em·phy·sem·a·tous (em-fi-sem′ă-tŭs). Relating to or affected with emphysema.

em·pir·ic (em-pir′ik). **1.** SYN empirical. **2.** A member of a school of Graeco-Roman physicians, late BC to early AD, who placed their confidence in and based their practice purely on experience, avoiding all speculation, theory, or abstract reasoning; they were little concerned with causes or with correlating symptoms in order to gain a true understanding of a disease, even holding basic knowledge, physiology, pathology, and anatomy in low esteem and of no value in practice. **3.** Modern: testing a hypothesis by careful observation, hence rationally based on experience. [see empirical]

em·pir·i·cal (em-pir′i-kăl). **1.** Founded on practical experience, rather than on reasoning alone, but not established scientifically, in contrast to rational (1). **2.** Relating to an empiric (2). **3.** Based on careful observational testing of a hypothesis; rational. SYN empiric (1). [G. *empeirikos;* fr. *empeiria,* experience, fr. *en,* in, + *peira,* a trial]

em·pir·i·cism (em-pir′i-sizm). A looking to experience as a guide to practice or to the therapeutic use of any remedy.

em·por·i·at·rics (em-pōr-ē-at′riks). The specialty of travel medicine, dealing with diseases that travelers can acquire, especially in the tropics. [G. *emporion,* market, fr. *emporos,* traveler, merchant, + *(technē) iatrikē,* medical art]

em·pros·thot·o·nos (em′pros-thot′ō-nŭs). A tetanic contraction of the flexor muscles, curving the back with concavity forward. [G. *emprosthen,* forward, + *tonos,* tension]

em·py·ec·to·my (em-pī-ek′tō-mē). Resection of an empyema and its capsule.

em·py·e·ma (em-pī-ē′mă, -pi-ē′mă). Pus in a body cavity; when used without qualification, refers specifically to pyothorax. [G. *empyēma,* suppuration, fr. *en,* in, + *pyon,* pus]

e. benig′num, SYN latent e.

e. of gallbladder, severe acute cholecystitis with purulent inflammation of the gallbladder.

latent e., the presence of pus in a cavity, especially one of the accessory sinuses, unattended by subjective symptoms. SYN e. benignum.

loculated e., pyothorax in which pleural adhesions form one or more pockets containing pus.

mastoid e., SYN mastoiditis.

e. necessita′tis, e. necessitans, a form of pyothorax in which the pus burrows to the outside, producing a subcutaneous abscess that finally ruptures through the skin; it may result in spontaneous recovery without requiring an operation.

e. of the pericardium, SYN purulent *pericarditis.*

pneumococcal e., infection of the pleural cavity by *Streptococcus pneumoniae,* the pneumococcus, with pus formation.

pulsating e., a large, tense collection of pus in the pleural cavity through which the cardiac pulsations are transmitted to the chest wall.

streptococcal e., purulent exudation into the pleural cavity caused by infection with *Streptococcus hemolyticus.*

em·py·e·mic (em-pī-ē′mik). Relating to empyema.

em·py·e·sis (em-pī-ē′sis). A pustular eruption. [G. suppuration]

em·py·o·cele (em′pī-ō-sēl). A suppurating hydrocele; a collection of pus in the scrotum. [G. *en,* in, + *pyon,* pus, + *kēlē,* tumor]

em·py·reu·ma (em-pī-roo′mă). Characteristic odor given off by organic substances when charred or subjected to destructive distillation in closed vessels. [G. a banked fire]

emu Abbreviation for electromagnetic *unit.*

emul·gent (ē-mŭl′jent). Denoting a straining, extracting, or purifying process. [L. *e- mulgeo,* pp. *-mulsus,* to milk out, drain out]

emul·si·fi·er (ē-mŭl′si-fī-er). An agent, such as gum arabic or the yolk of an egg, used to make an emulsion of a fixed oil. Soaps, detergents, steroids, and proteins can act as emulsifiers; they stabilize 2-phase systems of oil and aqueous phases.

emul·si·fy (ē-mŭl′si-fī). To make in the form of an emulsion.

emul·sin (ē-mŭl′sin). **1.** A preparation or ferment derived from almonds, that contains β-glucosidase. **2.** Sometimes used as a synonym for β-glucosidase.

emul·sion (ē-mŭl′shŭn). A system containing two immiscible liquids in which one is dispersed, in the form of very small globules (internal phase), throughout the other (external phase) (e.g., oil in water (milk) or water in oil (mayonnaise)). [Mod. L. fr. *e-mulgeo,* pp. *-mulsus,* to milk or drain out]

emul·sive (ē-mŭl′siv). **1.** Denoting a substance that can be made into an emulsion. **2.** Denoting a substance, such as a mucilage, by which a fat or resin can be emulsified. **3.** Making soft or pliant. **4.** Yielding a fixed oil on pressure.

emul·soid (ē-mŭl′soyd). A colloidal dispersion in which the dispersed particles are more or less liquid and exert a certain attraction on and absorb a certain quantity of the fluid in which they are suspended. SYN emulsion colloid, hydrophil colloid, hydrophilic colloid, lyophilic colloid.

em·u·re·sis (em-ū-rē′sis). A condition in which urinary excretion and intake of water act to produce an absolute hydration of the body. SEE ALSO ecuresis. [G. *en (em),* in, + *ourēsis,* urination]

emyl·ca·mate (ĕ-mil′kă-māt, em-il-kam′āt). A mild sedative, used to control tension and anxiety and to relieve pain and muscular spasm.

⌂**en-.** In; appears as em- before b, p, or m. [G.]

en·al·a·pril·at (ē-nal′ă-pril-āt). The active metabolite of enalapril, an ACE inhibitor used to treat hypertension and congestive heart failure.

enal·a·pril ma·le·ate (e-nal′ă-pril). A prodrug for enalaprilat, an angiotensin converting enzyme inhibitor used as an anti-hypertensive agent and in the treatment of congestive heart failure.

enam·el (ē-nam′ĕl) [TA]. The hard glistening substance covering the exposed portion of the tooth. In its mature form, it is composed of an inorganic portion made up of 90% hydroxyapatite and 6-8% calcium carbonate, calcium fluoride, and magnesium carbonate, the remainder comprising an organic matrix of protein and glycoprotein; structurally, it is made up of oriented rods each of which consists of a stack of rodlets encased in an organic prism sheath. SYN enamelum [TA], substantia adamantina, substantia vitrea. [M.E., fr. Fr. *enamailer,* to apply enamel, fr. *en,* on, + *amail,* enamel, fr. Germanic]

dwarfed e., SYN nanoid e.

interrod e., e. occupying the space between e. rods and serving to bind them together.

mottled e., alterations in e. structure due to excessive fluoride ingestion during tooth formation; varies in appearance from small white opacities to yellow and black spotting.

nanoid e., a condition of abnormal thinness of the e. SYN dwarfed e.

whorled e., e. in which the rods assume a spiral or twisting course.

en·am·el·ins. A class of proteins that form the organic matrix of mature tooth enamel. [enamel + -in]

enam·el·o·blast (en-am′el-ō-blast). SYN ameloblast.

enam·el·o·gen·e·sis (ē-nam′ĕl-ō-jen′ĕ-sis). SYN amelogenesis.

e. imperfec′ta, SYN *amelogenesis* imperfecta.

enam·el·o·ma (ē-nam-ĕl-ō′mă). A developmental anomaly in which there is a small nodule of enamel below the cementoenamel junction, usually at the bifurcation of molar teeth. SYN enamel drop, enamel nodule, enamel pearl.

enam·e·lum (ē-nam′ĕ-lŭm) [TA]. SYN enamel.

enan·thal (ē-nan′thăl). SYN heptanal.

enan·thate (e-nan′thāt). USAN-approved contraction for heptanoate, $CH_3(CH_2)_5COO^-$.

en·an·them, en·an·the·ma (en-an′them, en-an-thē′mă). A mucous membrane eruption, especially one occurring in connection with one of the exanthemas. [G. *en,* in, + *anthēma,* bloom, eruption, fr. *antheō,* to bloom]

⌂**enantio-.** Combining form meaning opposite or reversed. [G. *enantios,* opposite]

en·an·ti·o·mer (ē-nan′tē-ō-mer). One of a pair of molecules that are nonsuperimposable mirror images of each other; neither mole-

en

cule has an internal plane of symmetry. SYN optic antipode. [enantio- + G. *meros,* part]

en·an·ti·o·mer·ic (ē-nan′tē-ō-mer′ik). Pertaining to enantiomerism.

en·an·ti·om·er·ism (ē-nan-tē-om′er-izm). In chemistry, isomerism in which the molecules in their configuration are related to one another like an object and its mirror image (enantiomers) and, consequently, are not superimposable; e. entails optical activity, both enantiomers (in identical amounts) rotating the plane of polarized light equally, but in opposite directions.

en·an·ti·o·morph (ē-nan′tē-ō-mōrf). An enantiomer in crystal form.

en·an·ti·o·mor·phic (ē-nan′tē-ō-mōr′fik). **1.** Relating to two objects, each of which is the mirror image of the other. **2.** In chemistry, relating to isomers, the optical activities of which are equal in magnitude but opposite in sign. SYN enantiomorphous. [enantio- + G. *morphē,* form]

en·an·ti·o·mor·phism (ē-nan′tē-ō-mōr′fizm). The relation of two objects similar in form but not superimposable, as the two hands or an object and its mirror image. [enantio- + G. *morphē,* form]

en·an·ti·o·mor·phous (ē-nan′tē-ō-mōr′fŭs). SYN enantiomorphic.

en·ar·thro·di·al (en-ar-thrō′dē-al). Relating to an enarthrosis.

en·ar·thro·sis (en-ar-thrō′sis). ☆ official alternate term for ball and socket *joint.* [G. *en-arthrōsis,* a jointing where the ball is deep set in the socket]

en bloc (ăhn blok). In a lump; as a whole; used to refer to autopsy techniques in which visceral organs are removed in large blocks allowing the prosector to retain a continuity in organ architecture during the subsequent dissection. [Fr., in a lump]

en·cai·nide hy·dro·chlo·ride (en-kā′nīd). An anti-arrhythmic.

en·cap·su·lat·ed (en-kap′soo-lā-ted). Enclosed in a capsule or sheath. SYN encapsuled.

en·cap·su·la·tion (en-kap-soo-lā′shŭn). Enclosure in a capsule or sheath. [L. *in* + capsula, dim. of *capsa,* box]

en·cap·suled (en-kap′soold). SYN encapsulated.

en·car·di·tis (en-kar-dī′tis). SYN endocarditis.

en·ce·li·tis, en·ce·li·i·tis (en-sē-lī′tis, -lē-ī′tis). Obsolete term for inflammation of any of the abdominal viscera. [G. *en,* in, + *koilia,* belly, + *-itis,* inflammation]

△**encephal-.** SEE encephalo-.

en·ceph·a·lal·gia (en-sef-ă-lal′jē-ă). SYN headache. [encephalo- + G. *algos,* pain]

en·céph·ale iso·lé (ahn-sāf-al′ ē-sō-lā′). An animal with its caudal medulla transected and its respiration maintained artificially; it remains alert, has sleep-wake cycles, normal pupillary reactions, and a normal electroencephalogram. Cf. cerveau isolé. [Fr. isolated brain]

en·ceph·a·le·mia (en-sef-ă-lē′mē-ă). SYN brain *congestion.* [encephalo- + G. *haima,* blood]

en·ce·phal·ic (en′se-fal′ik). Relating to the brain, or to the structures within the cranium.

en·ceph·a·lit·ic (en-sef-ă-lit′ik). Relating to encephalitis.

en·ceph·a·li·tis, pl. **en·ceph·a·lit·i·des** (en-sef-ă-lī′tis, en-sef-ă-lit′i-dēz). Inflammation of the brain. [G. *enkephalos,* brain, + *-itis,* inflammation]

acute hemorrhagic e., e. of apoplectoid character due to blood extravasation. SYN e. hemorrhagica.

acute inclusion body e., SYN herpes simplex e.

acute necrotizing e., an acute form of e., characterized by destruction of brain parenchyma; caused by herpes simplex and other viruses.

Australian X e., SYN Murray Valley e.

bacterial e., e. of bacterial etiology. SYN e. pyogenica, purulent e., suppurative e.

bunyavirus e., e. of abrupt onset, with severe frontal headache and low-grade to moderate fever, caused by members of the genus Bunyavirus (Bunyaviridae family); infections also occur in rodents, lagomorphs, and domestic animals. SYN California e.

California e., SYN bunyavirus e.

coxsackie e., a viral e., seen mainly in infants and involving principally the gray matter of the medulla and cord, caused by Enterovirus human coxsackie B.

Dawson e., SYN subacute sclerosing *panencephalitis.*

epidemic e., a viral e. occurring epidemically, such as in Japanese B e., St. Louis e., and lethargic e.

equine e., SYN equine *encephalomyelitis.*

experimental allergic e. (EAE), SYN experimental allergic *encephalomyelitis.*

Far East Russian e., tick-borne e. (Eastern subtype).

e. hemorrhag′ica, SYN acute hemorrhagic e.

herpes e., SYN herpes simplex e.

herpes simplex e., the most common acute encephalitis, caused by HSV-1; affects persons of any age; preferentially involves the inferomedial portions of the temporal lobe and the orbital portions of the frontal lobes; pathologically, severe hemorrhagic necrosis is present along with, in the acute stages, intranuclear eosinophilic inclusion bodies in the neurons and glial cells. SYN acute inclusion body e., herpes e.

hyperergic e., e. as a result of an immunologic allergic reaction of the nervous system to antigenic stimuli.

Ilhéus e., an e. caused by the Ilhéus virus (genus Flavivirus) and endemic to eastern Brazil and other parts of South and Central America; transmitted by mosquitoes.

inclusion body e., SYN subacute sclerosing *panencephalitis.*

Japanese B e., an epidemic e. or encephalomyelitis of Japan, Siberian Russia, and other parts of Asia; due to the Japanese B e. virus (genus Flavivirus) and transmitted by mosquitoes; can occur as a symptomless, subclinical infection but may cause an acute meningoencephalomyelitis. SYN e. japonica, Russian autumn e.

e. japon′ica, SYN Japanese B e.

lead e., SYN lead *encephalopathy.*

e. lethar′gica, SYN von Economo *disease.*

Mengo e., an e. occurring in Africa, due to the Mengo strain of encephalomyocarditis virus, a member of the Picornaviridae.

Murray Valley e., a severe e. with a high mortality rate occurring in the Murray Valley of Australia; the disease is most severe in children and is characterized by headache, fever, malaise, drowsiness or convulsions, and rigidity of the neck; extensive brain damage may result; it is caused by the Murray Valley encephalitis virus (genus Flavivirus). SYN Australian X disease, Australian X e.

necrotizing e., any e. in which extensive brain necrosis occurs, e.g., acute necrotizing hemorrhagic encephalomyelitis.

e. neonato′rum, e. of the newborn, described by R. Virchow as marked by the presence of fat-laden cells in the brain.

e. periaxia′lis concen′trica, e. that is clinically similar to adrenoleukodystrophy, but pathologically characterized by concentric globes or circles of demyelination of cerebral white matter separated by normal tissue. SYN Baló disease.

e. periaxialis diffusa, SYN Schilder *disease.*

postvaccinal e., SYN postvaccinal *encephalomyelitis.*

Powassan e., an acute disease of children varying clinically from undifferentiated febrile illness to e.; caused by the Powassan virus, a member of the Flaviviridae family, and transmitted by ixodid ticks; most frequently seen in Canada.

purulent e., SYN bacterial e.

e. pyogen′ica, SYN bacterial e.

rasmussen e., e. in which antibodies to a stimulatory glutamate receptor in the CNS are found; perhaps autoimmune. SYN Rasmussen syndrome.

Russian autumn e., SYN Japanese B e.

Russian spring-summer e. (Eastern subtype), a tick-borne e. virus belonging to the family Flaviviridae.

Russian spring-summer e. (Western subtype), SYN tick-borne e. (Central European subtype).

Russian tick-borne e., SYN tick-borne e. (Eastern subtype).

secondary e., collective term for postinfectious, postexanthem, and postvaccinal encephalitides.

subacute inclusion body e., SYN subacute sclerosing *panencephalitis.*

e. subcortical'is chron'ica, SYN Binswanger *disease.*

suppurative e., SYN bacterial e.

tick-borne e. (Central European subtype), tick-borne meningo-encephalitis caused by a flavivirus closely related to the virus causing the Far Eastern type; it is transmitted by *Ixodes ricinus,* also by infected raw milk, especially that of goats. SYN biundulant meningoencephalitis, Central European tick-borne fever, diphasic milk fever, Russian spring-summer e. (Western subtype).

tick-borne e. (Eastern subtype), a severe form of e. caused by a flavivirus (Flaviviridae family), and transmitted by ticks (*Ixodes pertulcatus* and *I. ricinus*). SYN Russian tick-borne e.

van Bogaert e., SYN subacute sclerosing *panencephalitis.*

varicella e., e. occurring as a complication of chickenpox.

vernal e., tick-borne e. (Eastern subtype).

woodcutter's e., tick-borne e. (Eastern subtype).

en·ceph·a·li·to·gen (en-sef'ă-lī'tō-jen). An agent which evokes encephalitis, particularly with reference to the antigen which produces experimental allergic encephalomyelitis. [encephalitis + G. -gen, producing]

en·ceph·a·li·to·gen·ic (en-sef'ă-li-tō-jen'ik). Producing encephalitis; typically by hypersensitivity mechanisms. SEE encephalitogen.

En·ceph·a·li·to·zo·on (en-sef'ă-li-tō-zō'on). A genus of protozoan parasites, formerly considered part of the family Toxoplasmatidae, class Sporozoea, but now recognized as a member of the protozoan phylum Microspora, family Nosematidae. *E. cuniculi* is considered the primary microsporan parasite of mammals, commonly found in the brain and kidney tubules of rodents and carnivores and causing nosematosis in rabbits. [encephalitis + G. zōon, animal]

E. cuniculi, a common cryptic infection of most mammals and some birds, transmitted in urine-contaminated food and by transplacental transmission. Disseminated human infection has been reported among immunosuppressed individuals. Latent infection seen by serodiagnosis suggests widespread nonsymptomatic infection in tropical regions.

E. hellem, a species of E. described from human ophthalmic infections causing punctate keratopathy and corneal ulceration in AIDS patients.

E. intestinale, a diarrheogenic microsporidian described in HIV-infected patients; disease may be localized to the gastrointestinal tract or may disseminate intravascularly.

E. intestinalis, a species of E. described from human muscle; very few cases have been reported. Formerly called *Septata intestinale.*

en·ceph·a·li·za·tion (en-sef'ă-li-zā'shŭn). SYN corticalization.

⌂**encephalo-, encephal-.** The brain. Cf. cerebro-. [G. *en-kephalos*, brain]

en·ceph·a·lo·cele (en-sef'ă-lō-sēl). A congenital gap in the skull with herniation of brain substance. SYN craniocele, cranium bifidum, bifid cranium. [encephalo- + G. kēlē, hernia]

basal e., a defect in the skull floor with the herniation of brain tissue sometimes associated with *coloboma* of optic nerve.

en·ceph·a·lo·cys·to·cele. SYN hydrencephalocele.

en·ceph·a·lo·dur·o·ar·te·ri·o·syn·an·gi·o·sis (en-sef'a-lō-door-ō-ar-tēr'ē-ō-sin-anj-ē-ō'sis). SYN duraencephalosynangiosis.

en·ceph·a·lo·dyn·ia (en-sef'ă-lō-din'ē-ă). SYN headache. [encephalo- + G. odynē, pain]

en·ceph·a·lo·dys·pla·sia (en-sef'ă-lō-dis-plā'zē-ă). Any congenital abnormality of the brain. [encephalo- + G. dys, bad, + plastos, formed]

en·ceph·a·lo·gram (en-sef'ă-lō-gram). The record obtained by encephalography. [encephalo- + G. gramma, a drawing]

en·ceph·a·log·ra·phy (en-sef-ă-log'ră-fē). Obsolete technique of radiographic representation of the brain. SEE pneumoencephalography. [encephalo- + G. graphō, to write]

gamma e., imaging of the encephalon by the administration of small amounts of gamma-emitting radiopharmaceuticals; term may be used to refer to any number of particular studies (e.g., cerebral perfusion scintigraphy, cerebral neuroreceptor imaging) depending on the radiopharmaceutical used.

en·ceph·a·loid (en-sef'ă-loyd). Resembling brain substance; de-noting a carcinoma of soft, brainlike consistency, with reference to gross features. [encephalo- + G. *eidos*, resemblance]

en·ceph·a·lo·lith (en-sef'ă-lō-lith). A concretion in the brain or one of its ventricles. SYN cerebral calculus. [encephalo- + G. lithos, stone]

en·ceph·a·lol·o·gy (en-sef-ă-lol'ō-jē). The branch of medicine dealing with the brain in all its relations. [encephalo- + G. logos, study]

en·ceph·a·lo·ma (en-sef-ă-lō'mă-lā'shē-ă). Herniation of brain substance. SYN cerebroma.

en·ceph·a·lo·ma·la·cia (en-sef'ă-lō-mă-lā'shē-ă). Abnormal softness of the cerebral parenchyma often due to ischemia or infarction. SYN cerebromalacia. [encephalo- + G. malakia, softness]

en·ceph·a·lo·men·in·gi·tis (en-sef'ă-lō-men-in-jī'tis). SYN meningoencephalitis. [encephalo- + G. mēninx, membrane, + -itis, inflammation]

en·ceph·a·lo·me·nin·go·cele (en-sef'ă-lō-me-ning'gō-sēl). SYN meningoencephalocele. [encephalo- + G. mēninx, membrane, + kēlē, hernia]

en·ceph·a·lo·men·in·gop·a·thy (en-sef'ă-lō-men-in-gop'ă-thē). SYN meningoencephalopathy.

en·ceph·a·lo·mere (en-sef'ă-lō-mēr). SYN neuromere. [encephalo- + G. meros, a part]

en·ceph·a·lom·e·ter (en-sef-ă-lom'ĕ-ter). An apparatus for indicating on the skull the location of the cortical centers. [encephalo- + G. metron, measure]

en·ceph·a·lo·my·e·li·tis (en-sef-ă-lō-mī'ĕ-lī'tis). Inflammation of the brain and spinal cord. [encephalo- + G. myelon, marrow, + -itis, inflammation]

acute disseminated e., an acute demyelinating disorder of the central nervous system, in which focal demyelination is present throughout the brain and spinal cord. This process is common to postinfectious, postexanthem, and postvaccinal encephalomyelitis.

acute necrotizing hemorrhagic e., a fulminating demyelinating disorder of the central nervous system that affects mainly children and young adults. Almost always preceded by a respiratory infection, characterized by the abrupt onset of fever, headache, confusion, and nuchal rigidity, soon followed by focal seizures, hemiplegia, or quadriplegia, brainstem findings, and coma; the CSF shows evidence of an inflammatory process; due to the massive destruction of the white matter of one or both hemispheres, often accompanied by similar destruction of the white matter of the brainstem and cerebellar peduncles; of unknown etiology. SYN acute hemorrhagic leukoencephalitis, acute necrotizing hemorrhagic leukoencephalitis, Hurst disease.

e. associated with carcinoma, SYN paraneoplastic *encephalomyelopathy.*

benign myalgic e., SYN epidemic *neuromyasthenia.*

eastern equine e. (EEE), a form of mosquito-borne equine e. seen in the eastern U.S. and caused by the eastern equine e. virus, a species of Alphavirus, which belongs to the family Togaviridae; initial fever and viremia are followed by signs of central nervous system involvement (excitement, then somnolence, paralysis, and death); the incidence of clinical infection in humans is low but case fatality may be high.

epidemic myalgic e., SYN epidemic *neuromyasthenia.*

equine e., an acute, often fatal, virus disease of horses and mules transmitted by mosquitoes and characterized by central nervous system disturbances; in the U.S., this disease is typically caused by one of three alphaviruses, and their resulting diseases are designated western equine, eastern equine and Venezuelan equine e.; these viruses belong to the family Togaviridae and can also cause neurologic disease in humans. SYN equine encephalitis.

experimental allergic e., a demyelinating allergic e. produced by the injection of brain tissue, usually with an adjuvant. SYN experimental allergic encephalitis.

granulomatous e., an e. in which granulomas occur.

herpes B e., a frequently lethal disease of humans caused by infection with a normally latent monkey herpesvirus.

mouse e., e. due to the mouse encephalomyelitis virus (a species of Enterovirus) which is not pathogenic in monkeys or in man, but attacks mouse colonies and causes a flaccid paralysis, usually of the hind limbs.

postvaccinal e., a severe type of encephalomyelitis that can follow the rabies vaccination. SYN postvaccinal encephalitis.

Venezuelan equine e. (VEE), a form of mosquito-borne equine e. found in parts of South America, Panama, and Trinidad, caused by the Venezuelan equine e. virus (a species of Alphavirus in the family Togaviridae), and characterized by less central nervous system involvement than occurs in either eastern or western equine e.; fever, diarrhea, and depression are common; in humans, there is fever and severe headache after an incubation period of 2–5 days, and in a few cases there has been central nervous system involvement.

viral e., virus e., an e. due to a neurotropic virus.

western equine e. (WEE), an equine e. found in the western U.S. and parts of South America, transmitted by mosquitoes and caused by the western equine e. virus (a species of Alphavirus in the family Togaviridae); the infection is similar to but milder than eastern equine e. in humans and is, as a rule, inapparent, but some cases with central nervous system involvement have been fatal.

zoster e., inflammation of the brain and spinal cord caused by varicella-zoster virus, a member of the family Herpesviridae.

en·ceph·a·lo·my·e·lo·cele (en-sef'ă-lō-mī'ĕ-lō-sēl). Congenital defect in the skull, usually in the occipital region, and cervical vertebrae with herniation of the meninges and neural tissue. [G. *enkephalos,* brain, + *myelon,* marrow, + *kēlē,* hernia]

en·ceph·a·lo·my·e·lo·neu·rop·a·thy (en-sef'ă-lō-mī'ĕ-lō-noo-rop'ă-thē). A disease involving the brain, spinal cord, and peripheral nerves.

en·ceph·a·lo·my·e·lop·a·thy (en-sef'ă-lō-mī-ĕ-lop'ă-thē). Any disease of both brain and spinal cord. [G. *enkephalos,* brain, + *myelon,* marrow, + *pathos,* suffering]

carcinomatous e., SYN paraneoplastic e.

epidemic myalgic e., a disease superficially resembling poliomyelitis, characterized by diffuse involvement of the nervous system associated with myalgia.

necrotizing e. [MIM*256000], SYN Leigh *disease.*

paracarcinomatous e., SYN paraneoplastic e.

paraneoplastic e., an encephalomyelopathy as a remote effect of carcinoma, most often oat cell carcinoma of the lung; characterized by extensive nerve cell loss, which may be diffuse, but often predominates in particular portions of the central nervous system, particularly the limbic lobes, medulla, cerebellum, and gray matter of the spinal cord. SYN carcinomatous e., encephalomyelitis associated with carcinoma, paracarcinomatous e.

subacute necrotizing e. (SNE), a rare fatal disorder, primarily of children, being both acute and chronic in onset, manifested primarily as brainstem dysfunction, with ataxia, cranial nerve palsies, pseudobulbar palsy, hemi- or quadriplegia, mental deterioration, and involuntary movements; deficiencies of pyruvate dehydrogenase or cytochrome C oxidase have been found in some patients; pathologically, there is widespread symmetric necrosis involving much of the brainstem; these changes are similar to those seen with Wernicke encephalopathy.

en·ceph·a·lo·my·e·lo·ra·dic·u·li·tis (en-sef'ă-lō-mī'ĕ-lō-ră-dik'ū-lī-tis). SYN encephalomyeloradiculopathy.

en·ceph·a·lo·my·e·lo·ra·dic·u·lop·a·thy (en-sef'ă-lō-mī'ĕ-lō-ră-dik'ū-lop-ă-thē). A disease process involving the brain, spinal cord, and spinal roots. SYN encephalomyeloradiculitis.

en·ceph·a·lo·my·o·car·di·tis (en-sef'ă-lō-mī'ō-kar-dī'tis). Associated encephalitis and myocarditis; often caused by a viral infection such as in poliomyelitis.

en·ceph·a·lon, pl. **en·ceph·a·la** (en-sef'ă-lon, lă) [TA]. That portion of the cerebrospinal axis contained within the cranium, composed of the prosencephalon, mesencephalon, and rhombencephalon. [G. *enkephalos,* brain, fr. *en,* in, + *kephalē,* head]

en·ceph·a·lo·path·ia (en-sef'ă-lō-path'ē-ă). SYN encephalopathy.

en·ceph·a·lop·a·thy (en-sef'ă-lop'ă-thē). Any disorder of the brain. SYN cerebropathia, cerebropathy, encephalopathia, encephalosis. [encephalo- + G. *pathos,* suffering]

bilirubin e., SYN kernicterus.

Binswanger e., SYN Binswanger *disease.*

bovine spongiform e. (BSE), a disease of cattle first reported in 1986 in Great Britain; characterized clinically by apprehensive behavior, hyperesthesia, and ataxia, and histologically by spongiform changes in the gray matter of the brain stem; caused by a prion, like spongiform e.'s of other animals (e.g., scrapie) and human beings (Creutzfeldt-Jakob disease). SEE Creutzfeldt-Jakob *disease.* SYN mad cow disease.

In the middle 1990s, an unusual number of cases of Creutzfeldt-Jakob disease (CJD) were reported in persons under 30 years of age in Great Britain. These patients displayed typical clinical features but not the EEG changes characteristic of CJD, and autopsy specimens showed unusual amyloid plaques resembling those of kuru but not previously observed in CJD. These cases of variant Creutzfeldt-Jakob disease (V-CJD) were speculatively associated with an epizootic of bovine spongiform encephalopathy (mad cow disease) that killed more than 150,000 cattle in Britain between 1986 and 1996. Although the link between BSE and V-CJD cannot be confirmed on the basis of existing data, the mere possibility of such a link has already led to the development of recommendations to help reduce or prevent the occurrence of BSE in cattle worldwide. There is no evidence from U.S. surveillance activities or from scientific studies to indicate that BSE exists in the U.S. Since 1990, laboratory testing of brain specimens from cattle with CNS signs has shown no evidence of BSE. Since July 1989 the importation of cattle and cattle products from the U.K. has been banned by the U.S. Department of Agriculture. According to mortality statistics, the annual incidence of CJD in the U.S. remained stable at approximately 1 case per million persons between 1979 and 1994. WHO consultants have condemned the practice of feeding ruminant-derived meat-and-bone meal to cattle and urged the adoption of measures to ensure that no part of any animal that shows signs of a spongiform encephalopathy enters any human or animal food chain. Milk, dairy products, gelatin, and lard are considered safe.

demyelinating e., extensive idiopathic loss of myelin sheaths in the brain, as occurs in leukodystrophy.

hepatic e., SYN portal-systemic e.

HIV e., SYN AIDS dementia *complex.*

hypernatremic e., subarachnoid and subdural effusions in infants with hypernatremic dehydration.

hypertensive e., a metabolic e. caused by diffuse cerebral edema; follows an abrupt elevation of blood pressure in a long-term hypertensive patient.

hypoxic-hypercarbic e., SYN hypoventilation *coma.*

hypoxic ischemic e., permanent brain injury due to a lack of oxygen or adequate blood flow to the brain.

lead e., a metabolic e., caused by the ingestion of lead compounds and seen particularly in early childhood; it is characterized pathologically by extensive cerebral edema, status spongiosus, neurocytolysis, and some reactive inflammation; clinical manifestations include convulsions, delirium, and hallucinations. SEE ALSO lead *poisoning.* SYN lead encephalitis, saturnine e.

metabolic e., coma or its precursors resulting from a diffuse abnormality of cerebral neuronal or glial cell metabolism. Primary metabolic e. is due to any of the degenerative cerebral disorders that culminate in coma; secondary metabolic e. results when brain metabolism is disturbed by extracerebral disorders causing intoxication, electrolyte imbalances, or nutritional deficiencies, e.g., hepatic or renal disease or exogenous poisons.

necrotizing e., SYN Leigh *disease.*

palindromic e., a relatively mild form that tends to recur.

pancreatic e., a metabolic e. associated with extensive pancreatic necrosis.

portal-systemic e., an e. associated with cirrhosis of the liver, attributed to the passage of toxic nitrogenous substances from the portal to the systemic circulation; cerebral manifestations may include coma. SYN hepatic e.

progressive subcortical e., SYN progressive multifocal *leukoencephalopathy.*

pulmonary e., SYN hypoventilation *coma.*

recurrent e. [MIM*130950], a progressive form of e. occurring in young members of the same family; characterized by headache, vertigo, truncal ataxia, drowsiness and stupor, speech impairments, choreic-athetoid movements, and sometimes convulsions; probably autosomal dominant inheritance.

saturnine e., SYN lead e.

severe postanoxic e., SYN delayed *coma* after hypoxia.

spongiform e., an e. characterized by vacuolation within nerve and glial cells.

subacute spongiform e., a form of spongiform e. that is associated with a "slow virus," which to date has not been adequately described, is transmissible, and has a rapidly progressive, fatal course; e.g., Creutzfeldt-Jakob disease, kuru, Gerstmann-Sträussler syndrome, scrapie. SEE prion.

subcortical arteriosclerotic e., SYN Binswanger *disease.*

thyrotoxic e., a metabolic e. arising in severe cases of thyrotoxicosis.

traumatic e., an e. resulting from structural brain injury.

traumatic progressive e., chronic progressive brain damage resulting from multiple brain injuries, e.g., dementia pugilistica.

Wernicke e., SYN Wernicke *syndrome.*

Wernicke-Korsakoff e., SEE Wernicke *syndrome,* Korsakoff *syndrome.*

en·ceph·a·lo·py·o·sis (en-sef′ă-lō-pī-ō′sis). Archaic term for purulent inflammation of the brain. [encephalo- + G. *pyōsis,* suppuration]

en·ceph·a·lor·rha·chid·i·an (en-sef′ă-lō-ră-kid′ē-an). SYN cerebrospinal. [encephalo- + G. *rhachis,* spine]

en·ceph·a·los·chi·sis (en-sef-ă-los′ki-sis). Developmental failure of closure of the rostral part of the neural tube. [encephalo- + G. *schisis,* fissure]

en·ceph·a·lo·scle·ro·sis (en-sef′ă-lō-sklēr-o′sis). A sclerosis, or hardening, of the brain. SEE ALSO cerebrosclerosis. [encephalo- + G. *sklērōsis,* hardening]

en·ceph·a·lo·scope (en-sef′ă-lō-skōp). Any instrument used to view the interior of a brain abscess or other cerebral cavity through an opening in the skull. [encephalo- + G. *skopeō,* to view]

en·ceph·a·los·co·py (en-sef-ă-los′kŏ-pē). Examination of the brain or the cavity of a cerebral abscess by direct inspection.

en·ceph·a·lo·sis. SYN encephalopathy.

en·ceph·a·lo·spi·nal (en-sef′ă-lō-spī′năl). SYN cerebrospinal.

en·ceph·a·lo·tome (en-sef′ă-lō-tōm). An instrument for use in performing encephalotomy.

en·ceph·a·lot·o·my (en-sef-ă-lot′ō-mē). Dissection or incision of the brain. [encephalo- + G. *tomē,* incision]

en·chon·dral (en-kon′drăl). SYN intracartilaginous.

en·chon·dro·ma (en-kon-drō′mă). A benign cartilaginous growth starting within the medullary cavity of a bone originally formed from cartilage; e.'s may distend the cortex, especially of small bones, and may be solitary or multiple (endochondromatosis). [Mod. L. fr. G. *en,* in, + *chondros,* cartilage, + *-oma,* tumor]

en·chon·dro·ma·to·sis (en-kon′drō-ma-tō′sis) [MIM*166000 *225795]. A rare disorder characterized by hamartomatous proliferation of cartilage in the metaphyses of several bones, most commonly of the hands and feet, causing distorted growth in length and pathological fractures; chondrosarcoma may develop. When e. is associated with hemangiomas in the cutaneous or visceral regions, the condition is called Maffucci *syndrome.* Most cases are sporadic but a few instances demonstrate autosomal dominant inheritance with reduced penetrance. SYN asymmetric chondrodystrophy, dyschondroplasia, hereditary deforming chondrodystrophy (2), Ollier disease.

en·chon·drom·a·tous (en-kon-drō′mă-tŭs). Relating to or having the elements of enchondroma.

en·clave (en-klāv, ahn-klahv′). An enclosure; a detached mass of tissue enclosed in tissue of another kind; seen especially in the case of isolated masses of gland tissue detached from the main gland. [Fr. fr. L. *clavis,* key]

en·cod·ing (en-kōd′ing). The first stage in the memory process, followed by storage and retrieval, involving processes associated with receiving or briefly registering stimuli through one or more of the senses and modifying that information; a decay process or loss of this information (a type of forgetting) occurs rapidly unless the next two stages, storage and retrieval, are activated.

en·cop·re·sis (en-kō-prē′sis). The repeated, generally involuntary passage of feces into inappropriate places (e.g., clothing). [G. *enkopros,* full of manure]

en·cra·ni·al (en-krā′nē-ăl). SYN endocranial.

en·cra·ni·us (en-krā′nē-ŭs). In conjoined twins, a form of fetal inclusion in which the smaller parasite lies partly or wholly within the cranial cavity of the larger autosite. [G. *en,* in, + *kranion,* skull]

encu Acronym for *equivalent normal child unit,* that amount of information from any source (linkage analysis, parental, and collateral phenotypes, biochemistry of the carrier state, etc.) that will have the same impact on the probability as one usual progeny does that a consultand is a carrier for an autosomal dominant trait; e.g., each normal child contributes one encu. Cf. ensu.

en·cyst·ed (en-sis′ted). Encapsulated by a membranous bag. [G. *kystis,* bladder]

en·cyst·ment (en-sist′ment). The condition of being or becoming encysted.

end. An extremity, or the most remote point of an extremity.

acromial e. of clavicle [TA], the flattened lateral end of the clavicle that articulates with the acromion and is anchored to the coracoid process by the conoid and trapezoid ligaments. SYN extremitas acromialis claviculae [TA], acromial extremity of clavicle.

distal e., the posterior extremity of a dental appliance. SYN heel (3) [TA].

fixed e. [TA], for a given movement, the e. of a bone that is held stationary (as a consequence of attachment or muscular fixation) while the other e. of the bone (the mobile end) moves in response to muscle activity or gravity. SYN punctum fixa [TA].

mobile e. [TA], for a given movement, the e. of a bone that moves in response to muscle activity or gravity while the other e. of the bone (the fixed e.) is held stationary (as a consequence of attachment or muscular fixation). SYN punctum mobile [TA].

sternal e. of clavicle [TA], the enlarged medial end of the clavicle that articulates with the manubrium sterni. SYN extremitas sternalis claviculae [TA], sternal extremity of clavicle.

end-. SEE endo-.

end·a·del·phos (end′ă-del′fos). Unequal conjoined twins in which the parasitic member is included in the body of the host. [end- + G. *adelphos,* brother]

End·a·moe·ba (end′ă-mē′bă). A genus of amebae parasitic in invertebrates; originally described from cockroaches. [endo- + G. *amoibē,* change]

end·an·gi·i·tis, end·an·ge·i·tis (end-an-jē-ī′tis). Inflammation of the intima of a blood vessel. SYN endoangiitis, endovasculitis. [endo- + G. *angeion,* vessel, + *-itis,* inflammation]

e. oblit′erans, inflammation of the intima of a vessel with resulting occlusion of its lumen.

end·a·or·ti·tis (end′ā-ōr-tī′tis). Inflammation of the intima of the aorta. SYN endo-aortitis.

end·ar·ter·ec·to·my (end-ar-ter-ek′tō-mē). Excision of atheromatous deposits along with the diseased endothelium and media or most of the media of an artery so as to leave a smooth lining, mostly consisting of adventitia. [endo- + artery + G. *ektomē,* excision]

carotid e., excision of occluding material, including intima and most of the media, from the carotid a.

coronary e., excision of occluding material, including intima and most of the media, from the coronary artery.

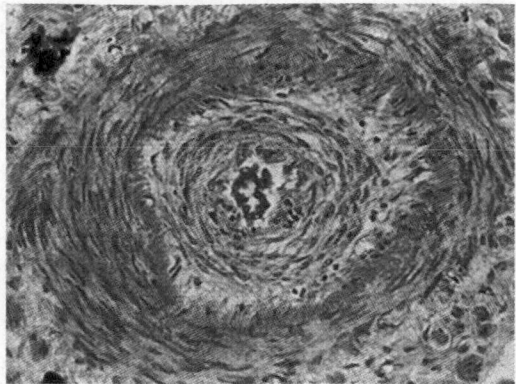
endangiitis: note narrowing of lumen of vessel by fibrous thickening

end·ar·te·ri·tis (end′ar-ter-ī′tis). Inflammation of the intima of an artery. SYN endoarteritis.

bacterial e., implantation and growth of bacteria with formation of vegetations on the arterial wall, such as may occur in a patent ductus arteriosus or arteriovenous fistula.

e. defor′mans, e. with atheromatous patches and calcareous deposits.

e. oblit′erans, obliterating e., an extreme degree of e. proliferans closing the lumen of the artery. SYN arteritis obliterans, obliterating arteritis.

e. prolif′erans, proliferating e., chronic e. accompanied by a marked increase of fibrous tissue in the intima.

end·au·ral (end-aw′răl). Within the ear. [endo- + L. *auris,* ear]

end·brain. SYN telencephalon.

end·brush (end′brŭsh). SYN telodendron.

end·bulb. SEE end *bulb.*

end-di·a·stol·ic (end′dī-ă-stol′ik). **1.** Occurring at the end of diastole, immediately before the next systole, as in end-diastolic pressure. **2.** Interrupting the final moments of diastole, barely premature, as in end-diastolic extrasystole.

endectocide. A drug effective against both endoparasites and ectoparasites, e.g., the macrolide antibiotic avermectin. SEE ALSO ivermectin. [*endo*parasite + *ecto*parasite + -cide]

en·de·mia (en-dē′mē-ă). Obsolete term for an endemic disease.

en·dem·ic (en-dem′ik). Denoting a temporal pattern of disease occurrence in a population in which the disease occurs with predictable regularity with only relatively minor fluctations in its frequency over time. Cf. epidemic, sporadic. [G. *endēmos,* native, fr. *en,* in, + *dēmos,* the people]

en·dem·o·ep·i·dem·ic (en-dem′ō-ep-i-dem′ik). Denoting a temporary large increase in the number of cases of an endemic disease.

end·er·gon·ic (en-der-gon′ik). Referring to a chemical reaction that takes place with absorption of energy from its surroundings (i.e., a positive change in Gibbs free energy). Cf. exergonic. [endo- + G. *ergon,* work]

en·der·mic, en·der·mat·ic (en-der′mik, en-der-mat′ik). In or through the skin; denoting a method of treatment, as by inunction; the remedy produces its constitutional effect when absorbed through the skin surface to which it is applied. [G. *en,* in, + *derma* (*dermat*-), skin]

en·der·mo·sis (en-der-mō′sis). Any eruptive disease of the mucous membrane.

end-feet. SYN axon *terminals,* under *terminal.*

end·gut. SYN hindgut.

end·ing. **1.** A termination or conclusion. **2.** A nerve e.

annulospiral e., one of two types of sensory nerve e. associated with a neuromuscular spindle (the other being the flower-spray e.); after entering the muscle spindle, the fiber divides into two flat, ribbonlike branches that wind themselves in rings or spirals about the intrafusal muscle fibers. SYN annulospiral organ.

calyciform e., caliciform e., a synaptic e. in relation to certain neuroepithelial hair cells of the inner ear.

epilemmal e., a nerve e. in close relation to the outer surface of the sarcolemma.

flower-spray e., one of the two types of sensory nerve e. associated with the neuromuscular spindle (the other being the annulospiral e.); in this type, the fiber branches spread out upon the surface of the intrafusal fibers like a spray of flowers. SYN flower-spray organ of Ruffini.

free nerve e.'s, a form of peripheral ending of sensory nerve fibers in which the terminal filaments end freely in the tissue. SYN terminationes nervorum liberae.

grape e.'s, an autodescriptive term applied to synaptic terminals at the ends of short, stalklike axon branches.

hederiform e., a type of free sensory ending in the skin.

nerve e., any one of the specialized terminations of peripheral sensory or motor nerve fibers. SEE motor *endplate,* corpuscle, bulb.

sole-plate e., SYN motor *endplate.*

synaptic e.'s, SYN axon *terminals,* under *terminal.*

Endo, Shigeru, Japanese bacteriologist, 1869–1937. SEE E. *agar, medium.*

endo-, end-. Prefixes indicating within, inner, absorbing, or containing. SEE ALSO ento-. [G. *endon,* within]

en·do·ab·dom·i·nal (en′dō-ab-dom′i-năl). Within the abdomen.

en·do·am·y·lase (en′dō-am′il-ās). A glucanohydrolase acting on internal glycosidic bonds (e.g., α-amylase).

en·do·an·eu·rys·mo·plas·ty (en′dō-an-ū-riz′mō-plas-tē). SYN aneurysmoplasty.

en·do·an·eu·rys·mor·rha·phy (en′dō-an-ū-riz-mōr′ă-fē). SYN aneurysmoplasty. [endo- + G. *aneurysma,* aneurysm, + *rhaphē,* suture]

en·do·an·gi·i·tis (en′dō-an-jē-ī′tis). SYN endangiitis.

en·do·a·or·ti·tis (en′dō-ā-ōr-tī′tis). SYN endaortitis.

en·do·ap·pen·di·ci·tis (en′dō-ă-pen-di-sī′tis). Simple catarrhal inflammation, limited more or less strictly to the mucosal surface of the vermiform appendix.

en·do·ar·te·ri·tis (en′dō-ar-ter-ī′tis). SYN endarteritis.

en·do·aus·cul·ta·tion (en′dō-aws-kŭl-tā′shŭn). Auscultation of the thoracic organs, especially the heart, by means of a stethoscopic tube passed into the esophagus or into the heart.

en·do·bag. SYN endosac.

en·do·ba·si·on (en′dō-bā′sē-on). A cephalometric and craniometric point located in the midline at the most posterior point of the anterior border of the foramen magnum on the contour of the foramen; it is slightly posterior and internal to basion.

en·do·bi·ot·ic (en-dō-bī-ot′ik). Living as a parasite within the host.

en·do·bron·chi·al (en-dō-brong′kē-ăl). SYN intrabronchial.

en·do·car·di·ac, en·do·car·di·al (en-dō-kar′dē-ak, -dē-ăl). **1.** SYN intracardiac. **2.** Relating to the endocardium.

en·do·car·di·og·ra·phy (en′dō-kar-dē-og′ră-fē). Electrocardiography with the exploring electrode within the chambers of the heart. SEE ALSO intracardiac *catheter.*

en·do·car·dit·ic (en′dō-kar-dit′ik). Relating to endocarditis.

en·do·car·di·tis (en′dō-kar-dī′tis). Inflammation of the endocardium. SYN encarditis.

abacterial thrombotic e., SYN nonbacterial thrombotic e.

acute bacterial e., a type of severe bacterial endocarditis caused by pyogenic organisms such as hemolytic streptococci or staphylococci.

atypical verrucous e., SYN Libman-Sacks e.

bacterial e., e. caused by the direct invasion of bacteria and leading to deformity and destruction of the valve leaflets. Two types are acute bacterial endocarditis and subacute bacterial endocarditis.

cachectic e., SYN nonbacterial thrombotic e.

e. chorda′lis, e. affecting particularly the chordae tendineae.

constrictive e., thickening of the endocardium due to inflammation of any origin that restricts the diastolic relaxation of one or both ventricles producing diastolic ventricular failure, e.g., Löffler fibroplastic e.

infectious e., infective e., e. due to infection by microorganisms.

isolated parietal e., fibrous thickening of the endocardium of the left ventricle without valvular involvement.

Libman-Sacks e., verrucous e. sometimes associated with disseminated lupus erythematosus. SYN atypical verrucous e., Libman-Sacks syndrome, nonbacterial verrucous e.

Löffler e., fibroplastic constrictive parietal e. with eosinophilia, an e. of obscure cause characterized by progressive congestive heart failure, multiple systemic emboli, and eosinophilia. SYN Löffler disease, Löffler syndrome (2).

Löffler parietal fibroplastic e., sclerosis of the endocardium in the presence of a high eosinophile count.

malignant e., acute bacterial e., usually secondary to suppuration elsewhere and running a fulminating course. SYN septic e.

marantic e., nonbacterial thrombotic e. associated with cancer and other debilitating diseases. Cf. terminal e.

mural e., inflammation of the endocardium involving the walls of the chambers of the heart.

mycotic e., e. due to infection by fungi.

nonbacterial thrombotic e., verrucous endocardial lesions occurring in the terminal stages of many chronic infectious and wasting diseases. SYN abacterial thrombotic e., cachectic e., terminal e., thromboendocarditis.

nonbacterial verrucous e., SYN Libman-Sacks e.

polypous e., bacterial e. with the formation of pedunculated masses of fibrin, or thrombi, attached to the ulcerated valves.

rheumatic e., endocardial involvement as part of rheumatic heart disease, recognized clinically by valvular involvement; in the acute stage, there may be tiny fibrin vegetations along the lines of closure of the valve leaflets, with subsequent fibrous thickening and shortening of the leaflets.

septic e., SYN malignant e.

subacute bacterial e. (SBE), e. of less acuity than acute bacterial e.

terminal e., SYN nonbacterial thrombotic e.

valvular e., inflammation confined to the endocardium of the valves.

▣ **vegetative e., verrucous e.,** e. associated with the presence of fibrinous clots (vegetations) forming on the ulcerated surfaces of the valves.

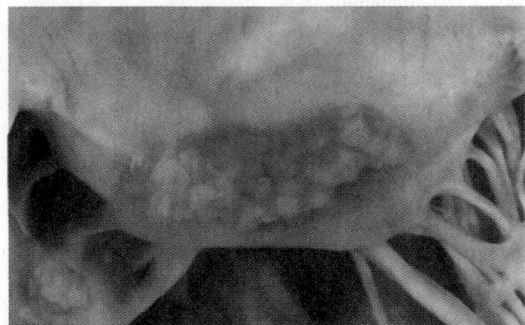

vegetative endocarditis: (shown here on the mitral valve)

en·do·car·di·um, pl. **en·do·car·dia** (en-dō-kar′dē-ŭm, -ē-ă) [TA]. The innermost tunic of the heart, which includes endothelium and subendothelial connective tissue; in the atrial wall, smooth muscle and numerous elastic fibers also occur. [endo- + G. *kardia*, heart]

en·do·ce·li·ac (en-dō-sē′lē-ak). Within one of the body cavities. [endo- + G. *koilia*, cavity, ventricle]

en·do·cer·vi·cal (en′dō-ser′vi-kăl). 1. Within any cervix, specifically within the cervix of the uterus. SYN intracervical. 2. Relating to the endocervix.

en·do·cer·vi·ci·tis (en′dō-ser-vi-sī′tis). Inflammation of the columnar epithelium cervix uteri.

en·do·cer·vix (en-dō-ser′viks). The mucous membrane of the cervical canal.

en·do·chon·dral (en-dō-kon′drăl). SYN intracartilaginous. [endo- + G. *chondros*, cartilage]

en·do·co·ag·u·la·tion (en-dō-kō-ag-oo-lā′shun). SYN thermocoagulation.

en·do·co·li·tis (en′dō-kō-lī′tis). Simple catarrhal inflammation of the colon.

en·do·cra·ni·al (en-dō-krā′nē-ăl). 1. Within the cranium. 2. Relating to the endocranium. SYN encranial, entocranial.

en·do·cra·ni·um (en′dō-krā′nē-ŭm). The lining membrane of the cranium, or dura mater of the brain. SYN entocranium.

▣ **en·do·crine** (en′dō-krin). 1. Secreting internally, most commonly into the systemic circulation; of or pertaining to such secretion. Cf. paracrine. 2. The internal or hormonal secretion of a ductless gland. 3. Denoting a gland that furnishes an internal secretion. [endo- + G. *krinō*, to separate]

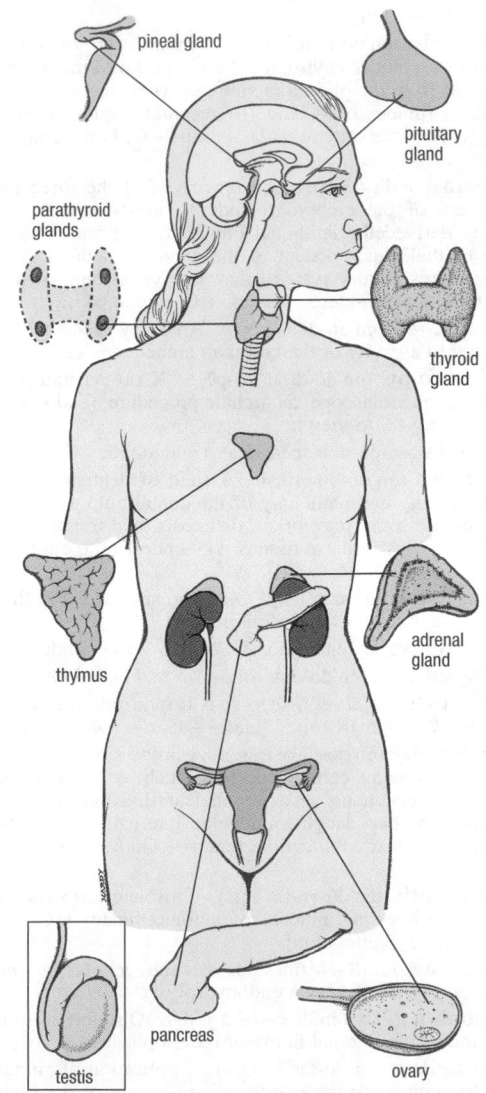

endocrine system: showing various endocrine organs

en·do·cri·nol·o·gist (en′dō-kri-nol′ō-jist). One who specializes in endocrinology.

en·do·cri·nol·o·gy (en'dō-kri-nol'ō-jē). The science and medical specialty concerned with the internal or hormonal secretions and their physiologic and pathologic relations. [endocrine + G. *logos*, study]

en·do·cri·no·ma (en'dō-kri-nō'mă). Obsolete term for a tumor with endocrine tissue that retains the function of the parent organ, usually to an excessive degree.

en·do·crin·o·path·ic (en'dō-kri-nō-path'ik). Relating to or suffering from an endocrinopathy.

en·do·cri·nop·a·thy (en'dō-kri-nop'ă-thē). A disorder in the function of an endocrine gland and the consequences thereof. [endocrine + G. *pathos*, disease]

en·do·cri·no·ther·a·py (en'dō-kri-nō-thār'ă-pē). Treatment of disease by the administration of extracts of endocrine glands. [endocrine + G. *therapeia*, medical treatment]

en·do·cy·clic (en-dō-sī'klik, -sik'lik). Within a cycle or ring; e.g., the six carbon atoms of the benzene ring in toluene. Cf. exocyclic.

en·do·cyst (en'dō-sist). The inner layer of a hydatid cyst.

en·do·cys·ti·tis (en'dō-sis-tī'tis). Obsolete term for inflammation of the epithelial lining of the bladder. [endo- + G. *kystis*, bladder, + *-itis*, inflammation]

en·do·cy·to·sis (en'dō-sī-tō'sis). Internalization of substances from the extracellular environment through the formation of vesicles formed from the plasma membrane. There are two forms: (a) fluid phase (pinocytosis), and (b) receptor mediated. SEE ALSO phagocytosis. Cf. exocytosis (2). [endo- + G. *kytos*, cell, + *-osis*, condition]

en·do·derm (en'dō-derm). The innermost of the three primary germ layers of the embryo (ectoderm, mesoderm, endoderm); from it is derived the epithelial lining of the primitive gut tract and the epithelial component of the glands and other structures (e.g., lower respiratory system) that develop as outgrowths from the gut tube. SYN entoderm. [endo- + G. *derma*, skin]

en·do·di·a·scope (en'dō-dī'ă-skōp). An x-ray tube that may be placed within a cavity of the body; an archaic device.

en·do·di·as·co·py (en'dō-dī-as'kŏ-pē). X-ray visualization by means of an endodiascope; an archaic procedure. [endo- + G. *dia*, through, + *skopeō*, to view]

en·do·don·tia (en-dō-don'shē-ă). SYN endodontics.

en·do·don·tics (en-dō-don'tiks). A field of dentistry concerned with the biology and pathology of the dental pulp and periapical tissues, and with the prevention, diagnosis, and treatment of diseases and injuries in these tissues. SYN endodontia, endodontology. [endo- + G. *odous*, tooth]

en·do·don·tist (en-dō-don'tist). One who specializes in the practice of endodontics. SYN endodontologist.

en·do·don·tol·o·gist (en'dō-don-tol'ō-jist). SYN endodontist.

en·do·don·tol·o·gy (en'do-don-tol'ō-jē). SYN endodontics.

en·do·dy·o·cyte (en'dō-dī'ō-sīt). **1.** A trophozoite formed by endodyogeny. **2.** SYN merozoite. [endo- + G. *dys*, two, + *kytos*, cell]

en·do·dy·og·e·ny (en'dō-dī-oj'ě-nē). A process of asexual development seen among certain coccidia, such as *Toxoplasma* and *Frenkelia*, in which no separate nuclear division occurs, as in schizogony; the two daughters develop internally within the parent, without nuclear conjugation. [endo- + G. *dys*, two, + *genesis*, creation]

en·do·en·ter·i·tis (en'dō-en-ter-ī'tis). Obsolete term for inflammation of the intestinal mucous membrane. [endo- + G. *enteron*, intestine, *-itis*, inflammation]

en·do·en·zyme (en-dō-en'zīm). **1.** SYN intracellular *enzyme*. **2.** An enzyme that catalyzes an endohydrolysis.

en·do·e·soph·a·gi·tis (en'dō-ē-sof-ă-jī'tis). Obsolete term for inflammation of the internal lining of the esophagus.

en·do·far·a·dism (en-dō-far'ă-dizm). Application of an alternating electric current to the interior of any cavity of the body. SEE fulguration.

en·do·gal·va·nism (en-dō-gal'van-izm). Application of a direct electric current to the interior of any cavity of the body. SEE fulguration.

en·dog·a·my (en-dog'ă-mē). Reproduction by conjugation between sister cells, the descendants of one original cell. [endo- + G. *gamos*, marriage]

en·do·gas·tric (en-dō-gas'trik). Within the stomach.

en·do·gas·tri·tis (en'dō-gas-trī'tis). Obsolete term for inflammation of the mucous membrane of the stomach. [endo- + G. *gastēr*, stomach, + *-itis*, inflammation]

en·do·gen·ic (en-dō-jen'ik). SYN endogenous.

en·do·ge·note (en-dō-jē'nōt). In microbial genetics, the recipient cell's genome. [endo- + genote]

en·dog·e·nous (en-doj'ě-nŭs). Originating or produced within the organism or one of its parts. SYN endogenic. [endo- + G. *-gen*, production]

endo·glin (en'dō-glin). A protein on the surface of endothelial cells that binds to transforming growth factor-β.

en·do·gnath·i·on (en-dog-nath'ē-on, en-dō-nā'thē-on). The medial of the two segments constituting the incisive bone. SEE mesognathion. [endo- + G. *gnathos*, jaw]

en·do·her·ni·ot·o·my (en'dō-her-nē-ot'ō-mē). An obsolete procedure for closure, by sutures, of the interior lining of a hernial sac.

en·do·in·tox·i·ca·tion (en'dō-in-tok-si-kā'shŭn). Poisoning by an endogenous toxin.

en·do·la·ryn·ge·al (en'dō-lă-rin'jē-ăl). Within the larynx.

En·do·li·max (en-dō-lī'maks). A genus of small nonpathogenic amebae parasitic in the large intestine of humans and other animals. [endo- + G. *leimax*, a meadow or garden]

en·do·lith (en'dō-lith). A calcified body found in the pulp chamber of a tooth; may be composed of irregular dentin (true denticle) or due to ectopic calcification of pulp tissue (false denticle). SYN denticle (1), pulp calcification, pulp calculus, pulp nodule, pulp stone. [endo- + G. *lithos*, stone]

en·do·lymph (en'dō-limf) [TA]. The fluid contained within the membranous labyrinth of the inner ear; endolymph resembles intracellular fluid in composition (potassium is the main positively-charged ion). SYN endolympha [TA], Scarpa fluid, Scarpa liquor.

en·do·lym·pha (en'dō-lim'fă) [TA]. SYN endolymph. [endo- + L. *lympha*, a clear fluid]

en·do·lym·phic (en-dō-lim'fik). Relating to the endolymph.

en·do·me·rog·o·ny (en'dō-me-rog'ō-nē). Production of merozoites in the asexual reproduction of sporozoan protozoa by a process originating in the interior of the schizont (as contrasted with ectomerogony); observed in species of *Eimeria*. [endo- + G. *meros*, part, + *gonē*, generation]

en·do·me·tria (en-dō-mē'trē-ă). Plural of endometrium.

en·do·me·tri·al (en-dō-mē'trē-ăl). Relating to or composed of endometrium.

en·do·me·tri·oid (en-dō-mē'trē-oyd). Microscopically resembling endometrial tissue.

en·do·me·tri·o·ma (en-dō-mē-trē-ō'mă). Circumscribed mass of ectopic endometrial tissue in endometriosis. [endometrium + *-oma*, tumor]

en·do·me·tri·o·sis (en'dō-mē-trē-ō'sis). Ectopic occurrence of endometrial tissue, frequently forming cysts containing altered blood. SYN endometrial implants. [endometrium + *-osis*, condition]

en·do·me·tri·tis (en'dō-mē-trī'tis). Inflammation of the endometrium. [endometrium + *-itis*, inflammation]

  decidual e., inflammation of the decidual mucous membrane of the gravid uterus.

  e. dis'secans, e. with ulceration and exfoliation of the mucous membrane.

en·do·me·tri·um, pl. **en·do·me·tria** (en'dō-mē'trē-ŭm, -trē-ă) [TA]. The mucous membrane comprising the inner layer of the uterine wall; it consists of a simple columnar epithelium and a lamina propria that contains simple tubular uterine glands. The structure, thickness, and state of the endometrium undergo marked change with the menstrual cycle. SYN tunica mucosa uteri [TA]. [endo- + G. *mētra*, uterus]

  Swiss cheese e., SYN simple endometrial *hyperplasia*.

en·do·me·tro·pic (en′dō-mē-trop′ik). Denoting an external stimulus capable of producing a response of the uterus, specifically the endometrium. [endo- + G. *mētra,* uterus, + *tropē,* a turning]

en·do·mi·to·sis (en′dō-mī-tō′sis). SYN endopolyploidy.

en·do·morph (en′dō-mōrf). A constitutional body type or build (biotype or somatotype) in which tissues that originated in the endoderm prevail; from a morphological standpoint, the trunk predominates over the limbs. SYN brachytype. [endo- + G. *morphē,* form]

en·do·mor·phic (en′dō-mōr′fik). Relating to, or having the characteristics of, an endomorph.

en·do·mo·tor·sonde (en′dō-mō′tŏr-sond′). Radiotelemetering capsule for studying the interior of the gastrointestinal tract. [endo- + L. *motor,* mover, + Fr. *sonde,* sounding line]

En·do·my·ce·ta·les (en′dō-mī-sē-tā′lēz). An order of Ascomycota that includes the yeasts. SYN Saccharomycetales.

en·do·my·o·car·di·al (en′dō-mī-ō-kar′dē-ăl). Relating to the endocardium and the myocardium.

en·do·my·o·car·di·tis (en-dō-mī′ō-kar-dī′tis). Inflammation of both endocardium and myocardium; endemic in East Africa.

en·do·my·o·me·tri·tis (en′dō-mī-ō-mē-trī′tis). Sepsis involving the tissues of the uterus. [endo- + G. *mys,* muscle, + *mētra,* uterus, + *-itis,* inflammation]

en·do·mys·i·um (en′dō-miz′ē-ŭm, -mis′ē-ŭm) [TA]. The fine connective tissue sheath surrounding a muscle fiber. [endo- + G. *mys,* muscle]

en·do·neu·ri·um (en-dō-noo′rē-ŭm) [TA]. The innermost connective tissue supportive structure of nerve trunks, that surrounds both myelinated and unmyelinated nerve fibers; consists principally of ground substance, collagen, and fibroblasts; with the perineurium and epineurium, comprises the peripheral nerve stroma. SYN Henle sheath, sheath of Key and Retzius. [endo- + G. *neuron,* nerve]

en·do·nu·cle·ase (en-dō-noo′klē-ās). An enzyme (phosphodiesterase) that cleaves the internal phosphodiester bonds in a DNA molecule, thus producing DNA fragments of varying size. Cf. exonuclease.

micrococcal e., an enzyme, produced by a member of the genus *Micrococcus,* that cleaves nucleic acids to oligonucleotides terminating in 3′-phosphates. SYN micrococcal nuclease, spleen e., spleen phosphodiesterases.

nucleate e., SYN endonuclease *Serratia marcescens.*

restriction e., one of many e.'s isolated from bacteria that cleave or hydrolyze (cut) foreign double-stranded DNA chains at specific recognition sites defined by DNA sequences; these e.'s have become standard laboratory devices for making specific cuts in DNA as a first step in deducing sequences and are sometimes referred to as a "chemical knife"; usually named by a three- or four-letter abbreviation of the name of the organism from which isolated (e.g., EcoB from *Escherichia coli,* strain B). SYN restriction enzyme.

single-stranded nucleate e., endonuclease S₁ *Aspergillus.*

spleen e., SYN micrococcal e.

en·do·nu·cle·ase S₁ As·per·gil·lus. An enzyme cleaving RNA or DNA to 5′-ended mono- or oligonucleotides; prefers single-stranded polynucleic acids. SYN deoxyribonuclease S₁.

en·do·nu·cle·ase Ser·ra·tia mar·ces·cens. A nuclease (a nucleate oligonucleotidohydrolase) that forms oligonucleotides ending in 5′-phosphates from RNA and DNA; hydrolyzes both double-stranded and single-stranded polynucleic acids. SYN nucleate endonuclease.

en·do·nu·cle·o·lus (en′dō-noo-klē′ō-lŭs). A minute unstainable spot near the center of a nucleolus.

en·do·par·a·site (en-dō-par′ă-sīt). A parasite living within the body of its host.

en·do·pep·ti·dase (en-dō-pep′ti-dās). An enzyme catalyzing the hydrolysis of a peptide chain at points well within the chain, not near termini; e.g., pepsin, trypsin. Cf. exopeptidase. SYN proteinase.

en·do·per·i·ar·te·ri·tis (en′dō-pār′i-ar-ter-ī′tis). SYN panarteritis. [endo- + G. *peri,* around, + arteritis]

en·do·per·i·car·di·ac (en′dō-pār-ē-kar′dē-ak). SYN intrapericardiac.

en·do·per·i·my·o·car·di·tis (en′dō-pār′i-mī′ō-kar-dī′tis). Simultaneous inflammation of the heart muscle and of the endocardium and pericardium. SYN pancarditis. [endo- + G. *peri,* around, + *mys,* muscle, + *kardia,* heart, + *-itis,* inflammation]

en·do·per·i·to·ni·tis (en′dō-pār′i-tō-nī′tis). Superficial inflammation of the peritoneum.

en·do·per·ox·ide (en′dō-per-ok′sīd). A peroxide (–O–O–) group that bridges two atoms that are both parts of a larger molecule.

en·do·phle·bi·tis (en′dō-fle-bī′tis). Inflammation of the intima of a vein. [endo- + G. *phleps (phleb-),* vein, + *-itis,* inflammation]

en·doph·thal·mi·tis (en-dof-thal-mī′tis). Inflammation of the tissues within the eyeball. [endo- + G. *ophthalmos,* eye, + *-itis,* inflammation]

granulomatous e., a diffuse, chronic inflammation of intraocular tissues.

e. ophthal′mia nodo′sa, e. due to intraocular caterpillar hairs. SEE *ophthalmia nodosa.*

e. phacoanaphylac′tica, inflammation of the uveal tract as a result of sensitization by the lens cortex; simulates sympathetic ophthalmia.

en·doph·thal·mo·do·nes·is (en′dof-thal-mō-dō-nē′sis). Tremulousness of any intraocular structure, especially of an implanted lens (pseudophakodonesis). [endo- + ophthalmo- + G. *doneō,* to shake]

en·do·phyte (en′dō-fīt). A plant parasite living within another organism. [endo- + G. *phyton,* plant]

en·do·phyt·ic (en-dō-fit′ik). **1.** Pertaining to an endophyte. **2.** Referring to an infiltrative, invasive tumor.

en·do·plasm (en′dō-plazm). The inner or medullary part of the cytoplasm, as opposed to the ectoplasm, containing the cell organelles. SYN entoplasm.

en·do·plas·mic (en′dō-plas′mik). Referring to the endoplasm.

en·do·plast (en′dō-plast). Former name for endosome. [endo- + G. *plastos,* formed]

en·do·plas·tic (en-dō-plas′tik). Relating to the endoplasm.

en·do·po·lyg·e·ny (en′dō-pō-lij′ĕ-nē). Asexual reproduction in which more than two offspring are formed within the parent organism and in which two or possibly more nuclear divisions occur before merozoite formation begins; a form of internal budding observed in *Toxoplasma gondii.* Cf. endodyogeny. [endo- + G. *polys,* many, + *genesis,* creation]

en·do·pol·y·ploid (en-dō-pol′ē-ployd). Relating to endopolyploidy.

en·do·pol·y·ploi·dy (en-dō-pol′ē-ploy-dē). The process or state of duplication of the DNA content of the nuclei without accompanying spindle formation or cytokinesis, resulting in a polyploid nucleus. SYN endomitosis. [endo- + polyploidy]

en·do·re·du·pli·ca·tion (en′dō-rē-doo′pli-kā′shŭn). A form of polyploidy or polysomy by redoubling of chromosomes, giving rise to four-stranded chromosomes at prophase and metaphase.

en·dor·phin·er·gic (en′dōr-fin-er′jik). Relating to nerve cells or fibers that employ an endorphin as their neurotransmitter. [endorphin + G. *ergon,* work]

en·dor·phins (en′dōr-finz). Opioid peptides originally isolated from the brain but now found in many parts of the body; in the nervous system, e.'s bind to the same receptors that bind exogenous opiates. A variety of e.'s (e.g., α, β, and γ) that vary not only in their physical and chemical properties but also in physiologic action have been isolated. SEE ALSO enkephalins. [fr. *endogenous morphine*]

en·dor·rha·chis (en-dō-rā′kis). SYN spinal *dura mater.* [endo- + G. *rhachis,* the spine]

en·do·sac (en′dō-sak). A sac or bag used in laparoscopic surgery in which tissue is placed to facilitate removal or morcellation. SYN endobag.

en·do·sal·pin·gi·o·sis (en′dō-sal-pin-jē-ō′sis). Aberrant mucous membrane in the ovary or elsewhere consisting of ciliated tubal mucosa without stroma of endometrial type.

en

en·do·sal·pin·gi·tis (en'dō-sal-pin-jī'tis). Inflammation of the lining membrane of the eustachian or the fallopian tube. [endo- + G. *salpinx* (*salping-*), tube, + *-itis,* inflammation]

en·do·sal·pinx (en'dō-sal'pinks). The mucosa of the fallopian tube. [endo + G. *salpinx,* tube]

en·do·sarc (en'dō-sark). The endoplasm of a protozoan. SYN entosarc. [endo- + G. *sarx* (*sark-*), flesh]

en·do·scope (en'dō-skōp). An instrument for the examination of the interior of a canal or hollow viscus. [endo- + G. *skopeō,* to examine]

flexible e., an optical instrument that transmits light and carries images back to the observer through a flexible bundle of small (about 10 μm) transparent fibers. It is used to inspect interior portions of the body. These instruments are generally equipped with mechanisms for steering and may have additional ports for allowing sampling and/or operative instruments along their axis to the internal site. SEE ALSO fiberoptics. SYN fiberscope.

en·dos·co·pist (en-dos'kŏ-pist). A specialist trained in the use of an endoscope.

en·dos·co·py (en-dos'kŏ-pē). Examination of the interior of a canal or hollow viscus by means of a special instrument, such as an endoscope. [see endoscope]

peroral e., visual examination of interior sections of the body by introduction of an instrument (an endoscope) through the mouth; examples include esophagoscopy, gastroscopy, bronchoscopy.

virtual e., computed tomographic data reconstructed in 3 dimensions to give information similar to that obtained with endoscopy.

en·do·skel·e·ton (en-dō-skel'ĕ-tŏn). The internal bony framework of the body; the skeleton in its usual context as distinguished from exoskeleton.

en·do·some (en'dō-sōm). A more or less central body in the vesicular nucleus of certain Feulgen-negative (DNA-) protozoa (e.g., trypanosomes, parasitic amebae, and phytoflagellates), with the chromatin (DNA₊) lying between the nuclear membrane and the e. Cf. nucleolus. [endo- + G. *sōma,* body]

en·do·son·og·ra·phy (en'dō-sō-nog'ră-fē). Ultrasonography performed using an ultrasound transducer mounted on or passed through a fiberoptic endoscope.

en·do·so·nos·co·py (en-dō-son'ŏ-skŏ-pē). A sonographic study carried out by transducers inserted into the body as miniature probes in the esophagus, urethra, bladder, vagina, or rectum.

en·do·sperm (en'dō-sperm). A storage tissue found in many seeds that nourishes the embryo of a plant.

en·do·spore (en'dō-spōr). **1.** A resistant body formed within the vegetative cells of some bacteria, particularly those belonging to the genera *Bacillus* and *Clostridium.* **2.** A fungus spore borne within a cell or within the tubular end of a sporophore as in the spherule of *Coccidioides immitis.* [endo- + G. *sporos,* seed]

en·dos·te·al (en-dos'tē-ăl). Relating to the endosteum.

en·dos·te·i·tis, en·dos·ti·tis (en'dos-tē-ī'tis, en'dos-tī'tis). Inflammation of the endosteum or of the medullary cavity of a bone. SYN central osteitis (2), perimyelitis. [endo- + G. *osteon,* bone, + *-itis,* inflammation]

en·dos·te·o·ma (en-dos'tē-ō'mă). A benign neoplasm of bone tissue in the medullary cavity of a bone. SYN endostoma. [endo- + G. *osteon,* bone, + *-ōma,* tumor]

en·do·steth·o·scope (en-dō-steth'ō-skōp). A stethoscopic tube used in endoauscultation. [endo- + G. *stēthos,* chest, + *skopeō,* to examine]

en·dos·te·um (en-dos'tē-ŭm) [TA]. A layer of cells lining the inner surface of bone in the central medullary cavity. SYN medullary membrane, perimyelis. [endo- + G. *osteon,* bone]

en·dos·to·ma (en-dō-stō'mă). SYN endosteoma.

en·do·ten·din·e·um (en'dō-ten-din'ē-ŭm). The fine connective tissue surrounding secondary fascicles of a tendon. [endo- + L. *tendon,* tendon, + *-eus,* adj.; the whole, in its neuter form, used substantively]

en·do·the·li·a (en-dō-thē'lē-ă). Plural of endothelium.

en·do·the·li·al (en-dō-thē'lē-ăl). Relating to the endothelium.

en·do·the·lin. A 21-amino acid peptide originally derived from endothelial cells. It is an extremely potent vasoconstrictor. Three different gene products have been identified, endothelin 1, endothelin 2, and endothelin 3; they are found in brain, kidney, and endothelium (endothelin 1), intestine (endothelin 2), and intestine and adrenal gland (endothelin 3).

en·do·the·li·o·cyte (en-dō-thē'lē-ō-sīt). SYN endothelial *cell.*

en·do·the·li·oid (en-dō-thē'lē-oyd). Resembling endothelium.

en·do·the·li·o·ma (en'dō-thē-lē-ō'mă). Generic term for a group of neoplasms, particularly benign tumors, derived from the endothelial tissue of blood vessels or lymphatic channels; e.'s may be benign or malignant. [endothelium + *-oma,* tumor]

en·do·the·li·o·sis (en'dō-thē-lē-ō'sis). Proliferation of endothelium.

en·do·the·li·um, pl. **en·do·the·li·a** (en-dō-thē'lē-ŭm, -lē-ă) [TA]. A layer of flat cells lining especially blood and lymphatic vessels and the heart. [endo- + G. *thēlē,* nipple]

e. of anterior chamber [TA], a single layer of large, squamous cells that covers the posterior surface of the cornea. SYN e. posterius corneae [TA], e. camerae anterioris.

e. cam'erae anterio'ris, SYN e. of anterior chamber.

e. posterius corneae [TA], SYN e. of anterior chamber.

en·do·ther·mic (en-dō-ther'mik). Denoting a chemical reaction during which heat (enthalpy) is absorbed. Cf. exothermic (1). [endo- + G. *thermē,* heat]

en·do·thrix (en'dō-thriks). Fungal spores (conidia) invading the interior of a hair shaft; there is no conspicuous external sheath of spores, as there is with ectothrix. [endo- + G. *thrix,* hair]

en·do·tox·e·mia (en'dō-tok-sē'mē-ă). Presence in the blood of endotoxins, which, if derived from Gram-negative rod-shaped bacteria, may cause a generalized Shwartzman phenomenon with shock.

en·do·tox·ic (en-dō-tok'sik). Denoting an endotoxin.

en·do·tox·i·co·sis (en'dō-tok-si-kō'sis). Poisoning by an endotoxin.

en·do·tox·in (en-dō-tok'sin). **1.** A bacterial toxin not freely liberated into the surrounding medium, in contrast to exotoxin. **2.** The complex phospholipid-polysaccharide macromolecules that form an integral part of the cell wall of a variety of relatively avirulent as well as virulent strains of Gram-negative bacteria. The toxins are relatively heat-stable, are less potent than most exotoxins, are less specific, and do not form toxoids; on injection, they may cause a state of shock and, in smaller doses, fever and leukopenia followed by leukocytosis; they have the capacity of eliciting the Shwartzman and the Sanarelli-Shwartzman phenomena. SYN intracellular toxin.

en·do·tra·che·al (en'dō-trā'kē-ăl). Within the trachea.

en·do·u·rol·o·gy (en-dō-ūr-ol'ō-jē). Genitourinary operative procedures (diagnostic and therapeutic) performed through instruments. These may be cystoscopic, pelviscopic, celioscopic, laparoscopic, percutaneous, or ureteroscopic.

en·do·vac·ci·na·tion (en'dō-vak-si-nā'shŭn). Oral administration of vaccines.

en·do·vas·cu·li·tis (en'dō-vas'kū-lī'tis). SYN endangiitis.

hemorrhagic e., endothelial and medial hyperplasia of placental blood vessels with thrombosis, fragmentation, and diapedesis of red blood cells resulting in stillbirth or fetal developmental disorders.

en·do·ve·nous (en-dō-vē'nŭs). SYN intravenous.

end-piece. The terminal part of the tail of a spermatozoon consisting of the axoneme and the flagellar membrane.

end·plate, end-plate (end'plāt). The ending of a motor nerve fiber in relation to a skeletal muscle fiber.

motor e., the large and complex end-formation by which the axon of a motor neuron establishes synaptic contact with a striated muscle fiber (cell); several terminal branches of a motor axon end in irregular, club-shaped synaptic end-formations that are bedded in a single troughlike depression of the muscle fiber's surface; the postsynaptic membrane, the sarcolemma that forms the bottom of the trough, is greatly increased in surface area by deep infoldings protruding into the underlying cytoplasm of the muscle fiber; the subsynaptic interval between the plasma membrane of the axon terminals and the sarcolemma is filled with an amorphous substance; the trough is closed off toward the surface by the Schwann sheath, which peels away from the axons as the latter enter the trough and thus forms a lid over the trough; the slight bulge of this closure plate corresponds to Doyère eminence. SYN sole-plate ending.

end·tid·al (end-tī′dăl). At the end of a normal expiration.

en·dy·ma (en′di-mă). SYN ependyma. [G. a garment]

E.N.E. Abbreviation for ethylnorepinephrine.

⌂-ene. Suffix applied to a chemical name indicating the presence of a carbon-carbon double bond; e.g., propene (unsaturated propane, $CH_3–CH=CH_2$). [G. ēnē, feminine adjectival suffix]

ene·di·ol (ēn-dī′ōl). The atomic arrangement $–C(OH)=C(OH)–$ produced by proton migration from the CH of a –CHOH group that is attached to a –CO– group to the oxygen of the –CO– group (usually induced by alkali), giving rise to doubly bonded carbon atoms (the -ene group), each bearing a –CHOH group (a diol); a special case of enolization.

en·e·ma (en′ĕ-mă). A rectal injection for clearing out the bowel, or administering drugs or food. [G.]

    air contrast e., a radiographic double contrast e. in which air is introduced after coating of the colon with a dense barium suspension. SYN air contrast barium e., double contrast e.

    air contrast barium e., SYN air contrast e.

    analeptic e., an e. of a pint of lukewarm water with one-half teaspoonful of table salt.

    barium e., a type of contrast enema; administration of barium sulfate suspension, a radiopaque medium, for radiographic and fluoroscopic study of the lower intestinal tract.

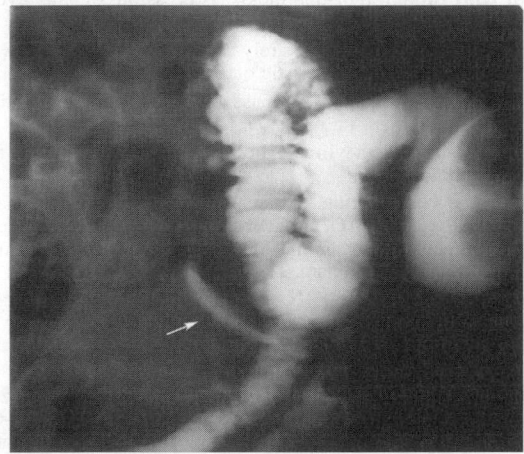

barium enema: radiograph of colon showing ruptured diverticulum (arrow)

    blind e., the introduction into the rectum of a rubber tube to facilitate the expulsion of flatus.

    contrast e., e. using barium sulfate or a water-soluble contrast medium.

    double contrast e., SYN air contrast e.

    flatus e., an e. of magnesium sulfate in glycerin and warm water.

    high e., an e. instilled high up into the colon. SYN enteroclysis (1).

    Hypaque e., e. with water-soluble radiographic contrast material, whether diatrizoate or other.

    nutrient e., a rectal injection of predigested food.

    oil retention e., a rectal injection of mineral oil, introduced at low pressure and retained for several hours before expelling, to soften feces.

    small bowel e., radiographic examination of the small intestine, by retrograde filling from the contrast-filled large bowel. Cf. enteroclysis, small bowel *series.*

    soapsuds e., an e. of shredded or powdered soap in warm water.

    turpentine e., an e. of turpentine and olive oil in soapsuds.

en·e·ma·tor (en-ĕ-mā′ter, -tōr). An appliance used to give an enema.

en·e·mi·a·sis (en-ĕ-mī′ă-sis). The use of enemas.

en·er·get·ics (en-er-jet′iks). The study of the energy changes involved in physical and chemical reactions and in overall systems.

en·er·gy (en′er-jē). The exertion of power; the capacity to do work, taking the forms of kinetic e., potential e., chemical e., electrical e., etc. SYN dynamic force. [G. energeia, fr. en, in, + ergon, work]

    e. of activation (E_a)**,** e. that must be added to that already possessed by a molecule or molecules in order to initiate a reaction; usually expressed in the Arrhenius equation relating a rate constant to absolute temperature.

    binding e., e. that would be released if a particular atomic nucleus were formed through the combination of individual protons and neutrons. SYN fusion e.

    chemical e., e. liberated or absorbed by a chemical reaction, e.g., oxidation of carbon, or absorbed in the formation of a chemical compound.

    free e. (F)**,** a thermodynamic function symbolized as F, or G (Gibbs free e.), $= H – TS$, where H is the enthalpy of a system, T the absolute temperature, and S the entropy; chemical reactions proceed spontaneously in the direction that involves a net decrease in the free e. of the system (i.e., $\Delta G < 0$).

    fusion e., SYN binding e.

    Gibbs e. of activation, the Gibbs e. that must be added to that already possessed by a molecule or molecules in order to initiate a reaction.

    Gibbs free e. (G)**,** SEE free e.

    Helmholtz e. (A)**,** e. equivalent to the internal energy minus the entropy contribution (TS).

    internal e. (U)**,** e. of a system measured by the heat absorbed from the system's surroundings and the amount of work done on the system by its surroundings.

    kinetic e. (K)**,** the e. of motion.

    latent e., SYN potential e.

    nuclear e., e. given off in the course of a nuclear reaction or stored in the formation of an atomic nucleus.

    nutritional e., SYN trophodynamics.

    e. of position, SYN potential e.

    potential e., the e., existing in a body by virtue of its position or state of existence, which is not being exerted at the time. SYN e. of position, latent e.

    psychic e., in psychoanalysis, a hypothetical mental force, analogous to the physical concept of e., which enables and vitalizes an individual's psychological activity. SEE ALSO libido. SYN psychic force.

    radiant e., e. contained in light rays or any other form of radiation.

    solar e., e. derived from sunlight.

    total e., the sum of kinetic and potential e.'s.

en·flu·rane (en-floor′ān). A potent volatile inhalation anesthetic that is nonflammable and nonexplosive.

ENG Abbreviation for electronystagmography.

en·gage·ment (en-gāj′ment). In obstetrics, the mechanism by which the biparietal diameter of the fetal head enters the plane of the inlet.

en·gas·tri·us (en-gas′trē-ŭs). Unequal conjoined twins in which the smaller parasite is wholly or partly within the abdomen of the larger autosite. [G. en, in, + gastēr, belly]

Engelmann, Guido, German surgeon, *1876. SEE E. *disease.*

Engelmann, Theodor W., German physiologist, 1843–1909. SEE E. basal *knobs,* under *knob.*

en·gi·neer·ing (en-jin-ēr′ing). The practical application of physical, mechanical, and mathematical principles.

    biomedical e., application of e. principles to obtain solutions to biomedical problems.

    dental e., application of e. principles to dentistry.

    genetic e., internal manipulation of basic genetic material of an

en

organism to modify biologic heredity or to produce peptides of high purity, such as hormones or antigens.

Englisch, Josef, Austrian physician, 1835–1915. SEE E. *sinus.*

en·globe (en-glōb′). To take in by a spheroidal body; said of the ingestion of bacteria and other foreign bodies by the phagocytes.

en·globe·ment (en-glōb′ment). The process of inclusion by a spheroidal body, such as by a phagocyte.

en·gorged (en-gōrjd′). Absolutely filled; distended with fluid. SEE ALSO congested, hyperemic. [O. Fr. fr. Mediev. L. *gorgia,* throat, narrow passage, fr. L. *gurges,* a whirlpool]

en·gorge·ment (en-gōrj′ment). Distention with fluid or other material. SEE ALSO congestion, hyperemia.

en·gram (en′gram). In the mnemic hypothesis, a physical change or memory trace made on the central nervous system of an organism as a result of experience or the repetition of stimuli. [G. *en,* in, + *gramma,* mark]

en·graph·ia (en-graf′ē-ă). The formation of engrams.

en grappe (ahn-grap′). Denoting the grapelike cluster arrangement of microconidia of certain dermatophytes. [Fr. *en,* in, + *grappe,* bunch of grapes]

en·hance·ment (en-hans′ment). **1.** The act of augmenting. **2.** In immunology, the prolongation of a process or event by suppressing an opposing process.

acoustic e., a manifestation of increased echo amplitude returning from regions beyond an object, such as a fluid-filled cyst, which causes little or no attenuation of the ultrasound beam. Cf. acoustic *shadow.*

contrast e., the intravenous administration of water-soluble iodinated contrast material, which increases the CT number of the vascular pool, as well as some lesions (particularly in the brain), due to abnormal leakage into the interstitium; the property of showing increased radiopacity from concentration of contrast medium.

edge e., using analogue or digital image processing to increase the contrast of each interface; equivalent to using a high-pass filter.

immunologic e., SYN immunoenhancement.

ring e., in computed tomography, when a bright circle appears on an image made after injection of contrast medium, characteristic of localization of the contrast in the wall of an abscess.

en·hanc·ers. Genetic elements important in the function of a specific promoter. [M.E. *enhauncen,* raise, increase, fr. O. Fr. *enhaucier,* fr. L.L. *inalto,* fr. *altus,* high, + *-er,* agent suffix]

en·keph·a·lin·er·gic (en-kef′ă-lin-er′jik). Relating to nerve cells or fibers that employ an enkephalin as their neurotransmitter. [enkephalin + G. *ergon,* work]

en·keph·a·lins (en-kef′ă-linz). Pentapeptide endorphins, found in many parts of the brain, that bind to specific receptor sites, some of which may be pain-related opiate receptors; hypothesized as endogenous neurotransmitters and nonaddicting analgesics. Met-enkephalin is Tyr–Gly–Gly–Phe–Met; leuenkephalin has Leu in place of Met; proenkephalin has Pro in place of Met.

en·large·ment (en-larj′ment) [TA]. **1.** An increase in size; an anatomic swelling, enlargement, or prominence. **2.** An intumescence or swelling. SYN intumescentia [TA], intumescence (1).

cervical e. [TA], a spindle-shaped swelling of the spinal cord extending from the third cervical to the second thoracic vertebra, with maximum thickness opposite the fifth or sixth cervical vertebra, consequential to the innervation of the upper limb. SYN intumescentia cervicalis [TA], cervical e. of spinal cord.

cervical e. of spinal cord, SYN cervical e.

choroid e. [TA], the enlarged portion of the choroid plexus located in the atrium of the lateral ventricle; may become partially calcified with age. SEE ALSO choroid *glomus.* SYN glomus choroideum [TA], choroid glomus, choroid skein.

gingival e., an overgrowth (localized or diffuse) of gingival tissue, nonspecific in nature. SEE ALSO gingival *hyperplasia.*

lumbosacral e. [TA], a spindle-shaped swelling of the spinal cord beginning at the level of the tenth thoracic vertebra and tapering into the medullary cone, with maximum thickness opposite the last thoracic vertebra, consequential to the innervation of the

lower limb. SYN intumescentia lumbosacralis [TA], lumbosacral e. of spinal cord.

lumbosacral e. of spinal cord, SYN lumbosacral e.

tympanic e. [TA], a swelling, not ganglionic, on the tympanic branch of the glossopharyngeus nerve; it is regarded as possibly similar to the carotid glomus. SEE ALSO tympanic *ganglion.* SYN intumescentia tympanica [TA], tympanic intumescence.

e. of the vestibular aqueduct, recessive hereditary hearing impairment associated with a large vestibular aqueduct.

△**-enoic.** Suffix indicating an unsaturated acid. [-ene + -ic]

enol (ē′nol). A compound possessing a hydroxyl group (alcohol) attached to a doubly bonded (ethylenic) carbon atom (–CH=CH-(OH)–); properly italicized when attached as a prefix or infix to an otherwise complete name; e.g., *enol* pyruvate; phospho*enol*pyruvate; usually in equilibrium with its keto tautomer. [-ene + -ol]

eno·lase (ē′nol-ās). An enzyme catalyzing the reversible dehydration of 2-phospho-D-glycerate to phospho*enol*pyruvate and water; a step in both glycolysis and gluconeogenesis; several isozymes exist; requires magnesium ion and is inhibited by F⁻. SYN phosphopyruvate hydratase.

neuron-specific e., an isoenzyme of e. present in neurons and glial cells; stains for this enzyme are frequently used in the differential diagnosis of neuronal or neuroendocrine tumors.

eno·li·za·tion (ē′nol-i-zā′shŭn). Conversion of a keto to an enol form; e.g., CH_3–CO–COOH → CH_2=C(OH)COOH.

enol py·ru·vate (ē-nol-pī′roo-vāt). CH_2=C(OH)–COO⁻, the form of pyruvate encountered in the biologically important phospho-*enol*pyruvate (*enol* pyruvate phosphate), not in the free form.

en·oph·thal·mia (en-of-thal′mē-ă). SYN enophthalmos.

en·oph·thal·mos (en′of-thal′mos). Recession of the eyeball within the orbit. SYN enophthalmia. [G. *en,* in, + *ophthalmos,* eye]

en·or·gan·ic (en-ōr-gan′ik). Rarely used term denoting that which occurs as an innate characteristic of an organism.

en·os·to·sis (en-os-tō′sis). A mass of proliferating bone tissue within a bone. [G. *en,* in, + *osteon,* bone, + *-osis,* condition]

en·o·yl (ēn′ō-il). The acyl radical of an unsaturated aliphatic acid. [-ene + -oyl]

en·o·yl-ACP re·duc·tase. An enzyme catalyzing hydrogenation of acyl-ACP (where ACP is acyl carrier protein) complexes to 2,3-dehydroacyl-ACP′s, with NAD⁺ as hydrogen acceptor; important in fatty acid metabolism. SYN crotonyl-ACP reductase.

en·o·yl-ACP re·duc·tase (NADPH). An enzyme carrying out the same reaction as enoyl-ACP (where ACP is acyl carrier protein) reductase, but with NADP⁺ as hydrogen acceptor. SYN acyl-ACP dehydrogenase, acyl-ACP reductase.

en·o·yl-CoA hy·dra·tase. Δ²-eEoyl-CoA hydratase; an enzyme catalyzing a reversible reaction between an L-3-hydroxyacyl-CoA and a 2,3- (or 3,4-) *trans*-enoyl-CoA in fatty acid degradation. SYN crotonase, enoyl hydrase.

eno·yl-CoA re·duc·tase. SYN *acyl-CoA* dehydrogenase (NADPH).

2-en·o·yl-CoA re·duc·tase. Acyl-CoA dehydrogenase (NADP⁺).

en·o·yl hy·drase. SYN enoyl-CoA hydratase.

E.N.S. Abbreviation for ethylnorepinephrine.

en·si·form (en′si-fōrm). SYN xiphoid. [L. *ensis,* sword, + *forma,* appearance]

en·sis·ter·num (en′sis-ter′nŭm). SYN xiphoid *process.* [L. *ensis,* sword, + sternum]

ensu Acronym for *e*quivalent *n*ormal *s*on *u*nit, that amount of information from any source (linkage, carrier, phenotype, etc.) that will have the same impact on the conditional probability that a female consultand is a carrier for an X-linked trait as one normal son does; each normal son contributes one ensu. Cf. encu.

ENT Abbreviation for ears, nose, and throat. SEE otorhinolaryngology.

△**ent-.** SEE ento-.

en·tac·tin (ent-ak′tin). A glycoprotein that binds to laminin and type IV collagen in the basal lamina of the renal glomerulus and is a major cell attachment factor; e. is a sulfated calcium-binding protein. SYN nidogen.

en·tad. Toward the interior. [G. *entos,* within, + L. *ad,* to]

en·tal (en'tăl). Relating to the interior; inside. [G. *entos,* within]

ent·am·e·bi·a·sis (ent-ă-mē-bī'ă-sis). Infection with *Entamoeba histolytica.* SEE amebiasis, amebic *dysentery.*

Ent·a·moe·ba (ent-ă-mē'bă). A genus of ameba parasitic in the oral cavity, cecum, and large bowel of humans and other primates and in many domestic and wild mammals and birds; with the exception of *E. histolytica,* members of the genus appear to be relatively harmless inhabitants of the host. [G. *entos,* within + *amoibē,* change]

E. bucca'lis, former name for *E. gingivalis.*

E. chattoni, a species that does not produce symptoms; most commonly found in monkeys but occasionally has been identified in humans; cysts are uninucleate.

E. co'li, nonpathogenic species of ameba that occurs in the large intestine of man, other primates, dogs, and possibly pigs; often confused with *E. histolytica,* but distinguished by nuclear details and by the number of nuclei and the form of chromatoidals in the cyst.

E. dispar, nonpathogenic species that occurs in the large intestine of humans; formerly considered *E. histolytica, E. dispar* is now considered a separate species; it is nonpathogenic and is not associated with symptomatic amebiasis in humans. Morphologically it resembles *E. histolytica;* however, the trophozoites are never found to contain ingested red blood cells.

E. gingiva'lis, a species of ameba found in the oral cavity of man, other primates, dogs, and cats; in humans, it is frequently associated with poor oral hygiene and its resultant diseases.

E. hartman'ni, a species of ameba found in the large intestine of humans, other primates, and dogs; now considered to be a distinct species that is nonpathogenic and smaller than *E. histolytica* but otherwise indistinguishable from it; formerly called the "small race" of *E. histolytica.*

i *E. histoly'tica,* a species of ameba that is the only distinct pathogen of the genus, the so-called "large race" of *E. histolytica,* causing tropical or amebic dysentery in humans and also in dogs (humans are the reservoir for canine infections). In humans, the organism may penetrate the epithelial tissues of the colon, causing ulceration (amebic dysentery); in a small proportion of these cases, the organism may reach the liver by the portal bloodstream and produce abscesses (hepatic amebiasis); in a fraction of these cases it may then spread to other organs, such as the lungs, brain, kidney, or skin and frequently be fatal. SEE ALSO *E. dispar.*

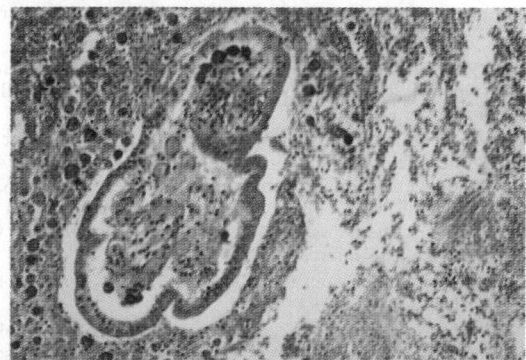

Entamoeba histolytica: many trophozoites are seen in an ulcerative colonic lesion; periodic acid–Schiff stain; × 80

E. moshkov'skii, a species of ameba very similar to *E. histolytica,* probably not infective to man, but a cause of diagnostic difficulties since it has been recovered from human sewage and may be responsible for false-positive results in tests of sewage plant effluents.

E. polecki, a species of ameba commonly found in the intestines of pigs; also parasitizes monkeys, cattle, goats, sheep and dogs;

also found in humans, where it does not produce symptoms; clinical importance lies in the possibility of confusing the organism with *E. histolytica.*

△**enter-.** SEE entero-.

en·ter·al (en'ter-ăl). Within, or by way of, the intestine or gastrointestinal tract, especially as distinguished from parenteral. [G. *enteron,* intestine]

en·ter·al·gia (en-ter-al'jē-ă). Enterdynia; severe abdominal pain accompanying spasm of the bowel. SYN enterdynia, enterodynia. [entero- + G. *algos,* pain]

en·ter·a·mine (en-ter-am'ēn). SYN serotonin.

en·ter·dy·nia (en-ter-din'ē-ă). SYN enteralgia.

en·ter·ec·ta·sis (en-ter-ek'tă-sis). Obsolete term for dilation of the bowel. [entero- + G. *ektasis,* a stretching]

en·ter·ec·to·my (en-ter-ek'tō-mē). Resection of a segment of the intestine. [entero- + G. *ektomē,* excision]

en·ter·el·co·sis (en-ter-el-kō'sis). Obsolete term for ulceration of the bowel. [entero- + G. *helkos,* ulcer]

en·ter·ic (en-ter'ik). Relating to the intestine. [G. *enterikos,* from *entera,* bowels]

en·ter·i·tis (en-ter-ī'tis). Inflammation of the intestine, especially of the small intestine. [entero- + G. *-itis,* inflammation]

e. anaphylac'tica, a hemorrhagic and necrotizing inflammation developing in the ileum (and also the colon) of sensitized dogs when they are fed a second dose of the sensitizing material. SYN chronic anaphylaxis.

chronic cicatrizing e., SYN regional e.

diphtheritic e., e. with the formation of a membrane or a false membrane. SEE ALSO pseudomembranous *enterocolitis.*

granulomatous e., SYN regional e.

human eosinophilic e., segmental eosinophilic inflammation of the gastrointestinal tract in humans; suspect etiologic agent is *Ancylostoma caninum;* laboratory indicators are eosinophilia and increased IgE.

mucomembranous e., an affection of the intestinal mucous membrane characterized by constipation or diarrhea (sometimes alternating), colic, and the passage of pseudomembranous shreds or incomplete casts of the intestine. SYN mucoenteritis (2).

e. necrot'icans, e. with necrosis of the bowel wall caused by *Clostridium welchii.*

phlegmonous e., severe acute inflammation of the intestine, with edematous bowel wall infiltrated with pus.

e. polypo'sa, e. associated with polyp formation.

pseudomembranous e., SYN pseudomembranous *enterocolitis.*

regional e., a subacute chronic e., of unknown cause, involving the terminal ileum and less frequently other parts of the gastrointestinal tract; characterized by patchy deep ulcers that may cause fistulas, and narrowing and thickening of the bowel by fibrosis and lymphocytic infiltration, with noncaseating tuberculoid granulomas that also may be found in regional lymph nodes; symptoms include fever, diarrhea, cramping abdominal pain, and weight loss. SYN chronic cicatrizing e., Crohn disease, distal ileitis, regional ileitis, terminal ileitis, granulomatous e.

tuberculous e., enteric tuberculosis may be caused by bovine tuberculosis contracted through drinking of unpasteurized milk or swallowing of tubercle bacilli expectorated from cavitary lesions in the lung; may occur in the absence of obvious pulmonary t.

△**entero-, enter-.** The intestine. [G. *enteron,* intestine]

en·ter·o·a·nas·to·mo·sis (en'ter-ō-an-as-tō-mō'sis). SYN entero-enterostomy.

en·ter·o·an·the·lone (en-ter-ō-an'thē-lōn). SYN enterogastrone.

En·ter·o·bac·ter (en'ter-ō-bak'ter). A genus of aerobic, facultatively anaerobic, nonsporeforming, motile bacteria (family Enterobacteriaceae) containing Gram-negative rods. The cells are peritrichous, and some strains have encapsulated cells. Glucose is fermented with the production of acid and gas. The Voges-Proskauer test is usually positive. Gelatin is slowly liquefied by the most commonly occurring forms (*E. cloacae*). These organisms occur in the feces of humans and other animals and in sewage, soil, water, and dairy products; recognized as an agent of common nosocomial infections of the urinary tract, lungs, or

en

blood; somewhat resistant to antibiotics. This genus characteristically acquires resistance rapidly in part because of the presence of inducible β-lactamases; the type species is *E. cloacae.*

E. aerog'enes, a bacterial species found in water, soil, sewage, dairy products, and the feces of humans and other animals. Organisms previously identified as motile strains of *Aerobacter aerogenes* are now placed in this species. SYN *Klebsiella mobilis.*

E. cloa'cae, a bacterial species found in the feces of humans and other animals and in sewage, soil, and water; it is occasionally found in urine and pus and in other pathologic materials from animals; it is the type species of the genus *E.* A serious cause of nosocomial infection.

E. sakazakii, a bacterial species especially associated with nursery-acquired neonatal meningitis.

en·ter·o·bac·te·ria (en'ter-ō-bak-tēr'ē-ă). Plural of enterobacterium.

En·ter·o·bac·te·ri·a·ce·ae (en'ter-ō-bak-tēr-ē-ā'sē-ē). A family of aerobic, facultatively anaerobic, nonsporeforming bacteria (order Eubacteriales) containing Gram-negative rods. Some species are nonmotile, and nonmotile variants of motile species occur; the motile cells are peritrichous. These organisms grow well on artificial media. They reduce nitrates to nitrites and utilize glucose fermentatively with the production of acid or acid and gas. Indophenol oxidase is not produced by these organisms. They do not liquefy alginate, and pectate is liquefied only by members of one genus, *Pectobacterium.* This family includes many animal parasites and some plant parasites causing blights, galls, and soft rots. Some of these organisms occur as saprophytes which decompose carbohydrate-containing plant materials. The type genus is *Escherichia.*

en·ter·o·bac·te·ri·um, pl. **en·ter·o·bac·te·ria** (en'ter-ō-bak-tēr' ē-ŭm, -ă). A member of the family Enterobacteriaceae.

en·ter·o·bi·a·sis (en'ter-ō-bī'ă-sis). Infection with *Enterobius vermicularis,* the human pinworm.

En·te·ro·bi·us (en-ter-ō'bī-ŭs). A genus of nematode worms, formerly included with the genus *Oxyuris,* which includes the pinworms (*E. vermicularis*) of humans and other primates. [entero- + G. *bios,* life]

en·ter·o·cele (en'ter-o-sēl). **1.** A hernial protrusion through a defect in the rectovaginal or vesicovaginal pouch. [entero- + G. *kēlē,* hernia] **2.** SYN abdominal *cavity.* [entero- + G. *koilia,* a hollow] **3.** An intestinal hernia. [see 1]
partial e., SYN parietal *hernia.*

en·ter·o·cen·te·sis (en'ter-ō-sen-tē'sis). Puncture of the intestine with a hollow needle (trocar and cannula) to withdraw substances. [entero- + G. *kentēsis,* puncture]

en·ter·o·cho·le·cys·tos·to·my (en'ter-ō-kō-lē-sis-tos'tō-mē). SYN cholecystenterostomy. [entero- + G. *cholē,* bile, + *kystis,* bladder, + *stoma,* mouth]

en·ter·o·cho·le·cys·tot·o·my (en'ter-ō-kō-lē-sis-tot'ō-mē). SYN cholecystenterotomy. [entero- + G. *cholē,* bile, + *kystis,* bladder, + *tomē,* a cutting]

enterocidal (en'ter-ō-sī'dal). An agent that kills parasites residing in the gastrointestinal tract.

en·ter·o·clei·sis (en-ter-ō-klī'sis). Occlusion of the lumen of the alimentary canal. [entero- + G. *kleisis,* a closing]
omental e., use of omentum to aid closure of an opening in the intestine.

en·ter·o·cly·sis (en-ter-o-k'li-sis). **1.** SYN high *enema.* **2.** In radiography of the small intestine, filling by introduction of contrast medium through a catheter advanced into the duodenum or jejunum from above. [entero- + G. *klysis,* a washing out]
radiologic e., method of imaging the duodenum and small intestine by intubation of the duodenum and instillation of dilute barium; also known as small bowel enema.

en·ter·o·coc·cem·ia (en'ter-ō-kok-sēm'ē-ah). A blood-borne disease, occasionally leading to septicemia, caused by members of the group D streptococci, *Enterococcus faecalis* or *Enterococcus faecium.*

En·ter·o·coc·cus (en'ter-ō-kok'ŭs). Genus of facultatively anaerobic, generally nonmotile, nonsporeforming, Gram-positive bacteria (family Streptococcaceae), formerly classified as part of the genus *Streptococcus.* Found in the intestinal tract of humans and animals, enterococci cause intraabdominal, wound, and urinary tract infections. Type species is *E. faecalis. E. faecium* is also clinically significant, because of its propensity to develop antibiotic resistance.

E. faecalis, a bacterial species found in human feces and in the intestines of many warm-blooded animals; occasionally found in urinary infections and in blood and heart lesions in cases of subacute endocarditis; a major cause of nosocomial infection, especially in association with Gram-negative pathogens. SYN *Streptococcus faecalis.*

E. faecium, the second most common species of this genus recovered in human infection; this species has low-level resistance to ampicillin, and in the U.S. and other countries where vancomycin is used frequently, resistant strains have been rapidly appearing as causes of nosocomial infections; in cases of septicemia in immunocompromised patients, fatality rates can be over 50%.

en·ter·o·coc·cus, pl. **en·ter·o·coc·ci** (en'ter-ō-kok'ŭs, -kok'sī). A streptococcus that inhabits the intestinal tract. [entero- + G. *kokkos,* a berry]

en·ter·o·co·li·tis (en'ter-ō-kō-lī'tis). Inflammation of the mucous membrane of a greater or lesser extent of both small and large intestines. SYN coloenteritis. [entero- + G. *kolon,* colon, + *-itis,* inflammation]
antibiotic e., e. caused by oral administration of broad spectrum antibiotics, resulting from overgrowth of antibiotic-resistant staphylococci or yeasts and fungi, when the normal fecal Gram-negative organisms are suppressed, resulting in diarrhea or pseudomembranous e.
necrotizing e., extensive ulceration and necrosis of the ileum and colon in premature infants in the neonatal period; possibly due to perinatal intestinal ischemia and bacterial invasion.
pseudomembranous e., e. with the formation and passage of pseudomembranous material in the stools; occurs most commonly as a sequel to antibiotic therapy; caused by a necrolytic exotoxin made by *Clostridium difficile.* SYN pseudomembranous colitis, pseudomembranous enteritis.
regional e., the changes of regional enteritis involving both the colon and the small intestine.

en·ter·o·co·los·to·my (en'ter-ō-kō-los'tō-mē). Establishment of a new communication between the small intestine and the colon. [entero- + G. *kōlon,* colon, + *stoma,* mouth]

en·ter·o·cyst (en'ter-ō-sist). A cyst of the wall of the intestine. SYN enterocystoma. [entero- + G. *kystis,* bladder]

en·ter·o·cys·to·cele (en'ter-ō-sis'tō-sēl). A hernia of both intestine and bladder wall. [entero- + G. *kystis,* bladder, + *kēlē,* hernia]

en·ter·o·cys·to·ma (en'ter-ō-sis-tō'mă). SYN enterocyst.

En·ter·o·cy·to·zo·on (en'ter-ō-sī'tō-zō'on). A genus in the protozoan phylum Microspora, all of which are obligate intracellular spore-forming parasites.

E. bieneusi, agent of microsporidian infection, primarily infecting the small intestine, especially in immunocompromised individuals. It is the microsporidian most frequently reported in AIDS patients, in whom it has been implicated in chronic diarrhea and weight loss; suggested treatment has been with octreotide with albendazole. SEE ALSO microsporidia.

en·ter·o·dyn·ia (en'ter-ō-din'ē-ă). SYN enteralgia. [entero- + G. *odynē,* pain]

en·ter·o·en·ter·os·to·my (en'ter-ō-en-ter-os'tō-mē). Establishment of a new communication between two segments of intestine. SYN enteroanastomosis, intestinal anastomosis.

en·ter·o·gas·tri·tis (en'ter-ō-gas-trī'tis). SYN gastroenteritis. [entero- + G. *gastēr,* belly, + *-itis,* inflammation]

en·ter·o·gas·trone (en'ter-ō-gas'trōn). A hormone, obtained from intestinal mucosa, that inhibits gastric secretion and motility; secretion of e. is stimulated by exposure of duodenal mucosa to dietary lipids. Some of the effects attributed to e. may be due to glucose-dependent insulinotropic peptide. SYN anthelone E, enteroanthelone.

en·ter·og·e·nous (en-ter-oj'ĕ-nŭs). Of intestinal origin. [entero- + G. *-gen,* producing]

en·ter·o·graph (en'ter-ō-graf). An instrument designed for use in enterography.

en·ter·og·ra·phy (en-ter-og'ră-fē). The making of a graphic record delineating the intestinal muscular activity. [entero- + G. *graphō*, to write]

en·ter·o·hep·a·ti·tis (en'ter-ō-hep-ă-tī'tis). Inflammation of both the intestine and the liver. [entero- + G. *hēpar* (*hēpat-*), liver, + -*itis*, inflammation]

en·ter·o·hep·a·to·cele (en'ter-ō-hep'ă-tō-sēl). Congenital umbilical hernia containing intestine and liver. SEE omphalocele. [entero- + G. *hēpar* (*hēpat-*), liver, + *kēlē*, hernia]

en·ter·oi·dea (en-ter-oy'dē-ă). Fevers due to infection caused by any of the intestinal bacteria, including the enteric fevers (typhoid and paratyphoid A and B) and the parenteric fevers. [entero- + G. *eidos*, resemblance]

en·ter·o·ki·nase (en'tēr-ō-kī'nās). SYN enteropeptidase.

en·ter·o·ki·ne·sis (en'ter-ō-ki-nē'sis). Muscular contraction of the alimentary canal. SEE ALSO peristalsis. [entero- + G. *kinēsis*, movement]

en·ter·o·ki·net·ic (en'ter-ō-ki-net'ik). Relating to, or producing, enterokinesis.

en·ter·o·lith (en'ter-ō-lith). An intestinal calculus formed of layers of soaps and earthy phosphates surrounding a nucleus of some hard body such as a swallowed fruit stone or other indigestible substance. [entero- + G. *lithos*, stone]

en·ter·o·li·thi·a·sis (en'ter-ō-li-thī'ă-sis). Presence of calculi in the intestine.

en·ter·ol·o·gy (en-ter-ol'ō-jē). The branch of medical science concerned especially with the intestinal tract. [entero- + G. *logos*, study]

en·ter·ol·y·sis (en-ter-ol'i-sis). Division of intestinal adhesions. [entero- + G. *lysis*, dissolution]

en·ter·o·meg·a·ly, en·ter·o·me·ga·lia (en'ter-ō-meg'ă-lē,; -ō-me-gā'lē-ă). SYN megaloenteron. [entero- + G. *megas*, great]

en·ter·o·me·nia (en-ter-ō-mē'nē-ă). Vicarious menstruation due to presence of tissue sensitive to effects of estrogen/progesterone in the intestine. [entero- + G. *emmēnos*, monthly]

en·ter·o·mer·o·cele (en'ter-ō-mēr'ō-sēl). Rarely used term for femoral *hernia*. [entero- + G. *mēros*, thigh, + *kēlē*, hernia]

en·ter·om·e·ter (en-ter-om'ĕ-ter). An instrument used in measuring the diameter of the intestine. [entero- + G. *metron*, measure]

En·te·ro·mo·nas (en'ter-ō-mō'nas, en-ter-om'ŏ-nas). A genus of flagellate protozoa, one species of which, *E. hominis*, is found as a rare nonpathogenic resident in the human large intestine. [entero- + G. *monas*, monad]

en·ter·o·my·co·sis (en'ter-ō-mī-kō'sis). An intestinal disease of fungal origin. [entero- + G. *mykēs*, fungus, + -*osis*, condition]

en·ter·o·pa·re·sis (en'ter-ō-pă-rē'sis, -par'i-sis). Rarely used term for a state of diminished or absent peristalsis with flaccidity of the muscles of the intestinal walls. [entero- + G. *paresis*, slackening, relaxation]

en·ter·o·path·o·gen (en'ter-ō-path'ō-jen). An organism capable of producing disease in the intestinal tract.

en·ter·o·path·o·gen·ic (en'ter-ō-path-ō-jen'ik). Capable of producing disease in the intestinal tract.

en·ter·op·a·thy (en-ter-op'ă-thē). An intestinal disease. [entero- + G. *pathos*, suffering]

gluten e., SYN celiac *disease*.

protein-losing e., increased fecal loss of serum protein, especially albumin, causing hypoproteinemia.

en·ter·o·pep·ti·dase (en'ter-ō-pep'ti-dās). An intestinal proteolytic glycoenzyme from the duodenal mucosa that converts trypsinogen into trypsin (removes a hexapeptide from trypsinogen). SYN enterokinase.

en·ter·o·pex·y (en'ter-ō-pek-sē). Fixation of a segment of the intestine to the abdominal wall. [entero- + G. *pēxis*, fixation]

en·ter·o·ple·gia (en'ter-ō-plē'jē-ă). Rarely used term for adynamic *ileus*. [entero- + G. *plēgē*, stroke]

en·ter·o·proc·tia (en'ter-ō-prok'shē-ă). Rarely used term for the presence of an artifical anus, as by a colostomy. [entero- + G. *prōktos*, anus]

en·ter·op·to·sis, en·ter·op·to·sia (en'ter-ō-tō'sis, -tō'sē-ă). Abnormal descent of the intestines in the abdominal cavity, usually associated with falling of the other viscera. [entero- + G. *ptōsis*, a falling]

en·ter·op·tot·ic (en'ter-ō-tot'ik). Relating to or suffering from enteroptosis.

en·ter·o·re·nal (en'ter-ō-rē'năl). Relating to both the intestines and the kidneys.

en·ter·or·rha·gia (en-ter-ō-rā'jē-ă). Bleeding within the intestinal tract. [entero- + G. *rhēgnymi*, to burst forth]

en·ter·or·rha·phy (en-ter-ōr'ă-fē). Suture of the intestine. [entero- + G. *rhaphē*, suture]

en·ter·or·rhex·is (en'ter-ō-rek'sis). Rarely used term for rupture of the gut or bowel. [entero- + G. *rhēxis*, rupture]

en·ter·o·scope (en'ter-ō-skōp). A speculum for inspecting the inside of the intestine in operative cases. [entero- + G. *skopeō*, to view]

en·ter·o·sep·sis (en'ter-ō-sep'sis). Sepsis occurring in or derived from the alimentary canal. [entero- + G. *sēpsis*, putrefaction]

en·ter·o·spasm (en'ter-ō-spazm). Increased, irregular, and painful peristalsis. [entero- + G. *spasmos*, spasm]

en·ter·o·sta·sis (en-ter-os'tă-sis). Intestinal stasis; a retardation or arrest of the passage of the intestinal contents. SYN intestinal stasis. [entero- + G. *stasis*, a standing]

en·ter·o·ste·no·sis (en'ter-ō-sten-ō'sis). Narrowing of the lumen of the intestine. [entero- + G. *stenōsis*, narrowing]

en·ter·os·to·my (en-ter-os'tō-mē). A connection between segments of the intestine or a fistula into the intestine through the abdominal wall. [entero- + G. *stoma*, mouth]

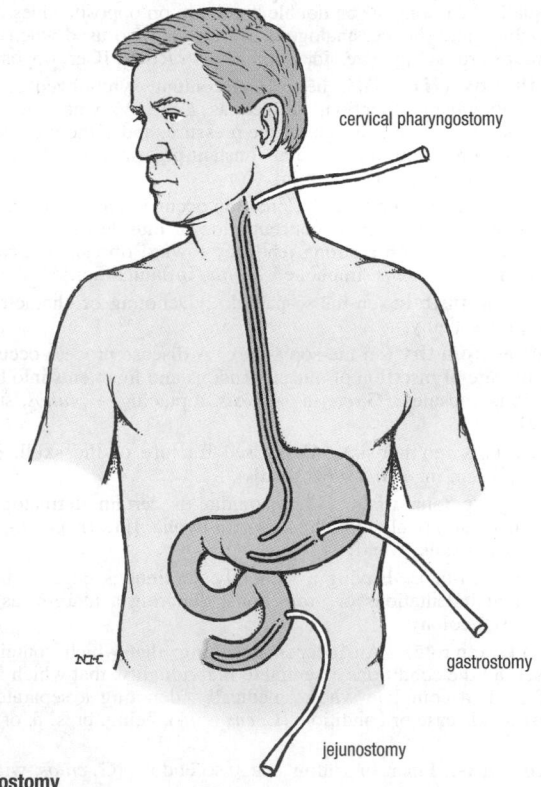

cervical pharyngostomy

gastrostomy

jejunostomy

enterostomy

double e., e. in which both proximal and distal openings of divided intestine are sutured to the abdomen wall.

en·ter·o·tome (en'ter-ō-tōm). An instrument for incising the intestine, especially in the creation of an artificial anus. [entero- + G. *tomē,* a cutting]

en·ter·ot·o·my (en-ter-ot′ō-mē). Incision into the intestine.

en·ter·o·tox·i·ca·tion (en′ter-ō-tok-si-kā′shŭn). SYN autointoxication.

en·ter·o·tox·i·gen·ic (en′ter-ō-tok-si-jen′ik). Denoting an organism containing or producing a toxin specific for cells of the intestinal mucosa.

en·ter·o·tox·in (en′ter-ō-tok′sin). A cytotoxin specific for the cells of the intestinal mucosa.

Clostridium perfringens e., a toxin produced by *Clostridium perfringens* that alters membrane permeability.

cytotonic e., an e. which morphologically changes, but does not kill, the target cell.

Escherichia coli e., e. produced by certain strains (serotypes) of *Escherichia coli,* seemingly associated with a transferable plasmid.

staphylococcal e., a soluble exotoxin produced by some strains of *Staphylococcus aureus,* and a cause of food poisoning.

en·ter·o·tox·ism (en′ter-ō-tok′sizm). SYN autointoxication.

en·ter·o·tro·pic (en′ter-ō-trop′ik). Attracted by or affecting the intestine. [entero- + G. *tropikos,* turning]

En·te·ro·vi·rus (en′ter-ō-vī′rŭs). A large and diverse group of viruses (family Picornaviridae) that includes poliovirus types 1 to 3, Coxsackievirus A and B, echoviruses, and the enteroviruses identified since 1969 and assigned type numbers. They are transient inhabitants of the alimentary canal and are stable at low pH.

en·ter·o·zo·ic (en′ter-ō-zō′ik). Relating to an enterozoon.

en·ter·o·zo·on (en′ter-ō-zō′on). An animal parasite in the intestine. [entero- + G. *zōon,* animal]

ent·ge·gen (*E*) (ent′ge-gen). Term used when the two higher ranking groups, attached to the different atoms in a double bond, usually a carbon-carbon double bond; are on opposite sides of the double bond (hence, analogous to *trans-*). Also used when those groups are on opposite sides of a ring structure. [Ger. opposite]

en·thal·py (*H*) (en′thal-pē). Heat content, symbolized as *H;* a thermodynamic function, defined as $E + PV$, where *E* is the internal energy of a system, *P* the pressure, and *V* the volume; the heat of a reaction, measured at constant pressure, is ΔH. SYN heat (4). [G. *enthalpō,* to warm in]

en·the·si·tis (en-thĕ-sī′tis). Condition occurring at the insertion of muscles where recurring concentration of muscle stress provokes inflammation with a strong tendency toward fibrosis and calcification. [G. *enthetos,* implanted, + *-itis,* inflammation]

en·the·so·path·ic (en-thē-sō-path′ik). Denoting or characteristic of enthesopathy.

en·the·sop·a·thy (en-thē-sop′ă-thē). A disease process occurring at the site of insertion of muscle tendons and ligaments into bones or joint capsules. [G. *en,* in, + *thesis,* a placing, + *pathos,* suffering]

en·thla·sis (en′thlă-sis). Depressed fracture of the skull. [G. a dent, fr. *en,* in, + *thlaō,* to crush]

en thyrse (ahn tirs′). Microconidia of certain dermatophytes arranged singly along both sides of a hypha. [Fr., fr. G. *en-,* in, + *thyrsos,* a stalk, wand]

en·tire (en-tīr′). Having a smoothly continuous edge or border without indentations or projections; denoting a margin, as of a bacterial colony.

en·ti·ty (en′ti-tē). An independent thing; that which contains in itself all the conditions essential to individuality; that which forms of itself a complete whole; medically, denoting a separate and distinct disease or condition. [L. *ens* (*ent-*), being, pres. p. of *esse,* to be]

△**ento-, ent-.** Inner, or within. SEE ALSO endo-. [G. *entos,* within]

en·to·blast (en′tō-blast). Cell nucleolus. [ento- + G. *blastos,* germ]

en·to·cele (en′tō-sēl). An internal hernia. [ento- + G. *kēlē,* hernia]

en·to·cho·roi·dea (en′tō-kō-roy′dē-ă). SYN capillary *lamina* of choroid. [ento- + G. *chorioeidēs,* choroid]

en·to·cone (en-tō-kōn). The mesiolingual cusp of a maxillary molar tooth. [ento- + G. *kōnos,* cone]

en·to·co·nid (en-tō-kō′nid). The inner posterior cusp of a mandibular molar tooth. [ento- + G. *kōnos,* cone]

en·to·cor·nea (en-tō-kōr′nē-ă). SYN posterior limiting *lamina* of cornea.

en·to·cra·ni·al (en′tō-krā′nē-ăl). SYN endocranial.

en·to·cra·ni·um (en′tō-krā′nē-ŭm). SYN endocranium.

en·to·derm (en′tō-derm). SYN endoderm. [ento- + G. *derma,* skin]

en·to·ec·tad (en-tō-ek′tad). From within outward. [G. *entos,* within, + *ektos,* without, + L. *ad,* to]

En·to·lo·ma si·nu·a·tum (en-tō-lō′mă sī-nū-ā′tum). A species of mushroom capable of producing mycetismus gastrointestinalis.

en·to·mi·on (en-tō′mē-on). The tip of the mastoid angle of the parietal bone. [G. *entomē,* notch]

en·to·mol·o·gy (en-tō-mol′ō-jē). The science concerned with the study of insects. [G. *entomon,* insect, + *logos,* study]

en·to·mo·pho·bia (en′tō-mō-fō′bē-ă). Morbid fear of insects. [G. *entomon,* insect, + *phobos,* fear]

Entomophthora (en-tō-mof′thor-ă). ?AU: please provide def. for this genus

E. coronata, a fungal genus reclassified as *Conidiobolus,* the cause of conidiobolomycosis.

Entomophthorales (en-tō-mof′thor-al′ēz). An order of the fungal class Zygomycetes. The genera include *Conidiobolus,* which causes a chronic granulomatous inflammation of a nasal and paranasal sinus mucosa (conidiobolomycosis) and *Basidiobolus,* which causes a chronic subcutaneous granuloma (basidiobolomycosis). When conidiobolomycosis and basidiobolomycosis are considered together, they are called entomophthoramycosis.

en·to·moph·tho·ra·my·co·sis (en-tō-mof′thō-ră-mī-kō′sis). A disease caused by fungi of the genera *Basidiobolus* or *Conididiobolus;* subcutaneous or paranasal tissues are invaded by broad nonseptate hyphae that become surrounded by eosinophilic material. A form of zygomycosis. SEE zygomycosis. [Entomophthorales (order name) + G. *mykēs,* fungus + -osis, condition]

e. basidiobo′lae, a subcutaneous phycomycosis due to the fungus *Basidiobolus ranarum,* characterized by the development of flat, firm subcutaneous fibrotic granulomas which do not ulcerate; occasionally, lesions may extend to muscles and lymph nodes and other deep tissues; the disease is found in Indonesia and in Uganda and other tropical African countries, but has not been seen in tropical America; a form of zygomycosis. SYN subcutaneous phycomycosis.

e. conidiobo′lae, a zygomycosis caused by *Conidiobolus coronatus,* characterized by large nasal polyps and granulomas of the nasal cavity; it has been reported from Texas, the West Indies, Africa, and South America; a form of zygomycosis.

En·to·mo·pox·vi·rus (en′tē-mō-poks-vī′rŭs). The genus of viruses (family Poxviridae) that comprises the poxviruses of insects; they seem not to multiply in vertebrates. [G. *entomon,* insect]

en·top·ic (en-top′ik). Placed within; occurring or situated in the normal place; opposed to ectopic. [G. *en,* within, + *topos,* place]

en·to·plasm (en′tō-plasm). SYN endoplasm.

ent·op·tic (en-top′tik). Within the eyeball. Often used to describe visual phenomena generated by mechanical or electrical stimulations of the retina. [ento- + G. *optikos,* relating to vision]

en·to·ret·i·na (en-tō-ret′i-nă). The layers of the retina from the outer plexiform to the nerve fiber layer inclusive. SYN Henle nervous layer.

en·to·sarc (en′tō-sark). SYN endosarc.

En·to·zoa (en-tō-zō′ă). A nontaxonomic name for the branch of the kingdom Animalia, whose members possess a digestive cavity or tract; includes all vertebrates and higher invertebrate forms. [ento- + G. *zōon,* animal]

en·to·zo·al (en-tō-zō′ăl). Relating to entozoa.

en·to·zo·on, pl. **en·to·zoa** (en-tō-zō′on, -ă). An animal parasite whose habitat is any of the internal organs or tissues. [ento- + G. *zōon,* animal]

en·trails (en′trālz). The viscera of an animal.

en·tro·pi·on, en·tro·pi·um (en-trō′pē-on, -pē-ŭm). **1.** Inversion or turning inward of a part. **2.** The infolding of the margin of an eyelid. [G. *en,* in, + *tropē,* a turning]

    atonic e., e. that follows loss of tone of the orbicularis oculi muscle or elasticity of the skin.

    cicatricial e., e. that follows scarring of the palpebral conjunctiva.

    spastic e., e. that arises from excessive contracture of the orbicularis oculi muscle.

en·tro·pi·on·ize (en-trō′pē-on-īz). To invert a part.

en·tro·py (*S*) (en′trō-pē). That fraction of heat (energy) content not available for the performance of work, usually because (in a chemical reaction) it has been used to increase the random motion of the atoms or molecules in the system; thus, e. is a measure of randomness or disorder. E. occurs in the Gibbs free energy (*G*) equation: $\Delta G = \Delta H - T\Delta S$ (ΔH, change in enthalpy or heat content; T, absolute temperature; ΔS, change in entropy). SEE ALSO second *law* of thermodynamics. [G. *entropia,* a turning toward]

en·ty·py (en′ti-pē). A type of gastrulation seen in some early mammalian embryos in which the endoderm covers the embryonic and amniotic ectoderm; part of the preplacental trophoblast may also be covered. [G. *entypē,* pattern]

enu·cle·ate (ē-noo′klē-āt). To remove entirely; to shell like a nut, as in the removal of an eye from its capsule or a tumor from its compressed surrounding tissue.

enu·cle·a·tion (ē-noo-klē-ā′shŭn). **1.** Removal of an entire structure (such as an eyeball or tumor), without rupture, as one shells the kernel of a nut. **2.** Removal or destruction of the nucleus of a cell. [L. *enucleo,* to remove the kernel, fr. *e,* out, + *nucleus,* nut, kernel]

en·u·re·sis (en-ū-rē′sis). Involuntary discharge or leakage of urine. [G. *en-oureō,* to urinate in]

    diurnal e., urinary accidents during wakefulness.

    nocturnal e., urinary incontinence during sleep. SYN bed-wetting.

en·ve·lope (en′vĕ-lōp). In anatomy, a structure that encloses or covers.

    corneocyte e., an electron-dense, 10–15 nm thick layer of highly cross-linked protein on the cytoplasmic surface of the cell membrane of epidermal corneocytes; it is highly resistant to proteolytic agents. SYN subplasmalemmal dense zone.

    nuclear e., the double membrane at the boundary of the nucleoplasm; it has regularly spaced pores covered by a disklike nuclear pore complex and a space or cisterna about 150 Å wide between the two layers; the outer membrane is continuous at intervals with the endoplasmic reticulum. SYN caryotheca, karyotheca, nuclear membrane.

    viral e., the outer structure or coat that encloses the nucleocapsids of some viruses that mature by budding through the membrane cell; may contain lipoprotein.

en·ven·om·a·tion (en-ven-ō-mā′shŭn). The act of injecting a poisonous material (venom) by sting, spine, bite, or other venom apparatus.

en·vi·ron·ment (en-vī′ron-ment). The milieu; the aggregate of all of the external conditions and influences affecting the life and development of an organism. It can be divided into physical, biological, social, cultural, etc., any or all of which can influence the health status of the population. [Fr. *environ,* around]

en·vy (en′vē). One's feeling of discontent or jealousy resulting from comparison with another person.

    penis e., the psychoanalytic concept in which a female envies male characteristics or capabilities, especially the possession of a penis.

en·zo·ot·ic (en-zō-ot′ik). SYN endemic. [G. *en,* in, + *zōon,* animal]

en·zy·got·ic (en-zī-got′ik). Derived from a single fertilized ovum; denoting twins so derived. [G. *eis* (*en*), one, + zygote]

en·zy·mat·ic (en-zī-mat′ik). Relating to an enzyme. SYN enzymic.

en·zyme (en′zīm). A protein that acts as a catalyst to induce chemical changes in other substances, itself remaining apparently unchanged by the process. E.'s, with the exception of those dis-

covered long ago (e.g., pepsin, emulsin), are generally named by adding -ase to the name of the substrate on which the e. acts (e.g., glucosidase), the substance activated (e.g., hydrogenase), and/or the type of reaction (e.g., oxidoreductase, transferase, hydrolase, lyase, isomerase, ligase or synthetase—these being the six main groups in the Enzyme Nomenclature Recommendations of the International Union of Biochemistry). For individual enzymes not listed below, see the specific name. SYN organic catalyst (1). [G. + L. *en,* in + *zymē,* leaven]

    acetyl-activating e., SYN *acetyl-CoA* ligase.

    acyl-activating e., (**1**) SYN long-chain fatty acid-CoA ligase; (**2**) SYN butyrate-CoA ligase.

    adaptive e., SYN induced e.

    allosteric e., an e. that exhibits the property of allosterism.

    amino acid activating e., SYN *aminoacyl-tRNA* synthetases.

    angiotensin-converting e. (ACE), SYN peptidyl dipeptidase A.

    antitumor e., an e. that stimulates the degradation of a particular metabolite that cannot be synthesized by tumor cells, inhibits the synthesis of a metabolite needed by tumor cells, or inhibits tumor-specific DNA utilization; e.g., asparaginase.

    autolytic e., an e. capable of causing lysis of the cell forming it.

    branching e., SYN 1,4-α-D-glucan-branching enzyme.

    β-carotene-cleavage e., SYN β-carotene 15,15′-dioxygenase.

    citrate-cleavage e., SYN ATP *citrate* (*pro-3S*)-lyase.

    cold-sensitive e., an e. that loses its stability as the temperature is lowered.

    condensing e., SYN *citrate* synthase.

    constitutive e., an e. that is constantly produced by the cell, regardless of the growth conditions. Cf. induced e.

    cooperative e., an e. that exhibits the property of cooperativity.

    D e., SYN 4-α-D-glucanotransferase.

    deamidizing e.'s, SYN amidohydrolases.

    deaminating e.'s, SYN deaminases.

    debranching e.'s, e.'s that bring about destruction of branches in glycogen; formerly considered to be one enzyme, now known to be a mixture of transferases (4-α-D-glucanotransferase) and hydrolases (amylo-1,6-glucosidase). SYN debranching factors.

    digestive e.'s, (**1**) e.'s that are utilized in the digestive system; (**2**) e.'s that are hydrolases of macromolecules (e.g., amylases, proteinases).

    disproportionating e., SYN 4-α-D-glucanotransferase.

    extracellular e., an e. performing its functions outside a cell; e.g., the various digestive e.'s. SYN exoenzyme.

    heat-stable e., SYN thermostable e.

    hydrolyzing e.'s, SYN hydrolases.

    immobilized e., an e. that has been bound, usually covalently, to an insoluble organic or inorganic matrix or has been encapsulated.

    induced e., inducible e., (**1**) an e. that can be detected in a growing culture of a microorganism, after the addition of a particular substance (inducer) to the culture medium, but was not detectable prior to the addition and can act on the inducer. A prototype is the β-galactosidase of *Escherichia coli,* synthesized upon the addition of various galactosides, whether or not these are good substrates. Cf. constitutive e; (**2**) any e. that has its rate of biosynthesis increased due to the presence of the substrate or some other molecular entity. SYN adaptive e.

    intracellular e., an e. that performs its functions within the cell that produces it; most e.'s are intracellular e.'s. SYN endoenzyme (1).

    Kornberg e., dNA polymerase I from *Escherichia coli.*

    malate-condensing e., SYN *malate* synthase.

    malic e., SYN *malate* dehydrogenase.

    marker e., an e. that is used to identify a specific cell type, cell organelle, or cell component.

    membrane e., an e. present or embedded in a biomembrane.

    methionine-activating e., SYN *methionine* adenosyltransferase.

    new yellow e., a former name for the D-amino-acid oxidase found in yeast, a flavoenzyme; so-called to distinguish it from Warburg old yellow e. Cf. *amino acid* oxidases.

    old yellow e., SYN *NADPH* dehydrogenase.

en

the major digestive enzymes

enzyme	enzyme source	digestive action
action of enzymes that digest carbohydrates		
ptyalin (salivary amylase)	salivary glands	starch → dextrin, maltose, glucose
amylase	pancreas	starch → dextrin, maltose, glucose dextrin → maltose, glucose
maltase	intestinal mucosa	maltose → glucose
sucrase	intestinal mucosa	sucrose → glucose, fructose
lactase	intestinal mucosa	lactose → glucose, galactose
action of enzymes that digest protein		
pepsin	gastric mucosa	protein → polypeptides
trypsin	pancreas	proteins and polypetides → polypeptides, dipeptides, amino acids
aminopeptidase	intestinal mucosa	polypeptides → dipeptides, amino acids
dipeptidase	intestinal mucosa	dipeptides → amino acids
action of enzymes that digest fat (triglyceride)		
pharyngeal lipase	pharyngeal mucosa	triglycerides → fatty acids, diglycerides, monoglycerides
steapsin	gastric mucosa	triglycerides → fatty acids, diglycerides, monoglycerides
pancreatic lipase	pancreas	triglycerides → fatty acids, diglycerides, monoglycerides

P e., SYN phosphorylase.

pantoate-activating e., SYN *pantothenate* synthetase.

phosphorylase-rupturing e. (PR e.), SYN *phosphorylase* phosphatase.

photoreactivating e. (PR e.), SYN deoxyribodipyrimidine photolyase.

PR e., abbreviation for phosphorylase-rupturing e.; photoreactivating e.

Q e., 1,4-α-glucan branching e. in plants.

R e., SYN α-dextrin endo-1,6-α-glucosidase.

reducing e., SYN reductase.

repair e., an e. that can catalyze the repair of damaged DNA; e.g., DNA ligase.

repressible e., an e. that is produced continuously unless production is repressed by excess of an inhibitor (corepressor). SEE ALSO inactive *repressor.*

respiratory e., a tissue e. that is part of an oxidation-reduction system accomplishing the conversion of substrates to CO_2 and H_2O and the transfer of the electrons removed to O_2.

restriction e., SYN restriction *endonuclease.*

RNA e., SYN ribozyme.

Schardinger e., SYN *xanthine* oxidase.

splitting e.'s, e.'s that, like aldolases, catalyze the conversion of a molecule into two smaller molecules without the addition or subtraction of any atoms.

T e., 1,4-α-D-glucan 6-α-D-glucosyltransferase.

terminal addition e., SYN DNA nucleotidylexotransferase.

thermostable e., an e. that is not readily subject to destruction or alteration by heat. SYN heat-stable e.

thiol e., an e. whose activity depends on a free thiol group.

transferring e.'s, SYN transferases.

Warburg old yellow e., SYN *NADPH* dehydrogenase; SEE ALSO new yellow e., yellow e.

Warburg respiratory e., SYN Atmungsferment.

yellow e., SYN flavoenzyme; SEE ALSO Warburg old yellow e., new yellow e.

En·zyme Com·mis·sion. SEE EC.

en·zy·mic (en-zī′mik). SYN enzymatic.

en·zy·mol·o·gist (en-zī-mol′ŏ-jist). A specialist in enzymology.

en·zy·mol·o·gy (en-zī-mol′ŏ-jē). The branch of chemistry concerned with the properties and actions of enzymes. [enzyme + G. *logos,* study]

en·zy·mol·y·sis (en-zī-mol′i-sis). **1.** The splitting or cleavage of a substance into smaller parts by means of enzymatic action. **2.** Lysis by the action of an enzyme. [enzyme + G. *lysis,* dissolution]

en·zy·mop·a·thy (en-zī-mop′ă-thē). Any disturbance of enzyme function, including genetic deficiency or defect in specific enzymes. [enzyme + G. *pathos,* disease]

EOG Abbreviation for electrooculography; electroolfactogram.

eo·sin (ē′ō-sin). A derivative of fluorescein used as a fluorescent acid dye for cytoplasmic stains and counterstains in histology and in Romanovsky-type blood stains. [G. *ēōs,* dawn]

e. B, the disodium salt of 4′,5′-dibromo-2′,7′-dinitrofluorescein. SYN acid red 91, e. I bluish. [C.I. 45400]

e. I bluish, SYN e. B.

e. y, e. Y, the disodium salt of 2′,4′,5′,7′-tetrabromofluorescein. SYN acid red 87, e. yellowish. [C.I. 45380]

e. yellowish, SYN e. y.

eo·sin·o·cyte (ē-ō-sin′ō-sīt). SYN eosinophilic *leukocyte.*

eo·sin·o·pe·nia (ē′ō-sin-ō-pē′nē-ă). The presence of eosinophils in an abnormally small number in the peripheral bloodstream. SYN hypoeosinophilia. [eosino(phil) + G. *penia,* poverty]

🔲 eo·sin·o·phil, eo·sin·o·phile (ē-ō-sin′ō-fil, -fīl). SYN eosinophilic *leukocyte.* [eosin + G. *philos,* fond]

eo·sin·o·phil·ia (ē′ō-sin-ō-fil′ē-ă). SYN eosinophilic *leukocytosis.*

simple pulmonary e., pulmonary infiltrates seen as transient migratory shadows on the chest x-ray, accompanied by blood e.; often symptomless, but there may be cough, fever, and breathlessness; most cases are due to worm infestation, especially by *Ascaris lumbricoides;* a few cases follow administration of drugs. SYN Löffler syndrome (1).

tropical e., e. associated with cough and asthma, caused by occult filarial infection without evidence of microfilaremia, occurring most frequently in India and Southeast Asia.

eo·sin·o·phil·ic (ē-ō-sin-ō-fil′ik). Staining readily with eosin dyes; denoting such cell or tissue elements.

eo·sin·o·phil·u·ria (ē-ō-sin′ō-fil-ū′rē-ă). Presence of eosinophils in the urine.

eo·sin·o·tac·tic (ē′ō-sin-ō-tak′tik). Exerting a force of attraction or repulsion on eosinophile cells. [eosino(phile) + G. *taktikos,* in orderly arrangement]

eo·sin·o·tax·is (ē′ō-sin-ō-tak′sis). Movement of eosinophils with reference to a stimulus which attracts or repels them.

eo·so·pho·bia (ē-ō-sō-fō′bē-ă). Morbid dread of the dawn. [G. *ēōs,* dawn, + *phobos,* fear]

EP Abbreviation for endogenous *pyrogen.*

epac·tal (ē-pak′tăl). SYN supernumerary. [G. *epaktos,* imported, fr. *epagō,* to bring on or in]

ep·am·ni·ot·ic (ep′am-nē-ot′ik). Upon or above the amnion. [G. *epi,* upon, + amnion]

ep·ar·te·ri·al (ep′ar-tēr-ē-ăl). Upon or superior to an artery. [G. *epi,* upon, + *artēia,* artery]

ep·ax·i·al (ep-ak′sē-ăl). Above or behind any axis, such as the spinal axis or the axis of a limb. [G. *epi,* upon, + L. *axis,* axis]

EPEC. Abbreviation for enteropathogenic *Escherichia coli.*

ep·en·dy·ma (ep-en′di-mă) [TA]. The cellular membrane lining the central canal of the spinal cord and the brain ventricles. SYN endyma. [G. *ependyma,* an upper garment]

ep·en·dy·mal (ep-en′di-măl). Relating to the ependyma.

ep·en·dy·mi·tis (ep-en-di-mī′tis). Inflammation of the ependyma.

ep·en·dy·mo·blast (ep-en′di-mō-blast). An embryonic ependymal cell. [ependyma + G. *blastos,* germ]

ep·en·dy·mo·blas·to·ma (ep-en′di-mō-blas-tō′mă). A glial neoplasm of the central nervous system, occurring typically in childhood; the prototype tumor cells resemble ependymoblasts. [ependymoblast + G. *-ōma,* tumor]

ep·en·dy·mo·cyte (ep-en′di-mō-sīt). An ependymal cell. [ependyma + G. *kytos,* cell]

ep·en·dy·mo·ma (ep-en-di-mō′mă). A glioma derived from relatively undifferentiated ependymal cells, comprising approximately 1–3% of all intracranial neoplasms; e.'s occur in all age groups and may originate from the lining of any of the ventricles or, more commonly, from the central canal of the spinal cord; histologically, the neoplastic cells tend to be arranged radially about blood vessels, to which they are attached by means of fibrillary processes.

myxopapillary e., a slow-growing e. of the filum terminale, occurring most often in young adults, consisting of cuboidal cells in papillary arrangement around a mucinous vascular core.

eph·apse (ef′aps). A place where two or more nerve cell processes (axons, dendrites) touch without forming a typical synaptic contact; some form of neural transmission may occur at such nonsynaptic contact sites. [G. *ephapsis,* contact]

eph·ap·tic (e-fap′tik). Relating to an ephapse.

ephe·bic (ĕ-fē′bik). Rarely used term relating to the period of puberty or to a youth. [G. *ephēbikos,* relating to youth, fr. *hēbē,* youth]

eph·e·bol·o·gy (ef-ĕ-bol′ō-jē). Rarely used term for the study of the morphologic and other changes incidental to puberty. [G. *ephēbos,* puberty, + *logos,* study]

ephed·ra (ē-fed′răh). *Ephedra equisetina* (family Gnetaceae). Ma Huang; the plant source for the alkaloid ephedrine. Indigenous to China and India, it is 0.75 to over 1% ephedrine; also contains some pseudoephedrine.

ephed·rine (ĕ-fed′rin, ef′ĕ-drin). An alkaloid from the leaves of *Ephedra equisetina,* E. sinica, and other species (family Gnetaceae), or produced synthetically; an adrenergic (sympathomimetic) agent with actions similar to those of epinephrine; used as a bronchodilator, mydriatic, pressor agent, and topical vasoconstrictor. Generally used salts are e. hydrochloride and e. sulfate.

ephe·lis, pl. **ephe·li·des** (ef-ē′lis, ef-ē′li-dēz). SYN freckle. [G.]

epi-. Upon, following, or subsequent to. [G.]

ep·i·an·dros·ter·one (ep′i-an-dros′ter-ōn). Inactive isomer (3β instead of 3α) of androsterone; found in urine and in testicular and ovarian tissue. SYN isoandrosterone.

ep·i·bati·dine (ep′ĭ-băt′tĭ-dīn). A toxic alkaloid extracted from the skin of a South American frog, *Epipedobates tricolor.* Apparently derived from particular insects consumed in the Amazon basin. The crude extract has been used as an arrow poison by native hunters; exerts analgesia by a mechanism other than activation of opiate receptors or cyclooxygenase inhibition.

ep·i·blast (ep′i-blast). Gives rise to the ectoderm, mesoderm, and endoderm of the embryo proper. [epi- + G. *blastos,* germ]

ep·i·blas·tic (ep-i-blas′tik). Relating to epiblast.

ep·i·bleph·a·ron (ep′i-blef′ă-ron). A congenital horizontal skin fold near the margin of the eyelid, caused by abnormal insertion of muscle fibers. In the upper lid, it simulates blepharochalasis; in the lower lid, it causes a turning inward of the lashes. [epi- + G. *blepharon,* eyelid]

epib·o·ly, epib·o·le (ē-pib′ō-lē). 1. A process involved in gastrulation of telolecithal eggs in which, as a result of differential growth, some of the cells of the protoderm move over the surface toward the lips of the blastopore. 2. Growth of epithelium in an organ culture to surround the underlying mesenchymal tissue. [G. *epibolē,* a throwing or laying on]

ep·i·bul·bar (ep-i-bŭl′bar). Upon a bulb of any kind; specifically, upon the eyeball.

ep·i·can·thus (ep-i-kan′thŭs). SYN palpebronasal *fold.* [epi- + G. *kanthos,* canthus]

e. inver′sus, a crescentic upward fold of skin from the lower eyelid at the inner canthus; frequent in congenital blepharoptosis.

e. palpebra′lis, e. arising from the upper lid above the tarsal portion and extending to the lower portion of the orbit.

e. supracilia′ris, e. arising from the region of the eyebrows and extending toward the tear sac.

e. tarsa′lis, e. arising from the tarsal fold and disappearing in the skin close to the inner canthus.

ep·i·car·dia (ep-i-kar′dē-ă). SYN abdominal *part* of esophagus. [epi- + G. *kardia,* heart]

ep·i·car·di·al (ep-i-kar′dē-ăl). 1. Relating to the epicardia. 2. Relating to the epicardium.

ep·i·car·di·um (ep-i-kar′dē-ŭm). ★official alternate term for visceral *layer* of serous pericardium. [epi- + G. *kardia,* heart]

ep·i·chord·al (ep-i-kōr′dăl). On the dorsal side of the notochord; applicable particularly to that part of the brain developing dorsal to the cephalic part of the notochord. [epi- + G. *chordē,* a chord]

ep·i·cil·lin (ep-ĭ-sil′in). Semisynthetic beta-lactam antibiotic related to penicillin; an antibacterial.

ep·i·co·mus (ep-i-kō′mŭs, ē-pik′ō-mŭs). Unequal conjoined twins in which the smaller parasite is joined to the larger autosite at the top of the head. SEE conjoined *twins,* under *twin.* [epi- + G. *komē,* hair of the head]

ep·i·con·dy·lal·gia (ep′i-kon-di-lal′jē-ă). Pain in an epicondyle of the humerus or in the tendons or muscles originating therefrom. [epicondyle + G. *algos,* pain]

e. exter′na, SYN tennis *elbow.*

ep·i·con·dyle (ep-i-kon′dīl) [TA]. A projection from a long bone near the articular extremity above or upon the condyle. SYN epicondylus [TA]. [epi- + G. *kondylos,* a knuckle]

lateral e. of femur [TA], the e. located proximal to the lateral condyle. SYN epicondylus lateralis femoris [TA], epicondylus lateralis ossis femoris, lateral femoral tuberosity.

lateral e. of humerus [TA], the e. situated at the lateral side of the distal end of the bone. SYN epicondylus lateralis humeri [TA].

medial e. of femur [TA], the e. located proximal to the medial condyle. SYN epicondylus medialis ossis femoris, medial femoral tuberosity.

medial e. of humerus [TA], the e. situated proximal and medial to the condyle. SYN epicondylus medialis humeri [TA], epitrochlea.

ep·i·con·dy·li (ep-i-kon′di-lī). Plural of epicondylus.

ep·i·con·dyl·i·an (ep-i-kon-dil′ē-an). SYN epicondylic.

ep·i·con·dyl·ic (ep-i-kon-dil′ik). Relating to an epicondyle or to the part above a condyle. SYN epicondylian.

ep·i·con·dy·li·tis (ep′i-kon-di-lī′tis). Inflammation of an epicondyle.

lateral humeral e., SYN tennis *elbow.*

ep·i·con·dy·lus, pl. **ep·i·con·dy·li** (ep-i-kon′di-lŭs, -lī) [TA]. SYN epicondyle. [L.]

e. lateralis femoris [TA], SYN lateral *epicondyle* of femur.

e. latera′lis hu′meri [TA], SYN lateral *epicondyle* of humerus.

e. latera′lis os′sis fem′oris, SYN lateral *epicondyle* of femur.

e. medialis femoris [TA],

e. media′lis hu′meri [TA], SYN medial *epicondyle* of humerus.

e. media′lis os′sis fem′oris, SYN medial *epicondyle* of femur.

ep·i·cor·a·coid (ep-i-kōr′ă-koyd). Upon or above the coracoid process.

ep·i·cra·ni·al. Relating to the epicranium.

ep·i·cra·ni·um (ep-i-krā′nē-ŭm). The muscle, aponeurosis, and skin covering the cranium. [epi- + G. *kranion,* skull]

ep·i·cra·ni·us. SEE epicranius (*muscle*).

ep·i·cri·sis (ep-i-krī′sis). A secondary crisis; a crisis terminating a recrudescence of morbid symptoms following a primary crisis.

ep·i·crit·ic (ep-i-krit′ik). That aspect of somatic sensation which permits the discrimination and the topographical localization of the finer degrees of touch and temperature stimuli. Cf. protopathic. [G. *epikritikos,* adjudicatory, fr. *epi,* on, + *krinō,* to separate, judge]

ep·i·cys·ti·tis (ep′i-sis-tī′tis). Inflammation of the cellular tissue around the bladder. [epi- + G. *kystis,* bladder, + *-itis,* inflammation]

ep·i·cyte (ep′i-sīt). A cell membrane, especially of protozoa; the external layer of cytoplasm in gregarines. [epi- + G. *kytos,* cell]

ep·i·dem·ic (ep-i-dem′ik). The occurrence in a community or region of cases of an illness, specific health-related behavior, or other health-related events clearly in excess of normal expectancy; the word also is used to describe outbreaks of disease in animals or plants. Cf. endemic, sporadic. [epi- + G. *dēmos,* the people]

behavioral e., an e. originating in behavioral patterns (in contrast to invading microorganisms); examples include medieval dancing mania, episodes of crowd panic.

point e., an e. where a pronounced clustering of cases of disease occurs within a very short period of time (within a few days or even hours) due to exposure of persons or animals to a common source of infection such as food or water.

ep·i·de·mic·i·ty (ep'i-dem-is'i-tē). The state of prevailing disease in epidemic form.

ep·i·de·mi·og·ra·phy (ep'i-dem-ē-og'ră-fē). A descriptive treatise of epidemic diseases or of any particular epidemic. [G. *epidēmios,* epidemic, + *graphē,* a writing]

ep·i·de·mi·ol·o·gist (ep-i-dē-mē-ol'ō-jist). An investigator who studies the occurrence of disease or other health-related conditions, states, or events in specified populations; one who practices epidemiology; the control of disease is usually also considered to be a task of the epidemiologist.

ep·i·de·mi·ol·o·gy (ep-i-dē-mē-ol'ō-jē). The study of the distribution and determinants of health-related states or events in specified populations, and the application of this study to control of health problems. [G. *epidēmios,* epidemic, + *logos,* study]

clinical e., the field concerned with applying epidemiological principles in a clinical setting.

genetic e., the branch of e. that studies the role of genetic factors and their interactions with environmental factors in the occurrence of disease in various populations.

molecular e., the use in epidemiologic studies of techniques of molecular biology such as DNA typing.

ep·i·derm, ep·i·der·ma (ep'i-derm, ep-i-der'mă). SYN epidermis.

ep·i·der·mal, ep·i·der·mat·ic (ep-i-der'măl, -der-mat'ik). Relating to the epidermis. SYN epidermic.

ep·i·der·mal·i·za·tion (ep-i-der'mal-i-zā'shŭn). SYN squamous *metaplasia*.

ep·i·der·mic (ep-i-der'mik). SYN epidermal.

ep·i·der·mi·do·sis (ep'i-der-mi-dō'sis). SYN epidermosis.

ep·i·der·mis, pl. **ep·i·derm·i·des** (ep-i-derm'is, -derm'i-dēz) [TA]. **1.** The superficial epithelial portion of the skin (cutis). The thick e. of the palms and soles contains the following strata from the surface: stratum corneum (keratin layer), stratum lucidum (clear layer), stratum granulosum (granular layer), stratum spinosum (prickle cell layer), and stratum basale (basal cell layer); in other parts of the body, the stratum lucidum may be absent. **2.** In botany, the outermost layer of cells in leaves and the young parts of plants. SYN cuticle (3), cuticula (2), epiderm, epiderma. [G. *epidermis,* the outer skin, fr. *epi,* on, + *derma,* skin]

ep·i·der·mi·tis (ep-i-der-mī'tis). Inflammation of the epidermis or superficial layers of the skin.

ep·i·der·mo·dys·pla·sia (ep-i-der'mō-dis-plā'zē-ă). Faulty growth or development of the epidermis. [epidermis + G. *dys-,* bad, + *plasis,* a molding]

e. verrucifor'mis [MIM*226400], a rare inherited disease with numerous flat warts on the hands and feet, in patients with inherited defects in cell-mediated immunity and increased susceptibility to human papilloma virus infections; skin carcinoma sometimes develops. There is a genetic component in the etiology, but the inheritance pattern is uncertain at present.

ep·i·der·moid (ep-i-der'moyd). **1.** Resembling epidermis. **2.** A cholesteatoma or other cystic tumor arising from aberrant epidermal cells. [epidermis + G. *eidos,* appearance]

ep·i·der·mol·y·sis (ep'i-der-mol'i-sis). A condition in which the epidermis is loosely attached to the corium, readily exfoliating or forming blisters. [epidermis + G. *lysis,* loosening]

e. bullo'sa [MIM*131800], a group of inherited chronic noninflammatory skin diseases in which large bullae and erosions result from slight mechanical trauma; a form localized to the hands and feet is called Weber-Cockayne *syndrome,* of autosomal dominant inheritance caused by mutation in either the gene encoding kera-

tin-5 (KRT5) on chromosome 12q or the gene for keratin-14 (KRT14) on 17q. SYN mechanobullous disease.

e. bullosa, dermal type, SYN e. bullosa dystrophica.

e. bullo'sa dystroph'ica [MIM*131705], a form of e. bullosa in which scarring develops after separation of the entire epidermis with blistering; it is inherited as an autosomal dominant (appearing in infancy or childhood) or recessive (present at birth or appearing in early infancy) trait, the latter including lethal and nonlethal types; both dominant and recessive forms are caused by mutation in the gene for type VII collagen (COL7A1) on chromosome 3p. SYN dermolytic bullous dermatosis, e. bullosa, dermal type.

e. bullosa, epidermal type (bu'lō-să), SYN e. bullosa simplex.

e. bullosa, junctional type, SYN e. bullosa lethalis.

e. bullo'sa letha'lis [MIM*226700], a form of e. bullosa characterized by persistent and nonhealing perioral and perinasal crusted lesions with bullae often present in the oral mucosa and trachea, but not on the palms and soles, complicated by dermal sepsis and serum protein and electrolyte loss leading to death; autosomal recessive inheritance, caused by mutation in any one of the three distinct polypeptides of laminin-5; alpha-3 (LAMA3) on chromosome 18q, beta-3 (LAMB3) and gamma-2 (LAMC2) on 1q or the gene encoding integrin, beta-4 (ITGB4) on 17q. SYN e. bullosa, junctional type, Herlitz syndrome.

e. bullo'sa sim'plex [MIM*131900], e. bullosa in which lesions heal rapidly without scarring; bulla formation is intraepidermal and microscopy reveals basal cell vacuolation and dissolution of tonofibrils; occurs most frequently on the feet of adults after unaccustomed trauma such as long marches; autosomal dominant inheritance caused by mutation in the keratin-5 gene (KRT5) on chromosome 12q or in the keratin-14 gene (KRT14) on 17q. SYN e. bullosa, epidermal type.

Ep·i·der·mo·phy·ton (ep'i-der-mof'i-ton, -der'mō-fī'ton). A genus of fungi, separated by Sabouraud from *Trichophyton* on the basis that it never invades the hair follicles, whose macroconidia are clavate and smooth walled. The only species, *E. floccosum,* is an anthropophilic species that is a common cause of tinea pedis and tinea cruris. [epidermis + G. *phyton,* plant]

ep·i·der·mo·sis (ep-i-der-mō'sis). A skin disease affecting only the epidermis. SYN epidermidosis.

ep·i·der·mot·ro·pism (ep-i-der-mot'rō-pizm). Movement towards the epidermis, as in the migration of T lymphocytes into the epidermis in mycosis fungoides. [epidermis + G. *tropē,* a turning]

ep·i·di·a·scope (ep-i-dī'ă-skōp). A projector by which images are reflected by a mirror through a lens, or lenses, onto a screen, using reflected light for opaque objects and transmitted light for translucent or transparent ones. SYN overhead projector. [epi- + G. *dia,* through, + *skopeō,* to view]

ep·i·did·y·mal (ep-i-did'i-măl). Relating to the epididymis.

ep·i·did·y·mec·to·my (ep'i-did-i-mek'tō-mē). Operative removal of the epididymis. [epididymis + G. *ektomē,* excision]

ep·i·did·y·mis, gen. **ep·i·did·y·mi·dis,** pl. **ep·i·did·y·mi·des** (ep-i-did'i-mis, -di-dim'i-dis, -di-dim'i-dēz) [TA]. An elongated structure connected to the posterior surface of the testis, consisting of the head, body, and tail, which turns sharply upon itself to become the ductus deferens; the main component is the very convoluted duct of the e. which in the tail and the beginning of the ductus deferens is a reservoir for spermatozoa. The e. transports, stores, and matures spermatozoa between testis and ductus deferens (vas deferens). SYN parorchis. [Mod. L. fr. G. *epididymis,* fr. *epi,* on, + *didymos,* twin, in pl. testes]

ca'put e., SYN *head* of epididymis.

cau'da e., SYN *tail* of epididymis.

cor'pus e., body of e.

ep·i·did·y·mi·tis, pl. **epididymiditides** (ep-i-did-i-mī'tis). Inflammation of the epididymis.

ep·i·did·y·mo·or·chi·tis (ep-i-did'i-mō-ōr-kī'tis). Simultaneous inflammation of epididymis and testis. [epididymis + G. *orchis,* testis]

ep·i·did·y·mo·plas·ty (ep-i-did'i-mō-plas-tē). Surgical repair of the epididymis. [epididymis + G. *plastos,* formed]

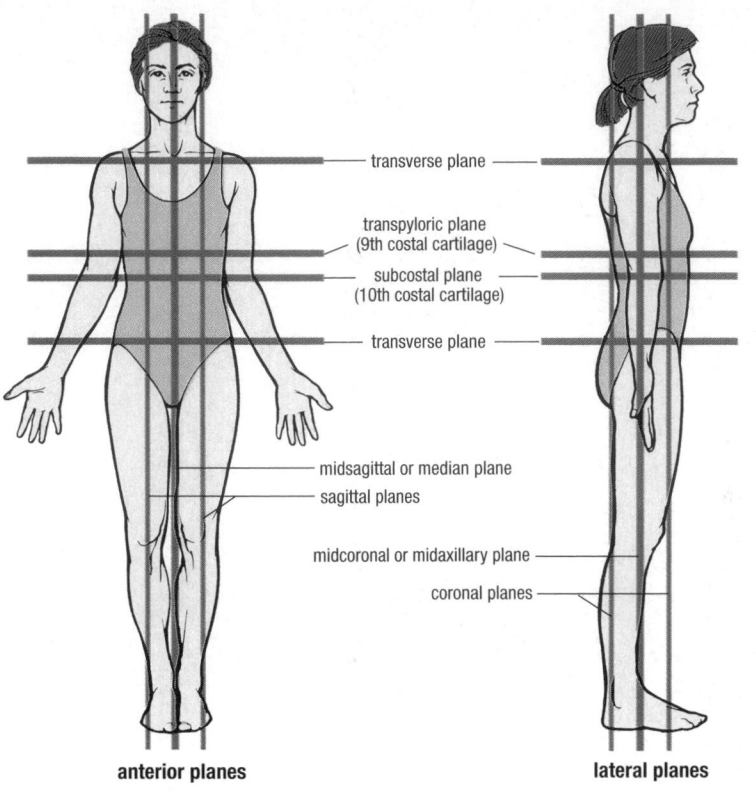

transverse plane

transpyloric plane
(9th costal cartilage)

subcostal plane
(10th costal cartilage)

transverse plane

midsagittal or median plane

sagittal planes

midcoronal or midaxillary plane

coronal planes

anterior planes

lateral planes

Anatomic Planes

Longitudinal plane:	made by cutting along long (longitudinal) axis of body or body part; in erect position, this plane is termed *vertical* and is perpendicular to horizontal
Transverse plane:	made by cutting across body or body part cross-wise (at a right angle to long axis); if patient is erect, this plane is termed *horizontal* (parallel to horizon)
Midsagittal or median plane:	longitudinal plane made by cutting from front (anterior) to back (posterior) along median line of body and along sagittal suture of skull
Sagittal plane:	longitudinal plane made by cutting from front (anterior) to back (posterior) on either side of sagittal suture and parallel to midsagittal or median plane
Coronal plane:	longitudinal plane made by cutting lengthwise from side to side through head and body (or body part) along coronal suture of skull or parallel to it
Transpyloric plane:	transverse plane made by cutting across from one side to the other at level of 9th costal cartilages; the name of this plane reflects the fact that it should cut across pylorus of stomach
Midcoronal (midaxillary) plane:	longitudinal plane made by cutting through head and body along the coronal suture of head and extending cut down the body

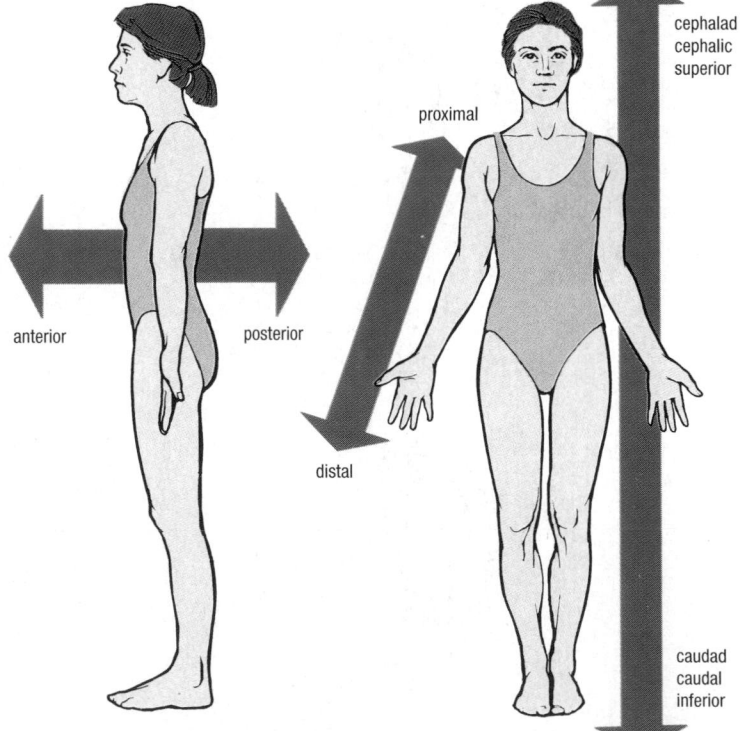

proximal

anterior

posterior

distal

cephalad
cephalic
superior

caudad
caudal
inferior

Body Part Terminology

Anterior:	in front of (toward front of body or a structure within it); sometimes referred to as *ventral*
Posterior:	in back of (toward back of body or a structure within it); sometimes referred to as *dorsal*
Proximal:	closer to point of attachment or origin; in extremities, closest to the trunk
Distal:	farther from point of attachment or origin; in extremities, farthest from the trunk
Cephalad, cephalic, superior	toward head or upper part of a structure
Caudad, caudal, inferior	away from head or the upper part of a structure (literally means "toward the tail")

Diagnostic Imaging

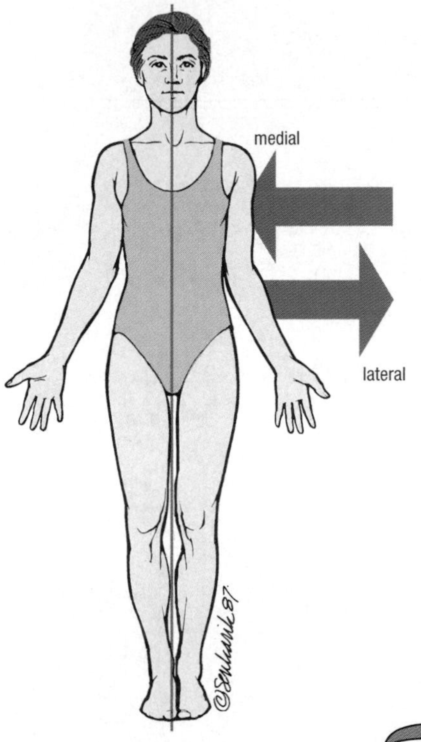

medial

lateral

supinate

pronate

Body Part Terminology (*continued*)

Medial: toward midline of body

Lateral: away from midline of body (to the side)

Body Movement

Abduction: movement of a limb or body part further away from midline of body

Adduction: movement of a limb or body part closer to or toward midline of body

Extension: straightening of a joint or extremity so that angle between contiguous (adjoining) bones is increased

Flexion: bending of a joint or extremity so that angle between contiguous (adjoining) bones is decreased

Eversion: movement of turning a body part outward (away from midline)

Inversion: movement of turning a body part inward (toward the midline)

Pronation: movement of turning a body part to face downward or turning hand so that palm is facing downward

Supination: movement of turning a body part to face upward or turning hand so that palm is facing upward

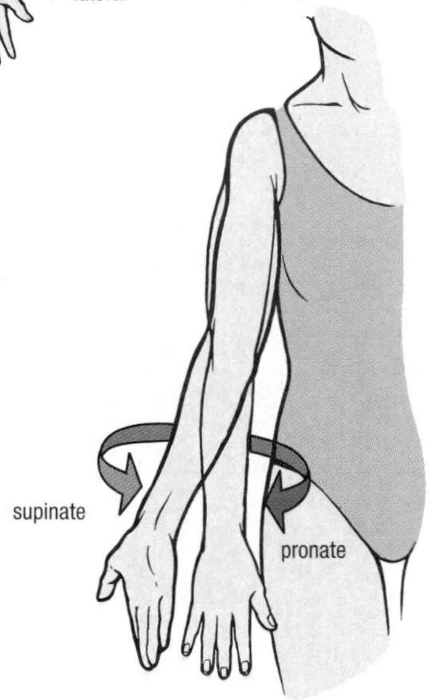

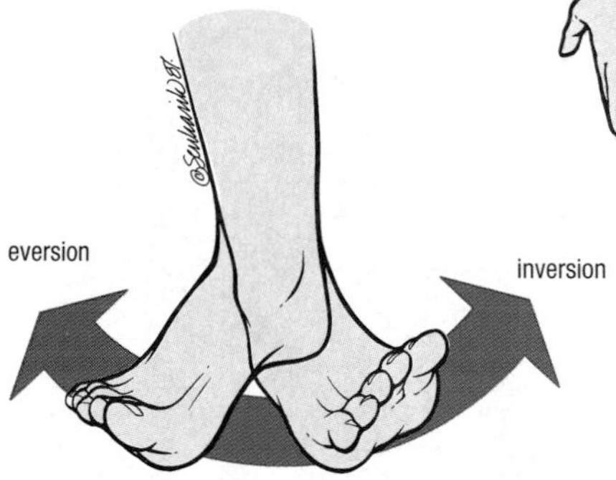

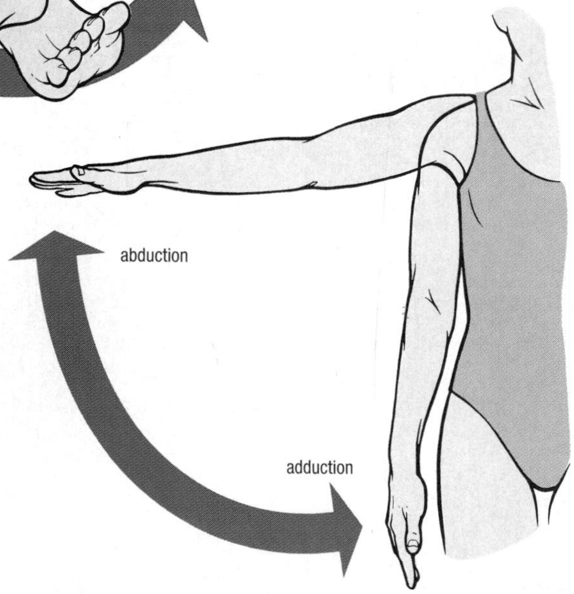

eversion

inversion

abduction

adduction

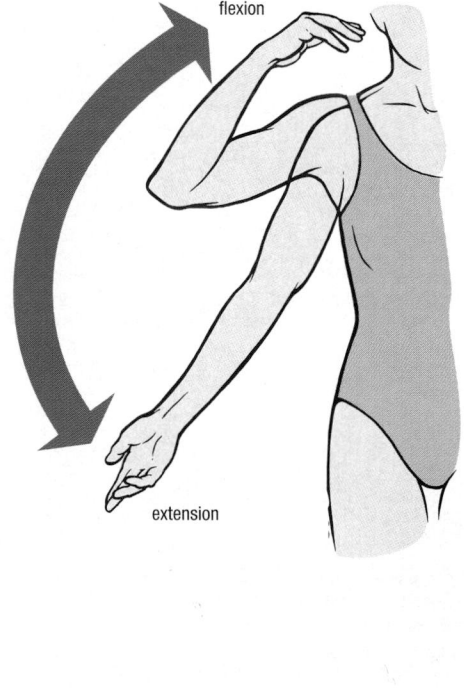

flexion

extension

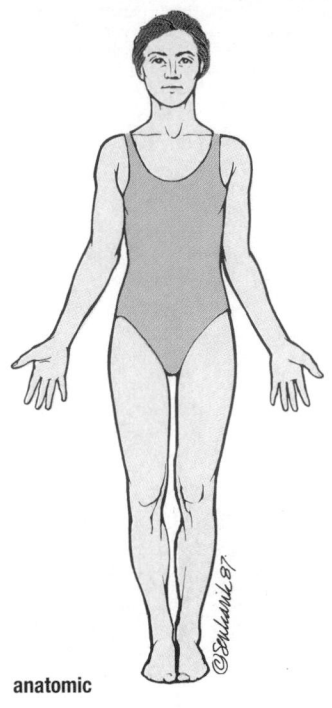

anatomic

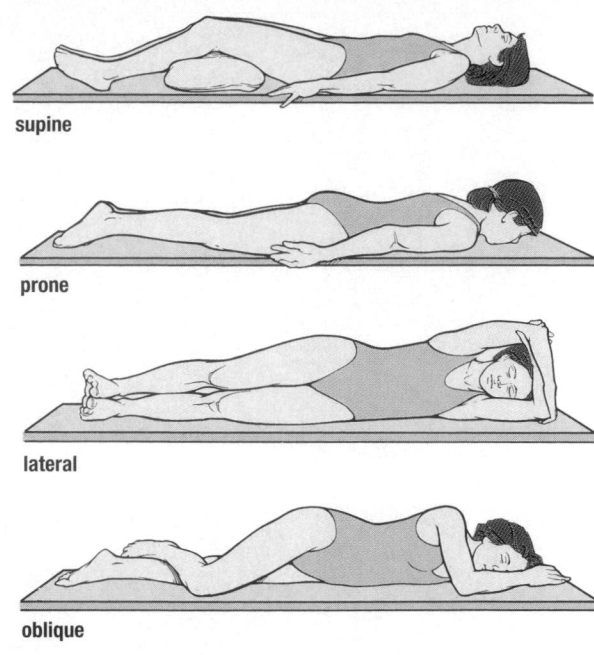

supine

prone

lateral

oblique

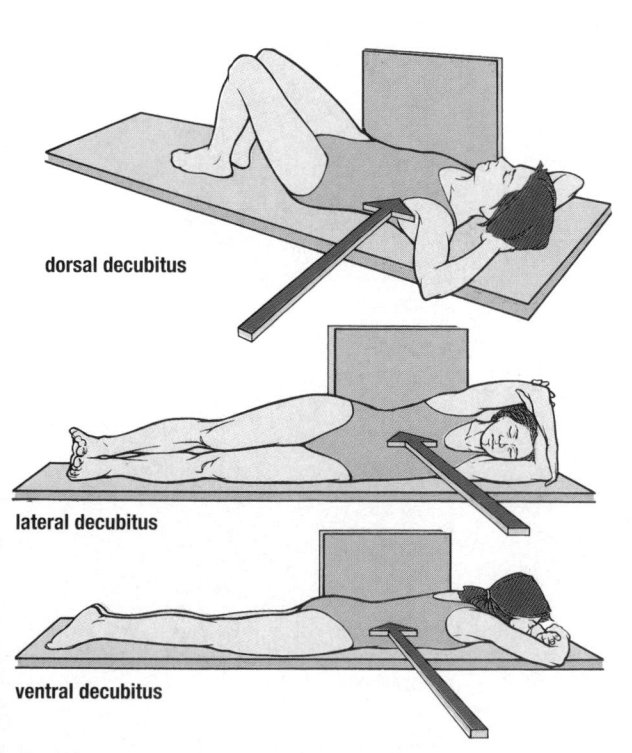

dorsal decubitus

lateral decubitus

ventral decubitus

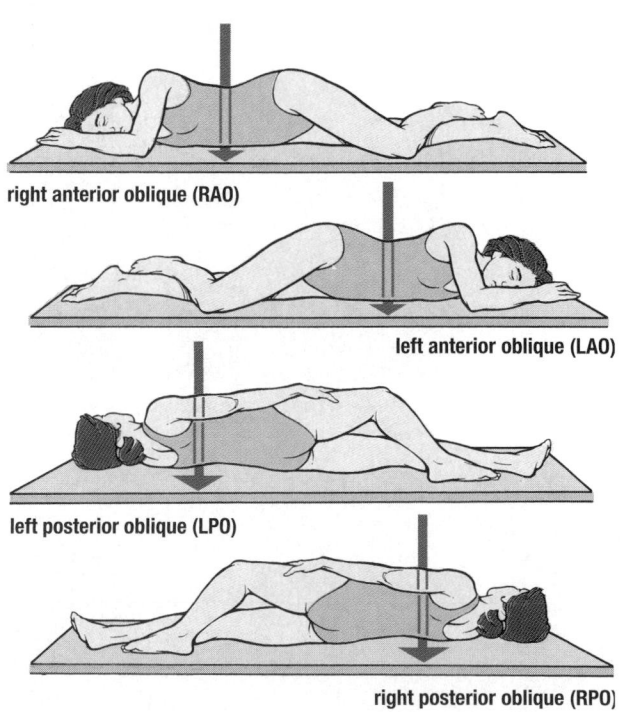

right anterior oblique (RAO)

left anterior oblique (LAO)

left posterior oblique (LPO)

right posterior oblique (RPO)

Diagnostic Imaging

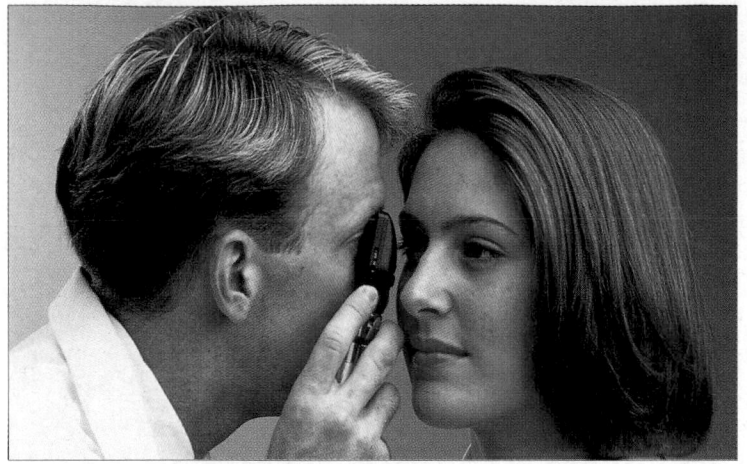

doctor examining patient using ophthalmoscope

ophthalmoscope

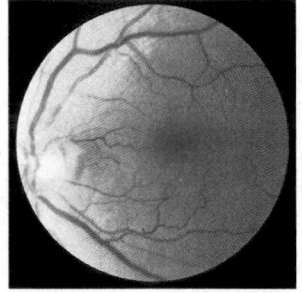

normal fundus

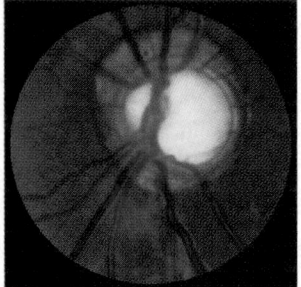

glaucomatous cupping of disc

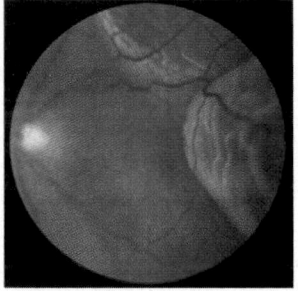

retinal detachment

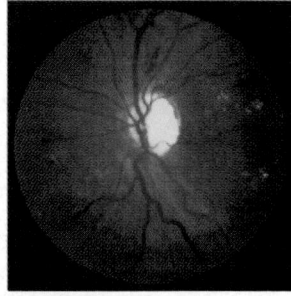

nonproliferative diabetic retinopathy

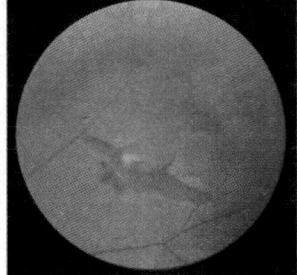

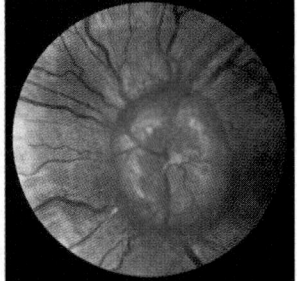

hypertensive retinopathy

retinal tear

papilledema

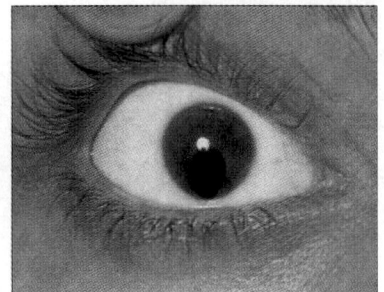

coloboma

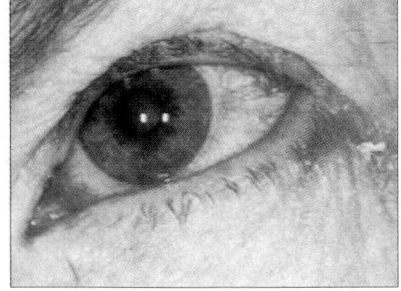

blepharitis angularis *(Staphylococcus aureus)*

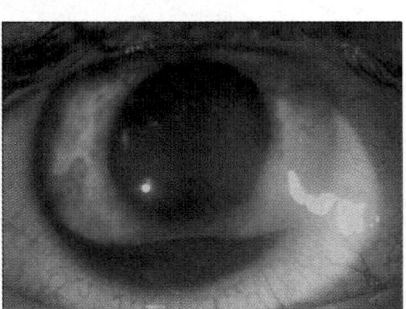

hyphema

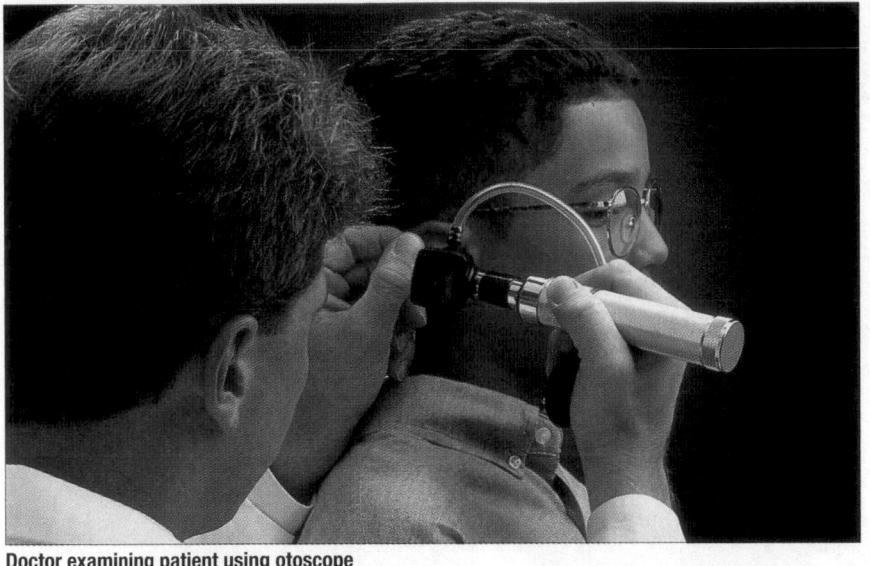

Doctor examining patient using otoscope

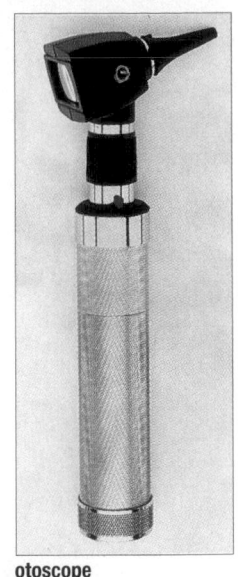

otoscope

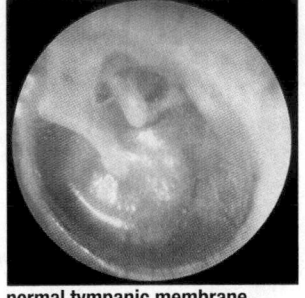

normal tympanic membrane

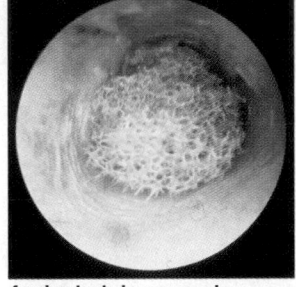

foreign body in ear canal

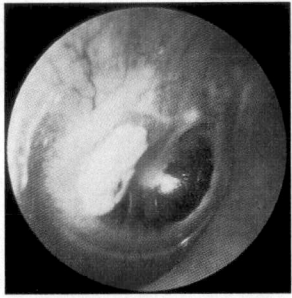

tympanosclerosis

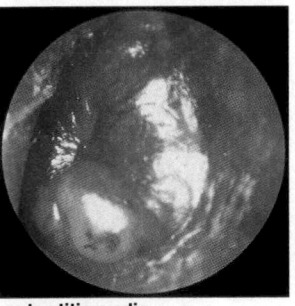

acute otitis media

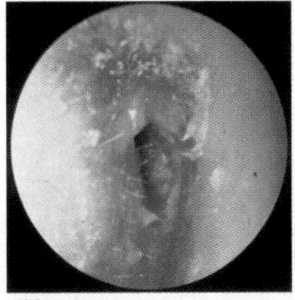

otitis externa

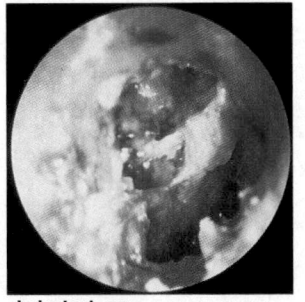

cholesteatoma

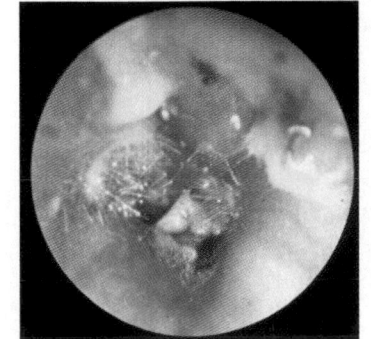

otomycosis

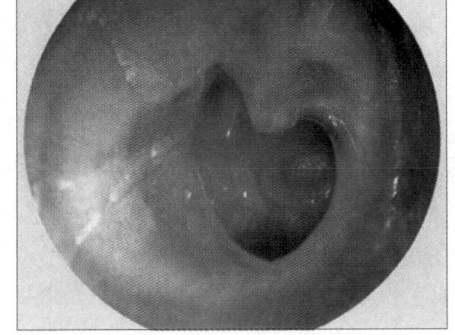

perforation

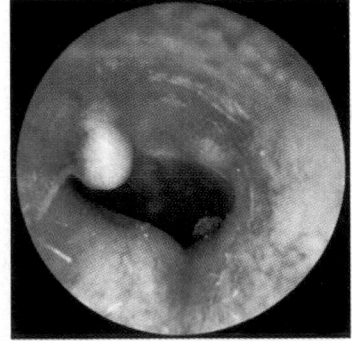

exostosis

Diagnostic Imaging

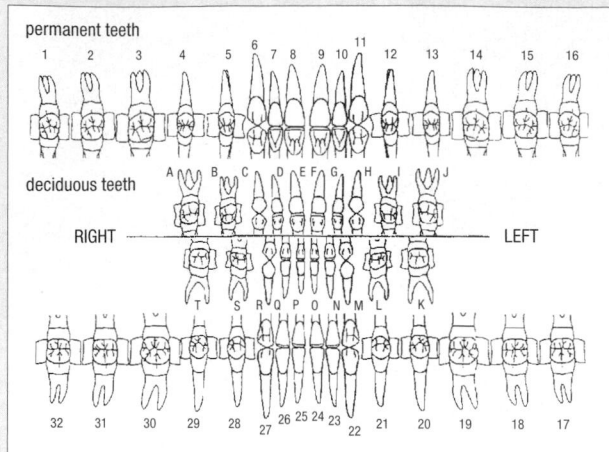

dental chart: showing all surfaces of the permanent and deciduous teeth; teeth numbered 1-16 are maxillary permanent teeth, 17-32 are mandibular permanent teeth; teeth designated A-J and K-T are, respectively, maxillary and mandibular deciduous teeth

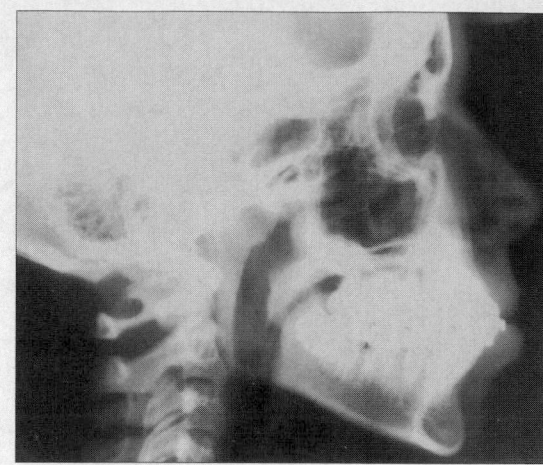

cephalometric radiograph: showing bony structures and overlying soft tissues

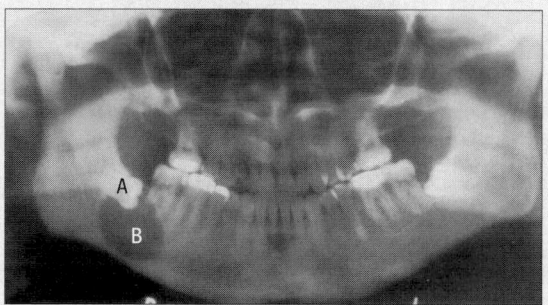

panoramic radiograph: adult dentition; unerupted mandibular third molar (A), and large cyst in mandibular bone around crown of molar (B)

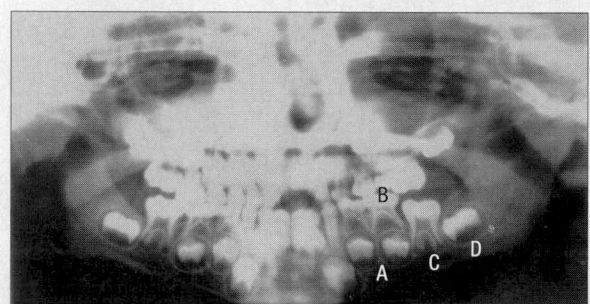

panoramic radiograph: mixed dentition; partially formed permanent mandibular molars (A) erupting below deciduous molars (B); erupted permanent first molar with incompletely formed roots (C); crown of incompletely formed, unerupted, second permanent molar (D)

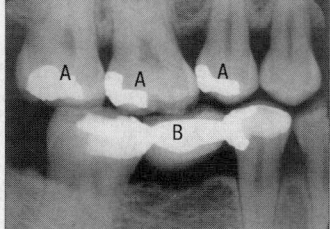

amalgam restorations (A) and fixed bridge (B); bitewing radiograph

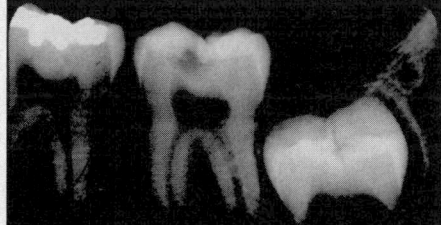

unerupted 3rd molar: the crown is formed but the roots are incomplete

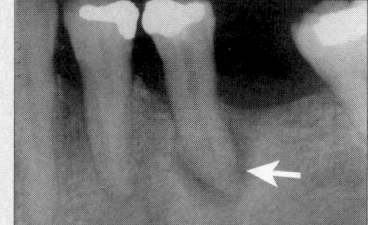

radiolucent area (arrow) around root of mandibular premolar indicating pathological process

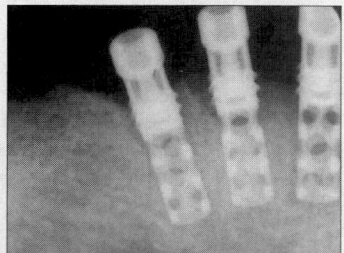

endosteal implants: in alveolar bone; crowns not yet in place

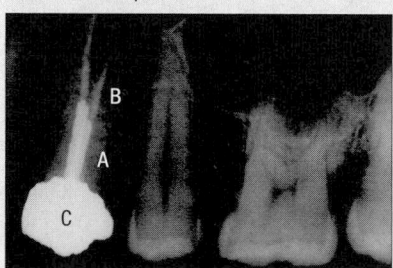

root canal filling (A), posts for retention (B) for metal-lined replacement crown (C)

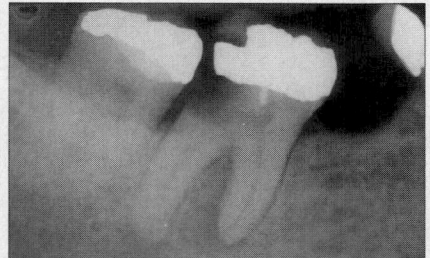

recurrent decay under a metal restoration in a molar

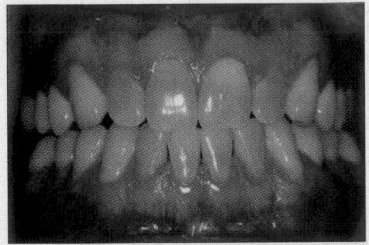
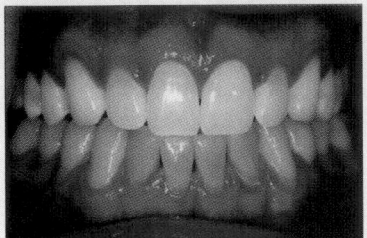

vital bleaching: of teeth to remove tetracycline stains; (top) before, (bottom) after

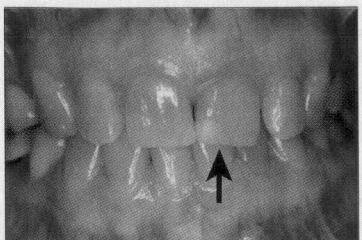
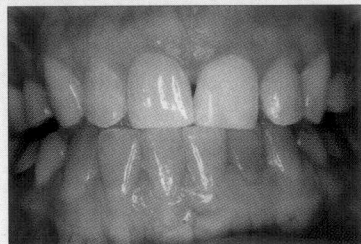

mismatched restoration (arrow top): maxillary teeth have been bleached (bottom) to remove tetracycline stains and restoration replaced

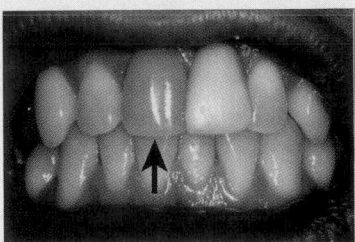
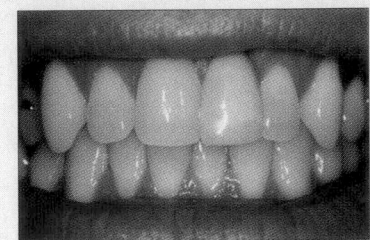

nonvital discolored central incisor (arrow top): bleached for esthetic appearance (bottom)

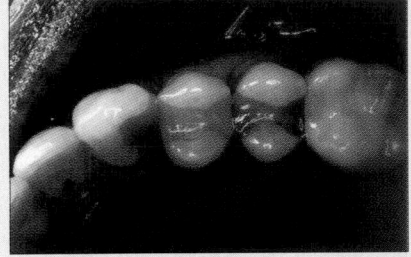
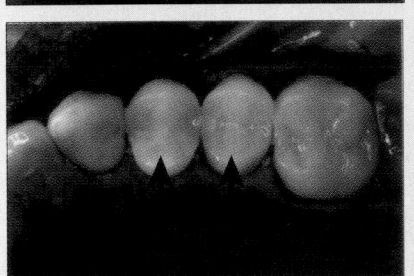

resin restorations: in premolar and cuspid teeth (top); unsightly restorations replaced with esthetic resin restorations (arrows in bottom image)

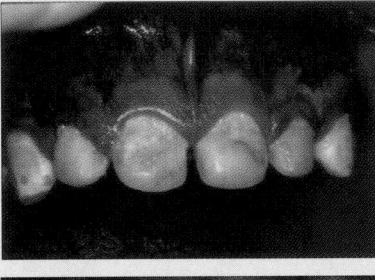
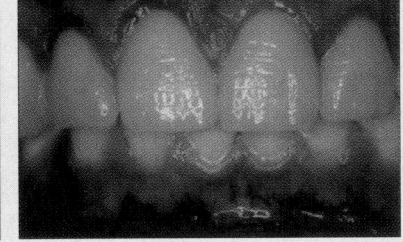

veneers: hypoplastic, stained teeth (top); esthetically restored with veneers (bottom)

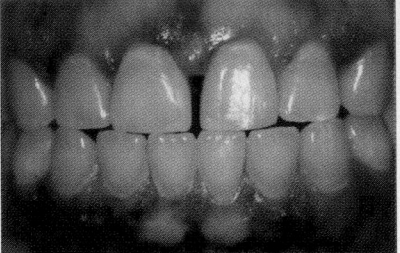
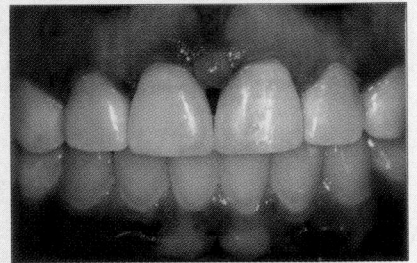

diastema (above): between teeth closed by resin composite veneers (bottom)

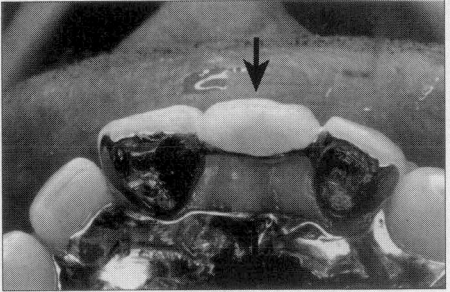
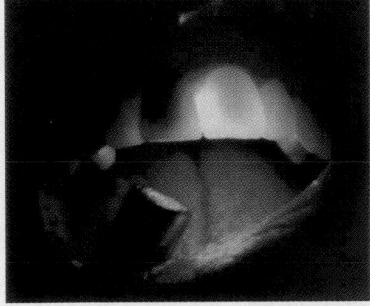

resin-bonded esthetic bridge: (far left) metal framework is bonded to natural, uncrowned, abutment teeth and holds replacement tooth (arrow)

porcelain crowns: (left) transilluminated demonstrating how crowns may be made to retain natural translucency

Diagnostic Imaging

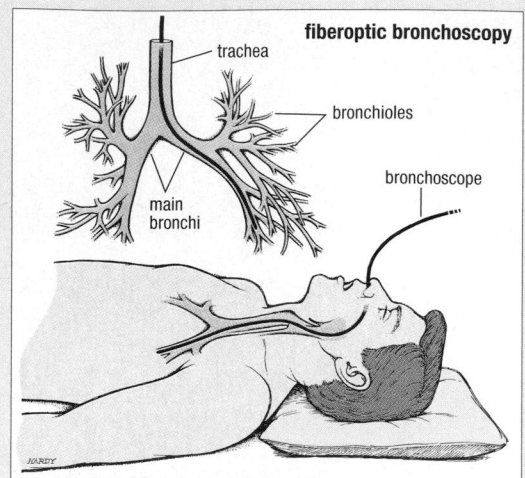

fiberoptic bronchoscopy

trachea

bronchioles

bronchoscope

main bronchi

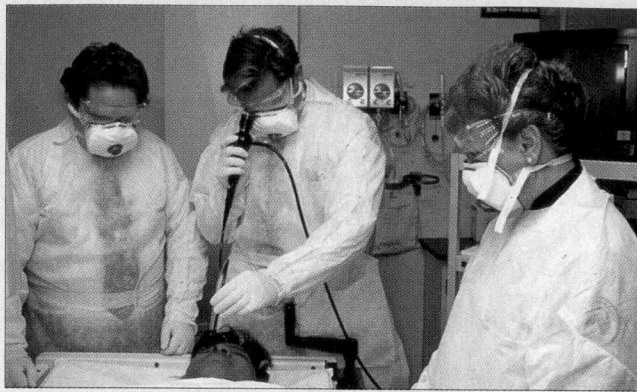

bronchoscopy team performing procedure

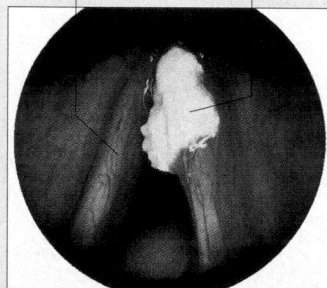

vocal fold   carcinoma

laryngeal carcinoma

bronchoscopy is the examination of the respiratory apparatus with a flexible bronchoscope for diagnostic or treatment purposes; the bronchoscope is introduced nasally and slowly led down the trachea until the desired level is reached; the photographs on this page were taken with a camera that attaches to the examiner's end of the instrument

carina

entire trachea and the carina

carina

right main bronchus

left main bronchus

carina

B^1

B^2

B^3

right upper lobe bronchus

left vocal fold

right vocal fold

glottis

vocal folds

esophagogastroduodenoscopy is the examination of the esophagus, stomach and upper small intestine using a flexible esophagogastroduodeno-scope; fiber optics in the instrument conduct bright, cool light along a curved path, allowing illumination of tissues and structures within the body; the scope often contains small instruments such as biopsy snares

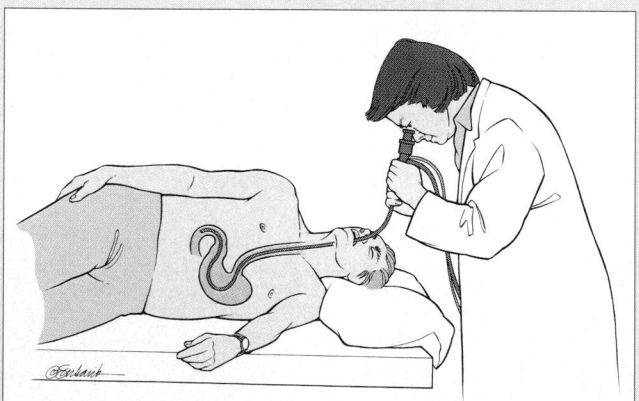

esophagoduodenoscope is introduced nasally or orally and led slowly down the esophagus and gastrointestinal tract until the disired level is reached

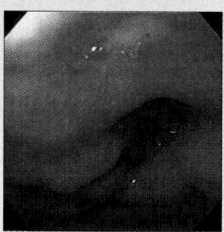

gastritis

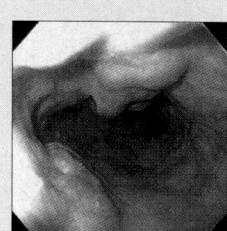

esophageal varices

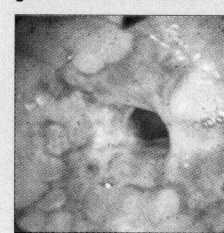

Barrett esophagus: tight esophageal stricture

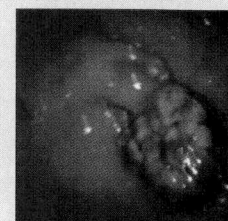

pedunculated hyperplastic **gastric polyp**

cystoscopy is the inspection of the inside of the bladder using a cystoscope, a flexible tube containing fiberoptics and small instruments; the cystoscope is introduced though the urethra and slowly advanced until the bladder is reached; cystoscopy can be used in diagnosis and in minor operative procedures as seen in the two cystoscopic images below

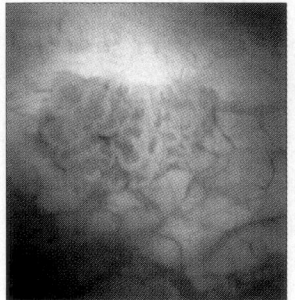

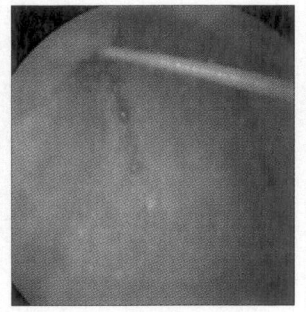

bladder tumor: on inside surface of bladder

cystoscopic view of a catheter being passed into a ureter

intraoperative cholangiography: a clean cut is being made into the lateral wall of the cystic duct so that a catheter can be inserted

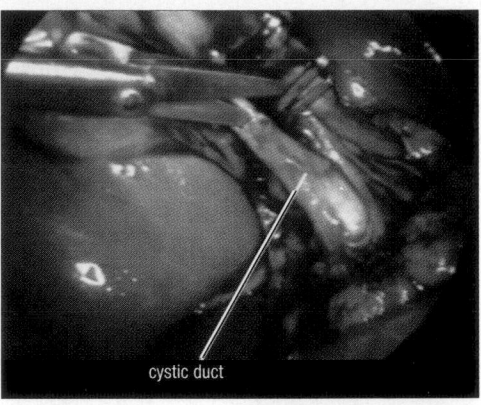

cystic duct

laparoscopy involves inserting a laparoscope into the peritoneal cavity through a 2-cm incision below the umbilicus to allow visualization of the pelvic structures (below left); indications for laparoscopy are diagnostic; laparoscopy can also facilitate minor operative procedures such as tubal ligation, ovarian biopsy, and lysing adhesions; a forceps is inserted through the scope to, in this case, grasp the uterine tube; insufflation of gas creates an air pocket (pneumoperitoneum), and the pelvis is elevated which forces the intestines higher in the abdomen

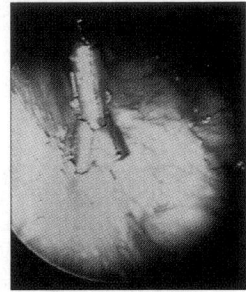

laparoscopic biopsy

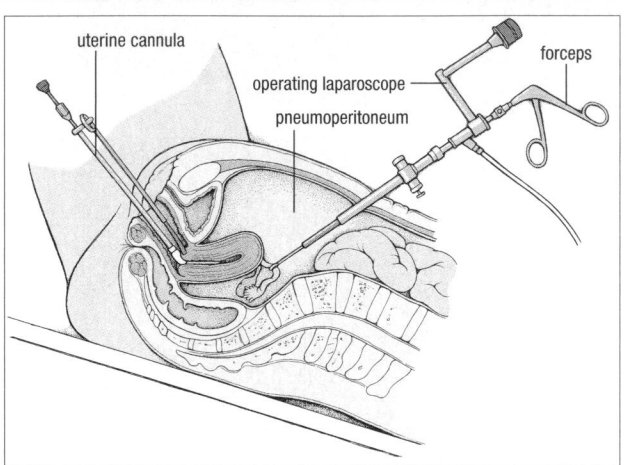

uterine cannula

operating laparoscope

pneumoperitoneum

forceps

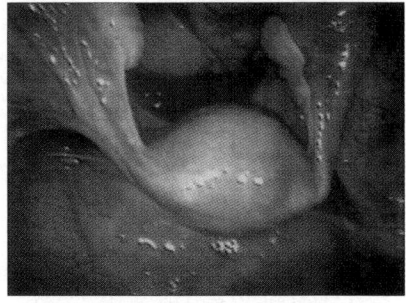

laparoscopic view of **normal pelvis**

thoracoscopy is a diagnostic procedure in which the pleural cavity is examined with an endoscope (right); small incisions are made into the pleural cavity in an intercostal space; the use of fiberoptic instruments and miniature video equipment permits visualization of thoracic structures; tissue can be excised for biopsy, and treatment of some thoracic conditions can be conducted

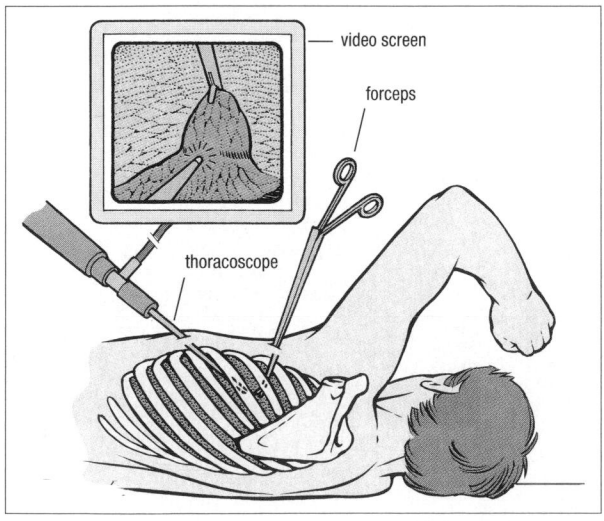

video screen

forceps

thoracoscope

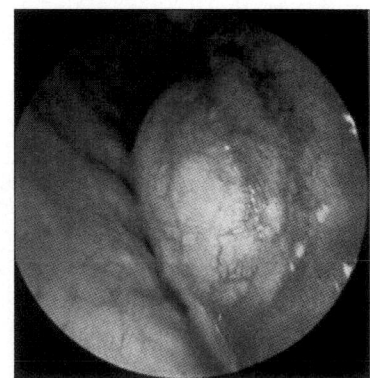

pleural cavity: thoracoscopic view; intercostal vessels can be seen on left and medially retracted pleura on right

Diagnostic Imaging

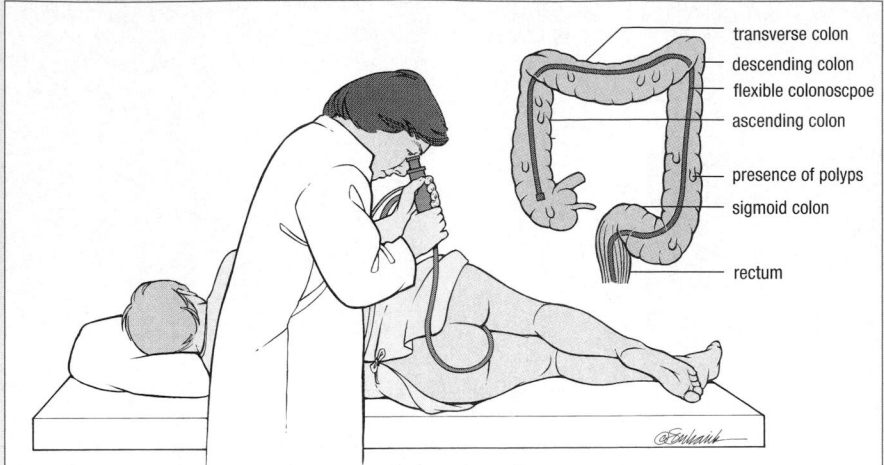

transverse colon
descending colon
flexible colonoscpoe
ascending colon
presence of polyps
sigmoid colon
rectum

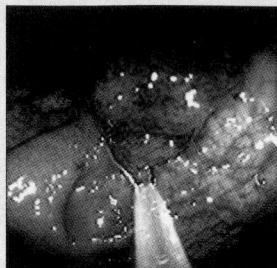

colon polypectomy

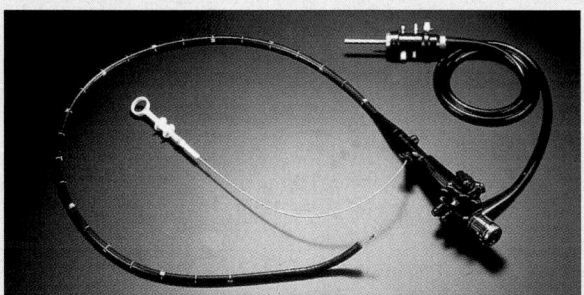

colonoscope

colonoscopy is the examination and diagnosis of conditions of the colon; the flexible colonoscope passes through the rectum and sigmoid colon into the descending, transverse, and ascending colon (above); small instruments can be passed through the colonoscope and used to facilatate minor operative procedures; the images to the right were taken by a camera attached to the colonoscope

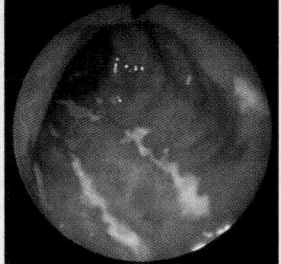

ulcerative colitis

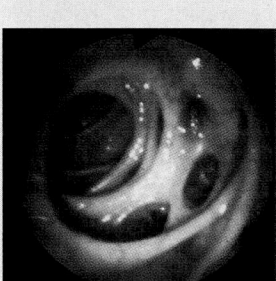

diverticulosis

arthroscopy is the endoscopic examination of the interior of a joint; tiny incisions, known as portals, are made for the insertion of the arthroscope and other instruments; the arthroscope contains fiber optics and a miniature video camera that projects the anatomy and procedure onto a video monitor (right); a second cannula contains instruments and motorized equipment used to repair structures and remove damaged tissue; saline solution is often introduced through a third cannula to expand the joint and rinse away any blood or debris; the images below were captured using an arthroscopic camera

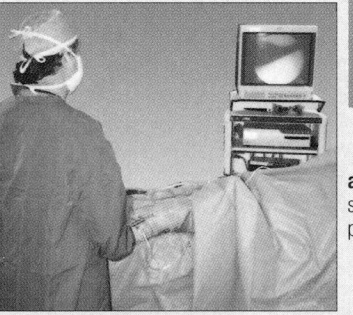

arthroscopic knee procedure: surgeon uses video monitor to view progress

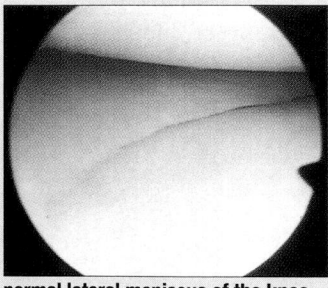

normal lateral meniscus of the knee

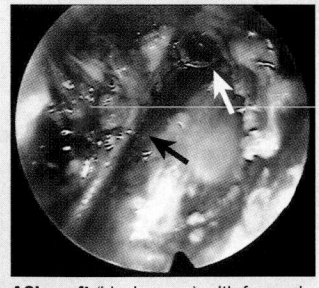

ACL graft (black arrow) with femoral interference screw visable (white arrow)

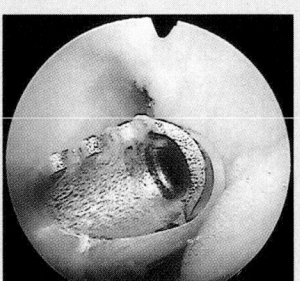

trimming of a torn lateral meniscus

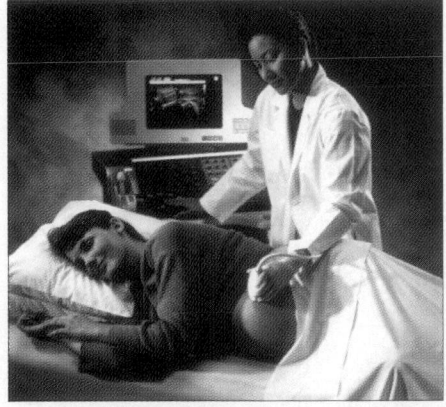

during **sonography** (right) energy in the form of sound waves is reflected off internal organs or, during pregnancy, the fetus, and is transformed into an image on a TV-type monitor; in the case of obstetrical sonography (left) an ultrasound image of the pregnant uterus is created in order to determine fetal development

obstetrical sonography performed on a pregnant woman

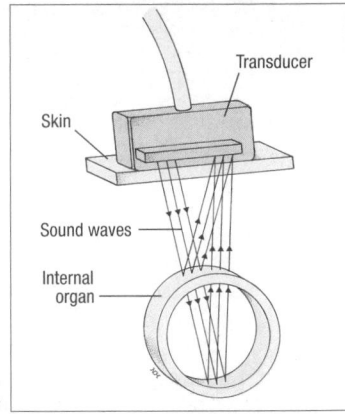

principle of sonography

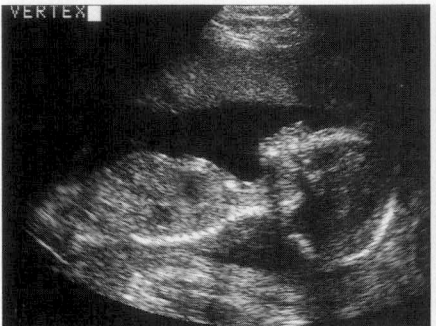

fetus in breech position: sagittal view

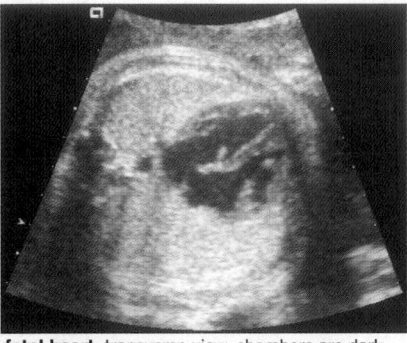

fetal heart: transverse view, chambers are dark areas surrounded by the lungs

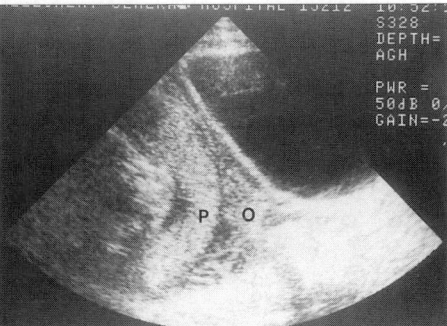

placenta previa: longitudinal scan shows the placenta (P) lying just above the cervical os (O)

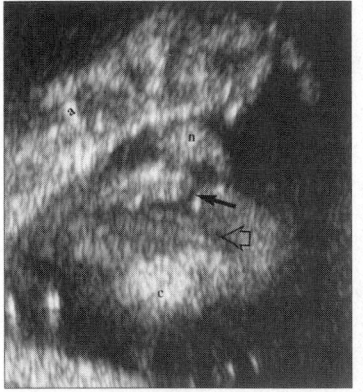

cleft lip: coronal view of fetal face reveals a cleft (arrow) in the left lip extending into left naris; mouth (open arrow), nose (n), chin (c)

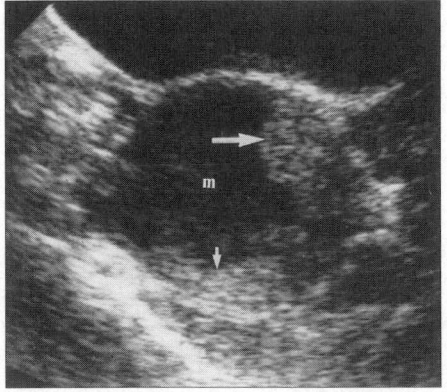

ovarian carcinoma: US of an adnexal mass (m) shows it to be predominantly cystic but with a thick wall (small arrow) and a prominent solid nodule (large arrow)

during **Doppler sonography** an instrument emits an ultrasonic beam into the body; the ultrasound reflected from moving structures changes its frequency (Doppler effect); Doppler sonography is often used in diagnosing peripheral vascular and cardiac disease

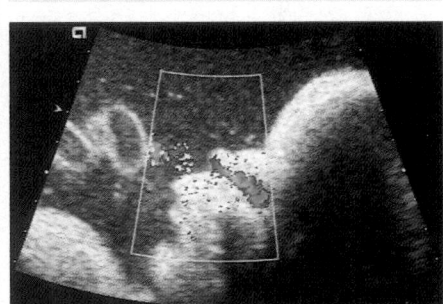

Doppler flow sonogram showing the flow of amniotic fluid into the nasal cavity of the fetus

echocardiography is the use of ultrasound in the investigation of the heart and great vessels and diagnosis of vascular lesions (left and far left)

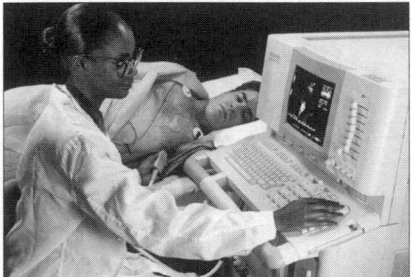

echocardiography technique

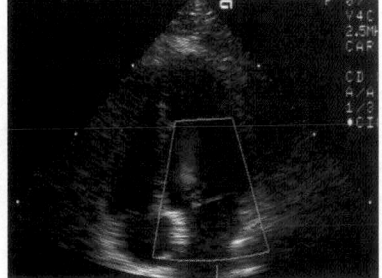

echocardiogram: normal, two dimensional, apical four-chamber view

Diagnostic Imaging

radiography or **roentgenography** is the examination of any part of the body for diagnostic purposes by means of x-rays with the record of findings usually impressed upon a photographic film

as shown in the graphic below, differential absorption of x-rays depends on the composition of various tissues; denser tissue (such as bone) absorbs more x-rays, less dense tissue (such as subcutaneous fat) transmits more x-rays; greater absorption produces less darkening on the film while lesser absorption produces more darkening; the resultant radiographic image is essentially a "shadowgram"

the **plain chest radiology** images on these two pages show various pathological conditions of the chest and respiratory system

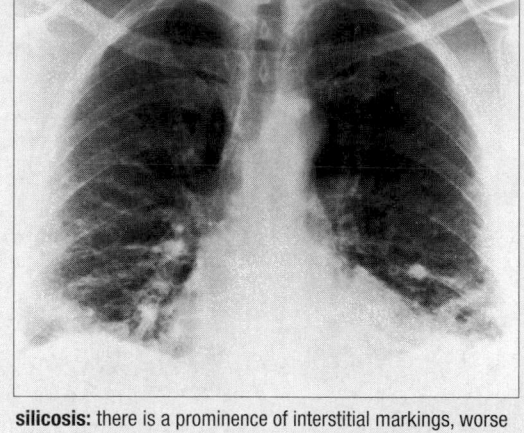

silicosis: there is a prominence of interstitial markings, worse in the lung bases

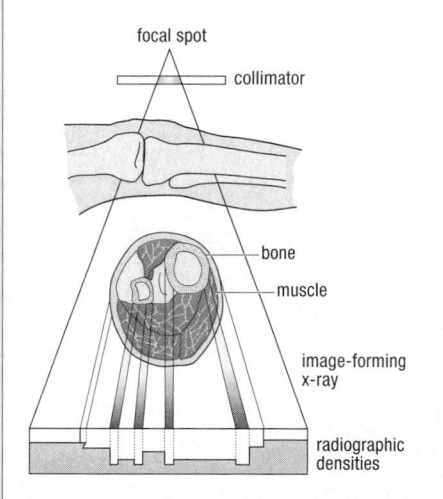

x-rays pass through body part with the denser structures absorbing more x-rays resulting in the lighter areas on the radiograph

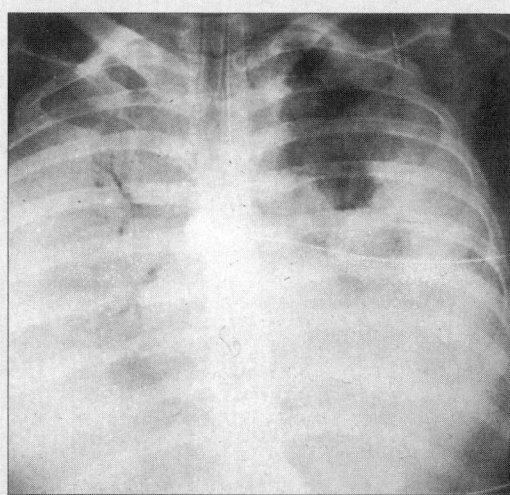

adult respiratory distress syndrome (ARDS)

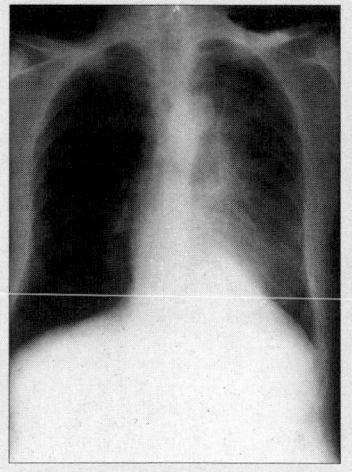
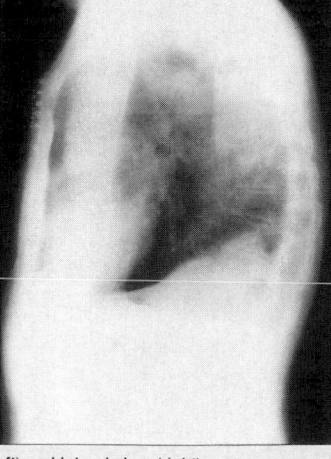

left upper lobe collapse: posteroanterior (left) and lateral view (right)

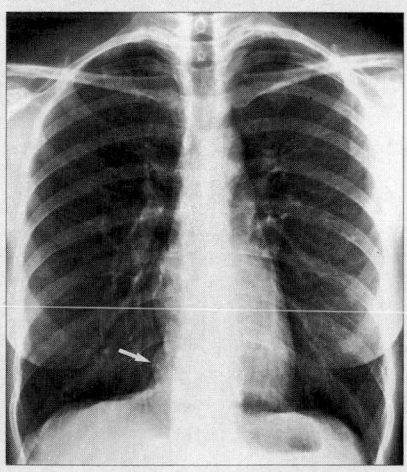

pericardial cyst: (arrow)

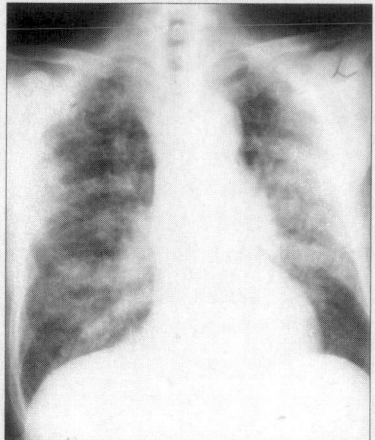

interstitial lung disease

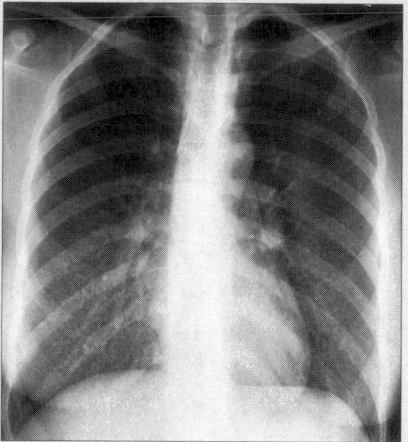

miliary tuberculosis: in patient with AIDS showing fine diffuse nodular pattern throughout both lower lobes

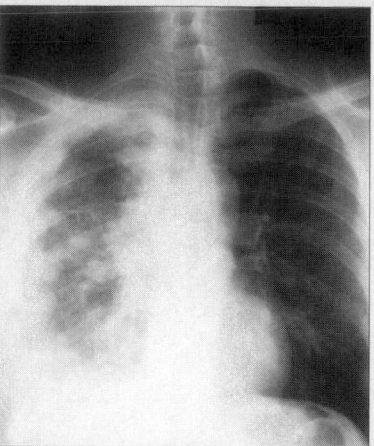

malignant mesothelioma: note lobulated right pleural thickening encompassing the right lung

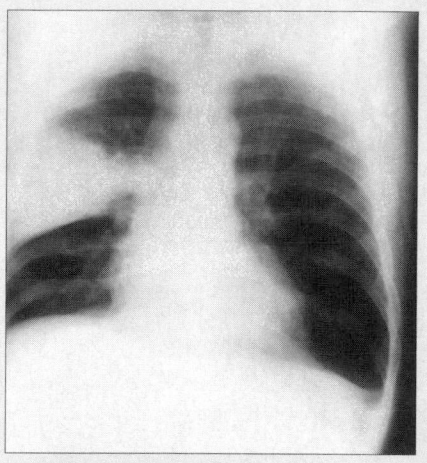

bacterial pneumonia: in right upper lobe

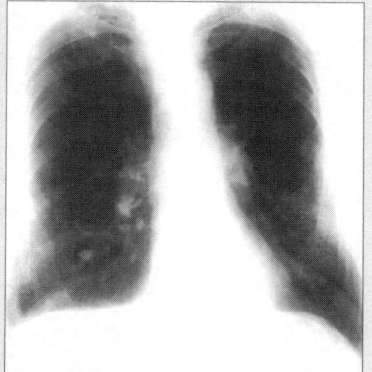

Ranke complex: with Ghon focus in right side secondary to healed tuberculosis

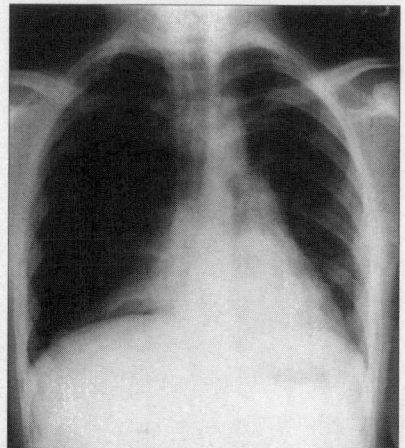

right sided pneumothorax: with evidence of medistinal shift (tension)

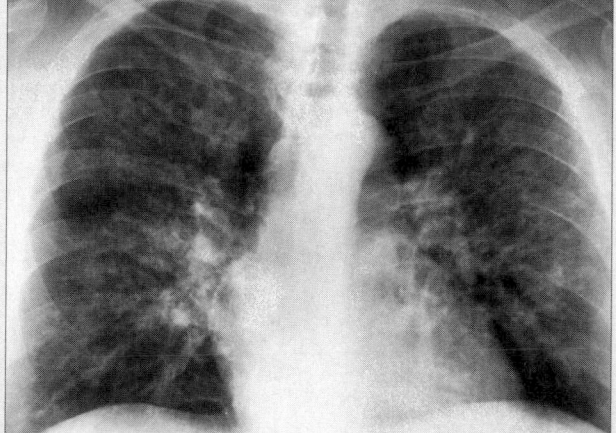

***Pneumocystis carinii* pneumonia (PCP):** in AIDS patient showing bilateral pneumonic densities

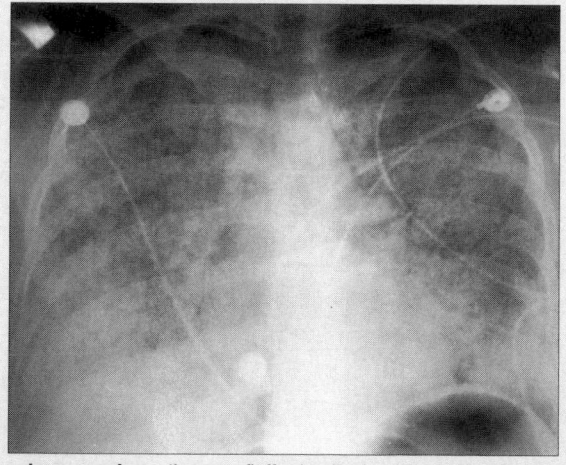

pulmonary edema: there are fluffy alveolar densities throught both lungs

Diagnostic Imaging

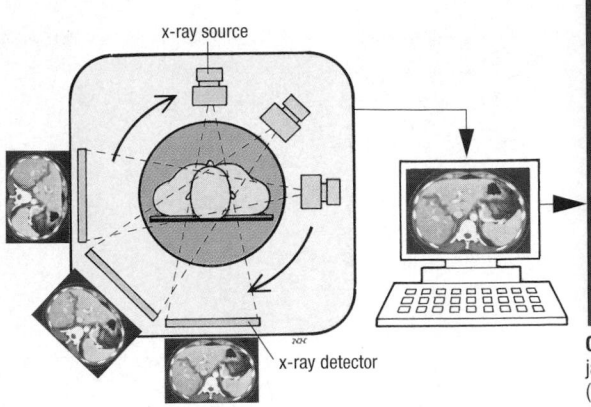

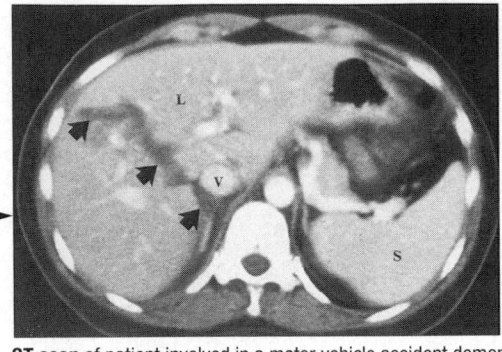

CT scan of patient involved in a motor vehicle accident demonstrates a jagged laceration (arrows) extending from posterior to inferior vena cava (V) through right lobe of the liver (L); (S), spleen

computed tomography (CT) is a radiologic procedure using a machine called a scanner to examine a body site by taking a series of cross-sectional images one slice at a time in a full circle rotation; a computer then calculates and converts the rates of absorption and density of the x-rays into a picture on a screen

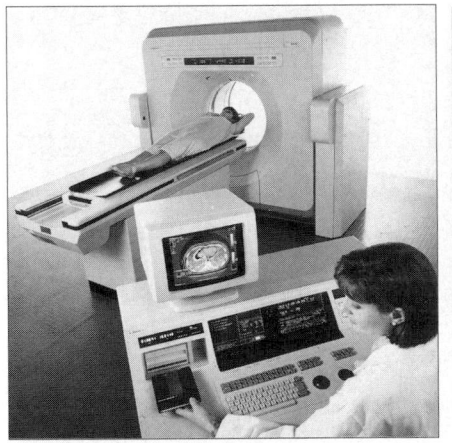

computed tomography apparatus

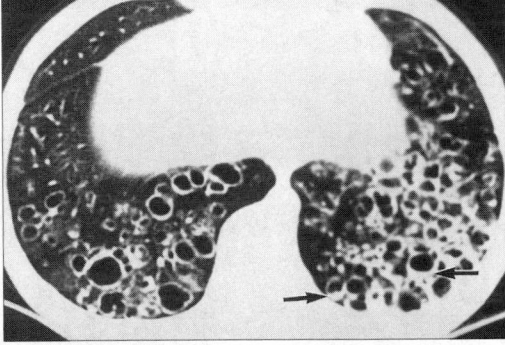

cystic bronchiectasis: note chronic dilation of bronchi and bronchioles (arrows)

acute epidural hematoma: note lentiform shape to the hematoma (arrows)

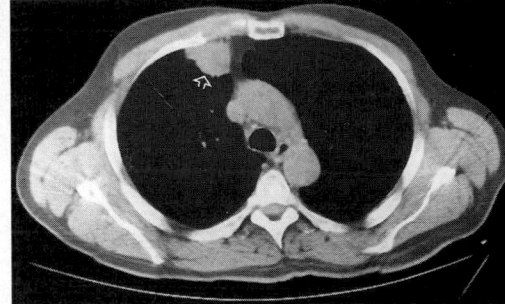

lung carcinoma: CT section shows mass to be located in anterior segment of right upper lobe (arrow) adjacent to pleura

mammography is the imaging examination of the breast by means of x-rays, ultrasound, and nuclear magnetic resonance, used for the screening and diagnosis of breast disease; x-ray mammography has proved to have the greatest efficacy for detecting occult breast cancer

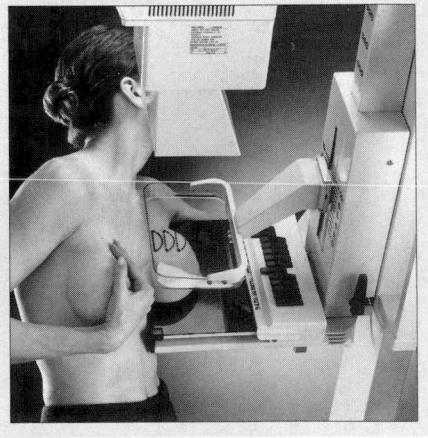

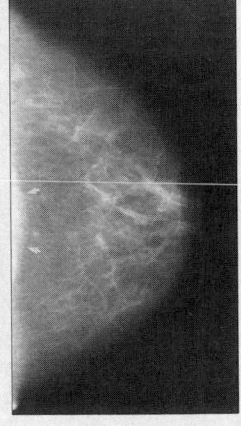

patient positioning for a MLO view (far left)

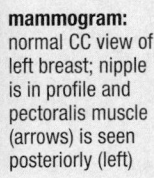

mammogram: normal CC view of left breast; nipple is in profile and pectoralis muscle (arrows) is seen posteriorly (left)

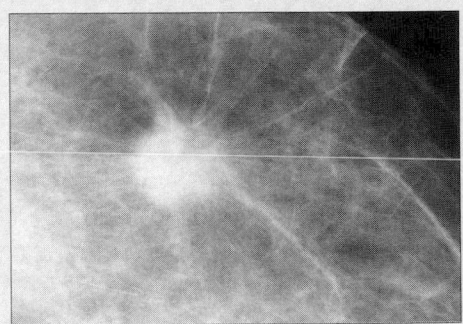

classic breast carcinoma: this spiculated breast mass is an infiltrating duct carcinoma

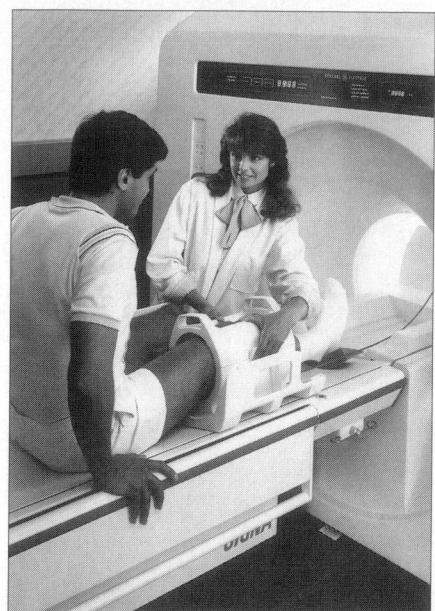

MRI unit

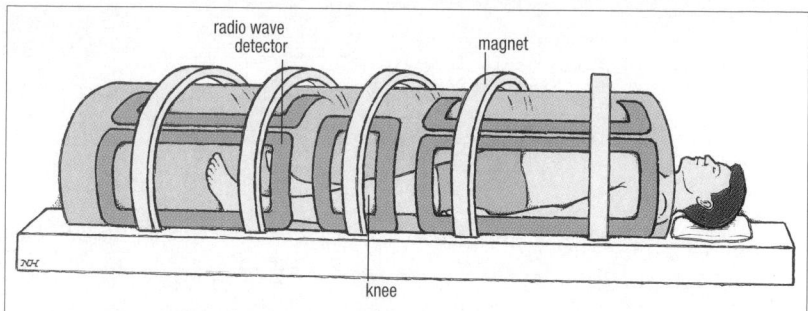

radio wave detector

magnet

knee

magnetic resonance imaging (MRI) is a nonionizing (non-x-ray) technique using magnetic fields and radiofrequency waves to visualize anatomic structures--useful in detecting joint, tendon, and vertebral disorders; the patient is positioned within a magnetic field (above) as radiowave signals are conducted through the selected body part; energy is absorbed by tissues and then released

computer processes the released energy and formulates image

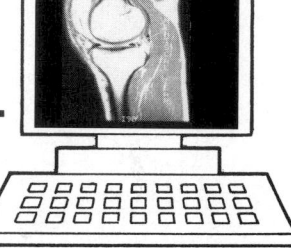

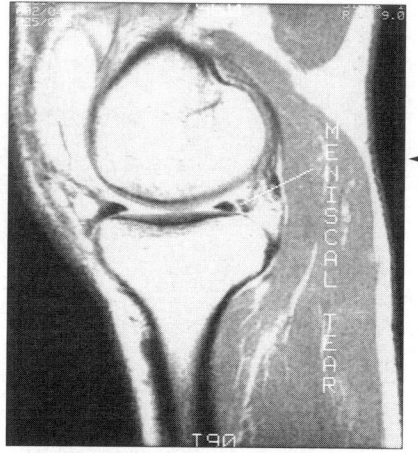

magnetic resonance image of knee (lateral view) identifying a torn meniscus

MENISCAL TEAR

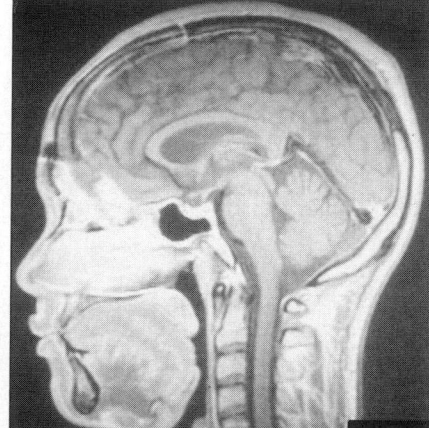

MRI image of normal brain: sagittal section

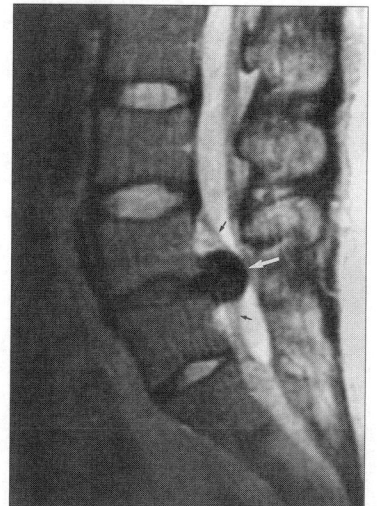

herniated nucleus pulposus: sagittal MRI shows a large posterior herniation (arrows) at the L4 disc space; note the posterior displacement of the thecal sac (small arrows)

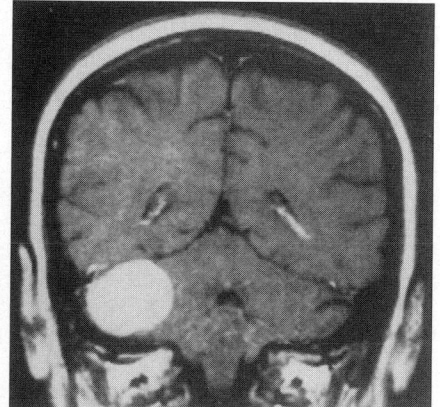

meningioma in the cerebellum

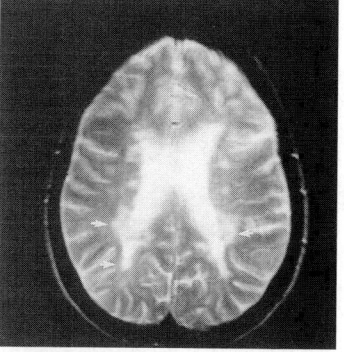

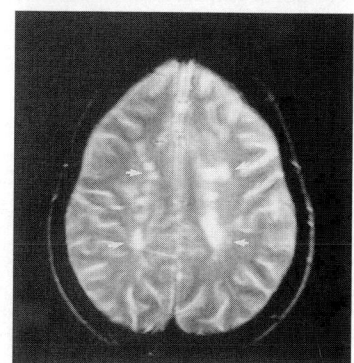

multiple sclerosis: contiguous T2-weighted MR images, show areas of ventricular plaques of high signal (arrows)

Diagnostic Imaging

nuclear medicine imaging is a diagnostic imaging technique using injected or ingested radioactive isotopes and a gamma-camera for determining size, shape, location, and function of various body parts

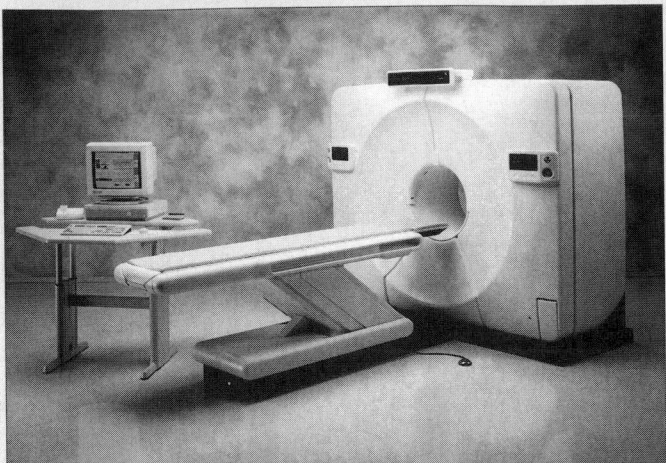

positron emission tomography (PET) combines nuclear medicine and computed tomography to produce images of brain anatomy and corresponding physiology-used to study conditions such as stroke, Alzheimer disease (right), epilepsy, metabolic brain disorders, and chemistry of neural function

warm colors (red and yellow) indicate a higher rate of metabolism and brain activity in the normal brain (A) when compared to the brain of a patient with Alzheimer disease (B)

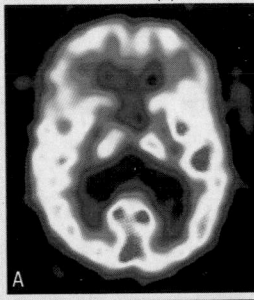

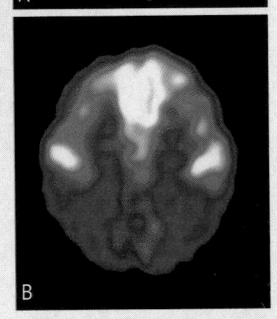

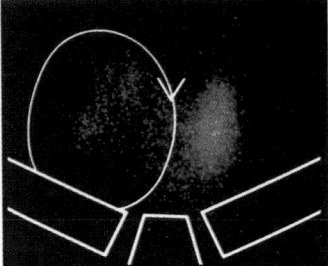

thyroid uptake and image is a nuclear image involving scanning of the thyroid gland to visualize radioactive accumulation of previously injected isotopes to detect thyroid nodules or tumors

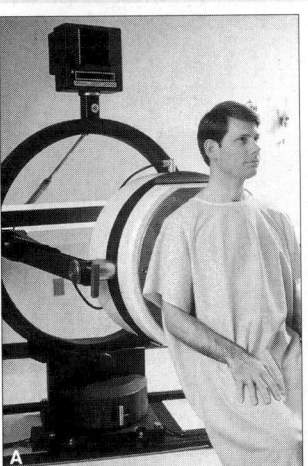

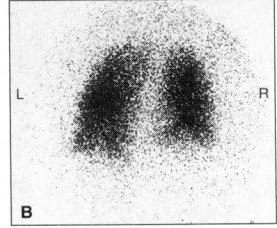

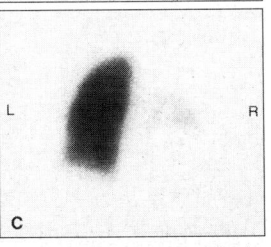

nuclear lung scan is used to detect abnormalities of perfusion (blood flow) or ventilation (respiration); commonly called a V / Q (ventilation / perfusion) scan; (A) gamma-camera used to produce lung scan; in this patient a posterior lung scan shows an embolus in the right lung; ventilation scan (B) shows a normal pattern; absence of blood flow to the right lung is apparent on perfusion scan (C)

DEXA scan (upper right) of a femur to test for bone density; warmer colors (yellows, reds) indicate areas of low density

liver scan (scintiscan): (right) showing normal results

bone scan: nuclear scan of bone tissue to detect abnormalities such as tumors malignancies; below is an example of of a full-body bone scan

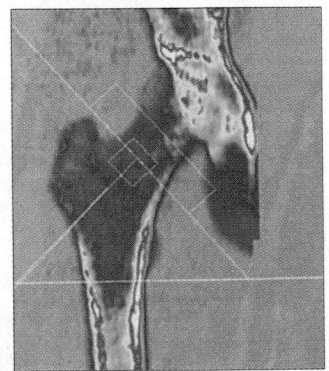

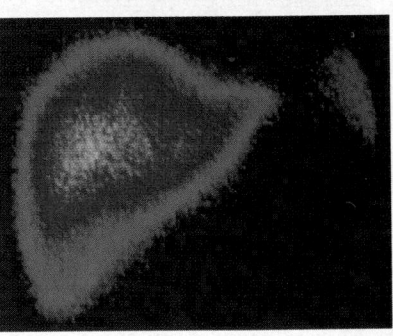

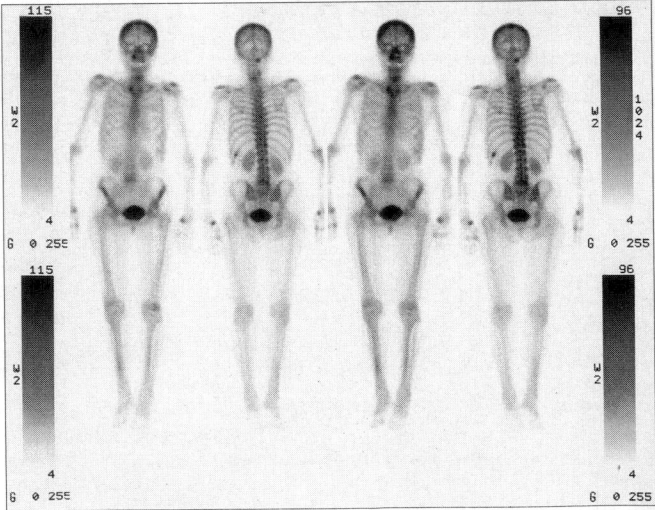

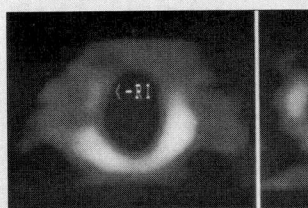

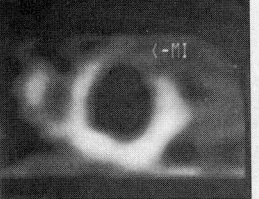

myocardial perfusion stress scan is a nuclear scan of the heart taken before and after controlled physical exercise (treadmill or bicycle) or a pharmaceutical agent that produces the effect of exercise stress in patients unable to ambulate

ep·i·did·y·mot·o·my (ep′i-did-i-mot′ō-mē). Incision into the epididymis, as in preparation for epididymovasostomy or for drainage of purulent material. [epididymis + G. *tomē*, a cutting]

ep·i·did·y·mo·vas·ec·to·my (ep-i-did′i-mō-va-sek′tō-mē). Surgical removal of the epididymis and vas deferens, usually proximal to its entry into the inguinal canal. [epididymis + vasectomy]

ep·i·did·y·mo·va·sos·to·my (ep-i-did′i-mō-va-sos′tō-mē). Surgical anastomosis of the vas deferens to the epididymis. [epididymis + vasostomy]

ep·i·du·ral (ep-i-doo′răl). Upon (or outside) the dura mater. SYN peridural.

ep·i·du·rog·ra·phy (ep-i-doo-rog′ră-fē). Radiographic visualization of the epidural space following the regional instillation of a radiopaque contrast medium; obsolete technique.

ep·i·es·tri·ol (ep-i-es′trē-ol). SEE estriol.

ep·i·fas·cial (ep-i-fash′ē-ăl). Upon the surface of a fascia, denoting a method of injecting drugs in which the solution is put on the fascia lata instead of injected into the substance of the muscle.

ep·i·gas·tral·gia (ep′i-gas-tral′jē-ă). Pain in the epigastric region. [epigastrium + G. *algos*, pain]

ep·i·gas·tric (ep-i-gas′trik). Relating to the epigastrium.

ep·i·gas·tri·um (ep-i-gas′trē-ŭm) [TA]. SYN epigastric *region*, epigastric *region*. [G. *epigastrion*]

ep·i·gas·tri·us (ep-i-gas′trē-ŭs). Unequal conjoined twins in which the smaller parasite is attached to the larger autosite in the epigastric region. SEE conjoined *twins*, under *twin*.

ep·i·gen·e·sis (ep-i-jen′ĕ-sis). **1.** Development of offspring from a zygote. Cf. preformation *theory*. **2.** Regulation of the expression of gene activity without alteration of genetic structure. [epi- + G. *genesis*, creation]

ep·i·ge·net·ic (ep′i-jĕ-net′ik). Relating to epigenesis.

ep·i·glot·tic, ep·i·glot·tid·e·an (ep-i-glot′ik, ep-i-glo-tid′ē-an). Relating to the epiglottis.

ep·i·glot·ti·dec·to·my (ep′i-glot-i-dek′tō-mē). Excision of the epiglottis. [epiglottis + G. *ektomē*, excision]

ep·i·glot·ti·di·tis (ep′i-glot-i-dī′tis). SYN epiglottitis.

ep·i·glot·tis (ep-i-glot′is) [TA]. A leaf-shaped plate of elastic cartilage, covered with mucous membrane, at the root of the tongue, which serves as a diverter valve over the superior aperture of the larynx during the act of swallowing; it stands erect when liquids are being swallowed, but is passively bent over the aperture by solid foods being swallowed. [G. *epiglōttis*, fr. *epi*, on, + *glōttis*, the mouth of the windpipe]

bifid e., congenital malformation in which the right and left sides of the e. are not joined; associated with stridor and aspiration in the newborn due to the rotation of the two sides of the e. into the glottis.

ep·i·glot·ti·tis (ep-i-glot-ī′tis). Inflammation of the epiglottis, which may cause respiratory obstruction, especially in children; frequently due to infection by *Haemophilus influenzae* type b. SYN epiglottiditis.

epig·na·thus (e-pig′nă-thŭs). Unequal conjoined twins in which the smaller, incomplete parasite is attached to the larger autosite at the lower jaw. SEE conjoined *twins*, under *twin*. [epi- + G. *gnathos*, jaw]

ep·i·hy·al (ep-i-hī′ăl). Above the hyoid arch.

ep·i·hy·oid (ep-i-hī′oyd). Upon the hyoid bone; denoting certain accessory thyroid glands lying above the geniohyoid muscle.

ep·i·ker·a·to·phak·ia (ep′i-ker′ă-tō-phak′ē-ă). Modification of refractive error by application of a donor cornea to the anterior surface of the patient's cornea from which epithelium has been removed. SYN epikeratophakic keratoplasty. [epi- + G. *keras*, horn, + *phakos*, lens]

ep·i·ker·a·to·pros·the·sis (ep′i-ker′ă-tō-pros′thē-sis). A contact lens attached to the corneal stroma to replace the epithelium. [epi- + G. *keras*, horn, + *prosthesis*, an addition]

ep·i·la·mel·lar (ep′i-lă-mel′ăr). Upon or above a basement membrane. [epi- + L. *lamella*, dim. of *lamina*, a thin metal plate]

ep·i·late (ep′i-lāt). To extract a hair; to remove the hair from a part by forcible extraction, electrolysis, or loosening at the root by chemical means. Cf. depilate. [L. *e*, out, + *pilus*, a hair]

ep·i·la·tion (ep-i-lā′shŭn). The act or result of removing hair. SYN depilation.

epil·a·to·ry (e-pil′ă-tō-rē). **1.** Having the property of removing hair; relating to epilation. SYN depilatory (1), psilotic (2). SEE ALSO decalvant. **2.** SYN depilatory (2).

ep·i·lem·ma (ep-i-lem′ă). The connective tissue sheath of nerve fibers near their termination. [epi- *lemma*, husk]

ep·i·lep·i·do·ma (ep′i-lep-i-dō′mă). A tumor resulting from hyperplasia of tissue derived from the true epiblast. [epi- + G. *lepis*, rind, + *-ōma*, tumor]

ep·i·lep·sia (ep-i-lep′sē-ă). SYN epilepsy. [G.]

e. partia′lis contin′ua, (1) a form of epilepsy marked by repetitive clonic muscular contractions with or without major convulsions; (2) simple partial motor status epilepticus of the rolandic cortex, often with myoclonic features; (3) a seizure type seen commonly with Rasmussen encephalitis. SYN Kojewnikoff epilepsy.

ep·i·lep·sy (ep′i-lep′sē). A chronic disorder characterized by paroxysmal brain dysfunction due to excessive neuronal discharge, and usually associated with some alteration of consciousness. The clinical manifestations of the attack may vary from complex abnormalities of behavior including generalized or focal convulsions to momentary spells of impaired consciousness. These clinical states have been subjected to a variety of classifications, none universally accepted to date and, accordingly, the terminologies used to describe the different types of attacks remain purely descriptive and nonstandardized; they are variously based on 1) the clinical manifestations of the seizure (motor, sensory, reflex, psychic or vegetative), 2) the pathologic substrate (hereditary, inflammatory, degenerative, neoplastic, traumatic, or cryptogenic), 3) the location of the epileptogenic lesion (rolandic, temporal, diencephalic regions), and 4) the time of life at which the attacks occur (nocturnal, diurnal, menstrual, etc.). SYN convulsive state, epilepsia, falling sickness. [G. *epilēpsia*, seizure]

anosognosic e., epilepsy characterized by attacks of which the person is unaware. SYN anosognosic seizures.

automatic e., SYN psychomotor e.

autonomic e., episodes of autonomic dysfunction presumably due to diencephalic irritation. SYN diencephalic e., vasomotor e., vasovagal e.

benign childhood e. with centrotemporal spikes, a specific epilepsy syndrome beginning in childhood and remitting in adolescence, characterized by nocturnal simple partial motor seizures or generalized tonic-clonic seizures. EEG shows centrotemporal spikes that are activated by sleep and an otherwise normal EEG background.

centrencephalic e., an imprecise term referring to e. characterized electroencephalographically by bilateral synchronous discharges, and clinically by absence or generalized tonic-clonic seizures.

childhood absence e., a generalized e. syndrome characterized by the onset of absence seizures in childhood, typically at age six or seven years. There is a strong genetic predisposition and girls are affected more often than boys. EEG reveals generalized 3-Hz spike-wave activity on a normal background. Prognosis for remission is good if the patient does not also have generalized tonic-clonic seizures. SEE ALSO absence. SYN petit mal e., pyknolepsy.

childhood e. with occipital paroxysms, a benign e. syndrome characterized by frequent occipital spikes often activated by eye closure. It has a seizure semiology that includes visual manifestations; not always remitting later in life.

complex precipitated e., a form of reflex e. initiated by specialized sensory stimuli, e.g., certain visual patterns.

cortical e., SYN focal e.

cryptogenic e., SYN generalized tonic-clonic *seizure*.

diencephalic e., SYN autonomic e.

early posttraumatic e., seizures beginning within one week after severe head injury.

eating e., epileptic, often generalized, seizures provoked by eating; a type of reflex e.

ep

focal e., e. of various etiologies characterized by focal seizures or secondarily generalized tonic-clonic seizures. Ictal symptoms are often related to the brain region where the seizure begins focally. SYN cortical e., local e., localization-related e. (2), partial e.

frontal lobe e., a localization-related e. with seizures originating in the frontal lobe. A variety of clinical syndromes exist depending on the exact localization of seizures and clinical semiology of the seizure type. Frontal lobe epilepsies have been divided into several specific syndromes including the syndrome of supplementary motor seizures, cingulate seizures, anterior frontal polar region seizures, orbital frontal seizures, dorsolateral seizures, opercular seizures, and seizures of the motor cortex.

generalized e., a major category of e. syndromes characterized by one or more types of generalized seizures.

generalized tonic-clonic e., SYN generalized tonic-clonic *seizure.*

grand mal e., older term for e. characterized by generalized tonic-clonic *seizure.*

idiopathic e., (1) an e. without evident cause; term often used to describe the genetic e.'s; **(2)** SYN generalized tonic-clonic *seizure.*

intractable e., e. not adequately controlled by medication. SYN pharmacoresistent e.

jacksonian e., SYN jacksonian *seizure.*

juvenile absence e., a generalized e. syndrome with onset around puberty, characterized by absence seizures and generalized tonic-clonic seizures. EEG often shows a greater than 3 Hz generalized spike wave pattern.

juvenile myoclonic e., an e. syndrome typically beginning in early adolescence, and characterized by early morning myoclonic jerks that may progress into a generalized tonic-clonic seizure. A genetic disorder: some families have had gene linkage to chromosome-6. The EEG is characterized by generalized polyspike and wave discharges at 4–6 Hz.

Kojewnikoff e., SYN *epilepsia* partialis continua.

laryngeal e., a form of reflex e. precipitated by coughing.

local e., SYN focal e.

localization-related e., (1) SYN myoclonus e; **(2)** SYN focal e.

major e., SYN generalized tonic-clonic *seizure.*

masked e., a form of e. characterized by a paroxysmal disturbance, such as headache or vomiting, associated with an epileptic electroencephalographic pattern.

matutinal e., a form of e. which occurs on awakening.

myoclonic astatic e., a petit mal variant characterized by atonic (drop attacks) and tonic or tonic-clonic attacks in neurologically disabled (hemiplegic, ataxic, etc.) children with mental retardation; characterized in EEG by 2/sec spike and wave discharges; usually progresses in spite of medication.

myoclonus e. [MIM*159800 and MIM*220300], a clinically diverse group of epilepsy syndromes, some benign, some progressive. Many are hereditary with mendelian and nonmendelian mitochondrial inheritance. All are characterized by the occurrence of myoclonus, which may be limited or predominate in the condition. Specific syndromes include cherry red spot myoclonus syndrome, ceroid lipofuscinosis, myoclonic e. with ragged red fibers, and Baltic myoclonus. SYN localization-related e. (1).

nocturnal e., an e. syndrome characterized by nocturnal seizures only.

occipital lobe e., a localization-related e. where seizures originate from the occipital lobe. Symptoms commonly include visual abnormalities during seizures.

parietal lobe e., a localization-related e. where seizures originate within the parietal lobe. Seizure semiology may involve abnormalities of sensation.

partial e., SYN focal e.

pattern-sensitive e., a form of reflex e. precipitated by viewing certain patterns.

petit mal e., SYN childhood absence e.

pharmacoresistent e., SYN intractable e.

photogenic e., a form of reflex e. precipitated by light.

posttraumatic e., a convulsive state following and causally related to head injury; with brain damage either manifested clinically or ascertained by special examinations such as computed tomog-

raphy. To assume causal relationship, the individual must have had no previous epilepsy, no cerebral disease, and no other brain trauma. The attacks should have started, depending on the severity of the wounding, within 3 months to 2 years of the alleged trauma and be of a type compatible with the site of injury and the EEG abnormalities.

primary generalized e., e. without evidence of focal or multifocal central nervous system disease. Seizures are generalized from onset, both by EEG and clinical criteria. Often a pure genetic form of e. SEE ALSO generalized tonic-clonic *seizure.*

procursive e., a psychomotor attack initiated by whirling or running.

psychomotor e., attacks with elaborate and multiple sensory, motor, and/or psychic components, the common feature being a clouding or loss of consciousness and amnesia for the event; clinical manifestations may take the form of automatisms; emotional outbursts of temper, anger or show of fear; motor or psychic disturbances; or may be related to any sphere of human activity. Electroencephalographically, the attack is characterized by spike discharges in the temporal lobe, especially in sleep. SEE ALSO procursive e., visceral e., uncinate e. SYN automatic e.

reflex e., seizures which are induced by peripheral stimulation; e.g., audiogenic, laryngeal, photogenic, or other stimulation. SYN sensory precipitated e.

rolandic e., a benign, autosomal dominant form of e. occurring in children, characterized clinically by arrest of speech, muscular contractions of the side of the face and arm, and epileptic discharges electroencephalographically. [Luigi *Rolando*]

secondary generalized e., a group of e. syndromes of diverse etiologies with diffuse or multifocal cerebral involvement. Patients typically have a variety of generalized seizure types, including tonic, atonic, myoclonic, atypical absence, and generalized tonic-clonic seizures. Partial seizures may also occur. One classic syndrome is the Lennox-Gastaut syndrome. SYN symptomatic e.

sensory e., focal e. initiated by a somatosensory phenomenon.

sensory precipitated e., SYN reflex e.

sleep e., incorrect term for narcolepsy.

somnambulic e., postictal automatism in which the patient walks or runs about exhibiting natural behavior of which he or she has no subsequent remembrance.

startle e., a form of reflex e. precipitated by sudden noises.

supplementary motor area e., a localization-related epilepsy syndrome in which seizures originate from the supplementary motor area of the mesial frontal lobe. Typical seizure semiology includes sudden bilateral tonic movements, vocalization, and preservation of consciousness. Attacks are often nocturnal.

symptomatic e., SYN secondary generalized e.

temporal lobe e., a localization-related e. with seizures originating from the temporal lobe, most commonly the mesial temporal lobe. The most common pathology is hippocampal sclerosis. SYN uncinate fit.

tonic e., an attack in which the body is rigid.

tornado e., a type of focal e. or partial seizure with an aura of severe vertigo and a feeling of being drawn up into space.

uncinate e., a form of psychomotor e. or complex partial seizure initiated by a dreamy state and hallucinations of smell and taste, usually the result of a medial temporal lesion. SYN uncinate attack.

vasomotor e., SYN autonomic e.

vasovagal e., SYN autonomic e.

visceral e., e., usually psychomotor, in which the attacks are initiated by visceral symptoms or sensations; most cases have their focus in the temporal lobe.

e. with grand mal seizures on awakening, generalized e. syndrome characterized by onset in the second decade of life, typically with generalized tonic-clonic seizures, of which most occur shortly after awakening (regardless of the time of day) and are exacerbated by sleep deprivation. There is a genetic predisposition and EEG shows one of several generalized patterns of interictal discharges; photosensitivity is common.

e. with myoclonic absences, a form of generalized e. characterized by absence seizures, severe bilateral rhythmic clonic jerks often associated with tonic contraction, and an EEG 3 Hz spike and wave pattern. Age of onset is usually around seven years and males are more often affected.

ep·i·lep·tic (ep-i-lep′tik). Relating to, characterized by, or suffering from epilepsy.

ep·i·lep·ti·form (ep-i-lep′ti-fōrm). SYN epileptoid.

ep·i·lep·to·gen·ic, ep·i·lep·tog·e·nous (ep-i-lep-tō-jen′ik, ep-i-lep-toj′ĕ-nŭs). Causing epilepsy.

ep·i·lep·toid (ep-i-lep′toyd). Resembling epilepsy; denoting certain convulsions, especially of functional nature. SYN epileptiform. [G. *epilēpsia,* seizure, epilepsy, + *eidos,* resemblance]

ep·i·loia (ep-i-loy′ă). SYN tuberous *sclerosis.*

ep·i·man·dib·u·lar (ep-i-man-dib′ū-lăr). Upon the lower jaw. [epi- + L. *mandibulum,* mandible]

ep·i·mas·ti·cal (ep-i-mast′i-kăl). Increasing steadily until an acme is reached, then declining; said of a fever. [G. *epakmastikos,* coming to a height]

ep·i·mas·ti·gote (ep-i-mas′ti-gōt). Term replacing "crithidial stage," to avoid confusion with the insect-parasitizing flagellates of the genus *Crithidia.* In the e. stage the flagellum arises from the kinetoplast alongside the nucleus and emerges from the anterior end of the organism; an undulating membrane is present. [epi- + G. *mastix,* whip]

ep·i·men·or·rha·gia (ep-i-men-ō-rā′jē-ă). Prolonged and profuse menstruation occurring at any time, but most frequently at the beginning and end of menstrual life.

ep·i·men·or·rhea (ep-i-men-ō-rē′ă). Too frequent menstruation, occurring at any time, but particularly at the beginning and end of menstrual life.

ep·i·mer (ep′i-mer). One of two molecules (having more than one chiral center) differing only in the spatial arrangement about a single chiral atom; e.g., α-D-glucose and α-D-galactose (with respect to carbon-4). SEE sugars. Cf. anomer. [epi- + G. *meros,* part]

ep·i·mer·ase (ep′i-mer-ās) [EC 5.1]. A class of enzymes catalyzing epimeric changes.

ep·i·mere (ep′i-mēr). The dorsal part of the myotome. SEE myotome (3). [epi- + G. *meros,* part]

ep·im·er·ite (ep-i-mēr′īt). The hooklike anchoring structure at the anterior end of a cephaline gregarine sporozoan; it is left embedded in tissues when the rest of the cephalont is freed in the lumen of the intestine of the invertebrate host. [epi- + G. *meros,* part]

ep·i·mi·cro·scope (ep-i-mī′krō-skōp). A microscope with a condenser built around the objective; used for the investigation of opaque, or only slightly translucent, minute specimens. SYN opaque microscope.

ep·i·mor·pho·sis (ep′i-mōr-fō′sis). Regeneration of a part of an organism by growth at the cut surface. [epi- + G. *morphē,* shape]

ep·i·mys·i·ot·o·my (ep′i-mis-ē-ot′ō-mē). Incision of the sheath of a muscle. [epimysium + G. *tomē,* a cutting]

ep·i·mys·i·um (ep-i-mis′ē-ŭm) [TA]. The fibrous connective tissue envelope surrounding a skeletal muscle. SYN perimysium externum. [epi- + G. *mys,* muscle]

ep·i·neph·rine (ep′i-nef′rin). A catecholamine that is the chief neurohormone of the adrenal medulla of most species; also secreted by neurons. The L-isomer is the most potent stimulant (sympathomimetic) of adrenergic α- and β-receptors, resulting in increased heart rate and force of contraction, vasoconstriction or vasodilation, relaxation of bronchiolar and intestinal smooth muscle, glycogenolysis, lipolysis, and other metabolic effects; used in the treatment of bronchial asthma, acute allergic disorders, open-angle glaucoma, cardiac arrest, and heart block, and as a topical and local vasoconstrictor. Generally used salts are e. hydrochloride and e. bitartrate, the latter most frequently used in topical preparations. SYN adrenaline. [epi- + G. *nephros,* kidney, + -ine]

ep·i·neph·ros (ep-i-nef′ros). SYN suprarenal *gland.* [epi- + G. *nephros,* kidney]

ep·i·neu·ral (ep-i-noo′răl). On a neural arch of a vertebra.

ep·i·neu·ri·al (ep-i-noo′rē-ăl). Relating to the epineurium.

ep·i·neu·ri·um (ep-i-noo′rē-ŭm) [TA]. The outermost supporting structure of peripheral nerve trunks, consisting of a condensation of areolar connective tissue; subdivided into those layers that surround the whole nerve trunk (epifascicular e.), and those layers which extend between the nerve fascicles (interfascicular e.). With the endoneurium and perineurium, the e. composes the peripheral nerve stroma. [epi- + G. *neuron,* nerve]

epifascicular e., the portion of the e. which surrounds the whole nerve trunk, in contrast to interfascicular e., which passes down between the nerve fascicles.

ep·i·o·nych·i·um (ep-i-ō-nik′ē-ŭm). SYN eponychium.

ep·i·ot·ic (ep′i-ot′ik, -ō′tik). One of the components of the otic capsule of some vertebrates; in the mammal the petrosal or petrous temporal bone incorporates the various otic elements seen in lower vertebrates. [epi- + G. *ous,* ear]

ep·i·pas·tic (ep-i-pas′tik). 1. Usable as a dusting powder. 2. A dusting powder. [G. *epi-passō,* to sprinkle over]

ep·i·per·i·car·di·al (ep′i-per-i-kar′dē-ăl). Upon or about the pericardium.

ep·i·phar·ynx (ep′i-far′ingks). SYN nasopharynx. [G. *epi,* on, over, + pharynx]

ep·i·phe·nom·e·non (ep′i-fĕ-nom′ĕ-non). A symptom appearing during the course of a disease, not of usual occurrence, and not necessarily associated with the disease.

epiph·o·ra (ē-pif′ō-ră). An overflow of tears upon the cheek, due to imperfect drainage by the tear-conducting passages. SYN tearing, watery eye (1). [G. a sudden flow, fr. *epi,* on, + *pherō,* to bear]

atonic e., e. arising from weakness of the orbicularis oculi muscle.

ep·i·phren·ic, ep·i·phre·nal (ep′i-fren′ik, -frē′năl). Upon or above the diaphragm. [epi- + G. *phrēn,* diaphragm]

ep·i·phys·i·al, epiph·y·se·al (ep-i-fiz′ē-ăl). Relating to an epiphysis.

epiph·y·si·od·e·sis (ep′i-fiz-ē-od′ĕ-sis). 1. Premature union of the epiphysis with the diaphysis, resulting in cessation of growth. 2. An operative procedure that partially or totally destroys an epiphysis and may incorporate a bone graft to produce fusion of the epiphysis or premature cessation of its growth; generally undertaken to equalize leg length. [epiphysis + G. *desis,* binding]

epiph·y·si·ol·y·sis (ep-i-fiz-ē-ol′i-sis). Loosening or separation, either partial or complete, of an epiphysis from the metaphysis of a bone. [epiphysis + G. *lysis,* loosening]

ep·i·phys·i·op·a·thy (ep-i-fiz-ē-op′ă-thē). Any disorder of an epiphysis of the long bones. [epiphysis + G. *pathos,* suffering]

epiph·y·sis, pl. **epiph·y·ses** (e-pif′i-sis, -sēz) [TA]. A part of a long bone developed from a center of ossification distinct from that of the shaft and separated at first from the latter by a layer of cartilage. [G. an excrescence, fr. *epi,* upon, + *physis,* growth]

atavistic e., a bone that is independent phylogenetically but is now fused with another bone, e.g., the coracoid process of the scapula.

e. cer′ebri, SYN pineal *body.*

pressure e., a secondary center of ossification in the articular end of a long bone.

stippled e., SYN *chondrodysplasia* punctata.

traction e., a secondary center of ossification at the site of attachment of a tendon.

epiph·y·si·tis (e-pif-i-sī′tis). Inflammation of an epiphysis.

ep·i·pi·al (ep′i-pī′ăl). On the pia mater.

△**epiplo-.** Omentum. SEE ALSO omento-. [G. *epiploon*]

epip·lo·cele (e-pip′lō-sēl). Rarely used term for hernia of the omentum. [epiplo- + G. *kēlē,* hernia]

ep·i·plo·ic (ep′i-plō′ik). SYN omental.

epip·lo·on (e-pip′lō-on). SYN greater *omentum.* [G.]

epipodophyllotoxin (ĕp-ē-pō-dō-   fī′lō-toks′in, -fil′ō-toks′in). Natural product that inhibits topoisomerase II. SEE ALSO etoposide. [epi- + *Podophyllum,* genus name of botanical source, + toxin]

ep·i·pter·ic (ep′i-ter′ik). In the neighborhood of the pterion.

ep·i·py·gus (ep-i-pī′gŭs). Unequal conjoined twins in which the smaller, incomplete parasite is attached to the buttock of the larger autosite. SEE pygomelus, conjoined *twins,* under twin. [epi- + G. *pygē,* buttocks]

D-**ep·i·rham·nose** (ep-i-ram′nōz). 6-Deoxy-D-glucose; occurs in plants and bacteria in combination with diacylglycerol and is often sulfated (at C-6) in glycolipids. SYN quinovose.

ep·i·scle·ra (ep′i-sklēr′ă). The connective tissue between the sclera and the conjunctiva. [epi- + sclera]

ep·i·scle·ral (ep-i-sklēr′ăl). **1.** Upon the sclera. **2.** Relating to the episclera.

▊**ep·i·scle·ri·tis** (ep-i-skle-rī′tis). Inflammation of the episcleral connective tissue. SEE ALSO scleritis.

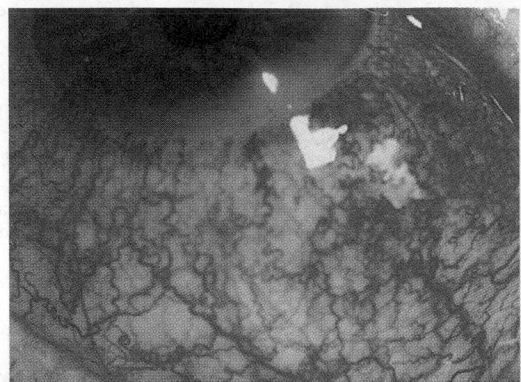

episcleritis: in rheumatoid arthritis

e. multinodula′ris, e. with numerous nodules near the corneoscleral limbus.

nodular e., e. with localized inflammation foci in episcleral tissues.

e. periodi′ca fu′gax, diffuse transient e., with a tendency to recur at regular intervals. SYN subconjunctivitis.

⬙**episio-.** The vulva. SEE ALSO vulvo-. [G. *episeion,* pubic region]

ep·i·si·o·per·i·ne·or·rha·phy (e-piz′ē-ō-per′i-nē-ōr′ă-fē, e-pis′). Repair of an incised or a ruptured perineum and lacerated vulva or repair of a surgical incision of the vulva and perineum. [episio- + G. *perinaion,* perineum, + *rhaphē,* a stitching]

ep·i·si·o·plas·ty (e-piz′ē-ō-plas-tē, e-pis′). Plastic surgery of the vulva. [episio- + G. *plastos,* formed]

ep·i·si·or·rha·phy (e-piz-i-ōr′ră-fē, e-pis-). Repair of a lacerated vulva or an episiotomy. [episio- + G. *rhaphē,* a stitching]

ep·i·si·o·ste·no·sis (e-piz′i-ō-stě-nō′sis, e-pis′). Narrowing of the vulvar orifice. [episio- + G. *stenōsis,* narrowing]

▊**ep·i·si·ot·o·my** (e-piz-ē-ot′ō-mē, e-pis-). Surgical incision of the vulva to prevent laceration at the time of delivery or to facilitate vaginal surgery. SYN vaginoperineotomy. [episio- + G. *tomē,* incision]

ep·i·so·de (ep′i-sōd). An important event or series of events taking place in the course of continuous events e.g., an episode of depression.

acute schizophrenic e., SYN acute *schizophrenia.*

e. of care, all services provided to a patient with a medical problem within a specific period of time across a continuum of care in an integrated system.

manic e., manifestation of a major mood disorder in which there is a distinct period during which the predominant mood of the individual is either elevated, expansive, or irritable, and there are associated symptoms of the excited or manic phase of the bipolar disorder. SEE affective *disorders,* under *disorder,* endogenous *depression.*

ep·i·some (ep′i-sōm). An extrachromosomal element (plasmid) that may either integrate into the bacterial chromosome of the host or replicate and function stably when physically separated from the chromosome. [epi- + G. *sōma,* body (chromosome)]

resistance-transferring e.'s, SYN resistance *plasmids,* under *plasmid.*

ep·i·spa·di·as (ep-i-spā′dē-ăs). A malformation in which the urethra opens on the dorsum of the penis; frequently associated with exstrophy of the bladder. [epi- + G. *spaō,* to tear or gouge]

balanitic e., excessively proximal position of meatus on dorsum of glans penis.

coronal e., excessively proximal position of meatus in coronal sulcus.

penile e., proximal position of urethral meatus on the dorsum of the penile shaft.

penopubic e., position of the urethral meatus at junction of base of penis and lower abdominal wall.

ep·i·spi·nal (ep-i-spī′năl). Upon the vertebral column or spinal cord, or upon any structure resembling a spine.

ep·i·sple·ni·tis (ep-i-splē-nī′tis). Inflammation of the capsule of the spleen.

epis·ta·sis (e-pis′tă-sis). **1.** The formation of a pellicle or scum on the surface of a liquid, especially as on standing urine. **2.** Phenotypic interaction of non-allelic genes. **3.** A form of gene interaction whereby one gene masks or interferes with the phenotypic expression of one or more genes at other loci; the gene whose phenotype is expressed is said to be "epistatic," while the phenotype altered or suppressed is then said to be "hypostatic." SYN epistasy. [G. scum; epi- + G. *stasis,* a standing]

epis·ta·sy (e-pis′tă-sē). SYN epistasis.

ep·i·stat·ic (ep-is-tat′ik). Relating to epistasis.

ep·i·stax·is (ep′i-stak′sis). Bleeding from the nose. SYN nasal hemorrhage, nosebleed. [G. fr. *epistazō,* to bleed at the nose, fr. *epi,* on, + *stazō,* to fall in drops]

renal e., hematuria occurring without a detectable lesion.

epis·te·mol·o·gy (ĕ-pis′tō-mol′ō-gē). The study of knowledge and rules of evidence involved. Traditionally a branch of philosophy, it is now coming to be used also as a discipline incorporated in, and in some respects peculiar to, individual fields of scholarship (medicine, science, history, etc.).

epis·te·mo·phil·ia (ĕ-pis′tē-mō-fil′ē-ă). Love, especially excessive, of knowledge. [G. *epistēmē,* knowledge, + *philos,* fond]

ep·i·ster·nal (ep-i-ster′năl). **1.** Over or on the sternum. **2.** Relating to the episternum.

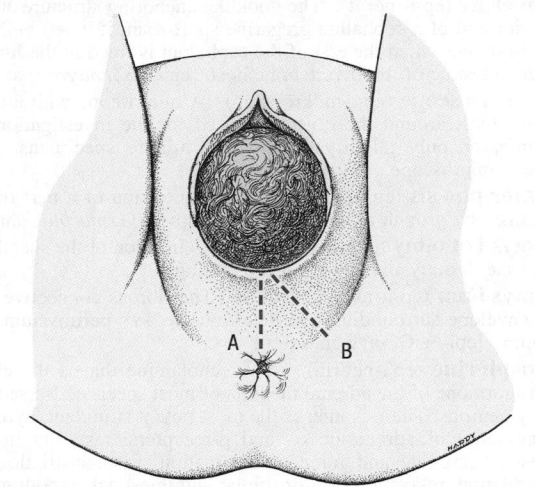

episiotomy: (A) median and (B) mediolateral

ep·i·ster·num (ep-i-ster′nŭm). SYN *manubrium* of sternum. [epi- + L. *sternum,* chest]

ep·i·stro·phe·us (ep-i-strō′fē-ŭs). SYN axis (5). [G. the pivot]

ep·i·tar·sus (ep-i-tar′sŭs). A fold of conjunctiva arising on the tarsal surface of the lid and losing itself in the skin close to the medial angle of the eye. [epi- + G. *tarsos,* flat mat, edge of eyelid]

ep·i·taxy (ep-i-tak′sē). The growth of one crystal in one or more specific orientations on the substrate of another kind of crystal, with a close geometric fit between the networks in contact; seen in the alternating layers of different composition in stones from the kidney and gallbladder, indicating an abrupt change of composition during formation. [epi- + G. *taxis,* arrangement]

ep·i·ten·din·e·um (ep'i-ten-din'ē-ŭm). The white fibrous sheath surrounding a tendon. SYN epitenon. [L.]

epit·e·non (ĕ-pit'ĕ-non, ep-i-ten'on). SYN epitendineum.

17-ep·i·tes·tos·ter·one (ep'i-tes-tos'ter-ōn). 17α-Epimer of testosterone; a biologically inactive steroid found in testes and ovaries; may be a metabolite of 4-androstene-3,17-dione and a precursor of 17α-estradiol.

ep·i·thal·a·mus (ep'i-thal'ă-mŭs) [TA]. A small dorsomedial area of the thalamus corresponding to the habenula and its associated structures, the stria medullaris of the thalamus, pineal gland, and habenular commissure. [epi- + thalamus]

ep·i·tha·lax·i·a (ep'i-thă-lak'sē-ă). Shedding of any surface epithelium, but especially of that lining the intestine. [epithelium + G. *allaxis,* exchange]

ep·i·the·lia (ep-i-thē'lē-ă). Plural of epithelium.

ep·i·the·li·al (ep-i-thē'lē-ăl). Relating to or consisting of epithelium.

ep·i·the·li·al·i·za·tion (ep-i-thē'lē-ăl-i-zā'shŭn). Formation of epithelium over a denuded surface. SYN epithelization.

ep·i·the·li·o·cyte (ep-i-thē'lē-ō-sīt). An in vitro tissue culture epithelial cell. [epithelium + G. *kytos,* cell]

ep·i·the·li·o·fi·bril (ep-i-thē'lē-ō-fī'bril). SYN tonofibril.

ep·i·the·li·o·glan·du·lar (ep-i-thē'lē-ō-glan'dū-lăr). Relating to glandular epithelium.

ep·i·the·li·oid (ep-i-thē'lē-oyd). Resembling or having some of the characteristics of epithelium. [epithelium + G. *eidos,* resemblance]

ep·i·the·li·o·lyt·ic (ep-i-thē'lē-ō-lit'ik). Destructive to epithelium.

ep·i·the·li·o·ma (ep'i-thē-lē-ō'mă). **1.** An epithelial neoplasm or hamartoma of the skin, especially of skin appendage origin. **2.** Obsolete term for a carcinoma of the skin derived from squamous, basal, or adnexal cells. [epithelium + G. *-ōma,* tumor]

e. adenoi'des cys'ticum, SYN trichoepithelioma.

basal cell e., SYN basal cell *carcinoma.*

Borst-Jadassohn type intraepidermal e., precancerous lesions clinically suggestive of actinic or seborrheic keratosis, with nests of immature or abnormal keratinocytes within the epidermis.

e. cunicula'tum, verrucous carcinoma occurring uncommonly on the sole of the foot, forming a slowly growing warty mass that may invade deeply but which rarely metastasizes.

Malherbe calcifying e., SYN pilomatrixoma.

malignant ciliary e., malignant hyperplasia of ciliary epithelium with frequent involvement of the pigmented layer. SYN adult medulloepithelioma.

multiple self-healing squamous e. [MIM*132800], multiple skin tumors, most frequently on the head, each resembling a well-differentiated squamous carcinoma or keratoacanthoma; individual tumors resolve spontaneously after several months, leaving deep-pitted scars with irregular crenellated borders, and are usually replaced by additional new tumors; autosomal dominant inheritance.

sebaceous e., a benign tumor of the sebaceous gland epithelium in which small basaloid or germinative cells predominate.

ep·i·the·li·om·a·tous (ep-i-thē-lē-ō'mă-tŭs). Pertaining to epithelioma.

ep·i·the·li·op·a·thy (ep'i-thē-lē-op'ă-thē). Disease involving epithelium. [epithelium + G. *pathos,* suffering]

acute multifocal placoid pigment e., an acute disease manifested by rapid loss of vision, and multifocal, cream-colored placoid lesions of the retinal pigment *epithelium;* resolves with restoration of vision.

ep·i·the·li·o·sis (ep-i-thē-lē-ō'sis). Proliferation of epithelial cells, as seen in ducts of the breast in fibrocystic disease.

ep·i·the·li·o·tro·pic (ep-ē-thē'lē-ō-trō'pik). Having an affinity for epithelium.

ⓘep·i·the·li·um, pl. **ep·i·the·lia** (ep-i-thē'lē-ŭm, -ă) [TA]. The purely cellular avascular layer covering all free surfaces, cutaneous, mucous, and serous, including the glands and other structures derived therefrom. [G. *epi,* upon, + *thēlē,* nipple, a term applied originally to the thin skin covering the nipples and the papillary layer of the border of the lips]

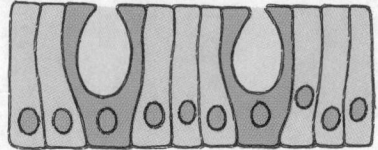
columnar epithelium
of intestines

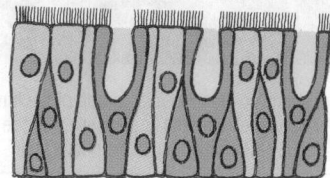
pseudostratified ciliated
columnar epithelium

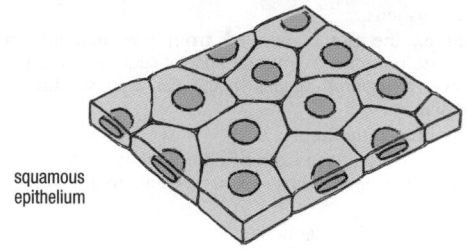
simple cuboidal
epithelium

squamous
epithelium

types of epithelium

anterior e. of cornea, the stratified squamous e. covering the outer surface of the cornea; it is smooth, consists usually of five layers of cells, and contains numerous free nerve endings. SYN e. anterius corneae.

e. ante'rius cor'neae, SYN anterior e. of cornea.

Barrett e., columnar esophageal e. seen in Barrett *syndrome.*

ⓘciliated e., any e. having motile cilia on the free surface.

columnar e., e. formed of a single layer of prismatic cells taller than they are wide. SYN cylindrical e.

crevicular e., the stratified squamous e. lining the inner aspect of the soft tissue wall of the gingival sulcus. SYN sulcular e.

cuboidal e., simple e. with cells appearing as cubes in a vertical section but as polyhedra in surface view.

cylindrical e., SYN columnar e.

e. duc'tus semicircula'ris, SYN e. of semicircular duct.

enamel e., the several layers of the enamel organ remaining on the enamel surface after formation of enamel is completed. SYN reduced enamel e.

external dental e., external enamel e., the cuboidal cells of the outer layer of the odontogenic organ of a developing tooth.

germinal e., a cuboidal layer of peritoneal e. covering the gonads, once thought to be the source of germ cells.

gingival e., a stratified squamous e. that undergoes some degree of keratinization and covers the free and attached gingiva.

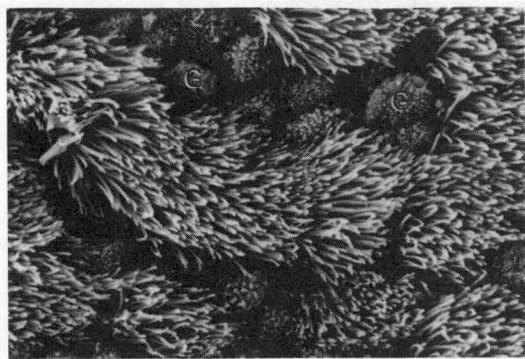

ciliated epithelium: scanning electron micrograph of the luminal surface of a bronchus; the nonciliated cells are the goblet cells, (G); the cilia of the many ciliated cells occupy the remainder of the micrograph

glandular e., e. composed of secretory cells.

inner dental e., inner enamel e., the columnar epithelial layer of enamel matrix of the odontogenic organ of a developing tooth that develops into the enamel-producing ameloblasts.

junctional e., a collar of epithelial cells attached to the tooth surface and subepithelial connective tissue found at the base of the gingival crevice. SYN epithelial attachment of Gottlieb, epithelial attachment.

laminated e., SYN stratified e.

e. of lens, the layer of cuboidal cells lying on the anterior surface of the crystalline lens inside the lens capsule. At the equator the cells elongate and give rise to the lens fibers. SYN e. lentis.

e. lentis, SYN e. of lens.

mesenchymal e., the flat e. derived from mesenchymal cells found lining certain connective tissue spaces such as the anterior chamber of eye, perilymph spaces in the ear, and subdural and subarachnoid spaces.

muscle e., SYN myoepithelium.

olfactory e., an e. of the pseudostratified type that contains olfactory, receptor, nerve cells whose axons extend to the olfactory bulb of the brain.

pavement e., SYN simple squamous e.

pigment e., e. composed of cells containing granules of pigment or melanin, as in the retinal or iris pigment layer.

pigment e. of optic retina, SEE retina.

pseudostratified e., an e. that gives a superficial appearance of being stratified because the cell nuclei are at different levels, but in which all cells reach the basement membrane, hence it is classed as a simple e.

reduced enamel e., SYN enamel e.

respiratory e., the pseudostratified ciliated e. that lines the conducting portion of the airway, including part of the nasal cavity and larynx, the trachea, and bronchi.

e. of semicircular duct, the simple squamous e. of the semicircular ducts. SYN e. ductus semicircularis.

seminiferous e., the e. lining the convoluted tubules of the testis where spermatogenesis and spermiogenesis occur.

simple e., an e. having one layer of cells.

simple squamous e., e. composed of a single layer of flattened scalelike cells, such as mesothelium, endothelium, and that in the pulmonary alveoli. SYN pavement e.

stratified e., a type of e. composed of a series of layers, the cells of each varying in size and shape. It is named more specifically according to the type of cells at the surface, e.g., stratified squamous e., stratified columnar e., stratified ciliated columnar e. SYN laminated e.

stratified ciliated columnar e., an e. consisting of several layers of cells with the deeper cells being polyhedral in form and the surface ones columnar with motile cilia, such as that which lines the fetal esophagus.

stratified squamous e., an e. consisting of several layers of keratin containing cells in which the surface cells are flattened and scale-like and the deeper cells are polyhedral in form. Keratin filaments become progressively more abundant toward the surface, which on the dry surfaces of the body may consist of a layer of dead corneocytes.

sulcular e., SYN crevicular e.

surface e., (1) a layer of celomic epithelial cells covering the gonadal ridges; (2) the mesothelial covering of the definitive ovary.

transitional e., a highly distensible pseudostratified e. with large polyploid superficial cells that are cuboidal in the relaxed state but broad and squamous in the distended state; occurs in the kidney, ureter, and bladder.

ep·i·the·li·za·tion (ep-i-thē-li-zā′shŭn). SYN epithelialization.

ep·i·them (ep′i-them). An external application, such as a poultice, but not a plaster or ointment. [G. epithēma, a cover]

ep·i·thet (ep′i-thet). Characterizing term or name. [G. epithetos, added, fr. epi- + tithēmi, to place]

specific e., in bacteriology, the second part of the name of a species; it is not, by itself, a name; the name of a bacterial species consists of two parts, the generic name and the specific e.

ep·i·thi·a·zide (ep-i-thī′ă-zīd). A diuretic.

ep·i·tope (ep′i-tōp). The simplest form of an antigenic determinant, on a complex antigenic molecule, which can combine with antibody or T cell receptor. [epi- + -tope]

shared e., SYN susceptibility cassette.

ep·i·tox·oid (ep-i-tok′soyd). A toxoid that has less affinity for specific antitoxin than that manifested by the toxin.

ep·i·trich·i·al (ep-i-trik′ē-ăl). Relating to the epitrichium.

ep·i·trich·i·um (ep-i-trik′ē-ŭm). SYN periderm. SEE dome cell. [epi- + G. trichion, dim. of thrix, (trich-), hair]

ep·i·troch·lea (ep-i-trok′lē-ă). SYN medial epicondyle of humerus. [epi- + L. trochlea, a pulley, block, contr. fr. G. trochilia]

ep·i·troch·le·ar (ep-i-trok′lē-ăr). Relating to the epitrochlea.

ep·i·tu·ber·cu·lo·sis (ep′i-too-ber-kū-lō′sis). The occurrence of lymph node swelling or pulmonary infiltration in an area near a focus of pulmonary tuberculosis or of enlarged bronchial glands.

ep·i·tym·pan·ic (ep-i-tim-pan′ik). Above, or in the upper part of, the tympanic cavity or membrane.

ep·i·tym·pa·num (ep′i-tim′pă-nŭm). SYN epitympanic recess.

ep·i·typh·li·tis (ep′ĭ-tif-lī′tis). Inflammation of tissues around or near the cecum. SEE appendicitis. [epi- + G. typhlon, cecum, + -itis, inflammation]

ep·i·zo·ic (ep-i-zō′ik). Living as a parasite on the skin surface.

ep·i·zo·ol·o·gy (ep′i-zō-ol′ō-jē). SYN epizootiology. [epi- + G. zōon, animal, + logos, study]

ep·i·zo·on, pl. **ep·i·zoa** (ep-i-zō′on, -zō′ă). An animal parasite living on the body surface. [epi- + G. zōon, animal]

ep·i·zo·ot·ic (ep′i-zō-ot′ik). **1.** Denoting a temporal pattern of disease occurrence in an animal population in which the disease occurs with a frequency clearly in excess of the expected frequency in that population during a given time interval. **2.** An outbreak (epidemic) of disease in an animal population. [epi- + G. zōon, animal]

ep·i·zo·ot·i·ol·o·gy (ep′i-zō-ot′ē-ol′ō-jē). Epidemiology of disease in animal populations. SYN epizoology. [epi- + G. zōon, animal, + logos, study]

éplu·chage (ā-ploo-shazh′). Rarely used term for the removal of all contaminated tissue in infected wounds. [F. picking, cleaning]

EPN. A sulfur-containing organophosphate-anticholinsterase used as an insecticide and acaricide.

EPO Abbreviation for exclusive provider organization.

epo·e·tin al·fa (ē-pō′ĕ-tin). Recombinant human erythropoietin, a powerful stimulator of red blood cell synthesis. Often used in patients with anemia and in those undergoing renal transplants and AZT treatment.

ep·o·nych·ia (ep-ō-nik′ē-ă). Infection involving the proximal nail fold.

ep·o·nych·i·um (ep-ō-nik′ē-ŭm) [TA]. **1.** The thin, condensed, eleidin-rich layer of epidermis that precedes and initially covers the nail plate in the embryo. It normally degenerates by the eighth month except at the nail base where it remains as the cuticle of the nail. **2** [NA]. The corneal layer of epidermis overlapping and in direct contact with the nail root proximally or the sides of the nail plate laterally, forming the undersurface of the nail wall or nail folds. SYN hidden nail skin, perionychium. **3.** The thin skin adherent to the nail at its proximal portion. SYN epionychium. [G. *epi,* upon, + *onyx* (*onych-*), nail]

ep·o·nym (ep′ō-nim). The name of a disease, structure, operation, or procedure, usually derived from the name of the person who discovered or described it first. [G. *epōnymos,* named after]

ep·o·nym·ic (ep-ō-nim′ik). **1.** Relating to an eponym. **2.** An eponym.

ep·o·oph·o·ron (ep′ō-of′ŏ-ron). A collection of rudimentary tubules in the mesosalpinx between the ovary and the uterine tube; composed of two portions, the longitudinal duct of epoöphoron and the transverse ductules of epoöphoron, they are the vestiges of tubules of the middle portion of the mesonephros and the homologue of the aberrant ductules and proximal duct of epididymis in the male. SYN corpus pampiniforme, organ of Rosenmüller, pampiniform body. [epi- + G. *ōophoros,* egg-bearing]

epo·prost·en·ol, epo·prost·en·ol so·di·um (e-pō-prost′en-ol). SYN prostacyclin.

epor·nit·ic (ep′or-nit′ik). Referring to an outbreak of disease in a bird population. [epi- + G. *ornithos,* bird + -ic]

ep·ox·y (ē-pok′sē). Chemical term describing an oxygen atom bound to two linked carbon atoms

$$-CH-CH-$$
$$\backslash O /$$

Generally, any cyclic ether, but commonly applied to a 3-membered ring; specifically, a three-membered ring is an oxirane, a four-membered ring is an oxetane, a five-membered ring is an oxolane, and a six-membered ring is an oxane; oxiranes are commonly produced from peracids acting on alkenes. E.'s are important chemical intermediates and the basis of e. resins (polymers) formed from e. monomers.

2,3-epox·y·squa·lene (ĕ-pok′sē-skwā′lēn). An oxirane derivative of squalene; a precursor to all of the steroids.

Epple, August, Associate of Leonard S. Fosdick. SEE Fosdick-Hansen-E. *test.*

EPR Abbreviation for electron paramagnetic *resonance.*

EPS Abbreviation for exophthalmos-producing *substance.*

ep·si·lon (ep′si-lon). Fifth letter of the Greek alphabet, ε.

EPSP Abbreviation for excitatory postsynaptic *potential.*

Epstein, Michael Anthony, English virologist, *1921. SEE E.-Barr *virus.*

Epstein, Alois, German pediatrician, 1849–1918. SEE E. *disease, pearls,* under *pearl, sign, symptom.*

epu·lis (ep-ū′lis). A nonspecific exophytic gingival mass. [G. *epoulis,* a gumboil]

congenital e. of newborn, a congenital benign nodular tumor of the alveolar ridge, of unknown histogenesis; histologically, it is composed of large cells with a granular cytoplasm similar to that of a granular cell tumor (myoblastoma).

e. fissura′tum, SYN inflammatory fibrous *hyperplasia.*

giant cell e., SYN giant cell *granuloma.*

e. gravida′rum, a gingival pyogenic granuloma that develops during pregnancy.

pigmented e., SYN melanotic neuroectodermal *tumor* of infancy.

ep·u·loid (ep′ū-loyd). A gingival mass that resembles an epulis.

Eq, eq Abbreviation for equivalent.

equa·tion (ē-kwā′zhŭn). A statement expressing the equality of two things, usually with the use of mathematical or chemical symbols. [L. *aequare,* to make equal]

alveolar gas e., the e. defining the steady state relation of the alveolar oxygen pressure to the barometric pressure, inspired gas composition, alveolar carbon dioxide pressure, and respiratory exchange ratio; the e. is used in various forms depending upon which simplifying assumptions are acceptable for different applications.

Arrhenius e., an e. relating chemical reaction rate (k) to the absolute temperature (T) by the e.: $d(\ln k)/dT) = \Delta E_a/RT^2$ where E_a is the activation energy and R is the universal gas constant.

Bohr e., an e. to calculate the respiratory dead space from the fact that gas expired from the lungs is a mixture of gas from the dead space and gas from the alveoli, i.e., the dead space volume divided by the tidal volume equals the difference between alveolar and mixed expired gas composition, divided by the difference between alveolar and inspired gas composition; gas composition can be expressed in any consistent units of concentration or partial pressure of oxygen or carbon dioxide.

chemical e., an e. on one side of which are the reactants and on the other side of which are the products of a chemical reaction; the two halves may be separated by an equals sign or by arrows.

constant field e., SYN Goldman e.

Einthoven e., SYN Einthoven *law.*

Gay-Lussac e., the overall chemical e. for alcoholic fermentation; $C_6H_{12}O_6 = 2CO_2 + 2CH_3CH_2OH$.

Gibbs-Helmholtz e., (1) an e. expressing the relationship in a galvanic cell between the chemical energy transformed and the maximal electromotive force obtainable. (2) $\Delta G = \Delta H = T(\partial \Delta G/\partial T)_P$, where ΔG is the change in Gibbs free energy, ΔH is the change in enthalpy, T is the absolute temperature, and P is the pressure.

Goldman e., an e. derived to predict membrane potentials in terms of the membrane's permeability to ions and their concentrations on either side. SYN constant field e., Goldman-Hodgkin-Katz e., GHK e.

Goldman-Hodgkin-Katz e., GHK e., SYN Goldman e.

Henderson-Hasselbalch e., a formula relating the pH value of a solution to the pK_a value of the acid in the solution and the ratio of the acid and the conjugate base concentrations: $pH = pK_a + \log([A^-]/[HA])$, where $[A^-]$ is the concentration of the conjugate base and $[HA]$ is the concentration of the protonated acid. For the bicarbonate buffer system in blood, $pH = pK' + \log([HCO_3^-]/[CO_2])$. The value of pK' for blood plasma is 6.10 and includes the first dissociation constant of H_2CO_3, the relation between $[H_2CO_3]$ and $[CO_2]$ and other corrections. The partial pressure of CO_2 multiplied by its solubility in plasma at 38°C (0.0301 mM/mm Hg) is commonly substituted for $[CO_2]$; e.g., when the plasma bicarbonate concentration is 24 mEq/L and the P_{CO_2} is 40 mm Hg, the pH value is $6.10 + \log(24/0.0301 \times 40) = 7.40$.

Henri-Michaelis-Menten e., SYN Michaelis-Menten e.

Hill e., the e. $y(1 - y) = [S]^n/K_d$, where y is the fractional degree of saturation, $[S]$ is the binding ligand concentration, n is the Hill coefficient, and K_d is the dissociation constant for the ligand. The Hill coefficient is a measure of the cooperativity of the protein; the larger the value, the higher the cooperativity. This coefficient cannot be higher than the number of binding sites. For the oxygen binding curve of hemoglobin, an association constant, K_a, is used and the e. becomes $y/(1 - y) = K_a[S]^n$. For human hemoglobin, $n = 2.5$. Cf. Hill *plot.*

Hüfner e., an e. expressing the relationship between myoglobin dissociation and oxygen partial pressure: $([MBO_2]/[Mb]) = (K \times pO_2)$.

Lineweaver-Burk e., a rearrangement of the Michaelis-Menten e., $1/v = 1/V_{max} + (K_m/V_{max})(1/[S])$, where v is the velocity of the reaction, V_{max} is the maximum velocity, K_m is the Michaelis constant; and $[S]$ is the substrate concentration. Cf. double-reciprocal *plot.*

Michaelis-Menten e., an initial-rate e. for a single-substrate noncooperative enzyme-catalyzed reaction relating the initial velocity to the initial substrate concentration; $v = V_{max} [S]/(K_m + [S])$, where v is the initial velocity of the reaction, V_{max} is the maximum velocity, $[S]$ is the initial substrate concentration, and K_m is the Michaelis constant. Similar equations can be derived for conditions in which the product is present and for multisubstrate enzymes. SYN Henri-Michaelis-Menten e.

Nernst e., the e. relating the equilibrium potential of electrodes to ion concentrations; the e. relating the electrical potential and concentration gradient of an ion across a permeable membrane at equilibrium: $E = [RT / nF] [\ln (C_1/C_2)]$, where E = potential, R =

eq

equation 612 **equivalent**

absolute gas constant, T = absolute temperature, n = valence, F = the Faraday, ln = the natural logarithm, and C_1 and C_2 are the ion concentrations on the two sides; in nonideal solutions, concentration should be replaced by activity. SEE ALSO activity (2).

personal e., a slight error in judgment, perceptual response, or action peculiar to the individual and so constant that it is usually possible to allow for it in accepting the person's statements or conclusions, thus arriving at approximate exactness; observed in persons whose work involves readings of events in time, such as navigators and air traffic controllers.

rate e., a mathematical expression for a chemical, radiochemical, or enzyme-catalyzed reaction.

Rayleigh e., a ratio of red to green required by each observer to match spectral yellow. SYN Rayleigh test.

Svedberg e., SEE sedimentation *constant*.

van't Hoff e., (1) e. for osmotic pressure of dilute solutions. SEE van't Hoff *law*; **(2)** for any reaction, $d(\ln K_{eq})/d(1/T)$ equals $-\Delta H/R$ where K_{eq} is the equilibrium constant, T the absolute temperature, R the universal gas constant, and ΔH the change in enthalpy; thus, plotting $\ln K_{eq}$ vs. $1/T$ allows the determination of ΔH.

equa·tor (ē-kwā′ter) [TA]. A line encircling a globular body, equidistant at all points from the two poles; the periphery of a plane cutting a sphere at the midpoint of, and at right angles to, its axis. [Mediev. L. *aequator*, fr. L. *aequo*, to make equal]

e. bul′bi oc′uli [TA], SYN e. of eyeball.

e. of eyeball [TA], an imaginary line encircling the globe of the eye equidistant from the anterior and posterior poles. SYN e. bulbi oculi [TA].

e. of lens [TA], the periphery of the lens lying between the two layers of the ciliary zonule. SYN e. lentis [TA].

e. len′tis [TA], SYN e. of lens.

equa·to·ri·al (ē-kwā-tō′rē-ăl). Situated, like the earth's equator, equidistant from each end.

equi·ax·i·al (ē′kwi-ak′sē-ăl). Having axes of equal length.

equi·ca·lor·ic (ē′kwi-kă-lōr′ik). Equal in heat value. SEE ALSO isodynamic. [L. *aequus*, equal, + *calor*, heat]

eq·ui·len·in (ek-wi-len′in). A weakly estrogenic steroid isolated from urine of pregnant mares. [L. *equa*, mare]

equil·i·bra·tion (ē′kwi-li-brā′shŭn, e-kwil-ĭ-). **1.** The act of maintaining an equilibrium or balance. **2.** The act of exposing a liquid, e.g., blood or plasma, to a gas at a certain partial pressure until the partial pressures of the gas within and without the liquid are equal. **3.** In dentistry, modification of occlusal forms of the teeth by grinding, with the intent of equalizing occlusal stress, producing simultaneous occlusal contacts, or harmonizing cuspal relations. **4.** In chromatography, the saturation of the stationary phase with the vapor of the elution solvent to be used.

equi·lib·ri·um (ē-kwi-lib′rē-ŭm). **1.** The condition of being evenly balanced; a state of repose between two or more antagonistic forces that exactly counteract each other. **2.** In chemistry, a state of apparent repose created by two reactions proceeding in opposite directions at equal speed; in chemical equations, sometimes indicated by two opposing arrows ($\leftrightarrow$) instead of the equal sign. SYN dynamic e. SEE ALSO equilibrium *constant*. [L. *aequilibrium*, a horizontal position, fr. *aequus*, equal, + *libra*, a balance]

acid-base e., SYN acid-base *balance*.

Donnan e., when a semipermeable membrane or its equivalent (e.g., a solid ion fexchanger) separates a nondiffusible substance, such as protein, from diffusible substances, the diffusible anions and cations are distributed on the two sides of the membrane so that 1) the products of their concentrations are equal, and 2) the sum of the diffusible and nondiffusible anions on either side of the membrane is equal to the sum of the concentrations of diffusible and nondiffusible cations; the unequal distribution of diffusible ions thus produced creates a potential difference across the membrane (membrane potential). SYN Gibbs-Donnan e.

dynamic e., SYN equilibrium (2).

genetic e., the condition of a dynamic genetic system in which the several rates of change between all possible pairs of parts are such that the composition is invariant.

Gibbs-Donnan e., SYN Donnan e.

Hardy-Weinberg e., that state in which the genetic structure of the population conforms to the prediction of the Hardy-Weinberg law; it is not a stable e., although for a large mating population it may be approximated. SYN random mating e.

homeostatic e., SEE homeostasis.

nitrogenous e., a condition in which the amount of nitrogen excreted from the body equals that taken in with the food; nutritive e. so far as protein is concerned.

nutritive e., condition in which there is a perfect balance between intake and excretion of nutritive material, so that there is no increase or loss in weight. SYN physiologic e.

physiologic e., SYN nutritive e.

radioactive e., a situation (not a true e.) in which a particular atom is being produced by the radioactive breakdown of a precursor while it is itself breaking down, the two breakdowns matching so that after a period of time the ratio of radioactivity of product and precursor is constant with time.

random mating e., SYN Hardy-Weinberg e.

secular e., a type of radioactive e. in which the half-life of the precursor (parent) radioisotope is so much longer than that of the product (daughter) that the radioactivity of the daughter becomes equal to that of the parent with time.

stable e., e. in which, after every small perturbation, the original state will tend to be restored.

transient e., a type of radioactive e. in which the half-life of the parent radioisotope is longer than that of the daughter so that the ratio of activities of parent and daughter become constant as they decrease with time.

unstable e., e. in which the response to a small perturbation will tend to make the perturbation greater (e.g., a logged feedback process of zero order).

eq·ui·lin (ek′wi-lin). An estrogenic steroid occurring in the urine of pregnant mares. [L. *equa*, mare]

equi·mo·lar (ē-kwi-mō′ler). Containing an equal number of moles or having the same molarity, as in two or more substances.

equi·mo·lec·u·lar (ē′kwi-mō-lek′ū-ler). Containing an equal number of molecules or molecular entities, as in two or more solutions.

e·quine (ē′kwīn). Relating to, derived from, or resembling the horse, mule, ass, or other members of the genus *Equus*. [L. *equinus*, fr. *equus*, horse]

equi·no·val·gus (ē-kwī-nō-val′gŭs, ek′wi-nō-). SYN *talipes* equinovalgus.

equi·no·var·us (ē-kwī-nō-vā′rŭs, ek′wi-nō-). SYN *talipes* equinovarus.

equi·tox·ic (ē-kwi-tok′sik). Of equivalent toxicity.

equiv·a·lence, equiv·a·len·cy (ē-kwiv′ă-lens, -len-sē). **1.** The property of an element or radical of combining with or displacing, in definite and fixed proportion, another element or radical in a compound. **2.** The point in a precipitin test at which antibody and antigen are present in optimal proportions. [L. *aequus*, equal, + *valentia*, strength (valence)]

equiv·a·lent (Eq, eq) (ē-kwiv′ă-lent). **1.** Equal in any respect. **2.** That which is equal in size, weight, force, or any other quality to something else. **3.** Having the capability to counterbalance or neutralize each other. **4.** Having equal valencies. **5.** SYN gram e. [see equivalence]

combustion e., the heat value of a gram of carbohydrate or fat oxidized outside the body.

gold e., a unit of power of the protective colloids; the number of milligrams of protective colloid just sufficient to prevent the precipitation of 10 ml of a 0.0053–0.0058% gold solution by the action of 1 ml of a 10% sodium chloride solution. SYN gold number.

gram e., **(1)** the weight in grams of an element that combines with or replaces 1 g of hydrogen; **(2)** the atomic or molecular weight in grams of an atom or group of atoms involved in a chemical reaction divided by the number of electrons donated, taken up, or shared by the atom or group of atoms in the course of that reaction; **(3)** the weight of a substance contained in 1 L of 1 N solution; a variant of (1). SYN combining weight, equivalent weight, equivalent (5).

Joule e. (J), the dynamic e. of heat; the amount of work converted to heat that will raise the temperature of 1 pound of water 1°F is 778 foot-pounds; in metric units, 1 calorie, which raises 1 g of water 1°C, equals 4.184×10^7 dyne-centimeters, or 4.184 J.

lethal e., (1) a combination of selective effects that on average have the same impact on the composition of the gene pool as one death; e.g., two carriers at 50% risk of dying would be the lethal e. of one carrier at 100% risk; **(2)** in the population genetics of recessive traits lethal e. is expressed as twice the sum of the expected number of deaths ascribable to the genetic load. **(3)** expression used of the genetic load of recessive genes in heterozygous state that if in homozygous state would cause death or carry a risk of death. The expected number of deaths from all such genes is expressed in e. equivalent.

metabolic e. (MET), the oxygen cost of energy expenditure measured at supine rest (1 MET = 3.5 ml O_2 per kg of body weight per minute); multiples of MET are used to estimate the oxygen cost of activity, e.g., 3–5 METs for light work; more than 9 METs for heavy work.

nitrogen e., the nitrogen content of protein; used in calculating the protein breakdown in the body from the nitrogen excreted in the urine, 1 g of nitrogen considered as having originated in 6.25 g of protein catabolized.

starch e., the amount of oxygen consumed in the combustion of a given weight of fat as compared with that consumed in the combustion of an equal weight of starch; the figure is about 2.38, that for starch being taken as 1.

toxic e., the amount of toxin or other poison per kilogram of body weight necessary to kill an animal.

ER Abbreviation for endoplasmic *reticulum.*

Er Symbol for erbium.

erad·i·ca·tion. Referring to disease, the termination of all transmission of infection by extermination of the infectious agent through surveillance and containment; global eradication has been achieved for smallpox, regional eradication for malaria and perhaps in some places for measles.

Eranko, Eino, Finnish anatomist, 1924–1984. SEE E. fluorescence *stain.*

Erb, Wilhelm H., German neurologist, 1840–1921. SEE E. *disease, palsy, paralysis;* E.-Charcot *disease;* Duchenne-E. *paralysis.*

ERBF Abbreviation for effective renal blood *flow.*

er·bi·um (Er) (er′bē-ŭm). A rare earth (lanthanide) element, atomic no. 68, atomic wt. 167.26. [from Ytterby, a village in Sweden]

er·cal·cid·i·ol (er-kal-sid′ē-ol). SYN 25-hydroxyergocalciferol.

er·cal·ci·ol (er-kal′sē-ol). SYN ergocalciferol.

er·cal·cit·ri·ol (er-kal-sit′rē-ol). SYN 1,25-dihydroxyergocalciferol.

ERCP Abbreviation for endoscopic retrograde *cholangiopancreatography.*

Erdheim, Jakob, Austrian physician, 1874–1937. SEE E. *disease, tumor.*

Erdmann, Hugo, German chemist, 1862–1910. SEE E. *reagent.*

erec·tile (ē-rek′tīl). Capable of erection.

erec·tion (ē-rek′shŭn). The condition of erectile tissue when filled with blood, which then becomes hard and unyielding; denoting especially this state of the penis. [L. *erectio,* fr. *erigo,* pp. *erectus,* to set up]

erec·tor (ĕrek′tŏr, -tōr). **1.** One who or that which raises or makes erect. **2.** Denoting specifically certain muscles having such action. SYN arrector. [Mod. L.]

er·e·mo·pho·bia (er′ē-mō-fō′bē-ă). Morbid fear of deserted places or of solitude. [G. *erēmia,* solitude, + *phobos,* fear]

er·eu·tho·pho·bi·a (er′oo-thō-fō′bē-ă). Morbid fear of blushing. [G. *ereuthos,* blushing, + *phobos,* fear]

ERG Abbreviation for electroretinogram.

erg. The unit of work in the CGS system; the amount of work done by 1 dyne acting through 1 cm, 1 g cm^2 s^{-2}; in the SI system, 1 erg equals 10^{-7} J. [G. *ergon,* work]

er·ga·sia (er-gā′zē-ă). **1.** Any form of activity, especially mental. **2.** The total of functions and reactions of an individual. [G. work]

er·ga·si·o·pho·bia (er-gas′ē-ō-fō′bē-ă). Aversion to work of any kind. [G. *ergasia,* work, + *phobos,* fear]

er·gas·the·nia (er-gas-thē′nē-ă). Rarely used term for debility or any morbid symptoms due to overexertion. [G. *ergasia,* work, + *astheneia,* weakness, disease]

er·gas·to·plasm (er-gas′tō-plazm). SYN granular endoplasmic *reticulum.* [G. *ergastēr,* a workman, + *plasma,* something formed]

erg·ine (erg′ēn). SYN *lysergic acid* amide.

⌂ergo-. Work. [G. *ergon*]

er·go·ba·sine (er-gō-bā′sēn). SYN ergonovine.

er·go·cal·cif·er·ol (er′gō-kal-sif′er-ol). Activated ergosterol, the vitamin D of plant origin; it arises from ultraviolet irradiation of ergosterol, which is cleaved at the 9,10 bond and develops a double bond between C-10 and C-19; used in prophylaxis and treatment of vitamin D deficiency. SYN calciferol, ercalciol, viosterol, vitamin D_2.

er·go·cor·nine (er-gō-kōr′nēn). An alkaloid isolated from ergot.

er·go·cris·tine (er′gō-kris′tēn). An alkaloid isolated from ergot.

er·go·cryp·tine (er-gō-krip′tēn). An alkaloid isolated from ergot.

er·go·dy·nam·o·graph (er′gō-dī-nam′ō-graf). An instrument for recording both the degree of muscular force and the amount of the work accomplished by muscular contraction. [ergo- + G. *dynamis,* force, + *graphō,* to write]

er·go·es·the·si·o·graph (er′gō-es-thē′zē-ō-graf). An apparatus for recording graphically muscular aptness as shown in the ability to counterbalance variable resistances. [ergo- + G. *aisthēsis,* sensation, + *graphō,* to record]

er·go·gen·ic (er-gō-jen′ik). Tending to increase work.

er·go·graph (er′gō-graf). An instrument for recording the amount of work done by muscular contractions, or the amplitude of contraction. [ergo- + G. *graphō,* to write]

Mosso e., an instrument consisting of pulleys, weights, and a recording lever, which is used to obtain a graphic record of flexion of a finger, hand, or arm.

er·go·graph·ic (er-gō-graf′ik). Relating to the ergograph and the record made by it.

er·go·lines (er′gō-linz). A class of drugs with prominent agonistic or antagonistic actions on dopamine receptors. Agents belonging to this group include bromocriptine, pergolide, and lisuride.

er·gom·e·ter (er-gom′ĕ-ter). SYN dynamometer. [ergo- + G. *metron,* measure]

er·go·met·rine (er-gō-met′rēn). SYN ergonovine.

e. maleate, SYN *ergonovine* maleate.

er·go·nom·ics (er-gō-nom′iks). A branch of ecology concerned with human factors in the design and operation of machines and the physical environment. [ergo- + G. *nomos,* law]

er·go·no·vine (er-gō-nō′vēn, -vin). An alkaloid from ergot; on hydrolysis it yields D-lysergic acid and L-2-aminopropanol; stimulates uterine contractions. SYN ergobasine, ergometrine, ergostetrine.

e. maleate, a powerful oxytocic agent; this action is more prominent, and other actions of ergot (vasoconstriction, central nervous system stimulation, adrenergic blockade, etc.) are less prominent than for other ergot alkaloids; effective orally and parenterally. SYN ergometrine maleate.

er·go·sine (er′gō-sēn, -sin). An alkaloid from ergot with actions similar to those of ergotamine.

er·gos·ter·in (er-gos′ter-in). SYN ergosterol.

er·gos·ter·ol (er-gos′ter-ol). The most important of the provitamins D_2; ultraviolet irradiation converts e. to lumisterol, tachysterol, and ergocalciferol; main sterol in yeast, ergot, and molds. SYN ergosterin.

er·go·stet·rine (er-gō-stet′rēn, -rin). SYN ergonovine.

er·got (er′got). The resistant, overwintering stage of the parasitic ascomycetous fungus *Claviceps purpurea,* a pathogen of rye grass that transforms the seed of rye into a compact spurlike mass of

er

fungal pseudotissue (the sclerotium) containing five or more optically isomeric pairs of alkaloids. The levorotary isomers induce uterine contractions, control bleeding, and alleviate certain localized vascular disorders (migraine headaches). SEE ALSO ergotism. SYN rye smut. [O. Fr. *argot*, cock's spur]

corn e., SYN *Ustilago maydis.*

er·got·a·mine (er-got′ă-mēn). $C_{33}H_{35}N_5O_5$; an alkaloid from ergot, used for the relief of migraine; it is a potent stimulant of smooth muscle, particularly of the blood vessels and the uterus, and produces adrenergic blockade (chiefly of the alpha receptors); hydrogenated e., dihydroergotamine, is less toxic and has fewer side effects. Also available as e. tartrate.

er·got·am·i·nine (er-got-am′i-nēn). An isomer of ergotamine but practically inert.

er·go·thi·o·ne·ine (er′gō-thī-ō-nē′in). The betaine of a sulfur-containing derivative of histidine, present in blood and other mammalian tissue and in ergot. SYN thiolhistidylbetaine, thioneine.

er·got·ism (er′got-izm). Poisoning by a toxic substance contained in the sclerotia of the fungus, *Claviceps purpura*, growing on rye grass; characterized by necrosis of the extremities (gangrene) due to contraction of the peripheral vascular bed. SEE ALSO ergot *poisoning*. SYN Saint Anthony fire (1).

er·go·tox·ine (er′gō-tok′sēn, -sin). A mixture of alkaloids obtained from ergot, consisting of 1:1:1 ergocristine, ergocornine and ergocryptine, more toxic than other natural and semisynthetic ergot alkaloids; a potent stimulant of smooth muscle, particularly of the blood vessels and uterus, and produces adrenergic blockade (chiefly of the alpha receptors). SYN ecboline.

er·go·tro·pic (er′gō-trop′ik). The term introduced by W.R. Hess to denote those mechanisms and the functional status of the nervous system that favor the organism's capacity to expend energy, as distinguished from the trophotropic mechanisms promoting rest and reconstitution of energy stores. In general, the balance between ergotropic and trophotropic nervous mechanisms corresponds in large part to that between the sympathetic and parasympathetic subdivisions of the autonomic nervous system. [ergo- + G. *tropos*, a turning]

er·i·o·dic·ty·on (ār′ē-ō-dik′tē-on). The dried leaves of *Eriodictyon californicum* (family Hydrophyllaceae); the fluidextract and the syrup have been used as an expectorant and flavoring agent to mask the taste of bitter substances. SYN mountain balm, yerba santa.

eris·o·phake (e-ris′ō-fāk). A surgical instrument designed to hold the lens by suction in cataract extraction; now seldom used. [G. *erysis*, a drawing, + *phakos*, lentil]

Erlenmeyer, Emil, German chemist, 1825–1909. SEE E. *flask*, flask *deformity.*

erode (ē-rōd′). 1. To cause, or to be affected by, erosion. 2. To remove by ulceration. [L. *erodo*, to gnaw away]

erog·e·nous (ĕ-roj′ĕ-nŭs). Capable of producing sexual excitement when stimulated. [G. *eros*, love, + *genos*, birth]

eros (ē′ros, ār′os). In psychoanalysis, the life principle representing all instinctual tendencies toward procreation and life. See also entries under instinct. Cf. thanatos. [G. love]

erose (ē-rōs′). Denoting an edge or margin which is irregularly notched or indented, as if gnawed away; used especially in reference to bacterial colonies. [L. *erodo*, pp. *erosus*, to gnaw away]

■**ero·sion** (ē-rō′zhŭn). 1. A wearing away or a state of being worn away, as by friction or pressure. Cf. corrosion. 2. A shallow ulcer; in the stomach and intestine, an ulcer limited to the mucosa, with no penetration of the muscularis mucosa. 3. The wearing away of a tooth by chemical action or abrasive; when the cause is unknown, it is referred to as idiopathic e. SYN odontolysis. [L. *erosio*, fr. *erodo*, to gnaw away]

Dieulafoy e., acute ulcerative gastroenteritis complicating pneumonia, possibly caused by overproduction of adrenal steroid hormones.

recurrent corneal e., repeated vesiculation followed by exfoliation of the corneal epithelium.

ero·sive (ē-rō′siv). 1. Having the property of eroding or wearing away. 2. An eroding agent.

erot·ic (ĕ-rot′ik). Lustful; relating to sexual passion; able to produce sexual arousal. [G. *erōtikos*, relating to love, fr. *eros*, love]

er·o·tism, erot·i·cism (er′ō-tizm, ĕ-rot′i-sizm). A condition of sexual excitement.

anal e., pleasurable experience centered around defecation and related activities associated with the anal zone, especially during the anal phase in 1- to 3-year-old children.

er·o·ti·za·tion (er′ō-ti-zā′shŭn). A process in which an object or action is rendered sexually exciting. SYN libidinization.

ero·to·gen·e·sis (er′ō-tō-jen′ĕ-sis). The origin or genesis of sexual impulses. [G. *eros*, love, + *genesis*, origin]

ero·to·gen·ic (er′ō-tō-jen′ik). Capable of causing sexual excitement or arousal. [G. *eros*, love, + -*gen*, production]

ero·to·ma·nia (er′ō-tō-mā′nē-ă). 1. Excessive or morbid inclination to erotic thoughts and behavior. 2. The delusional belief that one is involved in a relationship with another, generally of unattainable status. [G. *eros*, love, + *mania*, frenzy]

ero·to·path·ic (er′ō-tō-path′ik). Relating to erotopathy.

er·o·top·a·thy (er-ō-top′ă-thē). Any abnormality of the sexual impulse. [G. *eros*, love, + *pathos*, suffering]

ero·to·pho·bia (er′ō-tō-fō′bē-ă). Morbid aversion to the thought of sexual love and to its physical expression. [G. *eros*, love, + *phobos*, fear]

ERP Abbreviation for early receptor *potential.*

ERPF Abbreviation for effective renal plasma *flow.*

er·rat·ic (ĕ-rat′ik). 1. SYN eccentric (1). 2. Denoting symptoms that vary in intensity, frequency, or location. [L. *erro*, pp. *erratus*, to wander]

er·ror (er′ōr). 1. A defect in structure or function. 2. In biostatistics: 1) a mistaken decision, as in hypothesis testing or classification by a discriminant function; 2) the difference between the true value and the observed value of a variate, ascribed to randomness or misreading by an observer. 3. False positive and false negative results in a dichotomous trial. 4. A false or mistaken belief; in biomedical and other sciences, there are many varieties of e., for example due to bias, inaccurate measurements, or faulty instruments.

alpha e., SYN e. of the first kind.

beta e., SYN e. of the second kind.

experimental e., the total e. of measurement ascribed to the conduct of an empirical observation. It is commonly expressed as the standard deviation of replicated experiments. There may be many components, including those in the sampling procedure, the measurements, injudicious choice of a model, observer bias, etc.

e. of the first kind, in a Neyman-Pearson test of a statistical hypothesis the probability of rejecting the null hypothesis when it is true. SYN alpha e., type I e.

inborn e.'s of metabolism, a group of disorders, each of which involves a disorder of a single unique enzyme, genetic in origin and operating from birth; effects are ascribable to accumulation of the substrate on which the enzyme normally acts (e.g., phenylketonuria), to deficiency of the product of the enzyme (e.g., albinism), or to forcing metabolism through an auxiliary pathway (e.g., oxaluria).

interobserver e., the differences between interpretations of two or more individuals making observations of the same phenomenon.

intraobserver e., the differences between interpretations of an individual making observations of the same phenomenon at different times.

residual e., the estimated discrepancy between the actual measured datum and the value for that value computed after a model has been fitted to the set of the data by an estimator.

e. of the second kind, in a Neyman-Pearson test of a statistical hypothesis, the probability of accepting the null hypothesis when it is false; the complement of the power of the test. SYN beta e., type II e.

technical e., that component of experimental e. that is due to the conduct of the experiment and in principle estimated by replicate determinations on aliquots from the same specimen.

type I e., SYN e. of the first kind.

type II e., SYN e. of the second kind.

er·ta·cal·ci·ol (er-tă-kal'sē-ol). SEE tachysterol.

er·u·bes·cence (er-oo-bes'ens). A reddening of the skin. [L. *erubescere,* to redden]

eru·cic ac·id (ĕ-roo'sik). A 22-carbon unsaturated fatty acid present in the seeds of nasturtium (Indian cress) and of several *Cruciferae* species (rape, mustard, and wallflower); thought to be toxic to cardiac muscle.

eruc·ta·tion (ē-rŭk-tā'shŭn). The voiding of gas or of a small quantity of acid fluid from the stomach through the mouth. SYN belching, ructus. [L. *eructo,* pp. *-atus,* to belch]

erup·tion (ē-rŭp'shŭn). **1.** A breaking out, especially the appearance of lesions on the skin. **2.** A rapidly developing dermatosis of the skin or mucous membranes, especially when appearing as a local manifestation of one of the exanthemata; an e. is characterized, according to the nature of the lesion, as macular, papular, vesicular, pustular, bullous, nodular, erythematous, etc. **3.** The passage of a tooth through the alveolar process and perforation of the gums. [L. *e-rumpo,* pp. *-ruptus,* to break out]

accelerated e., a dental e. pattern which is chronologically advanced in comparison with the average pattern of dental e.; e. of the first tooth occurs at an earlier age than the average, and the intervals of time between subsequent dental e.'s are shorter than the average.

butterfly e., SYN butterfly (2).

clinical e., development of the crown of a tooth that can be observed clinically.

continuous e., the e. of a tooth into the mouth and its continuous movement in a vertical direction.

creeping e., SYN cutaneous *larva migrans.*

delayed e., a dental e. pattern which is chronologically late in comparison with the average pattern of dental e.; e. of the first tooth occurs at a later age than the average, and the intervals of time between subsequent dental e.'s are longer than the average.

◼**drug e.,** any e. caused by the ingestion, injection, or inhalation of a drug, most often the result of allergic sensitization; reactions to drugs applied to the cutaneous surface are not generally designated as drug e., but as contact-type dermatitis. SYN dermatitis medicamentosa, dermatosis medicamentosa, medicinal e.

feigned e., SYN *dermatitis* artefacta.

fixed drug e., a type of drug e. that recurs at the same site (or sites) following the administration of a particular drug; the lesions usually consist of intensely erythematous and purplish, sharply demarcated macules, and occasionally of herpetic vesicles; the affected areas undergo gradual involution, but flare and enlarge on readministration of the offending drug and may become hyperpigmented.

iodine e., an acneform or follicular e. or granulomatous lesion caused by a reaction to systemic iodine or iodide administration.

Kaposi varicelliform e., a now rare complication of either herpes simplex or vaccinia superimposed on atopic dermatitis, with generalized vesicles and vesicopapules and high fever.

medicinal e., SYN drug e.

passive e., the apparent continued e. of the teeth, actually the result of regression of the gingivae and crestal bone.

◼**polymorphous light e.,** a common pruritic papular e. appearing in a few hours and lasting up to several days on skin exposed to shortwave ultraviolet light (UVB); subepidermal edema and deep perivascular lymphocytic infiltration is seen microscopically.

seabather's e., pruritic rash believed to result from hypersensitivity to the venom of the larval thimble jellyfish (*Linuche unguiculata*).

e. sequestrum (sē'kwes-trum), spicule of bone overlying the central occlusal fossa of an erupting permanent molar.

serum e., urticaria seen in serum sickness.

surgical e., the uncovering of an unerupted tooth to permit its further e. into the oral cavity by surgically removing overlying soft tissue, bone, and sometimes teeth.

erup·tive (ē-rŭp'tiv). Characterized by eruption.

ERV Abbreviation for expiratory reserve *volume.*

◼**er·y·sip·e·las** (er-i-sip'ĕ-las). A specific, acute, superficial cutane-

ous cellulitis caused by β-hemolytic streptococci and characterized by hot, red, edematous, brawny, and sharply defined eruptions; usually accompanied by severe constitutional symptoms. [G., fr. *erythros,* red + *pella,* skin]

ambulant e., SYN e. migrans.

e. inter'num, an erysipelatous eruption in the vagina, uterus, and peritoneum, occurring in the puerperium.

e. mi'grans, a widely spreading form involving the entire face and body surface. SYN ambulant e., wandering e.

e. per'stans facie'i, chronic, dusky red eruption of erysipelas on the face.

phlegmonous e., a form marked by invasion of the subcutaneous tissues, with the formation of deep-seated abscesses.

e. pustulo'sum, development of pustules over the area of e.

surgical e., e. caused by infection of the wound following a surgical procedure.

swine e., a destructive disease of swine, occurring in both acute and chronic forms, caused by *Erysipelothrix rhusiopathiae.*

wandering e., SYN e. migrans.

er·y·sip·e·loid (er-i-sip'ĕ-loyd). A specific, usually self-limiting, cellulitis of the hand caused by *Erysipelothrix rhusiopathiae;* appears as a dusky erythema with diamondlike configuration of the skin at the site of a wound sustained in handling fish or meat and may become generalized, with plaques of erythema and bullae, and occasionally, severe toxemia. SYN blubber finger, crab hand, pseudoerysipelas, seal fingers, whale fingers. [G. *erysipelas* + *eidos,* resemblance]

Er·y·sip·e·lo·thrix (ār-i-sip'ĕ-lō-thriks, -si-pel'ō-thriks). A genus of bacteria (family Corynebacteriaceae) containing nonmotile, Gram-positive, rod-shaped organisms that have a tendency to form long filaments; older cells tend to become Gram-negative. They produce acid but no gas from glucose. They are facultatively anaerobic and catalase-negative. Members of this genus infect mammals, birds, and fish. The type species is *E. rhusiopathiae.* [erysipelas + G. *thrix,* hair]

E. insidio'sa, SYN *E. rhusiopathiae.*

E. rhusiopath'iae, a species that causes swine erysipelas, human erysipeloid, nonsuppurative polyarthritis in lambs, and septicemia in mice, and commonly infects fish handlers; it is the type species of the genus *E.* SYN *E. insidiosa.*

er·y·sip·e·lo·tox·in (ār-i-sip'ĕ-lō-tok'sin). A toxin produced by types of *Streptococcus pyogenes* (group A hemolytic streptococci), the bacterial cause of erysipelas.

er·y·the·ma (er-ĭ-thē'mă). Redness due to capillary dilation. [G. *erythēma,* flush]

e. ab ig'ne, a reticulated, pigmented, macular eruption that occurs, often on the shins, in bakers, stokers, and others exposed to radiant heat. SYN dermatitis calorica, e. caloricum, toasted shins.

acrodynic e., SYN acrodynia (2).

e. annula're, rounded or ringed lesions.

e. annula're centrif'ugum, a chronic, expanding, recurring erythematous eruption consisting of small and large annular lesions, with a scant marginal scale and central clearing, usually of unknown cause. SYN e. figuratum perstans.

e. annula're rheumat'icum, a variant of e. multiforme associated with rheumatic fever.

e. arthrit'icum epidem'icum, SYN Haverhill *fever.*

e. calor'icum, SYN e. ab igne.

e. chron'icum mi'grans, a raised erythematous ring with advancing indurated borders and central clearing, radiating from the site of a tick bite and persisting for 2–16 weeks; the characteristic skin lesion of Lyme disease, due to the spirochete *Borrelia burgdorferi,* which may be identified by PCR in biopsies.

e. circina'tum, e. multiforme in which the lesions are grouped in more or less circular fashion.

cold e., rash characterized by redness and itching, brought on by exposure to cold.

e. dyschro'micum per'stans, variously sized gray or red, slightly elevated macular lesions that tend to coalesce on the trunk and proximal extremities, commonly in dark-skinned Latin Americans; of unknown cause. SYN ashy dermatosis.

er

e. **eleva′tum diu′tinum,** a rare chronic symmetrical eruption of flattened nodules of a pinkish or purplish color, occurring in plaques on the buttocks; Achilles tendons; and extensors of wrists, elbows, and knees, becoming fibrotic and finally scarring. Early lesions show necrotizing vasculitis with fibrinoid or lipid deposits in vessel walls.

e. **exfoliati′va,** SYN *keratolysis* exfoliativa.

e. **figura′tum per′stans,** SYN e. annulare centrifugum.

e. **gyra′tum,** e. circinatum in which the various ringed lesions overlap each other.

e. **indura′tum,** recurrent hard subcutaneous nodules that frequently break down and form necrotic ulcers, usually on the calves and less frequently on the thighs or arms of middle-aged women; they are associated with erythrocyanotic changes in cold weather; although microscopically granulomatous and necrotizing, the lesions are sterile; but tuberculin skin tests are usually positive and polymerase chain reaction amplification is frequently positive for *Mycobacterium tuberculosis* complex DNA. SYN Bazin disease, nodular tuberculid.

e. **infectio′sum,** a mild infectious exanthema of childhood characterized by an erythematous maculopapular eruption, resulting in a lacelike facial rash or "slapped cheek" appearance. Fever and arthritis may also accompany infection; caused by Parvovirus B 19. SYN fifth disease.

e. **intertri′go,** SEE intertrigo.

e. **kerato′des,** keratodermia with an erythematous border.

macular e., SYN roseola.

e. **margina′tum,** a variant of e. multiforme seen in rheumatic fever; occasionally has a configuration to suggest the designation e. migrans (geographic tongue).

e. **multifor′me,** an acute eruption of macules, papules, or subepidermal vesicles presenting a multiform appearance, the characteristic lesion being the target or iris lesion over the dorsal aspect of the hands and forearms; its origin may be allergic, including drug sensitivity, or it may be caused by herpes simplex infection; the eruption, although usually self-limited (e.g., multiforme minor), may be recurrent or may run a severe course, sometimes with fatal termination (e.g., multiforme major or Stevens-Johnson syndrome).

e. **multifor′me bullo′sum,** SYN Stevens-Johnson *syndrome*.

e. **multifor′me exudati′vum,** SYN Stevens-Johnson *syndrome*.

e. **multifor′me ma′jor,** SYN Stevens-Johnson *syndrome*.

necrolytic migratory e., an erythematous, scaling, and sometimes bullous and erosive dermatitis occurring irregularly in plaques chiefly on the lower trunk, buttocks, perineum, and thighs; associated with weight loss, anemia, stomatitis, and elevation of plasma glucagon in islet cell tumor (glucagonoma) of the pancreas. SEE ALSO glucagonoma *syndrome*.

e. **neonato′rum,** SYN e. toxicum neonatorum.

e. **nodo′sum,** a panniculitis marked by the sudden formation of painful nodes on the extensor surfaces of the lower extremities, with lesions that are self-limiting but tend to recur; associated with arthralgia and fever; may be the result of drug sensitivity or associated with sarcoidosis and various infections. Deep biopsies show a septal panniculitis with infiltration by lymphocytes and scattered multinucleated giant cells. SYN nodal fever.

e. **nodo′sum lepro′sum,** an acute type of lepromatous reaction with generalized systemic involvement and tender deep cutaneous and subcutaneous nodules of the face, thighs, and arms; usually seen in undiagnosed, untreated, or neglected cases of leprosy. Immune complexes and scanty, fragmented lepra bacilli may be seen in the lesions.

e. **nodo′sum mi′grans,** SYN subacute migratory *panniculitis*.

e. **nuchae,** SYN Unna *nevus*.

e. **palma′re heredita′rium** [MIM*133000], a hereditary condition, which may be precipitated by pregnancy, characterized by asymptomatic symmetrical redness of the palms; autosomal dominant inheritance. SYN Lane disease.

e. **papula′tum,** the papular form of e. multiforme.

e. **paratrim′ma,** e. due to stasis over pressure points.

e. **per′nio,** SYN chilblain.

e. **per′stans,** probably a chronic form of e. multiforme in which the relapses recur so persistently that the eruption is almost permanent.

scarlatiniform e., e. scarlatinoi′des, an erythematous macular eruption accompanied by slight constitutional symptoms and followed by desquamation.

e. **sim′plex,** blushing or redness of the skin caused by a toxic reaction or a neurovascular phenomenon.

e. **sola′re,** SYN sunburn.

symptomatic e., a general term applied to various e.'s associated with systemic disease, fevers, allergic states, etc.

e. **tox′icum,** an innocuous, self-limited rash of unknown cause that occurs in newborn infants.

e. **tox′icum neonato′rum,** a common transient idiopathic eruption of erythema, small papules, and occasionally pustules filled with eosinophilic leukocytes overlying hair follicles of the newborn. SYN e. neonatorum.

e. **tubercula′tum,** e. multiforme in which the papules are of large size.

er·y·them·a·tous (er-i-them′ă-tŭs, -thē′mă-tŭs). Relating to or marked by erythema.

er·y·ther·mal·gia (er′i-ther-mal′jē-ă). SYN erythromelalgia.

△**erythr-.** SEE erythro-.

er·y·thral·gia (ār-i-thral′jē-ă). Painful redness of the skin. SEE ALSO erythromelalgia. [erythro- + G. *algos,* pain]

ery·thras·ma (er-i-thraz′mă). An eruption of well-circumscribed reddish brown patches, in the axillae and groins especially, due to the presence of *Corynebacterium minutissimum* in the stratum corneum. [G. *erythrainō,* to redden]

eryth·re·de·ma (ě-rith-rē-dē′mă). SYN acrodynia (2). [erythro- + G. *oidēma,* swelling]

er·y·thre·mia (er-i-thrē′mē-ă). SYN *polycythemia* vera. [erythro- + G. *haima,* blood]

altitude e., SYN chronic mountain *sickness*.

er·y·thris·tic (er-i-thris′tik). SYN rufous.

er·y·thrite (ě-rith′rīt). SYN erythritol.

eryth·ri·tol (ě-rith′ri-tol). The 4-carbon sugar alcohol obtained by the reduction of erythrose, notable for its sweetness (twice that of sucrose); found in lichens, algae, and fungi. SYN erythrite, erythrol.

eryth·ri·tyl tet·ra·ni·trate (ě-rith′ri-til tet-ră-nī′trāt). A vasodilator used in angina pectoris and hypertension. SYN erythrol tetranitrate, tetranitrol.

△**erythro-, erythr-.** 1. Combining form denoting red or red blood cell; corresponds to L. rub-. 2. Indicates the structure of erythrose in a larger sugar; used as such, it is italicized (e.g., 2-deoxy-D-*erythro*-pentose). [G. *erythros,* red]

eryth·ro·blast (ě-rith′rō-blast). Originally, a term denoting all forms of human red blood cells containing a nucleus, both pathologic (i.e., megaloblastic) and normal (e.g., normoblastic). The pathologic or megaloblastic series is observed in pernicious anemia in relapse. The term megaloblast is also used to indicate the first generation of cells in the red blood cell series that can be distinguished from precursor endothelial cells; hence with this usage, megaloblast denotes both a normal and an abnormal cell. In the *erythrobastic series* of maturation four stages of development can be recognized: 1) proerythroblast, 2) basophilic erythroblast, 3) polychromatic erythroblast, and 4) orthochromatic erythroblast. In the *megaloblastic series* of maturation, stages similar to those found in the normoblastic series are seen: 1) promegaloblast, 2) basophilic megaloblast, 3) polychromatic megaloblast, and 4) orthochromatic megaloblast. In the *normal series* of maturation, after loss of the nucleus, young erythrocytes are called *reticulocytes;* these cells may be recognized with supravital stains such as brilliant cresyl blue; ultimately the reticulocytes become erythrocytes, or mature red blood cells. SYN erythrocytoblast. [erythro- + G. *blastos,* germ]

eryth·ro·blas·te·mia (ě-rith′rō-blas-tē′mē-ă). The presence of nucleated red cells in the peripheral blood. [erythroblast + G. *haima,* blood]

eryth·ro·blas·to·pe·nia (ě-rith′rō-blas-tō-pē′nē-ă). A primary deficiency of erythroblasts in bone marrow, seen in aplastic anemia. [erythroblast + G. *penia,* poverty]

transient e. of childhood, a disorder of unknown cause with severe but transient normocytic, normochromic anemia that typically occurs between 6 months and 3 years of age; often follows a viral illness and usually resolves in 1–2 months.

eryth·ro·blas·to·sis (ĕ-rith′rō-blas-tō′sis). The presence of erythroblasts in considerable number in the blood. [erythroblast + -*osis,* condition]

fetal e., SYN e. fetalis.

e. feta′lis, a grave hemolytic anemia that, in most instances, results from development in an Rh-negative mother of anti-Rh antibody in response to the Rh factor in the (Rh-positive) fetal blood; it is characterized by many erythroblasts in the circulation, and often generalized edema (hydrops fetalis) and enlargement of the liver and spleen; the disease is sometimes caused by antibodies for antigens other than Rh. SYN anemia neonatorum, congenital anemia, fetal e., hemolytic anemia of newborn, hemolytic disease of newborn, neonatal anemia, Rh antigen incompatibility.

eryth·ro·blas·tot·ic (ĕ-rith′rō-blas-tot′ik). Pertaining to erythroblastosis, especially erythroblastosis fetalis.

eryth·ro·ca·tal·y·sis (ĕ-rith′rō-kă-tal′i-sis). Phagocytosis of the red blood cells. [erythro- + G. *katalysis,* dissolution]

eryth·ro·chro·mia (ĕ-rith′rō-krō′mē-ă). A red coloration or staining. [erythro- + G. *chrōma,* color]

eryth·ro·cla·sis (er-i-throk′lă-sis). Fragmentation of the red blood cells. [erythro- + G. *klasis,* a breaking]

eryth·ro·clas·tic (ĕ-rith′rō-klas′tik). Pertaining to erythroclasis; destructive to red blood cells.

eryth·ro·cu·pre·in (ĕ-rith′rō-koo′prē-in). SYN cytocuprein.

eryth·ro·cy·a·no·sis (ĕ-rith′rō-sī-ă-nō′sis). A condition seen in girls and young women in which exposure of the limbs to cold causes them to become swollen and dusky red; it results from direct exposure to cold, but not freezing, temperatures. [erythro- + G. *kyanos,* blue, + -*osis,* condition]

▣eryth·ro·cyte (ĕ-rith′rō-sīt). A mature red blood cell. SYN red blood cell, red corpuscle. [erythro- + G. *kytos,* cell]

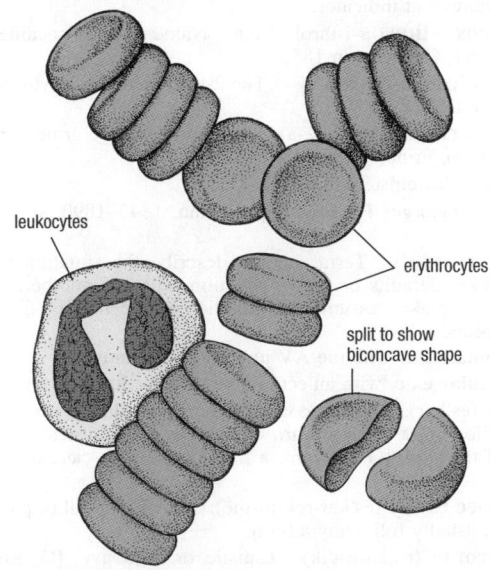

leukocytes

erythrocytes

split to show biconcave shape

erythrocytes: red blood cells grouped in rouleaux (like stacks of coins)

eryth·ro·cy·the·mia (ĕ-rith′rō-sī-thē′mē-ă). SYN polycythemia. [erythro- + G. *kytos,* cell, + *haima,* blood]

eryth·ro·cyt·ic (ĕ-rith-rō-sit′ik). Pertaining to an erythrocyte.

eryth·ro·cy·to·blast (ĕ-rith-rō-sī′tō-blast). SYN erythroblast. [erythro- + G. *kytos,* cell, + *blastos,* germ]

eryth·ro·cy·tol·y·sin (ĕ-rith′rō-sī-tol′i-sin). SYN hemolysin (1).

eryth·ro·cy·tol·y·sis (ĕ-rith′rō-sī-tol′i-sis). SYN hemolysis. [erythrocyte + G. *lysis,* loosening]

eryth·ro·cy·tom·e·ter (ĕ-rith′rō-sī-tom′ĕ-ter). An instrument for counting the red blood cells; Hayden used this term to denote an instrument to measure the diameter of red blood cells. [erythrocyte + G. *metron,* measure]

eryth·ro·cy·to·pe·nia (ĕ-rith′rō-sī-tō-pē′nē-ă). SYN erythropenia.

eryth·ro·cy·to·poi·e·sis (ĕ-rith′rō-sī′tō-poy-ē′sis). SYN erythropoiesis.

eryth·ro·cy·tor·rhex·is (ĕ-rith′rō-sī-tō-rek′sis). A partial erythrocytolysis in which particles of protoplasm escape from the red blood cells, which then become crenated and deformed. SYN erythrorrhexis. [erythrocyte + G. *rhēxis,* rupture]

eryth·ro·cy·tos·chi·sis (ĕ-rith′rō-sī-tos′ki-sis). A breaking up of the red blood cells into small particles that morphologically resemble platelets. [erythrocyte + G. *schisis,* a splitting]

eryth·ro·cy·to·sis (ĕ-rith′rō-sī-tō′sis). Polycythemia, especially that which occurs in response to some known stimulus.

eryth·ro·cy·tu·ria (ĕ-rith′rō-sī-too′rē-ă). Red blood cells in urine.

eryth·ro·de·gen·er·a·tive (ĕ-rith′rō-de-jen′er-ă-tiv). Pertaining to or characterized by degeneration of the red blood cells.

eryth·ro·der·ma (ĕ-rith-rō-der′mă). A nonspecific designation for intense and usually widespread reddening of the skin from dilation of blood vessels, often preceding, or associated with exfoliation. SYN erythrodermatitis. [erythro- + G. *derma,* skin]

bullous congenital ichthyosiform e. (ik-thē-os′ē-form), diffusely red, eroded skin at birth, with subsequent scaling, tending to improve in later life, characterized by generalized epidermolytic hyperkeratosis and autosomal dominant inheritance. SEE ALSO epidermolytic *hyperkeratosis.* SYN generalized epidermolytic hyperkeratosis, ichthyismus hystrix, ichthyosis hystrix.

congenital ichthyosiform e., a genodermatosis characterized by diffuse chronic erythema and scale formation which may be separated into bullous and nonbullous forms.

e. desquamati′vum, severe, extensive seborrheic dermatitis with exfoliative dermatitis, generalized lymphadenopathy, and diarrhea in the newborn; frequently occurs in undernourished, cachectic children. SYN Leiner disease.

nonbullous congenital ichthyosiform e., e. or a collodion membrane at birth, usually without improvement during childhood, characterized by proliferation of epidermal keratinocytes with lipid accumulation; autosomal recessive inheritance.

e. psoriat′icum, extensive exfoliative dermatitis simulating psoriasis.

Sézary e., SYN Sézary *syndrome.*

eryth·ro·der·ma·ti·tis (ĕ-rith′rō-der-mă-tī′tis). SYN erythroderma.

eryth·ro·dex·trin (ĕ-rith′rō-deks′trin). A partially digested form of dextrin identified by its color reaction with iodine (i.e., turning red).

eryth·ro·don·tia (ĕ-rith-rō-don′shē-ă). Reddish discoloration of the teeth, as may occur in porphyria. [erythro- + G. *odous,* tooth]

eryth·ro·gen·e·sis im·per·fec·ta (ĕ-rith-rō-jen′ĕ-sis im-per-fek′tă). SYN congenital hypoplastic *anemia.*

eryth·ro·gen·ic (ĕ-rith-rō-jen′ik). **1.** Producing red, as causing an eruption or a red color sensation. **2.** Pertaining to the formation of red blood cells. [erythro- + -*gen,* producing]

eryth·ro·go·ni·um, pl. **eryth·ro·go·nia** (ĕ-rith-rō-gō′nē-ŭm, -nē-ă). The precursor of an erythrocyte; occasionally refers to the erythropoietic tissue as a whole. [erythro- + G. *gonē,* generation]

er·y·throid (er′i-throyd, ĕ-rith′royd). Reddish in color.

er·y·throid·in (er′i-thrōy′din). A nicotinic cholinergic antagonist which unlike most members of this group of agents, is a tertiary amine and hence enters the central nervous system.

eryth·ro·ker·a·to·der·mi·a (ĕ-rith′rō-kār-ă-tō-der′mē-ă) [MIM* 133190]. A neurocutaneous syndrome characterized by papulosquamous erythematous plaques with onset shortly after birth; ataxia, nystagmus, dysarthria, and decreased tendon reflexes appear later in life; symmetrical progressive e. is inherited as an autosomal dominant disorder and does not involve the palms and soles. [erythro- + G. *keras,* horn, + *derma,* skin, + *-ia,* condition]

e. varia′bilis [MIM*133200], a dermatosis characterized by hyperkeratotic plaques of bizarre, geographic configuration, associated with erythrodermic areas that may vary remarkably in size, shape, and position from day to day; hair, nares, and teeth are not affected; onset is usually in the first year of life; autosomal dominant or recessive inheritance, caused by mutation in the connexin gene encoding gap junction protein beta-3 (GJB3) on 1p.

eryth·ro·ki·net·ics (ĕ-rith′rō-ki-net′iks). A consideration of the kinetics of erythrocytes from their generation to destruction; erythrokinetic studies are sometimes made in cases of anemia to evaluate the balance between erythrocyte production and destruction. [erythro- + G. *kinēsis,* movement]

er·y·throl (er′i-throl). SYN erythritol.

e. tetranitrate, SYN erythrityl tetranitrate.

eryth·ro·leu·ke·mia (ĕ-rith′rō-loo-kē′mē-ă). Simultaneous neoplastic proliferation of erythroblastic and leukoblastic tissues.

eryth·ro·leu·ko·sis (ĕ-rith′rō-loo-kō′sis). A condition resembling leukemia in which the erythropoietic tissue is affected in addition to the leukopoietic tissue.

er·y·throl·y·sin (er-i-throl′i-sin). SYN hemolysin (1).

er·y·throl·y·sis (er-i-throl′i-sis). SYN hemolysis.

eryth·ro·mel·al·gia (ĕ-rith′rō-mel-al′jē-ă). **1.** A rare disorder most common in middle age, characterized by paroxysmal attacks of severe burning pain, reddening, hyperalgesia, and sweating, involving one or more extremities, usually both feet; the attacks can be triggered by warmth, and are usually relieved by cold and limb elevation. **2.** Paroxysmal throbbing and burning pain in the skin often precipitated by exertion or heat, affecting the hands and feet, accompanied by a dusky mottled redness of the parts with increased skin temperature; associated with and often preceding myeloproliferative and other disorders. SYN erythermalgia, Gerhardt-Mitchell disease. [erythro- + G. *melos,* limb, + *algos,* pain]

eryth·ro·me·lia (ĕ-rith-rō-mē′lē-ă). Diffuse idiopathic erythema and atrophy of the skin of the lower limbs. [erythro- + G. *melos,* limb]

eryth·ro·my·cin (ĕ-rith-rō-mī′sin). A macrolide antibiotic agent obtained from cultures of a strain of *Streptomyces erythraeus* found in soil; it is active against *Corynebacterium diphtheriae* and several other species of *Corynebacterium,* Group A hemolytic streptococci, *Streptococcus pneumoniae,* and *Bordetella pertussis;* Gram-positive bacteria are in general more susceptible to its action than are Gram-negative bacteria, although *Neisseria* and *Brucella* are susceptible to its action. Available as the estolate, ethylcarbonate, ethylsuccinate, gluceptate, lactobionate, stearate, and salts; active against *Legionella* and *Mycoplasma pneumoniae.* Often used as a substitute antibiotic in penicillin-allergic patients.

e. estolate, a salt of the macrolide antibiotic, erythromycin.

e. glucoheptonate, a salt of the macrolide antibiotic, erythromycin.

e. propionate, a salt of the macrolide antibiotic, erythromycin.

e. stearate, a salt of the macrolide antibiotic, erythromycin.

er·y·thron (er′i-thron). The total mass of circulating red blood cells, and that part of the hematopoietic tissue from which they are derived.

eryth·ro·ne·o·cy·to·sis (ĕ-rith′rō-nē-ō-sī-tō′sis). The presence in the peripheral circulation of regenerative forms of red blood cells. [erythrocyte + G. *neos,* new, + *kytos,* cell, + *-osis,* condition]

eryth·ro·pe·nia (ĕ-rith-rō-pē′nē-ă). Deficiency in the number of red blood cells. SYN erythrocytopenia. [erythrocyte + G. *penia,* poverty]

eryth·ro·pha·gia (ĕ-rith-rō-fā′jē-ă). Phagocytic destruction of red blood cells. [erythrocyte + G. *phagō,* to eat, + -ia]

eryth·ro·phag·o·cy·to·sis (ĕ-rith′rō-fag′ō-sī-tō′sis). Phagocytosis of erythrocytes.

eryth·ro·phil (ĕ-rith′rō-fil). **1.** Staining readily with red dyes. SYN erythrophilic. **2.** A cell or tissue element that stains red. [erythro- + G. *philos,* fond]

eryth·ro·phil·ic (ĕ-rith-rō-fil′ik). SYN erythrophil (1).

eryth·ro·phore (ĕ-rith′rō-fōr). A chromatophore containing

granules of a red or brown pigment. SYN allophore. [erythro- + G. *phoros,* bearing]

eryth·ro·pla·kia (ĕ-rith-rō-plā′kē-ă). A red, velvety, plaquelike lesion of mucous membrane that often represents malignant change. [erythro- + G. *plax,* plate]

eryth·ro·pla·sia (ĕ-rith-rō-plā′zē-ă). Erythema and dysplasia of the epithelium. [erythro- + G. *plassō,* to form]

e. of Queyrat, obsolete term for carcinoma in situ of the glans penis.

eryth·ro·poi·e·sis (ĕ-rith′rō-poy-ē′sis). The formation of red blood cells. SYN erythrocytopoiesis. [erythrocyte + G. *poiēsis,* a making]

eryth·ro·poi·et·ic (ĕ-rith′rō-poy-et′ik). Pertaining to or characterized by erythropoiesis.

eryth·ro·poi·e·tin (ĕ-rith-rō-poy′ĕ-tin). A sialic acid-containing protein that enhances erythropoiesis by stimulating formation of proerythroblasts and release of reticulocytes from bone marrow; it is formed by the kidney and liver, and possibly by other tissues, and can be detected in human plasma and urine. SYN erythropoietic hormone (2), hematopoietin, hemopoietin.

eryth·ro·pros·o·pal·gia (ĕ-rith′rō-pros-ō-pal′jē-ă). A disorder similar to erythromelalgia, but with the pain and redness occurring in the face. [erythro- + G. *prosōpon,* face, + *algos,* pain]

eryth·rop·sia (ĕ-rith-rop′sē-ă). An abnormality of vision in which all objects appear to be tinged with red. SYN red vision. [erythro- + G. *ōps,* eye]

eryth·ro·pyk·no·sis (ĕ-rith′rō-pik-nō′sis). Alteration of red blood cells to develop the so-called "brassy bodies," under the influence of the malarial parasite. [erythro- + G. *pyknos,* dense]

er·y·thror·rhex·is (er′i-thrō-rek′sis, ĕ-rith-rō-rek′sis). SYN erythrocytorrhexis. [erythrocyte + G. *rhēxis,* rupture]

er·y·throse (ĕ-rith′rōs). An aldotetrose epimeric with threose. The D-isomer plays a role in intermediary metabolism.

e. 4-phosphate, a phosphorylated derivative of e. that serves as an important intermediate in the pentose phosphate pathway.

eryth·ro·sin B (ĕ-rith′rō-sin) [C.I. 45430]. Tetraiodofluorescein, a fluorescent red acid dye, used as a counterstain in histology and as a fluorescent indicator.

er·y·throx·y·line (er-i-throk′si-lēn). Name given to cocaine by its discoverer, Gaedeke, in 1855.

eryth·ru·lose (ĕ-rith′roo-lōs). The 2-keto analog of erythrose; the only ketotetrose.

er·y·thru·ria (er-i-throo′rē-ă). The passage of red urine. [erythro- + G. *ouron,* urine]

Es Symbol for einsteinium.

Esbach, Georges H., French physician, 1843–1890. SEE E. *reagent.*

es·cape (es-kāp′). Term used to describe the situation when a pacemaker defaults or AV conduction fails and another, usually lower pacemaker, assumes the function of pacemaking for one or more beats.

junctional e., e. with the AV junction as pacemaker.

ventricular e., e. with an ectopic ventricular focus as pacemaker.

es·char (es′kar). A thick, coagulated crust or slough which develops following a thermal burn or chemical or physical cauterization of the skin. [G. *eschara,* a fireplace, a scab caused by burning]

es·char·ec·to·my (es′kar-rek-tō-mē). Excision of all or part of an eschar, usually following a burn.

es·cha·rot·ic (es-kă-rot′ik). Caustic or corrosive. [G. *escharōtikos*]

es·cha·rot·o·my (es-kă-rot′ō-mē). Surgical incision in an eschar (necrotic dermis) to lessen constriction, especially after a circumferential third degree burn of an extremity or the thorax. [eschar + G. *tomē,* incision]

Esch·e·rich·ia (esh-ĕ-rik′ē-ă). A genus of aerobic, facultatively anaerobic bacteria containing short, motile or nonmotile, Gram-negative rods. Motile cells are peritrichous. Glucose and lactose are fermented with the production of acid and gas. These organisms are found in feces; some are pathogenic to humans, causing enteritis, peritonitis, cystitis, etc. It is the type genus of the family Enterobacteriaceae. The type species is *E. coli.* [T. *Escherich,* German pediatrician and bacteriologist, 1857–1911]

⊞*E. co'li,* a species that occurs normally in the intestines of humans and other vertebrates, is widely distributed in nature, and is a frequent cause of infections of the urogenital tract and of neonatal meningitis and diarrhea in infants; enteropathogenic strains (serovars) of *E. coli* cause diarrhea due to enterotoxin, the production of which seems to be associated with a transferable episome; the type species of the genus. SYN colibacillus, colon bacillus.

enterohemorrhagic *E. coli* (EHEC), enterohemorrhagic strains of *E. coli,* commonly of the serotype 0157:H7; produces a toxin resembling that produced by *Shigella;* associated with damage to the epithelium, ischemia of the bowel, and necrosis of the colon. Apparently responsible for a hemorrhagic form of colitis without fever, which can be very severe; spread primarily by contaminated beef and poultry. May also cause microangiopathic hemolytic anemia, renal failure, and the hemolytic uremic syndrome.

enteroinvasive *E. coli* (EIEC), enteroinvasive strain of *E. coli* penetrates gut mucosa and multiplies in colon epithelial cells, resulting in shigellosislike changes of the mucosa. This strain produces a severe diarrheal illness that can resemble shigellosis except for the absence of vomiting and shorter duration of illness.

enteropathogenic *E. coli* (EPEC), enteropathogenic strain of *E. coli;* organisms adhere to small bowel mucosa and produce characteristic changes in the microvilli. This strain produces symptomatic, sometimes serious, gastrointestinal illnesses, especially severe in neonates and young children; typically it produces toxins, one of which is heat-labile, resembling that produced by *Vibrio cholerae,* the other heat-stable.

enterotoxigenic *E. coli* (ETEC), enterotoxigenic strain of *E. coli;* attaches to the duodenum or proximal small intestine mucosa, where it forms heat-stable and heat-labile toxins that activate adenylate cyclase, causing watery diarrhea. Responsible for 40–70% of traveler's diarrhea; chiefly waterborne via human feces. Most important cause of diarrhea among infants living in tropical areas.

E. freun'dii, former name for *Citrobacter freundii.*

es·cor·cin, es·cor·cin·ol (es-kōr′sin, -sin-ol). A brown powder derived from esculetin, a substance derived from esculin; used for the detection of defects in the cornea and conjunctiva, which it marks by a red coloration.

es·cu·la·pi·an (es-kū-lā′pē-ăn). SYN aesculapian.

es·cu·lent (es′kū-lent). Edible; fit for eating. [L. *esculentus,* edible]

es·cu·lin (es′kū-lin). A glucoside from horse-chestnut bark; used as a sunburn protective. SYN aesculin. [L. *aesculus,* the Italian oak]

es·er·i·dine (es-er′i-dēn). An alkaloid from the seed of *Physostigma;* a parasympathomimetic agent. SYN eserine aminoxide, eserine oxide.

es·er·ine (es′er-ēn). SYN physostigmine.

  e. aminoxide, SYN eseridine.

  e. oxide, SYN eseridine.

  e. salicylate, SYN *physostigmine* salicylate.

⌂**-esis.** Condition, action, or process. [G. *-esis,* condition or process]

Esmarch, Johann F.A. von, German surgeon, 1823–1908. SEE E. *tourniquet.*

es·mo·lol hy·dro·chlo·ride (es′mō-lol). A β-adrenergic blocking agent with brief duration of action.

es·o·de·vi·a·tion (es′ō-dē-vē-ā′shŭn). **1.** SYN esophoria. **2.** SYN esotropia.

es·od·ic (es-sod′ik). SYN afferent. [G. *esō,* inward, + *hodos,* way]

esoph·a·gal·gia (ē-sof-ă-gal′jē-ă). Rarely used term for pain in the esophagus. SYN esophagodynia. [esophagus + G. *algos,* pain]

esoph·a·ge·al (ē-sof′ă-jē′ăl, ē′-sŏ-faj′ē-ăl). Relating to the esophagus.

e·soph·a·gec·to·my (ē-sof-ă-jek′tō-mē). Excision of all or any part of the esophagus. [esophagus + G. *ektomē,* excision]

Ivor Lewis e., commonly used approach for e. via laparotomy and right thoracotomy, with intrathoracic anastomosis.

three-incision e., e. via laparotomy, right chest and cervical incisions.

transhiatal e., resection of the esophagus from a cervical incision from above and transhiatal approach through an abdominal incision from below.

transthoracic e., resection of the esophagus through a thoracotomy incision.

esoph·a·gi (ē-sof′ă-jī, -gī). Plural of esophagus.

esoph·a·gism (ē-sof′ă-jizm). Esophageal spasm causing dysphagia. SYN dysphagia nervosa, nervous dysphagia.

esoph·a·gi·tis (ē-sof-ă-jī′tis). Inflammation of the esophagus.

  reflux e., peptic e., inflammation of the lower esophagus from regurgitation of acid gastric contents, usually due to malfunction of the lower esophageal sphincter; symptoms include substernal pain, "heartburn," and regurgitation of acid juice.

esoph·a·go·car·di·o·plas·ty (ē-sof′ă-gō-kar′dē-ō-plas-tē). A revisional procedure of the esophagus and cardiac end of the stomach.

esoph·a·go·cele (ē-sof′ă-gō-sēl). Protrusion of the mucous membrane of the esophagus through a tear in the muscular coat. [esophagus + G. *kēlē,* hernia]

esoph·a·go·dyn·ia (ē-sof′ă-gō-din′ē-ă). SYN esophagalgia. [esophagus + G. *odynē,* pain]

esoph·a·go·en·ter·os·to·my (ē-sof′ă-gō-en-ter-os′tō-mē). Surgical formation of a direct communication between the esophagus and intestine. [esophagus + G. *enteron,* intestine, + *stoma,* mouth]

esoph·a·go·gas·trec·to·my (ē-sof′ă-gō-gas-trek′tō-mē). Removal of a portion of the lower esophagus and proximal stomach.

esoph·a·go·gas·tro·a·nas·to·mo·sis (ē-sof′ă-gō-gas′trō-ă-nas-tō-mō′sis). SYN esophagogastrostomy.

esoph·a·go·gas·tro·du·o·de·nos·co·py (EGD) (ē-sof′ă-gō-gas′trō-doo′ō-den-os-kō-pē). Endoscopic examination of the esophagus, stomach and duodenum usually performed using a fiberoptic instrument.

esoph·a·go·gas·tro·my·ot·o·my (ē-sof′ă-gō-gas′trō-mī-ot′ō-mē). SYN esophagomyotomy.

esoph·a·go·gas·tro·plas·ty (ē-sof′ă-gō-gas′trō-plas-tē). SYN cardioplasty.

esoph·a·go·gas·tros·to·my (ē-sof′ă-gō-gas-tros′tō-mē). Anastomosis of esophagus to stomach, usually following esophagogastrectomy. SYN esophagogastroanastomosis, gastroesophagostomy. [esophagus + G. *gastēr,* stomach, + *stoma,* mouth]

esoph·a·go·gram (e-sof′ă-gō-gram). SYN esophagram.

esoph·a·gog·ra·phy (ē-sof-ă-gog′ră-fē). Radiography of the esophagus using swallowed or injected radiopaque contrast media; the technique of obtaining an esophagram. [esophagus + G. *graphō,* to write]

esoph·a·gol·o·gy (ē-sof′ă-gol′ō-gē). Study of the structure, physiology, and diseases of the esophagus. [esophagus + G. *logos,* study]

esoph·a·go·ma·la·cia (ē-sof′ă-gō-mă-lā′shē-ă). Softening of the walls of the esophagus. [esophagus + G. *malakia,* softness]

esoph·a·go·my·ot·o·my (ē-sof′ă-gō-mī-ot′ō-mē). Longitudinal division of the muscular layer down to the submucosa of the lowest part of the esophageal wall; some muscle fibers of the cardia may also be divided. SYN cardiomyotomy, esophagogastromyotomy. [esophagus + G. *mys,* muscle, + *tomē,* incision]

esoph·a·go·plas·ty (ē-sof′ă-gō-plas-tē). A revisional surgical procedure of the wall of the esophagus. [esophagus + G. *plastos,* formed]

esoph·a·go·pli·ca·tion (ē-sof′ă-gō-pli-kā′shŭn). Reduction in size of a dilated esophagus or of a pouch in it by making longitudinal folds or tucks in its wall. [esophagus + L. *plico,* to fold]

esoph·a·go·pto·sis, esoph·a·go·pto·sia (ē-sof′ă-gō-tō′sis, -tō′sē-ă). Relaxation and downward displacement of the walls of the esophagus. [esophagus + G. *ptōsis,* a falling]

esoph·a·go·scope (ē-sof′ă-gō-skōp). An endoscope for inspect-

es

ing the interior of the esophagus. [esophagus + G. *skopeō*, to examine]

esoph·a·gos·co·py (ē-sof-ă-gos′kŏ-pē). Inspection of the interior of the esophagus by means of an endoscope. [esophagus + G. *skopeō*, to examine]

esoph·a·go·spasm (ē-sof′ă-gō-spazm). Spasm of the walls of the esophagus.

esoph·a·go·ste·no·sis (ē-sof′ă-gō-stē-nō′sis). Stricture or a general narrowing of the esophagus. [esophagus + G. *stenōsis*, a narrowing]

esoph·a·go·sto·mi·a·sis (ē-sof′ă-gō-stō-mī′ă-sis). SYN oesophagostomiasis. [esophagus + G. *stoma*, mouth, + *-iasis*, condition]

esoph·a·gos·to·my (ē-sof-ă-gos′tō-mē). Surgical formation of an opening directly into the esophagus from without. [esophagus + G. *stoma*, mouth]

esoph·a·got·o·my (ē-sof-ă-got′ō-mē). An incision through the wall of the esophagus. [esophagus + G. *tomē*, an incision]

esoph·a·gram (ē-sof′ă-gram). A radiographic record of contrast esophagography or barium swallow. SYN esophagogram.

▣**esoph·a·gus**, pl. **esoph·a·gi** (ē-sof′ă-gŭs, -gī; -jī) [TA]. The portion of the digestive canal between the pharynx and stomach. It is about 25 cm long and consists of three parts: the cervical part, from the cricoid cartilage to the thoracic inlet; the thoracic part, from the thoracic inlet to the diaphragm; and the abdominal part, below the diaphragm to the cardiac opening of the stomach. [G. *oisophagos*, gullet]

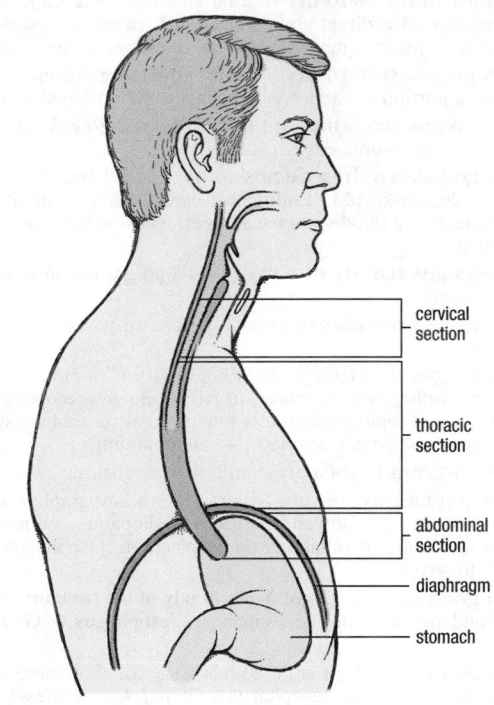

cervical section

thoracic section

abdominal section

diaphragm

stomach

esophagus

▣**Barrett e.,** SYN Barrett *syndrome*.

es·o·pho·ria (es-ō-fō′rē-ă). A tendency for the eyes to turn inward, prevented by binocular vision. SYN esodeviation (1). [G. *esō*, inward, + *phora*, a carrying]

es·o·phor·ic (es-ō-fōr′ik). Relating to or marked by esophoria.

es·o·tro·pia (es-ō-trō′pē-ă). The form of strabismus in which the visual axes converge; may be paralytic or concomitant, monocular or alternating, accommodative or nonaccommodative. SYN convergent squint, convergent strabismus, esodeviation (2), internal squint. [G. *esō*, inward, + *tropē*, turn]

A-pattern e., convergent strabismus greater in upward than in downward gaze.

basic e., SYN nonaccommodative e.

consecutive e., e. that follows surgical correction of exotropia.

cyclic e., periodic convergent strabismus often occurring every 48 hours. SYN alternate day strabismus.

mixed e., that type of e. in which both accommodative and nonaccommodative factors are present.

nonaccommodative e., that type of e. not influenced by correction of refractive error. SYN basic e.

nonrefractive accommodative e., that type of e. in which an abnormality of the accommodative-convergence mechanism is not eliminated by correction of refractive error.

refractive accommodative e., that type of e. eliminated by correction of hypermetropic refractive error.

V-pattern e., convergent strabismus greater in downward than in upward gaze.

X-pattern e., decreasing convergence from the primary position in both upward and downward gaze.

es·o·tro·pic (es-ō-trop′ik). Relating to or marked by esotropia.

ESP Abbreviation for extrasensory *perception*.

es·pun·dia (es-poon′dē-ă). A type of American leishmaniasis caused by *Leishmania braziliensis* that affects the mucous membranes, particularly in the nasal and oral region, resulting in grossly destructive changes; particularly common in Brazil, where a significant proportion of persons infected with *L. braziliensis* develop this condition; may develop metastatically from sores originally found elsewhere on the body. SYN Breda disease, bubas braziliana. [Sp., fr. L. *spongia*, sponge]

es·qui·nan·cea (es-kwi-nan′sē-ă). Sense of suffocation caused by an inflammatory swelling in the throat, as in suppurative tonsillitis or pharyngitis. [Fr. *esquinancie*, quinsy]

ESR Abbreviation for erythrocyte sedimentation *rate*; electron spin *resonance*.

es·sence (es′ens). **1.** The true characteristic or substance of a body. **2.** An element. **3.** A fluidextract. **4.** An alcoholic solution, or spirit, of the volatile oil of a plant. **5.** Any volatile substance responsible for odor or taste of the organism (usually a plant) producing it; by extension, synthetic perfumes or flavors. [L. *essentia*, fr. *esse*, to be]

essence of rose, SYN oil of rose.

es·sen·tial (ĕ-sen′shăl). **1.** Necessary, indispensable, (e.g., e. amino acids, e. fatty acids). **2.** Characteristic of. **3.** Determining. **4.** Of unknown etiology. **5.** Relating to an essence (e.g., e. oil). **6.** SYN intrinsic.

Esser, Johannes F.S., Dutch surgeon, 1877–1946.

Essick, C., 20th century U.S. anatomist. SEE E. cell *bands*, under *band*.

Essig splint. See under splint.

es·taz·o·lam (ĕs-taz′-ō-lam). A benzodiazepine compound with sedative/hypnotic properties.

es·ter (es′ter). An organic compound containing the grouping, –X(O)–O–R (X = carbon, sulfur, phosphorus, etc.; R = radical of an alcohol), formed by the elimination of H_2O between the –OH of an acid group and the –OH of an alcohol group; usually written as in ethyl acetate (from acetic acid and ethyl alcohol), $CH_3CO-OC_2H_5$ or $CH_3COOC_2H_5$.

carboxylic acid e., specifically, an e. derived from a carboxylic acid and an alcohol; R–CO–R′

Cori e., SYN D-glucose 1-phosphate.

Embden e., hexose phosphate; a mixture of D-glucose 6-phosphate and D-fructose 6-phosphate; significant in the understanding of sugar metabolism.

Harden-Young e., D-fructose 1,6-bisphosphate; important intermediate in sugar metabolism.

Neuberg e., SYN fructose 6-phosphate.

Robison e., SYN D-glucose 6-phosphate.

Robison-Embden e., SYN D-glucose 6-phosphate.

sugar e., e. of a sugar with an organic or inorganic acid; e.g., D-glucose 6-phosphate.

thiol e., an e. formed from a carboxylic acid and a thiol (i.e., RCO–SR′), e.g., acetyl-coenzyme A.

es·ter·ase (es'ter-ās). A generic term for enzymes (EC class 3.1, hydrolases) that catalyze the hydrolysis of esters.

C1 e., subunit of the first component of complement (C1) involved in the activation of the classical pathway.

es·ter·i·fi·ca·tion (es'ter'i-fi-kā'shŭn). The process of forming an ester, as in the reaction of ethanol and acetic acid to form ethyl acetate.

Estes, William L., Jr., U.S. surgeon, 1885–1940. SEE E. *operation.*

es·the·ma·tol·o·gy (es-thē-mă-tol'ō-jē). The science concerned with the senses and sense organs. [G. *aisthēma,* perception, + *logos,* study]

es·the·sia (es-thē'zē-ă). **1.** SYN perception. **2.** SYN sensitivity (2). [G. *aisthēsis,* sensation]

es·the·sic (es-thē'sik). Relating to the mental perception of the existence of any part of the body. [G. *aisthēsis,* sensation]

esthesio-. **1.** Sensation, perception. [G. *aesthēsis,* sense perception]

es·the·si·od·ic (es-thē-zē-od'ik). Conveying sensory impressions. SYN esthesodic. [esthesio- + G. *hodos,* way]

es·the·si·o·gen·e·sis (es-thē'zē-ō-jen'ĕ-sis). The production of sensation, especially of nervous erethism. [esthesio- + G. *genesis,* origin]

es·the·si·o·gen·ic (es-thē-zē-ō-jen'ik). Producing a sensation.

es·the·si·og·ra·phy (es-thē-zē-og'ră-fē). **1.** A description of the organs of sense and of the mechanism of sensation. **2.** Mapping out on the skin the areas of tactile and other forms of sensibility. [esthesio- + G. *graphē,* a writing]

es·the·si·ol·o·gy (es-thē-zē-ol'ō-jē). The science concerned with sensory phenomena. [esthesio- + G. *logos,* study]

es·the·si·om·e·ter (es-thē-zē-om'ĕ-ter). An instrument for determining the state of tactile and other forms of sensibility. SYN tactometer. [esthesio- + G. *metron,* measure]

es·the·si·om·e·try (es-thē-zē-om'ĕ-trē). Measurement of the degree of tactile or other sensibility.

es·the·si·o·neu·ro·blas·to·ma (es-thē'zē-ō-noor'ō-blas-tō'mă). A neoplasm of immature, poorly differentiated neuronal cells believed to arise from neuroepithelial precursors. [esthesio- + neuroblastoma]

olfactory e., SYN olfactory *neuroblastoma.*

es·the·si·o·neu·ro·cy·to·ma (es-thē'zē-ō-nur'ō-sī-tō'mă). A neoplasm composed of nearly mature neuronlike cells believed to arise from a spinal or cranial ganglia. [esthesio- + neurocytoma]

es·the·si·o·phys·i·ol·o·gy (es-thē'zē-ō-fiz-ē-ol'ō-jē). The physiology of sensation and the sense organs.

es·the·si·os·co·py (es-thē-zē-os'kŏ-pē). Examination into the degree and extent of tactile and other forms of sensibility. [esthesio- + G. *skopeō,* to view]

es·the·sod·ic (es'thē-zod'ik). SYN esthesiodic.

es·thet·ic (es-thet'ik). **1.** Pertaining to the sensations. **2.** Pertaining to esthetics (i.e., beauty). [G. *aisthēsis,* sensation]

es·thet·ics (es-thet'iks). The branch of philosophy concerned with art and beauty, especially with the components thereof.

denture e., **(1)** the cosmetic effect produced by a dental prosthesis; **(2)** the qualities involved in the appearance of a given restoration.

es·ti·mate (es'tĭ-māt). **1.** A measurement or a statement about the value of some quantity that is known, believed, or suspected to incorporate some degree of error. **2.** The result of applying any estimator to a random sample of data. It is not a random variable but a realization of one, a fixed quantity, and it has no variance although commonly it also furnishes an estimate of what the variance of the estimator is. (Not to be confused with an estimator, which is a prescription for obtaining an estimate.) [L. *aestimo,* pp. *aestimatum,* to appraise]

Kaplan-Meier estimate, nonparametric method of compiling life tables or survival tables that combines calculated probabilities of survival with estimates to allow for censored (missing) observations; used mainly in survival studies of cancer and similar long-term diseases.

es·ti·ma·tion (es-tĭ-mā-shun). Any nontrivial statistical procedure that assigns to an unknown quantity (parameter) a plausible value on the basis of appropriate and pertinent data collected in a proper random sample.

es·ti·ma·tor (es'tĭ-mā-tor). A prescription for obtaining an estimate from a random sample of data. An e. is a procedure, not a result, and therefore is a random variable and has a variance. For instance an e. of the mean weight in adult men may consist of the prescription "Add up the weights of 100 men and divide by 100." The actual outcome (the estimate) will vary from sample to sample, but one answer will not be a random variable.

least squares e., the prescription "Assign to the unknown parameter the value that minimizes the mean of the squares of the residual errors."

maximum likelihood e., the prescription "Assign to the unknown parameter that value that maximizes the likelihood for the sample." For many problems this procedure is an optimal one.

es·ti·val (es'ti-văl). Relating to or occurring in the summer. SYN aestival. [L. *aestivus,* summer (adj.)]

es·ti·va·tion (es-ti-vā'shŭn). Living through the summer in a quiescent, torpid state. Cf. hibernation.

es·ti·vo·au·tum·nal (es'ti-vō-aw-tŭm'năl). Relating to or occurring in summer and autumn. [L. *aestivus,* summer (adj.), + *autumnalis,* autumnal]

Estlander, Jakob A., Finnish surgeon, 1831–1881. SEE E. *flap.*

es·tra·di·ol (E₂) (es-tră-dī'ol). β-Estradiol; 17β-estradiol; the most potent naturally occurring estrogen in mammals, formed by the ovary, placenta, testis, and possibly the adrenal cortex; therapeutic indications for e. are those typical of an estrogen. α-Estradiol (17α-estradiol), exhibits considerably less biologic activity. E. is used in the treatment of menstrual disorders, menopause problems, etc. SYN estrogenic hormone, oestradiol.

e. benzoate, fatty acid esters of 17β-estradiol usually dissolved in oil for injection purposes; such esters exhibit a longer duration of action than does the unesterified steroid.

e. cypionate, has the same actions and uses as e. but a prolonged duration of action; administered in oil by intramuscular injection.

e. dipropionate, an esterified natural estrogen for parenteral use.

ethinyl e., SYN ethynyl e.

ethynyl e., a semisynthetic derivative of 17β-estradiol; active by mouth, with a long half-life, it is among the most potent of known estrogenic compounds; used in oral contraceptive preparations. SYN ethinyl e.

e. undecylate, an esterified natural estrogen for parenteral use.

e. valerate, same actions and uses as e., but with a prolonged duration of action; administered in sesame oil by intramuscular injection.

es·tra·gon oil (es'tră-gon). SYN tarragon oil.

es·tra·mus·tine phos·phate so·di·um (es-tră-mŭs'tēn). An antineoplastic agent that combines the actions of estrogen and nitrogen mustard in the treatment of carcinoma of the prostate.

es·trane (es'trān). Hypothetical parent hydrocarbon of the (steroid) estrogenic compounds whose names begin with "estr-" (estradiol, estrone, estriol); conceived to establish a systematic nomenclature.

es·tra·tri·ene (es-tră-trī'ēn). The hypothetical triply unsaturated estrane that is the nucleus of most naturally occurring estrogenic steroids in animals.

es·trin (es'trin). SYN estrogen.

es·tri·ol (es'trē-ol). An estrogenic metabolite of estradiol, usually the predominant estrogenic metabolite found in urine (especially during pregnancy); epimers at C-16, C-17, or both, are known as 16-epiestriol, etc. SYN folliculin hydrate, oestriol, trihydroxyestrin.

es·tro·die·nol (es-trō-dē'nol). SYN dienestrol.

es·tro·gen (es'trō-jen). Generic term for any substance, natural or synthetic, that exerts biologic effects characteristic of estrogenic hormones such as 17β-estradiol. E.'s are formed by the ovary, placenta, testes, and possibly the adrenal cortex, as well as by certain plants; they stimulate secondary sexual characteristics, and exert systemic effects, such as growth and maturation of long bones, and are used therapeutically in any disorder attributable to e. deficiency or amenable to e. therapy, such as menstrual disorders and menopausal problems. They control the course of the menstrual cycle. Used in certain treatments of coronary disorders in women. SYN estrin, oestrogen. [G. *oistrus*, estrus, + *-gen*, producing]

catechol e., any 2-hydroxylated derivative of an e.; they, with their methylated derivatives, can account for up to one-half of all excreted e. metabolites.

conjugated e., an amorphous preparation of naturally occurring, water-soluble, conjugated forms of mixed e.'s obtained from the urine of pregnant mares (conjugated equine e.); the principal e. present is sodium estrone sulfate; suitable for parenteral, oral, and topical administration, and used in conditions responsive to e. therapy.

esterified e.'s, a mixture of the sodium salts of sulfate esters of estrogenic substances; used for oral e. therapy.

es·tro·gen·ic (es-trō-jen'ik). **1.** Causing estrus in animals. **2.** Having an action similar to that of an estrogen.

es·trone (E_1) (es'trōn). A metabolite of 17β-estradiol, commonly found in urine, ovaries, and placenta; has considerably less biologic activity than the parent hormone. SYN follicular hormone, folliculin, ketohydroxyestrin, oestrone.

es·trous (es'trŭs). Pertaining to estrus. SYN estrual.

es·tru·al (es'troo-ăl). SYN estrous.

es·trus (es'trŭs). That portion or phase of the sexual cycle of female animals characterized by willingness to permit coitus; readily detectable behavioral and other signs are exhibited by animals during this period. SYN heat (3). [G. *oistros,* mad desire]

postpartum e., e. with ovulation and corpus luteum production that occurs in some animals (e.g., the fur seal) immediately following the birth of the young.

esu Abbreviation for electrostatic *unit.*

ESWL Abbreviation for electrohydraulic shock wave *lithotripsy*; extracorporeal shock wave *lithotripsy*

es·y·late (es'ī-lāt). USAN-approved contraction for ethanesulfonate, $CH_3CH_2SO_3^-$.

Et Abbreviation for ethyl.

eta (āt'a). The seventh letter of the Greek alphabet. **1.** In chemistry, denotes the position seven atoms from the carboxyl group or other primary functional group. **2.** Symbol for viscosity.

et·a·fed·rine hy·dro·chlo·ride (et-ă-fed'rēn). A sympathomimetic drug.

etaf·e·none (e-taf'ĕ-nōn). A coronary vasodilator.

etam·sy·late (e-tam'si-lāt). SYN ethamsylate.

état (ā-tah'). A condition or state. [Fr. state]

e. criblé (ā-tah'kri-blā), in neuropathology, a term describing perivascular atrophy of cerebral tissue, producing lacunae. [Fr. sieve]

e. mamelonné, obsolete term for the condition of the gastric mucous membrane in chronic inflammation, when it presents numerous nodular projections. [Fr. knobby, tubercular]

ETEC Abbreviation for enterotoxigenic *Escherichia coli.*

eth·ac·ri·dine lac·tate (eth-ak'ri-dēn). An antiseptic for treatment of wounds. SYN acrinol.

eth·a·cry·nate so·di·um (eth-ă-krī'nāt). Sodium salt of ethacrynic acid for parenteral use.

eth·a·cryn·ic ac·id (eth-ă-krin'ik). An unsaturated ketone derivative of aryloxyacetic acid; a potent loop diuretic and a weak antihypertensive;

eth·a·di·one (eth-ă-dī'ōn). An anticonvulsant.

eth·am·bu·tol hy·dro·chlo·ride (eth-am'boo-tol). A tuberculostatic, effective against organisms resistant to other tuberculostatic drugs; a serious reaction is visual impairment which, however, appears to be reversible. Used in combination with other antitubercular drugs to delay or prevent emergence of resistant strains of the tuberculosis bacilli.

etha·mi·van (eth-am'i-van). A central nervous system stimulant and analeptic, once used as an adjunctive agent in the treatment of severe respiratory depression due to barbiturates and carbon dioxide retention.

eth·a·mox·y·tri·phe·tol (eth-ă-moks'ē-trī-fē'tol). The prototype antiestrogen that inhibits the effects of estrogen at its specific

cellular receptors; the two most widely structurally related antiestrogens are clomiphene citrate and tamoxifen.

etham·sy·late (e-tham'si-lāt). A hemostatic agent. SYN cyclonamine, etamsylate.

eth·a·nal (eth'ă-nal). SYN acetaldehyde.

eth·ane (eth'ān). CH_3CH_3; a constituent of natural and "bottled" gases.

eth·ane·di·a·mine (eth-ān-dī'ă-mēn). SYN ethylenediamine.

eth·a·no·ic ac·id (eth-ă-nō'ik). SYN acetic acid.

eth·a·nol (eth'an-ol). SYN alcohol (2).

eth·a·nol·a·mine (eth-an-ol'ă-mēn). Used to prepare e. oleate, a sclerosing agent.

eth·a·nol·a·mine·phos·pho·trans·fer·ase (eth-ă-nol'ă-mēn-fos-fō-trans'fer-ās). A transferase that catalyzes the reaction of CDP-ethanolamine with a 1,2-diacylglycerol to yield CMP and a phosphatidylethanolamine; a key step in phospholipid biosynthesis. SYN phosphorylethanolamine glyceridetransferase.

eth·av·e·rine hy·dro·chlo·ride (eth-av'ĕ-rēn, eth-ă-ver'ēn). A smooth muscle relaxant. SYN ethylpapaverine hydrochloride.

eth·chlor·vy·nol (eth-klōr'vī-nol). An obsolete hypnotic.

eth·en·yl (eth'en-il). SYN vinyl.

eth·en·yl·ben·zene (eth-en-il-ben'zēn). SYN styrene.

eth·en·yl·ene (eth-en'il-ēn). SYN vinylene.

ether (ē'ther). **1.** Any organic compound in which two carbon atoms are independently linked to a common oxygen atom, thus containing the group –C–O–C–. SEE ALSO epoxy. **2.** Loosely used to refer to diethyl e. or an anesthetic e., although a large number of e.'s have anesthetic properties. For individual e.'s, see the specific name. [G. *aithēr,* the pure upper air]

anesthetic e., general designation for many e.'s.

glycol e.'s, chemicals such as ethylene glycol monomethyl e. and ethylene glycol monoethyl e.; they are teratogens which induce testicular atrophy in animals.

solvent e., a fairly pure form of e. ($C_4H_{10}O$) but not sufficiently pure for anesthesia; used as a solvent.

xylostyptic e., SYN styptic *collodion.*

ethe·re·al (ē-thēr'ē-ăl). **1.** Relating to or containing ether. **2.** Dissolved in an ether. [G. *aitherios,* etherial, fr. *aithēr,* the upper air]

ether·i·fi·ca·tion (ē-ther'i-fi-kā'shŭn). Conversion of an alcohol into an ether.

ether·i·za·tion (ē'ther-i-zā'shŭn). Administration of diethyl ether to produce anesthesia.

ethi·a·zide (e-thī'ă-zīd). A diuretic.

eth·i·cal (eth'i-kăl). Relating to ethics; in conformity with the rules governing personal and professional conduct.

eth·ics (eth'iks). The branch of philosophy that deals with the distinction between right and wrong, with the moral consequences of human actions. [G. *ethikos,* arising from custom, fr. *ethos,* custom]

medical e., the principles of proper professional conduct concerning the rights and duties of the physician, patients, and fellow practitioners, as well as the physician's actions in the care of patients and in relations with their families.

eth·i·dene (eth'i-dēn). SYN ethylidene.

ethid·i·um (eth-id'ē-ŭm). SYN homidium bromide.

ethid·i·um bro·mide (ĕ-thid'ē-ŭm). A sensitive fluorochrome that binds to DNA; used in cytochemistry and electrophoresis.

ethin·drone (e-thin'drōn). SYN ethisterone.

eth·i·nyl (e-thī'nil). SYN ethynyl.

e. trichloride, SYN trichloroethylene.

eth·i·nyl·es·tre·nol (eth'i-nil-es'tre-nol). SYN lynestrenol.

eth·i·o·dized oil (eth-ī'ō-dīzd). A radiopaque medium formerly used for lympangiography and hysterosalpingography.

eth·i·on·am·ide (ĕ-thī'on-ă-mīd). A second-line antituberculosis drug. Side effects are common, the most common manifestations are gastrointestinal.

ethi·o·nine (e-thī'ō-nēn). A methionine analog and antagonist, differing in the presence of an *S*-ethyl group in place of the *S*-methyl group.

ethis·ter·one (e-this'ter-ōn). An orally effective semisynthetic steroid that has biological effects similar to those of progesterone. SYN ethindrone, pregneninolone.

ethmo-. Combining form denoting: **1.** Ethmoid. **2.** The ethmoid bone. [G. *ēthmos*, sieve]

eth·mo·cra·ni·al (eth-mō-krā'nē-ăl). Relating to the ethmoid bone and the cranium as a whole.

eth·mo·fron·tal (eth-mō-fron'tăl). Relating to the ethmoid and the frontal bones.

eth·moid (eth'moyd) [TA]. SEE ethmoid *bone*. SYN os ethmoidale [TA]. [G. *ēthmos*, sieve, + *eidos*, resemblance]

eth·moi·dal (eth-moy'dăl). Resembling a sieve.

eth·moi·da·le (eth-moy-da'lē). A cephalometric point in the anterior cranial fossa located at the lowest sagittal point of the cribriform plate of the ethmoid bone.

eth·moi·dec·to·my (eth-moy-dek'tō-mē). Removal of all or part of the mucosal lining and bony partitions between the ethmoid sinuses. [ethmo- + G. *ektomē*, excision]

eth·moid·i·tis (eth-moy-dī'tis). Inflammation of the ethmoid sinuses.

eth·mo·lac·ri·mal (eth-mō-lak'ri-măl). Relating to the ethmoid and the lacrimal bones.

eth·mo·max·il·lary (eth-mō-mak'si-lā-rē). Relating to the ethmoid and the maxillary bones.

eth·mo·na·sal (eth-mō-nā'săl). Relating to the ethmoid and the nasal bones.

eth·mo·pal·a·tal (eth-mō-pal'ă-tăl). Relating to the ethmoid and the palate bones.

eth·mo·sphe·noid (eth-mō-sfē'noyd). Relating to the ethmoid and sphenoid bones.

eth·mo·tur·bi·nals (eth-mō-ter'bi-nalz). The conchae of the ethmoid bone; the superior and middle conchae; occasionally a third, the supreme concha, exists.

eth·mo·vo·mer·ine (eth'mō-vō'mer-in). Relating to the ethmoid bone and the vomer.

eth·nic group (eth'nik). A social group characterized by a distinctive social and cultural tradition maintained from generation to generation, a common history and origin and a sense of identification with the group; members of the group have distinctive features in their way of life, shared experiences and often a common genetic heritage; these features may be reflected in their experience of health and disease.

eth·no·cen·trism (eth-nō-sen'trizm). The tendency to evaluate other groups according to the values and standards of one's own ethnic group, especially with the conviction that one's own ethnic group is superior to the other groups. [G. *ethnos*, race, tribe, + *kentron*, center of a circle]

eth·nol·o·gy (eth-nol'ŏ-jē). The science that compares human culture and/or races; cultural anthropology.

eth·no·phar·ma·col·o·gy (eth'nō-farm-ă-kol'ō-jē). The study of differences in response to drugs based on varied ethnicity; pharmacogenetics.

eth·o·hep·ta·zine cit·rate (eth-ō-hep'tă-zēn). An obsolete analgesic.

eth·o·hex·a·di·ol (eth'ō-hek-să-dī'ol, -hek-sā'dī-ol). Used as an insect repellent.

ethol·o·gist (ē-thol'ŏ-jist). A specialist in ethology.

ethol·o·gy (ē-thol'ŏ-jē). The study of animal behavior. [G. *ethos*, character, habit, + *logos*, study]

eth·o·mox·ane (eth-ō-mok'sān). An antianxiety agent. SYN ethoxybutamoxane.

eth·o·phar·ma·col·o·gy (eth'ō-far-mă-kol'ō-jē). The study of drug effects on behavior, relying on observation and description of species-specific elements (acts and postures during social encounters). SEE ALSO pharmacogenetics. [G. *ethos*, character, habit, + pharmacology]

eth·o·pro·pa·zine hy·dro·chlo·ride (eth-ō-prō'pă-zēn). An an-

ticholinergic agent with some antihistaminic and ganglionic blocking activity. SYN profenamine hydrochloride.

eth·o·sux·i·mide (eth-ō-sŭk'si-mīd). An anticonvulsant used in the control of absence (petit mal) epilepsy; bone marrow damage and aplastic anemia may occasionally occur.

eth·o·to·in (eth-ō-tō'in). An anticonvulsant used in the treatment of generalized tonic clonic epilepsy.

eth·o·tri·mep·ra·zine (eth'ō-trī-mep'ră-zēn). SYN etymemazine.

ethox·a·zene hy·dro·chlo·ride (e-thok'să-zēn). An azo compound.

eth·oxy (e-thok'sē). The monovalent radical, $CH_3CH_2O–$.

eth·ox·y·bu·ta·mox·ane (eth-ok'si-bū-tă-mok'sān). SYN ethomoxane.

eth·ox·y·zol·a·mide (eth-ok-sē-zol'ă-mīd). A diuretic related chemically and pharmacologically to acetazolamide.

eth·yl (Et) (eth'il). The hydrocarbon radical, $CH_3CH_2–$.

e. alcohol, SYN alcohol (2).

e. aminobenzoate, SYN benzocaine.

e. biscoumacetate, an anticoagulant chemically related to bishydroxycoumarin and warfarin.

e. butyrate, used in perfumery.

e. carbamate, SYN urethan.

e. chloride, a very volatile explosive liquid (under increased pressure); when sprayed on the skin, produces local anesthesia by superficial freezing, but also is a potent inhalation anesthetic. SYN chloroethane.

e. formate, a volatile, flammable liquid used as a fumigant, agricultural larvicide, and fungicide; also used as a flavor.

e. oleate, an alternative vehicle in injections of deoxycorticosterone acetate, menaphthone, etc.

e. oxide, SYN diethyl ether.

e. salicylate, the salicylic acid ester of e. alcohol, with the same action as methyl salicylate.

eth·yl·ate (eth'i-lāt). A compound in which the hydrogen of the hydroxyl group of ethanol is replaced by a metallic atom, usually sodium or potassium; e.g., C_2H_5ONa, sodium ethylate.

eth·yl·benz·tro·pine (eth'il-benz-trō'pēn). An anticholinergic agent.

eth·yl·cel·lu·lose (eth-il-sel'ū-lōs). An ethyl ether of cellulose, used as a tablet binder.

eth·yl·di·chlo·ro·ar·sine (ED) (eth'il-dī-klōr-ō-ar'sēn). $C_2H_5AsCl_2$; a blister agent used in World War I; irritating to the respiratory tract.

eth·yl·ene (eth'i-lēn). An explosive constituent of ordinary illuminating gas; hastens ripening of fruit.

e. oxide, a fumigant, used for cold sterilization of surgical instruments. SYN oxirane.

e. tetrachloride, SYN tetrachlorethylene.

eth·yl·ene·di·a·mine (eth'i-lēn-dī'ă-mēn). A volatile colorless liquid of ammoniacal odor and caustic taste; the dihydrochloride is used as a urinary acidifier. Combined with theophylline to make aminophylline, a water-soluble salt suitable for intravenous or rectal administration. SYN ethanediamine.

eth·yl·ene·di·a·mine·tet·ra·a·ce·tic ac·id (EDTA) (eth'il-ēn-dī'ă-mēn-tet-ră-ă-sē'tik). A chelating agent used to remove multivalent cations from solution as chelates, and used in biochemical research to remove Mg^{2+}, Fe^{2+}, etc., from reactions affected by such ions. As the sodium salt, used as a water softener, to stabilize drugs rapidly decomposed in the presence of traces of metal ions, and as an anticoagulant; as the sodium calcium salt, used to remove radium, lead, strontium, plutonium, and cadmium from the hard tissue, forming stable un-ionized soluble compounds that are excreted by the kidneys. Cf. EGTA. SYN edathamil, edetic acid.

eth·yl·ene di·bro·mide. Compound used in antiknock gasolines. Severe skin irritant; may cause blistering. Inhalation causes delayed pulmonary lesions. Prolonged exposure may also result in liver and kidney injury. May be a human carcinogen.

eth·yl·ene gly·col. SEE glycol (2).

eth·yl·es·tre·nol (eth-il-es'tre-nol). A semisynthetic orally effective anabolic steroid.

eth·yl ether. SYN diethyl ether.

eth·yl green. SYN brilliant green.

eth·yl·i·dene (eth-il'i-dēn). The radical CH₃CH=. SYN ethidene.

eth·yl·i·dyne (eth-il'i-dīn). The radical CH₃C≡.

eth·yl·mor·phine hy·dro·chlo·ride (eth-il-mōr'fēn). The ethyl ether of morphine; an antispasmodic, antitussive, and narcotic analgesic, used locally as an irritant lymphagogue in chronic catarrhal middle ear disease, atrophic rhinitis, and painful ocular diseases (iritis, corneal ulcer, etc.).

eth·yl·nor·ep·i·neph·rine (E.N.E., E.N.S.) (eth'il-nōr-ep-i-nef'rin). A sympathomimetic, used in asthma; it does not raise the blood pressure.

eth·yl·pa·pav·er·ine hy·dro·chlo·ride (eth'il-pa-pav'er-ēn). SYN ethaverine hydrochloride.

eth·yl·par·a·ben (eth-il-par'ă-ben). An antifungal preservative.

eth·yl·phen·yl·eph·rine hy·dro·chlo·ride (eth'il-fen-il-ef'rēn). SYN etilefrine hydrochloride.

eth·yl·stib·a·mine (eth-il-stib'ă-mēn). A synthetic organic compound of antimony.

ethy·no·di·ol (ĕ-thī-nō-dī'ōl). A semisynthetic orally effective steroid with biological effects that largely resemble those of progesterone; in addition, it is weakly estrogenic and androgenic; administered in combination with an estrogen as an oral contraceptive.

  e. diacetate, an antifertility agent, usually used in combination with mestranol.

ethy·nyl (e-thī'nil). The monovalent radical HC≡C–. SYN acetenyl, ethinyl.

eti·do·caine (e-tī'dō-kān). A local anesthetic.

eti·dro·nate di·so·di·um (e-ti-drō'nāt). A drug that affects bone resorption, used in the treatment of Paget disease, heterotopic ossification, and hypercalcemia of malignancy.

eti·dron·ic ac·id (e-ti-dron'ik). Used as a calcium regulator, usually as the salt etidronate disodium.

et·il·ef·rine hy·dro·chlo·ride (et-il-ef'rin). A sympathomimetic amine vasopressor agent. SYN ethylphenylephrine hydrochloride.

etio-. **1.** Prefix used with (for example) cholane to indicate replacement of the C-17 side chain by H; thus, etiocholane is the 5β isomer of androstane. **2.** Combining form meaning cause. [G. *aitia,* cause]

eti·o·cho·lan·o·lone (ē'tē-ō-kō-lan'ō-lōn). A metabolite of adrenocortical and testicular hormones, and an important urinary 17-ketosteroid; produces fever when given to human beings.

eti·o·gen·ic (ē'tē-ō-jen'ik). Of a causal nature. [G. *aitia,* cause, + *genesis,* production]

eti·o·lat·ed (ē'tē-ō-lāt-ed). Subjected to, or characterized by, etiolation.

eti·o·la·tion (ē-tē-ō-lā'shŭn). **1.** Paleness or pallor resulting from absence of light, as in persons confined because of illness or imprisonment, or in plants bleached by being deprived of light. **2.** The process of blanching, bleaching, or making pale by withholding light. [Fr. *étioler,* to blanch]

eti·o·log·ic (ē'tē-ō-loj'ik). Relating to etiology.

eti·ol·o·gy (ē-tē-ol'ō-jē). **1.** The science and study of the causes of disease and their mode of operation. Cf. pathogenesis. **2.** The science of causes, causality; in common usage, cause. [G. *aitia,* cause, + *logos,* treatise, discourse]

eti·o·path·ic (ē'tē-ō-path'ik). Relating to specific lesions concerned with the cause of a disease. [G. *aitia,* cause, + *pathos,* disease]

eti·o·pa·thol·o·gy (ē'tē-ō-pa-thol'ō-jē). Consideration of the cause of an abnormal state or finding. [G. *aitia,* cause, + pathology]

eti·o·por·phy·rin (ē'tē-ō-pōr'fi-rin). A porphyrin derivative characterized by the presence on each of the four pyrrole rings of one methyl group and one ethyl group; four isomeric forms are thus possible.

eti·o·tro·pic (ē'tē-ō-trop'ik). Directed against the cause; denoting

a remedy that attenuates or destroys the causal factor of a disease. [G. *aitia,* cause, + *tropē,* a turning]

eto·fam·ide (ē-tō'fă-mīd). An intraluminal amebicide similar to teclozan and diloxanide.

etom·i·date (ē-tom'i-dāt). A potent intravenous hypnotic used in anesthesia.

eto·po·side (e-tō-pō'sīd). A semisynthetic derivative of podophyllotoxin; a mitotic inhibitor used in the treatment of refractory testicular tumors, small cell lung cancer, and other cancers.

etor·phine (et-ōr'fēn). A narcotic analgesic, having a potency about 1,000 times greater than morphine; used in tranquilizer darts.

et·o·zo·lin (et-ō-zō'lin). A diuretic.

ETP Abbreviation for electron transport *particles,* under *particle.*

etret·i·nate (e-tret'i-nāt). A retinoid used in the treatment of severe recalcitrant psoriasis.

et·y·mem·a·zine (et-i-mem'ă-zēn). An antihistaminic. SYN ethotrimeprazine.

Eu Symbol for europium.

eu-. Good, well; opposite of dys-, caco-. [G.]

eu·al·leles (ū'ă-lēlz). Genes having different nucleotide substitutions at the same position. Cf. heteroalleles.

Eu·bac·te·ri·a·les (ū'bak-tē-rē-ā'lēz). An obsolete name for an order of bacteria that contained simple, undifferentiated, rigid cells which were either spheres or straight rods. It contained motile (peritrichous) and nonmotile, Gram-negative and Gram-positive, and sporeforming and nonsporeforming species. The order contained 13 families: Achromobacteriaceae, Azotobacteriaceae, Bacillaceae, Bacteroidaceae, Brevibacteriaceae, Brucellaceae, Corynebacteriaceae, Enterobacteriaceae, Lactobacillaceae, Micrococcaceae, Neisseriaceae, Propionibacteriaceae, and Rhizobacteriaceae.

Eu·bac·te·ri·um (ū'bak-tēr'ē-ŭm). A genus containing more than 40 species of anaerobic, nonsporeforming, nonmotile bacteria containing straight or curved Gram-positive rods which usually occur singly, in pairs, or in short chains. Usually these organisms attack carbohydrates. They may be pathogenic, and rarely are associated with intraabdominal sepsis in humans. The type species is *E. limosum.*

E. aerofa'ciens, a bacterial species infrequently found in human intestines; pathogenic for mice.

E. combe'si, a bacterial species from forest soil found in an area then called French West Africa; it is not pathogenic for guinea pigs or mice. Formerly called *Cillobacterium combesi.*

E. contor'tum, a bacterial species found in cases of putrid, gangrenous appendicitis and in the intestines.

E. crispa'tum, former name for *Lactobacillus crispatus.*

E. filamento'sum, former name for *Clostridium ramosum.*

E. len'tum, a bacterial species occurring commonly in the feces of normal persons; occasional cause of septicemia and nosocomial infections.

E. limo'sum, a bacterial species that occurs in human feces and presumably in the feces of other warm-blooded animals. The type species of the genus.

E. minu'tum, a bacterial species that occurs infrequently in the intestines of breast-fed infants; it was originally found in a case of infant diarrhea; it is pathogenic for mice.

E. monilifor'me, a bacterial species found rarely in the human respiratory system; it is pathogenic for guinea pigs, causing death in eight days. Formerly called *Cillobacterium moniliforme.*

E. par'vum, a bacterial species found in the large intestine of a horse and in a case of acute appendicitis; it occurs infrequently in the intestines of foals and of humans, and is not pathogenic for laboratory animals.

E. poeciloi'des, a bacterial species infrequently found in human intestines; originally found in a case of intestinal occlusion; it is pathogenic for guinea pigs and rabbits.

E. pseudotortuo'sum, a bacterial species found in a case of purulent, acute appendicitis; occurs uncommonly in the intestines.

E. quar'tum, a bacterial species found in cases of infantile diarrhea; occurs in the intestines of children, but is rather uncommon.

E. quin'tum, a bacterial species found in cases of infantile diarrhea; pathogenic for guinea pigs.

E. recta'le, a bacterial species found in association with a rectal ulcer; occurs in the rectum.

E. ten'ue, a bacterial species isolated from dog feces; its pathogenicity is unknown; formerly called *Cillobacterium tenue.*

E. tortuo'sum, a bacterial species found infrequently in the intestines of humans.

eu·bi·ot·ics (ū-bī-ot'iks). The science of hygienic living. [eu- + G. *biotikos,* relating to life]

eu·caine (ū'kān). A local anesthetic.

eu·ca·lyp·tol (ū-kă-lip'tol). SYN cineole.

eu·ca·lyp·tus (ū-kă-lip'tŭs). The dried leaves of *Eucalyptus globulus* (family Myrtaceae), the blue gum or Australian fever tree.

e. oil, the volatile oil distilled with steam from the fresh leaf of *Eucalyptus globulus* or some other species of *Eucalyptus;* contains not less than 70% of eucalyptol; used as an antiseptic and expectorant in cough lozenges and in vaporizer aromatics.

eu·cap·nia (ū-kap'nē-ă). A state in which the arterial carbon dioxide pressure is optimal. SEE ALSO normocapnia. [eu- + G. *kapnos,* vapor]

eu·car·y·ote (ū-kar'ē-ōt). SYN eukaryote. [eu- + G. *karyon,* kernel, nut]

eu·car·y·ot·ic (ū-kar-ē-ot'ik). SYN eukaryotic.

eu·ca·sin (ū-kā'sin). Ammonium caseinate prepared by passing ammonia gas over finely powdered dry casein; added as a concentrated food to bouillon, chocolate, etc.

eu·cat·ro·pine hy·dro·chlo·ride (ū-kat'rō-pēn). It produces no anesthesia, pain, or increased intraocular pressure.

Eu·ces·to·da (ū-ses-tō'dă). SYN Cestoda.

eu·chlor·hy·dria (ū-klōr-hi'drē-ă). A condition in which free hydrochloric acid exists in normal amount in the gastric juice. [eu- + cholohydric (acid) + -ia]

eu·cho·lia (ū-kō'lē-ă). A normal state of the bile as regards quantity and quality. [eu- + G. *cholē,* bile]

eu·chro·mat·ic (ū-krō-mat'ik). **1.** SYN orthochromatic. **2.** Characteristic of euchromatin.

eu·chro·ma·tin (ū-krō'mă-tin). The parts of chromosomes that, during interphase, are uncoiled dispersed threads and not stained by ordinary dyes; metabolically active, in contrast to the inert heterochromatin.

eu·chro·mo·some (ū-krō'mō-sōm). SYN autosome.

Eucoleus (ū-kō'lē-us). One of three trichurid nematode genera, commonly referred to as *Capillaria.*

eu·cor·ti·cal·ism (ū-kōr'ti-kăl-izm). Normal functioning of the adrenal cortex.

eu·cra·sia (ū-krā'zhē-ă). **1.** Obsolete term for homeostasis. **2.** Obsolete term for a condition of reduced susceptibility to the adverse effects of certain drugs, articles of diet, etc. [G. *eukrasia,* good temperament, fr. *eu,* well, + *krasis,* a mixing]

eu·cu·pine (ū'koo-pēn). SYN euprocin hydrochloride.

eu·di·a·pho·re·sis (ū-dī'ă-fō-rē'sis). Normal free sweating. [eu- + G. *diaphorēsis,* perspiration]

eu·dip·sia (ū-dip'sē-ă). Ordinary mild thirst. [eu- + G. *dipsa,* thirst]

Eu·flag·el·la·ta (ū-flaj'ĕ-lā'tă). Former term for the protozoan flagellates now included in the subphylum Mastigophora.

eu·gen·ic (ū-jen'ik). Relating to eugenics.

eu·gen·ic ac·id. SYN eugenol.

eu·gen·ics (ū-jen'iks). **1.** Practices and policies, as of mate selection or of sterilization, that tend to better the innate qualities of progeny and human stock. **2.** Practices and genetic counseling directed to anticipating genetic disability and disease. SYN orthogenics. [G. *eugeneia,* nobility of birth, fr. *eu,* well, + *genesis,* production]

eu·gen·ism (ū'jen-izm). The belief that the human species can be improved through selective breeding.

eu·ge·nol (ū'je-nol). Obtained from oil of cloves; used in dentistry with zinc oxide as an analgesic and as a base for impression materials; also used in perfumery as a substitute for oil of cloves. SYN eugenic acid.

Eu·gle·na (ū-glē'nă). A widespread genus of photosynthesizing free-living fresh water flagellates (family Euglinidae). [eu- + G. *glēnē,* eyeball]

E. grac'ilis, an abundant species sometimes used in assaying vitamin B_{12} concentrations of serum and urine in various types of anemia.

E. vir'idis, a species that inhabits stagnant pools, often in great numbers.

Eu·gle·ni·dae (ū-glē'ni-dē). A family of green (phytomonad) flagellates (subphylum Mastigophora, class Phytomastigophorea).

eu·glob·u·lin (ū-glob'ū-lin). That fraction of the serum globulin that is soluble in isotonic salt solutions and less soluble in $(NH_4)_2SO_4$ solution than the pseudoglobulin fraction.

eu·gly·ce·mia (ū-glī-sē'mē-ă). A normal blood glucose concentration. SYN normoglycemia. [eu- + G. *glykys,* sweet, + *haima,* blood]

eu·gly·ce·mic (ū-glī-sē'mik). Denoting, characteristic of, or promoting euglycemia. SYN normoglycemic.

eu·gna·thia (ū-nā'thē-ă, -nath'ē-ă). An abnormality that is limited to the teeth and their immediate alveolar supports. SYN eugnathic anomaly. [eu- + G. *gnathos,* jaw]

eu·gno·sia (ū-nō'sē-ă). Normal ability to synthesize sensory stimuli. [eu- + G. *gnōsis,* perception]

eu·gon·ic (ū-gon'ik). A term used to indicate that the growth of a bacterial culture is rapid and relatively luxuriant; used especially in reference to the growth of cultures of the human tubercle bacillus (*Mycobacterium tuberculosis*). SEE ALSO dysgonic. [G. *eugonos,* productive, fr. *eu,* well, + *gonos,* seed, offspring]

Eu·gre·ga·rin·i·da (ū'greg-ă-rin'i-dă). An order of gregarines (subclass Gregarinia), reproducing only by sporogony, in which schizogony is absent; they are parasites of annelids and arthropods. [eu- + L. *gregarius,* gregarious]

eu·hy·dra·tion (ū-hī-drā'shŭn). Normal state of body water content; absence of absolute or relative hydration or dehydration.

Eu·kar·y·o·tae, Eu·car·y·o·tae (ū-kar-ē-ō'tē). A superkingdom of organisms characterized by eukaryotic cells; acellular members (kingdom Protoctista) are characterized by a single eukaryotic unit; more complex (multicellular) members have been assigned to the kingdoms Fungi, Plantae, and Animalia.

eu·kar·y·ote (ū-kar'ē-ōt). **1.** A cell containing a membrane-bound nucleus with chromosomes of DNA, RNA, and proteins, mostly large (10–100 μm), with cell division involving a form of mitosis in which mitotic spindles (or some microtubule arrangement) are involved; mitochondria are present, and, in photosynthetic species, plastids are found; undulipodia (cilia or flagella) are of the complex 9+2 organization of tubulin and various proteins. Possession of a. type of cell characterizes the four kingdoms above the Monera or prokaryote level of complexity: Protoctista, Fungi, Plantae, and Animalia, combined into the superkingdom Eukaryotae. **2.** Common name for members of the Eukaryotae. SYN eucaryote. [eu- + G. *karyon,* kernel, nut]

eu·kar·y·ot·ic (ū'kar-ē-ot'ik). Pertaining to or characteristic of a eukaryote. SYN eucaryotic.

eu·ker·a·tin (ū-kār'ă-tin). Hard keratin present in hair, wool, horn, nails, etc.

eu·ki·ne·sia (ū-ki-nē'zē-ă). Normal movement. [eu- + G. *kinēsis,* movement]

Eulenburg, Albert, German neurologist, 1840–1917. SEE E. *disease.*

eu·mel·a·nin (ū-mel'ă-nin). The most abundant type of human melanin, found in brown and black skin and hair; cross-linked polymers of 5,6-dihydroxyindoles, usually linked to proteins; levels are decreased in certain types of albinism. [eu- + G. *melos* (*melan-*), black]

eu·mel·a·no·some (ū-mel'ă-nō-sōm). SYN melanosome.

eu·me·tria (ū-mē'trē-ă). Graduation of the strength of nerve impulses to match the need. [G. moderation, goodness of meter]

eu·mor·phism (ū-mōr'fizm). Preservation of the natural form of a cell. [eu- + G. *morphē,* shape]

eu

eu·my·cetes (ū-mī-sē'tēz). The true fungi. [eu- + G. *mykēs*, fungus]

eumycetoma (oo-mī-set-ō'ma). Mycetoma caused by fungi. Cf. actinomycetoma.

Eu·my·ce·to·zo·ea (ū'mī-sē-tō-zō'ē-ă). Microscopic animal forms, frequently known as slime animals, that consist of an irregular semifluid mass of multinucleated ameboid protoplasm; although grouped as a class of the superclass Rhizopoda (subphylum Sarcodina), some of the mycetozoan forms closely resemble certain species of pseudomycetes and are sometimes classified as members of the Myxomycetes, the slime molds. SEE ALSO Proteomyxidia. [eu- + G. *mykēs* (*mykēt-*), fungus, + *zōon*, animal]

eu·nuch (ū'nŭk). A male individual whose testes have been removed or have never developed. [G. *eunouchos*, chamberlain, fr. *eunē*, bed, + *echmacr;o*, to have]

eu·nuch·ism (ū'nŭk-izm). 1. The state of being a eunuch; absence of the testes or failure of the gonads to develop or function with consequent lack of reproductive and sexual function and of development of secondary sex characteristics. 2. SYN eunuchoidism.

eu·nuch·oid (ū'nŭ-koyd). Resembling, or having the general characteristics of, a eunuch; usually indicating the physical habitus of a male in whom hypogonadism occurred before puberty. [G. *eunouchos*, eunuch, + *eidos*, resembling]

eu·nuch·oid·ism (ū'nŭ-koyd-izm). A state in which testes are present but fail to function normally; may be of gonadal or pituitary origin. SYN eunuchism (2), male hypogonadism.

hypergonadotropic e., e. of gonadal origin, commonly accompanied by enhanced levels of pituitary gonadotropins in the blood and urine, as in Klinefelter *syndrome*.

hypogonadotropic e., SYN hypogonadotropic *hypogonadism*.

eu·os·mia (ū-oz'mē-ă). 1. A pleasant odor. 2. Normal olfaction. [eu- + G. *osmē*, smell]

eu·pan·cre·a·tism (ū-pan'krē-ă-tizm). The state of normal pancreatic digestive function.

eu·pa·ral (ū'pa-răl). A medium for mounting histologic specimens, composed of sandarac, eucalyptol, paraldehyde, camphor, and phenyl salicylate.

Eu·pa·ryph·i·um (ū-pa-rif'ē-ŭm). A genus of nonpathogenic flukes (family Echinostomatidae), several species of which have been reported from the intestines of humans. [eu- + G. *paryphē*, a border]

eu·pav·er·in (ū-pav'ĕ-rin). A smooth muscle relaxant.

eu·pep·sia (ū-pep'sē-ă). Good digestion. [G., fr. *eu*, well, + *pepsis*, digestion]

eu·pep·tic (ū-pep'tik). Digesting well; having a good digestion.

eu·pep·tide (ū-pep'tīd). A peptide containing normal peptide bonds (between α-carboxyl groups and α-amino groups). Cf. isopeptide, peptide. [G. *eu-*, normal, usual + peptide]

eu·phen·ics (ū-fē'niks). Modification of the internal or external environment of an individual so as to prevent or modify the phenotypic expression of a genetic defect, without changing the genotype or the inheritance. [eu- + G. *phainō*, to show forth]

Eu·phor·bia pi·lu·lif·e·ra (ū-fōr'bē-ă pil-ŭ-lif'er-ă). A species of plant (family Euphorbiaceae); the dried herb used in asthma, coryza and other respiratory affections, in angina pectoris, and as an antispasmodic. SYN asthma-weed (2).

eu·pho·ret·ic (ū-fō-ret'ik). SYN euphoriant.

eu·pho·ria (ū-fōr'ē-ă). A feeling of well-being, commonly exaggerated and not necessarily well founded. [eu- + G. *pherō*, to bear]

eu·pho·ri·ant (ū-fōr'ē-ant). 1. Having the capability to produce a sense of well-being. 2. An agent with such a capability. SYN euphoretic.

eu·pla·sia (ū-plā'zē-ă). The state of cells or tissue that is normal or typical for that particular type. [eu- + G. *plassō*, form]

eu·plas·tic (ū-plas'tik). 1. Relating to euplasia. 2. Healing readily and well. [G. *euplastos*, easily molded; *eu*, well, + *plastos*, formed]

eu·ploid (ū'ployd). Relating to euploidy.

eu·ploidy (ū'ploy-dē). The state of a cell containing whole haploid sets. [eu- + G. *-ploos*, -fold]

eup·nea (ūp-nē'ă). Easy, free respiration; the type observed in a normal individual under resting conditions. [G. *eupnoia*, fr. *eu*, well, + *pnoia*, breath]

eu·prax·ia (ū-prak'sē-ă). Normal ability to perform coordinated movements. [eu- + G. *praxis*, a doing]

eu·pro·cin hy·dro·chlo·ride (ū'prō-sin). A derivative of quinine. SYN eucupine.

Eu·proc·tis (ū-prok'tis). A genus of moths. The hairs of the cocoon and caterpillar of the species *E. chrysorrhoea*, the browntail moth, cause caterpillar dermatitis. [eu- + G. *prōktos*, rump]

eu·rhyth·mia (ū-rith'mē-ă). Harmonious body relationships of the separate organs. [eu- + G. *rhythmos*, rhythm]

eu·ro·pi·um (Eu) (ū-rō'pē-ŭm). An element of the rare earth (lanthanide) group, atomic no. 63, atomic wt. 151.965. [L. *Europa*, Europe]

♻**eury-.** Broad, wide; opposite of steno-. [G. *eurys*, wide]

euryblepharon (ū-rē-blef'ă-ron). A congenital anomaly characterized by sagging of the lateral aspect of the lower eyelid away from the eye. [eury- + G. *blepharon*, eyelid]

eu·ry·ce·phal·ic, eu·ry·ceph·a·lous (ū'rē-se-fal'ik, -sef'ă-lŭs). Having an abnormally broad head; sometimes used in reference to a brachycephalic head. [eury- + G. *kephalē*, head]

eu·ryg·nath·ic (ū-rig-nath'ik). Having a wide jaw. SYN eurygnathous.

eu·ryg·na·thism (ū-rig'nă-thizm). The condition of having a wide jaw. [eury- + G. *gnathos*, jaw]

eu·ryg·na·thous (ū-rig'nă-thŭs). SYN eurygnathic.

eu·ry·on (ū'rē-on). The extremity, on either side, of the greatest transverse diameter of the head; a point used in craniometry. [G. *eurys*, broad]

eu·ry·op·ic (ū-rē-ŏp'ik). Wide-eyed. SEE blepharodiastasis. [eury- + G. *ops*, eye]

eu·ry·so·mat·ic (ū'rē-sō-mat'ik). Having a thick-set body. [eury- + G. *soma*, body]

eu·scope (ū'skōp). An instrument for showing on a screen an enlarged image from a microscope. [eu- + G. *skopeō*, to view]

Eu·sim·u·li·um (ū-si-mū'lē-ŭm). SYN *Simulium*. [eu- + L. *simulo*, to simulate]

eu·sta·chi·an (ū-stā'shŭn, ū-stā'kē-ăn). Described by or attributed to Eustachio.

Eustachio, Bartolommeo E., Italian anatomist, 1524–1574. SEE eustachian *catheter*, eustachian *cushion*, eustachian *tonsil*, *tuba* eustachiana, eustachian *tube*, eustachian *tuber*, eustachian *valve*.

eu·sta·chi·tis (ū-stā-kī'tis). Inflammation of the mucous membrane of the eustachian tube.

eus·the·nia (ū-sthē'nē-ă). Normal strength. [eu- + G. *sthenos*, strength]

eu·stron·gyl·oi·des (ū-stron-jil'oy-dēz). Nematode found in fish, amphibians, and reptiles; human infections, manifested by gastrointestinal symptoms, are rare and related to consumption of raw fish; larvae are pinkish red.

Eu·stron·gy·lus (ū-stron'ji-lŭs). Former name for *Dioctophyma*. [eu- + G. *strongylos*, rounded]

eu·sys·to·le (ū-sis'tō-lē). A condition in which the cardiac systole is normal in force and time. [eu- + systole]

eu·sys·tol·ic (ū-sis-tol'ik). Relating to eusystole.

eu·tec·tic (ū-tek'tik). 1. Easily melted; denoting specifically mixtures of certain chemical compounds that have a lower melting point than any of their individual ingredients; e.g., a solid, such as menthol, that when triturated with another solid of the same class, such as camphor, unites with it to form a liquid, the mixture having a lower melting point than either of its components. 2. The alloy that freezes at a constant temperature; the lowest of the series. [eu- + G. *tēxis*, a melting away]

eu·tha·na·sia (ū-thă-nā'zē-ă). 1. A quiet, painless death. 2. The intentional putting to death of a person with an incurable or painful disease intended as an act of mercy. [eu- + G. *thanatos*, death]

eu·then·ics (ū-then'iks). The science concerned with establishing optimum living conditions for plants, animals, or humans, especially through proper provisioning and environment. [G. *eutheneō*, to thrive]

eu·ther·a·peu·tic (ū'thār-ă-pū'tik). Having excellent curative properties.

Eu·the·ria (ū-thē'rē-ă). A subclass of mammals, excluding monotremes and marsupials, having a placenta through which the young are nourished. [eu- + G. *thērion*, animal]

eu·ther·mic (ū-ther'mik). At an optimal temperature. [eu- + G. *thermos*, warm]

eu·thy·mia (ū-thī'mē-ă). 1. Joyfulness; mental peace and tranquility. 2. Moderation of mood, not manic or depressed. [eu- + G. *thymos*, mind]

eu·thy·mic (ū-thī'mik). Relating to, or characterized by, euthymia.

eu·thy·roid·ism (ū-thī'roy-dizm). A condition in which the thyroid gland is functioning normally, its secretion being of proper amount and constitution.

eu·thy·scope (ū'thi-skōp). A modified ophthalmoscope, now seldom used, with which the site of excentric fixation may be dazzled by a bright light while the true fovea is simultaneously shielded by an opaque disk; used in pleoptics. [G. *euthys*, straight, + *skopeō*, to view]

eu·thys·co·py (ū-this'kŏ-pē). Examination with the euthyscope.

eu·ton·ic (ū-ton'ik). SYN normotonic (1). [eu- + G. *tonos*, tone]

eu·tri·cho·sis (ū-tri-kō'sis). A normal growth of healthy hair. [eu- + G. *thrix*, hair]

eu·tro·phia (ū-trō'fē-ă). A state of normal nourishment and growth. SYN eutrophy. [G. fr. *eu*, well, + *trophē*, nourishment]

eu·tro·phic (ū-trof'ik). Relating to, characterized by, or promoting eutrophia.

eu·tro·phy (ū'trō-fē). SYN eutrophia.

eu·vo·lia (ū-vō'lē-ă). Normal water content or volume of a given compartment; e.g., extracellular e.

eV, ev Abbreviation for electron-volt.

evac·u·ant (ē-vak'ū-ant). 1. Promoting an excretion, especially of the bowels. 2. An agent that increases excretion, especially a cathartic.

evac·u·ate (ē-vak'ū-āt). To accomplish evacuation. [L. *e-vacuo*, pp. *-vacuatus*, to empty out]

evac·u·a·tion (ē-vak-ū-ā'shŭn). 1. Removal of material, especially wastes from the bowels by defecation. 2. SYN stool (2). 3. Removal of air from a closed vessel; production of a vacuum.

evac·u·a·tor (ē-vak'ū-ā-tŏr). A mechanical evacuant; an instrument for the removal of fluid or small particles from a body cavity, or of impacted feces from the rectum.

Ellik e., a special instrument with glass receptacle, latex or plastic bulb, and flexible tubing, used to evacuate tissue fragments, blood clots, or calculi from the urinary bladder.

evag·i·na·tion (ē-vaj-i-nā'shŭn). Protrusion of some part or organ from its normal position. [L. *e*, out, + *vagina*, sheath]

eval·u·a·tion. Systematic, objective assessment of the relevance, effectiveness, and impact of activities in the light of specified objectives.

ev·a·nes·cent (ev-ă-nes'ent). Of short duration. [L. *e*, out, + *vanesco*, to vanish]

Evans, Herbert M., U.S. anatomist and physiologist, 1882–1971. SEE Evans blue.

Evans, Robert S., U.S. physician, 1912–1974. SEE E. *syndrome*.

Evans blue [C.I. 23860]. A diazo dye used for the determination of the blood volume on the basis of the dilution of a standard solution of the dye in the plasma after its intravenous injection; it binds to proteins and is also used as a vital stain for following diffusion through blood vessel walls. SYN azovan blue.

e·vap·o·rate (ē-vap'ōr-āt). To cause or undergo evaporation. SYN volatilize.

evap·o·ra·tion (ē-vap-ŏ-ra'shŭn). 1. A change from liquid to vapor form. 2. Loss of volume of a liquid by conversion into vapor. SYN volatilization. [L. *e*, out, + *vaporo*, to emit vapor]

eva·sion (ē-vā'zhŭn). The act of escaping, avoiding, or feigning.
macular e., SYN *horror* fusionis.

event.
sentinel e., a type of clinical indicator used to monitor and appraise the quality of care, indluding events that require immediate attention.

even·tra·tion (ē'ven-trā'shŭn). 1. Protrusion of omentum and/or intestine through an opening in the abdominal wall. SYN evisceration (4). 2. Removal of the contents of the abdominal cavity. [L. *e*, out, + *venter*, belly]
e. of the diaphragm, extreme elevation of a half or part of the diaphragm, which is usually atrophic and abnormally thin.

ever·sion (ē-ver'zhŭn). A turning outward, as of the eyelid or foot. [L. *e-everto*, pp. *-versus*, to overturn]

evert (ē-vert'). To turn outward. [L. *e-verto*, to overturn]

ev·i·ra·tion (ev-i-rā'shŭn, ē-vī-rā'shŭn). 1. SYN emasculation. 2. Loss or absence of the masculine, with acquisition of feminine characteristics; a type of effemination. 3. Delusional belief of a man that he has become a woman. [L. *e*, out, + *vir*, man]

evis·cer·a·tion (ē-vis-er-ā'shŭn). 1. SYN exenteration. 2. The process wherein tissue or organs that usually reside within a body cavity are displaced outside that cavity usualy through a traumatic disruption of the wall of the cavity; e.g., e. of bowel. 3. Removal of the contents of the eyeball, leaving the sclera and sometimes the cornea. 4. SYN eventration (1). [L. *eviscero*, to disembowel]

evis·cer·o·neu·rot·o·my (ē-vis'er-ō-noo-rot'ō-mē). Evisceration of the eye with division of the optic nerve. [L. *eviscero*, to disembowel, + G. *neuron*, nerve, + *tomē*, a cutting]

evo·ca·tion (ev-ō-kā'shŭn, ē-vō-kā'shŭn). Induction of a particular tissue produced by the action of an evocator during embryogenesis. [L. *evoco*, pp. *evocatus*, to call forth, evoke]

evo·ca·tor (ev'ō-kā-ter, -tōr). A factor in the control of morphogenesis in the early embryo.

ev·o·lu·tion (ev-ō-loo'shŭn). 1. A continuing process of change from one state, condition or form to another. 2. A progressive distancing between the genotype and the phenotype in a line of descent. 3. The liberation of a gas or heat in the course of a chemical or enzymatic reaction. [L. *e-volvo*, pp. *-volutus*, to roll out]

biologic e., the doctrine that all forms of animal or plant life have been derived by gradual changes from simpler forms and ultimately unicellular organisms. SYN organic e.

chemical e., the theory of the process by which life arose from inorganic matter.

coincidental e., SYN concerted e.

concerted e., the ability of two related genes to evolve together as though constituting a single locus. SYN coincidental e.

convergent e., the evolutionary development of similar structures in two or more species, often widely separated phylogenetically, in response to similarities of environment; for example, the winglike structures in insects, birds, and flying mammals.

darwinian e., the proposition that the phylogeny of all species is wholly ascribable to the combined effects of random variation (mutation) in genotypes of the members of a stock as a result of the operation of undirected accidents with consequences to their phenotypes and the operation of preferential (but by no means certain) survival of those resulting phenotypes most suited to survive in the contemporary environment. The proposed system survives largely because of genetic factors that avidly conserve the ontogeny of the stock.

divergent e., the process by which a species or gene product gives rise to two or more different products.

emergent e., appearance of a property in a complex system e.g., organism that could have been predicted only with difficulty, or perhaps not at all, from a knowledge and understanding of the individual genotype changes taken separately.

organic e., SYN biologic e.

saltatory e., the theory that e. of a new species from an older one may occur as a large jump, such as a major repatterning of chromosomes, rather than by gradual accumulation of small steps or mutations. Cf. emergent e.

ev

spontaneous e., the unaided delivery of the fetus from a transverse lie.

evul·sion (ē-vŭl′shŭn). A forcible pulling out or extraction. Cf. avulsion. [L. *evulsio,* fr. *e-vello,* pp. *-vulsus,* to pluck out]

Ewart, William, English physician, 1848–1929. SEE E. *procedure, sign.*

Ewing, James, U.S. pathologist, 1866–1943. SEE E. *sarcoma, tumor.*

Ewing, James H., pathologist, 1798–1827. SEE E. *sign.*

Ewin·gel·la (oo′ing-el′ah). Newly named genus of bacteria (family Enterobacteriaciae) that are usually motile, produce acid but not gas from glucose, use citrate as a carbon source, and do not produce hydrogen sulfide on triple sugar; the type species is *E. americana,* found in the human respiratory tract and recovered from cases of septicemia, usually in association with polymicrobial sepsis.

△**ex-.** Out of, from, away from. [L. and G. out of]

△**exa- (E).** Prefix used in the SI and metric system to signify a multiple of one quintillion (10^{18}).

ex·ac·er·ba·tion (eg-zas-er-bā′shŭn, -ek-sas-). An increase in the severity of a disease or any of its signs or symptoms. [L. *exacerbo,* pp. *-atus,* to exasperate, increase, fr. *acerbus,* sour]

ex·al·ta·tion (eks′al-tā′-shŭn). An utterance, discourse, or address conveying a marked level of joy, glee, and happiness.

ⓘex·am·i·na·tion (eg-zam-i-nā′shŭn). Any investigation or inspection made for the purpose of diagnosis; usually qualified by the method used.

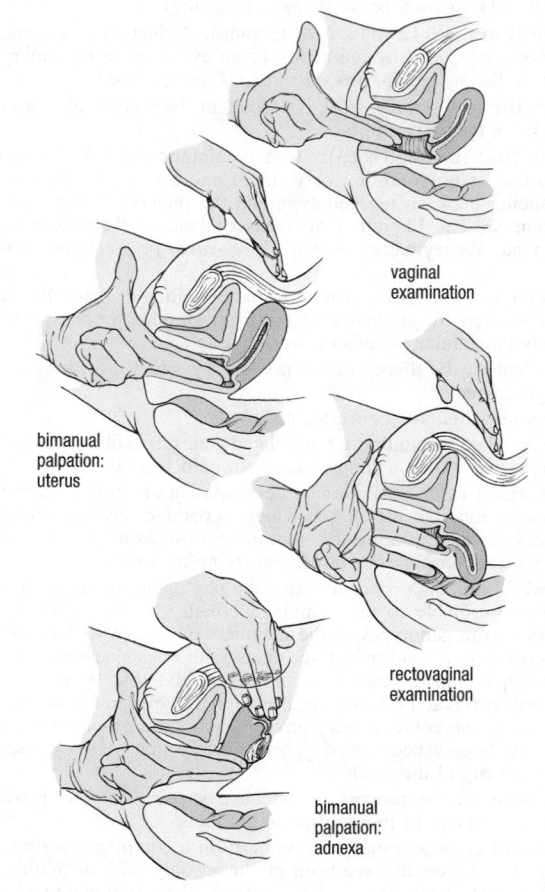

vaginal examination

bimanual palpation: uterus

rectovaginal examination

bimanual palpation: adnexa

pelvic examination

cytologic e., microscopic examination of cells, especially for diagnosis of disease.

direct wet mount e., microscopic review at low (100×) and high

dry (400×) total magnifications of a saline and fresh fecal specimen to detect parasites, including motile protozoan trophozoites.

EMG e., (1) needle electrode examination portion of the electrodiagnostic examination (limited sense); **(2)** synonym for entire electrodiagnostic examination, including not only the needle electrode examination (electromyogram proper), but the nerve conduction studies as well (expanded sense).

fecal e., microscopic review of direct wet mounts, concentration methods, and permanent stained smears to recover and identify parasites from stool specimens.

ova and parasite e., a comprehensive review of a fecal specimen, using direct wet mounts, concentration wet mounts, and permanent stained smears, for the recovery and identification of protozoan and helmintic parasite stages such as trophozoites, cysts, oocysts, spores, eggs, and larvae.

Papanicolaou e., SEE Pap *test.*

permanent stained smear e., microscopic review at oil immersion (1000×) magnification of fecal specimens stained with trichrome, iron-hematoxylin, and such stains; primarily used for protozoan trophozoites, cysts, oocysts, and spores.

physical e., e. by means such as visual inspection, palpation, percussion, and auscultation to collect information for diagnosis.

postmortem e., SYN autopsy.

ex·am·in·er (eg-zam′in-er). One who performs an examination. [L. *examino,* to weigh, examine]

medical e., (1) a physician who examines a person and reports upon that person's physical condition to the company or individual at whose request the examination was made. **(2)** in states or municipalities where the office of coroner has been abolished, a physician appointed to investigate all cases of sudden, violent, or suspicious death.

ex·an·them (eg-zan′them). SYN exanthema.

ex·an·the·ma (eg-zan-thē′mǎ). A skin eruption occurring as a symptom of an acute viral or coccal disease, as in scarlet fever or measles. SYN exanthem. [G. efflorescence, an eruption, fr. *anthos,* flower]

Boston e., a viral disease resembling e. subitum, with the e., if it develops, appearing after the fever has subsided; it is caused by strain 16 of ECHO virus. [after the city in which an epidemic occurred]

epidemic e., SYN epidemic *polyarthritis.*

keratoid e., a symptom occurring in the secondary stage of yaws: patches of fine, light colored, furfuraceous desquamation, scattered irregularly over limbs and trunk.

e. su′bitum, a disease of infants and young children caused by herpesvirus-6, marked by sudden onset with fever lasting several days (sometimes with convulsions) and followed by a fine macular (sometimes maculopapular) rash that appears within a few hours to a day after the fever has subsided. SYN Dukes disease, fourth disease, pseudorubella, roseola infantilis, roseola infantum, sixth disease.

ex·an·them·a·tous (eg-zan-them′ǎ-tŭs). Relating to an exanthema.

ex·an·the·sis (eg-zan-thē′sis). **1.** A rash or exanthem. **2.** The coming out of a rash or eruption. [G.]

e. arthro′sia, SYN dengue.

ex·an·thrope (ek′zan-thrōp). An external cause of disease, one not originating in the body. [G. *ex,* out of, + *anthrōpos,* man]

ex·an·throp·ic (ek-zan-throp′ik). Originating outside of the human body.

ex·ar·te·ri·tis (eks-ar-ter-ī′tis). SYN periarteritis.

ex·cal·a·tion (eks-kǎ-lā′shŭn). Absence, suppression, or failure of development of one of a series of structures, as of a digit or vertebra. [G. *ex,* from, + *chalaō,* to abate, release]

ex·ca·va·tio (eks-kǎ-vā′shē-ō). SYN excavation (1). [L. fr. *ex-cavo,* pp. *-cavatus,* to hollow out, fr. *ex,* out, + *cavus,* hollow]

e. dis′ci [TA], SYN *depression* of optic disk.

e. papil′lae, SYN *depression* of optic disk.

e. rectouteri′na [TA], SYN rectouterine *pouch.*

e. rectovesica′lis [TA], SYN rectovesical *pouch.*

e. vesicouteri′na [TA], SYN vesicouterine *pouch.*

ex·ca·va·tion (eks-kă-vā′shŭn). **1.** A natural cavity, pouch, or recess; a sunken or depressed area. SYN depression (2) [TA], excavatio. **2.** A cavity formed artificially or as the result of a pathologic process.
  atrophic e., an exaggeration of the normal or physiologic cupping of the optic disk caused by atrophy of the optic nerve.
  glaucomatous e., SYN glaucomatous *cup.*
  e. of optic disk, SYN *depression* of optic disk.
  physiologic e., SYN *depression* of optic disk.

ex·ca·va·tor (eks′că-vā-tŏr, -tōr). **1.** An instrument like a large sharp spoon or scoop, used in scraping out pathologic tissue. **2.** In dentistry, an instrument, generally a small spoon or curette, for cleaning out and shaping a carious cavity preparatory to filling.
  hatchet e., SEE hatchet.
  hoe e., a single-beveled dental e., with the blade at an angle to the axis of the handle and the cutting edge perpendicular to the plane of the angle.

ex·ce·men·to·sis (ek′sē-men-tō′sis). A nodular outgrowth of cementum on the root surface of a tooth.

ex·cen·tric (ek-sen′trik). Alternative spelling for eccentric (2, 3).

ex·cess (ek′ses). That which is more than the usual or specified amount.
  antibody e., in a precipitation test, the presence of antibody in an amount greater than that required to combine with all of the antigen present. SEE prozone.
  antigen e., (1) in a precipitation test, the presence of uncombined antigen above that required to combine with all of the antibody; precipitation may be inhibited because the presence of excess antigen gives rise to soluble antigen-antibody complexes; **(2)** in vivo the resultant antigen-antibody interaction in such an antigen e. may give rise to immune complexes, which have a potential to induce cellular damage; could be tolerogenic.
  base e., a measure of metabolic alkalosis, usually predicted from the Siggaard-Andersen nomogram; the amount of strong acid that would have to be added per unit volume of whole blood to titrate it to pH 7.4 while at 37°C and at a carbon dioxide pressure of 40 mm Hg.
  convergence e., that condition in which an esophoria or esotropia is greater for near vision than for far vision.
  negative base e., a measure of metabolic acidosis, usually predicted from the Siggaard-Andersen nomogram; the amount of strong alkali that would have to be added per unit volume of whole blood to titrate it to pH 7.4 while at 37°C and at a carbon dioxide pressure of 40 mm Hg.

ex·change (eks-chānj′). To substitute one thing for another, or the act of such substitution.
  sister chromatid e., the e. during mitosis of homologous genetic material between sister chromatids; increased as a result of inordinate chromosomal fragility due to genetic or environmental factors. SEE recombination.

ex·cip·i·ent (ek-sip′ē-ent). A more or less inert substance added in a prescription as a diluent or vehicle or to give form or consistency when the remedy is given in pill form; e.g., simple syrup, vegetable gums, aromatic powder, honey, and various elixirs. [L. *excipiens;* pres. p. of *ex- cipio,* to take out]

ex·cise (ek-sīz′). To cut out. SEE ALSO resect.

ex·ci·sion (ek-sizh′ŭn). **1.** The act of cutting out; the surgical removal of part or all of a structure or organ. SYN resection (3). **2.** In molecular biology, a recombination event in which a genetic element is removed. SYN exeresis. [L. *excido,* to cut out]

  loop e., a diagnostic and therapeutic gynecological surgical technique for removing dysplastic cells from the cervix. SYN loop electrosurgical excision procedure, loop resection.

  In this office procedure, a small wire loop is used to excise visible zones of abnormal epithelium from the uterine cervix. Like cautery, cryosurgery, and CO_2 laser procedures, loop excision is a simple and inexpensive way of removing dysplastic cells. Unlike these procedures, it provides a specimen so that the lesion can be studied histologically and the completeness of its removal assessed.

The cervix is first prepared with acetic acid and iodine solutions to enhance the demarcation of abnormal areas. Under local anesthesia and with colposcopic visualization, lesions are quickly undercut with a disposable loop electrode. The risk of complications (bleeding, severe postoperative pain, infection, cervical stenosis) is low. The success rate of the loop electrosurgical excision procedure, as defined by the absence of cytologic, histologic, or colposcopic evidence of abnormality 4–48 months after therapy, is 80–90%. Although loop excision does not cure human papilloma virus (HPV) infection, it offers excellent prognosis in HPV-induced dysplasias by removing transformation zone epithelium, which is most susceptible to such changes. The procedure is not appropriate for severe dysplasia or carcinoma in situ, which are treated by cervical conization.

ex·cit·a·bil·i·ty (ek-sī′tă-bil′i-tē). Having the capability of being excitable.
  supranormal e., at the end of phase three of the cardiac action potential, the successful stimulation threshold falls below (i.e., less negative than) the level necessary to produce excitation during the rest of the phase of diastole, so that an ordinary subthreshold stimulus becomes effective. Cf. supranormal *conduction.*

ex·cit·a·ble (ek-sī′tă-bl). **1.** Capable of quick response to a stimulus; having potentiality for emotional arousal. Cf. irritable. **2.** In neurophysiology, referring to a tissue, cell, or membrane capable of undergoing excitation in response to an adequate stimulus.

ex·cit·ant (ek-sī′tănt). SYN stimulant. [L. *excito,* pp. *-atus,* pres. p. *-ans,* to arouse]

ex·ci·ta·tion (ek-sī-tā′shŭn). **1.** The act of increasing the rapidity or intensity of the physical or mental processes. **2.** In neurophysiology, the complete all-or-none response of a nerve or muscle to an adequate stimulus, ordinarily including propagation of e. along the membranes of the cell or cells involved. SEE ALSO stimulation.
  anomalous atrioventricular e., ectopic atrial beat conducted to the ventricle.

ex·cit·a·to·ry (ek-sī′tă-tō-rē). Tending to produce excitation.

ex·cite·ment (ek-sīt′ment). An emotional state sometimes characterized by its potential for impulsive or poorly controlled activity.
  catatonic e., an excited catatonic state seen in one of the schizophrenic disorders. SEE catatonia.
  manic e., an excited mental state seen in a bipolar (manic-depressive) disorder characterized by hyperactivity, talkativeness, flight of ideas, pressured speech, grandiosity, and, occasionally, grandiose delusions. SEE mania, manic-depressive. SYN acute mania.

ex·ci·to·glan·du·lar (ek-sī′tō-glan′dū-lăr). Increasing the secretory activity of a gland.

ex·ci·to·met·a·bol·ic (ek-sī′tō-met-ă-bol′ik). Increasing the activity of the metabolic processes.

ex·ci·to·mo·tor (ek-sī′tō-mō′ter). Causing or increasing the rapidity of motion. SYN centrokinetic (2).

ex·ci·to·mus·cu·lar (ek-sī′tō-mŭs′kū-lăr). Causing muscular activity.

ex·ci·tor (ek-sī′ter, -tōr). SYN stimulant (2).

ex·ci·to·se·cre·to·ry (ek-sī′tō-sē-krē′tō-rē). Stimulating to secretion.

ex·ci·to·tox·ic (ek-sī′-tō-tok-sik). Possessing the property of exciting and then poisoning cells or tissues; examples include nerve injury and death produced by glutamate. [excite + G. *toxikon,* poison]

ex·ci·to·tox·ins (ek-sī′tō-toks′ins). Toxins that bind to certain receptors (e.g., certain glutamate receptors) and may cause neuronal cell death; e.'s may be involved in brain damage associated with strokes.

ex·clave (eks-klāv′). An outlying, detached portion of a gland or other part, such as the thyroid or pancreas; an accessory gland. [L. *ex,* out, + *-clave* (in enclave)]

ex·clu·sion (eks-kloo′zhŭn). A shutting out; disconnection from the main portion. [L. *ex- cludo,* pp. *-clusus,* to shut out]
  allelic e., in each cell of an individual heterozygous at an autoso-

ex

mal locus, the non-preferential suppression of the phenotypic manifestation of one or other of the alleles; the phenotype of the body is thus mosaic. Cf. lyonization.

e. of pupil, SYN seclusion of *pupil*.

exclusive provider organization (EPO). A managed care plan in which enrollees must receive their care from affiliated providers; treatment provided outside the approved network must be paid for by the patients. SEE ALSO managed *care*.

ex·con·ju·gant (eks-kon'joo-gant). A member of a conjugating pair of protozoan ciliates after separation and prior to the subsequent mitotic division of each of the e.'s. SEE ALSO conjugant, conjugation (3). [ex- + L. *conjugo,* to join]

ex·co·ri·ate (eks-kō'rē-āt). To scratch or otherwise strip off the skin by physical means.

ex·co·ri·a·tion (eks-kō'rē-ā'shŭn). A scratch mark; a linear break in the skin surface, usually covered with blood or serous crusts. [L. *excorio,* to skin, strip, fr. *corium,* skin, hide]

neurotic e., repeated self-induced e., with or without underlying skin lesions, associated with compulsive or neurotic behavioral problems.

ex·cre·ment (eks'krĕ-ment). Waste matter or any excretion cast out of the body; e.g., feces. [L. *ex- cerno,* pp. *-cretus,* to separate]

ex·cre·men·ti·tious (eks'krē-men-tish'ŭs). Relating to any excrement.

ex·cres·cence (eks-kres'ens). Any outgrowth from a surface. [L. *ex- cresco,* pp. *-cretus,* to grow forth]

Lambl e.'s, small pointed projections from the edges of the aortic cusps of unknown significance.

ex·cre·ta (eks-krē'tă). SYN excretion (2). [L. neut. pl. of *excretus,* pp. of *ex-cerno,* to separate]

ex·crete (eks-krēt'). To separate from the blood and cast out; to perform excretion.

ex·cre·tion (eks-krē'shŭn). **1.** The process whereby the undigested residue of food and the waste products of metabolism are eliminated, material is removed to regulate the composition of body fluids and tissues, or substances are expelled to perform functions on an exterior surface. **2.** The product of a tissue or organ that is material to be passed out of the body. SYN excreta. Cf. secretion. [see excrement]

ex·cre·to·ry (eks'krē-tō-rē). Relating to excretion.

ex·cur·sion (eks-ker'zhŭn). Any movement from one point to another, usually with the implied idea of returning again to the original position.

lateral e., movement of the mandible to the right or left side.

protrusive e., movement of the mandible to a position forward of the centric position.

retrusive e., the slight backward and return movement of the mandible between the position of closure and a slightly posterior position.

ex·cy·clo·duc·tion (ek-sī-klō-dŭk'shŭn). A cycloduction in which the upper pole of the cornea is rotated outward (laterally). [ex- + cyclo- + L. *duco,* pp. *ductus,* to lead]

ex·cy·clo·pho·ria (ek-sī-klō-fō'rē-ă). A cyclophoria in which the upper poles of each cornea tend to rotate laterally. [ex- + cyclo- + G. *phora,* a carrying]

ex·cy·clo·tor·sion (eks'sī-klō-tōr'shun). SYN extorsion (1). [ex- + cyclo- + L. *torqueo,* pp. *torsus,* to twist]

ex·cy·clo·tro·pia (eks'sī-klō-trō'pē-a). A cyclotropia in which the upper poles of the corneas are rotated outward (laterally) relative to each other. [ex- + cyclo- + G. *tropē,* a turning]

ex·cy·clo·ver·gence (ek-sī-klō-ver'jens). Rotation of the upper pole of each cornea outwards. [ex- + cyclo- + L. *vergo,* to bend, incline]

ex·cys·ta·tion (ek-sis-tā'shŭn). Removal from a cyst; denoting the action of certain encysted organisms in escaping from their envelope.

ex·duc·tion (eks-duk'shun). SYN lateroduction. [ex- + L. *duco,* pp. *ductus,* to lead]

ex·e·mia (ek-sē'mē-ă). A condition, as in shock, in which a considerable portion of the blood is removed from the main circu-

lation but remains within blood vessels in certain areas where it is stagnant. [G. *ex,* out of, + *haima,* blood]

ex·en·ce·pha·lia (eks'en-se-fā'lē-ă). SYN exencephaly.

ex·en·ce·phal·ic (eks'en-se-fal'ik). Relating to exencephaly. SYN exencephalous.

ex·en·ceph·a·lo·cele (eks'en-sef'ă-lō-sēl). Herniation of the brain. [ex, out, + G. *enkephalos,* brain, + *kēlē,* tumor]

ex·en·ceph·a·lous (eks-en-sef'ă-lŭs). SYN exencephalic.

ex·en·ceph·a·ly (eks-en-sef'ă-lē). Condition in which the skull is defective with the brain exposed or extruding. SYN exencephalia. [G. *ex,* out, + *enkephalos,* brain]

ex·en·ter·a·tion (eks-en-ter-ā'shŭn). Removal of internal organs and tissues, usually radical removal of the contents of a body cavity. SYN evisceration (1). [G. *ex,* out, + *enteron,* bowel]

anterior pelvic e., removal of the urinary bladder, lower parts of the ureter, vagina, uterus, adnexa, and adjacent lymph nodes; a urinary diversion is necessary.

orbital e., removal of the entire contents of the orbit.

pelvic e., removal of all of the organs and adjacent structures of the pelvis; usually performed to surgically ablate cancer involving urinary bladder, uterine cervix, and rectum.

posterior pelvic e., removal of the vagina, uterus, adnexa, rectum, anus, and adjacent lymph nodes; a colostomy is necessary.

total pelvic e., removal of the urinary bladder, lower parts of the ureter, vagina, uterus, adnexa, rectum, anus, and adjacent lymph nodes; a colostomy and urinary diversion are necessary. SYN Brunschwig operation.

ex·en·ter·i·tis (eks-en-ter-ī'tis). Inflammation of the peritoneal covering of the intestine. [G. *exō,* on the outside, + enteritis]

ex·er·cise (ek'ser-sīz). **1.** *Active:* bodily exertion for the sake of restoring the organs and functions to a healthy state or keeping them healthy. **2.** *Passive:* motion of limbs without effort by the patient.

isometric e., e. consisting of muscular contractions without movement of the involved parts of the body.

isotonic e., SYN isotonic *contraction*.

Kegel e.'s, alternate contraction and relaxation of perineal muscles for treatment of urinary stress incontinence.

ex·er·e·sis (ek-ser'ĕ-sis). SYN excision. [G. *exairesis,* a taking out, fr. *haireō,* to take, grasp]

ex·er·gon·ic (ek-ser-gon'ik). **1.** Referring to a chemical reaction that takes place with a negative charge in Gibbs free energy. Cf. endergonic. **2.** Any process that can produce work. [exo- + G. *ergon,* work]

ex·flag·el·la·tion (eks-flaj-ĕ-lā'shŭn). The extrusion of rapidly waving flagellum-like microgametes from microgametocytes; in the case of human malaria parasites, this occurs in the blood meal taken by the proper anopheline vector within a few minutes after ingestion of the infected blood by the mosquito. SYN polymitus.

ex·fo·li·a·tion (eks-fō-lē-ā'shŭn). **1.** Detachment and shedding of superficial cells of an epithelium or from any tissue surface. **2.** Scaling or desquamation of the horny layer of epidermis, which varies in amount from minute quantities to shedding the entire integument. **3.** Loss of deciduous teeth following physiological loss of root structure. [Mod. L. fr. L. *ex,* out, + *folium,* leaf]

e. of lens, sheetlike separation of the capsule of the lens; it may occur if the eyes are exposed to intense heat.

ex·fo·li·a·tive (eks-fō'lē-ā-tiv). Marked by exfoliation, desquamation, or profuse scaling. [Mod. L. *exfoliativus*]

ex·ha·la·tion (eks-hă-lā'shŭn). **1.** Breathing out. SYN expiration (1). **2.** The giving forth of gas or vapor. **3.** Any exhaled or emitted gas or vapor. [L. *ex-halo,* pp. *-halatus,* to breathe out]

ex·hale (eks'hāl). **1.** To breathe out. SYN expire (1). **2.** To emit a gas or vapor or odor.

ex·haus·tion (eg-zos'chŭn). **1.** Extreme fatigue; inability to respond to stimuli. **2.** Removal of contents; using up of a supply of anything. **3.** Extraction of the active constituents of a drug by treating with water, alcohol, or other solvent. [L. *ex-haurio,* pp. *-haustus,* to draw out, empty]

heat e., a form of reaction to heat, marked by prostration, weakness, and collapse, resulting from severe dehydration.

ex·hi·bi·tion·ism (ek-si-bish′ŭn-izm). A morbid compulsion to expose a part of the body, especially the genitals, with the intent of provoking sexual interest in the viewer.

ex·hi·bi·tion·ist (ek-si-bish′ŭn-ist). One who engages in exhibitionism.

ex·hil·a·rant (eg-zil′ar-ant). Mentally stimulating. [L. *ex-hilaro*, pp. *-atus*, pres. p. *-ans*, to gladden]

ex·is·ten·tial (eg-zi-sten′shăl). Pertaining to a branch of philosophy, existentialism, concerned with the search for the meaning of one's own existence, that has been extended into existential *psychotherapy*. [L. *existentia*, existence]

ex·i·tus (eks′i-tŭs). An exit or outlet; death. [L. fr. *ex-eo*, pp. *-itus*, to go out]

Exner, Siegmund, Austrian physiologist, 1846–1926. SEE Call-E. *bodies*, under *body;* E. *plexus.*

exo-. Exterior, external, or outward. SEE ALSO ecto-. [G. *exō*, outside]

ex·o·am·y·lase (ek-sō-am′il-ās). A glucanohydrolase acting on a glycosidic bond near an end of the polysaccharide; e.g., β-amylase.

ex·o·an·ti·gen (ek-sō-an′ti-jen). SYN ectoantigen.

ex·o·car·dia (ek-sō-kar′dē-ă). SYN ectocardia.

ex·o·crine (ek′sō-krin). **1.** Denoting glandular secretion delivered to an apical or luminal surface. SYN eccrine (1). **2.** Denoting a gland that secretes outwardly through excretory ducts. [exo- + G. *krinō*, to separate]

ex·o·cy·clic (ek-sō-sī′klik, -sik′lik). Relating to atoms or groups attached to a cyclic structure but not themselves cyclic; e.g., the methyl group of toluene. Cf. endocyclic.

ex·o·cy·to·sis (ek′sō-sī-tō′sis). **1.** The appearance of migrating inflammatory cells in the epidermis. **2.** The process whereby secretory granules or droplets are released from a cell; the membrane around the granule fuses with the cell membrane, which ruptures, and the secretion is discharged. SYN emeiocytosis, emiocytosis. Cf. endocytosis. [exo- + G. *kytos*, cell, + *-osis*, condition]

ex·o·de·vi·a·tion (ek′sō-dē-vē-ā′shŭn). **1.** SYN exophoria. **2.** SYN exotropia.

ex·o·don·tia (ek-sō-don′shē-ă). The branch of dental practice concerned with the extraction of teeth. [exo- + G. *odous*, tooth]

ex·o·don·tist (ek-sō-don′tist). One who specializes in the extraction of teeth.

ex·o·en·zyme (ek-sō-en′zīm). SYN extracellular *enzyme.*

ex·og·a·my (ek-sog′ă-mē). Sexual reproduction by means of conjugation of two gametes of different ancestry, as in certain protozoan species. [exo- + G. *gamos*, marriage]

ex·o·gas·tru·la (eks-ō-gas′troo-lă). An abnormal embryo in which the primitive gut has been everted.

ex·o·ge·net·ic (ek′sō-je-net′ik). SYN exogenous.

ex·o·ge·note (ek-sō-jē′nōt). In microbial genetics, the fragment of genetic material that has been transferred from a donor to the recipient and, being homologous for a region of the recipient's original genome (endogenote), produces in the homologous region a condition analogous to diploidy. [exo + genote]

ex·og·e·nous (eks-oj′ĕ-nŭs). Originating or produced outside of the organism. SYN ectogenous, exogenetic. [exo- + G. *-gen*, production]

exo-1,4-α-D-glu·co·si·dase. A hydrolase removing terminal α-1,4-linked D-glucose residues from nonreducing ends of chains, with release of β-D-glucose. SYN acid maltase, amyloglucosidase, γ-amylase, glucoamylase.

ex·o·lev·er (ek′sō-lē′ver). A modified elevator for the extraction of tooth roots. [exo- + L. *levare*, to raise]

ex·om·pha·los (eks-om′fă-lŭs). **1.** Protrusion of the umbilicus. SYN exumbilication (1). **2.** SYN umbilical *hernia.* **3.** SYN omphalocele. [G. *ex*, out, + *omphalos*, umbilicus]

ex·on (ek′son). A portion of a DNA that codes for a section of the mature messenger RNA from that DNA, and is therefore expressed ("translated" into protein) at the ribosome. [ex- + on]

ex·on shuf·fle. The variation in the patterns by which RNA may produce diverse sets of exons from a single gene.

ex·o·nu·cle·ase (ek-sō-noo′klē-ās). A nuclease that releases one nucleotide at a time, serially, beginning at one end of a polynucleotide (nucleic acid); several have been prepared from *Escherichia coli*, designated e. I, e. II, etc.; e. III, which removes nucleotides from 3′ ends of DNA, is used in DNA sequencing. Cf. endonuclease.

ex·o·pep·ti·dase (ek-sō-pep′ti-dās). An enzyme that catalyzes the hydrolysis of the terminal amino acid of a peptide chain; e.g., carboxypeptidase. Cf. endopeptidase.

Ex·o·phi·a·la (ek-sō-fī′ă-lă). A genus of pathogenic fungi having dematiaceous conidiophores with one- or two-celled annelloconidia. They cause mycetoma or phaeohyphomycosis; in cases of mycetoma, black granules develop in subcutaneous abscesses; in cases of phaeohyphomycosis, hyaline or brownish hyphae are found in tissues. [exo + G. *phialē*, a broad flat vessel]

E. jeansel′mei, a fungal species found in cases of mycetoma or phaeohyphomycosis.

E. wernec′kii, a fungal species that causes tinea nigra. SYN *Cladosporium werneckii.*

ex·o·pho·ria (ek′so-fō′rē-ă). Tendency of the eyes to deviate outward when fusion is suspended. SYN exodeviation (1). [exo- + G. *phora*, a carrying]

ex·o·phor·ic (ek-sō-fōr′ik). Relating to exophoria.

ex·oph·thal·mic (ek-sof-thal′mik). Relating to exophthalmos; marked by prominence of the eyeball.

ex·oph·thal·mom·e·ter (ek-sof-thal-mom′ĕ-ter). An instrument to measure the distance between the anterior pole of the eye and a fixed reference point, often the zygomatic bone. SYN orthometer, proptometer, statometer. [exophthalmos + G. *metron*, measure]

ex·oph·thal·mos, ex·oph·thal·mus (ek-sof-thal′mos). Protrusion of one or both eyeballs; can be congenital and familial, or due to pathology, such as a retroorbital tumor (usually unilateral) or thyroid disease (usually bilateral). SYN proptosis. [G. *ex*, out, + *ophthalmos*, eye]

endocrine e., e. associated with thyroid gland disorders. SEE Graves *ophthalmopathy*, Graves *orbitopathy.*

malignant e., relentless, progressive protrusion of the eyeballs.

ex·o·phyte (ek′sō-fīt). An exterior or external plant parasite. [exo- + G. *phyton*, plant]

ex·o·phyt·ic (ek-sō-fit′ik). **1.** Pertaining to an exophyte. **2.** Denoting a neoplasm or lesion that grows outward from an epithelial surface.

ex·o·plasm (ek′sō-plazm). SYN ectoplasm.

ex·o·se·ro·sis (ek′sō-se-rō′sis). Serous exudation from the skin surface, as in eczema or abrasions.

ex·o·skel·e·ton (ek-sō-skel′ĕ-tŏn). **1.** Hard parts, such as hair, teeth, nails, feathers, hooves, scales, etc., developed from the epidermis in vertebrates. SYN dermoskeleton. **2.** Outer chitinous envelope of an insect, or the chitinous or calcareous covering of certain Crustacea and other invertebrates.

ex·o·spore (ek′sō-spōr). An exogenous spore, not encased in a sporangium. [exo- + G. *sporos*, seed]

ex·o·spo·ri·um (ek-sō-spō′rē-um). The outer envelope of a spore.

ex·os·tec·to·my (ek-sos-tek′tō-mē). Removal of an exostosis. SYN exostosectomy. [exostosis + G. *ektomē*, excision]

ex·os·to·sec·to·my (ek-sos-tō-sek′tō-mē). SYN exostectomy.

ex·os·to·sis, pl. **ex·os·to·ses** (eks-os-tō′sis, -sēz). A cartilage-capped bony projection arising from any bone that develops from cartilage. SEE ALSO osteochondroma. SYN hyperostosis (2), poroma (2). [exo- + G. *osteon*, bone, + *-osis*, condition]

e. bursa′ta, an e. arising from the joint surface of a bone and covered with cartilage and a synovial sac.

e. cartilagin′ea, an ossified chondroma arising from the epiphysis or joint surface of a bone.

hereditary multiple exostoses [MIM*133700], a disturbance of enchondral bone growth in which multiple, generally benign osteochondromas of long bones appear during childhood, commonly with shortening of the radius and fibula; the skull is not involved;

ex

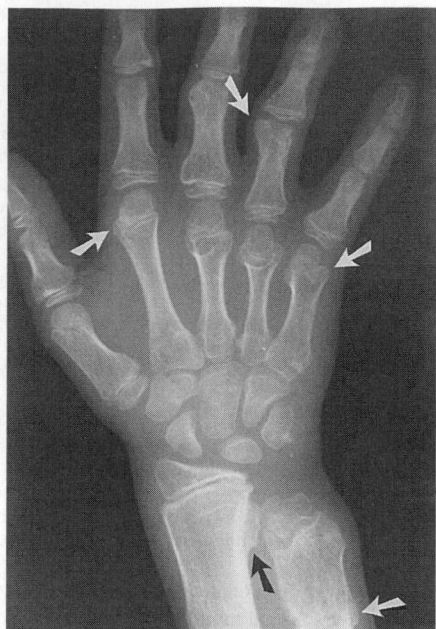

exostosis: several small osteochondromas (arrows)

the ill effects are usually mechanical but malignant change is rare; autosomal dominant inheritance with genetic heterogeneity of which some cases are due to mutation in the exostosis-1 gene (EXT1) on 8q. SYN hereditary deforming chondrodystrophy (1), multiple e., osteochondromatosis.

ivory e., a small, rounded, eburnated tumor arising from a bone, usually one of the cranial bones.

multiple e., SYN hereditary multiple exostoses.

solitary osteocartilaginous e., SYN osteochondroma.

subungual e., painful osseous outgrowths that elevate the nail of the great toe or fingers in young people.

ex·o·ter·ic (ek-sō-tār′ik). Of external origin; arising outside the organism. [G. *exōterikos*, outer]

ex·o·ther·mic (ek-sō-ther′mik). **1.** Denoting a chemical reaction during which heat (i.e., enthalpy) is emitted. Cf. endothermic. **2.** Relating to the external warmth of the body. [exo- + G. *thermē*, heat]

ex·o·tox·ic (ek-sō-tok′sik). **1.** Relating to an exotoxin. **2.** Relating to the introduction of an exogenous poison or toxin.

ex·o·tox·in (ek-sō-tok′sin). A specific, soluble, antigenic, usually heat labile, injurious substance elaborated by certain Gram-positive or Gram-negative bacteria; it is formed within the cell, but is released into the environment where it is rapidly active in extremely small amounts; most e.'s are protein in nature (MW 70,000–900,000) and can have the toxic portion of the molecule destroyed by heat, prolonged storage, or chemicals; the nontoxic but antigenic form is a toxoid. SYN ectotoxin, extracellular toxin.

ex·o·tro·pia (ek-sō-trō′pē-ă). That type of strabismus in which the visual axes diverge; may be paralytic or concomitant, monocular or alternating, constant or intermittent. SYN divergent squint, divergent strabismus, exodeviation (2), external squint, wall-eye (1). [exo- + G. *tropē*, turn]

A-pattern e., divergent strabismus greater in downward than in upward gaze.

basic e., e. in which the strabismus is the same for near and far vision.

divergence excess e., e. in which the strabismus is notably greater for far vision than for near vision.

divergence insufficiency e., e. in which the strabismus is notably greater for near vision than for far vision.

V-pattern e., divergent strabismus greater in upward than in downward gaze.

X-pattern e., increasing divergence from primary position in both upward and downward gaze.

ex·pan·sion (eks-pan′shŭn). **1.** An increase in size as of chest or lungs. **2.** The spreading out of any structure, as a tendon. **3.** An expanse; a wide area. [L. *ex-pando*, pp. *-pansus*, to spread out]

clonal e. (klō′nal), production of daughter cells all arising originally from a single cell.

extensor e., SYN extensor digital e.

extensor digital e., a triangular tendinous aponeurosis including the tendon of the extensor digitorum centrally, interosseus tendons on each side, and a lumbrical tendon laterally. It covers the dorsal aspect of the metacarpophalangeal joint and the proximal phalanx. SYN dorsal hood, extensor aponeurosis, extensor e.

hygroscopic e., (1) e. due to the absorption of moisture; (2) in dental casting, the addition of water to the surface of the casting investment during setting to increase the size of the mold.

perceptual e., development of an ability to recognize and interpret sensory stimuli through associations with past similar stimuli; perceptual e. by relaxation of defenses is a goal of psychotherapy.

setting e., the dimensional increase that occurs concurrently with the hardening of various materials, such as plaster of Paris.

wax e., in dentistry, a method of expanding wax patterns to compensate for the shrinkage of gold during the casting process.

ex·pan·sive·ness (ek-span′siv-nes). A state of optimism, loquacity, and reactivity.

ex·pec·ta·tion. In probability theory and statistics the true mean or average (of a sample distribution).

ex·pec·ta·tion of life. The average number of years of life an individual of a given age is expected to live if current mortality rates continue to apply; a statistical abstraction based on existing age-specific death rates.

e. o. l. at age x, the average number of additional years a person aged x would live if current mortality trends continue to apply, based on the age-specific death rates for a given year.

e. o. l. at birth, average number of years of life a newborn baby can be expected to live if current mortality trends continue.

ex·pect·ed. In probability theory and statistics, interchangeable with mean or average; it need not be a probable or even possible value. For instance, the expected number of children in completed families may be 2.53, but that is not a possible size of any actual family.

ex·pec·to·rant (ek-spek′tō-rănt). **1.** Promoting secretion from the mucous membrane of the air passages or facilitating its expulsion. **2.** An agent that increases bronchial secretion and facilitates its expulsion. [L. *ex*, out, + *pectus*, chest]

ex·pec·to·rate (ek-spek′tō-rāt). To spit; to eject saliva, mucus, or other fluid from the mouth.

ex·pec·to·ra·tion (ek-spek-tō-rā′shŭn). **1.** Mucus and other fluids formed in the air passages and upper food passages (the mouth), and expelled by coughing. SEE ALSO sputum (1). **2.** The act of spitting; the expelling from the mouth of saliva, mucus, and other material from the air or upper food passages. SYN spitting.

prune-juice e., SYN prune-juice *sputum*.

ex·pe·ri·ence (ek-spēr′ē-ens). The feeling of emotions and sensations, as opposed to thinking; involvement in what is happening rather than abstract reflection on an event or interpersonal encounter. [L. *experientia*, fr. *experior*, to try]

corrective emotional e., reexposure under favorable circumstances to an emotional situation with which one could not cope in the past.

ex·per·i·ment (eks-per′i-ment). **1.** A study in which the investigator intentionally alters one or more factors under controlled conditions in order to study the effects of doing so. **2.** In nuclear magnetic resonance, the term applied to a pulse sequence. [L. *experimentum*, fr. *experior*, to test, try]

Carr-Purcell e., in magnetic resonance, the multiple spin echo technique.

control e., an e. used to check another, to verify the result, or to demonstrate what would have occurred had the factor under study been omitted. SEE ALSO control, control *animal*.

delayed reaction e., a method of measuring memory: a stimulus is presented and removed before the organism is permitted to respond to it; the interval during which the stimulus is absent, providing the organism responds correctly, is an indication of the length of memory.

double blind e., an e. conducted with neither experimenter nor subjects knowing which e. is the control; prevents bias in recording results. SEE ALSO double-masked e.

double-masked e., a double-blind study conducted so neither the subject nor the observer knows the identity of the control or variable.

factorial e.'s, an experimental design in which two or more series of treatments are tried in all combinations.

hertzian e.'s, e.'s demonstrating that electromagnetic induction is propagated in waves, analogous to waves of light but not affecting the retina.

Mariotte e., an e. in which one looks fixedly with one eye (the other being closed), at a black dot on a card, on which is also marked a black cross; as the card is moved to or from the eye, at a certain distance the cross becomes invisible but appears again as the card is moved further; this proves the absence of photoreceptors where the optic nerve enters the eye.

pulse-chase e., an e. in which an enzyme, a metabolic pathway, a culture of cells, etc., interacts with a brief addition (pulse) of a labeled compound followed by its removal and replacement (chase) by an excess of unlabeled compound.

Scheiner e., a demonstration of accommodation; through two minute holes in a card, separated from each other by less than the diameter of the pupil, one looks at a pin; at a short distance from the eye the pin appears double; as it is moved from the eye a point is found where it appears single, and beyond which it remains single for the emmetropic eye, but for the myopic eye it soon again becomes double.

ex·pi·ra·tion (eks-pi-rā'shŭn). **1.** SYN exhalation (1). **2.** A death. [L. *expiro* or *ex-spiro,* pp. *-atus,* to breathe out]

ex·pi·ra·to·ry (eks-spī'ră-tō-rē). Relating to expiration.

ex·pire (ek-spīr'). **1.** SYN exhale (1). **2.** To die.

ex·plant (eks'plant). Living tissue transferred from an organism to an artificial medium for culture.

ex·plan·ta·tion (eks-plan-tā'shŭn). The act of transferring an explant.

ex·plo·ra·tion (eks-plōr-ā'shŭn). An active examination, usually involving a surgical procedure, to ascertain conditions present within a body cavity as an aid in diagnosis. [L. *ex-ploro,* pp. *-ploratus,* to explore]

ex·plor·a·to·ry (eks-plōr'ă-tōr-ē). Relating to, or with a view to, exploration.

ex·plor·er (ek'splōr'er). A sharp pointed probe used to investigate natural or restored tooth surfaces in order to detect caries or other defects.

ex·plo·sion (eks-plō'zhŭn). A sudden and violent increase in volume accompanied by noise and release of energy, as from a chemical change, nuclear reaction, or escape of gases or vapors under pressure. [L. *explosio,* fr. *explodo,* to drive away by clapping]

ex·pose (eks-pōz'). To perform or undergo exposure. [O. Fr. *exposer,* fr. L. *ex-pono,* pp. *ex-positum,* to set out, expose]

ex·po·sure (eks-pō'zhoor). **1.** A displaying, revealing, exhibiting, or making accessible. **2.** In dentistry, loss of hard tooth structure covering the dental pulp due to caries, dental instrumentation, or trauma. **3.** Proximity and/or contact with a source of a disease agent in such a manner that effective transmission of the agent or harmful effects of the agent may occur. **4.** The amount of a factor to which a group or individual was exposed, in contrast to the dose, the amount that enters or interacts with the organism.

ex·press (eks-pres'). To press or squeeze out. [L. *ex-premo,* pp. *-pressus,* to press out]

ex·pres·sion (eks-presh'ŭn). **1.** Squeezing out; expelling by pressure. **2.** Mobility of the features giving a particular emotional significance to the face. SYN facies (3) [TA]. **3.** Any act by an individual. **4.** Something that manifests something else. **5.** The act of allowing information to become manifest. **6.** A mathematical

function consisting of a combination of constants, variables, other functions, and mathematical operations.

differential gene e., gene e. that responds to signals or triggers; a means of gene regulation; e.g., effects of certain hormones on protein biosynthesis.

gene e., **(1)** the detectable effect of a gene. **(2)** appearance of an inherited trait; for many genetic (e.g., recessiveness, hypostasis, parastasis) and environmental (the absence of pertinent challenges) reasons, a gene may not be expressed at all. In those circumstances, it will have no impact on Darwinian evolution.

integrated rate e., an equation of a chemical or enzyme-catalyzed reaction for the entire progress curve.

e. library, a collection of plasmid or phage containing a representative sample of cDNA or genomic fragments that are constructed in such a way that they will be transcribed and translated by the host organism (usually bacteria).

ex·pres·siv·i·ty (eks-pres-siv'i-tē). In clinical genetics, the degree of severity in which a gene is manifested.

ex·pul·sive (eks-pŭl'siv). Tending to expel. [L. *ex-pello,* pp. *-pulsus,* to drive out]

ex·qui·site (eks-kwiz'it). Extremely intense, keen, sharp; said of pain or tenderness in a part. [L. *exquiro,* pp. *exquisitus,* to search out]

ex·san·gui·nate (ek-sang'gwi-nāt). **1.** To remove or withdraw the circulating blood; to make bloodless. **2.** SYN exsanguine. [L. *ex,* out, + *sanguis* (*-guin*), blood]

ex·san·gui·na·tion (ek-sang'gwi-nā'shŭn). Removal of blood; making exsanguine.

ex·san·guine (ek-sang'gwin). Deprived of blood. SYN exsanguinate (2).

ex·sect (ek-sekt'). Rarely used term for excise. [L. *ex- seco,* pp. *-sectus,* to cut out]

ex·sec·tion (ek-sek'shŭn). Rarely used term for excision.

Exserohilum (eks'er-ō-hī'lum). A genus of fungi; a cause of human phaeohyphomycosis.

ex·sic·cant (ek-sik'ant). SYN desiccant.

ex·sic·cate (ek'si-kāt). SYN desiccate.

ex·sic·ca·tion (ek-si-kā'shŭn). **1.** SYN desiccation. **2.** The removal of water of crystallization. SYN dehydration (3). [L. *ex sicco,* pp. *siccatus,* to dry up]

ex·so·ma·tize (ek-sō'mă-tīz). To remove from the body. [G. *ex,* out of, + *sōma,* body]

ex·sorp·tion (ek-sōrp'shŭn). Movement of substances from the blood into the lumen of the gut. [L. *ex,* out, + *sorbeo,* to suck]

ex·stro·phy (ek'strō-fē). Congenital eversion of a hollow organ. SYN ecstrophe. [G. *ex,* out, + *strophē,* a turning]

e. of the bladder, a congenital gap in the anterior wall of the bladder and the abdominal wall in front of it, the posterior wall of the bladder being exposed. SYN ectopia vesicae.

cloacal e., congenital anomaly with two exstrophied bladder units separated by an exstrophied segment of intestine, which is usually cecum, receiving ileum superiorly and continuing distally to blind ending microcolon. A number of variants of anatomic disarray can occur. SYN ectopia cloacae.

ex·tend (eks-tend'). To straighten a limb, to diminish or extinguish the angle formed by flexion; to place the distal segment of a limb in such a position that its axis is continuous with that of the proximal segment. [L. *ex- tendo,* pp. *-tensus,* to stretch out]

ex·ten·sion (eks-ten'shŭn) [TA]. **1.** The act of bringing the distal portion of a joint in continuity (though only parallel) with the long axis of the proximal portion. **2.** A pulling or dragging force exerted on a limb in a distal direction. **3.** Obsolete term for traction. [L. *extensio,* a stretching out]

Buck e., SYN Buck traction.

primer e., a technique for determining the 5′-untranslated region of a specific mRNA molecule. Uses an oligonucleotide complementary to the known RNA sequence as a primer for cDNA synthesis via reverse transcriptase.

ridge e., an intraoral surgical operation for deepening the labial, buccal, and/or lingual sulci; it is performed to increase the intraoral height of the alveolar ridge in order to assist denture retention.

skeletal e., SYN skeletal *traction.*

ex·ten·sor (eks-ten′ser, -sōr) [TA]. A muscle the contraction of which causes movement at a joint with the consequence that the limb or body assumes a more straight line, or so that the distance between the parts proximal and distal to the joint is increased or extended; the antagonist of a flexor. SEE muscle. [L. one who stretches, fr. *ex-tendo,* to stretch out]

ex·te·ri·or (eks-tē′rē-ōr). Outside; external. [L.]

ex·te·ri·or·ize (eks-tēr′ē-ōr-īz). **1.** To direct a patient's interests, thoughts, or feelings into a channel leading outside the self, to some definite aim or object. **2.** To expose an organ temporarily for observation, or permanently for purposes of experiment. **3.** Fixation of a segment of bowel with blood supply intact to the outer aspect of the abdominal wall.

ex·tern (eks′tern). An advanced student or recent graduate who assists in the medical or surgical care of hospital patients; formerly, one who lived outside of the institution. [F. *externe,* outside, a day scholar]

ex·ter·nal (eks-ter′năl) [TA]. On the outside or farther from the center; often incorrectly used to mean lateral. SYN externus [TA]. [L. *externus*]

ex·ter·nus (eks-ter′nŭs) [TA]. SYN external.

ex·ter·o·cep·tive (eks′ter-ō-sep′tiv). Relating to the exteroceptors; denoting the surface of the body containing the end organs adapted to receive impressions or stimuli from without. [L. *exterus,* outside, + *capio,* to take]

ex·ter·o·cep·tor (eks′ter-ō-sep′ter, -tōr). One of the peripheral end organs of the afferent nerves in the skin or mucous membrane, which respond to stimulation by external agents. [L. *exterus,* external, + *receptor,* receiver]

ex·tinc·tion (eks-tingk′shŭn). **1.** In behavior modification or classical or operant conditioning, a progressive decrease in the frequency of a response that is not positively reinforced; the withdrawal of reinforcers known to maintain an undesirable behavior. SEE conditioning. **2.** SYN absorbance. [L. *extinguo,* to quench]

specific e., SYN specific absorption *coefficient.*

visual e., SYN pseudo-*hemianopia.*

ex·tin·guish (eks-ting′gwish). **1.** To abolish; to quench, as a flame; to cause loss of identity; to destroy. **2.** In psychology, to progressively abolish a previously conditioned response. SEE conditioning. [L. *extinguo,* to quench]

ex·tir·pa·tion (eks-tir-pā′shŭn). Partial or complete removal of an organ or diseased tissue. [L. *extirpo,* to root out, fr. *stirps,* a stalk, root]

Exton, William G., U.S. physician, 1876–1943. SEE E. *reagent.*

ex·tor·sion (eks-tōr′shŭn). **1.** Conjugate rotation of the upper poles of each cornea outward. SYN excyclotorsion. **2.** Outward rotation of a limb or of an organ. [L. *extorsio,* fr. *ex-torqueo,* to twist out]

ex·tor·tor (eks-tōr′ter, -tōr). An outward rotator.

⌂ex·tra-. Without, outside of. [L.]

ex·tra·ar·tic·u·lar (eks-tră-ar-tik′ū-lăr). Outside of a joint.

ex·tra·ax·i·al (eks-tră-aks′ē-ăl). Off the axis; applied to intracranial lesions that do not arise from the brain itself.

ex·tra·buc·cal (eks-tră-bŭk′ăl). Outside or not part of the cheek.

ex·tra·bul·bar (eks-tra-bul′bar). Outside of or unrelated to any bulb, such as the bulb of the urethra, or the medulla oblongata.

ex·tra·cal·i·ce·al (eks′tră-kă-lis′ē-ăl). Outside of a calix.

ex·tra·cap·su·lar (eks′tră-kap′soo-lăr). Outside of the capsule of a joint.

ex·tra·car·pal (eks-tră-kar′păl). **1.** Outside of, having no relation to, the carpus. **2.** On the outer side of the carpus.

ex·tra·cel·lu·lar (eks-tră-sel′ū-lăr). Outside the cells.

ex·tra·chro·mo·som·al (eks′tră-krō-mō-sōm′ăl). Outside or separated from, a chromosome.

ex·tra·cor·po·re·al (eks′tră-kōr-pō′rē-ăl). Outside of, or unrelated to, the body or any anatomic "corpus."

ex·tra·cor·pus·cu·lar (eks′tră-kōr-pŭs′kū-lăr). Outside the corpuscles, especially the blood corpuscles.

ex·tra·cra·ni·al (eks-tră-krā′nē-ăl). Outside of the cranial cavity.

ex·tract. **1** (ek′strakt). A concentrated preparation of a drug obtained by removing the active constituents of the drug with suitable solvents, evaporating all or nearly all of the solvent, and adjusting the residual mass or powder to the prescribed standard. **2** (ek-strakt′). To remove part of a mixture with a solvent. **3.** To perform extraction. [L. *ex-traho,* pp. *-tractus,* to draw out]

alcoholic e., a solid e. obtained by extracting the alcohol-soluble principles of a drug, followed by the evaporation of the alcohol.

allergenic e., e. (usually containing protein) from various sources, e.g., food, bacteria, pollen, and the like, suspected of specific action in stimulating manifestations of allergy; may be used for skin testing or desensitization. SYN allergic e.

allergic e., SYN allergenic e.

belladonna e., a powdered e. from the leaves and/or roots of *Atropa belladonna;* used to formulate various pharmaceutical dosage forms. Contains the alkaloids of belladonna (atropine and scopolamine) and has been used in the treatment of ulcers, diarrhea, and parkinsonism.

Büchner e., a cell-free e. of yeast, such as was prepared by Eduard and Hans Büchner and observed to catalyze alcoholic fermentation; this observation essentially eliminated "vitalism" as being responsible for biologic chemical reactions and initiated the beginnings of modern biochemistry (enzymology).

equivalent e., a fluidextract of the same strength, weight for weight, as the original drug. SYN valoid.

fluid e., SEE fluidextract.

hydroalcoholic e., a solid e. obtained by extracting the soluble principles of the drug with alcohol and water, followed by evaporation of the solution.

liquid e., SYN fluidextract.

pollen e., liquid obtained by extracting the protein from the pollen of plants used for diagnostic testing or treatment.

ex·tract·ant (ek-strak′tant). An agent used to isolate or extract a substance from a mixture or combination of substances, from the tissues, or from a crude drug.

ex·trac·tion (ek-strak′shŭn). **1.** Luxation and removal of a tooth from its alveolus. **2.** Partitioning of material (solute) into a solvent. **3.** The active portion of a drug; the making of an extract. **4.** Surgical removal by pulling out. **5.** Removal of the fetus from the uterus or vagina at or near the end of pregnancy, either manually or with instruments. **6.** Removal by suction of the product of conception before a menstrual period has been missed. [L. *ex-traho,* pp. *-tractus,* to draw out]

Baker pyridine e., hot pyridine treatment of tissues fixed in dilute Bouin fixative, used to extract phospholipids from tissues as a control in the histochemical staining of this material.

breech e., obstetrical e. of the baby by the buttocks.

partial breech e., assisted breech delivery by the obstetrician with spontaneous delivery of the fetus to the level of the umbilicus.

podalic e., obstetrical e. of the baby by the feet.

serial e., the selective e. of certain deciduous or permanent teeth, or both, during the early years of dental development, usually with the eventual e. of the first, or occasionally the second, premolars, to encourage autonomous adjustment of moderate to severe crowding of anterior teeth; it may or may not require subsequent orthodontic treatment.

spontaneous breech e., delivery of a fetus in the breech presentation without e. by the obstetrician.

total breech e., delivery of a fetus in breech presentation with complete e. of the entire fetal body from the uterus.

ex·trac·tives (ek-strak′tivs). Substances present in vegetable or animal tissue that can be separated by successive treatment with solvents and recovered by evaporation of the solution.

ex·trac·tor (ek-strak′ter, tōr). Instrument for use in drawing or pulling out any natural part, as a tooth, or a foreign body.

vacuum e., device for producing traction upon the head of a fetus by means of a soft cup held by a vacuum.

ex·tra·cys·tic (eks-tră-sis′tik). Outside of, or unrelated to, the gallbladder or urinary bladder or any cystic tumor.

ex·tra·du·ral (eks-tră-doo′răl). **1.** On the outer side of the dura mater. **2.** Unconnected with the dura mater.

ex·tra·em·bry·on·ic (eks′tră-em-brē-on′ik). Outside the embryonic body; e.g., those membranes involved with the embryo's protection and nutrition which are discarded at birth without being incorporated in its body.

ex·tra·ep·i·phy·si·al (eks′tră-ep-i-fiz′ē-ăl). Not relating to, or connected with, an epiphysis.

ex·tra·gen·i·tal (eks′tră-jen′i-tăl). Outside of, away from, or unrelated to, the genital organs.

ex·tra·he·pat·ic (eks-tră-he-pat′ik). Outside of, or unrelated to, the liver.

ex·tra·lig·a·men·tous (eks-tră-lig-ă-men′tŭs). Outside of, or unconnected with, a ligament.

ex·tra·mal·le·o·lus (eks-tră-mal-ē′ŏ-lŭs). SYN lateral *malleolus.*

ex·tra·med·ul·lary (eks-tră-med′ū-lār-ē). Outside of, or unrelated to, any medulla, especially the medulla oblongata.

ex·tra·mi·to·chon·dri·al (eks-tră-mī-tō-kon′drē-al). Outside of the mitochondria.

ex·tra·mu·ral (eks-tră-mū′răl). Outside, not in the substance of, the wall of a part. [extra- + L. *murus,* wall]

ex·tra·ne·ous (eks-tră′nē-ŭs). Outside of the organism and not belonging to it. [L. *extraneus*]

ex·tra·nu·cle·ar (eks-tră-noo′klē-er). Located outside, or not involving, a cell nucleus.

ex·tra·oc·u·lar (eks-tră-ok′ū-lăr). Adjacent to but outside the eyeball.

ex·tra·o·ral (eks-tră-ō′răl). Outside of the oral cavity; external to the oral cavity. In its usual use it also includes anything external to the lips and cheeks.

ex·tra·ov·u·lar (eks-tră-ov′ū-lăr, -ōv′ū-lăr). Outside the egg; existence after hatching from the egg, as in reptiles and birds.

ex·tra·pap·il·lary (eks-tră-pap′i-lā-rē). Unconnected with any papillary structure.

ex·tra·pa·ren·chy·mal (eks′tră-pă-reng′kī-măl). Unrelated to the parenchyma of an organ.

ex·tra·per·i·ne·al (eks-tră-per-i-ne′al). Not connected with the perineum.

ex·tra·per·i·os·te·al (eks-tră-per-ē-os′tē-ăl). Not connected with, or unrelated to, the periosteum.

ex·tra·per·i·to·ne·al (eks-tră-per-i-tō-nē′ăl). Outside of the peritoneal cavity.

ex·tra·phys·i·o·log·ic (eks′tră-fiz-ē-ō-loj′ik). Outside of the domain of physiology; more than physiologic, therefore pathologic.

ex·tra·pla·cen·tal (eks-tră-pla-sen′tăl). Unrelated to the placenta.

ex·tra·pros·tat·ic (eks-tră-pros-tat′ik). Outside of, or independent of, the prostate.

ex·tra·psy·chic (eks-tră-fiz′ik). Denoting the psychological dynamics that occur in the mind in association with the individual's exchanges with other persons or events. Cf. intrapsychic.

ex·tra·pul·mo·nary (eks-tră-pŭl′mō-nār-ē). Outside of, or having no relation to, the lungs.

ex·tra·py·ram·i·dal (eks-tră-pi-ram′i-dăl). Other than the pyramidal tract. SEE extrapyramidal motor *system.*

ex·tra·sen·so·ry (eks-tră-sen′sōr-ē). Outside or beyond the ordinary senses; not limited to the senses, as in extrasensory *perception.*

ex·tra·se·rous (eks-tră-sē′rŭs). Outside a serous cavity.

ex·tra·so·mat·ic (eks-tră-sō-mat′ik). Outside of, or unrelated to, the body.

ex·tra·sys·to·le (eks′tră-sis′tō-lē). A nonspecific word for an ectopic beat from any source in the heart. SYN premature beat, premature systole.

atrial e., premature complex of the heart arising from an ectopic atrial focus. SYN auricular e.

atrioventricular e., SYN junctional e.

auricular e., SYN atrial e.

interpolated e., a ventricular or atrial e. which, instead of being

followed by a compensatory or noncompensatory pause, is sandwiched between two consecutive sinus cycles.

junctional e., a premature beat arising from the AV junction and leading to a simultaneous or almost simultaneous contraction of atria and ventricles. SYN atrioventricular e.

return e., a form of reciprocal rhythm in which the impulse having arisen in the ventricle ascends toward the atria, but before reaching the atria is reflected back to the ventricles to produce a second ventricular contraction.

supraventricular e., an e. arising from a center above the ventricle, i.e., arising from the atrium or AV junction.

ventricular e., a premature ventricular complex.

ex·tra·tar·sal (eks-tră-tar′săl). **1.** Outside, having no relation to, the tarsus. **2.** On the outer side of the tarsus.

ex·tra·tra·che·al (eks-tră-trā′kē-ăl). Outside of the trachea.

ex·tra·tub·al (eks-tră-too′băl). Outside of any tube; specifically, not in the auditory (eustachian) or uterine (fallopian) tubes.

ex·tra·u·ter·ine (eks-tră-ū′ter-in). Outside of the uterus.

ex·tra·vag·i·nal (eks-tră-vaj′i-năl). Outside of the vagina.

ex·trav·a·sate (eks-trav′ă-sāt). **1.** To exude from or pass out of a vessel into the tissues, said of blood, lymph, or urine. **2.** The substance thus exuded. SYN extravasation (2), suffusion (4). [L. *extra,* out of, + *vas,* vessel]

ex·trav·a·sa·tion (eks-trav′ă-sā′shŭn). **1.** The act of extravasating. **2.** SYN extravasate (2). [extra- + L. *vas,* vessel]

ex·tra·vas·cu·lar (eks-tră-vas′kū-lăr). Outside of the blood vessels or lymphatics or of any special blood vessel.

ex·tra·ven·tric·u·lar (eks-tră-ven-trik′ū-lăr). Outside of any ventricle, especially of one of the ventricles of the heart.

ex·tra·ver·sion (eks-tră-ver′zhŭn, -shŭn). SYN extroversion.

ex·tra·vert (eks′-tră-vert). SYN extrovert.

ex·tra·vi·su·al (ek-stră-vizh′oo-ăl). Outside the field of vision, or beyond the visible spectrum.

ex·trem·i·tal (eks-trem′i-tăl). Relating to an extremity. SEE ALSO distal.

ex·trem·i·tas (eks-trem′i-tas) [TA]. SYN extremity. SEE limb. [L. fr. *extremus,* last, outermost]

e. acromia′lis clavic′ulae [TA], SYN acromial *end* of clavicle.

e. ante′rior splenica [TA], SYN anterior *extremity* of spleen.

e. infe′rior [TA], SYN inferior *pole.*

e. infe′rior ren′is [TA], SYN inferior *pole* of kidney.

e. infe′rior tes′tis [TA], SYN lower *pole* of testis.

e. poste′rior splenica [TA], SYN posterior *extremity* of spleen.

e. sterna′lis clavic′ulae [TA], SYN sternal *end* of clavicle.

e. supe′rior [TA], SYN superior *pole.*

e. supe′rior ren′is [TA], SYN superior *pole* of kidney.

e. supe′rior tes′tis [TA], SYN upper *pole* of testis.

e. tuba′ria ovar′ii [TA], SYN tubal *extremity* of ovary.

e. uteri′na ovar′ii [TA], SYN uterine *extremity* of ovary.

ex·trem·i·ty (eks-trem′i-tē) [TA]. One of the ends of an elongated or pointed structure. Incorrectly used to mean limb. SEE ALSO limb, end, pole. SYN extremitas [TA].

acromial e. of clavicle, SYN acromial *end* of clavicle.

anterior e. of caudate nucleus, SYN *head* of caudate nucleus.

anterior e. of spleen [TA], the anterior end of the spleen (extremitas anterior splenis [NA]). SYN extremitas anterior splenica [TA].

inferior e., (1) ☆official alternate term for inferior *pole;* **(2)** incorrectly, but commonly used for lower *limb.*

inferior e. of kidney, ☆official alternate term for inferior *pole* of kidney.

lower e., SYN lower *limb.*

posterior e. of spleen [TA], the posterior end of the spleen (extremitas posterior splenis [NA]). SYN extremitas posterior splenica [TA].

sternal e. of clavicle, SYN sternal *end* of clavicle.

superior e., (1) ☆official alternate term for superior *pole;* **(2)** incorrectly, but commonly used term for upper *limb.*

superior e. of kidney, ☆official alternate term for superior *pole* of kidney.

ex

tubal e. of ovary [TA], the rounded lateral end of the ovary, usually directed toward the infundibulum of the uterine tube. SYN extremitas tubaria ovarii [TA], lateral pole.

upper e., SYN upper *limb*.

upper e. of fibula, SYN *head* of fibula.

uterine e. of ovary [TA], the rounded medial end of the ovary, usually directed toward the uterus. SYN extremitas uterina ovarii [TA], medial pole of ovary.

ex·trin·sic (eks-trin′sik). Originating outside of the part where found or upon which it acts; denoting especially a muscle, such as extrinsic muscles of hand. [L. *extrinsecus,* from without]

ex·tro·gas·tru·la·tion (eks′trō-gas-troo-lā′shŭn). Evagination of the primitive gut material during gastrulation instead of the normal invagination, as the result of some natural or experimental manipulation of the developing embryo or its environment.

ex·tro·ver·sion (eks′trō-ver′zhŭn, -shŭn). **1.** A turning outward. **2.** A trait involving social intercourse, as practiced by an extrovert. Cf. introversion. SYN extraversion. [incorrectly formed fr. L. *extra,* outside, + *verto,* pp. *versus,* to turn]

ex·tro·vert (eks′trō-vert). A gregarious person whose chief interests lie outside the self, and who is socially self-confident and involved in the affairs of others. Cf. introvert. SYN extravert.

ex·trude (eks-trood′). To thrust, force, or press out.

ex·tru·sion (eks-troo′zhŭn). **1.** A thrusting or forcing out of a normal position. **2.** The overeruption or migration of a tooth beyond its normal occlusal position.

e. of a tooth, elongation of a tooth; movement of a tooth in an occlusal or incisal direction.

ex·tu·bate (eks′too-bāt). To remove a tube.

ex·tu·ba·tion (eks′too-bā′shŭn). Removal of a tube from an organ, structure, or orifice; specifically, removal of the tube after intubation. [L. *ex,* out, + *tuba,* tube]

ex·u·ber·ant (ek-zoo′ber-ănt). Denoting excessive proliferation or growth, as of a tissue or granulation. [L. *exubero,* to abound, be abundant]

ex·u·date (eks′oo-dāt). Any fluid that has exuded out of a tissue or its capillaries, more specifically because of injury or inflammation (e.g., peritoneal pus in peritonitis, or the e. that forms a scab over a skin abrasion) in which case it is characteristically high in protein and white blood cells. Cf. transudate. SYN exudation (2). [L. *ex,* out, + *sudo,* to sweat]

ex·u·da·tion (eks-oo-dā′shŭn). **1.** The act or process of exuding. **2.** SYN exudate.

ex·ud·a·tive (eks-oo′dă-tiv). Relating to the process of exudation or to an exudate.

ex·ude (ek-zood′). In general, to ooze or pass gradually out of a body structure or tissue; more specifically, restricted to a fluid or semisolid that so passes and may become encrusted or infected, because of injury or inflammation. [L. *ex,* out, + *sudo,* to sweat]

ex·ul·cer·ans (eks-ŭl′ser-anz). Ulcerating.

ex·um·bil·i·ca·tion (eks′ŭm-bil-i-kā′shŭn). **1.** SYN exomphalos (1). **2.** SYN umbilical *hernia*. **3.** SYN omphalocele. [L. *ex,* out, + *umbilicus,* navel]

ex vi·vo (ex vē′vō). Referring to the use or positioning of a tissue or cell after removal from an organism while the tissue or cells remain viable. [L. from the living]

■eye (ī) [TA]. **1.** The organ of vision that consists of the eyeball and the optic nerve; SYN oculus [TA]. **2.** The area of the eye, including lids and other accessory organs of the eye; the contents of the orbit (common). [A.S. *ēage*]

amaurotic cat e., a yellow reflex from the pupil in cases of retinoblastoma or pseudoglioma.

aphakic e., the e. from which the lens is absent.

artificial e., a curved disk of opaque glass or plastic, containing an imitation iris and pupil in the center, inserted beneath the eyelids and supported by the orbital contents after evisceration or enucleation; it may be ready-made (stock) or custom-made.

black e., ecchymosis of the lids and their surroundings.

blear e., blepharitis accompanied by a viscid discharge that tends to cause the lid edges to cling together. SYN lippitude, lippitudo.

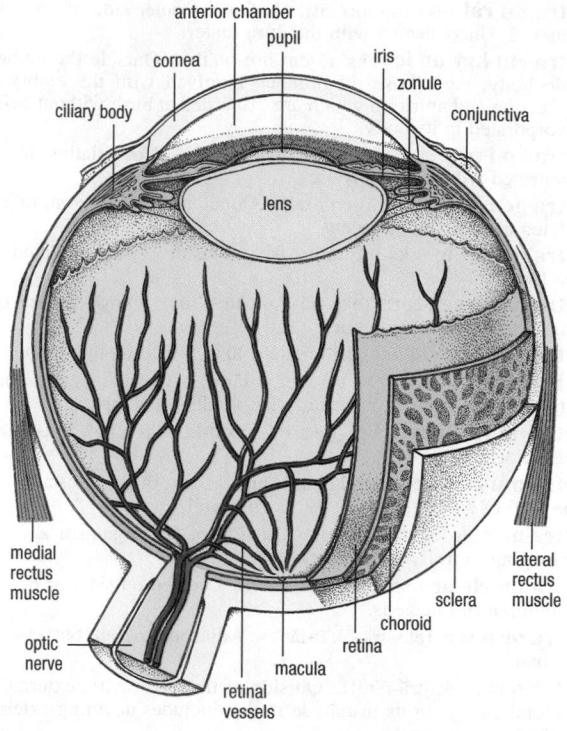

eye

bleary e., sore, runny, watery e. with an associated lackluster appearance and, by extension, dimness of vision.

compound e., the eye of arthropods, most highly developed in insects and crustaceans; the e. consists of a group of functionally related visual elements (ommatidia) whose corneal surfaces collectively form a segment of a sphere.

crossed e.'s, SYN strabismus.

cyclopian e., cyclopean e., SEE cyclopia.

dark-adapted e., an e. that has been in darkness or semidarkness and has undergone regeneration of rhodopsin (visual purple), which renders it more sensitive to reduced illumination. SYN scotopic e.

dominant e., the e. that is customarily used for monocular tasks. SYN master e.

epiphysial e., SYN pineal e.

exciting e., the injured e. in sympathetic ophthalmia.

fixing e., the e., in cases of strabismus, that is directed toward the object of regard.

hare's e., SYN lagophthalmia.

light-adapted e., an e. that has been exposed to light, with bleaching of rhodopsin (visual purple) and insensitivity to low illumination. SYN photopic e.

Listing reduced e., a representation that simplifies calculations of retinal imagery: radius of anterior refracting surface, 5.1 mm; total length, 20 mm; distance of nodal point to retina, 15 mm.

master e., SYN dominant e.

parietal e., SYN pineal e.

phakic e., an e. containing the natural lens.

photopic e., SYN light-adapted e.

pineal e., a non–image-forming, photoreceptive e. in or near the median line in certain crustacea and lower vertebrates; homologue of pineal gland in higher forms. SYN epiphysial e., parietal e.

raccoon e.'s, bilateral ecchymosis in the periorbital region; suggests a basilar skull fracture and may also be seen in neuroblastoma. SYN bilateral medial orbital ecchymoses.

reduced e., a simplified design of the ocular optical system, represented as having a single refracting surface and a uniform index of refraction; a model based on this concept is used in retinoscopy and ophthalmoscopy.

schematic e., the representation of the optical system of an ideal normal eye in which are listed the curvatures and indices of refraction of the refracting elements and their intervening distances.

scotopic e., SYN dark-adapted e.

shipyard e., SYN epidemic keratoconjunctivitis *virus*.

squinting e., the e., in cases of strabismus, that is not directed toward the object of regard.

accommodation of eye	
age-related decrease in accommodative power (in diopters [Δ]) for persons with normal vision	
8 years – 13.8 Δ	40 years – 5.8 Δ
16 years – 12.0 Δ	48 years – 2.5 Δ
24 years – 10.2 Δ	56 years – 1.25 Δ
32 years – 8.2 Δ	64 years – 1.1 Δ

sympathizing e., the uninjured e. in sympathetic ophthalmia that becomes involved later in the disease process.

watery e., (1) SYN epiphora; **(2)** excessive lacrimation.

web e., SYN pterygium (1).

eye·ball (ī′bawl) [TA]. The eye proper without the appendages. SYN bulbus oculi [TA], bulb of eye, globe of eye.

eye bank. A place where corneas of eyes removed after death are preserved for subsequent keratoplasty.

eye·brow [TA]. The crescentic line of hairs at the superior edge of the orbit. SYN supercilium.

eye·glass·es. SYN spectacles.

eye·grounds (ī′growndz). The fundus of the eye as seen with the ophthalmoscope.

eye·lash. One of the stiff hairs projecting from the margin of the eyelid. SYN cilium (1).

ectopic e., the condition in which the e.'s grow from the eyelid at a site other than the lid margin. SYN canities poliosis.

piebald e., an isolated bundle of white e.'s among normally pigmented e.'s. SYN canities circumscripta, ciliary poliosis.

eye·lid [TA]. One of the two movable folds covering the front of the eyeball when closed; formed of a fibrous core (tarsal plate) and the palpebral portions of the orbicularis oculi muscle covered with skin on the superficial, anterior surface and lined with conjunctiva on the deep, posterior surface; rapid contraction of the contained muscle fibers produces blinking; they each have fixed (orbital) and free margins, the latter separated centrally by the palpebral fissure, united at the lateral and medial palpebral commissures, and bearing eyelashes, the openings of tarsal and ciliary glands and (medially) the lacrimal puncta. SYN palpebra [TA], blepharon, lid.

inferior e. [TA], the inferior, smaller and less mobile of the two e.'s; a check ligament from the inferior rectus muscle extends into it, pulling the lid inferiorly when the gaze is directed downward. SYN palpebra inferior [TA], lower e.☆, lower lid.

lower e., ☆official alternate term for inferior e.

superior e. [TA], the superior, larger and more mobile of the two e.'s which covers most of the anterior surface of the eyeball, including the cornea, when closed; a portion of the lacrimal gland and the aponeurosis of the levator palpebrae superioris muscle extend into it, the muscle opening the closed eye and providing additional elevation when the gaze is directed upward. SYN palpebra superior [TA], upper e.☆, upper lid.

third e., SYN *plica* semilunaris of conjunctiva (2).

upper e., ☆official alternate term for superior e.

eye·piece (ī′pēs). The compound lens at the end of the microscope tube nearest the eye; it magnifies the image made by the objective.

eye·spot. **1.** A colored spot or plastid (chromatophore) in a unicellular organism. **2.** SYN ocellus (1).

eye·stone. A small smooth shell or other object that is inserted beneath the eyelid for the purpose of removing a foreign body.

eye·strain. SYN asthenopia.

eye·wash. A soothing solution used for bathing the eye.

F 1. Symbol for fractional concentration, followed by subscripts indicating location and chemical species; Fahrenheit; farad; fertility; visual *field*; fluorine; folate; filial *generation*, followed by subscript numerals indicating specified matings; phenylalanine; variance *ratio*. **2.** Abbreviation for focus (1); French *scale*.

F Symbol for faraday, Faraday *constant*, force; free *energy*.

f Symbol for femto-; respiratory *frequency*; fugacity; formyl; fumarose form (usually following the symbol for the monosaccharide).

F.A.A.N. Abbreviation for Fellow of the American Academy of Nursing.

FAB Abbreviation for French-American-British (classification of acute leukemias). SEE FAB *classification*.

Fab. SEE Fab *fragment*.

fa·bel·la (fa-bel′lă). A sesamoid bone in the tendon of the lateral head of the gastrocnemius muscle. [Mod. L. dim. of *faba,* bean]

Faber, Knud H., Danish physician, 1862–1956. SEE F. *anemia, syndrome*.

fa·bism (fā′bizm). SYN favism. [L. *faba,* bean]

fab·ri·ca·tion (fab-ri-kā′shŭn). Telling false tales as true; e.g., the malingering of symptoms or illness or feigning an incorrect response or calculation during a psychological or mental status examination.

Fabricius (Fabrizzi), Girolamo (Hieronymus ab Aquapendente), Italian anatomist and embryologist, 1537–1619. SEE *bursa* fabricii; F. *ship*.

Fabry, Johannes, German dermatologist, 1860–1930. SEE F. *disease*.

F.A.C.C.P. Abbreviation for Fellow of the American College of Chest Physicians.

F.A.C.D. Abbreviation for Fellow of the American College of Dentists.

face (fās) [TA]. **1.** The front portion of the head; the visage including eyes, nose, mouth, forehead, cheeks, and chin; excludes ears. SYN facies (1) [TA]. **2.** SYN surface.

bird f., SYN brachygnathia.

cow f., SYN *facies* bovina.

dish f., SYN *facies* scaphoidea.

frog f., the appearance caused by broadening of the nose, which occurs in certain cases of nasal polyps.

hippocratic f., SYN hippocratic *facies*.

masklike f., SYN Parkinson *facies*.

moon f., the round, usually red face, with large jowls, seen in Cushing disease or in exogenous hyperadrenocorticalism.

moon shaped f., moon *facies*.

superolateral f. of cerebral hemisphere [TA], SYN superolateral *surface* of cerebrum.

face-bow. A caliper-like device used to record the relationship of the jaws to the temporomandibular joints; the record may then be used to orient a cast or model of the maxilla to the opening and closing axis of the articulator. SYN hinge-bow.

adjustable axis f., a f. whose caliper ends can be adjusted to permit location of the axis of rotation of the mandible. SYN kinematic f.

kinematic f., SYN adjustable axis f.

face-lift. SYN rhytidectomy.

fac·et, fa·cette (fas′et, fă-set′) [TA]. **1.** A small smooth area on a bone or other firm structure. **2.** A worn spot on a tooth, produced by chewing or grinding. [Fr. *facette*]

acromial f. of clavicle [TA], a small oval facet on the lateral end of the clavicle for articulation with the acromion. SYN facies articularis acromialis claviculae [TA], acromial articular facies of clavicle, acromial articular surface of clavicle.

articular f., a relatively small articular surface of a bone, especially a vertebra.

articular f. of head of fibula [TA], the flat circular surface on the head of the fibula for articulation with the corresponding facet on the lateral condyle of the tibia. SYN facies articularis capitis fibulae [TA].

articular f. of head of rib [TA], an articular surface on the head of a rib that articulates with the body of a vertebra. SYN facies articularis capitis costae [TA].

articular f. of lateral malleolus [TA], the surface on the medial aspect of the lateral malleolus that articulates with the talus. SYN facies articularis malleoli lateralis fibulae [TA], malleolar articular surface of fibula.

articular f. of medial malleolus [TA], the articular facet on the lateral surface of the medial malleolus for articulation with the side of the talus; it is continuous with the inferior articular surface of the tibia. SYN facies articularis malleoli medialis tibiae [TA], malleolar articular surface of tibia.

articular f. of radial head [TA], the depression on the top (superior surface) of the head of the radius for articulation with the capitulum of the humerus. SYN fovea articularis capitis radii [TA], articular pit of head of radius, fovea of radial head.

articular f. of tubercle of rib [TA], an oval facet on the inferomedial part of the tubercle of a rib for articulation with a facet on the transverse process of a vertebra. SYN facies articularis tuberculi costae [TA].

f. (of atlas) for dens [TA], a circular facet on the posterior (inner) surface of the anterior arch of the atlas which articulates with the dens of the axis. SYN fovea dentis atlantis [TA], pit of atlas for dens.

clavicular f., SYN clavicular *notch* of sternum.

clavicular articular f. of acromion [TA], a small oval facet on the medial border of the acromion for articulation with the lateral end of the clavicle. SYN facies articularis clavicularis acromii [TA], articular surface of acromion.

corneal f., a corneal depression following loss of stroma.

costal f.'s, articular surface on a vertebra for articulation with a rib.

fibular articular f. of tibia [TA], the flat circular articular facet on the inferior and lateral aspect of the lateral condyle of the tibia for articulation with the head of the fibula. SYN facies articularis fibularis tibiae [TA], fibular articular surface of tibia.

inferior articular f. of atlas, SYN inferior articular *surface* of atlas.

inferior costal f. [TA], demifacet on the lower edge of the body of a vertebra articulating with the head of a rib. SYN fovea costalis inferior [TA], inferior costal pit.

lateral malleolar f. of talus [TA], that surface of the trochlea of the talus that articulates with the lateral malleolus of the fibula. SYN facies malleolaris lateralis tali [TA], lateral malleolar surface of talus.

Lenoir f., the medial articular surface of the patella.

locked f.'s, SYN *dislocation* of articular processes.

medial malleolar f. of talus [TA], the surface of the trochlea of the talus that articulates with the medial malleolus of the tibia. SYN facies malleolaris medialis tali [TA].

f. (on talus) for calcaneonavicular part of bifurcate ligament [TA], small f. at the lateral edge of the navicular articular surface that lies in contact with the medial surface of the medial part of the bifurcate ligament. SYN facies articularis partis calcaneonavicularis ligamenti bifurcati tali [TA].

f. (on talus) for plantar calcaneonavicular ligament [TA], inferiormost portion of the articular surface of the head of the talus

---

⟲ **Combining Forms**	☆ **Official alternate Terminologia Anatomica term**
🔲 **Indicates term is illustrated, see Illustration Index**	
SYN Synonym	**[MIM]** Mendelian Inheritance in Man
Cf. Compare	**C.I.** Colour Index
[NA] Nomina Anatomica	
[TA] Terminologia Anatomica	**High Profile Term**

that contacts (rests on) the plantar calcaneonavicular ligament. SYN facies ligamenti calcaneonavicularis plantaris tali [TA].

posterior articular f. of dens [TA], the facet on the posterior surface of the dens of the axis that articulates with the transverse ligament of the atlas. SYN facies articularis posterior dentis [TA], posterior articular surface of dens.

sternal f. of clavicle [TA], the oval surface on the sternal end of the clavicle that articulates with the fibrocartilaginous disk of the sternoclavicular joint. SYN facies articularis sternalis claviculae [TA], sternal articular surface of clavicle.

superior articular f. of atlas, SYN superior articular *surface* of atlas.

superior costal f. [TA], a demifacet on the upper edge of the body of a vertebra articulating with the head of a rib; a single rib articulates with the inferior costal f. and superior costal f. of the adjacent vertebrae. SYN fovea costalis superior [TA], superior costal pit.

superior f. of trochlear of talus [TA], the surface of the trochlea of the talus in contact with the inferior articular surface of the tibia. SYN facies superior tali [TA], superior surface of talus.

transverse costal f. [TA], a facet on the transverse process of a vertebra for articulation with the tubercle of a rib. SYN fovea costalis processus transversi [TA], costal pit of transverse process.

fac·e·tec·to·my (fas-ĕ-tek′tō-mē). Excision of a facet. [facet + G. *ektomē,* excision]

fa·cial (fā′shăl). Relating to the face. SYN facialis.

fa·ci·a·lis (fā-shē-ā′lis). SYN facial, facial. [L.]

△**-facient.** Causing; one who or that which brings about. [L. *facio,* to make]

FACIES

fa·ci·es, pl. **fa·ci·es** (fā′shē-ēz, fash′-ēz) [TA]. **1** [TA]. SYN face (1). **2** [NA]. SYN surface. **3.** SYN expression (2). [L.]

acromial articular f. of clavicle, SYN acromial *facet* of clavicle.

adenoid f., the open-mouthed and often dull appearance in children with adenoid hypertrophy, associated with a pinched nose.

f. antebrachia′lis ante′rior, SYN anterior *region* of forearm.

f. antebrachia′lis poste′rior, SYN posterior *region* of forearm.

f. ante′rior [TA], SYN anterior *surface.*

f. ante′rior antebra′chii, SYN anterior *region* of forearm.

f. ante′rior bra′chii, SYN anterior *region* of arm.

f. ante′rior cor′neae [TA], SYN anterior *surface* of cornea.

f. ante′rior cor′poris maxil′lae [TA], SYN anterior *surface* of maxilla.

f. ante′rior cru′ris, SYN anterior *region* of leg.

f. ante′rior glan′dulae suprarena′lis [TA], SYN anterior *surface* of suprarenal gland.

f. ante′rior ir′idis [TA], SYN anterior *surface* of iris.

f. ante′rior latera′lis cor′poris hu′meri, SYN anterolateral *surface* of (shaft of) humerus.

f. ante′rior len′tis [TA], SYN anterior *surface* of lens.

f. ante′rior media′lis cor′poris hu′meri, SYN anteromedial *surface* of shaft of humerus.

f. ante′rior mem′bri inferio′ris [TA], SYN anterior *surface* of lower limb.

f. ante′rior palpebra′rum, SYN anterior surface of eyelids.

f. ante′rior par′tis petro′sae os′sis tempora′lis [TA], SYN anterior *surface* of petrous part of temporal bone.

f. ante′rior patel′lae [TA], SYN anterior *surface* of patella.

f. ante′rior pros′tatae [TA], SYN anterior *surface* of prostate.

f. ante′rior ra′dii [TA], SYN anterior *surface* of radius.

f. ante′rior re′nis [TA], SYN anterior *surface* of kidney.

f. ante′rior ul′nae [TA], SYN anterior *surface* of ulna.

f. anterior uteri [TA], SYN anterior *surface* of uterus.

f. anteroinfe′rior corporis pancrea′tis [TA], SYN anteroinferior *surface* of pancreas.

f. anterolateralis cartilaginis arytenoideae [TA], SYN anterolateral *surface* of arytenoid cartilage.

f. anterolatera′lis cor′poris hu′meri [TA], SYN anterolateral *surface* of (shaft of) humerus.

f. anteromedia′lis cor′poris hu′meri [TA], SYN anteromedial *surface* of shaft of humerus.

f. anterosuperioris corporis pancrea′tis [TA], SYN anterosuperior *surface* of body of pancreas.

f. antoni′na, a facial expression due to alteration in the eyelids and anterior segment of the eye; found in leprosy.

aortic f., the pale sallow complexion of one suffering from incompetence of the aortic valve; nonspecific.

f. approxima′lis de′ntis, SYN approximal *surface* of tooth.

f. articular′is [TA], SYN articular *surface.*

f. articula′ris acromia′lis clavic′ulae [TA], SYN acromial *facet* of clavicle.

f. articula′ris ante′rior den′tis [TA], SYN anterior articular *surface* of dens.

f. articula′ris arytenoi′dea cricoi′deae [TA], SYN arytenoidal articular *surface* of cricoid.

f. articula′ris calca′nea ta′li [TA], SYN calcaneal articular *surface* of talus.

f. articula′ris cap′itis cos′tae [TA], SYN articular *facet* of head of rib.

f. articula′ris cap′itis fib′ulae [TA], SYN articular *facet* of head of fibula.

f. articula′ris car′pi ra′dii [TA], SYN carpal articular *surface* of radius.

f. articula′ris cartila′ginis arytenoi′deae [TA], SYN articular *surface* of arytenoid cartilage.

f. articula′ris clavicularis acro′mii [TA], SYN clavicular articular *facet* of acromion.

f. articula′ris cuboi′dea ossis calca′nei [TA], SYN articular *surface* on calcaneus for cuboid bone.

f. articula′ris fibula′ris tib′iae [TA], SYN fibular articular *facet* of tibia.

f. articula′ris fossae mandibularis os′sis tempora′lis [TA], SYN articular *surface* of mandibular fossa of temporal bone.

f. articula′ris infe′rior atlan′tis [TA], SYN inferior articular *surface* of atlas.

f. articula′ris infe′rior tib′iae [TA], SYN inferior articular *surface* of tibia.

f. articula′ris malle′oli latera′lis fib′ulae [TA], SYN articular *facet* of lateral malleolus.

f. articula′ris malle′oli medialis tib′iae [TA], SYN articular *facet* of medial malleolus.

f. articula′ris navicula′ris ta′li [TA], SYN navicular articular *surface* of talus.

f. articularis partis calcaneonavicularis ligamenti bifurcati tali [TA], SYN *facet* (on talus) for calcaneonavicular part of bifurcate ligament.

f. articula′ris patel′lae [TA], SYN articular *surface* of patella.

f. articula′ris poste′rior den′tis [TA], SYN posterior articular *facet* of dens.

f. articula′ris sterna′lis clavic′ulae [TA], SYN sternal *facet* of clavicle.

f. articula′ris supe′rior atlan′tis [TA], SYN superior articular *surface* of atlas.

f. articula′ris supe′rior tib′iae [TA], SYN superior articular *surface* of tibia.

f. articula′ris talaris ante′rior calcanei [TA], SYN anterior talar articular *surface* of calcaneus.

f. articula′ris tala′ris calca′nei [TA], SYN talar articular *surfaces* of calcaneus, under *surface.*

f. articula′ris talaris media calcanei [TA], SYN middle talar articular *surface* of calcaneus.

f. articularis talaris posterior calca′nei [TA], SYN posterior talar articular *surface* (of calcaneus).

fa

f. articula′ris thyroi′dea cricoi′deae [TA], SYN thyroid articular *surface* of cricoid (cartilage).

f. articula′ris tuber′culi cos′tae [TA], SYN articular *facet* of tubercle of rib.

f. auricula′ris os′sis il′ii [TA], SYN auricular *surface* of ilium.

f. auricula′ris os′sis sac′ri [TA], SYN auricular *surface* of sacrum.

f. bovi′na, the cowlike face of ocular hypertelorism; typical of craniofacial dysostosis. SYN cow face.

f. brachia′lis ante′rior, SYN anterior *region* of arm.

f. brachia′lis poste′rior, SYN posterior *region* of arm.

f. cerebra′lis, SYN cerebral *surface*.

cherubic f., the characteristic child-like f. seen in cherubism; also seen in glycogenosis, particularly type 2.

f. co′lica sple′nis [TA], SYN colic *impression* of spleen.

f. contac′tus den′tis, SYN approximal *surface* of tooth.

Corvisart f., the characteristic f. seen in cardiac insufficiency or aortic regurgitation; a swollen, purplish, cyanotic face with shiny eyes and puffy eyelids; nonspecific.

f. costa′lis [TA], SYN costal *surface*.

f. costa′lis pulmo′nis [TA], SYN costal *surface* of lung.

f. costa′lis scap′ulae [TA], SYN costal *surface* of scapula.

f. crura′lis ante′rior, SYN anterior *region* of leg.

f. crura′lis poste′rior, SYN posterior *region* of leg.

f. cubita′lis ante′rior, SYN anterior *region* of elbow.

f. cubita′lis poste′rior, SYN posterior *region* of elbow.

f. diaphragmat′ica [TA], SYN diaphragmatic *surface*.

f. digita′lis dorsa′lis (manus et pedis) [TA], SYN dorsal *surface* of digit (of hand or foot).

f. digita′lis palma′ris, SYN palmar *surfaces* of fingers, under *surface*.

f. digita′lis planta′ris, SYN plantar *surface* of toe.

f. digita′lis ventra′lis, SYN palmar *surfaces* of fingers, under *surface*.

f. dista′lis den′tis [TA], SYN distal *surface* of tooth.

f. doloro′sa, facial expression of an unhappy person or one sick or in pain.

f. dorsa′lis [TA], SYN dorsal *surface*.

f. dorsa′lis os′sis sac′ri [TA], SYN dorsal *surface* of sacrum.

f. dorsa′lis scap′ulae, SYN posterior *surface* of scapula.

elfin f., f. characterized by a short, upturned nose, wide mouth, widely spaced eyes, and full cheeks; it may be associated with hypercalcemia, supravalvar aortic stenosis, and mental retardation.

f. exter′na [TA], SYN external *surface*.

f. exter′na os′sis fronta′lis [TA], SYN external *surface* of frontal bone.

f. exter′na os′sis parieta′lis [TA], SYN external *surface* of parietal bone.

f. facia′lis den′tis, SYN vestibular *surface* of tooth.

f. femora′lis ante′rior, SYN anterior *region* of thigh.

f. femora′lis poste′rior, SYN posterior *region* of thigh.

f. gas′trica sple′nis [TA], SYN gastric *impression* on spleen.

f. glu′tea os′sis il′ii [TA], SYN gluteal *surface* of ilium.

hippocratic f., f. hippocra′tica, a pinched expression of the face, with sunken eyes, concavity of cheeks and temples, relaxed lips, and leaden complexion; observed in one close to death after severe and prolonged illness. SYN hippocratic face.

hound-dog f., the facial appearance in cutis laxa, with loose facial skin hanging in folds.

Hutchinson f., the peculiar facial expression produced by the drooping eyelids and motionless eyes in external ophthalmoplegia.

f. infe′rior hemispherii cer′ebri [TA], SYN inferior *surface* of cerebellar hemisphere.

f. infe′rior lin′guae [TA], SYN inferior *surface* of tongue.

f. infe′rior par′tis petro′sae os′sis tempora′lis [TA], SYN inferior *surface* of petrous part of temporal bone.

f. inferolatera′lis pros′tatae [TA], SYN inferolateral *surface* of prostate.

f. infratemporalis alaris majoris ossis sphenoidalis [TA], SYN infratemporal *surface* of greater wing of sphenoid.

f. infratempora′lis corporis maxil′lae [TA], SYN infratemporal *surface* of (body of) maxilla.

f. interloba′res pulmo′nis, SYN interlobar *surfaces* of lung, under *surface*.

f. inter′na [TA], SYN internal *surface*.

f. inter′na os′sis fronta′lis [TA], SYN internal *surface* of frontal bone.

f. inter′na os′sis parieta′lis [TA], SYN internal *surface* of parietal bone.

f. intestina′lis u′teri [TA], SYN intestinal *surface* of uterus.

f. latera′lis [TA], SYN lateral *surface*.

f. latera′lis bra′chii, SYN lateral *surface* of arm.

f. latera′lis cru′ris, SYN lateral *surface* of leg.

f. latera′lis dig′iti ma′nus, SYN lateral *surface* of finger.

f. latera′lis dig′iti pe′dis, SYN lateral *surface* of toe.

f. latera′lis fib′ulae, SYN lateral *surface* of fibula.

f. latera′lis mem′bri inferior′is, SYN lateral *surface* of lower limb.

f. latera′lis os′sis zygomat′ici, SYN lateral *surface* of zygomatic bone.

f. latera′lis ova′rii [TA], SYN lateral *surface* of ovary.

f. latera′lis tes′tis [TA], SYN lateral *surface* of testis.

f. latera′lis tib′iae [TA], SYN lateral *surface* of tibia.

leonine f., SYN leontiasis.

f. ligamenti calcaneonavicularis plantaris tali [TA], SYN *facet* (on talus) for plantar calcaneonavicular ligament.

f. lingua′lis den′tis [TA], SYN lingual *surface* of tooth.

f. luna′ta acetab′uli [TA], SYN lunate *surface* of acetabulum.

f. malleola′ris latera′lis ta′li [TA], SYN lateral malleolar *facet* of talus.

f. malleola′ris media′lis ta′li [TA], SYN medial malleolar *facet* of talus.

f. masticato′ria, SYN denture occlusal *surface*.

f. maxilla′ris alaris majoris ossis sphenoidalis [TA], SYN maxillary *surface* of greater wing of sphenoid bone.

f. maxilla′ris os′sis palati′ni, SYN maxillary *surface* of palatine bone.

f. media′lis [TA], SYN medial *surface*.

f. media′lis cartilag′inis arytenoi′deae [TA], SYN medial *surface* of arytenoid cartilage.

f. media′lis dig′iti pe′dis [TA], SYN medial *surface* of toes.

f. media′lis fib′ulae [TA], SYN medial *surface* of fibula.

f. media′lis hemispherii cer′ebri [TA], SYN medial *surface* of cerebral hemisphere.

f. media′lis ova′rii [TA], SYN medial *surface* of ovary.

f. media′lis pulmo′nis, SYN mediastinal *surface* of lung.

f. media′lis tes′tis, SYN medial surface of testis.

f. media′lis tib′iae, SYN medial surface of tibia.

f. media′lis ul′nae, SYN medial surface of ulna.

f. mediastinalis pulmonis [TA], SYN mediastinal *surface* of lung.

f. mesia′lis den′tis [TA], SYN mesial *surface* of tooth.

mitral f., the pink, slightly flushed cheeks of patients with mitral valve disease; nonspecific.

moon f., roundness of the face due to increased fat deposition laterally seen in patients with hyperadrenocorticalism, either of endogenous (e.g., Cushing disease) or exogenous origin, such as the use of cortisone-like drugs as therapy.

myasthenic f., the facial expression in myasthenia gravis, caused by drooping of the eyelids and corners of the mouth, and weakness of the muscles of the face.

myopathic f., facial appearance of some patients with myopathies and with myasthenia gravis, consisting of bilateral ptosis and inability to elevate the corners of the mouth, due to muscle weakness.

f. nasa′lis maxil′lae [TA], SYN nasal *surface* of maxilla.

f. nasa′lis os′sis palati′ni [TA], SYN nasal *surface* of palatine bone.

f. occlusa′lis den′tis [TA], SYN denture occlusal *surface*.

f. orbita′lis [TA], SYN orbital *surface*.

f. palati′na la′minae horizonta′lis os′sis pala′tini [TA], SYN palatine *surface* of horizontal plate of palatine bone.

f. palmares digitorum [TA], SYN palmar *surfaces* of fingers, under *surface*.

f. pancreatica splenica [TA],

Parkinson f., the expressionless or masklike f. characteristic of parkinsonism (1). SYN masklike face.

f. patella′ris fem′oris [TA], SYN patellar *surface* of femur.

f. pelvi′ca os′sis sa′cri [TA], SYN pelvic *surface* of sacrum.

f. poplit′ea fem′oris [TA], SYN popliteal *surface* of femur.

f. poste′rior [TA], SYN posterior *surface*.

f. poste′rior cartilag′inis arytenoi′deae [TA], SYN posterior *surface* of arytenoid cartilage.

f. poste′rior cor′neae [TA], SYN posterior *surface* of cornea.

f. poste′rior corporis hu′meri [TA], SYN posterior *surface* of shaft of humerus.

f. poste′rior cru′ris, SYN posterior *region* of leg.

f. poste′rior fib′ulae [TA], SYN posterior *surface* of fibula.

f. poste′rior glan′dulae suprarena′lis [TA], SYN posterior *surface* of suprarenal gland.

f. poste′rior ir′idis [TA], SYN posterior *surface* of iris.

f. poste′rior len′tis [TA], SYN posterior *surface* of lens.

f. poste′rior mem′bri inferio′ris, SYN posterior *surface* of lower limb.

f. poste′rior palpebra′rum [TA], SYN posterior *surface* of eyelids.

f. poste′rior pancrea′tis [TA], SYN posterior *surface* of pancreas.

f. poste′rior par′tis petro′sae os′sis tempora′lis [TA], SYN posterior *surface* of petrous part of temporal bone.

f. poste′rior pros′tatae [TA], SYN posterior *surface* of prostate.

f. poste′rior ra′dii [TA], SYN posterior *surface* of radius.

f. poste′rior re′nis [TA], SYN posterior *surface* of kidney.

f. posterior scapulae [TA],

f. poste′rior tib′iae [TA], SYN posterior *surface* of tibia.

f. poste′rior ul′nae [TA], SYN posterior *surface* of ulna.

Potter f., characteristic f. seen in bilateral renal agenesis and other severe renal malformations, exhibiting ocular hypertelorism, low-set ears, receding chin, and flattening of the nose. SEE ALSO Potter *syndrome*. SYN Potter disease.

f. pulmona′les cor′dis dextra/sinistra, SYN right/left pulmonary *surfaces* of heart, under *surface*.

f. pulmonales cordis dextra/sinistra,

f. rena′lis glan′dulae suprarena′lis [TA], SYN renal *surface* of suprarenal gland.

f. rena′lis lie′nis, ⭐official alternate term for renal *impression* of spleen.

f. rena′lis sple′nis [TA], SYN renal *impression* of spleen.

f. sacropelvi′na os′sis il′ii [TA], SYN sacropelvic *surface* of ilium.

f. scaphoi′dea, a facial malformation characterized by protuberant forehead, depressed nose and maxilla, and prominent chin. SYN dish face.

f. sternocosta′lis cor′dis [TA], SYN sternocostal *surface* of heart.

f. supe′rior hemisphe′rii cerebel′li, SYN superior *surface* of cerebellar hemisphere.

f. supe′rior ta′li [TA], SYN superior *facet* of trochlear of talus.

f. superolatera′lis hemispherii cer′ebri [TA], SYN superolateral *surface* of cerebrum.

f. symphysia′lis [TA], SYN symphysial *surface* of pubis.

f. tempora′lis [TA], SYN temporal *surface*.

f. urethra′lis pe′nis [TA], SYN urethral *surface* of penis.

f. vesica′lis u′teri [TA], SYN vesical *surface* of uterus.

f. vestibula′ris den′tis [TA], SYN vestibular *surface* of tooth.

f. viscera′lis hep′atis [TA], SYN visceral *surface* of liver.

f. viscera′lis sple′nis [TA], SYN visceral *surface* of the spleen;

SEE ALSO colic *impression* of spleen, gastric *impression* on spleen, renal *impression* of spleen.

fa·cil·i·ta·tion (fă-sil′i-tā′shŭn). Enhancement or reinforcement of a reflex or other nervous activity by the arrival at the reflex center of other excitatory impulses. [L. *facilitas,* fr. *facilis,* easy]

    Wedensky f., the arrival of an impulse at a blocked zone, enhancing the excitability of the nerve beyond the block and indicating that the neuromuscular preparation distal to the block has been changed even though the enhancing stimulus is not conducted through the blocked zone.

fac·ing (fās′ing). A tooth-colored material (usually plastic or porcelain) used to hide the buccal or labial surface of a metal crown to give the outward appearance of a natural tooth.

⬦**facio-.** The face. SEE ALSO prosopo-. [L. *facies*]

fa·ci·o·lin·gual (fā′shē-ō-ling′gwăl). Relating to the face and the tongue, often denoting a paralysis affecting these parts.

facioplasty (fā′shē-ō-plas-tē). Plastic surgery involving the face. [facio- + G. *plastos,* formed]

fa·ci·o·ple·gia (fā′shē-ō-plē′jē-ă). SYN facial *paralysis*. [facio- + G. *plēgē,* a stroke]

F.A.C.N.M. Abbreviation for Fellow of the American College of Nuclear Medicine.

F.A.C.N.P. Abbreviation for Fellow of the American College of Nuclear Physicians.

F.A.C.O.G. Abbreviation for Fellow of the American College of Obstetricians and Gynecologists.

F.A.C.P. Abbreviation for Fellow of the American College of Physicians, or of Prosthodontists.

F.A.C.R. Abbreviation for Fellow of the American College of Radiology.

FACS Abbreviation for fluorescence-activated cell sorter.

F.A.C.S. Abbreviation for Fellow of the American College of Surgeons.

F.A.C.S.M. Abbreviation for Fellow of the American College of Sports Medicine.

F-ac·tin. See under actin.

fac·ti·tious (fak-tish′ŭs). Artificial; self-induced; not naturally occurring. [L. *factitius,* made by art, fr. *facio,* to make]

FACTOR

fac·tor (fak′ter). **1.** One of the contributing causes in any action. **2.** One of the components that by multiplication makes up a number or expression. **3.** SYN gene. **4.** A vitamin or other essential element. **5.** An event, characteristic, or other definable entity that brings about a change in a health condition. **6.** A categoric independent variable, used to identify, by means of numeric codes, membership in a qualitatively identifiable group; for example, overcrowding is a factor in disease transmission. [L. maker, causer, fr. *facio,* to make]

    f. I, in the clotting of blood a f. that is converted to fibrin through the action of thrombin. SEE ALSO fibrinogen.

    f. II, a glycoprotein converted in the clotting of blood to thrombin by factor Xa, platelets, calcium ions, and factor V. SEE ALSO prothrombin.

    f. IIa, SYN thrombin.

    f. III, in the clotting of blood, tissue f. or thromboplastin; it initiates the extrinsic pathway by reacting with f. VII and calcium to form f. VIIa. SEE thromboplastin.

    f. IV, in the clotting of blood, calcium ions.

    f. V, in the clotting of blood, also known as: proaccelerin (Owren), labile or plasma labile f. (Quick), plasma accelerator globulin (Ware and Seegars), thrombogene (Nolf), prothrombokinase (Milstone), plasmin prothrombins conversion f. (Stefanini), component A of prothrombin (Quick), prothrombin accelerator

(Fantl and Nance), cofactor of thromboplastin (Honorato), and accelerator f. F. V does not have enzymatic action itself but participates in the common pathway of coagulation by binding f. Xa to platelet surfaces. Deficiency of this f. leads to a rare hemorrhagic tendency known as parahemophilia or hypoproaccelerinemia, with autosomal recessive inheritance; heterozygous individuals are recognized by reduced levels of f. V but have no bleeding tendency. SYN accelerator f., labile f., plasma accelerator globulin, plasma labile f., plasmin prothrombins conversion f., proaccelerin, prothrombokinase, thrombogene.

f. V_{1a}, SYN cobyric acid.

f. V_a, in the clotting of blood, accelerin.

f. VII, in the clotting of blood, also known as: proconvertin (Owren), convertin, serum prothrombin conversion accelerator (de Vries, Alexander), stable f. (Stefanini), cofactor V (Owren), prothrombinogen (Quick), cothromboplastin (Mann and Hurn), serum accelerator (Jacox). F. VII forms a complex with tissue thromboplastin and calcium to activate f. X. F. VII is known to be involved in: 1) the congenital deficiency of f. VII, with purpura and bleeding from mucous membranes, autosomal recessive inheritance; 2) the acquired deficiency of f. VII in association with a deficiency of vitamin K, the neonatal period, and the administration of prothrombinopenic drugs; 3) the acquired excess of f. VII in some patients with thromboembolism. It accelerates the conversion of prothrombin to thrombin, in the presence of tissue thromboplastin, calcium, and f. V. SYN proconvertin, prothrombinogen, stable f.

f. VIII, in the clotting of blood, also known as: antihemophilic f. A (Brinkhous), antihemophilic globulin (1) (Patek and Taylor), antihemophilic globulin A (Cramer), plasma thromboplastin f. (Ratnoff), plasma thromboplastin f. A (Aggeler), thromboplastic plasma component (Shinowara), thromboplastinogen (Quick), prothrombokinase (Feissly), platelet cofactor (Johnson), plasmokinin (Laki), thrombokatilysin (Leggenhager), and proserum prothrombin conversion accelerator. F. VIII participates in the clotting of the blood by forming a complex with f. IXa, platelets, and calcium and enzymatically catalyzing the activation of f. X. Deficiency of f. VIII is associated with classic hemophilia A. **F. VIII:C** is the coagulant component of f. VIII which, in normal persons, circulates in the plasma complexed with **f. VIIIR** (von Willebrand f.), the plasma f. VIII–related protein, a large glycoprotein component that is synthesized by endothelial cells and megakaryocytes, and circulates in the plasma where it binds to arteries that have lost their endothelial cell linings, creating a surface to which platelets adhere. Disorders involving f. VIIIR form a heterogenous group of abnormalities called von Willebrand disease. A deficiency of f. can lead to impaired blood coagulation. SYN antihemophilic f. A, antihemophilic globulin A, antihemophilic globulin (1), plasma thromboplastin f., platelet cofactor I, prothrombokinase.

f. IX, in the clotting of blood, also known as: Christmas f. (Biggs and Macfarlane), plasma thromboplastin component (Aggeler), antihemophilic globulin B (Cramer), plasma thromboplastin f. B (Aggeler), plasma f. X (Shulman), antihemophilic f. B, and platelet cofactor II. F. IX is required for the formation of intrinsic blood thromboplastin and affects the amount formed (rather than the rate). Its active form, f. IXa (EC 3.4.21.22) is a serine proteinase converting f. X to f. Xa by cleaving an arginine-isoleucine bond. Deficiency of f. IX causes hemophilia B. SYN antihemophilic f. B, antihemophilic globulin B, Christmas f., plasma f. X, plasma thromboplastin component, plasma thromboplastin f. B, platelet cofactor II.

f. X, in the clotting of blood, also known as: Stuart f., Stuart-Prower f., prothrombase, and prothrombinase. Its active form, f. Xa (EC 3.4.21.6), is formed from f. X by limited proteolysis and assists in the conversion of prothrombin to thrombin. A deficiency of f. X will lead to impaired blood coagulation. SYN prothrombinase, Stuart f., Stuart-Prower f.

f. X for *Haemophilus*, SYN hemin.

f. XI, in the clotting of blood, also known as plasma thromboplastin antecedent, a component of the contact system which is absorbed from plasma and serum by glass and similar surfaces. Its active form, f. XIa (EC 3.4.21.27), is a serine proteinase converting f. IX to f. IXa. Deficiency of f. XI results in a hemorrhagic

tendency and is caused by an autosomal recessive gene. SYN plasma thromboplastin antecedent.

f. XII, in the clotting of blood, also known as glass f. and Hageman f. When activated by glass or otherwise to its active form, f. XIIa (EC 3.4.21.38), a serine proteinase, it activates f.'s VII and XI and converts f. XI to its active form, f. XIa. Deficiency of f. XII results in great prolongation of the clotting time of venous blood, but only rarely in a hemorrhagic tendency; deficiency is caused by an autosomal recessive gene. SYN glass f., Hageman f.

f. XIII, in the clotting of blood, also known as: fibrin-stabilizing f., Laki-Lorand f., and L-L f. It is catalyzed by thrombin into its active form, f. XIIIa, which cross-links subunits of the fibrin clot to form insoluble fibrin. SYN fibrin-stabilizing f., L-L f., Laki-Lorand f.

f. 3, (1) operational name given to an incompletely characterized selenium-containing natural product which, in minute amounts, prevents liver damage in rats due to deficiency of vitamin E; **(2)** f. III in the vitamin B_{12} series, 5-hydroxybenzimidazole, analogue of the usual B_{12} nucleotide components.

ABO f.'s, see Blood Groups appendix.

accelerator f., SYN f. V.

acetate replacement f., SYN lipoic acid.

adrenal weight f., a postulated substance of adenohypophysial origin responsible for maintenance of the weight of the adrenal cortex.

adrenocorticotropic releasing f., hormone produced by hypothalamus that causes pituitary to secrete adrenocorticotropic hormone.

angiogenesis f., a substance of 2000–20,000 MW which is secreted by macrophages and stimulates neovascularization in healing wounds or in the stroma of tumors.

animal protein f. (APF), SYN *vitamin* B_{12}.

antialopecia f., SYN inositol.

antianemic f., SYN *vitamin* B_{12}.

antiangiogenesis f., one of several molecules capable of inhibiting angiogenesis.

antiberiberi f., SYN thiamin.

anti–black-tongue f., SYN nicotinic acid.

anticomplementary f., a f. that interferes with the action or function of its complement.

antidermatitis f., SYN pantothenic acid.

antihemophilic f. A (AHF), SYN f. VIII.

antihemophilic f. B, SYN f. IX.

antihemorrhagic f., SYN *vitamin* K.

antineuritic f., SYN thiamin.

antinuclear f. (ANF), a f., usually antibodies, present in serum with strong affinity for certain nuclear proteins and detected by fluorescent antibody technique; present in lupus erythematosus, rheumatoid arthritis, and certain other autoimmune conditions; may also be present at lower levels in normal individuals.

antipellagra f., SYN nicotinic acid.

antipernicious anemia f. (APA), (1) SYN *vitamin* B_{12}; **(2)** specifically, cyanocobalamin.

antisterility f., SYN *vitamin* E (2).

atrial natriuretic f. (ANF), an early name given to a natriuretic f. derived from cardiac atria. Because the f. is now known to be a peptide, the term is no longer used.

f. B, SEE *complement* pathways.

B_T f., SYN carnitine.

bacteriocin f.'s, SYN bacteriocinogenic *plasmids*, under *plasmid*.

B cell differentiating f., SYN interleukin-4.

B cell differentiation/growth f.'s, various substances, usually obtained from the supernatant of T cell cultures, such as interleukin 4, 5, and 6. These substances are necessary for B cell growth, maturation, and differentiation into plasma cells or B memory cells.

B cell stimulatory f. 2, SYN interleukin-6.

bifidus f., an unidentified substance associated with *Lactobacillus bifidus* subsp. *pennsylvanicus*, present in mammalian milk.

biotic f.'s, environmental f.'s or influences resulting from the activities of living organisms, as contrasted to those resulting from climatic, geological, or other f.'s.

Bittner milk f., SYN mammary tumor *virus* of mice.

branching f., 1,4-α-glucan-branching enzyme.

C f.'s, SYN coupling f.'s.

CAMP f., SEE CAMP *test*.

capillary permeability f., SYN *vitamin P*.

Castle intrinsic f., SYN intrinsic f.

Christmas f., SYN f. IX.

citrovorum f. (CF), SYN folinic acid.

clearing f.'s, lipoprotein lipases that appear in plasma during lipemia and catalyze hydrolysis of triglycerides only when the latter are bound to protein and when an acceptor (e.g., serum albumin) is present, thus "clearing" the plasma.

clotting f., any of the various plasma components involved in the clotting process. SYN coagulation f.

coagulation f., SYN clotting f.

cobra venom f., a component of cobra venom that can activate the alternative pathway of complement.

coenzyme f., SYN dihydrolipoamide dehydrogenase.

colony-stimulating f.'s (CSF), a group of glycoprotein growth f.'s regulating differentiation of myeloid cells. These substances act in either paracrine or autocrine fashion on marrow cells, appear to act synergistically in complex and poorly understood ways; each appears to have the ability to exert action on several lines of progenitor cells, and to influence end cell function.

complement chemotactic f., the activated complex of the fifth, sixth, and seventh components of complement C 5a, C 3a, C 5b, 6, 7 which induces chemotaxis in the case of polymorphonuclear leukocytes.

complement f. I, a heterodimeric glycoprotein; a deficiency results in uncontrolled activation of C3.

corticotropin-releasing f. (CRF), SYN corticotropin-releasing *hormone*.

coupling f.'s, proteins that restore phosphorylating ability to mitochondria that have lost it, i.e., have become "uncoupled" so that oxidation and electron transport no longer produce ATP. Usually termed coupling factor F_1, F_2, etc. SYN C f.'s.

f. D, SEE *complement* pathways.

debranching f.'s, SYN debranching *enzymes*, under *enzyme*.

decapacitation f., a f., postulated to be present in epididymal fluid and seminal plasma, that prevents the capacitation of spermatozoa.

diabetogenic f., rarely used term for a f. in crude extracts of the anterior lobe of the hypophysis that produces degenerative changes in the islet cells of the pancreas and causes permanent diabetes.

diffusing f., SYN hyaluronidase (1).

direct lytic f. of cobra venom, SYN cobrotoxin.

Duran-Reynals permeability f., Duran-Reynals spreading f., SYN hyaluronidase (1).

elongation f., proteins that catalyze the elongation of peptide chains during protein biosynthesis. SYN transfer f. (3).

endothelial relaxing f. (en′dō-thē′li-al), nitric oxide, which functions as a neurotransmitter and is produced by activated macrophages. It is capable of killing tumor cells, parasites, and intracellular bacteria.

endothelium-derived relaxing f. (EDRF), a diffusible substance produced by endothelial cells that cause vascular smooth muscle relaxation; nitric oxide (NO).

eosinophil chemotactic f. of anaphylaxis (ECF-A), a peptide (MW 500 to 600) that is chemotactic for eosinophilic leukocytes and is released from disrupted mast cells.

epidermal growth f. (EGF), a heat-stable antigenic protein isolated from the submaxillary glands of male mice; when injected into newborn animals, it accelerates eyelid opening and tooth eruption, stimulates epidermal growth and keratinization, and, in larger doses, inhibits body growth and hair development and produces fatty livers.

erythrocyte maturation f., SYN *vitamin* B_{12}.

essential food f.'s, those substances required in the diet: certain amino acids and unsaturated fatty acids, vitamins, essential minerals, etc.

extrinsic f., dietary vitamin B_{12}.

fermentation *Lactobacillus casei* **f.,** SYN pteropterin.

fertility f., SYN F *plasmid*.

fibrin-stabilizing f., SYN f. XIII.

filtrate f., former term for pantothenic acid.

Fitzgerald f., SYN high molecular weight *kininogen*.

Flaujeac f., SYN high molecular weight *kininogen*.

Fletcher f., SYN prekallikrein.

G f., (1) the single common variance or f. that is common to (i.e., empirically intercorrelates with) different intelligence tests (general); (2) a substance required for the growth of a specific organism.

glass f., SYN f. XII.

glucose tolerance f., a water-soluble complex containing chromium and nicotinate needed for normal glucose tolerance.

f. Gm, a f. that determines certain of the allotypes of human immunoglobulins; found only on the γ chains of IgG (γ-globulin).

gonadotropin-releasing f., SYN gonadoliberin (1).

granulocyte colony-stimulating f. (G-CSF) (gran′oo-lō-sīt), glycoproteins that are synthesized by a variety of cells that stimulate the production of neutrophils from hematopoietic stem cells. SEE ALSO colony-stimulating f.'s.

granulocyte-macrophage colony-stimulating f. (GM-CSF) (gran′oo-lō-sīt-mak′rō-fāj), a glycoprotein secreted by macrophages or bone stromal cells that functions as a growth factor for myeloid progenitor cells such as granulocytes, macrophages, and eosinophils. SEE ALSO colony-stimulating f.'s.

growth f.'s, natural substances produced by the body (hormones) or obtained from food (vitamins, minerals) that promote growth and development by directing cell maturation and differentiation and by mediating maintenance and repair of tissues; abnormalities in growth factors may be involved in benign and malignant neoplasia.

growth hormone-releasing f. (GHRF, GH-RF), SYN somatoliberin.

f. H, (1) former designation for biotin; (2) vitamin B_{12} analogue or precursor; (3) a glycoprotein that regulates the activity of complement factor C3b; a deficiency results in the lack of inhibition of the alternative hemolytic pathway leading to continuous activation and consumption of factor C3 (hemolytic uremic syndrome).

Hageman f., SYN f. XII.

HG f., SYN glucagon.

histamine-releasing f., a lymphokine produced from antigen-stimulated lymphocytes that induces the release of histamine from basophils.

human antihemophilic f., a lyophilized concentrate of f. VIII, obtained from fresh normal human plasma; used as a hemostatic agent in hemophilia. SYN antihemophilic globulin (2), human antihemophilic fraction.

hyperglycemic-glycogenolytic f. (HGF), SYN glucagon.

impact f., mathematical expression of frequency with which a particular medical journal's original articles are cited in other medical journals.

inhibition f., SYN migration-inhibitory f.

initiation f. (IF), one of several soluble proteins involved in the initiation of protein or RNA synthesis.

insulinlike growth f. (IGF), (formerly termed somatomedin C), is the most important somatomedin for postnatal growth; it is produced in the liver, kidney, muscle, pituitary, the gastrointestinal tract, and chondrocytes. IGF-I is a basic protein (7600 MW) that circulates bound to six distinct IGF binding proteins (IGF-BPs), which increase the half-life of circulating IGF-I to 3–18 h, as compared with the half-life of 20–30 min for unbound hormone. Local tissue generation of IGF-I/SM-C, particularly in bone, may play an important role in growth mediation through its paracrine effects. SYN somatomedins.

intrinsic f. (IF), a relatively small mucoprotein (MW about 50,000) secreted by the neck cell of the gastric glands and re-

fa

quired for adequate absorption of vitamin B_{12} and othe rcobalamins; deficiency results in pernicious anemia. SYN Castle intrinsic f.

f. Inv, obsolete term for Km allotypes on a f. of human immunoglobulins; found on the κ chains.

ischemia-modifying f.'s, various factors that play a role in determining the extent of necrosis with cerebral stroke; these include blood viscosity and osmolality, the blood pressure, and the anatomy of the neck and intracranial arteries.

labile f., SYN f. V.

Lactobacillus bulgaricus **f. (LBF),** SYN pantetheine.

Lactobacillus casei **f.,** SYN folic acid (2).

Laki-Lorand f., SYN f. XIII.

LE f.'s, antinuclear immunoglobulins in plasma of persons with disseminated lupus erythematosus, associated with positive LE tests.

lethal f., SEE genetic *lethal*.

leukemia inhibitory f., a lymphokine that inhibits the migration of neutrophils.

leukocytosis-promoting f., a substance obtained by Menkin from inflammatory exudates; it stimulates leukocytosis.

leukopenic f., a principle obtained by Menkin from inflammatory exudates; it causes leukopenia when injected into normal animals.

lipotropic f., SYN choline.

liver filtrate f., former term for pantothenic acid.

liver *Lactobacillus casei* **f.,** SYN folic acid (2).

L-L f., SYN f. XIII.

luteinizing hormone/follicle-stimulating hormone-releasing f. (LH/FSH-RF), SYN gonadoliberin (2).

luteinizing hormone-releasing f. (LH-RF, LRF), former name for luteinizing hormone-releasing *hormone*.

lymph node permeability f. (LNPF), a substance, released by lymphocytes when stimulated or damaged, that increases capillary permeability and the accumulation of mononuclear cells.

macrophage-activating f. (MAF) (mak′rō-fāj), a primarily $CD4^+$ T cell–derived lymphokine that induces macrophage activation. The major macrophage–activating f. is interferon gamma. In the mouse, interleukin-4 is also an MAF.

macrophage colony-stimulating f. (M-CSF), a glycoprotein growth f. that causes the committed cell line to proliferate and mature into macrophages. SEE ALSO colony-stimulating f.'s.

maize f., SYN zeatin.

mammotropic f., SYN prolactin.

maturation f., SYN *vitamin* B_{12}.

megakaryocyte growth and development f., SYN thrombopoietin.

melanotropin-releasing f. (MRF), SYN melanoliberin.

mesodermal f., a protein that can induce the formation of kidney and muscle primordia in embryos.

migration-inhibitory f. (MIF), a soluble, nondialyzable substance that is produced by sensitized lymphocytes (i.e., lymphocytes from a sensitized animal) when exposed to the specific antigen, and that causes adherence and inhibition of migration of macrophages. SYN inhibition f.

milk f., SYN mammary tumor *virus* of mice.

monocyte-derived neutrophil chemotactic f. (MDNCF), SYN interleukin-8.

mouse antialopecia f., SYN inositol.

müllerian inhibiting f., SYN müllerian inhibiting *substance*.

müllerian regression f., müllerian duct inhibitory f., a nonsteroidal substance of fetal testicular origin that acts unilaterally to inhibit development of the paramesonephric (müllerian) ducts and acts with testosterone to promote development of the vas deferens and related structures.

multicolony-stimulating f. (multi-CSF), SYN interleukin-3.

myocardial depressant f. (MDF), a toxic f. in shock that impairs cardiac contractility; probably a peptide released with underperfusion of the splanchnic area at the release of proteolytic enzymes from the pancreas.

natural killer cell stimulating f., obsolete term for interleukin-12.

nephritic f., a serum protein (possibly an IgG autoantibody), found in some patients with membranoproliferative glomerulonephritis and hypocomplementemia, which, together with the cofactors of the alternate pathway of complement activation, cleaves the third component of complement (C3).

nerve growth f. (NGF), a protein (MW about 26,000) that controls the development of sympathetic postganglionic neurons and possibly also sensory (dorsal root) ganglion cells in mammals; similar, but not identical, factors have been isolated from the venoms of several species of snakes; it has been isolated from the submaxillary glands of male mice, and when injected into newborn animals, sympathetic ganglia become hyperplastic and hypertrophic; stimulates synthesis of nucleic acids and protein.

neural f., a protein that can induce the formation of notochord tissue in embryos.

neutrophil-activating f., SYN interleukin-8.

neutrophil chemotactant f. (noo′trō-fil kē′mō-tak-tant), SYN interleukin-8.

nuclear f.-κB, an transcription f. associated with cytokine production.

osteoclast activating f., a lymphokine that stimulates bone resorption and inhibits bone-collagen synthesis.

ψ f., SYN psi f.

f. P, a chemical (postulated by T. Lewis), formed in ischemic skeletal or cardiac muscle, held to be responsible for the pain of intermittent claudication and angina pectoris. SYN P substance of Lewis.

P f., see P blood group, Blood Groups appendix.

pellagra-preventing f. (p-p f.), SYN nicotinic acid.

plasma labile f., SYN f. V.

plasma thromboplastin f. (PTF), SYN f. VIII.

plasma thromboplastin f. B, SYN f. IX.

plasma f. X, SYN f. IX.

plasmin prothrombins conversion f. (PPCF), SYN f. V.

platelet f. 3, a blood coagulation factor derived from platelets; chemically, a phospholipid lipoprotein that acts with certain plasma thromboplastin f.'s to convert prothrombin to thrombin.

platelet-activating f. (PAF), SYN platelet-aggregating f.

platelet-aggregating f. (PAF), phospholipid mediator of platelet aggregation, inflammation, and anaphylaxis. Produced in response to specific stimuli by a variety of cell types, including neutrophils, basophils, platelets, and endothelial cells. Several molecular species of PAF have been identified which vary in the length of the *O*-alkyl side chain. It is an important mediator of bronchoconstriction. SYN platelet-activating f.

platelet-derived growth f. (PDGF), a f. in platelets that is mitogenic for cells at the site of a wound, e.g., causing endothelial proliferation; cationic glycoprotein mitogen for fibroblasts, smooth muscle cells, and glial cells. Principal f. in serum required for the growth and proliferation of mesenchymal-derived cells in tissue culture.

platelet tissue f., SYN thromboplastin.

p-p f., abbreviation for pellagra-preventing f.

predisposing f.'s, attitudinal, personality, and related f.'s that motivate and guide an individual to take certain health actions.

prolactin-inhibiting f., dopamine, a substance that inhibits secretion of prolactin by the anterior pituitary gland.

properdin f. B, a normal serum protein (MW 95,000) and a component of the properdin system, which combines with C3b to form the C3 convertase of the alternative pathway.

properdin f. D, a normal serum α-globulin (MW about 25,000) required in the properdin system to cleave factor B into Bb and Ba. Bb combines with C3b to form the C3 convertase of the alternative complement pathway.

protein f., the f. (6.25) by which the nitrogen content of a protein is multiplied to give the amount of protein.

psi f., a protein responsible for the specific initiation of the RNA polymerase-catalyzed reaction at the promoter sites of genes. SYN ψ f.

pyruvate oxidation f., SYN lipoic acid.

quality f. (QF), a f. by which absorbed radiation doses are multiplied to obtain, for radiation protection purposes, a quantity that expresses the approximate biologic effectiveness of the absorbed dose. Cf. RBE, relative biologic *effectiveness*.

ρ **f.,** SYN rho f.

R f.'s, SYN resistance *plasmids*, under *plasmid*.

radiation weighting f., in radiation protection, a f. weighting the absorbed dose of radiation of a specific type and energy for its effect on tissue. SEE equivalent *dose*, relative biologic *effectiveness*, quality f.

releasing f. (RF), (1) substances, usually of hypothalamic origin, capable of accelerating the rate of secretion of a given hormone by the anterior pituitary gland; **(2)** f.'s required in the termination phase of either RNA biosynthesis or protein biosynthesis. SYN termination f. SYN liberins, releasing hormone, statins.

resistance f.'s, SYN resistance *plasmids*, under *plasmid*.

resistance-inducing f. (RIF), an agent from normal chick embryos that interferes with multiplication of the avian sarcoma virus, and is a leukosis virus antigenically related to the avian sarcoma virus.

resistance-transfer f., the portion of the plasmid that contain genes that confer resistance to e.g., antibiotics.

Rh f., the antigen of the Rh blood group system. See Blood Groups Appendix. SYN Rhesus f.

Rhesus f., see Blood Groups Appendix. SYN Rh f.

rheumatoid f.'s (RF), antibodies in the serum of individuals with rheumatoid arthritis. These f.'s are autoantibodies of the classes IgM, IgG, and IgA. The most common f. is IgM and is the one usually measured. Rheumatoid f.'s also occur in other autoimmune and certain infectious diseases.

rho f., a termination f. that releases RNA from the DNA template; a bacterial protein that is an ATP-dependent helicase. SYN ρ f.

risk f., a characteristic statistically associated with, although not necessarily causally related to, an increased risk of morbidity or mortality e.g., smoking as a risk f. for heart disease.

σ **f.,** SYN sigma f.

S f., the individual variables, or empirically most minute subclusters of intercorrelations or common variance, found in different intelligence tests (specific).

secretor f., the capacity to secrete antigens of the ABO blood group in saliva and other body fluids, controlled by a pair of allelic genes designated *Se* and *se* (or *S* and *s*), with the *Se* phenotype dominant to *se;* the saliva of genotypes *SeSe* and *Sese* contains the blood group substances A, B, or H found in their erythrocytes; the saliva of nonsecretors (genotype *sese*) contains no blood group substance; tests for ABH secretion are useful in genetic linkage and population studies; the secretor phenomenon is also closely associated with the Lewis blood group.

sex f., SYN F *plasmid*.

sigma f., a f. that inhibits the nonspecific DNA binding of RNA polymerase, as well as helping to identify the starting point of transcription; it promotes attachment of the RNA polymerase to specific initiation sites. SYN σ f.

slow-reacting f. of anaphylaxis (SRF-A), SYN slow-reacting *substance*.

SLR f., *Streptococcus lactis* **R f.,** SYN rhizopterin.

somatotropin release-inhibiting f. (SRIF, SIF), SYN somatostatin.

somatotropin-releasing f. (SRF), SYN somatoliberin.

spreading f., SYN hyaluronidase (1).

stable f., SYN f. VII.

stem cell f., a cytokine that promotes growth and differentiation of hematopoietic stem cells into a variety of cell lineages.

stringent f., the gene product (an enzyme) that is crucial to the cellular response of decreased ribosome production as a result of amino acid starvation. SEE ALSO stringent *response*.

Stuart f., Stuart-Prower f., SYN f. X.

sun protection f. (SPF), the ratio of the minimal ultraviolet dose required to produce erythema with and without a sunscreen; highly effective sunscreens have an SPF of 15 or more.

T-cell growth f., obsolete term for interleukin-2.

T-cell growth f.-1, obsolete term for interleukin-2.

T-cell growth f.-2, obsolete term for interleukin-4.

termination f., SYN releasing f. (2).

testis-determining f. (TDF), the product of a gene on the short arm of the Y chromosome that is responsible for production of testes.

thymic lymphopoietic f., a glycoprotein (MW about 12,000) that has been extracted from thymus; this thymus-produced hormone(s) confers immunological competence on thymus-dependent cells and induces lymphopoiesis.

thyroid-stimulating hormone-releasing f. (TSH-RF), SYN thyroliberin.

thyrotropin-releasing f. (TRF), former name for thyrotropin-releasing *hormone*.

tissue f., SYN thromboplastin.

tissue weighting f., in radiation protection, a f. weighting the equivalent dose in a particular tissue or organ in terms of its relative contribution to the total deleterious effects resulting from uniform irradiation of the whole body. SEE effective *dose*.

transfer f., (1) the transfer gene of a conjugative plasmid, especially of the resistance plasmid; **(2)** a dialyzable extract that is obtained from the leukocytes of a person with a delayed-type sensitivity and that, following injection into the skin of a nonsensitive person, transfers the specific sensitivity to the recipient; **(3)** SYN elongation f.

transforming f., the DNA responsible for bacterial transformation.

transforming growth f.'s (TGF), two polypeptide growth f.'s; TGF-α stimulates growth of many epidermal and epithelial cells and is obtained from conditioned media of transformed or tumor cells; TGF-β is obtained from kidney and platelets and controls proliferation and differentiation in many cell types.

transforming growth f. α **(TGFα),** a cytokine made by tumor and transformed cells that is associated with growth and differentiation. It is also made in normal tissues during embryogenesis and in certain adult tissues.

transforming growth f. β **(TGFβ),** a regulatory cytokine that has multifunctional properties that can enhance or inhibit many cellular functions, including interfering with the production of other cytokines and enhancing collagen deposition. It exists in multiple subtypes and is produced by platelets and macrophages but can be made by many other cell types.

transmethylation f., SYN choline.

tumor angiogenic f. (TAF), a substance released by solid tumors which induces formation of new blood vessels to supply the tumor.

tumor necrosis f. (TNF), SYN cachectin.

tumor necrosis f.-α, a pleiotropic cytokine synthesized widely throughout the female reproductive tract.

tumor necrosis f.-β, a cytokine that is produced by CD4 and CD8 T cells after exposure to an antigen.

uncoupling f.'s, SYN uncouplers.

von Willebrand f., SEE f. VIII.

W f., SYN biotin.

Williams f., SYN high molecular weight *kininogen*.

fac·to·ri·al (fak-tōr′ē-ăl). **1.** Pertaining to a statistical factor or factors. **2.** Of an integer, that integer multiplied by each smaller integer in succession down to one; e.g., 5! equals $5 \times 4 \times 3 \times 2 \times 1 = 120$.

fac·ul·ta·tive (fak-ŭl-tā′tiv). Able to live under more than one specific set of environmental conditions; possessing an alternative pathway.

fac·ul·ty (fak′ŭl-tē). A natural or specialized power of a living organism.

FAD Abbreviation for *flavin* adenine dinucleotide.

Faget, Jean C., French physician, 1818–1884. SEE F. *sign*.

Fahr, Theodore, German physician, 1877–1945. SEE F. *disease*.

Fahraeus, Robert (Robin) Sanno, Swedish pathologist, 1888–1968. SEE F.-Lindqvist *effect*.

Fahrenheit (F), Gabriel D., German-Dutch physicist, 1686–1736. SEE Fahrenheit *scale.*

fail·ure (fāl′ūr). The state of insufficiency or nonperformance.

backward heart f., a concept (formerly considered mutually exclusive with forward heart f.) that maintains that the phenomena of congestive heart f. result from passive engorgement of the veins caused by a "backward" rise in pressure proximal to the failing cardiac chambers. Cf. forward heart f.

cardiac f., SYN heart f. (1).

congestive heart f., SYN heart f. (1).

coronary f., acute coronary insufficiency.

electrical f., f. in which cardiac inadequacy is secondary to disturbance of the electrical impulse.

forward heart f., a concept (formerly considered mutually exclusive with backward heart f.) that maintains that the phenomena of congestive heart f. result from the inadequate cardiac output, and especially from the consequent inadequacy of renal blood flow with resulting retention of sodium and water. Cf. backward heart f.

heart f., (1) inadequacy of the heart so that as a pump it fails to maintain the circulation of blood, with the result that congestion and edema develop in the tissues; SYN cardiac f., cardiac insufficiency, congestive heart f., myocardial insufficiency. SEE ALSO forward heart f., backward heart f., right ventricular f., left ventricular f; **(2)** resulting clinical syndromes include shortness of breath or nonpitting edema, enlarged tender liver, engorged neck veins, and pulmonary rales in various combinations.

high output f., heart f. in which, despite relative myocardial insufficiency and consequent congestive heart f., the cardiac output is maintained at normal or supernormal levels, as is sometimes seen in emphysema, thyrotoxicosis, etc.

left-sided heart f., inability of the left heart to maintain its circulatory load, with corresponding rise in pressure in the pulmonary circulation usually with pulmonary congestion and ultimately pulmonary edema. SYN left ventricular f.

left ventricular f., SYN left-sided heart f.

low output f., heart f. in which the cardiac output is subnormal, as is usually seen in f. due to coronary, hypertensive, or valvular heart disease.

pacemaker f., f. of an artificial pacemaker to generate or deliver effective stimuli to the myocardium.

power f., SYN pump f.

premature ovarian f., SYN premature *menopause.*

pump f., a term used to emphasize mechanical default of the heart as a pump; in acute myocardial infarction, pump f. signifies congestive heart failure, pulmonary edema, or cardiogenic shock. Cf. electrical f. SYN power f.

pure autonomic f., a degenerative, sporadic neurologic disorder of adult onset, manifested principally as orthostatic hypotension and syncope, with no neurologic defects other than autonomic nervous system dysfunction evident; probably caused by selective degeneration of neurons in the sympathetic ganglia, with denervation of smooth muscle vasculature and the adrenal glands. SYN Bradbury-Eggleston syndrome.

renal f., loss of renal function, either acute or chronic, that results in azothemia and syndrome of uremia.

respiratory f., loss of pulmonary function either acute or chronic that results in hypoxemia or hypercarbia; final common pathway for myriad respiratory disorders.

right ventricular f., congestive heart f. manifested by distention of the neck veins, enlargement of the liver, and dependent edema due to pump f. of the right ventricle.

secondary f., (1) f. of the function of an organ as a result of antecedent pathology elsewhere; **(2)** decreasing responsiveness to a drug after an initial satisfactory response, usually occurring several months after initiation of treatment.

f. to thrive, a condition in which an infant's weight gain and growth are far below usual levels for age.

faint (fānt). **1.** Extremely weak; threatened with syncope. **2.** An episode of syncope. SEE ALSO syncope. [M.E., fr. O. Fr. *feindre,* to feign]

fal·cate (fal′kāt). SYN falciform.

fal·ces (fal′sēz). Plural of falx.

fal·cial (fal′shăl). Relating to the falx cerebelli or falx cerebri. SYN falcine.

fal·ci·form (fal′si-fōrm). Having a crescentic or sickle shape. SYN falcate. [L. *falx,* sickle, + *forma,* form]

fal·cine (fal′sēn). SYN falcial.

fal·cu·la (fal′kū-lă). SYN *falx* cerebelli. [L. dim. of *falx*]

fal·cu·lar (fal′kū-lăr). **1.** Resembling a sickle or falx. **2.** Relating to the falx cerebelli or cerebri.

fal·lo·pi·an (fa-lō′pē-an). Described by or attributed to Fallopius.

Fallopio, SEE Fallopius.

Fallopius (Fallopio), Gabriele, Italian anatomist, 1523–1562. SEE fallopian *aqueduct;* fallopian *arch;* fallopian *canal;* fallopian *hiatus;* fallopian *ligament;* fallopian *neuritis;* fallopian *pregnancy;* fallopian *tube; aqueductus* fallopii; *tuba* fallopiana; fallopian *tube.*

Fallot, Étienne-Louis A., French physician, 1850–1911. SEE *pentalogy* of F.; F. *tetrad, triad; trilogy* of F.

false neg·a·tive (fawls neg′ă-tiv). **1.** A test result that erroneously excludes an individual from a specific diagnostic or reference group. **2.** An individual whose test results exclude him or her from a particular diagnostic group to which the individual may truly belong. **3.** Term used to denote a false-negative *result.*

false pos·i·tive (fawls pos′i-tiv). **1.** A test result that erroneously assigns an individual to a specific diagnostic or reference group, due particularly to insufficiently exact methods of testing. **2.** An individual whose test results include him or her in a particular diagnostic group to which the individual may not truly belong. **3.** Term used to denote a false-positive *result.*

fal·set·to (fal-set′tō). Descriptive of phonation at an unnaturally high frequency. [It., fr. *falso,* false, + *-etto,* dim. suffix]

fal·si·fi·ca·tion (fawl′si-fi-kā′shŭn). The deliberate act of misrepresentation so as to deceive. SEE Munchausen *syndrome.* [L. *falsus,* false, + *facio,* to make]

retrospective f., unconscious distortion of past experience to conform to present psychological needs.

falx, pl. **fal·ces** (falks, fal′sēz) [TA]. A sickle-shaped structure. [L. sickle]

f. aponeurot′ica, SYN inguinal f.

cerebellar f., *☆*official alternate term for f. cerebelli.

f. cerebel′li [TA], a short process of dura mater projecting forward from the internal occipital crest below the tentorium; it occupies the posterior cerebellar notch and the vallecula, and bifurcates below into two diverging limbs passing to either side of the foramen magnum. SYN cerebellar f.*☆*, falcula.

cerebral f., *☆*official alternate term for f. cerebri.

f. cer′ebri [TA], the scythe-shaped fold of dura mater in the longitudinal fissure between the two cerebral hemispheres; it is attached anteriorly to the crista galli of the ethmoid bone and caudally to the upper surface of the tentorium. SYN cerebral f.*☆*.

inguinal f. [TA], common tendon of insertion of the transversus and internal oblique muscles into the crest and tubercle of the pubis and iliopectineal line; it is frequently largely muscular rather than aponeurotic and may be poorly developed; forms posterior wall of medial inguinal canal. SYN f. inguinalis [TA], conjoint tendon*☆*, tendo conjunctivus*☆*, conjoined tendon, f. aponeurotica, inguinal aponeurotic fold.

f. inguina′lis [TA], SYN inguinal f.

f. sep′ti, SYN *valve* of foramen ovale.

fa·mil·i·al (fa-mil′ē-ăl). Affecting more members of the same family than can be accounted for by chance, usually within a single sibship; commonly but incorrectly used to mean genetic. [L. *familia,* family]

fa·mil·i·al neu·ro·vis·cer·o·lip·i·do·sis. SYN infantile, generalized G_{M1} *gangliosidosis.*

fam·i·ly (fam′i-lē). **1.** A group of two or more persons united by blood, adoptive, or marital ties, or the common law equivalent. **2.** In biologic classification, a taxonomic grouping at the level intermediate between the order and the tribe or genus. **3.** A group of substances closely related structurally. **4.** A group of proteins with characteristic sequence, pharmacologic, and/or signaling profiles. [L. *familia*]

alu f., a set of dispersed sequences in the human genome having Alu cleavage sites at each end.

alu-equivalent f., a set of sequences in a mammalian genome that is related to the human Alu f.

cancer f., a group of blood relatives of whom several have had cancer; the mode of aggregation may be genetic and homogeneous, as in familial polyposis of the colon; diverse as in neurofibromatosis; or due to common exposure to a carcinogenic or oncogenic agent, such as a virus.

extended f., a group of persons comprising members of several generations united by blood, adoptive, marital, or equivalent ties.

gene f., group of genes related by sequence similarity.

nuclear f., in genetics, two parents and their progeny in common.

fa·mo·ti·dine (fă-mō′ti-dēn). A histamine H₂ antagonist used in the treatment of duodenal ulcers to reduce hydrochloric acid secretion.

fam·o·tine hy·dro·chlo·ride (fam′ō-tēn). An antiviral agent.

Fañanás, J., Spanish physician. SEE F. *cell.*

Fanconi, Guido, Swiss pediatrician, 1892–1979. SEE F. *anemia, pancytopenia, syndrome.*

fang. 1. A long tooth or tusk, usually a canine. **2.** The hollow tooth of a snake through which the venom is ejected. [A.S. *fōhan,* to seize]

fan·go (fang′gō). Mud from the Battaglio thermal springs in Italy, applied externally in the treatment of rheumatism and other diseases of the joints and muscles. [It. mud]

Fan·nia (fan′ē-ă). A genus of flies of the family Muscidae. Species include *F. canicularis* (the lesser housefly), commonly observed in kitchens or near food, which resembles *Musca domestica* (the common housefly) but is somewhat smaller and has three brown stripes on the thorax, and *F. scalaris* (the latrine fly), which commonly lays eggs in liquid feces of humans and animals and is distinguished from *F. canicularis* by two brown stripes on its thorax.

fan·ta·sy (fan′tă-sē). Imagery that is more or less coherent, as in dreams and daydreams, yet unrestricted by reality. SYN phantasia. [G. *phantasia,* idea, image]

FAP Abbreviation for familial adenomatous *polyposis.*

Farabeuf, Louis H., French surgeon, 1841–1910. SEE F. *amputation, triangle.*

far·ad (F) (fa′rad). A practical unit of electrical capacity; the capacity of a condenser having a charge of 1 coulomb under an electromotive force of 1 V. [M. *Faraday*]

Faraday, Michael, English physicist and chemist, 1791–1867. SEE farad; faraday; F. *constant, laws,* under *law.*

far·a·day (F), Fa·ra·day (fa′ră-dā). 96,485.309 coulombs per mole, the amount of electricity required to reduce one equivalent of a monovalent ion. [M. *Faraday*]

far·a·dism (fa′ră-dizm). Faradic (induction) electricity.

surging f., a current of gradually increasing and decreasing amplitude obtained by interposing a rhythmic resistance to the alternating current produced by the induction coil.

far·a·di·za·tion (fa′rad-i-zā′shŭn). Therapeutic application of the faradic (induced) electrical current.

fa·ra·do·con·trac·til·i·ty (fa′ră-dō-kon′trak-til′i-tē). Contractility of muscles under the stimulus of a faradic (induced) electric current.

fa·ra·do·mus·cu·lar (fa′ră-dō-mŭs′kū-lăr). Denoting the effect of applying a faradic (induced) electric current directly to a muscle.

far·a·do·pal·pa·tion (fa′ră-dō-pal-pā′shŭn). Esthesiometry by means of a sharp-pointed electrode through which a feeble alternating current passes to an indifferent electrode.

far·a·do·ther·a·py (fa′ră-dō-thār′ă-pē). Treatment of disease or paralysis by means of faradic (induced) electric current.

Farber, Sidney, U.S. pediatric pathologist, 1903–1973. SEE F. *disease, syndrome.*

far·cy (far′sē). **1.** A lymphatic disease of cattle caused by *Nocardia farcinica.* **2.** The skin form of glanders. [L. *farcio,* to stuff]

far·del (far′del). The total measurable penalty that is incurred as a result of the occurrence of a genetic disease in one individual; one of two major quantitative considerations in the prognostic aspects of genetic counseling, the other being risk of occurrence. The f. roughly measures the duration and the severity of the penalty, i.e., the integral of the total time-intensity function; e.g., color blindness has a low intensity of penalty throughout life, anencephaly causes intense distress for a brief time, Alzheimer disease is intermediate in both respects but the f. is greater. [M.E., fr. O. Fr., fr. Ar. *fardah,* bundle]

far·fa·ra (far′far-ă). The dried leaves of *Tussilago farfara* (family Compositae); a demulcent. [L. *farfarus,* coltsfoot]

fa·ri·na (fă-rē′nă). Flour or meal, as prepared from cereal grains such as *Avena sativa* (oats) or *Triticum sativum* (wheat); used as a starchy food. [L.]

f. avenae (fă-rē′nă ă-vē-nă), oatmeal flour.

f. tritici (fă-rē′nă trit′ĭ-sē), wheat flour.

far·i·na·ceous (far-i-nā′shŭs). **1.** Relating to farina or flour. **2.** Starchy.

α-far·ne·sene (far′nĕ-sēn). A straight open-chain hydrocarbon built up of three isoprene units; one of the four isomeric forms occurs in the natural coating of apples.

β-far·ne·sene. One of the two isomers (*trans*) that occurs in the alarm pheromone of some aphids and also in various essential oils.

far·ne·sene al·co·hol. SYN farnesol.

far·ne·sol (far′nĕ-sol). A difarnesyl group that occurs in the side chain of vitamin K₂ and constitutes squalene; found in oil of citronella; a sesquiterpene alcohol. SYN farnesene alcohol.

far·nes·yl py·ro·phos·phate (far′nĕ-sil pī′rō-fos′făt). The pyrophosphoryl derivative of farnesol; a key intermediate in the synthesis of steroids, dolichol, ubiquinone, prenylated proteins, and heme a.

far·no·qui·none (far′nō-kwin′ōn). SYN menaquinone-6.

Farnsworth, Dean, U.S. naval officer, 1902–1959. SEE F.-Munsell color *test.*

Farr, William, English medical statistician, 1807–1883. SEE F. *laws,* under *law.*

Farrant mount·ing flu·id. See under fluid.

Farre, Arthur, English obstetrician and gynecologist, 1811–1887. SEE F. *line.*

far·sight·ed·ness (far′sīt′ed-nes). SYN hyperopia.

Fas. A receptor present in cells that binds with f. ligand to induce apoptosis. SEE ALSO Fas *ligand.*

FASCIA

fas·cia, pl. **fas·ci·ae, fas·ci·as** (fash′ē-ă, -ē-ē) [TA]. A sheet of fibrous tissue that envelops the body beneath the skin; it also encloses muscles and groups of muscles, and separates their several layers or groups. [L. a band or fillet]

f. abdominalis parietalis, ☆official alternate term for extraperitoneal f.

Abernethy f., a layer of subperitoneal areolar tissue in front of the external iliac artery. SEE iliac f.

f. adhe′rens, a broad intercellular junction in the intercalated disk of cardiac muscle that anchors actin filaments.

anal f., SYN inferior f. of pelvic diaphragm.

antebrachial f. [TA], it is continuous with the brachial f.; in the region of the wrist it forms two thickened bands, the extensor and flexor retinacula. SYN f. antebrachii [TA], deep f. of forearm, f. of forearm.

f. antebra′chii [TA], SYN antebrachial f.

f. axilla′ris [TA], SYN axillary f.

axillary f. [TA], the perforated f. that forms the floor of the axilla. It is continuous with the pectoral and clavipectoral f. anteriorly, with the brachial f. laterally, and with the f. of the latissimus dorsi and serratus anterior muscles posteriorly and medially. SYN f. axillaris [TA].

bicipital f., SYN bicipital *aponeurosis*.

brachial f. [TA], the deep f. of the arm; it is continuous proximally with the pectoral f. and the f. covering the deltoid; distally it is continuous with the antebrachial f. SYN f. brachii [TA], deep f. of arm.

f. bra′chii [TA], SYN brachial f.

broad f., SYN deep f. of thigh.

f. buc′copharyn′gea [TA], SYN buccopharyngeal f.

buccopharyngeal f. [TA], the f. that covers the muscular layer of the pharynx and is continued forward onto the buccinator muscle. SYN f. buccopharyngea [TA].

Buck f., SYN f. of penis.

f. bul′bi, SYN fascial *sheath* of eyeball.

Camper f., SYN fatty *layer* of subcutaneous tissue of abdomen.

f. cervica′lis [TA], SYN (deep) cervical f.

f. cervicalis profunda, SYN (deep) cervical f.

f. cine′rea, SYN fasciolar *gyrus*.

clavipectoral f. [TA], a f. that extends between the coracoid process, the clavicle, and the thoracic wall. It includes the muscular f. which envelops the subclavius and pectoralis minor muscles and the strong membrane (costocoracoid membrane) formed in the interval between them, and the suspensory ligament of the axilla. The clavipectoral fascia (and the muscles it envelopes) constitute the deep anterior wall of the axilla. SYN f. clavipectoralis [TA].

f. clavipectora′lis [TA], SYN clavipectoral f.

f. clitor′idis [TA], SYN f. of clitoris.

f. of clitoris [TA], fibrous tissue comparable to the f. of the penis. SYN f. clitoridis [TA].

Colles f., SYN subcutaneous *tissue* of perineum.

Cooper f., SYN cremasteric f.

cremasteric f. [TA], intermediate coverings of the spermatic cord, formed of delicate connective tissue and of muscular fibers derived from the internal oblique muscle (cremaster muscle). SEE ALSO *aponeurosis* of internal oblique muscle. SYN f. cremasterica [TA], Cooper f., Scarpa sheath.

f. cremaster′ica [TA], SYN cremasteric f.

cribriform f. [TA], the part of the superficial f. of the thigh that covers the saphenous opening. SYN f. cribrosa [TA], Hesselbach f.

f. cribro′sa [TA], SYN cribriform f.

crural f., SYN deep f. of leg.

f. cru′ris [TA], SYN deep f. of leg.

Cruveilhier f., SYN subcutaneous *tissue* of perineum.

dartos f. [TA], a layer of smooth muscular tissue in the integument of the scrotum. SEE ALSO *dartos* muliebris, dartos *muscle*. SYN tunica dartos [TA], superficial f. of scrotum✩, membrana carnosa, tunica carnea.

deep f., a thin fibrous membrane, devoid of fat, that invests the muscles, separating the several groups and the individual muscles, forms sheaths for the nerves and vessels, becomes specialized around the joints to form or strengthen ligaments, envelops various organs and glands, and binds all the structures together into a firm compact mass. Terminologia Anatomica [TA] has recommended that the terms "superficial fascia" and "deep fascia" not be used generically in an unqualified way because of variation in their meanings internationally. The recommended terms are "subcutaneous tissue [TA] (tela subcutanea)" for the former superficial fascia, and "muscular fascia" or "visceral fascia" (fascia musculorum or fascia viscera[is]) in place of deep fascia. SYN f. profunda.

deep f. of arm, SYN brachial f.

(deep) cervical f. [TA], f. of the neck; it is divided into an external or investing layer (superficial lamina) that surrounds the neck and encloses the trapezius and sternocleidomastoid muscles, a middle or pretracheal layer in relation to the infrahyoid muscles, and a deep or prevertebral layer applied to the vertebrae and axial muscles. SYN f. cervicalis [TA], deep f. of neck, f. cervicalis profunda.

deep f. of forearm, SYN antebrachial f.

deep f. of leg [TA], f. of the leg; it is continuous with the f. lata and is attached proximally to the patella, ligamentum patellae, the tubercle and condyles of the tibia, and the head of the fibula; distally it is thickened to form the flexor and extensor retinacula. SYN f. cruris [TA], crural f., f. of leg.

deep f. of neck, SYN (deep) cervical f.

deep f. of penis, SYN f. of penis.

deep perineal f., ✩official alternate term for perineal f.

deep f. of thigh, the strong deep f. of the thigh, enveloping the muscles of the thigh and thickened laterally as the iliotibial track. SYN f. lata [TA], broad f.

f. denta′ta hippocam′pi, SYN dentate *gyrus*.

dentate f., SYN dentate *gyrus*.

f. diaphrag′matis pel′vis infe′rior [TA], SYN inferior f. of pelvic diaphragm.

f. diaphrag′matis urogenita′lis infe′rior, obsolete term for perineal *membrane*.

dorsal f. of foot [TA], the f. that encloses the extensor tendons of the toes and blends with the inferior extensor retinaculum. SYN f. dorsalis pedis [TA].

dorsal f. of hand [TA], the deep f. of the back of the hand continuous proximally with the extensor retinaculum. SYN f. dorsalis manus [TA].

f. dorsa′lis ma′nus [TA], SYN dorsal f. of hand.

f. dorsa′lis pe′dis [TA], SYN dorsal f. of foot.

Dupuytren f., SYN palmar *aponeurosis*.

endoabdominal f. [TA], (1) SYN extraperitoneal f; (2) term used generically to include not only the parietal extraperitoneal fascia hut also the visceral fascia in the abdominopelvic cavity. SYN f. endoabdominalis [TA].

f. endoabdominalis [TA], SYN endoabdominal f.

endopelvic f., ✩official alternate term for parietal pelvic f.

f. endopelvina, ✩official alternate term for parietal pelvic f.

endothoracic f. [TA], the extrapleural f. that lines the wall of the thorax; it extends over the cupula of the pleura as the suprapleural membrane and also forms a thin layer between the diaphragm and pleura (phrenicopleura f.) This loose areolar layer provides an extrapleural surgical plane. SYN f. endothoracica [TA].

f. endothora′cica [TA], SYN endothoracic f.

external spermatic f. [TA], the outer fascial covering of the spermatic cord; it is continuous at the superficial inguinal ring with the f. covering the external oblique muscle. SEE ALSO *aponeurosis* of external oblique muscle. SYN f. spermatica externa [TA].

f. of extraocular muscles, SYN muscular f. of extraocular muscle.

extraperitoneal f. [TA], fascial plane of mainly loose areolar tissue between the parietal peritoneum and the internal muscular (iliopsoas and inner lamina of thoracolumbar f.) and transversalis f. of the body wall; its quality and quantity vary considerably, being very thick and fatty posteriorly, as pararenal f. around the kidneys, but thin and fibrous anteriorly, deep to the linea alba of the anterior abdominal wall. SYN endoabdominal f. (1) [TA], parietal abdominal f. [TA], f. abdominalis parietalis✩, f. subperitonealis, subperitoneal f.

f. extraperitonealis [TA],

f. of forearm, SYN antebrachial f.

Gallaudet f., SYN perineal f.

Gerota f., SYN renal f.

Godman f., an extension of the pretracheal f. into the thorax and on to the pericardium.

Hesselbach f., SYN cribriform f.

hypothenar f., thinner, ulnar portion of the palmar f. overlying the hypothenar muscles, forming a roof for the hypothenar compartment of the palm. SEE ALSO palmar f.

iliac f. [TA], the f. covering the iliacus and psoas muscles, continuous with transversalis fascia anterolaterally and with femoral sheath inferiorly. SYN pars iliaca fasciae iliopsoaticae [TA], f. iliaca.

f. ili′aca, SYN iliac f.

iliopectineal f., a f. formed by the union of the fasciae covering the iliacus and pectinus muscles which cover the floor of the iliopectineal fossa. SEE iliopectineal *arch*.

inferior f. of pelvic diaphragm [TA], the f. that covers the inferior aspect of the levator ani and coccygeus muscles. SYN f. diaphragmatis pelvis inferior [TA], anal f.

inferior f. of urogenital diaphragm, obsolete term for perineal *membrane*.

f. in'fraspina'ta, SYN infraspinous f.

infraspinatus f., SYN infraspinous f.

infraspinous f. [TA], the f. attached to the borders of the infraspinous fossa and covering the infraspinatus muscle; it is continuous with the f. covering the deltoid. SYN f. infraspinata, infraspinatus f.

infundibuliform f., SYN internal spermatic f.

intercolumnar fasciae, SYN intercrural *fibers* of superficial ring, under *fiber*.

internal spermatic f. [TA], the inner covering of the spermatic cord, continuous above the deep inguinal ring with f. transversalis. SYN f. spermatica interna [TA], infundibuliform f., tunica vaginalis communis.

interosseous f., the f. covering the interosseous muscles of the hand or foot; it consists of a dorsal layer and a palmar or plantar layer.

f. investiens [TA], SYN investing *layer*.

f. investiens perinei superficialis, ✰official alternate term for perineal f.

investing f., SYN investing *layer* of cervical fascia.

lacrimal f., that part of the periorbita that bridges across the fossa or lacrimal sac.

f. la'ta [TA], SYN deep f. of thigh.

f. of leg, SYN deep f. of leg.

lumbodorsal f., SYN thoracolumbar f.

masseteric f. [TA], the f. that covers the lateral surface of the masseter muscle. SYN f. masseterica [TA].

f. massete'rica [TA], SYN masseteric f.

middle cervical f., SYN pretracheal *layer* of cervical fascia.

muscular f. [TA], a relatively thin fibrous membrane, devoid of fat, that invests the muscles, directly on their surfaces, separating the several groups and the individual muscles. Terminologia Anatomica [TA] has recommended that the terms "superficial fascia" and "deep fascia" not be used generically in an unqualified way because of variation in their meanings internationally. The recommended terms are "subcutaneous tissue [TA] (tela subcutanea)" for the former superficial fascia, and "muscular fascia" or "visceral fascia" (fascia musculorum or fascia viscera[is]) in place of deep fascia.

muscular f. of extraocular muscle [TA], muscular f.; the part of the orbital f. that envelops the extraocular muscles; it is thin posteriorly but becomes thicker where it is continuous with the bulbar sheath; the fascial sheaths of the four rectus muscles are connected by an intermuscular membrane. SYN f. muscularis musculorum bulbi [TA], f. of extraocular muscles, fascial sheaths of extraocular muscles.

f. muscula'ris musculo'rum bul'bi [TA], SYN muscular f. of extraocular muscle.

f. musculi quadrati lumborum, ✰official alternate term for anterior *layer* of thoracolumbar fascia.

f. nu'chae [TA], SYN nuchal f.

nuchal f. [TA], the f. that encloses the posterior muscles of the neck. SYN f. nuchae [TA].

obturator f. [TA], the portion of the pelvic f. that covers the obturator internus muscle. SYN f. obturatoria [TA], f. of obturator internus.

f. obturato'ria [TA], SYN obturator f.

f. of obturator internus, SYN obturator f.

orbital fasciae, the fascial structures of the orbit consisting of periorbita, orbital septum, muscular f., and fascial sheath of eyeball. SYN fasciae orbitales.

fas'ciae orbita'les, SYN orbital fasciae.

palmar f., the deep fascia of the palm of the hand, the thinner

lateral and medial portions of which are the thenar and hypothenar f., and the thick central portion, which roofs the central compartment of the palm, is the palmar aponeurosis. SEE ALSO palmar *aponeurosis*.

parietal abdominal f. [TA], SYN extraperitoneal f.

parietal pelvic f. [TA], including the obturator f., covers the muscles that pass from the interior of the pelvis to the thigh. SYN f. pelvis parietalis [TA], endopelvic f.✰, f. endopelvina✰.

parotid f. [TA], the part of the investing cervical f. that ensheaths the parotid gland and is fixed above to the zygomatic arch. SYN f. parotidea [TA], fibrous capsule of parotid gland, parotid sheath.

f. parotid'ea [TA], SYN parotid f.

parotideomasseteric f., a dense membrane covering both the lateral and medial surfaces of the parotid gland, continuous anteriorly with the f. covering the masseter muscle. SEE parotid f., masseteric f. SYN f. parotideomasseterica.

f. parotideomasseter'ica, SYN parotideomasseteric f.

pectoral f. [TA], the f. that covers the pectoralis major muscle; it is attached to the sternum and to the clavicle; laterally and below it is continuous with the f. of the shoulder, axilla, and thorax. SYN f. pectoralis [TA].

f. pectora'lis [TA], SYN pectoral f.

pelvic f. [TA], it includes parietal and visceral components: fascia pelvis parietalis and fascia pelvis visceralis. SYN f. pelvis [TA], f. pelvica✰.

f. pelvica, ✰official alternate term for pelvic f.

f. pel'vis [TA], SYN pelvic f.

f. pel'vis parieta'lis [TA], SYN parietal pelvic f.

f. pel'vis viscera'lis [TA], SYN visceral pelvic f.

f. pe'nis [TA], SYN f. of penis.

f. of penis [TA], a deep layer which surrounds the three erectile bodies of the penis. SYN f. penis [TA], Buck f., deep f. of penis, f. penis profunda.

f. pe'nis profun'da, SYN f. of penis.

f. pe'nis superficia'lis, SYN subcutaneous *tissue* of penis.

perineal f. [TA], f. that intimately invests the superficial perineal muscles (ischiocavernosus, bulbospongiosus, and superficial transverse perineal muscles); anteriorly it is fused to the suspensory ligament of the penis/clitoris, and is continuous with the deep f. covering the external oblique muscle of the abdomen and the rectus sheath. SYN f. perinei [TA], deep perineal f.✰, f. investiens perinei superficialis✰, superficial investing f. of perineum✰, Gallaudet f.

f. perine'i [TA], SYN perineal f.

f. perine'i superficia'lis, SYN subcutaneous *tissue* of perineum.

perirenal f., SYN renal f.

pharyngobasilar f. [TA], the fibrous coat of the pharyngeal wall situated between the mucous and muscular coats; it is attached above to the basilar part of the occipital bone, and the petrous part of the temporal bone. This layer and the mucosa which lines it forms the wall of the non-muscular pharynx (pharyngeal vault) above the superior pharyngesl constrictor muscle. SYN f. pharyngobasilaris [TA], aponeurosis pharyngea, tela submucosa pharyngis.

f. pharyngobasila'ris [TA], SYN pharyngobasilar f.

phrenicopleural f. [TA], the thin layer of endothoracic f. intervening between the diaphragmatic pleura and the diaphragm. SYN f. phrenicopleuralis [TA].

f. phrenicopleura'lis [TA], SYN phrenicopleural f.

plantar f., deep fascia of the sole of the foot; includes thick central part, the plantar aponeurosis, covering the central compartment of the sole of the foot, and thinner medial and lateral parts covering the hallucis and digit minimi muscles (compartments), respectively.

popliteal f., the f. that covers the popliteal fossa, continuous with fascia lata superiorly and crural fascia inferiorly.

Porter f., SYN pretracheal *layer* of cervical fascia.

prececocolic f. [TA], inconstant portion of endoabdominal f. crossing anterior to the cecum, sometimes extending superiorly onto a portion of the ascending colon. SYN f. prececocolica [TA].

f. prececocolica [TA], SYN prececocolic f.

presacral f. [TA], layer of endopelvic f. passing between sacrum and rectum, forming the anterior boundary of the presacral (retrorectal) fascial space, in which the hypogastric nervous plexus is embedded. SYN f. presacralis [TA], lamina retrorectalis fasciae endopelvicae, retrorectal lamina of endopelvic fascia, retrorectal lamina of hypogastric sheath.

f. presacra'lis [TA], SYN presacral f.

pretracheal f., SYN pretracheal *layer* of cervical fascia.

prevertebral f., SYN prevertebral *layer* of cervical fascia.

f. profun'da, SYN deep f.

f. pros'tatae [TA], SYN f. of prostate.

f. of prostate, the condensation of pelvic visceral f. that encloses the prostate gland. SYN f. prostatae [TA].

rectosacral f. [TA], fusion of the visceral f. of the rectum and the presacral endopelvic f. on the posterior aspect of the rectum. SYN f. rectosacralis [TA], mesoprocton.

f. rectosacra'lis [TA], SYN rectosacral f.

rectovesical f., SYN rectovesical *septum.*

renal f. [TA], the condensation of the fibroareolar tissue and fat surrounding the kidney to form a sheath for the organ. SYN f. renalis [TA], Gerota capsule, Gerota f., perirenal f.

f. rena'lis [TA], SYN renal f.

Scarpa f., SYN membranous *layer* of subcutaneous tissue of abdomen.

semilunar f., SYN bicipital *aponeurosis.*

Sibson f., SYN suprapleural *membrane.*

f. spermat'ica exter'na [TA], SYN external spermatic f.

f. spermat'ica inter'na [TA], SYN internal spermatic f.

subperitoneal f., SYN extraperitoneal f.

f. subperitonea'lis, SYN extraperitoneal f.

subsartorial f., SYN anteromedial intermuscular *septum.*

superficial f., SYN subcutaneous *tissue.*

superficial investing f. of perineum, *✗*official alternate term for perineal f.

f. superficia'lis, SYN subcutaneous *tissue.*

superficial f. of penis, SYN subcutaneous *tissue* of penis.

superficial f. of perineum, SYN subcutaneous *tissue* of perineum.

superficial f. of scrotum, *✗* official alternate term for dartos f.

f. supe'rior diaphrag'matis pel'vis [TA], SYN superior f. of pelvic diaphragm.

superior f. of pelvic diaphragm [TA], the f. on the superior aspect of the levator ani and coccygeus muscles. SYN f. superior diaphragmatis pelvis [TA].

temporal f. [TA], the f. covering the temporal muscle; it is composed of two layers, lamina superficialis and lamina profunda; both attach above to the superior temporal line but diverge inferiorly to attach to the lateral and medial surfaces of the zygomatic arch. SYN f. temporalis [TA], temporal aponeurosis.

f. tempora'lis [TA], SYN temporal f.

f. thoracolumba'lis [TA], SYN thoracolumbar f.

thoracolumbar f. [TA], gives origin to internal oblique and transversus abdominis muscles; exhibits three layers: posterior, middle, and anterior—the posterior and middle layers surround erector spinae muscles and the middle and anterior layers surround quadratus lumborum muscle. SYN f. thoracolumbalis [TA], lumbodorsal f., thoracolumbar aponeurosis.

Toldt f., continuation of Treitz f. behind the body of the pancreas.

f. transversa'lis [TA], SYN transversalis f.

transversalis f. [TA], the lining f. of the anterolateral abdominal wall, between the inner surface of the abdominal musculature and the peritoneum. SYN f. transversalis [TA].

Treitz f., f. behind the head of the pancreas.

triangular f., SYN reflected inguinal *ligament.*

f. triangula'ris abdom'inis, SYN reflected inguinal *ligament.*

Tyrrell f., SYN rectovesical *septum.*

umbilical f. [TA], the thin fascial layer interposed between the transversalis f. and the umbilicovesical f. It extends between the medial umbilical ligaments from the umbilicus downward in front of the bladder, forming the posterior boundary of the retropubic space. SYN umbilical prevesical f.

f. umbilicalis [TA],

umbilical prevesical f., SYN umbilical f.

umbilicovesical f., a thin fascial layer that extends between the medial umbilical ligaments and is continuous with f. enclosing the bladder.

vastoadductor f., SYN anteromedial intermuscular *septum.*

visceral f. [TA], a thin, fibrous membrane that envelops various organs and glands, binding structures together in some cases and forming partitions between them in other cases. Terminologia Anatomica [TA] has recommended that the terms "superficial fascia" and "deep fascia" not be used generically in an unqualified way because of variation in their meanings internationally. The recommended terms are "subcutaneous tissue [TA] (tela subcutanea)" for the former superficial fascia, and "muscular fascia" or "visceral fascia" (fascia musculorum or fascia viscera[is]) in place of deep fascia.

visceral pelvic f. [TA], covers the pelvic organs and surrounds vessels and nerves in the subperitoneal space. SYN f. pelvis visceralis [TA].

Zuckerkandl f., the posterior layer of the renal f.

---

fas·cial (fash'ē-ăl). Relating to any fascia.

fas·ci·cle (fas'i-kl). A band or bundle of fibers, usually of muscle or nerve fibers; a nerve fiber tract. SYN fasciculus (1) [TA].

anterior f. of palatopharyngeus (muscle) [TA], thicker portion of the muscle of the palatopharyngeal arch that passes forward between the levator and tensor veli palatini muscles to attach to the posterior border of the hard palate and the palatine aponeurosis; in so doing, some fibers cross the midline and interdigitate with fibers of the contralateral muscle. SYN fasciculus anterior musculi palatopharyngei [TA].

muscle f., a bundle of muscle fibers surrounded by perimysium.

nerve f., a bundle of nerve fibers surrounded by perineurium.

posterior f. of palatopharyngeus muscle [TA], thinner portion of the muscle of the palatopharyngeal arch, originating in the region of the midline where its fibers interdigitate with the contralateral partner, then passing posterior to the levator veli palatini muscle to join the longitudinal layer of pharyngeal musculature; acts as a sort of sphincter, reducing the caliber of the isthmus of fauces at the palatopharyngeal arch. SYN fasciculus posterior musculi palatopharyngei [TA], musculus sphincter palatopharyngeus*✗*, palatopharyngeal sphincter*✗*, pharyngeal ridge, sphincter of the pharyngeal isthmus, velopharyngeal sphincter.

fas·cic·u·lar (fa-sik'ū-lăr). Relating to a fasciculus; arranged in the form of a bundle or collection of rods. SYN fasciculate, fasciculated.

fas·cic·u·late, fas·cic·u·lat·ed (fa-sik'ū-lāt, -lā-ted). SYN fascicular.

fas·cic·u·la·tion (fa-sik-ū-lā'shŭn). **1.** An arrangement in the form of fasciculi. **2.** Involuntary contractions, or twitchings, of groups (fasciculi) of muscle fibers, a coarser form of muscular contraction than fibrillation.

fas·cic·u·li (fa-sik'ū-lī). Plural of fasciculus.

FASCICULUS

---

fas·cic·u·lus, gen. and pl. **fas·cic·u·li** (fă-sik'ū-lŭs, fă-sik'ū-lī) [TA]. **1.** SYN fascicle. **2.** SYN cord. **3.** SYN bundle. [L. dim. of *fascis,* bundle]

f. anterior musculi palatopharyngei [TA], SYN anterior *fascicle* of palatopharyngeus (muscle).

anterior f. proprius [TA], SYN fasciculi proprii.

anterior pyramidal f., SYN anterior corticospinal *tract.*

arcuate f., (1) SYN superior longitudinal f; **(2)** SYN unciform f.

f. at'rioventricula'ris [TA], SYN atrioventricular *bundle.*

Burdach f., SYN cuneate f.

calcarine f., a group of short association fibers beneath the calcarine fissure of the occipital lobe of the cerebrum.

central tegmental f., SYN central tegmental *tract.*

f. cir'cumoliva'ris pyram'idis, an anomalous bundle of nerve fibers on the anterior surface of the medulla oblongata that emerges from the pyramid and curves forward and dorsally over the lower pole of the olive; it is variously interpreted as an aberrant bundle of pontocerebellar fibers or corticopontine fibers.

f. corticospina'lis ante'rior, SYN anterior corticospinal *tract.*

f. corticospina'lis latera'lis, SYN lateral corticospinal *tract.*

cuneate f. [TA], the larger lateral subdivision of the posterior funiculus. SYN f. cuneatus [TA], Burdach column, Burdach f., Burdach tract, cuneate funiculus, wedge-shaped f.

f. cunea'tus [TA], SYN cuneate f.

dorsal longitudinal f. [TA], a bundle of thin, poorly myelinated nerve fibers reciprocally connecting the periventricular zone of the hypothalamus with ventral parts of the central gray substance of the midbrain. SYN f. longitudinalis posterior [TA], Schütz bundle, tract of Schütz.

dorsolateral f. [TA], a longitudinal bundle of thin, unmyelinated, and poorly myelinated fibers capping the apex of the posterior horn of the spinal gray matter, composed of posterior root fibers and short association fibers that interconnect neighboring segments of the posterior horn. SYN f. posterolateral tract [TA], tractus dorsolateralis [TA], tractus posterolateralis [TA], dorsolateral tract*, f. dorsolateralis, f. marginalis, Lissauer bundle, Lissauer column, Lissauer f., Lissauer marginal zone, Lissauer tract, marginal f., Spitzka marginal tract, Spitzka marginal zone, Waldeyer tract, Waldeyer zonal layer.

f. dorsolatera'lis, SYN dorsolateral f.

Flechsig fasciculi, f. proprius anterior [TA] and f. proprius lateralis [TA]. SEE fasciculi proprii.

Foville f., SYN terminal *stria.*

fronto-occipital f., SYN occipitofrontal f.

gracile f. [TA], the smaller medial subdivision of the posterior funiculus. SYN f. gracilis [TA], funiculus gracilis, Goll column, posterior pyramid of the medulla, slender f., tract of Goll.

f. grac'ilis [TA], SYN gracile f.

hooked f., SYN unciform f.

inferior longitudinal f. [TA], a well-marked bundle of long association fibers running the whole length of the occipital and temporal lobes of the cerebrum, in part parallel with the inferior horn of the lateral ventricle. SYN f. longitudinalis inferior [TA].

inferior occipitofrontal f. [TA], SEE occipitofrontal f.

interfascicular f. [TA], SYN semilunar f.

f. interfascicularis, SYN semilunar f.

intersegmental fasciculi, SYN fasciculi proprii.

f. latera'lis plex'us brachia'lis [TA], SYN lateral *cord* of brachial plexus.

lateral f. proprius [TA], SYN fasciculi proprii.

lateral pyramidal f., SYN lateral corticospinal *tract.*

lenticular f. [TA], the pallidal efferent fibers that cross the internal capsule and are insinuated between the subthalamic nucleus and zona incerta; they join in the formation of the thalamic fasciculus. SEE ALSO lenticular *loop.* SYN f. lenticularis [TA].

f. lenticula'ris [TA], SYN lenticular f.

Lissauer f., SYN dorsolateral f.

fasci'culi longitudina'les ligamen'ti crucifor'mis atlan'tis [TA], SYN longitudinal *bands* of cruciform ligament of atlas, under *band.*

fascic'uli longitudina'les pon'tis, SYN longitudinal pontine fasciculi.

f. longitudina'lis infe'rior [TA], SYN inferior longitudinal f.

f. longitudina'lis media'lis [TA], SYN medial longitudinal f.

f. longitudina'lis posterior [TA], SYN dorsal longitudinal f.

f. longitudina'lis supe'rior [TA], SYN superior longitudinal f.

longitudinal pontine fasciculi, the massive bundles of corticofugal fibers passing longitudinally through the ventral part of pons; they are composed of corticoreticular, tectopontine, corticopontine, corticonuclear (corticobulbar), and corticospinal fibers. SYN fasciculi longitudinales pontis, longitudinal pontine bundles.

macular f., the collection of fibers in the optic nerve directly connected with the macula lutea. SYN f. macularis.

f. macula'ris, SYN macular f.

mammillotegmental f. [TA], a small bundle of fibers that passes dorsalward from the mamillary body for a short distance with the mamillothalamic tract, then turns down the brainstem to reach the dorsal and ventral tegmental nuclei of the mesencephalon. SYN f. mammillotegmentalis [TA].

f. mammillotegmenta'lis [TA], SYN mammillotegmental f.

mammillothalamic f. [TA], a compact, thick bundle of nerve fibers that passes dorsalward from the mamillary body on either side to terminate in the anterior nucleus of the thalamus. SYN f. mammillothalamicus, f. thalamomammillaris, mammillothalamic tract, Vicq d'Azyr bundle.

f. mammillothalamicus, SYN mammillothalamic f.

marginal f., SYN dorsolateral f.

f. margina'lis, SYN dorsolateral f.

f. media'lis plex'us brachia'lis [TA], SYN medial *cord* of brachial plexus.

f. medialis telencephali [TA], SYN medial forebrain *bundle.*

medial longitudinal f. [TA], a longitudinal bundle of fibers extending from the upper border of the mesencephalon into the cervical segments of the spinal cord, located close to the midline and ventral to the central gray matter; it is composed largely of fibers from the vestibular nuclei ascending to the motor neurons innervating the external eye muscles (abducens, trochlear, and oculomotor nuclei), and descending to spinal cord segments innervating the musculature of the neck. SYN f. longitudinalis medialis [TA], Collier tract, medial longitudinal bundle, posterior longitudinal bundle.

f. of Meynert, SYN retroflex f.

oblique pontine f., a bundle of fibers in the ventral surface of the pons running from the anterior mesial portion outward and backward. SYN f. obliquus pontis, oblique bundle of pons.

f. obli'quus pon'tis, SYN oblique pontine f.

occipitofrontal f., association fibers consisting of upper (superior occipitofrontal fasciculus [TA]) and lower (inferior occipitofrontal fasciculus [TA]) bundles that extend from occipital to frontal lobes of the cerebral hemisphere. SYN fronto-occipital f.

f. occip'itofronta'lis, SEE occipitofrontal f.

f. occipitofrontalis inferior [TA], SEE occipitofrontal f.

f. occipitofrontalis superior [TA], SEE occipitofrontal f.

oval f., SEE semilunar f.

f. pedun'culomammilla'ris, SYN *peduncle* of mammillary body.

pedunculomammillary f., SYN *peduncle* of mammillary body.

perpendicular f., a bundle of association fibers running vertically and interconnecting regions of the temporal, occipital, and parietal lobes.

f. posterior musculi palatopharyngei [TA], SYN posterior *fascicle* of palatopharyngeus muscle.

f. poste'rior plex'us brachia'lis [TA], SYN posterior *cord* of brachial plexus.

posterior f. proprius [TA], SYN fasciculi proprii.

proper fasciculi, SYN fasciculi proprii.

fascic'uli pro'prii, (fasciculus proprius anterior [TA], fasciculus proprius lateralis [TA], fasciculus proprius posterior [TA]); ascending and descending spinospinal association fiber systems of the spinal cord that lie in the anterior, lateral, and posterior funiculi at the gray matter-white matter interface. SYN anterior f. proprius [TA], lateral f. proprius [TA], posterior f. proprius [TA], ground bundles, intersegmental fasciculi, lateral proprius bundle, proper fasciculi.

f. pro'prius ante'rior [TA], the ground bundle of the anterior column of the spinal cord. SEE fasciculi proprii. SYN anterior ground bundle.

f. pro'prius latera'lis [TA], SEE fasciculi proprii.

f. pyramida'lis ante'rior, SYN anterior corticospinal *tract.*

f. pyramida'lis latera'lis, SYN lateral corticospinal *tract.*

retroflex f. [TA], a compact bundle of fibers arising in the habenula and passing ventralward to the interpeduncular nucleus at the base of the midbrain; part of its fibers bypass this nucleus and

fa

terminate in the raphe nuclei of the caudal mesencephalic tegmentum. SYN f. retroflexus [TA], habenulointerpeduncular tract, habenulopeduncular tract [TA], tractus habenulointerpeduncularis [TA], f. of Meynert, habenulopeduncular tract, retroflex bundle of Meynert.

f. retroflex′us [TA], SYN retroflex f.

f. rotun′dus, SYN solitary *tract.*

round f., SYN solitary *tract.*

rubroreticular fasciculi, bundles of fibers that connect the red nucleus to the pontine and midbrain reticular nuclei. SYN fasciculi rubroreticulares.

fasciculi rubroreticula′res, SYN rubroreticular fasciculi.

semilunar f. [TA], a compact bundle composed of descending branches of posterior root fibers located near the border between the fasciculi gracilis and cuneatus of the cervical and thoracic spinal cord; it corresponds to the septomarginal f., Hoche tract, or oval area of Flechsig in the lumbar, and to the triangle of Philippe-Gombault in the sacral spinal segments; like these, it can be demonstrated only in cases of demyelination resulting from dorsal root lesions. SYN f. interfascicularis [TA], interfascicular f. [TA], f. semilunaris✫, comma bundle of Schultze, comma tract of Schultze.

f. semiluna′ris, ✫official alternate term for semilunar f; SEE semilunar f.

septomarginal f. [TA], septomarginal f. or tract. SEE semilunar f. SYN f. septomarginalis [TA].

f. septomargina′lis [TA], SYN septomarginal f.

slender f., SYN gracile f.

f. solita′rius, SYN solitary *tract.*

solitary f., SYN solitary *tract.*

subcallosal f., a bundle of thin nerve fibers running longitudinally beneath the corpus callosum in the angle between the latter and the caudate nucleus; it forms an anterior continuation of the tapetum of the temporal lobe and appears to consist largely of fibers projecting from the cerebral cortex to the caudate nucleus. SYN f. subcallosus for superior occipitofrontal fasciculus✫.

f. subcallo′sus for superior occipitofrontal fasciculus, ✫official alternate term for subcallosal f.

subthalamic f. [TA], nerve fibers crossing the internal capsule between the subthalamic nucleus and the globus pallidus; this f. contains pallidosubthalamic and subthalamopallidal fibers. SYN f. subthalamicus [TA].

f. subthalam′icus [TA], SYN subthalamic f.

superior longitudinal f. [TA], long association fiber bundle lateral to the centrum ovale of the cerebral hemisphere, connecting the frontal, occipital, and temporal lobes; the fibers pass from the frontal lobe through the operculum to the posterior end of the lateral sulcus where many fibers radiate into the occipital lobe and others turn downward and forward around the putamen and pass to anterior portions of the temporal lobe. SYN f. longitudinalis superior [TA], arcuate f. (1).

superior occipitofrontal f. [TA], SEE occipitofrontal f.

thalamic f. [TA], nerve fibers forming a composite bundle containing cerebellothalamic (crossed) and pallidothalamic (uncrossed) fibers that is insinuated between the thalamus and zona incerta. SEE ALSO *fields* of Forel, under *field.* SYN f. thalamicus [TA].

f. thalam′icus [TA], SYN thalamic f.

f. thal′amomammilla′ris, SYN mammillothalamic f.

transverse fasciculi [TA], SYN fasciculi transversi.

fascic′uli transver′si [TA], the transversely directed fibers in the distal portions of the palmar and plantar aponeuroses. SYN transverse fasciculi [TA].

unciform f., uncinate f. [TA], a band of long association fibers reciprocally connecting the frontal and temporal lobes of the cerebrum, running caudally through the white matter of the frontal lobe, sharply curving ventrally under the stem of the sylvian fissure, and then fanning out to the cortex of the anterior half of the superior and middle temporal gyri. SYN f. uncinatus [TA], arcuate f. (2), frontotemporal tract, hooked f., temporofrontal tract.

uncinate f. of cerebellum [TA], fastigial efferent fibers that cross

within the cerebellum and descend over the lateral surface of the superior cerebellar peduncle; these fibers largely terminate in the vestibular nuclei and the reticular formation of the pons and medulla. SYN f. uncinatus cerebelli [TA], hooked bundle of Russell, uncinate bundle of Russell, uncinate f. of Russell.

uncinate f. of Russell, SYN uncinate f. of cerebellum.

f. uncina′tus [TA], SYN unciform f.

f. uncinatus cerebelli [TA], SYN uncinate f. of cerebellum.

wedge-shaped f., SYN cuneate f.

---

fas·ci·ec·to·my (fash-ē-ek′tō-mē). Excision of strips of fascia. [fascia + G. *ektomē,* excision]

fas·ci·i·tis (fas-ē-ī′tis, fash-). **1.** Inflammation in fascia. **2.** Reactive proliferation of fibroblasts in fascia. SYN fascitis.

eosinophilic f., induration and edema of the connective tissues of the extremities, usually appearing following exertion; associated with elevated sedimentation rate, elevated IgG, and eosinophilia. SYN Shulman syndrome.

---

group A streptococcal necrotizing f., a severe and often fulminant toxic complication of infection with group A β-hemolytic streptococci in which superficial fascia and underlying muscle tissue are rapidly destroyed.

During the past decade there has been a rise in the incidence of acute systemic disease due to toxin-producing strains of *Streptococcus pyogenes.* Like staphylococcal toxic shock syndrome (TSS), toxin-mediated streptococcal syndromes are marked by rapid progression, shock, and multisystem toxicity that is out of proportion to local evidence of infection. The incidence of necrotizing fasciitis due to streptococci increased markedly in 1994 in both the United States and Europe. This disease is believed to be the same as the "malignant scarlet fever" of a century ago. In necrotizing fasciitis, streptococci in a skin wound, usually on an extremity, invade and destroy underlying muscles and other soft tissues. The skin of the affected extremity shows erythema, bulla formation, and often anesthesia due to destruction of sensory nerves. Rapid spread of infection along fascial planes and widespread liquefactive necrosis are accompanied by high fever, intense local pain, shock, and other evidence of systemic toxicity. The goals of therapy in streptococcal necrotizing fasciitis are to inhibit and destroy pathogens, reverse shock and systemic toxicity, and conserve structure and function. Treatment includes intravenous hydration and aggressive supportive measures as well as administration of penicillin, clindamycin, or other antibiotics as appropriate. (Antibiotic resistance has not been a problem with streptococcal TSS.) In necrotizing fasciitis, debridement or amputation may be life-saving. Throat cultures of contacts are recommended, to identify possible sources of further infection with virulent toxigenic streptococci.

---

necrotizing f., a rare soft-tissue infection primarily involving the superficial fascia and resulting in extensive undermining of surrounding tissues; progress is often fulminant and may involve all soft-tissue components, including the skin; usually occurs postoperatively, after minor trauma, or after inadequate care of abscesses or cutaneous ulcers. SEE ALSO group A streptococcal necrotizing f.

nodular f., a rapidly growing tumorlike proliferation of fibroblasts, not thought to be neoplastic, with mild inflammatory exudation occurring in fascia; the fibrosis may infiltrate surrounding tissue but does not progress indefinitely or metastasize. SYN pseudosarcomatous f.

parosteal f., a rare form of nodular f. arising from the periosteum, and which may be associated with reactive cortical bone formation.

plantar f., inflammation of the plantar fascia causing foot or heel pain.

proliferative f., a benign rapidly-growing subcutaneous nodule characterized by proliferation of fibroblasts and basophilic giant cells slightly resembling ganglion cells.

pseudosarcomatous f., SYN nodular f.

⚬**fascio-.** A fascia. [L. *fascia,* a band or fillet]

fas·ci·od·e·sis (fas-ē-od'ĕ-sis, fas-). Surgical attachment of a fascia to another fascia or a tendon. [fascio- + G. *desis,* a binding together]

Fas·ci·o·la (fa-sē'ō-lă, fa-sī'ō-lă). A genus of large, leaf-shaped, digenetic liver flukes (family Fasciolidae, class Trematoda) of mammals. [L. dim. of *fascia,* a band]

F. gigan'tica, a species, resembling *F. hepatica* but of larger size, found in herbivores, especially in Africa, where it also infects humans.

F. hepat'ica, the common liver fluke inhabiting the bile ducts of sheep and cattle; the intermediate hosts are aquatic snails, *Lymnaea* or related genera; after the cercariae escape, they become encysted on water plants by which they gain access to the intestinal canal; rarely, this fluke is reported from humans, in whom it may cause considerable biliary damage.

fas·ci·o·la, pl. **fas·ci·o·lae** (fa-sē'ō-lă, fa-sī'ō-lă; -ō-lē). A small band or group of fibers. [L. dim. of *fascia,* band, fillet]

f. cine′rea, SYN fasciolar *gyrus.*

fas·ci·o·lar (fa-sē'ō-lăr, fa-sī'). Relating to the gyrus fasciolaris.

fas·ci·o·li·a·sis (fas'ē-ō-lī'ă-sis, fa-sī'ō-lī'ă-sis). Infection with a species of *Fasciola.*

fas·ci·o·lid (fa-sē'ō-lid, fa-sī'). A member of the family Fasciolidae.

fas·ci·o·lop·si·a·sis (fas'ē-ō-lop-sī'ă-sis, fa-sī'o-). Parasitization by any of the flukes of the genus *Fasciolopsis.*

Fas·ci·o·lop·sis (fas'ē-ō-lop'sis, fa-sī'ō-). A genus of very large intestinal fasciolid flukes. [*Fasciola* + G. *opsis,* form, appearance]

F. bus'ki, the large intestinal fluke, a species found in the intestine of humans in eastern and southern Asia; transmitted via ingestion of water chestnuts or other vegetation contaminated with infective metacercariae.

F. rathoui'si, a species reported from China in a few cases in the intestine or liver; possibly the same as *F. buski.*

fas·ci·or·rha·phy (fash-ē-ōr'ă-fē). Suture of a fascia or aponeurosis. SYN aponeurorrhaphy. [fascio- + G. *rhaphē,* suture]

fas·ci·ot·o·my (fash-ē-ot'ō-mē). Incision through a fascia; used in the treatment of certain disorders and injuries when marked swelling is present or anticipated which could compromise blood flow; f. may be combined with embolectomy in the treatment of acute arterial embolism. [fascio- + G. *tomē,* incision]

fas·ci·tis (fa-sī'tis). SYN fasciitis.

fast. **1.** Durable; resistant to change; applied to stained microorganisms which cannot be decolorized. SEE ALSO acid-fast. **2.** Not eating. [A.S. *foest,* firm, fixed]

fast green FCF [C.I. 42053]. An acid arylmethane dye widely used in histology and cytology and less subject to fading than light green FCF which it has replaced in many procedures; used as a quantitative cytochemical stain for histones at alkaline pH after acid extraction of DNA, and also in electrophoresis as a protein stain.

fas·tid·i·ous (fas-tid'ē-ŭs). In bacteriology, having complex nutritional requirements.

fas·ti·ga·tum (fas-ti-gā'tŭm). SYN fastigial *nucleus.* [L. *fastigatus,* pointed]

fas·tig·i·um (fas-tij'ē-ŭm). **1** [TA]. Apex of the roof of the fourth ventricle of the brain, an angle formed by the anterior and posterior medullary vela extending into the substance of the vermis. **2.** The acme or period of full development of a disease. [L. top, as of a gable; a pointed extremity]

fast·ness (fast'nes). The state of tolerance exhibited by bacteria to a drug or other agent. SEE fast.

fat. **1.** SYN adipose *tissue.* **2.** Common term for obese. **3.** A greasy, soft-solid material, found in animal tissues and many plants, composed of a mixture of glycerol esters; together with oils they make up the homolipids. **4.** A triacylglycerol or a mixture of triacylglycerols. [A.S. *faet*]

brown f., thermogenic tissue that is composed of cells containing numerous small fat droplets; lobular masses are found in the interscapular and mediastinal regions and other locations; although found most frequently in certain hibernating animals, it is also found in pigs, rodents, and the newborn of humans. SYN brown adipose tissue, hibernating gland, interscapular gland, interscapular hibernoma, multilocular adipose tissue, multilocular f.

multilocular f., SYN brown f.

neutral f., a triester of fatty acids and glycerol (i.e., triacylglycerol).

paranephric f. [TA], the perirenal fat. SYN adipose capsule, capsula adiposa renis, fatty renal capsule, perirenal fat capsule.

retrobulbar f. [TA], the mass of fat contained in the orbit that contributes to the support of the eyeball. SYN corpus adiposum orbitae [TA], orbital fat body☆, fat body of orbit, orbital fat-pad.

saturated f., SEE saturated *fatty acid.*

split f., free fatty acids, as reduced by the action of lipases, neutral f.'s, or phospholipids.

unilocular f., adipose tissue in which the fat is present in a single droplet within the fat cells. SYN white f. (2).

unsaturated f., SEE unsaturated *fatty acid.*

white f., (1) SYN adipose *tissue;* (2) SYN unilocular f.

fa·tal (fā'tăl). Pertaining to or causing death; denoting especially inevitability or inescapability of death. [L. *fatalis,* of or belonging to fate]

fa·tal·i·ty (fā-tal'i-tē). **1.** A condition, disease, or disaster ending in death. **2.** An individual instance of death.

fate. The ultimate outcome.

prospective f., the normal development by any part of the egg or embryo without interference.

fat·i·ga·bil·i·ty (fat'i-gă-bil'i-tē). A condition in which fatigue is easily induced.

fa·ti·ga·ble (fat'i-gă-bl). Tiring on very slight exertion. [L. *fatigabilis,* easily tired, fr. *fatigo,* to tire]

fa·tigue (fă-tēg'). **1.** That state, following a period of mental or bodily activity, characterized by a lessened capacity for work and reduced efficiency of accomplishment, usually accompanied by a feeling of weariness, sleepiness, or irritability; may also supervene when, from any cause, energy expenditure outstrips restorative processes and may be confined to a single organ. **2.** Sensation of boredom and lassitude due to absence of stimulation, monotony, or lack of interest in one's surroundings. [Fr., fr. L. *fatigo,* to tire]

auditory f., temporary shift of threshold sensitivity following exposure to sound.

battle f., a term used to denote psychiatric illness consequent to the stresses of battle. SYN shell shock.

functional vocal f., SYN phonasthenia.

fat-pad [TA]. An accumulation of somewhat encapsulated adipose tissue. SYN corpus adiposum [TA], fat body☆.

Bichat f.-p., SYN buccal f.-p.

buccal f.-p., an encapsuled mass of fat in the cheek on the outer side of the buccinator muscle, especially marked in the infant; supposed to strengthen and support the cheek during the act of sucking. SYN corpus adiposum buccae [TA], Bichat f.-p., Bichat protuberance, fat body of cheek, sucking cushion, sucking pad, suctorial pad.

Imlach f.-p., fat surrounding the round ligament of the uterus in the inguinal canal.

infrapatellar f.-p. [TA], the fatty mass that occupies the area between the patellar ligament and the infrapatellar synovial fold of the knee joint. SYN corpus adiposum infrapatellare [TA], infrapatellar fat body.

ischiorectal f.-p., SYN fat *body* of ischioanal fossa.

orbital f.-p., SYN retrobulbar *fat.*

fat·ty (fat'ē). Oily or greasy; relating in any sense to fat.

fat·ty ac·id. Any acid derived from fats by hydrolysis (e.g., oleic, palmitic, or stearic acids); any long-chain monobasic organic acid; they accumulate in disorders associated with the peroxisomes.

activated f. a., a fatty acyl-coenzyme A thiol ester.

diethenoid f. a., a f. a. containing two double bonds, e.g., linoleic acid.

fa

essential f. a., a f. a. that is nutritionally essential; e.g., linoleic acid, linolenic acid.

ω-3 f. a.'s, a class of f. a.'s that have a double bond three carbons from the methyl moiety; reportedly, they play a role in lowering cholesterol and LDL levels. SYN omega-3 f. a.'s.

omega-3 f. a.'s, SYN ω-3 f. a.'s.

saturated f. a., a f. a., the carbon chain of which contains no ethylenic or other unsaturated linkages between carbon atoms (e.g., stearic acid and palmitic acid); called saturated because it is incapable of absorbing any more hydrogen.

f. a. synthase complex, the multienzyme complex that catalyzes the formation of palmitate from acetyl-coenzyme A, malonyl-coenzyme A, and NADPH.

f. a. thiokinase, (1) long-chain: long-chain fatty acid–CoA ligase; **(2)** medium-chain: butyrate-CoA ligase.

unesterified free f. a. (FFA, UFA), free f. a.'s which occur in plasma as a result of lipolysis in adipose tissue or when plasma triacylglycerols are taken into tissues.

unsaturated f. a., a f. a., the carbon chain of which possesses one or more double or triple bonds (e.g., oleic acid, with one double bond in the molecule, and linoleic acid, with two); called unsaturated because it is capable of absorbing additional hydrogen.

fau·ces, gen. **fau·ci·um** (faw′sēz, faw′sē-ŭm) [TA]. The space between the cavity of the mouth and the pharynx, bounded by the soft palate and the base of the tongue. SEE ALSO *isthmus* of fauces. SYN oropharyngeal passage. [L. the throat]

fau·cial (faw′shăl). Relating to the fauces.

fau·na (faw′nă). The animal forms of a continent, district, locality, or habitat. [Mod. L. application of *Fauna,* sister of *Faunus,* a rural deity]

fa·ve·o·late (fā-vē′ō-lāt). Pitted.

fa·ve·o·lus, pl. **fa·ve·o·li** (fā-vē′ō-lŭs, -ō-lī). A small pit or depression. [Mod. L. dim. of *favus,* honeycomb]

fa·vic chan·de·liers (fā′vik shan-dĕ-lērz′). Specialized fungal hyphae that are curved, branched, and antlerlike in appearance, formed by the pathogens *Trichophyton schoenleinii* and *T. concentricum.*

fa·vid (fā′vid). An allergic reaction in the skin observed in patients who have favus.

fa·vism (fā′vizm). An acute condition seen chiefly in Italy, following the ingestion of certain species of beans, e.g., *Vicia faba,* or inhalation of the pollen of its flower; characterized by fever, headache, abdominal pain, severe anemia, prostration, and coma; it occurs in certain individuals with genetic erythrocytic deficiency of glucose 6-phosphate dehydrogenase. Chance exposure to the *Vicia faba,* by its impact on the phenotype of glucose-6-phosphate dehydrogenase, impinges on the expression or the gene, an example of incomplete penetrance. SYN fabism. [Ital. *favismo,* from *fava,* bean]

Favre, Maurice J., French physician, 1876–1954. SEE Gamna-F. *bodies,* under *body;* Nicolas-F. *disease.*

Favre, Maurice Jules, French physician, 1876–1954. SEE Goldmann-Favre *syndrome.* SEE ALSO Goldmann-Favre *syndrome.*

Favre dys·tro·phy. See under dystrophy.

fa·vus (fā′vŭs, fah′vŭs). A severe, unremitting type of chronic ringworm of the scalp and nails, with scarring and formation of crusts called scutula, caused by three dissimilar dermatophytes, *Trichophyton schoenleinii* (most commonly), *T. violaceum,* and *Microsporum gypseum;* it occurs more frequently in the Mediterranean countries, southeastern Europe, southern Asia, and northern Africa. SYN crusted ringworm, honeycomb ringworm, tinea favosa. [L. honeycomb]

Fc. SEE Fc *fragment.*

F.C.A.P. Abbreviation for Fellow of the College of American Pathologists.

F.C.C.P. Abbreviation for Fellow of the College of Chest Physicians.

Fd Abbreviation for ferredoxin.

FDA Abbreviation for Food and Drug Administration of the United States Department of Health and Human Services.

FDNB Abbreviation for fluoro-2,4-dinitrobenzene.

FDP Abbreviation for fibrin/fibrinogen degradation *products,* under *product.*

Fe Symbol for iron. [L. *ferrum,* iron]

^{52}Fe Symbol for iron-52.

^{55}Fe Symbol for iron-55.

^{59}Fe Symbol for iron-59.

fear (fēr). Apprehension; dread; alarm; by having an identifiable stimulus, f. is differentiated from anxiety which has no easily identifiable stimulus. [A.S. *faer*]

fea·tures (fē′choorz). The various parts of the face, forehead, eyes, nose, mouth, chin, cheeks, and ears, that give to it its individuality and character. [through O. Fr., fr. L. *factura,* a making, fr. *facio,* to do]

feb·ri·cant (feb′ri-kant). SYN febrifacient.

fe·bric·u·la (fē-brik′ū-lă). A simple continued fever; a mild fever of short duration, of indefinite origin, and without any distinctive pathology. [L. dim. of *febris,* fever]

feb·ri·fa·cient (feb-ri-fā′shĕnt). **1.** Causing or favoring the development of fever. SYN febriferous, febrific. **2.** Anything that produces fever. SEE ALSO pyrogenic. SYN febricant. [L. *febris,* fever, + *facio,* to make]

fe·brif·er·ous (fē-brif′er-ŭs). SYN febrifacient (1). [L. *febris,* fever, + *fero,* to bear, + *-ous*]

fe·brif·ic (fē-brif′ik). SYN febrifacient (1).

fe·brif·u·gal (fē-brif′ū-găl). SYN antipyretic (1).

feb·ri·fuge (feb′ri-fūj). SYN antipyretic (2). [L. *febris,* fever, + *fugo,* to put to flight]

feb·rile (feb′ril, fē′brīl). Denoting or relating to fever. SYN feverish (1), pyrectic, pyretic.

fe·bris (fē′bris). SYN fever. [L.]

f. melitensis (fē′bris mel-ĭ-ten′sis), infection with *Brucella melitensis;* SEE ALSO *Brucella melitensis.*

f. undulans (fē′bris ŭn-doo-lanz′), SYN brucellosis.

fe·cal (fē′kăl). Relating to feces.

fe·ca·lith (fē′kă-lith). A hard mass consisting of inspissated feces. SYN coprolith, stercolith. [L. *faeces,* feces, + G. *lithos,* stone]

fe·cal·oid (fē′kă-loyd). Resembling feces. [L. *faeces,* feces, + G. *eidos,* resemblance]

fe·ca·lo·ma (fē′kă-lō-mă). An accumulation of inspissated feces in the colon or rectum giving the appearance of an abdominal tumor. SYN coproma, fecal tumor, scatoma, stercoroma.

fe·ca·lu·ria (fē-kă-loo′rē-ă). The commingling of feces with urine passed from the urethra in persons with a fistula connecting the intestinal tract and lower urinary tract, often noticed most dramatically by the passage of flatus through the urethra. [L. *faeces,* feces, + G. *ouron,* urine]

fe·ces (fē′sēz). The matter discharged from the bowel during defecation, consisting of the undigested residue of food, epithelium, intestinal mucus, bacteria, and waste material from the food. SYN stercus. [L., pl. of *faex* (*faec-*), dregs]

Fechner, Gustav T., German physicist, 1801–1887. SEE Weber-F. *law;* F.-Weber *law.*

fec·u·lent (fek′ū-lent). Foul. [L. *faeculentus,* full of excrement, fr. *faeces,* dregs, feces]

fe·cund (fē′kŭnd, fek′ŭnd). SYN fertile (1). [L. *fecundus,* fruitful]

fec·un·date (fē′kŭn-dāt). To impregnate; to make fertile. [L. *fecundo,* pp. *-atus,* to make fruitful, fertilize]

fec·un·da·tion (fē-kŭn-dā′shŭn). The act of rendering fertile. SEE ALSO fertilization, impregnation.

fe·cun·di·ty (fē-kŭn′di-tē). The ability to produce live offspring.

Fede, Francesco, Italian physician, 1832–1913. SEE Riga-F. *disease.*

feed·back (fēd′bak). **1.** In a given system, the return, as input, of some of the output, as a regulatory mechanism; e.g., regulation of a furnace by a thermostat. **2.** An explanation for the learning of motor skills: sensory stimuli set up by muscle contractions modulate the activity of the motor system. **3.** The feeling evoked by another person's reaction to oneself. SEE biofeedback.

auditory f., the unwanted sound that occurs in an amplification system when the microphone picks up the sound from the speaker; a major problem in the use of hearing aids.

negative f., that which occurs if the sign or sense of the returned signal results in reduced amplification.

positive f., that which occurs when the sign or sense of the returned signal results in increased amplification or leads to instability.

tubuloglomerular f., a blood flow control mechanism operating in the kidneys that limits changes in glomerular filtration rate.

feed·ing (fēd′ing). Giving food or nourishment.

fictitious f., SYN sham f.

forced f., forcible f., (1) giving liquid food through a nasal tube passed into the stomach; **(2)** forcing a person to eat more food than desired. SYN forced alimentation.

gastric f., giving of nutriment directly into the stomach by means of a tube inserted via the nasopharynx and esophagus or directly through the abdominal wall.

nasal f., the giving of nourishment through a flexible tube passed through the nasal passages into the stomach.

sham f., a procedure used in the study of the psychic phase of gastric secretion: in experiments on dogs, the food, after being eaten, does not enter the stomach but issues from an esophageal fistula made in the neck; the chewing and swallowing of food causes an abundant secretion of gastric juice. SYN fictitious f.

feel·ing (fēl′ing). **1.** Any kind of conscious experience of sensation. **2.** The mental perception of a sensory stimulus. **3.** A quality of any mental state or mood, whereby it is recognized as pleasurable or the reverse. **4.** A bodily sensation that is correlated with a given emotion.

Feer, Emil, Swiss pediatrician, 1864–1955. SEE F. *disease.*

FEF Abbreviation for forced expiratory *flow.*

Fehling, Hermann von, German chemist, 1812–1885. SEE F. *reagent, solution.*

Feil, André, French physician, *1884. SEE Klippel-F. *syndrome.*

Feiss, Henry O., 20th century American orthopedic surgeon. SEE F. *line.*

FEL Abbreviation for familial erythrophagocytic lymphohistiocytosis.

fel·bam·ate (fel′bă-māt). An anticonvulsant/antiepileptic agent chemically related to meprobamate; useful in complex partial seizures.

Feldberg, Wilhelm, British physiologist, 1900–1993. SEE Dale-F. *law.*

Feldman, Harry Alfred, U.S. epidemiologist, 1914–1986. SEE Sabin-F. dye *test.*

Fe·li·dae (fē′li-dē). A family of Carnivora embracing domestic and wild cats such as lions and tigers. [L. *felis,* cat]

fe·line (fē′līn). Pertaining or relating to cats. [L. *felis,* cat]

Felix, Arthur, Polish bacteriologist, 1887–1956. SEE Weil-F. *reaction, test.*

fel·la·tio (fĕ-lā′shē-ō). Oral stimulation of the penis; a type of oral-genital sexual activity; contrasted with cunnilingus, which is the oral stimulation of the vulva or clitoris. SYN irrumation. [L.]

fel·o·dip·ine (fĕ-lō′dĭ-pēn). A calcium blocking agent of the dihydropyridine class resembling nifedipine.

fel·on (fel′ŏn). SYN whitlow. [M.E. *feloun,* malignant]

Fel·son. Benjamin, U.S. radiologist, 1913–1988. SEE silhouette *sign* of Felson.

felt·work. **1.** A fibrous network. **2.** A close plexus of nerve fibrils. SEE neuropil.

Felty, Augustus R., U.S. physician, 1895–1963. SEE F. *syndrome.*

fel·y·pres·sin (fel-i-pres′in). [Phe^2,Lys^8]Vasopressin; lysine vasopressin with L-phenylalanine at position 2. SYN octapressin.

fe·male (fē′māl). In zoology, denoting the gender that bears the young or the ovum.

genetic f., (1) an individual with a normal female karyotype, including two X chromosomes; **(2)** an individual whose cell nuclei contain Barr sex chromatin bodies, which are normally absent in males.

XO f., the genetic f. in Turner syndrome, where the criterion is the macroscopic appearance of the external genitals.

XXX f., SEE triple X *syndrome.*

fem·i·ni·za·tion (fem′i-ni-zā′shŭn). Development of what are superficially external female characteristics by a male.

testicular f., SYN complete androgen insensitivity syndrome. SEE testicular feminization *syndrome.*

fem·o·ral (fem′ŏ-răl). Relating to the femur or thigh.

fem·o·ro·cele (fem′ŏ-rō-sēl). SYN femoral *hernia.* [L. *femur,* thigh, + G. *kēlē,* hernia]

fem·o·ro·tib·i·al (fem′ŏ-rō-tib′ē-ăl). Relating to the femur and the tibia.

⬦**femto- (f).** Prefix used in SI and metric system to signify a submultiple of one-quadrillionth (10^{-15}). [Danish and Norwegian *femten,* fifteen]

fe·mur, gen. **fe·mo·ris,** pl. **fem·o·ra** (fē′mŭr, fem′ŏ-ris, -ă) [TA]. **1.** SYN thigh. **2.** The long bone of the thigh, articulating with the hip bone proximally and the tibia and patella distally. [L. thigh]

fen·bu·fen (fen-boo′fen). A nonsteroidal anti-inflammatory agent resembling ibuprofen.

fen·ca·mine (fen′kă-mēn). A central nervous system stimulant.

fen·clo·fen·ac (fen-klō′fen-ak). A nonsteroidal anti-inflammatory drug used in the treatment of joint disorders; similar to diclofenac.

fen·clo·nine (fen′klō-nēn). A serotonin inhibitor.

Fendt, H., 19th century Austrian dermatologist. SEE cutaneous *pseudolymphoma;* Spiegler-F. *sarcoid.*

fe·nes·tra, pl. **fe·nes·trae** (fe-nes′tră, -trē) **1** [TA]. An anatomic aperture, often closed by a membrane. **2.** An opening left in a plaster of Paris cast or other form of fixed dressing in order to permit access to a wound or inspection of the part. **3.** The opening in one of the blades of an obstetric forceps. **4.** A lateral opening in the sheath of an endoscopic instrument that allows lateral viewing or operative maneuvering. **5.** Openings in the wall of a tube, catheter, or trocar designed to promote better flow of air or fluids. SYN window (1) [TA]. [L. window]

f. of the cochlea, SYN round *window.*

f. coch′leae [TA], SYN round *window.*

f. nov-ova′lis, artificial opening through the otic capsule into the lateral semicircular canal, connecting the membranous labyrinth with the mastoid cavity produced during fenestration surgery.

f. ova′lis, SYN oval *window.*

f. rotun′da, SYN round *window.*

f. of the vestibule, SYN oval *window.*

f. vestib′uli [TA], SYN oval *window.*

fen·es·trat·ed (fen′es-trā′ted). Having fenestrae or windowlike openings.

fen·es·tra·tion (fen-es-trā′shŭn). **1.** The presence of openings or fenestrae in a part. **2.** Making openings in a dressing to allow inspection of the parts. **3.** In dentistry, a surgical perforation of the mucoperiosteum and alveolar process to expose the root tip of a tooth to permit drainage of tissue exudate.

optic nerve sheath f., the cutting of a window in the dura of the optic nerve sheath to relieve papilledema and prevent further loss of optic nerve fibers.

tracheal f., a surgical procedure to create an epithelialized mucocutaneous opening from the neck into the trachea.

fen·eth·yl·line hy·dro·chlo·ride (fen-eth′ĭ-lēn). An analeptic.

fen·flur·a·mine hy·dro·chlo·ride (fen-floo′ră-mēn). An anorexigenic agent.

Fenn, Wallace Osgood, U.S. physiologist, 1893–1971. SEE F. *effect.*

fen·nel (fen′l). Fennel seed, the dried ripe fruit of cultivated varieties of *Foeniculum vulgare* (family Umbelliferae), an herb native to southern Europe and Asia, a diaphoretic and carminative; a volatile oil distilled from the fruit is used as a flavoring. [through O. Fr., fr. L. *faeniculum,* fennel, dim. of *faenum,* hay]

fen·o·pro·fen cal·ci·um (fen-ō-prō′fen). An anti-inflammatory analgesic used for treatment of mild to moderate pain and for osteoarthritis; similar to ibuprofen.

fen·o·ter·ol (fen′ō-ter′ol). A β_2 agonist inhalation bronchodilator.

fe

fen·pip·ra·mide (fen-pip′ră-mīd). An antispasmodic.

fen·ta·nyl cit·rate (fen′tă-nil). A short-acting narcotic analgesic about 100 times more potent than morphine used as a supplementary analgesic in general anesthesia.

fen·ti·clor (fen′ti-klōr). A topical anti-infective agent.

fen·u·greek (fen′ū-grēk). An annual plant indigenous to western Asia and cultivated in Africa and parts of Europe; the mucilaginous seeds are used as food and in the preparation of culinary spices (curry). [L. *faenum graecum*, fenugreek, fr. *faenum*, hay, + *Graecus*, Greek]

Fenwick, Edwin Hurry, British urologist, 1856–1944. SEE F.-Hunner *ulcer*.

fer·al (fer′il). Denoting an animal that is wild and untamed.

Féréol, Louis Felix Henri, French physician, 1825–1891.

Ferguson, J.K.W., 20th century obstetrician. SEE F. *reflex*.

Fergusson, Sir William, Scottish surgeon, 1808–1877. SEE F. *incision*.

fer·ment (fer-ment′). **1.** To cause or to undergo fermentation. **2.** An agent that causes fermentation. [L. *fermentum*, leaven]

fer·ment·a·ble (fer-ment′ă-bl). Capable of undergoing fermentation.

fer·men·ta·tion (fer-men-tā′shŭn). **1.** A chemical change induced in a complex organic compound by the action of an enzyme, whereby the substance is split into simpler compounds. **2.** In bacteriology, the anaerobic dissimilation of substrates with the production of energy and reduced compounds; the mechanism of f. does not involve a respiratory chain or cytochrome, hence oxygen is not the final electron acceptor as it is in oxidation. [L. *fermento*, pp. -*atus*, to ferment, from L. *fermentum*, yeast]

acetic f., acetous f., f., as of wine or beer, whereby the alcohol is oxidized to acetic acid (vinegar).

alcoholic f., the anaerobic formation of ethanol and CO_2 from D-glucose. Cf. Gay-Lussac *equation*.

amylic f., f. of potato or corn mash, or other starchy material, by which fusel oil is produced.

lactic acid f., the production of lactic acid in milk, or other carbohydrate-containing media, caused by the presence of any one of a number of lactic acid bacteria.

fer·ment·a·tive (fer-ment′ă-tiv). Causing or having the ability to cause fermentation.

fer·ment·er (fer-ment′er). A large container used in cultures of microorganisms.

fer·mi·um (Fm) (fer′mē-ŭm). Radioactive element, artificially prepared in 1955, atomic no. 100, atomic wt. 257.095; ^{257}Fm has the longest known half-life (100.5 days) of this transuranium element. [E. *Fermi*, It.-U.S. physicist and Nobel laureate, 1901–1954]

Fernandez re·ac·tion. See under reaction.

Fernbach, Auguste, French microbiologist, 1860–1939. SEE F. *flask*.

fern·ing. A term used to describe the pattern of arborization produced by cervical mucus, secreted at midcycle, upon crystallization, which resembles somewhat a fern or a palm leaf.

fer·ra·tin (fer′ă-tin). A hematinic.

fer·re·dox·ins (fer-ĕ-dok′sinz). Proteins containing iron-sulfur complexes, displaying electron-carrier activity but no classical enzyme function. F.'s are found in green plants, algae, anaerobic bacteria, and in mitochondria from the adrenal cortex and heart muscle. They are involved in several oxidation-reduction reactions in living organisms (e.g., nitrogen fixation).

Ferrein, Antoine, French anatomist, 1693–1769. SEE F. *canal*, *cords*, under *cord*, *foramen*, *ligament*, *pyramid*, *tube*, *vasa* aberrantia, under *vas*; *processus* ferreini.

ferri-. Prefix designating the presence of a ferric ion in a compound. [L. *ferrum*, iron]

fer·ric (fer′ik). Relating to iron, especially denoting a salt containing iron in its higher (triad) valence, Fe^{3+}.

fer·ric am·mo·ni·um cit·rate. A compound used in hypochromic anemia; it is relatively free of astringent and irritant action.

fer·ric am·mo·ni·um cit·rate, green. A compound used in hypochromic anemia.

f. a. c. am·mo·ni·um sul·fate. An astringent and styptic. SYN ammonium ferric sulfate, ferric alum, iron alum.

fer·ric chlo·ride. An astringent and styptic.

fer·ric fruc·tose. A potassium-iron-fructose; a hematinic drug.

fer·ric glyc·er·o·phos·phate. A tonic and a source of iron.

fer·ric hy·drox·ide. A compound previously used, freshly prepared, as an antidote to arsenic poisoning.

fer·ric ox·ide. A compound used as a coloring material.

fer·ric phos·phate. A compound used as a feed and as a food supplement.

soluble f. p., f. p. with sodium citrate; a hematinic.

fer·ric sul·fate. Iron persulfate, tersulfate, or sesquisulfate; an astringent and styptic.

fer·ri·cy·a·nide (fe-rī-sī′ă-nīd, fer-ē-). The anion $Fe(CN)_6^{3-}$.

fer·ri·cy·to·chrome (fe-rī-sī′tō-krōm, fer-ē-). A cytochrome containing oxidized (ferric) iron.

fer·ri·heme (fe′rī-hēm, fer′ē-). SYN hematin.

f. chloride, SYN hemin.

fer·ri·he·mo·glo·bin (fer′ī-hē-mō-glō′bin, fer′ē-). SYN methemoglobin.

fer·ri·por·phy·rin (fe-rī-pōr′fi-rin, fer-ē-). The compound formed between a ferric ion and a porphyrin; e.g., ferriprotoporphyrin (hemin).

f. chloride, SYN hemin.

fer·ri·pro·to·por·phy·rin (fer′i-prō-tō-pōr′fi-rin, fer′ē-). SYN hemin.

fer·ri·tin (fer′ĭ-tin, fer′ă-). An iron-protein complex, containing up to 23% iron, formed by the union of ferric ions with apoferritin; it is found in the intestinal mucosa, spleen, bone marrow, reticulocytes, and liver, and regulates iron storage and transport from the intestinal lumen to plasma.

ferro-. Prefix designating the presence of metallic iron or of the divalent ion Fe^{2+}. [L. *ferrum*, iron]

fer·ro·che·la·tase (fār-ō-kē′lă-tās). A lyase that catalyzes the reversible acid hydrolysis of heme, forming protoporphyrin IX and free ferrous iron; inhibited by lead; a deficiency of f. results in erythropoietic protoporphyria.

fer·ro·cho·li·nate (fār′ō-kō′li-nāt). Iron choline citrate chelate, used for oral administration in the treatment and prevention of iron deficiency anemias.

fer·ro·cy·a·nide (fār-ō-sī′ă-nīd). A compound containing the anion $Fe(CN)_6^{4-}$.

fer·ro·cy·to·chrome (fār-ō-sī′tō-krōm). A cytochrome containing reduced (ferrous) iron.

fer·ro·heme (fār′ō-hēm). SYN heme.

fer·ro·ki·net·ics (fār-ō-ki-net′iks). The study of iron metabolism using radioactive iron. [L. *ferrum*, iron, + G. *kinēsis*, movement]

fer·ro·por·phy·rin (fār-ō-pōr′fi-rin). The compound formed between a ferrous ion and a porphyrin; e.g., ferroprotoporphyrin (heme).

fer·ro·pro·teins (fār-ō-prō′tēnz). Proteins containing iron in a prosthetic group; e.g., heme, cytochromes.

fer·ro·pro·to·por·phy·rin (fār′ō-prō-tō-pōr′fi-rin). SYN heme.

fer·ro·so·fer·ric (fār-ō′sō-fār′ik). Denoting a combination of a ferrous compound with a ferric compound, as in Fe_3O_4.

fer·ro·ther·a·py (fār′ō-thār′ă-pē). Therapeutic use of iron. [L. *ferrum*, iron]

fer·rous (fār′ŭs). Relating to iron, especially denoting a salt containing iron in its lowest valence state, Fe^{2+}. [L. *ferreus*, made of iron]

fer·rous cit·rate. A compound that occurs in several forms, two of which are monoferrous acid citrate monohydrate and triferrous dicitrate decahydrate; a hematinic.

fer·rous fu·ma·rate. Iron fumarate, a hematinic.

fer·rous glu·co·nate. Iron gluconate; a hematinic.

fer·rous lac·tate. Iron lactate; a hematinic.

fer·rous suc·ci·nate. Iron succinate; a hematinic.

fer·rous f. s.. SYN iron *sulfate*.

dried f. s., exsiccated iron sulfate; a hematinic.

fer·ru·gi·na·tion (fe-roo′ji-nā′shŭn). Deposition of mineral deposits including iron in the walls of small blood vessels and at the site of a dead neuron. [L. *ferrugo,* iron-rust]

fer·ru·gi·nous (fe-roo′ji-nŭs). **1.** Iron-bearing; associated with or containing iron. **2.** Of the color of iron rust. [L. *ferrugineus,* iron rust, rust-colored]

fer·rule (fer′ool). A metal band or ring used around the crown or root of a tooth. [corrupted through O. Fr. and Medieval L., fr. L. *viriola,* a small bracelet]

Ferry, Erwin S., U.S. physicist, 1868–1956. SEE F.-Porter *law.*

fer·tile (fer′til). **1.** Fruitful; capable of conceiving and bearing young. SYN fecund. **2.** Impregnated; fertilized. [L. *fertilis,* fr. *fero,* to bear]

fer·til·i·ty (fer-til′i-tē). The actual production of live offspring, i.e., does not include stillbirths.

fer·til·i·za·tion (fer′til-i-zā′shŭn). The process beginning with penetration of the secondary oocyte by the spermatozoon and completed by fusion of the male and female pronuclei.

in vitro **f. (IVF),** a process whereby (usually multiple) ova are placed in a medium to which sperm are added for fertilization, the zygote thus produced then being introduced into the uterus and allowed to develop to term.

in vivo **f.,** f. of a ripe egg within the distal fallopian tube of a fertile donor female (rather than in an artificial medium), for subsequent nonsurgical transfer to an infertile recipient.

fer·til·i·zin (fer-til′i-zin). An acid polysaccharide-amino acid complex associated with the female gamete membrane of several organisms; provides receptor groups that agglutinate sperm and bind them to ova.

Fer·u·la (făr′oo-lă). A genus of plants of the family Umbelliferae. *F. assa-foetida, F. rubricaulis* and *F. foetida* furnish asafetida; *F. galbaniflua* and *F. rubricaulis,* galbanium; and *F. sumbul,* sumbul. [L. giant plant]

fer·ves·cence (fer-ves′ens). An increase of fever. [L. *fervesco,* to begin to boil, fr. *ferveo,* to boil]

FESS Abbreviation for functional endoscopic sinus *surgery.*

fes·ter. 1. To form pus or putrefy. **2.** To make inflamed. [L. *fistula*]

fes·ti·nant (fes′ti-nant). Rapid; hastening; accelerating. [L. *festino,* to hasten]

fes·ti·na·tion (fes-ti-nā′shŭn). SYN festinating *gait.* [L. *festino,* to hasten]

fes·toon (fes-toon′). **1.** A carving in the base material of a denture that simulates the contours of the natural tissue that is being replaced by the denture. **2.** A distinguishing characteristic of certain hard tick species, consisting of small rectangular areas separated by grooves along the posterior margin of the dorsum of both males and females. [thr. Fr. fr. L. *festum,* festival, hence festive decorations]

gingival f., an arcuate enlargement of the marginal gingiva.

fes·toon·ing (fes-toon′ing). Undulating, like the pattern of dermal papillae beneath a subepidermal blister.

FET Abbreviation for forced expiratory *time.*

fe·tal (fē′tăl). **1.** Relating to a fetus; **2.** In utero development after the eighth week.

fe·tal·ism (fē′tăl-izm). Presence of certain fetal structures or characteristics in the body after birth.

fe·tal re·tic·u·la·ris (fē′tăl re-tik-ū-lā′ris). **1.** SYN fetal adrenal *cortex.* **2.** SYN androgenic *zone* (2). **3.** SYN X *zone* (2).

fe·ta·tion (fē-tā′shŭn). SYN pregnancy.

fe·ti·cide (fē′ti-sīd). Destruction of the embryo or fetus in the uterus. [L. *fetus* + *caedo,* to kill]

fet·id (fet′id, fē′tid). Foul-smelling. [L. *foetidus*]

fet·ish (fet′ish, fē′tish). An inanimate object or nonsexual body part that is regarded as endowed with magic or erotic qualities. [Fr. *fétiche,* fr. L. *factitius,* made by art, artificial]

fet·ish·ism (fet′ish-izm, fē′tish-). The act of worshipping or using for sexual arousal and gratification that which is regarded as a fetish.

fe·to·glob·u·lins (fē-tō-glob′ū-linz). One of a number of proteins of unknown function found in fetal blood. α-F. occurs in small amounts in normal adults and in larger amounts in the fetus and pregnant mother, especially in the second trimester; elevated levels are also detected in adult patients with liver disease and neoplasms.

fe·tog·ra·phy (fē-tog′ră-fē). Radiography of the fetus *in utero,* using contrast medium; an obsolete technique. Cf. amniography. [L. *fetus* + G. *graphō,* to write]

fe·tol·o·gy (fē-tol′ō-jē). SYN maternal-fetal *medicine.* [L. *fetus* + G. *logos,* study]

fe·tom·e·try (fē-tom′e-trē). Estimation of the size of the fetus, especially of its head, prior to delivery. [L. *fetus* + G. *metron,* measure]

fe·top·a·thy (fē-top′ă-thē). SYN embryopathy. [L. *fetus* + G. *pathos,* suffering, disease]

diabetic f., f. resulting from maternal diabetes, which may cause macrosomia and fetal death.

fe·to·pla·cen·tal (fē′tō-pla-sen′tăl). Relating to the fetus and its placenta.

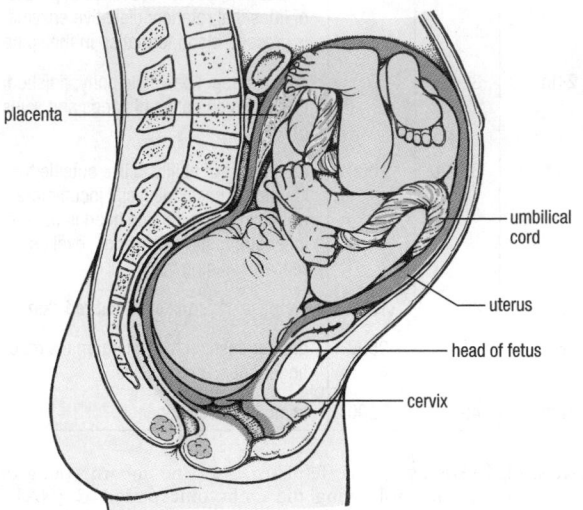

placenta

umbilical cord

uterus

head of fetus

cervix

fetus: (prior to delivery)

fe·to·pro·teins (fē-tō-prō′tēnz). Fetal proteins found in small amounts in adults in the following forms: α-f. (AFP) increases in maternal blood during pregnancy and, when detected by amniocentesis, is an important indicator of open neural tube defects and is also used as a tumor marker in adults (see definition below); β-f., although a fetal liver protein, has been detected in adult patients with liver disease; γ-f. occurs in various neoplasms. SEE ALSO fetoglobulins.

α **f.,** a protein normally produced during the 12th to 15th week of gestation, decreasing thereafter, but appearing in the blood in certain tumors, such as embryonal carcinomas of the testis and ovary, hepatoma, and less often in patients with carcinomas of the pancreas, stomach, colon, or lung. When present, a useful marker in following the course of a tumor.

fe·tor (fē′tōr). A very offensive odor. [L. an offensive smell, fr. *feteo,* to stink]

f. hepat′icus, a peculiar odor to the breath in persons with severe liver disease; caused by volatile aromatic substances that accumulate in the blood and urine due to defective hepatic metabolism. SYN liver breath.

f. o′ris, SYN halitosis.

fe

fe·to·scope (fē′tō-skōp). **1.** A fiberoptic endoscope used in fetology. **2.** A stethoscope designed for listening to fetal heart sounds.

fe·tos·co·py (fē-tos′kŏ-pē). Use of a fiberoptic endoscope to view the fetus and the fetal surface of the placenta transabdominally, and also for collection of fetal blood from the umbilical vein for antenatal diagnosis of fetal disorders.

fe·tu·in (fē-too′in). A low molecular-weight globulin that constitutes nearly the total globulin in fetal blood. [fetus + -in]

development of the fetus			
week of pregnancy	length (in cm)	weight (in g)	particular changes noted
12th	7.5–10		stump-formed extremities, sexual differences outwardly visible; anal opening, eyebrows present
16th	16		body fully shaped; eyelids fused shut; skin crab-red; down on forehead and chin; beginning of skeletal articulation, dental structures, blood formation in the liver
20th	25		vernix caseosa on forehead and chin; meconium; cecum descends in process of intestinal rotation; digestive enzyme is present, blood formation in the spine
24th	30–32		down (lanugo) on whole body; finished epidermis on palms of hands and soles of feet
28th	35–40	1000	attainment of ability to live outside the womb; fat cushioning still incomplete; grimacing face, hair on head is 0.5 cm in length; testicle descends, eyelids reopen, whining voice
32nd	46	1800	increase of vernix caseosa, red skin
36th	51	2500	greater cushion of fat; fingernails reach finger ends; strong voice
40th	49–53	3200	completely developed

fe·tus, pl. **fe·tus·es** (fē′tŭs, fē′tŭs-ez). **1.** The unborn young of a viviparous animal following the embryonic period. **2** [NA]. In humans, the product of conception from the end of the eighth week to the moment of birth. [L. offspring]

f. in fe′tu, condition in which a small, imperfectly formed fetus is contained within a fetus.

harlequin f., a severe autosomal recessive form of collodion baby in a newborn, usually premature, infant; i.e., a form of ichthyosiform erythroderma characterized by encasement of the body in grayish brown, often fissured plaques resembling plates of armor and by grotesque deformity of the face with eclabium and gangrene of terminal phalanges; usually fatal within a few days, although treatment with 13-*cis*-retinoic acid has been successful in some cases. SYN ichthyosis fetalis (1).

impacted f., a f. which, because of its large size or narrowing of the pelvic canal, has become wedged and incapable of spontaneous advance or recession.

f. papyra′ceus, one of twin fetuses that has died and been pressed flat against the uterine wall by the growth of the living f.

f. sanguinolentis (san-gwi′nō-len′tis), dead f. that has become macerated.

Feulgen, Robert, German nucleic acid biochemist and cytochemist, 1884–1955. First to detect DNA in cells by a specific cytochemical test. SEE Feulgen *cytometry*.

FEV Abbreviation for forced expiratory *volume*, with subscript indicating time interval in seconds.

FEVER

fe·ver (fē′ver). A complex physiologic response to disease mediated by pyrogenic cytokines and characterized by a rise in core temperature, generation of acute phase reactants, and activation of immune systems. SYN febris, pyrexia. [A.S. *fefer*]

absorption f., an elevation of temperature often occurring, without other untoward symptoms, shortly after childbirth, assumed to be due to absorption of uterine discharges through abrasions of the vaginal wall.

acclimating f., elevated temperature with malaise that occurs upon working in a very hot environment.

Aden f., SYN dengue.

aestivoautumnal f., SYN falciparum *malaria*.

African hemorrhagic f., hemorrhagic f. associated with the morphologically similar but antigenically distinct Marburg and Ebola viruses as well as numerous other viruses that cause similar diseases. SEE ALSO viral hemorrhagic f.

African tick f., SYN Crimean-Congo hemorrhagic f.

African tick-bite f., a febrile disease caused by the bacterium *Rickettsia africae* in southern Africa and characterized by taches noires at the sites of bites by infected *Amblyomma* ticks and lymphadenopathy.

algid pernicious f., a pernicious malarial attack in which the patient presents symptoms of collapse and shock.

ardent f., a term sometimes applied to hyperpyrexia occurring in intermittent malarial f. SYN heat apoplexy (2).

Argentinean hemorrhagic f., a form of hemorrhagic f. observed in South America, seemingly transmitted by contact from rodents to humans and caused by the Junin virus, a member of the family Arenaviridae.

artificial f., SYN pyretotherapy.

aseptic f., f. accompanied by malaise due to absorption of dead but not infected tissue following an injury.

Assam f., SYN visceral *leishmaniasis*.

Australian Q f., a variety of Q f. occurring in Australia; an acute infectious rickettsial infection caused by *Coxiella burnetii* and transmitted by ticks, enzootic in animals in Australia, especially bandicoots.

autumn f., (1) a f. resembling dengue occurring at the end of the summer in India; SYN seven-day f. (1). (2) SYN hasamiyami.

benign tertian f., SYN vivax *malaria*.

bilious remittent f., (1) old term for relapsing f.; (2) malarial "bilious" vomiting associated with marked increase of serum bilirubin.

black f., SYN Rocky Mountain spotted f.

blackwater f., hemoglobinuria resulting from severe hemolysis occurring in falciparum malaria. SYN malarial *hemoglobinuria*.

blue f., SYN Rocky Mountain spotted f.

Bolivian hemorrhagic f., a disease similar to Argentinian hemorrhagic f. but caused by the Machupo virus, a member of the family Arenaviridae.

bouquet f., SYN dengue.

boutonneuse f., SYN Mediterranean spotted f.

brass founder's f., an occupational disease, characterized by malaria-like symptoms, due to inhalation of particles and fumes of metallic oxides. Fumes are formed by evaporation at very high temperature and condensation in air into fine particles. SYN brass founder's ague, foundryman's f., metal fume f., zinc fume f.

Brazilian hemorrhagic f., SYN Brazilian spotted f.

Brazilian purpuric f., SYN Brazilian spotted f.

Brazilian spotted f., fulminating sepsis, usually beginning with conjunctivitis, characterized by purpuric skin lesions, a high fatality rate; thought to be due to *Haemophilus aegyptius*. SYN Brazilian hemorrhagic f., Brazilian purpuric f.

breakbone f., SYN dengue.

Bunyamwera f., a febrile illness of humans in Africa caused by the Bunyamwera virus (family Bunyaviridae) and transmitted by culicine mosquitoes.

Burdwan f., SYN visceral *leishmaniasis*.

Bwamba f., a febrile illness of humans in Africa caused by a virus of the family Bunyaviridae and transmitted by mosquitoes.

cachectic f., SYN visceral *leishmaniasis*.

camp f., (1) any epidemic febrile illness affecting troops in an encampment; **(2)** obsolete term for typhus.

canicola f., a disease of humans caused by the *canicola* serovar of *Leptospira interrogans* and transmitted by infective urine, usually from dogs but rarely from cattle and swine.

catarrhal f., old term for the group of respiratory tract diseases including the common cold, influenza, and lobular and lobar pneumonia.

cat-bite f., SYN cat-bite *disease*.

catheter f., SYN urinary f.

catscratch f., SYN catscratch *disease*.

Central European tick-borne f., SYN tick-borne *encephalitis* (Central European subtype).

cerebrospinal f., SYN meningococcal *meningitis*.

Charcot intermittent f., f., chills, right upper quadrant pain, and jaundice associated with intermittently obstructing common duct stones.

childbed f., SYN puerperal f.

Colorado tick f., an infection caused by Colorado tick f. virus and transmitted to humans by *Dermacentor andersoni;* the symptoms are mild, there is no rash, the temperature is not excessive, and the disease is rarely, if ever, fatal.

Congolian red f., SYN murine *typhus*.

continued f., obsolete term for a continual febrile illness without intermittency as with malaria. Many cases were typhoid f., but included many types of febrile illnesses.

cotton-mill f., SYN byssinosis.

Crimean f., SYN Mediterranean spotted f.

Crimean-Congo hemorrhagic f., a form of hemorrhagic f. distinct from Omsk hemorrhagic f., occurring in central Russia, transmitted by species of the tick *Hyalomma*, and caused by Crimean-Congo hemorrhagic f. virus, a member of the Bunyaviridae family; horses are the chief reservoir of human infection; characterized by abrupt onset, high f., headache, myalgia, widespread petechial hemorrhagic lesions, gastrointestinal bleeding, high fatality rate. SYN African tick f.

dandy f., SYN dengue.

date f., SYN dengue.

deer-fly f., SYN tularemia.

dehydration f., SYN thirst f.

dengue f., SYN dengue.

dengue hemorrhagic f., SYN dengue.

desert f., SYN primary *coccidioidomycosis*.

digestive f., a slight rise of body temperature occurring during the period of digestion.

diphasic milk f., SYN tick-borne *encephalitis* (Central European subtype).

double quotidian f., malaria in which two paroxysms of f. occur daily.

drug f., f. resulting from an allergic reaction to a drug that clears rapidly on discontinuation of the drug.

Dumdum f., SYN visceral *leishmaniasis*.

Dutton relapsing f., SYN Dutton *disease*.

Ebola hemorrhagic f., SYN hemorrhagic f.

elephantoid f., lymphangitis and an elevation of temperature marking the beginning of endemic elephantiasis (filariasis).

enteric f., (1) SYN typhoid f; **(2)** the group of typhoid and paratyphoid f.'s.

entericoid f., a f., neither paratyphoid nor typhoid, resembling the latter.

ephemeral f., a febrile episode lasting no more than a day or two.

epidemic hemorrhagic f., a condition characterized by acute onset of headache, chills and high f., sweating, thirst, photophobia, coryza, cough, myalgia, arthralgia, and abdominal pain with nausea and vomiting; this phase lasts from 3–6 days and is followed by capillary and renal interstitial hemorrhages, edema, oliguria, azotemia, and shock; most varieties are caused by numerous viruses including togaviruses, arenaviruses, flaviviruses, and bunyaviruses, and are rodent-borne. SYN hemorrhagic f. with renal syndrome, Songo f.

epimastical f., a f. increasing steadily until its acme is reached, then declining by crisis or lysis.

eruptive f., SYN Mediterranean spotted f.

essential f., f. without known infectious disease.

exanthematous f., fever associated with an exanthem.

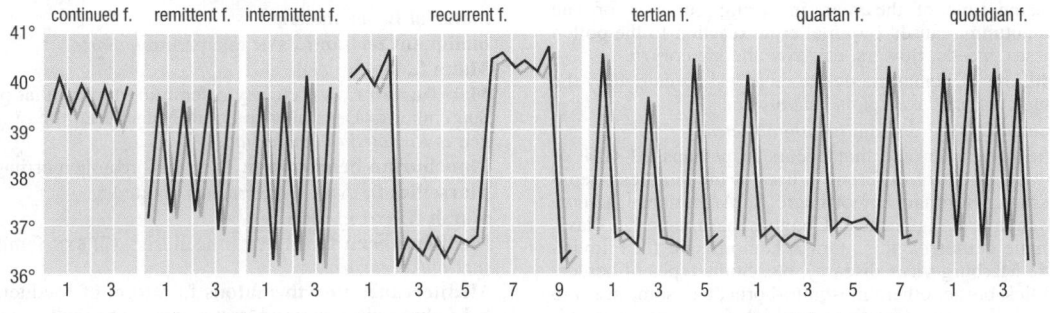

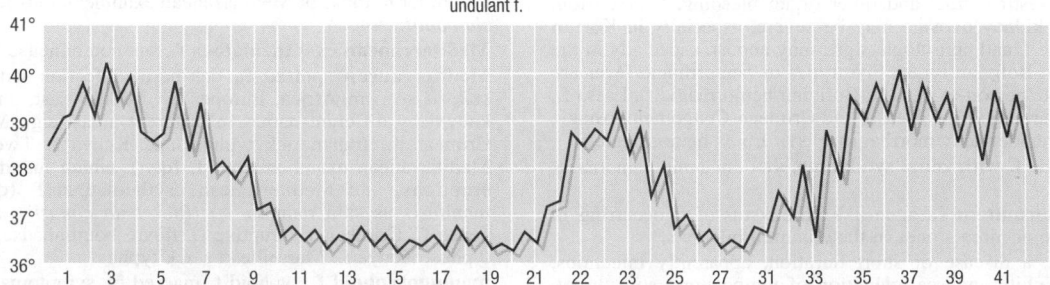

fever: units along horizontal axis represent days

exsiccation f., SYN thirst f.

falciparum f., SYN falciparum *malaria.*

familial Mediterranean f., SYN familial paroxysmal *polyserositis.*

Far East hemorrhagic f., tick-borne infection with *Rickettsia sibirica,* seen primarily in Siberia and Mongolia.

fatigue f., an elevation of the body temperature, lasting sometimes several days, following excessive and long continued muscular exertion.

field f., a leptospirosis caused by *leptospira.*

five-day f., SYN trench f.

Flinders Island spotted f., a febrile disease caused by the bacterium *Rickettsia honei* in southeastern Australia and characterized by headache, myalgia, and maculopapular rash. [named after Flinders Island in Tasmania, Australia, from which the first cases of the disease were identified]

flood f., SYN tsutsugamushi *disease.*

food f., a disorder seen primarily in childhood, consisting of a sudden rise of temperature accompanied by marked digestive disturbances, which lasts from a few days to several weeks; believed to be a form of food poisoning.

Fort Bragg f., SYN pretibial f.

foundryman's f., SYN brass founder's f.

Gambian f., an irregular relapsing f., lasting 1–4 days with intermissions of 2–5 days, marked by enlargement of the spleen, rapid pulse, and breathing; due to the presence in the blood of *Trypanosoma brucei gambiense,* the pathogenic microorganism of Gambian or West African sleeping sickness.

glandular f., SYN infectious *mononucleosis.*

Haverhill f., an infection by *Streptobacillus moniliformis* marked by initial chills and high f. (gradually subsiding), by arthritis usually in the larger joints and spine, and by a rash occurring chiefly over the joints and on the extensor surfaces of the extremities; "Haverhill f." is used to indicate *Streptobacillus moniliformis* infections not associated with rat bite but resulting from contaminated food or water. SYN erythema arthriticum epidemicum. [*Haverhill,* MA, where an epidemic occurred in 1926]

hay f., a form of atopy characterized by an acute irritative inflammation of the mucous membranes of the eyes and upper respiratory passages accompanied by itching and profuse watery secretion, usually without temperature elevation, followed occasionally by bronchitis and asthma; the episode recurs annually at the same or nearly the same time of the year, in spring, summer, or late summer and autumn, caused by an allergic reaction to the pollen of trees, grasses, weeds, flowers, etc. SYN allergic coryza.

hematuric bilious f., hematuria due to renal lesions caused by the malarial hematozoon, *Plasmodium falciparum.*

hemoglobinuric f., SYN malarial *hemoglobinuria.*

hemorrhagic f., a syndrome that occurs in perhaps 20–40% of infections by a number of different viruses of the families Arenaviridae (Lassa f., Bolivian hemorrhagic f., Argentinean hemorrhagic f.), Bunyaviridae (Crimean-Congo hemorrhagic f.), Flaviviridae (Dengue hemorrhagic f., Omsk hemorrhagic f.), Filoviridae (Ebola f., Marburg virus disease), etc. Some types of hemorrhagic f. are tick-borne, others mosquito-borne, and some seem to be zoonoses; clinical manifestations are high f., scattered petechiae, gastrointestinal tract and other organ bleeding, hypotension, and shock; kidney damage may be severe, especially in Korean hemorrhagic f. and neurologic signs may appear, especially in the Argentinean-Bolivian types. Five types of hemorrhagic fever are transmissible person-to-person: Bolivian hemorrhagic f., Lassa f., Ebola f., Marburg virus disease, and Crimean-Congo hemorrhagic f. SEE ALSO epidemic hemorrhagic f. SYN Ebola hemorrhagic f.

hemorrhagic f. with renal syndrome, SYN epidemic hemorrhagic f.

hepatic intermittent f., ague-like paroxysms of f. occurring in cases of one or more stones in the common bile duct.

herpetic f., a disease of short duration, apparently infectious, marked by chills, nausea, elevation of temperature, sore throat, and a herpetic eruption on the face and other areas; primary infection is with herpes simplex virus.

hospital f., SYN epidemic *typhus.*

icterohemorrhagic f., infection with the variety of *Leptospira interrogans* serotype known as icterohemorrhagiae, characterized by fever, jaundice, hemorrhagic lesions, azotemia, and central nervous system manifestations. SYN leptospirosis icterohemorrhagica.

Ilhéus f., a febrile illness caused by the Ilhéus virus, a Flavivirus, and transmitted by a mosquito. SEE ALSO Ilhéus *encephalitis.*

inanition f., SYN thirst f.

induced f., SYN pyretotherapy.

intermittent malarial f., SEE intermittent *malaria.*

inundation f., SYN tsutsugamushi *disease.*

island f., SYN tsutsugamushi *disease.*

jail f., SYN typhus.

Japanese river f., SYN tsutsugamushi *disease.*

Japanese spotted f., a febrile disease caused by the bacterium *Rickettsia japonica* and characterized by headache and exanthema; found in Japan.

jungle f., SYN malaria.

jungle yellow f., a form occurring in South America, transmitted by *Aedes leucocelaenus* and various treetop mosquitoes of the *Haemagogus* complex; transmitted normally to primates, occasionally by chance to humans to set off a human outbreak of classical yellow fever transmitted by *Aedes aegypti.*

Katayama f., SYN Katayama *disease.*

kedani f., SYN tsutsugamushi *disease.*

Kenya f., SYN Mediterranean spotted f.

Kew Gardens f., SYN rickettsialpox. [*Kew Gardens,* area in Queens, NYC, where first reported]

Kinkiang f., SYN *schistosomiasis* japonica.

Korean hemorrhagic f., a form of epidemic hemorrhagic f. caused by the Hantaan virus. SYN Manchurian hemorrhagic f.

Lassa f., a severe form of epidemic hemorrhagic f. which is highly fatal. It was first recognized in Lassa, Nigeria, is caused by the Lassa virus, a member of the Arenaviridae family, and is characterized by high f., sore throat, severe muscle aches, skin rash with hemorrhages, headache, abdominal pain, vomiting, and diarrhea; the multimammate rat *Mastomys natalensis* serves as reservoir, but person-to-person transmission also is common. SYN Lassa hemorrhagic f.

Lassa hemorrhagic f., SYN Lassa f.

laurel f., an affection of the same nature as hay f., occurring at the time of flowering of laurel.

malarial f., SEE malaria.

malignant tertian f., SYN falciparum *malaria.*

Malta f., SYN brucellosis.

Manchurian f., a f. closely resembling typhus that prevails from September to December in South Manchuria; the probable pathogen is *Rickettsia manchuriae.*

Manchurian hemorrhagic f., SYN Korean hemorrhagic f.

Marseilles f., SYN Mediterranean spotted f.

marsh f., SYN malaria.

Mediterranean f., (1) SYN brucellosis; (2) SYN familial paroxysmal *polyserositis.*

Mediterranean erythematous f., a form of Mediterranean spotted f. that causes skin redness; its course and other symptoms may be similar to those of Mediterranean exanthematous f. SEE *Rickettsia conorii.*

Mediterranean exanthematous f., SEE boutonneuse f.

Mediterranean spotted f., tick-borne infection with *Rickettsia conorii* seen in Africa, Europe, the Middle East, and India and known by different names in different areas, e.g., Marseilles f., Crimean f., Indian tick typhus, and Kenya f. Two forms are Mediterranean exanthematous f. (q.v.), which manifests as skin eruptions, and Mediterranean erythematous f. (q.v.), which manifests as skin redness. SEE *Rickettsia conorii.* SYN boutonneuse f., Crimean f., eruptive f., fièvre boutonneuse, Indian tick typhus, Kenya f., Marseilles f., tick typhus.

meningotyphoid f., typhoid f. marked by symptoms of irritation or inflammation of the cerebral or spinal meninges.

metal fume f., SYN brass founder's f.

Mexican spotted f., SYN Rocky Mountain spotted f.

miliary f., (1) an infectious disease characterized by profuse sweating and the production of sudamina, occurring formerly in severe epidemics; **(2)** SYN miliaria.

milk f., (1) a slight elevation of temperature following childbirth, said to be due to the establishment of the secretion of milk, but probably the same as absorption f.; **(2)** an afebrile metabolic disease, occurring shortly after parturition in dairy cattle, characterized by hypocalcemia and manifested by loss of consciousness and general paralysis.

mill f., SYN byssinosis.

miniature scarlet f., a reaction consisting of f., nausea, vomiting, and a transient scarlatiniform rash that appears in a susceptible person when injected with the toxin of *Streptococcus pyogenes.* [L. *minio,* pp. *atus,* to color with *minium,* red-lead]

monoleptic f., a continued f. having but one paroxysm. Cf. polyleptic f.

Mossman f., a f., noted especially among sugar-cane cutters in the Mossman District of North Queensland, caused by a leptospira.

mud f., a leptospirosis caused by the *grippotyphosa* serovar of *Leptospira interrogans;*

mumu f., samoan term for elephantoid f.

nanukayami f., a form of leptospirosis known in Japan and caused by a leptospira normally found in the field mouse or vole. SYN nanukayami.

nine mile f., SYN Q f.

nodal f., SYN *erythema* nodosum.

North Queensland tick f., a mild form of tick-borne typhus with eschar, adenopathy, rash, and fever, caused by *Rickettsia australis* and thought to be transmitted by the tick, *Ixodes holocyclus.*

Omsk hemorrhagic f., a form of epidemic hemorrhagic fever found in central Russia, caused by the Omsk hemorrhagic f. virus, a member of the family Flaviviridae, and transmitted by *Dermacentor* ticks; associated with gastrointestinal symptoms and hemorrhages but little or no central nervous system involvement.

o'nyong-nyong f., a denguelike disease caused by the o'nyong-nyong virus, a member of the family Togaviridae, and transmitted by a mosquito, characterized by joint pains and notable lymphadenopathy followed by a maculopapular eruption of the face which extends to the trunk and extremities but fades in several days without desquamation.

Oropouche f., acute febrile illness caused by a species of Bunyavirus.

Oroya f., a generalized, acute, febrile, endemic, and systemic form of bartonellosis; marked by high fever, rheumatic pains, progressive, severe anemia, and albuminuria. SYN Carrión disease.

Pahvant Valley f., SYN tularemia.

paludal f., SYN malaria.

pappataci f., SYN phlebotomus f.

paratyphoid f., an acute infectious disease with symptoms and lesions resembling those of typhoid f., though milder in character; associated with the presence of the paratyphoid organism of which at least three varieties (types A, B, and C) have been described. SYN paratyphoid.

parenteric f., one of a group of f.'s clinically resembling typhoid and paratyphoid A and B, but caused by bacteria differing specifically from those of either of these diseases.

parrot f., SYN psittacosis.

Pel-Ebstein f., the remittent fever common in Hodgkin disease. SYN Pel-Ebstein disease.

periodic f., an obsolete term introduced to describe the intermittent febrile episodes seen in disease later recognized and named familial Mediterranean f.

Persian relapsing f., a tick-borne relapsing f., occurring in the Middle East, caused by *Borrelia persica* and transmitted by *Ornithodoros tholozani* and possibly by *Ornithodoros lahorensis.*

pharyngoconjunctival f., a disease usually occurring in epidemic form characterized by fever, pharyngitis, and conjunctivitis, and caused by several types of adenoviruses.

Philippine hemorrhagic f., severe arbovirus infection with hemorrhagic manifestations, considerable mortality, probably due to mosquito borne dengue *virus*; seen in tropical and subtropical urban areas of southeast Asia, South Pacific, Australia, Central and South America, and the Caribbean islands.

phlebotomus f., an infectious but not contagious disease occurring in the Balkan Peninsula and other parts of southern Europe, caused by several viruses in the family Bunyaviridae apparently introduced by the bite of the sandfly, *Phlebotomus papatasii;* symptoms resemble those of dengue but are less severe and of shorter duration. SYN dog disease, pappataci f., Pym f., sandfly f., three-day f.

pinta f., a term used in Mexico for Rocky Mountain spotted f.

polka f., SYN dengue.

polyleptic f., a f. occurring in two or more paroxysms; e.g., smallpox, relapsing f., intermittent f. Cf. monoleptic f.

polymer fume f., an occupational disease marked by f., pain in the chest, and cough caused by the inhalation of fumes given off by a plastic, polytetrafluorethylene, when heated.

pretibial f., a mild disease first observed among military personnel at Fort Bragg, North Carolina, characterized by f., moderate prostration, splenomegaly, and a rash on the anterior aspects of the legs; due to the *autumnalis* serovar of *Leptospira interrogans.* SYN Fort Bragg f.

protein f., f. produced by the injection of foreign protein, such as milk.

puerperal f., postpartum sepsis with a rise in f. after the first 24 hours following delivery, but before the eleventh postpartum day. SYN childbed f., puerperal sepsis.

Pym f., SYN phlebotomus f.

pyogenic f., SYN pyemia.

Q f., a disease caused by the rickettsia *Coxiella burnetii,* which is propagated in sheep and cattle, where it produces no symptoms; human infections occur as a result of contact not only with such animals but also with other infected humans, air and dust, wild reservoir hosts, and other sources. SYN nine mile f. [*Q,* for "query," so named because etiologic agent was unknown]

quartan f., SYN malariae *malaria.*

quintan f., SYN trench f.

quotidian f., SYN quotidian *malaria.*

rabbit f., SYN tularemia.

rat-bite f., a single designation for two bacterial diseases associated with rat bites, one caused by *Streptobacillus moniliformis* (e.g., Haverhill f.), the other by *Spirillum minus* (e.g., sodoku); both diseases are characterized by relapsing f., chills, headache, arthralgia, lymphadenopathy, and a maculopapular rash on the extremities. SYN rat-bite disease, sodoku, sokosho.

recrudescent typhus f., SYN Brill-Zinsser *disease.*

recurrent f., SYN relapsing f.

red f., red f. of the Congo, SYN murine *typhus.*

relapsing f., an acute infectious disease caused by any one of a number of strains of *Borrelia,* marked by a number of febrile attacks lasting about 6 days and separated from each other by apyretic intervals of about the same length; the microorganism is found in the blood during the febrile periods but not during the intervals, the disappearance being associated with specific antibodies and previously evoked antibodies. There are two epidemiologic varieties: 1) the louse-borne variety, occurring chiefly in Europe, northern Africa, and India, and caused by strains of *B. recurrentis;* 2) the tick-borne variety, occurring in Africa, Asia, and North and South America, caused by various species of *Borrelia,* each of which is transmitted by a different species of the soft tick, *Ornithodoros.* SYN bilious typhoid of Griesinger, recurrent f., spirillum f., typhinia.

remittent f., a f. pattern in which temperature varies during each 24 hour period, but never reaches normal. Most f.'s are remittent and the pattern is not characteristic of any disease, although in the 19th century it was considered a diagnostic term.

remittent malarial f., SEE remittent *malaria.*

rheumatic f., a subacute febrile syndrome occurring after group A β-hemolytic streptococcal infection (usually pharyngitis) and mediated by an immune response to the organism; most often seen in children and young adults; features include f., myocarditis

fe

(causing tachycardia and sometimes acute cardiac failure), endocarditis (with valvular incompetence, followed after healing by scarring), and migratory polyarthritis; less often, subcutaneous nodules, erythema marginatum, and Syndenham chorea; relapses can occur after reinfection with streptococci.

Criteria for diagnosis of acute rheumatic fever were published by Jones in 1944. Regimens for prevention of initial and recurring attacks, and guidelines for treatment, have remained essentially unchanged for decades. Although acute rheumatic fever has ceased to be a major public health problem in the U.S., the incidence is still high in developing countries. In India, for example, where medical services have failed to keep pace with urbanization and industrialization, 250,000 new cases are diagnosed in school children annually. The incidence of rheumatic fever in the U.S., which had declined steadily for several decades after antibiotic treatment of streptococcal pharyngitis (strep throat) became standard, began rising again in the late 1980s and 1990s, with some urban clusters showing a 10-fold increase in incidence. Historically, rheumatic fever is a disease of children in lower socioeconomic strata. In a number of recent clusters, most of the victims were adults, and when children have been involved, they have often belonged to middle- and upper-class families. As many as 75% of patients denied any history of recent sore throat, and some of those who had been diagnosed with preceding strep throat had been treated with antibiotics. Cardiac and articular manifestations of rheumatic fever are considered autoimmune phenomena, due to a postulated rheumatogenic factor that has never been isolated. Pathogenicity in streptococci is known to be associated with the presence of an M protein in the cell membrane, which is also responsible for the appearance of a surface fuzz on microscopic examination of organisms, and the production of mucoid colonies on blood agar. Organisms implicated in several recent clusters of rheumatic fever have belonged to mucoid strains, particularly serotypes M 3 and M 18. Widespread antibiotic use in recent years, not all of it appropriate or justified by current medical knowledge, may have led to the resurgence of rheumatic fever by favoring the rise and spread of virulent strains of streptococcus, or by reducing the ability of certain populations to mount an immune response against them. Infectious disease authorities are currently reevaluating the diagnosis and management of streptococcal infection, particularly with respect to rapid slide tests and to drug regimens approved for use in the treatment of acute streptococcal pharyngitis and hence in the prophylaxis of rheumatic fever. See Jones *criteria*, under *criterion*.

rice-field f., a febrile illness affecting workers in rice fields, reported in Po valley in Italy and in Sumatra, caused by infection with a species of *Leptospira*.

Rift Valley f., a fatal endemic disease of sheep, caused by Rift Valley f. virus, a member of the family Bunyaviridae, which is also pathogenic for humans and cattle, producing in humans f. of an undifferentiated type; transmitted by mosquitoes and direct contact. [*Rift Valley* in Kenya]

Rocky Mountain spotted f., an acute infectious disease of high mortality, characterized by frontal and occipital headache, intense lumbar pain, malaise, a moderately high continuous f., and a rash on wrists, palms, ankles, and soles from the second to the fifth day, later spreading to all parts of the body; it occurs in the spring of the year primarily in the southeastern U.S. and the Rocky Mountain region, although it is also endemic elsewhere in the U.S., in parts of Canada, in Mexico, and in South America; the pathogenic organism is *Rickettsia rickettsii*, transmitted by two or more tick species of the genus *Dermacentor;* in the U.S. it is spread by *D. andersoni* in the western states and *D. variabilis* (a dog tick) in the eastern states. SYN black f., black measles (2), blue disease, blue f., Mexican spotted f., São Paulo f., Tobia f.

Roman f., malignant tertian, falciparum, or aestivoautumnal f., formerly prevalent in the Roman Campagna and in the city of Rome; caused by *Plasmodium falciparum*.

Ross River f., SYN epidemic *polyarthritis*.

sakushu f., SYN hasamiyami.

Salinem f., infection with *Leptospira pyrogenes*, reported in Salinem. SYN Salinem infection.

salt f., elevated temperature in an infant, following a rectal injection of a salt solution. SEE ALSO thirst f.

sandfly f., SYN phlebotomus f.

San Joaquin f., SYN primary *coccidioidomycosis*.

San Joaquin Valley f., SYN primary *coccidioidomycosis*.

São Paulo f., SYN Rocky Mountain spotted f.

scarlet f., SYN scarlatina.

Schamberg f., SYN progressive pigmentary *dermatosis*.

Sennetsu f., a disease of humans in western Japan caused by the rickettsia *Ehrlichia sennetsu* and characterized by fever, malaise, anorexia, backache, and lymphadenopathy.

septic f., SYN septicemia.

seven-day f., (1) SYN autumn f. (1); **(2)** SYN hasamiyami.

shin bone f., SYN trench f.

ship f., SYN typhus.

shoddy f., febrile disease occurring in workers in shoddy factories, with cough, dyspnea and headache, caused by inhalation of dust.

simian hemorrhagic f., a highly fatal disease of macaque monkeys caused by the simian hemorrhagic f. virus and characterized by fever, facial edema, anorexia, adipsia, skin petechiae, diarrhea, hemorrhages, and death.

Sindbis f., a febrile illness of humans in Africa, Australia, and other countries, characterized by arthralgia, rash, and malaise; caused by the Sindbis virus, a member of the family Togaviridae, and transmitted by culicine mosquitoes.

slime f., leptospiral infection with jaundice, presumably infection by *Leptospira icterohemorrhagica*.

slow f., a continued f. of long duration.

smelter's f., metal fume f., occurring in workers in zinc smelters. SYN smelter's chills, smelter's shakes.

snail f., SYN schistosomiasis.

solar f., (1) SYN dengue; **(2)** SYN sunstroke.

Songo f., SYN epidemic hemorrhagic f.

South African tick-bite f., a typhuslike f. of South Africa caused by *Rickettsia rickettsii* and usually characterized by primary eschar and regional adenitis, rigors, and maculopapular rash on the fifth day, often with severe central nervous system symptoms.

spirillum f., SYN relapsing f.

spotted f., tick typhus caused by *Rickettsia rickettsii* in North and South America and Siberia.

steroid f., f. presumably caused by elevated plasma concentrations of certain pyrogenic steroids; can be produced by administration of etiocholanolone.

symptomatic f., SYN traumatic f.

syphilitic f., the elevation of temperature often present in the early roseolous stage of secondary syphilis.

tertian f., SYN vivax *malaria*.

therapeutic f., SYN pyrotherapy.

thermic f., SYN heatstroke.

thirst f., an elevation of temperature in infants after reduction of fluid intake, diarrhea, or vomiting; probably caused by reduced available body water, with reduced heat loss by evaporation; an analogous condition in adults is seen when exertion is continued in the face of dehydration. SYN dehydration f., exsiccation f., inanition f.

three-day f., SYN phlebotomus f.

Tobia f., SYN Rocky Mountain spotted f.

traumatic f., elevation of temperature following an injury. SYN symptomatic f., wound f.

trench f., an uncommon rickettsial f. caused by *Bartonella quintana* and transmitted by the louse *Pediculus humanus*, first appearing as an epidemic during the trench warfare of World War I; characterized by the sudden onset of chills and f., myalgia (especially of the back and legs), headache, and general malaise that typically lasts 5 days but may recur. SYN five-day f., quintan f., shin bone f.

trypanosome f., the febrile stage of sleeping sickness.

tsutsugamushi f., SYN tsutsugamushi *disease.*

typhoid f., an acute infectious disease caused by *Salmonella typhi* and characterized by a continued f. rising in a steplike curve the first week, severe physical and mental depression, an eruption of rose-colored spots on the chest and abdomen, tympanites, early constipation, diarrhea, and sometimes intestinal hemorrhage or perforation of the bowel; average duration is 4 weeks, although aborted forms and relapses are not uncommon; the lesions are located chiefly in the lymph follicles of the intestines (Peyer patches), the mesenteric glands, and the spleen; antibody titer of the Widal test rises during the infection, and early positive blood and urine cultures become negative, usually results in immunity. SYN abdominal typhoid, enteric f. (1), typhoid (2).

undifferentiated type f.'s, a term applied to illnesses resulting from infection by any virus, that was formerly in the arbovirus group, pathogenic for humans, in which the only constant manifestation is f.; rash, lymphadenopathy, or arthralgia (alone or in combination) may occur in some individuals but not in others; some viruses may induce infections in which undifferentiated type f. is the only manifestation, whereas other viruses may induce in some persons only undifferentiated f., and in other persons similar f. followed by secondary manifestations, e.g., a hemorrhagic f. or encephalitis.

undulant f., SYN brucellosis. [referring to the wavy appearance of the long temperature curve]

undulating f., SYN brucellosis.

f. of unknown origin, the presence of f. (temperature >101°F or 38.3°C) of unknown cause after intensive investigation. Exact criteria for use of term vary, especially regarding duration of f. and extent of clinical investigation; generally a duration of greater than 1 week (some authors require 2–3 weeks) and thorough inpatient investigation or at least three outpatient visits, including a careful history, physical examination, and laboratory tests such as cultures, serologic studies, and invasive procedures for biopsy and/or culture, as indicated by clinical clues or epidemiological considerations.

urethral f., SYN urinary f.

urinary f., an elevation of temperature, usually slight and transitory, following catheterization of the urethra, or the passage of blood clots, gravel, or a calculus. SYN catheter f., urethral f.

urticarial f., SYN *schistosomiasis* japonica.

uveoparotid f., chronic enlargement of the parotid glands and inflammation of the uveal tract accompanied by a long-continued f. of low degree; now recognized as a form of sarcoidosis. SYN Heerfordt disease.

Uzbekistan hemorrhagic f., a viral f. in central Asia probably transmitted by *Hyalomma anatolicum.*

valley f., SYN primary *coccidioidomycosis.*

Venezuelan hemorrhagic f., a febrile disease caused by the Guanarito virus in Venezuela and characterized by headache, arthralgia, pharyngitis, leukopenia, thrombocytopenia, and hemorrhagic manifestations.

viral hemorrhagic f., an epidemic disease, and associated with fever, malaise, muscular pain, respiratory tract symptoms, vomiting, and diarrhea; epistaxis, hemoptysis, hematemesis, and subconjunctival hemorrhages occur in severe cases, and body rash and tremors occur in some instances; a disease caused by a number of different viruses in the families Arenoviridae, Bunyaviridae, Flaviviridae, Filoviridae, etc. SEE ALSO hemorrhagic f.

vivax f., SYN vivax *malaria.*

Wesselsbron f., a mosquito-borne disease of sheep and humans caused by the F. disease virus, a member of the family Flaviviridae, and characterized by abortion and lamb mortality in sheep and by fever, headache, muscular pains, and mild rash in humans. SYN Wesselsbron disease. [*Wesselsbron,* town in South Africa where causative agent first isolated]

West African f., SYN malarial *hemoglobinuria.*

West Nile f., a febrile illness caused by West Nile virus, a member of the family Flaviviridae, and characterized by headache, fever, maculopapular rash, myalgia, lymphadenopathy, and leukopenia; spread by *Culex* mosquitoes from a reservoir in birds.

wound f., SYN traumatic f.

Yangtze Valley f., SYN *schistosomiasis* japonica.

yellow f., a tropical mosquito-borne viral hepatitis, due to yellow f. virus, a member of the family Flaviviridae, with an urban form transmitted by *Aedes aegypti,* and a rural, jungle, or sylvatic form from tree-dwelling mammals by various mosquitoes of the *Haemagogus* species complex; characterized clinically by fever, slow pulse, albuminuria, jaundice, congestion of the face, and hemorrhages, especially hematemesis; used to occur in epidemics mainly in port cities, especially in late summer, with 20–40% case fatality rates; immunity to reinfection accompanies recovery.

Zika f., an acute disease, probably transmitted by mosquitoes, clinically resembling dengue; caused by *Zika* virus, a member of the family Flaviviridae.

zinc fume f., SYN brass founder's f.

fe·ver·ish (fē′ver-ish). **1.** SYN febrile. **2.** Having a fever.

FF Abbreviation for filtration *fraction.*

FFA Abbreviation for unesterified free *fatty acid.*

FFP Abbreviation for fresh frozen *plasma.*

F.F.R. Abbreviation for Fellow of the Faculty of Radiologists (United Kingdom).

FGAR Abbreviation for *N*-formylglycinamide ribotide.

FH₄ Abbreviation for tetrahydrofolic acid. SEE 5,6,7,8-tetrahydrofolate dehydrogenase, tetrahydrofolate methyltransferase.

FIBER

fi·ber (fī′ber) [TA]. A slender thread or filament. **1.** Extracellular filamentous structures such as collagenic or elastic connective tissue f.'s. **2.** The nerve cell axon with its glial cell or Schwann cell envelope. **3.** Elongated, hence threadlike, cells such as muscle cells and the epithelial cells composing the major part of the eye lens. **4.** Nutrients in the diet that are not digested by gastrointestinal enzymes. SYN fibra [TA], fibre. [L. *fibra*]

A f.'s, myelinated nerve f.'s in somatic nerves, measuring 1–22 μm in diameter, conducting nerve impulses at a rate of 6–120 m/sec.

accelerator f.'s, postganglionic sympathetic nerve f.'s originating in the superior, middle, and inferior cervical ganglia of the sympathetic trunk, conveying nervous impulses to the heart that increase the rapidity and force of the cardiac pulsations. SYN augmentor f.'s.

adrenergic f.'s, nerve f.'s's that transmit nervous impulses to other nerve cells (or smooth muscle or gland cells) by the medium of the adrenalinelike transmitter substance norepinephrine (noradrenaline).

afferent f.'s, those that convey impulses to a ganglion or to a nerve center in the brain or spinal cord.

alpha f.'s, large somatic motor or proprioceptive nerve f.'s with conducting impulses at rates of 80–120 m/sec.

anastomosing f.'s, anastomotic f.'s, individual f.'s passing from one nerve trunk or muscle bundle to another.

anterior external arcuate f.'s [TA], SEE external arcuate f.'s.

arcuate f.'s, nervous or tendinous f.'s passing in the form of an arch from one part to another. SEE arcuate f.'s of cerebrum, external arcuate f.'s, internal arcuate f.'s.

arcuate f.'s of cerebrum [TA], short association fibers that connect adjacent gyri in the cerebral cortex. SYN fibrae arcuatae cerebri [TA].

argyrophilic f.'s, reticular connective tissue f.'s that react with silver salts and appear black microscopically.

association f.'s, nerve f.'s interconnecting subdivisions of the cerebral cortex of the same hemisphere or different segments of the spinal cord on the same side. SYN endogenous f.'s, intrinsic f.'s.

astral f.'s, f.'s (fibrils) radiating from the centrosphere toward the periphery of the cell as seen with a light microscope; revealed as microtubules under the electron microscope. Cf. kinetochore f.'s, polar f.'s.

augmentor f.'s, SYN accelerator f.'s.

autonomic nerve f.'s [TA], any of the pre- and/or postsynaptic nerve f.'s that collectively comprise the sympathetic and parasympathetic parts of the autonomic division of the peripheral nervous system. SYN neurofibrae autonomicae [TA], visceral motor f.'s.

B f.'s, myelinated f.'s autonomic nerves, with a diameter of 2 µm or less, conducting at a rate of 3–15 m/sec.

Bergmann f.'s, filamentous glia f.'s traversing the cerebellar cortex perpendicular to the surface.

beta f.'s, nerve f.'s that have conduction velocities of 40–70 m/sec.

bulbar corticonuclear f.'s [TA], nerve f.'s projecting from the motor and somatic sensory cortices to motor and sensory relay nuclei of the medulla oblongata, such as the hypoglossal nucleus, accessory nucleus and gracile and cuneate nuclei. SEE corticonuclear f.'s. SYN fibrae corticonucleares bulbi [TA].

C f.'s, unmyelinated f.'s, 0.4–1.2 µm in diameter, conducting nerve impulses at a velocity of 0.7–2.3 m/sec.

cerebellohypothalamic f.'s, nerve f.'s originating from cells of the cerebellar nuclei and projecting, via the superior cerebellar peduncle, to the contralateral hypothalamus, mainly its dorsal, lateral, and posterior areas and dorsomedial nucleus.

cerebelloolivary f.'s [TA], axons that arise from neurons in the cerebellar nuclei, exit via the superior cerebellar peduncle, cross in its decussation, and descend in association with the central tegmental tract. Depending of their origin, these fibers terminate in the accessory and principal olivary nuclei; anterior and posterior interposed nuclei to the dorsal accessory and medial accessory olivary nuclei respectively, the medial cerebellar nucleus to the medial accessory olivary nucleus, and the lateral cerebellar nucleus to the principal olivary nucleus. SYN fibrae cerebelloolivares [TA].

cerebellospinal f.'s, f.'s that originate from the fastigial and interposed (primarily the posterior) cerebellar nuclei and descend to the contralateral side of the spinal cord. SEE fastigiospinal f.'s; SEE ALSO fastigiospinal f.'s.

cholinergic f.'s, nerve f.'s that transmit impulses to other nerve cells, muscle fibers, or gland cells by the medium of the transmitter substance acetylcholine.

chromatic f., SYN chromonema.

circular f.'s, the circular f.'s of the ciliary muscle. SYN fibrae circulares [TA], Müller f.'s (1), Müller muscle (2), Rouget muscle.

climbing f.'s, nerve f.'s in the cerebellar cortex that synapse upon smooth branchlets of Purkinje cell dendrites.

collagen f., collagenous f., an individual f. that varies in diameter from less than 1 µm to about 12 µm and is composed of fibrils; the f.'s' which are usually arranged in bundles, undergo some branching and are of indefinite length; chemically the f. is a glycoprotein, collagen, which yields gelatin upon boiling; they make up the principal element of irregular connective tissue, tendons, aponeuroses, and most ligaments, and occur in the matrix of cartilage and osseous tissue. SYN white f. (2).

commissural f.'s, nerve f.'s crossing the midline and connecting two corresponding parts or regions of the nervous system.

cone f., a part of the cone cell of the retina; the **inner cone f.** is a slender axon-like part of the cone extending from the cell body to the pedicle located in the outer plexiform layer of the retina; in the outer fovea, where the cones are much elongated, they narrow to an **outer cone f.,** located between the inner segment and the cell body.

corticobulbar f.'s, term formerly used to describe projections of the motor and sensory cortices to nuclei of the rhombencephalon innervating the musculature of the face, tongue, and jaws and some f.'s to rhombencephalic relay nuclei; replaced by bullar corticonuclear f.'s (to medulla), pontine corticonuclear f.'s (to

pons), mesencephalic corticonuclear f.'s (to midbrain). See these individual entries.

corticomesencephalic f.'s [TA], axons that originate in the cerebral cortex and terminate in mesencephalic structures such as the tectum, substantia nigra, or tegmentum. SYN fibrae corticomesencephalicae [TA].

corticonuclear f.'s, descriptive term connoting f.'s from a cortical structure (cerebral or cerebellar) passing to subcortical cell groups; f.'s comprising the fibrae corticonucleares bulbi [TA], fibrae corticonucleares pontis [TA] and fibrae corticonucleares mesencephali [TA]; cerebellar corticonuclear f.'s (Purkinje cell axons to the cerebellar nuclei). SYN fibrae corticonucleares [TA].

corticopontine f.'s [TA], the f.'s that compose the corticopontine *tract.* SYN fibrae corticopontinae [TA].

corticoreticular f.'s [TA], corticofugal f.'s distributed to the reticular formation of the mesencephalon and rhombencephalon. SEE ALSO corticonuclear f.'s. SYN fibrae corticoreticulares [TA].

corticorubral f.'s [TA], nerve f.'s projecting from the cerebral cortex (primarily precentral and premotor regions) to the red nucleus of the midbrain. SYN fibrae corticorubrales [TA].

corticospinal f.'s [TA], SYN pyramidal f.'s.

corticothalamic f.'s, a general term designating nerve f.'s originating from any area of the cerebral cortex and terminating in the nuclei of the thalamus.

cuneocerebellar f.'s [TA], SYN cuneocerebellar *tract.*

cuneospinal f.'s [TA], axons that originate in the cuneate nucleus of the medulla oblongata and descend ipsilaterally in the cuneate fasciculus to terminate primarily in the posterior horn of the spinal cord in cervical and upper thoracic levels. SYN fibrae cuneospinales [TA].

delta f.'s, nerve f.'s with conduction velocities in the range of 8–30 m/sec.

dentatorubral f.'s, nerve f.'s arising in the dentate nucleus of the cerebellum and projecting, via the superior cerebellar peduncle and its decussation, to the contralateral red nucleus of the midbrain. SYN fibrae dentatorubrales.

dentatothalamic f.'s, nerve f.'s projecting from the dentate nucleus of the cerebellum to the contralateral thalamus via the superior cerebellar peduncle (and its decussation); enter the thalamus as one component of the thalamic fasciculus.

dentinal f.'s, dental f.'s, (1) the processes of the pulpal cells, the odontoblasts, which extend in radial fashion through the dentin to the dentoenamel junction and are contained within the dentinal tubules; SYN Tomes f.'s. **(2)** the intertubular fine collagenous f.'s that with the dentinal ground substance infiltrated with calcium salts constitutes the dentinal matrix.

depressor f.'s, sensory nerve f.'s having pressure-sensitive nerve endings in the wall of certain arteries capable of activating blood pressure-lowering brainstem mechanisms when stimulated by an increase in intraarterial pressure.

dietary f., the plant polysaccharides and lignin that are resistant to hydrolysis by the digestive enzymes in humans.

efferent f.'s, those f.'s conveying impulses to effector tissues (muscle: smooth, cardiac or striated; or glands) in the periphery; those f.'s exiting a specific cell group (i.e., efferent fibers of the basilar pons), used in reference to a cell group.

elastic f.'s, f.'s that are 0.2–2 µm in diameter but may be larger in some ligaments; they branch and anastomose to form networks and fuse to form fenestrated membranes; the f.'s and membranes consist of microfibrils about 10 nm wide and an amorphous substance containing elastin. SYN yellow f.'s.

enamel f.'s, SYN *prismata* adamantina, under *prisma.*

endogenous f.'s, SYN association f.'s.

exogenous f.'s, nerve f.'s by which a given region of the central nervous system is connected with other regions; the term applies to both afferent and efferent fiber connections.

external arcuate f.'s, they include: 1) posterior external arcuate f.'s [TA] that arise from cells in the accessory or lateral cuneate nucleus and pass to the cerebellum; 2) anterior external arcuate f.'s [TA] that arise from the arcuate nuclei at the base of the medulla oblongata and pass around the lateral surface of the medulla; both enter the cerebellum as components of the restiform portion of the inferior cerebellar peduncle. SYN fibrae arcuatae externae.

fastigiobulbar f.'s, nerve f.'s projecting from the fastigial nuclei of the cerebellum to the brainstem; crossed and uncrossed f.'s that terminate mainly in the vestibular and reticular nuclei, and in the medial accessory olivary nucleus.

fastigiospinal f.'s, crossed descending f.'s originating in the fastigial nucleus of the cerebellum and ending in the spinal cord gray matter at cervical, and possibly lower, levels.

frontopontine f.'s [TA], a large group of f.'s arising from the frontal lobe of the cerebral hemisphere, especially the precentral gyrus, descending in the internal capsule, farther caudally composing the medial part of the crus cerebri through which they extend caudalward to end in the gray matter (pontine nuclei) of the ventral part of the pons. SEE ALSO corticopontine *tract*. SYN fibrae frontopontinae [TA].

gamma f.'s, nerve f.'s that have a conduction rate of 15–40 m/sec. SEE ALSO gamma *efferent*.

Gerdy f.'s, SYN superficial transverse metacarpal *ligament*.

gracilespinal f.'s [TA], axons that arise from neurons of the gracile nucleus of the medulla oblongata and descend ipsilaterally in the gracile fasciculus to terminate primarily in the posterior horn of the spinal cord in lower thoracic and lumbosacral levels. SYN fibrae gracilispinales [TA].

Gratiolet f.'s, SYN optic *radiation*.

gray f.'s, SYN unmyelinated f.'s.

hypothalamocerebellar f.'s, nerve f.'s originating from cells in the hypothalamus and projecting to the cerebellar cortex and nuclei.

hypothalamospinal f.'s [TA], a group of f.'s that originates primarily from the paraventricular nucleus and lateral and posterior hypothalamic areas, descends ipsilaterally through the ventrolateral brainstem and into the lateral funiculus of the spinal cord, and terminates in relation to neurons of the intermediolateral nucleus. SYN fibrae hypothalamospinales [TA].

inhibitory f.'s, nerve f.'s that inhibit the activity of the nerve cells with which they have synaptic connections, or of the effector tissue (smooth muscle, heart muscle, glands) in which they terminate.

intercolumnar f.'s, SYN intercrural f.'s of superficial ring.

intercrural f.'s of superficial ring [TA], horizontal arched fibers that pass from the inguinal ligament across the medial and lateral crura of the superficial inguinal ring. SYN fibrae intercrurales anuli inguinalis superficialis [TA], intercolumnar fasciae, intercolumnar f.'s.

internal arcuate f.'s [TA], f.'s that arise in the cuneate and gracile nuclei, pass in a curving course across the midline of the medulla oblongata, and form the contralateral medial lemniscus; may also designate other f.'s such as those of the olivocerebellar tract that arch through the substance of the medulla and may traverse the sensory decussation. SYN fibrae arcuatae internae [TA].

intrafusal f.'s, muscle f.'s present within a neuromuscular spindle.

intrathalamic f.'s [TA], f.'s that arise in one nucleus of the dorsal thalamus and terminate in another. SYN fibrae intrathalamicae [TA].

intrinsic f.'s, SYN association f.'s.

James f.'s, atrio-His bundle connections thought to be the basis for the short P-R interval syndrome; these f.'s should be distinguished from the controversial internodal tracts of the atrium, sometimes referred to as "James tracts." SYN James tracts.

kinetochore f.'s, f.'s of the mitotic spindle attached to the centromere and extending toward the poles. Cf. astral f.'s, polar f.'s.

Korff f.'s, argyrophilic f.'s that pass between odontoblasts at the periphery of the dental pulp and fan out into the dentin.

Kühne f., artificial muscle f. made by filling the intestine of an insect with a growth of myxomycetes; used to demonstrate the contractility of protoplasm.

f.'s of lens, the elongated cells of ectodermal origin forming the substance of the crystalline lens of the eye. SYN fibrae lentis.

long association f.'s [TA], nerve f.'s interconnecting lobes or gyri of the cerebral cortex of the same hemisphere that are not immediately adjacent to each other; nerve fibers connecting noncontiguous segments of the spinal cord on the same side; fibers that interconnect distant points. SYN fibrae associationes longae [TA].

longitudinal pontine f.'s [TA], SEE longitudinal pontine *fasciculi*, under *fasciculus*. SYN fibrae pontis longitudinales [TA].

Mahaim f.'s, paraspecific f.'s originating from the A-V node, the His bundle, or the bundle branches and inserting into the ventricular myocardium; they are potential pathways for reentrant dysrhythmias. SYN nodoventricular f.'s.

medullated nerve f., SYN myelinated nerve f.

meridional f.'s of ciliary muscle [TA], the longitudinal fibers of the ciliary muscle. SYN fibrae meridionales muscularis ciliaris [TA].

mesencephalic corticonuclear f.'s [TA], nerve f.'s projecting primarily from the motor cortex to motor nuclei of the mesencephalon such as the oculomotor and trochlear; these inputs are relayed via nuclei located adjacent to these motor nuclei. SEE corticonuclear f.'s. SYN fibrae corticonucleares mesencephali [TA].

mossy f.'s, highly branched nerve f.'s in the cerebellar cortex that terminate in rosette formations and synapse upon granule cell dendrites.

motor f.'s, nerve f.'s that transmit impulses that activate effector cells, e.g., in muscle or gland tissue.

Müller f.'s, (1) SYN circular f.'s; (2) sustentacular neuroglial cells of the retina, running through the thickness of the retina from the internal limiting membrane to the bases of the rods and cones where they form a row of junctional complexes. SYN Müller radial cells, sustentacular f.'s of retina.

myelinated nerve f., an axon enveloped by a myelin sheath formed by oligodendroglia cells (in brain and spinal cord) or Schwann cells (in peripheral nerves). SYN medullated nerve f.

Nélaton f.'s, SYN Nélaton *sphincter*.

nerve f., the axon of a nerve cell, ensheathed by oligodendroglia cells in brain and spinal cord, and by Schwann cells in peripheral nerves.

nodoventricular f.'s, SYN Mahaim f.'s.

nonmedullated f.'s, SYN unmyelinated f.'s.

nuclear bag f., the largest type of intrafusal muscle f.'s in a neuromuscular spindle, containing a central aggregation of nuclei (nuclear bag).

nuclear chain f., the shortest and most numerous type of intrafusal muscle f.'s in a neuromuscular spindle, containing a single row of centrally positioned nuclei.

nucleocortical f.'s, general term for projections from a nucleus to an overlying cortical structure; specifically used to designate axons of cerebellar nuclear cells that project to the cerebellar cortex (cerebellar nucleocortical f.'s) where they end as mossy f.'s.

oblique f.'s of muscular layer of stomach [TA], the smooth muscle fibers of the innermost layer of the muscular coat of the stomach; the fibers occur chiefly at the cardiac end of the stomach and spread over the anterior and posterior surfaces. SYN fibrae obliquae tunicae muscularis [TA].

occipitopontine f.'s [TA], a group of f.'s originating in the occipital lobe of the cerebral hemisphere and descending in the internal capsule and lateral part of the crus cerebri to the pontine nuclei of the basilar part of the pons. SEE ALSO corticopontine *tract*. SYN fibrae occipitopontinae [TA].

occipitotectal f.'s [TA], f.'s originating in visual regions of the occipital lobe and passing, via the retrolenticular limb of the internal capsule, to the tectum where they end mainly in the superior colliculus. SYN fibrae occipitotectales [TA].

olivocochlear f.'s, SEE olivocochlear *tract*.

olivospinal f.'s, a slender bundle of nerve f.'s in the peripheral zone of the lateral funiculus of the spinal cord, composed, more likely, of spinoolivary fibers than of olivospinal fibers. SYN fibrae olivospinales [TA], Helwig bundle.

osteocollagenous f.'s, fine collagenous f.'s in the matrix of osseous tissue.

fi

osteogenetic f.'s, the f.'s in the osteogenetic layer of the periosteum.

parietopontine f.'s [TA], a system of f.'s originating in the parietal lobe of the cerebral hemisphere that descend in the internal capsule and lateral part of the crus cerebri to terminate in the pontine nuclei in the ventral part of the pons. SEE ALSO corticopontine *tract.* SYN fibrae parietopontinae [TA].

pectinate f.'s, SYN pectinate *muscles,* under *muscle.*

perforating f.'s, bundles of collagenous f.'s that pass into the outer circumferential lamellae of bone or the cementum of teeth. SYN Sharpey f.'s.

periodontal f., ☆official alternate term for desmodentium.

periodontal ligament f.'s, SYN desmodentium.

periventricular f.'s [TA], a heterogeneous system of thin nerve f.'s in the periventricular gray matter of the hypothalamus; the dorsal longitudinal fasciculus is a caudal continuation of the system. SYN fibrae periventriculares [TA].

pilomotor f.'s, nerve f.'s that innervate the erector muscles of hair follicles responsible for piloerection.

polar f.'s, those f.'s of the mitotic spindle extending from the two poles of the spindle toward the equator. Cf. astral f.'s, kinetochore f.'s.

pontine corticonuclear f.'s [TA], nerve f.'s projecting from the motor and sensory cortices to motor and sensory relay nuclei in the pontine tegmentum such as the facial, abducens, and trigeminal nuclei; f.'s may be direct or relayed via the adjacent reticular nuclei. SEE corticonuclear f.'s. SYN fibrae corticonucleares pontis [TA].

pontocerebellar f.'s [TA], f.'s arising from the nuclei of the basilar pons and primarily crossing the midline (there is a modes uncrossed projection), centering the cerebellum via the middle cerebellar peduncle and terminating as mossy fibers in the cerebellar cortex. SYN fibrae pontocerebellares [TA].

postcommissural f.'s [TA], f.'s in the column of fornix that pass caudal (posterior) to the anterior commissure to enter the mammillary nuclei; the largest part of the column of fornix. SYN fibrae postcommissurales [TA].

posterior external arcuate f.'s [TA], SEE external arcuate f.'s.

postganglionic f.'s, a f. whose cell body is located in an autonomic (motor) ganglion and whose peripheral process will terminate on smooth muscle, cardiac muscle, or glandular epithelium; associated with sympathetic or parasympathetic parts of the autonomic nervous system.

postganglionic nerve f. [TA], SEE postganglionic.

precollagenous f.'s, immature, argyrophilic f.'s.

precommissural f.'s [TA], f.'s in the column of fornix that pass rostral (anterior) to the anterior commissure to enter primarily the septal nuclei. SYN fibrae precommissurales [TA].

preganglionic f.'s, a f. whose cell body is located in an autonomic nucleus in the spinal cord or brain stem and whose axon terminates in an autonomic (motor) ganglion; found in nerves conveying sympathetic or parasympathetic f.'s.

preganglionic nerve f.'s, SEE preganglionic. SYN neurofibrae preganglionicae.

pressor f.'s, sensory nerve f.'s whose stimulation causes vasoconstriction and rise of blood pressure.

pretectoolivary f.'s [TA], f.'s originating from the pretectal nuclei and projecting primarily to the ipsilateral medial accessory olivary nucleus. SYN fibrae pretectoolivares [TA].

projection f.'s, nerve f.'s connecting the cerebral cortex with other centers in the brain or spinal cord; fibers arising from cells in the central nervous system that pass to distant loci.

Prussak f.'s, elastic and connective tissue f.'s bounding the pars flaccida membranae tympani.

Purkinje f.'s, SYN subendocardial *branches* of atrioventricular bundles, under *branch.*

pyramidal f.'s, the f.'s that compose the corticospinal *tract.* SEE ALSO corticospinal *tract.* SYN corticospinal f.'s [TA], fibrae corticospinales [TA], fibrae pyramidales.

raphespinal f.'s, nerve f.'s originating from cells of the nuclei raphe magnus, pallidus, and obscurus of the pons and medulla and terminating in the spinal cord gray matter; f.'s involved in the descending inhibition of nociceptive input in the dorsal (posterior) horn; they contain serotonin.

red f.'s, red striated muscle f.'s that are rich in sarcoplasm, myoglobin, and mitochondria; they are smaller in diameter and contract more slowly than white f.'s.

Reissner f., a rodlike, highly refractive f. running caudally from the subcommissural organ throughout the length of the central canal of the brainstem and spinal cord.

Remak f.'s, SYN unmyelinated f.'s.

reticular f.'s, the collagen (type III) f.'s forming the distinctive loose connective tissue stroma of embryonic tissues, mesenchyme, red pulp of the spleen, cortex and medulla of lymph nodes, and the hematopoietic compartments of bone marrow and accounting for a substantial portion of the collagen f.'s of the skin, blood vessels, synovial membrane, uterine tissue, and granulation tissue; characterized by organization as a reticular meshwork of fine filaments and by an affinity for silver and for periodic acid-Schiff stains.

Retzius f.'s, stiff f.'s in Deiters cells.

rod f., a part of the rod cell of the retina that extends to either side of the cell body; the inner rod f. terminates in the spherule, a synaptic ending located in the outer plexiform layer.

Rosenthal f., an oval or elongated eosinophilic mass believed to represent a modified process of an astrocyte; seen in large numbers in certain slowly growing astrocytomas and areas of chronic reactive gliosis.

rubroolivary f.'s [TA], axons that arise from cells of the parvocellular part of the red nucleus, descend ipsilaterally as one

nerve fiber groups				
diameter of fiber thickness	histology	fiber groups	conduction speed	function
1–22 µm		α	80–120 m/sec	motor impulses, afferent impulses from muscle spindles and tendon organs
		β	60 m/sec	tactile impulses of the skin
3–20 µm	thick fibers with relatively thick myelin sheaths	A γ	40 m/sec	efferent impulses to the contractile portions of intrafusal muscle fibers
		δ	20 m/sec	mechanoreceptor impulses; cold, warm, and painful sensations of the skin (fast)
1–3 µm	thin fibers or thin myelin sheaths	B	10 m/sec	preganglionic vegetative fibers
1 µm	fibers without sheaths	C	1 m/sec	postganglionic vegetative fibers and afferent fibers of the sympathetic trunk, impulses of mechanoreceptors, cold and warm receptors (slow)

component of the central tegmental tract, and terminate primarily in the principal olivary nucleus. SYN fibrae rubroolivares [TA].

Sappey f.'s, nonstriated muscular f.'s in the check ligaments of the eyeball.

Sharpey f.'s, SYN perforating f.'s.

short association f.'s [TA], nerve f.'s that may interconnect adjacent lobes or gyri of the cerebral cortex of the same hemisphere or contiguous segments of the spinal cord on the same side; fibers that interconnect close or adjacent points. SYN fibrae associationes breves [TA].

skeletal muscle f.'s, multinucleated contractile cells varying from less than 10 to 100 μm in diameter and from less than 1 mm to several centimeters in length; the f. consists of sarcoplasm and cross-striated myofibrils, which in turn consist of myofilaments; human skeletal muscles are a mixture of red, white, and intermediate type f.'s.

somatic nerve f.'s [TA], afferent or efferent f.'s distributed outside the body cavities, i.e., to the parietes; the majority of somatic afferent fibers conduct impulses centrally stimulating conscious sensation; all somatic efferent fibers stimulate somatic (voluntary/striated/skeletal) muscle. SYN neurofibrae somaticae [TA].

spindle f., SEE mitotic *spindle*.

spinocuneate f.'s, axons that originate from cells in the posterior horn of cervical and upper thoracic spinal levels, ascend ipsilaterally in the cuneate fasciculus, and terminate in the cuneate nucleus. These are part of the postsynaptic–dorsal column system. SYN fibrae spinocuneatae [TA].

spinogracile f.'s [TA], axons that originate from neurons in the posterior horn of lower thoracic and lumbosacral spinal cord levels, ascend ipsilaterally in the gracile fasciculus, and terminate in the gracile nucleus. These are part of the postsynaptic–dorsal column system. SYN fibrae spinograciles [TA].

spinohypothalamic f.'s [TA], axons that originate in the spinal cord gray matter, ascend as part of the anterolateral system, and terminate in the hypothalamus SYN fibrae spinohypothalamicae [TA].

spinomesencephalic f.'s [TA], a composite group of f.'s traveling in the spinal lemniscus (anterolateral system) and ending in the mesencephalon; includes spinotectal fibers [TA] to the deeper layers of the superior colliculus and spinoperiaqeductal fibers [TA] that terminate in the periaqueductal gray matter. SYN fibrae spinomesencephalicae [TA].

spinoolivary f.'s [TA], f.'s that arise in the spinal cord and ascend primarily on the ipsilateral side to terminate in the accessory nuclei of the inferior olivary complex. SYN fibrae spinoolivares [TA].

spinoperiaqueductal f.'s [TA], axons originating from cell bodies of the posterior horn, ascending as part of the contralateral anterolateral system, and terminating in the periaqueductal gray of the mesencephalon; involved in descending pathways for pain suppression. SEE ALSO spinomesencephalic f.'s. SYN fibrae spinoperiaqueductales [TA].

spinoreticular f.'s [TA], nerve f.'s originating from the spinal cord and terminating in the reticular formation of the brainstem; some ascend as part of the anterolateral system. SYN fibrae spinoreticulares [TA], spinoreticular tract [TA].

spinotectal f.'s [TA], axons originating from cell bodies in the posterior horn, crossing in the anterior white commissure, ascending as part of the anterolateral system, and primarily terminating in the deeper layers of the superior colliculus. SEE ALSO spinomesencephalic f.'s. SYN fibrae spinotectales [TA].

stress f.'s, long bundles of microfilaments made up of actin; believed to be involved in the attachment of cultured cells to a substratum and also in the determination of the shape of cells such as fibroblasts; may be involved in cellular mobility.

striatonigral f.'s, SYN strionigral f.'s.

strionigral f.'s, nerve f.'s originating from cells of the caudate and putamen and terminating mainly in the pars reticulata of the substantia nigra; they utilize GABA and substance P. SYN striatonigral f.'s.

sudomotor f.'s, postganglionic and cholinergic sympathetic nerve f.'s that innervate the sweat glands.

sustentacular f.'s of retina, SYN Müller f.'s (2).

T f., a f. that branches at right angles to the right and left; term used to describe the branching patterns of granular cell axons in the molecular layer of the cerebellum.

tautomeric f.'s, nerve f.'s of the spinal cord that do not extend beyond the limits of the spinal cord segment in which they originate.

tectoolivary f.'s [TA], f.'s that originate in the deep layers of the superior colliculus and project primarily to the contralateral medial accessory olivary nucleus. SYN fibrae tectoolivares [TA].

tectopontine f.'s [TA], f.'s arising in the tectum of the mesencephalon and terminating in the ipsilateral nuclei of the basilar pons and in the reticulotegmental nucleus. SYN fibrae tectopontinae [TA].

tectoreticular f.'s [TA], f.'s that originate in the superior colliculus and project bilaterally to the reticular formation, primarily that of the midbrain. SYN fibrae tectoreticulares [TA].

temporopontine f.'s [TA], a f. group originating in the cerebral cortex of the temporal lobe, particularly the superior and middle temporal gyri, following the sublenticular limb of the internal capsule into the lateral margin of the crus cerebri in which it descends to its termination in the pontine nuclei in the basilar part of the pons. SEE ALSO corticospinal *tract*. SYN fibrae temporopontinae [TA].

thalamocortical f.'s, a general term identifying nerve f.'s arising from nuclei of the thalamus and projecting to, and terminating in, the cerebral cortex.

Tomes f.'s, SYN dentinal f.'s (1).

transseptal f.'s, nonelastic f.'s running from tooth to tooth over the crest of the alveolus.

transverse pontine f.'s [TA], f.'s arising from the pontine nuclei, decussate and pass into the cerebellum as the middle cerebellar peduncles. SYN fibrae pontis transversae [TA].

unmyelinated f.'s, a f. having no myelin covering (CNS); a naked axon; in the PNS represented by all axons lying in troughs in a single Schwann cell (Schwann cell unit); a slow conducting f. SYN gray f.'s, nonmedullated f.'s, Remak f.'s.

vasomotor f.'s, postganglionic visceral efferent f.'s innervating the smooth muscles of vessel walls.

visceral motor f.'s, SYN autonomic nerve f.'s.

Weitbrecht f.'s, SYN *retinaculum* of articular capsule of hip.

white f., (1) white mammalian muscle f.'s; larger in diameter than red f.'s they have less myoglobin, sarcoplasm, and mitochondria, and contract more quickly; **(2)** SYN collagen f.

yellow f.'s, SYN elastic f.'s.

zonular f.'s [TA], delicate fibers that pass from the equator of the lens to the ciliary body, collectively known as the ciliary zonule. SYN fibrae zonulares [TA].

---

fi·ber·op·tic (fī-ber-op′tik). Pertaining to fiberoptics.

fi·ber·op·tics (fī-ber-op′tiks). optical system in which the image is conveyed by a compact bundle of small-diameter, flexible, transparent fibers.

fi·ber·scope (fī′ber-skōp). SYN flexible *endoscope*.

fibr-. SEE fibro-.

fi·bra, pl. **fi·brae** (fī′bră, fī′brē) [TA]. SYN fiber, fiber. [L.]

fi′brae arcua′tae cer′ebri [TA], SYN arcuate *fibers* of cerebrum, under *fiber*.

fi′brae arcua′tae exter′nae, SYN external arcuate *fibers*, under *fiber*.

fibrae arcuatae externae anteriores [TA], SEE external arcuate *fibers*, under *fiber*.

fibrae arcuatae externae posteriores [TA], SEE external arcuate *fibers*, under *fiber*.

fi′brae arcua′tae inter′nae [TA], SYN internal arcuate *fibers*, under *fiber*.

fibrae associationes breves [TA], SYN short association *fibers*, under *fiber*.

fibrae associationes longae [TA], SYN long association *fibers*, under *fiber*.

fibrae cerebelloolivares [TA], SYN cerebelloolivary *fibers*, under *fiber*.

fi′brae circula′res [TA], SYN circular *fibers*, under *fiber*.

fibrae corticomesencephalicae [TA], SYN corticomesencephalic *fibers*, under *fiber*.

fi′brae corticonuclea′res [TA], SYN corticonuclear *fibers*, under *fiber*.

fibrae corticonucleares bulbi [TA], SYN bulbar corticonuclear *fibers*, under *fiber*.

fibrae corticonucleares mesencephali [TA], SYN mesencephalic corticonuclear *fibers*, under *fiber*.

fibrae corticonucleares pontis [TA], SYN pontine corticonuclear *fibers*, under *fiber*.

fi′brae corticopon′tinae [TA], SYN corticopontine *fibers*, under *fiber*.

fi′brae corticoreticula′res [TA], SYN corticoreticular *fibers*, under *fiber*.

fibrae corticorubrales [TA], SYN corticorubral *fibers*, under *fiber*.

fi′brae corticospina′les [TA], SYN pyramidal *fibers*, under *fiber*.

fibrae cuneocerebellares [TA], SYN cuneocerebellar *tract*.

fibrae cuneospinales [TA], SYN cuneospinal *fibers*, under *fiber*.

fi′brae dentatorubra′les, SYN dentatorubral *fibers*, under *fiber*. SEE dentatorubral *fibers*, under *fiber*.

fibrae frontopontinae [TA], SYN frontopontine *fibers*, under *fiber*.

fibrae gracilispinales [TA], SYN gracilespinal *fibers*, under *fiber*.

fibrae hypothalamospinales [TA], SYN hypothalamospinal *fibers*, under *fiber*.

fi′brae intercrura′les anuli inguinalis superficialis [TA], SYN intercrural *fibers* of superficial ring, under *fiber*.

fibrae intrathalamicae [TA], SYN intrathalamic *fibers*, under *fiber*.

fi′brae len′tis, SYN *fibers* of lens, under *fiber*.

fi′brae meridiona′les muscularis ciliaris [TA], SYN meridional *fibers* of ciliary muscle, under *fiber*.

fi′brae obli′quae tunicae muscularis [TA], SYN oblique *fibers* of muscular layer of stomach, under *fiber*.

fibrae occipitopontinae [TA], SYN occipitopontine *fibers*, under *fiber*.

fibrae occipitotectales [TA], SYN occipitotectal *fibers*, under *fiber*.

fibrae olivospinales [TA], SYN olivospinal *fibers*, under *fiber*.

fibrae parietopontinae [TA], SYN parietopontine *fibers*, under *fiber*.

fi′brae periventricula′res [TA], SYN periventricular *fibers*, under *fiber*.

fibrae pontis longitudinales [TA], SYN longitudinal pontine *fibers*, under *fiber*; SEE longitudinal pontine *fasciculi*, under *fasciculus*.

fi′brae pon′tis transver′sae [TA], SYN transverse pontine *fibers*, under *fiber*.

fibrae pontocerebellares [TA], SYN pontocerebellar *fibers*, under *fiber*.

fibrae postcommissurales [TA], SYN postcommissural *fibers*, under *fiber*.

fibrae precommissurales [TA], SYN precommissural *fibers*, under *fiber*.

fibrae pretectoolivares [TA], SYN pretectoolivary *fibers*, under *fiber*.

fi′brae pyramida′les, SYN pyramidal *fibers*, under *fiber*.

fibrae rubroolivares [TA], SYN rubroolivary *fibers*, under *fiber*.

fibrae spinocuneatae [TA], SYN spinocuneate *fibers*, under *fiber*.

fibrae spinograciles [TA], SYN spinogracile *fibers*, under *fiber*.

fibrae spinohypothalamicae [TA], SYN spinohypothalamic *fibers*, under *fiber*.

fibrae spinomesencephalicae [TA], SYN spinomesencephalic *fibers*, under *fiber*.

fibrae spinoolivares [TA], SYN spinoolivary *fibers*, under *fiber*.

fibrae spinoperiaqueductales [TA], SYN spinoperiaqueductal *fibers*, under *fiber*.

fibrae spinoreticulares [TA], SYN spinoreticular *fibers*, under *fiber*.

fibrae spinotectales [TA], SYN spinotectal *fibers*, under *fiber*.

fibrae tectoolivares [TA], SYN tectoolivary *fibers*, under *fiber*.

fibrae tectopontinae [TA], SYN tectopontine *fibers*, under *fiber*.

fibrae tectoreticulares [TA], SYN tectoreticular *fibers*, under *fiber*.

fibrae temporopontinae [TA], SYN temporopontine *fibers*, under *fiber*.

fi′brae zonula′res [TA], SYN zonular *fibers*, under *fiber*.

fibrates (fī′brāts). SYN fibric acids.

fi·bre (fī′ber). SYN fiber.

fi·bre·mia (fī-brē′mē-ă). An obsolete term for the presence of formed fibrin in the blood, causing thrombosis or embolism. SYN inosemia (2). [fibrin + G. *haima*, blood]

fibric acids. Drugs structurally related to clofibrate, used to treat hypercholesterolemia and hypertriglyceridemia. SYN fibrates.

fi·bril (fī′bril). A minute fiber or component of a fiber. SYN fibrilla. [Mod. L. *fibrilla*]

anchoring f.'s, collagen f.'s that insert in to the basal lamina of the epidermis and bind it down to the underlying dermis.

collagen f.'s, SYN unit f.'s.

muscular f., SYN myofibril.

subpellicular f., SYN subpellicular *microtubule*.

unit f.'s, the f.'s that comprise a collagen fiber, ranging from 20–200 nm and averaging about 100 nm in diameter (substantially larger in tendons), with cross-striations averaging 64 nm. SYN collagen f.'s.

fi·bril·la, pl. **fi·bril·lae** (fī-bril′ă, -ē). SYN fibril. [Mod. L. dim. of L. *fibra*, a fiber]

fi·bril·lar, fi·bril·lary (fī′bri-lăr, -lar-ē). **1.** Relating to a fibril. **2.** Denoting the fine rapid contractions or twitchings of fibers or of small groups of fibers in skeletal or cardiac muscle. SYN filar (1).

fi·bril·late (fī′bri-lāt). **1.** To make or to become fibrillar. **2.** SYN fibrillated. **3.** To be in a state of fibrillation (3).

fi·bril·lat·ed (fī′bri-lā-ted). Composed of fibrils. SYN fibrillate (2).

fi·bril·la·tion (fī-bri-lā′shŭn, fib-rĭ-). **1.** The condition of being fibrillated. **2.** The formation of fibrils. **3.** Exceedingly rapid contractions or twitching of muscular fibrils, but not of the muscle as a whole. **4.** Vermicular twitching, usually slow, of individual muscular fibers; commonly occurs in atria or ventricles of the heart as well as in recently denervated skeletal muscle fibers.

atrial f., auricular f., f. in which the normal rhythmical contractions of the cardiac atria are replaced by rapid irregular twitchings of the muscular wall; the ventricles respond irregularly to the dysrhythmic bombardment from the atria. SYN ataxia cordis.

ventricular f., coarse or fine, rapid, fibrillary movements of the ventricular muscle that replace the normal contraction.

fi·bril·lin (fī′bril-in). A microfibrillar protein in connective tissue with a wide distribution in the body; molecular weight about 350,000. There is good evidence that Marfan syndrome is due to mutations of f. [MIM*134797]. [Mod. L. *fibrilla*, fibril, + -in]

fi·bril·lo·flut·ter (fib′ril-ō-flut′er). SYN impure *flutter*.

fi·bril·lo·gen·e·sis (fī′bril-ō-jen′ĕ-sis). The development of fine fibrils (as seen with the electron microscope) normally present in collagenous fibers of connective tissue.

fi·brin (fī′brin). An elastic filamentous protein derived from fibrinogen by the action of thrombin, which releases fibrinopeptides A and B from fibrinogen in the coagulation of blood; a component of thrombi, vegetations, and acute inflammatory exudates such as in diphtheria and lobar pneumonia. [L. *fibra*, fiber]

fi·brin·ase (fī′brin-ās). **1.** Former term for *factor* XIII. **2.** SYN plasmin.

♻**fibrino-.** Fibrin. [L. *fibra*, fiber]

fi·bri·no·cel·lu·lar (fī′bri-nō-sel′ū-lăr). Composed of fibrin and cells, as in certain types of exudates resulting from acute inflammation.

fi·brin·o·gen (fī-brin′ō-jen). A globulin of the blood plasma that is converted into fibrin by the action of thrombin in the presence of ionized calcium to produce coagulation of the blood; the only coagulable protein in the blood plasma of vertebrates; it is absent in afibrinogenemia and is defective in dysfibrinogenemia.

human f., f. prepared from normal human plasma; a coagulant (clotting factor), used as an adjunct in the management of acute, congenital, or acquired chronic hypofibrinogenemia.

fi·brin·og·e·nase (fī-brin′ō-je-nās). SYN thrombin.

fi·brin·o·ge·ne·mia (fī-brin′ō-jĕ-nē′mē-ă). SYN hyperfibrinogenemia.

fi·bri·no·gen·e·sis (fī′bri-nō-jen′ĕ-sis). Formation or production of fibrin.

fi·bri·no·gen·ic, fi·bri·nog·e·nous (fī′brin-ō-jen′ik, fī′bri-noj′ĕ-nŭs). **1.** Pertaining to fibrinogen. **2.** Producing fibrin.

fi·brin·o·gen·ol·y·sis (fī-brin′ō-jen-ol′i-sis). The inactivation or dissolution of fibrinogen in the blood. [fibrinogen + G. *lysis,* dissolution]

fi·brin·o·gen·o·pe·nia (fī-brin′ō-jen-ō-pē′nē-ă). A concentration of fibrinogen in the blood that is less than the normal. [fibrinogen + G. *penia,* poverty]

fi·brin·oid (fī′bri-noyd). **1.** Resembling fibrin. **2.** A deeply or brilliantly acidophilic, homogeneous, proteinaceous material that: 1) is frequently formed in the walls of blood vessels and in connective tissue of patients with such diseases as disseminated lupus erythematosus, polyarteritis nodosa, scleroderma, dermatomyositis, and rheumatic fever; 2) is sometimes observed in healing wounds, chronic peptic ulcers, the placenta, necrotic arterioles of malignant hypertension, and other unrelated conditions. [fibrin + G. *eidos,* resemblance]

fi·bri·no·ki·nase (fī′brin-ō-kī′nās). Name proposed for the enzyme that converts plasminogen to plasmin; subsequently called urokinase, but now called plasminogen *activator.* SYN fibrinolysokinase.

fi·bri·nol·y·sin (fī-brin-ō-lī′sin). SYN plasmin.

streptococcal f., SYN streptokinase.

fi·bri·nol·y·sis (fī-bri-nol′i-sis). **1.** Hydrolysis of fibrin. **2.** The process of dissolution of fibrin in blood clots. [fibrino- + G. *lysis,* dissolution]

fi·bri·no·ly·so·ki·nase (fī′brin-ō-lī-sō-kī′nās). SYN fibrinokinase.

fi·bri·no·lyt·ic (fī-brin-ō-lit′ik). Denoting, characterized by, or causing fibrinolysis.

fi·brin·o·pep·tide (fī′brin-ō-pep′tīd). One of two pairs of peptides (A and B) released from the amino-terminal ends of 2α- (or Aα-) and 2β- (or Bβ-)chains of fibrinogen by the action of thrombin to form fibrin; they have a vasoconstrictive effect.

fi·bri·no·pu·ru·lent (fī′bri-nō-pū′roo-lent). Pertaining to pus or suppurative exudate that contains a relatively large amount of fibrin.

fi·bri·nos·co·py (fī-bri-nos′kŏ-pē). The chemical and physical examination of the fibrin of exudates, blood clots, etc. [fibrino- + G. *skopeō,* to view]

fi·brin·ous (fī′brin-ŭs). Pertaining to or composed of fibrin.

fi·bri·nu·ria (fī-bri-noo′rē-ă). The passage of urine that contains fibrin. [fibrin + G. *ouron,* urine]

⚲**fibro-, fibr-.** Fiber. [L. *fibra*]

fi·bro·ad·e·no·ma (fī′brō-ad-ĕ-nō′mă). A benign neoplasm derived from glandular epithelium, in which there is a conspicuous stroma of proliferating fibroblasts and connective tissue elements; commonly occurs in breast tissue.

giant f., a massive benign f. seen mostly in adolescent girls.

intracanalicular f., a f. of the breast consisting of nodules of fibrous tissue which invaginate and compress the ducts.

pericanalicular f., a f. of the breast consisting of an increased number of small ducts surrounded by concentric bands of fibrous tissue.

fi·bro·ad·i·pose (fī-brō-ad′i-pōz). Relating to or containing both fibrous and fatty structures. SYN fibrofatty.

fi·bro·a·re·o·lar (fī′brō-ă-rē′ō-lăr). Denoting connective tissue that is both fibrous and areolar in character.

fi·bro·blast (fī′brō-blast). A stellate or spindle-shaped cell with cytoplasmic processes present in connective tissue, capable of forming collagen fibers; an inactive f. is sometimes called a fibrocyte.

fi·bro·blas·tic (fī-brō-blas′tik). Relating to fibroblasts.

fi·bro·car·ti·lage (fī-brō-kar′ti-lij). A variety of cartilage that contains visible type I collagen fibers; appears as a transition between tendons or ligaments or bones. SYN fibrocartilago.

basilar f., SYN basilar *cartilage.*

circumferential f., a ring of f. around the articular end of a bone, serving to deepen the joint cavity. SEE ALSO acetabular *labrum,* glenoid *labrum* of scapula.

external semilunar f., SYN lateral *meniscus.*

interarticular f., SYN articular *disk.*

internal semilunar f. of knee joint, SYN medial *meniscus.*

interpubic f., ⋆official alternate term for interpubic *disk.*

semilunar f., SEE lateral *meniscus,* medial *meniscus.*

stratiform f., a layer of f. in the bottom of a groove in a bone through which a tendon runs.

fi·bro·car·ti·lag·i·nous (fī′brō-kar-ti-laj′i-nŭs). Relating to or composed of fibrocartilage.

fi·bro·car·ti·la·go (fī′brō-kar-ti-lā′gō). SYN fibrocartilage.

f. basa′lis, SYN basilar *cartilage.*

f. interarticula′ris, SYN articular *disk.*

f. interpubica, ⋆official alternate term for interpubic *disk.*

f. intervertebra′lis, SYN intervertebral *disk.*

fi·bro·cel·lu·lar (fī-brō-sel′ū-lăr). Both fibrous and cellular.

fi·bro·chon·dri·tis (fī′brō-kon-drī′tis). Inflammation of a fibrocartilage.

fi·bro·chon·dro·ma (fī′brō-kon-drō′mă). A benign neoplasm of cartilaginous tissue, in which there is a relatively unusual amount of fibrous stroma.

fi·bro·con·ges·tive (fī′brō-kon-jes′tiv). Term sometimes used to indicate the general condition of an organ or tissue in which acute or chronic, persistent congestion has resulted in degeneration and necrosis of cells and replacement with connective tissue elements, as in chronic congestive splenomegaly.

fi·bro·cys·tic (fī-brō-sis′tik). Pertaining to or characterized by the presence of fibrocysts.

fi·bro·cyte (fī′brō-sīt). Designation sometimes applied to an inactive fibroblast. [fibro- + G. *kytos,* cell]

fi·bro·dys·pla·sia (fī′brō-dis-plā′zē-ă). Abnormal development of fibrous connective tissue.

f. ossif′icans progressi′va [MIM*135100], a generalized disorder of connective tissue in which there is ectopic ossification with bone replacing tendons, fasciae, and ligaments; a lethal genetic disorder of autosomal dominant inheritance. SEE ALSO fibrous *dysplasia* of bone.

fi·bro·e·las·tic (fī′brō-ē-las′tik). Composed of collagen and elastic fibers.

fi·bro·e·las·to·sis (fī′brō-ē-las-tō′sis). Excessive proliferation of collagenous and elastic fibrous tissue.

endocardial f., endomyocardial f., (1) a congenital condition characterized by thickening of the left ventricular wall endocardium (chiefly due to fibrous and elastic tissue), thickening and malformation of the cardiac valves, subendocardial changes in the myocardium, and hypertrophy of the heart; chief symptoms are cyanosis, dyspnea, anorexia, and irritability; (2) SYN endomyocardial *fibrosis.*

fi·bro·ep·i·the·li·o·ma (fī′brō-ep-i-thē-lē-ō′mă). A skin tumor composed of fibrous tissue intersected by thin anastomosing bands of basal cells of the epidermis, enclosing keratin cysts; may give rise to basal cell carcinoma of the nodular type. SYN Pinkus tumor.

fi·bro·fat·ty (fī-brō-fat′ē). SYN fibroadipose.

fi·bro·fol·lic·u·lo·ma (fī′brō-fŏ-lik-ū-lō′mă). Small papular hamartomas of the fibrous sheath of the hair follicle, with solid extensions of the epithelium of the follicular infundibulum; multiple f.'s may be familial.

fi

fi·bro·gen·e·sis (fī-brō-jen'ĕ-sis). The production or development of fibers.

fi·bro·gli·o·sis (fī'brō-glī-ō'sis). A cellular reaction within the brain, usually in response to a penetrating injury, in which both astrocytes and fibroblasts participate and which culminates in a fibrous and glial scar. [fibro- + G. *glia,* glue, + *-osis,* condition]

fi·broid (fī'broyd). 1. Resembling or composed of fibers or fibrous tissue. 2. Old term for certain types of leiomyoma, especially those occurring in the uterus. 3. SYN fibroleiomyoma. [fibro- + G. *eidos,* resemblance]

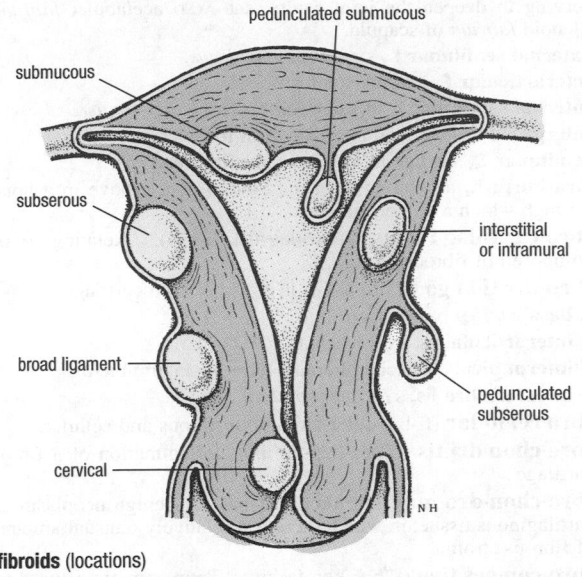

pedunculated submucous

submucous

subserous

broad ligament

cervical

interstitial or intramural

pedunculated subserous

fibroids (locations)

fi·broid·ec·to·my (fī-broy-dek'tō-mē). SYN myomectomy. [fibroid + G. *ektomē,* excision]

fi·bro·in (fī'brō-in). A white insoluble protein forming the primary constituent (70%) of cobweb and silk.

fi·bro·lei·o·my·o·ma (fī'brō-lī'ō-mī-ō'mă). A leiomyoma containing non-neoplastic collagenous fibrous tissue, which may make the tumor hard; f. usually arises in the myometrium, and the proportion of fibrous tissue increases with age. SYN fibroid (3), leiomyofibroma.

fi·bro·li·po·ma (fī'brō-li-pō'mă). A lipoma with an abundant stroma of fibrous tissue. SYN lipoma fibrosum.

fi·bro·ma (fī-brō'mă). A benign neoplasm derived from fibrous connective tissue. [fibro- + G. *-oma,* tumor]

ameloblastic f., a benign mixed odontogenic tumor characterized by neoplastic proliferation of both epithelial and mesenchymal components of the tooth bud without the production of dental hard tissue; presents clinically as a slow-growing painless radiolucency occurring most commonly in the mandible of children and adolescents.

aponeurotic f., a calcifying recurrent non-metastasizing but infiltrating f. seen most frequently on the palms of young people as a small firm nodule not attached to the overlying skin.

cementoossifying f., a form of f. with cementicles and bone rimmed with osteoblasts in moderately cellular stroma.

central ossifying f., a painless, slow-growing, expansile, sharply circumscribed benign fibro-osseus tumor of the jaws that is derived from cells of the periodontal ligament; presents initially as a radiolucency that becomes progressively more opaque as it matures.

chondromyxoid f., an uncommon benign bone tumor, occurring most frequently in the tibia of adolescents and young adults, composed of lobulated myxoid tissue with scanty chondroid foci. SYN chondrofibroma, chondromyxoma.

concentric f., a benign neoplasm, actually a leiomyoma, that occupies the entire circumference of the wall of the uterus.

desmoplastic f., a benign fibrous tumor of bone affecting children and young adults; cortical destruction may result.

giant cell f., a tumor of the oral mucosa composed of fibrous connective tissue with large stellate and multinucleate fibroblasts; shares a similar histology with the retrocuspid papilla, fibrous papule of the nose, pearly penile papule, and the ungual fibroma.

irritation f., a slow-growing nodule on the oral mucosa, composed of fibrous tissue covered by epithelium, resulting from mechanical irritation by dentures, fillings, cheek biting, etc.

f. mol'le, SYN skin *tag.*

f. mol'le gravida'rum, skin tags or polyps that develop on women during pregnancy and often disappear at term.

f. myxomato'des, SYN myxofibroma.

nonossifying f., a loculated osteolytic focus of cellular fibrous tissue, slightly expanding a bone, usually near the end of a long bone in older children; similar to fibrous cortical *defect,* although larger.

nonosteogenic f., SYN fibrous cortical *defect.*

odontogenic f., a rare odontogenic tumor found in soft tissue or as a central bony lesion. The tumor is composed of fibrous connective tissue, odontogenic epithelium, and sometimes calcification.

peripheral ossifying f., a reactive focal gingival overgrowth derived histogenetically from cells of the periodontal ligament and usually developing in response to local irritants (plaque and calculus) on associated teeth; consists microscopically of a hyperplastic cellular fibrous stroma supporting deposits of bone, cementum, or dystrophic calcification.

periungual f., multiple smooth firm nodules formed at the nail folds, often over 10 mm in length, which appear at or after puberty in some patients with tuberous sclerosis.

rabbit f., SYN Shope f.

recurring digital f. of childhood, multiple fibrous flesh-colored nodules on the extensor aspect of the terminal phalanges of adjacent digits of infants and young children that often recur after attempted excision, do not metastasize, and may spontaneously regress in two to three years; composed of spindle cells containing cytoplasmic inclusions believed to be derived from myofibrils. SYN infantile digital fibromatosis.

Shope f., a connective tissue tumor of cottontail rabbits caused by a poxvirus of the genus Leporipoxvirus and found by Shope to be transmissible with cellular suspensions or Berkefeld filtrates; it is related to myxomatosis and is used in Europe as a source of vaccine to protect against the myxoma virus. SYN rabbit f.

telangiectatic f., a benign neoplasm of fibrous tissue in which there are numerous small and large, frequently dilated vascular channels. SYN angiofibroma.

fi·bro·ma·toid (fī-brō'mă-toyd). A focus, nodule, or mass (of proliferating fibroblasts) that resembles a fibroma but is not regarded as neoplastic.

fi·bro·ma·to·sis (fī'brō-mă-tō'sis). 1. A condition characterized by multiple fibromas, with relatively widespread distribution. 2. Abnormal hyperplasia of fibrous tissue.

abdominal f., SYN desmoid (2).

aggressive infantile f., a childhood counterpart of abdominal or extra-abdominal desmoid tumors, characterized by firm subcutaneous nodules that grow rapidly in any part of the body that invade locally and recur but do not metastasize.

f. col'li, a fibrous mass in the midportion of the sternocleidomastoid muscle; the mass may be a hematoma resulting from a birth injury and may cause torticollis.

congenital generalized f. [MIM*228550], multiple subcutaneous and visceral fibrous tumors present at birth; a rare disorder often fatal in the first week of life, although sometimes undergoing spontaneous remission; probable autosomal recessive inheritance.

gingival f., f. that may be associated with trichodiscomas. Several genetic forms are known, all autosomal dominant [MIM*135300, *135400, *135500, *135550].

infantile digital f., SYN recurring digital *fibroma* of childhood.

juvenile hyalin f. [MIM*228600], a rare recessively inherited deforming disorder of head, neck, and generalized cutaneous nodules or tumors in children with normal mentality; the lesions consist of fibroblasts separated by an eosinophilic hyalin stroma composed mostly of glycosaminoglycans. SYN systemic hyalinosis.

juvenile palmo-plantar f., f. that occurs in children from birth to adolescence as a single poorly demarcated nodule of the thenar or hypothenar eminence or overlying the calcaneus of the mid-sole.

palmar f., nodular fibroplastic proliferation in the palmar fascia of one or both hands, preceding or associated with Dupuytren contracture.

penile f., SYN Peyronie *disease.*

plantar f., nodular fibroblastic proliferation in plantar fascia of one or both feet; rarely associated with contracture. SYN Dupuytren disease of the foot.

fi·bro·ma·tous (fī-brō′mă-tŭs). Pertaining to, or of the nature of, a fibroma.

fi·bro·mec·to·my (fī-brō-mek′tō-mē). SYN myomectomy.

fi·brom·e·ter (fī′brō-mē′ter). An instrument that measures clot formation (as in tests for blood clotting in vitro) by mechanical detection of the clot by a moving probe.

fi·bro·mus·cu·lar (fī′brō-mŭs′kū-lăr). Both fibrous and muscular; relating to both fibrous and muscular tissues.

fi·bro·my·al·gia (fī-brō-mī-al′ja). A syndrome of chronic pain of musculoskeletal origin but uncertain cause. The American College of Rheumatology has established diagnostic criteria that include pain on both sides of the body, both above and below the waist, as well as in an axial distribution (cervical, thoracic, or lumbar spine or anterior chest); additionally there must be point tenderness in at least 11 of 18 specified sites. SYN fibromyalgia syndrome.

fi·bro·my·ec·to·my (fī′brō-mī-ek′tō-mē). Excision of a fibromyoma.

fi·bro·my·o·ma (fī′brō-mī-ō′mă). A leiomyoma that contains a relatively abundant amount of fibrous tissue.

fi·bro·my·o·si·tis (fī′brō-mī-ō-sī′tis). Chronic inflammation of a muscle with an overgrowth, or hyperplasia, of the connective tissue. [fibro- + G. *mys,* muscle, + *-itis,* inflammation]

fi·bro·myx·o·ma (fī′brō-mik-sō′mă). A myxoma that contains a relatively abundant amount of mature fibroblasts and connective tissue. [fibro- + G. *myxa,* mucus, + *-ōma,* tumor]

fi·bro·nec·tins (fī-brō-nek′tins). High molecular weight multifunctional glycoproteins found on cell surface membranes and in blood plasma and other body fluids. Fibronectins are thought to function as adhesive ligandlike molecules that play a role in contact inhibition; also known as large external transformation sensitive protein (LETS), which is reduced after cells become transformed. SYN zetaprotein. [L. *fibra,* fiber, + *nexus,* interconnection]

plasma f., a circulating α_2-glycoprotein that functions as an opsonin, mediating reticuloendothelial and macrophage clearance of fibrin microaggregates, collagen debris, and bacterial particulates, protecting microvascular perfusion and lymphatic drainage.

fi·bro·neu·ro·ma (fī′brō-noo-rō′mă). SYN neurofibroma.

fi·bro·os·te·o·ma (fī′brō-os-tē-ō′mă). An osteoma in which the neoplastic bone-forming cells are situated within a relatively abundant stroma of fibrous tissue.

fi·bro·pap·il·lo·ma (fī′brō-pap-i-lō′mă). A papilloma characterized by a conspicuous amount of fibrous connective tissue at the base and forming the cores upon which the neoplastic epithelial cells are massed.

fi·bro·pla·sia (fī-brō-plā′zē-ă). Production of fibrous tissue, usually implying an abnormal increase of nonneoplastic fibrous tissue. [fibro- + G. *plasis,* a molding]

retrolental f., SYN *retinopathy* of prematurity.

fi·bro·plas·tic (fī-brō-plas′tik). Producing fibrous tissue. [fibro- + G. *plastos,* formed]

fi·bro·plate (fī′brō-plāt). SYN articular *disk.*

fi·bro·pol·y·pus (fī-brō-pol′i-pŭs). A polyp composed chiefly of fibrous tissue.

fi·bro·re·tic·u·late (fī′brō-re-tik′ū-lāt). Relating to or consisting of a network of fibrous tissue.

fi·bro·sa.

pericardium fibrosa [TA], SEE pericardium.

fi·bro·sar·co·ma (fī′brō-sar-kō′mă). A malignant neoplasm derived from deep fibrous tissue, characterized by bundles of immature proliferating fibroblasts arranged in a distinctive herringbone pattern with variable collagen formation, which tends to invade locally and metastasize by the bloodstream.

ameloblastic f., a rapidly growing, painful, destructive, radiolucent odontogenic tumor that usually arises through malignant change in the mesenchymal component of a pre-existing ameloblastic fibroma. SYN ameloblastic sarcoma.

Earle L f., a transplantable f. derived from subcutaneous tissue of a mouse of C3H strain, grown in tissue culture to which 20-methylcholanthrene had been added.

infantile f., a rapidly growing but infrequently metastasizing f. which usually appears on the extremities in the first year of life.

fi·brose (fī-brōs′). To form fibrous tissue.

fi·bro·se·rous (fī-brō-sē′rŭs). Composed of fibrous tissue with a serous surface; denoting any serous membrane.

fi·bro·sis (fī-brō′sis). Formation of fibrous tissue as a reparative or reactive process, as opposed to formation of fibrous tissue as a normal constituent of an organ or tissue.

African endomyocardial f., f. of the inner layers of the myocardium, often including the endocardium, causing diastolic restriction of the heart; indigenous to East Africa.

congenital f. of the extraocular muscles [MIM*135700], an autosomal dominant disorder associated with blepharoptosis and absence of eye movements.

▣ **cystic f., cystic f. of the pancreas** [MIM*219700], a congenital metabolic disorder in which secretions of exocrine glands are abnormal; excessively viscid mucus causes obstruction of passageways (including pancreatic and bile ducts, intestines, and bronchi), and the sodium and chloride content of sweat are increased throughout the patient's life; symptoms usually appear in childhood and include meconium ileus, poor growth despite good appetite, malabsorption and foul bulky stools, chronic bronchitis with cough, recurrent pneumonia, bronchiectasis, emphysema, clubbing of the fingers, and salt depletion in hot weather. Detailed genetic mapping and molecular biology have been accomplished by the methods of reverse genetics; autosomal recessive inheritance, caused by mutation in the cystic f. conductance regulator gene (CFTR) on chromosome 7q. SYN Clarke-Hadfield syndrome, fibrocystic disease of the pancreas, mucoviscidosis, viscidosis.

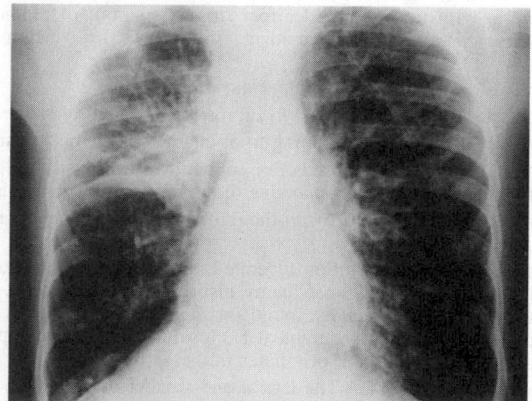

cystic fibrosis: characteristic changes of end-stage cystic fibrosis are seen, including bronchial wall thickening, bronchiectasis, and persistent atelectasis

endocardial f., scarring or collagenosis of the endocardium. SYN endocardial sclerosis.

endomyocardial f., thickening of the ventricular endocardium by f., involving the subendocardial myocardium, and sometimes the atrioventricular valves, with mural thrombosis, leading to progressive right and left ventricular failure with mitral and tricuspid insufficiency; occurs in adults and is endemic in parts of Africa.

fi

SYN Davies disease, endocardial fibroelastosis (2), endomyocardial fibroelastosis.

idiopathic interstitial f., SYN idiopathic pulmonary f.

idiopathic pulmonary f. (IPF), an acute to chronic inflammatory process or interstitial f. of the lung of unknown etiology. with collagen-vascular diseases. SYN chronic fibrosing alveolitis, cryptogenic fibrosing alveolitis, fibrosing alveolitis, Hamman-Rich syndrome, idiopathic interstitial f.

interstitial pulmonary f., includes both idiopathic pulmonary f. and pulmonary f. associated with connective tissue disease and other known primary diseases.

leptomeningeal f., a fibrous reaction within the subarachnoid space; sometimes a sequel to infectious or chemical meningitis. SEE ALSO adhesive *arachnoiditis*.

mediastinal f., f. that may obstruct the superior vena cava, pulmonary arteries, veins, or bronchi; most common cause is histoplasmosis; less commonly tuberculosis or unknown. SYN fibrosing mediastinitis, idiopathic fibrous mediastinitis.

nodular subepidermal f., SEE dermatofibroma.

oral submucous f., a precancerous condition of the oral mucosa and upper aerodigestive tract characteristically in a native of India.

pericentral f., f. occurring around the central veins in the hepatic lobules.

perimuscular f., f. in the outer media of arteries, usually the renal arteries of young women, where it causes segmental stenosis and hypertension; a variety of fibromuscular dysplasia. SYN subadventitial f.

pipestem f., a characteristic pipe-shaped f. formed around hepatic portal veins in some cases of long-continued heavy infection with *Schistosoma mansoni;* thought to be induced by the presence of large numbers of schistosome eggs in the hepatic tissues. SYN Symmers clay pipestem f., Symmers f.

replacement f., the formation of fibrous tissue that occupies sites where various other cells and tissues have become atrophied, or degenerated and necrotic.

retroperitoneal f., f. of retroperitoneal structures and connective tissue commonly involving and obstructing the ureters; the cause is usually unknown. SYN idiopathic fibrous retroperitonitis, Ormond disease, periureteritis plastica.

subadventitial f., SYN perimuscular f.

Symmers clay pipestem f., Symmers f., SYN pipestem f.

fi·bro·si·tis (fī-brō-sī′tis). **1.** Inflammation of fibrous tissue. **2.** Term used to denote generalized muscle aching, soreness, or stiffness, with multiple tender foci (trigger points); of unknown etiology. SYN muscular rheumatism. [fibro- + G. -itis, inflammation]

cervical f., SYN posttraumatic neck *syndrome*.

fi·bro·tho·rax (fī-brō-thō′raks). Fibrosis of the pleural space.

fi·brot·ic (fī-brot′ik). Pertaining to or characterized by fibrosis.

fi·brous (fī′brŭs). Composed of or containing fibroblasts, and also the fibrils and fibers of connective tissue formed by such cells.

fi·bro·xan·tho·ma (fī′brō-zan-thō′mă). A fibrohistiocytic neoplasm.

atypical f., a solitary, often ulcerated, small, cutaneous, usually benign, tumor composed of foamy histiocytes, spindle cells, and bizarre giant cells; usually found on the exposed skin of older people; microscopically, atypical f. closely resembles malignant fibrous histiocytoma, but originates in the dermis.

fib·u·la (fib′ū-lă) [TA]. The lateral and smaller of the two bones of the leg; it is not-weight bearing and articulates with the tibia above and the tibia and talus below. SYN calf bone, calf-bone (1), perone, peroneal bone. [L. *fibula* (contr. fr. *figibula*), that which fastens, a clasp, buckle, fr. *figo,* to fix, fasten]

fib·u·lar (fib′ū-lăr). Relating to the fibula. SYN fibularis, peroneal. [L. *fibularis*]

fib·u·la·ris (fib-ū-lā′ris). SYN fibular, fibular. [Mod. L.]

fib·u·lo·cal·ca·ne·al (fib′ū-lō-kal-kā′nē-ăl). Relating to the fibula and the calcaneus.

fi·cain (fī-kān). SYN ficin (2).

fi·cin (fī′sin). **1.** A cysteine endopeptidase isolated from figs

(*Ficus carica, globata,* and *doliaria*); used in industry as a protein digestant; f. has a wide specificity for protein substrates; an anthelmintic. **2.** The crude dried latex from *Ficus* spp. SYN ficain.

Fick, Adolf, German physician, 1829–1901. SEE F. *method, principle.*

FID Abbreviation for free induction *decay.*

Fiedler, Carl L.A., German physician, 1835–1921. SEE F. *myocarditis.*

field (fēld). A definite area of plane surface, considered in relation to some specific object. [A.S. *feld*]

auditory f., the space included within the limits of hearing of a definite sound, as of a tuning fork.

Broca f., SYN Broca *center.*

Cohnheim f., SYN Cohnheim *area.*

f. of consciousness, SEE field of *consciousness.*

f. of fixation, in ophthalmology, the angular distance around which the line of fixation can be turned.

f.'s of Forel, three circumscript, myelin-rich regions of the subthalamus known as H fields (from Haubenfelder); 1) field H_1, corresponding to the thalamic fasciculus, a horizontal fiber stratum at the junction of the subthalamus and the overlying thalamus, is composed of pallidothalamic and cerebellothalamic fibers (brachium conjunctivum) and is separated by the zona incerta from the more ventrally placed field H_2; 2) field H_2, formed by the lenticular fasciculus and arching over the dorsal border of the subthalamic nucleus, is composed largely of pallidothalamic fibers; 3) field H_3 or prerubral field, is a large field of intermingling gray and white matter immediately rostral to the red nucleus, uniting fields H_1 and H_2 around the medial margin of the zona incerta; its gray matter forms the prerubral nucleus. SEE ALSO lenticular *loop.* SYN campi foreli, tegmental f.'s of Forel.

free f., a f. (three-dimensional space) in a homogeneous, isotropic medium free from boundaries; in practice, a f. in which boundary effects are negligible.

H f.'s, SEE f.'s of Forel.

individuation f., the f. within which an organizer can bring about the rearrangement of primordial tissues in such a manner that a complete embryo is formed.

involved f., in radiation treatment, the area of the tumor itself.

magnetic f., the sphere of influence of a magnet.

microscopic f., the area within which objects are visible with microscope oculars and objectives of various magnifying powers.

nerve f., the regional distribution of nerve terminals.

prerubral f., SEE f.'s of Forel.

sound f., the environment in which sound waves are propagated. SYN acoustical surround.

tegmental f.'s of Forel, SYN f.'s of Forel.

visual f. (F), the area simultaneously visible to one eye without movement; often measured by means of a bowl perimeter located 330 mm from the eye.

Wernicke f., SYN Wernicke *center.*

Fielding, George H., British anatomist, 1801–1871. SEE F. *membrane.*

Field rap·id stain. See under stain.

field-vole (fēld-vōl). A species of field mouse (*Microtus montebelloi*), normal host of *Leptospira hebdomadis,* the cause of a type of leptospirosis resembling infectious mononucleosis.

Fiessinger, Noël Armand, French physician, 1881–1946. SEE F.-Leroy-Reiter *syndrome.*

fièv·re (fē-evr′) French term for fever.

f. boutonneuse (fē-evr′ boo-ton-nŭz′), SYN Mediterranean spotted *fever.*

fig. Ficus, the partially dried fruit of *Ficus carica* (family Moraceae); used as a nutrient, mild laxative, and demulcent. [L. *ficus;* A.S. *fic*]

FIGLU Abbreviation for formiminoglutamic acid.

fig·u·ra·tus (fig-ū-rā′tŭs). Figured; a term descriptive of certain skin lesions. [L. *figuro,* pp. *-atus,* to form, fashion]

fig·ure (fig′ūr). **1.** A form or shape. **2.** A person representing the essential aspects of a particular role (e.g., relating to one's male

figure 673 **Filarioidea**

boss as a father figure or to one's female teacher as a mother figure). **3.** A form, shape, outline, or representation of an object or person. [L. *figura,* fr *fingo,* to shape, fashion]

authority f., a real or projected person in a position of power; one's parents, police, and boss are authority figures to some people; during the transference phase of psychoanalysis, the psychoanalyst becomes an authority f.

flame f., a small area of dermal or subcutaneous necrosis with intense eosinophil staining of collagen bundles; seen in the lesions of eosinophilic cellulitis.

fortification f.'s, SYN fortification *spectrum.*

mitotic f., the microscopic appearance of a cell undergoing mitosis; a cell of which the chromosomes are visible by the light microscope.

myelin f., a rolled-up or scroll-like arrangement of a lipid bilayer within a cell, superficially resembling the myelin sheath of nerves; observed with the electron microscope in the cytoplasm or as inclusion in mitochondria and autophagic vacuoles where they may represent artifacts of lipid fixation. SYN myelin body.

Purkinje f.'s, shadows of the retinal vessels, seen as dark lines on a reddish field when a light enters the eye through the sclera and not the pupil.

fig·ure and ground. That aspect of perception wherein the perceived is separated into at least two parts, each with different attributes but influencing one another. Figure is the most distinct; ground the least formed; e.g., a bird or tree (figure) seen against the sky (ground).

fi·la (fī′lă). Plural of filum. [L.]

fi·la·ceous (fī-lā′shŭs). SYN filamentous. [L. *filum,* a thread]

fil·ag·grin (fil-ag′grin). A major protein of the keratohyalin granule, composed mostly of L-histidyl, lysyl, and arginyl residues (stratum corneum basic proteins). It aggregates keratin intermediate filaments and promotes disulfide bond formation. [*fil*ament + *aggre*gating]

fil·a·men, filamin (fil′ă-men). A high molecular weight, actin-binding protein that is part of the intracellular filamentous structure of fibroblastic cells; its distribution in cells is derived from its interaction with polymerized actin.

fil·a·ment (fil′ă-ment). **1.** SYN filamentum. **2.** In bacteriology, a fine threadlike form, unsegmented or segmented without constrictions. [L. *filamentum,* fr. *filum,* a thread]

actin f., one of the contractile elements in muscular fibers and other cells; in skeletal muscle, the actin f.'s are about 5 nm wide and 100 μm long, and attach to the transverse Z f.'s. SYN thin f.

axial f., the central f. of a flagellum or cilium; with the electron microscope it is seen as a complex of nine peripheral diplomicrotubules and a central pair of microtubules. SYN axoneme (2).

cytokeratin f.'s, SYN keratin f.'s.

intermediate f.'s, a class of tough protein f.'s (including keratin f.'s, neurofilaments, desmin, and vimentin) that measure 8–10 nm in thickness and comprise part of the cytoskeleton of the cytoplasm of most eukaryotic cells; so named because they are intermediate in thickness between actin f.'s and microtubules.

keratin f.'s, a class of intermediate f.'s that form a network within epithelial cells and anchor to desmosomes, thus imparting tensile strength to the tissue. SYN cytokeratin f.'s.

myosin f., one of the contractile elements in skeletal, cardiac, and smooth muscle fibers; in skeletal muscle, the f. is about 10 nm thick and 1.5 μm long. SYN thick f.

parabasal f., term formerly used for rhizoplast.

pial f., ✩official alternate term for pial *part* of filum terminale.

root f.'s, SYN radicular *fila,* under *filum.*

spermatic f., a spermatozoon, especially the tail of a spermatozoon.

thick f., SYN myosin f.

thin f., SYN actin f.

Z f., the thin zig-zag structure at the Z line of striated muscle fibers to which the actin f.'s attach.

fil·a·men·tous (fil-ă-men′tŭs). **1.** Threadlike in structure. SYN

filiform (1). **2.** Composed of filaments or threadlike structures. SYN filaceous, filar (2).

fil·a·men·tum, pl. **fil·a·men·ta** (fil-ă-men′tŭm, -tă). A fibril, fine fiber, or threadlike structure. SYN filament (1). [L.]

fi·lar (fī′lăr). **1.** SYN fibrillar. **2.** SYN filamentous. [L. *filum,* a thread]

ℹ️ *Fi·lar·ia* (fī-lar′ē-ă). Former genus of nematodes now classified in several genera and species of the family Onchocercidae; e.g., *Wuchereria bancrofti* (*F. bancrofti, F. diurna,* or *F. nocturna*), *Brugia malayi* (*F. malaya*), *Onchocerca volvulus* (*F. volvulus*), *Mansonella perstans* (*F. perstans* or *F. sanguinis hominis*), *M. streptocerca, M. ozzardi* (*F. demarquayi* or *F. ozzardi*), *Loa loa* (*F. extraocularis, F. lentis, F. loa,* or *F. oculi humani*), and *Dracunculus medinensis* (*F. medinensis*) SEE ALSO filaria.

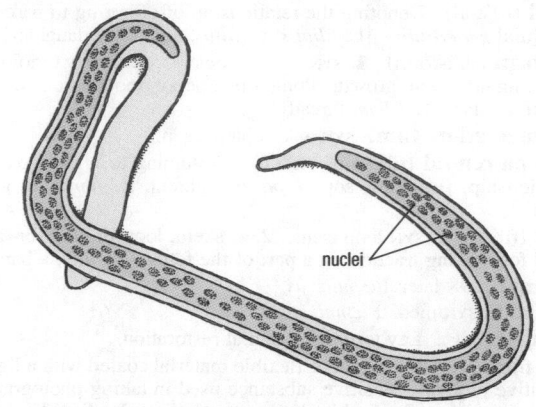

filaria (microfilaria of *Wuchereria bancrofti*)

fil·ar·ia, pl. **fil·ar·i·ae** (fi-lar′ē-ă, -ē-ē). Common name for nematodes of the family Onchocercidae, which live as adults in the blood, tissue fluids, tissues, or body cavities of many vertebrates. The females lay partially embryonated eggs, the embryos uncoil and circulate in blood or tissue fluids as microfilariae; if ingested by an appropriate bloodsucking arthropod, larval stages develop; later, infective larvae may be deposited on another vertebrate host's skin when the arthropod seeks another blood meal. [L. *filum,* a thread]

fil·ar·i·al (fi-lā′rē-ăl). Pertaining to a filaria (or filariae), including the microfilaria stage.

fil·a·ri·a·sis (fil-ă-rī′ă-sis). Presence of filariae in the tissues of the body or in blood (microfilaremia) or tissue fluids (microfilariasis), occurring in tropical and subtropical regions; living worms cause minimal tissue reaction, which may be asymptomatic, but death of the adult worms leads to granulomatous inflammation and permanent fibrosis causing obstruction of the lymphatic channels from dense hyalinized scars in the subcutaneous tissues; the most serious consequence is elephantiasis or pachyderma.

bancroftian f., f. caused by *Wuchereria bancrofti.*

Brug f., infection with filarial organism *Brugia malayi,* which causes adenitis, fever, lymphangitis, and sometimes elephantiasis; occurs primarily in southeast Asia, India, Indonesia, China, Japan, Korea, and the Philippines.

periodic f., a form of f. in which microfilariae appear in the peripheral blood at regular 24-hr intervals; usually refers to the nocturnal periodicity of bancroftian filariasis.

fil·ar·i·ci·dal (fil-lar-i-sī′dăl). Fatal to filariae.

fil·ar·i·cide (fi-lar′i-sīd). An agent that kills filariae. [filaria + L. *caedo,* to kill]

fil·ar·i·form (fi-lar′i-fōrm). **1.** Resembling filariae or other types of small nematode worms. SEE ALSO filariform *larva.* **2.** Thin or hairlike.

Fil·a·ri·i·cae (fi-lar′ē-i-sē). SYN Filarioidea.

Fil·ar·i·oi·dea (fil-lar′ē-oy′dē-ă). A superfamily of filarial nematodes parasitic in many animal species, including man; includes the families Filariidae, Diplotraenidae, Onchocercidae, and Stephanofilariidae. SEE *Filaria*. SEE ALSO *Dipetalonema, Dirofilaria, Loa loa, Mansonella, Onchocerca, Wuchereria, Brugia*. SYN *Filariicae*.

Filatov, Vladimir P., Russian ophthalmologist, 1875–1956. SEE F. *flap;* F.-Gillies *flap*.

Filatov, Nil F., Russian pediatrician, 1847–1902. SEE F. *disease*.

file (fīl). A tool for smoothing, grinding, or cutting.

Hedström f., a coarse root canal f. similar to a rasp.

periodontal f., an instrument with a series of ridges or points arranged in rows on its surface, used for scaling or removing dental calculus from the teeth.

root canal f., a pointed, flexible, steel intracanal instrument used in rasping canal walls.

fil·i·al (fil′ē-ăl). Denoting the relationship of offspring to parents. SEE filial *generation*. [L. *filialis*, fr. *filius*, son, *filia*, daughter]

fi·li·form (fil′i-fōrm). **1.** SYN filamentous (1). **2.** In bacteriology, denoting an even growth along the line of inoculation, either stroke or stab. [L. *filum*, thread]

fi·li·form ad·na·tum. SYN ankyloblepharon.

fil·i·o·pa·ren·tal (fil′ē-ō-pă-ren′tăl). Pertaining to a child-parent relationship. [L. *filius*, son, + *parens*, parent, fr. *pario*, to give birth]

fil·let (fil′et). **1.** SYN lemniscus. **2.** A skein, loop of cord, or tape used for making traction on a part of the fetus. [Fr. *filet*, a band]

lateral f., SYN lateral *lemniscus*.

medial f., SYN medial *lemniscus*.

fill·ing (fil′ing). Lay term for a dental restoration.

film (film). **1.** A thin sheet of flexible material coated with a light-sensitive or x-ray–sensitive substance used in taking photographs or radiographs. **2.** A thin layer or coating. **3.** A radiograph (colloq.).

absorbable gelatin f., a sterile, nonantigenic, absorbable, water-insoluble, thin sheet of gelatin prepared by drying a gelatin-formaldehyde solution on plates; used in the closure and repair of defects in membranes such as the dura mater or the pleura; it undergoes absorption over a period of 1–6 months.

bitewing f., a special packaging of radiographic f. that allows an appendage of the f. package to be held between the occlusal surfaces of the teeth.

decubitus f., a radiograph exposed with the subject in the decubitus position, named for the side that is dependent. SYN right or left lateral decubitus f.

horizontal beam f., a radiograph made with the central axis of the x-ray beam parallel to the floor, able to show an air-fluid level.

latitude f., SYN wide-latitude f.

panoramic x-ray f., in dentistry, a radiograph taken to give a panoramic view of the entire upper and lower dental arch as well as the temporomandibular joints.

plain f., a radiograph made without use of a contrast medium.

precorneal f., a protective f., 7 to 9 nm thick, consisting of external oily, intermediate watery, and deep mucoprotein layers. SYN tear f.

right or left lateral decubitus f., SYN decubitus f.

scout f., a radiograph exposed before contrast medium is given, such as the preliminary film for an angiogram, urogram, or barium contrast gastrointestinal examination. SYN scout radiograph.

f. speed, the relative sensitivity of f. emulsion to light or radiation exposure; speed is inversely related to detail resolution.

spot f., a radiograph made during the course of an examination under fluoroscopic control, with a device attached to the fluoroscope.

tear f., SYN precorneal f.

wide-latitude f., f. that does not show large contrast differences with differences in exposure; the slope of the H and D *curve* is low. SYN latitude f.

film chang·er. A device that moves film for radiographic studies that require rapid serial x-ray exposures, such as angiography. SYN rapid f. c., serial f. c.

rapid f. c., SYN film changer.

serial f. c., SYN film changer.

Fil·mer, David L., U.S. biochemist, *1932. SEE Adair-Koshland-Némethy-Filmer *model;* Koshland-Némethy-Filmer *model*.

fil·o·po·dia (fil-ō-pō′dē-ă). Plural of filopodium.

fil·o·po·di·um, pl. **fil·o·po·dia** (fī-lō-pō′dē-ŭm, -ă). A slender filamentous pseudopodium of certain free-living amebae. [L. *filum*, thread, + G. *pous*, foot]

fi·lo·pres·sure (fī-lō-presh′ŭr). Temporary pressure on a blood

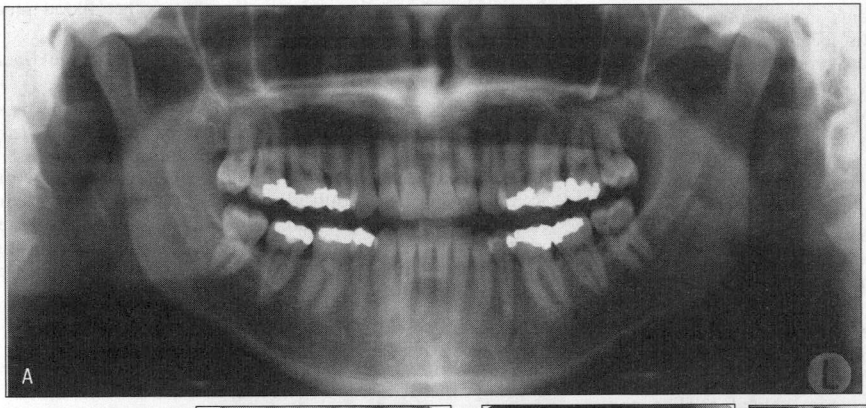
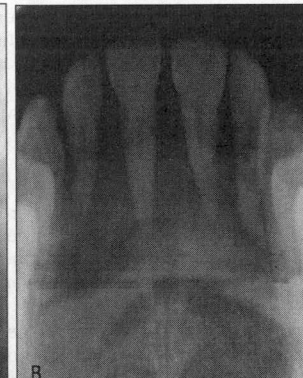
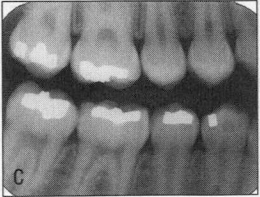
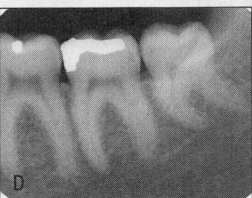
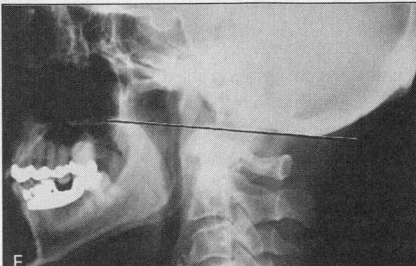

dental film techniques: (A) panoramic, (B) occlusal, (C) bitewing, (D) periapical, (E) cephalometric

vessel by a ligature, which is removed when the flow of blood has ceased. [L. *filum*, thread]

fi·lo·var·i·co·sis (fī′lō-var-ē-kō′sis). A series of swellings along the course of the axon of a nerve fiber. [L. *filum*, thread, + *varix*, dilation of vein]

Fil·o·vi·ri·dae (fī′lō-vī′rā-dā). A family of filamentous, single-stranded, negative sense RNA viruses with an enveloped nucleocapsid. These viruses were formerly classified with the Rhabdoviridae and are associated with hemorrhagic fever. The natural reservoir of these viruses is unknown. SEE Ebola *virus*. [L. *filum*, thread, + virus]

Fil·o·vi·rus (fī′lō-vī′rŭs). A genus in the family Filoviridae that includes Marburg and Ebola viruses.

fil·ter (fil′ter). **1.** A porous substance through which a liquid or gas is passed in order to separate it from contained particulate matter or impurities to sterilize. SYN filtrum. **2.** To use or to subject to the action of a f. **3.** In diagnostic or therapeutic radiology, a plate made of one or more metals such as aluminum and copper which, placed in the x- or gamma ray beam, permits passage of a greater proportion of higher-energy radiation and attenuation of lower-energy and less desirable radiation, raising the average energy or hardening the beam. **4.** A device used in spectrophotometric analysis to isolate a segment of the spectrum. **5.** A mathematical algorithm applied to image data for the purpose of enhancing image quality, usually by suppression or enhancement of high spatial frequencies. **6.** A passive electronic circuit or device that selectively permits the passage of certain electrical signals. **7.** A device placed in the inferior vena cava to prevent pulmonary embolism from low extremity clot. There are many variants. [Mediev. L. *filtro*, pp. -*atus*, to strain through felt, fr. *filtrum*, felt]

bandpass f., a device that allows a limited range of frequencies to pass.

Berkefeld f., a bacterial f. used in 1891, made of earth known as Kieselguhr taken from the name of the mine in Hanover, Germany, from which the earth was found. Ground water at this mine had a clear blue color suggesting the use of the earth as a filter. [Berkefeld, name of owner of the mine]

bird's nest f., a wire mesh inferior vena cava f.

Greenfield f., a multistrutted, spring-style vena cava f.

high-pass f., a device or material that allows high frequency signals to pass while attenuating other signals.

low-pass f., a device or material with the opposite effect from a high-pass f.; most tissues act as low-pass f.'s of ultrasound signals.

nitinol f., a vena cava f. made with a metal that springs into shape when warmed to body heat by the blood after catheter insertion.

vena cava f., a f. used for interruption of inferior vena cava to prevent pulmonary embolism; e.g., Greenfield f. SYN venocaval f.

venocaval f., SYN vena cava f.

fil·tra·ble, fil·ter·a·ble (fil′tră-bl, fil′ter-ă-bl). Capable of passing a filter; frequently applied to smaller viruses and some bacteria.

fil·trate (fil′trāt). That which has passed through a filter.

fil·tra·tion (fil-trā′shŭn). **1.** The process of passing a liquid or gas through a filter. **2.** In radiology, the process of attenuating and hardening a beam of x- or gamma rays by interposing a filter (3) between the radiation source and the object being irradiated; inherent f. is that which is caused by the apparatus itself, such as the glass of an x-ray tube, without addition of a filter. SYN percolation (1).

gel f., separation of molecular sizes by passage of a mixture through columns of beads of cross-linked dextrans or similar relatively inert material of a well-defined pore size range; the larger the molecule, the less time it spends in the interior of the beads, thus emerging earlier from the column than smaller molecules.

fil·trum (fil′trŭm). SYN filter (1). [Mediev. L.]

Merkel f. ventric′uli, SYN f. ventriculi.

f. ventric′uli, a groove between the two prominences, in each lateral wall of the vestibule of the larynx, formed by the cuneiform and the arytenoid cartilages. SYN Merkel f. ventriculi.

fi·lum, pl. **fi·la** (fī′lŭm, -lă) [TA]. A structure of filamentous or threadlike appearance. [L. thread]

f. du′rae ma′tris spina′lis, SYN dural *part* of filum terminale.

fi′la olfacto′ria [TA], SYN olfactory *nerves* [CN I], under *nerve*.

olfactory fila, SYN olfactory *nerves* [CN I], under *nerve*.

radicular fi′la, the small, individual fiber fascicles into which the roots of all of the spinal nerves and several cranial nerves (hypoglossus, vagus, oculomotorius) divide in fanlike fashion before entering or leaving the spinal cord or brainstem; the spinal dorsal root may divide into 8–12 such rootlets. SYN fila radicularia [TA], root filaments.

fi′la radicula′ria [TA], SYN radicular fila.

f. of spinal dura mater, SYN dural *part* of filum terminale.

terminal f., a long connective tissue (pia mater) strand extending from the extremity of the medullary cone to the inner aspect of the spinal dural sac (pial part of filum terminale [TA], filum terminale internum [TAalt]; stout strands of connective tissue attaching the spinal dural sac to the coccyx (dural part of filum terminale [TA], coccygeal ligament [TAalt], filum terminale externum [TAalt]. SYN f. terminale [TA], nervus impar, terminal thread.

f. termina′le [TA], SYN terminal f.

f. terminale externum, ✠official alternate term for dural *part* of filum terminale.

f. terminale internum, ✠official alternate term for pial *part* of filum terminale.

fim·bria, pl. **fim·bri·ae** (fim′brē-ă, -brē-ē). **1** [TA]. Any fringelike structure. SYN fringe. **2.** SYN pilus (2). [L. fringe]

f. hippocam′pi [TA], a narrow sharp-edged crest of white fiber matter, continuous with the alveus hippocampi, attached to the medial border of the hippocampus; composed of efferent fibers of the hippocampus that form the fornix, fibers of the hippocampal commissure, and septohippocampal fibers. SYN f. of hippocampus [TA], corpus fimbriatum (1), tenia hippocampi.

f. of hippocampus [TA], SYN f. hippocampi.

ovarian f. [TA], the longest of the fimbriae of the uterine tube; it extends from the infundibulum to the ovary. SYN f. ovarica [TA], infundibulo-ovarian ligament.

f. ova′rica [TA], SYN ovarian f.

fim′briae tu′bae uteri′nae [TA], SYN fimbriae of uterine tube.

fim′briae of uterine tube [TA], the irregularly branched or fringed processes surrounding the ampulla at the abdominal opening of the uterine tube; most of the lining epithelial cells have cilia that beat toward the uterus. SYN fimbriae tubae uterinae [TA], laciniae tubae.

fim·bri·ate, fim·bri·at·ed (fim′brē-āt, -ā-ted). Having fimbriae.

fim·bri·ec·to·my (fim′brē-ek′tō-mē). Excision of fimbriae. [L. *fimbria*, fringe, + G. *ektomē*, excision]

fim·brin (fim′brin). An actin-binding protein that cross-links adjacent filaments tightly to form parallel actin fibers in vertebrate cells. It assists in maintaining cell polarity and development. [L. *fimbriae*, threads, fibers, + -in]

fim·bri·o·cele (fim′brē-ō-sēl). Hernia of the corpus fimbriatum of the oviduct. [L. *fimbria*, fringe, + G. *kēlē*, hernia]

fim·bri·o·plas·ty (fim′brē-ō-plas-tē). Corrective operation upon the tubal fimbriae. [L. *fimbria*, fringe, + G. *plastos*, formed]

finasteride. A competitive inhibitor of steroid 5α-reductase, an intracellular enzyme that converts testosterone into 5α-dihydrotestosterone, a potent androgen; used in the treatment of benign prostatic hyperplasia; also used to treat male pattern baldness and to regrow hair.

Finckh, Johann, German psychiatrist, *1873. SEE F. *test*.

find·ing. A clinically significant observation, usually used in relation to one found on physical examination or laboratory test.

fine·ness (fīn′nes). A designator used to indicate the precious metal content of an alloy, 1000 fine being 24-carat or pure gold.

fin·ger (fing′ger) [TA]. One of the digits of the hand. SYN digitus manus [TA]. [A.S.]

baseball f., an avulsion, partial or complete, of the long finger extensor from the base of the distal phalanx. SYN drop f., hammer f., mallet f.

fi

blubber f., SYN erysipeloid.

clubbed f.'s, SEE clubbing.

dead f.'s, SYN acroasphyxia.

drop f., SYN baseball f.

fifth f., SYN little f.

first f., SYN thumb.

fourth f., SYN ring f.

hammer f., SYN baseball f.

hippocratic f.'s, SEE clubbing.

index f. [TA], the second f. (the thumb being counted as the first). SYN digitus (manus) secundus [II]☆, forefinger, index (1), second f.

jerk f., SYN trigger f.

little f. [TA], the little or fifth finger. SYN digitus (manus) minimus [TA], digitus auricularis, digitus (manus) quintus [V], fifth f.

lock f., SYN trigger f.

mallet f., SYN baseball f.

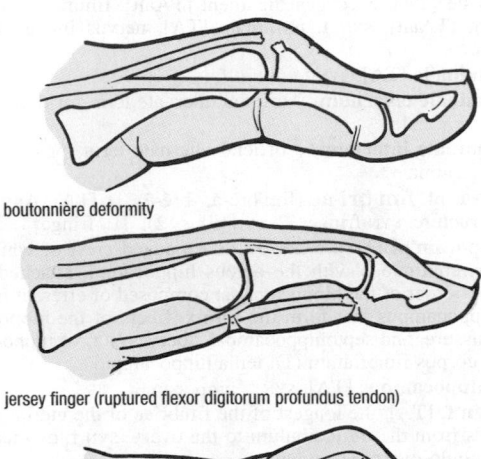

boutonnière deformity

jersey finger (ruptured flexor digitorum profundus tendon)

mallet finger

finger: deformities and fractures

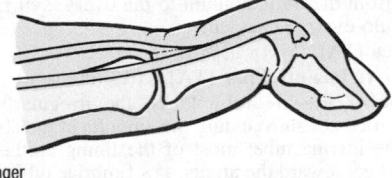

middle f. [TA], third finger. SYN digitus (manus) medius [TA], digitus (manus) tertius [III]☆, third f.

ring f. [TA], fourth finger. SYN digitus anularis [TA], digitus (manus) quartus IV☆, fourth f.

sausage f.'s, the thick, short f.'s of acromegaly; symmetric, diffusely swollen f.'s; an early change in systemic sclerosis.

seal f.'s, SYN erysipeloid.

second f., SYN index f.

snap f., SYN trigger f.

spade f.'s, the course, thick f.'s of acromegaly or myxedema.

spider f., SYN arachnodactyly.

spring f., SYN trigger f.

stuck f., SYN trigger f.

third f., SYN middle f.

trigger f., a condition in which the movement of the f. is arrested for a moment in flexion or extension and then continues with a jerk; results from localized swelling of the tendon that interferes with its gliding through the pulleys in the palm of the hand. SYN jerk f., lock f., snap f., spring f., stuck f.

waxy f.'s, SYN acroasphyxia.

webbed f.'s, two or more f.'s united and enclosed in a common sheath of skin.

whale f.'s, SYN erysipeloid.

white f.'s, an occupational disease occurring in operators of pneumatic hammers who are exposed to cold.

zinc f., a zinc-binding domain in a protein structure often seen in certain gene regulatory proteins, e.g., transcription factors.

fin·ger·nail (fing′ger-nāl). SEE nail.

fin·ger·print (fing′ger-print′). **1.** An impression of the inked bulb of the distal phalanx of a finger, showing the configuration of the surface ridges, used as a means of identification. SEE ALSO dermatoglyphics, Galton system of classification of f.'s. **2.** Term, sometimes used informally, referring to any analytic method capable of making fine distinctions between similar compounds or gel patterns; e.g., the pattern of an infrared absorption curve or of a two-dimensional paper chromatograph. **3.** In genetics, the analysis of DNA fragments to determine the identity of an individual or the paternity of a child. SYN genetic f.

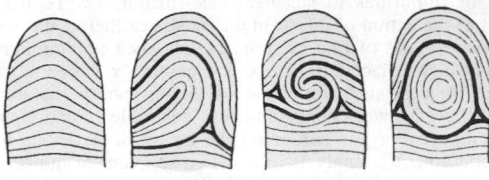

human fingerprints: schematic view, from right to left: whorls, double loops, loop, arch

Galton system of classification of f.'s, a system of classification based on the variations in the patterns of the ridges, which are grouped into arches, loops, and whorls (A.L.W. or arch-loop-whorl system). "Arches are formed when the ridges run from one side to the other of the bulb of the digit, without making any backward turn, but no twist; whorls, when there is a turn through at least one complete circle; they are also considered to include all duplex spirals." The abbreviations used in making a record of f.'s are: *a*, arch; *l*, loop; *w*, whorl; *i*, loop with an inner (thumb side) slope; *o*, loop with an outer (little-finger side) slope. The ten digits are registered in four groups as follows, distinguished by capital letters: *A*, the fore, middle, and ring fingers of the right hand; *B*, the fore, middle, and ring fingers of the left hand; *C*, the thumb and little finger of the right hand; *D*, the thumb and little finger of the left hand. SEE ALSO dermatoglyphics.

genetic f., SYN fingerprint (3).

fin·ger spel·ling. A system of communication with a profoundly hearing impaired person by spelling words in which the letters of the alphabet are represented by positions of the fingers.

Fink, R.P., 20th century U.S. anatomist. SEE F.-Heimer *stain*.

Finkeldey, Wilhelm, 20th century German pathologist. SEE Warthin-F. *cells*, under *cell*.

Finney, John M.T., U.S. surgeon, 1863–1942. SEE F. *operation*, *pyloroplasty*.

fire (fīr). In dentistry, the fusing of water and a powder containing kaolin, feldspar, and other substances to produce porcelain used in restorations and artificial teeth.

fire·damp (fīr′damp). Methane or other light hydrocarbons forming an explosive mixture when mixed with 7 or 8 volumes of air.

first aid. Immediate assistance administered in the case of injury or sudden illnes by a bystander or other lay person, before the arrival of trained medical personnel.

Fischer, Louis, U.S. pediatrician, 1864–1945. SEE F. *sign*, *symptom*.

Fischer, Emil, German chemist and Nobel laureate, 1852–1919. SEE F. projection formulas of *sugars*; Kiliani-Fischer *synthesis*; Kiliani-Fischer *reaction*.

Fishberg, Arthur M., U.S. physician, *1898. SEE F. concentration *test*.

fish ber·ry. The seeds of *Anamirta paniculata* which contain the amaroid, picrotoxin; a CNS and respiratory stimulant, used in veterinary medicine as an antidote to barbiturates. Name derived from the use of bruised berries thrown into streams to poison or incapacitate fish.

Fisher, Ronald A., British medical statistician and geneticist, 1890–1962; invented many statistical tests.

Fisher, C. Miller, U.S. neurologist, *1910. SEE F. *syndrome.*

Fishman-Lerner unit. See under unit.

fis·sion (fish′ŭn). **1.** The act of splitting, e.g., amitotic division of a cell or its nucleus. **2.** Splitting of the nucleus of an atom. [L. *fissio,* a cleaving, fr. *findo,* pp. *fissus,* to cleave]

binary f., simple f. in which the two new cells are approximately equal in size.

bud f., SYN gemmation.

multiple f., division of the nucleus, simultaneously or successively, into a number of daughter nuclei, followed by division of the cell body into an equal number of parts, each containing a nucleus.

simple f., division of the nucleus and then the cell body into two parts. SEE ALSO binary f.

fis·si·par·i·ty (fis-i-par′i-tē). SYN schizogenesis. [L. *fissio,* cleaving, fr. *findo,* to cleave, + *pario,* to bring forth]

fis·sip·a·rous (fi-sip′ă-rŭs). Reproducing or propagating by fission. [L. *findo,* pp. *fissus,* split, + *pario,* to produce]

fissula (fiz-ū-la). Diminutive of fissure; a small fissure or cleft.

f. ante fenestram [TA], minute, slitlike passage in the labyrinthine wall of the tympanic cavity, extending obliquely from the region of the cochleaform process to the vestibule of the bony labyrinth, anterior to the oval window; it is considered to be an extension of the perilymphatic space, but is occupied by a small band of connective tissue that is continuous with the mucosa of the tympanic cavity.

FISSURA

fis·su·ra, pl. **fis·su·rae** (fi-soo′ră, -soo′rē) [TA]. **1.** SYN fissure. **2.** In neuroanatomy, a particularly deep sulcus of the surface of the brain or spinal cord. [L. fr. *findo,* to cleave]

f. antitragohelici′na [TA], a fissure in the auricular cartilage between the cauda helicis and the antitragus. SYN antitragohelicine fissure.

f. calcari′na, SYN calcarine *sulcus.*

fissu′rae cerebel′li [TA], SYN cerebellar *fissures,* under *fissure.*

f. cer′ebri latera′lis, SYN lateral *sulcus.*

f. choroi′dea [TA], SYN optic *fissure.*

f. collatera′lis, SYN collateral *sulcus.*

f. denta′ta, SYN hippocampal *sulcus.*

f. hippocam′pi, SYN hippocampal *sulcus.*

f. horizonta′lis [TA], SYN horizontal *fissure* [TA] of cerebellum.

f. horizonta′lis pulmo′nis dex′tri [TA], SYN transverse *fissure* of the right lung.

f. intersemilunaris [TA], SYN ansoparamedian *fissure.*

f. intraculminalis [TA], SYN intraculminate *fissure.*

f. ligamen′ti tere′tis hepatis [TA], SYN *fissure* for ligamentum teres.

f. ligamen′ti veno′si [TA], SYN *fissure* for ligamentum venosum.

f. longitudina′lis cer′ebri [TA], SYN longitudinal cerebral *fissure.*

f. media′na ante′rior medul′lae oblonga′tae [TA], SYN anterior median *fissure* of medulla oblongata.

f. media′na ante′rior medul′lae spina′lis [TA], SYN anterior median *fissure* of spinal cord.

f. obli′qua pulmon′is [TA], SYN oblique *fissure* of lung.

f. orbita′lis infe′rior [TA], SYN inferior orbital *fissure.*

f. orbita′lis supe′rior [TA], SYN superior orbital *fissure.*

f. parietooccipita′lis, SYN parietooccipital *sulcus.*

f. petro-occipita′lis [TA], SYN petrooccipital *fissure.*

f. petrosquamo′sa [TA], SYN petrosquamous *fissure.*

f. petrotympan′ica [TA], SYN petrotympanic *fissure.*

f. posterior superior [TA], SYN posterior superior *fissure.*

f. posterolatera′lis [TA], SYN posterolateral *fissure.*

f. precentralis [TA], SYN precentral *fissure.*

f. preculminalis [TA], SYN preculminate *fissure.*

f. prepyramidalis [TA], SYN prepyramidal *fissure.*

f. pri′ma cerebel′li [TA], SYN primary *fissure* of cerebellum.

f. pterygoid′ea, SYN pterygoid *notch.*

f. pterygomaxilla′ris [TA], SYN pterygomaxillary *fissure.*

f. pterygopalati′na, SYN pterygomaxillary *fissure.*

f. puden′di, SYN pudendal *cleft.*

f. secun′da cerebel′li [TA], SYN secondary *fissure* [TA] of cerebellum.

f. sphenopetro′sa [TA], SYN petrosphenoidal *fissure.*

f. transver′sa cerebel′li, SYN transverse *fissure* of cerebellum.

f. transver′sa cer′ebri [TA], SYN transverse cerebral *fissure.*

f. tympanomastoid′ea [TA], SYN tympanomastoid *fissure.*

f. tympanosquamo′sa [TA], SYN tympanosquamous *fissure.*

fis·sur·al (fish′ŭ-răl). Relating to a fissure.

fis·su·ra·tion (fish′ŭ-rā′shŭn). State of being fissured.

FISSURE

fis·sure (fish′ŭr) [TA]. **1.** A deep furrow, cleft, or slit. (For most of the brain fissures, see entries under sulcus). **2.** In dentistry, a developmental break or fault in the tooth enamel. SYN fissura (1) [TA]. [L. *fissura*]

abdominal f., congenital failure of the ventral body wall to close. SEE ALSO celosomia, gastroschisis.

Ammon f., a round opening in the sclera during early embryogenesis.

anal f., a crack or slit in the mucous membrane of the anus, very painful and difficult to heal.

ansoparamedian f. [TA], the f. separating lobule HVIIA, crus II of the ansiform lobule, from lobule HVIIB, the paramedian lobule, of the posterior lobe of the cerebellum. SYN fissura intersemilunaris [TA], intersemilunar f.

anterior median f. of medulla oblongata [TA], the longitudinal groove in the midline of the anterior aspect of the medulla oblongata; it is the medullary equivalent of the anterior median f. of the spinal cord and ends at the foramen cecum posterius; its caudal part is obliterated by the decussation of the pyramids. SYN fissura mediana anterior medullae oblongatae [TA], anteromedian groove (1).

anterior median f. of spinal cord [TA], a deep median f. on the anterior surface of the spinal cord. SYN fissura mediana anterior medullae spinalis [TA], anteromedian groove (2), sulcus ventralis.

antitragohelicine f., SYN *fissura* antitragohelicina.

ape f., obsolete term for lunate *sulcus* [TA] of occipital lobe.

auricular f., SYN tympanomastoid f.

azygos f., the four-layered pleural fold that separates an azygos lobe from the rest of the right upper lobe of the lung, seen as an oblique line curving down from the right apex toward the mediastinal shadow on a chest radiograph. The azygos vein is projected as a teardrop shadow at the inferior end of the azygos f.

Bichat f., the nearly circular f. corresponding to the medial margin of the cerebral (pallial) mantle, marking the hilus of the cerebral hemisphere, consisting of the callosomarginal f. and choroidal f. along the hippocampus, both of which are continuous with the stem of the f. of Sylvius at the anterior extremity of the temporal lobe.

branchial f., a persistent branchial cleft.

Broca f., the f. surrounding Broca convolution.

calcarine f., SYN calcarine *sulcus.*

callosomarginal f., SYN cingulate *sulcus.*

caudal transverse f., SYN *porta* hepatis.

cerebellar f.'s, the deep furrows which divide the lobules of the cerebellum. SEE ALSO postcentral f., primary f. of cerebellum, secondary f. [TA] of cerebellum. SYN fissurae cerebelli [TA].

cerebral f.'s, the variously named fissures of the cerebral hemispheres. SEE ALSO *sulci* cerebri, under *sulcus*.

choroid f., SYN optic f.

choroidal f. [TA], **(1)** SYN optic f; **(2)** the narrow cleft along the medial wall of the lateral ventricle along the margins of which the choroid plexus is attached; it lies between the upper surface of the thalamus and lateral edge of the fornix in the central part of the ventricle and between the terminal stria and fimbria hippocampi in the inferior horn;

Clevenger f., SYN inferior temporal *sulcus*.

collateral f., SYN collateral *sulcus*.

decidual f., a cleft in the decidua basalis or placenta.

dentate f., SYN hippocampal *sulcus*.

Duverney f.'s, SYN *notch* in cartilage of acoustic meatus.

Ecker f., SYN petrooccipital f.

enamel f., a deep cleft between adjoining cusps affording retention to caries-producing agents.

glaserian f., SYN petrotympanic f.

great horizontal f., SYN horizontal f. [TA] of cerebellum.

great longitudinal f., SYN longitudinal cerebral f.

Henle f.'s, minute spaces filled with connective tissue between the muscular fasciculi of the heart.

hippocampal f., SYN hippocampal *sulcus*.

horizontal f. of right lung, SYN transverse f. of the right lung.

horizontal f. [TA] of cerebellum, horizontal f. that divides the ansiform lobule into its major parts, crus I (superior semilunar lobule) and crus II (inferior semilunar lobule). SYN fissura horizontalis [TA], great horizontal f.

inferior accessory f., the f. that commonly separates the medial basal segment of the right lower lobe of the lung from the other basal segments, occasionally seen as an oblique line near the right heart border on chest radiographs.

inferior orbital f. [TA], a cleft between the greater wing of the sphenoid and the orbital plate of the maxilla, through which pass the maxillary division and the orbital branch of the trigeminal nerve, fibers from the pterygopalatine (Meckel) ganglion, and the infraorbital vessels. SYN fissura orbitalis inferior [TA], sphenomaxillary f.

intersemilunar f. [offalt TA], SYN ansoparamedian f.

intraculminate f. [TA], the f. located within the culminate lobule separating lobule IV from lobule V in the anterior lobe of the cerebellum and extending to the lateral margin of the cerebellum. SYN fissura intraculminalis [TA].

lateral cerebral f., SYN lateral *sulcus*.

left sagittal f., a sagittal groove on the undersurface of the liver formed by the fissure for round ligament anteriorly and the fissure for ligamentum venosum posteriorly.

f. for ligamentum teres [TA], a cleft on the inferior surface of the liver, running from the inferior border to the left extremity of the porta hepatis; it lodges the round ligament of the liver. SYN fissura ligamenti teretis hepatis [TA], f. for round ligament of liver*, fossa venae umbilicalis, umbilical f., umbilical fossa.

f. for ligamentum venosum [TA], a deep cleft extending from the porta hepatis and the inferior vena cava between the left lobe and the caudate lobe; it lodges the ligamentum venosum and is thus a vestige of the fossa of the ductus venosus. SYN fissura ligamenti venosi [TA], f. of venous ligament.

linguogingival f., a f. sometimes occurring on the lingual surface of one of the upper incisors and extending into the cementum.

f.'s of liver, SEE left sagittal f., right sagittal f., *porta* hepatis, f. for ligamentum teres, f. for ligamentum venosum.

longitudinal cerebral f. [TA], the deep cleft separating the two hemispheres of the cerebrum. SYN fissura longitudinalis cerebri [TA], great longitudinal f.

lunate f. [TA], SYN lunate *sulcus*.

f.'s of lung, SEE transverse f. of the right lung, oblique f. of lung.

major f., SYN oblique f. of lung.

minor f., SYN transverse f. of the right lung.

oblique f., SYN oblique f. of lung.

oblique f. of lung [TA], the deep fissure in each lung that runs obliquely downward and forward. It divides the upper and lower lobes of the left lung and separates the upper and middle lobes from the lower lobe of the right lung. SYN fissura obliqua pulmonis [TA], major f., oblique f.

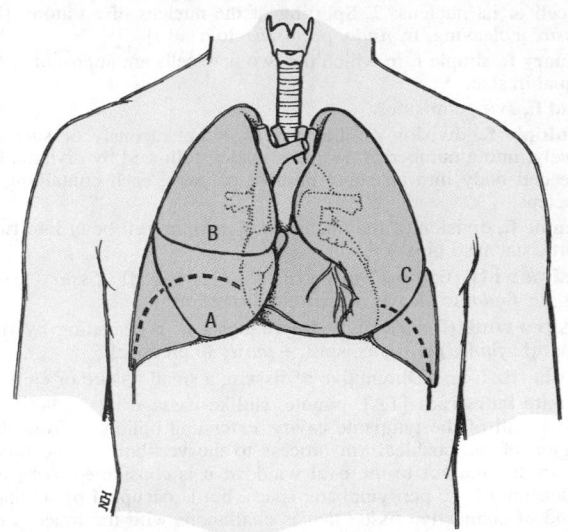

fissures of the lung: (A) oblique and (B) horizontal fissures of the right lung, (C) oblique fissure of the left lung

optic f., in the embryo, the temporary gap in the ventral margin of the developing optic cup. SYN choroidal f. (1) [TA], fissura choroidea [TA], choroid f.

oral f. [TA], the mouth slit; the aperture of the mouth. SYN rima oris [TA], oral opening*.

palpebral f. [TA], the lid slit, or fissure between the eyelids. SYN rima palpebrarum [TA].

Pansch f., a cerebral f. (sulcus) running from the lower extremity of the central f. (sulcus) nearly to the end of the occipital lobe.

paracentral f., SEE paracentral *sulcus*.

parietooccipital f., SYN parietooccipital *sulcus*.

petrooccipital f. [TA], a fissure between the petrous part of the temporal bone and the basilar part of the occipital bone that extends anteromedially from the jugular foramen; includes the jugular foramen (at its posterior end). SYN fissura petro-occipitalis [TA], Ecker f.

petrosphenoidal f. [TA], highly variable opening between the medial portion of the posterior border of the greater wing of the sphenoid bone (posterior to foramen ovale) and the medial portion of the anterior border of the petrous part of the temporal bone; it may be seen as a wide, lateral extension of the foramen lacerum in the dry skull, or it may be closed, especially laterally, taking the form of a petrosphenoidal suture rather than a fissure. SYN fissura sphenopetrosa [TA], sphenopetrosal f.

petrosquamous f. [TA], a shallow fissure indicating externally the line of fusion of the petrous and squamous portions of the temporal bone. SYN fissura petrosquamosa [TA].

petrotympanic f. [TA], a fissure between the tympanic and petrous portions of the temporal bone; it transmits the chorda tympani nerve through a small patent portion, the anterior canaliculus of the chorda tympani. SYN fissura petrotympanica [TA], glaserian f.

portal f., SYN *porta* hepatis.

postcentral f., a f. on the superior surface of the cerebellum separating the culmen from the central lobule.

posterior median f. of the medulla oblongata, SYN posterior median *sulcus* of medulla oblongata.

posterior median f. of spinal cord, SYN posterior median *sulcus* of spinal cord.

posterior superior f. [TA], the f. located between lobules VI and VII of the posterior lobe of the cerebellum and extending to the lateral margin of the cerebellum. SYN fissura posterior superior [TA].

posterolateral f. [TA], the earliest f. to appear in the development of the cerebellum; it separates the flocculus and nodulus from the uvula and tonsil. SYN fissura posterolateralis [TA], prenodular f.

posthippocampal f., SYN calcarine *sulcus.*

postlingual f., a transverse f. on the superior vermis of the cerebellum separating the lingula from the central lobule.

postlunate f., a transverse f. on the superior vermis of the cerebellum separating the posterior lunate lobule in front from the ansiform lobule behind.

postpyramidal f., a f. that separates the pyramid of the cerebellum from the tuber.

postrhinal f., a f. separating the hippocampal from the collateral gyrus.

precentral f. [TA], the f. located between the anterior and posterior parts (lobules II and III) of the central lobule of the anterior lobe of the cerebellum; extends from the vermis to the cerebellar margin; precentral fissure a is found between lobule I and lobule II, the latter of which forms the anterior part of the central lobule. SYN fissura precentralis [TA].

preculminate f. [TA], the f. located between lobules III and IV of the anterior lobe of the cerebellum, representing the f. between the central lobule and culmen; extends from the vermis to the cerebellar margin. SYN fissura preculminalis [TA].

prenodular f., SYN posterolateral f.

prepyramidal f. [TA], the f. located between lobules VIIB and VIII of the posterior lobe of the cerebellum; continues from the vermis into the hemisphere where it separates lobule HVIIB from HVIIIA. SYN fissura prepyramidalis [TA].

primary f. of cerebellum [TA], the deepest f. of the cerebellum; demarcates the division of anterior and posterior lobes of the cerebellum; second to appear embryologically. SYN fissura prima cerebelli [TA].

pterygoid f., SYN pterygoid *notch.*

pterygomaxillary f. [TA], the narrow gap between the lateral pterygoid plate and the infratemporal surface of the maxilla through which the infratemporal fossa communicates with the pterygopalatine fossa; gives passage to the third part of the maxillary artery and the posterior superior alveolar arteries, veins and nerves. SYN fissura pterygomaxillaris [TA], fissura pterygopalatina.

rhinal f., SYN rhinal *sulcus.*

right sagittal f., a sagittal groove on the undersurface of the liver formed by the fossa for gallbladder anteriorly and the groove for vena cava posteriorly.

f. of Rolando, SYN central *sulcus.*

f. for round ligament of liver, ✫official alternate term for f. for ligamentum teres.

Santorini f.'s, SYN *notch* in cartilage of acoustic meatus.

secondary f. [TA] **of cerebellum,** a f. that separates the uvula of the inferior vermis of the cerebellum from the pyramid. SYN fissura secunda cerebelli [TA].

simian f., SYN lunate *sulcus.*

sphenoidal f., SYN superior orbital f.

sphenomaxillary f., SYN inferior orbital f.

sphenopetrosal f., SYN petrosphenoidal f.

squamotympanic f., SYN tympanosquamous f.

superior orbital f. [TA], a cleft between the greater and the lesser wings of the sphenoid establishing a channel of communication between the middle cranial fossa and the orbit, through which pass the oculomotor and trochlear nerves, the ophthalmic division of the trigeminal nerve, the abducens nerve, and the ophthalmic veins. SYN fissura orbitalis superior [TA], foramen lacerum anterius, sphenoidal f.

superior temporal f., SYN superior temporal *sulcus.*

sylvian f., f. of Sylvius, SYN lateral *sulcus.*

transverse f. of cerebellum, the cleft caused by the protrusion of the anterior lobe of the cerebellum over the superior and middle cerebellar peduncles. SYN fissura transversa cerebelli.

transverse cerebral f. [TA], the triangular space between the corpus callosum and fornix above and the dorsal surface of the thalamus below, which is bounded laterally by the choroid f. of the lateral ventricle, lined by pia mater, and opens caudally into the cistern of the great cerebral vein of the subarachnoid space. SYN fissura transversa cerebri [TA].

transverse f. of the right lung [TA], the deep f. that separates the upper and middle lobes of the right lung. SYN fissura horizontalis pulmonis dextri [TA], horizontal f. of right lung, minor f.

tympanomastoid f. [TA], a fissure separating the tympanic portion from the mastoid portion of the temporal bone; it transmits the auricular branch of the vagus nerve. SYN fissura tympanomastoidea [TA], auricular f., tympanomastoid suture.

tympanosquamous f. [TA], the f. separating the tympanic part of the temporal bone from the squamous part; it is continuous medially with the petrotympanic f. and the petrosquamous f. SYN fissura tympanosquamosa [TA], squamotympanic f.

umbilical f., SYN f. for ligamentum teres.

f. of venous ligament, SYN f. for ligamentum venosum.

vestibular f. of cochlea, a fine f. in the lower part of the first turn of the cochlea, formed by a spiral lamina which projects from the outer wall of the cochlea but does not quite reach the osseous spiral lamina, thus leaving a narrow gap.

zygal f., a figure formed by two nearly parallel cerebral f.'s connected by a short f. at right angles, forming an H.

FISTULA

fis·tu·la, pl. **fis·tu·lae, fis·tu·las** (fis′tū-lă, -tū-lē, -tū-lăs). An abnormal passage from one epithelial surface to another epithelial surface. [L. a pipe, a tube]

abdominal f., a fistulous passage connecting one of the abdominal viscera to the external surface.

amphibolic f., amphibolous f., a complete anal f. opening both externally and internally.

anal f., a f. opening at or near the anus; usually, but not always, opening into the rectum above the internal sphincter.

arteriovenous f., an abnormal connection, either spontaneous or surgically created, between an artery and a vein.

f. au′ris congen′ita, a congenital f. anterior to the root of the helix resulting from a defect in the formation of the auricle of the ear.

biliary f., a f. leading to some portion of the biliary tract.

f. bimuco′sa, a complete f., both ends of which open on the mucous surface.

blind f., a f. that ends in a cul-de-sac, being open at one extremity only. SYN incomplete f.

BP f., SYN bronchopleural f.

branchial f., a congenital f. in the neck resulting from incomplete closure of a branchial cleft or pouch.

Brescia-Cimino f., a direct, surgically created, arteriovenous f.; used to facilitate chronic hemodialysis.

bronchobiliary f., communication between a bronchus and the biliary system, e.g., after a ruptured hepatic abscess.

bronchocavitary f., a communication between the bronchus and a lung abscess cavity.

bronchoesophageal f., communication between a bronchus and the esophagus; may occur in association with either infection or tumors involving a bronchus or the esophagus.

bronchopleural f., communication between a bronchus and the pleural cavity; usually caused by necrotizing pneumonia or empyema; also may follow pulmonary surgery or irradiation. SYN BP f.

bronchopleural-cutaneous f., a communication between the tracheobronchial tree and the skin that traverses the pleural space.

carotid-cavernous f., a fistulous communication, of spontaneous or traumatic origin, between the cavernous sinus and the traversing internal carotid artery; a pulsating unilateral exophthalmos and a detectable cranial bruit are common manifestations.

cholecystoduodenal f., an abnormal communication between gallbladder and duodenum, often secondary to severe cholecystitis with perforation and abscess formation; when stones are present in the gallbladder they may erode through the adjacent duodenal wall; if large stones pass into the duodenum, they may cause gallstone ileus.

chyle f., a leak of chyle from a lymph vessel to the skin surface; a complication of radical neck dissection when the thoracic duct is injured.

coccygeal f., a fistulous opening of a dermoid cyst in the coccygeal region.

colocutaneous f., a fistulous passage connecting the colon and the skin.

coloileal f., a fistulous passage connecting the colon and the ileum.

colonic f., (1) internal, a fistulous passage connecting the colon and a hollow viscus; (2) external, a fistulous passage connecting the colon and the skin.

colovaginal f., a fistulous passage connecting the colon and vagina.

colovesical f., a fistulous passage connecting the colon and urinary bladder. SYN vesicocolic f.

complete f., a f. that is open at both ends.

congenital pulmonary arteriovenous f., abnormal congenital communication between pulmonary arteries and veins usually found in the lung parenchyma.

dental f., SYN gingival f.

duodenal f., an opening through the duodenal wall and into another epithelial lined organ or through the abdominal wall.

dural cavernous sinus f., a vascular shunt between the meningeal branches of the internal or external carotid *arteries*, under *artery* and the cavernous *sinus*.

Eck f., transposition of the portal circulation to the systemic by making an anastomosis between the vena cava and portal vein and then ligating the latter close to the liver.

enterocutaneous f., a fistulous passage connecting the intestine and skin of the abdomen.

enterovaginal f., a fistulous passage connecting the intestine and the vagina.

enterovesical f., a fistulous passage connecting the intestine and the bladder.

ethmoidal-lacrimal f., a fistulous communication between the lacrimal sac and the ethmoidal sinus. SYN internal lacrimal f.

external f., a fistulous pasage connecting a hollow viscus and the skin.

fecal f., SYN intestinal f.

gastric f., a fistulous passage connecting the stomach to the abdominal wall.

gastrocolic f., a fistulous passage connecting the stomach and the colon.

gastrocutaneous f., a fistulous passage connecting the stomach and the skin.

gastroduodenal f., a fistulous passage connecting the stomach to the duodenum.

gastrointestinal f., a fistulous passage connecting the stomach with the intestine.

genitourinary f., a fistulous opening into the urogenital tract. SYN urogenital f.

gingival f., a sinus tract originating in a peripheral abscess and opening into the oral cavity on the gingiva. SYN dental f.

hepatic f., a fistulous passage leading to the liver.

hepatopleural f., a fistulous passage connecting the liver and the pleural space.

horseshoe f., an anal f. partially encircling the anus and opening at both extremities on the cutaneous surface.

H-type f., a rare form of congenital tracheoesophageal f. in which there is no esophageal atresia, manifest as aspiration pneumonias. SYN H-type tracheoesophageal f.

H-type tracheoesophageal f., SYN H-type f.

incomplete f., SYN blind f.

internal f., a fistulous passage connecting hollow viscera.

internal lacrimal f., SYN ethmoidal-lacrimal f.

intestinal f., a tract leading from the lumen of the intestine to the exterior. SYN fecal f.

labyrinthine f., a f. between a fluid-filled compartment of the inner ear and another fluid-filled compartment in the inner ear (internal) or a space external to the inner ear as the middle ear or mastoid air cells or subarachnoid space (external); it may result in auditory and vestibular disturbances, depending on its location.

lacrimal f., f. lacrima′lis, an abnormal opening into a tear duct or the lacrimal sac.

lacteal f., a fistulous opening into one of the lactiferous ducts. SYN mammary f.

lymphatic f., a congenital f. in the neck connecting with a lymphatic vessel and giving exit to lymph.

mammary f., SYN lacteal f.

Mann-Bollman f., a f. used in experimental investigations; a loop of ileum is isolated, the distal (aboral) end is anastomosed laterally to the duodenum or the small intestine, and the open proximal (oral) end is sutured to the abdominal wall; peristaltic waves travel from oral to aboral end, with leakage to the exterior thus reduced to a minimum.

metroperitoneal f., SYN uteroperitoneal f.

oroantral f., a pathologic communication between the oral cavity and the maxillary sinus, most commonly a complication of maxillary or molar tooth extraction.

orofacial f., a pathologic communication between the oral cavity and the face.

oronasal f., a pathologic communication between the oral cavity and the nasal cavity.

parietal f., a f., either blind or complete, opening on the wall of the thorax or abdomen. SYN thoracic f.

perilymphatic f., a f. between the vestibule of the inner ear and the middle ear through which perilymph can leak, resulting in auditory and vestibular disturbances; common sites for perilymphatic f. are the oval window through or around the footplate of the stapes or the round window through the round window membrane.

perineovaginal f., a fistulous passage connecting the perineum and the vagina.

pilonidal f., SYN pilonidal *sinus*.

pulmonary f., a parietal f. communicating with the lung.

rectolabial f., a fistulous passage connecting the rectum to the surface of a labium majus. SYN rectovulvar f.

rectourethral f., a fistulous passage connecting the rectum and the urethra.

rectovaginal f., a fistulous passage connecting the rectum and the vagina.

rectovesical f., a fistulous passage connecting the rectum and the bladder.

rectovestibular f., a fistulous passage connecting the rectum and the vestibule of the vagina.

rectovulvar f., SYN rectolabial f.

reverse Eck f., side-to-side anastomosis of the portal vein with the inferior vena cava and ligation of the latter above the anastomosis but below the hepatic veins; the blood from the lower part of the body is thus directed through the hepatic circulation.

salivary f., a pathologic communication between a salivary duct or gland and the cutaneous surface.

sigmoidovesical f., a fistulous passage connecting the sigmoid colon and urinary bladder.

spermatic f., a f. communicating with the testis or any of the seminal passages.

T-E f., SYN tracheoesophageal f.

Thiry f., an artificial f. for collecting the intestinal secretions of an animal for experimental purposes; a loop of intestine is isolated, its vascular and nervous connections are preserved, after the continuity of the intestinal tract is restored by an end-to-end anastomosis; one end of the isolated segment is closed, the other attached to the skin of the abdomen.

Thiry-Vella f., experimental isolation of a segment of intestine in an animal; a loop of intestine is isolated, its vascular and nervous connections are preserved, and continuity of the intestinal tract is restored by an end-to-end anastomosis, each end of the isolated segment is connected to an independent opening in the abdominal wall. SYN Vella f.

thoracic f., SYN parietal f.

tracheobiliary fistula, a rare congenital anastomosis between an accessory bronchus and aberrant biliary duct system.

tracheoesophageal f., fistulous passage connecting the trachea and esophagus; often associated with esophageal atresia; may also be acquired; in the adult, etiology is similar to that of bronchoesophageal f. SYN T-E f.

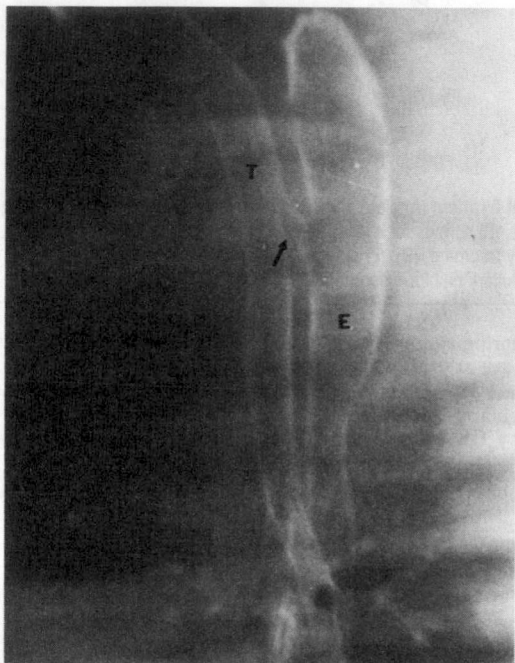

tracheoesophageal fistula: trachea (T) and esophagus (E) are connected by a fistula (arrow)

umbilical f., a fistulous passage connecting the intestine or urachus at the umbilicus.

urachal f., a fistulous passage connecting the urachus with a hollow organ.

ureterocutaneous f., a f. between the ureter and the skin.

ureterovaginal f., a f. between the lower ureter and vagina.

urethrocutaneous f., f. between urethra and penile skin; most likely a complication of hypospadias repair.

urethrovaginal f., a f. between the urethra and the vagina.

urinary f., a f. resulting in abnormal drainage of urine to the skin or into another organ.

urogenital f., SYN genitourinary f.

uteroperitoneal f., fistulous passage connecting the cavity of the uterus with the peritoneal cavity. SYN metroperitoneal f.

Vella f., SYN Thiry-Vella f.

vesical f., a fistulous passage from the urinary bladder.

vesicocolic f., SYN colovesical f.

vesicocutaneous f., a f. between the bladder and the skin.

vesicointestinal f., a fistulous passage connecting the urinary bladder and the small intestine.

vesicouterine f., a f. between the bladder and the uterus.

vesicovaginal f., f. between the bladder and the vagina.

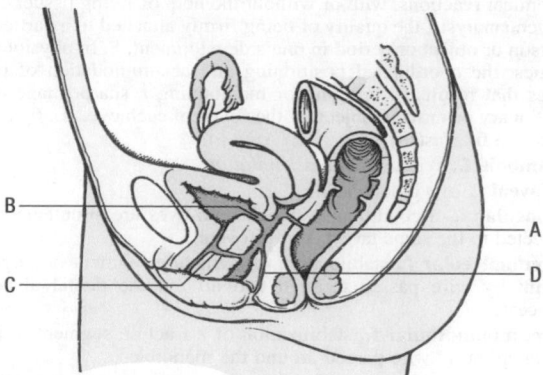

fistula: (A) rectovaginal, (B) vesicovaginal, (C) urethrovaginal, (D) vaginoperineal

vesicovaginorectal f., a fistulous passage connecting the vagina, the bladder, and rectum.

vitelline f., a f. between the umbilicus and the terminal ileum along the course of a persistent vitelline cord. SEE Meckel *diverticulum.*

fis·tu·la·tion, fis·tu·li·za·tion (fis-tū-lā'shŭn, -tū-li-zā'shŭn). Formation of a fistula in a part; becoming fistulous.

fis·tu·la·tome (fis'tū-lă-tōm). A long, thin-bladed, probe-pointed knife for slitting open a fistula. SYN fistula knife, syringotome. [fistula + G. *tomē,* a cutting]

fis·tu·lec·to·my (fis-tū-lek'tō-mē). Excision of a fistula. SYN syringectomy. [fistula + G. *ektomē,* excision]

fis·tu·lo·en·ter·os·to·my (fis'tū-lō-en-ter-os'tō-mē). An operation connecting a fistula with the intestine. [fistula + G. *enteron,* intestine, + *stoma,* mouth]

fis·tu·lot·o·my (fis-tū-lot'ō-mē). Incision or surgical enlargement of a fistula. SYN syringotomy. [fistula + G. *tomē,* incision]

fis·tu·lous (fis'tū-lŭs). Relating to or containing a fistula.

fit. 1. An attack of an acute disease or the sudden appearance of some symptom, such as coughing. **2.** A convulsion. **3.** (plural) epilepsy **4.** In dentistry, the adaptation of any dental restoration, e.g., of an inlay to the cavity preparation in a tooth, or of a denture to its basal seat. [A.S. *fitt*]

induced f., a conformational change in a macromolecule (e.g., protein) as a result of multiple weak interactions with a ligand or substrate.

uncinate f., SYN temporal lobe *epilepsy.*

FITC Abbreviation for fluorescein isothiocyanate.

fit·ness (fit'nes). **1.** Well-being. **2.** Suitability. **3.** In population genetics, a measure of the relative survival and reproductive success of a given individual or phenotype, or of a population subgroup. **4.** A set of attributes, primarily respiratory and cardiovascular, relating to ability to perform tasks requiring expenditure of energy.

clinical f., absence of frank disease or of subclinical precursors.

evolutionary f., the probability that the line of descent from an individual with a specific trait will not eventually die out.

genetic f., in a phenotype, the mean number of surviving offspring that it generates in its lifetime, usually expressed as a fraction or percentage of the average genetic f. of the population.

physical f., a state of well-being in which performance is optimal.

Fitz-Hugh, T., Jr., U.S. physician, 1894–1963. SEE Fitz-Hugh and Curtis *syndrome.*

fix·a·tion (fik-sā'shŭn). **1.** The condition of being firmly attached or set. **2.** In histology, the rapid killing of tissue elements and their preservation and hardening to retain as nearly as possible the same relations they had in the living body. SYN fixing. **3.** In chemistry, the conversion of a gas into solid or liquid form by

fi

chemical reactions, with or without the help of living tissue. **4.** In psychoanalysis, the quality of being firmly attached to a particular person or object or period in one's development. **5.** In physiologic optics, the coordinated positioning and accommodation of both eyes that results in bringing or maintaining a sharp image of a stationary or moving object on the fovea of each eye. [L. *figo*, pp. *fixus*, to fix, fasten]

ammonia f., SYN ammonia *assimilation.*

bifoveal f., SYN binocular f.

binocular f., a condition in which both eyes are simultaneously directed to the same target. SYN bifoveal f.

circumalveolar f., stabilization of a fracture segment or surgical splint by wire passed through and around the dental alveolar process.

circummandibular f., stabilization of a fracture segment or surgical splint by wire passed around the mandible.

circumzygomatic f., stabilization of a fracture segment or surgical splint by wire passed around the zygomatic arch.

complement f., f. of complement in a serum by an antigen-antibody combination whereby it is rendered unavailable to complete a reaction in a second antigen-antibody combination for which complement is necessary; the second system usually serves as an indicator (red blood cells plus specific hemolysin); if complement is fixed with the first antigen-antibody union, hemolysis does not occur, but, if complement is not so removed, it causes hemolysis in the second system; this technique is the basis for complement fixation tests, which are widely used in laboratories for the detection of antigens or antibodies. SEE ALSO Bordet-Gengou *phenomenon*, Wassermann *test.* SYN CF test, complement binding assay.

craniofacial f., stabilization of facial fractures to the cranial base by direct wiring or by external skeletal pin fixation.

crossed f., in convergent strabismus, the use of the right inturned eye to look at objects to the left and the left inturned eye to look at objects to the right, in order to avoid ocular rotation.

eccentric f., a monocular condition in which the line of sight connects the object and an extrafoveal retinal area.

elastic band f., the stabilization of fractured segments of the jaws by means of intermaxillary elastics applied to splints or appliances.

external f., f. of fractured bones by splints, plastic dressings, or transfixion pins.

external pin f., in oral surgery, stabilization of fractures of the mandible, maxilla, or zygoma by pins or screws drilled into the bony part through the overlying skin and connected by a metal bar.

external pin f., biphase, pin f. by replacing the rigid metal bar connector with an acrylic bar adapted at the time of reduction of the fracture.

freudian f., SEE fixation (4).

genetic f., the increase of the frequency of a gene by genetic drift until no other allele is preserved in a specific finite population.

intermaxillary f., f. of fractures of the mandible or maxilla by applying elastic bands or stainless steel wire between the maxillary and mandibular arch bars or other types of splint. SYN mandibulomaxillary f., maxillomandibular f.

internal f., stabilization of fractured bony parts by direct f. to one another with surgical wires, screws, pins, rods, or plates. SYN intraosseous f.

intraosseous f., SYN internal f.

mandibulomaxillary f., SYN intermaxillary f.

maxillomandibular f., SYN intermaxillary f.

nasomandibular f., mandibular immobilization, especially for edentulous jaws, with maxillomandibular splints, attached by connecting a circum-mandibular wire with an intraoral interosseous wire passed through a hole drilled into the anterior nasal spine of the maxillae.

nitrogen f., process in which atmospheric nitrogen is converted to ammonia.

fix·a·tive (fik′să-tiv). **1.** Serving to fix, bind, or make firm or stable. **2.** A substance used for the preservation of gross and histologic specimens of tissue, or individual cells, usually by

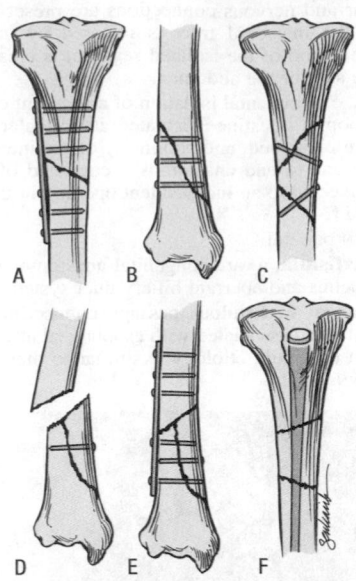

internal fixation: (A) plate and six screws for a transverse or short oblique fracture, (B) screws for a long oblique or spiral fracture, (C) screws for a long butterfly fragment, (D), (E) plate and six screws for a short butterfly fragment, (F) medullary nail for a segmental fracture

denaturing and precipitating or cross-linking the protein constituents. SEE ALSO fluid, solution.

acetone f., acetone used at low temperatures to fix enzymes, particularly phosphatases; it removes fat and glycogen.

AFA f., a combination of alcohol, formalin, and acetic acid used for the fixation of nematodes, trematodes, and cestodes.

alcohol-glycerin f., alcohol (70%) with 5% glycerin; suitable for most nematodes.

Altmann f., a bichromate-osmic acid f.

Bouin f., a solution of glacial acetic acid, formalin, and picric acid, useful for soft and delicate tissues (as those of embryos) and small pieces of tissues; it preserves glycogen and nuclei and permits brilliant staining, but penetrates slowly, distorts kidney tissue and mitochondria, and does not permit Feulgen stain for DNA.

Carnoy f., ethanol, chloroform, and acetic acid (6:3:1) or ethanol and acetic acid (3:1), an extremely rapid f. used for glycogen preservation and as a nuclear f.

Champy f., a mixture of potassium bichromate, chromic acid, and osmic acid, considered an excellent cytologic f. with advantages and disadvantages similar to those of Flemming's f.; it differs from Flemming f. in substituting bichromate for acetic acid.

Flemming f., a mixture of chromic acid, osmic acid, and acetic acid that makes an excellent cytoplasmic and chromosomal f., especially when acetic acid is omitted; disadvantages are that it penetrates poorly, requires lengthy washing, and deteriorates rapidly.

formaldehyde f., a widely used fixing agent for pathologic histology; the commercial solution is 37–40% formaldehyde and is known as 100% formalin or formol; a common impurity is formic acid, which must be neutralized or the f. made in buffer solution; tissues fixed may have a pigment artifact precipitated.

formol-calcium f., a f. for preservation of lipids.

formol-Müller f., Müller f. containing 2% commercial formalin.

formol-saline f., a general f. for histologic and histochemical preparations.

formol-Zenker f., Zenker f. in which glacial acetic acid has been replaced by formalin.

glutaraldehyde f., a f. used in phosphate or cacodylate buffer for electron microscopy, and as a chromatin and enzyme f.; may be used preceding osmic acid as a second f. to add membrane preservation for electron microscopy.

Golgi osmiobichromate f., an osmic-bichromate mixture used to demonstrate nerve cells and their processes.

Helly f., a combination of potassium dichromate, mercuric chloride, formaldehyde, and distilled water, used as a microanatomic f. for cytoplasmic granules and nuclear staining; has the same disadvantages as Zenker f.

Hermann f., a hardening f. of glacial acetic acid, osmic acid, and platinum chloride.

Kaiserling f., a method of preserving histologic and pathologic specimens without altering the color, by immersing them in an aqueous solution of potassium nitrate, potassium acetate, and formalin.

Luft potassium permanganate f., a f. useful in electron microscopy for cytologic preservation of lipoprotein complexes in membranes and myelin, because of its oxidative properties.

Marchi f., a mixture of Müller f. with osmium tetroxide, with potassium chlorate substituted for the potassium dichromate of Müller f. for better results; used to demonstrate degenerating myelin. SEE ALSO Marchi *stain.*

methanol f., a f. used with dry blood films, and often incorporated into the stain used.

Müller f., a hardening f. composed of potassium dichromate, sodium sulfate, and distilled water, similar to Regaud f.

neutral buffered formalin f., a general histologic f. less likely to leave formalin deposits in tissue than formol-saline f.

Newcomer f., a f. containing isopropanol, propionic acid, and dioxane, recommended as a substitute for Carnoy f. in preservation of chromatin; also useful for fixing polysaccharides; small pieces of tissue must be used, although excessive shrinkage may still occur.

Orth f., formalin added to Müller f., used for bringing out chromaffin, studying early degenerative processes and necrosis, and for demonstrating rickettsiae and bacteria.

osmic acid f., a f. used alone in buffer or as a postfixative after a glutaraldehyde f. in electron microscopy; an excellent membrane f. but a poor preservative of chromatin.

Park-Williams f., a f. for spirochetes, comprised of a 2% solution of osmic acid to the fumes of which the bacteria are exposed for a few seconds.

picroformol f., a f. containing formalin and picric acid.

PVA f., schaudinn f. using either a mercuric chloride, zinc sulfate, or copper sulfate base; contains polyvinyl alcohol plastic powder that is used as an adhesive for fecal specimens in the preparation of permanent smears for subsequent staining.

Regaud f., a f. containing formaldehyde and sodium dichromate, used to preserve mitochondria but not fat; requires afterchroming and extensive washing.

SAF f., sodium acetate-acetic acid-formalin mixture used to fix fecal specimens for subsequent concentration and staining of smears.

Schaudinn f., a solution of mercuric chloride, sodium chloride, alcohol, and glacial acetic acid, used on wet smears for cytologic fixation.

single vial f.'s, proprietary and commercially available solutions used for stool fixation; from the single vial, a concentration, permanent stain, and some immunoassay procedures can be performed.

Thoma f., nitric acid in 95% alcohol, used for decalcifying bone in the preparation of histologic specimens.

Zenker f., a rapid f. consisting of mercuric chloride, potassium dichromate, sodium sulfate, glacial acetic acid, and water, useful for trichrome stains; must be washed to remove potassium dichromate and treated with iodine solution to remove mercuric chloride; tissues tend to become brittle if left in the f. for more than 24 hours.

fix·a·tor (fĭk-sā′ter). A device providing rigid immobilization through external skeletal fixation by means of rods (f.'s) attached to pins which are placed in or through the bone.

fix·ing (fĭk′sing). SYN fixation (2).

flac·cid (flak′sid, flas′id). Relaxed, flabby, or without tone. [L. *flaccidus*]

flac·cid·i·ty (flă-sid′i-tē). The condition or state of being flaccid.

Flack, Martin W., British physiologist, 1882–1931. SEE F. *node;* Keith and F. *node.*

fla·gel·la (flă-jel′ă). Plural of flagellum.

fla·gel·lar (fla-jel′ăr). Relating to a flagellum or to the extremity of a protozoan.

Flag·el·la·ta (flaj′ě-lā′tă). Former name for Mastigophora.

flag·el·late (flaj′ě-lāt). **1.** Possessing one or more flagella. **2.** Common name for a member of the class Mastigophora.

collared f., SYN choanomastigote.

flag·el·lat·ed (flaj′ě-lā-ted). Possessing one or more flagella.

flag·el·la·tion (flaj′ě-lā′shŭn). **1.** Whipping either one's self or another as a means of arousing or heightening sexual feeling. **2.** The pattern of formation of flagella. [L. *flagellatus,* fr. *flagello,* to whip or scourge]

fla·gel·lin (flaj′ě-lin). Any member of a class of proteins containing the amino acid, ε-*N*-methyllysine; this class represents the main protein component of the flagella of bacteria.

flag·el·lo·sis (flaj′ě-lō′sis). Infection with flagellated protozoa in the intestinal or genital tract, e.g., trichomoniasis.

fla·gel·lum, pl. **fla·gel·la** (flă-jel′ŭm, -ă). A whiplike locomotory organelle of constant structural arrangement consisting of nine double peripheral microtubules and two single central microtubules; it arises from a deeply staining basal granule, often connected to the nucleus by a fiber, the rhizoplast. Though characteristic of the protozoan class Mastigophora, comparable structures are commonly found in many other groups, e.g., in spermatozoa. [L. dim. of *flagrum,* a whip]

flam·ma·ble (flam′ă-bl). The property of burning readily and quickly. SYN inflammable. [L. *flamma,* flame]

flange (flanj). That part of the denture base which extends from the cervical ends of the teeth to the border of the denture.

buccal f., the portion of the f. of a denture that occupies the buccal vestibule of the mouth.

denture f., (1) the essentially vertical extension from the body of the denture into one of the vestibules of the oral cavity; also, on the lower denture, the essentially vertical extension along the lingual side of the alveololingual sulcus; **(2)** the buccal and labial vertical extension of the upper or lower denture base, and the lingual vertical extension of the lower one; the buccal and labial denture f.'s have two surfaces: the buccal or labial surface and the basal seat surface; the lower lingual f. also has two surfaces: the basal seat surface and the lingual surface.

labial f., the portion of the f. of a denture which occupies the labial vestibule of the mouth.

lingual f., the portion of the f. of a mandibular denture that occupies the space adjacent to the tongue.

flank [TA]. The area of the abdomen on each side of the umbilical region between transpyloric plane and intertubercular or interspinous plane. SYN latus [TA], lateral abdominal region✲, lateral region of abdominal region✲, regio abdominis lateralis✲, regio lateralis abdominis✲.

flap. 1. Tissue for transplantation, vascularized by a pedicle; f. SEE ALSO local f., distant f. **2.** An uncontrolled movement, as of the hands. SEE asterixis. [M.E. *flappe*]

Abbe f., middle portion of the lower lip transferred into the upper lip and vascularized by the labial artery.

advancement f., SYN bipedicle f.

arterial f., a f. with an identifiable nutrient artery and draining veins. Cf. random pattern f.

axial pattern f., a f. that includes a direct specific artery within its longitudinal axis.

bipedicle f., a f. with two pedicles, one at each end. SYN advancement f., double pedicle f.

bone f., portion of cranium removed but left attached to overlying muscle-fascial blood supply; term is often used incorrectly for a completely detached cranial section, i.e., a bone graft.

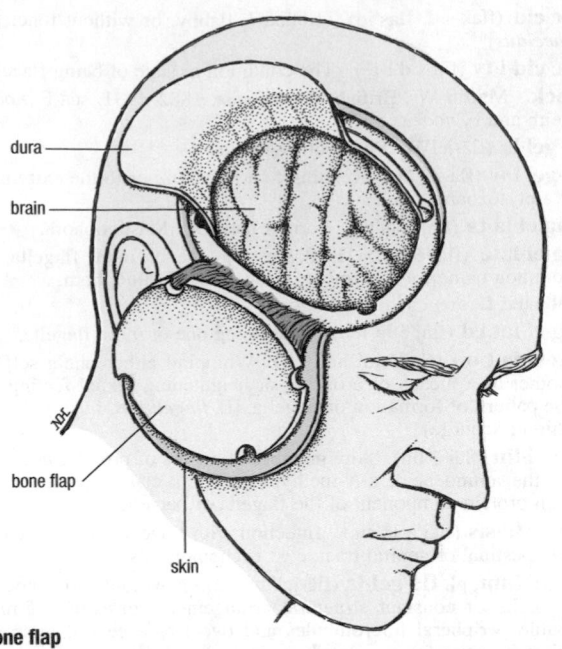

bone flap

buried f., a f. denuded of surface epithelium and superficial dermis and transferred into the subcutaneous tissues.

Byars f., skin f. made of dorsal prepuce to resurface the ventral penis in patients with chordee and/or hypospadias.

composite f., compound f., a f. of 2 or more tissue elements incorporating skin, subcutaneous muscle, bone, or cartilage.

cross f., a skin f. transferred from one part of the body to a corresponding part, as from one arm to the other.

delayed f., a f. incised and/or raised in its donor area in two or more stages to increase its chances of survival after transfer.

deltopectoral f., an axial pattern skin f. of the deltoid and pectoral regions, based on the internal mammary vessels.

direct f., a f. raised completely and transferred at the same stage.

distant f., a f. in which the donor site is distant from the recipient area. In the past this required multiple stages; now distant f.'s are transferred by microvascular anastomosis of artery and vein.

double pedicle f., SYN bipedicle f.

Eloesser f., a surgically created open skin-lined tract for chronic drainage of an empyema, often following pneumonectomy. SEE ALSO Eloesser *procedure*.

envelope f., a mucoperiosteal f. retracted from a horizontal incision along the free gingival margin.

Estlander f., a full-thickness f. of the lip, transferred from the side of one lip to the same side of the other lip. Other eponymous variations of this principle are the Sabbatini, Stein, and Abbe flaps.

Filatov f., SYN tubed f.

Filatov-Gillies f., SYN tubed f.

free f., f. in which the donor vessels are severed, the tissue is transported to another area, and the f. is revascularized by anastomosis of vessels in the recipient bed to the artery and vein(s) of the f.

free bone f., portion of cranium removed and detached from overlying soft tissue structures.

full-thickness f., a f. of the full thickness of mucosa and submucosa or of skin and subcutaneous tissues.

gingival f., a portion of the gingiva whose coronal margin is surgically detached from the tooth and the alveolar process.

hinged f., a turnover f. transferred by lifting it over as though the pedicle were a hinge.

Indian f., f. from a contiguous area, such as cheek or forehead, used to rebuild the nose.

interpolated f., f. that is rotated over intact skin into an adjoining area.

island f., a f. in which the pedicle consists solely of the supplying artery and vein(s), and sometimes a nerve.

Italian f., f. from a distant area; usually used in reference to a f. from the upper arm to rebuild a nose.

jump f., a distant f. transferred in stages via an intermediate carrier; e.g., an abdominal f. is attached to the wrist, and at a later stage the wrist is brought to the face.

lined f., a f. covered with epithelium on both sides; e.g., a folded skin f.

liver f., SEE asterixis.

local f., a f. transferred to an adjacent area, with intact pedicle.

mucoperichondrial f., a f. composed of mucous membrane and perichondrium, as from the nasal septum.

mucoperiosteal f., a f. composed of mucous membrane and periosteum, as from the hard palate or gingiva.

musculocutaneous f., SYN myocutaneous f.

myocutaneous f., a pedicled skin f., often an island f., with attached subjacent muscle, investments, and blood supply. SYN musculocutaneous f., myodermal f.

myodermal f., SYN myocutaneous f.

neurovascular f., a f. containing a sensory nerve; used to restore sensation to the recipient area.

omental f., a segment of omentum, with its supplying blood vessels, transplanted either with an intact pedicle or as free tissue to a distant area and revascularized by arterial and venous anastomoses.

osteoplastic bone f., vascularized tissue that includes living bone, usually with attached muscle and fascia, which can be attached by its pedicle or transferred by microvascular anastomosis from one site to another.

pedicle f., in periodontal surgery, a f. used to increase the width of attached gingiva, or to cover a root surface, by moving the attached gingiva, which remains joined at one side, to an adjacent position and suturing the free end.

pericoronal f., a f. of gingiva covering an unerupted tooth, especially the lower third molar.

pharyngeal f., a f. of mucosa and muscle raised from the posterior wall of the pharynx and attached to the soft palate, used to obturate the velopharyngeal passage to correct nasal air escape; for patients with velopharyngeal dysfunction, usually following repair of cleft palate.

random pattern f., a f. in which the pedicle blood supply is derived randomly from the network of vessels in the area, rather than from a single longitudinal artery as in an axial pattern f.

rotation f., a pedicle f. that is rotated from the donor site to an adjacent recipient defect.

skin f., a f. composed of skin and its subjacent subcutaneous tissue.

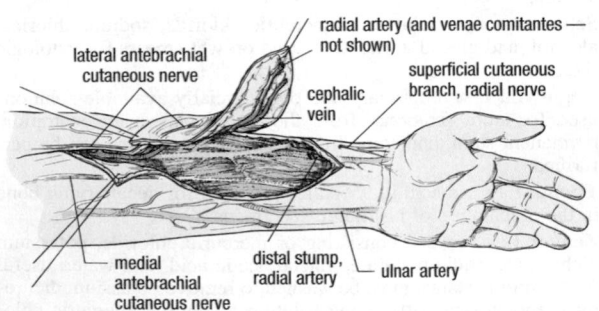

radial forearm flap

subcutaneous f., a pedicle f. in which the pedicle is denuded of epithelium and buried in the subcutaneous tissue of the recipient area.

tubed f., an old technique for transfer of skin in which a rectangular f. is elevated, sutured side to side, and the end of the tube inserted into another location. SYN Filatov f., Filatov-Gillies f., tubed pedicle f.

tubed pedicle f., SYN tubed f.

V-Y f., a f. in which the incision is made in a V shape and sutured in a Y shape to gain additional length of tissue. SYN V-Y plasty.

flare (flār). **1.** A gradual tapering or spreading outward. **2.** A diffuse redness of the skin extending beyond the local reaction to the application of an irritant; it is due to dilation of the arterioles and capillaries; depends upon an axon reflex set up by the liberation of a histamine-like substance in skin when injured. SEE ALSO triple *response*.

aqueous f., Tyndall phenomenon observed in the fluid of the anterior chamber of the eye.

flash. 1. A sudden and brief burst of light or heat. **2.** Excess material extruded between the sections of a flask in the process of molding denture bases or other dental restorations.

hot f., colloquialism for one of the vasomotor symptoms of the climacteric that may involve the whole body as a f. of heat; also used interchangeably with hot *flush*.

flash·back. An involuntary recurrence of some aspect of a hallucinatory experience or perceptual distortion occurring some time after ingestion of the hallucinogen that produced the original effect and without subsequent ingestion of the substance.

flask. A small receptacle, usually of glass, used for holding liquids, powder, or gases. [M.E. keg, fr. Fr. *flasque*, fr. Germanic]

casting f., SYN refractory f.

crown f., SYN denture f.

denture f., a sectional metal boxlike case in which a sectional mold is made of plaster of Paris or artificial stone for the purpose of compressing and curing dentures or other resinous restorations. SYN crown f.

Dewar f., a glass vessel, often silvered, with two walls, the space between which is evacuated; used for maintaining materials at constant temperature or, more usually, at low temperature. SYN vacuum f.

Erlenmeyer f., a f. with a broad base, conical body, and narrow neck; so shaped that its liquid content can be shaken laterally without spilling.

Fernbach f., a f. used in microbial fermentations where a large surface area of the liquid substrate is required.

Florence f., a globular long-necked bottle of thin glass used for holding water or other liquid in laboratory work.

hatching f., a f. painted a dark color so that only a small area of dechlorinated water at the top is exposed to light in simulation of pond water conditions, which stimulate hatching of any live schistosome eggs in fresh stool and urine sediment added to the f.; the released miracidium larvae will be searching for appropriate snail intermediate hosts.

injection f., a denture f. designed so as to permit the forced flow of denture base material from a reservoir into the mold after the flask is closed and during curing.

refractory f., a metal tube in which a refractory mold is made for casting metal dental restorations or appliances. SYN casting f., casting ring.

vacuum f., SYN Dewar f.

volumetric f., a narrow-necked f. calibrated to contain or to deliver a definite amount of liquid.

flask·ing. The process of investing the cast and a wax denture in a flask preparatory to molding the denture-base material into the form of the denture.

Flatau, Edward, Polish neurologist, 1869–1932. SEE F. *law*.

flat·foot (flat'fut). SYN *pes* planus.

flat·u·lence (flat'ū-lens). Presence of an excessive amount of gas in the stomach and intestines. [Mod. L. *flatulentus*, fr. L. *flatus*, a blowing, fr. *flo*, pp. *flatus*, to blow]

flat·u·lent (flat'ū-lent). Relating to or suffering from flatulence.

fla·tus (flā'tŭs). Gas or air in the gastrointestinal tract which may be expelled through the anus. [L. a blowing]

f. vagina'lis, expulsion of gas from the vagina.

flat·worm (flat'werm). A member of the phylum Platyhelminthes, including the parasitic tapeworms and flukes.

fla·ve·do (fla-vē'dō). Yellowness or sallowness of the skin. [L. *flavus*, yellow]

fla·vi·an·ic ac·id (flā-vē-an'ik) [C.I. 10316]. A naphthol derivative dye, useful in the precipitation (and subsequent determination) of arginine and other basic substances.

fla·vin, fla·vine (flā'vin, -vēn, flav'in, -ēn). **1.** SYN riboflavin. **2.** A yellow acridine dye, preparations of which are used as antiseptics. [L. *flavus*, yellow]

f. adenine dinucleotide (FAD), a condensation product of riboflavin and adenosine 5′-diphosphate; the coenzyme of various aerobic dehydrogenases, e.g., D-amino acid oxidase and aldehyde dehydrogenase; strictly speaking, FAD is not a dinucleotide since it contains a sugar alcohol; the coenzyme is reversibly reduced to $FADH_2$.

electron transfer f., flavoproteins that participate in the electron transport pathway.

f. mononucleotide (FMN), riboflavin 5′-phosphate; the coenzyme of a number of oxidation-reduction enzymes; e.g., NADH dehydrogenase. Strictly speaking, FMN is not a nucleotide since it contains a sugar alcohol instead of a sugar; the coenzyme is reversibly reduced to $FMNH_2$. SYN riboflavin 5′-phosphate.

Fla·vi·vi·ri·dae (flā'vī-vī'rā-dā). A family of enveloped single-stranded positive sense RNA viruses 40–60 mm in diameter formerly classified as the "group B" arboviruses, including yellow fever and dengue viruses; maintained in nature by transmission from arthropod vectors to vertebrate hosts.

Fla·vi·vi·rus (flā'vi-vī-rŭs). A genus in the family Flaviviridae that includes yellow fever, dengue, and St. Louis encephalitis viruses. [L. *flavus*, yellow, + virus]

Fla·vo·bac·te·ri·um (flā-vō-bak-tēr'ē-ŭm). A genus of aerobic to facultatively anaerobic, nonsporeforming, motile and nonmotile bacteria (family Achromobacteraceae) containing Gram-negative rods; motile cells are peritrichous. These organisms characteristically produce yellow, orange, red, or yellow-brown pigments. They are found in soil and fresh and salt water. Some species are pathogenic. The type species is *F. aquatile*. [L. *flavus*, yellow]

F. aqua'tile, a species found in water containing a high percentage of calcium carbonate; it is the type species of *F*.

F. bre've, a species found in sewage; pathogenic for laboratory animals.

F. meningisepticum, among the normal flora of the human respiratory tract, this bacterial species is an occasional cause of nosocomial infection, including neonatal meningitis.

F. piscici'da, former name for *Pseudomonas piscicida*.

fla·vo·en·zyme (flā-vō-en'zīm). Any enzyme that possesses a flavin nucleotide as coenzyme; e.g., xanthine oxidase, succinate dehydrogenase. SYN yellow enzyme.

fla·vo·ki·nase (flā-vō-kī'nās). SYN *riboflavin* kinase.

fla·vone (flā'vōn). **1.** A plant pigment that is the basis of the flavonoids; it is a potent inhibitor of prostaglandin biosynthesis. **2.** One of a class of compounds based on f. (1).

fla·vo·noids (flā'vō-noydz). **1.** Substances of plant origin containing flavone in various combinations (anthoxanthins, apigenins, flavones, quercitins, etc.) and with varying biologic activities. **2.** Derviatives of flavone.

fla·vo·nol (flā'vō-nol). **1.** Reduced flavone. **2.** flavone (1) hydroxylated at position 3; a member of a class of vascular pigments. **3.** Any hydroxylated flavone.

fla·vo·pro·tein (flā'vō-prō'tēn). A compound protein possessing a flavin as prosthetic group. Cf. flavoenzyme.

fla·vor (flā'ver). **1.** The quality (influenced by odor) affecting the taste of any substance. **2.** A therapeutically inert substance added to a prescription to give an agreeable taste to the mixture. [M.E., fr. O. Fr., fr. L.L. *flator*, aroma, fr. *flo*, to blow]

fla·vox·ate hy·dro·chlo·ride (flā-vok'sāt). A smooth muscle relaxant for the urinary tract.

fla·vus (flā'vŭs). Latin for yellow. [L.]

flax·seed (flaks'sēd). SYN linseed.

f. oil, SYN *linseed* oil.

fl

flea (flē). An insect of the order Siphonaptera, marked by lateral compression, sucking mouthparts, extraordinary jumping powers, and ectoparasitic adult life in the hair and feathers of warm-blooded animals. Important f.'s include *Ctenocephalides felis* (cat f.), or *C. canis* (dog f.), *Pulex irritans* (human f.), *Tunga penetrans* (chigger, chigoe, or sand f.), *Echidnophaga gallinacea* (sticktight f.), *Xenopsylla* (rat f.), and *Ceratophyllus*. SEE ALSO Copepoda.

fle·cai·nide ac·e·tate (flĕ-kā′nīd). A member of the membrane-stabilizing group of antiarrhythmics, with local anesthetic activity, used in the treatment of refractory ventricular arrhythmias.

Flechsig, Paul E., German neurologist, 1847–1929. SEE F. *areas,* under *area,* ground *bundles,* under *bundle, fasciculi,* under *fasciculus, tract;* oval *area* of F.; semilunar *nucleus* of F.

Flegel, H., 20th century German dermatologist. SEE F. *disease.*

Fleisch, Alfred, Swiss physician and physiologist, 1892–1973. SEE F. *pneumotachograph.*

Fleischer, Bruno, German ophthalmologist, 1874–1965. SEE F. *ring, vortex;* Kayser-F. *ring;* Fleischer-Strümpell *ring.*

Fleischmann, Friedrich Ludwig, 19th century German anatomist. SEE sublingual *bursa.*

Fleischner, Felix, Austrian-American radiologist, 1893–1969. SEE F. *lines,* under *line.*

Fleitmann, Theodore, 19th century German chemist. SEE F. *test.*

Fleming, Sir Alexander, Scottish bacteriologist, 1881–1955, co-winner of the 1945 Nobel prize for the discovery of penicillin.

Flemming, Walther, German anatomist, 1843–1905. SEE intermediate *body* of F.; germinal *center* of F.; F. *fixative,* triple *stain.*

Flesch, Rudolf F., Austrian educator, *1911. SEE F. *formula.*

flesh (flĕsh). **1.** The meat of animals used for food. **2.** SYN muscular *tissue.* [A.S. *flaesc*]

  goose f., SYN *cutis* anserina.

  proud f., historic term for exuberant granulations in the granulation tissue on the surface of a wound.

flesh·flies (flesh′flīz). Members of the order Diptera, whose larvae (maggots) develop in putrefying or living tissues. Maggots of the latter group produce myiasis; these include screw-worms (both primary and secondary invaders); wool maggots of sheep; botflies or skin maggots of humans and domestic animals (including warble or heel flies); head or nasal botflies of sheep and goats, horses, camels, and deer; and horse botflies (or gadflies) whose larvae develop in the stomach, duodenum, or rectum of horses.

flex (fleks). To bend; to move a joint in such a direction as to approximate the two parts which it connects. [L. *flecto,* pp. *flexus,* to bend]

flex·i·bil·i·tas ce·rea (flek-si-bil′i-tas sē′rē-ă). The rigidity of catalepsy which may be overcome by slight external force, but which returns at once, holding the limb firmly in the new position. [L. waxy flexibility]

flex·im·e·ter (flek-sim′ĕ-ter). SYN goniometer (3).

flex·ion (flek′shŭn) [TA]. **1.** The act of flexing or bending, e.g., bending of a joint so as to approximate the parts it connects; bending of the spine so that the concavity of the curve looks forward. **2.** The condition of being flexed or bent. [L. *flecto,* pp. *flexus,* to bend]

  palmar f., bending the hand or fingers toward the palmar surface.

  plantar f., bending the foot or toes toward the plantar surface.

Flexner, Simon, U.S. pathologist, 1863–1946. SEE F. *bacillus.*

flex·or (flek′ser, -sōr) [TA]. A muscle the action of which is to flex a joint.

flex·u·ra, pl. **flex·u·′rae** (flek-shūr′ă, -shūr′ē) [TA]. SYN flexure. [L. a bending]

  f. anorectalis [TA], SYN anorectal *flexure.*

  f. colica splenica, ☆ official alternate term for left colic *flexure.*

  f. co′li dex′tra [TA], SYN right colic *flexure.*

  f. coli hepatis, SYN right colic *flexure.*

  f. co′li sinis′tra [TA], SYN left colic *flexure.*

  f. duode′ni infe′rior [TA], SYN inferior duodenal *flexure.*

  f. duode′ni supe′rior [TA], SYN superior duodenal *flexure.*

  f. duode′nojejuna′lis [TA], SYN duodenojejunal *flexure.*

  f. perinea′lis (canalis ani), ☆ official alternate term for anorectal *flexure.*

  f. sacra′lis rec′ti [TA], SYN sacral *flexure* of rectum.

  f. sigmoid′ea, SYN sigmoid *colon.*

flex·ur·al (flek′sher-ăl). Relating to a flexure.

flex·ure (flek′sher) [TA]. A bend, as in an organ or structure. SYN flexura [TA]. [L. *flexura*]

  anorectal f. [TA], the anteroposterior curve or angle, with convexity directed anteriorly, of the anorectal junction; tonus of the puborectalis (muscle) produces the angle for maintaining fecal continence; relaxation of the muscle allows the angle to be reduced for defecation. SYN flexura anorectalis [TA], flexura perinealis (canalis ani)☆, perineal f. of anal canal☆, anorectal angle, perineal f. of rectum.

  basicranial f., SYN pontine f.

  caudal f., the bend in the lumbosacral region of the embryo. SYN sacral f.

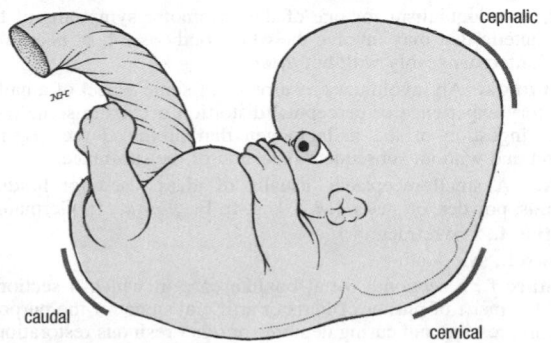

flexures: seen in a 6-week old embryo

  cephalic f., the sharp, ventrally concave bend in the developing midbrain of the embryo. SYN cerebral f., cranial f., mesencephalic f.

  cerebral f., SYN cephalic f.

  cervical f., the ventrally concave bend at the juncture of the brainstem and spinal cord in the embryo.

  cranial f., SYN cephalic f.

  dorsal f., a f. in the mid-dorsal region in the embryo.

  duodenojejunal f. [TA], an abrupt bend in the small intestine at the junction of the duodenum and jejunum. SYN flexura duodenojejunalis [TA], duodenojejunal angle.

  hepatic f., ☆ official alternate term for right colic f.

  inferior duodenal f. [TA], the bend at the junction of the descending and horizontal parts of the duodenum. Occasionally a bend, the left inferior duodenal flexure, occurs at the junction of the horizontal and ascending parts. SYN flexura duodeni inferior [TA].

  left colic f. [TA], the bend at the junction of the transverse and descending colon. SYN flexura coli sinistra [TA], flexura colica splenica☆, splenic f.☆.

  lumbar f., SYN lumbar *lordosis.*

  mesencephalic f., SYN cephalic f.

  perineal f. of anal canal, ☆ official alternate term for anorectal f.

  perineal f. of rectum, SYN anorectal f.

  pontine f., the dorsally concave curvature of the rhombencephalon in the embryo; appearance indicates division of rhombencephalon into myelencephalon and metencephalon. SYN basicranial f., transverse rhombencephalic f.

  right colic f. [TA], the bend of the colon at the juncture of its ascending and transverse portions. SYN flexura coli dextra [TA], hepatic f.☆, flexura coli hepatis.

  sacral f., SYN caudal f.

  sacral f. of rectum [TA], the anteroposterior curve with concavity anteriorward of the first portion of the rectum. SYN flexura sacralis recti [TA].

sigmoid f., SYN sigmoid *colon.*

splenic f., ⋆official alternate term for left colic f.

superior duodenal f. [TA], the flexure at the junction of the superior and descending parts of the duodenum. SYN flexura duodeni superior [TA].

telencephalic f., a f. appearing in the embryonic forebrain region.

transverse rhombencephalic f., SYN pontine f.

flick·er (flik′er). The visual sensation caused by stimulation of the retina by a series of intermittent light flashes occurring at a certain rate. SEE ALSO flicker *fusion,* critical flicker fusion *frequency.*

flicks (fliks). Rapid, involuntary fixation movements of the eye of 5–10 minutes of arc. SYN flick movements.

Flieringa, Henri J., Dutch ophthalmologist, *1891. SEE F. *ring.*

flight in·to dis·ease. Gain through falling ill or assuming the sick role. SEE primary *gain,* secondary *gain.*

flight in·to health. In dynamic psychotherapy, the early but often only temporary disappearance of the symptoms that ostensibly brought the patient into therapy; a defense against the anxiety engendered by the prospect of further psychoanalytic exploration of the patient's conflicts.

Flint, Austin, Jr., U.S. physiologist, 1836–1915. SEE F. *arcade.*

Flint, Austin, U.S. physician, 1812–1886. SEE Austin F. *murmur;* F. *murmur;* Austin F. *phenomenon.*

flip. A burn occurring on one side only of the entrance site in a gunshot wound of the soft parts.

flitter. SYN impure *flutter.*

float·er (flōt′er). An object in the field of vision that originates in the vitreous body. SEE ALSO muscae volitantes.

float·ing (flōt′ing). **1.** Free or unattached. **2.** Unduly movable; out of the normal position; denoting an occasional abnormal condition of certain organs, such as the kidneys, liver, spleen, etc.

floc (flok). A colloquial term for the product of a flocculation, i.e., the separation of the disperse phase of a colloidal suspension into discrete, usually visible particles, as in certain serologic precipitin tests.

floc·cil·la·tion (flok-si-lā′shŭn). An aimless plucking at the bedclothes, as if one were picking off threads or tufts of cotton. [Mod. L. *flocculus*]

floc·cose (flok′ōs). In bacteriology, applied to a growth of short, curving filaments or chains closely but irregularly disposed. [L. *floccus,* a flock of wool]

floc·cu·la·ble (flok′ū-lă-bl). Capable of undergoing flocculation.

floc·cu·lar (flok′ū-lăr). Relating to a flocculus of any sort; specifically to the flocculus of the cerebellum.

floc·cu·late (flok′ū-lāt). To become flocculent.

floc·cu·la·tion (flok-ū-lā′shŭn). Precipitation from solution in the form of fleecy masses; the process of becoming flocculent. SYN flocculence.

floc·cule (flok′ūl). SYN flocculus.

floc·cu·lence (flok′ū-lens). SYN flocculation.

floc·cu·lent (flok′ū-lent). **1.** Resembling tufts of cotton or wool; denoting a fluid, such as the urine, containing numerous shreds or fluffy particles of gray-white or white mucus or other material. **2.** In bacteriology, denoting a fluid culture in which there are numerous colonies either floating in the fluid medium or loosely deposited at the bottom.

floc·cu·lo·nod·u·lar (flok′ū-lō-nod′ū-lăr). SEE flocculonodular *lobe.*

floc·cu·lus, pl. **floc·cu·li** (flok′ū-lŭs, -lī). **1.** A tuft or shred of cotton or wool or anything resembling it. **2** [TA]. A small lobe of the cerebellum at the posterior border of the middle cerebellar peduncle anterior to the biventer lobule; it is associated with the nodulus of the vermis; together, these two structures compose the vestibular part of the cerebellum. SYN floccule. [Mod. L. dim. of L. *floccus,* a tuft of wool]

accessory f., an occasional small lobule of the cerebellum adjacent to the flocculus.

Flocks, Milton, U.S. ophthalmologist, *1914. SEE Harrington-F. *test.*

Flood, Valentine, Irish anatomist and surgeon, 1800–1847. SEE F. *ligament.*

flood (flŭd). **1.** To bleed profusely from the uterus, as after childbirth or in cases of menorrhagia. **2.** Colloquialism for a profuse menstrual discharge. [A.S. *flōd*]

flood·ing (flŭd′ing). **1.** Bleeding profusely from the uterus, especially after childbirth or in severe cases of menorrhagia. **2.** Profuse uterine hemorrhage. **3.** A type of behavior therapy; a therapeutic strategy at the beginning of therapy, in which the patients imagine the most anxiety-producing scene and fully immerse (flood) themselves in it. Cf. systematic *desensitization.*

floor (flōr) [TA]. The lower inner surface of an open space or hollow organ.

f. of orbit [TA], the floor of the orbit; the shortest of the four walls of the orbit, sloping upward from the orbital margin; it is comprised of the maxilla and orbital process of the palatine bone. SYN paries inferior orbitae [TA], inferior wall of orbit.

f. of tympanic cavity, ⋆official alternate term for jugular *wall* of middle ear.

flo·ra (flō′ră). **1.** Plant life, usually of a certain locality or district. **2.** The population of microorganisms inhabiting the internal and external surfaces of healthy conventional animals. SYN microbial associates. [L. *Flora,* goddess of flowers, fr. *flos (flor-),* a flower]

flor·an·ty·rone (flor-an′ti-rōn). An agent which increases the volume of bile without increasing the quantity of bile solids or stimulating evacuation of the gallbladder.

Florence, Albert, French physician, 1851–1927. SEE F. *crystals,* under *crystal.*

Florence flask. See under flask.

Florey, Sir Howard W., Australian-British pathologist and Nobel laureate, 1898–1968. SEE F. *unit.*

flor·id (flōr′id). **1.** Of a bright red color; denoting certain cutaneous lesions. **2.** Fully developed. [L. *floridus,* flowery]

Florschütz, Georg, German physician, *1859. SEE F. *formula.*

floss. **1.** SYN dental f. **2.** To use dental f. in oral hygiene.

dental f., an untwisted thread made from fine, short, silk or synthetic fibers, frequently waxed; used for cleansing interproximal spaces and between contact areas of the teeth. SYN floss silk, floss (1).

flo·ta·tion (flō-tā′shŭn). A process for separating solids by their tendency to float upon or sink into a liquid.

Flourens, Marie Jean Pierre, French physiologist, 1794–1867. SEE F. *theory.*

flow (flō) **1.** To bleed from the uterus less profusely than in flooding. **2.** The menstrual discharge. **3.** Movement of a liquid or gas; specifically, the volume of liquid or gas passing a given point per unit of time. In respiratory physiology, the symbol for gas flow is V̇ and for blood flow is Q̇, followed by subscripts denoting location and chemical species. **4.** In rheology, a permanent deformation of a body that proceeds with time. [A.S. *flōwan*]

Bingham f., the f. characteristics exhibited by a Bingham plastic.

Doppler color f., a computer-generated color image produced by Doppler ultrasonography in which different directions of f. are represented by different hues. SEE Doppler *ultrasonography.*

effective renal blood f. (ERBF), the amount of blood flowing to the parts of the kidney that are involved with production of constituents of urine.

effective renal plasma f. (ERPF), the amount of plasma flowing to the parts of the kidney that have a function in the production of constituents of urine; the clearance of substances such as iodopyracet and *p*-aminohippuric acid, assuming that the extraction ratio in the peritubular capillaries is 100%.

forced expiratory f. (FEF), expiratory f. during measurement of forced vital capacity; subscripts specify the exact parameter measured, e.g., peak instantaneous f., the instantaneous f. at some specified point on the curve of volume expired versus time, or on the flow-volume curve, the mean f. between two expired volumes.

gene f., changes over time in the genetic composition of a population as a result of migration rather than of mutation and selection.

laminar f., the relative motion of elements of a fluid along

fl

smooth parallel paths, which occurs at lower values of Reynolds number.

newtonian f., the type of f. characteristic of a newtonian fluid.

peak expiratory f., the maximum f. at the outset of forced expiration, which is reduced in proportion to the severity of airway obstruction, as in asthma.

shear f., a f. of a material in which parallel planes in the material are displaced in a direction parallel to each other.

Flower, Sir William H., English surgeon and anatomist, 1831–1899. SEE F. *bone*, dental *index*.

flow·er bas·ket of Bochdalek. Part of the choroid plexus of the fourth ventricle protruding through the foramen of Luschka and resting on the dorsal surface of the glossopharyngeal nerve.

flow·ers (flow′erz). A mineral substance in a powdery state after sublimation.

f. of antimony, SYN *antimony* trioxide.

f. of benzoin, SYN *benzoic* acid.

f. of sulfur, SYN sublimed *sulfur*.

f. of zinc, SYN *zinc* oxide.

flow·me·ter (flō′mē-ter). A device for measuring velocity or volume of flow of liquids or gases.

electromagnetic f., a f. in which a magnetic field is applied to a blood vessel to measure flow in terms of the voltage developed by the blood as a conductor moving through the magnetic field.

flox·a·cil·lin (flok′să-sil′in). A penicillin antibiotic resistant to β-lactamase (penicillinase).

flox·ur·i·dine (flok-soo′ri-dēn). The deoxynucleoside of fluorouracil; an antineoplastic agent. Fluorouracil is metabolized to f. and this, in turn, to 5-fluoro-2′-deoxyuridine 5′-monophosphate. The latter agent inhibits thymidylic synthetase; uridine phosphatase is also inhibited.

flu (floo). SYN influenza.

flu·an·i·sone (floo-an′i-sōn). An antianxiety agent.

flu·cry·late (floo′kri-lāt). A surgical tissue adhesive.

fluctuance. SYN fluctuation (2).

fluc·tu·ate (flŭk′tū-āt). **1.** To move in waves. **2.** To vary, to change from time to time, as in referring to any quantity or quality, e.g., height of blood pressure, concentration of substance in urine or blood, secretory activity, etc. [L. *fluctuo,* pp. *-atus,* to flow in waves]

fluc·tu·a·tion (flŭk-tū-ā′shŭn). **1.** The act of fluctuating. **2.** A wavelike motion felt on palpating a cavity with nonrigid walls, especially one containing fluid. SYN fluctuance.

flu·cy·to·sine (floo-sī′tō-sēn). An antifungal drug.

flu·dro·cor·ti·sone ac·e·tate (floo-drō-kōr′ti-sōn). A potent mineralocorticoid. SYN 9α-fluorocortisol, 9α-fluorohydrocortisone acetate.

flu·ence (*H*) (floo′ens). A measure of the quantity of x-radiation in a beam in diagnostic radiology, either particle f., the number of photons passing an aperture of unit cross-sectional area, or energy f., the sum of the energies of the photons passing through a unit area. Cf. flux. [L. *fluentia,* a flowing, fr. *fluo,* to flow]

flu·en·cy (floo′en-sē). The smooth flow of speech sounds in connected discourse, without interruptions or repetitions. [L. *fluentia,* a flowing, fr. *fluo,* to flow]

flu·ent (floo′ent). Relating to fluency.

flu·fen·am·ic ac·id (floo-fen-am′ik). An anti-inflammatory agent; resembles mefenamic acid.

flu·id (floo′id) [TA]. **1.** A nonsolid substance, such as a liquid or gas, that tends to flow or conform to the shape of the container. **2.** Consisting of particles or distinct entities that can readily change their relative positions; i.e., tending to move or capable of flowing. [L. *fluidus,* fr. *fluo,* to flow]

allantoic f., the f. within the allantoic cavity.

amnionic f., a liquid within the amnion that surrounds the fetus and protects it from mechanical injury. SYN liquor amnii.

Brodie f., an aqueous salt solution used in manometers designed for testing gas evolution or uptake, as in cell respiration.

bronchoalveolar f., a f. containing several lytic enzymes that

serves to remove inspired particulates from the pulmonary airways.

Callison f., a diluting f. for counting red blood cells, consisting of 1 ml of Loeffler alkaline methylene blue, 1 ml of formalin, 10 ml of glycerol, 1 g of neutral ammonium oxalate, and 2.5 g of sodium chloride added to 90 ml of distilled water, mixed well, and permitted to stand until the solids are dissolved and the reagent is clear; the preparation is filtered prior to use.

⬛**cerebrospinal f. (CSF)** [TA], a fluid largely secreted by the choroid plexuses of the ventricles of the brain, filling the ventricles and the subarachnoid cavities of the brain and spinal cord. SYN liquor cerebrospinalis [TA].

human cerebrospinal fluid	
(average measurements, mg/dL)	
volume	120–200 ml
specific gravity	1.006–1.008
reaction	pH ca. 7.5
freezing point depression	0.55°(0.52°–0.58°)
pressure (lumbar, subject reclining)	70–220 mm H_2O
protein	15–25
glucose	40–60 (up to 80)
phosphatidic acid	ca. 1.0
cholesterol	0.3–0.6
chloride	730–740
phosphate	3–5

crevicular f., SYN gingival f.

Dakin f., SYN Dakin *solution.*

dentinal f., the lymph or f. of dentin which appears on the surface of freshly cut dentin, especially in young teeth; it is a transudate of extracellular f., mainly cytoplasm of odontoblastic processes, from the dental pulp via the dentinal tubules. SYN dental lymph.

extracellular f. (ECF), (1) the interstitial f. and the plasma, constituting about 20% of the weight of the body; **(2)** sometimes used to mean all f. outside of cells, usually excluding transcellular f.

extravascular f., all f. outside the blood vessels, i.e., intracellular, interstitial, and transcellular f.'s; it constitutes about 48 to 58% of the body weight.

Farrant mounting f., an aqueous solution containing gum arabic, arsenic trioxide, glycerol, and water, used in mounting histologic sections directly from water; some modifications involve addition of potassium acetate to bring the pH up to neutrality and substitution of other preservatives like cresol or thymol for arsenic trioxide.

gingival f., f. containing plasma proteins, which is present in increasing amounts in association with gingival inflammation. SYN crevicular f., sulcular f.

infranatant f., clear f. that, after the settling out of an insoluble liquid or solid by the action of normal gravity or of centrifugal force, takes up the lower portion of the contents of a vessel.

interstitial f., the f. in spaces between the tissue cells, constituting about 16% of the weight of the body; closely similar in composition to lymph. SYN tissue f.

intracellular f. (ICF), the f. within the tissue cells, constituting about 30–40% of the body weight. SYN intracellular water.

intraocular f., SYN aqueous *humor.*

newtonian f., a f. in which flow and rate of shear are always proportional to the applied stress; such f. precisely obeys Poiseuille law. Cf. non-newtonian f.

non-newtonian f., a f. in which flow and rate of shear are not always proportional to the applied stress and which does not obey Poiseuille law. As in anomalous *viscosity*; Fahraeus-Lindqvist *effect*; Bingham *plastic.* Cf. newtonian f.

pleural f., the thin film of f. between the visceral and parietal pleurae. May significantly increase in disease states, when termed pleural effusion.

prostatic f., succus prostaticus; a whitish secretion that is one of the constituents of the semen.

pseudoplastic f., a f. which exhibits shear thinning.

Rees-Ecker f., an aqueous solution of sodium citrate, sucrose, and brilliant cresyl blue used in platelet counts.

Scarpa f., SYN endolymph.

seminal f., SYN semen (1).

sulcular f., SYN gingival f.

supernatant f., clear f. that, after the settling out of an insoluble liquid or solid by the action of normal gravity or of centrifugal force, takes up the upper portion of the contents of a vessel.

synovial f. [TA], a clear thixotropic fluid, the main function of which is to serve as a lubricant in a joint, tendon sheath, or bursa; consists mainly of mucin with some albumin, fat, epithelium, and leukocytes; synovial f. also helps to nourish the avascular articular cartilage. SYN synovia [TA], joint oil.

thixotropic f., a liquid that tends to turn into a gel when left standing, but which turns back into a liquid if agitated, as by vibrations or subjection to adequate shear.

tissue f., SYN interstitial f.

transcellular f.'s, the f.'s that are not inside cells, but are separated from plasma and interstitial f. by cellular barriers; e.g., cerebrospinal f., synovial f., pleural f.

ventricular f., the portion of the cerebrospinal f. that is contained in the ventricles of the brain.

flu·id·ex·tract (floo-id-eks′trakt). Pharmacopeial liquid preparation of vegetable drugs, made by percolation, containing alcohol as a solvent or as a preservative, or both, and so made that each milliliter contains the therapeutic constituents of 1 g of the standard drug that it represents. SYN liquid extract.

flu·id·glyc·er·ates (floo-id-glis′er-āts). Pharmaceutical preparations, formerly official in the NF, containing approximately 50% by volume of glycerin but no alcohol, and of the same drug strength as fluidextracts.

flu·id·ism (floo′i-dizm). SYN humoral *doctrine*.

flu·id·i·ty (floo-id′i-tē). The reciprocal of viscosity; unit: rhe = poise^{-1}.

flu·id·ounce (floo′id-owns′). A measure of capacity: 8 fluidrams. The imperial f. is a measure containing 1 avoirdupois ounce, 437.5 grains, of distilled water at 15.6°C, and equals 28.4 ml; the U.S. f. is $^{1}/_{128}$ gallon, contains 454.6 grains of distilled water at 25°C, and equals 29.57 ml.

flu·i·drachm, flu·i·dram (floo′i-dram′). A measure of capacity: $^{1}/_{8}$ of a fluidounce; a teaspoonful. The imperial f. contains 54.8 grains of distilled water, and equals 3.55 ml; the U.S. f. contains 57.1 grains of distilled water and equals 3.70 ml.

fluke (flook). Common name for members of the class Trematoda (phylum Platyhelminthes). All f.'s of mammals (subclass Digenea) are internal parasites in the adult stage and are characterized by complex digenetic life cycles involving a snail initial host, in which larval multiplication occurs, and the release of swimming larvae (cercariae), which directly penetrate the skin of the final host (as in schistosomes), encyst on vegetation (as in *Fasciola*), or encyst in or on another intermediate host (as in *Clonorchis* and other fish-borne f.'s). F.'s of lower vertebrates (order Monogenea), especially fish, are frequently monogenetic ectoparasites or gill parasites. Blood f.'s live in the mesenteric-portal bloodstream and associated vesical and pelvic venous plexuses; they include *Schistosoma haematobium* (the vesical blood f.), *S. mansoni* (Manson intestinal blood f.), and *S. japonicum* (the Oriental blood f.). Other important f.'s are *Paragonimus westermani* (bronchial or lung f.), *Opisthorchis felineus* (cat liver f.), *Clonorchis sinensis* (Chinese liver or Oriental f.), *Heterophyes heterophyes* (Egyptian or small intestinal f.), *Fasciolopsis buski* (large intestinal f.), *Dicrocoelium dendriticum* (lancet f.), *Fasciola hepatica* (liver or sheep liver f.), and *Paramphistomum* (rumen f.). [A.S. *flóc*, flatfish]

flu·maz·en·il (floo′mā-ze-nil). A benzodiazepine with antagonist properties at the benzodiazepine recognition site of the benzodiazepine-GABA-chloride channel complex. Used as a treatment

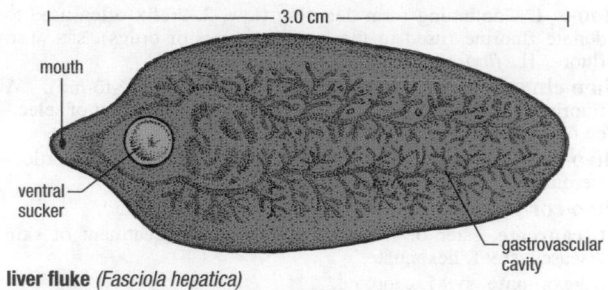
liver fluke *(Fasciola hepatica)*

for overdose with benzodiazepine-type central nervous system depressants.

flu·men, pl. **flu·mi·na** (floo′men, floo′min-ă). A flowing, or stream. SYN stream. [L.]

flumina pilo′rum, SYN hair *streams,* under *stream.*

flu·meth·a·sone (floo-meth′ă-sōn). The 21-pivalate salt and acetate are also available.

flu·me·thi·a·zide (floo′me-thī′ă-zīd). An orally effective diuretic agent, related chemically to chlorothiazide and with similar pharmacologic actions; it inhibits carbonic anhydrase.

flu·mi·na (floo′mi-nă). Plural of flumen.

flu·nar·i·zine (floo-nar′ĭ-zēn). A calcium-blocking agent with anticonvulsant properties.

flu·nis·o·lide (floo-nis′ō-lid). An anti-inflammatory corticosteroid used intranasally or by inhalation in the treatment of allergies and asthma.

fl

flu·ni·traz·e·pam (flū′nī-trāz′ĕ-pam). A benzodiazepine compound with sedative and hypnotic properties.

Flunitrazepam, said to be the most widely prescribed sedative and hypnotic in Europe although it is not licensed for sale in the U.S., has been the subject of increasing concern as illegal distribution and abuse of the drug have spread from southern states to other parts of this country. Abuse is particularly prevalent among high school and college youth. Used alone, flunitrazepam induces mild euphoria and sedation. It is often taken with other agents, for example, to enhance a heroin high or to ease coming down from a cocaine or crack high. Flunitrazepam and alcohol have a synergistic effect, producing disinhibition and amnesia when taken together. For this reason the drug may be surreptitiously added to alcoholic drinks to facilitate date rape. Part of the popularity of the drug arises from its low cost and the availability of legitimately manufactured, pure tablets. Flunitrazepam is marketed by Hoffman-La Roche under the brand name Rohypnol. Street names include "circles," "Mexican Valium," "la rocha," "R2," "rib," "roaches," "roachies," "Roche," "roofenol," "roofies," "rope," "rophies," and "ruffies." Being under the influence of the drug is referred to as being "roached out." The effects of flunitrazepam begin within 30 minutes after ingestion, peak within 2 hours, and may persist for 8 hours or more. Adverse effects include drowsiness, confusion, amnesia, paradoxic excitement or aggressiveness, visual disturbances, hypotension, gastrointestinal upset, and urinary retention. Lethal overdose has been uncommon. Continued use results in physical dependence. Withdrawal symptoms range from headache, muscle pain, restlessness, and confusion to loss of identity, hallucinations, delirium, convulsions, and cardiovascular collapse. Withdrawal seizures can occur a week or more after cessation of use. Phenobarbital has been used to ease medically supervised withdrawal. In 1997, in response to concerns about the use of flunitrazepam in date rape, Hoffman-LaRoche reformulated the tablets so that they dissolve more slowly in liquids and release a bright blue color to render detection more likely.

⌂**fluo-.** **1.** Combining form denoting flow. **2.** Prefix often used to denote fluorine (used in the generic names of drugs). SEE ALSO fluor-. [L. *fluo*, pp. *fluxus*, to flow]

flu·o·cin·o·lone ac·e·to·nide (floo-ō-sin′ō-lōn as′ĕ-tō-nīd). A fluorinated corticosteroid for topical use in the treatment of selected dermatoses.

flu·o·cin·o·nide (floo-ō-sin′ō-nīd). An anti-inflammatory corticosteroid used in topical preparations.

flu·o·cor·to·lone (floo-ŏ-kōr′tō-lōn). A glucocorticoid.

f. caproate, ester of f. used topically in the treatment of skin diseases. SYN f. hexanoate.

f. hexanoate, SYN f. caproate.

f. pivalate, an ester of f.

⌂**fluor-, fluoro-.** Fluorine.

flu·or·ap·a·tite (flōr-ap′ă-tīt). A naturally occurring fluorophosphate of calcium.

9*H*-**flu·o·rene** (flōr′ēn). Parent compound of 2-acetylaminofluorene; occurs in coal tar.

flu·o·res·ca·mine (flōr-es′ka-mēn). A nonfluorescent reagent that reacts with primary amines to form fluorescent compounds.

flu·o·resce (fluō-res′). To produce or exhibit fluorescence.

flu·o·res·ce·in (flōr-es′ē-in) [C.I. 45350]. An orange-red crystalline powder that yields a bright green fluorescence in solution, and is reduced to fluorescin; a nontoxic, water-soluble indicator used diagnostically to trace water flow. SYN resorcinol phthalic anhydride, resorcinolphthalein.

f. sodium, a dye used for diagnosis of certain ocular diseases, differentiation or delineation of organ parts in surgery, and determination of circulation time. SYN resorcinolphthalein sodium, uranin.

flu·o·res·ce·in iso·thi·o·cy·a·nate (FITC) (ī′sō-thī-ō-sī′ă-nāt). A fluorochrome dye frequently coupled to antibodies that are used to locate and identify specific antigens.

flu·o·res·cence (flōr-es′ens). Emission of a longer wavelength radiation by a substance as a consequence of absorption of energy from a shorter wavelength radiation, continuing only as long as the stimulus is present; distinguished from phosphorescence, which emission persists for a perceptible period of time after the stimulus has been removed. SEE photoelectric *effect*. [*fluor*spar + -*escence*, inchoative suffix]

flu·o·res·cence-ac·ti·vat·ed cell sort·er (FACS) (flōr-es′ens). A machine that can separate and analyze cells, such as lymphocytes, which are labeled with fluorochrome-conjugated antibody, by their fluorescence and light scattering patterns.

flu·o·res·cent (flōr-es′ent). Possessing the quality of fluorescence.

flu·o·res·cin (flōr′-es-in). Reduced fluorescein, with similar uses as fluorescein.

flu·o·ri·da·tion (flōr′i-dā′shŭn). Addition of fluorides to a community water supply, usually about 1 ppm, to reduce incidence of dental decay.

flu·o·ride (flōr′īd). **1.** A compound of fluorine with a metal, a nonmetal, or an organic radical. **2.** The anion of fluorine; inhibits enolase; found in bone and tooth apatite; f. has a cariostatic effect; high levels are toxic.

flu·o·ride num·ber. The percent inhibition of pseudocholinesterase produced by fluorides; used to differentiate normal from atypical pseudocholinesterases. SEE ALSO dibucaine number.

flu·o·ri·di·za·tion (flōr′i-di-zā′shŭn). Therapeutic use of fluorides to reduce the incidence of dental decay; sometimes used to refer to the topical application of fluoride agents to the teeth.

flu·o·rine (F) (flōr′ēn). A gaseous chemical element, atomic no. 9, atomic wt. 18.9984032; ^{18}F (half-life of 1.83 h) is used as a diagnostic aid in various tissue scans. [L. *fluere*, flow]

⌂**fluoro-.** SEE fluor-.

flu·o·ro·chrome (flōr′ō-krōm). Any fluorescent dye used to label or stain.

flu·or·o·chrom·ing (flōr′ō-krōm-ing). **1.** Tagging or "labeling" of antibody with a fluorescent dye so that it may be observed with a microscope (using ultraviolet light), as a means of studying the origin, distribution, and sites of reaction (with antigen) in tissues. **2.** Microscopic detection of cellular and tissue chemical components (DNA, RNA, proteins, polysaccharides) with the aid of fluorochromes bound to these components.

9α-flu·o·ro·cor·ti·sol (flōr-ō-kōr′ti-sol). SYN fludrocortisone acetate.

flu·o·ro·cyte (flōr′ō-sīt). Term used occasionally for a reticulocyte that exhibits fluorescence.

flu·o·ro-2,4-di·ni·tro·ben·zene (FDNB) (flōr′ō-dī-nī-trō-ben′zēn). A reagent used to combine with the free amino groups of aminoacyl residues in a peptide, thus marking those residues; the combined forms are known as DNP-proteins, Dnp-aminoacyl, etc., the fluorine having been replaced to leave a dinitrophenyl residue (DNP, Dnp, or N₂Ph–) attached to the NH₂ group. Hence, the *N*-terminal amino acid and lysine side chains will be covalently modified. SYN Sanger reagent.

flu·o·rog·ra·phy (flōr-og′ră-fē). SYN photofluorography.

9α-flu·o·ro·hy·dro·cor·ti·sone ac·e·tate (flōr′ō-hī-drō-kōr′ti-sōn). SYN fludrocortisone acetate.

flu·o·rom·e·ter (flōr-om′ĕ-ter). A device employing an ultraviolet source, monochromators for selection of wavelength, and a detector of visible light; used in fluorometry.

flu·o·ro·meth·o·lone (flōr-ō-meth′ŏ-lōn). A glucocorticoid for topical use.

flu·o·rom·e·try (flōr-om′ĕ-trē). An analytic method for detecting fluorescent compounds, using a beam of ultraviolet light that excites the compounds and causes them to emit visible light. [fluoro- + G. *metron*, measure]

flu·o·ro·pho·tom·e·try (flōr′ō-fō-tom′ĕ-trē). Photomultiplier tube measurement of fluorescence emitted from the interior of the eye after intravenous administration of fluorescein; used to measure the rate of formation of aqueous humor or integrity of the retinal vasculature.

fluoroquinolone (flōr-ō-kwin′ō-lōn). SYN quinolones.

flu·o·ro·quin·o·lones (flōr′ō-kwin′ō-lōnz). A class of antibiotics with a broad spectrum of antimicrobial activity; well-absorbed orally, with good tissue penetration and relatively long duration of effect.

The fluoroquinolones, introduced in the 1980s, are particularly useful in Gram-negative infections. Nalidixic acid, a nonfluorinated quinolone, has been used for several decades to treat urinary tract infections, but its value is limited by poor systemic distribution and rapid development of bacterial resistance. In contrast, the fluoroquinolones, which contain a fluorine atom, rapidly achieve therapeutic concentration in plasma, tissues, and urine after oral administration, and resistance develops slowly. The fluorine atom also broadens the spectrum of these agents, conferring activity against some Gram-positive bacteria. They are useful in susceptible infections of the respiratory tract, urinary tract, skin, and bone. Several of these agents are approved for single-dose oral treatment of uncomplicated gonorrhea. They are generally inactive against anaerobes and β-hemolytic streptococci. Fluoroquinolone antibiotics inhibit bacterial DNA gyrase, which is necessary for the replication of DNA as well as of plasmids involved in certain types of bacterial resistance. Elimination is primarily renal, and dosage must be adjusted for patients with renal failure. The fluoroquinolones are generally well tolerated. The most frequent side effects are nausea, abdominal distress, and dizziness. The drugs accumulate in articular cartilage and can cause severe damage during rapid growth of that tissue; hence they are contraindicated in persons under 18. Use during strenuous exercise may be hazardous to joints and can cause tendon rupture. These drugs may interfere with the hepatic biotransformation of theophylline and warfarin.

flu·o·ro·roent·gen·og·ra·phy (flōr′ō-rent-gen-og′ră-fē). SYN photofluorography.

flu·o·ro·scope (flōr′ō-skōp). An obsolete apparatus for rendering visible to the dark-adapted eye the patterns of x-rays that have passed through a body under examination, by interposing a glass plate coated with fluorescent materials, such as calcium tungstate; currently, image intensification and video display are used; to examine a patient using a fluoroscope, obsolete or modern. [fluorescence + G. *skopeō,* to examine]

flu·o·ro·scop·ic (flōr-ō-skop′ik). Relating to or effected by means of fluoroscopy (i.e., percutaneous biopsy).

flu·o·ros·co·py (flōr-os′kŏ-pē). Examination of the tissues and deep structures of the body by x-ray, using the fluoroscope or its successor, video f. (q.v.).

video f., f. using an image intensifier and television camera for image detection and a video monitor for display.

flu·o·ro·sis (flōr-ō′sis). **1.** A condition caused by an excessive intake of fluorides (2 or more p.p.m. in drinking water), characterized mainly by mottling, staining, or hypoplasia of the enamel of the teeth, although the skeletal bones are also affected. **2.** Chronic poisoning of livestock with fluorides that blacken and soften developing teeth and reduce bones to a chalky brittleness; most often caused by ingestion of forage contaminants near large aluminum plants.

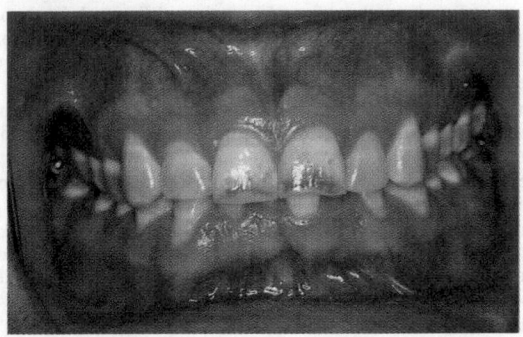

dental fluorosis: dentition exhibiting diffuse white and opaque enamel, with demonstrated areas of brown discoloration, in a patient with chronic ingestion of excess fluoride

chronic endemic f., f. caused by excessive fluorine in the natural water supply, as seen in parts of India; osteosclerosis with ankylosis of the spine may develop.

flu·o·ro·u·ra·cil (flōr-ō-ū′ră-sil). A pyrimidine analog; an antineoplastic effective in the treatment of some carcinomas; the cells of certain neoplasms incorporate uracil into ribonucleic acid more readily than do normal tissue cells. SEE ALSO floxuridine.

flu·o·sol-DA (flu′ō-sol). Experimental perfluorochemical solution under investigation as an artificial blood substitute.

flu·ox·e·tine hy·dro·chlo·ride (floo-oks′ĕ-tēn). An oral antidepressant; selectively prevents serotonin reuptake.

flu·ox·y·mes·ter·one (floo-ok-sē-mes′ter-ōn). An orally effective synthetic halogenated steroid, related in chemical structure and pharmacologic action to methyltestosterone, but more potent.

flu·pen·tix·ol (floo-pen-tik′sol). A neuroleptic.

flu·per·o·lone ac·e·tate (floo-per′ŏ-lōn). A synthetic corticosteroid.

flu·phen·a·zine (floo-fen′ă-zēn). A tranquilizer used as an antipsychotic and neuroleptic agent.

f. enanthate, a long-acting antipsychotic, used parenterally.

f. hydrochloride, an antipsychotic, used in the management of acute and chronic schizophrenia, involutional, senile, and toxic psychoses, and the manic phase of manic-depressive psychosis.

flu·pred·nis·o·lone (floo-pred-nis′ŏ-lōn). A glucocorticoid with anti-inflammatory activity and toxicity similar to those of cortisol.

flur·an·dren·o·lide (floor-an-dren′ŏ-līd). An anti-inflammatory glucocorticoid used in topical preparations.

flur·az·e·pam hy·dro·chlo·ride (floor-az′ĕ-pam). An oral hypnotic and sedative of the benzodiazepine series.

flur·bi·pro·fen (floor-bi′prō-fen). A nonsteroidal anti-inflamma-

tory agent with analgesic, anti-inflammatory, and antipyretic actions, similar to ibuprofen.

flur·o·ges·tone ac·e·tate (floor-ō-jes′tōn). A progestational agent.

flur·oth·yl (floor′ō-thil). An inhalant convulsant; produces grand mal convulsions.

flur·ox·ene (floor-ok′sēn). A volatile, halogenated inhalation anesthetic. SYN 2,2,2-trifluoroethyl vinyl.

flush (flŭsh). **1.** To wash out with a full stream of fluid. **2.** A transient erythema due to heat, exertion, stress, or disease. **3.** Flat, or even with another surface, as a f. stoma.

carcinoid f., periodic hyperemia (flushing) of the skin of the face and other parts of the body seen in patients with a carcinoid tumor; the tumors elaborate a variety of monoamines and peptide hormones, but the exact cause of the flush is uncertain; flush can be precipitated by alcohol, food, stress, or palpation of the liver.

hectic f., redness of the face associated with a rise of temperature in various fevers.

histamine f., vasodilation and erythema occurring as a result of release of histamine; thought to be a factor in genesis of f. of carcinoid syndrome.

hot f., colloquialism for a vasomotor symptom of the climacteric characterized by sudden vasodilation with a sensation of heat, usually involving the face and neck, and upper part of the chest. Cf. hot *flash.*

malar f., localized hectic f. and warmth of the malar eminences, often occurring in tuberculosis and sometimes seen in rheumatic fever or systemic lupus erythematosus.

flu·tam·ide (floo′tă-mīd). A nonsteroidal synthetic antiandrogen used in the treatment of prostatic cancer; antineoplastic (hormonal).

flut·ter (flŭt′er). Agitation; tremulousness. [A.S. *floterian,* to float about]

atrial f., auricular f., rapid regular atrial contractions occurring usually at rates between 250 and 330 per minute (Type I atrial f.) and often producing "saw-tooth" waves in the electrocardiogram, particularly leads II, III, and aVF. Type II atrial f. is at rates of 330–450 per minute. Unlike Type I, it cannot be terminated by overdrive pacing.

diaphragmatic f., rapid rhythmical contractions (average, 150 per minute) of the diaphragm, simulating atrial f. clinically and sometimes electrocardiographically.

impure f., mixture of atrial flutter (FF) waves and fibrillation (ff) waves in the electrocardiogram. SYN fibrilloflutter, flitter, flutter-fibrillation.

ocular f., a spontaneous, brief, intermittent, horizontal oscillation of the eyes occurring during fixation; it often coexists with ocular dysmetria in cerebellar syndromes.

ventricular f., a form of rapid ventricular tachycardia in which the electrocardiographic complexes assume a regular undulating pattern without distinct QRS and T waves.

flut·ter-fi·bril·la·tion. SYN impure *flutter.*

flux (flŭks). **1.** The discharge of a fluid material in large amount from a cavity or surface of the body. SEE ALSO diarrhea. **2.** Material discharged from the bowels. **3.** A material used to remove oxides from the surface of molten metal and to protect it when casting; serves a similar purpose in soldering operations. Also, an ingredient in dental porcelain that by its lower melting temperature helps to bond the silica particles. **4** (*J*). The moles of a substance crossing through a unit area of a boundary layer or membrane per unit of time. SYN flux density (1). **5.** Bidirectional movement of a substance at a membrane or surface. **6.** In diagnostic radiology, photon fluence per unit time. **7.** The strength of a field of force (e.g., magnetic) orthogonal to a unit area. **8.** The rate of chemical or physical transformation or translocation of a substance per unit time. [L. *fluxus,* a flow]

luminous f., the quantity of light emitted from a point source in a given time; its unit is the lumen.

net f., the difference between the two unidirectional f.'s.

unidirectional f., the f. of a substance from one surface of a boundary layer or membrane to the other, disregarding any coun-

fl

terbalancing f. in the other direction, as measured by tracer technique.

fly (flī). A two-winged insect in the order Diptera. Important f.'s include *Simulium* (black f.), *Calliphora* (bluebottle f.), *Piophila casei* (cheese f.), *Chrysops* (deer f.), *Siphona irritans* (horn f.), *Fannia scolaris* (latrine f.), *Oestrus ovis* and *Gasterophilus hemorrhoidalis* (nose f.), *Cochliomyia hominivorax* (primary screw-worm f.) and *C. macellaria* (secondary screw-worm f.), *Stomoxys calcitrans* (stable f.), *Glossina* (tsetse f.), and members of the insect order Trichoptera. For some types of flies not listed as subentries here (usually written as one word), see the full name (e.g., blowfly, botfly, gadfly, horsefly, housefly). [A.S. *fleóge*]

flesh f., genera of f.'s including *Wohlfahrtia*, *Sarcophaga*, and *Parasarcophaga* that feed on feces and decaying meat or fish; can cause human disease.

heel f., SEE botfly.

louse f.'s, pupiparous, dorsoventrally flattened dipterous ectoparasites of the family Hippoboscidae. SEE ALSO *Hippobosca*.

mangrove f., species of *Chrysops* in Africa, vectors of *Loa loa*; e.g., *Chrysops silacea*.

Russian f., Spanish f., SYN cantharis.

warble f., SEE botfly.

Flynn, P., U.S. physician. SEE F.-Aird *syndrome*; F. *phenomenon*.

Fm Symbol for fermium.

FMD Abbreviation for foot-and-mouth *disease*.

fMet Abbreviation for *N*-formylmethionine.

fMet-tRNA Abbreviation for formylmethionyl tRNA.

FMLH Abbreviation for familial hemophagocytic lymphohistiocytosis.

FMN Abbreviation for *flavin* mononucleotide.

FMR1. SYN fragile X *syndrome*.

FNA Abbreviation for fine needle aspiration biopsy.

foam (fōm). **1.** Masses of small bubbles on the surface of a liquid. **2.** To produce such bubbles. **3.** Masses of air cells in a solid or semisolid, as in f. rubber.

human fibrin f., a dry artificial sponge of human fibrin prepared by clotting with thrombin a f. of a solution of human fibrinogen; the clotted f. is dried from the frozen state and heated; used as a topical anticoagulant.

fo·cal (fō'kăl). **1.** Denoting a focus. **2.** Relating to a localized area.

fo·cal spot size. The measured size of a focal spot of an x-ray tube, a function of the actual size of the cathode and the angulation of the anode surface. SEE focal *spot*.

fo·ci (fō'sī). Plural of focus.

fo·cim·e·ter (fō-sim'ĕ-ter). SYN lensometer.

fo·cus, pl. **fo·ci** (fō'kŭs, fō'sī). **1 (F).** The point at which the light rays meet after passing through a convex lens. **2.** The center, or the starting point, of a disease process. [L. a hearth]

conjugate foci, two points so related to a lens or concave mirror that an image at one point is focused at the other, and vice versa.

Ghon f., SYN Ghon *tubercle*.

natural f. of infection, an ecosystem in which an infectious agent normally persists in nature; e.g., yellow fever virus in a jungle monkey-*Haemagogus* mosquito ecosystem.

principal f., the real or virtual meeting point of rays passing into a lens parallel to its axis.

real f., the point of meeting of convergent rays.

virtual f., the point from which divergent rays seem to proceed, or that at which they would meet if prolonged backward.

fo·drin (fō'drin). A spectrin-like protein that cross-links adjacent actin filaments in vertebrate cells.

Fogarty, Thomas J., U.S. thoracic surgeon, *1934. SEE F. embolectomy *catheter, clamp*.

fog·ging (fog'ing). A method of refraction in which accommodation is relaxed by overcorrection with a convex spherical lens.

fo·go sel·va·gem (fō'gō sel'vă-jem). A form of pemphigus foliaceus, occurring in southern Brazil, in which the lesions are bullous, appear localized to the face and upper trunk, become widespread, variegated, erythrodermic, and exfoliative, and are immunologically indistinguishable from pemphigus foliaceus or vulgaris. SYN Brazilian pemphigus, wildfire. [Pg. wild fire]

foil (foyl). An extremely thin pliable sheet of metal.

Foix, Charles, French neurologist, 1882–1927. SEE F.-Alajouanine *myelitis, syndrome;* F.-Cavany-Marie *syndrome*.

fo·late (fō'lāt). A salt or ester of folic acid.

FOLD

fold (fōld) [TA]. **1.** A ridge or margin apparently formed by the doubling back of a lamina. SYN plica. **2.** In the embryo, a transient elevation or reduplication of tissue in the form of a lamina.

adipose f.'s of the pleura, SYN fatty f.'s of pleura.

alar f.'s of intrapatellar synovial fold [TA], winglike fat-filled lateral and medial fringes or expansions of the infrapatellar synovial f. SYN plicae alares plicae synovialis infrapatellaris.

amnionic f., a f. of amnionic membrane enclosing the yolk stalk and extending from the point of insertion of the umbilical cord to the yolk sac; in reptiles and birds it is the reflected edge of the amnion where it folds over to cover the embryo during early development. SYN Schultze f.

ampullary f.'s of uterine tube, one of the f.'s of mucous membrane at the fimbriated extremity of the uterine tube. SYN plicae ampullares tubae uterinae.

anterior axillary f., bounds axilla anteriorly; formed by skin and fascia overlying inferior border of pectoralis major muscle.

aryepiglottic f. [TA], a prominent fold of mucous membrane stretching between the lateral margin of the epiglottis and the arytenoid cartilage on either side; it encloses the aryepiglottic muscle. SYN plica aryepiglottica [TA], arytenoepiglottidean f.

arytenoepiglottidean f., SYN aryepiglottic f.

axillary f., one of the folds of skin and muscular tissue bounding the axilla anteriorly and posteriorly. SYN plica axillaris.

caval f., a f. near the base on the right side of the dorsal mesentery, in which a primordial segment of the inferior vena cava develops between the right subcardinal vein and vessels within the liver.

cecal f.'s [TA], the two peritoneal folds that border the retrocecal fossa. SYN plicae cecales [TA].

f. of chorda tympani, the fold of mucosa that surrounds the chorda tympani nerve in its course through the tympanic cavity. SYN plica chordae tympani.

ciliary f.'s [TA], a number of low ridges in the furrows between the ciliary processes; together with the processes they constitute the corona ciliaris. SYN plicae ciliares [TA].

circular f.'s of small intestine [TA], the numerous folds of the mucous membrane of the small intestine, running transversely for about two-thirds of the circumference of the gut. SYN plicae circulares intestini tenuis [TA], Kerckring f.'s, Kerckring valves, valvulae conniventes.

Dennie-Morgan f., a f. or line below both lower eyelids caused by edema in atopic dermatitis. SYN Dennie line.

dinucleotide f., a structural domain in certain proteins that binds NAD^+ or $NADP^+$. SYN dinucleotide domain.

Douglas f., SYN rectouterine f.

Duncan f.'s, the f.'s on the peritoneal surface of the uterus immediately after delivery.

duodenojejunal f., ✕official alternate term for superior duodenal f.

duodenomesocolic f., ✕official alternate term for inferior duodenal f.

epicanthal f., SYN palpebronasal f.

epigastric f., SYN lateral umbilical f.

epiglottic f.'s, one of the three f.'s of mucous membrane passing between the tongue and the epiglottis, lateral glossoepiglottic f. on either side, and median glossoepiglottic f. centrally. SYN plicae epiglotticae.

falciform retinal f., a congenital f. from the disk to the ciliary region in the inferior temporal quadrant of the retina.

fatty f.'s of pleura, lobules of fat enveloped in the pleura, chiefly in the neighborhood of the costomediastinal sinus. SYN adipose f.'s of the pleura, plicae adiposae pleurae.

fimbriated f. of inferior surface of tongue [TA], one of several folds running outward from the frenulum on the undersurface of the tongue. SYN plica fimbriata faciei inferioris linguae [TA].

gastric f.'s [TA], characteristic folds of the gastric mucosa, especially evident when the stomach is contracted. SYN plicae gastricae [TA], gastric rugae☆, ruga gastrica, rugae of stomach.

gastropancreatic f.'s [TA], the folds of peritoneum in the omental bursa that encase the hepatic and left gastric arteries as these vessels pass toward their destinations. SYN plicae gastropancreaticae [TA].

genital f., SYN urogenital *ridge.*

giant gastric f.'s, enlarged gastric submucosal ridges covered by hyperplastic mucosa, as seen in Zollinger-Ellison syndrome, Ménétrièr disease, and hypertrophic hypersecretory gastropathy.

glossopalatine f., SYN palatoglossal *arch.*

gluteal f. [TA], a prominent f. that marks the upper limit of the thigh from the lower limit of the buttock; it coincides with the lower border of the gluteus maximus muscle; the furrow between the buttock and thigh. SYN sulcus gluteus [TA], gluteal furrow.

Guérin f., SYN *valve* of navicular fossa.

Hasner f., SYN lacrimal f.

head f., a ventral folding of the cephalic extremity in the embryonic disk, so that the brain lies rostrad to the mouth and pericardium.

Houston f.'s, SYN transverse f.'s of rectum.

ileocecal f. [TA], a fold of peritoneum bounding the ileocecal or ileoappendicular fossa. SYN plica ileocecalis [TA], Treves f.

incudal f., a variable fold of mucosa that passes from the roof of the tympanic cavity to the body and short limb of the incus. SYN plica incudis.

inferior duodenal f. [TA], a fold of peritoneum bounding the inferior duodenal recess. SYN plica duodenalis inferior [TA], duodenomesocolic f.☆, plica duodenomesocolica☆.

infrapatellar synovial f. [TA], a fold of synovial membrane extending from below the level of the articular surface of the patella to the anterior part of the intercondylar fossa. SYN plica synovialis infrapatellaris [TA], plica synovialis patellaris.

inguinal f., SYN *plica* inguinalis.

inguinal aponeurotic f., SYN inguinal *falx.*

interarytenoid f., the soft tissue between the arytenoid cartilages. SYN posterior commissure of the larynx.

interdigital f.'s, SYN *web* of fingers/toes.

interureteric f., SYN interureteric *crest.*

f.'s of iris [TA], numerous very fine, almost microscopic, radial folds on the posterior surface of the iris that extend around the pupillary margin. SYN plicae iridis [TA].

Kerckring f.'s, SYN circular f.'s of small intestine.

Kohlrausch f.'s, SYN transverse f.'s of rectum.

labioscrotal f.'s, lateral f.'s at either side of the embryonic cloacal membrane that develop into either the scrotum or the labia majora.

lacrimal f. [TA], a fold of mucous membrane guarding the lower opening of the nasolacrimal duct. SYN plica lacrimalis [TA], Hasner f., Huschke valve, Rosenmüller valve.

f. of laryngeal nerve, SYN f. of superior laryngeal nerve.

lateral f.'s, ventral foldings of the lateral margins of the embryonic disk, the development of which helps establish the definitive embryonic body form.

lateral glossoepiglottic f. [TA], the fold of mucous membrane that extends from the margin of the epiglottis to the pharyngeal wall and base of the tongue on each side, forming the lateral boundary of the epiglottic valleculae. SYN plica glossoepiglottica lateralis [TA], pharyngoepiglottic f.

lateral nasal f., SYN lateral nasal *prominence.*

lateral umbilical f. [TA], the ridge on the peritoneal surface of the anterior abdominal wall formed by the inferior epigastric vessels. SYN plica umbilicalis lateralis [TA], epigastric f., plica epigastrica.

f. of left vena cava [TA], a pericardial fold lying between the left oblique vein of the atrium and the left superior pulmonary vein containing the obliterated remains of the left superior vena cava. SYN plica venae cavae sinistrae [TA], Marshall vestigial f., vestigial f.

longitudinal f. of duodenum [TA], a fold of mucosa on the medial wall of the descending part of the duodenum above the major duodenal papilla, probably caused by the relation to the common bile duct. SYN plica longitudinalis duodeni [TA].

malar f., an ill-defined groove in the skin that extends downward and medially from the lateral canthus.

mallear f.'s [TA], two ligamentous bands, anterior and posterior, making folds on the tympanic side of the tympanic membrane extending from each extremity of the tympanic notch to the malleolar prominence; they mark the boundary between the tense and the flaccid portions of the tympanic membrane. SYN plicae malleares (anterior et posterior) [TA], plica membranae tympani.

mammary f., SYN mammary *ridge.*

Marshall vestigial f., SYN f. of left vena cava.

medial canthic f., ☆official alternate term for palpebronasal f.

medial nasal f., SYN medial nasal *prominence.*

medial umbilical f. [TA], a fold of peritoneum on the lower part of the anterior abdominal wall that covers the obliterated umbilical artery on either side of the urachus. SYN plica umbilicalis medialis [TA], plica hypogastrica.

median glossoepiglottic f. [TA], a fold of mucous membrane in the midline that extends from the back of the tongue to the epiglottis, forming the medial boundary of the epiglottic valleculae. SYN plica glossoepiglottica mediana [TA], frenulum epiglottidis, middle glossoepiglottic f.

median umbilical f. [TA], a fold of peritoneum on the anterior wall of the abdomen covering the urachus, or remains of the allantoic stalk. SYN middle umbilical f., plica urachi, urachal f.

medullary f.'s, SYN neural f.'s.

mesonephric f., SYN mesonephric *ridge.*

middle glossoepiglottic f., SYN median glossoepiglottic f.

middle transverse rectal f., SEE transverse f.'s of rectum.

middle umbilical f., SYN median umbilical f.

mongolian f., SYN palpebronasal f.

mucobuccal f., the line of flexure of the mucous membrane as it passes from the mandible or maxillae to the cheek.

mucosal f.'s of gallbladder [TA], the interlacing folds of the mucosa that produce a honeycomb appearance in the interior of the gallbladder. SYN plicae mucosae vesicae biliaris [TA], rugae of gallbladder☆, rugae vesicae biliaris☆.

nail f., SYN nail *wall.*

nasojugal f., a shallow groove in the skin that extends downward and laterally from the medial canthus.

Nélaton f., SEE transverse f.'s of rectum.

neural f.'s, the elevated margins of the neural groove. SYN medullary f.'s.

opercular f., tissue forming a bridge or an adhesion between the tonsil and the anterior pillar of the fauces.

palmate f.'s of cervical canal, the two longitudinal ridges, anterior and posterior, in the mucous membrane lining the cervix uteri, from which numerous secondary folds, or rugae, branch off. SYN plicae palmatae canalis cervicis uteri [TA], arbor vitae uteri, lyra uterina.

palpebronasal f. [TA], a fold of skin extending from the root of the nose to the medial termination of the eyebrow, overlapping the medial angle of the eye; its presence is normal in fetal life and in some Asians. SYN plica palpebronasalis [TA], medial canthic f.☆, epicanthal f., epicanthus, mongolian f.

paraduodenal f. [TA], a sickle-shaped fold of peritoneum sometimes found arching between the left side of the duodenojejunal flexure and the medial border of the left kidney; its right free edge contains the ascending branch of the left colic artery and inferior mesenteric vein; forms anterior boundary of the paraduodenal

fo

recess. SEE ALSO paraduodenal *recess.* SYN plica paraduodenalis [TA], Treitz arch.

pharyngoepiglottic f., SYN lateral glossoepiglottic f.

pleuropericardial f., a tissue f. jutting into the right or left embryonic pericardioperitoneal canal; it separates the developing pericardium from the pleural cavity and is formed by the growth of the common cardinal veins to the midline of the body. SYN pericardiopleural membrane, pleuropericardial membrane.

pleuroperitoneal f., a tissue f. jutting into the caudal portion of the embryonic pericardioperitoneal canal; it develops into the dorsal portion of the definitive diaphragm and is formed by the lungs growing caudally and the liver expanding cranially. SYN pleuroperitoneal membrane.

posterior axillary f., bounds axilla posteriorly; formed by skin and fascia overlying latissimus dorsi and teres major muscles and tendons of insertion.

presplenic f., a fan-shaped f. of peritoneum that passes from the gastrosplenic ligament near the lower end of the spleen to the phrenicocolic ligament with which it blends. It contains branches of the splenic or the left gastroepiploic artery.

rectal f.'s, SYN transverse f.'s of rectum.

rectouterine f. [TA], a fold of peritoneum, containing the rectouterine muscle, passing from the sacrum to the base of the broad ligament on either side, forming the lateral boundary of the rectouterine (Douglas) pouch. SYN plica rectouterina [TA], Douglas f., sacrouterine f.

rectovesical f., SYN sacrovesical f.

retinal f., a congenital or secondary f., consequent to membrane contraction, producing star-shaped, meridional, or circular f.'s on the retina.

retroauricular f., skin crease made by the junction of the pinna and the postauricular skin.

retrotarsal f., SYN conjunctival *fornix.*

Rindfleisch f.'s, semilunar f.'s of the serous surface of the pericardium, embracing the beginning of the aorta.

sacrogenital f.'s, peritoneal f.'s that extend backward from the sides of the bladder of the male or uterus of the female on either side of the rectum to the sacrum, forming the lateral boundaries of the rectovesical pouch. SEE sacrouterine f., sacrovesical f.

sacrouterine f., SYN rectouterine f.

sacrovaginal f., the lower part of the sacrouterine f. SYN plica rectovaginalis.

sacrovesical f., the f. of peritoneum in the male that bounds the rectovesical pouch laterally. SYN rectovesical f.

salpingopalatine f. [TA], a ridge of mucous membrane passing from the anterior border of the opening of the auditory (eustachian) tube to the palate. SYN plica salpingopalatina [TA], plica tubopalatina.

salpingopharyngeal f. [TA], a ridge of mucous membrane extending from the lower end of the tubal elevation along the wall of the pharynx overlying the salpingopharyngeus muscle. SYN plica salpingopharyngea [TA].

Schultze f., SYN amnionic f.

semilunar f. [TA], inconsistent curved fold connecting the palatoglossal arch and palatopharyngeal arch above the supratonsillar fossa; when present, it always contains lymphoid tissue. SYN plica semilunaris [TA].

semilunar f.'s of colon [TA], one of the folds of the wall of the colon between sacculations. SYN plicae semilunares coli [TA], plicae semilunares of colon.

semilunar conjunctival f., SYN *plica* semilunaris of conjunctiva.

spiral f. of cystic duct [TA], a series of crescentic folds of mucous membrane in the upper part of the cystic duct, arranged in a somewhat spiral manner. SYN plica spiralis ductus cystici [TA], Amussat valve, Heister valve, spiral valve of cystic duct, valvula spiralis.

stapedial f., SYN f. of stapes.

f. of stapes [TA], a reflection of the delicate mucous membrane from the posterior wall of the tympanic cavity that covers the stapes. SYN plica stapedialis, stapedial f.

sublingual f. [TA], an elevation in the floor of the mouth beneath the tongue, on either side, marking the site of the sublingual gland. SYN plica sublingualis [TA].

superior duodenal f. [TA], a fold of peritoneum bounding the superior duodenal recess. SYN plica duodenalis superior [TA], duodenojejunal f.✭, plica duodenojejunalis✭.

f. of superior laryngeal nerve [TA], the slight fold of mucosa in the piriform recess of the pharynx that encloses the superior laryngeal nerve. SYN plica nervi laryngei superioris [TA], f. of laryngeal nerve.

synovial f., a ridge or projection of the synovial membrane of a joint extending toward or between the two articular surfaces. SYN plica synovialis.

tail f., the ventral folding of the caudal extremity of the embryonic disk.

tarsal f., the f. marking the attachment of the levator palpebrae superioris muscle into the skin of the upper eyelid.

transverse palatine f. [TA], a masticatory vestige on the hard palate; one of several irregular, sometimes branching, crests of soft tissue that radiate from the region of the incisive papillae at their most anterior parts and extend a slight distance backward, crossing the hard palate and reaching laterally for variable distances. SYN plica palatina transversa [TA], ruga palatina, transverse palatine ridge.

transverse f.'s of rectum [TA], the three or four crescentic f.'s placed horizontally in the rectal mucous membrane; the superior rectal f. is situated near the beginning of the rectum on the left side; the middle rectal f. (Houston or Kohlrausch f.) is most prominent and consistent and projects from the right side about 8 cm above the anus (approximately the level of the floor of the rectouterine or rectovesical pouch); the inferior rectal f. is on the left side about 5 cm above the anus. SYN plicae transversales recti [TA], Houston f.'s, Kohlrausch f.'s, plicae recti, rectal f.'s, rectal valves.

transverse vesical f., a duplication of peritoneum passing over the empty bladder, but obliterated when the viscus is full. SYN plica vesicalis transversa.

Treves f., SYN ileocecal f.

triangular f. [TA], an inconstant f. of mucous membrane anterior to the palatine tonsil arising from the palatoglossal arch. SYN plica triangularis [TA].

urachal f., SYN median umbilical f.

ureteric f., SYN interureteric *crest.*

urorectal f., SYN urorectal *septum,* urorectal *membrane.*

f.'s of uterine tubes [TA], many longitudinal folds in the mucous membrane of the uterine (fallopian) tube. SYN plicae tubariae tubae uterinae [TA].

uterovesical f., SYN uterovesical *ligament.*

vascular f. of the cecum [TA], a peritoneal fold that arches over a branch of the ileocolic artery and bounds in front a narrow recess, the superior ileocecal (or ileocolic) recess. SYN plica cecalis vascularis [TA].

Vater f., a f. of mucous membrane in the duodenum just above the greater duodenal papilla.

ventricular f., SYN vestibular f.

vestibular f. [TA], one of the pair of folds of mucous membrane overlying the vestibular ligaments that stretch across the laryngeal cavity from the angle of the thyroid cartilage to the arytenoid cartilage; the right and left pair enclose a space called the rima vestibuli or false glottis, and form the superior boundary of the laryngeal ventricle. SYN plica vestibularis [TA], false vocal cord, plica ventricularis, ventricular band of larynx, ventricular f.

vestigial f., SYN f. of left vena cava.

vocal f. [TA], the sharp-edged fold of mucous membrane overlying the vocal ligament and stretching along either wall of the larynx from the angle between the laminae of the thyroid cartilage to the vocal process of the arytenoid cartilage; the vocal folds are the agents concerned in voice production. SYN plica vocalis [TA], chorda vocalis, Ferrein cords, labium vocale, true vocal cord, vocal cord, vocal shelf.

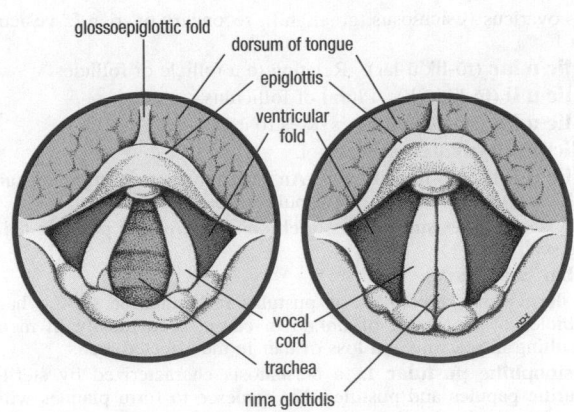

glossoepiglottic fold
dorsum of tongue
epiglottis
ventricular fold
vocal cord
trachea
rima glottidis

vocal cords: interior of the larynx, as seen with laryngoscope; (left) rima glottidis wide open, (right) rima glottidis closed

Foley, Frederic E.B., U.S. urologist, 1891–1966. SEE F. *catheter*, Y-plasty *pyeloplasty*.

fo·lia (fō'lē-ă). Plural of folium.

fo·li·a·ceous (fō-lē-ā'shŭs). SYN foliate.

fo·li·ar (fō'lē-ăr). SYN foliate.

fo·li·ate (fō'lē-āt). Pertaining to or resembling a leaf or leaflet. SYN foliaceous, foliar, foliose.

fo·lic ac·id (fō'lik). **1.** A collective term for pteroylglutamic acids and their oligoglutamic acid conjugates. A collective term for pteroylglutamic acids and their oligoglutamic acid conjugates. *N*-[p-[[(2-Amino-4-hydroxypteridin-6- yl)methyl]amino]benzoyl]-L(+)-glutamic acid; specifically, pteroylmonoglutamic acid; the growth factor for *Lactobacillus casei*, and a member of the vitamin B complex necessary for the normal production of red blood cells; present, with or without L(+)- glutamic acid moieties, in peptide linkages in liver, green vegetables, and yeast; used to treat folate deficiency and megaloblastic anemia. SEE ALSO homocysteine. **2.** The growth factor for *Lactobacillus casei*, and a member of the vitamin B complex necessary for the normal production of red blood cells. It is a hemopoietic vitamin present, with or without L-(+)-glutamic acid moieties, in peptide linkages in liver, green vegetables, and yeast; used to treat folate deficiency and megaloblastic anemia, and to assist in lowering homocysteine levels. SYN *Lactobacillus casei* factor, liver *Lactobacillus casei* factor, pteroylmonoglutamic acid. [L. *folium*, leaf, + -ic]

> Recent research has yielded a clearer understanding of the role of folic acid in human metabolism, identified health problems associated with dietary deficiency of folic acid, provided evidence of therapeutic benefits of folic acid supplementation, and suggested that dietary allowances of folic acid formerly recommended (200 µg/day for men and 180 µg/day for women) are insufficient for certain persons, including pregnant women. Natural sources of folic acid include whole-grain breads and cereals, orange juice, lentils, beans, yeast, liver, and green leafy vegetables such as broccoli, kale, and spinach. Folic acid and cobalamin (vitamin B_{12}) serve as components of coenzymes in 1-carbon reactions such as the methylation of homocysteine to methionine. Folic acid deficiency results in macrocytic anemia due to impairment of erythrocyte synthesis and is associated with elevation of plasma homocysteine levels, a risk factor for cardiovascular disease, including coronary atherosclerosis, stroke, and thromboembolism. Deficiency of folic acid in pregnancy is associated with an increased risk of neural tube defects such as spina bifida and anencephaly as well as an increased risk of preterm delivery and low birth weight. Persons with inherited deficiency of the enzyme 5,10 methylenetetrahydrofolic acid reductase have increased needs for dietary folic acid. The prevalence of the homozygous form of this deficiency may exceed 10% of the general population. Intake of folic acid, pyridoxine (vitamin B_6), and cobalamin above the current recommended dietary allowance has been associated with a substantially lower risk of coronary artery disease and of neural tube defects. Nutritionists recommend at least 400 µg/day of folic acid for all persons, and 1 mg/day or more for pregnant women and those with elevated plasma homocysteine levels. The Food and Drug Administration requires fortification of grains and cereals with folic acid.

fo·lie (fō-lē'). Old term for madness or insanity. [Fr. folly]

f. à deux (ă-du), identical or similar mental disorders, such as a paranoid fixation, usually affecting two members of the same family living together. SYN shared psychotic disorder. [Fr. two]

f. du doute (du-doot), an excessive doubting about all the affairs of life and a morbid scrupulousness concerning minutiae. [Fr. from doubt]

f. du pourquoi (poor-kwah'), a psychopathologic tendency to ask questions. [Fr. why]

f. gémellaire (zha-mel-ār'), a psychosis appearing simultaneously, or nearly so, in twins, who are not necessarily living together or intimately associated at the time. [Fr. relating to twins]

Folin, Otto K.O., U.S. biochemist, 1867–1934. SEE F. *reaction*, *test*; F.-Looney *test*.

fo·li·nate (fō'li-nāt). A salt or ester of folinic acid.

fo·lin·ic ac·id (fō-lin'ik). **1.** The active form of folic acid that acts as a formyl group carrier in transformylation reactions; the calcium salt, leucovorin calcium, has therapeutic use. **2.** The term is occasionally applied to other folates. SYN citrovorum factor, leucovorin.

fo·li·ose (fō'lē-ōs). SYN foliate.

fo·li·um, pl. **fo·lia** (fō'lē-ŭm, -lē-ă) [TA]. A broad, thin, leaflike structure. [L. a leaf]

fo'lia cerebel'li [TA], SYN folia of cerebellum.

folia of cerebellum [TA], the narrow, leaf-like gyri of the cerebellar cortex. SEE ALSO f. of vermis. SYN folia cerebelli [TA].

fo'lia lin'guae, SYN foliate *papillae*, under *papilla*.

f. ver'mis [TA], SYN f. of vermis.

f. of vermis [TA], a small posterior subdivision of the superior vermis of the cerebellum consisting of lobule VIIA. SYN f. vermis [TA].

Folli, Folius. Cecilio (Caesilius), Venetian anatomist, 1615–1660. SEE Folli *process*, follian *process*.

fol·li·cle (fol'i-kl) [TA]. **1.** A more or less spherical mass of cells usually containing a cavity. **2.** A crypt or minute cul-de-sac or lacuna, such as the depression in the skin from which the hair emerges. SYN folliculus [TA]. [L. *folliculus*, a small sac, dim. of *follis*, a pair of bellows]

aggregated lymphatic f.'s of small intestine, SYN aggregated lymphoid *nodules* of small intestine, under *nodule*.

aggregated lymphatic f.'s of vermiform appendix, SYN aggregated lymphoid *nodules*, under *nodule*.

anovular ovarian f., a f. that does not contain an ovum.

antral f., SYN vesicular ovarian f.

atretic ovarian f., a f. that degenerates before coming to maturity; great numbers of such atretic f.'s occur in the ovary before puberty; in the sexually mature woman, several are formed each month. SYN corpus atreticum.

dental f., the dental sac with its enclosed odontogenic organ and developing tooth.

gastric f.'s, SYN gastric *glands*, under *gland*.

graafian f., SYN vesicular ovarian f.

growing ovarian f., a f. having several layers of proliferating follicular cells surrounding the ovum, but separated from it by an extracellular glycoprotein layer (zona pellucida).

hair f. [TA], a tubelike invagination of the epidermis from which the hair shaft develops and into which the sebaceous glands open; the follicle is lined by a cellular inner and outer root sheath of epidermal origin and is invested with a fibrous sheath derived from the dermis. SYN folliculus pili [TA].

intestinal f.'s, SYN intestinal *glands*, under *gland*.

fo

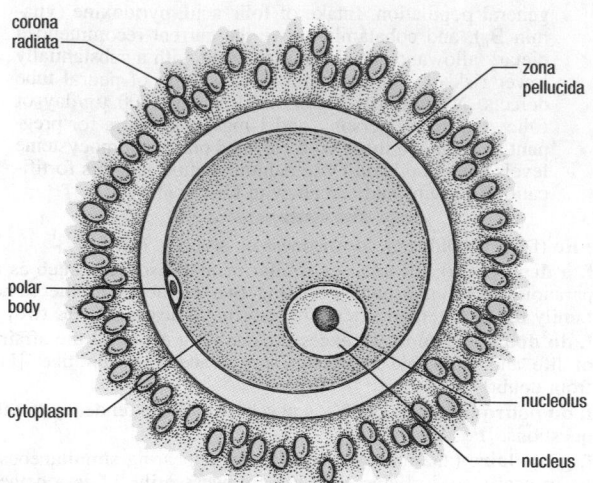

ovarian follicle: containing ovum

corona radiata — zona pellucida — polar body — cytoplasm — nucleolus — nucleus

Lieberkühn f.'s, SYN intestinal *glands,* under *gland.*

lingual f.'s, SYN *folliculi* linguales, under *folliculus.*

luteinized unruptured f., a f. that has undergone luteinization without prior rupture; once thought to cause infertility but now believed to occur equally often in fertile and infertile women.

lymphatic f.'s of larynx, SYN laryngeal lymphoid *nodules,* under *nodule.*

lymphatic f.'s of rectum, SYN *folliculi* lymphatici recti, under *folliculus.*

mature ovarian f., a f. ready for ovulation; in the human ovary its antrum attains a diameter of 6–8 mm and presents a surface bulge; a first maturation (meiotic) division of the ovum usually occurs just prior to the rupture of the f.

Montgomery f.'s, SYN areolar *glands,* under *gland.*

multilaminar primary f., a primary ovarian f. with two or more layers of cuboidal follicular cells investing the oocyte.

nabothian f., SYN nabothian *cyst.*

ovarian follicle, one of the spheroidal cell aggregations in the ovary containing an ovum.

polyovular ovarian f., a f. containing more than one ovum.

primary ovarian f., an ovarian f. before the appearance of an antrum; marked by developmental changes in the oocyte and follicular cells so that the latter form one or more layers of cuboidal or columnar cells; the f. becomes surrounded by a sheath of stroma, the theca. SYN folliculus ovaricus primarius.

primordial ovarian f., a f. in which the primordial oocyte is surrounded by a single layer of flattened follicular cells.

sebaceous f.'s, SYN sebaceous *glands,* under *gland.*

secondary ovarian f., SYN vesicular ovarian f.

solitary f.'s, SYN solitary lymphatic *nodules,* under *nodule.*

solitary lymphatic f.'s, SYN solitary lymphatic *nodules,* under *nodule.*

splenic lymph f.'s, small nodular masses of lymphoid tissue attached to the sides of the smaller arterial branches. SYN folliculi lymphatici lienales, malpighian bodies, malpighian corpuscles (2), malpighian glands, malpighian nodules, splenic corpuscles, splenic lymph nodules.

f.'s of thyroid gland, SYN *folliculi* glandulae thyroideae, under *folliculus.*

unilaminar primary f., a primary ovarian f. with a single layer of cuboidal follicular cells investing the oocyte.

vesicular f., SYN vesicular ovarian f.

vesicular ovarian f., a f. in which the oocyte attains its full size and is surrounded by an extracellular glycoprotein layer (zona pellucida) that separates it from a peripheral layer of follicular cells permeated by one or more fluid-filled antra; the theca of the f. develops into internal and external layers. SYN antral f., folliculus ovaricus vesiculosus, graafian f., secondary ovarian f., vesicular f.

fol·lic·u·lar (fŏ-lik'ū-lăr). Relating to a follicle or follicles.

fol·lic·u·li (fŏ-lik'ū-lī). Plural of folliculus.

fol·lic·u·lin (fō-lik'oo-lin). SYN estrone.

folliculin hydrate. SYN estriol.

fol·lic·u·li·tis (fŏ-lik-ū-lī'tis). An inflammatory reaction in hair follicles; the lesions may be papules or pustules.

f. absce'dens et suffo'diens, a chronic progressive pustular f. in the scalp.

f. bar'bae, SYN *tinea* barbae.

f. decal'vans, a papular or pustular inflammation of the hair follicles of the scalp, of unknown cause, seen mostly in men, resulting in scarring and loss of hair in the affected area.

eosinophilic pustular f., a dermatosis characterized by sterile pruritic papules and pustules that coalesce to form plaques with papulovesicular borders; spontaneous exacerbations and remissions may be accompanied by peripheral leukocytosis, eosinophilia, or both, and may result in eventual destruction of hair follicles and formation of eosinophilic abscesses. The disease has been reported in AIDS, and a possibly separate form of eosinophilic pustular f. occurs in infants. SYN Ofuji disease.

f. keloida'lis, SYN acne *keloid.*

f. na'res per'forans, inflammation of a hair follicle in the nose; the infection extends to, and perforates, the cutaneous surface.

perforating f., erythematous papules with a central keratin plug that are scattered on the arms, thighs, and buttocks; dermal fibers are seen in biopsies extending into the follicle; similar changes are seen especially in diabetics on hemodialysis. SEE ALSO *hyperkeratosis* follicularis et parafollicularis.

f. ulerythemato'sa reticula'ta, erythematous "ice-pick" or pitted scars on the cheeks; a scarring type of folliculitis, associated with keratosis pilaris and commonly inherited as an autosomal dominant trait.

fol·lic·u·lo·ma (fŏ-lik-ū-lō'mă). **1.** SYN granulosa cell *tumor.* **2.** Cystic enlargement of a graafian follicle.

fol·lic·u·lo·sis (fŏ-lik-ū-lō'sis). Presence of lymph follicles in abnormally great numbers.

fol·lic·u·lus, pl. **fol·lic·u·li** (fŏ-lik'ū-lŭs, -ū-lī) [TA]. SYN follicle. [L. a small sac, dim. of *follis,* bellows]

follic'uli glan'dulae thyroi'deae, the small spherical vesicular components of the thyroid gland lined with epithelium and containing colloid in varying amounts; the colloid serves for storage of the thyroid hormone precursor, thyroglobulin. SYN follicles of thyroid gland.

follic'uli lingua'les, collections of lymphoid tissue in the mucosa of the pharyngeal part of the tongue posterior to the terminal sulcus collectively forming the lingual tonsil. SYN lenticular papillae, lingual follicles.

follic'uli lymphat'ici aggrega'ti, SYN aggregated lymphoid *nodules* of small intestine, under *nodule.*

follic'uli lymphat'ici aggrega'ti appen'dicis vermifor'mis, SYN aggregated lymphoid *nodules,* under *nodule.*

folliculi lymphat'ici gas'trici, SYN gastric lymphoid *nodules,* under *nodule.*

follic'uli lymphat'ici laryn'gei, SYN laryngeal lymphoid *nodules,* under *nodule.*

follic'uli lymphat'ici liena'les, SYN splenic lymph *follicles,* under *follicle.*

follic'uli lymphat'ici rec'ti, scattered collections of lymphoid tissue in the wall of the rectum. SYN lymphatic follicles of rectum.

follic'uli lymphat'ici solita'rii, SYN solitary lymphatic *nodules,* under *nodule.*

f. lymphat'icus, SYN lymphoid *nodule.*

f. ovar'icus prima'rius, SYN primary ovarian *follicle.*

f. ovar'icus vesiculo'sus, SYN vesicular ovarian *follicle.*

f. pi'li [TA], SYN hair *follicle.*

Folling, Ivar A., Norwegian physician, 1888–1973. SEE F. *disease.*

fol·li·stat·in (fol-ĭ-stat-'n). A peptide synthesized by granulosa cells in response to FSH that suppresses FSH activity, probably by binding activins. [*follicle* + -*stat* + -*in*]

fol·li·tro·pin (fol-i-trō′pin). An acidic glycoprotein hormone of the anterior pituitary that stimulates the graafian follicles of the ovary and assists subsequently in follicular maturation and the secretion of estradiol; in the male, it stimulates the epithelium of the seminiferous tubules and is partially responsible for inducing spermatogenesis. SYN follicle-stimulating hormone, follicle-stimulating principle, gametokinetic hormone. [*follicle* + G. *tropē*, a turning, + -*in*]

Foltz, Jean C.E., French anatomist and ophthalmologist, 1822–1876. SEE F. *valvule.*

fo·men·ta·tion (fō-men-tā′shŭn). **1.** A warm application. SEE ALSO poultice, stupe. **2.** Application of warmth and moisture in the treatment of disease. [L. *fomento,* pp. -*atus,* to foment, fr. *fomentum,* a poultice, fr. *foveo,* to keep warm]

fo·mes, pl. **fom·i·tes** (fō′mēz, fōm′i-tēz). Objects, such as clothing, towels, and utensils that possibly harbor a disease agent and are capable of transmitting it; usually used in the plural. SYN fomite. [L. tinder, fr. *foveo,* to keep warm]

fo·mite (fō′mīt). SYN fomes. [L. *fomitis,* gen. of *fomes. See fomes.*]

fom·i·tes (fō′mi-tēz). Plural of fomes.

fo·na·zine mes·y·late (fō′nă-zēn). A serotonin inhibitor with muscle relaxant properties. SYN dimethothiazine mesylate.

Fonio, Anton, Swiss physician, 1881–1968. SEE F. *solution.*

Fonsecaea (fon-sē-sē′ă). A genus of fungi of which at least two species, *F. pedrosoi* and *F. compacta,* cause chromoblastomycosis.

Fontan, Francois M., French thoracic surgeon, *1929. SEE F. *procedure, operation.*

Fontana, Felice, Italian physiologist, 1730–1805. SEE F. *canal, spaces,* under *space.*

Fontana, Arturo, Italian dermatologist, 1873–1950. SEE F. *stain;* F.-Masson silver *stain;* Masson-F. ammoniac silver *stain.*

ℹ**fon·ta·nelle** (fon′tă-nel′) [NA]. One of several membranous intervals at the margins of the cranial bones in the infant. SEE cranial f.'s. SYN fonticulus. [Fr. dim. of *fontaine,* fountain, spring]

anterior f. [NA], a diamond-shaped membranous interval at the junction of the coronal, sagittal, and metopic sutures where the frontal angles of the parietal bones meet the two ununited halves of the frontal bone. SYN bregmatic f., fonticulus anterior, frontal f.

anterolateral f., SYN sphenoidal f.

bregmatic f., SYN anterior f.

Casser f., SYN mastoid f.

cranial f.'s [NA], the membranous intervals between the angles of the cranial bones in the infant; they include the midline anterior f. and posterior f., and the paired sphenoidal f. and mastoid f. SYN fonticuli cranii.

frontal f., SYN anterior f.

Gerdy f., SYN sagittal f.

mastoid f. [NA], the membranous interval on either side between the mastoid angle of the parietal bone, the petrous portion of the temporal bone, and the occipital bone. SYN fonticulus mastoideus [NA], fonticulus posterolateralis✩, Casser f., posterolateral f.

occipital f., SYN posterior f.

posterior f., a triangular interval at the union of the lambdoid and sagittal sutures where the occipital angles of the parietal bones meet the occipital. SYN fonticulus posterior, occipital f.

posterolateral f., SYN mastoid f.

sagittal f. [NA], an occasional f.-like defect in the sagittal suture in the newborn. SYN Gerdy f.

sphenoidal f. [NA], an irregularly shaped interval on either side where the frontal, sphenoidal angle of the parietal, squamous portion of the temporal and greater wing of the sphenoid meet. SYN fonticulus sphenoidalis [NA], fonticulus anterolateralis✩, anterolateral f.

fon·tic·u·lus, pl. **fon·tic·u·li** (fon-tik′ū-lŭs, -lī). SYN fontanelle. SEE cranial *fontanelles,* under *fontanelle.* [L. dim. of *fons* (font-), fountain, spring]

f. ante′rior, SYN anterior *fontanelle.*

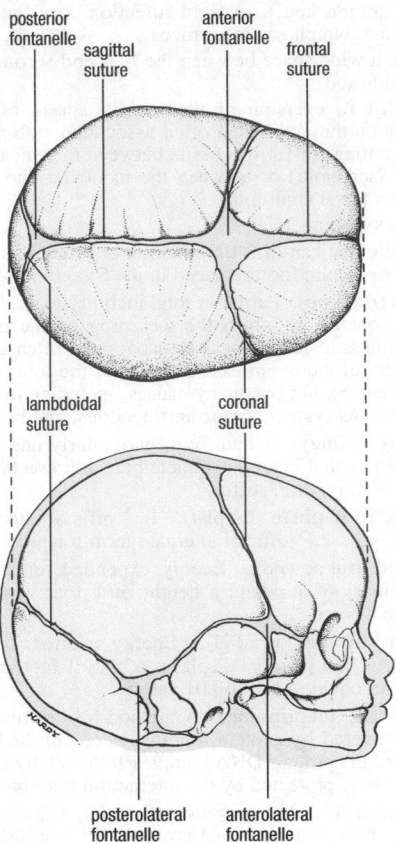

fontanelles and sutures of the fetal skull: (top) superior aspect, (bottom) lateral aspect

f. anterolatera′lis, ✩official alternate term for sphenoidal *fontanelle.*

fontic′uli cra′nii, SYN cranial *fontanelles,* under *fontanelle.*

f. mastoi′deus [NA], SYN mastoid *fontanelle.*

f. poste′rior, SYN posterior *fontanelle.*

f. posterolatera′lis, ✩official alternate term for mastoid *fontanelle.*

f. sphenoida′lis [NA], SYN sphenoidal *fontanelle.*

food (food). That which is eaten to supply necessary nutritive elements. [A.S. *fōda*]

Foot, N.C., 20th century U.S. pathologist. SEE F. reticulin impregnation *stain.*

foot (fut) [TA]. **1.** The lower, pedal, podalic, extremity of the leg. SYN pes (1). **2.** A unit of length, containing 12 inches, equal to 30.48 cm. [A.S. *fōt*]

athlete's f., SYN *tinea* pedis.

claw f., SEE clawfoot.

ℹ**club f.,** SEE *talipes* equinovarus.

contracted f., SYN *talipes* cavus.

drop f., SEE footdrop.

f. of hippocampus, the anterior thickened extremity of the hippocampus. SYN pes hippocampi [TA], digitationes hippocampi.

immersion f., a condition resulting from prolonged exposure to damp and cold; the extremity is initially cold and anesthetic, but on rewarming becomes hyperemic, paresthetic, and hyperhidrotic; recovery is often slow. SYN trench f.

Madura f., SYN mycetoma.

Morand f., a f. having eight toes.

mossy f., a profuse velvety papillomatous growth that develops large warty projections; caused by chronic lymphedema and stasis with maceration and associated infection. SYN lymphedematous keratoderma, lymphostatic verrucosis.

sandal f., a wide space between the first and second toes seen in Down syndrome.

spastic flat f., eversion of the f. with spasm of the muscles (peroneal) on the outer side; often associated with abnormal bars of bone cartilage or fibrous tissue between the calcaneum and the navicular (scaphoid) or between the navicular and the talus, resulting in a tarsal coalition.

trench f., SYN immersion f.

foot·can·dle (fut′kan-dl). Illumination or brightness equivalent to 1 lumen per square foot; replaced in the SI system by the candela.

foot·drop (fut′drop). Partial or total inability to dorsiflex the foot, as a consequence of which the toes drag on the ground during walking unless a steppage gait is used; most often ultimately due to weakness of the dorsiflexor muscles of the foot (especially the tibialis anterior), but has many causes, including disorders of the central nervous system, motor unit, tendons, and bones.

foot·ling (foot′ling). A fetal foot, particularly one that descends into the birth canal in an incomplete breech presentation. [foot, fr. A. S. *fot,* + *-ling,* dim. suffix]

foot·plate, foot-plate (fut′plāt). **1.** ✫official alternate term for *base* of stapes. **2.** ✫official alternate term for pedicel.

foot-pound (fut′pownd). Energy expended, or work done, in raising a mass of 1 pound a height of 1 foot vertically against gravitational force.

foot-pound·al (fut′pownd-ăl). Energy exerted, or work done, when a force of 1 poundal displaces a body 1 foot in the direction of the force; equal to about 0.01 calorie.

foot·print·ing (fŭt′print-ing). A method for determining the area of DNA covered by protein binding; accomplished by nuclease digestion of the protein-DNA complex followed by analysis of the region of DNA protected by the interaction with protein.

for·age (fōr-ahzh′). The operation of cutting a channel by surgical diathermy through an enlarged prostate. [Fr. boring]

FORAMEN

fo·ra·men, pl. **fo·ram·i·na** (fō-rā′men, fō-ram′i-nă) [TA]. An aperture or perforation through a bone or a membranous structure. SYN trema (1). [L. an aperture, fr. *foro,* to pierce]

foram′ina alveola′ria corporis maxillae [TA], SYN alveolar foramina of maxilla.

alveolar foramina of maxilla [TA], openings of the posterior dental canals on the infratemporal surface of the maxilla. SYN foramina alveolaria corporis maxillae [TA].

anterior condyloid f., SYN hypoglossal *canal.*

anterior palatine f., SYN greater palatine f.

aortic f., SYN aortic *hiatus.*

apical dental f., SYN apical f. of tooth.

apical f. of tooth [TA], the opening at the apex of the root of a tooth that gives passage to the nerve and blood vessels. SYN f. apicis dentis [TA], apical dental f., root f.

f. ap′icis den′tis [TA], SYN apical f. of tooth.

arachnoid f., SYN median *aperture* of fourth ventricle.

f. of Arnold, SYN f. petrosum.

blind f. of frontal bone, SYN f. cecum of frontal bone.

blind f. of the tongue, SYN f. cecum of tongue.

Bochdalek f., SYN pleuroperitoneal *hiatus.*

Botallo f., the orifice of communication between the two atria of the fetal heart. SEE ALSO f. ovale.

f. cae′cum medul′lae oblonga′tae [TA], a small triangular depression at the lower boundary of the pons between the pyramide that marks the upper limit of the anterior median fissure of the medulla oblongata. SYN f. caecum posterius, Vicq d'Azyr f.

carotid f., SYN *openings* of carotid canal, under *opening.*

cecal f. of frontal bone, SYN f. cecum of frontal bone.

cecal f. of the tongue, SYN f. cecum of tongue.

f. cecum of frontal bone [TA], blind or cecal f. of the frontal bone; the blind f. formed immediately anterior to the crista galli by a notch at the lower end of the frontal crest and its articulation with the ethmoid bone. It is insignificant postnatally, but gives passage to vessels during development. SYN f. cecum ossis frontalis [TA], blind f. of frontal bone, cecal f. of frontal bone.

f. ce′cum lin′guae [TA], SYN f. cecum of tongue.

f. ce′cum os′sis fronta′lis [TA], SYN f. cecum of frontal bone.

f. cae′cum poste′rius, SYN f. caecum medullae oblongatae.

f. cecum of tongue [TA], a median pit on the dorsum of the posterior part of the tongue, from which the limbs of a V-shaped furrow run forward and outward; it is the site of origin of the thyroid gland and subsequent thyroglossal duct in the embryo.

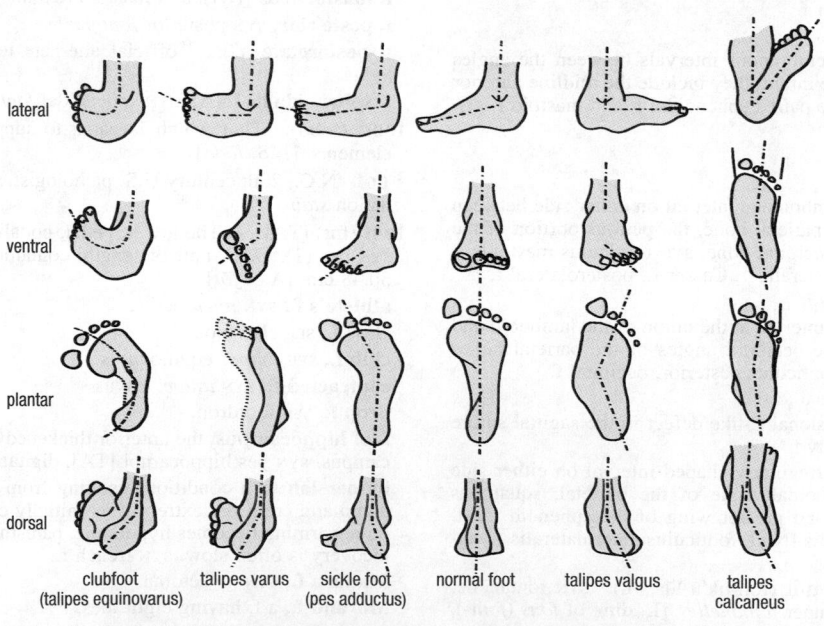

lateral

ventral

plantar

dorsal

clubfoot (talipes equinovarus)   talipes varus   sickle foot (pes adductus)   normal foot   talipes valgus   talipes calcaneus

foot deformities

SYN f. cecum linguae [TA], blind f. of the tongue, cecal f. of the tongue, Morgagni f. (1).

conjugate f., a f. formed by the notches of two bones in apposition.

f. costotransversa′rium [TA], SYN costotransverse f.

costotransverse f. [TA], an opening between the neck of a rib and the transverse process of a vertebra, occupied by the costotransverse ligament. SYN f. costotransversarium [TA].

cribriform foramina [TA], openings in the cribriform plate of the ethmoid bone, transmitting approximately 20 bundles of nerve fibers that collectively constitute the olfactory nerve (CN I). SYN foramina cribrosa [TA], olfactory f.

foramina cribrosa [TA], SYN cribriform foramina.

f. diaphrag′matis sel′lae, SYN f. of sellar diaphragm.

epiploic f., ⋆official alternate term for omental f.

f. epiplo′icum, ⋆official alternate term for omental f.

ethmoidal f. [TA], either of two foramina formed in the medial wall of the orbit by grooves on either edge of the ethmoidal notch of the frontal bone, and completed by similar grooves on the ethmoid bone: anterior ethmoidal f., located in an anterior position; posterior ethmoidal f. located in a posterior position. SYN f. ethmoidale (anterior et posterior) [TA].

f. ethmoida′le (anterior et posterior) [TA], SYN ethmoidal f.

external acoustic f., SYN external acoustic *pore*.

external auditory f., SYN external acoustic *pore*.

Ferrein f., SYN *hiatus* for greater petrosal nerve.

frontal f., an occasional small opening in the supraorbital margin of the frontal bone medial to the supraorbital foramen. SEE ALSO frontal *notch*. SYN f. frontale.

f. fronta′le, SYN frontal f.

great f., SYN f. magnum.

greater palatine f. [TA], an opening in the posterolateral corner of the hard palate opposite the last molar tooth, marking the lower end of the pterygopalatine canal. SYN f. palatinum majus [TA], anterior palatine f.

Huschke f., an opening in the floor of the bony part of the external acoustic meatus near the tympanic membrane, normally closed in the adult.

Hyrtl f., SYN *porus* crotaphytico-buccinatorius.

incisive f. [TA], one of several (usually four) openings of the incisive canals into the incisive fossa. SYN f. incisivum [TA], incisor f., Stensen f.

f. incisi′vum, [TA], SYN incisive f.

incisor f., SYN incisive f.

inferior dental f., SYN mandibular f.

infraorbital f. [TA], the external opening of the infraorbital canal, on the anterior surface of the body of the maxilla. SYN f. infraorbitale [TA].

f. infraorbita′le [TA], SYN infraorbital f.

▣**interatrial f. pri′mum,** (1) in the embryonic heart, the temporary opening between right and left atria situated between the lower margin of the septum primum and the atrioventricular canal cushions; (2) in an adult heart, the abnormal persistence of the so-named communication which is normal in young embryos. SYN f. subseptale, ostium primum, primary interatrial f.

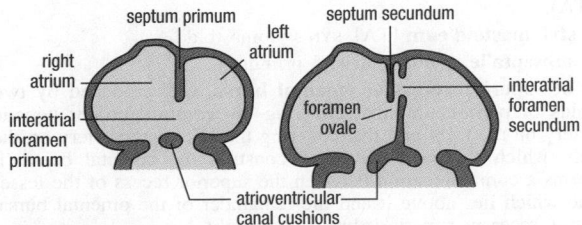

interatrial foramen primum and secundum: seen in the embryonic heart; (left) 5th week of pregnancy; (right) 6th week of pregnancy

interatrial f. secun′dum, a secondary opening appearing in the

upper part of the septum primum in the sixth week of embryonic life, just prior to the closure of the interatrial f. primum. SYN ostium secundum, secondary interatrial f.

f. intermesocolica transversa,

internal acoustic f., SYN internal acoustic *pore*.

internal auditory f., SYN internal acoustic *pore*.

interventricular f. [TA], the short, often slitlike passage that, on both the left and right side, connects the third brain ventricle (of the diencephalon) with the lateral ventricles (of the cerebral hemispheres); the passage is bounded anteriomedially by the column of fornix and posterolaterally by the anterior pole and anterior tubercle of the dorsal thalamus. SYN f. interventriculare [TA], Monro f., porta (2).

f. interventricula′re [TA], SYN interventricular f.

intervertebral f. [TA], one of a number of openings into the vertebral canal bounded by the pedicles of adjacent vertebrae above and below, the vertebral body (mostly of the superior vertebra) and intervertebral disk anteriorly, and the articular processes forming the zygapophysial joint posteriorly. SYN f. intervertebrale [TA].

f. intervertebra′le [TA], SYN intervertebral f.

f. ischiad′icum (anterior et posterior), SYN sciatic f.

f. ischiadicum majus et minor [TA], SYN sciatic f.

jugular f. [TA], a passage between the petrous portion of the temporal bone and the jugular process of the occipital, sometimes divided into two by the intrajugular processes; it contains the internal jugular vein, inferior petrosal sinus, the glossopharyngeal, vagus, and accessory nerves, and meningeal branches of the ascending pharyngeal and occipital arteries. SYN f. jugulare [TA], f. lacerum posterius.

f. jugula′re [TA], SYN jugular f.

f. of Key-Retzius, SYN lateral *aperture* of fourth ventricle.

lacerated f., SYN f. lacerum.

f. lac′erum [TA], an irregular aperture, filled with cartilage (basilar cartilage) in the living, located between the apex of the petrous part of the temporal bone, the body of the sphenoid, and the basilar part of the occipital bones. Several structures pass along the margins of the f. in a nearly horizontal direction but no structures pass through vertically. SYN f. lacerum medium, lacerated f., sphenotic f.

f. lac′erum ante′rius, SYN superior orbital *fissure*.

f. lac′erum me′dium, SYN f. lacerum.

f. lac′erum poste′rius, SYN jugular f.

Lannelongue foramina, SYN *openings* of smallest cardiac veins, under *opening*.

f. latera′lis ventric′uli quar′ti, SYN lateral *aperture* of fourth ventricle.

lesser palatine foramina [TA], openings on the hard palate of palatine canals passing vertically through the tuberosity of the palatine bone and transmitting the smaller palatine nerves and vessels. SYN foramina palatina minora [TA], posterior palatine foramina.

f. of Luschka, SYN lateral *aperture* of fourth ventricle.

f. of Magendie, SYN median *aperture* of fourth ventricle.

f. mag′num [TA], the large opening in the basal part of the occipital bone through which the spinal cord becomes continuous with the medulla oblongata. SYN great f.

malar f., SYN zygomaticofacial f.

f. mandib′ulae [TA], SYN mandibular f.

mandibular f. [TA], the opening into the mandibular canal on the medial surface of the ramus of the mandible giving passage to the inferior alveolar nerve, artery, and vein. SYN f. mandibulae [TA], inferior dental f.

mastoid f. [TA], an opening at the posterior portion of the mastoid process, transmitting the mastoid branch of the occipital artery to the dura and an emissary vein to the sigmoid sinus. SYN f. mastoideum [TA].

f. mastoi′deum [TA], SYN mastoid f.

mental f. [TA], the anterior opening of the mandibular canal on the body of the mandible lateral to and above the mental tubercle giving passage to the mental artery and nerve. SYN f. mentale [TA], mental canal.

f. menta'le [TA], SYN mental f.

Monro f., SYN interventricular f.

Morgagni f., (1) SYN f. cecum of tongue; **(2)** congenital defect in the fusion of sternal and costal elements of the diaphragmatic anlage that is the site of a retrosternal hernia.

nasal f., vascular f. opening on the outer surface of each nasal bone.

foram'ina nervo'sa [TA], the perforations along the tympanic lip of the spiral lamina giving passage to the cochlear nerves. SYN habenulae perforatae, zona perforata.

f. nutric'ium [TA], SYN nutrient f.

nutrient f. [TA], the external opening for the entrance of blood vessels in a bone. SYN f. nutricium [TA].

obturator f. [TA], a large, oval or irregularly triangular aperture in the hip bone, the margins of which are formed by the pubis and the ischium; it is closed in the natural state by the obturator membrane, except for a small opening for the passage of the obturator vessels and nerve. SYN f. obturatum [TA].

f. obtura'tum [TA], SYN obturator f.

olfactory f., SYN cribriform foramina.

omental f. [TA], the passage, below and behind the portal hepatis, connecting the two sacs of the peritoneum; it is bounded anteriorly by the hepatoduodenal ligament and posteriorly by a peritoneal fold over the inferior vena cava. SYN f. omentale [TA], epiploic f.⋆, f. epiploicum⋆, aditus ad saccum peritonei minorem, f. of Winslow.

f. omentale [TA], SYN omental f.

optic f., SYN optic *canal*.

f. op'ticum, SYN optic *canal*.

oval f. [TA], SYN f. ovale.

f. ova'le, (1) [TA], a large oval opening in the base of the greater wing of the sphenoid bone, transmitting the mandibular division of the trigeminal merge and a small meningeal artery; **(2)** valvular incompetence of the f. ovale of the heart; a condition contrasting with probe patency of the f. ovale in that the valvula foraminis ovalis has abnormal perforations in it, or is of insufficient size to afford adequate valvular action at the f. ovale prenatally, or effect a complete closure postnatally. SYN oval f. [TA].

f. ovale cordis, [TA] SYN f. ovale of heart.

f. ovale of heart, [TA] in the fetal heart, the oval opening at the free margin of the septum secundum; the persistent part of the septum primum acts as a valve for this interatrial communication during fetal life and normally postnatally becomes fused to the septum secundum to close it. SYN f. ovale cordis, oval f. of heart.

oval f. of heart, SYN f. ovale of heart.

foram'ina palati'na mino'ra [TA], SYN lesser palatine foramina.

f. palati'num ma'jus [TA], SYN greater palatine f.

foram'ina papilla'ria re'nis [TA], SYN *openings* of papillary ducts, under *opening*.

papillary foramina of kidney, SYN *openings* of papillary ducts, under *opening*.

parietal f. [TA], an inconstant f. in the parietal bone occasionally found bilaterally near the sagittal margin posteriorly; when present it transmits an emissary vein to the superior sagittal sinus. SYN f. parietale [TA].

f. parieta'le [TA], SYN parietal f.

petrosal f., SYN f. petrosum.

f. petro'sum [TA], an occasional opening in the greater wing of the sphenoid bone, between the f. spinosum and f. ovale, which transmits the lesser petrosal nerve. SYN canaliculus innominatus, f. of Arnold, petrosal f.

posterior condyloid f., SYN condylar *canal*.

posterior palatine foramina, SYN lesser palatine foramina.

postglenoid f., a small f. that is sometimes present in the temporal bone immediately in front of the external acoustic meatus.

primary interatrial f., SYN interatrial f. primum.

f. proces'sus transver'si, SYN transverse f.

f. quadra'tum, SYN caval *opening* of diaphragm.

f. recessus superioris bursae omentalis, SYN f. of superior recess of omental bursa.

f. of Retzius, SYN lateral *aperture* of fourth ventricle.

root f., SYN apical f. of tooth.

f. rotun'dum [TA], an opening in the base of the greater wing of the sphenoid bone, transmitting the maxillary nerve. SYN round f.

round f., SYN f. rotundum.

sacral foramina [TA], the openings between the fused sacral vertebrae transmitting the sacral nerves. The anterior sacral foramina transmit anterior (ventral) primary rami of the sacral nerves. The posterior sacral foramina give passage to posterior (dorsal) primary rami of the sacral nerves. The terms "anterior" and "posterior" are awkward with regard to the S1/S2 foramina especially since in the anatomic position the formina lie vertically, superior and inferior, to each other. SYN f. sacrale, foramina sacralia anterior et posterior.

f. sacra'le, SYN sacral foramina.

foramina sacralia anterior et posterior, SYN sacral foramina.

Scarpa foramina, two openings in the line of the intermaxillary suture; the anterior f. transmits the left nasopalatine nerve, the posterior the right.

sciatic f. [TA], either of two foramina formed by the sacrospinous and sacrotuberous ligaments crossing the sciatic notches of the hip bone: greater sciatic f. (f. ischiadicum majus) and lesser sciatic f. (f. ischiadicum minus). SYN f. ischiadicum majus et minor [TA], f. ischiadicum (anterior et posterior).

secondary interatrial f., SYN interatrial f. secundum.

f. of sellar diaphragm, a hole in the center of the diaphragm of the sella turcica giving passage to the infundibulum of the hypothalamus. SYN f. diaphragmatis sellae.

singular f., SYN f. singulare.

f. singula're [TA], a f. in the internal acoustic meatus, posterior to the cochlear area, that transmits the nerves to the ampulla of the posterior semicircular duct. SYN singular f.

foramina of the smallest veins of heart, SYN *openings* of smallest cardiac veins, under *opening*.

sphenoidal emissary f. [TA], a minute inconstant f. in the greater wing of the sphenoid bone, anterior and medial to the f. ovale, transmitting a small emissary vein from the cavernous sinus. SYN f. venosum [TA], venous f., Vesalius f.

sphenopalatine f. [TA], the f. formed from the sphenopalatine notch of the palatine bone in articulation with the sphenoid bone; it transmits the sphenopalatine artery and accompanying nerves. SYN f. sphenopalatinum [TA].

f. sphenopalati'num [TA], SYN sphenopalatine f.

sphenotic f., SYN f. lacerum.

f. spino'sum [TA], an opening in the base of the greater wing of the sphenoid bone, anterior to the spine of the sphenoid, transmitting the middle meningeal artery, and the meningeal branch (nervus spinosum) of the mandibular nerve.

Stensen f., SYN incisive f.

stylomastoid f. [TA], the distal or external opening of the facial canal on the inferior surface of the petrous portion of the temporal bone, between the styloid and mastoid processes; it transmits the facial nerve and stylomastoid artery. SYN f. stylomastoideum [TA].

f. stylomastoid'eum [TA], SYN stylomastoid f.

f. subsepta'le, SYN interatrial f. primum.

f. of superior recess of omental bursa, a f. produced by two folds of peritoneum, that covering the common/proper hepatic artery on the right and that covering the left gastric artery on the left, which encroach upon and constrict the omental bursa; it forms a communication between the superior recess of the lesser sac which lies above it and the remainder of the omental bursa. SYN f. recessus superioris bursae omentalis.

supraorbital f. [TA], a f. in the supraorbital margin of the frontal bone at the junction of the medial and intermediate thirds. SYN f. supraorbitale [TA].

f. supraorbita'le [TA], SYN supraorbital f; SEE ALSO supraorbital *notch*.

thebesian foramina, SYN *openings* of smallest cardiac veins, under *opening*.

thyroid f. [TA], an opening occasionally existing in one or both of the plates of the thyroid cartilage. SYN f. thyroideum [TA].

f. thyroid′eum [TA], SYN thyroid f.

f. transversa′rium [TA], SYN transverse f.

transverse f., f. processus transversus. SYN f. transversarium [TA], f. of transverse process, f. processus transversi, f. vertebroarteriale, vertebroarterial f.

f. of transverse process, SYN transverse f.

f. of vena cava, SYN caval *opening* of diaphragm.

vena caval f., SYN caval *opening* of diaphragm.

f. ve′nae ca′vae, SYN caval *opening* of diaphragm.

foramina of the venae minimae, SYN *openings* of smallest cardiac veins, under *opening*.

foram′ina vena′rum minima′rum cordis, SYN *openings* of smallest cardiac veins, under *opening*.

f. veno′sum [TA], SYN sphenoidal emissary f.

venous f., SYN sphenoidal emissary f.

vertebral f. [TA], the f. formed by the union of the vertebral arch with the body; in the articulated vertebral column, the vertebral f. collectively form the vertebral column. SYN f. vertebrale [TA].

f. vertebra′le [TA], SYN vertebral f.

vertebroarterial f., SYN transverse f.

f. vertebroarteria′le, SYN transverse f.

Vesalius f., SYN sphenoidal emissary f.

Vicq d'Azyr f., SYN f. caecum medullae oblongatae.

Vieussens foramina, SYN *openings* of smallest cardiac veins, under *opening*.

Weitbrecht f., an opening in the articular capsule of the shoulder joint, communicating with the subtendinous bursa of the subscapularis muscle.

f. of Winslow, SYN omental f.

zygomaticofacial f. [TA], the opening on the lateral surface of the zygomatic bone below the orbital margin that transmits the zygomaticofacial nerve. SYN f. zygomaticofaciale [TA], malar f.

f. zygomaticofacia′le [TA], SYN zygomaticofacial f.

zygomatico-orbital f. [TA], the common opening on the orbital surface of the zygomatic bone of the canals transmitting the zygomaticofacial and zygomaticotemporal nerves; sometimes each of these canals has a separate opening on the orbital surface. SYN f. zygomatico-orbitale [TA].

f. zygomat′ico-orbita′le [TA], SYN zygomatico-orbital f.

zygomaticotemporal f. [TA], the opening, on the temporal surface of the zygomatic bone, of the canal that gives passage to the zygomaticotemporal nerve. SYN f. zygomaticotemporale [TA].

f. zygomat′icotempora′le [TA], SYN zygomaticotemporal f.

---

fo·ram·i·na (fō-ram′i-nă). Plural of foramen.

Fo·ram·i·nif·e·ra (fō-ram-i-nif′er-ă, for′ă-mi-nif′er-ă). A subclass of Rhizopoda possessing anastomosing pseudopodia; these form a network around the cell which usually develops into a complex calcareous shell; an important component of the ocean bottom and of rockbeds overlying oil deposits. [L. *foramen,* aperture, + *fero,* to carry]

fo·ram·i·nif·er·ous (fō-ram-i-nif′er-ŭs, fōr′ă-mi-nif′er-ŭs). **1.** Possessing openings or foramina. **2.** Relating to the Foraminifera.

for·am·i·not·o·my (fōr′am-i-not′ō-mē). An operation upon an aperture, usually to open it, e.g., surgical enlargement of the intervertebral foramen. [L. *foramen,* aperture, + G. *tomē,* a cutting]

fo·ra·min·u·lum, pl. **fo·ra·min·u·la** (fōr′ă-min′ū-lŭm, ū-lă). A very minute foramen. [Mod. L. dim. of *foramen*]

Forbes, A.P., 20th century U.S. physician. SEE F.-Albright *syndrome*.

Forbes, Gilbert B., U.S. pediatrician, *1915. SEE F. *disease*.

force (*F*) (fōrs). That which tends to produce motion in a body. [L. *fortis,* strong]

animal f., muscular power.

chewing f., SYN f. of mastication.

dynamic f., SYN energy.

electromotive f. (EMF), the f. (measured in volts) that causes the flow of electricity from one point to another.

G f., inertial f. produced by accelerations or gravity, expressed in gravitational units; one G is equal to the pull of gravity at the earth's surface at sea level and 45° North latitude (32.1725 ft/sec^2; 980.621 cm/sec^2). SEE ALSO *g*.

f. of mastication, the motive f. created by the dynamic action of the muscles during the physiologic act of mastication. SYN biting strength, chewing f., masticatory f.

masticatory f., SYN f. of mastication.

occlusal f., the result of muscular f. applied on opposing teeth.

psychic f., SYN psychic *energy*.

reciprocal f.'s, in dentistry, f.'s whereby the resistance of one or more teeth is utilized to move one or more opposing teeth.

reserve f., the energy residing in the organism or any of its parts above that required for its normal functioning.

van der Waals f.'s, first postulated by van der Waals in 1873 to explain deviations from ideal gas behavior seen in real gases; the attractive f.'s between atoms or molecules other than electrostatic (ionic), covalent (sharing of electrons), or hydrogen bonding (sharing a proton); generally ascribed to dipolar and dispersion effects, π-electrons, etc.; these relatively nondescript f.'s contribute to the mutual attraction of organic molecules.

vital f., SEE vitalism.

force plat·form. A device used to measure the strength, symmetry, and latency of compensatory postural movements when visual, vestibular, and somatosensory stimuli are varied.

for·ceps (fōr′seps). **1.** An instrument to grasp a structure, for compression or traction. Cf. clamp. **2** [TA]. Bands of white fibers in the brain, major f. and minor f. [L. a pair of tongs]

Adson f., a small thumb f. with two teeth on one tip and one tooth on the other.

alligator f., a long f. with a small hinged jaw on the end.

Allis f., a straight grasping f. with serrated jaws, used to forcibly grasp or retract tissues or structures.

f. anterior, SYN minor f.

Arruga f., f. for the intracapsular extraction of a cataract.

arterial f., a locking f. with sloping blades for grasping the end of a blood vessel until a ligature is applied.

axis-traction f., obstetrical f. provided with a second handle so attached that traction can be made in the line in which the head must move in the axis of the pelvis.

Barton f., an obstetrical f. with one fixed curved blade and a hinged anterior blade for application to a high transverse head.

bayonet f., f. with offset blades, such as those for use through an otoscope.

bone f., a strong f. used for seizing or removing fragments of bone.

Brown-Adson f., an Adson f. with about 16 delicate teeth on each tip.

bulldog f., a soft-bladed f. for occluding a blood vessel.

bullet f., a f. with thin curved blades with serrated grasping surfaces, for extracting a bullet from tissues.

capsule f., f. used for removing the capsule of the lens in extracapsular extraction of a cataract.

Chamberlen f., the original obstetrical f., without a curvature.

clamp f., a f. with pronged jaws designed to engage the jaws of a rubber dam clamp so that they may be separated to pass over the widest buccolingual contour of a tooth. SYN rubber dam clamp f.

clip f., a small f. with spring catch to occlude the end of a bleeding vessel.

cup biopsy f., a slender flexible f. with movable cup-shaped jaws, used to obtain biopsy specimens by introduction through a specially designed endoscope.

cutting f., SYN labitome.

DeBakey f., nontraumatic f. used to pick up blood vessels; also known as "magics." SYN magic f.

fo

dental f., f. used to luxate teeth and remove them from the alveolus. SYN extracting f.

dressing f., a thumb f. for general use in dressing wounds, removing fragments of necrotic tissue, small foreign bodies, etc.

extracting f., SYN dental f.

frontal f., ⋆official alternate term for minor f.

f. frontalis, ⋆official alternate term for minor f.

Graefe f., a small thumb f. with one horizontal row of six or eight delicate teeth across each tip.

hemostatic f., a f. with a catch for locking the blades, used for seizing the end of a blood vessel to control hemorrhage.

jeweller f., a small thumb f. with very fine pointed blades, used to grasp tissues in microsurgical procedures.

Kjelland f., an obstetrical f. having a sliding lock, and little pelvic curve.

Lahey f., thyroid f. used to deliver the uterus in vaginohysterectomy.

Laplace f., a f. for approximating intestines during surgical anastomosis.

Levret f., a modification of the Chamberlen f., curved to correspond to the curve of the parturient passage.

lion-jaw bone-holding f., a sturdy f. with strong sharp teeth in the jaws, used for holding bone fragments.

Löwenberg f., f. with short curved blades ending in rounded grasping extremities devised for the removal of adenoid growths in the nasopharynx.

magic f., SYN DeBakey f.

Magill f., a bent blunt f. used to facilitate nasotracheal intubation.

f. ma′jor [TA], SYN major f.

major f. [TA], occipital radiation of the corpus callosum; that part of the fiber radiation of the corpus callosum which bends sharply backward into the occipital lobe of the cerebrum. SYN f. major [TA], occipital f.⋆, f. occipitalis, f. posterior, occipital part of corpus callosum, pars occipitalis corporis callosi.

f. mi′nor [TA], SYN minor f.

minor f. [TA], frontal radiation of the corpus callosum; that part of the fiber radiation of the corpus callosum which bends forward toward the frontal pole of the cerebrum. SYN f. minor [TA], f. frontalis⋆, frontal f.⋆, f. anterior, frontal part of corpus callosum, pars frontalis corporis callosi.

mosquito f., SYN mosquito *clamp*.

mouse-tooth f., a f. with one or two fine points at the tip of each blade, fitting into hollows between the points on the opposite blade.

needle f., SYN needle-holder.

nonfenestrated f., obstetrical f. without openings in the blades, thus facilitating rotation of the head.

obstetrical f., f. used for grasping and applying traction to or for rotation of the fetal head; the blades are introduced separately into the genital canal, permitting the fetal head to be grasped firmly but with minimal compression, and then are articulated after being placed in correct position.

occipital f., ⋆official alternate term for major f.

f. occipitalis, SYN major f.

O'Hara f., two slender clamp f.'s held together by a serrefine, once used in intestinal anastomosis; now obsolete.

Piper f., obstetrical f. used to facilitate delivery of the head in breech presentation.

f. poste′rior, SYN major f.

Randall stone f., a f. with variably curved slender blades and serrated jaws, used to extract calculi from the renal pelvis or calices.

rubber dam clamp f., SYN clamp f.

Simpson f., an obstetrical f.

speculum f., a tubular f. for use through a speculum.

Tarnier f., a type of axis-traction f.

tenaculum f., a f. with jaws armed each with a sharp, straight hook like a tenaculum.

thumb f., a spring f. used by compression with thumb and forefinger.

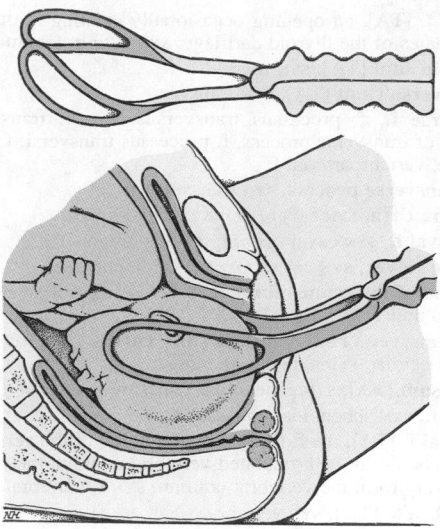

obstetrical forceps

tubular f., a long slender f. intended for use through a cannula or other tubular instrument.

Tucker-McLean f., a type of axis-traction f.

tying f., an instrument with flat, smooth tips used in ophthalmic surgery, particularly for tying sutures.

vulsella f., vulsellum f., a f. with hooks at the tip of each blade. SYN volsella, vulsella, vulsellum.

Willett f., obsolete term for a traction f. used to treat placenta previa by pulling the fetal head down against the placenta.

Forchheimer, Frederick, U.S. physician, 1853–1913. SEE F. *sign*.

for·ci·pate (fōr′si-pāt). Shaped like a forceps.

for·ci·pres·sure (fōr′si-presh-ŭr). A method of arresting hemorrhage by compressing a blood vessel with forceps.

Fordyce, John A., U.S. dermatologist, 1858–1925. SEE F. *angiokeratoma, disease, granules,* under *granule, spots,* under *spot;* Fox-F. *disease.*

fore·arm (fōr′arm) [TA]. The segment of the upper limb between the elbow and the wrist. SYN antebrachium [TA].

fore·brain (fōr′brān). ⋆official alternate term for prosencephalon.

fore·con·scious (fōr′kon-shŭs). Denoting memories, not at present in the consciousness, which can be evoked from time to time, or an unconscious mental process which becomes conscious only on the fulfillment of certain conditions. Cf. preconscious.

fore·fin·ger (fōr′fing′ger). SYN index *finger*.

fore·gut (fōr′gŭt). The cephalic portion of the primitive digestive tube in the embryo. From its endoderm arises the epithelial lining of the pharynx, trachea, lungs, esophagus, and stomach, the first part and cranial half of the second part of the duodenum, and the parenchyma of the liver, gallbladder, and pancreas. SYN headgut.

fore·head (fōr′ed, fōr′hed) [TA]. The part of the face between the eyebrows and the hairy scalp. SYN frons [TA], sinciput⋆, brow (2).

olympian f., the abnormally prominent, high, and broad f. in hereditary syphilis.

fore·kid·ney (fōr′kid-nē). SYN pronephros.

Forel, Auguste H., Swiss neurologist, 1848–1931. SEE F. *decussation; fields* of F., under *field; tegmental fields* of F. under *field.*

fore·lock (fō′lok). The lock of hair that grows just above the forehead.

white forelock, a triangular or diamond-shaped depigmented macule with white hairs, usually located in the anterior midline of the scalp, seen in piebaldism.

fore·milk (fōr'milk). SYN colostrum.

fo·ren·sic (fō-ren'sik). Pertaining or applicable to personal injury, murder, and other legal proceedings. [L. *forensis,* of a forum]

fore·play (fōr'plā). Stimulative sexual activity preceding sexual intercourse.

fore·pleas·ure (fōr'plezh·er, plā'zher). Sexual pleasure resulting from the foreplay that precedes the genital-orgastic pleasure in sexual intercourse.

fore·skin (fōr'skin). ⋆official alternate term for prepuce.

f. of penis [TA], SYN *prepuce* of penis.

Forestier, Jacques, French rheumatologist, 1890–1978. SEE F. *disease.*

fore·stom·ach (fōr'stŭm'ŭk). SYN cardiac *antrum.*

fore·wa·ters (fōr'wah-terz). Colloquialism for the bulging fluid-filled amniotic membrane presenting in front of the fetal head.

for·get·ting. Being unable to retrieve or recall information that was once registered, learned, and stored in short- or long-term memory.

fork (fōrk). **1.** A pronged instrument used for holding or lifting. **2.** An instrument resembling a f. in that it has tines or prongs.

bite f., SYN face-bow f.

face-bow f., that part of the face-bow assemblage used to attach the maxillary trial base to the face-bow proper. SYN bite f.

tuning f., a steel or magnesium-alloy instrument roughly resembling a two-pronged f., the vibrations of the prongs of which, when struck, produce a pure tone and overtones; used to test the hearing and vibratory sensation.

form (fōrm). Shape; mold. [L. *forma*]

accolé f.'s (ak-ōlā'), SYN appliqué f.'s.

appliqué f.'s (ap-li-kā'), a term applied to the manner in which the ring stage of *Plasmodium falciparum* parasitizes the marginal portion of erythrocytes. SYN accolé f.'s.

arch f., the shape and contour of the dental arch, or of an orthodontic wire formed to the shape of that arch.

boat f., the less stable of two conformations assumed by 6-membered cyclic sugars (pyranoses) or cyclohexane derivatives, as opposed to chair f. SEE ALSO Haworth conformational formulas of cyclic *sugars.*

cavity preparation f., the configuration or shape of a cavity preparation.

chair f., the more stable of two conformations assumed by 6-membered cyclic sugars (e.g., the pyranoses) or cyclohexane derivatives, as opposed to boat f. SEE ALSO Haworth conformational formulas of cyclic *sugars.*

convenience f., the changes needed outside the basic outline f. to enable proper instrumentation for the cavity preparation and insertion of a dental restoration.

extension f., the extension of the cavity preparation outline f. to include areas of incipient carious lesions; this extension provides a dental restoration with margins that are self-cleansing or easily cleaned.

face f., **(1)** the outline f. of the face; **(2)** the outline f. of the face from an anterior view.

half-chair f., SEE Haworth conformational formulas of cyclic *sugars.*

involution f., an irregular or atypical bacterial cell produced as a result of exposure to unfavorable conditions.

L f., SEE L-phase *variants,* under *variant.*

occlusal f., the f. of the occlusal surface of a tooth or a row of teeth. SYN occlusal pattern.

outline f., the shape of the area of the tooth surface included within the cavosurface margins of the cavity preparation of a dental restoration.

posterior tooth f., the distinguishing contours of the occlusal surface of the various posterior teeth.

replicative f. (RF), (1) an intermediate stage in the replication of either DNA or RNA viral genomes that is usually double-strand-

ed; **(2)** the altered, double-stranded f. to which single-stranded coliphage DNA is converted after infection of a susceptible bacterium, formation of the complementary ("minus") strand being mediated by enzymes that were present in the bacterium before entrance of the viral ("plus") strand.

resistance f., the shape given to a cavity preparation that enables the dental restoration to withstand masticatory forces.

retention f., the shape of a cavity preparation that prevents displacement of the dental restoration by lateral or tipping forces as well as masticatory forces.

sickle f., SYN malarial *crescent.*

skew f., SEE Haworth conformational formulas of cyclic *sugars.*

tooth f., the characteristics of the curves, lines, angles, and contours of various teeth which permit their identification and differentiation.

twist f., SEE Haworth conformational formulas of cyclic *sugars.*

wave f., SEE waveform. SYN waveshape.

wax f., SYN wax *pattern.*

△**-form.** In the form, shape of; equivalent to -oid. SEE morpho-. [L. *-formis*]

Formad, Henry, U.S. physician, 1847–1892. SEE F. *kidney.*

for·mal·de·hyde (fōr-mal'dĕ-hīd). A pungent gas, HCHO; used as an antiseptic, disinfectant, and histologic fixative. SYN formic aldehyde, methyl aldehyde. [form(ic) + aldehyde]

active f., (1) a hydroxymethyl derivative of tetrahydrofolate or thiamin pyrophosphate; **(2)** N^5,N^{10}-methylenetetrahydrofolate.

for·ma·lin (fōr'mă-lin). A 37% aqueous solution of formaldehyde. SYN formol.

for·ma·lin·ize (fōr-mă-li-nīz'). To add formalin solution to inactivate vaccines without destroying their immunizing power.

for·mam·i·dase (fōr-mam'i-dās). An enzyme catalyzing the hydrolysis of N-formyl-L-kynurenine to L-kynurenine and formate, a reaction of significance in L-tryptophan catabolism. SYN formylase, kynurenine formamidase.

5-for·mam·i·do·im·id·a·zole-4-car·box·im·ide ri·bo·tide. An intermediate in purine biosynthesis.

for·mant (fōr'mant). Tones and their overtones resulting from the production of vowel phonemes.

for·mate (fōr'māt). A salt or ester of formic acid; i.e., the monovalent radical HCOO– or the anion HCOO⁻.

active f., N^{10}-formyltetrahydrofolate or an equivalent oxidation product of tetrahydrofolate.

for·ma·tio, pl. **for·ma·ti·o·nes** (fōr-mā'shē-ō, -ō'nēz) [TA]. **1.** SYN formation. **2.** A structure of definite shape or cellular arrangement. [L. fr. *formo,* pp. *-atus,* to form]

f. hippocampa'lis, hippocampal formation. SEE hippocampus.

f. reticula'ris [TA], SYN reticular *formation.*

for·ma·tion (fōr-mā'shŭn) [TA]. **1.** A formation; a structure of definite shape or cellular arrangement. **2.** That which is formed. **3.** The act of giving form and shape. SYN formatio (1) [TA].

concept f., in psychology, the learning to conceive and respond in terms of abstract ideas based upon an action or object.

personality f., the life history associated with the development of individual patterns and of one's individuality.

reaction f., in psychoanalysis, a postulated defense mechanism in which attitudes and behaviors that are adopted are the opposites of that which the individual would ordinarily be expected to express and actually feel at an unconscious level.

reticular f. (RF), a massive but vaguely delimited neural apparatus composed of closely intermingled gray and white matter and extending throughout the central core of the brainstem and into the diencephalon; the term refers to the large neuronal population of the brainstem that does not compose motoneuronal cell groups or cell groups forming part of specific sensory conduction systems; its neurons generally have long dendrites and heterogeneous afferent connections, the reason why the f. is often called "nonspecific"; the reticular f. has complex, largely polysynaptic ascending and descending connections that play a role in the central control of autonomic (respiration, blood pressure, thermoregulation, etc.) and endocrine functions, as well as in bodily posture, skeletomuscular reflex activity, and general behavioral states such

fo

as alertness and sleep. SYN formatio reticularis [TA], reticular substance (2), substantia reticularis (2).

rouleaux f., the arrangement of red blood cells in fluid blood (or in diluted suspensions) with their biconcave surfaces in apposition, thereby forming groups that resemble stacks of coins. SYN pseudoagglutination (2). [Fr. pl. of *rouleau,* a roll]

symptom f., SYN symptom *substitution.*

for·ma·ti·o·nes (fōr-mā′shē-ō′nēz). Plural of formatio.

for·ma·zan (fōr′mă-zan). A water-insoluble colored compound of the general structure, RNH—N=CR′—N=NR″, formed by reduction of a tetrazolium salt in the histochemical demonstration of oxidative enzymes; the R's are usually phenyl groups; examples include neotetrazolium, blue tetrazolium, and nitro blue tetrazolium.

form·board (fōrm′bōrd). A board containing cut-outs in various shapes, into which blocks of corresponding shape are to be fitted; a neuropsychological test of which the Tactual Performance Test of the Halstead-Reitan Battery is an example. SEE Halstead-Reitan *battery.*

forme fruste, pl. **formes frustes** (fōrm′ froost′). A partial, arrested, or inapparent form of disease. [Fr. unfinished form]

for·mic (fōr′mik). **1.** Pertaining to f. acid. **2.** Relating to ants. [L. *formica,* ant]

for·mic ac·id. HCOOH; the smallest carboxylic acid; a strong caustic, used as an astringent and counterirritant.

for·mic al·de·hyde. SYN formaldehyde.

for·mi·ca·tion (fōr-mi-kā′shŭn). A form of paresthesia or tactile hallucination; a sensation as if small insects are creeping under the skin. [L. *formica,* ant]

for·mim·i·no·glu·tam·ic ac·id (FIGLU) (fōr-mim′i-nō-gloo-tam′ik). An intermediate metabolite in L-histidine catabolism in the conversion of L-histidine to L-glutamic acid, with the formimino group being transferred to tetrahydrofolate; it may appear in the urine of patients with folic acid or vitamin B_{12} deficiency, or liver disease.

N-for·mim·i·no·tet·ra·hy·dro·fo·late (for-mim′i-nō-tet′ră-hī-drō-fō′lāt). A derivative of one-carbon tetrahydrofolate formed via L-histidine catabolism.

formin (for′min). A family of proteins that participates in cell polarization, cytokinesis, and vertebrate limb formation. [L. *forma,* form, + -in]

for·mo·cre·sol (fōr-mō-krē′sol). An aqueous solution containing cresol, formaldehyde, and glycerine, used in vital primary teeth needing coronal pulpotomy.

for·mol (fōr′mol). SYN formalin.

for·mo·sul·fa·thi·a·zole (fōr′mō-sŭl-fă-thī′ă-zol). An antimicrobial agent for treatment of intestinal infections.

FORMULA

for·mu·la, pl. **for·mu·las, for·mu·lae** (fōr′mū-lă, -lăz, -lē). **1.** A recipe or prescription containing directions for the compounding of a medicinal preparation. **2.** In chemistry, a symbol or collection of symbols expressing the number of atoms of the element or elements forming one molecule of a substance, together with, on occasion, information concerning the arrangement of the atoms within the molecule, their electronic structure, their charge, the nature of the bonds within the molecule, etc. **3.** An expression by symbols and numbers of the normal order or arrangement of parts or structures. **4.** A mathematic relationship or principle, typically provided via an equation. [L. dim. of *forma,* form]

Arneth f., the normal, approximate ratio of polymorphonuclear neutrophils, based on the number of lobes in the nuclei, as follows: 1 lobe, 5%; 2 lobes, 35%; 3 lobes, 41%; 4 lobes, 17%; 5 lobes, 2%.

Bazett f., a f. for correcting the observed QT interval in the electrocardiogram for cardiac rate (R-R interval): corrected QT =

Q-T sec/√RR sec.

Bernhardt f., a f. used to calculate the ideal weight, in kilograms, for an adult; it is the height in centimeters times the chest circumference in centimeters divided by 240.

Black f., a translation of Pignet f. into British measurements: $F = (W + C) - H$; F is the empirical factor, W is the weight in pounds, C the chest girth in inches at full inspiration, and H the height in inches; a man is classed as very strong when F is over 120, strong between 110 and 120, good 100 to 110, fair 90 to 100, weak 80 to 90, very weak under 80.

Broca f., a fully developed man (30 years old) should weigh as many kilograms as he is centimeters in height over and above 1 meter.

chemical f., a statement of the structure of a molecule expressed in chemical symbols.

Christison f., SYN Häser f.

constitutional f., SYN structural f.

Demoivre f., an obsolete f. for calculating life expectancy.

dental f., a statement in tabular form of the number of each kind of teeth in the jaw; the dental f. for man is, for the deciduous teeth:

$$\text{i. } \frac{2\text{-}2}{2\text{-}2}, \text{ c. } \frac{1\text{-}1}{1\text{-}1}, \text{ m. } \frac{2\text{-}2}{2\text{-}2} = 20$$

for the permanent teeth:

$$\text{i. } \frac{2\text{-}2}{2\text{-}2}, \text{ c. } \frac{1\text{-}1}{1\text{-}1}, \text{ bic. } \frac{2\text{-}2}{2\text{-}2}, \text{ m. } \frac{3\text{-}3}{3\text{-}3} = 32.$$

Dreyer f., an obsolete f. indicating relationship between vital capacity and body surface area.

DuBois f., a f. for predicting a man's surface area from weight and height: $A = 71.84 W^{0.425} H^{0.725}$, where A = surface area in cm^2, W = weight in kg, and H = height in cm.

electrical f., a graphic representation by means of symbols of the reaction of a muscle to an electrical stimulus.

empirical f., in chemistry, a f. indicating the kind and number of atoms in the molecules of a substance, or its composition, but not the relation of the atoms to each other or the intimate structure of the molecule. SYN molecular f.

Fischer projection formulas, SEE Fischer projection formulas of *sugars.*

Flesch f., a method of determining the difficulty of a written passage by a formulation that provides an estimate of how many people in the U.S. would be able to read and understand the passage; used in determining patient comprehension of hospital consent forms.

Florschütz f., the correct relation of height to the abdominal circumference: $L : (2B - L)$, L representing the individual's height, and B the circumference of the abdomen; the normal value so determined would be 5, and any below that would indicate obesity.

Gorlin f., a f. for calculating the area of the orifice of a cardiac valve, based on flow across the valve and the mean pressures in the chambers on either side of the valve.

graphic f., SYN structural f.

Hamilton-Stewart f., SYN Hamilton-Stewart *method.*

Häser f., a f. to determine the number of grams of urinary solids per liter, obtained by multiplying 2.33 by the last two figures of the specific gravity of the urine. SYN Christison f., Trapp f., Trapp-Häser f.

Haworth perspective and conformational formulas, SEE Haworth perspective formulas of cyclic *sugars.*

Jellinek f., a method of estimating the prevalence of alcoholism in a nation's population, based on the assumption that a predictable proportion of persons addicted to alcohol die of cirrhosis of the liver.

Ledermann f., a f. to calculate alcohol dependancy levels. Ledermann showed empirically that the distribution of alcohol consumption in a population is log normal; the formula used this observation to estimate the prevalence of various degrees of alcohol dependency. Some questions have been raised about the validity of Ledermann observations.

Long f., a f. for estimating from the specific gravity of a specimen of urine the approximate amount of solids in grams per liter; the last two figures of the value for specific gravity are multiplied by 2.6. SYN Long coefficient.

Mall f., a f. for determining the age (in days) of a human embryo; calculated as the square root of its length (measured from vertex to breech) in millimeters multiplied by 100.

Meeh f., SYN Meeh-Dubois f.

Meeh-Dubois f., a f. for predicting surface area, assuming that it is proportional to the $\frac{2}{3}$ power of the body weight. SYN Meeh f.

molecular f., SYN empirical f.

official f., a f. contained in the Pharmacopeia or the National Formulary.

Pignet f., SEE Black f.

Poisson-Pearson f., a f. to determine the statistical error in calculating the endemic index of malaria: let N = total number of children under 15 years in a locality; n = total number examined for the spleen-rate; x = number found with enlarged spleen; $(x/n)100$ = spleen-rate; $e\%$ = percentage of error; the percentage error will be, by this f.:

$$e\% = \frac{200}{n}\sqrt{\frac{2x(n-x)}{n}}\sqrt{1 - \frac{n-1}{N-1}}.$$

Ranke f., A = grams of albumin per liter of a serous fluid: then, A = (sp. gr. − 1000) × 0.52 − 5.406.

rational f., in chemistry, a f. that indicates the constitution as well as the composition of a substance.

Reuss f., a means of estimating the approximate amount of albumin in a transudate or exudate; $\frac{3}{8}$ (sp. gr. - 1.000) − 2.8 results in a value that is a practicable indication of the percentage of albumin in the fluid.

Runeberg f., a f. for estimating the percentage of albumin in a serous fluid, similar to Reuss f. except that, instead of 2.8, 2.73 is subtracted in the instance of a transudate, and 2.88 in that of an inflammatory exudate.

spatial f., SYN stereochemical f.

stereochemical f., a chemical f. in which the arrangement of the atoms or atomic groupings in space are indicated. SYN spatial f.

structural f., a f. in which the connections of the atoms and groups of atoms, as well as their kind and number, are indicated. SYN constitutional f., graphic f.

Toronto f. for pulmonary artery banding, a technique that provides a general guide for the size of the band relative to the patient's weight.

Trapp f., SYN Häser f.

Trapp-Häser f., SYN Häser f.

Van Slyke f., SYN standard urea *clearance*.

vertebral f., a f. indicating the number of vertebrae in each segment of the spinal column; for humans it is C. 7, T. 12, L. 5, S. 5, Co. 4 = 33, the letters standing for cervical, thoracic, lumbar, sacral, and coccygeal.

---

for·mu·lary (fōr′mū-lā-rē). A collection of formulas for the compounding of medicinal preparations. SEE National Formulary, Pharmacopeia.

hospital f., a continually revised compilation of approved pharmaceuticals, plus important ancillary information, that reflects the current clinical judgment of the institution's medical staff.

for·myl (f) (fōr′mil). The radical, HCO–.

active f., the f. group taking part in transformylation reactions with a folic acid derivative in the role of carrier.

formyl-methionyl-f., SYN initiation tRNA.

for·my·lase (fōr′mi-lās). SYN formamidase.

N**-for·myl·gly·cin·a·mide ri·bo·tide (FGAR).** An intermediate in purine biosynthesis.

N**-for·myl·ky·nur·e·nine** (en-fōr′mil-ki-noor′ĕ-nēn). The product of the oxidative cleavage of the indole ring in L-tryptophan; the intermediate first formed in L-tryptophan catabolism.

N**-for·myl·me·thi·o·nine (fMet)** (fōr′mil-me-thī′ō-nēn). Methionine acylated on the NH_2 group by a formyl (–CHO) group. This is the starting amino acid residue for virtually all bacterial polypeptides. It is also observed in mitochondria and chloroplasts of eukaryotes. SEE ALSO initiating *codon*.

for·myl·me·thi·o·nyl-tRNA. Initiation tRNA in certain organisms.

N^{10}**-for·myl·tet·ra·hy·dro·fo·late.** A formyl derivative of tetrahydrofolate that serves as a one-carbon source in metabolism.

Forney, William R., U.S. pediatrician, *1931.

for·ni·cate (fōr′ni-kāt). **1.** Vaulted or arched; resembling a fornix. [L. *fornicatus,* arched, fr. *fornix,* vault, arch] **2.** To have sexual intercourse. [see fornication]

for·ni·ca·tion (fōr-ni-kā′shŭn). Sexual intercourse, especially between unmarried partners. [L. *fornicatio,* an arched or vaulted basement (brothel)]

for·ni·ces (fōr′ni-sēz). Plural of fornix.

for·nix, gen. **for·ni·cis,** pl. **for·ni·ces** (fōr′niks, -ni-sis, -ni-sēz) [TA]. **1** [TA]. In general, an arch-shaped structure; often the arch-shaped roof (or roof portion) of an anatomic space. **2** [TA]. The compact, white fiber bundle by which the hippocampus of each cerebral hemisphere projects to the contralateral hippocampus and to the septum, anterior nucleus of the thalamus, and mamillary body. Arising from pyramidal cells of Ammon horn, the fibers of the f. form the alveus hippocampi and the fimbria hippocampi, and in their further course compose, sequentially, the commissure of the fornix [TA], also called the hippocampal commissure [TA] (commissura hippocampi [TA]), the crus of fornix [TA] (crus fornicis [TA]), the body of fornix [TA] (corpus fornicis [TA]), and the column of fornix [TA] (columna fornicis [TA]), which divides into a smaller portion of precommissural fibers [TA] that pass anterior to the anterior commissure to the septal area and a larger portion of postcommissural fibers [TA] that pass posterior to the anterior commissure to end mainly in the mamillary nuclei and to a lesser extent in the anterior thalamic nucleus. SYN trigonum cerebrale. SYN cerebral trigone. [L. arch, vault]

f. conjuncti′vae, SYN conjunctival f.

conjunctival f. [TA], the space formed by the junction of the bulbar and palpebral portions of the conjunctiva, that of the upper lid being the superior conjunctival f. and that of the lower lid, the inferior conjunctival f. SYN conjunctival cul-de-sac, f. conjunctivae, retrotarsal fold.

f. gastricus [TA], SYN f. of stomach.

f. of lacrimal sac [TA], fornix of the lacrimal sac; the upper, blind end of the lacrimal sac that extends above the openings of the lacrimal canaliculi. SYN f. sacci lacrimalis [TA].

pharyngeal f., SYN *vault* of pharynx.

f. pharyn′gis [TA], SYN *vault* of pharynx.

f. sac′ci lacrima′lis [TA], SYN f. of lacrimal sac.

f. of stomach [TA], formerly considered to be a synonym of the official Nomina Anatomica term "fundus of stomach" (used more commonly than fundus in radiology), Terminologia Anatomica lists fornix and fundus of stomach separately, considering that all stomachs have a fundus, being the uppermost portion of the body of the stomach, the mucosa of which includes the greatest density of fundic cells; fornix is now reserved for the domed or pocket-like portion of the stomach that lies superior to and to the left of the cardial orifice, in which, in the upright position, gas is often contained. SYN f. gastricus [TA].

transverse f., SYN *commissura* fornicis.

f. u′teri, SYN vaginal f.

f. vagi′nae [TA], SYN vaginal f.

vaginal f. [TA], the recess at the vault of the vagina; it is divided into an anterior part, posterior part, and lateral part with respect to its relation to the cervix of the uterus. The posterior part is clinically significant as the site for culdocentesis and culdoscopy. The proximity of the ureter (below) and the uterine artery (above) adjacent to the lateral fornix is important clinically. SYN f. vaginae [TA], f. uteri.

forsk·o·lin (fōr′skŏ-lin). A phorbol ester that binds to and activates protein kinase C, thus mimicking the actions of diacylglycerol. [fr. *Coleus forskohlii,* taxonomic name of botanical source]

Forssman, John, Swedish bacteriologist and pathologist, 1868–1947. SEE F. *antibody, antigen, reaction,* antigen-antibody *reaction.*

Fo

Forssman, Hans, Swedish physician, *1912. SEE Börjeson-F.-Lehmann *syndrome.*

Förster, Richard, German ophthalmologist, 1825–1902. SEE F. *uveitis.*

fos·car·net (fos-kar′net). A pyrophosphate analog antiviral drug.

Fosdick, Leonard S., U.S. chemist, 1903–1969. SEE F.-Hansen-Epple *test.*

Foshay, Lee, U.S. bacteriologist, 1896–1961. SEE F. *test.*

FOSSA

fos·sa, gen. and pl. **fos·sae** (fos′ă, fos′ē) [TA]. A depression usually more or less longitudinal in shape below the level of the surface of a part. [L. a trench or ditch]

acetabular f. [TA], a depressed area in the floor of the acetabulum superior to the acetabular notch. SYN f. acetabuli [TA].

f. acetab′uli [TA], SYN acetabular f.

adipose fossae, subcutaneous spaces containing accumulations of fat in the breast.

amygdaloid f., SYN tonsillar f.

anconal f., SYN olecranon f.

anterior cranial f. [TA], the portion of the internal base of the skull, anterior to the sphenoidal ridges and limbus, in which the frontal lobes of the brain rest. SYN f. cranii anterior [TA], anterior cranial base.

f. anthel′icis, SYN f. antihelica.

f. of anthelix, SYN f. antihelica.

f. antihelica [TA], the depression on the medial surface of the auricle that corresponds to the anthelix. SYN f. anthelicis, f. of anthelix, periconchal sulcus.

articular f. of temporal bone, SYN mandibular f.

f. axilla′ris, SYN axilla.

axillary f., SYN axilla.

Bichat f., SYN pterygopalatine f.

Biesiadecki f., SYN iliacosubfascial f.

Broesike f., SYN parajejunal f.

f. cani′na [TA], SYN canine f.

canine f. [TA], a depression on the anterior surface of the maxilla below the infraorbital foramen and on the lateral side of the canine eminence. SYN f. canina [TA].

f. carot′ica, SYN carotid *triangle.*

cerebellar f. [TA], the large concave impressions on the inner surface of the occipital bone on either side of the foramen magnum and internal occipital crest, housing the cerebellar hemispheres; a part of the posterior cranial f. SYN f. cerebellaris [TA].

f. cerebellaris [TA], SYN cerebellar f.

Claudius f., SYN ovarian f.

condylar f. [TA], a depression behind the condyle of the occipital bone in which the posterior margin of the superior facet of the atlas lies in extension. SYN f. condylaris [TA].

f. condyla′ris [TA], SYN condylar f.

f. coronoi′dea humeri [TA], SYN coronoid f. of humerus.

coronoid f. of humerus [TA], a hollow on the anterior surface of the distal end of the humerus, just above the trochlea, in which the coronoid process of the ulna rests when the elbow is flexed. SYN f. coronoidea humeri [TA].

f. cra′nii ante′rior [TA], SYN anterior cranial f.

f. cra′nii me′dia [TA], SYN middle cranial f.

f. cra′nii poste′rior [TA], SYN posterior cranial f.

crural f., SYN femoral f.

Cruveilhier f., SYN scaphoid f. of sphenoid bone.

cubital f. [TA], the f. in front of the elbow, bounded laterally and medially by the humeral origins of the extensors and flexors of the forearm, respectively, and superiorly by an imaginary line connecting the humeral condyles. SYN f. cubitalis [TA], antecubital space, chelidon, triangle of elbow.

f. cubita′lis [TA], SYN cubital f.

digastric f. [TA], a hollow on the posterior surface of the base of the mandible, on either side of the median plane, giving attachment to the anterior belly of the digastric muscle. SYN f. digastrica [TA].

f. digas′trica [TA], SYN digastric f.

digital f., (1) SYN trochanteric f; (2) SYN f. of lateral malleolus.

f. duc′tus veno′si, SYN f. of ductus venosus.

f. of ductus venosus, a wide groove located posteriorly on the undersurface of the fetal liver between the caudate and left lobes; it lodges the ductus venosus and becomes the fissure of the ligamentum venosum in the adult. SYN f. ductus venosi.

duodenal fossae, SEE inferior duodenal f., superior duodenal f.

duodenojejunal f., SYN superior duodenal f.

epigastric f. [TA], the slight depression in the midline just inferior to the xiphoid process of the sternum. (TA lists this term as synonymous with epigastric *region*). SYN f. epigastrica [TA], pit of stomach, scrobiculus cordis.

f. epigas′trica [TA], SYN epigastric f.

femoral f., a depression on the peritoneal surface of the abdominal wall, inferior to the inguinal ligament, corresponding to the situation of the femoral ring. SYN crural f., fovea femoralis.

floccular f., SYN subarcuate f.

gallbladder f., SYN f. for gallbladder.

f. for gallbladder [TA], a depression on the visceral surface of the liver anteriorly, between the quadrate and the right lobes, lodging the gallbladder. SYN f. vesicae biliaris [TA], f. vesicae felleae*, gallbladder f.

Gerdy hyoid f., SYN carotid *triangle.*

f. glan′dulae lacrima′lis [TA], SYN f. for lacrimal gland.

glenoid f., (1) SYN glenoid *cavity* of scapula; (2) SYN mandibular f.

greater supraclavicular f. [TA], formerly considered a synonym for omoclavicular triangle (a subdivision of the posterior triangle of the neck); Terminologica Anatomica reserves this term for the surface feature that overlies the omoclavicular triangle: a depressed area above the middle of the clavicle, lateral to the sternocleidomastoid. SYN f. supraclavicularis major [TA].

Gruber-Landzert f., SYN inferior duodenal f.

f. of helix, SYN scapha (1).

hyaloid f. [TA], a depression on the anterior surface of the vitreous body in which lies the lens. SYN f. hyaloidea [TA], lenticular f., patellar f. of vitreous.

f. hyaloi′dea [TA], SYN hyaloid f.

hypophysial f. [TA], f. of the sphenoid bone housing the pituitary gland. SEE ALSO *sella* turcica. SYN f. hypophysialis [TA], pituitary f.

f. hypophysia′lis [TA], SYN hypophysial f.

iliac f. [TA], the smooth inner surface of the ilium above the arcuate line, giving attachment to the iliacus muscle. SYN f. iliaca [TA].

f. ili′aca [TA], SYN iliac f.

iliacosubfascial f., a peritoneal recess between the psoas muscle and the crest of the ilium. SYN Biesiadecki f., f. iliacosubfascialis.

f. iliacosubfascia′lis, SYN iliacosubfascial f.

iliopectineal f., a hollow between the iliopsoas and pectineus muscles in the center of the femoral triangle, lodging the femoral vessels and nerve.

f. incisi′va [TA], SYN incisive f.

incisive f. [TA], the depression in the midline of the bony palate behind the central incisors into which the incisive canals open. SYN f. incisiva [TA].

incudal f., SYN f. of incus.

f. incu′dis, SYN f. of incus.

f. of incus [TA], a small depression in the lower and posterior part of the epitympanic recess that lodges the short limb of the incus. SYN f. incudis, incudal f.

inferior duodenal f. [TA], the variable peritoneal recess which lies behind the inferior duodenal fold and along the ascending part of the duodenum. SYN recessus duodenalis inferior [TA], Gruber-Landzert f., inferior duodenal recess.

infraclavicular f. [TA], a triangular depression bounded by the clavicle and the adjacent borders of the deltoid and pectoralis major muscles. SYN f. infraclavicularis [TA], deltoideopectoral trigone, infraclavicular triangle, Mohrenheim f., Mohrenheim space, regio infraclavicularis.

f. infraclavicula´ris [TA], SYN infraclavicular f.

infraduodenal f., SYN retroduodenal *recess*.

f. infraspina´ta [TA], SYN infraspinous f.

infraspinous f. [TA], the hollow on the dorsal aspect of the scapula inferior to the spine, giving attachment chiefly to the infraspinatus muscle. SYN f. infraspinata [TA].

infratemporal f. [TA], the cavity on the side of the skull bounded laterally by the zygomatic arch and ramus of the mandible, medially by the lateral pterygoid plate, anteriorly by the zygomatic process of the maxilla and infratemporal surface of the maxilla, posteriorly by the tympanic plate and styloid and mastoid processes of the temporal bone, and superiorly by the infratemporal surface of the greater wing of the sphenoid bone. SYN f. infratemporalis [TA], zygomatic f.

f. infratempora´lis [TA], SYN infratemporal f.

inguinal f., SEE lateral inguinal f., medial inguinal f.

f. inguina´lis latera´lis [TA], SYN lateral inguinal f.

f. inguina´lis media´lis [TA], SYN medial inguinal f.

f. innomina´ta, SYN innominate f.

innominate f., a shallow depression between the false vocal cord and the aryepiglottic fold on either side. SYN f. innominata.

intercondylar f. [TA], the deep f. between the femoral condyles in which the cruciate ligaments are attached. SYN f. intercondylaris [TA], intercondyloid f. (2), intercondylic f., intercondyloid notch, popliteal notch.

f. intercondyla´ris [TA], SYN intercondylar f.

intercondyloid f., intercondylic f., (1) SEE *area* intercondylaris anterior tibiae, *area* intercondylaris posterior tibiae; **(2)** SYN intercondylar f.

f. intermesocol´ica transver´sa, SYN transverse intermesocolic f.

interpeduncular f. [TA], deep depression on the inferior surface of the mesencephalon, between the crura cerebri, the floor of which is formed by the posterior perforated substance. SEE interpeduncular *cistern*. SYN f. interpeduncularis [TA].

f. interpeduncula´ris [TA], SYN interpeduncular f.

intrabulbar f., the dilated commencement of the spongy part of the male urethra lying within the bulb of the penis.

ischioanal f. [TA], a wedge-shaped space with its base toward the perineum and lying between the tuberosity of the ischium and the obturator internus muscle laterally and the external anal sphincter and the levator ani muscle medially. SYN f. ischioanalis [TA], f. ischiorectalis, ischiorectal f., Velpeau f.

f. ischioana´lis [TA], SYN ischioanal f.

ischiorectal f., SYN ischioanal f.

f. ischiorecta´lis, SYN ischioanal f.

Jobert de Lamballe f., the hollow just above the knee formed by the adductor magnus and the sartorius and gracilis.

Jonnesco f., SYN superior duodenal f.

jugular f. [TA], an oval depression near the posterior border of the petrous portion of the temporal bone, medial to the styloid process, in which lies the beginning of the internal jugular vein (jugular bulb); SYN f. jugularis [TA].

f. jugula´ris [TA], SYN jugular f.

lacrimal f., ☆official alternate term for f. for lacrimal gland.

f. for lacrimal gland [TA], a hollow in the orbital plate of the frontal bone, formed by the overhanging margin and zygomatic process, lodging the lacrimal gland. SYN f. glandulae lacrimalis [TA], lacrimal f.☆.

f. for lacrimal sac [TA], a f. formed by the lacrimal bone and the frontal process of the maxilla, lodging the lacrimal sac. SYN f. sacci lacrimalis [TA].

Landzert f., a f. formed by two peritoneal folds, enclosing the left colic artery and the inferior mesenteric vein, respectively, at the side of the duodenum; it is smaller than the paraduodenal recess which is sometimes found in the same region.

lateral f. of brain, SYN lateral cerebral f.

lateral cerebral f. [TA], the deep depression of the basal surface of the forebrain that corresponds in position to the anterior perforated substance. Bounded medially by the optic tract and rostrally by the orbital surface of the frontal lobe, it extends laterally around the overhanging pole of the temporal lobe into the Sylvian fissure (sulcus lateralis). SYN f. lateralis cerebri [TA], f. of Sylvius, lateral f. of brain, vallecula sylvii.

lateral inguinal f. [TA], a depression on the peritoneal surface of the anterior abdominal wall lateral to the ridge formed by the inferior epigastric artery; it corresponds to the position of the deep inguinal ring, and is the site of an indirect inguinal hernia. SYN f. inguinalis lateralis [TA].

f. latera´lis cer´ebri [TA], SYN lateral cerebral f.

f. of lateral malleolus [TA], a large rough depression on the medial aspect of the lower end of the fibula just behind the articular facet for the talus giving attachment to the posterior talofibular and the transverse tibiofibular ligaments. SYN f. malleoli lateralis [TA], digital f. (2), f. malleoli fibulae.

lenticular f., SYN hyaloid f.

lesser supraclavicular f. [TA], a triangular space between the two heads of origin of the sternocleidomastoid muscle. SYN f. supraclavicularis minor [TA].

little f. of the cochlear window, SYN f. of round window.

little f. of the oval (vestibular) window, SYN f. of oval window.

Malgaigne f., SYN carotid *triangle*.

f. malle´oli fib´ulae, SYN f. of lateral malleolus.

f. malle´oli latera´lis [TA], SYN f. of lateral malleolus.

mandibular f. [TA], a deep hollow in the squamous portion of the temporal bone at the root of the zygoma, in which rests the condyle of the mandible. SYN f. mandibularis [TA], articular f. of temporal bone, cavitas glenoidalis, glenoid cavity, glenoid f. (2), glenoid surface.

f. mandibula´ris [TA], SYN mandibular f.

mastoid f., f. mastoi´dea, SYN suprameatal *triangle*.

medial inguinal f. [TA], a depression on the peritoneal surface of the anterior abdominal wall between the ridges formed by the inferior epigastric artery and the medial umbilical ligament; it corresponds to the position of the superficial inguinal ring and is the site of a direct inguinal hernia. SYN f. inguinalis medialis [TA], fovea inguinalis interna.

Merkel f., a groove in the posterolateral wall of the vestibule of the larynx between the corniculate and cuneiform cartilages.

mesentericoparietal f., SYN parajejunal f.

middle cranial f. [TA], a butterfly-shaped portion of the internal base of the skull posterior to the sphenoidal ridges and limbus and anterior to the crests of the petrous part of the temporal bones and dorsum sellae; it lodges the temporal lobes of the brain in the lateral portions, and the hypophysis centrally. SYN f. cranii media [TA].

Mohrenheim f., SYN infraclavicular f.

Morgagni f., SYN navicular f. of urethra.

mylohyoid f., SYN mylohyoid *groove*.

f. navicula´ris auric´ulae, SYN triangular f. of auricle.

f. navicula´ris au´ris, outmoded term for scapha (1).

f. navicula´ris Cruveil´hier, SYN scaphoid f. of sphenoid bone.

f. navicula´ris ure´thrae [TA], SYN navicular f. of urethra.

f. navicula´ris vestib´ulae vagi´nae, SYN vestibular f.

navicular f. of urethra [TA], the terminal dilated portion of the urethra in the glans penis. SYN f. navicularis urethrae [TA], f. terminalis urethrae, Morgagni f., Morgagni fovea.

f. olecra´ni [TA], SYN olecranon f.

olecranon f. [TA], a hollow on the dorsum of the distal end of the humerus, just above the trochlea, in which the olecranon process of the ulna rests when the elbow is extended. SYN f. olecrani [TA], anconal f.

oval f., ☆official alternate term for f. ovalis (1).

f. ova´lis, (1) [NA], an oval depression on the lower part of the septum of the right atrium; it is a vestige of the foramen ovale, and its floor corresponds to the septum primum of the fetal heart; SYN oval f.☆. **(2)** SYN saphenous *opening*.

f. of oval window [TA], a depression on the medial wall of the middle ear that has the oval window (fenestra vestibulae) in its lower portion. SYN fossula fenestrae vestibuli [TA], Huguier sinus, little f. of the oval (vestibular) window.

ovarian f. [TA], a depression in the parietal peritoneum of the pelvis; it is bounded in front by the occluded part of the umbilical artery, and behind by the ureter and the uterine vessels; it lodges the ovary. SYN f. ovarica [TA], Claudius f.

f. ova′rica [TA], SYN ovarian f.

paraduodenal f., SYN paraduodenal *recess.*

parajejunal f., a peritoneal f. that has been seen in a few cases in which the jejunum has no mesentery but is attached to the posterior parietal peritoneum; the f. begins at the point where the mesentery ends, and is seen on raising up the knuckle of free intestine. SYN Broesike f., f. parajejunalis, mesentericoparietal f., mesentericoparietal recess.

f. parajejuna′lis, SYN parajejunal f.

pararectal f. [TA], a peritoneal depression on either side of the rectum formed by peritoneal (sacrogenital) folds passing from the posterolateral pelvic wall to the central pelvic viscera. The f. is a lateral extension of the male rectovesical pouch or the female rectouterine pouch. SYN f. pararectalis [TA], pararectal pouch.

f. pararectalis [TA], SYN pararectal f.

paravesical f. [TA], a peritoneal depression formed by the reflection of the peritoneum from the lateral pelvic wall onto the roof of the bladder; in the female, it is the lateral portion of the uterovesical pouch, and is separated from the pararectal pouch, which lies posteriorly, by the broad ligament. SYN f. paravesicalis [TA], paracystic pouch, paravesical pouch.

f. paravesica′lis [TA], SYN paravesical f.

patellar f. of vitreous, SYN hyaloid f.

peritoneal fossae, depressions or pouches formed between various peritoneal folds; they may be the sites of internal hernias.

petrosal f., SYN petrosal *fossula.*

piriform f. [TA], a recess in the anterolateral wall of the nasopharynx on each side of the vestibule of the larynx separated from it by the aryepiglottic folds. SYN recessus piriformis [TA], piriform recess☆, piriform sinus.

pituitary f., SYN hypophysial f.

f. poplit′ea [TA], SYN popliteal f.

popliteal f. [TA], the diamond-shaped space posterior to the knee joint bounded superficially by the diverging biceps femoris and semimembranosus muscles above and inferiorly by the two heads of the gastrocnemius muscle; deeply, the f. is bound superiorly by the diverging supracondylar lines of the femur and the soleal line of the tibia inferiorly. Contents: tibial nerve, popliteal artery, vein, fat. SYN f. poplitea [TA], ham (1), poples, popliteal region, popliteal space, popliteus (2).

posterior cranial f. [TA], the internal base of the skull posterior to the crest of the petrous part of the temporal bones and the dorsum sellae and anterior to the grooves for the transverse sinuses, where the cerebellum, pons, and medulla oblongata rest. SYN f. cranii posterior [TA].

f. provesica′lis, SYN Hartmann *pouch.*

pterygoid f. [TA], the f. formed by the divergence posteriorly of the plates of the pterygoid process of the sphenoid bone; it lodges the origin of medial pterygoid and the tensor palati muscles. SYN f. pterygoidea [TA].

f. pterygoi′dea [TA], SYN pterygoid f.

pterygomaxillary f., SYN pterygopalatine f.

f. pterygopalati′na [TA], SYN pterygopalatine f.

pterygopalatine f. [TA], sphenomaxillary f., a small pyramidal space, housing the pterygopalatine ganglion, between the pterygoid process, the maxilla, and the palatine bone. SYN f. pterygopalatina [TA], Bichat f., pterygomaxillary f., sphenomaxillary f.

radial f. of humerus [TA], a shallow depression on the anterior aspect of the distal humerus, superior to the capitulum of the humerus and lateral to the coronoid fossa, in which the margin of the head of the radius rests when the elbow is in extreme flexion. SYN f. radialis humeri [TA].

f. radia′lis hu′meri [TA], SYN radial f. of humerus.

retroduodenal f., SYN retroduodenal *recess.*

retromandibular f., the depression inferior to the auricle and posterior to the ramus and angle of the mandible. SYN f. retromandibularis.

f. retromandibula′ris, SYN retromandibular f.

retromolar f. [TA], a triangular depression in the mandible posterior to the third molar tooth. SYN f. retromolaris [TA].

f. retromolaris [TA], SYN retromolar f.

rhomboid f. [TA], the floor of the fourth ventricle of the brain, formed by the ventricular surface of the rhombencephalon. SYN f. rhomboidea [TA].

f. rhomboi′dea [TA], SYN rhomboid f.

Rosenmüller f., SYN pharyngeal *recess.*

f. of round window [TA], a depression on the medial wall of the middle ear which has the round window (fenestra cochleae) in its lower portion. SYN fossula fenestrae cochleae [TA], fossula rotunda, little f. of the cochlear window.

f. sac′ci lacrima′lis [TA], SYN f. for lacrimal sac.

scaphoid f. [TA], a boat-shaped hollow. SEE ALSO scaphoid f. of sphenoid bone. SYN f. scaphoidea [TA].

f. scaphoidea [TA], SYN scaphoid f.

f. scaphoid′ea ossis sphenoidalis, SYN scaphoid f. of sphenoid bone.

scaphoid f. of sphenoid bone, a longitudinal hollow on the posterior surface of the superior portion (root) of the medial pterygoid plate; it gives origin to the tensor veli palati muscle. SYN f. Cruveilhier f., f. navicularis Cruveilhier, f. scaphoidea ossis sphenoidalis.

f. scar′pae ma′jor, SYN femoral *triangle.*

sigmoid f., SYN *groove* for sigmoid sinus.

sphenomaxillary f., SYN pterygopalatine f.

f. subarcua′ta [TA], SYN subarcuate f.

subarcuate f. [TA], an irregular depression on the posterior surface of the petrous portion of the temporal bone just below its crest and above and lateral to the internal acoustic meatus. In the fetus, the flocculus of the cerebellum rests here; in the adult, a small vein enters the bone here. SYN f. subarcuata [TA], floccular f., hiatus subarcuatus.

subcecal f., an inconstant depression in the peritoneum extending posterior to the cecum. SYN Treitz f.

subinguinal f., the depression on the anterior surface of the thigh beneath the groin.

sublingual f. [TA], a shallow depression on either side of the mental spine, on the inner surface of the body of the mandible, superior to the mylohyoid line, lodging the sublingual gland. SYN fovea sublingualis [TA], sublingual pit.

submandibular f. [TA], the depression on the medial surface of the body of the mandible inferior to the mylohyoid line in which the submandibular gland is lodged. SYN fovea submandibularis [TA], f. submandibularis, fovea submaxillaris, submaxillary f.

f. submandibula′ris, SYN submandibular f.

submaxillary f., SYN submandibular f.

subscapular f. [TA], the concave ventral aspect of the body of the scapula giving origin to the subscapularis muscle. SYN f. subscapularis [TA].

f. subscapula′ris [TA], SYN subscapular f.

superior duodenal f. [TA], a peritoneal recess extending upward behind the superior duodenal fold. SYN recessus duodenalis superior [TA], superior duodenal recess☆, duodenojejunal f., duodenojejunal recess, Jonnesco f.

f. supraclavicularis major [TA], SYN greater supraclavicular f.

f. supraclavicula′ris mi′nor [TA], SYN lesser supraclavicular f.

supramastoid f., SYN suprameatal *triangle.*

f. supraspina′ta [TA], SYN supraspinous f.

supraspinous f. [TA], the hollow on the dorsal aspect of the scapula above the spine, lodging the supraspinatus muscle. SYN f. supraspinata [TA].

supratonsillar f. [TA], the interval between the palatoglossal and palatopharyngeal arches above the tonsil, most obvious after the tonsil has regressed in the adult. SYN f. supratonsillaris [TA], supratonsillar recess, Tourtual sinus.

f. supratonsilla′ris [TA], SYN supratonsillar f.

supravesical f. [TA], the depression on the peritoneal surface of the anterior abdominal wall above the bladder and between the median and medial umbilical folds. Its level, relative to the pubis, changes with filling of the bladder. SYN f. supravesicalis [TA], f. supravesicalis.

f. supravesica′lis [TA], SYN supravesical f.

f. of Sylvius, SYN lateral cerebral f.

temporal f. [TA], the space on the side of the cranium bounded by the temporal lines and terminating below at the level of the zygomatic arch. SYN f. temporalis [TA].

f. tempora′lis [TA], SYN temporal f.

f. termina′lis ure′thrae, SYN navicular f. of urethra.

tonsillar f. [TA], the depression between the palatoglossal and palatopharyngeal arches occupied by the palatine tonsil. SYN f. tonsillaris [TA], amygdaloid f., sinus tonsillaris.

f. tonsilla′ris [TA], SYN tonsillar f.

transverse intermesocolic f., a f. occupying the position of the superior duodenal recess but extending transversely from right to left for a few cms. SYN f. intermesocolica transversa.

Treitz f., SYN subcecal f.

triangular f. of auricle [TA], the depression at the upper part of the auricle between the two crura of the antihelix. SYN f. triangularis auriculae [TA], f. navicularis auriculae.

f. triangula′ris auriculae [TA], SYN triangular f. of auricle.

trochanteric f., a depression at the root of the neck of the femur beneath the curved tip of the great trochanter; it gives attachment to the tendon of the obturator externus. SYN digital f. (1), f. trochanterica.

f. trochanter′ica, SYN trochanteric f.

trochlear f., SYN trochlear *fovea*.

f. trochlea′ris, SYN trochlear *fovea*.

umbilical f., SYN *fissure* for ligamentum teres.

Velpeau f., SYN ischioanal f.

f. ve′nae ca′vae, SYN *sulcus* for vena cava.

f. ve′nae umbilica′lis, SYN *fissure* for ligamentum teres.

f. veno′sa, SYN paraduodenal *recess*.

vermian f., a small depression near the lower part of the internal occipital crest that lodges part of the inferior vermis of the cerebellum.

f. vesi′cae bilia′ris [TA], SYN f. for gallbladder.

f. vesicae felleae, ☆official alternate term for f. for gallbladder.

vestibular f. [TA], the portion of the vestibule of the vagina between the frenulum of the labia minora and the posterior labial commissure of the vulva. SYN f. vestibuli vaginae [TA], f. navicularis vestibulae vaginae, f. of vestibule of vagina.

f. of vestibule of vagina, SYN vestibular f.

f. vestib′uli vagi′nae [TA], SYN vestibular f.

Waldeyer fossae, SEE inferior duodenal f., superior duodenal f.

zygomatic f., SYN infratemporal f.

---

fos·sette (fo-set′). **1.** SYN fossula. **2.** A seldom-used term for corneal ulcer of small diameter. [Fr. dim. of *fosse,* a ditch]

fos·su·la, pl. **fos·su·lae** (fos′ū-lă, -lē) [TA]. **1** [NA]. A small fossa. **2.** A minor fissure or slight depression on the surface of the cerebrum. SYN fossette (1). [L. dim. of *fossa,* ditch]

f. fenes′trae coch′leae [TA], SYN *fossa* of round window.

f. fenes′trae vestib′uli [TA], SYN *fossa* of oval window.

f. petro′sa [TA], SYN petrosal f.

petrosal f. [TA], a small and often only faintly marked depression on the inferior surface of the petrous portion of the temporal bone, between the jugular fossa and the opening of the carotid canal; here opens the canaliculus tympanicus transmitting the tympanic nerve. SYN f. petrosa [TA], petrosal fossa, receptaculum ganglii petrosi.

f. post fenestram, the small passage filled with connective tissue posterior to the oval window of the cochlea; a site of predilection for otosclerosis.

f. rotun′da, SYN *fossa* of round window.

tonsillar fossulae [TA], the small pits at the openings of the tonsillar crypts onto the external surface of the tonsil. They occur as palatine and pharyngeal tonsils. SYN fossulae tonsillarum (palatini et pharyngealis) [TA].

fos′sulae tonsilla′rum (palatini et pharyngealis) [TA], SYN tonsillar fossulae.

fos·su·late (fos′ū-lāt). Grooved; containing a fossula or small fossa; hollowed out.

Foster frame. See under frame.

Foster Kennedy. SEE Kennedy.

Fothergill, John, English physician, 1712–1780. SEE F. *disease, neuralgia, sign.*

Fothergill, William E., English gynecologist, 1865–1926. SEE F. *operation.*

Fouchet, A., French physician, *1894. SEE F. *reagent, stain.*

fou·lage (foo-lahzh′). Kneading and pressure of the muscles, constituting a form of massage. [Fr. impression]

foun·da·tion (fown-dā′shŭn). A base; a supporting structure.

denture f., that portion of the oral structures which is available to support a denture. SEE ALSO denture foundation *area,* denture foundation *surface,* mean foundation *plane.*

found·er (fown′der). A person who contributes to the initial genetic structure of a population and is liable to contribute to a large proportion of the genes in the descendants from it.

four·chette (foor-shet′). ☆official alternate term for *frenulum* of labia minora. [Fr. dim. of *fourché,* fr. L. *furca,* fork]

Fou·ri·er, J.B.J., French mathematician and administrator, 1768–1830. SEE Fourier *analysis,* Fourier *transform,* Fourier *transfer.*

Fourneau, Ernest F.A., French chemist and pharmacologist, 1872–1949. SEE F. 710, 933.

Fourneau 710. A synthetic quinoline; an antimalarial agent. [Ernest F.A. *Fourneau*]

Fourneau 933. SYN piperoxan hydrochloride. [Ernest F.A. *Fourneau*]

Fournier, Jean A., French syphilographer, 1832–1914. SEE F. *disease, gangrene; syphiloma* of F.

fo·vea, pl. **fo·ve·ae** (fō′vē-ă, fō′vē-ē) [TA]. Any natural depression on the surface of the body, such as the axilla, or on the surface of a bone. Cf. dimple. SYN pit (1). [L. a pit]

f. ante′rior, SYN superior f.

anterior f., SYN superior f.

f. articula′ris cap′itis ra′dii [TA], SYN articular *facet* of radial head.

f. articula′ris infe′rior atlan′tis, SYN inferior articular *surface* of atlas.

f. articula′ris supe′rior atlan′tis, SYN superior articular *surface* of atlas.

f. cap′itis fem′oris [TA], SYN f. for ligament of head of femur.

f. cardi′aca, anterior intestinal portal; the opening of the foregut into the midgut. SEE ALSO epigastric *fossa.* SYN anterior intestinal portal.

f. centra′lis maculae luteae [TA], SYN central retinal f.

central retinal f. [TA], a depression in the center of the macula retinae containing only cones and lacking blood vessels. SYN f. centralis maculae luteae [TA], central pit.

f. costa′lis infe′rior [TA], SYN inferior costal *facet.*

f. costa′lis proces′sus transver′si [TA], SYN transverse costal *facet.*

f. costa′lis supe′rior [TA], SYN superior costal *facet.*

f. den′tis atlan′tis [TA], SYN *facet* (of atlas) for dens.

f. ellip′tica, SYN elliptical *recess* of bony labyrinth.

f. ethmoida′lis, the roof of the ethmoid air cells.

f. of the femoral head, SYN f. for ligament of head of femur.

f. femora′lis, SYN femoral *fossa.*

f. hemiellip′tica, SYN elliptical *recess* of bony labyrinth.

f. hemisphe′rica, SYN spherical *recess* of bony labyrinth.

f. infe′rior [TA], SYN inferior f.

inferior f. [TA], a small depression in the limiting sulcus of the rhomboidal fossa below the medullary striae of either side, gener-

fo

ally lateral to the hypoglossal and vagal trigones. SYN f. inferior [TA].

f. inguina'lis inter'na, SYN medial inguinal *fossa.*

f. for ligament of head of femur [TA], a depression on the extremity of the head of the femur giving attachment to the ligamentum teres femoris. SYN f. capitis femoris [TA], f. of the femoral head, pit of head of femur.

Morgagni f., SYN navicular *fossa* of urethra.

f. oblon'ga cartilag'inis arytenoid'eae [TA], SYN oblong f. of arytenoid cartilage.

oblong f. of arytenoid cartilage [TA], a broad shallow depression on the anterolateral surface of the arytenoid cartilage, for attachment of the thyroarytenoid muscle. SYN f. oblonga cartilaginis arytenoideae [TA], oblong pit of arytenoid cartilage.

pterygoid f. [TA], a depression on the antero-medial side of the neck of the condylar process of the mandible, giving attachment to the lateral pterygoid muscle. SYN f. pterygoidea [TA], pterygoid depression, pterygoid pit.

f. pterygoid'ea [TA], SYN pterygoid f.

f. of radial head, SYN articular *facet* of radial head.

f. sphe'rica, SYN spherical *recess* of bony labyrinth.

f. sublingua'lis [TA], SYN sublingual *fossa.*

f. submandibula'ris [TA], SYN submandibular *fossa.*

f. submaxilla'ris, SYN submandibular *fossa.*

f. supe'rior, SYN superior f.

superior f. [TA], a slight depression in the limiting sulcus on either side of the rhomboidal fossa, above the medullary striae and lateral to the facial colliculus. SYN f. superior [TA], anterior f., f. anterior.

f. supravesica'lis, SYN supravesical *fossa.*

triangular f. of arytenoid cartilage [TA], a deep depression in the upper portion of the anterolateral surface of the arytenoid cartilage, lodging glands. SYN f. triangularis cartilaginis arytenoideae [TA], triangular pit of arytenoid cartilage.

f. triangula'ris cartilag'inis arytenoid'eae [TA], SYN triangular f. of arytenoid cartilage.

trochlear f. [TA], a shallow depression in the roof of the orbit close to the medial margin to which is attached the pulley for the superior oblique tendon. SYN f. trochlearis [TA], fossa trochlearis, trochlear fossa, trochlear pit.

f. trochlea'ris [TA], SYN trochlear f.

fo·ve·ate, fo·ve·at·ed (fō'-vē-āt, -ā-ted). Pitted; having foveas or depressions on the surface.

fo·ve·a·tion (fō-vē-ā'shŭn). Pitted scar formation, as in smallpox, chickenpox, or vaccinia. [L. *fovea,* a pit]

fo·ve·o·la, pl. **fo·ve·o·lae** (fō-vē'ō-lă, -lē) [TA]. A minute fovea or pit. [Mod. L. dim. of L. *fovea,* pit]

f. coccy'gea [TA], SYN coccygeal f.

coccygeal f. [TA], a depression in the skin over the coccyx caused by the caudal retinaculum. SYN f. coccygea [TA], coccygeal dimple, postanal dimple.

f. gas'trica [TA], SYN gastric *pit.*

granular foveolae [TA], pits on the inner surface of the skull, along the course of the superior sagittal sinus, in which are lodged the arachnoidal granulations. SYN foveolae granulares [TA], granular pits, pacchionian depressions.

foveolae granula'res [TA], SYN granular foveolae.

f. ocula'ris, SYN f. of retina.

f. papilla'ris, the minute depression sometimes seen at the apex of a papilla of the kidney where a papillary duct opens into a calix.

f. of retina [TA], the central portion of the central retinal fovea that contains cones only. SYN f. retinae [TA], f. ocularis.

f. retinae [TA], SYN f. of retina.

f. suprameatalis, SYN suprameatal *triangle.*

f. supramea'tica [TA], SYN suprameatal *triangle.*

fo·ve·o·lar (fō-vē'ō-lăr). Pertaining to a foveola.

fo·ve·o·late (fō'vē-ō-lāt, fō-vē'ō-lăt). Having minute pits (foveolae) or small depressions on the surface.

Foville, Achille L., French neurologist, 1799–1878. SEE F. *fasciculus, syndrome.*

Fowler, George R., U.S. surgeon, 1848–1906. SEE F. *position.*

Fox, George H., U.S. dermatologist, 1846–1937. SEE F.-Fordyce *disease.*

Fox, Lewis, U.S. periodontist, *1903. SEE Goldman-F. *knives,* under *knife.*

fox·glove (foks'glŭv). SYN *Digitalis.*

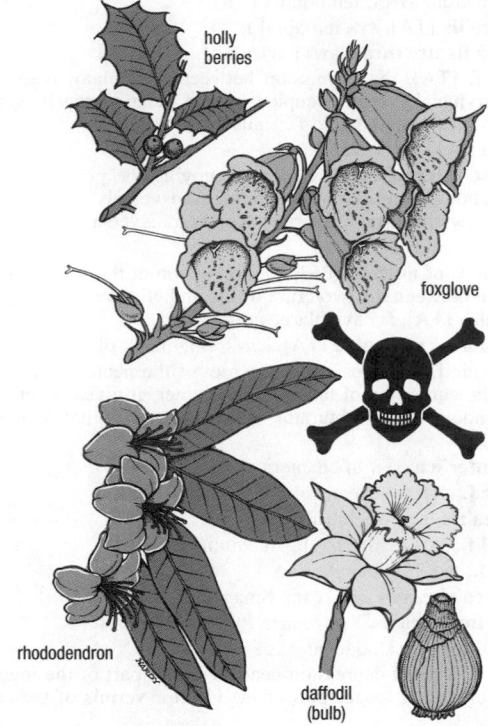

foxglove and other poisonous plants

FPLC Abbreviation for fast protein liquid chromatography.

FPS, fps Abbreviation for foot-pound-second. SEE foot-pound-second *system,* foot-pound-second *unit.*

Fr 1. Symbol for francium.

Fraccaro, Marco, Italian ophthalmologist, *1926. SEE Schmid-F. *syndrome.*

Fraccaro, M., Italian physician. SEE Parenti-Fraccaro *syndrome.*

F.R.A.C.P. Abbreviation for Fellow of the Royal Australasian College of Physicians.

fractals (frak'talz). Mathematical patterns developed by Benoit Mandelbrot in 1977, in which small parts have the same shape as the whole. Blood vessels and the bronchial tree behave as f.; some infections and neoplasms also behave as f. [Fr., fr. L. *fractus,* broken, pp. of *frango,* to break, + -al]

frac·tion (frak'shŭn). **1.** The quotient of two quantities. **2.** An aliquot portion or any portion. **3.** As a verb, to separate into portions.

amorphous f. of adrenal cortex, noncrystalline residue of an acetone extract of the adrenal cortex after crystalline steroids, e.g., corticosterone, deoxycorticosterone, etc., have been isolated.

blood plasma f.'s, portions of the blood plasma as separated by electrophoresis or other technique.

f. collector, a device used to collect the eluate from a column in column chromatography.

dried human plasma protein f., freeze-dried human plasma protein f.

ejection f., the f. of the blood contained in the ventricle at the end of diastole that is expelled during its contraction, i.e., the stroke

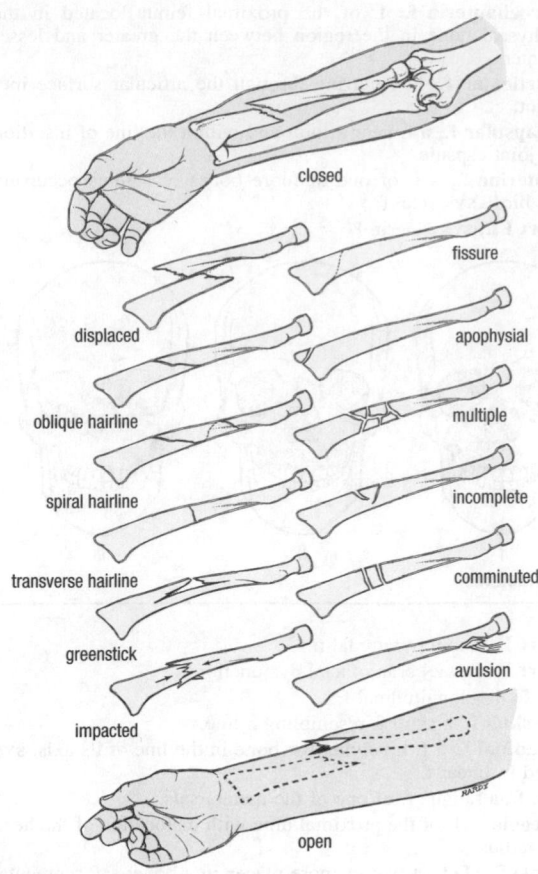

closed

fissure

displaced

apophysial

oblique hairline

multiple

spiral hairline

incomplete

transverse hairline

comminuted

greenstick

avulsion

impacted

open

types of fractures

volume divided by end-diastolic volume, normally 0.55 (by electrocardiogram) or greater; with the onset of congestive heart failure, the ejection f. decreases, sometimes to 0.10 or even less in severe cases.

filtration f. (FF), the f. of the plasma entering the kidney that filters into the lumen of the renal tubules, determined by dividing the glomerular filtration rate by the renal plasma flow; normally, it is around 0.17.

human antihemophilic f., SYN human antihemophilic *factor*.

human plasma protein f., a sterile solution of selected proteins derived from the blood plasma of adult human donors, containing 4.5 to 5.5 g of protein per 100 ml, of which 83 to 90% is albumin and the remainder is α- and β-globulins; used as a blood volume supporter.

mole f., the ratio of the moles of one component of a system to the total moles of all the components present.

radionuclide ejection f., a nuclear medicine study for determination of ejection f. of either ventricle; supersedes multiple-gated acquisition *scan* in some centers. SEE ALSO multiple-gated acquisition *scan*.

recombination f., the proportion of progeny of a mating pair of specific genotype and coupling phase that are recombinant; there must be no differential selection among the possible types of progeny, and the recombination f. should be the same regardless of the alleles involved or their coupling phase.

regurgitant f., the amount of blood regurgitated into a cardiac chamber divided by the stroke output; normally, no blood regurgitates; in patients with severe valvular lesions such as mitral or aortic insufficiency, regurgitant f. can approach 80%; this f. affords a quantitative measure of the severity of the valvular lesion.

frac·tion·a·tion (frak-shŭn-ā′shŭn). **1.** To separate components of a mixture. **2.** The administration of a course of therapeutic

radiation of a neoplasm in a planned series of fractions of the total dose, most often once a day for several weeks, in order to minimize radiation damage of contiguous normal tissues.

FRACTURE

frac·ture (frak′choor). **1.** To break. **2.** A break, especially the breaking of a bone or cartilage. [L. *fractura,* a break]

apophysial f., separation of apophysis from bone.

articular f., a f. involving the joint surface of a bone.

avulsion f., a f. that occurs when a joint capsule, ligament, or muscle insertion of origin is pulled from the bone as a result of a sprain dislocation or strong contracture of the muscle against resistance; as the soft tissue is pulled away from the bone, a fragment (or fragments) remains attached to the soft tissue of the bone. SYN strain f.

Barton f., f. of the distal radius with volar subluxation or dislocation of the radiocarpal joint.

basal skull f., a f. involving the base of the cranium.

bending f., an injury in which a long bone or bones, usually the radius and ulna, are bent (i.e., angulated) due to multiple microfractures, none of which can be seen by x-ray imaging.

Bennett f., f. dislocation of the first metacarpal bone at the carpal-metacarpal joint.

bimalleolar f., SYN Pott f.

birth f., f. occurring during the trauma of delivery or, occasionally, before delivery in infants with osteogenesis imperfecta.

blow-out f., a f. of the floor of the orbit, without a fracture of the rim, produced by a blow on the globe with the force being transmitted via the globe to the orbital floor.

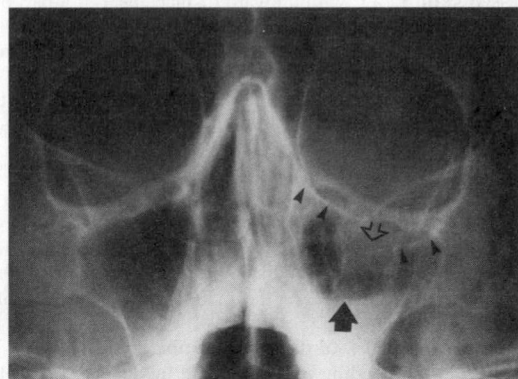

orbital floor blow-out fracture: Waters view on plain film shows major findings associated with an orbital floor blow-out injury: disruption of orbital floor (arrowheads), soft-tissue mass in the superior aspect of maxillary sinus (open arrow), and maxillary sinus fluid level (closed arrow)

boxer's f., f. of the neck of a metacarpal bone—typically of the fifth metacarpals.

capillary f., SYN hairline f.

Chance f., a transverse f., usually in the thoracic or lumbar spine, through the body of the vertebra extending posteriorly through the pedicles and the spinous process.

clay shoveler's f., an avulsion f. of the base of spinous processes of C-7, C-6, or T-1 (in order of prevalence).

closed f., a f. in which skin is intact at site of f. SYN simple f.

closed skull f., f. with intact overlying scalp and/or mucous membranes. SYN simple skull f.

Colles f., a f. of the distal radius with displacement and/or angulation of the distal fragment dorsally.

comminuted f., a f. in which the bone is broken into more than two fragments.

comminuted skull f., a f. of the skull with fragmentation of bone.

complex f., a f. with significant soft tissue injury.

compound f., f. in which the skin is perforated and there is an open wound down to the site of the f. SYN open f.

compound skull f., SYN open skull f.

f. by contrecoup, skull f. at a point distant from the site of impact.

cough f., a f. of a rib or cartilage, usually the fifth or seventh, from vigorous coughing.

craniofacial dysjunction f., a complex f. in which the facial bones are separated from the cranial bones. SYN Le Fort III craniofacial dysjunction, Le Fort III f., transverse facial f.

dentate f., a f. in which the opposing surfaces are rough, with toothed or serrate projections fitting into corresponding indentations.

depressed f., SYN depressed skull f.

depressed skull f., a f. with inward displacement of a part of the calvarium; may or may not be associated with disruption of the underlying dura or cerebral cortex. SYN depressed f.

derby hat f., regular cranial concavity in infants; may or may not be associated with f. SYN dishpan f.

diastatic skull f., (1) separation of cranial bones at a suture; (2) f. with marked separation of bone fragments.

direct f., a f., especially of the skull, occurring at the point of injury.

dishpan f., SYN derby hat f.

dislocation f., a f. of a bone near an articulation with a concomitant dislocation of the adjacent.

double f., SYN segmental f.

Dupuytren f., f. of lower part of fibula, with dislocation of ankle.

epiphysial f., epiphyseal f., separation of the epiphysis of a long bone, caused by trauma. SEE Salter-Harris *classification* of epiphysial plate injuries.

expressed skull f., a f. with outward displacement of a part of the cranium.

extracapsular f., a f. near a joint, but outside of the line of attachment of the joint capsule.

fatigue f., f. that occurs in bone subjected to repetitive stress, most often transverse in configuration. SYN stress f.

fetal f., SYN intrauterine f.

fissured f., SYN longitudinal f.

folding f., SYN torus f.

freeze f., a procedure for preparing cells or other biological samples for electron microscopy in which the sample is frozen quickly and then broken with a sharp blow. SYN cryofracture.

Galeazzi f., f. of the shaft of the radius with dislocation of the distal radioulnar joint.

Gosselin f., v-shaped f. of distal end of tibia.

greenstick f., the bending of a bone with incomplete f. involving the convex side of the curve only.

growing f., linear skull f. in a young child which increases in size, usually as the result of an associated dural tear and arachnoid cyst formation within the f. line.

Guérin f., a f. of the facial bones in which there is a horizontal f. at the base of the maxillae above the apices of the teeth. SYN horizontal f., Le Fort I f.

gutter f., a long, narrow, depressed f. of the skull.

hairline f., a f. without separation of the fragments, the line of break being hairlike, as seen sometimes in the skull. SYN capillary f.

hangman's f., a f. of the cervical spine through the pedicles of C2; may be associated with an anterior dislocation of the C2 vertebral body with respect to C3.

horizontal f., SYN Guérin f.

impacted f., a f. in which one of the fragments is driven into the cancellous bone of the other fragment.

incomplete f., a f. in which the line of f. does not completely traverse the bone.

indirect f., a f., especially of the skull, that occurs at a point not at the site of impact.

intertrochanteric f., f. of the proximal femur located in the metaphyseal bone in the region between the greater and lesser trochanters.

intraarticular f., f. occurring through the articular surface into the joint.

intracapsular f., a f. near a joint and within the line of insertion of the joint capsule.

intrauterine f., a f. of one or more bones of a fetus occurring before birth. SYN fetal f.

Le Fort I f., SYN Guérin f.

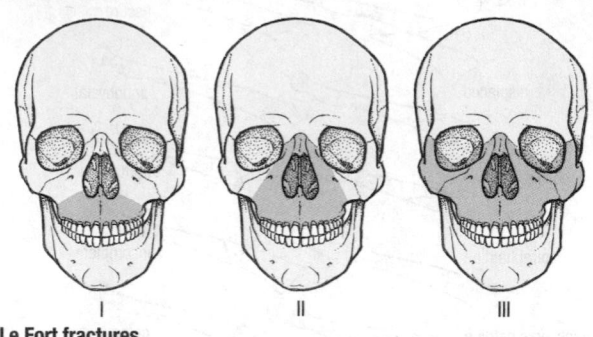

Le Fort fractures

Le Fort II f., SYN pyramidal f.

Le Fort III f., SYN craniofacial dysjunction f.

linear f., SYN longitudinal f.

linear skull f., a skull f. resembling a line.

longitudinal f., a f. involving the bone in the line of its axis. SYN fissured f., linear f.

march f., a fatigue f. of one of the metatarsals.

Monteggia f., f. of the proximal ulna with dislocation of the head of the radius.

multiple f., (1) f. at two or more places in a bone; SEE segmental f; (2) f. of several bones occurring simultaneously.

neurogenic f., a f. in bone weakened by disease of the nerve supply.

oblique f., a f. the line of which runs obliquely to the longitudinal axis of the bone.

occult f., a condition in which there are clinical signs of f. but no radiographic evidence; after 2 to 4 weeks, radiographic imaging shows new bone formation; magnetic resonance imaging frequently confirms the fracture before changes are evident on radiography; commonly seen in the navicular bone of the wrist.

open f., SYN compound f.

open skull f., a f. with laceration of overlying scalp and/or mucous membrane. SYN compound skull f.

parry f., obsolete term for Monteggia f.

pathologic f., a f. occurring at a site weakened by preexisting disease, especially neoplasm or necrosis, of the bone.

pertrochanteric f., a f. through the intertrochanteric region of the femur; a form of extracapsular hip f.

pilon f., a f. of the distal metaphysis of the tibia extending into the ankle joint.

ping-pong f., SEE derby hat f.

pond f., a circular depressed skull f.

Pott f., f. of the lower part of the fibula and of the malleolus of the tibia, with outward displacement of the foot. SYN bimalleolar f.

pyramidal f., a f. of the midfacial skeleton with the principal f. lines meeting at an apex at or near the superior aspect of the nasal bones. SYN Le Fort II f.

segmental f., a f. in two parts of the same bone. SYN double f.

Shepherd f., a f. of the external tubercle (posterior process) of the talus, sometimes mistaken for a displacement of the os trigonum.

silver-fork f., a Colles f. of the wrist in which the deformity has the appearance of a fork in profile.

simple f., SYN closed f.

simple skull f., SYN closed skull f.

Skillern f., obsolete term for f. of distal radius with greenstick f. of neighboring portion of ulna.

skull f., a break of the cranium resulting from trauma.

Smith f., reversed Colles f.; f. of the distal radius with displacement of the fragment toward the palmar (volar) aspect.

spiral f., a f. the line of which is helical in the bone; usually results from a twisting injury.

splintered f., a comminuted f. in which the fragments are long and sharp-pointed.

spontaneous f., a f. occurring without any external injury.

sprain f., an avulsion f. in which a small portion of adjacent bone has been pulled off.

stable f., a f. that does not tend to displace once it has been reduced and immobilized.

stellate f., a f. in which the lines of break radiate from a central point.

stellate skull f., a skull f. with multiple linear fractures radiating from the site of impact.

strain f., SYN avulsion f.

stress f., SYN fatigue f.

subcapital f., an intracapsular f. of the neck of the femur, at the point where the neck of the femur joins the head.

subperiosteal f., a f. occurring beneath the periosteum, and without displacement.

supracondylar f., a f. of the distal end of the humerus or femur located above the condylar region.

toddler's f., a spiral f. of the tibia seen frequently in children 1–2 years of age.

torsion f., a f. resulting from twisting of the limb.

torus f., a bone deformity in children in which the bone bends and buckles but does not fracture; it occurs commonly in the radius or ulna or both. This fracture occurs only in children because their bones are softer than adults. SYN folding f.

transcervical f., a f. through the neck of the femur.

transcondylar f., a f. through condyles of the humerus or femur.

transverse f., a f., the line of which forms a right angle with the longitudinal axis of the bone.

transverse facial f., SYN craniofacial dysjunction f.

trimalleolar f., a f. of the ankle through the lateral malleolus of the fibula and the medial malleolus and posterior process of the tibia.

tripod f., a facial f. involving the three supports of the malar prominence, the arch of the zygomatic bone, the zygomatic process of the frontal bone, and the zygomatic process of the maxillary bone.

unstable f., a f. with an intrinsic tendency to displace after reduction.

ununited f., a f. in which union between the ends of the bone fails to occur.

Fraenkel, Albert, German physician, 1848–1916. SEE F. *pneumococcus*.

fra·gil·i·tas (frǎ-jil′i-tas). SYN fragility. [L.]

f. crin′ium, brittleness of the hair; a condition in which the hair of the head or face tends to split or break off.

f. san′guinis, SYN osmotic *fragility*.

fra·gil·i·ty (frǎ-jil′i-tē). Brittleness; liability to break, burst, or disintegrate. SYN fragilitas. [L. *fragilitas*]

f. of the blood, SYN osmotic f.

capillary f., the susceptibility of capillaries to breakage and extravasation of red cells under conditions of increased stress.

osmotic f., the susceptibility of erythrocytes to hemolyze when exposed to increasingly hypotonic saline solutions. SYN fragilitas sanguinis, f. of the blood.

fra·gil·o·cyte (fra-jil′ō-sīt). A red blood cell that is unusually fragile when subjected to a hypotonic salt solution. [L. *fragilis*, brittle, + G. *kytos*, hollow (cell)]

fra·gil·o·cy·to·sis (fra-jil′ō-sī-tō′sis). A condition of the blood in which the red blood cells are abnormally fragile.

frag·ment (frag′ment). A small part broken from a larger entity.

acentric f., SYN acentric *chromosome*.

Brimacombe f., a ribonucleoprotein f. obtained by mild ribonuclease treatment of ribosomes.

butterfly f., a broad triangular f. that is commonly present in comminuted fractures of the diaphysis.

Fab f., the antigen-binding f. of an immunoglobulin molecule, consisting of both a light chain and part of a heavy chain. SYN Fab piece.

Fc f., the crystallizable f. of an immunoglobulin molecule composed of part of the heavy chains and responsible for binding to antibody receptors (Fc receptor) on cells and the Clq component of complement. SYN Fc piece.

Klenow f., carboxyl terminal fragment of DNA polymerase I, contains polymerase as well as $3' \rightarrow 5'$ exonuclease activity to edit out mismatches.

Okazaki f., a relatively short (100–2000 bp in *Escherichia coli* and 100–200 bp in mammals) fragment of DNA that is later joined by DNA ligase to allow for $3' \rightarrow 5'$ overall chain growth during replication.

one-carbon f., the formyl group or the methyl group that takes part in transformylation or transmethylation reactions; by means of these reactions, a group containing a single carbon atom is added to a compound being biosynthesized, adding a methyl group (as in thymidine formation), adding a hydroxymethyl group (as in serine biosynthesis), or closing a ring (as in purine formation).

two-carbon f., the acetyl group (CH_3CO-) that takes part in transacetylation reactions with coenzyme A as carrier; commonly referred to as acetate or acetic acid, from which it is derived.

frag·men·ta·tion (frag-men-tā′shŭn). The breaking of an entity into smaller parts. SYN spallation (1).

f. of the myocardium, a transverse rupture of the muscular fibers of the heart, especially those of the papillary muscles.

fraise (frāz). A burr in the shape of a hemispherical button with cutting edges, used to enlarge a trephine opening in the skull or to cut osteoplastic flaps; the smooth convexity of the button prevents injury to the dura. [Fr. strawberry]

Fraley, Elwin E., U.S. urologist, *1934. SEE F. *syndrome*.

fram·be·sia tro·pi·ca (fram-ē′zē-ă trop′ĭ-kǎ). SYN yaws. [Fr. *framboise*, raspberry]

fram·be·si·form (fram-bē′zi-fōrm). Resembling the lesion of yaws.

fram·be·si·o·ma (fram-bē-zē-ō′mǎ). SYN mother *yaw*. [frambesia + -*oma*, tumor]

frame (frām). A structure made of parts fitted together.

Balkan f., an overhead f., supported on uprights attached to the bedposts or to a separate stand, from which a splinted limb is slung in the treatment of fracture or joint disease. SYN Balkan beam, Balkan splint.

Bradford f., an oblong rectangular f. made of pipe, over which are stretched transversely two strips of canvas; permits trunk and lower extremities of a bed-ridden patient to move as a unit; now rarely used.

Deiters terminal f.'s, platelike structures in the organ of Corti uniting the outer phalangeal cells with Hensen cells.

Foster f., a reversible bed similar to a Stryker f.

occluding f., SYN articulator.

Stryker f., a f. that holds the patient and permits turning in various planes without individual motion of parts.

trial f., a type of spectacle f. with variable adjustments, for holding trial lenses during refraction.

Whitman f., a f. similar to the Bradford f., but with curved sides.

frame·shift (frām′shift). As used in genetics: a mutation that causes a sequence such that the reading frame groups of three bases in mRNA become out of register; the insertion or deletion of one or two bases, for example, would lead to an altered grouping of three bases causing incorrect amino acid residues to be incorporated into growing polypeptide chains, or would signal premature chain termination.

frame·work (frām'wŏrk). **1.** SEE stroma. **2.** In dentistry, the skeletal prosthesis (usually metal) around which and to which are attached the remaining portions of the prosthesis to produce the finished appliance (partial denture).

Franceschetti, Adolphe, Swiss ophthalmologist, 1896–1968. SEE F. *syndrome;* F.-Jadassohn *syndrome.*

Francisella (fran'si-sel'lă). A genus of nonmotile, nonsporeforming, aerobic bacteria that contain small, Gram-negative cocci and rods. Capsules are rarely produced and the cells may show bipolar staining. These organisms are highly pleomorphic; they do not grow on plain agar or in liquid media without special enrichment; they are pathogenic and cause tularemia in humans. The type species is *F. tularensis.*

F. tularen'sis, a bacterial species that causes tularemia in humans, transmitted from wild animals by bloodsucking insects or by contact with infected animals such as ticks; main sources of infection are rabbits and ticks; it can penetrate unbroken skin to cause infection, and if inhaled can cause a rapidly fatal pneumonia; type species of the genus *F.* SYN *Pasteurella tularensis.*

fran·ci·um (Fr) (fran'sē-ŭm). Radioactive element of the alkali metal series; atomic no. 87; half-life of most stable known isotope, ^{223}Fr, is 21.8 min. [*France,* native country of Mlle. M. Perey (1909–1975), the discoverer]

Francke, Karl E., German physician, 1859–1920. SEE F. *needle.*

François, Jules, contemporary Belgian ophthalmologist. SEE central cloudy corneal *dystrophy* of François. SEE ALSO central cloudy corneal *dystrophy* of François.

fran·gu·la (frang'goo-lă). The bark of *Rhamnus frangula* (family Rhamnaceae); a laxative or cathartic.

fran·gu·lic ac·id (frang'ū-lik). SYN emodin. [see frangula]

fran·gu·lin (frang'ū-lin). A glycoside from frangula; has been used as a purgative. SYN rhamnoxanthin.

Frank, Otto, German physiologist, 1865–1944. SEE F.-Starling *curve.*

frank. Unmistakable; manifest; clinically evident.

Frankenhäuser, Ferdinand, German gynecologist, 1832–1894. SEE F. *ganglion.*

Frankfort (frank'fert). SEE Frankfort horizontal *plane,* Frankfort-mandibular incisor *angle.* [*Frankfurt*-am-Main, Germany]

frank·in·cense (frangk'in-sens). SYN olibanum. [Mediev. L. *francum incensum,* pure incense]

Franklin, Benjamin, U.S. physicist and statesman, 1706–1790. SEE franklinic; F. *spectacles.*

Franklin, Edward C., U.S. physician and immunologist, *1928. SEE F. *disease.*

frank·lin·ic (frank'lin-ik). Denoting static or frictional electricity. [B. *Franklin*]

Fräntzel (frănt'zel), Oscar Maximilian Victor, German physician, 1838–1894. SEE Fräntzel *murmur.*

Fraser, Alexander, Canadian pathologist, 1869–1939. SEE F.-Lendrum *stain* for fibrin.

Fraser, George R., 20th century British geneticist. SEE F. *syndrome.*

Fraumeni, Joseph F., Jr., epidemiologist, *1933. SEE Li-F. cancer *syndrome.*

Fraunhofer, Joseph von, German optician, 1787–1826. SEE F. *lines,* under *line.*

Frazier, Charles H., U.S. surgeon, 1870–1936. SEE F. *needle;* F.-Spiller *operation.*

FRC Abbreviation for functional residual *capacity.*

F.R.C.P. Abbreviation for Fellow of the Royal College of Physicians (of England).

F.R.C.P.(C) Abbreviation for Fellow of the Royal College of Physicians (Canada).

F.R.C.P.(E), F.R.C.P.(Edin) Abbreviation for Fellow of the Royal College of Physicians (Edinburgh).

F.R.C.P.(I) Abbreviation for Fellow of the Royal College of Physicians (Ireland).

F.R.C.S. Abbreviation for Fellow of the Royal College of Surgeons (of England).

F.R.C.S.(C) Abbreviation for Fellow of the Royal College of Surgeons (Canada).

F.R.C.S.(E), F.R.C.S.(Edin) Abbreviation for Fellow of the Royal College of Surgeons (Edinburgh).

F.R.C.S.(I) Abbreviation for Fellow of the Royal College of Surgeons (Ireland).

freck·le (frek'l). Yellowish or brownish macules developing on the exposed parts of the skin, especially in persons of light complexion; the lesions increase in number on exposure to the sun; the epidermis is microscopically normal except for increased melanin. SEE ALSO lentigo. SYN ephelis. [O. E. *freken*]

Hutchinson f., SYN *lentigo* maligna.

iris f.'s, small, pigmented clusters of uveal melanocytes on the surface of the iris.

melanotic f., SYN *lentigo* maligna.

Fredet, Pierre, French surgeon, 1870–1946. SEE F.-Ramstedt *operation.*

Freeman, Ernest A., †1975. SEE F.-Sheldon *syndrome.*

freeze-dry·ing (frēz'drī-ing). SYN lyophilization.

freez·ing (frē'zing). Congealing, stiffening, or hardening by exposure to cold.

gastric f., formerly used treatment for peptic ulcer designed to reduce or eliminate the production of acid gastric juice by freezing the secretory cells with a supercooled fluid introduced into a balloon positioned in the stomach.

Frei, Wilhelm S., German dermatologist, 1885–1943. SEE F. *test;* F.-Hoffmann *reaction.*

Freiberg, Albert Henry, U.S. surgeon, 1869–1940. SEE F. *disease.*

Frejka, Bedrich, Czech orthopedist, 1890–1972. SEE F. pillow *splint.*

fré·mis·se·ment cat·taire (frā-mēs'mon kat'air). SEE fremitus.

frem·i·tus (frem'i-tŭs). A vibration imparted to the hand resting on the chest or other part of the body. SEE ALSO thrill. [L. a dull roaring sound, fr. *fremo,* pp. *-itus,* to roar, resound]

bronchial f., adventitious pulmonary sounds or voice sounds perceptible to the hand resting on the chest, as well as by the ear.

hydatid f., SYN hydatid *thrill.*

pericardial f., vibration in the chest wall produced by the friction of opposing roughened surfaces of the pericardium. SEE ALSO pericardial *rub.*

pleural f., vibration in the chest wall produced by a friction rub resulting from the rubbing together of the roughened inflamed opposing surfaces of the pleura.

rhonchal f., f. produced by vibrations from the passage of air in the bronchial tubes partially obstructed by mucous secretion.

subjective f., vibration felt within the chest by the patient himself, when humming with the mouth closed; or f. felt when there is a rough, pericardial or pleural friction rub, particularly when pain is minimal.

tactile f., vibration felt with the hand on the chest during vocal f.

tussive f., a form of f. similar to the vocal, produced by a cough.

vocal f., the vibration in the chest wall, felt on palpation, produced by the spoken voice.

fre·na (frē'nă). Plural of frenum.

fre·nal (frē'năl). Relating to any frenum.

French. SEE French *scale.*

fre·nec·to·my (frē-nek'tō-mē). Removal of any frenum. [frenum + G. *ektomē,* excision]

fre·no·plas·ty (frē'nō-plas-tē). Correction of an abnormally attached frenum by surgically repositioning it. [frenum + G. *plastos,* formed]

fre·not·o·my (frē-not'ō-mē). Division of any frenum or frenulum, especially that of the tongue. [frenum + G. *tomē,* a cutting]

fren·u·lum, pl. **fren·u·la** (fren'ū-lŭm, -lă) [TA]. A small frenum or bridle. SEE ALSO frenum. SYN habenula (1) [TA]. [Mod. L. dim. of L. *frenum,* bridle]

cerebellar f., SYN f. of superior medullary velum.

f. cerebell′i, SYN f. of superior medullary velum.

f. clitor′idis [TA], SYN f. of clitoris.

f. of clitoris [TA], the line of union of the inner-laminae portions of the labia minora on the undersurface of the glans clitoridis. SYN f. clitoridis [TA], f. preputii clitoridis.

f. epiglot′tidis, SYN median glossoepiglottic *fold*.

f. of foreskin, ✩official alternate term for f. of prepuce.

f. of Giacomini, SYN uncus *band* of Giacomini.

f. of ileal orifice [TA], a fold, more evident in cadavers, running from the junction of the two commissures of the ileocecal valve on either side along the inner wall of the cecocolic junction. SYN f. ostii ilealis [TA], f. of ileocecal valve, f. of Morgagni, f. valvae ileocecalis, Morgagni frenum, Morgagni retinaculum.

f. of ileocecal valve, SYN f. of ileal orifice.

f. of labia minora [TA], the fold connecting the two labia minora posteriorly. SYN f. labiorum pudendi [TA], fourchette✩, f. labiorum minorum, f. of pudendal lips, f. pudendi.

f. la′bii inferio′ris, f. la′bii superio′ris [TA], SYN f. of lower lip.

f. labio′rum mino′rum, SYN f. of labia minora.

f. labio′rum puden′di [TA], SYN f. of labia minora.

f. lin′guae [TA], SYN f. of tongue.

lingual f., SYN f. of tongue.

f. of lower lip, f. of upper lip [TA], the folds of mucous membrane extending from the gingiva to the midline of the lower and upper lips, respectively. SYN f. labii inferioris, f. labii superioris [TA].

f. of M'Dowel, tendinous fasciculi passing from the tendon of the pectoralis major muscle across the bicipital groove.

f. of Morgagni, SYN f. of ileal orifice.

f. ostii ilealis [TA], SYN f. of ileal orifice.

f. of prepuce [TA], a fold of mucous membrane passing from the undersurface of the glans penis to the deep surface of the prepuce. SYN f. preputii [TA], f. of foreskin✩, vinculum preputii.

f. prepu′tii [TA], SYN f. of prepuce.

f. prepu′tii clitor′idis, SYN f. of clitoris.

f. of pudendal lips, SYN f. of labia minora.

f. puden′di, SYN f. of labia minora.

f. of superior medullary velum, a band passing from the longitudinal groove between the quadrigeminal bodies on to the superior medullary velum. SYN f. veli medullaris superioris [TA], cerebellar f., f. cerebelli.

synovial frenula, SYN *vincula* tendinea of digits of hand and foot, under *vinculum*.

f. of tongue [TA], a fold of mucous membrane extending from the floor of the mouth to the midline of the undersurface of the tongue. SYN f. linguae [TA], lingual f., vinculum linguae.

f. val′vae ileoceca′lis, SYN f. of ileal orifice.

f. ve′li medulla′ris superio′ris [TA], SYN f. of superior medullary velum.

fre·num, pl. **fre·na, fre·nums** (frē′nŭm, -nă, -nŭmz). **1.** A narrow reflection or fold of mucous membrane passing from a more fixed to a movable part, serving to check undue movement of the part. **2.** An anatomical structure resembling such a fold. SYN bridle (1). [L. a bridle, curb]

Morgagni f., SYN *frenulum* of ileal orifice.

synovial frena, SYN *vincula* tendinea of digits of hand and foot, under *vinculum*.

fren·zy (fren′zē). Extreme mental or emotional excitement. [thr. Old Fr. and L. fr. G. *phrenēsis,* inflammation of the brain, fr. *phrēn,* mind]

fre·quen·cy (ν) (frē′kwen-sē). The number of regular recurrences in a given time, e.g., heartbeats, sound vibrations. [L. *frequens,* repeated, often, constant]

best f., SYN characteristic f.

characteristic f., f. at which a given neuron responds to the least sound intensity. SYN best f.

critical flicker fusion f., the minimal number of flashes of light per second at which an intermittent light stimulus no longer stimulates a continuous visual sensation.

f. domain, the expression of a function by its amplitude and phase at each component f., usually as determined by Fourier analysis.

dominant f., the f. occurring most often in an electroencephalogram.

f. encoding, in magnetic resonance imaging, a method of varying the magnetic field strength by location to encode the location of each voxel uniquely in one direction.

fundamental f., (1) the principal component of a sound wave, which has the greatest wavelength; **(2)** tone produced by the vibration of the vocal folds before the air reaches any cavities.

gene f., (1) the probability that a gene picked at random from a defined population is of a particular type; **(2)** epidemiologically, the proportion of genes in a population that are of the particular type; **(3)** statistically, the estimate of either of the foregoing two quantities.

Larmor f., in magnetic resonance, the precessional f., n_0, of magnetic nuclei in a plane perpendicular to the direction of the external magnetic field; $\nu_0 = \gamma B_0/2\pi$, where B_0 is the magnetic field strength and γ is the magnetogyric ratio.

f. of micturition, micturition at short intervals; it may result from increased urine formation, decreased bladder capacity, or lower urinary tract irritation.

mutational f., the proportions of mutations in a population.

nearest neighbor f., the f. by which certain types of entities or structures are immediately adjacent to a given structure.

resonant f., the f. at which individual magnetic nuclei absorb or emit radiofrequency energy in magnetic resonance studies. SYN resonance (6).

respiratory f. (f), the number of breaths per minute.

Frerichs, Friedrich T. von, German pathologist and clinician, 1819–1885. SEE F. *theory.*

fresh·en·ing (fresh′ĕn-ing). Preparation of an open, partially healed wound for secondary closure by removal of fibrin, granulations, and early scar tissue.

Fresnel, Augustin Jean, French physicist, 1788–1827. SEE F. *lens, prism.*

fress·re·flex (fres′rē-fleks). Sucking and chewing movements elicited by stimulation of the face and lips. [Ger fr. *fressen,* to feed, said of animals]

fret·ting (fret′ing). Abrasive polishing and wear of two metallic surfaces at their interface due to repetitive motion. [M.E., fr. O.E. *fretan,* to devour]

fre·tum, pl. **fre·ta** (frē′tŭm, -tă). A strait; a constriction. [L.]

Freud, Sigmund, Austrian neurologist and psychiatrist, 1856–1939, founder of psychoanalysis. SEE freudian; freudian *fixation;* freudian *psychoanalysis; freudian* slip; F. *theory.*

freud·i·an (froyd′ē-ăn). Relating to or described by Sigmund Freud (1856–1939).

f. slip, a mistake in speech or deed that presumably suggests some underlying motive, often sexual or aggressive in nature.

Freund, Jules, U.S. bacteriologist, 1891–1960. SEE F. complete *adjuvant,* incomplete *adjuvant.*

Freund, Wilhelm A., German gynecologist, 1833–1918. SEE F. *anomaly, operation.*

Frey, Max von, German physician, 1852–1932. SEE F. *hairs,* under *hair.*

Frey, Lucie, Polish physician, 1852–1932. SEE F. *syndrome.*

FRH Abbreviation for follitropin-releasing hormone.

fri·a·ble (frī′ă-bl). **1.** Easily reduced to powder. **2.** In bacteriology, denoting a dry and brittle culture falling into powder when touched or shaken. [L. *friabilis,* fr. *frio,* to crumble]

fric·a·tive (frik′ă-tiv). Speech sound made by forcing the air stream through a narrow orifice, created by apposition of the teeth, tongue, and lips in producing consonant phonemes such as f, v, s, and z.

fric·tion (frik′shŭn). **1.** The act of rubbing the surface of an object against that of another; especially rubbing the limbs of the body to aid the circulation. **2.** The force required for relative motion of two bodies that are in contact. [L. *frictio,* fr. *frico,* to rub]

dynamic f., the force that must be overcome to maintain steady

fr

motion of one body relative to another because they remain in contact. Cf. starting f.

starting f., the force that must be overcome to initiate the motion of one body relative to another because they have been resting in contact. Cf. dynamic f. SYN static f.

static f., SYN starting f.

Friderichsen, Carl, Danish physician, *1886. SEE Waterhouse-F. *syndrome;* Friderichsen-Waterhouse *syndrome.*

Friedländer, Carl, German pathologist, 1847–1887. SEE F. *bacillus, pneumonia, stain* for capsules.

Friedman, Emanuel A., U.S. obstetrician, *1926. SEE Friedman *curve.*

Friedreich, Nikolaus, German neurologist, 1825–1882. SEE F. *ataxia, phenomenon, sign.*

Friend, Charlotte, U.S. microbiologist, 1921–1987. SEE F. *disease, virus,* leukemia *virus.*

frig·id (frij'id). **1.** SYN cold. **2.** Temperamentally, especially sexually, cold or irresponsive. [L. *frigidus,* cold]

fri·gid·i·ty (fri-jid'i-tē). **1.** Impotence in the female. **2.** The state of being frigid (2); female sexual inadequacy ranging from the freudian concept of inability to achieve orgasm to any degree of sexual response considered unsatisfactory by either the female or her partner.

frig·o·rif·ic (frig-ō-rif'ik). Producing cold. [L. *frigus,* cold, + *facio,* to make]

frig·o·rism (frig'ō-rizm). SYN cryopathy. [L. *frigus,* cold]

fringe (frinj). SYN fimbria (1).

costal f., an irregularly disposed collection of visible veins seen in the skin of people usually of or past middle age; it has no specific connection with any deep structure, such as the diaphragm, and no necessary connection with underlying visceral disease. SYN zona corona.

synovial f., SYN synovial *villi,* under *villus.*

frit (frit). **1.** The material from which the glaze for artificial teeth is made. **2.** A powdered pigment material used in coloring the porcelain of artificial teeth. [Fr. *frit,* fried]

Fritsch, Heinrich, German gynecologist, 1844–1915. SEE Bozeman-F. *catheter.*

Froehde, A., 19th century German chemist. SEE F. *reagent.*

frog (frŏg). An amphibian in the order Anura, which includes the toads; the commonest frog genera are *Rana* (grass frogs) and *Hyla* (tree frogs). [A.S. *frogge*]

Fröhlich, Alfred, Austrian neurologist and pharmacologist, 1871–1953. SEE F. *dwarfism, syndrome.*

Frohn, Damianus, German physician, *1843. SEE F. *reagent.*

Froin, Georges, French physician, 1874–1932. SEE F. *syndrome.*

frôle·ment (frol-mon'). **1.** Light friction or massage with the palm of the hand. **2.** A rustling sound heard in auscultation. [Fr.]

Froment, Jules, Lyon physician, 1878–1946. SEE F. *sign.*

Frommel, Richard, German gynecologist, 1854–1912. SEE Chiari-F. *syndrome.*

frons, gen. **fron·tis** (fronz, fron'tis) [TA]. SYN forehead. [L.]

front (frŭnt). The position of the leading edge of the solvent in chromatography.

front·ad (frŭn'tad). Toward the front.

fron·tal (frŭn'tăl) [TA]. **1.** In front; relating to the anterior part of a body. **2.** Referring to the frontal (coronal) plane or to the frontal bone or forehead. SYN frontalis [TA].

fron·ta·lis (frŭn-tā'lis) [TA]. SYN frontal. [L.]

fron·to·ma·lar (frŭn'tō-mā'lăr). SYN frontozygomatic.

fron·to·max·il·lary (frŭn'tō-mak'si-lā-rē). Relating to the frontal and the maxillary bones.

fron·to·na·sal (frŭn'tō-nā'zăl). Relating to the frontal and the nasal bones.

fron·to·oc·cip·i·tal (frŭn'tō-ok-sip'i-tăl). Relating to the frontal and the occipital bones, or to the forehead and the occiput.

fron·to·pa·ri·e·tal (frŭn'tō-pa-rī'ĕ-tăl). Relating to the frontal and the parietal bones.

fron·to·tem·po·ral (frŭn-tō-tem'pŏ-răl). Relating to the frontal and the temporal bones.

fron·to·tem·po·ra·le (frŭn'tō-tem-pō-rā'lē). A craniometric point located at the most anterior point of the temporal line on the frontal bone.

fron·to·zy·go·mat·ic (frŭn'tō-zī'gō-mat'ik). Relating to the frontal and zygomatic bones. SYN frontomalar.

Froriep, August von, German anatomist, 1849–1917. SEE F. *ganglion.*

frost. A deposit resembling that of frozen vapor or dew.

urea f., uremic f., powdery deposits on the skin, especially the face, including urea and uric acid salts, due to excretion of nitrogenous compounds in the sweat; seen in severe uremia. SYN uridrosis crystallina.

Frost, Albert D., U.S. ophthalmologist, 1889–1945. SEE F. *suture.*

Frost, Wade H., U.S. epidemiologist, 1880–1938. SEE Reed-F. *model.*

Frost, William A., English ophthalmologist, 1853–1935.

frost·bite (frost'bīt). Local tissue destruction resulting from exposure to extreme cold; in mild cases, it results in superficial, reversible freezing followed by erythema and slight pain (frostnip); in severe cases, it can be painless or paresthetic and result in blistering, persistent edema, and gangrene. F. is currently treated by rapid rewarming.

frot·tage (frō-tahzh'). **1.** The rubbing movement in massage. **2.** Production of sexual excitement by rubbing against someone. [F. a rubbing]

frot·teur (frō-tuhr'). One who gets sexual excitement through frottage.

FRS Abbreviation for first rank *symptoms,* under *symptom.*

F.R.S. Abbreviation for Fellow of the Royal Society.

F.R.S.C. Abbreviation for Fellow of the Royal Society (Canada).

Fru Symbol for fructose.

fruc·tan (frŭk'tan). SYN fructosan (1).

△**fructo-.** Chemical prefix denoting the fructose configuration. [L. *fructus,* fruit]

fruc·to·fu·ra·nose (frŭk-tō-foor'ă-nōs, fruk-). Fructose in furanose form.

β-fruc·to·fu·ran·o·sid·ase (frŭk'tō-foor-ă-nō-sīd'ās, fruk-). β-*h*-Fructosidase; an enzyme hydrolyzing β-D-fructofuranosides and releasing free D-fructose; if the substrate is sucrose, the product is D-glucose plus D-fructose (invert sugar); invert sugar is more easily digestible than sucrose. SYN invertase, invertin, saccharase.

fruc·to·ki·nase (frŭk-tō-kī'nās, fruk-). A liver enzyme that catalyzes the reaction of ATP and D-fructose to form fructose 6-phosphate and ADP; deficient in individuals with essential fructosuria (hepatic f. deficiency).

fruc·tol·y·sis (fruk-to'li-sis). The conversion of fructose to lactate; analogous to glycolysis.

fruc·to·san (frŭk'tō-san, fruk-). **1.** A polysaccharide of fructose (e.g., inulin) containing small amounts of other sugars; present in certain tubers. SYN fructan, levan, levulan, levulin, levulosan, polyfructose. **2.** 2,6-Anhydrofructofuranose.

fruc·tose (Fru) (frŭk'tōs, fruk-). The D-isomer (also referred to as fruit sugar, levoglucose, levulose, and D-*arabino*-2-hexulose) is a 2-ketohexose that is physiologically the most important of the ketohexoses and one of the two products of sucrose hydrolysis; it is metabolized or converted to glycogen in the absence of insulin. [L. *fructus,* fruit, + -ose]

fruc·tose-bis·phos·pha·tase. A hydrolase that catalyzes conversion of fructose 1,6-bisphosphate to D-fructose 6-phosphate and orthophosphate in gluconeogenesis; AMP is an allosteric inhibitor; f.-b. deficiency results in problems with impaired gluconeogenesis; there is a similar enzyme that acts on fructose 2,6-bisphosphate.

fruc·tose 1,6-bis·phos·phate. A key intermediate in glycolysis and gluconeogenesis. SYN hexosebisphosphatase, hexosediphosphatase.

fruc·tose 2,6-bis·phos·phate. An analog of fructose 1,6-bisphosphate that plays a key role in the regulation of glycolysis and gluconeogenesis; activates phosphofructokinase and inhibits fructose 1,6-bisphosphatase.

fruc·tose-bis·phos·phate al·dol·ase.   Fructose-1,6-bisphosphate triophosphate-lyase; an enzyme reversibly cleaving fructose 1,6-bisphosphate to dihydroxyacetone phosphate and glyceraldehyde 3-phosphate; also acts on certain ketose 1-phosphates; deficient in individuals with hereditary fructose intolerance (aldolase B); a deficiency of aldolase A leads to erythrocyte aldolase deficiency with nonspherocytic hemolytic anemia. Cf. hereditary fructose *intolerance.*   SYN 1-phosphofructaldolase, fructose-diphosphate aldolase.

fruc·tose-di·phos·phate al·dol·ase.   SYN fructose-bisphosphate aldolase.

fruc·to·se·mia (frŭk-tō-sē′mē-ă, fruk-).   Presence of fructose in the circulating blood. SEE ALSO hereditary fructose *intolerance.* SYN levulosemia.

fruc·tose 1-phos·phate.   A fructose derivative that accumulates in individuals with hereditary fructose intolerance.

fruc·tose 6-phos·phate.   An intermediate in glycolysis and in transketolation of erythrose 4-phosphate. SYN Neuberg ester.

fruc·to·side (frŭk′tō-sīd, fruk′).   Fructose in –C–O– linkage where the –C–O– group is the original 2-group of the fructose.

fruc·to·su·ria (frŭk-tō-soo′rē-ă, fruk-).   Excretion of fructose in the urine. SYN levulosuria. [fructose + G. *ouron,* urine]

benign f., SYN essential f.

essential f. [MIM*229800], a benign, asymptomatic inborn error of metabolism due to deficiency of fructokinase, the first enzyme in the specific fructose pathway; fructose appears in the blood and urine, but is simply excreted unchanged; autosomal recessive inheritance. A fructokinase deficiency. SEE ALSO hereditary fructose *intolerance.* SYN benign f., fructokinase deficiency.

△**fructosyl-.**   Chemical prefix indicating fructose in –C–R– (not –C–O–R–) linkage through its carbon-2 (R is usually C).

fru·se·mide (froo′sĕ-mīd).   SYN furosemide.

frus·tra·tion (frŭs′trā′shŭn).   A psychologic or psychiatric term indicating the thwarting of or inability to gratify a desire or to satisfy an urge or need. [L. *frustro,* pp. *-atus,* to deceive, disappoint, fr. *frustra* (adv.), in vain]

FSH   Abbreviation for follicle-stimulating *hormone.*

ft.   Abbreviation for L. *fiat,* let it be done (made); abbreviation for foot or feet.

FTA-ABS.   Abbreviation for fluorescent treponemal antibody absorption. SEE fluorescent treponemal antibody-absorption *test.*

FTI   Abbreviation for free thyroxine *index.*

Fuc   Abbreviation for fucose.

Fuchs,   Ernst, Austrian ophthalmologist, 1851–1930. SEE F. *adenoma;* angle of F.; F. heterochromic *cyclitis, coloboma,* endothelial *dystrophy,* black *spot, spur, stomas,* under *stoma, syndrome, uveitis;* Dalen-F. *nodules,* under *nodule.*

fuch·sin (fuk′sin).   A nonspecific term referring to any of several red rosanilin dyes used as stains in histology and bacteriology. [Leonhard *Fuchs,* German botanist, 1501–1506]

acid f. [C.I. 42685], a mixture of the sodium salts bi- and trisulfonic acids of rosanilin and pararosanilin; used as an indicator dye and for staining of cytoplasm and collagen. SYN rubin S, rubine.

aldehyde f., a stain developed by Gomori, utilizing basic f. paraldehyde and hydrochloric acid; it produces violet staining of elastic fibers, mast cell granules, gastric chief cells, beta cells of the pancreatic islets, and certain hypophyseal beta granules; other pituitary granules and cells stain in other colors. SEE ALSO Gomori aldehyde fuchsin *stain.*

aniline f., a mixture of aniline and basic f. in 30% ethanol with a trace of phenol, as in Goodpasture stain.

basic f. [C.I. 42500], a triphenylmethane dye whose dominant component is pararosanilin; an important stain in histology, histochemistry, and bacteriology. SYN diamond f.

carbol f., SEE carbol-fuchsin *paint,* Ziehl *stain.*

diamond f., SYN basic f.

fuch·sin·o·phil (fuk′si-nō-fil).   **1.** Staining readily with fuchsin

dyes. SYN fuchsinophilic.   **2.** A cell or histologic element that stains readily with fuchsin. [fuchsin + G. *philos,* fond]

fuch·sin·o·phil·ia (fuk′si-nō-fil′ē-ă).   The property of staining readily with fuchsin.

fuch·sin·o·phil·ic (fuk′si-nō-fil′ik).   SYN fuchsinophil (1).

fu·cose (Fuc) (fū′kōs).   6-Deoxygalactose; a methylpentose, the L-configuration of which occurs in the mucopolysaccharides of the blood group substances, in human milk (as a polysaccharide), and elsewhere in nature. The D-configuration has been found in certain antibiotics and in certain plant glycosides. SYN rhodeose.

α-fu·co·si·dase (fū-kōs′i-dās).   An enzyme that catalyzes the hydrolysis of an an α-L-fucoside, producing an alcohol and L-fucose; a deficiency of the lysosomal enzyme will result in fucosidosis.

fu·co·si·do·sis (fū′kō-sī-dō′sis) [MIM*230000].   A metabolic storage disease characterized by accumulation of fucose-containing glycolipids and deficiency of the enzyme α-fucosidase; progressive neurologic deterioration begins after the first year of life, accompanied by spasticity, tremor, and mild skeletal changes; autosomal recessive inheritance, caused by mutation in the α-1-fucosidase gene on chromosome 1.

FUDR   Abbreviation for fluorodeoxyuridine. SEE floxuridine.

fu·gac·i·ty (f) (foo-gas′i-tē).   The tendency of the molecules in a fluid, as a result of all forces acting on them, to leave a given site in the body; the escaping tendency of a fluid, as in diffusion, evaporation, etc. [L. *fuga,* flight]

△**-fugal.**   Movement away from the part indicated by the main portion of the word. [L. *fugio,* to flee]

△**-fuge.**   Flight, denoting the place from which flight takes place or that which is put to flight. [L. *fuga* a running away]

fu·gi·tive (fū′ji-tiv).   **1.** Temporary; transient.   **2.** Fleeting; denoting certain inconstant symptoms. [L. *fugitivus,* fleeing, fr. *fugio,* pp. *fugitus,* to flee]

fugue (fūg).   A condition in which an individual suddenly abandons a present activity or lifestyle and starts a new and different one for a period of time, often in a different city; afterward, the individual alleges amnesia for events occurring during the f. period, although earlier events are remembered and habits and skills are usually unaffected. [Fr. fr. L. *fuga,* flight]

fu·gu·tox·in (foo′goo-tok-sin).   The potent poison derived from the ovaries and skin of the Pacific pufferfish. SEE ALSO tetrodotoxin.

Fukase,   Masaichi. SEE Crow-f. *syndrome.*

ful·crum, pl. **ful·cra, ful·crums** (ful′krŭm, -kră, -krŭmz).   A support or the point thereon on which a lever turns. [L. a bedpost, fr. *fulcio,* to prop up]

ful·gu·rant (ful′gŭ-rănt).   Sharp and piercing. Cf. fulminant. SYN fulgurating (1). [L. *fulgur,* flashing lightning]

ful·gu·rat·ing (ful′gŭ-rā-ting).   **1.** SYN fulgurant.   **2.** Relating to fulguration.

ful·gu·ra·tion (ful-gŭ-rā′shŭn).   Destruction of tissue by means of a high-frequency electric current: **direct f.** utilizes an insulated electrode with a metal point, which is connected to the uniterminal of the high-frequency apparatus, from which a spark of electricity is allowed to impinge on the area to be treated; **indirect f.** involves directly connecting the patient by a metal handle to the uniterminal and utilizing an active electrode to complete an arc from the patient. [L. *fulgur,* lightning stroke]

ful·mi·nant (ful′mi-nănt).   Occurring suddenly, with lightning-like rapidity, and with great intensity or severity; applied to certain pains, e.g., those of tabes dorsalis. Cf. fulgurant. [L. *fulmino,* pp. *-atus,* to hurl lightning, fr. *fulmen,* lightning]

ful·mi·nat·ing (ful′mi-nā′ting).   Running a rapid course, worsening quickly.

fu·ma·rase (fū′mă-rās).   SYN fumarate hydratase.

fu·ma·rate hy·dra·tase (fū′mă-rāt).   An enzyme catalyzing the reversible interconversion of fumarate and water to malate, a reaction of importance in the tricarboxylic acid cycle. A deficiency will lead to mental retardation. SYN fumarase.

fu·ma·rate re·duc·tase (NADH).   SYN *succinate* dehydrogenase.

fu·mar·ic ac·id (fū-mar′ik).   *trans*-Butanedioic acid; an unsaturated dicarboxylic acid occurring as an intermediate in the tricarboxylic acid cycle.

fu·mar·ic ac·i·de·mia. Elevated levels of fumarate in blood plasma; due to a decrease in activity of fumarate hydratase.

fu·mar·ic am·i·nase. SYN *aspartate* ammonia-lyase.

fu·mar·ic hy·dro·gen·ase. SYN *succinate* dehydrogenase.

fum·ar·yl·ac·e·to·ac·e·tate (fū-mă′ril-as-ē′tō-ăs-ē-tāt). An intermediate in phenylalanine and tyrosine catabolism; elevated in tyrosinemia IA.

f. hydrolase, an enzyme that catalyzes the hydrolysis of f. to fumarate and acetoacetate; a deficiency indicates tyrosinemia IA.

fu·mi·gant (fū′mi-gănt). A substance utilized in fumigation.

fu·mi·gate (fū′mi-gāt). To expose to the action of smoke or of fumes of any kind as a means of disinfection or eradication. [L. *fumigo* pp. -*atus,* to fumigate, fr. *fumus,* smoke, + *ago,* to drive]

fu·mi·ga·tion (fū-mi-gā′shŭn). The act of fumigating; the use of a fumigant.

fum·ing (fūm′ing). Giving forth a visible vapor, a property of concentrated nitric, sulfuric, and hydrochloric acids, and certain other substances. [L. *fumus,* smoke]

func·tio lae·sa (fŭngk′shē-ō lē′să). Impaired function; a fifth sign of inflammation added by Galen to those enunciated by Celsus (rubor, tumor, calor, and dolor). [L.]

func·tion (fŭngk′shŭn). **1.** The special action or physiologic property of an organ or other part of the body. **2.** To perform its special work or office, said of an organ or other part of the body. **3.** The general properties of any substance, depending on its chemical character and relation to other substances, according to which it may be grouped among acids, bases, alcohols, esters, etc. **4.** A particular reactive grouping in a molecule; e.g., a functional group, such as the –OH group of an alcohol. **5.** A quality, trait, or fact that is so related to another as to be dependent upon and to vary with this other. **6.** A mathematical variable or expression. [L. *functio,* fr. *fungor,* pp. *functus,* to perform]

allomeric f., the combined f. of the several segments of the spinal cord and medulla, communicating with each other by means of the white matter.

arousal f., the ability of a sensory event to arouse the cortex to vigilance or readiness.

atrial transport f., the role of the atria in filling and stretching the ventricles by their presystolic contraction, without which the force of ventricular contraction and hence the cardiac output may significantly decrease.

discriminant f., a particular combination of continuous variable test results designed to achieve separation of groups; e.g., a single number representing a combination of weighted laboratory test results designed to discriminate between clinical classes.

isomeric f., the individual f. of an isolated segment of the spinal cord.

line spread f. (LSF), a measure of the ability of a system to form sharp images; in radiology, determined by measuring the spatial density distribution on film of the x-ray image of a narrow slit in a dense metal, such as uranium; from this can be calculated the modulation transfer f.

modulation transfer f. (MTF), in testing radionuclide detectors or radiographic systems, the efficiency, at each spatial frequency, of reproducing the variation (contrast) in the object density or signal in the image; it is an expression of spatial resolution and is used to evaluate imaging systems and their components; the integral of the line spread function; also known as the frequency response function or contrast transmission f.; usually given as a plot of percentage amplitude response versus frequency in cycles per millimeter.

func·tion·al (fŭnk′shŭn-ăl). **1.** Relating to a function. **2.** Not organic in origin; denoting a disorder with no known or detectable organic basis to explain the symptoms. SEE neurosis.

func·tion·al·ism (fŭnk′shŭn-ăl-izm). A branch of psychology concerned with the function of mental processes in humans and animals, especially the role of the mind, intellect, emotions, and behavior in an individual's adaptation to the environment. Cf. structuralism.

func·tion cor·rec·tor. A removable orthodontic appliance utilizing oral and facial muscle forces to move teeth and possibly change the relationship of the dental arches.

fun·da·ment (fŭn′dă-ment). **1.** A foundation. **2.** The anus. [L. *fundamentum,* foundation, fr. *fundus,* bottom]

fun·dec·to·my (fŭn-dek′tō-mē). SYN fundusectomy. [fundus + G. *ektomē,* excision]

fun·dic (fŭn′dik). Relating to a fundus.

fun·di·form (fŭn′di-fōrm). Looped; sling-shaped. [L. *funda,* a sling, + *forma,* shape]

fun·do·pli·ca·tion (fŭn′dō-pli-kā′shŭn). Suture of the fundus of the stomach completely or partially around the gastroesophageal junction to treat gastroesophageal reflux disease; can be performed by open abdominal or thoracic operation, but increasingly by laparoscopy. [fundus + L. *plico,* to fold]

Belsey f., partial (270°) f. performed via thoracotomy. SYN Belsey Mark operation, Belsey procedure.

Collis-Belsey f., SYN Collis-Nissen f.

Collis-Nissen f., operation for f. in the presence of a shortened esophagus; the esophagus is lengthened by tubular stapling of the gastric cardia, and the f. is then performed around this neoesophagus. SYN Collis-Belsey f., Collis-Belsey procedure.

Dor f., a partial (180°) and anterior f., popular in Europe and South America and most often used along with a myotomy for the treatment of achalasia.

Nissen f., complete (360°) f.; can be done via abdominal or thoracic approach; currently most often performed laparoscopically. SYN Nissen operation.

Toupet f., a partial posterior f., in which the stomach edge is secured to the esophagus; modifications of Toupet f. are commonly used for laparoscopic f.

fun·dus, pl. **fun·di** (fŭn′dŭs, dī) [TA]. The bottom or lowest part of a sac or hollow organ; that part farthest removed from the opening or exit; occasionally a broad cul-de-sac. [L. bottom]

f. albipuncta′tus [MIM*136880], a nonprogressive disorder of the retinal pigment epithelium characterized by numerous discrete, white dots; night blindness is a feature; autosomal dominant and recessive forms have been suggested.

f. of bladder [TA], the f. is formed by the posterior wall that is somewhat convex. SYN f. vesicae urinariae [TA], bas-fond, base of bladder, f. of urinary bladder.

f. diabet′icus, SYN diabetic *retinopathy.*

f. flavimacula′tus [MIM*228980], a genetic disorder of the pigment epithelium of the retina manifested by yellowish white flecks; some loss of central vision is involved; probably autosomal recesssive.

f. of gallbladder [TA], the wide closed end of the gallbladder situated at the inferior border of the liver. SYN f. vesicae biliaris [TA], f. vesicae felleae⋆.

f. gas′tricus [TA], SYN f. of stomach.

f. of internal acoustic meatus [TA], lateral end of the internal acoustic meatus, the wall of which is formed by the thin cribriform plate of bone separating the cochlea and vestibule from the internal acoustic meatus; a transverse crest divides the f. into two regions; in the superior region are located the facial nerve area and the superior vestibular area; in the inferior region are located the cochlear area, inferior vestibular area, and singular foramen. SYN f. meatus acustici interni [TA], f. of internal auditory meatus.

f. of internal auditory meatus, SYN f. of internal acoustic meatus.

leopard f., SYN tessellated f.

f. mea′tus acus′tici inter′ni [TA], SYN f. of internal acoustic meatus.

mosaic f., SYN tessellated f.

f. oc′uli, the portion of the interior of the eyeball around the posterior pole, visible through the ophthalmoscope. SEE eyegrounds.

pepper and salt f., ophthalmoscopic appearance of the f. caused by choriocapillaris atrophy and pigment proliferation.

f. polycythe′micus, the engorged, dilated veins, with cyanotic retina, occurring in erythremia.

f. of stomach [TA], the portion of the stomach that lies above the cardiac notch. SYN f. gastricus [TA], f. ventriculi, greater cul-de-sac.

tessellated f., a normal f. to which a deeply pigmented choroid gives the appearance of dark polygonal areas between the choroidal vessels, especially in the periphery. SYN f. tigré, leopard f., leopard retina, mosaic f., tigroid f., tigroid retina.

f. tigré, SYN tessellated f.

tigroid f., SYN tessellated f.

f. tym′pani, SYN jugular *wall* of middle ear.

f. of urinary bladder, SYN f. of bladder.

f. u′teri [TA], SYN f. of uterus.

f. of uterus [TA], the upper rounded extremity of the uterus above the openings of the uterine (fallopian) tubes. SYN f. uteri [TA].

f. ventric′uli, SYN f. of stomach.

f. vesi′cae biliar′is [TA], SYN f. of gallbladder.

f. vesicae felleae, ✩official alternate term for f. of gallbladder.

f. vesi′cae urina′riae [TA], SYN f. of bladder.

fun·du·scope (fŭn′dŭs-skōp). SYN ophthalmoscope. [L. *fundus,* bottom, + G. *skopeō,* to view]

fun·dus·co·py (fŭn-dŭs′kŏ-pē). SYN ophthalmoscopy.

fun·du·sec·to·my (fŭn-dŭ-sek′tō-mē). Excision of the fundus of an organ. SYN fundectomy. [L. *fundus,* + G. *ektomē,* excision]

fun·gal (fŭng′găl). SYN fungous.

fun·gate (fŭng′gāt). To grow exuberantly like a fungus or spongy growth.

fun·ge·mia (fŭn-jē′mē-ă). Fungal infection disseminated by way of the bloodstream.

Fun·gi (fŭn′jī). A division of eukaryotic organisms that grow in irregular masses, without roots, stems, or leaves, and are devoid of chlorophyll or other pigments capable of photosynthesis. Each organism (thallus) is unicellular to filamentous, and possesses branched somatic structures (hyphae) surrounded by cell walls containing glucan or chitin or both, and containing true nuclei. They reproduce sexually or asexually (spore formation), and may obtain nutrition from other living organisms as parasites or from dead organic matter as saprobes (saprophytes). [L. *fungus,* a mushroom]

fun·gi (fŭn′jī). Plural of fungus.

fun·gi·ci·dal (fŭn-ji-sī′dăl). Having a killing action on fungi. [fungus + L. *caedo,* to kill]

fun·gi·cide (fŭn′ji-sīd). Any substance that has a destructive killing action upon fungi. SYN mycocide.

fun·gi·ci·din (fŭn-ji-sī′din). SYN nystatin.

fun·gi·form (fŭn′ji-fōrm). Shaped like a fungus or mushroom; applied to any structure with a broad, often branched, free portion and a narrower base. SYN fungilliform.

Fun·gi Im·per·fec·ti (fŭn′jī im-per-fek′tī). A phylum of fungi in which sexual reproduction is not known or in which one of the mating types has not yet been discovered. Formerly, most fungi causing disease in humans were considered asexual and were placed in this class, but studies have revealed that many are not imperfect and that in their sexual forms they can be classified as ascomycetes or basidiomycetes.

fun·gil·li·form (fŭn-jil′i-fōrm). SYN fungiform. [Mod L. *fungillus,* dim. of L. *fungus*]

fun·gi·stat (fŭn′ji-stat). An agent having fungistatic action.

fun·gi·stat·ic (fŭn-ji-stat′ik). Having an inhibiting action upon the growth of fungi. SYN mycostatic. [fungus + G. *statos,* standing]

fun·gi·tox·ic (fŭn-ji-tok′sik). Poisonous or in any way deleterious to the growth of fungi.

fun·gi·tox·ic·i·ty (fŭn′ji-tok-sis′i-tē). The property of being fungitoxic.

fun·goid (fŭng′goyd). Resembling a fungus; denoting an exuberant morbid growth on the surface of the body.

fun·gous (fŭng′gŭs). Relating to a fungus. SYN fungal.

fun·gus, pl. **fun·gi** (fŭng′gŭs, fŭn′jī). A general term used to encompass the diverse morphologic forms of yeasts and molds. Originally classified as primitive plants without chlorophyll, the fungi are placed in the kingdom Fungi and some in the kingdom Protista, along with the algae (all but the blue-green algae), the protozoa, and the slime molds. Fungi share with bacteria the important ability to break down complex organic substances of almost every type (cellulose) and are essential to the recycling of carbon and other elements in the cycle of life. Fungi are important as foods and to the fermentation process in the development of substances of industrial and medical importance, including alcohol, the antibiotics, other drugs, and foods. Relatively few fungi are pathogenic for humans, whereas most plant diseases are caused by fungi. [L. *fungus,* a mushroom]

f. cer′ebri, an ulcerated cerebral hernia with granulation tissue protruding from scalp wound.

dematiaceous fungi (de-măt′ē-ā-cē-ous), dark f. that form melanin. [Mod. L. *Dematium* (genus name), fr. g. *demation,* fine strand, fr. *dema,* band, fr. *deō,* to bind + suffix *-aceous,* characterized by]

imperfect f., a f. in which the means of sexual reproduction is not yet recognized; these fungi generally reproduce by means of conidia.

perfect f., a f. possessing both sexual and asexual means of reproduction, and in which both mating forms are recognized.

ray f., a bacterium of the order Actinomycetales.

thrush f., SYN *Candida albicans.*

umbilical f., a mass of granulation tissue on the stump of the umbilical cord in the newborn.

yeast f., obsolete term for *Saccharomyces.*

fu·nic (few′nik). Relating to the funis, or umbilical cord. SYN funicular (2).

fu·ni·cle (fū′ni-kl). SYN cord.

fu·nic·u·lar (fū-nik′ū-lăr). **1.** Relating to a funiculus. **2.** SYN funic.

fu·nic·u·li·tis (fū-nik′ū-lī′tis). **1.** Inflammation of a funiculus, especially of the spermatic cord. **2.** Inflammation of the umbilical cord usually associated with chorioamnionitis. [funiculus + G. *-itis,* inflammation]

endemic f., SYN filarial f.

filarial f., cellulitis of the spermatic cord due to filariasis; occurs endemically in Sri Lanka and Egypt, and probably elsewhere in the East. SYN endemic f.

fu·nic·u·lus, pl. **fu·nic·u·li** (fū-nik′ū-lŭs, -lī) [TA]. SYN cord. [L. dim. of *funis,* cord]

anterior f. [TA], anterior white column of spinal cord, a column or bundle of white matter on either side of the anterior median fissure, between that and the anterolateral sulcus. SYN f. anterior [TA], ventral f.✩.

f. ante′rior [TA], SYN anterior f.

cuneate f., SYN cuneate *fasciculus.*

dorsal f., ✩official alternate term for posterior f.

f. dorsa′lis, SYN posterior f.

f. gra′cilis, SYN gracile *fasciculus.*

lateral f. [TA], the lateral white column of the spinal cord between the lines of exit and entrance of the anterior and posterior nerve roots. SYN f. lateralis [TA], anterolateral column of spinal cord, lateral f. of spinal cord.

f. latera′lis [TA], SYN lateral f.

lateral f. of spinal cord, SYN lateral f.

funic′uli medu′llae spina′lis [TA], the three major white columns of the spinal cord.

posterior f., posterior white column of the spinal cord, the large wedge-shaped fiber bundle lying between the posterior gray column and the posterior median septum, and composed largely of dorsal root fibers. SYN f. posterior [TA], dorsal f.✩, f. dorsalis.

f. poste′rior [TA], SYN posterior f.

f. sep′arans [TA], an oblique ridge in the floor of the fourth ventricle of the brain, separating the area postrema from the vagal trigone.

f. solita′rius, SYN solitary *tract.*

f. spermat′icus [TA], SYN spermatic *cord.*

f. te′res, SYN medial *eminence.*

f. umbilica′lis, SYN umbilical *cord.*

fu

ventral f., ✩official alternate term for anterior f.

fu·ni·form (fū′ni-fōrm). Ropelike. [L. *funis,* cord, + *forma,* shape]

fu·ni·punc·ture (fū-nē-pŭnk-chŭr). SYN cordocentesis. [L. *funis,* cord, + puncture]

fu·nis (fū′nis). **1.** SYN umbilical *cord.* **2.** A cordlike structure. [L. a rope, cord]

funisitis (fū-nē-sī-tis). Inflammation of the umbilical cord. [funis + -itis]

fun·nel (fŭn′ĕl). **1.** A hollow conical vessel with a tube of variable length proceeding from its apex, used in pouring fluids from one container to another, in filtering, etc. **2.** In anatomy, an infundibulum.

Büchner f., a porcelain f. that contains a perforated porcelain plate upon which filter paper can be laid.

Martegiani f., the funnel-shaped dilation on the optic disk that indicates the beginning of the hyaloid canal. SYN Martegiani area.

pial f., the pia-lined channel in which each blood vessel entering the brain lies suspended; essentially, the pial f.'s are perivascular extensions of the subarachnoid space.

FUO Abbreviation for fever of unknown origin.

fur (fer). **1.** The coat of soft, fine hair of some mammals. **2.** A layer of epithelial debris and fungal elements on the dorsum of the tongue. It is related more to neglected oral hygiene than to an underlying disease process. [M.E. *furre,* fr. O.Fr., fr. Germanic]

fura-2 (foo′ra). A fluorescent indicator which binds calcium; it is excited at longer wavelengths when free of calcium than when calcium is bound; the ratio of fluorescence intensity at two excitation wavelengths provides a measure of free calcium ion concentration; may be injected into cells to monitor moment-to-moment changes in intracellular free calcium ion concentration. SEE ALSO aequorin.

fu·ral·ta·done (fū-ral′tă-dōn). An antibacterial agent.

fu·ran (fūr′an). **1.** A cyclic compound found, usually in saturated form, in those sugars with an oxygen bridge between carbon atoms 1 and 4, or 2 and 5, or 3 and 7, for which reason they are known as furanoses. **2.** Oxa-2,4-cyclopentadiene.

fu·ra·nose (fūr′ă-nōs). A saccharide unit or molecule containing the furan cyclic structure; specific examples are preceded by prefixes indicating the configuration, e.g., fructofuranose, ribofuranose. [furan + -ose(1)]

fu·ra·zol·i·done (fū-ră-zol′i-dōn). Has antibacterial and antiprotozoal activity against enteric organisms; used in the treatment of bacterial enteritis and diarrhea.

fur·cal (fer′kăl). Forked.

fur·ca·tion (fŭr-kā′shŭn). **1.** A forking, or a forklike part or branch. **2.** In dental histology, the region of a multirooted tooth at which the roots divide. [L. *furca,* fork]

fur·cu·la (fer′kū-lă). **1.** The fused clavicles, which form the V-shaped bone (wishbone) of the bird's skeleton. **2.** In the embryo, an inverted U-shaped elevation that appears on the ventral wall of the pharynx, being formed by the two linear ridges and the caudal part of the hypobranchial eminence; the depression enclosed by the U is the laryngotracheal groove. [L. a forked prop, dim. of *furca,* a fork]

fur·fur, pl. **fur·fu·res** (fer′fer, fer′fū-rēz). An epidermal scale; e.g., dandruff. [L. bran]

fur·fu·ra·ceous (fer-fū-rā′shŭs). Branny, or composed of small scales; denoting a form of desquamation. SYN pityroid. [L. *furfuraceus,* fr. *furfur,* bran]

fur·fu·ral (fer′fūr-ăl). C_4H_3O–CHO; a colorless, aromatic, irritating fluid obtained in the distillation of bran with dilute sulfuric acid; used in the manufacture of medicinal agents.

fur·fu·rol (fer′fūr-ol). Misnomer for furfural and furfuryl alcohol.

fur·fu·ryl (fer′fū-ril). The monovalent radical derived from f. alcohol by loss of the OH group.

f. alcohol, 2-furanmethanol; 2-hydroxymethylfuran; a solvent and wetting agent.

fur·nace (fŭr′năs). A stovelike apparatus containing a chamber for heating, melting, or fusing.

dental f., **(1)** a f. used to eliminate the wax pattern from the investment mold prior to casting in metal; **(2)** a f. used to fuse and glaze dental porcelains.

muffle f., **(1)** an electric f. heated by direct transfer of heat from a resistant muffle; **(2)** a dental f. heated by a muffle.

fu·ro·se·mide (fū-rō′sĕ-mid, -mīd). A diuretic used in edematous states and hypertension. SYN frusemide.

fur·row (fer′rō). A groove or sulcus. [A.S. *furh*]

digital f., SYN digital *crease.*

genital f., a groove on the genital tubercle in the embryo, appearing toward the end of the second month.

gluteal f., SYN gluteal *fold.*

mentolabial f., SYN mentolabial *sulcus.*

primitive f., SYN primitive *groove.*

skin f.'s, SYN skin *sulci,* under *sulcus.*

fu·run·cle (fū′rŭng-kl). A localized pyogenic infection, most frequently by *Staphylococcus aureus,* originating deep in a hair follicle. SYN boil, furunculus. [L. *furunculus,* a petty thief]

▯ fu·run·cu·lo·sis (fū-rŭng-kū-lō′sis). A condition marked by the presence of furuncles, often chronic and recurrent.

fu·run·cu·lus, pl. **fu·run·cu·li** (fū-rŭng′kū-lŭs, -lī). SYN furuncle. [L. a petty thief, a boil, dim. of *fur,* a thief]

Fu·sar·i·um (fū-zā′rē-ŭm). A genus of rapidly growing fungi producing characteristic sickle-shaped, multiseptate macroconidia which can be mistaken for those produced by some dermatophytes. Usually saprobic, a few species such as *F. oxysporum, F. solani,* and *F. moniliforme* can produce corneal ulcers; some species may cause disseminated infection. [L. *fusus,* spindle]

fu·seau (fĕ-zō). A fusiform or spindle-shaped, multiseptate macroconidium. [Fr. *spindle* fr. L. *fusus*]

fu·si·date so·di·um (fū′si-dāt). The sodium salt of fusidic acid; has antibacterial properties. SYN sodium fusidate.

fu·sid·ic ac·id (fū-sid′ik). A fermentation product of *Fusidium coccineum,* a parasitic fungus on the plant *Veronica;* inhibits protein synthesis and the accumulation of ppGpp. SEE fusidate sodium. SYN ramycin.

fu·si·form (fū′zi-fōrm, fū′si-). Spindle-shaped; tapering at both ends. [L. *fusus,* a spindle, + *forma,* form]

Fu·si·for·mis (fū-si-fōr′mis). An obsolete generic name sometimes used for the anaerobic fusiform bacteria found in the human mouth; these organisms are closely related to the anaerobic organisms found in the human intestine and have been placed in the genus *Fusobacterium.* [see fusiform]

fu·si·mo·tor (fū′zē-mō′ter). Pertaining to the efferent innervation of intrafusal muscle fibers by gamma motor neurons. SEE ALSO neuromuscular *spindle.* [L. *fusus,* spindle, + *moveo,* to move]

fusin (fū′zin). A G protein–linked receptor present on certain human cells that is thought to be required for HIV fusion with a target cell. [fuse, fr. L. *fundo,* pp. *fusum,* to melt, + -in]

fu·sion (fū′zhŭn). **1.** Liquefaction, as by melting by heat. **2.** Union, as by joining together; e.g., bone fusion. **3.** The blending of slightly different images from each eye into a single perception. **4.** The joining of two or more adjacent teeth during their development by a dentinal union. SEE ALSO concrescence. **5.** Joining of two genes, often neighboring genes. **6.** The joining of two bones into a single unit, thereby obliterating motion between the two. **7.** The process in which two membranes are joined together. [L. *fusio,* a pouring, fr. *fundo,* pp. *fusus,* to pour]

bone block f., a method of fusing two bones in which a block of bone graft is placed between the two surfaces to obtain f. and correct preexisting deformity.

cell f., the merging of the contents of two cells by artificial means without the destruction of either, resulting in a heterokaryon that, for at least a few generations, will reproduce its kind; an important method in assignment of loci to chromosomes.

centric f., SYN robertsonian *translocation.*

flicker f., SEE critical flicker fusion *frequency.*

nuclear f., the formation of more complex atomic nuclei from less complex nuclei with release of energy, as in the formation of helium nuclei from hydrogen nuclei (hydrogen f.).

spinal f., spine f., an operative procedure to accomplish bony ankylosis between two or more vertebrae. SYN spondylosyndesis, vertebral f.

splenogonadal f., the formation of a mass consisting of splenic and testicular or ovarian tissue.

vertebral f., SYN spinal f.

Fu·so·bac·te·ri·um (fū′zō-bak-tēr′ē-ŭm). A genus of bacteria (family Bacteroidaceae) containing Gram-negative, non-sporeforming, nonmotile, obligately anaerobic rods that produce butyric acid as a major metabolic product. These organisms are found in cavities of humans and other animals; some species are pathogenic. The type species is *F. nucleatum.* [L. *fusus,* a spindle, + bacterium]

F. morti′ferum, Sphaerophorus mortiferus; a bacterial species found in the gastrointestinal tract and associated with abdominal infections in humans.

F. necro′phorum, Sphaerophorus necrophorus; an unusually pleomorphic species causing or associated with several necrotic conditions in animals, such as calf diphtheria, labial necrosis of rabbits, necrotic rhinitis of pigs, foot rot of cattle, sheep, and goats, and occasionally necrotic lesions in humans. SYN necrosis bacillus.

F. nuclea′tum, a bacterial species (probably Plaut or Vincent bacillus) found in the mouth and in infections of the upper respiratory tract, pleural cavity, and occasionally the lower intestinal tract; it is the most common cause of human fusobacterium infection, and is the type species of the genus *F.*

fu·so·cel·lu·lar (fū′zō-sel′ū-lăr). Spindle-celled.

fu·so·spi·ro·chet·al (fū-zō-spī-rō-kē′tăl). Referring to the associated fusiform and spirochetal organisms such as those found in the lesions of Vincent angina.

fus·tic (fŭs′tik). A complex of natural dyes derived from certain West Indian, Central, and South American trees, *Rhus cotinus* and *Chlorophora tinctoria;* used as mordant dyes for textiles. An important dye in the complex is morin, which is associated with the dye maclurin.

fus·ti·ga·tion (fŭs′ti-gā′shŭn). A form of massage consisting of beating the surface with light rods. [L. *fustigo,* pp. *-atus,* to beat with a cudgel]

Futcher, Palmer Howard, U.S.-Canadian physician, *1910.

FVC Abbreviation for forced vital *capacity.*

Fy blood group. See Duffy blood group, Blood Groups Appendix.

γ **1.** Third letter in the Greek alphabet, gamma. **2.** In chemistry, denotes the third in a series, the fourth carbon in an aliphatic acid, or position 2 removed from the α position in the benzene ring. **3.** Symbol for 10^{-4} gauss; surface *tension*; activity *coefficient*; microgram. **4.** Symbol for photon. For terms having this prefix, see the specific term.

G Abbreviation or symbol for gravitational *units*, under *unit*; gap (3); gauss; giga-; D-glucose, as in UDPG; guanosine, as in GDP; glycine; guanine.

G Symbol for Newtonian *constant* of gravitation; Gibbs free *energy*; G_{act} or $G^{\ddagger}$, Gibbs *energy* of activation.

g Abbreviation for gram; gaseous state.

g Unit of acceleration based on the acceleration produced by the earth's gravitational attraction, where 1 *g* = 980.621 cm/sec^2 (about 32.1725 ft/sec^2) at sea level and 45° latitude. At 30° latitude, *g* equals 979.329 cm/sec^2.

G1. Symbol for gap$_1$ *period*.

G2. Symbol for *gap* 2.

Ga Symbol for gallium.

^{67}**Ga** Symbol for gallium-67.

^{68}**Ga** Symbol for gallium-68.

GABA Abbreviation for γ-aminobutyric acid.

G ac·id. 2-Naphthol-6,8-disulfonic acid.

G-ac·tin. See under actin.

GAD Abbreviation for *glutamate* decarboxylase.

Gaddum, John H., English pharmacologist, 1900–1965. SEE G. and Schild *test*.

gad·fly (gad′flī). SEE *Tabanus*.

gad·o·di·am·ide (gad-ō-dī′ă-mid). A nonionic structural analog of gadolinium DPTA; used as a paramagnetic contrast medium in magnetic resonance imaging.

gad·o·le·ic ac·id (gad-ō-lē′ik). A *cis*-unsaturated fatty acid from cod liver oil and other sources. SYN 9-eicosenoic acid.

gad·o·lin·i·um (Gd) (gad-ō-lin′ē-ŭm). An element of the lanthanide group, atomic no. 64, atomic wt. 157.25. The paramagnetic properties of this element are used in contrast media for magnetic resonance imaging. [mineral, gadolinite, from Johan *Gadolin*, Finnish chemist, 1760–1852]

gad·o·pen·te·tate (gad-ō-pen′tĕ-tāt). (NMG)2, dimeglumine diethylenetriaminepentaacetatogadolinate (III); the methylglucamine salt of dianionic gadolinium DPTA, an acyclic chelate; used as a paramagnetic contrast medium in magnetic resonance imaging.

gad·o·ter·i·dol (gad-ō-ter′i-dol). GdHP-DO3A; a gadolinium (III) chelate of 10-(2-hydroxypropyl)-1,4,7,10-tetraaza-cyclododecane-1,4,7-triacetic acid; a nonionic macrocyclic analog of gadolinium DOTA; used as a paramagnetic contrast medium in magnetic resonance imaging.

Gaenslen, Frederick J., U.S. surgeon, 1877–1937. SEE G. *sign*.

Gaffky, Georg T.A., German hygienist, 1850–1918. SEE G. *scale*, *table*.

GAG Abbreviation for glycosaminoglycan.

gag. 1. To retch; to cause to retch or heave. **2.** To prevent from talking. **3.** An instrument adjusted between the teeth to keep the mouth from closing during operations in the mouth or throat.

Crowe-Davis mouth g., instrument used for opening the mouth, depressing the tongue, maintaining the airway, and transmitting volatile anesthetics during tonsillectomy or other oropharyngeal surgery.

gage (gāj). SYN gauge.

gain (gān). **1.** Profit; advantage. **2.** The ratio of output to input of an amplifying system, generally expressed in decibels in ultrasound. [M.E. *gayne*, booty, fr. O.Fr., fr. Germanic]

primary g., interpersonal, social, or financial advantages from the conversion of emotional stress directly into demonstrably organic illnesses (e.g., hysterical blindness or paralysis). Cf. secondary g.

secondary g., interpersonal or social advantages (e.g., assistance, attention, sympathy) gained indirectly from organic illness. Cf. primary g.

time-compensated g., SYN time-gain *compensation*.

time compensation g. (TCG), SYN time-gain *compensation*.

time-varied g. (TVG), SYN time-gain *compensation*.

Gairdner, Sir William T., Scottish physician, 1824–1907. SEE G. *disease*.

Gaisböck, Felix, German physician, 1868–1955. SEE G. *syndrome*.

gait (gāt). Manner of walking.

antalgic g., a characteristic g. resulting from pain on weightbearing in which the stance phase of g. is shortened on the affected side.

ataxic g., SYN cerebellar g.

calcaneal g., a g. disturbance, characterized by walking on heel, due to paralysis of the calf muscles, seen following poliomyelitis and in some other neurologic diseases.

cerebellar g., wide-based gait with lateral veering, unsteadiness, and irregularity of steps; often with a tendency to fall to one or other side, forward or backward. SYN ataxic g.

Charcot g., the g. of hereditary ataxia.

circumduction g., SYN hemiplegic g.

equine g., SYN high-steppage g.

festinating g., g. in which the trunk is flexed, legs are flexed at the knees and hips, but stiff, while the steps are short and progressively more rapid; characteristically seen with parkinsonism (1) and other neurologic diseases. SYN festination.

gluteus maximus g., compensatory backward propulsion of trunk to maintain center of gravity over the supporting lower extremity.

gluteus medius g., compensatory list of body (or throw of trunk) to the weak gluteal side, to place the center of gravity over the supporting lower extremity.

helicopod g., a g., seen in some conversion reactions or hysterical disorders, in which the feet describe half circles. SYN helicopodia.

hemiplegic g., g. in which the leg is stiff, without flexion at knee and ankle, and with each step is rotated away from the body, then towards it, forming a semicircle. SYN circumduction g., spastic g.

high-steppage g., a g. in which the foot is raised high to avoid catching a drooping foot and brought down suddenly in a flapping manner; often seen in peroneal nerve palsy (i.e., foot-drop) and tabes. SYN equine g.

hysterical g., a variety of bizarre g.'s seen with hysteria-conversion reaction; usually the foot is dragged or pushed ahead, instead of lifted, while walking; frequently the foot is held dorsiflexed and inverted.

scissor g., g. in which each leg swings medially as well as forward on walking; usually due to bilateral lower extremity spasticity, the result of cerebral palsy.

spastic g., SYN hemiplegic g.

steppage g., a g. in which the advancing foot is lifted higher than usual so that it can clear the ground, because it cannot be dorsiflexed. Seen with peroneal neuropathies and other disorders causing foot dorsiflexion weakness. SEE high-steppage g. SYN steppage.

toppling g., a g. in which the steps are uncertain and hesitant, and the patient totters and sometimes falls; probably due to a balance disorder; may be seen in elderly patients after a stroke.

Trendelenburg g., SYN Trendelenburg *sign*.

waddling g., rolling g. in which the weight-bearing hip is not stabilized; it bulges outward with each step, while the opposite side of the pelvis drops, resulting in alternating lateral trunk movements; due to gluteus medius muscle weakness, and seen with muscular dystrophies, among other disorders. SYN waddle.

Gal Symbol for galactose.

⊙**galact-.** SEE galacto-.

ga·lac·ta·cra·sia (gă-lak′tă-krā′zē-ă). Abnormal composition of mother's milk. [galact- + G. *akrasia*, bad mixture, fr. *a-* priv. + *krasis*, a mixing]

ga·lac·ta·gogue (gă-lak′tă-gog). An agent that promotes the secretion and flow of milk. [galact- + G. *agōgos*, leading]

ga·lac·tans (gă-lak′tanz). Polymers of galactose occurring naturally, along with galacturonans and arabans, in pectins; e.g., agar. SYN galactosans.

ga·lac·tic (gă-lak′tik). Pertaining to milk; promoting the flow of milk.

ga·lac·ti·dro·sis (gă-lak-ti-drō′sis). Sweating of a milky fluid. [galact- + G. *hidrōs*, sweat, + *-osis*, condition]

ga·lac·ti·tol (gă-lak′ti-tol). A sugar alcohol derived from galactose; g. accumulates in transferase deficiency galactosemia.

⊙**galacto-, galact-.** Milk. Cf. lact-. [G. *gala*]

ga·lac·to·blast (gă-lak′tō-blast). SYN colostrum *corpuscle*. [galacto- + *blastos*, germ]

ga·lac·to·cele (gă-lak′tō-sēl). Retention cyst caused by occlusion of a lactiferous duct. SYN lactocele. [galacto- + G. *kēlē*, tumor]

ga·lac·to·gen (gă-lak′tō-jen). A polysaccharide containing galactose in various forms. [galacto- + G. *-gen*, producing]

ga·lac·to·ki·nase (gă-lak-tō-kī′nās). An enzyme (phosphotransferase) that, in the presence of ATP, catalyzes the phosphorylation of D-galactose to D-galactose L-phosphate, the first step in the metabolism of D-galactose; g. is deficient in one form of galactosemia.

ga·lac·tom·e·ter (gal′ak-tom′ĕ-ter). A form of hydrometer for determining the specific gravity of milk as an indication of its fat content. SYN lactometer. [galacto- + G. *metron*, measure]

gal·ac·toph·a·gous (gal′ak-tof′ă-gŭs). Subsisting on milk. [galacto- + G. *phagō*, to eat]

ga·lac·to·phore (gă-lak′tō-fōr). SYN lactiferous *ducts*, under *duct*. [galacto- + G. *phoros*, bearing]

ga·lac·to·pho·ri·tis (gă-lak′tō-fō-rī′tis). Inflammation of the milk ducts. [galacto- + G. *phoros*, carrying, + *-itis*, inflammation]

gal·ac·toph·o·rous (gal-ak-tof′ŏ-rŭs). Conveying milk.

ga·lac·to·poi·e·sis (gă-lak′tō-poy-ē′sis). Milk production. [galacto- + G. *poiēsis*, forming]

ga·lac·to·poi·et·ic (gă-lak′tō-poy-et′ik). Pertaining to galactopoiesis.

ga·lac·to·pyr·a·nose (gă-lak-tō-pir′ă-nōs). Galactose in pyranose form.

ga·lac·tor·rhea (gă-lak-tō-rē′ă). **1.** Any white discharge from the nipple that is persistent and looks like milk. **2.** Continued discharge of milk from the breasts between intervals of nursing or after the child has been weaned. SYN incontinence of milk, lactorrhea. [galacto- + G. *rhoia*, a flow]

ga·lac·tos·a·mine (gă-lak-tō-sam′ēn). The 2-amino-2-deoxy derivative of galactose, in which the NH$_2$ replaces the 2-OH group; the D-isomer occurs in various mucopolysaccharides, notably of chondroitin sulfuric acid and of B blood group substance; usually found as the *N*-acetyl derivative.

ga·lac·tos·am·i·no·gly·can (gă-lak′tōs-am-i-nō-glī′kan). SEE mucopolysaccharide.

ga·lac·to·sans (gă-lak′tō-sanz). SYN galactans.

ga·lac·to·scope (gă-lak′tō-skōp). An instrument for judging of the richness and purity of milk by the translucency of a thin layer. SYN lactoscope. [galacto- + G. *skopeō*, to examine]

ga·lac·tose (Gal) (gă-lak′tōs). An aldohexose found (in D form) as a constituent of lactose, cerebrosides, gangliosides, mucoproteins, etc., in galactoside or galactosyl combination; an epimer of D-glucose.

ga·lac·to·se·mia (gă-lak-tō-sē′mē-ă). **1** [MIM*230400]. An inborn error of galactose metabolism due to congenital deficiency

of the enzyme galactosyl-1-phosphate uridylyltransferase, resulting in tissue accumulation of galactose 1-phosphate; manifested by nutritional failure, hepatosplenomegaly with cirrhosis, cataracts, mental retardation, galactosuria, aminoaciduria, and albuminuria that regress or disappear if galactose is removed from the diet; autosomal recessive inheritance; caused by mutation in the galactose-1-phosphate uridyltransferase gene (GALT) on 9p. SEE ALSO galactokinase *deficiency*. **2.** An inborn error in metabolism other than a deficiency in galactosyl-1-phosphate uridyltransferase (see subentries below). SYN galactose diabetes. [galactose + G. *haima*, blood]

epimerase deficiency g., an inborn error in metabolism in which there is a deficiency of uridine diphosphate galactose 4-epimerase; galactose 1-phosphate accumulates.

galactokinase deficiency g., an autosomal recessive disorder resulting in an accumulation of galactose and galactitol.

transferase deficiency g., an autosomal recessive disorder in which there is a deficiency of galactose-1-phosphate uridylyltransferase (see main entry for g.).

ga·lac·tose-1-phos·phate. A phosphorylated derivative of galactose that is key in galactose metabolism; accumulates in certain types of galactosemia.

g.-1-p. uridylyltransferase, an enzyme catalyzing the reaction of UTP and α-D-g.-1-p. to form UDP galactose and pyrophosphate, the second and most important step in the metabolism of D-galactose; a deficiency of this enzyme results in an accumulation of galactose, g.-1-p., and galactitol.

ga·lac·tose-6-sul·fa·tase. An enzyme that eliminates sulfur from the galactose 6-sulfate residues of certain mucopolysaccharides, producing 3,6-anhydrogalactose residues; it is absent in Morquio syndrome type A. SYN galactose-6-sulfurase.

ga·lac·tose-6-sul·fu·rase. SYN galactose-6-sulfatase.

α-D-ga·lac·to·sid·ase (gă-lak-tō-sīd′ās). An enzyme catalyzing the hydrolysis of α-D-galactosides to release free D-galactose. A deficiency of type A α-D-galactosidase is associated with Fabry disease. SYN melibiase.

β-ga·lac·to·sid·ase (ga-lak′tō-si′dās). An enzyme that hydrolyzes the beta galactoside linkage in lactose-producing glucose and galactose; also hydrolyzes the chromogenic substrate IPTG (isopropylthiogalactoside) and thus is used as an indicator of fused genes and gene expression.

β-D-ga·lac·to·sid·ase. A sugar-splitting enzyme that catalyzes the hydrolysis of lactose into D-glucose and D-galactose, and that of other β-D-galactosides; it also catalyzes galactotransferase reactions; a deficiency of β-D-galactosidase leads to problems in the intestinal digestion of lactose; used in the production of milk products for adults who do not have the intestinal enzyme; a defect of one isozyme of β-D-galactosidase is associated with Morquio syndrome type B. Cf. lactase *persistence*, lactase *restriction*. SYN lactase.

ga·lac·to·side (gă-lak′tō-sīd). A compound in which the H of the OH group on carbon-1 of galactose is replaced by an organic moiety.

ga·lac·to·sis (gal-ak-tō′sis). Formation of milk by the lacteal glands. [galacto- + G. *-osis*, condition]

ga·lac·tos·u·ria (gă-lak-tō-soo′rē-ă). The excretion of galactose in the urine. [galactose + G. *ouron*, urine]

ga·lac·to·syl (gă-lak′tō-sil). The galactose portion of a galactoside.

β-ga·lac·to·syl·cer·am·i·dase. An enzyme that participates in the catabolism of certain ceramides; a deficiency of β-galactosylceramidase is associated with Krabbe disease.

ga·lac·to·syl·cer·a·mide (gă-lak′tō-sil-ser′ă-mīd). A sphingolipid that accumulates in individuals with Krabbe disease.

ga·lac·to·ther·a·py (gă-lak′tō-thār′ă-pē). Treatment of disease by means of an exclusive or nearly exclusive milk diet. SYN lactotherapy.

ga·lac·tur·o·nan (gă-lak′toor-ō-nan). A polysaccharide that yields galacturonic acid on hydrolysis; a constituent of some pectins.

D-ga·lac·tu·ron·ic ac·id (gă-lak-toor-on′ik). The D-isomer is an oxidation product of D-galactose, in which the 6-CH$_2$OH group

ga

has become a –COOH group; occurs in many natural products (e.g., pectins) and cell walls. SYN pectic acid.

ga·lan·gal, ga·lan·ga (ga-lan′găl, -gă). The rhizome of *Alpinia offcinarum* (family Zingiberaceae); an aromatic stimulant and carminative. SYN Chinese ginger. [Mediev. L. *galanga,* mild ginger, fr. Chinese]

Galant, Nikolay Fedorovich, Russian hygienist, *1893. SEE G. *reflex.*

ga·lan·tha·mine (gă-lan′thă-mēn). An alkaloid derived from Caucasian snowdrops (a white flower of early spring) *Galanthus woronowii* (family Amaryllidaceae); from *Narcissus* spp. An alkaloid with anticholinesterase properties; enjoys use in Eastern Europe.

ga·lea (gā′lē-ă). **1** [NA]. A structure shaped like a helmet. **2.** SYN epicranial *aponeurosis.* **3.** A form of bandage covering the head. **4.** SYN caul (1). [L. a helmet]

g. aponeurot′ica [TA], SYN epicranial *aponeurosis.*

Galeati, Domenico, Italian physician, 1686–1775. SEE G. *glands,* under *gland.*

ga·le·at·o·my (gā-lē-at′ō-mē). Incision of the galea aponeurotica. [galea + G. *tomē,* incision]

Galeazzi, Riccardo, Italian surgeon, 1886–1952. SEE G. *fracture.*

Galen (Galenius, Galenos), Claudius, Greek physician and medical scientist in Rome, *c.* 130–201 A.D. SEE G. *anastomosis, nerve; veins* of G., under *vein;* great *vein* of G.

ga·le·na (gă-lē′nă). SYN *lead* sulfide. [L.]

ga·len·ic (gă-len′ik). Relating to Galen or to his theories.

ga·len·i·cals (gă-len′i-kălz). **1.** Herbs and other vegetable drugs, as distinguished from the mineral or chemical remedies. **2.** Crude drugs and the tinctures, decoctions, and other preparations made from them, as distinguished from the alkaloids and other active principles. **3.** Remedies prepared according to an official formula. [Claudius *Galen*]

gall (gawl). **1.** SYN bile. **2.** An excoriation or erosion. **3.** SYN nutgall. [A.S. *gealla*]

gal·la (gal′ă). SYN nutgall. [L.]

gal·la·mine tri·eth·i·o·dide (gal′ă-mēn trī-eth-ī′ō-dīd). A triple quaternary ammonium compound with action comparable to that of curarine.

Gallavardin, Louis, French physician, 1875–1957. SEE G. *phenomenon.*

gall·blad·der (gawl′blad-er) [TA]. A pear-shaped receptacle on the inferior surface of the liver, in a hollow between the right lobe and the quadrate lobe; it serves as a storage reservoir for bile. SYN vesica biliaris [TA], vesica fellea⋆, bile cyst, cholecyst, cholecystis, cystis fellea, gall bladder, vesicula fellis.

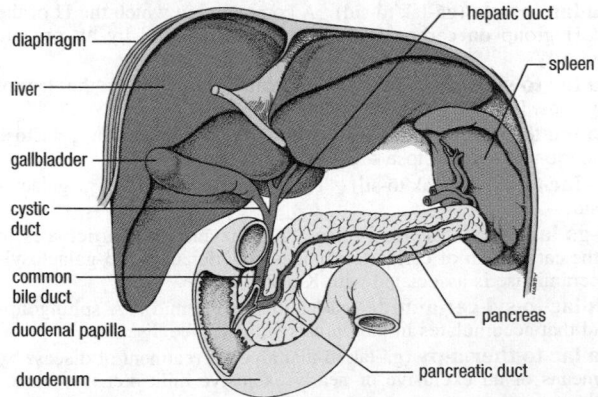

- hepatic duct
diaphragm
- spleen
liver
gallbladder
cystic duct
common bile duct
duodenal papilla
- pancreas
duodenum
- pancreatic duct

gallbladder, liver and biliary system

Courvoisier g., an enlarged, often palpable g. in a patient with carcinoma of the head of the pancreas. It is associated with jaun-

dice due to obstruction of the common bile duct. SEE Courvoisier *law.*

porcelain g., intramural calcification of the g. commonly associated with g. cancer.

sandpaper g., a roughened condition of the mucous membrane of the g., associated usually with the presence of gallstones.

strawberry g., a g. of which the mucosa is dotted with yellowish cholesterol deposits contrasting with the red hyperemic background.

Gallego dif·fer·en·ti·at·ing so·lu·tion. See under solution.

gal·le·in (gal′ē-in). Structurally related to fluorescein and used as an aniline dye indicator, turning rose red above pH 6.6, yellowish brown below pH 4. SYN pyrogallolphthalein.

gal·lic ac·id (gal′ik). Usually made from tannic acid or nutgalls; used locally as an astringent, for the same purpose as tannic acid.

Gallie, William E., Canadian surgeon, 1882–1959. SEE G. *transplant.*

Gal·li·for·mes (gal-i-fōr′mēz). An order of birds embracing the pheasant, turkey, and chicken. [L. *gallus,* a cock, + *forma,* form]

gal·li·na·ceous (gal-i-nā′shŭs). Pertaining to the order Galliformes. [L. *gallinaceus,* fr. *gallina,* a hen]

gal·li·um (Ga) (gal′ē-ŭm). A rare metal, atomic no. 31, atomic wt. 69.723. [L. *Gallia,* France]

gal·li·um-67 (^{67}Ga). A cyclotron-produced radionuclide with a half-life of 3.260 days and major gamma ray emissions of 93, 185, and 300 keV; used in the citrate form as a tumor- and inflammation-localizing radiotracer.

gal·li·um-68 (^{68}Ga). A positron emitter with a radioactive half-life of 1.130 h.

gal·lo·cy·a·nin, gal·lo·cy·a·nine (gal-ō-sī′ă-nin, ă-nēn) [C.I. 51030]. A blue phenoxazin dye used as a stain for nucleic acids after boiling with chrome alum, which is applicable for quantitative cytophotometric determination of these moieties.

gal·lon (gal′ŭn). A measure of U.S. liquid capacity containing 4 quarts, 231 cu. in., or 8.3293 pounds of distilled water at 20°C; it is the equivalent of 3.785412 L. The British imperial g. contains 277.4194 cu. in. [O.Fr. *galon*]

gal·lop (gal′op). A triple cadence to the heart sounds; due to an abnormal third or fourth heart sound being heard in addition to the first and second sounds, and usually indicative of serious disease. SYN bruit de galop, cantering rhythm, gallop rhythm, Traube bruit.

atrial g., SYN presystolic g.

presystolic g., g. cadence in which the g. sound in late diastole is an audible fourth heart sound due to forceful ventricular filling following atrial systole. SYN atrial g.

protodiastolic g., g. rhythm in which the g. sound occurs in early diastole and is an abnormal third heart sound.

S$_3$ g., SYN summation g.

summation g., g. rhythm in which the g. sound is due to superimposition of third and fourth heart sounds; sometimes heard in normal subjects with tachycardia, but usually indicative of myocardial disease. SYN S$_7$ g., S$_7$.

systolic g., obsolete term for a triple cadence to the heart sounds in which the extra sound occurs during systole, usually in the form of a systolic "click."

gall·stone (gawl′stōn). A concretion in the gallbladder or a bile duct, composed chiefly of a mixture of cholesterol, calcium bilirubinate, and calcium carbonate, occasionally as a pure stone composed of just one of these substances. SYN biliary calculus, cholelith.

opacifying g.'s, g.'s becoming roentgenographically opaque after prolonged exposure to cholecystographic contrast mediums.

silent g.'s, g.'s that cause no symptoms and are discovered by radiographic or ultrasound examination at the time of operation or autopsy.

Gal·lus (gal′ŭs). A genus of gallinaceous birds including *G. domestica,* the domestic chicken. [L. *gallus,* a cock]

GALT Abbreviation for gut-associated lymphoid *tissue.*

Galton, Sir Francis, English scientist, 1822–1911. SEE G. *delta,* system of classification of *fingerprints,* under *fingerprint, law, whistle.*

gal·to·ni·an (gahl-tō′nē-ăn). Attributed to or described by Sir Francis Galton.

Gal·vani, Luigi, Italian physician and anatomist, 1737-1798. SEE galvanism.

gal·van·ic (gal-van′ik). Pertaining to galvanism. SYN voltaic.

gal·va·nism (gal′vă-nizm). **1.** Direct current electricity produced by chemical action, as by a battery. **2.** Oral manifestations of direct current electricity occurring when dental restorations with dissimilar electric potentials (such as silver and gold) are placed in the mouth; characterized by pain or development of small areas of leukoplakia. SYN voltaism.

gal·va·ni·za·tion (gal′va-ni-zā′shŭn). Application of direct current (galvanic) electricity, as in galvanizing (electroplating).

⚠**galvano-.** Prefix denoting electrical, primarily direct current. [see galvanism]

gal·va·no·cau·tery (gal′vă-nō-kaw′ter-ē). A form of electrocautery using a wire heated by a galvanic current.

gal·va·no·con·trac·til·i·ty (gal′vă-nō-kon-trak-til′i-tē). The capability of a muscle of contracting under the stimulus of a galvanic (direct) current.

gal·va·no·far·a·di·za·tion (gal′vă-nō-far′ă-di-zā′shŭn). Simultaneous application of a galvanic and a faradic current.

gal·va·nom·e·ter (gal′vă-nom′ĕ-ter). An instrument for measuring the strength of an electric current.

d'Arsonval g., a sensitive g. consisting of a moving coil suspended in a permanent magnetic field between delicate metallic wires or ribbons that serve as both torsion springs and conductors; a mirror on the coil deflects a beam of light along the scale.

Einthoven string g., the original instrument on which Einthoven developed the first electrocardiogram.

gal·va·no·mus·cu·lar (gal′vă-nō-mŭs′kū-lăr). Denoting the effect of the application of a galvanic (direct) current to a muscle.

gal·va·no·pal·pa·tion (gal′vă-nō-pal-pā′shŭn). Esthesiometry by means of a sharp-pointed electrode through which a feeble direct current passes to the cathode applied to an indifferent part.

gal·va·no·scope (gal′vă-nō-skōp). An instrument for detecting the presence of a galvanic current. [galvano- + G. skopeō, to view]

gal·va·no·sur·gery (gal′vă-nō-ser′jer-ē). An operation in which direct electric current is utilized.

gal·va·no·tax·is (gal′vă-nō-tak′sis). SYN electrotaxis.

gal·va·no·ther·a·py (gal′van-ō-thăr′ă-pē). Treatment of disease by application of direct (galvanic) current.

gal·va·not·o·nus (gal-vă-not′ō-nŭs). **1.** SYN electrotonus. **2.** Tonic muscular contraction in response to a galvanic stimulus. [galvano- + G. tonos, tension]

gal·va·not·ro·pism (gal-vă-not′rō-pizm). SYN electrotaxis. [galvano- + G. tropē, a turning]

gam·a·bu·fa·gin (gam-ă-boo′fă-jin). SYN gamabufotalin.

gam·a·bu·fo·gen·in (gam-ă-boo′fō-jen-in). SYN gamabufotalin.

gam·a·bu·fo·tal·in (gam-ă-boo′fō-tal-in). A trihydroxybufadienolide, present in the venoms of toads (family Bufonidae), which chemically and pharmacologically resembles digitalis. SYN gamabufagin, gamabufogenin.

gam·bir (gam′bēr). An extract from the leaves of *Uncaria* (*Ourouparia*) *gambier* (family Rubiaceae); an astringent. Commercial g. is known as terra japonica.

game (gām). A contest, physical or mental, conducted according to set rules, played for amusement or for a stake. [M.E. fr. O.E. *gamen*]

language g., in philosophy, all the operations and behaviors contained in and expressed by symbols, language rules, and the social customs concerning language use.

model g., the use of g.'s, especially of g.'s of strategy, for the explanation of human behavior (both normal and abnormal).

ga·me·tan·gi·um (gam′ĕ-tan′jē-ŭm). A structure in which gametes are produced.

gam·ete (gam′ēt). **1.** One of two haploid cells that can undergo karyogamy. **2.** Any germ cell, whether ovum or spermatozoon. [G. *gametēs*, husband; *gametē*, wife]

joint g., the haploid set of (nonallelic) genes inherited in a single germinal cell.

⚠**gameto-.** A gamete. [G. *gametēs*, husband, *gametē*, wife, fr. *gameō*, to marry]

ga·me·to·cide (gă-mē′tō-sīd). An agent destructive of gametes, specifically the malarial gametocytes. [gameto- + L. *caedo,* to kill]

ga·me·to·cyst (ga-mē′tō-sist). A cyst formed around a pair of united gregarine gamonts in which gametes are produced. [gameto- + G. *kystis,* bladder]

ga·me·to·cyte (gă-mē′tō-sīt). A cell capable of dividing to produce gametes, e.g., a spermatocyte or oocyte. SYN gamont. [gameto- + G. *kytos,* cell]

ga·me·to·gen·e·sis (gam′ĕ-tō-jen′ĕ-sis). The process of formation and development of gametes. [gameto- + G. *genesis,* production]

ga·me·to·go·nia (gam′ĕ-tō-gō′nē-ă). SYN gametogony.

gam·e·tog·o·ny (gam-ĕ-tog′ō-nē). A stage in the sexual cycle of sporozoans in which gametes are formed, often by schizogony. SYN gametogonia, gamogony. [gameto- + G. *gonē,* a begetting]

gam·e·toid (gam′ĕ-toyd). Pertaining to certain biologic features that resemble those characteristic of gametes or reproductive cells.

ga·me·to·ki·net·ic (gam′ĕ-tō-ki-net′ik). Promoting or causing karyogamy or true conjugation. [gameto- + G. *kinēsis,* movement]

gam·e·to·pha·gia (gam′ĕ-tō-fā′jē-ă). The disappearance of the male or female element in zygosis. SYN gamophagia. [gameto- + G. *phagō,* to eat]

Gamgee, Joseph Sampson, British surgeon, 1828–1886. SEE Gamgee *tissue.*

gam·ic (gam′ik). Relating to or derived from sexual union; usually used as a suffix. [G. *gamikos,* pert. to marriage]

gam·ma (gam′ă). **1.** Third letter of the Greek alphabet, γ. **2.** A unit of magnetic field intensity equal to 10^{-9} T. [G.]

gam·ma ben·zene hex·a·chlo·ride (GBH). One of the purified isomers of hexachlorobenzene which is used as a scabicide and pediculicide applied topically to the skin in various lotions, creams, and shampoos; GBH can be absorbed through the skin. Resembles DDT in its actions but is less persistent. SYN hexachlorocyclohexane.

gam·ma·cism (gam′ă-sizm). Mispronunciation of, or trouble articulating, the "g" sound. [G. *gamma,* equivalent of the letter g]

gam·ma·gram (gam′ă-gram). Archaic term for scintiscan.

Gam·ma·her·pes·vir·i·nae (gam′ă-her′pez-vir′ĭ-nē). A subfamily of Herpesviridae containing Epstein-Barr virus and others that cause lymphoproliferation.

gam·mop·a·thy (gă-mop′ă-thē). A primary disturbance in immunoglobulin synthesis.

benign monoclonal g., SYN monoclonal g. of undetermined significance.

biclonal g., a g. in which the serum contains two distinct monoclonal immunoglobulins.

monoclonal g., any one of a group of disorders due to proliferation of a single clone of lymphoid or plasma cells and characterized by the presence of monoclonal immunoglobulin in serum or urine (visible on electrophoresis as a single peak).

monoclonal g. of undetermined significance, a paraproteinemia (an abnormal gammaglobulin, typically with λ light chain component) of less than 3 g/100 ml, which at the time of discovery, is without apparent cause; specifically, there is no evidence of multiple myeloma or other malignant disorders. SYN benign monoclonal g.

monoclonal g. of unknown significance (MGUS), a g. diagnosed by electrophoresis of serum of asymptomatic elderly persons who have no other evidence of plasma cell neoplasia; in 20% of cases it evolves into plasma cell malignancy.

polyclonal g., a g. in which there is a heterogeneous increase in immunoglobulins involving more than one cell line; may be caused by any of a variety of inflammatory, infectious, or neoplastic disorders.

Gamna, Carlos, Italian physician, 1896–1950. SEE G. *disease;*

Ga

G.-Favre *bodies*, under *body;* Gandy-G. *bodies*, under *body;* G.-Gandy *bodies*, under *body*, *nodules*, under *nodule*.

gam·o·gen·e·sis (gam-ō-jen′ĕ-sis). SYN sexual *reproduction*. [G. *gamos*, marriage, + *genesis*, production]

gam·og·o·ny (gam-og′ō-nē). SYN gametogony.

gam·ont. SYN gametocyte. [G. *gamos*, marriage, + *ōn* (*ont*-), being]

gam·o·pha·gia (gam-ō-fā′jē-ă). SYN gametophagia.

gam·o·pho·bia (gam-ō-fō′bē-ă). Morbid fear of marriage. [G. *gamos*, marriage, + *phobos*, fear]

gan·ci·clo·vir (gan-sī′klō-vir). An antiviral agent used in the treatment of opportunistic cytomegalovirus infections.

Gandy, Charles, French physician, *1872. SEE Gamna-G. *bodies*, under *body*, *nodules*, under *nodule;* G.-Gamna *bodies*, under *body;* G.-Nanta *disease*.

gan·ga (gang′gă). An extract of the flowers of *Cannabis sativa* (Indian hemp or hashish) which grows in India, Persia, and Arabia. SEE ALSO cannabis.

gan·glia (gang′glē-ă). Plural of ganglion.

gan·gli·al (gang′glē-ăl). SYN ganglionic.

gan·gli·ate, gan·gli·at·ed (gang′glē-āt, gang′glē-ă-ted). Having ganglia. SYN ganglionated.

gan·gli·form (gang′glē-fōrm). Having the form or appearance of a ganglion. SYN ganglioform.

gan·gli·i·tis (gang-glē-ī′tis). SYN ganglionitis.

gan·gli·o·blast (gang′glē-ō-blast). An embryonic cell from which develop ganglion cells. [ganglion + G. *blastos*, germ]

gan·gli·o·cyte (gang′glē-ō-sīt). SYN ganglion *cell*.

gan·gli·o·cy·to·ma (gang′glē-ō-sī-tō′mă). A rare lesion that contains neuronal (ganglion) cells in a sparse glial stoma. SYN central ganglioneuroma. [ganglion + G. *kytos*, cell, + *-oma*, tumor]

gan·gli·o·form (gang′glē-ō-fōrm). SYN gangliform.

gan·gli·o·gli·o·ma (gang′glē-ō-glē-ō′mă). A rare tumor composed of a glioma component and an atypical neuronal (ganglion) cell component; in younger patients often associated with seizures.

gan·gli·ol·y·sis (gang-glē-ol′i-sis). The dissolution or breaking up of a ganglion.

percutaneous radiofrequency g., g. produced by radiofrequency currents applied to a ganglion by a needle passed through the skin.

gan·gli·o·ma (gang-glē-ō′mă). SYN ganglioneuroma.

GANGLION

---

gan·gli·on, pl. **gan·glia, gan·gli·ons** (gang′glē-on, -glē-ă, -glē-onz). **1** [TA]. Originally, any group of nerve cell bodies in the central or peripheral nervous system; currently, an aggregation of nerve cell bodies located in the peripheral nervous system. SYN nerve g., neural g., neuroganglion. **2.** A cyst containing mucopolysaccharide-rich fluid within fibrous tissue or, occasionally, muscle bone or a semilunar cartilage; usually attached to a tendon sheath in the hand, wrist, or foot, or connected with the underlying joint. SYN myxoid cyst, peritendinitis serosa, synovial cyst. [G. a swelling or knot]

aberrant g., a collection of nerve cells sometimes found on a posterior spinal nerve root between the spinal g. and the spinal cord.

acousticofacial g., a primordial ganglionic cell mass in young embryos which later separates into the acoustic or spiral g. of the vestibulocochlear (eighth cranial) nerve and the geniculate g. of the facial (seventh cranial) nerve.

Acrel g., **(1)** pseudoganglion on the posterior interosseous nerve on the dorsal aspect of the wrist joint; **(2)** a cyst on a tendon of an extensor muscle at the level of the wrist.

Andersch g., SYN inferior g. of glossopharyngeal nerve.

aorticorenal ganglia [TA], a semidetached portion of the celiac ganglia, at the origin of each renal artery; contains the postsynaptic sympathetic neurons innervating the vasculature of the kidney. SYN ganglia aorticorenalia [TA].

gang′lia aorticorena′lia [TA], SYN aorticorenal ganglia.

Arnold g., SYN otic g.

auditory g., SYN cochlear g.

Auerbach ganglia, collections of postsynaptic parasympathetic nerve cells in the myenteric plexus. SEE myenteric (nervous) *plexus*.

auricular g., SYN otic g.

autonomic ganglia, visceral ganglia. SEE autonomic *division* of nervous system.

ganglia of autonomic plexuses, autonomic ganglia lying in plexuses of autonomic fibers, e.g., the celiac and inferior mesenteric ganglia of the sympathetic, and the small parasympathetic ganglia of the myenteric plexus. SYN ganglia plexuum autonomicorum [TA].

basal ganglia, originally, all of the large masses of gray matter at the base of the cerebral hemisphere; currently, the striate body (caudate and lentiform nuclei) and cell groups functionally associated with the striate body, such as the subthalamic nucleus and substantia nigra. SEE ALSO basal *nuclei*, under *nucleus*.

Bezold g., an aggregation of nerve cells in the interatrial septum.

Bochdalek g., a g. of the plexus of the dental nerve lying in the maxilla just above the root of the canine tooth.

Bock g., SYN carotid g.

Böttcher g., g. on the cochlear nerve in the internal acoustic meatus.

cardiac ganglia [TA], parasympathetic ganglia of the cardiac plexus lying between the arch of the aorta and the bifurcation of the pulmonary artery and of the plexus extension onto the atria and atrioventricular groove. One such g. is commonly found adjacent to the ligamentum arteriosum; the ganglia send postsynaptic parasympathetic fibers to the nodal tissue and periarterial plexuses of the coronary arteries. SYN ganglia cardiaca [TA], Wrisberg ganglia.

gang′lia cardi′aca [TA], SYN cardiac ganglia.

carotid g., a small ganglionic swelling on filaments from the internal carotid plexus, lying on the undersurface of the carotid artery in the cavernous sinus. SYN Bock g., Laumonier g.

celiac ganglia [TA], the largest and highest group of prevertebral sympathetic ganglia, located on the superior part of the abdominal aorta, on either side of the origin of the celiac artery; contains postsynaptic sympathetic neurons whose unmyelinated postganglionic axons innervate the stomach, liver, gallbladder, spleen, kidney, small intestine, and ascending and transverse colon. SYN ganglia coeliaca [TA], solar ganglia, Vieussens ganglia, Willis centrum nervosum.

g. cervica′le infe′rius [TA], SYN inferior cervical g.

g. cervica′le me′dium [TA], SYN middle cervical g.

g. cervica′le supe′rius [TA], SYN superior cervical g.

cervicothoracic g. [TA], a sympathetic trunk g. lying posterior to the subclavian artery near the origin of the vertebral artery, it is formed by the fusion of the inferior cervical ganglion, at the level of the seventh cervical vertebra, with the first thoracic g. SYN g. cervicothoracicum [TA], g. stellatum✶, stellate g.✶.

g. cervicothoracicum [TA], SYN cervicothoracic g.

chain ganglia, SYN g. of sympathetic trunk.

g. cilia′re [TA], SYN ciliary g.

ciliary g. [TA], a small parasympathetic g. lying in the orbit between the optic nerve and the lateral rectus muscle; it receives presynaptic fibers from the Edinger-Westphal nucleus by way of the oculomotor nerve (CN III) and in turn gives rise to postsynaptic fibers that innervate the ciliary muscle and the sphincter of the iris (sphincter pupillae muscle). SYN g. ciliare [TA], lenticular g., Schacher g.

coccygeal g., SYN g. impar.

cochlear g. [TA], an elongated g. of bipolar sensory nerve cell bodies on the cochlear part of the vestibulocochlear nerve in the spiral canal of the modiolus; each g. cell gives rise to a peripheral process that passes between the layers of the bony spiral lamina to the organ of Corti, and a central axon that enters the hindbrain as a component of the inferior (cochlear) root of the eighth nerve, which conveys auditory sensation. SYN g. cochleare [TA], spiral g. of cochlea [TA], g. spirale cochleae⋆, auditory g., Corti g., spiral cochlear g.

g. cochleare [TA], SYN cochlear g.

gang′lia coeli′aca [TA], SYN celiac ganglia.

Corti g., SYN cochlear g.

gang′lia craniospinal′ia sensoria [TA], SYN craniospinal sensory ganglia.

craniospinal sensory ganglia [TA], a term collectively designating the sensory ganglia on the dorsal (posterior) roots of spinal nerves and on those cranial nerves that contain general sensory and taste fibers; also called encephalospinal ganglia. SYN ganglia craniospinalia sensoria [TA].

diffuse g., a cystic swelling due to inflammatory effusion into one or several adjacent tendon sheaths.

dorsal root g., ⋆official alternate term for spinal g.

Ehrenritter g., SYN superior g. of glossopharyngeal nerve.

extracranial ganglia, SYN inferior g. of glossopharyngeal nerve.

g. extracrania′le, SYN inferior g. of glossopharyngeal nerve.

g. of facial nerve, SYN geniculate g.

Frankenhäuser g., SYN uterovaginal (nervous) plexus.

Froriep g., a temporary collection of nerve cells on the dorsal aspect of the hypoglossal nerve in the embryo; it represents a rudimentary sensory g.

gasserian g., SYN trigeminal g.

geniculate g. [TA], a g. of the nervus intermedius fibers conveyed by the facial nerve, located within the facial canal at the genu of the canal and containing the sensory neurons innervating the taste buds on the anterior two-thirds of the tongue and a small area on the external ear. SYN g. geniculi [TA], g. geniculatum⋆, g. of facial nerve, g. of intermediate nerve, g. of nervus intermedius, intumescentia ganglioformis.

g. geniculatum, ⋆official alternate term for geniculate g.

g. genic′uli [TA], SYN geniculate g.

Gudden g., SYN interpeduncular nucleus.

g. haben′ulae, SYN habenular nuclei, under nucleus.

hypogastric ganglia, SYN pelvic ganglia.

g. im′par [TA], the most inferior, unpaired g. of the sympathetic trunk; inconstant. SYN coccygeal g., Walther g.

inferior cervical g. [TA], inferior-most of the three ganglia of the cervical portion of the sympathetic trunk, occurring at the C7 vertebral level. Most commonly, it is fused to the first thoracic sympathetic ganglion to form a cervicothoracic (stellate) ganglion. SYN g. cervicale inferius [TA].

inferior g. of glossopharyngeal nerve [TA], the lower, more significant, of two sensory ganglions on the glossopharyngeal nerve immediately inferior to its exit from the jugular foramen. The unipolar neurons comprising the ganglia convey taste and general sensation from the posterior third of the tongue, and general sensation only from the fauces, soft palate, and oropharynx. SYN g. inferius nervi glossopharyngei [TA], Andersch g., extracranial ganglia, g. extracraniale, petrosal g., petrous g.

inferior mesenteric g. [TA], the lowest of the sympathetic prevertebral ganglia, located at the origin of the inferior mesenteric artery from the aorta and containing the postsynaptic sympathetic neurons innervating the descending and sigmoid colon. SYN g. mesentericum inferius [TA].

inferior g. of vagus nerve [TA], a large sensory g. of the vagus, anterior to the internal jugular vein. SYN g. inferius nervi vagi [TA], g. of trunk of vagus, nodose g.

g. infe′rius ner′vi glossopharyn′gei [TA], SYN inferior g. of glossopharyngeal nerve.

g. infe′rius ner′vi va′gi [TA], SYN inferior g. of vagus nerve.

intercrural g., SYN interpeduncular nucleus.

gang′lia interme′dia [TA], SYN intermediate ganglia.

intermediate ganglia [TA], small sympathetic ganglia most commonly found on the communicating branches in the cervical and lumbar region. SYN ganglia intermedia [TA].

g. of intermediate nerve, SYN geniculate g.

interpeduncular g., SYN interpeduncular nucleus.

intervertebral g., SYN spinal g.

intracranial g., SYN superior g. of glossopharyngeal nerve.

g. isth′mi, SYN interpeduncular nucleus.

jugular g., (1) SYN superior g. of glossopharyngeal nerve; **(2)** SYN superior g. of vagus nerve.

Laumonier g., SYN carotid g.

Lee g., SYN uterovaginal (nervous) plexus.

lenticular g., SYN ciliary g.

Lobstein g., SYN thoracic splanchnic g.

Ludwig g., a small collection of parasympathetic nerve cells in the interatrial septum.

gang′lia lumba′lia [TA], SYN lumbar ganglia.

lumbar ganglia [TA], four or more ganglia on the medial border of the psoas major muscle on either side; they form, with the sacral and coccygeal ganglia and their interganglionic branches, the abdominopelvic part of the sympathetic trunk. SYN ganglia lumbalia [TA].

Meckel g., SYN pterygopalatine g.

g. mesenter′icum infe′rius [TA], SYN inferior mesenteric g.

g. mesenter′icum supe′rius [TA], SYN superior mesenteric g.

middle cervical g. [TA], a sympathetic g., of small size and sometimes absent; located at the level of the cricoid cartilage. SYN g. cervicale medium [TA].

nasal g., SYN pterygopalatine g.

nerve g., neural g., SYN ganglion (1).

g. of nervus intermedius, SYN geniculate g.

nodose g., SYN inferior g. of vagus nerve.

otic g. [TA], an autonomic g. situated inferior to the foramen ovale medial to the mandibular nerve; its postsynaptic parasympathetic fibers are secretomotor fibers distributed to the parotid gland. SYN g. oticum [TA], Arnold g., auricular g., otoganglion.

g. o′ticum [TA], SYN otic g.

parasympathetic ganglia [TA], those ganglia of the autonomic nervous system composed of cholinergic neurons receiving presynaptic fibers from visceral motor neurons in either the brainstem or the middle sacral spinal segments (S2 to S4); on the basis of their location with respect to the organs they innervate, most parasympathetic ganglia, at least outside the head, can be categorized as juxtamural or intramural ganglia (i.e., located in or on the viscus being innervated). SEE ALSO autonomic division of nervous system. SYN ganglia parasympathetica [TA].

ganglia parasympathetica [TA], SYN parasympathetic ganglia.

paravertebral ganglia, SYN g. of sympathetic trunk.

pelvic ganglia [TA], the parasympathetic ganglia scattered through the pelvic plexus of either side. SYN ganglia pelvica [TA], hypogastric ganglia.

gang′lia pel′vica [TA], SYN pelvic ganglia.

periosteal g., a flattened subperiosteal cavity containing clear, yellow, viscous, synovial-like fluid.

petrosal g., petrous g., SYN inferior g. of glossopharyngeal nerve.

phrenic ganglia [TA], several small autonomic ganglia contained in the plexuses accompanying the inferior phrenic arteries. SYN ganglia phrenica [TA].

gang′lia phren′ica [TA], SYN phrenic ganglia.

gang′lia plex′uum autonomico′rum [TA], SYN ganglia of autonomic plexuses.

prevertebral ganglia, the sympathetic ganglia (celiac, aorticorenal, superior and inferior mesenteric) lying in front of the vertebral column, as distinguished from the ganglia of the sympathetic trunk (paravertebral ganglia); these ganglia occur mostly around the origin of the major branches of the abdominal aorta; all are in the abdominopelvic cavity; the neurons comprising the ganglia send postsynaptic sympathetic fibers to abdominopelvic viscera via periarterial plexuses.

pterygopalatine g. [TA], a small parasympathetic g. in the upper part of the pterygopalatine fossa whose secretomotor postsynaptic fibers supply the lacrimal, nasal, palatine, and pharyngeal glands. SYN g. pterygopalatinum [TA], Meckel g., nasal g., sphenopalatine g.

ga

g. pterygopalati'num [TA], SYN pterygopalatine g.

Remak ganglia, (1) groups of nerve cells in the wall of the venous sinus where it joins the right atrium of the heart; (2) autonomic ganglia in nerves of the stomach.

renal ganglia [TA], small scattered sympathetic ganglia along the renal plexus. SYN ganglia renalia [TA].

gang'lia rena'lia [TA], SYN renal ganglia.

Ribes g., a small sympathetic g. situated on the anterior communicating artery of the brain.

sacral ganglia [TA], three or four ganglia on either side constituting, with the g. impar and the interganglionic branches, the pelvic part of the sympathetic trunk. SYN ganglia sacralia [TA].

gang'lia sacra'lia [TA], SYN sacral ganglia.

Scarpa g., SYN vestibular g.

Schacher g., SYN ciliary g.

semilunar g., SYN trigeminal g.

g. sensorium nervi spinalis [TA], SYN spinal g.

sensory g., a cluster of primary sensory neurons forming a usually visible swelling in the course of a peripheral nerve or its dorsal root; such nerve cells establish the sole afferent neural connection between the sensory periphery (skin, mucous membranes of the oral and nasal cavities, muscle tissue, tendons, joint capsules, special sense organs, blood vessel walls, tissues of the internal organs) and the central nervous system; they are the cells of origin of all sensory fibers of the peripheral nervous system.

Soemmerring g., SYN substantia nigra.

solar ganglia, SYN celiac ganglia.

sphenopalatine g., SYN pterygopalatine g.

ⓘ **spinal g.** [TA], the g. of the posterior (dorsal) root of each spinal segmental nerve (commonly with the exception of the first cervical spinal nerve); contains the cell bodies of the pseudounipolar primary sensory neurons whose peripheral axonal branches become part of the mixed segmental nerve, while the central axonal branches enter the spinal cord as a component of the sensory posterior root. SYN g. sensorium nervi spinalis [TA], dorsal root g.✶, g. spinale, intervertebral g.

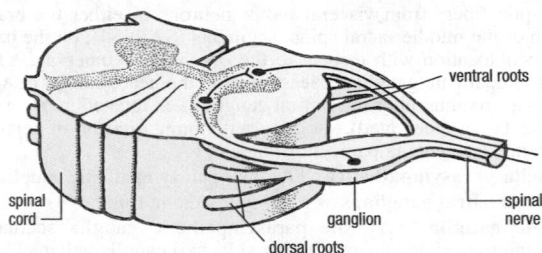

spinal cord — ventral roots — ganglion — dorsal roots — spinal nerve

spinal (dorsal root) ganglion

g. spina'le, SYN spinal g.

spiral g. of cochlea [TA], SYN cochlear g.

spiral cochlear g., SYN cochlear g.

g. spira'le coch'leae, ✶official alternate term for cochlear g.

stellate g., ✶official alternate term for cervicothoracic g.

g. stella'tum, ✶official alternate term for cervicothoracic g.

sublingual g. [TA], a tiny parasympathetic g. occasionally found anterior to the submandibular g., of which it is a displaced portion; its postsynaptic fibers are secretomotor to the sublingual gland. SYN g. sublinguale [TA].

g. sublingua'le [TA], SYN sublingual g.

submandibular g. [TA], a small parasympathetic g. suspended from the lingual nerve; its postsynaptic fibers are secretomotor to the submandibular and sublingual glands; its presynaptic fibers come from the superior salvatory nucleus by way of the chorda tympani. SYN g. submandibulare [TA], submaxillary g.

g. submandibula're [TA], SYN submandibular g.

submaxillary g., SYN submandibular g.

superior cervical g. [TA], the superior-most and largest of the ganglia of the sympathetic trunk, lying near the base of the skull

between the internal carotid artery and the internal jugular vein. All postsynaptic sympathetic fibers distributed to the head and upper neck are derived from the cell bodies that constitute this g. SYN g. cervicale superius [TA].

superior g. of glossopharyngeal nerve [TA], the upper, smaller, and less significant of two ganglia on the glossopharyngeal nerve as it traverses the jugular foramen; it is usually regarded as a detached part of the inferior g. SYN g. superius nervi glossopharyngei [TA], Ehrenritter g., intracranial g., jugular g. (1).

superior mesenteric g. [TA], an often paired sympathetic g. located at the origin of the superior mesenteric artery from the aorta. The neurons comprising the g. send postsynaptic fibers to the portions of the small and large intestines supplied by the superior mesenteric artery. SYN g. mesentericum superius [TA].

superior g. of vagus nerve [TA], a small sensory g. on the vagus as it traverses the jugular foramen. SYN g. superius nervi vagi [TA], jugular g. (2).

g. supe'rius ner'vi glossopharyn'gei [TA], SYN superior g. of glossopharyngeal nerve.

g. supe'rius ner'vi va'gi [TA], SYN superior g. of vagus nerve.

sympathetic ganglia, those ganglia of the autonomic nervous system that receive efferent fibers originating from preganglionic visceral motor neurons in the intermediolateral cell column of thoracic and upper lumbar spinal segments (T1–L2). On the basis of their location, the sympathetic ganglia can be classified as paravertebral ganglia (ganglia trunci sympathici) and prevertebral ganglia (ganglia celiaca). SEE ALSO autonomic division of nervous system.

g. of sympathetic trunk [TA], the clusters of postsynaptic neurons located at intervals along the sympathetic trunks, including the superior cervical, middle cervical, and cervicothoracic (stellate) g., the thoracic, lumbar, and sacral ganglia, and the g. impar. SYN ganglia trunci sympathici [TA], chain ganglia, paravertebral ganglia.

terminal g. [TA], (1) one of the cells located along the terminal nerves; SYN g. terminale [TA]. (2) one of the scattered postsynaptic autonomic neurons located in or close to the wall of the organ innervated; they are usually parasympathetic.

g. termina'le [TA], SYN terminal g. (1).

thoracic ganglia [TA], sympathetic ganglia, 11 or 12 on either side, at the level of the head of each rib, constituting with the interganglionic branches the thoracic part of the sympathetic trunk. SYN ganglia thoracica [TA].

gang'lia thorac'ica [TA], SYN thoracic ganglia.

thoracic splanchnic g., a small sympathetic g. often present in the course of the greater splanchnic nerve. SYN g. thoracicum splanchnicum, Lobstein g.

g. thoracicum splanch'nicum, SYN thoracic splanchnic g.

trigeminal g. [TA], the large flattened sensory g. of the trigeminal nerve lying adjacent to the cavernous sinus along the medial part of the middle cranial fossa in the trigeminal cave (cavity) of the dura mater. SYN g. trigeminale [TA], gasserian g., semilunar g.

g. trigemina'le [TA], SYN trigeminal g.

Troisier g., historic term for a lymph node immediately above the clavicle, especially on the left side, that is palpably enlarged as the result of a metastasis from a malignant neoplasm; the presence of such a node indicates that the probable site of primary involvement is in an abdominal organ. SEE ALSO signal node. SYN Troisier node.

gang'lia trun'ci sympath'ici [TA], SYN g. of sympathetic trunk.

g. of trunk of vagus, SYN inferior g. of vagus nerve.

tympanic g., a small g. on the tympanic nerve during its passage through the petrous portion of the temporal bone. SYN g. tympanicum✶.

g. tympan'icum, ✶official alternate term for tympanic g.

Valentin g., a g. on the superior alveolar nerve.

vertebral g. [TA], an inconstant, small g. located along the cervical part of the sympathetic trunk or one of the interganglionic branches connecting the middle cervical g. and the cervicothoracic g.; it usually lies near the vertebral artery. SYN g. vertebrale [TA].

g. vertebra'le [TA], SYN vertebral g.

vestibular g. [TA], a collection of bipolar sensory nerve cell bodies concerned with equilibration and forming a swelling on the vestibular part of the eighth cranial nerve in the fundus of the internal acoustic meatus; consists of a superior part and an inferior part connected by a narrow isthmus. SYN g. vestibulare [TA], Scarpa g.

g. vestibula′re [TA], SYN vestibular g.

Vieussens ganglia, SYN celiac ganglia.

Walther g., SYN g. impar.

Wrisberg ganglia, SYN cardiac ganglia.

---

gan·gli·on·at·ed (gang′glē-ō-nā′ted). SYN gangliate.

gan·gli·on·ec·to·my (gang′glē-ō-nek′tō-mē). Excision of a ganglion. [ganglion + G. *ektomē*, excision]

ganglioneuroblastoma (gang′lē-ō-noor-ō-blas-tō′ma). A tumor of mixed cellular type, with elements of neuroblastoma and ganglioneuroma.

gan·glio·neu·ro·ma (gang′glē-ō-noo-rō′mă). A benign neoplasm composed of mature ganglionic neurons, in varying numbers, scattered singly or in clumps within a relatively abundant and dense stroma of neurofibrils and collagenous fibers; usually found in the posterior mediastinum and retroperitoneum, sometimes in relation to the adrenal glands. SYN ganglioma. [ganglion + G. *neuron*, nerve, + *-oma*, tumor]

central g., SYN gangliocytoma.

dumbbell g., a g. in which the gross configuration resembles a dumbbell, e.g., two spheroidal masses connected by a narrow portion, usually the result of the neoplasm being somewhat molded by a resistant structure such as two ribs.

gan·glio·neu·ro·ma·to·sis (gang′glē-ō-noor′ō-mă-tō′sis). The condition of having many widespread ganglioneuromas.

gan·gli·on·ic (gang-glē-on′ik). Relating to a ganglion. SYN ganglial.

gan·gli·on·i·tis (gang′glē-ō-nī′tis). 1. Inflammation of a lymphatic ganglion. 2. Inflammation of a nerve ganglion. SYN gangliitis.

gan·gli·o·nos·to·my (gang′glē-ō-nos′tō-mē). Making an opening into a ganglion (2). [ganglion + G. *stoma*, mouth]

gan·gli·o·ple·gic (gang′glē-ō-plē′jik). A pharmacologic compound that paralyzes an autonomic ganglion, usually for a relatively short period of time. [ganglion + G. *plēgē*, stroke, shock]

gan·gli·os·i·a·li·do·sis (gang′glē-ō-sī-al-ē-dō′sis). SYN gangliosidosis.

gan·gli·o·side (gang′glē-ō-sīd). A glycosphingolipid chemically similar to cerebrosides but containing one or more sialic (*N*-acetylneuraminic or *N*-glycolylneuraminic) acid residues; found principally in nerve tissue, spleen, and thymus; G_{M1} accumulates in generalized gangliosidosis; G_{M2} accumulates in Tay-Sachs disease. SYN sialoglycosphingolipid.

gan·gli·o·si·do·sis (gang′glē-ō-si-dō′sis). Any disease characterized, in part, by the abnormal accumulation within the nervous system of specific gangliosides, e.g., G_{M2} gangliosidosis, Tay-Sachs disease, caused by hexosaminidase A enzyme deficiency with accumulation of G_{M2} ganglioside. SYN gangliosialidosis, ganglioside lipidosis.

G_{M1} **g.,** three forms exist: infantile, generalized; juvenile; and adult; g. characterized by accumulation of a specific monosialoganglioside, G_{M1}; due to deficiency of G_{M1}-β-galactosidase. SYN generalized g.

G_{M2} **g.,** one of the hereditary metabolic disorders; several forms exist, including Tay-Sachs *disease*, Sandhoff *disease*, AV variant and adult onset; characterized by accumulation of a specific metabolite, G_{M2} ganglioside, due to deficiency of hexosaminidase A or B, or G_{M2} activator factor.

generalized g., SYN G_{M1} g.

infantile G_{M2} g., SYN Tay-Sachs *disease*.

infantile, generalized G_{M1} g., one of the hereditary metabolic diseases of infancy; resembles Tay-Sachs *disease*, except other organ systems (bone, liver, kidney) are affected. SYN familial neuroviscerolipidosis, pseudo-Hurler disease, Type 1 G_{M1} g.

Type 1 G_{M1} g., SYN infantile, generalized G_{M1} g.

gan·go·sa (gang-gō′să). A destructive ulceration beginning on the soft palate and extending thence to the hard palate, nasopharynx, and nose, resulting in mutilating cicatrices. The disease, so far as is known, occurs only in certain portions of the tropics, especially the islands of the Pacific, and is generally regarded as a sequel to yaws. [Sp. *gangoso,* snuffling]

gan·grene (gang′grēn). 1. Necrosis due to obstruction, loss, or diminution of blood supply; it may be localized to a small area or involve an entire extremity or organ (such as the bowel), and may be wet or dry. SYN mortification. 2. Extensive necrosis from any cause, e.g., gas gangrene. [G. *gangraina*, an eating sore, fr. *graō*, to gnaw]

arteriosclerotic g., dry g. resulting from sclerotic changes in the arteries, with subsequent occlusion, as in the aged.

cold g., SYN dry g.

cutaneous g., g. of the skin characterized by sloughing; may occur in shingles or in any acute infection that interferes with superficial circulation.

decubital g., SYN decubitus *ulcer*.

diabetic g., g. resulting from arteriosclerosis associated with diabetes.

disseminated cutaneous g., SYN *dermatitis* gangrenosa infantum.

dry g., a form of g. in which the involved part is dry, sharply demarcated, and shriveled; usually due to slowly occlusive vascular disease. SYN cold g., mummification (1).

embolic g., g. resulting from obstruction of an artery by an embolus.

emphysematous g., SYN gas g.

Fournier g., SYN Fournier *disease*.

gas g., g. occurring in a wound infected with various anaerobic sporeforming bacteria, especially *Clostridium perfringens* and *C. novyi*, which cause rapidly advancing crepitation of the surrounding tissues, due to gas liberated by bacterial fermentation, and constitutional toxic and septic symptoms including cytotoxic damage to kidney, liver, and other organs. SYN clostridial myonecrosis, emphysematous g., gangrenous emphysema, progressive emphysematous necrosis.

hemorrhagic g., (1) SYN hemorrhagic *infarct*; **(2)** g. occurring rarely in advanced meningococcal septicemia.

hospital g., SYN decubitus *ulcer*.

hot g., g. following inflammation of the part.

Meleney g., SYN Meleney *ulcer*.

moist g., SYN wet g.

presenile spontaneous g., g. occurring in middle life as a result of thromboangiitis obliterans.

pressure g., SYN decubitus *ulcer*.

progressive bacterial synergistic g., SYN Meleney *ulcer*.

senile g., dry g. occurring in the aged in consequence of occlusion of an artery, particularly affecting the extremities.

spontaneous g. of newborn, g. due to vascular occlusion of unknown cause, usually in marasmic or dehydrated infants.

static g., moist g. due to obstruction in the return circulation. SYN venous g.

symmetrical g., g. affecting the extremities of both sides of the body; it is seen particularly in severe arteriosclerosis, myocardial infarction, and ball-valve thrombus.

thrombotic g., g. due to occlusion of an artery by a thrombus.

trophic g., SYN trophic *ulcer*.

venous g., SYN static g.

wet g., ischemic necrosis of an extremity with bacterial putrefaction, producing cellulitis adjacent to the necrotic areas. SYN moist g.

white g., death of a part accompanied by the formation of grayish white sloughs. SYN leukonecrosis.

gan·gre·nous (gang′grĕ-nŭs). Relating to or affected with gangrene.

gan·o·blast (gan′o-blast). SYN ameloblast.

Ganong, William F., U.S. physiologist, *1924. SEE Lown-G.-Levine *syndrome*.

Ga

Ganser, Siegbert J.M., German psychiatrist, 1853–1931. SEE G. *commissure, syndrome; nucleus* basalis of G.

Gant, Samuel G., U.S. surgeon, 1869–1944. SEE G. *clamp.*

gan·try (gan'trē). A frame housing the x-ray tube, collimators, and detectors in a CT machine, with a large opening into which the patient is inserted; a mechanical support for mounting a device to be moved in a circular path. [M.E., fr. O.Fr., fr. L. *cantherius,* wooden frame, fr. G. *kanthēlia,* pack saddle, fr. *kanthos,* pack ass]

Gantzer, Carol F.L., 17th century German anatomist. SEE G. accessory *bundle, muscle.*

Ganz, William, U.S. cardiologist, *1919. SEE Swan-G. *catheter.*

gap. **1.** A hiatus or opening in a structure. **2.** An interval or discontinuity in any series or sequence. **3 (G).** A period in the cell cycle.

g. 1 (G1), in the somatic cell cycle, the g. that follows mitosis and is followed by synthesis in preparation for the next cycle.

g. 2 (G2), in the somatic cell cycle, a pause between completion of synthesis and the onset of cell division.

air-bone g., the difference between the threshold for hearing by bone conduction and by air conduction.

anion g., the difference between the sum of the measured cations and anions in the plasma or serum calculated as follows: $(Na + K) - (Cl + HCO_3) = < 20$ MMOL/L. Elevated values may occur in diabetic or lactic acidosis; normal or low values occur in bicarbonate-losing metabolic acidoses. SYN cation-anion difference.

auscultatory g., the period during which Korotkoff sounds indicating true systolic pressure fade away and reappear at a lower pressure point; responsible for errors made in recording falsely low systolic blood pressure, especially in hypertensive patients, of up to 25 mm Hg, and avoided by pumping the cuff 30 mm Hg beyond palpable systolic pressure. SYN silent g.

Bochdalek g., SYN lumbocostal *triangle* of diaphragm.

chromosomal g., a localized area of thinning in a chromatid which may simulate a complete break.

DNA g., a localized loss of one of the two strands in the double helix of DNA.

excitable g., SYN gap *phenomenon.*

interocclusal g., SYN freeway *space.*

silent g., SYN auscultatory g.

Garbe, William, Canadian dermatologist, *1908. SEE Sulzberger-G. *disease, syndrome.*

Gardner, F.H. SEE G.-Diamond *syndrome.*

Gardner, Eldon J., U.S. geneticist, *1909. SEE G. *syndrome.*

Gard·ner·el·la (gărd'ner-el'ă). A genus of facultatively anaerobic, oxidase- and catalase-negative, nonsporeforming, nonencapsulated, nonmotile, pleomorphic bacteria with Gram-variable rods.

G. vaginalis, a species that is an etiologic agent of bacterial vaginosis in humans.

gar·gle (gar'gl). **1.** To rinse the fauces with fluid in the mouth through which expired breath is forced to produce a bubbling effect while the head is held far back. **2.** A medicated fluid used for gargling; a throat wash. [O. Fr. fr. L. *gurgulio,* gullet, windpipe]

Gariel, Maurice, French physician, 1812–1878. SEE G. *pessary.*

Garland, Hugh G., British neurologist 1903–1967. SEE Marinesco-Garland *syndrome.*

Garland, M., U.S. physician, 1848–1926. SEE G. *triangle.*

gar·lic (gar'lik). SYN allium.

g. oil, a volatile oil from the bulb or entire plant of *Allium sativum* (family Liliaceae); contains diallyl disulfide and allyl propyl disulfide; has been used as an anthelmintic and rubefacient.

Garré, Carl, Swiss surgeon, 1857–1928. SEE G. *disease;* Garré *osteomyelitis.*

Gärtner, August, German physician, 1848–1934. SEE G. *method,* vein *phenomenon, tonometer.*

Gartner, Herman T., Danish anatomist and surgeon, 1785–1827. SEE G. *canal, cyst, duct.*

GAS Abbreviation for group A *streptococci,* under *streptococcus.*

gas. **1.** A thin fluid, like air, capable of indefinite expansion but convertible by compression and cold into a liquid and, eventually, a solid. **2.** In clinical practice, a liquid entirely in its vapor phase at one atmosphere of pressure because ambient temperature is above its boiling point. [coined by J.B. van Helmont, Flemish chemist and physician, 1577–1644]

alveolar g. (symbol subscript A), the g. in the pulmonary alveoli, where O_2-CO_2 exchange with pulmonary capillary blood occurs. SYN alveolar air.

anesthetic g., SEE inhalation *anesthetic.*

blood g.'s, a clinical expression for the determination of the partial pressures of oxygen and carbon dioxide in blood.

carbonic acid g., SYN *carbon* dioxide.

expired g., **(1)** any g. that has been expired from the lungs; **(2)** often used synonymously with mixed expired g.

hemolytic g., a poisonous g., such as arsine, inhalation of which causes hemolysis with hemoglobinuria, jaundice, gastroenteritis, and nephritis.

ideal alveolar g., the uniform composition of g. that would exist in all alveoli for a given total respiratory exchange if all alveoli had identical ventilation-perfusion ratios and achieved perfect equilibrium with the blood leaving the pulmonary capillaries.

inert g.'s, SYN noble g.'s.

inspired g. (I) (symbol subscript I), **(1)** any g. that is being inhaled; **(2)** specifically, that g. after it has been humidified at body temperature.

laughing g., a historical term for nitrous oxide. [so called because its inhalation sometimes excites a hilarious delirium preceding insensibility]

marsh g., SYN methane.

mixed expired g., one or more complete breaths of expired g. coming thoroughly mixed from the dead space and the alveoli.

mustard g. (HD), a poisonous vesicating gas introduced in World War I; it is the progenitor of the so-called nitrogen mustards; used in chemical warfare; a known carcinogen. SYN di(2-chloroethyl)-sulfide, mustard (2), sulfur mustard.

noble g.'s, elements in the zero group in the periodic series: helium, neon, argon, krypton, xenon, and radon. SYN inert g.'s.

sewer g., g., probably mostly methane, resulting from decomposition of organic matter in sewers; potentially explosive and toxic.

sneezing g., SYN sternutator.

suffocating g., a g., such as chlorine or phosgene, that causes intense irritation of the bronchial tubes and lungs, resulting in pulmonary edema.

tear g., a g., such as acetone, benzene bromide, and xylol, that causes irritation of the conjunctiva and profuse lacrimation. SEE ALSO lacrimator.

vesicating g., a g., such as mustard g., which upon contact with the skin causes vesication and sloughing; inhalation may result in bronchopneumonia.

vomiting g., a g., such as chloropicrin, that can cause vomiting and gastrointestinal disorders such as colic and diarrhea.

water g., an illuminating and fuel g. produced by passing steam over red-hot coal; consists chiefly of hydrogen, hydrocarbons, and carbon monoxide.

gas·e·ous (gas'ē-ŭs). Of the nature of gas.

Gaskell, Walter H., English physiologist, 1847–1914. SEE G. *bridge, clamp.*

gas·om·e·ter (gas-om'ĕ-ter). A calibrated instrument or vessel for measuring the volumes of gases. SEE ALSO spirometer.

gas·o·met·ric (gas-ō-met'rik). Relating to gasometry.

gas·om·e·try (gas-om'ĕ-trē). Measurement of gases; determination of the relative proportion of gases in a mixture.

Gass, John D.M., U.S. ophthalmologist, *1928. SEE Irvine-G. *syndrome.*

Gasser (Gas·ser·i·o), Johann L., Austrian anatomist, 1723–1765. SEE gasserian *ganglion.*

gas·ser·i·an (ga-ser'ē-an). Relating to or described by Johann L. Gasser.

gas·sing (gas'ing). Poisoning by irrespirable or otherwise noxious gases.

Gastaut, Henri, French biologist, *1915. SEE Lennox-G. *syndrome.*

gas·ter (gas′ter) [TA]. **1.** SYN stomach. **2.** Prominent part of wasp or ant abdomen, separated from the other body parts by a thin connecting segment. [G. *gastēr,* belly]

Gas·ter·o·phil·i·dae (gas′ter-ō-fil′i-dē). A family of botflies (or warble flies) that produce enteric myiasis in members of the horse family (genus *Gasterophilus*), in rhinoceroses (genus *Gyrostigma*), and in elephants (genera *Cobboldia, Platycobboldia,* and *Rodhainomyia*). SYN Gastrophilidae. [G. *gastēr,* belly, stomach, + *philos,* fond]

△**gastr-.** SEE gastro-.

gas·tral·gia (gas-tral′jē-ă). SYN stomach *ache.* [gastr- + G. *algos,* pain]

gas·trec·ta·sis, gas·trec·ta·sia (gas-trek′tă-sis, gas-trek-tā′zē-ă). Dilation of the stomach. [gastr- + G. *ektasis,* extension]

gas·trec·to·my (gas-trek′tō-mē). Excision of a part or all of the stomach. [gastr- + G. *ektomē,* excision]

Hofmeister g., hofmeister operation in which a portion of the stomach is removed and a retrocolic gastrojejunostomy is constructed in an end-to-side fashion to only the greater curvature portion of the transected stomach.

Pólya g., operation in which a portion of the stomach is removed and a retrocolic gastrojejunostomy is constructed in an end-to-side fashion to the entire cut end of the stomach. SYN Pólya operation.

gas·tric (gas′trik). Relating to the stomach. SYN gastricus.

gas·tric car·dia (gas′trik kar′dē-ă). SYN cardia.

gas·tric·sin (gas-trik′sin). An alternative term for a human peptidase now termed pepsin C. It is present in the gastric juices of most vertebrates.

gas·tri·cus (gas′tri-kŭs). SYN gastric. [L.]

gas·trin·o·ma (gas-tri-nō′mă). A gastrin-secreting tumor associated with the Zollinger-Ellison syndrome.

gas·trins (gas′trinz). Hormones secreted in the pyloric-antral mucosa of the mammalian stomach that stimulate secretion of HCl by the parietal cells of the gastric glands; there are three main types: big gastrin (34 amini acyl residues), little gastrin (17 residues), and minigastrin (14 residues), as well as sulfated derivatives. The C-terminal pentapeptide is also seen in cholecystokinin and cerulein. [G. *gastēr,* stomach, + -in]

⊞**gas·tri·tis** (gas-trī′tis). Inflammation, especially mucosal, of the stomach. [gastr- + G. *-itis,* inflammation]

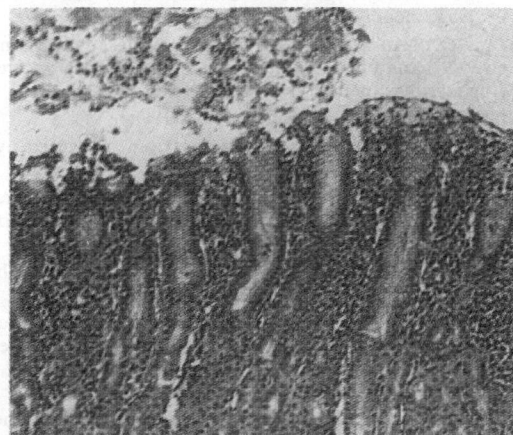

acute gastritis: with epithelial damage and inflammation of the gastric glands

alkaline reflux g., an inflammation of the gastric mucosa believed to be caused by irritating factors that reflux from the intestine into the stomach; most common after a procedure that resects or ablates the pylorus. SYN bile g.

atrophic g., chronic g. with atrophy of the mucous membrane and destruction of the peptic glands, sometimes associated with pernicious anemia or gastric carcinoma; also applied to gastric atrophy without inflammatory changes.

bile g., SYN alkaline reflux g.

catarrhal g., g. with excessive secretion of mucus.

g. cys′tica polypo′sa, large sessile mucosal polyps arising in the stomach proximal to an old gastroenterostomy.

eosinophilic g., SYN eosinophilic *gastroenteritis.*

exfoliative g., g. with excessive shedding of mucosal epithelial cells.

hypertrophic g., SYN Ménétrier *disease.*

interstitial g., inflammation of the stomach involving the submucosa and muscle coats.

polypous g., a form of chronic g., in which there is irregular atrophy of the mucous membrane with cystic glands giving rise to a knobby or polypous appearance of the surface.

pseudomembranous g., g. characterized by the formation of a false membrane.

sclerotic g., a fibrous thickening of the walls of the stomach with diminution in the capacity of the organ.

△**gastro-, gastr-.** The stomach, abdomen. [G. *gastēr,* the belly]

gas·tro·a·ceph·a·lus (gas′trō-ă-sef′ă-lŭs). Unequal conjoined twins in which an acephalous parasite is attached to the abdomen of the autosite. SEE conjoined *twins,* under *twin.* [gastro- + G. *a*-priv. + *kephalē,* head]

gas·tro·al·bum·or·rhea (gas′trō-al-bū-mō-rē′ă). Loss of albumin into the stomach. [gastro- + albumin, + G. *rhoia,* flow]

gas·tro·a·mor·phus (gas′trō-ă-mōr′fŭs). An included amorphous parasitic twin within the abdomen of the autosite. [gastro- + G. *amorphos,* unshapely]

gas·tro·a·nas·to·mo·sis (gas′trō-an-as-tō-mō′sis). SYN gastrogastrostomy.

gas·tro·a·to·nia (gas′trō-ă-tō′nē-ă). Obsolete term for loss of tone in the stomach musculature. [gastro- + G. *atonia,* languor]

gas·tro·blen·nor·rhea (gas′trō-blen-ō-rē′ă). Excessive proliferation of mucus by the stomach. [gastro- + blennorrhea]

gas·tro·car·di·ac (gas′trō-kar′dē-ak). Relating to both the stomach and the heart.

gas·tro·cele (gas′trō-sēl). Hernia of a portion of the stomach. [gastro- + G. *kēlē,* hernia]

gas·tro·chron·or·rhea (gas′trō-kron-ō-rē′ă). Excessive continuous gastric secretion. [gastro- + G. *chronos,* time (chronic), + *rhoia,* a flow]

gas·troc·ne·mi·us (gas-trok-nē′mē-ŭs). SYN gastrocnemius (*muscle*). [G. *gastroknēmia,* calf of the leg, fr. *gaster* (*gastr*-), belly, + *knēmē,* leg]

gas·tro·co·lic (gas′trō-kol′ik). Relating to the stomach and the colon.

gas·tro·co·li·tis (gas′trō-kō-lī′tis). Inflammation of both stomach and colon.

gas·tro·co·lop·to·sis (gas′trō-kō-lō-tō′sis). Displacement downward of stomach and colon. [gastro- + G. *kōlon,* colon, + *ptōsis,* a falling]

gas·tro·co·los·to·my (gas′trō-kō-los′tō-mē). Establishment of a communication between stomach and colon usually secondary to gastric ulcer disease or a malignant process in either the colon or stomach. [gastro- + G. *kōlon,* colon, + *stoma,* mouth]

gas·tro·cys·to·plas·ty (gas′trō-sis′tō-plas-tē). Augmentation of the bladder by a piece of vascularized stomach.

gas·tro·di·al·y·sis (gas′trō-dī-al′i-sis). Dialysis across the mucous membrane of the stomach.

Gas·tro·dis·coi·des hom·i·nis (gas′trō-dis-koy′dēz hom′i-nis). A species of trematode sometimes found in the intestinal canals of humans in India, Southeast Asia, and China; its normal host is the pig. SYN *Gastrodiscus hominis.* [gastro- + G. *diskos,* disk; L. *homo,* gen. *hominis,* man]

Gas·tro·dis·cus hom·i·nis (gas-trō-dis′kŭs). SYN *Gastrodiscoides hominis.*

gas·tro·du·o·de·nal (gas′trō-doo′ō-dē′năl, -du-od′ĕ-nal). Relating to the stomach and duodenum.

ga

gas·tro·du·o·de·ni·tis (gas'trō-doo-ō-dē-nī'tis). Inflammation of both stomach and duodenum.

gas·tro·du·o·de·nos·co·py (gas'trō-doo-ō-dě-nos'kŏ-pē). Visualization of the interior of the stomach and duodenum by a gastroscope. [gastro- + duodenum, + G. *skopeō,* to view]

gas·tro·du·o·de·nos·to·my (gas'trō-doo-ō-dě-nos'tō-mē). Establishment of a communication between the stomach and the duodenum. [gastro- + duodenum + G. *stoma,* mouth]

gas·tro·dyn·ia (gas-trō-din'ē-ă). SYN stomach *ache*. [gastro- + G. *odynē,* pain]

gas·tro·en·ter·ic (gas'trō-en-ter'ik). SYN gastrointestinal.

gas·tro·en·ter·i·tis (gas'trō-en-ter-ī'tis). Inflammation of the mucous membrane of both stomach and intestine. SYN enterogastritis. [gastro- + G. *enteron,* intestine, + *-itis,* inflammation]

acute infectious nonbacterial g., SYN epidemic nonbacterial g.

endemic nonbacterial infantile g., an endemic viral g. of young children (6 mos–12 yrs) that is especially widespread during winter, caused by strains of rotavirus (family Reoviridae); the incubation period is 2–4 days, with symptoms lasting 3–5 days, including abdominal pain, diarrhea, fever, and vomiting. SYN infantile g.

eosinophilic g., gastroenteritis with abdominal pain, malabsorption, often obstructive symptoms, associated with peripheral eosinophilia and areas of eosinophilic infiltration of the stomach, small intestine and/or colon with eosinophiles. May be an allergic etiology and responds to elimination diet in some patients; corticosteroid therapy is also effective. SYN eosinophilic gastritis.

epidemic nonbacterial g., an epidemic, highly communicable but rather mild disease of sudden onset, caused by the epidemic gastroenteritis virus (especially Norwalk agent), with an incubation period of 16–48 hours and a duration of 1–2 days, which affects all age groups; infection is associated with some fever, abdominal cramps, nausea, vomiting, diarrhea, and headache, one or another of which may be predominant. SYN acute infectious nonbacterial g.

infantile g., SYN endemic nonbacterial infantile g.

viral g., SEE endemic nonbacterial infantile g., epidemic nonbacterial g.

gas·tro·en·ter·o·a·nas·to·mo·sis (gas'trō-en-ter-ō-an-as-tō-mō'sis). SYN gastroenterostomy.

gas·tro·en·ter·o·co·li·tis (gas'trō-en'ter-ō-kō-lī'tis). Inflammatory disease involving the stomach and intestines. [gastro- + G. *enteron,* intestine, + *kōlon,* colon, + *-itis,* inflammation]

gas·tro·en·ter·o·co·los·to·my (gas'trō-en-ter-ō-kō-los'tō-mē). Formation of direct communication between the stomach and the large and small intestines, usually secondary to gastric ulcer disease or a malignant process in either the colon or stomach. [gastro- + G. *enteron,* intestine, + *kōlon,* colon + *stoma,* mouth]

gas·tro·en·ter·ol·o·gist (gas'trō-en-ter-ol'ō-jist). A specialist in gastroenterology.

gas·tro·en·ter·ol·o·gy (gas'trō-en-ter-ol'ō-jē). The medical specialty concerned with the function and disorders of the gastrointestinal tract, including stomach, intestines, and associated organs. [gastro- + G. *enteron,* intestine, + *logos,* study]

gas·tro·en·ter·op·a·thy (gas'trō-en-ter-op'ă-thē). Any disorder of the alimentary canal. [gastro- + G. *enteron,* intestine, + *pathos,* suffering]

gas·tro·en·ter·o·plas·ty (gas'trō-en-ter-ō-plas'tē). Operative repair of defects in the stomach and intestine. [gastro- + G. *enteron,* intestine, + *plassō,* to form]

gas·tro·en·ter·op·to·sis (gas'trō-en-ter-ō-tō'sis). Downward displacement of the stomach and a portion of the intestine. [gastro- + G. *enteron,* intestine, + *ptōsis,* a falling]

[]gas·tro·en·ter·os·to·my (gas'trō-en-ter-os'tō-mē). Establishment of a new opening between the stomach and the intestine, either anterior or posterior to the transverse colon. SYN gastroenteroanastomosis. [gastro- + G. *enteron,* intestine, + *stoma,* mouth]

gas·tro·en·ter·ot·o·my (gas'trō-en-ter-ot'ō-mē). Section into both stomach and intestine. [gastro- + G. *enteron,* intestine, + *tomē,* incision]

gas·tro·ep·i·plo·ic (gas'trō-ep'i-plō'ik). Relating to the stomach and the greater omentum (epiploon).

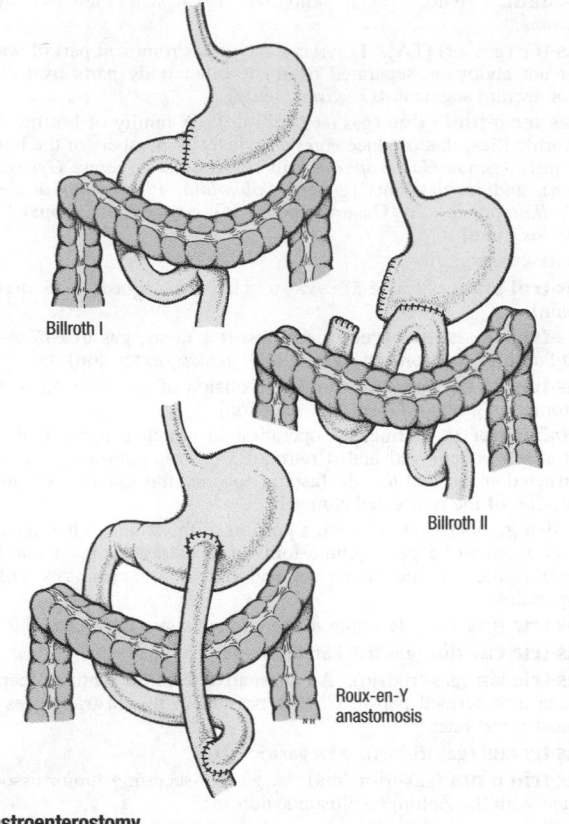

Billroth I

Billroth II

Roux-en-Y anastomosis

gastroenterostomy

gas·tro·e·soph·a·ge·al (gas'trō-ē-sof'ă-jē'ăl). Relating to both stomach and esophagus. [gastro- + G. *oisophagos,* gullet (esophagus)]

gas·tro·e·soph·a·gi·tis (gas'trō-ē-sof-ă-jī'tis). Inflammation of the stomach and esophagus.

gas·tro·e·soph·a·gos·to·my (gas'trō-ē-sof-ă-gos'tō-mē). SYN esophagogastrostomy. [gastro- + G. *oisophagos,* gullet (esophagus), + *stoma,* mouth]

gas·tro·gas·tros·to·my (gas'trō-gas-tros'tō-mē). Anastomosis between two parts of the stomach usually to bypass an area of narrowing. SYN gastroanastomosis.

gas·tro·ga·vage (gas-trō-gă-vahzh'). SYN gavage (1).

gas·tro·gen·ic (gas-trō-jen'ik). Deriving from or caused by the stomach.

gas·tro·graph (gas'trō-graf). An instrument for recording graphically the movements of the stomach. SYN gastrokinesograph. [gastro- + G. *graphē,* a writing]

gas·tro·he·pat·ic (gas'trō-he-pat'ik). Relating to the stomach and the liver. [gastro- + G. *hēpar* (*hēpat-*), liver]

gas·tro·hy·dror·rhea (gas'trō-hī-drō-rē'ă). Excretion into the stomach of a large amount of watery fluid containing neither hydrochloric acid, chymosin nor pepsin ferments. [gastro- + G. *hydōr,* water, + *rhoia,* a flow]

gas·tro·il·e·i·tis (gas'trō-il-ē-ī'tis). Inflammation of the alimentary canal in which the stomach and ileum are primarily involved.

gas·tro·il·e·os·to·my (gas'trō-il-ē-os'tō-mē). A surgical joining of stomach to ileum; most commonly used in the treatment of severe obesity.

gas·tro·in·tes·ti·nal (GI) (gas'trō-in-tes'tin-ăl). Relating to the stomach and intestines. SYN gastroenteric.

gas·tro·je·ju·no·co·lic (gas'trō-jē-joo'nō-kol'ik). Referring to the stomach, jejunum, and colon.

gas·tro·je·ju·nos·to·my (gas'trō-jē-joo-nos'tō-mē). Establishment of a direct communication between the stomach and the jejunum. SYN gastronesteostomy. [gastro- + jejunum G. *stoma*, mouth]

gas·tro·ki·ne·so·graph (gas'trō-ki-nē'sō-graf). SYN gastrograph. [gastro- + G. *kinēsis*, motion, + *graphē*, a writing]

gas·tro·la·vage (gas-trō-lă-vahzh'). Lavage of the stomach.

gas·tro·li·e·nal (gas-trō-lī'ē-năl). SYN gastrosplenic. [gastro- + L. *lien*, spleen]

gas·tro·lith (gas'trō-lith). A concretion in the stomach. SYN gastric calculus. [gastro- + G. *lithos*, stone]

gas·tro·li·thi·a·sis (gas'trō-li-thī'ă-sis). Presence of one or more calculi in the stomach. [gastro- + G. *lithos*, stone + *-iasis*, condition]

gas·trol·o·gist (gas-trol'ō-jist). A specialist in gastrology.

gas·trol·o·gy (gas-trol'ō-jē). The branch of medicine concerned with the stomach and its diseases. [gastro- + G. *logos*, study]

gas·trol·y·sis (gas-trol'i-sis). Division of perigastric adhesions. [gastro- + G. *lysis*, loosening]

gas·tro·ma·la·cia (gas'trō-mă-lā'shē-ă). Softening of the walls of the stomach. [gastro- + G. *malakia*, softness]

gas·tro·meg·a·ly (gas'trō-meg'ă-lē). 1. Enlargement of the stomach. 2. Enlargement of the abdomen. [gastro- + G. *megas* (*megal-*), large]

gas·trom·e·lus (gas-trom'ĕ-lŭs). A condition in which an individual has a supernumerary limb attached to the abdomen. SEE conjoined *twins*, under *twin*. [gastro- + G. *melos*, a limb]

gas·tro·myx·or·rhea (gas'trō-mik-sō-rē'ă). Excessive secretion of mucus in the stomach. SYN myxorrhea gastrica. [gastro- + G. *myxa*, mucus, + *rhoia*, a flow]

gas·tro·ne·ste·os·to·my (gas'trō-nes-tē-os'tō-mē). SYN gastrojejunostomy. [gastro- + G. *nēstis*, jejunum, + *stoma*, mouth]

gas·trop·a·gus (gas-trop'ă-gŭs). Conjoined twins united at the abdomen. SEE conjoined *twins*, under *twin*. [gastro- + -pagus]

gas·tro·pa·ral·y·sis (gas'trō-pă-ral'i-sis). Paralysis of the muscular coat of the stomach.

gas·tro·par·a·si·tus (gas'trō-par-ă-sī'tŭs). Unequal conjoined twins in which the incomplete parasite is attached to, or within, the abdomen of the autosite. SEE conjoined *twins*, under *twin*.

gas·tro·pa·re·sis (gas'trō-pă-rē'sis, -par'ĕ-sis). Weakness of gastric peristalsis, which results in delayed emptying of the bowels. [gastro- + G. *paresis*, a letting go, paralysis]

g. diabetico'rum, dilation of the stomach with gastric retention in diabetics, commonly seen in association with severe acidosis or coma.

gas·tro·path·ic (gas-trō-path'ik). Denoting gastropathy.

gas·trop·a·thy (gas-trop'ă-thē). Any disease of the stomach. [gastro- + G. *pathos*, disease]

hypertrophic hypersecretory g., nodular thickenings of gastric mucosa with acid hypersecretion and frequently peptic ulceration, not associated with a gastrin-secreting tumor.

gas·tro·pex·y (gas'trō-pek-sē). Attachment of the stomach to the abdominal wall or diaphragm. [gastro- + G. *pēxis*, fixation]

Gas·tro·phil·i·dae (gas-trō-fil'i-dē). SYN Gasterophilidae.

gas·tro·phren·ic (gas'trō-fren'ik). Relating to the stomach and the diaphragm. [gastro- + G. *phrēn*, diaphragm]

gas·tro·plas·ty (gas'trō-plas-tē). 1. Operative treatment of a defect in the stomach or the production of a gastric tube at the lower esophagus that uses the stomach wall for the reconstruction. 2. The producing of a staple line across the upper portion of the stomach to limit intake, used in severe obesity. [gastro- + G. *plastos*, formed]

Collis g., a technique for lengthening a "short" esophagus; a full-thickness incision of the gastric cardia is made parallel to the lesser curvature, usually with a staple line to lengthen the esophagus by making a tube of the upper part of the stomach.

vertical banded g., a g. for treatment of morbid obesity in which an upper gastric pouch is formed by a vertical staple line, with a band applied at the outlet into the main pouch to prevent dilation.

gas·tro·pli·ca·tion (gas'trō-pli-kā'shŭn). An operation for reducing the size of the stomach by suturing a longitudinal fold with

the peritoneal surfaces in apposition. SYN gastroptyxis, gastrorrhaphy (2), stomach reefing. [gastro- + L. *plico*, to fold]

gas·tro·pneu·mon·ic (gas'trō-noo-mon'ik). SYN pneumogastric. [gastro- + G. *pneumōn*, lung]

gas·tro·pod (gas'trō-pod). Common name for members of the class Gastropoda.

Gas·trop·o·da (gas-trop'ŏ-dă). A class of the phylum Mollusca that includes the snails, whelks, slugs, and limpets. [gastro- + G. *pous* (*pod-*), foot]

gas·trop·to·sis, gas·trop·to·sia (gas-trō-tō'sis, -tō'sē-ă). Downward displacement of the stomach. SYN bathygastry, descensus ventriculi, ventroptosis, ventroptosia. [gastro- + G. *ptosis*, a falling]

gas·tro·ptyx·is (gas-trō-tik'sis). SYN gastroplication. [gastro- + G. *ptyxis*, a fold]

gas·tro·pul·mo·nary (gas-trō-pŭl'mo-nar-ē). SYN pneumogastric.

gas·tro·py·lor·ic (gas'trō-pī-lōr'ik). Relating to the stomach as a whole and to the pylorus.

gas·tror·rha·gia (gas-trō-rā'jē-ă). Hemorrhage from the stomach. SYN gastric hemorrhage. [gastro- + G. *rhēgnymi*, to burst forth]

gas·tror·rha·phy (gas-trōr'ă-fē). 1. Suture of a perforation of the stomach. 2. SYN gastroplication. [gastro- + G. *rhaphē*, a stitching]

gas·tror·rhea (gas-trō-rē'ă). Excessive secretion of gastric juice or of mucus (gastromyxorrhea) by the stomach. [gastro- + G. *rhoia*, a flow]

gas·tror·rhex·is (gas'trō-rek'sis). A tear or bursting of the stomach. [gastro- + G. *rhēxis*, a bursting]

gas·tros·chi·sis (gas-tros'ki-sis). A congenital fissure in the abdominal wall not involving the umbilical cord; usually accompanied by protrusion of viscera. [gastro- + G. *schisis*, a fissure]

gas·tro·scope (gas'trō-skōp). An endoscope for inspecting the interior of the stomach. [gastro- + G. *skopeō*, to examine]

fiberoptic g., instrument using fiberoptics for inspection of the interior of the stomach.

gas·tro·scop·ic (gas-trō-skop'ik). Relating to gastroscopy.

▣ **gas·tros·co·py** (gas-tros'kŏ-pē). Inspection of the interior of the stomach through an endoscope.

gas·tro·spasm (gas'trō-spazm). Spasmodic contraction of the walls of the stomach.

gas·tro·splen·ic (gas-trō-splen'ik). Relating to the stomach and the spleen. SYN gastrolienal.

gas·tro·stax·is (gas'trō-stak'sis). Rarely used term for oozing of blood from the mucous membrane of the stomach. [gastro- + G. *staxis*, trickling]

gas·tro·ste·no·sis (gas-trō-ste-nō'sis). Diminution in size of the cavity of the stomach. [gastro- + G. *stenōsis*, narrowing]

gas·tros·to·ga·vage (gas-tros'tō-gă-vahzh'). SYN gavage (1).

gas·tros·to·la·vage (gas-tros'tō-lă-vahzh'). Lavage of the stomach through a gastric fistula.

gas·tros·to·my (gas-tros'tō-mē). Establishment of a new opening into the stomach. [gastro- + G. *stoma*, mouth]

percutaneous endoscopic g., a g. performed without opening the abdominal cavity; usually involves gastroscopy, insufflation of the stomach, puncture of stomach and abdominal wall, followed by placement of a special tube.

gas·tro·tho·ra·cop·a·gus (gas'trō-thōr-ă-kop'ă-gŭs). Conjoined twins united at thorax and abdomen. SEE conjoined *twins*, under *twin*. [gastro- + G. *thōrax*, chest, + *pagos*, something fixed]

gas·tro·tome (gas'trō-tōm). A knife for incising the stomach.

gas·trot·o·my (gas-trot'ō-mē). Incision into the stomach. [gastro- + G. *tomē*, incision]

gas·tro·to·nom·e·ter (gas'trō-tō-nom'ĕ-ter). An apparatus used in gastrotonometry.

gas·tro·to·nom·e·try (gas'trō-tō-nom'ĕ-trē). The measurement of intragastric pressure. [gastro- + G. *tonos*, tension, + *metron*, measure]

gas·tro·tox·ic (gas-trō-tok'sik). Poisonous to the stomach.

ga

gas·tro·tox·in (gas-trō-tok′sin). A cytotoxin specific for the cells of the mucous membrane of the stomach.

gas·tro·tro·pic (gas-trō-trop′ik). Affecting the stomach. [gastro- + G. *tropikos,* turning]

gas·trox·ia (gas-trok′sē-ă). Rarely used term for gastroxynsis. [gastro- + G. *oxys,* keen, acid]

gas·trox·yn·sis (gas-trok-sin′sis). Rarely used term for intermittent excessive secretion of the gastric juice. [gastro- + G. *oxynō,* to make sharp, acid]

gas·tru·la (gas′troo-lă). The embryo in the stage of development following the blastula; in lower forms with minimal yolk, it is a simple double-layered structure consisting of ectoderm and endoderm enclosing the archenteron, which opens to the outside by way of the blastopore; in forms with considerable yolk, the configuration of the g. is greatly modified owing to the persistence of the yolk throughout the gastrulation process. SYN invaginate planula. [Mod. L. dim. of G. *gastēr,* belly]

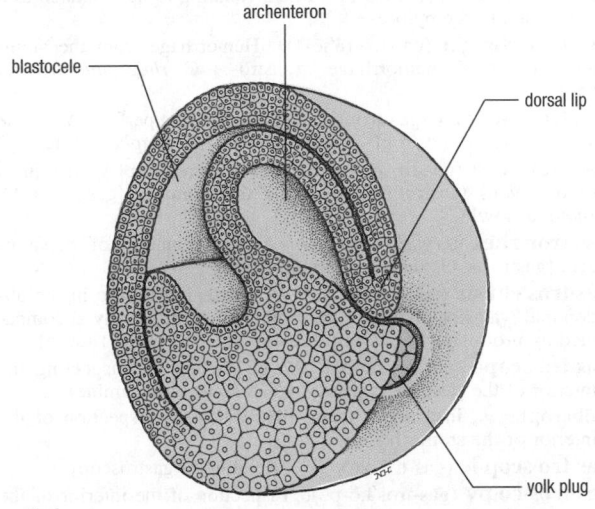

gastrula

gas·tru·la·tion (gas-troo-lā′shŭn). Transformation of the blastula into the gastrula; the development and invagination of the embryonic germ layers.

Gatch, Willis D., U.S. surgeon, 1878–1961. SEE G. *bed.*

gate (gāt). **1.** To close an ion channel by electrical (e.g., membrane potential) or chemical (e.g., neurotransmitter) action. **2.** Action of a special nerve fiber to block the transmission of impulses through a synapse, e.g., gating of pain impulses at synapses in the dorsal horns. **3.** A device which can be switched electronically to control the passage of a signal. **4.** To use a physiological signal, such as an ECG, to trigger an event such as an x-ray exposure or to partition continuously collected data. SEE gated radionuclide *angiocardiography.* SEE ALSO cardiac *gating.* [O.E. *geat*]

gate·keep·er (gāt′kēp-er). A health professional, typically a physician or nurse, who has the first encounter with a patient and who thus controls the patient's entry into the health care system.

gat·ing (gāt′ing). **1.** In a biologic membrane, the opening and closing of a channel, believed to be associated with changes in integral membrane proteins. **2.** A process in which electrical signals are selected by a gate, which passes such signals only when the gate pulse is present to act as a control signal, or passes only the signals that have certain characteristics. SEE gate.

cardiac gating, using an electronic signal from the cardiac cycle to trigger an event, such as in imaging separate phases of cardiac contraction.

respiratory gating, any technique that derives a signal from breathing to trigger an electronic circuit, such as for data collection during expiration. SEE ALSO navigator *echo.*

Gaucher, Philippe C.E., French physician, 1854–1918. SEE G. *cells,* under *cell, disease;* pseudo-G. *cell.*

Gauer, Otto Hans, German physiologist, 1909–1979. SEE Henry-G. *response.*

gauge (gāj). A measuring device. SYN gage.

bite g., SYN gnathodynamometer.

Boley g., a caliper-type g. graduated in millimeters used to measure the thickness of various dental materials.

catheter g., a metal plate with holes of graduated diameter used to determine the size of a catheter.

strain g., a device, employing the Wheatstone bridge principle, used for accurate measurement of forces such as strain, stress, or pressure.

undercut g., a device, used with a surveyor, to precisely locate areas for the placement of the retentive components of clasps when designing removable partial dentures.

gaul·the·ria oil (gawl-thēr′ē-ă). SYN methyl salicylate.

gaul·the·rin (gawl′thĕ-rin). A glycoside from the bark of several species of *Betula* (birch); it yields methyl salicylate, D-glucose, and D-xylose on hydrolysis.

gaunt·let (gawnt′let). A glove. SEE bandage.

Gauss, Johann K.F., German physicist, 1777–1855. SEE gauss, gaussian *curve,* gaussian *distribution.*

Gauss, Karl J., German gynecologist, 1875–1957. SEE G *sign.*

gauss (G) (gows). A unit of magnetic field intensity, equal to 10^{-4} T. [J.K.F. *Gauss*]

Gaussel, Amans, French physician, 1871–1937. SEE Grasset-G. *phenomenon.*

gaus·si·an (gows′ē-ăn). Relating to or described by Johann K.F. Gauss. SEE gaussian *curve.*

gauze (gawz). A bleached cotton cloth of plain weave, used for dressings, bandages, and absorbent sponges; petrolatum g. is saturated with petrolatum. [Fr. *gaze,* fr. Ar. *gazz,* raw silk]

ga·vage (gă-vahzh′). **1.** Forced feeding by stomach tube. SYN gastrogavage, gastrostogavage. **2.** Therapeutic use of a high-potency diet administered by stomach tube. [Fr. *gaver,* to gorge fowls]

Gavard, Hyacinthe, French anatomist, 1753–1802. SEE G. *muscle.*

Gay, Alexander H., Russian anatomist, 1842–1907. SEE G. *glands,* under *gland.*

gay (gā). **1.** A homosexual, especially male. **2.** Denoting a homosexual individual or the male homosexual lifestyle. SEE lesbian.

Gay-Lussac, Joseph L., French naturalist, 1778–1850. SEE Gay-Lussac *equation;* Gay-Lussac *law.*

gaze (gāz). The act of looking steadily at an object.

conjugate g., movement of both eyes with the visual axes parallel.

dysconjugate g., failure of the eyes to turn together in the same direction.

G-band·ing. SEE G-banding *stain.*

GBG Abbreviation for gonadal steroid-binding *globulin.*

GBH Abbreviation for gamma benzene hexachloride.

GC Abbreviation for the guanine and cytosine base pair in polynucleic acids.

G-CSF Abbreviation for granulocyte colony-stimulating *factor.*

Gd Symbol for gadolinium.

GDP Abbreviation for guanosine 5′-diphosphate.

GDPman·nose phos·pho·ryl·ase. SYN mannose-1-phosphate guanylyltransferase (GDP).

Ge Symbol for germanium.

Ge·doel·stia (ge-del′stē-ă). A genus of nasal botflies (family Oestridae) that includes the species *G. cristata* and *G. haessleri* which parasitize wildebeest, hartebeeste, and other African antelopes, and may also cause an ophthalmomyiasis in sheep and humans.

ge·doel·sti·o·sis (ge-del-sti-ō′sis). Infection of herbivores and, rarely, humans with larvae of flies of the genus *Gedoelstia,* causing ophthalmomyiasis in humans. SYN bulging eye disease.

Gehrig, Henry Louis, U.S. baseball player; 1903–1941, victim of Lou Gehrig *disease*. SEE Lou Gehrig *disease*.

Geigel, Richard, German physician, 1859–1930. SEE G. *reflex*.

Geiger, Hans, German physicist, 1882–1945. SEE G.-Müller *counter*, *tube*.

gel (jel). **1.** A jelly, or the solid or semisolid phase of a colloidal solution. SYN gelatum. **2.** To form a g. or jelly; to convert a sol into a g. [Mod. L. *gelatum*]

colloidal g., a colloid that has developed resistance to flow because of chemical or thermal change.

pharmacopeial g., a suspension, in a water medium, of an insoluble drug in hydrated form wherein the particle size approaches or attains colloidal dimensions.

gel·ate (jel′āt). SYN gelatinize.

gel·a·tin (jel′ă-tin). A derived protein formed from the collagen of tissues by boiling in water; it swells up when put in cold water, but dissolves only in hot water; used as a hemostat, plasma substitute, and protein food adjunct in malnutrition. [L. *gelo*, pp. *gelatus*, to freeze, congeal]

glycerinated g., a preparation made of equal parts of g. and glycerin; a firm mass liquefying at gentle heat; it is used as a vehicle for suppositories and urethral bougies. SYN glycerin jelly, glycerogelatin, glycogelatin.

Irish moss g., g. extracted from Irish moss; used to make the mucilage of Irish moss that is used as a substitute for gum arabic in making emulsions.

vegetable g., a substance similar to g., obtained from gluten.

zinc g., SYN *zinc* gelatin.

gel·a·tin·ase (jel′ă-tin-ās). Pepsin B; a metalloproteinase that hydrolyzes gelatin and a number of types of collagen. SEE pepsin.

ge·la·ti·nif·er·ous (jel′ă-ti-nif′er-ŭs). Producing or containing gelatin or having a gel-like quality. [gelatin + L. *fero*, to bear]

ge·lat·i·ni·za·tion (jĕ-lat′i-ni-zā′shŭn). Conversion into gelatin or a substance resembling it.

ge·lat·i·nize (jĕ-lat′i-nīz). **1.** To convert into gelatin. **2.** To become gelatinous. SYN gelate.

ge·lat·i·noid (jĕ-lat′i-noyd). SYN gelatinous (2).

ge·lat·i·nous (jĕ-lat′i-nŭs). **1.** Pertaining to or characteristic of gelatin. **2.** Jellylike or resembling gelatin. SYN gelatinoid.

ge·la·tion (jĕ-lā′shŭn). **1.** In colloidal chemistry, the transformation of a sol into a gel. **2.** The solidification of a liquid by cold temperatures.

ge·la·tum (jĕ-lā′tŭm). SYN gel (1). [Mod. L.]

Gélineau, Jean Baptiste Edouard, French physician, 1859–1906. SEE G. *syndrome*.

Gell, Philip G.H., British immunologist. SEE G. and Coombs *reactions*, under *reaction*.

Gellé, Marie-Ernst, French otologist, 1834–1923. SEE G. *test*.

Gellerstedt, Nils, *1896. SEE Ceelen-G. *syndrome*.

ge·lo·sis (jĕ-lō′sis). An extremely firm mass in tissue (especially in a muscle), with a consistency resembling that of frozen tissue. [L. *gelo*, to freeze, congeal, + G. *-osis*, condition]

gel·se·mine (jel′sĕ-mēn). A crystallizable alkaloid derived from gelsemium (yellow jasmine); a mydriatic and central nervous system stimulant. [Mod. L. *gelsemium*, fr. Pers. *yāsmin*, jasmine]

gel·so·lin (jel-sol′in). An actin-binding protein; a Ca^{2+}-triggered actin-filament-severing protein; hence, it has roles in locomotion, secretion, and endocytosis.

Gély, Jules A., French surgeon, 1806–1861. SEE G. *suture*.

△**gem-.** Prefix denoting twin substitutions on a single atom; e.g., the *gem*-dimethyl substitution on carbon-4 of lanosterol. [L. *geminus*, twin]

Ge·mel·la (jĕ-mel′ă). A genus of motile, aerobic, facultatively anaerobic, coccoid bacteria (family Streptococcaceae) that occur singly or in pairs, with flattened adjacent sides. They are Gram-indeterminate but have a cell wall like that of Gram-positive bacteria, and are parasitic on mammals. The type species is *G. haemolysans*, which is found in bronchial secretions and in mucus from the respiratory tract. [L. dim. of *geminus*, twin]

G. morbillorum, a microaerophilic bacterium, formerly called *Streptococcus morbillorum*, that fails to produce β-hemolysis of blood agar and lacks distinguishing serogroup antigens; causes serious infections in some patients similar to those seen with viridans streptococci.

ge·mel·lol·o·gy (jem-el-ol′ō-jē). The study of twins and the phenomenology of twinning. [L. *gemellus*, twin-born, + G. *logos*, study]

ge·mel·lus (jĕ-mel′ŭs). SYN inferior gemellus (*muscle*), superior gemellus (*muscle*). [L. dim. of *geminus*, twin]

gem·fi·bro·zil (jem-fī′brō-zil). An antihyperlipidemic agent.

gem·i·nate (jem′i-nāt). Occurring in pairs. SYN geminous. [L. *gemino*, pp. *-atus*, to double, fr. *geminus*, twin]

gem·i·na·tion (jem-i-nā′shŭn). Embryologic partial division of a primordium. For example, g. of a single tooth germ results in two partially or completely separated crowns on a single root. [L. *geminatio*, a doubling]

gem·i·nous (jem′i-nŭs). SYN geminate.

ge·mis·to·cyte (jĕ-mis′tō-sīt). SYN gemistocytic *astrocyte*. [G. *gemistos*, loaded, fr. *gemizō*, to fill, + -cyte]

ge·mis·to·cy·to·ma (jĕ-mis′tō-sī-tō′mă). SYN gemistocytic *astrocytoma*.

gem·ma (jem′ă). Any budlike or bulblike body, especially a taste bud or end bulb. [L. bud]

gem·ma·tion (jem-ā′shŭn). A form of fission in which the parent cell does not divide, but puts out a small budlike process (daughter cell) with its proportionate amount of chromatin; the daughter cell then separates to begin independent existence. SYN bud fission, budding. [L. *gemma*, a bud]

gem·mule (jem′ūl). **1.** A small bud that projects from the parent cell, and finally becomes detached, forming a cell of a new generation. **2.** SYN dendritic *spines*, under *spine*. [L. *gemmula*, dim. of *gemma*, bud]

Hoboken g.'s, SYN Hoboken *nodules*, under *nodule*.

△**gen-.** Being born, producing, coming to be. [G. *genos*, birth]

△**-gen.** Suffix denoting "precursor of." SEE ALSO pro- (2).

ge·na (jē′nă). SYN cheek. [L.]

ge·nal (jē′năl). Relating to the gena, or cheek.

gen·der (jen′der). Category to which an individual is assigned by self or others, on the basis of sex. Cf. sex, gender *role*.

gene (jēn). A functional unit of heredity that occupies a specific place (locus) on a chromosome, is capable of reproducing itself exactly at each cell division and directs the formation of an enzyme or other protein. The g. as a functional unit consists of a discrete segment of a giant DNA molecule containing the purine (adenine and guanine) and pyrimidine (cytosine and thymine) bases in the correct sequence to code the sequence of amino acids of a specific peptide. Protein synthesis is mediated by molecules of messenger-RNA formed on the chromosome with the g. acting as a template. The RNA then passes into the cytoplasm and becomes oriented on the ribosomes where it in turn acts as a template to organize a chain of amino acids to form a peptide. In organisms reproducing sexually, normally occur in pairs in all cells except gametes, as a consequence of the fact that all chromosomes are paired except the sex chromosomes (X and Y) of the male. SYN factor (3). [G. *genos*, birth]

allelic g., SEE allele, *dominance* of traits.

autosomal g., a g. located on any chromosome other than the sex chromosomes (X or Y).

BRCA1 g., a tumor suppressor g. on chromosome 17 at locus 17q21, isolated in 1994; encodes p53 protein, which prevents cells with damaged DNA from dividing; carriers of germline mutations in BRCA1 are predisposed to develop both breast and ovarian cancer. SEE ALSO BRCA2 g., *carcinoma* of the breast.

BRCA2 g., a tumor suppressor g. identified in 1995 on chromosome 13 at locus 13q12–q13; a large g. consisting of 27 exons distributed over 70kb, encoding a protein of 3418 amino acids; carriers of germline mutations in BRCA2 have an increased risk, similar to that of those with BRCA1 mutations, of developing breast cancer and a moderately increased risk of ovarian cancer; BRCA2 families also exhibit an increased incidence of male

ge

breast, pancreatic, prostate, laryngeal, and ocular cancers. SEE ALSO BRCA1 g., *carcinoma* of the breast.

Familial clustering of breast cancer has long been recognized. Familial breast cancers are characterized by onset before age 45 and by clustering in 3 or more close relatives and in members of more than 1 generation. About 5% of all breast cancers are due to the inheritance of dominant susceptibility genes, particularly BRCA1 and BRCA2. Whereas spontaneous mutations of the BRCA genes are uncommon, hundreds of inherited mutations have been discovered on each gene. The clinical significance of many of these is unknown. Since these are autosomal chromosomes, men as well as women can inherit and pass on the BRCA mutations. The histology of breast cancer in women with BRCA1 and BRCA2 mutations differs from that of sporadic cases. The proportion of medullary carcinomas is higher among BRCA1-associated breast cancers than among all breast cancers. BRCA1 and BRCA2 are tumor suppressor genes, inhibiting tumor development when functioning normally. Both are large genes encoding large negatively charged proteins. Inactivating mutations identified to date are distributed throughout both genes, with a predominance of 2 distinct mutations for BRCA1 and 1 for BRCA2. Despite the high penetrance of the mutant gene, not all carriers develop cancer. Hormonal, environmental, reproductive, and other genetic factors may influence penetrance. Estradiol increases cell proliferation and production of the BRCA1 gene product in vitro, while the estrogen antagonist tamoxifen inhibits both cell proliferation and BRCA1 gene expression. Observed mutations are distributed throughout the gene; most are insertions, deletions, or nonsense mutations. Two common changes (185delAG and 5382insC, in exons 2 and 20, respectively) account for approximately 19% of BRCA1 mutations. The former of these is present in about 1% of Ashkenazic Jews and is responsible for about 32% of familial breast cancer in Jews. It is also found in 13% of ovarian cancer patients with no family history of breast or ovarian cancer, and in 30% of those with family histories suggesting inherited disease. BRCA1 mutations cause a 3-fold increase in the risk of prostate cancer in males and a 4-fold increase in the risk of colon cancer in persons of both sexes. The BRCA2 6174delT mutation is estimated to be present in 1.3% of Ashkenazic Jews. Earlier estimates of the risk that a women with a BRCA1 or BRCA2 gene mutation would develop breast cancer at some time in her life ranged from 10–90%. These figures were based on intensive study of families known to be at risk. Current estimates are that the risk of breast cancer may be no higher than 30%. In addition, 15–20% percent of women with the BRCA1 mutation will develop ovarian cancer. Although testing for BRCA genetic mutations is commercially available, most authorities do not recommend routine screening except in women with a strong family history of cancer. Women found to have BRCA genetic mutations have been advised to begin breast self-examination at age 18 and regular annual physician examinations and mammograms at age 25. The benefit of radiologic screening must be weighed against the possible effect of radiation on the BRCA1 or BRCA2 allele. In addition, mammograms are often difficult to interpret in young women because of the density of breast tissue. BRCA2 carriers are also advised to begin ovarian cancer surveillance, consisting of annual or semiannual screening using transvaginal ultrasound (TVS) with color flow Doppler and morphology index, and determination of serum CA-125 levels, at age 25–35. Support for prophylactic mastectomy and oophorectomy is waning as it becomes evident that these drastic procedures cannot altogether abolish cancer risk. Tamoxifen has been shown to reduce the risk of breast cancer in genetically predisposed women by as much as 45%.

C g., the g. coding for the constant regions of immunoglobulin chains.

codominant g., a set of two or more alleles, each expressed phenotypically in the presence of the other.

control g., SEE operator g., regulator g.

dominant g., SEE *dominance* of traits.

extrachromosomal g., a g. located outside of the nucleus (e.g., mitochondrial genes).

H g., SYN histocompatibility g.

histocompatibility g., in laboratory animals, a g. which can elicit an immune response and thereby cause rejection of a homograft when tissue is transplanted from one individual to another; in humans, histocompatibility g.'s control HLA antigens. SYN H g.

holandric g., SYN Y-linked g.

homeotic g.'s, a group of g.'s that regulate the development of the body parts by defining the boundaries of the several regions.

housekeeping g.'s, g.'s that are generally always expressed and thought to be involved in routine cellular metabolism.

immune response g.'s, g.'s in the HLA-D region of the histocompatibility complex of human chromosome 6 which control the immune response to specific antigens.

jumping g., a g. associated with transposable elements. SEE transposon.

lethal g., a g. that produces a genotype that leads to death of the organism before reproduction is possible or that precludes reproduction; for a recessive g. the homozygous or hemizygous state is lethal.

microophthalmia transcription factor g., g. that when mutated causes Waardenburg syndrome type 2 and Tietz syndrome in at least some subsets of families with these autosomal dominant inherited syndromes.

mimic g.'s, nonallelic (independent) g.'s with closely similar effects, e.g., elliptocytosis.

mitochondrial g., a functioning g. located not in the nucleus of a cell but in the mitochondrial chromosome.

modifier g., a nonallelic g. that controls or changes the manifestation of a g. by interfering with its transcription.

mutant g., a g. that has been changed from an ancestral type, not necessarily in the current generation. SEE ALSO mutant, mutation.

operator g., a g. with the function of activating the production of messenger RNA by one or more adjacent structural loci; part of the feedback system for determining the rate of production of an enzyme.

pleiotropic g., a g. that has multiple, apparently unrelated, phenotypic manifestations. SYN polyphenic g.

polyphenic g., SYN pleiotropic g.

regulator g., a g. that produces a repressor substance that inhibits an operator g. when combined with it. It thus prevents production of a specific enzyme. When the enzyme is again in demand, a specific regulatory metabolite inhibits the repressor substance.

repressor g., a g. that prevents a nonallele from being transcribed.

SOS g.'s, a group of g.'s involved in DNA repair, often induced by damage severe enough to cause stoppage of DNA synthesis.

g. splicing, SYN splicing (1).

split g.'s, g.'s where the genomic sequences are interrupted by intervening sequences (introns) that are spliced out of the mRNA prior to translation.

structural g., a g. that codes for a specific protein or peptide.

transfer g.'s, g.'s carried by a conjugative plasmid, essential for fertility and establishment of the bacterial donor state.

transforming g., SYN oncogene.

tumor suppressor g., a gene that encodes a protein involved in controlling cellular growth; inactivation of this type of gene leads to deregulated cellular proliferation, as in cancer. SEE ALSO oncogene. SYN antioncogene.

In a person born with 2 normal copies of a tumor suppressor gene, both copies must be inactivated by spontaneous point mutation, deletion, or failure of expression before tumor formation occurs. An inherited mutation in a tumor suppressor gene is the basis of most familial predispositions to cancer. In a person so predisposed, malignant cellular proliferation does not occur until the remaining intact copy of the gene is inactivated by deletion of part or all of its chromosome. Of many tumor suppressor genes thus far identified, the p53 gene on chromosome 17, which encodes a phosphoprotein that suppresses cell proliferation, appears to be the most important. Mutations of p53 have been found in the DNA of more than half of all human cancers studied. Li-Fraumeni syndrome, characterized by early-onset carcinomas and sarcomas, is an inherited (autosomal dominant) mutation in the p53 tumor suppressor gene. BRCA1 and BRCA2, involved in familial early-onset breast cancer and ovarian cancer, are tumor suppressor genes.

V g., the g. coding for the major part of the variable region of an immunoglobulin chain.

X-linked g., a g. located on an X chromosome.

Y-linked g., a g. located on a Y chromosome. SYN holandric g.

Z g., the structural g. for β-galactosidase.

ge·ne·al·o·gy (jē-nē-awl′ō-jē). **1.** Heredity. **2.** The explicit assembly of the descent of a person or family; it may be of any length. [G. *genea*, descent, + *logos*, study]

gene li·brary. A haphazard assembly of cloned DNA fragments inside of a vector which may contain genetic information about a species.

gen·era (jen′er-ă). Plural of genus.

gen·er·al·ist (jen′er-ăl-ist). A general physician or family physician; a physician trained to take care of the majority of diseases not requiring surgery, sometimes including obstetrics.

gen·er·al·i·za·tion (jen′er-ăl-i-zā′shŭn). **1.** Rendering or becoming general, diffuse, or widespread, as when a primarily local disease becomes systemic. **2.** The reasoning by which a basic conclusion is reached, which applies to different items, each having some common factor.

  stimulus g., in Pavlovian conditioning, the eliciting of a conditioned response by stimuli never before experienced but which are similar to a particular conditioned stimulus. SEE conditioning, classical *conditioning*.

gen·er·al·ized (jen′er-ă-līzd). Involving the whole of an organ, as opposed to a focal or regional process.

gen·er·ate (jen′er-āt). **1.** To produce. **2.** To procreate. [L. *genero*, pp. *-atus*, to beget]

gen·er·a·tion (jen-er-ā′shŭn). **1.** SYN reproduction (1). **2.** A discrete stage in succession of descent; e.g., father, son, and grandson are three g.'s. [L. *generatio*, fr. *genero*, pp. *-atus*, to beget]

  asexual g., reproduction by fission, gemmation, or in any other way without union of the male and female cell, or conjugation. SEE ALSO parthenogenesis. SYN heterogenesis (2), nonsexual g.

  filial g. (F), the offspring of a genetically specified mating: first filial g. (symbol F₁), the offspring of parents of contrasting genotypes; second filial g. (F₂), the offspring of two F₁ individuals; third filial g. (F₃), fourth filial g. (F₄), etc., the offspring in succeeding g.'s of continued inbreeding of F₁ descendents.

  nonsexual g., SYN asexual g.

  parental g. (P₁), the parents of a mating, commonly experimental, involving contrasting genotypes; the original mating of a genetic experiment; parents of the F₁ g.

  sexual g., reproduction by conjugation, or the union of male and female cells, as opposed to asexual g.

  skipped g., a phenomenon of pedigrees in which a gene is transmitted from one affected person to another through a phenotypically unaffected person, as by recessivity (especially for X-linked traits), epistasis, variable expressivity, or absence of an environmental challenge such as a toxin. Except at a crass phenotypic level (e.g., clinical or commercial) this term becomes progressively less useful as the mechanisms are elucidated.

  spontaneous g., the false concept according to which living matter can arise by the vitalization of nonliving matter. SEE ALSO biogenesis. SYN heterogenesis (3).

  virgin g., SYN parthenogenesis.

gen·er·a·tion·al. Pertaining to generations, i.e., the discrete staging in genealogic descent.

gen·er·a·tive (jen′er-ă-tiv). Pertaining to the process of generating.

gen·er·a·tor (jen′er-ā-ter). An apparatus for conversion of chemical, mechanical, atomic, or other forms of energy into electricity. [*generator*, a begetter, producer]

  aerosol g., a device for producing airborne suspensions of small particles for inhalation therapy or experimental work; e.g., a La Mer g., spinning disk, or vibrating reed, each of which produces a monodisperse aerosol.

  asynchronous pulse g., a g. in which the rate of discharge is independent of the natural activity of the heart. SYN fixed rate pulse g.

  atrial synchronous pulse g., a ventricular stimulating pulse whose rate of discharge is directly determined by the atrial rate. SYN atrial triggered pulse g.

  atrial triggered pulse g., SYN atrial synchronous pulse g.

  demand pulse g., SYN ventricular inhibited pulse g.

  fixed rate pulse g., SYN asynchronous pulse g.

  pulse g., a device that produces an electrical discharge with a regular or rhythmic waveform in which the electromotive force varies in a specific pattern in relation to time; e.g., in an electronic pacemaker, it produces an electric discharge at regular intervals, and these intervals may be modified by a sensory circuit that can reset the time-base for subsequent discharge on the basis of other electrical activity, such as that produced by spontaneous cardiac beating.

  radionuclide g., a column containing a large amount of a particular radionuclide (mother radionuclide) that decays down to a second radionuclide of shorter physical half-life; the daughter radionuclide is separated from the parent by the process of elution and affords a continuing supply of relatively short-lived radionuclides for laboratory use; the elution is loosely termed "milking" with the generator referred to as a "radioactive cow."

  standby pulse g., SYN ventricular inhibited pulse g.

  ventricular inhibited pulse g., a g. which suppresses its output in response to natural ventricular activity but which, in the absence of such activity, functions as an asynchronous pulse g. SYN demand pulse g., standby pulse g.

  ventricular synchronous pulse g., a pulse which delivers its output synchronously with naturally occurring ventricular activity but which, in the absence of such activity, functions as an asynchronous pulse g. SYN ventricular triggered pulse g.

  ventricular triggered pulse g., SYN ventricular synchronous pulse g.

  x-ray g., the electronic device that controls production of x-rays in radiography; a key function is rectification of line voltage to produce a smooth direct current voltage to the x-ray tube.

ge·ner·ic (jĕ-nār′ik). **1.** Relating to or denoting a genus. **2.** General. **3.** Characteristic or distinctive. [L. *genus* (*gener-*), birth]

ge·ner·ic name. **1.** In chemistry, a noun that indicates the class or type of a single compound; e.g., salt, saccharide (sugar), hexose, alcohol, aldehyde, lactone, acid, amine, alkane, steroid, vitamin. "Class" is more appropriate and more often used than is "generic." **2.** In the pharmaceutical and commercial fields, a misnomer for nonproprietary name. **3.** In the biologic sciences, the first part of the scientific name (Latin binary combination or binomial) of an organism; written with an initial capital letter and in italics. In bacteriology, the species name consists of two parts (comprising one name): the g. n. and the specific epithet; in other biologic disciplines, the species name is regarded as being composed of two names: the g. n. and the specific name.

ge·ne·si·al (je-nē′sē-ăl). Relating to generation.

ge·ne·si·ol·o·gy (je-nē-sē-ol′ō-jē). The branch of science concerned with generation or reproduction. [G. *genesis*, generation, + *logos*, study]

gen·e·sis (jen′ĕ-sis). An origin or beginning process; also used as combining form in suffix position. [G.]

ge·net·ic (jĕ-net′ik). Pertaining to genetics; genetical.

ge

ge·net·i·cist (jĕ-net′i-sist). A specialist in genetics.

ge·net·ics (jĕ-net′iks). **1.** The branch of science concerned with the means and consequences of transmission and generation of the components of biologic inheritance. **2.** The genetic features and constitution of any single organism or set of organisms. [G. *genesis,* origin or production]

behavioral g., the study of heritable factors in behavioral patterns, as by pedigree analysis, biochemical abnormality, or karyotypic analysis.

biochemical g., the study of g. in terms of the chemical (biochemical) events involved, as in the manner in which DNA molecules replicate and control the synthesis of specific enzymes by the genetic code.

classical g., that body of method and analysis that perceives g. as the study of the transmission of genotype from parent to offspring; the study of multiple individuals is essential to it.

clinical g., g. applied to the diagnosis, prognosis, management, and prevention of genetic diseases. Cf. medical g.

epidemiologic g., the study of g. as a phenomenon of defined populations by the criteria, methods, and objectives of epidemiology rather than of population g.

galtonian g., the study of traits by analysis of the first two moments of metrical data; the preferred method for analysis of traits following the multivariate gaussian distribution.

Galtonian-Fisher g., the g. of measurable traits determined by multiple loci which make contributions that are independent, additive, and approximately equal. SYN multilocal g.

human g., the study of the genetic aspects of humans as a species. Cf. medical g.

mathematical g., the study of genetic traits by formal analysis, e.g., quantitative g., population dynamics, genetic epidemiology, modeling.

medical g., the study of the etiology, pathogenesis, and natural history of human diseases which are at least partially genetic in origin. Cf. clinical g., human g.

mendelian g., the study of the pattern of segregation of phenotypes under the control of genetic loci taken one at a time.

microbial g., the study of hereditary mechanisms of microbes.

modern g., that body of method and analysis that perceives g. as the study of the economy of nucleic acids and associated compounds.

molecular g., molecular biology applied to g.

multilocal g., SYN Galtonian-Fisher g.

population g., the study of genetic influences on the components of cause and effect in the somatic characteristics of populations.

quantitative g., the formal study of measurable genetic traits, traditionally but not necessarily confined to galtonian g.

reverse g., term referring to tracing of a gene responsible for a disease by learning its position in the human genome. This approach makes no claim of providing information about the gene product. SYN positional cloning.

somatic cell g., the study of the structure, organization, and function of a genome by the techniques of cell hybridization.

statistical g., the study of the applications of principles of statistics to problems in genetics.

transplantation g., g. as applied to the transplanting of tissues from one animal to another.

ge·net·o·tro·phic (jĕ-net-ō-trof′ik). Relating to inherited individual distinctions in nutritional requirements. [G. *genesis,* origin, + *trophē,* nourishment]

Ge·ne·va Con·ven·tion. An international agreement formed at meetings in Geneva, Switzerland, in 1864 and 1906, relating (among medical subjects) to the safeguarding of the wounded in battle, of those having the care of them, and of the buildings in which they are being treated. The direct outcome of the first of these meetings was the establishment of the Red Cross Society.

Ge·ne·va lens mea·sure. See under measure.

Gengou, Octave, French bacteriologist, 1875–1957. SEE G. *phenomenon;* Bordet-G. potato blood *agar, bacillus, phenomenon;* Bordet and G. *reaction.*

ge·ni·al, ge·ni·an (jĕ-nī′ăl, -nī′an). SYN mental (2). [G. *geneion,* chin]

△**-genic.** Producing, forming; produced, formed by. [G. *genos,* birth]

ge·nic·u·la (je-nik′ū-lă). Plural of geniculum.

ge·nic·u·lar (je-nik′ū-lăr). Commonly used to mean genual.

ge·nic·u·late (je-nik′ū-lāt). **1.** Bent like a knee. SYN geniculated. **2.** Referring to the geniculum of the facial nerve, denoting the ganglion there present. **3.** Denoting the lateral or medial geniculate body. [L. *geniculo,* pp. -*atus,* to bend the knee, fr. *genu,* knee]

ge·nic·u·lat·ed (je-nik′ū-lā-ted). SYN geniculate (1).

ge·nic·u·lum, pl. **ge·nic·u·la** (je-nik′ū-lŭm, -lă). **1** [TA]. A small genu or angular kneelike structure. **2.** A knotlike structure. [L. dim. of *genu,* knee]

g. cana′lis facia′lis [TA], SYN g. of facial canal.

g. of facial canal [TA], the bend in the facial canal linking the medial and lateral crura of the horizontal port of the canal and corresponding to the location of the geniculate ganglion of the facial nerve. SYN g. canalis facialis [TA], genu of facial canal.

g. of facial nerve [TA], **(1)** a sharp bend in the facial nerve in the facial canal where it turns posteriorly from its previously anterior course to run in the medial wall of the middle ear (external g.); **(2)** complex loop of facial nerve fibers around the abducens nucleus (internal g.). SYN g. nervus facialis [TA].

g. ner′vus facia′lis [TA], SYN g. of facial nerve.

△**-genin.** Suffix used to denote the basic steroid unit of the toxic substance, usually a steroid glycoside (e.g., the aglycon portion).

ge·ni·o·glos·sus (jĕ-nī-ō-glos′ŭs). SYN genioglossus (*muscle*). [G. *geneion,* chin, + *glōssa,* tongue]

ge·ni·o·hy·oid (jĕ-nī′ō-hī′oyd). SYN geniohyoid (*muscle*).

ge·ni·o·hy·oi·de·us (jĕ-nī′ō-hī-oyd′ē-ŭs). SYN geniohyoid (*muscle*). [G. *geneion,* chin, + *hyoeidēs,* y-shaped, hyoid]

ge·ni·on (jĕ-nī′on). The tip of the mental spine, a point in craniometry. [G. *geneion,* chin]

ge·ni·o·plas·ty (jĕ′nī-ō-plas-tē). Surgical correction of the bony contour of the chin. [G. *geneion,* chin, cheek, + *plastos,* formed]

gen·i·tal (jen′i-tăl). **1.** Relating to reproduction or generation. **2.** Relating to the primary female or male sex organs or genitals. **3.** Relating to or characterized by genitality. [L. *genitalis,* pertaining to reproduction, fr. *gigno,* to bring forth]

gen·i·ta·lia (jen′i-tā′lē-ă) [TA]. The organs of reproduction or generation, external and internal. SYN organa genitalia [TA], genital organs, genitals. [L. neut. pl. of *genitalis,* genital]

ambiguous g., SYN genital *ambiguity.*

ambiguous external g., SYN genital *ambiguity.*

external g., the vulva in the female, and the penis and scrotum in the male.

female external g. [TA], the external feminine genital organs, the vulva and clitoris. SYN external female genital organs, organa genitalia feminina externa.

female internal g. [TA], the internal feminine genital organs, the ovaries, uterine tubes, uterus, and vagina. SYN internal female genital organs, organa genitalia feminina interna.

indifferent g., reproductive organs of the embryo before definitive sex formation.

male external g. [TA], the external masculine genital organs, the penis and scrotum. SYN external male genital organs, organa genitalia masculina externa.

male internal g. [TA], the internal masculine genital organs, the testes, epididymides, deferent ducts, seminal vesicles, prostate, and bulbourethral glands. SYN internal male genital organs, organa genitalia masculina interna.

gen·i·tal·i·ty (jen-i-tal′i-tē). In psychoanalysis, a term referring to the genital components of sexuality (i.e., the penis and vagina), as opposed, for example, to orality and anality.

gen·i·tals (jen′i-tălz). SYN genitalia. [see genitalia]

gen·i·to·cru·ral (jen′i-tō-kroo′răl). SYN genitofemoral.

gen·i·to·fem·o·ral (jen′i-tō-fem′ŏ-răl). Relating to the genitalia and the thigh; denoting the g. nerve. SYN genitocrural.

gen·i·to·u·ri·nary (GU) (jen′i-tō-ū′ri-nar-ē). Relating to the organs of reproduction and urination. SYN urinogenital, urinosexual, urogenital.

ge·nius (jēn′yŭs, jēn′ē-ŭs). **1.** Markedly superior intellectual or artistic abilities or exceptional creative power. **2.** A person so endowed. **3.** In psychology, an individual who ranks in the top 1% of all individuals on a test of intelligence. [L.]

ge·nius ep·i·dem·i·cus (ep-i-dem′i-kŭs). The influence, atmospheric, telluric, or cosmic, or the combination of any two or three, regarded by the ancients as the cause of epidemic and endemic diseases. [Mod. L.]

Gennari, Francesco, Italian anatomist, 1750–1795. SEE G. *band, stria; line* of G.; *stripe* of G.

gen·o·blast (jen′ō-blast). The nucleus of the fertilized ovum.

gen·o·copy (jen′ō-kop-e). A genotype at one locus that produces a phenotype which at some levels of resolution is indistinguishable from that produced by another genotype; e.g., two types of elliptocytosis that are g.'s of each other, but are distinguished by the fact that one is linked to the Rh blood group locus and the other is not.

ge·no·der·ma·tol·o·gy (jen′ō-der-mă-tol′ō-jē). Study of the hereditary aspects of cutaneous disorders. [G. *genos,* birth, descent, + *derma,* skin, + *logos,* theory]

ge·no·der·ma·to·sis (jen′ō-der-mă-tō′sis). A skin condition of genetic origin.

ge·nome (je′nōm, -nom). **1.** A complete set of chromosomes derived from one parent, the haploid number of a gamete. **2.** The total gene complement of a set of chromosomes found in higher life forms (the haploid set in a eukaryotic cell), or the functionally similar but simpler linear arrangements found in bacteria and viruses. SEE ALSO Human Genome Project. [gene + chromosome]

ge·nom·ic (jĕ-nom′ik). Relating to a genome.

genomics (jen-ōm-′ks). Study of the structure of the genome of particular organisms, including mapping and sequencing.

 functional g., the study of expressed genes in organisms, including the identity of the genes and the factors that control differential expression.

ge·no·spe·cies (jē′nō-spē-sēz, jen′). A group of organisms in which interbreeding is possible, as evidenced by genetic transfer and recombination.

ge·note (je′nōt). In microbial genetics, an element of recombination in which one of the pair is not a complete chromosome; commonly used as a suffix (e.g., endogenote, exogenote, F genote). [gene + G. -*ōtēs,* toponymic suffix]

ge·no·tox·ic (jē-nō-toks′ik). Denoting a substance that by damaging DNA may cause mutation or cancer. [gene + toxic]

gen·o·type (jen′ō-tūp). **1.** The genetic constitution of an individual. **2.** Gene combination at one specific locus or any specified combination of loci. For specific blood group genotypes, see Blood Groups appendix. [G. *genos,* birth, descent, + *typos,* type] **ZZ g.,** individuals who have a deficiency of α₁-antitrypsin and have emphysema.

gen·o·typ·ic (jen′ō-tip-ik). SYN genotypical.

gen·o·typ·i·cal (jen-ō-tip′i-kăl). Relating to the genotype. SYN genotypic.

gen·ta·mi·cin (jen-tă-mī′sin). A broad spectrum antibiotic of the aminoglycoside class, obtained from *Micromonospora purpurea* and *M. echinospora,* that inhibits the growth of both Gram-positive and Gram-negative bacteria; the sulfate salt is used medicinally.

gen·tian, gen·tian root (jen′shŭn). The dried rhizome and roots of *Gentiana lutea* (family Gentianaceae), an herb of southern and central Europe; a simple bitter.

gen·tian·o·phil, gen·tian·o·phile (jen′shŭn-o-fil, -fīl). Staining readily with gentian violet. SYN gentianophilous. [gentian + G. *philos,* fond]

gen·tian·oph·i·lous (jen-shŭn-of′i-lŭs). SYN gentianophil.

gen·tian·o·pho·bic (jen′shŭn-ō-fō′bik). Not taking a gentian violet stain, or taking it poorly. [gentian + G. *phobos,* fear]

gen·tian root. SEE gentian.

gen·tian vi·o·let. An unstandardized dye mixture of violet rosanilins: it is also used topically as an antiinfective. SEE crystal violet.

gen·ti·o·bi·ase (jen′shi-ō-bī′ās). SYN β-D-glucosidase.

gen·ti·o·bi·o·se (jen′tē-ō-bī′ōs). A disaccharide containing two D-glucopyranose molecules linked β-1,6; a structural moiety in many compounds (e.g., amygdalin). SYN amygdalose.

gen·tis·ic ac·id (jen-tis′ik). This compound is chemically related to salicylate and aspirin (acetylsalicylate) and shares with the latter agent analgesic and anti-inflammatory properties. A metabolite of aspirin.

genu, gen. **ge·′nus,** pl. **gen·ua** (jē′noo, jē′nŭs, jen′oo-ă) [TA]. **1.** The place of articulation between the thigh and the leg. SYN knee (1) [TA]. SEE ALSO knee *joint,* geniculum. **2.** Any structure of angular shape resembling a flexed knee. [L.]

 g. cap′sulae inter′nae [TA], SYN g. of internal capsule.

 g. cor′poris callo′si [TA], SYN g. of corpus callosum.

 g. of corpus callosum [TA], the anterior extremity of the corpus callosum that folds downward and backward on itself, terminating in the rostrum. SYN g. corporis callosi [TA].

 g. of facial canal, SYN *geniculum* of facial canal.

 g. of facial nerve [TA], the curve which the fibers of the root of the facial nerve describe around the abducens nucleus in the pontine tegmentum; the internal g. of the facial nerve. SYN g. nervi facialis [TA].

 g. of internal capsule [TA], the obtuse angle, opening laterally in the horizontal plane, formed by the union of the two limbs (crus anterius and crus posterius) of the internal capsule. SYN g. capsulae internae [TA].

 g. ner′vi facia′lis [TA], SYN g. of facial nerve.

 g. recurva′tum, hyperextension of the knee, the lower extremity having a forward curvature. SYN back-knee.

 g. val′gum, a deformity marked by lateral angulation of the leg in relation to the thigh. SYN knock-knee, tibia valga.

 g. va′rum, a deformity marked by medial angulation of the leg in relation to the thigh; an outward bowing of the legs. SYN bandyleg, bowleg, bow-leg, tibia vara.

gen·u·al (jen′ū-ăl). Relating to the knee. [L. *genu,* knee]

ge·nus, pl. **gen·era** (jē′nŭs, jen′er-ă). In natural history classification, the taxonomic level of division between the family, or tribe, and the species; a group of species alike in the broad features of their organization but different in detail, and incapable of fertile mating. [L. birth, descent]

gen·y·an·trum (jen-ē-an′trŭm). SYN maxillary *sinus.* [G. *genys,* cheek, + *antron,* cave]

△**geo-.** The earth, soil. [G. *gē,* earth]

ge·ode (jē′ōd). A cystlike space (or spaces) with or without an epithelial lining, observed radiologically in subarticular bone, usually in arthritic disorders. [Fr., fr. L. *geodes,* precious stone, fr. G. *gē,* earth, + -*ōdēs,* appearance]

ge·o·med·i·cine (jē-ō-med′i-sin). The science concerned with the influence of climatic and environmental conditions on health and disease. SYN nosochthonography, nosogeography.

ge·o·pa·thol·o·gy (jē′ō-pă-thol′ō-jē). The study of disease in relation to regions, climates, and other environmental influences.

ge·o·pha·gia, ge·oph·a·gism, ge·oph·a·gy (jē-ō-fā′jē-ă, jē-of′ă-jizm, -of′ă-jē). The practice of eating dirt or clay. SYN dirt-eating. [geo- + G. *phagō,* to eat]

ge·o·phil·ic. Terrestrial, soil inhabiting. [geo- + G. *philos,* love, attraction, + -ic]

Ge·oph·i·lus (jē-of′i-lŭs). A genus of centipedes, characterized by very large numbers of legs (47–67 pairs); includes *G. californius, G. rubens,* and *G. umbraticus,* in the U.S.

Georgi, Walter, German bacteriologist, 1889–1920. SEE Sachs-G. *test.*

ge·o·tax·is (jē-ō-tak′sis). A form of positive barotaxis in which there is a tendency to growth or movement toward or into the earth. SYN geotropism. [geo- + G. *taxis,* orderly arrangement]

ge·ot·ri·cho·sis (jē′ō-tri-kō′sis). An opportunistic systemic hyalohyphomycosis caused by *Geotrichum candidum;* ascribed symp-

ge

toms are diverse and suggestive of secondary or mixed infections. [geo- + G. *thrix,* hair, + -*osis,* condition]

Ge·ot·ri·chum (jē-ot'ri-kŭm). A genus of yeastlike fungi that produce arthroconidia but rarely blastoconidia. *G. candidum* was once thought to cause infection in humans.

ge·ot·ro·pism (jē-ot'rō-pizm). SYN geotaxis. [geo- + G. *tropē,* a turning]

gephyrin (je-fir'in). A protein in the ataxia telangiectasia mutation–related family, essential for glycine receptor clustering on neuronal membranes.

geph·y·ro·pho·bia (jĕ-fī-rō-fō'bē-ă). Fear of crossing a bridge. [G. *gephyra,* bridge, + *phobos,* fear]

gep·i·rone (jē-pī'rōn). A nonbenzodiazepine anxiolytic which resembles buspirone both chemically and pharmacologically. Acts on serotonergic receptors rather than benzodiazepine receptors. Lacks dependence-producing properties and tolerance of benzodiazepine-type agents.

ge·ran·i·ol (jĕ-ra'nē-ol). An olefinic terpene alcohol that is the principal constituent of oil of rose and oil of palmarosa; also found in many other volatile oils, such as citronella and lemon grass. An isomer of linalool; an oily liquid with sweet rose odor used in perfumery. Also used as an insect attractant.

ger·a·nyl·ger·a·nyl py·ro·phos·phate (jer'a-nil-jer-a-nil pī-rō-fos'fāt). A key intermediate in the biosynthesis of many terpenes; the key substrate for introducing the geranylgeranyl group into proteins.

ger·a·nyl py·ro·phos·phate (jer'a-nil-pī-rō-fos'fāt). A key intermediate in the biosynthesis of sterols, dolichols, ubiquinone, and prenylated proteins.

ger·a·tol·o·gy (jār-ă-tol'ō-jē). SYN gerontology.

Gerbich an·ti·gen. See under antigen.

Gerbode, Frank, U.S. cardiothoracic surgeon, 1907–1984. SEE Gerbode *defect.*

GERD Abbreviation for gastroesophageal reflux *disease.*

Gerdy, Pierre N., French surgeon, 1797–1856. SEE G. *fibers,* under *fiber, fontanelle,* hyoid *fossa, ligament,* interatrial *loop, tubercle.*

Gerhardt, Carl A.C.J., German physician, 1833–1902. SEE G. *reaction, test* for acetoacetic acid; Gerhardt-Mitchell *disease.*

Gerhardt, Charles F., French chemist, 1816–1856. SEE G. *test* for urobilin in the urine.

ger·i·at·ric (jār-ē-at'rik). Relating to old age or to geriatrics.

ger·i·at·rics (jār-ē-at'riks). The branch of medicine concerned with the medical problems and care of the aged. [G. *gēras,* old age, + *iatrikos,* healing]

dental g., treatment of dental problems peculiar to advanced age. SYN gerodontics, gerodontology.

Gerlach, Joseph, German anatomist, 1820–1896. SEE G. annular *tendon, tonsil; valve* of vermiform appendix; G. *valvula.*

Gerlier, Felix, Swiss physician, 1840–1914. SEE G. *disease.*

germ (jerm). **1.** A microbe; a microorganism. **2.** A primordium; the earliest trace of a structure within an embryo. [L. *germen,* sprout, bud, germ]

dental g., SYN tooth g.

enamel g., the enamel organ of a developing tooth; one of a series of knoblike projections from the dental lamina, later becoming bell-shaped and receiving in its hollow the dental papilla.

reserve tooth g., enamel organ and papilla of a permanent tooth.

tooth g., the enamel organ and dentin papilla, constituting the developing tooth. SYN dental g.

wheat g., the embryo of wheat; contains thiamine, riboflavin, and other vitamins.

ger·ma·ni·um (Ge) (jer-mān'ē-ŭm). A metallic element, atomic no. 32, atomic wt. 72.61. [L. *Germania,* Germany]

ger·mi·ci·dal (jer-mi-sī'dăl). SYN germicide (1).

ger·mi·cide (jer'mi-sīd). **1.** Destructive to germs or microbes. SYN germicidal. **2.** An agent with this action. [germ + L. *caedo,* to kill]

ger·mi·nal (jer'mi-năl). Relating to a germ or, in botany, to germination.

ger·mine (jer'mīn). An alkaloid that occurs in *Veratrum* and *Zygandenus* species. The drug, like veratrine and veratridine, induces repetitive discharges in nerve cells, seemingly because of derangements in sodium channel function. Often used as the acetate or diacetate derivative.

ger·mi·no·ma (jer-mi-nō'mă). A neoplasm of the germinal tissue of gonads, mediastinum, or pineal region such as seminoma. [L. *germen,* bud, + -*oma,* tumor]

△**gero-, geront-, geronto-.** Old age. SEE ALSO presby-. [G. *gerōn,* old man]

ger·o·der·ma (jār-ō-der'mă). **1.** The atrophic skin of the aged. **2.** Any condition in which the skin is thinned and wrinkled, resembling the integument of old age. [gero- + G. *derma,* skin]

ger·o·don·tics, ger·o·don·tol·o·gy (jār-ō-don'tiks, -don-tol'ō-jē). SYN dental *geriatrics.* [gero- + G. *odous,* tooth]

ger·o·ma·ras·mus (jār'ō-mă-raz'mŭs). SYN senile *atrophy.* [gero- + G. *marasmos,* a wasting]

ge·ron·tal (jār-on'tăl). Relating to old age.

ger·on·tine (jār'on-tēn). SYN spermine.

△**geronto-.** SEE gero-.

ger·on·tol·o·gist (jār-on-tol'ō-jist). One who specializes in gerontology.

ger·on·tol·o·gy (jār-on-tol'ō-jē). The scientific study of the process and problems of aging. SYN geratology. [geronto- + G. *logos,* study]

ge·ron·to·phil·ia (jār'on-tō-fil'ē-ă). Morbid love for old persons. [geronto- + G. *philos,* fond]

ge·ron·to·pho·bia (jār'on-tō-fō'bē-ă). Morbid fear of old persons. [geronto- + G. *phobos,* fear]

ge·ron·to·ther·a·peu·tics (jār-on'tō-thār-ă-pū'tiks). The science concerned with treatment of the aged.

ge·ron·to·ther·a·py (jār-on'tō-thār-ă-pē). Treatment of disease in the aged. SYN geriatric therapy.

ger·on·tox·on (jār'on-tok'son). SYN arcus senilis. [geronto- + G. *toxon,* bow]

Gerota, Dimitru, Roumanian anatomist and surgeon, 1867–1939. SEE G. *capsule, fascia, method.*

Gersh, Isidore, U.S. histologist, *1907. SEE Altmann-G. *method.*

Gerstmann, Josef, Austrian neurologist, 1887–1969. SEE G. *syndrome;* G.-Sträussler-Scheinker *syndrome.*

ges·ta·gen (jes'tă-jen). Inclusive term used to denote any one of several gestagenic substances, which are usually steroid hormones. SYN gestin, progestin (3).

ges·ta·gen·ic (jes-tă-jen'ik). Inducing progestational effects in the uterus.

ge·stalt (ge-stahlt). A perceived entity so integrated as to constitute a functional unit with properties not derivable from its parts. SEE gestaltism. [Ger. shape]

ge·stalt·ism (ge-stahlt'izm). The theory in psychology that the objects of mind come as complete forms or configurations which cannot be split into parts; e.g., a square is perceived as such rather than as four discrete lines. [see gestalt]

ges·ta·tion (jes-tā'shŭn). SYN pregnancy. [L. *gestatio,* from *gesto,* pp. *gestatus,* to bear]

ges·tin (jes'tin). SYN gestagen.

ges·to·sis, pl. **ges·to·ses** (jes-tō'sis, -sēz). Any disorder of pregnancy. [L. *gesto,* to carry, to bear, + G. -*osis,* condition]

ges·ture (jes'chŭr). **1.** Any movement expressive of an idea, opinion, or emotion. **2.** An act. [L. *gestus,* movement, gesture]

suicide g., an apparent attempt at suicide by someone wishing to attract attention, gain sympathy, or achieve some goal other than self-destruction.

Gey, George O., U.S. physician and researcher, 1899–1970. SEE G. *solution.*

GFR Abbreviation for glomerular filtration *rate.*

GH Abbreviation for growth *hormone.*

GHB Abbreviation for γ-hydroxybutyrate.

ghee (gē). A clarified butter in India made from cow or buffalo milk that has been coagulated before churning; used as an emollient, a dressing for wounds, and a food. [Eng. spelling of Hind. *ghi*]

Ghon, Anton, Czechoslovakian pathologist, 1866–1936. SEE G. *complex, focus,* primary *lesion, tubercle.*

ghost (gōst). A hemoglobin-depleted erythrocyte that has also lost most, if not all, of its internal proteins.

GHRF, GH-RF Abbreviation for growth hormone-releasing *factor.*

GHRH, GH-RH Abbreviation for growth *hormone*-releasing *hormone.*

GHz Abbreviation for gigahertz, equal to one billion (10^9) hertz; used in ultrasound.

GI Abbreviation for gastrointestinal; Gingival Index.

Giacomini, Carlo, Italian anatomist, 1841–1898. SEE *band* of G.; *frenulum* of G.; uncus *band* of G.

Giannuzzi, Italian anatomist, 1839–1876. SEE G. *crescents,* under *crescent, demilunes,* under *demilune.*

Gianotti, F., 20th century Italian dermatologist. SEE G.-Crosti *syndrome.*

gi·ant·ism (jī'an-tizm). SYN gigantism.

Gi·ar·dia (jē-ar'dē-ă). A genus of parasitic flagellates that parasitize the small intestine of many mammals, including most domestic animals and humans; e.g., *G. bovis* in cattle, *G. canis* in dogs, and *G. cati* in cats. Many species have been described, but recent workers have suggested that these should be reduced to only two or three. [Alfred *Giard,* Fr. biologist, 1846–1908]

G. intestinalis, SYN *G. lamblia.*

G. lam'blia, a flattened, heart-shaped organism (10–20 μm in length) with 8 flagella; it attaches itself to the intestinal mucosa by means of a pair of sucking organs; it is usually asymptomatic except in heavy infections, when it may interfere with absorption of fats and produce flatulence, steatorrhea, and acute discomfort; it is the common species of *G.* in man, but is also found in pigs. SYN *G. intestinalis.*

gi·ar·di·a·sis (jē-ar-dī'ă-sis). Infection with the protozoan parasite *Giardia; Giardia lamblia* may cause diarrhea, dyspepsia, and occasionally malabsorption in humans. SYN lambliasis.

gib·ber·el·lic ac·id (jib'er-el-ik). An auxin, i.e., a plant hormone which stimulates growth; most prominent of the plant-growth-promoting metabolites of *Gibberella fujikuroi.* Used as a plant growth regulator and promoter, especially the growth of seedlings. Used also as a food additive in the malting of barley.

gib·ber·el·lins. A class of plant growth hormones (auxins) of which over 60 are known; these were first isolated in 1938 from cultures of *Gibberella fujikuroi,* the fungus causing Bakanese disease in rice. Also found in higher plants; diterpenoid acids available commercially.

gib·bon (gib'on). A genus of anthropoid apes, *Hylobates,* of the superfamily Hominoidea. [Fr.]

gib·bous (gib'ŭs). Humped; humpbacked; denoting a sharp angle in the flexion of the spine. [L. *gibbosus*]

Gibbs, Josiah W., U.S. mathematician and physicist, 1839–1903. SEE G.-Donnan *equilibrium;* G.-Helmholtz *equation;* Helmholtz-G. *theory;* G. *theorem,* free *energy, energy* of activation.

gib·bus (gib'ŭs). Extreme kyphosis, hump, or hunch; a deformity of spine in which there is a sharply angulated segment, the apex of the angle being posterior. [L. a hump]

Gibney, Virgil P., U.S. orthopedist, 1847–1927. SEE G. fixation *bandage, boot.*

Gibson, George A., Scottish physician, 1854–1913. SEE G. *murmur.*

Gibson, Kasson C., U.S. dentist, 1849–1925. SEE G. *bandage.*

Giemsa, Gustav, German bacteriologist, 1867–1948. SEE G. *stain,* chromosome banding *stain.*

Gierke, Edgar von, German pathologist, 1877–1945. SEE G. *disease;* von G. *disease.*

Gierke, Hans P.B., German anatomist, 1847–1886. SEE G. respiratory *bundle.*

Gifford, Harold, U.S. ophthalmologist, 1858–1929. SEE G. *reflex.*

GIFT Abbreviation for gamete intrafallopian *transfer.*

giga- (G). Prefix used in the SI and metric system to signify multiples of one billion (10^9). [G. *gigas,* giant]

gi·gan·tism (jī'gan-tizm). A condition of abnormal size or overgrowth of the entire body or of any of its parts. SYN giantism. [G. *gigas,* giant]

acromegalic g., a form of pituitary g. in which the signs of acromegaly accompany abnormal height.

cerebral g., a syndrome characterized by increased birth weight and length (above 90th percentile), accelerated growth rate for the first 4 or 5 years without elevation of serum growth hormone levels, and then reversion to normal growth rate; characteristic facies include prognathism, hypertelorism, antimongoloid slant, and dolichocephalic skull; moderate mental retardation and impaired coordination are also associated. SEE Sotos *syndrome.*

eunuchoid g., g. with deficient development of sexual organs; may be of pituitary or gonadal origin; g. accompanied by body proportions typical of hypogonadism during adolescence.

fetal g., excessive fetal or newborn size, e.g., cerebral g. and infants of diabetic mothers.

pituitary g., a form of g. caused by hypersecretion of pituitary growth hormone; a rare disorder commonly the result of a pituitary adenoma.

primordial g., unusually large size from birth due to familial or genetic factors or intrauterine environment (e.g., maternal prediabetic state) and not to hyperpituitarism.

giganto-. Huge, gigantic. [G. *gigas,* one of the race of giants]

gi·gan·to·mas·tia (jī-gan'tō-mas'tē-ă). Massive hypertrophy of the breast. [giganto- + G. *mastos,* breast]

Gi·gan·to·rhyn·chus (ji-gan'to-ring'kŭs). A genus of very large acanthocephalan worms. SEE ALSO *Macracanthorhynchus, Moniliformis.* [giganto- + G. *rhynchos,* snout]

Gigli, Leonardo, Italian gynecologist, 1863–1908. SEE G. *saw.*

GIH Abbreviation for growth *hormone*-inhibiting *hormone.*

Gi·la mon·ster (hē'lă). A large poisonous lizard, *Heloderma suspectum* of New Mexico, Arizona, and northern Mexico. [*Gila,* a river in Arizona]

Gilbert, Nicholas A., French physician, 1858–1927. SEE G. *disease, syndrome.*

Gilbert, Walter, U.S. microbiologist and Nobel laureate, *1932. SEE Maxim-G. *sequencing.*

gil·bert. The unit of magnetomotive force or magnetic potential. [W. *Gilbert,* English physicist, 1544–1603]

Gilchrist, Thomas C., U.S. physician, 1862–1927. SEE G. *disease.*

Gilford, Hastings, English physician, 1861–1941. SEE Hutchinson-G. *disease, syndrome.*

Gilles de la Tourette, Georges, French physician, 1857–1904. SEE G. de la T. *disease, syndrome;* Tourette *disease;* Tourette *syndrome.*

Gillespie, Frank, U.S. ophthalmologist, *1927. SEE G. *syndrome.*

Gillette, Eugène P., French surgeon, 1836–1886. SEE G. suspensory *ligament.*

Gilliam, David Tod, U.S. gynecologist, 1844–1923. SEE G. *operation.*

Gillies, Sir Harold D., British plastic surgeon, 1882–1960. SEE G. *operation;* Filatov-G. *flap.*

Gillmore nee·dle. See under needle.

Gilman, Alfred G., *1941, co-winner of the 1994 Nobel Prize for work related to G proteins, q.v.

Gilmer, Thomas L., U.S. oral surgeon, 1849–1931. SEE G. *wiring.*

Gil-Vernet, Jose Maria Vila, Spanish urologist, *1922. SEE Gil-Vernet *operation.*

Gimbernat, Antonio de, Spanish anatomist and surgeon, 1734–1816. SEE G. *ligament.*

gin·ger (jin'jer). The dried rhizome of *Zingiber officinale* (family Zingiberaceae), known in commerce as Jamaica g., African g., and Cochin g. The outer cortical layers are often either partially or completely removed; used as a carminative and flavoring agent. SYN zingiber.

gi

Chinese g., SYN galangal.

Indian g., SYN *Asarum* canadense.

g. oleoresin, a carminative, stimulant, and flavoring agent.

wild g., SYN *Asarum* canadense.

gin·gi·li oil (jin′ji-lē). SYN *sesame* oil.

gin·gi·va, gen. and pl. **gin·gi·vae** (jin′ji-vă, -vē) [TA]. The dense fibrous tissue and overlying mucous membrane, which envelop the alveolar processes of the upper and lower jaws and surrounds the necks of the teeth. SYN gum (2)✝. [L.]

alveolar g., gingival tissue applied to the alveolar bone.

attached g., that part of the oral mucosa which is firmly bound to the tooth and alveolar process.

buccal g., that portion of the g. that covers the buccal surfaces of the teeth and alveolar process.

free g., that portion of the g. that surrounds the tooth and is not directly attached to the tooth surface; the outer wall of the gingival sulcus.

labial g., that portion of the g. that covers the labial surfaces of the teeth and the alveolar process.

lingual g., that portion of the g. that covers the lingual surfaces of the teeth and the alveolar process.

septal g., that portion of the g. that covers the interdental septum.

gin·gi·val (jin′ji-văl). Relating to the gums.

Gin·gi·val In·dex (GI). An index of periodontal disease based upon the severity and location of the lesion.

Gin·gi·val-Per·i·o·don·tal In·dex (GPI). An index of gingivitis, gingival irritation, and advanced periodontal disease.

gin·gi·vec·to·my (jin-ji-vek′tō-mē). Surgical resection of unsupported gingival tissue. SYN gum resection. [gingiva + G. *ektomē,* excision]

gin·gi·vi·tis (jin-ji-vī′tis). Inflammation of the gingiva as a response to bacterial plaque on adjacent teeth; characterized by erythema, edema, and fibrous enlargement of the gingiva without resorption of the underlying alveolar bone. [gingiva + G. *-itis,* inflammation]

acute necrotizing ulcerative g. (ANUG), SEE necrotizing ulcerative g.

atypical g., SYN plasma cell g.

chronic desquamative g., a clinical term for a gingival condition of unknown etiology, usually encountered in middle-aged and older women, characterized by erythema, mucosal atrophy, and desquamation, and usually accompanied by a burning sensation and pain; diagnosis is usually made by biopsy and direct immunofluorescence. SYN gingivosis.

diabetic g., g. in which the host response to bacterial plaque is presumably modified by the metabolic alterations encountered in the uncontrolled diabetic patient.

dilantin g., SYN diphenylhydantoin g.

diphenylhydantoin g., g. exacerbated by long-term therapy with diphenylhydantoin; the host response to bacterial plaque is characterized by marked hyperplasia of the fibrous connective tissue and, to a lesser degree, of the surface epithelium, resulting in gross enlargement of interdental papillae which may coalesce and obscure the clinical crowns of the teeth. SYN dilantin g.

fusospirochetal g., SYN necrotizing ulcerative g.

hormonal g., g. in which the host response to bacterial plaque is presumably exacerbated by hormonal alterations occurring during puberty, pregnancy, oral contraceptive use, or menopause. SYN pregnancy g.

hyperplastic g., g. of long-standing duration in which the gingiva becomes enlarged and firm due to proliferation of fibrous connective tissue.

leukemic hyperplastic g., enlarged gingiva due to infiltration of leukemic cells and infection from local factors in the face of diminshed host response.

marginal g., g. in which the clinical alterations are confined to the marginal gingiva and do not involve the attached gingiva.

necrotizing ulcerative g. (NUG), an acute or recurrent g. of young and middle-aged adults characterized clinically by gingival erythema and pain, fetid odor, and necrosis and sloughing of interdental papillae and marginal gingiva which gives rise to a

gray pseudomembrane; fever, regional lymphadenopathy, and other systemic manifestations also may be present. A fusiform bacillus and *Treponema vincentii* can be isolated from the gingival tissues in large numbers and are felt to play a significant but poorly defined role in the pathogenesis. SYN fusospirochetal g., trench mouth, ulceromembranous g., Vincent disease, Vincent infection.

plasma cell g., intense hyperemic edema and inflammation of the gingiva resulting from a hypersensitivity reaction. A dense plasma cell infiltrate is seen in the lamina propria. SYN atypical g.

pregnancy g., SYN hormonal g.

proliferative g., inflammatory changes in the gingiva characterized by proliferation of the gingival components.

suppurative g., g. in which a purulent exudate can be expressed from the gingival surface.

ulceromembranous g., SYN necrotizing ulcerative g.

△**gingivo-.** The gingivae, the gums of the mouth. [L. *gingiva*]

gin·gi·vo·ax·i·al (jin′ji-vō-ak′sē-ăl). Pertaining to the line angle formed by the gingival and axial walls of a cavity.

gin·gi·vo·glos·si·tis (jin′ji-vō-glos-sī′tis). Inflammation of both the gingival tissues and tongue. SEE ALSO stomatitis.

gin·gi·vo·la·bi·al (jin′ji-vō-lā′bē-ăl). Referring to the line angle formed by the junction of the gingival and labial walls of a (class III or IV) cavity.

gin·gi·vo·lin·guo·ax·i·al (jin′ji-vō-ling′gwo-ak′sē-ăl). Referring to the point angle formed by the gingival, lingual, and axial walls of a cavity.

gin·gi·vo·os·se·ous (jin′ji-vō-os′ē-ŭs). Referring to the gingiva and its underlying bone.

gin·gi·vo·plas·ty (jin′ji-vō-plas-tē). A surgical procedure that reshapes and recontours the gingival tissue in order to attain esthetic, physiologic, and functional form.

gin·gi·vo·sis (jin-ji-vō′sis). SYN chronic desquamative *gingivitis.*

gin·gi·vo·sto·ma·ti·tis (jin′ji-vō-stō′mă-tī′tis). Inflammation of the gingiva and other oral mucous membranes. [gingivo- + G. *stoma,* mouth, + *-itis,* inflammation]

primary herpetic g., SYN primary herpetic *stomatitis.*

gin·gly·form (jing′gli-fōrm, ging-). SYN ginglymoid. [G. *ginglymos,* a hinge joint, + L. *forma,* form]

gin·glym·o·ar·thro·di·al (jing′gli-mō-ar-thrō′dē-ăl, ging-). Denoting a joint having the form of both ginglymus and arthrodia, or hinge joint and sliding joint.

gin·gly·moid (jing′gli-moyd, ging-). Relating to or resembling a hinge joint. SYN ginglyform. [G. *ginglymos,* a hinge joint, + *eidos,* resembling]

gin·gly·mus (jing′gli-mŭs, ging-) [TA]. SYN hinge *joint.* [G. *ginglymos*]

helicoid g., SYN pivot *joint.*

lateral g., SYN pivot *joint.*

Ginkgo biloba. A tall ornamental deciduous tree of the family Ginkgoaceae with distinctive bilobed fan-shaped leaves; female trees bear edible seeds surrounded by a fleshy covering that when ripe smells strongly of butyric acid; native to China, but extinct in the wild, surviving only in cultivation; extracts of the leaves contain ginkgoheterosides and terpene lactones and are used medicinally in cerebral and peripheral vascular disease. SYN maidenhair tree.

The leaves of the ginkgo tree have been used in Chinese and Japanese traditional medicine for many centuries in diseases of the brain, heart, and lungs. Several well-controlled studies have shown that ginkgo extracts enhance both cerebral and peripheral blood flow in some vascular insufficiency syndromes. They have relieved symptoms in dementia, vertigo, and tinnitus of vascular origin and in intermittent claudication and premenstrual syndrome. Ginkgo extracts also inhibit platelet aggregation and scavenge free radicals. The usual dosage is 120–240 mg/day in 2–3 divided doses. Administration for several weeks may be required before beneficial effects are noted. Although *G. biloba* is promoted as a "smart pill" by purveyors of herbal remedies, it does not improve mental function in persons without cerebrovascular disease. Side effects are uncommon and include gastrointestinal upset, headache, and rash. A few cases of subarachnoid hemorrhage and hyphema have been reported, particularly in persons also taking aspirin. Administration of ginkgo extract should be discontinued before surgery.

gin·seng (jin'seng). The roots of several species of *Panax* (family Araliaceae), esteemed as of great medicinal virtue by the Chinese, used extensively as a "nutriceutical"; alleged to improve mental and physical functions. [Ch.]

Giordano-Giovannetti di·et. See under diet.

GIP Abbreviation for gastric inhibitory *polypeptide*; gastric inhibitory *peptide*.

Girard, Alfred C., Swiss-born U.S. surgeon, 1841–1914. SEE G. *reagent*.

gir·dle (ger'dl) [TA]. A belt; a zone. A structure that has the form of a belt or girdle. SYN cingulum (1) [TA]. [A.S. *gyrdel*]

   Hitzig g., SYN tabetic *cuirass*.

   Neptune g., a wet pack applied around the abdomen.

   pectoral g. [TA], the incomplete bony ring, formed by the clavicles and the scapulae, that supports the upper limb, attaching its appendicular skeleton to the axial skeleton (manubrium sterni). SYN cingulum pectorale [TA], cingulum membri superioris★, shoulder g.★, thoracic g.

   pelvic g. [TA], the right and left hip bones, joined at the pubic symphysis, by which the appendicular skeleton of the lower limbs is attached to the axial skeleton (sacrum), which in so doing forms a bony ring; the bony pelvis. SYN cingulum pelvici [TA], cingulum membri inferioris★.

   shoulder g., ★official alternate term for pectoral g.

   thoracic g., SYN pectoral g.

   white limbal g. of Vogt, symmetric arcuate yellow-white deposits in the peripheral cornea often seen in patients over age forty.

Girdlestone, Gathorne Robert, British orthopedist, 1881–1950. SEE G. *procedure*.

gi·tal·in (jit'ǎ-lin). An extract of *Digitalis purpurea* containing a mixture of glycosides and aglycons, with action and uses similar to those of digitalis.

gith·a·gism (gith'ǎ-jizm). A disease similar to lathyrism, believed to be due to poisoning by seeds of the corn cockle, *Lychnis githago*. [L. *gith*, a plant, Roman coriander, + *ago*, to drive]

gi·tog·e·nin (jit'ō-jen-in). The genin of gitonin; a cardiotonic agent.

gi·to·nin (jit'ō-nin). A gitogenin tetraglycoside composed of two galactoses, one glucose, and one xylose; F-gitogenin has one galactose, two glucoses, and one xylose. Both are cardiotonic agents.

gi·tox·i·gen·in (ji-toks'ē-jen-in). The aglycon of gitoxin.

gi·tox·in (ji-tok'sin). A secondary cardiac glycoside from *Digitalis purpurea* and *D. lanata*. SYN anhydrogitalin, bigitalin, pseudodigitoxin.

git·ter·zel·le (git'er-zel-e). SYN gitter *cell*. [Ger. fr. *Gitter*, lattice, + *Zelle*, cell]

Gla Abbreviation for 4-carboxyglutamic acid.

gla·bel·la (glǎ-bel'ǎ) [TA]. **1.** A smooth prominence, most marked in the male, on the frontal bone above the root of the nose. **2.** The most forward projecting point of the forehead in the midline at the level of the supraorbital ridges. SYN mesophryon. SEE ALSO antinion. SYN intercilium. [L. *glabellus*, hairless, smooth, dim. of *glaber*]

gla·bel·lad (glǎ-bel'ad). Toward the glabella.

gla·brous, gla·brate (glā'brŭs, glā'brāt). Smooth or hairless; denoting areas of the body where hair does not normally grow, i.e., palms or soles. [L. *glaber*, smooth]

glad·i·ate (glad'ē-āt). SYN xiphoid. [L. *gladius*, a sword]

glad·i·o·lus (glǎ-dī'ō-lŭs, glad'ē-ō'lŭs). SYN body of sternum. [L. dim. of *gladius*, a sword]

GLAND

🔲**gland** [TA]. An organized aggregation of cells functioning as a secretory or excretory organ. SYN glandula (1) [TA]. [L. *glans*, acorn]

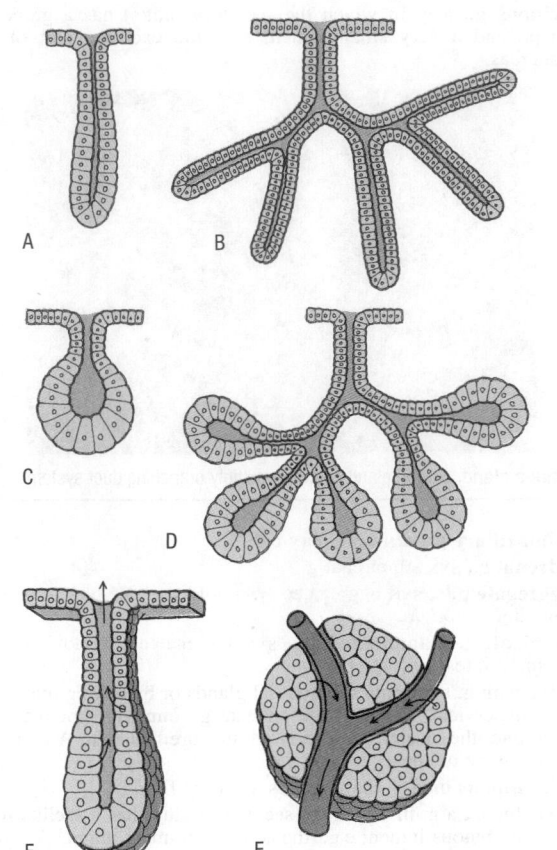

types of **glands:** (A) tubular, (B) compound tubular, (C) acinous, (D) compound acinous, (E) exocrine, (F) endocrine

   accessory g., a small mass of glandular structure, detached from but lying near another and larger g., to which it is similar in structure and probably in function.

   accessory lacrimal g.'s [TA], small, compound, branched, tubular glands located sometimes in the middle part of the lid (Wolfring glands, 1872, or Ciaccio glands, 1874) or along the superior and inferior fornices of the conjunctival sac (Krause g.'s, 1854). These accessory g.'s are ectopic portions of the lacrimal tissue; all of them produce the same kind of tears, secreting onto the conjunctival surface. Henle and Baumgarten "glands" are in fact not g.'s at all, but mere epithelial invaginations. SYN glandulae lacrimales accessoriae [TA].

   accessory parotid g. [TA], an occasional islet of parotid tissue separate from the mass of the gland, lying anteriorly just above the commencement of the parotid duct. SYN glandula parotidea accessoria [TA], admaxillary g., glandula parotis accessoria, socia parotidis.

   accessory suprarenal g.'s [TA], isolated, often minute, masses of suprarenal tissue sometimes found near the main glands or in the broad ligament or the epididymis. SYN glandulae suprarenales accessoriae [TA].

   accessory thyroid g. [TA], an isolated mass, or one of several

gl

such masses, of thyroid tissue, sometimes present in the side of the neck, or ranging in position from just superior to the hyoid bone (suprahyoid accessory thyroid gland) to the arch of the aorta inferiorly. SYN glandula thyroidea accessoria [TA], accessory thyroid, prehyoid g., suprahyoid g., thyroidea accessoria, thyroidea ima, Wölfler g.

acid g., one of the gastric g.'s secreting the hydrochloric acid of the gastric juice. SYN oxyntic g.

acinotubular g., SYN tubuloacinar g.

acinous g., a g. in which the secretory unit(s) has a grapelike shape and a very small lumen; e.g., the exocrine part of the pancreas.

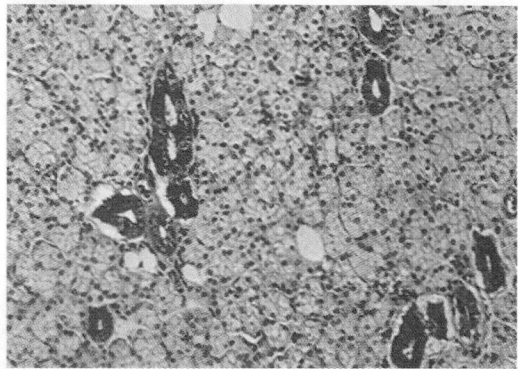

acinous gland: parotid gland showing multiply branching duct system

admaxillary g., SYN accessory parotid g.

adrenal g., SYN suprarenal g.

aggregate g.'s, SYN aggregated lymphoid *nodules* of small intestine, under *nodule.*

agminate g.'s, agminated g.'s, SYN aggregated lymphoid *nodules* of small intestine, under *nodule.*

Albarran g.'s, minute submucosal glands or branching tubules in the subcervical region of the prostate g., emptying for the most part into the posterior portion of the urethra. SYN Albarran y Dominguez tubules.

albuminous g., a g. that secretes a watery fluid.

alveolar g., a g. in which the secretory unit(s) has a saclike form and an obvious lumen; e.g., the active mammary gland.

anal g., (1) one of a number of large sudoriferous g.'s in the mucous membrane of the anus; **(2)** an incorrect synonym for anal sac.

anterior lingual g., one of the small mixed glands deeply placed near the apex of the tongue on each side of the frenulum. SYN apical g., Bauhin g., Blandin g., glandula lingualis anterior, Nuhn g.

apical g., SYN anterior lingual g.

apocrine g., a g. whose secretory product includes an apical portion of the secretory cell such as the secretion of lipid droplets in lactation.

apocrine sweat g.'s, sudoriferous g.'s that develop in association with hair follicles and undergo enlargement and secretory development at puberty; they secrete a viscous and odorless sweat that supports the growth of bacteria leading to an acrid odor; secretion is by an eccrine, not apocrine, mechanism. SYN axillary sweat g.'s.

areolar g.'s [TA], a number of larger sebaceous glands forming small rounded projections from the surface of the areola of the breast; they enlarge with pregnancy and during lactation secrete a substance presumed to resist chapping. SYN glandulae areolares [TA], Montgomery follicles, Montgomery g.'s.

arteriococcygeal g., SYN coccygeal *body.*

arytenoid g.'s, SYN laryngeal g.'s.

Aselli g., a single large lymph node ventral to the abdominal aorta that receives all the lymph from the intestines in many smaller mammals. SYN Aselli pancreas.

g.'s of auditory tube, SYN tubal g.'s of pharyngotympanic tube.

axillary g.'s, SYN axillary *lymph nodes,* under *lymph node.*

axillary sweat g.'s, SYN apocrine sweat g.'s.

Bartholin g., SYN greater vestibular g.

basal g., SYN pituitary g.

Bauhin g., SYN anterior lingual g.

Baumgarten g.'s, SYN Henle g.'s.

biliary g.'s, ✕ official alternate term for g.'s of (common) bile duct.

g.'s of biliary mucosa, small, mucous, tubuloalveolar glands in the mucosa of the larger bile ducts and especially in the neck of the gallbladder. SYN glandulae mucosae biliosae, Luschka cystic g.'s, Theile g.'s.

Blandin g., SYN anterior lingual g.

Bowman g., SYN olfactory g.'s. SEE olfactory g.'s.

brachial g., one of the lymph nodes of the arm.

bronchial g.'s [TA], mucous and seromucous glands whose secretory units lie outside the muscle of the bronchi. SYN glandulae bronchiales [TA].

Bruch g.'s, lymph nodes in the palpebral conjunctiva. SYN trachoma g.'s.

Brunner g.'s, SYN duodenal g.'s.

buccal g.'s [TA], numerous racemose, mucous, or serous glands in the submucous tissue of the cheeks. SYN glandulae buccales [TA], genal g.'s.

bulbourethral g. [TA], one of two small compound racemose glands, that produce a mucoid secretion, lying side by side along the membranous urethra just above the bulb of the penis; they discharge through a small duct into the spongy part of the urethra. SYN glandula bulbourethralis [TA], Cowper g., Méry g.

cardiac g., a coiled tubular g. located in the cardiac region of the stomach; secretes primarily mucus.

cardiac g.'s, SYN cardiac g.'s of stomach.

cardiac g.'s of esophagus, SYN cardiac g.'s of stomach.

cardiac g.'s of stomach [TA], g.'s located in the lamina propria of the uppermost and lowermost levels of the esophagus; they resemble cardiac g.'s of the stomach in that they are branched tubules of mucous cells, which secrete a neutral mucus assumed to afford protection against acid reflux. SYN cardiac g.'s of esophagus, cardiac g.'s.

ceruminous g.'s, apocrine sudoriferous glands in the external acoustic meatus. SYN glandulae ceruminosae (1).

cervical g.'s, SYN glandulae cervicales uteri [TA]. SYN cervical g.'s of uterus.

cervical g.'s of uterus [TA], branched mucus-secreting glands in the mucosa of the cervix. SYN cervical g.'s.

Ciaccio g.'s, SEE accessory lacrimal g.'s.

ciliary g.'s [TA], a number of modified apocrine sudoriferous glands in the eyelids, with ducts that usually open into the follicles of the eyelashes. SYN glandulae ciliares [TA], Moll g.'s.

circumanal g.'s, large apocrine sweat glands surrounding the anus. SYN Gay g.'s, glandulae circumanales.

coccygeal g., SYN coccygeal *body.*

coil g., a g. whose secretory part is convoluted. SYN convoluted g.

g.'s of (common) bile duct [TA], mucin-secreting tubuloalveolar g.'s, arranged in clusters, along the walls of the (common) bile duct. SYN glandulae ductus choledochi [TA], biliary g.'s ✕, glandulae ductus biliaris ✕.

compound g., a g. whose larger excretory ducts branch repeatedly into smaller ducts, which ultimately drain secretory units.

conjunctival g.'s [TA], clusters of mucous cells in the conjunctival epithelium, most numerous on the bulbar conjunctiva. SYN glandulae conjunctivales [TA], Terson g.'s.

convoluted g., SYN coil g.

Cowper g., SYN bulbourethral g.

cutaneous g.'s [TA], any of the glands of the skin. SYN glandulae cutis [TA].

ductless g.'s, SYN endocrine g.'s.

duodenal g.'s [TA], small, branched, coiled tubular glands that occur mostly in the submucosa of the first third of the duodenum; they secrete an alkaline mucoid substance that serves to neutralize gastric juice. SYN glandulae duodenales [TA], Brunner g.'s, Wepfer g.'s.

Duverney g., SYN greater vestibular g.

Ebner g.'s, serous g.'s of the tongue opening in the bottom of the trough surrounding the circumvallate papillae.

eccrine g., a coiled tubular sweat g. (other than apocrine g.'s) that occurs in the skin on almost all parts of the body.

ecdysial g.'s, insect structures that originate from the ectoderm of the ventrocaudal part of the head and serve as a source of ecdysone. SYN peritracheal g.'s, prothoracic g.'s, thoracic g.'s, ventral g.'s.

Eglis g.'s, small, inconstant mucous g.'s of the ureter and renal pelvis.

endocrine g.'s [TA], glands that have no ducts, their secretions being absorbed directly into the blood. SYN glandulae endocrinae [TA], ductless g.'s, endocrine system, g.'s of internal secretion, glandulae sine ductibus.

esophageal g.'s, a variable number of small compound mucous glands in the submucosa of the esophagus. SYN glandulae esophageae.

g.'s of eustachian tube, SYN tubal g.'s of pharyngotympanic tube.

excretory g., a g. separating excrementitious or waste material from the blood.

exocrine g., a g. from which secretions reach a free surface of the body by ducts.

external salivary g., SYN parotid g.

g.'s of the female urethra, SYN urethral g.'s of female.

follicular g., a g. consisting of follicles.

fundic g.'s, SYN gastric g.'s.

Galeati g.'s, SYN intestinal g.'s.

gastric g.'s [TA], branched tubular glands lying in the mucosa of the fundus and body of the stomach; such glands contain parietal cells that secrete hydrochloric acid, zymogen cells that produce pepsin, and mucous cells. SYN glandulae gastricae [TA], fundic g.'s, gastric follicles, Wasmann g.'s.

Gay g.'s, SYN circumanal g.'s.

genal g.'s, SYN buccal g.'s.

genital g., (**1**) SYN testis; (**2**) SYN ovary.

Gley g.'s, SEE parathyroid g.

glomiform g.'s, SYN glomus (2).

greater vestibular g. [TA], one of two mucoid-secreting tubulo-alveolar glands on either side of the lower part of the vagina, the equivalent of the bulbourethral glands in the male; ensheathed with vestibular bulbs by ischiocavernosus muscles. Thus erection and concurrent muscle contraction cause secretion into vestibule of vagina. SYN glandula vestibularis major [TA], Bartholin g., Duverney g., Tiedemann g., vulvovaginal g.

Guérin g.'s, SYN urethral g.'s of female.

hemal g., SYN hemal node.

hematopoietic g., a blood-forming organ, such as the spleen.

hemolymph g., SYN hemal node.

Henle g.'s, formerly considered accessory lacrimal g.'s, these epithelial invaginations are located near the fornices in the medial part of the palpebral conjunctiva; they open on the conjunctival surface. SEE ALSO accessory lacrimal g.'s. SYN Baumgarten g.'s.

hibernating g., SYN brown fat.

holocrine g., a g. whose secretion consists of disintegrated cells of the g. itself, e.g., a sebaceous g., in contrast to a merocrine g.

internal salivary g., the sublingual and submandibular g.'s regarded as one.

g.'s of internal secretion, SYN endocrine g.'s.

interscapular g., SYN brown fat.

interstitial g., SEE interstitial cells, under cell.

intestinal g.'s [TA], the tubular glands in the mucous membrane of the small and large intestines. SYN glandulae intestinales [TA], crypts of Lieberkühn, Galeati g.'s, intestinal follicles, Lieberkühn follicles, Lieberkühn g.'s.

intraepithelial g.'s, accumulations of glandular cells that lie within an epithelium, as those of the urethra.

jugular g., SYN signal lymph node.

Knoll g.'s, g.'s in the ventricular folds of the larynx (false vocal cords).

Krause g.'s, (**1**) SEE accessory lacrimal g.'s; (**2**) g.'s in the mucous membrane of the tympanic cavity. SEE accessory lacrimal g.'s.

labial g.'s [TA], mucous glands in the submucous tissue of the lips. SYN glandulae labiales [TA].

lacrimal g. [TA], the gland that secretes tears; it consists of 6–12 separate compound tubuloalveolar serous glands, located in the upper lateral part of the orbit, and is partially divided into a smaller palpebral part (pars palpebralis) and a larger orbital part (pars orbitalis) by the aponeurosis of the levator palpebrae muscle. SYN glandula lacrimalis [TA].

lactiferous g., SYN mammary g.

g.'s of large intestine [TA], tubules of mucosal epithelium, perpendicular to the luminal surface that appears sievelike because of the abundance of gland openings; g.'s are lined with short columnar epithelial cells—mostly goblet cells with interspersed water-absorbing and fewer enteroendocrine cells; the g.'s of the large intestine are longer (deeper), more abundant, more closely apposed and have a higher density of goblet cells (but no Paneth cells) compared with g.'s of the small intestine. SEE ALSO g.'s of small intestine. SYN glandulae intestini crassi [TA], crypts of Lieberkühn of large intestine.

laryngeal g.'s [TA], a large number of mixed glands in the mucous membrane of the larynx; they are called, according to their situation, anterior, middle, and posterior. SYN glandulae laryngeae [TA], arytenoid g.'s.

lesser vestibular g.'s [TA], a number of minute mucous glands opening on the surface of the vestibule between the orifices of the vagina and urethra. SYN glandulae vestibulares minores [TA].

Lieberkühn g.'s, SYN intestinal g.'s.

Littré g.'s, SYN urethral g.'s of male.

Luschka g., (**1**) SYN pharyngeal tonsil; (**2**) former name for corpus coccygeum.

Luschka cystic g.'s, SYN g.'s of biliary mucosa.

lymph g., SYN lymph node.

major salivary g.'s [TA], a category of salivary g.'s's that includes the three largest g.'s of the oral cavity that also secrete most of the saliva: the parotid, submandibular, and sublingual g.'s. SYN glandulae salivariae majores [TA].

g.'s of the male urethra, SYN urethral g.'s of male.

malpighian g.'s, SYN splenic lymph follicles, under follicle.

mammary g. [TA], the potential and active compound, alveolar, apocrine, milk-secreting gland that lies within the breast. It consists of 15–24 lobes, each consisting of many lobules, separated by adipose tissue and fibrous septa; the parenchyma of the resting postpubertal female gland consists of ducts; the alveoli develop only during pregnancy, remaining active until weaning. Normally, the gland remains rudimentary (undistinguishable from that of childhood) in men. SEE ALSO breast. SYN glandula mammaria [TA], lactiferous g., milk g.

marrow-lymph g., a type of hemal node, resembling the bone marrow in structure and probable function.

master g., SYN pituitary g.

maxillary g., SYN submandibular g.

meibomian g.'s, SYN tarsal g.'s.

merocrine g., a g. that releases only an acellular secretory product, in contrast to a holocrine g.

Méry g., SYN bulbourethral g.

mesenteric g.'s, SEE mesenteric lymph nodes, under lymph node.

milk g., SYN mammary g.

minor salivary g.'s [TA], the smaller, largely mucus-secreting, exocrine g.'s of the oral cavity, consisting of the labial, buccal, molar, lingual, and palatine g.'s. SYN glandulae salivariae minores [TA].

mixed g., (**1**) a g. that contains both serous and mucous secretory units; (**2**) a g. that is both exocrine and endocrine, e.g., the pancreas.

molar g.'s [TA], four or five large buccal glands in the neighborhood of the last molar tooth. SYN glandulae molares [TA].

gl

Moll g.'s, SYN ciliary g.'s.

Montgomery g.'s, SYN areolar g.'s.

g.'s of mouth [TA], glands that empty into the oral cavity. SYN glandulae oris [TA].

mucilaginous g., obsolete term for one of the synovial villi, supposed by Havers to secrete the synovia.

muciparous g., SYN mucous g.

mucous g., a gland that secretes mucus. SYN glandula mucosa, muciparous g.

mucous g.'s of auditory tube, SYN tubal g.'s of pharyngotympanic tube.

nasal g.'s [TA], seromucous glands in the respiratory region of the nasal mucous membrane. SYN glandulae nasales [TA].

Nuhn g., SYN anterior lingual g.

odoriferous g., (1) a g., such as Tyson g., the secretion of which has a strong odor; **(2)** SEE sweat g.'s.

oil g.'s, SYN sebaceous g.'s.

olfactory g.'s [TA], branched tubuloalveolar serous secreting glands (of Bowman) in the mucous membrane of the olfactory region of the nasal cavity. SYN glandulae olfactoriae [TA], Bowman g.

oxyntic g., SYN acid g.

pacchionian g.'s, SYN arachnoid *granulations,* under *granulation.*

palatine g.'s [TA], a number of racemose mucous glands in the posterior half of the submucous tissue covering the hard palate. SYN glandulae palatinae [TA].

palpebral g.'s, SYN tarsal g.'s.

parathyroid g. [TA], one of two small paired endocrine glands, superior and inferior, usually found embedded in the connective tissue capsule on the posterior surface of the thyroid gland; they secrete parathyroid hormone that regulates the metabolism of calcium and phosphorus. The parenchyma is composed of chief and oxyphilic cells arranged in anastomosing cords. Inadvertent removal of all parathyroid g.'s, as during thyroidectomy, produces tetany and may be fatal in the absence of hormone replacement therapy. SYN glandula parathyroidea [TA], epithelial body, parathyroid (2).

paraurethral g.'s, SYN urethral g.'s of female.

parotid g. [TA], the largest of the salivary glands, one of the bilateral compound acinous glands situated inferior and anterior to the ear, on either side, extending from the angle of the jaw inferiorly, to the zygomatic arch superiorly, posteriorly to the sternocleidomastoid muscle, and medially into the infratemporal fossa, deep to the ramus of the mandible; it is subdivided into a superficial part (pars superficialis) and a deep part (pars profunda) by emerging branches of the facial nerve, and discharges through the parotid duct. SYN glandula parotidea [TA], external salivary g., glandula parotis.

pectoral g.'s, SEE axillary *lymph nodes,* under *lymph node.*

peptic g., a pepsin-secreting g. SEE gastric g.'s.

peritracheal g.'s, SYN ecdysial g.'s.

perspiratory g.'s, SYN sweat g.'s.

Peyer g.'s, SYN aggregated lymphoid *nodules* of small intestine, under *nodule.*

pharyngeal g.'s [TA], racemose mucous glands beneath the mucous membrane of the pharynx. SYN glandulae pharyngeales [TA].

Philip g.'s, enlarged deep g.'s just above the clavicle, found in children with pulmonary tuberculosis and occasionally in others.

pileous g., a sebaceous g. emptying into the hair follicle.

pineal g. [TA], SYN pineal *body.*

pituitary g. [TA], an unpaired compound gland suspended from the base of the hypothalamus by a short extension of the infundibulum, the infundibular or pituitary stalk. The g. consists of two major subdivisions: 1) the neurohypophysis, comprising the infundibulum and its bulbous termination, the neural part or infundibular process (posterior lobe), which is composed of neuroglialike pituicytes, blood vessels, and unmyelinated nerve fibers of the hypothalamohypophyseal tract whose cell bodies reside in the supraoptic and paraventricular nuclei of the hypothalamus, and convey to the lobe for storage and release the neurosecretory hormones oxytocin and antidiuretic hormone; 2) the adenohy-

pophysis, comprising the larger distal part, a sleevelike extension of this lobe (infundibular part) that invests the infundibular stalk, and a thin intermediate part (poorly developed in humans) between the anterior and posterior lobes; the anterior lobe consists of cords of cells of several different types interspersed with capillaries of the hypothalamohypophysial portal system; secretion of somatotropins, prolactin, thyroid-stimulating hormone, gonadotropins, adrenal corticotropin, and other related peptides in the adenohypophysis is regulated by releasing and inhibiting factors elaborated by neurons in the hypothalamus that are taken up by a primary plexus of capillaries in the median eminence and transported via portal vessels in the infundibular part and infundibular stem to a secondary plexus of capillaries in the distal part. SYN hypophysis [TA], glandula pituitaria☆, basal g., glandula basilaris, hypophysis cerebri, master g.

Poirier g., a lymph node on the uterine artery where it crosses the ureter.

prehyoid g., SYN accessory thyroid g.

preputial g.'s [TA], sebaceous glands of the corona and neck of the glans penis, which produce an odoriferous substance called smegma. SYN glandulae preputiales [TA], Tyson g.'s.

prostate g., SYN prostate.

prothoracic g.'s, SYN ecdysial g.'s.

pyloric g.'s [TA], the coiled, tubular glands of the pylorus whose cells secrete mucus. SYN glandulae pyloricae [TA].

racemose g., a g. that has the appearance of a bunch of grapes if viewed as a three-dimensional reconstruction; e.g., a compound acinous or alveolar g.

Rivinus g., SYN sublingual g.

Rosenmüller g., SYN proximal deep inguinal *lymph node.*

saccular g., a single alveolar g.

salivary g. [TA], any of the saliva-secreting exocrine glands of the oral cavity. SEE ALSO major salivary g.'s, minor salivary g.'s. SYN glandula salivaria [TA].

sebaceous g.'s [TA], numerous holocrine glands in the dermis that usually open into the hair follicles and secrete an oily semifluid, sebum. SYN glandulae sebaceae [TA], oil g.'s, sebaceous follicles.

seminal g. [TA], one of two folded, sacculated, glandular structures that is a diverticulum of the ductus deferens; its secretion is one of the components of the semen; it normally does not store spermatozoa as was thought historically. SYN glandula vesiculosa [TA], glandula seminalis☆, seminal vesicle☆, vesicula seminalis☆, gonecyst, gonecystis, seminal capsule.

sentinel g., a single enlarged lymph node in the omentum that may be an indication of an ulcer opposite to it in the greater or lesser curvature of the stomach.

seromucous g., (1) a gland in which some of the secretory cells are serous and some mucous; **(2)** a gland whose cells secrete a fluid intermediate between a watery and a viscous mucoid substance. SYN glandula seromucosa.

serous g., a gland that secretes a watery substance that may or may not contain an enzyme. SYN glandula serosa.

Serres g.'s, epithelial cell rests found in the subepithelial connective tissue in the palate of the newborn, similar to those found in the gingivae.

sexual g., SEE testis, ovary.

Skene g.'s, SYN urethral g.'s of female.

g.'s of small intestine [TA], parallel, tubular, epithelial pits (crypts) with openings at the bases of the intestinal villi; their thin walls are formed by columnar epithelial cells: mostly undifferentiated stem and intermediate cells and an increasing number of goblet cells as the small intestine proceeds distally, all of which migrate out of the glands onto the villi, but also protein- (enzyme-) secreting Paneth cells which remain in the glands. SEE ALSO g.'s of large intestine. SYN glandulae intestini tenuis [TA], crypts of Lieberkühn of small intestine.

solitary g.'s, SYN solitary lymphatic *nodules,* under *nodule.*

sublingual g. [TA], one of two salivary glands in the floor of the mouth beneath the tongue, discharging through the sublingual ducts; most of the secretory units in the human gland are mucus-secreting with serous demilunes. SYN glandula sublingualis [TA], Rivinus g.

submandibular g. [TA], one of two salivary glands in the neck, located in the space bounded by the two bellies of the digastric muscle and the angle of the mandible; it discharges through the submandibular duct; the secretory units are predominantly serous although a few mucous alveoli, some with serous demilunes, occur. SYN glandula submandibularis [TA], maxillary g., submaxillary g.

submaxillary g., SYN submandibular g.

sudoriferous g.'s, SYN sweat g.'s.

suprahyoid g., SYN accessory thyroid g.

suprarenal g. [TA], a flattened, roughly triangular body positioned in relation to the superior end of each kidney but attached primarily to the diaphragmatic crura; it is one of the endocrine (ductless) glands furnishing internal secretions (epinephrine and norepinephrine from the medulla and steroid hormones from the cortex). SYN glandula suprarenalis [TA], adrenal body, adrenal capsule, adrenal g., atrabiliary capsule, epinephros, glandula atrabiliaris, paranephros, suprarenal body, suprarenal capsule.

Suzanne g., a small mucous g. in the floor of the mouth.

sweat g.'s [TA], the coil glands of the skin that secrete the sweat to enable evaporative cooling in a hot environment, or in response to emotion. SYN glandulae sudoriferae [TA], perspiratory g.'s, sudoriferous g.'s.

target g., the effector that functions when stimulated by the internal secretion of another gland or by some other stimulus.

tarsal g.'s [TA], sebaceous glands embedded in the tarsal plate of each eyelid, discharging at the edge of the lid near the posterior border. Their secretions create a lipid barrier along the margin of the eyelids which contains the normal secretions in the conjunctival sac by preventing the watery fluid from spilling over the barrier when the eye is open. SYN glandulae tarsales [TA], meibomian g.'s, palpebral g.'s.

Terson g.'s, SYN conjunctival g.'s.

Theile g.'s, SYN g.'s of biliary mucosa.

thoracic g.'s, SYN ecdysial g.'s.

thymus g., SYN thymus.

thyroid g. [TA], an endocrine (ductless) gland, consisting of irregularly spheroidal follicles, lying in front and to the sides of the upper part of the trachea, and of horseshoe shape, with two lateral lobes connected by a narrow central portion, the isthmus; occasionally an elongated offshoot, the pyramidal lobe, passes upward from the isthmus in front of the trachea. It is supplied by branches from the external carotid and subclavian arteries, and its nerves are derived from the middle cervical and cervicothoracic ganglia of the sympathetic system. It secretes thyroid hormone and calcitonin. SYN glandula thyroidea [TA], thyroid body, thyroidea.

Tiedemann g., SYN greater vestibular g.

tracheal g.'s [TA], numerous tubuloalveolar mixed glands located principally in the submucosa of the trachea; they open into the tracheal lumen through short ducts. SYN glandulae tracheales [TA].

trachoma g.'s, SYN Bruch g.'s.

tubal g.'s of pharyngotympanic tube [TA], glands located principally near the pharyngeal end of the auditory tube. SYN g.'s of auditory tube, g.'s of eustachian tube, glandulae tubariae, mucous g.'s of auditory tube.

tubular g., a g. composed of one or more tubules ending in a blind extremity.

tubuloacinar g., a g. whose secretory elements are elongated acini. SYN acinotubular g.

tubuloalveolar g., a g. that has secretory units of short tubules.

tympanic g., one of the mucous g.'s in the mucosa of the tympanic cavity. SYN tympanic body.

Tyson g.'s, SYN preputial g.'s.

unicellular g., a single secretory cell such as a mucous goblet cell.

urethral g.'s, SEE urethral g.'s of female, urethral g.'s of male.

urethral g.'s of female [TA], numerous mucous g.'s in the wall of the female urethra. SYN glandulae urethrales femininae [TA],

g.'s of the female urethra, Guérin g.'s, paraurethral g.'s, Skene g.'s.

urethral g.'s of male [TA], numerous mucous glands in the wall of the penile urethra. SYN glandulae urethrales masculinae [TA], g.'s of the male urethra, Littré g.'s.

uterine g.'s [TA], numerous simple tubular glands in the uterine mucosa that secrete a glycogen-rich mucous fluid during the luteal phase of the menstrual cycle. SYN glandulae uterinae [TA].

vaginal g., one of the mucous g.'s in the mucous membrane of the vagina.

vascular g., SYN hemal *node*.

ventral g.'s, SYN ecdysial g.'s.

vesical g., one of a number of mucous follicles, not true g.'s, in the mucous membrane near the neck of the bladder.

vestibular g.'s, SEE greater vestibular g., lesser vestibular g.'s.

vulvovaginal g., SYN greater vestibular g.

Waldeyer g.'s, coil g.'s near the margins of the eyelids.

Wasmann g.'s, SYN gastric g.'s.

Weber g.'s, muciparous g.'s at the border of the tongue on either side posteriorly.

Wepfer g.'s, SYN duodenal g.'s.

Wölfler g., SYN accessory thyroid g.

Wolfring g.'s, SEE accessory lacrimal g.'s.

Zeis g.'s, sebaceous g.'s opening into the follicles of the eyelashes.

---

glan·ders (glan′derz). A chronic debilitating disease of horses and other equids, as well as some members of the cat family, caused by *Pseudomonas mallei* and transmissible to humans. It attacks the mucous membranes of the nostrils of the horse, producing an increased and vitiated secretion and discharge of mucus, and enlargement and induration of the glands of the lower jaw. [O. Fr. *glandres,* glands]

glan·des (glan′dēz). Plural of glans.

glan·di·lem·ma (glan-di-lem′ă). The capsule of a gland. [L. *glandula,* gland, + G. *lemma,* sheath]

glan·du·la, pl. **glan·du·lae** (glan′doo-lă, -lē) [TA]. **1** [NA]. SYN gland. **2.** SYN glandule. [L. gland, dim. of *glans,* acorn]

glan′dulae areola′res [TA], SYN areolar *glands,* under *gland.*

g. atrabilia′ris, SYN suprarenal *gland.*

g. basila′ris, SYN pituitary *gland.*

glandulae bronchiales [TA], SYN bronchial *glands,* under *gland.*

glan′dulae bucca′les [TA], SYN buccal *glands,* under *gland.*

g. bulbourethra′lis [TA], SYN bulbourethral *gland.*

glan′dulae cerumino′sae, (1) SYN ceruminous *glands,* under *gland*; **(2)** tubuloalveolar glands of the external auditory meatus believed to be modified apocrine sweat glands; they secrete the waxy substance cerumen.

glan′dulae cervica′les uteri [TA], SYN cervical *glands,* under *gland.*

glan′dulae cilia′res [TA], SYN ciliary *glands,* under *gland.*

glan′dulae circumana′les, SYN circumanal *glands,* under *gland.*

glan′dulae conjunctiva′les [TA], SYN conjunctival *glands,* under *gland.*

glan′dulae cu′tis [TA], SYN cutaneous *glands,* under *gland.*

glandulae ductus biliaris, ✩official alternate term for *glands* of (common) bile duct, under *gland.*

glandulae ductus choledochi [TA], SYN *glands* of (common) bile duct, under *gland.*

glan′dulae duodena′les [TA], SYN duodenal *glands,* under *gland.*

glan′dulae endocri′nae [TA], SYN endocrine *glands,* under *gland.*

glan′dulae esopha′geae, SYN esophageal *glands,* under *gland.*

glan′dulae gas′tricae [TA], SYN gastric *glands,* under *gland.*

glan′dulae glomifor′mes, (1) SYN glomus (2); **(2)** tubular glands of the skin, the blind extremity of which is coiled in the form of a ball or glomerulus; collective term for small eccrine and large apocrine sweat glands.

glan′dulae intestina′les [TA], SYN intestinal *glands,* under *gland.*

glandulae intestini crassi [TA], SYN *glands* of large intestine, under *gland.*

glandulae intestini tenuis [TA], SYN *glands* of small intestine, under *gland.*

glan'dulae labia'les [TA], SYN labial *glands,* under *gland.*

glan'dulae lacrima'les accesso'riae [TA], SYN accessory lacrimal *glands,* under *gland.*

g. lacrima'lis [TA], SYN lacrimal *gland.*

glan'dulae laryn'geae [TA], SYN laryngeal *glands,* under *gland.*

g. lingua'lis ante'rior, SYN anterior lingual *gland.*

g. mamma'ria [TA], SYN mammary *gland.*

glan'dulae mola'res [TA], SYN molar *glands,* under *gland.*

g. muco'sa, SYN mucous *gland.*

glan'dulae muco'sae bilio'sae, SYN *glands* of biliary mucosa, under *gland.*

glan'dulae nasa'les [TA], SYN nasal *glands,* under *gland.*

glan'dulae olfacto'riae [TA], SYN olfactory *glands,* under *gland.*

glan'dulae o'ris [TA], SYN *glands* of mouth, under *gland.*

glan'dulae palati'nae [TA], SYN palatine *glands,* under *gland.*

g. parathyroi'dea [TA], SYN parathyroid *gland.*

g. parotid'ea [TA], SYN parotid *gland.*

g. parotid'ea accesso'ria [TA], SYN accessory parotid *gland.*

g. paro'tis, SYN parotid *gland.*

g. paro'tis accesso'ria, SYN accessory parotid *gland.*

glan'dulae pharyngea'les [TA], SYN pharyngeal *glands,* under *gland.*

g. pinealis [TA], SYN pineal *body.*

g. pituita'ria, ✫official alternate term for pituitary *gland.*

glan'dulae preputia'les [TA], SYN preputial *glands,* under *gland.*

g. prosta'tica, SYN prostate.

glan'dulae pylor'icae [TA], SYN pyloric *glands,* under *gland.*

g. saliva'ria [TA], SYN salivary *gland.*

glandulae salivariae majores [TA], SYN major salivary *glands,* under *gland.*

glandulae salivariae minores [TA], SYN minor salivary *glands,* under *gland.*

glan'dulae seba'ceae [TA], SYN sebaceous *glands,* under *gland.*

g. semina'lis, ✫official alternate term for seminal *gland,* seminal *gland.*

g. seromuco'sa, SYN seromucous *gland.*

g. sero'sa, SYN serous *gland.*

glan'dulae sine duc'tibus, SYN endocrine *glands,* under *gland.*

g. sublingua'lis [TA], SYN sublingual *gland.*

g. submandibula'ris [TA], SYN submandibular *gland.*

glan'dulae sudorif'erae [TA], SYN sweat *glands,* under *gland.*

glan'dulae suprarena'les accesso'riae [TA], SYN accessory suprarenal *glands,* under *gland.*

g. suprarena'lis [TA], SYN suprarenal *gland.*

glan'dulae tarsa'les [TA], SYN tarsal *glands,* under *gland.*

g. thyroi'dea [TA], SYN thyroid *gland.*

g. thyroi'dea accesso'ria, pl. **glan'dulae thyroi'deae accesso'riae** [TA], SYN accessory thyroid *gland.*

glan'dulae trachea'les [TA], SYN tracheal *glands,* under *gland.*

glan'dulae tuba'riae, SYN tubal *glands* of pharyngotympanic tube, under *gland.*

glan'dulae urethra'les femini'nae [TA], SYN urethral *glands* of female, under *gland.*

glan'dulae urethra'les masculi'nae [TA], SYN urethral *glands* of male, under *gland.*

glan'dulae uteri'nae [TA], SYN uterine *glands,* under *gland.*

g. vesiculosa [TA], SYN seminal *gland.*

glan'dulae vestibula'res mino'res [TA], SYN lesser vestibular *glands,* under *gland.*

g. vestibula'ris ma'jor [TA], SYN greater vestibular *gland.*

glan·du·lar (glan'doo-lăr). Relating to a gland. SYN glandulous.

glan·dule (glan'dool). A small gland. SYN glandula (2) [TA]. [L. *glandula*]

glan·du·lous (glan'doo-lŭs). SYN glandular.

glans, pl. **glan·des** (glanz, glan'dēz) [TA]. A conical acorn-shaped structure. [L. acorn]

g. clitor'idis [TA], SYN g. of clitoris.

g. of clitoris [TA], a small mass of highly-sensitized erectile tissue capping the body of the clitoris. SYN g. clitoridis [TA].

g. pe'nis [TA], the conical expansion of the corpus spongiosum which forms the head of the penis. SYN balanus.

glan·u·lar (glan'ū-lar). Pertaining to the glans penis. [irreg. fr. *glans,* by analogy with *glandular*]

Glanzmann, Eduard, Swiss clinician, 1887–1959. SEE G. *disease, thrombasthenia.*

gla·phen·ine (gla-fen'ēn). An anti-inflammatory agent with analgesic properties.

glare (glār). A sensation caused by brightness within the visual field that is sufficiently greater than the luminance to which the eyes are adapted; results in annoyance, discomfort, and decreased visual performance.

blinding g., g. resulting from excessive illumination. SYN veiling g.

dazzling g., g. produced by excessive illumination in the peripheral field.

peripheral g., g. occurring when the surrounding brightness is greater than the brightness of the object of attention.

specular g., g. arising from specularly reflected light.

veiling g., SYN blinding g.

gla·rom·e·ter (glā-rom'ĕ-ter). An instrument that measures sensitivity to central glare from the headlights of an approaching vehicle.

Glaser (Glaserius), Johann H., Swiss anatomist, 1629–1675. SEE glaserian *artery;* glaserian *fissure.*

gla·se·ri·an (gla-ser'ē-an). Relating to or described by Johann H. Glaser.

Glasgow, William C., U.S. physician, 1845–1907. SEE G. *sign.*

Glasgow co·ma scale. SEE coma *scale.*

glass (glas). A transparent substance composed of silica and oxides of various bases. [A.S. *glaes*]

cover g., a thin g. disk or plate covering an object examined under the microscope. SYN coverslip.

Crookes g., a spectacle lens combined with metallic oxides to absorb ultraviolet or infrared rays.

crown g., a compound of lime, potash, alumina, and silica; commonly used in lenses; has a low dispersion (52.2) relative to index of refraction (1.523).

cupping g., a g. vessel, from which the air has been exhausted by heat or a special suction apparatus, formerly applied to the skin in order to draw blood to the surface. SEE ALSO cupping, cup. SYN cup (2).

flint g., g. that contains lead oxide instead of lime to increase index of refraction; used in reading segments of fused bifocal lenses.

object g., SYN objective (1).

quartz g., a transparent, colorless crystal, made by fusing pure quartz sand, which transmits ultraviolet light.

soluble g., a silicate of potassium or sodium, soluble in hot water but solid at ordinary temperatures; used for fixed dressings. SYN water g.

vita g., a specially prepared g. that is transparent to ultraviolet rays of the spectrum.

water g., SYN soluble g.

Wood g., a g. containing nickel oxide, used in Wood lamp.

glass·es (glas'ez). **1.** SYN spectacles. **2.** Lenses for correcting refractive errors in the eyes.

Glauber, Johann R., German chemist, 1604–1670. SEE G. *salt.*

glau·cine (glaw'sēn). *d*-Form prevalent in nature. Found in *Glaucium flavum,* (*G. luteum scop.*), *Papaveraceae* and in *Dicentra* and *Corydalis* species, family *Fumariceae.* Antitussive agent. SYN boldine dimethyl ether.

glau·co·ma (glaw-kō'mă). A disease of the eye characterized by increased intraocular pressure, excavation, and atrophy of the optic nerve; produces defects in the field of vision. [G. *glaukōma,* opacity of the crystalline lens, fr. *glaukos,* bluish green]

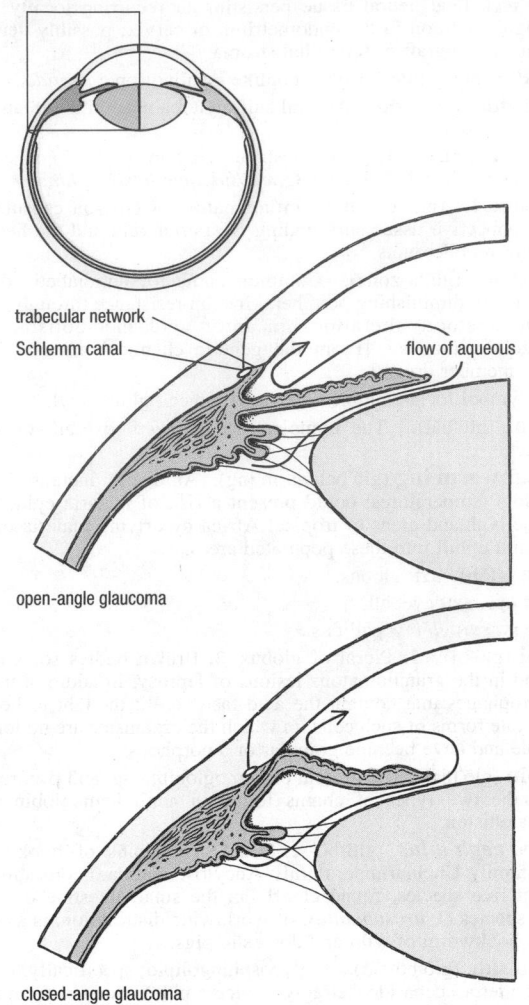

trabecular network
Schlemm canal
flow of aqueous

open-angle glaucoma

closed-angle glaucoma

glaucoma

absolute g., the final stage of blindness in g.

acute g., SYN angle-closure g.

angle-closure g., primary g. in which contact of the iris with the peripheral cornea excludes aqueous humor from the trabecular drainage meshwork. SYN acute g., closed-angle g., narrow-angle g.

aphakic g., g. following cataract removal.

chronic g., SYN open-angle g.

α-chymotrypsin-induced g., transient secondary g. following the use of α-chymotrypsin in cataract extraction.

closed-angle g., SYN angle-closure g.

combined g., g. with angle-closure and open-angle mechanisms in the same eye.

compensated g., SYN open-angle g.

congenital g., SYN buphthalmia.

corticosteroid-induced g., g. caused by a hereditary predisposition in which local instillation of eyedrops containing corticosteroid causes increased intraocular pressure.

g. ful′minans, acute angle-closure g. rapidly followed by blindness.

ghost cell g., g. occurring after vitrectomy, arising from erythrocyte membranes blocking outflow channels of aqueous humor.

hemorrhagic g., secondary g. after formation of new blood vessels in the iris.

hypersecretion g., g. caused by excessive formation of the aqueous humor.

low-tension g., optic nerve atrophy and excavation with typical field defects of g. but without abnormal increase in intraocular pressure. SYN normal-tension g.

malignant g., secondary g. caused by forward displacement of the iris and lens, obliterating the anterior chamber; usually follows a filtering operation for primary glaucoma.

narrow-angle g., SYN angle-closure g.

neovascular g., g. occurring in rubeosis iridis.

normal-tension g., SYN low-tension g.

open-angle g., primary g. in which the aqueous humor has free access to the trabecular meshwork. SYN chronic g., compensated g., simple g., g. simplex.

phacogenic g., SYN phacomorphic g.

phacolytic g., g. secondary to hypermature cataract and occlusion of the trabecular drainage meshwork by lens material.

phacomorphic g., secondary g. caused by either excessive size or spherical shape of the lens. SYN phacogenic g.

pigmentary g., g. associated with erosion of pigment from the posterior iris, and with an accumulation of pigment particles in the trabecular meshwork.

pseudoexfoliative g., g. occurring in association with widespread deposition of cellular organelles on the lens capsule, ocular blood vessels, iris, and ciliary body. SEE ALSO *pseudoexfoliation* of lens capsule.

pupillary block g., g. secondary to failure of the aqueous humor to pass through the pupil to the anterior chamber.

secondary g., g. occurring as a sequel of preexisting ocular disease or injury.

simple g., g. sim′plex, SYN open-angle g.

glau·co·ma·to·cy·clit·ic (glaw-kō′mă-tō-si-klit′ik). Denoting increased intraocular pressure associated with evidences of cyclitis. SEE ALSO glaucomatocyclitic *crisis.*

ⓘ glau·co·ma·tous (glaw-kō′mă-tŭs). Relating to glaucoma.

glau·co·su·ria (glaw′kō-soo′rē-ă). Obsolete term for indicanuria. [G. *glaukos,* bluish green, + *ouron,* urine]

GLC Abbreviation for gas-liquid *chromatography.*

Glc, GlcA, GlcN, GlcNAc, GlcUA Symbols for the radicals of D-glucose, gluconic and glucuronic acid, glucosamine, *N*-acetylglucosamine, and glucuronic acid, respectively.

Gleason, Donald F., U.S. pathologist, *1920. SEE G. tumor *grade, score.*

gleet (glēt). Obsolete term for a chronic urethral discharge following gonorrhea. [M.E. *glet,* slime, fr. O.Fr. *glette,* fr. L. *glittus,* sticky]

Glenn. William W., *1914. SEE Glenn *shunt.*

Glenner, George B., U.S. pathologist and histologist, *1927. SEE G.-Lillie *stain* for pituitary.

gle·no·hu·mer·al (glē′nō-hū′mer-ăl). Relating to the glenoid cavity and the humerus.

gle·noid (glē′noyd, glen′oyd). Resembling a socket; denoting the articular depression of the scapula entering into the formation of the shoulder joint. [G. *glēnoeidēs,* fr. *glēnē,* pupil of eye, socket of joint, honeycomb, + *eidos,* appearance]

Gley, Marcel E., French physiologist, 1857–1930. SEE G. *glands,* under *gland.*

glia (glī′ă). SYN neuroglia. [G. glue]

gli·a·cyte (glī′ă-sīt). A neuroglia cell. SEE neuroglia. [G. *glia,* glue, + *kytos,* cell]

gli·a·din (glī′ă-din). A class of protein, separable from wheat and rye glutens; a member of the prolamins (proline-rich proteins), which are insoluble in water, absolute alcohol, and neutral solvents, but soluble in 50–90% alcohol.

gli·al (glī′ăl). Pertaining to glia or neuroglia.

gli·cla·zide (glī′klă-zīd). A sulfonylurea oral antidiabetic agent used for the treatment of type II diabetes mellitus. The drug releases endogenous insulin from beta cells of the islands of Langerhans located in the pancreas; resembles glipizide and tolbutamide.

gl

glide (glīd). A smooth, or effortless, continuous movement.

mandibular g., the side-to-side, protrusive, and intermediate movement of the mandible occurring when the teeth or other occluding surfaces are in contact.

glide-wire (glīd′wīr). A hydrophilic or lubricated guidewire, generally used in the urinary tract. SEE ALSO guidewire.

⟁**glio-.** Glue, gluelike (relating specifically to the neuroglia). [G. *glia,* glue]

gli·o·blast (glī′ō-blast). An early neural cell developing, like the neuroblast, from the early ependymal cell of the neural tube; gives rise to neuroglial and ependymal cells, astrocytes, and oligodendrocytes. SEE ALSO spongioblast. [glio- + G. *blastos,* germ]

🔲**gli·o·blas·to·ma multiforme** (glī′ō-blas-tō′mă). A glioma consisting chiefly of undifferentiated anaplastic cells of astrocytic origin that show marked nuclear pleomorphism, necrosis, and vascular endothelial proliferation; frequently, tumor cells are arranged radially about an irregular focus of necrosis; these neoplasms grow rapidly, invade extensively, and occur most frequently in the cerebrum of adults. [G. *glia,* glue, + *blastos,* germ, + *-oma,* tumor]

giant cell g. m., a histologic form of glioblastoma with large, often multinucleated, bizarre, tumor cells. SYN giant cell monstrocellular sarcoma of Zülch, gigantocellular glioma.

gli·o·blas·to·sis ce·re·bri. SYN *gliomatosis* cerebri.

gli·o·ma (glī-ō′mă). Any neoplasm derived from one of the various types of cells that form the interstitial tissue of the brain, spinal cord, pineal gland, posterior pituitary gland, and retina. [G. *glia,* glue, + *-oma,* tumor]

brainstem g., a g., generally an astrocytoma, arising in the medulla, pons, or midbrain.

gigantocellular g., SYN giant cell *glioblastoma multiforme.*

mixed g., a glioma composed of two or more malignant elements, most frequently astrocytoma and oligodendroglioma.

nasal g., term for a lesion that is probably not a true neoplasm, but a teratoma consisting of glial tissue with reactive astrocytes, ganglionic neurons, and ependymal cells in small nodules at the dorsum of the nose, often with intracranial connections.

g. of optic chiasm, a slow-growing tumor, usually an astrocytoma, of the optic chiasm in children.

optic nerve g., a g., generally an astrocytoma, involving the optic nerve or chiasm.

g. of the spinal cord, a glial tumor of the spinal cord, commonly an ependymoma; neoplasms of the spinal cord are relatively rare, but g.'s constitute approximately one-fourth of the total.

telangiectatic g., g. telangiecto′des, a g. in which the stroma has numerous, conspicuous, frequently dilated small blood vessels and capillaries, as well as large, endothelium-rimmed lakes of blood.

gli·o·ma·to·sis (glī-ō-mă-tō′sis). Neoplastic growth of neuroglial cells in the brain or spinal cord; the term is used especially with reference to a relatively large neoplasm or to multiple foci. SYN neurogliomatosis.

g. cerebri, (glī′ō-blas-tō′sis ser′ĕ-brī), a diffuse intracranial neoplasm of astrocytic origin. SYN astrocytosis cerebri, glioblastosis cerebri.

gli·o·ma·tous (glī-ō′mă-tŭs). Pertaining to or characterized by a glioma.

gli·o·myx·o·ma (glī′ō-mik-sō′mă). A myxoma that contains a considerable amount of proliferating glial cells and fibers.

gli·o·neu·ro·ma (glī′ō-noo-rō′mă). A ganglioneuroma derived from neurons, with numerous glial cells and fibers in the matrix.

gli·o·sar·co·ma (glī′ō-sar-kō′mă). A glioblastoma multiforme with an associated malignant mesenchymal component. Sometimes used as a term for a malignant neoplasm derived from connective tissue (e.g., that associated with blood vessels in the brain) in which there are proliferating glial cells.

gli·o·sis (glī-ō′sis). Overgrowth of the astrocytes in an area of damage in the brain or spinal cord.

isomorphous g., a gliosis in which there is a regular and ordered arrangement of glial fibers.

piloid g., an area of chronic, reactive astrocytosis composed of thin, hairlike cells in vaguely parallel array.

g. u′teri, fetal neural tissue persisting or recurring locally as a benign condition in the endometrium or cervix; possibly derived from a homograft of fetal glial stroma.

GLIP Abbreviation for glucagonlike insulinotropic *peptide.*

glip·i·zide (glip′i-zīd). An oral sulfonylurea used in the treatment of type II diabetes.

Glisson, Francis, English physician, anatomist, physiologist and pathologist, 1597–1677. SEE G. *capsule, cirrhosis, sphincter.*

glis·so·ni·tis (glis-ŏ-nī′tis). Inflammation of Glisson capsule, or the connective tissue surrounding the portal vein and the hepatic artery and bile ducts.

glitazones (glī′ta-zonz). Common name for antidiabetic drugs that act by diminishing peripheral insulin resistance through poorly understood alterations in fatty acid metabolism. SYN thiazolidinediones. [From the generic chemical names of the class member drugs.]

Gln Symbol for glutamine or its acyl radical, glutaminyl.

glob·al (glō′băl). The complete, generalized, overall, or total aspect.

glo·bal warm·ing (glō′bal warm′ing). An overall increase in the world's temperatures; could present a risk of malaria epidemics in the highland areas of tropical Africa by driving malaria transmission uphill into these populated areas.

globe (glōb). SYN globus.

g. of eye, SYN eyeball.

pale g., SYN *globus* pallidus.

glo·bi (glō′bī). **1.** Plural of globus. **2.** Brown bodies sometimes found in the granulomatous lesions of leprosy, in addition to the macrophages that contain the acid-fast bacilli; thought to be degenerate forms of such cells, in which the organisms are no longer viable and have become granular or amorphous.

glo·bin (glō′bin). The protein of hemoglobin; α-g. and β-g. represent the two types of chains found in adult hemoglobin. SYN hematohiston.

Glo·bo·ceph·a·lus (glō-bō-sef′ă-lŭs). A genus of hookworm (subfamily Uncinariinae, family Ancylostomatidae) consisting of about five species, found chiefly in the small intestine of pigs. The species G. *urosubalatus,* of worldwide distribution, is a common hookworm of wild and domestic pigs.

glo·bo·side (glō′bō-sīd). A glycosphingolipid; specifically, a ceramide tetrasaccharide (tetraglycosylceramide), isolated from kidney and erythrocytes; accumulates in individuals with Sandhoff disease.

glo·bo·tri·a·o·syl·cer·a·mide (glō′bō-trī-ă-ō-sil-ser-a-mīd). A sphingolipid containing three sugar moieties that accumulates in individuals with Fabry disease. SYN trihexosylceramide.

glob·ule (glob′ūl). **1.** A small spherical body of any kind. **2.** A fat droplet in milk. SYN globulus. [L. *globulus,* dim. of *globus,* a ball]

dentin g., calcospherites formed by calcification or mineralization of the dentin occurring in globular areas.

Morgagni g.'s, vesicles beneath the capsule and between lens fibers in early cataract. SYN Morgagni spheres.

polar g., SYN polar *body.*

glob·u·lif·er·ous (glob-ū-lif′er-ŭs). Containing globules or corpuscles, especially red blood cells. [L. *globulus,* globule, + *fero,* to bear]

glob·u·lin (glob′ū-lin). Name for a family of proteins precipitated from plasma (or serum) by half-saturation with ammonium sulfate (i.e., addition of an equal volume of saturated ammonium sulfate). G.'s may be further fractionated by solubility, electrophoresis, ultracentrifugation, and other separation methods into many subgroups. The main groups are α-, β-, and γ-g., which contains most antibodies. [L. *globulus,* globule]

accelerator g. (AcG, ac-g), g. in serum that promotes the conversion of prothrombin to thrombin in the presence of thromboplastin and ionized calcium. SEE *factor* V_a, *factor* V, serum accelerator g.

antihemophilic g. (AHG), (1) SYN *factor* VIII; **(2)** SYN human antihemophilic *factor.*

antihemophilic g. A, SYN *factor* VIII.

antihemophilic g. B, SYN *factor* IX.

antihuman g., serum from a rabbit or other animal previously immunized with purified human g. to prepare antibodies directed against human immunoglobulin, some of which may be used in the direct and indirect Coombs tests. SYN Coombs serum.

antilymphocyte g. (ALG), SYN antilymphocyte *serum.*

β₁c g., globulin fraction of serum that contains the third component (C3) of complement. SEE *component* of complement.

chickenpox immune g. (human), g. fraction of serum from persons recently recovered from herpes zoster infection; used to prevent infection of high-risk children. SYN chickenpox immunoglobulin.

corticosteroid-binding g. (CBG), SYN transcortin.

gonadal steroid-binding g. (GBG), a protein that transports 65% of the testosterone in plasma. SYN sex steroid-binding g.

human gamma g., a preparation of the proteins of liquid human serum, containing the antibodies (primarily IgG) of normal adults; it is obtained from pooled liquid human serum from a number of donors and may be prepared by precipitation under controlled conditions of pH, ionic strength, and temperature. SYN human normal immunoglobulin.

immune serum g., a sterile solution of g.'s that contains many antibodies normally present in adult human blood; a passive immunizing agent frequently used for prophylaxis against hepatitis A and for treatment of Kawasaki disease, idiopathic thrombocytopenic purpura, and some immunodeficiencies.

measles immune g. (human), a sterile solution of g.'s derived from the blood plasma of adult human donors with elevated titers to measles: it is prepared from immune serum g. that complies with the measles antibody reference standard; a passive immunizing agent. SYN measles immunoglobulin.

pertussis immune g., a sterile solution of g.'s derived from the plasma of adult human donors who have been immunized with pertussis vaccine; used both prophylactically and therapeutically. SYN pertussis immunoglobulin.

plasma accelerator g., SYN *factor* V.

poliomyelitis immune g. (human), a sterile solution of g.'s that contains antibodies normally present in adult human blood with elevated titers to poliomyelitis and confers temporary but significant protection against paralytic polio. SYN poliomyelitis immunoglobulin.

rabies immune g. (human), g. fraction of pooled plasma of high anti-rabies virus titer from immunized persons. SYN rabies immunoglobulin.

RH₀(D) immune g., a g. fraction of antibody, derived from human donors, specific for the most common antigen, Rh₀(D), of the Rh group; used to prevent Rh-sensitization of an Rh-negative woman after delivery of an Rh-positive fetus. SYN anti-D immunoglobulin, Rh₀(D) immunoglobulin.

serum accelerator g., a substance in serum that accelerates the conversion of prothrombin to thrombin in the presence of thromboplastin and calcium; produced by the action of traces of thrombin upon plasma accelerator g.

sex hormone-binding g. (SHBG), a plasma β-g., produced by the liver, that binds testosterone and, with a weaker affinity, estrogen; serum levels of SHBG in women are twice the levels seen in men; serum concentrations are increased in certain types of liver disease and in hyperthyroidism but are decreased with advancing age, by androgens, and in hypothyroidism. SYN testosterone-estrogen-binding g.

sex steroid-binding g., SYN gonadal steroid-binding g.

specific immune g. (human), g. fraction of pooled serums (or plasma) selected for high titer of antibodies specific for a particular antigen, or from persons specifically immunized.

testosterone-estrogen-binding g., SYN sex hormone-binding g.

tetanus immune g., a sterile solution of g.'s derived from the blood plasma of adult human donors who have been immunized with tetanus toxoid; a passive immunizing agent. SYN tetanus immunoglobulin.

thyroxine-binding g. (TBG), an α-globulin of blood with a strong binding affinity for thyroxine; triiodothyronine is bound to

it much less firmly; a deficiency or excess of this protein may occur as a rare benign X-linked disorder. SYN thyroxine-binding protein (1).

zoster immune g., a g. fraction of pooled plasma from individuals who have recovered from herpes zoster; used prophylactically for immunosuppressed children exposed to varicella and therapeutically to ameliorate varicella infection.

glob·u·li·nu·ria (glob′ū-li-noo′rē-ă). The excretion of globulin in the urine, usually, if not always, in association with serum albumin.

glob·u·lus (glob′ū-lŭs). SYN globule. [L.]

glo·bus, pl. **glo·bi** (glō′bŭs, -bī). **1** [TA]. A round body; ball. **2.** SEE globi. SYN globe. [L.]

g. hyster′icus, difficulty in swallowing; a sensation as of a ball in the throat or as if the throat were compressed; a symptom of conversion *disorder.*

g. ma′jor, SYN *head* of epididymis.

g. mi′nor, SYN *tail* of epididymis.

g. pal′lidus [TA], the inner and lighter gray portion of the lentiform nucleus; composed of a lateral segment (g. pallidus lateralis [TA]) and a medial segment (g. pallidus medialis [TA]) separated by a vertically oriented lamina of fibers, the lamina medullaris medialis [TA] (medial medullary lamina [TA]). The medial segment may also be incompletely divided into a lateral part [TA] (pars lateralis [TA]) and a medial part [TA] (pars medialis [TA]) by the accessory medullary lamina [TA] (lamina medullaris accessoria [TA]). SEE ALSO paleostriatum. SYN pallidum [TA], pale globe.

glo·mal (glō′măl). Relating to or involving a glomus.

glo·man·gi·o·ma (glō-man-jē-ō′mă). A variant of glomus *tumor,* characterized often by multiple tumors resembling cavernous hemangioma q.v., lined by glomus cells. SEE ALSO glomus.

glo·man·gi·o·sis (glō-man-jē-ō′sis). The occurrence of multiple complexes of small vascular channels, each resembling a glomus.

pulmonary g., g. occurring within small pulmonary arteries in severe pulmonary hypertension and congenital heart disease.

glome (glōm). SYN glomus.

glo·mec·to·my (glō-mek′tō-mē). Excision of a glomus tumor. [L. *glomus* + G. *ektomē,* cutting out]

glom·era (glom′er-ă). Plural of glomus.

glom·era aor·ti·ca. ✭official alternate term for paraaortic *bodies,* under *body.*

glo·mer·u·lar (glō-mār′ū-lăr). Relating to or affecting a glomerulus or the glomeruli. SYN glomerulose.

glom·er·ule (glom′er-ūl). SYN glomerulus.

glo·mer·u·li·tis (glō-mār′ū-lī′tis). Inflammation of a glomerulus, specifically of the renal glomeruli, as in glomerulonephritis.

glo·mer·u·lo·ne·phri·tis (glō-mār′ū-lō-nef-rī′tis). Renal disease characterized by diffuse inflammatory changes in glomeruli that are not the acute response to infection of the kidneys. SYN glomerular nephritis. [glomerulus + G. *nephros,* kidney, + *-itis,* inflammation]

acute g., g. that frequently occurs as a late complication of pharyngitisor or skin infection, due to a nephritogenic strain of β-hemolytic streptococci, characterized by abrupt onset of hematuria, edema of the face, oliguria, and variable azotemia and hypertension; the renal glomeruli usually show cellular proliferation or infiltration by polymorphonuclear leukocytes. SYN acute hemorrhagic g., acute nephritis, acute poststreptococcal g.

acute crescentic g., SYN rapidly progressive g.

acute hemorrhagic g., SYN acute g.

acute poststreptococcal g., SYN acute g.

anti–basement membrane g., g. resulting from anti-basement membrane antibodies, characterized by smooth linear deposits of IgG and C3 along glomerular capillary walls; includes rapidly progressive g. and g. in Goodpasture syndrome.

Berger focal g., SYN focal g.

chronic g., g. that presents with persisting proteinuria, chronic renal failure, and hypertension, of insidious onset or as a late sequel of acute g.; the kidneys are symmetrically contracted and

gl

granular, with scarring and loss of glomeruli and the presence of tubular atrophy and interstitial fibrosis. SYN chronic nephritis.

diffuse g., g. affecting most of the renal glomeruli; it may lead to azotemia.

exudative g., g. with infiltration of glomeruli by polymorphonuclear leukocytes, occurring in acute g.

focal g., g. affecting a small proportion of renal glomeruli which commonly presents with hematuria and may be associated with acute upper respiratory infection in young males, not usually due to streptococci; associated with IgA deposits in the glomerular mesangium and may also be associated with systemic disease, as in Henoch-Schönlein purpura. SYN Berger disease, Berger focal g., focal nephritis, IgA nephropathy.

focal embolic g., g. associated with subacute bacterial endocarditis, frequently producing microscopic hematuria without azotemia.

hypocomplementemic g., SYN membranoproliferative g.

immune complex g., immune complexes are deposited in the renal glomerulus where they bind complement and initiate an inflammatory process attracting neutrophils and macrophages resulting in an alteration of the basement layer of the kidney. The disease state can lead to ultimate destruction of the glomerulus and renal failure.

lobular g., SYN membranoproliferative g.

local g., SYN segmental g.

membranoproliferative g., chronic g. characterized by mesangial cell proliferation, increased lobular separation of glomeruli, thickening of glomerular capillary walls and increased mesangial matrix, and low serum levels of complement; occurs mainly in older children, with a variably slow progressive course, episodes of hematuria or edema, and hypertension. It is classified into three types: type 1, the commonest, in which there are subendothelial electron-dense deposits; type 2, dense-deposit disease, in which the lamina densa is greatly thickened by extremely electron-dense material; type 3, in which there are both subendothelial and subepithelial deposits. SYN hypocomplementemic g., lobular g., mesangiocapillary g.

membranous g., g. characterized by diffuse thickening of glomerular capillary basement membranes, due in part to subepithelial deposits of immunoglobulins separated by spikes of basement membrane material, and clinically by an insidious onset of the nephrotic syndrome and failure of disappearance of proteinuria; the disease is most commonly idiopathic but may be secondary to malignant tumors, drugs, infections, or systemic lupus erythematosus.

mesangial proliferative g., g. characterized clinically by the nephrotic syndrome and histologically by diffuse glomerular increases in endocapillary and mesangial cells and in mesangial matrix; in some cases, there are mesangial deposits of IgM and complement. SYN diffuse mesangial proliferation, IgM nephropathy.

mesangiocapillary g., SYN membranoproliferative g.

proliferative g., g. with hypercellularity of glomeruli due to proliferation of endothelial or mesangial cells, occurring in acute g. and membranoproliferative g.

rapidly progressive g., g. usually presenting insidiously, without preceding streptococcal infection, with increasing renal failure leading to uremia within a few months; at autopsy the kidneys are normal in size, numerous glomerular capsular epithelial crescents are present, and antiglomerular basement membrane antibodies are frequently found. SYN acute crescentic g.

segmental g., g. affecting only part of a glomerulus or glomeruli. SYN local g.

subacute g., undesirable term for g. with proteinuria, hematuria and azotemia persisting for many weeks; renal changes are variable, including those of rapidly progressive and membranoproliferative g. SYN subacute nephritis.

glo·mer·u·lop·a·thy (glō-mār-ū-lop'ă-thē). Glomerular disease of any type. [glomerulus + G. *pathos*, suffering]

focal sclerosing g., focal, segmental glomerulosclerosis reported in adults and children with normal serum complement, progressing to chronic glomerulonephritis.

glo·mer·u·lo·scle·ro·sis (glo-mār'ū-lō-sklĕ-rō'sis). Hyaline deposits or scarring within the renal glomeruli, a degenerative process occurring in association with renal arteriosclerosis or diabetes. SYN glomerular sclerosis. [glomerulus + G. *sklērōsis*, hardness]

diabetic g., proteinuria and ultimately, renal failure occuring in long standing diabetes and characterized by rounded hyaline or laminated nodules in the periphery of the glomeruli with capillary basement membrane thickening and increased mesangial matrix. SYN intercapillary g.

focal segmental g., segmental collapse of glomerular capillaries with thickened basement membranes and increased mesangial matrix; seen in some glomeruli of patients with nephrotic syndrome or mesangial proliferative glomerulonephritis.

intercapillary g., SYN diabetic g.

glo·mer·u·lose (glō-mār'ū-lōs). SYN glomerular.

glo·mer·u·lus, pl. **glo·mer·u·li** (glō-mār'ū-lŭs, -ū-lī). **1.** A plexus of capillaries. **2.** A tuft formed of capillary loops at the beginning of each nephric tubule in the kidney; this tuft with its capsule (Bowman capsule) constitutes the corpusculum renis (malpighian body). SYN malpighian g., malpighian tuft. **3.** The twisted secretory portion of a sweat gland. **4.** A cluster of dendritic ramifications and axon terminals forming a complex synaptic relationship and surrounded by a glial sheath. SYN glomerule. [Mod. L. dim. of L. *glomus*, a ball of yarn]

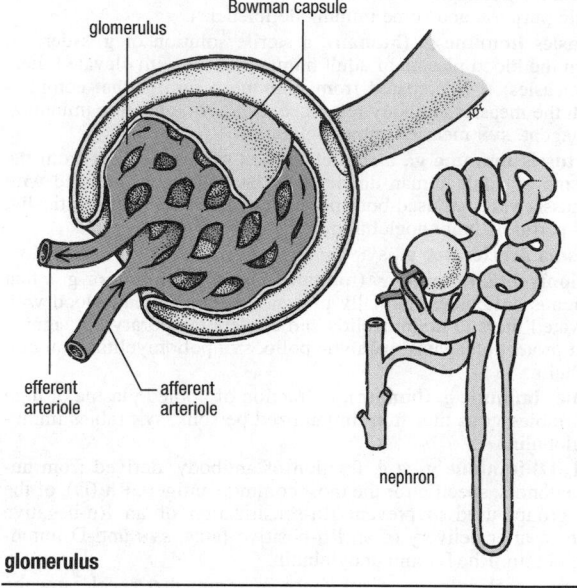

glomerulus

juxtamedullary g., a g. close to the medullary border.

malpighian g., SYN glomerulus (2).

g. of mesonephros, one of the tufts of capillary vessels within the mesonephros derived from a lateral branch of the primary aorta; each g. is connected to a tubule.

olfactory g., one of the small spherical territories in the olfactory bulb in which dendrites of mitral and tufted cells synapse with axons of olfactory receptor cells.

g. of pronephros, one of the tufts of capillary vessels in the pronephros derived from a lateral branch of the aorta.

glo·mus, pl. **glom·era** (glō'mŭs, glom'er-ă). **1** [TA]. A small globular body. **2.** A highly organized arteriolovenular anastomosis forming a tiny nodular focus in the nailbed, pads of the fingers and toes, ears, hands, and feet and many other organs of the body. The afferent arteriole enters the connective tissue capsule of the g., becomes devoid of an internal elastic membrane, and develops a relatively thick epithelioid muscular wall and small lumen; the anastomosis may be branched and convoluted, richly innervated with sympathetic and myelinated nerves, and connected with a short, thin-walled vein that drains into a periglomic vein and then into one of the veins of the skin. The g. functions as a shunt- or bypass-regulating mechanism in the flow of blood, temperature, and conservation of heat in the part as well as in the indirect control of the blood pressure and other functions of the circulatory system. SYN glandulae glomiformes (1), glomiform glands, glomus body. SYN glome. [L. *glomus,* a ball]

aortic glomera, ☆official alternate term for paraaortic *bodies,* under *body.*

g. aorticum [TA], SYN paraaortic *bodies,* under *body.*

g. carot′icum [TA], SYN carotid *body.*

choroid g., SYN choroid *enlargement.*

g. choroi′deum [TA], SYN choroid *enlargement.*

g. coccy′geum, SYN coccygeal *body.*

intravagal g., a minute collection of chemoreceptor cells on the auricular branch of the vagus nerve. A tumor of this g. may cause deafness and tinnitus. SYN g. intravagale.

g. intravaga′le, SYN intravagal g.

jugular g., a microscopic collection of chemoreceptor tissue in the adventitia of the jugular bulb; a tumor of this g. may cause paralysis of the vocal cords, attacks of dizziness, blackouts, and nystagmus. SYN g. jugulare.

g. jugula′re, SYN jugular g.

g. pulmona′le, SYN pulmonary g.

pulmonary g., a structure similar to the carotid body, found in relation to the pulmonary artery. SYN g. pulmonale.

⌂**gloss-.** SEE glosso-.

glos·sa (glos′ă). SYN tongue (1). [G.]

glos·sag·ra (glos-ag′ră). Glossalgia of gouty origin. [gloss- + G. *agra,* a seizure]

glos·sal (glos′ăl). SYN lingual (1).

glos·sal·gia (glos-al′jē-ă). SYN glossodynia. [gloss- + G. *algos,* pain]

glos·sec·to·my (glo-sek′tō-mē). Resection or amputation of the tongue. SYN elinguation, glossosteresis. [gloss- + G. *ektomē,* excision]

Glos·si·na (glo-sī′nă). A genus of bloodsucking Diptera (tsetse flies) confined to Africa; they serve as vectors of the pathogenic trypanosomes that cause various forms of African sleeping sickness in humans and in domestic and wild animals. [G. *glōssa,* tongue]

G. mor′sitans, a species originally thought to be the sole transmitter of *Trypanosoma brucei brucei,* the cause of nagana in central Africa; this species transmits this disease in some regions, but it is not the sole or even always the principal transmitting agent; it is the vector of *T. brucei rhodesiense,* one of the pathogenic agents of East African, Rhodesian, or acute sleeping sickness.

G. pallid′ipes, a species that is the principal transmitter of nagana; it also transmits *Trypanosoma brucei rhodesiense.*

G. palpa′lis, a species of *G.* that transmits *Trypanosoma brucei gambiense,* one of the pathogenic parasites of West African, Gambian, or chronic sleeping sickness.

glos·si·tis (glo-sī′tis). Inflammation of the tongue. [gloss- + G. *-itis,* inflammation]

g. area′ta exfoliati′va, SYN geographic *tongue.*

atrophic g., an erythematous, edematous, and painful tongue which appears smooth due to loss of the filiform and sometimes the fungiform papillae secondary to certain nutritional deficiencies, especially B-vitamin deficencies, as seen in pellagra, thiamin deficiency, and disorders such as pernicious anemia (Hunter or Moeller g.). SYN bald tongue.

benign migratory g., SYN geographic *tongue.*

g. desic′cans, a painful affection of the tongue, of unknown origin, in which the surface becomes raw and fissured.

Hunter g., SEE atrophic g.

median rhomboid g., an asymptomatic, ovoid or rhomboid, macular, erythematous area with absence of papillae on the median portion of the dorsum of the tongue just anterior to the circumvallate papillae; thought to represent a persistent tuberculum impar.

Moeller g., SEE atrophic g.

⌂**glosso-, gloss-.** Language; corresponds to L. linguo-. Cf. linguo-. [G. *glōssa,* tongue]

glos·so·cele (glos′ō-sēl). Swelling and protrusion of the tongue from the mouth. SEE ALSO macroglossia. [glosso- + G. *kēlē,* tumor, hernia]

glos·so·cin·es·thet·ic (glos′ō-sin-es-thet′ik). SYN glossokinesthetic.

glos·so·don·to·tro·pism (glos-ō-don′tō-trō-pizm). A manifestation of tension or anxiety in which the tongue is attracted to the teeth or to dental faults. [glosso- + G. *odous (odont-),* tooth, + *tropē,* a turning]

glos·so·dy·na·mom·e·ter (glos′ō-dī-nă-mom′ĕ-ter). An apparatus for estimating the contractile force of the tongue muscles. [glosso- + G. *dynamis,* power, + *metron,* measure]

glos·so·dyn·ia (glos′ō-din′ē-ă). A condition characterized by burning or painful tongue. SYN burning tongue, glossalgia, glossopyrosis. [glosso- + G. *odynē,* pain]

glos·so·dyn·i·o·tro·pism (glos-ō-din′ē-ō-trō-pizm). Apparent satisfaction from subjecting the tongue to a pain-inducing dental fault; considered by some to be a masochistic behavior or manifestation. [glosso- + G. *odynē,* pain, + *tropē,* a turning]

glos·so·ep·i·glot·tic, glos·so·ep·i·glot·tid·e·an (glos′ō-ep-i-glot′ik, glos′ō-ep-i-glo-tid′ē-an). Relating to the tongue and the epiglottis.

glos·so·graph (glos′ō-graf). An instrument for recording the movements of the tongue in speaking. [glosso- + G. *graphō,* to write]

glos·so·hy·al (glos-ō-hī′ăl). SYN hyoglossal.

glos·so·kin·es·thet·ic (glos′ō-kin-es-thet′ik). Denoting the subjective sensation of the movements of the tongue. SYN glossocinesthetic. [glosso- + G. *kinēsis,* movement, + *aisthētikos,* perceptive]

glos·so·la·lia (glos-ō-lā′lē-ă). Rarely used term for unintelligible jargon or babbling. [glosso- + G. *lalia,* talk, chat]

glos·sol·o·gy (glos-ol′ō-jē). The branch of medical science concerned with the tongue and its diseases. SYN glottology. [glosso- + G. *logos,* study]

glos·son·cus (glos-ong′kŭs). Any swelling involving the tongue, including neoplasms. [glosso- + G. *onkos,* mass, tumor]

glos·so·pal·a·ti·nus (glos′ō-pal-ă-tī′nŭs). SYN palatoglossus (*muscle*). [glosso- + Mod. L. *palatinus,* fr. L. *palatum,* palate]

glos·sop·a·thy (glos-op′ă-thē). A disease of the tongue. [glosso- + G. *pathos,* suffering]

glos·so·pha·ryn·ge·al (glos′ō-fă-rin′jē-ăl). Relating to the tongue and the pharynx.

glos·so·pha·ryn·ge·us (glos′ō-fă-rin′jē-ŭs). SEE superior pharyngeal constrictor (*muscle*).

glos·so·plas·ty (glos′ō-plas-tē). Plastic surgery of the tongue. [glosso- + G. *plastos,* formed]

glos·so·ple·gia (glos-ō-plē′jē-ă). Paralysis of the tongue. [glosso- + G. *plēgē,* stroke]

glos·sop·to·sis, glos·sop·to·sia (glos-op-tō′sis, -op-tō′sē-ă). Downward displacement of the tongue toward the pharynx. [glosso- + G. *ptōsis,* a falling]

glos·so·py·ro·sis (glos-ō-pī-rō′sis). SYN glossodynia. [glosso- + G. *pyrōsis,* a burning]

glos·sor·rha·phy (glo-sōr′ă-fē). Suture of a wound of the tongue. [glosso- + G. *rhaphē,* suture]

glos·so·spasm (glos′ō-spazm). Spasmodic contraction of the tongue.

glos·so·ste·re·sis (glos′ō-ste-rē′sis). SYN glossectomy.

glos·sot·o·my (glo-sot′ō-mē). Any cutting operation on the tongue, usually to obtain access to further reaches of the pharynx. [glosso- + G. *tomē,* incision]

glos·so·trich·ia (glos-ō-trik′ē-ă). SYN hairy *tongue.* [glosso- + G. *thrix,* hair]

glot·tal (glot′ăl). Relating to the glottis.

glot·tal·iz·a·tion (glot′al-ĭ-zā′shun). SYN vocal fry.

glot·tic (glot′ik). Relating to (1) the tongue or (2) the glottis.

gl

glot·ti·do·spasm (glot′i-dō-spazm). SYN laryngospasm.

glot·tis, pl. **glot·ti·des** (glot′is, glot′i-dēz) [TA]. The vocal apparatus of the larynx, consisting of the vocal folds of mucous membrane investing the vocal ligament and vocal muscle on each side, the free edges of which are the vocal cords, and of a median fissure, the rima glottidis. [G. *glōttis,* aperture of the larynx]
  false g., SYN rima vestibuli.
  g. respirato′ria, SYN intercartilaginous *part* of rima glottidis.
  g. spu′ria, SYN *rima vestibuli.*
  true g., SYN *rima glottidis.*
  g. ve′ra, SYN *rima glottidis.*
  g. voca′lis, SYN intermembranous *part* of rima glottidis.

glot·ti·tis (glo-tī′tis). Inflammation of the glottic portion of the larynx.

glot·tol·o·gy (glo-tol′ō-jē). SYN glossology. [G. *glōssa, glōtta,* tongue, + *logos,* study]

GLP-1 Abbreviation for glucagonlike *peptide.*

Glp Abbreviation for 5-oxoproline.

Glu Symbol for glutamic acid or its acyl radical, glutamyl.

glu·ca·gon (gloo′kă-gon). A hormone consisting of a straight-chain polypeptide of 29 amino acyl residues, extracted from pancreatic alpha cells. Parenteral administration of 0.5–1 mg results in prompt mobilization of hepatic glycogen, thus elevating blood glucose concentration. It activates hepatic phosphorylase, thereby increasing glycogenolysis, decreases gastric motility and gastric and pancreatic secretions, and increases urinary excretion of nitrogen and potassium; it has no effect on muscle phosphorylase. As the hydrochloride, it is used in the treatment of glycogen storage disease (von Gierke) and hypoglycemia, particularly hypoglycemic coma due to exogenously administered insulin. SYN HG factor, hyperglycemic-glycogenolytic factor, pancreatic hyperglycemic hormone. [glucose + G. *agō,* to lead]
  gut g., a substance of intestinal origin that is secreted into the blood following ingestion of glucose and is a potent stimulus to the secretion of insulin; its chemical structure and the biologic effects that it produces are different from those of g., and it cross-reacts with antibodies to g.

glu·ca·gon·o·ma (gloo′kă-gon-ō′mă). A glucagon-secreting tumor, usually derived from pancreatic islet cells.

glu·cal (gloo′kăl). SYN glycal.

glu·can (gloo′kan). SYN glucosan.

1,4-α-D-glu·can-branch·ing en·zyme. Amylo-(1,4→1,6)-transglucosylase or transglucosidase; an enzyme in muscle and in plants (Q enzyme) that cleaves α-1,4 linkages in glycogen or starch, transferring the fragments into α-1,6 linkages, creating branches in the polysaccharide molecules; in plants, it converts amylose to amylopectin; this enzyme is deficient in individuals with glycogen storage disease type IV. SYN α-glucan-branching glycosyltransferase, amylo-1,4:1,6-glucantransferase, amylo-(1,4→1,6)-transglucosidase, amylo-(1,4→1,6)-transglucosylase, branching enzyme.

α-glu·can-branch·ing gly·co·syl·trans·fer·ase. SYN 1,4-α-D-glucan-branching enzyme.

1,4-α-D-glu·can 6-α-D-glu·co·syl·trans·fer·ase. A glucosyltransferase that transfers an α-glucosyl residue in a 1,4-α-glucan to the primary hydroxyl group of glucose in a 1,4-α-glucan. SEE ALSO 1,4-α-D-glucan-branching enzyme. SYN oligoglucan-branching glycosyltransferase.

4-α-D-glu·can·o·trans·fer·ase. Dextrin transglycosylase or glycosyltransferase; a 4-glycosyltransferase converting maltodextrins into amylose and glucose by transferring parts of 1,4-glucan chains to new 4-positions on glucose or other 1,4-glucans. SYN amylomaltase, D enzyme, dextrin glycosyltransferase, dextrin transglycosylase, disproportionating enzyme.

α-glu·can phos·pho·ryl·ase. SYN phosphorylase.

glu·cep·tate (gloo-sep′tat). USAN-approved contraction for glucoheptonate.

glu·ci·phore (gloo′si-fōr). Term coined for chemical groups believed to be responsible for sweet taste. [G. *glykys,* sweet, + *phoros,* bearing]

gluco-. Combining form denoting relationship to glucose. SEE ALSO glyco-. [G. *gleukos,* sweet new wine, sweetness]

glu·co·am·y·lase (gloo-kō-am′i-lās). SYN exo-1,4-α-D-glucosidase.

glu·co·a·scor·bic ac·id (gloo′kō-as-kōr′bik). A compound resembling ascorbic acid but with an additional –CHOH– between C-5 and C-6 of ascorbic acid; shows toxic effects on addition to diet that apparently are not caused by ascorbic acid antagonism.

β-glu·co·cer·e·bro·sid·ase (gloo′kō-ser′ĕ-brō-sīd-ās). An enzyme that hydrolyzes β-glucosides in cerebrosides; a deficiency of this enzyme results in Gaucher disease.

glu·co·cer·e·bro·side (gloo-kō-ser′ĕ-brō-sīd). SYN glucosylceramide.

glu·co·cor·ti·coid (gloo-kō-kōr′ti-koyd). **1.** Any steroid-like compound capable of significantly influencing intermediary metabolism such as promotion of hepatic glycogen deposition, and of exerting a clinically useful anti-inflammatory effect. Cortisol (hydrocortisone) is the most potent of the naturally occurring g.'s; most semisynthetic g.'s are cortisol derivatives. **2.** Denoting this type of biologic activity. SYN glycocorticoid.

glu·co·cor·ti·co·tro·phic (gloo′kō-kōr′ti-kō-trōf′ik). Denoting a principle postulated to be present in the anterior hypophysis, that stimulates the production of glucocorticoid hormones of the adrenal cortex; no hormone exerting only this effect has been identified, but ACTH does stimulate adrenal corticoid production.

glu·co·cy·a·mine (gloo-kō-sī′ă-mēn). SYN glycocyamine.

glu·co·fu·ra·nose (gloo-kō-foor′ă-nōs). Glucose in furanose form.

glu·co·gen·e·sis (gloo-kō-jen′ĕ-sis). Formation of glucose. [gluco- + G. *genesis,* production]

glu·co·gen·ic (gloo-kō-jen′ik). Giving rise to or producing glucose. SYN glucoplastic.

glu·co·in·vert·ase (gloo-kō-in′ver-tās). SYN α-D-glucosidase.

glu·co·ki·nase (gloo-kō-kī′nās). Phosphotransferase that catalyzes the conversion of D-glucose and ATP to D-glucose 6-phosphate and ADP; the liver enzyme has a higher K_m value for D-glucose than does hexokinase and is not strongly inhibited by the product D-glucose 6-phosphate.

glu·co·ki·net·ic (gloo′kō-ki-net′ik). Tending to mobilize glucose; usually evidenced by a reduction of the glycogen stores in the tissues to produce an increase in the concentration of glucose circulating in the blood.

glu·co·lip·ids (gloo-kō-lip′idz). Lipids that contain D-glucose.

glu·col·y·sis (gloo-kol′i-sis). SYN glycolysis.

glu·co·ne·o·gen·e·sis (gloo′kō-nē-ō-jen′ĕ-sis). The formation of glucose from noncarbohydrates, such as protein or fat. SYN glyconeogenesis (2).

glu·con·ic ac·id (gloo-kon′ik). The hexonic (aldonic) acid derived from glucose by oxidation of the –CHO group to –COOH.

glu·con·o·lac·to·nase (gloo′kon-o-lak′tō-nās). An enzyme catalyzing the hydrolysis of D-glucono-δ-lactone to D-gluconic acid. SYN lactonase.

glu·co·pe·ni·a (gloo-kō-pē′nē-ă). SYN hypoglycemia. [gluco- + G. *penia,* poverty]

glu·co·plas·tic. SYN glucogenic.

glu·co·pro·tein (gloo-kō-prō′tēn). A glycoprotein in which the sugar is glucose.

glu·co·pyr·a·nose (gloo-kō-pir′ă-nōs). Glucose in its pyranose form.

glu·co·sa·mine (gloo′kō-să-mēn). An amino sugar found in chitin, cell membranes, and mucopolysaccharides generally; used as a pharmaceutic aid.

glu·cos·a·mi·no·gly·cans (gloo-kōs-ă-mē′nō-glī′kans). Glycosaminoglycans (or mucopolysaccharides) in which all of the constituent sugar amines are glucosamines.

glu·co·san (gloo′kō-san). A polysaccharide yielding glucose upon hydrolysis; e.g., callose, cellulose, glycogen, starch, dextrins. SYN glucan.

D-glu·cose (G, Glc) (gloo′kōs). Dextrose; a dextrorotatory monosaccharide (hexose) found in the free state in fruits and other parts of plants, and combined in glucosides, disaccharides (often with fructose in sugars), oligosaccharides, and polysaccharides; it is the product of complete hydrolysis of cellulose, starch, and glycogen. Free g. also occurs in the blood, where it is a principal energy source for use by body tissues (normal human concentration, 70–110 mg per 100 mL); in diabetes mellitus, it appears in the urine. The epimers of D-g. are D-allose, D-mannose, D-galactose, and L-idose. Dextrose should not be confused with the L-isomer, which is sinistrose. SYN cellohexose.

activated g., a nucleoside diphosphoglucose such as UDPglucose.

g. dehydrogenase, converts β-D-glucose to D-glucono-δ-lactone, transferring hydrogen to NAD$^+$ or NADP$^+$. Cf. g. oxidase.

liquid g., a pharmaceutic aid consisting of dextrose, dextrins, maltose, and water, obtained by the incomplete hydrolysis of starch.

g. oxidase, an antibacterial flavoprotein enzyme, obtained from *Penicillum notatum* and other fungi, which is antibacterial only in the presence of glucose and oxygen, its effect being due to the oxidation of D-glucose to D-glucono-δ-lactone, with the coconversion of O_2 to H_2O_2; used in the preservation of food and in assays for glucose levels. SYN g. oxyhydrase, microcide.

g. oxyhydrase, SYN g. oxidase.

g. phosphomutase, SYN phosphoglucomutase.

D-glu·cose 1,6-bis·phos·phate. A bisphosphorylated derivative of D-glucose that is a required intermediate in the interconversion of D-glucose 1-phosphate and D-glucose 6-phosphate.

glu·cose-6-phos·pha·tase. A liver enzyme catalyzing the hydrolysis of D-glucose 6-phosphate to D-glucose and orthophosphate; this enzyme is deficient in glycogen storage disease Ia.

glu·cose 6-phos·phate. An ester of glucose with phosphoric acid; made in the course of glucose metabolism by mammalian and other cells; a normal constituent of resting muscle, probably always existing in equilibrium with fructose 6-phosphate.

D-glu·cose 1-phos·phate. An important intermediate in glycogenesis and glycogenolysis. SYN Cori ester.

D-glu·cose 6-phos·phate. A key intermediate in glycolysis, glycogenolysis, pentose phosphate shunt, etc.; elevated levels inhibit brain hexokinase and glycolysis. SYN Robison ester, Robison-Embden ester.

glu·cose-6-phos·phate de·hy·dro·gen·ase. An NADP$^+$ enzyme catalyzing the dehydrogenation of D-glucose 6-phosphate to 6-phospho-D-glucono-δ-lactone, this reaction initiating the pentose shunt. A deficiency of this enzyme can lead to severe hemolytic anemia and favism. A deficiency of the leukocyte enzyme prevents neutrophils expressing respiratory burst. SYN Robison ester dehydrogenase, Zwischenferment.

glu·cose-phos·phate isom·er·ase. An enzyme that catalyzes the reversible interconversion of D-fructose 6-phosphate and D-glucose 6-phosphate; a part of glycolysis and gluconeogenesis; g.-p. i. deficiency is an inherited disorder resulting in liver glycogenesis and hemolytic anemia. SYN hexosephosphate isomerase, phosphohexomutase, phosphohexose isomerase.

glu·cose-1-phos·phate ki·nase. SYN phosphoglucokinase.

glu·cose-1-phos·phate phos·pho·dis·mu·tase. A phosphotransferase catalyzing the reversible transfer of a phosphate residue from one D-glucose 1-phosphate to another, yielding D-glucose 1,6-bisphosphate and D-glucose. This enzyme provides a crucial intermediate needed for glucose-phosphate isomerase.

glu·cose-6-phos·phate trans·lo·case. A transport protein in the membrane of the endoplasmic reticulum; a deficiency of this protein is associated with glycogen storage disease type Ib.

glu·cose-1-phos·phate uri·dyl·yl·trans·fer·ase. An enzyme that activates D-glucose by reacting D-glucose 1-phosphate with UTP, producing pyrophosphate and UDPglucose; a crucial step in glycogen biosynthesis.

α-D-glu·co·si·dase (gloo′kō-si-dās). Maltase; a glucohydrolase removing terminal nonreducing 1,4-linked α-glucose residues by hydrolysis, yielding α-glucose; a deficiency of the lysosomal enzyme is associated with glycogen storage disease type II. There are at least five isozymes of maltase. SYN glucoinvertase.

β-D-glu·co·si·dase. A glucohydrolase similar to α-D-glucosidase,

but attacking β-glucosides and releasing β-D-glucose. SYN amygdalase, cellobiase, gentiobiase.

glu·co·si·das·es (gloo′kō-sid-ās-ez). Enzymes that hydrolyze glucosides.

glu·co·side (gloo′kō-sīd). A compound of glucose with an alcohol or other R–OH compound involving loss of the H atom of the 1-OH (hemiacetal) group of the glucose, yielding a –C–O–R link from the C-1 of the glucose; a glycoside of glucose.

glucosinolates. A group of secondary plant metabolites occurring in cruciferous plants, especially Brassica vegetables (such as cabbage); hydrolyzed into wide range of biologically active compounds, including isothiocyanates, which show anticarcinogenic activity.

glu·co·sone (gloo′kō-sōn). A 2-dehydrogenation (2-keto) product of glucose; a possible intermediate in the formation of glucosamine from glucose. [glucose + -one]

glu·co·sul·fone so·di·um (gloo-kō-sŭl′fōn). A chemotherapeutic agent used in the treatment of leprosy; parenteral administration is better tolerated than oral administration.

glu·cos·u·ria (gloo-kō-soo′rē-ă). The urinary excretion of glucose, usually in enhanced quantities. SYN glycosuria (1), glycuresis (1). [glucose + G. *ouron,* urine]

glu·co·syl (gloo′kō-sil). The radical of glucose that has lost its hemiacetal (C-1) OH.

glu·co·syl·cer·a·mide (gloo′kō-sil-ser′ă-mīd). A neutral glycolipid containing equimolar amounts of fatty acid, glucose, and sphingosine (or a derivative thereof); accumulates in individuals with Gaucher disease. SYN glucocerebroside.

glu·co·syl·trans·fer·ase (gloo′kō-sil-trans′fer-ās). Any enzyme transferring glucosyl groups from one compound to another; g.'s are in EC subclass 2.4 (glycosyltransferases). SYN transglucosylase.

glu·cu·ro·nate (gloo-koor′ō-nāt). A salt or ester of glucuronic acid.

glu·cu·rone (gloo′koo-rōn). SYN D-glucuronolactone.

glu·cu·ron·ic ac·id (gloo-koo-ron′ik). The uronic acid of glucose in which C-6 is oxidized to a carboxyl group; the D-isomer detoxicates or inactivates various substances (e.g., benzoic acid, phenol, camphor, and the female sex hormones) undergoing conjugation with such substances in the liver, the glucuronides so formed being excreted in the urine.

β-D-glu·cu·ron·i·dase (gloo-koo-ron′i-dās). An enzyme catalyzing the hydrolysis of various β-D-glucuronides, liberating free D-glucuronic acid and an alcohol; a deficiency of this enzyme is associated with Sly syndrome. SYN glusulase, glycuronidase.

glu·cu·ro·nide (gloo-koo′rōn-īd). A glycoside of glucuronic acid; many foreign chemicals, as well as catabolic products of normal body constituents (e.g., steroid hormones), are commonly excreted in the urine as D-g.'s, the conjugation taking place in the liver. SYN glucuronoside.

D-glu·cu·ron·o·lac·tone (gloo′kŭ-rō′nō-lak′tōn). Used as a means of orally administering glucuronic acid in the management of collagen and joint diseases. SYN glucurone.

glu·cu·ro·no·side (gloo-koo-ron′ō-sīd). SYN glucuronide.

glu·cu·ron·o·syl·trans·fer·ase (gloo-koo-koo-ron′ō-sil-trans′fer-ās). Any of a family of enzymes that transfer D-glucuronate to the acceptor named, forming glucuronosides; e.g., UDPglucuronate-bilirubin glucuronosyltransferase.

glue-sniff·ing (gloo′snif-ing). Inhalation of fumes from plastic cements; the solvents, which include toluene, xylene, and benzene, induce central nervous system stimulation followed by depression. SEE ALSO solvent *inhalation.*

Gluge, Gottlieb, German histologist, 1812–1898. SEE G. *corpuscles,* under *corpuscle.*

glu·sul·ase (gloo′sŭl-ās). SYN β-D-glucuronidase.

glu·ta·con·ic ac·id (gloo′ta-kon-ik). Dicarboxylic acid that accumulates in individuals with glutaric acidemia type I.

glu·ta·mate (gloo′tă-māt). A salt or ester of glutamic acid.

g. acetyltransferase, (1) an enzyme catalyzing transfer of an acetyl group from N^2-acetylornithine to L-g. forming L-ornithine and *N*-acetyl-L-glutamate, an activator of the urea cycle; **(2)** an enzyme that catalyzes the transfer of an acetyl group from acetyl-CoA to L-g. to form coenzyme A and *N*-acetyl-L-g., which is an activator of the urea cycle. SYN ornithine acetyltransferase.

g. decarboxylase (GAD), a carboxy-lyase converting L-g. to 4-aminobutyrate and CO_2 as well as L-aspartate to 3-aminopropanoate and CO_2; a defect in the binding of this protein's coenzyme is believed to be the cause of pyridoxine dependency with seizures. SYN aspartate 1-decarboxylase.

g. dehydrogenases, enzymes that catalyze the reaction of L-g., H_2O, and NAD^+ (or $NADP^+$ in some cases) producing α-ketoglutarate (2-oxoglutarate), ammonia, and NADH; in mammals, this is the prime contributor to oxidative deamination. SYN glutamic acid dehydrogenases.

g. formiminotransferase, an enzyme that catalyzes the transfer of the formimino moiety of *N*-formimino-L-glutamate to tetrahydrofolate; a deficiency of this enzyme will lead to elevated formiminoglutamate levels.

g. γ-semialdehyde, an intermediate in L-proline and L-ornithine metabolism; becomes elevated in type II hyperprolinemia.

g. synthase, an enzyme that converts L-glutamine, α-ketoglutarate, and NADH (in some cases, NADPH) to two L-g.'s and NAD^+ (or $NADP^+$); apparently, a nonmammalian enzyme. In some plants this is a ferredoxin-dependent reaction.

γ-glu·ta·mate (glu·ta·mate γ-) car·box·y·pep·ti·dase. SYN γ-glutamyl hydrolase.

glu·tam·ic ac·id (E, Glu) (gloo-tam'ik). An amino acid; the sodium salt is monosodium glutamate. Cf. glutamate.

g. a. dehydrogenases, SYN *glutamate* dehydrogenases.

g. a. hydrochloride, a gastric acidifier alleged to aid in digestion; also used for gastric HCl replacement therapy.

glu·tam·ic-as·par·tic trans·am·i·nase. SYN *aspartate* aminotransferase.

glu·tam·ic-ox·a·lo·ace·tic trans·am·i·nase (GOT). SYN *aspartate* aminotransferase.

glu·tam·ic-py·ru·vic trans·am·i·nase (GPT). SYN alanine aminotransferase.

glu·ta·min·ase (gloo-tam'in-ās). An enzyme in kidney and other tissues that catalyzes the hydrolysis of L-glutamine to ammonia and L-glutamic acid; an important enzyme for urinary ammonia formation.

glu·ta·min·ate (gloo-tam'in-āt). The anion form of glutamine.

glu·ta·mine (Gln, Q) (gloo'tă-mēn, -tă-min, gloo-tam'in). The δ-amide of glutamic acid, derived by oxidation from proline in the liver or by the combination of glutamic acid with ammonia; the L-isomer is present in proteins and in blood and other tissues, and is an important source of urinary ammonia, being broken down in the kidney by the action of the enzyme glutaminase; nonenzymatically, it is converted to 5-oxoproline.

g. aminotransferase, an enzyme that reversibly reacts L-glutamine with α-ketoglutarate to produce α-ketoglutaramate and L-glutamate; α-ketoglutaramate is elevated in certain cases of hepatocoma. SYN g. transaminase.

g. synthetase, an enzyme that catalyzes the reaction of L-glutamic acid, ammonia, and ATP to g., ADP, and orthophosphate; one of the few known mammalian enzymes that uses ammonium ion as a substrate under physiological conditions.

g. transaminase, SYN g. aminotransferase.

glu·tam·i·nyl (Gln, Glx, Q) (gloo-tam'i-nil). The acyl radical of glutamine.

glu·tam·o·yl (gloo-tam'ō-il). The radical of glutamic acid from which both α- and δ-hydroxyl groups have been removed.

glu·tam·yl (E, Glu, Glx) (gloo-tam'il, gloo'tă-mil). The radical of glutamic acid from which either the α- or the δ-hydroxyl group has been removed.

γ-glu·tam·yl car·box·yl·ase. An enzyme that catalyzes the formation of γ-carboxyglutamyl residues in many proteins, several appearing in the blood clotting cascade.

γ-glu·ta·myl·cys·teine (gloo'tă-mil-sis'te-in). A necessary precursor in the biosynthesis of glutathione; contains an isopeptide rather than a eupeptide bond.

γ-g. synthetase, an enzyme that catalyzes the first step in glutathi-

one biosynthesis, reacting L-glutamate, L-cysteine, and ATP to form γ-g., ADP, and orthophosphate; inhibited by thiols such as glutathione.

γ-glu·tam·yl hy·dro·lase. An enzyme cleaving L-glutamyl residues from pteridine oligoglutamates; used in certain antitumor treatments. SYN carboxypeptidase G, γ-glutamate (glutamate γ-) carboxypeptidase.

γ-glu·tam·yl·trans·fer·ase (gloo-tam'il-trans'fer-ās). An enzyme that catalyzes the transfer of a γ-glutamyl group from a γ-glutamyl peptide (usually glutathione) to another peptide, certain amino acids, or water; a deficiency of this enzyme will result in glutathionuria. SYN γ-glutamyl transpeptidase.

γ-glu·tam·yl trans·pep·ti·dase. SYN γ-glutamyltransferase.

glu·ta·ral (gloo'tă-ral). SYN glutaraldehyde.

glu·tar·al·de·hyde (gloo-tă-ral'dĕ-hīd). A dialdehyde used as a fixative for electron microscopy, especially for nuclear morphology and for localization of enzyme activity; also used as a germicidal agent for disinfection and sterilization of instruments or equipment that cannot be heat sterilized. SYN glutaral.

glu·tar·ic ac·id (gloo-tar'ik). Pentanedioic acid; an intermediate in tryptophan catabolism; accumulates in glutaric acidemia.

glu·ta·ryl-CoA (gloo'tă-ril). The mono thiol ester of coenzyme A and glutaric acid; an intermediate in L-lysine and L-tryptophan catabolism.

g.-CoA dehydrogenase, an enzyme that catalyzes the reaction of g.-CoA with an acceptor to form crotonoyl-CoA, CO_2, and the reduced acceptor; a deficiency of this enzyme will lead to either glutaric acidemia type I or hyperoxaluria type II.

g.-CoA synthetase, an enzyme similar to acyl-CoA synthetase, but which splits ATP, GTP, or ITP to the nucleoside diphosphate and orthophosphate in acting on glutarate, thus forming g.-CoA.

glu·ta·thi·one (GSH) (gloo-tă-thī'ōn). A tripeptide of glycine, L-cysteine, and L-glutamate, with L-glutamate having an isopeptide bond with the amino moiety of L-cysteine. G. has a wide variety of roles in a cell; it is the most prevalent non-protein thiol. G. disulfide (GSSG) consists of two g.'s linked via a disulfide bridge; the term oxidized g. for GSSG should be avoided since it includes the sulfones and sulfoxides. The term reduced g. is not necessary since g. is the thiol form. A deficiency of g. can cause hemolysis with oxidative stress. It is also used in the course of intermediary metabolism as a donor of thiol (SH) groups and is essential for detoxification of acetaminophen. SEE ALSO oxidized g., reduced g., g. reductase.

oxidized g., (1) g. acting in cells as a hydrogen acceptor; reduced by g. reductase; glutathione disulfide; **(2)** sulfones or sulfoxides of glutathione or glutathione disulfide.

g. peroxidase, an enzyme that catalyzes the reaction of two g.'s with H_2O_2 forming GSSG and two water molecules; a crucial enzyme in hydrogen peroxide detoxification.

reduced g., g. acting as a hydrogen donor; glutathione.

g. reductase, an enzyme that catalyzes the reaction of GSSG with NADH (or NADPH) forming two g.'s and NAD^+ (or $NADP^+$); involved in many redox reactions; a deficiency can cause hemolysis with oxidative stress.

g. synthetase, an enzyme that catalyzes the formation of g., ADP, and orthophosphate from γ-glutamylcysteine, ATP, and glycine; a deficiency will lead to metabolic acidosis and progressive brain dysfunction.

g. *S*-transferase, a class of enzymes that catalyze the reaction of g. with an acceptor molecule (e.g., an arene oxide) to form an *S*-substituted g.; a key step in detoxification of many substances; start of the mercapturic acid pathway. SYN ligandin.

glu·ta·thi·o·nu·ria (gloo-tă-thī'ō-nur-ē-ă). Elevated glutathione and/or glutathione disulfide levels in the urine.

glu·te·al (gloo'tē-ăl). Relating to the buttocks. [G. *gloutos*, buttock]

glu·te·lins (gloo'tĕ-linz). A class of simple proteins occurring in the seeds of grain; soluble in dilute acids and bases, but not in neutral solutions (e.g., glutenin from wheat and orycenin in rice). They have glutamin-rich domains and serve as storage proteins.

glu·ten (gloo'tĕn). The insoluble protein (prolamines) constituent of wheat and other grains; a mixture of gliadin, glutenin, prolamins, and other proteins; the presence of g. allows flour to rise. SYN wheat gum. [L. *gluten,* glue]

g. casein, a protein resembling casein, present in g.

glu·te·nin (gloo'tĕ-nin). Any glutelin in the endosperm of wheat seeds; believed to be responsible for the viscoelastic properties of wheat dough.

glu·te·o·fem·o·ral (gloo'tē-ō-fem'ō-răl). Relating to the buttock and the thigh.

glu·te·o·in·gui·nal (gloo'tē-ō-ing'gwi-năl). Relating to the buttock and the groin.

glu·teth·i·mide (gloo-teth'i-mīd). A central nervous system depressant used as a hypnotic in simple insomnia and formerly as a daytime sedative.

glu·te·us (gloo-tē'ŭs). SEE gluteus maximus (*muscle*), gluteus medius (*muscle*), gluteus minimus (*muscle*).

glu·ti·noid (gloo'ti-noyd). SYN albuminoid (3).

glu·ti·nous (gloo'tin-ŭs). Sticky.

glu·ti·tis (gloo-tī'tis). Inflammation of the muscles of the buttock. [G. *gloutos,* buttock, + *-itis,* inflammation]

Glx Symbol for glutamyl (Glu), glutaminyl (Gln), and/or any substance that would yield glutamate upon acid hydrolysis of a peptide (e.g., 5-oxoproline, 4-carboxyglutamate) to denote the uncertainty between them.

Gly Symbol for glycine or its acyl radical, glycyl.

gly·bu·ride (glī'bū-rīd). An oral hypoglycemic drug used in the treatment of type II diabetes.

gly·cal (glī'kăl). An unsaturated sugar derivative in which the adjacent hydroxyl groups are removed, one of which is that upon the carbon-1 of the aldose (or carbon-2 of the ketose), yielding a CH=CH between these two positions. SYN glucal.

gly·can (glī'kan). SYN polysaccharide. SEE ALSO heteroglycan, homoglycan.

gly·can·o·hy·dro·las·es (glī'kan-ō-hī'drō-lā-sez) [EC 3.2.1.x]. Hydrolases acting on glycans; e.g., chitinase, hyaluronoglucosidase.

gly·cate (glī'kāt). The product of the nonenzymic reaction between a sugar and the free amino group(s) of proteins in which it is not known if the sugar is attached by a glycosyl or a glycoside linkage, or has formed a Schiff base.

gly·ca·tion (glī-kā'shŭn). The nonenzymic reaction that forms a glycate.

gly·ce·mia (glī-sē'mē-ă). The presence of glucose in the blood. [G. *glykys,* sweet, + *haima,* blood]

glyc·er·al·de·hyde (glis-er-al'dĕ-hīd). A triose and the simplest optically active aldose; the dextrorotatory isomer is taken as the structural reference point for all D compounds, the levorotatory isomer for all L compounds. SYN glyceric aldehyde.

glyc·er·al·de·hyde 3-phos·phate. An intermediate in the glycolytic breakdown of D-glucose; one of the products of the splitting of fructose 1,6-bisphosphate under the catalytic influence of fructose-bisphosphate aldolase.

gly·cer·ic ac·id (gli-ser'ik, glis'er-ik). The fatty acid analog of glycerol; occurs particularly in the form of phosphorylated derivatives as an intermediate in glycolysis.

D-gly·cer·ic ac·i·dur·i·a (gli-ser'ik as-id-oo-rē-a). **1.** Elevated levels of D-glyceric acid in the urine. **2.** An inborn error in metabolism resulting in D-glyceric aciduria (1).

L-gly·cer·ic ac·i·du·ria. Excretion of L-glyceric acid in the urine; a primary metabolic error due to deficiency of D-glyceric dehydrogenase resulting in excretion of L-glyceric and oxalic acids, leading to the clinical syndrome of oxalosis with frequent formation of oxalate renal calculi.

gly·cer·ic al·de·hyde. SYN glyceraldehyde.

glyc·er·i·das·es (glis'er-ĭ-dās-ez). General term for enzymes catalyzing the hydrolysis of glycerol esters (glycerides); e.g., triacylglycerol lipase.

glyc·er·ide (glis'er-id, -īd). An ester of glycerol. The term is usually used in combination with phospho- (phosphoglyceride). The use of mono-, di-, and triglyceride is being replaced by the more precise terms mono-, di-, and triacylglycerol, respectively.

mixed g.'s, g.'s which, on hydrolysis, yield more than one variety of fatty acid.

glyc·er·in (glis'er-in). SYN glycerol.

g. jelly, SYN glycerinated *gelatin.*

glyc·er·ite (glis'er-īt). **1.** SYN glycerol. **2.** A pharmaceutical preparation made by triturating the active medicinal substance with glycerol.

starch g., a preparation containing 100 g of starch, 2 g of benzoic acid, 200 ml of purified water, and 700 g of glycerin in each 1000 g; a topical emollient.

tannic acid g., g. of tannin, containing tannic acid, sodium citrate, exsiccated sodium sulfite, and glycerin; an astringent.

glyc·er·o·gel·a·tin (glis'er-ō-jel'ă-tin). SYN glycerinated *gelatin.*

glyc·er·o·ki·nase (glis'er-ō-kī'nās). SYN glycerol kinase.

glyc·er·ol (glis'er-ol). A sweet viscous fluid obtained by the saponification of fats and fixed oils; used as a solvent, as a skin emollient, by injection or in the form of suppository for constipation, and as a vehicle and sweetening agent. SYN 1,2,3-propanetriol, glycerin, glycerite (1), glyceryl alcohol.

iodinated g., a form of organically bound iodine which liberates iodine systemically. Has been used as a medicinal source of iodine and as an expectorant in place of inorganic iodides such as potassium iodide. SYN iodopropylidene glycerol, organidin.

g. kinase, an enzyme that catalyzes a reaction between ATP and glycerol to yield sn-glycerol 3-phosphate and ADP; in adipose tissue, the first and rate-limiting step in the synthesis of triacylglycerols; deficiency results in the disruption of adrenal, muscle, and/or liver and brain function. SYN glycerokinase.

g. phosphate, the anion of a phosphoric ester of g.; the 3-derivative is the central component of phosphatidates (R-glycerol 3-phosphate). SYN glycerophosphate.

glyc·er·ol-3-phos·phate ac·yl·trans·fer·ase. An enzyme that participates in phospholipid biosynthesis, catalyzing the transfer of an acyl group from a fatty acyl-CoA to sn-glycerol-3-phosphate, producing coenzyme A and lysophosphatidic acid.

glyc·er·ol-3-phos·phate de·hy·dro·gen·ase (NAD⁺). α-Glycerol phosphate dehydrogenase; 3-phosphoglycerol dehydrogenase; a flavoenzyme that catalyzes the interconversion of dihydroxyacetone phosphate and sn-glycerol 3-phosphate, with the participation of NAD⁺; its action provides the glycerol moiety from carbohydrate during lipogenesis.

gly·cer·one. The IUPAC recommended name for dihydroxyacetone.

glyc·er·o·phos·phate (glis'er-ō-fos'fāt). SYN glycerol phosphate.

glyc·er·o·phos·pho·cho·line (glis'er-ō-fos-fō-kō'lēn). A component of phosphatidylcholines (lecithins), in which the two OH's of g. are esterified with fatty acids. SYN glycerophosphorylcholine.

glyc·er·o·phos·phor·ic ac·id (glis'er-ō-fos-fōr'ik). A phosphoric ester of glycerol. SEE ALSO *glycerol* phosphate.

glyc·er·o·phos·pho·ryl·cho·line (glis'er-ō-fos'fōr-il-kō'lēn). SYN glycerophosphocholine.

glyc·er·ul·ose (glis-er'ul-ōse). SYN dihydroxyacetone.

glyc·er·yl (glis'er-il). **1.** The trivalent radical, $C_3H_5^{3-}$, of glycerol; often used in error for glycero- or glycerol. **2.** Any group derived from glycerol by removing one or more of the hydroxyl groups.

g. alcohol, SYN glycerol.

g. borate, SYN boroglycerin.

g. guaiacolate, SYN guaifenesin.

g. iodide, an organic form of iodine which slowly liberates iodine in the body after oral administration. Used primarily as an expectorant/mucolytic. SYN 3-iodo-1,2-propanediol, γ-iodopropyleneglycol.

g. monostearate, the ester of glycerol and one molecule of stearic acid; used in the manufacture of cosmetic creams and dermatologic preparations.

g. triacetate, SYN triacetin.

g. tributyrate, SYN tributyrin.

g. tricaprate, SYN caprin.

g. trinitrate, SYN nitroglycerin.

gl

gly·cin·am·ide ri·bo·nu·cle·o·tide (glī-sin′a-mīd). SEE glycineamide ribonucleotide.

gly·cin·ate (glī′sin-āt). **1.** A salt of glycine. **2.** Glycine anion.

gly·cine (G, Gly) (glī′sēn). The simplest amino acid; a major component of gelatin and silk fibroin; used as a nutrient and dietary supplement, and in solution for irrigation; used in the treatment of sweaty feet syndrome. SYN gelatin sugar.

g. acyltransferase, an enzyme catalyzing the reversible transfer of an acyl group from acyl-CoA to g., producing free coenzyme A and N-acylglycine; a step in a detoxification pathway.

g. amidinotransferase, an enzyme catalyzing the transfer of an amidine group from L-arginine to glycine, forming guanidinoacetate and L-ornithine; an important reaction in creatine biosynthesis; it can also act on canavanine. SYN g. transamidinase.

g. betaine, SYN betaine.

g. cleavage complex, a complex of several proteins that catalyze the reversible reaction of g. with tetrahydrofolate to produce CO_2, NH_3, and N^5,N^{10}-methylenetetrahydrofolate; a deficiency of this enzyme (or one of its subunits) will result in nonketotic hyperglycinemia. SYN g. synthase.

g. dehydrogenases, enzymes that catalyze the conversion of glycine to glyoxylate and ammonia, using either NAD^+ or ferricytochrome c.

g. synthase, SYN g. cleavage complex.

g. transamidinase, SYN g. amidinotransferase.

gly·cine·a·mide ri·bo·nu·cle·o·tide, gly·cin·am·ide ri·bo·nu·cle·o·tide (glī′sin-ă-mīd, glī-sin′a-mīd). An intermediate in purine biosynthesis, in which the amide nitrogen of glycineamide is linked to the C-1 of a ribosyl moiety.

gly·cin·in (glī-sen′in). The chief protein of soybeans; a globulin that is structurally similar to arachin, edestin, and excelsin.

gly·ci·ni·um (glī-sen-ē-um). Glycine cation.

gly·ci·nu·ria (glī-si-noo′rē-ă). The excretion of glycine in the urine. [glycine + G. ouron, urine]

familial g. [MIM*138500], a metabolic disorder believed to be due to defective renal glycine reabsorption; it may or may not be accompanied by oxalate urolithiasis; may be the heterozygous state of iminoglycinuria; autosomal dominant inheritance.

⌂**glyco-.** Combining form denoting relationship to sugars (e.g., glycogen) or to glycine (e.g., glycocholate). SEE ALSO gluco-. [G. glykys, sweet]

gly·co·bi·ar·sol (glī-kō-bī′ar-sol). A pentavalent arsenical containing bismuth; used in the treatment of milder forms of intestinal amebiasis or as subsequent therapy.

gly·co·ca·lyx (glī-kō-kā′liks). A PAS-positive filamentous coating on the apical surface of certain epithelial cells, composed of carbohydrate moieties of proteins that protrude from the free surface of the plasma membrane. [glyco- + G. kalyx, husk, shell]

gly·co·cho·late (glī-kō-kō′lāt). A salt or ester of glycocholic acid.

g. sodium, a normal constituent of bile of humans and herbivores; g. sodium from herbivores is purified and used as a choleretic and cholagogue.

gly·co·cho·lic ac·id (glī-kō-kō′lik). N-Cholylglycine; one of the major bile acid conjugates, formed by condensation of the –COOH group of cholic acid and the amino group of glycine; water-soluble and a powerful detergent.

gly·co·con·ju·gates (glī-kō-kon′joo-gātz). A general class of sugar-containing macromolecules of the body including glycolipids, glycoproteins, and proteoglycans.

gly·co·cor·ti·coid (glī′kō-kōr′ti-koyd). SYN glucocorticoid.

gly·co·cy·a·mine (glī-kō-sī′ă-mēn). 2-Guanidinoacetic acid; formed by the transfer of the amidine group from L-arginine to glycine. SYN glucocyamine.

gly·co·gel·a·tin (glī-kō-jel′ă-tin). SYN glycerinated gelatin.

gly·co·gen (glī′kō-jen). A glucosan of high molecular weight, resembling amylopectin in structure [with α(1,4) linkages] but with even more highly branched [α(1,6) linkages, as well as a small number of α(1,3) linkages], found in most of the tissues of the body, especially those of the liver and muscle; as the principal carbohydrate reserve, it is readily converted into glucose. SYN animal dextran, animal starch, hepatin, liver starch.

g. phosphorylase, SYN phosphorylase.

g. synthase, g. starch synthase, a glucosyltransferase catalyzing the incorporation of D-glucose from UDP-D-glucose into 1,4-α-D-glucosyl chains. A deficiency of the liver enzyme may lead to a type of hypoglycemia.

gly·co·ge·nase (gli′kō-jĕ-nās). SYN α-amylase, β-amylase.

gly·co·gen·e·sis (glī-kō-jen′ĕ-sis). Formation of glycogen from D-glucose by means of glycogen synthase and dextrin dextranase; the first enzyme catalyzes formation of a polyglucose with α-1,4 links from UDPglucose, the second cleaves fragments from one chain and transfers them to an α-1,6 linkage in another. [glyco- + G. genesis, production]

gly·co·ge·net·ic (glī′kō-jĕ-net′ik). Relating to glycogenesis. SYN D-glycogenous.

gly·co·gen·ic (glī-ko-gen′ik). Giving rise to or producing glycogen.

gly·co·gen·ol·y·sis (glī′kō-jĕ-nol′i-sis). The hydrolysis of glycogen to glucose.

🔲**gly·co·ge·no·sis** (glī′kō-jĕ-nō′sis). Any of the glycogen deposition diseases characterized by accumulation of glycogen of normal or abnormal chemical structure in tissue; there may be enlargement of the liver, heart, or striated muscle, including the tongue, with progressive muscular weakness. Seven types (Cori classification) are recognized, depending on the enzyme deficiency involved, all of autosomal recessive inheritance, but with a different gene for each enzyme deficiency. [MIM designations: 1, *232200; *232220; *232240; 2, *232300; 3, *232400; 4, *232500; 5, *232600; 6, *232700; 7, *232800]. SYN dextrinosis, glycogen-storage disease.

brancher deficiency g., SYN brancher glycogen storage *disease*.

generalized g., SYN type 2 g.

glucose-6-phosphatase hepatorenal g., SYN type 1 g.

hepatophosphorylase deficiency g., SYN type 6 g.

myophosphorylase deficiency g., SYN type 5 g.

type 1 g., g. due to glucose 6-phosphatase deficiency, resulting in accumulation of excessive amounts of glycogen of normal chemical structure, particularly in liver and kidney. SYN Gierke disease, glucose-6-phosphatase hepatorenal g., von Gierke disease.

type 2 g., g. due to lysosomal α-1,4-glucosidase deficiency, resulting in accumulation of excessive amounts of glycogen of normal chemical structure in heart, muscle, liver, and nervous system. SYN generalized g., Pompe disease.

type 3 g., g. due to amylo-1,6-glucosidase deficiency, resulting in accumulation of abnormal glycogen with short outer chains in liver and muscle. SYN Cori disease, debranching deficiency limit dextrinosis, limit dextrinosis, Forbes disease.

type 4 g., familial cirrhosis of the liver with storage of abnormal glycogen; g. due to deficiency of 1,4-α-glucan branching enzyme, resulting in accumulation of abnormal glycogen with long inner and outer chains in liver, kidney, muscle, and other tissues. SYN Andersen disease.

type 5 g., g. due to muscle glycogen phosphorylase deficiency, resulting in accumulation of glycogen of normal chemical structure in muscle. SYN McArdle disease, McArdle syndrome, McArdle-Schmid-Pearson disease, myophosphorylase deficiency g.

type 6 g., g. due to hepatic glycogen phosphorylase deficiency, resulting in accumulation of glycogen of normal chemical structure in liver and leukocytes. SYN hepatophosphorylase deficiency g., Hers disease.

type 7 g., phosphofructokinase deficiency of muscle resulting in muscle cramps and myoglobinuria on extreme exertion. The clinical picture resembles type 5 g.

D-gly·cog·e·nous (glī-koj′ĕ-nŭs). SYN glycogenetic.

gly·co·geu·sia (glī-kō-goo′sē-ă). A subjective sweet taste. [glyco- + G. geusis, taste]

gly·co·gly·ci·nu·ria (glī′kō-glī-si-noo′rē-ă) [MIM*138070]. A metabolic disorder characterized by glucosuria and hyperglycinuria; autosomal dominant inheritance.

gly·co·his·to·chem·is·try (glī-kō-his-tō-kem′-is-trē). Study of specific sugar moieties in tissue.

lectin glycohistochemistry, technique for measuring the endogenous ligands for specific sugar moieties, such as peanut agglutinin, wheat germ agglutinin, and gores seed agglutinin, in characterization of surface epithelium.

gly·col (glī′kol). **1.** A compound containing two alcohol groups. **2.** Ethylene g., $HOCH_2CH_2OH$, the simplest g.

gly·col·al·de·hyde (glī-kol-al′dĕ-hīd). $HOCH_2CHO$; the simplest (2-carbon) sugar; the aerobic deamination product of ethanolamine. SYN diose.

active g., 2-(1,2-dihydroxyethyl)thiamin pyrophosphate; a derivative formed in carbohydrate metabolism.

gly·col·al·de·hyde·trans·fer·ase (glī-kol-al′dĕ-hīd-trans′fer-ās). SYN transketolase.

gly·co·late (glī-kō′lāt). A salt or ester of glycolic acid.

gly·co·leu·cine (glī′kō-loo-sin). SYN norleucine.

gly·col·ic ac·id (glī-kol′ik). An intermediate in the interconversion of glycine and ethanolamine. SYN hydroxyacetic acid.

gly·col·ic ac·i·du·ria. Excessive excretion of glycolic acid in the urine; a primary metabolic defect due to deficiency of 2-hydroxy-3-oxoadipate carboxylase, resulting in excretion of glycolic and oxalic acids, leading to the clinical syndrome of oxalosis.

gly·co·lip·id (glī-kō-lip′id). A lipid with one or more covalently attached sugars.

gly·co·lyl (glī′kō-lil). $HOCH_2CO-$; the acyl radical of glycolic acid, replacing acetyl in some sialic acids; the products are called N-glycolylneuraminic acids.

gly·co·lyl·u·rea (glī′kō-lil-ū-rē′ă). SYN hydantoin.

gly·col·y·sis (glī-kol′i-sis). The energy-yielding conversion of D-glucose to lactic acid (instead of pyruvate oxidation products) in various tissues, notably muscle, when sufficient oxygen is not available (as in an emergency situation); since molecular oxygen is not consumed in the process, this is frequently referred to as "anaerobic g." Cf. Embden-Meyerhof-Parnas *pathway.* SYN glucolysis. [glyco- + G. *lysis,* a loosening]

gly·co·lyt·ic (glī-kō-lit′ik). Relating to glycolysis.

gly·co·ne·o·gen·e·sis (glī′kō-nē-ō-jen′ĕ-sis). **1.** The formation of glycogen from noncarbohydrates, such as protein or fat, by conversion of the latter to D-glucose. SEE ALSO glycogenesis. **2.** SYN gluconeogenesis. [glyco- + G. *neos,* new, + *genesis,* production]

gly·con·ic ac·ids (glī-kon′ik). SYN aldonic acids.

gly·co·pe·nia (glī-kō-pē′nē-ă). A deficiency of any or all sugars in an organ or tissue. [glyco- + G. *penia,* poverty]

gly·co·pep·tide (glī-kō-pep′tīd). A compound containing sugar(s) linked to amino acids (or peptides), with the latter preponderant, as in bacterial cell walls. Cf. peptidoglycan.

Gly·co·pha·gus (glī-kof′ă-gŭs). A common genus of grain mites, frequently implicated in dermatitis among food handlers. SEE ALSO *Tyrophagus putrescentiae.* [glyco- + G. *phagō,* to eat]

gly·co·phil·ia (glī-kō-fil′ē-ă). A condition in which there is a distinct tendency to develop hyperglycemia, even after the ingestion of a relatively small quantity of glucose. [glyko- + G. *phileō,* to love]

gly·co·pho·rins (glī-kō-fōr′ins). A group of glycoproteins found in erythrocyte membranes; certain glycophorins are associated with blood group antigens; glycophorin A is the major glycophorin; a deficiency of glycophorin C is observed in type 4 hereditary elliptocytosis.

gly·co·pro·tein (glī-kō-prō′tēn). **1.** One of a group of proteins containing covalently linked carbohydrates, among which the most important are the mucins, mucoid, and amyloid. **2.** Sometimes restricted to proteins containing small amounts of carbohydrate, in contrast to mucoids or mucoproteins, usually measured as hexosamine; such conjugated proteins are found in many places, notably γ-globulins, α_1-globulins, α_2-globulins, transferrin, etc., and are contained in mucus and mucins. SEE ALSO mucoprotein.

α_1-acid g., SYN orosomucoid.

gly·co·pty·a·lism (glī-kō-tī′ă-lizm). SYN glycosialia. [glyco- + G. *ptyalon,* saliva]

gly·co·pyr·ro·late (glī-kō-pī′rō-lāt). A parasympatholytic compound (like atropine) used as premedication prior to general anesthesia, as an antagonist to the bradycardic effects of neostigmine during curare reversal, and as an adjunct in the treatment of peptic ulcer.

gly·cor·rha·chia (glī-kō-rā′kē-ă, -rak-ē-ă). Presence of sugar in the cerebrospinal fluid. [glyco- + G. *rhachis,* spine]

gly·cor·rhea (glī-kō-rē′ă). A discharge of sugar from the body, as in glucosuria, especially in unusually large quantities. [glyco- + G. *rhoia,* a flow]

gl

	types of glycogenoses			
type	glycogenosis	deficient enzyme	biochemical diagnosis	clinical symptoms
1	hepatorenal g., Gierke disease	glucose-6-phosphatase	normal glycogen; excessive amounts in liver and kidneys	hypoglycemia, hyperlipemia, ketosis, hyperuricemia, hepatomegaly, dwarfism
2	generalized, malignant g.; Pompe disease; cardiomegalia glycogenica	α-1.4-glucosidase	normal glycogen, excessive in all organs	muscle hypotonia, heart failure, neurologic symptoms, infant death
3	hepatomuscular, benign g.; Cori disease, Forbes disease (with subvariants 3b through f)	amylo-1.6-glucosidase	abnormal glycogen, with short outer chains, in liver and (more rarely) in muscles	hepatomegaly, hypoglycemia; mild course of disease
4	liver, cirrhotic, reticuloendothelial g.; Anderson disease; amylopectinosis	α-1.4-glucan: α-1.4-glucan-6-glycosyltransferase	abnormal glycogen, with long outer chains, in liver, spleen, and lymph nodes	cirrhosis of the liver; hepatosplenomegaly
5	muscular g., McArdle-Schmid-Pearson disease	α-glucanphosphorylase of the muscle	normal glycogen, excessive amounts in muscle	generalized myasthenia and myalgia, myoglobinuria
6	hepatic g., Hers disease	α-glucanphosphorylase I of the liver	normal glycogen, excessive amounts in liver	hepatomegaly, relatively benign
7	muscular g.; Tarui disease	phosphofructokinase of the muscle	normal glycogen, in the skeletal muscle	muscle cramping, myoglobinuria
8	hepatic g.; X-chromosome inheritance	phosphorylase-b kinase of the liver	normal glycogen, in the liver	clinically mild manifestation, hepatomegaly, hypoglycemia

gly·cos·am·i·no·gly·can (GAG) (glī'kōs-am-i-nō-glī'kan). SEE mucopolysaccharide.

gly·co·se·cre·to·ry (glī'kō-sē-krē'tō-rē). Causing or involved in the secretion of glycogen.

gly·co·si·a·lia (glī'kō-sī-al'ē-ă, -ā'lē-ă). The presence of sugar in the saliva. SYN glycoptyalism. [glyco- + G. *sialon*, saliva]

gly·co·si·a·lor·rhea (glī'kō-sī'ă-lō-rē'ă). An excessive secretion of saliva that contains glucose. [glyco- + G. *sialon*, saliva, + *rhoia*, a flow]

gly·cos·i·dases (glī-kō-sīd-ās'ez). (glī-kō-sīd-ās'ez;) A class of hydrolytic enzymes that act on glycosides; α-glycosidases act on α-glycosidic linkages (e.g., α-amylase) while β-glycosidases act on β-glycosidic linkages (e.g., β-glucosidase). They can be further divided into those enzymes that act on *O*-glycosyl, *N*-glycosyl, or *S*-glycosyl compounds.

gly·co·side (glī'kō-sīd). Condensation product of a sugar with any other radical involving the loss of the OH of the hemiacetal or hemiketal of the sugar, leaving the anomeric carbon as the link; thus, the condensation through the carbon with an alcohol, which loses its hydrogen on its hydroxyl group, yields an alcohol-glycoside (or a glycosido-alcohol); links with a purine or pyrimidine –NH– group yield glycosyl (or *N*-glycosyl) compounds.

cardiac g.'s, generic term for a large number of drugs with the capacity to increase the force of contraction of the failing heart. Examples include digitalis (foxglove) extracts as well as those obtained from other plant and animal sources.

cyanogenic g., a g. capable of generating CN⁻ upon metabolism (e.g., amygdalin).

N-**gly·co·side.** Misnomer for glycosyl.

gly·co·sid·ic (glī-kō-sid'ik). Referring to or denoting a glycoside or glycoside linkage.

gly·co·sphin·go·lip·id (glī'kō-sfing-gō-lip'id). A ceramide linked to one or more sugars via the terminal OH group; included as g.'s are cerebrosides, gangliosides, and ceramide oligosaccharides (oligoglycosylceramides). The prefix glyc- may be replaced by gluc-, galact-, lact-, etc. SYN ceramide saccharide.

gly·co·stat·ic (glī-kō-stat'ik). Indicating the property of certain extracts of the anterior hypophysis that permits the body to maintain its glycogen stores in muscle, liver, and other tissues.

gly·cos·ur·ia (glī-kō-soo'rē-ă). **1.** SYN glucosuria. **2.** Urinary excretion of carbohydrates. SYN glycuresis (2). [glyco- + G. *ouron*, urine]

alimentary g., g. developing after the ingestion of a moderate amount of sugar or starch, which normally is disposed of without appearing in the urine, because rate of intestinal absorption exceeds capacity of the liver and the other tissues to remove the glucose, thus allowing blood glucose levels to become high enough for renal excretion to occur. SYN alimentary diabetes, digestive g.

benign g., g. not associated with diabetes mellitus but resulting from a low renal threshold for sugar.

digestive g., SYN alimentary g.

nondiabetic g., SYN nonhyperglycemic g.

nonhyperglycemic g., presence of glucose in the urine without hyperglycemia due to abnormality in renal tubular reabsorption of filtered glucose. SYN nondiabetic g., orthoglycemic g.

normoglycemic g., SYN renal g.

orthoglycemic g. (ōr-thō-glī'cēm-ik), SYN nonhyperglycemic g.

pathologic g., chronic excretion of relatively large amounts of sugar in the urine.

phlorizin g., phloridzin g., the presence of sugar in the urine after the experimental administration of phlorizin, which results in a lower renal threshold for glucose reabsorption of glucose. SYN phlorizin diabetes.

renal g., the recurring or persistent excretion of glucose in the urine, in association with blood glucose levels that are in the normal range; results from the failure of proximal renal tubules to reabsorb glucose at a normal rate from the glomerular filtrate (low renal threshold); defect in the glucose carrier in the nephron. SYN normoglycemic g., renal diabetes.

gly·co·syl (glī'kō-sil). The radical resulting from detachment of

the OH of the hemiacetal or hemiketal of a saccharide. Cf. glycoside.

gly·co·sy·la·tion (glī'kō-si-lā'shŭn). Formation of linkages with glycosyl groups, as between D-glucose and the hemoglobin chain to form the fraction hemoglobin A_{Ic}, whose level rises in association with the raised blood D-glucose concentration in poorly controlled or uncontrolled diabetes mellitus. SEE ALSO glycosylated *hemoglobin*.

gly·co·syl·trans·fer·ase (glī'kō-sil-trans'fer-ās). Any enzyme (EC subclass 2.4) transferring glycosyl groups from one compound to another. SYN transglycosylase.

gly·co·tro·pic, gly·co·tro·phic (glī-kō-trop'ik, -trof'ik). Pertaining to a principle in extracts of the anterior lobe of the pituitary that antagonizes the action of insulin and causes hyperglycemia. [glyco- + G. *trophē*, nourishment; *tropē*, a turning]

glyc·u·re·sis (glī-koo-rē'sis). **1.** SYN glucosuria. **2.** SYN glycosuria (2). [glyco- + G. *ourēsis*, urination]

gly·cu·ron·ate (glī-koor'on-āt). A salt or ester of a glycuronic acid.

gly·cu·ron·ic ac·id (glī-koor-on'ik). The uronic acid of a sugar in which the terminal carbon is oxidized to a carboxyl group.

gly·cu·ron·i·dase (glī-koor-on'i-dās). SYN β-D-glucuronidase.

gly·cu·ro·nide (glī-koor'on-īd). A glycoside of a uronic acid; e.g., glucuronide.

gly·cu·ro·nu·ria (glī-koo-rō-noo'rē-ă). The presence of glucuronic acid in the urine.

gly·cy·cla·mide (glī-sī'klă-mīd). An oral hypoglycemic agent. SYN cyclamide, tolcyclamide, tolhexamide.

gly·cyl (Gly) (glī'sil). The acyl radical of glycine.

glyc·yr·rhi·za (glis-ĭ-rī'ză). The dried rhizome and root of *Glycyrrhiza glabra* (family Leguminoseae) and allied species; a demulcent, mild laxative, and expectorant; also used to disguise the taste of other remedies; its action appears to depend upon glycyrrhizic acid, a salt-retaining glycoside that mimics the action of aldosterone. SYN licorice, liquorice. [G. fr. *glykys*, sweet, + *rhiza*, root]

gly·ox·al (glī-oks'ăl). OHC–CHO; the simplest dialdehyde. SYN oxalaldehyde.

gly·ox·a·lase (glī-oks'ă-lās). An enzyme, lactoylglutathione lyase (g. I) or hydroxyacylglutathione hydrolase (g. II), in red cells and other tissues that converts glyoxal and substituted glyoxals bound to glutathione into the corresponding free hydroxy acids (g. II) or glyoxals (g. I).

gly·ox·y·late trans·a·cet·y·lase (glī-oks'i-lāt). SYN *malate* synthase.

gly·ox·yl·di·u·reide (glī-oks-il-dī'ū-rīd). SYN allantoin.

gly·ox·yl·ic ac·id (glī-oks-il'ik). OHC–COOH; produced by the action of glycine dehydrogenases upon glycine or sarcosine, or from allantoic acid by allantoicase or via alanine:glyoxylate aminotransferase. SYN oxoacetic acid.

gm Former abbreviation for gram.

GM-CSF Abbreviation for granulocyte-macrophage colony-stimulating *factor*.

Gmelin, Leopold, German physiologist and chemist, 1788–1853. SEE G. *test;* Rosenbach-G. *test.*

GMP Abbreviation for guanylic acid.

GMP re·duc·tase Abbreviation for *guanylic acid* reductase.

GMP syn·the·tase Abbreviation for *guanylic acid* synthetase.

GMS Abbreviation for Gomori methenamine-silver *stain*, under *stain*.

gnash·ing (nash'ing). The grinding together of the teeth as a nonmasticatory function; sometimes associated with emotional tension. SEE ALSO bruxism.

gnat (nat). A midge; general term applied to several species of minute insects, including species of *Simulium* (buffalo g.) and *Hippelates* (eye g.). British authors sometimes include mosquitoes in this group, but this is not done in the U.S. [A.S. *gnaet*]

△gnath-. SEE gnatho-.

gnath·ic (nath'ik). Relating to the jaw or alveolar process. [G. *gnathos*, jaw]

gnath·i·on (nath'ē-on). The most inferior point of the mandible in the midline. In cephalometrics, it is the midpoint between the most anterior and inferior point on the bony chin, measured at the intersection of the mandibular baseline and the nasion-pogonion line. [G. *gnathos,* jaw]

gnatho-, gnath-. The jaw. [G. *gnathos*]

gnath·o·ceph·a·lus (nath-ō-sef'ă-lŭs). A fetal malformation with little of the head formed except the jaws. [gnatho- + G. *kephalē,* head]

gnath·o·dy·nam·ics (nath'ō-dī-nam'iks). The study of the relationship of the magnitude and direction of the forces developed by and upon the components of the masticatory system during function. [gnatho- + G. *dynamis,* power]

gnath·o·dy·na·mom·e·ter (nath'ō-dī-nă-mom'ĕ-ter). A device for measuring biting pressure. SYN bite gauge, occlusometer. [gnatho- + dynamometer]

gnath·og·ra·phy (nă-thog'ră-fē). The recording of the action of the masticatory apparatus in function.

gnath·o·log·ic·al (nath-ō-loj'i-kăl). Pertaining to gnathodynamics.

gnath·ol·o·gy (nă-thol'ō-jē). The science of the masticatory system, including physiology, functional disturbances, and treatment.

gnath·os·chi·sis (nă-thos'ki-sis). Cleft of the jaw. [gnatho- + G. *schisis,* a cleaving]

gnath·o·stat·ics (nath-ō-stat'iks). In orthodontic diagnosis, a technical procedure for orienting the dentition to certain cranial landmarks. [gnatho- + G. *statikos,* causing to stand]

Gna·thos·to·ma (nă-thos'tō-mă). A genus of spiruroid nematode worms (family Gnathostomatidae) characterized by several rows of cuticular spines about the head and by multiple-host aquatic life cycles; it includes pathogenic parasites of cats, cattle, and swine. [gnatho- + G. *stoma,* mouth]

G. doloresi, nematode species found in domestic and wild pigs; human infections (cutaneous larva migrans) reported in Japan.

G. hispidum, nematode species found in domestic and wild pigs; human infections (cutaneous larva migrans) reported in Japan.

G. nipponicum, nematode species found in weasels; human infections (cutaneous larva migrans) reported in Japan.

G. siamen'se, invalid name for *G. spinigerum.*

G. spinig'erum, a parasite of cats, dogs, and wild carnivores, it has occasionally been found in humans in the Far East; it is transmitted via copepods and fish; human infection is usually confined to the skin, but several cases have been reported of eye or brain infection with wandering larvae of this species.

gna·thos·to·mi·a·sis (nath-ō-stō-mī'ă-sis). A migrating edema, or creeping eruption, caused by cutaneous infection by larvae of *Gnathostoma spinigerum.* SYN Yangtze edema.

gnos·co·pine (nos'kō-pēn). An opium alkaloid, $C_{22}H_{23}NO_7$, obtained by racemization of noscapine; an antitussive. SYN *dl*-narcotine.

gno·sia (nō'sē-ă). The perceptive faculty enabling one to recognize the form and the nature of persons and things; the faculty of perceiving and recognizing. [G. *gnōsis,* knowledge]

gno·to·bi·ol·o·gy (nō'tō-bī-ol'ō-jē). The study of animals in the absence of contaminating microorganisms; i.e., of "germ-free" animals. [G. *gnotos,* known, + *bios,* life, + *logos,* study]

gno·to·bi·o·ta (nō'tō-bī-ō'tă). Living colonies or species, assembled from pure isolates. [G. *gnotos,* known, + Mod. L. *biota,* fr. G. *bios,* life]

gno·to·bi·ote (nō-tō-bī'ōt). An individual organism from a group assembled from pure isolates (gnotobiota).

gno·to·bi·ot·ic (nō'tō-bī-ot'ik). Denoting germ-free or formerly germ-free organisms in which the composition of any associated microbial flora, if present, is fully defined. [see gnotobiota]

GnRH Abbreviation for gonadotropin-releasing *hormone.*

goal (gōl). In psychology, any object or objective that an organism seeks to attain or achieve. [M.E. *gol*]

Godélier, Charles P., French physician, 1813–1877. SEE G. *law.*

Godman, John D., U.S. anatomist, 1794–1830. SEE G. *fascia.*

Godwin, John T., U.S. pathologist, *1917. SEE G. *tumor.*

Goeckerman, William H., U.S. dermatologist, 1884–1954. SEE G. *treatment.*

Gofman, Moses, German physician, *1887. SEE G. *test.*

Goggia, Carlo P., 20th century Italian physician. SEE G. *sign.*

gog·gle (gog'gl). **1.** A screen cover for the eye. **2.** A type of spectacle with auxiliary shields for protecting the eyes. [M.E. *gogelen,* to squint]

plethysmographic g., a specially designed g. to serve as an ophthalmodynamometer while permitting subjective visual and objective ocular changes during transient increased intraocular pressure.

goi·ter (goy'ter). A chronic enlargement of the thyroid gland, not due to a neoplasm, occurring endemically in certain localities, especially regions where glaciation occurred and the soil is low in iodine, and sporadically elsewhere. SYN struma (1). [Fr. from L. *guttur,* throat]

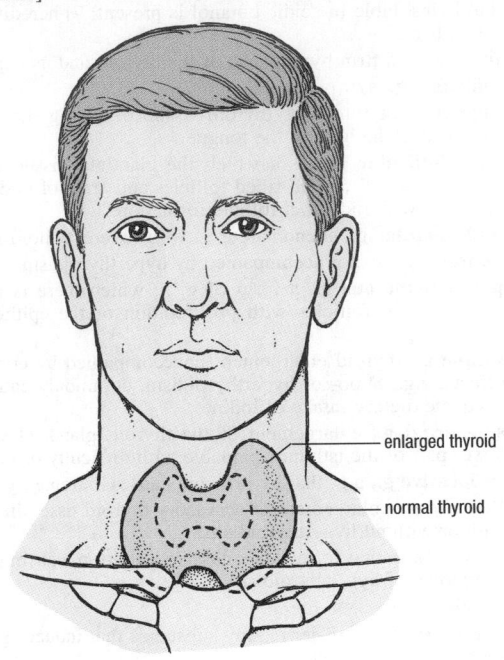

— enlarged thyroid

— normal thyroid

goiter

go

aberrant g., enlargement of a supernumerary thyroid gland. SYN struma aberrata.

acute g., a g. that develops very rapidly.

adenomatous g., an enlargement of the thyroid gland due to the growth of one or more encapsulated adenomas or multiple nonencapsulated colloid nodules within its substance.

Basedow g., colloid g. which becomes hyperfunctional after the ingestion of excess iodine, the Jod-Basedow *phenomenon.*

cabbage g., g. due to ingestion of cabbage or other goitrogenic foodstuff.

colloid g., a form of g. in which the contents of the follicles increase greatly, causing pressure atrophy of the epithelium so that the gelatinous matter predominates in the tumor. SYN struma colloides.

cystic g., an enlargement in the thyroid region due to the presence of one or more cysts within the gland.

diffuse g., g. in which the morbid process involves the whole gland, as opposed to nodular g. or thyroid adenoma.

diving g., a freely movable g. that is sometimes above and sometimes below the sternal notch. SYN wandering g.

endemic g., g., usually of simple type, prevalent in certain regions where dietary intake of iodine is suboptimal.

exophthalmic g., any of the various forms of hyperthyroidism in which the thyroid gland is enlarged and exophthalmos is present.

familial g., a group of heritable thyroid disorders in which g. is commonly apparent first during childhood; often associated with skeletal and/or mental retardation, and with other signs of hypothyroidism that may develop with age. Various types of familial g. have been identified: 1) iodide transport defect [MIM*274400]; of autosomal recessive inheritance caused by mutation in the sodium iodide symporter gene (SLC5A5) on 19p, in which the gland is unable to concentrate iodide; 2) organification defect [MIM*274500 and *274600], in which the iodination of tyrosine is defective; 3) Pendred *syndrome* [MIM*274600]; autosomal recessive inheritance caused by mutation in the Pendred syndrome gene (PDS) on 7q; 4) coupling defect, in which cretinism results from defective coupling of iodotyrosines to form iodothyronines [MIM*274700]; 5) iodotyrosine deiodinase defect, in which deiodination of iodotyrosine is defective, considerable glandular loss of these hormonal precursors occurs, and cretinism may be present [MIM*274800]; 6) plasma iodoprotein disorder [MIM*274900], in which an abnormal iodinated serum protein that is insoluble in acidic butanol is present; 7) hereditary hyperthyroidism.

fibrous g., a firm hyperplasia of the thyroid and its capsule.

follicular g., SYN parenchymatous g.

lingual g., a tumor of thyroid tissue involving the embryonic rudiment at the base of the tongue.

microfollicular g., g. in which the glandular tissue consists of unusually small colloid filled follicles and areas of undifferentiated tissue with indistinct follicle formation.

multinodular g., adenomatous g. with several colloid nodules.

nontoxic g., g. not accompanied by hyperthyroidism.

parenchymatous g., a form of g. in which there is a great increase in the follicles with proliferation of the epithelium. SYN follicular g.

simple g., thyroid enlargement unaccompanied by constitutional effects, e.g., hypo- or hyperthyroidism, commonly caused by inadequate dietary intake of iodine.

substernal g., enlargement of the thyroid gland, chiefly of the lower part of the isthmus, palpable with difficulty or not at all.

suffocative g., a g. that by pressure causes extreme dyspnea.

thoracic g., enlargement of accessory thyroid tissue in the thorax with or without hyperthyroidism.

toxic g., a g. that forms an excessive secretion, causing signs and symptoms of hyperthyroidism.

wandering g., SYN diving g.

goi·tro·gen (goy′trō-jen). Any substance that induces goiter, e.g., cabbage, rapeseed, etc.

goi·tro·gen·ic (goy-trō-jen′ik). Causing goiter.

goi·trous (goy′trŭs). Denoting or characteristic of a goiter.

gold (Au). A yellow metallic element, atomic no. 79, atomic wt. 196.96654; ^{198}Au (half-life of 2.694 days) is used in the treatment of certain tumors, for radiation synovectomy, and in imaging. SYN aurum.

cohesive g., nearly pure g. so treated as to be free of adsorbed surface gases and impurities so that it will weld under pressure at room temperature; in dentistry, used as a restorative material placed directly into a prepared cavity and welded by pressure.

colloidal radioactive g., SYN radiogold colloid.

mat g., powdered g. formed by electrolytic precipitation, compressed into strips, and sintered.

noncohesive g., g. that will not weld because gases adsorb to the surface; some forms may be made cohesive by heat treatment; in dentistry, used as a direct filling material.

powdered g., g. formed by atomizing or by chemical precipitation, lightly precondensed, and wrapped with g. foil so as to form pellets.

g. sodium thiomalate, used in the treatment of rheumatoid arthritis. SYN sodium aurothiomalate.

g. sodium thiosulfate, used in the treatment of lupus erythematosus and some cases of rheumatoid arthritis. SYN sodium aurothiosulfate.

g. standard, term used to describe a method or procedure that is widely recognized as the best available. [jargon]

g. thioglucose, SYN aurothioglucose.

Goldblatt, Harry, U.S. pathologist, 1891–1977. SEE G. *hypertension, kidney, hypertension.*

Gol·den, Ross, U.S. radiologist, 1889–1975. SEE S *sign* of Golden.

Goldenhar, Maurice, 20th century American physician. SEE G. *syndrome.*

gold·en seal (gold′n sēl). SYN hydrastis.

Goldflam, Samuel V., Polish neurologist, 1852–1932. SEE G. *disease.*

gold foil. Pure gold rolled into extremely thin sheets; used in the restoration of carious or fractured teeth. SEE ALSO cohesive *gold,* noncohesive *gold.*

Goldie, James H., 20th century Canadian epidemiologist. SEE G.-Coldman *hypothesis.*

Goldman, Henry M., U.S. periodontist, 1911–1980. SEE G.-Fox *knives,* under *knife.*

Goldman, David E., U.S. physiologist, *1910. SEE G. *equation;* G.-Hodgkin-Katz *equation.*

Goldmann, Hans, Swiss ophthalmologist, 1899–1991. SEE G. *perimeter,* applanation *tonometer.*

Goldscheider, Johannes K.A.E., German neurologist, 1858–1935. SEE G. *test.*

Goldstein, Hyman I., U.S. physician, 1887–1954. SEE G. toe *sign.*

Golgi, Camillo, Italian histologist and Nobel laureate, 1843–1926. SEE G. *apparatus, complex, corpuscle,* tendon *organ,* internal *reticulum, zone, cells,* under *cell,* osmiobichromate *fixative, stain;* G.-Mazzoni *corpuscle;* Holmgrén-G. *canals,* under *canal.*

gol·gi·o·ki·ne·sis (gol′jē-ō-ki-nē′sis). In mitosis, the process of division of the Golgi apparatus and its distribution to the two daughter cells.

Goll, Friedrich, Swiss anatomist, 1829–1903. SEE G. *column;* nucleus of G.; *tract* of G.

Goltz, Robert W., U.S. dermatologist, *1923. SEE G. *syndrome.*

Gombault, Albert F., French neurologist and pathologist, 1844–1904. SEE G. *triangle.*

go·me·nol (gō′mĕ-nol). An ethereal oil obtained from a plant, *Melaleuca viridiflora;* the chief constituent is cineole. It has germicidal action, is free from irritating properties, and has been used in chronic inflammations of the pulmonary mucous membranes and as a vermifuge. SYN oleogomenol. [*Gomen,* a locality in New Caledonia, + L. *oleum,* oil]

gom·i·to·li (gō-mē′tō-lē). Intricately coiled and looped capillary vessels present largely in the upper infundibular stem of the stalk of the pituitary gland; they make up a portion of the pituitary portal circulation. [It. *gomitolo,* coil]

gom·mel·in (gom′mē-lin). A form of dextrin.

Gomori, George, Hungarian histochemist in the U.S., 1904–1957. SEE Grocott-G. methenamine-silver *stain;* G. nonspecific alkaline phosphatase *stain,* one-step trichrome *stain,* silver impregnation *stain,* chrome alum hematoxylin-phloxine *stain.* See entries under stain.

Gompertz, Benjamin, English actuary, 1779–1865. SEE G. *hypothesis, law.*

gom·pho·sis (gom-fō′sis) [TA]. A form of fibrous joint in which a peglike process fits into a hole, as the root of a tooth into the socket in the alveolus. SYN articulatio dentoalveolaris, dentoalveolar joint, gompholic joint, peg-and-socket articulation, peg-and-socket joint, socket. [G. *gomphos,* bolt, nail, + *-osis,* condition]

go·nad (gō′nad). An organ that produces sex cells; a testis or an ovary. [Mod. L. fr. G. *gonē,* seed]

female g., SYN ovary.

indifferent g., the primordial organ in an embryo before its differentiation into testis or ovary. SEE indifferent *genitalia.*

male g., SYN testis.

streak g., SYN gonadal *streak.*

△**gonad-.** SEE gonado-.

go·nad·al (gō-nad′ăl). Relating to a gonad.

go·nad·ec·to·my (gō-nad-ek′tō-mē). Excision of ovary or testis.

SEE ALSO castration, orchiectomy, ovariectomy. [gonado- + G. *ektomē*, excision]

△**gonado-, gonad-.** The gonads. [G. *gonē*, seed]

go·nad·o·blas·to·ma (gō-nad-ō-blas-tō′ma). Benign neoplasm composed of germ cells, sex cord, stromal cells; appears in cases of mixed or pure gonadal dysgenesis; usually small (1–3 cm) and partially calcified, but may give rise to malignant germ-cell tumors, most often seminoma/dysgerminoma or embryonal.

go·nad·o·crins (gō-nad′ō-krinz). Peptides that stimulate release of both follicle-stimulating hormone and luteinizing hormone from the pituitary; found in ovarian follicular fluid in rats. [gonad + G. *krinō*, to secrete]

go·nad·o·lib·er·in (gō′nad-ō-lib′er-in). **1.** A hypothalamic substance causing the release of gonadotropin. SYN gonadotropin-releasing factor, gonadotropin-releasing hormone. **2.** A decapeptide from pig hypothalami that induces release of both lutropin and follitropin in constant proportions and thus acts as both luliberin and folliberin. SYN luteinizing hormone/follicle-stimulating hormone-releasing factor. [gonad + L. *libero*, to free, + -in]

gon·a·dop·athy (gon-ă-dop′ă-thē). Disease affecting the gonads. [gonado- + G. *pathos*, suffering]

go·nad·o·rel·in hy·dro·chlo·ride (gō-nad-ō-rel′in). $C_{55}H_{75}N_{17}O_{13} \cdot x$HCl; a gonadotropin-releasing hormone obtained from sheep, pigs, or other animals and used to evaluate the functional capacity of the gonadotrophs of the anterior pituitary. [*go-nad*otropin-*rel*easing + -in]

go·nad·o·troph (gō-nad′ō-trof, -gon′ă-dō-). An endocrine cell of the adenohypophysis that affects certain cells of the ovary or testis.

go·nad·o·tro·phic (gō′nad-o-trōf′ik, gon′ă-dō-). SYN gonadotropic. [gonado- + G. *trophē*, nourishment]

go·nad·o·tro·phin (gō′nad-ō-trō′fin, gon′ă-dō-). SYN gonadotropin. [for gonadotrophin, fr. gonad + G. *trophē*, nourishment]

go·nad·o·tro·pic (gō′nad-ō-trōp′ik, gon′ă-dō-). **1.** Descriptive of or relating to the actions of a gonadotropin. **2.** Promoting the growth and/or function of the gonads. SYN gonadotrophic. [gonado- + G. *tropē*, a turning]

go·nad·o·tro·pin (gō′nad-ō-trō′pin, gon′ă-dō-). **1.** A hormone capable of promoting gonadal growth and function; such effects, as exerted by a single hormone, usually are limited to discrete functions or histologic components of a gonad, such as stimulation of follicular growth or of androgen formation; most g.'s exert their effects in both sexes, although the effect of a given g. will differ in males and females. **2.** Any hormone that stimulates gonadal function. **3.** Any substance that has the combined effects of follicle-stimulating hormone and luteinizing hormone. SYN gonadotrophin, gonadotropic hormone.

anterior pituitary g., any g. of hypophysial origin; formerly used to designate a single hormone, because it was thought that the anterior hypophysis secreted only one g. SYN pituitary gonadotropic hormone.

chorionic g. (CG), a glycoprotein with a carbohydrate fraction composed of D-galactose and hexosamine, extracted from the urine of pregnant women and produced by the placental trophoblastic cells; its most important role appears to be stimulation, during the first trimester, of ovarian secretion of the estrogen and progesterone required for the integrity of conceptus; it appears to play no significant role in the last two trimesters of pregnancy, as the estrogen and progesterone are then formed by the placenta. SYN β-HCG, choriogonadotropin, chorionic gonadotropic hormone, chorionic gonadotrophic hormone, placenta g., placentagonadotropin.

human chorionic g. (HCG, hCG), SEE chorionic g.

β-human chorionic g., a 145-amino acid subunit unique to HCG, which has the same α-chain as FSH, LH, and TSH. Pregnancy tests specific for β-HCG are more sensitive since there is no confusion with other gonadotropins secreted by the pituitary.

human menopausal g. (HMG, hMG), a hormone of pituitary originally obtained from the urine of postmenopausal women now produced synthetically; used to induce ovulation. SEE ALSO menotropins.

placenta g. (plă-sen′tă-gō′nad-ō-trō-pin), SYN chorionic g.

gon·a·duct (gon′ă-dŭkt). **1.** SYN seminal *duct*. **2.** SYN uterine *tube*. [gonado- + duct]

go·nal·gia (gō-nal′jē-ă). Obsolete term for pain in the knee. [G. *gony*, knee, + *algos*, pain]

gon·ane (gon′ān). The hypothetical parent (17-carbon) hydrocarbon molecule of gonadal steroid hormones, such as estrane or androstane, which was conceived to achieve forms of systematic nomenclature.

gon·ar·thri·tis (gon-ar-thrī′tis). Inflammation arthritis of the knee joint. [G. *gony*, knee, + *arthron*, joint, + *-itis*, inflammation]

gon·e·cyst, gon·e·cys·tis (gon′ĕ-sist, gon-ĕ-sis′tis). SYN seminal *gland*. [G. *gonē*, seed, + *kystis*, bladder]

Gon·gy·lo·ne·ma (gon′ji-lō-nē′mă). A genus of spiruroid nematodes that parasitize the alimentary canal of birds and mammals; transmitted via various insects, especially beetles, carrying the encysted infective larvae. Several species are of veterinary importance, and one is also known to parasitize humans. [Gr. *gongylos*, round, + *nēma*, thread]

G. pul′chrum, the gullet worm of cattle; a species that penetrates the submucosa of the esophagus or rumen of many domestic and wild ruminants, pigs, bears, and humans (human cases are chiefly caused by immature worms); it is transmitted by coprophagous beetles and is of worldwide distribution.

gon·gy·lo·ne·mi·a·sis (gon′ji-lō-nē-mī′ă-sis). Infection of animals and, rarely, humans with nematodes of the genus *Gongylonema*.

go·nia (gō′nē-ă). Plural of gonion.

△**gonio-.** Angle. [G. *gōnia*]

go·ni·o·cra·ni·om·e·try (gō′nē-ō-krā-nē-om′ĕ-trē). Measurement of the angles of the cranium. [G. *gōnia*, angle, + *kranion*, skull, + *metron*, measure]

go·ni·o·dys·gen·e·sis (gō′nē-ō-dis-jen′ĕ-sis). Developmental aberration of the anterior ocular segment. [G. *gōnia*, angle, + dysgenesis]

▯**go·ni·om·e·ter** (gō-nē-om′ĕ-ter). **1.** An instrument for measuring angles. **2.** An appliance for the static test of labyrinthine disease, which consists of a plank, one end of which may be raised to any desired height; as one end of the plank is gradually raised, the point at which a patient loses balance is noted. **3.** A calibrated device designed to measure the arc or range of motion of a joint. SYN arthrometer, fleximeter, pronometer. **4.** Device used to measure the amount of head turn in strabismus or nystagmus. [G. *gōnia*, angle, + *metron*, measure]

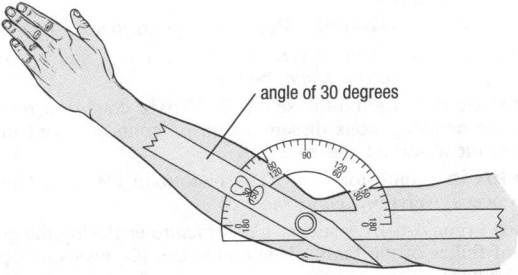

angle of 30 degrees

goniometer: used to measure degrees of joint motion, this example shows 30 degrees of flexion at the elbow

go·ni·on, pl. **go·nia** (gō′nē-on, gō′nē-ă) [TA]. The lowest posterior and most outward point of the angle of the mandible. In cephalometrics, it is measured by bisecting the angle formed by the tangents to the lower and the posterior borders of the mandible; when the angles of both sides of the mandible appear on the lateral radiograph, a point midway between the right and left side is used. [G. *gōnia*, an angle]

go·ni·o·punc·ture (gō′nē-ō-pŭnk-choor). An operation for congenital glaucoma in which a puncture is made in the filtration angle of the anterior chamber.

go·ni·o·scope (gō′nē-ō-skōp). A lens designed to study the angle

go

of the anterior chamber of the eye. [G. *gōnia,* angle, + *skopeō,* to examine]

go·ni·os·co·py (gō-nē-os'kŏ-pē). Examination of the angle of the anterior chamber of the eye with a gonioscope or with a contact prism lens.

go·ni·o·syn·ech·ia (gŏ'nē-ō-si-nek'ē-ă). Adhesion of the iris to the posterior surface of the cornea in the angle of the anterior chamber; associated with angle-closure glaucoma. SYN peripheral anterior synechia. [G. *gōnia,* angle, + *synechis,* holding together]

go·ni·ot·o·my (gō-nē-ot'ō-mē). Surgical opening of the trabecular meshwork in congenital glaucoma. [G. *gōnia,* angle, + *tomē,* incision]

gon·o·cho·rism, gon·o·cho·ris·mus (gon-ok'ō-rizm, -ō-riz'mŭs). Normal gonadal differentiation appropriate to the sex. [G. *gonē,* seed, sex, + *chōrizō,* to separate]

gon·o·cide (gon'ō-sīd). **1.** Destructive to the gonococcus. **2.** An agent that kills gonococci. SYN gonococcicide.

gon·o·coc·cal (gon'ō-kok'ăl). Relating to the gonococcus. SYN gonococcic.

gon·o·coc·ce·mia (gon'ō-kok-sē'mē-ă). The presence of gonococci in the circulating blood. [gonococcus + G. *haima,* blood]

gon·o·coc·ci (gon-ō-kok'sī). Plural of gonococcus.

gon·o·coc·cic (gon'ō-kok'sik). SYN gonococcal.

gon·o·coc·ci·cide (gon-ō-kok'si-sīd). SYN gonocide. [gonococcus + L. *caedo,* to kill]

gon·o·coc·cus, pl. **gon·o·coc·ci** (gon-ō-kok'ŭs, -sī). SYN *Neisseria gonorrhoeae.* [G. *gonē,* seed, + *kokkos,* berry]

gon·o·cyte (gon'ō-sīt). SYN primordial germ *cell.* [G. *gonē,* seed, + *kytos,* hollow (cell)]

gon·o·he·mia (gon-ō-hē'mē-ă). Obsolete term for gonococcemia.

gon·o·op·so·nin (gon-ō-op'sŏ-nin). A specific gonococcal opsonin.

gon·o·phage (gon'ō-fāj). A gonocidal bacteriophage.

gon·o·phore, gon·oph·o·rus (gon'ŏ-fōr, gō-nof'ŏ-rŭs). Any structure serving to store up or conduct the sexual cells; oviduct, spermatic duct, uterus, or seminal vesicle; an accessory generative organ. [G. *gonē,* seed, + *phoros,* bearing]

gon·or·rhea (gon-ō-rē'ă). A contagious catarrhal inflammation of the genital mucous membrane, transmitted chiefly by coitus and due to *Neisseria gonorrhoeae;* may involve the lower or upper genital tract, especially the urethra, endocervix, and uterine tubes, or spread to the peritoneum and rarely to the heart, joints, or other structures by way of the bloodstream. [G. *gonorrhoia,* fr. *gonē,* seed, + *rhoia,* a flow]

gon·or·rhe·al (gon-ō-rē'ăl). Relating to gonorrhea.

gon·o·some (gon'ō-sōm). SYN sex *chromosomes,* under *chromosome.* [G. *gonē,* seed + *sōma,* body]

gon·o·tox·e·mia (gon'ō-tok-sē'mē-ă). Toxic condition resulting from the hematogenous dissemination of gonococci and the effects of the absorbed endotoxin.

gon·o·tox·in (gon-ō-tok'sin). The endotoxin elaborated by the gonococcus, *Neisseria gonorrhoeae.*

gon·o·tyl (gon'ō-til). A sucker-like structure enclosing the genital pore of flukes of the family Heterophyidae. [G. *gonos,* offspring, + *tylē,* knob]

Go·ny·au·lax cat·a·nel·la (gon-ē-aw'laks kat-ă-nel'ă). A marine dinoflagellate protozoan that produces a powerful toxin that accumulates in the tissues of mussels and other filter-feeding shellfish and may cause fatal mussel poisoning in humans. [G. *gony,* knee, + *aulakos,* a furrow]

go·ny·camp·sis (gon-ē-kamp'sis). Obsolete term for ankylosis or any abnormal curvature of the knee. [G. *gony,* knee, + *kampsis,* a bending or curving]

Goodell, William, U.S. gynecologist, 1829–1894. SEE G. *sign.*

good·ness of fit. Degree of agreement between an empirically observed distribution and a mathematical or theoretical distribution.

Goodpasture, Ernest W., U.S. pathologist, 1886–1960. SEE G. *stain, syndrome.*

Goormaghtigh, Norbert, Belgian physician, 1890–1960. SEE G. *cells,* under *cell.*

goose·flesh (goos'flesh). SYN *cutis* anserina.

Gopalan, C., 20th century Indian biochemist. SEE G. *syndrome.*

Gordius (gōr'dē-ŭs). An old name for the nematode genus *Dracunculus,* properly applied to members of the phylum Nematomorpha, commonly called the gordian or horsehair worms, hair worms, or hair snakes. [L., fr. G. *Gordios,* king of Gordium in Phrygia; an allusion to the knotlike twistings of these worms]

Gordon, Alfred, U.S. neurologist, 1869–1953. SEE G. *reflex, sign, symptom.*

Gor·dona (gor'dō-na). A genus of aerobic bacteria that are Gram-positive or Gram-variable actinomycetes found in the human respiratory tract; some species are associated with bronchiectasis and with mixed flora pulmonary abscesses; the type species is *Gordona bronchialis.*

Gordon and Sweet stain. See under stain.

gor·get (gōr'jet). A director or guide with wide groove for use in lithotomy.

probe g., a g. with a probe-pointed tip.

Gorham, Lemuel W., U.S. physician, 1885–1968. SEE G. *disease;* Gorham *syndrome.*

Goriaew rule. See under rule.

Gorlin, Richard, U.S. physiologist and cardiologist, *1926. SEE G. *formula.*

Gorlin, Robert J., U.S. oral pathologist, *1923. SEE G. *sign, syndrome;* G.-Chaudhry-Moss *syndrome.*

go·ron·dou (gō-ron'doo). SYN goundou.

goserelin (gos'er-ĕ-lin). A synthetic decapeptide agonist analog of the LHRH (GnRH). It inhibits pituitary gonadotropin secretion and is used in the treatment of prostate cancer, breast cancer, endometriosis, and for prethinning the endometrium before endometrial ablation or resection.

Gosselin, Léon Athanese, French surgeon, 1815–1887. SEE G. *fracture.*

Gosset, William Sealy, British statistician and chemist who used the pseudonym Student, 1876–1937.

gos·sy·pol (gos'i-pol). A toxic principle isolated from the seed of the cotton plant (*Gossypium*) that reduces sperm count; used in China as an oral male contraceptive.

gos·sy·pose (gos'i-pōs). SYN raffinose.

GOT Abbreviation for glutamic-oxaloacetic transaminase.

Göthlin, Gustaf F., Swedish physiologist, 1874–1949. SEE G. *test.*

Gottlieb, Bernard, Austrian dentist, 1885–1950 SEE epithelial *attachment* of Gottlieb.

gouge (gowj). A strong curved chisel used in operations on bone.

Gougerot, Henri, French dermatologist, 1881–1955. SEE G. and Blum *disease;* G.-Sjögren *disease;* G.-Carteaud *syndrome.*

Gould, Sir Alfred P., English surgeon, 1852–1922. SEE G. *suture.*

Gouley, John W.S., U.S. urologist, 1832–1920. SEE G. *catheter.*

goun·dou (goon'doo). A disease, endemic in West Africa, characterized by exostoses from the nasal processes of the maxillary bones, producing a symmetrical swelling on each side of the nose; believed to be an osteitis connected with yaws. SYN anákhré, dog nose, gorondou, henpuye. [native name]

gout (gowt). A disorder of purine metabolism, occurring especially in men, characterized by a raised but variable blood uric acid level and severe recurrent acute arthritis of sudden onset resulting from deposition of crystals of sodium urate in connective tissues and articular cartilage; most cases are inherited, resulting from a variety of abnormalities of purine metabolism. The familial aggregation is for the most part galtonian with a threshold of expression determined by the solubility of uric acid. However, g. is also a feature of the Lesch-Nyhan *syndrome* an X-linked disorder [MIM*308000]. [L. *gutta,* drop]

abarticular g., rarely used term for g. involving structures other than the joints.

articular g., the usual form of g. attacking one or more of the joints.

calcium g., SYN pseudogout.

idiopathic g., acute episodes of crystal-induced synovitis due to abnormality of purine metabolism; lower than normal urinary excretion of urate leading to hyperuricemia and acute episodes of joint inflammation. SYN primary g.

interval g., an asymptomatic phase between acute attacks of g.

latent g., hyperuricemia without symptoms of gout. Often used synonymously with interval g. SYN masked g.

lead g., SYN saturnine g.

masked g., SYN latent g.

primary g., SYN idiopathic g.

retrocedent g., obsolete term for the occurrence of severe gastric, cardiac, or cerebral symptoms during an attack of g., especially when the joint and other symptoms suddenly subside at the same time.

saturnine g., g. occurring in a person with lead poisoning. SYN lead g.

secondary g., g. resulting from increased serum uric acid levels as a result of an antecedent disease, such as a proliferative disease of the blood and bone marrow, lead poisoning, or prolonged chronic renal failure (on dialysis).

tophaceous g., g. in which deposits of uric acid and urates occur as gouty tophi.

gouty (gow′tē). Relating to or characteristic of gout.

Gowers, Sir William R., English neurologist, 1845–1915. SEE G. *column, contraction, disease, syndrome, tract.*

GPI Abbreviation for Gingival-Periodontal Index.

GPT Abbreviation for glutamic-pyruvic transaminase.

gr Abbreviation for grain (3).

Graaf, Reijnier de, Dutch physiologist and histologist, 1641–1673. SEE graafian *follicle.*

graafian. Relating to or described by R. de Graaf.

grac·i·lis (gras′i-lis). **1.** Slender; denoting a thin or slender structure. **2.** SYN gracilis (*muscle*). [L.]

grad. Abbreviation for L. *gradatim,* by degrees, gradually.

grade (grād). **1.** A rank, division, or level on the scale of a value system. **2.** In cancer pathology, a classification of the degree of malignancy or differentiation of tumor tissue; e.g., well, moderately well, or poorly differentiated, and undifferentiated or anaplastic. **3.** In exercise testing, the measurement of a vertical rise or fall as a percent of the horizontal distance traveled. [L. *gradus,* step]

Gleason tumor g., a classification of adenocarcinoma of the prostate by evaluation of the pattern of glandular differentiation; the tumor g., known as Gleason score, is the sum of the dominant and secondary patterns, each numbered on a scale of 1 to 5.

Heath-Edwards g.'s, a system that describes the pathology of hypertensive pulmonary vascular disease.

Gradenigo, Giuseppe, Italian otologist, 1859–1926. SEE G. *syndrome.*

gra·di·ent (grā′dē-ent). Rate of change of temperature, pressure, magnetic field, or other variable as a function of distance, time, etc.

atrioventricular g., the diastolic pressure difference between the atrium and ventricle.

concentration g., SYN density g.

density g., a solution in which the concentration (density) of a solute increases in a continuous fashion from top to bottom, or end to end, of a container (e.g., the centrifuge tube in density-gradient centrifugation). SYN concentration g.

electrochemical g., a measure of the tendency of an ion to move passively from one point to another, taking into consideration the differences in its concentration and in the electrical potentials between the two points; commonly expressed as the additional voltage needed to achieve equilibrium.

g. encoding, SYN *phase* encoding.

field g., SYN magnetic field g.

magnetic field g., in magnetic resonance imaging, a magnetic field that varies with location, superimposed on the uniform field

of the magnet, to alter the resonant frequency of nuclei and allow calculation of their spatial position. SYN field g.

mitral g., the diastolic pressure difference between the left atrium and left ventricle.

systolic g., the difference in pressure during systole between two communicating cardiovascular chambers, e.g., between the left ventricle and aorta in aortic stenosis.

ventricular g., the algebraic sum of (i.e., the net electrical difference between) the area enclosed within the QRS complex and that within the T wave in the electrocardiogram.

grad·u·ate (grad′ū-ăt). A vessel, usually of glass and suitably marked, used for measuring the volume of liquids; g. cylinder. [Mediev. L. *graduatus,* fr. L. *gradus,* step]

grad·u·at·ed (grad′ū-āt′ed). **1.** Marked by lines or in other ways to denote capacity, degrees, percentages, etc. **2.** Divided or arranged in levels, grades, or successive steps.

Graefe, Albrecht von, German ophthalmologist, 1828–1870. SEE G. *forceps, knife, operation, sign;* pseudo-G. *phenomenon;* G. *sign;* von G. *sign.*

Graefenberg, Ernst, German gynecologist in America, 1881–1957. SEE G. *ring.*

Graffi, Arnold, German pathologist, *1910. SEE G. *virus.*

GRAFT

▣ **graft** (graft). **1.** Any tissue or organ for transplantation. **2.** To transplant such structures. SEE ALSO flap, implant, transplant. [A.S. *graef*]

allogeneic g., SYN allograft.

animal g., SYN zoograft.

autogeneic g., SYN autograft.

autologous g., SYN autograft.

autoplastic g., SYN autograft.

bone g., bone transplanted from a donor site to a recipient site, without anastomosis of nutrient vessels; bone can be transplanted within the same individual (i.e., autogeneic graft) or between different individuals (i.e., allogeneic graft). SEE ALSO osteoplasty.

chorioallantoic g., transplanting of living material to the chorioallantoic membrane of the embryonic chick.

composite g., a g. composed of several tissues, such as skin and cartilage or a full-thickness segment of the ear.

corneal g., SYN keratoplasty.

Davis g., "pinch grafts," i.e., small pieces (2–3 mm) of full-thickness skin g.'s.

delayed g., delaying application of a skin g. for several days until recipient bed is clean or no longer bleeding.

dermal g., a g. of dermis, made from skin by cutting away the epidermis.

dermal-fat g., a dermal g. with attached subcutaneous fat.

dowel g., in orthopedic surgery, a specific type of bone g. characterized by a circular shape usually obtained with special instruments used as a structural bone g. to obtain fusion between two adjacent vertebrae. SYN dowel (4).

fascia g., a g. of fibrous tissue, usually the fascia lata.

fascicular g., a nerve g. in which each bundle of fibers is approximated and sutured separately.

fat g., a free g. of fat.

free g., a g. transplanted without its normal attachment (a pedicle) from one site to another.

full-thickness g., a g. of the full thickness of mucosa and submucosa or of skin and subcutaneous tissue.

funicular g., a nerve g. in which each funiculus (composed of two or more fasciculi) is approximated and sutured separately.

H g., SYN H shunt.

heterologous g., SYN xenograft.

heteroplastic g., SYN xenograft.

heterotopic g., transplantation of a tissue or organ into a position it normally does not occupy.

homologous g., SYN allograft.

homoplastic g., SYN allograft.

inlay g., a skin g. wrapped (raw side out) around a firm supporting material and inserted into a prepared surgical pocket. SYN epithelial inlay.

isogeneic g., SYN syngraft.

isologous g., SYN syngraft.

isoplastic g., SYN syngraft.

Krause g., a full-thickness skin g. SYN Krause-Wolfe g.

Krause-Wolfe g., SYN Krause g.

mesh g., split-thickness g. incised with multiple staggered vertical cuts to allow expansion; used to cover problematic wounds or when donor skin is lacking.

mucosal g., a g. of mucous membrane, usually the full thickness of the lining of the cheek or lower lip.

nerve g., a nerve, or part of a nerve, used as a g.

Ollier g., a thin split-thickness g. SYN Ollier-Thiersch g.

Ollier-Thiersch g., SYN Ollier g.

onlay g., a bone g. applied on the outside of the recipient bone(s).

orthotopic g., transplantation of a tissue or organ into its normal anatomic position.

osteoperiosteal g., a g. of bone with its attached periosteum.

partial-thickness g., SYN split-thickness g.

pedicle g., SEE pedicle *flap*.

periosteal g., a g. of periosteum.

pinch g., old technique in which small bits of skin, of partial or full thickness, removed from a healthy area and seeded onto an open wound. SYN Reverdin g.

porcine g., a split-thickness g. from a pig, applied to a raw area on a human as a temporary dressing.

primary skin g., a skin g. transferred immediately after the creation of a raw area.

punch g.'s, small full-thickness g.'s of the scalp, removed with a circular punch and transplanted to a bald area to grow hair.

Reverdin g., SYN pinch g.

skin g., a piece of skin transplanted from one part of the body to another to cover a denuded area.

sleeve g., a g. for repairing a severed nerve by connecting central and peripheral ends with a sleevelike structure, commonly, a segment of vein.

split-skin g., SYN split-thickness g.

split-thickness g., a g. of the upper portions of the skin, i.e., the epidermis and part of the dermis, or of the mucosa and submucosa. SYN partial-thickness g., split-skin g.

Stent g., an inlay skin g., or a skin g. held in place by sutures tied over a conforming/immobilizing dressing.

syngeneic g., SYN syngraft.

tendon g., a g. of tendon, as in tendon transplantation.

Thiersch g., old term for split-thickness g., SEE Ollier-Thiersch g.

Wolfe g., a full-thickness skin g. without subcutaneous fat. SYN Wolfe-Krause g.

Wolfe-Krause g., SYN Wolfe g.

xenogeneic g., SYN xenograft.

zooplastic g., SYN zoograft.

graft·ing. The process of applying a graft.

Graham, Evarts Ambrose, U.S. surgeon, 1883–1957. Reported with W. H. Cole the first successful cholecystography in 1924; In

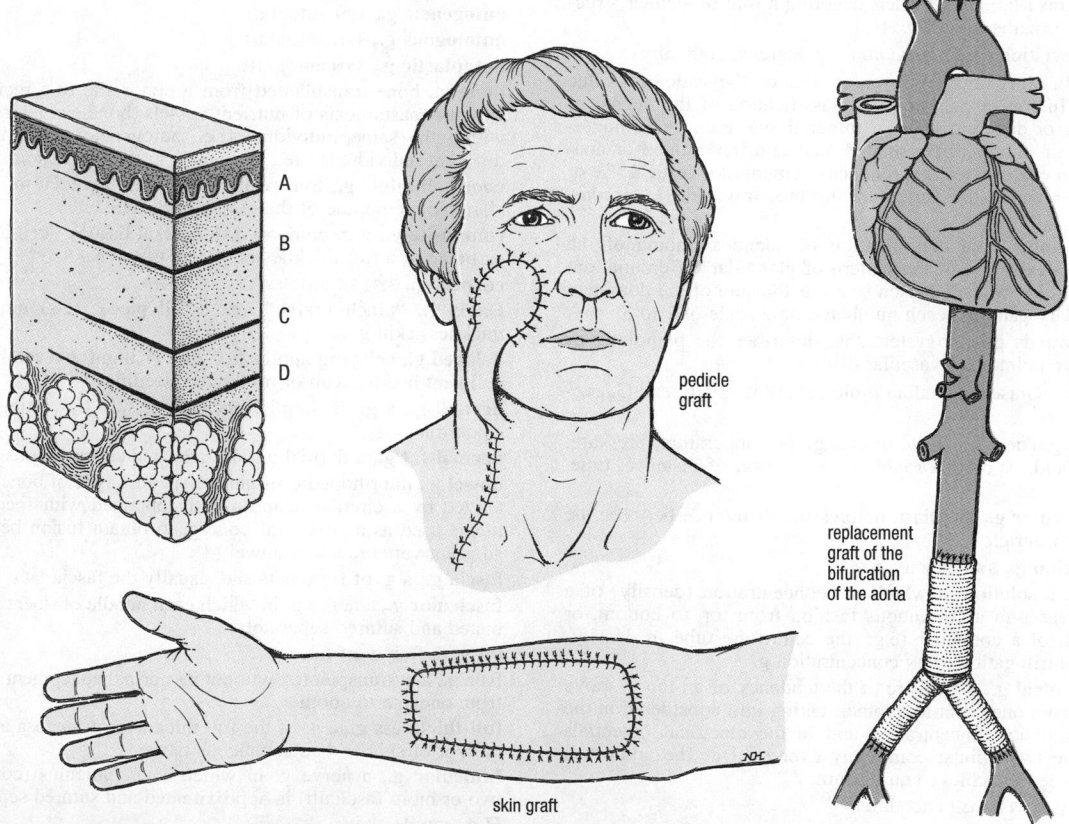

graft types: (A, B, C) split-thickness grafts, (D) full-thickness graft

pedicle graft

replacement graft of the bifurcation of the aorta

skin graft

1933, with J. J. Singer, reported first successful removal of a lung for cancer in one stage. SEE Graham-Cole *test*.

Graham, Thomas, English chemist, 1805–1869. SEE G. *law*.

Gra·ha·mel·la (grā-am-el′ă). A former genus of aerobic, nonmotile bacteria that are now reclassified as members of the genus *Bartonella*. [G. S. *Graham-Smith*]

Graham Steell, SEE Steell.

grain (grān). **1.** Cereal plants, such as corn, wheat, or rye, or a seed of one of them. **2.** A minute, hard particle of any substance, as of sand. **3 (gr).** A unit of weight, $\frac{1}{60}$ dram (apoth. or troy), $\frac{1}{437.5}$ avoirdupois ounce, $\frac{1}{480}$ troy ounce, $\frac{1}{5760}$ troy pound, $\frac{1}{7000}$ avoirdupois pound; the equivalent of 0.064799 g. **4.** A macroscopically visible cluster of organisms living in tissue of patients with actinomycosis or mycetoma. [L. *granum*]

grains (grānz). Parakeratotic nuclei within the horny layer of the epidermis, found in keratosis follicularis.

Gram, Hans C.J., Danish bacteriologist, 1853–1938. SEE G. *iodine, stain;* G.-chromotrope *stain;* Weigert-G. *stain*.

gram (g, gm). A unit of weight in the metric or centesimal system, the equivalent of 15.432358 gr or 0.03527 avoirdupois ounce.

△**-gram.** A recording, usually by an instrument. Cf. -graph. [G. *gramma,* character, mark]

gram·cen·ti·me·ter. The energy exerted, or work done, when a mass of 1 g is raised a height of 1 cm; equal to 9.807×10^{-5} J or newton-meters.

gram·i·ci·din (gram-i-sī′din). One of a group of polypeptide antibiotics produced by *Bacillus brevis* that are primarily bacteriostatic in action against Gram-positive cocci and bacilli. Commercial preparations contain several g.'s known as g. A, B, C, and D; g. S (for Soviet) is cyclic, the others are linear.

gram·i·on. The weight in grams of an ion that is equal to the sum of the atomic weights of the atoms making up the ion.

gram·me·ter. A unit of energy equal to 100 gram-centimeters.

gram·mol·e·cule. See under molecule.

Gram-neg·a·tive. Refers to the inability of a bacterium to resist decolorization with alcohol after being treated with Gram crystal violet. However, following decolorization, these bacteria can be readily counterstained with safranin, imparting a pink or red color to the bacterium when viewed by light microscopy. This reaction is usually an indication that the outer structure of the bacterium consists of a cytoplasmic (inner) membrane surrounded by a relatively thin peptidoglycan layer, which in turn, is surrounded by an outer membrane. SEE Gram *stain*.

Gram-pos·i·tive. Refers to the ability of a bacterium to resist decolorization with alcohol after being treated with Gram crystal violet stain, imparting a violet color to the bacterium when viewed by light microscopy. This reaction is usually an indication that the outer structure of the bacterium consists of a cytoplasmic membrane surrounded by a thick, rigid bacterial cell wall composed of peptidoglycan. SEE Gram *stain*.

gra·na (grā′nă). Bodies within the chloroplasts of plant cells that contain layers composed of chlorophyll and phospholipids. [pl. of L. *granum,* grain]

gra·na·tum (gra-nā′tum). SYN pomegranate. [L. *granatus,* having many seeds]

gran·di·ose (gran′dē-ōs). Pertaining to feelings of great importance, expansiveness, or delusions of grandeur. [It. *grandioso,* fr. L. *grandis,* large]

Granger, Amedee, U.S. radiologist, 1879–1939. SEE G. *line*.

Granit, Ragnar A., Finnish-Swedish neurophysiologist and Nobel laureate, 1900–1991 SEE G. *loop*.

gran·u·lar (gran′ū-lăr). **1.** Composed of or resembling granules or granulations. **2.** Particles with strong affinity for nuclear stains, seen in many bacterial species.

gra·nu·la·tio, pl. **gran·u·la·ti·o·nes** (gran-ū-lā′shē-ō, -shē-o′ nēz). SYN granulation. [L.]

granulatio′nes arachnoideae [TA], SYN arachnoid *granulations,* under *granulation;* SEE ALSO arachnoid *villi,* under *villus*.

gran·u·la·tion (gran′ū-lā′shŭn). **1.** Formation into grains or gran-

ules; the state of being granular. **2.** A granular mass in or on the surface of any organ or membrane; or one of the individual granules forming the mass. **3.** The formation of minute, rounded, fleshy connective tissue projections on the surface of a wound, ulcer, or inflamed tissue surface in the process of healing; one of the fleshy granules composing this surface. SEE ALSO granulation *tissue.* **4.** In pharmacy, the formation of crystals by constant agitation of a supersaturated solution of a salt; product used in the manufacture of tablets for oral use. SYN granulatio. [L. *granulatio*]

arachnoid g.'s [TA], tufted prolongations of pia-arachnoid, composed of numerous arachnoid villi that penetrate dural venous sinuses and effect transfer of cerebrospinal fluid to the venous system. At advanced age these are more numerous and tend to calcify. SYN arachnoidal g.'s [TA], granulationes arachnoideae [TA], pacchionian bodies, pacchionian corpuscles, pacchionian glands, pacchionian g.'s.

arachnoidal g.'s [TA], SYN arachnoid g.'s.

pacchionian g.'s, SYN arachnoid g.'s.

gran·u·la·ti·o·nes (gran-ū-lā-shē-ō′nēz). Plural of granulatio.

gran·ule (gran′ūl). **1.** A grainlike particle; a granulation; a minute discrete mass. **2.** A very small pill, usually gelatin or sugar coated, containing a drug to be given in a small dose. **3.** A colony of the bacterium or fungus causing a disease or simply colonizing the tissues of the patient. In immunocompromised patients the differentiation is difficult. **4.** A small particle that can be seen by electron microscopy; contains stored material. [L. *granulum,* dim. of *granum,* grain]

α g.'s, large, rodlike, or filamentous g.'s found in several types of cells, especially platelets where they are the most numerous type of g.; contain secretory proteins, including fibrinogen, fibronectin, fibrospondin, von Willebrand factor (collectively known as adhesive proteins) and other proteins (platelet factor 4, platelet-derived growth factor, coagulation factor V, etc.).

acidophil g., a g. that stains with an acid dye such as eosin. SYN oxyphil g.

acrosomal g., the single glycoprotein rich g. within an acrosomal vesicle, which results from the coalescence of proacrosomal g.'s.

alpha g., a g. of an alpha cell that was named as the first of several kinds or because it was acidophilic.

Altmann g., (1) SYN fuchsinophil g; (2) SYN mitochondrion.

amphophil g., a g. that stains with both acid and basic dyes.

argentaffin g.'s, g.'s that reduce silver ions from an ammoniac silver nitrate staining solution.

azurophil g., a g. that stains a reddish purple color with an azure dye; such g.'s are seen in dry smears of certain mature and developing blood cells, and are membrane-bound primary lysosomes containing enzymes. SYN kappa g.

basal g., SYN basal *body*.

basophil g., a g. that stains readily with a basic dye.

Bensley specific g.'s, g.'s in the cells of the islands of Langerhans in the pancreas.

beta g., a g. of a beta cell.

Birbeck g., SYN Langerhans g.

Bollinger g.'s, (1) relatively small, but frequently microscopically visible, pale yellow or yellow-white g.'s observed in the granulomatous lesion, or the exudate, in botryomycosis; the g.'s consist of irregular aggregates or colonizations of Gram-positive cocci, usually staphylococci; (2) term sometimes incorrectly used synonymously with Bollinger bodies.

chromatic g., SYN chromophil g. (2).

chromophil g., (1) any readily stainable g.; (2) a g. of chromophil (Nissl) substance. SYN chromatic g.

chromophobe g.'s, g.'s that do not stain or stain poorly with the ordinary dyes; such g.'s are present in some cells in the anterior lobe of the pituitary.

cone g., nucleus of a retinal cell connecting with one of the cones.

Crooke g.'s, lumpy masses of basophilic material in the basophil cells of the anterior lobe of the pituitary, associated with Cushing disease, or following the administration of ACTH.

delta g., a g. of a delta cell.

elementary g., a particle of blood dust, or hemoconia.

eosinophil g., a g. that stains with eosin.

Fordyce g.'s, SYN Fordyce *spots,* under *spot.*

fuchsinophil g., a g. that has an affinity for fuchsin. SYN Altmann g. (1).

glycogen g., glycogen occurring in cells as beta g.'s which average about 300 Å in diameter, or as alpha g.'s which are aggregates measuring 900 Å of smaller particles.

iodophil g., a g. that stains brown with iodine; found in many of the polymorphonuclear leukocytes in pneumonia, erysipelas, scarlet fever, and various other acute diseases.

juxtaglomerular g.'s, osmophilic secretory g.'s present in the juxtaglomerular cells, thought to contain renin.

kappa g., SYN azurophil g.

keratohyalin g.'s, irregularly shaped basophilic g.'s in the cells of the stratum granulosum of the epidermis.

lamellar g., SYN keratinosome.

Langerhans g., a small tennis racket-shaped membrane-bound g. with characteristic cross-striated internal ultrastructure; first reported in Langerhans cells of the epidermis. SYN Birbeck g.

Langley g.'s, g.'s in serous secreting cells.

membrane-coating g.'s, SYN keratinosome.

metachromatic g.'s, (1) g.'s that stain a color different from that of the dye used; SEE ALSO metachromasia; (2) term sometimes used as a synonym for volutin.

mucinogen g.'s, g.'s that produce mucin, as in cells of the salivary glands and in the gastric and intestinal mucosae.

Neusser g.'s, tiny basophilic g.'s sometimes observed in an indistinct zone about the nucleus of a leukocyte.

neutrophil g., a g. stainable with the neutral component of stains, e.g., the Romanovsky-type blood stains.

Nissl g.'s, SYN Nissl *substance.*

oxyphil g., SYN acidophil g.

Palade g., SYN ribosome.

proacrosomal g.'s, small carbohydrate-rich g.'s appearing in vesicles of the Golgi apparatus of spermatids; they coalesce into a single acrosomal g. contained within an acrosomal vesicle.

prosecretion g.'s, g.'s in the cytoplasm of a cell indicative of a preliminary step in the formation of a secretory product.

rod g., the nucleus of a retinal cell connecting with one of the rods.

Schüffner g.'s, SYN Schüffner *dots,* under *dot.*

secretory g., a membrane-bound particle, usually protein, formed in the granular endoplasmic reticulum and the Golgi complex.

seminal g., one of the minute granular bodies present in the semen.

specific g.'s, the distinctive g.'s of basophilic, eosinophilic, and neutrophilic leukocytes, as opposed to their nonspecific azurophilic g.'s.

volutin g.'s, SYN volutin.

Zimmermann g., obsolete term for platelet.

zymogen g., secretory g. in pancreatic acinar cells.

⟁**granulo-.** Granular, granules. [L. *granulum,* a small grain.]

gran·u·lo·blast (gran′ū-lō-blast). Rarely used term for an immature hematopoietic cell capable of giving rise to granulocytes. [granulo- + G. *blastos,* germ]

gran·u·lo·cyte (gran′ū-lō-sīt). A mature granular leukocyte, including neutrophilic, acidophilic, and basophilic types of polymorphonuclear leukocytes, i.e., respectively, neutrophils, eosinophils, and basophils. [granulo- + G. *kytos,* cell]

   immature g., an immature neutrophil; it may be neutrophilic, acidophilic, or basophilic in character.

gran·u·lo·cy·to·pe·nia (gran′ū-lō-sī-tō-pē′nē-ă). Less than the normal number of granular leukocytes in the blood. SYN granulopenia, hypogranulocytosis. [granulocyte + G. *penia,* poverty]

gran·u·lo·cy·to·poi·e·sis (gran′ū-lō-sī′tō-poy-ē′sis). SYN granulopoiesis.

gran·u·lo·cy·to·poi·et·ic (gran′ū-lō-sī′tō-poy-et′ik). SYN granulopoietic. [granulocyte + G. *poieō,* to make]

gran·u·lo·cy·to·sis (gran′ū-lō-sī-tō′sis). A condition character-

---

ized by more than the normal number of granulocytes in the circulating blood or in the tissues.

GRANULOMA

gran·u·lo·ma (gran-ū-lō′mă). Term applied to nodular inflammatory lesions, usually small or granular, firm, persistent, and containing compactly grouped modified phagocytes such as epithelioid cells, giant cells, and other macrophages. SEE ALSO granulomatosis. [granulo- + G. -*oma,* tumor]

actinic g., an annular eruption on sun-exposed skin which microscopically shows phagocytosis of dermal elastic fibers by giant cells and histiocytes. SYN Miescher g.

amebic g., SYN ameboma.

g. annula′re, a chronic or recurrent, usually self-limited papular eruption that tends to develop on the distal portions of the extremities and over prominences, although the condition may be generalized; waxy papules tend to form annular lesions characterized microscopically by foci of dermal necrosis with mucin deposits, bordered by histiocytes with palisaded nuclei.

apical g., SYN periapical g.

beryllium g., a sarcoid-like granulomatous reaction to exposure to inhaled beryllium, or to skin cuts by fluorescent lamp glass.

bilharzial g., SYN schistosome g.

Capillaria **g.,** granulomatous lesions found in the liver and lung are a tissue response at the site of eggs or worms.

cholesterol g., g. with prominent clefts of cholesterol surrounded by foreign-body giant cells found in chronic otitis media and sinusitis.

coccidioidal g., SYN secondary *coccidioidomycosis.*

cutaneous leishmaniasis g., lymphocytic g.'s with necrotic centers found during the healing process.

dental g., SYN periapical g.

Enterobius **g.,** lesions containing dead worms and eggs of this nematode; have been found in vagina, cervix, fallopian tubes, omentum, peritoneum, liver, kidneys, and lungs.

eosinophilic g., a form of Langerhans histiocytosis predominately involving the bones of young people; may be solitary or multiple; histologically composed of Langerhans cells and eosinophils.

g. facia′le, persistent, well-demarcated, reddish-brown nodules of unknown cause that usually appear on the face in middle age and consist of a dense dermal infiltrate of eosinophils and neutrophils, separated from the epidermis and hair follicles, with fibrinoid vasculitis of unknown cause.

fish-tank g., SYN swimming pool g.

foreign body g., a g. caused by the presence of foreign particulate material in tissue, characterized by a histiocytic reaction with foreign body giant cells.

g. gangrenes′cens, SYN lethal midline g.

giant cell g., a nonneoplastic lesion characterized by a proliferation of granulation tissue containing numerous multinucleated giant cells; it occurs on the gingiva and alveolar mucosa (occasionally on other soft tissues) where it presents as a soft red-blue hemorrhagic nodular swelling; it also occurs within the mandible or maxilla as a unilocular or multilocular radiolucency; microscopically similar lesions occur in the tubular bones of the hands and feet, are considered neoplastic, and may have a malignant course. Identical bony lesions may be seen in hyperparathyroidism and cherubism. SEE ALSO giant cell *tumor* of bone. SYN giant cell epulis, reparative giant cell g.

g. gravida′rum, a pyogenic g. developing on the gingiva during pregnancy; thought to be related to hormonally altered response of the oral mucous membranes to local irritants such as bacterial plaque on adjacent teeth. SYN pregnancy tumor.

infectious g., any granulomatous lesion known to be caused by a living agent; e.g., bacteria, fungi, helminths.

g. inguina′le, a specific g., classified as a venereal disease and caused by *Calymmatobacterium granulomatis* observed in macrophages as Donovan bodies; the ulcerating granulomatous lesions occur in the inguinal regions and the genitalia; peripheral extension of the lesions produces extensive destruction. SYN g. venereum.

laryngeal g., a polypoid projection of granulomatous tissue into the lumen of the larynx, commonly following a traumatic tracheal intubation.

lethal midline g., (1) destruction of the nasal septum, hard palate, lateral nasal walls, paranasal sinuses, skin of the face, orbit and nasopharynx by an inflammatory infiltrate with atypical lymphocytic and histiocytic cells; a form of lymphoma in most cases. **(2)** obsolete term for polymorphic *reticulosis*. SYN g. gangrenescens, malignant g., midline malignant reticulosis granuloma.

lipoid g., g. characterized by aggregates or accumulations of fairly large mononuclear phagocytes that contain lipid.

lipophagic g., a lesion formed as a result of the inflammatory reaction provoked by foci of necrosis in subcutaneous fat, as in certain types of traumatic injury; the central focus of necrotic material is surrounded by an irregular zone of numerous macrophages, many of which become laden with tiny globules of lipid.

lymphatic filariasis g., granulomatous lesion often found surrounding dead microfilariae.

Majocchi g.'s, inflammatory ringworm of the glabrous skin. SYN tinea profunda.

malignant g., SYN lethal midline g.

Miescher g., SYN actinic g.

g. multifor'me, a chronic granulomatous annular eruption of the skin on the upper body in older adults in central Africa; of unknown cause.

ocular larva migrans g., eosinophilic granulomata found surrounding dead worms (generally, *Toxocara* spp.) in the eye; may mimic retinoblastoma.

oily g., reaction to inclusion of a bulky, insoluble liquid (often an oily substance) which occurs several months, but sometimes years, after injection of the material.

paracoccidioidal g., SYN paracoccidioidomycosis.

Paragonimus **g.,** lesions caused by adult worms and eggs of the lung fluke trapped in the pulmonary parenchyma.

periapical g., a proliferation of granulation tissue surrounding the apex of a nonvital tooth and arising in response to pulpal necrosis. SYN apical g., dental g., root end g.

pulse g., SYN giant cell hyaline *angiopathy*.

pyogenic g., g. pyogen'icum, an acquired small rounded mass of highly vascular granulation tissue, frequently with an ulcerated surface, projecting from the skin, especially of the face, or oral mucosa; histologically, the mass is a lobular capillary hemangioma. SYN lobular capillary hemangioma.

reparative g., complication of stapedectomy in which a g. forms in the oval window around the prosthesis; it results in a sensory hearing loss.

reparative giant cell g., SYN giant cell g.

root end g., SYN periapical g.

sarcoidal g., a non-necrotizing epithelioid cell g. similar to those seen in sarcoidosis.

schistosome g., a granulomatous lesion formed around schistosome eggs embedded in tissues in cases of schistosomiasis (bilharziasis); typically these granulomata are found in intestinal tissues (*Schistosoma japonicum* or *S. mansoni* infection), bladder tissue (*S. haematobium*), and hepatic tissue (all human schistosomes). SYN bilharzial g.

sea urchin g., granulomatous nodules, either foreign-body type or composed of epithelioid cells, from the retention of the spine of the sea urchin, occurring several months after the wounding of the skin.

silica g., eruption of granulomatous lesions due to traumatic inoculation of the skin with sand, or materials that contain silica; this condition may follow dermabrasion using sandpaper technique.

silicotic g., granulomatous nodule resulting from deposition of silica particles, usually occurring in lung.

swimming pool g., a chronic, verrucous lesion most commonly seen on the knees; due to infection by *Mycobacterium marinum*. SYN fish-tank g.

trichinosis g., lesions caused by cell death after penetration of migrating newborn nematode larvae.

g. trop'icum, SYN yaws.

umbilical g., moist granulation tissue at the center of the umbilicus in neonates.

g. vene'reum, SYN g. inguinale.

zirconium g., g. from zirconium salts, usually occurring in the axillae, from antiperspirants containing this material, or from the application of hydrous zirconium oxide to poison ivy lesions.

gran·u·lo·ma·to·sis (gran'ū-lō-mă-tō'sis). Any condition characterized by multiple granulomas.

allergic g., SYN Churg-Strauss *syndrome*.

lipid g., lipoid g., SYN xanthomatosis.

lymphomatoid g., angiocentric malignant lymphoma of the lung; may involve the upper respiratory tract and other parts of the body. SEE ALSO polymorphic *reticulosis*.

g. siderot'ica, a form in which firm, brown foci that contain iron pigment (Gamna bodies) are present in an enlarged spleen.

Wegener g., a disease, occurring mainly in the fourth and fifth decades, characterized by necrotizing granulomas and ulceration of the upper respiratory tract, with purulent rhinorrhea, nasal obstruction, and sometimes with otorrhea, hemoptysis, pulmonary infiltration and cavitation, and fever; exophthalmos, involvement of the larynx and pharynx, and glomerulonephritis may occur; the underlying condition is a vasculitis affecting small vessels, and is possibly due to an immune disorder. SEE ALSO lymphomatoid g.

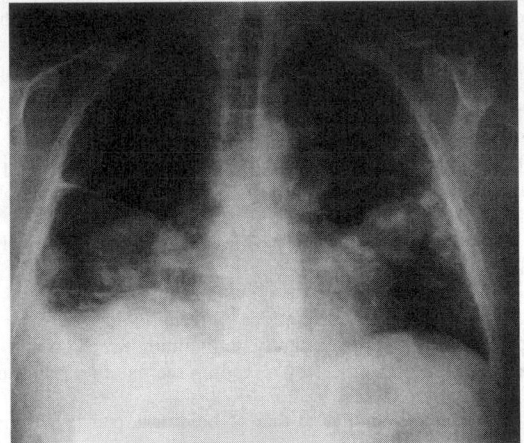

Wegener granulomatosis (radiograph): granulomas in both lungs

gran·u·lom·a·tous (gran-ū-lom'ă-tŭs). Having the characteristics of a granuloma.

gran·u·lo·mere (gran'ū-lō-mēr). The central part of a blood platelet. SYN chromomere (2). [granulo- + G. *meros*, a part]

gran·u·lo·pe·nia (gran'ū-lō-pē'nē-ă). SYN granulocytopenia.

gran·u·lo·plasm (gran'ū-lō-plazm). The inner substance of an ameba, or other unicellular organism, within the ectoplasm and surrounding the nucleus.

gran·u·lo·plas·tic (gran'ū-lō-plas'tik). Forming granules.

gran·u·lo·poi·e·sis (gran'ū-lō-poy-ē'sis). Production of granulocytes. In adults, granulocytes are produced chiefly in the red bone marrow of flat bones. SYN granulocytopoiesis. [granulo(cyte) + G. *poiēsis*, a making]

gran·u·lo·poi·et·ic (gran'ū-lō-poy-et'ik). Pertaining to granulopoiesis. SYN granulocytopoietic.

gran·u·lo·sa (gran-ū-lō'să). SYN *stratum* granulosum folliculi ovarici vesiculosi.

gran·u·lo·sis (gran-ū-lō'sis). A mass of minute granules of any character.

g. ru'bra na'si, erythema, papules, and occasional vesicles of the tip of the nose and extending upward and laterally to the cheeks, resulting from occlusion and chronic inflammation of sweat ducts.

gra·num (grā′nŭm). Singular of grana.

gran·zymes (gran′zīmz). Proteases with serine esterase activities that represent most of the granule content of T cytotoxic cells. It is not known if these enzymes are required for killing by the T cytotoxic cell. [granule + -zyme]

graph (graf). **1.** A line or tracing denoting varying values of commodities, temperatures, urinary output, etc.; more generally, any geometric or pictorial representation of measurements that might otherwise be expressed in tabular form. **2.** Visual display of the relationship between two variables, in which the values of one are plotted on the horizontal axis, the values of the other on the vertical axis; three-dimensional g.'s that show relationships between three variables can be depicted and comprehended visually in two dimensions. [G. graphō, to write]

△**-graph. 1.** Something written, as in monograph, radiograph. **2.** The instrument for making a recording, as in kymograph. Cf. -gram. [G. graphō, to write]

graph·an·es·the·sia (graf′an-es-thē′zē-ă). Tactual inability to recognize figures or letters written on the skin; may be due to spinal cord or brain disease. [G. graphē, writing + anaisthēsia, fr. an- priv. + aisthēsis, perception]

graph·es·the·sia (graf-es-thē′zē-ă). Tactual ability to recognize writing on the skin. [G. graphē, writing, + aisthēsis, perception]

graph·ite (graf′īt). A crystallizable soft black form of carbon. SYN black lead, plumbago.

△**grapho-.** A writing, description. [G. graphō, to write]

gra·phol·o·gy (gră-fol′ō-jē). The study of handwriting as an indication of temperament, character, or personality. [grapho- + G. logos, study]

graph·o·ma·nia (graf-ō-mā′ne-ă). Morbid and excessive impulse to write. [grapho- + G. mania, insanity]

graph·o·mo·tor (graf-ō-mō′ter). Relating to the movements used in writing. [grapho- + L. motus, fr. movere, to move]

graph·o·pa·thol·o·gy (graf′ō-path-ol′ō-jē). Interpretation of personality disorders from a study of handwriting. SEE graphology. [grapho- + pathology]

graph·o·pho·bia (graf-ō-fō′bē-ă). Morbid fear of writing. [grapho- + G. phobos, fear]

graph·o·spasm (graf′ō-spazm). SYN writer's cramp.

△**-graphy.** A writing, a description. [G. graphō, to write]

grasp. The act of taking securely and holding firmly.

palm g., holding an object by wrapping the palm and the fingers around it.

pen g., a method, similar to that of holding a pen in writing, of grasping an instrument.

GRASS Abbreviation for gradient-recalled *acquisition* in the steady state.

Grasset, Joseph, French physician, 1849–1918. SEE G. *law, phenomenon, sign;* G.-Gaussel *phenomenon;* Landouzy-G. *law.*

Gratiolet, Louis P., French anatomist, physiologist, and physician, 1815–1865. SEE G. *fibers,* under *fiber, radiation.*

grat·tage (gră-tazh′). Scraping or brushing an ulcer or surface with sluggish granulations to stimulate the healing process. [Fr. scraping]

grave (grāv). Denoting symptoms of a serious or dangerous character. [L. gravis, heavy, grave]

grav·el (grav′l). Small concretions, usually of uric acid, calcium oxalate, or phosphates, formed in the kidney and passed through the ureter, bladder, and urethra. SYN urocheras (1), uropsammus (1). [M.E., fr. O.Fr.]

Graves, Robert James, Irish physician remembered for his description of exophthalmic goiter in 1835, 1796–1853. SEE G. *disease, ophthalmopathy, orbitopathy.*

grav·id. SYN pregnant.

grav·i·da (grav′i-dă). A pregnant woman. Gravida followed by a roman numeral or preceded by a Latin prefix (primi-, secundi-, etc.) designates the pregnant woman by number of pregnancies; e.g., **gravida I,** primigravida; a woman in her first pregnancy;

gravida II, secundigravida; a woman in her second pregnancy. Cf. para. [L. gravidus (adj.), fem. gravida, fr. gravis, heavy]

gra·vid·ic (grav-id′ik). Relating to pregnancy or a pregnant woman.

grav·id·ism (grav′id-izm). SYN pregnancy.

gra·vid·i·tas (grav-vid′i-tas). SYN pregnancy. [L.]

   g. examnia′lis, SYN extraamniotic *pregnancy.*

   g. exochoria′lis, SYN extrachorial *pregnancy.*

gra·vid·i·ty (gră-vid′i-tē). The number of pregnancies (complete or incomplete) experienced by a woman. [L. graviditas, pregnancy]

gra·vim·e·ter (gră-vim′ĕ-ter). SYN hydrometer. [L. gravis, heavy, + G. metron, measure]

grav·i·met·ric (grav-i-met′rik). Relating to or determined by weight.

grav·i·re·cep·tors (grav′i-rē-sep′terz). Highly specialized receptor organs and nerve endings in the inner ear, joints, tendons, and muscles that give the brain information about body position, equilibrium, direction of gravitational forces, and the sensation of "down" or "up." [L. gravis, heavy, + receptor]

grav·i·ta·tion (grav-i-tā′shŭn). The force of attraction between any two bodies in the universe, varying directly as the product of their masses and inversely as the square of the distance between their centers; expressed as $F = Gm_1m_2 l^{-2}$, where G (Newtonian constant of gravitation) = 6.67259×10^{-11} m^3 kg^{-1} s^{-2}, m_1 and m_2 are the masses (in kg) of the two bodies, and l is the distance separating them in meters. [L. gravitas, weight]

grav·i·ty (grav′i-tē). The attraction toward the earth that makes any mass exert downward force or have weight. Strictly speaking, g. is the algebraic sum of the gravitational attraction of the earth and the opposing centrifugal effect of the mass's rotation around the earth. Thus, gravitational attraction at the north and south poles is larger than at the equator. A satellite in a stable orbit has zero gravity because the centrifugal effect of orbital motion exactly balances the gravitational attraction of the earth. [L. gravitas]

specific g. (sp. gr.), the weight of any body compared with that of another body of equal volume regarded as the unit; usually the weight of a liquid compared with that of distilled water.

zero g., SEE zero gravity.

Grawitz, Paul, German pathologist, 1850–1932. SEE G. *basophilia, tumor.*

gray (Gy) (grā). The SI unit of absorbed dose of ionizing radiation, equivalent to 1 J/kg of tissue; 1 Gy = 100 rad. SYN griseus. [Louis H. *Gray,* British radiologist, 1905–1965]

Greeff, Richard, German ophthalmologist, 1862–1938. SEE Prowazek-G. *bodies,* under *body.*

green (grēn). A color between blue and yellow in the spectrum. For individual green dyes, see specific names.

Scheele g., SYN cupric arsenite.

Greenfield. L., American surgeon who designed the Greenfield filter. SEE Greenfield *filter.*

greg·a·loid (greg′ă-loyd). Denoting a loose colony of protozoa formed by the chance union of independent cells, especially among sarcodines with pseudopodial adherence. [L. grex (greg-), a flock]

Greg·a·ri·na (greg-ă-rī′nă). A genus of sporozoan protozoa (phylum Apicomplexa, subclass Gregarinia), parasitic in annelids and arthropods, and lacking schizogony and endodyogeny in the life cycle. [L. gregarius, gregarious, fr. grex (greg-), a flock]

greg·a·rine (greg′ă-rēn). A member of the subclass Gregarinia.

Greg·a·ri·nia (greg′ă-rin′i-ă). A sporozoan subclass consisting of a number of parasites of the body cavity and intestinal tract of invertebrates, especially annelids and arthropods; typical genera include *Gregarina* in insects and *Monocystis* in earthworms.

greg·a·ri·no·sis (greg′ă-ri-nō′sis). A disease due to the presence of gregarines.

Greig, David M., Scottish physician, 1864–1936. SEE G. *syndrome.*

gres·sion (gres'shŭn). Displacement of a tooth backward. [L. *grador,* pp. *gressus,* to walk, fr. *gradus,* a step]

grey mat·ter. SEE gray *matter.*

Grey Turner, SEE Turner.

GRH Abbreviation for gonadotropin-releasing *hormone.*

grid (grid). **1.** A chart with horizontal and perpendicular lines for plotting curves. **2.** In x-ray imaging, a device formed of lead or aluminum strips for preventing scattered radiation from reaching the x-ray film. [M.E. *gridel,* fr. L. *craticula,* lattice]

Amsler g., SYN Amsler *chart.*

focused g., a g. (2) in which the divergent beam of x-rays from a particular distance range will be parallel to the lead strips.

Wetzel g., chart of growth, plotting height, weight, physical fitness and related aspects of young and adolescent children during growth.

Gridley, Mary F., U.S. medical technologist, 1908–1954. SEE G. *stain, stain* for fungi.

grief (grēf). A normal emotional response to an external loss; distinguished from a depressive disorder since it usually subsides after a reasonable time.

Griesinger, Wilhelm, German neurologist, 1817–1868. SEE G. *disease;* bilious *typhoid* of G.; G. *sign.*

grin·de·lia (grin-dē'lē-ă). The dried leaves and flowering tops of *G. camporum, G. humilius,* and *P. squarrosa* (family Compositae); used as an expectorant; a fluid extract has been used externally in the treatment of rhus poisoning. [David H. *Grindel,* German botanist, 1776–1836]

grind·ing (grīnd'ing). SYN abrasion (3).

selective g., the modification of the occlusal forms of teeth by g. according to a plan or by g. at selected places marked by articulating ribbon or paper.

grind·ing-in. A term used to denote the act of correcting occlusal disharmonies by grinding the natural or artificial teeth.

grip. 1. SYN influenza. **2.** SEE grasp.

devil g., SYN epidemic *pleurodynia.*

grippe (grip). SYN influenza. [Fr. *gripper,* to seize]

gris·e·o·ful·vin (gris'ē-ō-fŭl'vin). A fungistatic antibiotic produced by *Penicillium griseofulvin, P. patulum,* and *P. janczewskii;* used in the systemic treatment of superficial fungal infections caused by the dermatophytes *Microsporum, Trichophyton,* and *Epidermophyton;* inhibits microtubule assembly.

gris·e·us (gris'ē-ŭs). SYN gray. [L.]

Gri·so·nel·la ra·tel·li·na (gri-sŏ-nel'ă ra-te-li'nă). A South American weasel, a reservoir host of *Trypanosoma cruzi.*

gris·tle (gris'l). SYN cartilage. [A.S.]

Gritti, Rocco, Italian surgeon, 1828–1920. SEE G. *operation;* G.-Stokes *amputation.*

Grocco, Pietro, Italian physician, 1857–1916. SEE G. *sign, triangle;* Orsi-G. *method.*

Grocott-Gomori meth·en·a·mine-sil·ver stain. See under stain.

Groenouw, Arthur, German ophthalmologist, 1862–1945. SEE G. corneal *dystrophy.*

groin (groyn) [TA]. **1.** Topographic area of the inferior abdomen related to the inguinal canal, lateral to the pubic region. SYN inguen [TA], inguinal region⋆, regio inguinalis⋆, iliac region. **2.** Sometimes used to indicate just the crease in the junction of the thigh with the trunk.

Grönblad, Ester E., Swedish ophthalmologist, *1898. SEE G.-Strandberg *syndrome.*

GROOVE

groove (groov) [TA]. A narrow, elongate depression or furrow on any surface. SEE ALSO sulcus.

alveolobuccal g., the upper and lower half of the buccal vestibule

on each side. SYN alveolobuccal sulcus, gingivobuccal g., gingivobuccal sulcus.

alveololabial g., (1) the upper and lower half of the labial vestibule; **(2)** in the embryo, the g. formed by the deepening of the labial sulcus; its inner wall becomes incorporated with the alveolar process of the mandible or the maxilla, and its outer wall with the lips and cheeks. SYN alveololabial sulcus, gingivolabial g., gingivolabial sulcus.

alveololingual g., (1) that part of the oral cavity proper, on each side of the frenulum linguae, between the tongue and the mandibular alveolar process or ridge; **(2)** in the embryo, the g. on each side between the lingual primordium and the alveolar elevations of the mandible. SYN alveololingual sulcus, gingivolingual g., gingivolingual sulcus.

ampullary g. [TA], the groove on the external surface of the ampulla of each semicircular duct where the nerve enters the ampullary crest. SYN sulcus ampullaris [TA], ampullary sulcus.

anterior auricular g., SYN anterior *notch* of auricle.

anterior intermediate g., SYN anterior intermediate *sulcus.*

anterior interventricular g., SYN anterior interventricular *sulcus.*

anterolateral g., SYN anterolateral *sulcus.*

anteromedian g., (1) SYN anterior median *fissure* of medulla oblongata; **(2)** SYN anterior median *fissure* of spinal cord.

g. for arch of aorta, a broad, deep sulcus arching superiorly over the hilus on the mediastinal surface of the left lung formed in the cadaver as a result of the aortic arch impressing or indenting the lung.

arterial g.'s [TA], branching grooves on the interior surface of the cranial vault in which the meningeal arteries course, the most prominent of which are related to branches of the middle meningeal artery. SYN sulci arteriosi [TA].

atrioventricular g., SYN coronary *sulcus.*

g. for auditory tube, SYN *sulcus* for pharyngotympanic tube.

auriculoventricular g., SYN coronary *sulcus.*

bicipital g., ⋆official alternate term for intertubercular *sulcus.*

branchial g., an external embryonic g. between contiguous branchial arches. SEE ALSO branchial *clefts,* under cleft.

carotid g., SYN cavernous g.

carpal g. [TA], the concavity on the anterior surface of the arch formed by the carpal bones. SYN sulcus carpi [TA], carpal canal (2).

cavernous g. [TA], the groove on the body of the sphenoid bone in which the internal carotid artery lies in its course through the cavernous sinus. SYN sulcus caroticus [TA], carotid g., carotid sulcus.

chiasmatic g., SYN prechiasmatic *sulcus.*

coronary g., SYN coronary *sulcus.*

costal g. [TA], a groove in the lower inner border of the rib, lodging the intercostal vessels and nerve. SYN sulcus costae [TA], subcostal g.

g. of crus of helix [TA], a transverse fissure on the cranial surface of the auricle corresponding to the crus of the helix. SYN sulcus cruris helicis [TA].

dental g., a transitory depression in the gingival surface of the embryonic jaw along the line of ingrowth of the dental lamina.

g. for the descending aorta, a broad, deep, vertical sulcus immediately posterior to the hilus on the mediastinal surface of the cadaveric left lung, formed as a result of the descending aorta impressing or indenting the lung.

developmental g.'s, fine lines found in the enamel of a tooth that mark the junction of the lobes of the crown in its development. SYN developmental lines.

digastric g., SYN mastoid *notch.*

ethmoidal g. [TA], a groove on the inner surface of each nasal bone, lodging the external nasal branch of the anterior ethmoid nerve. SYN sulcus ethmoidalis [TA].

g. of first rib for subclavian artery [TA], a groove immediately posterior to the scalene tubercle on the upper surface of the first rib across which the subclavian artery passes. SYN sulcus arteriae subclaviae costae primae [TA], sulcus costae arteriae subclaviae.

gr

frontal g.'s, SEE inferior frontal *sulcus*, middle frontal *sulcus*, superior frontal *sulcus*.

gingival g., SYN gingival *sulcus*.

gingivobuccal g., SYN alveolobuccal g.

gingivolabial g., SYN alveololabial g.

gingivolingual g., SYN alveololingual g.

greater palatine g. [TA], a groove on both the body of the maxilla and the perpendicular plate of the palatine bone; when the bones are articulated the grooves form the greater palatine canal. SYN sulcus palatinus major [TA], pterygopalatine g., sulcus for greater palatine nerve, sulcus pterygopalatinus.

g. for greater petrosal nerve [TA], the groove on the anterior surface of the petrous part of the temporal bone that lodges the greater petrosal nerve. SYN sulcus nervi petrosi majoris [TA].

Harrison g., a deformity of the ribs which results from the pull of the diaphragm on ribs weakened by rickets or other softening of the bone.

inferior petrosal g., SYN g. for inferior petrosal sinus.

g. for inferior petrosal sinus [TA], a groove lodging the inferior petrosal sinus, formed by union of similarly named grooves in the petrous part of the temporal bone and the basilar part of the occipital bone. SYN sulcus sinus petrosi inferioris [TA], inferior petrosal g., inferior petrosal sulcus.

g. for inferior venae cava, SYN *sulcus* for vena cava.

infraorbital g. [TA], a gradually deepening groove on the orbital surface of the maxilla, which leads to the infraorbital canal. SYN sulcus infraorbitalis [TA].

interosseous g., (**1**) SYN calcaneal *sulcus*; (**2**) SYN *sulcus* tali.

interosseous g. of calcaneus, SYN calcaneal *sulcus*.

interosseous g. of talus, SYN *sulcus* tali.

intertubercular g. [TA], SYN intertubercular *sulcus*.

interventricular g.'s, SEE anterior interventricular *sulcus*, posterior interventricular *sulcus*.

lacrimal g. [TA], (2) the groove in the nasal surface of the maxilla which, together with the lacrimal bone, forms the fossa for the lacrimal sac. SYN sulcus lacrimalis [TA].

laryngotracheal g., the depression in the floor of the caudal end of the pharynx, continued downward on the ventral wall of the foregut; from it are developed the lower part of the larynx and the trachea, bronchi, and lungs. SYN tracheobronchial g.

lateral bicipital g. [TA], the groove along the lateral side of the arm separating the biceps brachii and brachialis muscles. SYN sulcus bicipitalis lateralis [TA], sulcus bicipitalis radialis☆.

g. of lesser petrosal nerve [TA], the groove on the anterior surface of the petrous part of the temporal bone that accommodates the lesser petrosal nerve in its course to the otic ganglion. SYN sulcus nervi petrosi minoris [TA].

linguogingival g., a g. separating the embryonic mandibular portion of the tongue from the remainder of the mandibular process.

Lucas g., SYN *stria* spinosa.

g. of lung for subclavian artery, a sulcus on the surface of the cadaveric lung just below the apex, corresponding to the course of the subclavian artery. SYN sulcus subclavius.

major g., in a detailed analysis of DNA structure, there are two types of g.'s that can be seen; the major g. has the nitrogen and oxygen atoms of the base pairs pointing inward toward the helical axis, while in the minor g., the nitrogen and oxygen atoms point outwards; important because the major g. is more dependent on base composition and may be the site for protein recognition of specific DNA sequences or regions.

malleolar g. [TA], a broad groove on the posterior surface of the medial malleolus, through which the tendon of the tibialis posterior muscle runs. SYN sulcus malleolaris [TA], g. for tibialis posterior tendon, malleolar sulcus.

mastoid g., SYN mastoid *notch*.

medial bicipital g. [TA], the groove along the medial side of the arm separating the biceps brachii and brachialis muscles. SYN sulcus bicipitalis medialis [TA], sulcus bicipitalis ulnaris☆.

median g. of tongue, SYN median *sulcus* of tongue.

medullary g., SYN neural g.

middle meningeal artery g., a narrow g. on the inner table of the

calvarium, seen on lateral radiographs as a thin dark line, which may be mistaken for a skull fracture. SEE *sulci* arteriosi, under *sulcus*.

g. for middle temporal artery [TA], a vertical groove located above the external acoustic meatus on the external surface of the squamous part of the temporal bone. SYN sulcus arteriae temporalis mediae [TA], sulcus for middle temporal artery.

minor g., SEE major g.

musculospiral g., SYN radial g.

mylohyoid g. [TA], a groove on the medial surface of the ramus of the mandible beginning at the lingula; it lodges the mylohyoid artery and nerve. SYN sulcus mylohyoideus [TA], mylohyoid fossa.

g. of nail matrix, SYN *sulcus* matricis unguis.

nasolabial g., SYN nasolabial *sulcus*.

nasopalatine g., a g. on the vomer lodging the nasopalatine nerve.

nasopharyngeal g., an indistinct line marking the boundary between the nasal cavities and the nasopharynx.

neural g., the gutterlike g. formed in the midline of the embryo's dorsal surface by the progressive elevation of the lateral margins of the neural plate; the ultimate dorsal fusion of the margins results in the formation of the neural tube. SYN medullary g.

obturator g. [TA], a deep groove on the inner surface of the superior ramus of the pubis. SYN sulcus obturatorius [TA].

occipital g. [TA], a narrow groove medial to the mastoid notch of the temporal bone that lodges the occipital artery. SYN sulcus arteriae occipitalis [TA], sulcus of occipital artery.

olfactory g., SYN olfactory *sulcus*.

olfactory g. of nasal cavity [TA], the narrow groove in the nasal cavity above the agger nasi that leads from the atrium to the olfactory area. SYN sulcus olfactorius cavi nasi [TA], olfactory sulcus of nasal cavity.

optic g., SYN prechiasmatic *sulcus*.

palatine g.'s [TA], a number of grooves on the lower surface of the palatine process of the maxilla in which the palatine vessels and nerves lie. SYN sulci palatini [TA].

palatovaginal g. [TA], a furrow on the inferior aspect of the vaginal process of the sphenoid bone that is bridged below by the sphenoidal process of the palatine bone to form the palatovaginal canal. SYN sulcus palatovaginalis [TA].

paraglenoid g., SYN preauricular g.

pharyngeal g.'s, embryonic endodermal or ectodermal g.'s between successive pharyngeal arches.

pharyngotympanic g., SYN *sulcus* for pharyngotympanic tube.

pontomedullary g., SYN medullopontine sulcus [TA].

popliteal g., SYN g. for popliteus.

g. for popliteus [TA], a g. on the lateral condyle of the femur between the epicondyle and the articular margin. Its anterior end gives origin to the popliteus muscle; its posterior end lodges the tendon of the muscle when the knee is fully flexed. SYN sulcus popliteus [TA], popliteal g.

posterior auricular g. [TA], the g. between the antitragus and cauda helicis overlying the antitragicohelicine fissure. SYN sulcus posterior auriculae [TA].

posterior intermediate g., SYN posterior intermediate *sulcus*.

posterior interventricular g., SYN posterior interventricular *sulcus*.

posterolateral g., SYN posterolateral *sulcus*.

preauricular g., a g. on the pelvic surface of the ilium just lateral to the auricular surface; it is more pronounced in the female. SYN paraglenoid g., paraglenoid sulcus, preauricular sulcus, sulcus paraglenoidalis.

primary labial g., SYN labial *sulcus*.

primitive g., the median depression in the primitive streak flanked by the primitive ridges. SYN primitive furrow.

g. of promontory of labyrinthine wall of tympanic cavity [TA], a narrow branched groove running vertically over the surface of the promontory in the middle ear, lodging the tympanic plexus. SYN sulcus promontorii cavitatis tympanicae [TA], sulcus of promontory of tympanic cavity.

g. for pterygoid hamulus [TA], a groove at the base of the pterygoid hamulus that forms a pulley for the tendon of the tensor veli palatini muscle. SYN sulcus hamuli pterygoidei [TA], sulcus of pterygoid hamulus.

g. of pterygoid hamulus [TA], the notch or fissure between the tuberosity of the maxilla and the pterygoid hamulus of the sphenoid bone. SYN hamular notch, pterygomaxillary notch.

pterygopalatine g., SYN greater palatine g.

pulmonary g. [TA], the deep recess on either side of the vertebral column formed by the posterior sweep of the curvature of the ribs. SYN sulcus pulmonalis [TA], paravertebral gutter, pulmonary sulcus.

radial g. [TA], the shallow groove that passes around the shaft of the humerus; it lodges the radial nerve and deep brachial artery. SYN sulcus nervi radialis [TA], g. for radial nerve ⭐, musculospiral g., spiral g.

g. for radial nerve, ⭐official alternate term for radial g.

retention g., one of the g.'s forming opposing vertical constrictions in a tooth to aid in retention of a dental restoration.

rhombic g.'s, seven pairs of transverse furrows in the floor of the embryonic hindbrain.

sagittal g., SYN g. for superior sagittal sinus.

Sibson g., a g. occasionally seen on the outer side of the thorax formed by the prominent lower border of the pectoralis major muscle.

sigmoid g., SYN g. for sigmoid sinus.

g. for sigmoid sinus [TA], a broad groove in the posterior cranial fossa, first situated on the lateral portion of the occipital bone, then curving around the jugular process on to the mastoid portion of the temporal bone, and finally turning sharply on the posterior inferior angle of the parietal bone and becoming continuous with the transverse groove; it lodges the transverse sinus. SYN sulcus sinus sigmoidei [TA], sigmoid fossa, sigmoid g., sigmoid sulcus.

skin g.'s, SYN skin sulci, under sulcus.

g. for spinal nerve [TA], the laterally directed groove on the superior surface of the transverse processes of typical cervical vertebrae between the anterior and posterior tubercles along which the emerging spinal nerve passes. SYN sulcus nervi spinalis [TA].

spiral g., SYN radial g.

subclavian g. [TA], a groove on the inferior surface of the body of the clavicle to which is attached the subclavius muscle. SYN sulcus musculi subclavii [TA], g. for subclavius ⭐, subclavian sulcus, sulcus subclavianus.

g. for subclavian vein [TA], a groove just anterior to the scalene tubercle of the first rib marking the course of the subclavian vein across the rib. SYN sulcus venae subclaviae [TA].

g. for subclavius, ⭐official alternate term for subclavian g.

subcostal g., SYN costal g.

g. for superior petrosal sinus [TA], a groove on the crest of the petrous portion of the temporal bone in which rests the superior petrosal sinus. SYN sulcus sinus petrosi superioris [TA], superior petrosal sulcus.

g. for superior sagittal sinus, the groove in the midline of the inner table of the calvaria lodging the superior sagittal sinus. SYN sagittal g., sagittal sulcus, sulcus sinus sagittalis superioris, superior longitudinal sulcus.

g. for superior vena cava, a g. on the surface of the cadaveric right lung, above the hilum, in which runs the superior vena cava. SYN sulcus venae cavae cranialis.

supplemental g., a curvilinear depression normally found on each side of a triangular ridge (crista triangularis).

supra-acetabular g. [TA], a groove, posterosuperior to the acetabulum, that is the attachment for the reflected head of the rectus femoris muscle. SYN sulcus supraacetabularis [TA], supraacetabular sulcus.

g. for tendon of fibularis longus [TA], **(1)** the g. below the peroneal trochlea of the calcaneus; **(2)** the g. distal to the tuberosity of the cuboid bone. SYN sulcus tendinis musculi fibularis longi [TA], g. for tendon of peroneus longus ⭐, sulcus tendinis musculi peronei longi (1) ⭐.

g. for tendon of flexor hallucis longus [TA], a vertical g. on the posterior process of the talus continuous with another groove (of the same name) on the underside of the sustentaculum tali of the calcaneus. SYN sulcus tendinis musculi flexoris hallucis longi [TA].

g. for tendon of peroneus longus, ⭐official alternate term for g. for tendon of fibularis longus.

g. for tibialis posterior tendon, SYN malleolar g.

tracheobronchial g., SYN laryngotracheal g.

transverse anthelicine g., a deep groove on the cranial surface of the auricle separating the eminences of the triangular fossa and of the concha. SYN sulcus anthelicis transversus.

transverse nasal g., SYN stria nasi transversa.

g. for transverse sinus [TA], the groove on the inner surface of the occipital bone marking the course of the transverse sinus; the tentorium is attached to its margins. SYN sulcus sinus transversi [TA], sulcus for transverse sinus.

tympanic g., SYN tympanic sulcus.

g. for ulnar nerve [TA], a furrow on the posterior surface of the medial epicondyle of the humerus, lodging the ulnar nerve. SYN sulcus nervi ulnaris [TA].

urethral g., the g. on the ventral surface of the embryonic penis which ultimately is closed to form the penile portion of the urethra.

venous g.'s [TA], grooves occasionally found on the internal surface of the parietal bone, in which veins lie. SYN sulci venosi [TA].

vertebral g., the depression bounded by the spinous processes and laminae of the vertebrae, in which lie the deep muscles of the back.

g. for vertebral artery [TA], the g. on the superior aspect of the posterior arch of the atlas that transmits the vertebral artery medially toward the foramen magnum. SYN sulcus arteriae vertebralis [TA], sulcus for vertebral artery.

vomeral g., SYN vomerine g.

vomerine g. [TA], the groove on the anterior border of the vomer that receives the septal cartilage. SYN sulcus vomeris [TA], sulcus vomeralis, vomeral g., vomeral sulcus.

vomerovaginal g. [TA], a g. on the inferior aspect of the vaginal process of the sphenoid bone that, together with ala of the vomer, forms the vomerovaginal canal. SYN sulcus vomerovaginalis [TA].

Gross, Ludwik, U.S. oncologist, *1904. SEE G. virus, leukemia virus.

gross (gros). Coarse or large; large enough to be visible to the naked eye; macroscopic. [L. grossus, thick]

group (groop). **1.** A number of similar or related objects. **2.** In chemistry, a radical. For individual chemical groups, see the specific name.

blood g., SEE blood group.

characterizing g., a g. of atoms in a molecule that distinguishes the class of substances in which it occurs from all other classes; thus carbonyl (CO) is the characterizing g. of ketones; COOH, of organic acids, etc.

connective tissue g., a collective name for mucous tissue, dentin, bone, cartilage, and ordinary connective tissue, all derived from the mesenchyme.

control g., a g. of subjects participating in the same experiment as another g. of subjects, but which is not exposed to the variable under investigation. SEE ALSO experimental g.

cytophil g., the part of an antibody that binds it to the cell.

determinant g., SYN antigenic determinant.

diagnosis-related g. (DRG), a scheme for billing for medical and especially hospital services by combining diseases into g.'s according to the resources needed for care, arranged by diagnostic category. A dollar value is assigned to each g. as the basis of payment for all cases in that group, without regard to the actual cost of care or duration of hospitalization of any individual case, as a mechanism to motivate health-care providers to economize.

encounter g., a form of psychological sensitivity training that emphasizes the experiencing of individual relationships within the g. and minimizes intellectual and didactic input; the g. focuses on

gr

the present rather than concerning itself with the past or outside problems of its members. SEE ALSO sensitivity training g.

experimental g., a g. of subjects exposed to the variable of an experiment, as opposed to the control g.

functional g., SEE function (4).

HACEK g., a group of Gram-negative bacteria that includes *Haemophilus* spp., *Actinobacillus actinomycetemcomitans, Cardiobacterium hominis, Eikenella corrodens*, and *Kingella kingae.* Bacteria in this group have in common a culture requirement of an enhanced carbon dioxide atmosphere and ability to infect human heart valves.

linkage g., a set of two or more loci that have been shown by linkage analysis to be physically close in the genome but that have not yet been assigned to specific chromosomes. It is rapidly becoming an outmoded term.

matched g.'s, a method of experimental control in which subjects in one g. are matched on a one-to-one basis with subjects in other g.'s concerning all organism variables (e.g., age, sex, height, weight) which the experimenter believes could influence the variable being investigated.

prosthetic g., a non-amino acid compound attached to a protein, often in a reversible fashion, that confers new properties upon the conjugated protein thus produced. SEE ALSO coenzyme.

sensitivity training g., a g., more popular in the 1960s and 1970s, in which members seek to develop self-awareness and an understanding of g. processes rather than to obtain therapy for an emotional disturbance. SEE ALSO encounter g., personal growth *laboratory.*

symptom g., SEE syndrome, complex (1).

T g., abbreviation for training g.

therapeutic g., any g. of patients meeting together for mutual psychotherapeutic, personal development, and life change goals.

training g. (T g.), any g. emphasizing training in self-awareness and group dynamics. SEE sensitivity training g.

Grover, Ralph W., U.S. dermatologist, *1920. SEE G. *disease.*

growth (grōth). The increase in size of a living being or any of its parts occurring in the process of development.

accretionary g., g. by an increase of intercellular material.

appositional g., g. accomplished by the addition of new layers on those previously formed; e.g., the addition of lamellae in the formation of bone; it is the characteristic method of g. when rigid materials are involved.

auxetic g., g. by increase in the size of component cells. SYN intussusceptive g.

bacterial g., g. of a bacterial culture either by increase in cell material or cell number.

differential g., different rates of g. in associated tissues or structures; used especially in embryology when the differences in g. rates result in changing the original proportions or relations.

exponential g., SEE logarithmic *phase.*

interstitial g., g. from a number of different centers within an area; in contrast with appositional g., it can occur only when the materials involved are nonrigid.

intussusceptive g., SYN auxetic g.

multiplicative g., g. by an increase in the number of cells.

new g., SYN neoplasm.

grub (grŭb). Wormlike larva or maggot of certain insects, particularly in the orders Coleoptera, Diptera, and Hymenoptera, and the genus *Hypoderma.*

Gruber, George B., German physician, 1884–1977. SEE Meckel-G. *syndrome;* Martin-G. *anastomosis.*

Gruber, Josef, Austrian otologist, 1827–1900. SEE G. *method.*

Gruber, Max von, German hygienist, 1853–1927. SEE G. *reaction;* G.-Widal *reaction.*

Gruber, Wenzel (Wenaslaus) L., Russian anatomist, 1814–1890. SEE G. *cul-de-sac;* G.-Landzert *fossa.*

gru·el (groo'ĕl). A semiliquid food of oatmeal or other cereal boiled in water; thin porridge. [thru O. Fr., fr. Mediev. L. *grutum,* meal]

gru·mous (groo'mŭs). Thick and lumpy, as clotting blood. [L. *grumus,* a little heap]

Grunert spur. See under spur.

Grunstein-Hogness as·say. See under assay.

Grünwald. SEE May-Grünwald *stain.*

Grütz, O., German dermatologist, *1886. SEE Bürger-G. *syndrome.*

Grynfeltt, Joseph C., French surgeon, 1840–1913. SEE G. *triangle.*

gry·o·chrome (grī'ō-krōm). A term applied by Nissl to nerve cells in which the stainable portion is present in the form of minute granules without definite arrangement. [G. *gry,* something insignificant, + *chrōma,* color]

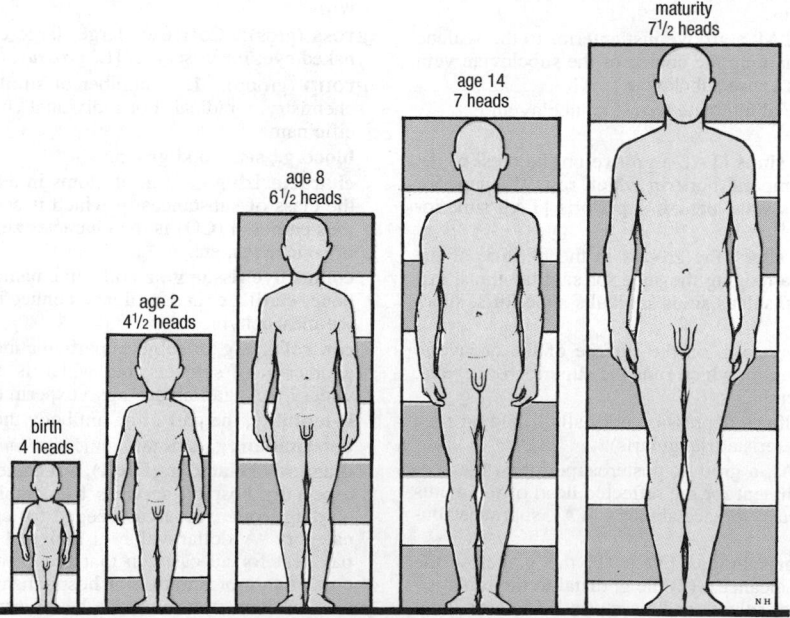

growth: proportions at various ages

gry·po·sis (gri-pō'sis). An abnormal curvature. [G. *grypos,* hooked, + *-osis,* condition]

GSH Abbreviation for glutathione.

GSR Abbreviation for galvanic skin *response.*

GSSG Abbreviation for glutathione disulfide.

G-stro·phan·thin. SEE ouabain.

gt. Abbreviation for gutta.

g-tol·er·ance. The tolerance of a person or a piece of equipment to forces that develop as a result of acceleration or deceleration.

GTP Abbreviation for guanosine 5'-triphosphate.

gtt. Abbreviation for guttae.

GU Abbreviation for genitourinary.

Gua Abbreviation for guanine.

guai·ac (gwī'ak). The resin of *Guaiacum officinale* or *G. sanctum* (family Zygophyllaceae); a nauseant, diaphoretic, stimulant, and reagent in testing for occult blood. SYN guaiac gum. [Sp. *guayaco,* imitating the native Carib name]

guai·a·cin (gwī'ă-sin). Guaiac saponin, a constituent of guiac used as a reagent for oxidases, with which it gives a blue color.

guai·a·col (gwī'ă-kol). Has been used as an expectorant and intestinal disinfectant; also available as g. carbonate.

  g. glyceryl ether, SYN guaifenesin.

  g. phosphate, phosphoric guaiacyl ether, a white crystalline powder, insoluble in water; used as an intestinal antiseptic and in fever.

guai·fen·e·sin (gwī-fen'ĕ-sin). An expectorant that allegedly reduces the viscosity of sputum, thus facilitating its elimination. SYN glyceryl guaiacolate, guaiacol glyceryl ether.

guan·a·benz ac·e·tate (gwahn-ă-benz). A centrally acting antiadrenergic antihypertensive similar in action to clonidine.

gua·na·cline sul·fate (gwahn'ă-klēn). An antihypertensive.

gua·na·drel sul·fate (gwahn'ă-drel). An antihypertensive drug similar in action to guanethidine.

gua·nase (gwahn'ās). SYN *guanine* deaminase.

guanazolo (gwahn-ă-zōl'ō). SYN 8-azaguanine.

gua·neth·i·dine sul·fate (gwahn-eth'i-dēn). A potent antihypertensive agent. It appears to interfere with the release of the chemical mediator (norepinephrine) at the sympathetic neuroeffector junction; it does not produce ganglionic or parasympathetic blockade with recommended doses. In ophthalmology, it is used topically for the treatment of glaucoma and to counteract eyelid retraction in Graves disease.

guan·fa·cine (gwan'fă-sēn). An antihypertensive agent which is an α$_2$-adrenergic agonist acting in the central nervous system to reduce the output of the sympathetic nervous system; resembles clonidine in its pharmacologic profile.

gua·ni·dine (gwahn'i-dēn, -din). A strongly basic compound, usually found (in some plants and lower animals) as the hydrochloride; a constituent of creatine and arginine; administered as a cholinergic striated muscle stimulant.

guan·id·i·ni·um (gwahn'i-din-ē-um). Referring to a guanidine moiety in a molecule (e.g., in arginine).

gua·ni·di·no·ac·e·tate (gwahn'i-din-ō-ăs-ē-tāt). An intermediate in creatine biosynthesis.

gua·ni·di·no·ac·e·tate N-meth·yl·trans·fer·ase. The enzyme catalyzing the transfer of a methyl group from *S*-adenosyl-L-methionine ("active methionine") to guanidinoacetate (glycocyamine), forming creatine and *S*-adenosyl-L-homocysteine.

gua·nine (Gua, G) (gwahn'ēn, -in). 2-Amino-6-oxypurine; one of the two major purines (the other being adenine) occurring in all nucleic acids.

  g. aminase, SYN g. deaminase.

  g. deaminase, a deaminase of the liver that catalyzes the hydrolysis of guanine into xanthine and ammonia; the first step in purine degradation. SYN guanase, g. aminase.

  g. deoxyribonucleotide, SYN deoxyguanylic acid.

  g. ribonucleotide, SYN guanylic acid.

gua·no·chlor sul·fate (gwahn'ō-klōr). Used as an α-adrenergic blocking agent for the treatment of essential hypertension.

gua·no·sine (G, Guo) (gwahn'ō-sēn, -sin). 9-β-D-Ribosylguanine (guanine combined through its N-9 with the C-1 of β-D-ribose); a major constituent of RNA and of guanine nucleotides. SYN 9-β-D-ribofuranosylguanine.

  cyclic g. 3',5'-monophosphate (cGMP), an analog of cAMP; a second messenger for atrial natriuretic factor. SYN cyclic GMP.

gua·no·sine 5'-di·phos·phate (GDP). Guanosine esterified at its 5' position with diphosphoric acid; bound tightly in microtubules.

gua·no·sine 5'-monophos·phate. SYN guanylic acid.

gua·no·sine 5'-tri·phos·phate (GTP). An immediate precursor of guanine nucleotides in RNA; similar to ATP; has a crucial role in microtubule formation.

  GTP cyclohydrolase, an enzyme that catalyzes the reaction of GTP and H$_2$O forming formate and a precursor of tetrahydrobiopterin; a deficiency of this enzyme will result in one form of malignant hyperphenylalaninemia.

guan·ox·an sul·fate (gwahn-ok'san). An antihypertensive agent.

gua·nyl (gwahn'il). The radical of guanine.

  g. cyclase, SYN guanylate cyclase.

guan·y·late cy·clase (gwahn'i-lāt). Analogous to adenylate (adenylyl) cyclase, but cyclizing guanosine 5'-triphosphate to guanosine 3':5'-cyclic monophosphate and also producing pyrophosphate; activated by nitric oxide. SYN guanyl cyclase, guanylyl cyclase.

gua·nyl·ic ac·id (GMP) (gwă-nil'ik). A major component of ribonucleic acids. SYN guanine ribonucleotide, guanosine 5'-monophosphate.

  g. a. reductase (GMP reductase), an enzyme that catalyzes the reaction of GMP with NADPH, producing IMP, NH$_3$, and NADP$^+$; a part of the purine salvage pathway.

  g. a. synthetase (GMP synthetase), an enzyme catalyzing the reaction of L-glutamine, XMP, and ATP to produce GMP, L-glutamate, AMP, and pyrophosphate; a key step in purine biosynthesis.

gua·nyl·o·ri·bo·nu·cle·ase (gwahn'i-lō-rī-bō-noo'klē-ās). SYN RNase T$_1$. See entries under ribonuclease.

gua·nyl·yl (gwahn'i-lil). The radical of guanylic acid.

  g. cyclase, SYN guanylate cyclase.

gua·ra·na (gwah-rah-nah'). A dried paste of the crushed seeds of *Paullinia cupana* (family Sapindaceae), a vine extensively cultivated in Brazil. It contains guaranine (caffeine), saponin, a volatile oil, and paullinitannic acid. Has been used for the relief of headache. [Native Brazilian word]

gua·ra·nine (gwahr'ă-nēn). SYN caffeine.

guard·ing (gard'ing). A spasm of muscles to minimize motion or agitation of sites affected by injury or disease.

  abdominal g., a spasm of abdominal wall muscles, detected on palpation, to protect inflamed abdominal viscera from pressure; usually a result of inflammation of the parietal peritoneal surface as in appendicitis, diverticulitis, or generalized peritonitis.

  involuntary g., abdominal muscle spasm, caused by retroperitoneal inflammation, which cannot be willfully suppressed.

  voluntary g., abdominal muscle spasm that can be willfully suppressed.

Guarnieri, Giuseppi, Italian physician, 1856–1918. SEE G. *bodies,* under *body.*

gu·ber·nac·u·lum (goo'ber-nak'ū-lŭm) [TA]. A fibrous cord connecting two structures. A mesenchymal column of tissue that connects the fetal testis to the developing scrotum; it appears to play a role in testicular descent. SYN g. testis. [L. a helm]

  g. den'tis, a connective tissue band uniting the tooth sac with the gum.

  Hunter g., obsolete term for g. testis.

  g. tes'tis, SYN gubernaculum.

Gubler, Adolphe, French physician, 1821–1879. SEE G. *line, paralysis, syndrome;* Millard-G. *syndrome.*

Gudden, Bernhard A. von, German neurologist, 1824–1886. SEE G. *commissure, ganglion,* tegmental *nuclei,* under *nucleus.*

Gu

Guedel, Arthur Ernest, U.S. anesthesiologist, 1883–1956. SEE G. *airway.*

Guéneau de Mussy, Noël F.O., French physician, 1813–1885. SEE G. de M. *point.*

Guérin, Camille, French bacteriologist, 1872–1961. SEE bacille Calmette-Guérin; bacillus Calmette-Guérin *vaccine;* Calmette *test;* Calmette-Guérin *bacillus;* Calmette-Guérin *vaccine.*

Guérin, Alphonse F.M., French surgeon, 1816–1895. SEE G. *fold, fracture, glands,* under *gland, sinus, valve.*

guid·ance (gī′dăns). 1. The act of guiding. 2. A guide.

condylar g., the mechanical device on an articulator which is intended to produce g. in articulator movement, similar to those produced by the paths of the condyles in the temporomandibular joints. SEE ALSO condylar guidance *inclination.* SYN condylar guide.

incisal g., the influence on mandibular movements caused by the contacting surfaces of the mandibular and maxillary anterior teeth during eccentric excursions. SYN incisal path.

guide (gīd). 1. To lead in a set course. 2. Any device or instrument by which another is led into its proper course, e.g., a grooved director, a catheter g. [M.E., fr. O.Fr. *guier,* to show the way, fr. Germanic]

anterior g., SYN incisal g.

catheter g., a flexible metallic wire or thin sound over which a catheter is passed to advance it into its proper position, as in a blood vessel or the urethra. SEE ALSO stylet.

condylar g., SYN condylar *guidance.*

incisal g., in dentistry, that part of an articulator on which the anterior g. pin rests to maintain the vertical dimension of occlusion and the incisal g. angle as established by the incisal guidance; may be adjustable, with a superior surface that may be changed to provide variations in the incisal g. angle, or customized, being individually formed in plastic to allow other than straight line incisal guidance in eccentric movements. SYN anterior g.

mold g., a g. used to specify the shape of artificial teeth, or of an artificial tooth.

guide·line (gīd′līn). A marking in the form of a line that serves as a guide or reference.

clasp g., SYN survey *line.*

clinical practice g.'s, a formal statement about a defined task or function in clinical practice, such as desirable diagnostic tests or the optimal treatment regimen for a specific diagnosis; generally based on the best available evidence, e.g., randomized controlled trials that have been assessed by a Cochrane collaborating group. SEE ALSO Cochrane *collaboration.*

Cummer g., SYN survey *line.*

practice g.'s, recommendations developed by groups of clinicians for delivery of care based on various indications. SYN practice parameters.

guide·wire (gīd′wīr). A wire or spring used as a guide for placement of a larger device or prosthesis, such as a catheter or intramedullary pin.

Guillain, Georges, French neurologist, 1876–1961. SEE G.-Barré *reflex, syndrome;* Landry-G.-Barré *syndrome.*

guil·lo·tine (gil′ŏ-tēn, gē′ō-tēn). An instrument in the shape of a metal ring through which runs a sliding knifeblade, used in excising a tonsil. [Fr. an instrument for execution by decapitation]

guin·ea green B (gin′ē) [C.I. 42085]. An acid diaminotriphenylmethane dye, used as an indicator for H-ion determinations (changing at pH 6.0 from magenta to green) and as a fiber cytoplasmic stain in certain Masson trichrome staining procedures.

guin·ea pig (gin′ē). SYN *Cavia* porcellus.

Guldberg, C., Norwegian chemist, 1862–1902. SEE G.-Waage *law.*

gul·let (gŭl′et). SYN throat (1). [L. *gula,* throat]

Gullstrand, Allvar, Swedish ophthalmologist and Nobel laureate, 1862–1930. SEE biomicroscope.

L-gu·lon·ic ac·id (goo-lon′ik). Reduction product of glucuronic acid (–CHO → –CH₂OH); oxidation product of L-gulose (–CHO

→ –COOH); a precursor (except in certain primates, guinea pigs, certain fishes, and the Indian fruit bat) of ascorbic acid via L-gulonolactone.

L-gu·lon·o·lac·tone (goo-lon′ō-lak-tōn). The immediate precursor of ascorbic acid in those animals capable of ascorbic acid biosynthesis. SYN dihydroascorbic acid, L-gulono-γ-lactone.

L-g. oxidase, the enzyme catalyzing the conversion of L-g. and O₂ to H₂O₂ and L-*xylo*-hexulonolactone, a precursor of ascorbic acid; absent in humans.

L-gul·o·no-γ-lac·tone. SYN L-gulonolactone.

gu·lose (goo′lōs). One of the eight pairs (D and L) of aldoses; D-g. is an epimer of D-galactose.

gum (gŭm). 1. The dried exuded sap from a number of trees and shrubs, forming an amorphous brittle mass; it usually forms a mucilaginous solution in water and is often used as a suspending agent in liquid preparations of insoluble drugs. [L. *gummi*] 2. ✶official alternate term for gingiva. [A.S. *goma,* jaw] 3. Water-soluble glycans, often containing uronic acids, found in many plants.

g. arabic, SYN acacia; SEE ALSO arabin.

Bassora g., a g. from Iran and Turkey, resembling tragacanth, acacia, and the gummy exudate of cherry and plum trees; used in making storax.

g. benjamin, g. benzoin, SYN benzoin.

British g., a form of dextrin.

eucalyptus g., a dried gummy exudation from *Eucalyptus rostrata* and other species of *Eucalyptus* (family Myrtaceae); used as an astringent (in gargles and troches) and as an antidiarrheal agent. SYN red g.

ghatti g., SYN Indian g.

guaiac g., SYN guaiac.

guar g., the ground endosperms of *Cyamopsis tetragonolobus;* used in pharmaceutical jelly formulations.

Indian g., an exudation from *Anogeisus latifolia* (family Combrettaceae); the mucilage is used as a substitute for acacia mucilage. SYN ghatti g.

karaya g., SYN sterculia g.

locust g., SYN algaroba.

g. opium, SYN opium.

red g., SYN eucalyptus g.

senegal g., the g. of *Acacia senegal.* SEE acacia.

starch g., SYN dextrin.

sterculia g., the dried gummy exudation from *Sterculia urens, S. villosa, S. tragacantha,* or other species of *Sterculia,* or from *Cochlospermum gossypium* or other species of *Cochlospermum* (family Bixaceae); used as a hydrophilic laxative and in the manufacture of lotions and pastes. SYN karaya g.

wheat g., SYN gluten.

gum·boil (gŭm′boyl). SYN gingival *abscess.*

gum·ma, pl. **gum·ma·ta, gum·mas** (gŭm′ă, ă-tă, -z). An infectious granuloma that is characteristic of tertiary syphilis, but does not always develop, and that may be solitary (as large as 8–10 cm in diameter) or multiple and diffusely scattered (1 mm or less in diameter). Gummas are characterized by an irregular central portion that is firm, sometimes partially hyalinized, and consisting of coagulative necrosis in which "ghosts" of structures may be recognized; a poorly defined middle zone of epithelioid cells, with occasional multinucleated giant cells; and a peripheral zone of fibroblasts and numerous capillaries, with infiltrated lymphocytes and plasma cells. As gummas become older, an irregular scar or rounded fibrous nodule persists. SYN syphiloma. [L. *gummi,* gum, fr. G. *kommi*]

Gumprecht, Ferdinand A., German physician, 1864–1941. SEE Klein-Gumprecht shadow *nuclei,* under *nucleus;* G. *shadows,* under *shadow.*

Gunn, Robert Marcus, British ophthalmologist, 1850–1909. SEE G. *phenomenon, dots,* under *dot, sign, syndrome;* Marcus G. *pupil.*

Günning, Jan W., Dutch chemist, 1827–1901. SEE G. *reaction.*

Gunning, Thomas B., U.S. dentist, 1813–1889. SEE G. *splint.*

Günz, Justus W., German anatomist, 1714–1815. SEE G. *ligament.*

Günzberg, Alfred, German physician, *1861. SEE G. *reagent, test.*

Guo Symbol for guanosine.

gur·ney (gŭr′nē). A stretcher or cot with wheels used to transport patients. [Sir Goldsworthy *Gurney,* British physician and inventor, 1793–1875]

gush·er (gush′er). An abundant flow of fluid.

perilymphatic g., abnormal flow of perilymph when the footplate of the stapes is perforated; occurs in X-linked mixed deafness (DFN 3) due to a mutation of the POU3F4 gene and in other conditions.

Gussenbauer, Carl, German surgeon, 1842–1903. SEE G. *suture.*

gus·ta·tion (gŭs-tā′shŭn). 1. The act of tasting. 2. The sense of taste. [L. *gustatio,* fr. *gusto,* pp. -*atus,* to taste]

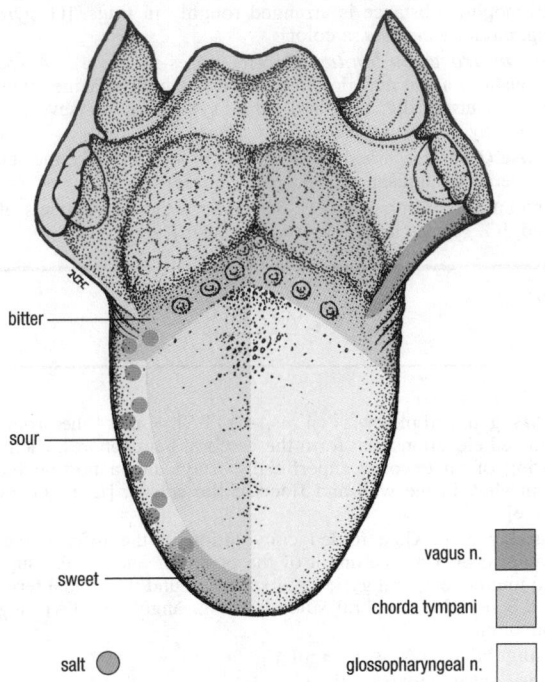

bitter

sour

sweet

salt ●

vagus n.

chorda tympani

glossopharyngeal n.

gustation: regions of taste perception and their gustatory nerves

gus·ta·to·ry (gŭs′tă-tōr-ē). Relating to gustation, or taste.

gust·duc·in (gŭst-dus-in). A protein messenger in taste buds that is activated in response to sweet tastes; gustducin is a G-protein α-subunit. [L. *gustus,* taste, + *duco,* to lead, induce, + -in]

gut (gŭt). 1. SYN intestine. 2. Embryonic digestive tube. 3. Abbreviated term for catgut. SEE ALSO suture. [A.S.]

blind g., SYN cecum (1).

postanal g., an extension of the hindgut caudal to the point at which the anal opening is formed. SYN postcloacal g., tailgut.

postcloacal g., SYN postanal g.

preoral g., SYN Seessel *pocket.*

primitive g., a flat sheet of intraembryonic endoderm that will change into a tubular g. due to the folding of embryonic body— head, tail and lateral body folds. SYN archenteron, celenteron, endodermal canal, subgerminal cavity.

Guthrie, George J., English ophthalmologist, 1785–1856. SEE G. *muscle.*

Guthrie, Robert, U.S. pediatrician, 1916–1995. SEE G. *test.*

Gutmann, Carl, German physician, *1872. SEE Michaelis-G. *body.*

gut·ta (gt.), pl. **gut·tae (gtt.)** (gŭt′ă, -ē). 1. A drop. 2. A rubber-like polyterpene found in gutta-percha. Cf. chicle, gutta-percha. [L.]

g. sere′na, former term for blindness of unknown etiology; the "serena" suggested that the anterior segment of the eye was clear and tranquil, that there was no visible cause for the blindness, no corneal scar, no inflammation, no cataract. Thus, g. serena became the code word for blindness due to some unfathomable posterior cause, some damage to retina, optic nerve, or brain. This was the name given to John Milton's blindness. With the opthalmoscope, in 1851, the diagnosis of g. serena suddenly became old-fashioned and inadequate.

gut·tae. Plural of gutta. [L.]

gut·ta-per·cha (gŭt′ă-per′chă). The coagulated, purified, dried, milky juice of trees of the genera *Palaguium* and *Payena* (family Sapotaceae); used as a filling material in dentistry, and in the manufacture of splints and electrical insulators; a solution is used as a substitute for collodion, as a protective, and to seal incised wounds. Cf. chicle, gutta. [Malay *gatah,* gum, + *percha,* the name of a tree]

guttat. Abbreviation for L. *guttatim,* drop by drop.

gut·tate (gŭt′tāt). Of the shape of, or resembling, a drop, characterizing certain cutaneous lesions.

gut·ter [TA]. Deep recess or grooves.

paracolic gutters [TA], the grooves between the lateral aspect of the ascending or descending colon and the abdominal wall. SYN sulci paracolici [TA], paracolic recesses.

paravertebral gutter, SYN pulmonary *groove.*

Guttman, L.L., 20th century U.S. epidemiologist. SEE G. *scale.*

gut·tur·al (gŭt′er-ăl). Relating to the throat.

gut·tur·o·tet·a·ny (gŭt′er-ō-tet′ă-nē). Laryngeal spasm causing a temporary stutter. [L. *guttur,* throat, + G. *tetanos,* convulsive tension]

Gutzeit, Max A.G., German chemist, 1847–1915. SEE G. *test.*

Guyon, Jean C.F., French surgeon, 1831–1920. SEE G. *amputation, isthmus, sign;* Guyon tunnel *syndrome.*

GVH Abbreviation for graft versus host.

GVHR Abbreviation for graft versus host *reaction.*

Gy Abbreviation for gray.

gym·di·ol. SEE gym-*diol.*

Gym·na·moe·bi·da (jim-nă-mē′bi-dă). An order of naked amebae lacking a shell (testa), although there may be an enveloping layer of condensed ectoplasm; includes the genus *Amoeba.* [G. *gymnos,* naked, + *amoibē,* change (ameba)]

gym·nas·tics (jim-nas′tiks). Muscular exercise, performed indoors, as distinguished from athletics, and usually by means of special apparatus. [G. *gymnos,* naked]

Swedish g., SYN Swedish *movements,* under *movement.*

Gym·no·as·ca·ce·ae (jim′nō-as-kā′sē-ē). A family of fungi that includes the ascomycetous state of many of the dermatophytes and several of the systemic pathogens for humans (*Histoplasma capsulatum, Blastomyces dermatitidis,* etc.). Until the sexual forms were recognized, these pathogens were classified with Fungi Imperfecti.

Gymnodinium (jim-nō-din′ē-um). Genus of marine dinoflagellates that includes the unicellular organism that causes red tide.

G. breve, a species of microscopic algae that causes red tide; it produces a toxin that affects the central nervous system of fish, paralyzing and killing them.

gym·no·phal·loi·des (jim-nōfal-oy′dēz). Small trematode (family Gymnophallidae) normally found in birds; often reported in human intestine in Korea; the intermediate host is presumed to be a marine oyster or clam.

g. seoi, trematode found in inhabitants of an island southwest of Korean peninsula; infection produces vague intestinal symptoms; it is a human parasite under natural conditions, not accidental infections, and bivalves are intermediate hosts.

gym·no·pho·bia (jim-nō-fō′bē-ă). Morbid dread of the sight of a naked person or of an uncovered part of the body. [G. *gymnos,* naked, + *phobos,* fear]

gym·no·the·ci·um (jim′nō-the′sē-um). An ascomycetous fruiting

gy

body composed of loosely interwoven hyphae. [G. *gymnos*, naked, + *thēkion*, case, dim. fr. *thēkē*, box]

GYN Abbreviation for gynecology.

△**gyn-, gyne-, gyneco-, gyno-.** Female. [G. *gynē*, woman]

gy·nan·drism (ji-nan′drizm, gī′nan-drizm). A developmental abnormality characterized by hypertrophy of the clitoris and union of the labia majora, simulating in appearance the penis and scrotum. SEE hermaphroditism, female *pseudohermaphroditism*. [gyn- + G. *anēr* (*andr*-), man]

gy·nan·dro·blas·to·ma (ji-nan′drō-blas-tō′mă, gī-). **1.** SYN Sertoli-Leydig cell *tumor*. **2.** A rare variety of arrhenoblastoma of the ovary, containing granulosa or theca cell elements and producing simultaneous androgenic and estrogenic effects.

gy·nan·droid (gī-nan′droyd, jĭ-). An individual exhibiting gynandrism. [gyn- + G. *anēr* (*andr*-), man, + *eidos*, resemblance]

gy·nan·dro·mor·phism (gī-nan-drō-mōr′fizm, jĭ-). **1.** An abnormal combination of male and female characteristics. **2.** The presence of male and female sex chromosome complements in different tissues; sex chromosome mosaicism. [gyn- + G. *anēr* (*andr*-), a male human, + *morphē*, form]

gy·nan·dro·mor·phous (gī-nan-drō-mōr′fŭs, jĭ-). Having both male and female characteristics.

gy·na·tre·sia (gī-nă-trē′zē-ă, jĭ-). Occlusion of some part of the female genital tract, especially occlusion of the vagina by a thick membrane. [gyn- + G. *a-* priv. + *trēsis*, a hole]

△**gyne-.** SEE gyn-.

gy·ne·cic (gī-nē′sik, jĭ-). Pertaining to or associated with women.

gy·ne·co·gen·ic (gī′nĕ-kō-jen′ik, jin′ĕ-). **1.** Giving birth predominantly to females. **2.** Obsolete term meaning productive of female characteristics.

gy·ne·coid (gī′nĕ-koyd, jin′ĕ-). Resembling a woman in form and structure. [gyneco- + G. *eidos*, resemblance]

gy·ne·co·log·ic, gy·ne·co·log·i·cal (gī′nĕ-kō-loj′ik, jin′ĕ-; -loj′i-kăl). Relating to gynecology.

gy·ne·col·o·gist (gī-nĕ-kol′ō-jist, jĭ-nĕ-). A physician specializing in gynecology.

gy·ne·col·o·gy (GYN) (gī-nĕ-kol′ō-jē, jin-ĕ-). The medical specialty concerned with diseases of the female genital tract, as well as endocrinology and reproductive physiology of the female. [gyneco- + G. *logos*, study]

gy·ne·co·ma·nia (gī′nĕ-kō-mā′nē-ă, jin′ĕ-). Morbid or excessive desire for women. [gyneco- + G. *mania*, frenzy]

gy·ne·co·mas·tia, gy·ne·co·mas·ty (gī′nĕ-kō-mas′tē-ă, jin′ĕ-; -mas′tē). Excessive development of the male mammary glands, due mainly to ductal proliferation with periductal edema; frequently secondary to increased estrogen levels, but mild g. may occur in normal adolescence. [gyneco- + G. *mastos*, breast]

refeeding g., temporary breast enlargement seen in male patients who have been starving, when nutritional repletion is occurring. It probably represents an imbalance in endocrine function, as some systems increase function before others; seen most notably when concentration camp inmates and Allied prisoners of war were freed at the end of World War II.

gy·ne·pho·bia (gī-nĕ-fō′bē-ă, jin-ĕ-). Morbid fear of women or of the female sex. [gyne- + G. *phobos*, fear]

gy·ni·at·rics (gī-nē-at′riks, jin-ē-). Treatment of the diseases of women. SYN gyniatry. [gyn- + G. *iatrikos*, of medicine or surgery]

gy·ni·at·ry (gī-nē-at′rē, jin-ē). SYN gyniatrics.

△**gyno-.** SEE gyn-.

gy·no·car·dia oil (gī-nō-kar′dē-ă). SYN chaulmoogra oil.

gy·no·gen·e·sis (gī-nō-jen′ĕ-sis, jin-ō-). Egg development activated by a spermatozoon, but to which the male gamete contributes no genetic material. [gyno- + G. *genesis*, production]

gy·nop·a·thy (gī-nop′ă-thē, jĭ-). Any disease peculiar to women. [gyno- + G. *pathos*, suffering]

gynoplasty (gī′nō-plas-tiks). Reparative or plastic surgery of the female genital organs. [gyno- + G. *plassō*, to form]

gyp·sum (jip′sŭm). The natural hydrated form of calcium sulfate;

a component of the stones, plasters, and investments used in dentistry. [L. fr. G. *gypsos*]

gy·rase (gī′ras). The procaryotic topoisomerase II that utilizes ATP to generate negative supercoils of DNA. [L. *gyro*, to turn in a circle, fr. *gyrus*, G. *gyros*,]

gy·rate (jī′rāt). **1.** Of a convoluted or ring shape. **2.** To revolve. [L. *gyro*, pp. *gyratus*, to turn round in a circle, *gyrus*]

gy·ra·tion (jī-rā′shŭn). **1.** A circular motion or revolution. **2.** Arrangement of convolutions or gyri in the cerebral cortex.

gy·rec·to·my (jī-rek′tō-mē). Excision of a cerebral gyrus. [G. *gyros*, ring, + *ektomē*, excision]

gyr·en·ce·phal·ic (jī′ren-sĕ-fal′ik). Denoting brains, such as that of humans, in which the cerebral cortex has convolutions, in contrast to the lissencephalic (smooth) brains of small mammals such as the rodents. [G. *gyros*, ring (gyrus), + *enkaphalē*, brain]

gy·ri (jī′rī). Plural of gyrus. [L.]

gy·ro·chrome (jī′rō-krōm). Denoting a nerve cell in which the chromophil substance is arranged roughly in rings. [G. *gyros*, a ring, circle, + *chrōma*, a color]

Gy·ro·mi·tra es·cu·len·ta (gī-rō-mē′tră es-kū-len′tă). A species of mushroom that may produce a monomethylhydrazine toxin that causes nausea, diarrhea, and other symptoms; in severe cases death may occur. SYN *Helvella esculenta*.

gy·rose (jī′rōs). Marked by irregular curved lines like the surface of a cerebral hemisphere. [G. *gyros*, circle]

gy·ro·spasm (jī′rō-spazm). Spasmodic rotary movements of the head. [G. *gyros*, circle, + *spasmos*, spasm]

GYRUS

gy·rus, gen. and pl. **gy·′ri** (jī′rŭs, -rī) [TA]. One of the prominent rounded elevations that form the cerebral hemispheres, each consisting of an exposed superficial portion and a portion hidden from view in the wall and floor of the sulcus. [L. fr. G. *gyros*, circle]

angular g. [TA], a folded convolution in the inferior parietal lobule formed by the union of the posterior ends of the superior and middle temporal gyri; a g. located around the caudal terminus of the superior temporal sulcus. SYN g. angularis [TA], angular convolution.

g. angula′ris [TA], SYN angular g.

annectent g., SYN transitional g.

anterior central g., SYN precentral g.

anterior paracentral g. [TA], the anterior portion of the paracentral lobule; the medial continuation of the primary somatomotor cortex (precentral gyrus) in which the thigh, leg, and foot are represented. SYN g. paracentralis anterior [TA].

anterior piriform g., SYN prepiriform g.

anterior transverse temporal g. [TA], SEE transverse temporal gyri. SYN g. temporalis transversus anterior [TA].

ascending frontal g., SYN precentral g.

ascending parietal g., SYN postcentral g.

gy′ri bre′ves in′sulae [TA], SYN short gyri of insula.

callosal g., SYN cingulate g.

central gyri, the precentral and postcentral gyri.

cerebral gyri [TA], SYN gyri cerebri.

gy′ri cer′ebri [TA], the gyri or convolutions of the cerebral cortex. SYN cerebral gyri [TA].

cingulate g. [TA], a long, curved convolution of the medial surface of the cortical hemisphere, arched over the corpus callosum from which it is separated by the deep sulcus of corpus callosum; together with the parahippocampal g., with which it is continuous behind the corpus callosum, it forms the fornicate g. SYN g. cinguli [TA], callosal convolution, callosal g., cingulate convolution, falciform lobe, lobus falciformis.

g. cin′guli [TA], SYN cingulate g.

deep transitional g., the transverse g. of the embryo which in

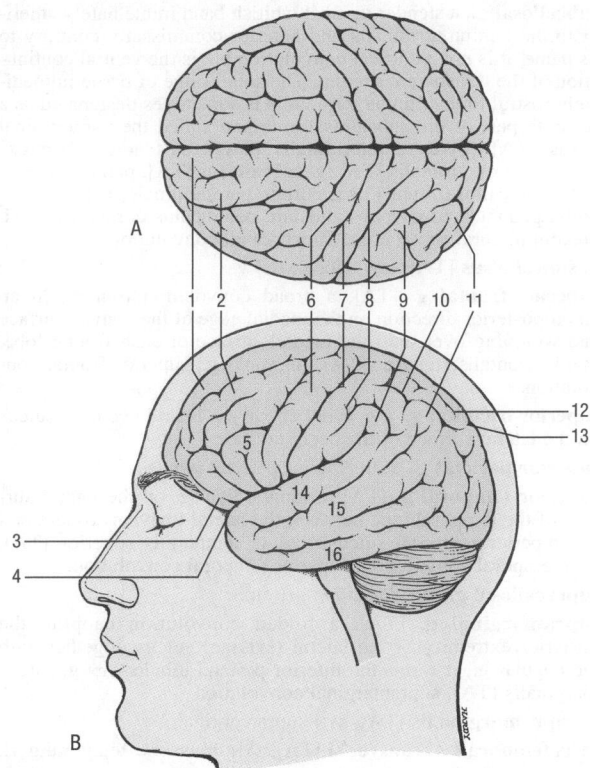

gyrus: (A) superior, (B) lateral views of brain. (1) sup. frontal gyrus; (2) middle frontal gyrus, (3) orbital gyri, (4) lateral cerebral fossa; (5) inferior frontal gyrus, (6) precentral gyrus; (7) central sulcus; (8) postcentral gyrus; (9) supramarginal gyrus; (10) intraparietal sulcus; (11) inferior parietal lobule; (12) intraparietal sulcus; (13) superior parietal lobule; (14) superior temporal gyrus; (15) middle temporal gyrus; (16) inferior temporal gyrus

development becomes buried in the depth of the central sulcus of the cerebral hemisphere.

dentate g. [TA], one of the two interlocking gyri composing the hippocampus, the other one being the Ammon horn. SYN g. dentatus [TA], dentate fascia, fascia dentata hippocampi.

g. denta'tus [TA], SYN dentate g.

fasciolar g. [TA], a small paired band that passes around the splenium of the corpus callosum from the lateral longitudinal stria to the dentate g. SYN g. fasciolaris [TA], fascia cinerea, fasciola cinerea.

g. fasciola'ris [TA], SYN fasciolar g.

fornicate g., the horseshoe-shaped cortical convolution bordering the hilus of the cerebral hemisphere; its upper limb is formed by the cingulate g., its lower by the parahippocampal g.; SYN g. fornicatus (1).

g. fornica'tus, (1) SYN fornicate g; **(2)** used previously to refer to the entire limbic system.

g. fronta'lis infe'rior [TA], SYN inferior frontal g.

g. frontalis medialis [TA], SYN medial frontal g.

g. fronta'lis me'dius [TA], SYN middle frontal g.

g. fronta'lis supe'rior [TA], SYN superior frontal g.

fusiform g., an extremely long convolution extending lengthwise over the inferior aspect of the temporal and occipital lobes, demarcated medially by the collateral sulcus from the lingual g. and the anterior part of the parahippocampal g., laterally by the inferior temporal sulcus from the inferior temporal g. SYN g. occipitotemporalis lateralis [TA], lateral occipitotemporal g. [TA], g. fusiformis, lobulus fusiformis.

g. fusifor'mis, SYN fusiform g.

Heschl gyri, SYN transverse temporal gyri.

hippocampal g., SYN parahippocampal g.

inferior frontal g. [TA], a broad convolution on the convexity of the frontal lobe of the cerebrum between the inferior frontal sulcus and the sylvian fissure; divided by branches of the sylvian fissure into three parts: opercular part [TA] (pars opercularis [TA]), triangular part [TA] (pars triangularis [TA]), and orbital part [TA] (pars orbitalis [TA]); the first two constitute a portion of the frontal operculum. SYN g. frontalis inferior [TA], inferior frontal convolution.

inferior occipital g., a g. situated below the lateral occipital sulcus on the lower part of the lateral surface of the occipital lobe.

inferior parietal g., SYN inferior parietal *lobule.*

inferior temporal g. [TA], a sagittal convolution on the inferolateral border of the temporal lobe of the cerebrum, separated from the middle temporal g. by the inferior temporal sulcus. On the inferior surface of the temporal lobe it is separated from the medial occipitotemporal g. by the occipitotemporal sulcus. It includes the lateral occipitotemporal g. SYN g. temporalis inferior [TA], inferior temporal convolution, third temporal convolution.

gy'ri in'sulae [TA], SYN insular gyri.

insular gyri [TA], the short gyri of insula and long g. of insula. SYN gyri insulae [TA].

interlocking gyri, several small gyri in the walls of the central sulcus of the hemisphere; the opposed gyri interlock with one another.

lateral occipitotemporal g. [TA], SYN fusiform g.

lateral olfactory g. [TA], superficial layers of cells located adjacent to the lateral olfactory stria; poorly developed in microsmatic animals but well developed in macrosmatic animals. SYN g. olfactorius lateralis [TA].

lingual g. [TA], a relatively short horizontal convolution on the inferomedial aspect of the occipital and temporal lobes, demarcated from the lateral occipitotemporal or fusiform g. by the deep collateral sulcus, from the cuneus by the calcarine sulcus; its anterior extreme abuts the isthmus of the parahippocampal g.; the medial or upper strip of the g. forming the lower bank of the calcarine sulcus corresponds to the inferior half of the striate area or primary visual cortex and represents the contralateral upper quadrant of the binocular field of vision. SYN g. lingualis [TA], g. occipitotemporalis medialis [TA], medial occipitotemporal g. [TA].

g. lingua'lis [TA], SYN lingual g.

long g. of insula [TA], the most posterior and longest of the slender straight gyri that compose the insula. SYN g. longus insulae [TA].

g. lon'gus in'sulae [TA], SYN long g. of insula.

marginal g., SYN superior frontal g.

medial frontal g. [TA], term sometimes used to designate the part of the superior frontal gyrus that wraps over, and is located on, the medial surface of the frontal lobe. SYN g. frontalis medialis [TA].

medial occipitotemporal g. [TA], SYN lingual g.

medial olfactory g. [TA], layers of cells located adjacent to the medial olfactory stria; well developed in macrosmatic animals but poorly developed in microsmatic animals. SYN g. olfactorius medialis [TA].

middle frontal g., a convolution on the convexity of each frontal lobe of the cerebrum running in an anteroposterior direction between the superior and inferior frontal sulci. SYN g. frontalis medius [TA], middle frontal convolution.

middle temporal g. [TA], a longitudinal g. on the lateral surface of the temporal lobe, between the superior and inferior temporal sulci. SYN g. temporalis medius [TA], middle temporal convolution, second temporal convolution.

occipital gyri, SEE inferior occipital g., superior occipital g.

g. occip'itotempora'lis latera'lis [TA], SYN fusiform g.

g. occip'itotempora'lis media'lis [TA], SYN lingual g.

g. olfactorius lateralis [TA], SYN lateral olfactory g.

g. olfactorius medialis [TA], SYN medial olfactory g.

orbital gyri [TA], a number of small, irregular convolutions occupying the concave inferior surface of each frontal lobe of the cerebrum. SYN gyri orbitales [TA].

gy

gy'ri orbita'les [TA], SYN orbital gyri.

g. paracentralis anterior [TA], SYN anterior paracentral g.

g. paracentralis posterior [TA], SYN posterior paracentral g.

parahippocampal g. [TA], a long convolution on the medial surface of the temporal lobe, forming the lower part of the fornicate g., extending from behind the splenium corporis callosi forward along the dentate g. of the hippocampus from which it is demarcated by the hippocampal fissure. The anterior extreme of the g. curves back upon itself, forming the uncus, the major location of the olfactory cortex. SEE ALSO entorhinal *area*. SYN g. parahippocampalis [TA], hippocampal convolution, hippocampal g.

g. par'ahippocampa'lis [TA], SYN parahippocampal g.

paraterminal g. [TA], SYN subcallosal g.

g. paratermina'lis [TA], SYN subcallosal g.

postcentral g. [TA], the anterior convolution of the parietal lobe, bounded in front by the central sulcus (fissure of Rolando) and posteriorly by the interparietal sulcus. SYN g. postcentralis [TA], ascending parietal convolution, ascending parietal g., posterior central convolution, posterior central g.

g. postcentra'lis [TA], SYN postcentral g.

posterior central g., SYN postcentral g.

posterior paracentral g. [TA], the posterior part of the paracentral lobule; the medial continuation of the primary somatosensory cortex (postcentral gyrus) in which sensory input from the thigh, leg, and foot are represented. SYN g. paracentralis posterior [TA].

posterior transverse temporal g. [TA], posterior portion of the primary auditory cortex when two gyri are present. SEE ALSO transverse temporal gyri. SYN g. temporalis transversus posterior [TA].

precentral g. [TA], bounded posteriorly by the central sulcus and anteriorly by the precentral sulcus. SYN g. precentralis [TA], anterior central convolution, anterior central g., ascending frontal convolution, ascending frontal g.

g. precentra'lis [TA], SYN precentral g.

prepiriform g., a g. covering deeply placed amygdaloid nucleus; concerned with olfactory function. SYN anterior piriform g.

g. rec'tus [TA], SYN straight g.

Retzius g., the intralimbic g. in the cortical portion of the rhinencephalon.

short gyri of insula [TA], several short, radiating gyri converging toward the base of the insula, composing approximately the anterior two-thirds of the insular cortex. SYN gyri breves insulae [TA].

splenial g., the band of cortex on the medial surface of the cerebral hemisphere which passes around the splenium of the corpus callosum, narrowing anteriorly and finally blending with the indusium griseum.

straight g. [TA], a g. running along the medial part of the orbital surface of the frontal lobe of the cerebral hemisphere. It is bounded laterally by the olfactory sulcus. SYN g. rectus [TA].

subcallosal g., a slender vertical whitish band immediately anterior to the lamina terminalis and anterior commissure; contrary to its name, it is not a cortical convolution but is the ventral continuation of the transparent septum. The small ridge of tissue immediately rostral to the lamina terminalis is sometimes designated as a separate part of the subcallosal area and called the paraterminal gyrus [TA] (gyrus paraterminalis [TA]). SYN area subcallosa [TA], g. paraterminalis [TA], g. subcallosus [TA], paraterminal g. [TA], subcallosal area [TA], corpus paraterminale, paraterminal body, peduncle of corpus callosum, pedunculus corporis callosi, precommissural septal area, Zuckerkandl convolution.

g. subcallo'sus [TA], SYN subcallosal g.

superior frontal g. [TA], a broad convolution running in an anteroposterior direction on the medial edge of the convex surface and wrapping over onto the medial surface of each frontal lobe. SYN g. frontalis superior [TA], marginal g., superior frontal convolution.

superior occipital g., a g. lying above the lateral occipital sulcus on the lateral surface of the occipital lobe.

superior parietal g., SYN superior parietal *lobule*.

superior temporal g. [TA], a longitudinal g. on the lateral surface of the temporal lobe between the lateral (sylvian) fissure and the superior temporal sulcus. SYN g. temporalis superior [TA], first temporal convolution, superior temporal convolution.

supracallosal g., SYN *indusium* griseum.

supramarginal g. [TA], a folded convolution capping the posterior extremity of the lateral (sylvian) sulcus; together with the angular g., it forms the inferior parietal lobule. SYN g. supramarginalis [TA], supramarginal convolution.

g. supramargina'lis [TA], SYN supramarginal g.

gy'ri tempora'les transver'si [TA], SYN transverse temporal gyri.

g. tempora'lis infe'rior [TA], SYN inferior temporal g.

g. tempora'lis me'dius [TA], SYN middle temporal g.

g. tempora'lis supe'rior [TA], SYN superior temporal g.

g. temporalis transversus anterior [TA], SYN anterior transverse temporal g; SEE transverse temporal gyri.

g. temporalis transversus posterior [TA], SYN posterior transverse temporal g.

transitional g., a small convolution connecting two lobes or two main gyri in the depth of a sulcus. SYN annectent g., transitional convolution.

transverse temporal gyri [TA], two or three convolutions running transversely on the upper surface of the temporal lobe bordering on the lateral (sylvian) fissure, separated from each other by the transverse temporal sulci. SYN gyri temporales transversi [TA], Heschl gyri, transverse temporal convolutions.

uncinate g., SYN uncus (2).

H Abbreviation or symbol for hydrogen; hyperopia; hyperopic; horizontal; Hauch; Holzknecht *unit*; henry, unit of electrical inductance; the Fraunhofer line at λ 3968 due to calcium; histidine; magnetic field strength; heroin; histone; histamine.

H⁺ Symbol for hydrogen *ion*, the proton.

¹H Symbol for hydrogen-1.

²H Symbol for hydrogen-2.

³H Symbol for hydrogen-3.

H Symbol for enthalpy, heat content, in the equation for free energy; fluence; magnetic field strength.

h Symbol for hecto-; height; hour.

hν. Symbol for photon, and represents photon energy, where h = Planck's constant and ν = frequency of electromagnetic wave.

h Symbol for Planck *constant*; h = h/2π.

HAA Abbreviation for hepatitis-associated *antigen.*

Haab, Otto, Swiss ophthalmologist, 1850–1931.

Haase rule. See under rule.

ha·be·na, pl. **ha·be·nae** (hă-bē′nă, -bē′nē). **1.** A frenum or restricting fibrous band. **2.** A restraining bandage. **3.** SYN habenula (2). [L. strap]

hab·e·nal, ha·be·nar (hab′ĕ-năl, hă-bē′năr). Relating to a habena.

ha·ben·u·la, pl. **ha·ben·u·lae** (ha-ben′ū-lă, -lē) [TA]. **1.** SYN frenulum. **2** [TA]. In neuroanatomy, the term originally denoted the stalk of the pineal gland (pineal habenula; pedunculus of pineal body), but gradually came to refer to a neighboring group of nerve cells with which the pineal gland was believed to be associated, the habenular nucleus. Currently, the TA term refers exclusively to this circumscript cell mass in the caudal and dorsal aspect of the dorsal thalamus, embedded in the posterior end of the medullary stria from which it receives most of its afferent fibers. By way of the retroflex fasciculus (habenulointerpeduncular tract) it projects to the interpeduncular nucleus and other paramedian cell groups of the midbrain tegmentum. Despite its proximity to the pineal stalk, no habenulopineal fiber connection is known to exist. It is a part of the epithalamus. SYN habena (3). [L.]

h. of cecum, extension of the mesocolic tenia, dorsal or ventral to the terminal ileum.

Haller h., rarely used term for the cordlike remains of the vaginal process of the peritoneum. SYN Scarpa h.

haben′ulae perfora′tae, SYN *foramina* nervosa, under *foramen.*

pineal h., the peduncle or stalk of the pineal gland. SEE habenula (2).

Scarpa h., SYN Haller h.

h. urethra′lis, one of two fine, whitish lines running from the meatus urethrae to the clitoris in girls and young women; the vestiges of the anterior part of the corpus spongiosum.

ha·ben·u·lar (hă-ben′ū-lăr). Relating to a habenula, especially the stalk of the pineal body.

Haber, Henry, British dermatologist, 1900–1962. SEE H. *syndrome.*

Habermann, R., German dermatologist, 1884–1941. SEE Mucha-H. *disease.*

hab·it. 1. An act, behavioral response, practice, or custom established in one's repertoire by frequent repetition of the same act. SEE ALSO addiction. **2.** A basic variable in the study of conditioning and learning used to designate a new response learned either by association or by being followed by a reward or reinforced event. SEE conditioning, learning. [L. *habeo,* pp. *habitus,* to have]

ha·bit·u·a·tion (ha-bit-choo-ā′shŭn). **1.** The process of forming a habit, referring generally to psychological dependence on the continued use of a drug to maintain a sense of well-being, which can result in drug addiction. **2.** The method by which the nervous system reduces or inhibits responsiveness during repeated stimulation.

hab·i·tus (hab′i-tŭs). The physical characteristics of a person. [L. habit]

fetal h., relationship of one fetal part to another. SYN fetal attitude.

gracile h., small stature, frail, underweight appearance.

Hab·ro·ne·ma (ha-brō-nē′mă). A genus of spiruroid nematodes inhabiting the stomach of horses. The larvae develop in housefly and stable fly maggots living in manure, become infective when the fly larvae pupate, and are carried by adult flies to open wounds on horses, where they are left and cause cutaneous habronemiasis; reinfection of the horse's stomach by H. occurs by accidental ingestion of infected flies or from licking wounds in which infective larvae are found. [G. *habros,* graceful, delicate, + *nēma,* a thread]

H. ma′jus, one of two species (the other being *H. microstoma*) similar in appearance, hosts, distribution, and life cycle to *H. muscae;* the intermediate host is the stable fly, *Stomoxys calcitrans.*

H. megas′toma, a species that causes tumors in gastric mucosa containing large numbers of the small nematodes; the larvae cause cutaneous habronemiasis; the intermediate host is the common housefly, *Musca domestica.*

H. micros′toma, SEE H. majus.

H. mus′cae, a species that occurs in the stomach of the horse, mule, ass, or zebra; the intermediate host is the common housefly, *Musca domestica,* or related flies.

hack·ing (hak′ing). A chopping stroke made with the edge of the hand in massage.

Hadfield, Geoffrey, British physician, 1889–1968. SEE Clarke-H. *syndrome.*

Ha·dru·rus (hă-droo′rŭs). A genus of scorpions found in the southwestern U.S., characterized by numerous setae on the stinger; the commonest species is *H. arizonensis,* the olive hairy scorpion. SEE ALSO Scorpionida. [G. *hadros,* thick, stout, + *ouro,* tail]

Haeckel, Ernst H.P.A., German naturalist, 1834–1919. SEE H. gastrea *theory, law.*

⌂**haem-.** SEE hem-.

Hae·ma·dip·sa cey·lon·i·ca (hē-mă-dip′să să-lon′i-kă). A species of land leech found in Sri Lanka; it attaches itself to the skin of animals or humans. Its bite is painful, and numerous bites may cause anemia. [G. *haima,* blood, + *dipsa,* thirst]

Hae·ma·moe·ba (hē-mă-mē′bă). Old term for ameboid protozoa now classified in the suborder Haemosporina, blood parasites that include the genus *Plasmodium.* [G. *haima,* blood, + *amoibē,* change]

Hae·ma·phy·sa·lis (hē-mă-fĭ′să-lis). A genus of small, eyeless, inornate ticks. As larvae and nymphs, they are found chiefly on small mammals and birds; as adults, they are found on larger mammals and some birds. They are important as vectors of protozoa and viruses, (e.g., Kyasanur Forest disease virus). [G. *haima,* blood, + *physaleos,* full of wind]

H. cinnabari′na, a tick that occurs chiefly in the dry district of British Columbia; this species can cause tick paralysis in both humans and animals. [G. *kinnabarinos,* like cinnabar, vermilion]

H. concin′na, common rodent tick species of the area formerly known as the U.S.S.R. that is a vector and reservoir of tick typhus.

H. leach′i, a species of Africa, Asia, and Australia that occurs on domestic and wild carnivores, on small rodents, and occasionally on cattle; it transmits canine babesiosis and boutonneuse fever.

H. spinige′ra, a tropical forest species in India that is a vector of

Ha

⌂ Combining Forms	☆ Official alternate Terminologia Anatomica term
🔲 Indicates term is illustrated, see Illustration Index	
	[MIM] Mendelian Inheritance in Man
SYN Synonym	
Cf. Compare	C.I. Colour Index
[NA] Nomina Anatomica	
[TA] Terminologia Anatomica	**High Profile Term**

Kyasanur Forest disease; various rodents and insectivores serve as hosts of immature ticks of this species, which carry an arbovirus of the Russian spring-summer B group complex; monkeys act as reservoirs of human infection.

Hae·ma·to·pi·nus (hē'mă-tō-pī'nŭs). An important genus of sucking lice (family Haematopinidae) affecting swine and other domestic and wild animals; it is normally nonpathogenic. *H. asini* affects horses, mules, and asses; *H. eurysternus* and *H. quadripertusus*, cattle; and *H. suis*, swine. [G. *haima*, blood, + L. *pinus*, pine tree]

Hae·mo·coc·cid·i·um (hē'mō-kok-sid'ē-ŭm). Old name for *Plasmodium* species. [G. *haima*, blood, + *kokkos*, berry]

Hae·mo·dip·sus ven·tri·co·sus (hē-mō-dip'sŭs ven-tri-kō'sŭs). The rabbit louse, a transmitter of *Francisella tularensis*. [G. *haima*, blood, + *dipsos*, thirst; L. *venter* (*ventr*-), belly]

Hae·mo·greg·a·ri·na (hē'mō-greg-ă-rī'nă). A sporozoan coccidian genus (order Eucoccidiida, family Haemogregarinidae) that parasitizes the blood cells of cold-blooded animals and the digestive system of invertebrate primary hosts in an obligatory two-host cycle. [G. *haima*, blood, + L. *grex*, a flock]

Hae·mon·chus (hē-mong'kŭs). An economically important genus of nematode parasites (family Trichostrongylidae) occurring in the abomasum of ruminant animals and causing severe anemia, especially in younger or previously unexposed animals. Some significant species are *H. placei* (in cattle, sheep, and goats), *H. similis* (in cattle and sheep), and *H. contortus*, the stomach, barberpole, or twisted wire worm of cattle, sheep, goats, and other ruminants, of which a few cases have been reported from humans; accidental parasite of humans. [G. *haima*, blood, + *onchos*, spear]

Hae·moph·i·lus (hē-mof'i-lŭs). A genus of aerobic to facultatively anaerobic, nonmotile bacteria (family Brucellaceae) containing minute, Gram-negative, rod-shaped cells that sometimes form threads and are pleomorphic. These organisms are strictly parasitic, growing best, or only, on media containing blood. They may or may not be pathogenic. They occur in various lesions and secretions, as well as in normal respiratory tracts, of vertebrates. The type species is *H. influenzae*. [G. *haima*, blood, + *philos*, fond]

H. actinomycetemcomi'tans, SYN *Actinobacillus actinomycetemcomitans.*

H. aegyp'tius, a bacterial species that causes acute or subacute infectious conjunctivitis in warm climates. SYN Koch-Weeks bacillus.

H. aphroph'ilus, a bacterial species found in the blood and, rarely, on the heart valve as a cause of endocarditis.

H. ducrey'i, a bacterial species that causes the sexually transmitted soft chancre (chancroid). SYN Ducrey bacillus.

H. haemolyt'icus, a bacterial species that is usually nonpathogenic but which, on rare occasions, causes subacute endocarditis.

H. influen'zae, a bacterial species found in the respiratory tract that causes acute respiratory infections, including pneumonia, acute conjunctivitis, otitis, and purulent meningitis in children (rarely in adults in whom it contributes to sinusitis and chronic bronchitis). Originally considered to be the cause of influenza, it is the type species of the genus *H.* SYN influenza bacillus, Weeks bacillus.

H. influenzae Type b, the most virulent serotype (there are six, a–f, based on antigenic typing of the polysaccharide capsule); species responsible for meningitis and respiratory infections in young children.

nontypeable *H. influenzae*, bacterial species that is a major pathogen in acute otitis media.

H. parahaemoly'ticus, a bacterial species found in the upper respiratory tract and associated frequently with pharyngitis; occasionally causes subacute endocarditis.

H. parainfluen'zae, a bacterial species that is usually nonpathogenic but which occasionally causes subacute endocarditis.

H. paratropicalis, a relatively nonpathogenic bacterial species that has been associated with human infection, including cases of endocarditis.

H. segnis, a usually saprophytic bacterial species that occasion-

ally causes endocarditis, meningitis, and other infections in humans.

Hae·mo·pro·te·us (hē'mō-prō'tē-ŭs). A genus of sporozoa (suborder Haemosporina) parasitic in birds and reptiles, combined with *Leucocytozoon, Hepatocystis*, and other genera in the family Haemoproteidae. Schizogony occurs in endothelial cells of blood vessels, especially in the lungs of the host, while halter-shaped gametocytes are found in the red blood cells. Infection is transmitted by pupiparous Diptera, such as louse flies (Hippoboscidae) and by bloodsucking midges (*Culicoides*) [G. *haima*, blood, + *Proteus*, a sea god who had the power of assuming different shapes]

Hae·mo·spo·ri·na (hē'mō-spō-rī'nă). A suborder of coccidia (class Sporozoea) that lack syzygy, with separate development of macrogamete and microgamont, the latter producing eight flagellated microgametes; heteroxenous with merogany in vertebrates and sporogony in bloodsucking insects; includes the genera *Haemoproteus, Leucocytozoon*, and *Plasmodium*. [G. *haima*, blood, + *sporos*, seed]

Haens·zel, William M., U.S. epidemiologist/statistician, 1910–1998. SEE Mantel-Haenszel *test.*

Haffkine, Waldemar M.W., Russian physician, 1860–1930. SEE H. *vaccine.*

Haf·nia (haf'nē-ah). Genus in the family Enterobacteriaceae; found in human feces, a rare cause of nosocomial infection; associated with diarrheal disease of undefined mechanism. There is a single species, *Hafnia alvei.*

haf·ni·um (Hf) (haf'nē-ŭm). A rare chemical element, atomic no. 72, atomic wt. 178.49. [L. *Hafnia,* Copenhagen]

Hagedorn, Hans Christian, Danish physician, *1888. SEE NPH *insulin.*

Hagedorn, Werner, German surgeon, 1831–1894. SEE H. *needle.*

Hageman. Surname of person in whom deficiency of Hageman *factor* was first observed.

hag·i·o·ther·a·py (hag'ē-ō-thār'ă-pē). Treatment of the sick by contact with relics of the saints, visits to shrines, and other religious observances. [G. *hagios,* sacred]

Haglund, S.E. Patrik, Swedish orthopedist, 1870–1937. SEE H. *deformity, disease.*

Hahnemann, Christian F.S., German physician and founder of homeopathy, 1755–1843. SEE hahnemannian.

hah·ne·man·ni·an (hah-ně-mahn'ē-an). Relating to homeopathy as taught by Hahnemann.

Hahn ox·ine re·a·gent. See under reagent.

Haidinger, Wilhelm von, Austrian mineralogist, 1795–1871. SEE H. *brushes,* under *brush.*

Hailey, Hugh E., U.S. dermatologist, *1909. SEE H.-H. *disease.*

Hailey, W. Howard, U.S. dermatologist, 1898–1967. SEE H.-H. *disease.*

▉hair (hār) [TA]. **1.** One of the fine, keratinized filamentous epidermal growths arising from the skin of the body of mammals except the palms, soles, and flexor surfaces of the joints; the full length and texture of hair varies markedly in different body sites. SYN pilus (1) [TA]. **2.** One of the fine, hairlike processes of the auditory cells of the labyrinth, and of other sensory cells, called auditory h., sensory h., etc. SYN thrix [TA]. [A.S. *haer*]

auditory h.'s, cilia on the free surface of the auditory cells.

axillary h.'s [TA], h. of the armpit. SYN hircus (2).

bamboo h., h. with regularly spaced nodules along the shaft caused by intermittent fractures with invagination of the distal h. into the proximal portion, with intervening lengths of normal h., giving the appearance of bamboo; seen in Netherton syndrome; autosomal recessive trait. SYN trichorrhexis invaginata.

bayonet h., a spindle-shaped developmental defect occurring at the tapered end of the h.

beaded h., SYN monilethrix.

burrowing h.'s, SYN ingrown h.'s.

club h., a h. in resting state, prior to shedding, in which the bulb has become a club-shaped mass.

downy h. [TA], fine, soft, lightly pigmented fetal hair with min-

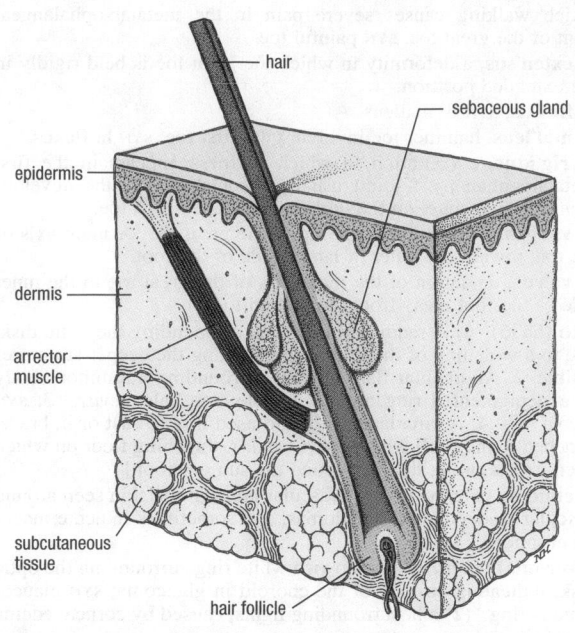

hair

sebaceous gland

epidermis

dermis

arrector muscle

subcutaneous tissue

hair follicle

hair: with associated anatomic structures

ute shafts and large papillae; it appears toward the end of the third month of gestation. SYN lanugo [TA], primary h.☆, lanugo h.

exclamation point h., the type of dystrophic anagen h. found at margins of patches of alopecia areata; the bulb is absent.

Frey h.'s, short h.'s of varying degrees of stiffness, set at right angles into the end of a light wooden handle; used for assessing sensation.

h.'s of head [TA], a hair of the scalp of the head. SYN scalp h.

ingrown h.'s, h.'s that grow at more acute angles than is normal, and in all directions; they incompletely clear the follicle, turn back in, and cause pseudofolliculitis. SYN burrowing h.'s.

kinky h., tightly curled or bent h. SEE kinky-hair *disease*.

lanugo h., SYN downy h.

moniliform h., SYN monilethrix.

nettling h.'s, sharp-pointed barbed h.'s of certain caterpillars which cause a dermatitis when brought in contact with the skin.

primary h., ☆ official alternate term for downy h.

pubic h. [TA], one of the pubic hairs; the hair of the pubic region just above the external genitals. SYN pubes (1) [TA].

ringed h., a rare condition in which the h. shows alternate pigmented and bright segments, the latter due to air cavities within the cortex. SYN pili annulati.

scalp h., SYN h.'s of head.

Schridde cancer h.'s, thick lusterless h.'s scattered in the beard and the temporal region, said to occur in cancerous patients but found also in persons with other cachectic conditions.

spun glass h., SYN uncombable hair *syndrome*.

stellate h., h. split in several strands at the free end.

taste h.'s, hairlike projections of gustatory cells of taste buds; electron micrographs show them to be clusters of microvilli.

terminal h., a mature pigmented, coarse h.

h.'s of tragus [TA], hairs growing from the tragus of the auricle.

twisted h.'s, SYN pili torti, under *pilus*.

vellus h., colorless, soft, fine postnatal to adult h.

h.'s of vestibule of nose [TA], one of the hairs growing at the nares, or vestibule of the nose. SYN vibrissa [TA].

woolly h., tightly coiled h., oval in cross-section, with the texture of wool.

hair·pin (hār'pin). **1.** The structure formed by a polynucleic acid by base-pairing between neighboring complementary sequences of a single strand of either DNA or RNA. **2.** The structure seen in

a prostaglandin where two segments of the molecule fold back on one another.

hair·worm (hār'werm). SEE *Trichostrongylus, Gordius*.

hairy (hār'ē). **1.** Of or resembling hair. **2.** Covered with hair. SEE ALSO hirsutism. SYN pilar, pilary, pilose.

ha·la·tion (hă-lā'shŭn). Blurring of the visual image by glare.

hal·a·zone (hal'ă-zōn). A chloramine used for the sterilization of drinking water.

Halbeisen, William A., U.S. physician, *1915. SEE Stryker-H. *syndrome*.

Halberstaedter, Ludwig, German physician, 1876–1949. SEE Halberstaedter-Prowazek *bodies*, under *body*.

Haldane, John B.S., English biochemist and geneticist, 1892–1964. SEE H. *relationship*.

Haldane, John S., Scottish physiologist at Oxford, 1860–1936. SEE H. *apparatus, effect, transformation, tube;* H.-Priestley *sample*.

Hale col·loi·dal iron stain. See under stain.

Hales, Stephen, English physiologist, 1677–1761. SEE H. *piesimeter*.

half-hap·ten (haf-hap'ten). A substance that elicits an antigen-antibody reaction, but no precipitation.

half-life (haf'līf). The period in which the radioactivity or number of atoms of a radioactive substance decreases by half; similarly applied to any substance, such as a drug in serum, whose quantity decreases exponentially with time. Cf. half-time.

biologic h.-l., the time required for one-half of an amount of a substance to be lost through biologic processes.

effective h.-l., the time required for the body burden of an administered quantity of radioactivity to decrease by half through a combination of radioactive decay and biologic elimination.

physical h.-l., the time required for half the atoms of a radionuclide to undergo disintegration.

half-moon (haf'moon). SYN lunule of nail.

red h.-m., irregular red discoloration of the usually pale demilune at the base of the fingernail; may be seen in congestive failure, malignant disease, or liver disease, but not specific for any of these.

half-time (haf'tīm). The time, in a first-order chemical (or enzymic) reaction, for half of the substance (substrate) to be converted or to disappear. Cf. half-life.

half·way house (haf'wā hows). A facility for individuals who no longer require the complete facilities of a hospital or institution but are not yet prepared to return to independent living.

hal·i·but liv·er oil (hal'i-bŭt). The fixed oil obtained from the fresh or suitably preserved livers of halibut species of the genus *Hippoglossus* (family Pleuronectidae); a supplementary source of vitamins A and D.

hal·ide (hal'īd). A salt of a halogen.

hal·i·pha·gia (hal-i-fā'jē-ă). Ingestion of an excessive quantity of a salt or salts, especially of sodium chloride, calcium, magnesium, or potassium salts, or of sodium bicarbonate. [G. *hals*, salt, + *phagō*, to eat]

hal·i·ste·re·sis (hă-lis-ter-ē'sis). A deficiency of lime salts in the bones. SYN halosteresis. [G. *hals*, salt, + *sterēsis*, privation, fr. *stereō*, to deprive]

hal·i·ste·ret·ic (hă-lis-ter-et'ik). Relating to or marked by halisteresis.

hal·i·to·sis (hal-i-tō'sis). A foul odor from the mouth. SYN fetor oris, ozostomia, stomatodysodia. [L. *halitus*, breath, + G. *-osis*, condition]

hal·i·tus (hal'i-tŭs). Any exhalation, as of a breath or vapor. [L., fr. *halo*, to breathe]

hal·la·chrome (hal'ă-krōm). A quinone intermediate, derived from L-dopa, in the formation of melanin from L-tyrosine.

Hallé, Adrien J.M.N., French physician, 1859–1947. SEE H. *point*.

Haller, Albrecht von, Swiss physiologist, 1708–1777. SEE H. *ansa, anulus, arches*, under *arch, circle, cones*, under *cone, habenula, insula, line, plexus, rete*, vascular *tissue, tripod, tunica vasculosa, unguis, vas* aberrans.

Ha

Hallermann, Wilhelm, German ophthalmologist, 1901–1976. SEE H.-Streiff *syndrome;* Hallermann-Streiff-François *syndrome.*

Hallervorden, Julius, German neurologist, 1882–1965. SEE H. *syndrome;* H.-Spatz *disease, syndrome.*

hal·lex, pl. **hal·li·ces** (hal'eks, hal'i-sēz). SYN great *toe* I. [L.]

Hallgren, Bertil, 20th century Swedish geneticist. SEE H. *syndrome.*

Hallopeau, François H., French dermatologist, 1842–1919. SEE H. *disease.*

Hallpike, C.S., 20th century British otologist. SEE Dix-H. *maneuver.*

hal·lu·cal (hal'oo-kăl). Relating to the hallux.

hal·lu·ci·na·tion (ha-loo'si-nā'shŭn). The apparent, often strong subjective perception of an object or event when no such stimulus or situation is present; may be visual, auditory, olfactory, gustatory, or tactile. [L. *alucinor,* to wander in mind]

auditory h., a symptom frequently observed in a schizophrenic disorder consisting, in the absence of an external source, of hearing a voice or other auditory stimulus that other individuals do not perceive.

command h., a symptom, usually auditory but sometimes visual, consisting of a message, from no external source, to do something.

formed visual h., h. composed of scenes, often landscapes.

gustatory h., the sensation of taste in the absence of a gustatory stimulus; may be seen in temporal lobe epilepsy.

haptic h., the sensation of touch in the absence of stimuli; may be seen in alcoholic delirium tremens.

hypnagogic h., h. occurring when going to sleep in the period between wakefulness and sleep; one of the components of narcolepsy.

hypnopompic h., vivid hallucinations that occur when wakening from sleep; occurs with narcolepsy, but grouped with hypnagogic h.

kinesthesia h., the sense of movement of one or more muscles, when no movement is taking place.

lilliputian h., h. of reduced size of objects or persons.

mood-congruent h., h. in which the content is mood appropriate.

mood-incongruent h., h. that is not consistent with external stimuli; content is not consistent with either manic or depressed mood.

olfactory h., false perception in smell.

stump h., SYN phantom limb *pain.*

tactile h., false perception of movement or sensation, as from an amputated limb, or crawling sensation on the skin.

unformed visual h., h. composed of sparks, lights, or bursting spheres of light.

hal·lu·ci·no·gen (ha-loo'si-nō-jen). A mind-altering chemical, drug, or agent, specifically a chemical whose most prominent pharmacologic action is on the central nervous system (e.g., mescaline); in normal subjects, it elicits optical or auditory hallucinations, depersonalization, perceptual disturbances, and disturbances of thought processes. SYN psychedelic drug, psychodysleptic drug, psycholytic drug, psychotomimetic drug. [L. *alucinor,* to wander in mind, + G. -*gen,* producing]

hal·lu·ci·no·gen·e·sis (ha-loo'si-nō-jen'ĕ-sis). The process of producing an hallucination.

hal·lu·ci·no·gen·ic (ha-loo'si-nō-jen'ik). SYN psychedelic.

hal·lu·ci·no·sis (ha-loo-si-nō'sis). A syndrome, usually of organic origin, characterized by more or less persistent hallucinations e.g., alcoholic h.

organic h., the state of experiencing a false sensory perception in the absence of external stimulus observed in individuals with one of the organic mental disorders (e.g., the frightening sensations experienced in alcoholic hallucinosis or by a person who has ingested LSD or another of the mind-altering drugs). SEE hallucination.

hal·lus (hal'ŭs). SYN great *toe* I.

hal·lux, pl. **hal·lu·ces** (hal'ŭks, hal'ū-sēz) [TA]. SYN great *toe* I. [a Mod. L. form for L. *hallex* (*hallic*-), great toe]

h. doloro'sus, a condition, usually associated with flatfoot, in which walking causes severe pain in the metatarsophalangeal joint of the great toe. SYN painful toe.

h. exten'sus, a deformity in which the great toe is held rigidly in the extended position.

h. flex'us, SYN h. malleus.

h. mal'leus, hammer toe involving the first toe. SYN h. flexus.

h. rig'idus, a condition in which stiffness appears in the first metatarsophalangeal joint; usually associated with the development of bone spurs on the dorsal surface. SYN stiff toe.

h. val'gus, a deviation of the tip of the great toe, or main axis of the toe, toward the outer or lateral side of the foot.

h. va'rus, deviation of the main axis of the great toe to the inner side of the foot away from the second toe.

ha·lo (hā'lō). **1.** A reddish yellow ring surrounding the optic disk, due to a widening of the scleral ring making the deeper structures visible. **2.** An annular flare of light surrounding a luminous body or a depigmented ring around a mole. SEE halo *nevus.* **3.** SYN areola (4). **4.** A circular metal band used in a h. cast or h. brace, attached to the skull with pins. [G. *halōs,* threshing floor on which oxen trod a circle; the halo round the sun or moon]

anemic h., pale, relatively avascular areas in the skin seen around vascular spiders, cherry angiomas, and sometimes in acute macular eruptions.

glaucomatous h., (1) a yellowish white ring surrounding the optic disk, indicating atrophy of the choroid in glaucoma; SYN glaucomatous ring. (2) a h. surrounding lights, caused by corneal edema in glaucoma. SYN rainbow symptom.

senile h., circumpapillary h. seen in choroidal atrophy of the aged.

hal·o·al·kyl·a·mines (hal-ō-al-kil'ă-mēnz). A class of drugs, including phenoxybenzamine and diabenamine, which binds so as to alkylate α-adrenergic receptors so that they are irreversibly inactivated.

hal·o·gen (hal'ō-jen). One of the chlorine group (fluorine, chlorine, bromine, iodine, astatine) of elements; h.'s form monobasic acids with hydrogen, and their hydroxides (fluorine forms none) are also monobasic acids. [G. *hals,* salt, + -*gen,* producing]

hal·o·gen·a·tion (hal'ō-jě-nā'shŭn). Incorporation of one or more halogen atoms into a molecule.

hal·o·gen·o·der·ma (hal-ō-gen'ō-der-mă). Dermatosis caused by ingestion or injection of halogens, most notably bromides and iodides. [halogen + G. *derma,* skin]

Hal·o·ge·ton (hal-ō-jē'ton). A genus of plants (family Chenopodiaceae) on range lands in the western U.S. and other arid regions of the world; it causes poisoning in cattle and sheep because of the presence of soluble oxalates.

ha·lom·e·ter (hal-om'ě-ter). An instrument used to measure the diffraction halo of a red blood cell; based on the premise that the halo of the large erythrocyte of pernicious anemia is smaller than that of the normal cell; the hazy colorless halo of normal size is characteristic of secondary anemia.

hal·o·phil, hal·o·phile (hal'ō-fil, -fīl). A microorganism whose growth is enhanced by or dependent on a high salt concentration. [G. *hals,* salt, + *philos,* fond]

hal·o·phil·ic (hal-ō-fil'ik). Requiring a high concentration of salt for growth.

hal·o·ste·re·sis (hă-los-tě-rē'sis). SYN halisteresis.

hal·o·thane (hal'ō-thān). A widely used potent nonflammable and nonexplosive inhalation anesthetic, with rapid onset and reversal; side effects include respiratory and cardiovascular depression, and sensitization to epinephrine-induced arrhythmias. Often used in children, as the odor is less pungent than some other anesthetic agents.

Halstead, Ward C., U.S. psychologist, 1908–1968. SEE H.-Reitan *battery.*

Halsted, William Stewart, U.S. surgeon, 1852–1922. SEE H. *law, operation, suture.*

Hal·te·rid·i·um (hawl-tě-rid'ē-ŭm). Former name for *Haemoproteus.* [G. *haltēres,* weights held in the hand in leaping]

hal·zoun (hal'zŭn). Local name of a buccopharyngeal infection occurring in Lebanon, probably caused by pentastomid larvae of the dog tongue worm, *Linguatula serrata*, which wander into the throat of the human host after ingestion of infected raw sheep, or goat liver or lymph nodes. [Ar., snail]

Ham, Thomas Hale, U.S. physician, 1905–1987. SEE H. *test.*

ham. 1. SYN popliteal *fossa.* **2.** The buttock and back part of the thigh. [A.S.]

HAMA Abbreviation for human antimouse *antibody.*

ham·a·me·lis (ham'ă-mē'lis). A shrub or small tree, *Hamamelis virginiana* (family Harmarmelidaceae), whose bark and dried leaves have been used externally as an application to contusions and other injuries, in headache, and for the cure of noninflammatory hemorrhoids; the water, popularly known as "extract of witch hazel," is made from the bark and contains 14% alcohol. SYN witch hazel. [Mod. L., fr. G. *hama- mēlis,* fr. *hama,* together with, + *mēlon,* apple]

ha·mar·tia (ham-ar'shē-ă). A localized developmental disturbance characterized by abnormal arrangement and/or combinations of the tissues normally present in the area. [G. *hamartion,* a bodily defect]

ham·ar·to·blas·to·ma (hă-mar'tō-blas-tō'mă). A malignant neoplasm of undifferentiated anaplastic cells thought to be derived from a hamartoma. [hamartoma + blastoma]

ham·ar·to·chon·dro·ma·to·sis (ham-ar'tō-kon'drō-mă-tō'sis). Neoplasm-like foci of cartilaginous tissue in sites where cartilage is a normal constituent, but in which the growth of cartilage cells is out of proportion to the other elements of the organ. [G. *hamartion,* bodily defect, + *chondros,* cartilage, + *-osis,* condition]

ham·ar·to·ma (ham-ar-tō'mă). A focal malformation that resembles a neoplasm, grossly and even microscopically, but results from faulty development in an organ; composed of an abnormal mixture of tissue elements, or an abnormal proportion of a single element, normally present in that site, which develop and grow at virtually the same rate as normal components, and are not likely to result in compression of adjacent tissue (in contrast to a neoplasm). [G. *hamartion,* a bodily defect, + *-oma,* tumor]

fibrous h. of infancy, a tumor appearing usually in the upper arm or shoulder in the first two years of life and consisting of cellular fibrous tissue infiltrating the subcutis.

pulmonary h., h. of the lung, producing a coin lesion composed primarily of cartilage and bronchial epithelium.

ham·ar·tom·a·tous (ham-ar-tō'mă-tŭs). Relating to hamartoma.

ham·ar·to·pho·bia (ham'ar-tō-fō'bē-ă). Morbid fear of error or sin. [G. *hamartia,* fault, + *phobos,* fear]

ha·mate. SEE hamate (*bone*).

ha·ma·tum (ha-mā'tŭm). SYN hamate (*bone*). [L. neut. of *hamatus,* hooked, fr. *hamus,* a hook]

Hamburger, Hartog J., Dutch physiologist, 1859–1924. SEE H. *phenomenon.*

Hamman, Louis, U.S. physician, 1877–1946. SEE H. *disease, murmur, sign, syndrome;* Hamman-Rich *syndrome.*

Hammarsten, Olof, Swedish physiological chemist, 1841–1932. SEE H. *reagent.*

ham·mer (ham'er). SYN malleus.

Hammerschlag, Albert, Austrian physician, 1863–1935. SEE H. *method.*

Hammond, William A., U.S. neurologist, 1828–1900. SEE H. *disease.*

Hampton, Aubrey Otis, U.S. radiologist, 1900–1955. SEE H. *line, maneuver, technique, hump.*

ham·ster. Any of four genera (subfamily Cricetinae, family Muridae) of small rodents widely used in research and as pets: *Cricetus, Cricetulus, Mesocricetus,* and *Phodopus.* All hamsters are seed and plant feeders, store food, hibernate in winter, and breed throughout the year under laboratory conditions.

ham·string. 1. One of the tendons bounding the popliteal space on either side; the **medial h.** comprises the tendons of the semimembranosus and semitendinosus muscles; the **lateral h.** is the tendon of the biceps femoris muscle. H. muscles (a) have origin from the ischial tuberosity, (b) act across (at) both the hip and knee joints (producing extension and flexion, respectively), and (c) are innervated by the tibial portion of the sciatic nerve. The medial h. contributes to medial rotation of the leg at the flexed knee joint, while the lateral h. contributes to lateral rotation. **2.** In domestic animals, the combined tendons of the superficial digital flexor, triceps surae, biceps femoris, and semitendinosus muscles which are referred to as the common calcanean tendon (tendo calcaneus communis); it is attached to the tuber calcis of the hock.

ham·u·lar (ham'ū-lăr). Hook-shaped; unciform. [L. *hamulus, q.v.*]

ham·u·lus, gen. and pl. **ham·u·li** (ham'ū-lŭs, -lī) [TA]. Any hooklike structure. SYN hook (2)⭐. [L. dim. of *hamus,* hook]

h. coch'leae, SYN h. of spiral lamina.

lacrimal h. [TA], the hooklike lower end of the lacrimal crest, curving between the frontal process and orbital surface of the maxilla to form the upper aperture of the bony portion of the nasolacrimal canal. SYN h. lacrimalis [TA], hamular process of lacrimal bone.

h. lacrima'lis [TA], SYN lacrimal h.

h. lam'inae spira'lis [TA], SYN h. of spiral lamina.

h. os'sis hama'ti [TA], SYN hook of hamate.

pterygoid h. [TA], the inferior, hook-shaped extremity of the medial plate of the pterygoid process, which serves as a pulley (trochlea) for the tendon of the tensor veli palati muscle. SYN hamular process of sphenoid bone, h. pterygoideus.

h. pterygoid'eus, SYN pterygoid h.

h. of spiral lamina [TA], the upper hooklike termination of the bony spiral lamina at the apex of the cochlea. SYN h. laminae spiralis [TA], h. cochleae, hook of spiral lamina.

Hancock, Henry, English surgeon, 1809–1880. SEE H. *amputation.*

Hand, Alfred, U.S. pediatrician, 1868–1949. SEE H.-Schüller-Christian *disease.*

hand [TA]. The portion of the upper limb distal to the radiocarpal joint, comprising the wrist, palm, and fingers. SYN manus [TA], main. [A.S.]

accoucheur h., position of the h. in tetany or in muscular dystrophy; the fingers are flexed at the metacarpophalangeal joints and extended at the phalangeal joints, with the thumb flexed and adducted into the palm; in resemblance to the position of the physician's hand in making a vaginal examination. SYN obstetric h.

ape h., a deformity marked by extension of the thumb in the same plane as the palm and fingers. SYN monkey h., monkey-paw.

claw h., SEE clawhand.

cleft h., a congenital deformity in which the division between the fingers, especially between the third and fourth, extends into the metacarpal region. SEE ALSO lobster-claw *deformity.* SYN split h.

club h., congenital or acquired angulation deformity of h. associated with partial or complete absence of radius or ulna; usually with intrinsic deformities of the h. in congenital variants.

crab h., SYN erysipeloid.

dorsum of h. [TA], the back of the hand. SYN dorsum manus [TA].

drop h., SYN wrist-drop.

ghoul h., a condition seen in African blacks, probably a manifestation of tertiary yaws, marked by depigmentation of the palms and contraction of the skin which give a clawlike and corpselike appearance to the h.'s.

Marinesco succulent h., edema of the h. with coldness and lividity of the skin, observed in syringomyelia. SYN main succulente.

monkey h., SYN ape h.

obstetric h., SYN accoucheur h.

opera-glass h., a deformity of the h. seen in chronic absorptive arthritis, the fingers and wrists being shortened and the covering skin wrinkled into transverse folds; the phalanges appear to be retracted into one another like an opera glass or miniature telescope.

simian h., deformity in which there is flattening of the thenar eminence, and the thumb lies adducted and extended; usually due to a median nerve lesion.

skeleton h., extension of fingers with atrophy of tissues; occurs in progressive muscular atrophy.

ha

spade h., the coarse, thick, square h. of acromegaly or myxedema.

split h., SYN cleft h.

trident h., a h. in which the fingers are of nearly equal length and deflected at the first interphalangeal joint, so as to give a forklike shape; seen in achondroplasia.

writing h., a contraction of the h. muscles in parkinsonism, bringing the fingers somewhat into the position of holding a pen.

hand·ed·ness (hand′ed-nes). Preference for the use of one hand, most commonly the right, associated with dominance of the opposite cerebral hemisphere; may also be the result of training or habit.

hand·i·cap (hand′i-kap). **1.** A physical, mental, or emotional condition that interferes with an individual's normal functioning. **2.** Reduction in a person's capacity to fulfill a social role as a consequence of an impairment, inadequate training for the role, or other circumstances. SEE ALSO disability. [fr. *hand in cap,* (game)]

hand·piece (hand′pēs). A powered dental instrument held in the hand, used to hold rotary cutting, grinding, or polishing implements while they are being revolved.

hand·shapes (hand′shāps). Manual symbols of speech sounds used in cued speech.

HANE Acronym for hereditary angioneurotic *edema.*

hang·nail (hang′nāl). A loose triangular tag of skin attached proximally in the medial or lateral nail fold.

Hanhart, Ernst, Swiss internist, 1891–1973. SEE H. *syndrome.*

Hanks, Horace Tracy, U.S. surgeon, 1837–1900. SEE H. *dilators.*

Hanks so·lu·tion. See under solution.

Hanlon, C. Rollins, U.S. cardiovascular and thoracic surgeon, *1915. SEE Blalock-H. *operation.*

Hannover, Adolph, Danish anatomist, 1814–1894. SEE H. *canal.*

Hanot, Victor C., French physician, 1844–1896. SEE H. *cirrhosis.*

Hansen, Gerhard A., Norwegian physician, 1841–1912. SEE H. *bacillus, disease.*

Han·ta·vi·rus (han′tā-vā-rŭs). A genus of Bunyaviridae responsible for pneumonia and hemorrhagic fevers. At least 7 members of the genus are thus far recognized: Hantaan, Puumala, Seoul, Prospect Hill, Thailand, Thottapalayam, and Sin Nombre virus. A number of other species have not been classified as yet. Hantaan virus causes Korean hemorrhagic fever. Various rodent species are the asymptomatic carriers of these viruses, which are shed in saliva, urine, and feces. Human infection is direct, or by the respiratory route from contaminated specimens; person-to-person spread is thought to be rare. An outbreak of hantavirus infection, the Hantavirus Pulmonary Syndrome (HPS), causing severe and often fatal pulmonary symptoms was identified in the Four-Corners region of the western U.S. in 1993 and the agent was subsequently named Sin Nombre virus.

hap·a·lo·nych·ia (hap′ă-lō-nik′ē-ă). Thinning of nails resulting in bending and breaking of the free edge, with longitudinal fissures. SYN egg shell nail. [G. *hapalos,* soft + G. *onyx (onych-),* nail]

haph·al·ge·sia (haf-al-jē′zē-ă). Pain or an extremely disagreeable sensation caused by the merest touch. SYN Pitres sign (1). [G. *haphē,* touch, + *algēsis,* sense of pain]

hap·haz·ard. Lacking any coherent system, organization, or objective; not to be confused with random or chaotic.

haph·e·pho·bia (haf-ē-fō′bē-ă). A morbid dislike or fear of being touched. [G. *haphē,* touch, + *phobos,* fear]

△**haplo-.** Simple, single. [G. *haplous*]

hap·lo·dont (hap′lō-dont). Having molar teeth with simple crowns, i.e., simple conical teeth without ridges or tubercles. [haplo- + G. *odous,* tooth]

hap·loid (hap′loyd). Denoting the number of chromosomes in sperm or ova, which is half the number in somatic (diploid) cells; the h. number in normal human beings is 23. SYN monoploid. [G. *haplos,* simple, + *eidos,* appearance]

hap·lol·o·gy (hap-lol′ō-jē). The omission of syllables because of excessive speed of utterance. [haplo- + G. *logos,* study]

hap·lo·pro·tein (hap-lō-prō′tēn). The functional complex between an apoprotein and the prosthetic group that together are responsible for biologic activity.

hap·lo·scope (hap′lō-skōp). An instrument for presenting separate views to each eye so that they may be seen as one. [haplo- + G. *skopeō,* to view]

mirror h., a h. using mirrors to displace the field of view of the two eyes, as in Worth amblyoscope and the synoptophore.

hap·lo·scop·ic (hap-lō-skop′ik). Relating to a haploscope.

Hap·lo·spo·rid·ia (hap′lō-spō-rid′ē-ă). An order of sporozoans, now placed in the protozoan phylum Ascetospora, class Stellatosporea, that reproduce asexually by schizogony and produce spores but no flagella, though pseudopodia may be present. [haplo- + G. *sporos,* seed]

hap·lo·type (hap′lō-tīp). **1.** The genetic constitution of an individual with respect to one member of a pair of allelic genes; individuals are of the same h. (but of different genotypes) if alike with respect to one allele of a pair but different with respect to the other allele of a pair. **2.** In immunogenetics, that portion of the phenotype determined by a set of closely linked genes inherited from one parent (i.e., genes located on one of the pair of chromosomes). [haplo- + G. *typos,* impression, model]

hap·ten (hap′-ten). A molecule that is incapable, alone, of causing the production of antibodies but can, however, combine with a larger antigenic molecule called a carrier. A h.-carrier complex can stimulate production of antibodies, some of which combine with the h. portion of the complex. SEE ALSO hapten *inhibition* of precipitation. SYN incomplete antigen, partial antigen. [G. *haptō,* to fasten, bind]

conjugated h., a h. that may cause the production of antibodies when it has been covalently linked to protein. SYN conjugated antigen.

Forssman h., a glycolipid from mammalian organs; it is a ceramide pentasaccharide. Cf. Forssman *antibody,* Forssman *antigen.*

half h., SEE half-hapten.

hap·to·dys·pho·ria (hap′tō-dis-fō′rē-ă). An unpleasant sensation derived from touching certain objects. [G. *haptō,* to touch, + dysphoria]

hap·to·glo·bin (HP) (hap-tō-glō′bin) [MIM*140100 & MIM* 140210]. A group of α_2-globulins in human serum, so called because of their ability to combine with hemoglobin, preventing loss in the urine; variant types form a polymorphic system, with α- and β-polypeptide chains controlled by separate genetic loci. Levels are decreased in hemolytic disorders and increased in inflammatory conditions or with tissue damage. [G. *haptō,* to grasp, + hemoglobin]

hap·tom·e·ter (hap-tom′ĕ-ter). Instrument for measuring sensitivity to touch. [G. *haptō,* to touch, + *metron,* measure]

Har Abbreviation for homoarginine.

Harada, Einosuke, Japanese surgeon, 1892–1947. SEE H. *disease, syndrome;* Harada-Ito *procedure.*

Harada, T., 20th century Japanese pathologist. SEE H.-Mori filter paper strip *culture.*

Harden, Sir Arthur, English biochemist and Nobel laureate, 1865–1940. SEE H.-Young *ester.*

hardening (har′den-ing). **1.** A condition of lessened reactions to allergens from repeated or prolonged nontherapeutic exposure, similar to hyposensitization. **2.** Any procedure in tissue preparation for examinations, such as sectioning for microscopy, that renders the tissue firmer.

har·di·ness (har′di-nes). A health-enhancing behavior trait believed to increase one's resistance to illness, characterized by a high level of personal control, commitment, and action in responding to events of daily life. [M.E., fr. O.Fr. *hardi,* fr. Germanic]

Harding, Harold E., 20th century British pathologist. SEE H.-Passey *melanoma.*

hard·ness (hard′nes). **1.** The degree of firmness of a solid, as determined by its resistance to deformation, scratching, or abrasion. SEE ALSO hardness *scale,* number. **2.** The relative penetrating power of a beam of x-rays, used both within the diagnostic range of energy and in radiation therapy; expressed in terms of half-value layer.

indentation h., a number related to the size of the impression made by an indenter (or tool) of specific size and shape under a known load.

hard·ware. The electronic component of a computer.

Hardy, George H., English mathematician, 1877–1947. SEE H.-Weinberg *equilibrium, law.*

Hardy, LeGrand H., U.S. ophthalmologist, 1894–1954. SEE H.-Rand-Ritter *test.*

hare·lip (hār′lip). SYN cleft *lip.*

har·ma·line (har′mă-līn). An amine oxidase inhibitor and a central nervous system stimulant; obtained from the seeds of *Peganum harmala* (family Zygophyllaceae) and from *Banisteria caapi* (family Malpighiaceae); has been used in parkinsonism. SYN harmidine.

har·mi·dine (har′mi-dēn). SYN harmaline.

har·mine (har′mēn). A central nervous system stimulant and potent monoamine oxidase inhibitor obtained from *Peganum harmala* (family Zygophyllaceae) and *Banisteria caapi* (family Malpighiaceae); psychic effects resemble those of LSD, but sedative and depressive qualities may predominate over hallucinatory manifestations. SYN banisterine, leucoharmine, telepathine. [G. *harmala,* harmal, fr. Ar. *harmalah,* + -ine]

har·mo·nia (har-mō′nē-ă). SYN plane *suture.* [L. and G. a joining]

har·mon·ic (har-mon′ik). A component of complex sound, the frequency of which is a multiple of the fundamental frequency. The fundamental frequency is called the first harmonic; the second harmonic has twice the frequency of the fundamental, and so forth.

har·mo·ny (har′mō-nē). Denoting, in a complex sound, a mathematical relationship among the frequencies of the fundamental tone and its overtones so that the frequencies of the overtones are whole number multiples or partials of the frequency of the fundamental tone; the resulting auditory effect has a musical or pleasant quality, as opposed to noise. [G., L. *harmonia,* agreement, articulation, fr. *harmos,* joint]

functional occlusal h., such occlusal relationship of opposing teeth in all functional ranges and movements as will provide the greatest masticatory efficiency without causing undue strain or trauma upon the supporting tissues, teeth, and muscles.

occlusal h., occlusion without deflective or interceptive occlusal contacts in centric jaw relation as well as eccentric movements.

har·pax·o·pho·bia (har′paks-ō-fō′bē-ă). Morbid fear of robbers. [G. *harpax,* robber, + *phobos,* fear]

har·poon (har-poon′). A small, sharp-pointed instrument with a barbed head used for extracting bits of tissue for microscopic examination.

Harrington, David O., U.S. ophthalmologist, *1904. SEE H.-Flocks *test.*

Harris, Henry A., English anatomist, 1886–1968. SEE H. *lines,* under *line.*

Harris, Henry F., U.S. physician, 1867–1926. SEE H. *hematoxylin.*

Harris, R.I., 20th century Canadian orthopedist. SEE Salter-H. *classification* of epiphysial plate injuries.

Harris, Seale, U.S. physician, 1870–1957, investigated food conditions and nutritional diseases. SEE Harris *syndrome.*

Harris, Wilfred, English neurologist, 1869–1960. SEE H. *migraine.*

Harrison, Edward, English physician, 1766–1838. SEE H. *groove.*

Harris and Ray test. See under test.

Hartel, Fritz, German surgeon. SEE H. *technique.*

Hartman, LeRoy L., U.S. dentist, 1893–1951. SEE H. *solution.*

Hartmann, Alexis F., U.S. pediatrician, 1898–1964. SEE H. *solution;* Shaffer-H. *method.*

Hartmann, Arthur, German laryngologist, 1849–1931. SEE H. *curette.*

Hartmann, Henri A.C.A., French surgeon, 1860–1952. SEE H. *operation, pouch.*

Hart·man·nel·la (hart-mă-nel′ă). A common free-living ameba found in soil, sewage, and water, known to invade invertebrates (snails, grasshoppers, oysters); suspected but not established as an agent of human primary amebic meningoencephalitis.

Hartnup. Surname of British family in which the disease was first described. SEE Hartnup *disease,* Hartnup *syndrome.*

harts·horn (harts′hōrn). A mixture of ammonium bicarbonate and ammonium carbamate obtained from ammonium sulfate and calcium carbonate by sublimation; used as an expectorant and in smelling salts; so called because originally obtained from deer antlers.

har·vest bug. The larva of *Trombicula* species.

Harvey, William, 1578–1657. English anatomist, physiologist, and physician who first described the circulation of the blood in 1628. He understood that the interventricular septum is not porous so blood cannot pass through it. He demonstrated the volume of blood that passes unidirectionally through a segment of a peripheral vein exceeds the volume of blood within the body, so blood must recirculate. He described the organization of the fetal circulation and the transition to the postnatal organization.

has·a·mi·ya·mi (has′ă-mē-yah′mē). A fever occurring in Japan in the autumn; resembles Weil disease, but is milder and is caused by the *autumnalis* serovar of *Leptospira interrogans.* SYN akiyami, autumn fever (2), sakushu fever, seven-day fever (2).

Häser, Heinrich, German physician, 1811–1884. SEE H. *formula;* Trapp-H. *formula.*

Hashimoto, Japanese surgeon, 1881–1934. SEE H. *disease,* struma, *thyroiditis.*

hash·ish (hash′ish). A form of cannabis that consists largely of resin from the flowering tops and sprouts of cultivated female plants; contains the highest concentration of cannabinols among the preparations derived from cannabis. [Ar. hay]

Hasner, Joseph Ritter von, Czechoslovakian ophthalmologist, 1819–1892. SEE H. *fold.*

Hassall, Arthur, British physician, 1817–1894. SEE H. *bodies,* under *body,* concentric *corpuscle,* under *corpuscle;* H.-Henle *bodies,* under *body;* Virchow-H. *bodies,* under *body.*

Hasselbalch, Karl, Danish biochemist and physician, 1874–1962. SEE Henderson-H. *equation.*

hatch·et. A dental instrument with an end cutting blade set at an angle to the axis of the handle and having one or two bevels; in the former case, made as right and left pairs called enamel h.'s; used for removing enamel and dentin on teeth.

Haubenfelder (how′ben-fel′der). SEE *fields* of Forel, under *field.* [Ger.]

Hauch (H) (howkh). A term used to designate the flagellar antigen of bacteria. SEE ALSO H *antigen.* [Ger. breath]

Haudek, Martin, Austrian roentgenologist, 1880–1931. SEE H. *niche.*

Hauser, G.A., 20th century German gynecologist. SEE Mayer-Rokitansky-Küster-H. *syndrome;* Rokitansky-Küster-H. *syndrome.*

haus·to·ri·um, pl. **haus·to·ria** (haw-stō′rē-ŭm, -stō′rē-ă). An organ for the absorption of nutriment. [Mod. L. fr. L. *haustus,* a drinking]

haus·tra (haw′stră). Plural of haustrum. [L.]

haus·tral (hos′trăl). Relating to a haustrum.

haus·tra·tion (hos′trā′shŭn). 1. The process of formation of a haustrum. 2. An increase in prominence of the haustra.
h.'s of colon, SYN *haustra* of colon, under *haustrum.*

haus·trum, pl. **haus·tra** (hos′trŭm, haw′stră) [TA]. One of a series of saccules or pouches, so called because of a fancied resemblance to the buckets on a water wheel. [L. a machine for drawing water, fr. *haurio,* pp. *haustus,* to draw up, drink up]
haus′tra co′li [TA], SYN haustra of colon.
haustra of colon [TA], the sacculations of the colon, caused by the teniae, or longitudinal bands, which are slightly shorter than the gut so that the latter is thrown into tucks or pouches. SYN

ha

haustra coli [TA], cellulae coli, haustrations of colon, sacculation of colon.

haus·tus (haws'tŭs). A potion or medicinal draft. [L. a drink, draft]

HAV Abbreviation for hepatitis A *virus*.

Ha·ver·hil·lia mul·ti·for·mis (ha-ver-hil'ē-ă mŭl-ti-fōr'mis). SEE *Streptobacillus moniliformis.*

Havers, Clopton, British anatomist, 1650–1702. SEE haversian *canals,* under *canal;* haversian *lamella;* haversian *spaces,* under *space;* haversian *system.*

ha·ver·si·an (ha-ver'shan). Relating to Clopton Havers and the various osseous structures described by him.

Hawley, C.A., U.S. orthodontist. SEE H. *appliance, retainer.*

Haworth, Sir Walter Norman, British chemist and Nobel laureate, 1883–1950. SEE H. conformational formulas of cyclic *sugars,* perspective formulas of cyclic *sugars.*

Hayem, Georges, French physician, 1841–1933. SEE H. *hematoblast, solution;* H.-Widal *syndrome.*

Hayflick, Leonard, U.S. microbiologist, *1928. SEE H. *limit.*

Haygarth, John, English physician, 1740–1827. SEE H. *nodes,* under *node.*

ha·zel·wort (hā'zel-wōrt). SYN *Asarum* europaeum.

Hb Abbreviation for hemoglobin.

HbChesapeake Abbreviation for *hemoglobin* Chesapeake.

HB_eAb Abbreviation for antibody to the hepatitis B e *antigen*.

HB_cAb Abbreviation for antibody to the hepatitis B core *antigen*.

HB_sAb Abbreviation for antibody to the hepatitis B surface *antigen*.

HB_cAg Abbreviation for hepatitis B core *antigen*.

HB_sAg Abbreviation for hepatitis B surface *antigen*.

HbCO Abbreviation for carboxyhemoglobin.

HBE Abbreviation for His bundle *electrogram*.

HBe, HB_eAg Abbreviation for hepatitis B e *antigen*.

HbO₂ Abbreviation for oxyhemoglobin.

Hb S Abbreviation for sickle cell *hemoglobin*.

HBV Abbreviation for hepatitis B *virus*.

HCC Abbreviation for 25-hydroxycholecalciferol.

HCFA Abbreviation for Health Care Financing Administration.

HCG, hCG Abbreviation for human chorionic *gonadotropin*.

β-HCG. SYN chorionic *gonadotropin.*

H chain. SYN heavy *chain.*

HCS Abbreviation for human chorionic somatomammotropic *hormone*; human chorionic *somatomammotropin*.

Hct Abbreviation for hematocrit.

HCV Abbreviation for hepatitis C *virus*.

Hcy Abbreviation for homocysteine.

HD Abbreviation for mustard *gas*.

h.d. Abbreviation for L. *hora decubitus,* at bedtime.

HDCV Abbreviation for human diploid cell *vaccine*; human diploid cell rabies *vaccine*.

HDL Abbreviation for high density lipoprotein. SEE lipoprotein.

HDV Abbreviation for hepatitis delta *virus*.

He Symbol for helium.

³He, ⁴He Symbols for helium-3 and helium-4, respectively.

Head, Sir Henry, English neurologist, 1861–1940. SEE H. *areas,* under *area, lines,* under *line, zones,* under *zone.*

■**head** (hed) [TA]. **1** [TA]. The upper or anterior extremity of the animal body, containing the brain and the organs of sight, hearing, taste, and smell. **2** [TA]. The upper, anterior, or larger extremity, expanded or rounded, of any body, organ, or other anatomic structure. **3.** The rounded extremity of a bone. **4.** That end of a muscle that is attached to the less movable part of the skeleton. SYN caput [TA]. [A.S. *heáfod*]

bulldog h., the broad h. with high vault occurring in achondroplasia.

h. of caudate nucleus [TA], the head or anterior extremity of the caudate nucleus projecting into the anterior horn of the lateral ventricle. SYN caput nuclei caudati [TA], anterior extremity of caudate nucleus.

clavicular h. of pectoralis major muscle [TA], SEE pectoralis major (*muscle*). SYN pars clavicularis musculi pectoralis majoris [TA], clavicular part of pectoralis major (muscle).

deep h. of flexor pollicis brevis [TA], the head of short flexor of the thumb that arises from the trapezoid and capitate bones and transverse carpal ligaments. It is innervated by the deep ulnar nerve, and considered by many to be the first palmar interosseous muscle. SYN caput profundum musculi flexoris pollicis brevis [TA].

h. of epididymis [TA], the upper and larger extremity of the epididymis. SYN caput epididymidis [TA], caput epididymis, globus major.

h. of femur [TA], the hemispheric articular surface at the upper extremity of the thigh bone. SYN caput femoris [TA], caput ossis femoris, h. of thigh bone.

h. of fibula [TA], the superior extremity of the fibula, which articulates by a facet with the undersurface of the lateral condyle of the tibia. SYN caput fibulae [TA], upper extremity of fibula.

hourglass h., in congenital syphilis, a skull with depressed coronal suture.

humeral h. [TA], the name applied to the heads of forearm muscles that attach to the humerus. Terminologia Anatomica lists humeral heads (caput humerale ...) of the following: 1) flexor carpli ulnaris (... musculi flexoris carpi ulnaris [TA]); 2) pronator teres (... musculi pronatoris teretis [TA]); and 3) extensor carpi ulnaris (...musculi extensoris carpi ulnaris [TA]). SYN caput humerale [TA].

humeroulnar h. of flexor digitorum superficialis muscle [TA], the head of the superficial flexor of the digits that attaches to both the humerus and the ulna. SYN caput humeroulnare musculi flexoris digitorum superificialis [TA].

h. of humerus [TA], the upper rounded extremity fitting into the glenoid cavity of the scapula. SYN caput humeri [TA].

lateral h. [TA], h. of origin farthest from the midline. Terminologia Anatomica lists lateral h.'s (caput laterale ...) of the following: 1) triceps brachii (... musculi tricipitis brachii [TA]); 2) gastrocnemius (... musculi gastrocnemii [TA]); and 3) flexor hallucis brevis (...musculi flexoris hallucis brevis [TA]). SYN caput laterale [TA].

little h. of humerus, SYN *capitulum* of humerus.

long h. [TA], the head that has the more proximal origin. Terminologia Anatomica lists long h.'s (caput longum ...) of the following: 1) biceps brachii (... musculi bicipitis brachii [TA]); 2) biceps femoris (... musculi bicipitis femoris [TA]); and 3) triceps brachii (... musculi tricipitis brachii [TA]). SYN caput longum [TA].

h. of malleus [TA], the rounded portion of the malleus articulating with the body of the incus. SYN caput mallei [TA].

h. of mandible [TA], the expanded articular portion of the condylar process of the mandible. SYN caput mandibulae [TA].

medial h. [TA], the h. of origin closest to the midline. Terminologia Anatomica lists medial h. (caput mediale) of the following: 1) triceps brachii (... musculi tricipitis brachii [TA]); 2) gastrocnemius (... musculi gastrocnemii [TA]); and 3) flexor hallucis brevis (... musculi flexoris hallucis brevis [TA]). SYN caput mediale [TA].

Medusa h., SYN *caput* medusae.

h. of metacarpal [TA], the expanded distal end of a metacarpal that articulates with the proximal phalanx of the same digit. SYN caput ossis metacarpalis [TA].

h. of metatarsal [TA], the expanded distal end of a metatarsal bone that articulates with the proximal phalanx of the same digit. SYN caput ossis metatarsalis [TA].

oblique h. [TA], h. of origin which is diagonally situated. Terminologia Anatomica lists oblique h.'s (caput obliquum ...) of the following: 1) adductor hallucis (... musculi adductoris hallucis [TA]); and 2) adductor pollicis (... musculi adductoris pollicis [TA]). SYN caput obliquum [TA].

optic nerve h., SYN optic *disk.*

h. of pancreas [TA], that portion of the pancreas lying in the concavity of the duodenum. SYN caput pancreatis [TA].

h. of phalanx (of hand or foot) [TA], the rounded articular surface at the distal end of the proximal and middle phalanx of each finger and toe. SYN caput phalangis (manus et pedis) [TA].

h. of radius [TA], the disk-shaped upper extremity articulating with the capitulum of the humerus. SYN caput radii [TA].

h. of rib [TA], the rounded medial extremity of a rib that, except for ribs 1, 10, 11, and 12, articulates by two facets with the bodies of two contiguous vertebrae. SYN caput costae [TA].

saddle h., SYN clinocephaly.

short h. [TA], for a muscle with two heads of origin (a "biceps" muscle), the head originating nearest the insertion. SEE short h. of biceps brachii, short h. of biceps femoris. SYN caput breve [TA].

short h. of biceps brachii [TA], h. of biceps brachii originating from coracoid process of scapula. SYN caput breve musculi bicipitis brachii [TA].

short h. of biceps femoris [TA], part of biceps femoris originating from linea aspera of distal half of femur. SYN caput breve musculi bicipitis femoris [TA].

h. of stapes [TA], the portion of the stapes that articulates with the lenticular process of the incus. SYN caput stapedis [TA].

sternocostal h. of pectoralis major (muscle) [TA], portion of pectoralis major (muscle) originating from the sternum and ribs; acting alone the ternocostal part extends the arm at the shoulder joint; acting with the clavicular head it adducts the arm. SEE pectoralis major (*muscle*). SYN pars sternocostalis musculi pectoralis majoris [TA], sternocostal part of pectoralis major muscle.

superficial h. of flexor pollicis brevis [TA], the head of the short flexor of the thumb that arises from the transverse carpal ligament (flexor retinaculum) and the trapezium. It is innervated by the recurrent branch of the median nerve. SYN caput superficiale musculi flexoris pollicis brevis [TA].

h. of talus [TA], the rounded anterior portion of the talus articulating with the navicular bone. SYN caput tali [TA].

h. of thigh bone, SYN h. of femur.

transverse h. [TA], h. of origin of a muscle that is transversely situated. Terminologia Anatomica lists transverse h.'s (caput transversum ...) of the following: 1) adductor hallucis (... musculi adductoris hallucis [TA]); and 2) adductor pollicis (... musculi adductoris pollicis [TA]). SYN caput transversum [TA].

h. of ulna [TA], the small rounded distal extremity of the ulna articulating with the ulnar notch of the radius and the articular disk. SYN caput ulnae [TA].

ulnar h. [TA], the name applied to a h. of origin of a forearm muscle arising from the ulna. Terminologia Antomica lists ulnar h.'s (caput ulnare ...) of the following: 1) flexor carpi ulnaris (... musculi flexoris carpi ulnaris [TA]); 2) pronator teres (... musculi pronatoris teritis [TA]); and 3) extensor carpi ulnaris (... musculi extensoris carpi ulnaris [TA]). SYN caput ulnare [TA].

head·ache (hed'āk). Pain in various parts of the head, not confined to the area of distribution of any nerve. SEE ALSO cephalodynia. SYN cephalalgia, encephalalgia, encephalodynia.

benign exertional h., h. occurring with exertion or straining in the absence of any intracranial disease.

bilious h., SYN migraine.

blind h., SYN migraine.

cluster h., possibly due to a hypersensitivity to histamine; characterized by recurrent, severe, unilateral orbitotemporal h.'s associated with ipsilateral photophobia, lacrimation, and nasal congestion. SYN histaminic cephalalgia, histaminic h., Horton cephalalgia, Horton h.

coital h., a form of benign exertional h. occurring during sexual activity. SYN benign coital cephalalgia.

fibrositic h., h. centered in the occipital region due to fibrositis of the occipital muscles; tender areas are present and, commonly, tender nodules are found in the scalp in the lower occipital region.

histaminic h., SYN cluster h.

Horton h., SYN cluster h.

ice pick h., SYN idiopathic stabbing h.

idiopathic stabbing h., brief repetitive sharp pains in the temporal-parietal area of the head. SYN ice pick h.

migraine h., SEE migraine.

muscle contraction h., SYN tension h.

nodular h., radiating pain in the head accompanied by nodular swellings in the splenius, frontalis, trapezius, and other muscles.

organic h., h. due to intracranial disease.

posttraumatic h., h. following trauma to the head or neck.

reflex h., SYN symptomatic h.

sick h., SYN migraine.

spinal h., h., usually frontal or occipital, that follows lumbar puncture; precipitated by patient's sitting or standing, and relieved by lying down; due to leakage of cerebrospinal (CSF) fluid through the puncture site, with resulting reduction in CSF pressure and traction on the dural and cerebral vessels. SYN post–lumbar puncture syndrome.

symptomatic h., a h. secondary to another organic condition. SYN reflex h.

tension h., h. associated with nervous tension, anxiety, etc., often related to chronic contraction of the scalp muscles. SEE ALSO posttraumatic neck *syndrome*. SYN muscle contraction h., tension-type h.

tension-type h., SYN tension h.

thunderclap h., sudden severe nonlocalizing head pain not associated with any abnormal neurological findings; of varied etiology, including subarachnoid hemorrhage, migraine, carotid or vertebral artery dissection, cavernous sinus thrombosis, and idiopathic.

vacuum h., h. due to closure of the frontal sinus.

vascular h., SYN migraine.

head·gear (hed'gēr). A removable extraoral appliance used as a source of traction to apply force to the teeth and jaws.

head·gut (hed'gŭt). SYN foregut.

head·nod·ding (hed'nod-ing). Head movements associated with congenital nystagmus, spasmus nutans, and miner's nystagmus. SYN head tremors.

head·tilt (hed'tilt). An abnormal position of the head adopted to prevent double vision resulting from underaction of the vertical ocular muscles.

heal (hēl). **1.** To restore to health, especially to cause an ulcer or wound to cicatrize or unite. **2.** To become well, to be cured; to cicatrize or close, said of an ulcer or wound. [A.S. *healan*]

heal·er (hē'ler). **1.** A physician; one who heals or cures. **2.** One who claims to cure by prayer, mysticism, new thought, or other form of suggestion.

heal·ing (hēl'ing). **1.** Restoring to health; promoting the closure of wounds and ulcers. **2.** The process of a return to health. **3.** Closing of a wound. SEE ALSO union.

faith h., a treatment utilized since antiquity based upon prayer and a profound belief in divine intervention in human affairs.

h. by first intention, h. by fibrous adhesion, without suppuration or granulation tissue formation. SYN primary adhesion, primary union.

h. by second intention, delayed closure of two granulating surfaces. SYN secondary adhesion, secondary union.

h. by third intention, the slow filling of a wound cavity or ulcer by granulations, with subsequent cicatrization.

health (helth). **1.** The state of the organism when it functions optimally without evidence of disease or abnormality. **2.** A state of dynamic balance in which an individual's or a group's capacity to cope with all the circumstances of living is at an optimum level. **3.** A state characterized by anatomic, physiologic, and psychologic integrity, ability to perform personally valued family, work, and community roles; ability to deal with physical, biologic, psychologic, and social stress; a feeling of well-being; and freedom from the risk of disease and untimely death. [A.S. *haelth*]

behavioral h., an interdisciplinary field dedicated to promoting a philosophy of h. that stresses individual responsibility in the application of behavioral and biomedical science knowledge and techniques to the maintenance of h. and prevention of illness and dysfunction by a variety of self-initiated individual and shared activities.

h. education, process by which individuals and groups learn to

he

behave in a manner conducive to promotion, maintenance, or restoration of health.

mental h., emotional, behavioral, and social maturity or normality; the absence of a mental or behavioral disorder; a state of psychological well-being in which one has achieved a satisfactory integration of one's instinctual drives acceptable to both oneself and one's social milieu; an appropriate balance of love, work, and leisure pursuits.

public h., the art and science of community health, concerned with statistics, epidemiology, hygiene, and the prevention and eradication of epidemic diseases; an effort organized by society to promote, protect, and restore the people's health; public h. is a social institution, a service, and a practice.

Health Care Fi·nanc·ing Ad·min·is·tra·tion (HCFA). The federal agency that determines reimbursement for federal programs.

health cen·ter. An institution or group of institutions providing all types of medical care and preventive services to a population.

Health Resources and Services Administration (HRSA). A federal agency responsible for managing national data banks, such as the National Practitioner Data Bank, as well as other health care programs.

healthy (helth′ē). Well; in a state of normal functioning; free from disease.

Heaney, Noble Sproat, U.S. gynecological surgeon and obstetrician, 1880–1955. SEE H. *operation*.

hear (hēr). To perceive sounds; denoting the function of the ear. [A.S. *hēran*]

hear·ing (hēr′ing). The ability to perceive sound; the sensation of sound as opposed to vibration. SYN audition.

color h., a subjective perception of color produced by certain sounds. SEE ALSO pseudochromesthesia. SYN chromatic audition.

normal h., SYN acusis.

hear·ing aid (hēr′ing ād). An electronic amplifying device designed to bring sound into the ear; it consists of a microphone, amplifier, and receiver. SYN hearing instrument.

behind-the-ear h. a., h. a. that rests on the medial aspect of the pinna.

completely in the canal h. a. (CIC), a h. a. that fits entirely in the external auditory canal and is not visible at the surface of the body.

digital h. a., programmable h. a. that can be customized to the extent of the user's hearing loss.

in-the-canal h. a., h. a. that is placed in the external auditory canal but is still visible.

in-the-ear h. a., h. a. that fits into the shell of the ear.

HEARING IMPAIRMENT

◾**hear·ing im·pair·ment, hear·ing loss.** A reduction in the ability to perceive sound; may range from slight inability to complete deafness. SEE ALSO deafness, threshold *shift*.

acoustic trauma hearing loss, sensory hearing loss due to exposure to high-intensity noise.

Alexander h. i. [MIM*203500], high frequency h. i. due to membranous cochlear dysplasia.

boilermaker's hearing loss, SYN noise-induced h. i.

conductive h. i., a form of h. i. due to a lesion in the external auditory canal or middle ear.

functional h. i., SYN psychogenic h. i.

hereditary h. i., h. i. occurring in syndromic forms (in which there are other anomalies in addition to the hearing impairment) and nonsyndromic forms (in which hearing impairment is the only unusual finding) with autosomal dominant and recessive, X-linked, and mitochondrial modes of transmission; may be congenital, of early onset in childhood, or late onset in mid-life and advanced age.

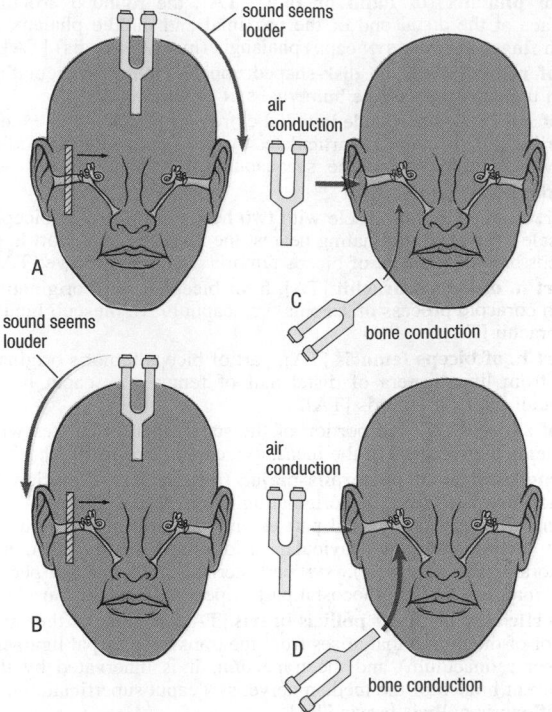

hearing loss: (A) sensorineural hearing loss demonstrated by the Weber test; (B) conductive hearing loss demonstrated by Weber test; (C) Rinne test: with normal hearing or sensorineural hearing loss, sound seems louder by air conduction than by bone conduction; (D) Rinne test: with conductive hearing loss, sound seems louder by bone conduction

high-frequency h. i., selective loss of hearing for high frequencies, usually associated with sensory damage; common in acoustic trauma and noise-induced hearing loss.

hysterical h. i., SYN psychogenic h. i.

industrial hearing loss, SYN noise-induced h. i.

low-tone hearing loss, inability to hear low notes or frequencies.

mixed h. i., combination of conductive and sensorineural hearing loss.

Mondini h. i., the hearing impairment resulting from the structural aberration of Mondini dysplasia.

neural h. i., form of sensorineural hearing loss due to a lesion in the auditory division of the 8th cranial nerve.

noise-induced h. i., sensory hearing loss due to exposure to intense impulse or continuous sound. SYN boilermaker's hearing loss, industrial hearing loss, occupational hearing loss.

occupational hearing loss, SYN noise-induced h. i.

organic h. i., h. i. due to a pathologic process or an organic cause, as opposed to psychogenic h. i.

perceptive h. i., former term for sensorineural h. i.

psychogenic h. i., h. i. without evidence of organic cause; often follows severe psychic shock. SYN functional h. i., hysterical h. i.

retrocochlear h. i., term for sensorineural h. i.; suggesting a lesion proximal to the cochlea.

Scheibe h. i., h. i. due to cochleosaccular dysplasia; usually autosomal recessive inheritance.

sensorineural h. i., a form of hearing loss due to a lesion of the auditory division of the 8th cranial nerve or the inner ear.

sensory h. i., form of sensorineural h. i. caused by a lesion in the inner ear.

◾**heart** (hart) [TA]. A hollow muscular organ that receives the blood from the veins and propels it into the arteries. In mammals it is divided by a musculomembranous septum into two halves—right or venous and left or arterial—each of which consists of a receiving chamber (atrium) and an ejecting chamber (ventricle). SYN cor [TA], coeur. [A.S. *heorte*]

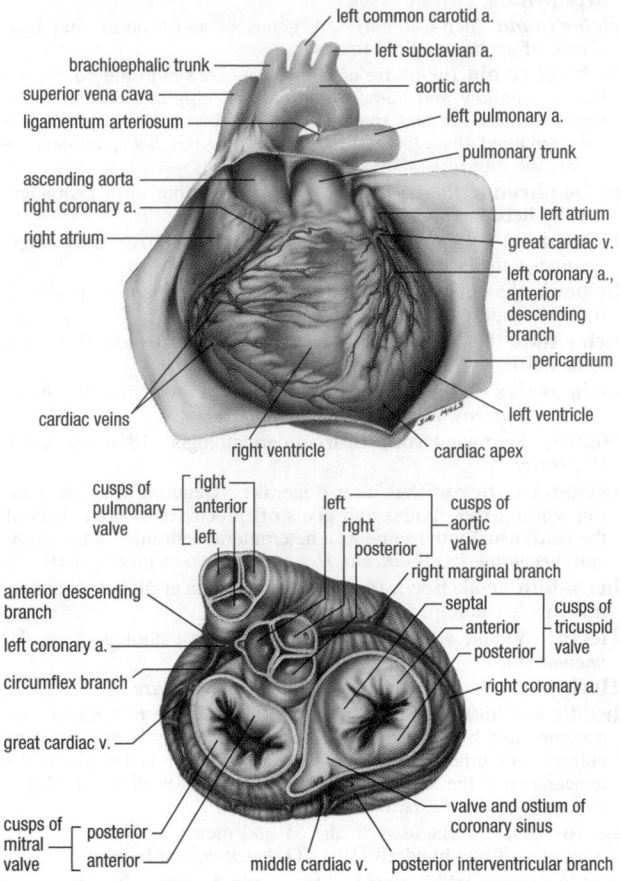

left common carotid a.
left subclavian a.
brachioephalic trunk
aortic arch
superior vena cava
ligamentum arteriosum
left pulmonary a.
pulmonary trunk
ascending aorta
right coronary a.
left atrium
right atrium
great cardiac v.
left coronary a., anterior descending branch
pericardium
cardiac veins
icing h.
left ventricle
right ventricle
cardiac apex

cusps of pulmonary valve — right anterior, left
left, right, posterior — cusps of aortic valve
anterior descending branch
right marginal branch
left coronary a.
septal, anterior, posterior — cusps of tricuspid valve
circumflex branch
right coronary a.
great cardiac v.
cusps of mitral valve — posterior, anterior
valve and ostium of coronary sinus
middle cardiac v.   posterior interventricular branch

human heart: (top) a ventral view with pericardium opened, (bottom) transverse section at the level of the valves

armor h., extensive to complete calcification (rarely ossification) of the pericardium usually producing constrictive pericarditis.

armored h., calcareous deposits in the pericardium due to subacute or chronic pericarditis. SYN panzerherz.

artificial h., a mechanical pump used to replace the function of a damaged heart, either temporarily or as a permanent prosthesis.

athlete's h., a more or less loose designation for cardiac findings in healthy athletes that would be or could be abnormal in patients with disease, including atrioventricular blocks, left ventricular hypertrophy and, sometimes, benign arrhythmias and atrioventricular blocks.

athletic h., hypertrophy of the h. supposedly due to systematic athletic conditioning.

beer h., SYN alcoholic *cardiomyopathy.*

beriberi h., h. disease due to thiamine deficiency that may be epidemic or sporadic as characterized by cardiac metabolic damage and myocardial failure, often of the "high output" type, with edema (except in "dry" shoshin beriberi) and polyneuritis. The term is derived from Singhalese, "I am unable."

bony h., the presence of extensive calcareous patches in the pericardium and walls of the h., some of which chronically develop bony changes.

chaotic h., apparently totally uncoordinated cardiac action or rhythm.

crisscross h., an anomaly in which the ventricular relationships are not as expected for the given atrioventricular connection.

drop h., SYN cardioptosia.

fatty h., (**1**) fatty degeneration of the myocardium; (**2**) accumulation of adipose tissue on the external surface of the h. with occasional infiltration of fat between the muscle bundles of the h. wall. SYN cor adiposum.

frosted h., hyaloserositis involving the pericardium. SYN icing h.

globular h., SYN round h.

hairy h., SYN fibrinous *pericarditis.*

Holmes h., a variant of double inlet left ventricle where the ventricular-arterial connection is concordant and the right ventricle is rudimentary.

horizontal h., description of the h.'s electrical position; recognized in the electrocardiogram when the QRS in lead aVL resembles that in V_6 and QRS in aVF resembles that in V_1; also, loosely, when the electrical axis lies between $-30°$ and $+30°$.

hyperthyroid h., response of the h. to hyperthyroidism, essentially the result of sympathetic stimulation producing rapid h. rates and ultimately cardiac failure and atrial fibrillation if untreated.

hypoplastic h., a small h., as seen in Addison disease.

icing h., SYN frosted h.

intermediate h., loosely, description of the h.'s electrical axis when this is directed at approximately between $+30°$ and $+60°$. For cardiac position, recognized in the electrocardiogram when the QRS complexes in both lead aVL and aVF resemble that in V_6.

Jarvik artificial h., a pneumatic artificial heart.

left h., the left atrium and left ventricle.

mechanical h., term loosely applied to any mechanical circulatory assist device.

movable h., SYN cor mobile.

myxedema h., the enlarged h. associated with untreated severe hypothyroidism, often accompanied by pericardial effusion; rare in modern medicine.

ox h., a very large h., due to chronic hypertension or, more often, to aortic valve disease, especially regurgitation. SYN bucardia, cor bovinum.

parchment h., a congenital or acquired condition in which there is thinning of the right ventricular myocardium. SEE Uhl *anomaly.* SYN right ventricular hypoplasia.

pendulous h., SYN cor pendulum.

pulmonary h., the right atrium and ventricle, receiving the venous blood and propelling it to the lungs. SEE ALSO cor pulmonale.

right h., the right atrium and right ventricle.

round h., abnormally smooth arcuate contours of the heart on imaging due either to disease of the ventricles or to a false cardiac appearance produced by excessive pericardial fluid. SYN globular h.

sabot h., SYN *coeur* en sabot.

semihorizontal h., loosely refers to the h.'s electrical axis when this is directed at approximately $0°$. As a cardiac electrical position, recognized in the electrocardiogram when the QRS complex in lead aVL resembles V_6 while that in aVF is small algebraically or absolutely.

semivertical h., loosely descriptive of the h.'s electrical axis when this is directed at approximately $+60°$. As a cardiac electrical position, recognized in the electrocardiogram when the QRS complex in lead aVF resembles V_6 while that in aVL is small algebraically or absolutely.

stone h., SYN ischemic *contracture* of the left ventricle.

systemic h., the left atrium and ventricle, receiving the aerated blood from the lungs and propelling it throughout the body.

three-chambered h., congenital abnormality in which there may be a single atrium with two ventricles or a single ventricle with two atria. Rudimentary parts of the atrial and ventricular septa may be present but are incompetent to prevent a virtual single chamber in either case.

tiger h., a fatty degenerated h. in which the fat is disposed in the form of broken stripes in the subendocardial myocardium.

tobacco h., cardiac irritability marked by irregular action, palpita-

he

tion, and sometimes pain, believed to occur as a result of the heavy use of tobacco.

univentricular h., an anomaly in which all blood flows through one ventricle or in which the arterioventricular valves are committed to empty into only one chamber in the ventricular mass.

venous h., the right side, including both the atrium and ventricle, of the h.

vertical h., loosely descriptive of the h.'s electrical axis when this is directed at approximately +90°. As a cardiac electrical position, recognized in the electrocardiogram when the QRS complex in lead aVL resembles V_1 while that in aVF resembles V_6.

wooden-shoe h., SYN *coeur* en sabot.

heart·beat (hart'bēt). A single complete cycle of contraction and dilation of heart muscle.

heart·burn (hart'bern). SYN pyrosis.

heart·worm. SYN *Dirofilaria immitis.*

heat (q) (hēt). **1.** A high temperature; the sensation produced by proximity to fire or an incandescent object, as opposed to cold. **2.** The kinetic energy of atoms and molecules, as well as rotation and vibration. **3.** SYN estrus. **4.** SYN enthalpy. [A.S. *haete*]

atomic h., the amount of h. required to raise an atom from 0° to 1°C; approximately the same for all elements (about 25 kJ/g-atom).

h. of combustion, the quantity of h. liberated per gram-molecular weight when a substance undergoes complete oxidation.

h. of compression, h. produced when a gas is compressed.

conductive h., h. transmitted by direct contact, as by an electric pad or hot-water bottle.

convective h., h. conveyed by a warm medium, such as air or water, in motion from its source.

conversive h., h. produced in a body by the absorption of waves that are not in themselves hot, such as the sun's rays or infrared radiation.

h. of crystallization, the quantity of h. liberated or absorbed per mol when a substance passes into the crystalline state.

h. of dissociation, the h. (expressed in calories or joules) expended in the dissociation of 1 mol of a substance into specified products.

h. of evaporation, the h. absorbed in the evaporation of water, sweat or other liquid; for water it amounts to 540 cal/g at 100°C. SYN h. of vaporization.

h. of formation, the h. (expressed in calories or joules) absorbed or liberated during the (hypothetical) reaction in which a mole of a compound is formed from the necessary elements, in elemental form.

initial h., the first burst of h. produced after the beginning of a muscle twitch, described by A. V. Hill.

innate h., in ancient Greek medicine, the h. of the heart sustained by the pneuma and distributed by the arteries throughout the body.

latent h., the amount of h. that a substance may absorb without an increase in temperature, as in conversion from solid to liquid state (ice to water at 0°C), or from liquid to gaseous state (water to steam at 100°C). Cf. sensible h.

molecular h., the product of the specific h. of a body multiplied by its molecular weight.

prickly h., SYN *miliaria* rubra.

radiant h., h. given off from any body in the form of infrared waves.

sensible h., the amount of h. that, when absorbed by a substance, causes a rise in temperature. Cf. latent h.

h. of solution, the quantity of h. absorbed or evolved when a solid is dissolved in a liquid.

specific h., the amount of h. required to raise any substance through 1°C of temperature, compared with that raising the same volume of water 1°C.

h. of vaporization, SYN h. of evaporation.

heat-la·bile (hēt'lā'bl). Destroyed or altered by heat.

heat-sta·ble (hēt'stā'bl). SYN thermostabile.

heat·stroke (hēt'strōk). A severe and often fatal illness produced by exposure to excessively high temperatures, especially when

accompanied by marked exertion; characterized by headache, vertigo, confusion, hot dry skin, and a slight rise in body temperature; in severe cases, very high fever, vascular collapse, and coma develop. SYN heat apoplexy (1), heat hyperpyrexia, malignant hyperpyrexia, thermic fever.

Heb·e·lo·ma (heb-ĕ-lō'mă). A genus of mushrooms that is a source of gastrointestinal toxins.

he·be·phre·nia (hē-bĕ-frē'nē-ă, heb'ē-). A syndrome characterized by shallow and inappropriate affect, giggling, and silly, regressive behavior and mannerisms; a subtype of schizophrenia now renamed disorganized *schizophrenia*. [G. *hēbē*, puberty, + *phrēn*, the mind]

he·be·phren·ic (hē-bĕ-frēn'ik, heb-ē-). Relating to or characterized by hebephrenia.

Heberden, William, English physician, 1710–1801. SEE H. *angina, nodes,* under *node;* Rougnon-H. *disease.*

he·bet·ic (hē-bet'ik). Pertaining to youth. [G. *hēbētikos,* youthful, fr. *hēbē,* youth]

heb·e·tude (heb'ĕ-tood). SYN moria (1). [L. *hebetudo,* fr. *hebeo,* to be dull]

he·bi·at·rics (hē-bē-at'riks). SYN adolescent *medicine.* [G. *hēbē,* youth, + *iatrikos,* relating to medicine]

Hebra, Ferdinand von, Austrian dermatologist, 1816–1880. SEE H. *prurigo.*

hec·a·ter·o·mer·ic (hek'ă-ter-ō-mer'ik). Denoting a spinal neuron whose axon divides and gives off processes to both sides of the cord; usually the same as a heteromeric neuron. SYN hecatomeral, hecatomeric. [G. *hekateros,* each of two, + *meros,* part]

hec·a·tom·er·al, hec·a·to·mer·ic (hek'ă-tom'er-ăl, hek'ă-tō-mer'ik). SYN hecateromeric.

Hecht, Victor, early 20th century Austrian pathologist. SEE H. *pneumonia.*

Heck, John W., U.S. dentist, *1923. SEE H. *disease.*

hec·tic (hek'tik). Denoting a daily afternoon rise of temperature, accompanied by a flush on the cheeks, occurring in active tuberculosis and other infections; use of the term is based on the appearance of the temperature chart. [G. *hektikos,* habitual, hectic, consumptive, fr. *hexis,* habit]

◊**hecto- (h).** Prefix used in the SI and metric system to signify multiples of one hundred (10^2). [G. *hekaton,* one hundred]

hec·to·gram (hek'tō-gram). One hundred grams, the equivalent of 1543.7 grains.

hec·to·li·ter (hek'tō-lē-ter). One hundred liters, the equivalent of 105.7 quarts or 26.4 American (22 imperial) gallons.

hed·e·o·ma (he-dē-ō'mă). SEE pennyroyal.

hed·er·i·form (hed'er-i-fōrm). Ivy-shaped; a term used for certain sensory endings in the skin. [L. *hedera,* ivy, + *forma,* shape]

he·do·no·pho·bia (hē'dŏ-nō-fō'bē-ă). Morbid fear of pleasure. [G. *hēdonē,* delight, + *phobos,* fear]

Hedström, Gustav, Swedish endodontist. SEE H. *file.*

heel (hēl) [TA]. **1.** Proximal portion of the plantar surface of the foot. **2.** SYN calx (2). **3.** SYN distal *end.* [A.S. *hēla*]

black h., SYN calcaneal *petechiae.*

cracked h., SYN *keratoderma* plantare sulcatum.

painful h., a condition in which bearing weight on the h. causes pain of varying severity. SYN calcaneodynia.

prominent h., a condition marked by a tender swelling on the os calcis due to a thickening of the periosteum or fibrous tissue covering the back of the os calcis.

Heerfordt, Christian Frederick, Danish ophthalmologist, *1871. SEE H. *disease.*

Hegar, Alfred, German gynecologist, 1830–1914. SEE H. *dilators,* under *dilator, sign.*

Hegglin, Robert M.P., Swiss physician, 1907–1970. SEE H. *anomaly, syndrome;* May-H. *anomaly.*

Hehner, Otto, British chemist, 1853–1924. SEE H. *number.*

Heidenhain, Rudolph P.H., German histologist and physiologist, 1834–1897. SEE H. *crescents,* under *crescent, demilunes,* under *demilune, law,* azan *stain,* iron hematoxylin *stain, pouch;* Biondi-H. *stain.*

height (h) (hīt). Vertical measurement.

anterior facial h. (AFH), in cephalometrics, the linear measurement from the nasion to the menton.

h. of contour, the line encircling a tooth or other structure at its greatest bulge or diameter. It relates to a selected path of insertion of a dental appliance or device.

cusp h., (1) the shortest distance between the tip of a cusp and its base plane; **(2)** the shortest distance between the deepest part of the central fossa of a posterior tooth and a line connecting the points of the cusps of the tooth.

facial h., the linear dimension in the midline from the hairline to the menton.

nasal h., the distance between the nasion and the lower border of the nasal aperture.

orbital h., the distance between the midpoints of the upper and lower margins of the orbit.

Heilbronner, Karl, Dutch physician, 1869–1914. SEE H. *thigh.*

Heim, Ernst L., German physician, 1747–1834. SEE H.-Kreysig *sign.*

Heimlich, Henry J., U.S. thoracic surgeon, *1920. SEE H. *maneuver.*

Heine, Leopold, German ophthalmologist, 1870–1940.

Heineke, Walter, German surgeon, 1834–1901. SEE H.-Mikulicz *pyloroplasty.*

Heinz, Robert, German pathologist, 1865–1924. SEE H. body *anemia, bodies,* under *body,* body *test;* H.-Ehrlich *body;* H. body *anemia.*

Heister, Lorenz, German anatomist, 1683–1758. SEE H. *diverticulum, valve.*

HeLa (hē'la). Referring to cells of the first continuously cultured (human cervical) carcinoma strain. [*Henrietta Lacks* (d. 1951), whose cervical carcinoma was the source of the cell line]

hel·co·me·nia (hel-kō-mē'nē-ă). Occurrence of ulcers at the time of a menstruation. [G. *helkos,* ulcer, + *emmēnos,* monthly]

Held, Hans, German anatomist, 1866–1942. SEE H. *bundle, decussation.*

he·li·an·thine (hē-li-an'thin). SYN methyl orange.

hel·i·cal (hel'i-kăl). **1.** Relating to a helix. SYN helicine (2). **2.** SYN helicoid. [G. *helix,* a coil]

hel·i·ces (hel'i-sēz). Plural of helix.

hel·i·cine (hel'i-sēn). **1.** Coiled. **2.** SYN helical (1). [G. *helix,* a coil]

Hel·i·co·bac·ter (hel'ĭ-kō-bak'ter). A genus of helical, curved, or straight microaerophilic bacteria with rounded ends and multiple sheathed flagella (unipolar or bipolar and lateral) with terminal bulbs. Form nonpigmented, translucent colonies, 1–2 mm in diameter. Catalase and oxidase positive. Found in gastric mucosa of primates, including human beings and ferrets. Some species are associated with gastric and peptic ulcers and predispose to gastric carcinoma. The type species is *Helicobacter pylori.*

H. cinaedi, a bacterial species associated with cases of proctitis and colitis in homosexual men.

H. fennelliae, a bacterial species reported associated with proctitis and colitis in homosexual men.

H. heilmannii, species observed in gastric mucosa. This agent has a low prevalence (less than 1% in patients), has not been cultured in vitro, and is of unknown pathogenic significance.

H. pylo'ri, a bacterial species that produces urease and causes gastritis and is involved in most cases of peptic ulcer disease of the stomach and duodenum; infection with this organism also plays an etiologic role (probably along with dietary cofactors) in dysplasia and metaplasia of gastric mucosa, distal gastric adenocarcinoma, and non-Hodgkin lymphoma of the stomach. SYN *Campylobacter pylori.*

The organism was first observed in 1982 by Robin Warren and Barry J. Marshall at Royal Perth Hospital in Western Australia in biopsy specimens from patients with chronic gastritis. Originally believed to be a species of *Campylobacter,* the organism was reclassified as *Helicobacter py-lori* in 1989. *Helicobacter pylori,* a curved or spiral, flagellated Gram-negative bacillus, colonizes the gastric mucosa, attaching itself to the surface of mucus-secreting columnar cells. The ability of the organism to survive in an acid medium is due to its production of urease, which converts urea to ammonia and alkalizes the film of mucus in which it resides. Infection with *Helicobacter pylori* is common worldwide, and the incidence of infection increases with age, reaching about 50% among persons aged 60. Transmission is believed to be from person to person by the fecal-oral route. Familial clustering of infection and a higher incidence among blacks and Hispanics have been attributed to social rather than genetic factors. Once infection occurs, it typically remains for life unless treated with antibiotics. Newly acquired infection results in extensive damage to parietal cells, with acute gastritis accompanied by impairment of acid production, which may be transitory. Most people infected have no symptoms (possibly because some strains of *Helicobacter pylori* do not produce cytotoxins) but about 1% of *Helicobacter pylori*–infected adults each year develop peptic ulcer. The risk of progression to peptic ulcer disease is increased by cigarette smoking and long-term use of nonsteroidal antiinflammatory agents. About 70% of all people with gastric ulcers and 90% of those with duodenal ulcers are found to be infected with *Helicobacter pylori.* In the U.S., about 500,000 new cases of peptic ulcer disease occur each year. The disease is responsible for 3–4 million physician visits and approximately 16,000 deaths annually. *Helicobacter pylori* infection has not been associated with nonulcer dyspepsia or inflammatory disorders of the digestive tract other than peptic ulceration. However, the incidence of both gastric adenocarcinoma and gastric lymphoma is higher in infected persons. In addition, the organism has been implicated in some cases of cholecystitis and autoimmune thyroiditis, and some studies have suggested that gastric infection with *Helicobacter pylori* may be a factor, by an unknown mechanism, in some cases of sudden infant death syndrome (SIDS). Diagnosis of *Helicobacter pylori* infection can be confirmed by identification of the organism in stained sections of gastric biopsy material, by culture from biopsy material, by testing biopsy material for urease activity, by identification of bacterial antigen in stool, by finding IgG antibody to the organism in the serum (the method of choice to confirm infection in a previously untreated patient), or by detection of urease activity with various biochemical tests. The urea breath test is more useful than serologic testing to confirm eradication of *Helicobacter pylori* after a course of treatment, since IgG antibody may remain elevated for more than 1 year after eradication. Eradication of the organism with antibiotic therapy does not yield faster healing of a peptic ulcer than treatment with antisecretory agents, but it greatly reduces the likelihood of ulcer recurrence. Recommended regimens for eradication of *Helicobacter pylori* include combinations of bismuth subsalicylate with 2 antibiotics (metronidazole or clarithomycin and tetracycline or amoxicillin). Acquired resistance of *Helicobacter pylori* to the macrolide and imidazole antibiotics is a growing problem. It is estimated that about 30% of strains of the organism in the U.S. are resistant to metronidazole and that almost 10% are resistant to macrolides. A major factor in the emergence of resistant strains appears to be an inadequate or failed first course of treatment. Active vaccination by oral administration of an enzymatically inactive recombinant subunit of Helicobacter pylori urease combined with a mucosal adjuvant (labile toxin of *Escherichia coli*) has elicited microbiologic and clinical cure of *Helicobacter pylori* infection in animal studies and limited human trials.

hel·i·coid (hel'i-koyd). Resembling a helix. SYN helical (2). [G. *helix,* a coil, + *eidos,* resemblance]

hel·i·co·po·dia (hel'i-kō-pō'dē-ă). SYN helicopod *gait*. [G. *helix*, a coil, + *pous*, foot]

hel·i·co·tre·ma (hel'i-kō-trē'mă) [TA]. A semilunar opening at the apex of the cochlea through which the scala vestibuli and the scala tympani of the cochlea communicate with one another. SYN Breschet hiatus, Scarpa hiatus. [G. *helix*, a spiral, + *trēma*, a hole]

Helie, Louis T., French gynecologist, 1804–1867. SEE H. *bundle.*

he·li·en·ceph·a·li·tis (hē-lē-en-sef-ă-lī'tis). Inflammation of the brain following sunstroke. [G. *helios*, sun, + *enkephalos*, brain, + *-itis*, inflammation]

△**helio-.** The sun. [G. *hēlios*]

he·li·o·aer·o·ther·a·py (hē'lē-ō-ār-ō-thār'ă-pē). Treatment of disease by exposure to sunshine and fresh air.

he·li·op·a·thy (hē-lē-op'ă-thē). Injury from exposure to sunlight. [helio- + G. *pathos*, suffering]

he·li·o·pho·bia (hē'lē-ō-fō'bē-ă). Morbid fear of exposure to the sun's rays. [helio- + G. *phobos*, fear]

he·li·o·sis (hē-lē-ō'sis). SYN sunstroke. [helio- + G. *-osis*, condition]

he·li·o·tax·is (hē-lē-ō-tak'sis). A form of phototaxis, and perhaps of thermotaxis, in which there is a tendency to growth or movement toward (positive h.) or away from (negative h.) the sun or the sunlight. SYN heliotropism. [helio- + G. *taxis*, orderly arrangement]

he·li·ot·ro·pism (hē-lē-ot'rō-pizm). SYN heliotaxis. [helio- + G. *tropē*, a turning]

He·li·o·zo·ea (hē'lē-ō-zō'ē-ă). A class of protozoans (subphylum Sarcodina) distinguished by stiff radiating axopodia on all sides, usually naked, though some have a skeleton of siliceous scales and spines, but without a central capsule. They are mostly fresh water dwellers, and colonial forms are common. [helio- + G. *zōon*, animal]

he·li·um (He) (hē'lē-ŭm). A gaseous element present in minute amounts in the atmosphere (0.000524% of dry volume); atomic no. 2, atomic wt. 4.002602; used as a diluent of medicinal gases; used as a diluent of oxygen principally in nonmedical applications, and in its liquid form as the coolant for super-conducting magnets (as in magnetic resonance imaging). [G. *hēlios*, the sun]

he·li·um-3. The rare stable isotope of helium (1.37 parts per million of ordinary helium); produced by the beta decay of tritium.

he·li·um-4. The common helium isotope, making up 99.999% of natural helium; it is emitted in the form of alpha rays (which are helium nuclei), from a variety of radionuclides.

he·lix, pl. **hel·i·ces** (hē'liks, hel'i-sēz) [TA]. **1** [NA]. The margin of the auricle; a folded rim of cartilage forming the upper part of the anterior, the superior, and the greater part of the posterior edges of the auricle. **2.** A line in the shape of a coil (or a spring, or the threads on a bolt), each point being equidistant from a straight line that is the axis of the cylinder in which each point of the h. lies; often, mistakenly, applied to a spiral. [L. fr. G. *helix*, a coil]

3_{10} **h.,** a type of right-handed h. found in small pieces in a number of proteins; has three amino acid residues per turn.

3.6$_{13}$ h., SYN α h.

α **h.,** the helical (commonly right-handed) form present in many proteins, deduced by Pauling and Corey from x-ray diffraction studies of proteins such as α-keratin; the h. is stabilized by hydrogen bonds between, e.g., $R_2C=O$ and HNR_2' groups (symbolized by the center dot in $R_2CO \cdot HNR_2'$) of different eupeptide bonds. In a true α h., there are 3.6 amino acid residues per turn of the h. and a rise of 1.5 Å per residue. SYN 3.6$_{13}$ h., Pauling-Corey h.

collagen h., an extended left-handed h. resulting from the high levels of glycine, L-proline, and L-hydroxyproline present in the collagens. There are 3.3 amino acids per turn of the helix. Three of those left-handed helices form a triple superhelix that is right-handed.

DNA h., SYN Watson-Crick h.

double h., SYN Watson-Crick h.

π **h.,** a rare right-handed h. found only in small portions of certain proteins. Stabilized by similar hydrogen bonds as in an α h.; there are 4.3 amino acid residues per turn of this h.

Pauling-Corey h., SYN α h.

triple h., the superhelix formed (right-handed) from three individual collagen helices (each being left-handed).

twin h., SYN Watson-Crick h.

Watson-Crick h., the helical structure assumed by two strands of deoxyribonucleic acid, held together throughout their length by hydrogen bonds between bases on opposite strands, referred to as Watson-Crick base pairing. SEE base *pair.* SYN DNA h., double h., twin h.

hel·le·bore (hel'ĕ-bōr). A plant of the genus *Helleborus*, especially *H. niger* (black h.). SEE ALSO *Veratrum album, Veratrum viride.* [G. *helleboros*]

false h., SYN adonis.

hel·leb·o·rin (hĕ-leb'o-rin, hel-ĕ-bō'rin). A toxic glycoside from *Veratrum viride* (green hellebore); a narcotic.

hel·le·bor·ism (hel'ĕ-bōr-izm). A condition resulting from poisoning by *Veratrum Helleborus.*

hel·leb·o·rus (he-leb'ŏ-rŭs). Black hellebore, the dried rhizome and roots of *Helleborus niger* (family Ranunculaceae); used as a cardiac and arterial tonic, diuretic, and cathartic. [G. *helleboros*]

Heller, Arnold L.G., German pathologist, 1840–1913. SEE H. *plexus.*

Heller, Ernst, German surgeon, 1877–1964. SEE H. *operation.*

Hellin, Dyonizy (Dionys), Polish pathologist, 1867–1935. SEE H. *law.*

Helly, Konrad, Swiss pathologist, *1875. SEE H. *fixative.*

Helmholtz, Hermann L.F. von, German physician, physicist, and physiologist, 1821–1894. SEE H. axis *ligament, energy, theory* of accommodation, *theory* of color vision, *theory* of hearing; H.-Gibbs *theory;* Gibbs-H. *equation;* Young-H. *theory* of color vision.

hel·minth (hel'minth). An intestinal vermiform parasite, primarily nematodes, cestodes, trematodes, and acanthocephalans. [G. *helmins*, worm]

hel·min·tha·gogue (hel-minth'ă-gog). SYN anthelmintic (1). [G. *helmins*, worm, + *agōgos*, leading]

hel·min·them·e·sis (hel-min-them'ĕ-sis). The vomiting or expulsion through the mouth of intestinal worms. [G. *helmins*, a worm, + *emesis*, vomiting]

hel·min·thi·a·sis (hel-min-thī'ă-sis). The condition of having intestinal vermiform parasites. SYN helminthism, invermination.

hel·min·thic (hel-min'thik). **1.** Helmintic. **2.** SYN anthelmintic (1).

hel·min·thism (hel'min-thizm). SYN helminthiasis.

hel·min·thoid (hel-min'thoyd). Wormlike. [G. *helminthōdes*, wormlike, fr. *helmins*, worm, + *eidos*, resemblance]

hel·min·thol·o·gy (hel-min-thol'ō-jē). The branch of science concerned with worms; especially the branch of zoology and of medicine concerned with intestinal vermiform parasites. SYN scolecology. [G. *helmins*, worm, + *logos*, study]

hel·min·tho·ma (hel-min-thō'mă). A discrete nodule of granulomatous inflammation (including the healed stage) caused by a helminth or its products, so termed on the basis of certain gross resemblances to a neoplasm. [G. *helmins*, worm, + *-oma*, tumor]

hel·min·tho·pho·bia (hel'min-thō-fō'bē-ă). Morbid fear of worms. [G. *helmins*, worm, + *phobos*, fear]

Hel·min·tho·spo·ri·um (hel-min-thō-spōr'ē-ŭm). A saprobic fungus that is usually isolated in clinical laboratories; it has determinant parallel-walled conidiophores; commonly misapplied to isolates of *Drechslera.*

hel·min·tic (hel-min'tik). **1.** Relating to or infected with parasitic worms. **2.** SYN anthelmintic (1).

He·lo·der·ma (hē-lō-der'mă). The only genus of poisonous lizards, such as the Gila monster, so named because of the tubercular scales which cover their bodies. They are native to Mexico and the southwestern U.S. [G. *hēlos*, nail, + *derma*, skin]

Hel·vel·la es·cu·len·ta (hel-vel'ă es-kū-len'tă). SYN *Gyromitra esculenta.*

Helweg, Hans K.S., Danish physician, 1847–1901. SEE H. *bundle.*

Helweg-Larssen, Helweg-Larssen, Hans F., 20th century Danish dermatologist. SEE Helweg-Larssen *syndrome.*

⌂**hem-, hema-.** Blood. SEE ALSO hemat-, hemato-, hemo-. [G. *haima*]

he·ma·chrome (hē′mă-krōm, hem′ă-). The coloring matter of the blood, hemoglobin or hematin. [hema- + G. *chrōma,* color]

he·ma·cy·tom·e·ter (hē′mă-sī-tom′ĕ-ter, hem′ă-). SYN hemocytometer.

he·ma·cy·to·zo·on (hē′mă-sī-tō-zō′on, hem′ă). SYN hemocytozoon.

he·ma·do·ste·no·sis (hē′mă-dō-ste-nō′sis, hem′ad-ŏ). Contraction of the arteries. [G. *haimas (haimad-),* a stream of blood, + *stenōsis,* a narrowing]

he·mad·sorp·tion (hē′mad-sōrp-shŭn, hem′ad-). A phenomenon manifested by an agent or substance adhering to or being adsorbed on the surface of a red blood cell.

he·ma·fa·ci·ent (hē-mă-fā′shē-ent, hem-ă-). SYN hemopoietic.

he·mag·glu·ti·na·tion (hē-mă-gloo′ti-nā′shŭn). The agglutination of red blood cells; may be immune as a result of specific antibody either for red blood cell antigens per se or other antigens which coat the red blood cells, or may be nonimmune as in h. caused by viruses or other microbes. SYN hemoagglutination.

passive h., a kind of passive agglutination in which erythrocytes, usually modified by mild treatment with tannic acid or other chemicals, are used to adsorb soluble antigen onto their surface, and which then agglutinate in the presence of antiserum specific for the adsorbed antigen. SYN indirect hemagglutination test.

reverse passive h., a diagnostic technique for virus infection using agglutination by viruses of red blood cells that previously have been coated with antibody specific to the virus.

viral h., the nonimmune agglutination of suspended red blood cells by certain of a wide range of otherwise unrelated viruses, usually by the virion itself but in some instances by products of viral growth (e.g., subunits), the species of erythrocyte agglutinated differing with the different viruses. SEE ALSO hemagglutination *inhibition.*

he·mag·glu·ti·nin (hē′mă-gloo′ti-nin, hem-). A substance, antibody or other, that causes hemagglutination. SYN hemoagglutinin.

he·ma·gog·ic (hē-mă-goj′ik, hem-ă-). Promoting a flow of blood.

he·mal (hē′măl). **1.** Relating to the blood or blood vessels. **2.** Referring to the ventral side of the vertebral bodies or their precursors, where the heart and great vessels are located, as opposed to neural (2). [G. *haima,* blood]

he·mal·um (hē-mal′ŭm, hem-). A solution of hematoxylin and alum used as a nuclear stain in histology, especially with eosin as a counterstain.

he·mam·e·bi·a·sis (hē′mă-mē-bī′ă-sis, hem′ă-). Any infection with ameboid forms of parasites in red blood cells, as in malaria.

he·ma·nal·y·sis (hē-mă-nal′ĭ-sis, hem-). Analysis of the blood; an examination of the blood, especially with reference to chemical methods. [G. *haima,* blood, + analysis]

he·man·gi·ec·ta·sis, he·man·gi·ec·ta·sia (hē-man-jē-ek′tăsis, hem-an-; -ek-tā′zē-ă). Dilation of blood vessels. [G. *haima,* blood, + *angeion,* vessel, + *ektasis,* a stretching]

⌂**hemangio-.** The blood vessels. [G. *haima,* blood, + *angeion,* vessel]

he·man·gi·o·blast (he-man′jē-ō-blast). A primitive embryonic cell of mesodermal origin producing cells from which are derived vascular endothelium, reticuloendothelial elements, and blood-forming cells of all types. [hemangio- + G. *blastos,* germ]

he·man·gi·o·blas·to·ma (he-man′jē-ō-blas-tō′mă). A benign neoplasm frequently arising in the cerebellum composed of capillary vessel–forming endothelial cells and stromal cells; a slowly growing tumor that affects, primarily, middle-aged individuals; increased incidence in von Hippel-Lindau disease. SYN angioblastoma, Lindau tumor.

he·man·gi·o·en·do·the·li·o·blas·to·ma (he-man′jē-ō-en-dō-thē′-lē-ō-blastō′mă). Hemangioendothelioma in which the endothelial cells seem to be especially immature forms. [hemangio- + endothelium + G. *blastos,* germ, + *-oma,* tumor]

he·man·gi·o·en·do·the·li·o·ma (he-man′jē-ō-en-dō-thē-lē-ō′mă). A neoplasm derived from blood vessels, characterized by numerous prominent endothelial cells that occur singly, in aggregates,

and as the lining of congeries of vascular tubes or channels; in the elderly, may be malignant (angiosarcoma or hemangiosarcoma), but in children are benign and probably represent a growing stage of capillary hemangioma. [hemangio- + endothelium + G. *-oma,* tumor]

h. tubero′sum mul′tiplex, an eruption of pinkish papules, caused by hyperplasia of the endothelium of the superficial blood vessels.

he·man·gi·o·fi·bro·ma (he-man′jē-ō-fī-brō′mă). A hemangioma with an abundant fibrous tissue framework.

juvenile h., SYN juvenile *angiofibroma.*

he·man·gi·o·ma (he-man′jē-ō′mă). A congenital anomaly, in which proliferation of blood vessels leads to a mass that resembles a neoplasm; it can occur anywhere in the body but is most frequently noticed in the skin and subcutaneous tissues; most h.'s undergo spontaneouos regression. SEE ALSO nevus. [hemangio- + G. *-oma,* tumor]

capillary h., an overgrowth of capillary blood vessels, seen most commonly in the skin, at or soon after birth, as a soft bright red to purple nodule or plaque that usually disappears by the fifth year. The most common type of h. SYN capillary angioma, capillary h. of infancy, nevus vascularis, nevus vasculosus, superficial angioma.

capillary h. of infancy, SYN capillary h.

ℹ️ **cavernous h.,** old term for deep cutaneous hemangioma that manifests spontaneous involution. Also used incorrectly for venous malformation.

lobular capillary h., SYN pyogenic *granuloma.*

racemose h., SYN cirsoid *aneurysm.*

sclerosing h., (1) a benign lung or bronchial lesion, often subpleural, sometimes multiple, which forms hyalinized connective tissue. **(2)** SYN dermatofibroma.

senile h., red papules caused by weakening of dermal capillary walls, that do not blanch on pressure, seen mostly in persons over 30 years of age. SYN cherry angioma, De Morgan spots.

spider h., SYN spider *angioma.*

strawberry h., hyperproliferation of immature capillary vessels, usually on the head and neck, present at birth or within the first 2–3 months postnatally, which commonly regresses without scar formation.

verrucous h., incorrect term for cutaneous vascular malformation comprised of abnormal capillaries and lymphatics.

he·man·gi·o·ma·to·sis (he-man′jē-ō-mă-tō′sis). A condition in which there are numerous hemangiomas.

he·man·gi·o·per·i·cy·to·ma (he-man′jē-ō-per′i-sī-tō′mă). An uncommon vascular, usually benign, neoplasm composed of round and spindle cells that are derived from the pericytes and surround endothelium-lined vessels; malignant h.'s are difficult to distinguish microscopically from the benign. [hemangio- + pericyte + G. *-oma,* tumor]

he·man·gi·o·sar·co·ma (he-man′jē-ō-sar-kō′mă). A rare malignant neoplasm characterized by rapidly proliferating, extensively infiltrating, anaplastic cells derived from blood vessels and lining irregular blood-filled or lumpy spaces.

he·ma·phe·ic (hē-mă-fē′ik, hem-ă-). Pertaining to or containing hemaphein.

he·ma·phe·in (hē-mă-fē′in, hem-ă-). A brown pathologic pigment derived from hemoglobin; said to be a combination of indican and urobilin. [G. *haima,* blood, + *phaios,* dusky]

he·ma·phe·ism (hē-mă-fē′izm, hem-ă-). The presence of hemaphein in the blood plasma and urine.

he·mar·thro·sis (hē′mar-thrō′sis, hem′ar-). Blood in a joint. [G. *haima,* blood, + *arthron,* joint]

he·ma·stron·ti·um (hē-mă-stron′shē-ŭm, hem-ă-). A stain made by adding strontium chloride to a solution of hematein and aluminum chloride in citric acid and alcohol; used in histology.

⌂**hemat-.** Blood. SEE ALSO hem-, hemato-, hemo-. [G. *haima (haimat-)*]

he·ma·ta·chom·e·ter (hē′mă-tă-kom′ĕ-ter, hem′ă-). SYN hematachometer.

he·mat·ap·os·te·ma (hē′mat-ă-pos-tē′mă, hem′at-). An abscess into which blood has effused. [hemat- + G. *apostēma,* abscess]

he

he·ma·te·in (hē-mă-tē'in, hem-ă). An oxidation product of hematoxylin.

Baker acid h., an acidic solution of oxidized hematoxylin used on frozen sections for staining phospholipids.

he·ma·tem·e·sis (hē-mă-tem'ĕ-sis, hem-ă-). Vomiting of blood. SYN vomitus cruentes. [hemat- + G. *emesis*, vomiting]

he·mat·en·ceph·a·lon (hē'mat-en-sef'ă-lon, hem'at-). SYN cerebral *hemorrhage*. [hemat- + G. *enkephalos*, brain]

he·ma·ther·a·py (hē'mă-thār'ă-pē, hem'ă-). SYN hemotherapy.

he·ma·therm (hē'mă-therm, hem'ă-). SYN homeotherm. [G. *haima*, blood, + *thermos*, warm]

he·ma·ther·mal (hē-mă-ther'măl, hem-ă-). SYN homeothermic. [G. *haima*, blood, + *thermos*, warm]

he·ma·ther·mous (hē-mă-ther'mŭs, hem-ă-). SYN homeothermic.

he·ma·tho·rax (hē-mă-thōr'aks, hem-ă-). SYN hemothorax.

he·mat·ic (hē-mat'ik). 1. Relating to blood. SYN hemic. 2. SYN hematinic (2).

he·ma·tid (hē'mă-tid, hem'a-). 1. Obsolete term for a red blood cell. 2. Obsolete term for a cutaneous eruption presumed to be caused by a substance in the circulating blood. [hemat- + -*id*]

he·ma·ti·dro·sis (hē'mat-i-drō'sis, hem'at-). Excretion of blood or blood pigment in the sweat; an extremely rare disorder. [hemat- + G. *hidrōs*, sweat]

he·ma·tim·e·ter (hē-mă-tim'ĕ-ter, hem-ă-). SYN hemocytometer.

hem·a·tin (hē'mă-tin, hem'ă-). Heme in which the iron is Fe(III) (Fe^{3+}); the prosthetic group of methemoglobin. SYN ferriheme, hematosin, hydroxyhemin, oxyheme, oxyhemochromogen, phenodin.

h. chloride, SYN hemin.

reduced h., SYN heme.

he·ma·ti·ne·mia (hē'mă-ti-nē'mē-ă, hem'ă-). The presence of heme in the circulating blood. [hematin + G. *haima*, blood]

hem·a·tin·ic (hē-mă-tin'ik, hem-a-). 1. Improving the condition of the blood. 2. An agent that improves the quality of blood by increasing the number of erythrocytes and/or the hemoglobin concentration. SYN hematic (2). SYN hematonic.

△**hemato-.** Combining form denoting blood. SEE ALSO hem-, hemat-, hemo-. [G. *haima* (*haimat-*)]

he·ma·to·bil·ia (hē'mă-tō-bil'ē-ă, hem'ă-). SYN hemobilia.

he·ma·to·bi·um (hē-mă-tō'bē-ŭm, hem-ă-). Any microorganism that is parasitic in the blood, especially an animal form or hemozoon. [hemato- + G. *bios*, life]

he·ma·to·blast (hē'mă-tō-blast, hem'ă-). A primitive, undifferentiated form of blood cell from which erythroblasts, lymphoblasts, myeloblasts, and other immature blood cells are derived; probably identical or closely similar to hemocytoblast and hemohistioblast; in normal bone marrow, present only in small numbers and difficult to identify in smears, inasmuch as h.'s are fragile and easily disintegrated; when marrow is hyperplastic, they may be observed in small groups. [hemato- + G. *blastos*, germ]

Hayem h., obsolete term for platelet.

he·ma·to·cele (hē'mă-tō-sēl, hem'ă-). 1. SYN hemorrhagic *cyst*. 2. Effusion of blood into a canal or a cavity of the body. 3. Swelling due to effusion of blood into the tunica vaginalis testis. [hemato- + G. *kēlē*, tumor]

pelvic h., intraperitoneal effusion of blood into the pelvis.

pudendal h., effusion of blood into the labium majus.

hem·a·to·ceph·a·ly (hē'mă-tō-sef'ă-lē, hem'ă-). Intracranial effusion of blood, commonly in a fetus. [hemato- + G. *kephalē*, head]

he·ma·to·che·zia (hē'mă-tō-kē'zē-ă, hem'ă-). Passage of bloody stools, in contradistinction to melena, or tarry stools. [hemato- + G. *chezō*, to go to stool]

he·ma·to·chlo·rin (hē'mă-tō-klō'rin, hem'ă). A green coloring matter derived from hemoglobin obtained from the placenta. [hemato- + G. *chlōros*, light green + -*in*]

he·ma·to·chy·lu·ria (hē'mă-tō-kī-loo'rē-ă, hem'a-). Presence of blood as well as chyle in the urine. [hemato- + G. *chylos*, juice, + *ouron*, urine]

he·ma·to·col·po·me·tra (hē'mă-tō-kol'pō-mē'tră). Accumulation of blood in the uterus and vagina resulting from an imperfo-rate hymen or other lower vaginal obstruction. [hemato- + G. *kolpos*, vagina, + *mētra*, womb]

he·ma·to·col·pos (hē'mă-tō-kol'pos, hem'ă-). An accumulation of menstrual blood in the vagina in consequence of imperforate hymen or other obstruction. SYN retained menstruation. [hemato- + G. *kolpos*, vagina]

he·mat·o·crit (Hct) (hē'mă-tō-krit, hem'ă-). 1. Percentage of the volume of a blood sample occupied by cells. Cf. plasmacrit. 2. Obsolete term for a centrifuge or device for separating the cells and other particulate elements of the blood from the plasma. [hemato- + G. *krinō*, to separate]

he·ma·toc·ry·al (hē-mă-tok'rē-ăl, hem-ă-). SYN poikilothermic. [hemato- + G. *kryos*, cold]

he·ma·to·cyst (hē'mă-tō-sist, hem'ă-). SYN hemorrhagic *cyst*.

he·ma·to·cys·tis (hē'mă-tō-sis'tis, hem'ă-). Presence of blood in the bladder. [hemato- + G. *kystis*, bladder]

he·ma·to·cyte (hē'mă-tō-sīt, hem'ă-). SYN hemocyte.

he·ma·to·cy·to·blast (hē'mă-tō-sī'tō-blast, hem'ă-). SYN hemocytoblast.

he·ma·to·cy·tol·y·sis (hē'mă-tō-sī-tol'ē-sis, hem'ă-). SYN hemocytolysis.

he·ma·to·cy·tom·e·ter (hē'mă-tō-sī-tom'ĕ-ter, hem'ă-). SYN hemocytometer.

he·ma·to·cy·to·zo·on (hē'mă-tō-sī'tō-zō'on, hem'ă-). SYN hemocytozoon.

he·ma·to·dys·cra·sia (hē'mă-tō-dis-krā'zē-ă, hem'ă-). SYN hemodyscrasia.

he·ma·to·dys·tro·phy (hē'mă-tō-dis'trō-fē, hem'ă-). SYN hemodystrophy.

he·ma·to·gen·e·sis (hē'mă-tō-jen'ĕ-sis, hem'ă-). SYN hemopoiesis. [hemato- + G. *genesis*, production]

he·ma·to·gen·ic, he·ma·tog·e·nous (hē'mă-tō-jen'ik, hem'ă-; hem-ă-toj'en-ŭs). 1. SYN hemopoietic. 2. Pertaining to anything produced from, derived from, or transported by the blood.

he·ma·to·his·ti·o·blast (hē'mă-tō-his'tē-ō-blast, hem'ă-). SYN hemohistioblast.

he·ma·to·his·ton (hē'mă-tō-his'tŏn, hem'ă-). SYN globin.

he·ma·toi·din (hē-mă-toy'din). A pigment derived from hemoglobin that contains no iron but is closely related to or identical to bilirubin. H. is formed intracellularly, presumably within reticuloendothelial cells, but is often found extracellularly after 5–7 days in foci of previous hemorrhage. It occurs as refractile, yellow-brown and orange-red granules, but more characteristically as rhomboid plates arranged in a radial pattern, so-called h. burrs. SYN blood crystals, hematoidin crystals. [hemato- + G. *eidos*, resemblance, + -*in*]

he·ma·tol·o·gist (hē-mă-tol'ō-jist, hem-ă-). A physician trained and experienced in hematology, i.e., skilled in performing diagnostic examinations of blood and bone marrow, or in treatment of such diseases, or both.

he·ma·tol·o·gy (hē-mă-tol'ō-jē, hem-ă-). The medical specialty that pertains to the anatomy, physiology, pathology, symptomatology, and therapeutics related to the blood and blood-forming tissues. SYN hemology. [hemato- + G. *logos*, study]

he·ma·to·lymph·an·gi·o·ma (hē'mă-tō-limf'an-jē-ō'-mă). A congenital anomaly consisting of numerous, closely packed, variably sized lymphatic vessels and larger channels, in association with a moderate number of blood vessels of a similar type.

he·ma·tol·y·sis (hē-mă-tol'ĭ-sis, hem-ă-). SYN hemolysis.

he·ma·to·lyt·ic (hē'ma-tō-lit'ik, hem'ă). SYN hemolytic.

he·ma·to·ma (hē-mă-tō'mă, hem-ă-). A localized mass of extravasated blood that is relatively or completely confined within an organ or tissue, a space, or a potential space; the blood is usually clotted (or partly clotted), and, depending on how long it has been there, may manifest various degrees of organization and decolorization. [hemato- + G. -*oma*, tumor]

communicating h., SYN pseudoaneurysm.

corpus luteum h., SYN *corpus* hemorrhagicum.

ℹ**epidural h.,** SYN extradural *hemorrhage*.

intracranial h., SEE intracranial *hemorrhage*.

intramural h., a h. in the wall of a structure, such as the bowel or bladder, usually resulting from trauma or excessive anticoagulation.

pulsatile h., SYN pseudoaneurysm.

subdural h., SYN subdural *hemorrhage.*

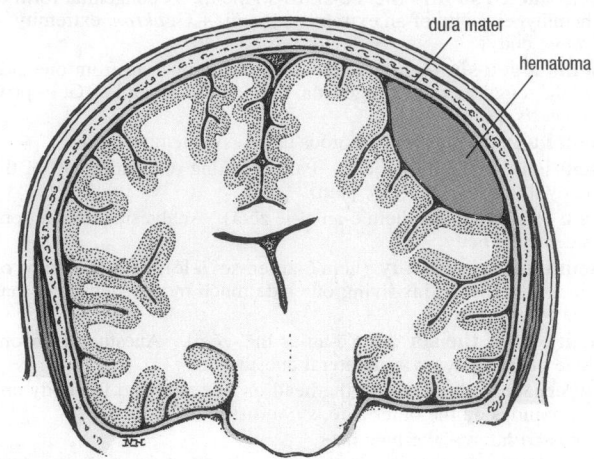

dura mater

hematoma

subdural hematoma: showing frontal section of brain

---

he·ma·to·me·tra (hē′mă-tō-mē′tră, hem′ă-). A collection or retention of blood in the uterine cavity. SYN hemometra. [hemato- + G. *mētra,* uterus]

he·ma·tom·e·try (hē-mă-tom′ĕ-trē, hem-ă). Examination of the blood in order to determine any or all of the following: 1) the total number, types, and relative proportions of various blood cells; 2) the number or proportion of other formed elements; 3) the percentage of hemoglobin. In some instances, h. is used to include a determination of blood pressure. SYN hemometry. [hemato- + G. *metron,* measure]

he·mat·om·pha·lo·cele (hē′mat-om-fal′ō-sēl, hem′at-). Umbilical hernia into which an effusion of blood has taken place. [hemato- + G. *omphalos,* umbilicus, + *kēlē,* hernia]

he·ma·to·my·e·lia (hē′mă-tō-mē′ē-lē-ă). Hemorrhage into the substance of the spinal cord; it is usually a posttraumatic lesion but may also be encountered in instances of spinal cord capillary telangiectases. SYN hematorrhachis interna, myelapoplexy, myelorrhagia. [hemato- + G. *myelos,* marrow]

he·ma·to·my·e·lo·pore (hē′mă-tō-mī′ĕ-lō-pōr). Formation of porosities in the spinal cord as a result of hemorrhages. [hemato- + G. *myelos,* marrow, + *poros,* a pore]

he·ma·ton·ic (hē-mă-ton′ik, hem-ă-). SYN hematinic.

he·ma·to·pa·thol·o·gy (hē′mă-tō-path-ol′ō-jē, hem′ă-). The division of pathology concerned with diseases of the blood and of hemopoietic and lymphoid tissues. SYN hemopathology. [hemato- + G. *pathos,* suffering, + *logos,* study]

he·ma·top·a·thy (hē-mă-top′ă-thē, hem-ă-). SYN hemopathy.

he·ma·to·pe·nia (hē′mă-tō-pē′nē-ă, hem′ă-). Deficiency of blood, including hypocytosis or cytopenia. [hemato- + G. *penia,* poverty]

he·ma·to·pha·gia (hē′mă-tō-fā′jē-ă, hem′ă-). Living on the blood of another animal, as does the vampire bat or a leech. SYN hemophagia. [hemato- + G. *phagō,* to eat]

he·ma·toph·a·gous (hē′mă-tof′ă-gŭs, hem′ă-). Subsisting on blood. [hemato- + G. *phagō,* to eat]

he·ma·toph·a·gus (hē′mă-tof′ă-gŭs, hem′ă-). A blood eater, especially bloodsucking insects. [hemato- + G. *phagō,* to eat]

he·ma·to·plas·tic (hē′mă-tō-plas′tik, hem′ă). SYN hemopoietic. [hemato- + G. *plassō,* to form]

he·ma·to·poi·e·sis (hē′mă-tō-poy-ē′sis, hem′ă-). SYN hemopoiesis.

he·ma·to·poi·et·ic (hē′mă-tō-poy-et′ik). SYN hemopoietic.

he·ma·to·poi·e·tin (hē′mă-tō-poy′ĕ-tin, hem′ă-). SYN erythropoietin.

he·ma·to·por·phyr·ia (hē′mă-tō-pōr-fir′ē-ă, hem′ă-). Obsolete term for any disorder of porphyrin metabolism, regardless of the cause. [hemato- + G. *porphyra,* purple]

he·ma·to·por·phy·rin (hē′mă-tō-pōr′fi-rin, hem′ă-). A dark red, almost purple, porphyrin resulting from the decomposition of hemoglobin; chemical composition is that of heme with the iron removed and the two vinyl ($-CH=CH_2$) groups hydrated to hydroxyethyl ($-CH(OH)-CH_3$). SYN hemoporphyrin.

he·ma·to·por·phy·ri·ne·mia (hē′mă-tō-pōr′fī-ri-nē′mē-ă, hem′ă-). Older term used to designate the occurrence of hematoporphyrin in the circulating blood.

he·ma·to·por·phy·rin·u·ria (hē′mă-tō-pōr′fī-ri-noo′rē-ă, hem′ă-). Older term used to designate enhanced urinary excretion of porphyrins.

he·ma·top·sia (hē-mă-top′sē-ă, hem-ă-). SYN hemophthalmia. [hemato- + G. *opsis,* vision]

he·ma·tor·rha·chis (hē-mă-tōr′ă-kis, hem-ă-). A spinal hemorrhage. [hemato- + G. *rhachis,* spine]

h. exter′na, hemorrhage into the spinal canal external to the cord, either within or outside the dura. SYN extradural h., subdural h.

extradural h., SYN h. externa.

h. inter′na, SYN hematomyelia.

subdural h., SYN h. externa.

he·ma·to·sal·pinx (hē′mă-tō-sal′pinks, hem′ă-). Collection of blood in a tube, often associated with a tubal pregnancy. SYN hemosalpinx. [hemato- + G. *salpinx,* a trumpet]

he·ma·to·sep·sis (hē′mă-tō-sep′sis, hem′ă). Obsolete term for septicemia.

he·ma·to·sin (hē-mă-tō′sin, hem-ă-). SYN hematin.

he·ma·to·sis (hē-mă-tō′sis, hem-ă-). **1.** SYN hemopoiesis. **2.** Oxygenation of the venous blood in the lungs.

he·ma·to·spec·tro·scope (hē′mă-tō-spek′trō-skōp, hem′ă-). A spectroscope especially adapted to examination of the blood.

he·ma·to·spec·tros·co·py (hē′mă-tō-spek-tros′kō-pē, hem′ă-). Examination of the blood by means of a spectroscope.

he·ma·to·sper·mat·o·cele (hē′mă-tō-sper′mă-tō-sēl, hem′ă-). A spermatocele that contains blood.

he·ma·to·sper·mia (hē′mă-tō-sper′mē-ă, hem′ă-). SYN hemospermia.

he·ma·to·stat·ic (hē′mă-tō-stat′ik, hem′ă-). **1.** Variant of hemostatic. **2.** Due to stagnation or arrest of blood in the vessels of the part.

he·ma·to·stax·is (hē′mă-tō-stak′sis, hem′ă-). Spontaneous bleeding due to a disease of the blood. [hemato- + G. *staxis,* a dripping]

he·ma·tos·te·on (hē-mă-tos′tē-on, hem-ă-). Bleeding in the medullary cavity of a bone. [hemato- + G. *osteon,* bone]

he·ma·to·ther·mal (hē′mă-tō-ther′măl, hem′ă-). SYN homeothermic.

he·ma·to·tox·in (hē′mă-tō-toks′in, hem′ă-). SYN hemotoxin.

he·ma·to·tro·pic (hē′mă-tō-trop′ik, hem′ă-). SYN hemotropic.

he·ma·to·tym·pa·num (hē′mă-tō-tim′pan-ŭm, hem′ă-). SYN hemotympanum.

he·ma·tox·in (hē-mă-toks′in, hem-ă). SYN hemotoxin.

he·ma·tox·y·lin (hē-mă-toks′i-lin, hem-ă-) [C.I. 75290]. A crystalline compound, containing the coloring matter of *Haematoxylon campechianum* (logwood), from which it is obtained by extraction with ether. It is used as a dye in histology, especially for cell nuclei and chromosomes, muscle cross-striations, and enterochromaffin cells; its staining properties depend upon its oxidation to hematein and mordanting with chrome and iron alums. It is also used as an indicator (red to yellow at pH 0.0 to 1.0, yellow to violet at pH 5.0 to 6.0).

Boehmer h., an alum type of h. in which natural ripening occurs in about 8 to 10 days, and the solution is good for many months.

Delafield h., an alum type of h. used in histology; natural ripening takes about 2 months and the solution is good for years.

Harris h., an alum type of h. similar to Delafield h., but which uses chemical ripening to produce oxidation of h. for immediate use.

iron h., unique ferric lakes of hematein that produce deep blue-black stains; useful for studies of cytologic detail, such as chromosomes, spindle fibers, Golgi apparatus, myofibrils, and mitochrondria; also useful to demonstrate *Entamoeba histolytica*. SEE ALSO Heidenhain iron hematoxylin *stain*, Weigert iron hematoxylin *stain*.

phosphotungstic acid h. (PTAH), a stain with broad application in cytology and histology; nuclei, mitochrondria, fibrin, neuroglial fibrils, and cross-striations of skeletal and cardiac muscle stain blue; cartilage ground substance, bone reticulum, and elastin appear in shades of yellow-orange and brownish red; also useful for demonstrating abnormal or diseased astrocytes, often in combination with periodic acid-Schiff stain and Luxol fast blue. SYN Mallory phosphotungstic acid hematoxylin stain.

he·ma·to·zo·ic (hē′ma-tō-zō′ik, hem′ă). SYN hemozoic.

he·ma·to·zo·on (hē′ma-tō-zō′on, hem′ă-). SYN hemozoon.

he·ma·tu·ria (hē-mă-too′-rē-ă, hem-ă-). Presence of blood or red blood cells in the urine. [hemato- + G. *ouron*, urine]

Egyptian h., SYN *schistosomiasis* haematobium.

endemic h., SYN *schistosomiasis* haematobium.

false h., SYN pseudohematuria.

gross h., the presence of blood in the urine in sufficient quantity to be visible to the naked eye.

initial h., the presence of blood only in the first fraction of voided urine, usually indicating a urethral or prostatic source of bleeding.

microscopic h., presence of blood cells in urine, visible only under the microscope.

painful h., h. associated with dysuria, usually indicating the coexistence of infection, trauma, calculi, or foreign bodies within the lower urinary tract.

painless h., h. not associated with dysuria, often connoting a vascular or neoplastic etiology.

renal h., h. resulting from extravasation of blood into the glomerular spaces, or tubules, or pelves of the kidneys.

terminal h., the presence of blood only in the last fraction of voided urine, usually indicating a prostatic source of bleeding.

total h., blood throughout all fractions of the voided urine, commonly indicating an upper or mid-urinary tract source of bleeding.

urethral h., h. in which the site of bleeding is in the urethra.

vesical h., h. in which the site of bleeding is in the urinary bladder.

heme (hēm). **1.** The porphyrin chelate of iron in which the iron is Fe(II) (or Fe^{2+}); the oxygen-carrying, color-furnishing, prosthetic group of hemoglobin. **2.** Iron complexed with nonporphyrins but related tetrapyrrole structures (e.g., biliverdin heme). **3.** Iron chelated with any porphyrin, irrespective of the valence state of the iron atom. SYN ferroheme, ferroprotoporphyrin, reduced hematin. [G. *haima*, blood]

h. a, a derivative of h. found in cytochrome aa_3.

h. c, a derivative of h. found in cytochromes c, b_4, and f.

hem·er·a·lo·pia (hem′er-al-ō′pē-ă). Inability to see as distinctly in a bright light as in reduced illumination; seen in patients with impaired cone function. SYN day blindness, hemeranopia, night sight. [G. *hēmera*, day, + *alaos*, obscure, + *ōps*, eye]

hem·er·a·no·pia (hem′er-ă-nō′pē-ă). SYN hemeralopia. [G. *hemera*, day, + *an-*, priv., + *ōps*, eye]

he·me·ryth·rins (hē-mĕ-rith′rinz, hem-ĕ-). Iron-containing, oxygen-binding proteins in certain invertebrates, with molecular weights approximately that of hemoglobin but differing from hemoglobin in that the molecules do not contain porphyrin groups. Oxygenated h. is oxyhemerythrin. [G. *haima*, blood, + G. *erythros*, red, + -in]

⚠**hemi-.** One-half. Cf. semi-. [G.]

hem·i·a·car·di·us (hem′ē-ă-kar′dē-ŭs). One of twin fetuses, in which only a part of the circulation is effected by its own heart, the rest by the heart of the other twin. [hemi- + G. *a-* priv. + *kardia*, heart]

hem·i·ac·e·tal (hem′ē-as′e-tăl). RCH(OH)OR′, a product of the addition of an alcohol to an aldehyde (an acetal is formed by the addition of an alcohol to a hemiacetal). In the aldose sugars, the h. formation is internal and labile, brought about by the 4-OH or 5-OH attack on the carbonyl O, yielding the furanose or pyranose structures; the h. forms of the sugars are involved in all polysaccharides, as glycosyls or glycosides. SEE ALSO hemiketal, acetal.

hem·i·ac·ro·so·mia (hem′ē-ak-rō-sō′mē-ă). A congenital form of hemihypertrophy of an extremity. [hemi- + G. *akron*, extremity, + *sōma*, body]

hem·i·a·geu·sia (hem′ē-ă-goo′sē-ă). Loss of taste from one side of the tongue. SYN hemiageustia, hemigeusia. [hemi- + G. *a-* priv. + *geusis*, taste]

hem·i·a·geus·tia (hem′ē-ă-goos′tē-ă). SYN hemiageusia.

hem·i·al·gia (hem-ē-al′jē-ă). Pain affecting one entire half of the body. [hemi- + G. *algos*, pain]

hem·i·an·al·ge·sia (hem′ē-an′al-jē′zē-ă). Analgesia affecting one side of the body.

hem·i·an·en·ceph·a·ly (hem′ē-an-en-sef′ă-lē). Anencephaly on one side only, or involving one side much more extensively than the other.

hem·i·an·es·the·sia (hem′ē-an-es-thē′-zē-ă). Anesthesia on one side of the body. SYN unilateral anesthesia.

alternate h., h. affecting the head on one side and the body and extremities on the other side. SYN crossed h.

crossed h., SYN alternate h.

hem·i·a·no·pia (hem′ē-ă-nō′pē-ă). Loss of vision for one half of the visual field of one or both eyes. SYN hemianopsia.

absolute h., h. in which the affected field is totally insensitive to all visual stimuli. SYN complete h.

altitudinal h., a defect in the visual field in which the upper or lower half is lost; may be unilateral or bilateral.

binasal h., blindness in the nasal field of vision of both eyes.

bitemporal h., blindness in the temporal field of vision of both eyes.

complete h., SYN absolute h.

congruous h., h. in which the visual field defects in both eyes are completely symmetric in extent and intensity.

crossed h., SYN heteronymous h.

heteronymous h., attitudinal h. involving the upper field of one eye and the lower field of the other; or a binasal or bitemporal h. SYN crossed h.

homonymous h., blindness in the corresponding (right or left) field of vision of each eye.

incomplete h., h. involving less than half the visual field of each eye.

incongruous h., an incomplete or asymmetric homonymous h.

pseudo-h., a condition in which individual stimuli are seen correctly, but when the nasal visual field of one eye and the temporal visual field of the fellow eye are stimulated simultaneously, one field is blind. SYN visual extinction.

quadrantic h., SYN quadrantanopia.

unilateral h., loss of sight in one-half of the visual field of one eye only. SYN uniocular h.

unilocular h., SYN unilateral h.

hem·i·a·nop·ic (hem′ē-an-op′ik). Pertaining to hemianopia.

hem·i·a·nop·sia (hem′ē-an-op′sē-ă). SYN hemianopia. [hemi- + G. *an-* priv. + *opsis*, vision]

hem·i·an·os·mia (hem′ē-an-oz′mē-ă). Loss of the sense of smell on one side. [hemi- + G. *an-* priv. + *osmē*, smell]

hem·i·a·pla·sia (hem′ē-ă-plā′zē-ă). Absence of one lobe of a bilobed organ; used especially with reference to the thyroid gland. [hemi- + aplasia]

hem·i·a·prax·ia (hem′ē-ă-prak′sē-ă). Apraxia affecting one side of the body.

hem·i·ar·thro·plas·ty (hem-ē-ar′thrō-plas-tē). Arthroplasty in which one joint surface is replaced with artificial material, usually metal.

hem·i·a·sy·ner·gia (hem′ē-ă-sin-er′jē-ă). Asynergia affecting one side of the body.

hem·i·a·tax·ia (hem′ē-ă-tak′sē-ă). Ataxia affecting one side of the body.

hem·i·ath·e·to·sis (hem′ē-ath′ĕ-tō′sis). Athetosis affecting one hand, or one hand and foot, only.

hem·i·at·ro·phy (hem-ē-at′rō-fē). Atrophy of one lateral half of a part or of an organ, as the face or tongue.

  facial h., atrophy, usually progressive, affecting the tissues of one side of the face. SYN facial h. of Romberg, Romberg disease, Romberg syndrome.

  facial h. of Romberg, SYN facial h.

  lingual h., atrophy of one lateral half of the tongue.

hem·i·bal·lism (hem-ē-bal′izm). SYN hemiballismus. [hemi- + G. *ballismos,* jumping about]

hem·i·bal·lis·mus (hem-ē-bal-iz′mŭs). Ballism involving one side of the body. SYN hemiballism. [hemi- + G. *ballismos,* jumping about]

hem·i·block (hem′ē-blok). SYN divisional *block.*

he·mic (hē′mik). SYN hematic (1).

hem·i·car·dia (hem-ē-kar′dē-ă). **1.** Either lateral half, including atrium and ventricle, of the heart. **2.** A congenital malformation of the heart in which only two of the usual four chambers are formed. [hemi- + G. *kardia,* heart]

  h. dex′tra, right side of the heart.

  h. sinis′tra, left side of the heart.

hem·i·cel·lu·lose (hem-ē-sel′ū-lōs). Plant cell-wall polysaccharides closely associated with cellulose, such as xylans, mannans, and galactans. SYN cellulosan.

hem·i·cen·trum (hem′ē-sen′trŭm). One of the two lateral halves of the body of the vertebra. [hemi- + G. *kentron,* center]

hem·i·ceph·a·lal·gia (hem′ē-sef′ă-lal′jē-ă). The unilateral headache characteristic of typical migraine. SYN hemicrania (2). [hemi- + G. *kephalē,* head, + *algos,* pain]

hem·i·ce·pha·lia (hem-ē-se-fā′lē-ă). Congenital failure of the cerebrum to develop normally; usually the cerebellum and basal ganglia are represented at least in rudimentary form. SYN partial anencephaly. [hemi- + G. *kephalē,* head]

hem·i·cer·e·brum (hem′ē-ser′ĕ-brŭm). A cerebral hemisphere.

hem·i·cho·lin·i·um (hem′ē-kō-lin′ē-ŭm). A chemical which interferes with the synthesis of acetylcholine in cholinergic nerve terminals.

Hem·i·chor·da (hem-ē-kōr′dă). SYN Hemichordata.

Hem·i·chor·da·ta (hem-ē-kōr-dā′tă). A phylum composed of soft-bodied, bilaterally symmetric wormlike marine animals with gill-slits to the pharynx and a conical proboscis; a ciliated larval stage resembles that of echinoderms. SYN Hemichorda. [hemi- + Mod. L. *chordata,* having a notochord, fr. G. *chordē,* string]

hem·i·cho·rea (hem′ē-kōr-ē′ă). Chorea involving the muscles on one side only. SYN hemilateral chorea.

hem·i·col·ec·to·my (hem′ē-kō-lek′tō-mē). Removal of the right or left side of the colon. [hemi- + G. *kolon,* colon, + *ektomē,* excision]

hem·i·cor·po·rec·to·my (hem′ē-kōr-pō-rek′tō-mē). Surgical removal of the lower half of the body, including the lower extremities, bony pelvis, genitalia, and various of the pelvic contents including the lower part of the rectum and the anus. [hemi- + L. *corpus,* body, + G. *ektomē,* excision]

hem·i·cra·nia (hem-ē-krā′nē-ă). **1.** SYN migraine. **2.** SYN hemicephalalgia. [hemi- + G. *kranion,* skull]

hem·i·cra·ni·ec·to·my (hem′ē-krā-nē-ek′tōmē). SYN hemicraniotomy. [hemi- + G. *kranion,* skull, + *ektomē,* excision]

hem·i·cra·ni·o·sis (hem′ē-krā-nē-ō′sis). Enlargement of one side of the cranium.

hem·i·cra·ni·ot·o·my (hem′ē-krā-nē-ot′ō-mē). Separation and reflection of the greater part or all of one half of the cranium, as a preliminary to an operation upon the brain. SYN hemicraniectomy. [hemi- + G. *kranion,* skull, + *tomē,* cut]

hem·i·des·mo·somes (hem-ē-des′mō-sōmz). Half desmosomes that occur on the basal surface of the stratum basalis of stratified squamous epithelium.

hem·i·di·a·pho·re·sis (hem′ē-dī-ă-fō-rē′sis). Diaphoresis, or sweating, on one side of the body. SYN hemidrosis, hemihidrosis.

hem·i·dro·sis (hem-i-drō′sis). SYN hemidiaphoresis.

hem·i·dys·es·the·sia (hem′ē-dis-es-thē′-zē-ă). Dysesthesia affecting one side of the body.

hem·i·dys·tro·phy (hem-ē-dis′trō-fē). Underdevelopment of one lateral half of the body. [hemi- + G. *dys-,* ill, + *trophē,* nourishment, growth]

hem·i·ec·tro·me·lia (hem′ē-ek-trō-mē′lē-ă). Defective development of the limbs on one side of the body. [hemi- + ectromelia]

hem·i·fa·cial (hem-ē-fā′shăl). Pertaining to one side of the face.

hem·i·gas·trec·to·my (hem′ē-gas-trek-tō-mē). Excision of the distal one-half of the stomach.

hem·i·geu·sia (hem′ē-goo′sē-ă). SYN hemiageusia.

hem·i·glos·sal (hem′ē-glos′ăl). SYN hemilingual. [hemi- + G. *glōssa,* tongue]

hem·i·glos·sec·to·my (hem-ē-glos-ek′tō-mē). Surgical removal of one-half of the tongue. [hemi- + G. *glōssa,* tongue, + *ektomē,* excision]

hem·i·glos·si·tis (hem′ē-glos-ī′tis). A vesicular eruption on one side of the tongue and the corresponding inner surface of the cheek, probably herpetic. [hemi- + G. *glōssa,* tongue, + -*itis,* inflammation]

hem·i·gna·thia (hem-ē-nath′ē-ă). Defective development of one side of the mandible. [hemi- + G. *gnathos,* jaw]

hem·i·hep·a·tec·to·my (hem′ē-hep-ă-tek′tō-mē). Surgical removal of one-half or a lobe of the liver.

hem·i·hi·dro·sis (hem′ē-hī-drō′sis). SYN hemidiaphoresis.

hem·i·hy·dran·en·ceph·a·ly (hem-ē-hī′dran-en-sef′ă-lē). A unilateral form of hydranencephaly.

hem·i·hyp·al·ge·sia (hem′ē-hī-pal-je′zē-ă). Hypalgesia affecting one side of the body.

hem·i·hy·per·es·the·sia (hem′ē-hī′per-es-thē′zē-ă). Hyperesthesia, or increased tactile and painful sensibility, affecting one side of the body.

hem·i·hy·per·hi·dro·sis (hem′ē-hī-per-hī-drō′sis). Excessive sweating confined to one side of the body. [hemi- + G. *hyper,* over, + *hidrōsis,* sweating]

hem·i·hy·per·to·nia (hem′ē-hī-per-tō′nē-ă). Exaggerated muscular tonicity on one side of the body. [hemi- + G. *hyper,* over, + *tonos,* tone]

hem·i·hy·per·tro·phy (hem′ē-hī-per′trō-fē). Muscular or osseous hypertrophy of one side of the face or body.

hem·i·hyp·es·the·sia (hem′ē-hī-pes-thē′zē-ă). Diminished sensibility in one side of the body. SYN hemihypoesthesia. [hemi- + G. *hypo,* under, + *aesthēses,* sensation]

hem·i·hy·po·es·the·sia (hem′ē-hī-pō-es-thē′zē-ă). SYN hemihypesthesia. [hemi- + G. *hypo,* under, + *aisthēses,* sensation]

hem·i·hy·po·to·nia (hem′ē-hī-pō-tō′nē-ă). Partial loss of muscular tonicity on one side of the body. [hemi- + G. *hypo,* under, + *tonos,* tone]

hem·i·kar·y·on (hem-i-kar′i-on). A cell nucleus containing a haploid set of chromosomes. [hemi- + G. *karyon,* nut (nucleus)]

hem·i·ke·tal (hem′ē-kē-tăl). RC(R′)(OH)OR″, a product of the addition of an alcohol to a ketone. In the ketose sugars, the h. formation is from an attack by an internal OH on the ketone carbonyl leading to intramolecular cyclization (furanose or pyranose); the h. forms of the sugars are involved in polysaccharide formation, as glycosyls or glycosides. SEE ALSO hemiacetal, ketal.

hem·i·lam·i·nec·to·my (hem′ē-lam-i-nek′tō-mē). Removal of a portion of a vertebral lamina, usually performed for exploration of, access to, or decompression of the intraspinal contents. [hemi- + L. *lamina,* layer, + G. *ektomē,* excision]

hem·i·lar·yn·gec·to·my (hem′ē-lar-in-jek′tō-mē). Excision of one lateral half of the larynx. [hemi- + G. *larnyx (laryng-),* larynx, + *ektomē,* excision]

hem·i·lat·er·al (hem-ē-lat′er-ăl). Relating to one lateral half.

hem·i·le·sion (hem-ē-lē′zhŭn). A unilateral lesion.

hem·i·lin·gual (hem-ē-ling′gwăl). Relating to one lateral half of the tongue. SYN hemiglossal. [hemi- + L. *lingua,* tongue]

hem·i·mac·ro·glos·sia (hem′ē-mak′rō-glos′ē-ă). Enlargement of half the tongue. [hemi- + G. *makros,* large, + *glōssa,* tongue]

hem·i·man·dib·u·lec·to·my (hem'ē-man-dib'ū-lek'tō-mē). Resection of one-half of the mandible.

hemimelia (hem-ē-mēl'ē-ă). Congenital partial absence of a part of an extremity; for example, absence of the fibula and presence of the tibia. [hemi- + G. *melos,*limb, + -ia]

hem·i·me·tab·o·lous (hem'ē-me-tab'ŏ-lŭs). Pertaining to a member of the series of insect orders, the Hemimetabola, in which simple or incomplete metamorphosis is found. [hemi- + G. *metabolē,* change]

he·min (hēm'in). **1.** Chloride of heme in which Fe^{2+} has become Fe^{3+}. H. crystals are called Teichmann *crystals,* under *crystal.* **2.** Any coordination complex of chloro(porphyrinato)iron(III). SYN chlorohemin, factor X for *Haemophilus,* ferriheme chloride, ferriporphyrin chloride, ferriprotoporphyrin, hematin chloride.

hem·i·o·pal·gia (hem'ē-ō-pal'jē-ă). Pain in one eye, usually accompanied by hemicrania. [hemi- + G. *ōps,* eye, + *algos,* pain]

hem·ip·a·gus (hem-ip'ă-gŭs). Conjoined twins that are united laterally at the thorax; the zone of union may also involve the neck and jaws. SEE conjoined *twins,* under *twin.* [hemi- + G. *pagos,* something fixed]

hem·i·pan·cre·at·ec·to·my (hem'ē-pan'-krē-ă- tek'tō-mē). Surgical resection of half of the pancreas.

hem·i·pa·re·sis (hem-ē-pa-rē'sis, -par'ē-sis). Weakness affecting one side of the body.

hem·i·pel·vec·to·my (hem'ē-pel-vek'tō-mē). Amputation of an entire lower extremity together with a portion of the ipsilateral pelvis. SYN hindquarter amputation, Jaboulay amputation. [hemi- + L. *pelvis,* basin (pelvis), + G. *ektomē,* excision]

hem·i·ple·gia (hem-ē-plē'jē-ă). Paralysis of one side of the body. [hemi- + G. *plēgē,* a stroke]
  alternating h., h. on one side with contralateral cranial nerve palsies. SYN crossed h., crossed paralysis.
  contralateral h., paralysis occurring on the side opposite to the causal central lesion.
  crossed h., SYN alternating h.
  double h., SYN diplegia.
  facial h., paralysis of one side of the face, the muscles of the extremities being unaffected.
  infantile h., acute hemiparesis that occurs in infancy and is usually caused by a vascular accident such as cerebral infarction or thrombosis; frequently associated with seizures.
  spastic h., a h. with increased tone in the antigravity muscles of the affected side.

hem·i·ple·gic (hem-ē-plē'jik). Relating to hemiplegia.

He·mip·ter·a (hem-ip'ter-ă). An arthropod order of the class Insecta that includes many plant lice and other true bugs; those of the subfamily Triatominae are bloodsuckers and of medical importance. The best known species is *Cimex lectularius,* the common bedbug. [hemi- + G. *pteron,* wing]

hem·i·sec·tion (hem-ē-sek'shŭn). Surgical removal of a root and its related coronal portion of a multirooted tooth.

hem·i·sen·so·ry (hem'ē-sen'sōr-ē). Loss of sensation on one side of the body. Cf. hemianesthesia.

hem·i·sep·tum (hem-ē-sep'tŭm). A lateral half of any septum.

hem·i·spasm (hem'ē-spazm). A spasm affecting one or more muscles of one side of the face or body.

hem·i·sphere (hem'i-sfēr) [TA]. Half of a spherical structure. SYN cerebral h. (1) [TA]. [hemi- + G. *sphaira,* ball, globe]
  h. of bulb of penis, one of the lateral halves of the bulb of the penis that are separated by a median groove on the posterior part of the undersurface. SYN hemispherium bulbi urethrae.
  h. of cerebellum, SYN h. of cerebellum HII–HX.
  h. of cerebellum HII–HX, the large part of the cerebellum lateral to the vermis cerebelli. SYN hemispherium cerebelli [HII–HX] [TA], hemispherium (2) [TA], h. of cerebellum, hemisphericum cerebelli HII–HX, hemisphericum.
  cerebral h. [TA], **(1)** SYN hemisphere; **(2)** the large mass of the telencephalon, on either side of the midline, consisting of the cerebral cortex and its associated fiber systems, together with the deeper-lying subcortical telencephalic nuclei (i.e., basal ganglia

[nuclei]). SYN hemispherium cerebri [TA], hemispherium (1) [TA].
  dominant h., that cerebral hemisphere containing the representation of speech and controlling the arm and leg used preferentially in skilled movements; usually the left hemisphere.

hem·i·spher·ec·to·my (hem'ē-sfēr-ek'tō-mē). Excision of one cerebral hemisphere; undertaken for malignant tumors, intractable epilepsy usually associated with infantile hemiplegia due to birth injury, and other cerebral conditions.

hem·i·spher·i·cum. SYN *hemisphere* of cerebellum HII–HX.
  hemisphericum cerebelli HII–HX, SYN *hemisphere* of cerebellum HII–HX.

hem·i·sphe·ri·um (hem'i-sfēr'ē-ŭm) [TA]. **1.** SYN cerebral *hemisphere.* **2.** SYN *hemisphere* of cerebellum HII–HX. [G. *hemisphairion*]
  h. bul'bi ure'thrae, SYN *hemisphere* of bulb of penis.
  h. cerebel'li [HII–HX] [TA], SYN *hemisphere* of cerebellum HII–HX.
  h. cer'ebri [TA], SYN cerebral *hemisphere.*

Hem·i·spo·ra (hem'ē-spō'ră). Generic name for certain species of *Fungi Imperfecti* in which chains of conidia develop from tubular structures that form as the result of a constriction at the end of each of a series of short hyphal branches; close septations divide the contents of the tube into relatively square, thick-walled, deeply staining segments that eventually separate and become rounded, thick-walled spores with rough surfaces. *H.* organisms occur fairly frequently as contaminants in cultures for other fungi; they are usually regarded as nonpathogenic forms, but there are a few reported instances in which they were apparently the causal agents of disease. [hemi- + G. *sporos,* seed]

hem·i·stru·mec·to·my (hem'ē-stroo-mek'tō-mē). Rarely used term for excision of approximately one-half of a goiter. [hemi- + L. *struma,* + G. *ektomē,* excision]

hem·i·sub·stance (hem'ē-sŭb'stans). An amorphous substance found in cell walls.

hem·i·syn·drome (hem'ē-sin-drōm). **1.** A condition in which one-half of the body is atrophied or hypertrophied. **2.** Unilateral lesion of the spinal cord.

hem·i·ter·pene (hem-ē-ter'pēn). Isoprene or a derivative of a single isoprene.

hem·i·ther·mo·an·es·the·sia (hem'ē-ther'mō-an-es-thē'zē-ă). Loss of sensibility to heat and cold affecting one side of the body.

hem·i·tho·rax (hem-ē-thō'raks). One side of the thorax.

hem·i·trem·or (hem'ē-trem'er, -trē'mer). Tremor affecting the muscles of one side of the body.

hem·i·trun·cus (hem'ē-trunk'us). A variant truncus arteriosus in which only one pulmonary artery originates from the truncal artery.

hem·i·ver·te·bra (hem-ē-ver'tĕ-bră). A congenital defect of the spine in which one side of a vertebra fails to develop completely.

hem·i·zy·gos·i·ty (hem'i-zī-gos'i-tē). The state of being hemizygous.

hem·i·zy·gote (hem-i-zī'gōt). An individual hemizygous with respect to one or more specified loci; e.g., a normal male is a h. with respect to the gene for all X-linked or Y-linked genes in his genome. [hemi- + G. *zygōtos,* yoked]

hem·i·zy·got·ic (hem'i-zī-got'ik). SYN hemizygous.

hem·i·zy·gous (hem-i-zī'gŭs). Having unpaired genes in an otherwise diploid cell; males are normally h. for genes on both sex chromosomes. SYN hemizygotic.

hem·lock (hem'lok). SYN conium.

△**hemo-.** Combining form denoting blood. SEE ALSO hem-, hemat-, hemato-. [G. *haima*]

he·mo·ag·glu·ti·na·tion (hē'mō-ă-gloo'ti-nā'shŭn). SYN hemagglutination.

he·mo·ag·glu·ti·nin (hē'mō-ă-gloo'ti-nin). SYN hemagglutinin.

he·mo·an·ti·tox·in (hē'mō-an-ti-tok'sin). An antibody that neutralizes the effects of a hemotoxin, such as the hemolytic material in cobra venom.

he·mo·bil·ia (hē-mō-bil'ē-ă). Bleeding into the biliary passages, usually as a result of hepatic trauma or a neoplasm in the liver or biliary tract. SYN hematobilia.

he·mo·blast (hēm′ō-blast). SYN hemocytoblast.

lymphoid h. of Pappenheim, obsolete term for pronormoblast. SEE ALSO erythroblast.

he·mo·blas·to·sis (hē′mō-blas-tō′sis). A proliferative condition of the hematopoietic tissues in general.

he·mo·ca·thar·sis (hē′mō-kă-thar′sis). Cleansing the blood. [hemo- + G. *katharsis,* a cleansing]

he·mo·cath·e·re·sis (hē′mō-kath-e-rē′sis). Destruction of the blood cells, especially of erythrocytes (hemocytocatheresis). [hemo- + G. *kathairesis,* destruction]

he·mo·cath·e·re·tic (hē′mō-kath-ĕ-ret′ik). Pertaining to or characterized by hemocatheresis.

he·mo·cele (hē′mō-sēl). The system of blood-containing spaces pervading the body in arthropods. [hemo- + G. *koilōma,* cavity]

he·mo·cho·le·cys·ti·tis (hē′mō-kō′lē-sis-tī′tis). Hemorrhagic cholecystitis.

he·mo·chro·ma·to·sis (hē′mō-krō-mă-tō′sis). A disorder of iron metabolism characterized by excessive absorption of ingested iron, saturation of iron-binding protein, and deposition of hemosiderin in tissue, particularly in the liver, pancreas, and skin; cirrhosis of the liver, diabetes (bronze diabetes), bronze pigmentation of the skin, and, eventually heart failure may occur; also can result from administration of large amounts of iron orally, by injection, or in forms of blood transfusion therapy. [hemo- + G. *chrōma,* color, + *-osis,* condition]

exogenous h., hemosiderosis due to repeated blood transfusions; it can progress to pigmentary cirrhosis.

primary h. [MIM*235200], a specific inherited metabolic defect with increased absorption and accumulation of iron on a normal diet; autosomal recessive inheritance caused by a mutation in the hemochromatosis gene (HFE) on 6p, less florid in females; juvenile h. may represent a homozygous state of the same gene.

secondary h., increased intake and accumulation of iron secondary to known cause, such as oral iron therapy or multiple transfusions.

he·mo·chrome (hē′mō-krōm). SYN hemochromogen.

he·mo·chro·mo·gen (hē-mō-krō′mō-jen). Term originally used for combinations of ferro- or ferriporphyrins with 2 mol of a nitrogenous base or protein, e.g., pyridine ferroporphyrin. SYN hemochrome. [hemo- + G. *chrōma,* color, + *-gen,* producing]

he·moc·la·sis, he·mo·cla·sia (hē-mok′lă-sis, hē′mō-klā′zē-ă). Rupture, dissolution (hemolysis), or other type of destruction of red blood cells. [hemo- + G. *klasis,* a breaking]

he·mo·clas·tic (hē′mō-klas′tik). Pertaining to hemoclasis.

he·mo·con·cen·tra·tion (hē′mō-kon-sen-trā′shŭn). Decrease in the volume of plasma in relation to the number of red blood cells; increase in the concentration of red blood cells in the circulating blood.

he·mo·co·nia (hē-mō-kō′nē-ă). An obsolete term for small refractive particles in the circulating blood, probably lipid material associated with fragmented stroma from red blood cells. SYN blood dust, blood motes, dust corpuscles. [hemo- + G. *konis,* dust]

he·mo·co·ni·o·sis (hē′mō-kō-nē-ō′sis). A condition in which there is an abnormal amount of hemoconia in the blood.

he·mo·cry·os·co·py (hē′mō-krī-os′kŏ-pē). Determination of the freezing point of blood. [hemo- + G. *kryos,* cold, + *skopeō,* to examine]

he·mo·cu·pre·in (hē-mō-koo′prē-in). SYN cytocuprein.

he·mo·cy·a·nin (hē-mō-sī′ă-nin). An oxygen-carrying pigment (molecular weights between 0.45 and 13×10^6) of lower sea animals (including molluscs and crustacea) and arthropods; copper is an essential component, but it contains no heme; used as an experimental antigen.

he·mo·cyte (hē′mō-sīt). Any cell or formed element of the blood. SYN hematocyte. [hemo- + G. *kytos,* a hollow (cell)]

he·mo·cy·to·blast (hē′mō-sī′tō-blast). A blood cell derived from embryonic mesenchyme, characterized by basophilic cytoplasm and a relatively large nucleus with a spongy, loose network of chromatin and several nucleoli; mitochondria are extremely fine and delicate. H.'s represent the primitive stem cells of the monophyletic theory of the origin of blood and have the potentiality of developing into erythroblasts, young forms of the granulocytic series, megakaryocytes, etc. SYN hematocytoblast, hemoblast. [hemo- + G. *kytos,* cell, + *blastos,* germ]

he·mo·cy·to·ca·ther·e·sis (hē′mō-sī′tō-kă-ther′ē-sis). Hemolysis, or other type of destruction of red blood cells. [hemo- + G. *kytos,* a hollow (cell), + *kathairesis,* destruction]

he·mo·cy·tol·y·sis (hē′mō-sī-tol′i-sis). The dissolution of blood cells, including hemolysis. SYN hematocytolysis. [hemo- + G. *kytos,* cell, + *lysis,* dissolution]

he·mo·cy·tom·e·ter (hē′mō-sī-tom′ě-ter). An apparatus for estimating the number of blood cells in a quantitatively measured volume of blood; it consists of a glass pipette with an ampulla for collecting and diluting the blood, and a counting chamber marked in squares. SYN hemacytometer, hematimeter, hematocytometer. [hemo- + G. *kytos,* cell, + *metron,* measure]

he·mo·cy·tom·e·try (hē′mō-sī-tom′ě-trē). The counting of red blood cells.

he·mo·cy·to·trip·sis (hē′mō-sī-tō-trip′sis). Fragmentation or disintegration of blood cells by means of mechanical trauma, e.g., compression between hard surfaces. [hemo- + G. *kytos,* + *tripsis,* a grinding]

he·mo·cy·to·zo·on (hē′mō-sī-tō-zō′on). A protozoon parasite of the blood cells. SYN hemacytozoon, hematocytozoon. [hemo- + G. *kytos,* cell, + *zōon,* animal]

he·mo·di·ag·no·sis (hē′mō-dī-ag-nō′sis). Diagnosis by means of examination of the blood.

🔲 **he·mo·di·al·y·sis** (hē′mō-dī-al′i-sis). Dialysis of soluble substances and water from the blood by diffusion through a semipermeable membrane; separation of cellular elements and colloids from soluble substances is achieved by pore size in the membrane and rates of diffusion.

he·mo·di·a·lyz·er (hē-mō-dī′ă-lī-zer). A machine for hemodialysis in acute or chronic renal failure; toxic substances in the blood are removed by exposure to dialyzing fluid across a semipermeable membrane. SYN artificial kidney.

ultrafiltration h., a h. that uses fluid pressure differentials to bring about loss (usually) of protein-free fluid from the blood to the bath.

he·mo·di·a·stase (hē-mō-dī′as-tās). Blood amylase.

he·mo·di·lu·tion (hē′mō-di-loo′shŭn). Increase in the volume of plasma in relation to red blood cells; reduced concentration of red blood cells in the circulation.

he·mo·dy·nam·ic (hē′mō-dī-nam′ik). Relating to the physical aspects of the blood circulation.

he·mo·dy·nam·ics (hē′mō-dī-nam′iks). The study of the dynamics of the blood circulation. [hemo- + G. *dynamis,* power]

he·mo·dys·cra·sia (hē′mō-dis-krā′zē-ă). Any abnormal condition or disorder of the blood and hemopoietic tissue, used especially with reference to those resulting in changes in the formed elements. SYN hematodyscrasia. [hemo- + G. *dyscrasia,* bad temperament]

he·mo·dys·tro·phy (hē-mō-dis′trō-fē). Any disease or abnormal condition of the blood and hemopoietic tissues, exclusive of simple transitory changes. SYN hematodystrophy.

he·mo·fil·tra·tion (hē′mō-fil-trā′shŭn). A process, similar to hemodialysis, by which blood is dialyzed using ultrafiltration, and usually to remove a specific product of fluid volume.

he·mo·flag·el·lates (hē-mō-flaj′ě-lāts). Protozoan flagellates in the family Trypanosomatidae that are parasitic in the blood of many species of domestic and wild animals and birds, and of humans; they include the genera *Leishmania* and *Trypanosoma,* several species of which are important pathogens. [hemo- + L. *flagellum,* dim. of *flagrum,* a whip]

he·mo·fus·cin (hē-mō-fŭs′in). A brown pigment derived from hemoglobin that occurs in urine occasionally along with hemosiderin, usually indicative of increased red blood cell destruction; occurs also in the liver with hemosiderin in cases of hemochromatosis.

he

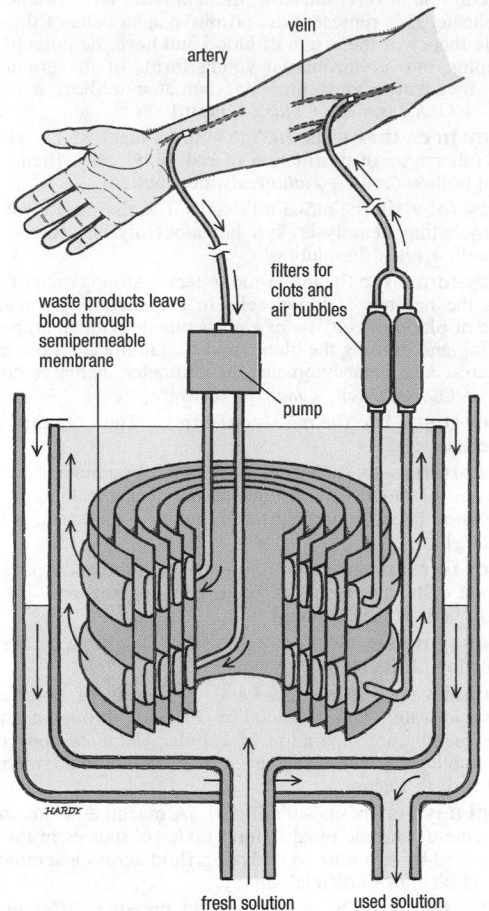

waste products leave blood through semipermeable membrane

artery
vein

filters for clots and air bubbles

pump

HARDY

fresh solution   used solution

hemodialysis

he·mo·gen·e·sis (hē-mō-jen′ĕ-sis). SYN hemopoiesis.
he·mo·gen·ic (hē-mō-jen′ik). SYN hemopoietic.

HEMOGLOBIN

▣**he·mo·glo·bin (Hb)** (hē-mō-glō′bin) [MIM*141800–142310]. The red respiratory protein of erythrocytes, consisting of approximately 3.8% heme and 96.2% globin, with a molecular weight of 64,450, which as oxyhemoglobin (HbO_2) transports oxygen from the lungs to the tissues where the oxygen is readily released and HbO_2 becomes Hb. When Hb is exposed to certain chemicals, its normal respiratory function is blocked; e.g., the oxygen in HbO_2 is easily displaced by carbon monoxide, thereby resulting in the formation of fairly stable carboxyhemoglobin (HbCO), as in asphyxiation resulting from inhalation of exhaust fumes from gasoline engines. When the iron in Hb is oxidized from the ferrous to ferric state, as in poisoning with nitrates and certain other chemicals, a nonrespiratory compound, methemoglobin (MetHb), is formed.

In humans there are at least five kinds of normal Hb: two embryonic Hb's (Hb Gower-1, Hb Gower-2), fetal (Hb F), and two adult types (Hb A, Hb A_2). There are two α globin chains containing 141 amino acid residues, and two of another kind (β, γ, δ, ϵ, or ζ), each containing 146 amino acid residues in four of the Hb's. Hb Gower-1 has two ζ chains and two ϵ chains. The

production of each kind of globin chain is controlled by a structural gene of similar Greek letter designation; normal individuals are homozygous for the normal allele at each locus. Substitution of one amino acid for another in the polypeptide chain can occur at any codon in any of the five loci and have resulted in the production of many hundreds of abnormal Hb types, most of no known clinical significance. In addition, deletions of one or more amino acid residues are known, as well as gene rearrangements due to unequal crossing over between homologous chromosomes.

The Hb types below are the main abnormal types known to be of clinical significance. Newly discovered abnormal Hb types are first assigned a name, usually the location where discovered, and a molecular formula is added when determined. The formula consists of Greek letters to designate the basic chains, with subscript 2 if there are two identical chains; a superscript letter (^{A} if normal for adult Hb, etc.) is added, or the superscript may designate the site of amino acid substitution (numbering amino acid residues from the N-terminus of the polypeptide) and specifying the change, using standard abbreviations for the amino acids. There is an exhaustive listing of variant h.'s in MIM where a composite numbering system is used.

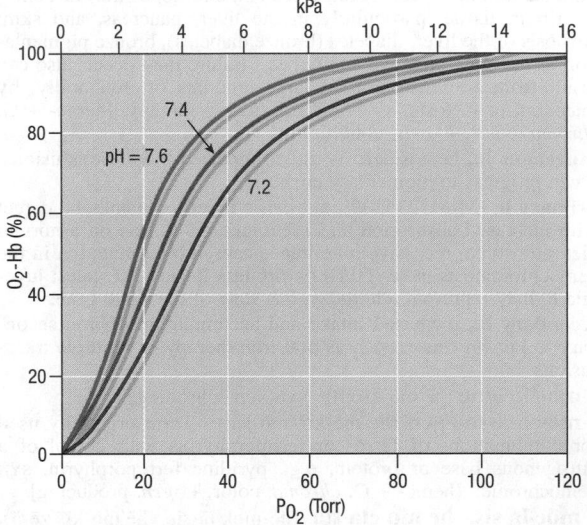

oxygen dissociation curves of hemoglobin: *ordinates,* oxygen saturation; *abscissae,* oxygen pressure of alveolar air

h. A [MIM*141800], normal adult Hb (Hb A) with formula $\alpha_2^A\beta_2^A$ or $\alpha_2\beta_2$.

h. A_2 [MIM*141850], the normal Hb (Hb A_2) of the formula $\alpha_2^A\delta_2$ or $\alpha_2\delta_2$, which makes up approximately 2.5% of the total adult h. concentration. At least 18 mutant variants of the δ chain have been reported.

h. A_{Ic}, the major fraction of glycosylated h.

aberrant h., a mutant Hb that functions abnormally. Cf. variant h.

h. anti-Lepore, a group of abnormal h.'s similar to h. Lepore. These h.'s have normal α chains, but the non-α chain consists of the N-terminal portion of the β chain joined to the C-terminal portion of the δ chain. This is the opposite crossing over pattern observed in h. Lepore. Examples of h. anti-Lepore include Hb_{Miyada}, Hb P_{Congo}, Hb $P_{Nilotic}$, and $Hb_{Lincoln Park}$. There is also one variant that is both h. Lepore and h. anti-Lepore ($Hb_{Parchman}$). Cf. h. Lepore.

h. Bart [MIM*142309], a Hb homotetramer (all four polypeptides identical) of formula γ_4, found in the early embryo and in α-thalassemia 2; not effective in oxygen transport; does not display a Bohr effect.

bile pigment h., SYN choleglobin.

h. C [MIM*141900.0038], an abnormal Hb with substitution of lysyl residue for glutamyl at the 6th position of the β chain, of formula $\alpha_2 2^A\beta_2^{6Glu\rightarrow Lys}$, this type reduces the normal plasticity of erythrocytes. Heterozygotes: Hb C trait, about 28–44% of total Hb is Hb C, no anemia. Homozygotes: nearly all Hb is Hb C, moderate normocytic hemolytic anemia. Individuals heterozygous for both Hb C and Hb S (Hb SC disease) and for Hb C and thalassemia are known, and have atypical hemolytic anemias; sickling is enhanced in Hb SC disease.

h. C$_{Georgetown}$, h. C$_{Harlem}$ [MIM*141900.0039], two abnormal Hb's, both with the substitution of a valyl residue for a glutamyl residue at the 6th position of the β chain as in Hb S, and in addition, each has a second substitution of an asparaginyl residue for an aspartyl residue at position 73 of the β chain; both types cause sickling of erythrocytes similar to Hb S.

carbon monoxide h., SYN carboxyhemoglobin.

h. Chesapeake (Hb$_{Chesapeake}$) [MIM*141800.0018], an abnormal hemoglobin with a single α chain substitution, molecular formula $\alpha_2^{92Arg\rightarrow Leu}\beta_2^A$; heterozygotes have polycythemia, apparently to compensate for the increased oxygen affinity of this Hb, resulting in decreased liberation of oxygen in the tissues.

h. Constant Spring, an abnormal hemoglobin having an extended polypeptide chain (31 additional amino acyl residues) on the α chain (thus, the α chain is 172 amino acids long); approximately 20% of the individuals with Hb H disease also have this defect.

h. D$_{Punjab}$ [MIM*141900.0065], an abnormal Hb with a single β chain substitution, molecular formula $\alpha_2^A\beta_2^{121Glu\rightarrow Gln}$; heterozygotes are asymptomatic, homozygotes have mild hemolytic anemia; there is an increase in O_2 affinity; identical to h. D$_{Los\ Angeles}$, h. D$_{North\ Carolina}$, h. D$_{Portugal}$, h. D$_{Chicago}$, and h. Oak Ridge.

h. E [MIM*141900.0071], an abnormal Hb with a single β chain substitution, molecular formula $\alpha_2^A\beta_2^{26Glu\rightarrow Lys}$, common in Southeast Asia, especially Thailand; heterozygotes are asymptomatic with 35–45% Hb E; homozygotes have mild to moderate hemolytic anemia with 90–100% Hb E and the remainder Hb F.

embryonic h., SEE h. Gower-1, h. Gower-2.

h. F [MIM*142200], normal fetal Hb (Hb F) of molecular formula $\alpha_2^A\gamma_2^F$, which is the major Hb component during intrauterine life, decreasing rapidly during infancy to reach a concentration of less than 0.5% in normal children and adults; the concentration of Hb F is increased in some hemoglobinopathies and in some cases of hypoplastic anemia, pernicious anemia, and leukemia; Hb F has a weaker affinity for 2,3-bisphosphoglycerate than does Hb A. More than 50 mutant variants of the γ chain have been reported. SYN fetal h.

fetal h., SYN h. F.

h. F (hereditary persistence of) [MIM*142200.0026], a condition due to an allele that depresses synthesis of β and δ chains (as in thalassemia), but this is fully compensated by increased γ chain synthesis and there is no anemia; there are 3 types: 1) African type, no β or δ chain synthesis by the chromosome with the abnormal gene, heterozygotes have 20–30% Hb F and Hb A$_2$ slightly decreased, homozygotes form no Hb A or Hb A$_2$; 2) Greek type, reduced β and δ chain synthesis, heterozygotes have 10–20% Hb F and normal Hb A$_2$; 3) Swiss type, heterozygotes have only 1 to 3% Hb F and normal Hb A$_2$.

glycosylated h., any one of four h. A fractions (A$_{Ia1}$, A$_{Ia2}$, A$_{Ib}$, or A$_{Ic}$) to which D-glucose and related monosaccharides are covalently linked; concentrations are increased in the erythrocytes of patients with diabetes mellitus and can be used as a retrospective index of glucose control over time in such patients.

h. Gower-1, a Hb of molecular formula $\zeta_2\varepsilon_2$, found as a minor Hb in the early embryo; disappears by the third month of pregnancy in favor of h. Gower-2 and h. Portland and then by Hb F; the ζ chain has 141 amino acid residues. Synthesis of the ζ chain is deficient in cases of hydrops fetalis. Cf. h. Gower-2, h. Portland.

h. Gower-2, a normal Hb of molecular formula $\alpha_2\varepsilon_2$, which is a major Hb component of the early embryo; production of ε chains normally ceases at about the third month of fetal development and is replaced by Hb F. Cf. h. Gower-1, h. Portland.

green h., SYN choleglobin.

h. H [MIM*142309], a homotetramer of Hb (all four polypeptides identical) of molecular formula β_4, found only when α chain synthesis is depressed and not effective in oxygen transport. Hb H disease (α-thalassemia intermedia) is a thalassemialike syndrome in individuals heterozygous for both severe and mild genes for α-

thalassemia; moderate anemia and red cell abnormalities with 25–35% Hb Bart at birth, but with Hb Bart later replaced by Hb H and with Hb A$_2$ decreased. Hb H shows no cooperativity with O_2 binding and does not exhibit a Bohr effect.

h. I [MIM*141800.0055], an abnormal Hb with a single α chain substitution, molecular formula $\alpha_2^{16Lys\rightarrow Glu}\beta_2^A$; a thalassemialike syndrome has been found in persons heterozygous for both Hb I and α-thalassemia genes, with formation of about 70% Hb I.

h. J$_{Capetown}$ [MIM*141800.0063], an abnormal Hb with a single α chain substitution, molecular formula $\alpha_2^{92Arg\rightarrow Gln}\beta_2^A$; heterozygotes have polycythemia because of increased oxygen affinity of this Hb.

h. Kansas [MIM*141900.0145], an abnormal Hb of molecular formula $\alpha_2^A\beta_2^{102Asn\rightarrow Thr}$; found in association with familial cyanosis due to decreased oxygen affinity of this Hb.

h. Lepore [MIM 142000-various], a group of abnormal Hb's with normal α chains, but the non-α chains consist of the N-terminal portion of the δ chain joined to the C-terminal portion of the β chain, apparently as the result of nonhomologous pairing and crossing over between the genes for β and δ chains. The major types are Hb Lepore$_{Boston}$ (identical to Hb Lepore$_{Washington}$), Hb Lepore$_{Hollandia}$, and Hb Lepore$_{Baltimore}$, which differ in the region of crossing over (δ87–β116, δ22–β50, and δ50–β86, respectively). Heterozygotes form about 10% Hb Lepore, normal amounts of Hb A$_2$, and moderately increased amounts of Hb F and usually have mild anemia, microcytosis, and hypochromia; homozygotes form only Hb Lepore and Hb F and have severe anemia. Cf. h. anti-Lepore.

h. M [MIM*142310 & various], a group of abnormal Hb's in which a single amino acid substitution favors the formation of methemoglobin in spite of normal quantities of methemoglobin reductase. Strictly speaking, Hb's M are h.'s with mutations at the proximal or distal histidyl residues. Other Hb's M tend to favor the Fe(III) state. Heterozygotes have congenital methemoglobinemia; the homozygous state of these genes is unknown and is presumably lethal. Specific types include: Hb M$_{Iwate}$, $\alpha^{87His\rightarrow Tyr}$ (α chain, position 87, histidine replaced by tyrosine); Hb M$_{Hyde\ Park}$, $\beta^{92His\rightarrow Tyr}$; Hb M$_{Boston}$, $\alpha^{58His\rightarrow Tyr}$; Hb M$_{Saskatoon}$, $\beta^{63His\rightarrow Tyr}$; Hb M$_{Milwaukee-1}$, $\beta^{67Val\rightarrow Glu}$.

mean corpuscular h. (MCH), the h. content of the average red cell, calculated from the h. therein and the red cell count, in erythrocyte indices.

muscle h., SYN myoglobin.

oxygenated h., SYN oxyhemoglobin.

h. Portland, a form of embryonic h. containing the ζ chains of h. Gower-1 and the γ chains of Hb F, thus having the formula $\zeta_2\gamma_2$; essentially disappears by the third month of pregnancy. Cf. h. Gower-1, h. Gower-2.

h. Rainier [MIM*141900-0232], an abnormal Hb of the molecular formula $\alpha_2^A\beta_2^{145Tyr\rightarrow Cys}$; heterozygotes have polycythemia because of increased oxygen affinity of this Hb.

reduced h., the form of Hb in red blood cells after the oxygen of oxyhemoglobin is released in the tissues.

h. S [MIM*141900], an abnormal Hb with substitution of valine for glutamic acid at the 6th position of the β chain; the formula is $\alpha_2^A\beta_2^S$, or, more specifically, $\alpha_2^A\beta_2^{6Glu\rightarrow Val}$. Heterozygous state: sickle cell trait, no anemia, Hb S 20–45% of total, the rest Hb A. Homozygous state: sickle cell anemia, Hb S 75–100% of total, the rest Hb F or Hb A$_2$. SYN sickle cell h.

sickle cell h. (Hb S), SYN h. S.

unstable h.'s, a group of rare Hb's with amino acid substitutions (or amino acid deletions in three types) that alter the three-dimensional shape of the globin in a manner that renders the molecule unstable; they have an increased but variable tendency to autooxidation and Heinz body formation and are associated with congenital nonspherocytic hemolytic anemia. The unstable β-chain abnormalities include Hb's Genova, Gun Hill, Hammersmith, Köln, Philly, Sabine, Santa Ana, Sydney, Wien, and Zürich; unstable α-chain abnormalities include Hb's Bibba, Sinai, and Torino.

variant h., a harmless mutant form of Hb.

h. Yakima [MIM*141900-0301], an abnormal Hb of the molecu-

he

lar formula $\alpha_2{}^A\beta_2{}^{99Asp\rightarrow His}$; heterozygotes have polycythemia because of increased oxygen affinity of this Hb.

---

he·mo·glo·bi·ne·mia (hē′mō-glo-bi-nē′mē-ă). The presence of free hemoglobin in the blood plasma, as when intravascular hemolysis occurs.

paroxysmal nocturnal h., an acquired hematopoietic stem cell disorder characterized by formation of defective platelets, granulocytes, erythrocytes, and possibly lymphocytes. The red cell abnormality causes complement-mediated intravascular lysis, which may be expressed in an irregular or even occult manner.

puerperal h., SYN postparturient *hemoglobinuria.*

he·mo·glo·bi·no·cho·lia (hē′mō-glō′bi-nō-kō′lē-ă). The presence of hemoglobin in the bile. [hemoglobin + G. *cholē,* bile]

he·mo·glo·bi·nol·y·sis (hē′mō-glō-bi-nol′i-sis). Destruction or chemical splitting of hemoglobin. SYN hemoglobinopepsia. [hemoglobin + G. *lysis,* dissolution]

he·mo·glo·bi·nop·a·thy (hē′mō-glō-bi-nop′ă-thē). A disorder or disease caused by or associated with the presence of abnormal hemoglobins in the blood, e.g., sickle cell disease, hemoglobin C, D, E, H, or I disorders. Occasionally, combinations of abnormal hemoglobins are seen in hemoglobinopathies. [hemoglobin + G. *pathos,* disease]

he·mo·glo·bi·no·pep·sia (hē-mō-glō′bi-nō-pep′sē-ă). SYN hemoglobinolysis. [hemoglobin + G. *pepsis,* digestion]

he·mo·glo·bi·no·phil·ic (hē′mō-glō′bi-nō-fil′ik). Denoting certain microorganisms that cannot be cultured except in the presence of hemoglobin. [hemoglobin + G. *phileō,* to love]

he·mo·glo·bi·nu·ria (hē′mō-glō-bi-noo′rē-ă). The presence of hemoglobin in the urine, including certain closely related pigments that are formed from slight alteration of the hemoglobin molecule; when present in sufficient quantities, they result in the urine being colored varying shades from light red-yellow to fairly dark red. [hemoglobin + G. *ouron,* urine]

epidemic h., the presence of hemoglobin, or of pigments derived from it, in the urine of young infants, attended with cyanosis, jaundice, and other conditions; may be due to secondary methemoglobinemia; also called Winckel disease.

intermittent h., recurrent episodic attacks of h. characteristic of paroxysmal nocturnal h. or paroxysmal cold h.

malarial h., a condition, now uncommon, resulting from *Plasmodium falciparum* infection (malignant tertian malaria with severe hemolysis); seen in whites after interrupted treatment. SYN blackwater fever, hemoglobinuric fever, West African fever.

march h., a form occurring after marathon races, protracted marching, or heavy physical exercise.

paroxysmal cold h., a rare disorder in which acute severe hemolysis follows exposure to cold.

paroxysmal nocturnal h., an infrequent disorder with insidious onset (usually in the third or fourth decade) and chronic course, characterized by episodes of hemolytic anemia, hemoglobinuria (chiefly at night), pallor, icterus or bronzing of the skin, a moderate degree of splenomegaly, and sometimes hepatomegaly; red blood cells are usually macrocytic and vary considerably in size, but there is no evidence of spherocytosis, erythrophagocytosis, or abnormal leukocytes. The disorder is a result of an abnormality of the red cell membrane which makes the red cell unusually sensitive to lysis by complement. SYN Marchiafava-Micheli anemia, Marchiafava-Micheli syndrome.

postparturient h., a sudden, severe hemolytic disease that appears sporadically in well-nourished dairy cows 2–4 weeks after calving, and usually occurs in stabled animals in the winter and early spring; the cause is not known, although the disease is often associated with hypophosphatemia. SYN puerperal hemoglobinemia.

toxic h., h. occurring after the ingestion of various poisons, in certain blood diseases, and in certain infections.

he·mo·glo·bi·nu·ric (hē′mō-glō-bi-noo′rik). Relating to or marked by hemoglobinuria.

he·mo·gram (hē′mō-gram). A complete detailed record of the findings in a thorough examination of the blood, especially with reference to the numbers, proportions, and morphologic features of the formed elements. [hemo- + G. *gramma,* a drawing]

he·mo·his·ti·o·blast (hē′mō-his′tē-ō-blast). A primitive mesenchymal cell believed to be capable of developing into all types of blood cells, including monocytes, and into histiocytes. SYN Ferrata cell, hematohistioblast. [hemo- + G. *histion,* web, + *blastos,* germ]

he·mo·la·mel·la (hē′mō-lă-mel′ă). Obsolete term for platelet.

he·mo·li·pase (hē-mō-lip′ās). Blood lipase.

he·mo·lith (hē′mō-lith). A concretion in the wall of a blood vessel. [hemo- + G. *lithos,* stone]

he·mol·o·gy (hē-mol′ō-jē). SYN hematology.

he·mo·lymph (hē′mō-limf). **1.** The blood and lymph, in the sense of a "circulating tissue." **2.** The nutrient fluid of certain invertebrates. [hemo- + L. *lympha,* clear water]

he·mol·y·sate (hē-mol′i-sāt). Preparation resulting from the lysis of erythrocytes.

he·mo·ly·sin (hē-mol′i-sin). **1.** Any substance elaborated by a living agent and capable of causing lysis of red blood cells and liberation of their hemoglobin. SYN erythrocytolysin, erythrolysin. **2.** A sensitizing (complement-fixing) antibody that combines with red blood cells of the antigenic type that stimulated formation of the h., a fixing complement with the antibody-cell union resulting in lysis of the cells.

α' **h.,** SEE α' *hemolysis.*

β **h.,** SEE β *hemolysis.*

bacterial h., any hemolytic agent elaborated by various species of bacteria, or by certain strains within a species.

cold h., SYN Donath-Landsteiner cold *autoantibody.*

heterophil h., a sensitizing antibody that can combine with red blood cells of various species (in addition to those used as the antigen in stimulating the formation of the h.), resulting in hemolysis when the proper amount of complement is present.

immune h., a sensitizing, complement-fixing, hemolytic antibody formed in an animal as the result of parenteral administration of red blood cells or whole blood from another species; immune h. may also be formed in human beings who are transfused with human blood that is antigenic in the recipient, e.g., the formation of anti-Rh antibody in an Rh-negative person who is treated with Rh-positive red blood cells.

natural h., h. occurring in the plasma of an animal of one species, e.g., a dog, which fixes complement with the red blood cells of some other species, e.g., a rabbit, thereby causing hemolysis of the cells of the rabbit, although the dog was not previously exposed to antigenic stimulation with such cells.

specific h., a sensitizing, complement-fixing, hemolytic antibody that reacts totally or completely with red blood cells of the antigenic type used to stimulate the formation of the h.

warm-cold h., h. which combines with red blood cells at temperatures below 20°C and are eluted at warmer temperatures, e.g., 30–37°C. SEE Donath-Landsteiner cold *autoantibody*, hemagglutinating cold *autoantibody*.

he·mo·ly·sin·o·gen (hē′mō-lī-sin′ō-jen). The antigenic material in red blood cells that stimulates the formation of hemolysin.

he·mol·y·sis (hē-mol′i-sis). Alteration, dissolution, or destruction of red blood cells in such a manner that hemoglobin is liberated into the medium in which the cells are suspended, e.g., by specific complement-fixing antibodies, toxins, various chemical agents, tonicity, alteration of temperature. SYN erythrocytolysis, erythrolysis, hematolysis. [hemo- + G. *lysis,* destruction]

α' **h.,** h. observed in blood agar cultures of occasional strains of pneumococci or streptococci; the zone of h. about the colony is greenish caused by a partial decomposition of hemoglobin.

β **h.,** complete or "true" h. observed in blood agar cultures of various bacteria, especially hemolytic streptococci and staphylococci; virtually all of the erythrocytes are destroyed in a relatively wide, regularly circumscribed, circular zone about the colony, thereby resulting in a clear "halo" of transparent agar; the zone of h. is frequently much wider than the diameter of the colony; the degree of change varies with species of erythrocytes.

biologic h., h. caused by materials elaborated by various living organisms.

conditioned h., SYN immune h.

γ **h.,** a term sometimes used to indicate that there is no h. in relation to bacterial colonies in or on blood agar; thus, nonhemolytic organisms may be referred to as producing γ h.

immune h., h. caused by complement when erythrocytes have been sensitized by specific complement-fixing antibody. SYN conditioned h.

phenylhydrazine h. (fen′il-hī′-dră-zin), an in vitro test for glucose-6-phosphate dehydrogenase (G6PD) deficiency; h. resulting from in vitro addition of phenylhydrazine to blood with red cells which are deficient in G6PD, with the appearance of Heinz-Ehrlich bodies.

venom h., that caused by hemolytic material in the venom of various species of snakes or other venomous animals.

viridans h., SEE α′ h.

he·mo·lyt·ic (hē-mō-lit′ik). Destructive to blood cells, resulting in liberation of hemoglobin. SYN hematolytic, hemotoxic (2), hematotoxic, hematoxic.

he·mo·ly·za·tion (hē′mol-i-zā′shŭn). The production or occurrence of hemolysis.

he·mo·lyze (hē′mō-līz). To produce hemolysis or liberation of the hemoglobin from red blood cells.

he·mo·me·di·as·ti·num (hē′mō-mē-dē-ă-stī′nŭm). Blood in the mediastinum.

he·mo·me·tra (hē-mō-mē′tră). SYN hematometra.

he·mom·e·try (hē-mom′ĕ-trē). SYN hematometry.

he·mo·pa·thol·o·gy (hē′mō-pa-thol′ō-jē). SYN hematopathology.

he·mop·a·thy (hē-mop′ă-thē). Any abnormal condition or disease of the blood or hemopoietic tissues. SYN hematopathy. [hemo- + G. *pathos,* suffering]

he·mo·per·fu·sion (hē′mō-per-fū′zhŭn). Passage of blood through columns of adsorptive material, such as activated charcoal, to remove toxic substances from the blood. [hemo- + L. *perfusio,* to pass through]

he·mo·per·i·car·di·um (hē′mō-pār′-i-kar′dē-ŭm). Blood in the pericardial sac.

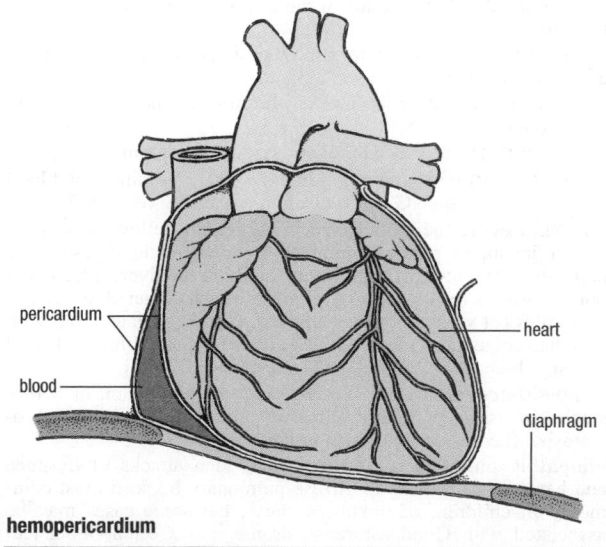

pericardium

blood

heart

diaphragm

hemopericardium

he·mo·per·i·to·ne·um (hē′mō-pār-i-tō-nē′ŭm). Blood in the peritoneal cavity.

he·mo·pex·in (hēm-ō-peks′in). A serum glycoprotein related to β-globulins, with molecular weight around 57,000, containing 22% carbohydrate; important in binding heme and porphyrins, preventing excretion, and perhaps regulating heme in drug metabolism. [hemo- + G. *pēxis,* fixation, + -in]

he·mo·pha·gia (hē-mō-fā′jē-ă). SYN hematophagia. [hemo- + G. *phagein,* to eat]

he·mo·phag·o·cy·to·sis (hē′mō-fag′ō-sī-tō′sis). The process of engulfment (and usually destruction) of blood cells by the various types of phagocytic cells; used especially with reference to the engulfment of erythrocytes and others of the erythroid series.

he·mo·phil, he·mo·phile (hē′mō-fil, -fīl). A microorganism growing preferably in media containing blood. [hemo- + G. *philos,* fond]

he·mo·phil·ia (hē-mō-fil′ē-ă). An inherited disorder of blood coagulation characterized by a permanent tendency to hemorrhages, spontaneous or traumatic, because of a defect in the blood coagulating mechanism. [hemo- + G. *philos,* fond]

h. A [MIM*306700-various], h. due to deficiency of factor VIII; an X-linked recessive condition, occurring almost exclusively in human males and also affecting several breeds of dogs, characterized by prolonged clotting time, decreased formation of thromboplastin, and diminished conversion of prothrombin. SYN classic h.

h. B [MIM*306900-various], a clotting disorder resembling h. A, caused by hereditary deficiency of factor IX; also seen as an X-linked recessive condition in the Cairn terrier breed of dogs. SYN Christmas disease.

h. C, h. due to deficiency of factor XI; clinically resembles h. A and B but is transmitted as an autosomal dominant inheritance; occurs primarily in persons of Jewish ancestry.

classic h., SYN h. A.

he·mo·phil·i·ac (hē-mō-fil′ē-ak). A person suffering from hemophilia.

he·mo·phil·ic (hē-mō-fil′ik). Relating to hemophilia.

he·mo·phil·o·sis (hē-mō-fil-ō′sis). Any disease caused by bacteria of the genus *Haemophilus.*

he·mo·pho·bia (hē-mō-fō′bē-ă). Morbid fear of blood or of bleeding. [hemo- + G. *phobos,* fear]

he·mo·pho·re·sis (hē′mō-fō-rē′sis). Blood convection or irrigation of tissues. [hemo- + G. *phoreō,* to bear]

he·moph·thal·mia, he·moph·thal·mus (hē-mof-thal′mē-ah, -mof-thal′mŭs). A blood-filled eye. SYN hematopsia. [hemo- + G. *ophthalmos,* eye]

he·moph·thi·sis (hē-mof′thi-sis, hē-mof-thī′sis). An obsolete term for anemia resulting from abnormal degeneration or destruction, or a deficiency in the formation of red blood cells. [hemo- + G. *phthisis,* a wasting away]

he·mo·plas·tic (hē-mō-plas′tik). SYN hemopoietic.

he·mo·plas·ty (hē′mō-plas-tē). Formation or elaboration of blood by the hemopoietic tissues. [hemo- + G. *plassō,* to form]

he·mo·pneu·mo·per·i·car·di·um (hē′mō-noo′mō-pār-i-kar′dē-ŭm). Concurrence of blood and air in the pericardium. SYN pneumohemopericardium. [hemo- + G. *pneuma,* air, + pericardium]

he·mo·pneu·mo·tho·rax (hē′mō-noo-mō-thō′raks). Accumulation of air and blood in the pleural cavity. SYN pneumohemothorax. [hemo- + G. *pneuma,* air, + thorax]

he·mo·poi·e·sis (hē′mō-poy-ē′sis). The process of formation and development of the various types of blood cells and other formed elements. SYN hematogenesis, hematopoiesis, hematosis (1), hemogenesis, sanguification. [hemo- + G. *poiēsis,* a making]

he·mo·poi·et·ic (hē′mō-poy-et′ik). Pertaining to or related to the formation of blood cells. SYN hemafacient, hematogenic (1), hematogenous, hematoplastic, hematopoietic, hemogenic, hemoplastic, sanguifacient.

he·mo·poi·e·tin (hē-mō-poy′ĕ-tin). SYN erythropoietin.

he·mo·por·phy·rin (hē-mō-pōr′fi-rin). SYN hematoporphyrin.

he·mo·pre·cip·i·tin (hē′mō-prē-sip′i-tin). An antibody that combines with and precipitates soluble antigenic material from erythrocytes.

he·mo·pro·tein (hē-mō-prō′tēn). Protein linked to a metal-porphyrin compound (e.g., cytochromes, myoglobin, catalase).

he·mop·ty·sis (hē-mop′ti-sis). Spitting of blood derived from the lungs or bronchial tubes as a result of pulmonary or bronchial hemorrhage. SYN bronchostaxis. [hemo- + G. *ptysis,* a spitting]

he

endemic h., SYN parasitic h.

parasitic h., the clinical expression of paragonimiasis, marked by a cough and spitting of blood from the lungs. SYN endemic h.

he·mo·py·el·ec·ta·sis, he·mo·py·el·ec·ta·sia (hē′mō-pī′ĕ-lek′tă-sis, -lek-tā′zē-ă). Obsolete term for dilation of the pelvis of the kidney with blood and urine. [hemo- + pyelectasia]

he·mo·re·pel·lant (hē′mō-rē-pel′ant). **1.** A substance or surface that discourages the adherence of blood. **2.** Having such an action.

he·mo·rhe·ol·o·gy (he′mō-rē-ol′ō-jē). The science of the flow of blood in relation to the pressures, flow, volumes, and resistances in blood vessels, especially in terms of blood viscosity and red cell deformation in the microcirculation. [hemo- + G. *rheos,* stream, flow, + *logos,* study]

hem·or·rhage (hem′ŏ-rij). **1.** An escape of blood from the intravascular space. **2.** To bleed. [G. *haimorrhagia,* fr. *haima,* blood, + *rhēgnymi,* to burst forth]

brainstem h., h. into the pons or mesencephalon, often secondary to brainstem distortion by transtentorial herniations due to rapidly expanding intracranial lesions.

cerebral h., h. into the substance of the cerebrum, usually in the region of the internal capsule by the rupture of the lenticulostriate artery. SYN hematencephalon, intracerebral h.

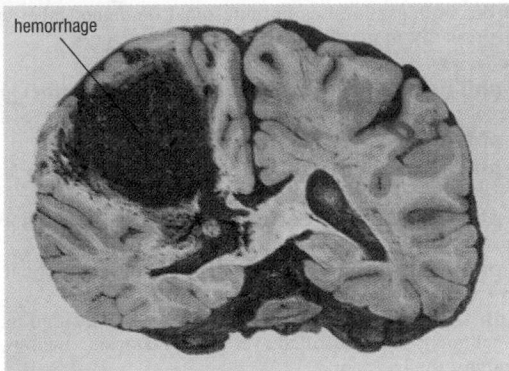

hemorrhage

hemorrhage: autopsy specimen showing massive hemorrhage in the left cerebral hemisphere

concealed h., SYN internal h.

Duret h., small brainstem h. resulting from brainstem distortion secondary to transtentorial herniation.

extradural h., an accumulation of blood between the skull and the dura mater. SYN epidural hematoma.

gastric h., SYN gastrorrhagia.

intermediate h., h. that is recurrent.

internal h., bleeding into organs or cavities of the body. SYN concealed h.

intracerebral h., SYN cerebral h.

intracranial h., bleeding within the cranial vault; includes cerebral h. and subarachnoid h.

intrapartum h., h. occurring in the course of normal labor and delivery.

intraventricular h., extravasation of blood into the ventricular system of the brain.

nasal h., SYN epistaxis.

parenchymatous h., bleeding into the substance of an organ.

h. per rhex′is, h. due to the rupture of a blood vessel.

petechial h., capillary h. into the skin that forms petechiae. SYN punctate h.

pontine h., h. occurring in the substance of the pons, typically in hypertensive patients.

postpartum h., h. from the birth canal in excess of 500 ml after a vaginal delivery or 1000 mL after a cesarean delivery during the first 24 hours after birth.

primary h., h. immediately after an injury or operation, as distinguished from intermediate or secondary h.

punctate h., SYN petechial h.

renal h., hematuria, of which the kidney is the source.

secondary h., h. at an interval after an injury or an operation.

serous h., obsolete term for a profuse transudation of plasma through the walls of the capillaries.

splinter h.'s, tiny longitudinal subungual h.'s typically seen in but not diagnostic of bacterial endocarditis, trichinosis, etc.

subarachnoid h., extravasation of blood into the subarachnoid space, often due to aneurysm rupture and usually spreading throughout the cerebrospinal fluid pathways.

subdural h., extravasation of blood between the dural and arachnoidal membranes; acute and chronic forms occur; chronic hematomas may become encapsulated by neomembranes. SYN subdural hematoma.

subgaleal h., collection of blood beneath the galea aponeurotica.

syringomyelic h., h. into a syringomyelic cavity.

hem·or·rhag·ic (hem-ŏ-raj′ik). Relating to or marked by hemorrhage.

hem·or·rhag·ins (hem-ŏ-raj′inz, -rā′jins). Cytolysins found in certain venoms and poisonous material from some plants, e.g., rattlesnake venom and ricin; h. cause degeneration and lysis of endothelial cells in capillaries and small vessels, thereby resulting in numerous small hemorrhages in the tissues. [hemorrhage + -in]

hem·or·rhoid (hem′ŏ-royd). Denoting one of the tumors or varices constituting hemorrhoids.

hem·or·rhoi·dal (hem-ŏ-roy′dăl). **1.** Relating to hemorrhoids. **2.** Formerly applied to certain arteries and veins supplying the region of the rectum and anus, currently described by "anal" or "rectal."

hem·or·rhoid·ec·to·my (hem′ŏ-roy-dek′tō-mē). Surgical removal of hemorrhoids; usually accomplished by excision of hemorrhoidal tissues by sharp dissection, or by application of elastic ligature at the base of the hemorrhoidal bundles to produce ischemic necrosis and ultimate ablation of the h. [hemorrhoids + G. *ektomē,* excision]

hem·or·rhoids (hem′ŏ-roydz). A varicose condition of the external hemorrhoidal veins causing painful swellings at the anus. SYN piles. [G. *haimorrhois,* pl. *haimorrhoides,* veins likely to bleed, fr. *haima,* blood, + *rhoia,* a flow]

cutaneous h., hyperplasia of the connective tissue in one or more of the normal radiating folds of the skin immediately surrounding the anus.

external h., dilated veins forming tumors at the outer side of the external sphincter.

internal h., dilated veins beneath the mucous membrane within the sphincter.

he·mo·sal·pinx (hē′mō-sal′pinks). SYN hematosalpinx.

he·mo·si·al·em·e·sis (hē′mō-sī-ăl-em′ĕ-sis). Vomiting of blood and saliva. [hemo- + G. *sialon,* saliva, + *emesis,* vomiting]

he·mo·sid·er·in (hē-mō-sid′er-in). A golden yellow or yellow-brown insoluble protein produced by phagocytic digestion of hematin; found in most tissues, especially in the liver, spleen, and bone marrow, in the form of granules much larger than ferritin molecules (of which they are believed to be aggregates), but with a higher content, as much as 37%, of iron; stains blue with Perl Prussian blue stain. [hemo- + G. *sideros,* iron, + -in]

he·mo·sid·er·o·sis (hē′mō-sid-er-ō′sis). Accumulation of hemosiderin in tissue, particularly in liver and spleen. SEE hemochromatosis. [hemosiderin + -osis, condition]

idiopathic pulmonary h., repeated sudden attacks of dyspnea and hemoptysis leading to diffuse pulmonary h., seen most commonly in children; of unknown cause, but some cases may be associated with Goodpasture syndrome. SYN Ceelen-Gellerstedt syndrome.

nutritional h., a disease that results from ingestion of iron in foodstuffs prepared in iron vessels.

he·mo·sper·mia (hē′mō-sper′mē-ă). Presence of blood in the seminal fluid. SYN hematospermia. [hemo- + G. *sperma,* seed]

h. spu′ria, h. occurring in the prostatic urethra.

h. ve′ra, h. from the seminal vesicles.

he·mo·spo·rid·i·um (hē′mō-spō-rid′ē-ŭm). A blood parasite of the order Haemosporidia. [hemo- + Mod. L. dim. of G. *sporos,* seed]

he·mo·spo·rines (hē'mō-spō-rēnz). Common term for members of the order Haemosporidia.

he·mo·sta·sia (hē-mō-stā'zē-ă). SYN hemostasis.

he·mo·sta·sis (hē'mō-stā-sis, hē-mos'tă-sis). **1.** The arrest of bleeding. **2.** The arrest of circulation in a part. **3.** Stagnation of blood. SYN hemostasia. [hemo- + G. *stasis,* a standing]

he·mo·stat (hē'mō-stat). **1.** Any agent that arrests, chemically or mechanically, the flow of blood from an open vessel. **2.** An instrument for arresting hemorrhage by compression of the bleeding vessel.

he·mo·stat·ic (hē-mō-stat'ik). **1.** Arresting the flow of blood within the vessels. **2.** SYN antihemorrhagic.

he·mo·styp·tic (hē-mo-stip'tik). SYN styptic (2). [hemo- + G. *styptikos,* astringent]

he·mo·suc·cus pan·cre·a·ti·cus. Bleeding into the pancreatic duct, usually as a result of trauma, tumor, inflammation, or pseudoaneurysm associated with pseudocyst.

he·mo·ta·cho·gram (hē-mō-ta'chō-gram). The record produced by hemotachometer. [hemo + tachos + G. *gramma,* something written]

he·mo·ta·chom·e·ter (hē'mō-tă-kom'ĕ-ter). An instrument for measuring the rapidity of the flow of blood in the arteries. SYN hematachometer. [hemo- + G. *tachos,* swiftness, + *metron,* measure]

he·mo·ther·a·py, he·mo·ther·a·peu·tics (hē'mō-thār'ă-pē, thār-ă-pū'tiks). Treatment of disease by the use of blood or blood derivatives, as in transfusion. SYN hematherapy.

he·mo·tho·rax (hē-mō-thōr'aks). Blood in the pleural cavity. SYN hemathorax.

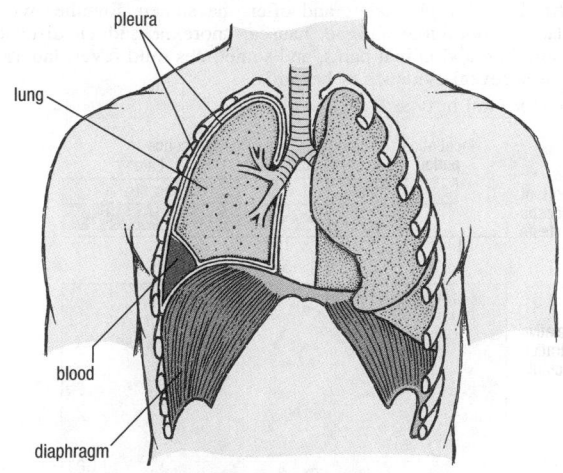

hemothorax: in the right lung cavity

---

he·mo·tox·ic, he·ma·to·tox·ic, he·ma·tox·ic (hē-mō-tok'sik; hē'mă-tō-toks'ik, hem'ă-; hē-mă-toks'ik, hem-ă-). **1.** Causing blood poisoning. **2.** SYN hemolytic.

he·mo·tox·in (hē-mō-tok'sin). Any substance that causes destruction of red blood cells, including various hemolysins; usually used with reference to substances of biologic origin, in contrast to chemicals. SYN hematotoxin, hematoxin.

cobra h., the constituent in cobra venom that hemolyzes the red blood cells of various species.

he·mo·troph, he·mot·ro·phe (hēm'ō-trof). The nutritive materials supplied to the embryos of placental mammals through the maternal bloodstream. Cf. embryotroph, histotroph. [hemo- + G. *trophē,* food]

he·mo·tro·pic (hē-mō-trop'ik). Pertaining to the mechanism by which a substance in or on blood cells, especially the erythrocytes, attracts phagocytic cells; the latter change direction and

migrate toward the h. cells. SYN hematotropic. [hemo- + G. *tropos,* direction (or *tropē,* a turning)]

he·mo·tym·pa·num (hē'mō-tim'pă-nŭm). The presence of blood in the middle ear. SYN hematotympanum.

he·mo·zo·ic (hē-mō-zō'ik). Parasitic in the blood of vertebrates; denoting certain protozoa. SYN hematozoic.

he·mo·zo·on (hē-mō-zō'on). A blood-dwelling parasitic animal such as the trypanosomes or microfilariae of *Wuchereria* or *Brugia.* SYN hematozoon. [hemo- + G. *zōon,* animal]

HEMPAS Abbreviation for *h*ereditary *e*rythroblastic *mu*ltinuclearity associated with *p*ositive *a*cidified *s*erum. SEE HEMPAS *cells,* under *cell.*

hen·bane (hen'bān). SYN hyoscyamus.

Henderson, Lawrence J., U.S. biochemist, 1878–1942. SEE H.-Hasselbalch *equation.*

Hendersonula toruloidea. SYN *Nattrassia mangiferae.*

Henke, Wilhelm, German anatomist, 1834–1896. SEE H. *space.*

Henle, Friedrich G.J., German anatomist, pathologist, and histologist, 1809–1885. SEE *crypts* of H., under *crypt; H. ampulla, ansa, glands,* under *gland, fissures,* under *fissure, layer,* fiber *layer,* nervous *layer, loop, membrane,* fenestrated elastic *membrane, reaction, sheath, spine, tubules,* under *tubule, warts,* under *wart;* Hassall-H. *bodies,* under *body.*

hen·na (hen'ă). The leaves of the Egyptian privet, *Lawsonia inermis;* used as a cosmetic and hair dye. [Ar. *hennā*]

Hen·ne·bert. Camille, Belgian otologist, 1867–1958. SEE Hennebert *sign.*

Henoch, Eduard H., German pediatrician, 1820–1910. SEE H. *chorea, purpura;* H.-Schönlein *purpura, syndrome;* Schönlein-H. *syndrome.*

hen·pu·ye (hen-poo'yē). SYN goundou. [native term on the Gold Coast (Ghana) meaning "dog-nose"]

Hen·ri, Victor, French 20th-century biochemist. SEE Michaelis-Menten *equation;* H.-Michaelis-Menten *equation.*

Henry, James Paget, U. S. physiologist, *1914. SEE H.-Gauer *response.*

Henry, Joseph, U.S. physicist, 1797–1878. SEE Dalton-H. *law.*

Henry, William, British chemist, 1774–1836. SEE H. *law.*

hen·ry (H) (hen'rē). The unit of electrical inductance, when 1 V is induced by a change in current of 1 A/sec. [Joseph *Henry*]

Henseleit, K., German internist, *1907. SEE Krebs-H. *cycle.*

Hensen, Victor, German anatomist and physiologist, 1835–1924. SEE H. *canal, cell, disk, duct, knot, line, node, stripe.*

Hensing, Friedrich W., German anatomist, 1719–1745. SEE H. *ligament.*

He·pad·na·vi·ri·dae (hē-pa'd'nă-vī'rā-dā). A family of lipid-containing icosahedral DNA-containing viruses 42 mm in diameter whose genome consists of a single molecule of noncovalently closed, circular DNA that is partially single-stranded and partially double-stranded; associated with hepatitis in a number of animal species. The principal genus ortho Hepadnavirus is associated with hepatitis B in mammals and the genus Avihepadnavirus with disease in birds; persistant infection is common and is associated with chronic disease and liver cancer. [*hepatitis* + DNA + virus]

he·par, gen. **hep·a·tis** (hē'par, hē'pah-tis) [TA]. SYN liver. [L. borrowed fr. G. *hēpar,* gen. *hēpatos,* the liver]

h. loba'tum, a fissured liver, from the scars of healed syphilitic gummas.

hep·a·ran *N*-sul·fa·tase (hep'ă-ran). An enzyme that participates in the stepwise degradation of heparan sulfate; heparan *N*-sulfatase hydrolyzes the sulfate moiety attached to the amino group of the glucosamine residue of heparan sulfate; a deficiency of this enzyme is associated with mucopolysaccharidose IIIA (Sanfilippo syndrome A).

hep·a·ran sul·fate. SYN heparitin sulfate.

hep·a·rin (hep'ă-rin). An anticoagulant principle that is a component of various tissues (especially liver and lung) and mast cells in humans and several mammalian species; its principal and active constituent is a glycosaminoglycan composed of D-glucuronic acid and D-glucosamine, both sulfated, in 1,4-α linkage, of molecular weight 6,000–20,000. In conjunction with a serum protein cofactor (the so-called heparin cofactor), h. acts as an antithrombin and an antiprothrombin. Synthetic preparations are commonly used in therapeutic anticoagulation. It also enhances activity of "clearing factors" (lipoprotein lipases). SYN heparinic acid.

h. eliminase, SYN h. lyase.

h. lyase, an enzyme eliminating Δ-4,5-D-glucuronate residues from heparin and similar 1,4-linked polyglucuronates. SYN h. eliminase, heparinase.

h. sodium, a mixture of active principles (usually obtained from various tissues of domestic animals) having the properties of prolonging the clotting time of human blood.

hep·a·rin·ase (hep′ă-rin-ās). SYN *heparin* lyase.

hep·a·ri·ne·mia (hep′ă-ri-nē′mē-ă). The presence of demonstrable levels of heparin in the circulating blood.

hep·a·rin·ic ac·id (hep-ă-rin′ik). SYN heparin.

hep·a·rin·ize (hep′ă-rin-īz). To perform therapeutic administration of heparin.

hep·a·rit·in sul·fate (hep′ă-rit-in). A heteropolysaccharide that has the same repeating disaccharide as heparin but with fewer sulfates and more acetyl groups; accumulates in individuals with certain types of mucopolysaccharidosis. SYN heparan sulfate.

⚠**hepat-, hepato-.** The liver. [G. *hēpar* (*hēpat-*)]

hep·a·ta·tro·phia, hep·a·tat·ro·phy (hep′ă-tă-trō′fē-ă, hep-ă-tat′rō-fē). Atrophy of the liver.

hep·a·tec·to·my (hep-ă-tek′tō-mē). Removal of the liver, whole or in part. [hepat- + G. *ektomē*, excision]

he·pa·tic (he-pat′ik). Relating to the liver. [G. *hēpatikos*]

he·pat·i·co·do·chot·o·my (he-pat′i-kō-dō-kot′ō-mē). Combined hepaticotomy and choledochotomy.

he·pat·i·co·du·o·de·nos·to·my (he-pat′i-kō-doo′ō-de-nos′tō-mē). Establishment of a communication between the hepatic ducts and the duodenum. SYN hepatoduodenostomy. [hepatico- + duodenostomy]

he·pat·i·co·en·ter·os·to·my (he-pat′i-kō-en-ter-os′tō-mē). Establishment of a communication between the hepatic ducts and the intestine. SYN hepatocholangioenterostomy. [hepatico- + enterostomy]

he·pat·i·co·gas·tros·to·my (he-pat′i-kō-gas-tros′tō-mē). Establishment of a communication between the hepatic duct and the stomach. [hepatico- + gastrostomy]

he·pat·i·co·li·thot·o·my (he-pat′i-kō-li-thot′ō-mē). Removal of a stone from a hepatic duct. [hepatico- + G. *lithos*, stone, + *tomē*, a cutting]

he·pat·i·co·lith·o·trip·sy (he-pat′i-kō-lith′ō-trip-sē). The crushing or fragmentation of a biliary calculus in a hepatic duct. [hepatico- + G. *lithos*, stone, + *tripsis*, a rubbing]

he·pat·i·co·pul·mo·nary (he-pat′i-kō-pul′mŏ-nār-ē). SYN hepatopneumonic.

he·pat·i·cos·to·my (he-pat-i-kos′tō-mē). Establishment of an opening into the hepatic duct. [hepatico- + G. *stoma*, mouth]

he·pat·i·cot·o·my (he-pat-i-kot′ō-mē). Incision into the hepatic duct. [hepatico- + G. *tomē*, incision]

hep·a·tin (hep′ă-tin). SYN glycogen.

hep·a·tit·ic (hep-ă-tit′ik). Relating to hepatitis.

ℹ**hep·a·ti·tis** (hep-ă-tī′tis). Inflammation of the liver, due usually to viral infection but sometimes to toxic agents. [hepat- + -itis]

> Previously endemic throughout much of the developing world, viral hepatitis now ranks as a major public health problem in industrialized nations. The 3 most common types of viral hepatitis (A, B, and C) afflict millions worldwide. Acute viral hepatitis is characterized by varying degrees of fever, malaise, weakness, anorexia, nausea, and abdominal distress. Hepatocellular damage causes bilirubin retention, often with jaundice, and a rise in serum levels of certain enzymes (particularly transaminases). Hepatitis A, caused by an enterovirus, is spread by the fecal-oral route, most often through ingestion of contaminated food or water. The case fatality rate is less than 1%,

and recovery is complete. The presence of antibody to hepatitis A virus indicates prior infection, noninfectivity, and immunity to future attacks. Hepatitis B, due to a small DNA virus, is transmitted through sexual contact, sharing of needles by IV drug abusers, needlestick injuries among health care workers, and from mother to fetus. The annual incidence in the U.S. is 300,000 cases. The incubation period is 6–24 weeks. Some patients become carriers, and in some an immune response to the virus induces a chronic phase leading to cirrhosis, hepatic failure, and risk of hepatocellular carcinoma. Hepatitis B surface antigen (HBsAg) is detectable early in serum; its persistence correlates with chronic infection and infectivity. Core antigen (HBcAg) appears later and also indicates infectivity. Hepatitis C is the principal form of transfusion-induced hepatitis; a chronic active form often develops. Acute infection with hepatitis B or C has a higher mortality rate than hepatitis A. Effective vaccines are available for active immunization against hepatitis A and hepatitis B. Interferon-alpha brings about clinical remission in some cases of hepatitis B and hepatitis C. Hepatitis D is due to an RNA virus capable of causing disease only in persons previously infected with hepatitis B. Hepatitis E, which occurs chiefly in the tropics, resembles hepatitis A in that it is transmitted by the fecal-oral route and does not become chronic or lead to a carrier state, but it has a much higher mortality rate.

h. A, SYN viral h. type A.

acute parenchymatous h., SYN acute massive liver *necrosis.*

anicteric h., h. without jaundice.

anicteric virus h., a relatively mild h., without jaundice, due to a virus; the principal physical signs and symptoms are enlargement of the liver, lymph nodes, and often the spleen, together with headache, continuous fatigue, nausea, anorexia, sudden distaste for smoking, abdominal pains, and sometimes mild fever; laboratory tests reveal evidence of hepatitis.

ℹ**h. B,** SYN viral h. type B.

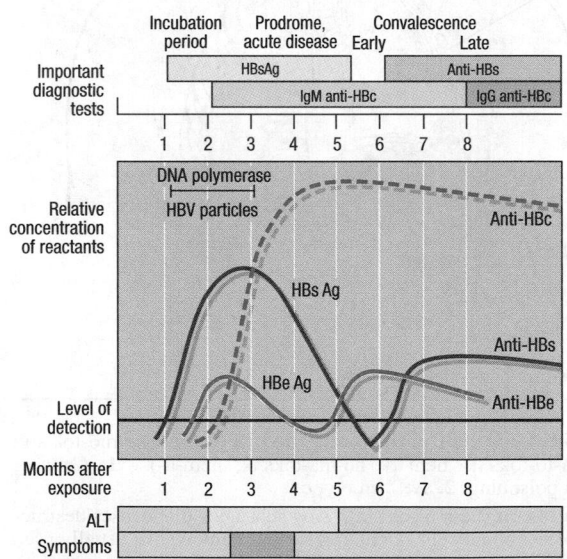

hepatitis B virus infection: clinical and serologic events

ℹ**h. C,** SYN viral h. type C.

cholangiolitic h., h. with inflammatory changes around small bile ducts, producing mainly obstructive jaundice; may be due to viral or bacterial infection ascending biliary tree because of obstruction.

cholestatic h., jaundice with bile stasis in inflamed intrahepatic bile ducts; usually due to toxic effects of a drug.

chronic h., any of several types of h. persisting for more than six months, often progressing to cirrhosis. SYN chronic active liver disease.

chronic active h., h. with chronic portal inflammation that extends into the parenchyma, with piecemeal necrosis and fibrosis which usually progresses to a coarsely nodular postnecrotic cirrhosis. SYN juvenile cirrhosis, posthepatitic cirrhosis, subacute h.

chronic interstitial h., obsolete term for cirrhosis of the liver.

chronic persistent h., SYN chronic persisting h.

chronic persisting h., a form of chronic h. that is usually benign, not progressing to cirrhosis, and usually asymptomatic without physical findings but with continuing abnormalities of tests of liver status. SYN chronic persistent h.

h. D, SYN viral h. type D.

delta h., SYN viral h. type D.

drug-induced h., hepatocellular damage produced by a drug.

h. E, SYN viral h. type E.

epidemic h., SYN viral h. type A.

h. exter'na, SYN perihepatitis.

h. F, a disease caused by an as yet poorly characterized DNA virus.

fulminant h., severe, rapidly progressive loss of hepatic function due to viral infection or other cause of inflammatory destruction of liver tissue.

h. G, a disease caused by an RNA virus similar to h. virus.

giant cell h., SYN neonatal h.

halothane h., hepatocellular damage said to result from the administration of halothane anesthesia.

infectious h. (IH), SYN viral h. type A.

long incubation h., outdated name for h. B based on the longer incubation period (range 30–180 days, usually 60–90) compared with h. A (15–45 days, mean 30).

lupoid h., jaundice with evidence of liver cell damage and positive antinuclear antibody or LE cell tests, but without evidence of systemic lupus erythematosus; liver biopsies usually show chronic active h. with infiltration by plasma cells, or postnecrotic cirrhosis; serum is negative for h. B antigen. SYN plasma cell h.

MS-1 h., SYN viral h. type A.

NANB h., SYN non-A, non-B h.

NANBNC h., abbreviation for non-A, non-B, non-C h.

neonatal h., h. in the neonatal period presumed to be due to any of a variety of causes, chiefly viral; characterized by direct and indirect bilirubinemia, hepatocellular degeneration, and appearance of multinucleated giant cells; may be difficult to distinguish from biliary atresia, but is more likely to end with recovery, although cirrhosis may develop. SYN giant cell h.

non–A-E h., an acute h. not caused by any of the identified viral agents A through E.

non-A, non-B h., h. caused by any number of infectious agents not detectable by methods that reveal the presence of h. viruses A and B. SYN NANB h.

non-A, non-B, non-C h. (NANBNC h.), h. caused by viral organisms other than h. viruses A, B, or C.

peliosis h., a rare condition in which the liver contains very numerous small blood-filled spaces, sometimes lined with endothelium; it may be found incidentally or rupture may cause intraperitoneal hemorrhage.

plasma cell h., SYN lupoid h.

serum h. (SH), SYN viral h. type B.

short incubation h., SYN viral h. type A.

subacute h., SYN chronic active h.

suppurative h., h. with abscess formation; often amebic in origin.

transfusion h., SYN viral h. type B.

viral h., (1) h. caused by any one of at least 7 immunologically unrelated viruses: h. A virus, h. B virus, h. C virus, h. D virus, h. E virus, h. F virus, h. G virus; (2) h. caused by a viral infection, including that by Epstein-Barr virus and cytomegalovirus. SYN virus h.

viral h. type A, a virus disease with a short incubation period (usually 15–50 days), caused by h. A virus, a member of the

nomenclature of hepatitis antigens and the corresponding antibodies

disease	component of system	definition
Hepatitis A	HAV	Hepatitis A virus. Etiologic agent of infectious hepatitis. A picornavirus, the prototype of a new genus, *Hepatovirus.*
	Anti-HAV	Antibody to HAV. Detectable at onset of symptoms; lifetime persistence.
	IgM anti-HAV	IgM class antibody to HAV. Indicates recent infection with hepatitis A; positive up to 4–6 months after infection.
Hepatitis B	HBV	Hepatitis B virus. Etiologic agent of serum hepatitis (long-incubation hepatitis). A hepadnavirus.
	HBsAG	Hepatitis B surface antigen. Surface antigens of HBV detectable in large quality in serum; several subtypes identified.
	HBcAG	Hepatitis B core antigen.
	Anti-HBS	Antibody to HBsAg. Indicates past infection with and immunity to HBV, presence of passive antibody from HBIG, or immune response from HBV vaccine.
	Anti-HBc	Antibody to HBeAg. Presence in serum of HBsAG carrier suggests lower titer of HBV.
	Anti-HBc	Antibody to HBcAg. Indicates infection with HBV at some undefined time in the past.
	IgM anti-HBc	IgM class antibody to HBcAG. Indicates recent infection with HBV; positive for 4–6 months after infection.
Hepatitis C	HCV	Hepatitis C virus, a common etiologic agent of posttransfusion hepatitis. A flavivirus.
	Anti-HCV	Antibody to HCV
Hepatitis D	HDV	Hepatitis D virus. Etiologic agent of D hepatitis; causes infection only in presence of HBV.
	HDAg	Delta antigen (delta-Ag). Detectable in early acute HDV infection.
	Anti-HDV	Antibody to delta-Ag (anti-delta). Indicates past or present infection with HDV.
Hepatitis E	HEV	Hepatitis E virus. Enterically transmitted hepatitis virus. Causes large epidemics in Asia and North Africa.; fecal-oral or waterborne transmission. Perhaps a calicivirus.
Immune globulins	IG	Immune globulin USP. Contains antibodies to HAV; no antibodies to HBsAg, HCV, or HIV.
	HBIG	Hepatitis B immune globulin. Contains high titers of antibodies to HBV.

he

family Picornaviridae, often transmitted by fecal-oral route; may be inapparent, mild, severe, or occasionally fatal and occurs sporadically or in epidemics, commonly in school-age children and young adults; necrosis of periportal liver cells with lymphocytic and plasma cell infiltration is characteristic and jaundice is a common symptom. SYN epidemic h., h. A, infectious h., MS-1 h., short incubation h., virus A h.

viral h. type B, a virus disease with a long incubation period (usually 50–160 days), caused by a hepatitis B virus, a DNA virus and member of the family Hepadnaviridae, usually transmitted by injection of infected blood or blood derivatives or by use of contaminated needles, lancets, or other instruments; clinically and pathologically similar to viral h. type A, but there is no cross-protective immunity; HB$_s$Ag is found in the serum and the hepatitis delta virus occurs in some patients. SYN h. B, serum h., transfusion h., virus B h.

viral h. type C, (NANB); principal cause of non-A, non-B post-transfusion h. caused by an RNA virus that is classified with the Flaviviridae family. The incubation period is 6–8 weeks with about 75% of infections subclinical and giving rise to chronic persistent infection. A high percentage of these develop chronic liver disease leading to cirrhosis and possible hepatocellular carcinoma. SYN h. C, virus C h.

viral h. type D, acute or chronic h. caused by a satellite virus, the h. deltavirus, a defective RNA virus requiring HBV for replication since it uses HB$_s$Ag as its own coat. The acute type occurs in two forms: 1) coinfection, the simultaneous occurrence of h. B virus and h. delta virus infections, which usually is self-limiting; 2) superinfection, the appearance of h. delta virus infection in a h. B virus carrier, which often leads to chronic h. The chronic type appears to be more severe than other types of viral h. SYN delta h., h. D.

viral h. type E, h. caused by a nonenveloped, single-stranded, positive-sense RNA virus 27–34 nm in diameter, unrelated to other h. and belonging to the family Caliciviridae; it is the principal cause of enterically transmitted, waterborne, epidemic NANB hepatitis occurring primarily in Asia, Africa and South America. SYN h. E.

virus h., SYN viral h.

virus A h., SYN viral h. type A.

virus B h., SYN viral h. type B.

virus C h., SYN viral h. type C.

hep·a·ti·za·tion (hep′ă-ti-zā′shŭn). Conversion of a loose tissue into a firm mass like the substance of the liver macroscopically, denoting especially such a change in the lungs in the consolidation of pneumonia.

gray h., the second stage of h. in pneumonia, when the exudate is beginning to degenerate prior to breaking down; the color is a yellowish gray or mottled.

red h., the first stage of h. in which the exudate is blood-stained.

yellow h., the final stage of h. in which the exudate is becoming purulent.

△**hepato-.** SEE hepat-.

he·pa·to·blas·to·ma (hep′ă-tō-blas-tō′mă). A malignant neoplasm occurring in young children, primarily in the liver, composed of tissue resembling embryonal or fetal hepatic epithelium, or mixed epithelial and mesenchymal tissues.

he·pa·to·car·ci·no·ma (hep′ă-tō-kar-si-nō′mă). SYN hepatocellular carcinoma.

he·pa·to·cele (hep′ă-tō-sēl, he-pat′ō-sēl). Protrusion of part of the liver through the abdominal wall or the diaphragm. [hepato- + G. kēlē, hernia]

he·pa·to·chol·an·gi·o·en·ter·os·to·my (hep′ă-tō-kō-lan′jē-ō-en-ter-os′tō-mē). SYN hepaticoenterostomy. [hepato- + G. cholē, bile, + angeion, vessel, + enteron, intestine, + stoma, mouth]

he·pa·to·chol·an·gi·o·je·ju·nos·to·my (hep′ă-tō-kō-lan′jē-ō-jē-joo-nos′tō-mē). Union of the hepatic duct to the jejunum. [hepato- + G. cholē, bile, + angeion, vessel, + jejunostomy]

he·pa·to·chol·an·gi·os·to·my (hep′ă-tō-kō-lan-jē-os′tō-mē). Creation of an opening into the common bile duct to establish drainage.

he·pa·to·chol·an·gi·tis (hep′ă-tō-kō-lan-jī′tis). Inflammation of the liver and biliary tree.

he·pa·to·cu·pre·in (hep′ă-tō-koo′prē-in). SYN cytocuprein.

he·pa·to·cys·tic (hep′ă-tō-sis′tik). Relating to the gallbladder, or to both liver and gallbladder. [hepato- + G. kystis, bladder]

He·pa·to·cys·tis (hep′ă-tō-sis′tis). A genus of blood-parasitizing hemosporines (family Plasmodiidae) with gametocytes in red cells and cystlike exoerythrocytic schizonts in the liver parenchyma; parasitic in Old World primates, bats, and squirrels, but not in domestic animals or in the western hemisphere. The species *H. kochi*, a common parasite of African baboons and other monkeys, is transmitted by the biting midge, *Culicoides*. [hepato- + G. kystis, bladder]

he·pa·to·cyte (hep′ă-tō-sīt). A parenchymal liver cell.

he·pa·to·du·o·de·nos·to·my (hep′ă-tō-doo-ō-de-nos′tō-mē). SYN hepaticoduodenostomy.

he·pa·to·dys·en·ter·y (hep′ă-tō-dis′en-ter-ē). Dysentery associated with liver disease.

he·pa·to·en·ter·ic (hep′ă-tō-en-tĕr′ik). Relating to the liver and the intestine. [hepato- + G. enteron, intestine]

hep·a·to·fu·gal (hep′ă-tō-fū′găl). Away from the liver, usually referring to portal blood flow.

he·pa·to·gas·tric (hep′ă-tō-gas′trik). Relating to the liver and the stomach.

he·pa·to·gen·ic, he·pa·tog·e·nous (hep-ă-tō-jen′ik, -toj′en-ŭs). Of hepatic origin; formed in the liver.

he·pa·tog·ra·phy (hep-ă-tog′ră-fē). Radiography of the liver. [hepato- + G. graphē, a writing]

he·pa·to·he·mia (hep′ă-tō-hē′mē-ă). Rarely used term for congestion of the liver. [hepato- + G. haima, blood]

he·pa·toid (hep′ă-toyd). Resembling or like the liver. [hepato- + G. eidos, resemblance]

he·pa·to·jug·u·la·rom·e·ter (hep′ă-tō-jŭg′ū-lă-rom′ĕ-ter). An apparatus for the quantitative control and measurement of the pressure and force applied over the liver to test the hepatojugular reflux. [hepato- + L. jugulum, throat, + G. metron, measure]

he·pa·to·li·en·og·ra·phy (hep′ă-tō-lī-en-og′ră-fē). SYN hepatosplenography. [hepato- + L. lien, spleen, + G. graphē, a writing]

he·pa·to·li·en·o·meg·a·ly (hep′ă-tō-lī′ĕ-nō-meg′ă-lē). SYN hepatosplenomegaly.

he·pa·to·lith (hep′ă-tō-lith). A concretion in the liver. [hepato- + G. lithos, stone]

he·pa·to·li·thec·to·my (hep′ă-tō-li-thek′tō-mē). Removal of a calculus from the liver. [hepato- + G. lithos, stone, + ektomē, excision]

he·pa·to·li·thi·a·sis (hep′ă-tō-li-thī′ă-sis). Presence of calculi in the liver. [hepato- + G. lithiasis, presence of a calculus]

he·pa·tol·o·gist (hep-ă-tol′ō-jist). A specialist in hepatology.

he·pa·tol·o·gy (hep-ă-tol′ō-jē). The branch of medicine concerned with diseases of the liver. [hepato- + G. logos, study]

he·pa·tol·y·sin (hep-ă-tol′i-sin). A cytolysin that destroys parenchymal cells of the liver.

he·pa·to·ma (hep-ă-tō′mă). SEE malignant h. [hepato- + G. -oma, tumor]

malignant h., SYN hepatocellular *carcinoma*.

he·pa·to·ma·la·cia (hep′ă-tō-mă-lā′shē-ă). Softening of the liver. [hepato- + G. malakia, softening]

he·pa·to·meg·a·ly, he·pa·to·me·ga·lia (hep′ă-tō-meg′ă-lē, -mĕ-gā′lē-ă). Enlargement of the liver. [hepato- + G. megas, large]

he·pa·to·mel·a·no·sis (hep′ă-tō-mel′ă-nō′sis). Heavy pigmentation of the liver. [hepato- + G. melas, black, + -osis, condition]

he·pa·tom·pha·lo·cele (hep′ă-tom-fal′ō-sēl, hep-ă-tom′fă-lō-sēl). Umbilical hernia with involvement of the liver. SYN hepatomphalos. [hepato- + omphalocele]

he·pa·tom·pha·los (hep-ă-tom′fă-lōs). SYN hepatomphalocele.

he·pa·to·ne·cro·sis (hep′ă-tō-ne-krō′sis). Death of liver cells.

he·pa·to·neph·ric (hep′ă-tō-nef′rik). SYN hepatorenal.

he·pa·to·neph·ro·meg·a·ly (hep′ă-tō-nef′rō-meg′ă-lē). Enlargement of both liver and kidney or kidneys. [hepato- + G. *nephros*, kidney, + *megas*, great]

he·pa·to·path·ic (hep′ă-tō-path′ik). Damaging the liver.

he·pa·top·a·thy (hep-ă-top′ă-thē). Disease of the liver. [hepato- + G. *pathos*, suffering]

he·pa·to·per·i·to·ni·tis (hep′ă-tō-pār′i-tō-nī′tis). SYN perihepatitis.

hep·a·to·pet·al (hep′ă-tō-pet′al). Toward the liver, usually referring to the normal direction of portal blood flow.

he·pa·to·pex·y (hep′ă-tō-pek-sē). Anchoring of the liver to the abdominal wall. [hepato- + G. *pēxis*, fixation]

he·pa·to·phy·ma (hep′ă-tō-fī′mă). Rounded or nodular tumor of the liver. [hepato- + G. *phyma*, tumor]

he·pa·to·pneu·mon·ic (hep′ă-tō-noo-mon′ik). Relating to the liver and the lungs. SYN hepaticopulmonary, hepatopulmonary. [hepato- + G. *pneumonikos*, pulmonary]

he·pa·to·por·tal (hep′ă-tō-pōr′tăl). Relating to the portal system of the liver.

he·pa·to·pto·sis (hep′ă-top-tō′sis, tō-tō′sis). A downward displacement of the liver. SYN wandering liver. [hepato- + G. *ptōsis*, a falling]

he·pa·to·pul·mo·nary (hep′ă-tō-pŭl′mō-nār′ē). SYN hepatopneumonic.

he·pa·to·re·nal (hep-ă-tō-rē′năl). Relating to the liver and the kidney. SYN hepatonephric. [hepato- + L. *renalis*, renal, fr. *renes*, kidneys]

he·pa·tor·rha·gia (hep′ă-tō-rā′jē-ă). Hemorrhage into or from the liver. [hepato- + G. *rhēgnymi*, to burst forth]

he·pa·tor·rha·phy (hep-ă-tōr′ă-fē). Suture of a wound of the liver. [hepato- + G. *rhaphē*, a suture]

he·pa·tor·rhex·is (hep′ă-tō-rek′sis). Rupture of the liver. [hepato- + G. *rhēxis*, rupture]

he·pa·tos·co·py (hep-ă-tos′kŏ-pē). Examination of the liver. [hepato- + G. *skopeō*, to examine]

he·pa·to·sple·ni·tis (hep′ă-tō-splē-nī′tis). Inflammation of the liver and spleen.

he·pa·to·sple·nog·ra·phy (hep′ă-tō-splē-nog′ră-fē). The use of a contrast medium to outline or depict the liver and spleen radiographically. SYN hepatolienography.

he·pa·to·splen·o·meg·a·ly (hep′ă-tō-splē-nō-meg′ă-lē). Enlargement of the liver and spleen. SYN hepatolienomegaly. [hepato- + G. *splēn*, spleen, + *megas*, large]

he·pa·to·sple·nop·a·thy (hep′ă-tō-splē-nop′ă-thē). Disease of the liver and spleen.

he·pa·tos·to·my (hep-ă-tos′tō-mē). Establishment of a fissure into the liver. [hepato- + G. *stoma*, mouth]

he·pa·to·ther·a·py (hep′ă-tō-thār′ă-pē). Rarely used term for: **1.** Treatment of disease of the liver. **2.** Therapeutic use of liver extract or of the raw substance of the liver.

he·pa·tot·o·my (hep-ă-tot′ō-mē). Incision into the liver. [hepato- + G. *tomē*, incision]

he·pa·to·tox·e·mia (hep′ă-tō-tok-sē′mē-ă). Autointoxication assumed to be due to improper functioning of the liver. [hepato- + G. *toxikon*, poison, + *haima*, blood]

he·pa·to·tox·ic (hep′ă-tō-tok′sik). Relating to an agent that damages the liver, or pertaining to any such action.

he·pa·to·tox·ic·i·ty. The capacity of a drug, chemical, or other exposure to produce injury in the liver. Agents with recognized hepatotoxicity include carbon tetrachloride, alcohol, dantrolene sodium, valproic acid, isonicotinic acid hydrazide.

he·pa·to·tox·in (hep′ă-tō-tok′sin). A toxin that is destructive to parenchymal cells of the liver.

He·pa·to·zo·on (hep′ă-tō-zō′on). A genus of coccidian parasites (family Haemogregarinidae), in which schizogony occurs in the visceral organs, gametogony in the leukocytes or erythrocytes of vertebrate animals, and sporogony in certain ticks and other blood-sucking invertebrates. *H. canis* occurs in dogs, cats, jackals, and hyenas, but is most pathogenic in dogs, in which it may cause serious disease and death; other species have been described from rats, mice, rabbits, and squirrels. [hepato- + G. *zōon*, animal]

HEPES. A compound lacking in pharmacologic effects and widely used as a biological buffer in *in vitro* experiments.

△**hepta-.** Prefix denoting seven. Cf. septi-, sept-. [G. *hepta*]

hep·ta·chlor (hep′tă-klōr). A chlorinated hydrocarbon insecticide for control of cotton boll weevil. It is a poison which may enter the body via skin contamination, inhalation or ingestion. Because of human toxicity concerns, this chemical has only limited application.

hep·tad (hep′tad). A septivalent chemical element or radical.

hep·ta·nal (hep′tă-năl). Obtained from the ricinoleic acid of castor oil by chemical means; used in the manufacture of ethyl oenanthate, a constituent of many artificial essences (flavors). SYN enanthal, oenanthal.

hep·ta·pep·tide (hep-tă-pep′tīd). A peptide containing seven amino acids.

hep·tose (hep′tōs). A sugar with seven carbon atoms in its molecule; e.g., sedoheptulose.

hep·tu·lose (hep′too-lōs). SYN ketoheptose.

D-*altro*-2-**hep·tu·lose.** SYN sedoheptulose.

D-*manno*-**hep·tu·lose.** A ketoheptose of the mannose configuration, occurring in the urine of individuals who have eaten a large quantity of avocados.

n-**hep·tyl·pen·i·cil·lin** (hep′til-pen-ĭ-sil′in). Penicillin K.

Herbert, Herbert, English ophthalmic surgeon, 1865–1942.

her·biv·o·rous (her-biv′ŏ-rŭs). Feeding on plants. [L. *herba*, herb, + *voro*, to devour]

herd (hĕrd). A group of people or animals in a given area. [O.E. *heord*]

he·red·i·tary (hĕ-red′i-ter-ē). Transmissible from parent to offspring by information encoded in the parental germ cell. [L. *hereditarius;* fr. *heres* (*hered*-), an heir]

he·red·i·ty (hĕ-red′i-tē). **1.** The transmission of characters from parent to offspring by information encoded in the parental germ cells. **2.** Genealogy. [L. *hereditas*, inheritance, fr. *heres* (*hered*-), heir]

△**heredo-.** Heredity. [L. *heres*, an heir]

her·e·do·path·ia atac·ti·ca pol·y·neu·ri·ti·for·mis (her′ĕ-dō-path′ē-ă ă-tak′ti-kă pol′ē-noo-rī-ti-fōr′mis). SYN Refsum *disease*.

her·e·do·tax·ia. SYN Friedreich *ataxia*.

Herelle, Felix H. SEE d'Herelle.

He·rel·lea (hĕ-rel′ē-ă). A bacterial generic name which has been officially rejected because its type species, *H. vaginicola*, is a member of the genus *Acinetobacter*.

Hering, Karl E.K., German physiologist, 1834–1918. SEE H. *test*, *theory* of color vision; *canal* of H.; Traube-H. *curves*, under *curve*, *waves*, under *wave;* Semon-Hering *theory*.

Hering, Heinrich Ewald, German physiologist, 1866–1948. SEE sinus *nerve* of H.; H.-Breuer *reflex;* Traube-H. *curves*, under *curve*.

her·i·ta·bil·i·ty (her′i-tă-bil′i-tē). **1.** In psychometrics, a statistical term used to denote the extent of variance of an individual's total score or response that is attributable to a presumed genetic component, in contrast to an acquired component. **2.** In genetics, a statistical term used to denote the proportion of phenotypic variance due to variance in genotypes that is genetically determined, denoted by the traditional symbol h^2. [see heredity]

h. in the broad sense, the proportion of the total phenotypic variance that can be ascribed to genetic factors of any kind (additive, those due to dominance effects, epistasis and hypostasis, and interactions of all kinds).

h. in the narrow sense, the proportion of the total phenotypic variance that can be ascribed to additive genetic variance alone. It reflects the similarity between parent and offspring, and is related to the commercial breeding value.

her·i·tage (her′i-tij). The total of all the inherited characters. [O. Fr.]

Herlitz, Gillis, Swedish pediatrician, *1902. SEE H. *syndrome*.

Herman. E., 20th century U.S. histologist. SEE Padykula-Herman *stain* for myosin ATPase. SEE Padykula-Herman *stain* for myosin ATPase.

He

Hermann, Friedrich, German anatomist, 1859–1920. SEE H. *fixative*.

Hermansky, Frantisek, 20th century Czech physician. SEE H.-Pudlak *syndrome*.

her·maph·ro·dism (her-maf′rō-dizm). SYN hermaphroditism.

her·maph·ro·dite (her-maf′rō-dīt). A person with hermaphroditism. [G. *Hermaphroditos,* the son of *Hermēs,* Mercury, + *Aphroditē,* Venus]

her·maph·ro·dit·ism (her-maf′rō-dīt-izm). The presence in one individual of both ovarian and testicular tissue; i.e., true h. SYN hermaphrodism.

adrenal h., altered appearance of the genitalia due to disorders of adrenocortical function, most often female virilization; not an example of true h.

bilateral h., true h. with an ovotestis on both sides.

dimidiate h., SYN lateral h.

false h., SYN pseudohermaphroditism.

female h., ambiguity of reproductive organs so that the sex of the individual is neither exclusively male or female, but predominantly female h. in which only ovaries are present.

lateral h., a form in which a testis is present on one side and an ovary on the other. SYN dimidiate h.

male h., more correctly designated as male pseudohermaphroditism, as the term is commonly used; however, it may designate an instance of true h. in which overt bodily characteristics are predominantly male h. in which only testes are present.

transverse h., pseudohermaphroditism in which the external genitalia are characteristic of one sex and the gonads are characteristic of the other sex.

true h., h. in which both ovarian and testicular tissue are present. Somatic characteristics of both sexes are present; also called true intersex.

unilateral h., h. in which the doubling of sex characteristics occurs on one side only: ovotestis on one side and either ovary or testis on the other.

her·met·ic (her-met′ik). Airtight; denoting a vessel closed or sealed in such a way that air can neither enter it nor issue from it.

HERNIA

her·nia (her′nē-ă). Protrusion of a part or structure through the tissues normally containing it. SYN rupture (1). [L. rupture]

abdominal h., a h. protruding through or into any part of the abdominal wall. SYN laparocele.

Barth h., a loop of intestine between a persistent vitelline duct and the abdominal wall.

Béclard h., a h. through the opening for the saphenous vein.

bilocular femoral h., SYN Cooper h.

h. of the broad ligament of the uterus, a coil of intestine contained in a pouch projecting into the substance of the broad ligament.

cecal h., a h. containing cecum.

cerebral h., protrusion of brain substance through a defect in the skull.

Cloquet h., a femoral h. perforating the aponeurosis of the pectineus and insinuating itself between this aponeurosis and the muscle, lying therefore behind the femoral vessels.

complete h., an indirect inguinal h. in which the contents extend into the tunica vaginalis.

concealed h., a h. not found on inspection or palpation.

congenital diaphragmatic h., (1) absence of the left pleuroperitoneal membrane; **(2)** SYN Morgagni foramen h.

Cooper h., a femoral h. with two sacs, the first being in the femoral canal, and the second passing through a defect in the superficial fascia and appearing immediately beneath the skin. SYN bilocular femoral h., Hey h.

crural h., SYN femoral h.

diaphragmatic h., protrusion of abdominal contents into the chest through a weakness in the respiratory diaphragm; a common type is the hiatal h.

direct inguinal h., SEE inguinal h.

double loop h., SYN "w" h.

dry h., a h. with adherent sac and contents.

duodenojejunal h., a h. in the subperitoneal tissues. SYN retroperitoneal h., Treitz h.

h. en bissac, SYN properitoneal inguinal h.

epigastric h., h. through the linea alba above the navel.

extrasaccular h., SYN sliding h.

fascial h., a bulging of muscle through a defect in its fascia.

fat h., a h. in which the tissue protruding out of its normal location is composed only of fat.

fatty h., SYN pannicular h.

femoral h., h. through the femoral ring. SYN crural h., femorocele.

foramen of Bochdalek h., SYN Morgagni foramen h.

gastroesophageal h., a hiatal h. into the thorax.

gluteal h., SYN sciatic h.

Hesselbach h., h. with diverticula through the cribriform fascia, presenting a lobular outline.

Hey h., SYN Cooper h.

hiatal h., hiatus h., h. of a part of the stomach through the esophageal hiatus of the diaphragm; they are classified as sliding (esophagogastric junction above the diaphragm) or paraesophageal (esophagogastric junction below the diaphragm).

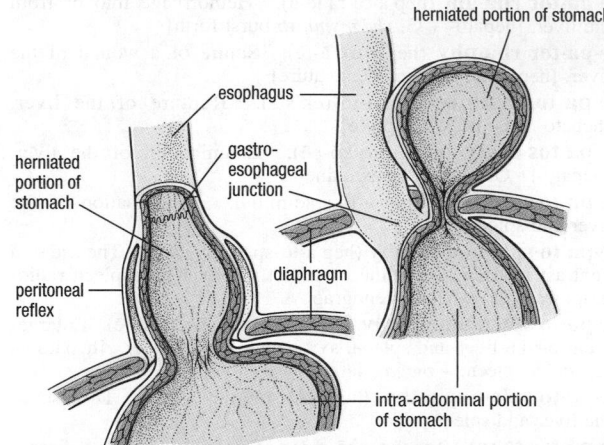

sliding esophageal and paraesophageal hernias: in sliding esophageal hernias (left) the upper stomach and cardioesophageal junction slide in and out of thorax; in paraesophageal hernias (right) all or part of the stomach pushes through diaphragm next to gastroesophageal junction

Holthouse h., inguinal h. with extension of the loop of intestine along Poupart ligament.

iliacosubfascial h., a h. the sac of which passes through the iliac fascia and lies in the iliac fossa in contact with the iliacus muscle.

incarcerated h., SYN irreducible h.

incisional h., h. occurring through a surgical incision or scar.

indirect inguinal h., SEE inguinal h.

infantile h., a h. in which an intestinal loop descends behind the tunica vaginalis, having, therefore, three peritoneal layers in front of it.

inguinal h., a h. at the inguinal region: direct inguinal h. involves the abdominal wall between the deep epigastric artery and the edge of the rectus muscle; indirect inguinal h. involves the internal inguinal ring and passes into the inguinal canal.

inguinocrural h., inguinofemoral h., a bilocular or double h., both inguinal and femoral.

inguinolabial h., an inguinal h. descending into the labium.

inguinoscrotal h., an inguinal h. descending into the scrotum.

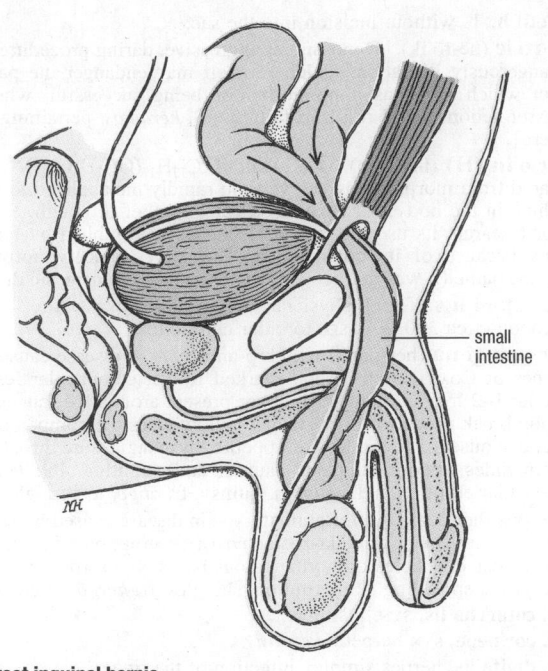

small intestine

indirect inguinal hernia

inguinosuperficial h., an inguinal h. that has turned cephalad away from the scrotum and lies subcutaneously on the abdominal wall.

internal h., protrusion of an intraperitoneal viscus into a compartment or under a constricting band within the abdominal cavity.

intersigmoid h., a h. into the intersigmoid fossa on the under surface of the root of the mesosigmoid near the inner border of the psoas magnus muscle.

interstitial h., a h. in which the protrusion is between any two of the layers of the abdominal wall.

intraepiploic h., a coil of intestine incarcerated in an omental sac.

intrailiac h., an interstitial h. projecting from the internal inguinal ring.

intrapelvic h., an interstitial h. projecting into the pelvis from the internal inguinal ring.

irreducible h., that cannot be reduced without operation. SYN incarcerated h.

ischiatic h., a h. through the sacrosciatic foramen.

Krönlein h., SYN properitoneal inguinal h.

labial h., h. through the canal of Nuck.

lateral ventral h., SYN spigelian h.

Laugier h., a h. passing through an opening in the lacunar ligament.

levator h., SYN perineal h.

Littré h., (1) SYN parietal h; **(2)** h. of Meckel diverticulum.

lumbar h., a h. between the last rib and the iliac crest where the aponeurosis of the transversus muscle is covered only by the latissimus dorsi.

Malgaigne h., infantile inguinal h. prior to the descent of the testis.

meningeal h., herniation of meninges through a spina bifida or cranioschesis.

mesenteric h., h. through a hole in the mesentery.

Morgagni foramen h., a congenital anterior, retrosternal h. of abdominal contents, most often only omentum but occasionally stomach, usually through the right retrosternal Morgagni foramen, through which the internal mammary artery passes to become the superior epigastric artery; often asymptomatic. SYN congenital diaphragmatic h. (2), foramen of Bochdalek h., parasternal h., retrosternal h.

obturator h., h. through the obturator foramen.

orbital h., displacement of orbital fat through a defect in the orbital septum or Tenon capsule into the subcutaneous tissues of the eyelid or subconjunctivally.

pannicular h., the escape of subcutaneous fat through a gap in a fascia or an aponeurosis. SYN fatty h.

pantaloon h., an inguinal h. that involves both an indirect and a direct component.

paraduodenal h., a type of internal h., resulting from abnormal or incomplete midgut rotation, which involves one of several paraduodenal spaces.

paraesophageal h., a h. through or adjacent to the esophageal hiatus of the diaphragm in which the esophagogastric junction remains below the diaphragm and the stomach rolls up into the chest.

parahiatal h., a h. through the diaphragm that occurs at a point separate from the esophageal hiatus.

paraperitoneal h., a vesical h. in which only a part of the protruded organ is covered by the peritoneum of the sac.

parasaccular h., SYN sliding h.

parasternal h., SYN Morgagni foramen h.

parietal h., a h. in which only a portion of the wall of the intestine is engaged. SYN Littré h. (1), partial enterocele, Richter h.

perineal h., a h. protruding through the pelvic diaphragm. SYN levator h., pudendal h.

Petit h., lumbar h., occurring in Petit triangle.

posterior vaginal h., downward displacement of Douglas pouch.

properitoneal inguinal h., a complicated h. having a double sac, one part in the inguinal canal, the other projecting from the internal inguinal ring in the subperitoneal tissues. SYN h. en bissac, Krönlein h.

pudendal h., SYN perineal h.

reducible h., a h. in which the contents of the sac can be returned to their normal location.

retrograde h., a double loop h. the central loop of which lies in the abdominal cavity.

retroperitoneal h., SYN duodenojejunal h.

retropubic h., a h. projecting downward, in the subperitoneal tissues, from the internal inguinal ring.

retrosternal h., SYN Morgagni foramen h.

Richter h., SYN parietal h.

Rokitansky h., a separation of the muscular fibers of the bowel allowing protrusion of a sac of the mucous membrane.

sciatic h., protrusion of intestine through the great sacrosciatic foramen. SYN gluteal h., ischiocele.

scrotal h., complete inguinal h., located in the scrotum.

sliding h., a h. in which an abdominal viscus forms part of the sac. SYN extrasaccular h., parasaccular h., slipped h.

sliding esophageal hiatal h., displacement of the cardioesophageal junction and the stomach through the esophageal hiatus into the mediastinum. SYN sliding hiatal h.

sliding hiatal h., SYN sliding esophageal hiatal h.

slipped h., SYN sliding h.

spigelian h., abdominal h. through the semilunar line. SYN lateral ventral h.

strangulated h., an irreducible h. in which the circulation is arrested; gangrene occurs unless relief is prompt.

synovial h., protrusion of a fold of the stratum synoviale through a rent in the stratum fibrosum of a joint capsule.

Treitz h., SYN duodenojejunal h.

umbilical h., a h. in which bowel or omentum protrudes through the abdominal wall under the skin at the umbilicus. SEE ALSO omphalocele. SYN exomphalos (2), exumbilication (2).

h. uteri inguinale, SYN persistent müllerian duct syndrome.

Velpeau h., femoral h. in which the intestine is in front of the blood vessels.

ventral h., an abdominal incisional h.

vesicle h., protrusion of a segment of the bladder through the abdominal wall or into the inguinal canal and into the scrotum.

vitreous h., prolapse of the vitreous humor into the anterior

he

chamber; may follow removal or displacement of the lens from the lenticular space.

"w" h., the presence of two loops of intestine in a hernial sac. SYN double loop h.

---

her·nial (her′nē-ăl). Relating to hernia.

her·ni·at·ed (her′nē-ā-ted). Denoting any structure protruded through a hernial opening.

her·ni·a·tion (her-nē-ā′shŭn). Protrusion of an anatomic structure (e.g., intervertebral disk) from its normal anatomic position.

caudal transtentorial h., displacement of medial temporal structures through the incisura, with or without rostrocaudal brainstem shift. SYN uncal h.

cingulate h., displacement of the cingulate gyrus beneath the falx.

contained disk h., herniated disk material that remains covered by a thin layer of posterior annulus fibrosus or posterior longitudinal ligament; a disk protrusion is an example of a contained disk h.

disk h., extension of disk material beyond the posterior annulus fibrosus and posterior longitudinal ligament and into the spinal canal.

foraminal h., displacement of cerebellar tonsils through the foramen magnum.

noncontained disk h., herniated disk material that comes directly in contact with the anterior epidural space through a complete defect in the posterior annulus fibrosus and posterior longitudinal ligament; of two main types: (1) extrusions, herniated material that is in continuity with the disk space, but extends completely into the epidural space and (2) sequestered, material that has lost continuity with the disk space and becomes a free fragment in the epidural space.

rostral transtentorial h., displacement of anterior cerebellar structures through the incisura, with or without caudorostral brainstem shift.

sphenoidal h., displacement of ventral frontal lobar tissue over the sphenoid ridge.

subfalcial h., h. beneath the falx cerebri; usually of the cingulate gyrus.

tonsillar h., h. of the cerebellar tonsils through the foramen magnum.

transtentorial h., h. into the incisura, either from above (rostral transtentorial h.) or below (caudal transtentorial h.).

uncal h., SYN caudal transtentorial h.

△**hernio-.** A hernia. [L. *hernia,* rupture]

her·ni·o·en·ter·ot·o·my (her′nē-ō-en-ter-ot′ō-mē). Incision of the intestine following the reduction of a hernia.

her·ni·og·ra·phy (her-nē-og′ră-fē). Radiographic examination of a hernia following injection of a contrast medium into the hernial sac. [hernia + G. *graphō,* to write]

her·ni·oid (her′nē-oyd). Resembling hernia. [hernio- + G. *eidos,* resemblance]

her·ni·o·lap·a·rot·o·my (her′nē-ō-lap-ă-rot′ō-mē). Laparotomy for correction of hernia.

her·ni·o·punc·ture (her′nē-ō-pŭnk′choor). Insertion of a hollow needle into a hernia in order to reduce the size of the tumor by withdrawing gas or liquid.

her·ni·or·rha·phy (her′nē-ōr′ă-fē). Surgical repair of a hernia. [hernio- + G. *rhaphē,* a seam]

Bassini h., an h. for an indirect inguinal hernia repair; after reduction of the hernia, the sac is twisted, ligated, and cut off, then a new inguinal floor is made by uniting the edge of the internal oblique muscle to the inguinal ligament, placing on this the cord, and covering the latter by the external oblique muscle. SYN Bassini operation.

her·ni·o·tome (her′nē-ō-tōm). SYN hernia *knife.*

Cooper h., a slender bistoury with short cutting edge for dividing the constricting tissues at the neck of a hernial sac.

her·ni·ot·o·my (her-nē-ot′ō-mē). Surgical division of the constriction or strangulation of a hernia, often followed by herniorrhaphy. [hernio- + G. *tomē,* a cutting]

Petit h., h. without incision into the sac.

he·ro·ic (hē-rō′ik). Denoting an aggressive, daring procedure in a dangerously ill patient which in itself may endanger the patient but which also has a possibility of being successful, whereas lesser action would result in failure. [G. *hērōikos,* pertaining to a hero]

her·o·in (H) (her′ō-in). An alkaloid, $C_{17}H_{17}(OC_2H_3O)_2ON$, prepared from morphine by acetylation; rapidly metabolized to morphine in the body; formerly used for the relief of cough. Except for research, its use in the United States is prohibited by federal law because of its potential for abuse. SYN diacetylmorphine. [trade name (it was marketed as the "heroine" of analgesic drugs)]

He·roph·i·lus. Greek physician and anatomist of the Alexandrian school, circa 300 B.C. SEE torcular herophili.

her·pan·gi·na (her-pan′ji-nă, herp-an-jī′nă). A disease caused by types of Coxsackievirus and marked by vesiculopapular lesions about 1–2 mm in diameter that are present around the fauces and soon break down to form grayish yellow ulcers; accompanied by sudden onset of fever, loss of appetite, dysphagia, sore throat, and sometimes abdominal pain, nausea, and vomiting. [G. *herpēs,* vesicular eruption, + L. *angina,* quinsy, fr. *ango,* to strangle]

her·pes (her′pēz). An inflammatory skin disease caused by herpes simplex *virus* or varicella-zoster *virus;* an eruption of groups of deep-seated vesicles on erythematous bases. SYN serpigo (2). [G. *herpēs,* a spreading skin eruption, shingles, fr. *herpō,* to creep]

h. catarrha′lis, SYN h. simplex.

h. cor′neae, SYN herpetic *keratitis.*

h. digita′lis, herpes simplex infection of the finger.

h. facia′lis, SYN h. simplex.

h. febri′lis, SYN h. simplex.

h. generalisa′tus, generalized h. simplex virus infection.

h. genita′lis, genital h., herpes simplex infection on the genitals, most commonly herpes simplex-2 virus.

h. gestatio′nis, a polymorphous, bullous eruption, more common on the extremities and abdomen than on the upper trunk, with the appearance of pemphigoid or dermatitis herpetiformis; beginning in the second or third trimester, flaring about the time of delivery and subsequently resolving; usually recurrent during subsequent pregnancy. Linear C3 is shown in the epidermal basement membrane by direct immunofluorescence. Not caused by viral infection.

h. gladiato′rum, h. simplex infection associated with trauma to cutaneous tissue.

h. labia′lis, SYN h. simplex.

neonatal h., herpes simplex virus type 1 or 2 infection transmitted from the mother to the newborn infant, often during passage through an infected birth canal; severity varies from mild to fatal generalized infection, the latter especially with primary maternal genital h.

h. progenita′lis, genital h. infection caused by h. simplex virus.

h. sim′plex, a variety of infections caused by herpesvirus types 1 and 2; type 1 infections are marked most commonly by the eruption of one or more groups of vesicles on the vermilion border of the lips or at the external nares, type 2 by such lesions on the genitalia; both types often are recrudescent and reappear during other febrile illnesses or even physiologic states such as menstruation. The viruses frequently become latent and may not be expressed for years. SYN h. catarrhalis, h. facialis, h. febrilis, h. labialis, Simplexvirus.

traumatic h., h. simplex infection at the site of trauma or of a burn, sometimes accompanied by temperature elevation and malaise.

h. whitlow, h. simplex inflammation at base of fingernail.

h. zos′ter, an infection caused by a herpesvirus (varicella-zoster virus), characterized by an eruption of groups of vesicles on one side of the body following the course of a nerve due to inflammation of ganglia and dorsal nerve roots resulting from activation of the virus, which in many instances has remained latent for years following a primary chickenpox infection; the condition is self-limited but may be accompanied by or followed by severe postherpetic pain. SEE ALSO varicella. SYN zona (2) [TA], shingles, zoster.

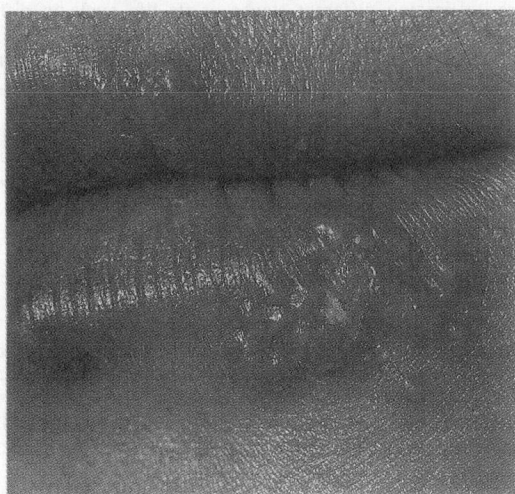

herpes simplex: of the lip

h. zos'ter ophthal'micus, a herpetic involvement of the ophthalmic branch of the trigeminal nerve, which may lead to corneal ulceration.

h. zos'ter o'ticus, a painful varicella virus infection presenting with a vesicular eruption on the pinna, with or without facial nerve paralysis. SYN geniculate zoster, Ramsay Hunt syndrome (2).

h. zos'ter varicello'sus, h. zoster associated with disseminated varicelliform lesions.

Her·pes·vir·i·dae (her′pĕs-vir′i-dē). A heterogeneous family of morphologically similar viruses, all of which contain double-stranded DNA and which infect man and a wide variety of other vertebrates. Infections produce type A inclusion bodies; in many instances, infection may remain latent for many years, even in the presence of specific circulating antibodies. Virions are enveloped, ether-sensitive, and vary up to 200 nm in diameter; the nucleocapsids are 100 nm in diameter and of icosahedral symmetry, with 162 capsomeres. The family is subdivided into 3 subfamilies Alphaherpesvirinae, Betaherpesvirinae, and Gammaherpesvirinae, and includes herpes simplex virus, varicella-zoster virus, cytomegalovirus, and EB virus (all of which infect humans), pseudorabies virus of swine, equine rhinopneumonitis virus, infectious bovine rhinotracheitis virus, canine herpesvirus, B virus of Old World monkeys, several viruses of New World monkeys, virus III of rabbits, infectious laryngotracheitis virus of fowl, Marek disease virus of chickens, Lucké tumor virus of frogs, and many others.

her·pes·vi·rus (her′pēz-vī′rŭs). Any virus belonging to the family Herpesviridae.

cercopithecrine h., an h., in the family Herpesviridae, affecting Old World monkeys, that is very similar morphologically to herpes simplex h.; fatal infection may occur in humans following the bite of an infected monkey, although other modes of transmission have also been documented. SYN B virus.

human h. 1, herpes simplex virus, type 1. SEE *herpes* simplex.

human h. 2, herpes simplex virus, type 2. SEE *herpes* simplex.

human h. 3, SYN varicella-zoster *virus.*

human h. 4, SYN Epstein-Barr *virus.*

human h. 5, a highly species-specific h. (Cytomegalovirus) with particular affinity for the salivary gland tissue. SYN salivary gland virus, salivary virus.

human h. 6, a human h. that was found in certain lymphoproliferative disorders, replicates in a number of different types of leukocytes, and is associated with the childhood disease roseola (exanthema subitum).

human h. 7, virus found in association with human T lymphocytes and is shed in the saliva of most adults; however, a causal relationship to any known disease has not been determined.

human h. 8, a linear double-stranded DNA virus that induces Kaposi sarcoma (KS) in immunodeficient persons. DNA sequences unique to this virus are regularly found in KS specimens from HIV-negative persons as well. The virus is also associated with several uncommon lymphoproliferative syndromes in AIDS patients, including multicentric Castleman disease and primary effusion lymphoma (body cavity–based lymphoma).

Among persons with AIDS, Kaposi sarcoma occurs in 15–25% of male homosexuals but only in 1–3% of persons who acquire AIDS by nonsexual routes (e.g., hemophiliacs and other transfusion recipients). These facts support the hypothesis that the virus is sexually transmitted. KS is characterized histologically by abnormal vascularization and the presence of proliferating endothelial cells, fibroblasts, infiltrating leukocytes, and spindle-shaped tumor cells. Replication of HHV8 occurs only in a small subset of spindle cells, but the majority of such cells are latently infected. Spindle cell proliferation is apparently triggered by growth factors released from HIV-infected cells. Spindle cells, in turn, produce factors that promote angiogenesis. HHV8 DNA can also be found in circulating CD19 B lymphocytes in 40–50% of AIDS patients with KS. Serologic assays are available for anti-HHV8 antibodies, most of them using viral antigen from cell lines derived from body cavity–based lymphomas. Viral replication is insensitive to acyclovir, but is inhibited by ganciclovir, foscarnet, cidofovir, and interferon alpha.

h. saimiri, an ubiquitous infection of squirrel monkeys that is highly oncogenic when injected into other monkey species.

suid h., the causative agent of pseudorabies.

her·pet·ic (her-pet′ik). **1.** Relating to or characterized by herpes. **2.** Relating to or caused by a herpesvirus.

her·pet·i·form (her-pet′i-fōrm). Resembling herpes.

		examples		biologic properties	
subfamily	**genus**	**official name**	**common name**	**cytopathology**	**latent infections**
Alphaherpesvirinae	*Simplexvirus*	human herpesvirus 1	herpes simplex virus type 1	cytolytic	neurons
		human herpesvirus 2	herpes simplex virus type 2		
	Varicellovirus	human herpesvirus 3	varicella-zoster virus		
Betaherpesvirinae	*Cytomegalovirus*	human herpesvirus 5	cytomegalovirus	cytomegalic	glands, kidneys
	Roseolovirus	human herpesvirus 6	human herpesvirus 6	lymphoproliferative	lymphoid tissue
		human herpesvirus 7	human herpesvirus 7		
Gammaherpesvirinae	*Lymphocryptovirus*	human herpesvirus 4	Epstein-Barr virus	lymphoproliferative	lymphoid tissue
	Rhadinovirus	human herpesvirus 8	Kaposi sarcoma–associated herpesvirus		

classification of human herpesviruses

he

her·pe·tol·o·gist (her-pet-ol′ō-jist). One who specializes in herpetology.

her·pe·tol·o·gy (her-pet-ol′ō-jē). The branch of zoology concerned with the study of reptiles and amphibians.

Her·pe·to·mo·nas (her-pĕ-tom′ŏ-nas). A genus of asexual monogenetic flagellates (family Trypanosomatidae) that are strictly insect parasites, with a variety of body forms including promastigote (leptomad), epimastigote (crithidial), amastigote (leishmanial), and trypomastigote (trypanosome-like); infective forms are passed in the host feces. *H. muscae domesticae,* the type species, is found in the common housefly. [G. *herpeton,* a reptile (fr. *herpō,* to creep), + *monas,* unit (one of the *Monadidae*)]

Her·pet·o·vir·i·dae. Obsolete term for Herpesviridae.

her·pe·to·vi·rus (her′pĕ-tō-vī′rŭs). Obsolete name for a virus belonging to the family Herpesviridae. SEE ALSO herpesvirus.

Herring, Percy T., English physiologist, 1872–1967. SEE H. *bodies,* under *body.*

Herrmann, C., Jr., 20th century. SEE H. *syndrome.*

Hers, G., French biochemist. SEE H. *disease.*

her·sage (ār-sahzh′). Separating the individual fibers of a nerve trunk. [Fr. (from L. *hirpex,* a large rake), a harrowing]

Hertwig, Wilhelm A.O., German embryologist, 1849–1922. SEE H. *sheath.*

Hertwig, Richard, German zoologist, 1850–1937. SEE Magendie-H. *sign, syndrome.*

Hertz, Heinrich R., German physicist, 1857–1894. SEE hertz; hertzian *experiments,* under *experiment.*

hertz (Hz) (herts). A unit of frequency equivalent to 1 cycle/sec; this term should not be used for radial (circular) frequency or for angular velocity, in which cases the term sec^{-1} should be used. [H.R. *Hertz*]

hertz·i·an (hert′zē-an). Attributed to or described by Heinrich R. Hertz.

Herxheimer, Karl, German dermatologist, 1861–1944. SEE H. *reaction;* Jarisch-H. *reaction.*

herz·stoss (hārz′stos). Cardiac systole producing a diffuse precordial heave with or without any definite point of maximal impulse. [Ger. heart thrust]

Heschl, Richard L., Austrian pathologist, 1824–1881. SEE H. *gyri,* under *gyrus.*

hes·i·tan·cy (hez′i-tăn-sē). An involuntary delay or inability in starting the urinary stream.

hes·i·tant (hez′ĭ-tant). Term used to descibe the state of RNA polymerase when it is susceptible to pause, arrest or termination signals. SEE ALSO overdrive, antitermination.

hes·per·i·din (hes-per′i-din). A flavone diglycoside obtained from unripe citrus fruit, which reputedly possesses vitamin P activity. SYN cirantin.

Hess, Carl von, German ophthalmologist, 1860–1923. SEE H. *screen.*

Hess, Walter R., Swiss physiologist and Nobel laureate, 1881–1973. SEE trophotropic *zone* of H.

Hesselbach, Franz K., German anatomist and surgeon, 1759–1816. SEE H. *fascia, hernia, ligament, triangle.*

het·a·starch (het′ă-starch). A carbohydrate starch derivative used as a cryoprotective agent for erythrocytes. Also used as an extender of blood plasma volume.

⌂**heter-.** SEE hetero-.

het·er·a·del·phus (het-er-ă-del′fŭs). Unequal conjoined twins in which the smaller incomplete parasite is attached to the larger, more nearly normal autosite. SEE conjoined *twins,* under *twin.* [heter- + G. *adelphos,* brother]

het·er·a·li·us (het-er-ā′lē-ŭs). Unequal conjoined twins in which the parasite appears as little more than an excrescence on the autosite. SEE conjoined *twins,* under *twin.* [heter- + G. *halios,* useless]

het·er·ax·i·al (het-er-ak′sē-ăl). Having mutually perpendicular axes of unequal length.

het·er·e·cious (het-er-ē′shŭs). Having more than one host; said of a parasite passing different stages of its life cycle in different animals. SYN metoxenous. [heter- + G. *oikion,* home]

het·er·e·cism (het′er-ē-sizm). The occurrence, in a parasite, of two cycles of development passed in two different hosts. SYN metoxeny (1). [heter- + G. *oikion,* home]

het·er·es·the·sia (het-er-es-thē′zē-ă). A change occurring in the degree (either plus or minus) of the sensory response to a cutaneous stimulus as the latter crosses a certain line on the surface. [heter- + G. *aisthēsis,* sensation]

⌂**hetero-, heter-.** The other, different; opposite of homo- [G. *heteros,* other]

het·er·o·ag·glu·ti·nin (het′er-ō-ă-gloo′ti-nin). A form of hemagglutinin, one that agglutinates the red blood cells of species other than that in which the h. occurs. SEE ALSO hemagglutinin.

het·er·o·al·leles (het′er-ō-ă-lēlz′). Genes that have undergone mutation at different nucleotide positions and therefore result from different mutational events. Cf. eualleles.

het·er·o·an·ti·body (het′er-ō-an′ti-bod-ē). Antibody that is heterologous with respect to antigen, in contradistinction to isoantibody.

het·er·o·an·ti·se·rum (het′er-ō-an′ti-sē-rŭm). Antiserum developed in one animal species against antigens or cells of another species.

het·er·o·at·om (het′er-ō-at′ŏm). An atom, other than carbon, located in the ring structure of an organic compound, as the N in pyridines or pyrimidines (heterocyclic compounds).

het·er·o·blas·tic (het-er-ō-blas′tik). Developing from more than a single type of tissue. [hetero- + G. *blastos,* germ]

het·er·o·cel·lu·lar (het′er-ō-sel′ū-lăr). Formed of cells of different kinds.

het·er·o·cen·tric (het-er-ō-sen′trik). **1.** Having different centers; said of rays that do not meet at a common focus. Cf. homocentric. **2.** SYN allocentric. [hetero- + G. *kentron,* center]

het·er·o·ceph·a·lus (het-er-ō-sef′ă-lŭs). Conjoined twins with heads of unequal size. SEE conjoined *twins,* under *twin.* [hetero- + G. *kephalē,* head]

het·er·o·chei·ral, het·er·o·chi·ral (het-er-ō-kī′răl). Relating to or referred to the other hand. [hetero- + G. *cheir,* hand]

het·er·o·chro·mat·ic (het′er-ō-krō-mat′ik). Characteristic of heterochromatin.

het·er·o·chro·ma·tin (het′er-ō-krō′mă-tin). The part of the chromonema that remains tightly coiled and condensed during interphase and thus stains readily. SYN heteropyknotic chromatin.

constitutive h., repetitive h. that lies in secondary constrictions in the nucleolar organizers.

facultative h., nonrepetitive h. that comprises translatable sequences of DNA.

satellite-rich h., h. that codes for 18 S and 28 S components of ribosomal RNA and is located close to the centromeres of certain chromosomes.

het·er·o·chro·mia (het′er-ō-krō′mē-ă). A difference in coloration in two structures which are normally alike in color. [hetero- + G. *chrōma,* color]

atrophic h., h. iridis after trauma or inflammation, or in old age.

binocular h., an increase or decrease in pigmentation of one eye, with or without extraocular pigmentary defects.

h. i′ridis, h. of iris, a difference in coloration of the irides. SEE binocular h.

monocular h., SYN *iris* bicolor.

simple h., h. iridis appearing as a developmental defect, without any innervation defect.

sympathetic h., h. iridis occurring after lesions of the cervical sympathetic nerves.

het·er·o·chro·mous (het′er-ō-krō′mŭs). Having an abnormal difference in coloration.

het·er·o·chron (het′er-ō-kron). Having varying chronaxies. [hetero- + G. *chronos,* time]

het·er·o·chro·nia (het-er-ō-krō′nē-ă). Origin or development of tissues or organs at an unusual time or out of the regular sequence. Cf. synchronia. [hetero- + G. *chronos,* time]

het·er·o·chron·ic (het-er-ō-kron′ik). SYN heterochronous.

het·er·och·ro·nous (het-er-ok′rŏ-nŭs). Relating to heterochronia. SYN heterochronic.

het·er·o·clad·ic (het′er-ō-klad′ik). Denoting an anastomosis between branches of different arterial trunks, as distinguished from homocladic. [hetero- + G. *klados*, a twig]

het·er·o·crine (het′er-ō-krin). Denoting the secretion of two or more kinds of material. [hetero- + G. *krinō*, to separate]

het·er·o·cri·sis (het′er-ō-krī′sis). Rarely used term for an irregular crisis, one occurring at an abnormal time or with unusual symptoms.

het·er·o·cy·to·tro·pic (het′er-ō-sī′tō-trop′ik). Having an affinity for cells of a different species. [hetero- + G. *kytos*, cell, + *tropē*, a turning toward]

het·er·o·dis·perse (het′er-ō-dis-pers′). Of varying size; describing aerosols whose particles are not uniform in size.

het·er·o·dont (het′er-ō-dont). Having teeth of varying shapes, such as those of humans and the majority of mammals, in contrast to homodont. [hetero- + G. *odous*, tooth]

Het·er·o·dox·us spi·ni·ger (het-er-ō-dok′sŭs spī′ni-ger). A biting louse of the dog, sometimes called the kangaroo louse.

het·er·od·ro·mous (het-er-ōd′rŏ-mŭs). Moving in the opposite direction. [hetero- + G. *dromos*, running]

❚het·er·o·du·plex (het′er-ō-doo′pleks). 1. A DNA molecule, the two constitutive strands of which derive from distinct sources and hence are likely to be somewhat mismatched. 2. A DNA-RNA hybrid. [hetero- + L. *duplex*, two-fold]

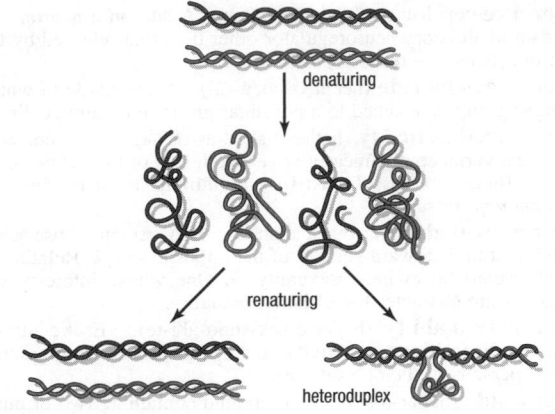

heteroduplex formation: schematic

het·er·od·y·mus (het-er-od′i-mŭs). Unequal conjoined twins in which the incomplete parasite, consisting of head and neck and, to some extent, thorax, is attached to the anterior surface of the autosite. SEE conjoined *twins*, under *twin*. [hetero- + G. *didymos*, twin]

het·er·o·e·rot·i·cism (het′er-ō-ē-rot′ĭ-sism). A condition of sexual excitement brought about by congress with a person of the opposite sex.

het·er·o·ga·met·ic (het′er-ō-gă-met′ik). Having sex gametes of contrasting types; human males are h. SYN digametic. [hetero- + G. *gametikos*, connubial]

het·er·og·a·mous (het-er-og′ă-mŭs). Relating to heterogamy.

het·er·og·a·my (het-er-og′ă-mē). 1. Conjugation of unlike gametes. 2. Bearing different types of flowers. 3. Reproduction by indirect methods of pollination. [hetero- + G. *gamos*, marriage]

het·er·o·ge·ne·i·ty (het′er-ō-jĕ-nē′i-tē). Heterogeneous state or quality.

genetic h., the character of a phenotype produced by mutation at more than one gene or by more than one genetic mechanism. SEE genocopy.

het·er·o·ge·neous (het′er-ō-jē′nē-ŭs). Comprising elements with various and dissimilar properties.

het·er·o·gen·e·sis (het′er-ō-jen′ĕ-sis). 1. Alternation of generations. 2. SYN asexual *generation*. 3. SYN spontaneous *generation*. [hetero- + G. *genesis*, production]

het·er·o·ge·net·ic (het′er-ō-jĕ-net′ik). Relating to heterogenesis.

het·er·o·gen·ic, het·er·o·ge·ne·ic (het′er-ō-jen′ik, -jĕ-nē′ik). Having different gene constitutions, especially in diverse species.

het·er·o·ge·note (het′er-ō-jĕ′nōt). In microbial genetics, an organism that contains exogenous genetic material that differs somewhat from the corresponding region of its own original genome, but in a very limited way resembles a heterozygote.

het·er·og·e·nous (het′er-oj′ĕ-nŭs). Of foreign origin. Commonly confused with heterogeneous.

het·er·o·gly·can (het′er-ō-glī′kan). SYN heteropolysaccharide.

het·er·o·graft (het′er-ō-graft). SYN xenograft.

het·er·o·kar·y·on (het′er-ō-kar′ē-on). A cell containing diverse nuclei inside a common cytoplasm, usually resulting from the artificial fusion of two cells from different species. [hetero- + G. *karyon*, kernel, nut]

het·er·o·kar·y·ot·ic (het′er-ō-kar-ē-ot′ik). Exhibiting the properties of a heterokaryon.

het·er·o·ker·a·to·plas·ty (het′er-ō-ker′ă-tō-plas-tē). Keratoplasty in which the cornea from one species of animal is grafted to the eye of another species.

het·er·o·ki·ne·sia (het′er-ō-ki-nē′zē-ă). Executing movements the reverse of those one is told to make. SYN heterokinesis (2). [hetero- + G. *kinēsis*, movement]

het·er·o·ki·ne·sis (het′er-ō-ki-nē′sis). 1. Differential distribution of X and Y chromosomes during meiotic cell division. 2. SYN heterokinesia. [hetero- + G. *kinēsis*, movement hetero- + G. *kinēsis*, movement]

het·er·o·lat·er·al (het′er-ō-lat′er-ăl). SYN contralateral. [hetero- + L. *latus*, side]

het·er·o·lip·ids (het′er-ō-lip′idz). 1. Lipids containing N and P atoms in addition to the usual C, H, and O. 2. Any complex lipids. Cf. homolipids.

het·er·o·lit·er·al (het′er-ō-lit′er-ăl). Substitution of one letter for another in the pronunciation of certain words. [hetero- + L. *littera*, letter]

het·er·ol·o·gous (het-er-ol′ō-gŭs). 1. Pertaining to cytologic or histologic elements occurring where they are not normally found. SEE ALSO xenogeneic. 2. Derived from an animal of a different species, as the serum of a horse is h. for a rabbit. [hetero- + G. *logos*, ratio, relation]

het·er·ol·o·gy (het-er-ol′ō-jē). A departure from the normal in structure, arrangement, or mode or time of development.

het·er·o·ly·sin (het-er-ol′i-sin). A lysin that is formed in one species of animal and manifests lytic activity on the cells of a different species.

het·er·ol·y·sis (het-er-ol′i-sis). Dissolution or digestion of cells or protein components from one species by a lytic agent from a different species. [hetero- + G. *lysis*, a loosening]

het·er·o·lyt·ic (het′er-ō-lit′ik). Pertaining to heterolysis or to the effect of a heterolysin.

het·er·o·mas·ti·gote (het-er-ō-mas′ti-gōt). A flagellate having two flagella, one anterior and one posterior. [hetero- + G. *mastix*, a whip]

het·er·om·er·al (het′er-om′er-ăl). SYN heteromeric (2).

het·er·o·mer·ic (het′er-ō-mār′ik). 1. Having a different chemical composition. 2. Denoting spinal neurons that have processes passing over to the opposite side of the cord. SYN heteromeral, heteromerous. [hetero- + G. *meros*, part]

het·er·om·er·ous (het′er-om′er-ŭs). SYN heteromeric (2).

het·er·o·me·tab·o·lous (het′er-ō-me-tab′ō-lŭs). Pertaining to a member of the Heterometabola, a superorder sometimes used for a series of insect orders in which incomplete metamorphosis is found. [hetero- + G. *metabolē*, change]

het·er·o·met·a·pla·sia (het′er-ō-met-ă-plā′zē-ă). Tissue transformation resulting in production of a tissue foreign to the part where produced.

he

het·er·o·met·ric (het′er-ō-met′rik). Involving or depending upon a change in size. [hetero- + G. *metron,* measure]

het·er·o·me·tro·pia (het′er-ō-me-trō′pē-ă). A condition in which the refraction is different in the two eyes. [hetero- + G. *metron,* measure, + *ōps,* eye]

het·er·o·mor·phism (het′er-ō-mōrf′izm). In cytogenetics, a difference of shape or size in metaphase between the two homologous chromosomes. [hetero- + G. *morphē,* shape]

het·er·o·mor·pho·sis (het′er-ō-mōr-fō′sis). 1. Development of one tissue from a tissue of another kind or type. 2. Embryonic development of tissue or an organ inappropriate to its site. [hetero- + G. *morphōsis,* a molding]

het·er·o·mor·phous (het′er-ō-mōr′fŭs). Differing from the normal form.

het·er·on·o·mous (het-er-on′ō-mŭs). 1. Different from the type; abnormal. 2. Subject to the direction or control of another; not self-governing. Cf. autonomous. [hetero- + G. *nomos,* law]

het·er·on·o·my (het-er-on′ō-mē). The condition or state of being heteronomous. [hetero- + G. *nomos,* law]

het·er·o·nu·cle·ar (het′er-ō-noo′klē-er). Denoting a heterokaryon that has lost some of the nuclear material of which the cell line was originally constituted.

het·er·on·y·mous (het-er-on′i-mŭs). Having different names or expressed in different terms. [G. *heterōnymos,* having a different name, fr. *onyma,* or *onoma,* name]

het·er·op·a·gus (het-er-op′ă-gŭs). Unequal conjoined twins in which the imperfectly developed parasite is attached to the ventral portion of the autosite. SEE conjoined *twins,* under *twin.* SEE ALSO epigastrius. [hetero- + G. *pagos,* fixed]

het·er·op·a·thy (het′er-op′ă-thē). 1. Abnormal sensitivity to stimuli. 2. SYN allopathy. [hetero- + G. *pathos,* suffering]

het·er·oph·a·gy (het-er-of′ă-jē). Digestion within a cell of an exogenous substance phagocytosed from the cell's environment. [hetero- + G. *phago,* to eat]

het·er·o·phil, het·er·o·phile (het-er-ō-fil, -fīl). 1. Pertaining to heterogenetic or cross-reacting antigens occurring in different species or to antibodies directed against such antigens. 2. The neutrophilic leukocyte in man; in some animals the granules vary in size and staining reaction. [hetero- + G. *philos,* fond]

het·er·o·pho·nia (het′er-ō-fō′nē-ă). 1. The change of voice at puberty. 2. Any abnormality in the voice sounds. SYN heterophthongia. [hetero- + G. *phōnē,* voice]

het·er·o·pho·ria (het′er-ō-fō′rē-ă). A tendency for deviation of the eyes from parallelism, prevented by binocular vision. [hetero- + G. *phora,* movement]

het·er·oph·thal·mus (het′er-of-thal′mŭs). A seldom-used term for a difference in the appearance of the two eyes, usually due to heterochromia iridis. SYN allophthalmia. [hetero- + G. *ophthalmos,* eye]

het·er·oph·thon·gia (het-er-of-thon′jē-ă). SYN heterophonia. [G. *heterophthongos,* fr. *heteros,* different, + *phthongos,* sound, voice]

Het·er·o·phy·es (het-er-of′i-ēz). A genus of digenetic flukes (family Heterophyidae) parasitic in fish-eating birds and mammals, including man; cercariae from infected snails penetrate and encyst in fish, which are eaten by the final hosts. [hetero- + G. *phyē,* stature, form]

H. brevicae′ca, a species reported in humans in the Philippines and implicated in heart lesions caused by the eggs of this minute fluke, carried from the intestinal mucosa to obstruct coronary capillaries.

H. heteroph′yes, the Egyptian intestinal or small intestinal fluke, a species infecting the small intestine and cecum in humans and other fish-eating mammals in Egypt and the Far East.

H. katsura′dai, a species, somewhat smaller than *H. heterophyes,* found in Japan.

het·er·o·phy·i·a·sis (het′er-ō-fī-ī′ă-sis). Infection with a heterophyid trematode, particularly *Heterophyes heterophyes.* SYN heterophyidiasis.

het·er·o·phy·id (het′er-o-fī′id). Common name for a member of the family Heterophyidae.

Het·er·o·phy·i·dae (het′er-ō-fī′i-dē). A family of tiny fish-borne trematodes, including the genus *Heterophyes* and its common human parasite, *H. heterophyes.*

het·er·o·phy·id·i·a·sis (het′er-ō-fī-id-ī′ă-sis). SYN heterophyiasis.

het·er·o·pla·sia (het′er-ō-plā′zē-ă). 1. Development of cytologic and histologic elements that are not normal for the organ or part in question, as the growth of bone in a site where there is normally fibrous connective tissue. 2. Malposition of tissue or a part that is otherwise normal, as a ureter that develops at the lower pole of a kidney. SYN alloplasia. [hetero- + G. *plasis,* a forming]

het·er·o·plas·tic (het′er-ō-plas′tik). 1. Pertaining to or manifesting heteroplasia. 2. Relating to heteroplasty.

het·er·o·plas·tid (het′er-ō-plas′tid). The graft in heteroplasty.

het·er·o·ploid (het′er-ō-ployd). Relating to heteroploidy.

het·er·o·ploi·dy (het′er-ō-ploy′dē). The state of a cell possessing some number of complete haploid sets other than the normal. [hetero- + G. *ploides,* in form]

het·er·o·pol·y·sac·cha·ride (het′er-ō-pol-ē-sak′ă-rīd). A polysaccharide composed of two or more different types of monosaccharides. Cf. glycan, homoglycan. SYN heteroglycan.

het·er·o·pro·te·ose (het′er-ō-prō′tē-ōs). SEE primary *proteose.*

het·er·o·pyk·no·sis (het′er-ō-pik-nō′sis). Any state of variable density or condensation, usually in different chromosomes or between different regions of the same chromosome; a region may be attentuated (**negative h**) or accentuated (**positive h**). [hetero- + G. *pyknos,* dense]

het·er·o·pyk·not·ic (het′er-ō-pik-not′ik). Relating to or characterized by heteropyknosis.

het·er·o·re·cep·tor (het′er-ō-rē-sep′ter). A site on a neuron that binds a modulatory neuroregulator other than that released by the neuron. [hetero- + receptor]

het·er·o·sac·cha·ride (het′er-ō-sak′ă-rīd). A glycoside in which a sugar group is attached to a nonsugar group; e.g., amygdalin.

het·er·o·sced·as·tic·i·ty (het′er-ō-skĕd-as-tis′ĭ-tē). Non-constancy of the variance of a measure over the levels of the factor under study. [hetero + G. *skedastikos,* pertaining to scattering, fr. *skedannumi,* to scatter]

het·er·o·sex·u·al (het′er-ō-sek′shoo-ăl). 1. A person whose sexual orientation is toward persons of the opposite sex. 2. Relating to or characteristic of heterosexuality. 3. One whose interests and behavior are characteristic of heterosexuality.

het·er·o·sex·u·al·i·ty (het′er-ō-sek-shoo-al′i-tē). Erotic attraction, predisposition, or activity, including sexual congress between persons of the opposite sex.

het·er·o·side (het′er-ō-sīd). A compound containing two or more different carbohydrate residues that are covalently linked to a noncarbohydrate moiety.

het·er·o·sis (het-er-ō′sis). The beneficial effect on the phenotype of crossing (hybridization) upon growth, vigor, and physical or mental qualities in a strain of plants or in animal stock, as measured by the difference between the midparent mean phenotype and that of F₁; also referred to as hybrid vigor. [hetero- + -ōsis, condition]

het·er·os·mia (het′er-os′mē-a). SYN allotriosmia.

het·er·o·some (het′er-ō-sōm). In genetics, the chromosome pair that is different in the two sexes. SEE sex *chromosomes,* under *chromosome.* [hetero- + G. *sōma,* body]

het·er·o·spe·cif·ic (het′er-ō-spe-sif′ik). Heterologous, as pertains to grafts.

het·er·o·sug·ges·tion (het′er-ō-sŭg-jes′chŭn). A rarely used term for hypnotic suggestion received from another person; opposed to autosuggestion.

het·er·o·tax·ia (het′er-ō-taks′ē-ă). Abnormal arrangement of organs or parts of the body in relation to each other. SYN heterotaxis, heterotaxy. [hetero- + G. *taxis,* arrangement]

    cardiac h., SEE dextrocardia.

het·er·o·tax·ic (het-er-ō-taks′ik). Abnormally placed or arranged.

het·er·o·tax·is, het·er·o·taxy (het-er-ō-taks′is, het′er-ō-taks-ē). SYN heterotaxia.

het·er·o·thal·lic (het′er-ō-thal′ik). In fungi, denoting a kind of sexual reproduction in which a sexual spore is produced only by fusion with a nucleus of another mating type. Cf. homothallic. [hetero- + G. *thallos,* a young shoot]

het·er·o·therm (het′er-ō-therm). A heterothermic animal.

het·er·o·ther·mic (het′er-ō-ther′mik). Having partial regulation of body temperature; between poikilothermic and homeothermic.

het·er·ot·ic (het-er-ot′ik). Relating to heterosis.

het·er·o·to·nia (het′er-ō-tō′nē-ă). Abnormality or variation in tension or tonus. [hetero- + G. *tonos,* tension]

het·er·o·to·pia (het-er-ō-tō′pē-ă). 1. SYN ectopia. 2. In neuropathology, displacement of gray matter, typically into the deep cerebral white matter. [hetero- + G. *topos,* place]

h. mac′ulae, SYN *ectopia* maculae.

het·er·o·top·ic (het-er-ō-top′ik). 1. SYN ectopic (1). 2. Relating to heterotopia (2). [hetero- + *topos,* place, + suffix *-ic,* pertaining to]

het·er·ot·o·pous (het-er-ot′ō-pŭs). Heterotopic, especially in reference to teratomas composed of tissues that are out of place in the region where found.

het·er·o·trans·plan·ta·tion (het′er-ō-tranz-plan-tā′shŭn). Transfer of a heterograft (xenograft).

het·er·o·tri·cho·sis (het′er-ō-tri-kō′sis). A condition characterized by hair growth of variegated color. [hetero- + G. *trichōsis,* growth of hair]

het·er·o·troph (het′er-ō-trof, -trōf). A microorganism that obtains its carbon, as well as its energy, from organic compounds. SEE ALSO autotroph. [hetero- + G. *trophē,* nourishment]

het·er·o·tro·phic (het′er-ō-tro-fik). 1. Relating to or exhibiting the properties of heterotrophy. 2. Relating to a heterotroph.

het·er·ot·ro·phy (het′er-ō-trō-fē). The ability or requirement to synthesize all metabolites from organic compounds.

het·er·o·tro·pia, het·er·ot·ro·py (het′er-ō-trō′pē-ă, het-er-ot′rō-pē). SYN strabismus. [hetero- + G. *tropē,* a turning]

het·er·o·typ·ic (het′er-ō-tip′ik). Of a different or unusual type or form.

het·er·o·xan·thine (het′er-ō-zan′thin). 7-Methylxanthine; one of the alloxuric bases in urine, representing end products of purine metabolism.

het·er·ox·e·nous (het-er-oks′ĕ-nŭs). SYN digenetic (1). [hetero- + G. *xenos,* stranger]

het·er·o·zo·ic (het-er-ō-zō′ik). Relating to another animal or another species of animal. [hetero- + G. *zōikos,* relating to an animal]

het·er·o·zy·gos·i·ty, het·er·o·zy·go·sis (het′er-ō-zī-gos′i-tē, -zī-gō′sis). The state of being heterozygous. [hetero- + G. *zygon,* a yoke]

het·er·o·zy·gote (het′er-ō-zī′gōt). A heterozygous individual. [hetero- + G. *zygotos,* yoked]

compound h., in medical genetics, the presence of two different mutant alleles at the same loci. SYN genetic compound.

manifesting h., an organism heterozygous for what is ordinarily a recessive condition which, as a result of special mechanisms (such as lyonization, allelic exclusion, or a deletion in the homologous chromosome), has phenotypic manifestations. SYN manifesting carrier.

het·er·o·zy·gous (het′er-ō-zī′gŭs). Having different alleles at one locus regarding a specific character; heterotic.

doubly h., in the analysis of linkage between two loci, denoting that genotype in which a parent is h. at both loci, the state that on average contains the maximum information about the linkage.

Heubner, Johann O.L., German pediatrician, 1843–1926. SEE *artery* of H.; H. *arteritis.*

Heurenius, Johannes. SEE van Horne.

Heuser, Chester H., U.S. embryologist, 1885–1965. SEE H. *membrane.*

HEV Abbreviation for hepatitis E *virus.*

⊿**hexa-, hex-.** Prefix denoting six. [G. *hex*]

hex·a·canth (hek′să-kanth). The motile six-hooked first-stage larva of cyclophyllidean cestodes; it emerges from the egg and actively claws its way through the intermediate host's intestine prior to development into the next larval stage; e.g., the h. of

Taenia saginata, which penetrates the intestine of a cow that ingested the egg, then forms a cysticercus in the muscles of the intermediate host. SYN oncosphere. [hexa- + G. *akantha,* hook or thorn]

hex·a·chlo·ro·cy·clo·hex·ane (hek-să-klō′rō-sī-klō-hek′sān). SYN gamma benzene hexachloride.

hex·a·chlo·ro·phane (hek-să-klō′rō-fān). SYN hexachlorophene.

hex·a·chlo·ro·phene (hek-să-klo′rō-fēn). An antibacterial; formerly widely used in soaps and detergents to inhibit bacterial growth; excessive use causes neurologic lesions; currently limited use. SYN hexachlorophane.

hex·a·co·sa·no·ic ac·id (heks′ă-kō′sān-ō-ik). Systemic name for cerotinic acid.

hex·a·co·sa·nol (heks-ă-kō′să-nol). SEE ceryl.

hex·a·co·syl (heks-ă-kō′sil). SYN ceryl.

hex·ad (heks′ad). A sexivalent element or radical.

hex·a·dac·ty·ly, hex·a·dac·tyl·ism (hek′să-dak′ti-lē, -lizm). The presence of six fingers or six toes on one or both hands or feet. [hexa- + G. *daktylos,* finger]

hex·a·dec·a·no·ic ac·id (hek′să-dek-ă-nō′ik). SYN palmitic acid.

1-hex·a·dec·a·nol (hek-să-dek′ă-nol). SYN *cetyl* alcohol.

hex·a·flu·o·ren·i·um bro·mide (hek′să-floo-rēn′ē-ŭm). A potentiator for succinylcholine in anesthesiology by producing a mild nondepolarizing neuromuscular blockade; also inhibits plasma cholinesterase.

hex·a·mer (hek′să-mer). 1. A group of six protein subunits that form a capsomere on the surface of an icosohedral virus. 2. A complex or compound containing six subunits or moieties (e.g., a protein complex with six polypeptide chains or an oligopeptide with six amino acid residues). [hexa- + G. *meros,* part]

hex·a·mer·ic (heks′ă-mer-ik). Containing six subunits or moieties.

hex·a·met·a·zime (HMPAO). A lipophilic substance that readily crosses the blood-brain barrier; combined with ^{99m}Tc to produce a radiopharmaceutical for SPECT imaging or cerebral blood flow estimates. SYN hexamethylpropyleneamine oxime.

hex·a·meth·yl·prop·yl·ene·a·mine ox·ime (heks-ă-meth′il-prō′pi-lēn- ă-mēn oks′ēm). SYN hexametazime.

hex·am·i·dine is·e·thi·o·nate (hek-sam′i-dēn). A topical antiseptic.

hex·a·mine (hek′să-mēn). SYN methenamine.

hex·ane (hek′sān). A saturated hydrocarbon, C_6H_{14}, of the paraffin series (typically *n*-h., $CH_3–(CH_2)_4–CH_3$).

hex·a·no·ate (hek-să-nō-āt). SYN caprolyate.

***n*-hex·a·no·ic ac·id** (hek-să-nō′ik). SYN *n*-caproic acid.

hex·a·no·yl (hek′să-nō-il). SYN caproyl.

hex·a·pep·tide (heks′a-pep′tīd). A peptide containing six amino acid residues.

hex·a·ploi·dy (heks′ă-ploy-dē). SEE polyploidy.

Hex·a·po·da (hek-sap′ō-dă). SYN Insecta. [hexa- + G. *pous,* foot]

hex·es·trol (hek-ses′trol). A synthetic *meso*-compound with estrogenic activity.

hex·i·tol (heks′i-tol). The polyol (sugar alcohol) obtained on the reduction of a hexose (e.g., D-sorbitol).

hex·o·ki·nase (heks-ō-kī′nās). A phosphotransferase present in yeast, muscle, brain, and other tissues that catalyzes the ATP-dependent phosphorylation of D-glucose and other hexoses to form D-glucose 6-phosphate (or other hexose 6-phosphates); the first step in glycolysis; a deficiency of h. can result in hemolytic anemia and impaired glycolysis.

hex·on (heks′on). One of a group of six protein units (hexamer unit) on the triangular face of an icosohedral capsomere on certain viruses. [hex- + -on]

hex·on·ic ac·id (heks-on′ik). The aldonic acid obtained on the oxidation of the aldehyde group of an aldohexose to a carboxylic acid (e.g., gluconic acid from glucose).

hex·os·a·mine (heks′ō-sam′ēn). The amine derivative (NH_2 replacing OH) of a hexose; e.g., glucosamine.

hex·os·a·min·i·dase (hek′sō-sa-min′i-dās). General term for en-

he

zymes cleaving *N*-acetylhexose (e.g., *N*-acetylglucosamine) residues from gangliosidelike oligosaccharides. At least four specific enzymes carrying out this type of reaction are known: α-*N*-acetyl-D-galactosaminidase, α-*N*-acetyl-D-glucosaminidase, β-*N*-acetyl-D-hexosaminidase, and β-*N*-acetyl-D-galactosaminidase, each being specific for the configuration and type of sugar included in the name.

h. A, a hydrolytic enzyme that acts on ganglioside G_{M2}, producing *N*-acetyl-D-galactosamine and ganglioside G_{M3}; a deficiency of this enzyme is associated with Tay-Sachs disease.

h. B, a hydrolytic enzyme that acts on ganglioside G_{M1}, producing ganglioside G_{M1} and galactose, as well as on globoside, producing *N*-acetylgalactosamine and trihexosylceramide; a deficiency of this enzyme is associated with Sandhoff disease.

hex·o·sans (hek′sō-sanz). Polysaccharides with the general formula $(C_6H_{10}O_5)_x$ that, on hydrolysis, yield hexoses; included are glucosans (glucans), mannans, galactans, and fructosans (fructans). SYN polyhexoses.

hex·ose (hek′sōs). A monosaccharide containing six carbon atoms in the molecule $(C_6H_{12}O_6)$; D-glucose is the principal h. in nature.

hex·ose·bis·phos·pha·tase, hex·ose·di·phos·pha·tase (hek′sōs-bis-fos′fă-tās, -dī-). SYN fructose 1,6-bisphosphate.

hex·ose phos·pha·tase (hek′sōs fos′fa-tāz). An enzyme catalyzing the hydrolysis of a hexose phosphate to a hexose (e.g., glucose-6-phosphatase).

hex·ose·phos·phate isom·er·ase (hek-sōs-fos′fāt). SYN glucosephosphate isomerase.

hex·ose-1-phos·phate uri·dyl·yl·trans·fer·ase. SYN UDPglucose-hexose-1-phosphate uridylyltransferase.

hex·u·lose (hek′sū-lōs). SYN ketohexose.

hex·u·ron·ic ac·id (hek-sūr-on′ik). The uronic acid of a hexose.

hex·yl (hek′sil). The radical of hexane, $CH_3(CH_2)_4CH_2-$.

hex·yl·res·or·cin·ol (hek′sil-re-sōr′si-nol). A broad spectrum anthelmintic and antiseptic.

Hey, William, English surgeon, 1736–1819. SEE H. *amputation, hernia,* ligament.

Heyer, W.T., U.S. scientist, *1902. SEE H.-Pudenz *valve.*

Hf Symbol for hafnium.

Hg Symbol for mercury (hydrargyrum).

HGE Abbreviation for human granulocytic *ehrlichiosis.*

HGF Abbreviation for hyperglycemic-glycogenolytic *factor.*

HGH Abbreviation for human growth hormone. SEE somatotropin.

HGPRT Abbreviation for *hypoxanthine* guanine phosphoribosyltransferase.

HGSIL Abbreviation for high-grade squamous intraepithelial *lesion.*

HGV Abbreviation for hepatitis G *virus.*

HHV Abbreviation for human herpesvirus.

hi·a·tal (hī-ā′tăl). Relating to a hiatus.

hi·a·tus (hī-ā′tŭs) [TA]. An aperture, opening, or foramen. [L. an aperture, fr. *hio,* pp. *hiatus,* to yawn]

adductor h. [TA], the aperture in the aponeurotic insertion of the adductor magnus that transmits the femoral artery and vein from the adductor canal to the popliteal space. SYN h. adductorius [TA], femoral opening, h. tendineus, tendinous opening.

h. adducto′rius [TA], SYN adductor h.

aortic h. [TA], the opening in the diaphragm bounded by the two crura, the vertebral column, and the median arcuate ligament, through which pass the aorta and thoracic duct. SYN h. aorticus [TA], aortic foramen, aortic opening.

h. aor′ticus [TA], SYN aortic h.

Breschet h., SYN helicotrema.

h. cana′lis facia′lis, SYN h. for greater petrosal nerve.

h. cana′lis ner′vi petro′si majo′ris [TA], SYN h. for greater petrosal nerve.

h. cana′lis ner′vi petro′si mino′ris [TA], SYN h. for lesser petrosal nerve.

esophageal h. [TA], the opening in the right crus of the diaphragm, between the central tendon and the h. aorticus, through

which pass the esophagus and the two vagus nerves. SYN h. esophageus [TA], esophageal opening.

h. esopha′geus [TA], SYN esophageal h.

h. ethmoida′lis, SYN semilunar h.

h. of facial canal, SYN h. for greater petrosal nerve.

fallopian h., SYN h. for greater petrosal nerve.

h. for greater petrosal nerve [TA], the opening on the anterior aspect of the petrous part of the temporal bone that leads to the facial canal and gives passage to the greater petrosal nerve. SYN h. canalis nervi petrosi majoris [TA], fallopian h., Ferrein foramen, h. canalis facialis, h. of facial canal.

h. for lesser petrosal nerve [TA], the small opening in the petrous bone lateral to the h. for greater petrosal nerve that gives passage to the lesser petrosal nerve. SYN h. canalis nervi petrosi minoris [TA], Arnold canal, canalis nervi petrosi superficialis minoris.

h. maxilla′ris [TA], SYN maxillary h.

maxillary h. [TA], the large opening into the maxillary sinus on the nasal surface of the maxilla. SYN h. maxillaris [TA].

pleuropericardial h., an opening connecting the pleural and pericardial cavities; usually the result of incomplete development of the pleuropericardial fold of the embryo.

pleuroperitoneal h., an opening through the diaphragm, connecting pleural and peritoneal cavities, usually the result of defective development of the pleuroperitoneal membrane in the embryo; if the defect is extensive there may be herniation of digestive organs into the pleural cavity. SEE ALSO diaphragmatic *hernia.* SYN Bochdalek foramen.

sacral h. [TA], a normally occurring gap at the lower end of the sacrum, exposing the vertebral canal, due to failure of the laminae of the last sacral segment to coalesce. It is closed by the sacrococcygeal ligament, and provides cannular access to the sacral epidural space for administration of anesthetics (caudal nerve blocks). SYN h. sacralis [TA].

h. sacra′lis [TA], SYN sacral h.

saphenous h., SYN saphenous *opening.*

h. saphe′nus [TA], SYN saphenous *opening.*

scalene h., triangular gap bounded by the scalenus anterior and scalenus medius muscles and the first rib to which the muscles attach; the h. provides passage for the subclavian artery and the roots of the brachial plexus. Compression of the structures passing through the h. by any means is manifest as "thoracic outlet syndrome." SYN interscalene triangle.

Scarpa h., SYN helicotrema.

semilunar h. [TA], a deep, narrow groove in the lateral wall of the middle meatus of the nasal cavity, into which the maxillary sinus, the frontonasal duct, and the middle ethmoid cells open. SYN h. semilunaris [TA], h. ethmoidalis.

h. semiluna′ris [TA], SYN semilunar h.

h. subarcua′tus, SYN subarcuate *fossa.*

h. tendin′eus, SYN adductor h.

h. tota′lis sacra′lis, developmental clefting in all sacral vertebrae; may also involve adjacent lumbar vertebrae.

hi·ber·na·tion (hī-ber-nā′shŭn). A torpid condition in which certain animals pass the cold months. True hibernators, such as woodchucks, ground squirrels, dormice, and some others, have body temperatures reduced to near the freezing point, with a very slow heartbeat, low metabolism, and infrequent respirations. Partial hibernators, such as bears, skunks, and raccoons, have reduced physiologic activity during the cold months, but they are not comatose. Cf. estivation. SYN winter sleep. [L. *hibernus,* relating to winter]

hi·ber·no·ma (hī′ber-nō′mă). A rare type of benign neoplasm in humans, consisting of brown fat that resembles the fat in certain hibernating animals; individual tumor cells contain multiple lipid droplets. SEE ALSO brown *fat.* [L. *hibernus,* pertaining to winter, + G. -*ōma,* tumor]

interscapular h., SYN brown *fat.*

hic·cup, hic·cough (hik′ŭp). A diaphragmatic spasm causing a sudden inhalation that is interrupted by a spasmodic closure of the glottis, producing a noise. SYN singultus.

epidemic h., a persistent h. occurring as a complication of influenza.

Hickman, Robert o., 20th century U.S. pediatric surgeon. SEE H. *catheter.*

Hicks, SEE Braxton Hicks.

HIDA Abbreviation for dimethyl iminodiacetic acid.

⬭**hidr-.** SEE hidro-.

hi·drad·e·ni·tis (hī-drad′ĕ-nī′tis). Inflammation of the sweat glands. SYN hydradenitis. [G. *hidrōs,* sweat, + *adēn,* gland, + *-itis,* inflammation]

h. suppurati′va, chronic suppurative folliculitis of apocrine sweat-gland–bearing skin of the perianal, axillary, and genital areas or under the breasts, developing after puberty and producing abscesses or sinuses with scarring.

neutrophilic eccrine h., an inflammatory condition occuring in patients receiving chemotherapy, with deep eccrine gland neutrophil infiltration.

hi·drad·e·no·ma (hī-drad-ĕ-nō′mă). A benign neoplasm derived from epithelial cells of sweat glands. SYN hydradenoma. [G. *hidrōs,* sweat, + *adēn,* gland, + *-oma,* tumor]

clear cell h., a tumor derived from eccrine sweat glands, composed of glycogen-rich clear cells. SYN eccrine acrospiroma, nodular h.

nodular h., SYN clear cell h.

papillary h., a solitary benign tumor occurring in women usually in the labia majora, cystic and papillary, and composed of epithelium resembling that of apocrine glands. SYN apocrine adenoma, h. papilliferum.

h. papillife′rum, SYN papillary h.

⬭**hidro-, hidr-.** Sweat, sweat glands. Cf. sudor-. [G. *hidrōs*]

hi·droa (hī-drō′ă). SYN hydroa.

hi·dro·cys·to·ma (hī′drō-sis-tō′mă). A cystic form of hidradenoma, usually apocrine. SYN hydrocystoma (2), syringocystoma. [hidro- + G. *kystis,* bladder, + *-ōma,* tumor]

apocrine h., SYN sudoriferous *cyst.*

hi·dro·mei·o·sis (hī′drō-mī-ō′sis). A decline in the rate of sweating during exposure to heat, especially that from warm baths. [hidro- + G. *meiōsis,* a lessening]

hi·dro·poi·e·sis (hī′drō-poy-ē′sis, hid′rō-). The formation of sweat. [hidro- + G. *poiēsis,* formation]

hi·dros·che·sis (hī-dros′kē-sis, hid-ros′). Suppression of sweating. [hidro- + G. *schesis,* a checking]

hi·dro·sis (hi-drō′sis, hī-). The production and excretion of sweat. [G. *hidrōs,* sweat, + *-osis,* condition]

hi·drot·ic (hi-drot′ik, hī-). Relating to or causing hidrosis.

hi·er·ar·chy (hī′er-ar-kē, hī-rar′kē). **1.** Any system of persons or things ranked one above the other. **2.** In psychology and psychiatry, an organization of habits or concepts in which simpler components are combined to form increasingly complex integrations. [G. *hierarchia,* rule or power of the high priest]

dominance h., a social situation in which one organism dominates all below it, the next all below it, and so on down to the organism dominated by all; e.g., the pecking order in apes, seals, barnyard hens, and other species.

Maslow h., a ranking of needs which humans presumably fills successively in the order of lowest to highest: physiological needs, love and belonging, self-esteem, and self-actualization.

response h., alternative reactions or modes of adjustment to a given situation arranged in the probable order of prior effectiveness; e.g., a mother attempting to discipline an unruly child may first request, cajole, then plead, scold, and finally punish; her behaviors can be ordered along a response h. for further monitoring of effectiveness.

h. of terms, in radiology, the semantic concept of using different terms to describe anatomic or pathologic structures versus the resultant diagnostic images.

hi·er·o·pho·bia (hī′er-ō-fō′bē-ă). Morbid fear of religious or sacred objects. [G. *hieros,* holy, + *phobos,* fear]

hi·er·o·ther·a·py (hī′er-ō-thār′ă-pē). Treatment of disease by prayer and religious practices. [G. *hieros,* holy, + *therapeia,* therapy]

Higashi, Ototaka. Japanese physician. SEE Chédiak-H. *disease;* Chédiak-Steinbrinck-H. *anomaly, syndrome.*

Highmore, Nathaniel, British anatomist, 1613–1685. SEE *antrum* of H.; H. *body.*

Higoumenakia sign. See under sign.

hi·la (hī′lă). Plural of hilum.

hi·lar (hī′lăr). Pertaining to a hilum.

hi·li·tis (hī-lī′tis). Inflammation of the lining membrane of any hilus.

Hill, Archibald V., English biophysicist and Nobel laureate, 1886–1977. SEE H. *equation, plot;* initial *heat.*

Hill, Austin Bradford, British medical statistician, 1897–1991. SEE H.'s *criteria* of evidence, under *criterion.*

Hill, Harold A., 20th century U.S. radiologist. SEE H.-Sachs *lesion.*

Hill, Sir Leonard Erskine, English physiologist, 1866-1952. SEE H. *sign, phenomenon.*

Hill, Lucius D., U.S. thoracic surgeon, *1921. SEE H. *operation.*

Hill, Robert, British plant physiologist, *1899. SEE H. *reaction.*

Hillis, David S., U.S. obstetrician-gynecologist, 1873–1942. SEE H.-Müller *maneuver.*

hil·lock (hil′lok). In anatomy, any small elevation or prominence.

axon h., the conical area of origin of the axon from the nerve cell body; it contains parallel arrays of microtubules and is devoid of Nissl substance. SYN implantation cone.

facial h., SYN facial *colliculus.*

seminal h., SYN seminal *colliculus.*

Hilton, John, English surgeon, 1804–1878. SEE H. *law,* white *line, method, sac.*

hi·lum, pl. **hi·la** (hī′lŭm, hī′lă) [TA]. **1.** The part of an organ where the nerves and vessels enter and leave. SYN porta (1). **2.** A depression or slit resembling the h. in the olivary nucleus of the brain. [L. a small bit or trifle]

h. of dentate nucleus [TA], the mouth of the flasklike dentate nucleus of the cerebellum, directed inward, and giving exit to many of the fibers which compose the superior cerebellar peduncle or brachium conjunctivum. SYN h. nuclei dentati [TA].

h. of inferior olivary nucleus [TA], the medially oriented opening in the folded cell layer composing the inferior olivary nucleus through which the efferent fibers of the nucleus make their exit. SYN h. nuclei olivaris inferioris [TA].

h. of kidney [TA], the depression on the medial border of the kidney through which pass the segmental renal vessels and renal nerves and where the apex of the renal pelvis occurs. SYN h. renalis [TA], porta renis.

h. li′enis, ✕official alternate term for splenic h.

h. of lung [TA], a wedge-shaped depression on the mediastinal surface of each lung, where the bronchus, blood vessels, nerves, and lymphatics enter or leave the viscus. SYN h. pulmonis [TA], porta pulmonis.

h. of lymph node [TA], the depressed area of the surface of a lymph node through which the efferent lymphatics emerge from the medulla and through which blood vessels enter and leave the node. SYN h. nodi lymphatici [TA].

h. no′di lympha′tici [TA], SYN h. of lymph node.

h. nu′clei denta′ti [TA], SYN h. of dentate nucleus.

h. nu′clei oliva′ris inferioris [TA], SYN h. of inferior olivary nucleus.

h. ova′rii, SYN h. of ovary.

h. of ovary, the depression along the mesovarian margin, at the insertion of the mesovarium, where vessels and nerves enter or leave the ovary. SYN h. ovarii.

h. pulmo′nis [TA], SYN h. of lung.

h. rena′lis [TA], SYN h. of kidney.

h. of spleen, SYN splenic h.

splenic h. [TA], a fissure on the gastric surface of the spleen, giving passage to the splenic vessels and nerves. SYN h. splenicum [TA], h. lienis✕, h. of spleen, porta lienis.

hi

h. sple′nicum [TA], SYN splenic h.

hi·lus (hī′lŭs). Former incorrect designation for hilum. [an Eng. variant of L. *hilum*]

hi·man·to·sis (hī-man-tō′sis). An unusually long uvula. [G. *himas*, strap, + *-osis*, condition]

hind·brain (hīnd′brān) [TA]. SYN rhombencephalon.

hind·gut (hīnd′gŭt). **1.** The caudal or terminal part of the embryonic gut. **2.** Descending and sigmoid colon, rectum and anal canal; some include entire large intestine. SYN endgut.

hind·wa·ter (hīnd′wah-ter). Colloquialism for amniotic fluid *in utero* behind the presenting part of the fetus.

hinge-bow (hinj′bō). SYN face-bow.

Hinman, Frank, Jr., U.S. urologist, *1915. SEE H. *syndrome*.

Hinton, William A., U.S. physician, 1883–1959. SEE H. *test;* Mueller-H. *agar*.

hip. 1. The lateral prominence of the pelvis from the waist to the thigh. SYN coxa (1) [TA]. **2.** Head, neck, and greater and lesser trochanter of femur. It is this sense that is meant in the common phrases "hip fracture" or "hip replacement." **3.** More strictly, the hip joint. [A.S. *hype*]

snapping h., a condition in which the fascia lata or gluteus maximus muscle under tension, moving over the greater trochanter of the proximal end of the femur or the iliopsoas tendon moves over the lesser trochanter and causes a click.

hip·ber·ries. SYN *rose* hips.

Hippel, Eugen von. SEE von H.

Hip·pe·la·tes (hip-ĕ-lā′tēz). The eye gnats, a genus of flies in the family Chloropidae (fruit flies) that are attracted to the body secretions and fluids of animals and humans, particularly those in the eyes. *H.* is suspected of transmitting certain types of conjunctivitis (such as pinkeye), bovine mastitis, and yaws (frambesia tropica). [G. *hippelatēs*, driver of horses]

Hip·po·bos·ca (hip-ō-bos′kă). A genus of pupiparous louse flies (family Hippoboscidae) related to the tsetse flies; they are ectoparasites on birds and mammals. [G. *hippos*, horse, + *boskein*, to feed]

hip·po·cam·pal (hip-ō-kam′păl). Relating to the hippocampus.

hip·po·cam·pus (hip-ō-kam′pŭs) [TA]. The complex, internally convoluted structure that forms the medial margin ("hem") of the cortical mantle of the cerebral hemisphere, bordering the choroid fissure of the lateral ventricle, and composed of two gyri (Ammon horn and the dentate gyrus), together with their white matter, the alveus and fimbria hippocampi. In monkeys, apes, and humans the h. is confined to the temporal lobe by the massive development of the corpus callosum. Cytoarchitecturally a unique form of allocortex (archicortex), the h. forms part of the limbic system (formerly rhinencephalon). Its major afferent connections are with the entorhinal area of the parahippocampal gyrus, and transparent septum; by way of the fornix it projects to the septum, anterior nucleus of the thalamus, and mamillary body. SYN h. major, major h. [G. *hippocampos*, seahorse]

h. ma′jor, SYN hippocampus.

major h., SYN hippocampus.

h. mi′nor, SYN calcarine *spur*.

minor h., SYN calcarine *spur*.

Hippocrates of Cos. Greek physician, called the "Father of Medicine," circa 460–377 B.C. SEE hippocratic *facies*, hippocratic *fingers*, under *finger*, Hippocratic *nails*, under *nail*, hippocratic *school*, hippocratic *succussion*.

hip·po·crat·ic (hip-ŏ-krat′ik). Relating to, described by, or attributed to Hippocrates.

Hip·po·crat·ic Oath. An oath usually taken by physicians about to enter the practice of their profession, that, though usually attributed to Hippocrates of Cos, is probably an ancient oath of the Asclepiads. Its original form, now often revised, appears in a book of the Hippocratic collection as follows:

"I swear by Apollo the physician, by Aesculapius, Hygeia, and Panacea, and I take to witness all the gods, all the goddesses, to keep according to my ability and my judgment the following Oath:

To consider dear to me as my parents him who taught me this art; to live in common with him and if necessary to share my goods with him; to look upon his children as my own brothers, to teach them this art if they so desire without fee or written promise; to impart to my sons and the sons of the master who taught me and the disciples who have enrolled themselves and have agreed to the rules of the profession, but to these alone, the precepts and the instruction. I will prescribe regimen for the good of my patients according to my ability and my judgment and never do harm to anyone. To please no one will I prescribe a deadly drug, nor give advice which may cause his death. Nor will I give a woman a pessary to procure abortion. But I will preserve the purity of my life and my art. I will not cut for stone, even for patients in whom the disease is manifest; I will leave this operation to be performed by practitioners (specialists in this art). In every house where I come I will enter only for the good of my patients, keeping myself far from all intentional ill-doing and all seduction, and especially from the pleasures of love with women or with men, be they free or slaves. All that may come to my knowledge in the exercise of my profession or outside of my profession or in daily commerce with men, which ought not to be spread abroad, I will keep secret and will never reveal. If I keep this oath faithfully, may I enjoy my life and practice my art, respected by all men and in all times; but if I swerve from it or violate it, may the reverse be my lot."

hip·poc·ra·tism (hi-pok′ră-tizm). A system of medicine, attributed to Hippocrates and his disciples, based on the imitation of nature's processes in the therapeutic management of disease.

hip·pu·rate (hip′ū-rāt). A salt or ester of hippuric acid.

hip·pu·ria (hi-pū′rē-ă). The excretion of an abnormally large amount of hippuric acid in the urine.

hip·pu·ric ac·id (hi-pūr′ik). A detoxification and excretory product of benzoate found in the urine of humans and many herbivorous animals; used therapeutically in the form of its salts (hippurates of calcium and ammonium). [G. *hippos*, horse, + *ouron*, urine]

hip·pu·ri·case (hi-pūr′i-cās). SYN aminoacylase.

hip·pus (hip′ŭs). Intermittent pupillary dilation and constriction, independent of illumination, convergence, or psychic stimuli. [G. *hippos*, horse, from a fancied suggestion of galloping movements]

respiratory h., dilation of the pupils occurring during forced, voluntary inspiration, and contraction during expiration.

hir·ci. Plural of hircus.

hir·cis·mus (her-siz′mŭs). Offensive odor of the axillae. [L. *hircus,* goat]

hir·cus, gen. and pl. **hir·ci** (her′kŭs, her′sī). **1.** The odor of the axillae. **2** [TA]. SYN axillary *hairs*, under *hair*. **3.** SYN tragus (1). [L. he-goat]

Hirschberg, Julius, German ophthalmologist, 1843–1925. SEE H. *method*.

Hirschfeld, Isador, U.S. dentist, 1881–1965. SEE H. *canals*, under *canal*.

Hirsch-Peiffer stain. See under stain.

Hirschsprung, Harald, Danish physician, 1830–1916. SEE H. *disease*.

hir·sute (her-soot′). Relating to or characterized by hirsutism. [L. *hirsutus,* shaggy]

hir·su·ti·es (her-su′tē-ēz). SYN hirsutism. [Mod. L. fr. L. *hirsutus,* shaggy]

hir·sut·ism (her′soo-tizm). Presence of excessive bodily and facial hair, usually in a male pattern, especially in women; may be present in normal adults as an expression of an ethnic characteristic or may develop in children or adults as the result of androgen excess due to tumors or drugs, or nonandrogenetic drugs. SYN hirsuties, pilosis. [L. *hirsutus,* shaggy]

constitutional h., mild to moderate degree of h. present in an individual exhibiting otherwise normal endocrine and reproductive function.

idiopathic h., h. of uncertain origin in women, who may additionally exhibit menstrual abnormalities and infertility.

hir·tel·lous (hĭr′tĕ-lŭs). Having or resembling fine hairs; term describing the filamentous protein polysaccharide coating of microvilli. SEE glycocalyx. [L. *hirtus,* hairy, shaggy]

hir·u·di·cide (hi-roo′di-sīd). An agent that kills leeches. [L. *hirudo,* leech, + *caedo,* to kill]

hir·u·din (hir′ū-din). An antithrombin substance extracted from the salivary glands of the leech that has the property of preventing coagulation of the blood. [L. *hirudo,* leech]

Hir·u·din·ea (hir′oo-din′ē-ă). The leeches, a class of worms (phylum Annelida) with flat, segmented bodies, a sucker at the posterior end, and often a smaller sucker at the anterior end; they are predatory on invertebrate tissues, or feed on blood and tissue exudates of vertebrates. [L. *hirudo,* leech]

hir·u·di·ni·a·sis (hi-roo-di-nī′ă-sis). A condition resulting from leeches attaching themselves to the skin or being taken into the mouth or nose while drinking. [L. *hirudo,* leech, + G. *-iasis,* condition]

hir·u·din·i·za·tion (hir-roo′di-nī-zā′shŭn). **1.** The process of rendering the blood noncoagulable by the injection of hirudin. **2.** The application of leeches.

Hir·u·do (hi-roo′dō). A genus of leeches (class Hirudinea, family Gnathobdellidae). Species previously used in medicine are: *H. australis,* Australian leech; *H. decora,* American leech; *H. interrupta* or *H. troctina,* a leech of northern Africa; *H. medicinalis,* speckled, Swedish, or German leech, the species previously in most general use; *H. m. officinalis,* a variety of the preceding; *H. provincialis,* the green or Hungarian leech; *H. quinquestriata,* five-striped leech. [L. leech]

His, Wilhelm, Jr., German physician, 1863–1934. SEE H. *band, bundle,* bundle *electrogram, spindle;* Kent-H. *bundle;* H.-Tawara *system.*

His, Wilhelm, Sr., Swiss anatomist and embryologist in Germany, 1831–1904. SEE H. *copula, line,* perivascular *space; isthmus* of H.

His–, –His– Symbol for histidyl.

–His Symbol for histidino.

His Symbol for histidine.

Hiss, Philip, U.S. bacteriologist, 1868–1913. SEE H. *stain.*

his·ta·mi·nase (his-tam′i-nās). SYN *amine* oxidase (copper-containing).

his·ta·mine (H) (his′tă-mēn). A vasodepressor amine derived from histidine by histidine decarboxylase and present in ergot and in animal tissues. It is a powerful stimulant of gastric secretion, a constrictor of bronchial smooth muscle, and a vasodilator (capillaries and arterioles) that causes a fall in blood pressure. H., or a substance indistinguishable in action from it, is liberated in the skin as a result of injury. When injected intradermally in high dilution, it causes the triple response.

h. phosphate, used in the treatment of certain allergies, cephalalgia, and acute multiple sclerosis with varying results; also used to test gastric secretory function, in the diagnosis of pheochromocytoma and in the treatment of Ménière disease; also available as h. acid phosphate.

his·ta·mine-fast. Indicating the absence of the normal response to histamine, especially in speaking of true gastric anacidity.

his·ta·mi·ne·mia (his′tă-mi-nē′mē-ă). The presence of histamine in the circulating blood. [histamine + G. *haima,* blood]

his·ta·mi·nu·ria (his′tă-mi-noo′rē-ă). The excretion of histamine in the urine. [histidine + G. *ouron,* urine]

his·tan·gic (his-tan′jik). SYN histoangic.

his·ti·dase (his′ti-dās). SYN *histidine* ammonia-lyase.

his·ti·din·al (his′ti-din-ăl). The aldehyde analog of histidine (–CHO replacing –COOH).

his·ti·di·nase (his′ti-di-nās). SYN *histidine* ammonia-lyase.

his·ti·dine (H, His) (his′ti-dēn). α-Amino-β-(4-imidazolyl)-propionic acid; the L-isomer is a basic amino acid found in most proteins. It is a nutritionally essential amino acid in mammals.

h. ammonia-lyase, an enzyme catalyzing deamination of L-histidine to urocanate and ammonia; this enzyme is absent or deficient in individuals with histidinemia. SYN histidase, histidinase, h. deaminase.

h. deaminase, SYN h. ammonia-lyase.

histamine	
H₁ receptors	**H₂ receptors**
lung	
contraction of bronchial muscles (humans)	relaxation of bronchial muscles (sheep)
heart/circulatory system	
positive bathmotropic effect	positive inotropic effect
positive dromotropic effect	positive chronotropic effect
vasoconstriction (vessels < 80 μm)	
vasodilation (vessels > 80 μm)	
distribution of epinephrine	
endothelial contraction, and thereby increased permeability (edema of tissue)	
uterus	
contraction (guinea pig)	relaxation (rat)
intestine	
contraction	
stomach	
	increase of acid secretion

h. decarboxylase, an enzyme catalyzing the pyridoxal-phosphate-dependent decarboxylation of L-histidine to histamine and CO_2; thus, it plays a role in constriction of bronchial smooth muscle.

his·ti·di·ne·mia (his′ti-di-nē′mē-ă) [MIM*235800]. A metabolic disorder characterized by speech defects, growth deficiency, and mild mental retardation in some patients; associated with elevation of blood histidine level and excretion of histidine and related imidazole metabolites in urine due to deficiency of histidine ammonia lyase or histidinase; autosomal recessive inheritance, caused by mutation in the histidinase gene (HIS) on chromosome 12q. [histidine + G. *haima,* blood, + *-ia*]

his·ti·dino (–His) (his′ti-din-ō). The radical of histidine produced by removal of a hydrogen from a nitrogen atom; prefixed by N^α, N^τ, or N^π.

his·ti·di·nol (his′ti-di-nol). The alcohol analog of histidine (–COOH becomes –CH₂OH).

his·ti·di·nu·ria (his′ti-di-noo′rē-ă). Excretion of considerable amounts of histidine in the urine; frequently observed in later months of pregnancy, and in histidinemia.

his·ti·dyl (His–) (his′ti-dil). The acyl radical of histidine.

histio-. Tissue, especially connective tissue. [G. *histion,* web (tissue)]

his·ti·o·blast (his′tē-ō-blast). A tissue-forming cell. SYN histoblast. [histio- + G. *blastos,* germ]

his·ti·o·cyte (his′tē-ō-sīt). A tissue macrophage; the class includes hepatic Kupffer cells, alveolar macrophages, giant cells of granulomas, osteoclasts, and dermal Langerhans cells. These cells derive from precursors that normally reside in bone marrow but migrate through the bloodstream to egress into tissues for final differentiation. SYN histocyte. [histio- + G. *kytos,* cell]

cardiac h., a large mononuclear cell found in connective tissue of the heart wall in inflammatory conditions, especially in the Aschoff body. The ovoid nucleus contains a central chromatin mass appearing as a wavy bar in longitudinal section. SYN Anitschkow cell, Anitschkow myocyte, caterpillar cell.

sea-blue h., a h. containing cytoplasmic granules that stain bright blue with hematologic stains such as Wright-Giemsa; found in bone marrow and in the spleen, associated with hepatosplenomegaly and thrombocytopenic purpura and in other blood diseases.

his·ti·o·cy·to·ma (his′tē-ō-sī-tō′mă). A tumor composed of histiocytes. [histio- + G. *kytos,* cell, + *-ōma,* tumor]

hi

fibrous h., SYN dermatofibroma; SEE dermatofibroma.

generalized eruptive h., a rare recurring generalized eruption in adults of flesh colored or erythematous papules remaining localized to the skin and consisting of dermal nodules of mononuclear histiocytes that do not stain for lipid. SYN nodular non-X histiocytosis.

malignant fibrous h., a sarcoma of variable malignant potential, occurring most often in the extremities and retroperitoneum; often recurs locally after resection, less often metastasizes; shows partial fibroblastic and histiocytic differentiation with a variable storiform pattern, myxoid areas, and giant cells.

his·ti·o·cy·to·sis (his'tē-ō-sī-tō'sis). A generalized proliferation of histiocytes. SYN histocytosis.

Langerhans cell h., a set of closely related disorders unified by a common proliferating element, the Langerhans cell. Three overlapping clinical syndromes are recognized: a single site disease (eosinophilic granuloma), a multifocal unisystem process (Hand-Schuller-Christian syndrome), and a multifocal, multisystem histiocytosis (Letter-Siwe syndrome.) Formerly this process was known as histiocytosis X. SYN h. X.

lipid h., h. with cytoplasmic accumulation of lipid, either phospholipid (Niemann-Pick disease) or glucocerebroside (Gaucher disease).

malignant h., a rapidly fatal form of lymphoma, characterized by fever, jaundice, pancytopenia, and enlargement of the liver, spleen, and lymph nodes; the affected organs show focal necrosis and hemorrhage, with proliferation of histiocytes and phagocytosis of red blood cells.

nodular non-X h., SYN generalized eruptive *histiocytoma*.

nonlipid h., SYN Letterer-Siwe *disease*.

sinus h. with massive lymphadenopathy, a chronic disease occurring in children and characterized by massive painless cervical lymphadenopathy due to distension of the lymphatic sinuses by macrophages containing ingested lymphocytes, and by capsular and pericapsular fibrosis. SYN Rosai-Dorfman disease.

h. X, SYN Langerhans cell h.

h. Y, SYN verrucous *xanthoma*.

his·ti·o·gen·ic (his'tē-ō-jen'ik). SYN histogenous.

his·ti·oid (his'tē-oyd). SYN histoid.

his·ti·o·ma (his-tē-ō'mă). SYN histoma.

his·ti·on·ic (his-tē-on'ik). Relating to any tissue.

⌂**histo-.** Tissue. [G. *histos*, web (tissue)]

his·to·an·gic (his-tō-an'jik). Relating to the structure of blood vessels, especially in terms of their function. SYN histangic. [histo- + G. *angeion*, vessel]

his·to·blast (his'tō-blast). SYN histioblast.

his·to·chem·is·try (his'tō-kem'is-trē). SYN cytochemistry.

his·to·com·pat·i·bil·i·ty (his'tō-kom-pat-i-bil'i-tē). A state of immunologic similarity (or identity) that permits successful homograft transplantation.

his·to·cyte (his'tō-sīt). SYN histiocyte.

his·to·cy·to·sis (his'tō-sī-tō'sis). SYN histiocytosis.

his·to·dif·fer·en·ti·a·tion (his'tō-dif-er-en-shē-ā'shŭn). The morphologic appearance of tissue characteristics during development.

his·to·flu·o·res·cence (his-tō-flōr-es'ens). Fluorescence of the tissues under exposure to ultraviolet rays following the injection of a fluorescent substance or as a result of a natural fluorescing substance.

his·to·gen·e·sis (his-tō-jen'ĕ-sis). The origin of a tissue; the formation and development of the tissues of the body. SYN histogeny. [histo- + G. *genesis*, origin]

his·to·ge·net·ic (his-tō-jĕ-net'ik). Relating to histogenesis.

his·tog·e·nous (his-toj'ĕ-nŭs). Formed by the tissues; e.g., the h. cells in an exudate arising from proliferation of the fixed tissue cells. SYN histiogenic. [histo- + G. *-gen*, producing]

his·tog·e·ny (his-toj'ĕ-nē). SYN histogenesis.

his·to·gram (his'tō-gram). **1.** A graphic columnar or bar representation to compare the magnitudes of frequencies or numbers of items. **2.** Graphical representation of the frequency distribution of a variable, in which rectangles are drawn with their bases on a uniform linear scale representing intervals, and their heights are proportional to the values within each of the intervals. [histo- + G. *gramma*, a writing]

his·toid (his'toyd). **1.** Resembling in structure one of the tissues of the body. **2.** Sometimes used with reference to the histologic structure of a neoplasm derived from and consisting of a single, relatively simple type of neoplastic tissue that closely resembles the normal, as in certain fibromas and leiomyomas. SYN histioid. [histo- + G. *eidos*, resemblance]

his·to·in·com·pat·i·bil·i·ty (his'tō-in'kom-pat-i-bil'i-tē). A state of immunologic dissimilarity of tissues sufficient to cause rejection of a homograft when tissue is transplanted from one individual to another; implies a difference in histocompatibility genes in donor and recipient.

his·to·log·ic, his·to·log·i·cal (his-tō-loj'ik, i-kăl). Pertaining to histology.

his·tol·o·gist (his-tol'ō-jist). One who specializes in the science of histology. SYN microanatomist.

his·tol·o·gy (his-tol'ō-jē). The science concerned with the minute structure of cells, tissues, and organs in relation to their function. SEE microscopic *anatomy*. SYN microanatomy. [histo- + G. *logos*, study]

pathologic h., SYN histopathology.

his·tol·y·sis (his-tol'i-sis). Disintegration of tissue. [histo- + G. *lysis*, dissolution]

his·to·ma (his-tō'mă). A benign neoplasm in which the cytologic and histologic elements are closely similar to those of normal tissue from which the neoplastic cells are derived. SYN histioma. [histo- + G. *-oma*, tumor]

his·to·met·a·plas·tic (his'tō-met-ă-plas'tik). Exciting tissue metaplasia.

his·to·mor·phom·e·try (his'tō-mōr-fom'ĕ-trē). The quantitative measurement and characterization of microscopical images using a computer; manual or automated digital image analysis typically involves measurements and comparisons of selected geometric areas, perimeters, length angle of orientation, form factors, center of gravity coordinates, as well as image enhancement. [histo- + G. *morphē*, shape, + *metron*, measure]

his·tone (H) (his'tōn). One of a number of simple proteins (often found in the cell nucleus) that contains a high proportion of basic amino acids, are soluble in water, dilute acids, and alkalies, and are not coagulable by heat; e.g., the proteins associated with nucleic acids in the nuclei of plant and animal tissues. They constitute about half of the mass of the chromosomes of eukaryotic cells.

his·to·nec·to·my (his-tō-nek'tō-mē). SYN periarterial *sympathectomy*. [histo- + G. *ektomē*, excision]

his·to·neu·rol·o·gy (his-tō-noo-rol'ō-jē). SYN neurohistology.

his·ton·o·my (his-ton'ō-mē). A law of the development and structure of the tissues of the body. [histo- + G. *nomos*, law]

his·to·nu·ria (his-tō-noo'rē-ă). The excretion of histone in the urine, as observed in certain instances of leukemia, febrile illnesses, and wasting diseases. [histone + G. *ouron*, urine]

his·to·path·o·gen·e·sis (his'tō-path-ō-jen'ĕ-sis). Abnormal embryonic development or growth of tissue. [histogenesis + pathogenesis]

his·to·pa·thol·o·gy (his'tō-pa-thol'ō-jē). The science or study dealing with the cytologic and histologic structure of abnormal or diseased tissue. SYN pathologic histology.

his·to·phys·i·ol·o·gy (his'tō-fiz-ē-ol'ō-jē). The microscopic study of tissues in relation to their functions.

His·to·plas·ma cap·su·la·tum (his-tō-plaz'mă kap-soo-lā'tŭm). A dimorphic fungus species of worldwide distribution that causes histoplasmosis in humans and other mammals; its ascomycetous state is *Ajellomyces capsulatum*. The organism's natural habitat is soil fertilized with bird and bat droppings, where it grows as a mold, fragments of which, following inhalation, produce the primary pulmonary infection; within the mammalian host tissues, inhaled mycelial fragments grow as uninuclear yeasts that reproduce by budding. This parasitic form may also be induced in the laboratory by culturing the mycelial phase at 37°C on a blood-enriched medium; growth reverts to the mycelial form when the temperature is below 37°C. *H. c.* var. *duboisii* causes a clinically distinct disease, African histoplasmosis, in which large yeast cells with thicker walls are found in tissues, in contrast to the small yeast cells of *H. c.* var. *farciminosum*, which causes epizootic lymphangitis. [histo- + G. *plasma*, something formed]

his·to·plas·min (his'tō-plas'min). An antigenic extract of *Histoplasma capsulatum*, used in immunological tests for the diagnosis of histoplasmosis; also used in skin test surveys of populations to determine the geographic distribution of the fungus and to predict those that are endemic for histoplasmosis.

his·to·plas·mo·ma (his'tō-plaz-mō'mă). An infectious granuloma caused by *Histoplasma capsulatum*.

his·to·plas·mo·sis (his'tō-plaz-mō'sis). A widely distributed infectious disease caused by *Histoplasma capsulatum* and occurring occasionally in outbreaks; usually acquired by inhalation of spores of the fungus in soil dust and manifested by a self-limited pneumonia. In patients with emphysema, infection may be chronic and cause pulmonary fibrocavitary disease resembling tuberculosis; in immunosuppressed patients and, rarely, in normals, h. may cause disseminated disease of the reticuloendothelial system, which is manifested by fever, emaciation, splenomegaly, and leukopenia. SYN Darling disease.

acute h., caused by inhalation of microconidia, resulting in illness ranging from flulike to the acute diffuse pneumonitis seen with heavy exposure. Often, following illness, lesions heal, leaving calcified nodules.

African h., a form of h. caused by the fungus *Histoplasma capsulatum* var. *duboisii*, observed only in tropical Africa; infection is manifest as chronic granulomatous lesions in bone, skin, and other organs.

chronic h., disease usually seen in patients with underlying abnormal lung parenchyma, particularly emphysema and bullous lung disease. The disease is indolent, characterized by cough and sputum production, and radiographically by gradual loss of lung volume.

chronic mediastinal h., mediastinal fibrosis caused by lymph node involvement by h. Can cause a huge fibrotic mass involving many critical structures in the mediastinum.

disseminated h., widespread infection that involves many organs; occurs in infants and immunocompromised patients, such as those with AIDS.

presumed ocular h., subretinal neovascularization in the macular region associated with chorioretinal atrophy and pigment proliferation adjacent to the optic disk, and peripheral chorioretinal atrophy ("histo-spots").

his·to·ra·di·og·ra·phy (his'tō-rā-dē-og'ră-fē). Radiography of tissue, specifically microscopic sections; usually microradiography.

his·tor·rhex·is (his-tō-rek'sis). Breakdown of tissue by some agency other than infection. [histo- + G. *rhēxis*, rupture]

his·to·tome (his'tō-tōm). SYN microtome. [histo- + G. *tomē*, cut]

his·tot·o·my (his-tot'ō-mē). SYN microtomy.

his·to·tope (his'tō-tōp). That part of the Class II major histocompatibility molecule that interacts with the T cell receptor. [histo- + -tope]

his·to·tox·ic (his-tō-tok'sik). Relating to poisoning of the respiratory enzyme system of the tissues.

his·to·troph (his'tō-trof). The part of the nutrition of the embryo derived from cellular sources other than blood. Cf. embryotroph, hemotroph.

his·to·tro·phic (his-tō-trof'ik). Providing nourishment for or favoring the formation of tissue. [histo- + G. *trophē*, nourishment]

his·to·tro·pic (his-tō-trop'ik). Attracted toward the tissues; denoting certain parasites, stains, and chemical compounds. [histo- + G. *tropikos*, turning]

his·to·zo·ic (his-tō-zō'ik). Living in the tissues outside of a cell body; denoting certain parasitic protozoa. [histo- + G. *zōikos*, relating to an animal]

his·to·zyme (his'tō-zīm). SYN aminoacylase.

hitch·hik·er (hitch'hīk-er). A gene that has no selective advan-

tage, or may even be harmful, but that nevertheless temporarily becomes widespread because it is closely linked and coupled with a highly advantageous gene that is strongly selected.

Hitzig, Eduard, German psychiatrist, 1838–1907. SEE H. *girdle*.

HIV Abbreviation for human immunodeficiency *virus*.

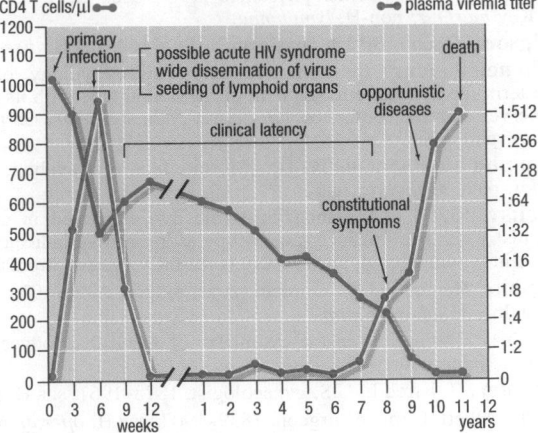

HIV infection: typical course: during early period after primary infection, there is widespread dissemination of virus and a sharp decrease in number of CD4 T cells in peripheral blood; an immune response to HIV ensues, with a decrease in detectable viremia followed by a prolonged period of clinical latency; sensitive assays for viral RNA show that virus is present in plasma at all times; CD4 T-cell count continues to decrease during following years until it reaches a critical level below which there is a substantial risk of opportunistic diseases

HIV-1 Abbreviation for human immunodeficiency virus-1.

HIV-2. Abbreviation for human immunodeficiency virus-2. SEE human immunodeficiency *virus*.

hives (hīvz). **1.** SYN urticaria. **2.** SYN wheal.

   giant h., SYN angioedema.

hK3. Abbreviation for human glandular *kallikrein* 3.

HL-7. Abbreviation for Health Level 7, a medical informatics standard that facilitates communication among different digital systems.

HLA Abbreviation for human leukocyte *antigens*, under *antigen*.

HMB-45. An antibody to a premelanosome glycoprotein found to be present in melanomas and other tumors derived from melanocytes.

HME Abbreviation for human monocytic *ehrlichiosis*.

HMG, hMG Abbreviation for human menopausal *gonadotropin*.

HMG-CoA Abbreviation for β-hydroxy-β-methylglutaryl-CoA.

HMO Abbreviation for hypothetical mean *organism*; health maintenance *organization*.

HMPAO Abbreviation for hexametazime or hexamethylpropyleneamine oxime.

HMS Abbreviation for hypothetical mean *strain*.

HN2 Symbol for nitrogen mustard. SEE nitrogen *mustards*, under *mustard*.

hnRNA Abbreviation for heterogeneous nuclear RNA.

Ho Symbol for holmium.

Hoagland sign. See under sign.

hoarse (hōrs). Having a noisy voice. [A.S. *hās*]

hoarse·ness (hōrs'nes). A noisy quality of the voice.

Hoboken, Nicholaus van, Dutch anatomist and physician, 1632–1678. SEE H. *gemmules*, under *gemmule*, *nodules*, under *nodule*, *valves*, under *valve*.

HOCA SYN HOCM.

Hoche, Alfred E., German psychiatrist, 1865–1943. SEE H. *bundle, tract*.

Ho

HOCM Abbreviation for high osmolar contrast medium. SYN HOCA.

Hodge, Hugh L., U.S. gynecologist, 1796–1873. SEE H. *pessary.*

Hodgkin, Alan L., British physiologist and Nobel laureate, *1914. SEE Goldman-H.-Katz *equation.*

Hodgkin, Thomas, British physician, 1798–1866. SEE H. *disease;* H.-Key *murmur;* non-H. *lymphoma.*

Hodgson, Joseph, British physician, 1788–1869. SEE H. *disease.*

ho·do·neu·ro·mere (hō-dō-noo'rō-mēr). In embryology, obsolete term for a metameric segment of the neural tube with its pair of nerves and their branches. [G. *hodos,* path, + *neuron,* nerve, + *meros,* part]

ho·do·pho·bia (hō-dō-fō'bē-ă). Morbid fear of traveling. [G. *hodos,* path, + *phobos,* fear]

HOECHST 33258. A bisbenzimidazole dye employed in cytochemistry and fluorescence microscopy as a sensitive indicator of DNA in chromosomes, specifically constitutive heterochromatin.

Hoeppli, Reinhard J.C., German parasitologist, 1893–1973. SEE Splendore-H. *phenomenon.*

hof (hōf). The hollow in the cytoplasm of a cell that lodges the nucleus. [Ger. court]

Hofbauer, J. Isfred I., U.S. gynecologist, 1878–1961. SEE H. *cell.*

Hoffa, Albert, German surgeon, 1859–1907. SEE H. *operation.*

Hoffman, August Wilhelm, German chemist, 1818–1892. SEE Frei-Hoffmann *reaction,* Hoffman *violet.*

Hoffmann, Friedrich (Fredericus), German physician, 1660–1742. Professor of Anatomy and Surgery at Halle, noted for clinical observations of a variety of infectious diseases.

Hoffmann, Johann, German neurologist, 1857–1919. SEE H. muscular *atrophy, phenomenon, reflex, sign;* Werdnig-H. *disease;* Werdnig-Hoffmann muscular *atrophy.*

Hoffmann, Moritz, German anatomist, 1622–1698. SEE H. *duct.*

Hofmann (Hofmann-Wellenhof), Georg von, Austrian bacteriologist, 1843–1890. SEE H. *bacillus.*

Hofmeister, Franz, German biochemist, 1850–1922. SEE H. *series, gastrectomy.*

Hofmeister, Franz von, German surgeon, 1867–1926. SEE H. *operation;* H.-Pólya *anastomosis.*

Hog·ben, Lawrence, British mathematician, *1895. SEE H. *number.*

Hogness, D.S., U.S. molecular biologist, *1925. SEE Grunstein-H. *assay;* H. *box.*

hol·an·dric (hol-an'drik). Related to genes located on the Y chromosome. [G. *holos,* entire, + *aner,* human male]

hol·ar·thrit·ic (hol-ar-thrit'ik). Relating to holarthritis.

hol·ar·thri·tis (hol-ar-thrī'tis). Inflammation of all or a great number of the joints. [G. *holos,* entire, + *arthron,* joint, + *-itis,* inflammation]

Holden, Luther, English anatomist, 1815–1905. SEE H. *line.*

Holder. SEE Virchow-Holder *angle.*

hole in ret·i·na. A break in the continuity of the sensory retina, permitting separation between the retinal pigment epithelium and sensory retina.

ho·lism (hō'lizm). **1.** The principle that an organism, or one of its actions, is not equal to merely the sum of its parts but must be perceived or studied as a whole. **2.** The approach to the study of a psychological phenomenon through the analysis of a phenomenon as a complete entity in itself. Cf. atomism. [G. *holos,* entire]

ho·lis·tic (hō-lis'tik). Pertaining to the characteristics of holism or h. psychologies.

Holl, Mortiz, Austrian surgeon, 1852–1920. SEE H. *ligament.*

Hollander, Franklin, U.S. physiologist, 1899–1966. SEE H. *test.*

Hollenhorst, Robert W., U.S. ophthalmologist, *1913. SEE H. *plaques,* under *plaque.*

Hol·li·day, R. SEE H. *junction, structure.*

hol·low (hol'ō). A concavity or depression.

Sebileau h., depression between the inferior aspect of the tongue and the sublingual glands.

Holmes, Sir Gordon M., English neurologist, 1876–1965. SEE H.-Adie *pupil, syndrome;* Stewart-H. *sign.*

Holmes, Oliver Wendell. American physician, 1809–1894, identified the mode of spread and control of puerperal fever,

Holmes, Thomas, U.S. psychiatrist, *1918. SEE H.-Rahe *questionnaire.*

Holmes, Walter Chapin, 1884–1932. SEE H. *stain.*

Holmgren, Alarik Frithiof, Swedish physiologist, 1831–1897. SEE H. wool *test.*

Holmgren, Emil A., Swedish histologist, 1866–1922. SEE Holmgrén-Golgi *canals,* under *canal.*

hol·mi·um (Ho) (hol'mē-ŭm). An element of the lanthanide group, atomic no. 67, atomic wt. 164.93032. [L. *Holmia,* for Stockholm]

△**holo-.** Whole, entire, complete. [G. *holos*]

hol·o·a·car·di·us (hol'ō-ă-kar'dē-ŭs). A separate, grossly defective twin lacking a heart of its own, its blood supply being dependent on a shunt from the placental circulation of a more nearly normal twin; a placental parasitic twin or omphalosite. Cf. acardius. [holo- + G. *a-* priv. + *kardia,* heart]

h. aceph'alus, a h. also lacking a head.

h. amor'phus, a h. in which the body of the parasite is represented by only a shapeless mass. SEE ALSO anideus.

ho·lo-ACP syn·thase. An enzyme catalyzing transfer of the 4'-phosphopantetheinyl residue from coenzyme A to a serine of apo-ACP (acyl carrier protein) to form holo-ACP, releasing adenosine 3',5'-bisphosphate; a required step if fatty acid biosynthesis is to function.

hol·o·a·cra·nia (hol'ō-ă-krā'nē-ă). A congenital skull defect in which bones of the vault are absent. [holo- + G. *a-* priv. + *kranion,* skull]

hol·o·an·en·ceph·a·ly (hol'ō-an-en-sef'ă-lē). Complete absence of cranium and brain. [holo- + G. *an-* priv. + *enkephalos,* brain]

hol·o·blas·tic (hol-ō-blas'tik). Denoting the involvement of the entire (isolecithal or moderately telolecithal) ovum in cleavage. [holo- + G. *blastos,* germ]

hol·o·car·box·y·lase syn·the·tase (hōl-ō-kar-boks'il-ās sen'thē-tās). One of several enzymes that biotinylate other proteins (e.g., carboxylases); a deficiency of h. s. will result in organic acidemia.

hol·o·ce·phal·ic (hol'ō-sĕ-fal'ik). Denoting a fetus with a complete head but having deficiencies in other body parts. [holo- + G. *kephalē,* head]

hol·o·cord (hol'ō-kōrd). Relating to the entire spinal cord, extending from the cervicomedullary junction to the conus medullaris.

hol·o·crine (hol'ō-krin). SEE holocrine *gland.* [holo- + G. *krinō,* to separate]

hol·o·di·a·stol·ic (hol'ō-dī-ă-stol'ik). Relating to or occupying the entire diastolic period.

hol·o·en·dem·ic (hol'ō-en-dem'ik). Endemic in the entire population, as trachoma in the villages of Saudi Arabia.

hol·o·en·zyme (hol-ō-en'zīm). A complete enzyme, i.e., apoenzyme plus coenzyme, cofactor, metal ion, and/or prosthetic group.

hol·o·gas·tros·chi·sis (hol'ō-gas-tros'ki-sis). A congenital malformation in which a cleft extends the entire length of the abdomen. [holo- + G. *gastēr,* belly, + *schisis,* cleaving]

hol·o·gram (hol'ō-gram). A three-dimensional image produced by wavefront reconstruction and recorded on a photographic plate. [holo- + G. *gramma,* something written]

hol·og·ra·phy (hō-log'ră-fē). The process of creating a hologram.

hol·o·gyn·ic (hol-ō-jin'ik). Related to characters manifest only in females. [holo- + G. *gynē,* woman]

hol·o·mas·ti·gote (hol-ō-mas'ti-gōt). Possessing flagella over the entire surface. [holo- + G. *mastix,* whip]

hol·o·me·tab·o·lous (hol'ō-me-tab'ŏ-lŭs). Pertaining to a member of the Holometabola, a series of insect orders in which complex or complete metamorphosis is found. [holo- + G. *metabolē,* change]

hol·o·mi·ant·ic (in·fec·tion) (hol'ōm-ī-an-tik). Infectious outbreak due to exposure of a group of persons to an agent that affects or is common to all members of the group. [holo + C. *miantos*, defiled, fr. *miainō*. to defile, + -ic]

hol·o·mor·pho·sis (hol'ō-mōr-fō'sis). Rarely used term for attainment or reestablishment of physical wholeness. [holo- + G. *morphosis*, shaping]

hol·o·phyt·ic (hol-ō-fit'ik). Having a plantlike mode of obtaining nourishment; denoting certain photosynthesizing protozoans, e.g., Euglena. [holo- + G. *phyton*, plant]

hol·o·pros·en·ceph·a·ly (hol'ō-pros-en-sef'ă-lē). Presence of a single forebrain hemisphere or lobe; cycloplia occurs in the severest form. It is often accompanied by a deficit in median facial development. [holo- + G. *prosō*, forward, + *enkephalos*, brain]

hol·o·pro·tein (hō-lō-prō-tēn). A complete protein; i.e., apoprotein plus metal ion and/or prosthetic group.

hol·o·ra·chis·chi·sis (hol'ō-ră-kis'ki-sis). Spina bifida of the entire spinal column. SYN araphia, rachischisis totalis. [holo- + G. *rhachis*, spine, + *schisis*, fissure]

hol·o·side (hōl'ō-sīd). A compound containing one or more identical, glycosidically linked carbohydrates.

hol·o·sys·tol·ic (hol'ō-sis-tol'ik). SYN pansystolic.

hol·o·tel·en·ceph·a·ly (hol'ō-tel-en-sef'ă-lē). Holoprosencephaly associated with arrhinencephaly. [holo- + telencephalon]

hol·o·thur·ins (hōl-ō-thu'rins). A class of highly toxic sulfated steroid glycosides secreted by sea cucumbers (*Holothurioidea*).

ho·lot·ri·chous (ho-lot'ri-kŭs). Possessing cilia over the entire surface. [holo- + G. *thrix*, hair]

hol·o·zo·ic (hol-ō-zō'ik). Animal-like in mode of obtaining nourishment, lacking photosynthetic capacity; denoting certain protozoans, in distinction to others that are holophytic. [holo- + G. *zōon*, animal]

Holt, Mary, 20th century English cardiologist. SEE H.-Oram *syndrome*.

Holter, Norman, U.S. biophysicist, 1914–1983. SEE H. *monitor*.

Holthouse, Carsten, British surgeon, 1810–1901. SEE H. *hernia*.

Holzknecht, Guido, Austrian radiologist, 1872–1931. SEE H. *unit*.

hom·a·lo·ceph·a·lous (hom'ă-lō-sef'ă-lŭs). Having a flattened head. [G. *homalos*, level, + *kephalē*, head]

Ho·ma·lo·my·ia (hom'ă-lō-mī'yă). A genus of flies the larvae of which sometimes infect human or animal intestines. [G. *homalos*, even, + *myia*, a fly]

hom·a·lu·ria (hom-ă-loo'rē-ă). Rarely used term for normal urine flow. [G. *homalos*, level, + *ouron*, urine]

Homans, John, U.S. surgeon, 1877–1954. SEE H. *sign*.

ho·mat·ro·pine (hō-mat'rō-pēn). An anticholinergic, mydriatic, and cycloplegic agent; available as the hydrobromide and the methylbromide. SYN mandelytropine, tropine mandelate.

hom·ax·i·al (hō-mak'sē-ăl). Having all the axes alike, as a sphere. [G. *homos*, the same, + axis]

Home, Sir Everard, English surgeon, 1756–1832. SEE H. *lobe*.

homeo-. The same, alike. SEE ALSO homo- (1). [G. *homoios*, similar]

ho·me·o·box. A highly conserved DNA sequence of about 180 base pairs near the 3' end of specific homeotic genes; it encodes a DNA-binding domain that allows the homeobox proteins to bind to and regulate gene expression in development. SYN homeodomain.

ho·me·o·do·main (hō'mē-ō-dō- mān'). SYN homeobox.

ho·me·o·met·ric (hō'mē-ō-met'rik). Without change in size. [homeo- + G. *metron*, measure]

ho·me·o·mor·phous (hō'mē-ō-mōr'fŭs). Of similar shape, but not necessarily of the same composition. [homeo- + G. *morphē*, shape]

ho·me·o·path (hō'mē-ō-path). SYN homeopathist.

ho·me·o·path·ic (hō'mē-ō-path'ik). 1. Relating to homeopathy. SYN homeotherapeutic (1). 2. Denoting an extremely small dose of a pharmacologic agent that theoreticaly mimics the symptoms produced by the condition being treated, such as might be used in homeopathy; more generally, a dose believed to be too small to produce the effect usually expected from that agent. An alterna-

tive form of medicine to allopathic, in which drugs antagonize the effects of the disease. Cf. pharmacologic (2), physiologic (4), supraphysiologic. [homeo- + G. *pathos*, disease]

ho·me·op·a·thist (hō-mē-op'ă-thist). A medical practitioner of homeopathy. SYN homeopath.

ho·me·op·a·thy (hō-mē-op'ă-thē). A system of therapy developed by Samuel Hahnemann based on the "law of similia," from the aphorism, *similia similibus curantur* (likes are cured by likes), which holds that a medicinal substance that can evoke certain symptoms in healthy individuals may be effective in the treatment of illnesses having similar symptoms, if given in very small doses [homeo- + G. *pathos*, suffering]

ho·me·o·pla·sia (hō'mē-ō-plā'zē-ă). The formation of new tissue of the same character as that already existing in the part. SYN homoioplasia. [homeo- + G. *plasis*, a molding]

ho·me·o·plas·tic (hō'mē-ō-plas'tik). Relating to or characterized by homeoplasia.

ho·me·or·rhe·sis (hō'mē-ō-rē'sis). The set of processes by which imbalances and other defects in ontogeny are corrected before development is completed. SYN ontogenic homeostasis, waddingtonian homeostasis. [homeo- + G. *rheos*, stream, current]

ho·me·o·sis (hō-mē-ō'sis). Formation of a body part having characteristics normally found in a related or homologous part at another location in the body. [homeo- + G. -*osis*, condition]

ho·me·o·sta·sis (hō'mē-ō-stā'sis, -os'tă-sis). 1. The state of equilibrium (balance between opposing pressures) in the body with respect to various functions and to the chemical compositions of the fluids and tissues. 2. The processes through which such bodily equilibrium is maintained. [homeo- + G. *stasis*, standing]
  Bernard-Cannon h., the set of mechanisms responsible for the cybernetic adjustment of physiologic and biochemical states in postnatal life. SYN physiologic h.
  genetic h., SYN Lerner h.
  Lerner h., the restorative mechanisms that tend to correct perturbations in the genetic composition of a population. SYN genetic h.
  ontogenic h., SYN homeorrhesis.
  physiologic h., SYN Bernard-Cannon h.
  waddingtonian h., SYN homeorrhesis.

ho·me·o·stat·ic (hō'mē-ō-stat'ik). Relating to homeostasis.

ho·me·o·ther·a·peu·tic (hō'mē-ō-thār-ă-pū'tik). 1. SYN homeopathic (1). 2. Relating to homeotherapy.

ho·me·o·ther·a·py, ho·me·o·ther·a·peu·tics (hō'mē-ō-thār'ă-pē, -thār-ă-pū'tiks). Treatment or prevention of a disease using the principles of homeopathy.

ho·me·o·therm (hō'mē-ō-therm). Any of the animals, including mammals and birds, that tend to maintain a constant body temperature. SYN hematherm, warm-blooded animal. [homeo- + G. *thermos*, warm]

ho·me·o·ther·mal (hō'mē-ō-ther'măl). SYN homeothermic.

ho·me·o·ther·mic (hō'mē-ō-ther'mik). Pertaining to, or having the essential characteristic of, homeotherms. Cf. poikilothermic, heterothermic. SYN hemathermal, hemathermous, hematothermal, homeothermal, homoiothermal, homothermal, warm-blooded.

ho·me·ot·ic (hō-mē-ot'ik). Pertaining to or characterized by homeosis.

ho·me·o·typ·i·cal (hō'mē-ō-tip'i-kăl). Of or resembling the usual type.

hom·er·gy (hom'er-jē). Obsolete term for normal metabolism and its results. [G. *homos*, same, + *ergon*, work]

hom·i·cid·al (hom-i-sī'dăl). Having a tendency toward homicide.

hom·i·cide (hom'i-sīd). The killing of one human being by another. [L. *homo*, man, + *caedo*, to kill]

ho·mid·i·um bro·mide (hō-mid'ē-ŭm). A trypanocide used in veterinary medicine. SYN ethidium.

Ho·min·i·dae (hō-min'i-dē). The primate family, which includes modern humans (*Homo sapiens*) and several fossil groups.

Ho·mi·noi·dea (hom-i-noy'dē-ă). A superfamily of the Primates including the anthropoid apes and humans. Divided into the fami-

Ho

lies Pongidae (anthropoid apes) and Hominidae (humans). [L. *homo* (*homin-*), man, + G. *eidos*, form]

Ho·mo (hō′mō). The genus of primates that includes humans. [L. man]

H. sa′piens, modern human beings. [L. wise man]

⚠**homo-.** **1.** Combining form meaning the same, alike; opposite of hetero-. SEE ALSO homeo-. **2.** In chemistry, prefix used to indicate insertion of one more carbon atom in a chain (i.e., insertion of a methylene moiety). [G. *homos*, the same]

ho·mo·ar·gi·nine (Har) (hō-mō-ar′ji-nēn). A homolog of arginine having an additional methylene group.

ho·mo·bi·o·tin (hō-mō-bī′ō-tin). A compound resembling biotin except for the substitution of an oxygen atom for the sulfur and the presence of an additional CH_2 group in the side chain; an active biotin antagonist.

ho·mo·blas·tic (hō-mō-blas′tik). Developing from a single type of tissue. [homo- + G. *blastos*, germ]

ho·mo·car·no·sine (hō-mō-kar′nō-sēn). N^2-(4-Aminobutyryl)-L-histidine; a constituent of the brain formed from L-histidine and γ-aminobutyric acid.

ho·mo·car·no·sin·o·sis (hō-mō-kar′nō-sēn-ō-sis). An inborn error in metabolism in which homocarnosine levels are elevated, particularly in the cerebral spinal fluid.

ho·mo·cen·tric (hō′mō-sen′trik). Having the same center; denoting rays that meet at a common focus. Cf. heterocentric (1).

ho·moch·ro·nous (hō-mōk′rō-nŭs). **1.** SYN synchronous. **2.** Occurring at the same age in each generation. [homo- + G. *chronos*, time]

ho·mo·cit·rul·li·nu·ria (hō-mō-sit′ru-lēn-oor′ē-ă). An inherited disorder associated with elevated urinary levels of homocitrulline.

ho·mo·clad·ic (hō-mō-klad′ik). Denoting an anastomosis between branches of the same arterial trunk, as distinguished from heterocladic. [homo- + G. *klados*, a branch]

ho·mo·cys·te·ine (Hcy) (hō-mō-sis′tē-ēn, - sis′tīn). $HSCH_2CH_2CH(NH_3)+COO-$; a homolog of cysteine, produced by the demethylation of methionine, and an intermediate in the biosynthesis of L-cysteine from L-methionine via L-cystathionine. Elevated levels of h. have been associated with certain forms of heart disease. SEE ALSO folic acid.

Elevation of the level of homocysteine in the plasma is an independent risk factor for cardiovascular disease (including myocardial infarction, stroke, thromboembolic disease, and intermittent claudication) and (in pregnant women) for fetal neural tube defects such as spina bifida and anencephaly. An increased plasma total homocysteine level has been reported to confer an independent risk of vascular disease similar to that of smoking or hyperlipidemia, and to compound the risk associated with smoking and hypertension. Approximately 25% of people with atherosclerosis are found to have elevation of plasma homocysteine above 15 mmol/L. Because homocysteine rises after myocardial infarction and remains elevated for months, some have questioned the causal role assigned to it in vascular disease. Several prospective studies have failed to establish a connection between homocysteine levels and coronary disease risk. Homocysteine appears to exert a direct toxic effect on the intima of arteries, besides inducing oxidation of low-density lipoproteins and predisposing to thrombus formation by activating platelets and coagulation factors. In animal reproduction studies it promotes neural tube defects, cardiac anomalies, and failure of ventral closure. Elevation of plasma homocysteine occurs in various conditions, including genetic disorders, nutritional deficiencies, and chronic diseases. The level is higher in men and tends to rise with advancing age. Premature cardiovascular disease was first linked to elevation of homocysteine in people with homocystinuria, a rare genetic disorder in which deficiency of the enzyme cystathionine β-synthase leads to elevation of homocysteine in plasma and of its oxidation product, homocystine, in urine. A more common genetic disorder associated with abnormally high levels of homocysteine results from mutation of the gene that encodes the enzyme methylene tetrahydrofolate reductase. The marked increase in homocysteine levels after menopause may play a role in the increased incidence of vascular disease, cancer, and osteoporosis in postmenopausal women. Dietary deficiency of folic acid, vitamin B_6 (pyridoxine), and vitamin B_{12} is also associated with elevation of homocysteine, as are chronic renal failure, hypothyroidism, and some malignancies. Lowering the serum concentration of homocysteine by administration of folic acid has been shown to reduce the risk of adverse cardiovascular events in people with homocystinuria. In animal studies, administration of folic acid prevents the teratogenic effect of homocysteine. Screening for elevated homocysteine levels is advised for people with coronary artery disease out of proportion to known risk factors, or for those with a family history of premature atherosclerotic disease. Administration of folic acid in a dose of 1 mg/day or more reduces homocysteine levels nearly to normal and protects against both vascular disease and birth defects.

ho·mo·cys·tine (hō-mō-sis′tēn). The disulfide resulting from the mild oxidation of homocysteine; an analog of cystine.

ho·mo·cys·ti·ne·mia (hō′mō-sis-ti-nē′mē-ă). Presence of an excess of homocystine in the plasma, as in homocystinuria.

ho·mo·cys·ti·nu·ria (hō′mō-sis-ti-noo′rē-ă) [MIM*236200]. A metabolic disorder characterized by sparse blond hair, long limbs, pectus excavatum, dislocation of lens, failure to thrive, mental retardation, psychiatric disturbances, and thromboembolic episodes; some patients have alleviation of symptoms with pyridoxine while others are not responsive; associated with increased urinary excretion of homocystine and methionine. Autosomal recessive inheritance, but carriers have an increased risk of occlusive vascular disease; caused by mutation in the cysthathione beta-synthase gene (CBS) on chromosome 21q. In addition, there are seven other causes of h.: (1) defect in vitamin B12 metabolism [MIM*277400], (2) deficiency of *N*-methylene-tetrahydrofolate reductase [MIM*236250], (3) selective intestinal malabsorption of vitamin B12 [MIM*261100], (4) vitamin B12 responsive h., cblE type [MIM*236270], (5) methylcobalamin deficiency, cblG type [MIM*250940], (6) vitamin B12 metabolic defect type 2 [MIM*277410], and (7) transcobalamin II deficiency [MIM*275350].

ho·mo·cy·to·tro·pic (hō′mō-sī′tō-trop′ik). Having an affinity for cells of the same or a closely related species. [homo- + G. *kytos*, cell, + *tropē*, a turning toward]

ho·mo·dont (hō′mō-dont). Having teeth all alike in form, as those of the lower vertebrates, in contrast to heterodont. [homo- + G. *odous*, tooth]

ho·mod·ro·mous (hō-mod′rō-mŭs). Moving in the same direction. [homo- + G. *dromos*, running]

⚠**homoeo-.** SEE homeo-.

ho·mo·er·ot·ism, ho·mo·e·rot·i·cism (hō-mō-er′ō-tizm, -ĕ-rot′i-sizm). SYN homosexuality. [homo- + G. *erōs*, love]

ho·mo·ga·met·ic (hō′mō-gă-met′ik). Producing only one type of gamete with respect to sex chromosomes; in humans and most animals, the female is h. SYN monogametic. [homo- + G. *gametikos*, connubial]

ho·mog·a·my (hō-mog′ă-mē). Similarity of husband and wife in a specific trait. [homo- + G. *gamos*, marriage]

ho·mog·e·nate (hŏ-moj′ĕ-nāt). Tissue ground into a creamy consistency in which the cell structure is disintegrated (so-called "cell-free"). Cf. brei.

ho·mo·ge·neous (hō-mō-jē′nē-ŭs). Of uniform structure or composition throughout. [homo- + G. *genos*, race]

ho·mo·gen·e·sis (hō-mō-jen′ĕ-sis). Production of offspring similar to the parents, in contrast to heterogenesis. SYN homogeny. [homo- + G. *genesis*, production]

ho·mog·e·ni·za·tion (hŏ-moj′ĕ-ni-zā′shŭn). The process by which a material is made homogeneous.

ho·mog·e·nize (hŏ-moj′ĕ-nīz). To make homogeneous.

ho·mog·e·nous (hō-moj'ĕ-nŭs). Having a structural similarity because of descent from a common ancestor. Commonly confused with homogeneous. [homo- + G. *genos,* family, kind]

ho·mo·gen·tis·ate 1,2-di·ox·y·gen·ase (hō-mō-jen'tis-āt). An iron-containing enzyme that catalyzes the oxidative cleavage of the benzene ring in homogentisic acid by O_2, forming 4-maleylacetoacetate; an absence or deficiency of this enzyme will result in alcaptonuria. SYN homogentisic acid oxidase.

ho·mo·gen·tis·ic ac·id (hō'mō-jen-tis'ik). Glycosuric acid; (2,5-dihydroxyphenyl)acetic acid; an intermediate in L-phenylalanine and L-tyrosine catabolism; if made alkaline, it oxidizes rapidly in air to a quinone that polymerizes to a melaninlike material; elevated levels are observed in individuals having alcaptonuria. SYN alcapton, alkapton.

h. a. oxidase, SYN homogentisate 1,2-dioxygenase.

ho·mog·e·ny (hō-moj'ĕ-ne). SYN homogenesis.

ho·mo·gly·can (hō-mō-glī'kan). A polysaccharide consisting of only one type of monosaccharide subunit (e.g., glucan). Cf. heteroglycan, glycan.

ho·mo·graft (hō'mō-graft). SYN allograft.

ho·moi·o·pla·sia (hō'moy-ō-plā'zē-ă). SYN homeoplasia.

ho·moi·o·ther·mal (hō-moy-ō-ther'măl). SYN homeothermic.

ho·mo·kar·y·on (hō-mō-kar'ē-on). Genetically identical multiple nuclei in a common cytoplasm, usually resulting from fusion of two cells from the same species. [homo- + G. *karyon,* kernel, nut]

ho·mo·kar·y·ot·ic (hō'mō-kar-ē-ot'ik). Exhibiting the properties of a homokaryon.

ho·mo·ker·a·to·plas·ty (hō'mō-ker'ă-tō-plas-tē). Corneal transplant between members of the same species.

ho·mo·lat·er·al (hō-mō-lat'er-ăl). SYN ipsilateral. [homo- + L. *latus,* side]

ho·mo·lip·ids (hō-mō-lip'idz). Lipids containing only C, H, and O. Cf. heterolipids. SYN simple lipids.

ho·mo·log, ho·mo·logue (hom'ō-log). A member of a homologous pair or series. [homo- + G. *logos,* word, ratio, relation]

ho·mol·o·gous (hŏ-mol'ō-gŭs). Corresponding or alike in certain critical attributes. **1.** In biology or zoology, denoting organs or parts corresponding in evolutionary origin and similar to some extent in structure, but not necessarily similar in function. **2.** In chemistry, denoting a single chemical series, differing by fixed increments. **3.** In genetics, denoting chromosomes or chromosome parts identical with respect to their construction and genetic content. **4.** In immunology, denoting serum or tissue derived from members of a single species, or an antibody with respect to the antigen that produced it. **5.** Proteins having identical or similar functions (particularly with respect to proteins from different species). [see homolog]

ho·mol·o·gy (hŏ-mol'ō-jē). The state of being homologous.

h. of chains, the degree of similarity between the base sequences of strands of two DNAs. SYN h. of strands.

DNA h., the degree (or percentage) of hybridization capable between the DNA of different microorganisms.

h. of strands, SYN h. of chains.

ho·mol·y·sin (hō-mol'i-sin). A sensitizing hemolytic antibody (hemolysin) formed as the result of stimulation by an antigen derived from an animal of the same species. [homo- + hemolysin]

ho·mol·y·sis (hō-mol'i-sis). Lysis of red blood cells by a homolysin and complement.

ho·mo·mor·phic (hō-mō-mōr'fik). Denoting two or more structures of similar size and shape. [homo- + G. *morphē,* shape, appearance]

ho·mon·o·mous (hō-mon'ō-mŭs). Denoting parts, having similar form and structure, arranged in a series, as the fingers or toes. [G. *homonomos,* under the same laws, fr. *homos,* same, + *nomos,* law]

ho·mon·o·my (hō-mon'ō-mē). The condition of being homonomous.

ho·mo·nu·cle·ar (hō-mō-noo'klē-er). Denoting a cell line that retains the original chromosome complement.

ho·mon·y·mous (hō-mon'i-mŭs). Having the same name or expressed in the same terms, e.g., the corresponding halves (right or left, superior or inferior) of the retinas. [G. *homōnymous,* of the same name, fr. *onyma,* name]

ho·mo·phenes (hō'mō-fēnz). Words in which the visible organs of speech behave the same, e.g., tug, tongue, tuck.

ho·mo·phil (hō'mō-fil). Denoting an antibody that reacts only with the specific antigen which induced its formation. [homo- + G. *philos,* fond]

homophobia (hō-mō-fō'bē-ă). Irrational fear of homosexual feelings, thoughts, behaviors, or persons.

internalized h., h. occurring in a homosexual person, often associated with self-loathing, self-censure, and self-censorship.

ho·mo·plas·tic (hō-mō-plas'tik). Similar in form and structure, but not in origin. [homo- + G. *plastos,* formed]

ho·mo·pol·y·mer (hō-mō-pol'i-mer). A polymer composed of a series of identical moieties; e.g., polylysine, poly(adenylic acid), polyglucose.

ho·mo·pro·line (hō-mō-prō'lēn). SYN pipecolic acid.

ho·mo·pro·to·cat·e·chu·ic ac·id (hō'mō-prō'tō-kat-ě-choo'ik). (3,4-Dihydroxyphenyl)acetic acid; an isomer of homogentisic acid found in urine; a degradation product of L-tyrosine, L-dopa, and hydroxytyramine.

hom·or·gan·ic (hom-ōr-gan'ik). Produced by the same organs, or by homologous organs.

ho·mo·sal·ate (hō-mō-sal'āt). An ultraviolet screening agent for topical application to the skin.

ho·mo·sced·as·tic·i·ty (hō'mō-skě-das-tis'ĭ-tē). Constancy of the variance of a measure over the levels of the factor under study.

ho·mo·ser·ine (hō-mō-ser'ēn). Amino-4-hydroxybutyric acid; a hydroxyamino acid differing from serine in the possession of an additional CH_2 group. An intermediate in the biosynthesis of cystathionine, threonine, and methionine.

h. deaminase, SYN cystathionine γ-lyase.

h. dehydratase, SYN cystathionine γ-lyase.

h. lactone, the cyclic ester (i.e., the δ-lactone) of h.; formed by the reaction of cyanogen bromide on methionyl residues in peptides and proteins.

ho·mo·sex·u·al (hō-mō-sek'shoo-ăl). **1.** Relating to or characteristic of homosexuality. **2.** One whose interests and behavior are characteristic of homosexuality. SEE gay, lesbian.

ho·mo·sex·u·al·i·ty (hō'mō-sek-shoo-al'i-tē). Erotic attraction or activity, including sexual congress, between individuals of the same sex, especially past puberty. SYN homoerotism, homoeroticism.

ego-dystonic h., a psychological or psychiatric disorder in which an individual experiences persistent distress associated with same-sex preference and a strong need to change the behavior or, at least, to alleviate the distress associated with the h.; no longer a DSM-recognized diagnosis; now included under sexual disorder, not otherwise specified.

female h., erotic predisposition, or activity, including sexual congress, between two women past the age of puberty.

latent h., an erotic inclination toward members of the same sex not consciously experienced or expressed in overt action, as opposed to overt h. Use of this term is disappearing because of both its potentially iatrogenic effect and the inability to validate the phenomenon by techniques outside of psychoanalytic theory. SYN unconscious h.

male h., erotic predisposition, or activity, including sexual congress, between two men, past the age of puberty.

overt h., homosexual inclinations consciously experienced and expressed in actual homosexual behavior.

unconscious h., SYN latent h.

D-ho·mo·ster·oid (hō-mō-stēr'oyd). A steroid in which the D ring is made up of six carbon atoms instead of the usual five.

ho·mo·ster·oid. A steroid that has had at least one of the rings in its structure expanded.

4-ho·mo·sul·fa·nil·a·mide (hō'mō-sŭl-fă-nil'ă-mīd). SYN mafenide.

ho·mo·thal·lic (hō-mō-thal'ik). In fungi, denoting a kind of sexual reproduction in which a nucleus of a thallus is capable of fusing

ho

with another nucleus from the same thallus or mating type. Cf. heterothallic. [homo- + G. *thallos,* a young shoot]

ho·mo·ther·mal (hō-mō-ther'măl). SYN homeothermic. [homo- + G. *thermē,* heat]

ho·mo·ton·ic (hō-mō-ton'ik). Of uniform tension or tonus.

ho·mo·top·ic (hō-mō-top'ik). Pertaining to or occurring at the same place or part of the body. [homo- + G. *topos,* place]

ho·mo·trans·plan·ta·tion (hō'mō-tranz-plan-tā'shŭn). SYN allotransplantation.

ho·mo·tro·pic (hō-mō-trō-pik). Referring to the binding of the same ligand to a macromolecule; e.g., the binding of four O_2 to hemoglobin is homotropic cooperativity.

ho·mo·type (hō'mō-tīp). Any part or organ of the same structure or function as another, especially as one on the opposite side of the body. [homo- + G. *typos,* type]

ho·mo·typ·ic, ho·mo·typ·i·cal (hō-mō-tip'ik, i-kăl). Of the same type or form; corresponding to the other one of two paired organs or parts.

ho·mo·va·nil·lic ac·id (HVA) (hō'mō-vă-nil'ik). 4-Hydroxy-3-methoxyphenylacetic acid; a phenol found in human urine; produced through the methylation of homoprotocatechuic acid on the *meta*-OH group. It is the principal urinary metabolite of dopa and dopamine.

ho·mo·zo·ic (hō-mō-zō'ik). Relating to the same animal or the same species of animal. [homo- + G. *zōikos,* relating to an animal]

ho·mo·zy·gos·i·ty, ho·mo·zy·go·sis (hō'mō-zī-gos'i-tē, -zī-gō'sis). The state of being homozygous. [homo- + G. *zygon,* yoke]

ho·mo·zy·gote (hō-mō-zī'gōt). A homozygous individual. [homo- + G. *zygōtos,* yoke]

ho·mo·zy·gous (hō-mō-zī'gŭs). Having identical alleles at one or more loci.

ho·mo·zy·gous by de·scent. Possessing two identical alleles at a given locus that are descended from a single source, as may occur in consanguineous mating.

ho·mun·cu·lus (hō-mŭngk'ū-lŭs). **1.** An exceedingly minute body which, according to the views of development held by some medical scientists of the 16th and 17th centuries, was contained in a sex cell. From this preformed but infinitely small structure the human body was thought to be developed. SEE ALSO preformation *theory,* animalcule. **2.** The figure of a human sometimes superimposed on pictures of the surface of the brain to represent the motor or sensory regions of the body represented there. [L. dim. of *homo,* man]

Hon·du·ras bark (hon-doo'răs). SYN *cascara* amara.

hon·ey (hŏn'ē). Clarified h., a saccharine substance deposited in the honeycomb by the honeybee, *Apis mellifera;* used as an excipient, as a flavor in gargles and cough remedies, and as a food. SYN mel (1). [A.S. *hunig*]

honk (hawnk). **1.** In medical terms, a sound that can be likened to the call of a goose. **2.** Sometimes specifically used to denote a sound of laryngeal origin made by vocal cords vibrating in a forced expiration because of a congenital vascular ring compressing the trachea. [echoic]

systolic h., a somewhat musical systolic murmur likened to the honking of a goose; sometimes of innocent but unexplained origin, at other times a sign of mitral insufficiency. SYN systolic whoop.

hood (hud). **1.** The anterior part of the integument of soft ticks (family Argasidae) that extends over the capitulum and forms the roof of the camerostome. **2.** An expanded, covering structure that resembles the hood of robe or cloak in shape or function, such as the extensor digital expansions that overly the dorsal aspect of the heads of the metacarpals. [O.E. *hōd,* hat]

dorsal h., SYN extensor digital *expansion.*

hook (huk). **1.** An instrument curved or bent near its tip, used for fixation of a part or traction. **2.** ☆ official alternate term for hamulus. [A.S. *hōk*]

calvarial h., an instrument used in prying off the top of the skull after it has been sawed around, at autopsies and dissections.

h. of hamate, a hooklike process on the distal and medial part of

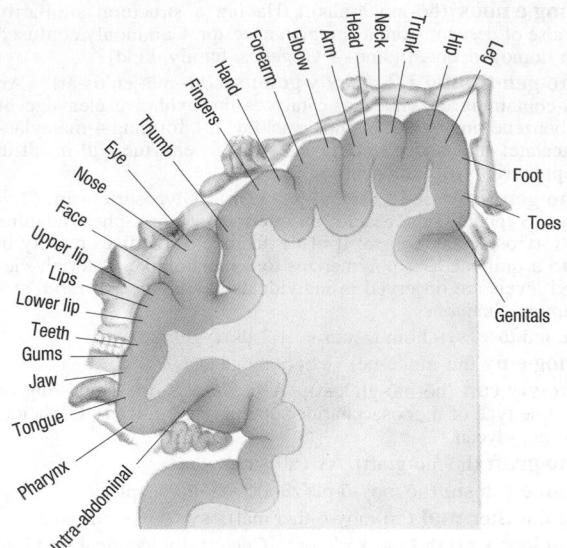

somatotopic projection of the body surface onto primary somatosensory cortex (homunculus): map is a cross-section through postcentral gyrus; neurons in each area are most responsive to parts of body illustrated above them

the palmar surface of the hamate bone. SYN hamulus ossis hamati [TA].

palate h., an instrument for pulling forward the soft palate in order to facilitate posterior rhinoscopy.

sliding h., a movable attachment used on an orthodontic wire for the application of elastic traction or headgear force.

h. of spiral lamina, SYN *hamulus* of spiral lamina.

squint h., a surgical instrument used to lift ocular muscles.

tracheotomy h., right-angled h. used in holding the trachea steady during tracheotomy.

Hooke, Robert, British experimental physicist, 1635–1703. SEE hookean *behavior;* H. *law.*

hook·lets (huk'letz). **1.** Clawlike, retractile chitinous hooks that encircle or line the rostellum of the scolex of certain taenioid tapeworms for attachment to the intestinal mucosa, with the additional aid of suckers; the h.'s can be withdrawn and the rostellum inverted when the tapeworm moves. Various arrangements and forms of the h.'s characterize the families of taenioid cestodes. **2.** H.'s of degenerated scoleces of *Echinococcus* species in the fluids of the hydatid cyst. **3.** The h.'s of the oncosphere, by which it claws out of its membrane sheath after hatching and penetrates the host gut wall; these h.'s can later be found in the cercomer of the procercoid or cysticercoid.

hook·worm (huk'werm). Common name for bloodsucking nematodes of the family Ancyclostomatidae, chiefly members of the genera *Ancylostoma* (the Old World hookworm), *Necator,* and *Uncinaria,* and including the species *A. caninum* (dog h.) and *N. americanus* (New World h.).

Hoover, Charles F., U.S. physician, 1865–1927. SEE H. *signs,* under *sign.*

Hopkins, H. H., 20th century Br. optical physicist. SEE H. rodlens *telescope.*

Hopkins, Sir Frederick G., English biochemist and Nobel laureate, 1861–1947. SEE Benedict-H.-Cole *reagent.*

Hop·lop·syl·lus anom·a·lus (hop-lō-sil'ŭs ă-nom'ă-lŭs). A species of flea parasitic on ground squirrels of the western U.S., and a vector of plague. [G. *hoplo,* tool, weapon, + *psyll,* flea]

Hopmann, Carl M., German rhinologist, 1849–1925. SEE H. *papilloma, polyp.*

hops. SYN humulus.

hor. decub. Abbreviation for L. *hora decubitus,* at bedtime.

hor·de·nine (hōr′den-ēn). A biogenic amine first isolated from barley; increases blood pressure. [L. *hordeum*, barley, + -in]

hor·de·o·lum (hōr-dē′ō-lŭm). A suppurative inflammation of a gland of the eyelid. [Mod. L., *hordeolus*, a sty in the eye, dim. of *hordeum*, barley]

h. exter′num, inflammation of the sebaceous gland of an eyelash. SYN sty, stye.

h. inter′num, an acute purulent infection of a meibomian (tarsal) gland. SYN acute chalazion, h. meibomianum, meibomian sty.

h. meibomia′num, SYN h. internum.

Horecker, Bernard L., U.S. biochemist, *1914. SEE Warburg-Dickens-Horecker *shunt*.

hore·hound, hoar·hound (hōr-hound). *Marrubium vulgare* (family Labitae); bitter principle is marrubium, a volatile oil. A compound alleged to have expectorant properties and often found in cough drops and other patent medicines. [O.E. *hār*, hoary, + *hūne*, herb]

hor·i·zon·ta·lis (hōr-i-zon-tā′lis). Horizontal, referring to the plane of the body, perpendicular to the vertical plane, at right angles both to the median and coronal planes, that separates the body into upper and lower parts. [L.]

hor·me·sis (hōr-mē′sis). The stimulating effect of subinhibitory concentrations of any toxic substance on any organism. [Gr. *hormēsis*, rapid motion]

hor·mi·on (hōr′mē-on). A craniometric point at the junction of the posterior border of the vomer with the sphenoid bone. [G. *hormos*, cord, chain, necklace]

hor·mo·gon·al (hōr-mō′gō-nal). Referring to a class of Cyanobacteria in which the cells grow in filaments.

hor·mo·nal (hōr-mōn′ăl). Pertaining to hormones.

HORMONE

hor·mone (hōr′mōn). A chemical substance, formed in one organ or part of the body and carried in the blood to another organ or part; depending on the specificity of their effects, h.'s can alter the functional activity, and sometimes the structure, of just one organ or tissue or various numbers of them. A number of h.'s are formed by ductless glands, but secretin, cholecystokinin, and pancreozymin, formed in the gastrointestinal tract, by definition are also h.'s. For h.'s not listed below, see specific names. [G. *hormōn*, pres. part. of *hormaō*, to rouse or set in motion]

adipokinetic h., SYN adipokinin.

adrenal androgen-stimulating h. (AASH), a putative pituitary h. that may be responsible for increased secretion of adrenal androgens at the time of puberty.

adrenocortical h.'s, h.'s secreted by the human adrenal cortex; e.g., cortisol, aldosterone, corticosterone.

adrenocorticotropic h. (ACTH), the h. of the anterior lobe of the hypophysis that governs the nutrition and growth of the adrenal cortex, stimulates it to functional activity, and also possesses extraadrenal adipokinetic activity; it is a polypeptide containing 39 amino acids, but exact structure varies from one species to another; sometimes prefixed by α to distinguish it from β-corticotropin. The first 13 amino acids at the *N*-terminal region are identical to α-melanotropin. SYN adrenocorticotropin, adrenotropic h., adrenotropin, corticotropic h., corticotropin (1).

adrenomedullary h.'s, h.'s produced by the adrenal medulla, particularly the catecholamines epinephrine and norepinephrine.

adrenotropic h., SYN adrenocorticotropic h.

androgenic h., any h. that produces a masculinizing effect; of the naturally occurring androgenic h.'s, testosterone is the most potent.

antidiuretic h. (ADH), SYN vasopressin.

anti-müllerian h., SYN müllerian inhibiting *substance*.

cardiac h., SYN herz h.

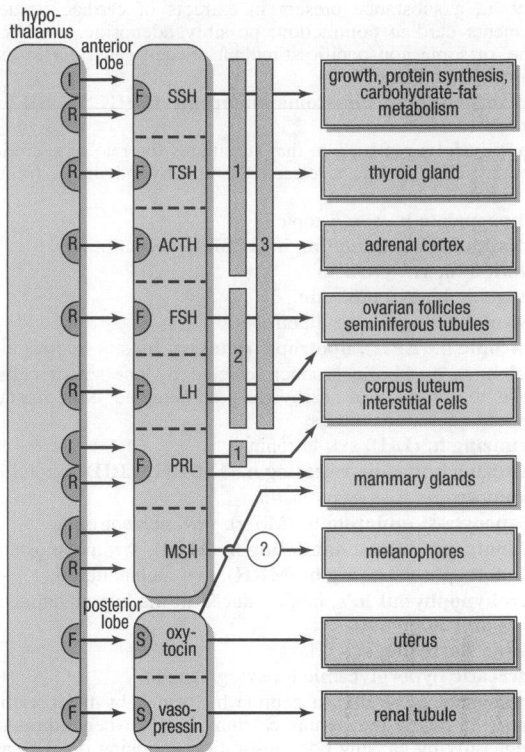

hypophyseal hormones: (I) inhibiting hormones, (R) releasing hormones, (F) formation, (S) storage, (1) metabolic hormones, (2) gonadotropins, (3) glandotropic hormones

chorionic gonadotropic h., chorionic gonadotrophic h., SYN chorionic *gonadotropin*.

chorionic "growth h.-prolactin" (CGP), SYN human placental *lactogen*.

cortical h.'s, steroid h.'s produced by the adrenal cortex.

corticotropic h., SYN adrenocorticotropic h.

corticotropin-releasing h. (CRH), a factor secreted by the hypothalamus that stimulates the pituitary to release adrenocorticotropic h. SYN corticotropin-releasing factor.

ectopic h., a h. formed by tissue outside the normal endocrine site of production; e.g., adrenocorticotropic h. produced by a bronchogenic carcinoma. SYN inappropriate h.

endocrine h.'s, h.'s produced by the endocrine system. Cf. tissue h.'s.

erythropoietic h., (1) generally, any h. that promotes the formation of red blood cells, e.g., testosterone; (2) SYN erythropoietin.

estrogenic h., SYN estradiol.

follicle-stimulating h. (FSH), SYN follitropin.

follicular h., SYN estrone.

galactopoietic h., SYN prolactin.

gametokinetic h., SYN follitropin.

gastrointestinal h., any secretion of the gastrointestinal mucosa affecting the timing and quantity of various digestive secretions (e.g., secretin) or causing enhanced motility of the target organ (e.g., cholecystokinin).

gonadal h.'s, SYN sex h.'s.

gonadotropic h., SYN gonadotropin.

gonadotropin-releasing h. (GnRH, GRH), SYN gonadoliberin (1).

growth h. (GH), SYN somatotropin.

growth h.-inhibiting h. (GIH), SYN somatostatin.

growth h.-releasing h. (GHRH, GH-RH), SYN somatoliberin.

heart h., SYN herz h.

ho

herz h., a substance present in extracts of cardiac tissue that augments cardiac contraction; possibly adenosine, a catecholamine, or some nonspecific stimulant present generally in tissues. SYN cardiac h., heart h.

human chorionic somatomammotropic h. (HCS), SYN human placental *lactogen.*

hypophysiotropic h., a h. that stimulates the rate of secretion of hypophysial h.'s; e.g., a releasing factor; hypothalamic (regulatory) factor.

inappropriate h., SYN ectopic h.

interstitial cell-stimulating h. (ICSH), SYN lutropin.

lactation h., SYN prolactin.

lactogenic h., SYN prolactin.

lipid-mobilizing h., SYN lipotropin.

lipotropic h. (LPH), lipotropic pituitary h., SYN lipotropin.

local h., a metabolic product secreted by one set of cells that affects the function of nearby cells; an autacoid; e.g., prostaglandins and neurotransmitters.

luteinizing h. (LH), SYN lutropin.

luteinizing hormone-releasing h. (LH-RH, LRH), SYN luliberin.

mammotropic h., SYN prolactin.

melanocyte-stimulating h. (MSH), SYN melanotropin.

melanotropin release-inhibiting h. (MIH), SYN melanostatin.

melanotropin-releasing h. (MRH), SYN melanoliberin.

neurohypophysial h.'s, h.'s produced in the hypothalamus; e.g., oxytocin, vasopressin.

ovarian hormone, SYN relaxin.

pancreatic hyperglycemic h., SYN glucagon.

parathyroid h. (PTH), a peptide h. formed by the parathyroid glands; it raises the serum calcium levels when administered parenterally by causing bone resorption, reducing renal clearance of calcium and increasing efficiency of calcium absorption in the intestine. It acts in conjunction with calcitonin and other hormones. SYN parathormone, parathyrin.

pituitary gonadotropic h., SYN anterior pituitary *gonadotropin.*

pituitary growth h., SYN somatotropin.

placental growth h., SYN human placental *lactogen.*

pregnancy h., SYN progesterone.

progestational h., SYN progesterone.

proparathyroid h., the immediate precursor of parathyroid h.; proparathyroid differs from parathyroid h. by an N-terminal hexapeptide extension.

releasing h. (RH), SYN releasing *factors.*

salivary gland h., SYN parotin.

sex h.'s, a general term covering those steroid h.'s that are formed by testicular, ovarian, and adrenocortical tissues, and that are androgens or estrogens. SYN gonadal h.'s.

somatotropic h. (STH), SYN somatotropin.

somatotropin release-inhibiting h. (SIH), SYN somatostatin.

somatotropin-releasing h. (SRH), SYN somatoliberin.

steroid h.'s, those h.'s possessing the steroid ring system; e.g., androgens, estrogens, adrenocortical h.'s.

sympathetic h., SYN sympathin.

thyroid-stimulating h. (TSH), SYN thyrotropin.

thyrotropic h., SYN thyrotropin.

thyrotropin-releasing h. (TRH), SYN thyroliberin.

tissue h.'s, h.'s synthesized by cells other than those in the endocrine system. Cf. endocrine h.'s.

tropic h.'s, trophic h.'s, those h.'s of the anterior lobe of the pituitary that affect the growth, nutrition, or function of other endocrine glands (e.g., TRH, ACTH).

vertebrate h.'s, h.'s synthesized in vertebrates.

---

hor·mo·no·gen·e·sis (hōr′mō-nō-jen′ĕ-sis). The formation of hormones. SYN hormonopoiesis.

hor·mo·no·gen·ic (hōr′mō-nō-jen′ik). Pertaining to the formation of a hormone. SYN hormonopoietic.

hor·mo·no·poi·e·sis (hōr′mō-nō-poy-ē′sis). SYN hormonogenesis. [hormone + G. *poiēsis,* production]

hor·mo·no·poi·et·ic (hōr′mō-nō-poy-et′ik). SYN hormonogenic.

hor·mo·no·priv·ia (hōr′mō-nō-priv′ē-ă). Obsolete term meaning partial or total deprivation of hormones. [hormone + G. *privus,* deprived of]

hor·mo·no·ther·a·py (hōr′mō-nō-thār′ă-pē). Treatment with hormones.

horn (hōrn) [TA]. Any structure resembling a horn in shape. SYN cornu (1). [A.S.]

Ammon h. [TA], one of the two interlocking gyri composing the hippocampus, the other being the dentate gyrus. Based on cytoarchitectural features, Ammon h. can be divided into region I [TA] (regio I cornus ammonis [TA]), region II [TA] (regio II cornus ammonis [TA]), region III [TA] (regio III cornus ammonis [TA]) and region IV [TA] (regio IV cornus ammonis [TA]). SYN cornu ammonis. [G. *Ammōn,* the Egyptian deity *Amūn*]

anterior h. [TA], (1) the frontal or anterior division of the lateral ventricle of the brain, extending forward from Monro interventricular foramen; SEE lateral *ventricle;* (2) the anterior h. or ventral gray column of the spinal cord as appearing in cross section. The anterior h. is composed of the spinal lamina VIII-IV [TA] of Rexed with portions of VII also extending into its geographical boundaries in lumbosacral and cervical levels. The nuclei of the anterior h. are the anterolateral nucleus [TA] or ventrolateral nucleus [TAalt] (nucleus anterolateralis [TA]), anterior nucleus [TA] (nucleus anterior [TA]), anteromedial nucleus [TA] or ventromedial nucleus [TAalt], (nucleus anteromedialis [TA]), posterolateral nucleus [TA] or dorsolateral nucleus [TAalt] (nucleus posterolateralis [TA]), retroposterior lateral nucleus [TA] or retrodorsal lateral nucleus [TAalt] (nucleus retroposterolateralis [TA]), posteromedial nucleus [TA] or dorsomedial nucleus [TAalt] (nucleus posteromedialis [TA]), central nucleus [TA] (nucleus centralis [TA]) and the accessory nucleus and phrenic nucleus, both found in cervical levels only. SEE ALSO anterior *column,* gray *columns,* under *column.* SYN cornu anterius [TA], ventral h.

cicatricial h., a keratinous h. projecting outward from a scar.

coccygeal h., SYN coccygeal *cornu.*

cutaneous h., a protruding keratotic growth of the skin; the base may show changes of actinic keratosis or carcinoma. SYN cornu cutaneum, warty h.

frontal h. [TA], SEE inferior h. of lateral ventricle, inferior h.

greater h. of hyoid bone [TA], the larger and more lateral of the two processes on either side of the hyoid bone. SYN cornu majus ossis hyoidei [TA].

h.'s of hyoid bone, SEE greater h. of hyoid bone, lesser h. of hyoid.

iliac h., bony spur of posterior part of ilium, often found in nail-patella syndrome.

inferior h., a lower or downward prolongation of a part or structure of the body. SYN cornu inferius [TA].

inferior h. of falciform margin of saphenous opening [TA], the lower part of the falciform margin of the opening in the fascia lata through which the greater saphenous vein passes. SYN cornu inferius marginis falciformis hiatus sapheni [TA], crus inferius marginis falciformis hiatus sapheni★.

inferior h. of lateral ventricle, the part of the lateral ventricle extending downward and forward into the medial part of the temporal lobe. SEE lateral *ventricle.* SYN cornu inferius ventriculi lateralis [TA], cornu temporale ventriculi lateralis [TA], temporal h. [TA].

inferior h. of thyroid cartilage [TA], one of the pair of downward prolongations at the back of the thyroid cartilage; it articulates on each side with the cricoid cartilage. SYN cornu inferius cartilaginis thyroideae [TA].

lateral h. [TA], the small lateral gray column of the spinal cord as appearing in transverse section containing the interomedial cell column. SEE ALSO gray *columns,* under *column.* SYN cornu laterale [TA].

lesser h. of hyoid [TA], the shorter and more medial of the two processes on either side of the hyoid. SYN cornu minus ossis hyoidei [TA], styloid cornu.

occipital h. [TA], SYN posterior h.

posterior h., (1) the occipital or posterior division of the lateral ventricle of the brain, extending backward into the occipital lobe; SEE ALSO posterior *column*; **(2)** [TA], the posterior h. or gray column of the spinal cord as appearing in cross section. The posterior horn [TA] or dorsal horn [TAalt] contains spinal laminae I-VI [TA] of Rexed. The nuclei of the posterior h. are the marginal nucleus [TA] (nucleus marginalis [TA]), gelatinous substance [TA] (substantia gelatinosa [TA]), nucleus proprius [TA], secondary visceral grey substance [TA] (substantia visceralis secundaria [TA]), internal basilar nucleus [TA] (nucleus basilar internus [TA]), medial cervical nucleus [TA] (nucleus cervicalis medialis [TA]), posterior nucleus of lateral funiculus [TA] (nucleus posterior funiculi lateralis [TA]) and the lateral cervical nucleus. SYN cornu posterius ventriculi lateralis [TA], cornu posterius [TA], occipital h. [TA], cornu of spinal cord.

pulp h., a prolongation of the pulp extending toward the cusp of a tooth.

sacral h., ☆official alternate term for sacral *cornu.*

h.'s of saphenous opening, SEE inferior h. of falciform margin of saphenous opening, superior h. of falciform margin of saphenous opening.

sebaceous h., a solid outgrowth from a sebaceous cyst.

superior h. of falciform margin of saphenous opening [TA], the upper part of the falciform margin of the opening in the fascia lata through which the greater saphenous vein passes. SYN cornu superius marginalis falciformis [TA], Burns falciform process, Burns ligament, crus superius marginis falciformis hiatus sapheni, Hey ligament.

superior h. of thyroid cartilage [TA], one of the pair of upward prolongations from the thyroid cartilage to which the lateral hyothyroid ligament attaches. SYN cornu superius cartilaginis thyroideae [TA].

temporal h. [TA], SYN inferior h. of lateral ventricle.

h.'s of thyroid cartilage, SEE inferior h. of thyroid cartilage, superior h. of thyroid cartilage.

uterine h., h. of uterus [TA], the portion of the uterus to which the intramural section of the uterine tube enters on either the right or left. SYN cornu uteri [TA].

ventral h., SYN anterior h.

warty h., SYN cutaneous h.

Horner, Johann F., Swiss ophthalmologist, 1831–1886. SEE H. *syndrome, pupil;* Bernard-H. *syndrome;* H.-Trantas *dots,* under *dot.*

Horner, William E., U.S. anatomist, 1793–1853. SEE H. *muscle, teeth,* under *tooth.*

horny (hōrn′ē). Of the nature or structure of horn. SYN keratinous (2).

🔳**ho·rop·ter** (hō-rop′ter). The sum of the points in space, the images of which for a given fixation point fall on corresponding retinal points. If the fixation point is 2 m., the horopter is a straight line; if less, a curve concave to the face; if more, a convex curve. [G. *horos,* limit, + *optēr,* spy, scout, fr. *oraō,* fut. *opsomai,* to see]

empirical h., an experimentally determined ellipse passing through the optical centers of two eyes by which points adjacent to the point of fixation, both lying on the ellipse, are perceived to be stimulating corresponding retinal points.

hor·rip·i·la·tion (ho-rip-i-lā′shŭn). Erection of the fine hairs on contraction of the arrectores pilorum. [L. *horreo,* to bristle, + *pilus,* hair]

hor·ror (hor′er). Dread; fear. [L.]

h. autotox′icus, a term introduced by Ehrlich, meaning that immunity is directed against foreign materials but not against the constituents of one's own body; exceptions to this concept are the autoallergic reactions and diseases. SYN self-tolerance. [L., dread of self-poisoning]

h. fusio′nis, simultaneous projection into consciousness of retinal images so different that fusion is impossible. SYN macular evasion. [L., dread of intermingling]

horse·fly (hōrs′flī). SEE *Tabanus, Anthomyia canicularis.*

horse·pow·er (hōrs′pow-er). A unit of power, 550 foot-pounds/sec, or 745.7 W.

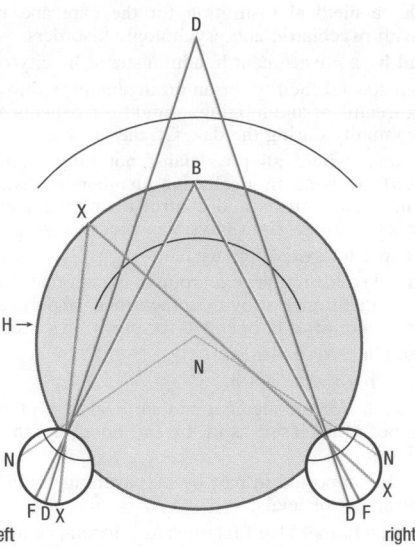

horopter plane: one fixation point (B) is imaged in fovea (F), while other fixation point (X) is imaged at same distance from fovea in both eyes; objects outside horopter plane (D) show a nasal disparity, while those inside it (N) show a temporal disparity

Horsfall, Frank L., Jr., U.S. physician, 1906–1971. SEE Tamm-H. *mucoprotein, protein.*

Horsley, Sir Victor A.H., English surgeon, 1857–1916. SEE H. bone *wax.*

hor. som. Abbreviation for L. *hora somni,* before sleep, at bedtime.

Hortega, Pio del Rio, Spanish neurohistologist in South America, 1882–1945. SEE H. *cells,* under *cell,* neuroglia *stain.*

Horton, Bayard T., U.S. physician, *1895. SEE H. *arteritis, cephalalgia, headache.*

hos·pice (hos′pis). An institution that provides a centralized program of palliative and supportive services to dying persons and their families, in the form of physical, psychological, social, and spiritual care; such services are provided by an interdisciplinary team of professionals and volunteers who are available at home and in specialized inpatient settings. [L. *hospitium,* hospitality, lodging, fr. *hospes,* guest]

hos·pi·tal (hos′pi-tăl). An institution for the treatment, care, and cure of the sick and wounded, for the study of disease, and for the training of physicians, nurses, and allied health personnel. [L. *hospitalis,* for a guest, fr. *hospes* (hospit-), a host, a guest]

base h., a h. unit located in a military or recreational encampment; usually of small size and limited facilities, for immediate care of illnesses and injuries. SYN camp h.

camp h., SYN base h.

closed h., a h. that restricts membership on its attending or consulting staff, sometimes to employed physicians or physicians on a selective membership list, thereby limits who may admit and treat patients.

day h., a special facility, or an arrangement within a h. setting, that enables the patient to come to the h. for treatment during the day and return home or to another facility at night. Cf. night h.

general h., any large civilian h. that is equipped to care for medical, surgical, maternity, and psychiatric cases, and usually has a resident medical staff.

government h., a h. administered by officials of the city, county, state, or nation. SYN public h.

group h., a private h. organized and controlled by a group of physicians and restricted to the reception and care of their own patients.

maternity h., a special h. for the care of women in childbirth.

ho

mental h., a medical institution for the care and treatment of persons with psychiatric and psychologic disorders.

municipal h., a government h. administered by city officials.

night h., a special facility, or an arrangement within a h. setting, providing treatment and lodging at night for patients able to work in the community during the day. Cf. day h.

open h., a h. where all physicians, not only members of the regular staff, or those on a selective membership list, are permitted to send their patients and control their treatment; extremely rare, as most hospitals limit physician access to some degree.

philanthropic h., SYN voluntary h.

private h., (1) a h. similar to a group h. except that it is controlled by a single practitioner or by the practitioner and the associates in his or her office; (2) a h. operated for profit. SYN proprietary h.

proprietary h., SYN private h.

public h., SYN government h.

special h., a h. for the medical and surgical care of patients with specific types of diseases, as of the ear, nose, and throat, eyes, or mental illness.

state h., a h. supported in part by taxpayers and administered by state government officials.

teaching h., a h. that also functions as a formal center of learning for the training of physicians, nurses, and allied health personnel.

Veterans Administration h., a h. operated at federal government expense and administered by the Veterans Administration for care of veterans of U.S. wars and retired military personnel.

voluntary h., a h. supported in part by voluntary contributions and under the control of a local, usually self-appointed, board of managers; a non-profit h. SYN philanthropic h.

weekend h., a special facility, or an arrangement within a h. setting, which enables a patient to work in the community during the work week and receive treatment in the hospital during the weekend.

hos·pi·tal·ist (hos′pit-al-ist). **1.** A physician whose professional activities are performed chiefly within a hospital, e.g., anesthesiologists, emergency department physicians, intensivists (intensive care specialists), pathologists, and radiologists. SYN hospital-based physician. **2.** A primary care physician (not a house officer) who assumes responsibility for the observation and treatment of hospitalized patients and returns them to the care of their private physicians when they are discharged from the hospital. [hospital + -ist]

> Hospitalists may be employees of a hospital or HMO, contractors, or private practitioners. Hospital-based primary care physicians free general practitioners from the need to make daily rounds to visit hospitalized patients. While the availability of physicians oriented to inpatient care improves the efficiency of health care delivery and shortens hospital stays, some have viewed it as a threat to the integrity of the traditional patient-physician relationship. Organized medicine has opposed contractual relationships, including managed-care arrangements, whereby private physicians are required to turn over to a hospitalist the care of all patients admitted to a hospital. While this arrangement bears many similarities to the British system of consultants and general practitioners, some have noted that limiting primary care physicians to office practice may lead to a weakening of critical diagnostic and therapeutic skills and a decline of prestige among both colleagues and the public. The impact of the hospitalist system on medical education and on the hospital staff system, whereby practitioners and consultants maintain staff "privileges" by providing inpatient care to their own patients in compliance with regulations or by-laws, has also raised concerns.

hos·pi·tal·i·za·tion (hos′pi-tăl-i-zā′shŭn). Confinement in a hospital as a patient for diagnostic study and treatment.

host. The organism in or on which a parasite lives, deriving its body substance or energy from the h. [L. *hospes,* a host]

accidental h., one that harbors an organism which usually does not infect it.

amplifier h., a h. in which infectious agents multiply rapidly to high levels, providing an important source of infection for vectors in vector-borne diseases.

dead-end h., a h. from which infectious agents are not transmitted to other susceptible h.'s.

definitive h., one in which a parasite reaches the adult or sexually mature stage. SYN final h.

final h., SYN definitive h.

intermediate h., intermediary h., (1) one in which larval or developmental stages occur; (2) a host through which a microorganism can pass or which contains an asexual stage of a parasite. SYN secondary h.

paratenic h., an intermediate h. in which no development of the parasite occurs, although its presence may be required as an essential link in the completion of the parasite's life cycle; e.g., the successive fish h.'s that carry the plerocercoid of *Diphyllobothrium latum,* the broad fish tapeworm, to larger food fish eventually eaten by humans or other final h.'s. SYN transport h.

reservoir h., the h. of an infection in which the infectious agent multiplies and/or develops, and upon which the agent is dependent for survival in nature; the h. essential for the maintenance of the infection during times when active transmission is not occurring.

secondary h., SYN intermediate h.

transport h., SYN paratenic h.

Hounsfield, Godfrey N., British electronics engineer, *1919. Developed first practical computed tomography device, the EMI scanner; received the Nobel prize in Medicine in 1979 jointly with physicist A. M. Cormack. SEE H. *unit, number.*

house·fly (hows′flī). SEE *Musca, Fannia.*

house of·fi·cer. A person with a medical degree employed by a hospital to provide service to patients while receiving training in a medical specialty.

Houssay, Bernardo A., Argentinian physiologist and Nobel laureate, 1887–1971. SEE H. *animal, phenomenon, syndrome.*

Houston, John, Irish physician, 1802–1845. SEE H. *folds,* under *fold, muscle.*

Hovius, Jacob, Dutch ophthalmologist, 1710–1786. SEE *canal* of H.

Howard, John Eager, U.S. internist and endocrinologist, 1902–1985. SEE H. *test;* Ellsworth-H. *test.*

Howell, William H., U.S. physiologist, 1860–1945. SEE H. *unit;* H.-Jolly *bodies,* under *body.*

Howship, John, British surgeon, 1781–1841. SEE H. *lacunae,* under *lacuna.*

Hoyer, Heinrich F., Polish anatomist and histologist, 1834–1907. SEE H. *anastomoses,* under *anastomosis, canals,* under *canal;* Sucquet-H. *canals,* under *canal.*

HP Abbreviation for haptoglobin.

HPL Abbreviation for human placental *lactogen.*

HPLC Abbreviation for high-pressure liquid chromatography; high-performance liquid *chromatography.*

HPV Abbreviation for human papillomavirus.

H_2Q Symbol for ubiquinol.

h.r.a. Abbreviation for health risk *assessment.*

HRCT Abbreviation for high-resolution computed *tomography.*

HRSA Abbreviation for Health Resources and Services Administration.

HRT Abbreviation for hormone replacement *therapy.*

h.s. Abbreviation for L. *hora somni,* before sleep, at bedtime.

HSIL Abbreviation for high-grade squamous intraepithelial *lesion.*

hsp Abbreviation for heat shock *proteins,* under *protein.*

HSV Abbreviation for herpes simplex *virus.*

5-HT Abbreviation for 5-hydroxytryptamine.

Ht Abbreviation for total *hyperopia.*

HTLV Abbreviation for human T-cell lymphoma/leukemia *virus.*

HTLV-I Abbreviation for T-cell lymphotrophic virus type I; human lymphotropic virus, type 1.

HTLV-II Abbreviation for T-cell lymphotrophic virus type II; human lymphotropic virus, type 2.

HTLV-III Old abbreviation for human T-cell lymphotropic virus type III. SEE human immunodeficiency *virus*.

hU, hu Abbreviation for dihydrouridine.

Hubrecht, Ambrosius A.W., Dutch zoologist and comparative anatomist, 1853–1915. SEE H. protochordal *knot*.

Hucker-Conn stain. See under stain.

Hudson, Arthur Cyril, British ophthalmologist, 1875–1962. SEE H.-Stähli *line*.

hue (hū). One of the three qualities of color; that property by which colors of the spectrum are distinguished from each other and from grays of similar brightness; determined by the wavelength or a combination of wavelengths of light.

Hueck, Alexander F., German anatomist, 1802–1842. SEE H. *ligament*.

Huët, G.J., Dutch physician, *1879. SEE Pelger-Huët nuclear *anomaly*.

Hueter, Karl, German surgeon, 1838–1882. SEE H. *maneuver*.

Hüfner, Carl Gustav von, German physician, 1840–1908. SEE H. *equation*.

Huguier, Pierre C., French surgeon, 1804–1873. SEE H. *canal*, *circle*, *sinus*.

Huhner, Max, U.S. urologist, 1873–1947. SEE H. *test*.

Hull, Edgar, U.S. cardiologist, *1904.

hum (hŭm). A low continuous murmur. [echoic]

venous h., brief or continuous noise originating from the neck veins that may be confused with cardiac murmurs, particularly with the continuous murmur of patent ductus arteriosus. SYN bruit de diable, nun's murmur.

Human Genome Initiative. SYN Human Genome Project.

Human Genome Project. A comprehensive effort by molecular biologists worldwide to map the human genome, which consists of about 100,000 genes, or 3 billion nucleotide base pairs. SYN Human Genome Initiative.

Initiated by Congress in 1990, the U.S. Human Genome Project is a 15-year multidisciplinary effort, jointly administered by the Department of Energy and the National Institutes of Health, to map and sequence the human genome. Similar undertakings have been launched by Great Britain, Japan, and other countries, as well as by privately funded organizations. If printed out, the entire human genome would fill 1000 large-city telephone books, each having 1000 pages. Sequencing the DNA in all 46 chromosomes is expected to take 15 years and cost $3 billion, even with the help of polymerase chain reactions, fluorescent in situ hybridization, cloning of DNA segments, and automated sequencing technology. The resulting map will be a highly idealized representation, like an illustration in an anatomy atlas, since no 2 persons, except (perhaps) identical twins, have exactly the same genetic makeup. Completion of the genomic map will broaden our understanding of human biology and facilitate the detection and treatment of genetic diseases. Projects also under way to study the genomes of bacteria, yeasts, crop plants, farm animals, and other organisms will foster advances in agriculture, environmental science, and industrial processes. About 5% of the budget of the Human Genome Project has been devoted to anticipating and resolving the ethical, legal, and social issues likely to arise from this research.

hu·man pap·il·lo·ma·vi·rus (HPV). an icosahedral DNA virus, 55 nm in diameter, of the genus *Papillomavirus*, family Papovaviridae; certain types cause cutaneous and genital warts; other types are associated with severe cervical intraepithelial neoplasia and anogenital and laryngeal carcinomas. Over 70 types have been characterized on the basis of DNA relatedness. SYN infectious papilloma virus.

Human papillomavirus infection is the most common sexually transmitted viral disease. The interval between exposure and clinical evidence of disease ranges from 3 weeks to 8 months. A single unprotected contact with an infected person carries a 60% risk of infection. At least 80% of cervical cancers are attributable to HPV infection, and 25% of all irregularities seen on Pap smears are believed to result from the presence of the virus, which is often otherwise asymptomatic. HPV typing in women with atypical squamous cells of undetermined significance (ASCUS) on cervical Pap smear helps to identify those in whom more intensive surveillance for premalignant change is warranted. Invasive cervical cancer is associated with types 16, 18, 31, 33, and others. Some 40% of HIV-positive women develop severe cervical dysplasia caused by HPV, which in many cases proceeds to fatal cancer with an aggressiveness not commonly seen among non–HIV-positive women. External genital warts (condylomata acuminata) are usually due to HPV type 6 or 11. Women with external genital warts are not at increased risk of cervical cancer and do not need colposcopy or other special surveillance if routine Pap smears are negative. About 20–30% of HPV infections regress spontaneously. Diagnosis of HPV infection is based on visual inspection (including colposcopy with application of acetic acid to the cervix), Pap smear, and biopsy, with detection of viral DNA in tissue. Treatment options include surgical excision, cryosurgery, laser ablation, loop electrosurgical excision, and intralesional injection of interferon. External genital warts usually respond to topical treatment of podofilox gel or to imiquimod (a cytokine-inducing agent), which can be applied by the patient. Subclinical HPV infection, detectable only by Pap smear or other laboratory methods, may prove impossible to eradicate. The virus cannot be cultured, and there is no test to confirm cure.

hu·mec·tant (hū-mek′tănt). **1.** Moistening. **2.** A substance used to obtain a moistening effect (e.g., glycerin solution).

hu·mec·ta·tion (hū-mek-tā′shŭn). **1.** Therapeutic application of moisture. **2.** Serous infiltration of the tissues. **3.** Soaking of a crude drug in water preparatory to the making of an extract. [L. *humecto*, pp. -*mectus*, to moisten, fr. *humeo*, to be damp]

hu·mer·al (hū′mer-ăl). Relating to the humerus.

hu·mer·o·ra·di·al (hū′mer-ō-rā′dē-ăl). Relating to both humerus and radius; denoting especially the ratio of length of one to the other.

hu·mer·o·scap·u·lar (hū′mer-ō-skap′ū-lăr). Relating to both humerus and scapula.

hu·mer·o·ul·nar (hū′mer-ō-ŭl′năr). Relating to both humerus and ulna; denoting especially the ratio of length of one to the other.

hu·mer·us, gen. and pl. **hu·meri** (hū′mer-ŭs, -ī) [TA]. The bone of the arm, articulating with the scapula above and the radius and ulna below. SYN arm bone. [L. shoulder]

hu·mid·i·ty (hū-mid′i-tē). Moisture or dampness, as of the air. [L. *humiditas,* dampness]

absolute h., the mass of water vapor actually present per unit volume of gas or air.

relative h., the actual amount of water vapor present in the air or in a gas, divided by the amount necessary for saturation at the same temperature and pressure; expressed as a percentage.

hu·min (hū′min). An insoluble brownish or blackish residue obtained upon acid hydrolysis of glycoproteins.

Hummelsheim, Eduard K.M.J., German ophthalmologist, 1868–1952. SEE H. *operation;* Hummelsheim *procedure*.

hu·mor, gen. **hu·mor·is** (hū′mer, hū-mōr′is) [TA]. **1** [NA]. Any clear fluid or semifluid hyaline anatomic substance. **2.** One of the elemental body fluids that were the basis of the physiologic and pathologic teachings of the hippocratic school: blood, yellow bile,

hu

black bile, and phlegm. SEE ALSO humoral *doctrine*. [L. correctly, *umor*, liquid]

aqueous h. [TA], the watery fluid that fills the anterior and posterior chambers of the eye. It is secreted by the ciliary processes within the posterior chambers and passes through the the pupil into the anterior chamber where it filters through the trabecular meshwork and is reabsorbed into the venous system at the iridocorneal angle by way of the sinus venosus of the sclera; SYN h. aquosus [TA], intraocular fluid.

h. aquo′sus [TA], SYN aqueous h.

Morgagni h., SYN Morgagni *liquor*.

ocular h., one of the two humors of the eye: aqueous and vitreous.

peccant humors, based on the historic humoral theory of disease, such humors or deranged fluids in the body were regarded as the direct causes of various illnesses.

vitreous h. [TA], the fluid component of the vitreous body, with which it is often erroneously equated. SYN h. vitreus [TA].

h. vit′reus [TA], SYN vitreous h.

hu·mor·al (hū′mōr-ăl). Relating to a humor in any sense.

hu·mor·al·ism, hu·mor·ism (hū′mŏr-ăl-izm, -mŏr-izm). SYN humoral *doctrine*. [L. *umor, humor*, moisture]

hump (hŭmp). A rounded protuberance or bulge.

buffalo h., SYN buffalo *type*.

dowager h., postmenopausal cervical kyphosis of older women due to osteoporosis and compression fractures of vertebra.

Hampton h., a juxtapleural pulmonary soft tissue density on a chest radiograph, convex toward the hilum, usually at the costophrenic angle; described as a manifestation of pulmonary infarction, due to pulmonary embolism.

hump·back (hŭmp′bak). Nonmedical term for kyphosis or gibbus.

Humphry, Sir George M., English surgeon, 1820–1896. SEE H. *ligament*.

hu·mu·lin (hū′moo-lin). SYN lupulin.

hu·mu·lus (hū′moo-lŭs). The dried fruits (strobiles) of *Humulus lupulus* (family Moraceae), a climbing herb of central and northern Asia, Europe, and North America; an aromatic bitter, mildly sedative, and a diuretic; primarily used in the brewing industry for giving aroma and flavor to beer. SYN hops. [Mediev. L.]

hunch·back (hŭnch′bak). Nonmedical term for kyphosis or gibbus.

Hünermann, Carl, German physician. SEE Conradi-Hünermann *disease*.

hun·ger (hŭn′ger). **1.** A desire or need for food. **2.** Any appetite, strong desire, or craving. [A.S.]

affect h., emotional h. for maternal love and feelings of protection and care implied in the mother-child relationship.

narcotic h., the physiological craving for narcotics.

Hunner, Guy L., U.S. surgeon, 1868–1957. SEE H. *ulcer;* Fenwick-H. *ulcer*.

Hunt, William E., U.S. neurosurgeon, *1921. SEE Tolosa-H. *syndrome*.

Hunt, James Ramsay, U.S. neurologist, 1872–1937. SEE H. *neuralgia*, paradoxic *phenomenon, syndrome;* Ramsay H. *syndrome*.

Hunter, William, Scottish anatomist and obstetrician, 1718–1783. SEE H. *ligament, line, membrane*.

Hunter, William, English pathologist, 1861–1937. SEE H. *glossitis*.

Hunter, Charles, Canadian physician, 1872–1955. SEE H. *syndrome*.

Hunter, John, Scottish surgeon, anatomist, physiologist and pathologist, 1728–1793. SEE H. *canal, gubernaculum, operation;* H.-Schreger *bands*, under *band, lines*, under *line*.

hunt·ing (hŭnt′ing). The oscillation of a controlled variable, such as the temperature of a thermostat, around its set point. SEE hunting *reaction*.

Huntington, George, U.S. physician, 1850–1916. SEE H. *chorea, disease*.

Hurler, Gertrud, Austrian pediatrician, 1889–1965. SEE H. *disease, syndrome;* Pfaundler-H. *syndrome*.

Hurst, Edward Weston, 20th century Australian physician. SEE H. *disease*.

Hurst, Sir Arthur Frederick (born Hertz), English physician, 1879–1944.

Hürthle, Karl W., German histologist, 1860–1945. SEE H. *cell*, cell *adenoma*, cell *carcinoma*.

Huschke, Emil, German anatomist, 1797–1858. SEE H. *cartilages*, under *cartilage, foramen*, auditory *teeth*, under *tooth, valve*.

Hutchinson, Sir Jonathan, British surgeon, 1828–1913. SEE H. *facies, freckle, mask*, crescentic *notch, patch, pupil, teeth*, under *tooth, triad;* H.-Gilford *disease, syndrome*.

Hutchison, Sir Robert, English pediatrician, 1871–1960. SEE H. *syndrome*.

Huxley, Thomas H., English biologist, physiologist, and comparative anatomist, 1825–1895. SEE H. *layer, membrane, sheath*.

Huygens, Christian, Dutch physicist, 1629–1695. SEE H. *ocular, principle*.

HV Abbreviation for half-value.

HVA Abbreviation for homovanillic acid.

HVL Abbreviation for half-value *layer*.

△**hyal-.** SEE hyalo-.

hy·a·lin (hī′ă-lin). A clear, eosinophilic, homogeneous substance occurring in cellular degeneration; e.g., in arteriolar walls in arteriolar sclerosis and in glomerular tufts in diabetic glomerulosclerosis. [G. *hyalos*, glass]

alcoholic h., SYN Mallory *bodies*, under *body*.

hy·a·line (hī′ă-lin, -lēn). Relating to transparent or colorless hyphae or other fungal structures. SYN hyaloid. [G. *hyalos*, glass]

hy·a·lin·i·za·tion (hī′ă-lin-i-zā′shŭn). The formation of hyalin.

hy·a·li·no·sis (hī′ă-li-nō′sis). hyaline *degeneration*, especially that of relatively extensive degree.

h. cutis et mucosae, SYN lipoid *proteinosis*.

systemic h., SYN juvenile hyalin *fibromatosis*.

hy·a·li·nu·ria (hī-ă-li-noo′rē-ă). The excretion of hyalin or casts of hyaline material in the urine. [hyalin + G. *ouron*, urine]

hy·a·li·tis (hī-ă-lī′tis). SYN vitreitis.

suppurative h., purulent vitreous humor due to exudation from adjacent structures, as in panophthalmitis.

△**hyalo-, hyal-.** Glassy, hyalin; vitreous. Cf. vitreo-. [G. *hyalos*, glass]

hy·a·lo·bi·u·ron·ic ac·id (hī′ă-lō-bī-ūr-on′ik). A disaccharide made up of D-glucuronic acid and *N*-acetyl-D-glucosamine in a β1,3 linkage; occurs in hyaluronic acid as the repeating unit.

hy·a·lo·cyte (hī′ă-lō-sīt). SYN vitreous *cell*. [hyalo- + G. *kytos*, cell]

hy·a·lo·gens (hī-al′ō-jenz). Substances similar to mucoids that are found in many animal structures (e.g., cartilage, vitreous humor, hydatid cysts) and yield sugars on hydrolysis.

hy·a·lo·hy·pho·my·co·sis (hī′ă-lō-hī′fō-mī-kō′sis). A general term for infection in tissue caused by a fungus with hyaline (colorless) mycelium. If the mold can be identified, disease should be given a specific name, such as aspergillosis or fusariosis. [hyalo- + G. *hyphē*, web, + *mykēs*, fungus, + *-osis*, condition]

hy·a·loid (hī′ă-loyd). SYN hyaline. [hyalo- + G. *eidos*, resemblance]

hy·al·o·mere (hī′ă-lō-mēr). The clear periphery of a blood platelet. [hyalo- + G. *meros*, part]

Hy·a·lom·ma (hī-ă-lom′ă). An Old World genus (about 21 species) of large ixodid ticks with submarginal eyes, coalesced festoons, an ornate scutum, and a long rostrum. Adults parasitize all domestic animals and a wide variety of wild animals; larvae or nymphs may parasitize small mammals, birds, and reptiles. Species harbor a great variety of pathogens of humans and animals, and also cause considerable mechanical injury. [hyalo- + G. *omma*, eye]

H. anato′licum, former name for *H. anatolicum anatolicum*.

H. anato′licum anato′licum, a subspecies infesting cattle, camels and horses in Asia, the Near and Middle East, southeastern Europe, and North Africa; it is a vector of bovine tropical theileriosis, of equine babesiosis, and of human Crimean-Congo hemorrhagic fever.

H. margina'tum, a particularly common species of tick carried by birds migrating between Europe and Asia and Africa, and the probable vector of the virus of Crimean hemorrhagic fever.

H. variega'tum, species of tick that is the vector of the viral agent of lymphocytic choriomeningitis in Ethiopia.

hy·a·lo·pha·gia, hy·a·loph·a·gy (hī'ă-lō-fā'jē-ă, hī-ă-lof'ă-jē). The eating or chewing of glass. [hyalo- + G. *phagō,* to eat]

hy·a·lo·pho·bia (hī'ă-lō-fō'bē-ă). Morbid fear of glass objects. SYN crystallophobia. [hyalo- + G. *phobos,* fear]

hy·al·o·plasm, hy·a·lo·plas·ma (hī'ă-lō-plazm, -plaz'mă). The protoplasmic fluid substance of a cell. [hyalo- + G. *plasma,* thing formed]

    nuclear h., SYN karyolymph.

hy·a·lo·se·ro·si·tis (hī'ă-lō-ser-ō-sī'tis). Inflammation of a serous membrane with a fibrinous exudate that eventually becomes hyalinized, resulting in a relatively thick, dense, opaque, glistening, white or gray-white coating; when the process involves the visceral serous membranes of various organs, the grossly apparent condition is sometimes colloquially termed icing liver, sugar-coated spleen, frosted heart, and so on, depending on the site. [hyalo- + Mod. L. *serosa,* serous membrane, + -*itis,* inflammation]

hy·a·lo·sis (hī-ă-lō'sis). Degenerative changes in the vitreous body. [hyalo- + G. -*osis,* condition]

    asteroid h., numerous small spherical bodies ("snowball" opacities) in the corpus vitreum, visible ophthalmoscopically; an age change, usually unilateral, and not affecting vision.

    punctate h., a condition marked by minute opacities in the vitreous.

hy·al·o·some (hī-al'ō-sōm). An oval or round structure within a cell nucleus that stains faintly but otherwise resembles a nucleolus. [hyalo- + G. *sōma,* body]

hy·a·lu·rate (hī-ă-loo'rāt). SYN hyaluronate.

hy·al·u·ro·nate (hī-ă-loo'ron-āt). A salt or ester of hyaluronic acid. SYN hyalurate.

    h. lyase, a lyase that catalyzes the cleavage of hyaluronic acids, producing a number of 3-(4-deoxy-β-D-gluc-4-enuronosyl)-N-acetyl-D-glucosamines (hyalobiuronic acid). SEE ALSO hyaluronidase (1), hyaluronoglucosaminidase. SYN hyaluronic lyase.

hy·al·u·ron·ic ac·id (hī'ă-loo-ron'ik). A mucopolysaccharide made up of alternating β1,4-linked residues of hyalobiuronic acid, forming a gelatinous material in the tissue spaces and acting as a lubricant and shock absorbant generally throughout the body; it is hydrolyzed to disaccharide or tetrasaccharide units by hyaluronidase.

hy·al·u·ron·ic ly·ase. SYN *hyaluronate* lyase.

hy·al·u·ron·i·dase (hī'ă-loo-ron'i-dās). **1.** Term used loosely for hyaluronate lyase, hyaluronoglucosaminidase, and hyaluronoglucuronidase, one or more of which are present in testis, sperm, other organs, bee and snake venoms, type II pneumonococci, certain hemolytic streptococci, etc. SYN diffusing factor, Duran-Reynals permeability factor, Duran-Reynals spreading factor, invasin, spreading factor. **2.** A soluble enzyme product prepared from mammalian testes; it is used to increase the effect of local anesthetics and to permit wider infiltration of subcutaneously administered fluids, is suggested in the treatment of certain forms of arthritis to promote resolution of redundant tissue, is used to speed the resorption of traumatic or postoperative edema and hematoma, is used in combination with collagenase to dissociate organs such as liver and heart into viable cell suspensions, and in histochemistry is used on tissue secretions to verify the presence of hyaluronic acid or chondroitin sulfates.

hy·al·u·ron·o·glu·cos·a·min·i·dase (hī-ă-loo'ron-ō-gloo'kō-să-min'i-dās). An enzyme hydrolyzing β1,4 linkages in hyaluronates. SEE ALSO hyaluronidase (1), *hyaluronate* lyase.

hy·al·u·ron·o·glu·cu·ron·i·dase (hī-ă-loo'ron-ō-gloo-kur-on'i-dās). An enzyme hydrolyzing β1,3 linkages in hyaluronates. SEE ALSO hyaluronidase (1).

hy·bar·ox·ia (hī-bă-rok'sē-ă). Oxygen therapy with pressures greater than 1 atmosphere or ambient oxygen pressure applied to the entire body in a chamber or room. [G. *hyper,* above, + *baros,* pressure, + *oxys,* acute]

hy·ben·zate (hī-ben'zāt). USAN-approved contraction for *o*-(4-hydroxybenzoyl)benzoate.

hy·brid (hī'brid). **1.** An individual (plant or animal) whose parents are different varieties of the same species or belong to different but closely allied species. **2.** Fused tissue culture cells, as in a hybridoma. **3.** A bond or valence orbital obtained by the linear combination of two or more different atomic orbitals. SYN crossbreed (1). [L. *hybrida,* offspring of a tame sow and a wild boar, fr. G. *hybris,* violation, wantonness]

    DNA-RNA h., double-stranded polynucleic acids in which one strand is DNA and the other strand is the complementary RNA; formed during transcription and during multiplication of oncogenic RNA viruses.

    SV40-adenovirus h., a virion consisting of SV40 genetic material encased in an adenovirus capsid.

hy·brid·ism (hī'brid-izm). The state of being hybrid.

hy·brid·i·za·tion (hī'brid-i-zā'shŭn). **1.** The process of breeding a hybrid. **2.** Crossing over between related but nonallelic genes. **3.** The specific reassociation of complementary strands of polynucleic acids; e.g., the formation of a DNA-RNA hybrid. **4.** The process or act of forming a macromolecular hybrid in which the subunits are obtained from different sources. SYN crossbreeding.

    cell h., fusion of two or more dissimilar cells, leading to formation of a synkaryon.

    cross h., annealing of a DNA probe to an imperfectly matching DNA molecule.

    DNA h., a technique used to determine the relatedness of microorganisms by the speed and efficiency of the reassociation of single-stranded DNA to form double-stranded DNA when one of the strands originates from one organism and the other strand from another organism; occurs when the base sequences are complementary or nearly so.

    fluorescence in situ h., SYN fluorescent in situ h.

    fluorescent in situ h., a method used to determine the chromosomal location or expression pattern of genomic DNA or cDNA fragments. The piece of DNA to be mapped (the "probe") is labeled with a fluorescent dye and hybridized to a chromosome preparation or to a tissue section. The probe anneals to complementary DNA or RNA sequences. Examination of the chromosomes or tissue section under a fluorescence microscope reveals the number, size, and location of the target sequences. SYN fluorescence in situ h.

    nucleic acid h., SYN anneal (5).

    overlap h., SYN *chromosome* walking.

    in situ h., a technique developed in 1969 for annealing nucleic acid probes to cellular DNA for detection by autoradiography. Under proper laboratory conditions, the binding process occurs spontaneously. In situ h. constitutes a key step in DNA fingerprinting. SYN in situ nucleic acid h.

    in situ nucleic acid h., SYN in situ h.

    somatic cell h., production of a heterokaryon.

hy·brid·o·ma (hī-brid-ō'mă). A tumor of hybrid cells used in the in vitro production of specific monoclonal antibodies; produced by fusion of an established tissue culture line of lymphocyte tumor cells (e.g., mouse plasmacytoma cells) and specific antibody-producing cells (e.g., splenocytes from specifically immunized mice); fusions are accomplished by use of polyethylene glycol or other methods. [G. *hybris,* violation, wantonness, + -*ōma,* tumor]

hy·clate (hī'klāt). USAN-approved contraction for monohydrochloride hemiethanolate hemihydrate, $HCl \cdot \frac{1}{2}C_2H_5OH \cdot \frac{1}{2}H_2O$.

hy·dan·to·in (hī-dan'tō-in). 2,4-Imidazolidinedione; derived from urea or from allantoin; the $NH–CH_2–CO$ group is prototypical of α-amino acids. H. derivatives are formed by the reaction of phenylisothiocyanate and a polypeptide. SYN glycolylurea.

hy·dan·to·in·ate (hī-dan-tō'in-āt). A salt of hydantoin.

hy·da·tid (hī′da-tid). **1.** SYN hydatid *cyst*. **2.** A vesicular structure resembling an *Echinococcus* cyst. [G. *hydatis,* a drop of water, a hyatid]

Morgagni h., SYN vesicular *appendages* of epoophoron, under *appendage*.

nonpedunculated h., SYN *appendix* of testis.

pedunculated h., SYN *appendix* of epididymidis.

sessile h., SYN *appendix* of testis.

stalked h., SYN vesicular *appendages* of epoophoron, under *appendage*.

hy·da·tid·i·form (hī-da-tid′i-form). Having the form or appearance of a hydatid.

hy·da·tid·o·cele (hī-da-tid′ō-sēl). A cystic mass composed of one or more hydatids formed in the scrotum. [hydatid + G. *kēlē,* tumor]

hy·da·tid·o·sis (hī′da-ti-dō′sis). The morbid state caused by the presence of hydatid cysts.

hy·da·ti·dos·to·my (hī′da-ti-dos′tō-mē). Surgical evacuation of a hydatid cyst. [hydatid + G. *stoma,* mouth]

Hy·da·tig·e·ra tae·ni·ae·for·mis (hī-da-tij′er-ă tē-ni-ē-fōr′mis). SYN *Taenia taeniaeformis.*

hy·da·toid (hī′da-toyd). **1.** The aqueous humor. **2.** The hyaloid membrane. **3.** Relating to the aqueous humor. **4.** Watery or resembling water. [G. *hydōr* (*hydat*-), water, + *eidos,* resemblance]

hyd·no·car·pus oil (hid-nō-kar′pŭs). SYN chaulmoogra oil.

△**hydr-.** SEE hydro-.

hy·drac·e·tin (hī-dras′ĕ-tin). Pure form of acetylphenylhydrazine.

hy·drad·e·ni·tis (hī′drad-ĕ-nī′tis). SYN hidradenitis.

hy·drad·e·no·ma (hī′drad-ĕ-nō′mă). SYN hidradenoma.

hy·dra·gogue (hī′dră-gog). Producing a discharge of watery fluid; denoting a class of cathartics that retain fluids in the intestine and aid in the removal of edematous fluids, e.g., saline cathartics. [hydr- + G. *agōgos,* drawing forth]

hy·dral·a·zine hy·dro·chlo·ride (hī-dral′ă-zēn). A vasodilating antihypertensive agent.

hy·dral·lo·stane (hī-dral′ō-stān). 11β,17α,21-Trihydroxy-5β-pregnane-3,20-dione; a metabolite of cortisole, reduced at the 4,5 double bond. SYN 4,5α-dihydrocortisol.

hy·dra·mi·tra·zine tar·trate (hī-dră-mī′tră-zēn). An intestinal antispasmodic.

hy·dram·ni·os, hy·dram·ni·on (hī-dram′nē-os, -nē-on). Presence of an excessive amount of amniotic fluid, usually over 2,000 mL. SYN polyhydramnios. [G. *hydōr,* water, + amnion]

hy·dran·en·ceph·a·ly (hī′dran-en-sef′ă-lē). Absence of cereberal hemispheres, which have been replaced by fluid-filled sacs, lined by leptomeninges. The skull and its brain cavities are normal. [hydr- + G. *an*- priv. + *enkephalos,* brain]

hy·drar·gyr·ia, hy·drar·gy·rism (hī-drar-jir′ē-ă, hī-drar′jir-izm). SYN mercury *poisoning*. [L. *hydrargyrum,* mercury]

hy·drar·gy·rum (hī-drar′ji-rŭm). SYN mercury. [G. *hydrargyros,* quicksilver, fr. *hydōr,* water, + *argyros,* silver]

hy·drar·thro·di·al (hī-drar-thrō′dē-ăl). Relating to hydrarthrosis.

hy·drar·thro·sis (hī-drar-thrō′sis). Effusion of a serous fluid into a joint cavity. [hydr- + G. *arthron,* joint]

intermittent h., a disorder characterized by a periodically recurring serous effusion into the cavity of a joint; the articulation may be the seat of a chronic arthritis or may apparently be normal in the intervals of the attacks.

hy·drase (hī′drās). Former name for hydratase.

hy·dras·tine (hī-dras′tēn). An alkaloid of hydrastis; an isoquinoline chemically related to narcotine. As the hydrochloride, was used locally in the treatment of catarrhal inflammation of the mucous membranes, and internally in the treatment of gastric inflammation, as a uterine stimulant, and to check uterine hemorrhage.

hy·dras·ti·nine (hī-dras′ti-nēn). A semisynthetic alkaloid prepared from hydrastine; the hydrochloride has been used in uterine hemorrhage and as an oxytocic; in large doses, it is a powerful depressant of the entire motor system (motor cortex, nerve, and muscle).

hy·dras·tis (hī-dras′tis). The dried rhizome of *Hydrastis canadensis* (family Ranunculaceae), a native of the eastern U.S.; formerly used in the treatment of chronic catarrhal states of the mucous membranes and in metrorrhagia. SYN golden seal, jaundice root, yellow root. [Mod. L. fr. G. *hydōr* (hydro-), water, + *draō,* to accomplish]

hy·dra·tase (hī′dră-tās). Trivial name applied, together with dehydratase, to certain hydro-lyases (EC 4.2.1.x) catalyzing hydration-dehydration; e.g., fumarate-malate interconversion by fumarate hydratase.

hy·drate (hī′drāt). An aqueous solvate (in older terminology, a hydroxide); a compound crystallizing with one or more molecules of water; e.g., $CuSO_4 \cdot 5H_2O$.

hy·drat·ed (hī′drāt-ed). Combined with water, forming a hydrate. SYN hydrous.

hy·dra·tion (hī-drā′shŭn). **1.** Chemically, the addition of water; differentiated from hydrolysis, where the union with water is accompanied by a splitting of the original molecule and the water molecule. SEE ALSO solvation. **2.** Clinically, the taking in of water; used commonly in the sense of reduced h. or dehydration. **3.** The formation of a shell of water molecules around a molecular entity.

absolute h., actual water excess as measured by a difference from the normal or from a given water content.

hy·dra·zide (hī′dră-zīd). An organic compound of the general formula RCO–NHNH$_2$; an acyl derivative of hydrazine.

hy·dra·zine (hī′dră-zēn). H$_2$N–NH$_2$, an oily liquid from which phenylhydrazine and similar products are derived. It is very toxic and possibly a carcinogen.

hy·dra·zine yel·low. SYN tartrazine.

hy·dra·zi·nol·y·sis (hī′dră-zi-nol′i-sis). Cleavage of chemical bonds by hydrazine; applied in protein and nucleic acid degradations.

hy·dra·zone (hī′dră-zōn). A substance derived from aldehydes and ketones by reaction with hydrazine or a hydrazine derivative to give the grouping R′R″C=N–NHR.

hy·dre·mia (hī-drē′mē-ă). A condition in which the blood volume is increased as a result of an increase in the water content of plasma, with or without a reduction in the concentration of protein; there is an excess of plasma in proportion to the cellular elements and a corresponding decrease in hematocrit. SYN dilution anemia, polyplasmia. [hydr- + G. *haima,* blood]

hy·dren·ceph·a·lo·cele (hī-dren-sef′ă-lō-sēl). Protrusion, through a cleft in the skull, of brain substance expanded into a sac containing fluid. SYN encephalocystocele, hydrocephalocele, hydroencephalocele. [hydr- + G. *enkephalos,* brain, + *kēlē,* tumor]

hy·dren·ceph·a·lo·me·nin·go·cele (hī′dren-sef′ă-lō-me-ning′gō-sēl). Protrusion, through a defect in the skull, of a sac containing meninges, brain substance, and cerebrospinal fluid.

hy·dren·ceph·a·lus (hī-dren-sef′ă-lŭs). Rarely used term for internal *hydrocephalus*. [hydr- + G. *enkephalos,* brain]

hy·dri·at·ric, hy·dri·a·tic (hī-drē-at′rik, -at′ik). Relating to the obsolete use of water to treat or cure disease. SYN hydrotherapeutic. [hydr- + G. *iatrikos,* relating to medicine]

hy·dric (hī′drik). Relating to hydrogen in chemical combination.

hy·dride (hī′drīd). A negatively charged hydrogen (i.e., H:⁻) or a compound of hydrogen in which it assumes a formal negative charge, e.g., sodium borohydride (NaBH$_4$).

hy·drin·dan·tin (hī-drin-dan′tin). The reduced form of ninhydrin. It is often used in conjunction with ninhydrin in the detection of amino or imino groups.

△**hydro-, hydr-.** **1.** Water, watery. **2.** Containing or combined with hydrogen. **3.** A hydatid. [G. *hydōr,* water]

hy·droa (hī-drō′ă). Any vesicular or bullous eruption. SYN hidroa. [hydro + G. *ōon,* egg]

h. aestiva′le, SYN h. vacciniforme.

h. puero′rum, SYN h. vacciniforme.

h. vaccinifor′me, a recurrent eruption of erythema evolving to umbilicated bullae, occurring on exposure to the sun and affecting chiefly male children with resolution before adult life. In severe cases, hand and face deformities and corneal opacity may develop. SYN h. aestivale, h. puerorum.

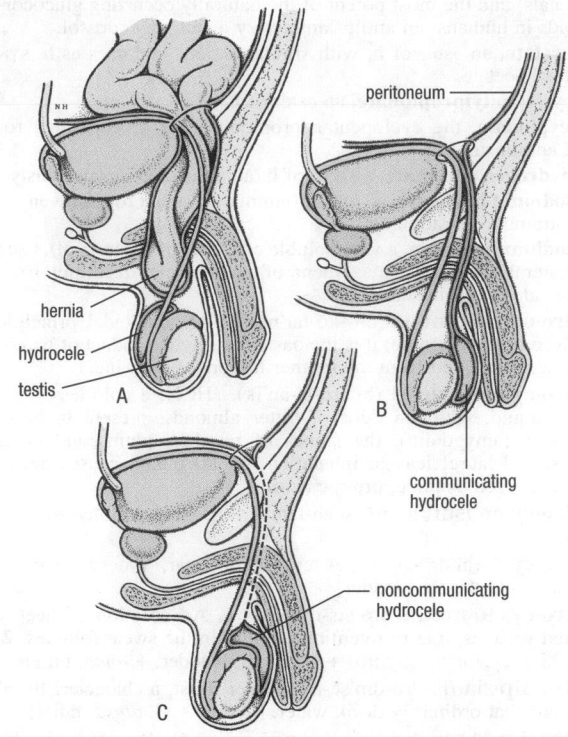

types of hydroceles: peritoneum shown in blue, hydroceles shown in light blue

---

hy·dro·a·dip·sia (hī′drō-ă-dip′sē-ă). Absence of thirst for water. [hydro- + G. *a-* priv. + *dipsa*, thirst]

hy·dro·ap·pen·dix (hī′drō-ă-pen′diks). Distention of the vermiform appendix with a serous fluid.

hy·dro·bil·i·ru·bin (hī′drō-bil-i-roo′bin). A dark brown-red pigment that may be formed when bilirubin is reduced.

hy·dro·bro·mate (hī-drō-brō′māt). A salt of hydrobromic acid.

hy·dro·bro·mic ac·id (hī-drō-brō′mik). An aqueous solution of hydrogen bromide (HBr); its salts are bromides.

hy·dro·cal·y·co·sis (hī′drō-kal-i-kō′sis). A usually symptomless anomaly of the renal calix that is dilated from obstruction of the infundibulum; usually discovered incidentally at pyelography or autopsy; may become infected. [hydro- + G. *kalyx,* cup of a flower]

hy·dro·car·bon (hī-drō-kar′bŏn). A compound containing only hydrogen and carbon.

Diels h., a phenanthrene derivative obtained by the dehydrogenation of various steroids.

saturated h., a h. that contains the greatest possible number of hydrogen atoms, so that the molecule contains neither rings nor multiple bonds.

hy·dro·cele (hī′drō-sēl). A collection of serous fluid in a sacculated cavity; specifically, such a collection in the space of the tunica vaginalis testis, or in a separate pocket along the spermatic cord. [hydro- + G. *kēlē*, hernia]

cervical h., a cyst formed by secretion into a persistent duct or fissure of the neck; when it involves lymph channels, it is usually a lymphangioma. SYN h. colli.

h. col′li, SYN cervical h.

communicating h., associated with patent processus vaginalis.

congenital h., a collection of fluid in the patent processus vaginalis leading from the abdominal cavity to the investing sac of the testis.

cord h., isolated h. of spermatic cord. SYN funicular h.

Dupuytren h., bilocular h. in which the sac fills the scrotum and also extends into the abdominal cavity beneath the peritoneum.

h. fem′inae, accumulation of serous fluid in the labium majus or in Nuck canal. SYN Nuck h.

filarial h., h. due to microfilaria (chiefly of *Wuchereria bancrofti*) in the tunica vaginalis.

funicular h., SYN cord h.

noncommunicating h., cord or scrotal hydrocele without communication to peritoneal cavity because processus vaginalis is not patent.

Nuck h., SYN h. feminae.

h. spina′lis, SYN *spina* bifida.

hy·dro·ce·lec·to·my (hī′drō-sē-lek′tō-mē). Excision of a hydrocele by drainage of its fluids and, sometimes partial excision of tunical vaginalis. [hydrocele + G. *ektomē*, excision]

hy·dro·ce·phal·ic (hī′drō-se-fal′ik). Relating to or suffering from hydrocephalus.

hy·dro·ceph·a·lo·cele (hī-drō-sef′ă-lō-sēl). SYN hydrencephalocele.

hy·dro·ceph·a·loid (hī-drō-sef′ă-loyd). **1.** Resembling hydrocephalus. **2.** A condition in infants suffering from diarrhea or other debilitating disease, in which there are dehydration and general symptoms resembling those of hydrocephalus without, however, any abnormal accumulation of cerebrospinal fluid.

hy·dro·ceph·a·lus (hī-drō-sef′ă-lŭs). A condition marked by an excessive accumulation of cerebrospinal fluid resulting in dilation of the cerebral ventricles and raised intracranial pressure; may also result in enlargement of the cranium and atrophy of the brain. SYN hydrocephaly. [hydro- + G. *kephalē*, head]

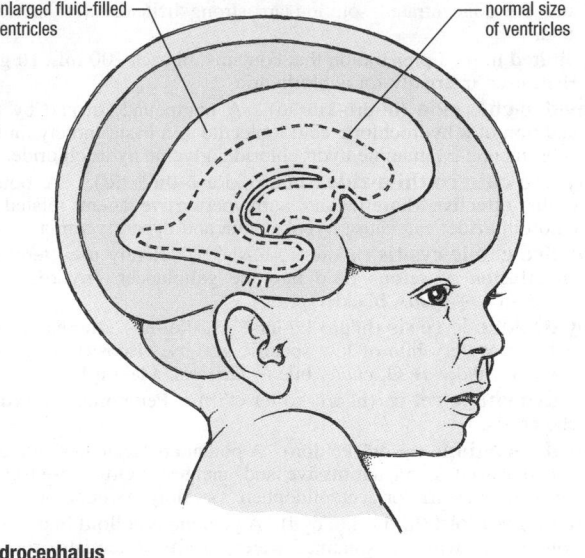

hydrocephalus

communicating h., type of h. in which there is an abnormality in cerebrospinal fluid absorption; there is no obstruction to cerebrospinal fluid flow in the ventricular system or where the cerebrospinal fluid passes into the spinal canal.

congenital h., h. due to a developmental defect of the brain. SYN primary h.

double compartment h., independent supra- and infratentorial h. usually due to a veil occlusion of the aqueduct of Sylvius.

external h., (1) accumulation of fluid in the subarachnoid spaces of the brain; (2) accumulation of fluid in the subdural space owing to a persistent communication between the subarachnoid and subdural spaces.

h. ex vac′uo, h. due to loss or atrophy of brain tissue; less commonly associated with raised intracranial pressure.

internal h., h. in which the accumulation of fluid is confined to the ventricles.

hy

noncommunicating h., SYN obstructive h.

normal pressure h., a type of h. developing usually in older people, due to failure of cerebrospinal fluid to be absorbed by the pacchionian granulations, and characterized clinically by progressive dementia, unsteady gait, urinary incontinence, and usually, a normal spinal fluid pressure. SYN occult h.

obstructive h., h. secondary to a block in cerebrospinal fluid flow in the ventricular system or between the ventricular system and spinal canal. SYN noncommunicating h.

occult h., SYN normal pressure h.

otitic h., a form of h. associated with otitis media and thrombosis of one or both sigmoid sinuses of the dura, characterized by marked increase in cerebrospinal fluid pressure.

postmeningitic h., ventricular dilation following meningitis and secondary to obstruction of cerebrospinal fluid pathways.

posttraumatic h., ventricular dilation following injury, due either to impaired circulation and/or absorption of cerebrospinal fluid or due to loss of brain substance (h. ex vacuo).

primary h., SYN congenital h.

secondary h., an accumulation of fluid in the cranial cavity, due to meningitis or obstruction to the venous flow.

thrombotic h., increase in cerebrospinal fluid and of intracranial pressure following thrombosis of the cerebral veins or sinuses; caused by septic infection, dehydration, tuberculosis, typhoid, leukemia, and other conditions.

toxic h., thrombotic h. associated with some general infection or toxic state.

hy·dro·ceph·a·ly (hī-drō-sef′ă-lē). SYN hydrocephalus.

hy·dro·chlo·ric ac·id (hī-drō-klōr′ik). HCl; the acid of gastric juice. The commercial product is used as an escharotic; the gas and the concentrated solution are strong irritants. SYN muriatic acid.

diluted h. a., a preparation that contains, in each 100 mL, 10 g of HCl; used internally for achlorhydria.

hy·dro·chlo·ride (hī-drō-klōr′īd). A compound formed by the addition of a hydrochloric acid molecule to a basic moiety on the substance; e.g., guanine hydrochloride, glycine hydrochloride.

hy·dro·chlo·ro·thi·a·zide (hī′drō-klōr-ō-thī′ă-zīd). A potent orally effective diuretic and antihypertensive agent related to chlorothiazide; can cause hypokalemia and hyperglycemia.

hy·dro·cho·le·cys·tis (hī′drō-kō-lē-sis′tis). Rarely used term for an effusion of serous fluid into the gallbladder. [hydro- + G. *cholē,* bile, + *kystis,* bladder]

hy·dro·cho·le·re·sis (hī′drō-kō-ler-ē′sis, -kol-er-). Increased output of a watery bile of low specific gravity, viscosity, and solid content. [hydro- + G. *cholē,* bile, + *hairesis,* a taking]

hy·dro·cho·le·ret·ic (hī′drō-kō-ler-et′ik). Pertaining to hydrocholeresis.

hy·dro·co·done (hī-drō-kō′dōn). A potent analgesic derivative of codeine used as an antitussive and analgesic. Often used combined with aspirin or acetaminophen. SYN dihydrocodeinone.

hy·dro·col·loid (hī-drō-kol′oyd). A gelatinous colloid in unstable equilibrium with its contained water, useful in dentistry for impressions because of its dimensional stability under controlled conditions.

irreversible h., a h. whose physical state is changed by an irreversible chemical reaction when water is added to a powder and an insoluble substance is formed.

reversible h., a h. composed of a base substance whose physical state may be changed from a solid or semisolid to a liquid by the application of heat and then changed to that of an elastic gel by cooling.

hy·dro·col·po·cele, hy·dro·col·pos (hī-drō-kol′pō-sēl, -kol′pos). Accumulation of mucus or other nonsanguineous fluid in the vagina. [hydro- + G. *kolpos,* bosom (vagina)]

hy·dro·cor·ta·mate hy·dro·chlo·ride (hī-drō-kōr′tă-māt). An ester-salt of hydrocortisone, used topically in the treatment of acute and chronic dermatoses.

hy·dro·cor·ti·sone (hī-drō-kōr′ti-sōn). A reduction product (at C-11) of cortisone; a steroid hormone secreted by the adrenal cortex (the active hormone secreted in the greatest quantity by the adrenals) and the most potent of the naturally occurring glucocorticoids in humans; an antiinflammatory agent. SYN cortisol.

h. acetate, an ester of h. with similar actions and uses as h. SYN cortisol acetate.

h. cyclopentylpropionate, an ester of h.

h. cypionate, the cyclopentanepropionic ester of cortisone, for oral administration.

h. hydrogen succinate, a form of h. administered intravenously.

h. sodium phosphate, an anti-inflammatory agent for intravenous or intramuscular administration.

h. sodium succinate, a very soluble ester salt of h. (cortisol), used parenterally in the management of emergencies resulting from acute adrenal insufficiency.

hy·dro·co·tar·nine (hī′drō-kō-tar′nēn). An alkaloidal principle derived from cotarnine; it is the basic hydrolytic product of narcotine; also obtained from the mother liquors of thebaine.

hy·dro·cy·an·ic ac·id (hī′drō-sī-an′ik). HCN; a colorless, very toxic liquid, with the odor of bitter almonds, present in bitter almonds (amygdalin), the stones of peaches, plums and other fruits, and laurel leaves; inhalation of 300 p.p.m. causes death. SYN hydrogen cyanide, prussic acid.

hy·dro·cy·an·ism (hī-drō-sī′an-izm). Poisoning with hydrocyanic acid.

hy·dro·cyst (hī′drō-sist). A cyst with clear, watery contents. [hydro- + G. *kystis,* bladder]

hy·dro·cys·to·ma (hī′drō-sis-tō′mă). **1.** An eruption of deeply seated vesicles, due to retention of fluid in the sweat follicles. **2.** SYN hidrocystoma. [hydro- + G. *kystis,* bladder, + *-ōma,* tumor]

hy·dro·dip·sia (hī-drō-dip′sē-ă). Water thirst, a characteristic of animals that ordinarily drink water. [hydro- + G. *dipsa,* thirst]

hy·dro·dip·so·ma·nia (hī′drō-dip′sō-mā′nē-ă). Periodic episodes of uncontrollable thirst, occasionally found in epileptic patients. [hydro- + G. *dipsa,* thirst, + *mania,* frenzy]

hy·dro·di·u·re·sis (hī′drō-dī-ū-rē′sis). Diuresis effected by water.

hy·dro·dy·nam·ics (hī′drō-dī-nam′iks). The branch of physics concerned with the flow of liquids. [hydro- + G. *dynamis,* force]

hy·dro·en·ceph·a·lo·cele (hī′drō-en-sef′ă-lō-sēl). SYN hydrencephalocele.

hy·dro·flu·o·ric ac·id (hī-drō-flōr′ik). A solution of hydrogen fluoride gas in water; a poisonous, caustic, foaming liquid that is used to clean metals and can etch glass; extremely irritating to skin and lungs.

hy·dro·gel (hī′drō-jel). A colloid in which the particles are in the external or dispersion phase and water in the internal or dispersed phase. Cf. hydrosol.

hy·dro·gen (H) (hī′drō-jen). **1.** A gaseous element, atomic no. 1, atomic wt. 1.00794. **2.** The molecular form (H_2) of the element. SYN dihydrogen. [hydro- + G. *-gen,* producing]

activated h., h. removed by a dehydrogenase, e.g., via a flavoprotein, from a metabolite for transference to another substance with which it combines.

arseniureted h., SYN arsine.

h. bromide, HBr; a colorless gas that has a very irritating odor and fumes in moist air; in aqueous solution, it is hydrobromic acid.

h. chloride, HCl; a very soluble gas which, in solution, forms hydrochloric acid.

h. cyanide, SYN hydrocyanic acid.

h. dehydrogenase, a flavoprotein catalyzing the conversion of NAD^+ to NADH by molecular hydrogen (H_2); i.e., $H_2 + NAD^+ \rightarrow H^+ + NADH$.

h. dioxide, SYN h. peroxide.

heavy h., SYN hydrogen-2.

h. peroxide, an unstable compound readily broken down to water and oxygen, a reaction catalyzed by various powdered metals and by the enzyme, catalase; a 3% solution is used as a mild antiseptic for skin and mucous membranes. SYN h. dioxide, hydroperoxide.

h. phosphide, SYN phosphine.

phosphureted h., SYN phosphine.

h. sulfide, H_2S; a colorless, flammable, toxic gas with a familiar "rotten egg" odor, formed in the decomposition of organic matter containing sulfur; used as a reagent, and in the manufacture of chemicals. SYN sulfureted h.

sulfureted h., SYN h. sulfide.

hy·dro·gen-1 (^{1}H). The common h. isotope, making up 99.985% of the h. atoms occurring in nature. SYN protium.

hy·dro·gen-2 (^{2}H). The isotope of h. of atomic wt. 2; the less common stable isotope of h., making up 0.015% of the h. atoms occurring in nature; the nucleus consists of a proton and a neutron. SYN deuterium, heavy hydrogen.

hy·dro·gen-3 (^{3}H). A hydrogen isotope of atomic wt. 3; weakly radioactive, emitting beta particles to become the stable helium-3; half-life, 12.32 years. SYN tritium.

hy·dro·gen·ase (hī′drō-je-nās, hī-droj′ĕ-nās). **1.** Any enzyme that removes a hydride ion (or H:⁻) from NADH (or NADPH). SYN hydrogenlyase. **2.** The enzyme that catalyzes the reaction of 2H⁺ with ferricytochrome or ferredoxin to generate H$_2$.

hy·dro·gen·a·tion (hī′drō-jĕ-nā′shŭn, hī-droj′ĕ-nā-shŭn). Addition of hydrogen to a compound, especially to an unsaturated fat or fatty acid; thus, soft fats or oils are solidified or "hardened."

hy·dro·gen ex·po·nent. The decadic logarithm of the hydrogen ion concentration in blood or other fluid; its negative is the pH of that fluid.

hy·dro·gen·ly·ase (hī′drō-gen-lī′ās). SYN hydrogenase (1).

hy·dro·ki·net·ic (hī′drō-ki-net′ik). Pertaining to the motion of fluids and the forces giving rise to such motion.

hy·dro·ki·net·ics (hī′drō-ki-net′iks). That branch of kinetics concerned with fluids in motion.

hy·dro·la·bile (hī-drō-lā′bil). Unstable in the presence of water.

hy·dro·la·bil·i·ty (hī′drō-lă-bil′i-tē). A state in which the fluid in the tissues readily changes in amount.

hy·dro·las·es (hī′drō-lās-ez). Enzymes (EC class 3) cleaving substrates with addition of H$_2$O at the point of cleavage; e.g., esterases, phosphatases, nucleases, peptidases. SYN hydrolyzing enzymes.

cysteine h., h. that utilize an active site cysteinyl residue for the catalytic event.

serine h., h. that utilize an active site seryl residue for the catalytic event.

hy·dro·ly·as·es (hī-drō-lī′ās-ĕz). A class of lyases (EC 4.2.1.x) comprising enzymes removing H and OH as water, leading to formation of new double bonds within the affected molecule; the trivial names usually contain dehydratase or hydratase.

hy·dro·lymph (hī′drō-limf). The circulating fluid in many of the invertebrates.

hy·drol·y·sate (hī-drol′i-sāt). A solution containing the products of hydrolysis.

hy·drol·y·sis (hī-drol′i-sis). A chemical process whereby a compound is cleaved into two or more simpler compounds with the uptake of the H and OH parts of a water molecule on either side of the chemical bond cleaved; h. is effected by the action of acids, alkalies, or enzymes. Cf. hydration. SYN hydrolytic cleavage. [hydro- + G. *lysis,* dissolution]

hy·dro·lyt·ic (hī-drō-lit′ik). Referring to or causing hydrolysis.

hy·dro·lyze (hī′drō-līz). To subject to hydrolysis.

hy·dro·ma (hī-drō′mă). SYN hygroma.

hy·dro·mas·sage (hī′drō-mă-sahzh). Massage produced by streams of water.

hy·dro·me·nin·go·cele (hī′drō-men-ing′gō-sēl). Protrusion of the meninges of brain or spinal cord through a defect in the bony wall, the sac so formed containing cerebrospinal fluid. [hydro- + G. *mēninx,* membrane, + *kēlē,* hernia]

hy·drom·e·ter (hī-drom′ĕ-ter). An instrument for determining the specific gravity or density of a liquid. SYN areometer, gravimeter. [hydro- + G. *mēron,* measure]

hy·dro·me·tra (hī-drō-mē′tră). Accumulation of thin mucus or other watery fluid in the cavity of the uterus. [hydro- + G. *mētra,* uterus]

hy·dro·met·ric (hī-drō-met′rik). Relating to hydrometry or the hydrometer.

hy·dro·me·tro·col·pos (hī′drō-mē-trō-kol′pos). Distention of uterus and vagina by fluid other than blood or pus. [hydro- + G. *mētra,* uterus, + *kolpos,* bosom (vagina)]

hy·drom·e·try (hī-drom′ĕ-trē). Determination of the specific gravity of a fluid by means of a hydrometer.

hy·dro·mi·cro·ceph·a·ly (hī′drō-mī-krō-sef′ă-lē). Microcephaly associated with an increased amount of cerebrospinal fluid.

hy·dro·mor·phone hy·dro·chlo·ride (hī-drō-mōr′fōn). A synthetic derivative of morphine, with analgesic potency about 10 times that of morphine. SYN dihydromorphinone hydrochloride.

hy·drom·pha·lus (hī-drom′fă-lŭs). A cystic tumor at the umbilicus, most commonly a vitellointestinal cyst. [hydro- + G. *omphalos,* umbilicus]

hy·dro·my·e·lia (hī-drō-mī-ē′lē-ă). An increase of fluid in the dilated central canal of the spinal cord, or in congenital cavities elsewhere in the cord substance. [hydro- + G. *myelos,* marrow]

hy·dro·my·e·lo·cele (hī-drō-mī′ĕ-lō-sēl). Protrusion of a portion of cord, thinned out into a sac distended with cerebrospinal fluid, through a spina bifida. [hydro- + G. *myelos,* marrow, + *kēlē,* tumor, hernia]

📖**hy·dro·ne·phro·sis** (hī′drō-ne-frō′sis). Dilation of the pelvis and calices of one or both kidneys. This may result from obstruction to the flow of urine, vesicoureteral reflux, or it may be a primary congenital deformity without an apparent cause. SYN pelvocaliectasis, pyeloureterectasis. [hydro- + G. *nephros,* kidney, + *-osis,* condition]

hydronephrosis (causes)
I. mechanical obstruction of urinary tract

a) changes inside the tract
      1. hyperplasia and carcinoma of the prostate
      2. tumors of the efferent urinary tract
      3. scarring in the ureter or the urethra
      4. formation of stones
      5. congenital or other deformities (nephroptosis)

b) changes outside the urinary tract
      1. tumors of the pelvis (cervical carcinoma)
      2. tumors and proliferative processes of the retroperitoneum
      3. retroperitoneal fibrosis
      4. pressure from aberrant renal arteries or aneurysms of the renal arteries
      5. pressure from adhesions

II. neuromuscular problems   spina bifida, paraplegia, tabes dorsalis, multiple sclerosis
III. pregnancy
IV. unknown causes   functional narrowing of the ureter, at the passage from the renal pelvis: megaloureter-megacystis syndrome

hy·dro·ne·phrot·ic (hī′drō-ne-frot′ik). Relating to hydronephrosis.

hy·dro·ni·um (hī-drō′nē-um). SEE hydronium *ion.*

hy·dro·par·a·sal·pinx (hī′drō-par-ă-sal′pinks). Accumulation of serous fluid in the accessory tubes of the oviduct. [hydro- + G. *para,* beside, + *salpinx,* trumpet]

hy·dro·path·ic (hī-drō-path′ik). Relating to hydropathy.

hy·drop·a·thy (hī-drop′ă-thē). The obsolete use of water to treat and cure disease.

hy·dro·pe·nia (hī-drō-pē′nē-ă). Reduction or deprivation of water. [hydro- + G. *penia,* poverty]

hy·dro·pe·nic (hī-drō-pē′nik). Pertaining to or characterized by hydropenia.

hy·dro·per·i·car·di·um (hī′drō-pār-i-kar′dē-ŭm). A noninflammatory accumulation of fluid in the pericardial sac.

hy·dro·per·i·to·ne·um, hy·dro·per·i·to·nia (hī′drō-pār-i-tō-nē′ŭm, -tō′nē-ă). SYN ascites. [hydro- + peritoneum]

hy·dro·per·ox·i·das·es (hī′drō-per-oks′i-dā-sez). Those oxidore-

hy

ductases that require H_2O_2 as hydrogen acceptors; e.g., peroxidases, catalase.

hy·dro·per·ox·ide (hī′drō-per-ok′sīd). SYN *hydrogen* peroxide.

hy·dro·phil, hy·dro·phile (hī′drō-fil, -fīl). A substance that is hydrophilic.

hy·dro·phil·ia (hī-drō-fil′ē-ă). A tendency of the blood and tissues to absorb fluid. [hydro- + G. *philos,* fond]

hy·dro·phil·ic (hī-drō-fil′ik). **1.** Denoting the property of attracting or associating with water molecules, possessed by polar radicals or ions, as opposed to hydrophobic (2). **2.** Tending to dissolve in water. **3.** Polar. SYN hydrophilous.

hy·droph·i·lous (hī-drof′i-lŭs). SYN hydrophilic.

hy·dro·pho·bia (hī-drō-fō′bē-ă). SYN rabies. [hydro- + G. *phobos,* fear; from reports of inability to swallow and resultant resistance to oral fluids in human and animal rabies]

hy·dro·pho·bic (hī-drō-fōb′ik). **1.** Relating to or suffering from hydrophobia. **2.** Lacking an affinity for water molecules, as opposed to hydrophilic. SYN apolar (2). **3.** Tending not to dissolve in water. **4.** Nonpolar.

hy·droph·thal·mia, hy·droph·thal·mos, hy·droph·thal·mus (hī′drof-thal′mē-ă, -thal′mos). SYN buphthalmia. [hydro- + G. *ophthalmos,* eye]

Hy·dro·phy·i·dae (hī-drō-fī′i-de). A family of snakes, the true sea snakes, characterized by a vertically compressed tail, giving it a paddle- or oarlike appearance; their fangs, like those of cobras, are small, grooved, and permanently erect. They are common in shallow waters along coastal margins in many regions of the Pacific basin and are important medically in western Malaysia and coastal Vietnam. There are numerous species, all venomous, but few bite humans.

hy·drop·ic (hī-drop′ik). Containing an excess of water or of watery fluid. SYN dropsical.

hy·dro·pneu·ma·to·sis (hī-drō-noo-mă-tō′sis). Combined emphysema and edema; the presence of liquid and gas in tissues. [hydro- + G. *pneuma,* breath, spirit]

hy·dro·pneu·mo·per·i·car·di·um (hī-drō-noo′mō-per-i-kar′dē-ŭm). The presence of a serous effusion and of gas in the pericardial sac. SYN pneumohydropericardium. [hydro- + G. *pneuma,* air, + pericardium]

hy·dro·pneu·mo·per·i·to·ne·um (hī-drō-noo′mō-pār-i-tō-nē′ŭm). The presence of gas and serous fluid in the peritoneal cavity. SYN pneumohydroperitoneum. [hydro- + G. *pneuma,* air, + peritoneum]

hy·dro·pneu·mo·tho·rax (hī′drō-noo-mō-thōr′aks). The presence of both gas and fluids in the pleural cavity. SYN pneumohydrothorax, pneumoserothorax. [hydro- + G. *pneuma,* air, + thorax]

hy·dro·po·sia (hī-drō-pō′zē-ă). Water-drinking, a characteristic of animals that ordinarily drink water. [hydro- + G. *posis,* drinking]

hy·drops (hī′drops). An excessive accumulation of clear, watery fluid in any of the tissues or cavities of the body; synonymous, according to its character and location, with ascites, anasarca, edema, etc. [G. *hydrōps*]

endolymphatic h., SYN Ménière *disease.*

fetal h., h. fetal′is, abnormal accumulation of serous fluid in the fetal tissues, as in erythroblastosis fetalis.

h. follic′uli, accumulation of fluid in a graafian follicle.

h. of gallbladder, accumulation of clear watery fluid in the gallbladder as a result of long-standing cystic duct obstruction.

immune fetal h., fetal edema and ascites secondary to maternal/fetal blood group incompatibility.

nonimmune fetal h., fetal edema and ascites unrelated to maternal/fetal blood group incompatibilities; multiple etiologies include fetal cardiac disease, fetal viral disease, and fetal structural anomalies.

h. ova′rii, SYN hydrovarium.

h. pericardii (hī′drops per-i-kar′dē-ī), an obsolete term for pericardial *effusion.*

h. tu′bae, SYN hydrosalpinx.

h. tu′bae pro′fluens, SYN intermittent *hydrosalpinx.*

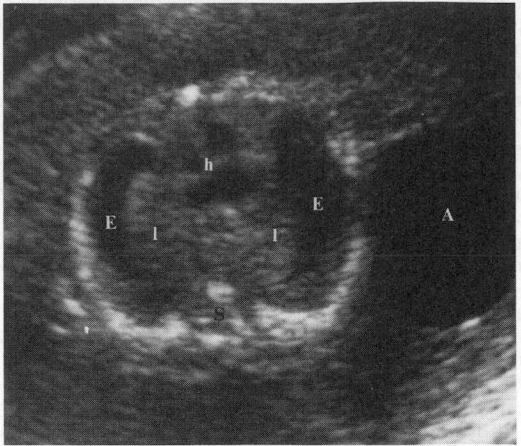

fetal hydrops: transverse image through the fetal thorax at level of heart (h) demonstrates bilateral pleural effusions (E) outlining lungs (l); fetal chest is viewed from above, with the spine (S) posterior; this fetus also had ascites; a pocket of amniotic fluid (A) is seen adjacent to right side of fetus

hy·dro·py·o·ne·phro·sis (hī′drō-pī′ō-ne-frō′sis). Presence of purulent urine in the pelvis and calices of the kidney following obstruction of the ureter. [hydro- + G. *pyon,* pus, + nephrosis]

hy·dro·quin·ol (hī-drō-kwin′ol). SYN hydroquinone.

hy·dro·qui·none (hī-drō-kwin′ōn). An antioxidant used in ointments. SYN hydroquinol, quinol.

hy·dror·chis (hī-drōr′kis). A collection of fluid (hydrocele) around the testis, as in the tunica vaginalis or along the spermatic cord. [hydro- + G. *orchis,* testicle]

hy·dro·rhe·o·stat (hī-drō-rē′ō-stat). A rheostat in which resistance to the flow of electric current is provided by water.

hy·dror·rhea (hī-drō-rē′ă). A profuse discharge of watery fluid from any part of the body. [hydro- + G. *rhoia,* flow]

h. grav′idae, h. gravida′rum, discharge of a watery fluid from the vagina during pregnancy.

hy·dro·sal·pinx (hī-drō-sal′pinks). Accumulation of serous fluid in the fallopian tube, often an end result of pyosalpinx. SYN hydrops tubae. [hydro- + G. *salpinx,* trumpet]

intermittent h., intermittent discharge of watery fluid from the oviduct. SYN hydrops tubae profluens.

hy·dro·sar·ca (hī-drō-sar′kă). SYN anasarca. [hydro- + G. *sarx,* flesh]

hy·dro·sar·co·cele (hī-drō-sar′kō-sēl). A chronic swelling of the testis complicated with hydrocele. [hydro- + G. *sarx,* flesh, + *kēlē,* tumor]

hy·dro·sol (hī′dro-sol). A colloid in aqueous solution, the particles being in the dispersed or internal phase and the water in the external or dispersion phase. Cf. hydrogel.

hy·dro·sphyg·mo·graph (hī-drō-sfig′mō-graf). A sphygmograph in which the pulse beat is transmitted to the recorder through a column of water.

hy·dro·stat (hī′drō-stat). A device for regulating water level. [hydro- + G. *statikos,* causing to stand]

hy·dro·stat·ic (hī-drō-stat′ik). Relating to the pressure of fluids or to their properties when in equilibrium.

hy·dro·su·dop·a·thy (hī′drō-soo-dop′ă-thē). SYN hydrosudotherapy. [hydro- + L. *sudor,* sweat, + G. *pathos,* suffering]

hy·dro·su·do·ther·a·py (hī′drō-soo′dō-thār′ă-pē). Hydrotherapy combined with induced sweating, as in the Turkish bath. SYN hydrosudopathy.

hy·dro·sy·rin·go·my·e·lia (hī′drō-sĭ-rin′gō-mī-ē′lē-ă). SYN syringomyelia. [hydro- + G. *hydōr,* water, + *syrinx,* a tube, + *myelos,* marrow]

hy·dro·tax·is (hī-drō-tak′sis). The movement of cells or organisms in relation to water. [hydro- + G. *taxis,* arrangement]

hy·dro·ther·a·peu·tic (hī′drō-thār′ă-pū′tik). SYN hydriatric.

hy·dro·ther·a·peu·tics (hī′drō-thār′ă-pū′tiks). SYN hydrotherapy.

hy·dro·ther·a·py (hī-drō-thār′ă-pē). Therapeutic use of water by external application, either for its pressure effect or as a means of applying physical energy to the tissues. SYN hydrotherapeutics. [hydro- + G. *therapeia*, therapy]

hy·dro·ther·mal (hī-drō-ther′măl). Relating to hot water. [hydro- + G. *thermē*, heat]

hy·dro·thi·o·ne·mia (hī′drō-thī-ō-nē′mē-ă). The presence of hydrogen sulfide in the circulating blood. [hydro- + G. *theion*, sulfur, + *haima*, blood]

hy·dro·thi·o·nu·ria (hī′drō-thī-ō-noo′rē-ă). The excretion of hydrogen sulfide in the urine. [hydro- + G. *theion*, sulfur, + *ouron*, urine]

hy·dro·tho·rax (hī-drō-thōr′aks). SYN pleural *effusion*.
chylous h., SYN chylothorax.

hy·drot·o·my (hī-drot′ō-mē). In histology, tearing apart the tissue elements by injection of water. [hydro- + G. *tomē*, a cutting]

hy·dro·tro·pism (hī-drō-trō′pizm, hī-drot′rō-pizm). The property in growing organisms of turning toward a moist surface (**positive h.**) or away from a moist surface (**negative h.**). [hydro- + G. *tropos*, a turning]

hy·dro·tu·ba·tion (hī′drō-too-bā′shŭn). Injection of a liquid medication or saline solution through the cervix into the uterine cavity and fallopian tubes for dilation and/or treatment of the tubes.

hy·dro·u·re·ter (hī′drō-ū-rē′ter, -ūr′ē-ter). SYN ureterectasia.

hy·dro·ure·ter·o·ne·phro·sis (hī-drō-ū-rē′ter-ō-net-rō′sis). SYN ureterohydronephrosis.

hy·drous (hī′drŭs). SYN hydrated.

hy·dro·va·ri·um (hī-drō-vā′rē-ŭm). A collection of fluid in the ovary. SYN hydrops ovarii.

hy·drox·am·ic ac·ids (hī-drok-sam′ik). R–CO–NH–OH ↔ RC(OH)=N–OH; hydroxylamine derivatives of carboxylic acids, including amino acids, formed by the action of hydroxylamine.

hy·drox·ide (hī-drok′sīd). **1.** A compound containing a potentially ionizable hydroxyl group; particularly a compound that liberates OH⁻ upon dissolving in water. **2.** The hydroxide anion, OH⁻.

hy·drox·o·co·bal·a·min (hī-drok′sō-kō-bal′ă-min). Vitamin B_{12b}, differing from cyanocobalamin (vitamin B_{12}) in the presence of a hydroxyl ion in place of the cyanide ion at the sixth coordinate position on the cobalt atom. SEE ALSO *vitamin* B_{12}. SYN hydroxocobemine.

hy·drox·o·co·be·mine (hī-drok′sō-kō-bĕ-mēn). SYN hydroxocobalamin.

hydroxy-. Prefix indicating addition or substitution of the –OH group to or in the compound whose name follows. SEE ALSO oxa-, oxo-, oxy-.

hy·drox·y·ace·tic ac·id (hī-drok′sē-a-sē′tik). SYN glycolic acid.

hy·drox·y ac·id (hī-drok′sē). An organic acid containing both OH and COOH groups; e.g., lactic acid.

3-hy·drox·y·ac·yl-CoA de·hy·dro·gen·ase (hī-drok′sē-as′il). β-Hydroxyacyl dehydrogenase; an enzyme catalyzing the oxidation of an L-3-hydroxyacyl-CoA to a 3-ketoacyl-CoA with the concomitant reduction of NAD⁺; one of the enzymes of the β oxidation of fatty acids. SYN β-ketohydrogenase, β-ketoreductase.

hy·drox·y·a·cyl·glu·ta·thi·one hy·dro·lase (hī-drok′sē-as′il-gloo-tă-thī′ōn). An enzyme with catalytic activity similar to that of lactoylglutathione lyase, but more general; catalyzes the hydrolysis of an *S*-2-hydroxyacylglutathione, producing glutathione and a 2-hydroxy acid anion. SEE ALSO glyoxalase.

3-hy·drox·y·anth·ran·il·ic ac·id (hī-drok′sē-anth-ra-nil′ik). A metabolite of tryptophan degradation that can serve as a precursor for the biosynthesis of NAD⁺.

hy·drox·y·ap·a·tite (hī-drok′sē-ap-ă-tīt). A natural mineral structure that the crystal lattice of bones and teeth (i.e., amorphous h.) closely resembles; used in chromatography of nucleic acids; also found in pathologic calcifications (e.g., atherosclerotic aortas). SYN hydroxylapatite.

amorphous h., containing ion contaminants (e.g., 6–8% CO_3^{2-}, 3–5% Mg^{2+}, F⁻, Cl⁻, etc.); found in mineralized connective tissue (e.g., bone, dentin, cementum). SYN poorly crystalline h.
poorly crystalline h., SYN amorphous h.

3-hy·drox·y·bu·ta·no·ic ac·id. SYN 3-hydroxybutyric acid.

γ-hydroxybutyrate (GHB) (gam′ă-hī-drok′sē- byu′tir-āt). a naturally occurring short-chain fatty acid, a metabolite of γ- aminobutyric acid (GABA) found in all body tissues, with the highest concentration in the brain; it affects levels of GABA, dopamine, 5-hydroxytryptamine, and acetylcholine, and may itself be a neurotransmitter; accumulation of GHB in people with an inherited disorder in the metabolism of GABA causes ataxia and mental retardation. Synthetic GHB, formerly used in anesthesia and in the treatment of narcolepsy and alcohol withdrawal, has been banned by the Food and Drug Administration because of severe neurologic, cardiovascular, respiratory, and gastrointestinal side effects. SYN 4-hydroxybutyrate.

Illicit use of GHB has become increasingly popular, particularly among body-builders, because it is easily and inexpensively manufactured in the home and is alleged to suppress appetite, relieve depression, enhance muscle mass by stimulating release of growth hormones, and improve sleep. It has also been used as a euphoriant and (because it is odorless and nearly tasteless and quickly induces sedation with retrograde amnesia) to facilitate date rape. Common street names for GHB include "grievous bodily harm," "liquid ecstasy," "liquid E," "liquid X," and "scoop." The drug is rapidly absorbed after oral administration and readily crosses the blood-brain barrier. It is primarily a CNS depressant, but also lowers body temperature, heart rate, and cardiac output. Acute toxicity may be manifested by drowsiness, confusion, combative and self-injurious behavior, nausea, tremors, seizures, and coma. The drug acts synergistically with alcohol, benzodiazepines, and narcotics to produce profound CNS and respiratory depression. Most toxic episodes occur in males aged 18–25 and involve alcohol as well. Habituation and severe withdrawal symptoms have been reported. Treatment of toxicity is purely supportive; there is no antidote. Because the industrial and household solvent γ-butyrolactone is metabolized to GHB, it has been marketed illicitly as a nutritional supplement alleged to have the same therapeutic effects as GHB. Its use has been associated with numerous reports of adverse events, including death.

4-hydroxybutyrate. SYN γ-hydroxybutyrate.

β-hy·drox·y·bu·tyr·ic ac·id. SYN 3-hydroxybutyric acid.

3-hy·drox·y·bu·tyr·ic ac·id (hī-drōk′sē-bū-tir′ik). The D-stereoisomer is one of the ketone bodies and is formed in ketogenesis; it is an important fuel for extrahepatic tissues; as an acyl derivative it is also an intermediate in fatty acid biosynthesis. The L-isomer is found as a coenzyme A derivative in β oxidation of fatty acids. SYN 3-hydroxybutanoic acid, β-hydroxybutyric acid.

D-3-h. a. dehydrogenase, an enzyme that reversibly catalyzes the interconversion of the two main ketone bodies, catalyzing acetoacetate + NADH + H⁺ ↔ D-3-hydroxybutyrate + NAD⁺.

4-hy·drox·y·bu·ty·ric ac·i·du·ria (hī-drok′sē-bū-tir′ik). Elevated levels of 4-hydroxybutyrate in the urine. An inherited disorder that can lead to hypotonia and mental retardation.

hy·drox·y·car·bam·ide (hī-drok′sē-kar′bă-mīd). SYN hydroxyurea.

hy·drox·y·chlo·ro·quine sul·fate (hī-drok′sē-klōr′ō-kwīn). A quinoline derivative; an antimalarial agent whose actions and uses resemble those of chloroquine phosphate; also used in the treatment of lupus erythematosus and rheumatoid arthritis.

25-hy·drox·y·cho·le·cal·cif·er·ol (HCC) (hī-drok′sē-kō′lē-kal-sif′er-ol). SYN calcidiol.

7α-hy·drox·y·cho·les·ter·ol (hī-droks′ē-kol-es-ter-ol). First intermediate in the conversion of cholesterol to the bile acids; formed in the principal rate-limiting step of bile acid biosynthesis.

hy

hy·drox·y·chro·man (hī-drok-sē-krō′man). SYN chromanol.

hy·drox·y·chro·mene (hī-drok-sē-krō′mēn). SYN chromenol.

hy·drox·y·eph·ed·rine (hī-drok′sē-ĕ-fed′rēn). A sympathomimetic agent for the treatment of shock.

25-hy·drox·y·er·go·cal·cif·er·ol (hī-drok′sēr′gō-kal-sif″er-ol). A biologically active and major circulatory metabolite of vitamin D₂. SYN ercalcidiol.

α-hy·drox·y·eth·yl·thi·a·min py·ro·phos·phate. SYN activated *acetaldehyde*.

hy·drox·y·fat·ty ac·id (hī-drok′sē-fat′te). A fatty acid that has a hydroxyl group covalently attached to it (e.g., in hydroxynervone).

3-hy·drox·y·glu·tar·ic ac·id (hī-drok′sē-gloo-tar′ik). A dicarboxylic acid that accumulates in individuals with glutaric acidemia type I.

hy·drox·y·he·min (hī-drok-sē-hē′min). SYN hematin.

β-hy·drox·y·i·so·bu·tyr·ic ac·id (hī-droks′ē-ī-sō-byu-ter-ik). An intermediate in the degradation of L-valine.

3-L-hy·drox·y·ky·nu·ren·ine (hī-drok′sē-ki-noo-rĕ-nēn). An intermediate in the catabolism of L-tryptophan and a precursor of xanthurenate; elevated in cases of a vitamin B₆ deficiency.

hy·drox·y·ky·nu·re·ni·nu·ria (hī-drok′sē-kī-noo′rĕ-ni-noo′rē-ă) [MIM*236800]. An abnormality in tryptophan metabolism, probably due to a defect in kynureninase, characterized by mild mental retardation, migraine-like headaches, and urinary excretion of large amounts of kynurenine, 3-hydoxykynurenine, and xanthurenic acid; autosomal recessive inheritance.

hy·drox·yl (hī-drok′sil). The radical or moiety, –OH.

hy·drox·yl·a·mine (hī-drok′sil-ă′mēn). **1.** NH₂OH; a partially oxidized derivative of ammonia; reacts with carbonyl groups to produce oximes; forms acid salts, e.g., h. hydrochloride. It is a chemical mutagen that causes deamination of cytosine residues in DNA. **2.** Any compound containing RNH–OH.

h. reductase, an enzyme catalyzing the reversible reduction of h. to ammonia with a variety of donors (e.g., methylene blue, flavin). SEE ALSO *NADH*-hydroxylamine reductase.

hy·drox·yl·a·mi·no (hī-drok′sil-am-i-nō). The monovalent group or moiety, –NH–OH.

hy·drox·yl·ap·a·tite (hī-drok′sil-ap-ă-tīt). SYN hydroxyapatite.

hy·drox·y·las·es (hī-drok′si-lā-sez). Enzymes catalyzing formation of hydroxyl groups by addition of an oxygen atom, hence oxidizing the substrate; most are found in EC subclass 1.14.

hy·drox·yl·a·tion (hī-drok-si-lā′shŭn). Placing of a hydroxyl group on a compound in a position where one did not exist before.

δ-hy·drox·y·ly·sine. SYN 5-hydroxylysine.

5-hy·drox·y·ly·sine (5Hyl). A hydroxylated amino acid found in certain collagens. The decreased ability to form 5-hydroxylysine is associated with Ehlers-Danlos syndrome type VI. SYN δ-hydroxylysine.

p-hy·drox·y·mer·cur·i·ben·zo·ate (hī-drok′sē-mer′kū-rē-ben′zō-āt). An organic mercurial formed spontaneously by hydrolysis of p-chloromercuribenzoate. SEE ALSO p-mercuribenzoate.

β-hy·droxy-β-meth·yl·glu·tar·yl-CoA (HMG-CoA). A key intermediate in the synthesis of ketone bodies, of steroids, and of farnesyl and geranyl derivatives. SYN 3-hydroxy-3-methylglutaryl-CoA.

β-h.-β-m.-CoA lyase, an enzyme, found primarily in liver and rumen epithelium that catalyzes the formation of acetyl-CoA and acetoacetate from β-h.-β-m.-CoA; a key step in ketogenesis; a deficiency of this enzyme leads to episodes of severe metabolic acidosis without ketosis.

β-h.-β-m.-CoA reductase, an enzyme that catalyzes the rate-limiting step of cholesterol biosynthesis: β-h.-β-m.-CoA + 2NADPH + 2H⁺ → (R)-mevalonate + 2NADP⁺ + CoA.

β-h.-β-m.-CoA synthase, an enzyme in mitochondria that catalyzes the reaction of acetyl-CoA with acetoacetyl-CoA and water to form (S)-β-h.-β-m.-CoA and coenzyme A, a step required for both ketogenesis and steroidogenesis to occur.

3-hy·droxy-3-meth·yl·glu·tar·yl-CoA. SYN β-hydroxy-β-methylglutaryl-CoA.

hy·drox·y·ner·vone (hī-drok-sē-ner′vōn). A cerebroside containing α-hydroxynervonic acid. SYN oxynervone.

hy·drox·y·ner·von·ic ac·id (hī-drok′sē-ner-von′ik). An important constituent of certain cerebrosides.

p-hy·drox·y·phe·nyl·ac·e·tate (hī-droks′ē-fen′il-as′e-tāt). A minor side product of L-tyrosine degradation that is elevated in the urine in cases of neonatal tyrosinemia and in Richner-Hanhart syndrome.

p-hy·drox·y·phe·nyl·lac·tate (hī-droks′ē-fen′il-lak′tāt). A metabolite in tyrosine degradation that is elevated in individuals with Richner-Hanhart syndrome.

p-hy·drox·y·phe·nyl·py·ru·vate (hī-droks′ē-fen′il-pī′roo-vāt). A metabolite formed by the transamination of tyrosine; elevated in the urine of individuals with tyrosinemia.

hy·drox·y·phen·yl·u·ria (hī-drok′sē-fen-il-oo′rē-ă). Urinary excretion of tyrosine and phenylalanine, as a result of ascorbic acid deficiency; occurs notably in those premature infants who lack this vitamin.

3α-hy·drox·y-5α-preg·nan-20-one. A catabolite of progesterone; found in the urine of pregnant women.

17α-hy·drox·y·pro·ges·ter·one (hī-drok′sē-prō-jes′ter-ōn). A steroid hormone with medical use similar to that of progesterone. The acetate is an orally effective derivative, useful in conditions in which parenterally administered progesterone or the caproate is indicated; it possesses some androgenic potency and may cause virilizing changes in a female fetus. The caproate or hexanoate has essentially the same actions and uses as progesterone, but is more potent and has a longer duration of action. A precursor of the androgens, estrogens, and adrenocortical hormones.

21-hy·drox·y·pro·ges·ter·one. SYN deoxycorticosterone.

3-hy·drox·y·pro·line (3Hyp) (hī-drok′sē-prō′lēn). A derivative of proline found in certain collagens, particularly basement membrane collagen. SYN 3-hydroxy-2-pyrrolidinecarboxylic acid.

4-hy·drox·y·pro·line (4Hyp, Hyp). 4-Hydroxy-2-pyrrolidine-carboxylic acid; the *trans*-L-isomer is a pyrrolidine found among the hydrolysis products of collagen; not found in proteins other than those of connective tissue. A vitamin C deficiency will result in impaired formation of h.

h. oxidase, (1) a flavoenzyme that catalyzes the conversion of h. to Δ′-pyrroline-3-hydroxy-5-carboxylate using FAD; this enzyme appears to be deficient in individuals with hyperhydroxyprolinemia; **(2)** an enzyme that catalyzes the reaction of h. with NAD⁺ to form NADH and 4-oxoproline. SYN 4-oxoproline reductase.

hy·drox·y·pro·li·ne·mia (hī-drok′sē-prō-li-nē′mē-ă) [MIM* 237000]. A metabolic disorder characterized by mental retardation and microscopic hematuria in some patients; associated with enhanced plasma concentration and urinary excretion of free hydroxyproline because of a deficiency of hydroxyproline oxidase; autosomal recessive inheritance.

β-hy·drox·y·pro·pi·o·nic ac·id (hī-drok′sē-prō′pē-on′ik). A minor intermediate in propionate and methylmalonate metabolism. SEE β-hydroxypropionic aciduria.

β-hy·drox·y·pro·pi·o·nic ac·i·du·ria. Elevated levels of β-hydroxypropionic acid in the urine; seen in defects in methylmalonic acid and propionate metabolism, as well as in ketotic hyperglycinemia syndrome.

15-hy·drox·y·pros·ta·glan·din de·hy·dro·gen·ase (hī-drok′sē-pros-tă-glan′din). An enzyme that catalyzes the oxidation of prostaglandins, rendering them inactive, by converting the 15-hydroxyl group to a keto group using NAD⁺.

6-hy·drox·y·pu·rine. SYN hypoxanthine.

3-hy·droxy-2-pyr·ro·li·di·ne·car·box·yl·ic ac·id. SYN 3-hydroxyproline.

8-hy·drox·y·quin·o·line (hī-drok-sē-kwin′ō-lin). A fungistat and chelating agent. SYN quinolinol.

3β-hy·drox·y·ste·roid sul·fa·tase (hī-drok′sē-stēr′ōid). An enzyme, found in most mammalian tissues, that is capable of hydrolyzing the sulfate ester bonds of a variety of sulfated sterols; a deficiency of this enzyme will result in X-linked ichthyosis.

hy·drox·y·stil·bam·i·dine is·e·thi·o·nate (hī-drok′sē-stil-bam′i-dēn). An antifungal and antiprotozoan agent used in the treatment of the nonprogressive cutaneous form of blastomycosis.

hy·drox·y·to·lu·ic ac·id (hī-drok′sē-tō-loo′ik). SYN mandelic acid.

5-hy·drox·y·tryp·ta·mine (5-HT) (hī-drok-sē-trip′tă-mēn). SYN serotonin.

hy·drox·y·tryp·to·phan de·car·box·yl·ase (hī-drok-sē-trip′tō-fan). SYN aromatic D-amino acid decarboxylase.

3-hy·drox·y·ty·ra·mine (hī-drok-sē-tī′ră-mēn). SYN dopamine.

hy·drox·y·u·rea (hī-drok′sē-ū-rē′ă). An oral antineoplastic agent that inhibits DNA synthesis; used in the treatment of a variety of malignancies including melanoma, chronic myelocytic leukemia, and carcinoma of the ovary. SYN hydroxycarbamide.

hy·drox·y·zine (hī-drok′si-zēn). A mild sedative and minor tranquilizer used in neuroses; available as the hydrochloride and pamoate. Often used to prevent nausea and to enhance the effects of narcotics.

Hy·dro·zoa (hī-drō-zō′ă). A class of coelenterates or jellyfishes, including *Hydra*, a freshwater polyp, *Physalia*, the "Portuguese man-of-war," *Millepora*, a stinging coral, and the sea wasps, *Chironex heckeri* and *Chiropsalmus quadrigatus*, whose stings can cause severe wheals, pain, and skin necrosis, and occasionally rapid death from respiratory and cardiac depression. [hydro- + G. *zōon*, animal]

hy·giei·ol·o·gy (hī-jē-yol′ō-jē). The science of hygiene and sanitation, and the practice thereof. [G. *hygieia*, health, + *-logia*]

hy·gie·ist (hī′jē-ist). SYN hygienist. [G. *hygieia*, health]

hy·giene (hi′jēn). **1.** The science of health and its maintenance. **2.** Cleanliness that promotes health and well being, especially of a personal nature. [G. *hygieinos*, healthful, fr. *hygiēs*, healthy]

criminal h., obsolete term for the branch of mental h. or penology devoted to the study of the causes and prevention of criminality and the treatment of criminals.

industrial h., practices adopted by an industrial concern to minimize occupation-related disease and/or injury.

mental h., the science and practice of maintaining and restoring mental health; a branch of early twentieth century psychiatry that has become an interdisciplinary field including subspecialties in psychology, nursing, social work, law, and other professions.

oral h., the cleaning of the mouth by means of brushing, flossing, irrigating, massaging, or the use of other devices. SEE ALSO oral *physiotherapy*.

hy·gien·ic (hī-jen′ik, hī-jē-en′ik). Healthful; relating to hygiene; tending to maintain health.

hy·gien·ist (hī-jē′nist, hī′jē-en-ist). One who is skilled in the science of health and its maintenance. SYN hygieist.

dental h., a licensed, professional auxiliary in dentistry who is both an oral health educator and clinician, and who uses preventive, therapeutic, and educational methods for the control of oral diseases.

△**hygr-.** SEE hygro-.

hy·gric (hī′grik). Relating to moisture. [G. *hygros*, moist]

hy·gric ac·id. *N*-Methylproline, the methylbetaine of which is stachydrine.

△**hygro-, hygr-.** Moisture, humidity; opposite of xero-. [G. *hygros*, moist]

hy·gro·ma (hī-grō′mă). A cystic swelling containing a serous fluid, such as housemaid's knee, etc. SYN hydroma. [hygro- + G. *-oma*, tumor]

h. axilla′re, h. of the axillary region.

cervical h., a benign cystic overgrowth of lymphatics of the neck, present at birth, which may form a large tumor-like mass. SYN h. colli cysticum.

h. col′li cys′ticum, SYN cervical h.

cystic h., fetal malformation of fluid accumulations, usually around the neck and shoulders; may be simple or complex; often associated with Turner syndrome.

subdural h., accumulation in the subdural space of proteinaceous fluid, usually derived from serum, or of cerebrospinal fluid due to a tear in the arachnoid membrane.

hy·grom·e·ter (hī-grom′ĕ-ter). Any device for measuring the water vapor in the atmosphere, usually indicating relative humidity directly. [hygro- + G. *metron*, measure]

hy·grom·e·try (hī-grom′ĕ-trē). SYN psychrometry.

hy·gro·pho·bia (hī-grō-fō′bē-ă). Morbid fear of dampness or moisture. [hygro- + G. *phobos*, fear]

hy·gro·scop·ic (hī-grō-skop′ik). Denoting a substance capable of readily absorbing and retaining moisture; e.g., NaOH, $CaCl_2$.

hy·gro·sto·mia (hī′grō-stō′mē-ă). SYN sialorrhea. [hygro- + G. *stoma*, mouth]

Hyl Symbol for hydroxylysine or hydroxylysyl (5Hyl specifically refers to 5-hydroxylysine).

5Hyl Abbreviation for 5-hydroxylysine.

hy·la (hī′lă). A lateral extension of the cerebral (or sylvian) aqueduct. [G. *hylē*, wood]

hy·le·pho·bia (hī-lĕ-fō′bē-ă). Morbid fear of forests. [G. *hylē*, forest, + *phobos*, fear]

hy·men (hī′men) [TA]. A thin membranous fold highly variable in appearance which partly occludes the ostium of the vagina prior to its rupture (which may occur for a variety of reasons). It is frequently absent (even in virgins) although remnants are commonly present as hymenal caruncula tags. [G. *hymēn*, membrane]

h. bifenestra′tus, h. bifo′ris, a h. in which there are two openings separated by a wide septum. Cf. septate h.

cribriform h., a h. with a number of small perforations.

denticulate h., a h. with markedly serrated edges.

imperforate h., a h. in which there is no opening, the membrane completely occluding the vagina.

infundibuliform h., a projecting, funnel-shaped h. with a central opening with sloping edges.

h. sculpta′tus, a h. with markedly uneven and ragged edges.

septate h., a h. in which there are two openings separated by a narrow band of tissue. Cf. h. bifenestratus.

h. subsep′tus, a h. in which the opening is partly closed by a septum.

vertical h., a h. in which the opening is perpendicular.

hy·men·al (hī′men-ăl). Relating to the hymen.

hy·me·nec·to·my (hī-me-nek′tō-mē). Excision of the hymen. [G. *hymēn*, membrane, + *ektomē*, excision]

hy·me·ni·tis (hī-me-nī′tis). Inflammation of the hymen.

hy·men·oid (hī′men-oyd). **1.** SYN membranous. **2.** Resembling the hymen.

hy·me·no·le·pi·a·sis (hī′me-nō-lĕ-pī′ă-sis). Illness produced by infection with tapeworms of the genus *Hymenolepis*.

hy·me·no·lep·i·did (hī′men-ō-lep′i-did). Common name for tapeworms of the family Hymenolepididae.

Hy·men·o·lep·i·di·dae (hī′men-ō-lep′i-did-ē). A family of tapeworms (order Cyclophyllidea) that includes the medically important genus *Hymenolepis*. [G. *hymēn*, membrane, + *lepis*, rind]

Hy·me·nol·e·pis (hī-me-nol′ĕ-pis). The largest genus (family Hymenolepididae) of tapeworms in the order Cyclophyllidea; especially common parasites of rodents, shrews, and aquatic birds. [G. *hymēn*, membrane, + *lepis*, rind]

H. diminu′ta, a tapeworm species of rats and mice, rarely found in man; its cysticercoid larvae are harbored by beetles, fleas, caterpillars, and other insects.

H. lanceola′ta, a tapeworm of aquatic birds, rarely found in humans.

H. na′na, the dwarf or dwarf mouse tapeworm; a small tapeworm of man, sometimes found in great numbers in the intestine; the cysticercoid can develop by two pathways: in the final host, with the egg from one human directly infective to another human host, in which both larval and adult stages occur, or through two hosts, an insect (or crustacean) intermediate and a vertebrate final host, the obligate two-host cycle of most cyclophylidean cestodes; in addition, *H. nana* can internally reinfect the same human or rodent host, producing a massive reinfection.

H. na′na, var. *frater′na,* a race, strain, or subspecies of *H. nana* adapted to mice, although infectivity to humans may remain; the

Hy

human form, *H. nana*, presumably is derived from the rodent strain.

hy·me·nol·o·gy (hī-mĕ-nol′ō-jē). The branch of anatomy and physiology concerned with the membranes of the body. [G. *hymēn*, membrane, + *logos*, study]

Hy·me·nop·tera (hī-me-nop′ter-ă). An order of insects, including bees, wasps, and ants, characterized by locked pairs of membranous wings and high development of social or colonial behavior. [G. *hymēn*, membrane, + *pteron*, wing]

hy·me·nor·rha·phy (hī-me-nōr′ă-fē). Obsolete procedure of suturing the hymen in order to close the vagina. [G. *hymēn*, membrane, + *raphē*, a suture]

hy·men·ot·o·my (hī-me-not′ō-mē). Surgical division of a hymen. [G. *hymēn*, membrane, + *tomē*, incision]

Hynes, Wilfred, British plastic surgeon, *1903.

△**hyo-.** U-shaped, hyoid. [G. *hyoeides*, shaped like the letter upsilon, υ]

hy·o·ep·i·glot·tic (hī′ō-ep-i-glot′ik). Relating to the hyoid bone and the epiglottis; denoting the elastic h. ligament connecting the two structures. SYN hyoepiglottidean.

hy·o·ep·i·glot·tid·e·an (hī′ō-ep-i-glo-tid′ē-an). SYN hyoepiglottic.

hy·o·glos·sal (hī′ō-glos′ăl). Relating to the hyoid bone and the tongue. SYN glossohyal.

hy·o·glos·sus (hī′ō-glos′ŭs). SYN hyoglossus (*muscle*).

hy·oid (hī′oyd). U-shaped or V-shaped; denoting the hyoid *bone* and the hyoid *apparatus*. [G. *hyoeidēs*, shaped like the letter upsilon, υ]

hy·o·pha·ryn·ge·us (hī′ō-far′in-jē′ŭs). SEE middle constrictor (*muscle*) of pharynx.

hy·o·scine (hī′ō-sēn). SYN scopolamine.

   h. hydrobromide, SYN *scopolamine* hydrobromide.

hy·o·scy·a·mine (hī-ō-sī′ă-mēn). An alkaloid found in hyoscyamus, belladonna, duboisine, and stramonium; the levorotatory component of the racemic mixture, atropine; used as an antispasmodic, analgesic, and sedative; h. hydrobromide is used for the same purposes. SYN daturine.

   h. sulfate, an antispasmodic, hypnotic, and sedative, also used in parkinsonism to relieve tremor, rigidity, and excessive salivation.

dl-**hy·o·scy·a·mine.** SYN atropine.

hy·o·scy·a·mus (hī-ō-sī′ă-mŭs). The leaves and flowering tops of *Hyoscyamus niger* (family Solanaceae); it contains hyoscyamine and hyoscine (scopolamine); an anticholinergic and antispasmodic. SYN henbane. [G. *hyoskyamos*, henbane or hog's bean, fr. *hys*, gen. *hyos*, a hog, + *kyamos*, a bean]

hy·o·thy·roid (hī′ō-thī′royd). SEE thyrohyoid *membrane*.

Hyp Abbreviation for hypoxanthine; hydroxyproline (3Hyp and 4Hyp specifically refer to 3-hydroxyproline and 4-hydroxyproline, respectively).

3Hyp Abbreviation for 3-hydroxyproline.

4Hyp Abbreviation for 4-hydroxyproline.

△**hyp-.** Variation of the prefix hypo-, often used before a vowel. Cf. sub-.

hyp·a·cu·sia (hī′pă-koo′zē-ă, hip′ă-). SYN hypacusis.

hyp·a·cu·sis (hī′pă-koo′sis, hip′ă-). Hearing impairment of a conductive or sensorineural nature. SYN hypacusia, hypoacusis. [hypo- + G. *akousis*, hearing]

hyp·al·bu·mi·ne·mia (hī′pal-bū-mi-nē′mē-ă, hip′al-). SYN hypoalbuminemia. [G. *hypo*, under, + albuminemia]

hyp·al·ge·sia (hī′pal-jē′zē-ă, hīp′al-). Decreased sensibility to pain. SYN hypoalgesia. [G. *hypo*, under, + *algēsis*, sense of pain]

hyp·al·ge·sic, hyp·al·get·ic (hī′pal-jē′sik, hip′al-; -jet′ik). Relating to hypalgesia; having diminished sensitiveness to pain.

hyp·am·ni·on, hyp·am·ni·os (hī-pam′nē-on, -nē-os) SYN oligohydramnios.

hyp·an·a·ki·ne·sia, hyp·an·a·ki·ne·sis (hī-pan′ă-ki-nē′sē-ă, -kin-ē′sis). Diminution in the normal gastric or intestinal movements. [G. *hypo*, under, + *anakinēsis*, a to-and-fro movement]

hyp·ar·te·ri·al (hī′par-tēr′ē-ăl, hip′ar-). Below or beneath an artery. [G. *hypo*, beneath, + *artēria*, artery]

hyp·ax·i·al (hī-pak′sē-ăl, hip-ak′). Below any axis, such as the spinal axis or the axis of a limb. SEE hypomere. [G. *hypo*, beneath, + axis]

hyp·az·o·tu·ria (hī′paz-ō-too′rē-ă). SYN hypoazoturia.

hyp·en·ceph·a·lon (hī′pen-sef′ă-lon). The midbrain, pons, and medulla. [G. *hypo*, under, + *enkephalos*, brain]

hyp·en·gy·o·pho·bia (hī-pen′gī-ō-fō′bē-ă). Morbid fear of responsibility. [G. *hypengyos*, responsible, + *phobos*, fear]

△**hyper-.** Excessive, above normal; opposite of hypo-. [G. *hyper*, above, over]

hy·per·ab·duc·tion. SYN superabduction.

hy·per·a·cid·i·ty (hī′per-a-sid′i-tē). An abnormally high degree of acidity, as of the gastric juice.

hy·per·ac·tiv·i·ty (hī′per-ak-tiv′i-tē). **1.** SYN superactivity. **2.** General restlessness or excessive movement such as that characterizing children with attention deficit disorder or hyperkinesis.

hy·per·a·cu·sis, hy·per·a·cu·sia (hī′per-ă-koo′sis, -koo′sē-ă). Abnormal hearing sensitivity. SYN auditory hyperesthesia. [hyper- + G. *akousis*, a hearing]

hy·per·ad·e·no·sis (hī′per-ad-ĕ-nō′sis). Glandular enlargement, especially of the lymphatic glands. [hyper- + G. *adēn*, gland, + *-ōsis*, condition]

hy·per·ad·i·po·sis, hy·per·ad·i·pos·i·ty (hī′per-ad-i-pō′sis, -pos′i-tē). An extreme degree of adiposis or fatness.

hy·per·ad·re·nal·cor·ti·cal·ism (hī′per-ă-drē′năl-kōr′ti-kăl-izm). SYN hypercorticoidism.

hy·per·a·dre·no·cor·ti·cal·ism (hī′per-ă-drē′nō-kōr′ti-kăl-izm). SYN hypercorticoidism.

hy·per·al·a·nine·mia (hī′per-al′ă-nēn-ē′mē-ă). Elevated levels of alanine in the serum.

hy·per-β-al·a·nine·mia (hī′per-bā′ta-al′ă-nen-ē′mē-a). Elevated levels of β-alanine in the serum; believed to be due to a deficiency of β-alanine:pyruvate aminotransferase; leads to impaired CNS function.

hy·per·al·do·ste·ron·ism (hī′per-al-dos′ter-on-izm). SYN aldosteronism.

hy·per·al·ge·sia (hī-per-al-jē′zē-ă). Extreme sensitivity to painful stimuli. [hyper- + G. *algos*, pain]

hy·per·al·ge·sic, hy·per·al·get·ic (hī′per-al-jē′sik, -jet′ik). Relating to hyperalgesia.

hy·per·al·i·men·ta·tion (hī′per-al′i-men-tā′shŭn). Administration or consumption of nutrients beyond minimum normal requirements, in an attempt to replace nutritional deficiencies. SYN superalimentation, suralimentation.

   enteral h., h. by the administration of elemental nutrients via a catheter placed within the intestinal tract; usually used in patients with at least a portion of functional small intestine.

   parenteral h., h. of nutrients via central venous catheter in patients who cannot consume adequate nutrition by the enteral route.

hy·per·al·lan·to·in·u·ria (hī′per-ă-lan′tō-i-noo′rē-ă). Increased excretion of allantoin in the urine.

hy·per·al·pha·lip·o·pro·tei·ne·mia (hi′per-ăl′fa-lip-ō-prō′tēn-ē′mē-ă). An inherited defect that results in elevated levels of high-density lipoproteins in the serum.

hy·per·a·mi·no·ac·i·du·ria (hī′per-am′i-nō-as-i-doo′rē-ă). SYN aminoaciduria.

hy·per-β-ami·no·iso·bu·ty·ric ac·i·du·ria. Elevated levels of β-aminoisobutyric acid in the urine; believed to be due to a deficiency of liver β-aminoisobutyrate:pyruvate aminotransferase.

hy·per·am·mo·ne·mia (hī′per-am-ō-nē′mē-ă). SYN ammonemia.

hy·per·am·y·la·se·mia (hī′per-am′i-lā-sē′mē-ă). Elevated serum amylase, usually seen as one of the manifestations of acute pancreatitis. [hyper- + amylase, + G. *haima*, blood]

hy·per·an·a·ci·ne·sia, hy·per·an·a·ci·ne·sis (hī′per-an-ă-si-nē′zē-ă, -nē′sis). SYN hyperanakinesia.

hy·per·an·a·ki·ne·sia, hy·per·an·a·ki·ne·sis (hī′per-an-ă-ki-nē′

zē-ă, -ki-nē′sis). Excessive to-and-fro movement, e.g., of the stomach or intestine. SYN hyperanacinesia, hyperanacinesis. [hyper- + G. *anakinēsis,* to-and-fro movement]

hy·per·a·phia (hī′per-ā′fē-ă). Extreme sensitivity to touch. SYN oxyaphia, tactile hyperesthesia. [hyper- + G. *haphē,* touch]

hy·per·aph·ic (hī-per-af′ik). Marked by hyperaphia.

hy·per·ar·gi·ni·ne·mia (hī′per-ar-jen-in-ē-mē-a). Elevated levels of arginine in the blood plasma; usually associated with a deficiency of arginase.

hy·per·bar·ic (hī-per-bar′ik). **1.** Pertaining to pressure of ambient gases greater than 1 atmosphere. **2.** Concerning solutions, more dense than the diluent or medium; e.g., in spinal anesthesia, a h. solution has a density greater than that of spinal fluid. [hyper- + G. *baros,* weight]

hy·per·bar·ism (hī-per-bar′izm). Disturbances in the body resulting from the pressure of ambient gases at greater than 1 atmosphere; e.g., nitrogen narcosis, oxygen toxicity, bends. [hyper- + G. *baros,* weight]

hy·per·be·ta·lip·o·pro·tein·e·mia (hī′per-bet-ă-lip′ō-prō-tē-nē′mē-ă). Enhanced concentration of β-lipoproteins in the blood.

familial h., SEE type II familial *hyperlipoproteinemia.*

familial h. and hyperprebetalipoproteinemia, SYN type III familial *hyperlipoproteinemia.*

hy·per·bil·i·ru·bi·ne·mia (hī′per-bil′i-roo-bi-nē′mē-ă). An abnormally large amount of bilirubin in the circulating blood, resulting in clinically apparent icterus or jaundice when the concentration is sufficient.

neonatal h., serum bilirubin greater than 12.9 mg/dl (220 μol/L) or rising at a rate greater than 5 mg/dl per day; also applied to a nonphysiologic pattern of h., i.e., jaundice in the first 24 hours of life or extending beyond the first week of life in term infants.

hy·per·brach·y·ceph·a·ly (hī′per-brak-ē-sef′ă-lē). An extreme degree of brachycephaly, with a cephalic index of over 85. [hyper- + G. *brachys,* short, + *kephalē,* head]

hy·per·cal·ce·mia (hī′per-kal-sē′mē-ă). An abnormally high concentration of calcium compounds in the circulating blood; commonly used to indicate an elevated concentration of calcium ions in the blood.

humoral h. of benignancy, h. induced by parathyroid hormone-like protein of benign tumor.

idiopathic h. of infants, persistent h. of unknown cause in very young children, associated with osteosclerosis, renal insufficiency, and sometimes hypertension; also may be associated with supravalvular aortic stenosis, elfin facies, and mental retardation.

hy·per·cal·ci·nu·ria (hī′per-kal-si-noo′rē-ă). SYN hypercalciuria.

hy·per·cal·ci·u·ria (hī′per-kal-sē-yu′rē-ă). Excretion of abnormally large amounts of calcium in the urine, as in hyperparathyroidism and types of hereditary hypophosphatemic rickets. SYN calcinuric diabetes, hypercalcinuria, hypercalcuria.

hy·per·cal·cu·ria (hī′per-kal-kū′rē-ă). SYN hypercalciuria.

hy·per·cap·nia (hī-per-kap′nē-ă). Abnormally increased arterial carbon dioxide tension. SYN hypercarbia. [hyper- + G. *kapnos,* smoke, vapor]

hy·per·car·bia (hī-per-kar′bē-ă). SYN hypercapnia.

hy·per·car·dia (hī-per-kar′dē-ă). Hypertrophy of the heart. [hyper- + G. *kardia,* heart]

hy·per·cat·a·bol·ic (hī′per-kat-ă-bol′ik). Pertaining to hypercatabolism.

hy·per·cat·ab·o·lism (hī′per-kă-tab′ō-lizm). Excessive metabolic breakdown of a specific substance or of body tissue in general, leading to weight loss and wasting.

hy·per·ca·thar·sis (hī′per-kă-thar′sis). Excessive and frequent defecation. [hyper- + G. *katharsis,* a cleansing]

hy·per·ca·thex·is (hī′per-kă-thek′sis). In psychoanalysis, an individual's excessive investment of libido or interest in an object, person, or idea. [hyper- + G. *kathexis,* a holding in, retention]

hy·per·ce·men·to·sis (hī′per-sē-men-tō′sis). Excessive deposition of secondary cementum on the root of a tooth, which may be caused by localized trauma or inflammation, excessive tooth eruption, or osteitis deformans, or may occur idiopathically. SYN cementum hyperplasia. [hyper- + L. *caementum,* a rough quarry stone, + *-osis,* condition]

hy·per·chlor·e·mia (hī′per-klō-rē′mē-ă). An abnormally large amount of chloride ions in the circulating blood. SYN chloremia (2).

hy·per·chlor·hy·dria (hī′per-klōr-hī′drē-ă). Presence of an excessive amount of hydrochloric acid in the stomach. SYN chlorhydria, hyperhydrochloria. [hyper- + chlorhydric (acid)]

hy·per·chlor·u·ria (hī′per-klōr-ū′rē-ă). Increased excretion of chloride ions in the urine.

hy

differential diagnosis of hypercalcemia

malignancy	familial hypocalciuric hypercalcemia

with skeletal involvement
  direct tumor erosion of the bone
  local tumor production of bone-resorbing agents
    (i.e., prostaglandin E_2)
	idiopathic hypercalcemia of infancy

	vitamin overdose
	  vitamin D
	  vitamin A

no skeletal involvement (humoral hypercalcemia of malignancy)
  parathyroid hormone–related protein
  growth factor(s) (tumor growth factor, epidermal growth factor,
    platelet-derived growth factor)
	granulomatous disease
	  sarcoidosis
	  tuberculosis
	  berylliosis
	  coccidioidomycosis

hematologic malignancy
  cytokinase (interleukin-1, tumor necrosis factor, lymphotoxin)
  1,25-dihydroxyvitamin D (lymphoma)
  coexistent primary hyperparathyroidism
	renal failure
	  chronic renal failure
	  acute renal failure—diuretic phase
	  post renal transplantation

primary hyperparathyroidism
  adenoma, hyperplasia, carcinoma
  familial
  multiple endocrine neoplasia type I with pituitary and pancreatic tumors
  multiple endocrine neoplasia type II with medullary thyroid carcinoma
    and pheochromocytoma
	chlorothiazide diuretics

	lithium therapy
	milk-alkali syndrome

other endocrine disorders
  hyperthyroidism
  hypothyroidism
  acromegaly
  acute adrenal insufficiency
  pheochromocytoma
	immobilization

	increased serum proteins
	  hemoconcentration
	  hyperglobulinemia due to multiple myeloma

hy·per·cho·les·ter·e·mia (hī′per-kō-les′ter-ē′mē-ă). SYN hypercholesterolemia.

hy·per·cho·les·ter·in·e·mia (hī′per-kō-les′ter-i-nē′mē-ă). SYN hypercholesterolemia.

hy·per·cho·les·ter·ol·e·mia (hī′per-kō-les′ter-ol-ē′mē-ă). The presence of an abnormally large amount of cholesterol in the blood. SYN hypercholesteremia, hypercholesterinemia.

familial h., SEE type II familial *hyperlipoproteinemia.*

familial h. with hyperlipemia, SYN type III familial *hyperlipoproteinemia.*

hy·per·cho·les·ter·o·lia (hī′per-kō-les′ter-ō′lē-ă). The presence of an abnormally large quantity of cholesterol in the bile.

hy·per·cho·lia (hī-per-kō′lē-ă). A condition in which an abnormally large amount of bile is formed in the liver. [hyper- + G. *cholē,* bile]

hy·per·chro·maf·fin·ism (hī′per-krō′maf-in-izm). Presence of a functioning pheochromocytoma.

hy·per·chro·ma·sia (hī′per-krō-mā′zē-ă). SYN hyperchromatism.

hy·per·chro·mat·ic (hī′per-krō-mat′ik). **1.** Abnormally highly colored, excessively stained, or overpigmented. SYN hyperchromic (1). **2.** Showing increased chromatin. [hyper- + G. *chrōma,* color]

hy·per·chro·ma·tism (hī′per-krō′mă-tizm). **1.** Excessive pigmentation. **2.** Increased staining capacity, especially of cell nuclei for hematoxylin. **3.** An increase in chromatin in cell nuclei. SYN hyperchromasia, hyperchromia. [hyper- + G. *chrōma,* color]

hy·per·chro·mia (hī-per-krō′mē-ă). SYN hyperchromatism.

macrocytic h., hyperchromatic macrocythemia; a misnomer inasmuch as the red blood cells are larger than normal, the total amount of hemoglobin per cell is increased, but the percentage of hemoglobin per cell is usually in the normochromic range.

hy·per·chro·mic (hī-per-krōm′ik). **1.** SYN hyperchromatic (1). **2.** Denoting increased light absorption. **3.** Denoting more highly colored than normal. **4.** Describing erythrocytes that contain, or appear to contain, more hemoglobin than normal.

hy·per·chy·lia (hī-per-kī′lē-ă). Excessive secretion of gastric juice. [hyper- + G. *chylos,* juice]

hy·per·chy·lo·mi·cro·ne·mia (hī′per-kī′lō-mī-krō-nē′mē-ă). Increased plasma concentrations of chylomicrons.

familial h., SYN type I familial *hyperlipoproteinemia.*

familial h. with hyperprebetalipoproteinemia, SYN type V familial *hyperlipoproteinemia.*

hy·per·ci·ne·sis, hy·per·ci·ne·sia (hī′per-si-nē′sis, -si-nē′zē-ă). SYN hyperkinesis.

hy·per·co·ag·u·la·bil·i·ty (hī′per-kō-ag′oo-lă-bil-i-tē). Abnormally increased coagulability.

hy·per·co·ag·u·la·ble (hī′-per-kō-ag′oo-lă-bl). Characterized by abnormally increased coagulation.

hy·per·cor·ti·coid·ism (hī′per-kōr′ti-koyd-izm). Excessive secretion of one or more steroid hormones of the adrenal cortex; sometimes used also to designate the state produced by therapeutic administration of large quantities of steroids having glucocorticoid activity, e.g., hydrocortisone. SEE ALSO Cushing *syndrome.* SYN adrenalism, hyperadrenalcorticalism, hyperadrenocorticalism.

hy·per·cor·ti·sol·ism (hī′per-kōr′ti-sol-izm). SEE hyperadrenocorticalism.

hy·per·cry·al·ge·sia (hī′per-krī-al-jē′zē-ă). SYN hypercryesthesia. [hyper- + G. *kryos,* cold, + *algēsis,* the sense of pain]

hy·per·cry·es·the·sia (hī′per-krī-es-thē′zē-ă). Extreme sensibility to cold. SYN hypercryalgesia. [hyper- + G. *kryos,* cold, + *aisthēsis,* sensation]

hy·per·cu·pre·mia (hī′per-koo-prē′mē-ă). An abnormally high level of plasma copper. [hyper- + L. *cuprum,* copper, + G. *haima,* blood]

hy·per·cy·a·not·ic (hī′per-sī-ă-not′ik). Marked by extreme cyanosis.

hy·per·cy·e·sis, hy·per·cy·e·sia (hī′per-sī-ē′sis, -ē′zē-ă). SYN superfetation. [hyper- + G. *kyēsis,* pregnancy]

hy·per·cy·the·mia (hī′per-sī-thē′mē-ă). The presence of an abnormally high number of red blood cells in the circulating blood.

SYN hypererythrocythemia. [hyper- + G. *kytos,* cell, + *haima,* blood]

hy·per·cy·to·chro·mia (hī′per-sī-tō-krō′mē-ă). Increased intensity of staining of a cell, especially of blood cells. [hyper- + G. *kytos,* cell, + *chrōma,* color]

hy·per·cy·to·sis (hī′per-sī-tō′sis). Obsolete term for any condition in which there is an abnormal increase in the number of cells in the circulating blood or the tissues; frequently used synonymously with leukocytosis.

hy·per·di·crot·ic (hī′per-dī-krot′ik). Pronouncedly dicrotic. SYN superdicrotic.

hy·per·di·cro·tism (hī-per-dik′rō-tizm, -dī′krō-tizm). Extreme dicrotism.

hy·per·dip·loid (hī′per-dip′loid). Having a chromosome number greater than the diploid number.

hy·per·dip·sia (hī-per-dip′sē-ă). Intense thirst that is relatively temporary. [hyper- + G. *dipsa,* thirst]

hy·per·dis·ten·tion (hī′per-dis-ten′shŭn). Extreme distention. SYN superdistention.

hy·per·ech·o·ic (hī′per-ĕ-kō′ik). **1.** In ultrasonography, pertaining to material that produces echoes of higher amplitude or density than the surrounding medium. **2.** Denoting a region in an ultrasound image in which the echoes are stronger than normal or than surrounding structures.

hyperekplexia (hī′per-ek-pleks′ē-ă) [MIM#149400]. A hereditary disorder in which there are pathologic startle responses, i.e., protective reactions to unanticipated, potentially threatening, stimuli of any type, particularly auditory; the stimuli induce often widespread and violent sudden contractions of the head, neck, spinal, and sometimes limb musculature, resulting in involuntary shouting, jerking, jumping, and falling; autosomal dominant and recessive inheritance forms, with the responsible gene localized to chromosome 5q; probably the result of lack of inhibitory neurotransmitters, glycine, or GABA. SYN kok disease, startle disease. [hyper- + G. *ekplēxia,* sudden shock, fr. *ekplēssō,* to startle]

hy·per·em·e·sis (hī-per-em′ĕ-sis). Excessive vomiting. [hyper- + G. *emesis,* vomiting]

h. gravida′rum, pernicious vomiting in pregnancy.

h. lacten′tium, vomiting by nursing infants with pyloric stenosis.

hy·per·e·met·ic (hī′per-ĕ-met′ik). Marked by excessive vomiting.

hy·per·e·mia (hī-per-ē′mē-ă). The presence of an increased amount of bloodflow in a part or organ. SEE ALSO congestion. [hyper- + G. *haima,* blood]

active h., h. due to an increased afflux of arterial blood into dilated capillaries. SYN arterial h., fluxionary h.

arterial h., SYN active h.

Bier h., obsolete term for h. produced by Bier *method* (2).

collateral h., increased blood flow through abundant collateral channels when the circulation through the main artery to a part is arrested.

fluxionary h., SYN active h.

passive h., h. due to an obstruction in the flow of blood from the affected part, the venous radicles becoming distended. SYN venous h.

peristatic h., SYN peristasis.

reactive h., h. following the arrest and subsequent restoration of the blood supply to a part.

venous h., SYN passive h.

hy·per·e·mic (hī-per-ē′mik). Denoting hyperemia.

hy·per·en·ceph·a·ly (hī′per-en-sef′ă-lē). A fetal developmental deficiency of the vault of the cranium, exposing the poorly formed brain. [hyper- + G. *enkephalos,* brain]

hy·per·e·o·sin·o·phil·ia (hī′per-ē-ō-sin-ō-fil′ē-ă). A greater degree of abnormal increase in the number of eosinophilic granulocytes in the circulating blood or the tissues; e.g., in diseases where the degree of eosinophilia usually ranges from 10–30%, an increase to 50 or 60% (or more) might be regarded as h.

hy·per·er·gia (hī′per-er′jē-ă). An allergic hypersensitivity. SYN hypergia.

hy·per·er·gic (hī-per-er′jik). Relating to hyperergia. SYN hypergic.

hy·per·e·ryth·ro·cy·the·mia (hī′per-ē-rith′rō-sī-thē′mē-ă). SYN hypercythemia.

hy·per·es·o·pho·ria (hī′per-es-ō-fō′rē-ă). A tendency of one eye to deviate upward and inward, prevented by binocular vision. [hyper- + G. *esō*, inward, + *phora*, movement]

hy·per·es·the·sia (hī′per-es-thē′zē-ă). Abnormal acuteness of sensitivity to touch, pain, or other sensory stimuli. [hyper- + G. *aisthēsis*, sensation]

auditory h., SYN hyperacusis.

cervical h., the hypersensitivity of teeth in the cervical area due to exposure of the dentin.

gustatory h., SYN hypergeusia.

muscular h., sensitiveness of the muscles to pressure.

olfactory h., h. olfacto′ria, SYN hyperosmia.

h. op′tica, extreme sensitivity of the eyes to light. SEE photophobia, photosensitivity.

tactile h., SYN hyperaphia.

hy·per·es·thet·ic (hī′per-es-thet′ik). Marked by hyperesthesia.

hy·per·eu·ry·pro·so·pic (hī′per-ū′ri-prō-sop′ik). Pertaining to or characterized by a very low and wide face. [hyper- + G. *eurys*, wide, + *prosōpon*, face]

hy·per·ex·o·pho·ria (hī′per-ek-sō-fō′rē-ă). A tendency of one eye to deviate upward and outward, prevented by binocular vision. [hyper- + G. *exō*, outward, + *phora*, movement]

hy·per·ex·ten·sion (hī′per-eks-ten′shŭn). Extension of a limb or part beyond the normal limit. SYN overextension, superextension.

hy·per·fer·re·mia (hī′per-fer-ē′mē-ă). High serum iron level; found in hemochromatosis.

hy·per·fi·brin·o·ge·ne·mia (hī′per-fī-brin′ō-jĕ-nē′ē-ă). An increased level of fibrinogen in the blood. SYN fibrinogenemia.

hy·per·fi·bri·nol·y·sis (hī′per-fī-brin-ol′i-sis). Markedly increased fibrinolysis, as in subdural hematomas.

hy·per·flex·ion (hī-per-flek′shŭn). Flexion of a limb or part beyond the normal limit. SYN superflexion.

hy·per·fruc·to·se·mia (hī′per-frŭk-tō-sē-mē-ă). Elevated serum fructose levels.

hy·per·gal·ac·to·sis (hī′per-ga-lak-tō′sis). Excessive secretion of milk. [hyper- + G. *gala*, milk, + *-ōsis*, condition]

hy·per·gam·ma·glob·u·lin·e·mia (hī′per-gam-ă-glob′ū-li-li-nē′mē-ă). An increased amount of the γ-globulins in the plasma, such as that frequently observed in chronic infectious diseases.

hy·per·gan·gli·on·o·sis (hī-per-ga′ng-glē-ō-nō′sis). SYN neuronal *hyperplasia*.

hy·per·gen·e·sis (hī-per-jen′ĕ-sis). Excessive development or redundant production of parts or organs of the body. [hyper- + G. *genesis*, production]

hy·per·ge·net·ic (hī-per-jĕ-net′ik). Relating to hypergenesis.

hy·per·gen·i·tal·ism (hī-per-jen′i-tăl-izm). Abnormal overdevelopment of genitalia.

hy·per·geu·sia (hī-per-goo′sē-ă, -joo′sē-ă). Abnormal acuteness of the sense of taste. SYN gustatory hyperesthesia. [hyper- + G. *geusis*, taste]

hy·per·gia (hī-per′jē-ă). SYN hyperergia.

hy·per·gic (hī-per′jik). SYN hyperergic.

hy·per·glan·du·lar (hī-per-glan′dyŭ-lăr). Characterized by overactivity or increased size of a gland.

hy·per·glob·u·lia, hy·per·glob·u·lism (hī′per-glob-ū′lē-ă, -glob′ū-lizm). Old term for polycythemia. [hyper- + L. *globulus*, globule]

hy·per·glob·u·lin·e·mia (hī′per-glob′ū-lin-ē′mē-ă). An abnormally high concentration of globulins in the circulating blood plasma.

hy·per·gly·ce·mia (hī′per-glī-sē′mē-ă). An abnormally high concentration of glucose in the circulating blood, seen especially in patients with diabetes mellitus. SYN hyperglycosemia. [hyper- + G. *glykys*, sweet, + *haima*, blood]

ketotic h., an inborn error of glycine metabolism characterized by lethargy, vomiting, convulsions, hypertonia, and difficulty breathing; milk protein and casein induce attacks; autosomal recessive inheritance.

nonketotic h., SYN hyperosmolar (hyperglycemic) nonketotic *coma*.

posthypoglycemic h., SYN Somogyi *phenomenon*.

hy·per·glyc·er·i·de·mia (hī′per-glis′er-i-dē′mē-ă). Elevated plasma concentration of glycerides.

endogenous h., type IV familial hyperlipoproteinemia or, more commonly, a nonfamilial sporadic variety.

exogenous h., persistent h. due to retarded rate of removal from plasma of chylomicrons of dietary origin; occurs in alcoholism, hypothyroidism, insulinopenic diabetes mellitus, types I and V hyperlipoproteinemia, and during acute pancreatitis.

hy·per·gly·ci·ne·mia (hī′per-glī-si-nē′mē-ă). Elevated plasma glycine concentration.

ketotic h., an inherited metabolic defect which results from a deficiency of propionyl Coenzyme A carboxylase, the enzyme that converts propionate to methylmalonate; the enzyme requires biotin as a cofactor; clinically, affected infants have overwhelming illness, with lethargy, metabolic acidosis with ketosis, hypotonia; coma and seizures typically develop with early death; propionic acid is markedly elevated in plasma and urine; there is also hyperammonemia, and elevated levels of other metabolites as well, including glycine, hence the original name for the syndrome. SYN methylmalonic acidemia, propionic acidemia.

nonketotic h. [MIM*238300], an inborn error of glycine metabolism, due to a deficiency of glycine dicarboxylase P protein (GCSP), a component of glycine cleavage system; characteristically overwhelming disease in the newborn period, with coma, seizures and death, or, less often, gradual onset with failure to thrive, focal seizures, and mental retardation; there is massive elevation of plasma glycine, with increased levels in cerebrospinal fluid and urine; plasma hyperosmolality, severe dehydration occur without ketoacidosis; autosomal recessive inheritance; caused by mutation in the GCSP gene on chromosome 9p.

hy·per·gly·ci·nu·ria (hī′per-glī-si-noo′rē-ă). Enhanced urinary excretion of glycine.

hy·per·gly·co·gen·ol·y·sis (hī′per-glī′kō-jĕ-nol′i-sis). Excessive glycogenolysis. [hyper- + glycogen + G. *lysis*, loosening]

hy·per·gly·cor·rha·chia (hī′per-glī-kō-rak′ē-ă). Excessive sugar in the cerebrospinal fluid. [hyper- + G. *glykys*, sweet, + *rhachis*, spine]

hy·per·gly·co·se·mia (hī′per-glī-kō-sē′mē-ă). SYN hyperglycemia.

hy·per·gly·co·su·ria (hī′per-glī-kō-soo′rē-ă). Persistent excretion of unusually large amounts of glucose in the urine; i.e., an extreme degree of glucosuria.

hy·per·gly·ox·yl·e·mia (hī′per-glī-ok′si-lē′mē-ă). Enhanced plasma (and possibly tissue) concentrations of glyoxylate; may develop during thiamine deficiency.

hy·per·gno·sis (hī-per-nō′sis). **1.** Projection of inner conflicts into the environment. **2.** Exaggerated perception, such as the expansion of an isolated thought. [hyper- + G. *gnōsis*, knowledge]

hy·per·go·nad·ism (hī-per-gō′nad-izm). A clinical state resulting from enhanced secretion of gonadal hormones.

hy·per·go·nad·o·tro·pic (hī′per-gō′nă-dō-trop′ik). Indicating an increased production or excretion of gonadotropic hormones.

hy·per·gran·u·lo·sis (hī′per-gran-ū-lō′sis). Increased thickness of the granular layer of the epidermis, associated with hyperkeratosis. [hyper- + (stratum) granulosum + *-osis*, condition]

hy·per·guan·i·di·ne·mia (hī′per-gwan′i-di-nē′mē-ă). A condition in which there is an abnormally large amount of guanidine in the circulating blood.

hy·per·gy·ne·cos·mia (hī′per-gī-nĕ-koz′mē-ă). Overdevelopment of secondary sex characteristics of the mature female or their precocious development in the young girl. [hyper- + G. *gyne*, woman, + *kosmeō*, to decorate]

hy·per·he·do·nia, hy·per·he·do·nism (hī′per-hē-dō′nē-ă, -hē′don-izm). The feeling of an abnormally great pleasure in any act or from any happening. [hyper- + G. *hēdonē*, pleasure]

hy

hy·per·he·mo·glo·bi·ne·mia (hī′per-hē′mō-glō-bi-nē′mmē-ă). An unusually large amount of hemoglobin in the circulating blood plasma; i.e., much more than that ordinarily observed in most examples of hemoglobinemia.

hy·per·hep·a·ri·ne·mia (hī′per-hep′ar-in-ē′mē-ă) [MIM* 144050]. Elevated plasma concentrations of heparin; believed to be the cause of a heritable bleeding tendency; probably autosomal dominant inheritance.

hy·per·hi·dro·sis (hī′per-hī-drō′sis). Excessive or profuse sweating. SYN polyhidrosis, sudorrhea. [hyper- + hidrosis]

gustatory h., excessive sweating of the lips, nose, and forehead after eating certain foods; it is physiologic in many persons, but sometimes occurs after parotid surgery or as a result of damage to the parasympathetic or sympathetic nerves of the head and neck.

hy·per·hy·dra·tion (hī′per-hī-drā′shŭn). Excess water content of the body; may result from the intravenous administration of unduly large amounts of glucose solution. SYN overhydration.

hy·per·hy·dro·chlo·ria (hī′per-hī-drō-klōr′ē-ă). SYN hyperchlorhydria.

hy·per·hy·dro·chlo·rid·i·a (hī′-per-hī′drō-chlōr-id-ē-ă). Excessive acid secretion by the stomach; associated with peptic ulcer disease. [hyper + hydrochloric, acid + -ia]

hy·per·hy·dro·pexy, hy·per·hy·dro·pex·is (hī-per-hī′drō-pek-sē, hī′per-hī-drō-pek′sis). Increased fixation of water in tissues. [hyper- + G. hydōr, water, + pēgnymi, to fasten]

hy·per·hy·drox·y·pro·line·mia (hī′per-hī-drok′sē-prō-lēn-ē-mē-a). SEE hydroxyprolinemia.

hy·per·im·i·do·di·pep·ti·du·ria (hī′per-im′i-dō-dī-pep′tīd-oor-ē-ă). Elevated levels of imidodipeptides (e.g., Xaa–Pro) in the urine; due to a deficiency of prolidase.

hy·per·im·mune (hī′per-im-mum′). Having large quantities of specific antibodies in the serum from repeated immunizations or infections.

hy·per·im·mu·ni·ty (hī′per-i-mu′-ni-tē). A high degree of immunity.

hy·per·im·mu·ni·za·tion (hī′per-im-oo-nī-zăshŭn). **1.** The induction of a heightened state of immunity by the administration of repeated doses of antigen, often used in allergy desensitization. **2.** Passively acquired immunity by the injection of hyperimmune gamma globulin.

hy·per·in·di·can·e·mia (hī′per-in′di-kan-ē′mē-ă). An unusually large amount of indican in the circulating blood; i.e., greater than that observed in most instances of indicanemia.

hy·per·in·fec·tion (hī′per-in-fek′shŭn). Infection by very large numbers of organisms as a result of immunologic deficiency. Cf. superinfection.

hyperinflation (hī-per-in-flā′shun). Overdistention of airways and alveoli, sometimes leading to emphysema, caused by obstructive lung disease; occurs reversibly with asthma, and can occur locally with aspiration of a foreign body with a subsequent ball-valve phenomenon. [hyper- + inflation]

hy·per·i·no·se·mia (hī′per-i′nō-sē′mē-ă, hī′per-in′ō-). A greatly increased quantity of fibrinogen in the circulating blood; under certain conditions, unusually large amounts of fibrin may be formed, thereby resulting in a greater degree of coagulability of the blood. SYN hyperinosis. [hyper- + G. is (in-), fiber, + haima, blood]

hy·per·i·no·sis (hī-per-i-nō′sis). SYN hyperinosemia.

hy·per·in·su·li·ne·mia (hī′per-in′soo-lin-ē′mē-ă). SYN hyperinsulinism.

hy·per·in·su·lin·ism (hī′per-in′soo-lin-izm). Increased levels of insulin in the plasma due to increased secretion of insulin by the beta cells of the pancreatic islets; decreased hepatic removal of insulin is a cause in some patients, although h. usually is associated with insulin resistance and is commonly found in obesity in association with varying degrees of hyperglycemia. SYN hyperinsulinemia.

alimentary h., elevated levels of insulin in the plasma following ingestion of meals by individuals with abnormally rapid gastric emptying (e.g., following gastroenterostomy or vagotomy); rapid glucose absorption leads to excessive insulin release which in turn can lead to a marked fall in blood glucose to hypoglycemic levels.

hy·per·in·vo·lu·tion (hī′per-in′vō-loo′shŭn). SYN superinvolution.

hy·per·i·so·ton·ic (hī′per-ī-sō-ton′ik). SYN hypertonic.

hy·per·ka·le·mia (hī′per-kă-lē′mē-ă). A greater than normal concentration of potassium ions in the circulating blood. SYN hyperkaliemia, hyperpotassemia. [hyper- + Mod. L. kalium, potash, + G. haima, blood]

hy·per·kal·i·e·mia (hī′per-kal-i-ē′mē-ă). SYN hyperkalemia.

hy·per·kal·u·re·sis (hī′per-kal-ū-rē′sis). Excessive urinary excretion of potassium. [hyper- + Mod. L. kalium, potassium, + G. oureō, to urinate]

hy·per·ker·a·tin·i·za·tion (hī′per-ker′at-i-ni-zā′shŭn). SYN hyperkeratosis.

hy·per·ker·a·to·sis (hī′per-ker-ă-tō′sis). Thickening of the horny layer of the epidermis or mucous membrane. SEE ALSO keratoderma, keratosis. SYN hyperkeratinization.

h. congen′ita, SYN ichthyosis vulgaris.

diffuse h. of palms and soles, an autosomal dominant disorder with onset in early infancy; characterized by hyperkeratotic, scaling plaques and often hyperhidrosis on the palms and soles. SYN Unna-Thost syndrome.

epidermolytic h. [MIM*144200], characterized by localized lesions, keratosis palmaris and plantaris, and elevated IgE, associated with hyperkeratosis, hypergranulosis, and reticular degeneration in the upper epidermis; autosomal dominant inheritance, caused by mutation in the epidermolytic palmoplantar keratoderma gene (EPPK) on chromosome 17q. Generalized epidermolytic h. is present in bullous congenital ichthyosiform erythroderma. SYN porcupine skin.

h. follicula′ris et parafollicula′ris, discrete and confluent horny follicular plugs on a crateriform base, often occurring on the arms and legs in diabetics with renal failure; possibly a severe form of perforating folliculitis. SEE ALSO perforating folliculitis. SYN Kyrle disease.

generalized epidermolytic h., SYN bullous congenital ichthyosiform erythroderma.

h. lenticula′ris per′stans [MIM*144150], small hyperkeratotic papules on the dorsa of the feet and legs and occasionally elsewhere, with pinpoint keratotic papules of the palms and soles; onset in the third and fourth decades; an autosomal dominant trait. SYN Flegel disease.

hy·per·ke·to·ne·mia (hī′per-kē′tō-nē′mē-ă). Elevated concentrations of ketone bodies in the blood.

hy·per·ke·ton·u·ria (hī′per-kē′tō-noo′rē-ă). Increased urinary excretion of ketonic compounds.

hy·per·ki·ne·mia (hī′per-ki-nē′mē-ă). Increased circulation rate; increased volume flow through the circulation; supernormal cardiac output. [hyper- + G. kineō, to move, + haima, blood]

hy·per·ki·ne·sis, hy·per·ki·ne·sia (hī′per-ki-nē′sis, -nē′zē-ă). **1.** Excessive motility. **2.** Excessive muscular activity. SYN hypercinesis, hypercinesia, supermotility. [hyper- + G. kinēsis, motion]

hy·per·ki·net·ic (hī′per-ki-net′ik). Pertaining to or characterized by hyperkinesia.

hy·per·lac·ta·tion (hī′per-lak-tā′shŭn). SYN superlactation.

hy·per·leu·ko·cy·to·sis (hī′per-loo′kō-sī-tō′sis). An unusually great increase in the number and proportion of leukocytes in the circulating blood or the tissues; i.e., much more than that ordinarily observed in most instances of leukocytosis.

hy·per·lex·ia (hī-per-lek′sē-ă). In mentally retarded children, the presence of relatively advanced reading ability. [hyper- + G. lexis, word, phrase]

hy·per·li·pe·mia (hī′per-li-pē′mē-ă). Elevated levels of lipids in the blood plasma. There are several types of h. One is associated with a deficiency of δ-aminoadipic semialdehyde synthase. SEE ALSO lipemia.

carbohydrate-induced h., SYN type III familial hyperlipoproteinemia, type IV familial hyperlipoproteinemia.

combined fat- and carbohydrate-induced h., SYN type V familial hyperlipoproteinemia.

familial combined h., SEE familial *hyperlipoproteinemia.*
familial fat-induced h., SYN type I familial *hyperlipoproteinemia.*
idiopathic h., SYN type I familial *hyperlipoproteinemia.*
mixed h., SYN type V familial *hyperlipoproteinemia.*

hy·per·lip·id·e·mia (hī′per-lip-i-dē′mē-ă). SYN lipemia.
mixed h., SYN mixed hyperlipoproteinemia familial, type 5 h.

mixed hyperlipoproteinemia familial, type 5 h., elevations of VLDL and chylomicrons found in plasma. SYN mixed h.

hy·per·lip·oi·de·mia (hī′per-lip-oy-dē′mē-ă). SYN lipemia.

hy·per·lip·o·pro·tein·e·mia (hī′per-lip′ō-prō′tē-in-ē′mē-ă, -prō′ tēn-). An increase in the lipoprotein concentration of the blood.

acquired h., nonfamilial h. that develops as a consequence of some primary disease, such as thyroid deficiency.

familial h., a group of diseases characterized by changes in concentration of β-lipoproteins and pre-β-lipoproteins and the lipids associated with them. SEE type I familial h., type II familial h., type III familial h., type IV familial h., type V familial h.

lipoprotein(a) h., elevated levels of lipoprotein(a) in the serum; associated with an increased risk of coronary disease.

type I familial h. [MIM*238600], h. characterized by the presence of large amounts of chylomicrons and triglycerides in the plasma when the patient has a normal diet, and their disappearance on a fat-free diet; low α- and β-lipoproteins on a normal diet, with increase on a fat-free diet; decreased plasma postheparin lipolytic activity; and low tissue lipoprotein lipase activity. It is accompanied by bouts of abdominal pain, hepatosplenomegaly, pancreatitis, and eruptive xanthomas; autosomal recessive inheritance; caused by mutation in the lipoprotein lipase gene (LPL) on chromosome 8p. SEE ALSO familial lipoprotein lipase *inhibitor.* SYN Bürger-Grütz syndrome, familial fat-induced hyperlipemia, familial hyperchylomicronemia, familial hypertriglyceridemia (1), idiopathic hyperlipemia.

type II familial h. [MIM*143890 and MIM*144400], h. characterized by increased plasma levels of β-lipoproteins and cholesterol, elevated or normal levels of triglycerides; heterozygotes have mild lipid changes and are susceptible to atherosclerosis in middle age, but homozygotes have severe changes—often with generalized xanthomatosis, xanthelesma, corneal arcus, and frank clinical atherosclerosis as young adults. This disorder is divided into two classes, both inherited as autosomal dominant with homozygotes more severely affected than heterozygotes: 1) type IIA, which is characterized by elevated LDL but normal triglycerides and is due to a deficiency of the LDL receptor, a defect of the receptor or a modified LDL-apolipoprotein B-100, caused by mutation in the LDL receptor (LDLR) gene on chromosome 19p. SYN familial hypercholesterolemia; 2) type IIB has elevated LDL, cholesterol, and triglycerides, due to dysregulation of 3-hydroxy-3-methylglutaryl coenzyme A reductase (HMG CoA reductase), the rate-controlling enzyme in cholesterol biosynthesis. SYN familial hyperbetalipoproteinemia, familial hypercholesterolemic xanthomatosis.

type III familial h. [MIM*107741], h. characterized by increased plasma levels of LDL, β-lipoproteins, pre-β-lipoproteins, cholesterol, phospholipids, and triglycerides; hypertriglyceridemia induced by a high carbohydrate diet, and glucose tolerance is abnormal; frequent eruptive xanthomas and atheromatosis, particularly coronary artery disease; biochemical defect lies in apolipoproteins; there are many varieties; one variety is caused by mutation in the APOE gene on chromosome 19q. SYN carbohydrate-induced hyperlipemia, dysbetalipoproteinemia, familial hyperbetalipoproteinemia and hyperprebetalipoproteinemia, familial hypercholesterolemia with hyperlipemia.

type IV familial h. [MIM*144600], plasma levels of VLDL, pre-β-lipoproteins and triglycerides are increased on a normal diet, but β-lipoproteins, cholesterol, and phospholipids are normal; hypertriglyceridemia is induced by a high carbohydrate diet; may be accompanied by abnormal glucose tolerance and susceptibility to ischemic heart disease; probably autosomal dominant inheritance but genetic heterogeneity is a possibility. SYN carbohydrate-induced hyperlipemia, familial hyperprebetalipoproteinemia, familial hypertriglyceridemia (2).

type V familial h. [MIM*144650], h. characterized by increased plasma levels of chylomicrons, VLDL, pre-β-lipoproteins, and triglycerides, and slight rise of cholesterol on a normal diet, with β-lipoproteins normal; may be accompanied by bouts of abdominal pain, hepatosplenomegaly, susceptibility to atherosclerosis, and abnormal glucose tolerance; probably autosomal recessive inheritance. SYN combined fat- and carbohydrate-induced hyperlipemia, familial hyperchylomicronemia with hyperprebetalipoproteinemia, mixed hyperlipemia.

hy·per·li·po·sis (hī′per-li-pō′sis). **1.** Excessive adiposity. **2.** An extreme degree of fatty degeneration. [hyper- + G. *lipos,* fat]

hy·per·li·thu·ria (hī′per-li-thu′rē-ă). An excessive excretion of uric (lithic) acid in the urine.

hy·per·lo·gia (hī-per-lō′jē-ă). Morbid verbosity or loquacity. SEE logorrhea. [hyper- + G. *logios,* eloquent]

hy·per·lor·do·sis (hī′per-lōr-dō′sis). Extreme lordosis.

hy·per·lu·cent (hī′-per-loo′sent). A region on a chest film showing greater than normal film blackening from increased transmission of x-rays. SEE unilateral hyperlucent *lung.* [hyper- + L. *lucens,* shining, fr. *luceo,* to shine]

hy·per·ly·si·ne·mia (hī′per-lī-si-nē′mē-ă) [MIM*238700]. A metabolic disorder characterized by mental retardation, convulsions, anemia, and asthenia; associated with an abnormal increase of the amino acid lysine in the circulating blood due to a deficiency of lysine-ketoglutarate reductase. One variant [MIM*268700] is associated with a deficiency of α-aminoadipic semialdehyde synthase, resulting in hyperlysinemia and saccharopinemia.

hy·per·ly·si·nu·ria (hī′per-lī-si-noo′rē-ă). The presence of abnormally high concentrations of lysine in the urine; a form of aminoaciduria that occurs in cystinuria, hepatolenticular degeneration, and the Fanconi syndrome.

hy·per·mag·ne·se·mia (hī′per-mag-ně-sē′mē-ă). An abnormally large concentration of magnesium in the blood serum.

hy·per·mas·tia (hī-per-mas′tē-ă). **1.** SYN polymastia. **2.** Excessively large mammary glands. [hyper- + G. *mastos,* breast]

hy·per·men·or·rhea (hī′per-men-ō-rē′ă). Excessively prolonged or profuse menses. SYN menorrhagia. [hyper- + G. *mēn,* month, + *rhoia,* flow]

hy·per·me·tab·o·lism (hī′per-me-tab′ŏ-lizm). Heat production by the body above normal, as in thyrotoxicosis.

extrathyroidal h., a state of increased metabolic rate with normal levels of thyroid hormone production.

hy·per·met·a·mor·pho·sis (hī′per-met-ă-mōr′fŏ-sis). Excessive and rapid change of ideas occurring in a mental disorder. SEE mania, manic-depressive, manic *excitement.* [hyper- + G. *metamorphōsis,* transformation]

hy·per·me·thi·o·nine·mia (hī-per-meth-ī-ō-mēn-ē-mē-ă). Elevated levels of methionine in the sera.

hy·per·me·tria (hī-per-mē′trē-ă). Ataxia characterized by overreaching a desired object or goal; usually seen with cerebellar disorders. Cf. hypometria. [hyper- + G. *metron,* measure]

hy·per·me·trope (hī-per-met′rōp). SYN hyperope.

hy·per·me·tro·pia (hī′per-me-trō′pē-ă). SYN hyperopia. [hyper- + G. *metron,* measure, + *ōps,* eye]

index h., h. arising from decreased refractivity of the lens.

hy·perm·ne·sia (hī-per-nē′zē-ă). **1.** Extreme power of memory. **2.** A capacity under hypnosis for immediate registration and precise recall of many more individual items than is thought possible under ordinary circumstances. Cf. hypomnesia. [hyper- + G. *mnēmē,* memory]

hy·per·mo·bil·i·ty (hī′per-mō-bil′i-tē). Increased range of movement of joints, and joint laxity, occurring normally in children and adolescents or as a result of disease, e.g., Marfan or Ehlers-Danlos syndrome.

hy·per·morph (hī′per-mōrf). **1.** Person whose sitting height is low in proportion to the standing height, owing to excessive length of limb. Cf. hypomorph, ectomorph. **2.** A mutant gene that causes an increase in the activity controlled by the gene. Cf. hypomorph. [hyper- + G. *morphē,* form]

hy·per·my·ot·ro·phy (hī′per-mī-ot′rō-fē). Muscular hypertrophy. [hyper- + G. *mys,* muscle, + *trophē,* nourishment]

hy·per·na·tre·mia (hī′per-nă-trē′mē-ă). An abnormally high

hy

plasma concentration of sodium ions. [hyper- + natrium, + G. *haima*, blood]

hy·per·ne·o·cy·to·sis (hī′per-nē′ō-sī-tō′sis). Hyperleukocytosis in which there are considerable numbers of immature and young cells (especially in the granulocytic series); i.e., a "shift to the left" in the hemogram. SYN hyperskeocytosis. [hyper- + G. *neos*, new, + *kytos*, cell, + *-osis*, condition]

hy·per·neph·roid (hī-per-nef′royd). Resembling or of the type of the adrenal gland. [hyper- + G. *nephros*, kidney, + *eidos*, appearance]

hy·per·noia (hī-per-noy′ă). **1.** Great rapidity of thought. **2.** Excessive mental activity or imagination of the type seen in the manic phase of manic depression. SEE depression. [hyper- + G. *noeō*, to think]

hy·per·nom·ic (hī-per-nom′ik). Controlled to excess. [hyper- + G. *nomos*, law]

hy·per·nu·tri·tion (hī′per-noo-trish′ŭn). SYN supernutrition.

hy·per·on·cot·ic (hī′per-on-kot′ik). Indicating an oncotic pressure higher than normal, e.g., of blood plasma.

hy·per·o·nych·ia (hī′per-ō-nik′ē-ă). Hypertrophy of the nails. [hyper- + G. *onyx*, (*onych-*), nail]

hy·per·ope (hī′per-ōp). One suffering from hyperopia. SYN hypermetrope.

hy·per·o·pia (H) (hī-per-ō′pē-ă). Longsightedness; that optical condition in which only convergent rays can be brought to focus on the retina. SYN far sight, farsightedness, hypermetropia, long sight. [hyper- + G. *ōps*, eye]

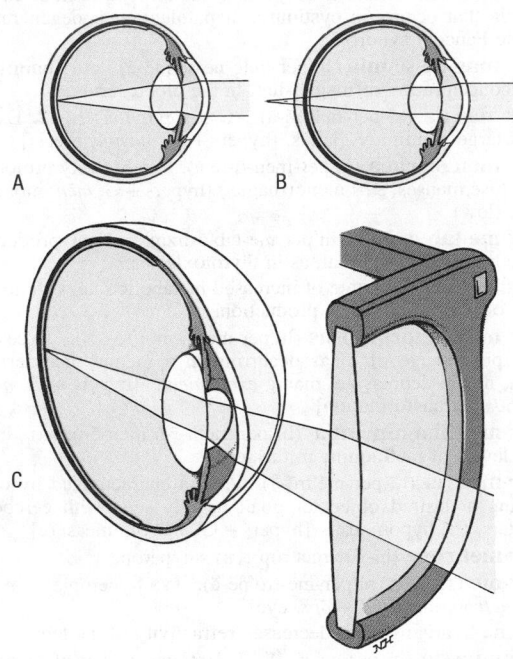

A   B

C

hyperopia: (A) normal (20/20) vision, light rays focus sharply on retina; (B) hyperopic (farsighted) vision, light rays from close objects come to sharp focus behind the retina; (C) hyperopia corrected by eyeglasses with convex lenses

absolute h., manifest h. that cannot be overcome by an effort of accommodation.

axial h., h. due to shortening of the anteroposterior diameter of the globe of the eye.

curvature h., h. due to decreased refraction of the anterior ocular segment.

facultative h., SYN manifest h.

latent h., the difference between total and manifest h.

manifest h., h. that can be compensated by accommodation. SYN facultative h.

total h. (Ht), that which can be determined after complete paralysis of accommodation by means of a cycloplegic.

hy·per·o·pic (H) (hī-per-ō′pik). Pertaining to hyperopia.

hy·per·o·ral·i·ty (hī′per-ō-ral′i-tē). A condition in which inappropriate objects are placed in the mouth. [hyper- + L. *os* (*or-*), mouth]

hy·per·o·rex·ia (hī′per-ō-rek′sē-ă). SYN *bulimia* nervosa. [hyper- + G. *orexis*, appetite]

hy·per·or·ni·thi·ne·mia (hī′per-ōrn′a-thēn-ē-mē-ă). Elevated levels of ornithine in the serum; sometimes associated with hyperammonemia and homocitrullinuria.

hy·per·or·tho·cy·to·sis (hī′per-ōr′thō-sī-tō′sis). Hyperleukocytosis in which the relative percentages of the various types of white blood cells are within the normal range and immature forms are not observed. [hyper- + G. *orthos*, correct, + *kytos*, cell, + *-osis*, condition]

hy·per·os·mia (hī-per-oz′mē-ă). An exaggerated or abnormally acute sense of smell. SYN olfactory hyperesthesia, hyperesthesia olfactoria. [hyper- + G. *osmē*, sense of smell]

hy·per·os·mo·lal·i·ty (hī′per-oz-mō-lal′i-tē). Increased osmotic concentration of a solution expressed as osmoles of solute per kilogram of serum water.

hy·per·os·mo·lar·i·ty (hī′per-oz-mō-lar′i-tē). An increase in the osmotic concentration of a solution expressed as osmoles of solute per liter of solution.

hy·per·os·mot·ic (hī′per-oz-mot′ik). **1.** Having an osmolality greater than another fluid, ordinarily assumed to be plasma or extracellular fluid. **2.** Relating to increased osmosis.

hy·per·os·te·oi·do·sis (hī′per-os-tē-oy-dō′sis). Excessive formation of osteoid, as seen in rickets and osteomalacia.

hy·per·os·to·sis (hī′per-os-tō′sis). **1.** Hypertrophy of bone. **2.** SYN exostosis. [hyper- + G. *osteon*, bone, + *-ōsis*, condition]

ankylosing h., SYN diffuse idiopathic skeletal h.

h. cortica′lis defor′mans [MIM*239000], marked irregular thickening of the skull and bone cortex, with thickening and widening of the shafts of long bones and high serum alkaline phosphatase; autosomal recessive inheritance.

diffuse idiopathic skeletal h. (DISH), a generalized spinal and extraspinal articular disorder characterized by calcification and ossification of ligaments, particularly of the anterior longitudinal ligament; distinct from ankylosing spondylitis or degenerative joint disease. SYN ankylosing h., Forestier disease, hyperostotic spondylosis.

flowing h., SYN rheostosis.

h. fronta′lis inter′na, abnormal deposition of bone on the inner aspect of the os frontale, visible by x-ray; may be a part of Morgagni syndrome.

generalized cortical h., SYN van Buchem *syndrome*.

infantile cortical h. [MIM*114000], neonatal subperiosteal bone formation over many bones, especially the mandible, clavicles, and the shafts of long bones; it follows fever, usually appearing before 6 months of age and disappearing during childhood; familial cases are inherited as autosomal dominant. SYN Caffey disease, Caffey syndrome, Caffey-Silverman syndrome.

streak h., SYN rheostosis.

hy·per·o·var·i·an·ism (hī′per-ō-vā′rē-an-izm). Sexual precocity in young girls due to premature maturation of the hypotholomic-pituitary axis and development of ovaries accompanied by the secretion of ovarian hormones. SYN true precocious puberty.

hy·per·ox·al·u·ria (hī′per-ok-să-loo′rē-ă). Presence of an unusually large amount of oxalic acid or oxalates in the urine; renal stones may occur. SYN oxaluria.

primary h. and oxalosis [MIM*259900 & MIM*260000], a metabolic disorder, usually evident clinically in the first decade of life, characterized by calcium oxalate nephrocalcinosis and nephrolithiasis, extrarenal oxalosis, and increased urinary output of oxalic and glycolic acids, leading to progressive renal failure and uremia. Type I is due to a deficiency in alanine-glyoxylate aminotransferase and type II to a deficiency in D-glycerate dehydrogenase; the latter is a milder disease with a better long-term prognosis for renal function. Both types are inherited as autosomal recessive, caused by mutation in the alanine-glyoxylate aminotransferase gene (AGXT) on 2q.

hy·per·ox·ia (hī-per-ok′sē-ă). **1.** An increased amount of oxygen in tissues and organs. **2.** A greater oxygen tension than normal, such as that produced by breathing air or oxygen at pressures greater than 1 atmosphere.

hy·per·ox·i·da·tion (hī′per-oks-i-dā′shŭn). Excessive oxidation.

hy·per·pan·cre·a·tism (hī′per-pan′krē-ă-tizm). A condition of increased activity of the pancreas, trypsin being in excess among the enzymes.

hy·per·par·a·site (hī-per-par′ă-sīt). A secondary parasite capable of development within a previously existing parasite.

hy·per·par·a·sit·ism (hī-per-par′ă-sīt-izm). A condition in which a secondary parasite develops within a previously existing parasite. SYN biparasitism.

hy·per·par·a·thy·roid·ism (hī′per-par-ă-thī′royd-izm). A condition due to an increase in the secretion of the parathyroids, causing elevated serum calcium, decreased serum phosphorus, and increased excretion of both calcium and phosphorus, calcium stones and sometimes generalized osteitis fibrosa cystica.

primary h., h. due to neoplasms or idiopathic hyperplasia of the parathyroid glands.

secondary h., h. that arises as a result of disordered metabolism producing hypocalcemia, as in chronic uremia due to renal disease, malabsorption, rickets, or osteomalacia; associated with hyperplasia of the parathyroid glands.

hy·per·pa·rot·i·dism (hī′per-pa-rot′i-dizm). Increased activity of the parotid glands.

hy·per·path·ia (hī-per-path′ē-ă). Exaggerated subjective response to painful stimuli, with a continuing sensation of pain after the stimulation has ceased. [hyper- + G. *pathos,* suffering]

hy·per·pep·sia (hī-per-pep′sē-ă). **1.** Abnormally rapid digestion. **2.** Impaired digestion with hyperchlorhydria. [hyper- + G. *pepsis,* digestion]

hy·per·pep·sin·ia (hī′per-pep-sin′ē-ă). An excess of pepsin in the gastric juice.

hy·per·per·i·stal·sis (hī′per-per-i-stal′sis). Excessive rapidity of the passage of food through the stomach and intestine.

hy·per·pha·gia (hī-per-fā′jē-ă). Gluttony; overeating. [hyper- + G. *phagein,* to eat]

hy·per·pha·lan·gism (hī′per-fă-lan′jizm). Presence of a supernumerary phalanx in a finger or toe. SYN polyphalangism.

hy·per·phen·yl·al·a·ni·ne·mia (hī′per-fen′il-al-ă-ni-nē′mē-ă). The presence of abnormally high blood levels of phenylalanine, which may or may not be associated with elevated tyrosine levels, in newborn infants (premature and full-term), associated with the heterozygous state of phenylketonuria, maternal phenylketonuria, or transient deficiency of phenylalanine hydroxylase or *p*-hydroxyphenylpyruvic acid oxidase.

malignant h., (1) dHPR-deficient form; an inherited disorder in which there is an absence or deficiency of dihydropteridine reductase (DHPR); this results in impaired regeneration of tetrahydrobiopterin, causing an elevation in phenylalanine levels; (2) gTP-CH form; an inherited disorder in which there is a deficiency of guanosine triphosphate cyclohydrolase, an enzyme used in the biosynthesis of tetrahydrobiopterin; (3) 6-PTS form; an inherited disorder in which there is a deficiency of 6-pyruvoyl tetrahydropterin synthase, an enzyme that participates in the biosynthesis of tetrahydrobiopterin. SYN nonclassical phenylketonuria.

non-PKU h., a benign phenotype in which phenylalanine monooxygenase is deficient but is greater than 1% of normal levels.

hy·per·pho·ne·sis (hī′per-fō-nē′sis). An increase in the percussion sound or of the voice sound in auscultation. [hyper- + G. *phōnēsis,* a sounding]

hy·per·pho·nia (hī-per-fō′nē-ă). Excessive effort in voice production characterized by loudness and undue tension of the vocal muscles. [hyper- + G. *phōnē,* sound, voice]

hy·per·pho·ria (hī-per-fō′rē-ă). A tendency of the visual axis of one eye to deviate upward, prevented by binocular vision. [hyper- + G. *phora,* motion]

hy·per·phos·pha·ta·se·mia (hī′per-fos′fă-tă-sē′mē-ă). Abnormally high content of alkaline phosphatase in the circulating blood. SEE ALSO hyperphosphatasia.

hy·per·phos·pha·ta·sia (hī′per-fos-fă-tā′zē-ă) [MIM*239000 and MIM*239300]. A skeletal dysplasia characterized by dwarfism, macrocranium, expansion of the diaphyses of tubular bones with multiple fractures, patchy osteosclerosis, leg bowing, and occasionally mental retardation; serum alkaline phosphatase is elevated; autosomal recessive inheritance.

hy·per·phos·pha·te·mia (hī′per-fos-fă-tē′mē-ă). Abnormally high concentration of phosphates in the circulating blood.

hy·per·phos·pha·tu·ria (hī′per-fos-fă-too′rē-ă). An increased excretion of phosphates in the urine.

hy·per·phre·nia (hī-per-frē′nē-ă). Rarely used term for an excessive degree of intellectual activity; a form of mania. [hyper- + G. *phrēn,* mind]

hy·per·pi·e·sis, hy·per·pi·e·sia (hī′per-pī-ē′sis, -pī-ē′zē-ă). SYN hypertension. [hyper- + G. *piesis,* pressure]

hy·per·pi·et·ic (hī-per-pī-et′ik). Relating to or marked by high blood pressure.

hy·per·pig·men·ta·tion (hī′per-pig-men-tā′shŭn). An excess of pigment in a tissue or part.

hy·per·pip·e·co·la·te·mia (hī-per-pip′ě-kō-lă-tē′mē-ă). A metabolic disorder in which serum concentration of pipecolic acid is greatly increased; characterized by hepatomegaly and progressive, generalized demyelination of the nervous system. SYN hyperpipecolic acidemia.

hy·per·pip·e·co·lic ac·i·de·mia (hī′per-pī′pē-ko-lik). SYN hyperpipecolatemia.

hy·per·pi·tu·i·ta·rism (hī′per-pi-too′i-tă-rizm). Excessive production of anterior pituitary hormones, especially growth hormone; may result in gigantism or acromegaly.

hy·per·pla·sia (hī-per-plā′zhē-ă). An increase in number of normal cells in a tissue or organ, excluding tumor formation, whereby the bulk of the part or organ may be increased. SEE ALSO hypertrophy. SYN numerical hypertrophy, quantitative hypertrophy. [hyper- + G. *plasis,* a molding]

adenomatous h., SYN complex endometrial h.

angiofollicular mediastinal lymph node h., SYN benign giant lymph node h.

angiolymphoid h. with eosinophilia, solitary or multiple small benign cutaneous erythematous nodules, occurring mainly on the head and neck in young adults, characterized by dermal proliferation of blood vessels with vacuolated histiocytoid endothelial cells and with a varied infiltrate of eosinophils, lymphocytes which may form follicles, and histiocytes. SYN Kimura disease.

atypical endometrial h., increase in the number of glands, which have little, if any, stroma separating them but retain an orderly architecture distinguishing them from adenocarcinoma.

atypical melanocytic h., proliferation of melanocytes showing nuclear atypicality, especially as scattered single cells high in the epidermis; interpreted by some pathologists as malignant melanoma in situ.

basal cell h., increase in the number of cells in an epithelium resembling the basal cells.

benign giant lymph node h., solitary masses of lymphoid tissue containing concentric perivascular aggregates of lymphocytes, occurring usually in the mediastinum or hilar region of young adults; similar changes have been reported outside the mediastinum and, if associated with interfollicular sheets of plasma cells, may progress to lymphoma or plasmacytoma. SYN angiofollicular mediastinal lymph node h., Castleman disease.

benign prostatic h., progressive enlargement of the prostate due to h. of both glandular and stromal components, typically beginning in the fifth decade and sometimes causing obstructive or irritative symptoms, or both; does not evolve into cancer.

cementum h., SYN hypercementosis.

complex endometrial h., closely packed endometrial glands, with a single layer of cells with slightly enlarged nuclei that are generally basally located. SYN adenomatous h.

congenital adrenal h., a group of autosomal recessively inherited

hy

disorders associated with a deficiency of one of the enzymes involved in cortisol biosynthesis, resulting in elevation of ACTH levels and overproduction and accumulation of cortisol precursors proximal to the block; androgens are produced in excess, causing virilization. The most common disorder is the 21-hydroxylase deficiency, caused by mutation in the cytochrome P450 21-hydroxylase gene (CYP21) on chromosome 6p. There are four major types with some clinical similarities but distinctive genetic and biochemical differences: 1) the salt-losing form [MIM*201710, MIM*201810, and MIM*201910], 2) the hypertensive form [MIM*202010 and MIM*202110], 3) the simple virilizing form [MIM*201910], and 4) the pseudohermaphrodite form [MIM*201810 and MIM*202110].

congenital virilizing adrenal h., a series of inherited inborn errors of metabolism with h. of the adrenal cortex and overproduction of virilizing hormones. Most common forms are due to partial or complete 21-hydroxylase deficiency, leading to increased ACTH production by the pituitary, stimulating adrenal growth and function. Severe form is characterized by salt-losing state.

cystic h., formation of multiple retention cysts from obstruction of ducts or glands by h. of the lining epithelium, as in fibrocystic disease of the breast and metropathia hemorrhagica.

cystic h. of the breast, SYN fibrocystic *condition* of the breast.

denture h., SYN inflammatory fibrous h.

ductal h., h. characterized by intraductal proliferation of epithelial cells, e.g., in the breast.

endometrial h., increase in the number of endometrial glands, usually secondary to hyperestrinism; classified as simple h., complex h., or complex h. with atypia; the latter may progress to adenocarcinoma.

fibromuscular h., thickening of arterial media by fibrosis and muscular h., usually involving the renal arteries and causing multifocal stenosis and hypertension; a variety of fibromuscular dysplasia.

focal epithelial h., multiple soft nodular lesions of the lips, buccal mucosa, tongue, and other oral sites in children and adolescents; lesions spontaneously regress after a period of several months, and have been attributed to papovaviruses. SYN Heck disease.

gingival h., gingival enlargement due to proliferation of fibrous connective tissue. SYN gingival proliferation.

inflammatory fibrous h., overgrowth of tissue in the mucobuccal or labial fold, induced by chronic trauma from ill-fitting dentures. SYN denture h., epulis fissuratum.

inflammatory papillary h., closely arranged papules of the palatal mucosa underlying an ill-fitting denture. SYN palatal papillomatosis.

intravascular papillary endothelial h., a benign florid papillary endothelial proliferation within the veins of the skin or subcutis, less often in visceral blood vessels.

neuronal h., increased numbers of ganglion cells with myenteric plexus h. and increased acetylcholinesterase activity in nerves of the mucosa and submucosa. Clinically, neuronal h. mimics Hirschsprung disease. Similar findings are seen in patients with multiple endocrine neoplasia syndrome, type IIB, and in neurofibromatosis. SYN hyperganglionosis, neuronal intestinal dysplasia.

nodular h. of prostate, glandular and stromal h. occurring very commonly in the transition zone and anterior fibromuscular stroma of older men, forming nodules that may increasingly obstruct the urethra.

nodular regenerative h., SYN nodular *transformation* of the liver.

pseudoepitheliomatous h., pseudocarcinomatous h., a benign marked increase and downgrowth of epidermal cells, observed in chronic inflammatory dermatoses and over some dermal neoplasms and nevi; microscopically, it resembles well-differentiated squamous cell carcinoma.

senile sebaceous h., h. of mature sebaceous glands, forming a nodule on the skin of the face or forehead in elderly persons.

simple endometrial h., increase in the amount of endometrial tissue, with glands separated by abundant stroma. SYN Swiss cheese endometrium.

squamous cell h., increase in the number of cells in a squamous epithelium. SYN hypertrophic dystrophy.

verrucous h., h. of the oral mucosa, occurring in the elderly, characterized by sharp or blunt upward papillary projections of squamous epithelium.

hy·per·plas·tic (hī-per-plas'tik). Relating to hyperplasia.

hy·per·pnea (hī-per-nē'ă, hī-perp'nē-ă). Breathing that is deeper and more rapid than is normal at rest. [hyper- + G. *pnoē*, breathing]

hy·per·po·lar·i·za·tion (hī'per-pō'lăr-i-zā'shŭn). An increase in polarization of membranes of nerves or muscle cells; the reverse change from that associated with excitatory action.

hy·per·po·tas·se·mia (hī'per-pō-tas-ē'mē-ă). SYN hyperkalemia.

hy·per·pre·be·ta·lip·o·pro·tein·e·mia (hī'per-prē-bā'tă-lip-ō-prō'tē-in-ē'mē-ă, -prō'tēn-). Increased concentrations of pre-β-lipoproteins in the blood.

familial h., SYN type IV familial *hyperlipoproteinemia*.

hy·per·pro·chor·e·sis (hī'per-prō-kōr-ē'sis). Rarely used term for hyperperistalsis. [hyper- + G. *pro-chōreō*, to go forward]

hy·per·pro·in·su·li·ne·mia (hī'per-prō-in'sŭl-i-nē'mē-ă). Elevated plasma levels of proinsulin or proinsulin-like material.

hy·per·pro·lac·ti·ne·mia (hī'per-prō-lak-ti-nē'mē-ă). Elevated levels of prolactin in the blood, which is a normal physiological reaction during lactation, but pathological otherwise; prolactin may also be elevated in cases of certain pituitary tumors, and amenorrhea is often present.

hy·per·pro·li·ne·mia (hī'per-prō-li-nē'mē-ă) [MIM*239500 & MIM*239510]. A metabolic disorder characterized by enhanced plasma proline concentrations and urinary excretion of proline, hydroxyproline, and glycine; autosomal recessive inheritance. Type I h. is associated with a deficiency of proline oxidase and renal disease; Type II h. is associated with a deficiency of Δ-pyrroline-5-carboxylate dehydrogenase, mental retardation, and convulsions and is caused by mutation in the δ-pyrroline 5 carboxylate gene (P5CD) on 1p.

hy·per·pro·tein·e·mia (hī'per-prō'tē-in-ē'mē-ă, -prō'tēn-). An abnormally large concentration of protein in plasma.

hy·per·pro·te·o·sis (hī'per-prō-tē-ō'sis). The condition due to an excessive amount of protein in the diet.

hy·per·py·ret·ic (hī'per-pī-ret'ik). Relating to hyperpyrexia. SYN hyperpyrexial.

hy·per·py·rex·ia (hī'per-pī-rek'sē-ă). Extremely high fever. [hyper- + G. *pyrexis*, feverishness]

fulminant h., SYN malignant *hyperthermia*.

heat h., SYN heatstroke.

malignant h., SYN heatstroke.

hy·per·py·rex·i·al (hī'per-pī-rek'sē-ăl). SYN hyperpyretic.

hy·per·re·flex·ia (hī'per-rē-flek'sē-ă). A condition in which the deep tendon reflexes are exaggerated.

detrusor h., SYN detrusor *instability*.

hy·per·res·o·nance (hī-per-rez'ō-nans). **1.** An extreme degree of resonance. **2.** Resonance increased above the normal, and often of lower pitch, on percussion of an area of the body; occurs in the chest due to overinflation of the lung as in emphysema or pneumothorax and in the abdomen over distended bowel.

hy·per·sal·e·mia (hī'per-sal-ē'mē-ă). Obsolete term for an increase in the salt content of the circulating blood.

hy·per·sa·line (hī-per-sā'lēn, -sā'līn). Marked by increased salt concentrations in a saline solution.

hy·per·sal·i·va·tion (hī'per-sal-i-vā'shŭn). Increased salivation.

hy·per·sar·co·si·ne·mia (hī'per-sar-kō-si-nē'mē-ă). SYN sarcosinemia.

hy·per·se·cre·tion (hī'per-sē-krē'shŭn). Excessive secretion of any tissue or gland.

gastric h., excessive formation of gastric juice, especially the acid component.

hy·per·seg·men·ta·tion. Excessive division of a tissue or part into segments.

hereditary hypersegmentation of neutrophils, an autosomal dominant condition characterized by neutrophil hypersegmentation; affected persons are asymptomatic.

◨ hy·per·sen·si·tiv·i·ty (hī′per-sen-si-tiv′i-tē). Abnormal sensitivity, a condition in which there is an exaggerated response by the body to the stimulus of a foreign agent. SEE allergy.

contact h., (1) SYN contact *dermatitis*; **(2)** SYN delayed *reaction*.

delayed h., (1) SYN cell-mediated *immunity*; **(2)** SYN delayed *reaction*; **(3)** a cell-mediated response that occurs in immune individuals peaking in 24–48 hours after challenge with the same antigen used in an initial challenge. The interaction of T-helper I lymphocytes with MHC class II positive antigen-presenting cells initiates the response. This interaction induces the T helper 1 and macrophages at the site to secrete cytokines, which are the major players in the reaction. Called tuberculin-type h.

immediate h., an exaggerated immune response mediated by antibodies occurring within minutes after exposing a sensitized individual to the approximate antigen; also called Type I h. Clinical symptoms include atopic allergy and systemic anaphylaxis. The antigen induces IgE antibodies, which bind to most cells and basophils. Subsequent exposure to antigen causes binding with the cytophilic IgE resulting in the release of mediators. SEE allergy.

tuberculin-type h., SYN delayed *reaction*.

hy·per·sen·si·ti·za·tion (hī′per-sen′si-ti-zā′shŭn). The immunological process by which hypersensitivity is induced.

hy·per·se·ro·to·ne·mia (hī′per-sēr′ō-tō-nē′mē-ă). Unusually large amounts of serotonin in the circulating blood; probable cause of some of the symptoms and signs in the carcinoid syndrome.

hy·per·ske·o·cy·to·sis (hī′per-skē′ō-sī-tō′sis). SYN hyperneocytosis. [G. *skaios*, left, + *kytos*, cell, + *-osis*, condition]

hy·per·so·ma·to·tro·pism (hī′per-sō′mă-tō-trō′pizm). A state characterized by abnormally enhanced secretion of pituitary growth hormone (somatotropin).

hy·per·som·nia (hī-per-som′nē-ă). A condition in which sleep periods are excessively long, but the person responds normally in the intervals; distinguished from somnolence. [hyper- + L. *somnus*, sleep]

hy·per·son·ic (hī-per-son′ik). Pertaining to or characterized by supersonic speeds of Mach 5 or greater. While any speed above the speed of sound may be referred to as supersonic, speeds of Mach 5 or greater are specifically referred to as h. [hyper- + L. *sonus*, sound]

hy·per·sphyx·ia (hī-per-sfik′sē-ă). A condition of high blood pressure and increased circulatory activity. [hyper- + G. *sphyxis*, pulse]

hy·per·splen·ism (hī-per-splēn′izm). Any of a group of conditions in which the cellular components of the blood or platelets are removed at an abnormally high rate by the spleen, resulting in low circulating levels.

hy·per·ste·a·to·sis (hī′per-stē-ă-tō′sis). Excessive sebaceous secretion.

hy·per·sthe·nia (hī-per-sthē′nē-ă). Excessive tension or strength. [hyper- + G. *sthenos*, strength]

hy·per·sthen·ic (hī-per-sthen′ik). Pertaining to or marked by hypersthenia.

hy·per·sthen·u·ria (hī′per-sthen-ū′rē-ă). Excretion of urine of unusually high specific gravity and concentration of solutes, resulting usually from loss or deprivation of water. [hyper- + G. *sthenos*, strength, + *ouron*, urine]

hy·per·sus·cep·ti·bil·i·ty (hī′per-sŭ-sep-ti-bil′i-tē). Increased susceptibility or response to an infective, chemical, or other agent.

hy·per·sys·to·le (hī-per-sis′tō-lē). Abnormal force or duration of the cardiac systole.

hy·per·sys·tol·ic (hī′per-sis-tol′ik). Relating to or marked by hypersystole.

hy·per·tel·or·ism (hī-per-tel′ōr-izm). Abnormal distance between two paired organs. [hyper- + G. *tēle*, far off, + *horizō*, to separate, fr. *horos*, a boundary]

Bixler type h., accompanying features are microtia and clefting of the lip, palate, and nose, mental deficiency, atresia of the auditory canals, ectopic kidneys, and thenar hypoplasia; autosomal recessive inheritance

canthal h., SYN telecanthus.

ocular h. [MIM*145400], increased width between the eyes due to an arrest in development of the greater wings of the sphenoid, thus fixing the orbits in the widely separated fetal position; autosomal dominant inheritance. Ocular h. is a feature of many syndromes. A distinct form [MIM*145410] shows other congenital defects such as hypospadias and esophageal anomalies. SEE ALSO faciodigitogenital *dysplasia*. SYN Greig syndrome, Opitz BBB syndrome, Opitz G syndrome.

hy·per·ten·sin (hī-per-ten′sin). Former name for angiotensin.

hy·per·ten·sin·o·gen (hī′per-ten-sin′ō-jen). Former name for angiotensinogen.

hy·per·ten·sion (hī′per-ten′shŭn). High blood pressure; transitory or sustained elevation of systemic arterial blood pressure to a level likely to induce cardiovascular damage or other adverse consequences. H. has been arbitrarily defined as a systolic blood pressure above 140 mm Hg or a diastolic blood pressure above 90 mm Hg. Consequences of uncontrolled h. include retinal vascular damage (Keith-Wagener-Barker changes), cerebrovascular disease and stroke, left ventricular hypertrophy and failure, myocardial infarction, dissecting aneurysm, and renovascular disease. An underlying disorder (e.g., renal disease, Cushing syndrome, pheochromocytoma) is identified in fewer than 10% of all cases of h. The remainder, traditionally labeled "essential" h., probably arise from a variety of disturbances in normal pressure-regulating mechanisms (which involve baroreceptors, autonomic influences on the rate and force of cardiac contraction and vascular tone, renal retention of salt and water, formation of angiotensin II under the influence of renin and angiotensin-converting enzyme, and other factors known and unknown), and most are probably genetically conditioned. SYN hyperpiesis, hyperpiesia. [hyper- + L. *tensio*, tension]

> Because of its wide prevalence and its impact on cardiovascular health, hypertension is a major cause of disease and death in industrialized societies. It is estimated that 50–70 million Americans, including about 50% of all people over age 60, have hypertension, but that only about one-third of these are aware of their condition and are under appropriate treatment. Hypertension causes 35,000 deaths annually in the U.S., and is a contributing factor in a further 180,000 deaths. It is associated with a 3-fold increase in the risk of heart attack and a 7- to 10-fold increase in the risk of stroke. The prevalence of hypertension and the incidence of nonfatal and fatal consequences are substantially higher in African-Americans. Although people with extremely high diastolic pressure may experience headache, dizziness, and even encephalopathy, uncomplicated hypertension seldom causes symptoms. Hence the diagnosis of hypertension is usually made by screening apparently healthy persons or those under treatment for another condition. Risk factors for hypertension include a family history of hypertension, African-American race, advancing age, the postmenopausal state, excessive dietary sodium, obesity, excessive use of alcohol, sedentary lifestyle, and chronic emotional stress. Treatment options include lifestyle changes (maintenance of healthful weight; at least 30 minutes of aerobic exercise several days a week; limitation of sodium intake to 2.4 g daily and of ethanol to 1 oz daily; consumption of adequate potassium, calcium, and magnesium; and avoidance of excessive emotional stress) and a broad range of drugs, including diuretics, beta-blockers, calcium channel blockers, angiotensin-converting enzyme inhibitors, angiotensin II receptor antagonists, α_1-adrenergic antagonists, centrally acting alpha-agonists, and others. In recent decades, early detection and aggressive treatment of hypertension have reduced associated morbidity and mortality. Current practice standards call for still more diligent management, including prevention through avoidance of known risk factors, particularly in persons with a family history of hypertension, and control of cofactors known to increase the risk of cardiovascular damage in persons with hypertension (smoking, hypercholesterolemia, diabetes mellitus).

hy

Some studies suggest that the goal of treatment should be a diastolic blood pressure of 80 or lower.

—————

accelerated h., h. advancing rapidly with increasing blood pressure and associated with acute and rapidly worsening signs and symptoms.

adrenal h., h. due to an adrenal medullary pheochromocytoma or to hyperactivity or functioning tumor of the adrenal cortex.

benign h., h. that runs a relatively long and symptomless course.

borderline h., by consensus, that blood pressure zone between highest acceptable "normal" blood pressure and hypertensive blood pressure. The Framingham Heart Study defines this as pressures between 140 and 160 mm Hg systolic and 90 and 95 mm Hg diastolic.

episodic h., h. manifest intermittently, triggered by anxiety or emotional factors. SYN paroxysmal h.

essential h., h. without known cause. SYN idiopathic h., primary h.

gestational h., h. during pregnancy in a previously normotensive woman or aggravation of h. during pregnancy in a hypertensive woman. SYN pregnancy-induced h.

Goldblatt h., increased blood pressure following obstruction of blood flow to one kidney.

idiopathic h., SYN essential h.

labile h., frequently changing levels of elevated blood pressure.

malignant h., severe h. that runs a rapid course, causing necrosis of arteriolar walls in kidney, retina, etc.; hemorrhages occur, and death most frequently is caused by uremia or rupture of a cerebral vessel.

pale h., h. with pallor of the skin, a severe form with pronounced constriction of peripheral vessels.

paroxysmal h., SYN episodic h.

portal h., h. in the portal system as seen in cirrhosis of the liver and other conditions causing obstruction to the portal vein.

postpartum h., increased blood pressure immediately following the completion of labor.

pregnancy-induced h., SYN gestational h.

primary h., SYN essential h.

pulmonary h., h. in the pulmonary circuit; may be primary, or secondary to pulmonary or cardiac disease, e.g., fibrosis of the lung or mitral stenosis.

renal h., h. secondary to renal disease.

renovascular h., h. produced by renal arterial obstruction.

secondary h., arterial h. produced by a known cause, e.g., hyperthyroidism, kidney disease, etc., in contrast to primary h. that is of unknown cause.

systemic venous h., increased pressure in the veins ultimately leading to the right atrium nearly always due to disease of the right heart or pericardium but occasionally due to blockade of one or both venae cavae.

hy·per·ten·sive (hī-per-ten′siv). **1.** Marked by an increased blood pressure. **2.** Denoting a person suffering from high blood pressure.

hy·per·ten·sor (hī-per-ten′ser, -sōr). SYN pressor.

hy·per·tes·toid·ism (hī-per-tes′toyd-izm). Hypergonadism in the male, characterized by proliferation of Leydig cells with excessive production of testosterone.

hy·per·the·co·sis (hī′per-thē-kō′sis). Diffuse hyperplasia of the theca cells of the graafian follicles.

stromal h., condition in which luteinized cells are present in ovarian stroma at a distance from follicular structures.

hy·per·the·lia (hī-per-thē′lē-ă). SYN polythelia. [hyper- + G. thēlē, nipple]

hy·per·ther·mal·ge·sia (hī′per-ther-măl-jē′zē-ă). Extreme sensitiveness to heat. [hyper- + G. thermē, heat, + algēsis, pain]

hy·per·ther·mia (hī-per-ther′mē-ă). Therapeutically induced hyperpyrexia. [hyper- + G. thermē, heat]

malignant h., rapid onset of extremely high fever with muscle rigidity, precipitated by exogenous agents in genetically susceptible persons, especially by halothane or succinylcholine. Cf. futile cycle. SYN fulminant hyperpyrexia.

hy·per·ther·mo·es·the·sia (hī-per-ther′mō-es-the′zē-ă). Extreme sensitiveness to heat. [hyper- + G. thermē, heat, + aisthēsis, feeling]

hy·per·throm·bi·ne·mia (hī′per-throm-bi-nē′mē-ă). An abnormal increase of thrombin in the blood, frequently resulting in a tendency to intravascular coagulation.

hy·per·thy·mia (hī-per-thī′mē-ă). State of overactivity, greater than average and less than the overactivity of the manic state of manic-depressive disorder. [hyper- + G. thymos, soul, thought]

hy·per·thy·mic (hī-per-thī′mik). **1.** Pertaining to hyperthymia. **2.** Pertaining to hyperthymism.

hy·per·thy·mism (hī-per-thī′mizm). Excessive activity of the thymus gland; formerly postulated to be a causal factor in certain instances of unexpected and sudden death, such as status thymicolymphaticus. SYN hyperthymization.

hy·per·thy·mi·za·tion (hī′per-thī-mi-zā′shŭn). SYN hyperthymism.

hy·per·thy·rea (hī′per-thī-rē′ă). SYN hyperthyroidism.

hy·per·thy·roid·ism (hī-per-thī′royd-izm). An abnormality of the thyroid gland in which secretion of thyroid hormone is usually increased and is no longer under regulatory control of hypothalamic-pituitary centers; characterized by a hypermetabolic state, usually with weight loss, tremulousness, elevated plasma levels of thyroxin and/or triiodothyronine, and sometimes exophthalmos; may progress to severe weakness, wasting, hyperpyrexia, and other manifestations of thyroid storm; often associated with exophthalmos (Graves disease). SEE ALSO thyrotoxicosis. SYN hyperthyrea, thyroidism (1), thyrointoxication.

hereditary h., a rare inherited (autosomal dominant) disorder with constitutive stimulation of the thyrocytes.

iodine-induced h., SYN Jod-Basedow phenomenon.

masked h., h. occurring without the usual manifestations, especially lack of hyperactivity and eye findings, often with hypoactivity, even somnolence. Manifestation can be limited to heart failure.

ophthalmic h., SYN Graves disease.

primary h., h. due to a disorder originating within the thyroid gland, in contrast to one of pituitary origin; may be due to generalized overactivity of the gland, to a localized hyperactive nodule, or to circulating antibody, which stimulates the gland (long-acting thyroid stimulator).

secondary h., h. due to stimulation of the thyroid gland by an excess of thyrotrophin secreted by the pituitary gland.

hy·per·thy·rox·i·ne·mia (hī′per-thī-rok-si-nē′mē-ă). An elevated thyroxine concentration in the blood.

hy·per·to·nia (hī-per-tō′nē-ă). Extreme tension of the muscles or arteries. SYN hypertonicity (1). [hyper- + G. tonos, tension]

h. polycythe′mica, a form of polycythemia without a prominent degree of splenomegaly, but with increased blood pressure.

sympathetic h., overfunction of the sympathetic nervous system, often experienced as anxiety.

hy·per·ton·ic (hī-per-ton′ik). **1.** Having a greater degree of tension. SYN spastic (1). **2.** Having a greater osmotic pressure than a reference solution, which is ordinarily assumed to be blood plasma or interstitial fluid; more specifically, refers to a fluid in which cells shrink. SYN hyperisotonic.

hy·per·to·nic·i·ty (hī′per-tō-nis′i-tē). **1.** SYN hypertonia. **2.** An increased effective osmotic pressure of body fluids.

hy·per·tri·chi·a·sis (hī′per-tri-kī′ă-sis). SYN hypertrichosis.

hy·per·trich·o·phry·dia (hī′per-trik-ō-fri′dē-ă). Excessively thick eyebrows. [hyper- + G. thrix, hair, + ophrys, eyebrow]

hy·per·tri·cho·sis (hī′per-tri-kō′sis). Growth of hair in excess of the normal. SEE ALSO hirsutism. SYN hypertrichiasis. [hyper- + G. trichōsis, being hairy]

h. lanugino′sa, excessive growth of lanugo hair associated with internal malignancy.

nevoid h., congenital growth of hair abnormal for its site, texture, color, or length; often associated with congenital melanocytic nevi.

h. partia′lis, abnormally excessive hair growth in patches in unusual areas.

h. universa·lis, generalized excessive hair growth.

hy·per·tri·glyc·er·i·de·mia (hī′per-trī-glis′er-i-dē′mē-ă). Elevated triglyceride concentration in the blood.

familial h., (1) SYN type I familial *hyperlipoproteinemia*; **(2)** SYN type IV familial *hyperlipoproteinemia*.

hy·per·troph (hī′per-trof). A microorganism that requires living cells to supply the enzyme systems necessary for growth and reproduction.

hy·per·tro·phia (hī-per-trō′fē-ă). SYN hypertrophy.

hy·per·tro·phic (hī-per-trof′ik). Relating to or characterized by hypertrophy.

hy·per·tro·phy (hī-per′trō-fē). General increase in bulk of a part or organ, not due to tumor formation. Use of the term may be restricted to denote greater bulk through increase in size, but not in number, of cells or other individual tissue elements. Cf. hyperplasia. SYN hypertrophia. [hyper- + G. *trophē,* nourishment]

adaptive h., thickening of the walls of a hollow organ, like the urinary bladder, when there is obstruction to outflow.

benign prostatic h., erroneous term that is often considered a synonym of nodular *hyperplasia* of prostate.

compensatory h., increase in size of an organ or part of an organ or tissue, when called upon to do additional work or perform the work of destroyed tissue or of a paired organ.

compensatory h. of the heart, thickening of the walls of the heart in response to vascular, valvular, other heart disease, or athletic conditioning.

complementary h., increase in size or expansion of part of an organ or tissue to fill the space left by the destruction of another portion of the same organ or tissue.

concentric h., thickening of the walls of the heart or any cavity with apparent diminution of the capacity of the cavity.

eccentric h., thickening of the wall of the heart or other cavity, with dilation.

endemic h., enlargement of the calcaneus preceded by fever and pain in the heel, reported from the Gold Coast (now Ghana) and in Taiwan among the indigenous population.

false h., SYN pseudohypertrophy.

functional h., SYN physiologic h.

giant h. of gastric mucosa, SYN Ménétrier *disease.*

hemangiectatic h., SYN Klippel-Trenaunay-Weber *syndrome.*

lipomatous h., SYN lipomatous *infiltration.*

numerical h., SYN hyperplasia.

physiologic h., temporary increase in size of an organ or part to provide for a natural increase of function, such as the kind that occurs in the walls of the uterus and in the mammae during pregnancy. SYN functional h.

quantitative h., SYN hyperplasia.

simple h., increase in size of cells.

simulated h., increased size of a part due to continued growth unrestrained by attritions, as is seen in the case of the teeth of certain animals when the opposing teeth have been destroyed.

true h., an increase in size involving all the different tissues composing the part.

vicarious h., h. of an organ following failure of another organ because of a functional relationship between them; e.g., enlargement of the pituitary gland, after destruction of the thyroid.

hy·per·tro·pia (hī′per-trō′pē-ă). An ocular deviation with one eye higher than the other. [hyper- + G. *tropē,* a turn]

hy·per·ty·ro·si·ne·mia (hī′per-tī′rō-si-nē′mē-ă). SYN tyrosinemia.

hy·per·ura·cil thy·mi·nu·ria (hī′per-oor′a-sil). An inherited disorder in which there are elevated levels of uracil and thymine in the urine; associated with a deficiency of dihydropyrimidine dehydrogenase and resultant impaired CNS function.

hy·per·u·ri·ce·mia (hī′per-ū-rē-sē′mē-ă). Enhanced blood concentrations of uric acid.

hy·per·u·ri·ce·mic (hī′per-ū-ri-sē′mik). Relating to or characterized by hyperuricemia.

hy·per·u·ri·cu·ria (hī′per-ū-ri-kū′rē-ă). Increased urinary excretion of uric acid.

hy·per·vac·ci·na·tion (hī′per-vak-si-nā′shŭn). Repeated inoculation of an individual already immunized; used as a means of preparing a highly potent antiserum.

hy·per·val·i·ne·mia (hī′per-val-i-nē′mē-ă). Abnormally high plasma concentrations of valine, a common finding in maple syrup urine disease.

hy·per·vas·cu·lar (hī′per-vas′kū-ler). Abnormally vascular; containing an excessive number of blood vessels. [hyper- + L. *vas,* a vessel]

hy·per·ven·ti·la·tion (hī′per-ven-ti-lā′shŭn). Increased alveolar ventilation relative to metabolic carbon dioxide production, so that alveolar carbon dioxide pressure decreases to below normal. SYN overventilation.

hy·per·vi·ta·min·o·sis (hī′per-vī′tă-mi-nō′sis). A condition resulting from the ingestion of an excessive amount of a vitamin preparation, symptoms varying according to the particular vitamin implicated; serious effects may be caused by overdosage with fat-soluble vitamins, especially A or D, and rarely with water-soluble vitamins.

hy·per·vo·le·mia (hī′per-vō-lē′mē-ă). Abnormally increased volume of blood. SYN plethora (1), repletion. [hyper- + L. *volumen,* volume, + G. *haima,* blood]

hy·per·vo·le·mic (hī′per-vō-lē′mik). Pertaining to or characterized by hypervolemia.

hy·per·vo·lia (hī-per-vō′lē-ă). Augmented water content or volume of a given compartment; e.g., cellular h.

hyp·es·the·sia (hī-pes-thē′zē-ă). Diminished sensitivity to stimulation. SYN hypoesthesia. [G. *hypo,* under, + *aisthēsis,* feeling]

olfactory h., SYN hyposmia.

hy·pha, pl. **hy·phae** (hī′fă, hī′fē). A branching tubular cell characteristic of the filamentous fungi (molds). In most species the hyphae are divided by cross-walls (septa) into multicellular hyphae; intercommunicating hyphae constitute a mycelium, the visible colony on natural substrates or artificial laboratory media. The terms hypha and mycelium often are used interchangeably. [G. *hyphē,* a web]

racquet h., a vegetative h. with distal ends of successive cells inflated, resembling a string of elongated snowshoes or tennis racquets; seen in many mycelial fungi, e.g., many dermatophyte species in culture.

spiral hyphae, hyphae that end in a flat or helical coil, as in laboratory colonies of *Trichophyton mentagrophytes.*

hyp·he·do·nia (hīp-hē-dō′nē-ă). A habitually lessened or attenuated degree of pleasure from that which should normally give great pleasure. [G. *hypo,* under, + *hēdonē,* pleasure]

hy·phe·ma (hī-fē′mă). Blood in the anterior chamber of the eye. [G. *hyphaimos,* suffused with blood]

hy·phe·mia (hī-fē′mē-ă). SYN hypovolemia. [hypo- + G. *haima,* blood]

intertropical h., tropical h., SYN ancylostomiasis.

Hy·pho·my·ces des·tru·ens (hī-fō-mī′sēs des′troo-enz). Older name for *Pythium insidiosum.*

Hy·pho·my·ce·tes (hī′fō-mī-sē′tēs). A class of fungi that includes all of the filamentous members of the Fungi Imperfecti that form neither acervuli nor pycnidia. No sexual reproduction occurs; most members of this group produce asexual spores. [G. *hyphe,* web, + *mykēs,* fungus]

hy·pho·my·co·sis (hī′fō-mī-kō′sis). A disease of horses and mules (rarely of humans) caused by the fungus *Pythium insidiosum* (*Hyphomyces destruens*), characterized by granulomatous and necrotic lesions that appear on the head and lower legs, ulcerate, and enlarge by subcutaneous extension.

hypn-. SEE hypno-.

hyp·na·gog·ic (hip-nă-goj′ik). Denoting a transitional state, related to the hypnoidal, preceding sleep; applied also to various hallucinations that may manifest themselves at that time. SEE hypnoidal. [hypno- + G. *agōgos,* leading]

hypno-, hypn-. Sleep, hypnosis. [G. *hypnos,*]

hyp·no·a·nal·y·sis (hip′nō-ă-nal′i-sis). Psychoanalysis or other psychotherapy which employs hypnosis as an adjunctive technique.

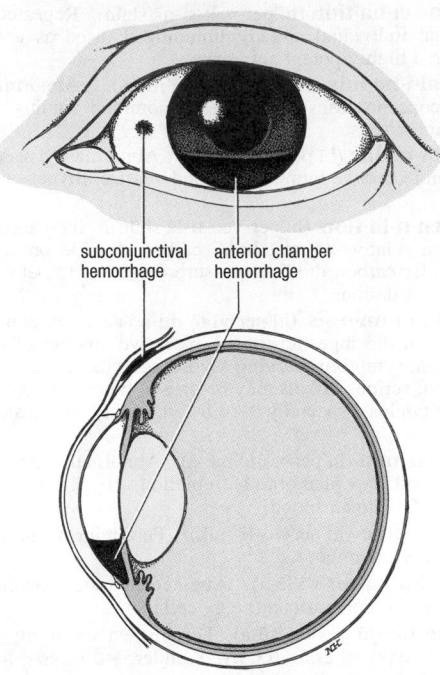

subconjunctival hemorrhage

anterior chamber hemorrhage

hyphema (anterior chamber hemorrhage) and subconjunctival hemorrhage

hyp·no·an·a·lyt·ic (hip′nō-an-ă-lit′ik). Pertaining to hypnoanalysis.

hyp·no·ca·thar·sis (hip′nō-kă-thar′sis). Ventilation of suppressed or repressed emotional tension, conflicts, and anxiety under hypnosis. [hypno- + G. *katharsis,* purification]

hyp·no·cyst (hip′nō-sist). A quiescent or "sleeping" cyst; an encysted protozoon, the reproductive activity of which is in abeyance. [hypno- + G. *kystis,* bladder (cyst)]

hyp·no·gen·e·sis (hip-nō-jen′ĕ-sis). The induction of sleep or of the hypnotic state. [hypno- + G. *genesis,* production]

hyp·no·gen·ic, hyp·nog·e·nous (hip-nō-jen′ik, -noj′ĕ-nŭs). **1.** Relating to hypnogenesis. **2.** An agent capable of inducing a hypnotic state. SEE hypnosis.

hypnoid. SYN hypnoidal.

hyp·noi·dal (hip-noy′dăl). Resembling hypnosis; denoting the subwaking state, a mental condition intermediate between sleeping and waking. SEE hypnagogic. SYN hypnoid. [hypno- + G. *eidos,* resemblance]

hyp·no·pho·bia (hip-nō-fō′bē-ă). Morbid fear of falling asleep. [hypno- + G. *phobos,* fear]

hyp·no·pom·pic (hip-nō-pom′pik). Denoting the occurrence of visions or dreams during the drowsy state following sleep. [hypno- + G. *pompē,* procession]

hyp·no·sis (hip-nō′sis). An artificially induced trancelike state, resembling somnambulism, in which the subject is highly susceptible to suggestion, oblivious to all else, and responds readily to the commands of the hypnotist; its scientific validity has been accepted and rejected through several cycles during the past two centuries. SEE mesmerism. SYN hypnotic sleep, hypnotic state. [G. *hypnos,* sleep, + *-osis,* condition]

lethargic h., the deep sleep following major h. SYN trance coma.

major h., a state of extreme suggestibility in h. in which the subject is insensible to all outside impressions except the commands of the hypnotist.

minor h., an induced state resembling normal sleep in which the subject is susceptible to suggestion, though not to the extent of catalepsy or somnambulism.

hyp·no·ther·a·py (hip-nō-thār′ă-pē). **1.** Psychotherapeutic treatment by means of hypnotism. **2.** Treatment of disease by inducing a trance-like sleep.

hyp·not·ic (hip-not′ik). **1.** Causing sleep. **2.** An agent that promotes sleep. SYN soporific (2). **3.** Relating to hypnotism. [G. *hypnōtikos,* causing one to sleep]

hyp·no·tism (hip′nō-tizm). **1.** The process or act of inducing hypnosis. SYN somnolism. **2.** The practice or study of hypnosis. SEE mesmerism. [G. *hypnos,* sleep]

hyp·no·tist (hip′nō-tist). One who practices hypnotism.

hyp·no·tize (hip′nō-tīz). To induct one into hypnosis.

hyp·no·zo·ite (hip-nō-zō′īt). Exoerythrocytic schizozoite of *Plasmodium vivax* or *P. ovale* in the human liver, characterized by delayed primary development; thought to be responsible for malarial relapse.

△**hypo-.** **1.** Prefix denoting deficient, below normal. SEE ALSO hyp-. Cf. sub-. **2.** In chemistry, denoting the lowest, or least rich in oxygen, of a series of chemical compounds. [G. *hypo,* under]

hy·po·a·cid·i·ty (hī′pō-a-sid′i-tē). A lower than normal degree of acidity, as of the gastric juice.

hy·po·a·cu·sis (hī′pō-ă-koo′sis). SYN hypacusis.

hy·po·a·de·nia (hī-pō-ă-dē′nē-ă). Any deficiency in the function of a glandular organ or tissue. [hypo- + G. *adēn,* gland]

hy·po·a·dre·nal·ism (hī′pō-ă-drē′năl-izm). Reduced adrenocortical function.

hy·po·al·bu·mi·ne·mia (hī′pō-al-boo-mi-nē′mē-ă). An abnormally low concentration of albumin in the blood. SYN hypalbuminemia.

hy·po·al·dos·ter·on·ism (hī′pō-al-dos′ter-on-izm). A condition due to deficient secretion of aldosterone; can occur in two forms: 1) as part of generalized adrenocortical insufficiency; 2) as a selective deficiency caused by a primary defect of the adrenal gland or a defect in control of aldosterone secretion.

hyporeninemic h., selective aldosterone deficiency resulting from low renin production.

isolated h., SYN selective h.

selective h., aldosterone deficiency without a concomitant deficiency of glucocorticoid hormones. SYN isolated h.

hy·po·al·do·ster·on·u·ria (hī′pō-al-dos′ter-on-oo′rē-ă). Abnormally low levels of aldosterone in the urine.

hy·po·al·ge·sia (hī-pō-al-jē′zē-ă). SYN hypalgesia. [hypo- + G. *algēsis,* a sense of pain]

hy·po·al·i·men·ta·tion (hī′pō-al-i-men-tā′shŭn). SYN subalimentation.

hy·po·az·o·tu·ria (hī′pō-az-ō-too′rē-ă). Excretion of abnormally small quantities of nonprotein nitrogenous material (especially urea) in the urine. SYN hypazoturia. [hypo- + Fr. *azote,* nitrogen, + G. *ouron,* urine]

hy·po·bar·ia (hī-pō-bar′ē-ă). SYN hypobarism.

hy·po·bar·ic (hī-pō-bar′ik). **1.** Pertaining to pressure of ambient gases below 1 atmosphere. **2.** With respect to solutions, less dense than the diluent or medium; e.g., in spinal anesthesia, a h. solution has a density lower than that of spinal fluid. [hypo- + G. *baros,* weight]

hy·po·bar·ism (hī-pō-bar′izm). Dysbarism resulting from decreasing barometric pressure on the body without hypoxia; gas in body cavities tends to expand, and gases dissolved in body fluids tend to come out of solution as bubbles. Cf. decompression *sickness.* SYN hypobaria.

hy·po·ba·rop·a·thy (hī′pō-ba-rop′ă-thē). Sickness produced by reduced barometric pressure; not always distinguished from hypobarism and altitude sickness. [hypo- + G. *baros,* weight, + *pathos,* suffering]

hy·po·be·ta·lip·o·pro·tein·e·mia (hī′pō-bā′tă-lip′ō-prō′tēn-ē′mē-ă) [MIM*107730]. Abnormally low levels of β-lipoproteins in the plasma, occasionally with acanthocytosis and neurological signs; autosomal dominant inheritance; caused by mutation in the apolipoprotein B gene (APOB) on 2p. SEE ALSO abetalipoproteinemia.

familial h., a disorder similar to abetalipoproteinemia; chylomicron formation still occurs, but LDL levels are typically low.

h. with apo B-37, a disorder in which LDL levels are very low, there is a mild fat malabsorption, and a truncated apolipoprotein B-37 is formed.

hy·po·blast (hī′pō-blast). Cell layer adjacent to the yolk sac cavity and subjacent to the epiblast of a bilayered embryo. [hypo- + G. *blastos,* germ]

hy·po·blas·tic (hī-pō-blas′tik). Relating to or derived from the hypoblast.

hy·po·bran·chi·al (hī-pō-brang′kē-ăl). Located beneath the branchial apparatus.

hy·po·bro·mite (hī-pō-brō′mīt). A salt of hypobromous acid.

hy·po·bro·mous ac·id (hī-pō-brō′mŭs). An acid, HOBr, the aqueous solution of which possesses oxidizing and bleaching properties.

hy·po·cal·ce·mia (hī′pō-kal-sē′mē-ă). Abnormally low levels of calcium in the circulating blood; commonly denotes subnormal concentrations of calcium ions.

differential diagnosis of hypocalcemia
hypoalbuminemia
chronic renal failure
magnesium deficiency
hypoparathyroidism
pseudohypoparathyroidism
osteomalacia and rickets due to vitamin D deficiency or resistance
acute hemorrhagic and edematous pancreatitis
healing phase of bone disease of treated hyperparathyroidism, hyperthyroidism, and hematologic malignancies (hungry bone syndrome)

hy·po·cal·ci·fi·ca·tion (hī′pō-kal-si-fi-kā′shŭn). Deficient calcification of bone or teeth.

enamel h. [MIM*104500], a defect of enamel maturation, characterized by soft opaque or yellowish white lusterless enamel. A variety of amelogenesis imperfecta. Autosomal dominant, autosomal recessive, and X-linked recessive forms exist.

hy·po·cap·nia (hī-pō-kap′nē-ă). Abnormally decreased arterial carbon dioxide tension. SYN hypocarbia. [hypo- + G. *kapnos,* smoke, vapor]

hy·po·car·bia (hī-pō-kar′bē-ă). SYN hypocapnia.

hy·po·ce·lom (hī-pō-sē′lom). Rarely used term for the ventral portion of the celom, or body cavity, of the embryo. [hypo- + G. *koilos,* hollow]

hy·po·chlor·e·mia (hī′pō-klō-rē′mē-ă). An abnormally low level of chloride ions in the circulating blood.

hy·po·chlor·e·mic (hī′pō-klō-rē′mik). Pertaining to or characterized by hypochloremia.

hy·po·chlor·hy·dria (hī′pō-klōr-hī′drē-ă, -hid′rĭ-ah). Presence of an abnormally small amount of hydrochloric acid in the stomach. SYN hypohydrochloria.

hy·po·chlo·rite (hī-pō-klōr′īt). A salt of hypochlorous acid.

hy·po·chlo·rous ac·id (hī-pō-klōr′ŭs). An acid, HOCl, having oxidizing and bleaching properties.

hy·po·chlor·u·ria (hī′pō-klōr-ū′rē-ă). Excretion of abnormally small quantities of chloride ions in the urine.

hy·po·cho·les·ter·e·mia (hī′pō-kō-les-tĕ-rē′mē-ă). SYN hypocholesterolemia.

hy·po·cho·les·ter·in·e·mia (hī′pō-kō-les′tĕ-ri-nē′mē-ă). SYN hypocholesterolemia.

hy·po·cho·les·ter·ol·e·mia (hī′pō-kō-les′ter-ol-ē′mē-ă). The presence of abnormally small amounts of cholesterol in the circulating blood. SYN hypocholesteremia, hypocholesterinemia.

hy·po·cho·lia (hī-pō-kō′lē-ă). Rarely used term for oligocholia.

hy·po·chon·dria (hī-pō-kon′drē-ă). SYN hypochondriasis.

hy·po·chon·dri·ac (hī-pō-kon′drē-ak). **1.** A person with a somatic overconcern, including morbid attention to the details of bodily functioning and exaggeration of any symptoms no matter how insignificant. **2.** A person manifesting hypochondriasis. **3.** Beneath the ribs; relating to the hypochondrium.

hy·po·chon·dri·a·cal (hī′pō-kon-drī′ă-kăl). Relating to or suffering from hypochondriasis.

hy·po·chon·dri·a·sis (hī′pō-kon-drī′ă-sis). A morbid concern about one's own health and exaggerated attention to any unusual bodily or mental sensations; a delusion that one is suffering from some disease for which no physical basis is evident. SYN hypochondria, hypochondriacal neurosis. [fr. hypochondrium, regarded as the site of hypochondria, + G. *-iasis,* condition]

hy·po·chon·dri·um, pl. **hy·po·chon·dria** (hī-pō-kon′drē-ŭm, -ă) [TA]. SYN hypochondriac *region.* [L. fr. G. *hypochondrion,* abdomen, belly, from *hypo,* under, + *chondros,* cartilage (of ribs)]

hy·po·chon·dro·pla·sia (hī′pō-kon-drō-plā′zē-ă) [MIM* 146000]. A skeletal dysplasia characterized by dwarfism with features similar to but much milder than achondroplasia; the skull and facies are normal; features not clinically evident until midchildhood. Autosomal dominant inheritance, caused in some cases by mutation in the fibroblast growth factor receptor 3 (FGFR3) gene on chromosome 4p. [hypo- + G. *chondros,* cartilage, + *plasis,* a molding]

hy·po·chord·al (hī-pō-kōr′dăl). On the ventral side of the spinal cord. [hypo- + G. *chordē,* cord]

hy·po·chro·ma·sia (hī′pō-krō-mā′zē-ă). SYN hypochromia.

hy·po·chro·mat·ic (hī′-pō-krō-mat′ik). Containing a small amount of pigment, or less than the normal amount for the individual tissue. SYN hypochromic (1). [hypo- + G. *chrōma,* color]

hy·po·chro·ma·tism (hī-pō-krō′mă-tizm). **1.** The condition of being hypochromatic. **2.** SYN hypochromia.

hy·po·chro·mia (hī-pō-krō′mē-ă). An anemic condition in which the percentage of hemoglobin in the red blood cells is less than the normal range. SYN hypochromasia, hypochromatism (2), hypochrosis. [hypo- + G. *chrōma,* color]

hy·po·chro·mic (hī-pō-krō′mik). **1.** SYN hypochromatic. **2.** Denoting decrease in light absorption with a shift in wavelength to a lower wavelength.

hy·po·chro·sis (hī-pō-krō′sis). SYN hypochromia. [hypo- + G. *chrōsis,* a tinting]

hy·po·chy·lia (hī-pō-kī′lē-ă). Rarely used term for oligochylia. [hypo- + G. *chylos,* juice]

hy·po·ci·ne·sis, hy·po·ci·ne·sia (hī′pō-si-nē′sis, -nē′zē-ă). SYN hypokinesis.

hy·po·cit·ra·tur·ia (hī′pō-si-trā-toor′ē-ă). Abnormally low concentration of citrate in the urine.

hy·po·com·ple·men·te·mia (hī′pō-kom′plĕ-men-tē′mē-ă). A condition in which one or another component of complement is lacking or reduced in amount; associated with immune complex diseases and cases of membranoproliferative glomerulonephritis in which nephritic factor is present. Various autosomal forms are known, domimant [MIM*120550 and MIM*120980] and recessive [MIM*216950 and MIM*217070].

hy·po·cone (hī′pō-kōn). The distolingual cusp of an upper molar tooth. [hypo- + G. *kōnos,* pine cone]

hy·po·con·id (hī-pō-kon′id). The distobuccal cusp of a lower molar tooth.

hy·po·con·ule (hī-pō-kon′ūl). The distal, or fifth, cusp of an upper molar tooth. [hypo- + Mod. L. dim. of L. *conus,* cone]

hy·po·con·u·lid (hī-pō-kon′ū-lid). The distal, or fifth, cusp of a lower molar tooth. [hypo- + Mod. L. dim. of L. *conus,* cone]

hy·po·cor·ti·coid·ism (hī-pō-kōr′ti-koyd-izm). SYN adrenocortical *insufficiency.*

hy·po·cu·pre·mia (hī′pō-koo-prē′mē-ă). Reduced copper content of the blood; found in Wilson disease because ceruloplasmin is depressed, even though serum albumin-attached copper is increased. [hypo- + L. *cuprum,* copper, + G. *haima,* blood]

hy·po·cy·cloi·dal (hī′-pō-sī-kloy′dăl). A tricyclic motion used by mechanical tomography units to optimize blurring and reduce artifacts. [hypo- + G. *kuklos,* circle, + *-oeidēs,* appearance]

hy·po·cys·tot·o·my (hī′pō-sis-tot′ō-mē). Perineal cystotomy.

hy

hy·po·cy·the·mia (hī′pō-sī-thē′mē-ă). Hypocytosis of the circulating blood, such as that observed in aplastic anemia. [hypo- + G. *kytos,* cell, + *haima,* blood]

hy·po·cy·to·sis (hī′pō-sī-tō′sis). Varying degrees of abnormally low numbers of red and white cells and other formed elements of the blood; in some instances, the term is also used to indicate a paucity of component cells of any tissue. SEE ALSO cytopenia, pancytopenia. [hypo- + G. *kytos,* cell, + *-osis,* condition]

hy·po·dac·ty·ly, hy·po·dac·tyl·ia, hy·po·dac·tyl·ism (hī′pō-dak′ti-lē, -dak-til′ē-ă, -dak′til-izm). Less than the full normal complement of digits. [hypo- + G. *daktylos,* finger]

hy·po·derm (hī′pō-derm). SYN subcutaneous *tissue.* [hypo- + G. *derma,* skin]

Hy·po·der·ma (hī-pō-der′mă). A genus of botflies whose larvae are the cause of a tropical form of myiasis linearis (cutaneous larva migrans) of man; occasionally they invade the interior of the eye. Two species, *H. bovis* and *H. lineatum,* are botflies of cattle. The ova of *H. bovis* are deposited on hairs of the legs, and the larvae penetrate the skin and migrate through the tissues to the skin of the back, where they appear during late winter as the common warbles; these ulcerate to the surface and mature larvae escape in early summer, fall to the ground, pupate, and give rise to a new generation of flies. [hypo- + G. *derma,* skin]

hy·po·der·mat·oc·ly·sis (hī′pō-der-mă-tok′li-sis). Rarely used spelling of hypodermoclysis.

hy·po·der·mat·o·my (hī′pō-der-mat′ō-mē). Subcutaneous division of a structure. [hypo- + G. *derma,* skin, + *tomē,* incision]

hy·po·der·ma·to·sis (hī′pō-der-mă-tō′sis). Infection of herbivores and humans with larvae of flies of the genus *Hypoderma.*

hy·po·der·mic (hī′pō-der′mik). **1.** SYN subcutaneous. **2.** SYN hypodermic *injection.* **3.** SYN hypodermic *syringe.*

hy·po·der·mis (hī-pō-der′mis). ✩official alternate term for subcutaneous *tissue.*

hy·po·der·moc·ly·sis (hī′pō-der-mok′li-sis). Subcutaneous injection of a saline or other solution. [hypo- + G. *derma,* skin, + *klysis,* a washing out]

hy·po·dip·loid (hī′-pō-dip′loid). Having a chromosome number less than the diploid number.

hy·po·dip·sia (hī-pō-dip′sē-ă). A physiologic condition, perhaps caused by hypertonicity of body fluids, insufficient to initiate drinking but at times sufficient to sustain drinking when started; loosely, oligodipsia. SYN insensible thirst, subliminal thirst. [hypo- + G. *dipsa,* thirst]

hy·po·don·tia (hī-pō-don′shē-ă). A condition of having fewer than the normal complement of teeth, either congenital or acquired. SYN oligodontia, partial anodontia. [hypo- + G. *odous,* tooth]

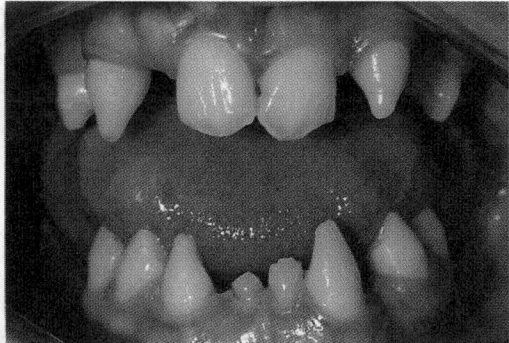

hypodontia: dentition demonstrating retained deciduous teeth and the absence of numerous permanent teeth that never developed

hy·po·dy·nam·ia (hī′pō-dī-nā′mē-ă, -dī-nam′ē-ă). Diminished power. [hypo- + G. *dynamis,* force]
　h. cor′dis, diminished force of cardiac contraction.

hy·po·dy·nam·ic (hī′pō-dī-nam′ik). Possessing or exhibiting subnormal power or force.

hy·po·ec·cri·sis (hī′pō-ek′ri-sis). Reduced excretion of waste matter. [hypo- + G. *eccrisis,* separation]

hy·po·ec·crit·ic (hī′pō-ĕ-krit′ik). Characterized by hypoeccrisis.

hy·po·ech·o·ic (hī′pō-e-kō′ik). A region in an ultrasound image in which the echoes are weaker or fewer than normal or in the surrounding regions. [hypo- + echo + -ic]

hy·po·e·o·sin·o·phil·ia (hī′pō-ē′ō-sin-ō-fil′ē-ă). SYN eosinopenia.

hy·po·es·o·pho·ria (hī′pō-es-ō-fō′rē-ă). A tendency of the visual axis of one eye to deviate downward and inward, prevented by binocular vision. [hypo- + G. *esō,* within, + *phoros,* bearing]

hy·po·es·the·sia (hī′pō-es-thē′zē-ă). SYN hypesthesia.

hy·po·ex·o·pho·ria (hī′pō-ek-sō-fō′rē-ă). A tendency of the visual axis of one eye to deviate downward and outward, prevented by binocular vision. [hypo- + G. *exō,* without, + *phoros,* bearing]

hy·po·fer·re·mia (hī′pō-fer-ē′mē-ă). A deficiency of iron in the circulating blood.

hy·po·fi·brin·o·ge·ne·mia (hī′pō-fī-brin′ō-jě-nē′mē-ă). Abnormally low concentration of fibrinogen in the circulating blood plasma.

hypofrontality (hī′pō-fron-tal′i-tē). A decrease in the neuronal activity of various areas of the frontal lobes, arising from various etiologies and associated with a number of clinical symptoms or disorders.

hy·po·func·tion (hī′pō-fŭnk-shŭn). Reduced, low, or inadequate function.

hy·po·ga·lac·tia (hī′pō-ga-lak′shē-ă). Less than normal milk secretion. [hypo- + G. *gala,* milk]

hy·po·ga·lac·tous (hī′pō-ga-lak′tŭs). Producing or secreting a less than normal amount of milk.

hy·po·gam·ma·glo·bi·ne·mia (hī′pō-gam′ă-glō′bi-nē′mē-ă). SYN hypogammaglobulinemia.

hy·po·gam·ma·glob·u·lin·e·mia (hī′pō-gam′ă-glob′ū-li-nē′mē-ă). Decreased quantity of the gamma fraction of serum globulin; sometimes used loosely to denote decreased quantity of immunoglobulins in general; associated with increased susceptibility to pyogenic infections. SYN hypogammaglobinemia.
　acquired h., SYN common variable *immunodeficiency.*
　primary h., h. due to a primary immunodeficiency of immunoglobulin-forming cells (B-lymphocytes).
　secondary h., SYN secondary *immunodeficiency.*
　transient h. of infancy, a type of primary immunodeficiency that occurs in infants of both sexes, usually before the sixth month of life, probably resulting from immaturity of lymphoid tissue. SYN transient agammaglobulinemia.
　X-linked h., X-linked infantile h., a congenital, primary immunodeficiency characterized by decreased numbers (or absence) of circulating B lymphocytes with corresponding decrease in immunoglobulins of the five classes; associated with marked susceptibility to infection by pyogenic bacteria (notably, pneumococci and *Haemophilus influenzae*) beginning after loss of maternal antibodies; X-linked recessive inheritance caused by mutation in the Bruton tyrosine kinase gene (BTK) on Xq.
　X-linked h. with growth hormone deficiency, h. combined with a reduced number of B cells; characterized by short stature, delayed puberty, and recurrent infections.

hy·po·gan·gli·o·no·sis (hī′pō-gang-lē-on-ō′sis). A reduction in the number of ganglionic nerve cells.

hy·po·gas·tric (hī-pō-gas′trik). Relating to the hypogastrium.

hy·po·gas·tri·um (hī′pō-gas′trē-ŭm) [TA]. SYN pubic *region,* pubic *region.* [G. *hypogastrion,* lower belly, fr. *hypo,* under, + *gastēr,* belly]

hy·po·gas·tro·cele (hī′pō-gas′trō-sēl). Hernia of the lower part of the abdomen. [hypogastrium + G. *kēlē,* hernia]

hy·po·gas·trop·a·gus (hī′pō-gas-trop′ă-gŭs). Twins joined at the hypogastrium. SEE conjoined *twins,* under *twin.* [hypogastrium + G. *pagos,* fr. *pēgnynai,* to fasten]

hy·po·gas·tros·chi·sis (hī′pō-gas-tros′ki-sis). Congenital fissure of the abdominal wall in the hypogastric region. [hypogastrium + G. *schisis,* cleaving]

hy·po·gen·e·sis (hī′pō-jen′ě-sis). Congenital defect of growth with underdevelopment of parts or organs of the body. [hypo- + G. *genesis,* origin]

polar h., a less than normal degree of development at the cephalic or caudal extremity of the embryo.

hy·po·ge·net·ic (hī′pō-jĕ-net′ik). Relating to hypogenesis.

hy·po·gen·i·tal·ism (hī-pō-jen′i-tăl-izm). Partial or complete failure of maturation of the genitalia; commonly, a consequence of hypogonadism.

hy·po·geu·sia (hī-pō-gū′sē-ă). Diminished sense of taste. It may be: 1) general to all tastants, partial to some tastants, or specific to one or more tastants; 2) due to transport disorders (in access to the interior of the taste bud) or to sensorineural disorders (affecting the gustatory sensory cells or nerves or the central gustatory neural pathways); and 3) hereditary or acquired. [hypo- + G. *geusis,* taste]

hy·po·glob·u·lia (hī′pō-glo-bū′lē-ă). Obsolete term for abnormally low numbers of red blood cells in the circulating blood; also used infrequently with reference to abnormally decreased proportions of erythroid elements in the bone marrow. [hypo- + G. *globulus,* globule]

hy·po·glos·sal (hī-pō-glos′ăl). 1. Below the tongue. 2. Relating to the twelfth cranial nerve, nervus hypoglossus. SYN hypoglossus. [L. *hypoglossus* fr. hypo- + *glossus,* tongue]

hy·po·glos·sis (hī-pō-glos′is). SYN hypoglottis.

hy·po·glos·sus (hī′pō-glos′ŭs). SYN hypoglossal, hypoglossal. [L.]

hy·po·glot·tis (hī′pō-glot′is). The undersurface of the tongue. SYN hypoglossis. [G. *hypoglōssis,* or *-glōttis,* undersurface of tongue, fr. *hypo,* under, + *glōssa,* tongue]

hy·po·gly·ce·mia (hī′pō-glī-sē′mē-ă). 1. Symptoms resulting from low blood glucose (normal glucose range 60–100 mg/dL (3.3 to 5.6 mmol/L)) which are either autonomic or neuroglycopenic. Autonomic symptoms include sweating, trembling, feelings of warmth, anxiety, and nausea. Neuroglycopenic symptoms include feelings of dizziness, confusion, tiredness, difficulty speaking, headache and inability to concentrate. 2. Organic disease more often leads to neuroglycopenic symptoms, functional disorders to autonomic symptoms. Functional hypoglycemia is of doubtful existence; the so-called post-prandial hypoglycemic syndrome has not been confirmed by blood sugar measurements. No convincing evidence has been found of the existence of early-diabetes hypoglycemia, or alimentary hypoglycemia. SYN glucopenia.

fasting h., excessively low blood glucose in association with fasting; can be seen in patients with hyperinsulinism but also occurs without definable disease.

ketotic h., the most common form of childhood h. after the neonatal period; it usually presents between the ages of 18 months and 5 years, and resolves spontaneously by late childhood; manifested by hypoglycemic episodes usually occurring during minor illnesses that cause decreased appetite; probably due to a defect in gluconeogenesis and limited glycogen stores.

leucine h., reduction in blood glucose concentration produced by administration of leucine; believed to reflect the ability of this amino acid to stimulate insulin secretion.

leucine-induced h., rare cause of h. occurring following ingestion of leucine. Seen especially in infants. SYN leucine-sensitive h.

leucine-sensitive h., SYN leucine-induced h.

mixed h., h. due to more than one cause.

neonatal h. [MIM*240900], familial onset of symptomatic h. during infancy, with persistently low blood glucose; a variant form [MIM*240800] is leucine-induced with hyperinsulinism and variable mental retardation.

hy·po·gly·ce·mic (hī′pō-glī-sē′mik). Pertaining to or characterized by hypoglycemia.

hy·po·gly·co·gen·ol·y·sis (hī′pō-glī′kō-jĕ-nol′i-sis). Deficient glycogenolysis.

hy·po·gly·cor·rha·chia (hī′pō-glī-kō-rak′ē-ă). Depressed concentration of glucose in the cerebrospinal fluid; a characteristic of bacterial, fungal, and tuberculous meningitis. [hypo- + G. *glykys,* sweet, + *rhachis,* spine]

hy·pog·na·thous (hī′pō-nath′ŭs, hī-pog′na-thŭs). Having a congenitally defectively developed small lower jaw. [hypo- + G. *gnathos,* jaw]

hy·pog·na·thus (hī′pō-nath′ŭs, hī-pog′na-thŭs). Unequal conjoined twins in which the rudimentary parasite is attached to the mandible of the autosite. SEE conjoined *twins,* under *twin.* [hypo- + G. *gnathos,* jaw]

hy·po·go·nad·ism (hī′pō-gō′nad-izm). Inadequate gonadal function, as manifested by deficiencies in gametogenesis and/or the secretion of gonadal hormones; results in atrophy or deficient development of secondary sexual characteristics and, when occurring in prepubertal males, in altered body habitus characterized by a short trunk and long limbs.

familial hypogonadotropic h. [MIM*312100 & MIM*307300], a group of disorders characterized by failure of sexual development, owing to inadequate secretion of pituitary gonadotropins; perhaps X-linked, but probably autosomal dominant and recessive modes of inheritance also exist.

hypergonadotropic h., defective gonadal development or function of the gonads, resulting from elevated levels of gonadotropins.

hypogonadotropic h., defective gonadal development or function, or both, resulting from inadequate secretion of pituitary gonadotropins. SYN hypogonadotropic eunuchoidism, secondary h.

male h., SYN eunuchoidism.

primary h., defective gonadal development or function, or both, due to abnormality or loss of the gonad itself.

secondary h., SYN hypogonadotropic h.

h. with anosmia, failure of sexual development secondary to inadequate secretion of pituitary gonadotrophins, associated with anosmia due to agenesis of the olfactory lobes of the brain. Autosomal dominant [MIM*147950], autosomal recessive [MIM*244200], and X-linked recessive [MIM*308700] forms exist; the X-linked form is caused by mutation in the Kallmann gene (KAL1) on Xp. SYN Kallmann syndrome.

hy·po·go·nad·o·tro·pic (hī′pō-gon′ă-dō-trop′ik). Indicating inadequate secretion of gonadotropins and its consequences.

hy·po·gran·u·lo·cy·to·sis (hī′pō-gran′ū-lō-sī-tō′sis). SYN granulocytopenia.

hy·po·he·pat·ia (hī′pō-hĕ-pat′ē-ă). Rarely used term for underfunctioning of the liver. [hypo- + G. *hēpar,* liver]

hy·po·hi·dro·sis (hī′pō-hī-drō′sis). Diminished perspiration.

hy·po·hy·dre·mia (hī′pō-hī-drē′mē-ă). Any deficiency in the amount of fluid in the blood. [hypo- + G. *hydōr,* water, + *haima,* blood]

hy·po·hy·dro·chlo·ria (hī′pō-hī-drō-klōr′ē-ă). SYN hypochlorhydria.

hy·po·i·so·ton·ic (hī′pō-ī-sō-ton′ik). SYN hypotonic.

hy·po·ka·le·mia (hī′pō-ka-lē′mē-ă). The presence of an abnormally small concentration of potassium ions in the circulating blood; occurs in familial periodic paralysis and in potassium depletion due to excessive loss from the gastrointestinal tract or kidneys. The changes of h. may include vacuolation of renal tubular epithelial cytoplasm with impairment of urinary concentrating power and acidification, flattening of the T wave of the electrocardiogram, and muscle weakness. SYN hypopotassemia. [hypo- + Mod. L. *kalium,* potassium, + G. *haima,* blood]

hy·po·ki·ne·mia (hī′pō-ki-nē′mē-ă). Reduced circulation rate; reduced volume flow through the circulation; subnormal cardiac output. [hypo- + G. *kineo,* to move, + *haima,* blood]

hy·po·ki·ne·sis, hy·po·ki·ne·sia (hī′pō-ki-nē′sis, -nē′zē-ă). Diminished or slow movement. SYN hypocinesis, hypocinesia, hypomotility. [hypo- + G. *kinēsis,* movement]

hy·po·ki·net·ic (hī′pō-ki-net′ik). Relating to or characterized by hypokinesis.

hy·po·leu·ke·mia (hī′pō-loo-kē′mē-ă). SYN subleukemic *leukemia.*

hy·po·ley·dig·ism (hī-pō-lī′dig-izm). Subnormal secretion of androgens by the interstitial (Leydig) cells of the testes.

hy

hy·po·lip·o·pro·teine·mia (hī′pō-lip′ō-prō-tēn-ē-mē-ă). Decreased levels of a lipoprotein in the serum.

hy·po·li·po·sis (hī′pō-li-pō′sis). Presence of an abnormally small amount of fat in the tissues.

hy·po·lo·gia (hī′pō-lō′jē-ă). Lack of ability for speech. [hypo- + G. *logos,* word]

hy·po·lym·phe·mia (hī′pō-lim-fē′mē-ă). Abnormally small numbers of lymphocytes in the circulating blood.

hy·po·mag·ne·se·mia (hī′pō-mag-nē-sē′mē-ă). Subnormal blood serum concentration of magnesium; may cause convulsions and concurrent hypocalcemia.

hy·po·ma·nia (hī′pō-mā′nē-ă). A mild degree of mania.

hy·po·mas·tia (hī′pō-mas′tē-ă). Atrophy or congenital smallness of the breasts. [hypo- + G. *mastos,* breast]

hy·po·mel·an·cho·lia (hī′pō-mel-an-kō′lē-ă). A mild degree of mental depression.

hy·po·mel·a·no·sis (hī′pō-mel-ă-nō′sis). SYN leukoderma.
h. of Ito [MIM*146150 and MIM*308300], not a specific entity but rather represents features of many different forms of mosaicism; characterized by unilateral or bilateral hypopigmented macules in whorls, streaks, and patches in a "marble-cake" pattern, variably associated with epidermal nevi, alopecia, and ocular, skeletal, and neural abnormalities. SEE ALSO *incontinentia* pigmenti. SYN incontinentia pigmenti achromians.

hy·po·me·lia (hī-pō-mē′lē-ă). General term for hypoplasia of some or all parts of one or more limbs. [hypo- + G. *melos,* limb]

hy·po·men·or·rhea (hī′pō-men-ō-rē′ă). Diminution of the flow or a shortening of the duration of menstruation. [hypo- + G. *mēn,* month, + *rhoia,* flow]

hy·po·mere (hī′pō-mēr). **1.** The portion of the myotome that extends ventrolaterally to form body-wall and limb muscle, innervated by the primary ventral ramus of a spinal nerve. SEE hypaxial. **2.** Less commonly, the somatic and splanchnic layers of the lateral mesoderm which give rise to the lining of the celom. [hypo- + G. *meros,* part]

hy·po·me·tab·o·lism (hī′pō-me-tab′ō-lizm). Reduced metabolism. SEE ALSO hypometabolic *state.*
euthyroid h., an unusual condition resembling myxedema but with an apparently normal thyroid gland.

hy·po·met·ria (hī-pō-mē′trē-ă). Ataxia characterized by underreaching an object or goal; seen with cerebellar disease. Cf. hypermetria. [hypo- + G. *metron,* measure]

hy·pom·ne·sia (hī-pō-nē′zē-ă). Impaired memory. Cf. hypermnesia. [hypo- + G. *mnēmē,* memory]

hy·po·morph (hī′pō-mōrf). **1.** A person whose standing height is short in proportion to the sitting height, owing to shortness of the limbs. Cf. hypermorph, endomorph. **2.** A mutant gene that causes a partial decrease in the activity controlled by the gene. Cf. hypermorph. [hypo- + G. *morphē,* form]

hy·po·mo·til·i·ty (hī′pō-mō-til′i-tē). SYN hypokinesis.

hy·po·my·e·li·na·tion, hy·po·my·e·lin·o·gen·e·sis (hī′pō-mī′ĕ-lin-ā-shun, -ō-jen′ĕ-sis). Defective formation of myelin in the spinal cord and brain; the basis for a number of demyelinating diseases.

hy·po·my·o·to·nia (hī′pō-mī-ō-tō′nē-ă). A condition of diminished muscular tonus. [hypo- + G. *mys (myo-)* muscle, + *tonos,* tension]

hy·po·myx·ia (hī′pō-mik′sē-ă). A condition in which the secretion of mucus is diminished. [hypo- + G. *myxa,* mucus]

hy·po·na·tre·mia (hī′pō-nă-trē′mē-ă). Abnormally low concentrations of sodium ions in the circulating blood. [hypo- + natrium, + G. *haima,* blood]
depletional h., decreased serum sodium concentration associated with loss of sodium from the circulating blood via the GI tract, kidney, skin, or into "third space." Accompanied by hypovolemic and hypotonic state.

hy·po·ne·o·cy·to·sis (hī′pō-nē′ō-sī-tō′sis). Leukopenia associated with the presence of immature and young leukocytes (especially in the granulocytic series), i.e., a "shift to the left" in the hemo-

gram. SYN hyposkeocytosis. [hypo- + G. *neos,* new, + *kytos,* cell, + *-osis,* condition]

hy·po·noia (hī′pō-noy′-ă). Deficient or sluggish mental activity or imagination. [hypo- + G. *noeō,* to think]

hy·po·nych·i·al (hī′pō-nik′ē-ăl). **1.** SYN subungual. **2.** Relating to the hyponychium.

hy·po·nych·i·um (hī′pō-nik′ē-ŭm) [TA]. The epithelium of the nail bed, particularly its proximal part in the region of the nailroot and lunula, forming the nail matrix. [hypo- + G. *onyx,* nail]

hy·pon·y·chon (hī-pon′i-kon). Subungual hemorrhage. [hypo- + G. *onyx,* nail]

hy·po·on·cot·ic (hī′pō-on-kot′ik). Indicating an oncotic pressure less than normal, e.g., of blood plasma.

hy·po·or·tho·cy·to·sis (hī′pō-ōr′thō-sī-tō′sis). Leukopenia in which the relative numbers of the various types of white blood cells are within the normal range, and no immature cells are found in the circulating blood. [hypo- + G. *orthos,* correct, + *kytos,* cell, + *-osis,* condition]

hy·po·o·var·i·an·ism (hī′pō-ō-vā′rē-an-izm). Inadequate ovarian function, commonly referring to reduced secretion of ovarian hormones. SYN hypovarianism.

hy·po·pan·cre·a·tism (hī′pō-pan′krē-ă-tizm). A condition of diminished activity of digestive enzyme secretion by the pancreas.

hy·po·pan·cre·or·rhea (hī′pō-pan′krē-ō-rē′ă). Reduced delivery of pancreatic digestive enzyme secretions. [hypo- + pancreas + G. *rhoia,* flow]

hy·po·par·a·thy·roid·ism (hī′pō-par-ă-thī′royd-izm). A condition due to diminution or absence of the secretion of the parathyroid hormones, with low serum calcium and tetany, and sometimes with increased bone density. SEE ALSO pseudohypoparathyroidism. SYN parathyroid insufficiency.
familial h., inherited isolated h. characterized by hypocalcemia, hyperphosphatemia, cataracts, intracerebral calcifications, and tetany; all three mendelian forms (sex-linked, autosomal dominant and recessive) of inheritance are known [MIM*146200, MIM*241400, and MIM*307700]. The autosomal dominant form is caused by mutation in either the parathyroid hormone gene (PTH) on chromosome 11p or the calcium sensing receptor gene (CASR) on 3q.

hy·po·pep·sia (hī-pō-pep′sē-ă). Impaired digestion, especially that due to a deficiency of pepsin. SYN oligopepsia. [hypo- + G. *pepsis,* digestion]

hy·po·per·i·stal·sis (hī′pō-per-i-stal′sis). Reduced or inadequate peristalsis.

hy·po·pha·lan·gism (hī′pō-fă-lan′jizm). Congenital absence of one or more of the phalanges of a finger or toe.

hy·po·phar·ynx (hī′pō-far′inks). ☆official alternate term for laryngopharynx.

hy·po·pho·ne·sis (hī′pō-fō-nē′sis). In percussion or auscultation, a sound that is diminished or fainter than usual. [hypo- + G. *phōnēsis,* a sounding]

hy·po·pho·nia (hī′pō-fō′nē-ă). An abnormally weak voice due to incoordination of the muscles concerned in vocalization. SYN leptophonia, microphonia, microphony. [hypo- + G. *phōnē,* voice]

hy·po·pho·ria (hī′pō-fō′rē-ă). A tendency of the visual axis of one eye to deviate downward, prevented by binocular vision. [hypo- + G. *phora,* motion]

hy·po·phos·pha·ta·se·mia (hī′pō-fos′fă-tă-sē′mē-ă). SYN hypophosphatasia.

hy·po·phos·pha·ta·sia (hī′pō-fos′fă-tā′zē-ă). An abnormally low content of alkaline phosphatase in the circulating blood. SYN hypophosphatasemia.
adult h., an autosomal dominant trait with early loss of teeth, bowing, and beaten-copper skull; there is evidence that the basic defect is in liver alkaline phosphatase.
childhood h., a relatively mild autosomal recessive form of h.; it may be allelic with congenital h.
congenital h. [MIM*241500], a rare disorder associated with a low level of serum alkaline phosphatase, hyperphosphaturia, hypercalcemia, skeletal abnormalities, pathologic fractures, craniostenosis, premature loss of teeth, and often early death; eyes may

show blue sclerae, lid retraction, band-shaped keratopathy, cataracts, papilledema, and optic atrophy; autosomal recessive inheritance, caused by mutation in the liver alkaline phosphatase gene (ALPL) on chromosome 1p.

hy·po·phos·pha·te·mia (hī′pō-fos-fă-tē′mē-ă). Abnormally low concentrations of phosphates in the circulating blood. See also entries under rickets.

hy·po·phos·pha·tu·ria (hī′pō-fos′fă-too′rē-ă). Reduced urinary excretion of phosphates.

hy·po·phos·pho·rous ac·id (hī-pō-fos′fō-rŭs). An aqueous solution containing 31% HPH_2O_2; used as a stabilizing reducing agent in pharmaceutical preparations.

hy·po·phra·sia (hī′pō-frā′zē-ă). Slowness or lack of speech associated with a psychosis or brain injury. [hypo- + G. *phrasis,* speaking]

hy·po·phy·se·al (hī′pō-fiz′ē-ăl). SYN hypophysial.

hy·po·phy·sec·to·mize (hī′pof-i-sek′tō-mīz). To remove the pituitary gland.

hy·poph·y·sec·to·my (hī′pof-i-sek′tō-mē). Surgical removal of the hypophysis or pituitary gland.

hy·po·phys·e·o·priv·ic (hī′pō-fiz′ē-ō-priv′ik). SYN hypophysioprivic.

hy·po·phys·e·o·tro·pic (hī′pō-fiz′ē-ō-trop′ik). SYN hypophysiotropic.

hy·po·phy·si·al (hī′pō-fiz′ē-ăl). Relating to a hypophysis. SYN hypophyseal.

hy·poph·y·sin (hī-pof′i-sin). An aqueous extract of the posterior lobe of the fresh hypophysis of cattle; contains oxytocin and vasopressin.

hy·po·phys·i·o·priv·ic (hī′pō-fiz′ē-ō-priv′ik). Denoting the condition in which the pituitary gland may be functionally inactive or may be absent, as after hypophysectomy. SYN hypophyseoprivic. [hypophysis + L. *privus,* deprived of]

hy·po·phys·i·o·tro·pic (hī′pō-fiz′ē-ō-trop′ik). Denoting a stimulatory hormone that acts on the pituitary gland (hypophysis). SYN hypophyseotropic.

hy·poph·y·sis (hī-pof′i-sis) [TA]. SYN pituitary *gland.* SEE ALSO hypothalamus. [G. an undergrowth]

h. cere′bri, SYN pituitary *gland.*

pharyngeal h., residual tissue derived from the hypophysial diverticulum that lies in the lamina propria of the nasopharynx; its cells and their arrangement are identical with those of the pars distalis. SYN pars pharyngea hypophyseos.

h. sic′ca, SYN posterior *pituitary.*

hy·poph·y·si·tis (hī-pof-i-sī′tis). Inflammation of the hypophysis.

lymphocytic h., an acute anterior pituitary lymphocytic reaction characterized clinically by signs and symptoms of anterior pituitary insufficiency; probably an autoimmune disorder because antipituitary antibodies are present in the serum. SYN lymphoid h.

lymphoid h., SYN lymphocytic h.

hy·po·pi·e·sis (hī′pō-pī-ē′sis). SYN hypotension (1). [hypo- + G. *piesis,* pressure]

orthostatic h., SYN orthostatic *hypotension.*

hypopigmentation (hī′pō-pig-men-tā′shun). Deficiency of cutaneous melanin relative to surrounding skin. SEE albinism. [hypo- + pigmentation]

hy·po·pi·tu·i·ta·rism (hī′pō-pi-too′i-tă-rizm). A condition due to diminished activity of the anterior lobe of the hypophysis, with inadequate secretion, to varying degrees, of one or more anterior pituitary hormones.

hy·po·pla·sia (hī′pō-plā′zē-ă). **1.** Underdevelopment of a tissue or organ, usually due to a deficiency in the number of cells. **2.** Atrophy due to destruction of some of the elements and not merely to their general reduction in size. [hypo- + G. *plasis,* a molding]

cartilage-hair h. [MIM*250250 & MIM*250460], a skeletal dysplasia prevalent among the Amish, characterized by short-limb dwarfism, sparse, light-colored hair, T-cell immunologic defect rendering them susceptible to infections, and radiographic findings of metaphyseal dysplasia. Autosomal recessive inheritance, the gene maps to 9p. SYN McKusick metaphyseal dysplasia.

enamel h., a developmental disturbance of teeth characterized by deficient or defective enamel matrix formation; may be hereditary, as in amelogenesis imperfecta, or acquired, as encountered in dental fluorosis, local infection, childhood fevers, and congenital syphilis.

focal dermal h. [MIM*305600], inherited as an X-linked dominant with in utero lethality in males; characterized by linear areas of dermal atrophy or hypoplasia, herniation of fat through the dermal defects, and papillomata of the mucus membranes or skin; may be associated with digital, ocular, and oral anomalies; mental retardation; and bony striations. SYN Goltz syndrome.

optic nerve h., congenitally small optic disk resulting from a reduced number of retinal ganglion cells and, therefore, a reduced number of axons; visual impairment may be marked. SEE de Morsier *syndrome.*

renal h., an abnormally small kidney that is morphologically normal but has either a reduced number of nephrons or smaller nephrons.

h. of right ventricle, failure of development of the right ventricle resulting in its having little muscle and much connective tissue instead of the reverse.

right ventricular h., SYN parchment *heart.*

thymic h., SYN DiGeorge *syndrome.*

hy·po·plas·tic (hī′pō-plas′tik). Pertaining to or characterized by hypoplasia.

hy·po·pnea (hī-pop′nē-ă). Breathing that is shallower, and/or slower, than normal. SYN oligopnea. [hypo- + G. *pnoē,* breathing]

hy·po·po·sia (hī′pō-pō′sē-ă). Hypodipsia, primarily due to reduced tendency to drink rather than the reduced sensation of thirst. [hypo- + G. *posis,* drinking]

hy·po·po·tas·se·mia (hī′pō-pō-ta-sē′mē-ă). SYN hypokalemia.

hy·po·pro·ac·cel·er·i·ne·mia (hī′pō-prō-ak-sel′er-i-nē′mē-ă). Abnormally low concentration of blood-clotting factor V, i.e., proaccelerin, in the circulating blood.

hy·po·pro·con·ver·ti·ne·mia (hī′pō-prō-kon-ver′ti-nē′mē-ă). Abnormally low concentration of blood-clotting factor VII, i.e., proconvertin, in the circulating blood; a deficiency causes a quantitative prolongation of the prothrombin time.

hy·po·pro·tein·e·mia (hī′pō-prō′tē-in-ē′mē-ă, -prō-tēn-). Abnormally small amounts of total protein in the circulating blood plasma.

hy·po·pro·tein·o·sis (hī′pō-prō′tē-in-o′sis, -prō′tēn-). A condition, especially in children, due to a dietary deficiency of protein; characterized by anorexia, vomiting, retardation of growth, anemia, and increased susceptibility to infections.

hy·po·pro·throm·bin·e·mia (hī′pō-prō-throm′bin-ē′mē-ă). Abnormally small amounts of prothrombin in the circulating blood. SYN prothrombinopenia.

hy·pop·ty·a·lism (hī′pō-tī′ă-lizm). SYN hyposalivation. [hypo- + G. *ptyalon,* saliva]

hy·po·py·on (hī-pō′pi-on). The presence of leukocytes in the anterior chamber of the eye. [hypo- + G. *pyon,* pus]

recurrent h., SYN Behçet *syndrome.*

hy·po·re·flex·ia (hī′pō-rē-flek′sē-ă). A condition in which the reflexes are weakened.

hy·po·ren·i·ne·mia (hī′pō-ren-i-nē′mē-ă). Low levels of renin in the circulating blood.

hy·po·ren·i·nem·ic (hī′pō-ren-i-nē′mik). Denoting or characterized by hyporeninemia.

hy·po·ri·bo·fla·vin·o·sis (hī′pō-rī′bō-flā-vi-nō′sis). A more correct term than the more commonly used ariboflavinosis, *q.v.*

hy·po·sal·i·va·tion (hī′pō-sal′i-vā′shŭn). Reduced salivation. SYN hypoptyalism.

hy·pos·che·ot·o·my (hī-pos-kē-ot′ō-mē). Incision or puncture into a hydrocele at its most dependent point. [hypo- + G. *oscheon,* scrotum, + *tomē,* incision]

hy·po·scle·ral (hī-pō-sklēr′ăl). Beneath the sclerotic coat of the eyeball.

hy

hy·po·sen·si·tiv·i·ty (hī′pō-sen-si-tiv′i-tē). A condition of subnormal sensitivity, in which the response to a stimulus is unusually delayed or lessened in degree.

hy·po·sen·si·ti·za·tion. SYN desensitization.

hy·po·ske·o·cy·to·sis (hī′pō-skē′ō-sī-tō′sis). SYN hyponeocytosis. [hypo- + *skaios,* left, + *kytos,* cell, + *-osis,* condition]

hy·pos·mia (hī-poz′mē-ă). Diminished sense of smell. It may be: 1) general to all odorants, partial to some odorants, or specific to one or more odorants; 2) due to transport disorders (in nasal obstruction) or to sensorineural disorders (affecting the olfactory neuroepithelium or the central olfactory neural pathways); and 3) hereditary or acquired. SYN olfactory hypesthesia. [hypo- + G. *osmē,* smell]

hy·pos·mo·sis (hī-pos-mō′sis). A reduction in the rapidity of osmosis.

hy·pos·mot·ic (hī-pos-mot′ik). Having an osmolality less than another fluid, ordinarily assumed to be plasma or extracellular fluid.

hy·po·so·ma·to·tro·pism (hī′pō-sō′mă-tō-trō′pizm). A state characterized by deficient secretion of pituitary growth hormone (somatotropin).

hy·po·so·mia (hī′pō-sō′mē-ă). Inadequate development of the body. [hypo- + G. *sōma,* body]

hy·po·som·ni·ac (hī′pō-som′nē-ak). A person with a reduction in sleep time. [hypo- + L. *somnus,* sleep]

hy·po·spa·di·ac (hī′pō-spā′dē-ak). Relating to hypospadias.

hy·po·spa·di·as (hī′pō-spā′dē-ăs). A developmental anomaly characterized by a defect on the ventral surface of the penis so that the urethral meatus is proximal to its normal glanular location; may be associated with chordee; also a similar defect in the female in which the urethra opens into the vagina. Cf. epispadias. SYN urogenital sinus anomaly. [hypo- + G. *spaō,* to tear or gouge]

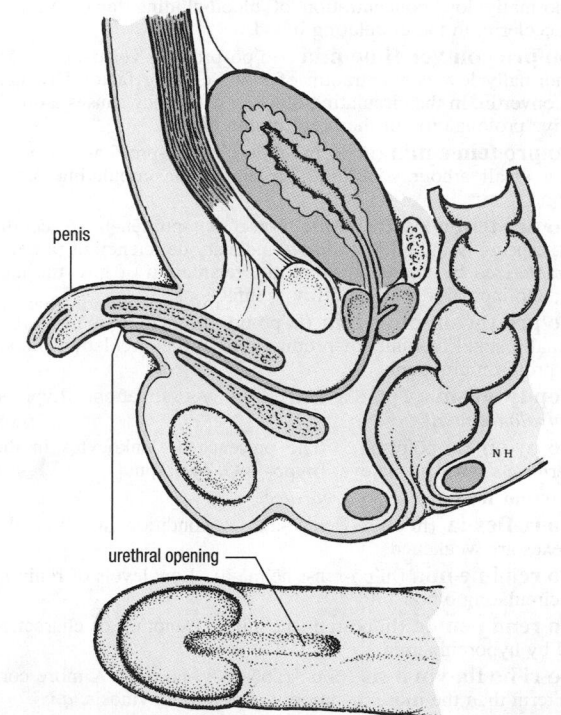

penis

urethral opening

N H

hypospadius: (top) midsagittal view, (bottom) ventral view of penis

balanic h., SYN glanular h.

coronal h., ventral and proximal malposition of meatus in the coronal sulcus.

glanular h., ventral and proximal glanular malposition of urethral meatus in a male. SYN balanic h.

penile h., malposition of the urethral meatus on the ventral penile shaft.

penoscrotal h., malposition of the urethral opening at the junction of the penis and scrotum.

perineal h., h. in which the urethral meatus opens in the perineum near the anus; the scrotum is usually cleft.

scrotal h., h. with the urethral opening on the scrotal surface.

subcoronal h., malposition of the meatus in the coronal sulcus.

hy·po·sphyg·mia (hī′pō-sfig′mē-ă). Abnormally low blood pressure with sluggishness of the circulation. [hypo- + G. *sphyxis,* pulse]

hy·po·splen·ism (hī′pō-splēn′izm). Absent or reduced splenic function, usually due to surgical removal, congenital aplasia, tumor replacement, or splenic vascular accident. Red cell abnormalities, including the presence of inclusions, nucleated erythrocytes, and target cells, are commonly present. Patients with h. are at increased risk of bacterial sepsis, especially due to pneumococcus.

hy·pos·ta·sis (hi-pos′tă-sis). 1. Formation of a sediment at the bottom of a liquid. 2. SYN hypostatic *congestion.* 3. The phenomenon whereby the phenotype that would ordinarily be manifested at one locus is obscured by the genotype at another epistatic locus; e.g., in humans, the phenotype for the ABO blood group locus can be expressed only in the presence of its precursor, H substance. The Bombay factor in the homozygous state blocks H formation and obscures the ABO phenotype. [G. *hypo-stasis,* a standing under, sediment]

postmortem h., SYN postmortem *livedo.*

pulmonary h., hydrostatic congestion of the lung.

hy·po·stat·ic (hī-pō-stat′ik). 1. Sedimentary; resulting from a dependent position. 2. Relating to hypostasis.

hy·pos·the·nu·ria (hī′pos-thĕ-noo′rē-ă). Excretion of urine of low specific gravity, due to inability of the tubules of the kidneys to produce a concentrated urine; also occurs following excessive water ingestion in diabetes insipidus. [hypo- + G. *sthenos,* strength, + *ouron,* urine]

hy·po·stome (hī′pō-stōm). The central unpaired holdfast organ of the tick capitulum; the h. is covered with recurved spines that enable it to serve as an anchoring device while the tick feeds. [hypo- + G. *stoma,* mouth]

hy·po·sto·mia (hī′pō-stō′mē-ă). A form of microstomia in which the oral opening is a small vertical slit. [hypo- + G. *stoma,* mouth]

hyp·os·to·sis (hīp-os-tō′sis). Deficient development of bone. [hypo- + G. *osteon,* bone, + *-osis,* condition]

hy·po·supra·dren·al·ism (hī′pō-soo′pră-ă-drē′nal-izm). SYN chronic adrenocortical *insufficiency.*

hy·po·sys·to·le (hī′pō-sis′tō-lē). A weak or incomplete cardiac systole.

hy·po·tel·or·ism (hī-pō-tel′ōr-izm). Abnormal closeness of eyes. [hypo- + G. *tēle,* far off, + *horizō,* to separate, fr. *horos,* boundary]

hy·po·ten·sion (hī′pō-ten′shŭn). 1. Subnormal arterial blood pressure. SYN hypopiesis. 2. Reduced pressure or tension of any kind. [hypo- + L. *tensio,* a stretching]

arterial h., SEE hypotension (1).

idiopathic orthostatic h., the tendency for blood pressure to drop for unknown reasons on assuming upright posture.

induced h., controlled h., deliberate acute reduction of arterial blood pressure to reduce operative blood loss by pharmacologic means during anesthesia and surgery.

intracranial h., subnormal pressure of cerebrospinal fluid; most commonly following lumbar puncture and associated with headache, nausea, vomiting, stiffness of the neck, and sometimes fever; may also result from dehydration.

orthostatic h., a form of low blood pressure that occurs in a standing posture. SYN orthostatic hypopiesis, postural h.

postural h., SYN orthostatic h.

hy·po·ten·sive (hī′pō-ten′siv). Characterized by low blood pressure or causing reduction in blood pressure.

hy·po·ten·sor (hī-pō-ten′ser, -sōr). SYN depressor (4).

hy·po·thal·a·mo·hy·po·phy·si·al (hī′pō-thal′ă-mō-hī′pō-fiz′ē-ăl). Relating to both the hypothalamus and the hypophysis.

hy·po·thal·a·mus (hī′pō-thal′ă-mŭs) [TA]. The ventral and medial region of the diencephalon forming the walls of the ventral half of the third ventricle; it is delineated from the thalamus by the hypothalamic sulcus, lying medial to the internal capsule and subthalamus, continuous with the precommissural septum anteriorly and with the mesencephalic tegmentum and central gray substance posteriorly. Its ventral surface is marked by, from before backward, the optic chiasma, the unpaired infundibulum that extends by way of the infundibular stalk into the posterior lobe of the hypophysis, and the paired mamillary bodies. The h. consists of the anterior hypothalamic area [TA], dorsal hypothalamic area [TA], intermediate hypothalamic area [TA], lateral hypothalamic area [TA], and posterior hypothalamic area [TA], each of these containing specific nuclei. It has afferent fiber connections with the mesencephalon, limbic system, cerebellum, and efferent fiber connections with the same structures and with the posterior lobe of the hypophysis; its functional connection with the anterior lobe of the hypophysis is established by the hypothalamohypophysial portal system. The h. is prominently involved in the functions of the autonomic (visceral motor) nervous system and, through its vascular link with the anterior lobe of the hypophysis, in endocrine mechanisms; it also appears to play a role in neural mechanisms underlying moods and motivational states. SEE ALSO pituitary *gland*. [hypo- + thalamus]

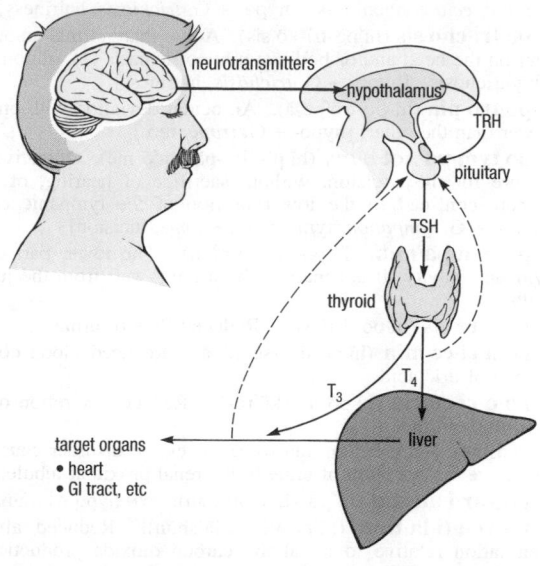

hypothalamic-pituitary-thyroid axis: thyroid-releasing hormone (TRH) from the hypothalamus stimulates the pituitary gland to secrete thyroid-stimulating hormone (TSH). TSH acts to produce thyroid hormone (T_3 and T_4). High circulating levels of T_3 and T_4 inhibit further TSH secretion and thyroid hormone production through a negative feedback mechanism (dashed lines)

hy·po·the·nar (hī′pō-thē′nar, hī-poth′ĕ-nar) [TA]. **1** [NA]. SYN hypothenar *eminence*. **2.** Denoting any structure in relation with the hypothenar eminence or its underlying collective components. [hypo- + G. *thenar*, the palm]

hy·po·ther·mal (hī-pō-ther′măl). Denoting hypothermia.

hy·po·ther·mia (hī′pō-ther′mē-ă). A body temperature significantly below 98.6°F (37°C). [hypo- + G. *thermē*, heat]

accidental h., unintentional decrease in body temperature, especially in the newborn, infants, and elderly, particularly during operations.

moderate h., a body temperature of 23–32°C. induced by surface cooling.

profound h., a body temperature of 12–20°C.

regional h., reduction of the temperature of an extremity or organ by external cold or perfusion with cold blood or solutions.

total body h., the deliberate reduction of total body temperature, in order to reduce tissue metabolism.

hy·poth·e·sis (hī-poth′ĕ-sis). A conjecture advanced for heuristic purposes, cast in a form that is amenable to confirmation or refutation by the conductance of definable experiments and the critical assembly of empiric data; not to be confused with assumption, postulation, or unfocused speculation. SEE ALSO postulate, theory. [G. foundation, assumption fr. *hypotithenai*, to lay down]

adaptor h., a h., proposed by F.H.C. Crick, that an adaptor molecule must be present between the information-containing DNA and the protein being synthesized.

alternative h., in Neyman-Pearson testing of a h., the h. or family of hypotheses about the numerical value of a parameter if and only if the null h. is rejected as untenable.

autocrine h., that tumor cells containing viral oncogenes may have encoded a growth factor, normally produced by other cell types, and thereby produce the factor autonomously, leading to uncontrolled proliferation.

Avogadro h., SYN Avogadro *law*.

Bayesian h., an array of surmised values of a parameter to be severally explored in the light of a current set of data, with logical symmetry being preserved among all. The merits of each h. entertained are based on quantity, the prior probability. The probability of the data conditional on the h. is computed as the conditional probability for each; the product of the two for each h. is the joint probability, and the ratio of each joint probability to the sum of all the joint probabilities is the posterior probability for that h. Unlike the Neyman-Pearson test of hypotheses, the answer is a statement about the h., not about the sample conditional on the h. No h. is preferred or prevails by default. The procedure may be applied recursively any number of times, as the data becomes available.

frustration-aggression h., the theory that frustration may lead to aggression, but that aggression is always the result of some form of frustration.

gate-control h., SYN gate-control *theory*.

Goldie-Coldman h., a mathematic model that predicts that tumor cells mutate to a resistant phenotype at a rate dependent on their intrinsic genetic instability. The probability that a cancer would contain drug-resistant clones depends on the mutation rate and the size of the tumor. According to this h., even the smallest detectable cancers would contain at least 1 drug-resistant clone; therefore, the best chance of cure would be to use all effective chemotherapy drugs; in practice, this has meant using 2 different non–cross-resistant chemotherapy regimens in alternating cycles.

Gompertz h., a theory that the force of mortality increases in geometrical progression, being based on the assumption that the average exhaustion of an individual's power to avoid death is such that at the end of equal infinitely small intervals of time the individual loses equal proportions of the power to oppose destruction that were available at the commencement of each of these intervals.

insular h., obsolete theory of the origin of diabetes mellitus from destruction or loss of function of the islets of Langerhans in the pancreas.

Knudsen h., an explanation for the bilateral (and earlier) occurrence of hereditary retinoblastoma; if one tumor suppressor gene is mutated by inheritance, only one somatic mutation is needed inactivate the other allele. In the sporadic form, 2 mutations, which inactivate each allele, are necessary.

Lyon h., SYN lyonization.

Makeham h., a development of Gompertz h. as to the force of mortality following some mathematical law. Makeham assumed that death was the consequence of two generally coexisting causes: 1) chance; 2) a deterioration or increased inability to withstand destruction. The first of these is constant, the second is an increasing geometrical progression.

Michaelis-Menten h., a h. that a complex is formed between an enzyme and its substrate (also known as the O'Sullivan-Tompson h.), which complex then decomposes to yield free enzyme and the reaction products (also referred to as the Brown h.), the latter step being the rate-determining step for the overall rate of substrate-

hy

product conversion. SEE ALSO Michaelis-Menten *constant*, Michaelis-Menten *equation*.

mnemic h., the theory that stimuli or irritants leave definite traces (engrams) on the protoplasm of the animal, and when these stimuli are regularly repeated they induce a habit which persists after the stimuli cease. SYN mnemic theory, mnemism, Semon-Hering theory.

monoamine h., the classical theory of the neurochemical basis of depression linking it to a deficiency of at least one of three monoamine neurotransmitters, norepinephrine, serotonin, or dopamine.

Neyman-Pearson statistical h., a formal conjecture about the numerical value of a parameter to be tested exclusively in the light of an immediate set of data without attention to prior knowledge or convictions and ignoring other sets of evidence treated in a similar fashion. The answer is a statement not about whether the h. is true but whether it is an acceptable explanation of the data or should be rejected in favor of another h.

Norton-Simon h., h. that a tumor is composed of populations of faster-growing cells, which are sensitive to therapy, and slower-growing, more resistant cells. Since only therapy that completely eradicates all tumor cells will be curative, this is most likely to occur with sequential, non–cross-resistant regimens. The initial regimen must be effective enough to result in a low residual tumor burden and is followed by one or more non–cross-resistant treatments to eradicate the remainder of the cancer.

null h., the statistical hypothesis that one variable has no association with another variable or set of variables, or that two or more populations do not differ from each other; the statement that results do not differ from those that might be expected by the operation of chance alone; if rejected, it increases confidence in the h.

sequence h., that the amino acid sequence of a protein is determined by a particular sequence of nucleotides (the cistron) in the DNA of the organism producing the protein.

sliding filament h., the theory that the contracting muscle shortens because two sets of filaments slide past each other.

Starling h., the principle that net filtration through capillary membranes is proportional to the transmembrane hydrostatic pressure difference minus the transmembrane oncotic pressure difference; although well established, it is called Starling h. to distinguish it from Starling law of the heart.

upregulation/downregulation h., a theory of the neurochemical basis of depression (an elaboration of the monoamine h.) linking it to an increase in number (upregulation) of postsynaptic monoamine receptors, which are then effectively decreased in number (downregulation) as a result of antidepressant activity. SEE ALSO monoamine h.

wobble h., SEE wobble *base*, wobble.

zwitter h., that an amphoteric molecule (e.g., an amino acid) has, at its isoelectric point, equal numbers of positive and negative charges, thus becoming a zwitterion.

hy·po·throm·bi·ne·mia (hī′pō-throm-bin-ē′mē-ă). Abnormally small amounts of thrombin in the circulating blood, resulting in bleeding tendency.

hy·po·throm·bo·plas·ti·ne·mia (hī′pō-throm′bō-plas-ti-nē′mē-ă). Abnormally small amounts of thromboplastin in the blood, as a result of deficient quantities being released from the tissues.

hy·po·thy·mia (hī′pō-thī′mē-ă). Depression of spirits; the "blues." [hypo- + G. *thymos*, mind, soul]

hy·po·thy·mic (hī-pō-thē′mik). Denoting or characteristic of hypothymia.

hy·po·thy·mism (hī′pō-thī′mizm). Obsolete term for inadequate function of the thymus.

hy·po·thy·roid (hī′pō-thī′royd). Marked by reduced thyroid function.

hy·po·thy·roid·ism (hī′pō-thī′royd-izm). Diminished production of thyroid hormone, leading to clinical manifestations of thyroid insufficiency, including low metabolic rate, tendency to weight gain, somnolence and sometimes myxedema. SYN athyrea (1). [hypo- + G. *thyreoeidēs*, thyroid]

congenital h., lack of thyroid secretion. SEE infantile h.

infantile h., can be due to endemic congenital goiter, nonendemic cases are usually due to defective thyroidal embryogenesis, defective hypothalamic-pituitary function, congenital defects in thyroid hormone synthesis or action, or intrauterine exposure to goitrogenic agents. SYN Brissaud infantilism, congenital myxedema, dysthyroidal infantilism, hypothyroid dwarfism, hypothyroid infantilism, infantile myxedema, myxedematous infantilism.

secondary h., h. that arises as a consequence of inadequate thyrotropin secretion by the anterior pituitary gland.

hy·po·thy·rox·i·ne·mia (hī′pō-thī-rok-sin-ē′mē-ă). A subnormal thyroxine concentration in the blood.

hy·po·to·nia (hī′pō-tō′nē-ă). **1.** Reduced tension in any part, as in the eyeball. **2.** Relaxation of the arteries. **3.** A condition in which there is a diminution or loss of muscular tonicity. SYN hypotonicity (1), hypotonus, hypotony. [hypo- + G. *tonos,* tone]

benign congenital h., nonprogressive h. of unknown etiology in infants and children; other known causes of h. must be excluded.

hy·po·ton·ic (hī-pō-ton′ik). **1.** Having a lesser degree of tension. **2.** Having a lesser osmotic pressure than a reference solution, which is ordinarily assumed to be blood plasma or interstitial fluid; more specifically, refers to a fluid in which cells would swell. SYN hypoisotonic.

hy·po·to·nic·i·ty (hī′pō-tō-nis′i-tē). **1.** SYN hypotonia. **2.** A decreased effective osmotic pressure.

hy·po·to·nus, hy·pot·o·ny (hī′pō-tō′nŭs, hī-pot′ō-nē). SYN hypotonia.

hy·po·tri·chi·a·sis (hī′pō-tri-kī′ă-sis). **1.** SYN hypotrichosis. **2.** SYN *alopecia* congenitalis. [hypo- + G. *trichiasis,* hairiness]

hy·po·tri·cho·sis (hī′pō-tri-kō′sis). A less than normal amount of hair on the head and/or body. SYN hypotrichiasis (1), oligotrichia, oligotrichosis. [hypo- + G. *trichōsis,* hairiness]

hy·po·tro·pia (hī-pō-trō′pē-ă). An ocular deviation with one eye lower than the other. [hypo- + G. *trope,* turn]

hy·po·tym·pa·not·o·my (hī′pō-tim-pă-not′ō-mē). Operative procedure for the excision, without sacrifice of hearing, of small tumors confined to the lower portion of the tympanic cavity. [hypo- + G. *tympanon,* tympanum, + *tome,* incision]

hy·po·tym·pa·num (hī′pō-tim′pă-nŭm). The lower part of the tympanic cavity. It is separated by a bony wall from the jugular bulb.

hy·po·u·re·sis (hī′pō-ū-rē′sis). Reduced flow of urine.

hy·po·u·ri·ce·mia (hī′pō-ū-ri-sē′mē-ă). Reduced blood concentration of uric acid.

hy·po·u·ri·cu·ria (hī′pō-ū′ri-kū′rē-ă). Reduced excretion of uric acid in the urine.

hereditary renal h., an autosomal recessive disorder caused by defective reabsorption of urate in the renal proximal tubule.

hy·po·var·i·an·ism (hī′pō-vā′rē-an-izm). SYN hypoovarianism.

hy·po·ven·ti·la·tion (hī′pō-ven-ti-lā′shŭn). Reduced alveolar ventilation relative to metabolic carbon dioxide production, so that alveolar carbon dioxide pressure increases above normal. SYN underventilation.

hy·po·vi·ta·min·o·sis (hī′pō-vī′tă-min-ō′sis). A nutritional deficiency state characterized by relative insufficiency of one or more vitamins in the diet; manifested first by depletion of tissue levels, then by functional changes, and finally by appearance of morphologic lesions. Cf. avitaminosis.

hy·po·vo·le·mia (hī′pō-vō-lē′mē-ă). A decreased amount of blood in the body. SYN hyphemia. [hypo- + L. *volumen,* volume, + G. *haima,* blood]

hy·po·vo·le·mic (hī′pō-vō-lē′mik). Pertaining to or characterized by hypovolemia.

hy·po·vo·lia (hī-pō-vō′lē-ă). Diminished water content or volume of a given compartment; e.g., extracellular h. [hypo- + L. *volumen,* volume]

hy·po·xan·thine (Hyp) (hī-pō-zan′thin). 6-Oxypurine; purin-6(1*H*)-one; a purine present in the muscles and other tissues, formed during purine catabolism by deamination of adenine; elevated in molybdenum-cofactor deficiency. SYN 6-hydroxypurine.

h. guanine phosphoribosyltransferase (HGPRT), SYN h. phosphoribosyltransferase.

h. oxidase, SYN *xanthine* oxidase.

h. phosphoribosyltransferase, an enzyme present in human tissue that converts h. and guanine to their respective 5′ nucleotides, with 5-phosphoribose 1-diphosphate as the ribose-phosphate donor; a partial deficiency of this enzyme can result in elevated purine biosynthesis resulting in gout; another level of deficiency is associated with Lesch-Nyhan syndrome. SYN h. guanine phosphoribosyltransferase.

hy·po·xan·thin·o·sine (hī′pō-zan-thēn′ō-sēn). SYN inosine.

hy·pox·e·mia (hī-pok-sē′mē-ă). Subnormal oxygenation of arterial blood, short of anoxia. [hypo- + oxygen, + G. *haima*, blood]

hy·pox·ia (hī-pok′sē-ă). Decrease below normal levels of oxygen in inspired gases, arterial blood, or tissue, short of anoxia. [hypo- + oxygen]

anemic h., h. resulting from a decreased concentration of functional hemoglobin or a reduced number of erythrocytes; it is caused by hemorrhage or anemia of various types, or by poisoning with carbon monoxide, nitrites, or chlorates.

diffusion h., abrupt transient decrease in alveolar oxygen tension when room air is inhaled at the conclusion of a nitrous oxide anesthesia, because nitrous oxide diffusing out of the blood dilutes the alveolar oxygen.

hypoxic h., h. resulting from a defective mechanism of oxygenation in the lungs; may be caused by a low tension of oxygen, abnormal pulmonary function or respiratory obstruction, or a right-to-left shunt in the heart.

ischemic h., tissue h. characterized by tissue oligemia and caused by arterial or arteriolar obstruction or vasoconstriction.

oxygen affinity h., h. due to reduced ability of hemoglobin to release oxygen.

stagnant h., tissue h. characterized not by tissue oligemia (tissue blood volume being normal or even increased), but by intravascular stasis due to impairment of venous outflow or (in some instances) to decreased arterial inflow.

hy·pox·ic (hī-pok′sik). Denoting or characterized by hypoxia.

hyp·sa·rhyth·mia, hyp·sar·rhyth·mia (hip′să-rith′mē-ă). The abnormal and characteristically chaotic electroencephalogram commonly found in patients with infantile spasms. [G. *hypsi*, high, + *a*- priv. + *rhythmos*, rhythm]

hypsi-, hypso-. High, height. [G. *hypsos*, height]

hyp·si·brach·y·ce·phal·ic (hip-sē-brak′ē-sě-fal′ik). Having a high broad head. [hypsi- + G. *brachys*, broad, + *kephalē*, head]

hyp·si·ceph·a·ly (hip-si-sef′ă-lē). SYN oxycephaly. [hypsi- + G. *kephalē*, head]

hyp·si·con·chous (hip-si-kon′kŭs). Having a high orbit, with an orbital index above 85. [hypsi- + G. *konchos*, a shell, the upper part of the skull]

hyp·si·loid (hip′si-loyd). Y-shaped; U-shaped. SYN upsiloid, ypsiliform. [G. *upsilon (ypsilon)*]

hyp·si·sta·phyl·ia (hip′si-stă-fil′ē-ă). A condition in which the palate is high and narrow. [hypsi- + G. *staphylē*, uvula]

hyp·si·sten·o·ce·phal·ic (hip-si-sten′ō-sě-fal′ik). Having a high, narrow head. [hypsi- + G. *stenos*, narrow, + *kephalē*, head]

hypso-. SEE hypsi-.

hyp·so·ceph·a·ly (hip-sō-sef′ă-lē). SYN oxycephaly. [hypso- + G. *kephalē*, head]

hyp·so·chro·mic (hip-sō-krōm′ik). Denoting the shift of an absorption spectrum maximum to a shorter wavelength (greater energy). [hypso- + G. *chroma*, color]

hyp·so·dont (hip′sō-dont). Having long teeth. [hypso- + G. *odous*, tooth]

hy·pur·gia (hī-per′jē-ă). A rarely used term for any minor factor(s) modifying the course of a disease for good or for ill, especially the former. [G. *hypourgia*, help, service, fr. *hypo*, + *ergon*, work]

Hyrtl, Joseph, Austrian anatomist, 1811–1894. SEE H. *anastomosis, foramen, loop*, epitympanic *recess, sphincter*.

hyster-. SEE hystero-.

hys·ter·al·gia (his′ter-al′jē-ă). Pain in the uterus. SYN hysterodynia, metrodynia. [hystero- + G. *algos*, pain]

hys·ter·a·tre·sia (his′ter-ă-trē′zē-ă). Atresia of the uterine cavity, usually resulting from inflammatory endocervical adhesions.

hys·ter·ec·to·my (his-ter-ek′tō-mē). Removal of the uterus; unless otherwise specified, usually denotes complete removal of the uterus (corpus and cervix). [hystero- + G. *ektomē*, excision]

abdominal h., removal of the uterus through an incision in the abominal wall. SYN abdominohysterectomy.

abdominovaginal h., a combined vaginal and abdominal surgical approach that allows partial or complete removal of vagina, vulva, rectum, and perineum (abdominoperineal approach), as well as pelvic organs; usually done in cases of advanced pelvic cancer.

cesarean h., cesarean section followed by h. SYN Porro h.

laparoscopic-assisted vaginal h., vaginal h. in which the ovarian pedicle, broad ligament, and uterosacral ligaments are surgically severed using laparoscopic instruments and the procedure completed through a colpotomy done in the typical fashion.

modified radical h., an extended h. in which a portion of the upper vagina is removed; the ureters are exposed and pulled back laterally without dissection from the ureteral bed. SYN TeLinde operation.

Porro h., SYN cesarean h.

radical h., complete removal of the uterus, upper vagina, and parametrium.

hy

signs and symptoms of systemic hypoxia			
organ/function	mild	moderate	severe
mental	euphoria, disorientation	visual disturbances, anxiety	dizziness delirium, coma
gastrointestinal tract	nausea	retching	vomiting
subjective symptoms	headache	precordial pain	
respirations	rate and depth increased	apnea after O$_2$ administration	depressed, irregular, Cheyne-Stokes breathing, apnea
blood pressure	slight elevation (systolic and diastolic)	elevation	abrupt drop
pulse	rapid, becoming irregular	slow, bounding, irregular	very faint, irregular, failing
muscular system	incoordination	spasms, rigidity, convulsions	weakness, paralysis
skin			
with normal Hb	cyanotic (depending on Hb) warm, moist	deeply cyanotic, warm, damp	deeply cyanotic, clammy
in anemia	bluish, dry	slate gray, damp to diaphoretic	gray, clammy
pupils	irregular	dilating	maximally dilated and fixed
central venous pressure	slight elevation	marked elevation	falling

subtotal h., SYN supracervical h.

supracervical h., removal of the fundus of the uterus, leaving the cervix in situ. SYN subtotal h.

vaginal h., removal of the uterus through the vagina without incising the wall of the abdomen. SYN colpohysterectomy, vaginohysterectomy.

hys·ter·e·sis (his-ter-ē'sis). **1.** Failure of either one of two related phenomena to keep pace with the other; or any situation in which the value of one depends upon whether the other has been increasing or decreasing. **2.** The lag of a magnetic effect behind its cause. SYN magnetic inertia. **3.** The temperature differential that exists when a substance, such as reversible hydrocolloid, melts at one temperature and solidifies at another. **4.** The basis of a type of cooperativity observed in many enzyme-catalyzed reactions in which the degree of cooperativity is associated with a slow conformational change of the enzyme. Cf. allosterism, cooperativity. [G. *hysterēsis,* a coming later]

static h., the difference in the value reached by a dependent variable at a particular constant value of the independent variable, depending on whether the latter value had been approached from above or below; e.g., in measuring the pressure volume relations of the lungs, if one completely expires and then inspires to a particular volume and holds it constant, the transpulmonary pressure required to maintain that lung volume is greater than if one had completely inspired and then expired to the same volume and held it constant.

hys·te·ria (his-ter'ē-ă, his-tēr'). A somatoform (psychoneurotic or psychosomatic) disorder in which there is an alteration or loss of physical functioning that suggests a physical disorder such as paralysis of an arm or disturbance of vision, but that is instead apparently an expression of a psychological conflict or need; a diagnostic term, referable to a wide variety of psychogenic symptoms involving disorder of function, which may be mental, sensory, motor, or visceral. SEE somatoform *disorder.* [G. *hystera,* womb, from the original notion of womb-related disturbances in women]

anxiety h., h. characterized by manifest anxiety.

conversion h., h. characterized by the substitution, through psychic transformation, of physical signs or symptoms for anxiety; generally restricted to such major symptoms as blindness, deafness, and paralysis, or lesser ones such as blurred vision and numbness. SYN conversion hysteria neurosis, conversion neurosis, conversion reaction.

dissociative h., an unconscious process sometimes seen in patients with multiple personalities, or in h., in which a group of mental processes is separated from the rest of the thinking processes, resulting in an independent functioning of these processes and a loss of the usual relationships among them.

epidemic h., SYN mass h.

mass h., (1) spontaneous, en masse development of identical physical and/or emotional symptoms among a group of individuals, as seen in a classroom of schoolchildren; (2) a socially contagious frenzy of irrational behavior in a group of people as a reaction to an event. SYN epidemic h., mass sociogenic illness.

hys·ter·i·cal, hys·ter·ic (his-ter'ē-kăl, -ter'ik). Relating to or characterized by hysteria.

hys·ter·ics (his-ter'iks). An expression of emotion accompanied often by crying, laughing, and screaming.

⌂**hystero-, hyster-. 1.** The uterus. SEE ALSO metr-, utero-. [G. *hystera,* womb (uterus)] **2.** Hysteria. [G. *hystera,* womb (uterus)] **3.** Later, following. [G. *hysteros,* later]

hys·ter·o·cat·a·lep·sy (his'ter-ō-kat'ă-lep-sē). Hysteria with cataleptic manifestations.

hys·ter·o·cele (his'ter-ō-sēl). **1.** An abdominal or perineal hernia containing part or all of the uterus. **2.** Protrusion of uterine contents into a weakened, bulging area of uterine wall. [hystero- + G. *kēlē,* hernia]

hys·ter·o·clei·sis (his'ter-ō-klī'sis). Operative occlusion of the uterus. [hystero- + G. *kleisis,* closure]

hys·ter·o·col·po·scope (his'ter-ō-kol'pō-skōp). Instrument for inspection of the uterine cavity and vagina. [hystero- + G. *kolpos,* vagina, + *skopeō,* to view]

hys·ter·o·cys·to·pexy (his'ter-ō-sis'tō-pek-sē). Attachment of both uterus and bladder to the abdominal wall to correct prolapse. [hystero- + G. *kystis,* bladder, + *pēxis,* fixation]

hys·ter·o·dyn·ia (his'ter-ō-din'ē-ă). SYN hysteralgia. [hystero- + G. *odynē,* pain]

hys·ter·o·gen·ic, hys·ter·og·en·ous (his-ter-ō-jen'ik, his-ter-oj' ĕ-nŭs). Causing hysterical symptoms or reactions. [hysteria + G. *-gen,* producing]

hys·ter·o·gram (his'ter-ō-gram). **1.** X-ray examination of the uterus, usually using a contrast medium. **2.** A recording of the strength of uterine contractions.

hys·ter·o·graph (his'ter-ō-graf). Apparatus for recording the strength of uterine contractions.

hys·ter·og·ra·phy (his-ter-og'ră-fē). **1.** Radiographic examination of the uterine cavity filled with a contrast medium. **2.** Graphic procedure used to record uterine contractions. [hystero- + G. *graphō,* to write]

hys·ter·oid (his'ter-oyd). Resembling or simulating hysteria. [hystero- + G. *eidos,* resemblance]

hys·ter·ol·y·sis (his-ter-ol'i-sis). Breaking up of adhesions between the uterus and neighboring parts. [hystero- + G. *lysis,* dissolution]

hys·ter·om·e·ter (his-ter-om'ĕ-ter). A graduated sound for measuring the depth of the uterine cavity. SYN uterometer. [hystero- + G. *metron,* measure]

hys·ter·o·my·o·mec·to·my (his'ter-ō-mī-ō-mek'tō-mē). SYN myomectomy. [hysteromyoma + G. *ektomē,* excision]

hys·ter·o·my·ot·o·my (his'ter-ō-mī-ot'ō-mē). Incision into the muscles of the uterus. [hystero- + G. *mys,* muscle, + *tomē,* incision]

hys·ter·o·ooph·o·rec·to·my (his'ter-ō-ō'of-ō-rek'tō-mē). Surgical removal of the uterus and ovaries. [hystero- + G. *ōon,* egg, + *phoros,* bearing, + *ektomē,* excision]

hys·ter·op·a·thy (his-ter-op'ă-thē). Any disease of the uterus. [hystero- + G. *pathos,* suffering]

hys·ter·o·pex·y (his'ter-ō-pek-sē). Fixation of a displaced or abnormally movable uterus. SYN uterofixation, uteropexy. [hystero- + G. *pēxis,* fixation]

abdominal h., attachment of the uterus to the anterior abdominal wall.

hys·ter·o·plas·ty (his'ter-ō-plas-tē). SYN uteroplasty.

hys·ter·or·rha·phy (his-ter-ōr'ă-fē). Sutural repair of a lacerated uterus. [hystero- + G. *rhaphē,* suture]

hys·ter·o·sal·pin·gec·to·my (his'ter-ō-sal-pin-jek'tō-mē). Operation for the removal of the uterus and one or both uterine tubes. [hystero- + G. *salpinx,* a trumpet, + *ektomē,* excision]

hys·ter·o·sal·pin·gog·ra·phy (his'ter-ō-sal-ping-gog'ră-fē). Radiography of the uterus and fallopian tubes after the injection of radiopaque material. SYN hysterotubography, uterosalpingography, uterotubography. [hystero- + G. *salpinx,* a trumpet, + *graphō,* to write]

hys·ter·o·sal·pin·go-o·oph·o·rec·to·my (his'ter-ō-sal-ping'gō-ō-of-ō-rek'tō-mē). Excision of the uterus, oviducts, and ovaries. [hystero- + G. *salpinx,* trumpet, + *ōon,* egg, + *phoros,* bearing, + *ektomē,* excision]

hys·ter·o·sal·pin·go·sto·my (his'ter-ō-sal-ping-gos'tō-mē). Operation to restore patency of a uterine tube. [hystero- + G. *salpinx,* trumpet, + *stoma,* mouth]

hys·ter·o·scope (his'ter-ō-skōp). An endoscope used in direct visual examination of the uterine cavity. SYN uteroscope. [hystero- + G. *skopeō,* to view]

contact h., h. with a graded refractive index rod lens; it does not require distension for visualization and affords very short focal length views; suitable for localizing hemorrhages.

flexible h., steerable flexible h. of small diameter for operative or diagnostic procedures, that does not require an outer sheath, has fiberoptics for visualization, and must be used with a distending gas.

hys·ter·os·co·py (his-ter-os′kŏ-pē). Visual instrumental inspection of the uterine cavity. SYN uteroscopy.

hys·ter·o·spasm (his′ter-ō-spazm). Spasm of the uterus.

hys·ter·o·sys·to·le (his-ter-ō-sis′tō-lē). A delayed contraction of the heart; opposed to premature contraction or extrasystole. [G. *hysteros,* following, after, + *systolē,* a contracting]

hys·ter·o·ther·mom·e·try (his′ter-ō-ther-mom′ĕ-trē). Measurement of uterine temperature.

hys·ter·ot·o·my (his-ter-ot′ō-mē). Incision of the uterus. SYN metrotomy, uterotomy. [hystero- + G. *tomē,* incision]

  abdominal h., transabdominal incision into the uterus. SYN abdominohysterotomy.

  vaginal h., incision into the uterus via the vagina. SYN colpohysterotomy.

hys·ter·o·trach·e·lec·to·my (his′ter-ō-trak-el-ek′tō-mē). Removal of the cervix uteri. [hystero- + G. *trachēlos,* neck, + *ektomē,* excision]

hys·ter·o·trach·e·lo·plas·ty (his′ter-ō-trak′ĕ-lō-plas-tē). Plastic surgery of the cervix uteri. [hystero- + G. *trachēlos,* neck, + *plastos,* formed, shaped]

hys·ter·o·tra·che·lor·rha·phy (his′ter-ō-trak-ĕ-lōr′ă-fē). Sutural repair of a lacerated cervix uteri. [hystero- + G. *trachēlos,* neck, + *rhaphē,* a seam]

hys·ter·o·trach·e·lot·o·my (his′ter-ō-trak-ĕ-lot′ō-mē). Incision of the cervix uteri. [hystero- + G. *trachēlos,* neck, + *tomē,* incision]

hys·ter·o·tu·bog·ra·phy (his′ter-ō-too-bog′ră-fē). SYN hysterosalpingography.

Hz Abbreviation for hertz.

ι The ninth letter in the Greek alphabet, iota.

I 1. Symbol for iodine; luminous *intensity* or radiant *intensity*; ionic *strength* (in mol/L); isoleucine; inosine. **2.** Abbreviation (in italics) for intensity of electrical current, expressed in amperes. **3.** As a subscript, symbol for inspired *gas.* **4.** Designation for I blood group (see Blood Groups appendix).

^{123}**I** Symbol for iodine-123.

^{125}**I** Symbol for iodine-125.

^{127}**I** Symbol for iodine-127.

^{131}**I.** Symbol for iodine-131.

^{132}**I** Symbol for iodine-132.

⌂**-ia.** A suffix used to form terms for states or conditions, often abnormal. Cf. -ism. [G. *-ia,* an ancient noun-forming suffix]

IAHS Abbreviation for infection-associated hemophagocytic syndrome.

IANC Abbreviation for International Anatomical Nomenclature Committee. SEE Nomina Anatomica.

IAP Abbreviation for intermittent acute *porphyria.*

⌂**-iasis.** A condition or state, especially an unhealthy one; in medical neologisms it has the same value as, and is sometimes interchangeable with, -osis. [G. suffix forming nouns from verbs]

ia·tra·lip·tic (ī'ă-tră-lip'tik). Obsolete term denoting treatment by inunction. [G. *iatros,* physician, + *aleiptēs,* an anointer]

ia·tra·lip·tics (ī'ă-tră-lip'tiks). Method of treatment by inunction.

iat·ric (ī-at'rik). Pertaining to medicine or to a physician or healer. [G. *iatros,* physician]

⌂**iatro-.** Physicians, medicine, treatment. Cf. medico-. [G. *iatros,* physician]

iat·ro·chem·i·cal (ī-at-rō-kem'i-kăl). Denoting a school of medicine practicing iatrochemistry.

iat·ro·chem·ist (ī-at-rō-kem'ist). A member of the iatrochemical school.

iat·ro·chem·is·try (ī-at-rō-kem'is-trē). The study of chemistry in relation to physiologic and pathologic processes, and the treatment of disease by chemical substance as practiced by a school of medical thought in the 17th century.

iat·ro·gen·ic (ī-at-rō-jen'ik). Denoting response to medical or surgical treatment, induced by the treatment itself; usually used for unfavorable responses. [iatro- + G. *-gen,* producing]

ia·trol·o·gy (ī-a-trol'ō-jē). Rarely used term for medical science. [iatro- + G. *logos,* study]

iat·ro·math·e·mat·i·cal (ī-at'rō-math-ĕ-mat'i-kăl). SYN iatrophysical.

iat·ro·me·chan·i·cal (ī-at'rō-mĕ-kan'i-kăl). SYN iatrophysical.

iat·ro·phys·i·cal (ī-at'rō-fiz'i-kăl). Denoting a school of medical thought in the 17th century that explained all physiologic and pathologic phenomena by the laws of physics. SYN iatromathematical, iatromechanical.

iat·ro·phys·i·cist (ī-at'rō-fiz'-i-sist). A member of the iatrophysical school.

iat·ro·phys·ics (ī-at'rō-fiz'iks). Physics as applied to medicine.

iat·ro·tech·nique (ī-at'rō-tek-nēk'). Rarely used term for the art of medicine and surgery; the technique or mode of application of medical science. [iatro- + G. *technē,* art]

IBC Abbreviation for iron-binding *capacity.*

ibo·ga·ine (ī'bō-gān). Indole alkaloid of the *iboga* group. Obtained from several parts of the African shrub *Tabernanthe iboga* (family Apocynaceae). Used by African hunters to arrest movement of the hunter; hallucinogenic, antidepressant, and euphoric.

ibo·ten·ic ac·id (ī'bō-ten-ik). Chemical similar to kainic acid extracted from poisonous mushroom species *Amanita muscaria* and *A. pantherina* (family Agaricaceae). Exhibits substantial neuroexcitatory properties. Used in neuropharmacologic research.

ibu·pro·fen (ī-boo'prō-fen). A propionic acid–derived, nonsteroidal analgesic and anti-inflammatory agent.

⌂**-ic. 1.** Suffix denoting of, pertaining to. **2.** Chemical suffix denoting an element in a compound in one of its highest valencies. Cf. -ous (1). **3.** Suffix indicating an acid. [L. *-icus,* fr. G. *-ikos*]

ICAM-1 Abbreviation for intercellular adhesion *molecule*-1.

ic·co·somes (ī'kō-sōmz). Beaded cytoplasmic structure on follicular dendrite cells; thought to be a repository for antigens. [*im*mune *c*omplex *co*ated + -*some*]

ICD Abbreviation for *International Classification of Diseases of the World Health Organization.*

ICDA Abbreviation for *International Classification of Diseases, Adapted for Use in the United States;* includes a classification of surgical operations and other therapeutic and diagnostic procedures.

ice pack. A cold local application to limit or reduce swelling in recently traumatized tissues; usually in the form of a water-impervious container for ice. Improvised means for containing ice (plastic bags, towels, etc.) are often employed, as are chemical sacks that when struck allow the commingling of chemicals that react endothermically.

ICF Abbreviation for intracellular *fluid.*

ichor (ī'kōr). Rarely used term for a thin watery discharge from an ulcer or unhealthy wound. [G. *ichōr,* serum]

icho·re·mia (ī-kō-rē'mē-ă). SYN ichorrhemia.

icho·roid (ī'kō-royd). Denoting a thin purulent discharge. [G. *ichōr,* serum, + *eidos,* resemblance]

ichor·ous (ī'kōr-ŭs). Relating to or resembling ichor.

ichor·rhea (ī'kō-rē'ă). A profuse ichorous discharge. [G. *ichōr,* serum, + *rhoia,* a flow]

ichor·rhe·mia (ī-kō-rē'mē-ă). Sepsis resulting from infection accompanied by an ichorous discharge. SYN ichoremia. [G. *ichōr,* serum, + *rhoia,* a flow, + *haima,* blood]

ICHPPC Abbreviation for International Classification of Health Problems in Primary Care.

ich·tham·mol (ik'tham-mol). A viscous fluid, reddish brown to brownish black in color, with a strong, characteristic, empyreumatic odor, soluble in water and in glycerin; obtained by the destructive distillation of certain bituminous schists, sulfonating the distillate and neutralizing the product with ammonia. It is used in skin disorders; its beneficial effect is due to its mild irritant, stimulant, antiseptic, and analgesic action; has been used in 10 and 20 percent concentration in an ointment ("drawing salve"). SYN ammonium ichthosulfonate.

ich·thy·ism (ik'thi-izm). Poisoning by eating stale or otherwise unfit fish. SYN ichthyismus. [G. *ichthys,* fish]

ich·thy·is·mus (ik-thi-iz'mŭs). SYN ichthyism. [G. *ichthys,* fish]

i. exanthemat'icus, toxic erythematous eruption due to ingestion of spoiled fish.

i. hys'trix, SYN bullous congenital ichthyosiform *erythroderma.*

⌂**ichthyo-.** Fish. [G. *ichthys*]

ich·thy·o·a·can·tho·tox·ism (ik'thi-ō-ă-kan'thō-tok'sizm). Poisoning from the stings or spines of venomous fishes. [ichthyo- + G. *akantha,* thorn, + *toxikon,* poison]

ich·thy·o·col·la (ik-thē-ō-kol'ă). Fish gelatin obtained from sounds or swim bladders of fish such as the hake, cod, and sturgeon; used as a glue, a food substitute, and a clarifying agent. SYN isinglass. [ichthyo- + G. *kolla,* glue]

ich·thy·o·he·mo·tox·in (ik'thē-ō-hē'mō-tok'sin). The toxic substance in the blood of certain fishes. [ichthyo- + G. *haima,* blood, + *toxikon,* poison]

⌂ **Combining Forms**	☆ **Official alternate**
	Terminologia Anatomica
☷ **Indicates term is illustrated,**	**term**
see Illustration Index	
	[MIM] Mendelian Inheritance
SYN Synonym	**in Man**
Cf. Compare	**C.I.** Colour Index
[NA] Nomina Anatomica	
	High Profile Term
[TA] Terminologia Anatomica	

ich·thy·o·he·mo·tox·ism (ik′thē-ō-hē′mō-tok′sizm). Poisoning resulting from the ingestion of fish containing the toxic substance, ichthyohemotoxin.

ich·thy·oid (ik′thē-oyd). Fish-shaped. [ichthyo- + G. *eidos*, resemblance]

ich·thy·o·o·tox·in (ik′thē-ō-ō-tok′sin). Toxic substance restricted to the roe of fishes. [ichthyo- + G. *ōon*, egg, + *toxikon*, poison]

ich·thy·oph·a·gous (ik-thē-of′ă-gŭs). Fish-eating; subsisting on fish. [ichthyo- + G. *phagō*, to eat]

ich·thy·o·pho·bia (ik′thē-ō-fō′bē-ă). Morbid fear of fish. [ichthyo- + G. *phobos*, fear]

ich·thy·o·sar·co·tox·in (ik′thē-ō-sar′kō-tok′sin). Toxic substance found in the flesh or organs of fishes. [ichthyo- + G. *sarx*, flesh, + *toxikon*, poison]

ich·thy·o·sar·co·tox·ism (ik′thē-ō-sar′kō-tok′sizm). Poisoning caused by the toxic substance (ichthyosarcotoxin) in the flesh or organs of fish. [ichthyo- + G. *sarx*, flesh, + *toxikon*, poison]

ich·thy·o·sis (ik-thē-ō′sis). Congenital disorders of keratinization characterized by noninflammatory dryness and scaling of the skin, often associated with other defects and with abnormalities of lipid metabolism; distinguishable genetically, clinically, microscopically, and by epidermal cell kinetics. SYN alligator skin, fish skin, sauriasis. [ichthyo- + G. *-osis*, condition]

acquired i., a thickening and scaling of the skin associated with some malignant diseases (e.g., Hodgkin lymphoma), leprosy, and severe nutritional deficiencies.

i. congenita, SYN lamellar i.

i. congen′ita neonato′rum, generalized i. with parchmentlike skin seen in premature babies.

i. cor′neae, an ocular complication of a congenital abnormality of the skin with corneal keratinization, dryness, and scaling.

i. feta′lis, (1) SYN harlequin *fetus*; **(2)** recessive condition in Holstein and Norwegian red poll cattle resembling harlequin fetus in humans.

i. follicula′ris, a form of autosomal dominant type of i., with horny follicular plugging of the extensor surfaces of the extremities; onset in early childhood.

harlequin i. [MIM*242500], a fetal form of i. thought to be distinct from lamellar i., with plaques having a diamondlike shape resembling the suit of a harlequin clown; the keratinocytes contain increased amounts of tonofibrils, which are fibrillar structural proteins; autosomal recessive inheritance.

i. hys′trix, SYN bullous congenital ichthyosiform *erythroderma*. [G. *hystrix*, hedgehog]

lamellar i. [MIM*242300], a dry form of congenital ichthyosiform erythroderma, characterized by ectropion and large, coarse scales over most of the body with thickened palms and soles; may be fatal with complications of sepsis, protein, and electrolyte loss in the first year of life; histology shows hyperkeratosis, a prominent granular layer in the epidermis, slight acanthosis, many mitotic figures, and normal or reduced epidemal cell turnover. Autosomal recessive inheritance, caused by mutation in the gene encoding keratinocyte transglutaminase (TGM1) on chromosome 14q. SEE ALSO collodion *baby*, harlequin *fetus*. SYN i. congenita.

i. linea′ris circumflex′a, congenital or infantile migratory polycyclic erythema and scaling that shows a peripheral double margin; persists throughout life and may be associated with trichorrhexis invaginata in Netherton syndrome [MIM*256500]; autosomal recessive inheritance.

nacreous i., a variant of i. characterized by dry pearly scales.

i. palma′ris et planta′ris, SYN palmoplantar *keratoderma*.

i. scutula′ta, i. marked by diamond-shaped or shield-shaped lesions.

i. sim′plex, SYN i. vulgaris.

i. vulga′ris [MIM*146700], an autosomal dominant trait, with onset in childhood of scales on the trunk and extremities but not on the flexural areas, and associated with atopy and prominent palmar and plantar markings; histologically, there is hyperkeratosis, absence of a granular layer in the epidermis, and normal epidermal cell turnover. SYN hyperkeratosis congenita, i. simplex.

X-linked i. [MIM*308100], a form of i., with onset at birth or in early infancy and affecting males; characterized by scaling predominantly on the scalp, neck and trunk and progressing centripetally; the palms and soles are spared; histologic manifestations are hyperkeratosis, a granular layer in the epidermis, and normal epidermal cell turnover. X-linked recessive inheritance, caused by mutation in the steroid sulfatase gene (STS) on Xp. SYN steroid sulfatase deficiency.

ich·thy·ot·ic (ik-thē-ot′ik). Relating to ichthyosis.

ich·thy·o·tox·i·col·o·gy (ik′thē-ō-tok-si-kol′ō-jē). The study of the poisons produced by fishes, and their recognition, effects, and antidotes. [ichthyo- + G. *toxikon*, poison, + *logos*, study]

ich·thy·o·tox·i·con (ik-thē-ō-tok′si-kon). A toxic principle in certain fishes. SYN fish poison (1). [ichthyo- + G. *toxikon*, poison]

ich·thy·o·tox·in (ik′thē-ō-tok′sin). The hemolytic active principle of eel serum. [ichthyo- + G. *toxicon*, poison]

ich·thy·o·tox·ism (ik′thē-ō-tok′sizm). Poisoning by fish. [ichthyo- + G. *toxikon*, poison]

ICIDH Abbreviation for International Classification of Impairments, Disabilities and Handicaps.

ico·sa·he·dral (ī′kō-să-hē′drăl). Having 20 equilateral triangular surfaces and 12 vertices, as do most viruses with cubic symmetry. [G. *eikosi*, twenty, + *-edros*, having sides or bases]

***n*-ico·sa·no·ic ac·id** (ī′kō-să-nō′ik). SYN arachidic acid.

ICP Abbreviation for intracranial *pressure*.

ICRP Abbreviation for International Commission on Radiological Protection.

△-ics. Organized knowledge, practice, treatment. [-ic + -s]

ICSH Abbreviation of interstitial cell-stimulating *hormone*.

ic·tal (ik′tăl). Relating to or caused by a stroke or seizure. [L. *ictus*, a stroke]

ic·ter·ic (ik-ter′ik). Relating to or marked by jaundice. [G. *ikterikos*, jaundiced]

△ictero-. Icterus. [G. *ikteros*, jaundice]

ic·ter·o·a·ne·mia (ik′ter-ō-ă-nē′mē-ă). SYN acquired hemolytic *icterus*.

ic·ter·o·gen·ic (ik′ter-ō-jen′ik). Causing jaundice. [ictero- + G. *-gen*, producing]

ic·ter·o·he·ma·tu·ric (ik′ter-ō-hē′mă-too′rik). Denoting jaundice with the passage of blood in the urine. [ictero- + G. *haima*, blood, + *ouron*, urine]

ic·ter·o·he·mo·glo·bi·nu·ria (ik′ter-ō-hē′mō-glō-bi-noo′rē-ă). Jaundice with hemoglobin in the urine.

ic·ter·oid (ik′ter-oyd). Yellow-hued, or seemingly jaundiced. [ictero- + G. *eidos*, resemblance]

ic·ter·us (ik′ter-ŭs). SYN jaundice. [G. *ikteros*]

acquired hemolytic i., i. and anemia occuring in association with a moderate degree of splenomegaly, increased fragility of red blood cells, and increased amounts of urobilin in the urine. SYN icteroanemia.

benign familial i., SYN familial nonhemolytic *jaundice*.

cholestatic hepatosis i. gravidarum, SYN intrahepatic *cholestasis* of pregnancy.

chronic familial i., SYN hereditary *spherocytosis*.

congenital hemolytic i., SYN hereditary *spherocytosis*.

cythemolytic i., i. caused by absorption of bile produced in excess through stimulation by free hemoglobin caused by the destruction of red blood corpuscles.

i. gra′vis, jaundice associated with high fever and delirium; seen in severe hepatitis and other diseases of the liver with severe functional failure. SYN malignant jaundice.

infectious i., SYN Weil *disease*.

i. mel′as, a form in which the skin assumes a dirty dark brown color.

i. neonato′rum, SYN physiologic i. SYN physiologic *jaundice*.

physiologic i., SYN i. neonatorum.

i. prae′cox, a relatively innocent but rapidly developing type of jaundice with mild anemia in the newborn, most frequently caused by ABO incompatibility between mother and fetus.

ic·tom·e·ter (ik-tom′ĕ-ter). An apparatus for determining the force of the apex beat of the heart. [L. *ictus,* stroke, + G. *metron,* measure]

ic·tus (ik′tŭs). **1.** A stroke or attack. **2.** A beat. [L.]

i. cor′dis, SYN heart *beat.*

i. epilep′ticus, an epileptic convulsion.

i. paralyt′icus, a paralytic stroke.

i. so′lis, SYN sunstroke.

ICU Abbreviation for intensive care *unit.*

I.D. Abbreviation for infecting dose. SEE minimal infecting *dose.*

id. 1. In psychoanalysis, one of three components of the psychic apparatus in the freudian structural framework, the other two being the ego and superego. It is completely in the unconscious realm, is unorganized, is the reservoir of psychic energy or libido, and is under the influence of the primary processes. **2.** The total of all psychic energy available from the innate biologic hungers, appetites, bodily needs, drives and impulses, in a newborn infant; through socialization this diffuse undirected energy becomes channeled in less egocentric and more socially responsive directions (development of the ego from the id). [L. *id,* that]

⌂-id. 1. A state of sensitivity of the skin in which a part remote from the primary lesion reacts ("-id reaction") to substances of the pathogen, giving rise to a secondary inflammatory lesion; the lesion manifesting the reaction is designated by the use of -id as a suffix. [G. *-eidēs,* resembling, through Fr. *-ide*] **2.** Small, young specimen. [G. *-idion,* a diminutive ending]

IDA Abbreviation for iminodiacetate, whose derivatives are used in radiopharmaceuticals with a ^{99m}Tc label. SEE HIDA. SEE ALSO DISIDA.

IDDM Abbreviation for insulin-dependent *diabetes* mellitus.

⌂-ide. 1. Suffix denoting the more electronegative element in a binary chemical compound; formerly denoted by the qualification -ureted; e.g., hydrogen sulfide was sulfureted hydrogen. **2.** Suffix (in a sugar name) indicating substitution for the H of the hemiacetal OH; e.g., glycoside.

idea (ī-dē′ă). Any mental image or concept. [G. form, appearance, fr. *idein,* to have seen, fr. obs. *eidō,* to see]

autochthonous i.'s, thoughts that suddenly burst into awareness as if they are vitally important, often as if they have come from an outside source.

compulsive i., a fixed and repetitively recurring i.

dominant i., an i. that governs all one's actions and thoughts.

fixed i., (1) an exaggerated notion, belief, or delusion that persists, despite evidence to the contrary, and controls the mind; **(2)** the obstinate conviction of a psychotic person regarding the correctness of a delusion. SYN idée fixe, overvalued i.

flight of i.'s, an uncontrollable symptom of the manic phase of a bipolar depressive disorder in which streams of unrelated words and i.'s occur to the patient at a rate that is impossible to vocalize despite a marked increase in the individual's overall output of words. SEE ALSO mania.

overvalued i., SYN fixed i.

i. of reference, the misinterpretation that other people's statements or acts or neutral objects in the environment are directed toward one's self when, in fact, they are not.

ide·al (ī-dēl′). A standard of perfection.

ego i., the part of the personality that comprises the goals, aspirations, and aims of the self, usually growing out of the emulation of a significant person with whom one has identified.

ide·a·tion (ī-dē-ā′shŭn). The formation of ideas or thoughts.

ide·a·tion·al (ī-dē-ā′shŭn-ăl). Relating to ideation.

idée fixe (ē-dā′fēks′). SYN fixed *idea.* [Fr. obsession]

iden·ti·fi·ca·tion (ī-den′ti-fi-kā′shŭn). **1.** Act or process of determining classification or nature of. **2.** A sense of oneness, or psychic continuity with another person or group; one of the freudian defense mechanisms common to everyone whereby anxiety regarding one's personal identity or worth is dissipated via the mechanism of perceiving oneself as having characteristics in common with a person in the public eye, or in childhood identifying with a more powerful person such as a parent. SYN incorporation. [Mediev. L. *identicus,* fr. L. *idem,* the same, + *facio,* to make]

projective i., a defensive attribution of one's own psychic processes to another person.

synthetic sentence i., a test of central auditory pathway integrity in which a closed set of 10 syntactically incomplete sentences are presented with a competing message for identification.

iden·ti·ty (ī-den′ti-tē). A person's social role person and his or her perception of it.

ego i., the ego's sense of its own identity.

gender i., the consistency and persistence of one's individuality as male, female, or androgynous. Particularly as experienced in self-awareness; the internalized representation of gender role. Cf. gender *role,* sex *role.*

sense of i., one's sense of one's own identity or psychological selfhood.

⌂ideo-. Ideas; ideation Cf. idio-. [G. *idea,* form, notion]

ide·o·ki·net·ic (ī′dē-ō-ki-net′ik). SYN ideomotor.

ide·ol·o·gy (ī-dē-ol′ō-jē, id-ē-). The composite system of ideas, beliefs, and attitudes that constitutes an individual's or group's organized view of others. [ideo- + G. *logos,* study]

ide·o·mo·tion (ī-dē-ō-mō′shŭn). Muscular movement executed under the influence of a dominant idea, being practically automatic and not volitional.

ide·o·mo·tor (ī′dē-ō-mō′ter). Relating to ideomotion. SYN ideokinetic.

ide·o·pho·bia (ī′dē-ō-fō′bē-ă). Morbid fear of new or different ideas.

⌂idio-. Private, distinctive, peculiar to. Cf. ideo-. [G. *idios,* one's own]

id·i·o·ag·glu·ti·nin (id′ē-ō-ă-gloo′tin-in). An agglutinin that occurs naturally in the blood of a person or an animal, without the injection of a stimulating antigen or the passive transfer of antibody.

id·i·o·dy·nam·ic (id′ē-ō-dī-nam′ik). Independently active.

id·i·o·gen·e·sis (id′ē-ō-jen′ĕ-sis). Origin without evident cause; denoting especially that of an idiopathic disease. [idio- + G. *genesis,* production]

id·i·o·glos·sia (id′ē-ō-glos′ē-ă). An extreme form of lalling or vowel or consonant substitution, by which the speech of a child may be made unintelligible and appear to be another language to one who does not have the key to the literal changes. [idio- + G. *glōssa,* tongue, speech]

id·i·o·glot·tic (id′ē-ō-glot′ik). Relating to idioglossia.

id·i·o·gram (id′ē-ō-gram). **1.** SYN karyotype. **2.** Diagrammatic representation of chromosome morphology characteristic of a species or population. [idio- + G. *gramma,* something written]

id·i·o·graph·ic (id′ē-ō-graf′ik). Pertaining to the characteristics or behavior of a particular individual as an individual, as opposed to nomothetic. [idio- + G. *graphō,* to write]

id·i·o·het·er·o·ag·glu·ti·nin (id′ē-ō-het′er-ō-ă-gloo′tin-in). An idioagglutinin occurring in the blood of one animal, but capable of combining with the antigenic material from another species. [idio- + G. *heteros,* another, + agglutinin]

id·i·o·het·er·o·ly·sin (id′ē-ō-het-er-ol′i-sin). An idiolysin occurring in the blood of an animal of one species, but capable of combining with the red blood cells of another species, thereby causing hemolysis when complement is present.

id·i·o·hyp·no·tism (id′ē-ō-hip′nō-tizm). SYN autohypnosis.

id·i·o·i·so·ag·glu·ti·nin (id′ē-ō-ī′sō-ă-gloo′tin-in). An idioagglutinin occurring in the blood of an animal of a certain species, capable of agglutinating the cells from animals of the same species. [idio- + G. *isos,* equal, + agglutinin]

id·i·o·i·sol·y·sin (id′ē-ō-ī-sol′i-sin). An idiolysin occurring in the blood of an animal of a certain species, capable of combining with the red blood cells from animals of the same species, thereby causing hemolysis when complement is present.

id·i·o·la·lia (id′ē-ō-lā′lē-ă). Use of a language invented by the person himself. [idio- + G. *lalia,* talk]

id·i·ol·y·sin (id-ē-ol′i-sin). A lysin that occurs naturally in the blood of a person or an animal, without the injection of a stimulating antigen or the passive transfer of antibody.

id·i·o·mus·cu·lar (id′ē-ō-mŭs′kū-lăr). Relating to the muscles alone, independent of the nervous control.

id·i·o·nod·al (id′ē-ō-nō′dăl). Arising from the AV node itself; applied to the ventricular rhythm in complete S-A or AV block, or in other forms of AV dissociation, when the AV node rather than an ectopic ventricular focus controls the ventricles. More accurately idiojunctional, since it is usually impossible to more accurately locate an "AV nodal" rhythm; the AV node is part of the AV junction. SEE ALSO idioventricular.

id·i·o·pa·thet·ic (id′ē-ō-pă-thet′ik). Rarely used term for idiopathic.

id·i·o·path·ic (id′ē-ō-path′ik). Denoting a disease of unknown cause. SYN agnogenic. [idio- + G. *pathos,* suffering]

id·i·op·a·thy (id-ē-op′ă-thē). An idiopathic disease. [idio- + G. *pathos,* suffering]

id·i·o·phren·ic (id′ē-ō-fren′ik). Relating to, or originating in, the mind or brain alone, not reflex or secondary. [idio- + G. *phrēn,* mind]

id·i·o·psy·cho·log·ic (id′ē-ō-sī-kō-loj′ik). Relating to ideas developed within one's own mind, independent of suggestion from without.

id·i·o·re·flex (id-ē-ō-rē′fleks). A reflex due to a stimulus or irritation originating in the organ or part in which the reflex occurs.

id·i·o·some (id′ē-ō-sōm). The centrosome of a spermatid or of an oocyte. [idio- + G. *sōma,* body]

id·i·o·syn·cra·sy (id′ē-ō-sin′kră-sē). **1.** An individual mental, behavioral, or physical characteristic or peculiarity. **2.** In pharmacology, an abnormal reaction to a drug, sometimes specified as genetically determined. [G. *idiosynkrasia,* fr. *idios,* one's own, + *synkrasis,* a mixing together]

id·i·o·syn·crat·ic (id′ē-ō-sin-krat′ik). Relating to or marked by an idiosyncrasy.

id·i·o·tope (id′ē-ōtōp). Single antigenic determinant of an idiotype. SEE ALSO idiotypic antigenic *determinant.* SYN idiotypic antigenic determinant. [idio- + -tope]

set of idiotopes, (antigenic determinants) of either the immunoglobulin or T cell receptor variable regions.

id·i·ot-prod·i·gy (id′ē-ŏt prod′i-jē). SYN idiot-savant.

id·i·o·tro·phic (id′ē-ō-trof′ik). Capable of choosing its own food. [idio- + G. *trophē,* food]

id·i·o·tro·pic (id′ē-ō-trop′ik). Turning inward upon one's self. [idio- + G. *tropē,* a turning]

id·i·ot-sa·vant (ē-dē-ō′ sah-vahn′). A person of low general intelligence who possesses an unusual faculty for certain mental tasks of which most normal persons are incapable. SYN idiot-prodigy. [Fr.]

id·i·o·type (id′ē-ō-tīp). Collection of idiotopes within the variable region that confers on an immunoglobulin molecule an antigenic "individuality" and is frequently a unique attribute of a given antibody in a given animal. It is the product of a limited number of B lymphocyte clones; also found on the T-cell receptor. SEE idiotope. [idio- + G. *typos,* model]

id·i·o·ven·tric·u·lar (id-ē-ō-ven-trik′ū-lăr). Pertaining to or associated with the cardiac ventricles alone.

id·i·tol (ī′di-tol). Reduction product of the hexose idose.

IDL Abbreviation for intermediate density *lipoprotein.*

id·ose (ī′dōs). One of the aldohexoses, isomeric with galactose; L-i. is epimeric with D-glucose. SEE sugar.

idox·ur·i·dine (IDU) (ī-doks-ū′ri-dēn). A pyrimidine analogue that produces both antiviral and anticancer effects by interference with DNA synthesis; used locally in the eye for the treatment of keratitis from herpes simplex or vaccinia.

IDP Abbreviation for inosine 5′-diphosphate.

IDU Abbreviation for idoxuridine.

id·ur·o·nate (ī-door-on′āt). The salt or ester of iduronic acid.
i. sulfatase, an enzyme required for the desulfation of 2-sulfate i. residues in heparan sulfate. It is also required in dermatan sulfate degradation; Hunter syndrome is associated with a deficiency of this enzyme.

idur·on·ic ac·id (ī-door-on′ik). The uronic acid of idose; a constituent of dermatan sulfate.

α-L-id·ur·on·id·ase (ī-door-on′i-dās). An enzyme that hydrolyzes terminal desulfated α-L-iduronic acid residues of dermatan sulfate and of heparan sulfate; a deficiency of this enzyme is associated with Hurler syndrome and Scheie syndrome.

IEP Abbreviation for isoelectric *point.*

IF Abbreviation for initiation *factor;* intrinsic *factor.*

IFN Abbreviation for interferon.

IFN-α Abbreviation for *interferon* alpha.

IFN-β Abbreviation for *interferon* beta.

IFN-γ Abbreviation for *interferon* gamma.

Ig Abbreviation for immunoglobulin.

IgA Abbreviation for immunoglobulin A.

IgD Abbreviation for immunoglobulin D.

IgE Abbreviation for immunoglobulin E.

IGF Abbreviation for insulinlike growth *factor.*

IgG Abbreviation for immunoglobulin G.

IgM Abbreviation for immunoglobulin M.

ig·na·tia (ig-nā′shē-ă). The dried ripe seed of *Strychnos ignatii* (family Loganiaceae). It is similar in its properties to nux vomica and is a source of strychnine. [*St. Ignatius*]

ig·ni·pe·di·tes (ig′ni-pe-dī′tēz). Burning pain in the soles of the feet, in multiple neuritis. [L. *ignis,* fire, + *pes* (*ped-*), foot, + G. *itēs*]

ig·ni·punc·ture (ig′ni-pŭngk-choor). The original procedure of closing a retinal break in retinal separation by transfixation of the break with cautery. [L. *ignis,* fire, + puncture]

ig·no·tine (ig′nō-tēn). SYN carnosine.

IH Abbreviation for infectious *hepatitis.*

IJP Abbreviation for inhibitory junction *potential.*

iko·ta (ī-kō′tă). A neurosis, similar to latah, affecting married women among the Samoyeds of Siberia.

IL-1 Abbreviation for interleukin-1.

IL-2 Abbreviation for interleukin-2.

IL-3 Abbreviation for interleukin-3.

IL-4 Abbreviation for interleukin-4.

IL-5 Abbreviation for interleukin-5.

IL-6 Abbreviation for interleukin-6.

IL-7 Abbreviation for interleukin-7.

IL-8 Abbreviation for interleukin-8.

IL-9 Abbreviation for interleukin-9.

IL-10 Abbreviation for interleukin-10.

IL-11 Abbreviation for interleukin-11.

IL-12 Abbreviation for interleukin-12.

IL-13 Abbreviation for interleukin-13.

IL-14 Abbreviation for interleukin-14.

IL-15 Abbreviation for interleukin-15.

IL-16 Abbreviation for interleukin-16.

IL-17 Abbreviation for interleukin-17.

IL-18 Abbreviation for interleukin-18.

ILA Abbreviation for insulinlike *activity.*

il·e·ac (il′ē-ak). **1.** Relating to ileus. **2.** Relating to the ileum.

il·e·a·del·phus (il′ē-ă-del′fŭs). SYN *duplicitas* posterior.

il·e·al (il′ē-ăl). Of or pertaining to the ileum.

il·e·ec·to·my (il-ē-ek′tō-mē). Removal of the ileum. [ileum + G. *ektomē,* excision]

il·e·i·tis (il-ē-ī′tis). Inflammation of the ileum.
backwash i., involvement of the terminal ileum by the inflammatory and ulcerative changes seen in chronic ulcerative colitis; distinguished from involvement of ileum and proximal colon by regional (granulomatous) enteritis (e.g., Crohn disease of terminal ileum and proximal colon).
distal i., regional i., terminal i., SYN regional *enteritis.*

ileo-. The ileum. [New L. *ileum,* groin]

il·e·o·ce·cal (il′ē-ō-sē′kăl). Relating to both ileum and cecum.

il

il·e·o·ce·co·cys·to·plas·ty (il′ē-ō-sē′kō-sis′tō-plas-tē). Bladder reconstruction and augmentation with an isolated vascularized segment of ileocecum. [ileo- + ceco- + G. *kystis,* bladder, + *plastos,* formed]

il·e·o·ce·cos·to·my (il′ē-ō-sē-kos′tō′mē). Anastomosis of the ileum to the cecum. SYN cecoileostomy.

il·e·o·ce·cum (il-ē-ō-sē′kŭm). The combined ileum and cecum.

il·e·o·co·lic (il′ē-ō-kol′ik). Relating to the ileum and the colon. SYN ileocolonic.

il·e·o·co·li·tis (il′ē-ō-kō-lī′tis). Inflammation to a varying extent of the mucous membrane of both ileum and colon.

il·e·o·co·lon·ic (il′ē-ō-kō-lon′ik). SYN ileocolic.

il·e·o·co·los·to·my (il′ē-ō-kō-los′tō-mē). Anastomosis of the ileum to the colon. [ileo- + colostomy]

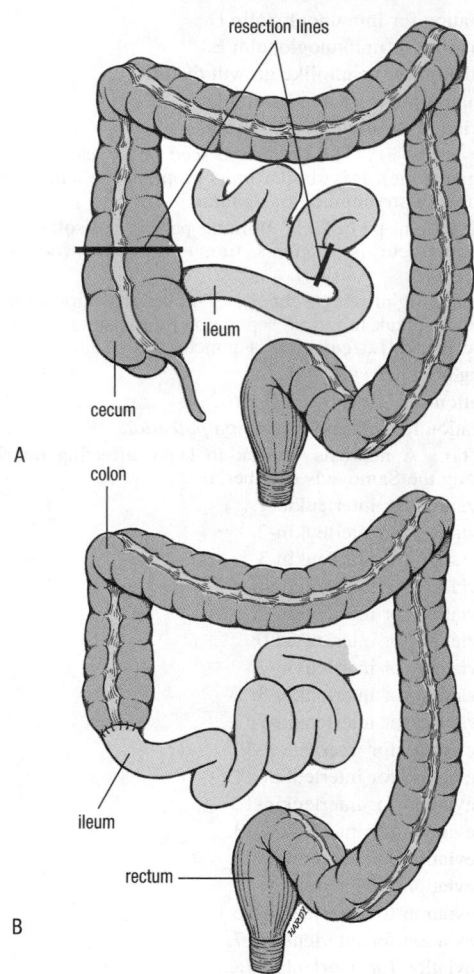

resection lines

ileum

cecum

A

colon

ileum

rectum

B

ileocolostomy: diseased portions of ileum and cecum resected (A) and resected ends anastomosed (B)

il·e·o·cys·to·plas·ty (il′ē-ō-sis′tō-plas-tē). Reconstruction of the bladder with an isolated vascularized segment of ileum to augment bladder capacity. [ileo- + G. *kystis,* bladder, + *plastos,* formed]

il·e·o·en·tec·tro·py (il′ē-ō-en-tek′trō-pē). Rarely used term for eversion of a segment of the ileum. [ileo- + G. *entos,* within, + *ek,* out, + *tropē,* a turning]

il·e·o·il·e·os·to·my (il′ē-ō-il-e-os′tō-mē). **1.** Anastomosis between two segments of the ileum. **2.** The opening so established. [ileum + ileum + G. *stoma,* mouth]

il·e·o·je·ju·ni·tis (il′ē-ō-je-joo-nī′tis). A chronic inflammatory

condition involving the jejunum and parts or most of the ileum; occurs in different forms: a granulomatous state resembling regional ileitis, pseudodiverticula, or cicatricial stenosis of the bowel.

il·e·o·pexy (il′ē-ō-pek′sē). Surgical fixation of ileum. [ileo- + G. *pēxis,* fixation]

il·e·o·proc·tos·to·my (il′ē-ō-prok-tos′tō-mē). Anastomosis between the ileum and the rectum. SYN ileorectostomy. [ileo- + G. *prōktos,* anus (rectum), + *stoma,* mouth]

il·e·o·rec·tos·to·my (il′ē-ō-rek-tos′tō-mē). SYN ileoproctostomy. [ileum + rectum + G. *stoma,* mouth]

il·e·or·rha·phy (il′ē-ōr′ă-fē). Suturing the ileum. [ileo- + G. *rhaphē,* suture]

il·e·o·sig·moid·os·to·my (il′ē-ō-sig′moyd-os′tō-mē). Anastomosis between the ileum and the sigmoid colon. [ileo- + sigmoid, + G. *stoma,* mouth]

il·e·os·to·my (il′ē-os′tō-mē). Establishment of a fistula through which the ileum discharges directly to the outside of the body. [ileo- + G. *stoma,* mouth]

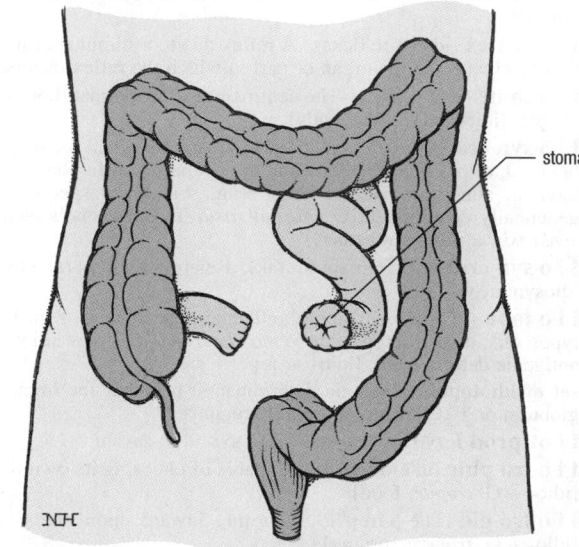

stoma

ileostomy

Brooke i., i. in which the divided proximal ileum, brought through the abdominal wall, is evaginated and its edge is sutured to the dermis; a 2-cm protrusion is the desired result of the procedure.

Kock i., SYN Kock *pouch.*

il·e·ot·o·my (il′ē-ot′ō-mē). Incision into the ileum. [ileo- + G. *tomē,* incision]

il·e·o·trans·ver·sos·to·my (il′ē-ō-tranz-vers-os′tō-me). Anastomosis of the ileum to the transverse colon. [ileum + transverse colon, + G. *stoma,* mouth]

il·e·um (il′ē-ŭm) [TA]. The third and longest portion of the small intestine, about 12 feet in length in humans, extending from an indistinct junction with the jejunum to the ileocecal opening. Overall, it is distinct from jejunum in being typically smaller in diameter with thinner walls, having smaller and less complex circular folds (plicae circulares), its mesentery having more fat and its arteries (ileal arteries) forming more tiers of arterial arcades with shorter vasa recta. [L. fr. G. *eileō,* to roll up, twist]

i. du′plex, tubular or cystic segmental duplications of alimentary tract.

il·e·us (il′ē-ŭs). Mechanical, dynamic, or adynamic obstruction of the bowel; may be accompanied by severe colicky pain, abdominal distention, vomiting, absence of passage of stool, and often fever and dehydration. [G. *eileos,* intestinal colic, from *eilō,* to roll up tight]

adynamic i., obstruction of the bowel due to paralysis of the bowel wall, usually as a result of localized or generalized peritonitis or shock. SYN paralytic i.

dynamic i., intestinal obstruction due to spastic contraction of a segment of the bowel. SYN spastic i.

gallstone i., obstruction of the small intestine produced by passage of a gallstone from the biliary tract (usually the gallbladder as a result of cholecystitis) into the intestinal tract (usually by means of a fistulous connection between the gallbladder and the small intestine); occurrence and site of obstruction depend upon size of the stone, but the usual location is at or near the ileocecal junction.

mechanical i., obstruction of the bowel due to some mechanical cause, e.g., volvulus, gallstone, adhesions.

meconium i., intestinal obstruction in the fetus and newborn following inspissation of meconium and caused by lack of trypsin; associated with cystic fibrosis.

occlusive i., complete mechanical blocking of the intestinal lumen.

paralytic i., SYN adynamic i.

spastic i., SYN dynamic i.

i. subpar′ta, obstruction of the large bowel by pressure of the pregnant uterus.

terminal i., obstruction of the lower part of the small bowel. SYN pars terminalis ilei [TA].

verminous i., obstruction due to masses of intestinal parasites.

il·i·ac (il′ē-ak). Relating to the ilium.

il·i·a·cus (il-ī′ă-kŭs). SEE iliacus (*muscle*).

il·i·a·del·phus (il′ē-ă-del′fŭs). SYN *duplicitas* posterior. [L. *ilium* + G. *adelphos,* brother]

ilio-. The ilium. [L. *ilium*]

il·i·o·coc·cyg·e·al (il′ē-ō-kok-sij′ē-ăl). Relating to the ilium and the coccyx.

il·i·o·co·lot·o·my (il′ē-ō-kō-lot′ō-mē). The operation of opening into the colon in the inguinal (iliac) region. [ilio- + G. *kolon,* colon, + *tomē,* incision]

il·i·o·cos·tal (il′ē-ō-kos′tăl). Relating to the ilium and the ribs; denoting muscles passing between the two parts.

il·i·o·cos·ta·lis (il′ē-ō-kos-tā′lis). SEE iliocostalis (*muscle*).

il·i·o·fem·o·ral (il′ē-ō-fem′ŏ-răl). Relating to the ilium and the femur.

il·i·o·fem·o·ro·plas·ty (il-ē-o-fem′ōr-ō-plas-tē). An obsolete method of securing a hip fusion by an extra-articular technique (a joint bypass procedure) in which a turned down bone flap from the ilium is placed into a split in the greater trochanter.

il·i·o·hy·po·gas·tric (il′ē-ō-hī-pō-gas′trik). Relating to the iliac and the hypogastric regions.

il·i·o·in·gui·nal (il′ē-ō-ing′gwi-năl). Relating to the iliac region and the groin.

il·i·o·lum·bar (il-ē-ō-lŭm′băr). Relating to the iliac and the lumbar regions.

il·i·op·a·gus (il-ē-op′ă-gŭs). Conjoined twins in which the fusion is restricted to the iliac region. SEE conjoined *twins,* under *twin*. [ilio- + G. *pagos,* something fixed]

il·i·o·pec·tin·e·al (il′ē-ō-pek-tin′ē-ăl). Relating to the ilium and the pubis.

il·i·o·pel·vic (il′ē-ō-pel′vik). Relating to the iliac region and the cavity of the pelvis.

il·i·o·sa·cral (il′ē-ō-sā′krăl). Relating to the ilium and the sacrum.

il·i·o·sci·at·ic (il′ē-ō-sī-at′ik). Relating to the ilium and the ischium.

il·i·o·spi·nal (il′ē-ō-spī′năl). Relating to the ilium and the spinal column.

il·i·o·tho·ra·cop·a·gus (il′ē-ō-thōr-ă-kop′ă-gŭs). Conjoined twins in which union occurs through the ilia and extends to involve the thoraces. SEE conjoined *twins,* under *twin*. SYN ischiothoracopagus. [ilio- + G. *thorax,* chest, + *pagos,* fixed]

il·i·o·tib·i·al (il′ē-ō-tib′ē-ăl). Relating to the ilium and the tibia.

il·i·o·tro·chan·ter·ic (il′ē-ō-trō-kan-ter′ik). Relating to the ilium and the greater trochanter of the femur.

il·i·o·xi·phop·a·gus (il′ē-ō-zī-fop′ă-gŭs). Conjoined twins in which the fusion extends from the xiphoid to the iliac region. SEE conjoined *twins,* under *twin*. [ilio- + xiphoid, + G. *pagos,* fixed]

il·i·um, pl. **il·i·a** (il′ē-ŭm, il′ē-ă) [TA]. The broad, flaring portion of the hip bone, distinct at birth but later becoming fused with the ischium and pubis; it consists of a body, which joins the pubis and ischium to form the acetabulum and a broad thin portion, called the ala or wing, bordered superiorly by a thicker crest. The body transmits the weight of the trunk to the femur, while the ala and crest provide for muscle attachment and protect abdominopelvic viscera. SYN os ilium [TA], flank bone, iliac bone, os iliacum. [L. groin, flank]

il·lic·i·um (il-lis′ē-ŭm). Chinese or star anise, the dried fruit of *Illhicium verum* (family Magnoliaceae), an evergreen shrub or small tree of southern China; used as a stimulating carminative. [L. an allurement, fr. *il-licio,* to allure]

il·lin·i·tion (il-in-ish′ŭn). The friction of a surface to facilitate absorption of an ointment. [L. *il-lino,* pp. -*litus,* to smear on (*in* + *lino*)]

ill·ness (il′nes). SYN disease (1).

environmental i., SYN multiple chemical *sensitivity*.

factitious i. by proxy, SYN Munchausen *syndrome* by proxy.

functional i., SYN functional *disorder*.

manic-depressive i., an older term for manic-depressive *disorder,* which is now called bipolar *disorder* in the current DSM.

mass sociogenic i., SYN mass *hysteria*.

mental i., (1) a broadly inclusive term, generally denoting one or all of the following: 1) a disease of the brain, with predominant behavioral symptoms, as in paresis or acute alcoholism; 2) a disease of the "mind" or personality, evidenced by abnormal behavior, as in hysteria or schizophrenia; also called mental or emotional disease, disturbance, or disorder, or behavior disorder; (**2**) any psychiatric illness listed in *Current Medical Information and Terminology* of the American Medical Association or in the *Diagnostic and Statistical Manual of Mental Disorders* of the American Psychiatric Association. SEE ALSO behavior *disorder*.

nonspecific building-related i.'s, a heterogeneous group of work- or domicile-related symptoms without clear objective physical or laboratory findings. Cf. specific building-related i.'s.

severity of i., the degree of i. and risk of disease manifested by patients, based either on clinical data from the medical records or on hospital discharge/billing data. Outcome comparisons usually are interpreted in terms of severity of i. to ensure meaningful data interpretations are made.

specific building-related i.'s, a group of infectious, allergic, and immunologic diseases with fairly homogeneous clinical signs whose causes can be traced to factors in buildings in which afflicted patients work or reside. Cf. nonspecific building-related i.'s.

il·lu·mi·na·tion (i-loo′mi-nā′shŭn). **1.** Throwing light on the body or a part or into a cavity for diagnostic purposes. **2.** Lighting an object under a microscope. [L. *il-lumino,* pp. -atus, to light up]

axial i., the transmission or reflection of light in the direction of the axis of an optical system. SYN central i.

central i., SYN axial i.

contact i., i. of the eye by means of an instrument in contact with the cornea or bulbar conjunctiva.

critical i., the precise focusing of the light source directly upon the object being examined.

dark-field i., a procedure in which a black circular shield is used to block the majority of the vertically directed rays of light (e.g., the field is dark), and a circumferential, suitably angled, mirrored surface is used to direct the peripheral rays horizontally against the object, thereby reflecting the light vertically through the objective lens and along the optical axis; thus, the object is well illuminated in a contrasting dark background. SYN dark-ground i.

dark-ground i., SYN dark-field i.

direct i., an i. in which the rays of light are directed downward, almost perpendicularly onto the upper surface of the object, which

il

reflects the rays upward into the optical system. SYN erect i., vertical i.

erect i., SYN direct i.

focal i., i. in which a beam of light is directed diagonally to an object so that it is brilliantly illuminated while the surrounding area is in shadow. SYN lateral i., oblique i.

Köhler i., a method of i. of microscopic objects in which the image of the light source is focused on the substage condenser diaphragm and the diaphragm of the light source is focused in the same plane with the object to be observed; maximizes both the brightness and uniformity of the illuminated field.

lateral i., SYN focal i.

oblique i., SYN focal i.

vertical i., SYN direct i.

il·lu·mi·nism (i-loo′mi-nizm). A psychotic state of exaltation in which one has delusions and hallucinations of communion with supernatural or exalted beings.

il·lu·sion (i-loo′zhŭn). A false perception; the mistaking of something for what it is not. [L. *illusio,* fr. *il- ludo,* pp. *-lusus,* to play at, mock]

i. of doubles, SYN Capgras *syndrome.*

i. of movement, successive stimulation of neighboring retinal points which causes the sensation of movement.

oculogravic i., apparent movement of the visual field when the body is subjected to acceleration; due to gravity.

oculogyral i., an i. occurring in angular acceleration in which the position of fixed light appears to drift.

optical i., a false interpretation of the color, form, size, or movement of a visual sensation.

il·lu·sion·al (i-loo′zhŭn-ăl). Relating to or of the nature of an illusion.

Ilosvay, Lajos de, Hungarian chemist, 1851–1936. SEE I. *reagent.*

IM Abbreviation for internal *medicine.*

I.M., i.m. Abbreviation for intramuscular, or intramuscularly.

ima (ī′mă). Lowest. SEE ALSO imus. [L.]

im·age (im′ij). **1.** Representation of an object made by the rays of light emanating or reflected from it. **2.** Representation produced by x-rays, ultrasound, tomography, thermography, radioisotopes, etc. **3.** To produce such representations. [L. *imago,* likeness]

accidental i., SYN afterimage.

body i., (1) the cerebral representation of all body sensation organized in the parietal cortex; (2) personal conception of one's own body as distinct from one's actual anatomic body or the conception other persons have of it. SYN body schema.

catatropic i., SYN Purkinje-Sanson i.'s.

direct i., SYN virtual i.

eidetic i., vivid mental i. in the form of a dream, fantasy, or an unusual power of memory and visualization of objects previously seen or imagined.

false i., the i. in the deviating eye in strabismus.

heteronymous i., a double i. in physiological diplopia, when fixation is directed beyond an object; the right i. arises from the left eye, while the left i. arises from the right eye; i.e., there is a crossed diplopia.

homonymous i.'s, double i.'s produced by stimuli arising from points proximal to the horopter. SYN homonymous diplopia, simple diplopia, uncrossed diplopia.

hypnagogic i., imagery occurring between wakefulness and sleep.

hypnopompic i., imagery occurring after the sleeping state and before complete wakefulness; similar to hypnagogic imagery except for the time of occurrence.

inverted i., SYN real i.

magnitude i., in magnetic resonance *imaging,* an i. formed from the amplitude of the signal, distinct from the phase information. SEE ALSO magnetic resonance *imaging.*

mental i., a picture of an object not present, produced in the mind by memory or imagination.

mirror i., a representation of an object or part thereof as its reflected i. in a mirror.

motor i., the i. of body movements.

negative i., SYN afterimage.

optical i., an i. formed by the refraction or reflection of light.

phase i., a magnetic resonance i. showing only phase shift information, to detect motion.

Purkinje i.'s, SYN Purkinje-Sanson i.'s.

Purkinje-Sanson i.'s, the two images formed by the anterior and posterior surfaces of the cornea and the two images formed by the anterior and posterior surfaces of the lens. SYN catatropic i., Purkinje i.'s, Sanson i.'s.

real i., an i. formed by the convergence of the actual rays of light from an object. SYN inverted i.

retinal i., a real i. formed on the retina.

Sanson i.'s, SYN Purkinje-Sanson i.'s.

sensory i., an i. based on one or more types of sensation.

specular i., i. of a source of light made visible by the reflection from a mirror.

tactile i., an i. of an object as perceived by the sense of touch.

unequal retinal i., SYN aniseikonia.

virtual i., an erect i. formed by projection of divergent rays from an optical system. SYN direct i.

visual i., a collection of foci corresponding to all the luminous points of an object.

im·age in·ten·si·fi·er. SYN image *amplifier.*

im·ag·e·ry (im′ij-rē). A technique in behavior therapy in which the client or patient is conditioned to substitute pleasant fantasies to counter the unpleasant feelings associated with anxiety.

imag·i·nal (ĭ-maj′i-năl). Relating to an image or to the process of imagining.

imag·ing (im′ă-jing). Production of a clinical image using x-rays, ultrasound, computed tomography, magnetic resonance, radionuclide scanning, and thermography; especially, cross-sectional imaging, such as ultrasonography, CT, or MRI. SEE image.

blood pool i., nuclear medicine study using a radionuclide that is confined to the vascular compartment.

exercise i., SEE stress *test.*

magnetic resonance i. (MRI), a diagnostic radiologic modality, using nuclear magnetic resonance technology, in which the magnetic nuclei (especially protons) of a patient are aligned in a strong, uniform magnetic field, absorb energy from tuned radiofrequency pulses, and emit radiofrequency signals as their excitation decays. These signals, which vary in intensity according to nuclear abundance and molecular chemical environment, are converted into sets of tomographic images by using field gradients in the magnetic field, which permits 3-dimensional localization of the point sources of the signals. SYN nuclear magnetic resonance i., NMR i., nuclear magnetic resonance tomography.

nuclear magnetic resonance i., NMR i., SYN magnetic resonance i.

pharmacologic stress i., SEE stress *test.*

through transfer i., SYN transfer i.

transfer i., the production of an ultrasound image by detection and analysis of sound on the opposite side of the body from the emitting transducer. SYN through transfer i.

imag·ing de·part·ment. The diagnostic radiology department. SEE imaging, radiology.

ima·go, pl. **imag·ines** (i-mā′gō, i-maj′i-nēz). **1.** The last stage of an insect after it has completed all its metamorphoses through the egg, larva, and pupa; the adult insect form. **2.** SYN archetype (2). [L. image]

im·bal·ance (im-bal′ans). **1.** Lack of equality between opposing forces. **2.** Lack of equality in some aspect of binocular vision, such as muscle balance, image size, and/or image shape. [L. *in-* neg. + *bi-lanx* (*-lanc-*), having two scales, fr. *bis,* twice, + *lanx,* dish, scale of a balance]

autonomic i., a lack of balance between sympathetic and parasympathetic nervous systems, especially in relation to the vasomotor disturbances. SYN vasomotor i.

occlusal i., an inharmonious relationship between the teeth of the maxilla and mandible during closing or functional movements of the jaw.

sex chromosome i., any abnormal pattern of sex chromosomes;

e.g., XXY in men with seminiferous tubule dysgenesis, XO in women with Turner syndrome; rarer patterns of i. are XXX, XXXY, and XYY. SEE ALSO isochromosome.

sympathetic i., SYN vagotonia.

vasomotor i., SYN autonomic i.

im·be·cile (im'bĕ-sil). An obsolete term for a subclass of mental *retardation* or the individual classified therein. [L. *imbecillus,* weak, silly]

im·bed. SYN embed.

im·bi·bi·tion (im-bi-bish'ŭn). **1.** Absorption of fluid by a solid body without resultant chemical change in either. **2.** Taking up of water by a gel, thereby increasing its size. [L. *im-bibo,* to drink in (*in* + *bibo*)]

im·bri·cate, im·bri·cat·ed (im'bri-kāt, im'bri-kā-ted). Overlapping like shingles. [L. *imbricatus,* covered with tiles]

im·bri·ca·tion (im'bri-kā'shŭn). The operative overlapping of layers of tissue in the closure of wounds or the repair of defects. [see imbricate]

eyelid i., an abnormality of eyelid position by which the upper eyelid overrides the lower eyelid on closure, leading to chronic ocular irritation.

im·id·a·zole (im-id-az'ōl). A five-membered heterocyclic compound occurring in L-histidine and other biologically important compounds.

i. alkaloids, alkaloids containing one or more i. moieties as part of its structure (e.g., pilocarpine).

4-im·id·a·zo·lone-5-pro·pi·on·ate (im-id-a-zō'lōn). An intermediate in histidine degradation; seen in reduced levels in urocanic aciduria.

im·id·az·o·lyl (im-id-az'ō-lil). The radical of imidazole. SYN iminazolyl.

im·ide (im'īd). The radical, group, or moiety, =NH, attached to two –CO– groups.

△**imido-.** Prefix denoting the radical of an imide, formed by the loss of the H of the =NH group.

im·i·do·di·pep·ti·dase (im'i-dō-dī-pep'ti-dās). SYN *proline* dipeptidase.

im·id·o·di·pep·ti·du·ria (im-idō-dī-pep'tīd-oor-ē-ă). Elevated levels of proline-containing dipeptides in the urine; associated with a deficiency of prolidase (peptidase D) resulting in impaired development.

im·i·dole (im'i-dōl). SYN pyrrole.

im·in·az·o·lyl (im-in-az'ō-lil). SYN imidazolyl.

△**-imine.** Suffix denoting the group =NH.

△**imino-.** Prefix denoting the group =NH.

im·i·no ac·ids (im'i-nō, i-mē'nō). Compounds with molecules containing both an acid group (usually the carboxyl, –COOH) and an imino group (=NH).

im·i·no·car·bon·yl (im'i-nō-kar'bon-il). SEE carboxamide.

im·i·no·di·pep·ti·dase (im'i-nō-dī-pep'ti-dās). SYN *prolyl* dipeptidase.

im·i·no·gly·ci·nu·ria (im'i-nō-glī-si-noo'rē-ă) [MIM*242600]. A benign inborn error of amino acid transport in renal tubule and intestine; glycine, proline, and hydroxyproline are excreted in the urine; probably autosomal recessive inheritance; genetic heterogeneity is suggested.

im·i·no·hy·dro·las·es (im'i-nō-hī'drō-lās-ez) [EC class 3.5.3]. Enzymes that hydrolyze imino groups; e.g., arginine deiminase. SYN deiminases.

im·in·os·til·benes (im'i-nō-stil'bēnz). A chemical class of agents of which carbamazepine, an antiepileptic drug, is the most prominent.

im·i·pen·em (im-i-pen'em). A thienamycin antibiotic with broad spectrum activity used, in combination with cilastin, to treat a variety of infections.

imip·ra·mine hy·dro·chlo·ride (im-ip'ră-mēn). A tricyclic antidepressant. Metabolized to form desipramine, another tricyclic antidepressant.

imiquimod. An immune response modifier used on the skin in the treatment of external genital and perianal warts.

IML Abbreviation for intermediolateral cell column of the spinal cord gray matter.

Imlach, Francis, Scottish anatomist and surgeon, 1819–1891. SEE I. *fat-pad.*

im·me·di·ca·ble (im-med'i-kă-bl). Obsolete term meaning not curable by medicinal remedies. [L. *in-* neg. + *medicabilis,* curable]

im·mer·sion (i-mer'zhŭn). **1.** The placing of a body under water or other liquid. **2.** In microscopy, filling the space between the objective lens and the top of the cover glass with a fluid, such as water or oil, to reduce spherical aberration and increase effective numerical aperture by elimination of refractive effects that result from an air-glass interface; the best resolution is achieved when the space between the condenser lens and the specimen slide is also filled with the fluid. [L. *immergo,* pp. *-mersus,* to dip in (*in* + *mergo*)]

homogeneous i., in i. microscopy, use of a fluid, such as oil, that has a refractive index virtually identical to that of glass, providing the highest possible numerical aperture.

oil i., water i., SEE immersion (2).

im·mis·ci·ble (i-mis'i-bl). Incapable of mutual solution; e.g., oil and water. [L. *im-misceo,* to mix in (*in* + *misceo*)]

immission (im-ish'in). Environmental concentration of a pollutant, resulting from a combination of imissions and dispersals; often synonymous with exposure. [L. *immissio,* introduction, fr. *im- mitto,* to introduce]

im·mit·tance (i-mit'ans). Measurement of middle ear impedance and compliance. SYN admittance. [L. *immitto,* to send in]

im·mo·bi·li·za·tion (i-mo'bi-li-zā'shŭn). The act of making immovable. [see immobilize]

im·mo·bi·lize (i-mō'bi-līz). To render fixed or incapable of moving. [L. *in-* neg. + *mobilis,* movable]

im·mor·tal·i·za·tion (i-mōr'tăl-i-zā'shŭn). Conferring on normal cells cultured in vitro the property of an infinite lifespan, as from spontaneous mutation, by exposure to chemical carcinogens, or by viral infection. I. of primary cells in culture is the first of several steps in the expression of transforming genes of DNA tumor viruses, of retrovirus oncogenes, and cellular oncogenes derived from human cancer cells.

im·mune (i-mūn'). **1.** Free from the possibility of acquiring a given infectious disease; resistant to an infectious disease. **2.** Pertaining to the mechanism of sensitization in which the reactivity is so altered by previous contact with an antigen that the responsive tissues respond quickly upon subsequent contact, or to in vitro reactions with antibody-containing serum from such sensitized individuals. [L. *immunis,* free from service, fr. *in,* neg., + *munus* (*muner-*), service]

im·mu·ni·fa·cient (im'ū-ni-fā'shent). Making immune after a specific disease. [L. *immunis,* exempt, + *faciens,* making, pr. part. of *facio*]

im·mu·ni·ty (i-mū'ni-tē). **1.** The status or quality of being immune (1). **2.** Protection against infectious disease. SYN insusceptibility. [L. *immunitas* (see immune)]

acquired i., resistance resulting from previous exposure of the individual in question to an infectious agent or antigen; it may be *active* and *specific,* as a result of naturally acquired (apparent or inapparent) infection or intentional vaccination (artificial active i.); or it may be *passive,* being acquired from transfer of antibodies from another person or from an animal, either naturally, as from mother to fetus, or by intentional inoculation (artificial passive i.), and, with respect to the particular antibodies transferred, it is *specific.* Passive, cell-mediated i. produced by the transfer of living lymphoid cells from an immune (allergic or sensitive) animal to a normal one is sometimes referred to as adoptive i.

active i., SEE acquired i.

adoptive i., SEE acquired i.

antiviral i., i. resulting from virus infection, either naturally acquired or produced by intentional vaccination; compared to some bacterial i.'s, it is of relatively long duration, but this may be the result of infection-immunity rather than being peculiar to virus infection per se, since it occurs also in bacterial i. after infections such as typhoid fever.

im

summary of nonspecific host defenses

type	mechanism
atomic barriers	
skin	mechanical barrier retards entry of microbes
	acidic environment (pH 3–5) retards growth of microbes
mucous membranes	normal flora compete with microbes for attachment sites and nutrients
	mucus entraps foreign microorganisms
	cilia propel microorganisms out of body
physiologic barriers	
temperature	body temperature inhibits growth of some pathogens
	fever response inhibits growth of some pathogens
low pH	acidic pH of stomach kills most ingested microorganisms
chemical mediators	lysozyme cleaves bacterial cell wall
	interferon induces antiviral state in uninfected cells
	complement lyses microorganisms or facilitates phagocytosis
phagocytic/endocytic barriers	
	various cells internalize (endocytose) and break down foreign macromolecules
	specialized cells (blood monocytes, neutrophils, tissue macrophages) phagocytize, kill, and digest whole microorganisms
inflammatory barriers	
	tissue damage and infection induce leakage of vascular fluid, containing serum proteins with antibacterial activity, and influx of phagocytic cells into the affected area

artificial active i., SEE acquired i.

artificial passive i., SEE acquired i.

bacteriophage i., the state induced in a bacterium by lysogeniza-tion, the lysogenic bacterium being insusceptible to further lyso-genization or to a lytic cycle by a superinfecting bacteriophage, in contradistinction to bacteriophage resistance.

cell-mediated i. (CMI), cellular i., immune responses that are initiated by an antigen-presenting cell interacting with and medi-ated by T lymphocytes (e.g., graft rejection, delayed-type hyper-sensitivity). SYN delayed hypersensitivity (1).

concomitant i., SYN infection i.

general i., i. associated with widely diffused mechanisms that tend to protect the body as a whole, as compared with local i.

group i., SYN herd i.

herd i., the resistance to invasion and spread of an infectious agent in a group or community, based on the resistance to infec-tion of a high proportion of individual members of the group; resistance is a product of the number susceptible and the probabil-ity that susceptibles will come into contact with an infected per-son. SYN group i.

humoral i., i. associated with circulating antibodies, in contradis-tinction to cellular i.

infection i., the paradoxical immune status in which resistance to reinfection coincides with the persistence of the original infection. SYN concomitant i.

innate i., resistance manifested by a species (or by races, families, and individuals in a species) that has not been immunized (sensi-tized, allergized) by previous infection or vaccination; much of it results from body mechanisms that are poorly understood, but are different from those responsible for the altered reactivity associat-ed with the specific nature of acquired i.; in general, innate i. is nonspecific and is not stimulated by specific antigens. SEE ALSO self. SYN natural i., nonspecific i.

local i., a natural or acquired i. to certain infectious agents, as manifested by an organ or a tissue, as a whole or in part.

maternal i., i. acquired by a fetus because of the presence of maternal IgG that passes through the placenta.

natural i., nonspecific i., SYN innate i.

passive i., SEE acquired i.

relative i., a modified, not completely effective resistance that results when there is a sort of "fluctuating equilibrium" between the defense mechanisms of the host and the infective agent.

specific i., the immune status in which there is an altered reactivi-ty directed solely against the antigenic determinants (infectious agent or other) that stimulated it. SEE acquired i.

specific active i., SEE acquired i.

specific passive i., SEE acquired i.

stress i., insusceptibility or resistance to the effects of emotional strain.

im·mu·ni·za·tion (im-mū'ni-zā'shun). Protection of susceptible individuals from communicable diseases by administration of a living modified agent (e.g., yellow fever vaccine), a suspension of killed organisms (e.g., pertussis vaccine), or an inactivated toxin (e.g., tetanus). SEE ALSO vaccination, allergization.

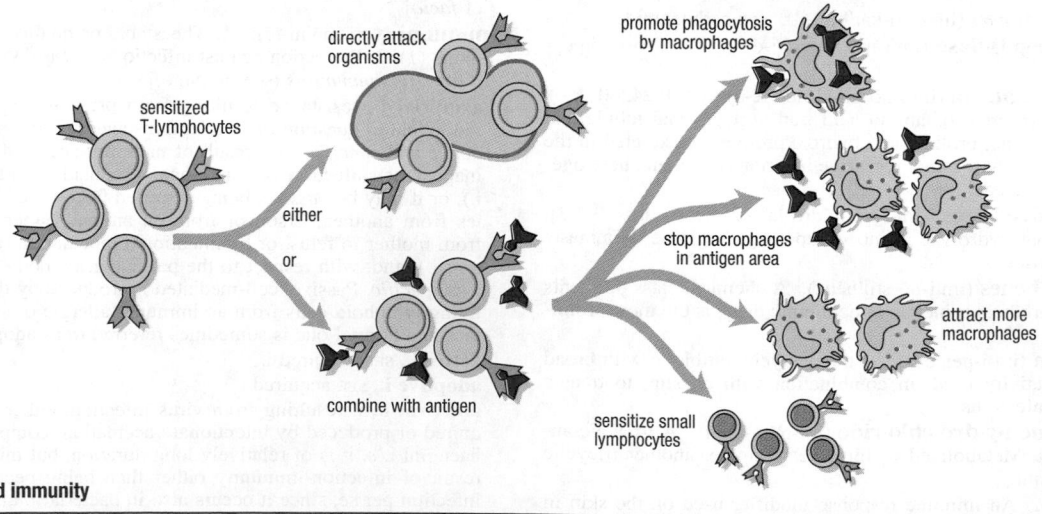

cell-mediated immunity

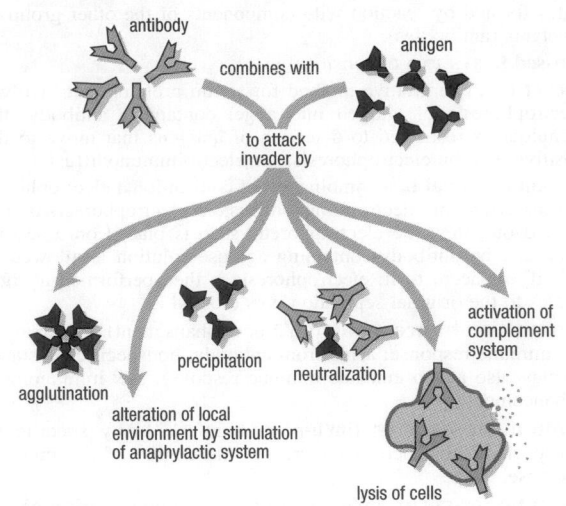

antibody

combines with

antigen

to attack invader by

activation of complement system

precipitation

neutralization

agglutination

alteration of local environment by stimulation of anaphylactic system

lysis of cells

humoral immunity

active i., the production of active immunity.

passive i., the production of passive immunity.

im·mu·nize (im′ū-nīz). **1.** To render immune. **2.** To administer immunization.

△**immuno-.** Immune, immunity. [L. *immunis,* immune]

im·mu·no·ad·ju·vant (im′ū-nō-ad′joo-vant). SEE adjuvant (2).

im·mu·no·ag·glu·ti·na·tion (im′ū-nō-ă-gloo-ti-nā′shŭn). Specific agglutination effected by antibody.

im·mu·no·as·say (im′ū-nō-as′ā, im-ū′nō). Detection and assay of substances by serological (immunological) methods; in most applications the substance in question serves as antigen, both in antibody production and in measurement of antibody by the test substance. SEE ALSO enzyme-linked immunosorbent *assay,* radioimmunoassay, radioimmunoelectrophoresis, immunologic pregnancy *test.* SYN immunochemical assay.

double antibody i., SYN double antibody *precipitation.*

enzyme i., any of several i. methods that use an enzyme covalently linked to an antigen or antibody as a label; the most common types are enzyme-linked immunosorbent assay (ELISA) and enzyme-multiplied immunoassay technique (EMIT). SEE ALSO enzyme-linked immunosorbent *assay,* enzyme-multiplied i. technique.

enzyme-multiplied i. technique (EMIT), a type of i. in which the ligand is labeled with an enzyme, and the enzyme-ligand-antibody complex is enzymatically inactive, allowing quantitation of unlabeled ligand. SEE ALSO competitive binding *assay,* enzyme-linked immunosorbent *assay.*

solid phase i., i. in which the antigen or serum is bound to a solid surface, such as a microplate wall or the sides of a tube, the other reactants being free in solution.

thin-layer i., a method for detection of antigen-antibody reactions, applicable to detection of either antigen or antibody, based on the fact that either reactant, when added to a polystyrene surface (such as a well in a polystyrene plate) is adsorbed as a thin layer and acts as an immunosorbent capable of binding with the second reactant.

im·mun·o·bi·ol·o·gy (im′ū-nō-bī-ōl-ō-ijē, im-oo′nō). The study of the immune factors that affect the growth, development, and health of biological organisms.

im·mu·no·blast (im′ū-nō-blast). An antigenically stimulated lymphocyte; a large cell with well-defined basophilic cytoplasm, a large nucleus with prominent nuclear membrane, distinct nucleoli, and clumped chromatin. SEE ALSO lymphoblast, lymphocyte *transformation.* [immuno- + G. *blastos,* germ]

im·mu·no·blot, im·mu·no·blot·ting (i′mū-nō-blot′). Process by which antigens can be separated by electrophoresis and allowed to adhere onto nitrocellulose sheets where they bind non-

specifically and then are subsequently identified by staining with appropriately labeled antibodies. SEE ALSO Western blot *analysis.*

im·mu·no·blot·ting. SEE immunoblot.

im·mu·no·chem·is·try (im′ū-nō-kem′is-trē). The field of chemistry concerned with chemical aspects of immunologic phenomena, e.g., chemical reactions related to antigen stimulation of tissues, chemical studies of antigens and antibody.

im·mu·no·com·pe·tence (im′ū-nō-kom′pĕ-tens). The ability to produce a normal immune response.

im·mu·no·com·pe·tent (im′ū-nō-kom′pĕ-tent). Possessing the ability to mount a normal immune response.

im·mu·no·com·plex. Complexes of antibody and antigen. SEE immune *complex.*

im·mu·no·com·pro·mised (im′ū-nō-kom′pro-mīzd). Denoting an individual whose immunologic mechanism is deficient either because of an immunodeficiency disorder or because it has been rendered so by immunosuppressive agents.

im·mu·no·con·glu·ti·nin (im′ū-nō-kon-gloo′ti-nin). An autoantibody-like immunoglobulin (IgM) formed in animals (or man) against their own complement following injection of complement-containing complexes or sensitized bacteria.

im·mu·no·cyte (im′ū-nō-sīt, im-oo′nō). An immunologically competent leukocyte capable, actively or potentially, of producing antibodies or reacting in cell-mediated immunity reactions. SEE ALSO I *cell.* [immuno- + G. *kytos,* cell]

im·mu·no·cy·to·ad·her·ence (im′ū-nō-sī′tō-ad-her′ens). A method for determining cell surface properties, in which immunoglobulin or receptors on the surface of one cell population cause cells with corresponding molecular configurations on their surface to adhere in rosettes around the cells.

im·mu·no·cy·to·chem·is·try (im′ū-nō-sī-tō-kem′is-trē). The study of cell constituents by immunologic methods, such as the use of fluorescent antibodies or immunoperoxidase staining..

⃞im·mu·no·de·fi·cien·cy (im′ū-nō-dē-fish′en-sē, im-ū′). A condition resulting from a defective immune mechanism; may be *primary* (due to a defect in the immune mechanism itself) or *secondary* (dependent upon another disease process), *specific* (due to a defect in either the B-lymphocyte or the T-lymphocyte system, or both) or *nonspecific* (due to a defect in one or another component of the nonspecific immune mechanism: the complement, properdin, or phagocytic system). SYN immune deficiency, immunity deficiency, immunologic deficiency.

cellular i. with abnormal immunoglobulin synthesis, an ill-defined group of sporadic disorders of unknown cause, occurring in both males and females and associated with recurrent bacterial, fungal, protozoal, and viral infections; there is thymic hypoplasia with depressed cellular (T-lymphocyte) immunity combined with defective humoral (B-lymphocyte) immunity, although immunoglobulin levels may be normal. SYN Nezelof syndrome.

combined i., i. of both the B-lymphocytes and T-lymphocytes.

common variable i., of unknown cause, and usually unclassifiable; usual onset after age 15 years but may occur at any age in either sex; the total quantity of immunoglobulin is commonly less than 300 mg/dL; the number of B lymphocytes is often within normal limits but there is a lack of plasma cells in lymphoid tissue; cellular (T-lymphocyte) immunity is usually intact; there is an increased susceptibility to pyogenic infection and often autoimmune disease. SYN acquired agammaglobulinemia, acquired hypogammaglobulinemia.

phagocytic dysfunction i., suppression in number or function of phagocytic cells such as in chronic granulomatous disease. SYN phagocytic dysfunction disorders i.

phagocytic dysfunction disorders i., SYN phagocytic dysfunction i.

secondary i., i. in which there is no evident defect in the lymphoid tissues, but rather hypercatabolism or loss of immunoglobulins such as occurs in familial idiopathic hypercatabolic hypoproteinemia or in defects associated with the nephrotic syndrome. SYN secondary agammaglobulinemia, secondary antibody deficiency, secondary hypogammaglobulinemia.

severe combined i. (SCID) [MIM*202500,MIM*300400, and MIM*312863], an i. in which there is absence of both humoral

im

and cellular immunity with lymphopenia (of both B-type and T-type lymphocytes); characterized by thymus atrophy, lack of delayed hypersensitivity, and marked susceptibility to infections by bacteria, viruses, fungi, protozoa, and live vaccines; although bone marrow transplants have been effective, death may occur in the first year of life. Both autosomal recessive and X-linked forms occur; about one-half of those with autosomal recessive SCID have adenosine deaminase deficiency. The X-linked form is caused by mutation in the interleukin-2 receptor gamma gene (IL2RG) on Xq. SYN Swiss type agammaglobulinemia.

i. with elevated IgM, i. with reduced IgG- and IgA-bearing cells; there is recurrent pyogenic infection; X-linked in some families.

i. with hypoparathyroidism, SYN DiGeorge *syndrome.*

im·mu·no·de·fi·cient (im′ū-nō-dē-fish′ent). Lacking in some essential function of the immune system.

im·mu·no·de·pres·sant (im′ū-nō-dē-pres′ănt). SYN immunosuppressant.

im·mu·no·de·pres·sor (im′ū-nō-dē-pres′ŏr, -ōr). SYN immunosuppressant.

im·mu·no·di·ag·no·sis (im′ū-nō-dī-ag-nō′sis). The process of determining specified immunologic characteristics of individuals or of cells, serum, or other biologic specimens.

im·mu·no·dif·fu·sion (im′ū-nō-di-fū′zhŭn,, im-ū′nō-). A technique to study antigen-antibody reactions by observing precipitates formed by antigen-antibody complexes, which are formed by combination of specific antigen and antibodies which have diffused in a gel in which they have been separately placed.

double i., SEE gel diffusion precipitin *tests* in two dimensions, under *test.*

radial i. (RID), SEE gel diffusion precipitin *tests* in one dimension, under *test.*

single i., SEE gel diffusion precipitin *tests* in one dimension, under *test,* gel diffusion precipitin *tests* in two dimensions, under *test.*

im·mu·no·e·lec·tro·pho·re·sis (im′ū-nō-ē-lek′trō-fō-rē′sis). A kind of precipitin test in which the components of one group of immunological reactants (usually a mixture of antigens) are first separated on the basis of electrophoretic mobility in agar or other medium, the separated components then being identified, by means of the technique of double diffusion, on the basis of precip-

itates formed by reaction with components of the other group of reactants (antibodies).

crossed i., SYN two-dimensional i.

rocket i., a quantitative method for serum proteins that involves electrophoresis of antigen into a gel containing antibody; the technique is restricted to detection of antigens that move to the positive pole on electrophoresis. SEE electroimmunodiffusion.

two-dimensional i., a combination of conventional electrophoretic separation and electroimmunodiffusion; electrophoresis is first carried out, then the electrophoretic strip is placed on a second slide and an antibody-containing agarose solution is allowed to solidify adjacent to it; electrophoresis is then performed at right angles to the original separation. SYN crossed i.

im·mu·no·en·hance·ment (im′ū-nō-en-hans′ment). Increasing the immune response; aside from antibody, nonspecific substances may also act to enhance immune response. SYN immunologic enhancement.

im·mu·no·en·hanc·er (im′ū-nō-en-hans′er). Any specific or nonspecific substance that increases the degree of the immune response.

im·mu·no·fer·ri·tin (im′ū-nō-fer′i-tin). Antibody-ferritin conjugate used to identify specific antigen by electron microscopy.

im·mu·no·flu·o·res·cence (im′ū-nō-flōr-es′ens, i-mū′nō-). An immunohistochemical technique using labeling of antibodies by a fluorescent dye to identify antigenic material specific for the labeled antibody; the specific binding of antibody can be determined microscopically through the production of a characteristic visible light by the application of ultraviolet rays to the preparation. SEE ALSO fluorescent antibody *technique.*

direct i., fluorescence microscopy of tissue from lesions after application of labeled antibodies. SEE ALSO fluorescent antibody *technique.*

indirect i., fluorescence *microscopy* of normal tissue after application of the patient's serum, to detect antibodies to normal tissue components (autoantibodies). SEE ALSO fluorescent antibody *technique.*

im·mu·no·gen (i-mū′nō-jen). SYN antigen.

im·mu·no·ge·net·ics (im′ū-nō-jě-net′iks, im-ū′nō-). The study of the genetics of transplantation and tissue rejection, histochemical

classification of primary immunodeficiency disorders			
antibody (B-cell) immunodeficiencies	**cellular (T-cell) immunodeficiencies**	**combined B-cell (antibody) and T-cell (cellular) deficiencies**	**phagocytic dysfunction diseases**
X-linked agammaglobulinemia	DiGeorge anomaly	severe combined immunodeficiency (including X-linked SCID, Nezelof syndrome, etc.)	neutropenic syndromes
transient hypogammaglobulinemia of infancy	chronic mucocutaneous candidiasis	combined immunodeficiency with T-cell membrane or signaling defects	chronic granulomatous disease
common variable immunodeficiency	biotin-dependent multiple cocarboxylase deficiency	Wiskott-Aldrich syndrome	leukocyte glucose-6-phosphate dehydrogenase deficiency
hyper-IgM immunodeficiency	natural killer cell deficiency	ataxia-telangiectasia	Chediak-Higashi syndrome
IgA deficiency	idiopathic CD4 lymphopenia	Nijmegen breakage syndrome	myeloperoxidase deficiency
IgM deficiency		immunodeficiency with short-limbed dwarfism, hypoplasia of cartilage and hair	specific granule deficiency
IgG subclass deficiencies		immunodeficiency with enzyme deficiency; adenosine deaminase or nucleoside	glycogen storage disease type 1b
polysaccharide unresponsiveness		graft-versus-host disease	hyper-IgE/Job syndrome
transcobalamin deficiency		bare lymphocyte syndrome	leukocyte adhesion defect
immunodeficiency with thymoma		Omenn syndrome	Schwachman syndrome
		reticular dysgenesis	tuftsin deficiency
		X-linked lymphoproliferative syndrome	periodontitis syndromes

SCID, severe combined immunodeficiency disease

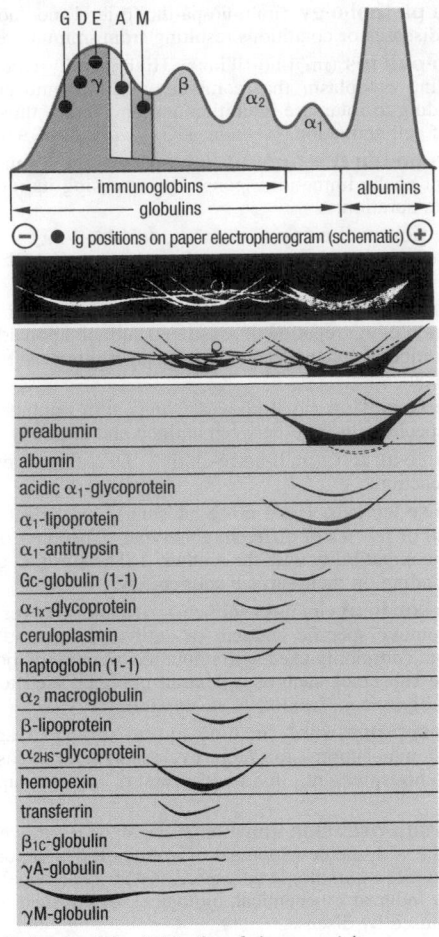

immunoelectrophoresis: distribution of plasma protein

loci, immunologic response, immunoglobulin structure, and immunosuppression.

im·mu·no·gen·ic (im′ū-nō-jen′ik). SYN antigenic.

im·mu·no·ge·nic·i·ty (im′ū-nō-jĕ-nis′i-tē). SYN antigenicity.

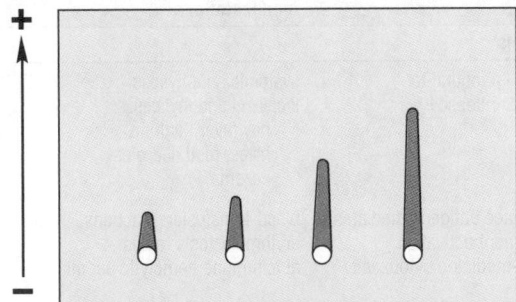

rocket immunoelectrophoresis: schematic view of electrophoresis of antigen in a gel containing antibody; the higher the concentration of antigen, the longer and denser the zone of precipitation

im·mu·no·glob·u·lin (Ig) (im′ū-nō-glob′ū-lin). One of a class of structurally related proteins, each consisting of two pairs of polypeptide chains, one pair of light (L) [low molecular weight] chains (κ or λ), and one pair of heavy (H) chains (γ, α, μ, δ, and ε), usually all four linked together by disulfide bonds. On the basis of the structural and antigenic properties of the H chains,

Ig's are classified (in order of relative amounts present in normal human serum) as IgG (7S in size, 80%), IgA (10–15%), IgM (19S, a pentamer of the basic unit, 5–10%), IgD (less than 0.1%), and IgE (less than 0.01%). All of these classes are homogeneous and susceptible to amino acid sequence analysis. Each class of H chain can associate with either κ or λ L chains. Subclasses of Ig's, based on differences in the H chains, are referred to as IgG1, etc.

When split by papain, IgG yields three pieces: the Fc piece, consisting of the C-terminal portion of the H chains, with no antibody activity but capable of fixing complement, and crystallizable; and two identical Fab pieces, carrying the antigen-binding sites and each consisting of an L chain bound to the remainder of an H chain.

Antibodies are Ig's, and all Ig's probably function as antibodies. However, Ig refers not only to the usual antibodies, but also to a great number of pathological proteins classified as myeloma proteins, which appear in multiple myeloma along with Bence Jones proteins, myeloma globulins, and Ig fragments.

From the amino acid sequences of Bence Jones proteins, it is known that all L chains are divided into a region of variable sequence (V_L) and one of constant sequence (C_L), each comprising about half the length of the L chain. The constant regions of all human L chains of the same type (κ or λ) are identical except for a single amino acid substitution, under genetic controls. H chains are similarly divided, although the V_H region, while similar in length to the V_L region, is only one-third or one-fourth the length of the C_H region. Binding sites are a combination of V_L and V_H protein regions. The large number of possible combinations of L and H chains make up the "libraries" of antibodies of each individual.

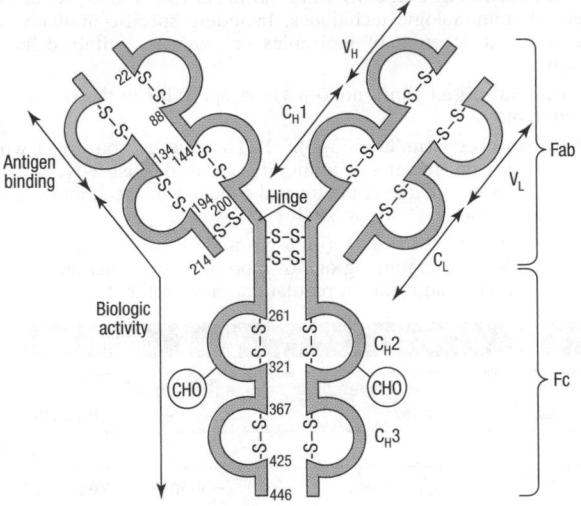

immunoglobulin (schematic structure)

anti-D i., SYN $RH_0(D)$ immune *globulin*.

chickenpox i., SYN chickenpox immune *globulin* (human).

i. domains, structural units of i. heavy or light chains that are composed of approximately 110 amino acids. Light chains of an i. are composed of one constant domain and one variable domain. Heavy chains are composed of either three or four constant domains and one variable domain.

i. G subclass deficiency, a rare inherited disorder in which there are reduced levels of one or more IgG subclasses resulting from defective heavy chain genes or an abnormality in the regulation of i. isotype switching.

human normal i., SYN human gamma *globulin*.

measles i., SYN measles immune *globulin* (human).

monoclonal i., a homogeneous i. resulting from the proliferation of a single clone of plasma cells and which, during electrophoresis of serum, appears as a narrow band or "spike"; it is characterized by heavy chains of a single class and subclass, and light

im

chains of a single type. SYN M protein (2), monoclonal protein, paraprotein (2).

pertussis i., SYN pertussis immune *globulin.*

poliomyelitis i., SYN poliomyelitis immune *globulin* (human).

rabies i., SYN rabies immune *globulin* (human).

Rh₀(D) i., SYN RH₀(D) immune *globulin.*

secretory i., usually IgA but may be IgM linked to a secretory component and found in mucous secretions.

secretory i. A, a subclass of IgA that is found primarily in secretions such as tears and colostrum. This form of IgA is protected from proteolytic degradation by the presence of a secretory component.

selective i. A deficiency, an inherited disorder in which there is a markedly reduced or absent IgA, resulting in immature IgA-bearing B cells.

tetanus i., SYN tetanus immune *globulin.*

thyroid-stimulating i.'s (TSI), in Graves disease, the antibodies to TSH receptors in the thyroid gland. These antibodies are produced by B-lymphocytes and stimulate the receptors, causing hyperthyroidism. Formerly known as LATS (long-acting thyroid *stimulator*).

im·mu·no·he·ma·tol·o·gy (im′ū-nō-hē-mă-tol′ō-jē, im-ū′nō-). That division of hematology concerned with immune, or antigen-antibody reactions and with related changes in the blood.

im·mu·no·his·to·chem·is·try (im′ū-nō-his′tō-kem′is-trē). Demonstration of specific antigens in tissues by the use of markers that are either fluorescent dyes or enzymes such as horseradish peroxidase.

im·mu·no·lo·cal·i·za·tion (im′ū-nō-lō′cal-ī-zā-shŭn). Refers to use of immunologic techniques, including specific antibody, to identify the location of molecules or structures within cells or tissues.

im·mu·nol·o·gist (im-ū-nol′ō-jist). A specialist in the science of immunology.

im·mu·nol·o·gy (im′ū-nol′ō-jē). **1.** The science concerned with the various phenomena of immunity, induced sensitivity, and allergy. **2.** Study of the structure and function of the immune system. [immuno- + G. *logos,* study]

im·mu·no·mod·u·la·to·ry (im′ū-nō-mod′ū-la-to-rē). **1.** Capable of modifying or regulating one or more immune functions. **2.** An immunological adjustment, regulation, or potentiation.

im·mu·no·pa·thol·o·gy (im′ū-nō-pă-thol′ō-jē, i-moo′nō-). The study of diseases or conditions resulting from immune reactions.

im·mu·no·phil·ins (im′ū-nō-fil′inz). High-affinity receptor proteins in the cytoplasm that combine with immunosuppressant drugs leading to rotamase inhibition and, in T cells, thus to interruption of cell activation. [immune + G. *philos,* fond, + in]

im·mu·no·po·ten·ti·a·tion (im′ū-nō-pō-ten-shē-ā′shŭn). Enhancement of the immune response by increasing its rate or prolonging its duration.

im·mu·no·po·ten·ti·a·tor (im′ū-nō-pō-ten′shē-ā-tŏr). Any of a wide variety of specific or nonspecific substances which on inoculation enhances or augments an immune response.

im·mu·no·pre·cip·i·ta·tion (im′ū-nō-prē-sip-i-tā′shŭn). The phenomenon of aggregation of sensitized antigen upon addition of specific antibody (precipitin) to antigen in solution. SYN immune precipitation.

⊞im·mu·no·re·ac·tion (im′ū-nō-rē-ak′shŭn). An immunologic reaction, especially in vitro between antigen and antibody.

im·mu·no·re·ac·tive (im′ū-nō-rē-ak′tiv). Denoting or exhibiting immunoreaction.

im·mu·no·se·lec·tion (im′ū-nō-se-lek′shŭn). **1.** Selective death or survival of fetuses of different genotypes depending on immunologic incompatibility with the mother. **2.** The survival of certain cells depending on their surface antigenicity.

im·mu·no·sor·bent (im′ū-nō-sōr′bent). An antibody (or antigen) used to remove specific antigen (or antibody) from solution or suspension; commonly used with reference to antibody bound to a particulate substance such as a dextran polymer used to remove soluble antigen (e.g., insulin) from solution.

im·mu·no·sup·pres·sant (im′ū-nō-sŭ-pres′ant). An agent that induces immunosuppression (e.g., cyclosporine, corticosteroids). SYN immunodepressant, immunodepressor, immunosuppressive (2).

im·mu·no·sup·pres·sion (im′ū-nō-sŭ-presh′ŭn). Prevention or interference with the development of immunologic response; may reflect natural immunologic unresponsiveness (tolerance), may be artificially induced by chemical, biological, or physical agents, or may be caused by disease.

im·mu·no·sup·pres·sive (im′ū-nō-sŭ-pres′iv). **1.** Denoting or inducing immunosuppression. **2.** SYN immunosuppressant.

im·mu·no·sur·veil·lance (im′ū-nō-ser-vā′lance). Theory that

	classification of hypersensitivity reactions			
type	descriptive name	initiation time	mechanism	typical manifestations
		immediate reactions		
type I	IgE-mediated hypersensitivity	2–30 min	Ag induces cross-linkage of IgE bound to mast cells and basophils with release of vasoactive mediators	systemic anaphylaxis localized anaphylaxis: hay fever, asthma hives, food allergies eczema
type II	antibody-mediated cytotoxic hypersensitivity	5–8 h	Ab directed against cell-surface antigens mediates cell destruction via complement activation or antibody-dependent cell-mediated cytotoxicity	blood-transfusion reactions erythroblastosis fetalis autoimmune hemolytic anemia
type III	immune complex–mediated hypersensitivity	2–8 h	Ag-Ab complexes deposited in various tissues induce complement activation and an ensuing inflammatory response	localized Arthus reaction generalized reactions: serum sickness, glomerulonephritis rheumatoid arthritis, systemic lupus erythematosus
		delayed reactions		
type IV	cell-mediated hypersensitivity	24–72 h	sensitized T_DTH cells release cytokines that activate macrophages or T_C cells, which mediate direct cellular damage	contact dermatitis tubercular lesions graft rejection

holds that the immune system eliminates aberrant or tumor cells that arise spontaneously.

im·mu·no·sym·pa·thec·to·my (im′ū-nō-sim′pă-thek′tō-mē). Inhibition of development of sympathetic ganglia induced in newborn animals by injection of antiserum specific for the protein which selectively enhances growth of sympathetic neurons.

im·mu·no·ther·a·py (im′ū-nō-thār′ă-pē). Originally, therapeutic administration of serum or immune globulin containing preformed antibodies produced by another individual; currently, i. includes nonspecific systemic stimulation, adjuvants, active specific i., and adoptive i. New forms of i. include the use of monoclonal antibodies. SYN biologic i.

This method has been widely adopted in oncology, particularly in cases that fail to respond to other treatment. Immunotherapy seeks to boost immune system function, as with the administration of interferons and interleukin-2, or to attack cancerous cells directly, as with the injection of monoclonal antibodies. Various immunotherapeutic techniques have also been used in the treatment of AIDS. In addition, a number of alternative medical practices are claimed to enhance immune function, and various over-the-counter substances have gained popularity for this supposed property.

adoptive i., passive transfer of immunity from an immune donor through inoculation of sensitized lymphocytes, or antibodies in serum or gamma globulin. Vaccination with plasmid DNA is currently under investigation.

biologic i., SYN immunotherapy.

im·mu·no·tol·er·ance (im′ū-nō-tol′er-ăns). SYN immunologic *tolerance.*

im·mu·no·trans·fu·sion (im′ū-nō-trans-fū′zhŭn, i-moo′nō-). An indirect transfusion in which the donor is first immunized by means of injections of an antigen prepared from microorganisms isolated from the recipient; later, the donor's blood is collected, defibrinated, and then administered to the patient; the latter is then presumably passively immunized by means of antibody formed in the donor, e.g., antibody that reacts with the microorganisms in the patient.

IMP Abbreviation for inosine 5′-monophosphate.

im·pact. **1** (im′pakt). The forcible striking of one body against another. **2** (im-pakt′). To press two bodies, parts, or fragments closely together so that the two parts move as a single unit. [L. *impingo,* pp. *-pactus,* to strike at (*in + pango*), fasten, drive in]

im·pact·ed (im-pak′ted). Wedged or pressed closely so as to move as a single unit.

im·pac·tion (im-pak′shŭn). The process or condition of being impacted.

dental i., confinement of a tooth in the alveolus and prevention of its eruption into normal position. SEE ALSO impacted *tooth.*

fecal i., an immovable collection of compressed or hardened feces in the colon or rectum.

food i., the forcible wedging of food between adjacent teeth during mastication, producing gingival recession and pocket formation.

mucus i., filling of the proximal bronchi, and also the bronchioles, with mucus.

im·pair·ment (im-pār′ment). A physical or mental defect at the level of a body system or organ. The official WHO definition is: any loss or abnormality of psychologic, physiologic, or anatomic structure or function.

mental i., a disorder characterized by the display of an intellectual defect, as manifested by diminished cognitive, interpersonal, social, and vocational effectiveness and quantitatively evaluated by psychological examination and assessment.

IMP-as·par·tate li·gase. SYN adenylosuccinate synthase.

im·pat·ent (im-pat′ent, im-pā′tent). Not patent; closed.

im·ped·ance (im-pē′dăns). **1.** Total opposition to flow. In electricity, when flow is steady, i. is simply the resistance, e.g., the driving pressure per unit flow; when flow is changing, i. also

includes the factors that oppose changes in flow. Thus, deviations of i., from simple ohmic resistance because of the effects of capacitance and inductance, become more important in alternating current as the frequency of oscillations increases. In fluid analogies (e.g., pulsatile flow of blood, to-and-fro flow of respiratory gas), i. depends not only on viscous resistance but also on compressibility, compliance, inertance, and the frequency of imposed oscillations. **2.** Resistance of an acoustic system to being set in motion.

acoustic i., the resistance that a material offers to the passage of a sound wave (colloquial); a property of a medium computed as the product of density and sound propagation speed (characteristic acoustic i.). Discontinuities in acoustic i. are responsible for the echoes on which ultrasound imaging is based. Unit: the rayl.

im·per·cep·tion (im-per-sep′shŭn). Inability to form a mental image of an object by combining the sensory data obtained therefrom. [L. *in-,* not, + *per-cipio,* pp. *-ceptus,* to perceive]

im·per·fo·rate (im-per′fōr-āt). SYN atretic.

im·per·fo·ra·tion (im-per-fōr-ā′shŭn). Condition of being atretic, occluded, or closed; indicated in compound words by the prefix *atreto-* or the suffix *-atresia.* [L. *im-* neg. + *per-foro,* pp. *-atus,* to bore through]

im·per·me·a·ble (im-per′mē-ă-bl). Not permeable; not permitting the passage of substances (e.g., liquids, gases) or heat through a membrane or other structure. SYN impervious. [L. *impermeabilis,* not to be passed through]

im·per·me·ant (im-per′mē-ant). Unable to pass through a particular semipermeable membrane. [L. *im-,* neg., + *permano,* to penetrate]

im·per·sis·tence (im-per-sis′tens). A transitory existence or occurrence, lasting only a short time. [L. *im-,* neg. + *persisto,* to persist]

motor i., inability to sustain a movement.

im·per·vi·ous (im-per′vē-ŭs). SYN impermeable.

im·pe·tig·i·ni·za·tion (im′pe-tij′i-ni-zā′shŭn). The occurrence of impetigo by infection of an area of preexisting dermatosis.

im·pe·tig·i·nous (im-pe-tij′i-nŭs). Relating to impetigo.

im·pe·ti·go (im-pe-tī′gō). A contagious superficial pyoderma, caused by *Staphylococcus aureus* and/or group A streptococci, that begins with a superficial flaccid vesicle that ruptures and forms a thick yellowish crust, most commonly occurring in children. SYN i. contagiosa, i. vulgaris. [L. a scabby eruption, fr. *im-peto (inp-),* to rush upon, attack]

Bockhart i., SYN follicular i.

i. bullo′sa, i. with lesions of large size, forming bullae.

bullous i. of newborn, usually, widely disseminated bullous lesions appearing soon after birth, caused by infection with *Staphylococcus aureus.* SYN i. neonatorum (2), pemphigus gangrenosus (2).

i. circina′ta, a ringlike configuration of bullous lesions of i. formed by confluence of several bullae or by the rupture of a single lesion with crusting of the periphery.

i. contagio′sa, SYN impetigo.

i. contagio′sa bullo′sa, discrete purulent skin lesions occasionally seen with streptococcal pyoderma.

follicular i., a superficial follicular pustular eruption involving the scalp or other hairy area. SYN Bockhart i.

i. herpetifor′mis, a rare pyoderma, which may be related to pustular psoriasis, occurring most commonly in pregnant women in the third trimester as an eruption of small, closely aggregated pustules developing upon an inflammatory base and accompanied by severe constitutional symptoms and fetal death; recurs with subsequent pregnancy.

i. neonato′rum, (1) SYN *dermatitis* exfoliativa infantum; **(2)** SYN bullous i. of newborn.

i. vulga′ris, SYN impetigo.

im·pe·tus (im′pe-tŭs). In psychoanalysis, the motor element of an instinct; the amount of force of the individual's energy which the instinctive impulse demands. [L. an onset, fr. *im-peto,* to attack]

im·plant. **1** (im-plant′). To graft or insert. **2.** Material inserted into nonliving tissues. SEE ALSO graft, transplant. **3** (im′plant). In

im

genitourinary surgery a device inserted to restore continence or potency. Also an injectable material to create a valvular competence of the ureterovesical junction or bladder outlet. SEE ALSO prosthesis. [L. *im-*, in, + *planto*, pp. *-atus*, to plant, fr. *planta*, a sprout, shoot]

carcinomatous i.'s, transference of carcinoma cells from a primary tumor to adjacent tissues where growth continues.

cochlear i., an electronic device consisting of a microphone, speech processor, and electrodes that are implanted in the inner ear to stimulate the remaining nerve fibers of the auditory division of the eighth cranial nerve in adults and children with profound hearing impairment and deafness. Many recipients of cochlear i.'s achieve high, open-set word recognition and can understand speech even over the telephone. SEE ALSO auditory *prosthesis*. SYN cochlear prosthesis.

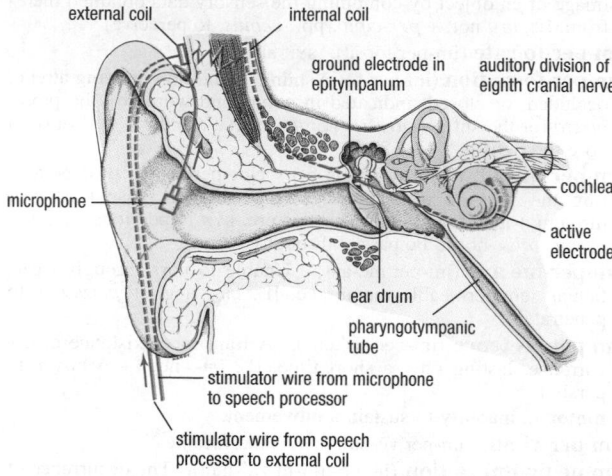

Labels: external coil; internal coil; ground electrode in epitympanum; auditory division of eighth cranial nerve; microphone; cochlea; active electrode; ear drum; pharyngotympanic tube; stimulator wire from microphone to speech processor; stimulator wire from speech processor to external coil

cochlear implant

dental i.'s, crowns, bridges, or dentures attached permanently to the jaw by means of metal anchors, most frequently titanium posts.

endometrial i.'s, fragments of endometrial mucosa implanted on pelvic structure following retrograde transference through the oviducts. SYN endometriosis.

endo-osseous i., an i. into alveolar bone inserted through the prepared root canal of a tooth in order to increase effective root length.

endosseous i., SYN endosteal i.

endosteal i., an i. that is inserted into the alveolar and/or basal bone and protrudes through the mucoperiosteum. SYN endosseous i.

inflatable i., an empty silicone rubber bag with an inlet tube and a valve inserted into or behind the breast, then inflated with a liquid to the desired size; used in augmentation mammaplasty, and breast reconstruction.

intracorneal i.'s, inserts placed within corneal pockets to alter the refractive power of the eye.

intraocular i., a plastic lens placed in the anterior or posterior chamber of the eye to substitute for the lens removed in cataract extraction.

magnetic i., a tissue-tolerated, magnetized metal placed within the bone to aid in denture retention; a similar magnet is placed in the overlying denture to complete the field.

orbital i., the glass, plastic, or metal device placed in the muscle cone after enucleation of an eye.

penile i., a rigid, flexible, or inflatable device surgically placed in the corpora cavernosa to produce an erection.

pin i., a type of dental i. usually rod-shaped, used in the area of the maxillary sinuses.

post i., that portion of a dental i. substructure that protrudes through the mucosa to connect with the restoration.

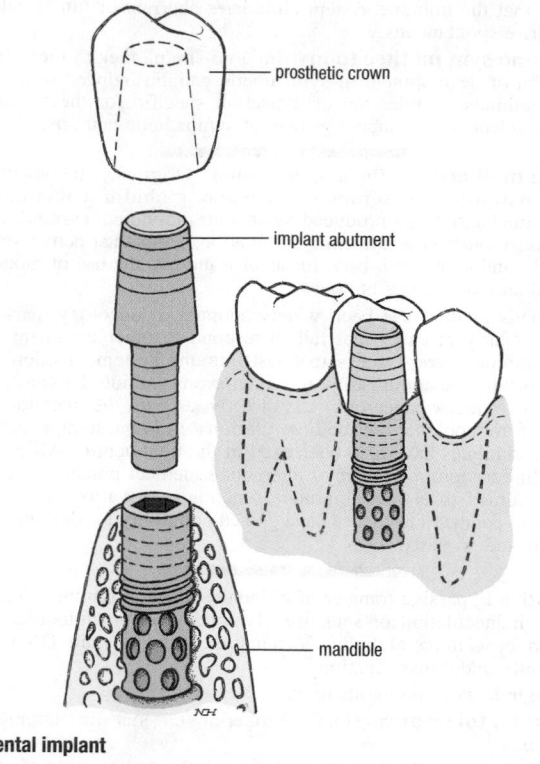

Labels: prosthetic crown; implant abutment; mandible

dental implant

root-form i., an i. shaped like the root of a tooth.

silicone i., i. composed of silicone; common form of breast i. for augmentation.

submucosal i., a dental i. resting beneath the mucosa. SEE ALSO implant *denture*.

subperiosteal i., an artificial dental metal appliance made to conform to the shape of a bone and placed on its surface beneath the periosteum. SEE implant denture *substructure*.

supraperiosteal i., an alloplastic graft inserted superficial to the periosteum to change the contour of an area.

testicular i., a device placed surgically in the scrotum in males with absence or severe hypoplasia of the testis. SYN testicular prosthesis.

threaded i., an i. with screwlike threads that is either screwed into bone previously threaded by a tap, or by self-tapping, the i. cutting threads in the bone as it is inserted into a predrilled hole.

triplant i., a combination of three pin i.'s to form a single abutment to support or retain a dental prosthesis.

im·plan·ta·tion (im-plan-tā′shŭn). **1.** Attachment of the fertilized ovum (blastocyst) to the endometrium, and its subsequent embedding in the compact layer, occurring 6 or 7 days after fertilization of the ovum in humans. **2.** The process of placing a device or substance within the body, e.g., placement of a saline-filled device beneath the breast mound. **3.** Insertion of a natural tooth into an artificially constructed alveolus. **4.** Tissue grafting. SEE ALSO transplantation.

central i., i. in which the blastocyst remains in the uterine cavity, as in carnivores, rhesus monkeys, and rabbits. SYN circumferential i., superficial i.

circumferential i., SYN central i.

collagen i., SYN collagen *injection*.

cortical i., i. of blastocyst in the ovarian cortex, causing an ovarian pregnancy. SEE ectopic *pregnancy*.

eccentric i., i. in which the blastocyst lies in a uterine crypt, as in the mouse, rat, and hamster.

interstitial i., i. in which the blastocyst lies within the substance of the endometrium, as in humans and guinea pigs.

nerve i., planting one nerve into the sheath of another nerve.

pellet i., intramuscular or subcutaneous insertion of an active therapeutic agent in pellet form to provide protracted absorption at a rate slower than subcutaneous or intramuscular injection and as a means of providing a sustained therapeutic effect without repeated administration.

periosteal i., insertion of a normal tendon into a periosteum as part of a tendon transplantation operation.

subcutaneous i., insertion of material under the skin.

superficial i., SYN central i.

im·plo·sion (im-plō'shŭn). **1.** A sudden collapse, as of an evacuated vessel, in which there is a bursting inward rather than outward as in an explosion. **2.** A type of behavior therapy, similar to flooding, during which the patient is given massive exposure to extreme anxiety-arousing stimuli by being asked to describe, and thus relive in imagination, those life events or situations typically producing these overwhelming emotional reactions. As the patient does so, the therapist attempts to extinguish the future influence of such unconscious material over the patient's behavior and feelings, and previous avoidance responses to the stimuli are replaced by more appropriate responses.

im·po·tence, im·po·ten·cy (im'pŏ-tens, -ten-sē). **1.** Weakness; lack of power. **2.** Specifically, inability of the male to achieve and/or maintain penile erection and thus engage in copulation; a manifestation of neurologic, vascular, or psychological dysfunction. [L. *impotentia,* inability, fr. *in-* neg. + *potentia,* power]

psychic i., that caused by psychologic factors.

vasculogenic i., i. due to alterations in the flow of blood to and from the penis.

im·preg·nate (im-preg'nāt). **1.** To fecundate; to cause to conceive. **2.** To diffuse or permeate with another substance. SEE ALSO saturate. [L. *im-,* in, + *praegnans,* with child]

im·preg·na·tion (im-preg-nā'shŭn). **1.** The act of making pregnant. **2.** The process of diffusing or permeating with another substance, as in metallic i. of tissue components with silver nitrate or ammoniacal silver. SEE ALSO saturation.

im·pres·sio, pl. **im·pres·si·o·nes** (im-pres'ē-ō, im-pres-ē-ō'nēz) [TA]. SYN impression. [L.]

i. aortica pulmonis sinistri, SYN aortic *impression* of left lung.

i. cardi'aca faciei diaphragmaticae hep'atis [TA], SYN cardiac *impression* of diaphragmatic surface of liver.

i. cardi'aca pulmo'nis, SYN cardiac *impression* on lung.

i. col'ica hepatis [TA], SYN colic *impression* on liver.

impressio'nes digita'tae, ☆ official alternate term for *impressions* of cerebral gyri.

i. duodena'lis hepatis [TA], SYN duodenal *impression* on liver.

i. esopha'gea hepatis [TA], SYN esophageal *impression* on liver.

i. gas'trica hepatis [TA], SYN gastric *impression* on liver.

impressiones gyrorum [TA], SYN *impressions* of cerebral gyri.

i. ligamen'ti costoclavicula'ris [TA], SYN *impression* for costoclavicular ligament.

i. petro'sa pal'lii, SYN petrosal *impression* of the pallium.

i. rena'lis hepatis [TA], SYN renal *impression* on liver.

i. suprarena'lis hepatis [TA], SYN suprarenal *impression* on liver.

i. trigemina'lis [TA], SYN trigeminal *impression.*

im·pres·sion (im-presh'ŭn). **1.** A mark seemingly made by pressure of one structure or organ on another, seen especially in cadaveric dissections. See also *groove* for the various impressions of the lungs, e.g., descending aorta, subclavian artery, and vena cavae. **2.** An effect produced upon the mind by some external object acting through the organs of sense. SYN mental i. **3.** An imprint or negative likeness; especially, the negative form of the teeth and/or other tissues of the oral cavity, made in a plastic material that becomes relatively hard or set while in contact with these tissues, made in order to reproduce a positive form or cast of the recorded tissues; classified, according to the materials of that they are made, as reversible and irreversible hydrocolloid i., modeling plastic i., plaster i., and wax i. SYN impressio [TA]. [L. *impressio,* fr. *im-* primo, pp. *-pressus,* to press upon]

aortic i. of left lung, a broad deep groove on the medial aspect of the left lung above and behind the hilum receiving the arch of the aorta and the thoracic aorta. SYN aortic sulcus, impressio aortica pulmonis sinistri, sulcus aorticus.

basilar i., an invagination of the base of the skull into the posterior fossa with compression of the brainstem and cerebellar structures into the foramen magnum. Cf. platybasia.

cardiac i. of diaphragmatic surface of liver [TA], a depression on the superior area of the diaphragmatic surface of the liver corresponding to the position of the heart. SYN impressio cardiaca faciei diaphragmaticae hepatis [TA].

cardiac i. on lung [TA], the depression on the medial surface of each lung produced by the presence of the heart. It is more pronounced on the left lung. SYN impressio cardiaca pulmonis.

i. of cerebral gyri [TA], the depressions on the inner surface of the skull which correspond to the convolutions of the brain. SYN impressiones gyrorum [TA], impressiones digitatae☆, juga cerebralia☆, digitate i.'s.

colic i. on liver [TA], a hollow on the visceral surface of the right lobe of the liver anteriorly, corresponding to the situation of the right flexure and beginning of the transverse colon. SYN impressio colica hepatis [TA].

colic i. of spleen [TA], the part of the visceral surface of the spleen in contact with the colon. SYN facies colica splenis [TA], colic surface of spleen.

complete denture i., (1) an i. of an edentulous arch made for the purpose of constructing a complete denture; (2) a negative registration of the entire denture-bearing, stabilizing area of either the maxillae or mandible; (3) a negative registration of the entire denture foundation and border seal areas present in the edentulous mouth.

i. for costoclavicular ligament [TA], an irregular pitted area on the inferior surface of the clavicle at its sternal end, giving attachment to the costoclavicular ligament. SYN impressio ligamenti costoclavicularis [TA], costal tuberosity, rhomboid i., tuberositas costalis.

deltoid i., SYN deltoid *tuberosity* (of humerus).

digitate i.'s, SYN i. of cerebral gyri.

direct bone i., an i. of denuded bone, used in the construction of subperiosteal denture implants.

duodenal i. on liver [TA], a hollow on the visceral surface of the right lobe of the liver alongside the gallbladder, marking the situation of the duodenum. SYN impressio duodenalis hepatis [TA].

esophageal i. on liver [TA], the marking of the esophagus on the back of the left lobe of the liver. SYN impressio esophagea hepatis [TA].

i.'s of esophagus, SYN esophageal *constrictions,* under *constriction.*

final i., in dentistry, the i. that is used to make the master cast.

gastric i. on liver [TA], a hollow on the visceral surface of the left lobe of the liver corresponding to the location of the stomach. SYN impressio gastrica hepatis [TA].

gastric i. on spleen [TA], the surface of the spleen in contact with the stomach. SYN facies gastrica splenis [TA], gastric surface of spleen.

mental i., SYN impression (2).

partial denture i., an i. or negative copy of all or a part of the partially edentulous dental arch or area, made for the purpose of designing or constructing a partial denture.

petrosal i. of the pallium, a shallow impression on the inferior surface of the cerebral hemisphere made by the superior margin of the petrous part of the temporal bone. SYN impressio petrosa pallii.

preliminary i., in dentistry, one made for the purpose of diagnosis or the construction of a tray. SYN primary i.

primary i., SYN preliminary i.

renal i. on liver [TA], a hollow on the visceral surface of the right lobe of the liver, in which lies the right kidney. SYN impressio renalis hepatis [TA].

renal i. of spleen [TA], the portion of the visceral surface of the spleen that contacts the left kidney. SYN facies renalis splenis [TA], facies renalis lienis☆, renal surface of spleen.

rhomboid i., SYN i. for costoclavicular ligament.

im

sectional i., an i. that is made in sections.

suprarenal i. on liver [TA], a hollow on the visceral surface of the right lobe of the liver, adjoining the groove for inferior venae cava, in which lies the right suprarenal gland. SYN impressio suprarenalis hepatis [TA].

trigeminal i. [TA], a depression on the anterior surface of the petrous portion of the temporal bone, near the apex, formed in relationship to the trigeminal ganglion. SYN impressio trigeminalis [TA].

im·print·ing. A particular kind of learning characterized by its occurrence in the first few hours of life, and which determines species-recognition behavior.

genomic i., epigenetic process that leads to inactivation of paternal or maternal allele of certain genes susceptible to epigenetic regulation; accounts, among others, for the Angelman and Prader-Willi syndromes.

im·pro·mi·dine (im'prō-mĭ-dēn). An agent which is an agonist at H_2-type histamine receptors. Causes gastric acid secretion and tachycardia. Actions can be blocked by agents such as cimetidine and ranitidine.

im·pulse (im'pŭls). **1.** A sudden pushing or driving force. **2.** A sudden, often unreasoning, determination to perform some act. **3.** The action potential of a nerve fiber. [L. *im-pello,* pp. *-pulsus,* to push against, impel (*inp-*)]

apex i., conventionally the lowermost, leftmost area of cardiac pulsation that is usually palpable.

cardiac i., movement of the chest wall produced by cardiac contraction.

ectopic i., an electrical i. from an area of the heart other than the sinus node.

escape i., one or more i.'s (atrial, junctional, or ventricular) arising as a result of delay in the formation or arrival of impulses from the prevailing pacemaker.

irresistible i., a compulsion to act such that one feels or claims it cannot be resisted.

morbid i., an i. that drives one to commit some act, usually of a deviant or forbidden nature, notwithstanding efforts to restrain oneself.

right parasternal i.'s, cardiac activity as palpable or recordable just to the right of the sternum.

im·pul·sion (im-pŭl'shŭn). An abnormal urge to perform a certain activity.

im·pul·sive (im-pŭl'siv). Relating to or actuated by an impulse, rather than controlled by reason or careful deliberation.

imus (ī'mŭs). Lowest; the most inferior or caudal of several similar structures. [L.]

IMV Abbreviation for intermittent mandatory *ventilation.*

IMViC Acronym for *i*ndole production, *m*ethyl red, *V*oges-Proskauer reaction, and ability to use *c*itrate as a sole source of carbon (*i* inserted for euphony); used primarily to differentiate *Escherichia coli* from *Enterobacter aerogenes* and related organisms.

In Symbol for indium; inulin.

[113m]**In** Abbreviation for indium-113m.

[111]**In** Symbol for indium-111.

△**in-.** **1.** Not, akin to G. a-, an-, or Eng. un-. **2.** In, within, inside. **3.** Very; appears as im- before b, p, or m. [L.]

△**-in.** A suffix widely used to form names of biochemical substances, including proteins (e.g., *globulin*), lipids (*lecithin*), hormones (*insulin*), botanical principles (*digoxin*), antibiotics (*streptomycin*), synthetic drugs (*aspirin*), dyes (*eosin*), and others; initially a variant of *-ine;* in a few terms (e.g., *dentin, thyroxin,* spellings with and without final *e* are both found. [G. *-inos,,* L. *-inus,* adj. suffixes]

in·ac·tion (in-ak'shŭn). Inactivity, rest, or lack of response to a stimulus.

in·ac·ti·vate (in-ak'ti-vāt). To destroy the biologic activity or the effects of an agent or substance, as the activity of complement is destroyed when serum is heated.

in·ac·ti·va·tion (in-ak-ti-vā'shŭn). The process of destroying or removing the activity or the effects of an agent or substance; e.g.,

the complementary effect of a serum may be destroyed by means of i. at 56°C for 30 min.

insertional i., a technique of recombinant DNA technology used to select bacteria that carry recombinant plasmids; a fragment of foreign DNA is inserted into a restriction site within a gene for antibiotic resistance, thus causing that gene to become nonfunctional.

X i., SEE lyonization.

in·an·i·mate (in-an'i-māt). Not alive. [L. *in-* neg. + *anima,* breath, soul]

in·a·ni·tion (in'ă-nish'ŭn). Severe weakness and wasting as occurs from lack of food, defect in assimilation, or neoplastic disease. [L. *inanis,* empty]

in·ap·par·ent (in'ă-pār'ent). Not apparent; beneath the threshold of clinical recognition, as an inapparent infection.

in·ap·pe·tence (in-ap'ĕ-tens). Lack of desire or of craving. [L. *in-* neg. + *ap-peto,* pp. *-petitus,* to strive after, long for (*adp-*)]

in·ar·tic·u·late (in-ar-tik'ū-lit). **1.** Not articulate in intelligible speech. **2.** Unable to express oneself satisfactorily in words.

in·as·sim·i·la·ble (in-ă-sim'il-ă-bl). Not assimilable; not capable of undergoing assimilation. SEE assimilation.

in·at·ten·tion (in-ă-ten'shŭn). Lack of attention; negligence.

selective i., an aspect of attentiveness in which a person attempts to ignore or avoid perceiving that which generates anxiety.

sensory i., the inability to feel a tactile stimulus when a similar stimulus, presented simultaneously in a homologous area of the body, is perceived.

visual i., the inability to perceive a photic stimulus in a visual field when a similar but perceived stimulus is presented simultaneously in the homologous field.

in·born (in'bōrn). Initiated during development in utero. In the specific context of i. error of metabolism, it connotes a genetic disruption of an enzyme. SEE inborn *errors* of metabolism, under *error.* SYN innate.

in·bred. Denoting populations (groups, genetic lines, etc.) descended over several generations almost exclusively from a small set of ancestors, and hence having a high rate of consanguinity, often occult.

in·breed·ing (in'brēd-ing). **1.** Mating between organisms that are genetically more closely related than organisms selected at random from the population. **2.** A practice of mating animals that are closely related. The term is clearly relative to how the population is defined; the higher the i. in the population, the less it will lie in the individual mating.

in·car·cer·at·ed (in-kar'ser-ā-ted). Confined; imprisoned; trapped. [L. *in,* in, + *carcero,* pp. *-atus,* to imprison, fr. *carcer,* prison]

in·car·nant (in-kar'nant). Promoting or accelerating the granulation of a wound. SYN incarnative. [L. *incarno,* fr. *in* + *caro* (*carn-*), flesh]

in·car·na·tive (in-kar'nă-tiv). SYN incarnant.

in·cen·di·a·rism (in-sen'di-ă-rizm). SYN pyromania. [L. *incendiarius,* causing a conflagration]

in·cen·tive (in-sen'tiv). In experimental psychology, an object or goal of motivated behavior. [LL. *incentivus,* provocative]

in·cer·tae se·dis (in-ser'tē sē'dis). Of uncertain or doubtful affiliation or doubtful position, said of organisms in taxonomic classifications. [L.]

in·cest (in'sest). **1.** Sexual relations between persons closely related by blood, especially between parents and children, brother and sister. **2.** The crime of sexual relations between persons related by blood, where such cohabitation is prohibited by law. [L. *incestus,* unchaste, fr. *in-,* not, + *castus,* chaste]

in·ces·tu·ous (in-ses'choo-ŭs). **1.** Pertaining to incest. **2.** Guilty of incest.

in·ci·dence (in'si-dens). **1.** The number of specified new events, e.g., persons falling ill with a specified disease, during a specified period in a specified population. **2.** In optics, intersection of a ray of light with a surface. [L. *incido,* to fall into or upon, to happen]

in·ci·dent (in'si-dent). Going toward; impinging upon, as incident rays. [L. *incido,* pp. *-casus,* to fall into, to meet with]

in·ci·dent·a·lo·ma (in'sĭ-den-tă-lō'mă). Mass lesion, usually of the adrenal gland, serendipitously noted during computerized tomographic examinations performed for other reasons. [incidental + -*oma*, tumor]

in·ci·sal (in-sī'zăl). Cutting; relating to the cutting edges of the incisor and cuspid teeth. [L. *incido*, pp. -*cisus*, to cut into]

in·cise (in-sīz'). To cut with a knife.

in·ci·sion (in-sizh'ŭn). A cut; a surgical wound; a division of the soft parts usually made with a knife. [L. *incisio*]

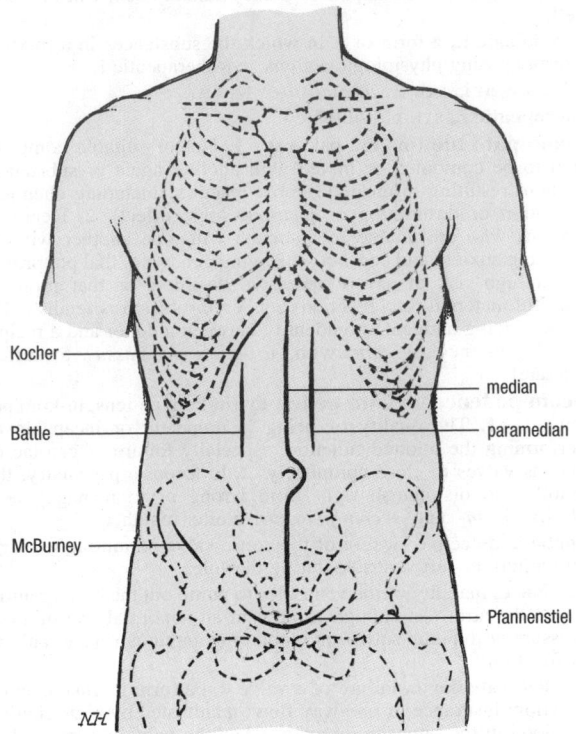

Kocher —
Battle —
McBurney —
median
paramedian
Pfannenstiel
NH

surgical incisions

bucket-handle i., a bilateral subcostal abdominal i.

celiotomy i., an i. through the abdominal wall.

chevron i., a bilateral subcostal i. in the abdomen, in the shape of an inverted "V"; used in upper abdominal procedures.

clamshell i., i. made up of bilateral submammary anterior thoracotomies connected by a transverse sternotomy and providing access similar to that of a standard sternotomy. SEE ALSO transverse *thoracosternotomy.* SYN clamshell thoracotomy.

collar i., a cervical incision, placed a few cm above the sternal notch, that is frequently used for thyroid or parathyroid procedures.

Deaver i., an i. in the right lower abdominal quadrant, with medial displacement of the rectus muscle.

Dührssen i.'s, three surgical i.'s of an incompletely dilated cervix, corresponding roughly to 2, 6, and 10 o'clock, used as a means of effecting immediate delivery of the fetus when there is an entrapped head during a breech delivery.

endaural i., i. through the external auditory canal, avoiding cartilage, to permit mastoid surgery.

Fergusson i., an i. used in maxillectomy, along the junction of the nose and cheek, and bisecting the upper lip.

flank i., an i. usually made near and parallel to the 12th rib between the iliac crest and the rib.

Kocher i., an i. several inches below and parallel with the right costal margin.

lumbotomy i., SYN posterior *nephrectomy.*

McBurney i., an i. parallel with the course of the external oblique muscle, one or two inches cephalad to the anterior superior spine of the ilium.

midline i., a vertical abdominal i. placed in the midline aponeurosis between the two sheaths of the rectus muscles of the abdomen.

paramedian i., an i. lateral to the midline.

Pfannenstiel i., an i. made transversely, and through the external sheath of the recti muscles, about an inch above the pubes, the muscles being separated at the midline in the direction of their fibers.

postauricular i., an i. parallel and a few millimeters posterior to the retroauricular fold, made to gain access to the mastoid cortex.

transmeatal i., an i. in the skin of the posterior external auditory canal that extends from just above the posterior malleolar fold to six o'clock inferiorly; for access to the posterior part of the middle ear.

transverse abdominal i., an abdominal i. that is placed perpendicular to the axis of the rectus muscles of the abdomen.

in·ci·sive (in-sī'siv). **1.** Cutting; having the power to cut. **2.** Relating to the incisor teeth.

in·ci·sor (in-sī'zŏr). SYN incisor *tooth.* [L. *incido*, to cut into]

central i., the first tooth in the maxilla and mandible on either side of the midsagittal plane of the head.

Hutchinson i.'s, SYN Hutchinson *teeth*, under *tooth.*

lateral i., SYN second i.

second i., second maxillary or mandibular permanent or deciduous tooth on either side of the midsagittal plane of the head. SYN lateral i.

INCISURA

in·ci·su·ra, pl. **in·ci·su·rae** (in'sī-soo'ră, in'si-soo'rē) [TA]. SYN notch. [L. a cutting into]

i. acetab'uli [TA], SYN acetabular *notch.*

i. angula'ris [TA], SYN angular *incisure.*

i. anterior auriculae [TA],

i. ante'rior au'ris, SYN anterior *notch* of auricle.

i. ap'icis cor'dis [TA], SYN *notch* of cardiac apex.

i. cardi'aca, SYN cardial *notch.*

i. cardi'aca pulmo'nis sinis'tri [TA], SYN cardiac *notch* of left lung.

i. cardialis [TA], SYN i. cardialis. SYN i. cardialis [TA].

i. cartilag'inis mea'tus acus'tici [TA], SYN *notch* in cartilage of acoustic meatus.

i. cerebel'li ante'rior, SYN anterior cerebellar *notch.*

i. cerebel'li poste'rior, SYN posterior cerebellar *notch.*

i. clavicula'ris [TA], SYN clavicular *notch* of sternum.

incisurae costa'les [TA], SYN costal *notches*, under *notch.*

i. ethmoida'lis [TA], SYN ethmoidal *notch.*

i. fibula'ris [TA], SYN fibular *notch.*

i. fronta'lis [TA], SYN frontal *notch.*

i. interarytenoi'dea [TA], SYN interarytenoid *notch.*

i. intertrag'ica [TA], SYN intertragic *notch.*

i. ischiad'ica ma'jor [TA], SYN greater sciatic *notch.*

i. ischiad'ica mi'nor [TA], SYN lesser sciatic *notch.*

i. jugula'ris os'sis occipita'lis [TA], SYN jugular *notch* of occipital bone.

i. jugula'ris os'sis tempora'lis [TA], SYN jugular *notch* of petrous part of temporal bone.

i. jugula'ris sterna'lis [TA], SYN jugular *notch* of sternum.

i. lacrima'lis [TA], SYN lacrimal *notch.*

i. ligamen'ti tere'tis hep'atis [TA], SYN *notch* for ligamentum teres.

i. mandib'ulae [TA], SYN mandibular *notch.*

i. mastoi'dea [TA], SYN mastoid *notch.*

i. nasa'lis [TA], SYN nasal *notch.*

in

i. pancrea′tis [TA], SYN pancreatic *notch*.

i. parieta′lis [TA], SYN parietal *notch*.

i. preoccipita′lis [TA], SYN preoccipital *notch*.

i. pterygoi′dea, SYN pterygoid *notch*.

i. radia′lis [TA], SYN radial *notch*.

i. rivi′ni, SYN tympanic *notch*.

i. santori′ni, SYN *notch* in cartilage of acoustic meatus.

i. scap′ulae, SYN suprascapular *notch*.

i. semiluna′ris ul′nae, SYN trochlear *notch*.

i. sphenopalati′na [TA], SYN sphenopalatine *notch*.

i. supraorbita′lis [TA], SYN supraorbital *notch*; SEE ALSO supraorbital *foramen*.

i. tento′rii [TA], SYN tentorial *notch*.

i. of tentorium, ☆official alternate term for tentorial *notch*.

i. terminalis auricularis [TA], SYN terminal *notch* of auricle.

i. termina′lis au′ris, SYN terminal *notch* of auricle.

i. thyroi′dea infe′rior [TA], SYN inferior thyroid *notch*.

i. thyroi′dea supe′rior [TA], SYN superior thyroid *notch*.

i. trag′ica, SYN intertragic *notch*.

i. trochlea′ris [TA], SYN trochlear *notch*.

i. tympan′ica [TA], SYN tympanic *notch*.

i. ulna′ris [TA], SYN ulnar *notch*.

i. umbilica′lis, SYN *notch* for ligamentum teres.

i. vertebra′lis [TA], SYN vertebral *notch*.

---

in·ci·sure (in-sī′zhoor). SYN notch. [L. *incisura*]

angular i. [TA], a sharp angular depression in the lesser curvature of the stomach at the junction of the body with the pyloric canal. SYN incisura angularis [TA], angular notch, sulcus angularis.

Lanterman i.'s, SYN Schmidt-Lanterman i.'s.

Rivinus i., SYN tympanic *notch*.

Santorini i.'s, SYN *notch* in cartilage of acoustic meatus.

Schmidt-Lanterman i.'s, funnel-shaped interruptions in the regular structure of the myelin sheath of nerve fibers, formerly interpreted as actual breaks in the sheath but shown by electron microscopy to correspond each to a strand of cytoplasm locally separating the two otherwise fused oligodendroglial (or, in peripheral nerves, Schwann cell) membranes composing the myelin sheath. SYN Lanterman i.'s, Schmidt-Lanterman clefts.

tympanic i., SYN tympanic *notch*.

in·cli·na·tio, pl. **in·cli·na·ti·o·nes** (in′kli-nā′shē-ō, -nā-shē-ō′nēz) [TA], SYN inclination. [L.]

i. pel′vis [TA], SYN pelvic *inclination*.

in·cli·na·tion (in-kli-nā′shŭn) [TA]. **1.** A leaning or sloping. **2.** In dentistry, deviation of the long axis of a tooth from the perpendicular. SYN inclinatio [TA], version (3). [L. *inclinatio,* a leaning]

condylar guidance i., the angle of i. of the condylar guidance to an accepted horizontal plane.

enamel rod i., the direction of the enamel rods with reference to the outer surface of the enamel of a tooth.

lateral condylar i., the direction of the lateral condyle path.

pelvic i. [TA], the angle that the plane of the superior pelvic aperture makes with the horizontal plane. SYN inclinatio pelvis [TA], i. of pelvis.

i. of pelvis, SYN pelvic i.

in·cli·nom·e·ter (in′kli-nom′ĕ-ter). Obsolete instrument for determining the direction of the ocular axes in astigmatism. [L. *inclino,* to incline, + G. *metron,* measure]

in·clu·sion (in-kloo′zhŭn). **1.** Any foreign or heterogeneous substance contained in a cell or in any tissue or organ, not introduced as a result of trauma. **2.** The process by which a foreign or heterogeneous structure is misplaced in another tissue. [L. *inclusio,* a shutting in, fr. *includo,* pp. *-clusis,* to close in]

cell i.'s, (1) the residual elements of the cytoplasm that are metabolic products of the cell, e.g., pigment granules or crystals; **(2)** storage materials such as glycogen or fat; **(3)** engulfed material such as carbon or other foreign substances. SEE ALSO inclusion *bodies,* under *body.*

Döhle i.'s, SYN Döhle *bodies,* under *body.*

fetal i., unequal conjoined twins in which the incompletely developed parasite is wholly enclosed in the autosite.

leukocyte i.'s, SYN Döhle *bodies,* under *body.*

in·co·her·ent (in-kō-hēr′ent). Not coherent; disjointed; confused; denoting a lack of connectedness or organization of parts during verbal expression. [L. *in-* neg. + *co-haereo,* pp. *-haesus,* to cling together, fr. *haereo,* to stick]

in·com·pat·i·bil·i·ty (in′kom-pat-i-bil′i-tē). **1.** The quality of being incompatible. **2.** A means of classifying bacterial plasmids; two plasmids are incompatible if they cannot coexist in one host cell.

physiologic i., a form of i. in which the substances in a mixture exert opposing physiologic actions. SYN therapeutic i.

Rh antigen i., SYN *erythroblastosis* fetalis.

therapeutic i., SYN physiologic i.

in·com·pat·i·ble (in-kom-pat′i-bl). **1.** Not of suitable composition to be combined or mixed with another agent or substance, without resulting in an undesirable reaction (including chemical alteration or destruction or pharmacologic effect). **2.** Denoting persons who are unable to associate with one another without resulting anxiety and conflict. **3.** Having genotypes that put progeny at high risk of severe recessive disorders or that promote harmful maternal-fetal reaction (e.g., erythroblastosis fetalis is Rh i.). **4.** Having antigenic nonidentity between a donor and a recipient. [L. *in-* neg., + *con-,* with, + *patior,* pp. *passus,* to suffer, tolerate]

in·com·pe·tence, in·com·pe·ten·cy (in-kom′pe-tens, in-kom′pĕ-ten-sē). **1.** The quality of being incompetent or incapable of performing the allotted function, especially failure of cardiac or venous valves to close completely. **2.** In forensic psychiatry, the inability to distinguish right from wrong or to manage one's affairs. [L. *in-,* neg. + *com-peto,* strive after together]

aortic i., defective closure of the aortic valve permitting regurgitation into the left ventricle during diastole.

cardiac i., inability of the ventricles to pump out the blood returning to the atria fast enough to prevent an abnormal rise in atrial pressure or to pump sufficient blood to maintain normal circulatory function.

cardiac valvular i., failure of a valve to perform its fundamental function: insurance of one-way flow; manifested by regurgitation of blood in the opposite direction when the valve is supposed to be closed.

mitral i., defective closure of the mitral valve permitting regurgitation into the left atrium during systole.

muscular i., imperfect closure of an anatomically normal cardiac valve, in consequence of defective action of its papillary muscles.

pulmonary i., pulmonic i., defective closure of the pulmonic valve permitting regurgitation into the right ventricle during diastole.

pyloric i., a patulous state or want of tone of the pylorus that allows the passage of food into the intestine before gastric digestion is completed.

relative i., imperfect closure of a cardiac valve, in consequence of excessive dilation of the corresponding cavity of the heart.

tricuspid i., defective closure of the tricuspid valve permitting regurgitation into the right atrium during systole.

valvular i., SYN valvular *regurgitation.*

in·con·stant (in-kon′stant). **1.** Irregular. **2.** In anatomy, denoting a structure, such as an artery, nerve, etc., that may or may not be present.

in·con·ti·nence (in-kon′ti-nens). **1.** Inability to prevent the discharge of any of the excretions, especially of urine or feces. **2.** Lack of restraint of the appetites, especially sexual. Cf. intemperance. SYN incontinentia. [L. *in-continentia,* fr. *in-* neg. + *con-tineo,* to hold together, fr. *teneo,* to hold]

fecal i., SYN i. of feces.

i. of feces, the involuntary voiding of feces into clothing or bedclothes, usually due to pathology affecting sphincter control or loss of cognitive functions. SYN fecal i.

i. of milk, SYN galactorrhea.

overflow i., involuntary loss of urine associated with overdistention of the bladder, with or without a detrusor contraction. SYN paradoxical i., passive i.

paradoxical i., SYN overflow i.

passive i., SYN overflow i.

i. of pigment, loss of melanin from the epidermis, and accumulation in melanophages in the upper dermis; seen in several inflammatory diseases of the skin and in incontinentia pigmenti.

reflex i., loss of urine due to unintended detrusor hyperreflexia.

stress urinary i. (SUI), leakage of urine as a result of coughing, straining, or some sudden voluntary movement, due to incompetence of the sphincteric mechanisms. SYN urinary exertional i.

urge i., urgency i., leakage of urine by unintended detrusor contraction with a strong desire to void.

urinary exertional i., SYN stress urinary i.

i. of urine, the involuntary voiding of urine into clothing or bedclothes. A common problem in elderly populations, especially those in nursing homes, it may be due to neurologic abnormalities, loss of sphincter function (especially common in multiparous women), chronic bladder outlet obstruction, or loss of cognitive functions.

in·con·ti·nent (in-kon′ti-nent). Denoting incontinence.

in·con·ti·nen·tia (in-kon′ti-nen′shē-ă). SYN incontinence. [L.]

i. pigmen′ti [MIM*146150, MIM*308300, and MIM*308310], a rare genodermatosis characterized by hyperpigmented lesions in linear, zebra stripe, and other bizarre configurations following the lines of Blaschko; occasionally accompanied by other developmental anomalies of the eyes, teeth, nails, skeleton, nails, heart. The dermatologic features involve four stages: stage I is characterized by erythema, vesicles, and pustules; stage II by papules, verrucous lesions, and hyperkeratosis; stage III by hyperpigmentation; and stage IV by pallor, atrophy, and scarring. Historically, there were thought to be two forms: 1) the sporadic type of i. pigmenti (IP1), which is now known to be *hypomelanosis* of Ito and 2) the familial type (IP2), which is X-linked dominant and a genetic lethal in males. SEE ALSO *hypomelanosis* of Ito. SYN Bloch-Sulzberger disease, Bloch-Sulzberger syndrome.

i. pigmen′ti achro′mians [MIM*146150], SYN *hypomelanosis* of Ito.

in·co·or·di·na·tion (in-kō-ōr-di-nā′shŭn). SYN ataxia. [L. *in*-neg. + coordination]

in·cor·po·ra·tion (in-kōr-pŏ-rā′shŭn). SYN identification. [L. *in*-, in, + *corporare,* pp. *corporatus,* to make into a body]

in·crease (in′krēs). Any growth in quantity.

absolute cell i., an actual i. in one of the types of leukocytes, the absolute number of leukocytes in 1 cu mm of blood being obtained by multiplying the total leukocyte count by the percentage of the cell types in question.

base i. at low levels, a hearing aid signal-processing strategy to increase gradually the amplification of low frequencies at low-intensity levels.

treble i. at low levels, a hearing aid signal-processing strategy to increase gradually the amplification of high-frequency sounds at low levels.

in·cre·ment (in′kre-ment). A change in the value of a variable; usually an increase, with "decrement" applied to a decrease, though "increment" can also correctly be applied to both. [L. *incrementum,* increase]

incretin. Generic term for all insulinotropic substances originating in the gastrointestinal tract that are released into the circulation by meals containing glucose. One is glucose-dependent insulinotropic polypeptide, which is released into the circulation from crypt cells in the proximal duodenum and jejunum after meals containing glucose or long-chain fatty acids. Another is proglucagon-derived polypeptide, cleavage product of glucagon, which is further processed into glucagonlike peptide-1 and then to glucagonlike insulinotropic peptide.

in·cre·tion (in-krē′shŭn). The functional activity of an endocrine gland. [in- + secretion]

in·crus·ta·tion (in′krŭs-tā′shŭn). 1. Formation of a crust or a scab. 2. A coating of some adventitious material or an exudate; a scab. [L. *in-crusto,* pp. *-atus,* to incrust, fr. *crusta,* crust]

in·cu·ba·tion (in′kū-bā′shŭn). 1. Act of maintaining controlled environmental conditions for the purpose of favoring growth or development of microbial or tissue cultures or to maintain optimal conditions for a chemical or immunologic reaction. 2. Maintenance of an artificial environment for an infant, usually a premature or hypoxic one, by providing proper temperature, humidity, and, usually, oxygen. 3. The development, without sign or symptom, of an infection from the time the infectious agent gains entry until the appearance of the first signs or symptoms. [L. *incubo,* to lie on]

in·cu·ba·tor (in′kū-bā′tōr). 1. A container in which controlled environmental conditions may be maintained; e.g., for culturing microorganisms. 2. An apparatus for maintaining an infant (usually premature) in an environment of proper oxygenation, humidity, and temperature.

in·cu·bus (in′koo-bŭs). Originally, an evil spirit that lay upon and oppressed sleeping persons; especially, a male spirit that copulated with sleeping women. Cf. succubus. [L. fr. *incubo,* to lie on]

in·cu·dal (in′koo-dăl). Relating to the incus.

in·cu·dec·to·my (in-koo-dek′tō-mē). Removal of the incus of the tympanum. [incus + G. *ektomē,* excision]

in·cu·des (in-koo′dēz). Plural of incus. [L.]

in·cu·di·form (in-koo′di-fōrm). Shaped like an anvil. [L. *incus* (*incud-*), anvil]

in·cu·do·mal·le·al (in-koo′dō-mal′lē-ăl). Relating to the incus and the malleus; denoting the articulation between the incus and the malleus in the middle ear. SYN ambomalleal.

in·cu·do·sta·pe·di·al (in-koo′dō-stā-pē′dē-ăl). Relating to the incus and the stapes; denoting the articulation between the incus and the stapes in the middle ear.

in·cur·a·ble (in-kūr′ă-bl). Denoting a disease or morbid process that is unresponsive to medical or surgical treatment.

in·cur·va·tion (in′ker-vā′shŭn). An inward curvature; a bending inward.

in·cus, gen. **in·cu·dis,** pl. **in·cu·des** (ing′kŭs, in-koo′dis, in-koo′dēz) [TA]. The middle of the three ossicles in the middle ear; it has a body and two limbs or processes (long crus of incus and short crus of incus); at the tip of the long crus is a small knob, the lenticular process, which articulates with the head of the stapes. SYN anvil. [L. anvil]

in·cy·clo·duc·tion (in-sī-klō-dŭk′shŭn). A cycloduction in which the upper pole of the cornea is rotated inward (medially). [in- + cyclo- + L. *duco,* pp. *ductus,* to lead]

in·cy·clo·pho·ria (in-sī′klō-fō′rē-ă). A cyclophoria in which the 12 o'clock position in the iris tends to twist medially. [L. in- + cyclo- + G. *phora,* a carrying]

in·cy·clo·tro·pia (in-sī-klō-trō′pē-ă). A cyclotropia in which the upper poles of the corneas are rotated inward (medially) to each other. [in- + cyclo- + G. *trope,* a turning]

in d. Abbreviation for L. *in dies,* daily.

in·dan·e·di·one de·riv·a·tives. Anticoagulants similar to warfarin in action. Anisindione and pheninindione are clinically used; diphenadione is very long acting and used as a rodenticide.

in·dan·e·di·ones (in′dan-dī-ōnz). A class of orally effective indirect-acting anticoagulants of which phenindione is representative.

in·de·cid·u·ate (in-dē-sid′ū-āt). Relating to the mammals (Indecidua) that do not shed any maternal uterine tissue when expelling the placenta at birth (e.g., horse, pig), in contrast to deciduate mammals (e.g., human, dog, rodent).

in·den·i·za·tion (in-den-i-zā′shŭn). SYN innidiation. [in- + denizen]

in·den·ta·tion (in-den-tā′shun). 1. The act of notching or pitting. 2. A notch. 3. A state of being notched. [Mediev. L. *indento,* pp. *-atus,* to make notches like teeth, fr. L. *dens* (*dent-*), tooth]

in·de·pen·dence. 1. The relationship between two or more events in which no information about any combination of some of them contains any information about any combination of the others. 2. The state of mutual detachment between or among autonomous units.

causal i., the state of systems that share no causes or effects.

in

stochastic i., i. of two or more events or variables; the state in which their joint probability or distribution is equal to the product of their marginal probabilities or distributions.

INDEX

in·dex, gen. **in·di·cis**, pl. **in·di·ces**, **in·dex·es** (in′deks, -di-sis, -di-sēz, -dek-sĕz). **1** [NA]. SYN index *finger*. **2.** A guide, standard, indicator, symbol, or number denoting the relation in respect to size, capacity, or function, of one part or thing to another. SEE ALSO quotient, ratio. **3.** A core or mold used to record or maintain the relative position of a tooth or teeth to one another and/or to a cast. **4.** A guide, usually made of plaster, used to reposition teeth, casts, or parts. **5.** In epidemiology, a rating scale. [L. one that points out, an informer, the forefinger, an index, fr. *in-dico*, pp. *-atus*, to declare]

absorbancy i., **(1)** SYN specific absorption *coefficient*; **(2)** SYN molar absorption *coefficient*.

alveolar i., **(1)** SYN gnathic i; **(2)** SYN basilar i.

amnionic fluid i., the sum of the diameters of the largest vertical pocket of amnionic fluid in each of the four quadrants of the uterus as obtained by ultrasound; a measure of fluid volume during pregnancy.

anesthetic i., ratio of the number of units of anesthetic required for anesthesia to the number of units of anesthetic required to produce respiratory or cardiovascular failure.

antitryptic i., an obsolete term for the relative retardation in loss of viscosity of a solution of casein incubated with trypsin, to which a drop of abnormal blood serum (as from a cancerous patient) has been added, compared with that in a similar solution to which normal serum has been added; if the former drips through the tube of the viscosimeter in 100 seconds, and the latter in 104 seconds, the antitryptic i. is 4.

apnea-hypopnea i., the number of apneic and hypopneic episodes combined per hour of sleep.

Arneth i., an expression based on adding the percentages of polymorphonuclear neutrophils with 1 or 2 lobes in their nuclei, plus one-half the percentage with 3 lobes; the normal value is 60%. SEE ALSO Arneth *formula*, Arneth *count*.

auricular i., relation of the width to the height of the auricle or pinna: (width of pinna × 100)/length of pinna.

Ayala i., the cerebrospinal i. when 10 ml of cerebrospinal fluid have been removed. SYN Ayala quotient, spinal quotient.

basilar i., ratio between the basialveolar line and the maximum length of the cranium, according to the formula: (basialveolar line × 100)/length of cranium. SYN alveolar i. (2).

Bödecker i., a modification of the DMF caries i.

body mass i., an anthropometric measure of body mass, defined as weight in kilograms divided by height in meters squared; a method of determining caloric nutritional status.

buffer i., SYN buffer *value*.

cardiac i., the amount of blood ejected by the heart in a unit of time divided by the body surface area; usually expressed in liters per minute per square meter.

centromeric i., the ratio of the length of the short arm of the chromosome to that of the total chromosome; ordinarily expressed as a percentage.

cephalic i., the ratio of the maximal breadth to the maximal length of the head, obtained by the formula: (breadth × 100)/length. SYN length-breadth i.

cephalo-orbital i., the ratio of the cubic content of the two orbits to that of the cranial cavity multiplied by 100.

cerebral i., the ratio of the transverse to the anteroposterior diameter of the cranial cavity multiplied by 100.

cerebrospinal i., the figure obtained by multiplying the pressure of the cerebrospinal fluid, after fluid has been withdrawn by spinal puncture, by the quantity of fluid withdrawn and then dividing by the original pressure.

chemotherapeutic i., the ratio of the minimal effective dose of a chemotherapeutic agent to the maximal tolerated dose. Originally used by Ehrlich to express the relative toxicity of a chemotherapeutic agent to a parasite and to its host.

chest i., SYN thoracic i.

cranial i., the ratio of the maximal breadth to the maximal length of the skull, obtained by the formula: (breadth × 100)/length.

Cumulative I. Medicus, collection of medical literature, published annually, which began in the US Army Surgeon General's office at the end of the Civil War. It has been taken over by the National Library of Medicine and has evolved into a database called MEDLINE.

Dean fluorosis i., an i. that measures the degree of mottled enamel (fluorosis) in teeth; used most often in epidemiological field studies.

def caries i., DEF caries i., an i. of past caries experience based upon the number of decayed, extracted, and filled deciduous (indicated by lower case letters) or permanent (indicated by capital letters) teeth.

degenerative i., the percentage of granulocytes that contain toxic granules in the cytoplasm, as compared with the total percentage of granulocytes.

dental i. (DI), (1) relation of the dental length (distance from the mesial surface of the first premolar to the distal surface of the third molar) to the basinasal (basion to nasion) length: (dental length ×100)/basinasal length; **(2)** a system of numbers for indicating comparative size of the teeth. SYN Flower dental i.

df caries i., DF caries i., an i. of past caries experience based upon the number of decayed and filled deciduous (indicated by lower case letters) or permanent (indicated by capital letters) teeth. SYN df, DF.

diet quality i., a measure of the quality of the diet using a composite of eight recommendations regarding the consumption of foods and nutrients from the National Academy of Sciences (NAS). Meeting the standard is assigned a value of 0, within 30% of goal a value of 1, differing by more than 30% a 2. The resulting index can be a figure of between 0–16, the lower the better. The NAS recommendations include : reducing total fat intake to 30% or less of total energy; reducing saturated fatty-acid intake to less than 10% of energy; reducing cholesterol intake to less than 300 mg daily; eating 5 or more servings daily of vegetables and fruits; increasing intake of starches and other complex carbohydrates by eating 6 or more servings daily of bread, cereal, and legumes; maintaining protein intake at moderate levels (levels lower than twice the RDA); limiting total daily intake of sodium to 2400 mg or less; and maintaining adequate calcium intake (approximately the RDA).

dmfs caries i., DMFS caries i., an i. of past caries experience based upon the number of decayed, missing, and filled surfaces of deciduous (indicated by lower-case letters) or permanent (indicated by capital letters) teeth.

effective temperature i., a composite i. of environmental comfort which is compared after exposure to different combinations of air temperature, humidity, and movement.

empathic i., the degree of emotional understanding or empathy experienced by a health services provider or other person concerning another person, more particularly of a sufferer from some emotional or somatic condition.

endemic i., the percentage of children infected with malaria or other endemic disease, in any given locality.

erythrocyte indices, calculations for determining the average size, hemoglobin content, and concentration of hemoglobin in red blood cells, specifically mean cell volume, mean cell hemoglobin, and mean cell hemoglobin concentration; results are commonly used in the classification and diagnosis of red cell disorders.

facial i., relation of the length of the face to its maximal width between the zygomatic prominences; to get **superior facial i.,** the length of the face is measured from the nasion to the alveolar point: (nasialveolar length × 100)/bizygomatic width; for **total facial i.,** length is measured from the nasion to the mental tubercle: (nasimental length × 100)/bizygomatic width.

Flower dental i., SYN dental i.

free thyroxine i. (FTI), an arbitrary value obtained by multiplying the triiodothyronine uptake by the serum thyroxine concentration; it largely corrects for variations in thyroid-bound globulin concentration by providing a clinically valid estimate of the physiologically active free thyroxine; direct assay or laboratory measurement of free serum thyroxine yields a more accurate value.

glycemic i., a ranking of the rise in serum glucose from various foodstuffs.

gnathic i., relation between the basialveolar (basion to alveolar point) and basinasal (basion to nasion) lengths: (basialveolar length × 100)/basinasal length; the result indicates the degree of projection of the maxilla or upper jaw. SYN alveolar i. (1).

health status i., set of measurements designed to detect short-term fluctuations in health of members of a population; the measurements usually include physical function, emotional well-being, activities of daily living, feelings, etc.

height-length i., SYN vertical i.

international sensitivity i. (ISI), the slope of the line of best fit relating the log prothrombin time obtained with a standard reagent to the log prothrombin time obtained with the working reagent for both normal and patients who receive stable oral anticoagulant therapy; the standard reagents used for this value assignment are reference preparations calibrated against the World Health Organization standard reagent. SEE ALSO international normalized *ratio*.

iron i., an obsolete i. of iron obtained by dividing the figure for the average content of iron in normal blood (42.74 mg) by the red cell count in millions; it normally varies between 8 and 9; in pernicious anemia, the i. is usually greater than 10, but it tends to be normal in chronic secondary anemia.

karyopyknotic i., an i. used to monitor the hormonal status of the patient as reflected by exfoliated vaginal cells and their morphology; an expression of the percentage of intermediate and superficial cells from squamous cells of vaginal epithelium which have pyknotic nuclei.

length-breadth i., SYN cephalic i.

length-height i., SYN vertical i.

leukopenic i., a significant decrease in the white blood count after ingestion of food to which a patient is hypersensitive, a count made during the normal fasting state being used as the basis for evaluation of the postprandial count.

maturation i., an i. indicating the degree of maturation attained by the vaginal epithelium as adjudged by the cell types being exfoliated; serves as an objective means of evaluating hormonal secretion or response; represents the percentage of parabasal cells/intermediate cells/superficials, in that order; "shift to the left" indicates more immature cells on the surface (atrophy), while "shift to the right" indicates more mature epithelium.

metacarpal i., the average ratio of length to breadth of metacarpals II to V; this ratio is increased in the Marfan syndrome.

mitotic i., the ratio of cells in a tissue that are undergoing mitosis, often expressed as either the number of cells in a specified area of tissue section or as a percentage of the total cell sample.

molar absorbancy i., SYN molar absorption *coefficient*.

nasal i., relation of the greatest width of the nasal aperture to the length of a line from the nasion to the lower border of the nasal aperture: (nasal width × 100)/nasal height.

nucleoplasmic i., the quotient of the nuclear volume divided by the cytoplasmic volume.

obesity i., body weight divided by body volume.

opsonic i., a value that indicates the relative content of opsonin in the blood of a person with an infectious disease, as evaluated in vitro in comparison with presumably normal blood; the opsonic i. is calculated from the following equation: phagocytic i. of normal serum ÷ phagocytic i. of test serum = 1 ÷ *x*, where *x* represents the opsonic i.

orbital i., relation of the height of the orbit to its width: (orbital height × 100)/orbital width.

orbitonasal i., the ratio of the width between the lateral angles of the eyes, measured with a tape measure passing over the root of the nose times 100, to the width between the lateral angles of the eyes measured with a caliper.

palatal i., palatine i., SYN palatomaxillary i.

palatomaxillary i., relation of the palatomaxillary width, mea-

sured between the outer borders of the alveolar arch just above the middle of the second molar tooth, and the palatomaxillary length, measured from the alveolar point to the middle of a transverse line touching the posterior borders of the two maxillae: (palatomaxillary width × 100)/palatomaxillary length; it notes the varying forms of the dental arcade and palate. SYN palatal i., palatine i.

Pearl i., the number of failures of a contraceptive method per 100 woman years of exposure.

pelvic i., the ratio of the conjugate of the pelvic inlet to the transverse diameters of the pelvis: (conjugate of pelvic inlet × 100)/transverse diameter.

phagocytic i., the average number of bacteria or other particles observed in the cytoplasm of polymorphonuclear leukocytes or other phagocytic cells after mixing and incubating, at 37°C. It may reflect either the average number of particles ingested or the rate at which particles are cleared from either the blood or a culture.

Pirquet i., an obsolete method of establishing the presence of malnutrition by dividing the weight (grams/10) by the sitting height (in cm); the cube root of the quotient if < 0.945 was considered as indicating malnutrition.

PMA i., an i. which measures the presence or absence of gingival inflammation as occurring on the papillae or the marginal or attached gingivae.

ponderal i., cube root of body weight times 100 divided by height in cm.

pressure-volume i., method of evaluating the cerebrospinal fluid hydrodynamics.

pulsatility i., calculation of Doppler measurements of systolic and diastolic velocities in the uterine, umbilical, or fetal circulations.

refractive i. (*n*), the relative velocity of light in another medium compared to the velocity in air; e.g., in the case of air to crown glass, *n* = 1.52; in the case of air to water, *n* = 1.33. SEE ALSO *law* of refraction.

Robinson i., an i. used to calculate heart work load. SEE double *product*.

Röhrer i., body weight in grams times 100 divided by the cube of height in centimeters.

root caries i., the ratio of the number of teeth with carious lesions of the root, and/or restorations of the root, to the number of teeth with exposed root surfaces.

sacral i., a ratio obtained by multiplying the greatest breadth of the sacrum by 100 and dividing by the length.

saturation i., an indication of the relative concentration of hemoglobin in the red blood cells, calculated as: grams of hemoglobin per 100 ml (expressed as percent of normal) ÷ hematocrit value (expressed as percent of normal) = saturation i. The normal i. for adults and infants is 0.97 to 1.02; in primary and secondary anemia, the i. is usually considerably less than 0.97.

Schilling i., SYN Schilling *blood count*.

shock i., the quotient of the cardiac rate divided by the systolic blood pressure; normally approximately 0.5, but in shock (e.g., rising pulse rate with falling blood pressure), the i. may reach 1.0.

short increment sensitivity i., a measure of the ability to detect small (1dB) increments in intensity; with cochlear lesions, this ability exceeds normal.

small increment sensitivity i., SEE SISI *test*.

spiro-i., SEE spiro-index.

splenic i., a rough indication of the salubrity, or the reverse, in regard to malaria of a particular district, judged by the relative absence or prevalence of enlarged spleens among the population.

staphyloopsonic i., the opsonic i. calculated in relation to a staphylococcal infection, with a young culture of *Staphylococcus aureus* or the strain of staphylococcus from the patient being used in the test.

stroke work i., a measure of the work done by the heart with each contraction, adjusted for body surface area; equal to the stroke volume of the heart multiplied by the arterial pressure and divided by body surface area; the normal stroke work i. does not exceed 40 g-m per m^2.

in

therapeutic i., the ratio of LD_{50} to ED_{50}, used in quantitative comparison of drugs.

thoracic i., anteroposterior diameter of the thorax times 100 divided by the transverse diameter of the thorax. SYN chest i.

tibiofemoral i., the ratio obtained by multiplying the length of the tibia by 100 and dividing by the length of the femur.

transversovertical i., SYN vertical i.

tuberculoopsonic i., the opsonic i. calculated in relation to tuberculous infection, with an actively growing culture of *Mycobacterium tuberculosis* or the strain of tubercle bacillus from the patient being used in the test.

ultraviolet i., a daily i. issued by the U.S. National Weather Service for many cities, forecasting the amount of dangerous ultraviolet light that will arrive at the earth's surface about noon the following day.

uricolytic i., the percentage of uric acid oxidized to allantoin before being secreted.

vertical i., the relation of the height to the length of the skull: (height × 100)/length. SYN height-length i., length-height i., transversovertical i.

vital i., the ratio of births to deaths within a population during a given time.

Volpe-Manhold i. (V-MI), an index for comparing the amount of dental calculus in individuals.

volume i., an indication of the relative size (e.g., volume) of erythrocytes, calculated as follows: hematocrit value, expressed as per cent of normal ÷ red blood cell count, expressed as per cent of normal = volume i.

zygomaticoauricular i., the ratio between the zygomatic and the auricular diameters of the skull or head.

---

in·di·can (in'di-kan). **1.** Indoxyl β-D-glucoside from *Indigofera* species and *Polygonium tinctorium;* a source of indigo. SYN plant i. **2.** 3-Indoxylsulfuric acid, a substance found (as its salts) in sweat and in variable amounts in urine; indicative, when in quantity, of protein putrefaction in the intestine (indicanuria). SYN metabolic i., uroxanthin.

metabolic i., SYN indican (2).

plant i., SYN indican (1).

in·di·can·i·dro·sis (in'di-kan-i-drō'sis). Excretion of indican in the sweat. [indican + G. *hidrōs,* sweat]

in·di·cant (in'di-kant). **1.** Pointing out; indicating. **2.** An indication; especially a symptom indicating the proper line of treatment. [L. *in-dico,* pres. p. *-ans (-ant),* to point out]

in·di·can·u·ria (in'di-kan-ū're-ă). An increased urinary excretion of indican, a derivative of indol formed chiefly in the intestine when protein is putrefied; indol is also formed during the putrefaction of protein in other sites.

in·di·ca·tion (in-di-kā'shŭn). The basis for initiation of a treatment for a disease or of a diagnostic test; may be furnished by a knowledge of the cause (**causal i.**), by the symptoms present (**symptomatic i.**), or by the nature of the disease (**specific i.**). [L. fr. *in-dico,* pp. *-atus,* to point out, fr. *dico,* to proclaim]

off label i., use of a medication for a purpose other than that approved by the FDA.

in·di·ca·tor (in'di-kā-ter, -tōr). **1.** In chemical analysis, a substance that changes color within a certain definite range of pH or oxidation potential, or in any way renders visible the completion of a chemical reaction; e.g., litmus, phenolsulfonphthalein. **2.** An isotope that is used as a tracer. **3.** The labeled substance whose distribution between reactants of a system is used to determine the amount of analyte present. [L. one that points out]

alizarin i., a solution consisting of 1 g sodium alizarin sulfonate dissolved in 100 mL distilled water; used as an i. for free acidity in gastric contents.

clinical i., a measure, process, or outcome used to judge a particular clinical situation and indicate whether the care delivered was appropriate.

health i., variable, susceptible to direct measurement, that reflects the state of health of persons in a community.

oxidation-reduction i., a substance that undergoes a definite color change at a specific oxidation potential. SYN redox i.

redox i., SYN oxidation-reduction i.

in·di·ces (in'di-sēz). Alternative plural of index.

In·di·el·la (in-dē-el'ă). Old name for *Madurella.*

in·dig·e·nous (in-dij'ĕ-nŭs). Native; natural to the country or region where found. [L. *indigenus,* born in fr. *indu,* within (old form of *in*), + G. *-gen,* producing]

in·di·ges·tion (in-di-jes'chŭn). Nonspecific term for a variety of symptoms resulting from a failure of proper digestion and absorption of food in the alimentary tract.

acid i., i. resulting from hyperchlorhydria; often used by the laity as a synonym for pyrosis.

fat i., SYN steatorrhea.

gastric i., SYN dyspepsia.

nervous i., i. caused by emotional upsets or stress.

in·di·go (in'dĭ-gō) [C.I. 73000]. A blue dyestuff obtained from *Indigofera tinctoria,* and other species of *Indigofera* (family Leguminosae); also made synthetically. SYN indigo blue, indigotin. [L. *indicum,* fr. G. *indikon,* indigo, ntr. of *Indikos,* Indian]

in·di·go blue. SYN indigo.

in·di·go car·mine [C.I. 73015]. A blue dye used for measurement of kidney function and as a special stain for Negri bodies. SYN sodium indigotin disulfonate.

in·dig·o·tin (in-dig'ō-tin, in-di-gō'tin). SYN indigo.

in·di·go·u·ria, in·di·gu·ria (in'dī-gō-ū're-ă, in-di-goo're-ă). The excretion of indigo in the urine.

in·dis·po·si·tion (in-dis-pō-zish'ŭn). Illness, usually slight; malaise. [L. *in* neg. + *dispositio,* an arrangement, fr. *dis-pono,* pp. *-positus,* to place apart]

in·di·um (In) (in'dē-ŭm). A metallic element, atomic no. 49, atomic wt. 114.82. [*indigo,* because of its blue line in the spectrum]

in·di·um-111 (^{111}In). A cyclotron-produced radionuclide with a half-life of 2.8049 days and with gamma ray emissions of 171.2 and 245.3 kiloelectron volts. In a chloride form, it is used as a bone marrow and tumor-localizing tracer; in a chelate form, as a cerebrospinal fluid tracer. It is also used as a white blood cell labeling agent and as an antibody label.

i. chloride, i. trichloride, Cl_3In; used in electron microscopy to stain nucleic acids in thin tissue sections.

in·di·um-113m (^{113m}In). A radioactive isomer of ^{113}In; it has a half-life of 1.658 hours; it has been used in cisternography and as a diagnostic aid in cardiac output.

in·di·vid·u·a·tion (in'di-vid-ū-ā'shŭn). **1.** Development of the individual from the specific. **2.** In jungian psychology, the process by which one's personality is differentiated, developed, and expressed. **3.** Regional activity in an embryo as a response to an organizer.

in·do·cy·a·nine green (in-dō-sī'ă-nēn). A tricarbocyanine dye that binds to serum albumin and is used in blood volume determinations and in liver function tests.

in·do·cy·bin (in-dō-sī'bin). SYN psilocybin.

in·dol·ac·e·tu·ria (in'dōl-as-ĕ-too're-ă). Excretion of an appreciable amount of indoleacetic acid in the urine; a manifestation of Hartnup disease, also seen in patients with carcinoid tumors.

in·dol·a·mine (in-dol'ă-mēn). General term for an indole or indole derivative containing a primary, secondary, or tertiary amine group (e.g., serotonin).

in·dole (in'dōl). **1.** 2,3-Benzopyrrole; basis of many biologically active substances (e.g., serotonin, tryptophan); formed in degradation of tryptophan. SYN ketole. **2.** Any of many alkaloids containing the i. (1) structure.

in·do·lent (in'dō-lent). Inactive; sluggish; painless or nearly so, said of a morbid process. [L. *in-* neg. + *doleo,* pr. p. *dolens (-ent-),* to feel pain]

in·dol·ic ac·ids (in-dōl'ik). Metabolites of L-tryptophan formed within the body or by intestinal microorganisms; the principal i. a. encountered in urine are indoleacetic acid, indoleacetylglutamine, 5-hydroxyindoleacetic acid, and indolelactic acid.

in·do·log·e·nous (in′dō-loj′ĕ-nŭs). Producing or causing the production of indole.

in·do·lu·ria (in-dō-loo′rē-ă). Excretion of indole in the urine; actual reference commonly is to indolic acids and indoxyl, as indole itself rarely appears in the urine.

in·do·lyl (in′dō-lil). The radical of indole.

in·do·meth·a·cin (in-dō-meth′ă-sin). An analgesic, antipyretic, and anti-inflammatory nonsteroidal agent used in the management of rheumatoid arthritis and in the treatment of osteoarthritis, ankylosing spondylitis, and gout. It is also used to produce closure of a patent ductus arteriosus in infants.

in·do·phe·nol·ase (in-dō-fē′nol-ās). SYN cytochrome *c* oxidase.

in·do·phe·nol ox·i·dase (in-dō-fē′nol). SYN cytochrome *c* oxidase.

in·dor·a·min (in-dor′ă-min). A selective competitive α_1-antagonist that has been used for the treatment of hypertension; also an antagonist at H_1-histamine receptors and 5-HT receptors.

in·dox·yl (in-dok′sil). The radical of 3-hydroxyindole; a product of intestinal bacterial degradation of indoleacetic acid, excreted in the urine as indoleaceturic acid (conjugated with glycine), as a sulfate (urinary indican), or as a glucuronide (glucosiduronate); increased amounts are excreted in phenylketonuria.

in·dox·yl·u·ria (in-dok-sil-ū′rē-ă). The excretion of indoxyl, especially indoxyl sulfate, in the urine; i. may be associated with indicanuria, inasmuch as hydrolysis of indican results in formation of indoxyl.

in·duce (in-doos′). To cause or bring about. SEE induction.

in·duc·er (in-doos′er). A molecule, usually a substrate of a specific enzyme pathway, that combines with and deactivates an active repressor (produced by a regulator gene); this allows an operator gene previously repressed to activate the structural genes controlled by it to result in enzyme production; a homeostatic mechanism for regulating enzyme production in an inducible enzyme system.
embryonal i., any compound that will effect differentiation in the early stages of development.
gratuitous i., an analog of a natural i. that is capable of inducing an operon while not serving as a substrate for the enzyme being induced.

in·duc·tance (L) (in-dŭk′tans). The coefficient of electromagnetic induction; the unit of inductance is the henry. [see induction]

in·duc·tion (in-dŭk′shŭn). 1. Production or causation. 2. Production of an electric current or magnetic state in a body by electricity or magnetism in another body close to the first body. 3. The period from the start of anesthesia to the establishment of a depth of anesthesia adequate for a surgical procedure. 4. In embryology, the influence exerted by an organizer or evocator on the differentiation of adjacent cells or on the development of an embryonic structure. 5. A modification imposed on the offspring by the action of environment on the germ cells of one or both parents. 6. In microbiology, the change from probacteriophage to vegetative phage that may occur spontaneously or after stimulation by certain physical and chemical agents. 7. In enzymology, the process of increasing the amount or the activity of a protein. SEE ALSO inducer. 8. A stage in the process of hypnosis. 9. Causal analysis; a method of reasoning in which an inference is made from one or more specific observations to a more general statement. Cf. deduction. [L. *inductio,* a leading in]
electromagnetic i., electromagnetic waves propagated by i. in an electromagnetic field.
lysogenic i., i. that occurs when prophage is transferred to a nonlysogenic bacterium by conjugation or by transduction.
spinal i., the manner in which one sensory stimulus lowers the threshold for another.

in·duc·tor (in-dŭk′ter, -tōr). 1. That which brings about induction. 2. In embryology, an evocator or an organizer.

in·duc·to·ri·um (in-dŭk-tō′rē-ŭm). An instrument formerly used in physiologic experiments to generate pulses of induced electricity for stimulating nerve or muscle.

in·duc·to·therm (in-dŭk′tō-therm). The apparatus used in inductothermy.

in·duc·to·ther·my (in-dŭk′tō-ther-mē). Artificial fever production by means of electromagnetic induction. [induction + G. *thermē,* heat]

in·du·lin (in′doo-lin) [C.I. 50400-50415]. A blue quinone-imine dye related to nigrosin; occasionally used as a stain in histology and bacteriology.

in·du·lin·o·phil, in·du·lin·o·phile (in-doo-lin′ō-fil, -fīl). Taking an indulin stain readily. [indulin + G. *philos,* fond]

in·du·rat·ed (in′doo-rāt-ed). Hardened, usually used with reference to soft tissues becoming extremely firm but not as hard as bone. [L. *in-duro,* pp. *-duratus,* to harden, fr. *durus,* hard]

in·du·ra·tion (in-doo-rā′shŭn). 1. The process of becoming extremely firm or hard, or having such physical features. 2. A focus or region of indurated tissue. SYN sclerosis (1). [L. *induratio* (see indurated)]
brown i. of the lung, a condition characterized by firmness of the lungs, and a brown color associated with hemosiderin-pigmented macrophages in alveoli, consequent upon long-continued congestion due to heart disease. SYN pigment i. of the lung.
cyanotic i., i. related to persistent, chronic venous congestion in an organ or tissue, frequently resulting in fibrous thickening of the walls of the veins and eventual fibrosis of adjacent tissue; the affected tissue becomes firmer than normal, and tends to have an unusual, red-blue color.
gray i., a condition occurring in lungs during and after pneumonic processes in which there is failure of resolution; there is a conspicuous increase in fibrous connective tissue in the walls of the alveoli, and also within the alveoli (e.g., fibrous organization of exudate); in contrast to brown i., there is usually not a prominent degree of pigmentation, unless chronic passive congestion is also present.
pigment i. of the lung, SYN brown i. of the lung.
plastic i., sclerosis of corpus cavernosum of penis.
red i., a condition observed in lungs in which there is an advanced degree of acute passive congestion, acute pneumonitis or a similar pathologic process.

in·du·ra·tive (in′doo-ră-tiv). Pertaining to, causing, or characterized by induration.

in·du·si·um, pl. **in·du·sia** (in-doo′zē-ŭm, -zē-ă). 1. A membranous layer or covering. 2. The amnion. [L. a woman's undergarment, fr. *induo,* to put on]
i. gris′eum [TA], a thin layer of gray matter on the dorsal surface of the corpus callosum in which the medial and lateral longitudinal striae lie embedded. The i. griseum is a rudimentary component of the hippocampus, continuous caudally around the splenium of the corpus callosum with the fasciolar gyrus, a slender convolution in turn continuous with the dentate gyrus of the hippocampus; rostrally the i. griseum curves around the genu and rostrum of the corpus callosum and extends ventralward to the olfactory trigone as the tenia tecta or rudimentum hippocampi, hidden in the depth of the posterior parolfactory sulcus that marks the anterior border of the subcallosal gyrus or precommissural septum. SYN supracallosal gyrus.

△-ine. 1. A suffix used to form the names of chemical substances, including halogens (e.g., *chlorine*), organic bases (*guanine*), amino acids (*glycine*), botanical principles (*caffeine*), pharmaceuticals (*meperidine*), and others. 2. General adj. suffix (e.g., *equine, uterine*). 3. Dim. suffix (e.g., *cholerine*). [G. *-inos,,* L. *-inus,* adj. suffixes]

in·e·bri·ant (in-ē′brē-ant). 1. Making drunk; intoxicating. 2. An intoxicant, such as alcohol. [see inebriety]

in·e·bri·a·tion (in-ē-brē-ā′shŭn). Intoxication, especially by alcohol. [see inebriety]

in·e·bri·e·ty (in-ē-brī′ĕ-tē). Habitual indulgence in alcoholic beverages in excessive amounts. [L. *in-* intensive + *ebrietas,* drunkenness]

In·er·mi·cap·si·fer (in-er-mi-cap′si-fer). Genus of tapeworm (order Cyclophyllidae) first recognized in humans in 1935; an arthropod is thought to be involved in transmission (rodent to human, human to human).
I. madagascariensis, cestode often seen as human infection in Cuba in children 1–3 yrs old, causing vague intestinal symptoms;

suspected arthropod vector; proglottids, eggs, and egg capsules resemble those of *Raillietina* spp.

in·ert (in-ert'). **1.** Slow in action; sluggish; inactive. **2.** Devoid of active chemical properties, as the inert gases. **3.** Denoting a drug or agent having no pharmacologic or therapeutic action. [L. *iners,* unskillful, sluggish, fr. *in,* neg. + *ars,* art]

in·er·tia (in-er'shē-ă, in-er'shăh). **1.** The tendency of a physical body to oppose any force tending to move it from a position of rest or to change its uniform motion. **2.** Denoting inactivity or lack of force, lack of mental or physical vigor, or sluggishness of thought or action. [L. want of skill, laziness]

magnetic i., SYN hysteresis (2).

psychic i., a psychiatric term denoting resistance to any change in ideas or to progress; fixation of an idea.

uterine i., absence of effective uterine contractions during labor; **primary uterine i., true uterine i.,** uterine i. that occurs when the uterus fails to contract with sufficient force to effect continuous dilation or effacement of the cervix or descent or rotation of the fetal head, and when the uterus is easily indentable at the acme of contraction; **secondary uterine i.,** uterine i. that occurs when the uterine contractions are initially vigorous but then decrease in vigor, and the progress of labor ceases.

in ex·tre·mis (in eks-trē'mis). At the point of death. [L. *extremus,* last]

in·fan·cy (in'fan-sē). Babyhood; the earliest period of extrauterine life; roughly, the first year of life.

in·fant. A child under the age of 1 year. [L. *infans,* not speaking]

i. Hercules, term applied to young children with precocious sexual and muscular development due to a virilizing adrenocortical disorder.

liveborn i., the product of a livebirth; an i. who shows evidence of life after birth; life is considered to be present after birth if any one of the following is observed: 1) if the infant breathes; 2) if the infant shows beating of the heart; 3) if pulsation of the umbilical cord occurs; or 4) if there is definite movement of voluntary muscles.

postmature i., a baby born after over 42 weeks of gestation, which puts the child at risk because of inadequate placental function. The infant usually shows wrinkled skin, sometimes more serious abnormalities.

postterm i., an i. with a gestational age of 42 completed weeks or more (294 days or more).

preterm i., an i. with gestational age of more than 20 weeks and less than 37 completed weeks (259 completed days).

stillborn i., an i. who has achieved 20 weeks of gestation and shows no evidence of life after birth. Cf. liveborn i.

term i., an i. with gestational age between 37 completed weeks (259 completed days) and 42 completed weeks (294 completed days).

in·fan·ti·cide (in-fan'ti-sīd). **1.** The killing of an infant. **2.** One who murders an infant. [infant + L. *caedo,* to kill]

in·fan·tile (in'făn-tīl). **1.** Relating to, or characteristic of, infants or infancy. **2.** Denoting childish behavior.

in·fan·ti·lism (in-fan'ti-lizm). **1.** A state marked by slow development of mind and body. SYN infantile dwarfism. **2.** Childishness, as characterized by a temper tantrum of an adolescent or adult. **3.** Underdevelopment of the sexual organs.

Brissaud i., SYN infantile *hypothyroidism.*

dysthyroidal i., SYN infantile *hypothyroidism.*

hepatic i., delayed development as a result of liver disease.

hypophysial i., growth hormone deficiency due to failure of hypothalamic growth hormone-releasing hormone (also known as somatocrinin.)

hypothyroid i., SYN infantile *hypothyroidism.*

idiopathic i., dwarfism generally associated with hypogonadism; may be caused by deficient secretion of anterior pituitary hormones. SYN Lorain disease, proportionate i., universal i.

Lorain-Lévi i., SYN pituitary *dwarfism.*

myxedematous i., SYN infantile *hypothyroidism.*

pancreatic i., i. associated with deficiency or absence of pancreatic secretion.

pituitary i., SYN pituitary *dwarfism.*

proportionate i., SYN idiopathic i.

renal i., SYN renal *rickets.*

sexual i., failure to develop secondary sexual characteristics after the normal time of puberty.

static i., a condition observed in young children resembling spastic spinal paralysis; it is marked by hypotonia of the muscles of the trunk and hypertonia of the muscles of the extremities.

tubal i., a term descriptive of a corkscrew-like fallopian tube as seen in fetal life.

universal i., SYN idiopathic i.

in·farct (in'farkt). An area of necrosis resulting from a sudden insufficiency of arterial or venous blood supply. SYN infarction (2). [L. *in-farcio,* pp. *-fartus* (*-ctus,* an incorrect form), to stuff into]

anemic i., an i. in which little or no bleeding into tissue spaces occurs when the blood supply is obstructed. SYN pale i., white i. (1).

bland i., an uninfected i.

bone i., an area of bone tissue that has become necrotic as a result of loss of its arterial blood supply.

Brewer i.'s, dark-red, wedge-shaped areas resembling i.'s, seen on section of a kidney in pyelonephritis.

embolic i., an i. caused by an embolus.

hemorrhagic i., an i. red in color from infiltration of blood from collateral vessels into the necrotic area. SYN hemorrhagic gangrene (1), red i.

pale i., SYN anemic i.

red i., SYN hemorrhagic i.

Roesler-Dressler i., myocardial infarction in dumbbell form involving the anterior and posterior left ventricle and the left side of the ventricular septum.

septic i., an area of necrosis resulting from vascular obstruction by emboli composed of clumps of bacteria or infected material.

thrombotic i., an i. caused by a thrombus.

uric acid i., precipitates of uric acid distending renal collecting tubules in the newborn; since there is no necrosis, the term infarct is a misnomer.

white i., (1) SYN anemic i; **(2)** in the placenta, intervillous fibrin with ischemic necrosis of villi.

Zahn i., a pseudoinfarct of the liver, consisting of an area of congestion with parenchymal atrophy but no necrosis; due to obstruction of a branch of the portal vein.

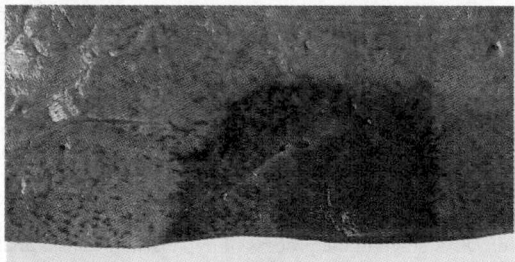

Zahn infarct: liver section

in·farc·tion (in-fark'shŭn). **1.** Sudden insufficiency of arterial or venous blood supply due to emboli, thrombi, mechanical factors, or pressure that produces a macroscopic area of necrosis; any organ can be affected. **2.** SYN infarct.

anterior myocardial i., i. involving the anterior wall of the left ventricle, and producing indicative electrocardiographic changes in the anterior chest leads and often in limb leads, I and aVL.

anteroinferior myocardial i., i. involving both anterior and inferior walls of the heart simultaneously.

anterolateral myocardial i., extensive anterior i. producing indicative changes across the precordium, often also on leads I and aVL.

anteroseptal myocardial i., an anterior i. in which indicative electrocardiographic changes are confined to the medial chest leads (V_1–V_4).

apical i., SYN inferolateral myocardial i.

cardiac i., SYN myocardial i.

diaphragmatic myocardial i., SYN inferior myocardial i.

Freiberg i., SYN Freiberg *disease*.

inferior myocardial i., i. in which the inferior or diaphragmatic wall of the heart is involved, producing indicative changes in leads II, III, and aVF in the electrocardiogram. SYN diaphragmatic myocardial i.

inferolateral myocardial i., i. involving the inferior and lateral surfaces of the heart and producing indicative changes in the electrocardiogram in leads II, III, aVF, V_5, and V_6. SYN apical i.

lateral myocardial i., i. involving only the lateral wall of the heart, producing indicative electrocardiographic changes confined to leads I, aVL, or V_5 and V_6.

myocardial i. (MI), i. of an segment of the heart muscle, usually as a result of occlusion of a coronary artery. SYN cardiac i., heart attack.

Myocardial infarction is the most common cause of death in the U.S. About 800,000 people annually sustain first heart attacks, with a mortality rate of 30%, and 450,000 people sustain recurrent heart attacks, with a mortality rate of 50%. The most common cause of MI is thrombosis of an atherosclerotic coronary artery. Less common causes are coronary artery anomalies, vasculitis, or spasm induced by cocaine, ergot derivatives, or other agents. Risk factors for MI include male gender, family history of MI, obesity, hypertension, cigarette smoking, and elevation of total cholesterol, LDL cholesterol, homocysteine, lipoprotein (a), or C-reactive protein. At least 80% of MIs occur in people without a prior history of angina pectoris, and 20% are not recognized, either because they cause no symptoms (silent infarction) or because symptoms are attributed to other causes. Some 20% of people sustaining MI die before reaching a hospital. The classical symptom of MI is crushing anterior chest pain radiating into the neck, shoulder, or arm, lasting more than 30 minutes, and not relieved by nitroglycerin; typically pain is accompanied by dyspnea, diaphoresis, weakness, and nausea. Significant physical findings, often absent, include an atrial gallop rhythm (4th heart sound) and a pericardial friction rub. The electrocardiogram shows ST segment elevation (later changing to depression) and T wave inversion in leads reflecting the area of infarction. Q waves indicate transmural damage and a poorer prognosis. Diagnosis is supported by acute elevation in serum levels of CK-MB, lactic dehydrogenase, the myoglobin isoenzyme of creatine kinase, and troponins. Unequivocal evidence of MI may be lacking during the first 6 hours in as many as 50% of patients. Death from acute MI is usually due to arrhythmia (ventricular fibrillation or asystole), shock (forward failure), congestive heart failure, or papillary muscle rupture. Other grave complications, which may occur during convalescence, include cardiorrhexis, ventricular aneurysm, and mural thrombus. Acute MI is treated (ideally under continuous ECG monitoring in the intensive care or coronary care unit of a hospital) with narcotic analgesics, oxygen by inhalation, intravenous administration of a thrombolytic agent, antiarrhythmic agents when indicated, and usually anticoagulants (aspirin, heparin), beta-blockers, and ACE inhibitors. Patients with evidence of persistent ischemia require angiography and may be candidates for balloon angioplasty. Data from the Framingham Heart Study show that a higher percentage of acute MIs are silent or unrecognized in women and the elderly. Several studies have shown that women and the elderly tend to wait longer before seeking medical care after the onset of acute coronary symptoms than men and younger persons. In addition, women seeking emergency treatment for symptoms suggestive of acute coronary disease are less likely than men with similar symptoms to be admitted for evaluation, and women are less frequently referred than are men for diagnostic tests such as coronary angiography. Other studies have shown important gender differences in the presenting symptoms and medical recognition of MI. Chest pain is the most common symptom reported by both men and women, but men are more likely to complain of diaphoresis, while women are more likely to experience neck, jaw, or back pain, nausea, vomiting, dyspnea, or cardiac failure, in addition to chest pain. The incidence rates of acute pulmonary edema and cardiogenic shock in MI are higher in women, and mortality rates at 28 days and 6 months are also higher.

	ECG changes:	strongly indicative	weakly indicative
anterior		I, aVL, V_2-V_5	II, V_1, V_6
anteroseptal		V_2, V_3	I, aVL, V_1, V_4
anterolateral		V_5, V_6	I, aVL, V_4
posterolateral		II, III, aVF, V_5, V_6, V_8 (2 intercostal spaces lower) D	aVL
posterior		III, aVF, V_8 (2 intercostal spaces lower)	II

myocardial infarction

nontransmural myocardial i. (NTMI), necrosis of heart muscle that fails to extend from the endocardium completely to the epicardium, often erroneously considered relatively benign.

posterior myocardial i., i. involving the posterior wall of the heart; also formerly used erroneously of i.'s involving the inferior or diaphragmatic surface of the heart.

silent myocardial i., i. that produces none of the characteristic symptoms and signs of myocardial i.

subendocardial myocardial i., i. that involves only the layer of muscle subjacent to the endocardium.

through-and-through myocardial i., SYN transmural myocardial i.

transmural myocardial i., i. that involves the whole thickness of the heart muscle from endocardium to epicardium. SYN through-and-through myocardial i.

watershed i., cortical i. in an area where the distribution of major cerebral arteries meet or overlap.

in·fect (in-fekt'). **1.** For a microorganism to enter, invade, or inhabit another organism, causing infection or contamination. **2.** To dwell internally, endoparasitically, as opposed to externally (infest). [L. *in-ficio,* pp. *-fectus,* to dip into, dye, corrupt, infect, fr. *in + facio,* to make]

in·fec·tion (in-fek'shŭn). Invasion of the body with organisms that have the potential to cause disease.

agonal i., SYN terminal i.

in

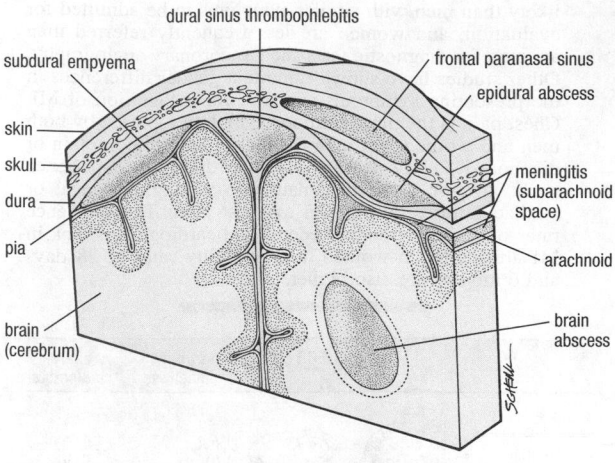

subdural empyema

dural sinus thrombophlebitis

frontal paranasal sinus

epidural abscess

skin

skull

dura

pia

meningitis (subarachnoid space)

arachnoid

brain (cerebrum)

brain abscess

intracranial infections secondary to paranasal sinusitis

airborne i., a mechanism of transmission of an infectious agent by particles, dust, or droplet nuclei suspended in the air.

apical i., implantation of microorganisms at the apex of a tooth, usually the result of the migration of microorganisms from the pulp canal through the apical foramen.

cross i., i. spread from one source to another, person to person, animal to person, person to animal, animal to animal.

cryptogenic i., bacterial, viral, or other i., the source of which is unknown.

disseminated gonococcal i., i. from *Neisseria gonorrhea* which is spread to distant parts of the body beyond the original portal of entry (usually the lower genital tract). Usually manifest by rash and arthritis.

droplet i., i. acquired through the inhalation of droplets or aerosols of saliva or sputum containing virus or other microorganisms expelled by another person during sneezing, coughing, laughing, or talking.

endogenous i., i. caused by an infectious agent already present in the body, the previous i. having been inapparent.

focal i., an old term that distinguishes local i.'s (focal) from generalized i.'s (sepsis).

inapparent i., presence of i. in a host without the occurrence of recognizable symptoms or signs.

latent i., an asymptomatic i. capable of manifesting symptoms under particular circumstances or if activated.

mass i., i. resulting from the entrance of a large number of pathogens into the circulation or tissues.

mixed i., i. by more than one variety of pathogenic microorganisms.

pyogenic i., i. characterized by severe local inflammation, usually with pus formation, generally caused by one of the pyogenic bacteria.

Salinem i., SYN Salinem *fever.*

scalp i., an i. external to the galea; e.g., folliculitis or cellulitis.

secondary i., an i., usually septic, occurring in a person or animal already suffering from an i. of another nature.

terminal i., an acute i., commonly pneumonic or septic, occurring toward the end of any disease and often the cause of death. SYN agonal i.

urinary tract i. (UTI), microbial i., usually bacterial, of any part of the urinary tract; can involve the parenchyma of the kidney, the renal pelvis, the ureter, the bladder, the urethra or combinations of these organs; often the entire urinary tract is affected; the most common organism causing such infection is *Escherichia coli.*

vector-borne i., class of i.'s transmitted by an insect or animal vector. The vector may merely be a passive carrier of the infectious agent, but many kinds of infectious agents undergo a stage in biological development in the vector, i.e., the vector, as well as the human host, is essential to the survival of the infectious agent.

Vincent i., SYN necrotizing ulcerative *gingivitis.*

zoonotic i., an i. shared in nature by humans and other species of animals.

in·fec·tion-im·mu·ni·ty. SEE infection *immunity.*

in·fec·ti·os·i·ty (in-fek-shē-os′i-tē). SYN infectiousness.

in·fec·tious (in-fek′shŭs). **1.** A disease capable of being transmitted from person to person, with or without actual contact. **2.** SYN infective. **3.** Denoting a disease due to the action of a microorganism.

in·fec·tious·ness (in-fek′shŭs-nes). The state or quality of being infectious. SYN infectiosity.

in·fec·tive (in-fek′tiv). Capable of transmitting an infection. SYN infectious (2).

in·fec·tiv·i·ty (in-fek-tiv′i-tē). **1.** The characteristic of a disease agent that embodies capability of entering, surviving in, and multiplying and causing disease in a susceptible host. **2.** The proportion of exposures in defined circumstances that result in infection.

in·fe·cun·di·ty (in-fē-kŭn′di-tē). SYN female *sterility.* [L. *infecunditas,* barrenness]

in·fer·ence (in′fer-ens). The logical process of passing from observations and axioms to generalizations; in statistics, the development of generalizations from sample data, usually with calculated degrees of uncertainty.

in·fe·ri·or (in-fē′rē-ōr). **1.** Situated below or directed downward. **2** [TA]. In human anatomy, situated nearer the soles of the feet in relation to a specific reference point; opposite of superior. **3.** Less useful or of poorer quality. SYN Lower. [L. lower]

in·fe·ri·or·i·ty (in-fēr-ē-ōr′i-tē). The condition or state of being or feeling inadequate or inferior, especially relative to one's peers or to others similarly situated.

in·fer·til·i·ty (in-fer-til′i-tē). Diminished or absent ability to produce offspring; in either the male or the female, not as irreversible as sterility. [L. *in-* neg. + *fertilis,* fruitful]

in·fest (in-fest′). To occupy a site and dwell ectoparasitically on external surface tissue, as opposed to internally (infect). [L. *infesto,* pp. *-atus,* to attack]

in·fes·ta·tion. Development on (rather than in) the body of a pathogenic agent, e.g., body lice. SYN ectoparasitism.

in·fib·u·la·tion (in-fib-oo-la′shun). Closure of the vaginal vestibule by creating a fusion of the labia majora; typically done after excision of the labia minora and clitoris and incision of the labia majora to create raw surfaces that can be surgically joined by pinning so that they will eventually grow together; done for cultural, not medical, reasons. SEE ALSO female *circumcision.* [L. *infibulo,* to pin or clasp together, to join surgically (Celsus), fr. *in-* + *fibula,* pin, clasp]

in·fil·trate (in′-fil-trāt, in-fil′trāt). **1.** To perform or undergo infiltration. **2.** SYN infiltration (2). **3.** A cellular infiltration (1) in the lung as inferred from appearance of a localized, ill-defined opacity on a chest radiograph; commonly used to describe a shadow on a radiograph. [L. *in* + Mediev. L. *filtro,* pp. *-atus,* to strain through felt, fr. *filtrum,* felt]

Assmann tuberculous i., SYN infraclavicular i.

infraclavicular i., an incipient lesion of tuberculous infection. SYN Assmann tuberculous i.

in·fil·tra·tion (in′fil-trā′shŭn). **1.** The act of permeating or penetrating into a substance, cell, or tissue; said of gases, fluids, or matter held in solution. **2.** The gas, fluid, or dissolved matter that has entered any substance, cell, or tissue. SYN infiltrate (2). **3.** Injection of solution into tissues, as in infiltration anesthesia. **4.** Extravasation of solutions intended for intravascular injection.

adipose i., growth of normal adult fat cells in sites where they are not usually present.

calcareous i., SYN calcification.

cellular i., migration of cells from their sources of origin, or direct extension of cells as a result of unusual growth and multiplication, thereby resulting in fairly well-defined foci, irregular accumulations, or diffusely distributed individual cells in the connective tissue and interstices of various organs and tissues; used especially with reference to such changes associated with inflammations and certain types of malignant neoplasms.

epituberculous i., an i. superimposed upon a tuberculous lesion.

fatty i., abnormal accumulation of fat droplets in the cytoplasm of cells, particularly of fat derived from outside the cells. SEE ALSO fatty *degeneration.*

gelatinous i., SYN gray i.

gray i., a term sometimes used for the relatively rapidly formed, semisolid, gray or gray-white exudate (chiefly necrotic cells and remnants of tissue, and macrophages) resulting from unusually acute, overwhelming, diffuse tuberculous infection in the lung. SYN gelatinous i.

lipomatous i., nonencapsulated adipose tissue forming a lipomalike mass, usually in the cardiac interatrial septum where it may cause arrhythmia and sudden death. SYN lipomatous hypertrophy.

paraneural i., SYN perineural i.

perineural i., i. adjacent to or along a nerve. SYN paraneural i.

in·fin·i·ty (in-fin′i-tē). SYN infinite *distance.*

in·firm (in-ferm′). Weak or feeble because of old age or disease. [L. *in-firmus,* fr. in- neg. + *firmus,* strong]

in·fir·ma·ry (in-fer′mă-rē). A clinic or small hospital, especially in a school or college. [L. *infirmarium;* see infirm]

in·fir·mi·ty (in-fer′mi-tē). A weakness; an abnormal, more or less disabling, condition of mind or body. [see infirm]

in·flam·ma·ble (in-flam′ă-bl). SYN flammable. [L. *in-,* intensive, + flamma, flame]

in·flam·ma·tion (in-flă-mā′shŭn). A fundamental pathologic process consisting of a dynamic complex of cytologic and chemical reactions that occur in the affected blood vessels and adjacent tissues in response to an injury or abnormal stimulation caused by a physical, chemical, or biologic agent, including: 1) the local reactions and resulting morphologic changes, 2) the destruction or removal of the injurious material, 3) the responses that lead to repair and healing. The so-called "cardinal signs" of i. are: *rubor,* redness; *calor,* heat (or warmth); *tumor,* swelling; and *dolor,* pain; a fifth sign, *functio laesa,* inhibited or lost function, is sometimes added. All of the signs may be observed in certain instances, but no one of them is necessarily always present. [L. *inflammo,* pp. *-atus,* fr. *in,* in, + *flamma,* flame]

active i., SYN acute i.

acute i., any i. that has a fairly rapid onset, quickly becomes severe, and is usually manifested for only a few days, but which may persist for even a few weeks; characterized histologically by edema, hyperemia, and infiltrates of polymorphonuclear leukocytes. SYN active i.

adhesive i., i. in which the amount of fibrin in the exudate is sufficient to result in a slight or moderate degree of adherence of adjacent tissues, as in healing by first intention.

allergic i., SEE allergic *reaction.*

alterative i., a local reaction to injury, occasionally observed in the walls of blood vessels and in parenchymal cells of various organs in reacting to certain chemicals, viruses, and other intracellular agents; the response is characterized by degenerative changes in the cytoplasm and nucleus, frequently resulting in necrosis, but exudation (if any) is ordinarily observed only in the wall of the affected vessel, or in the interstices immediately adjacent to the affected vessel or parenchymal cells. SYN degenerative i.

atrophic i., a form of chronic i. or repeated episodes of acute i. in which the continued or recurrent proliferation of fibroblasts results in the formation of fibrous tissue that eventually contracts and leads to compression and atrophy of parenchymal tissue. SYN fibroid i.

catarrhal i., obsolete term for an inflammatory process that is most frequent in the respiratory tract, but may occur in any mucous membrane, and is characterized by hyperemia of the mucosal vessels, edema of the interstitial tissue, enlargement of the secretory epithelial cells (which proliferate and form conspicuous globules of mucus), and an irregular layer of viscous, mucinous material on the surface; as exudation progresses, variable numbers of neutrophils migrate into the affected tissue and are included in

the exudate, along with fragments of degenerated and necrotic epithelial cells; such an i. may frequently become mucopurulent.

chronic i., an i. that may begin with a relatively rapid onset or in a slow, insidious, and even unnoticed manner, and which tends to persist for several weeks, months, or years and has a vague and indefinite termination; occurs when the injuring agent (or products resulting from its presence) persists in the lesion, and the host's tissues respond in a manner (or to a degree) that is not sufficient to overcome completely the continuing effects of the injuring agent; characterized histopathologically by infiltrates of lymphocytes, plasma cells, and histiocytes; fibrosis; and granuloma formation.

chronic active i., the coexistence of chronic i. and superimposed acute i.

degenerative i., SYN alterative i.

exudative i., i. in which the conspicuous or distinguishing feature is an exudate, which may be chiefly serous, serofibrinous, fibrinous, or mucous (e.g., relatively few cells are present), or may be characterized by relatively large numbers of neutrophils, eosinophils, lymphocytes, monocytes, or plasma cells, frequently with one or two types being predominant; it occurs not only as a separate and distinct pathologic process, but also frequently as a part of certain granulomatous i.'s.

fibrinopurulent i., a purulent i. in which the exudate contains an unusually large amount of fibrin; also, a fibrinous or serofibrinous i. in which the accumulation of large numbers of polymorphonuclear leukocytes results in liquefactive necrosis of tissue and the formation of pus with a relatively large quantity of fibrin.

fibrinous i., an exudative i. in which there is a disproportionately large amount of fibrin.

fibroid i., SYN atrophic i.

granulomatous i., a form of proliferative i. SEE ALSO granuloma.

hyperplastic i., SYN proliferative i.

immune i., SEE allergic *reaction.*

interstitial i., i. in which the inflammatory reaction occurs chiefly in the supportive fibrous connective tissue or stroma of an organ.

necrotic i., necrotizing i., usually an acute inflammatory reaction in which the predominant histologic change is fairly rapid necrosis that occurs diffusely or extensively in relatively large foci throughout the affected tissue, frequently with only little or no evidence of cells in the exudate.

productive i., a vague term ordinarily used with reference to proliferative i., with or without an exudate; also sometimes used to indicate any i. in which grossly visible exudate is formed.

proliferative i., an inflammatory reaction in which the distinguishing feature is an actual increase in the number of tissue cells, especially the reticuloendothelial macrophages, in contrast to cells exuded from blood vessels; in addition, exudates of various types are likely to be observed in granulomas and other forms of proliferative i., but the latter may occur without an exudate being formed (as in certain infections caused by virus). SYN hyperplastic i.

pseudomembranous i., a form of exudative i. that involves mucous and serous membranes; relatively large quantities of fibrin in the exudate result in a rather tenacious membrane-like covering that is fairly adherent to the underlying acutely inflamed tissue; the pseudomembrane usually contains (in addition to the dense network of fibrin) varying quantities of plasma protein, degenerated and necrotic elements from the affected tissue, polymorphonuclear leukocytes, bacteria, etc.

purulent i., an acute exudative i. in which the accumulation of polymorphonuclear leukocytes is sufficiently great that their enzymes cause liquefaction of the affected tissues, focally or diffusely; the purulent exudate is frequently termed pus, and consists of plasma and its constituents, end products of the enzymatic digestion of tissue, degenerated and necrotic cells and their debris, polymorphonuclear leukocytes and other white blood cells, the causal agent of the i., etc. SYN suppurative i.

sclerosing i., i. leading to extensive formation of fibrous and scar tissue.

serofibrinous i., i. in which the exudate consists chiefly of serous fluid with an unusually large proportion of fibrin.

in

serous i., an exudative i. in which the exudate is predominantly fluid (e.g., exuded from the blood vessels), with the protein, electrolytes, and other material contained therein; relatively few (if any) cells are observed.

subacute i., an i. that is intermediate in duration between that of an acute i. and that of a chronic i., usually persisting longer than 3 or 4 weeks.

suppurative i., SYN purulent i.

in·flam·ma·to·ry (in-flam′ă-tōr-ē). Pertaining to, characterized by, causing, resulting from, or becoming affected by inflammation.

in·fla·tion (in-flā′shŭn). Distention by a fluid or gas. [L. *inflatio,* fr. *in-flo,* pp. *-flatus,* to blow into, inflate]

in·fla·tor (in-flā′ter, -tŏr). An instrument for injecting air.

in·flec·tion, in·flex·ion (in-flek′shŭn). **1.** An inward bending. **2.** Obsolete term for diffraction. [L. *in-flecto,* pp. *-flexus,* to bend]

in·flu·en·za (in-floo-en′ză). An acute infectious respiratory disease, caused by influenza viruses, which are in the family Orthomyxoviridae, in which the inhaled virus attacks the respiratory epithelial cells of susceptible persons and produces a catarrhal inflammation; characterized by sudden onset, chills, fever of short duration (3–4 days), severe prostration, headache, muscle aches, and a cough that usually is dry and may be followed by secondary bacterial infections that can last up to 10 days. The disease commonly occurs in epidemics, sometimes in pandemics, which develop quickly and spread rapidly; mortality rate is usually low, but may be high in cases with secondary bacterial pneumonia, particularly in the elderly and those with underlying debilitating diseases; strain-specific immunity develops, but mutations in the virus are frequent, and the immunity usually does not affect antigenically different strains. SYN flu, grip (1), grippe. [It. influence (of planets or stars), fr. L. *influentia,* fr. *in-fluo,* to flow in]

i. A, the most common type of influenza. These strains have a high propensity for antigenic change resulting in mutations, partly because they can infect various animals where dual infections can occur, giving rise to new hybrid strains. The infections occur in epidemics, which may occur every 2–3 years and which vary in size and severity; perhaps the most important of the three types of i. (A, B, and C).

Asian i., a worldwide i., apparently originating in China in the summer of 1957, which produces a milder disease than that of the pandemic of 1917–1919.

i. B, i. caused by strains of influenza virus type B; outbreaks are usually more limited than those due to influenza virus type A, although infections by the two types are clinically indistinguishable; occasionally associated with Reye syndrome.

i. C, i. caused by strains of type C influenza virus; the disease is milder than that caused by types A and B and has become uncommon in recent years.

endemic i., i., usually of a less severe type, occurring with some degree of regularity during the winter season, especially in the larger cities of the world. SYN i. nostras.

Hong Kong i., influenza caused by a serotype of influenza virus type A and first identified in Hong Kong in 1968.

i. nos′tras, SYN endemic i.

Russian i., a pandemic of a strain i. A virus thought to have originated in Russia; occurred in 1978.

Spanish i., i. that caused several waves of pandemic in 1918–1919, resulting in more than 20 million deaths worldwide; it was particularly severe in Spain (hence the name), but now is thought to have originated in the U.S. as a form of swine i.

swine i., an acute respiratory disease of swine caused by strains of influenza virus type A; it is believed to have become adapted to swine in the United States during the great human pandemic in 1918; fatal cases, as in such cases of pandemic i. in humans, are commonly associated with secondary bacterial pneumonia.

in·flu·en·zal (in-floo-en′zăl). Relating to, marked by, or resulting from influenza.

In·flu·en·za vi·rus (in-floo-en′ză-vī-rŭs). The family of Orthomyxoviridae contains 3 genera: Influenzavirus A, B; Influenzavirus C; and "Thogoto-like viruses." Each type of virus has a stable nucleoprotein group antigen common to all strains of the type, but distinct from that of the other type; the genome is negative sense single-stranded RNA in 6–8 segments; each also has a mosaic of surface antigens (hemagglutinin and neuraminidase) that characterize the strains and that are subject to variations of two kinds: 1) a rather continual drift that occurs independently within the hemagglutinin and neuraminidase antigens; 2) after a period of years, a sudden shift (notably in type A virus of human origin) to a different hemagglutinin or neuraminidase antigen. The sudden major shifts are the basis of subdivisions of type A virus of human origin, which occur following infection of the animal host with 2 different strains at the same time, resulting in a hybrid virus. Strain notations indicate type, geographic origin, year of isolation, and, in the case of type A strains, the characterizing subtypes of hemagglutinin and neuraminidase antigens (e.g., A/Hong Kong/1/68 ($H_3 N_2$); B/Hong Kong/5/72).

in·fold (in-fōld′). To inclose within a fold, as in "infolding" an ulcer of the stomach, in which the walls on either side of the lesion are brought together and sutured.

informatics (in-for-mat′iks). **1.** The study of information and ways to process and handle it, especially by means of information technology, i.e., computers and other electronic devices for rapid transfer, processing, and analysis of large amounts of data. **2.** The science of arranging and organizing the product of genomic and functional genomic studies so that useful insight can result. SEE ALSO bioinformatics. [*inform*ation + -ics]

in·formed con·sent. Voluntary consent given by a person or a responsible proxy (e.g., a parent) for participation in a study, immunization program, treatment regimen, invasive procedure, etc., after being informed of the purpose, methods, procedures, benefits, and risks. The essential criteria of i. c. are that the subject has both knowledge and comprehension, that consent is freely given without duress or undue influence, and that the right of withdrawal at any time is clearly communicated to the subject. Other aspects of i. c. in the context of epidemiologic and biomedical research, and criteria to be met in obtaining it, are specified in *International Guidelines for Ethical Review of Epidemiologic Studies* (Geneva: CIOMS/WHO 1991) and *International Ethical Guidelines for Biomedical Research Involving Human Subjects* (Geneva: CIOMS/WHO 1993).

in·for·mo·fers (in-fōr′mō-fers). Name suggested for the protein particles that appear when RNA is removed from nucleoprotein particles. [information + -fer]

in·for·mo·somes (in-fōr′mō-sōmz). Name suggested for the bodies composed of messenger (informational) RNA and protein that are found in the cytoplasm of animal cells. [*inform*ation + G. *sōma,* body]

infra-. A position below the part denoted by the word to which it is joined. [L. below]

in·fra·ax·il·lary (in′fră-ak′si-lār-ē). SYN subaxillary.

in·fra·bulge (in′fră-bŭlj). **1.** That portion of the crown of a tooth gingival to the height of contour. **2.** That area of a tooth where the retentive portion of a clasp of a removable partial denture is placed.

in·fra·car·di·ac (in′fră-kar′dē-ak). Beneath the heart; below the level of the heart.

in·fra·ce·re·bral (in′fră-ser′e-brăl). Pertaining to that portion of the nervous system below the level of the cerebrum.

in·fra·cla·vic·u·lar (in′fră-kla-vik′ū-lăr). SYN subclavian (1).

in·fra·clu·sion (in-fră-kloo′zhŭn). The state wherein a tooth has failed to erupt to the maxillomandibular plane of interdigitation. SYN infraocclusion, infraversion (3).

in·fra·cor·ti·cal (in-fră-kōr′ti-kăl). Beneath the cortex of an organ, mainly the brain or kidney. SEE subcortical.

in·fra·cos·tal (in-fră-kos′tăl). SYN subcostal (1).

in·fra·cot·y·loid (in-fră-kot′i-loyd). Below the acetabulum or cotyloid cavity.

in·fra·cris·tal (in-fră-kris′tăl). Below the supraventricular crest of the right ventricle; usually used in reference to ventricular septal defect. [infra- + L. *crista,* crest]

in·frac·tion (in-frak′shŭn). Obsolete term for fracture; especially one without displacement. [L. *infractio*, a breaking, fr. *infringere*, to break]

in·fra·den·ta·le (in′fră-den-tā′lē). In craniometrics, the apex of the septum between the mandibular central incisors. SYN lower alveolar point.

in·fra·di·an (in-frā′dē-ăn). Relating to biologic variations or rhythms occurring in cycles less frequent than every 24 hours. Cf. circadian, ultradian. [infra- + L. *dies*, day]

in·fra·di·a·phrag·mat·ic (in′fră-dī′ă-frag-mat′ik). SYN subdiaphragmatic.

in·fra·duc·tion (in-fră-dŭk′shŭn). SYN deorsumduction.

in·fra·gle·noid (in′fră-glē′noyd). Inferior to the glenoid cavity of the scapula. SYN subglenoid.

in·fra·glot·tic (in-fră-glot′ik). Inferior to the glottis. SYN subglottic.

in·fra·he·pa·tic (in-fră-he-pat′ik). SYN subhepatic.

in·fra·hy·oid (in′fră-hī′oyd). Below the hyoid bone; denoting especially a group of muscles: the sternohyoideus, sternothyroideus, thyrohyoideus, and omohyoideus. SYN subhyoid, subhyoidean.

in·fra·mam·il·lary (in-fră-mam′ĭ-lār-ē). Relating to that which is situated below a nipple.

in·fra·mam·ma·ry (in-fră-mam′ă-rē). Inferior to the mammary gland. SYN submammary (2).

in·fra·man·dib·u·lar (in-fră-man-dib′ū-lăr). SYN submandibular.

in·fra·mar·gin·al (in-fră-mar′ji-năl). Below any margin or edge.

in·fra·max·il·lary (in-fră-mak′si-lā-rē). SYN mandibular.

in·fra·na·tant (in′fră-nā′tănt). **1.** SEE infranatant *fluid*. **2.** Lying below. [infra- + L. *natare*, to swim]

in·fra·oc·clu·sion (in′fră-ŏ-kloo′zhŭn). SYN infraclusion.

in·fra·or·bit·al (in′fră-ōr′bi-tăl). Below or beneath the orbit. SYN suborbital.

in·fra·pa·tel·lar (in-fră-pa-tel′ăr). Inferior to the patella; denoting especially a bursa, a pad of fat, or a synovial fold. SYN subpatellar (2).

in·fra·psy·chic (in-fră-sī′kik). Denoting ideas or actions originating below the level of consciousness.

in·fra·red (IR, ir) (in′fră-red). That portion of the electromagnetic spectrum with wavelengths between 730 and 1000 nm.

in·fra·scap·u·lar (in-fră-skap′ū-lăr). Inferior to the scapula. SYN subscapular (2).

in·fra·son·ic (in′fră-son′ik). Denoting those frequencies that lie below the range of human hearing. [infra- + L. *sonus*, sound]

in·fra·spi·na·tus (in-fră-spī-nā′tŭs). SEE infraspinatus (*muscle*).

in·fra·spi·nous (in-fră-spī′nŭs). Below a spine or spinous process; specifically, the fossa infraspinata. SYN subspinous (1).

in·fra·splen·ic (in′fră-splen′ik, -sple′nik). Beneath or below the spleen.

in·fra·ster·nal (in-fră-ster′năl). Inferior to the sternum. SYN substernal (2).

in·fra·sub·spe·cif·ic (in′fră-sŭb-spe-si′fik). Denoting a category of organisms of rank lower than subspecies.

in·fra·tem·po·ral (in-fră-tem′pŏ-răl). Below the temporal fossa.

in·fra·tho·rac·ic (in′fră-thō-ras′ik). Below or at the lower portion of the thorax.

in·fra·ton·sil·lar (in-fră-ton′si-lăr). Below the palatine tonsil or cerebellar tonsil.

in·fra·troch·le·ar (in′fră-trok′lē-ăr). Inferior to the trochlea or pulley of the superior oblique muscle of the eye.

in·fra·um·bil·i·cal (in′fră-ŭm-bil′i-kăl). Inferior to the umbilicus. SYN subumbilical.

in·fra·ver·sion (in′fră-ver′shŭn). **1.** A turning (version) downward. **2.** In physiologic optics, rotation of both eyes downward. **3.** SYN infraclusion.

in·fric·tion (in-frik′shŭn). The application of liniments or ointments combined with friction. [L. *in*, on, + *frictio*, a rubbing]

in·fun·dib·u·la (in-fŭn-dib′ū-lă). Plural of infundibulum.

in·fun·dib·u·lar (in-fŭn-dib′ū-lăr). Relating to an infundibulum.

in·fun·dib·u·lec·to·my (in′fŭn-dib′ū-lek′tō-mē). Excision of the infundibulum, especially of hypertrophied ventricular septal myocardium encroaching on the ventricular outflow tract in the tetralogy of Fallot. [infundibulum + G. *ektomē*, excision]

in·fun·dib·u·li·form (in-fŭn-dib′ū-li-fōrm). SYN choanoid. [L. *infundibulum*, funnel, + *forma*, form]

in·fun·dib·u·lin (in-fŭn-dib′ū-lin). A 20% solution of an extract of the posterior lobe of the hypophysis cerebri.

in·fun·dib·u·lo·ma (in-fŭn-dib′ū-lō′mă). A pilocytic astrocytoma arising in the neurohypophysis of the pituitary. [infundibulum + G. *-oma*, tumor]

in·fun·dib·u·lo-ovar·i·an (in-fŭn-dib′ū-lō-ō-vā′rē-an). Relating to the fimbriated extremity of a uterine tube and the ovary.

in·fun·dib·u·lo·pel·vic (in-fŭn-dib′ū-lō-pel′vik). Relating to any two structures called infundibulum and pelvis, such as the expanded portion of a calyx and the pelvis of the kidney, or the fimbriated extremity of the uterine tube and the pelvis.

in·fun·dib·u·lum, pl. **in·fun·dib·u·la** (in-fŭn-dib′ū-lŭm, -ū-lă). **1** [TA]. A funnel or funnel-shaped structure or passage. **2.** SYN i. of uterine tube. **3.** The expanding portion of a calyx as it opens into the renal pelvis. **4** [TA]. SYN *conus* arteriosus. **5.** Termination of a bronchiole in the alveolus. **6.** Termination of the cochlear canal beneath the cupola. **7** [TA]. The funnel-shaped, unpaired prominence of the base of the hypothalamus behind the optic chiasm, enclosing the infundibular recess of the third ventricle and continuous below with the stalk of the hypophysis. [L. a funnel]

ethmoid i., SYN ethmoidal i.

ethmoidal i. [TA], a passage from the middle meatus of the nose communicating with the anterior ethmoidal cells and frontal sinus. SYN i. ethmoidale [TA], ethmoid i.

i. ethmoida′le [TA], SYN ethmoidal i.

i. of gallbladder [TA], tapering portion of gallbladder, opposite the fundus, as the body of the gallbladder narrows to the neck (from which the cystic duct proceeds). SYN i. vesicae biliaris [TA], i. vesicae felleae✫.

i. hypophysis [TA],

i. hypothal′ami [TA], SYN i. of pituitary gland.

hypothalamic i., SYN i. of pituitary gland.

i. of lungs, in the embryo, one of the expanded extremities of the subdivisions of the lung buds; in later development minute pouches (the air sacs) appear in its wall.

i. of pituitary gland [TA], the apical portion of the tuber cinereum extending into the stalk of the hypophysis. SYN i. hypothalami [TA], hypothalamic i.

i. of right ventricle [TA],

i. tu′bae uteri′nae [TA], SYN i. of uterine tube.

i. of uterine tube [TA], the funnel-like expansion of the abdominal extremity of the uterine (fallopian) tube. SYN i. tubae uterinae [TA], infundibulum (2).

i. vesicae biliaris [TA], SYN i. of gallbladder.

i. vesicae felleae, ✫official alternate term for i. of gallbladder.

in·fu·si·ble (in-foo′zi-bl). **1.** Incapable of being melted or fused. **2.** Capable of being made into an infusion.

in·fu·sion (in-fū′zhŭn). **1.** The process of steeping a substance in water, either cold or hot (below the boiling point), in order to extract its soluble principles. **2.** A medicinal preparation obtained by steeping the crude drug in water. **3.** The introduction of fluid other than blood, e.g., saline solution, into a vein. [L. *infusio*, fr. *in-fundo*, pp. *-fusus*, to pour in]

In·fu·so·ria (in-foo-sō′rē-ă). Archaic term for Ciliophora. [Mod. L. pertaining to or found in an infusion, fr. *in-fundo*, pp. *in-fusus*, to pour in]

in·fu·so·ri·an (in-fū-sō′rē-an). Archaic term for a member of the class Infusoria, now the phylum Ciliophora.

Ingelfinger, Franz, U.S. nephrologist and editor, 1910–1980. SEE I. *rule*.

in·ges·ta (in-jes′tă). Solid or liquid nutrients taken into the body. [pl. of L. *ingestum*, ntr. pp. of *in-gero*, *-gestus*, to carry in]

in·ges·tion (in-jes′chŭn). **1.** Introduction of food and drink into the stomach. **2.** Incorporation of particles into the cytoplasm of a

in

phagocytic cell by invagination of a portion of the cell membrane as a vacuole. [L. *in-gero*, to carry in]

in·ges·tive (in-jes'tiv). Relating to ingestion.

Ingrassia, Giovanni F., Italian anatomist, 1510–1580. SEE I. *process.*

in·gra·ves·cent (in-gră-ves'ent). Increasing in severity. [L. *ingravesco,* to grow heavier, fr. *gravis,* heavy]

in·guen (ing'gwen) [TA]. SYN groin (1). [L.]

in·gui·nal (ing'gwi-năl). Relating to the groin.

in·gui·no·cru·ral (ing'gwi-nō-kroo'răl). Relating to the groin and the thigh.

in·gui·no·dyn·ia (ing'gwi-nō-din'ē-ă). Rarely used term for pain in the groin. [L. *inguen* (*inguin-*), groin, + G. *odynē,* pain]

in·gui·no·la·bi·al (ing'gwi-nō-lā'bē-ăl). Relating to the groin and the labium.

in·gui·no·per·i·to·ne·al (ing'gwi-nō-per'i-tō-nē'ăl). Relating to the groin and the peritoneum.

in·gui·no·scro·tal (ing'gwi-nō-skrō'tăl). Relating to the groin and the scrotum.

INH Abbreviation for isonicotinic acid hydrazide.

in·hal·ant (in-hā'lant). **1.** That which is inhaled; a remedy given by inhalation. **2.** A drug (or combination of drugs) with high vapor pressure, carried by an air current into the nasal passage, where it produces its effect. **3.** Group of products consisting of finely powdered or liquid drugs that are carried to the respiratory passages by the use of special devices such as low pressure aerosol containers. SYN insufflation (2). SEE ALSO inhalation, aerosol. [see inhalation]

in·ha·la·tion (in-hă-lā'shŭn). **1.** The act of drawing in the breath. SYN inspiration. **2.** Drawing a medicated vapor in with the breath. **3.** A solution of a drug or combination of drugs for administration as a nebulized mist intended to reach the respiratory tree. [L. *in-halo,* pp. *-halatus,* to breathe at or in]

solvent i., i. of volatile organic solvents used in glue, nail polish remover, lacquer thinners, cleaning fluid, lighter fluid, and gasoline, for the purpose of self-intoxication. SEE ALSO glue-sniffing.

in·hale (in-hāl'). To draw in the breath. SYN inspire.

in·hal·er (in-hāl'er). **1.** SYN respirator (2). **2.** An apparatus for administering pharmacologically active agents by inhalation.

▪metered-dose i., a device used to administer a defined dose of medication for inhalation; used frequently in the treatment of asthma and other respiratory conditions.

in·her·ent (in-her'ent). Occurring as a natural part or consequence; latent imminent; intrinsic. [L. *inhaerens,* sticking to, adhering]

in·her·i·tance (in-her'i-tans). **1.** Characters or qualities that are transmitted from parent to offspring by coded cytologic data; that which is inherited. **2.** Cultural or legal endowment. **3.** The act of inheriting. [L. *heredito,* inherit, fr. *heres* (*hered-*), an heir]

alternative i., **(1)** SYN mendelian i; **(2)** galton term for an assumed form in which all the characters are derived from one parent.

blending i., galton term for i. in which no component is conspicuous or obtrusive.

codominant i., i. in which two alleles are individually expressed in the presence of each other; there may be other alleles available at the locus that may or may not exhibit codominance.

collateral i., the appearance of characters in collateral members of a family group, as when an uncle and a niece show the same character inherited from a common ancestor; in recessive characters it may appear irregularly, in contrast to dominant characters transmitted directly from one generation to the next.

cytoplasmic i., transmission of characters dependent on self-perpetuating elements not nuclear in origin (e.g., mitochondrial DNA). SYN extranuclear i.

dominant i., SEE *dominance* of traits.

extrachromosomal i., transmission of characters dependent on some factor not connected with the chromosomes.

extranuclear i., SYN cytoplasmic i.

galtonian i., i. in which a measurable phenotype is generated by

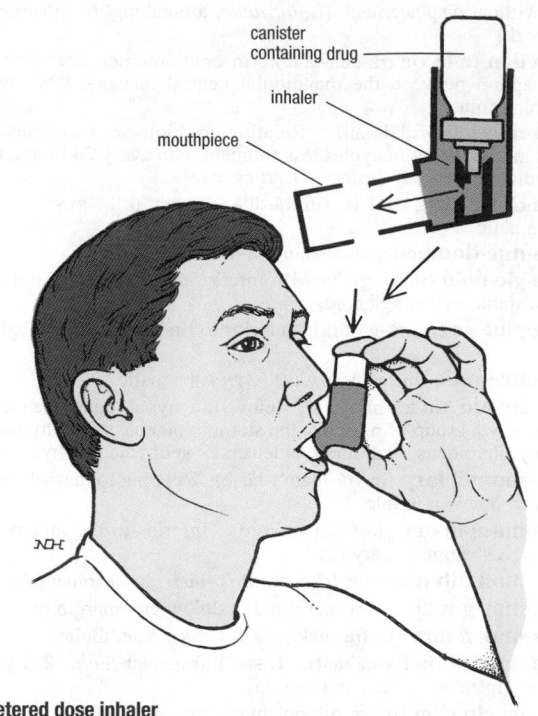

metered dose inhaler

many loci, the contributions of which are statistically independent, additive, and of about equal value. (The latter are in accordance with the classical central limit therein and justify the use of the multivariate normal distribution in galtonian genetics). SYN polygenic i.

holandric i., SYN Y-linked i.

hologynic i., transmission of a trait from mother to her daughters but to no sons, attributed to attached (partially fused) X chromosomes, to cytoplasmic i., or to sex limitation with abnormal segregation, e.g., hematocolpos.

maternal i., transmission of characters that are dependent on properties of the egg cytoplasm produced by nuclear genes or by mitochondrial genes or both.

▪mendelian i., i. in which stable and undecomposable characters controlled entirely or overwhelmingly by a single genetic locus are transmitted over many generations. SEE Mendel first *law, law* of segregation, *law* of independent assortment. SYN alternative i. (1).

mosaic i., i. in which the paternal influence is dominant in one group of cells and the maternal in another. Cf. lyonization.

multifactorial i., i. involving many factors, of which at least one is genetic but none is of overwhelming importance, as in the causation of a disease by multiple genetic and environmental factors. Cf. galtonian i.

polygenic i., SYN galtonian i.

recessive i., SEE *dominance* of traits.

sex-influenced i., i. that is autosomal but has a different intensity of expression in the two sexes, e.g., male pattern baldness.

sex-limited i., i. of a trait that can be expressed in one sex only, e.g., testicular feminization.

sex-linked i., the pattern of inheritance that may result from a mutant gene located on either the X or Y chromosome.

X-linked i., the pattern of i. that may result from a mutant gene on an X chromosome.

Y-linked i., the pattern of i. that may result from a mutant gene located on a Y chromosome. SYN holandric i.

in·her·it·ed (in-her'it-ed). Derived from a preformed genetic code present in the parents. Contrast with acquired.

in·hib·in (in-hib'in). One of several proteins that participate in differentiation and growth. Two glycoproteins, i. A and i. B, are secreted by Sertoli cells in the testis and granulosa cells in the ovary, inhibiting FSH secretion by direct action on the pituitary. [inhibit + -in]

in·hib·it (in-hib′it). To curb or restrain.

in·hib·i·tine (in-hib′i-tēn). SYN carnosine.

in·hi·bi·tion (in-hi-bish′ŭn). **1.** Depression or arrest of a function. SEE ALSO inhibitor. **2.** In psychoanalysis, the restraining of instinctual or unconscious drives or tendencies, especially if they conflict with one's conscience or with societal demands. **3.** In psychology, a generic term for a variety of processes associated with the gradual attenuation, masking, and extinction of a previously conditioned response. **4.** The reduction of the rate of a reaction or process. [L. *inhibeo,* pp. *-hibitus,* to keep back, fr. *habeo,* to have]

allogeneic i., i. or injury to allogeneic cells that occurs when lymphocytes are mixed and cultured with other cells of different genotypes in vitro.

central i., suppression or diminution of outgoing impulses from a reflex center.

competitive i., blocking of the action of an enzyme by a compound that binds to the free enzyme, preventing the substrate from binding and thus preventing the enzyme from acting on that substrate. The competitive inhibitor is often a substrate analog and binds at the active site; however, this is not an absolute requirement for competitive i. Saturating concentrations of substrate can remove the inhibition. Cf. isostery. SYN selective i.

contact i., cessation of replication of dividing cells that come into contact, as in the center of a healing wound.

end product i., SYN feedback i.

feedback i., i. of activity by an end product of the pathway of which that activity is a part; e.g., thyroliberin stimulates thyroglobulin production, and thyroglobulin decreases thyrotropin formation. SYN end product i., retroinhibition.

hapten i. of precipitation, i. of precipitation that occurs when the antibody has combined with hapten of the same specificity as the subsequently added antigen.

hemagglutination i., i. of nonimmune hemagglutination by antibody specific for the hemagglutinin; e.g., viral hemagglutination will not occur if antibody specific for the virus is added before addition of red blood cells. The i. is specific and is widely used for virus identification and for antibody determination.

noncompetitive i., a type of enzyme i. in which the inhibiting compound does not compete with the natural substrate for the active site on the enzyme, but inhibits the reaction by combining with the enzyme-substrate complex or with the free enzyme.

potassium i., arrest of the heart in the fully relaxed state as a result of potassium intoxication.

proactive i., a type of interference or negative transfer, observed in memory experiments and other learning situations, when something learned previously interferes with present learning or recall. Cf. retroactive i.

product i., i. of an enzyme activity by a product of the reaction catalyzed by that enzyme.

reciprocal i., (**1**) SYN reciprocal *innervation*; (**2**) SYN systematic *desensitization.*

reflex i., a situation in which sensory stimuli decrease reflex activity.

residual i., the i. or suppression of tinnitus by use of a sound-generating device (residual inhibitor) that masks the sounds of tinnitus and produces a residual sound-inhibiting effect when the device is turned off.

retroactive i., the partial or complete obliteration of memory by a more recent event, particularly new learning. Cf. proactive i.

selective i., SYN competitive i.

substrate i., i. of an enzyme activity by a substrate of the reaction catalyzed by that enzyme; often, this type of i. occurs at elevated substrate concentrations in which the substrate is binding to a second, non-active site on the enzyme.

uncompetitive i., an inhibitory effect on a metabolic function, such as an enzyme, not based on competition for the binding site of the naturally occurring substrate, but on a different effect on the molecule whose function is being inhibited.

Wedensky i., i. of muscle response resulting from application of a series of rapidly repeated stimuli to the motor nerve where slower frequency of stimulation results in muscle response.

in·hib·i·tor (in-hib′i-ter, -tōr). **1.** An agent that restrains or retards physiologic, chemical, or enzymatic action. **2.** A nerve, stimulation of which represses activity. SEE ALSO inhibition.

α-glucosidase i., an oral agent that aids in the control of diabetes mellitus by delaying the absorption of glucose from the digestive system.

α-Glucosidase inhibitors such as acarbose block the function of enzymes produced by mucosal cells of the proximal small bowel that normally break down complex dietary carbohydrates into simple sugars, including glucose. As a consequence, postprandial rises in blood glucose occur much more gradually. Administered before meals, acarbose can reduce peak postprandial glucose levels by as much as 75 mg/dL. Hence it permits reduction in the dose of oral antihyperglycemic agents or insulin. The drug is not absorbed into the circulation and acts only topically on intestinal lining cells. By itself it cannot induce hypoglycemia, but by reducing the need for insulin, it can increase the risk of hypoglycemia for a given dose of a sulfonylurea or insulin. It may cause flatulence, bloating, and diarrhea as complex carbohydrates reach the colon instead of being digested and absorbed.

angiotensin-converting enzyme i.'s (ACEI), a class of drugs used in the treatment of hypertension and congestive heart failure; they produce a reduction of peripheral arterial resistance, although the exact mechanism of action has not been fully determined; they block the conversion of angiotensin I to angiotensin II, a powerful vasoconstrictor.

aromatase i.'s, drugs, such as aminoglutethimide, that inhibit aromatase, an enzyme used in the synthesis of estrogens.

Bowman-Birk i., a polypeptide that will inhibit both trypsin and chymotrypsin.

carbonate dehydratase i., an agent, usually chemically related to the sulfonamides, that inhibits the activity of carbonate dehydratase, producing a general decrease in the formation of H_2CO_3 in the tissues. SEE ALSO acetazolamide, dichlorphenamide. SYN carbonic anhydrase i.

carbonic anhydrase i., SYN carbonate dehydratase i.

in

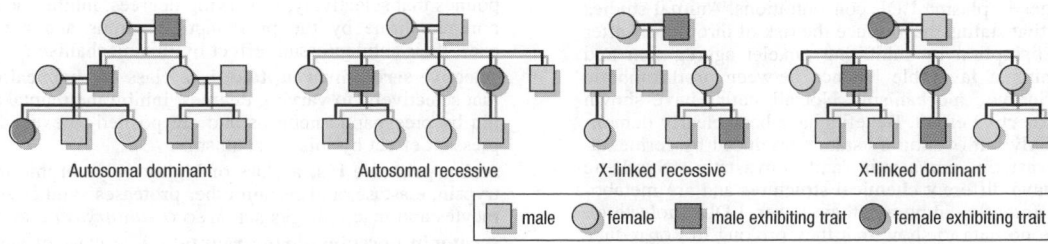

Autosomal dominant   Autosomal recessive   X-linked recessive   X-linked dominant

□ male   ○ female   ■ male exhibiting trait   ● female exhibiting trait

mendelian inheritance: major modes

C1 esterase i., an α_2-neuraminoglycoprotein that inhibits the enzymatic activity of C1 esterase, the activated first component of complement. A deficiency of this i. results in a lack of inhibition of C1r and C1s leading to uncontrolled activation of the complement cascade and edema.

cholinesterase i., a drug, such as neostigmine, which, by inhibiting biodegradation of acetylcholine, restores myoneural function in myasthenia gravis or after nondepolarizing neuromuscular relaxants have been administered.

familial lipoprotein lipase i., an i. found in certain individuals that inhibits lipoprotein lipase resulting in accumulation of chylomicrons, VLDL, and triacylglycerols; similar in symptoms to familial lipoprotein lipase deficiency.

glucosidase i.'s, agents such as acarbose that reduce gastrointestinal absorption of carbohydrates. This group of drugs has been known popularly as "starch blockers." They lower plasma glucose levels and tend to cause weight loss. A limiting side effect is flatulence.

HMG CoA-reductase i.'s, drugs that interfere with the biosynthesis of cholesterol; used to treat hyperlipidemia.

HMG-CoA reductase inhibitors, generically called statins, lower total cholesterol and LDL cholesterol in people with hyperlipidemia, delay progression of atherosclerosis, and decrease the risk of cardiovascular morbidity and mortality. In the synthesis of cholesterol in the liver, 3-hydroxy-3-methylglutaryl coenzyme A (HMG-CoA) is converted to mevalonic acid by the enzyme HMG-CoA reductase. Normally this enzyme is inhibited by a high dietary intake of cholesterol, and conversely a reduction of dietary cholesterol may increase HMG-CoA reductase activity. Drugs that block the action of HMG-CoA reductase are structural analogs of HMG-CoA and competitively inhibit the enzyme, preventing cholesterol synthesis. A decline in intracellular cholesterol levels promotes increased expression of cell surface LDL receptors and uptake of circulating LDL. Controlled studies have shown that in people with a history of angina pectoris or heart attack, lovastatin, pravastatin, and simvastatin substantially reduce cardiovascular mortality, conferring protection against unstable angina and lowering the risk of fatal and nonfatal myocardial infarction, the number and duration of hospitalizations, the need for revascularization procedures, and the incidence of transient ischemic attacks and strokes. Prospective studies on the use of these agents by people with normal cholesterol levels have shown substantial reduction in the risk of a major coronary event in postmenopausal women and in people of both sexes over 65. In contrast, studies in which cholesterol was lowered by diet alone or by other drugs (e.g., cholestyramine, gemfibrozil) have shown no consistent effect on the rate of either heart attacks or strokes. The beneficial effects of cholesterol lowering with statins are independent of concomitant medicines such as aspirin, beta-blockers, and calcium-channel blockers. Hence physical regression of atheroma may not be the principal mechanism by which cholesterol lowering alters cardiac risk. There is experimental evidence that statins affect immune function and the proliferation and metabolism of macrophages and endothelial cells independently of changes in plasma LDL concentrations. Animal studies suggest that statins may reduce the risk of thrombosis after plaque disruption by inhibiting platelet aggregation and maintaining a favorable balance between prothrombotic and fibrinolytic mechanisms. Not all statins have shown equal protective effect. Benefits have been clearly demonstrated only with "natural" statins produced by fermentation (lovastatin, pravastatin, and simvastatin). Synthetic statins have different chemical structures and are metabolized differently; although they lower LDL cholesterol, there are no data to show that they prolong life or reduce the risk of heart attack.

human α_1-protease i. (α_1PI), SYN α_1-*antitrypsin*.

β-lactamase i.'s, drugs such as clavulanic acid, which are used to inhibit bacterial β-lactamases; often used with a penicillin or cephalosporin to overcome drug resistance.

lipoprotein-associated coagulation i. (LACI), formerly known as anticonvertin; a protein that inhibits the extrinsic pathway of coagulation by binding to the tissue factor III-factor VII-Ca^{2+}-factor Xa complex.

mechanism-based i., SYN suicide *substrate*.

monoamine oxidase i. (MAOI), a class of chemical compounds that exert antidepressant effect by the reversible or irreversible inhibition of monoamine oxidase A.

ovulation i., a compound that inhibits ovulation; often found in oral contraceptives.

protease i., a newly developed class of synthetic drug used in the treatment of HIV infection, with a mode of action different from those of previously used antiretroviral agents including nucleoside analogs.

HIV-1 protease activity is critical for the terminal maturation of infectious virions. Protease *i.'s* specific for HIV-1 competitively inhibit this enzyme, thereby preventing the maturation of virions capable of infecting other cells. These agents can reduce the viral load (level of HIV RNA in the serum) below the measurable level in a patient with AIDS. Their use has been shown to reduce the risk of disease progression and mortality in patients with HIV infection. They have also been found to improve CD4 counts and reverse AIDS dementia in some patients. Protease *i.'s* are administered in combination with nucleoside analogs (nucleoside reverse transcriptase *i.'s*) in order to exploit the different modes of action of these 2 classes of antiviral drug. Because emergence of resistance to protease *i.'s* has already been a problem, combination regimens including 3 agents are standard. A few strains of HIV have shown resistance to all available protease *i.'s*. Significant side effects of protease *i.'s* include elevation of cholesterol and triglyceride levels, insulin resistance and emergence of frank diabetes mellitus, and cosmetically objectionable lipodystrophy (excessive accumulation of fat in the abdomen and breasts accompanied by fat wasting in the face, extremities, and buttocks). Protease *i.'s* currently in use include indinavir, nelfinavir, ritonavir, and saquinavir. Several others are in various stages of development and testing.

proton pump i., agents that block the transport of hydrogen ions into the stomach and hence are useful in the treatment of gastric hyperacidity, as observed in ulcer disease.

5α-reductase i.'s, Drugs that inhibit the action of 5α-reductase, resulting in lower levels of prostatic dihydrotestosterone, produced by the enzyme from testosterone as the primary androgen in the prostate.

residual i., a sound-generating device, worn in the ear, that inhibits or suppresses the sounds of tinnitus by masking, with a residual inhibitory effect when the device is turned off.

respiratory i., a compound that inhibits the respiratory chain. SYN respiratory poison.

selective norepinephrine reuptake i., a class of chemical compounds that selectively, to varying degrees, inhibit the reuptake of norepinephrine by the presynaptic neurons and are posited to exert their antidepressant effect by this mechanism.

selective serotonin reuptake i., a class of chemical compounds that selectively, to varying degrees, inhibit the reuptake of serotonin by presynaptic neurons and are posited to exert their antidepressant effect by this mechanism.

serine protease i.'s, a class of highly polymorphic inhibitors of trypsin, elastase, and certain other proteases synthesized by hepatocytes and macrophages SEE ALSO α_1-*antitrypsin*. SYN serpins.

serotonin norepinephrine reuptake i., a class of antidepressant drugs whose action is thought to result from inhibition of presynaptic reuptake of serotonin and norepinephrine.

suicide i., SYN suicide *substrate*.

trypsin i., (1) a peptide formed from trypsinogen via hydrolysis under the catalytic influence of enteropeptidase, with trypsin also produced as a result; so called because the peptide masks or inhibits the active site of the trypsin molecule; **(2)** one of the polypeptides, from various sources (e.g., human and bovine colostrum, soybeans, egg white), that inhibit the action of trypsin. Cf. Bowman-Birk i.

α_1-**trypsin i.,** SYN α_1-*antitrypsin.*

uncompetitive i., a type of enzyme i. in which the inhibiting compound only binds to the enzyme-substrate complex.

in·hib·i·to·ry (in-hib'i-tōr-ē). Restraining; tending to inhibit.

in·i·ac (in'ē-ak). Relating to the inion. SYN inial.

in·i·ad (in'ē-ad). In a direction toward the inion. [L. *ad,* to]

in·i·al (in'ē-ăl). SYN iniac.

in·i·en·ceph·a·ly (in'ē-en-sef'ă-lē). Malformation consisting of a cranial defect at the occiput, with the brain exposed; often in combination with a cervical rachischisis and retroflexion. [G. *inion,* back of the head, + *enkephalos,* brain]

in·i·on (in'ē-on) [TA]. A point located on the external occipital protuberance at the intersection of the midline with a line drawn tangent to the uppermost convexity of the right and left superior nuchal lines. [G. nape of the neck]

in·i·op·a·gus (in'ē-op'ă-gŭs). SYN *craniopagus* occipitalis. [inion + G. *pagos,* fixed]

in·i·ops (in'ē-ops). SYN *janiceps* asymmetrus. [inion + G. *ōps,* eye, face]

in·i·ti·a·tion (i-ni-shē-ā'shŭn). **1.** The first stage of tumor induction by a carcinogen; subtle alteration of cells by exposure to a carcinogenic agent so that they are likely to form a tumor upon subsequent exposure to a promoting agent (promotion). **2.** Starting point of replication or translation in macromolecule biosynthesis. **3.** Start of chemical or enzymatic reaction. **4.** The first step in a chain reaction.

in·i·tis (in-ī'tis). **1.** Inflammation of fibrous tissue. **2.** SYN myositis. [G. *is* (*in-*), fiber, + *-itis,* inflammation]

in·ject (in-jekt'). To introduce into the body; denoting a fluid forced beneath the skin or into a blood vessel. SEE ALSO injection. [L. *injicio,* to throw in]

in·ject·a·ble (in-jek'tă-bl). **1.** Capable of being injected into anything. **2.** Capable of receiving an injection.

in·ject·ed (in-jek'ted). **1.** Denoting a fluid introduced into the body. **2.** Denoting visible blood vessels distended with blood.

in·jec·tion (in-jek'shŭn). **1.** Introduction of a medicinal substance or nutrient material into the subcutaneous tissue (subcutaneous or hypodermic i.), the muscular tissue (intramuscular i.), a vein (intravenous i.), an artery (intraarterial i.), the rectum (rectal i. or enema), the vagina (vaginal i. or douche), the urethra, or other canals or cavities of the body. **2.** An injectable pharmaceutical preparation. **3.** Congestion or hyperemia. [L. *injectio,* a throwing in, fr. *in-jicio,* to throw in]

adrenal cortex i., obsolete treatment involving the parenteral administration of extract of the adrenal cortex; formerly used in treatment of Addison *disease.*

collagen i., correction of superficial soft tissue deformities, acne scars, or age-related skin changes by i. (implantation) of collagen; bovine collagen preparations are commonly used. Prior intradermal testing is necessary to exclude hypersensitivity. SYN collagen implantation.

depot i., an i. of a substance in a vehicle that tends to keep it at the site of i. so that absorption occurs over a prolonged period.

hypodermic i., the administration of a remedy in liquid form by i. into the subcutaneous tissues. SYN hypodermic (2).

insulin i., a preparation that usually contains 100 USP insulin units per ml; it is administered subcutaneously, occasionally intravenously, and has a rapid onset of action, has a brief duration (5 to 7 hours), and is compatible for mixing with long-acting insulin preparations; used in the treatment of diabetic acidosis and insulin coma. SYN regular insulin i.

intracytoplasmic sperm i., a procedure in which a single sperm cell is injected into the oocyte during in vitro fertilization.

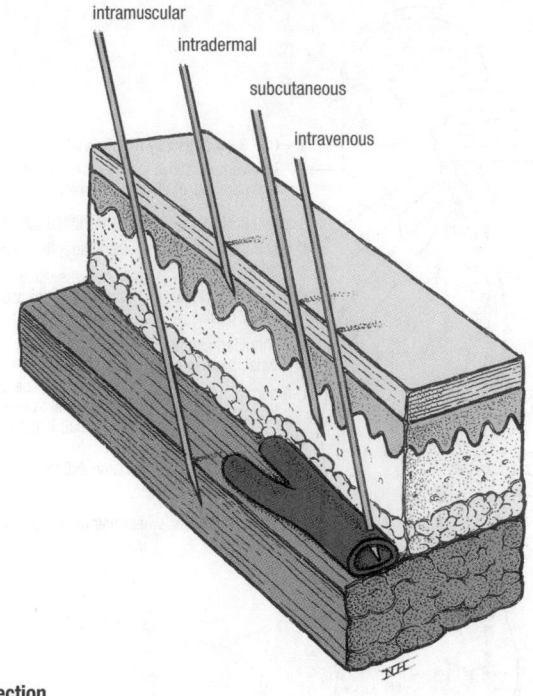

injection

intrathecal i., introduction of material for diffusion throughout the subarachnoid space by means of lumbar puncture.

intraventricular i., the introduction of materials for diffusion throughout the ventricular and subarachnoid space by means of ventricular puncture.

jet i., hypodermic i. of drugs by a jet injector.

lactated Ringer i., a sterile solution of calcium chloride, potassium chloride, sodium chloride, and sodium lactate in water for injection; used intravenously as a systemic alkalizer and a fluid and electrolyte replenisher.

regular insulin i., SYN insulin i.

Ringer i., a sterile solution of sodium chloride, potassium chloride, and calcium chloride, containing in each 100 ml between 820 and 900 mg of sodium chloride, between 25 and 35 mg of potassium chloride, and between 30 and 37 mg of calcium chloride; used intravenously as a fluid and electrolyte replenisher.

selective i., i. of contrast medium following selective catheterization of a branch artery or vein for angiography.

sensitizing i., an i. that sensitizes a person so that subsequent exposure to the antigen (allergen) evokes an allergic response.

test i., intravenous i. of a few milliliters of radiographic contrast medium to screen for allergic or idiosyncratic responses.

Z-tract i., a technique in which the skin and subcutaneous tissue are displaced laterally before inserting the needle intramuscularly; used to prevent leakage along the track of the needle and consequent tissue irritation.

in·jec·tor (in-jek'ter). A device for making injections.

jet i., an i. that uses high pressure to force a liquid through a small orifice at a velocity sufficient to penetrate skin or mucous membrane without the use of a needle.

power i., an i. for rapid contrast medium injection in angiography or computed tomography.

in·jure (in'jer). To wound, hurt, or harm.

in·ju·ry (in'jer-ē). The damage or wound of trauma. [L. *injuria,* fr. *in-* neg. + *jus (jur-),* right]

blast i., tearing of lung tissue or rupture of any tissue or organ without external i., as by the force of an explosion.

brachial plexus i., damage to the brachial plexus related to delivery; associated with excessive lateral stretching of the head, typi-

in

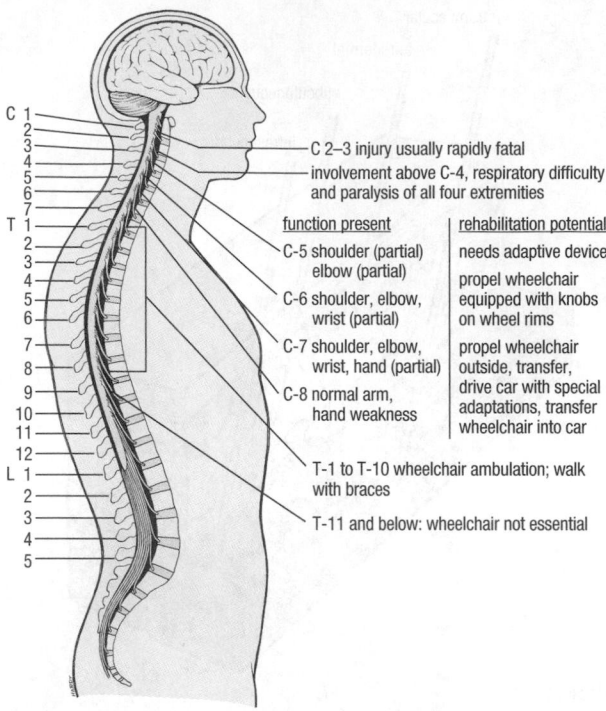

C 1
2
3 — C 2–3 injury usually rapidly fatal
4 — involvement above C-4, respiratory difficulty
5 and paralysis of all four extremities
6
7
T 1
2 **function present** | **rehabilitation potential**
3 — C-5 shoulder (partial) | needs adaptive devices
4 elbow (partial)
5 — C-6 shoulder, elbow, | propel wheelchair
6 wrist (partial) | equipped with knobs
on wheel rims
7 — C-7 shoulder, elbow, | propel wheelchair
8 wrist, hand (partial) | outside, transfer,
drive car with special
9 — C-8 normal arm, | adaptations, transfer
hand weakness | wheelchair into car
10
11
12
L 1 — T-1 to T-10 wheelchair ambulation; walk
2 with braces
3 — T-11 and below: wheelchair not essential
4
5

spinal cord injury: sequelae at various levels

cally in cases of shoulder dystocia or breech deliveries. SEE ALSO brachial birth *palsy*.

closed head i., a head i. in which continuity of the scalp and mucous membranes is maintained.

contrecoup i. of brain, an i. occurring beneath the skull opposite to the area of impact.

coup i. of brain, an i. occurring directly beneath the skull at the area of impact.

current of i., SEE *current* of injury.

degloving i., avulsion of the skin of a portion of the body (most commonly on the extremities) in which the part is skeletonized by removal of most or all of the skin and subcutaneous tissue.

egg-white i., SYN egg-white *syndrome*.

flexion-extension i., forceful application of a forward and backward movement of the unsupported head that may produce an injury to the cervical spine or the brain.

hyperextension-hyperflexion i., violence to the body causing the unsupported head to move rapidly backward and forward resulting in hyperextension and hyperflexion of the neck; does not imply any specific resultant trauma or pathology.

i. of intervertebral disk, SEE traumatic cervical *discopathy*.

open head i., a head i. in which there is a loss of continuity of scalp or mucous membranes; the term is sometimes used to indicate a communication between the exterior and the intracranial cavity. SEE ALSO penetrating *wound*.

pneumatic tire i., separation of the skin and subcutaneous tissue from the underlying fascia, classically occurring when an extremity is crushed and rolled over by the tire of a vehicle; however, it may be incurred through other mechanisms that produce shear forces; similar to a degloving i., except that the skin and subcutaneous tissue layers remain in continuity.

reperfusion i., myocardial impairment, usually with arrhythmia, following the opening of arterial blockage and considered to be due to oxygen-derived free radicals.

steering wheel i., trauma to the anterior chest wall caused by impact with the steering wheel during an automobile accident; can include fractured sternum and ribs, cardiac contusion, tear of the aorta or other great vessels, as well as lung injuries.

whiplash i., popular term for flexion-extension i.

in·lay (in′lā). **1.** In dentistry, a prefabricated restoration sealed in the cavity with cement. **2.** A graft of bone into a bone cavity. **3.** A graft of skin into a wound cavity for epithelialization. **4.** In orthopedics, an orthomechanical device inserted into a shoe; commonly called an "arch support."

epithelial i., SYN inlay *graft*.

gold i., a gold restoration fabricated by casting in a mold made from a wax pattern; the restoration is sealed in the prepared cavity with dental cement.

porcelain i., a fused porcelain restoration luted in a cavity prepared in a tooth.

in·let [TA]. A passage leading into a cavity. SYN aditus [TA].

laryngeal i. [TA], the aperture between the pharynx and larynx, bounded by the superior edges of the epiglottis (anteriorly), the aryepiglottic folds (laterally), and the mucosa between the arytenoids (posteriorly). SYN aditus laryngis [TA], laryngeal aditus [TA], i. of larynx, laryngeal aperture.

i. of larynx, SYN laryngeal i.

pelvic i. [TA], the upper opening of the true pelvis, bounded anteriorly by the pubic symphysis and the pubic crest on either side, laterally by the iliopectineal lines, and posteriorly by the promontory of the sacrum. SYN apertura pelvis superior [TA], aditus pelvis, first parallel pelvic plane, pelvic brim, pelvic plane of inlet, plane of inlet, superior pelvic aperture.

thoracic i., SYN superior thoracic *aperture*.

in·nate (i′nāt, i-nāt′). SYN inborn. [L. *in-nascor,* pp. *-natus,* to be born in, pp. as adj. inborn, innate]

in·ner·va·tion (in′er-vā′shŭn). The supply of nerve fibers functionally connected with a part. [L. *in,* in, + *nervus,* nerve]

reciprocal i., contraction in a muscle is accompanied by a loss of tone or by relaxation in the antagonistic muscle. SYN reciprocal inhibition (1).

in·nid·i·a·tion (i-nid-ē-ā′shŭn). The growth and multiplication of abnormal cells in another location to which they have been transported by means of lymph or blood stream, or both. SEE ALSO metastasis. SYN colonization (1), indenization. [L. *in,* in, + *nidus,* nest]

in·no·cent (in′ō-sent). **1.** Not apparently harmful. **2.** Free from legal or moral wrong. [L. *innocens (-ent-),* fr. *in,* neg., + *noceo,* to injure]

in·noc·u·ous (i-nok′ū-ŭs). Harmless. SYN innoxious. [L. *innocuus*]

in·nom·i·na·tal (i-nom′i-nā-tăl). Relating to the hip bone.

in·nom·i·nate (i-nom′i-nāt). Without name; a term formerly applied to the large vessels in the thorax (now called the brachiocephalic trunk and vein) and the hip bone. SYN anonyma. [L. *innominatus,* fr. *in-* neg. + *nomen (nomin-),* name]

in·nox·ious (i-nok′shŭs). SYN innocuous. [L. *in-noxius,* fr. *in,* neg. + *noceo,* to injure]

INO Acronym for internuclear *ophthalmoplegia*.

Ino Symbol for inosine.

ino-, in-. Fiber, fibrous. SEE ALSO fibro-. [G. *is (in-),* fiber]

in·oc·u·la·bil·i·ty (i-nok′ū-lă-bil′i-tē). The quality of being inoculable.

in·oc·u·la·ble (i-nok′ū-lă-bl). **1.** Transmissible by inoculation. **2.** Susceptible to a disease transmissible by inoculation.

in·oc·u·late (i-nok′ū-lāt). **1.** To introduce the agent of a disease or other antigenic material into the subcutaneous tissue or a blood vessel, or through an abraded or absorbing surface for preventive, curative, or experimental purposes. **2.** To implant microorganisms or infectious material into or upon culture media. **3.** To communicate a disease by transferring its virus. [L. *inoculo,* pp. *-atus,* to ingraft]

in·oc·u·la·tion (i-nok-ū-lā′shŭn). Introduction into the body of the causative organism of a disease. Also sometimes used, incorrectly, to mean immunization with any type of vaccine.

stress i., in clinical psychology, an approach intended to provide patients with cognitive and attitudinal skills that they can use to cope with stress.

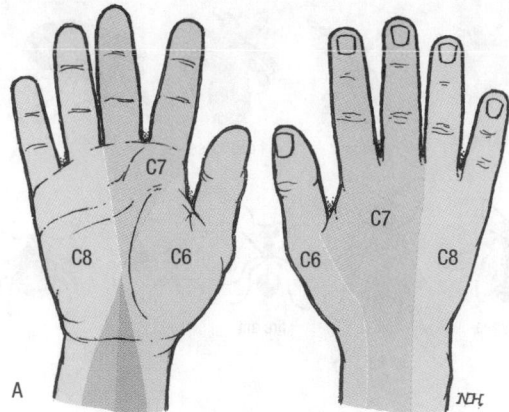

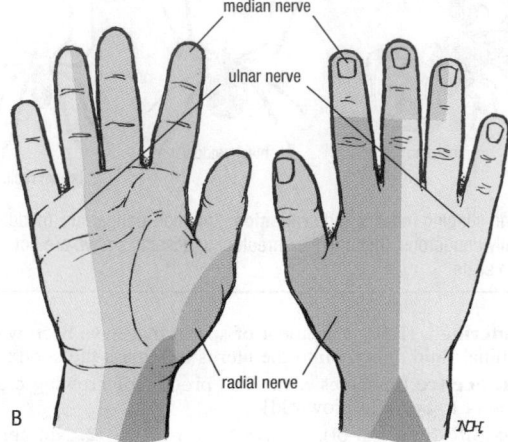

median nerve

ulnar nerve

radial nerve

innervation of the hand and wrist: (A) segmental dermatomes, (B) cutaneous nerve distribution

---

in·oc·u·lum (i-nok′ū-lŭm). The microorganism or other material introduced by inoculation.

In·o·cy·be (i-nŏ′sī-bē). A genus of mushrooms containing several species that have a high yield of muscarine.

in·o·pec·tic (in-ō-pek′tik). Relating to inopexia.

in·op·er·a·ble (in-op′er-ă-bl). Denoting that which cannot be operated upon, or a condition that cannot likely be cured by surgery.

in·o·pex·ia (in-ō-pek′sē-ă). A tendency toward spontaneous coagulation of the blood. [ino + G. *pexis*, fixation, + -ia]

in·or·gan·ic (in-ōr-gan′ik). **1.** Not organic; not formed by living organisms. **2.** SEE inorganic *compound*. **3.** Not containing carbon.

in·os·a·mine (in-ōs′ă-mēn). An inositol in which an –OH group is replaced by an –NH₂ group.

in·os·co·py (in-os′kŏ-pē). The microscopic examination of biologic materials (e.g., tissue, sputum, clotted blood) after dissecting or chemically digesting the fibrillary elements and strands of fibrin. [ino- + G. *skopeō*, to look at]

in·ose (in′ōs). SYN inositol.

in·o·se·mia (in-ō-sē′mē-ă). **1.** The presence of inositol in the circulating blood. **2.** SYN fibremia. [inose + G. *haima*, blood]

in·o·si·nate (in-ō′si-nāt). A salt or ester of inosinic acid.

in·o·sine (I, Ino) (in′ō-sēn). 9-β-D-Ribosylhypoxanthine; a nucleoside formed by the deamination of adenosine. SYN hypoxanthinosine.

in·o·sine 5′-di·phos·phate (IDP). Inosine esterified at its 5′ position with diphosphoric acid.

in·o·sine 5′-mon·o·phos·phate (IMP). SYN inosinic acid.

IMP dehydrogenase, an enzyme that catalyzes the reaction of IMP, water, and NAD⁺ to form NADH and xanthosine 5′-monophosphate (XMP), the immediate precursor of GMP.

in·o·sine pran·o·bex (in′ō-sēn pran′ō-beks). A 1:3 molar complex of 1-dimethylaminopropan-2-ol-4-acetamidobenzoate and inosine, used as an antiviral agent.

in·o·sine 5′-tri·phos·phate (ITP) (in′ō-sēn). Inosine with triphosphoric acid esterified at its 5′ position; participates in a number of enzyme-catalyzed reactions.

in·o·sin·ic ac·id (in-ō-sin′ik). A mononucleotide found in muscle and other tissues; a key intermediate in purine biosynthesis; also produced in relatively high levels in muscle. SYN inosine 5′-monophosphate.

in·o·sin·i·case (in-o-sin′-a-kās). An enzyme that functions in purine biosynthesis and catalyzes the ring closure reaction that produces inosinic acid from 5′-phosphoribosyl 5-formamidoimidazole-4-carboxamide.

in·o·sin·yl (in-ō′si-nil). The radical of inosinic acid.

in·o·site (in′ō-sīt). SYN inositol.

in·o·si·tide (in-ō′si-tīd). Term used for phosphatidylinositol or any inositol-containing phospholipid.

in·o·si·tol (in-ō′si-tōl, -tol). 1,2,3,4,5,6-Hexahydroxycyclohexane; a member of the vitamin B complex necessary for growth of yeast and of mice; absence from the diet causes alopecia and dermatitis in mice and "spectacle eyes" in rats. It occurs in a number of stereoisomeric forms: *cis-*, *epi-*, *allo-*, *neo-*, *myo-*, *muco-*, *chiro-*, and *scyllo-*inositols; the most abundant naturally occurring i. is *myo*-inositol (usually meant when "inositol" occurs without a prefix). SYN antialopecia factor, inose, inosite, liposital, mouse antialopecia factor.

i. niacinate, a peripheral vasodilator.

i. 1,3,4,5-tetraphosphate, a phosphorylated derivative of i. formed from inositol 1,4,5-trisphosphate that causes Ca²⁺ entry into the cytosol from the extracellular medium; inactivated by hydrolysis to form inositol 1,3,4-trisphosphate.

i. 1,4,5-trisphosphate (IP₃), a second messenger formed from phosphatidylinositol 4,5-bisphosphate; triggers the release of calcium ions from special vesicles of the endoplasmic reticulum; has a role in the activation of neutrophils.

***meso*-in·o·si·tol. 1.** Generic term for any isomer of *meso*-inositol in which the hydroxyl groups are so arranged that the molecule as a whole possesses a plane of symmetry and is optically inactive. **2.** Former name for *myo*-inositol.

***myo*-in·o·si·tol.** 1,2,3,5/4,6-Inositol; a constituent of various phosphatidylinositols and the most widely distributed form of inositol found in microorganisms, higher plants, and animals. In plants, it is found as phytic acid and as phytin; partially phosphorylated and free forms occur throughout nature and in many tissues.

in·o·si·tu·ria (in′ō-sī-too′rē-ă). The excretion of inositol in the urine. SYN inosuria (1). [inositol + G. *ouron*, urine]

in·o·su·ria (in-ō-soo′rē-a). **1.** SYN inosituria. **2.** The occurrence of fibrin in the urine.

in·o·tro·pic (in-ō-trop′ik). Influencing the contractility of muscular tissue. [ino- + G. *tropos*, a turning]

negatively i., weakening muscular action.

positively i., strengthening muscular action.

Ino·vir·i·dae (i-nō-vir′i-dē). A family of filamentous viruses that infect Gram-negative bacteria with a genome of single-stranded DNA (MW 1.9–2.7 × 10⁶). Coliphage fd, the type species of the fd phage group genus, adsorbs to the tips of pili of male enterobacteria and, after multiplication, particles are released without causing lysis of the host bacterium. [ino- + virus]

in phase. Moving in the same direction at the same time; a possible characteristic of two simultaneous oscillations of similar frequency.

in·quest (in′kwest). A legal inquiry into the cause of sudden, violent, or mysterious death. [L. *in,* in, + *quaero,* pp. *quaesitus,* to seek]

in·qui·line (in′kwi-līn, -lin). An animal that lives habitually in the

in

abode of some other species (an oyster crab within the shell of an oyster) causing little or no inconvenience to the host. SEE ALSO commensal. [L. *inquilinus,* an inhabitant of a place that is not his own, fr. *in,* in, + *colo,* to inhabit]

INR Abbreviation for international normalized *ratio.*

in·sa·lu·bri·ous (in-să-loo′brē-ŭs). Unwholesome; unhealthful; usually in reference to climate. [L. *in-salubris,* unwholesome]

in·sane (in-sān′). **1.** Of unsound mind; severely mentally impaired; deranged; crazy. **2.** Relating to insanity. [L. *in-* neg. + *sanus,* sound, sane]

in·san·i·tary (in-san′i-tār-ē). Injurious to health, usually in reference to an unclean or contaminated environment. SYN unsanitary. [L. *in-* neg. + *sanus,* sound]

in·san·i·ty (in-san′i-tē). **1.** An outmoded term referring to severe mental illness or psychosis. **2.** In law, that degree of mental illness which negates the individual's legal responsibility or capacity. [L. *in-* neg. + *sanus,* sound]

criminal i., in forensic psychiatry, a term that describes the degree of mental competence and that is defined by such currently applicable legal precedents as the American Law Institute rule, Durham rule, M'Naghten rule, and the New Hampshire rule.

i. defense, in forensic psychiatry, the use in the courtroom of i. as a mitigating factor in the defense of an individual on trial for a serious criminal offense. SEE criminal i.

in·scrip·tio (in-skrip′shē-ō). SYN inscription. [L. fr. *in-scribo,* pp. *-scriptus,* to write on]

i. tendin′ea, SYN tendinous *intersection.*

in·scrip·tion (in-skrip′shŭn). **1.** The main part of a prescription; that which indicates the drugs and the quantity of each to be used in the mixture. **2.** A mark, band, or line. SYN inscriptio. [L. *inscriptio*]

tendinous i., SYN tendinous *intersection.*

In·sec·ta (in-sek′tă). The insects, the largest class of the phylum Arthropoda and the largest major grouping of living things, chiefly characterized by flight, great adaptability, vast speciation in terrestrial and freshwater environments, and possession of three pairs of jointed legs and, usually, two pairs of wings. Some are parasitic, others serve as intermediate hosts for parasites, including those that cause many human diseases. Some are wingless; others, such as the Diptera, have only one pair of wings. Respiration is by tracheoles, cuticle-lined air tubes that pass air directly to the tissues. Development in higher forms is holometabolous and passes through distinctive egg, larval, pupal, and adult stages. SYN Hexapoda. [L. pl. of *insectus,* insect, fr. *in-seco,* pp. *-sectus,* to cut into]

in·sec·tar·i·um (in-sek-tā′rē-ŭm). Place for keeping and breeding insects for scientific purposes. [L.]

in·sec·ti·cide (in-sek′ti-sīd). An agent that kills insects. [insect + L. *caedō,* to kill]

in·sec·ti·fuge (in-sek′ti-fooj). A substance that drives off insects. [insect + L. *fugo,* to put to flight]

In·sec·tiv·o·ra (in-sek-tiv′ō-ră). An order of small, plantigrade, placental mammals that are extremely active and often highly predaceous; they feed mostly on insects and small rodents, although the jes or potomogale of Africa feeds on fish. Eight living families include the solenodons of Cuba and Haiti, tenrecs of Madagascar, hedgehog of Europe and Asia, and shrews and moles of the U.S., Africa, and Asia. [insect + L. *voro,* to devour]

in·sec·tiv·o·rous (in-sek-tiv′ŏ-rŭs). Insect-eating. [insect + L. *voro,* to devour]

in·se·cu·ri·ty (in-sē-kūr′i-tē). A feeling of unprotectedness and helplessness.

in·sem·i·na·tion (in-sem-i-nā′shŭn). Deposit of seminal fluid within the vagina, normally during coitus. SYN semination. [L. *in-semino,* pp. *-atus,* to sow or plant in, fr. *semen,* seed]

artificial i., the introduction of semen into the vagina other than by coitus.

donor i., SYN heterologous i.

heterologous i., artificial i. with semen from a donor who is not the woman's husband. SYN donor i.

homologous i., artificial i. with the husband's semen.

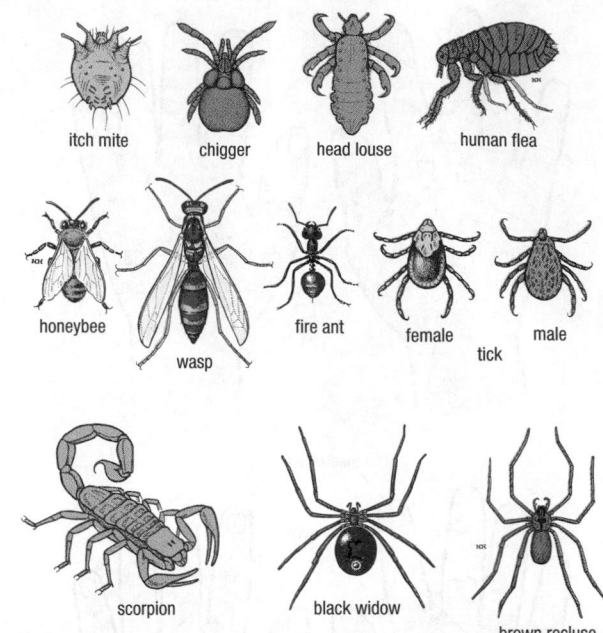

biting and stinging **insects** and **arachnids:** (top) non-dangerous, (middle) potentially dangerous, (bottom) life-threatening; insects shown are not drawn to scale

[image labels: itch mite, chigger, head louse, human flea, honeybee, wasp, fire ant, female, male, tick, scorpion, black widow, brown recluse]

intrauterine i. (IUI), placement of sperm that have been washed of seminal fluid directly into the uterus to bypass the cervix.

in·se·nes·cence (in-sĕ-nes′ens). The process of growing old. [L. *insenesco,* to begin to grow old]

in·sen·si·ble (in-sen′si-bl). **1.** SYN unconscious. **2.** Not appreciable by the senses. [L. *in-sensibilis,* fr. *in,* neg. + *sentio,* pp. *sensus,* to feel]

in·sert (in′sert). **1.** An additional length of base pairs in DNA that has been introduced into that DNA. **2.** An additional length of bases that has been introduced into RNA. **3.** An additional length of amino acids acyl residues that has been introduced into a protein.

in·ser·tion (in-ser′shŭn). **1.** A putting in. **2.** The usually more distal attachment of a muscle to the more movable part of the skeleton, as distinguished from origin. **3.** In dentistry, the intraoral placing of a dental prosthesis. **4.** Intrusion of fragments of any size from molecular to cytogenetic into the normal genome. [L. *insertio,* a planting in, fr. *insero, -sertus,* to plant in]

parasol i., SYN velamentous i.

velamentous i., a form of i. of the fetal blood vessels into the placenta, in which the vessels separate before reaching the placenta and develop toward it in a fold of amnion, somewhat like the ribs of an open parasol. SYN parasol i.

in·sheathed (in-shēthd′). Enclosed in a sheath or capsule.

in·sid·i·ous (in-sid′ē-ŭs). Treacherous; stealthy; denoting a disease that progresses gradually with inapparent symptoms. [L. *insidiosus,* cunning, fr. *insidiae* (pl.), an ambush]

in·sight (in′sīt). Self-understanding as to the motives and reasons behind one's own actions or those of another's.

in si·tu (in sī′too). In position, not extending beyond the focus or level of origin. [L. *in,* in, + *situs,* site]

in·so·la·tion (in-sō-lā′shŭn). **1.** Exposure to the sun's rays. **2.** SYN sunstroke. [L. *insolare,* to place in the sun]

in·sol·u·ble (in-sol′ū-bl). Not soluble.

in·som·nia (in-som′nē-ă). Inability to sleep, in the absence of external impediments, such as noise, a bright light, etc., during the period when sleep should normally occur; may vary in degree from restlessness or disturbed slumber to a curtailment of the normal length of sleep or to absolute wakefulness. SYN sleeplessness. [L. fr. *in*- priv. + *somnus*, sleep]

conditioned i., a form of insomnia resulting from conditioned behaviors that are incompatible with sleep, e.g., each time a person walks into his bedroom, his first thought is that he is not going to be able to sleep.

subjective i., a condition characterized by the subjective experience of greatly reduced sleep, in the context of relatively normal physiologic measures of sleep.

in·som·ni·ac (in-som'nē-ak). **1.** A sufferer from insomnia. **2.** Exhibiting, tending toward, or producing insomnia.

in·sorp·tion (in-sōrp'shŭn). Movement of substances from the lumen of the gut into the blood. [L. *in*, in, + *sorbeo*, to suck]

inspection.
visual i. with acetic acid, SYN acetowhitening, cervicoscopy.

in·sper·sion (in-sper'shŭn, -zhŭn). Sprinkling with a fluid or a powder. [L. *inspersio*, fr. *in-spergo*, pp. -*spersus*, to scatter upon, fr. *spargo*, to scatter]

in·spi·ra·tion (in-spi-rā'shŭn). SYN inhalation (1). [L. *inspiratio*, fr. *in-spiro*, pp. -*atus*, to breathe in]

crowing i., noisy breathing associated with respiratory obstruction, usually at the larynx.

in·spi·ra·to·ry (in-spī'ră-tō-rē). Relating to or timed during inhalation.

in·spire (in-spīr'). SYN inhale.

in·spi·rom·e·ter (in-spī-rom'ĕ-ter). An instrument for measuring the force, frequency, or volume of inspirations. [L. *in-spiro*, to breathe in, + G. *metron*, measure]

in·spis·sate (in-spis'āt). To perform or undergo inspissation.

in·spis·sa·tion (in-spi-sā'shŭn). **1.** The act of thickening or condensing, as by evaporation or absorption of fluid. **2.** An increased thickening or diminished fluidity. [L. *in*, intensive, + *spisso*, pp. -*atus*, to thicken]

in·spis·sa·tor (in-spis'ă-tŏr). An apparatus for evaporating fluids.

in·sta·bil·i·ty (in-stă-bil'i-tē). The state of being unstable, or lacking stability.

detrusor i., involuntary detrusor contractions that may occur at bladder volumes below capacity. SYN detrusor hyperreflexia.

spinal i., the inability of the spinal column, under physiologic loads, to maintain its normal configuration; may result in damage to the spinal cord or nerve roots or lead to the development of a painful spinal deformity.

in·star (in'stahr). Any of the successive nymphal stages in the metamorphosis of hemimetabolous insects (simple or incomplete metamorphosis), or the stages of larval change by successive molts that characterize the holometabolous insects (complex or complete metamorphosis). [L. *form*]

in·step. The arch, or highest part of the dorsum of the foot. SEE ALSO tarsus.

in·stil·la·tion (in-sti-lā'shŭn). Dropping of a liquid on or into a body part. [L. *instillatio*, fr. *in-stillo*, pp. -*atus*, to pour in by drops, fr. *stilla*, a drop]

in·stil·la·tor (in'sti-lā-ter). A device for performing instillation. SYN dropper.

in·stinct (in'stinkt). **1.** An enduring disposition or tendency of an organism to act in an organized and biologically adaptive manner characteristic of its species. **2.** The unreasoning impulse to perform some purposive action without an immediate consciousness of the end to which that action may lead. **3.** In psychoanalytic theory, the forces or drives assumed to exist behind the tension caused by the needs of the id. [L. *instinctus*, impulse]

aggressive i., SYN death i.

death i., an i. of living creatures toward self-destruction, death, or a return to the inorganic lifelessness from which they arose. SYN aggressive i.

ego i.'s, self-preservative needs and self-love, as opposed to object love; drives that are primarily erotic.

herd i., tendency or inclination to band together with and share the customs of others of a group, and to conform to the opinions and adopt the views of the group. SYN social i.

life i., the i. of self-preservation and sexual procreation; the basic urge toward preservation of the species. SYN sexual i.

sexual i., SYN life i.

social i., SYN herd i.

in·stinc·tive, in·stinc·tu·al (in-stink'tiv, -stink'choo-ăl). Relating to instinct.

in·stru·ment (in'stroo-ment). A tool or implement. [L. *instrumentum*]

diamond cutting i.'s, in dentistry, cylinders, disks, and other cutting i.'s to which numerous small diamond pyramids have been attached by a plating of metal.

hearing i., SYN hearing aid.

Krueger i. stop, a mechanical device limiting the insertion of a root canal i. into a canal.

plugging i., SYN plugger.

purse-string i., an intestinal clamp with jaws at an angle to the handle; when closed across the bowel, large grooved interdigitating serrations allow passage of a straight needle and suture through each side to form a purse-string suture, after which the clamp is removed.

Sabouraud-Noiré i., an obsolete device for measuring the quantity of x-rays by means of the change in color of a disk of barium platinocyanide which exposure to them produces; the unit used in this method is called tint B. SEE erythema dose.

stereotactic i., stereotaxic i., an apparatus attached to the head, used to localize precisely an area in the brain by means of coordinates related to intracerebral structures.

test handle i., a root canal i. the handle of which is similar to a collet chuck and which can be secured in position on the root canal i. to adjust its effective length.

in·stru·men·tar·i·um (in'stroo-men-tār'ē-ŭm). A collection of instruments and other equipment for an operation or for a medical procedure.

in·stru·men·ta·tion (in'stroo-men-tā'shŭn). **1.** The use of instruments. **2.** In dentistry, the application of armamentarium in a restorative procedure.

in·suc·ca·tion (in'sŭ-kā'shŭn). Maceration or soaking, especially of a crude drug to prepare it for further pharmaceutical operation. [L. *insuco*, pp. -*atus*, to soak in, fr. *in*, in, + *sucus*, juice, sap (improp. *succ*-)]

in·su·date (in'soo-dāt). Fluid swelling within an arterial wall (ordinarily serous), differing from an exudate in that it does not come to lie extramurally. [L. *in*, in, + *sudo*, pp. -*atus*, to sweat]

in·suf·fi·cien·cy (in-sŭ-fish'en-sē). Lack of completeness of function or power. SEE ALSO incompetence. [L. *in*-, neg. + *sufficientia*, fr. *sufficio* to suffice]

accommodative i., a lack of appropriate accommodation for near focus.

acute adrenocortical i., severe adrenocortical i. when an intercurrent illness or trauma causes an increased demand for adrenocortical hormones in a patient with adrenal insufficiency due to disease or use of relatively large amounts of similar hormones as therapy; characterized by nausea, vomiting, hypotension, and frequently hyperthemia, hyponatremia, hyperkalemia, and hypoglycemia; can be fatal if untreated. SYN addisonian crisis, adrenal crisis, Bernard-Sergent syndrome.

adrenocortical i., loss, to varying degrees, of adrenocortical function. SYN hypocorticoidism.

aortic i., SEE valvular *regurgitation*.

cardiac i., SYN heart *failure* (1).

chronic adrenocortical i., adrenocortical i. usually as the result of idiopathic atrophy or destruction of both adrenal glands by tuberculosis, an autoimmune process, or other diseases; characterized by fatigue, decreased blood pressure, weight loss, increased melanin pigmentation of the skin and mucous membranes, anorexia, and nausea or vomiting; without appropriate replacement therapy, it can progress to acute adrenocortical i. SYN Addison disease, addisonian syndrome, hyposupradrenalism, morbus Addisonii.

convergence i., that condition in which an exophoria or exotropia is more marked for near vision than for far vision.

in

coronary i., inadequate coronary circulation leading to anginal pain. SYN coronarism (1).

divergence i., that condition in which an esophoria or esotropia is more marked for far vision than for near vision.

exocrine pancreatic i., lack of exocrine secretions of pancreas, due to destruction of acini, usually by chronic pancreatitis; lack of digestive enzymes from pancreas results in diarrhea, usually fatty (steatorrhea) because of lack of pancreatic enzymes.

hepatic i., defective functional activity of the liver cells.

latent adrenocortical i., adrenocortical i. not clinically evident but which can become severe if a sudden stress, such as an intercurrent acute illness, develops.

mitral i., SEE valvular *regurgitation.*

muscular i., failure of any muscle to contract with its normal force, especially such failure of any of the eye muscles.

myocardial i., SYN heart *failure* (1).

parathyroid i., SYN hypoparathyroidism.

partial adrenocortical i., normal basal adrenocortical function with failure of adrenocortical reserve to respond to ACTH stimulation.

primary adrenocortical i., adrenocortical i. caused by disease, destruction, or surgical removal of the adrenal cortices.

pulmonary i., SEE valvular *regurgitation.*

pyloric i., patulousness of the pyloric outlet of the stomach, allowing regurgitation of duodenal contents into the stomach.

renal i., defective function of the kidneys, with accumulation of waste products (particularly nitrogenous) in the blood.

respiratory i., failure to adequately provide oxygen to the cells of the body and to remove excess carbon dioxide from them.

secondary adrenocortical i., adrenocortical i. caused by failure of ACTH secretion resulting from anterior pituitary disease or inhibition of ACTH production resulting from exogenous steroid therapy.

thyroid i., subnormal secretion of hormones by the thyroid gland. SEE ALSO hypothyroidism.

tricuspid i., SEE valvular *regurgitation.*

uterine i., atony of the uterine musculature.

valvular i., SYN valvular *regurgitation.*

velopharyngeal i., anatomical or functional deficiency in the soft palate or superior constrictor muscle of the pharynx, resulting in the inability to achieve velopharyngeal closure.

venous i., inadequate drainage of venous blood from a part, resulting in edema or dermatosis.

in·suf·flate (in-sŭf′lāt). To deliver air or gas under pressure to a cavity or chamber of the body as, e.g., the injection of carbon dioxide into the peritoneum to achieve pneumoperitoneum during laparoscopy and laparoscopic surgery. [L. *in-sufflo,* to blow on or into]

in·suf·fla·tion (in-sŭf-lā′shŭn). **1.** The act or process of insufflating. **2.** SYN inhalant (3).

perirenal i., an obsolete technique involving injection of air or carbon dioxide about the kidneys for radiography of the adrenal glands.

peritoneal i., the administration of a gas, usually carbon dioxide, within the peritoneal cavity to facilitate laparoendoscopic procedures.

in·suf·fla·tor (in′sŭf-lā-ter). An instrument used in insufflation.

in·su·la, gen. and pl. **in·su·lae** (in′soo-lă, -lē) [TA]. **1** [TA]. An oval region of the cerebral cortex overlying the extreme capsule, lateral to the lenticular nucleus, buried in the depth of the fissura lateralis cerebri (sylvian fissure), separated from the adjacent opercula by the circular sulcus of insula. SYN insular area, insular cortex, island of Reil. **2.** SYN island. **3.** Any circumscribed body or patch on the skin. [L. island]

Haller i., a doubling of the thoracic duct for part of its course through the thorax. SYN Haller anulus.

in·su·lar (in′soo-lăr). Relating to any insula, especially the island of Reil.

in·su·late (in′sŭ-lāt). To prevent the passage of electric or radiant energy by the interposition of a nonconducting substance. [L. *insulatus,* made like an island]

in·su·la·tion (in-sŭ-lā′shŭn). **1.** The act of insulating. **2.** The nonconducting substance so used. **3.** The state of being insulated.

in·su·la·tor (in′sŭ-lā-ter). A nonconducting substance used as insulation.

in·su·lin (in′sŭ-lin). A polypeptide hormone, secreted by beta cells in the islets of Langerhans, that promotes glucose utilization, protein synthesis, and the formation and storage of neutral lipids; available in a variety of preparations including genetically engineered human i., which is presently favored, i. is used parenterally in the treatment of diabetes mellitus. [L. *insula,* island, + -in]

insulin (metabolic effects)			
metabolic change	effect	mechanism	main organ
1. glucose transport	+	unknown	muscles, fatty tissue
2. amino acid transport	+	unknown	muscles, fatty tissue
3. potassium transport	+	unknown; sometimes in connection with glucose transport	liver, muscles
4. glucose oxidation	+	increased glucose transport into cells	muscles, fatty tissue
5. glycogen synthesis	+	increased glucose transport into cells; activation of glycogen synthetase through dephosphorylation of the enzyme	muscles, liver
6. fatty acid synthesis	+	as in 4; plus reduction of acyl-CoA, increased acetyl-CoA from glucose resulting from activation of pyruvate dehydrogenase, release of acetyl-CoA-carboxylase	fatty tissue, liver
7. lipid synthesis	+	as in 4; plus production of α-glycerophosphate from glucose	fatty tissue, liver, muscles
8. protein synthesis	+	activation of ribosomes (translation of messenger RNA)	muscles, fibroblasts
9. lipolysis	−	antagonistic to lipolytic hormones; inhibition of adenylate cyclase	fatty tissue, liver
10. ketogenesis	−	inhibition of fatty acid production through antilipolysis (see 9)	liver
11. gluco-neogenesis and glycogenolysis	−	inhibition of glucagon-stimulated glucose release; inhibition of adenylate cyclase	liver
12. proteolysis	−	unknown; inhibition of urea production in the liver, through reduced production of amino acids	liver, muscle

biphasic i., the specific antidiabetic principle of the pancreas of the ox in a solution of that from the pancreas of the pig.

globin i., SYN regular i.

globin zinc i., a sterile solution of i. modified by the addition of zinc chloride and globin; it contains 100 units per ml; duration of action is about 18 hours.

human i., a protein that has the normal structure of i. produced by the human pancreas, prepared by recombinant DNA techniques and by semisynthetic processes.

immunoreactive i., that portion of i. in blood measured by immunochemical methods for the hormone; presumed to represent the free (unbound) and biologically active fraction of total blood i.

isophane i., a modified form of i. composed of i., protamine, and zinc; an intermediately acting preparation used for the treatment of diabetes mellitus. SYN NPH i.

lente i., SYN insulin zinc *suspension.*

lispro i., a modified version of natural human i., synthesized by a genetically programmed strain of nonpathogenic *Escherichia coli,* in which the amino acids lysine (Lys) and proline (Pro) near the end of the B chain are transposed. This chemical alteration yields an i. with a much faster onset of action, which reaches its peak effect earlier than regular i. [Lys + Pro]

Lispro insulin, introduced in 1996, has the same molecular weight and the same biochemical functions as the natural hormone, and when administered intravenously its effects are virtually indistinguishable from those of regular insulin. However, when it is injected subcutaneously it reaches its peak serum level in 30–90 minutes, as compared to 50–120 minutes for regular insulin, and it also has a shorter half-life. While the original indication for lispro insulin was for use as a rapid-acting premeal insulin, clinical experience has shown that this agent improves postprandial glucose levels, reduces the incidence of severe hypoglycemia and nighttime hypoglycemia, and improves glucose control as measured by glycosylated hemoglobin, when appropriate adjustments are made to basal insulin, snacking, and exercise level. Unlike other insulins, lispro insulin is not available without a prescription. It is not recommended for use in pregnancy because its effects on the fetus have not been assessed.

NPH i., SYN isophane i. [*N*eutral *P*rotamine *H*agedorn]

protamine zinc i., i. modified by the addition of protamine and zinc chloride; it contains 100 units per ml.

regular i., a rapidly acting form of i. which is a clear solution and may be administered intravenously as well as subcutaneously; may be mixed with longer acting forms of i. to extend the duration of effect. Onset of effect occurs in ½ to 1 hour, peak effects are observed in 2 to 3 hours, and the duration of effect is about 5 to 7 hours. SYN globin i.

semilente i., SYN prompt insulin zinc *suspension.*

ultralente i., a form of zinc precipitated i. in suspension in which the particle size is large, and thus release into the bloodstream after subcutaneous injection is slow; it can be mixed with other i.'s having different particle sizes to achieve different durations of activity. Can be derived from porcine, bovine, or genetically engineered human type.

in·su·li·ne·mia (in′sŭ-li-nē′mē-ă). Literally, insulin in the circulating blood; usually connotes abnormally large concentrations of insulin in the circulating blood. [insulin + G. *haima,* blood]

in·su·lin·o·gen·e·sis (in′sŭ-lin-ō-jen′ĕ-sis). Production of insulin. [insulin + G. *genesis,* production]

in·su·lin·o·gen·ic, in·su·lo·gen·ic (in′sŭ-lin-ō-jen′ik, in′sŭ-lō-je-n′ik). Relating to insulinogenesis.

in·su·li·no·ma (in′sŭ-li-nō′mă). An islet cell adenoma that secretes insulin.

in·su·li·tis (in′sŭ-lī′tis). Inflammation of the islands of Langerhans, with lymphocytic infiltration which may result from viral infection and be the initial lesion of insulin-dependent diabetes mellitus. [L. *insula,* island, + *-itis,* inflammation]

in·sult (in′sŭlt). An injury, attack, or trauma. [LL. *insultus,* fr L. *insulto,* to spring upon]

insurance.

fee-for-service i., i. coverage that reimburses participants and providers following submission of a claim. Participants have few if any restrictions on which hospitals or doctors to use.

in·sus·cep·ti·bil·i·ty (in′sŭ-sep′ti-bil′i-tē). SYN immunity. [L. *suscipio,* pp. *-ceptus,* to take upon one, fr. *sub,* under, + *capio,* to take]

int. cib. Abbreviation for L. *inter cibos,* between meals.

in·te·gral (int′ē-gral). **1.** Constituent. **2.** Integrated. **3.** SEE integration (3).

in·te·gra·tion (in-tĕ-grā′shŭn). **1.** The state of being combined, or the process of combining, into a complete and harmonious whole. **2.** In physiology, the process of building up, as by accretion, anabolism, etc. **3.** In mathematics, the process of ascertaining a function from its differential. **4.** In molecular biology, a recombination event in which a genetic element is inserted. [L. *integro,* pp. *-atus,* to make whole, fr. *integer,* whole]

personality i., the effective organization of old and new experience, data, and emotional capacities into the personality; the harmonious organization of the personality.

in·te·grins (in-te′grinz). A family of cell membrane glycoproteins that are heterodimers composed of α- and β-chain subunits. They serve as extracellular matrix glycoprotein receptors involved in cell adhesion, e.g., the mediation of adhesion of neutrophils to endothelial cells. [L. *integer,* whole, intact, fr. *in-* + *tango,* to touch + *-in*]

in·teg·ri·ty (in-teg′ri-tē). Soundness or completeness of structure; a sound or unimpaired condition.

marginal i. of amalgam, the ability of a dental amalgam restoration to maintain its original marginal form at the cavosurface margins.

in·teg·u·ment (in-teg′ū-ment) [TA]. **1.** The enveloping membrane of the body; includes, in addition to the epidermis and dermis, all of the derivatives of the epidermis, e.g., hairs, nails, sudoriferous and sebaceous glands, and mammary glands. **2.** The rind, capsule, or covering of any body or part. SYN tegument (2). SYN integumentum commune [TA], integumentary system, tegument (1). [L. *integumentum,* a covering, fr. *intego,* to cover]

in·teg·u·men·ta·ry (in-teg-ū-men′tă-rē). Relating to the integument. SEE ALSO cutaneous, dermal.

in·teg·u·men·tum com·mune (in-teg-ū-men′tŭm kō-moo′nē) [TA]. SYN integument.

in·tel·lec·tu·al·i·za·tion (in-te-lek′choo-ăl-i-zā′shŭn). An unconscious defense mechanism in which reasoning, logic, or focusing on and verbalizing intellectual minutiae is used in an attempt to avoid confrontation with an objectionable impulse, affect, or interpersonal situation. [L. *intellectus,* perception, discernment]

in·tel·li·gence (in-tel′i-jens). **1.** An person's aggregate capacity to act purposefully, think rationally, and deal effectively with the environment, especially in relation to the extent of one's perceived effectiveness in meeting challenges. **2.** In psychology, a person's relative standing on two quantitative indices, measured i. and effectiveness of adaptive behavior; a quantitative score or similar index on both indices constitutes the operational definition of i. [L. *intelligentia*]

abstract i., the capacity to understand and manage abstract ideas and symbols.

artificial i., (1) a branch of computer science in which attempts are made to replicate human intellectual functions. One application is the development of computer programs for diagnosis. Such programs are often based on epidemiologic analysis of data in large numbers of medical records; (2) a machine that replicates human intellectual functions, although no machine (i.e., computer) can do this yet.

measured i., that i. which can be ranked relative to an age or peer group quantitative index by use of scores on i. tests.

mechanical i., the capacity to understand and manage technical mechanisms.

social i., the capacity to understand and manage one's human relations and social affairs.

in·tem·per·ance (in-tem′per-ăns). Lack of proper self-control, usually in reference to the use of alcoholic beverages. Cf. incontinence (2). [L. *intemperantia,* fr. *in-,* neg. + *temperantia,* moderation]

in·ten·si·ty (in-ten′si-tē). **1.** Marked tension; great activity; often used simply to denote a measure of the degree or amount of some quality. **2.** The magnitude of energy flux, field strength, or force. [L. *in- tendo,* pp. *-tensus,* to stretch out]

luminous i. (I), the luminous flux per unit solid angle in a given direction. SYN candle-power, radiant i.

in

performance i., the improvement in recognition of spoken words that occurs with increasing intensity of sound.

radiant i. (I), SYN luminous i.

i. of sound, the objective measurement of the amplitude of vibration of a sound wave.

in·ten·sive (in-ten'siv). Relating to or marked by intensity; denoting a form of treatment by means of very large doses or of substances possessing great strength or activity.

in·ten·tion (in-ten'shŭn). **1.** An objective. **2.** In surgery, a process or operation. [L. *intentio,* a stretching out; intention]

⟳inter-. Among, between. [L. *inter,* between]

in·ter·ac·i·nar (in-ter-as'i-nar). SYN interacinous.

in·ter·ac·i·nous (in-ter-as'i-nŭs). Between the acini of a gland. SYN interacinar.

in·ter·ac·tion (int'er-ak'shŭn). **1.** The reciprocal action between two entities in a common environment as in chemical i., ecological i., social i., etc. **2.** The effects when two entities concur that would not be observed with either in isolation. **3.** In statistics, pharmacology, and quantitative genetics, the phenomenon that the combined effects of two causes differ from the sum of the effects separately (as in synergism and antagonism). **4.** Independent operation of two or more causes to produce or prevent an effect. **5.** In statistics, the necessity for a product term in a linear model. **6.** The transfer of energy between elementary particles or between fields of energy.

apolar i., SYN hydrophobic i.

hydrophobic i., i. between uncharged substituents on different molecules without a sharing of electrons or protons; entropy-driven i. SYN apolar i.

in·ter·al·ve·o·lar (in'ter-al-vē'ō-lăr). Between any alveoli, especially the alveoli of the lungs.

in·ter·an·nu·lar (in-ter-an'ū-lăr). Between any two ringlike structures or constrictions. [inter- + L. *anulus,* ring]

in·ter·arch (in'ter-arch). SEE interarch *distance.*

in·ter·ar·tic·u·lar (in-ter-ar-tik'ū-lăr). **1.** Between two joints. Cf. intra-articular. **2.** Between two joint surfaces. [inter- + L. *articulus,* joint]

in·ter·ar·y·te·noid (in'ter-ăr'i-tē'noyd). Between the arytenoid cartilages.

in·ter·as·ter·ic (in-ter-ă-stē'rik). Between the two asteria. SEE asterion.

in·ter·a·tri·al (in-ter-ā'trē-ăl). Between the atria of the heart. SYN interauricular (1).

in·ter·au·ral (in-ter-aw'ral). Referring to differences between ears, particularly temporal events occurring in or emanating from the ears.

in·ter·au·ric·u·lar (in'ter-aw-rik'ū-lăr). **1.** SYN interatrial. **2.** Between the auricles or pinnae.

in·ter·bod·y (in'ter-bod'ē). Between the bodies of two adjacent vertebrae.

in·ter·ca·dence (in-ter-kā'dens). The occurrence of an extra beat between the two regular pulse beats. [inter- + L. *cado,* pr. p. *cadens* (*-ent-*), to fall]

in·ter·ca·dent (in-ter-kā'dent). Irregular in rhythm; characterized by intercadence.

in·ter·ca·lary (in-ter'kă-ler-ē, in-ter-kal'er-ē). **1.** Occurring between two others; as in a pulse tracing, an upstroke interposed between two normal pulse beats. **2.** In fungi, located in a hypha or between hyphal segments, not at a hyphal terminus. [L. *intercalarius,* concerning an insertion]

in·ter·ca·lat·ed (in-ter'kă-lā-ted). Interposed; inserted between two others. [L. *intercalatus*]

in·ter·ca·la·tion (in'ter-kă-lā-shun). The process of insertion between two other entities; e.g., insertion of a dye or drug between stacked bases in DNA.

in·ter·can·a·lic·u·lar (in-ter-kan-ă-lik'ū-lăr). Between canaliculi.

in·ter·cap·il·lary (in-ter-kap'i-lā-rē). Between or among capillary vessels.

in·ter·ca·rot·ic, in·ter·ca·rot·id (in-ter-ka-rot'ik, -id). Between the internal and external carotid arteries.

in·ter·car·pal (in-ter-kar'păl). Between the carpal bones.

in·ter·car·ti·lag·i·nous (in'ter-kar-ti-laj'i-nŭs). Between or connecting cartilages. SYN interchondral.

in·ter·cav·ern·ous (in'ter-kav'er-nŭs). Between two cavities.

in·ter·cel·lu·lar (in-ter-sel'ū-lăr). Between or among cells.

in·ter·cen·tral (in-ter-sen'trăl). Connecting or lying between two or more centers.

in·ter·ce·re·bral (in'ter-ser'ē-brăl). Between the cerebral hemispheres.

in·ter·chon·dral (in-ter-kon'drăl). SYN intercartilaginous. [inter- + L. *chondros,* cartilage]

in·ter·cil·i·um (in-ter-sil'ē-ŭm). SYN glabella. [inter- + L. *cilium,* eyelid]

in·ter·cla·vic·u·lar (in-ter-kla-vik'ū-lăr). Between or connecting the clavicles.

in·ter·coc·cyg·e·al (in'ter-kok-sij'ē-ăl). Situated between unfused segments of the coccyx.

in·ter·co·lum·nar (in-ter-kŏ-lŭm'nar). Between any two columns, as the columns or crura of the superficial inguinal ring.

in·ter·con·dy·lar, in·ter·con·dyl·ic, in·ter·con·dy·loid (in-ter-kon'di-lăr, -kon-dil'ik, -kon'di-loyd). Between two condyles.

in·ter·con·ver·sion (in-ter-kon-ver'shun). A mutual alteration of the physical or chemical nature of a substance or entity; e.g., i. of chemical compounds or of foodstuffs.

enzyme i., the reversible transformation of one enzyme form into another, typically with an alteration in the enzyme activity or regulation, e.g., phosphorylation of a glycogen phosphorylase.

in·ter·cos·tal (in-ter-kos'tăl). Between the ribs. [inter- + L. *costa,* rib]

in·ter·cos·to·hu·mer·al (in'ter-kos'tō-hū'mer-ăl). Relating to an intercostal space and the arm. SEE intercostobrachial *nerves,* under *nerve.*

in·ter·cos·to·hu·me·ra·lis (in-ter-kos'tō-hū-mer-ā'lis). SEE intercostobrachial *nerves,* under *nerve.*

in·ter·course (in'ter-kōrs). Communication or dealings between or among people. [L. *intercursus,* a running between]

sexual i., SYN coitus.

in·ter·cri·co·thy·rot·o·my (in-ter-krī'kō-thī-rot'ō-mē). SYN cricothyrotomy.

in·ter·crines (in'ter-krīnz). SYN chemokines. [inter- + G. *krinō,* to separate, secrete]

in·ter·cris·tal (in-ter-kris'tăl). Between two crests, as between the crests of the ilia, applied to one of the pelvic measurements.

in·ter·cross (in'ter-kros). A mating between two individuals both heterozygous at a specified locus or loci.

in·ter·cru·ral (in-ter-kroo'răl). Between two crura; e.g., the cerebral peduncles of the brain, etc .

in·ter·cur·rent (in-ter-ker'ent). Intervening; said of a disease attacking a person already ill of another malady. [inter- + L. *curro,* pr. p. *currens* (*-ent-*), to run]

in·ter·cus·pa·tion (in'ter-kŭs-pā'shun). **1.** The cusp-to-fossa relation of the maxillary and mandibular posterior teeth to each other. **2.** The interlocking or fitting together of the cusps of opposing teeth. SYN interdigitation (4). SYN intercusping.

in·ter·cusp·ing (in-ter-kŭs'ping). SYN intercuspation. [L. *inter,* among, mutually, + cusp]

in·ter·cu·ta·ne·o·mu·cous (in'ter-kū-tā'nē-ō-mŭ'kŭs). Between skin and mucous membrane, as in the cheek or lip or at the mucocutaneous border of the lips or anus.

in·ter·de·fer·en·tial (in-ter-def-er-en'shăl). Between the deferent ducts.

in·ter·den·tal (in-ter-den'tăl). **1.** Between the teeth. **2.** Denoting the relationship between the proximal surfaces of the teeth of the same arch. [inter- + L. *dens,* tooth]

in·ter·den·ti·um (in-ter-den'shē-ŭm). The interval between any two contiguous teeth.

in·ter·dig·it (in-ter-dij'it). That part of the hand or foot lying between any two adjacent fingers or toes.

in·ter·dig·i·tal (in-ter-dij'i-tăl). Between the fingers or toes.

in·ter·dig·i·ta·tion (in′ter-dij-i-tā′shŭn). **1.** The mutual interlocking of toothed or tonguelike processes. **2.** The processes thus interlocked. **3.** Infoldings or plicae of adjacent cell or plasma membranes. **4.** SYN intercuspation (2). [inter- + L. *digitus,* finger]

in·ter·dis·ci·pli·nary (in-ter-dis′i-pli-nār-ē). Denoting the overlapping interests of different fields of medicine and science. [inter- + L. *disciplina,* instruction, teaching]

in·ter·face (in′ter-fās). **1.** A surface that forms a common boundary of two bodies. **2.** The boundary between regions of different radiopacity, acoustic, or magnetic resonance properties; the projection of the i. between tissues of different such properties on an image.

crystalline i., in dentistry, a boundary between adjacent crystals.

dermoepidermal i., the line of meeting of the dermis and epidermis.

metal i., in dentistry, a boundary between metal and nonsolvent solder, or between metal and surface oxide.

structural i., in dentistry, a boundary between tooth and restorative material.

in·ter·fa·cial (in-ter-fā′shăl). Relating to an interface.

in·ter·fas·cic·u·lar (in′ter-fă-sik′ū-lăr). Between fasciculi.

in·ter·fem·o·ral (in-ter-fem′ŏ-răl). Between the thighs.

in·ter·fer·ence (in-ter-fēr′ens). **1.** The coming together of waves in various media in such a way that the crests of one series correspond to the hollows of the other, the two thus neutralizing each other; or so that the crests of the two series correspond, thus increasing the excursions of the waves. **2.** Collision within the myocardium of two waves of excitation at the junction of territories controlled by each, as is seen in AV dissociation. **3.** Also, in AV dissociation, the disturbance of the regular rhythm of the ventricles by a conducted impulse from the atria, e.g., by a ventricular capture (interference beat). **4.** The condition in which infection of a cell by one virus prevents superinfection by another virus, or in which superinfection prevents effects which would result from infection by either virus alone, even though both viruses persist. [inter- + L. *ferio,* to strike]

bacterial i., the condition in which colonization by one bacterial strain prevents colonization by another strain.

cuspal i., SYN deflective occlusal *contact.*

in·ter·fer·om·e·ter (in′ter-fe-rom′ĕ-ter). An instrument for measuring minute distances or movements through the interference of light waves thereby produced. [interfere + G. *metron,* measure]

electron i., an i. that employs an electron beam in place of a light beam.

in·ter·fer·o·me·try (in′ter-fe-rom′ĕ-trē). Measurement of minute distances or movements by interaction of waves of electromagnetic energy.

electron i., i. in which a beam of electrons is used instead of a beam of light.

■ **in·ter·fer·on (IFN)** (in-ter-fēr′on). A class of small protein and glycoprotein cytokines (15–28 kD) produced by T cells, fibroblasts, and other cells in response to viral infection and other biological and synthetic stimuli. I.'s bind to specific receptors on cell membranes; their effects include inducing enzymes, suppressing cell proliferation, inhibiting viral proliferation, enhancing the phagocytic activity of macrophages, and augmenting the cytotoxic activity of T lymphocytes. I.'s are divided into five major classes (alpha, beta, gamma, tau, and omega) and several subclasses (indicated by Arabic numerals and letters) on the basis of physicochemical properties, cells of origin, mode of induction, and antibody reactions. [interfere + -on]

> The discovery in 1957 that viral infection of human cells induces the formation of natural antiviral agents raised the hope that these substances might have therapeutic potential. Early studies showed that, unlike antibodies, interferons are active against a broad range of viruses, but progress in applying this knowledge to human medicine was retarded by the difficulty of producing interferons in sufficient quantity. In the 1980s the development of recombinant DNA technology overcame this obstacle, and interferons now play an important role in the treatment not

only of viral infections but also of certain malignancies. Commercially available interferons are produced by genetically altered colonies of *Escherichia coli* or Chinese hamster ovary cells, or are induced by controlled viral infection in pooled human leukocytes. Alpha interferons have found the widest application in medicine. (The spelling alpha is used with respect to naturally occurring interferons; in compliance with international conventions for generic drug names, the spelling alfa appears in names of pharmaceutical formulations.) Alpha interferons are used in the treatment of chronic hepatitis B and hepatitis C, hairy cell leukemia, chronic myelogenous leukemia, AIDS-related Kaposi sarcoma, malignant melanoma, condylomata acuminata and recurrent respiratory papillomatosis due to human papillomavirus, and infantile hemangiomatosis. About 50% of patients treated for chronic hepatitis B with interferon-alfa show disappearance of hepatitis B$_e$ antigen (HB$_e$Ag) and reversion of alanine aminotransferase to normal. The response rate in chronic hepatitis C is lower (15–25%), but better results are achieved by using more aggressive therapy (daily rather than thrice weekly administration) and continuing it longer (a minimum of 12 months). Modified formulations of interferon-alfa conjugated with polyethylene glycol (PEG), which have yielded promising results in hepatitis C with once-a-week dosing, are in phase III trials. Beta interferons reduce clinical recurrences and progression of myelin damage in multiple sclerosis. Gamma interferon is effective in retarding tissue changes in osteopetrosis and systemic scleroderma and in reducing the frequency and severity of infections in chronic granulomatous disease. Administration of interferons is parenteral (intravenous, intramuscular, subcutaneous, intranasal, intrathecal, or intralesional) and several weeks of treatment may be required before clinical response is noted. More than 50% of patients experience a flulike syndrome of fatigue, myalgia, and arthralgia. Gastrointestinal and CNS side effects are also common, and marrow suppression may occur with prolonged treatment.

FDA approved clinical uses of interferons	
alpha	
hairy cell leukemia	hepatitis B
condyloma acuminatum	hepatitis C
Kaposi sarcoma	malignant melanoma (postsurgical)
beta	**gamma**
multiple sclerosis	chronic granulomatous disease

i. alfa 2b, a water-soluble protein (MW 19,271) secreted by cells infected by virus; used to treat hairy cell leukemia, malignant melanoma, condylomata acuminata, AIDS-related Kaposi sarcoma, and chronic hepatitis C.

i. alpha (IFN-α), the major i. made by virus-induced leukocytes; a number of different subtypes exist that are elaborated by leukocytes in response to viral infection or to stimulation with double-stranded RNA. There are 14 genes on the short arm of chromosome 9 that code for these substances in humans. IFN-α-2A and -2B are protein products made by recombinant DNA techniques and are used as antineoplastic agents. SYN leukocyte i.

antigen i., SYN i. gamma.

i. beta (IFN-β), i. elaborated by fibroblasts and microphages in response to the same stimuli as i. alpha; only one gene codes for this i. SYN fibroblast i.

i. beta 1b, a purified protein containing 165 amino acids (MW approximately 18,500) with antiviral and immunomodulatory effects, used in the treatment of relapsing-remitting multiple sclerosis to reduce the frequency of clinical exacerbations.

fibroblast i., SYN i. beta.

i. gamma (IFN-γ), i. elaborated by T lymphocytes in response to

in

either specific antigen or mitogenic stimulation; only one gene codes for γ i. I. gamma behaves like a biological response modifies and is highly immunoregulatory. SYN antigen i., immune i.

immune i., SYN i. gamma.

leukocyte i., SYN i. alpha.

i.-omega, a form of i. known as interferon-alpha-2.

i.-tau, an i. secreted by bovine concepti, with potent antiretroviral activity; in experimental use. SYN trophoblast i., trophoblastin.

trophoblast i., SYN i.-tau.

type I i., antiviral interferons, including interferon-alpha; and interferon-beta;.

type II i., immune interferon, interferon-gamma;

in·ter·fer·on-β2. SYN interleukin-6.

in·ter·fi·bril·lar, in·ter·fi·bril·lary (in′ter-fī′bri-lăr, -fī′bri-lār-ē; -fī-bril′ăr). Between fibrils.

in·ter·fi·brous (in-ter-fī′brŭs). Between fibers.

in·ter·fil·a·men·tous (in′ter-fil-ă-men′tŭs). Between filaments.

in·ter·fron·tal (in-ter-fron′tăl). Between the unfused halves of the frontal bone; denoting a persistent suture there present. (anomalous)

in·ter·gan·gli·on·ic (in′ter-gang′lē-on′ik). Between or among or connecting ganglia.

in·ter·gem·mal (in′ter-jem′ăl). Between any two or more budlike or bulblike bodies such as the taste buds; denoting especially a nerve termination between two end bulbs. [inter- + L. *gemma,* bud]

in·ter·ge·nal (in-ter-jēn′al). Between different genes.

in·ter·glob·u·lar (in-ter-glob′ū-lăr). Between globules.

in·ter·glu·te·al (in-ter-gloo′tē-ăl). Between the buttocks. [inter- + G. *gloutos,* buttock]

in·ter·go·ni·al (in-ter-gō′nē-ăl). Between the two gonia. SEE gonion. [inter- + G. *gōnia,* angle]

in·ter·gy·ral (in-ter-jī′răl). Between the gyri or convolutions of the brain.

in·ter·hem·i·ce·re·bral (in′ter-hem′ē-ser′ē-brăl). Between the cerebral hemispheres.

in·ter·ic·tal (in-ter-ik′tăl). The period between convulsions. [inter- + L. *ictus,* stroke]

in·te·ri·or (in-tēr′ē-ōr). Relating to the inside; situated within.

in·ter·is·chi·ad·ic (in-ter-is-kē-ad′ik). Between the two ischia; especially, between the two tuberosities of the ischia. SYN inter8ciatic.

in·ter·ki·ne·sis (in′ter-ki-nē′sis). Period between the first and second divisions of meiosis; comparable to interphase of mitosis. [inter- + G. *kinēsis,* movement]

in·ter·la·mel·lar (in′ter-hem′ē-mel′ăr, -lam′ĕ-lăr). Between lamellae.

in·ter·leukin. The name given to a group of multifunctional cytokines once their amino acid structure is known. They are synthesized by lymphocytes, monocytes, macrophages, and certain other cells. SEE lymphokine, cytokine. [inter- + *leuk*ocyte + -in]

recombinant human i. 11, a drug that increases the number of blood platelets; useful in ameliorating severe thrombocytopenia resulting from cancer chemotherapy. SYN rhIL-11.

in·ter·leu·kin-1 (IL-1) (in-ter-loo′kin). A cytokine, derived primarily from mononuclear phagocytes, which enhances the proliferation of T helper cells and growth and differentiation of B cells. When secreted in larger quantities it is a mediator of inflammation, entering the bloodstream and causing fever, inducing synthesis of acute phase proteins, and initiating metabolic wasting. There are two distinct forms of IL-1: α and β, both of which perform the same functions, but represent different proteins.

in·ter·leu·kin-2 (IL-2). A cytokine derived from T helper lymphocytes that causes proliferation of T lymphocytes and activated B lymphocytes.

in·ter·leu·kin-3 (IL-3). A cytokine derived from activated CD4+ lymphocytes, fibroblasts, and endothelial cells that increases production of monocytes. It acts in hematopoiesis by controlling production and differentiation of granulocytes. SYN multicolony-stimulating factor.

in·ter·leu·kin-4 (IL-4). A cytokine derived from T4 lymphocytes that causes differentiation of B lymphocytes. Promotes Ig class switch. It stimulates DNA biosynthesis. SYN B cell differentiating factor.

in·ter·leu·kin-5 (IL-5). A cytokine derived from T lymphocytes that causes activation of B lymphocytes and differentiation of eosinophils.

in·ter·leu·kin-6 (IL-6). A cytokine derived from macrophages and endothelial cells that increases synthesis and secretion of immunoglobulins by B lymphocytes; also induces acute phase proteins. In hepatocytes, it induces acute-phase reactants. SYN B cell stimulatory factor 2, interferon-β2.

in·ter·leu·kin-7 (IL-7). A cytokine derived from bone marrow cells that causes proliferation of B and T lymphocytes.

in·ter·leu·kin-8 (IL-8). A cytokine (chemokine) derived from endothelial cells, fibroblasts, keratinocytes, macrophages, and monocytes which causes chemotaxis of neutrophils and T-cell lymphocytes. SYN anionic neutrophil-activating peptide, monocyte-derived neutrophil chemotactic factor, neutrophil chemotactant factor, neutrophil-activating factor.

in·ter·leu·kin-9 (IL-9). A cytokine derived from T cells that causes IL-2/Il-4-independent growth and proliferation of T cells.

in·ter·leu·kin-10 (IL-10). A cytokine derived from helper T-cell lymphocytes (TH₂) that inhibits γ-interferon (IFNγ) and IL-2 secretion by T cell lymphocytes (TH₁) and inhibits mononuclear cell inflammation.

in·ter·leu·kin-11 (IL-11). A cytokine and growth factor derived from bone marrow stromal cells (endothelial cells, macrophages, and preadipocytes) that stimulates increased plasma concentrations of acute phase proteins and is a growth factor with multiple hematopoietic effects.

in·ter·leu·kin-12 (IL-12). A cytokine derived from B lymphocytes and macrophages that induces γ-interferon (IFNγ) gene expression and IL-2 in T lymphocytes and NK cells and down regulates TH₂ cytokines.

in·ter·leu·kin-13 (IL-13). A cytokine derived from helper T cell lymphocytes that inhibits mononuclear cell inflammation and is considered a modulator or B cell responses.

in·ter·leu·kin-14 (IL-14). A cytokine derived from T cells that stimulates B cell proliferation and inhibits Ig secretion.

in·ter·leu·kin-15 (IL-15). A cytokine derived from T cells which stimulates T cell proliferation and NK cell activation.

in·ter·leu·kin-16 (IL-16). A cytokine made by T cells that is a potent chemotactant for CD4⁺ T cells.

in·ter·leu·kin-17 (IL-17). A proinflammatory cytokine made by T cells.

in·ter·leu·kin-18 (IL-18). A cytokine made by macrophages; a potent inducer of interferon-γ by T cells and NK cells.

in·ter·lo·bar (in-ter-lō′bar). Between the lobes of an organ or other structure.

in·ter·lo·bi·tis (in′ter-lō-bī′tis). Inflammation of the pleura separating two pulmonary lobes.

in·ter·lob·u·lar (in-ter-lob′ū-lăr). Between the lobules of an organ.

in·ter·mal·le·o·lar (in-ter-mal-ē′ō-lăr). Between the malleoli.

in·ter·mam·ma·ry (in-ter-mam′ă-rē). Between the breasts. [inter- + L. *mamma,* breast]

in·ter·mam·mil·lary (in-ter-mam′i-lā-rē). Between the breasts; between the nipples; denoting a line drawn between the two nipples. [inter- + L. *mammilla,* breast, nipple]

in·ter·mar·riage (in-ter-mar′ij). 1. Marriage of relatives. 2. Marriage of persons of different races or cultures.

in·ter·max·il·la (in-ter-maks-il′ă). SYN incisive *bone.*

in·ter·max·il·lary (in-ter-mak′si-lā-rē). Between the maxillae, or upper jaw bones.

in·ter·me·di·ary (in′ter-mē′dē-ār-ē). Occurring between. [L. *intermedius,* lying between, fr. *medius,* middle]

in·ter·me·di·ate (in′ter-mē′dē-it) [TA]. 1. Between two extremes; interposed; intervening. 2. A substance formed in the course of chemical reactions that then proceeds to participate in further reactions; such substances, when appearing in the course of the reactions involved in metabolism, are metabolic i.'s. **3.** In dentistry, a cement base. **4.** An element or organ between right and left (or lateral and medial) structures. SYN intermedius [TA].

replicative i., during the copying of the viral RNA of an RNA virus, the opposite sense strand that serves as a template for positive strand production.

in·ter·me·din (in-ter-mē′din). SYN melanotropin.

in·ter·me·di·o·lat·er·al (in-ter-mē′dē-ō-lat′er-ăl). Intermediate, and to one side, not central. Used especially to denote the intermediolateral cell column of spinal cord gray mattter, abbreviated IML, the location of all presynaptic sympathetic nerve cell bodies. SEE intermediolateral *nucleus.*

in·ter·me·di·us (in-ter-mē′dē-ŭs) [TA]. SYN intermediate (4). [L.]

in·ter·mem·bra·nous (in-ter-mem′bră-nŭs). Between membranes.

in·ter·me·nin·ge·al (in′ter-me-nin′jē-ăl). Between the meninges.

in·ter·men·stru·al (in-ter-men′stroo-ăl). Between two consecutive menstrual periods.

in·ter·met·a·car·pal (in-ter-met′ă-kar′păl). Between the metacarpal bones.

in·ter·met·a·mer·ic (in′ter-met′ă-mer′ik). Between two metameres; denoting especially the intervertebral disks.

in·ter·met·a·tar·sal (in-ter-met′ă-tar′săl). Between the metatarsal bones.

in·ter·met·a·tar·se·um (in-ter-met′ă-tar′sē-ŭm). SYN *os* intermetatarseum.

in·ter·mis·sion (in-ter-mish′ŭn). **1.** A temporary cessation of symptoms or of any action. **2.** An interval between two paroxysms of a disease, such as malaria. [L. *intermissio,* fr. *intermitto,* to leave off, intermit, fr. *mitto,* to send]

in·ter·mit. To cease for a time.

in·ter·mit·tence, in·ter·mit·ten·cy (in-ter-mit′ens, -en-sē). **1.** A condition marked by intermissions or interruptions in the course of a disease or other process or state or in any continued action; denoting especially a loss of one or more pulse beats. **2.** Complete cessation of symptoms between two periods of activity of a disease.

in·ter·mit·tent (in-ter-mit′ent). Marked by intervals of complete quietude between two periods of activity.

in·ter·mus·cu·lar (in-ter-mŭs′kū-lăr). Between the muscles.

in·tern (in′tern). An advanced student or recent graduate undertaking further education (usually the first postgraduate year) by assisting in the medical or surgical care of hospital patients, with supervision and instruction; formerly, one who resided within the institution. [F. *interne,* inside]

in·ter·nal (in-ter′năl) [TA]. Away from the surface; often incorrectly used to mean medial. SYN internus [TA]. [L. *internus*]

in·ter·nal·i·za·tion (in-ter′năl-i-zā′shŭn). Adopting as one's own the standards and values of another person or society.

in·ter·na·ri·al (in-ter-nā′rē-ăl). Between the nares or nostrils. SYN internasal.

in·ter·na·sal (in-ter-nā′săl). SYN internarial.

In·ter·na·tion·al Clas·si·fi·ca·tion of Dis·eases (ICD, ICDA). The classification of specific conditions and groups of conditions determined by an internationally representative expert committee that advises the World Health Organization, which publishes the complete list in a periodically revised book, the *Manual of the International Statistical Classification of Diseases, Injuries and Causes of Death.* The Tenth Revision (ICD-10) came into use in 1992; it has 20 chapters, each with a hierarchical arrangement of subdivisions (rubrics); some chapters are etiological, some relate to body systems, some to classes of conditions, some to procedures.

In·ter·na·tion·al Clas·si·fi·ca·tion of Health Prob·lems in Pri·ma·ry Care (ICHPPC). A classification of diseases, conditions and problems arranged for use in primary care where diagnostic precision is seldom possible.

In·ter·na·tion·al Clas·si·fi·ca·tion of Im·pair·ments, Dis·a·

bil·i·ties and Hand·i·caps (ICIDH). A WHO-sponsored numerical taxonomy of the impairments, disabilities and handicaps consequent upon injury and disease.

In·ter·na·tion·al Com·mit·tee of the Red Cross. A politically neutral Swiss organization serving as an intermediary between contending forces in armed conflict, in civil war, or internal strife, to help victims receive protection and other humanitarian assistance under the Geneva Conventions in accordance with the fundamental principles of the Red Cross.

In·ter·na·tion·al Sys·tem of Units (SI). A system of measurements, based on the metric system, adopted at the 11th General Conference on Weights and Measures of the International Organization for Standardization (1960) to cover both the coherent units (basic, supplementary, and derived units) and the decimal multiples and submultiples of these units formed by use of prefixes proposed for general international scientific and technological use. SI proposes seven basic units: meter (m), kilogram (kg), second (s), ampere (A), Kelvin (K), candela (cd), and mole (mol) for the basic quantities of length, mass, time, electric current, temperature, luminous intensity, and amount of substance, respectively; supplementary units proposed include the radian (rad) for plane angle and steradian (sr) for solid angle; derived units (e.g., force, power, frequency) are stated in terms of the basic units (e.g., velocity is in meters per second, $m\ s^{-1}$). Multiples (prefixes) in descending order are: exa- (E, 10^{18}), peta- (P, 10^{15}), tera- (T, 10^{12}), giga- (G, 10^{9}), mega- (M, 10^{6}), kilo- (k, 10^{3}), hecto- (h, 10^{2}), deca- (da, 10^{1}), deci- (d, 10^{-1}), centi- (c, 10^{-2}), milli- (m, 10^{-3}), micro- (μ, 10^{-6}), nano- (n, 10^{-9}), pico- (p, 10^{-12}), femto- (f, 10^{-15}), atto- (a, 10^{-18}). Proposed prefixes are zetta- (z, 10^{21}), yotta- (y, 10^{24}), zepto- (z, 10^{-21}), and yocto- (y, 10^{-24}). Those involving a multiple of 10^{3} are recommended; compounds of these are not recommended (e.g., mμ for n). [Fr. *Système International d'Unités*]

in·terne. Intern.

in·ter·neu·ro·mer·ic (in′ter-noor-ō-mer′ik). Between the neuromeres.

in·ter·neu·rons (in′ter-noo′ronz). Combinations or groups of neurons between sensory and motor neurons that govern coordinated activity.

in·tern·ist (in-ter′nist, in′ter-nist). A physician trained in internal medicine.

in·ter·nod·al (in-ter-nō′dăl). Between two nodes; relating to an internode.

in·ter·node (in′ter-nōd). SYN internodal *segment.*

in·ter·nu·cle·ar (in-ter-noo′klē-ăr). Between nerve cell groups in the brain or retina.

in·ter·nun·ci·al (in-ter-nun′sē-ăl). **1.** Indicating a neuron functionally interposed between two or more other neurons. **2.** Acting as a medium of communication between two organs. [L. *internuntius* (or *-nuncius*), a messenger between two parties, fr. *inter,* between, + *nuncius,* a messenger]

in·ter·nus (in-ter′nŭs) [TA]. SYN internal. [L.]

in·ter·oc·clu·sal (in′ter-ŏ-kloo′săl). Between the occlusal surfaces of opposing teeth.

in·ter·o·cep·tive (in′ter-ō-sep′tiv). Relating to the sensory nerve cells innervating the viscera (thoracic, abdominal and pelvic organs, and the cardiovascular system), their sensory end organs, or the information they convey to the spinal cord and the brain. [inter- + L. *capio,* to take]

in·ter·o·cep·tor (in′ter-ō-sep′ter). One of the various forms of small sensory end organs (receptors) situated within the walls of the respiratory and gastrointestinal tracts or in other viscera. [inter- + L. *capio,* to take]

in·ter·ol·i·vary (in-ter-ol′i-vār-ē). Between the left and right inferior olive of the medulla oblongata.

in·ter·or·bit·al (in-ter-ōr′bi-tăl). Between the orbits.

in·ter·os·se·al (in-ter-os′ē-ăl). SYN interosseous.

in·ter·os·sei (in-ter-os′ē-ī). Plural of interosseus.

in·ter·os·se·ous (in′ter-os′ē-ŭs). Lying between or connecting bones; denoting certain muscles and ligaments. SYN interosseal. [inter- + L. *os,* bone]

in

in·ter·os·se·us, pl. **in·ter·os·sei** (in′ter-os′ē-ŭs, -os′e-ī). SEE muscle.

in·ter·pal·pe·bral (in-ter-pal′pe-brăl). Between the eyelids.

in·ter·pa·ri·e·tal (in′ter-pă-rī′ĕ-tăl). Between the walls of a part, or between the parietal bones. [inter- + L. *paries,* wall]

in·ter·par·ox·ys·mal (in′ter-par-ok-siz′măl). Occurring between successive paroxysms of a disease.

in·ter·pe·dic·u·late (in-ter-pe-dik′ū-lāt). Between vertebral pedicles.

in·ter·pe·dun·cu·lar (in-ter-pe-dŭnk′ū-lăr). Between any two peduncles.

in·ter·per·son·al (in-ter-per′sŏn-ăl). Pertaining to relations and social exchanges between persons.

in·ter·pha·lan·ge·al (in′ter-fă-lan′jē-ăl). Between two phalanges; denoting the finger or toe joints.

in·ter·phase (in′ter-fāz). The stage between two successive divisions of a cell nucleus in which the biochemical and physiologic functions of the cell are performed and replication of chromatin occurs. SYN karyostasis.

in·ter·phy·let·ic (in′ter-fī-let′ik). Denoting the transitional forms between two kinds of cells during the course of metaplasia. [inter- + G. *phylē,* tribe]

in·ter·plant. The material transferred from donor to host in interplanting.

in·ter·plant·ing. In experimental embryology, the transferring of a primordial cell mass from an embryo to an indifferent environment in another embryo, as in chorioallantoic grafts or intraocular transplants.

in·ter·pre·ta·tion (in-ter-pre-tā′shŭn). **1.** In psychoanalysis, the characteristic therapeutic intervention of the analyst. **2.** In clinical psychology, drawing inferences and formulating the meaning in terms of the psychological dynamics inherent in an individual's responses to psychological tests or during psychotherapy.

in·ter·prox·i·mal (in-ter-prok′si-măl). Between adjoining surfaces.

in·ter·pu·bic (in-ter-pū′bik). Between the two pubic bones.

in·ter·pu·pil·lary (in-ter-pū′pi-lār-ē). Between the pupils.

in·ter·ra·di·al (in-ter-rā′dē-ăl). Situated between radii or rays.

in·ter·re·nal (in-ter-rē′năl). Between the two kidneys.

in·ter·scap·u·lar (in-ter-skap′ū-lăr). Between the scapulae.

in·ter·scap·u·lum (in-ter-skap′ū-lŭm). The part of the back between the shoulders, or that between the scapulae.

in·ter·sci·at·ic (in-ter-sī-at′ik). SYN interischiadic.

in·ter·sec·tio, pl. **in·ter·sec·ti·o·nes** (in′ter-sek′shē-ō, -sek-shē-ō′nēz) [TA]. SYN intersection. [L.]

intersectiones tendineae musculi recti abdominis [TA], SYN tendinous *intersections* of rectus abdominis, under *intersection.*

i. tendin′ea [TA], SYN tendinous *intersection.*

in·ter·sec·tion (in′ter-sek-shŭn) [TA]. The site of crossing of two structures. SYN intersectio [TA].

tendinous i. [TA], a tendinous band or partition running across a muscle. SYN intersectio tendinea [TA], inscriptio tendinea, tendinous inscription.

tendinous i.'s of rectus abdominis [TA], usually three but occasionally four transverse fibrous bands or partial bands occurring at intervals as interruptions of the fleshy, contractile portions of the rectus abdominis muscle; they usually occur at and superior to the umbilicus. SYN intersectiones tendineae musculi recti abdominis [TA].

in·ter·sec·ti·o·nes (in-ter-sek-shē-ō′nēz). Plural of intersectio.

in·ter·seg·men·tal (in-ter-seg-men′tăl). Between two segments, such as metameres or myotomes.

in·ter·sep·tal (in-ter-sep′tăl). Lying between two septa.

in·ter·sep·to·val·vu·lar (in′ter-sep-tō-val′vū-lăr). Between the embryonic septum primum and septum spurium.

in·ter·sep·tum (in-ter-sep′tŭm). SYN diaphragm (1). [L]

in·ter·sex·u·al (in-ter-seks′ū-ăl). Relating to or characterized by intersexuality.

in·ter·sex·u·al·i·ty (in′ter-seks-ū-al′i-tē). The condition of having both male and female characteristics; being intermediate between the sexes.

in·ter·space (in′ter-spās). Any space between two similar objects, such as a costal i. or interval between two ribs.

in·ter·spi·nal (in-ter-spī′năl). Between two spines, such as the spinous processes of the vertebrae. SYN interspinous.

in·ter·spi·na·lis (in-ter-spī-nā′lis). SEE interspinales (*muscles*), under *muscle.*

in·ter·spi·nous (in-ter-spī′nŭs). SYN interspinal.

in·ter·stice, pl. **in·ter·stic·es** (in-ter′stis, -sti-siz). SYN interstitium. [L. *interstitium,* fr. *sisto,* to stand]

in·ter·sti·tial (in-ter-stish′ăl). **1.** Relating to spaces or interstices in any structure. **2.** Relating to spaces within a tissue or organ, but excluding such spaces as body cavities or potential space. Cf. intracavitary.

in·ter·stit·i·um (in-ter-stish′ē-ŭm). A small area, space, or gap in the substance of an organ or tissue. SEE ALSO connective *tissue.* SYN interstice. [L.]

in·ter·tar·sal (in-ter-tar′săl). Denoting the articulations of the tarsal bones with each other. SYN tarsotarsal.

in·ter·tha·lam·ic (in-ter-thal′ă-mik). Between the thalami.

in·ter·trans·ver·sa·lis (in-ter-trans-ver-sā′lis). Intertransversarius. SEE muscle.

in·ter·trans·verse (in′ter-trans′vers). Between the transverse processes of the vertebrae.

in·ter·trig·i·nous (in-ter-trij′i-nŭs). Characterized by or related to intertrigo.

in·ter·tri·go (in-ter-trī′gō). Irritant dermatitis occurring between folds or juxtaposed surfaces of the skin, as between the buttocks, between the scrotum and the thigh, beneath pendulous breasts, etc.; caused by friction, sweat retention, moisture, warmth, and concomitant overgrowth of resident microorganisms; occurring in young children (see diaper *dermatitis*) and obese adults. [L. a galling of the skin, fr. *inter,* between, + *tero,* to rub]

in·ter·tro·chan·ter·ic (in′ter-trō-kan-tār′ik). Between the two trochanters of the femur.

in·ter·tu·bu·lar (in-ter-too′bū-lăr). Between or among tubules.

in·ter·u·re·ter·al (in′ter-ū-rē′ter-ăl). Between the two ureters. SYN interureteric.

in·ter·u·re·ter·ic (in-ter-ū-rē-tār′ik). SYN interureteral.

in·ter·val (in′ter-văl). A time or space between two periods or objects; a break in continuity. [L. *inter-vallum,* space between breastworks in a camp, an interval, fr. *vallum,* a rampart, wall]

a-c i., the interval between the onset of the a wave and that of the c wave of the jugular pulse.

AH i., the time from the initial rapid deflection of the atrial wave to the initial rapid deflection of the His bundle (H) potential; it approximates the conduction time through the AV node (normally 50–120 msec).

AN i., the time between onset of the atrial deflection and the nodal potential (normally 40–100 msec).

atrioventricular i., SYN auriculoventricular i.

auriculoventricular i., the time between depolarization of the atria and of the ventricle. SYN atrioventricular i.

AV i., the time from the beginning of atrial systole to the beginning of ventricular systole as measured from pressure pulses or cardiac volume curves in animals, or from the electrocardiogram in humans.

BH i., the duration of the His bundle deflections (normally 15–20 msec).

calibration i., the period of time or series of measurements during which calibration can be expected to remain stable within specified and documented limits.

cardioarterial i., c-a i., the time between the apex beat of the heart and the radial pulse beat.

confidence i., a range of values for a variable of interest, constructed so that this range has a specified probability of including the true value of the variable.

coupling i., the i., expressed in milliseconds, between a normal sinus beat and the ensuing premature beat.

escape i., the time between the last beat of the patient's basic rhythm (ectopic or sinus beat) and a beat from a spontaneous escape focus or the initial electronic pacemaker impulse (a preset i. in the circuitry); it may be either a shorter or a longer time period than the pulse i.

focal i., the distance between the anterior and posterior focal points of the eye.

HV i., the time from the initial deflection of the His bundle (H) potential and the onset of ventricular activity (normally 35–45 msec).

interectopic i., the distance between consecutive ectopic complexes in the electrocardiogram.

isovolumic i., time during which both an AV and a semilunar valve are closed.

lucid i., in psychoses or delirium, a rational period appearing in the course of the mental disorder.

PA i., the time from onset of the P wave to the initial rapid deflection of the A wave in the His bundle electrogram (normally 25–45 msec); it represents the intraatrial conduction time.

PJ i., the time elapsing from the beginning of the P wave to the end of the QRS complex (J for junction between QRS and T wave) in the electrocardiogram.

P-P i., the distance between consecutive P waves in the electrocardiogram.

PQ i., SYN PR i.

PR i., in the electrocardiogram, the time elapsing between the beginning of the P wave and the beginning of the next QRS complex; it corresponds to the a-c i. of the venous pulse and is normally 0.12–0.20 sec. SYN PQ i.

QR i., the time elapsing from the onset of the QRS complex to the peak of the R or the final R wave; measures the time of onset of the intrinsicoid deflection if determined in an appropriate unipolar lead tracing.

QRB i., the time between the onset of the Q wave of the QRS complex and the right bundle-branch potential (normally 15–20 msec).

QRS i., the duration of the QRS complex in the electrocardiogram.

QS₂ i., SYN electromechanical *systole*.

QT i., time from electrocardiogram Q wave to the end of the T wave corresponding to electrical systole.

R-R i., the time elapsing between two consecutive R waves in the electrocardiogram.

serial i., the period of time between analogous phases of an infectious illness in successive cases of a chain of infection that is spread from person to person. SEE ALSO mass action *principle*, infection transmission *parameter*.

sphygmic i., the period in the cardiac cycle when the semilunar valves are open and blood is being ejected from the ventricles into the arterial system. SYN ejection period.

Sturm i., the distance between the anterior and posterior focal lines in a spherocylindrical lens combination.

systolic time i.'s, SEE electromechanical *systole*, left ventricular ejection *time*, preejection *period*.

in·ter·vas·cu·lar (in-ter-vas′kū-lăr). Between blood or lymph vessels.

in·ter·ven·tion (in-ter-ven′shŭn). An action or ministration that produces an effect or that is intended to alter the course of a pathologic process. [L. *inter-ventio,* a coming between, fr *inter-venio,* to come between]

crisis i., a psychotherapeutic technique directed at counseling at the time of an acute life crisis and limited in aim to helping resolve the crisis.

in·ter·ven·tric·u·lar (in-ter-ven-trik′ū-lăr). Between the ventricles.

in·ter·ver·te·bral (in-ter-ver′te-brăl). Between two vertebrae.

interview.

Zarit burden i., a structured verbal interaction used to evaluate levels of stress in family members or caregivers of Alzheimer patients.

in·ter·vil·lous (in-ter-vil′ŭs). Between or among villi.

in·tes·ti·nal (in-tes′ti-năl). Relating to the intestine.

i. pseudo-obstruction, clinical manifestations falsely suggesting obstruction of the small intestine, usually occurring in patients with multiple jejunal diverticula.

in·tes·tine (in-tes′tin) [TA]. The digestive tube passing from the stomach to the anus. It is divided primarily into the intestinum tenue (small intestine) and the intestinum crassum (large intestine). SYN bowel, gut (1), intestinum (1). [L. *intestinum*]

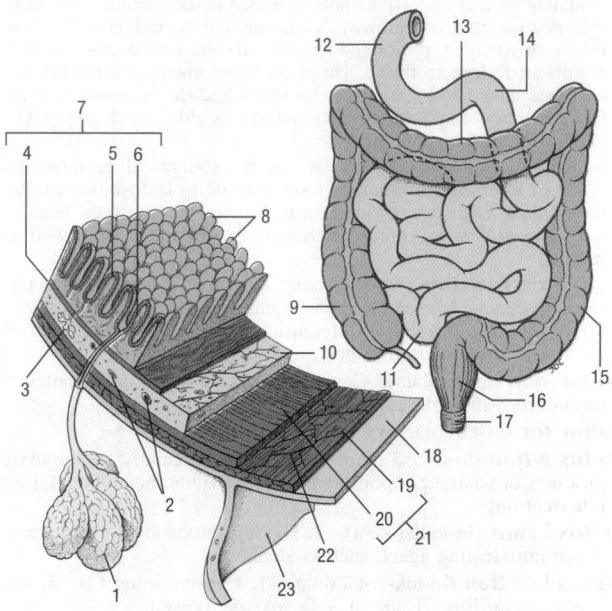

intestines: (bottom) diagram of four main layers of the wall of the digestive tube: mucosa, submucosa, muscularis, and serosa (below the diaphragm); (top) anterior view of the abdominal intestines; (1) gland outside gut but developing from it (liver), (2) blood vessels, (3) gland in submucosa, (4) muscularis mucosae, (5) epithelium, (6) lamina propria, (7) mucous membrane, (8) villi, (9) ascending colon, (10) submucosa, (11) ileum, (12) duodenum, (13) transverse colon, (14) jejunum, (15) descending colon, (16) rectum, (17) anus, (18) serosa, (19) circular muscle, (20) longitudinal muscle, (21) muscularis, (22) myenteric plexus, (23) mesentery

large i. [TA], the portion of the digestive tube extending from the ileocecal valve to the anus; it comprises the cecum, colon, rectum, and anal canal. SYN intestinum crassum [TA].

small i. [TA], the portion of the digestive tube between the stomach and the cecum or beginning of the large intestine; it consists of three portions: duodenum, jejunum, and ileum. SYN intestinum tenue [TA].

in·tes·ti·no·tox·in (in-tes′ti-nō-tok′sin). Obsolete term for enterotoxin.

in·tes·ti·num, pl. **in·tes·ti·na** (in-tes-tī′nŭm, -nă). **1** [TA]. SYN intestine. **2.** Inward; inner. [neuter of *intestinus*] [L. *intestinus,* internal, ntr. as noun, the entrails, fr. *intus,* within]

i. ce′cum, SYN cecum (1).

i. cras′sum [TA], SYN large *intestine*.

i. il′eum, twisted intestine. SEE ileum.

i. jeju′num, empty intestine. SEE jejunum.

i. rec′tum, straight intestine. SEE rectum.

i. ten′ue [TA], SYN small *intestine*.

i. ten′ue mesenteria′le, SYN mesenteric *portion* of small intestine.

in·ti·ma (in′ti-mă). Innermost. SEE *tunica* intima. [L. fem. of *intimus,* inmost]

in·ti·mal (in′ti-măl). Relating to the intima or inner coat of a vessel.

in·ti·mi·tis (in-ti-mī′tis). Inflammation of an intima, as in endangiitis. [intima + G. *-itis,* inflammation]

proliferative i., eruption characterized by dusky erythema and small ulcers due to proliferative changes in capillary bed.

in·toe (in′tō). SYN *metatarsus* adductus.

in·tol·er·ance (in-tol′er-ăns). Abnormal metabolism, excretion, or other disposition of a given substance; term often used to indicate impaired utilization or disposal of dietary constituents.

hereditary fructose i. [MIM*229600], a metabolic error due to deficiency of hepatic fructose 1,6-bisphosphate aldolase B (which also acts on fructose 1-phosphate), which is the second enzyme in the specific fructose pathway. Vomiting and hypoglycemia follow intake of fructose; prolonged fructose ingestion in young children results in failure to thrive, jaundice, hepatomegaly, albuminuria, aminoaciduria, and sometimes cachexia and death; autosomal recessive inheritance caused by mutation in aldolase B gene (AL-DOB) on chromosome 9q.

lactose i., a disorder characterized by abdominal cramps and diarrhea after consumption of food containing lactose (e.g., milk, ice cream); believed to reflect a deficiency of intestinal lactase; may appear first in young adults who had tolerated milk well as infants.

lysinuric protein i., an autosomal recessive disorder characterized by elevated levels of dibasic amino acids (e.g., L-lysine, L-arginine, and L-ornithine) in the urine; apparently due to a defect in dibasic amino acid transport.

in·tor·sion (in-tōr′shŭn). Conjugate rotation of the upper poles of each cornea inward. [L. *in-torqueo*, pp. *tortus*, to twist]

in·tor·tor (in-tōr′tōr). SYN medial *rotator*.

in·tox·a·tion (in-tok-sā′shŭn). Poisoning, especially by the toxic products of bacteria or poisonous animals, other than alcohol. [see intoxication]

in·tox·i·cant (in-tok′si-kant). **1.** Having the power to intoxicate. **2.** An intoxicating agent, such as alcohol.

in·tox·i·ca·tion (in-tok-si-kā′shŭn). **1.** SYN poisoning (2). **2.** SYN acute *alcoholism*. [L. *in*, in, + G. *toxikon*, poison]

acid i., poisoning by acid products (β-oxybutyric acid, diacetic acid, or acetone) formed as a result of faulty metabolism (e.g., uncontrolled diabetes mellitus) or by acids introduced from without; marked by epigastric pain, headache, loss of appetite, constipation, restlessness, and an odor of acetone in the breath, followed by air hunger, coma, and collapse.

anaphylactic i., i. following an anaphylactic reaction.

citrate i., a toxic condition that may develop during massive replacement therapy with transfused blood that contains citrate as an anticoagulant; the citrate combines with calcium ions and may result in tetany.

intestinal i., SYN autointoxication.

septic i., SYN septicemia.

water i., a metabolic encephalopathy resulting from severe overhydration.

△**intra-.** Inside, within; opposite of extra-. SEE ALSO endo-, ento-. [L. within]

in·tra·ab·dom·i·nal (in′tră-ab-dom′i-năl). Within the abdomen.

in·tra·ac·i·nous (in-tră-as′i-nŭs). Within an acinus.

in·tra·ad·e·noi·dal (in′tră-ad-ĕ-noy′dăl). Within the adenoids.

in·tra·ar·te·ri·al (in′tră-ar-tēr′ē-ăl). Within an artery or the arteries.

in·tra·ar·tic·u·lar (in′tră-ar-tik′ūlăr). Within the cavity of a joint. [intra- + L. *articulus*, joint]

in·tra·a·tri·al (in′tră-ā-trē-ăl). Within one or both of the atria of the heart.

in·tra·au·ral (in′tră-aw′răl). Within the ear. [intra- + L. *auris*, ear]

in·tra·au·ric·u·lar (in′tră-aw-rik′ū-lăr). Within an auricle (e.g., of the ear).

in·tra·bron·chi·al (in-tră-brong′kē-ăl). Within the bronchi or bronchial tubes. SYN endobronchial.

in·tra·buc·cal (in′tră-bŭk′ăl). **1.** Within the mouth. **2.** Within the substance of the cheek. [intra- + L. *bucca*, cheek]

in·tra·can·a·lic·u·lar (in′tră-kan-ă-lik′ū-lăr). Within a canaliculus or canaliculi.

in·tra·cap·su·lar (in′tră-kap′soo-lăr). Within a capsule, especially the capsule of a joint.

in·tra·car·di·ac (in′tră-kar′dē-ak). Within one of the chambers of the heart. SYN endocardiac (1), endocardial, intracordal. [intra- + G. *kardia*, heart]

in·tra·car·pal (in-tră-kar′păl). Within the carpus; among the carpal bones.

in·tra·car·ti·lag·i·nous (in′tră-kar-ti-laj′i-nŭs). Within a cartilage or cartilaginous tissue. SYN enchondral, endochondral.

in·tra·cath·e·ter (in′tră-kath′e-ter). A plastic tube, usually attached to the puncturing needle, inserted into a blood vessel for infusion, injection, or pressure monitoring.

in·tra·cav·i·tary (in′tră-cav′i-tār-ē). Within an organ or body cavity.

in·tra·ce·li·al (in′tră-sē′lē-ăl). Within any of the body cavities, especially within one of the ventricles of the brain. [intra- + G. *koilia*, cavity]

in·tra·cel·lu·lar (in-tră-sel′ū-lăr). Within a cell or cells.

in·tra·cer·e·bel·lar (in′tră-ser-ĕ-bel′ăr). Within the cerebellum.

in·tra·ce·re·bral (in′tră-ser′ē-brăl). Within the cerebrum.

in·tra·cer·e·bro·ven·tric·u·lar (in-tra-ser-ē′-brō-ven-trik′-ū-lar). The locus of administration of drugs or chemicals into the ventricular system of the brain. Often used in animal studies and occasionally for the introduction of antiinfectives that do not penetrate the blood-brain barrier into the brain in humans.

in·tra·cer·vi·cal (in′tră-ser′vi-kăl). SYN endocervical (1).

in·tra·cis·ter·nal (in′tră-sis-ter′năl). Within one of the subarachnoid cisternae; usually refers to the introduction of a cannula into the cerebellomedullary cistern for aspiration of cerebrospinal fluid or the injection of air into the ventricles of the brain.

in·tra·co·lic (in′tră-kol′ik). Within the colon.

in·tra·cor·dal (in′tră-kōr′dăl). SYN intracardiac. [intra- + L. *cor*, heart]

in·tra·cor·o·nal (in′tră-kōr′ŏ-năl). Within the crown portion of a tooth.

in·tra·cor·po·re·al (in′tră-kōr-po′rē-ăl). **1.** Within the body. **2.** Within any structure anatomically styled a corpus. [intra- + L. *corpus*, body]

in·tra·cor·pus·cu·lar (in′tră-kōr-pŭs′kū-lăr). Within a corpuscle, especially a red blood corpuscle. SYN intraglobular (2).

in·tra·cos·tal (in′tră-kos′tăl). On the inner surface of the ribs.

in·tra·cra·ni·al (in′tră-krā′nē-ăl). Within the skull.

intracrine (in′tră-krin). Denoting self-stimulation through cellular production of a factor that acts within the cell. [intra- + G. *krinō*, to separate, secrete]

in·trac·ta·ble (in′trak′tă-bl). **1.** SYN refractory (1). **2.** SYN obstinate (1). [L. *in-tractabilis*, fr. *in-* neg. + *tracto*, to draw, haul]

in·tra·cu·ta·ne·ous (in′tră-koo-tā′nē-ŭs). Within the substance of the skin, particularly the dermis. SYN intradermal, intradermic. [intra- + L. *cutis*, skin]

in·tra·cys·tic (in′tră-sis′tik). Within a cyst or the urinary bladder.

in·trad (in′trăd). Toward the inner part.

in·tra·der·mal, in·tra·der·mic (in′tră-der′măl, -der′mik). SYN intracutaneous. [intra- + G. *derma*, skin]

in·tra·duct (in′tră-dŭkt). Within the duct or ducts of a gland.

in·tra·du·ral (in′tră-doo′răl). Within or enclosed by the dura mater.

in·tra·em·bry·on·ic (in′tră-em-brē-on′ik). Within the embryonic body, e.g., the portion of the umbilical vein within the embryo (in contrast to the portion in the umbilical cord which is discarded at birth). Cf. extraembryonic.

in·tra·ep·i·der·mal (in′tră-ep-i-der′măl). Within the epidermis.

in·tra·ep·i·phys·i·al (in′tră-ep-i-fiz′ē-ăl). Within the epiphysis of a long bone.

in·tra·ep·i·the·li·al (in′tră-ep-i-thē′lē-ăl). Within or among the epithelial cells.

in·tra·far·a·di·za·tion (in′tră-fa-ră-di-zā′shŭn). Application of a faradic cauterizing current to the inner surface of a cavity or hollow organ.

in·tra·fas·cic·u·lar (in′tră-fă-sik′ū-lăr). Within the fasciculi of a tissue or structure (e.g., fasciculus intrafasciculus).

in·tra·fe·brile (in′tră-fē′bril, -feb′ril). Occurring during the febrile stage of a disease. SYN intrapyretic.

in·tra·fi·lar (in′tră-fī′lăr). Lying within the meshes of a network. [intra- + L. *filum,* thread]

in·tra·fu·sal (in′tră-fū′săl). Applied to structures within the muscle spindle.

in·tra·gal·va·ni·za·tion (in′tră-gal-van-i-zā′shŭn). Application of a galvanic cauterizing current to the interior of a cavity or hollow organ.

in·tra·gas·tric (in′tră-gas′trik). Within the stomach.

in·tra·gem·mal (in′tră-jem′ăl). Within any budlike or bulblike body; denoting especially a nerve termination within an end bulb or taste bud. [intra- + L. *gemma,* bud]

in·tra·ge·nal (in′tră-jēn′al). Within a gene.

in·tra·glan·du·lar (in′tră-glan′doo-lăr). Within a gland or glandular tissue.

in·tra·glob·u·lar (in′tră-glob′ū-lăr). **1.** Within a globule in any sense. **2.** SYN intracorpuscular.

in·tra·gy·ral (in′tră-jī′răl). Within a gyrus or convolution of the brain.

in·tra·he·pat·ic (in′tră-he-pat′ik). Within the liver.

in·tra·hy·oid (in′tră-hī′oyd). Within the hyoid bone; denoting certain accessory thyroid glands that lie in the hollow or within the substance of the hyoid bone.

in·tra·la·ryn·ge·al (in′tră-lă-rin′jē-ăl). Within the larynx.

in·tra·lig·a·men·tous (in′tră-lig-ă-men′tŭs). Within a ligament, especially the broad ligament of the uterus.

in·tra·lo·bar (in′tră-lō′bar). Within a lobe of any organ or other structure.

in·tra·lob·u·lar (in′tră-lob′ū-lăr). Within a lobule.

in·tra·loc·u·lar (in·tră-lok′ū-lăr). Within the loculi of any structure or part.

in·tra·lu·mi·nal (in-tră-loo′mi-năl). SYN intratubal.

in·tra·med·ul·lary (in′tră-med′ū-lār-ē). **1.** Within the bone marrow. **2.** Within the spinal cord. **3.** Within the medulla oblongata.

in·tra·mem·bra·nous (in′tră-mem′bră-nŭs). **1.** Within, or between the layers of, a membrane. **2.** Denoting a method of bone formation directly from mesenchymal cells without an intervening cartilage stage (occurring, for example, in the calvaria), as distinguished from intracartilaginous bone formation.

in·tra·me·nin·ge·al (in′tră-mĕ-nin′jē-ăl). Within or enclosed by the meninges of the brain or spinal cord.

in·tra·mi·to·chon·dri·al (in′tră-mī-tō-kon′drē-al). Within the mitochondria.

in·tra·mo·lec·u·lar (in′tră-mŏ-lek′ū-lăr). Referring to situations and events within a molecule.

in·tra·mu·ral (in′tră-mū′răl). Within the substance of the wall of any cavity or hollow organ. SYN intraparietal (1).

in·tra·mus·cu·lar (I.M., i.m.) (in′tră-mŭs′kū-lăr). Within the substance of a muscle.

in·tra·my·o·car·di·al (in′tră-mī′ō-kar′dē-ăl). Within the myocardium.

in·tra·my·o·me·tri·al (in′tră-mī′ō-mē′trē-ăl). Within the muscular coat of the uterus.

in·tra·na·sal (in′tră-nā′săl). Within the nasal cavity.

in·tra·na·tal (in′tră-nā′tăl). During or at the time of birth. [intra- + L. *natalis,* relating to birth]

in·tra·neu·ral (in′tră-noo′răl). Within a nerve. [intra- + G. *neuron,* nerve]

in·tra·nu·cle·ar (in′tră-noo′klē-ăr). Within the nucleus of a cell.

in·tra·oc·u·lar (in′tră-ok′ū-lăr). Within the eyeball.

in·tra·o·ral (in′tră-ō′răl). Within the mouth. [intra- + L. *os,* mouth]

in·tra·or·bit·al (in′tră-ōr′bi-tăl). Within the orbit.

in·tra·os·se·ous (in′tră-os′ē-ŭs). Within bone. SYN intraosteal. [intra- + L. *os,* bone]

in·tra·os·te·al (in′tră-os′tē-ăl). SYN intraosseous.

in·tra·o·var·i·an (in′tră-ō-vā′rē-an). Within the ovary.

in·tra·ov·u·lar (in′tră-ov′ū-lăr). Within the ovum.

in·tra·pa·ri·e·tal (in′tră-pă-rī′ĕ-tăl). **1.** SYN intramural. **2.** Denoting the intraparietal sulcus. SEE intraparietal *sulcus.*

in·tra·par·tum (in′tră-par′tŭm). During labor and delivery or childbirth. Cf. antepartum, postpartum. [intra- + L. *partus,* childbirth]

in·tra·pel·vic (in′tră-pel′vik). Within the pelvis.

in·tra·per·i·car·di·ac, in·tra·per·i·car·di·al (in′tră-per′ē-kar′dē-ak, -kar′dē-ăl). Within the pericardial cavity. SYN endopericardiac.

in·tra·per·i·to·ne·al (I.P., i.p.) (in′tră-per′i-tō-nē′ăl). Within the peritoneal cavity.

in·tra·per·son·al (in′tră-per′sŏn-ăl). SYN intrapsychic.

in·tra·pi·al (in′tră-pī′ăl). Within the pia mater.

in·tra·pleu·ral (in′tră-ploo′răl). Within the pleura or the pleural cavity.

in·tra·pon·tine (in′tră-pon′tīn). Within the pons of the brainstem.

in·tra·pros·tat·ic (in′tră-pros-tat′ik). Within the prostate gland.

in·tra·pro·to·plas·mic (in′tră-prō-tō-plas′mik). Within the protoplasm of a cell.

in·tra·psy·chic (in′tră-sī′kik). Denoting the psychological dynamics that occur inside the mind without reference to the individual's exchanges with other persons or events. SYN intrapersonal.

in·tra·pul·mo·nary (in′tră-pul′mo-nār-ē). Within the lungs.

in·tra·py·ret·ic (in′tră-pī-ret′ik). SYN intrafebrile. [intra- + L. *pyretos,* fever]

in·tra·rec·tal (in′tră-rek′tăl). Within the rectum.

in·tra·re·nal (in′tră-rē′năl). Within the kidney. [intra- + L. *ren,* kidney]

in·tra·ret·i·nal (in′tră-ret′i-năl). Within the retina.

in·trar·rha·chid·i·an, in·tra·ra·chid·i·an (in′tră-ră-kid′ē-an). SYN intraspinal. [intra- + G. *rachis,* spine]

in·tra·scro·tal (in′tră-skrō′tăl). Within the scrotum.

in·tra·spi·nal (in′tră-spī′năl). Within the vertebral canal or spinal cord. SYN intrarrhachidian, intrarachidian.

in·tra·splen·ic (in′tră-splen′ik). Within the spleen.

in·tra·stro·mal (in′tră-strō′măl). Within the stroma or foundation substance of any organ or part.

in·tra·syn·ov·i·al (in′tră-si-nō′vē-ăl). Within the synovial sac of a joint or a synovial tendon sheath.

in·tra·tar·sal (in′tră-tar′săl). Within the tarsus; among the tarsal bones.

in·tra·the·cal (in′tră-thē′kăl). **1.** Within a sheath. **2.** Within either the subarachnoid or the subdural space.

in·tra·tho·rac·ic (in′tră-thō-ras′ik). Within the cavity of the chest.

in·tra·ton·sil·lar (in′tră-ton-si-lăr). Within the substance of a tonsil.

in·tra·tub·al (in′tră-too′băl). Within any tube. SYN intraluminal.

in·tra·tu·bu·lar (in′tră-too′bū-lăr). Within any tubule.

in·tra·tym·pan·ic (in′tră-tim-pan′ik). Within the middle ear or tympanic cavity.

in·tra·u·ter·ine (in′tră-ū′ter-in). Within the uterus.

in·tra·vas·cu·lar (in′tră-vas′kū-lăr). Within the blood vessels or lymphatics.

in·tra·ve·nous (I.V., i.v.) (in′tră-vē′nŭs). Within a vein or veins. SYN endovenous.

in·tra·ven·tric·u·lar (I-V) (in′tră-ven-trik′ū-lăr). Within a ventricle of the brain or heart.

in·tra·ves·i·cal (in′tră-ves′i-kăl). Within a bladder, especially the urinary bladder.

in·tra·vi·tam (in′tră vī′tăm). During life. [L. *vita,* life]

in·tra·vi·tel·line (in′tră-vi-tel′in, -ēn). Within the vitellus yolk.

in·tra·vit·re·ous (in′tră-vit′rē-ŭs). Within the vitreous body.

in

in·trin·sic (in-trin′sik). **1.** Belonging entirely to a part. **2.** In anatomy, denoting those muscles whose origin and insertion are both within the structure under consideration, distinguished from the extrinsic muscles that have their origin outside of the structure under consideration; applied especially to the limbs but also to the ciliary muscle as distinguished from the recti and other orbital muscles which are outside the eyeball. SYN essential (6). [L. *intrinsecus,* on the inside]

⌂**intro-.** Inwardly, into; opposite of extra-. Cf. intra-. [L. *intro,* into]

in·tro·duc·er (in-trō-doos′er). An instrument, such as a catheter, needle, or endotracheal tube, for introduction of a flexible device. SYN intubator. [L. *intro-duco,* to lead into, introduce]

in·tro·flec·tion, in·tro·flex·ion (in′trō-flek′shun). A bending inward. [intro- + L. *flecto,* pp. *flectus,* to bend]

in·tro·gas·tric (in-trō-gas′trik). Leading or passed into the stomach. [intro- + G. *gastēr,* belly, stomach]

in·tro·i·tus (in-trō′i-tŭs). The entrance into a canal or hollow organ, as the vagina. [L. entrance, fr. *intro-eo,* to go into]
i. cana′lis, SYN i. of facial canal.
i. of facial canal, entrance to facial canal, through which the facial nerve passes, at end of internal acoustic meatus. SYN i. canalis.
vaginal i., SYN *vestibule* of vagina.

introject (in′trō-jekt). The dynamically endowed, enduring internal representation of an object.

in·tro·jec·tion (in-trō-jek′shun). A psychological defense mechanism involving appropriation of an external happening and its assimilation by the personality, making it a part of the self. [intro- + L. *jacto,* to throw]

in·tro·mis·sion (in-trō-mish′ŭn). The insertion or introduction of one part into another. [intro- + L. *mitto,* to send]

in·tro·mit·tent (in-trō-mit′ent). Conveying or sending into a body or cavity.

in·tron (in′tron). A portion of DNA that lies between two exons, is transcribed into RNA, but does not appear in that mRNA after maturation because the i. is removed and the exons spliced together, and so is not expressed (as protein) in protein synthesis. By customary usage, the term is extended to the corresponding regions in the primary transcript of mRNA prior to maturation. SYN intervening sequence. [inter- + -on]

in·tro·spec·tion (in-trō-spek′shun). Looking inward; self-scrutinizing; contemplating one's own mental processes. [intro- + L. *specto,* to look at, inspect]

in·tro·spec·tive (in-trō-spek′tiv). Relating to introspection.

in·tro·sus·cep·tion (in′trō-sŭs-sep′shun). SYN intussusception.

in·tro·ver·sion (in-trō-ver′zhŭn). **1.** The turning of a structure into itself. SEE ALSO intussusception, invagination. **2.** A trait of preoccupation with oneself, as practiced by an introvert. Cf. extraversion. [intro- + L. *verto,* pp. *versus,* to turn]

in·tro·vert. 1 (in′trō-vert). One who tends to be unusually shy, introspective, self-centered, and avoids becoming concerned with or involved in the affairs of others. Cf. extrovert. **2** (in-trō-vert′). To turn a structure into itself, to invert.

in·tu·bate (in′too-bāt). To insert a tube.

▯**in·tu·ba·tion** (in-too-bā′shun). Insertion of a tubular device into a canal, hollow organ, or cavity; specifically, passage of an oro- or nasotracheal tube for anesthesia or for control of pulmonary ventilation. [L. *in,* in, + *tuba,* tube]
altercursive i., rarely used term for diversion of secretion intermittently to the exterior from its normal destination, e.g., of the bile from the intestine.
aqueductal i., insertion of a tube in the sylvian aqueduct to relieve atresia or narrowing of the aqueduct.
blind nasotracheal i., passage of tube through the nose into the trachea without using a laryngoscope.
endotracheal i., passage of a tube through the nose or mouth into the trachea for maintenance of the airway during anesthesia or for ventilatory support or for maintenance of an imperiled airway. SYN intratracheal i.
intratracheal i., SYN endotracheal i.

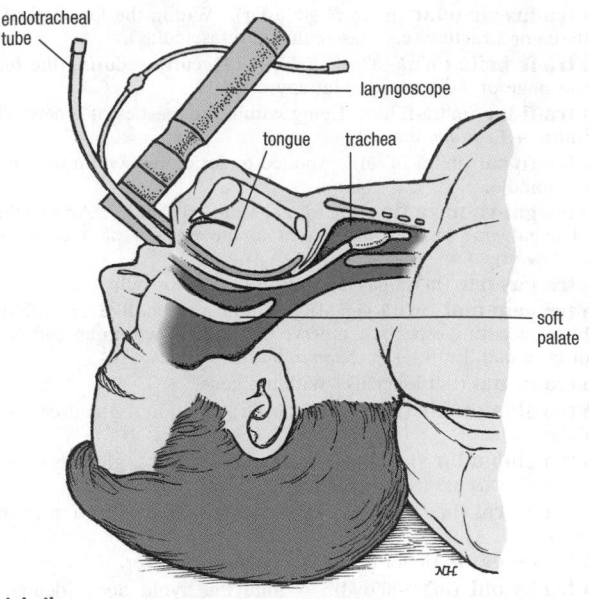

intubation

nasotracheal i., tracheal i. through the nose.
orotracheal i., tracheal i. through the mouth.
tracheal i., passage of a tube through the nose, mouth, or a tracheotomy into the trachea for maintenance of patency of the airway.

in·tu·ba·tor (in′too-bā-tŏr). SYN introducer.

in·tu·mesce (in-too-mes′). To swell up; to enlarge. [L. *in-tumesco,* to swell up, fr. *tumeo,* to swell]

in·tu·mes·cence (in-too-mes′ens). **1.** SYN enlargement. **2.** The process of enlarging or swelling; used to describe the spinal enlargements.
tympanic i., SYN tympanic *enlargement.*

in·tu·mes·cent (in-too-mes′ent). Enlarging; becoming enlarged or swollen.

in·tu·mes·cen·tia (in-too-mes-sen′shē-ă) [TA]. SYN enlargement. [Mod. L.]
i. cervica′lis [TA], SYN cervical *enlargement.*
i. gangliofor′mis, SYN geniculate *ganglion.*
i. lumbosacra′lis [TA], SYN lumbosacral *enlargement.*
i. tympan′ica [TA], SYN tympanic *enlargement.*

in·tus·sus·cep·tion (in′tŭs-sŭ-sep′shŭn). **1.** The taking up or receiving of one part within another, especially the enfolding of one segment of the intestine within another. SEE ALSO introversion, invagination. **2.** Often, specifically, the process of incorporation of new material in the growth of the cell wall. SYN introsusception. [L. *intus,* within, + *sus-cipio,* to take up, fr. *sub* + *capio,* to take]
colic i., the ensheathing of one portion of the colon into another.
double i., a second i. that involves the bowel above the first; the first i. is followed by contraction of the bowel wall around it, and the solid mass so formed is enveloped by the proximal portion of the bowel and is thus the cause of the second i.
ileal i., i. in which one portion of the ileum is ensheathed in another portion of the same division of the bowel.
ileocecal i., i. in which the lower segment of the ileum passes through the valve of the colon into the cecum.
ileocolic i., i. in which the lower portion of the ileum with the valve of the cecum passes into the ascending colon.
jejunogastric i., a rare complication following gastrojejunostomy in which the afferent or the efferent loop of bowel invaginates into the stomach.

retrograde i., the invagination of a lower segment of the bowel into one just above.

in·tus·sus·cep·tive (in′tŭs-sŭ-sep′tiv). Relating to or characterized by intussusception.

in·tus·sus·cep·tum (in′tŭs-sŭ-sep′tŭm). The inner segment in an intussusception; that part of the bowel which is received within the other part.

in·tus·sus·cip·i·ens (in′tŭs-sŭ-sip′ē-enz). The portion of the bowel, in intussusception, which receives the other portion. [L. *intus,* within, + *suscipiens,* pr. p. of *suscipio,* to take up]

in·u·lase (in′ū-lās). SYN inulinase.

in·u·lin (In) (in′ū-lin). A fructose polysaccharide from the rhizome of *Inula helenium* or *elecampane* (family Compositae) and other plants; used by intravenous injection, where it is filtered by the renal glomeruli but not re-absorbed and thus can be used to determine the rate of glomerular filtration; also used in bread for diabetics. Cf. inulin *clearance.* SYN alant starch, alantin, dahlin.

in·u·lin·ase (in′ū-lin-ās). An enzyme acting upon 2,1-β-D-fructoside links in inulin, releasing D-fructose. SYN inulase.

in·u·lol (in′ū-lol). SYN alantol.

in·unc·tion (in-ŭngk′shŭn). Administration of a drug in ointment form by rubbing to cause absorption of the active ingredient. [L. *inunctio,* an anointing, fr. *inunguo,* pp. *-unctus,* to smear on]

in·vac·ci·na·tion (in-vak-si-nā′shŭn). Obsolete term for accidental inoculation of some disease, e.g., syphilis, during vaccination.

in vac·uo (in vak′ū-ō). In a vacuum, e.g., under reduced pressure. [L.]

in·vag·i·nate (in-vaj′i-nāt). To ensheathe, infold, or insert a structure within itself or another. [L. *in,* in, + *vagina,* a sheath]

in·vag·i·na·tion (in-vaj′i-nā′shŭn). **1.** The ensheathing, enfolding, or insertion of a structure within itself or another. **2.** The state of being invaginated. SEE ALSO introversion, intussusception.

basilar i., SYN platybasia.

in·vag·i·na·tor (in-vag′i-nā-ter, -tōr). An instrument for pushing inward any tissue.

in·va·lid (in′vă-lid). **1.** Weak; sick. **2.** A person partially or completely disabled. [L. *in-* neg. + *validus,* strong]

in·va·lid·ism (in′vă-lid-izm). The condition of being an invalid.

in·va·sin (in-vā′sin). SYN hyaluronidase (1).

in·va·sion (in-vā′zhŭn). **1.** The beginning or incursion of a disease. **2.** Local spread of a malignant neoplasm by infiltration or destruction of adjacent tissue; for epithelial neoplasms, i. signifies infiltration beneath the epithelial basement membrane. **3.** Entrance of foreign cells into a tissue, such as polymorphonuclear leukocytes in inflammation. [L. *invasio,* fr. *in-vado,* pp. *-vasus,* to go into, attack]

in·va·sive (in-vā′siv). **1.** Denoting or characterized by invasion. **2.** Denoting a procedure requiring insertion of an instrument or device into the body through the skin or a body orifice for diagnosis or treatment.

in·ven·to·ry (in′ven-tōr-ē). A detailed, often descriptive, list of items.

Millon clinical multiaxial i. (MCMI), SYN Millon Clinical Multiaxial Inventory *test.*

Minnesota Multiphasic Personality I., SYN Minnesota Multiphasic Personality Inventory *test.*

personality i., a psychological test for evaluation of habitual modes of behavior, thinking, and feeling based on the comparable characteristics of individuals in one's peer group.

in·ver·mi·na·tion (in-ver-mi-nā′shŭn). SYN helminthiasis. [L. *in,* in, + *vermis* (*vermin-*), worm]

in·ver·sion (in-ver′zhŭn). **1.** A turning inward, upside down, or in any direction contrary to the existing one. **2.** Conversion of a disaccharide or polysaccharide by hydrolysis into a monosaccharide; specifically, the hydrolysis of sucrose to D-glucose and D-fructose; so called because of the change in optical rotation. **3.** Alteration of a DNA molecule made by removing a fragment, reversing its orientation, and putting it back into place. **4.** Heat-induced transition of silica, in which the quartz tridymite or cristobalite changes its physical properties as to thermal expansion. **5.**

Conversion of a chiral center into its mirror image. [L. *inverto,* pp. *-versus,* to turn upside down, to turn about]

i. of chromosomes, a chromosome aberration resulting from a double break in a segment of the chromosome, with end for end rotation of the fragment between the fracture lines, and refusion of the fragments; this results in reversal of the order of genes in that segment.

paracentric i., i. in a chromosome of a single segment in which the centromere is not included.

pericentric i., i. in a chromosome of a single segment that includes the centromere.

i. of the uterus, a turning of the uterus inside out, usually following childbirth.

visceral i., SYN *situs* inversus viscerum.

in·vert (in′vert). **1.** In chemistry, subjected to inversion, e.g., invert sugar. **2.** To reverse in direction, sequence, or effect. **3.** Rarely used term for a homosexual. SEE inversion.

in·vert·ase (in′ver-tās). SYN β-fructofuranosidase.

In·ver·te·bra·ta (in-ver-tĕ-brā′tă). A general category of the kingdom Animalia (multicellular animals) including those phyla whose members lack a notochord; i.e., all animals except vertebrates in the phylum Chordata.

in·ver·te·brate (in-ver′tĕ-brāt). **1.** Not possessed of a spinal or vertebral column. **2.** Any animal that has no spinal column.

in·vert·ed re·peat. A sequence of nucleotides that is repeated nearly without change except in the opposite direction, usually at some point distant from the original sequence; often associated with gene insertion.

in·ver·tin (in′ver-tin). SYN β-fructofuranosidase.

in·ver·tor (in-ver′ter, -tōr). A muscle that inverts or causes inversion or turns a part, such as the foot, inward. [see inversion]

in·vest·ing. **1.** In dentistry, covering or enveloping wholly or in part an object such as a denture, tooth, wax form, crown, etc., with a refractory investment material before curing, soldering, or casting. **2.** In psychoanalysis, allocating to or charging an object with psychic energy or cathexis.

vacuum i., the i. of a pattern utilizing a vacuum to remove trapped air from the investment material.

in·vest·ment. **1.** In dentistry, any material used in investing. **2.** In psychoanalysis, the psychic charge or cathexis invested in an object.

refractory i., an i. material which can withstand the high temperatures used in soldering or casting.

in·vet·er·ate (in-vet′er-āt). Long seated; firmly established; said of a disease or of confirmed habits. [L. *in-vetero,* pp. *-atus,* to render old, fr. *vetus,* old]

in·vis·ca·tion (in-vis-kā′shŭn). **1.** Smearing with mucilaginous matter. **2.** The mixing of the food, during mastication, with saliva. [L. *in,* in, on, + *viscum,* birdlime]

in vi·tro (in vē′trō). In an artificial environment, referring to a process or reaction occurring therein, as in a test tube or culture media. Cf. in vivo. [L. in glass]

in vi·vo (in vē′vō). In the living body, referring to a process or reaction occurring therein. Cf. in vitro. [L. in the living being]

in·vo·lu·cre (in′vō-loo-ker). SYN involucrum.

in·vo·lu·crin (in-vō-loo′krin). A non–keratin-soluble precursor of the highly cross-linked protein known as the corneocyte envelope. [fr. L. *involucrum,* a wrapper]

in·vo·lu·crum, pl. **in·vo·lu·cra** (in-vō-loo′krŭm, -loo′kră). **1.** An enveloping membrane, e.g., a sheath or sac. **2.** The sheath of new bone that forms around a sequestrum. SYN involucre. [L. a wrapper, fr. *in-volvo,* to roll up]

in·vol·un·tary (in-vol′ŭn-tār-ē). **1.** Independent of the will; not volitional. **2.** Contrary to the will. [L. *in-* neg. + *voluntarius,* willing, fr. *volo,* to wish]

in·vo·lu·tion (in-vō-loo′shŭn). **1.** Return of an enlarged organ to normal size. **2.** Turning inward of the edges of a part. **3.** In psychiatry, mental decline associated with advanced age. SYN catagenesis. [L. *in-volvo,* pp. *-volutus,* to roll up]

senile i., the retrogression of vital organs and psychological processes incident to aging.

in

i. of the uterus, the process of reduction of the uterus to its normal nonpregnant size and state following childbirth.

in·vo·lu·tion·al (in-vō-loo′shŭn-ăl). Relating to involution.

io·ben·zam·ic ac·id (ī-ō-ben-zam′ik). A radiographic contrast medium formerly used for oral cholecystography.

io·ce·tam·ic ac·id (ī′ō-sē-tam′ik). A radiographic contrast medium formerly used for oral cholecystography.

io·da·mide (ī-ō′dă-mīd). A radiographic contrast medium formerly used for oral cholecystography. SYN ametriodinic acid.

Iod·a·moe·ba (ī-od-ă-mē′bă). A genus of parasitic amebae in the superclass Rhizopoda, order Amoebida.

I. bütsch′lii, a parasitic ameba in the large intestine of man; trophozoites are usually 9–14 μm in diameter; the cysts are usually 8–10 μm in diameter, uninucleate and somewhat irregular in shape, with a thick wall and a large compact mass of glycogen that stains deeply with a solution of iodine; clinically recognizable amebiasis caused by this organism is rare, with symptoms resembling those of chronic disease caused by *Entamoeba histolytica;* it is also found in other primates and is the commonest ameba of pigs.

io·date (ī′ō-dāt). A salt of iodic acid.

iod·ic (ī-od′ik). **1.** Relating to, or caused by, iodine or an iodide. **2.** Denoting a compound of iodine in its pentavalent state.

iod·ic ac·id. Crystalline powder, soluble in water; used as an astringent, caustic, disinfectant, deodorant, and formerly as an intestinal antiseptic.

io·dide (ī′ō-dīd). **1.** The negative ion of iodine, I^-. **2.** Any salt of hydroiodic acid. **3.** Any compound containing an iodine atom linked to a carbon.

i. peroxidase, an oxidoreductase catalyzing reactions between iodine and water to yield iodide and H_2O_2; also catalyzes iodination and deiodination of tyrosine compounds; a deficiency of this enzyme leads to a loss of the iodotyrosine derivatives and iodine from the thyroid and results in goiter. SYN iodinase, iodotyrosine deiodase.

sodium i. iodine-131, prepared from radioactive iodine (^{131}I); nominally carrier-free, with a half-life of 8.1 days; used as a diagnostic agent in suspected thyroid disease and in the treatment of selected thyroid diseases.

io·dim·e·try (ī-ō-dim′ĕ-trē). SYN iodometry. [iodine + G. *metron,* measure]

io·di·nase (ī′ō-din-ās). SYN *iodide* peroxidase.

io·di·nate (ī′ō-di-nāt). To treat or combine with iodine.

io·dine (I) (ī′ō-dīn, -dēn). A nonmetallic chemical element, atomic no. 53, atomic wt. 126.90447; used in the manufacture of i. compounds and as a catalyst, reagent, tracer, constituent of radiographic contrast media, topical antiseptic, antidote for alkaloidal poisons, and in certain stains and solutions; formerly used for prophylaxis of iodine deficiency. [G. *iōdēs,* violet-like, fr. *ion,* a violet, + *eidos,* form]

butanol-extractable i. (BEI), i. that can be separated from plasma proteins by butanol or other extractable solvents; used to measure thyroid function.

Gram i., a solution containing i. and potassium iodide, used in Gram stain.

povidone i., a water soluble complex of i. with polyvinylpyrrolidone. Applied as an antiseptic in the form of solutions or ointments, it releases i. Used in cleansing and disinfecting the skin, preparing the skin preoperatively, and treating infections susceptible to i. SYN polyvinylpyrrolidone-iodine complex, povidone-iodine.

protein-bound i. (PBI), thyroid hormone in its circulating form, consisting of one or more of the iodothyronines bound to one or more of the serum proteins.

radioactive i., the i. radioisotopes ^{131}I, ^{125}I, or ^{123}I used as tracers in biology and medicine.

tamed i., SYN iodophor.

i. tincture, a hydroalcoholic solution containing 2% elemental i. and 2.4% potassium iodide to facilitate dissolution and 47% alcohol; used as an antiseptic/germicide on the skin surface for cuts and scratches. Has been used as a skin disinfectant before surgery but is now largely replaced by organic forms of i.

io·dine-123 (^{123}I). A radioisotope of iodine with a 159 keV gamma emission and a physical half-life of 13.2 h, used for studies of thyroid disease and of renal function.

io·dine-125 (^{125}I). Radioactive iodine isotope that decays by K-capture (internal conversion) with a half-life of 59.4 days; used as a label in immunoassay and in imaging; formerly used as a tracer in thyroid studies and as a label in imaging.

io·dine-127 (^{127}I). Stable, nonradioactive iodine, the most abundant iodide isotope found in nature; dietary deficiency causes simple goiter; used to block thyroid uptake of radioactive iodine released from nuclear accidents.

io·dine-131 (^{131}I). A radioactive iodine isotope; beta and gamma emitter with a half-life of 8.1 days; used as a tracer in thyroid studies, as therapy in hyperthyroidism and thyroid cancer, and as a label in immunoassay and imaging; formerly used as therapy in heart disease.

io·dine-132 (^{132}I). A beta- and gamma-emitting radioisotope of iodine with a half-life of 2.28 h, usually obtained from a tellurium-132 radionuclide generator; its clinical use has been supplanted by ^{131}I and ^{123}I.

io·dine-fast. Denoting hyperthyroidism unresponsive to iodine therapy, which develops frequently in most cases so treated.

io·din·o·phil, io·din·o·phile (ī-ō-din′ō-fil, -fīl). **1.** Staining readily with iodine. SYN iodinophilous. **2.** Any histologic element that stains readily with iodine. [iodine + G. *philos,* fond]

io·din·oph·i·lous (ī-ō-din-of′i-lŭs). SYN iodinophil (1).

io·dip·a·mide (ī-ō-dip′ă-mīd). An ionic, dimeric, water-soluble radiographic contrast medium for intravenous cholangiography; used as the sodium or methylglucamine salt. SYN Adipiodone.

methylglucamine i., a water-soluble organic iodine compound used for intravenous cholangiography and cholecystography.

io·dism (ī′ō-dizm). Poisoning by iodine, a condition marked by severe coryza, an acneform eruption, weakness, salivation, and foul breath; caused by the continuous administration of iodine or one of the iodides.

io·dix·an·ol (ī-ō-diks′ă-nol). 5,5′-[(2-Hydroxy-1,3-propane)bis-(acetylamino)]bis[*N,N*′-bis(2,3- dihydroxypropyl)-2,4,6- triiodo-1,3-benzenedicarboxamide]; a dimeric, nonionic, low osmolar, water-soluble radiographic contrast medium for intravascular use.

io·dize (ī′ō-dīz). To treat or impregnate with iodine.

i·o·dized oil (ī′ō-dīzd). An iodine addition product of vegetable oils, containing not less than 38% and not more than 42% of organically combined iodine; a radiopaque medium.

io·do·a·cet·a·mide (ī-ō′dō-ă-sē′tă-mīd). ICH_2-CONH_2; a chemical reacting readily with sulfhydryl groups and therefore a strong inhibitor of many enzymes.

io·do·al·phi·on·ic ac·id (ī-ō′dō-al-fē-on′ik). A radiographic contrast medium formerly used for cholecystography.

io·do·ca·sein (ī-ō-dō-kā′sēn). A compound of iodine with casein, in which the iodine is attached to tyrosine molecules; possesses thyroxine activity.

io·do·chlor·hy·drox·y·quin, io·do·chlo·ro·hy·drox·y·quin·o·line (ī′ō-dō-klōr′hī-drok′si-kwin, -klōr′ō-hī-drok′si-kwin′ō-lēn). Topical antiinfective. SYN chloriodoquin, clioquinol.

io·do·chlo·rol (ī′ō-dō-klōr′ol). SYN chloriodized oil.

io·do·der·ma (ī-ō′dō-der′mă). 1An eruption of follicular papules and pustules, or panniculitis, caused by iodine toxicity or sensitivity.

io·do·form (ī-ō′dō-fōrm). A topical antiseptic. SYN triiodomethane.

io·do·glob·u·lin (ī-ō′dō-glob′ū-lin). SYN thyroglobulin (1).

io·do·gor·go·ic ac·id (ī-ō′dō-gōr-gō′ik). 3,5-Diiodotyrosine; a precursor of thyroxine.

io·do·hip·pu·rate so·di·um (ī-ō′dō-hip′poo-rāt). A radiopaque compound formerly used intravenously, orally, or for retrograde urography. When tagged with iodine-131, it is used to measure effective renal plasma flow and to image the kidneys for radioisotopic renography.

io·do·meth·a·mate so·di·um (ī-ō′dō-meth′ă-māt). A high osmolar, ionic, water-soluble, radiographic contrast medium formerly used widely as the disodium salt for intravenous urography.

io·do·met·ric (ī-ō′dō-met′rik). Relating to iodometry.

io·dom·e·try (ī-ō-dom′ĕ-trē). Analytic techniques involving titrations in which visible form(s) of iodine is either formed or consumed, the sudden appearance or disappearance of iodine marking the end point. SYN iodimetry. [iodine + G. *metron*, measure]

io·do·pa·no·ic ac·id (ī-ō′dō-pa-nō′ik). SYN iopanoic acid.

io·do·phen·dyl·ate (ī-ō′dō-fen′dil-āt). SYN iophendylate.

io·do·phil·ia (ī-ō′dō-fil′ē-ă). An affinity for iodine, as manifested by some leukocytes in certain conditions. When treated with a solution of iodine and potassium iodide, normal polymorphonuclear leukocytes stain a fairly bright yellow; in certain pathologic conditions, the polymorphonuclear leukocytes frequently stain diffusely brown or yellow-brown; the reaction may be intracellular (as described) or extracellular, affecting the particles in the immediate vicinity of the leukocytes. [iodine + G. *phileō*, to love]

io·do·phor (ī-ō′dō-fōr). A combination of iodine with a surfactant carrier, usually polyvinylpyrrolidone. Commercial preparations generally contain 1% "available" iodine, which is slowly released to take effect against microorganisms; used as skin disinfectants, particularly for surgical scrubs. SYN tamed iodine. [iodine + G. *phora*, a carrying]

io·do·phtha·lein (ī-ō′dō-thal′ēn, -dof-thal′e-in). A radiographic contrast medium. The disodium salt was once used in radiography of the gallbladder. SYN tetraiodophenolphthalein sodium.

3-io·do-1,2-pro·pane·di·ol. SYN *glyceryl* iodide.

γ-io·do·pro·py·lene·gly·col. SYN *glyceryl* iodide.

io·do·pro·pyl·i·dene glyc·er·ol. SYN iodinated *glycerol.*

io·do·pro·teins (ī-ō′dō-prō′tēnz). Proteins containing iodine bound to tyrosyl groups.

io·dop·sin (ī-ō-dop′sin). Any of three visual pigments, composed of 11-*cis*-retinal bound to an opsin, found in the cones of the retina. SYN visual violet. [G. *ion*, violet, + *ōps*, eye, + -in]

io·do·py·ra·cet (ī-ō′dō-pī′ră-set). A radiographic contrast medium formerly used for intravenous urography; also used to determine the renal plasma flow and the renal tubular excretory mass. SYN diodone.

io·do·qui·nol (ī-ō′dō-kwin′ol). Drug used as an amebicide prepared by the action of iodine monochloride on 8-hydroxyquinoline.

io·do·ther·a·py (ī-ō-dō-thār′ă-pē). Treatment with iodine.

io·do·thy·ro·nines (ī-ō′dō-thī′rō-nēnz). Iodinated derivatives of thyronine.

io·do·ty·ro·sine (ī-ō′dō-tī′rō-sēn). An iodinated tyrosine.

i. deiodase, SYN *iodide* peroxidase.

io·dox·a·mate meg·lu·mine (ī-ō-doks′ă-māt). The methylglucamine salt of an ionic, water-soluble, dimeric, radiographic contrast medium; formerly used primarily for intravenous cholangiography.

io·du·ria (ī-ō-doo′rē-ă). Urinary excretion of iodine.

io·gly·cam·ic ac·id (ī′ō-glī-kam′ik). 3,3′-[oxybis(methylene carbonylimino)]bis[2,4,6-triiodobenzoic acid]; an ionic, water-soluble, dimeric, radiographic contrast medium, formerly used for intravenous cholangiography.

io·hex·ol (ī′ō-heks′ol). A monomeric, nonionic, water-soluble, low osmolar radiographic contrast medium for urography or angiography. Used intrathecally and intravascularly.

iom·e·ter (ī-om′ĕ-ter). An apparatus for measuring ionization. [ion + G. *metron*, measure]

ion (ī′on). An atom or group of atoms carrying an electric charge by virtue of having gained or lost one or more electrons. I.'s charged with negative electricity (anions) travel toward a positive pole (anode); those charged with positive electricity (cations) travel toward a negative pole (cathode). I.'s may exist in solid, liquid, or gaseous environments, although those in liquid (electrolytes) are more common and familiar. [G. *iōn*, going]

aquo-i., SEE aquo-ion.

dipolar i.'s, i.'s possessing both a negative charge and a positive charge, each localized at a different point in the molecule, which thus has both positive and negative "poles"; amino acids are the most notable dipolar i.'s, containing a positively charged NH_3^+ group and a negatively charged COO^- group at neutral pH. SYN amphions, zwitterions.

gram-i., SEE gram-ion.

hydride i., the H^- i., transferred to acceptor molecules in some biologic oxidations.

hydrogen i. (H^+), a hydrogen atom minus its electron and therefore carrying a unit positive charge (i.e., a proton); in water, it combines with a water molecule to form hydronium i., H_3O^+.

hydronium i., the hydrated proton, H_3O^+, a form in which hydrogen i. exists in aqueous solutions; also, $H_3O^+ \cdot H_2O$, $H_3O^+ \cdot 2H_2O$, etc. SYN oxonium i.

oxonium i., SYN hydronium i.

sulfonium i., a compound in which a sulfur atom has three single covalent bonds and therefore has a positive charge analogous to the nitrogen of an ammonium compound; e.g., *S*-adenosyl-L-methionine.

Ionescu, SEE Jonnesco.

ion ex·change (ī′on eks-chanj′). SEE anion exchange, cation exchange, ion exchange *chromatography.*

ion ex·chang·er (ī′on eks-chanj′er). SEE anion exchanger, cation exchanger.

ion·ic (ī-on′ik). Relating to an ion.

io·ni·um (ī-ō′nē-ŭm). Former term for thorium-230. [G. *iōn*, going]

ion·i·za·tion (ī′on-i-zā′shŭn). **1.** Dissociation into ions, occurring when an electrolyte is dissolved in water or certain liquids or when molecules are subjected to electrical discharge or ionizing radiation. **2.** Production of ions as a result of interaction of radiation with matter. **3.** SYN iontophoresis.

ion·ize (ī′on-īz). To separate into ions; to dissociate atoms or molecules into electrically charged atoms or radicals.

ion·o·gram (ī′on-ō-gram). SYN electropherogram.

io·none (ī′ō-nōn). One of two cyclic terpene ketones with an odor of violets or cedar wood, the α and β varieties of which differ in the location of the double bond in the ring: provitamins A and vitamin A have i. configuration in the ring portion; α-carotene contains one α- and one β-ionone moieties, β-carotene contains two β-ionone moieties, and γ-carotene contains one β-ionone moiety.

ion·o·pher·o·gram (ī′on-ō-fer′ō-gram). SYN electropherogram.

ion·o·phore (ī-on′ō-fōr). A compound or substance that forms a complex with an ion and transports it across a membrane. [ion + G. *phore*, a bearer]

ion·o·pho·re·sis (ī-on′ō-fōr-ē′sis). SYN electrophoresis. [ion + G. *phorēsis*, a carrying]

ion·o·pho·ret·ic (ī-on′ō-fōr-et′ik). SYN electrophoretic.

ion·to·pho·re·sis (ī-on′tō-fōr-ē′sis). The introduction into the tissues, by means of an electric current, of the ions of a chosen medicament. SYN ionic medication, ionization (3), iontotherapy. [ion + G. *phorēsis*, a carrying]

ion·to·pho·ret·ic (ī-on′tō-fōr-et′ik). Relating to iontophoresis.

ion·to·ther·a·py (ī-on′tō-thār′ă-pē). SYN iontophoresis.

io·pam·i·dol (ī′ō-pam′i-dol). A monomeric, nonionic, water-soluble, low osmolar radiographic contrast medium for urography or angiography.

io·pa·no·ic ac·id (ī′ō-pa-nō′ik). A water-insoluble radiographic contrast medium, once used widely for oral cholecystography. SYN iodopanoic acid.

io·pen·tol (ī′ō-pen′tol). *N,N*′-Bis(2,3-dihydroxypropyl)-5-[*N*-(2-hydroxy-3-methoxypropyl) acetamido]-2,4,6-triiodoisophthalamide; a nonionic, monomeric, low osmolar radiographic contrast medium for intravenous urography or angiography.

io·phen·dyl·ate (ī-ō-fen′dil-āt). A mixture of isomers of ethyl iodophenylundecylate, an iodized fatty acid of low viscosity; used for radiography of the spinal canal. SYN iodophendylate.

io·phe·no·ic ac·id (ī′ō-fen-ō-ik). SYN iophenoxic acid.

io

io·phen·ox·ic ac·id (ī′ō-fen-oks′ik). A radiographic contrast medium; formerly used for oral cholecystography. SYN iophenoic acid.

io·pho·bia (ī-ō-fō′bē-ă). Morbid fear of poisons. [G. *ios,* poison, + *phobos,* fear]

io·pro·mide (ī-ō′prō-mid). *N,N′*-Bis(2,3-dihydroxy propyl)-2,4-6-triiodo-5-(2-methoxyacetamido)-*N*-methyl isophthalamide; a monomeric, nonionic, water-soluble, low osmolar radiographic contrast medium for intravenous urography or angiography.

i·o·ta (ι) (ī-ōt′a). **1.** The ninth letter in the Greek alphabet. **2.** In chemistry, denotes the ninth in a series, or the ninth atom from a carboxyl group or other functional group. **3.** A tiny or minute amount.

io·ta·cism (ī-ō′tă-sizm). A speech defect marked by the frequent substitution of a long *e* sound (that of the Greek iota) for other vowels. [G. *iōta,* the letter ι]

io·tha·lam·ic ac·id (ī′ō-thă-lam′ik). An ionic, monomeric, water-soluble radiographic contrast medium, widely used as the sodium or methylglucamine salt (iothalamate) for intravenous urography and angiography.

io·thi·o·u·ra·cil so·di·um (ī′ō-thī-ō-ūr′ă-sil). The sodium salt of 5-iodo-2-thiouracil; an organic iodine derivative of thiouracil with the thyroid-involuting action of iodine and the capability of inhibiting thyroxine production.

io·trol (ī′ō-trol). SYN iotrolan.

io·tro·lan (ī-ō′trō-lan). 5,5′-[Malonylbis(methylimino)]bis[*N, N′*-bis[2,3-dihydroxy-1-(hydroxymethyl)propyl]-2,4,6-triiodoisophthalamide]; a dimeric, nonionic, water-soluble, low osmolar radiographic contrast medium, used for myelography and other nonvascular applications. SYN iotrol.

io·ver·sol (ī-ō-ver′sol). *N,N′*-Bis(2,3-dihydroxypropyl)-5-[*N*-[2-hydroxyethyl)glycolamido]-2,4,6-triiodoisophthalamide; a water-soluble, nonionic, low osmolar, radiographic contrast medium.

iox·ag·late (ī-oks-ag′lāt). A diagnostic radiopaque medium, usually a combination of i. meglumine ($C_{24}H_{21}I_6N_5O_8·C_7H_{17}NO_5$), and i. sodium ($C_{24}H_{20}I_6N_5NaO_8$); used in angiography, aortography, arteriography, venography, and urography.

iox·i·lan (ī-oks′ĭ-lan). *N*-(2,3-Dihydroxypropyl)-5-[*N*(2,3-dihydroxypropyl)acetamido]-*N′*-(2-hydroxyethyl)-2,4,6-triiodoisophthalamide; a monomeric, nonionic, water-soluble, low osmolar radiographic contrast medium for urography or angiography.

iox·i·thal·a·mate (ī-oks-ĭ-thal′ă-māt). 5-Acetamido-2,4,6-triiodo-*N*-(2-hydroxyethyl)isophthalamic acid; an ionic, monomeric, water-soluble radiographic contrast medium for urography and angiography.

I.P., i.p. Abbreviation for intraperitoneal or intraperitoneally; isoelectric *point.*

IP₃ Abbreviation for *inositol* 1,4,5-trisphosphate.

IPA Abbreviation for independent practice *association*; isopropyl alcohol.

ip·e·cac (ip′ē-kak). SYN ipecacuanha.

  powdered i., a form of i. used in the preparation of ipecac syrup.

ip·e·cac·u·a·nha (ip-ē-kak-ū-an′ă). The dried root of *Uragoga (Cephaelis) ipecacuanha* (family Rubiaceae), a shrub of Brazil and other parts of South America; contains emetine, cephaeline, emetamine, ipecacuanhic acid, psychotrine, and methylpsychotrine; has expectorant, emetic, and antidysenteric properties. SYN ipecac. [native Brazilian word]

  de-emetinized i., i. from which the emetic principle has been extracted; has been used as an antidysenteric agent.

  prepared i., a fine powder to contain 2% of the total alkaloids of i., calculated as emetine.

IPF Abbreviation for idiopathic pulmonary *fibrosis* or interstitial pulmonary *fibrosis.*

ipo·date (ī′pō-dāt). A radiographic contrast medium, given orally as the sodium or, more often, the calcium salt, for opacification of the gallbladder and central biliary tree.

ip·o·mea (ī-pō-mē′ă). The dried root of *Ipomoea orizabensis* (family Convolvulaceae). SEE ALSO ipomea *resin.* SYN orizaba jalap root. [G. *ips* (*ip*-), a worm, + *homoios,* like]

Ip·o·moea (ī-pō-mē′ă). A plant genus of the family Convolvulaceae including the morning glory. [L. ipomea]

  I. **rubrocoeru′lea** var. **prae′cox,** the seeds contain lysergic acid amide, isolysergic acid amide, chanoclavine, elymoclavine, and other ergot (indole) alkaloids; ingestion of the seeds produces hallucinatory and euphoric effects. SYN morning glory (1).

  I. **versico′lor,** a species whose seeds contain hallucinogenic ergot (indole) alkaloids.

IPPB Abbreviation for intermittent positive pressure *breathing.*

IPPV Abbreviation for intermittent positive pressure *ventilation.*

ipra·tro·pi·um (i-pră-trō′pē-ŭm). A synthetic quaternary ammonium compound, chemically related to atropine, that has anticholinergic activity and is a bronchodilator given by inhalation.

ipro·ni·a·zid (ī-prō-nī′ă-zid). An antituberculous and antidepressant agent similar to isoniazid, but more toxic and rarely used; it inhibits monoamine oxidase. The first antidepressant agent.

ipro·ver·a·tril (ī-prō-ver′ă-tril). SYN verapamil.

iPrSGal Abbreviation for isopropylthiogalactoside.

Ips Abbreviation for pipsyl.

ip·se·fact (ip′se-fakt). All parts or aspects of the environment that an individual, colony, population, or species of animal has modified chemically or physically by its own behavior (e.g., a nest or home, rodent or deer runs, excrement, pheromones). [L. *ipse,* self, + *factum,* a thing done]

ip·si·lat·er·al (ip-si-lat′er-ăl). On the same side, with reference to a given point, e.g., a dilated pupil on the same side as an extradural hematoma with contralateral limbs being paretic. SYN homolateral. [L. *ipse,* same, + *latus* (*later*-), side]

IPSP Abbreviation for inhibitory postsynaptic *potential.*

IPTG Abbreviation for isopropylthiogalactoside.

IPV Abbreviation for inactivated poliovirus *vaccine.* SEE poliovirus *vaccines,* under *vaccine.*

IQ Abbreviation for intelligence *quotient.*

IR, ir Abbreviation for infrared.

Ir Symbol for iridium.

IRB Abbreviation for institutional review *board.*

△**irid-.** SEE irido-.

ir·i·dal (ī′ri-dăl, ir′i-dăl). Relating to the iris. SYN iridial, iridian, iridic.

ir·i·dec·to·my (ir′i-dek′tō-mē). **1.** Excision of a portion of the iris. **2.** The hole in the iris produced by a surgical iridectomy. [irido- + G. *ektomē,* excision]

  buttonhole i., SYN peripheral i.

  optical i., i. performed for the purpose of improving vision by making an artificial pupil.

  peripheral i., in narrow-angle glaucoma, the surgical removal of a minute portion of the iris at its root; in intracapsular extraction of cataract, removal of one or more minute sections near the peripheral border, leaving the pupillary margin intact. SYN buttonhole i., stenopeic i.

  sector i., an i. in which a portion of the pupillary margin is excised.

  stenopeic i., SYN peripheral i.

  therapeutic i., an i. performed for the prevention or cure of disease, e.g., angle-closure glaucoma.

ir·i·den·clei·sis (ir′i-den-klī′sis). The incarceration of a portion of the iris by corneoscleral incision in glaucoma to effect filtration between the anterior chamber and subconjunctival space. [irido- + G. *enkleiō,* to shut in]

ir·i·der·e·mia (ir′i-der-ē′mē′ă, ī′rid-). Condition wherein the iris is so rudimentary as to appear to be absent. Cf. aniridia. [irido- + G. *erēmia,* absence]

ir·i·des (ir′i-dēz). Plural of iris. [G.]

ir·i·des·cent (ir-i-des′ent). Presenting multiple bright refractile colors, typically as a result of optical interference when incident white light is broken into its spectral components when reflected back through several thin-layered films. [G. *iris,* rainbow]

irid·e·sis (i-rid′e-sis, ī-ri-dē′sis). Ligature of a portion of the iris brought out through an incision in the cornea. [irido- + G. *desis,* a binding together]

irid·i·ai, irid·i·an, irid·ic (ī-rid′ē-al; ī-rid′ē-an; ī-rid′ik, i-rid′-). SYN iridal.

ir·i·din (ir′i-din). **1.** Irigenin 7-glucoside from orris root, *Iris florentina.* **2.** A resinoid from blue flag, *Iris versicolor;* used as a cholagogue and cathartic. SYN irisin.

irid·i·um (Ir) (i-rid′ē-ŭm). A white, silvery metallic element, atomic no. 77, atomic wt. 192.22; ^{192}Ir is a radioisotope (half-life of 73.83 days) that has been used in the interstitial treatment of certain tumors. [L. *iris,* rainbow]

⌂**irido-, irid-.** The iris. [G. *iris (irid-),* rainbow]

ir·i·do·a·vul·sion (ir′i-dō-ă-vŭl′shŭn). Avulsion, or tearing away, of the iris.

ir·i·do·cele (ir′i-dō-sēl). Herniation of a portion of the iris through a corneal defect. [irido- + G. *kēlē,* hernia]

ir·i·do·cho·roid·i·tis (ir′i-dō-kō-roy-dī′tis). Inflammation of both iris and choroid.

ir·i·do·col·o·bo·ma (ir′i-dō-ko-lō-bō′mă). A coloboma or congenital defect of the iris. [irido- + G. *kolobōma,* coloboma]

ir·i·do·cor·ne·al (ir′i-dō-kōr′nē-ăl). Relating to the iris and the cornea.

ir·i·do·cy·clec·to·my (ir′i-dō-sī-klek′tō-mē). Removal of the iris and ciliary body for excision of a tumor. [irido- + G. *kyklos,* circle (ciliary body), + *ektomē,* excision]

ir·i·do·cy·cli·tis (ir′i-dō-sī-klī′tis). Inflammation of both iris and ciliary body. SEE ALSO iritis, uveitis. [irido- + G. *kyklos,* circle (ciliary body), + *-itis,* inflammation]
 i. sep′tica, SYN Behçet *syndrome.*

ir·i·do·cy·clo·cho·roid·i·tis (ir′i-dō-sī′klō-kō-royd-ī′tis). Inflammation of the iris, involving the ciliary body and the choroid.

ir·i·do·cys·tec·to·my (ir′i-dō-sis-tek′tō-mē). An operation for making an artificial pupil when posterior synechiae follow extracapsular extraction of cataract; the border of the iris and a portion of the capsule of the lens are drawn out through an incision in the cornea and cut off. [irido- + G. *kystis,* bladder (capsule), + *ektomē,* excision]

ir·i·do·di·ag·no·sis (ir′i-dō-dī-ag-nō′sis). Diagnosis of systemic diseases by observation of changes in form and color of the iris.

ir·i·do·di·al·y·sis (ir′i-dō-dī-al′i-sis). A colobomatous defect of the iris caused by its separation from the scleral spur. [irido- + G. *dialysis,* loosening]

ir·i·do·di·la·tor (ir′i-dō-dī-lā′ter). Causing dilation of the pupil; applied to the musculus dilator pupillae.

ir·i·do·do·ne·sis (ir′i-dō-dō-nē′sis). Agitated motion of the iris. SYN tremulous iris. [irido- + G. *doneō,* to shake to and fro]

ir·i·do·ki·net·ic (ir′i-dō-ki-net′ik). Relating to the movements of the iris.

ir·i·dol·o·gy (ir-i-dol′ō-jē). A hypothetical non–evidence-based system of medicine based on an examination of the iris, using a chart on which certain areas of the iris are presumed diagnostically specific for particular organs, systems, and structures. [irido- + G. *logos,* study]

ir·i·do·ma·la·cia (ir′i-dō-mă-lā′shē-ă). Degenerative softening of the iris. [irido- + G. *malakia,* softness]

ir·i·do·mes·o·di·al·y·sis (ir′i-dō-mes′ō-dī-al′i-sis). Separation of adhesions around the inner margin of the iris. [irido- + G. *mesos,* middle, + *dialysis,* loosening]

ir·i·do·mo·tor (ir′i-dō-mō′tŏr). SYN pupillomotor.

ir·i·do·pa·ral·y·sis (ir′i-dō-pă-ral′i-sis). SYN iridoplegia.

ir·i·dop·a·thy (ir-i-dop′ă-thē). Pathologic lesions in the iris.

ir·i·do·ple·gia (ir′i-dō-plē′jē-ă). Paralysis of the musculus sphincter iridis. SYN iridoparalysis. [irido- + G. *plēgē,* stroke]
 complete i., paralysis of both the dilator and sphincter muscles of the iris.
 reflex i., absence of the pupillary light reflex, as in the Argyll Robertson pupil.
 sympathetic i., i. due to the paralysis of the sympathetically innervated dilator pupillae muscle.

ir·i·dop·to·sis (ir′i-dop-tō′sis). Prolapse of the iris. [irido- + G. *ptōsis,* a falling]

ir·i·dor·rhex·is (ir′i-dō-rek′sis). Deliberate, surgical tearing of the iris from the scleral spur in order to increase the breadth of a coloboma. [irido- + G. *rhēxis,* rupture]

ir·i·dos·chi·sis (ir-i-dos′ki-sis). Separation of the anterior layer of the iris from the posterior layer; ruptured anterior fibers float in the aqueous humor. [irido- + G. *schisma,* cleft]

ir·i·do·scle·rot·o·my (ir′i-dō-skle-rot′ō-mē). An incision involving both sclera and iris. [irido- + sclera, + G. *tomē,* incision]

ir·i·dot·o·my (ir-i-dot′ō-mē). Transverse division of some of the fibers of the iris, forming an artificial pupil. [irido- + G. *tomē,* incision]
 laser i., peripheral iridectomy as performed by laser.

Ir·i·do·vir·i·dae (ir′i-do-vir′i-dē). A family of viruses including iridescent viruses of insects (Iridovirus) and viruses that infect frogs and fish. These viruses are large, icosahedral (120–170 nm in diameter), and contain lipid. The genome is a single molecule of double-stranded DNA with molecular weight of 130–160 × 10^6.

Ir·i·do·vi·rus (ir′i-dō-vī′rŭs). A genus of viruses (family Iridoviridae) comprised of the iridescent insect viruses of which the type species is the tipula iridescent virus.

iri·gen·in (i-ri-jen′in). A trihydroxy trimethoxy isoflavone component of iridin.

iris, pl. **ir·i·des** (ī′ris, ir′i-dēz) [TA]. The anterior division of the vascular tunic of the eye, a diaphragm, perforated in the center (the pupil), attached peripherally to the scleral spur; it is composed of stroma and a double layer of pigmented retinal epithelium from which are derived the sphincter and dilator muscles of the pupil. SYN orris. [G. rainbow, the iris of the eye]
 i. bicolor, a variegated or two-colored i. SYN monocular heterochromia.
 i. bombé, a condition occurring in posterior annular synechia, in which an increase of fluid in the posterior chamber causes a forward bulging of the peripheral i.
 plateau i., in angle-closure glaucoma, a flat appearance of the i. rather than a forward convexity.
 tremulous i., SYN iridodonesis.

iris frill. SYN collarette.

iri·sin (ī′ri-sin). SYN iridin (2).

irit·ic (ī-rit′ik). Relating to iritis.

iri·tis (ī-rī′tis). Inflammation of the iris. SEE ALSO iridocyclitis, uveitis.
 fibrinous i., acute inflammation of the iris, with profuse exudate; occurs in uveitis of tertiary syphilis.
 follicular i., rarely used term for chronic i. with glassy nodules situated deep down between the anterior and posterior layers of the iris.
 i. glaucomato′sa, an outpouring of exudate and cells after control of angle-closure glaucoma.
 hemorrhagic i., i. with such severe hyperemia that hyphema occurs.
 nodular i., i. with aggregations of round cells in the iris.
 plastic i., i. with a fibrinous exudation.
 quiet i., i. without inflammatory signs such as redness or edema of the cornea.
 serous i., inflammation of the iris, with a serous exudate in the anterior chamber.
 sympathetic i., i. consecutive to a similar condition in the other eye.

iron (Fe) (ī′ern, ī′rŭn). A metallic element, atomic no. 26, atomic wt. 55.847, that occurs in the heme of hemoglobin, myoglobin, transferrin, ferritin, and iron-containing porphyrins, and is an essential component of enzymes such as catalase, peroxidase, and the various cytochromes; its salts are used medicinally. For individual salts not listed below, see ferric and ferrous entries. [A.S. *iren*]
 albuminized i., i. albuminate, a compound of i. oxide and albumin; rendered soluble by the presence of sodium citrate; occurs as

ir

reddish brown, lustrous granules, odorless or nearly so; used in anemia.

i. alum, SYN *ferric* ammonium sulfate.

i. filings, small packets of *Paragonimus* spp. eggs that can be seen in the sputum; the egg clumps tend to be yellow-brown.

i. protoporphyrin, a protoporphyrin to which an i. atom is complexed; e.g., heme.

i. pyri′tes, native sulfide of i.

iron-52 (^{52}Fe). A radioactive iron isotope; a cyclotron-produced positron emitter with a half-life of 8.28 h, used to study iron metabolism.

iron-55 (^{55}Fe). An iron isotope; a positron emitter with a half-life of 2.73 years; used (less often than ^{59}Fe) as a tracer in study of iron metabolism and in blood perfusion studies.

iron-59 (^{59}Fe). An iron isotope; a gamma and beta emitter with a half-life of 44.51 days; used as tracer in the study of iron metabolism, determination of blood volume, and in blood transfusion studies.

ir·ra·di·ate (i-rā′dē-āt). To apply radiation from a source to a structure or organism. [see irradiation]

ir·ra·di·a·tion (i-rā-dē-ā′shŭn). 1. The subjective enlargement of a bright object seen against a dark background. 2. Exposure to the action of electromagnetic radiation (e.g., heat, light, x-rays). 3. The spreading of nervous impulses from one area in the brain or cord, or from a tract, to another tract. SEE ALSO radiation. [L. *ir-radio, (in-r)*, pp. *-radi-atus*, to beam forth]

ir·ra·tion·al (i-rash′ŭn-ăl). Not rational; unreasonable (contrary to reason) or unreasoning (not exercising reason). [L. *irrationalis*, without reason]

ir·re·duc·i·ble (ir-rē-doo′si-bl, i-rē-). 1. Not reducible; incapable of being made smaller. 2. In chemistry, incapable of being made simpler, or of being replaced, hydrogenated, or reduced in positive charge.

ir·re·spir·a·ble (ir-rē-spīr′ă-bl). 1. Incapable of being inhaled because of irritation to the airway, resulting in breath-holding. 2. Denoting a gas or vapor either poisonous or containing insufficient oxygen. 3. Denoting an aerosol composed of particles with aerodynamic size larger than 10 µ.

ir·re·spon·si·bil·i·ty (ir′rē-spons-i-bil′i-tē). The state of not acting in a manner that is responsible, for conscious or unconscious reasons.

criminal i., the state, usually attributed to mental defect or disease, that renders a person not responsible for criminal conduct.

ir·re·sus·ci·ta·ble (ir′rē-sŭs′i-tă-bl). Incapable of being revived.

ir·re·vers·i·ble (ir-rē-ver′si-bl). Incapable of being reversed; permanent. [L. *in-* (*ir-*) neg. + *re-verto*, pp. *-versus*, to turn back]

ir·ri·gate (ir′i-gāt). To perform irrigation. [L. *ir-rigo*, pp. *-atus*, to irrigate, fr. *in, on*, + *rigo*, to water]

ir·ri·ga·tion (ir-i-gā′shŭn). The washing out of a body cavity, space, or wound with a fluid. [see irrigate]

ir·ri·ga·tor (ir′i-gā-ter). An appliance used in irrigation.

ir·ri·ta·bil·i·ty (ir′i-tă-bil′i-tē). The property inherent in protoplasm of reacting to a stimulus. [L. *irritabilitas*, fr. *irrito*, pp. *-atus*, to excite]

electric i., the response of a nerve or muscle to the passage of a current of electricity; in cases of degeneration in nerve or muscle this i. is altered or lost. SEE modal *alteration*, qualitative *alteration*, quantitative *alteration*.

myotatic i., the ability of a muscle to contract in response to the stimulus produced by a sudden stretching.

ir·ri·ta·ble (ir′i-tă-bl). 1. Capable of reacting to a stimulus. 2. Tending to react immoderately to a stimulus. Cf. excitable.

ir·ri·tant (ir′i-tant). 1. Irritating; causing irritation. 2. Any agent with this action.

primary i., a substance that causes inflammation and other evidence of irritation, particularly of the skin, on first contact or exposure, or as a reaction to cumulative contacts, not dependent on a mechanism of sensitization.

ir·ri·ta·tion (ir-i-tā′shŭn). 1. Extreme incipient inflammatory reaction of the tissues to an injury. 2. The normal response of nerve

or muscle to a stimulus. 3. The evocation of a normal or exaggerated reaction in the tissues by the application of a stimulus. [L. *irritatio*]

ir·ri·ta·tive (ir-i-tā′tiv). Causing irritation.

ir·ru·ma·tion (ir′oo-mā′shŭn). SYN fellatio. [L. *irrumo*, pp. *-atus*, to give suck]

ir·rup·tion (i-rŭp′shŭn). Act or process of breaking through to a surface. [L. *irruptio*, fr. *irrumpo*, to break in]

ir·rup·tive (i-rŭp′tiv). Relating to or characterized by irruption.

IRS-1 Abbreviation for insulin receptor *substrate*-1.

IRV Abbreviation for inspiratory reserve *volume*.

Irvine, A. Ray, Jr., U.S. ophthalmologist, *1917. SEE I.-Gass *syndrome*.

ISA Abbreviation for intrinsic sympathomimetic *activity*.

Is·a·mine blue (is′ă-mēn, ī′să-). SYN pyrrol blue.

is·aux·e·sis (ī-sawk-zē′sis). Growth of parts at the same rate as growth of the whole. [G. *isos*, even, + *auxēsis*, increase]

is·che·mia (is-kē′mē-ă). Local anemia due to mechanical obstruction (mainly arterial narrowing or disruption) of the blood supply. [G. *ischō*, to keep back, + *haima*, blood]

myocardial i., inadequate circulation of blood to the myocardium, usually as a result of coronary artery disease. SEE ALSO angina pectoris, myocardial *infarction*.

postural i., the reduced blood pressure and flow induced in a part, e.g., the leg or foot, by raising it above the heart level; used to reduce bleeding during surgical operations on the extremities.

i. ret′inae, diminished blood supply in the retina due to failure of the arterial circulation; it may occur as a result of arterial embolism or spasm; poisoning, as by quinine; or exsanguination from recurring profuse hemorrhages; bilateral transitory or permanent blindness may result.

silent i., myocardial i. without accompanying signs or symptoms of angina pectoris; can be detected by ECG and other lab techniques. SEE ALSO silent myocardial *infarction*.

is·che·mic (is-kē′mik). Relating to or affected by ischemia.

is·che·sis (is-kē′sis). Suppression of any discharge, especially of a normal one. [G. *ischō*, to hold back]

is·chia (is′kē-ă). Plural of ischium.

is·chi·ad·ic (is-kē-ad′ik). SYN sciatic (1).

is·chi·a·di·cus (is-kē-ad′i-kŭs). SYN sciatic. [L.]

is·chi·al (is′kē-ăl). SYN sciatic (1).

is·chi·al·gia (is-kē-al′jē-ă). 1. Obsolete term for pain in the hip; specifically, the ischium. SYN ischiodynia. 2. Obsolete term for sciatica. [G. *ischion*, hip, + *algos*, pain]

is·chi·at·ic (is-kē-at′ik). SYN sciatic (1).

ischio-. The ischium. [G. *ischion*, hip joint, haunch (ischium)]

is·chi·o·a·nal (is-kē-ō-ā′năl). Relating to the ischium and the anus.

is·chi·o·bul·bar (is-kē-ō-bŭl′bar). Relating to the ischium and the bulb of the penis.

is·chi·o·cap·su·lar (is-kē-ō-kap′soo-lăr). Relating to the ischium and the capsule of the hip joint; denoting that part of the capsule which is attached to the ischium.

is·chi·o·cav·er·no·sus. SEE ischiocavernous (*muscle*).

is·chi·o·cav·ern·ous (is-kē-ō-kav′er-nŭs). Relating to the ischium and the corpus cavernosum.

is·chi·o·cele (is′kē-ō-sēl). SYN sciatic *hernia*. [ischio- + G. *kēlē*, hernia]

is·chi·o·coc·cyg·e·al (is-kē-ō-kok-sij′ē-ăl). Relating to the ischium and the coccyx.

is·chi·o·coc·cyg·e·us (is-kē-ō-kok-sij′ē-ŭs). SYN coccygeus *muscle*. SEE muscle.

is·chi·o·dyn·ia (is′kē-ō-din′ē-ă). SYN ischialgia (1). [ischio- + G. *odynē*, pain]

is·chi·o·fem·o·ral (is-kē-ō-fem′ŏ-răl). Relating to the ischium, or hip bone, and the femur, or thigh bone.

is·chi·o·fib·u·lar (is′kē-ō-fib′ū-lăr). Relating to or connecting the ischium and the fibula.

is·chi·o·me·lus (is-ki-om′ĕ-lŭs). Unequal conjoined twins in which the parasite, often only an arm or a leg, arises from the pelvic region of the autosite. SEE conjoined *twins*, under *twin*. [ischio- + G. *melos*, limb]

is·chi·o·ni·tis (is′kē-ō-nī′tis). Inflammation of the ischium.

is·chi·op·a·gus (is-kē-op′ă-gŭs). Conjoined twins united in their ischial region. SEE conjoined *twins*, under *twin*. [ischio- + G. *pagos*, fixed]

is·chi·o·per·i·ne·al (is′kē-ō-per-i-nē′ăl). Relating to the ischium and the perineum.

is·chi·o·pu·bic (is′kē-ō-poo′bik). Relating to both ischium and pubis.

is·chi·o·rec·tal (is′kē-ō-rek′tăl). Relating to the ischium and the rectum.

is·chi·o·sa·cral (is′kē-ō-sā′krăl). Relating to the ischium and the sacrum.

is·chi·o·tho·ra·cop·a·gus (is′kē-ō-thōr-ă-kop′ă-gŭs). SYN iliothoracopagus.

is·chi·o·tib·i·al (is′kē-ō-tib′ē-ăl). Relating to or connecting the ischium and the tibia.

is·chi·o·vag·i·nal (is-kē-ō-vaj′i-năl). Relating to the ischium and the vagina.

is·chi·o·ver·te·bral (is-kē-ō-ver′tĕ-brăl). Relating to the ischium and the vertebral column.

is·chi·um, gen. **is·chii**, pl. **is·chia** (is′kē-ŭm, is′kē-ī, is′kē-ă) [TA]. The lower and posterior part of the hip bone, distinct at birth but later becoming fused with the ilium and pubis; it consists of a body, where it joins the ilium and superior ramus of the pubis to form the acetabulum, and a ramus joining the inferior ramus of the pubis. SYN os ischii [TA], ischial bone. [Mod. L. fr. G. *ischion*, hip]

is·cho·chy·mia (is-kō-kī′mē-ă). Retention of food in the stomach due to dilation of that organ. [G. *ischō*, to keep back, + *chymos*, juice]

is·chu·ret·ic (is-koo-ret′ik). **1.** Relating to or relieving ischuria. **2.** An agent that relieves retention or suppression of urine.

is·chu·ria (is-koo′rē-ă). Retention or suppression of urine. [G. *ischō*, to keep back, + *ouron*, urine]

is·e·thi·o·nate (ī-sĕ-thī′ō-nāt). A salt or ester of isethionic acid.

is·e·thi·on·ic ac·id (ī′sĕ-thī-on′ik). 2-Hydroxyethanesulfonic acid; a colorless viscous liquid, miscible with water and alcohols, that forms crystalline salts with organic acids.

Ishak, SEE Luna-Ishak *stain*.

Ishihara, Shinobu, Japanese ophthalmologist, 1879–1963. SEE I. *test*.

ISI Abbreviation for international sensitivity *index*.

isin·glass (ī′zing-glas). SYN ichthyocolla. [Old Ger. *huysenblas*, sturgeon's bladder]

is·land (ī′land). In anatomy, any isolated part, separated from the surrounding tissues by a groove, or marked by a difference in structure. SYN insula (2) [TA]. [A.S. *īgland*]

> **blood i.,** an aggregation of splanchnic mesodermal cells on the embryonic yolk sac, with the potentiality of forming vascular endothelium and primitive blood cells. SYN blood islet.

> **bone i.,** a macroscopic focus of cortical bone within medullary bone, commonly seen as a dense round or oval opacity on radiographs of the pelvis, femoral head, humerus, or ribs.

> **i.'s of Calleja,** dense clusters of very small nerve cells (granule cells) characteristic of the olfactory tubercle at the base of the forebrain.

> **epimyoepithelial i.'s** (ep′ē-mī-ō-ep′ē-thē′lī-al), proliferation of salivary gland ductal epithelium and myoepithelium. Characteristic of benign lymphoepithelial lesions and Sjögren syndrome.

> **Langerhans i.'s,** SYN *islets* of Langerhans, under *islet*.

> **pancreatic i.'s,** SYN *islets* of Langerhans, under *islet*.

> **i. of Reil,** SYN insula (1).

is·let (i′let). A small island.

> **blood i.,** SYN blood *island*.

> **i.'s of Langerhans,** cellular masses varying from a few to hundreds of cells lying in the interstitial tissue of the pancreas; they are composed of different cell types that comprise the endocrine

portion of the pancreas and are the source of insulin and glucagon. SYN islet tissue, Langerhans islands, pancreatic islands, pancreatic i.'s.

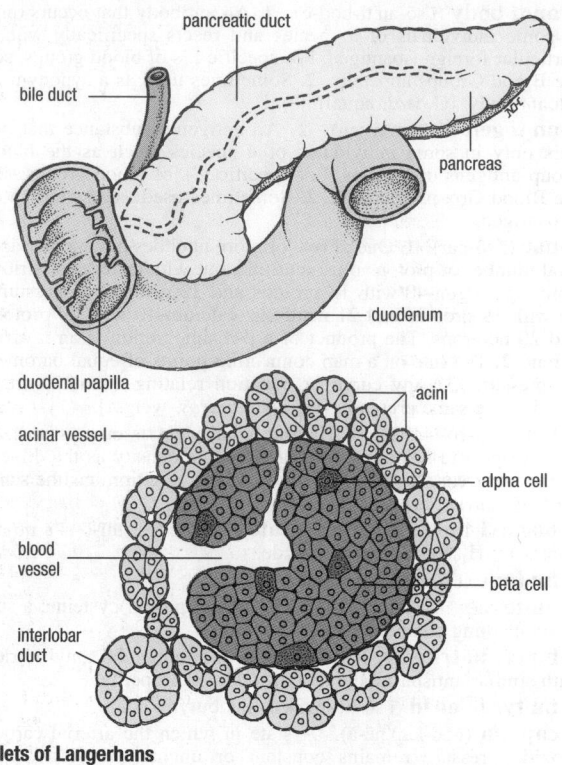

islets of Langerhans

pancreatic i.'s, SYN i.'s of Langerhans.

-ism. **1.** A condition, disease, or intoxication. **2.** A practice, doctrine. Cf. -ia, -ismus. [G. *-isma, -ismos,* noun-forming suffix]

-ismus. L. for -ism; customarily used to imply spasm, contraction. [L. fr. G. *-ismos,* suffix forming nouns of action]

iso-. **1.** Prefix meaning equal, like. **2.** In chemistry, prefix indicating "isomer of" (isomerism); e.g., isocyanate vs. cyanate. **3.** In immunology, prefix designating sameness with respect to species; in recent years, the meaning has shifted to sameness with respect to genetic constitution of individuals. [G. *isos,* equal]

iso·ac·cept·or tRNA (ī′sō-ak′sep-tor). Different tRNA species that bind to alternate codons for the same amino acid residue; can be one tRNA that recognizes the various codons that signify those for the particular amino acid residue.

iso·ag·glu·ti·na·tion (ī′sō-ă-gloo-ti-nā′shŭn). Agglutination of red blood cells as a result of the reaction between an isoagglutinin and specific antigen in or on the cells. SYN isohemagglutination. [iso- + L. *ad,* to, + *gluten,* glue]

iso·ag·glu·ti·nin (ī′sō-ă-gloo′ti-nin). An isoantibody that causes agglutination of cells of genetically different members of the same species. SYN isohemagglutinin.

iso·ag·glu·tin·o·gen (ī′sō-ă-gloo-tin′ō-jen). An isoantigen that induces agglutination of the cells to which it is attached upon exposure to its specific isoantibody.

iso·al·lele (ī′sō-ă-lēl′). One of a number of alleles that can be distinguished only by special analyses.

iso·al·lox·a·zine (ī′sō-ă-loks′ă-zēn). The heterocyclic compound that forms the structural foundation of riboflavin and other flavins.

iso·am·i·nile (ī-sō-am′i-nīl). An antitussive agent.

iso·am·yl (ī-sō-am′il). SEE amyl.

iso·am·y·lase (ī-sō-am′il-ās). A hydrolase that cleaves 1,6-α-D-glucosidic branch linkages in glycogen, amylopectin, and their β-limit dextrins; part of the complex known as debranching enzyme;

is

similar to α-dextrin endo-1,6-α-glucosidase but unable to act on pullulan.

iso·an·dros·ter·one (ī′sō-an-dros′ter-ōn). SYN epiandrosterone.

iso·an·ti·body (ī′sō-an′ti-bod-ē). **1.** An antibody that occurs only in some individuals of a species and reacts specifically with a particular foreign isoantigen. For specific i.'s of blood groups, see the Blood Groups appendix. **2.** Sometimes used as a synonym of alloantibody. [G. *isos*, equal]

iso·an·ti·gen (ī′sō-an′ti-jen). **1.** An antigenic substance that occurs only in some individuals of a species, such as the blood group antigens of humans. For specific i.'s of blood groups, see the Blood Groups appendix. **2.** Sometimes used as a synonym of alloantigen.

iso·bar (ī′sō-bar). **1.** One of two or more nuclides having the same total number of protons plus neutrons, but with different distribution; e.g., argon-40 with 18 protons and 22 neutrons, potassium-40 with 19 protons and 21 neutrons, calcium-40 with 20 protons and 20 neutrons. The product of a β-disintegration is an i. of its parent. **2.** The line on a map connecting points of equal barometric pressure. **3.** Any curve or equation relating quantities measured at the same pressure. [iso- + G. *baros*, weight]

iso·bar·ic (ī-sō-bar′ik). **1.** Having equal weights or pressures. **2.** With respect to solutions, having the same density as the diluent or medium; e.g., in spinal anesthesia, an i. solution has the same specific gravity as has spinal fluid.

iso·bor·nyl thi·o·cy·a·no·ac·e·tate (ī-sō-bōr′nil thī-ō-sī′ă-nō-as′ĕ-tāt). $C_{13}H_{19}NO_2S$; a pediculicide.

iso·bu·tane (ī′sō-bū′tān). SEE butane.

iso·bu·te·ine (ī-sō-bū′tē-ēn). *S*-(2-Carboxypropyl)cysteine; a sulfur-containing compound found in urine.

iso·bu·tyl ni·trite. A liquid present in commercial amyl nitrite, with similar antispasmodic and vasodilator properties.

iso·bu·tyr·ic ac·id (ī′sō-bū-tir′ik). SEE butyric acid.

iso·cap·nia (ī-sō-kap′nē-ă). A state in which the arterial carbon dioxide pressure remains constant or unchanged. [iso- + G. *kapnos*, vapor]

iso·cel·lu·lar (ī′sō-sel′ū-lăr). Composed of cells of equal size or of similar character. [iso- + L. *cellula*, dim. of *cella*, a storeroom]

iso·chor·ic (iī′sō-kōr′ik). SYN isovolumic. [iso- + G. *chōra*, space]

iso·chro·mat·ic (ī-sō-krō-mat′ik). **1.** Of uniform color. SYN isochroous. **2.** Denoting two objects of the same color. [iso- + G. *chrōma*, color]

iso·chro·mat·o·phil, iso·chro·mat·o·phile (ī′sō-krō-mat′ō-fil, fīl). Having an equal affinity for the same dye; said of cells or tissues. [iso- + G. *chrōma*, color, + *philos*, fond]

iso·chro·mo·some (ī′sō-krō′mō-sōm). A chromosomal aberration that arises as a result of transverse rather than longitudinal division of the centromere during meiosis; two daughter chromosomes are formed, each lacking one chromosome arm but with the other doubled.

iso·chro·nia (ī-sō-krō′nē-ă). **1.** The state of having the same chronaxie. **2.** Agreement, with respect to time, rate, or frequency, between processes. [iso- + G. *chronos*, time]

isoch·ro·nous (ī-sok′rŏ-nŭs). Occurring during the same time.

isoch·ro·ous (ī-sok′rŏ-ŭs). SYN isochromatic (1).

iso·cit·rase, iso·cit·ra·tase (ī-sō-sit′rās, -sit′ră-tās). SYN *isocitrate* lyase.

iso·ci·trate (ī-sō-sit′rāt). (ī-sīt′rāt) A salt or ester of isocitric acid.

i. dehydrogenase, one of two enzymes that catalyze the conversion of *threo*-D₈-isocitrate, the product of the action of both aconitase and isocitrate lyase, to α-ketoglutarate (2-oxoglutarate) and CO_2; one of the isozymes uses NAD^+ (participating in the tricarboxylic acid cycle), while the other uses $NADP^+$. SYN isocitric acid dehydrogenase, oxalosuccinic carboxylase.

i. lyase, an enzyme that catalyzes the reversible aldol condensation of glyoxylate and succinate, forming *threo*-D₈-isocitrate; participates in the glyoxylate cycle. SYN isocitrase, isocitratase, isocitritase.

iso·cit·ric ac·id (ī-sō-sit′rik). An intermediate in the tricarboxylic acid cycle.

i. a. dehydrogenase, SYN *isocitrate* dehydrogenase.

iso·cit·ri·tase (ī-sō-sit′ri-tās). SYN *isocitrate* lyase.

iso·cline (ī′sō-klīn). A line in a geographical region that joins all points at which in a population there is the same average frequency for the various alleles at a genetic locus. SEE ALSO cline. [iso- + G. *klinō*, to slope]

iso·con·a·zole (ī′sō-kō′nă-zōl). Antibacterial and antifungal related to ketoconazole and oxiconazole.

iso·co·ria (ī-sō-kō′rē-ă). Equality in the size of the two pupils. [iso- + G. *korē*, pupil]

iso·cor·tex (ī-sō-kōr′teks) [TA]. O. and C. Vogt term for the larger part of the mammalian cerebral cortex, distinguished from the allocortex by being composed of a larger number of nerve cells arranged in six layers. SEE ALSO cerebral *cortex*. SYN neocortex [TA], homotypic cortex, neopallium.

iso·cy·a·nate (ī-sō-sī′ă-nāt). The radical –N=C=O from isocyanic acid.

iso·cy·an·ic ac·id (ī-sō-sī′ă-nik). A highly reactive chemical, HNCO.

iso·cy·a·nide (ī-sō-sī′ă-nīd). The radical –NC; organic i.'s are called isonitriles.

iso·cy·tol·y·sin (ī′sō-sī-tol′i-sin). A cytolysin that reacts with the cells of certain other animals of the same species, but not with the cells of the individual that formed the i.

iso·dac·tyl·ism (ī-sō-dak′ti-lizm). Condition in which the fingers or toes are all approximately of equal length. [iso- + G. *daktylos*, finger]

iso·dense (ī′sō-dens). Denoting a tissue having a radiopacity (radiodensity) similar to that of another or adjacent tissue.

iso·des·mo·sine (ī-sō-des′mō-sēn). A cross-linking amino acid formed from lysyl residues; found in elastin.

isodose. Area of equivalent radiation dose. [iso- + dose]

iso·dul·cit (ī-sō-dŭl′sit). SYN L-rhamnose.

iso·dy·nam·ic (ī′sō-dī-nam′ik). **1.** Of equal force or strength. **2.** Relating to foods or other materials that liberate the same amount of energy on combustion. [iso- + G. *dynamis*, force]

iso·dy·na·mo·gen·ic (ī′sō-dī-nă-mō-jen′ik, -dī-nam′ō-). **1.** SYN isoenergetic. **2.** Producing equal nerve force. [iso- + G. *dynamis*, force, + -*gen*, producing]

iso·e·lec·tric (ī′sō-ē-lek′trik). Of equal electrical potential. Cf. isoelectric *point*. SYN isopotential.

i. focusing, electrophoresis of small molecules or macromolecules in a pH gradient.

iso·en·er·get·ic (ī′sō-en-er-jet′ik). Exerting equal force; equally active. SYN isodynamogenic (1).

iso·en·zyme (ī-sō-en′zīm). One of a group of enzymes that catalyze the same reaction but may be differentiated by variations in physical properties, such as isoelectric point, electrophoretic mobility, kinetic parameters, or modes of regulation; e.g., lactate dehydrogenase, a tetramer composed of varying amounts of α and β subunits (i.e., 4α, 3α + 1β, 2α + 2β, 1α + 3β, and 4β). SYN isozyme.

creatine kinase i.'s, the isoenzymes of creatine kinase. Creatine kinase is a dimer with M (muscle) and/or B (brain) subunits; it exists in three isoenzyme forms: CK-MM, the predominant form, found primarily in skeletal muscle; CK-MB, found in cardiac muscle, tongue, diaphragm, and in small amounts in skeletal muscle; and CK-BB found in the brain, smooth muscle, thyroid, lungs, and prostate. Elevations detected by electrophoresis or other methodologies can be used to help in the differential diagnosis of a variety of disease states, with CK-MB elevations as an important marker following myocardial infarctions, elevations in CK-MM an indicator of muscle disease, and increases in CK-BB an occasional finding following brain infarcts, bowel infarcts, or in the presence of certain malignancies.

iso·e·ryth·rol·y·sis (ī′sō-ĕ-rith-rol′i-sis). Destruction of erythrocytes by isoantibodies. [iso- + erythrocyte = G. *lysis*, dissolution] **neonatal i., (1)** i. in the newborn animal; **(2)** hemolytic icterus of the newborn.

iso·flu·or·phate (ī-sō-flōr′fāt). A toxic cholinergic agent that acts by irreversible inhibition of cholinesterase; an ophthalmic cholinergic agent used in the treatment of glaucoma; also used in biochemical research as an enzyme inhibitor. SYN diisopropyl fluorophosphate.

iso·flu·rane (ī-sō-floor'ān). A nonflammable, nonexplosive, halogenated ether with potent anesthetic action; an isomer of enflurane.

iso·ga·mete (ī-sō-gam'ēt). **1.** One of two or more similar cells that conjugate or fuse and subsequently divide, resulting in reproduction. **2.** A gamete of the same size as the gamete with which it unites. [iso- + G. *gametēs* or *gametē*, husband or wife]

isog·a·my (ī-sog'ă-mē). Conjugation between two equal gametes or two individual cells alike in all respects. [iso- + G. *gamos*, marriage]

iso·ge·ne·ic, iso·gen·ic (ī'sō-jĕ-nē'ik, -jen'ik). SYN syngeneic.

isog·e·nous (ī-soj'ĕ-nŭs). Of the same origin, as in development from the same tissue or cell. [iso- + G. *genos*, family, kind]

iso·gen·ti·o·bi·ose (ī'sō-jen-shi-ō-bī'ōs). SYN isomaltose.

iso·glu·ta·mine (ī-sō-gloo'tă-mēn). A glutamic amide.

iso·gna·thous (ī-sog'nā-thŭs). Having jaws of approximately the same width. [iso- + G. *gnathos*, jaw]

iso·graft (ī'sō-graft). SYN syngraft.

iso·he·mag·glu·ti·na·tion (ī'sō-hē'mă-gloo'ti-nā'shŭn). SYN isoagglutination. [iso- + G. *haima*, blood, + L. *ad*, to, + *gluten*, glue]

iso·he·mag·glu·ti·nin (ī'sō-hē'mă-gloo'ti-nin). SYN isoagglutinin.

iso·he·mo·ly·sin (ī'sō-hē-mol'i-sin). An isolysin that reacts with red blood cells.

iso·he·mol·y·sis (ī'sō-hē-mol'i-sis). A form of isolysis in which there is dissolution of red blood cells as a result of the reaction between an isolysin (isohemolysin) and specific antigen in or on the cells. [iso- + G. *haima*, blood, + *lysis*, dissolution]

iso·hy·dric (ī-sō-hī'drik). Denoting two substances possessing the same pH.

iso·hy·dru·ria (ī'sō-hī-droo'rē-ă). Fixation of the pH of the urine without the usual variation. [iso- + G. *hydor*, water, + *ouron*, urine, + -ia]

iso·im·mu·ni·za·tion (ī'sō-im'ū-nī-zā'shŭn). Development of a significant titer of specific antibody as a result of antigenic stimulation with material contained on or in the red blood cells of another individual of the same species; e.g., i. is likely to occur when an Rh-negative person is treated with a transfusion of Rh-positive blood from another human being, or an Rh-negative woman has a pregnancy in which the fetus inherits Rh-positive red blood cells.

iso·late (ī'sō-lāt). **1.** To separate, to set apart from others; that which is so treated. **2.** To free of chemical contaminants. **3.** In psychoanalysis, to separate ideas, experiences, or memories from the affects pertaining to them. **4.** In group psychotherapy, an individual who is not responded to by others in the group. **5.** Viable organisms separated on a single occasion from a sample taken from a host or culture system. **6.** A population that for geographic, linguistic, cultural, social, religious, or other reasons is subject to little or no gene flow. SYN genetic i. [It. *isolare*; Mediev. L. *insulo*, pp. *-atus*, to insulate, fr. L. *insula*, island]

genetic i., SYN isolate (6).

mating i., a population separated from its neighbors by any means so that all or most matings occur within the population group.

iso·la·tion. **1.** In microbiology, separation of an organism from others, usually by making serial cultures. **2.** Separation for the period of communicability of infected persons or animals from others, so as to prevent or limit the direct or indirect transmission of the infectious agent from those who are infected to those who are susceptible.

iso·lec·i·thal (ī-sō-les'i-thăl). Denoting an ovum in which there is a moderate amount of uniformly distributed yolk.

iso·leu·cine (I) (ī-sō-loo'sēn). 2-Amino-3-methylvaleric acid; the L-amino acid found in almost all proteins; an isomer of leucine and, like it, a dietary essential amino acid.

iso·leu·cyl (ī-sō-loo'sil). The acyl radical of isoleucine.

iso·leu·ko·ag·glu·ti·nin (ī'sō-loo'kō-ă-gloo'ti-nin). Abnormal

antibody in the blood of some persons, capable of agglutinating human leukocytes.

isol·o·gous (lī-sol'ō-gŭs). SYN syngeneic. [iso- + G. *logos*, ratio]

isol·y·sin (ī-sol'i-sin). An antibody that combines with, sensitizes, and results in complement-fixation and dissolution of cells that contain the specific isoantigen; i.'s occur in the blood of some members of a species and they react with the cells of that species, but not with the cells of the individual (or the same type) in which the i.'s are naturally formed.

isol·y·sis (ī-sol'i-sis). Lysis or dissolution of cells as a result of the reaction between an isolysin and specific antigen in or on the cells. SEE ALSO isohemolysis. [iso- + G. *lysis*, dissolution]

iso·lyt·ic (ī-sō-lit'ik). Pertaining to, characterized by, or causing isolysis.

iso·malt·ase (ī-sō-mal'tās). SYN oligo-α-1,6-glucosidase. SEE ALSO sucrose α-D-glucohydrolase.

iso·malt·ose (ī-sō-mal'tōs). A disaccharide in which two glucose molecules are attached by an α-1,6 link, rather than an α-1,4 link as in maltose. SYN isogentiobiose.

iso·mas·ti·gote (ī-sō-mas'ti-gōt). Denoting a protozoan having two or four flagella of equal length at one extremity. [iso- + G. *mastix*, whip]

iso·mer (ī'sō-mer). **1.** One of two or more substances displaying isomerism (q.v.); e.g., L-glucose and D-glucose or citrate and isocitrate. Cf. stereoisomer. **2.** One of two or more nuclides having the same atomic and mass numbers but differing in energy states for a finite period of time; e.g., ^{99m}Tc and ^{99}Tc. [iso- + G. *meros*, part]

geometric i., SEE geometric *isomerism*.

isom·er·ase (ī-som'er-ās). A class of enzymes (EC class 5) catalyzing the conversion of a substance to an isomeric form; e.g., glucosephosphate isomerase.

iso·mer·ic (ī-sō-mār'ik). Relating to or characterized by isomerism. SYN isomerous.

isom·er·ism (ī-som'er-izm). The existence of a chemical compound in two or more forms that are identical with respect to percentage composition but differ as to the positions of one or more atoms within the molecules, as well as in physical and chemical properties.

geometric i., a form of i. displayed by unsaturated or ring compounds where free rotation about a bond (usually a carbon-carbon bond) is restricted; e.g., the i. of a *cis*- or *trans*- compound as in oleic acid and elaidic acid. Cf. cis-, entgegen, trans-, zusammen.

optic i., stereoisomerism involving the arrangement of substituents about an asymmetric atom or atoms (usually carbon) so that there is a difference in the behavior of the various isomers with regard to the extent of their rotation of the plane of polarized light. Cf. stereoisomerism.

stereochemical i., SYN stereoisomerism.

structural i., i. involving the same atoms in different arrangements; e.g., the butyric acids, leucine and isoleucine, glucose and fructose.

isom·er·i·za·tion (ī-som'er-ī-zā'shŭn). A process in which one isomer is formed from another, as in the action of isomerases.

enzyme i., reversible changes in enzyme conformation.

isom·er·ous (ī-som'er-ŭs). SYN isomeric.

iso·meth·a·done (ī-sō-meth'ă-dōn). A narcotic analgesic.

iso·meth·ep·tene (ī'sō-meth-ep'ten). An unsaturated aliphatic sympathomimetic amine with antispasmodic and vasoconstrictor actions.

iso·met·ric (ī-sō-met'rik). **1.** Of equal dimensions. **2.** In physiology, denoting the condition when the ends of a contracting muscle are held fixed so that contraction produces increased tension at a constant overall length. Cf. auxotonic, isotonic (3), isovolumic. [iso- + G. *metron*, measure]

iso·me·tro·pia (ī'sō-me-trō'pē-ă). Equality in refraction in the two eyes. [iso- + G. *metron*, measure, + *ōps* (*ōp-*), eye]

iso·mor·phic (ī-sō-mōr'fik). SYN isomorphous.

iso·mor·phism (ī-sō-mōr'fizm). Similarity of form between two or more organisms or between parts of the body. [iso- + G. *morphē*, shape]

iso·mor·phous (ī-sō-mōr'fŭs). Having the same form or shape, or being morphologically equal. SYN isomorphic.

iso·naph·thol (ī-sō-naf'thol). SEE naphthol.

ison·cot·ic (ī-son-kot'ik). Of equal oncotic pressure.

iso·ni·a·zid (ī-sō-nī'ă-zid). Isonicotinic acid hydrazide; first-line and probably most commonly used antituberculosis drug. Organisms rapidly develop resistance against this drug if it is used alone in the treatment of active disease. Hepatic toxicity is the major side effect.

iso·nic·o·tin·ic ac·id (ī-sō-nik-ō-tin'ik). The substance of which the hydrazide is isoniazid.

iso·ni·trile (ī-sō-nī'tril). An organic isocyanide.

iso·ni·tro·so·ac·e·tone (ī'sō-nī-trō-sō-as'ĕ-tōn). A cholinesterase reactivator that can penetrate the blood-brain barrier readily and cause significant reactivation of phosphorylated acetylcholinesterase in the central nervous system; used to protect human beings and animals against otherwise lethal poisoning with organophosphorous anticholinesterase agents. SYN monoisonitrosoacetone, pyruvaldoxine.

iso·os·mot·ic (ī'sō-os-mot'ik). SYN isosmotic.

isop·a·thy (ī-sop'ă-thē). Treatment of disease by means of the causal agent or a product of the same disease; or treatment of a diseased organ by an extract of a similar organ from a healthy animal. SEE ALSO homeopathy. [iso- + G. *pathos,* suffering]

iso·pen·ten·yl·py·ro·phos·phate (ī-sō-pen-tēn-il'pī-rō-fos'fāt). An intermediate in the biosynthesis of steroids, terpenes, dolichol, and prenylated proteins.

iso·pen·tyl (ī-sō-pen'til). SEE amyl.

iso·pep·tide (ī-sō-pep'tīd). SEE isopeptide *bond.*

isoph·a·gy (ī-sof'ă-jē). SYN autolysis. [iso- + G. *phagō,* to eat]

iso·plas·sonts (ī-sō-plas'onts). Like-formed entities having certain features in common. [iso- + G. *plassō,* to form]

iso·plas·tic (ī-sō-plas'tik). SYN syngeneic. [iso- + G. *plassō,* to form]

iso·pleth (ī'sō-pleth). A line on a Cartesian nomogram consisting of all points that represent a particular value of a variable; e.g., an isobar is an i. for a particular pressure.

iso·po·ten·tial (ī'sō-pō-ten'chŭl). SYN isoelectric.

iso·pre·cip·i·tin (ī'sō-prē-sip'i-tin). An antibody that combines with and precipitates soluble antigenic material in the plasma or serum, or in an extract of the cells, from another member, but not all members, of the same species. [iso- + precipitin]

iso·pren·a·line hy·dro·chlo·ride (ī-sō-pren'ă-lēn). SYN isoproterenol hydrochloride.

iso·pren·a·line sul·fate. SYN isoproterenol sulfate.

iso·prene (ī'sō-prēn). 2-Methyl-1,3-butadiene; an unsaturated five-carbon hydrocarbon with a branched chain, which in the plant and animal kingdom is used as the basis for the formation of isoprenoids; e.g., terpenes, carotenoids and related pigments, rubber. Fat-soluble vitamins either are isoprenoid or have isoprenoid side chains; steroids are synthesized via isoprenoid intermediates as are ubiquinone, dolichol, and prenylated proteins.

iso·pre·noids (ī-sō-prēn'oydz). Polymers whose carbon skeletons consist in whole or in large part of isoprene units joined end to end; e.g., carotene, lycopene, vitamin A. Vitamins K and E and the coenzymes Q have isoprenoid side chains.

iso·pre·nyl·a·tion (ī-sō-pren'il-ā'shun). SEE prenylation.

iso·pro·pa·nol (ī-sō-prō'pă-nol). SYN isopropyl alcohol.

iso·pro·phen·a·mine hy·dro·chlo·ride (ī'sō-prō-fen'ă-mēn). SYN clorprenaline hydrochloride.

iso·pro·pyl al·co·hol (ī-sō-prō'pil). An isomer of propyl alcohol and a homologue of ethyl alcohol, similar in its properties, when used externally, to the latter, but more toxic when taken internally; used as an ingredient of various cosmetics and of medicinal preparations for external use; also available as isopropyl rubbing alcohol, which contains 68 to 72% of isopropyl alcohol (by volume) in water; used as a rubefacient. SYN dimethylcarbinol, isopropanol.

iso·pro·pyl·ar·te·re·nol hy·dro·chlo·ride (ī-sō-prō'pil-ar-ter'ĕ-nol). SYN isoproterenol hydrochloride.

iso·pro·pyl·car·bi·nol (ī'sō-prō-pil-kar'bin-ol). SEE *butyl* alcohol.

iso·pro·pyl myr·is·tate (ī-sō-prō'pil). A pharmaceutic aid used in topical medicinal preparations to promote absorption through the skin.

iso·pro·pyl·thi·o·ga·lac·to·side (iPrSGal, IPTG) (ī-sō-prō'pil-thī'ō-gă-lak'tō-sīd). An artificial galactoside capable of inducing β-galactosidase in *Escherichia coli* without being split, as are the natural substrates such as lactose.

iso·pro·te·re·nol hy·dro·chlo·ride (ī'sō-prō-ter'ĕ-nol). A sympathomimetic β-receptor stimulant possessing the cardiac excitatory, but not the vasoconstrictor, actions of epinephrine. Chemically it differs from epinephrine in having an isopropyl group replacing the methyl group attached to the nitrogen atom; used in the treatment of bronchial asthma and heart block, including Adams-Stokes attacks. SYN isoprenaline hydrochloride, isopropylarterenol hydrochloride.

iso·pro·te·re·nol sul·fate. Used for inhalation as an aerosol in the treatment of acute asthmatic attacks and chronic pulmonary emphysema; now rarely used because less toxic, more specific agents are preferred. SYN isoprenaline sulfate.

isop·ter (ī-sop'ter). A line of equal retinal sensitivity in the visual field. [iso- + G. *optēr,* observer]

iso·pyk·nic (ī-sō-pik'nik). Having the same density. [iso- + G. *phknos,* thick, dense, + -ic]

iso·py·ro·cal·cif·er·ol (ī-sō-pī'rō-cal-sif'er-ol). 9β-Ergosterol; a thermal decomposition product of calciferol; a stereoisomer of pyrocalciferol and ergosterol.

iso·quin·o·line (ī-sō-kwin'ō-lēn). **1.** Ring structure characteristic of the group of opium alkaloids represented by papaverine. **2.** A class of alkaloids containing the i. (1) ring structure.

iso·ri·bo·fla·vin (ī'sō-rī'bō-flā-vin). 8-Demethyl-6-methylriboflavin; a riboflavin antimetabolite, differing from riboflavin in that the methyl groups on the isoalloxazine nucleus are in the 6,7 positions rather than the 7,8.

isor·rhea (ī-sō-rē'ă). Equality of intake and output of water; maintenance of water equilibrium. [iso- + G. *rhoia,* a flow]

isos·best·ic (ī-sos-bes'tik). Denoting the wavelength of light at which two related compounds have identical extinction coefficients; e.g., the wavelength at which the absorption spectra of hemoglobin and oxyhemoglobin cross is their i. point. Spectrophotometry at that wavelength measures total concentration of hemoglobin, regardless of the extent to which it might be oxygenated. [Ger. *isosbestisch,* fr. G. *isos,* equal, + *sbestos,* extinguished]

iso·schiz·o·mer (ī-sō-skiz'ō-mer). A restriction endonuclease from different organisms that recognizes and hydrolyzes at the same DNA sequence. [jiso- + G. *schizō* to split, + -mer]

iso·sen·si·tize (ī-sō-sen'si-tīz). SYN autosensitize.

iso·sex·u·al (ī-sō-sek'shoo-ăl). Descriptive of an individual's somatic characteristics, or of processes occurring within, that are consonant with the sex of that individual.

is·os·mot·ic (ī'sos-mot'ik). Having the same total osmotic pressure or osmolality as another fluid (ordinarily intracellular fluid); such a fluid is not isotonic if it includes solutes that freely permeate cell membranes. SYN iso-osmotic.

iso·sor·bide. A compound with diuretic properties prepared by acid dehydration of D-glucitol.

iso·sor·bide di·ni·trate (ī-sō-sōr'bīd dī-nī'trāt). A coronary vasodilator that acts via the formation of nitric oxide.

Isos·po·ra (ī-sos'pō-ră). A genus of coccidia (family Eimeriidae, class Sporozoea), with species chiefly in mammals; the ripe oocysts contain two sporocysts, each of which contains four sporozoites. This genus is now known to be closely related to *Toxoplasma* and *Sarcocystis,* with a similar sexual phase in the life cycle and a similar apical complex. [iso- + G. *sporos,* seed]

I. bel'li, a relatively rare species occurring in the small intestine of man, most common in the tropics but probably of worldwide distribution; most infections are subclinical, but sometimes they may cause mucous diarrhea.

I. bigem'ina, a species that occurs in the small intestine of the dog, cat, fox, mink, and possibly other carnivores; the most pathogenic coccidium in dogs and cats, causing enteritis and diarrhea; the oocysts are usually sporulated when passed in the feces, but are indistinguishable from those of *Toxoplasma gondii*, so considerable question remains as to the status of these parasites.

I. ca′nis, a species of worldwide distribution that is mildly pathogenic in dogs and is not infective in cats.

I. fe′lis, a species found in the small intestine and sometimes the cecum and colon of cats, lions, and other felids; it is only slightly, if at all, pathogenic in cats and is not infective in dogs.

I. rivol′ta, a species that occurs in the small intestine of dogs, cats, dingos, and probably other wild carnivores; pathogenic capabilities are similar to those of *I. bigemina*.

I. su′is, a species that affects the small intestine of the pig, producing mild diarrhea.

isos·po·ri·a·sis (ī-sos-pō-rī′ă-sis). Disease caused by infection with a species of *Isospora,* such as *I. belli* of humans; human disease usually is mild except in cases of immunodeficiency, as in AIDS, where it may cause an intractable diarrhea.

iso·stere (ī′sō-stēr). One of two or more atoms or molecules having the same electron arrangement; e.g., N_2 and CO. [iso- + G. *stereos,* solid]

iso·stery (ī-sō-stēr′ē). Physiological enzyme or metabolic regulation via competitive inhibition by structural analogs of natural substrates.

isos·the·nu·ria (ī-sos′thē-noo′rē-ă, ī′sō-sthē-). A state in chronic renal disease in which the kidney cannot form urine with a higher or a lower specific gravity than that of protein-free plasma; specific gravity of the urine becomes fixed around 1.010, irrespective of the fluid intake. [iso- + G. *sthenos,* strength, + *ouron,* urine]

iso·suc·cin·ic ac·id (ī′sō-sŭk-sin′ik). SYN methylmalonic acid.

iso·sul·fan blue (ī-sō-sŭl′fan). A dye used as a radiographic adjunct to mark lymphatic vessels during lymphography.

iso·ther·mal (ī-sō-ther′măl). Having the same temperature. [iso- + G. *thermē,* heat]

iso·thi·o·cy·a·nate (ī′sō-thī-ō-sī′ă-nāt). The radical of isothiocyanic acid, –N=C=S.

iso·thi·pen·dyl (ī′sō-thī-pen′dil). An H_1 antihistaminic.

iso·tone (ī′sō-tōn). One of several nuclides having the same number of neutrons in their nuclei; e.g., $^{39}_{19}K$ and $^{40}_{20}Ca$ with 20 each, $^{56}_{26}Fe$ and $^{58}_{28}Ni$ with 30 each. [iso- + G. *tonos,* stretching, tension]

iso·to·nia (ī-sō-tō′nē-ă). A condition of tonic equality in which tension or osmotic pressure in two substances or solutions is the same. [iso- + G. *tonos,* tension]

iso·ton·ic (ī-sō-ton′ik). **1.** Relating to isotonicity or isotonia. **2.** Having equal tension; denoting solutions possessing the same osmotic pressure; more specifically, limited to solutions in which cells neither swell nor shrink. Thus, a solution that is isosmotic with intracellular fluid will not be i. if it includes solute, such as urea, that freely permeates cell membranes. **3.** In physiology, denoting the condition when a contracting muscle shortens against a constant load, as when lifting a weight. Cf. auxotonic, isometric (2).

iso·to·nic·i·ty (ī-sō-tō-nis′i-tē). **1.** The quality of possessing and maintaining a uniform tone or tension. **2.** The property of a solution being isotonic.

iso·tope (ī′sō-tōp). One of two or more nuclides that are chemically identical, having the same number of protons, yet differ in mass number, since their nuclei contain different numbers of neutrons; individual i.'s are named with the inclusion of their mass number in the superior position (^{12}C) and the atomic number (nuclear protons) in the inferior position ($_6C$). In former usage, the mass numbers follow the chemical symbol (C-12). [iso- + G. *topos,* part, place]

    daughter i., an element produced by radioactive decay of another. SEE radionuclide *generator,* cow.

    radioactive i., an i. with an unstable nuclear composition; such nuclei decompose spontaneously by emission of a nuclear electron (β particle) or helium nucleus (α particle) and radiation (γ rays), thus achieving a stable nuclear composition; used as tracers and as radiation and energy sources. SEE half-life.

stable i., a nonradioactive nuclide; an i. that shows no tendency to undergo radioactive decomposition.

iso·to·pic (ī-sō-top′ik). Of identical chemical composition but differing in some physical property, such as atomic weight.

iso·trans·plan·ta·tion (ī′sō-tranz-plan-tā′shŭn). Transfer of an isograft (syngraft).

iso·tret·i·noin (ī-sō-tret′i-noyn). A retinoid used for treatment of severe recalcitrant cystic acne; a known human teratogen.

iso·tro·pic, isot·ro·pous (ī-sō-trop′ik, ī-sot′rō-pŭs). Having properties that are the same in all directions. [iso- + G. *tropē,* a turn]

iso·type (ī′sō-tīp). An antigenic determinant (marker) that occurs in all members of a class or subclass in the heavy chains of an immunoglobulin or in the type and subtype of light chains of an immunoglobulin molecule. Whereas a given allotypic marker or determinant is thought to occur in only one subclass, an antigenic marker that is isotypic in one subclass may also occur as an allotypic marker in another subclass. [iso- + G. *typos,* model]

iso·typ·ic (ī-sō-tip′ik). Pertaining to an isotype.

iso·va·ler·ic ac·id (ī′so-vă-lār′ik, -lēr′ik). 3-Methylbutyric acid; a metabolic intermediate in oxidative processes; elevated in cases of isovaleric acidemia.

iso·va·ler·ic ac·i·de·mia [MIM*243500]. An inborn error of leucine metabolism characterized by psychomotor retardation, a specific odor reminiscent of sweaty feet, vomiting, acidosis, and coma; associated with excessive production of isovaleric acid upon protein ingestion or during infectious episodes and is due to a deficiency of isovaleryl-CoA dehydrogenase; severe metabolic acidosis results from the large quantities of acid formed. Autosomal recessive inheritance; two forms are known: 1) the acute neonatal form with fulminant metabolic acidosis and rapid death, and 2) the chronic form characterized by intermittent episodes of severe ketoacidosis. SYN sweaty feet syndrome.

iso·va·ler·yl-CoA (ī-sō-văl′er-il). The condensation product of isovaleric acid and coenzyme A; an intermediate in the catabolism of L-leucine. SYN isovalerylcoenzyme A.

    i.-CoA dehydrogenase, an enzyme that participates in the catabolism of L-leucine; it converts i.-CoA to 3-methylcrotonyl-CoA using FAD; a deficiency in this enzyme will result in isovaleric acidemia.

iso·va·ler·yl·co·en·zyme A. SYN isovaleryl-CoA.

iso·val·thine (ī-sō-val′thēn). A sulfur-containing compound found in urine.

iso·vol·ume (ī-sō-vol′ūm). At the same or equal volume. SEE ALSO isovolumic.

iso·vol·u·met·ric (ī′sō-vol-ū-met′rik). SYN isovolumic.

iso·vol·u·mic (ī′sō-vol-ū′mik). Occurring without an associated alteration in volume, as when, in early ventricular systole, the muscle fibers initially increase their tension without shortening so that ventricular volume remains unaltered. SEE ALSO isometric. SYN isochoric, isovolumetric.

isox·sup·rine hy·dro·chlo·ride (ī-soks′soo-prēn). Sympathomimetic amine with potent inhibitory effects on vascular, uterine, and other smooth muscles; used as a vasodilator in various vascular diseases and as a uterine relaxant.

iso·zyme (ī′sō-zīm). SYN isoenzyme.

is·sue (ish′ū). Archaic term for a discharge of pus, blood, or other matter. [Fr. a going out]

    nature-nurture i., a controversy concerning the relative importance of heredity (nature) and environment (nurture) in various aspects of individual development, such as intelligence, personality, or mental illness.

isth·mec·to·my (is-mek′tō-mē). Excision of the midportion of the thyroid. [G. *isthmos,* isthmus, + *ektomē,* excision]

isth·mic, isth·mi·an (is′mik, is′mē-an). Denoting an anatomical isthmus.

isth·mo·pa·ral·y·sis (is′mō-pă-ral′i-sis). Paralysis of the velum pendulum palati and the muscles forming the anterior pillars of the fauces. SYN faucial paralysis, isthmoplegia. [G. *isthmos,* isthmus, + paralysis]

is

isth·mo·ple·gia (is'mō-plē'jē-ă). SYN isthmoparalysis. [G. *isthmos,* isthmus, + *plēgē,* stroke]

isth·mus, pl. **isth·mi, isth·mus·es** (is'mŭs, -mī, -mŭs-ez) [TA]. **1.** A constriction in the embryonic neural tube delineating the anterior portion of the rhombencephalon, the future metencephalon, from the more rostrally located mesencephalon. **2.** SYN rhombencephalic i. [G. *isthmos*]

i. of aorta, SYN aortic i.

i. aor'tae [TA], SYN aortic i.

aortic i. [TA], a slight constriction of the aorta immediately distal to the left subclavian artery at the point of attachment of the ductus arteriosus. SYN i. aortae [TA], i. of aorta.

i. of auditory tube, SYN i. of pharyngotympanic tube.

i. of cartilage of ear, SYN i. of cartilaginous auricle.

i. of cartilaginous auricle [TA], a narrow bridge connecting the cartilage of the external acoustic meatus and the lamina of the tragus with the main portion of the cartilage of the auricle. SYN i. cartilaginis auris, i. of cartilage of ear.

i. cartilaginis auricularis [TA],

i. cartilag'inis au'ris, SYN i. of cartilaginous auricle.

i. of cingulate gyrus [TA], the narrowing of the cingulate gyrus, at its transition with the hippocampal gyrus behind and below the splenium of the corpus callosum, caused by the anterior extension of the conjoined parieto-occipital and calcarine sulci. SYN i. gyri cinguli [TA], i. of gyrus fornicatus, i. of limbic lobe.

i. of eustachian tube, SYN i. of pharyngotympanic tube.

i. of external acoustic meatus, the narrowest portion of this canal in the bony part near its deep termination. SYN i. meatus acustici externi.

i. of fauces [TA], the constricted and short space which establishes the connection between the cavity of the mouth and the oropharynx, bounded anteriorly by the palatoglossal folds and posteriorly by the palatopharyngeal folds; the lateral well is the tonsillar fossa. SYN i. faucium [TA], oropharyngeal i.

i. fau'cium [TA], SYN i. of fauces.

i. glan'dulae thyroid'eae [TA], SYN i. of thyroid gland.

Guyon i., SYN i. of uterus.

i. gy'ri cin'guli [TA], SYN i. of cingulate gyrus.

i. of gy'rus fornica'tus, SYN i. of cingulate gyrus.

i. of His, SYN rhombencephalic i.

Krönig i., the narrow straplike portion of the resonant field that extends over the shoulder, connecting the larger areas of resonance over the pulmonary apex in front and behind.

i. of limbic lobe, SYN i. of cingulate gyrus.

i. mea'tus acus'tici exter'ni, SYN i. of external acoustic meatus.

oropharyngeal i., SYN i. of fauces.

pharyngeal i., SYN i. of pharynx.

i. pharyngis, SYN i. of pharynx.

i. pharyngonasa'lis, SYN choanae.

i. of pharyngotympanic tube [TA], the narrowest portion of the auditory tube at the junction of the cartilaginous and bony portions. SYN i. tubae auditivae [TA], i. tubae auditoriae✩, i. of auditory tube, i. of eustachian tube.

i. of pharynx [TA], passage posterior to the soft palate by which the nasopharynx and oropharynx communicate (i.e., the junction of naso- and oropharynx), closed during swallowing by elevation of the soft palate and contraction of the posterior fascicle of palatopharyngeus (muscle), forming a Passavant cushion. SYN i. pharyngis, pharyngeal i.

pleural i., SYN mesopneumonium.

i. pros'tatae [TA], SYN i. of prostate.

i. of prostate [TA], the narrow middle part of the prostate anterior to the urethra. SYN i. prostatae [TA].

i. rhombenceph'ali, SYN rhombencephalic i.

rhombencephalic i., (1) a constriction in the embryonic neural tube delineating the mesencephalon from the rhombencephalon; (2) the anterior portion of the rhombencephalon connecting with the mesencephalon. SYN isthmus (2) [TA], i. of His, i. rhombencephali.

i. of thyroid gland [TA], the central part of the thyroid gland joining the two lateral lobes. SYN i. glandulae thyroideae [TA].

i. tu'bae auditi'vae [TA], SYN i. of pharyngotympanic tube.

i. tubae auditoriae, ✩official alternate term for i. of pharyngotympanic tube.

i. tu'bae uteri'nae [TA], SYN i. of uterine tube.

i. u'teri [TA], SYN i. of uterus.

i. of uterine tube [TA], the narrow portion of the uterine tube adjoining the uterus. SYN i. tubae uterinae [TA].

i. of uterus [TA], an elongated constriction at the junction of the body and cervix of the uterus. SYN i. uteri [TA], Guyon i., orificium internum uteri, os uteri internum, ostium uteri internum.

Vieussens i., SYN *limbus* fossae ovalis.

it·a·con·ic ac·id (it'ă-kon'ik). The decarboxylation product of *cis*-aconitic acid. SYN methylenesuccinic acid.

itch. 1. An irritating sensation in the skin that arouses the desire to scratch. SYN pruritus (2). **2.** Common name for scabies. [A.S. *gikkan*]

azo i., itching that occurs among workers in azo dyes.

baker i., an eruption on the hands and arms of bakers due to an allergic reaction to flour or other substances handled, or to the grain itch mite.

barber i., SYN *tinea* barbae.

bath i., SYN bath *pruritus.*

copra i., a dermatitis occurring in workers in copra mills, caused by the presence of a mite, *Tyrophagus putrescentiae.*

Cuban i., SYN alastrim.

frost i., SYN winter i.

grain i., a wheal-like cutaneous eruption occasionally noted in farmers and grain handlers, caused by the action of the mite *Pyemotes ventricosus.*

grocer i., a vesicular dermatitis seen in grocers and bakers who handle sugar or flour; caused by a mite of the genus *Glycophagus.*

ground i., SYN cutaneous *larva migrans.*

kabure i., SYN *schistosomiasis* japonica.

Norway i., SYN Norwegian *scabies.*

poultryman's i., eruption due to infestation with the mite, *Dermanyssus gallinae.*

rice i., SYN *schistosomiasis* japonica.

Saint Ignatius i., SYN pellagra.

straw i., straw-bed i., an urticarial eruption caused by the mite, *Pyemotes ventricosus,* which can infest straw used in mattresses. SYN dermatitis pediculoides ventricosus.

summer i., SYN *pruritus* aestivalis.

swimmer's i., SYN schistosomal *dermatitis.*

water i., (1) SYN cutaneous *larva migrans;* (2) SYN schistosomal *dermatitis.*

winter i., a recurrent eczema appearing with the advent of cold weather. SYN dermatitis hiemalis, frost i., pruritus hiemalis.

itch·ing. An uncomfortable sensation of irritation of the skin or mucous membranes that causes scratching or rubbing of the affected parts. SYN pruritus (1).

♾-ite. 1. Of the nature of, resembling. **2.** A salt of an acid that has the termination -ous. **3.** In comparative anatomy, a suffix denoting an essential portion of the part to the name of which it is attached. SEE ALSO -ites. [G. *-ītēs,* fem. *-itis*]

iter (ī'ter). A passage leading from one anatomic part to another. SEE ALSO canaliculus. [L. *iter* (*itiner-*), a way, journey]

i. chor'dae ante'rius, SYN anterior *canaliculus* of chorda tympani.

i. chor'dae poste'rius, SYN posterior *canaliculus* of chorda tympani.

i. den'tis, the route or routes by which one or more teeth erupt. SYN i. dentium.

i. den'tium, SYN i. dentis.

i. a ter'tio ad quar'tum ventric'ulum, SYN cerebral *aqueduct.* [L. path from the third to the fourth ventricle]

iter·al (ī'ter-ăl). Relating to an iter.

♾-ites. G. adjectival suffix attached to noun stems, corresponding to L. *-alis* or *-inus* or to Eng. -y or -like. An adjective formed with this suffix sometimes stands alone, representing a phrase from which a noun has been dropped (e.g., tympanites for *tympanitēs hydrōps*, drumlike swelling of the abdomen. SEE ALSO -ite, -itis. [G. *itēs*,]

△-**itides.** Plural of -itis.

△-**itis.** Feminine form of the G. adjectival suffix -ites. An adjective formed with this suffix sometimes stands alone, representing a phrase from which a noun has been droped e.g., nephritis for *nephritis nosos*, disease of the kidneys). Hence is has become in effect a noun suffix. Moreover, it so frequently occurs in terms for inflammatory disorders that it has acquired the denotation of inflammation. SEE ALSO -ites. [G. *-ites*]

Ito, Toshio, 20th century Japanese physician. SEE I. *cells*, under *cell*.

Ito, Minor, 20th century Japanese dermatologist. SEE Ito *nevus; hypomelanosis* of I.

ITP Abbreviation for idiopathic thrombocytopenic *purpura*; inosine 5′-triphosphate.

itra·min tos·yl·ate (ī′tră-min). A vasodilator.

IU Abbreviation for international *unit*.

IUB Abbreviation for International Union of Biochemistry.

IUCD Abbreviation for intrauterine contraceptive *devices*, under *device*.

IUD Abbreviation for intrauterine *devices*, under *device*.

IUI Abbreviation for intrauterine *insemination*.

IUPAC Abbreviation for International Union of Pure and Applied Chemistry.

I-V Abbreviation for intraventricular.

I.V., i.v. Abbreviation for intravenous, or intravenously.

IVB Abbreviation for intraventricular *block*.

IVC Abbreviation for inferior *vena* cava.

Ivemark, Björn, Swedish pathologist, *1925. SEE I. *syndrome*.

iver·mec·tin (ī-ver-mek′tin). A semisynthetic macrolide antibiotic effective in the treatment of filariasis. The drug destroys *Onchocerca microfilaria* and *Filaria bancrofti*. Also approved by the FDA for the treatment of scabies by topical administration.

IVF Abbreviation for *in vitro fertilization*.

IVF-ET. Abbreviation for in vitro fertilization and in vivo transfer of the embryo to the uterus, Fallopian tube, or the peritoneal cavity.

IVP Abbreviation for intravenous *pyelography* or pyelogram.

IVU Abbreviation for intravenous urogram; preferred to IVP. SEE intravenous *urography*.

Ivy, Robert H., U.S. oral and plastic surgeon, 1881–1974. SEE I. loop *wiring*, bleeding time *test*.

Ix·o·des (ik-sō′dēz). A genus of hard ticks (family Ixodidae), many species of which are parasitic on humans and animals; they are characterized by an anal groove surrounding the anus anteriorly, absence of eyes and festoons, and marked sexual dimorphism; about 40 species have been described from North America. [G. *ixōdēs*, sticky, like bird-lime, fr. *ixos*, mistletoe, + *eidos*, form]

I. cook′ei, a species that is a vector of Powassan virus in Canada.

I. damm′ini, a species that is a vector of Lyme disease (*Borrelia burgdorferi*) and human babesiosis (*Babesia microti*) in the U.S. Bites causing Lyme disease in humans are from nymphal ticks about the size of a pencil point, infected with *B. burgdorferi* from white-footed field mice. Adult ticks complete their two-year life cycle feeding on deer.

I. pacif′icus, the California black-legged tick, a species that is the vector of Lyme disease in the western U.S.

I. persulca′tus, the taiga tick, a Eurasian species that is a vector for Russian spring-summer encephalitis and Lyme disease.

I. redikorzevi, a Eurasian species that has caused human toxicosis in Israel.

I. rici′nus, the castor bean tick, a Eurasian species that infests cattle, sheep, and wild animals, and transmits the piroplasm *Babesia divergens*, the tick-borne encephalitis virus, and the Lyme disease bacterium.

I. scapula′ris, the black-legged or shoulder tick, a species found on animals in the southern and eastern U.S.; is the primary vector of Lyme disease in the U.S.

I. spinipal′pis, a species parasitic on wild rodents in British Columbia and the vector of Powassan virus in mice of the genus *Peromyscus*.

ix·o·di·a·sis (ik-sō-dī′ă-sis). Skin lesions caused by the bites of ixodid ticks.

ix·od·ic (ik-sod′ik). Relating to or caused by ticks.

ix·o·did (ik′sō-did). Common name for members of the family Ixodidae.

Ix·od·i·dae (ik-sod′i-dē). A family of ticks (order Acarina, suborder Ixodidea), the so-called "hard" ticks, characterized by rigid body form, presence of a dorsal shield, and an anteriorly projecting capitulum. It includes the genera *Ixodes, Hyalomma, Amblyomma, Boophilus, Margaropus, Dermacentor, Haemaphysalis,* and *Rhipicephalus,* species of which transmit many important human and animal diseases and cause tick paralysis; they occasionally attack humans, a few habitually so. [G. *ixōdēs*, sticky]

Ix·o·doi·dea (ik′sō-dō-id′ē-ă). Superfamily of the order Acarina that includes the families Ixodidae and Argasidae. [G. *ixōdēs*, sticky]

Ix

J Symbol for joule; Joule *equivalent*; electric current density.

J Symbol for flux (4); coupling constant.

Ja·bo·ran·di. SYN pilocarpus.

Jaboulay, Mathieu, French surgeon, 1860–1913. SEE J. *pyloroplasty, amputation.*

Jaccoud, François Sigismond, French physician, 1830–1913. SEE J. *arthritis, arthropathy.*

jack·et (jak′et). **1.** A fixed bandage applied around the body in order to immobilize the spine. **2.** In dentistry, a term commonly used in reference to an artificial crown composed of fired porcelain or acrylic resin. [M.E., fr. O.Fr. *jaquet,* dim. of *jaque,* tunic, fr. *Jacques,* nickname of Fr. peasants.]

Minerva j., a plaster of Paris body cast incorporating the head and trunk, usually for fracture of the cervical spine.

jack·screw (jak′skroo). A threaded device used in appliances for the separation of approximated teeth or jaws.

Jackson, Jabez N., U.S. surgeon, 1868–1935. SEE J. *membrane, veil.*

Jackson, John Hughlings, English neurologist, 1835–1911. SEE jacksonian *epilepsy;* J. *law, rule, sign.*

jack·so·ni·an (jak-sō′nē-an). Described by John Hughlings Jackson. SEE jacksonian *epilepsy,* jacksonian *seizure.*

Jacobaeus, Hans C., Swedish surgeon, 1879–1937. SEE J. *operation.*

Jacobson, Ludwig L., Danish anatomist, 1783–1843. SEE J. *anastomosis, canal, cartilage, nerve, organ, plexus, reflex.*

Jacquart, Henri, 19th century French physician. SEE J. facial *angle.*

Jacquemet, Marcel, French anatomist, 1872–1908. SEE J. *recess.*

Jacquemin, Emile, 19th century French chemist. SEE Jacquemin *test.*

Jacques, Paul, 19th century French physician. SEE J. *plexus.*

Jadassohn, Josef, German dermatologist in Switzerland, 1863–1936; introduced the patch *test* for contact dermatitis. SEE J. *nevus;* Borst-J. type intraepidermal *epithelioma;* J.-Pellizzari *anetoderma;* Franceschetti-J. *syndrome;* J.-Lewandowski *syndrome.*

Jaeger, Eduard, Ritter von Jaxthal, Austrian ophthalmologist, 1818–1884. SEE J. *test types.*

Jaffe, Max, German biochemist, 1841–1911. SEE J. *reaction, test.*

Jaffe, Henry L., U.S. pathologist, 1896–1979 SEE J.-Lichtenstein *disease.*

Jakob, Alfons M., German neuropsychiatrist, 1884–1931. SEE Creutzfeldt-Jakob *disease.*

jal·ap. The dried tuberous root of *Exogonium purga, E. jalapa,* or *Ipomoea purga* (family Convolvulaceae); used as a cathartic. [*Jalapa* or *Xalapa,* a Mexican city from where the drug was exported]

James, George C.W., U.S. radiologist, 1915–1972. SEE Swyer-J. *syndrome;* Swyer-J.-MacLeod *syndrome.*

James, Thomas N., U.S. cardiologist and physiologist, *1925. SEE J. *fibers,* under *fiber, tracts,* under *tract.*

James·town weed. SYN *Datura stramonium.*

Janet, Pierre M.F., French neurologist, 1859–1947. SEE J. *test.*

Janeway, Edward G., U.S. physician, 1841–1911. SEE J. *lesion.*

jan·i·ceps (jan′i-seps). Conjoined twins having their two heads fused together, with the faces looking in opposite directions. SEE conjoined *twins,* under *twin.* SEE ALSO craniopagus, syncephalus. [L. *Janus,* a Roman diety having two faces, + *caput,* head]

j. asym′metrus, a j. with one very small and imperfectly developed face. SYN iniops, syncephalus asymmetros.

j. parasit′icus, a j. in which one of the twins is a small and incompletely formed parasite attached to the more fully formed autosite.

Jansen, Albert, German otologist, 1859–1933. SEE J. *operation.*

Jansky, Jan, Czech physician, 1873–1921. SEE J.-Bielschowsky *disease;* J. *classification.*

Janus green B [C.I. 11050]. A basic dye used in histology and to stain mitochondria supravitally.

jar. **1.** To jolt or shake. **2.** A jolting or shaking.

heel j., the patient standing on tiptoe feels pain on suddenly bringing the heels to the ground: **(1)** in the spine in Pott disease or disk space infection; **(2)** in one lumbar region in renal calculus.

jar·gon (jar′gŏn). Language or terminology peculiar to a specific field, profession, or group. SEE ALSO paraphasia. [Fr. gibberish]

Jarisch, Adolf, Austrian dermatologist, 1850–1902. SEE J.-Herxheimer *reaction;* Bezold-J. *reflex.*

Jarman, Brian, 20th century British Primary Care physician. SEE J. *score.*

Jar·vik. Robert Koffler, U.S. cardiologist. SEE Jarvik artificial *heart.*

Ja·tro·pha (jat′rō-fă). A genus of plants of the family Euphorbiaceae; a poisonous plant found in eastern Africa and the West Indies. [G. *iatros,* physician, + *trophē,* nourishment]

J. cur′cas, barbados nut or physic-nut, the seed of which furnishes a purgative oil similar to croton oil. SYN *J. glandulifera.*

J. glandulif′era, SYN *J. curcas.*

J. u′rens, a species of South America; the macerated fresh leaves are used as a rubefacient and stimulating poultice; the seeds furnish a purgative oil.

jaun·dice (jawn′dis). A yellowish staining of the integument, sclerae, deeper tissues, and excretions with bile pigments, resulting from increased levels in the plasma. SYN icterus. [Fr. *jaune,* yellow]

acholuric j., j. with excessive amounts of unconjugated bilirubin in the plasma and without bile pigments in the urine.

anhepatic j., j. due to hemolysis, with normal function of the liver and biliary tract. SYN anhepatogenous j.

anhepatogenous j., SYN anhepatic j.

choleric j., j. with the presence of biliary derivatives in the urine; occurs in regurgitation hyperbilirubinemia.

cholestatic j., j. produced by inspissated bile or bile plugs in small biliary passages in the liver.

chronic acholuric j., SYN hereditary *spherocytosis.*

chronic familial j., SYN hereditary *spherocytosis.*

chronic idiopathic j., SYN Dubin-Johnson *syndrome.*

congenital hemolytic j., SYN hereditary *spherocytosis.*

familial nonhemolytic j. [MIM*143500], mild j. due to increased amounts of unconjugated bilirubin in the plasma without evidence of liver damage, biliary obstruction, or hemolysis; thought to be due to an inborn error of metabolism in which the excretion of bilirubin by the liver is defective, ascribed to decreased conjugation of bilirubin as a glucuronide or impaired uptake of hepatic bilirubin; autosomal dominant inheritance. SYN benign familial icterus, constitutional hepatic dysfunction, Gilbert disease, Gilbert syndrome.

hematogenous j., SYN hemolytic j.

hemolytic j., j. resulting from increased production of bilirubin from hemoglobin as a result of any process (toxic, genetic, or immune) causing increased destruction of erythrocytes. SYN hematogenous j., toxemic j.

hepatocellular j., j. resulting from diffuse injury or inflammation or failure of function of the liver cells, usually referring to viral or toxic hepatitis.

hepatogenous j., j. resulting from disease of the liver, as distinguished from that due to blood changes.

△ **Combining Forms**	☆ **Official alternate Terminologia Anatomica term**
⧯ **Indicates term is illustrated, see Illustration Index**	
SYN **Synonym**	**[MIM] Mendelian Inheritance in Man**
Cf. **Compare**	**C.I. Colour Index**
[NA] **Nomina Anatomica**	
[TA] **Terminologia Anatomica**	**High Profile Term**

homologous serum j., obsolete term for viral *hepatitis* type B.

human serum j., obsolete name for hepatitis transmitted parenterally, usually by blood or blood products; usually due to hepatitis B.

infectious j., (1) SYN Weil *disease*; **(2)** obsolete term for viral *hepatitis* type A.

infective j., acute onset of malaise, fever, myalgia, nausea, anorexia, abdominal pain, and icterus caused by members of the genus *Leptospira*.

leptospiral j., j. associated with infection by various species of *Leptospira*.

malignant j., SYN *icterus* gravis.

mechanical j., SYN obstructive j.

neonatal j., SYN physiologic j.

j. of the newborn, SYN physiologic j.

nonobstructive j., any j. in which the main biliary passages are not obstructed, e.g., hemolytic j. or j. due to hepatitis.

nuclear j., SYN kernicterus.

obstructive j., j. resulting from obstruction to the flow of bile into the duodenum, whether intra- or extrahepatic. SYN mechanical j.

painless j., j. not associated with abdominal pain; usually used for obstructive j. resulting from obstruction of the common bile duct at the head of the pancreas by a tumor or impaction of a stone.

physiologic j., a form of j. observed frequently in newborn infants in the first 1–2 weeks of life. It is caused by several factors, including a comparatively high red cell mass at birth compared with that of adults, shorter red cell life span, transiently impaired conjugation of bilirubin in the liver, and lack of gut flora (which are helpful in intestinal metabolism and excretion of bilirubin); is related to indirect (unconjugated) bilirubinemia that peaks at 2–3 days of age in normal, full-term infants and later with higher levels in preterm infants and is accentuated in breast-fed infants. SYN icterus neonatorum, j. of the newborn, neonatal j.

postarsphenamine j., liver toxicity, causing j., in a patient who has received arsphenamine.

recurrent j. of pregnancy, SYN intrahepatic *cholestasis* of pregnancy.

regurgitation j., j. due to biliary obstruction, the bile pigment having been conjugated and secreted by the hepatic cells and then reabsorbed into the bloodstream.

retention j., j. due to insufficiency of liver function or to an excess of bile pigment production; the bilirubin is unconjugated because it has not passed through the liver cells.

Schmorl j., kernicterus.

spherocytic j., hemolytic j. associated with spherocytosis.

spirochetal j., j. caused by infection with *Leptospira* species, usually *Leptospira icterohemorrhagica*.

toxemic j., SYN hemolytic j.

jaun·dice root. SYN hydrastis.

jaw. 1. One of the two bony structures, in which the teeth are set, forming the framework of the mouth. **2.** Common name for either the maxillae or the mandible. [A.S. *ceōwan*, to chew]

crackling j., chronic subluxation with clicking on motion.

Hapsburg j., prognathism and pouting lower lip, characteristic of the Hispano-Austrian imperial dynasty.

jaw winking, a paradoxical movement of eyelids associated with movements of the jaw.

lock-j., SYN trismus.

lower j., SYN mandible.

lumpy j., SYN actinomycosis.

parrot j., a condition caused by protrusion of incisor teeth.

upper j., SYN maxilla.

Jaworski, Walery, Polish physician, 1849–1924. SEE J. *bodies,* under *body.*

Jeanselme, Edouard, French dermatologist, 1858–1935. SEE J. *nodules,* under *nodule.*

Jeghers, Harold, U.S. physician, *1904. SEE Peutz-J. *syndrome;* J.-Peutz *syndrome.*

△**jejun-.** SEE jejuno-.

je·ju·nal (je-joo′năl). Relating to the jejunum.

je·ju·nec·to·my (je-joo-nek′tō-mē). Excision of all or a part of the jejunum. [jejunum + G. *ektomē,* excision]

je·ju·ni·tis (je-joo-nī′tis). Inflammation of the jejunum.

△**jejuno-, jejun-.** The jejunum, jejunal. [L. *jejunus,* empty]

je·ju·no·co·los·to·my (je-joo-nō-kō-los′tō-mē). An anastomosis between the jejunum and the colon. [jejuno- + colon + G. *stoma,* mouth]

je·ju·no·il·e·al (je-joo′nō-il′ē-ăl). Relating to the jejunum and the ileum.

je·ju·no·il·e·i·tis (je-joo′nō-il-ē-ī′tis). Inflammation of the jejunum and ileum.

je·ju·no·il·e·os·to·my (je-joo′nō-il-ē-os′tō-mē). An anastomosis between the jejunum and the ileum. [jejuno- + ileum + G. *stoma,* mouth]

je·ju·no·je·ju·nos·to·my (je-joo′nō-jĕ-joo-nos′tō-mē). An anastomosis between two portions of jejunum. [jejuno- + jejuno- + G. *stoma,* mouth]

je·ju·no·plas·ty (je-joo′nō-plas-tē). A corrective surgical procedure on the jejunum. [jejuno- + G. *plastos,* molded]

je·ju·nos·to·my (je-joo-nos′tō-mē). Operative establishment of a fistula from the jejunum to the abdominal wall, usually with creation of a stoma. [jejuno- + G. *stoma,* mouth]

je·ju·not·o·my (je-joo-not′ō-mē). Incision into the jejunum. [jejuno- + G. *tomē,* incision]

je·ju·num (jĕ-joo′nŭm) [TA]. The portion of small intestine, about 8 feet in length, between the duodenum and the ileum. The jejunum is distinct from the ileum in being more proximal, of larger diameter with a thicker wall, having larger, more highly developed plicae circulares, being more vascular (redder in appearance), with the jejunal arteries forming fewer tiers of arterial arcades and longer vasa recta. [L. *jejunus,* empty]

Jellinek, Edward J., British physician specializing in alcohol-related disorders, 1890–1963. SEE Jellinek *formula.*

jel·ly (jel′ē). **1.** A semisolid tremulous compound usually containing some form of gelatin in aqueous solution. **2.** SYN jellyfish. [L. *gelo,* to freeze]

box j., SYN *Chiropsalmus quadrumanus.*

cardiac j., term introduced by C.L. Davis for the gelatinous, noncellular material between the endothelial lining and the myocardial layer of the heart in very young embryos; later in development it serves as a substratum for cardiac mesenchyme.

interlaminar j., term introduced by B.M. Patten for the gelatinous material between ectoderm and endoderm that serves as the substrate on which mesenchymal cells migrate.

Wharton j., the mucous connective tissue of the umbilical cord.

jel·ly·fish (jel′ē-fish). Marine coelenterates (class Hydrozoa) including some poisonous species, notably *Physalia,* the Portuguese man-of-war; toxin is injected into the skin by nematocysts on the tentacles, causing linear wheals. SYN jelly (2).

Jendrassik, Ernö, Hungarian physician, 1858–1921. SEE J. *maneuver.*

Jenner, Edward, 1749–1823; English physician and naturalist who discovered the method of vaccinating against smallpox by inoculating susceptible persons with cowpox (vaccinia); Jenner method led directly to the eradication of smallpox worldwide in 1977, the greatest public health achievement ever.

Jenner, Harley D., Canadian physician, *1907. SEE J.-Kay *unit.*

Jenner, Louis, English physician, 1866–1904. SEE J. *stain.*

Jennings, E.R., 20th century U.S. statistcian. SEE Levey-J. *chart.*

Jensen, Edmund Z., Danish ophthalmologist, 1861–1950. SEE J. *disease.*

Jensen, Carl O., Danish veterinary surgeon and pathologist, 1864–1934. SEE J. *sarcoma.*

jerk. 1. A sudden pull. **2.** SYN deep *reflex.*

ankle j., SYN Achilles *reflex.*

chin j., SYN jaw *reflex.*

crossed j., SYN crossed *reflex.*

crossed adductor j., SYN crossed adductor *reflex.*

crossed knee j., SYN crossed knee *reflex.*

je

elbow j., SYN triceps *reflex.*

jaw j., SYN jaw *reflex.*

knee j., SYN patellar *reflex.*

supinator j., SYN brachioradial *reflex.*

jerks (pl.). Chorea or any form of tic.

Jervell, Anton, 20th century Norwegian cardiologist. SEE J. and Lange-Nielsen *syndrome.*

Jes·u·its bark. SYN cinchona.

jet. A region of very high blood velocity just downstream of a vessel stenosis.

jet lag. An imbalance of the normal circadian rhythm resulting from subsonic or supersonic travel through a varied number of time zones and leading to fatigue, irritability, and various functional disturbances.

Jeune, M., 20th century French pediatrician. SEE J. *syndrome.*

Jewett, Hugh J., U.S. urologist, 1903–1990. SEE J. *sound,* and Strong *staging.*

Jewett, Eugene Lyon, U.S. orthopaedic surgeon and inventor of many orthopedic instruments, *1900.

jig·ger. Common name for *Tunga penetrans.* SEE ALSO chigoe.

jim·son weed. SYN *Datura stramonium.*

Jk blood group. See Kidd blood group, Blood Groups appendix.

JNA Abbreviation for *Jena Nomina Anatomica,* 1935. SEE *Terminologia Anatomica.*

Jobert de Lamballe, Antoine J., French surgeon, 1799–1867. SEE J. de L. *fossa, suture.*

Jod-Basedow, jod·bas·e·dow (yod-bas′ĕ-dō). SEE Jod-Basedow *phenomenon.* [Ger. *Jod,* iodine, + K.A. von *Basedow*]

Joffroy, Alexis C., French physician, 1844–1908. SEE J. *reflex, sign.*

Johne, H. Albert, German physician, 1839–1910. SEE johnin.

joh·nin (yō′nin). A product used as a diagnostic agent, analogous to tuberculin but made from *Mycobacterium paratuberculosis* (the causative organism of Johne disease) grown in a broth medium containing *Mycobacterium phlei* (timothy hay bacillus); used as an allergen to provoke reactions in infected animals. [H. A. *Johne*]

Johnson, Frank B., U.S. pathologist, *1919. SEE Dubin-J. *syndrome.*

Johnson, Frank C., U.S. pediatrician, 1894–1934. SEE Stevens-J. *syndrome.*

Johnson, Harry B., U.S. dentist. SEE J. *method.*

Johnson, Treat Baldwin, U.S. chemist, 1875–1947. SEE Wheeler-J. *test.*

JOINT

joint (joynt) [TA]. In anatomy, the place of union, usually more or less movable, between two or more bones. J.'s between skeletal elements exhibit a great variety of form and function, and are classified into three general morphologic types: fibrous j.'s; cartilaginous j.'s; and synovial j.'s. SYN junctura (1) [TA], arthrosis (1), articulation (1), articulus. [L. *junctura;* fr. *jungo,* pp. *junctus,* to join]

acromioclavicular j. [TA], a plane synovial joint between the acromial end of the clavicle and the medial margin of the acromion. SYN articulatio acromioclavicularis [TA].

ankle j. [TA], a hinge synovial joint between the tibia and fibula above and the talus below. SYN articulatio talocruralis [TA], ankle (1), mortise j., talocrural articulation, talocrural j.

anterior intraoccipital j., SYN anterior intraoccipital *synchondrosis.*

arthrodial j., SYN plane j.

atlantoaxial j., compound j. between first and second cervical vertebrae.

atlanto-occipital j. [TA], a condylar synovial joint between the superior articular facets of the atlas and the condyles of the occipital bone. SYN articulatio atlanto-occipitalis [TA], atlanto-occipital articulation.

j.'s of auditory ossicles [TA], the joints of the ossicular chain consisting of incudomallear j., incudostapedeal j., and the tympanostapedeal syndesmosis. SYN articulationes ossiculorum auditus [TA], articulationes ossiculorum auditoriorum*, j.'s of ear bones.

ball and socket j., a multiaxial synovial joint in which a more or

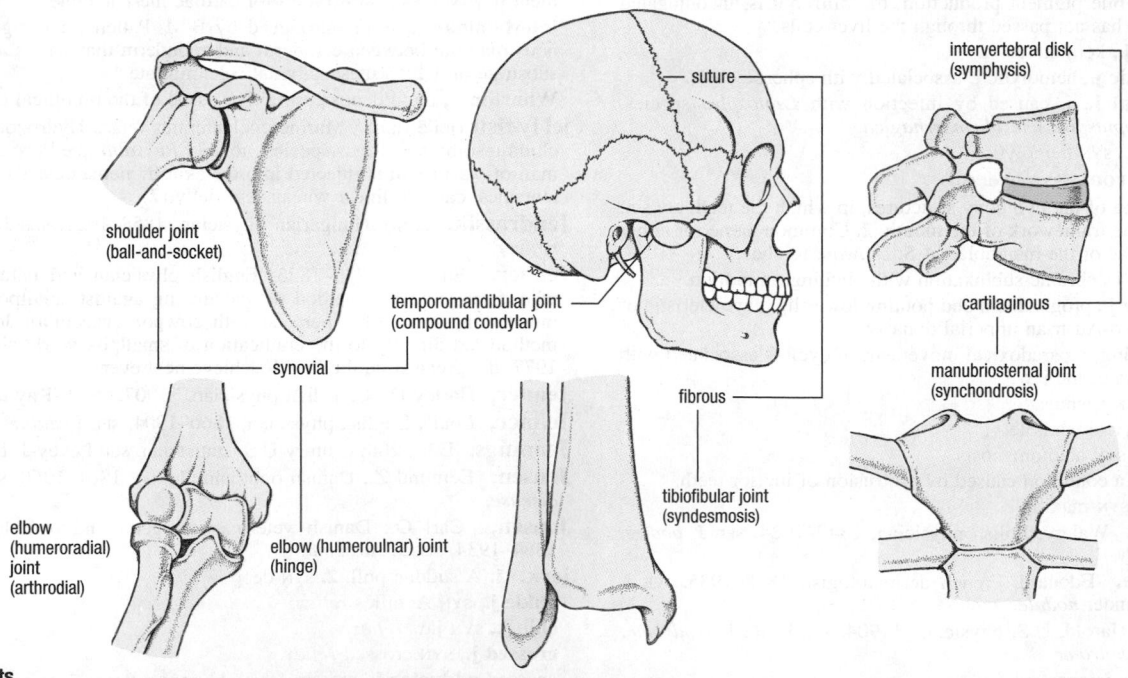

shoulder joint (ball-and-socket)

synovial

temporomandibular joint (compound condylar)

suture

intervertebral disk (symphysis)

cartilaginous

manubriosternal joint (synchondrosis)

elbow (humeroradial) joint (arthrodial)

elbow (humeroulnar) joint (hinge)

fibrous

tibiofibular joint (syndesmosis)

joints

less extensive sphere on the head of one bone fits into a rounded cavity in the other bone, as in the hip joint. SYN articulatio spheroidea [TA], enarthrosis✭, spheroidal j.✭, articulatio cotylica, cotyloid j., enarthrodial j., socket j., spheroid articulation.

biaxial j., one in which there are two principal axes of movement situated at right angles to each other; e.g., saddle j.'s.

bicondylar j. [TA], a synovial joint in which two more or less distinct, rounded surfaces of one bone articulate with shallow depressions on another bone. SYN articulatio bicondylaris [TA], bicondylar articulation.

bilocular j., one in which the intraarticular disk is complete, dividing the j. into two distinct cavities.

Budin obstetrical j., SYN posterior intraoccipital *synchondrosis.*

calcaneocuboid j. [TA], a somewhat saddle-shaped synovial joint between the anterior surface of the calcaneus and the posterior surface of the cuboid. This is the lateral element of the compound transverse tarsal joint. SYN articulatio calcaneocuboidea [TA].

capitular j., SYN j. of head of rib.

carpal j.'s [TA], the synovial joints between the carpal bones. SYN articulatio carpi [TA], articulationes carpi [TA], articulationes intercarpales✭, intercarpal j.'s✭.

carpometacarpal j.'s [TA], the synovial joints between the carpal and metacarpal bones; these are all plane joints except that of the thumb, which is saddle-shaped. SYN articulationes carpometacarpales [TA].

carpometacarpal j. of thumb [TA], the saddle-shaped synovial articulation between the trapezium and the base of the first metacarpal bone. SYN articulatio carpometacarpalis pollicis.

cartilaginous j. [TA], a joint in which the apposed bony surfaces are united by cartilage; they are divided into synchondroses and symphyses; in synchondroses, the cartilage connecting the apposed surfaces is, as a rule, ultimately converted to bone, as between epiphyses and diaphyses of long bones; exceptions are the sternal synchondroses and the cartilaginous union of the first rib and the manubrium of the sternum; in symphyses the bones are connected by a flat disk of fibrocartilage that remains unossified throughout life; e.g., the intervertebral disk and the symphysis pubis. SYN junctura cartilaginea [TA], articulatio cartilaginis, cartilaginous articulation, synarthrodial j. (2).

Charcot j., SYN neuropathic j.

Chopart j., SYN transverse tarsal j.

Clutton j.'s, symmetrical arthrosis, especially of the knee joints, in cases of congenital syphilis.

coccygeal j., SYN sacrococcygeal j.

cochlear j., a variety of hinge j. in which the elevation and depression, respectively, on the opposing articular surfaces form part of a spiral, flexion being then accompanied by a certain amount of lateral deviation. SYN screw j., spiral j.

complex j. [TA], a joint composed of three or more skeletal elements, or in which two anatomically separate joints function as a unit. For example, the telonavicular and calcaneocuboid joints act together as the compound transverse tarsal joint. SYN articulatio composita [TA], articulatio complexa, composite j., compound articulation, compound j.

composite j., SYN complex j.

compound j., SYN complex j.

condylar j. [TA], a modified ball-and-socket synovial joint in which the joint surfaces are elongated or ellipsoidal; it is a biaxial joint, i.e., two axes of motion at right angles to each other, the radiocarpal being an example. SYN articulatio ellipsoidea [TA], ellipsoidal j.✭, articulatio condylaris, condylar articulation.

costochondral j.'s [TA], the cartilaginous joints between the sternal end of ribs and the lateral ends of costal cartilages. SYN articulationes costochondrales [TA], costochondral junctions.

costotransverse j., the synovial articulation between the neck and tubercle of a rib and the transverse process of a vertebra. SYN articulatio costotransversaria.

costovertebral j.'s [TA], the synovial joints uniting ribs and vertebrae; they consist of the j. capitis costae and the j. costotransversaria. SYN articulationes costovertebrales [TA].

cotyloid j., SYN ball and socket j.

cranial synovial j.'s [TA], synovial j.'s of the head, composed of the temporomandibular j. (TMJ) and atlanto-occipital j. SYN articulationes cranii [TA].

cricoarytenoid j. [TA], the synovial joint between the base of each arytenoid cartilage and the upper border of the lamina of the cricoid cartilage. SYN articulatio cricoarytenoidea [TA], cricoarytenoid articulation.

cricothyroid j. [TA], the synovial articulation between the inferior horn of the thyroid cartilage and the side of the cricoid cartilage. SYN articulatio cricothyroidea [TA], cricothyroid articulation.

Cruveilhier j., SYN median atlantoaxial j.

cubital j., SYN elbow j.

cuboideonavicular j., a fibrous j. between adjacent parts of the cuboid and navicular bones; occasionally a synovial cavity is found here as an extension of the cuneonavicular j.

cuneocuboid j., the synovial articulation between the lateral surface of the lateral cuneiform and the anterior two-thirds of the medial surface of the cuboid.

cuneometatarsal j.'s, SYN tarsometatarsal j.'s.

cuneonavicular j., the synovial joint between the anterior surface of the navicular and the posterior surfaces of the three cuneiform bones. SYN articulatio cuneonavicularis [TA], cuneonavicular articulation.

cylindrical j. [TA], a class of freely movable j.'s that rotate about a single long axis, that includes pivot and hinge j.'s. SYN articulatio cylindrica [TA].

dentoalveolar j., SYN gomphosis.

diarthrodial j., SYN synovial j.

digital j.'s, SYN interphalangeal j.'s of hand.

DIP j.'s, SYN distal interphalangeal j.'s.

distal interphalangeal j.'s, the synovial j.'s between the middle and distal phalanges of the fingers and of the toes. SYN DIP j.'s.

distal radioulnar j. [TA], the pivot synovial joint between the head of the ulna and the ulnar notch on the radius; an articular disk passes across the distal part of the joint. SYN articulatio radioulnaris distalis [TA], distal radioulnar articulation, inferior radioulnar j.

distal tibiofibular j., SYN tibiofibular *syndesmosis.*

j.'s of ear bones, SYN j.'s of auditory ossicles.

elbow j. [TA], a compound hinge synovial joint between the humerus and the bones of the forearm; it consists of the j. humeroradialis and the j. humeroulnaris. SYN articulatio cubiti [TA], cubital j.

ellipsoidal j., ✭official alternate term for condylar j.

enarthrodial j., SYN ball and socket j.

facet j.'s, SYN zygapophysial j.'s.

false j., SYN pseudarthrosis.

femoropatellar j., the articulation of the facets on the articular surface of the patella with corresponding surfaces on the femoral condyles.

fibrous j. [TA], a union of two bones by fibrous tissue such that there is no joint cavity and almost no motion possible; the types of fibrous joints are sutures, syndesmoses, and gomphoses. SYN junctura fibrosa [TA], articulatio fibrosa, immovable j., synarthrodia, synarthrodial j. (1).

flail j., a j. with loss of function caused by loss of ability to stabilize the j. in any plane within its normal range of motion.

j.'s of foot [TA], j.'s including the talocrural, intertarsal, tarsometatarsal, intermetatarsal, metatarsophalangeal and interphalangeal joints. SYN articulationes pedis [TA], articulations of foot.

j.'s of free inferior limb, SYN synovial j.'s of free lower limb.

j.'s of free superior limb, SYN synovial j.'s of free upper limb.

ginglymoid j., SYN hinge j.

glenohumeral j. [TA], a ball-and-socket synovial joint between the head of the humerus and the glenoid cavity of the scapula. SYN articulatio humeri [TA], articulatio glenohumeralis✭, shoulder j.✭, glenohumeral articulation, humeral articulation.

gliding j., SYN plane j.

gompholic j., SYN gomphosis.

j.'s of hand [TA], these joints include the radiocarpal or wrist joint; intercarpal, carpometacarpal, intermetacarpal; metacarpo-

jo

phalangeal and interphalangeal joints. SYN articulationes manus [TA], articulations of hand.

j. of head of rib [TA], the synovial joint between a rib and bodies of two adjacent vertebrae; the joint cavity is divided by an intra-articular ligament which attaches to the intervertebral disk; the first, tenth, eleventh, and twelfth ribs articulate with only one vertebra. SYN articulatio capitis costae [TA], capitular j.

hemophilic j., chronic arthropathy due to repeated hemarthrosis in a hemophiliac.

hinge j. [TA], a uniaxial joint in which a broad, transversely cylindrical convexity on one bone fits into a corresponding concavity on the other, allowing of motion in one plane only, as in the elbow. SYN ginglymus [TA], ginglymoid j.

hip j. [TA], the ball-and-socket synovial joint between the head of the femur and the acetabulum. SYN articulatio coxae [TA], coxa (2) [TA], articulatio coxofemoralis ✩, thigh j.

humeroradial j. [TA], the portion of the elbow joint between the capitulum of the humerus and the head of the radius. SYN articulatio humeroradialis [TA], humeroradial articulation.

humeroulnar j. [TA], the portion of the elbow joint between the trochlea of the humerus and the trochlear notch of the ulna. SYN articulatio humeroulnaris [TA].

hysterical j., a simulation of j. disease, with symptoms of pain, possibly swelling, and impairment of motion.

immovable j., SYN fibrous j.

incudomalleolar j. [TA], the saddle synovial joint between the incus and the malleus. SYN articulatio incudomallearis [TA], incudomalleolar articulation.

incudostapedial j. [TA], the synovial joint between the lenticular process on the long crus of the incus and the head of the stapes. SYN articulatio incudostapedia [TA], incudostapedial articulation.

j.'s of inferior limb girdle, SYN j.'s of pelvic girdle.

inferior radioulnar j., SYN distal radioulnar j.

inferior tibiofibular j., SYN tibiofibular *syndesmosis*.

interarticular j.'s, SYN zygapophysial j.'s.

intercarpal j.'s, ✩ official alternate term for carpal j.'s.

interchondral j.'s [TA], the synovial joints between the contiguous surfaces of the fifth, sixth, seventh, eighth, ninth, and tenth costal cartilages, forming the costal arch. SYN articulationes interchondrales [TA], interchondral articulations.

intercuneiform j.'s [TA], the articulations between contiguous surfaces of the cuneiform bones. SEE ALSO intertarsal j.'s. SYN articulationes intercuneiformes [TA].

intermetacarpal j.'s [TA], the synovial joints between the bases of the second, third, fourth, and fifth metacarpal bones. SYN articulationes intermetacarpales [TA].

intermetatarsal j.'s [TA], the synovial joints between the bases of the five metatarsal bones. SYN articulationes intermetatarsales [TA], intermetatarsal articulations.

interphalangeal j.'s of foot [TA], the hinge synovial j.'s between the phalanges of the toes. SYN articulationes interphalangeae pedis [TA].

interphalangeal j.'s of hand [TA], the hinge synovial j.'s between the phalanges of the fingers. SYN articulationes interphalangeae manus [TA], digital j.'s, interphalangeal articulations, phalangeal j.'s.

intersternebral j.'s, SYN *synchondroses* intersternebrales, under *synchondrosis*.

intertarsal j.'s, the synovial joints which unite the tarsal bones. SYN articulationes intertarseae, intertarsal articulations, tarsal j.'s.

jaw j., SYN temporomandibular j.

knee j. [TA], a compound condylar synovial joint consisting of the joint between the condyles of the femur and the condyles of the tibia, articular menisci (semilunar cartilages) being interposed, and the articulation between femur and patella. SYN articulatio genus [TA].

lateral atlantoaxial j. [TA], a condylar synovial joint between the inferior articular facets of the atlas and the superior articular facets of the axis. SYN articulatio atlantoaxialis lateralis [TA], lateral atlantoepistrophic j.

lateral atlantoepistrophic j., SYN lateral atlantoaxial j.

Lisfranc j.'s, SYN tarsometatarsal j.'s.

lumbosacral j. [TA], the articulation of the fifth lumbar vertebra with the sacrum. SYN articulatio lumbosacralis [TA], junctura lumbosacralis.

Luschka j.'s, SYN uncovertebral j.'s.

mandibular j., SYN temporomandibular j.

manubriosternal j. [TA], the early union, by hyaline cartilage, of the manubrium and the body of the sternum, which later becomes a symphysial type of joint. SYN synchondrosis manubriosternalis [TA].

median atlantoaxial j. [TA], a pivot synovial joint between the dens of the axis and the ring formed by the anterior arch and the transverse ligament of the atlas. SYN articulatio atlantoaxialis mediana [TA], Cruveilhier j., middle atlantoepistrophic j.

metacarpophalangeal j.'s [TA], the condylar or ellipsoid synovial joints between the heads of the metacarpals and the bases of the proximal phalanges. The palmar aspects of the metacarpal heads are partially divided, so the joint is nearly bicondylar. SYN articulationes metacarpophalangeae [TA], metacarpophalangeal articulations, MP j.'s (1).

metatarsophalangeal j.'s [TA], the condylar or ellipsoid synovial joints between the heads of the metatarsals and the bases of the proximal phalanges of the toes. SYN articulationes metatarsophalangeae [TA], metatarsophalangeal articulations, MP j.'s (2).

midcarpal j. [TA], the synovial joint between the proximal and distal rows of carpal bones. SYN articulatio mediocarpalis [TA], middle carpal j.

middle atlantoepistrophic j., SYN median atlantoaxial j.

middle carpal j., SYN midcarpal j.

middle radioulnar j., SYN radioulnar *syndesmosis*.

midtarsal j., SYN transverse tarsal j.

mortise j., SYN ankle j.

movable j., SYN synovial j.

MP j.'s, (1) SYN metacarpophalangeal j.'s; **(2)** SYN metatarsophalangeal j.'s.

multiaxial j., one in which movement occurs in a number of axes. SEE ball and socket j. SYN polyaxial j.

neurocentral j., SYN neurocentral *synchondrosis*.

neuropathic j., destructive j. disease caused by diminished proprioceptive sensation, with gradual destruction of the j. by repeated subliminal injury, commonly associated with tabes dorsalis or diabetic neuropathy. SYN Charcot j., neuropathic arthropathy.

j.'s of pectoral girdle [TA], the joints uniting the scapulae and clavicles to each other and the latter to the sternum forming the superior limb girdle; these are the acromioclavicular and the sternoclavicular joints. SYN articulationes cinguli pectoralis ✩, articulationes cinguli membri superioris, j.'s of superior limb girdle, juncturae membri superioris.

peg-and-socket j., SYN gomphosis.

j.'s of pelvic girdle [TA], the j.'s that unite the sacrum and the two hip bones to form the pelvic girdle; these are the sacroiliac j.'s, the pubic symphysis, the sacrotuberal and sacrospinal ligaments, and the obturator membrane. SYN articulationes cinguli pelvici [TA], articulationes cinguli membri inferioris, j.'s of inferior limb girdle.

petrooccipital j., SYN petrooccipital *synchondrosis*.

phalangeal j.'s, SYN interphalangeal j.'s of hand.

PIP j.'s, SYN proximal interphalangeal j.'s.

pisiform j. [TA], the synovial joint between the pisiform and triquetrum; it is separate from the other intercarpal joints. SYN articulatio ossis pisiformis [TA], articulation of pisiform bone, pisotriquetral j.

pisotriquetral j., SYN pisiform j.

pivot j. [TA], a synovial joint in which a section of a cylinder of one bone fits into a corresponding cavity on the other, as in the proximal radioulnar joint. SYN articulatio trochoidea [TA], helicoid ginglymus, lateral ginglymus, rotary j., rotatory j., trochoid articulation, trochoid j.

plane j. [TA], a synovial joint in which the opposing surfaces are nearly planes and in which there is only a slight, gliding motion, as in the intermetacarpal joints. SYN articulatio plana [TA], arthrodia, arthrodial articulation, arthrodial j., gliding j.

polyaxial j., SYN multiaxial j.

posterior intraoccipital j., SYN posterior intraoccipital *synchondrosis*.

proximal interphalangeal j.'s, the synovial j.'s between the proximal and middle phalanges of the fingers and of the toes. SYN PIP j.'s.

proximal radioulnar j. [TA], the pivot synovial joint between the head of the radius and the ring formed by the radial notch of the ulna and the annular ligament. SYN articulatio radioulnaris proximalis [TA], proximal radioulnar articulation, superior radioulnar j.

proximal tibiofibular j., SYN tibiofibular j.

radiocarpal j., SYN wrist j.

rotary j., rotatory j., SYN pivot j.

sacrococcygeal j. [TA], the cartilaginous articulation of the coccyx with the sacrum. SYN articulatio sacrococcygea [TA], coccygeal j., junctura sacrococcygea, sacrococcygeal junction, symphysis sacrococcygea.

sacroiliac j. [TA], the synovial joint on either side between the auricular surface of the sacrum and that of the ilium. SYN articulatio sacroiliaca [TA], sacroiliac articulation.

saddle j. [TA], a biaxial synovial joint in which the double motion is effected by the opposition of two surfaces, each of which is concave in one direction and convex in the other; as in the carpometacarpal joint of the thumb. SYN articulatio sellaris [TA], articulatio ovoidalis.

schindyletic j., SYN schindylesis.

screw j., SYN cochlear j.

secondary cartilaginous j. [TA], SYN symphysis.

shoulder j., ⋆official alternate term for glenohumeral j.

simple j. [TA], one composed of two bones only. SYN articulatio simplex [TA].

socket j., SYN ball and socket j.

sphenooccipital j., SYN sphenooccipital *synchondrosis*.

spheroidal j., ⋆official alternate term for ball and socket j.

spiral j., SYN cochlear j.

sternal j.'s, SYN sternal *synchondroses*, under *synchondrosis*.

sternoclavicular j. [TA], the synovial articulation between the medial end of the clavicle and the manubrium of the sternum and cartilage of the first rib; an articular disk subdivides the joint into two cavities. SYN articulatio sternoclavicularis [TA].

sternocostal j.'s [TA], the joints between the cartilages of the first seven ribs and the sternum; synovial cavities are variable in occurrence in these joints. SYN articulationes sternocostales [TA], sternocostal articulations.

stress-broken j., SYN nonrigid *connector*.

subtalar j. [TA], a plane synovial joint between the inferior surface of the talus and the posterior articular surface of the calcaneus. The term is also used clinically to refer to the compound joint formed by the talcalcaneal and talocalcaneonavicular joints. SYN articulatio subtalaris [TA], articulatio talocalcanea⋆, talocalcaneal j.⋆.

j.'s of superior limb girdle, SYN j.'s of pectoral girdle.

superior radioulnar j., SYN proximal radioulnar j.

superior tibiofibular j., ⋆official alternate term for tibiofibular j.

suture j., SYN suture (1).

synarthrodial j., (1) SYN fibrous j; **(2)** SYN cartilaginous j.

synchondrodial j. [TA], SYN synchondrosis.

syndesmodial j., syndesmotic j., SYN syndesmosis.

synovial j. [TA], a joint in which the opposing bony surfaces are covered with a layer of hyaline cartilage or fibrocartilage; there is a joint cavity containing synovial fluid, lined with synovial membrane and reinforced by a fibrous capsule and ligaments; and there is some degree of free movement possible. SYN junctura synovialis [TA], articulatio⋆, diarthrosis⋆, articulatio synovialis, diarthrodial j., movable j., perarticulation.

synovial j.'s of free lower limb [TA], the joints uniting the bones of the free inferior limb to one another and to the pelvic girdle; they are the hip joint, knee joint, tibiofibular joints, and the joints

of the ankle and foot. SYN articulationes membri inferioris liberi [TA], j.'s of free inferior limb, juncturae membri inferioris liberi.

synovial j.'s of free upper limb [TA], the joints uniting the bones of the free superior limb girdle; they are the shoulder joint, elbow joint, radioulnar joints, and joints of the wrist and hand. SYN articulationes membri superioris liberi [TA], j.'s of free superior limb, juncturae membri superioris liberi.

synovial j.'s of thorax [TA], synovial j.'s of the thoracic skeleton, including the costovertebral, sternocostal, costochondral, and interchondral j.'s. SYN articulationes thoracis [TA].

talocalcaneal j., ⋆official alternate term for subtalar j.

talocalcaneonavicular j. [TA], a ball-and-socket synovial joint, part of which participates in the transverse tarsal joint, formed by the head of the talus articulating with the navicular bone and the anterior part of the calcaneus. SYN articulatio talocalcaneonavicularis [TA].

talocrural j., SYN ankle j.

talonavicular j., the part of the talocalcaneonavicular j. that forms the medial element of the compound transverse tarsal j.

tarsal j.'s, SYN intertarsal j.'s.

tarsometatarsal j.'s [TA], the three synovial joints between the tarsal and metatarsal bones, consisting of a medial joint between the first cuneiform and first metatarsal, an intermediate joint between the second and third cuneiforms and corresponding metatarsals, and a lateral joint between the cuboid and fourth and fifth metatarsals. SYN articulationes tarsometatarsales [TA], cuneometatarsal j.'s, Lisfranc j.'s.

▯ temporomandibular j. [TA], the synovial articulation between the head of the mandible and the mandibular fossa and articular tubercle of the temporal bone; a fibrocartilaginous articular disk divides the joint into two cavities. SYN articulatio temporomandibularis [TA], articulatio mandibularis, jaw j., mandibular j., temporomandibular articulation.

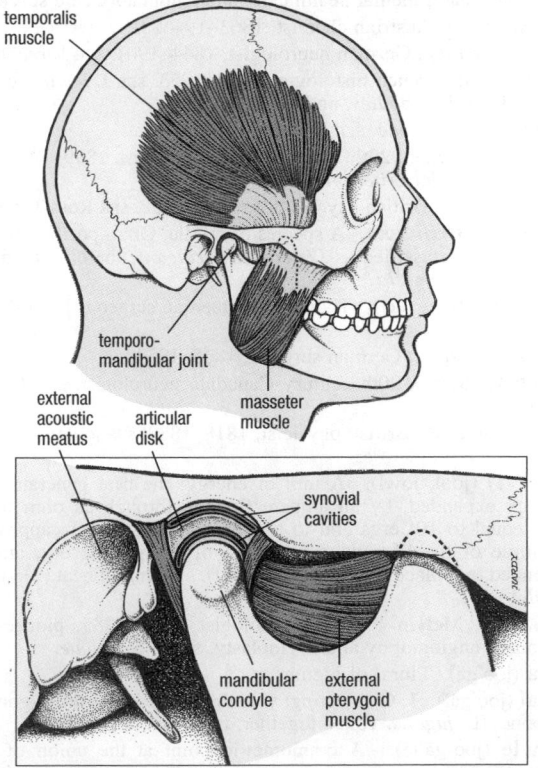

temporalis muscle

temporo-mandibular joint

external acoustic meatus

articular disk

masseter muscle

synovial cavities

mandibular condyle

external pterygoid muscle

temporomandibular joint

thigh j., SYN hip j.

tibiofibular j. [TA], the plane synovial joint between the lateral condyle of the tibia and the head of the fibula. SYN articulatio tibiofibularis [TA], superior tibiofibular j.✭, proximal tibiofibular j., superior tibial articulation, tibiofibular articulation (1).

transverse tarsal j. [TA], the synovial joints between the talus and navicular bone medially and the calcaneus and navicular bones laterally that act as a unit in allowing the front of the foot to pivot relative to the back of the foot about the longitudinal axis of the foot, contributing to the total inversion and eversion movements. SYN articulatio tarsi transversa [TA], Chopart j., midtarsal j., transverse tarsal articulation.

trochoid j., SYN pivot j.

uncovertebral j.'s, small synovial j.'s between adjacent lateral lips of the bodies of the lower cervical vertebrae. SYN Luschka j.'s.

uniaxial j., one in which movement is around one axis only.

unilocular j., one in which an intraarticular disk is incomplete or absent, the j. having but a single cavity.

wedge-and-groove j., SYN schindylesis.

wrist j. [TA], the synovial joint between the distal end of the radius and its articular disk and the proximal row of carpal bones with the exception of the pisiform bone. SYN articulatio radiocarpalis [TA], radiocarpal articulation, radiocarpal j.

xiphisternal j. [TA], the cartilaginous union between the xiphoid process and the body of the sternum. SYN symphysis xiphosternalis [TA], synchondrosis xiphosternalis.

zygapophysial j.'s [TA], the synovial joints between zygapophyses or articular processes of the vertebrae. SYN articulationes zygapophysiales [TA], facet j.'s, interarticular j.'s, juncturae zygapophysiales.

Joint Commission on Accreditation of Healthcare Organizations. A private, not-for-profit organization that evaluates and accredits health care organizations in the United States including hospitals and other organizations providing home care, long-term care, mental health care, and ambulatory care services.

Jolles, Adolf, Austrian chemist, 1863–1944. SEE J. test.

Jolly, Friedrich, German neurologist, 1844–1904. SEE J. reaction.

Jolly, Justin, French histologist, 1870–1953. SEE J. bodies, under body; Howell-J. bodies, under body.

Jones, Henry Bence. SEE Bence J.

Jones, T. Duckett, 20th century U.S. cardiologist, 1899–1954. SEE J. criteria, under criterion.

Jones, Ernest, British psychiatrist, 1879–1958. SEE Ross-J. test.

Jonesia dentrificans. A species of motile, Gram-positive bacteria formerly classified as LIsteria dendrificans; the only member of the genus Jonesia.

Jonnesco (Ionescu), Thomas, Roumanian surgeon, 1860–1926. SEE J. fossa.

Joseph, Jacques, German surgeon, 1865–1934.

Joubert, Marie, 20th century Canadian neurologist. SEE J. syndrome.

Joule, James P., British physicist, 1818–1889. SEE joule; J. equivalent.

joule (J) (jool, jowl). A unit of energy; the heat generated, or energy expended, by an ampere flowing through an ohm for 1 sec; equal to 10^7 ergs and to a newton-meter. It is an approved multiple of the SI fundamental unit of energy, the erg, and is intended to replace the calorie (4.184 J). SYN unit of heat (3). [J.P. Joule]

Judkins, Melvin P., U.S. radiologist, 1922–1985; pioneer in coronary angiography and angioplasty. SEE J. technique.

ju·ga (joo′gă). Plural of jugum.

ju·gal (joo′găl). **1.** Connecting; yoked. **2.** Relating to the zygomatic bone. [L. jugalis, yoked together, fr. jugum, a yoke]

ju·ga·le (joo-gā′lē). A craniometric point at the union of the temporal and frontal processes of the zygomatic bone. SYN jugal point.

ju·go·max·il·lary (joo′gō-mak′si-lār-ē). Relating to the zygomatic bone and the maxilla.

jug·u·lar (jŭg′ū-lar). **1.** Relating to the throat or neck. **2.** Relating to the j. veins. **3.** A j. vein. [L. jugulum, throat]

jug·u·lum (jŭg′ū-lŭm). SYN throat (2).

ju·gum, pl. **ju·ga** (joo′gŭm, -gă) [TA]. **1.** A ridge or furrow connecting two points. SYN yoke [TA]. **2.** A type of forceps. [L. a yoke]

juga alveola′ria [TA], SYN alveolar yokes, under yoke.

juga cerebralia, ✭official alternate term for impressions of cerebral gyri.

j. sphenoida′le [TA], a plane surface on the sphenoid bone, in front of the sella turcica, connecting the two lesser wings, and forming part of the anterior cranial fossa and especially later in life, the roof of the anteriormost portion of the sphenoidal sinus. SYN planum sphenoidale [TA], sphenoidal yoke✭.

juice (joos). **1.** The interstitial fluid of a plant or animal. **2.** A digestive secretion. [L. jus, broth]

appetite j., gastric j. secreted upon the sight or smell of food and at the time of eating, influenced by the attractiveness of the food and delight in the food ingested; a conditioned reflex.

gastric j., the digestive fluid secreted by the glands of the stomach; a thin colorless liquid of acid reaction containing primarily hydrochloric acid, chymosin, pepsinogen, and intrinsic factor plus mucus.

intestinal j., an alkaline straw-colored fluid secreted by the intestinal glands; its enzymes (peptidases, saccharases, nucleases, lecithinases, phosphatases, lipases) complete the hydrolysis of carbohydrates, proteins, and lipids.

pancreatic j., the external secretion of the pancreas; a clear alkaline fluid containing several enzymes: α-amylase, nucleases, trypsinogen, chymotrypsinogen, and triacylglycerol lipase.

Jukes (jooks). The pseudonym for a celebrated family, most of whose members were social misfits, feebleminded, and degenerate. the subject of arguments for now discredited theories of genetic superiority. SEE ALSO Kallikak.

junctio. ✭official alternate term for junction.

junctio anorectalis [TA], SYN anorectal junction.

junc·tion (jŭngk′shŭn) [TA]. The point, line, or surface of union of two parts, mainly bones or cartilages. SYN juncture. SYN junctura (2) [TA], junctio✭.

adhering j.'s, intercellular j.'s, including zonulae adherentes, hemidesmosomes, and desmosomes, that primarily serve to bind cells together physically.

amelodental j., amelodentinal j., rarely used terms for dentinoenamel j.

amnioembryonic j., the line of amnionic attachment to the periphery of the embryonic disk.

anorectal j. [TA], transition from rectum to anal canal; corresponds to the perineal flexure, or the level at which the gut perforates the pelvic diaphragm; here the rectal ampulla narrows abruptly into a narrow slip. SYN junctio anorectalis [TA].

AV j., imprecisely defined zone surrounding and including the AV node and the adjacent atrial and ventricular myocardium.

cardioesophageal j., SYN esophagogastric j.

cementodentinal j., the surface at which the cementum and dentin of the root of a tooth are joined. SYN dentinocemental j.

cementoenamel j., the surface at which the enamel of the crown and the cementum of the root of a tooth are joined. SEE ALSO cervical line.

choledochoduodenal j., that part of the duodenal wall traversed by the ductus choledochus, ductus pancreaticus, and ampulla.

communicating j., SYN gap j.

corneoscleral j., SYN corneal limbus.

costochondral j.'s, SYN costochondral joints, under joint.

dentinocemental j., SYN cementodentinal j.

dentinoenamel j., the surface at which the enamel and the dentin of the crown of a tooth are joined.

duodenojejunal j., point along the course of the gastrointestinal tract where the duodenum ends and the jejunum begins; occurs approximately at the level of the L2 vertebra, 2–3 cm to the left of the midline; usually takes the form of an acute angle, the duodenojejunal flexure, and is supported by the attachment of the suspensory muscle (ligament) of the duodenum. SEE ALSO duodenojejunal flexure.

electrotonic j., SYN gap j.

esophagogastric j., terminal end of esophagus and beginning of stomach at the cardiac orifice; site of the physiologic inferior esophageal sphincter. SYN cardioesophageal j.

gap j., (1) an intercellular j. formerly considered to be a tight, membrane-to-membrane j. (macula occludens) but now shown to have a 2-nm gap between apposed cell membranes; the gap is not void but contains subunits in the form of polygonal lattices; it occurs in epithelia, between certain nerve cells, and in smooth and cardiac muscle; it is believed to mediate electrotonic coupling which allows ionic currents to pass from one cell to another. SEE ALSO synapse; (2) areas of increased electrochemical communication between myometrial cells which aid in the propagation of the contractions of labor. SYN communicating j., electrotonic j., electrotonic synapse, macula communicans, nexus.

Holliday j., the cross-strand structure formed when two DNA duplexes cross in a recombination event. SYN Holliday structure.

ileocecal j., point along the course of the gastrointestinal tract where the small intestine (ileum) ends as it opens into the cecal portion of the large intestine; occurs usually within the iliac fossa, demarcated internally as the ileocecal orifice.

impermeable j., SYN *zonula* occludens.

intercellular j.'s, specializations of the cellular margins that contribute to the adhesion or allow for communication between cells; they include the macula adherens (desmosome), zonula adherens, zonula occludens, and nexus (gap junction).

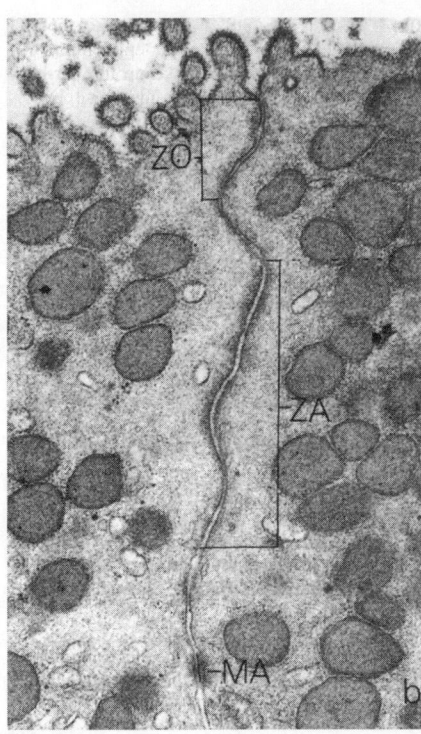

intercellular junction: electron micrograph of the apical portions of two adjoining epithelial cells of the gastric mucosa, showing the junctional complex; MA, macula adherens; ZA, zonula adherens; and ZO, zonula occludens; ×30,000

intermediate j., SYN *zonula* adherens.

j. of lips, SYN *commissure* of lips.

manubriosternal j., SYN sternal *angle.*

mucocutaneous j., the site of transition from epidermis to the epithelium of a mucous membrane.

muscle-tendon j., SYN muscle-tendon *attachment.*

myoneural j., the synaptic connection of the axon of the motor neuron with a muscle fiber. SEE motor *endplate.* SYN neuromuscular j.

neuroectodermal j., the margin of the embryonic neural plate separating it from the embryonic surface ectoderm; cells from this region form the neural crest. SYN neurosomatic j.

neuromuscular j., SYN myoneural j.

neurosomatic j., SYN neuroectodermal j.

rectosigmoid j., the site at which the sigmoid colon becomes the rectum; usually takes the form of an acute angle, demarcated externally by a discontinuation of appendices epiploicae, a spreading out of the teniae coli to completely encircle the rectum, and consequently, termination of the sacculations (haustrae) between the teniae.

right splicing j., boundary between the right end of an intron and the left end of the adjacent exon. SYN acceptor splicing site.

sacrococcygeal j., SYN sacrococcygeal *joint.*

sclerocorneal j., SYN corneal *limbus.*

squamocolumnar j., the site of transition from stratified squamous epithelium to columnar epithelium, usually characterized by stratified coboidal epithelium.

ST j., SYN J *point.*

sternomanubrial j., SYN manubriosternal *symphysis.*

tight j., SYN *zonula* occludens.

tympanostapedial j., SYN tympanostapedial *syndesmosis.*

ureteropelvic j. (UPJ), site of origin of the ureter from the renal pelvis, a common location for congenital or acquired obstruction.

ureterovesical j., the site of entry of the ureter into the bladder, with an oblique angulation through the detrusor to avoid reflux. SEE ALSO vesicoureteral *reflux.*

junc·tu·ra, pl. **junc·tu·rae** (jŭngk-too′ră, -rē) [TA]. **1.** SYN joint. **2.** SYN junction. [L. a joining]

j. cartilagi′nea [TA], SYN cartilaginous *joint.*

j. fibro′sa [TA], SYN fibrous *joint.*

j. lumbosacra′lis, SYN lumbosacral *joint.*

junctu′rae mem′bri inferio′ris li′beri, SYN synovial *joints* of free lower limb, under *joint.*

junctu′rae mem′bri superio′ris, SYN *joints* of pectoral girdle, under *joint.*

junctu′rae mem′bri superio′ris li′beri, SYN synovial *joints* of free upper limb, under *joint.*

junctu′rae os′sium, alternative name for articulationes. SEE articulatio.

j. sacrococcy′gea, SYN sacrococcygeal *joint.*

j. synovia′lis [TA], SYN synovial *joint.*

junctu′rae ten′dinum, SYN intertendinous *connections* of extensor digitorum, under *connection.*

junctu′rae zygapophysia′les, SYN zygapophysial *joints,* under *joint.*

junc·ture (jŭngk′choor). SYN junction.

Jung, Carl Gustav, Swiss psychiatrist and psychologist, 1875–1961. SEE jungian *psychoanalysis.*

Jung, Karl G., Swiss anatomist, 1793–1864. SEE J. *muscle.*

jung·i·an (yung′ē-an). The psychological system or the psychoanalytic form of treatment deriving from it; developed by Carl Gustav Jung.

Jüngling, Adolph O., German surgeon, 1884–1944. SEE J. *disease.*

ju·ni·per (joo′ni-per). The dried ripe fruit of *Juniperus communis* (family Pinaceae). [L. the juniper tree]

j. berry oil, SYN *oil* of juniper.

j. tar, the empyreumatic volatile oil obtained from the woody portion of *Juniperus oxycedrus;* used externally for skin diseases. SYN cade oil.

jur·is·pru·dence (joor-is-proo′dens). The science of law, its principles and concepts. [L. *juris prudentia,* knowledge of law]

dental j., SYN forensic *dentistry.*

medical j., SYN forensic *medicine.*

jus·tice. The ethical principle that persons who have similar circumstances and conditions should be treated alike; sometimes known as distributive justice. [L. *justitia,* fr. *jus,* right, law]

jus·to ma·jor (jus′tō mā′jer). SEE *pelvis* justo major.

ju

jus·to mi·nor (jus'tō mī'ner). SEE *pelvis* justo minor.

ju·ve·nile de·lin·quent. A minor who cannot be controlled by parental authority and commits antisocial or criminal acts, such as vandalism, violence, or robbery.

jux·ta·crine (juks'tă-krin). A mode of hormone action that requires the cell producing the effector to be in direct contact with the cell containing the appropriate receptor. [L. *juxta,* close to, + G. *krinō,* to separate]

jux·ta·ep·i·phys·i·al (jŭks'tă-ep-i-fiz'ē-ăl). Close to or adjoining an epiphysis.

jux·ta·glo·mer·u·lar (jŭks'tă-glŏ-mer'ū-lăr). Close to or adjoining a renal glomerulus.

jux·tal·lo·cor·tex (jŭks'tă-lō-kōr'teks). O. Vogt collective term for several regions of the cerebral cortex which occupy an intermediate position between the isocortex and the allocortex.

jux·ta·med·ul·lary (jŭks'tă-med'ŭ-lār-ē). Close to or adjoining the medullary border.

jux·ta·po·si·tion (jŭks-tă-pō-zish'ŭn). A position side by side. SEE ALSO apposition, contiguity. [L. *juxta,* near to, + *positio,* a placing, fr. *pono,* pp. *positus,* to place]

κ Symbol for kappa, the tenth letter in the Greek alphabet.

K 1. Symbol for potassium; kalium; phylloquinone; kelvin; lysine; lysyl. **2.** In optics, the coefficient of scleral rigidity. **3.** In contact lens fitting, the radius of curvature of the flattest meridian of the apical cornea.

^{39}**K** Symbol for potassium-39.

^{40}**K** Symbol for potassium-40.

^{42}**K** Symbol for potassium-42.

^{43}**K** Symbol for potassium-43.

K Symbol for dissociation *constant*; kinetic *energy*; luminous efficiency. SEE K_d.

K_a Symbol for dissociation *constant* of an acid; association *constant* (2) (often used with gases).

K_b Symbol for dissociation *constant* of a base.

K_d Symbol for dissociation *constant*.

K_{eq} Symbol for equilibrium *constant*.

K_i Symbol for the dissociation constant of an inhibitor; in enzyme kinetics, K_{ii} reflects the values of K_i that affect the intercept of a double-reciprocal plot, whereas K_{is} reflects the values of K_i that affect the slope of the same plot.

K_m Symbol for Michaelis *constant*; Michaelis-Menten *constant*.

K_w Symbol for autoprotolysis constant of water.

k Symbol for kilo-.

k Symbol for rate *constants*, under *constant* or velocity *constants*, under *constant*; Boltzmann constant.

k_{cat} The overall catalytic rate of an enzyme; symbol for turnover *number*; V_{max} divided by the total enzyme concentration.

ka·bu·re (kah-boo′rē). SYN *schistosomiasis* japonica.

Kaes, Theodor, German neurologist, 1852–1913. SEE *line* of K.; *band* of K.-Bechterew.

ka·fin·do (kă-fin′dō). SYN onyalai.

kai·nic ac·id (kā′in-ik). A glutamate analog that exhibits powerful and long-acting excitatory and toxic activity on neurons; used as a research tool in neurobiology to destroy neurons and as an activator of glutamate receptors. Has been used as an anthelmintic against nematodes.

kai·ro·mones (kī′rō-mōn). Chemical messengers that are emitted by organisms of one species but benefit or affect organisms of another species; for example, a flower scent used to attract or repel other species. Cf. pheromones, allomones.

Kaiserling, Karl, German pathologist, 1869–1942. SEE K. *fixative*.

⌂**kak-, kako-.** SEE caco-.

⌂**kal-, kali-.** Potassium; sometimes improperly written as kalio-. [L. *kalium*, potassium]

ka·la azar (kah′lah ah-zahr′). SYN visceral *leishmaniasis*. [Hind. *kala*, black, + *azar*, poison]

ka·le·mia (kă-lē′mē-ă). The presence of potassium in the blood.

ka·li·o·pe·nia (kā′lē-ō-pē′nē-ă). Insufficiency of potassium in the body. SEE ALSO hypokalemia. [Mod. L. *kalium*, potassium, + G. *penia*, poverty]

ka·li·o·pe·nic (kā′lē-ō-pē′nik). Relating to kaliopenia.

Kalischer, Siegfried, German physician, *1862. SEE Sturge-K.-Weber *syndrome*.

ka·li·um (K) (kā′lē-ŭm). SYN potassium. [Mod. L. fr. Ar. *quali*, potash]

ka·li·u·re·sis (kā′lē-ū-rē′sis). SYN kaluresis.

ka·li·u·ret·ic (kā′lē-ū-ret′ik). SYN kaluretic.

kal·li·din (kal′i-din). Bradykinin with a lysyl group attached to the amino terminus; this group can be removed by an aminopeptidase in the blood to yield bradykinin; a decapeptide vasodilator. SYN bradykininogen, k. 10, k. II, lysyl-bradykinin.

k. 9, SYN bradykinin.

k. 10, SYN kallidin.

k. I, SYN bradykinin.

k. II, SYN kallidin.

Kal·li·kak (kal′ĭ-kak). The pseudonym for a celebrated family with two lines of descendants, one of respectable citizens, the other of social misfits and criminals. SEE ALSO Jukes.

kal·li·kre·in (kal-i-krē′in). A group of enzymes (e.g., plasma, tissue, pancreatic, urinary, submandibular k.) that can convert kininogen by proteolysis to bradykinin or kallidin; trypsin and plasmin can also effect the conversion; plasma k. activates the Hageman factor and acts on kininogen. Tissue k. is a serine endopeptidase that can generate kallidin from kininogen. SYN kininogenase, kininogenin.

human glandular k. 3 (hK3), SYN prostate-specific *antigen*.

Kallmann, Franz Josef, U.S. medical geneticist and psychiatrist, 1897–1965. SEE K. *syndrome*.

kal·u·re·sis (kal-ū-rē′sis). The increased urinary excretion of potassium. SYN kaliuresis. [Mod. L. *kalium*, potassium, + G. *ourēsis*, urination]

kal·u·ret·ic (kal-ū-ret′ik). Relating to, causing, or characterized by kaluresis. SYN kaliuretic.

Kandori, Fumio, Japanese ophthalmologist, *1904. SEE fleck *retina* of Kandori.

Kanner, Leo, Austrian psychiatrist in U.S., 1894–1981. SEE K. *syndrome*.

kan·yem·ba (kan-yem′bă). SYN chiufa.

ka·od·ze·ra (kah′od-ze′rā). A disease prevalent in Zimbabwe (formerly Rhodesia), similar to sleeping sickness, caused by *Trypanosoma rhodesiense*. SEE ALSO Rhodesian *trypanosomiasis*.

ka·o·lin (kā′ō-lin). Hydrated aluminum silicate; when powdered and freed from gritty particles by elution, k. is used as a demulcent and adsorbent; in dentistry, it is used to add toughness and opacity to porcelain teeth. SYN aluminum silicate. [Ch. *kao lin*, High Ridge, name of a locality in China where the substance is found in abundance]

ka·o·lin·o·sis (kā′ō-lin-ō′sis). Pneumoconiosis caused by the inhalation of clay dust.

Kaposi, Moritz, (born Moritz Kohn), Hungarian dermatologist in Austria, 1837–1902. SEE K. varicelliform *eruption*, *sarcoma*.

kap·pa (κ) (kap′a). **1.** The tenth letter in the Greek alphabet. **2.** In chemistry, denotes the position of a substituent located on the tenth atom from the carboxyl or other functional group. **3.** A measure of the degree of nonrandom agreement between observers or measurements of the same categorical variable.

kap·pa·cism (kap′ă-sizm). Faulty pronunciation of the "k" sound. [G. *kappa*, the letter κ]

Karman can·nu·la. See under cannula.

Karmen, Albert, U.S. internist and clinical pathologist, *1930. SEE K. *unit*.

Karnofsky, David A., 20th century U.S. physician, †1970. SEE K. *scale*.

Kartagener, Manes, Swiss physician, 1897–1975. SEE K. *syndrome, triad*.

⌂**karyo-.** Nucleus. Cf. nucleo-. [G. *karyon*, nucleus]

kar·y·o·chrome (kar′ē-ō-krōm). A nerve cell body having little or no Nissl substance visible but a nucleus that stains intensely. [karyo- + G. *chroma*, color]

kar·y·oc·la·sis (kar-ē-ok′lă-sis). SYN karyorrhexis. [karyo- + G. *klasis*, a breaking]

⌂ **Combining Forms**	☆ **Official alternate Terminologia Anatomica term**
🄸 **Indicates term is illustrated, see Illustration Index**	
SYN Synonym	**[MIM] Mendelian Inheritance in Man**
Cf. Compare	**C.I. Colour Index**
[NA] Nomina Anatomica	
[TA] Terminologia Anatomica	**High Profile Term**

ka

kar·y·o·cyte (kar′ē-ō-sīt). A young, immature normoblast. [karyo- + G. *kytos,* cell]

kar·y·o·gam·ic (kar-ē-ō-gam′ik). Relating to or marked by karyogamy.

kar·y·og·a·my (kar-ē-og′ă-mē). Fusion of the nuclei of two cells, as occurs in fertilization or true conjugation. [karyo- + G. *gamos,* marriage]

kar·y·o·gen·e·sis (kar-ē-ō-jen′ĕ-sis). Formation of the nucleus of a cell. [karyo- + G. *genesis,* production]

kar·y·o·gen·ic (kar-ē-ō-jen′ik). Relating to karyogenesis; forming the nucleus.

kar·y·o·go·nad (kar′ē-ō-gō′nad). SYN micronucleus (2). [karyo- + G. *gonē,* generation, descent]

kar·y·o·gram (kar′ē-ō-gram). SYN karyotype.

kar·y·ol·o·gy (kar′ē-ol′o-jē). The branch of cytology that deals with the study of the cell nucleus, its organelles, structures, and functions. [karyo + -logy]

kar·y·o·lymph (kar′ē-ō-limf). The presumably fluid substance or gel of the nucleus in which stainable elements were believed to be suspended; much that was formerly considered to be k. is now known to be euchromatin. SYN nuclear hyaloplasm, nuclear sap, nucleochylema, nucleochyme. [karyo- + L. *lympha,* clear water]

kar·y·ol·y·sis (kar-ē-ol′i-sis). Apparent destruction of the nucleus of a cell by swelling and the loss of affinity of its chromatin for basic dyes. [karyo- + G. *lysis,* dissolution]

kar·y·o·lyt·ic (kar′ē-ō-lit′ik). Relating to karyolysis.

kar·y·o·mere (kar′ē-ō-mer′). A vesicle containing only a small part of the typical nucleus, usually following an abnormal mitosis. [karyo- + G. *meros,* part]

kar·y·o·mi·cro·some (kar-ē-ō-mī′krō-sōm). One of the minute particles or granules making up the substance of the cell nucleus. SYN nucleomicrosome. [karyo- + G. *mikros,* small, + *soma,* body]

kar·y·o·mi·to·me (kar′-ē-ōm-ī′-tom). The nuclear chromatin network. [karyo- + mitosis + -ome]

kar·y·o·mor·phism (kar′ē-ō-mōr′fizm). **1.** Development of the nucleus of a cell. **2.** Denoting the nuclear shapes of cells, especially leukocytes. [karyo- + G. *morphē,* form]

kar·y·on (kar′ē-on). SYN nucleus (1). [G. *karyon,* a nut, kernel]

kar·y·o·phage (kar′ē-ō-fāj). An intracellular parasite that feeds on the host nucleus. [karyo- + G. *phagō,* to devour]

kar·y·o·plasm (kar′ē-ō-plazm). Rarely used term for nucleoplasm.

kar·y·o·plas·mol·y·sis (kar′ē-ō-plaz-mol′i-sis). SYN achromatolysis.

kar·y·o·plast (kar′ē-ō-plast). A cell nucleus surrounded by a narrow band of cytoplasm and a plasma membrane. [karyo- + G. *plastos,* formed]

kar·y·o·plas·tin (kar′ē-ō-plas′tin). The achromatic nuclear material that forms the spindle apparatus.

kar·y·o·pyk·no·sis (kar′ē-ō-pik-nō′sis). Cytologic characteristics of the superficial or cornified cells of stratified squamous epithelium in which there is shrinkage of the nuclei and condensation of the chromatin into structureless masses. [karyo- + G. *pyknos,* thick, crowded, + *-osis,* condition]

kar·y·o·pyk·not·ic (kar′ē-ō-pik-not′ik). Pertaining to or causing karyopyknosis.

kar·y·or·rhex·is (kar-ē-ō-rak′sis). Fragmentation of the nucleus whereby its chromatin is distributed irregularly throughout the cytoplasm; a stage of necrosis usually followed by karyolysis. SYN karyoclasis. [karyo- + G. *rhexis,* rupture]

kar·y·o·some (kar′ē-ō-sōm). A mass of chromatin often found in the interphase cell nucleus representing a more condensed zone of chromatin filaments. SYN chromatin nucleolus, chromocenter, false nucleolus, net knot. [karyo- + G. *sōma,* body]

kar·y·os·ta·sis (kar-ē-os′tă-sis). SYN interphase. [karyo- + G. *stasis,* a standing still]

kar·y·o·the·ca (kar′ē-ō-thē′kă). SYN nuclear *envelope.* [karyo- + G. *thēkē,* box, sheath]

kar·y·o·type (kar′ē-ō-tīp). The chromosome characteristics of an individual cell or of a cell line, usually presented as a systema-

tized array of metaphase chromosomes from a photomicrograph of a single cell nucleus arranged in pairs in descending order of size and according to the position of the centromere. SYN idiogram (1), karyogram. [karyo- + G. *typos,* model]

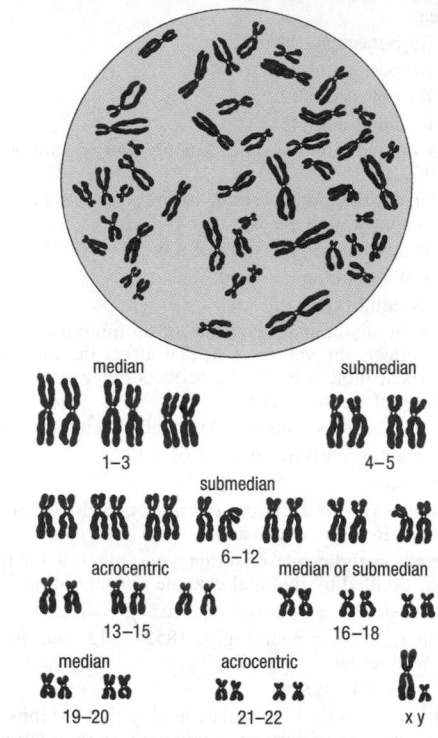

karyotype of a normal human cell

kar·y·o·zo·ic (kar′ē-ō-zō′ik). Denoting a parasite inhabiting the cell nucleus of its host. [karyo- + G. *zōon,* animal]

Kasabach, Haig H., U.S. physician, 1898–1943. SEE K.-Merritt *syndrome.*

Kasai, Morio, Japanese surgeon. SEE K. *operation.*

ka·sai (kă-sī′). A form of anemia occurring in the Congo River region, with associated edema of subcutaneous tissues, depigmented regions in the skin, and various gastrointestinal disturbances; thought to result from deficiencies in nutrition. SYN Belgian Congo anemia.

Kashin, Nikolai I., Russian orthopedist, 1825–1872. SEE K.-Bek *disease.*

Kasten, Frederick H., U.S. histochemist and cell biologist, *1927. SEE K. fluorescent Schiff *reagents,* under *reagent,* fluorescent Feulgen *stain,* fluorescent PAS *stain.*

kat Abbreviation for katal.

kata-. Alternative spelling for cata-; down. [G. *kata,* down]

kat·al (kat) (kat′ăl). Unit of catalytic activity equal to 1 mol of product formed (or substrate consumed) per second, as of the amount of enzyme that catalyzes transformation of 1 mol of substrate per second.

kat·a·ther·mom·e·ter (kat′ă-ther-mom′ĕ-ter). An alcohol-filled thermometer of specified design that is heated above ambient temperature and then allowed to cool; the time taken to cool between specified temperatures is a measure of the heat content of the environment that takes into account air movement as well as temperature. The bulb may be silvered to minimize radiation effects or blackened to maximize them.

Katayama, Kunika, Japanese physician, 1856–1931. SEE K. *fever, test.*

kathexis. A rare disorder characterized by bone marrow retention of myeloid elements leading to severe peripheral neutropenia;

neutrophils have a distinctly abnormal appearance; Gm-CSF levels are undetectable and administration of this substance is therapeutically effective. SYN myelokathexis.

Katz, Sir Bernard, German-British neurophysiologist and Nobel laureate, *1911. SEE Goldman-Hodgkin-K. *equation.*

ka·va (kah'vah). **1.** SYN methysticum. **2.** SYN yaqona. [Tongan and Marquesan, Litter]

Kawasaki, Tomisaku, 20th century Japanese pediatrician. SEE K. *disease, syndrome.*

Kay, Herbert D., British biochemist, *1893. SEE Jenner-K. *unit.*

Kayser, Bernhard, German physician, 1869–1954. SEE K.-Fleischer *ring.*

Kazanjian, Varaztad H., Armenian otorhinolaryngologist in the U.S., 1879–1974. SEE K. *operation.*

kb Abbreviation for kilobase.

K blood group, k blood group. See Kell blood group, Blood Groups appendix.

kc Abbreviation for kilocycle.

kcal Abbreviation for kilogram *calorie*; kilocalorie.

Kearns, Thomas P., U.S. ophthalmologist, *1922. SEE K.-Sayre *syndrome.*

Keating-Hart, Walter V., French physician, 1870–1922. SEE Keating-Hart *method.*

keel (kēl). Paratyphoid or salmonellosis of ducklings.

Keen, William W., U.S. surgeon, 1837–1932. SEE K. *operation.*

Kegel, A.H., 20th century U.S. gynecologist. SEE K. *exercises,* under *exercise.*

Kehr, Hans, German surgeon, 1862–1916. SEE K. *sign.*

Keith, Sir Arthur, Scottish anatomist, 1866–1955. SEE K. *bundle, node,* and Flack *node.*

ke·lec·tome (kē'lek-tōm). An instrument used, like the harpoon, to remove a specimen of tumor substance for examination. [G. *kēlē,* tumor, + *ektomē,* excision]

Kell blood group. See Blood Groups appendix.

Keller, William Lordan, U.S. surgeon, 1874–1959. SEE K. *bunionectomy.*

Kellie, George, 18th century Scottish anatomist. SEE Monro-K. *doctrine.*

Kelly, Howard A., U.S. gynecologist, 1858–1943. SEE K. *clamp, operation,* rectal *speculum.*

Kelly, Adam B., British otolaryngologist, 1865–1941. SEE Paterson-K. *syndrome;* Paterson-Brown-K. *syndrome.*

ke·loid (kē'loyd). A nodular, firm, movable, nonencapsulated, often linear mass of hyperplastic scar tissue, tender and frequently painful, consisting of wide irregularly distributed bands of collagen; occurs in the dermis and adjacent subcutaneous tissue, usually after trauma, surgery, a burn, or severe cutaneous disease such as cystic acne, and is more common in blacks. SYN cheloid. [G. *kēlē,* a tumor (or *kēlis,* a spot), + *eidos,* appearance]

acne k., a chronic eruption of fibrous papules that develop at the site of deep folliculitis, usually on the back of the neck at the hairline. SYN folliculitis keloidalis.

ke·loi·do·sis (kē'loy-dō'sis). Multiple keloids.

ke·lo·so·mia (kē-lō-sō'mē-ă). SYN celosomia.

Kelvin, Lord William Thomson, Scottish physicist, 1824–1907. SEE kelvin; K. *scale.*

kel·vin (K). A unit of thermodynamic temperature equal to 273.16^{-1} of the thermodynamic temperature of the triple point of water. SEE Kelvin *scale.* [Lord *Kelvin*]

Kendall, J., 20th century U.S. pathologist. SEE Abell-Kendall *method.*

Kendall. SEE Abell-Kendall *method.*

Kennedy, Edward, U.S. dentist, *1883. SEE K. *classification.*

Kennedy, Robert Foster, U.S. neurologist, 1884–1952. SEE K. *syndrome;* Foster K. *syndrome.*

Kennedy, William, U.S. neurologist. SEE Kennedy *disease.*

Kenny, Elizabeth, Australian nurse, 1880–1952. SEE K. *treatment.*

△**keno-.** SEE ceno- (3). [G. *kenos,* empty]

Kent, Albert F.S., English physiologist, 1863–1958. SEE K. *bundle;* K.-His *bundle.*

keph·a·lin (kef'ă-lin). SYN cephalin.

Kerandel, Jean F., French physician, 1873–1934. SEE Kerandel *sign.*

ker·a·sin (ker'ă-sin). Obsolete term for glucocerebroside. SYN cerasin.

△**kerat-.** SEE kerato-.

ker·a·tan sul·fate (ker'ă-tan). A type of sulfated mucopolysaccharide containing D-galactose in place of the uronic acid of hyaluronic acid or chondroitin; also containing unsulfated and 6-sulfated *N*-acetyl-D-glucosamine; found in cartilage, bone, connective tissue, the cornea, aorta, and in the intervertebral disks; accumulates in Morquio syndrome; k. s. I is abundant in cornea and is attached to a protein via an asparaginyl residue; k. s. II is found in loose connective tissue and bone and is linked to a seryl or threonyl residue. SYN keratosulfate.

ker·a·tec·ta·sia (ker-ă-tek-tā'zē-ă). SYN keratoectasia. [kerato- + G. *ektasis,* extrusion]

ker·a·tec·to·my (ker-ă-tek'tō-mē). An operation done to change the refraction of the cornea; a crescentic piece of corneal stroma is removed and the resultant corneal wound is sutured. This steepens the cornea and increases its power in that axis. SEE ALSO keratotomy. [kerato- + G. *ektomē,* excision]

automated lamellar k., resection of a disk of corneal tissue using a precise machine to alter the refractive power of the eye.

photorefractive k. (PRK), removal of part of the cornea with a laser to change its shape, and thus to modify the refractive error of the eye (reduce its myopia, for example).

phototherapeutic k. (PTK), ablation of diseased corneal tissue using an excimer *laser.*

ker·a·te·in (ker'ă-tē-in). The easily digested reduction product of keratin, in which the disulfide links are reduced to SH groups, the individual peptide chains being separated.

ker·a·tin (ker'ă-tin). Collective name for a group of proteins that form the intermediate filaments in epithelial cells. K.'s have a molecular weight between 40 kd and 68 kd, and are separated one from another by electrophoresis and isoelectric focusing; thus separated, they are sequentially numbered from 1–20, and also subdivided into low, intermediate, and high molecular weight proteins. According to their isoelectric mobility they are either acidic or basic. In general, each acidic k. protein has its basic equivalent with which it is paired to form the intermediate filaments; some k. proteins, however, occur unpaired. Various epithelial cells contain different k. proteins, in a tissue-specific manner. Antibodies to keratin proteins are widely used for histologic typing of tumors, and are especially useful for distinguishing carcinomas from sarcomas, lymphomas, and melanomas. SYN ceratin, cytokeratin. [G. *keras (kerat-),* horn, + -in]

ker·a·tin·as·es (ker'ă-tin-ās-ez). Hydrolases catalyzing the hydrolysis of keratin; each having slightly different specificities.

ker·a·tin·i·za·tion (ker'ă-tin-i-zā'shŭn). Keratin formation or development of a horny layer; may also apply to premature formation of keratin. SYN cornification.

ker·a·tin·ized (ker'ă-ti-nīzd). Having become horny. SYN cornified.

ke·rat·i·no·cyte (ke-rat'i-nō-sīt). A cell of the living epidermis and certain oral epithelium that produces keratin in the process of differentiating into the dead and fully keratinized cells of the stratum corneum.

ke·rat·i·no·phil·ic (ke-rat'i-nō-fil'ik). Denoting fungi that use keratin as a substrata, e.g., dermatophytes. [keratin + Gr. *philos,* love, attraction, + -ic]

ke·rat·i·no·some (ke-rat'i-nō-sōm). A membrane-bound granule, 100 to 500 nm in diameter, located in the upper layers of the stratum spinosum of certain stratified squamous epithelia. SYN lamellar granule, membrane-coating granule, Odland body.

ke·rat·i·nous (ke-rat'i-nŭs). **1.** Relating to keratin. **2.** SYN horny.

ker·a·ti·tis (ker-ă-tī'tis). Inflammation of the cornea. SEE ALSO keratopathy. [kerato- + G. *-itis,* inflammation]

ke

actinic k., a reaction of the cornea to ultraviolet light.

deep punctate k., sharply defined opacities in an otherwise clear cornea, occurring in syphilitic iritis.

dendriform k., dendritic k., a form of herpetic k.

diffuse deep k., SYN k. profunda.

Dimmer k., SYN k. nummularis.

disciform k., large disk-shaped infiltration of the central or paracentral corneal stroma. This lesion is deep and nonsuppurative and is seen in virus infections, particularly herpetic. SYN k. disciformis.

k. discifor′mis, SYN disciform k.

exposure k., inflammation of the cornea resulting from irritation caused by inability to close the eyelids. SYN lagophthalmic k.

fascicular k., a phlyctenular k. followed by the formation of a band or fascicle of blood vessels extending from the margin toward the center.

filamentary k., a condition characterized by the formation of epithelial filaments of varying size and length on the corneal surface. SYN k. filamentosa.

k. filamento′sa, SYN filamentary k.

geographic k., k. with coalescence of superficial lesions in herpes keratitis.

herpetic k., inflammation of the cornea (or cornea and conjunctiva) due to herpes simplex virus. SYN herpes corneae, herpetic keratoconjunctivitis.

interstitial k., an inflammation of the corneal stroma, often with neovascularization.

lagophthalmic k., SYN exposure k.

k. linea′ris mi′grans, a deep, linear corneal opacity stretching from limbus to limbus; associated with congenital syphilis.

marginal k., a corneal inflammation at the limbus.

metaherpetic k., a postinfectious corneal inflammation in herpetic k. leading to epithelial erosion; not due to virus replication.

mycotic k., an infection of the cornea of the eye caused by a fungus.

necrotizing k., severe inflammation and destruction of corneal tissue that may be seen in response to herpes infection.

neuroparalytic k., SYN neurotrophic k.

neurotrophic k., inflammation of the cornea after corneal anesthesia. SYN neuroparalytic k.

k. nummula′ris, coin-shaped or round, discrete, grayish areas 0.5 to 1.5 mm in diameter scattered throughout the various layers of the cornea. SYN Dimmer k.

phlyctenular k., an inflammation of the corneal conjunctiva with the formation of small red nodules of lymphoid tissue (phlyctenulae) near the corneoscleral limbus. SYN scrofulous k.

pneumococcal/suppurative k., SYN serpiginous k.

polymorphic superficial k., epithelial degeneration occurring in starvation.

k. profun′da, an inflammation of the posterior corneal stroma. SYN diffuse deep k.

punctate k., k. puncta′ta, SYN keratic *precipitates,* under *precipitate.*

sclerosing k., inflammation of the cornea complicating scleritis; characterized by opacification of the corneal stroma.

scrofulous k., SYN phlyctenular k.

serpiginous k., a severe, creeping, central, suppurative ulcer often due to pneumococci. SYN pneumococcal/suppurative k., serpent ulcer of cornea.

k. sic′ca, SYN *keratoconjunctivitis* sicca.

superficial linear k., spontaneous, painful k. with epithelial erosion and folds in Bowman membrane.

superficial punctate k., epithelial punctate k. associated with viral conjunctivitis. SYN Thygeson disease.

trachomatous k., SEE pannus, corneal *pannus.*

vascular k., superficial cellular infiltration of the cornea and neovascularization between Bowman membrane and the epithelium.

vesicular k., k. with coalescence of areas of epithelial corneal edema.

xerotic k., SYN keratomalacia.

△**kerato-, kerat-. 1.** The cornea. **2.** Horny tissue or cells. SEE ALSO cerat-, cerato-. [G. *keras,* horn]

▮**ker·a·to·ac·an·tho·ma** (ker′ă-tō-ak′an-thō′mă). A rapidly growing tumor that may be umbilicated, and usually occurs on exposed areas of the skin in elderly white men, which invades the dermis but remains localized and usually resolves spontaneously if untreated; microscopically, the nodule is composed of well-differentiated squamous epithelium with a central keratin mass that opens on the skin surface. [kerato- + G. *akantha,* thorn, +-*oma,* tumor]

ker·a·to·an·gi·o·ma (ker′ă-tō-an-jē-ō′mă). SYN angiokeratoma.

ker·a·to·cele (ker′ă-tō-sēl). Hernia of Descemet membrane through a defect in the outer layers of the cornea. [kerato- + G. *kēlē,* hernia]

ker·a·to·con·junc·ti·vi·tis (ker′ă-tō-kon-jŭngk′ti-vī′tis). Inflammation of the conjunctiva and of the cornea.

atopic k., a chronic papillary inflammation, of the conjunctiva showing Trantas dots in a patient with a history of atopy.

epidemic k., follicular conjunctivitis followed by subepithelial corneal infiltrates; often caused by adenovirus type 8, less commonly by other types. SYN virus k.

flash k., SYN ultraviolet k.

herpetic k., SYN herpetic *keratitis.*

microsporidian k., a form of k. often associated with immunosuppressed persons, such as those suffering from AIDS.

k. sic′ca, k. associated with decreased tears. SEE ALSO Sjögren *syndrome.* SYN dry eye syndrome, keratitis sicca.

superior limbic k., inflammatory edema of the superior corneoscleral limbus.

ultraviolet k., acute k. resulting from exposure to intense ultraviolet irradiation. SYN actinic conjunctivitis, arc-flash conjunctivitis, flash k., ophthalmia nivalis, snow conjunctivitis, welder's conjunctivitis.

vernal k., SYN vernal *conjunctivitis.*

virus k., SYN epidemic k.

▮**ker·a·to·co·nus** (ker′ă-tō-kō′nŭs). A conical protrusion of the cornea caused by thinning of the stroma; usually bilateral. SEE ALSO Fleischer *ring,* Munson *sign.* SYN conical cornea. [kerato- + G. *kōnos,* cone]

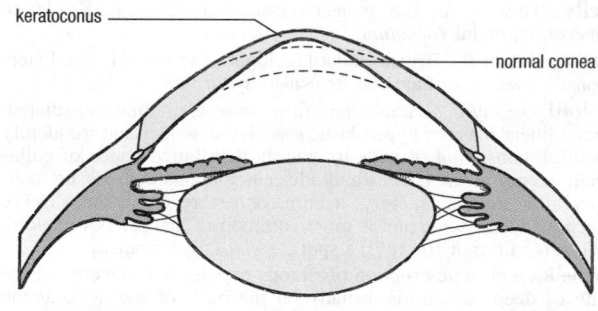

keratoconus

---

circumscribed posterior k., congenital corneal defect characterized by a craterlike defect on the posterior corneal surface.

ker·a·to·cri·coid (ker′ă-tō-krī′koyd). SYN ceratocricoid.

ker·a·to·cyst (ker′ă-tō-sist). Odontogenic cyst derived from remnants of the dental lamina and appearing as a unilocular or multilocular radiolucency which may produce jaw expansion; epithelial lining is characterized microscopically by a uniform thickness, a corrugated superficial layer of parakeratin, and a prominent basal layer composed of palisaded columnar cells; associated with the bifid rib basal cell nevus syndrome.

odontogenic k. (ke-rā′tō-sist), a cyst of dental lamina origin with a high recurrence rate and well-defined histologic criteria of a corrugated parakeratin surface, uniformly thin epithelium, and a palisaded basal layer. One manifestation of the basal cell nevus syndrome.

ker·a·to·cyte (ker′ă-tō-sīt). The fibroblastic stromal cell of the cornea.

ker·a·to·der·ma (ker′ă-tō-der′mă). **1.** Any horny superficial growth. **2.** A generalized thickening of the horny layer of the epidermis. [kerato- + G. *derma,* skin]

k. blennorrhag′ica, SYN *keratosis* blennorrhagica.

k. blennorrhagicum (blen-ō-raj′ĭ-kŭm), the scattered, thickened, hyperkeratotic skin lesions seen in Reiter syndrome.

lymphedematous k., SYN mossy *foot.*

mutilating k. [MIM*124500], diffuse k. of the extremities, with the development during childhood of constricting fibrous bands around the middle phalanx of the fingers or toes that may lead to spontaneous amputation; there may be congenital deafness; autosomal dominant inheritance, caused by mutation in the gene for loricrin (LOR), a component of the epidermal differentiation complex on 1q. SYN keratoma hereditarium mutilans, Vohwinkel syndrome.

k. palma′ris et planta′ris, SYN palmoplantar k.

palmoplantar k. [MIM*148600 & MIM*244850], the occurrence of symmetrical diffuse or patchy areas of hypertrophy of the horny layer of the epidermis on the palms and soles; a group of ectodermal dysplasias of considerable variety, and either autosomal dominant or recessive inheritance. SYN ichthyosis palmaris et plantaris, k. palmaris et plantaris, k. symmetrica, keratoma plantare sulcatum, keratosis palmaris et plantaris, tylosis palmaris et plantaris.

k. planta′re sulca′tum, hyperkeratosis and fissure formation on the soles. SYN cracked heel.

punctate k. [MIM*175860], horny papules over the palms, soles, and digits that develop central plugs; seen commonly in blacks; autosomal dominant inheritance. SYN keratoma disseminatum, keratosis punctata.

senile k., SYN actinic *keratosis.*

k. symmet′rica, SYN palmoplantar k.

type III punctate palmoplantar k., SYN acrokeratoelastoidosis.

ker·a·to·der·ma·ti·tis (ker′ă-tō-der-mă-tī′tis). Inflammation with proliferation of the horny layer of the skin. [kerato- + G. *derma,* skin, + *-itis,* inflammation]

ker·a·to·ec·ta·sia (ker′ă-tō-ek-tā′zē-ă). A bulging forward of the cornea. SYN corneal ectasia, keratectasia.

ker·a·to·elas·toid·o·sis (ker′ă-tō-ă-las′toy-dō-sis). Hyperkeratosis and degeneration of dermal elastic tissue. SEE ALSO acrokeratoelastoidosis. [kerato- + Mod. L. *elasticus,* elastic, fr. G. *elastikos,* propulsive, fr. *elaunō,* to drive + *eidos,* resemblance, + suffix *-ōsis,* condition]

k. marginalis (mar-gin-āl′is), hyperkeratosis and solar elastosis presenting as linear papules along the junction of the palms and dorsal surface of the hands in the elderly. [L. marginal]

ker·a·to·ep·i·the·li·o·plas·ty (ker′ă-tō-ep-i-thē′lē-ō-plas-tē). A surgical procedure for the repair of persistent corneal epithelial defects. All corneal epithelium is removed from the recipient cornea, and small pieces of donor cornea, with epithelium attached, are placed at the corneoscleral limbus. The donor corneal epithelium grows and spreads out to cover the recipient cornea. [kerato- + epithelio- + G. *plastos,* formed]

ker·a·to·gen·e·sis (ker′ă-tō-jen′ĕ-sis). Production or origin of horny cells or tissue. [kerato- + G. *genesis,* production]

ker·a·to·ge·net·ic (ker′ă-tō-jĕ-net′ik). Relating to keratogenesis.

ker·a·tog·e·nous (ker-ă-toj′ĕ-nŭs). Causing a growth of cells that produce keratin and result in the formation of horny tissue, such as fingernails, scales, feathers, etc.

ker·a·to·glo·bus (ker′ă-tō-glō′bŭs). Congenital anomaly consisting of an enlarged anterior segment of the eye. SYN anterior megalophthalmos, megalocornea. [kerato- + L. *globus,* ball]

ker·a·tog·ra·phy (ker′ah-tog′ra-fē). A record or portrayal of the cornea. SEE photokeratoscope, videokeratoscope. [kerato- + G. *graphō,* to write]

ker·a·to·hy·al (ker′ă-tō-hī′ăl). SYN ceratohyal.

ker·a·to·hy·a·lin (ker′ă-tō-hī′ă-lin). The substance in the large basophilic granules of the stratum granulosum of the epidermis rich in proline and sulfhydryl groups. [kerato- + hyalin]

ker·a·toid (ker′ă-toyd). Resembling corneal tissue. [kerato- + G. *eidos,* resemblance]

ker·a·to·lep·tyn·sis (ker′ă-tō-lep-tin′sis). **1.** SYN gutter *dystrophy* of cornea. **2.** An operation for removing the surface of the cornea and replacement by bulbar conjunctiva for cosmetic reasons. [kerato- + G. *leptynsis,* a making thin]

ker·a·to·leu·ko·ma (ker′ă-tō-loo-kō′mă). A white corneal opacity. [kerato- + G. *leukos,* white, + *-ōma,* growth]

ker·a·tol·y·sis (ker-ă-tol′i-sis). **1.** Separation or loosening of the horny layer of the epidermis. **2.** Specifically, a disease characterized by a shedding of the epidermis recurring at more or less regular intervals. SYN deciduous skin. [kerato- + G. *lysis,* loosening]

k. exfoliati′va [MIM*270300], familial continual noninflammatory skin peeling characterized by a separation of stratum corneum in leaflike flakes occurring everywhere except on the palms and soles; autosomal recessive inheritance. SYN erythema exfoliativa.

pitted k., noninflammatory Gram-positive bacterial infection of the plantar surfaces producing small depressions in the stratum corneum, associated frequently with humidity and hyperhidrosis. SYN k. plantare sulcatum.

k. planta′re sulca′tum, SYN pitted k.

ker·a·to·lyt·ic (ker′ă-tō-lit′ik). Relating to keratolysis.

ker·a·to·ma (ker-ă-tō′mă). **1.** SYN callosity. **2.** A horny tumor. [kerato- + G. *-oma,* tumor]

k. dissemina′tum, SYN punctate *keratoderma.*

k. heredita′rium mu′tilans, SYN mutilating *keratoderma.*

k. planta′re sulca′tum, SYN palmoplantar *keratoderma.*

senile k., SYN actinic *keratosis.*

ker·a·to·ma·la·cia (ker′ă-tō-mă-lā′shē-ă). Dryness with ulceration and perforation of the cornea, with absence of inflammatory reactions, occurring in cachectic children; results from severe vitamin A deficiency. SYN xerotic keratitis. [kerato- + G. *malakia,* softness]

ker·a·tome (ker′ă-tōm). A knife used for incising the cornea. SYN keratotome.

ker·a·tom·e·ter (ker-ă-tom′ĕ-ter). An instrument for measuring the curvature of the anterior corneal surface. SYN ophthalmometer. [kerato- + G. *metron,* measure]

ker·a·tom·e·try (ker-ă-tom′ĕ-trē). Measurement of the radii of corneal curvature.

ker·a·to·mi·leu·sis (ker′ă-tō-mī-loo′sis). Surgical alteration of refractive error by changing the shape of a deep layer of the cornea: the anterior lamella is peeled back, frozen, and recarved on its back surface on a lathe; or, some of the corneal stroma can be removed from the bed with a laser or a knife. [coinage, prob. fr. G. *keras* (*kerat-*), horn, cornea, + *smileusis,* carving]

laser-assisted in situ k. (LASIK), a refractive procedure to correct myopia by which a flap of cornea is made, excimer *laser* ablation of corneal stoma is performed, and the flap laid back in position.

ker·a·to·my·co·sis (ker-ă-tō-mī-kō′sis). Fungal infection of the cornea.

ker·a·to·no·sis (ker′ă-tō-nō′sis). Any abnormal noninflammatory, usually hypertrophic, affection of the horny layer of the skin. [kerato- + G. *-osis,* condition]

ker·a·to·pach·y·der·ma (ker′ă-tō-pak-i-der′mă). A syndrome of congenital deafness with development of hyperkeratosis of the skin of the palms, soles, elbows, and knees in childhood, and with bandlike constrictions of the fingers. [kerato- + G. *pachys,* thick, + *derma,* skin]

ker·a·to·path·i·a (ker′ă-tō-path′ē-ă). SYN keratopathy.

k. guttata, wartlike endothelial excrescence on the posterior surface of the cornea.

ker·a·top·a·thy (ker-ă-top′ă-thē). Any corneal disease, damage, dysfunction, or abnormality. SYN keratopathia. [kerato- + G. *pathos,* suffering, disease]

band-shaped k., a horizontal, gray, interpalpebral opacity of the cornea that begins at the periphery and progresses centrally; occurs in hypercalcemia, chronic iridocyclitis, and Still disease.

bullous k., edema of the corneal stroma and epithelium; occurs in

Fuchs endothelial dystrophy, advanced glaucoma, iridocyclitis, and sometimes after intraocular lens implantation.

chronic actinic k., SYN climatic k.

climatic k., a bilateral, symmetrical corneal dystrophy caused by prolonged exposure to extremes of heat or cold; nodular opacities are limited to the interpalpebral area and vision is only mildly affected. SYN chronic actinic k., climatic droplike k., Labrador k., spheroidal degeneration.

climatic droplike k., SYN climatic k.

filamentary k., formation of fine elongations of corneal epithelium in inflammation, edema, and degenerative states.

infectious crystalline k., fernlike, needle-shaped deposits that may be seen in bacterial keratitis, particularly that due to α-hemolytic *streptococci*, under *streptococcus*.

Labrador k., SYN climatic k.

lipid k., occurrence of fats in an area of corneal vascularization.

neuroparalytic k., corneal inflammation or ulceration associated with dysfunction of the ophthalmic branch of the trigeminal nerve.

striate k., corneal stromal edema with formation of criss-cross tracts.

vesicular k., corneal epithelial edema with formation of vacuoles.

ker·a·to·pha·kia (ker′ă-tō-fak′ē-ă). Implantation of a donor cornea or plastic lens within the corneal stroma to modify refractive error. SYN keratophakic keratoplasty. [kerato- + G. *phakos,* lens]

ker·a·to·plas·ia (ker′a-to-plā′zē-ă). The formation or renewal of a horny layer. [kerato- + G. *plassō*; to fashion]

ker·a·to·plas·ty (ker′ă-tō-plas-tē). Any surgical modification of the cornea; the removal of a portion of the cornea containing an opacity and the insertion in its place of a piece of cornea of the same size and shape removed from elsewhere. SYN corneal graft, corneal transplantation, corneal trepanation, trepanation of cornea, transplantation of cornea. [kerato- + G. *plassō,* to form]

allopathic k., corneal transplant with donor material of glass, plastic, or other inert material.

autogenous k., corneal transplant with donor material from the same individual.

epikeratophakic k., SYN epikeratophakia.

heterogenous k., corneal transplant with donor material from another species.

homogenous k., corneal transplant with donor material from another individual of the same species.

keratophakic k., SYN keratophakia.

lamellar k., layered k., SYN nonpenetrating k.

nonpenetrating k., k. in which only the anterior layer of the cornea is used (not a tectonic k.). SYN lamellar k., layered k.

optical k., transplantation of transparent corneal tissue to replace a leukoma or scar that impairs vision.

penetrating k., corneal transplant with replacement of all layers of the cornea, but retaining the peripheral cornea. SYN perforating k.

perforating k., SYN penetrating k.

refractive k., any procedure in which the shape of the cornea is modified, with the intent of changing the refractive error of the eye; for example, if the cornea is flattened, the eye becomes less myopic. SEE photorefractive *keratectomy,* keratophakia, lamellar k., thermokeratoplasty, keratomileusis, radial *keratotomy.* SYN keratorefractive surgery.

tectonic k., grafting to replace lost corneal tissue.

total k., corneal transplant in which the entire cornea is removed and replaced.

ker·a·to·pros·the·sis (ker′ă-tō-pros-thē′sis). Replacement of the central area of an opacified cornea by plastic. [kerato- + G. *prosthesis,* addition]

ker·a·to·rhex·is, ker·a·tor·rhex·is (ker′ă-tō-rek′sis). Rupture of the cornea, due to trauma or perforating ulcer. [kerato- + G. *rhēxis,* a bursting]

ker·a·to·rus (ker-a-tō′rŭs). Vaultlike corneal herniation with severe regular myopic astigmatism. [kerat- + L. *torus,* swelling, knot, bulge]

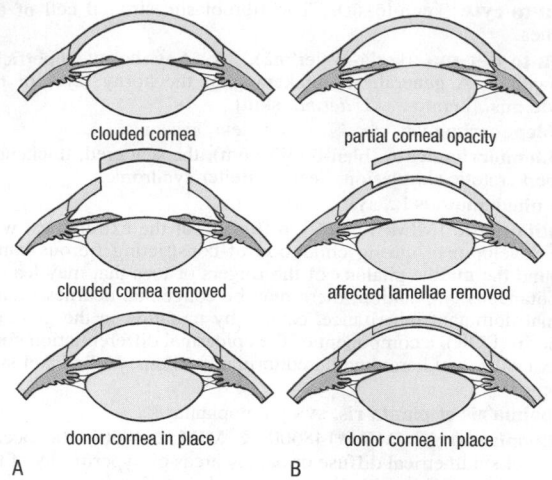

full and partial corneal transplantation: (A) penetrating keratoplasty: a full-thickness (7- to 8- mm) disk is removed from the host and replaced with a matching full-thickness button from the donor; (B) lamellar keratoplasty: a thin layer of corneal tissue is excised from the host eye, sparing the stroma and entire endothelium

ker·a·to·scle·ri·tis (ker′ă-tō-skle-rī′tis). Inflammation of both cornea and sclera.

ker·a·to·scope (ker′ă-tō-skōp). An instrument marked with lines or circles by means of which the corneal reflex can be observed. SYN Placido da Costa disk. [kerato- + G. *skopeō,* to examine]

ker·a·tos·co·py (ker-ă-tos′kŏ-pē). **1.** Examination of the reflections from the anterior surface of the cornea in order to determine the character and amount of corneal astigmatism. **2.** A term first applied by Cuignet to his method of retinoscopy. [kerato- + G. *skopeō,* to examine]

ker·a·to·sis, pl. **ker·a·to·ses** (ker-ă-tō′sis, -sēz). Any lesion on the epidermis marked by the presence of circumscribed overgrowths of the horny layer. [kerato- + G. *-osis,* condition]

actinic k., a premalignant warty lesion occurring on the sun-exposed skin of the face or hands in aged light-skinned persons; hyperkeratosis may form a cutaneous horn, and squamous cell carcinoma of low-grade malignancy may develop in a small proportion of untreated patients. SYN senile keratoderma, senile keratoma, senile k., k. senilis, senile wart, solar k., verruca plana senilis, verruca senilis.

arsenical k., multiple punctate keratoses, most commonly of the palms and soles but also of the fingers and proximal portions of the extremities, resulting from long-term arsenic ingestion; they resemble Bowen disease microscopically and may become squamous cell or basal cell carcinoma.

k. blennorrhag′ica, pustules and crusts associated with Reiter syndrome. SYN keratoderma blennorrhagica.

k. follicula′ris [MIM*124200], an autosomal dominant disorder characterized by eruption, beginning usually in late childhood, in which keratotic papules originating from both follicles and interfollicular epidermis of the trunk, face, scalp, and axillae become crusted and verrucous; the papules are often intensely pruritic. Microscopically, dyskeratotic cells termed corps ronds are seen in the epidermis. Longitudinal nail bands are frequent. SYN Darier disease.

inverted follicular k., a solitary benign epithelial tumor of infundibular hair follicle origin occurring on the face, consisting of a lobulated epidermal downgrowth of keratinizing squamous cells with a pattern of eddies or whorls.

k. labia′lis, thickening of stratum corneum on the lips.

lichenoid k., a solitary benign papule or plaque, with microscopic features resembling lichen planus, occurring on sun-exposed or unexposed skin. SYN lichen planus-like k.

lichen planus-like k., SYN lichenoid k.

k. obtu′rans, an accretion of epithelia in the external auditory canal. SYN laminated epithelial plug.

k. palma′ris et planta′ris, SYN palmoplantar *keratoderma.*

k. pilaris, a common benign eruption consisting of scaly papules of the follicles; primarily affects the extensor surfaces of the arms and thighs.

k. pila′ris atroph′icans facie′i, erythema and horny plugs of outer portions of the eyebrows with destruction of follicles; onset in early infancy.

k. puncta′ta, SYN punctate *keratoderma.*

◧**seborrheic k., k. seborrhe′ica,** superficial, benign, verrucous, often pigmented, greasy lesions consisting of proliferating epidermal cells, resembling basal cells, enclosing horn cysts; they usually occur after the third decade. SYN basal cell papilloma, seborrheic verruca.

senile k., k. seni′lis, SYN actinic k.

solar k., SYN actinic k.

tar k., warty lesions of the face and hands resulting from repeated, prolonged exposure to tar and pitch; also occurs as keratoacanthoma-like lesions that can become malignant, particularly on the scrotum.

ker·a·to·sul·fate (ker′ă-tō-sŭl-fāt). SYN keratan sulfate.

ker·a·to·tome (ker′ă-tō-tōm). SYN keratome.

ker·a·tot·o·my (ker′ă-tot′ŏ-mē). **1.** Any incision through the cornea. **2.** An operation making a partial thickness incision into the cornea to flatten it and reduce its refractive power in that meridian. [kerato- + G. *tomē,* incision]

delimiting k., incision in the cornea along the margin of an advancing ulcer.

radial k., a k. with radial incisions around a clear central zone. A form of refractive keratoplasty used in the treatment of myopia.

refractive k., modification of corneal curvature by means of corneal incisions to minimize hyperopia, myopia, or astigmatism.

ke·rau·no·pho·bia (kĕ-raw′nō-fō′bē-ă). Morbid fear of thunder and lightning. [G. *keraunos,* thunderbolt, + *phobos,* fear]

Kerckring (Kerckringius), Theodor, Dutch anatomist, 1640–1693. SEE K. *center, folds,* under *fold;* ossicle; K. *valves,* under *valve.*

ke·ri·on (kē′rē-on). A granulomatous secondarily infected lesion complicating fungal infection of the hair; typically, a raised boggy lesion. [G. *kērion,* honeycomb; a skin disease, fr. *kēros,* beeswax]

Kerley, Peter J., English radiologist, 1900–1979. SEE K. B *lines,* under *line.*

ker·nel (ker′nĕl). The central portion of the software expression of a mathematical algorithm, as in computed tomography. [O.E. *cyrnel,* a little corn]

ker·nic·ter·us (ker-nik′ter-ŭs). Jaundice associated with high levels of unconjugated bilirubin, or in small premature infants with more modest degrees of bilirubinemia; yellow staining and degenerative lesions are found chiefly in basal ganglia including in the lenticular nucleus, subthalamus, Ammon horn, and other areas; may occur with hemolytic disorder such as Rh or ABO erythroblastosis or G6PD deficiency as well as with neonatal sepsis or Crigler-Najjar syndrome; characterized early clinically by opisthotonus, high-pitched cry, lethargy, and poor sucking, as well as abnormal or absent Moro reflex, and loss of upward gaze; later consequences include deafness, cerebral palsy, other seninieural deficits, and mental retardation. SYN bilirubin encephalopathy, nuclear jaundice. [Ger. *Kern,* kernel (nucleus), + *Ikterus,* jaundice]

Kernig, Vladimir, Russian physician, 1840–1917. SEE K. *sign.*

Kernohan, James W., U.S. pathologist, 1896–1981. SEE K. *notch.*

ker·o·sene (ker′ō-sēn). A mixture of petroleum hydrocarbons, chiefly of the methane series; the fifth fraction in the distillation of petroleum, used as fuel for lamps and stoves, as a degreaser and cleaner, and in insecticides. Contact on human skin can lead to irritation and infection; inhalation may cause headache, drowsiness, coma; swallowing causes irritation, vomiting, and diarrhea. Vomiting should not be induced, as aspiration of vomitus causes pneumonitis. [G. *kēros,* wax, + -ene]

Kerr, Harry Hyland, U.S. surgeon, 1881–1963. SEE Parker-K. *suture.*

Kestenbaum, Alfred, U.S. ophthalmologist, 1890–1961. SEE Kestenbaum *sign,* Kestenbaum *number,* Kestenbaum *procedure.*

ke·tal (kē′tăl). RC(OR′)(R″)OR‴; a hydrated ketone in which both hydroxyl groups are esterified with alcohols.

ket·a·mine (kēt′ă-mēn). A parenterally administered anesthetic that produces catatonia, profound analgesia, increased sympathetic activity, and little relaxation of skeletal muscles; side effects include sialorrhea and occasional pronounced dysphoria, especially in adults; chemically related to phencyclidine (PCP), it can produce hallucinations.

ke·tan·ser·in (kēt-an′ser-in). Specific serotonin 5HT$_2$-receptor antagonist with antihypertensive properties; the drug also reduces platelet aggregation produced by serotonin.

ke·tene (kē′tēn). **1.** $CH_2=C=O$; a very reactive acetylating agent, used in chemical syntheses. **2.** Any substituted k.

ket·i·mine (kē′ta-mēn). R–N=C(R′)(R″); a tautomer of an aldimine, formed in many enzyme-catalyze reactions; e.g., aminotransferases.

♲**keto-.** Combining form denoting a compound containing a ketone group; replaced by oxo- in systematic nomenclature. [Ger.]

ke·to ac·id (kē′tō). An acid containing a ketone group (–CO–) in addition to the acid group(s); α-k. a. refers to a 2-oxo acid (e.g., pyruvic acid); β-k. a. refers to a 3-oxo acid (e.g., acetoacetic acid), etc. SYN oxo acid.

α-k. a. dehydrogenase, one of several distinct multienzyme complexes that catalyzes the formation of an acyl-CoA derivative, CO_2, and NADH from an α-keto acid, NAD$^+$, and coenzyme A; maple syrup urine disease results from several different inherited defects in the mitochondrial branched chain α-keto acid dehydrogenase complex.

3-ke·to·ac·id-CoA trans·fer·ase. SYN 3-oxoacid-CoA transferase.

ke·to·ac·id·e·mia (kē′tō-as-id-ē′mē-ă). SYN maple syrup urine *disease.*

ke·to·ac·i·do·sis (kē′tō-as-i-dō′sis). Acidosis, as in diabetes or starvation, caused by the enhanced production of ketone bodies.

ke·to·ac·i·du·ria (kē′tō-as-i-doo′rē-ă). Excretion of urine having an elevated content of keto acids.

branched chain k., SYN maple syrup urine *disease.*

β-ke·to·ac·yl-ACP re·duc·tase (kē-tō-as′il). SYN 3-oxoacyl-ACP reductase.

β-ke·to·ac·yl-ACP syn·thase. SYN 3-oxoacyl-ACP synthase.

3-ke·to·ac·yl-CoA thi·o·lase. SYN *acetyl-CoA* acyltransferase.

2-ke·to·a·dip·ic ac·id (kē′tō-a-dip′ik). An intermediate in L-tryptophan and L-lysine catabolism; 2-k. a. accumulates in certain inherited disorders, probably due to a deficiency of one of the proteins in the α-ketoadipate dehydrogenase complex; 2-oxoadipic acid; 2-oxohexadioic acid.

2-k. a. dehydrogenase complex, the multienzyme complex that reacts 2-k. a. with coenzyme A and NAD$^+$ to produce glutaryl-CoA, CO_2, and NADH + H$^+$ in L-lysine and L-tryptophan catabolism; a deficiency of one of the proteins in this complex results in 2-ketoadipic acidemia.

2-ke·to·a·dip·ic ac·i·de·mia (kē′tō-a-dip′ik). Elevated levels of 2-ketoadipic acid in the serum.

ke·to·con·a·zole (kē-tō-kō′nă-zōl). A broad spectrum antifungal agent used to treat systemic and topical fungal infections.

α-ke·to·de·car·box·y·lase (kē′tō-dē-kar-boks′i-lās). Formerly, the enzyme system converting pyruvate (a 2-oxoacid) to acetyl-CoA and CO_2, with reduction of NAD$^+$ to NADH and the participation of lipoamide and thiamin pyrophosphate; now known to involve at least three enzymes in succession: pyruvate dehydrogenase, dihydrolipoamide acetyltransferase, and dihydrolipoamide dehydrogenase. Cf. *pyruvate* dehydrogenase (lipoamide).

ke·to·gen·e·sis (kē-tō-jen′ĕ-sis). Metabolic production of ketones or ketone bodies.

ke·to·gen·ic (kē-tō-jen′ik). Giving rise to ketone bodies in metabolism.

α·ke·to·glu·tar·am·ic ac·id (kē′tō-gloo-tār-ik). A metabolite of glutamine formed by the action of glutamine aminotransferase; elevated in certain cases of hepatocoma. SYN 2-oxoglutaric acid.

α·ke·to·glu·tar·ate. A salt or ester of α-ketoglutaric acid.

α·k. dehydrogenase, an enzyme that catalyzes the oxidative decarboxylation of 2-ketoglutaric acid to succinyldihydrolipoate; the succinyl group is later transferred to CoA and the reduced lipoate is oxidized by NAD+; a complex that is a part of the tricarboxylic acid cycle. SYN 2-oxoglutarate dehydrogenase, α-ketoglutarate dehydrogenase complex.

ke·to·hep·tose (kē-tō-hep′tōs). A seven-carbon sugar possessing a ketone group. SYN heptulose.

ke·to·hex·ose (kē-tō-heks′ōs). A six-carbon sugar possessing a ketone group; e.g., fructose. SYN hexulose.

β·ke·to·hy·dro·gen·ase (kē-tō-hī′drō-jen-ās). SYN 3-hydroxyacyl-CoA dehydrogenase.

ke·to·hy·drox·y·es·trin (kē′tō-hī-drok-sē-es′trin). SYN estrone.

ke·tol (kē′tol). A ketone that has an OH group near the CO group. In an α-k., the OH is attached to a carbon atom that is attached to the CO carbon atom; in a β-k., one carbon atom intervenes.

ke·tole (kē′tōl). SYN indole (1).

ke·tole group. Carbons 1 and 2 of a 2-ketose (HOCH₂CO–); *trans*-ketolation from D-xylose 5-phosphate to C-1 of aldoses is important in various metabolic pathways involving carbohydrates (e.g., photosynthesis, Dickens shunt); the two-carbon unit is transferred as α,β-dihydroxyethylthiamin pyrophosphate.

ke·to·lyt·ic (kē-tō-lit′ik). Causing the dissolution of ketone or acetone substances, referring usually to oxidation products of glucose and allied substances.

ke·tone (kē′tōn). A substance with the carbonyl group

$$\begin{matrix} O \\ \| \\ -CO- \end{matrix}$$

linking two carbon atoms; the most important in medicine and the simplest k. is dimethyl k. (acetone).

ke·tone al·co·hol. A compound containing a carbonyl or ketone group as well as a hydroxyl group; e.g., dihydroxyacetone.

ke·tone-al·de·hyde mu·tase. SYN lactoylglutathione lyase.

ke·to·ne·mia (kē-tō-nē′mē-ă). The presence of recognizable concentrations of ketone bodies in the plasma. [ketone + G. *haima*, blood]

ke·ton·ic (kē-tōn′ik). Pertaining to, or possessing the characteristics of, a ketone.

ke·to·ni·za·tion (kē-tō-ni-zā′shŭn). Conversion into a ketone.

ke·ton·u·ria (kē-tōn-ū-noo′rē-ă). Enhanced urinary excretion of ketone bodies.
  branched chain k., SYN maple syrup urine *disease*.

ke·to·pan·to·ic ac·id (kē′tō-pan-tō′ik). Oxidized precursor of pantoic acid, intermediate on the synthetic pathway between α-ketoisovaleric acid and pantothenic acid.

ke·to·pen·tose (kē-tō-pen′tōs). A five-carbon sugar in which carbons 2, 3, or 4 make up part of a carbonyl group; e.g., ribulose.

β·ke·to·re·duc·tase (kē′tō-rē-dŭk′tās). SYN 3-hydroxyacyl-CoA dehydrogenase.

ket·or·o·lac. A pyrrolo-pyrrole nonsteroidal antiinflammatory agent with antipyretic and analgesic properties; similar in actions to ibuprofen but substantially more potent and capable of relieving severe pain. Often used by injection.

ke·tose (kē′tōs). A carbohydrate containing the characteristic carbonyl group of the ketones; i.e., a polyhydroxyketone; e.g., fructose, ribulose, sedoheptulose; the majority of the naturally occurring k.'s have the carbonyl group on the second carbon.

ke·tose-1-phos·phate al·dol·ase. Fructose bisphosphate aldolase.

ke·tose re·duc·tase. SYN D-sorbitol-6-phosphate dehydrogenase.

ke·to·sis (kē-tō′sis). A condition characterized by the enhanced production of ketone bodies, as in diabetes mellitus or starvation. [ketone + -*osis*, condition]
  bovine k., a common metabolic disease of cows which appears as a rule within a few weeks after parturition; characterized by

hypoglycemia, ketonuria, loss of appetite, lethargy, loss of milk production, and rapid emaciation.

17-ke·to·ste·roids (17-KS) (kē-tō-stĕr′oydz). Nominally, any steroid with a carbonyl group on C-17; commonly used to designate urinary C₁₉ steroidal metabolites of androgenic and adrenocortical hormones that possess this structural feature. SYN 17-oxosteroids.

α·ke·to·suc·ci·nam·ic ac·id (kē′tō-sŭk-si-nam′ik). The transamination product of asparagine; acted upon by ω-amidase.

ke·to·suc·ci·nic ac·id (kē-tō-sŭk′si-nik). SYN oxaloacetic acid.

ke·to·su·ria (kē′tō-su′rē-ă′). The presence of ketones in the urine.

ke·to·tet·rose (kē′tō-tet′rōs). A four-carbon sugar possessing a ketone group; e.g., erythrulose.

β·ke·to·thi·o·lase (kē-tō-thī′ō-lās). SYN *acetyl-CoA* acyltransferase.

ke·to·tic (kē′tot-ik). Pertaining to ketone bodies; presence of acidosis due to excess ketone body production such as occurs in uncontrolled insulin-dependent diabetes.

ke·to·tri·ose (kē-tō-trī′ōs). A three-carbon sugar possessing a ketone group; i.e., dihydroxyacetone.

keV. Abbreviation for kiloelectron volts, a unit of energy in diagnostic radiography and nuclear medicine, equivalent to the kinetic energy gained by an electron falling through a potential of 1 volt.

Key, Charles Alston, English physician, 1793–1849.

Key, Ernst A.H., Swedish anatomist and physician, 1832–1901. SEE *foramen* of K.-Retzius; *sheath* of K. and Retzius.

key·way (kē′wā). The female portion of a precision attachment.

kg Abbreviation for kilogram.

khat (kot). The tender fresh parts of *Catha edulis*.

khel·lin (kel′in). The active principle in extracts of *Ammi visnaga*, an umbelliferous plant growing in the Near East; used in angina pectoris and asthma. [Ar. *khella*]

KHN Abbreviation for Knoop hardness *number*.

kick (kik). A brisk mechanical stimulus.
  atrial k., the priming force contributed by atrial contraction immediately before ventricular systole to increase the efficiency of ventricular ejection due to acutely increased preload.
  idioventricular k., the increased contractility of the initially contracting ventricular fibers which, by stretching the later contracting fibers, increases their force of contraction.

Kidd blood group. See Blood Groups appendix.

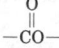 **kid·ney** (kid′nē). One of the paired organs that excrete urine. The k.'s are bean-shaped organs (about 11 cm long, 5 cm wide, and 3 cm thick) lying on either side of the vertebral column, posterior to the peritoneum, about opposite the twelfth thoracic and first three lumbar vertebrae. SYN nephros, ren. [A.S. *cwith*, womb, belly, + *neere*, kidney (L. *ren*, G. *nephros*)]
  amyloid k., a k. in which amyloidosis has occurred, usually in association with some chronic illness such as multiple myeloma, tuberculosis, osteomyelitis, or other chronic suppurative inflammation; such k.'s are moderately enlarged and grossly manifest a waxy appearance, with amyloid deposited beneath the endothelium in the glomerular loops and in the arterioles, apparently beginning as foci of thickening of the basement membranes. SYN waxy k.
  Armanni-Ebstein k., glycogen vacuolization of the loops of Henle, seen in diabetics before the introduction of insulin. SYN Armanni-Ebstein change.
  arteriolosclerotic k., a k. in which there is sclerosis of the arterioles, i.e., arteriolar nephrosclerosis resulting from long-standing benign hypertension. Such k.'s tend to be pale red-brown or relatively gray, moderately reduced in size, and firmer than normal organs; the capsular surfaces are uniformly finely granular. Most of the arterioles are thickened and hyalinized, thereby resulting in varying degrees of narrowing of the lumens, ischemia, and fibrosis in the interstitial tissue, leading to uniform contraction of the cortex.
  arteriosclerotic k., a k. in which there is sclerosis of arterial vessels larger than arterioles. Such k.'s are usually not significantly reduced in size, but are likely to be paler than usual; the

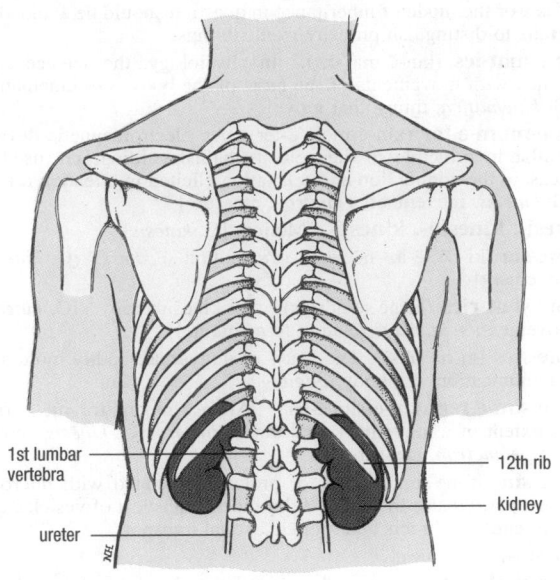

kidney: location

capsular surface may be marked by a few, possibly several, conical, relatively deep V-shaped scars that result from fibrosis and ischemic atrophy of the region supplied by the affected vessel.

artificial k., SYN hemodialyzer.

Ask-Upmark k., true renal hypoplasia with decreased lobules and deep transverse grooving of the cortical surfaces of the kidney.

atrophic k., a k. that is diminished in size because of inadequate circulation and/or loss of nephrons.

cake k., a solid, irregularly lobed organ of bizarre shape, usually situated in the pelvis toward the midline, produced by fusion of the renal anlagen.

contracted k., a diffusely scarred k. in which the relatively large amount of abnormal fibrous tissue and ischemic atrophy leads to a moderate or great reduction in the size of the organ, as in arteriolar nephrosclerosis and chronic glomerulonephritis.

cow k., a k. containing an abnormally large number of minor calices, resembling normal bovine renal anatomy.

crush k., acute oliguric renal failure following crushing injuries of muscle; k.'s show the changes of hypoxic tubular damage, plus pigment casts in renal tubules that contain myoglobin.

cystic k., a general term used to indicate a k. that contains one or more cysts, including polycystic disease, solitary cyst, multiple simple cysts, and retention cysts (associated with parenchymal scarring).

disk k., SYN pancake k.

duplex k., a k. in which two pelviocaliceal systems are present.

fatty k., a k. in which there is fatty metamorphosis of the parenchymal cells, especially fatty degeneration.

flea-bitten k., the k. seen at autopsy in some cases of bacterial endocarditis, the appearance being caused by diffuse petechial hemorrhages resulting from focal glomerulonephritis.

floating k., the abnormally mobile k. that frequently descends to the brim of the pelvis when the patient assumes the erect position; nephroptosis. SYN movable k., wandering k.

Formad k., an enlarged and deformed k. sometimes seen in chronic alcoholism.

fused k., a single, anomalous organ produced by fusion of the renal anlagen.

Goldblatt k., a k. whose arterial blood supply has been compromised, as a consequence of which arterial (renovascular) hypertension develops.

granular k., a k. in which fairly uniform, diffusely and evenly situated foci of scarring of the interstitial tissue of the cortex (and

sometimes scarring of glomeruli), and the associated slight degree of bulging of groups of dilated tubules, leads to the development of a minutely bosselated surface; such k.'s are seen in arteriolar nephrosclerosis or chronic glomerulonephritis. SYN sclerotic k.

head k., SYN pronephros (1).

hind k., SYN metanephros.

horseshoe k., union of the lower or occasionally the upper extremities of the two k.'s by a band of tissue extending across the vertebral column.

medullary sponge k., cystic disease of the renal pyramids associated with calculus formation and hematuria; differs from cystic disease of the renal medulla in that renal failure does not usually develop.

middle k., SYN mesonephros.

mortar k., SYN putty k.

movable k., SYN floating k.

pancake k., a disk-shaped organ produced by fusion of both poles of the contralateral k. anlagen. SYN disk k.

pelvic k., a congenital abnormality in which the kidney is in the pelvis; usually the arterial blood supply comes off the bifurcation of the aorta or the iliac artery.

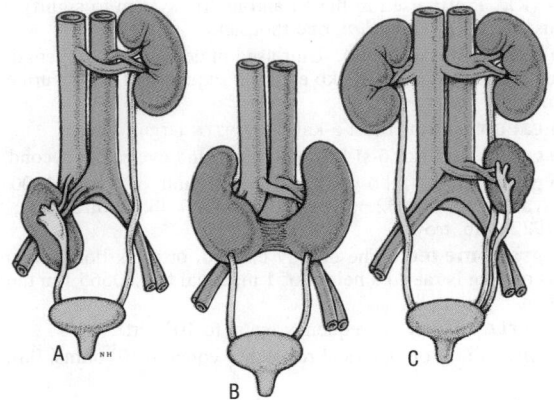

kidney anomalies: (A) pelvic kidney, (B) horseshoe kidney, (C) supernumerary kidney

polycystic k., a progressive disease characterized by formation of multiple cysts of varying size scattered diffusely throughout both k.'s, resulting in compression and destruction of renal parenchyma, usually with hypertension, gross hematuria, and uremia leading to progressive renal failure. There are two major types: 1) with onset in infancy or early childhood, usually of autosomal recessive inheritance [MIM*263200]; 2) with onset in adulthood, of autosomal dominant inheritance with genetic heterogeneity [MIM*173900, 173910, and 600666]; may be caused by mutation in either polycystin-1 gene on chromosome 16p, polycystin-2 gene on 4q, or gene(s) not identified yet. SYN polycystic disease of kidneys.

primordial k., SYN pronephros.

putty k., a k. containing caseous material trapped by stricture of the ureter due to tuberculous granulations in renal tuberculosis. SYN mortar k.

pyelonephritic k., a k. deformed by multiple scars as a result of chronic or recurrent renal infection.

Rose-Bradford k., a form of fibrotic k. of inflammatory origin found in young persons.

sclerotic k., SYN granular k.

sigmoid k., upper pole of one k. fused with the lower pole of the other.

supernumerary k., a k., in addition to the two usually present, developed from the splitting of the nephrogenic blastema or from a separate metanephric blastema, into which a partial or complete duplication of the ureteral stalk enters to form a separate, capsulated k.; in some cases, the separation of the duplicated organ is incomplete.

ki

thoracic k., ectopic k. that partially lies above the diaphragm in the posterior mediastinum.

wandering k., SYN floating k.

waxy k., SYN amyloid k.

Kiel clas·si·fi·ca·tion. See under classification.

Kielland. SEE Kjelland.

Kien, Alphonse M.J., 19th century German physician. SEE Kussmaul-K. *respiration.*

Kienböck, Robert, Austrian roentgenologist, 1871–1953. SEE K. *disease, dislocation, unit.*

Kiernan, Francis, English physician, 1800–1874. SEE K. *space.*

Kiesselbach, Wilhelm, German laryngologist, 1839–1902. SEE K. *area.*

Kikuchi, M, 20th century Japanese hematologist. SEE K. *disease.*

Kilian, Hermann F., German gynecologist, 1800–1863. SEE K. *line.*

Kiliani, H., chemist, 1855–1945. SEE Kiliani-Fischer *synthesis;* Kiliani-Fischer *reaction.*

Killian, Gustav J., German laryngologist, 1860–1921. SEE K. *bundle, operation, triangle.*

♲**kilo- (k).** Prefix used in the SI and metric system to signify one thousand (10^3). [G. *chilioi,* one thousand]

kil·o·base (kb) (kil′ō-bās). Unit used in designating the length of a nucleic acid sequence; 1 kb equals a sequence of 1000 purine or pyrimidine bases.

kil·o·cal·o·rie (kcal) (kil′ō-kal-ō-rē). SYN large *calorie.*

kil·o·cy·cle (kc) (kil′ō-sī-kl). One thousand cycles per second.

kil·o·gram (kg) (kil′ō-gram). The SI unit of mass, 1000 g; equivalent to 15,432.358 gr, 2.2046226 lb. avoirdupois, or 2.6792289 lb. troy.

kil·o·gram-me·ter. The energy exerted, or work done, when a mass of 1 kg is raised a height of 1 m; equal to 9.80665 J in the SI system.

kil·o·hertz. A unit of frequency equal to 10^3 hertz.

kil·ohm. A unit of electrical resistance equal to 10^3 ohms. [kilo + ohm]

kil·o·joule. A unit of energy, work, or quantity of heat equal to 10^3 joules. [kilo + joule]

kil·o·volt (kv) (kil′ō-vōlt). A unit of electrical potential, potential difference, or electromotive force, equal to 10^3 volts. [kilo + volt]

kil·o·volt-me·ter (kil′ō-vōlt-mē′ter). An instrument designed to measure electromotive force in kilovolts.

Kimmelstiel, Paul, German pathologist in the U.S., 1900–1970. SEE K.-Wilson *disease, syndrome.*

Kimura, T., 20th century Japanese pathologist. SEE K. *disease.*

♲**kin-, kine-.** Movement, motion. SEE ALSO cine-. [G. *kineo,* to move, set in motion]

kin·an·es·the·sia (kin-an-es-thē′ze-ă). A disturbance of deep sensibility in which there is inability to perceive either direction or extent of movement, the result being ataxia. SYN cinanesthesia. [G. *kinēsis,* motion, + *an-* priv. + *aisthēsis,* sensation]

ki·nase (kī′nās). 1. An enzyme catalyzing the conversion of a proenzyme to an active enzyme; e.g., enteropeptidase (enterokinase). 2. An enzyme catalyzing the transfer of phosphate groups. For individual k.'s, see specific name.

kinase II. SYN peptidyl dipeptidase A.

kind·ling. Long-lasting epileptogenic changes induced by daily subthreshold electrical brain stimulation without apparent neuronal damage.

kin·dred. An aggregate of genetically related persons; distinguished from pedigree, which is a stylized representation of a k. [O.E. *kynrēde,* fr. *cyn,* kin, + *rēde,* condition]

degree of k., degree of k. between two members of a pedigree, the minimum number of steps to be traced in going from the one to the other. First degree relatives are sibs, parents, and progeny; second degree are uncles, aunts, nephews, and nieces and so forth. The term is defined for legal purposes e.g., consanguineous marriages, and may be misleading in genetics. The use of groups constituted by lumping together "first degree relatives" regardless

of sex or the mode of inheritance in question should be avoided as it fails to distinguish progeny from siblings.

kin·e·mat·ics (kin-ĕ-mat′iks). In physiology, the science concerned with movements of the parts of the body. SYN cinematics. [G. *kinēmatica,* things that move]

kin·e·mom·e·ter (kin-ĕ-mom′ĕ-ter). An electromagnetic device, similar in principle to the velocity ballistocardiograph, used to measure the contraction and relaxation elicited in a tendon reflex. [G. *kinēsis,* movement, + *metron,* measure]

♲**kinesi-, kinesio-, kineso-.** Motion. [G. *kinēsis*]

ki·ne·sia (ki-nē′sē-ă, -nē′zē-). SYN motion *sickness.* [G. *kinēsis,* movement]

ki·ne·si·at·rics (ki-nē′sē-at′riks). SYN kinesitherapy. [G. *kinēsis,* movement, + *iatrikos,* relating to medicine]

ki·ne·sics (ki-nē′siks). The study of nonverbal, bodily motion in communication. SEE body *language.*

kin·e·sim·e·ter (kin-ĕ-sim′ĕ-ter). An instrument for measuring the extent of a movement. SYN kinesiometer. [G. *kinēsis,* movement, + *metron,* measure]

ki·ne·sin (ki-nē′sin). A motor protein associated with microtubules; participates in the ATP-dependent transport of vesicles and other entities; directs anterograde axonal transport.

♲**kinesio-.** SEE kinesi-.

ki·ne·si·ol·o·gy (ki-nē-sē-ol′ō-jē). The science or the study of movement, and the active and passive structures involved. [G. *kinēsis,* movement, + *-logos,* study]

ki·ne·si·om·e·ter (ki-nē-sē-om′ĕ-ter). SYN kinesimeter.

kin·e·sip·a·thist (kin-ĕ-sip′ă-thist). A nonmedical person who treats disease by movements of various kinds.

ki·ne·sis (ki-nē′sis). Motion. As a termination, used to denote movement or activation, particularly the kind induced by a stimulus. [G.]

ki·ne·si·ther·a·py (ki-nē-si-thār′ă-pē). Physical therapy involving motion and range of motion exercises. SEE movement. SYN kinesiatrics.

♲**kineso-.** SEE kinesi-.

ki·ne·so·pho·bia (ki-nē-sō-fō′bē-ă). Morbid fear of movement. [G. *kinēsis,* movement, + *phobos,* fear]

kin·es·the·sia (kin′es-thē′zē-ă). 1. The sense perception of movement; the muscular sense. 2. An illusion of moving in space. [G. *kinēsis,* motion, + *aisthēsis,* sensation]

kin·es·the·si·om·e·ter (kin′es-thē′zē-om′ĕ-ter). An instrument for determining the degree of muscular sensation. [kinesthesia, + G. *metron,* measure]

kin·es·the·sis (kin′es-thē-sēz). SEE kinesthesia.

kin·es·thet·ic (kin-es-thet′ik). 1. Relating to kinesthesia. 2. Used to describe a person who preferentially uses mental imagery of that which has been felt. SEE ALSO internal *representation.*

ki·net·ic (ki-net′ik). Relating to motion or movement. [G. *kinētikos,* of motion, fr. *kinētos,* moving]

ki·net·ics (ki-net′iks). The study of motion, acceleration, or rate of change.

chemical k., the study of the rates of chemical reactions.

enzyme k., the study of the rates, and alterations in those rates, of enzyme-catalyzed reactions; includes the reactions catalyzed by synzymes, abzymes, and ribozymes.

♲**kineto-.** Motion. [G. *kinētos,* moving, movable]

ki·ne·to·car·di·o·gram (ki-nē′tō-kar′dē-ō-gram, ki-net′ō-). One type of graphic recording of the vibrations of the chest wall produced by cardiac activity.

ki·ne·to·car·di·o·graph (ki-nē′tō-kar′dē-ō-graf, ki-net′ō-). A device for recording precordial impulses due to cardiac movement; the absolute displacement of a point on the chest wall is recorded relative to a fixed reference point above the recumbent patient.

ki·ne·to·chore (ki-nē′tō-kōr, ki-net′ō-). The structural portion of the chromosome to which microtubules attach. Cf. centromere. [kineto- + G. *chōra,* space]

ki·ne·to·chores (ki-nē′tō-korz). The protein-bound region of the centromere.

ki·ne·to·gen·ic (ki-nē-tō-jen′ik, ki-net-ō-). Causing or producing motion.

ki·ne·to·plasm (ki-nē′tō-plazm). **1.** The most contractile part of a cell. **2.** The cytoplasm of the droplet that covers the sperm head during maturation. SYN cinetoplasm, cinetoplasma, kinoplasm. [kineto- + G. *plasma,* a thing formed]

ki·ne·to·plast (ki-nē′tō-plast, ki-net′ō-). An intensely staining rod-, disc-, or spherical-shaped extranuclear DNA structure found in parasitic flagellates (family Trypanosomatidae) near the base of the flagellum, posterior to the blepharoplast, and often at right angles to the nucleus. Electron micrographs show it to be part of a single giant mitochondrion filling most of the cytoplasm of amastigote flagellates, the k. portion being visible by light microscopy. DNA of the k. is termed kDNA to distinguish it from nuclear DNA, or nDNA. The k. divides independently, along with the basal body, prior to nuclear division. The term k. formerly included parabasal body and blepharoplast in a locomotory apparatus, but is now recognized as a distinct organelle of most trypanosomatids. SEE ALSO parabasal *body.* [kineto- + G. *plastos,* formed]

ki·ne·to·scope (kĭ-ne′to-skōp). An apparatus for taking serial photographs to record movement. [kineto- + G. *skopeō,* to examine]

ki·net·o·some (ki-nē′tō-sōm, ki-net′ō-). SYN basal *body.* [kineto- + G. *sōma,* body]

King, Earl J., Canadian biochemist, 1901–1962. SEE K. *unit;* K.-Armstrong *unit.*

king·dom (king′dum). One of the four categories into which natural objects are usually classified: the animal kingdom, including all animals; the plant kingdom, including all plants; the mineral kingdom, including all objects and substances without life; and the protista, including all single-cell organisms. [A.S. *cyningdōm,* fr. *cyning,* king, + *-dom,* state, condition]

Kin·gel·la (kin-jel′ah). Genus in the family Neisseriaceae; members are medium-size, Gram-negative, aerobic and facultatively anaerobic, nonmotile cocci and coccobacilli in pairs or short chains, which may decolorize poorly with acetone-alcohol; they are oxidase positive, and ferment glucose with acid but not gas. The type species is *K. kingae.*

K. indolog′enes, former name for *Suttonella indologenes,* a bacterial species that is the causitive agent of eye infections and endocarditis on damaged (especially prosthetic) heart valves.

K. kin′gae, a β-hemolytic bacterial species that causes endocarditis, osteomyelitis, and septic arthritis in humans; formerly *Moraxella kingae.* SEE HACEK *group.* SYN *Moraxella kingae.*

king's evil. historic term for cervical tuberculous lymphadenitis (scrofula) which was formerly thought to be curable by the touch of a king.

Kingsley, Norman W., U.S. dentist, 1829–1913. SEE K. *splint.*

kin·ic ac·id (kin′ik). SYN quinic acid.

ki·nin (kī′nin). One of a number of widely differing substances having pronounced and dramatic physiologic effects. Some (e.g., kallidin and bradykinin) are polypeptides, formed in blood by proteolysis secondary to some pathological process, that stimulate visceral smooth muscle but relax vascular smooth muscle, thus producing vasodilation; others (e.g., kinetin) are plant growth regulators. [G. *kineō,* to move, + -in]

k. 9, SYN bradykinin.

ki·nin·o·gen (ki-nin′ō-jen). The globulin precursor of a (plasma) kinin.

high molecular weight k., a plasma protein of 110,000 molecular weight that normally exists in plasma in a 1:1 complex with prekallikrein. The complex is a cofactor in the activation of coagulation factor XII. The product of this reaction, XIIa, in turn activates prekallikrein to kallikrein. SYN Fitzgerald factor, Flaujeac factor, Williams factor.

low molecular weight k., a protein of 50,000 molecular weight that occurs in various normal tissues and which, upon cleavage by kallikrein or other k.'s, forms kallidin. Kallidin, in turn, is converted into bradykinin.

ki·nin·o·ge·nase (ki-nin′ō-jĕ-nās). SYN kallikrein.

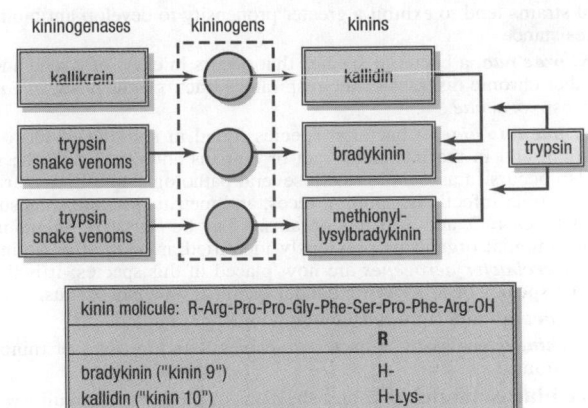

kinins

ki·nin·o·gen·in (ki-nin′ō-jen-in). SYN kallikrein.

kink. An angulation, bend, or twist.

Lane k., SYN Lane *band.*

kino-. Movement. [G. *kineō,* to move]

kin·o·cen·trum (kin-ō-sen′trŭm). SYN cytocentrum. [kino- + G. *kentron,* center]

ki·no·cil·i·um (kī-nō-sil′ē-ŭm). A cilium, usually motile, having nine peripheral double microtubules and two single central ones. [kino- + cilium]

kin·o·mom·e·ter (kin-ō-mom′ĕ-ter). An instrument for measuring degree of motion. [kino- + G. *metron,* measure]

kin·o·plasm (kin′ō-plazm, kī′nō). SYN kinetoplasm.

kin·o·plas·mic (kin-ō-plas′mik, kī-nō-). Relating to kinoplasm (kinetoplasm).

kin·ship. The state of being genetically related.

Kinyoun, Joseph J., U.S. physician, 1860–1919. SEE K. *stain.*

ki·on (kī′on). Obsolete term for uvula. See entries under cion- as a combining form of uvula. [G. *kiōn,* pillar, the uvula]

kion-, kiono-. The uvula. SEE uvulo-, uvul-. [G. *kiōn,* uvula]

Kirk, Norman Thomas, U.S. Army surgeon, 1888–1960. SEE K. *amputation.*

Kirkland, Olin, U.S. periodontist, 1876–1969. SEE K. *knife.*

Kirschner, Martin, German surgeon, 1879–1942. SEE K. *apparatus, wire.*

Kisch, Bruno, German physiologist, 1890–1966. SEE K. *reflex.*

Kitasato, Shibasaburo, Baron, Japanese bacteriologist, 1853–1931. SEE K. *bacillus.*

Kjeldahl, Johan G.C., Danish chemist, 1849–1900. SEE K. *apparatus, method;* macro-K. *method;* micro-K. *method.*

Kjelland (Kielland), Christian, Norwegian obstetrician, 1871–1941. SEE K. *forceps.*

Klatskin, Gerald, U.S. internist; (died 1988). SEE K. *tumor.*

Klebs, Theodor Albrecht Edwin, German physician, 1834–1913. SEE *Klebsiella;* K.-Loeffler *bacillus.*

Kleb·si·el·la (kleb-sē-el′ă). A genus of aerobic, facultatively anaerobic, nonmotile, nonsporeforming bacteria (family Enterobacteriaceae) containing Gram-negative, encapsulated rods which occur singly, in pairs, or in short chains. These organisms produce acetylmethylcarbinol and lysine decarboxylase or ornithine decarboxylase. They do not usually liquefy gelatin. Citrate and glucose are ordinarily used as sole carbon sources. These organisms may or may not be pathogenic. They occur in the respiratory, intestinal, and urogenital tracts of humans as well as in soil, water, and grain. The type species is *K. pneumoniae.* [E. *Klebs*]

K. mo′bilis, SYN *Enterobacter aerogenes.*

K. oxytoca, a species characterized by its ability to produce indole. Clinically it resembles *K. pneumoniae;* however, nosocomi-

Kl

al strains tend to exhibit a greater propensity to develop antibiotic resistance.

K. ozae′nae, a bacterial species that occurs in cases of ozena and other chronic diseases of the respiratory tract. SYN *K. pneumoniae* subsp. *ozaenae.*

K. pneumo′niae, a bacterial species found in soil and water, on grain, and in the intestinal tract of humans and other animals; it also occurs in association with several pathologic conditions, urinary tract infections, sputum, feces, and metritis in mares; capsular types 1, 2, and 3 of this organism may be causative agents in pneumonia; organisms previously identified as nonmotile strains of *Aerobacter aerogenes* are now placed in this species; it is the type species of *K.* SYN Friedländer bacillus, pneumobacillus.

K. pneumo′niae subsp. *ozae′nae,* SYN *K. ozaenae.*

K. rhinosclero′matis, a bacterial species found in cases of rhinoscleroma.

klee·blatt·schä·del (klā-blat-she′dl). SEE cloverleaf skull *syndrome.* [Ger. cloverleaf skull]

Kleffner, Frank, 20th century U.S. neurologist. SEE Landau-Kleffner *syndrome.*

Kleffner. SEE Landau-Kleffner *syndrome.*

Kleihauer. SEE Kleihauer *stain,* Betke-Kleihauer *test.*

Klein, Edward E., Hungarian histologist, 1844–1925. SEE K.-Gumprecht shadow *nuclei,* under *nucleus.*

Kleine, Willi, 20th century German neuropsychiatrist. SEE K.-Levin *syndrome.*

klep·to·ma·nia (klep-tō-mā′nē-ă). A disorder of impulse control characterized by a morbid tendency to steal. [G. *kleptō,* to steal, + *mania,* insanity]

klep·to·ma·ni·ac (klep-tō-mā′nē-ak). A person exhibiting kleptomania.

klep·to·pho·bia (klep-tō-fō′bē-ă). Morbid fear of stealing or of becoming a thief. [G. *kleptō,* to steal, + *phobos,* fear]

Klinefelter, Harry F., Jr., U.S. physician, *1912. SEE K. *syndrome.*

Klippel, Maurice, French neurologist, 1858–1942. SEE K.-Feil *syndrome;* K.-Trenaunay-Weber *syndrome.*

Klumpke, SEE Dejerine-K.

Klüver, Heinrich, German-born U.S. neurologist, 1897–1975. SEE K.-Barrera Luxol fast blue *stain;* K.-Bucy *syndrome.*

Kluy·ve·ra (klooy-ver′ah). Genus in family Enterobacteriaceae; organisms are motile, lactose fermenting, and differentiated from other genera by specific phenotypic profiles and DNA-DNA hybridization parameters; some species have been associated with human infection; the type species is *K. ascorbata.*

Knapp, Herman J., U.S. ophthalmologist, 1832–1911. SEE K. *streaks,* under *streak, striae,* under *stria.*

ℹ️**knee** (nē) [TA]. **1.** SYN genu (1). **2.** Any structure of angular shape resembling a flexed knee. [A.S. *cneōw*]

Brodie k., chronic hypertrophic synovitis of the k. SYN Brodie disease (1).

housemaid's k., an adventitious occupational bursitis occurring over the area of contact when kneeling; not to be confused with infrapatellar bursitis. SYN prepatellar bursitis.

locked k., a condition in which the k. lacks full extension and flexion because of internal derangement, usually the result of a torn meniscus.

runner's k., an overuse syndrome of anterior k. pain associated with excessive lateral motion of the patella during activity. SYN patellofemoral stress syndrome.

Wilbrand k., bundle of inferior nasal optic nerve fibers subserving the superior temporal visual field and crossing in the anterior optic *chiasm,* briefly entering the contralateral posterior optic *nerve* [CN II] before proceeding into the contralateral optic *tract.* Recent research indicates that this may be an artifact of retinal degeneration and not present in the normal anatomy.

knee·cap (nē′kap). SYN patella.

Kne·mi·do·kop·tes (nē′mi-dō-kop′tēz). A genus of microscopic burrowing sarcoptid mites that infect fowl and caged birds; spe-

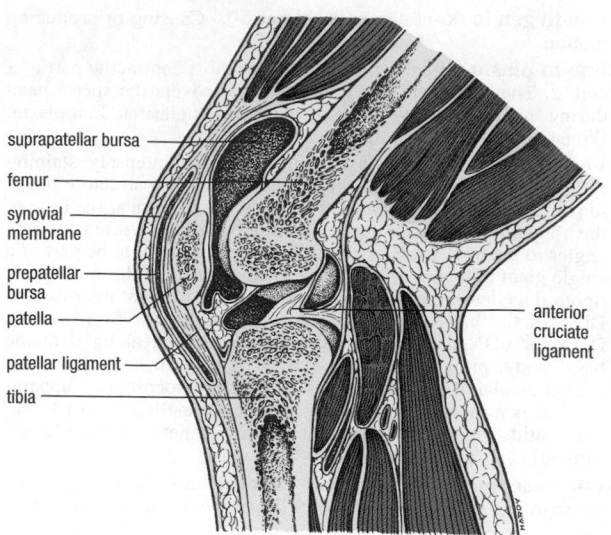

suprapatellar bursa
femur
synovial membrane
prepatellar bursa
patella
patellar ligament
tibia
anterior cruciate ligament

knee joint: sagittal section showing prepatellar and suprapatellar bursae

cies include *K. laevis* var. *gallinae,* the depluming mite, and *K. mutans,* the scaly leg mite. [G. *knēmē,* leg, + *koptō,* to cut]

KNF mod·el Abbreviation for Koshland-Némethy-Filmer *model.*

Kniest, Wilhelm, 20th century German pediatrician. SEE K. *syndrome.*

knife, pl. **knives** (nīf, nīvz). A cutting instrument used in surgery and dissection. [M.E. *knif,* fr. A.S. *cnif,* fr. O. Norse *knīfr*]

amputation k., a broad-bladed k. used primarily for transecting large muscles during major amputations.

Beer k., a triangular k. with a sharp point and one sharp edge, formerly used for incision for cataract.

cartilage k., SYN chondrotome.

cautery k., a k. that sears while cutting, to diminish bleeding.

chemical k., term sometimes used for restriction *endonuclease.*

electrode k., a blade-shaped electrical instrument used to cut tissues by means of a high-frequency electrical current.

fistula k., SYN fistulatome.

free-hand k., a manually operated k. or blade usually used to take split-thickness skin grafts; e.g., Blair-Brown k., Humby k. .

gamma k., a minimally invasive radiosurgical system used in the treatment of benign and malignant intracranial neoplasms and arteriovenous malformations. SEE ALSO radiosurgery.

> As a preliminary to use of the gamma knife, the lesion to be ablated is precisely located by imaging techniques such as MRI, CT, PET, and angiography. Beams of gamma rays from 200 cobalt-60 sources are then directed by a computer so that they converge on the lesion. A series of exposures are made during a period of about 1 hour. Lesions larger than about 3 cm cannot be treated. The mechanism is bulky and costly, but the procedure has shown a success rate of about 85% in the treatment of arteriovenous malformations and 50–95% for neoplasms. Besides avoiding the risks and complications of open surgery, the gamma knife permits treatment of lesions whose location prohibits any attempt at surgical removal. In addition, patient discomfort is minimal and most patients remain in the hospital for only 1 night; many return home, or even to work, on the day of treatment. The gamma knife is expected to prove useful in the treatment of other disorders, such as tumors of the eye and the pituitary gland, trigeminal neuralgia, epilepsy, parkinsonism, and other movement disorders.

Goldman-Fox knives, a set of knives used in periodontal surgery.

Graefe k., a narrow-bladed k. used in making a section of the cornea.

hernia k., a slender bladed k., with short cutting edge, for dividing the constricting tissues at the mouth of the hernial sac. SYN herniotome.

Kirkland k., a heart-shaped k. used in gingival surgery.

lenticular k., a scraper resembling a sharp spoon.

Liston knives, long-bladed knives of various sizes used in amputations.

Merrifield k., a long, narrow, triangularly shaped k. used in gingival surgery.

valvotomy k., a k. used in mitral or venous valvular surgery; also called valvulotome.

knis·mo·gen·ic (nis'mō-jen'ik). Causing a tickling sensation. [G. *knismos,* tickling, + *-gen,* production]

knit·ting (nit'ing). Nonmedical term denoting the process of union of the fragments of a broken bone or of the edges of a wound. [M.E., *knitten,* to knot, fr. A.S. *cnyttan*]

knob (nob). A protuberance; a mass; a nodule.

aortic k., the prominent shadow of the aortic arch on a frontal chest radiograph.

Engelmann basal k.'s, obsolete eponym for blepharoplast.

malarial k.'s, rounded protrusions of a red blood cell infected with *Plasmodium falciparum,* responsible for the adhesion of infected red cells to one another and to the endothelium of the blood vessels containing these infected cells; results in capillary blockage responsible for much of the pathology of malignant tertian malaria.

knock (nok). **1.** Colloquialism for a blow, especially a blow to the head. **2.** A sound simulating that of a blow or rap.

pericardial k., an early diastolic sound that is a variant of the third heart sound, but occurring distinctly earlier, due to rapid ventricular filling being abruptly halted by the restricting pericardium; a truly "knocking" quality is uncommon.

knock-knee (nok'nē). SYN *genu* valgum.

knock-out (nok'out). A genetically engineered organism in which the genome has been altered by site-directed recombination so that a gene is deleted.

Knoll, Philipp, Bohemian physiologist, 1841–1900. SEE K. glands, under gland.

Knoop, Hedwig, German physician, *1908. SEE K. theory.

Knoop hard·ness num·ber (KHN). See under number.

knot (not). **1.** An intertwining of the ends of two cords, tapes, or sutures, in such a way that they cannot easily become separated; or a similar twining or infolding of a cord in its continuity. **2.** In anatomy or pathology, a node, ganglion, or circumscribed swelling suggestive of a k. [A.S. *cnotta*]

false k.'s, false k.'s of umbilical cord, local increases in length or varicosity of the umbilical vein, causing markedly apparent twisting of the cord.

granny k., a double k. in which the free ends of the second loop are asymmetric and not in the same plane as the free ends of the first loop.

Hensen k., SYN primitive *node.*

Hubrecht protochordal k., SYN primitive *node.*

laparoscopic k., a k. placed intracorporally through a laparoscopic instrument. The k. itself may be tied extracorporally and passed into the body through a cannula or the k. may be both placed and tied intracorporally.

net k., SYN karyosome.

primitive k., SYN primitive *node.*

protochordal k., SYN primitive *node.*

square k., a double k. in which the free ends of the second loop are symmetric and in the same plane as the free ends of the first loop.

surgeon's k., the first loop of the k. has two throws rather than a single throw. The second loop has only one throw and that is placed in a square knot fashion leaving the free ends in the same plane as the first loop.

syncytial k., a localized aggregation of syncytiotrophoblastic nu-

clei in the villi of the placenta during early pregnancy. SYN syncytial bud, syncytial sprout.

true k., true k. of umbilical cord, actual intertwining of a segment of umbilical cord; circulation is usually not obstructed.

vital k., SYN noeud vital.

knuck·le (nŭk'l). **1.** A joint of a finger when the fist is closed, especially a metacarpophalangeal joint. **2.** A kink or loop of intestine, as in a hernia. [M.E. *knokel*]

aortic k., the contour of the aortic arch protruding from the mediastinal silhouette in an anteroposterior (AP) radiograph of the chest.

cervical aortic k., an anomalous aortic arch in which the aorta extends into the neck and forms an anteroposterior arch, which may be as high as the hyoid bone; the common carotid artery of one side is given off from the summit of the arch, and the common carotid of the other side arises from the more proximal part of the aorta; the pulsating arch may be mistaken for an aneurysm, but the radial pulses are equal.

Kobelt, Georg L., German physician, 1804–1857. SEE K. *tubules,* under *tubule.*

Kober, Philip A., U.S. chemist, *1884. SEE K. *test.*

Köbner, Heinrich, German dermatologist, 1838–1904. SEE K. *phenomenon.*

Koch, Robert, German bacteriologist and Nobel laureate, 1843–1910. SEE K. *bacillus, law,* old *tuberculin, phenomenon, postulates,* under *postulate;* K.-Weeks *bacillus.*

Koch, Walter, German surgeon, *1880. SEE K. *node, triangle.*

Kocher, Emil Theodor, Swiss surgeon and Nobel laureate, 1841–1917. SEE K. *clamp, incision, sign;* K.-Debré-Sémélaigne *syndrome.*

Kock, Nils G., 20th century Swedish surgeon. SEE K. *pouch.*

Koenig, Franz, German surgeon, 1832–1910. SEE K. *syndrome.*

Koerber, H., 20th century German ophthalmologist. SEE Koerber-Salus-Elschnig *syndrome.*

Koerte, Werner, German surgeon, 1853–1937. SEE K.-Ballance *operation.*

Koettstorfer, J., 19th century German chemist. SEE K. *number.*

Kogoj, Franjo, Yugoslavian physician, 1894–1983. SEE spongiform *pustule* of K.

Köhler, Alban, German roentgenologist, 1874–1947. SEE K. *disease.*

Köhler, August, German microscopist, 1866–1948. SEE K. *illumination.*

Kohlrausch, Otto L.B., German physician, 1811–1854. SEE K. *muscle, folds,* under *fold.*

Kohn, Hans N., German pathologist, *1866. SEE K. *pores,* under *pore.*

Kohnstamm, Oskar, German physician, 1871–1917. SEE K. *phenomenon.*

koi·lo·cyte (koy'lō-sīt). A squamous cell, often binucleated, showing a perinuclear halo; characteristic of human papillomavirus infection. [G. *koilos,* hollow, + *kytos,* cell]

koi·lo·cy·to·sis (koy'lō-sī-tō'sis). Perinuclear vacuolation. SEE ALSO koilocyte. [G. *koilos,* hollow, + *kytos,* cell, + *-osis,* condition]

koi·lo·nych·ia (koy-lō-nik'ē-ă). A malformation of the nails in which the outer surface is concave; often associated with iron deficiency or softening by occupational contact with oils. SYN spoon nail. [G. *koilos,* hollow, + *onyx (onych-),* nail]

koil·o·ster·nia (koy-lō-ster'nē-ă). SYN pectus excavatum. [G. *koilos,* hollow, + *sternon,* chest (sternum)]

Kojewnikoff (Kozhevnikov), Aleksei Y., Russian neurologist, 1836–1902. SEE K. *epilepsy.*

ko·jic ac·id (kō'jik). An antibiotic product of D-glucose catabolism in some molds; can be converted into flavor enhancers.

Kokoskin, Evelyn, 20th century Canadian pathologist. SEE K. *stain.*

ko·la (kō'lă). The dried cotyledons of *Cola nitida* or other species of *Cola* (family Sterculiaceae) which contains caffeine, theobromine, and a soluble principle, colatin; used as a cardiac and central nervous system stimulant. SYN cola (1).

ko

Kölliker, Rudolph A. von, Swiss histologist, 1817–1905. SEE K. *layer, reticulum.*

Kollmann, Arthur, 19th century German urologist. SEE K. *dilator.*

Kolmer, John A., U.S. pathologist, 1886–1962. SEE K. *test.*

Kolopp, P., 20th century French dermatologist. SEE Woringer-K. *disease.*

△**kolp-.** SEE colpo-.

ko·lyt·ic (kō-lit′ik). Denoting an inhibitory action. [G. *kolyō,* to hinder]

Kondoleon, Emmanuel, Greek surgeon, 1879–1939. SEE K. *operation.*

ko·ni·o·cor·tex (kō′nē-ō-kōr′teks). Regions of the cerebal cortex characterized by a particularly well developed inner granular layer (layer 4); this type of cerebral cortex is represented by the primary sensory area 17 of the visual cortex, areas 1 to 3 of the somatic sensory cortex, and area 41 of the auditory cortex. SEE ALSO cerebral *cortex.* [G. *konis,* dust, + L. *cortex,* bark]

konzo (kon′zō). A cyanide-caused upper motor neuron disease manifested principally as spastic paraplegia, seen in Africa, and resulting from the consumption of improperly prepared cassava roots, which contain high concentrations of cyanogenetic glucosides. [Yaka, tired legs]

Koplik, Henry, U.S. physician, 1858–1927. SEE K. *spots,* under *spot.*

kop·o·pho·bia (kop-ō-fō′bē-ă). Morbid fear of fatigue. [G. *kopos,* fatigue, + *phobos,* fear]

△**kopro-.** SEE copro-.

Korff, Karl von, 20th century German anatomist and histologist. SEE K. *fibers,* under *fiber.*

Kornberg, Arthur, U.S. biochemist and Nobel laureate, *1918. SEE K. *enzyme.*

Kornzweig, Abraham L., U.S. physician, *1900. SEE Bassen-K. *syndrome.*

ko·ro (kō′rō). An acute delusional state occurring in Macassars, natives of the Celebes, and other parts of the East, in which the subject experiences a sensation that his penis is shriveling or is being drawn into his abdomen. SYN shook jong.

ko·ro·ni·on (kŏ-rō′nē-on). SYN coronion.

Korotkoff, Nikolai S., Russian physician, 1874–1920. SEE K. *sounds,* under *sound, test.*

Korsakoff, Sergei S., Russian neurologist, 1853–1900. SEE K. *psychosis, syndrome;* Wernicke-K. *encephalopathy, syndrome.*

Koshland, Daniel E., U.S. biochemist, *1920. SEE Adair-K.-Némethy-Filmer *model;* K.-Némethy-Filmer *model.*

Kossa, SEE von Kossa.

Koyanagi, Yosizo, Japanese ophthalmologist, 1880–1954. SEE Vogt-K. *syndrome.*

Koyter. SEE Coiter.

Kr Symbol for krypton.

Krabbe, Knud H., Danish neurologist, 1885–1961. SEE K. *disease;* Christensen-K. *disease.*

krait (krīt). Elapid snake of the genus *Bungarus,* found in northern India, whose bite is associated with generalized anesthetic and paralytic effects, as opposed to local pain, discoloration, or edema; neurotoxic symptoms are similar to those induced by cobra venom. [Hindi *karait*]

Krantz, Kermit E., U.S. obstetrician-gynecologist, *1923. SEE Marshall-Marchetti-K. *operation.*

Kraske, Paul, German surgeon, 1851–1930. SEE K. *operation.*

krau·ro·sis vul·vae (kraw-rō′sis vŭl′vē). Atrophy and shrinkage of the epithelium of the vagina and vulva, often accompanied by a chronic inflammatory reaction in the deeper tissues; an outmoded term for lichen sclerosus et atrophicus of the vulva. SYN leukokraurosis. [G. *krauros,* dry, brittle]

Krause, Fedor, German surgeon, 1857–1937. SEE K. *graft;* Wolfe-K. *graft.*

Krause, Karl F.T., German anatomist, 1797–1868. SEE K. *glands,* under *gland, ligament.*

Krause, Wilhelm J.F., German anatomist, 1833–1910. SEE K. bone, end *bulbs,* under *bulb,* respiratory *bundle, valve.*

kreb·i·o·zen (krē′bē-oz′en). An extract from peach kernels, the composition of which has not been fully described but which gained notoriety in the 1960′s and 1970′s as a dubious but exploited remedy for cancer; currently not regarded as effective. [Ger. *Krebs,* crab, cancer]

Krebs, Edwin G., U.S. biochemist, *1918, joint winner of the 1992 Nobel Prize for the discovery of reversible protein phosphorylation as a biological regulatory mechanism.

Krebs, Sir Hans Adolph, German biochemist in England and Nobel laureate, 1900–1981. SEE K. *cycle;* K.-Henseleit *cycle;* K.-Ringer *solution.*

Kretschmann, Friederich, German otologist, 1858–1934. SEE K. *space.*

Kreysig, Friedrich L., German physician, 1770–1839. SEE K. *sign;* Heim-K. *sign.*

kriging (krī′jing). A method first used in the earth sciences to smooth data from spatially scattered point measurements, used in geographic epidemiology. [D. G. *Krige,* South African engineer]

krin·gle (krin′gle). A structural motif or domain seen in certain proteins in which a fold of large loops is stabilized by disulfide bonds; an important structural feature in blood coagulation factors. [Ger. *Kringel,* curl]

Krogh, August, Danish physiologist and Nobel laureate, 1874–1949. SEE K. *spirometer.*

Kronecker, Karl H., Swiss physiologist, 1839–1914. SEE K. *stain.*

Krönig, Georg, German physician, 1856–1911. SEE K. *isthmus, steps,* under *step.*

Krönlein, Rudolf U., Swiss surgeon, 1847–1910. SEE K. *operation, hernia.*

Krueger in·stru·ment stop. See under instrument.

Krukenberg, Adolph, German anatomist, 1816–1877. SEE K. *veins,* under *vein.*

Krukenberg, Friedrich, German pathologist, 1871–1946. SEE K. *amputation, spindle, tumor.*

Kruse, Walther, German bacteriologist, 1864–1943. SEE K. *brush;* Shiga-Kruse *bacillus.*

△**krymo-, kryo-.** SEE crymo-, cryo-.

kryp·ton (Kr) (krip′ton). One of the noble gases, present in small amounts in the atmosphere (1.14 ppm by dry volume); atomic no. 36, atomic wt. 83.80; ^{85}Kr (half-life of 10.73 years) has been used in studies of cardiac abnormalities. [G. *kryptos,* concealed]

17-KS Abbreviation for 17-ketosteroids.

KUB Abbreviation for kidneys, ureters, bladder; archaic term for a plain frontal supine radiograph of the abdomen.

ku·bi·sa·ga·ri, ku·bi·sa·ga·ru (koo-bi-sah-gah′rē, koo-bi-sah-gah′roo). SYN vestibular *neuronitis.* [Jap. *kubi,* head, neck, + *sagaru,* to hang down]

Kufs, Hugo, German psychiatrist, 1871–1955. SEE K. *disease.*

Kugel anastomotic ar·tery. See under artery.

Kugelberg, Eric, Swedish neurologist, 1913–1983. SEE K.-Welander *disease;* Wohlfart-K.-Welander *disease.*

Kühne, Wilhelm (Willy) F., German physiologist and histologist, 1837–1900. SEE K. *fiber, methylene blue, phenomenon, plate, spindle.*

Kuhnt, Hermann, German ophthalmologist, 1850–1925. SEE K. *spaces,* under *space.*

Kulchitsky, Nicholas, Russian histologist, 1856–1925. SEE K. *cells,* under *cell.*

Külz, Rudolph E., German physician, 1845–1895. SEE K. *cylinder.*

Küntscher, Gerhard, German surgeon, 1902–1972. SEE K. *nail.*

Kupffer, Karl W. von, German anatomist, 1829–1902. SEE K. *cells,* under *cell.*

kur·chi bark (ker′chē). SYN conessi.

Kürsteiner (Kuersteiner), W., 19th century German anatomist. SEE K. *canals,* under *canal.*

kur·to·sis (kur-tō'sis). The extent to which a unimodal distribution is peaked. [G., an arching]

ku·ru (koo'roo). A progressive, fatal form of spongiform encephalopathy endemic to Fore people in the highlands of New Guinea, initially attributed to a "slow virus" infection, but now known to be caused by prions. Transmission is believed to be effected by contamination and ingestion during ritual cannabalism. It is characterized by ataxia, tremors, lack of coordination and death; pathological lesions in the brain include neuronal loss, ostrocytosis and status spongiosus. SEE prion. [native dialect, to shiver from fear or cold]

Kurzrok-Ratner test. See under test.

Kussmaul, Adolph, German physician, 1822–1902. SEE K. *respiration, coma, disease, sign;* K.-Kien *respiration.*

Küster, Herman, early 20th century German gynecologist. SEE Mayer-Rokitansky-K.-Hauser *syndrome;* Rokitansky-K.-Hauser *syndrome.*

Küstner, Heinz, German gynecologist, *1897. SEE Prausnitz-K. *antibody, reaction;* reversed K. *reaction.*

kv Abbreviation for kilovolt.

Kveim, Morton A., Norwegian physician, *1892. SEE K. *antigen, test;* K.-Siltzbach *antigen, test;* Nickerson-K. *test.*

kVp Abbreviation for kilovolts peak, the highest instantaneous voltage across an x-ray tube, corresponding to the highest energy x-rays emitted.

kwa·shi·or·kor (kwah-shē-ōr'kōr). A disease seen originally in Africans, particularly children 1–3 years old, due to dietary deficiency, particularly of protein; characterized by marked hypoalbuminemia, anemia, edema, pot belly, depigmentation of the skin, loss of hair or change in hair color to red, and bulky stools containing undigested food; fatty changes in the cells of the liver, atrophy of the acinar cells of the pancreas, and hyalinization of the renal glomeruli are found postmortem. SYN infantile pellagra, malignant malnutrition. [Ga, a language of Ghana, red boy or displaced child]

marasmic k., severe protein-calorie malnutrition characterized by extreme weight loss, weakness, and features of k.

△**ky-.** For words beginning thus and not found below, see cy-.

ky·mo·gram (kī'mō-gram). The graphic curve made by a kymograph.

ky·mo·graph (kī'mō-graf). An obsolete instrument for recording wavelike motions or modulation, especially for recording variations in blood pressure; it consists of a drum usually revolved by clockwork and covered with smoked paper upon which the curve is inscribed by a stylet or other writing point. [G. *kyma,* wave, + *graphō,* to record]

ky·mog·ra·phy (kī-mog'ră-fē). Use of the kymograph.

ky·mo·scope (kī'mō-skōp). An apparatus once used for measuring the pulse waves, or the variation in blood pressure. [G. *kyma,* wave, + *skopeō,* to regard]

kyn·u·ren·ic ac·id (kin-ū-rē'nik, -ren'ik). A product of the metabolism of L-tryptophan; appears in human urine in states of marked pyridoxine deficiency.

kyn·u·ren·i·nase (kī-noo-ren'i-nās). A liver enzyme catalyzing the hydrolysis of the L-kynurenine side chain, with the formation of anthranilic acid and L-alanine, in L-tryptophan metabolism.

kyn·u·ren·ine (kī-noo'rĕ-nēn, -nin). A product of the metabolism of L-tryptophan, excreted in the urine in small amounts; elevated in cases of vitamin B_6 deficiency.

k. formamidase, SYN formamidase.

k. 3-hydroxylase, SYN k. 3-monooxygenase.

k. 3-monooxygenase, an enzyme catalyzing addition of a hydroxyl group to L-kynurenine, with the aid of NADPH and O_2, producing 3-hydroxy-L-kynurenine, $NADP^+$, and water; a step in the catabolism of L-tryptophan. SYN k. 3-hydroxylase.

ky·phos (kī'fos). A hump, the convex prominence in kyphosis. [G.]

ky·pho·sco·li·o·sis (kī-fō-skō'lē-ō-sis). Lateral and posterior curvature of the spine; severe congestive heart failure can be a late complication. SYN scoliokyphosis. [G. *kyphōsis,* kyphosis, + *scoliosis,* curved]

ky·pho·sis (kī-fō'sis). **1.** An anteriorly concave curvature of the vertebral column; the normal kyphoses of the thoracic and sacral regions are retained portions of the primary curvature (kyphosis) of the vertebral column. **2.** A forward (flexion) curvature of the spine; the thoracic spine normally has a mild kyphosis; excessive forward curvature of the thoracic spine may represent a pathologic condition. [G. *kyphōsis,* hump-back, fr. *kyphos,* bent, humpbacked]

juvenile k., SYN Scheuermann *disease.*

sacral k. [TA], the normal, anteriorly concave curvature of the sacrum (sacral segment of the vertebral column), in which the primary curvature of the fetal embryo is maintained into maturity. SYN k. sacralis TA] [TA].

k. sacralis TA [TA], SYN sacral k.

thoracic k. [TA], the normal, anteriorly concave curvature of the thoracic segment of the vertebral column, in which the primary curvature of the fetal embryo is maintained into maturity. SYN k. thoracica [TA].

k. thoracica [TA], SYN thoracic k.

ky·phot·ic (kī-fot'ik). Relating to or suffering from kyphosis.

Kyrle, Josef, German dermatologist, 1880–1926. SEE K. *disease.*

△**kyto-.** SEE cyto-.

ky

Λ 1. The 11th letter of the Greek alphabet, lambda. **2.** Symbol (λ) for Avogadro *number*; wavelength; radioactive *constant*; Ostwald solubility *coefficient*; molar conductivity of an electrolyte (Λ). **3.** In chemistry, denotes the position of a substituent located on the eleventh atom from the carboxyl or other functional group (λ).

L 1. Abbreviation for left (e.g., left eye); lumbar vertebrae (L1 to L5). **2.** Symbol for inductance; liter; leucine; leucyl. **3.** Abbreviation for limes; used with a lower case letter, plus sign, subscript letter, or subscript plus sign as a symbol for various doses of toxin. SEE dose.

L Symbol for linking *number*.

l Symbol for liter; liquid; length (in italics).

⬡*l-.* Levorotatory. Cf. *d-*. [L. *laevus,* on the left-hand side]

⬡**L-.** Prefix indicating a chemical compound to be structurally (sterically) related to L-glyceraldehyde. Cf. D-.

La Symbol for lanthanum.

Laband, Peter F., U.S. dentist, *1900. SEE L. *syndrome*.

Labbé, Leon, French surgeon, 1832–1916. SEE L. *triangle, vein*.

Labbé, Ernest M., French physician, 1870–1939.

la·bel. 1. To incorporate into a compound a substance that is readily detected, such as a radionuclide, whereby its metabolism can be followed or its physical distribution detected. **2.** The substance so incorporated.

la belle in·dif·fér·ence (lah bel an-dif-er-ahns'). A naive, inappropriate lack of emotion or concern for the perceptions by others of one's disability, typically seen in persons with conversion hysteria. [Fr.]

la·bet·a·lol hy·dro·chlo·ride (la-bet'ă-lol). An α-adrenergic and β-adrenergic blocking agent used in the treatment of hypertension.

la·bia (lā'bē-ă). Plural of labium.

la·bi·al (lā'bē-ăl). **1.** Relating to the lips or any labium. **2.** Toward a lip. **3.** One of the letters formed by means of the lips. [L. *labium,* lip]

la·bi·al·ism (lā'bē-ăl-izm). A form of stammering in which there is confusion in the use of the labial consonants.

la·bi·al·ly (lā'bē-ăl-ē). Toward the lips.

la·bile (lā'bīl, -bil). Unstable; unsteady, not fixed; denoting: **1.** An adaptability to alteration or modification, i.e., relatively easily changed or rearranged. **2.** Certain constituents of serum affected by increases in heat. **3.** An electrode that is kept moving over the surface during the passage of an electric current. **4.** In psychology or psychiatry, denoting free and uncontrolled mood or behavioral expression of the emotions. **5.** Easily removable; e.g., a l. hydrogen atom. [L. *labilis,* liable to slip, fr. *labor,* pp. *lapsus,* to slip]

la·bil·i·ty (lă-bil'i-tē). The state of being labile.

⬡**labio-.** The lips. SEE ALSO cheilo-. [L. *labium,* lip]

la·bi·o·cer·vi·cal (lā'bē-ō-ser'vi-kăl). Relating to a lip and a neck; specifically, to the labial or buccal surface of the neck of a tooth. [labio- + L. *cervix,* neck]

la·bi·o·cli·na·tion (lā'bē-ō-kli-nā'shŭn). Inclination of position more toward the lips than is normal; said of a tooth.

la·bi·o·den·tal (lā-bē-ō-den'tăl). Relating to the lips and the teeth; denoting certain letters the sound of which is formed by both lips and teeth. [labio- + L. *dens,* tooth]

la·bi·o·gin·gi·val (lā'bē-ō-jin'ji-văl). Relating to the point of junction of the labial border and the gingival line on the distal or mesial surface of an incisor tooth.

la·bi·o·glos·so·la·ryn·ge·al (lā'bē-ō-glos'ō-lă-rin'jē-ăl). Relating to the lips, tongue, and larynx; describing bulbar paralysis in which these parts are involved. [labio- + G. *glōssa,* tongue, + larynx]

la·bi·o·glos·so·pha·ryn·ge·al (lā'bē-ō-glos'ō-fă-rin'jē-ăl). Relating to the lips, tongue, and pharynx; describing bulbar paralysis involving these parts. [labio- + G. *glōssa,* tongue, + pharynx]

la·bi·o·graph (lā'bē-ō-graf). An instrument for recording the movements of the lips in speaking. [labio- + G. *graphō,* to record]

la·bi·o·men·tal (lā'bē-ō-men'tăl). Relating to the lower lip and the chin. [labio- + L. *mentum,* chin]

la·bi·o·na·sal (lā'bē-ō-nā'săl). **1.** Relating to the upper lip and the nose, or to both lips and the nose. **2.** Denoting a letter that is both labial and nasal in the production of its sound.

la·bi·o·pal·a·tine (lā'bē-ō-pal'ă-tīn). Relating to the lips and the palate.

la·bi·o·place·ment (lā'bē-ō-plās'ment). Positioning (e.g., of a tooth) more toward the lips than normal.

la·bi·o·plas·ty (lā'bē-ō-plas-tē). Plastic surgery of a lip. [labio- + G. *plastos,* formed]

la·bi·o·ver·sion (lā'bē-ō-ver-zhŭn). Malposition of an anterior tooth from the normal line of occlusion toward the lips.

lab·i·tome (lab'i-tōm). A forceps with sharp blades. SYN cutting forceps. [G. *labis,* pincers, + *tomē,* an incision]

la·bi·um, gen. **la·bii,** pl. **la·bia** (lā'bē-ŭm, -bē-ē, -bē-ă) [TA]. **1.** SYN lip. **2.** Any lip-shaped structure. [L.]

l. ante'rius os'tii u'teri [TA], SYN anterior *lip* of external os of uterus.

l. exter'num cris'tae ili'acae [TA], SYN outer *lip* of iliac crest.

l. infe'rius o'ris [TA], SYN lower *lip*.

l. inter'num cris'tae ili'acae [TA], SYN inner *lip* of iliac crest.

l. latera'le lin'eae as'perae [TA], SYN lateral *lip* of linea aspera.

l. lim'bi tympan'icum la'minae spira'lis ossei, SYN tympanic *lip* of spiral limbus.

l. limbi tympanicum limbi spiralis ossei [TA], SYN tympanic *lip* of spiral limbus.

l. lim'bi vestibula're la'minae spi'ralis ossei, SYN vestibular *lip* of spiral limbus.

l. limbi vestibulare limbi spiralis ossei [TA], SYN vestibular *lip* of spiral limbus.

l. ma'jus [TA], one of two rounded folds of integument forming the lateral boundaries of the pudendal cleft. The labia majora are the female homolog of the scrotum. SYN l. majus pudendi [TA], large pudendal lip.

l. ma'jus puden'di, pl. **la'bia majo'ra** [TA], SYN l. majus.

l. media'le lin'eae as'perae [TA], SYN medial *lip* of linea aspera.

l. mi'nus [TA], one of two narrow longitudinal folds of mucous membrane enclosed in the pudendal cleft within the labia majora; posteriorly, they gradually merge into the labia majora and join to form the frenulum labiorum pudendi (fourchette); anteriorly, each l. divides into two portions that unite with those of the opposite side in front of the glans clitoridis to form the prepuce. SYN l. minus pudendi, small pudendal lip.

l. mi'nus puden'di, pl. **la'bia mino'ra,** SYN l. minus.

la'bia o'ris [TA], SYN lips of mouth, under *lip*; SEE lip (1).

l. poste'rius os'tii u'teri [TA], SYN posterior *lip* of external os of uterus.

l. supe'rius o'ris [TA], SYN upper *lip*.

tympanic l. of limbus of spiral lamina, SYN tympanic *lip* of spiral limbus.

l. ure'thrae, one of the two lateral margins of the external urethral orifice of the female.

la'bia u'teri, SEE anterior *lip* of external os of uterus, posterior *lip* of external os of uterus.

vestibular l. of limbus of spiral lamina, SYN vestibular *lip* of spiral limbus.

l. voca'le, pl. **la'bia voca'lia,** SYN vocal *fold*.

⬡ Combining Forms	☆ Official alternate Terminologia Anatomica term
🔲 Indicates term is illustrated, see Illustration Index	
	[MIM] Mendelian Inheritance in Man
SYN Synonym	
Cf. Compare	C.I. Colour Index
[NA] Nomina Anatomica	
[TA] Terminologia Anatomica	**High Profile Term**

la·bor (lā'bŏr). The process of expulsion of the fetus and the placenta from the uterus. The **stages of l.** include: **first stage**, beginning with the onset of uterine contractions through the period of dilation of the os uteri; **second stage**, the period of expulsive effort, beginning with complete dilation of the cervix and ending with expulsion of the infant; **third s.** or **placental stage**, the period beginning at the expulsion of the infant and ending with the completed expulsion of the placenta and membranes. [L. toil, suffering]

active l., contractions resulting in progressive effacement and dilation of the cervix.

dry l., obsolete term for l. after spontaneous loss of the amniotic fluid.

false l., contractions which do not produce cervical dilation or effacement.

missed l., brief uterine contractions which do not lead to labor and expulsion of the infant, but which cease, resulting in the indefinite retention of the fetus (usually lifeless) either *in utero* or in the abdominal cavity.

precipitate l., very rapid l. ending in delivery of the fetus.

premature l., onset of labor after 20 weeks and before the 37th completed week of pregnancy dated from the last normal menstrual period.

trial of l. after cesarean section, the attempt to deliver vaginally after a cesarean section; carries some risk of rupture of the uterine scar.

lab·o·ra·to·ri·an (lab'ŏ-ră-tōr'ē-an). One who works in a laboratory; in the medical and allied health professions, one who examines or performs tests (or supervises such procedures) with various types of chemical and biologic materials, chiefly as an aid in the diagnosis, treatment, and control of disease, or as a basis for health and sanitation practices.

lab·o·ra·tory (lab'ŏ-ră-tō-rē, lab'ră-). A place equipped for the performance of tests, experiments, and investigative procedures and for the preparation of reagents, therapeutic chemical materials, and so on. [Mediev. L. *laboratorium,* a workplace, fr. L. *laboro,* pp. *-atus,* to labor]

personal growth l., a sensitivity training setting in which the primary emphasis is on each participant's potentialities for creativity, empathy, and leadership. SEE ALSO sensitivity training *group.*

la·bra (lā'bră). Plural of labrum. [L.]

la·bra·le in·fe·ri·us (lă-brā'lē in-fē'rē-ŭs). A point where the boundary of the vermilion border of the lower lip and the skin is intersected by the median plane.

la·bra·le su·pe·ri·us (lă-brā'lē soo-pē'rē-ŭs). The point on the upper lip lying in the median sagittal plane on a line drawn across the boundary of the vermilion border and skin.

lab·ro·cyte (lab'rō-sīt). SYN mast *cell.*

la·brum, pl. **la·bra** (lā'brŭm, lā'bră) [TA]. **1.** A lip. **2.** A lip-shaped structure. **3.** A fibrocartilaginous lip around the margin of the concave portion of some joints. SYN articular l., articular lip, l. articulare. [L.]

acetabular l. [TA], a fibrocartilaginous rim attached to the margin of the acetabulum of the hip bone. SYN l. acetabulare [TA], acetabular lip, circumferential cartilage (1), cotyloid ligament, ligamentum cotyloideum.

l. acetabula're [TA], SYN acetabular l.

articular l., SYN labrum (3).

l. articula're, SYN labrum (3).

l. glenoida'le scapulae [TA], SYN glenoid l. of scapula.

glenoid l. of scapula [TA], a ring of fibrocartilage attached to the margin of the glenoid cavity of the scapula to increase its depth. SYN l. glenoidale scapulae [TA], articular margin, circumferential cartilage (2), glenoid ligament (1), glenoidal lip, ligamentum glenoidale.

lab·y·rinth (lab'i-rinth) [TA]. Any of several anatomic structures with numerous intercommunicating cells or canals. **1.** The internal or inner ear, composed of the semicircular ducts, vestibule, and cochlea. **2.** Any group of communicating cavities, as in each lateral mass of the ethmoid bone. **3.** A group of upright test tubes

terminating below in a base of communicating, alternately ∪-shaped and ∩-shaped tubes, used for isolating motile from nonmotile organisms in culture, or a motile from a less motile organism (as the typhoid from the colon bacillus), the former traveling faster and farther through the tubes than the latter.

bony l. [TA], a series of cavities (cochlea, vestibule, and semicircular canals) contained within the otic capsule of the petrous portion of the temporal bone; the bony labyrinth is filled with perilymph, in which the delicate, endolymph-filled membranous labyrinth is suspended. SYN labyrinthus osseus [TA], osseous l.

cochlear l. [TA], the portion of the membranous labyrinth concerned with the sense of hearing (vs. the vestibular labyrinth, which is concerned with the sense of equilibration) and innervated by the cochlear nerve; it is located within the cochlea of the bony labyrinth, and consists of the cochlear duct, which contains the spiral organ. SYN labyrinthus cochlearis [TA], organ of hearing.

ethmoidal l. [TA], a mass of air cells with thin bony walls forming part of the lateral wall of the nasal cavity; the cells are arranged in three groups, anterior, middle, and posterior, and are closed laterally by the orbital plate which forms part of the wall of the orbit. SYN labyrinthus ethmoidalis [TA], ectethmoid, ectoethmoid, lateral mass of ethmoid bone.

Ludwig l., SYN convoluted *part* of kidney lobule.

membranous l. [TA], a complex arrangement of communicating membranous canaliculi and sacs, filled with endolymph and surrounded by perilymph, suspended within the cavity of the bony labyrinth; its chief divisions are the cochlear duct and the vestibular labyrinth. SYN labyrinthus membranaceus [TA].

osseous l., SYN bony l.

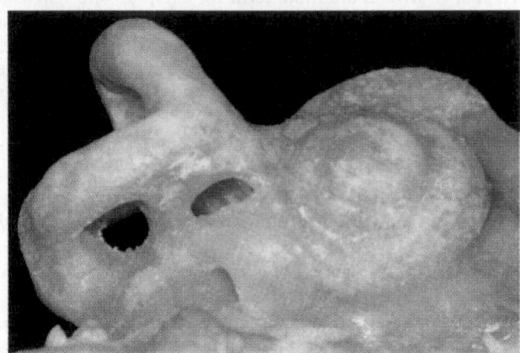

osseous labyrinth: removed from the petrous portion of the temporal bone

renal l., SYN convoluted *part* of kidney lobule.

Santorini l., SYN prostatic venous *plexus.*

vestibular l. [TA], the portion of the membranous labyrinth concerned with the sense of equilibration (vs. the cochlear labyrinth, which is concerned with the sense of hearing) and innervated by the vestibular nerve; it is located within the semicircular canals and vestibule of the bony labyrinth, and consists of the utricle, saccule, and the semicircular, utriculosaccular, and endolymphatic ducts. SYN labyrinthus vestibularis [TA], vestibular organ.

lab·y·rin·thec·to·my (lab-ĭ-rin-thek'tō-mē). Excision of the labyrinth; a destructive operation to destroy labyrinthine function. [labyrinth + G. *ektomē,* excision]

lab·y·rin·thine (lab-ĭ-rin'thin). Relating to any labyrinth.

lab·y·rin·thi·tis (lab'ĭ-rin-thī'tis). Inflammation of the labyrinth (the internal ear), sometimes accompanied by vertigo and deafness. SYN otitis interna.

lab·y·rin·thot·o·my (lab-ĭ-rin-thot'ō-mē). Incision into the labyrinth. [labyrinth + G. *tomē,* incision]

lab·y·rin·thus (lab-i-rin'thŭs). SYN convoluted *part* of kidney lobule. [L. fr. G. *labyrinthos,* labyrinth]

l. cochlea'ris [TA], SYN cochlear *labyrinth.*

l. ethmoida'lis [TA], SYN ethmoidal *labyrinth.*

l. membrana'ceus [TA], SYN membranous *labyrinth.*

l. os'seus [TA], SYN bony *labyrinth.*

la

l. vestibula′ris [TA], SYN vestibular *labyrinth*.

lac, gen. **lac·tis** (lak, lak′tis). **1.** SYN milk (1). **2.** Any whitish, milklike liquid. [L. milk]

l. sul′furis, SYN precipitated *sulfur*.

l. vacci′num, cow's milk.

lac·ca (lak′ă). SYN shellac.

lac·case (lak′ās). An enzyme oxidizing benzenediols to semiquinones with O_2. SYN monophenol monooxygenase (2), phenol oxidase, phenolase, polyphenol oxidase, urushiol oxidase.

lac·er·a·ble (las′er-ă-bl). Capable of being, or liable to be, torn. [L. *lacero,* to tear to pieces, fr. *lacer,* mangled]

lac·er·at·ed (las′er-ā-ted). Torn; rent; having a ragged edge. [L. *lacero,* pp. *-atus,* to tear to pieces]

lac·er·a·tion (las-er-a′shŭn). **1.** A torn or jagged wound, or an accidental cut wound. **2.** The process or act of tearing the tissues. [L. *lacero,* pp. *-atus,* to tear to pieces]

brain l., gross tearing of neural tissue.

scalp l., a tear of the dermis or underlying tissues and galea aponeurotica of the scalp.

through-and-through laceration, a l. that penetrates two surfaces of a structure, generally restricted to skin or mucosal surfaces, such as the cheek, lip, ala nasi, pinna, etc.

vaginal l., tearing of the vaginal wall. SYN colporrhexis.

la·cer·tus (lă-ser′tŭs) [TA]. **1** [TA]. A fibrous band, bundle, or slip related to a muscle. **2.** Originally the muscular part of the upper limb from shoulder to elbow. [L.]

l. cor′dis, one of the trabeculae carneae.

l. fibro′sus, ☆official alternate term for bicipital *aponeurosis.*

l. of lateral rectus muscle, the part of the tendon of origin of the lateral rectus muscle attaching to the greater wing of the sphenoid bone, lateral to the common tendinous ring; often incorrectly equated to the lateral check ligament of the eyeball. SYN l. musculi recti lateralis.

l. me′dius, SYN anterior longitudinal *ligament.*

l. mus′culi rec′ti latera′lis, SYN l. of lateral rectus muscle.

lach·ry·mal (lak′ri-măl). SYN lacrimal.

LACI Abbreviation for lipoprotein-associated coagulation *inhibitor.*

la·cin·i·ae tu·bae (la-sin′ē-ē too′bē). SYN *fimbriae* of uterine tube, under *fimbria.* [L. *lacinia,* fringe]

lac·ri·mal (lak′ri-măl). Relating to the tears, their secretion, the secretory glands, and the drainage apparatus. SYN lachrymal. [L. *lacrima,* a tear]

lac·ri·ma·tion (lak′ri-ma′shŭn). The secretion of tears, especially in excess. [L. *lacrimatio*]

lac·ri·ma·tor (lak′ri-mā-ter). An agent (such as tear gas) that irritates the eyes and produces tears. [L. *lacrima,* tear]

lac·ri·ma·to·ry (lak′ri-mă-tō-rē). Causing lacrimation.

lac·ri·mot·o·my (lak-ri-mot′ō-mē). The operation of incising the lacrimal duct or sac. [L. *lacrima,* tear, + G. *tomē,* incision]

△**lact-, lacti-, lacto-.** Milk. SEE ALSO galacto-. [L. *lac, lactis*]

lac·tac·i·de·mia (lak-tas-i-dē′mē-ă). SYN lactic acidemia.

lac·tac·i·do·sis (lak-tas-i-dō′sis). Acidosis due to increased lactic acid.

lac·tal·bu·min (lak-tal-bū′min). The albumin fraction of milk. It contains two proteins: α- and β-l.; the former, minor l., interacts with galactosyl transferase to form lactose synthase which synthesizes lactose from D-glucose and UDP-galactose in milk production; β-l. is the chief whey protein in bovine milk; α-l. is the most heat-stable of the whey proteins.

lac·tam, lac·tim (lak′tam, -tim). Contractions of "lactoneamine" and "lactoneimine," and applied to the tautomeric forms –NH–CO– and –N=C(OH)–, respectively, observed in many purines, pyrimidines, and other substances; the latter form accounts for the acidic properties of uric acid.

β**-lac·tam.** A class of broad-spectrum antibiotics that are structurally and pharmacologically related to the penicillins and cephalosporins.

lactamase (lak′ta-māz). SYN β-lactamase.

β**-lac·ta·mase** (lak′tă-mās). An enzyme produced by many species of bacteria that disrupts the four-membered β-lactam ring of penicillin and cephalosporin groups of antibiotics, destroying their antimicrobial activity. The ability of an organism to produce a β-lactamase may be chromosomal and constitutive or a plasmid-associated acquired property. SYN cephalosporinase, lactamase, penicillinase (1).

lac·tase (lak′tās). SYN β-D-galactosidase.

lac·tate (lak′tāt). **1.** A salt or ester of lactic acid. **2.** To produce milk in the mammary glands.

l. dehydrogenase (LDH), name for a number of enzymes, including: L-l. dehydrogenase (cytochrome), D-l. dehydrogenase (cytochrome), L-l. dehydrogenase, and D-l. dehydrogenase. The first two enzymes transfer hydrogen to ferricytochrome *c* or to cytochrome b_2, the last two enzymes transfer it to NAD^+, in catalyzing the oxidation of lactate to pyruvate; the isozyme distribution of heart and muscle l. dehydrogenase is of significant use in cases of myocardial infarction; a deficiency of a subunit will result in myoglobinuria after intense exercise. SYN lactic acid dehydrogenase.

excess l., the increase in l. concentration beyond what would be expected from the increase in pyruvate concentration resulting from a change in redox potential; used as an index of anaerobic carbohydrate metabolism.

Ringer l., SYN Ringer *solution.*

lac·tate 2-mon·o·ox·y·gen·ase. A flavoprotein oxidoreductase catalyzing oxidation (with O_2) of L-lactate to acetate plus CO_2 and water. SYN lactic acid oxidative decarboxylase.

lac·ta·tion (lak-tā′shŭn). **1.** Production of milk. **2.** Period following birth during which milk is secreted in the breasts. [L. *lactatio,* suckle]

lac·ta·tion·al (lak-tā′shŭn-ăl). Relating to lactation.

lac·te·al (lak′tē-ăl). **1.** Relating to or resembling milk; milky. **2.** A lymphatic vessel that conveys chyle. SYN chyle vessel, lacteal vessel.

central l., the blindly ending lymphatic capillary in the center of an intestinal villus.

lac·te·nin (lak′tĕ-nin). An antibacterial agent active against streptococci isolated from cow's milk.

lac·tes·cent (lak-tes′ent). Resembling milk; milky.

△**lacti-.** SEE lact-.

lac·tic (lak′tik). Relating to milk. [L. *lac* (*lact-*), milk]

lac·tic ac·id. A normal intermediate in the fermentation (oxidation, metabolism) of sugar. In pure form, a syrupy, odorless, and colorless liquid obtained by the action of the l. a. bacillus on milk or milk sugar; in concentrated form, a caustic used internally to prevent gastrointestinal fermentation. A culture of the bacillus, or milk containing it, is usually given in place of the acid. L-L. a. is also known as sarcolactic acid.

lac·tic ac·id de·hy·dro·gen·ase. SYN *lactate* dehydrogenase.

lac·tic ac·i·de·mia (lak′tik-as-i-dē′mē-ă). The presence of dextrorotatory lactic acid in the circulating blood. SYN lactacidemia. [lactic acid + G. *haima,* blood]

lac·tic ac·id ox·i·da·tive de·car·box·yl·ase. SYN lactate 2-mono-oxygenase.

lac·tif·er·ous (lak-tif′er-ŭs). Yielding milk. [lacti- + L. *fero,* to bear]

lac·tif·u·gal (lak-tif′ū-găl). SYN lactifuge (1).

lac·ti·fuge (lak′ti-fūj). **1.** Causing arrest of the secretion of milk. SYN lactifugal. **2.** An agent having such an effect. [lacti- + L. *fugo,* to drive away]

lac·tig·e·nous (lak-tij′ĕ-nŭs). Producing milk. [lacti- + *-gen,* producing]

lac·tim (-tim). SEE lactam.

lac·ti·mor·bus (lak-ti-mōr′bŭs). SYN milk *sickness.* [lacti- + L. *morbus,* disease]

lac·ti·nat·ed (lak′ti-nā-ted). Prepared with or containing milk sugar.

△**lacto-.** SEE lact-.

Lac·to·bac·il·la·ce·ae (lak′tō-bas′i-lā′sē-ē). A family of anaerobic to facultatively anaerobic, ordinarily nonmotile bacteria (order Eubacteriales) containing straight or curved, Gram-positive rods which usually occur singly or in chains; motile cells are peritrichous. These organisms have complex organic nutritional requirements; they produce lactic acid from carbohydrates. They are found in fermenting animal and plant products where carbohydrates are available; they are also found in the mouth, vagina, and intestinal tract of various warm-blooded animals, including humans. Only a few species are pathogenic. The type genus is *Lactobacillus*, which contains 56 species.

lac·to·ba·cil·li (lak-tō-bă-sil′ī). Plural of lactobacillus.

lac·to·ba·cil·lic ac·id (lak′tō-bă-sil′ik). A major constituent of the lipids of lactobacilli; notable for the presence of a cyclopropane ring in the molecule.

Lac·to·ba·cil·lus (lak-tō-bă-sil′ŭs). A genus of microaerophilic or anaerobic, nonsporeforming, ordinarily nonmotile bacteria (family Lactobacillaceae) containing Gram-positive curved or straight rods that vary from long and slender cells to short coccobacilli; chains are commonly produced especially in the later part of the logarithmic phase of growth. These organisms possess complex nutritional requirements, generally characteristic for each species; metabolism is fermentative and at least half of the end product is lactic acid. They are found in dairy products, effluents of grain and meat products, water, sewage, beer, wine, fruits and fruit juices, pickled vegetables, and in sourdough and mash, and are part of the normal flora of the mouth, intestinal tract, and vagina of many warm-blooded animals, including humans; as normal flora, they produce bacterocidins protective against pathogenic bacteria; rarely are they pathogenic. The type species is *L. delbrueckii*. [lacto- + bacillus]

L. acidoph′ilus, a bacterial species found in the feces of milk-fed infants and also in the feces of older persons on a high milk-, lactose-, or dextrin-containing diet.

L. bre′vis, a bacterial species widely distributed in nature, especially in plant and animal products; it is also found in the mouth and intestinal tract of humans and rats.

L. buch′neri, a bacterial species widely distributed in fermenting substances.

L. bulgar′icus, a bacterial species used in the production of yogurt.

L. ca′sei, a bacterial species found in milk and cheese.

L. catenafor′mis, an anaerobic bacterial species found in the intestines and pulmonary cavities of humans.

L. crispa′tus, a bacterial species found in pus from a dental abscess.

L. curva′tus, a bacterial species found in cow dung, dairy barn air, silage, milk, and in a case of endocarditis.

L. delbrueck′ii, a bacterial species found in fermenting vegetables and grain mashes; it is the type species of the genus *L.*

L. fermen′tum, a bacterial species found widely distributed in nature, especially in fermenting plant and animal products. Also found in the mouth of human beings.

L. jensen′ii, a bacterial species isolated from human sources such as vaginal discharge and blood clot.

L. planta′rum, a bacterial species found in dairy products and environments, fermenting plants, silage, sauerkraut, pickled vegetables, spoiled tomato products, sour dough, cow dung, and the human mouth, intestinal tract, and stools.

L. saliva′rius, a bacterial species found in the mouth and intestinal tract of the hamster, the mouth of humans, and the intestinal tract of the hen.

L. tricho′des, a bacterial species found in wines containing 20% ethanol and in lees in California, Australia, France, and Spain; in California this organism is commonly referred to as the hair bacillus, cottony bacillus, cottony mold, or Fresno mold.

lac·to·ba·cil·lus (lak-tō-bă-sil′ŭs). A vernacular term used to refer to any member of the genus *Lactobacillus*.

lactobezoar (lak′tō-bē′zōr). A bezoar attributed to enriched calcium or casein content in some formulas prepared for premature infants. [lacto- + bezoar]

lac·to·bu·ty·rom·e·ter (lak′tō-bū-ti-rom′ĕ-ter). A type of lactocrit. [lacto- + G. *boutyron,* butter, + *metron,* measure]

lac·to·cele (lak′tō-sēl). SYN galactocele. [lacto- + G. *kēlē,* tumor]

lac·to·chrome (lak′tō-krōm). SYN lactoflavin (1).

lac·to·crit (lak′tō-krit). An instrument used to estimate the amount of butterfat in milk. [lacto- + G. *krinō,* to separate]

lac·to·den·sim·e·ter (lak′tō-den-sim′ĕ-ter). A type of galactometer. [lacto- + L. *densus,* thick, + G. *metron,* measure]

lac·to·fer·rin (lak′tō-fār-in). A transferrin found in the milk of several mammalian species and thought to be involved in the transport of iron to erythrocytes; relatively high concentrations are found in human milk.

lac·to·fla·vin (lak′tō-flā-vin). 1. The flavin in milk. SYN lactochrome. 2. SYN riboflavin.

lac·to·gen (lak′tō-jen). An agent that stimulates milk production or secretion. [lacto- + G. *-gen,* producing]

human placental l. (HPL), l. isolated from human placentas and structurally similar to somatotropin; its biologic activity weakly mimics that of somatotropin and prolactin; secreted into maternal circulation; a deficiency of HPL during pregnancy leads to children having abnormal intrauterine and postnatal growth. SYN choriomammotropin, chorionic "growth hormone-prolactin", human chorionic somatomammotropic hormone, human chorionic somatomammotropin, placenta protein, placental growth hormone, purified placental protein.

lac·to·gen·e·sis (lak-tō-jen′ĕ-sis). Milk production. [lacto- + G. *genesis,* production]

lac·to·gen·ic (lak-tō-jen′ik). Pertaining to lactogenesis.

lac·to·glob·u·lin (lak-tō-glob′ū-lin). The globulin present in milk, making up 50–60% of bovine whey protein.

lac·tom·e·ter (lak-tom′ĕ-ter). SYN galactometer. [lacto- + G. *metron,* measure]

lac·to·nase (lak′tō-nās). SYN gluconolactonase.

lac·tone (lak′tōn). An intramolecular organic anhydride formed from a hydroxyacid by the loss of water between a hydroxyl and a –COOH group; a cyclic ester.

lac·to·per·ox·i·dase (lak′tō-per-oks′i-dās). A peroxidase obtained from milk. It also catalyzes the oxidation of iodide to iodine.

lac·to·pro·tein (lak-tō-prō′tēn). Any protein normally present in milk.

lac·tor·rhea (lak-tō-rē′ă). SYN galactorrhea. [lacto- + G. *rhoia,* a flow]

lac·to·scope (lak′tō-skōp). SYN galactoscope. [lacto- + G. *skopeō,* to view]

lac·tose (lak′tōs). A disaccharide present in mammalian milk, occurring naturally as α- and β-l.; obtained from cow's milk and used in modified milk preparation, in food for infants and convalescents, and in pharmaceutical preparations; large doses act as an osmotic diuretic and as a laxative. Human milk contains 6.7% l. SYN milk sugar, saccharum lactis.

l. synthase, the enzyme responsible for the synthesis of l., catalyzing the reaction between UDP-galactose and D-glucose to l. and UDP.

lac·tos·u·ria (lak′tō-soo′rē-ă). Excretion of lactose (milk sugar) in the urine; a common finding during pregnancy and lactation, and in newborns, especially premature babies. [lactose + G. *ouron,* urine, + -ia]

lac·to·ther·a·py (lak-tō-thār′ă-pē). SYN galactotherapy.

lactotrophic. Older term for prolactin-producing.

lac·to·tro·pin (lak-tō-trō′pin). SYN prolactin.

lac·to·veg·e·tar·i·an (lak′tō-vej-ĕ-tā′rē-ăn). 1. One who lives on a mixed diet of milk and milk products, eggs, and vegetables, but eschews meat. 2. A vegetarian who consumes milk and dairy products but not eggs or meats or seafood.

lac·to·yl·glu·ta·thi·one ly·ase (lak′tō-il-gloo-tă-thī′ōn). Glyoxalase I; a lyase cleaving *S*-D-lactoylglutathione to glutathione and methylglyoxal. SYN aldoketomutase, ketone-aldehyde mutase, methylglyoxalase.

lac·tu·lose (lak′too-lōs). A synthetic disaccharide used to treat hepatic encephalopathy and chronic constipation.

α-lac·tyl-thi·am·in py·ro·phos·phate. SYN active *pyruvate.*

la

la·cu·na, pl. **la·cu·nae** (lă-koo′nă, -koo′nē). **1** [TA]. A small space, cavity, or depression. **2.** A gap or defect. **3.** An abnormal space between strata or between the cellular elements of the epidermis. **4.** SYN corneal *space*. [L. a pit, dim. of *lacus*, a hollow, a lake]

cartilage l., a cavity within the matrix of cartilage, occupied by a chondrocyte. SYN cartilage space.

cerebral l., a small circumscribed loss of brain tissue caused by occlusion of one of the small penetrating arteries. SYN l. cerebri.

l. cer′ebri, SYN cerebral l.

Howship lacunae, tiny depressions, pits, or irregular grooves in bone that is being resorbed by osteoclasts. SYN resorption lacunae.

intervillous l., one of the blood spaces in the placenta into which the chorionic villi project.

lateral lacunae [TA], SYN lateral lacunae of superior sagittal sinus.

lacunae laterales [TA], SYN lateral lacunae of superior sagittal sinus.

lateral lacunae of superior sagittal sinus [TA], lateral expansions of the superior sagittal sinus of the dura mater, often increasing in width with advancing age until, in the very old, they may extend two cm lateral to the midline; the endothelium-lined lumens of the lacunae are usually reduced to a spongelike labyrinth by numerous arachnoid granulations and dural trabeculae. SYN lacunae laterales [TA], lateral lacunae [TA], lateral lakes, lateral venous lacunae, parasinoidal sinuses.

lateral venous lacunae, SYN lateral lacunae of superior sagittal sinus.

l. mag′na, a recess on the roof of the fossa navicularis of the penis, formed by a fold of mucous membrane, the valve of the navicular fossa.

Morgagni l., SYN urethral l.

muscular l., SYN muscular *space* of retroinguinal compartment.

l. musculo′rum, SYN muscular *space* of retroinguinal compartment.

l. musculorum retroinguinalis, SYN muscular *space* of retroinguinal compartment.

osseous l., a cavity in bony tissue occupied by an osteocyte.

pharyngeal l., a depression near the pharyngeal opening of the pharyngotympanic (auditory) tube. SYN l. pharyngis.

l. pharyn′gis, SYN pharyngeal l.

resorption lacunae, SYN Howship lacunae.

trophoblastic l., one of the spaces in the early syncytiotrophoblastic layer of the chorion before the formation of villi; in human embryos maternal blood enters these spaces by the 10th day; with the differentiation of the chorionic villi they become intervillous spaces, sometimes called intervillous lacunae.

urethral l. [TA], one of a number of little recesses in the mucous membrane of the spongy urethra into which empty the ducts of the urethral glands. SYN l. urethralis [TA], Morgagni l.

l. urethra′lis, pl. **lacu′nae urethra′les** [TA], SYN urethral l.

vascular l., SYN vascular *space* of retroinguinal compartment.

l. vasorum, SYN vascular *space* of retroinguinal compartment.

l. vasorum retroinguinalis [TA], SYN vascular *space* of retroinguinal compartment.

la·cu·nar (lă-koo′năr). Relating to a lacuna.

la·cu·nule (lă-koo′nool). A very small lacuna. [Mod. L. *lacunula*, dim. of L. *lacuna*]

la·cus, pl. **la·cus** (lā′kŭs) [TA]. SYN lake (1). [L. lake]

l. lacrima′lis [TA], SYN lacrimal *lake*.

l. semina′lis, SYN seminal *lake*.

LAD Abbreviation for leukocyte adhesion *deficiency*.

Ladd, William E., U.S. pediatric surgeon, 1880–1967. SEE L. *band, operation.*

Ladd-Franklin, Christine, U.S. psychologist, 1847–1930. SEE Ladd-Franklin *theory.*

Lae·laps echid·ni·nus (lē′laps ē-kid-nī′nŭs). The spiny rat mite, a common worldwide ectoparasite of the wild Norway rat and occasionally found on the house mouse, cotton rat, and other rodents; it is the natural vector of *Hepatozoon muris* and can

transmit the agent of tularemia experimentally. Junin virus has been isolated from this species in South America.

Laënnec, René T.H., French physician, 1781–1826. SEE L. *cirrhosis, pearls,* under *pearl.*

la·e·trile (lā′ĕ-tril). An allegedly antineoplastic drug consisting chiefly of amygdalin derived from apricot pits; its antitumor effect is unproven.

△**laev-.** SEE levo-.

Lafora, Gonzalo Rodriguez, Spanish neurologist, 1887–1971. SEE L. *body,* body *disease, disease.*

lag. 1. To move or progress more slowly than normal; to fall behind. **2.** The act or condition of falling behind. **3.** The time interval between a change in one variable and a consequent change in another variable.

anaphase l., slowing or arrest in the normal migration of chromosomes during anaphase, resulting in such chromosomes being excluded from one of the daughter cells.

homeostatic l., the interval in a homeostatic process between a change of the trait controlled and the appropriate response, due to afferent, efferent, and central components. The l. may be a pure random variable, e.g., the waiting time of an exponential process or the sum of several such processes taking any value greater than zero but with a mean considerably greater than zero; sometimes it may be deterministic or almost so and with a minimum sharply defined and greater than zero for anatomical reasons. For instance, the partial pressures of oxygen and carbon dioxide are controlled in the lungs but based on afferent information obtained from the carotid body that is already dated because of the circulation time of ten seconds or so between the two sites.

la·ge·na, pl. **la·ge·nae** (lă-jē′nă, -jē-nē). **1.** SYN cupular *cecum* of the cochlear duct. **2.** One of the three parts of the membranous labyrinth of the inner ear of lower vertebrates; in mammals, the l. becomes the cochlea. [L. flask]

lag·ging. Retarded or diminished ventilatory movement of the affected side of the chest due to pleural disease with muscle splinting or collapse of a lung.

lag·o·morph (lā′gō-mōrf). A member of the order Lagomorpha.

Lag·o·mor·pha (lā-gō-mōr′fă). An order of herbivorous mammals (class Eutheria) resembling rodents (order Rodentia) but having two pairs of upper incisors one behind the other; it includes the rabbits, hares, and pikas. [G. *lagōs,* hare, + *morphē,* form]

lag·oph·thal·mia (lag-of-thal′mē-ă). SEE lagophthalmos.

lag·oph·thal·mos, lag·oph·thal·mia (lag-of-thal′mŏs, lag-of-thal′mē-ă). A condition in which a complete closure of the eyelids over the eyeball is difficult or impossible. [G. *lagōs,* hare + *ophthalmos,* eye]

Lagrange, Pierre F., French ophthalmologist, 1857–1928.

Lahey, Frank H., U.S. surgeon, 1880–1935. SEE L. *forceps.*

LAK Abbreviation for lymphokine activated killer cells.

lake (lāk) [TA]. **1.** A small collection of fluid. SYN lacus [TA]. **2.** To cause blood plasma to become red as a result of the release of hemoglobin from the erythrocytes, as when the latter are suspended in water. SEE ALSO lacuna. [A.S. *lacu,* fr. L. *lacus,* lake]

capillary l., the total mass of blood contained in capillary vessels.

lacrimal l. [TA], the small cisternlike area of the conjunctiva at the medial angle of the eye, in which the tears collect after bathing the anterior surface of the eyeball and the conjunctival sac. SYN lacus lacrimalis [TA], lacrimal bay.

lateral l.'s, SYN lateral *lacunae* of superior sagittal sinus, under *lacuna.*

seminal l., the vault of the vagina after insemination. SYN lacus seminalis.

subchorial l., SYN subchorial *space.*

venous l.'s, (1) blue-purple, thin-walled, dilated blood vessels that blanch on pressure, found commonly in the ears and less often on the lips and on the face and neck of elderly sun-damaged men; (2) discontinuous venous cavities or channels; Cf. marginal *sinuses* of placenta, under *sinus;* (3) in skull radiography, round to oval radiolucent foci in the frontal or parietal bones caused by dilated diploic venous channels.

Laki-Lorand fac·tor. See under factor.

laky (lā'kē). Pertaining to the transparent bright red appearance of blood serum or plasma, developing as a result of hemoglobin being released from destroyed red blood cells.

la·li·a·try (lă-lī'ă-trē). The study and treatment of speech disorders. [G. *lalia,* speech, chatter, + *iatria,* cure]

lal·i·o·pho·bia (lal'ē-ō-fō'bē-ă). Morbid fear of speaking or stuttering. [G. *lalia,* speech, + *phobos,* fear]

Lallemand, Claude F., French surgeon, 1790–1853. SEE L. *bodies,* under *body;* Trousseau-L. *bodies,* under *body.*

lal·ling (lal'ing). A form of stammering in which the speech is almost unintelligible. [G. *laleō,* to chatter]

Lallouette, Pierre, French physician, 1711–1792. SEE L. *pyramid.*

lal·o·che·zia (lal-ō-kē'zē-ă). Emotional discharge gained by uttering indecent or filthy words. [G. *lalia,* speech, + *chezō,* to relieve oneself]

lal·og·no·sis (lal'og-nō'sis). Understanding and knowledge of speech. [G. *lalia,* speech, + *gnosis,* knowledge]

la·lo·ple·gia (la-lō-plē'jē-ă). Paralysis of the muscles concerned in the mechanism of speech. [G. *lalia,* speech, + *plēgē,* a stroke]

Lamarck, Jean-Baptiste P.A., French botanist, zoologist, and biologic philosopher, 1744–1829. SEE lamarckian *theory.*

Lamaze, Fernand, French obstetrician, 1890–1957. SEE L. *method.*

LAMB Acronym for *l*entigines, *a*trial myxoma, *m*ucocutaneous myxomas, and *b*lue nevi. SEE LAMB *syndrome.*

Lam B. Outer membrane protein of Gram-negative bacteria.

lamb·da (lam'dă). **1.** The 11th letter of the Greek alphabet, λ. **2.** The craniometric point at the junction of the sagittal and lambdoid sutures.

lamb·da·cism (lam'dă-sizm). **1.** Mispronunciation or disarticulation of the letter *l*. **2.** Substitution of the letter *l* for the letter *r*. [G. *lambda,* the letter L]

lamb·doid (lam'doyd). Resembling the Greek letter lambda (λ), as does the lambdoid suture. [lambda + G. *eidos,* resemblance]

Lambert, Edward H., U.S. physician, *1915. SEE L.-Eaton *syndrome;* Eaton-L. *syndrome.*

lam·bert (lam'bert). A unit of brightness; the brightness of a perfectly diffusing surface emitting or reflecting a total luminous flux of 1 lumen/sq cm of surface. [J.H. *Lambert,* German physicist and mathematician, 1728–1777]

Lamblia intestinalis (lam'blē-ă in-tes-ti-nā'lis). Old term for *Giardia lamblia,* still frequently used, especially by protozoologists in the former Soviet Union.

lam·bli·a·sis (lam-blī'ă-sis). SYN giardiasis.

lam·bo lam·bo (lam'bō-lam'bō). SYN tropical *pyomyositis.*

Lambrinudi, Constantine, British orthopedic surgeon, 1890–1943. SEE Lambrinudi *operation.*

la·mel·la, pl. **la·mel·lae** (lă-mel'ă, -mel'ē) [TA]. **1** [TA]. A thin sheet or layer (such as occurs in compact bone) or sublayer. **2.** A preparation in the form of a medicated gelatin disk, used as a means of making local applications to the conjunctiva in place of solutions. SYN discus [TA], disk (2) [TA]. [L. dim. of *lamina,* plate, leaf]

annulate lamellae, several pairs of parallel, smooth membranes, each pair containing regularly spaced pores resembling those of the nuclear envelope; they occur in germ cells, embryonic cells, and neoplastic cells.

articular l., the compact layer of bone on its articular surface that is firmly attached to the overlying articular cartilage.

l. of bone, a concentric, circumferential, or interstitial l.

circumferential l., a bony l. that encircles the outer or inner surface of a bone.

concentric l., one of the concentric tubular layers of bone surrounding the central canal in an osteon. SYN haversian l.

cornoid l., a narrow vertical column of parakeratosis in the epidermal stratum corneum; characteristic of porokeratosis.

elastic l., a thin sheet or membrane composed of elastic fibers; distinguished from elastic membrane, which usually refers to a condensed mass of fibers, as in an artery, whereas an elastic l.

may be a looser elastic layer such as found in a vein or the respiratory tract.

enamel l., an organic defect in enamel; a thin, leaflike structure that extends from the enamel surface toward the dentinoenamel junction.

glandulopreputial l., a layer of embryonic epithelial tissue that gives rise to the prepuce.

ground l., SYN interstitial l.

haversian l., SYN concentric l.

intermediate l., SYN interstitial l.

interstitial l., one of the lamellae of partially resorbed osteons occurring between newer, complete osteons. SYN ground l., intermediary system, intermediate l.

triangular l., SYN *tela* choroidea of third ventricle.

l. tympanica (laminae spiralis ossei) [TA], SYN tympanic l. (of osseous spiral lamina).

tympanic l. (of osseous spiral lamina) [TA], the thinner of two plates of bone, incompletely separated from each other by canals for peripheral fibers from the spiral (cochlear) ganglion, that together comprise the osseous spiral lamina; this plate lies on the side of the scala tympani, forming a portion of its wall. SYN l. tympanica (laminae spiralis ossei) [TA].

l. vestibularis (laminae spiralis ossei) [TA], SYN vestibular l. (of osseous spiral lamina).

vestibular l. (of osseous spiral lamina) [TA], the thicker of two plates of bone, incompletely separated from each other by canals for peripheral fibers from the spiral (cochlear) ganglion, that together comprise the osseous spiral lamina; this plate lies on the side of the scala vestibuli; a thickening of the periosteum, the spiral limbus, is attached to the vestibular lamella within the cochlear duct. SYN l. vestibularis (laminae spiralis ossei) [TA].

vitreous l., SYN *lamina* basalis choroideae.

lam·el·lar (lam'ĕ-lăr, lă-mel'ăr). **1.** Arranged in thin plates or scales. SYN lamellate, lamellated. **2.** Relating to lamellae.

lam·el·late, lam·el·lat·ed (lam'ĕ-lāt, -ed). SYN lamellar (1).

la·mel·li·po·di·um, pl. **la·mel·li·po·dia** (lă-mel-i-pō'dē-ŭm, -ă). A cytoplasmic veil produced on all sides of migrating polymorphonuclear leukocytes.

LAMINA

lam·i·na, pl. **lam·i·nae** (lam'i-nă, lam'i-nē) [TA]. SYN plate (1). SEE ALSO layer, stratum. [L]

l. affix'a [TA], that part of the medial ependymal wall of the lateral ventricle of the embryonic brain that in later development becomes adherent to the superior surface of the thalamus and thus comes to form the floor of the central part of the lateral ventricle; it covers the thalamostriate and choroidal veins.

l. ala'ris, SYN alar l. of neural tube.

alar l. of neural tube, the dorsal division of the lateral walls of the neural tube in the embryo; it gives rise to neurons relaying afferent impulses to higher centers; in the adult such neurons compose the sensory nuclei of the spinal cord and brainstem. SYN alar plate of neural tube, dorsolateral plate of neural tube, l. alaris, l. dorsalis, wing plate.

lam'inae al'bae cerebel'li, layers of white substance seen on section of the cerebellum. SYN laminae medullares cerebelli.

l. anterior fasciae thoracolumbalis [TA], SYN anterior *layer* of thoracolumbar fascia.

anterior limiting l. [TA], the periphery of the cornea marking the termination of Descemet membrane and the anterior border of the trabecular meshwork; an important landmark in gonioscopy. SYN l. limitans anterior [TA], anterior limiting ring, Schwalbe ring.

l. ante'rior vagi'nae mus'culi rec'ti abdo'minis, SYN anterior *layer* of rectus sheath.

l. ar'cus ver'tebrae [TA], SYN l. of vertebral arch.

basal l., (1) an amorphous extracellular layer applied to the basal

la

surface of epithelium and also investing muscle cells, fat cells, and Schwann cells; thought to be a selective filter and to serve both structural and morphogenetic functions. It is composed of a 20–100 nm network of file filaments called the l. densa which appears dense in the electron microscope, and on either side of this layer is a less dense layer called the l. rarae; SEE ALSO basement *membrane*, l. densa; **(2)** SYN l. densa.

basal l. of choroid [TA], SYN l. basalis choroideae.

basal l. of ciliary body [TA], the inner layer of the ciliary body, continuous with the basal layer of the choroid and supporting the pigment epithelium of the ciliary retina. SYN l. basilaris corporis ciliaris [TA], basal layer of ciliary body, l. basalis corporis ciliaris.

basal l. of cochlear duct [TA], the l. extending from the bony spiral l. to the basilar crest of the cochlea; it forms the greater part of the floor of the cochlear duct separating the latter from the scala tympani and it supports the organ of Corti. SYN l. basilaris ductus cochlearis [TA], basilar l., basilar membrane of cochlear duct, l. basilaris cochleae, membrana basilaris.

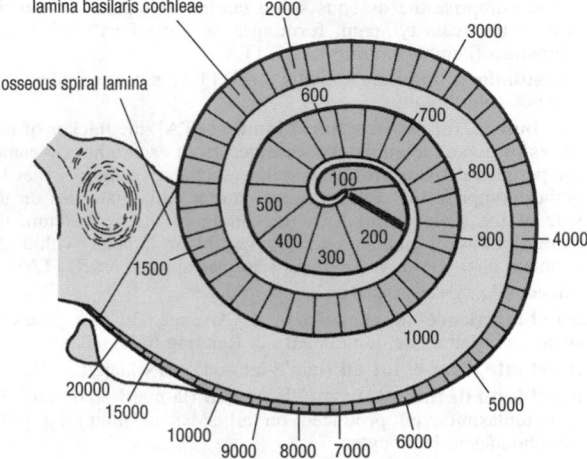

basilar membrane: figures indicate sound frequencies in Hz pertaining to each site

l. basalis, SYN basal l. of neural tube.

l. basa'lis choroi'deae [TA], the transparent, nearly structureless inner layer of the choroid in contact with the pigmented layer of the retina. SYN basal l. of choroid [TA], basal layer of choroid [TA], Bruch membrane, Henle membrane, l. vitrea, vitreous lamella, vitreous membrane (3).

l. basalis corporis ciliaris, SYN basal l. of ciliary body.

basal l. of neural tube, the ventral division of the lateral walls of the neural tube in the embryo; it contains neuroblasts giving rise to somatic and visceral motor neurons. SYN basal plate of neural tube, l. basalis, l. ventralis, ventral plate of neural tube.

basal l. of semicircular duct, SYN basal *membrane* of semicircular duct.

basement l., SYN basement *membrane.*

basilar l., SYN basal l. of cochlear duct.

l. basilaris cochleae, SYN basal l. of cochlear duct.

l. basilaris corporis ciliaris [TA], SYN basal l. of ciliary body.

l. basilaris ductus cochlearis [TA], SYN basal l. of cochlear duct.

boundary l., a basement membrane-like structure that invests muscle cells, fat cells, and Schwann cells. SEE ALSO basement *membrane,* basal l.

capillary l. of choroid [TA], the internal or deep portion of the choroidea of the eye, composed of a very close capillary network. SYN l. choroidocapillaris [TA], choriocapillaris, choriocapillary layer, entochoroidea, l. choriocapillaris, membrana choriocapillaris, Ruysch membrane.

l. cartilag'inis cricoi'deae [TA], SYN l. of cricoid cartilage.

l. cartilag'inis thyroi'deae [TA], SYN l. of thyroid cartilage.

l. choriocapilla'ris, SYN capillary l. of choroid.

l. choroi'dea, SYN epithelial l.

l. choroi'dea epithelia'lis, SYN epithelial l.

l. choroidocapilla'ris [TA], SYN capillary l. of choroid.

l. cine'rea, SYN l. terminalis of cerebrum.

l. cribro'sa os'sis ethmoida'lis [TA], SYN cribriform *plate* of ethmoid bone.

l. cribro'sa of sclera [TA], the portion of the sclera through which pass the fibers of the optic nerve. SYN l. cribrosa sclerae [TA], cribrous l., perforated layer of sclera.

l. cribro'sa scle'rae [TA], SYN l. cribrosa of sclera.

cribrous l., SYN l. cribrosa of sclera.

l. of cricoid cartilage [TA], a quadrate plate forming the posterior part of the cricoid cartilage. It resembles the shield of a signet ring, the arch of the cricoid representing the remainder of the ring. SYN l. cartilaginis cricoideae [TA].

deep l., SYN deep *layer.*

l. den'sa, (1) the electron-dense layer of the basal l. as seen in the electron microscope; SEE ALSO basement *membrane;* **(2)** the extraordinarily thick basal l. of the renal glomerulus. SYN basal l. (2).

dental l., SYN dental *ledge.*

l. denta'ta, SYN vestibular *lip* of spiral limbus.

dentogingival l., SYN dental *ledge.*

l. dorsa'lis, SYN alar l. of neural tube.

l. du'ra, the hard layer lining the dental alveoli.

l. elas'tica ante'rior, SYN anterior limiting *layer* of cornea.

l. elas'tica poste'rior, SYN posterior limiting l. of cornea.

elastic laminae of arteries, 1) external: the layer of elastic connective tissue lying immediately outside the smooth muscle of the tunica media; 2) internal: a fenestrated layer of elastic tissue of the tunica intima. SYN elastic layers of arteries, Henle fenestrated elastic membrane.

l. epiphysialis [TA], SYN epiphysial *plate.*

episcleral l., SYN episcleral *layer* of fibrous layer of eyeball.

l. episclera'lis [TA], SYN episcleral *layer* of fibrous layer of eyeball.

epithelial l., the layer of modified ependymal cells that forms the inner layer of the tela choroidea, facing the ventricle. SYN epithelial choroid layer, l. choroidea epithelialis, l. choroidea, l. epithelialis.

l. epithelialis, SYN epithelial l.

l. externa calvaria [TA], SYN external *table* of calvaria.

l. exter'na cra'nii, SYN external *table* of calvaria.

external medullary l. [TA], SEE medullary laminae of thalamus.

l. fibrocartilagin'ea interpu'bica, SYN interpubic *disk.*

l. fibroreticula'ris, a layer of the basement membrane in continuity with associated connective tissue; it is often discontinuous and may be lacking entirely in some cases.

l. fusca of sclera, SYN suprachoroid l. of sclera.

l. fusca sclerae [TA], SYN suprachoroid l. of sclera.

hepatic laminae, the plates of liver cells that radiate from the center of the liver lobule.

l. horizonta'lis os'sis palati'ni [TA], SYN horizontal *plate* of palatine bone.

l. interna calvariae [TA], SYN internal *table* of calvaria.

l. inter'na cra'nii, SYN internal *table* of calvaria.

internal medullary l. [TA], SEE medullary laminae of thalamus.

l. interna ossium cranii, SYN vitreous *table.*

iridopupillary l., embryonic precursor of the anterior stroma of the iris that forms the inner (posterior or deep) wall of the primary anterior chamber of the eye. Its central portion becomes attenuated as the pupillary membrane (membrana pupillaris [NA]).

labiogingival l., a band of ectodermal epithelial cells growing into the mesenchyme of the embryonic jaws between the developing lip and the growing gingival elevation; it later opens to form the labiogingival groove.

lateral l. of cartilage of pharyngotympanic (auditory) tube [TA], the narrow lateral portion of the cartilaginous part of the pharyngotympanic (auditory) tube. SYN l. lateralis cartilaginis tubae auditivae [TA], l. lateralis cartilaginis tubae auditoriae⭐, lateral cartilaginous plate, lateral plate of cartilaginous auditory tube.

l. latera′lis cartila′ginis tu′bae auditi′vae [TA], SYN lateral l. of cartilage of pharyngotympanic (auditory) tube.

l. latera′lis cartilag′inis tubae auditoriae, ⭐official alternate term for lateral l. of cartilage of pharyngotympanic (auditory) tube.

l. latera′lis proces′sus pterygoid′ei [TA], SYN lateral pterygoid *plate.*

lateral medullary l. [TA] of lentiform nucleus, a thin, sharply defined layer of fibers separating the putamen from the globus pallidus. SYN l. medullaris lateralis nuclei lentiformis [TA].

l. of lens, one of a series of concentric layers composed of the lens fibers that make up the substance of the lens.

l. limitans anterior [TA], SYN anterior limiting l.

l. lim′itans ante′rior cor′neae, SYN anterior limiting *layer* of cornea.

l. lim′itans poste′rior cor′neae, SYN posterior limiting l. of cornea.

l. lu′cida, the lightly staining layer of the basement membrane in contact with the plasmalemma of epithelial cells or other cells having an investment of basement membrane.

medial l. of cartilage of pharyngotympanic (auditory) tube [TA], the broad medial portion of the cartilaginous part of the pharyngotympanic (auditory) tube. SYN l. medialis cartilaginis tubae auditivae [TA], l. medialis cartilaginis tubae auditoriae⭐, medial cartilaginous plate, medial plate of cartilaginous auditory tube.

l. media′lis cartila′ginis tu′bae auditi′vae [TA], SYN medial l. of cartilage of pharyngotympanic (auditory) tube.

l. media′lis cartilag′inis tubae auditoriae, ⭐official alternate term for medial l. of cartilage of pharyngotympanic (auditory) tube, medial l. of cartilage of pharyngotympanic (auditory) tube.

l. media′lis proces′sus pterygoi′dei [TA], SYN medial pterygoid *plate.*

medial medullary l. [TA] of lentiform nucleus, a fiber layer separating the medial and lateral segments of the globus pallidus. SYN l. medullaris medialis nuclei lentiformis [TA].

lam′inae medulla′res cerebel′li, SYN laminae albae cerebelli.

lam′inae medulla′res thal′ami, SYN medullary laminae of thalamus.

l. medullaris lateralis [TA], SEE medullary laminae of thalamus.

l. medulla′ris latera′lis nuclei lentiformis [TA], SYN lateral medullary l. [TA] of lentiform nucleus.

l. medullaris medialis [TA], SEE medullary laminae of thalamus.

l. medulla′ris media′lis nuclei lentiformis [TA], SYN medial medullary l. [TA] of lentiform nucleus.

medullary laminae of thalamus, layers of myelinated fibers that appear on transverse sections of the thalamus; the l. medullaris lateralis [TA] (external medullary lamina [TA]) marks the ventral and lateral borders of the thalamus and delimits it from the subthalamus and reticular nucleus of thalamus; the l. medullaris medialis [TA] (internal medullary lamina [TA]) is interposed between the mediodorsal and ventral nuclei of the thalamus and encloses the intralaminar nuclei (centromedian, paracentral, and central lateral nuclei). SYN laminae medullares thalami, medullary layers of thalamus.

l. membrana′cea cartila′ginis tu′bae auditi′vae [TA], SYN membranous l. of cartilage of pharyngotympanic (auditory) plate.

l. membranacea cartilaginis tubae auditoriae, ⭐official alternate term for membranous l. of cartilage of pharyngotympanic (auditory) plate.

membranous l. of cartilage of pharyngotympanic (auditory) plate [TA], the connective tissue membrane that, with the lateral and medial laminae, completes the lateral and inferior walls of the cartilaginous part of the pharyngotympanic (auditory) tube. SYN l. membranacea cartilaginis tubae auditivae [TA], l. membranacea cartilaginis tubae auditoriae⭐, membranous layer.

l. of mesencephalic tectum, the roofplate of the mesencephalon formed by the quadrigeminal bodies. SYN l. tecti [TA], tectal plate

[TA], tectum mesencephali [TA], l. quadrigemina, quadrigeminal l., quadrigeminal plate, tectum of midbrain.

l. modi′oli cochleae [TA], SYN l. of modiolus of cochlea.

l. of modiolus of cochlea [TA], a bony plate, the continuation of the modiolus and of the septum between the convolutions of the spiral canal of the cochlea extending upward toward the cupola, forming with the hamulus the helicotrema. SYN l. modioli cochleae [TA], plate of modiolus.

l. molecularis corticis cerebri [TA], SYN molecular *layer* of cerebral cortex.

l. muscula′ris muco′sae, SYN *muscularis* mucosae.

nuclear l., a protein-rich layer lining the inner surface of the nuclear membrane in interphase cells.

orbital l. of ethmoid bone, SYN orbital *plate* of ethmoid bone.

l. orbita′lis os′sis ethmoida′lis [TA], SYN orbital *plate* of ethmoid bone.

osseous spiral l. [TA], a double plate of bone winding spirally around the modiolus dividing the spiral canal of the cochlea incompletely into two, scala tympani and scala vestibuli; between the two plates of this l., the fibers of the cochlear nerve reach the spiral organ (of Corti). SYN l. spiralis ossea [TA], spiral plate.

l. papyra′cea, SYN orbital *plate* of ethmoid bone.

l. parieta′lis [TA], SYN parietal *layer.*

l. parietalis pericar′dii serosi [TA], SYN parietal *layer* of serous pericardium.

l. parietalis tu′nicae vagina′lis tes′tis [TA], SYN parietal *layer* of tunica vaginalis of testis.

periclaustral l., SYN external *capsule.*

l. perpendicula′ris [TA], SYN perpendicular *plate.*

l. perpendicula′ris os′sis ethmoida′lis [TA], SYN perpendicular *plate* of ethmoid bone.

l. perpendicula′ris os′sis palati′ni [TA], SYN perpendicular *plate* of palatine bone.

posterior limiting l. of cornea [TA], a transparent homogeneous acellular layer between the substantia propria and the endothelial layer of the cornea; considered to be a highly developed basement membrane. SYN Descemet membrane, Duddell membrane, entocornea, hyaloid membrane, l. elastica posterior, l. limitans posterior corneae, membrana hyaloidea, membrana vitrea, posterior elastic layer, posterior limiting layer of cornea, tunica vitrea, vitreous membrane (1).

l. poste′rior vagi′nae mus′culi rec′ti abdo′minis [TA], SYN posterior *layer* of rectus sheath.

l. pretrachea′lis fasciae cervicalis [TA], SYN pretracheal *layer* of cervical fascia.

l. prevertebra′lis fasciae cervicalis [TA], SYN prevertebral *layer* of cervical fascia.

primary dental l., SYN dental *ledge.*

l. profun′da [TA], SYN deep *layer.*

l. profunda fas′ciae tempora′lis [TA], SYN deep *layer* of temporal fascia.

l. profunda fasciae thoracolumbalis, ⭐official alternate term for anterior *layer* of thoracolumbar fascia.

l. profunda mus′culi levato′ris pal′pebrae superio′ris, SYN deep *layer* of levator palpebrae superioris.

l. propria [TA], the layer of connective tissue underlying the epithelium of a mucous membrane. SYN l. propria mucosae.

l. pro′pria muco′sae, SYN l. propria.

pterygoid laminae, SEE lateral pterygoid *plate*, medial pterygoid *plate.*

l. quadrigem′ina, SYN l. of mesencephalic tectum.

quadrigeminal l., SYN l. of mesencephalic tectum.

l. ra′ra, the relatively electron-lucent layer on either side of the l. densa of the basement membrane.

reticular l., (1) a major component of the basement membrane, as seen by light microscopy; it consists largely of reticular fibers and ground substance. (2) the connective tissue plate in which the hair-bearing ends of the auditory sensory cells of the organ of Corti are embedded.

retrorectal l. of endopelvic fascia, SYN presacral *fascia.*

retrorectal l. of hypogastric sheath, SYN presacral *fascia.*

la

l. retrorectalis fasciae endopelvicae, SYN presacral *fascia*.

l. of Rexed, a division of the gray matter of the spinal cord into nine laminae (I–IX) and a gray area around the central canal (area X) based on cytoarchitectural features; the dorsal (posterior) horn is composed of laminae I–VI, the intermediate zone of lamina VII, and the ventral horn of laminae VIII and IX; general correlation of laminae with some of the major nuclei: I, posteromarginal nucleus; II, substantia gelatinosa; III and IV, nucleus proprius cornu dorsalis; V and VI, sometimes described as containing the spinal reticular formation; VII, Clarke nucleus, intermediolateral cell column; VIII, commissural nuclei, interneurons; IX, motor nuclei of ventral horn.

rostral l., a whitish line appearing on perfectly median sections of the brain as a thin bridge connecting the rostrum of the corpus callosum with the lamina terminalis; the rostral l. contains no commissural fibers; instead, it corresponds to the line along which the pia mater reflects from the medial surface of one hemisphere to that of the other. SYN l. rostralis, rostral layer, taeniola corporis callosi.

l. rostra′lis, SYN rostral l.

secondary spiral l. [TA], a ridge on the outer wall of the first turn of the cochlea opposite the spiral l. SYN l. spiralis secundaria [TA], secondary spiral plate.

l. sep′ti pellu′cidi, SYN l. of septum pellucidum.

l. of septum pellucidum, one of the two thin layers of the transparent septum, which extend from the corpus callosum to the fornix; often separated from each other by a space, the cavity of septum pellucidum. SYN l. septi pellucidi.

spinal l. II, ⋇official alternate term for gelatinous *substance*.

l. spinalis II, ⋇official alternate term for gelatinous *substance*.

l. spira′lis os′sea [TA], SYN osseous spiral l.

l. spira′lis secunda′ria [TA], SYN secondary spiral l.

successional l., an ectodermal bud on the labial side of the dental l. that develops into a permanent tooth.

superficial l., SYN superficial *layer*.

l. superficia′lis [TA], SYN superficial *layer*.

l. superficia′lis fas′ciae cervica′lis [TA], SYN investing *layer* of cervical fascia.

l. superficia′lis fas′ciae tempora′lis [TA], SYN superficial *layer* of temporal fascia.

l. superficia′lis mus′culi levato′ris pal′pebrae superio′ris, SYN superficial *layer* of the levator palpebrae superioris.

suprachoroid l. of sclera [TA], an exceedingly delicate layer of loose, pigmented connective tissue between the inner surface of the sclera and the outer surface of the choroid, connecting them; formerly, the l. fusca and suprachoroid l. were considered as two adjacent layers. SYN l. fusca sclerae [TA], brown layer, ectochoroidea, l. fusca of sclera, membrana fusca, suprachoroidea.

l. supraneuropor′ica, that part of the choroid membrane of the third ventricle that forms the roof of the foramen of Monro.

l. tec′ti [TA], SYN l. of mesencephalic tectum.

l. termina′lis [TA], SYN l. terminalis of cerebrum.

l. terminalis of cerebrum [TA], a thin plate passing upward from the optic chiasm and forming the rostral boundary of the third ventricle; membrane closing the rostral neuropore. SYN l. terminalis [TA], l. cinerea, terminal plate, velum terminale.

l. of thyroid cartilage [TA], one of the paired (right and left) thin quadrilateral plates of the thyroid cartilage that are joined anteriorly and form an open angle posteriorly. SYN l. cartilaginis thyroideae [TA].

tragal l. [TA], a longitudinal curved plate of cartilage, the beginning of the cartilaginous portion of the external acoustic meatus. SYN l. tragi [TA], l. of tragus.

l. tra′gi [TA], SYN tragal l.

l. of tragus, SYN tragal l.

vascular l. of choroid [TA], the external or superficial portion of the choroid of the eye containing the largest blood vessels. SYN l. vasculosa choroideae [TA], Haller vascular tissue, uvaeformis, vascular layer of choroid coat of eye, vascular layer.

l. vasculo′sa choroi′deae [TA], SYN vascular l. of choroid.

l. ventra′lis, SYN basal l. of neural tube.

l. of vertebral arch [TA], the flattened posterior portion of the vertebral arch extending between the pedicles and the midline, forming the dorsal wall of the vertebral foramen, and from the midline junction of which the spinous process extends. SYN l. arcus vertebrae [TA], neurapophysis.

l. viscera′lis [TA], SYN visceral *layer*.

l. viscera′lis pericar′dii, SYN visceral *layer* of serous pericardium.

l. viscera′lis tu′nicae vagina′lis tes′tis [TA], SYN visceral *layer* of tunica vaginalis of testis.

l. vit′rea, SYN l. basalis choroideae.

lam·i·na·gram (lam′i-nă-gram). An image made by laminagraphy (q.v.). SEE ALSO tomography.

lam·i·na·graph (lam′i-nă-graf). A device for laminagraphy; a laminagram.

lam·i·nag·ra·phy, lam·i·nog·ra·phy (lami-nahg′ră-fē, lam-i-nog′-ră-fē). Radiographic technique in which the images of tissues above and below the plane of interest are blurred out by reciprocal movement of the x-ray tube and film holder, to show a specific area more clearly. SEE ALSO tomography. [lamina + G. *graphē*, a writing]

lam·i·nar (lam′i-nar). **1.** Arranged in plates or laminae. SYN laminated. **2.** Relating to any lamina.

lam·i·nar·ia (lam-i-nā′rē-ă). Sterile rod made of kelp (genus *Laminaria*) which is hydrophilic, and, when placed in the cervical canal, absorbs moisture, swells, and gradually dilates the cervix. [L. *lamina*, a blade]

lam·i·nar·in (lam-i-nar′in). An algal polysaccharide, made up chiefly of β-D-glucose residues, obtained from *Laminaria* species (family Laminariaceae); variable proportions of the glucose chains contain at the potential reducing end a molecule of mannitol that can be sulfated.

l. sulfate, l. sulfated to varying degrees; two sulfate groups per glucose unit result in maximum stability and anticoagulant activity similar to that of heparin; l. with fewer sulfate groups has only antilipemic activity.

lam·i·nat·ed (lam′i-nāt-ed). SYN laminar (1).

lam·i·na·tion (lam-i-nā′shŭn). **1.** An arrangement in the form of plates or laminae. **2.** Embryotomy by removing the fetal head in slices.

lam·i·nec·to·my (lam′i-nek′tō-mē). Excision of a vertebral lamina; commonly used to denote removal of the posterior arch. [L. *lamina*, layer, + G. *ektomē*, excision]

lam·i·nin (lam′i-nin). A large multimeric glycoprotein component of the basement membrane; particularly its unstained laminae; a major protein component of the laminae of the renal glomerulus.

lam·i·ni·tis (lam-i-nī′tis). Inflammation of any lamina.

lam·i·nog·ra·phy (lam-i-nog′-ră-fē). SEE laminagraphy.

lam·i·not·o·my (lam-′i-not′ō-mē). Excision of a portion of a vertebral lamina in which the intervertebral foramen is enlarged by removal of a portion of the lamina. SYN rachiotomy. [L. *lamina*, layer, + G. *tomē*, incision]

lam·ins (lam′inz). Fibrous network associated with the inner membranes of cell nuclei, composed of polypeptides of varying molecular weights (60,000–80,000) and classified as A, B, C, etc. on the basis of physical properties; the phosphorylation of l. is associated with mitosis.

lam·o·tri·gine (lă-mō′trī-jēn). New structural class of antiepileptics; an anticonvulsant which appears in preclinical studies to resemble phenytoin.

lamp (lamp). Illuminating device; source of light. SEE ALSO light.

annealing l., an alcohol l. with a soot-free flame used in dentistry to drive off the protective NH_3 gas coating from the surface of cohesive gold foil.

Edridge-Green l., a lantern used to test recognition of colored signals; it displays a single light with color filters in rotating disks that can be modified to simulate conditions of weather and atmosphere. This test for color blindness was officially adopted in Great Britain in 1915 in place of the Holmgren wool test, but is now seldom used.

heat l., a l. that emits infrared light and produces heat; used to apply topical heat to the skin.

mercury vapor l., a l. in which the electric arc is in an ionized mercury vapor atmosphere; it produces ultraviolet light that can be used therapeutically or in diagnostic photometry.

mignon l., a minute electric light used in various endoscopic instruments.

slit l., a combination of a microscope and a narrow beam of collimated light, used to examine the eye.

spirit l., a l., used mainly for heating in laboratory work, in which alcohol is burned.

tungsten arc l., a l. having highly compressed tungsten elements.

ultraviolet l., a l. that emits rays in the ultraviolet band of the spectrum. SEE ALSO ultraviolet.

Wood l., an ultraviolet l. with a nickel oxide filter that only passes light with a maximal wavelength of about 3660 Å; used to detect by fluorescence hairs infected *Microsporum audouinii, M. canis,* var. *distortum,* or *M. ferrugineum,* producing greenish-yellow fluorescence.

Lamy, Maurice, French physician, 1895–1975. SEE Maroteaux-L. *syndrome.*

la·na, gen. and pl. **la·nae** (lan′ă, lan′ē). SYN wool. [L.]

la·nat·o·side D (lă-nat′ō-sīd). A digitalis glycoside from the leaves of *Digitalis lanata,* yielding the genin diginatigenin (12-hydroxygitoxigenin; 16-hydroxydigoxigenin).

la·nat·o·sides A, B, and C (lă-nat′ō-sīdz). Digilanides A, B, and C; the cardioactive precursor glycosides obtained from *Digitalis lanata.* Removal of the acetyl group yields desacetyllanatosides A, B, and C (purpurea glycosides A, B, and C, respectively); removal of the glucose from lanatosides A, B, and C yields acetyldigitoxin, acetylgitoxin, and acetyldigoxin, respectively; removal of glucose and the acetyl group yields digitoxin, gitoxin, and digoxin, respectively. SEE ALSO purpurea glycosides A.

lance (lans). **1.** To incise a part, as an abscess or boil. **2.** A lancet. [L. *lancea,* a slender spear]

Lancefield, Rebecca Craighill, U.S. bacteriologist, 1895–1981. SEE L. *classification.*

lan·cet (lan′set). A surgical knife with a short, wide, sharp-pointed, two-edged blade. [Fr. *lancette*]

gum l., a l. used for incising the gum over the crown of an erupting tooth.

spring l., a l. with a handle containing a blade that is activated by a spring.

thumb l., a l. with short flat blade that folds back, when closed, between two plates of the handle.

lan·ci·nat·ing (lan′si-nāt′ing). Denoting a sharp cutting or tearing pain. [L. *lancino,* pp. *-atus,* to tear]

Lancisi, Giovanni M., Italian physician, 1654–1720. SEE L. *sign; striae* lancisi, under *stria.*

Landau-Kleffner syn·drome. See under syndrome.

Landouzy, Louis T.J., French neurologist, 1845–1917. SEE L.-Dejerine *dystrophy;* L.-Grasset *law.*

Landry, Jean B.O., French physician, 1826–1865. SEE L. *paralysis, syndrome;* L.-Guillain-Barré *syndrome.*

Landschutz tu·mor. See under tumor.

Landsteiner, Karl, Austrian-U.S. pathologist and Nobel laureate, 1868–1943. SEE L.-Donath *test;* Donath-L. cold *autoantibody, phenomenon.*

Landström, John, Swedish surgeon, 1869–1910. SEE L. *muscle.*

Landzert, T., 19th century German anatomist. SEE L. *fossa;* Gruber-L. *fossa.*

Lane, Sir William Arbuthnot, English surgeon, 1856–1943. SEE L. *band, disease.*

Lang, Basil T., English ophthalmologist, 1880–1928.

Lange, Carl F.A., German biochemist, *1883. SEE L. *solution, test.*

Lange, Cornelia de. See under de Lange.

Langenbeck, Bernhard R.K. von, German surgeon, 1810–1887. SEE L. *triangle.*

Langendorff, Oscar, German physiologist, 1853–1908. SEE L. *method.*

Lange-Nielsen, F., 20th century Norwegian cardiologist. SEE Jervell and Lange-Nielsen *syndrome.*

Langer, Carl (Ritter von Edenberg), Austrian anatomist, 1819–1887. SEE L. *arch, lines,* under *line, muscle.*

Langer, Leonard O., American physician. SEE Langer-Saldino *syndrome.*

Langerhans, Paul, German anatomist, 1847–1888. SEE L. *cells,* under *cell, granule, islands,* under *island; islets* of L., under *islet.*

Langhans, Theodor, German pathologist, 1839–1915. SEE L. *cells,* under *cell;* L.-type giant *cells,* under *cell;* L. *layer, stria.*

Langley, John N., English physiologist, 1852–1925. SEE L. *granules,* under *granule.*

Langmuir, Irving, U.S. chemist and Nobel laureate, 1881–1957. SEE L. *trough.*

lan·guage (lang′gwij). The use of spoken, manual, written, and other symbols to express, represent, or receive communication. [L. *lingua*]

American Sign L. (ASL), the manual sign and gesture l. used by the deaf community in the United States. It is a l. distinct from English, with its own grammar and syntax, but no written form.

body l., (1) the expression of thoughts and feelings by means of nonverbal bodily movements, e.g., gestures, or via the symptoms of hysterical conversion; SEE kinesics; (2) communication by means of bodily signs.

lan·i·ary (lan′i-ār-ē). Adapted for tearing; in anatomy, sometimes applied to canine teeth, as l. teeth. [L. *lanio,* to tear to pieces]

lan·ka·my·cin (lăn′kă-mī-sin). Macrolide antibiotic produced by *Streptomyces violaceoniger* from the soil of Sri Lanka.

Lannelongue, Odilon M., French surgeon and pathologist, 1840–1911. SEE L. *foramina,* under *foramen, ligaments,* under *ligament.*

lan·o·lin (lan′ō-lin). SYN *adeps* lanae. [L. *lana,* wool, + *oleum,* oil]

anhydrous l., l. that contains not more than 0.25% of water; used as a water-adsorbable ointment base.

la·nos·ter·ol (lan-ō′stēr-ol). A zoosterol synthesized from squalene and a precursor to cholesterol.

Lanterman, A.J., 19th century U.S. anatomist in Strasbourg. SEE L. *incisures,* under *incisure, segments,* under *segment;* Schmidt-L. *clefts,* under *cleft, incisures,* under *incisure.*

lan·tha·nic (lan′thă-nik). Rarely used term denoting a disease process that produces no symptoms or clinical evidence of illness. [G. *lanthanō,* to lie hidden]

lan·tha·nides (lan′thă-nīdz). Those elements with atomic numbers 57–71 that closely resemble one another chemically and were once difficult to separate from one another. SYN rare earth elements. [*lanthanum,* first element of the series]

lan·tha·num (La) (lan′thă-nŭm). A metallic element, atomic no. 57, atomic wt. 138.9055; first of the rare earth elements (lanthanides). [G. *lanthanō,* to lie hidden]

l. nitrate, La(NO$_3$)$_3$; used in electron microscopy as a stain for extracellular mucopolysaccharides.

lan·thi·o·nine (lan-thī′ō-nēn). 3,3′-Thiodialanine; an amino acid obtained from wood that resembles cystine but has only one sulfur atom in the molecule rather than two; i.e., a sulfide rather than a disulfide.

la·nu·go (lă-noo′gō) [TA]. SYN downy *hair.* [L. down, wooliness, from *lana,* wool]

Lanz, Otto, Swiss surgeon in Amsterdam, 1865–1935. SEE L. *line.*

LAO Abbreviation for left anterior oblique projection, used in chest radiography, especially to assess the size of the left atrium and ventricle.

LAP Abbreviation for leukocyte alkaline phosphatase. SEE alkaline *phosphatase.*

laparo-. The loins (less properly, the abdomen in general). [G. *lapara,* flank, loins]

lap·a·ro·cele (lap′ă-rō-sēl). SYN abdominal *hernia.* [laparo- + G. *kēlē,* hernia]

la

laparoendoscopic (lap′ă-rō-en-dō-skop′ik). Having to do with the introduction of a laparoscope into the abdominal cavity for a variety of intracavitary procedures.

lap·a·ro·gas·tros·co·py (lap′ă-rō-gas-tros′kŏ-pē). Inspection of interior of the stomach after a gastrotomy. [laparo- + G. *gastēr*, stomach, + *skopeō*, to view]

lap·a·ro·my·o·si·tis (lap′ă-rō-mī′ō-sī′tis). Inflammation of the lateral abdominal muscles. [laparo- + G. *mys*, muscle, + *-itis*, inflammation]

lap·a·ror·rha·phy (lap′ă-rōr′ă-fē). SYN celiorrhaphy.

lap·a·ro·sal·pin·go-o·o·pho·rec·to·my (lap′ă-rō-sal′ping-gō-ō-of′ō-rek′tō-mē). Removal of the uterine tube and ovary through an abdominal incision.

lap·a·ro·scope (lap′ă-rō-skōp). An endoscope for examining the peritoneal cavity. SYN peritoneoscope. [laparo- + G. *skopeō*, to view]

▣**lap·a·ros·co·py** (lap-ă-ros′kŏ-pē). Examination of the contents of the abdominopelvic cavity with a laparoscope passed through the abdominal wall. SEE ALSO peritoneoscopy. SYN abdominoscopy.

Laparoscopy first became clinically practicable with the development of fiberoptics in the 1960s and of high-intensity, low-heat halogen bulbs in the 1970s. The technique has become standard, in selected cases, for many routine surgical procedures formerly requiring laparotomy, such as appendectomy, cholecystectomy, inguinal herniorrhaphy, oophorectomy, a second look after excision of an ovarian tumor, and diagnostic evaluation of endometriosis and female infertility. The peritoneal cavity is first inflated with CO_2 gas, and the laparoscope passed through a small incision in the abdominal wall. A second incision is usually required to provide surgical access to the area of interest. An elaborate armamentarium of surgical instruments has been developed to perform incision, drainage, excision, cautery, ligation, suturing, and other procedures with the laparoscope. The risk of intraoperative and postoperative complications, the cost of treatment, and hospitalization time are generally less with laparoscopic surgery than with traditional open procedures.

closed l., l. performed after insufflation of the abdominal cavity using a percutaneously placed needle.

open l., l. performed after insufflation of the abdomen using a trocar placed under direct vision after making a small celiotomy incision.

lap·a·rot·o·my (lap′ă-rot′ō-mē). **1.** Incision into the loin. **2.** SYN celiotomy. [laparo- + G. *tomē*, incision]

Lapicque, Louis, French physiologist, 1866–1952. SEE L. *law*.

lap·i·ni·za·tion (lap′i-ni-zā′shŭn). Serial passage of a virus or vaccine in rabbits. [Fr. *lapin*, rabbit]

lap·i·nized (lap′i-nīzd). Denoting viruses which have been adapted to develop in rabbits by serial transfers in this species. [Fr. *lapin*, rabbit]

Laplace, Ernest, U.S. surgeon, 1861–1924. SEE L. *forceps*.

Laplace, Pierre S. de, French mathematician, 1749–1827. SEE L. *law*.

Laquer, Ernst, German physiologist, *1910. SEE L. *stain* for alcoholic hyalin.

lard. SYN adeps (2). [L. *lardum*]

benzoinated l., used as a lubricant, in the manufacture of soap, for oiling wool, and as an illuminant. Formerly used as an ointment base.

lark·spur (lark′sper). SYN *Delphinium ajacis*.

Laron, Zvi, Israeli pediatric endocrinologist, *1927. SEE L. type *dwarfism*.

Laroyenne, Lucien, French surgeon, 1831–1902. SEE L. *operation*.

Larrey, Baron Dominique Jean de, French surgeon, 1766–1842. SEE L. *cleft*.

Larsen, Loren J., U.S. orthopedic surgeon, *1914. SEE L. *syndrome*.

Larsson, Tage Konrad Leopold, Swedish scientist, *1905. SEE Sjögren-L. *syndrome*.

lar·va, pl. **lar·vae** (lar′vă, lar′vē). **1.** The wormlike developmental stage or stages of an insect or helminth that are markedly different from the adult and undergo subsequent metamorphosis; a grub, maggot, or caterpillar. **2.** The second stage in the life cycle of a tick; the stage which hatches from the egg and, following engorgement, molts into the nymph. **3.** The young of fishes or amphibians which often differ in appearance from the adult. [L. a mask]

filariform l., infective third-stage l. of the hookworm, *Ascaris*, and other nematodes with penetrating larvae or with larvae that migrate through the body to reach the intestine.

rhabditiform l., early developmental larval stages (first and second) of soil-borne nematodes such as *Necator*, *Ancylostoma*, and *Strongyloides*, which precede the infectious third-stage filariform l.

lar·va·ceous (lar-vā′shŭs). SYN larvate.

lar·va cur·rens (lar′vă kŭr′enz). Cutaneous larva migrans caused by rapidly moving larvae of *Strongyloides stercoralis* (up to 10 cm per hr), typically extending from the anal area down the upper thighs and observed as a rapidly progressing linear urticarial trail; may also be caused by zoonotic species of *Strongyloides*. [L. *larva*, mask + *currens*, racing]

lar·val (lar′văl). **1.** Relating to larvae. **2.** SYN larvate.

▣**lar·va mi·grans** (lar′vă mī′granz). A larval worm, typically a nematode, that wanders for a period in the host tissues but does not develop to the adult stage; this usually occurs in unusual hosts that inhibit normal development of the parasite. [L. *larva*, mask, + *migro*, to transfer, migrate]

cutaneous l. m., a migratory serpiginous or netlike tunneling in the skin, with marked pruritus, caused by wandering hookworm larvae not adapted to intestinal maturation in humans; especially common in the eastern and southern coastal U.S. and other tropical and subtropical coastal areas; various hookworms of dogs and cats have been implicated, chiefly *Ancylostoma braziliense* of dog and cat feces from beaches and sandboxes in the U.S., but also *Ancylostoma caninum* of dogs, *Uncinaria stenocephala*, the European dog hookworm, and *Bunostomum phlebotomum*, the cattle hookworm; *Strongyloides* species of animal origin may also contribute to human cutaneous l. m. SYN ancylostoma dermatitis, creeping eruption, cutaneous ancylostomiasis, ground itch, water itch (1).

ocular l. m., visceral l. m. involving the eyes, primarily of older children; clinical symptoms include decreased visual acuity and strabismus.

spiruroid l. m., extraintestinal migration by nematode larvae of the order Spiruroidea, not adapted to maturation in the human intestine; caused chiefly by species of *Gnathostoma spinigerum* and *G. hispidum* in Japan and Thailand, following ingestion of uncooked fish infected with encapsulated third-stage infective larvae, and possibly by ingestion of infected copepods (the first intermediate host) in contaminated drinking water; the anteriorly spined larvae produce serpiginous tunnels in the skin or may cause subcutaneous or pulmonary abscess, or may invade the eye or brain.

visceral l. m., a disease, chiefly of children, caused by ingestion of infective ova of *Toxocara canis*, less commonly by other ascarid nematodes not adapted to humans, whose larvae hatch in the intestine, penetrate the gut wall, and wander in the viscera (chiefly the liver) for periods of up to 18–24 months; may be asymptomatic or may be marked by hepatomegaly (with granulomatous lesions caused by encapsulated larvae in the enlarged liver), pulmonary infiltration, fever, cough, hyperglobulinemia, and sustained high eosinophilia.

lar·vate (lar′vāt). Masked or concealed; applied to a disease with undeveloped, absent, or atypical symptoms. SYN larvaceous, larval (2). [L. *larva*, mask]

lar·vi·cid·al (lar-vi-sī′dăl). Destructive to larvae.

lar·vi·cide (lar'vi-sīd). An agent that kills larvae. [larva + L. *caedo*, to kill]

lar·vip·a·rous (lar-vip'ă-rŭs). Larvae-bearing; denoting passage of larvae, rather than eggs, from the body of the female, as in certain nematodes and insects. [larva + L. *pario*, to bear]

lar·vi·phag·ic (lar'vi-fā'jik). Consuming larvae; certain l. fish are used in mosquito control. [larva + G. *phagō*, to eat]

⚲**laryng-.** SEE laryngo-.

la·ryn·ge·al (lă-rin'jē-ăl). Relating in any way to the larynx.

lar·yn·gec·to·mee (lar-in-jek'tō-mē). A person who has had a laryngectomy.

la·ryn·gec·to·my (lar'in-jek'tō-mē). Excision of the larynx. [laryngo- + G. *ektomē*, excision]

  horizontal l., SYN partial l.

  partial l., incomplete resection of the larynx in which the supraglottic portion is removed preserving the vocal cords. SYN horizontal l., supraglottic l.

  supraglottic l., SYN partial l.

la·ryn·ges (lă-rin'jēz). Plural of larynx. [L.]

lar·yn·gis·mus (lar-in-jiz'mŭs). A spasmodic narrowing or closure of the rima glottidis. [L. fr. G. *larynx*, + *-ismos*, -ism]

  l. strid'ulus, a spasmodic closure of the glottis, causing noisy inspiration. Cf. *laryngitis* stridulosa. SYN pseudocroup, spasmus glottidis.

lar·yn·git·ic (lar-in-jit'ik). Relating to or caused by laryngitis.

lar·yn·gi·tis (lar-in-jī'tis). Inflammation of the mucous membrane of the larynx. [laryngo- + G. *-itis*, inflammation]

  chronic posterior l., a form of l. involving principally the interarytenoid area; thought to be caused by regurgitation of gastric contents.

  chronic subglottic l., SYN *chorditis* vocalis inferior.

  croupous l., inflammation of the subglottic larynx associated with respiratory infection and croupy or noisy breathing.

  membranous l., a form in which there is a pseudomembranous exudate on the vocal cords.

  l. sicca, l. characterized by dryness and crusting of the mucous membrane of the larynx.

  spasmodic l., SYN l. stridulosa.

  l. stridulo'sa, infectious inflammation of the larynx in children, accompanied by night attacks of spasmodic closure of the glottis, causing inspiratory stridor. SYN spasmodic l.

⚲**laryngo-, laryng-.** The larynx. [G. *larynx*]

la·ryn·go·cele (lă-ring'gō-sēl). An air sac communicating with the larynx through the ventricle, often bulging outward into the tissue of the neck, especially during coughing and playing of wind instruments. [laryngo- + G. *kēlē*, hernia]

la·ryn·go·fis·sure (lă-ring'gō-fish'er). Operative opening into the larynx, generally through the midline, commonly done for the excision of early carcinoma or the correction of laryngostenosis. SYN median laryngotomy, thyrofissure, thyroidotomy, thyrotomy (2).

la·ryn·go·graph (lă-ring'gō-graf). An instrument for making a tracing of the movements of the vocal folds. [laryngo- + G. *graphō*, to write]

la·ryn·gog·ra·phy (lă-rin-gog'ră-fē). Radiography of the larynx after coating mucosal surfaces with contrast material.

lar·yn·gol·o·gy (lar'ing-gol'ō-jē). The branch of medical science concerned with the larynx and the voice; the specialty of diseases of the larynx. [laryngo- + G. *logos*, study]

la·ryn·go·ma·la·cia (lă-ring'gō-mă-lā'shē-ă). SYN *chondromalacia* of larynx. [laryngo- + G. *malakia*, a softness]

la·ryn·go·pa·ral·y·sis (lă-ring'gō-pă-ral'i-sis). Paralysis of the laryngeal muscles. SYN laryngoplegia.

la·ryn·go·pha·ryn·ge·al (lă-ring'gō-fă-rin'jē-ăl). Relating to both larynx and pharynx or to the laryngopharynx.

la·ryn·go·phar·yn·gec·to·my (lă-ring'gō-far'in-jek'tō-mē). Resection or excision of both larynx and pharynx.

la·ryn·go·pha·ryn·ge·us (lă-ring'gō-făr'in-jē'ŭs). SYN inferior constrictor (*muscle*) of pharynx. [L.]

la·ryn·go·phar·yn·gi·tis (lă-ring'gō-far-in-jī'tis). Inflammation of the larynx and pharynx.

la·ryn·go·phar·ynx (lă-ring'gō-far-ingks) [TA]. The part of the pharynx lying below the aperture of the larynx and behind the larynx; it extends from the vestibule of the larynx to the esophagus at the level of the inferior border of the cricoid cartilage. SYN pars laryngea pharyngis [TA], hypopharynx✩, laryngeal part of pharynx, laryngeal pharynx.

la·ryn·go·phthi·sis (lă-ring'gō-thī'sis). Tuberculosis of the larynx. [laryngo- + G. *phthisis*, a wasting]

la·ryn·go·plas·ty (lă-ring'gō-plas-tē). Reparative or plastic surgery of the larynx. [laryngo- + G. *plassō*, to form]

la·ryn·go·ple·gia (lă-ring'gō-plē'jē-ă). SYN laryngoparalysis. [laryngo- + G. *plēgē*, stroke]

la·ryn·go·pto·sis (lă-ring-gō-tō'sis). An abnormally low position of the larynx, which may be congenital or acquired; does not impair the health of the neonate. Some degree of l. occurs with aging. [laryngo- + G. *ptōsis*, a falling]

la·ryn·go·scope (lă-ring'gō-skōp). Any of several types of tubes, equipped with electrical lighting, used in examining or operating upon the interior of the larynx through the mouth. [laryngo- + G. *skopeō*, to inspect]

la·ryn·go·scop·ic (lă-ring'gō-skop'ik). Relating to laryngoscopy.

lar·yn·gos·co·pist (lar'ing-gos'kŏ-pist). A person skilled in the use of the laryngoscope.

lar·yn·gos·co·py (lar'ing-gos'kŏ-pē). Inspection of the larynx by means of the laryngoscope.

  direct l., inspection of the larynx by means of either a hollow instrument or a fiberoptic cable.

  indirect l., inspection of the larynx by means of a reflected image on a mirror.

  suspension l., support of the laryngoscope by leverage from a supportive structure to provide maximum exposure of the pharyngeal cavity and larynx.

  transnasal fiberoptic l., l. performed with a fiberoptic endoscope introduced through the nose.

la·ryn·go·spasm (lă-ring'gō-spazm). Spasmodic closure of the glottic aperture. SYN glottidospasm, laryngospastic reflex.

la·ryn·go·ste·no·sis (lă-ring'gō-stĕ-nō'sis). Stricture or narrowing of the lumen of the larynx. [laryngo- + G. *stenōsis*, a narrowing]

lar·yn·gos·to·my (lar'ing-gos'tō-mē). The establishment of a permanent opening from the neck into the larynx. [laryngo- + G. *stoma*, mouth]

la·ryn·go·stro·bo·scope (lă-ring'gō-strō'bō-skōp, -strob'ō-skōp). Apparatus for observing the motion of the vocal folds during phonation with intermittent illumination. As the frequency of illumination approaches the frequency of opening and closing of the vocal cords, they appear to be still.

lar·yn·got·o·my (lar-ing-got'ō-mē). A surgical incision of the larynx. [laryngo- + G. *tomē*, incision]

  inferior l., SYN cricothyrotomy.

  median l., SYN laryngofissure.

  superior l., incision through the thyrohyoid membrane.

la·ryn·go·tra·che·al (lă-ring'gō-trā'kē-ăl). Relating to both larynx and trachea.

la·ryn·go·tra·che·i·tis (lă-ring'gō-trā-kē-ī'tis). Inflammation of both larynx and trachea.

la·ryn·go·tra·che·o·bron·chi·tis (lă-ring'gō-trā'kē-ō-brong-kī'tis). An acute respiratory infection involving the larynx, trachea, and bronchi. SEE croup.

lar·yn·go·tra·che·o·plas·ty (lar-ing'gō-trā'kē-ō-plas'tē). Operation to repair subglottic stenosis.

ℹ️**lar·ynx,** pl. **la·ryn·ges** (lar'ingks, lă-rin'jēz). The organ of voice production; the part of the respiratory tract between the pharynx and the trachea; it consists of a framework of cartilages and elastic membranes housing the vocal folds and the muscles which control the position and tension of these elements. [Mod. L. fr. G.]

  Cooper-Rand artificial l., an electronic device for vocal rehabili-

la

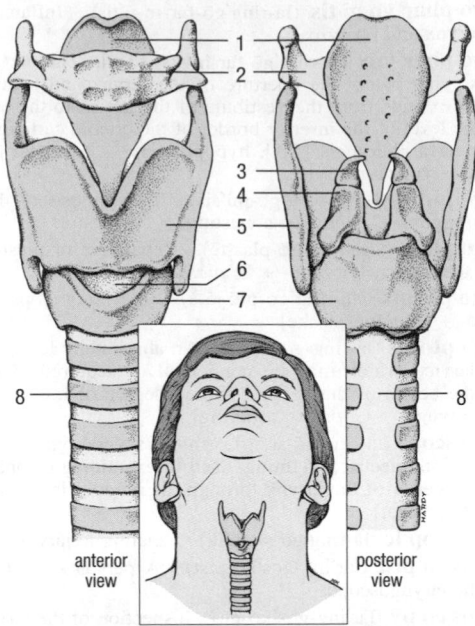

the laryngeal cartilages: (1) epiglottis, (2) hyoid bone, (3) corniculate cartilage, (4) arytenoid cartilage, (5) thyroid cartilage, (6) cricothyroid ligament, (7) cricoid cartilage, (8) trachea

tation after laryngectomy that produces an intraoral sound articulated into speech with the pharynx, palate, tongue, lips, and teeth.

lase (lāz). To cut, divide, or dissolve a substance, or to treat an anatomical structure, with a laser beam.

Lasègue, Ernest C., French physician, 1816–1883. SEE L. *sign, syndrome.*

la·ser (lā'zer). **1.** (noun) A device that concentrates high energies into an intense narrow beam of nondivergent monochromatic electromagnetic radiation; used in microsurgery, cauterization, and for a variety of diagnostic purposes. L.'s can be based on numerous chemical sources, gas, liquid, and solid, some of which are listed in chart. L.'s are widely used in printers of text or x-ray images. **2.** (verb) To treat a structure with a laser beam. [acronym coined from *l*ight *a*mplification by *s*timulated *e*mission of *r*adiation]

argon l., l. used for ophthalmic procedures, including retinal photocoagulation and trabeculoplasty, consisting of photons in the blue (488 nm) or green (514 nm) spectrum.

continuous wave l., a l. in which energy output is constant.

excimer l., l. used particularly for refractive procedures, consisting of photons in the ultraviolet spectrum emitted by unstable dimers of argon and fluoride. [*exci*ted di*mer*]

krypton l., l. used for ophthalmic procedures, particularly retinal photocoagulation in the presence of vitreous hemorrhage, consisting of photons in the red (647 nm) spectrum.

KTP l., l. in the blue-green to green (532 nm) spectrum, used for hemostasis; produced by doubling the frequency of an Nd:YAG l. by passing the beam through a KTP crystal. [*K* (potassium) *T*itanyl *P*hosphate]

Nd:YAG l., l. in the infrared spectrum (1064 nm), with a greater depth of penetration than other l.'s. [*Nd* (neodymium) + *Y*ttrium-*A*luminum-*Garnet*]

pulsed l., a l. in which energy output is pulsed, allowing short bursts of high energy.

pulsed dye l., extremely short bursts of focused yellow light absorbed by hemoglobin, used to treat hemangiomas without anesthesia in young children.

pumped l., a l. whose energy level is increased by the application

of separate sources of electrons or photons, which may themselves be primary lasers.

Q-switched l., (quality-switched); a l. in which the quality, or energy storage capacity is altered between a very high and a low value.

quasi-continuous wave l., a l. whose output can be controlled in milliseconds or similarly small increments by electronic control.

la·ser·ing (lā'zer-ing). The use of a laser beam to cut, divide, or dissolve a substance, or to treat an anatomical structure.

laser plume. The production of smoke with laser ablation; can cause respiratory difficulty for operative personnel. [L. *pluma,* feather]

Lash, Abraham Fae, U.S. obstetrician-gynecologist, *1898. SEE L. *operation.*

lash. An eyelash.

LASIK Acronym for laser-assisted in situ *keratomileusis.*

La·si·o·he·lea (las'ē-ō-hē'lē-ă). A genus of small bloodsucking gnats.

las·si·tude (las'i-tood). A sense of weariness. [L. *lassitudo,* fr. *lassus,* weary]

la·tah (lah'tah). One of the pathologic startle syndromes. A culture-bound disorder characterized by an exaggerated physical response to being startled or to unexpected suggestion, the subjects involuntarily uttering cries or executing movements in response to command or in imitation of what they hear or see in others. SEE ALSO jumping *disease.* [Malay, ticklish]

Latarget, André, French anatomist, 1877–1947. SEE L. *nerve, vein.*

lat·e·bra (lat'ē-bră). A flask-shaped region in large-yolked eggs extending from the animal pole to a dilated terminal portion near the center of the yolk; it contains the main bulk of the white yolk. [L. hiding place]

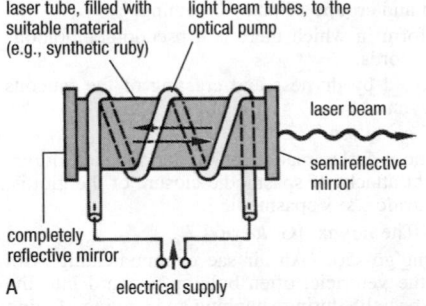

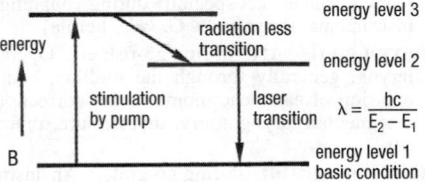

laser: (A) mode of operation, (B) energy levels of laser

la·ten·cy (lā'ten-sē). **1.** The state of being latent. **2.** In conditioning, or other behavioral experiments, the period of apparent inactivity between the time the stimulus is presented and the moment a response occurs. **3.** In psychoanalysis, the period of time from approximately age five to puberty.

la·tent (lā'tent). Not manifest, dormant, but potentially discernible. [L. *lateo,* pres. p. *latens* (*-ent-*), to lie hidden]

lat·er·ad (lat'er-ad). Toward the side. [L. *latus,* side, + *ad,* to]

lat·er·al (lat'er-ăl) [TA]. **1.** On the side. SYN lateralis [TA]. **2.** Farther from the median or midsagittal plane. SYN lateralis [TA]. **3.** In dentistry, a position either right or left of the midsagittal plane. **4.** A radiographic projection made with the film in the sagittal plane; especially, the second view of a chest series. SYN lateralis [TA]. [L. *lateralis,* lateral, fr. *latus,* side]

some common lasers used in medicine

continuous wave lasers	wavelength (nm)	some common uses
argon	488/514	trabeculoplasty; dental surface preparation
CO₂	10,600	dermatology; otologic surgery
He-Ne*	632.8	nephelometry; guide for invisible lasers
krypton	647	ophthalmic photocoagulation
quasicontinuous wave lasers		
copper vapor/bromide	510/578	pigmented or vascular skin lesions
dye argon	577/585	vascular skin lesions
KTP†	532	vascular skin lesions; otologic surgery
XeCl°	308	phacoablation
pulsed lasers		
erbium: YAG ‡	2940	skin resurfacing; ophthalmic procedures
flashlamp-pumped pulsed dye	585	vascular skin lesions
holmium: YAG	2100	urologic surgery
HF •	2900	dental surface preparation
q-switched lasers		
alexandrite	755	pigmented skin lesions
Nd: YAG	1064	dermatology; endotracheal surgery
ruby	694	pigmented skin lesions

* helium, neon
† potassium, titanyl, phosphate
° xenon, clorine
‡ yttrium, aluminum, garnet
• hydrogen fluoride

la·te·ra·lis (lat-er-ā′lis) [TA]. SYN lateral (1), lateral (2), lateral. [L.]

lat·er·al·i·ty (lat-er-al′i-tē). Referring to a side of the body or of a structure; specifically, the dominance of one side of the brain or the body.

crossed l., right dominance of some members, e.g., arm or leg, and left dominance of other members.

lat·er·al·i·za·tion (lat′er-al-ī-zā′shŭn). The process whereby certain embryological asymmetries of structure (such as the right-side location of the liver and the structure of the great vessels) and function (handedness) are ordained phylogenetically, coded genetically, and realized ontogenetically.

lat·er·i·flex·ion, lat·er·i·flec·tion (lat-er-i-flek′shŭn). SYN lateroflexion.

⟐**latero-.** Lateral, to one side. [L. *lateralis,* lateral, fr. *latus,* side]

lat·er·o·ab·dom·i·nal (lat′er-ō-ab-dom′i-năl). Relating to the sides of the abdomen, to the loins or flanks.

lat·er·o·de·vi·a·tion (lat′er-ō-dē-vē-ā′shŭn). A bending or a displacement to one side. [latero- + L. *devio,* to turn aside, fr. *via,* a way]

lat·er·o·duc·tion (lat′er-ō-dŭk′shŭn). A drawing to one side; denoting turning of the eyeball away from the midline. SYN exduction. [latero- + L. *duco,* pp. *ductus,* to lead]

lat·er·o·flex·ion, lat·er·o·flec·tion (lat′er-ō-flek′shŭn). A bending or curvature to one side. SYN lateriflexion, lateriflection. [latero- + L. *flecto,* pp. *flexus,* to bend]

lat·er·o·po·si·tion (lat′er-ō-pō-zish′ŭn). A shift to one side.

lat·er·o·pul·sion (lat′er-ō-pŭl′shŭn). An involuntary sidewise movement occurring in certain nervous affections. [latero- + L. *pello,* pp. *pulsus,* to push, drive]

lat·er·o·tor·sion (lat′er-ō-tōr′shŭn). A twisting to one side; denoting rotation of the eyeball around its anteroposterior axis, so that the top part of the cornea turns away from the sagittal plane. [latero- + L. *torsio,* a twisting]

lat·er·o·tru·sion (lat′er-ō-troo′zhŭn). The outward thrust given by the muscles of mastication to the rotating mandibular condyle during movement of the mandible. [latero- + L. *trudo,* pp. *trusus,* to thrust]

lat·er·o·ver·sion (lat′er-ō-ver′shŭn). Version to one side or the other, denoting especially a malposition of the uterus. [latero- + L. *verto,* pp. *versus,* to turn]

la·tex (lā′teks). **1.** An emulsion or suspension produced by some seed plants; it contains suspended microscopic globules of natural rubber. **2.** Similar synthetic materials such as polystyrene, polyvinyl chloride, etc. [L. liquid]

lathe (lādh). A motor-driven machine with a rotating shaft that can be fitted with various types of cutting instruments, grinding stones and polishing wheels; used in finishing and polishing dental appliances.

lath·y·rism (lath′i-rizm). A disease occurring in Ethiopia, Algeria, and India, characterized by various nervous manifestations, tremors, spastic paraplegia, and paresthesias; prevalent in districts where vetches, khasari (*Lathyrus sativus*), and allied species form the main food. Experimentally, a form of bone disease induced in laboratory animals by feeding *L. sativus* peas, or a principle derived from them, especially β-aminoproprionitrile. SYN lupinosis. [L. *lathyrus,* vetch]

lath·y·ro·gen (lath′ĭ-rō-jen). An agent or drug, occurring naturally or used experimentally, that induces lathyrism.

La·tin square. A statistical design for experiments that removes from experimental error the variation from two sources that may be identified with the rows and columns of a square. The allocation of experimental treatments is such that each treatment occurs exactly once in each row and column. For example, a design for a 5 × 5 square is as follows:

A	B	C	D	E
B	A	E	C	D
C	D	A	E	B
D	E	B	A	C
E	C	D	B	A

lat·i·tude (la′ti-tood). The range of light or x-ray exposure acceptable with a given photographic emulsion. SEE latitude *film.* SYN digital gray scale, gray scale. [L. *latitudo,* width, fr. *latus,* wide]

La·tro·dec·tus (lat-rō-dek′tŭs). A genus of relatively small spiders, the widow spiders, capable of inflicting highly poisonous, neurotoxic, painful bites; they are responsible, along with *Loxosceles* species (the brown spiders), for most of the severe reactions from spider envenomation. Medically important species are known from Australia, North and South America, South Africa, and New Zealand. Some venomous species, in addition to *L. mactans* (the black widow spider), are *L. bishopi* (the red-legged widow spider), *L. euracaviensis, L. geometricus,* and *L. tredecimguttatus.* [L. *latro,* servant, robber, + G. *dēktēs,* a biter]

L. mac′tans, the black widow spider, a venomous jet-black spider found in protected dark places; it is especially common in the southern U.S.; the full-grown female (slightly more than 1 cm long) has a brilliant red dumbbell- or hourglass-shaped mark on the ventral aspect of the abdomen, and her bite may be extremely painful, producing a syndrome mimicking an acute abdominal crisis; some deaths, though rare, have been reported, particularly in small children; the male spider lacks the hourglass mark and is not venomous.

LATS Abbreviation for long-acting thyroid *stimulator.*

lat·tice (lat′is). A regular arrangement of units into an array such that a plane passing through two units of a particular type or in a particular interrelationship will pass through an indefinite number of such units; e.g., the atom arrangement in a crystal.

la

la·tus, gen. **la·te·ris**, pl. **la·te·ra** (lā′tŭs, lat′er-is, lat′er-ă) [TA]. SYN flank. [L. side]

Latzko, Wilhelm, Austrian obstetrician, 1863–1945. SEE L. cesarean *section.*

laud·a·ble (law′dă-bl). A term from the past used to describe a quality of pus (thick and creamy) that suggested the wound would ultimately heal through granulation process and not be associated with sepsis and death. [L. *laudabilis,* praiseworthy]

lau·da·nine (law′dă-nēn). An isoquinoline alkaloid derived from the mother liquor of morphine; it causes tetanoid convulsions, with action similar to that of strychnine.

lau·da·no·sine (law′dă-nō-sēn). An isoquinoline alkaloid obtained from the mother liquor of morphine; it causes tetanic convulsions.

lau·da·num (law′dă-nŭm). A tincture containing opium. [G. *lēdanon,* a resinous gum]

Laugier, Stanislas, French surgeon, 1799–1872. SEE L. *hernia.*

Laumonier, Jean B.P.N.R., French surgeon, 1749–1818. SEE L. *ganglion.*

Launois, Pierre E., French physician, 1856–1914. SEE L.-Cléret *syndrome;* L.-Bensaude *syndrome.*

Laurence, John Zachariah, British ophthalmologist, 1830–1874. SEE L.-Moon *syndrome.*

Laurer, Johann F., German pharmacologist, 1798–1873. SEE L. *canal.*

lau·ric ac·id (law′rik). A fatty acid occurring in spermaceti, in milk, and in laurel, coconut, and palm oils as well as waxes and marine fats. SYN *n*-dodecanoic acid.

Lauth, Charles, English chemist, 1836–1913. SEE L. *violet.*

Lauth, Ernst A., German physician, 1803–1837. SEE L. *canal.*

Lauth, Thomas, German anatomist and surgeon, 1758–1826. SEE L. *ligament.*

Lauth vi·o·let. SYN thionine.

LAV Abbreviation for lymphadenopathy-associated *virus.*

la·vage (lă-vahzh′). The washing out of a hollow cavity or organ by copious injections and rejections of fluid. [Fr. from L. *lavo,* to wash]

antral l., irrigation of the maxillary sinus through its natural ostium or through a puncture of the inferior meatus.

bronchoalveolar l. (BAL), procedure for analyzing the cellular milieu of the alveoli (including microbiology, types of inflammatory cells) by use of a bronchoscope or other hollow tube through which saline is instilled into distal bronchi and then withdrawn.

Lavdovsky, Michail D., Russian histologist, 1846–1902. SEE L. *nucleoid.*

La·ver·an·ia (lav-er-ā′nē-ă). Old generic name for malaria-causing and other hematozoan protozoa. *L. falciparum* is a distinctive generic name for *Plasmodium falciparum,* and is preferred by some who believe that crescentic gametocytes should be the basis for classifying the causal agent of falciparum malaria in a separate genus. SEE *Plasmodium, Haemoproteus.* [C. *Laveran,* Fr. protozoologist and Nobel laureate, 1845–1922]

la·veur (lă-vŭr′). An instrument for irrigation or lavage. [Fr.]

LAW

law (law). **1.** A principle or rule. **2.** A statement of fact detailing a sequence or relation of phenomena that is invariable under given conditions. SEE ALSO principle, rule, theorem. [A.S. *lagu*]

Alexander l., states that a jerky *nystagmus* becomes worse when gazing in the direction of the fast component.

all or none l., SYN Bowditch l.

Ångström l., a substance absorbs light of the same wavelength as it emits when luminous.

Arndt l., obsolete l. stating that weak stimuli excite physiologic activity, moderately strong ones favor it, strong ones retard it, and very strong ones arrest it.

Arrhenius l., SYN Arrhenius *doctrine.*

l.'s of association, principles formulated by Aristotle to account for the functional relationships between ideas; the l. of contiguity (association) proved most useful to experimental psychologists, culminating in modern studies of respondent conditioning.

l. of average localization, visceral pain is most accurately localized in the least mobile viscera and least accurately in the most mobile.

Avogadro l., equal volumes of gases contain equal numbers of molecules, the conditions of pressure and temperature being the same. SYN Ampère postulate, Avogadro hypothesis, Avogadro postulate.

Baer l., the general organ characteristics found in all members of a group appear earlier in embryogenesis than the special organ characteristics that distinguish specific members of the group; this law is the predecessor of the recapitulation theory.

Baruch l., the effect of any hydriatic procedure is in direct proportion to the difference between the temperature of the water and that of the skin; when the temperature of the water is above or below that of the skin the effect is stimulating; when the two temperatures are the same the effect is sedative.

Beer l., the intensity of a color or of a light ray is inversely proportional to the depth of liquid through which it is transmitted; it is concluded that the absorption is dependent upon the number of molecules in the path of the ray. Cf. Beer-Lambert l.

Beer-Lambert l., the absorbance of light is directly proportional to the thickness of the media through which the light is being transmitted multiplied by the concentration of absorbing chromophore; i.e., $A = \varepsilon bc$ where A is the absorbance, ε is the molar extinction coefficient, b is the thickness of the solution, and c is the concentration.

Behring l., parenteral administration of serum from an immunized person provides a relative, passive immunity to that disease (i.e., prevents it, or favorably modifies its course) in a previously susceptible person.

Bell l., the ventral spinal roots are motor, the dorsal are sensory. SYN Bell-Magendie l., Magendie l.

Bell-Magendie l., SYN Bell l.

Bernoulli l., when friction is negligible, the velocity of flow of a gas or fluid through a tube is inversely related to its pressure against the side of the tube; i.e., velocity is greatest and pressure lowest at a point of constriction. SYN Bernoulli principle, Bernoulli theorem.

Berthollet l., salts in solution will always react with each other so as to form a less soluble salt, if possible.

biogenetic l., l. of biogenesis, SYN recapitulation *theory.*

Blagden l., the depression of the freezing point of dilute solutions is proportional to the amount of the dissolved substance.

Bowditch l., consistently total response to any effective stimulus. SYN all or none l.

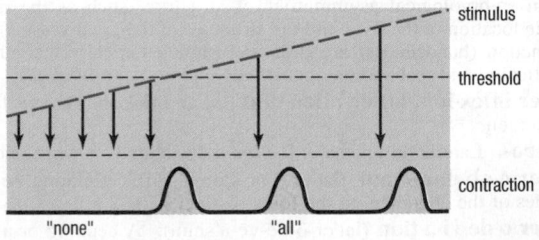

Bowditch law

Boyle l., at constant temperature, the volume of a given quantity of gas varies inversely with its absolute pressure. SYN Mariotte l.

Broadbent l., lesions of the upper segment of the motor tract cause less marked paralysis of muscles that habitually produce bilateral movements than of those that commonly act independently of the opposite side.

Bunsen-Roscoe l., in two photochemical reactions, e.g., the darkening of a photographic plate or film, if the products of the intensity of illumination and the time of exposure are equal, the quantities of chemical material undergoing change will be equal; the retina for short periods of exposure obeys this l. SYN reciprocity l., Roscoe-Bunsen l.

Charles l., all gases expand equally on heating, namely, $\frac{1}{273.16}$ of their 0°C volume for every additional degree Celsius. SYN Gay-Lussac l.

l. of constant numbers in ovulation, the number of ova discharged at each ovulation is nearly constant for any given species.

l. of contiguity, when two ideas or psychologically perceived events have once occurred in close association they are likely to so occur again, the subsequent occurrence of one tending to elicit the other; this l. figures prominently in modern theories of conditioning and learning.

l. of contrary innervation, SYN Meltzer l.

Coppet l., solutions having the same freezing point have equal concentrations of dissolved substances.

Courvoisier l., painless enlargement of the gallbladder with jaundice is likely to result from carcinoma of the head of the pancreas and not from a stone in the common duct, because in the latter the gallbladder is usually scarred from infection and does not distend. SYN Courvoisier sign.

Dale-Feldberg l., an identical chemical transmitter is liberated at all the functional terminals of a single neuron.

Dalton l., each gas in a mixture of gases exerts a pressure proportionate to the percentage of the gas and independent of the presence of the other gases present. SYN l. of partial pressures.

Dalton-Henry l., in dissolving a mixture of gases, a liquid will absorb as much of each gas in the mixture as if that were the only gas dissolved.

l. of definite proportions, the relative weights of the several elements forming a chemical compound are invariable. SYN Proust l.

l. of denervation, when a structure is denervated, its irritability to certain chemical agents is increased; e.g., the greater sensitivity of the pupil to acetylcholine after section and degeneration of the third nerve, and of the nictitating membrane to adrenaline after excision of the superior cervical ganglion.

Descartes l., SYN l. of refraction.

Donders l., the rotation of the eyeball is determined by the distance of the object from the median plane and the line of the horizon.

Draper l., a chemical change is produced in a photochemical substance only by those light rays that are absorbed by that substance.

Du Bois-Reymond l., SYN l. of excitation.

Dulong-Petit l., the specific heats of many solid elements are inversely proportional to their atomic weights.

Einthoven l., in the electrocardiogram the potential of any wave or complex in lead II is equal to the sum of its potentials in leads I and III. SYN Einthoven equation.

Elliott l., adrenaline acts upon those structures innervated by sympathetic nerve fibers.

l. of excitation, a motor nerve responds, not to the absolute value, but to the alteration of value from moment to moment, of the electric current; i.e., rate of change of intensity of the current is a factor in determining its effectiveness. SYN Du Bois-Reymond l.

Faraday l.'s, (1) the amount of an electrolyte decomposed by an electric current is proportional to the amount of the current; **(2)** when the same current is passed through several electrolytes, the amounts of the different substances decomposed are proportional to their chemical equivalents.

Farr l.'s, a set of mathematical formulae, axioms, and l.'s first enunciated in the annual reports submitted by William Farr to the Registrar General of England and Wales from 1839 to 1883. The l.'s deal with the relationship of incidence to prevalence, the natural history of epidemics, and mathematical features of common types of epidemic. [Derived from the writings of William Farr, British medical statistician]

Fechner-Weber l., SYN Weber-Fechner l.

Ferry-Porter l., the critical fusion is directly proportional to the logarithm of the light intensity.

Fick l.'s of diffusion, (1) the direction of movement of solutes by diffusion is always from a higher to a lower concentration and the diffusive flux J_A of solute A across a plane at x is proportional to the concentration gradient of A at x; i.e., $J_A = -D(C_A/x)$; **(2)** the increase of concentration of solute A with time, C_A/t, is directly proportional to the change in the concentration gradient, i.e., $C_A/t = D(fl^2/x^2)$.

Flatau l., a l. concerning the excentric position of the long spinal tracts; the greater the distance the nerve fibers run lengthwise in the cord, the more they tend to be situated toward its periphery.

Galton l., in a population mating at random, the progeny of a parent with an extreme value for a measurable phenotype will tend on average to have values nearer the population mean than in the extreme parent. SEE ALSO l. of regression to mean. SYN l. of regression to mean.

Gay-Lussac l., SYN Charles l.

Godélier l., tuberculosis of the peritoneum is always associated with tuberculosis of the pleura on one or both sides.

Gompertz l., the proportional relationship of mortality to age; after age 35–40, the increase in mortality with age tends to be logarithmic.

Graham l., the relative rapidity of diffusion of two gases varies inversely as the square root of their densities, i.e., their molecular weights.

Grasset l., SYN Landouzy-Grasset l.

l. of gravitation, SYN Newton l.

Guldberg-Waage l., SYN l. of mass action.

Haeckel l., SYN recapitulation *theory*.

Halsted l., transplanted tissue will grow only if there is a lack of that tissue in the host.

Hardy-Weinberg l., if mating occurs at random with respect to any one autosomal locus in a population in which the gene frequencies are equal in the two sexes, and the factors tending to change gene frequencies (mutation, differential selection, migration) are either absent or negligible, then in one generation the probabilities of all possible genotypes will on average equal the same proportions as if the genes were assembled at random. The l. does not apply to two or more loci jointly, nor to X-linked traits where the initial gene frequencies differ in the two sexes.

l. of the heart, the energy liberated by the heart when it contracts is a function of the length of its muscle fibers at the end of diastole. SYN Starling l.

Heidenhain l., glandular secretion is always accompanied by an alteration in the structure of the gland.

Hellin l., twins occur once in 89 births, triplets once in 89^2, and quadruplets once in 89^3. If the frequency of twins in a population is p, the frequency of triplets is p^2, and the frequency of quadruplets is p^3.

Henry l., at equilibrium, at a given temperature, the amount of gas dissolved in a given volume of liquid is directly proportional to the partial pressure of that gas in the gas phase (this is only true for gases that do not react chemically with the solvent).

Herring l., states that paired agonist muscles from each eye operating in the same field of gaze receive equal innervation while paired antagonist muscles receive equal inhibition.

Hess l., the amount of heat generated by a reaction is the same whether the reaction takes place in one step or several steps; i.e., ΔH values (and thus ΔG values) are additive.

Hilton l., the nerve supplying a joint supplies also the muscles which move the joint and the skin covering the articular insertion of those muscles.

Hooke l., the stress applied to stretch or compress a body is proportional to the strain, or change in length thus produced, so long as the limit of elasticity of the body is not exceeded.

l. of independent assortment, genes that are not alleles assort independently when the gametes are formed; traits at linked loci are an exception. SYN Mendel second l.

l. of intestine, SYN myenteric *reflex*.

inverse square l., as applied to point sources, the intensity of

la

radiation diminishes in proportion to the square of the distance from the source.

isodynamic l., for energy purposes, the different foodstuffs may replace one another in accordance with their caloric values when burned in a calorimeter.

Jackson l., loss of mental functions due to disease retraces in reverse order its evolutionary development.

Koch l., SYN Koch *postulates,* under *postulate.*

Lambert l., (1) each layer of equal thickness absorbs an equal fraction of the light that traverses it. Cf. Beer-Lambert l; (2) the illumination of a surface on which the light falls normally from a point source is inversely proportional to the square of the distance from the source.

Landouzy-Grasset l., in lesions of one hemisphere, the patient's head is turned to the side of the affected muscles if there is spasticity and to that of the cerebral lesion if there is paralysis. SYN Grasset l.

Lapicque l., the chronaxie is inversely proportional to the diameter of an axon.

Laplace l., the equilibrium relationship between transmural pressure difference (ΔP), wall tension (T), and radius of curvature (R) in a concave surface; for a sphere: $\Delta P = 2T/R$; for a cylinder: $\Delta P = T/R$.

Le Chatelier l., if external factors such as temperature and pressure disturb a system in equilibrium, adjustment occurs in such a way that the effect of the disturbing factors is reduced to a minimum. SYN Le Chatelier principle.

Listing l., when the eye leaves one object and fixes upon another, it revolves about an axis perpendicular to a plane cutting both the former and the present lines of vision.

Louis l., tuberculosis in any organ is associated with tuberculosis in the lung.

Magendie l., SYN Bell l.

Marey l., the pulse rate varies inversely with the blood pressure; i.e., the pulse is slow when the pressure is high; an expression of baroreceptor reflex influences on heart rate.

Marfan l., the healing of localized tuberculosis protects against subsequent development of pulmonary tuberculosis.

Mariotte l., SYN Boyle l.

mass l., SYN l. of mass action.

l. of mass action, the rate of a chemical reaction is proportional to the concentrations of the reacting substances; when the forward reaction rate equals the reverse reaction rate (i.e., at equilibrium) then, at constant temperature, the product of the concentrations of all the products divided by the product of the concentrations of all the reactants is itself a constant (K_{eq}). SYN Guldberg-Waage l., mass l.

Meltzer l., all living functions are continually controlled by two opposite forces: augmentation or action on the one hand, and inhibition on the other. SYN l. of contrary innervation.

Mendeléeff l., the properties of elements are periodical functions of their atomic weights; i.e., if the elements are arranged in the order of their atomic weights, every element in the series will be related in respect to its properties to the eighth in order before or after it. SYN periodic l.

Mendel first l., SYN l. of segregation.

Mendel second l., SYN l. of independent assortment.

l. of the minimum, growth and development of plants and animals are determined by the availability of that essential nutrient which is present in the smallest amount.

Müller l., each type of sensory nerve ending, however stimulated (electrically, mechanically, etc.), gives rise to its own specific sensation; moreover, each type of sensation depends not upon any special character of the different nerves but upon the part of the brain in which their fibers terminate. SYN l. of specific nerve energies.

l. of multiple proportions, SYN l. of reciprocal proportions.

Nasse l., an early statement of the pattern of X-linked recessive inheritance: hemophilia affects only boys but is transmitted through mothers and sisters.

Neumann l., in compounds of analogous chemical constitution,

the molecular heat, or the product of the specific heat and the atomic weight, is always the same.

Newton l., the attractive force between any two bodies is proportional to the product of their masses, and inversely proportional to the square of the distance between their centers. SYN l. of gravitation.

Nysten l., rigor mortis affects first the muscles of the head and spreads toward the feet.

Ochoa l., the content of the X-chromosome tends to be phylogenetically conserved.

Ohm l., in an electric current passing through a wire, the intensity of the current (I) in amperes equals the electromotive force (E) in volts divided by the resistance (R) in ohms: $I = E/R$.

l. of partial pressures, SYN Dalton l.

Pascal l., fluids at rest transmit pressure equally in every direction.

periodic l., SYN Mendeléeff l.

Pflüger l., SYN l. of polar excitation.

Plateau-Talbot l., when successive light stimuli follow each other sufficiently rapidly to become fused, their apparent brightness is diminished.

Poiseuille l., in laminar flow, the volume of a homogeneous fluid passing per unit time through a capillary tube is directly proportional to the pressure difference between its ends and to the fourth power of its internal radius, and inversely proportional to its length and to the viscosity of the fluid.

l. of polar excitation, a given segment of a nerve is irritated by the development of catelectrotonus and the disappearance of anelectrotonus, but the reverse does not hold; i.e., excitation occurs at the cathode when the circuit is closed and at the anode when it is opened. SYN Pflüger l.

l. of priority, use of the earliest published name (senior synonym) of two or more names of an organism as the correct name.

Profeta l., the subject of congenital syphilis is immune to the acquired disease.

Proust l., SYN l. of definite proportions.

Raoult l., the vapor pressure of a solution of a nonvolatile nonelectrolyte is that of the pure solvent multiplied by the molefraction of the solvent in the solution.

l. of recapitulation, SYN recapitulation *theory.*

l. of reciprocal proportions, the relative weights in which two substances form a chemical union singly with a third are the same as, or simple multiples of, those in which they unite with each other; a corollary of the law of definite proportions. SYN l. of multiple proportions.

reciprocity l., SYN Bunsen-Roscoe l.

l. of referred pain, pain arises only from irritation of nerves which are sensitive to those stimuli that produce pain when applied to the surface of the body.

l. of refraction, for two given media, the sine of the angle of incidence bears a constant relation to the sine of the angle of refraction. SYN Descartes l., Snell l.

l. of regression to mean, SYN Galton l.

Ribot l. of memory, in progressive dementias, remote memories tend to be preserved whereas recent memories are lost.

Ricco l., for small images, light intensity × area = constant for the threshold.

Roscoe-Bunsen l., SYN Bunsen-Roscoe l.

Rosenbach l., (1) in affections of the nerve trunks or nerve centers, paralysis of the flexor muscles appears later than that of the extensors; (2) in cases of abnormal stimulation of organs with rhythmical functional periodicity, there is often a grouping of the individual acts with corresponding lengthening of the pauses, in such a way that the proportion of total rest and activity remains nearly the same.

Rubner l.'s of growth, (1) the l. of constant energy consumption: the rapidity of growth is proportional to the intensity of the metabolic processes; (2) the l. of the constant growth quotient: in most young mammals, 24% of the entire food energy, or calories, is used for growth; in humans, only 5% is thus used.

Schütz l., SYN Schütz *rule.*

second l. of thermodynamics, the entropy of the universe moves toward a maximum; similarly, the entropy of any isolated microcosm (e.g., a chemical reaction) proceeds spontaneously only in that direction that yields an increase in entropy, entropy being maximal at equilibrium. To quote G.N. Lewis, "Every process that occurs spontaneously is capable of doing work; to reverse any such process requires the expenditure of work from the outside."

l. of segregation, factors that affect development retain their individuality from generation to generation, do not become contaminated when mixed in a hybrid, and become sorted out from one another when the next generation of gametes is formed. SYN Mendel first l.

Sherrington l., every dorsal spinal nerve root supplies a particular area of the skin, the dermatome (3), which is, however, invaded above and below by fibers from the adjacent spinal segments.

l. of similars, SEE similia similibus curantur.

Snell l., SYN l. of refraction.

Spallanzani l., the younger the individual the greater is the regenerative power of its cells.

l. of specific nerve energies, SYN Müller l.

Starling l., SYN l. of the heart.

Stokes l., (1) a muscle lying above an inflamed mucous or serous membrane is frequently the seat of paralysis; **(2)** a relationship of the rate of fall of a small sphere in a viscous fluid; applicable to centrifugation of macromolecules; **(3)** the wavelength of light emitted by a fluorescent material is longer than that of the radiation used to excite the fluorescence.

Tait l., an obsolete dictum that an exploratory laparotomy should be performed in every case of obscure pelvic or abdominal disease that threatens health or life.

Thoma l.'s, the development of blood vessels is governed by dynamic forces acting on their walls as follows: an increase in velocity of blood flow causes dilation of the lumen; an increase in lateral pressure on the vessel wall causes it to thicken; an increase in end-pressure causes the formation of new capillaries.

van't Hoff l., (1) in stereochemistry, all optically active substances have one or more multivalent atoms united to four different atoms or radicals so as to form in space an unsymmetrical arrangement; **(2)** the osmotic pressure exerted by any substance in very dilute solution is the same that it would exert if present as gas in the same volume as that of the solution; or, at constant temperature, the osmotic pressure of dilute solutions is proportional to the concentration (number of molecules) of the dissolved substance; i.e., the osmotic pressure, Π, in dilute solutions is $\Pi = RT\Sigma c_i$, where R is the universal gas constant, T is the absolute temperature, and c_i is the molar concentration of solute i; **(3)** the rate of chemical reactions increases between two- and three-fold for each 10°C rise in temperature.

Vogel l., when a phenotype may be transmitted by various modes of mendelian inheritance, the dominant will have the least deleterious phenotype, the recessive the most, and the X-linked intermediate between the two.

wallerian l., after section of the posterior root of a spinal nerve between the root ganglion and the spinal cord, the central portion degenerates; after division of the anterior root, the peripheral portion degenerates; the trophic center of the posterior root is therefore the ganglion, that of the anterior root the spinal cord.

Weber l., SYN Weber-Fechner l.

Weber-Fechner l., the intensity of a sensation varies by a series of equal increments (arithmetically) as the strength of the stimulus is increased geometrically; if a series of stimuli is applied and so adjusted in strength that each stimulus causes a just perceptible change in intensity of the sensation, then the strength of each stimulus differs from the preceding one by a constant fraction; thus, if a just perceptible change in a visual sensation is produced by the addition of 1 candle to an original illumination of 100 candles, 10 candles will be required to produce any change in sensation when the original illumination was one of 1000 candles. SYN Fechner-Weber l., Weber l.

Weigert l., the loss or destruction of a part or element in the organic world is likely to result in compensatory replacement and overproduction of tissue during the process of regeneration or repair (or both), as in the formation of callus when a fractured bone heals. SYN overproduction theory.

Williston l., as the vertebrate scale is ascended, the number of bones in the skull is reduced.

Wolff l., every change in the form and the function of a bone, or in its function alone, is followed by certain definite changes in its internal architecture and secondary alterations in its external conformation; these changes usually represent responses to alterations in weight-bearing stresses.

Lawrence, Robert D., English physician, 1892–1968. SEE L.-Seip *syndrome.*

law·ren·ci·um (Lr, Lw) (law-ren′sē-ŭm). An artificial transplutonium element; atomic no. 103; atomic wt. 262.11. [E.O. *Lawrence,* U.S. physicist and Nobel laureate, 1901–1958]

lax·a·tion (lak-sā′shŭn). Bowel movement, with or without laxatives. [see laxative]

lax·a·tive (lak′să-tiv). **1.** Mildly cathartic; having the action of loosening the bowels. **2.** A mild cathartic; a remedy that moves the bowels slightly without pain or violent action. [L. *laxativus,* fr. *laxo,* pp. *-atus,* to slacken, relax]

diphenylmethane l.'s, members of a chemical class of l. agents including phenolphthalein and bisacodyl.

LAYER

lay·er (lā′er) [TA]. A sheet of one substance lying on another and distinguished from it by a difference in texture or color or by not being continuous with it. SEE ALSO stratum, lamina. SYN panniculus.

ameloblastic l., the internal l. of the enamel organ. SYN enamel l.

anterior elastic l., SYN anterior limiting l. of cornea.

anterior limiting l. of cornea, a transparent homogeneous acellular layer, 6 to 9 μm thick, lying between the basal l. of the outer layer of stratified epithelium and the substantia propria of the cornea; considered to be a basement membrane. SYN anterior elastic l., Bowman l., Bowman membrane, lamina elastica anterior, lamina limitans anterior corneae.

anterior l. of rectus sheath [TA], the portion of the rectus sheath that lies anterior to the muscle, consisting in its upper two-thirds of contributions from the aponeuroses of the external and internal oblique muscles, and in its lower third (below the arcuate line) of contributions from the aponeuroses of all three muscles of the anterolateral abdominal wall. SYN lamina anterior vaginae musculi recti abdominis.

anterior l. of thoracolumbar fascia [TA], fascial membrane extending from transverse processes of lumbar vertebrae. SYN lamina anterior fasciae thoracolumbalis [TA], fascia musculi quadrati lumborum☆, lamina profunda fasciae thoracolumbalis☆, quadratus lumborum fascia☆.

bacillary l., SYN l. of rods and cones.

basal l., SYN *stratum* basale (1).

basal cell l., SYN *stratum* basale epidermidis.

basal l. of choroid [TA], SYN *lamina* basalis choroideae.

basal l. of ciliary body, SYN basal *lamina* of ciliary body.

l. of Bechterew, SYN *band* of Kaes-Bechterew.

blastodermic l.'s, the primordial cell l.'s on the yolk surface of a telolecithal egg; in the earliest stages they consist of protoderm, and then later differentiate into ectoderm, endoderm, and mesoderm.

Bowman l., SYN anterior limiting l. of cornea.

brown l., SYN suprachoroid *lamina* of sclera.

cambium l., (1) the inner osteogenic l. of the periosteum; **(2)** a highly cellular zone immediately beneath the epithelium covering a botryoid sarcoma.

l.'s of cerebellar cortex, SEE cerebellar *cortex.*

la

l.'s of cerebral cortex, SEE cerebral *cortex.*

cerebral l. of retina, the internal l. of the retina containing the neural elements, as distinguished from the outer leaf of the retina, or pigmented layer. SYN pars optica retinae [TA], neural l. of retina, stratum cerebrale retinae.

Chievitz l., in the developing retina of an embryo, a transitory zone between the inner and outer neuroblastic l.'s that is devoid of nuclei.

choriocapillary l., SYN capillary *lamina* of choroid.

circular l. of detrusor (muscle) of urinary bladder [TA], the substantial middle l. of three ill-defined, interlacing l.'s (the inner and outer l.'s being predominantly longitudinally oriented) of smooth (involuntary) muscle fibers constituting the muscle l. of the wall of the bladder. SYN stratum circulare musculi detrusoris vesicae [TA].

circular l. of muscle coat of small intestine [TA], the inner l. of smooth (involuntary) muscle of the muscle coat (muscularis externa) of the small intestine in which the muscle fibers encircle the lumen; it is claimed by some investigators that the orientation of the muscle fibers is a tight spiral or helix rather than being truly circular. SYN stratum circulare tunicae muscularis intestini tenuis [TA], short pitch helicoidal l.✲, stratum helicoidale brevis gradus✲.

circular l. of muscular coat [TA], the inner, circular l. of the smooth muscle of the muscular coat. Terminologia Anatomica lists circular l.'s of muscular coats (stratum circulare tunicae muscularis ...) of the following: 1) colon (... coli [TA]); 2) prostatic urethra (... urethrae prostaticae [TA]); 3) rectum (... recti [TA]); 4) small intestine (... intestini tenuis [TA]); 5) stomach (... gastricae [TA]); 6) urethra (... urethrae [TA]). SYN stratum circulare tunicae muscularis [TA].

circular l.'s of muscular tunics, SEE circular l. of muscular coat.

circular l. of tympanic membrane, SYN *stratum* circulare membranae tympani.

claustral l., the l. of subcortical gray matter between the external capsule and the white matter of the insula or extreme capsule.

clear l. of epidermis, SYN *stratum* lucidum.

columnar l., SYN *stratum* basale epidermidis.

conjunctival l. of bulb, SYN bulbar *conjunctiva.*

conjunctival l. of eyelids, SYN palpebral *conjunctiva.*

corneal l. of epidermis, SYN *stratum* corneum epidermidis.

cornified l. of nail, SYN *stratum* corneum unguis.

cutaneous l. of tympanic membrane, SYN *stratum* cutaneum membranae tympani.

deep l. [TA], in a stratified structure, the stratum which lies beneath all others, furthest from the surface. SEE deep l. of levator palpebrae superioris, deep l. of temporal fascia. SYN lamina profunda [TA], deep lamina.

deep gray l. of superior colliculus [TA], a l. of cell bodies in the superior colliculus located between the intermediate white l. and the deep white l. SYN stratum griseum profundum colliculis superioris [TA].

deep l. of levator palpebrae superioris, the deeper fibers of the levator muscle of the superior eyelid that are inserted into the superior tarsal plate. SYN lamina profunda musculi levatoris palpebrae superioris [TA].

deep l. of temporal fascia, the deep part of the temporal fascia attaching to the medial surface of the zygomatic arch. SYN lamina profunda fasciae temporalis [TA].

deep white l. of superior colliculus, a l. of neuron cell bodies in the superior colliculus located between the deep white l. and the intermediate white matter. SYN stratum medullare profundum [TA].

deep white l. [TA] of superior colliculus [TA], the innermost l. of the superior colliculus; a l. of myelinated fibers located internal to the deep gray l.

l.'s of dentate gyrus [TA], from the surface of the dentate gyrus, these layers are: the molecular layer [TA] (stratum moleculare [TA]), which contains dendrites of granular cells and some incoming axons from the perforant pathway, granular layer [TA] (stratum granulare [TA]), which contains the layer of small granular cells, and the multiform layer [TA] (stratum multiforme [TA]),

also sometimes called the polymorphic layer, which contains axons of granular cells and some afferent axons entering via the fornix. SYN strata gyri dentati [TA].

elastic l.'s of arteries, SYN elastic *laminae* of arteries, under *lamina.*

elastic l.'s of cornea, SEE anterior limiting l. of cornea, posterior limiting l. of cornea.

enamel l., SYN ameloblastic l.

ependymal l., an inner epithelial l. of cells bordering the lumen of the embryonic neural tube and brain, formed during the latter's stratification, and persisting in modified form throughout life. SYN ependymal zone, ventricular l.

episcleral l. of fibrous layer of eyeball [TA], the delicate moveable layer of loose connective tissue between the external surface of the sclera and the fascial sheath of the eyeball. SYN lamina episcleralis [TA], episcleral lamina.

epithelial l.'s, SEE epithelium.

epithelial choroid l., SYN epithelial *lamina.*

epitrichial l., the superficial flattened-cell l. of the epidermis of a young embryo before the definitive stratification has developed.

external nuclear l. of retina, SYN neuroepithelial l. of retina.

fatty l. of subcutaneous tissue, superficial portion of the subcutaneous tissue of certain areas of the body (e.g., inferior portion of anterior abdominal wall) which is specialized for fat storage and thus often has an abundance of fat, especially in the overnourished individual, compared with the deeper, fibrous portion of the subcutaneous tissue; in morbid obesity, this l. forms the core of a large, sagging apronlike fold. SEE ALSO fatty l. of subcutaneous tissue of abdomen. SYN panniculus adiposus [TA].

fatty l. of subcutaneous tissue of abdomen [TA], the more superficial, fatty part of the superficial fascia of the lower anterior abdominal wall. SYN panniculus adiposus telae subcutaneae abdominis [TA], Camper fascia, fatty l. of superficial fascia.

fatty l. of superficial fascia, SYN fatty l. of subcutaneous tissue of abdomen.

fibromusculocartilagenous l. of bronchi [TA], layer between submucosa and adventitia of bronchi which includes cartilages enclosed in perichondrium continuous between cartilages with a dense, fibrous membrane that includes smooth muscle and elastic fibers; this layer provides rigidity to the wall while allowing active reduction and passive increase in diameter of the bronchus. SYN tunica fibromusculocartilaginea bronchi [TA].

fibrous l., the outer dense connective tissue l. of the periosteum.

fibrous l. of eyeball [TA], the outer layer of the eyeball composed of the sclera and cornea. SYN tunica fibrosa bulbi [TA], fibrous tunic of eye, tunica externa oculi.

fibrous l. of joint capsule [TA], the outer fibrous part of the capsule of a synovial joint, which may in places be thickened to form capsular ligaments. SYN membrana fibrosa capsulae articularis [TA], fibrous layer of articular capsule✲, fibrous membrane of joint capsule✲, fibrous articular capsule, stratum fibrosum capsulae articularis.

fibrous l. in or on deep aspect of fatty layer of subcutaneous tissue [TA], fibrous tissue interspersed within or concentrated in the deeper portions of the otherwise fatty l. of subcutaneous tissue in a particular region, making it more substantial, but not organized into a uniform, membranous l. SYN stratum fibrosum panniculi adiposi telae subcutaneae [TA].

fillet l., SYN *stratum* lemnisci.

fusiform l., SYN multiform l. [TA] of cerebral cortex.

ganglionic l. [TA], the l. of the retina containing primarily the cell bodies of ganglion cells, although some amacrine cell bodies are also found. SEE ALSO ganglion *cells* of retina, under *cell.* SYN stratum ganglionicum [TA], ganglionic cell l. of retina.

ganglionic cell l. of retina, SYN ganglionic l.

ganglionic l. of cerebellar cortex, SYN Purkinje cell l.

ganglionic l. of cerebral cortex, l. 5 of the cortex cerebri.

ganglionic l. of optic nerve, obsolete term used to describe the multipolar neurons in the retina that give rise to the fibers of the optic nerve. SYN stratum ganglionare nervi optici.

▪ **germ l.,** one of the three primordial cell l.'s (ectoderm, endoderm, mesoderm) established in an embryo during gastrulation.

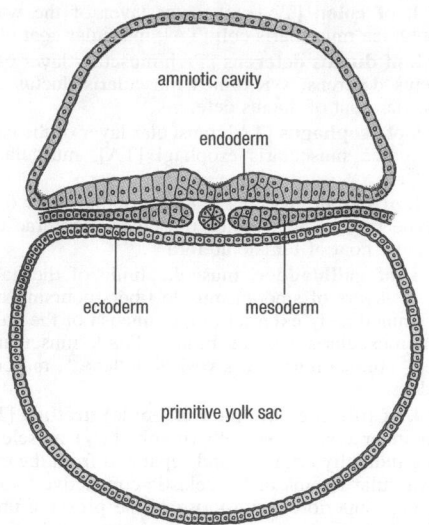

germ layers of the early embryo

Labels: amniotic cavity, endoderm, ectoderm, mesoderm, primitive yolk sac

---

germinative l., SYN *stratum* basale epidermidis.

germinative l. of nail, SYN *stratum* germinativum unguis.

glomerular l. of olfactory bulb, a l. composed of spherical bodies, called glomeruli, formed by the synapses of mitral cells with the olfactory nerve fibers derived from the cells of the olfactory epithelium.

granular l. [TA], SEE l.'s of dentate gyrus. SYN stratum granulare [TA].

granular l. of cerebellar cortex [TA], SYN granular l. of cerebellum.

granular l. of cerebellum [TA], the deepest of the three l.'s of the cortex; it contains large numbers of granule cells, the dendrites of which synapse with incoming mossy fibers in cerebellar glomeruli. Thin, unmyelinated axons of granule cells ascend perpendicularly into the molecular l. in which they bifurcate into fibers coursing parallel to the long axis of the cerebellar folia. Parallel fibers form numerous synapses with the dendrites of Purkinje cells, basket cells, and stellate cells. SYN granular l. of cerebellar cortex [TA], stratum granulosum corticis cerebelli [TA].

granular l.'s of cerebral cortex, l.'s 2 (outer) and 4 (inner) of the cortex cerebri.

granular l. of epidermis, a l. of somewhat flattened cells containing basophilic granules of keratohyalin and lying just above the stratum spinosum and deep to the stratum corneum. SYN stratum granulosum epidermidis.

granular l. of a vesicular ovarian follicle, SYN *stratum* granulosum folliculi ovarici vesiculosi.

gray l.'s of superior colliculus, term applied to any one of the three major l.'s of gray matter of the superior colliculus that alternate with l.'s composed chiefly of nerve fibers: 1) the superficial gray l. of superior colliculus, external to the largely white layer of the incoming fibers of the optic tract (optic l.); 2) the intermediate gray l. of superior colliculus, placed between the optic l. and a more deeply located l. of fibers, the l. lemnisci; 3) the deep gray l. of superior colliculus, between the l. lemnisci and the central gray substance surrounding the cerebral aqueduct, and containing the large nerve cells from which most of the colliculus descending connections (tectobulbar, tectopontine, and tectospinal tract) originate. SYN stratum cinereum colliculi superioris, stratum griseum colliculi superioris.

half-value l. (HVL), the thickness of a specific absorber (e.g., aluminum) that will reduce the intensity of a beam of radiation to one-half its initial value.

Henle l., the outer l. cells of the inner root sheath of the hair follicle.

Henle fiber l., the l. of inner cone fibers in the central area of the retina.

Henle nervous l., SYN entoretina.

l.'s of hippocampus [TA], four l.'s formed by cells and cell processes; they are, beginning at the alveus and ventricular surface: the oriens layer [TA] (stratum oriens [TA]) which contains basal dendrites and axon collaterals of the pyramidal cells, pyramidal layer [TA] (stratum pyramidale [TA]) which contains the sonata of the large pyramidal cells of the hippocampus, radiant layer [TA] (stratum radiatum [TA]) which contain the branching dendrites of the pyramidal cells and recurrent axon collaterals of the pyramidal cells, and the lacunar-molecular layer [TA] (stratum moleculare et substratum lacunosum [TA]) which contains the distal dendrites and some of the incoming axons of the preforant pathway. SYN strata hippocampi [TA].

horny l. of epidermis, SYN *stratum* corneum epidermidis.

horny l. of nail, SYN *stratum* corneum unguis.

Huxley l., a l. of cells interposed between Henle l. and the cuticle of the inner root sheath of the hair follicle. SYN Huxley membrane, Huxley sheath.

infragranular l., the cellular band deep to the inner granular l. of the developing human cerebral cortex, which differentiates into the ganglionic l. and multiform l. by the sixth fetal month.

inner l. of eyeball [TA], the third and deepest of the three l.'s of the eyeball, composed of the retina, intraocular part of the optic nerve, and the retinal blood vessels. SYN tunica interna bulbi [TA], nervous tunic of eyeball.

inner limiting layer [TA], the membranelike structure located immediately internal to the layer of nerve fibers; composed of the processes of the neuroglial cells (Müller cells) of the retina. SYN stratum limitans internum [TA].

inner nuclear l. [TA], the l. of the retina composed of the cell bodies of bipolar cells, horizontal cells, and some of the cell bodies of amacrine cells. SYN stratum nucleare internum [TA].

l. of inner and outer segments [TA], the l. of the retina located external to the outer limiting membrane and composed of the inner and outer segments of the rods and cones; the outer tips of the rod and cone segments are apposed to the pigmented l. SYN stratum segmentorum externorum et internorum [TA].

inner plexiform l. [TA], the l. of the retina composed of the processes of bipolar cells, ganglion cells, and amacrine cells; a layer containing synaptic contacts. SYN stratum plexiforme internum [TA].

intermediate l., SYN mantle l.

intermediate white l. [TA] of superior colliculus [TA], a l. of myelinated fibers located between the intermediate and deep gray layers of the superior colliculus. SYN stratum medullare intermedium [TA].

investing l. [TA], a fascial l. that ensheathes or intimately encloses a specific group of muscles. SYN fascia investiens [TA].

investing l. of cervical fascia [TA], the part of the cervical fascia investing the sternocleidomastoid and trapezius muscles and completely encircling the neck. SYN lamina superficialis fasciae cervicalis [TA], superficial l. of deep cervical fascia✫, investing fascia.

Kölliker l., the l. of connective tissue in the iris.

lacunar-molecular l. [TA], SEE l.'s of hippocampus. SYN stratum moleculare et substratum lacunosum [TA].

Langhans l., SYN cytotrophoblast.

latticed l., a cortical cell l. in the hippocampus.

limiting l.'s of cornea, SEE anterior limiting l. of cornea, posterior limiting *lamina* of cornea.

longitudinal l. of muscle coat of small intestine [TA], longitudinal layer of muscular coat of small intestine. SYN stratum longitudinale tunicae muscularis intestini tenuis [TA], stratum helicoidale longi gradus✫.

longitudinal l. of muscular coat [TA], the outer, longitudinal l. of the smooth muscle of the muscular coat. Terminologia Anatomica lists longitudinal l.'s of muscular coats (stratum longitudinale tunicae muscularis ...) of the following: 1) intermediate urethra (... urethrae intermediae [TA]); 2) colon (... coli [TA]); 3) prostatic urethra (... urethrae prostaticae [TA]); 4) rectum (... recti

la

[TA]); 5) small intestine (... intestini tenuis [TA]); 6) spongy urethra (... urethrae spongiosae [TA]); 7) stomach (... gastricae [TA]). SYN stratum longitudinale tunicae muscularis [TA].

longitudinal l.'s of muscular tunics, SEE longitudinal l. of muscular coat.

long pitch helicoidal l.,

malpighian l., SYN malpighian *stratum.*

mantle l., the nuclear zone of the developing neural tube between the marginal l. and the ependymal l.; forms the gray matter of the central nervous system. SYN intermediate l., mantle zone (1).

marginal l., the outer, nonnuclear l. of the embryonic neural tube; into its fibrous network grow the longitudinal nerve fibers that eventually become the white matter of the spinal cord and brainstem. SYN marginal zone (2).

medullary l.'s of thalamus, SYN medullary *laminae* of thalamus, under *lamina.*

membranous l., SYN membranous *lamina* of cartilage of pharyngotympanic (auditory) plate.

membranous l. of subcutaneous tissue of abdomen [TA], the deeper, membranous or lamellar part of the subcutaneous tissue of the lower abdominal wall; it is continuous with the superficial perineal (Colles) l. SYN membranous l. of superficial fascia of perineum (2), membranous l. of superficial fascia (2), Scarpa fascia.

membranous l. of superficial fascia, (1) SYN subcutaneous *tissue* of perineum; **(2)** SYN membranous l. of subcutaneous tissue of abdomen.

membranous l. of superficial fascia of perineum, (1) SYN subcutaneous *tissue* of perineum; **(2)** SYN membranous l. of subcutaneous tissue of abdomen.

meningeal l. of dura mater, SEE cranial *dura mater.*

Meynert l., SYN pyramidal cell l.

middle gray l. of superior colliculus, SEE gray l.'s of superior colliculus.

molecular l., term applied to any l. of brain tissue that contains few nerve-cell bodies and is composed largely of terminal arborizations of dendrites and axons; notable examples are the superficial l. (first l.) of the cerebral cortex and the molecular l. of cerebellum. SYN plexiform l., stratum moleculare.

molecular l. of cerebellar cortex [TA], the outer lamina of the cortex, containing the cell bodies (unless the Purkinje cell layer is designated as a separate layer) and dendrites of Purkinje cells, the axons of the granule cells, and the cell bodies, dendrites, and axons of basket cells. SYN stratum moleculare corticis cerebelli [TA], molecular l. of cerebellum.

molecular l. of cerebellum, SYN molecular l. of cerebellar cortex.

molecular l. of cerebral cortex [TA], l. 1 of the cortex cerebri. SYN lamina molecularis corticis cerebri [TA], plexiform l. of cerebral cortex.

molecular l.'s of olfactory bulb, the l.'s, composed mainly of nerve fibers, on the outer and inner sides of the l. of mitral cells of the bulb.

molecular l. of retina, name applied to each of the plexiform l.'s of the retina. SYN stratum moleculare retinae.

multiform l. [TA], SEE l.'s of dentate gyrus. SYN stratum multiforme [TA].

multiform l. [TA] **of cerebral cortex,** the innermost layer of the cerebral cortex, layer XI. SYN fusiform l., polymorphous l., spindle-celled l.

muscle l. in fatty layer of subcutaneous tissue [TA], l. of smooth or striated muscle embedded within the fatty subcutaneous tissue for contraction or to produce movement of the skin, e.g., facial muscles within subcutaneous tissue of face and neck, dartos muscle within the dartos fascia of scrotum. SYN stratum musculosum panniculi adiposi telae subcutaneae [TA].

muscular l. [TA], the muscular, usually middle, layer of a tubular structure; for most of the gastrointestinal tract, it consists of an outer longitudinal layer of muscle and an inner circular layer. SYN tunica muscularis [TA], muscular coat*.

muscular l. of bronchi, muscular layer of the bronchial wall. SYN tunica muscularis bronchiorum [TA], muscular coat of bronchi*.

muscular l. of colon [TA], muscular layer of the wall of the colon. SYN tunica muscularis coli [TA], muscular coat of colon*.

muscular l. of ductus deferens [TA], muscular layer of the wall of the ductus deferens. SYN tunica muscularis ductus deferentis [TA], muscular coat of ductus deferens*.

muscular l. of esophagus [TA], muscular layer of the esophageal wall. SYN tunica muscularis esophagi [TA], muscular coat of esophagus*.

muscular l. of female urethra [TA], muscular layer of the wall of the female urethra. SYN tunica muscularis urethrae femininae [TA], muscular coat of female urethra*.

muscular l. of gallbladder, muscular tunic of the gallbladder, consisting of layers of smooth muscle fibers coursing in various directions immediately external to the mucosa of the gallbladder. SYN tunica muscularis vesicae biliaris [TA], muscular coat of gallbladder*, tunica muscularis vesicae felleae*, muscular tunic of gallbladder.

muscular l. of intermediate part of (male) urethra [TA], relatively thin inner coat of smooth (involuntary) muscle bundles, mostly longitudinally arranged and separated from the epithelium by a thin vascular stroma of fibroelastic connective tissue, which are continuous superiorly with those of the prostatic urethra and peripherally with an outer, much more prominent l. of circularly oriented skeletal (voluntary) muscle fibers that forms the main, tubelike part of the external urethral sphincter. SEE ALSO external urethral *sphincter* of male. SYN tunica muscularis partis intermediae urethrae masculinae [TA], muscular coat of intermediate part of male urethra*.

muscular l. of large intestine [TA], muscular l. of the wall of all parts of the large intestine (cecum, colon, rectum, and anal canal) collectively. SYN tunica muscularis intestini crassi [TA], muscular coat of large intestine*.

muscular l. of male urethra [TA], muscular l. of the prostatic, intermediate, and spongy segments of the male urethra. SEE ALSO muscular l. of intermediate part of (male) urethra. SYN tunica muscularis urethrae masculinae [TA], muscular coat of male urethra.

muscular l. of mucosa, SYN *muscularis* mucosae.

muscular l. of pharynx [TA], muscular layer of the pharyngeal wall. In contrast with the muscular coats of the rest of the gastrointestinal tract (except anal canal), that of the pharynx has an outer circular layer and an inner longitudinal layer. SYN tunica muscularis pharyngis [TA], muscular coat of pharynx*.

muscular l. of prostatic urethra [TA], relatively thin inner coat of smooth (involuntary) muscle bundles, both circularly and longitudinally arranged and separated from the epithelium by a thin vascular stroma of fibroelastic connective tissue, which are continuous inferiorly with those of the intermediate urethra and peripherally with the fibromuscular tissue of the prostate, including a relatively thick, troughlike layer of skeletal (voluntary) muscle that ascends the anterior aspect of the prostatic urethra to the neck of the bladder as part of the external urethral sphincter; proximal (superior) to the seminal colliculus, which bears the openings of the ejaculatory ducts, the circular layer of smooth muscle is especially prominent as a continuation of the internal urethral sphincter of the intramural or preprostatic part of the urethra. SEE ALSO external urethral *sphincter* of male, internal urethral *sphincter.* SYN tunica muscularis partis prostaticae urethrae masculinae [TA], muscular coat of intermediate part of male urethra*, muscular coat of prostatic urethra.

muscular l. of rectum [TA], muscular layer of the wall of the rectum. SYN tunica muscularis recti [TA], muscular coat of rectum*.

muscular l. of renal pelvis [TA], middle l. (between outer adventitia and inner mucosa) composed of two morphologically and histochemically distinct types of smooth (involuntary) muscle fibers, one of which is identical and continuous with that of the ureters, while the other is unique to the calices and pelvis. SYN tunica muscularis pelvis renalis [TA].

muscular l. of seminal gland [TA], middle l. (between outer connective tissue and inner mucosa) of the seminal gland wall, composed of outer longitudinal and inner circular l.'s of smooth muscle. SYN tunica muscularis glandulae vesiculosae [TA].

muscular l. of small intestine [TA], muscular layer of the wall of the small intestine. SYN tunica muscularis intestini tenuis [TA], muscular coat of small intestine☆.

muscular l. of spongy (male) urethra [TA], relatively sparse l. of mostly longitudinally disposed smooth (involuntary) muscle fibers between the mucosa and the surrounding erectile tissue of the corpus spongiosum penis. SYN tunica muscularis partis spongiosae urethrae masculinae [TA], muscular coat of spongy part of male urethra☆.

muscular l. of stomach [TA], muscular tunic of the stomach, consisting of smooth muscles arranged in three fairly well-defined layers: an *outer longitudinal layer*, continuous with that of the esophagus but dividing at the cardia into two bands which run along the greater and lesser curvatures, leaving the middle areas of the anterior and posterior walls devoid of longitudinal fibers, and then coalescing in the pyloric region into a complete layer which is continuous with the longitudinal l. of the duodenum. The *middle circular layer* is most complete and strongest, continuous with the circular layer of the esophagus at the cardia; it thickens progressively toward the pylorus, ultimately forming the muscular ring of the pyloric sphincter. The *inner, oblique layer* is unique to the stomach and is most strongly developed in the fundic region and absent along the lesser curvature. This absence contributes to the formation of the "gastric canal." SYN tunica muscularis gastrica [TA], muscular coat of stomach☆, tunica muscularis ventriculi.

muscular l. of trachea [TA], muscular layer of the tracheal wall. SYN tunica muscularis tracheae [TA], muscular coat of trachea☆.

muscular l. of ureter [TA], muscular layer of the ureteric wall. SYN tunica muscularis ureteris [TA], muscular coat of ureter☆.

muscular l. of urinary bladder [TA], muscular layer of the wall of the urinary bladder. SYN tunica muscularis vesicae urinariae [TA], muscular coat of urinary bladder☆.

muscular l. of uterine tube [TA], muscular layer of the wall of the uterine tube. SYN tunica muscularis tubae uterinae [TA], muscular coat of uterine tube☆.

muscular l. of vagina [TA], muscular layer of the vaginal wall. SYN tunica muscularis vaginae [TA], muscular coat of vagina☆.

l. of nerve fibers [TA], the l. of the retina composed of the axonal processes of the ganglion cells; these processes converge to form the optic nerve. SYN stratum neurofibrarum [TA].

neural l. of optic part of retina, SEE retina.

neural l. of retina, SYN cerebral l. of retina.

neuroepithelial l. of retina, the outermost l. of the cerebral l. of retina, composed of the primary receptor cells of the retina; this area consists of two layers: 1) a layer of inner and outer segments [TA] made up of the rods and cones, the photosensitive processes of the receptor cells, and 2) the outer nuclear l. [TA] containing the cell bodies of these cells; the outer limiting membrane (outer limiting layer [TA]) forms a perforated supporting plate between the two sublayers; the name refers to the fact that the retinal receptor cells are a specialized form of (epithelial) ependyma cell and thus, in a sense, are comparable to the neuroepithelial cells (e.g., hair cells) of other sense organs. SYN external nuclear l. of retina, stratum neuroepitheliale retinae.

Nitabuch l., SYN Nitabuch *membrane.*

nuclear l.'s of retina, the outer nuclear l., l. 4, of the retina, neuroepithelial l. of retina, and the inner l., l. 6, of the retina, ganglionic layer of retina. SYN strata nuclearia externa et interna retinae.

odontoblastic l., a l. of mesenchymal cells at the periphery of the dental pulp of the tooth.

optic l. [TA], **(1)** a layer of white matter interspersed with nerve-cell bodies, immediately below the superficial gray l. of the superior colliculus, composed of myelinated fibers originating in the retina and striate cortex; **(2)** a rarely used term to describe the inner l. of the retina, consisting of the fibers originating from the cells of the ganglionic l. of the retina; in their further course these fibers combine to form the optic nerve. SYN stratum opticum [TA].

orbital l. of ethmoid bone, SYN orbital *plate* of ethmoid bone.

oriens l. [TA], SEE l.'s of hippocampus. SYN stratum oriens [TA].

osteogenetic l., the inner bone-forming l. of the periosteum.

outer limiting l. [TA], the membranelike structure located immediately internal to the l. of inner and outer segments; made up of processes of the neuroglial cells of the retina (Müller cells); penetrated by the portion of the rods and cones located between the inner and outer segments and the cell body. SYN stratum limitans externum [TA].

outer nuclear l. [TA], the l. of the retina containing the cell bodies of the rods and cones. SYN stratum nucleare externum [TA].

outer plexiform l. [TA], the l. of the retina composed of the processes of rods and cones, horizontal cells, and bipolar cells; a layer containing synaptic contacts. SYN stratum plexiforme externum [TA].

palisade l., SYN *stratum* basale epidermidis.

papillary l., SYN *stratum* papillare corii.

parietal l. [TA], the outer l. of an enveloping sac or bursa, usually lining the walls of the cavity or space occupied by the enveloped structure, the structure itself being covered with the inner or visceral layer of the enveloping sac; an actual or potential space is enclosed by the two continuous layers, intervening between parietal and visceral layers. The parietal l. is usually the more substantial l. SYN lamina parietalis [TA].

parietal l. of leptomeninges, SYN *arachnoid* mater.

parietal l. of serous pericardium [TA], the outer part of the serous pericardium suported by the fibrous pericardium. SYN lamina parietalis pericardii serosi [TA].

parietal l. of tunica vaginalis of testis [TA], the outer part of the tunica vaginalis testis supported by the internal spermatic fascia. SYN lamina parietalis tunicae vaginalis testis [TA].

perforated l. of sclera, SYN *lamina* cribrosa of sclera.

periosteal l. of dura mater, SEE cranial *dura mater.*

pigmented l. of ciliary body, SYN *stratum* pigmenti corporis ciliaris.

pigmented l. of iris, SYN *stratum* pigmenti iridis.

pigmented l. of retina [TA], the outer l. of the retina, consisting of pigmented epithelium. SYN ectoretina, stratum pigmenti bulbi, stratum pigmenti retinae, tapetum nigrum, tapetum oculi.

piriform neuron l., an obsolete term for the Purkinje cell l.

l. of piriform neurons, SYN Purkinje cell l.

plasma l., SYN still l.

plexiform l., SYN molecular l.

plexiform l. of cerebral cortex, SYN molecular l. of cerebral cortex.

plexiform l.'s of retina, l.'s of the retina where synapses occur; in the external l., processes of rods and cones synapse with bipolar neuron dendrites; in the internal l., axon terminals of bipolar cells synapse with ganglion cell dendrites. SEE retina. SYN stratum plexiforme internum [TA], stratum plexiforme externum.

polymorphous l., SYN multiform l. [TA] of cerebral cortex.

posterior elastic l., SYN posterior limiting *lamina* of cornea.

posterior limiting l. of cornea, SYN posterior limiting *lamina* of cornea.

posterior l. of rectus sheath [TA], the portion of the sheath of the rectus abdominis muscle that lies posterior to the muscle covering only its upper two-thirds; it is formed by contributions from the aponeuroses of the internal oblique and transversus abdominis muscles; its free inferior margin forms the arcuate line; it is deficient below this, the posterior aspect of the muscle being covered only by transversalis fascia and peritoneum. SYN lamina posterior vaginae musculi recti abdominis [TA].

pretracheal l. of cervical fascia [TA], the layer of fascia investing the infrahyoid muscles and contributing to the formation of the carotid sheath. SYN lamina pretrachealis fasciae cervicalis [TA], middle cervical fascia, Porter fascia, pretracheal fascia.

prevertebral l. of cervical fascia [TA], the part of the cervical fascia that covers the bodies of the cervical vertebrae and the muscles attaching to them and to the anterior parts of their transverse processes. SYN lamina prevertebralis fasciae cervicalis [TA], prevertebral fascia.

prickle cell l., SYN *stratum* spinosum epidermidis.

Purkinje cell l., the l. of large neuron cell bodies located at the

la

interface of molecular and granular layers in the cerebellar cortex; dendrites of these cells fan outward into the molecular l. in a plane transverse to the folium. SYN stratum purkinjense corticis cerebelli [TA], ganglionic l. of cerebellar cortex, l. of piriform neurons, Purkinje cells, Purkinje corpuscles.

pyramidal l. [TA], SEE l.'s of hippocampus. SYN stratum pyramidale [TA].

pyramidal cell l., l.'s 3 and 5 of the cortex cerebri. SYN Meynert l.

radiant l. [TA], SEE l.'s of hippocampus. SYN stratum radiatum [TA].

radiate l. of tympanic membrane, SYN *stratum* radiatum membranae tympani.

Rauber l., (1) the thinned-out trophoblastic membrane over the embryonic disk in developing carnivores and ungulates; **(2)** outermost cell layer which helps form the blastodisk; called blastodermic or primitive ectoderm.

reticular l. of corium, SYN *stratum* reticulare corii.

l.'s of retina, SEE retina.

l. of rods and cones, the l. of the retina next to the pigment l. and containing the visual receptors. SEE ALSO retina, neuroepithelial l. of retina. SYN bacillary l.

rostral l., SYN rostral *lamina*.

Sattler elastic l., the middle l. of the choroid.

serous l. of peritoneum, SYN *serosa* of peritoneum.

short pitch helicoidal l., ✭official alternate term for circular l. of muscle coat of small intestine.

l.'s of skin, SEE epidermis, dermis.

sluggish l., SYN still l.

somatic l., the external l. of the lateral mesoderm of the embryo, lying adjacent to the ectoderm and together with it constituting the somatopleure.

spindle-celled l., SYN multiform l. [TA] of cerebral cortex.

spinous l., SYN *stratum* spinosum epidermidis.

splanchnic l., the internal l. of the lateral mesoderm, lying adjacent to the endoderm and together with it forming the splanchnopleure.

spongy l. of female urethra [TA], inappropriate reference to the lamina propria of the mucous membrane of the female urethra, characterized by numerous, thin-walled veins that have in the past been falsely compared with erectile tissue. SYN tunica spongiosa urethrae femininae [TA].

spongy l. of vagina [TA], inappropriate collective reference to the abundant venous plexuses of the vagina, occurring within the mucosal and muscular layers (giving the rugae somewhat the character of erectile tissue) as well as in the adventitia (the laterally placed vaginal venous plexuses), falsely suggesting a discrete layer of erectile tissue. SYN tunica spongiosa vaginae [TA].

still l., the l. of the bloodstream in the capillary vessels, next to the wall of the vessel, that flows slowly and transports the white blood cells along the l. wall, while in the center the flow is rapid and transports the red blood cells. SYN plasma l., Poiseuille space, sluggish l.

subendocardial l., the loose connective tissue l. that joins the endocardium and myocardium; in the ventricles, it contains branches of the conducting system of the heart.

subendothelial l., the thin l. of connective tissue lying between the endothelium and elastic lamina in the intima of blood vessels.

subpapillary l., the vascular l. of the corium.

subserous l., ✭official alternate term for subserosa.

superficial l. [TA], in a stratified structure, the outermost or topmost of the strata; the stratum nearest the surface. SEE superficial l. of deep cervical fascia, superficial l. of the levator palpebrae superioris, superficial l. of temporal fascia. SYN lamina superficialis [TA], superficial lamina.

superficial l. of deep cervical fascia, ✭official alternate term for investing l. of cervical fascia.

superficial gray l. [TA] **of superior colliculus,** SEE gray l.'s of superior colliculus.

superficial l. of the levator palpebrae superioris [TA], the superficial fibers of the levator muscle of the superior eyelid

which are inserted into the skin of the superior eyelid. SYN lamina superficialis musculi levatoris palpebrae superioris.

superficial l. of temporal fascia [TA], the superficial part of the temporal fascia attaching to the lateral surface of the zygomatic arch. SYN lamina superficialis fasciae temporalis [TA].

suprachoroid l.,

Tomes granular l., a thin l. of dentin adjacent to the cementum, appearing granular in ground sections; the granules are small uncalcified spaces.

vascular l., SYN vascular *lamina* of choroid.

vascular l. of choroid coat of eye, SYN vascular *lamina* of choroid.

vascular l. of eyeball [TA], the vascular, pigmentary, or middle coat of the eye, comprising the choroid, ciliary body, and iris. SYN tunica vasculosa bulbi [TA], Haller tunica vasculosa, tunica vasculosa oculi, uvea, uveal tract, vascular tunic of eye.

vascular l. of testis [TA], innermost of three coats (with tunicae vaginalis and albuginea) investing the testis consisting of a vascular plexus in a delicate loose connective tissue matrix that covers the internal aspect of the tunica albuginea and extends deeply, covering the septa and therefore surrounding the lobules of the testis. SYN tunica vasculosa testis [TA].

ventricular l., SYN ependymal l.

visceral l. [TA], the inner l. of an enveloping sac or bursa which lines the outer surface of the enveloped structure, as opposed to the parietal layer which lines the walls of the occupied space or cavity. The visceral l. is usually thin, delicate and not apparent as being separate, but rather appears to be the outer surface of the structure itself. SEE ALSO serosa. SYN lamina visceralis [TA].

visceral l. of serous pericardium [TA], the inner part of the serous pericardium applied directly on the heart. SYN epicardium✭, lamina visceralis pericardii.

visceral l. of tunica vaginalis of testis [TA], the inner part of the tunica vaginalis testis applied directly to the testis and epididymis. SYN lamina visceralis tunicae vaginalis testis [TA].

Waldeyer zonal l., SYN dorsolateral *fasciculus*.

Weil basal l., the l. beneath the odontoblasts of the tooth; it contains reticular fibers but few if any cells. SYN Weil basal zone.

zonular l., (1) a thin l. of white substance covering the upper surface of the thalamus and forming part of the floor of the body of the lateral ventricle; **(2)** a l. of white substance on the surface of the superior colliculus. SYN stratum zonale [TA].

---

laz·a·ret, laz·a·ret·to (laz′ă-ret, -ret′ō). Obsolete term for: **1.** A hospital for the treatment of contagious diseases. **2.** A place of detention for persons in quarantine. [It. *lazzaretto,* fr. *lazzaro,* a leper]

lb. Abbreviation for pound.

LBF Abbreviation for *Lactobacillus bulgaricus factor.*

LCAT Abbreviation for lecithin-cholesterol acyltransferase.

l-cone. Long-wavelength–sensitive cone (red cone).

LD Abbreviation for lethal *dose.*

LDH Abbreviation for *lactate* dehydrogenase.

LDL Abbreviation for low density lipoprotein. See lipoprotein.

LE, L.E. Abbreviation for left eye; *lupus* erythematosus.

leach·ing (lēch′ing). **1.** Removal of the soluble constituents of a substance by running water through it. **2.** Solubilization of metals, typically from poor ores, using lithotrophic bacteria. [A.S. *leccan,* to wet]

lead (Pb) (led). A metallic element, atomic no. 82, atomic wt. 207.2. SYN plumbum.

l. acetate, has been used as an astringent in diarrhea, and in aqueous solution as a wet dressing in certain dermatoses. SYN sugar of lead.

black l., SYN graphite.

l. carbonate, a heavy white powder that is insoluble in water; occasionally, it is used to relieve irritation in dermatitis, but it is used largely in the manufacture of paint and in the arts and is thus productive of l. poisoning. SYN ceruse, white l.

l. chromate, SYN chrome yellow.

l. monoxide, has been used as an ingredient in external applications such as l. plaster. SYN l. oxide (yellow), litharge, massicot.

l. oxide (yellow), SYN l. monoxide.

red l., SYN l. tetroxide.

red oxide of l., SYN l. tetroxide.

l. sulfide, PbS; the native form in which l. is chiefly found. SYN galena.

l. tetraethyl, SYN tetraethyllead.

l. tetroxide, a bright orange-red powder that turns black when heated; used in ointments and plasters. SYN red l., red oxide of l.

white l., SYN l. carbonate.

lead (lēd). An electrocardiographic cable with connections within the electronics of the machine designated for an electrode placed at a particular point on the body surface.

ABC l.'s, the l.'s for recording one kind of vectorcardiogram utilizing the Arrighi triangle; supplanted by XYZ l.'s.

augmented l., electrocardiogram recorded between one limb and two other limbs. The augmented l.'s are designated aVF, aVL, and aVR for recordings made between the foot (left), left arm, and right arm, respectively, and the other two limbs.

bipolar l., a record obtained with two electrodes placed on different regions of the body, each electrode contributing significantly to the record; e.g., a standard limb l.

CB l., a bipolar chest l. with the negative electrode placed upon the subject's back.

CF l., a bipolar chest l. with the negative electrode placed on the subject's left leg.

chest l.'s, those in which the exploring electrode is on the chest overlying the heart or its vicinity. SYN precordial l.'s, semidirect l.'s.

CL l., a bipolar chest l. with the negative electrode placed on the subject's left arm.

CR l., a bipolar chest l. with the negative electrode placed on the subject's right arm.

direct l., in electrocardiography, a unipolar l. recorded with the exploring electrode placed directly on the surface of the exposed heart.

esophageal l., an electrocardiographic l. passed down the throat into the esophagus to record the electrocardiogram at various levels of the esophagus; especially useful for certain types of arrhythmias. Similarly, a transducer for echocardiography can be passed into the esophagus.

indirect l., SYN standard limb l.

intracardiac l., the record obtained when the exploring electrode is placed within one of the heart's chambers, usually by means of cardiac catheterization.

limb l., one of the three standard l.'s (l.'s I, II, III) or one of the unipolar limb l.'s (aVR, aVL, aVF).

precordial l.'s, SYN chest l.'s.

semidirect l.'s, SYN chest l.'s.

standard limb l., one of the three original bipolar limb l.'s of the clinical electrocardiogram, designated I, II, and III: l. I records the potential difference between the right and left arms; l. II the difference between right arm and the leg electrode; and l. III the difference between left arm and the leg electrode. SYN indirect l.

unipolar l.'s, those in which the exploring electrode is on the chest in the vicinity of the heart or on one of the limbs, while the other or indifferent electrode is the central terminal.

V l., a unipolar l. with the central terminal as the indifferent electrode; V is the symbol for unipolar (Latin "U").

leaf·let (lēf'let). **1.** A layer of phospholipid; thus, a bilayer has two leaflets. **2.** A thin flattened object or structure.

League of Red Cross So·ci·e·ties. The international federation of national Red Cross and similar societies.

learned help·less·ness. A laboratory model of depression involving both classical (respondent) and instrumental (operant) conditioning techniques; application of unavoidable shock is followed by failure to cope in situations where coping might otherwise be possible.

learn·ing (lern'ing). Generic term for the relatively permanent change in behavior that occurs as a result of practice. SEE ALSO conditioning, forgetting, memory.

incidental l., l. without a direct attempt. SYN passive l.

insight l., the grasp of the solution to a problem without the intervening series of the trial and error steps that are associated with most types of learning (e.g., a monkey housed behind the bars of a cage who, without proceeding through countless hours of futile attempts with one stick or the other, fits two sticks together to retrieve a banana outside the distance measured by either stick alone).

latent l., that l. which is not evident to the observer at the time it occurs, but which is inferred from later performance in which l. is more rapid than would be expected without the earlier experience.

passive l., SYN incidental l.

rote l., the l. of arbitrary relationships, usually by repetition of the l. procedure through memorization and without an understanding of the relationships.

state-dependent l., l. during a specific state of sleep or wakefulness, or during a chemically altered state, where retrieval of learned information (e.g., as measured by performance of a learned response) cannot be demonstrated unless the subject is restored to the state that originally existed during l.

least squares. A principle of estimation invented by Gauss in which the estimates of a set of parameters in a statistical model are the quantities that minimize the sum of squared differences between the observed values of the dependent variable and the values predicted by the model.

Le Bel, Joseph Achille, French chemist, 1847–1930. SEE Le B.-van't Hoff *rule.*

Leber, Theodor, German ophthalmologist, 1840–1917. SEE L. idiopathic stellate *neuroretinitis,* hereditary optic *atrophy, plexus; amaurosis* congenita of L.

Le Chatelier, Henri, French physical chemist, 1850–1936. SEE Le C. *law, principle.*

lec·i·thal (les'i-thăl). Having a yolk or pertaining to the yolk of any egg; used especially as a suffix. [G. *lekithos,* egg yolk]

lec·i·thin (les'i-thin). Traditional term for 1,2-diacyl-*sn*-glycero-3-phosphocholines or 3-*sn*-phosphatidylcholines, phospholipids that on hydrolysis yield two fatty acid molecules and a molecule each of glycerophosphoric acid and choline. In some varieties of l., both fatty acids are saturated, others contain only unsaturated acids (e.g., oleic, linoleic, or arachidonic acid); in others again, one fatty acid is saturated, the other unsaturated. L.'s are yellowish or brown waxy substances, readily miscible in water, in which they appear under the microscope as irregular elongated particles known as "myelin forms," and are found in nervous tissue, especially in the myelin sheaths, in egg yolk, and as essential constituents of animal and vegetable cells. [G. *lekithos,* egg yolk]

l. acyltransferase, SYN lecithin-cholesterol acyltransferase.

l.-cholesterol l., a plasma enzyme that catalyzes the uptake of cholesterol esters by intermediate-density lipoproteins formed by high density lipoproteins.

lec·i·thi·nase (les'i-thi-nās). SYN phospholipase.

l. A, SYN *phospholipase* A$_2$.

l. B, SYN lysophospholipase.

l. C, SYN *phospholipase* C.

l. D, SYN *phospholipase* D.

lec·i·thin-cho·les·ter·ol ac·yl·trans·fer·ase (LCAT). An enzyme that reversibly transfers an acyl residue from a lecithin to cholesterol, forming a 1-acylglycerophosphocholine (a lysolecithin) and a cholesteryl ester; a deficiency of this enzyme leads to an accumulation of unesterified cholesterol in plasma resulting in anemia, proteinuria, renal failure, and corneal opacities; LCAT is also low in individuals with fish eye disease. SYN lecithin acyl-transferase.

lec·i·tho·blast (les'i-thō-blast). One of the cells proliferating to form the yolk-sac endoderm. [G. *lekithos,* egg yolk, + *blastos,* germ]

lec·i·tho·pro·tein (les'i-thō-prō'tēn). A conjugated protein, with lecithin as the prosthetic group.

Leclef. SEE Denys-Leclef *phenomenon.*

Le

Le·cler·cia (le-clār′cē-a). A genus in the family Enterobacteriaceae that resembles the genus *Escherichia*, but is separable by metabolic and genetic classification. Isolated from the feces of humans and animals, it has been recovered clinically from blood, feces, sputum, urine, and wounds; its degree of pathogenicity is unclear.

lec·tin (lek′tin). Any of a group of glycoproteins of primarily plant (usually seed) origin that binds to glycoproteins on the surface of cells causing agglutination, precipitation, or other phenomena resembling the action of specific antibody; l.'s include plant agglutinins (phytoagglutinins, phytohemagglutinins), plant precipitins, and perhaps certain animal proteins; some have mitogenic properties and induce lymphocyte transformation. [L. *lego*, pp. *lectum*, to select, + -in]

mitogenic l., a l. that induces the replication of polynucleic acids and the proliferation of lymphocytes.

Ledermann, Sully, French psychiatrist. SEE Ledermann *formula*.

ledge (lej). In anatomy, a structure resembling a ledge. SEE ALSO shelf, lamina.

dental l., a band of ectodermal cells growing from the epithelium of the embryonic jaws into the underlying mesenchyme; local buds from the l. give rise to the primordia of the enamel organs of the teeth. SYN dental lamina, dental shelf, dentogingival lamina, enamel l., primary dental lamina.

enamel l., SYN dental l.

Lee, Robert, English physician, 1793–1877. SEE L. *ganglion*.

Lee, Roger I., U.S. physician, 1881–1967. SEE L.-White *method*.

leech (lēch). **1.** A bloodsucking aquatic annelid worm (genus *Hirudo*, class Hirudinea) sometimes used in medicine for local withdrawal of blood. For various *l.* species, see *Hirudo*. **2.** To treat medically by applying leeches. [A.S. *laece*, a physician; a leech, because of its therapeutic use]

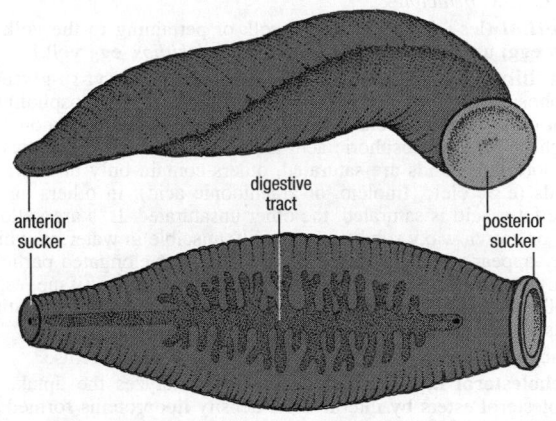

anterior sucker   digestive tract   posterior sucker

leech *(Hirudo medicinalis)*

leech·ing (lēch′ing). The former practice of applying leeches to the body to draw blood for therapeutic purposes.

Leede, Carl S., U.S. physician, *1882. SEE Rumpel-L. *sign*, *test;* L.-Rumpel *phenomenon.*

LEEP Abbreviation for loop electrocautery excision *procedure*; loop electrosurgical excision *procedure.*

Leeuwenhoek, Anton van, Dutch microscopist, 1632–1723. SEE L. *canals*, under *canal.*

Lefèvre, Paul, 20th century French dermatologist. SEE Papillon-L. *syndrome.*

Le Fort, Léon C., French surgeon and gynecologist, 1829–1893. SEE Le F. I *fracture*, II *fracture*, III *fracture*, *sound*, *amputation.*

left-foot·ed. SYN sinistropedal.

left-hand·ed. Denoting the habitual or more skillful use of the left hand for writing and for most manual operations. SYN sinistromanual.

left-sid·ed·ness. The normal left-sided location of certain unpaired organs, such as the spleen and most of the stomach.

bilateral l.-s., a syndrome in which normally unpaired organs develop more symmetrically in mirror image; two spleens, one on each side, are usually present, and cardiovascular anomalies are common. SYN polysplenia syndrome.

leg. 1 [TA]. Anatomically, the segment of the lower limb between the knee and the ankle; commonly used to mean the entire inferior limb. **2.** A structure resembling a leg. SYN crus (1) [TA].

l. of antihelix, SYN *crura* of antihelix, under *crus.*

bow-l., SEE *genu* varum.

elephant l., SYN elephantiasis.

restless l.'s, SYN restless legs *syndrome.*

rider's l., a strain of the adductor muscles of the thigh.

tennis l., a rupture of the gastrocnemius muscle at the musculotendinous junction, resulting from forcible contractions of the calf muscles; commonly seen in tennis players.

Legal, Emmo, German physician, 1859–1922. SEE L. *test.*

Legendre, Gaston J., French physician, *1887. SEE L. *sign.*

Legg, Arthur T., U.S. surgeon, 1874–1939. SEE L.-Calvé-Perthes *disease.*

-legia. Reading, as distinguished from the G. derivatives, -lexis and -lexy, which signify speech. [L. *lego*, to read]

Le·gion·el·la (lē-jŭ-nel′lă). A genus of aerobic, motile, nonacid-fast, nonencapsulated, Gram-negative bacilli (family Legionellaceae) that have a nonfermentative metabolism and require L-cysteine HCl and iron salts for growth; they are water-dwelling, airborne-spread, and pathogenic for humans. Over 40 species have been identified; the type species is *L. pneumophila.*

L. bozeman′ii, a bacterial species that causes human pneumonia.

L. dumoffii, a bacterial species implicated in pneumonia.

L. feeleii, a bacterial species implicated in pneumonia.

L. gormanii, a bacterial species implicated in pneumonia.

L. longbeachae, a bacterial species implicated in pneumonia.

L. micda′dei, a bacterial species that may be acid-fast, and that causes Pittsburgh pneumonia, a variant of Legionnaires disease. Accounts for approximately 60% of *Legionella* pneumonias other than those caused by *L. pneumophila.* SYN Pittsburgh pneumonia agent.

L. pneumo′phila, a bacterial species that is the primary etiologic agent of Legionnaires disease; believed to grow in plumbing systems or in standing water in ventilation systems. The type species of the genus *L.*

L. wadsworthii, a bacterial species implicated in pneumonia.

le·gi·o·nel·lo·sis (lē-jŭ-nel-ō′sis). SYN Legionnaires *disease.*

le·gu·min (lĕ-goo′min, leg′oo-min). SYN avenin.

le·gu·mi·niv·o·rous (le-goo-mi-niv′ŏ-rŭs). Feeding on beans, peas, and other legumes.

Lehmann, J.O. Orla, Swedish physician, *1927. SEE Börjeson-Forssman-L. *syndrome.*

Leigh, Denis, British psychiatrist, *1915. SEE L. *disease.*

Leiner, Karl, Austrian pediatrician, 1871–1930. SEE L. *disease.*

leio-. Smooth. [G. *leios*]

lei·o·my·o·fi·bro·ma (lī-ō-mī′ō-fī-brō′mă). SYN fibroleiomyoma.

lei·o·my·o·ma (lī′ō-mī-ō′mă). A benign neoplasm derived from smooth (nonstriated) muscle. [leio- + G. *mys*, muscle, + *-oma*, tumor]

l. cu′tis, cutaneous eruption of multiple small painful nodules composed of smooth muscle fibers; derived from arrector muscles of hair. Solitary, nonpainful l. cutis may arise from cutaneous blood vessels and genital skin. SYN dermatomyoma.

parasitic l., a uterine l. which has become detached from the uterus and adherent to another peritoneal surface from which it derives a blood supply.

vascular l., a markedly vascular l., apparently arising from the smooth muscle of blood vessels. SYN angioleiomyoma, angiomyofibroma, angiomyoma.

lei·o·my·o·ma·to·sis (lī′ō-mī′ō-mă-tō′sis). The state of having multiple leiomyomas throughout the body.

l. peritonealis disseminata, a benign condition characterized by multiple small nodules on abdominal and pelvic peritoneum grossly mimicking disseminated ovarian cancer but with histologic characteristics of benign myoma; often associated with recent pregnancy.

lei·o·my·o·mec·to·my (līʹō-mī-ō-mekʹtō-mē). Surgical resection of a leiomyoma, usually of the uterus.

lei·o·my·o·sar·co·ma (līʹō-mīʹō-sar-kōʹmă). A malignant neoplasm derived from smooth (nonstriated) muscle. [leio- + myosarcoma]

lei·ot·ri·chous (lī-otʹri-kŭs). Having straight hair. [leio- + G. *thrix,* hair]

leipo-. SEE lipo-.

Leipzig yel·low [C.I. 77600]. SYN chrome yellow.

Leishman, Sir William B., Scottish surgeon, 1865–1926. SEE *Leishmania; L.* chrome *cells,* under *cell, stain; L.*-Donovan *body.*

Leish·man·ia (lēsh-manʹē-ă). A genus of digenetic, asexual, protozoan flagellates (family Trypanosomatidae) that occur as amastigotes in the macrophages of vertebrate hosts, and as promastigotes in invertebrate hosts and in cultures. Species are largely indistinguishable morphologically, but may be separated by clinical manifestations, geographic distribution and epidemiology, developmental patterns of promastigotes in their sandfly hosts, virulence testing of clones in vivo, the effect of test sera on growth in culture, cross-immunity tests, and serotyping with promastigote excreted factors; strains also can be distinguished by various biochemical analyses. Such procedures have identified all of the recognized groups and confirmed the separation of New World leishmaniasis agents into two species complexes, *L. mexicana* and *L. braziliensis.* [W. B. *Leishman*]

L. aethio'pica, an African species of *L.* responsible for human cutaneous leishmaniasis in Ethiopia, with a reservoir of human infection in the rock hyraxes, *Procavia capensis* and *Heterohyrax brucei,* and in Kenya, with reservoirs in the tree hyrax, *Dendrohyrax arboreus,* and the giant rat, *Cricetomys gambianus;* vectors are the sandflies *Phlebotomus longipes* and *P. pedifer.* It causes a cutaneous leishmaniasis of three types: classical oriental sore, mucocutaneous leishmaniasis, and diffuse cutaneous leishmaniasis; ulceration is late or absent and healing takes one to three years.

L. brazilien'sis, a species that is the causal agent of mucocutaneous leishmaniasis, endemic in southern Mexico and Central and South America, and transmitted by various species of *Lutzomyia* (New World sandflies); forest rodents and other neotropical arboreal animals serve as reservoir hosts. *L. braziliensis* is currently divided into three clinically, epidemiologically, and biochemically distinct strains or subspecies: *L. b. braziliensis, L. b. guyanensis,* and *L. b. panamensis.*

L. brazilien'sis brazilien'sis, the type subspecies of *L. braziliensis* and the agent of mucocutaneous leishmaniasis. A natural reservoir of infection remains unknown, but the proven vector in Brazil is *Lutzomyia (Psychodopygus) wellcomei;* other sandflies may also transmit the infection.

L. brazilien'sis guyanen'sis, a subspecies within the *L. braziliensis* complex from Brazil and Guyana, and the cause of the cutaneous leishmaniasis condition locally known as "pian bois"; the reservoir host in Brazil is the sloth *Choloepus hoffmani* and the vector is the sandfly *Lutzomyia umbratilis.*

L. brazilien'sis panamen'sis, a subspecies of *L. braziliensis* found in Panama, Colombia, and neighboring regions; it causes ulcerating lesions of cutaneous leishmaniasis which do not heal spontaneously and often involve nearby lymphatic tissues, but nasopharyngeal involvement is rare. The sloth *Choloepus hoffmani* is the reservoir in Panama and Costa Rica; the sandfly *Lutzomyia trapidoi* has been proven to be a vector.

L. donova'ni, a species that is the causal agent of visceral leishmaniasis in Mediterranean and adjacent countries, the south central section of the former USSR, eastern India, northern China, Kenya, Ethiopia, and the Sudan; also found in Brazil, Argentina, Colombia, and Venezuela; in the Old World, it is transmitted by various species of *Phlebotomus;* New World vectors are species of *Lutzomyia;* dogs and other carnivores are known as reservoir hosts in some areas. The intracellular amastigote form multiplies in macrophages and produces a reticuloendothelial hyperplasia grossly affecting the spleen and liver, with other lymphoid tissues being involved as well, resulting in severe hepatosplenomegaly, which usually is fatal if untreated.

L. donova'ni archibal'di, SEE *L. donovani donovani.*

L. donova'ni chaga'si, a subspecies of *L.* found in South America, chiefly in Brazil, producing visceral leishmaniasis; infections have been found in domestic dogs and in foxes, though the primary reservoir host is unclear. The vector remains undiscovered, and the taxonomic status of this subspecies is uncertain.

L. donova'ni donova'ni, the type subspecies and agent of visceral leishmaniasis in Asia, Africa, and the Indian subcontinent; a few cases occur in the south central section of the former USSR, and in Iran, Iraq, and possibly Yemen; the dog and jackal are animal reservoirs. The form in Africa may be this subspecies, though the name *L. donovani archibaldi* is also used.

L. donova'ni infan'tum, a strain or subspecies of *L. donovani* that causes visceral leishmaniasis in young children in Mediterranean countries; the reservoir is the domestic dog.

L. furunculo'sa, former name for *L. tropica.*

L. ma'jor, a species responsible for zoonotic cutaneous leishmaniasis in a large area of the Mediterranean region and Asia Minor. The animal reservoirs are usually ground squirrels, such as *Rhombomys opimus* in the former USSR and elsewhere in south central Asia, and other rodents in northwest India, the Middle East, and northern Africa; proven sandfly vectors include *Phlebotomus papatasi, P. duboscqi,* and *P. salehi.* SYN *L. tropica major.*

L. mexica'na, the agent of many forms of cutaneous leishmaniasis, now considered a complex of several subspecies or possibly species, each with distinctive DNA and enzyme characteristics, distribution, and vector-reservoir host association, resulting in distinct manifestations of human leishmaniasis; reservoir hosts are extremely diverse and include a wide array of arboreal rodents as well as marsupials, primates, and small carnivores. Typical disease forms caused by this species are chiclero ulcer and diffuse cutaneous leishmaniasis, in contrast with mucocutaneous leishmaniasis, more characteristic of *L. braziliensis* infection. SYN *L. tropica mexicana.*

L. mexica'na amazonen'sis, a particularly widespread form of *L. mexicana* in the Amazon basin (Bolivia, Brazil, Colombia, Ecuador, and southern Venezuela), where it infects a variety of forest rodents, the reservoirs of human infection. The disease is rare in humans, but the single or multiple lesions, when induced, rarely heal spontaneously; the disseminated form is common, but nasopharyngeal involvement does not occur. The vector is the sandfly *Lutzomyia flaviscutellata.*

L. mexica'na garnha'mi, a subspecies of *L. mexicana,* found in western Venezuela, causing single or multiple lesions in humans that heal spontaneously in about six months; the probable sandfly vector is *Lutzomyia townsendi.*

L. mexica'na mexica'na, a species described from Mexico, Guatemala, and Belize; agent of a form of New World cutaneous leishmaniasis called chiclero ulcer, associated with chicle gum and mahogany forest workers. The New World sandfly, *Lutzomyia olmeca,* is a proven vector of this subspecies.

L. mexica'na pifa'noi, a strain of *L. mexicana* accorded species status by those who consider it responsible for the diffuse or disseminated form of cutaneous leishmaniasis. It is responsible for this condition in Venezuela, where it was described, but it is now recognized that several species and subspecies of *L.* cause similar disseminated forms of leishmaniasis in widely separated regions (*L. mexicana amazonensis, L. aethiopica*); absence or suppression of the cell-mediated immune response in the host is also an important factor in induction of diffuse cutaneous leishmaniasis. SYN *L. pifanoi.*

L. mexica'na venezuelen'sis, a recently described subspecies of *L. mexicana* from Venezuela that causes indolent, nodular, single lesions of cutaneous leishmaniasis to develop, sometimes with curable disseminated cutaneous leishmaniasis; infection has also been found in equines.

L. peruvia'na, species of *L.* found infecting humans in the high

Le

Andean valleys of Peru and Bolivia; cause of a distinct form of New World cutaneous leishmaniasis called uta.

L. pifa'noi, SYN *L. mexicana pifanoi.*

L. trop'ica, species that is the causal agent of anthroponotic cutaneous leishmaniasis; formerly endemic throughout the Mediterranean basin, the Middle East, parts of the southern section of the area formerly known as the USSR and elsewhere in Asia, and also reported from western Africa; it is transmitted by *Phlebotomus papatasi, P. sergenti,* and related species of sandflies; small rodents such as various ground squirrels serve as reservoir hosts.

L. trop'ica ma'jor, SYN *L. major.*

L. trop'ica mexica'na, SYN *L. mexicana.*

leishmania, pl. **leishmaniae** (lēsh-man'ē-ă). A member of the genus *Leishmania.*

leishmaniae. Plural of leishmania.

leish·man·i·a·sis (lēsh'mă-nī'ă-sis). Infection with a species of *Leishmania* resulting in a clinically ill-defined group of diseases traditionally divided into four major types: 1) visceral l. (kala azar); 2) Old World cutaneous l.; 3) New World cutaneous l.; 4) mucocutaneous l. Each is clinically and geographically distinct and each has in recent years been subdivided further into clinical and epidemiological categories. Transmission is by various sandfly species of the genus *Phlebotomus* or *Lutzomyia.* SEE tropical *diseases,* under *disease.* SYN leishmaniosis.

acute cutaneous l., SYN zoonotic cutaneous l.

American l., l. america'na, SYN mucocutaneous l.

anergic l., SYN diffuse cutaneous l.

anthroponotic cutaneous l., a form of Old World cutaneous l., usually with a prolonged incubation period and confined to urban areas. SYN chronic cutaneous l., dry cutaneous l., urban cutaneous l.

canine l., a mild infection of dogs, usually confined to the muzzle or ears, produced by human disease-causing species of *Leishmania;* dogs therefore are important reservoirs of human infection, such as with visceral l. in the Mediterranean region.

chronic cutaneous l., SYN anthroponotic cutaneous l.

cutaneous l., infection with promastigotes (leptomonads) of *Leishmania tropica* and of *L. major* inoculated into the skin by the bite of an infected sandfly, *Phlebotomus* (commonly *P. papatasi*); it is endemic in parts of Asia Minor, northern Africa, and India, and is known by innumerable names, including tropical sores, tropical ulcers, and other indications of locality (e.g., Aleppo, Baghdad, Delhi, or Jericho boil; Aden ulcer; Biskra button); the ulcer begins as a papule that enlarges to a nodule and then breaks down into an ulcer. Leishmanial cells are seen within histiocytes in hematoxylin and eosin–stained tissue sections. Two distinctive clinical and epidemiological diseases are recognized: the more common and widespread zoonotic rural disease with a moist acute form, caused by *L. major,* with reservoir rodent hosts, and an urban, anthroponotic, dry, chronic form of l. caused by *L. tropica,* without a reservoir host, and now largely controlled. SEE zoonotic cutaneous l., anthroponotic cutaneous l. SYN Old World l.

diffuse l., SYN diffuse cutaneous l.

diffuse cutaneous l., l. caused by several New and Old World species and strains of *Leishmania* (*L. mexicana amazonensis, L. m. pifanoi,* possibly *L. m. garnhami* and *L. m. venezuelensis;* in Ethiopia, *L. aethiopica,* and unidentified leishmanial agents in Namibia and Tanzania). The condition is associated with a suppressed cell-mediated immune response, so that the nonulcerating, nonnecrotizing cutaneous lesions can spread widely over the body; great numbers of parasite-filled macrophages are found in the dermal lesions. Healing does not appear to occur unless an acquired cellular hypersensitivity can develop. SYN anergic l., diffuse l., disseminated cutaneous l., l. tegumentaria diffusa, pseudolepromatous l.

disseminated cutaneous l., SYN diffuse cutaneous l.

dry cutaneous l., SYN anthroponotic cutaneous l.

infantile l., visceral l. in infants, from *Leishmania donovani infantum.*

lupoid l., SYN l. recidivans.

mucocutaneous l., a grave disease caused by *Leishmania brazili-*

ensis braziliensis, endemic in southern Mexico and Central and South America, except for the equatorial region of Chile; the organism does not invade the viscera, and the disease is limited to the skin and mucous membranes, the lesions resembling the sores of cutaneous l. caused by *L. mexicana* or *L. tropica;* the chancrous sores heal after a time, but some months or years later, fungating and eroding forms of ulceration may appear on the tongue and buccal or nasal mucosa; many variants of the disease exist, marked by differences in distribution, vector, epidemiology, and pathology, which suggest that it may in fact be caused by a number of closely related etiologic agents. SEE ALSO espundia. SYN American l., l. americana, bubas, nasopharyngeal l., New World l.

nasopharyngeal l., SYN mucocutaneous l.

New World l., SYN mucocutaneous l.

Old World l., SYN cutaneous l.

pseudolepromatous l., SYN diffuse cutaneous l.

l. recid'ivans, a partially healing leishmanial lesion caused by *Leishmania tropica* and characterized by an extreme form of cellular immune response, intense granuloma production, fibrinoid necrosis without caseation, and frequent development of satellite lesions that continue the production of granulomatous tissue without healing, sometimes over a period of many years; organisms are difficult to demonstrate but can be cultured. SYN lupoid l.

rural cutaneous l., SYN zoonotic cutaneous l.

l. tegumenta'ria diffu'sa, SYN diffuse cutaneous l.

urban cutaneous l., SYN anthroponotic cutaneous l.

visceral l., (**1**) a chronic disease, occurring in India, China, Pakistan, the Mediterranean littoral, the Middle East, South and Central America, Asia, and Africa caused by *Leishmania donovani* and transmitted by the bite of an appropriate species of sandfly of the genus *Phlebotomus* or *Lutzomyia;* the organisms grow and multiply in macrophages, eventually causing them to burst and liberate amastigote parasites which then invade other macrophages; proliferation of macrophages in the bone marrow causes crowding out of erythroid and myeloid elements, resulting in leukopenia, and anemia, splenomegaly, and hepatomegaly which are characteristic, along with enlargement of lymph nodes; fever, fatigue, malaise, and secondary infections also occur; different strains of *L. donovani* occur; *L. infantum* in Eurasia, *L. chagasi* in Latin America. (**2**) visceral l. caused by *Leishmania tropica,* cultured from bone marrow aspirates of some military patients following the Gulf War. SYN Assam fever, black sickness, Burdwan fever, cachectic fever, Dumdum fever, kala azar, tropical splenomegaly.

wet cutaneous l., SYN zoonotic cutaneous l.

zoonotic cutaneous l., a form of cutaneous l. characterized by rural distribution of human cases near infected rodents, particularly communal ground squirrels; characterized by acute rapidly developing dermal lesions that become severely inflamed, with moist necrotizing sores or ulcers that heal in 2–8-months after a 2–4-month incubation period; among nonimmune immigrants, multiple lesions may develop, which heal more slowly and leave disabling or disfiguring scars. A strong delayed hypersensitivity and involvement of immune complexes play a role in necrosis, which is part of the healing process and of the strong specific immunity that follows. SYN acute cutaneous l., rural cutaneous l., wet cutaneous l.

leish·man·i·o·sis (lēsh'man-ē-ō'sis). SYN leishmaniasis.

leish·man·oid (lēsh'mă-noyd). Resembling leishmaniasis.

dermal l., SYN post-kala azar dermal l.

post-kala azar dermal l., a chronic, progressive, granulomatous, nonulcerating hypopigmented nodular cutaneous eruption that may appear 6 months to 5 years after spontaneous or drug cure of visceral leishmaniasis (kala azar); this condition was first described in India and is most characteristic of kala azar in that country. SYN dermal l.

Leiter, Russell G., U.S. psychologist, *1901. SEE L. International Performance *Scale.*

Lejeune, Jerôme J.L.M., French cytogeneticist, 1926–1994. SEE L. *syndrome.*

Lembert, Antoine, French surgeon, 1802–1851. SEE L. *suture;* Czerny-L. *suture.*

le·mic (lē′mik). Relating to plague or any epidemic disease. [G. *loimos,* plague]

Le·min·or·ella (lem′in-ŏ-rel′ă). A genus in the family Enterobacteriaceae containing two species, *Leminorella grimontii* and *Leminorella richardii,* that have been isolated from clinical material, primarily from fecal samples; its clinical importance is unclear at present.

Lemli, Luc, 20th century U.S. pediatrician. SEE Smith-L.-Opitz *syndrome.*

lem·mo·blast (lem′ō-blast). In an embryo, a cell of neural crest origin capable of forming a cell of the neurilemma sheath. [G. *lemma,* husk, + *blastos,* germ]

lem·mo·cyte (lem′ō-sīt). One of the cells of the neurolemma. [G. *lemma,* husk, + *kytos,* cell]

lem·nis·cus, pl. **lem·nis·ci** (lem-nis′kŭs, -nis′ī) [TA]. A bundle of nerve fibers ascending from sensory relay nuclei to the thalamus. SYN fillet (1). [L. from G. *lēmniskos,* ribbon or fillet]

acoustic l., SYN lateral l.

auditory l., SYN lateral l.

gustatory l., the uncrossed secondary-sensory fiber system ascending from the rhombencephalic gustatory nucleus to the parabrachial nuclei (rostral pontine level) and directly to the thalamic gustatory nucleus (ventral postero-medial nucleus, pars parvicellularis).

lateral l. [TA], a bundle of ascending fibers that originate from the cochlear and auditory relay nuclei of the rhombencephalon, enter the trapezoid body, a transverse fiber stratum in which about half their number decussate, and from here turn rostrally along the lateral side of the spinothalamic tract; in the midbrain, it arches dorsally and enters the inferior colliculus in which all of its fibers terminate; the auditory pathway is transsynaptically extended from here by the brachium of the inferior colliculus to the medial geniculate body of the thalamus, from which in turn the auditory radiation leads to the auditory cortex; intercalated in the trapezoid body and along the ascending trajectory of the l. are several cell groups in which part of the fibers synapse. SYN l. lateralis [TA], acoustic l., auditory l., auditory tract, lateral fillet.

l. latera′lis [TA], SYN lateral l.

medial l. [TA], a band of white fibers originating from the gracile and cuneate nuclei and decussating in the lower medulla; thence it passes upward through the center of the medulla oblongata, close to the median raphe; on entering the pons it spreads out laterally to form a flat band ascending over the dorsal border of the pontine nuclei; in the mesencephalon it passes over the dorsal border of the substantia nigra and is displaced laterally by the red nucleus; passing medial to the medial geniculate body, the bundle enters and terminates in the ventral posterior nucleus of the thalamus. Throughout their course, the fibers retain a somatotopic order such that those originating from the gracile nucleus and representing the lower extremity lie lateral to those originating in the cuneate nucleus and representing the arm. The medial l. conveys somatic-sensory information involved in tactile discrimination (two-point discrimination), position sense, and vibration sense. SYN l. medialis [TA], medial fillet, Reil band (2), Reil ribbon.

l. media′lis [TA], SYN medial l.

spinal l. [TA], SYN spinothalamic *tract.*

l. spina′lis [TA], SYN spinothalamic *tract.*

trigeminal l. [TA], collective term denoting the fibers ascending from the sensory nuclei of the trigeminus; one such fiber system originates from the spinal trigeminal nucleus and from the principal sensory nucleus, decussates, and ascends as the anterior trigeminothalamic tract [TA] (ventral trigeminothalamic tract [TAalt]) in close association with the medial l. with which it enters the ventrobasal complex to terminate in the ventral posteromedial nucleus; a second, uncrossed, fiber group originating from the principal sensory nucleus that follows an ascending course through central parts of the mesencephalic tegmentum as the posterior trigeminothalamic tract [TA] (dorsal trigeminothalamic tract [TAalt]) also to terminate in the ventral posteromedial nucleus. The trigeminal l. conveys tactile, pain, and temperature impulses from the skin of the face, the mucous membranes of the nasal and oral cavities, and the eye, as well as proprioceptive information from the facial and masticatory muscles. SYN l. trigeminalis [TA].

l. trigemina′lis [TA], SYN trigeminal l.

lem·on (lem′ŏn). The fruit of *Citrus limon* (family Rutaceae); a source of citric and ascorbic acid; the freshly expressed juice of the ripe fruit is used as a refrigerant diuretic in fever, in the form of lemonade. SYN limon. [L. *limon*]

lem·on yel·low. SYN chrome yellow.

Lendrum, A.C., 20th century Scottish pathologist. SEE L. phloxine-tartrazine *stain;* Fraser-L. *stain* for fibrin.

Lenègre, Jean, 20th century French cardiologist. SEE L. *disease, syndrome.*

length (l). Linear distance between two points.

arch l., the amount of space required for the permanent teeth as measured from the mesial aspect of the first molar on one side to the mesial aspect of the first molar on the opposite side, as measured through the contact points along an imaginary line of the dental arch.

available arch l., the amount of space available for the permanent teeth around the dental arch from first permanent molar to first permanent molar.

crown-heel l. (CH, CHL), l. of an outstretched embryo or fetus from skull vertex to heel. SEE Streeter developmental horizon(s).

crown-rump l. (CR, CRL), a measurement from the skull vertex to the midpoint between the apices of the buttocks of an embryo or fetus, that permits approximation of embryonic or fetal age.

greatest l., measurement from the cranial to caudal end of the embryo prior to folding.

required arch l., the sum of the mesiodistal widths of the permanent teeth from first permanent molar to first permanent molar.

resting l., the length at rest from which a muscle develops maximum isometric tension.

spinal l. (SL), a measurement from the distal surface of the embryo where the plane passes through the developing eye (this is the cranial limit of the spinal cord) down to the rump.

Lenhossék, Michael (Mihály) von, Hungarian anatomist, 1863–1937. SEE L. *processes,* under *process.*

len·i·tive (len′i-tiv). **1.** Soothing; relieving discomfort or pain. **2.** Rarely used term for a demulcent. [L. *lenio,* pp. *lenitus,* to soften, fr. *lenis,* mild]

Lennert, Karl, *1921. SEE L. *lymphoma, classification.*

Lennox, William G., U.S. neurologist, 1884–1960. SEE L. *syndrome;* L.-Gastaut *syndrome.*

Lenoir, Camille A.H., French anatomist, *1867. SEE L. *facet.*

lens (lenz) [TA]. **1.** A transparent material with one or both surfaces having a concave or convex curve; acts upon electromagnetic energy to cause convergence or divergence of light rays. **2** [TA]. The transparent biconvex cellular refractive structure lying between the iris and the vitreous humor, consisting of a soft outer part (cortex) with a denser part (nucleus), and surrounded by a basement membrane (capsule); the anterior surface has a cuboidal epithelium, and at the equator the cells elongate to become lens fibers. SYN crystalline l. [L. a lentil]

achromatic l., a compound l. made of two or more l.'s having different indices of refraction, so correlated as to minimize chromatic aberration.

acoustic l., in ultrasonography, a l. used to focus or diverge a sound beam; may be simulated by electronic manipulation of signals.

aplanatic l., a l. designed to correct spherical aberration and coma (*q.v.*). SYN periscopic meniscus.

apochromatic l., a compound l. designed to correct both spherical and chromatic aberrations.

aspheric l., a l. with a paraboloidal surface that eliminates spherical aberration.

astigmatic l., SYN cylindrical l.

bandage contact l., a contact l. placed on the cornea to cover a defect.

le

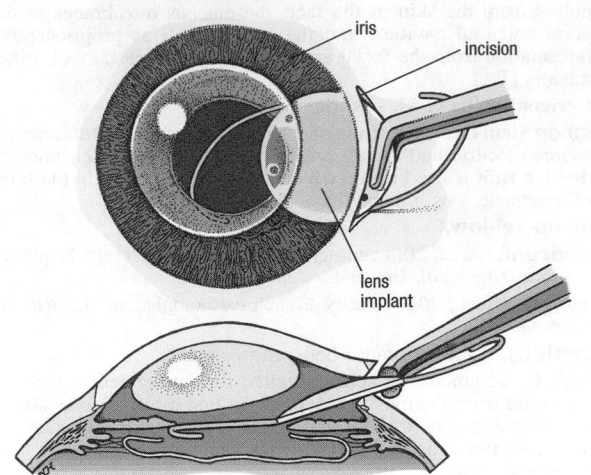

intraocular lens implant: being inserted into the anterior chamber of the eye

biconcave l., a l. that is concave on two opposing surfaces. SYN concavoconcave l., double concave l.

biconvex l., a l. with both surfaces convex. SYN convexoconvex l., double convex l.

bifocal l., a l. used in cases of presbyopia, in which one portion is suited for distant vision, the other for reading and close work in general; the reading addition may be cemented to the l., fused to the front surface, or ground in one-piece form; other bifocal l.'s are the flat-top Franklin type, or blended invisible.

cataract l., any l. prescribed for aphakia.

l. clock, SYN Geneva lens *measure.*

compound l., an optical system of two or more lenses.

concave l., a diverging minus power lens. SYN minus l.

concavoconcave l., SYN biconcave l.

concavoconvex l., a converging meniscus l. that is concave on one surface and convex on the opposite surface.

contact l., a l. that fits over the cornea and sclera or cornea only; used to correct refractive errors.

convex l., a converging l. SYN plus l.

convexoconcave l., a minus power l. having one surface convex and the opposite surface concave, with the latter having the greater curvature.

convexoconvex l., SYN biconvex l.

corneal l., contact l. of plastic without scleral portions.

crystalline l., SYN lens (2).

cylindrical l. (cyl., C), a l. in which one of the surfaces is curved in one meridian and less curved in the opposite meridian; e.g., a teaspoon or a football. SYN astigmatic l.

decentered l., a l. so mounted that the visual axis does not pass through the axis of the l.

dislocation of l., SYN *ectopia* lentis.

double concave l., SYN biconcave l.

double convex l., SYN biconvex l.

eye l., the upper of the two planoconvex l.'s of Huygens ocular. SYN ocular l.

field l., the lower of the two planoconvex l.'s of Huygens ocular.

foldable intraocular l., a l. often made of silicone or an acrylic polymer that may be doubled over for implantation into the eye following cataract removal.

Fresnel l., a l. with a surface consisting of a concentric series of zones that duplicate the power of a l. or prism but with less thickness. SYN lighthouse l.

Hruby l., a non–contact l. mounted on a slitlamp used for evaluating the retina.

immersion l., an objective (for a microscope) constructed in such a manner that the lower l. may be moved downward into direct contact with a fluid which is placed on the object being examined;

by using a fluid with a refractive index closely similar to that of glass, the loss of light is minimized.

lighthouse l., SYN Fresnel l.

meniscus l., a l. having a spherical concave curve on one side and a spherical convex curve on the other. SYN articular crescent, articular meniscus, intraarticular cartilage (2), meniscus articularis, meniscus (1).

minus l., SYN concave l.

multifocal l., a l. with segments providing two or more powers; commonly, a trifocal l.

ocular l., SYN eye l.

omnifocal l., a l. for near and distant vision in which the reading portion is a continuously variable curve.

orthoscopic l., a spectacle l. corrected for distortion and curvature of the periphery.

periscopic l., a lens with 1.25 D base curve.

photochromic l., a light-sensitive spectacle l. that reduces light transmission in sunlight and increases transmission in reduced light.

planoconcave l., a l. that is flat on one side and concave on the other.

planoconvex l., a l. that is flat on one side and convex on the other.

plus l., SYN convex l.

safety l., a l. that meets government specifications of impact resistance; the increased impact resistance required for safety l.'s is obtained by tempering, by an ion-exchange process, or by using laminated or plastic l.'s.

slab-off l., a spectacle l. with a base-up prism below; used in unequal myopia to equalize image displacement when reading.

spherical l. (S, sph.), a l. in which all refracting surfaces are spherical.

spherocylindrical l., a combined spherical and cylindrical l., one surface being spherical, the other cylindrical. SYN spherocylinder.

toric l., a lens in which both meridians are curved but not to the same degree.

trial l.'s, a series of cylindrical and spherical l.'s used in testing vision.

trifocal l., a l. with segments of three focal powers: distant, intermediate, and near.

lens clock. See under lens.

lens·ec·to·my (len-sek'tō-mē). Removal of the lens of the eye by an infusion-aspiration cutter; often done by puncture incision through the pars plana in the course of vitrectomy. [lens + G. *ektomē,* excision]

lens·om·e·ter (len-zom'ĕ-ter). An instrument to measure the power and cylindrical axis of a spectacle lens. SYN focimeter, vertometer. [lens + G. *metron,* measure]

lens·op·a·thy (lenz-op'ă-thē). The process by which tear proteins are deposited on a contact lens. [lens + G. *pathos,* suffering]

len·ti·co·nus (len-ti-kō'nŭs). Conical projection of the anterior or posterior surface of the lens of the eye, occurring as a developmental anomaly. [lens + L. *conus,* cone]

len·tic·u·la (len-tik'ū-lă). SYN lentiform *nucleus.* [L. dim. of *lens*]

len·tic·u·lar (len-tik'ū'lăr). **1.** Relating to or resembling a lens of any kind. **2.** Of the shape of a lentil. [L. *lenticula,* a lentil]

len·tic·u·lo-op·tic (len-tik'ū-lō-op'tik). Relating to the lentiform nucleus and the optic tract; specifically refers to branches of the middle cerebral artery considered to supply these structures.

len·tic·u·lo·pap·u·lar (len-tik'ū-lō-pap'ū-lăr). Indicating an eruption with dome-shaped or lens-shaped papules.

len·tic·u·lo·stri·ate (len-tik'ū-lō-strī'āt). Relating to the lenticular nucleus and the caudate nucleus; specifically refers to branches of the middle cerebral artery supplying these gray masses.

len·tic·u·lo·tha·lam·ic (len-tik'ū-lō-tha-lam'ik). Pertaining to the lentiform (lenticular) nucleus and the thalamus.

len·tic·u·lus, pl. **len·tic·u·li** (len-tik'ū-lŭs, -lī). Seldom-used term for an intraocular lens prosthesis placed in the anterior or posterior chamber of the eye, or attached to the iris after cataract extraction. SYN prosthetophacos, pseudophacos. [L. dim. of *lens, lentis,* a little lens]

len·ti·form (len'ti-fōrm). Lens-shaped.

len·tig·i·nes (len-tij'i-nēz). Plural of lentigo. [L.]

len·tig·i·no·sis (len-tij-i-nō'sis). Presence of lentigines in very large numbers or in a distinctive configuration.

  centrofacial l. [MIM*151000 & MIM*151001], uncommon autosomal dominant syndrome of small hyperpigmented macules in a horizontal band across the center of the face at one year, increasing in number up to ten years, and associated with skeletal and neural defects.

  generalized l., lentigines occurring singly or in groups from infancy onward.

len·ti·glo·bus (len-ti-glō'bŭs). Rare congenital anomaly with a spheroid elevation on the posterior surface of the lens of the eye. [lens + L. *globus,* sphere]

len·ti·go, pl. **len·tig·i·nes** (len-tī'gō, len-tij'i-nēz). A benign, acquired brown macule resembling a freckle except that the border is usually regular and microscopic elongation of rete ridges is present, with increased melanocytes and melanin pigment in the basal cell layer. SEE ALSO junction *nevus.* SYN l. simplex. [L. fr. *lens (lent-),* a lentil]

  l. maligna, a brown or black mottled, irregularly outlined, slowly enlarging lesion resembling a l. in which there are increased numbers of scattered atypical melanocytes in the epidermis, usually occurring on the face of older persons; after many years the dermis may be invaded and the lesion is then termed l. maligna melanoma. SYN Hutchinson freckle, melanotic freckle.

  senile l., a variably pigmented benign l. occurring on exposed skin of older white persons. SYN liver spot, solar l.

  l. simplex, SYN lentigo.

  solar l., SYN senile l.

Len·ti·vir·i·nae (len'ti-vir'i-nē). Term formerly used to describe a subfamily of nononcogenic viruses (family Retroviridae) that includes the slow viruses of sheep (visna virus and maedi virus) and human T-cell lymphotropic viruses, including human immunodeficiency viruses 1 and 2. The viruses resemble the C-type RNA tumor viruses (Oncovirinae) in many ways, including production of reverse transcriptase. [L. *lentus,* sluggish, slow]

len·ti·vi·rus (len'ti-vī-rŭs). A genus in the family Retroviridae containing 5 serogroups that reflect the host with which they are associated. Among the primate lentiviruses are human immunodeficiency viruses 1 and 2.

len·to·gen·ic (len-tō-jen'ik). Denoting the virulence of a virus capable of inducing lethal infection in embryonic hosts after a long incubation period and an inapparent infection in immature and adult hosts; the term is used in characterizing Newcastle disease virus, particularly strains used as vaccines administered in water or as sprays, i.e., mild or avirulent strains. [L. *lentus,* sluggish, inactive, + G. *-gen,* producing]

len·tu·la, len·tu·lo (len'tū-lă, -lō). A motorized, flexible, spiral wire instrument used in dentistry to apply paste filling material into the root canal(s) of a tooth. [L. *lentus,* pliant, flexible]

le·on·ti·a·sis (lē-on-tī'ă-sis). The ridges and furrows on the forehead and cheeks of patients with advanced lepromatous leprosy, giving a leonine appearance. SYN leonine facies. [G. *leōn (leont-),* lion]

  l. os'sea, SYN megacephaly.

LEOPARD [MIM*151100] Acronym for *l*entigines (multiple), *e*lectrocardiographic abnormalities, *o*cular hypertelorism, *p*ulmonary stenosis, *a*bnormalities of genitalia, *r*etardation of growth, and *d*eafness (sensorineural); of autosomal dominant inheritance.

leop·ard's bane. SYN arnica.

Leopold, Christian Gerhard, German physician, 1846–1911. SEE L. *maneuvers,* under *maneuver.*

Lepehne, Georg, German physician, *1887. SEE L.-Pickworth *stain.*

lep·er (lep'er). A person who has leprosy. [G. *lepra*]

le·pid·ic (lĕ-pid'ik). Relating to scales or a scaly covering layer. [G. *lepis (lepid-),* scale, rind]

Lep·i·dop·tera (lep-i-dop'ter-ă). An order of insects composed of

the moths and butterflies, characterized by wings covered with delicate scales. [G. *lepis,* scale, + *pteron,* wing]

Lep·or·i·pox·vi·rus (lep'ō-ri-poks'vī-rŭs). The genus of viruses (family Poxviridae) that comprises the fibroma and myxoma viruses of rabbits; unlike the orthopoxviruses, they are ether-sensitive. [L. *leporis,* gen. of *lepus,* a hare, + virus]

lep·o·thrix (lep'ō-thriks). SYN *trichomycosis* axillaris. [G. *lepos,* rind, husk, + *thrix,* hair]

lep·re·chaun·ism (lep'rĕ-kawn-izm) [MIM*246200]. A congenital form of dwarfism characterized by extreme growth retardation, endocrine disorders, and emaciation, with elfin facies and large, low-set ears; autosomal recessive inheritance; caused by mutation in the insulin receptor gene (INSR) on 19p. SYN Donohue disease, Donohue syndrome. [Irish *leprechaun,* elf]

lep·rid. Early cutaneous lesion of leprosy. [G. *lepra,* leprosy, + *-id* (1)]

le·pro·ma (lĕ-prō'mă). A fairly well-circumscribed discrete focus of granulomatous inflammation, caused by *Mycobacterium leprae,* which consists chiefly of an accumulation of large mononuclear phagocytic cells in which the cytoplasm seems finely vacuolated (i.e., foam cells); the foamlike character of the macrophages is related to the engulfing of numerous acid-fast organisms. [G. *lepros,* scaly, + *-oma,* tumor]

lep·rom·a·tous (lep-rō'mă-tŭs). Pertaining to, or characterized by, the features of a leproma.

lep·ro·min (lep'rō-min). An extract of tissue infected with *Mycobacterium leprae* used in skin tests to classify the stage of leprosy. SEE ALSO lepromin *reaction,* test.

lep·ro·sar·i·um (lep'rō-sar'ē-ŭm). A hospital especially designed for the care of those suffering from leprosy, especially those who need expert care.

lep·ro·sery (lep'rō-ser-ē). A leper home or colony.

lep·ro·stat·ic (lep-rō-stat'ik). **1.** Inhibiting to the growth of *Mycobacterium leprae.* **2.** An agent having this action.

lep·ro·sy (lep'rō-sē). **1.** A chronic granulomatous infection caused by *Mycobacterium leprae* affecting the cooler body parts, especially the skin, peripheral nerves, and testes. L. is classified into two main types, lepromatous and tuberculoid, representing extremes of immunologic response. **2.** A name used in the Bible to describe various cutaneous diseases, especially those of a chronic or contagious nature, which probably included psoriasis and leukoderma. SYN Hansen disease. [G. *lepra,* from *lepros,* scaly]

  anesthetic l., a form of l. chiefly affecting the nerves, marked by hyperesthesia succeeded by anesthesia, and by paralysis, ulceration, and various trophic disturbances, terminating in gangrene and mutilation. SYN Danielssen disease, Danielssen-Boeck disease, dry l., trophoneurotic l.

  borderline l., a form of l. that is very unstable immunologically; the cutaneous nerves frequently contain bacilli, but the lepromin test is usually negative; cutaneous lesions are composed of flat bands or plaques. SYN dimorphous l.

  dimorphous l., SYN borderline l.

  dry l., SYN anesthetic l.

  histoid l., a form of lepromatous l. with lesions microscopically resembling dermatofibroma or other spindle-celled tumors.

  indeterminate l., a transitory form of l. in which the immunologic status is not yet formed, and the histologic and clinical features are not yet characteristic of any of the major types of l.

  lepromatous l., a form of l. in which nodular cutaneous lesions are infiltrated, have ill-defined borders, and are bacteriologically positive; the lepromin test is negative, i.e., the immunologic mechanism of the patient is not responsive to the *Mycobacterium leprae* infection.

  Lucio l., an acute form occurring in pure diffuse lepromatous l. presenting irregularly shaped, intensely erythematous, tender plaques, especially of the legs, with tendency to ulceration and scarring. SYN Lucio leprosy phenomenon.

  macular l., a form of tuberculoid l. in which the lesions are small, hairless, and dry, and are erythematous in light skin and hypopigmented or copper-colored in dark skin.

  mutilating l., a late stage of anesthetic l.

le

nodular l., SYN tuberculoid l.

smooth l., SYN tuberculoid l.

trophoneurotic l., SYN anesthetic l.

tuberculoid l., a benign, stable, and resistant form of the disease in which the lepromin reaction is strongly positive and in which the lesions are erythematous, insensitive, infiltrated plaques with clear-cut edges. SYN nodular l., smooth l.

lep·rot·ic (lep-rot'ik). SYN leprous.

lep·rous (lep'rŭs). Relating to or suffering from leprosy. SYN leprotic.

⌂-lepsis, -lepsy. A seizure. [G. *lēpsis*]

lep·tan·dra (lep-tān'dră). Dried rhizome and roots of *Veronicastrum virginicum* (family Serophulariaceae). Indigenous to North America. Formerly used as a cathartic. SYN black root, Culver root.

lep·tin (lep'tin). A helical protein secreted by adipose tissue and acting on a receptor site in the ventromedial nucleus of the hypothalamus to curb appetite and increase energy expenditure as body fat stores increase. L. levels are 40% higher in women, and show a further 50% rise just before menarche, later returning to baseline levels; levels are lowered by fasting and increased by inflammation. [G. leptos, thin, + -in]

> Human genes encoding both leptin (locus 7q31.3) and the leptin receptor site (1p31) have been identified. Laboratory mice having mutations on the ob gene, which encodes leptin, become morbidly obese, diabetic, and infertile; administration of leptin to these mice improves glucose tolerance, increases physical activity, reduces body weight by 30%, and restores fertility. Mice with mutations of the db gene, which encodes the leptin receptor, also become obese and diabetic but do not improve with administration of leptin. Although mutations in both the leptin and leptin receptor genes have been found in a small number of morbidly obese human subjects with abnormal eating behavior, the majority of obese persons do not show such mutations, and have normal or elevated circulating levels of leptin. Leptin enhances insulin-mediated glucose transport into adipose cells in vitro. In preliminary trials, both lean and overweight persons have shown modest weight loss with daily subcutaneous injections of recombinant methionyl human leptin over several months. All subjects followed weight-reduction diets during the trial period. Weight loss in some subjects receiving leptin did not exceed that achieved by subjects receiving placebo, but when significant weight reduction occurred, it was proportionate to dosage. The immune deficiency seen in starvation may result from diminished leptin secretion. Mice lacking the gene for leptin or its receptor show impairment of T-cell function, and in laboratory studies leptin has induced a proliferative response in human CD4 lymphocytes.

⌂lepto-. Light, thin, frail. [G. *leptos,* slender, delicate, weak]

lep·to·ceph·a·lous (lep-tō-sef'ă-lŭs). Having an abnormally tall, narrow cranium. [lepto- + G. *kephalē,* head]

lep·to·ceph·a·ly (lep-tō-sef'ă-lē). A malformation characterized by an abnormally tall, narrow cranium. [lepto- + G. *kephalē,* head]

lep·to·chro·mat·ic (lep'tō-krō-mat'ik). Having a very fine chromatin network.

lep·to·cyte (lep'tō-sīt). A target or Mexican hat cell, i.e., an unusually thin or flattened red blood cell in which there is a central rounded area of pigmented material, a middle clear zone that contains no pigment, and an outer pigmented rim at the edge of the cell. L.'s are thought to be erythrocytes in which the cellular envelope or membrane is unusually large in proportion to its contents. [lepto- + G. *kytos,* cell]

lep·to·cy·to·sis (lep'tō-sī-tō'sis). The presence of leptocytes in the circulating blood, as in thalassemia, some instances of jaundice (even in the absence of anemia), occasional examples of hepatic disease (in the absence of jaundice), and some patients who have had the spleen removed.

lep·to·dac·ty·lous (lep-tō-dak'ti-lŭs). Having slender fingers. [lepto- + G. *daktylos,* finger]

lep·to·me·nin·ge·al (lep'tō-me-nin'jē-ăl). Pertaining to the leptomeninges.

lep·to·me·nin·ges, lep·to·me·ninx, sing. **lep·to·me·ninx** (lep-tō-me-nin'jēz, lep'tō-mē'ninks, lep'tō-mē'ninks) [TA]. SYN leptomeninx. [lepto- + G. *mēninx,* pl. *mēninges,* membrane]

lep·to·men·in·gi·tis (lep'tō-men-in-jī'tis). Inflammation of leptomeninges. SEE ALSO arachnoiditis. SYN pia-arachnitis.

basilar l., inflammation of the arachnoid at the base of the brain; often found in chronic meningitis of tuberculous, luetic, or mycotic origin.

lep·to·mere (lep'tō-mēr). A very minute particle of living matter; Asclepiades believed the body was composed of an aggregation of vast numbers of l.'s. [lepto- + G. *meros,* part]

lep·to·mo·nad (lep'tō-mō'nad, lep-tom'ŏ-nad). 1. Common name for a member of the genus *Leptomonas*. 2. SEE promastigote.

Lep·tom·o·nas (lep'tō-mō'nas, lep-tom'ŏ-nŭs). A genus of asexual, monogenetic, parasitic flagellates (family Trypanosomatidae) commonly found in the hindgut of insects. [lepto- + G. *monas,* unit]

lep·to·ne·ma (lep-tō-nē'mă). SYN leptotene. [lepto- + G. *nēma,* thread]

lep·to·pho·nia (lep'tō-fō'nē-ă). SYN hypophonia. [lepto- + G. *phōnē,* sound, voice]

lep·to·phon·ic (lep'tō-fon'ik). Weak-voiced.

lep·to·po·dia (lep-tō-pō'dē-ă). The condition of having slender feet. [lepto- + G. *pous,* foot]

lep·to·pro·so·pia (lep'tō-prō-sō'pē-ă). Narrowness of the face. [lepto- + G. *prosōpon,* face]

lep·to·pro·so·pic (lep'tō-prō-sō'pik). Having a thin, narrow face. Cf. leptosomatic.

lep·tor·rhine (lep'tō-rīn). Having a thin nose. Applied to a skull with a nasal index below 47 (Frankfort agreement) or 48 (Broca). [lepto- + G. *rhis,* nose]

lep·to·scope (lep'tō-skōp). An apparatus for measuring cell membranes.

lep·to·so·mat·ic, lep·to·som·ic (lep'tō-sō-mat'ik, -tō-sō'mik). Having a slender, light, or thin body. [lepto- + G. *sōma,* body]

Lep·to·spi·ra (lep'tō-spī'ră). A genus of motile aerobic bacteria (order Spirochaetales) containing thin, tightly coiled organisms 6–20 μm in length. They possess an axial filament, and one or both ends may be bent into a semicircular hook. They stain with difficulty except with Giemsa stain or silver impregnation. Associated with icterohemorrhagic fever. They include 7 pathogens and 3 nonpathogenic species; the type species is *L. interrogans*. [lepto- + G. *speira,* a coil]

L. inter'rogans, a species containing multiple named pathogenic serovars. Causative agent of leptospirosis. It is the type species of the genus *L*.

lep·to·spire (lep'tō-spīr). Common name for any organism belonging to the genus *Leptospira*.

lep·to·spi·ro·sis (lep'tō-spī-rō'sis). Infection with *Leptospira interrogans*.

anicteric l., infection with one of the species of the *Leptospira* group, usually mild, with limited liver and kidney involvement, as opposed to Weil *disease*.

l. icterohemorrhagica (ik'ter-ō-hem-ōr-aj'ĭ-kă), SYN icterohemorrhagic *fever*.

lep·to·spi·ru·ria (lep'tō-spī-roo'rē-ă). Presence of species of the genus *Leptospira* in the urine, as a result of leptospirosis in the renal tubules.

lep·to·tene (lep'tō-tēn). Early stage of prophase in meiosis in which the chromosomes contract and become visible as long filaments well separated from each other. SYN leptonema. [lepto- + G. *tainia,* band, tape]

lep·to·thri·co·sis (lep'tō-thri-kō'sis). Obsolete term for any disease caused by the now invalid genus *Leptothrix*.

Lep·to·thrix (lep′tō-thriks). A now invalid genus of sheathed organisms closely related to the genus *Sphaerotilus* found in fresh water.

Lep·to·trich·ia (lep-tō-trik′ē-ă). A genus of anaerobic, nonmotile bacteria containing Gram-negative, straight or slightly curved rods, 5–15 μm in length, with one or both ends rounded, often pointed. Granules are distributed evenly along the long axis, and one or more large granules may localize near the end of the cell. Branched or clubbed forms do not occur. Two or more cells join together and form septate filaments of varying length; in older cultures, filaments up to 200 μm may form and twist around each other; large, coccoid bodies may be found within a filament as a cell lyses. Carbon dioxide is essential for optimal growth. Lactic acid is produced from glucose. These organisms occur in the oral cavity of humans. The type species is *L. buccalis*. [lepto- + G. *thrix*, hair]

L. bucca′lis, a bacterial species found in the human mouth rarely found in the blood of immunocompromised patients; it is the type species of the genus *L.*

Lep·to·trom·bid·i·um (lep′tō-trom-bid′ē-ŭm). An important genus of trombiculid mites, formerly considered a subgenus of the genus *Trombicula*, which includes all of the vectors of scrub typhus (tsutsugamushi disease). Members of *L.* that serve as vectors of scrub typhus are within the *L. deliense* group: *L. akamushi* is the classical vector in Japan; *L. deliense* is the primary vector, extending from New Guinea, Australia, the Philippines, China, and Southeast Asia to western Pakistan; *L. fletcheri* is found in Malaysia, New Guinea, and the Philippines. Some eight other species have also been implicated in scrub typhus transmission in more limited areas.

L. akamu′shi, one of two species, the other being *L. deliensis* (*T. deliensis*), implicated in the transmission of *Rickettsia tsutsugamushi*, agent of tsutsugamushi disease in Japan and elsewhere in the Orient; the larvae of these species are characteristic parasites of rodents, which therefore are reservoirs of human infections, although the mites themselves are also reservoirs, as their rickettsial parasites are transovarially transmitted from generation to

generation (a requirement for transmission to humans as only larval mites feed parasitically and then only once in their lifetimes). SYN *Trombicula akamushi*.

ler·go·trile (ler′gō-trīl). A derivative of ergot which exerts agonistic properties on dopamine receptors; similar to bromocriptine and lisuride.

Leri, André, French orthopedic surgeon, 1875–1930. SEE L. *pleonosteosis, sign;* L.-Weill *disease, syndrome*.

Leriche, René, French surgeon, 1879–1955. SEE L. *operation, syndrome*.

Lermoyez, Marcel, French otolaryngologist, 1858–1929. SEE L. *syndrome*.

Lerner, I.M., U.S. population geneticist, 1910–1967. SEE L. *homeostasis*.

Leroy, Edgar August, French physician, *1883. SEE Fiessinger-L.-Reiter *syndrome*.

LES Acronym for lower esophageal *sphincter*; Lambert-Eaton *syndrome*.

les·bi·an (lez′bē-ăn). **1.** A female homosexual. **2.** Pertaining to homosexuality between women. SEE gay.

les·bi·an·ism (lez′bē-ăn-izm). Homosexuality between women. SYN sapphism. [G. *lesbios,* relating to the island of Lesbos]

Lesch, Michael, U.S. pediatrician, *1939. SEE L.-Nyhan *syndrome*.

Leser, Edmund, German surgeon, 1828–1916. SEE L.-Trélat *sign*.

le·sion (lē′zhŭn). **1.** A wound or injury. **2.** A pathologic change in the tissues. **3.** One of the individual points or patches of a multifocal disease. [L. *laedo,* pp. *laesus,* to injure]

Baehr-Lohlein l., SYN Lohlein-Baehr l.

Bankart l., a tear of the anterior glenoid labrum accompanying detachment of the inferior glenohumeral ligament.

benign lymphoepithelial l., benign tumor-like masses of lymphoid tissue in the parotid gland, containing scattered small, mainly solid islands of epithelial cells. SYN Godwin tumor.

Bracht-Wächter l., a focal collection of lymphocytes and mononuclear cells within the myocardium in bacterial endocarditis.

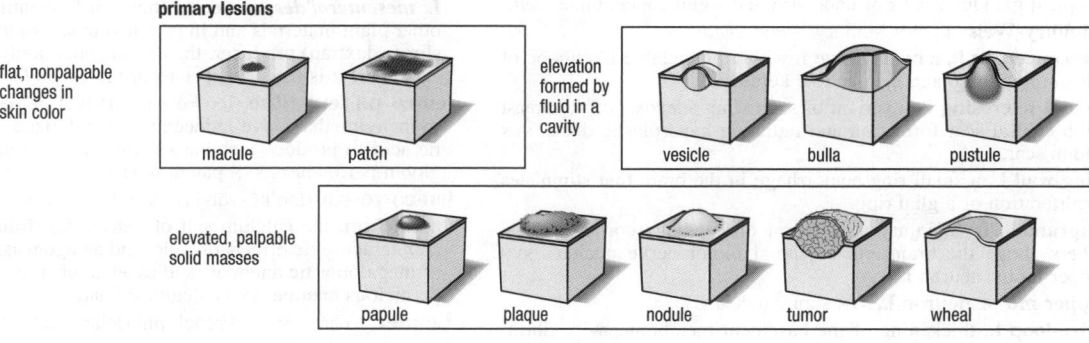

primary lesions

flat, nonpalpable changes in skin color — macule, patch

elevation formed by fluid in a cavity — vesicle, bulla, pustule

elevated, palpable solid masses — papule, plaque, nodule, tumor, wheal

secondary lesions

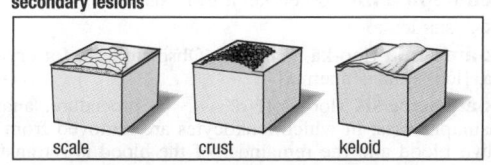

material on skin surface — scale, crust, keloid

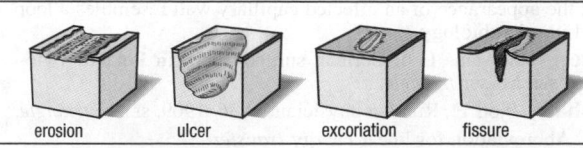

loss of skin surface — erosion, ulcer, excoriation, fissure

vascular lesions

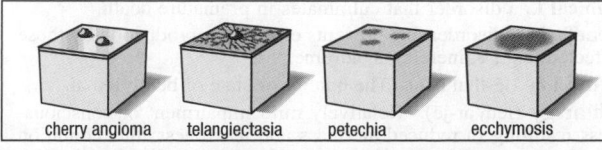

cherry angioma, telangiectasia, petechia, ecchymosis

lesions: types of primary, secondary, and vascular lesions

le

caviar l., a dilated vein or varicule existing in the venous collecting system under the tongue.

coin l. of lungs, SYN nodular *opacity.*

Dieulafoy l., an abnormally large submucosal artery located in the proximal stomach that may be the site of acute and recurrent episodes of massive hemorrhage.

Duret l., small hemorrhage(s) in the floor of the fourth ventricle or beneath the aqueduct of Sylvius.

Ghon primary l., SYN Ghon *tubercle.*

gross l., a l. plainly visible to the naked eye.

high-grade squamous intraepithelial l. (HSIL, HGSIL), term used in the Bethesda system for reporting cervical/vaginal cytologic diagnosis to describe a spectrum of noninvasive cervical epithelial abnormalities, including moderate and severe dysplasia, carcinoma in situ, and cervical intraepithelial neoplasia grades 2 and 3. SEE ALSO Bethesda *system,* ASCUS, atypical glandular *cells* of undetermined significance, under *cell,* low-grade squamous intraepithelial l.

Hill-Sachs l., an irregularity seen in the head of the humerus following anterior dislocation of the shoulder; caused by impaction of posterolateral portion of the head of the humerus against the anterior edge of the glenoid.

Janeway l., one of the stigmata of infectious endocarditis: irregular, erythematous, flat, painless macules on the palms, soles, thenar and hypothenar eminences of the hands, tips of the fingers, and plantar surfaces of the toes; rarely a diffuse rash. In acute endocarditis the lesions may be hemorrhagic or purple.

Lohlein-Baehr l., focal embolic glomerulonephritis occurring in bacterial endocarditis. SYN Baehr-Lohlein l.

lower motor neuron l., injury to motor cells in the brainstem or spinal cord, or of the axons derived from them.

low-grade squamous intraepithelial l. (LGSIL, LSIL), term used in the Bethesda system for reporting cervical/vaginal cytologic diagnosis to describe a spectrum of noninvasive cervical epithelial abnormalities; these l.'s include the cellular changes associated with human papilloma virus cytopathologic effect and mild dysplasia (cervical intraepithelial neoplasia grade 1). SEE ALSO Bethesda *system,* reactive *changes,* under *change,* ASCUS, atypical glandular *cells* of undetermined significance, under *cell.*

Mallory-Weiss l., SYN Mallory-Weiss *syndrome.*

precancerous l., a noninvasive l. with a predictable likelihood of becoming malignant; e.g., actinic keratosis.

radial sclerosing l., a variant of sclerosing adenosis of the breast with central scar formation and radiating hyperplastic ducts. SYN radial scar.

ring-wall l., a small ring hemorrhage in the brain that stimulates proliferation of a glial ring.

supranuclear l., injury to cerebral descending (corticonuclear) fibers above the brainstem or spinal motor nerve nucleus. SYN upper motor neuron l.

upper motor neuron l., SYN supranuclear l.

wire-loop l., thickening of the basement membrane, with fibrinoid staining, of scattered peripheral capillaries in renal glomeruli; characteristic of renal involvement in systemic lupus erythematosus; the appearance of an affected capillary wall resembles a loop used in microbiology.

Lesser, Ladislaus Leo, German surgeon born in Poland, 1846–1925. SEE Lesser *triangle.*

Lesshaft, Pjotr F., Russian physician, 1836–1909. SEE L. *triangle.*

LET Abbreviation for linear energy *transfer.*

le·thal (lē′thăl). Pertaining to or causing death; denoting especially the causal agent. [L. *letalis,* fr. *letum,* death]

clinical l., a disorder that culminates in premature death.

genetic l., a disorder that prevents effective reproduction by those affected; e.g., Klinefelter syndrome.

le·thal·i·ty (lē-thal′i-tē). The quality or state of being lethal.

leth·ar·gy (leth′ar-jē). Relatively mild impairment of consciousness resulting in reduced alertness and awareness; this condition has many causes but is ultimately due to generalized brain dysfunction. [G. *lēthargia,* drowsiness]

LETS Acronym for *l*arge, *e*xternal *t*ransformation-*s*ensitive fibronectin. SEE fibronectins.

Letterer, Erich, German pathologist, *1895. SEE L.-Siwe *disease.*

Leu Symbol for leucine; leucyl.

△**leuc-, leuco-.** White; white blood cell. SEE leuko-, leuk-. [G. *leukos,* white]

leu·cin (loo′sin). SYN leukin.

leu·cine (L, Leu) (loo′sēn). 2-Amino-4-methylvaleric acid; the L-isomer is one of the amino acids found in proteins; a nutritionally essential amino acid.

l. aminopeptidase, aminopeptidase (cytosol).

l. dehydrogenase, an enzyme that catalyzes the reaction of L-l., water, and NAD$^+$ to produce NADH, ammonia, and 4-methyl-2-oxopentanoate; used in the treatment of certain tumors.

l. zipper, a structural motif found in a number of proteins (e.g., some of the DNA-binding regulatory proteins) in which leucyl residues align along one edge of the helix and can interdigitate with a similar structure on another protein molecule. [Zipper, orig. a trademark for a fastening device with two rows of interlocking teeth]

leu·ci·no·sis (loo′si-nō′sis). A condition in which there is an abnormally large proportion of leucine in the tissues and body fluids.

leu·cin·u·ria (loo-si-noo′rē-ă). The excretion of leucine in the urine.

leu·co·har·mine (loo-kō-har′mēn). SYN harmine.

leu·co·line (loo′kō-lēn). SYN quinoline (1).

leu·co·meth·yl·ene blue (lu′kō-meth′i-lēn). The reduced and colorless form of methylene blue. SYN methylene white.

Leu·co·nos·toc (loo-kō-nos′tok). A genus of microaerophilic to facultatively anaerobic bacteria (family Lactobacillaceae) containing Gram-positive, spherical cells which may, under certain conditions, lengthen and become pointed and even form rods. Lactic and acetic acids are produced by these organisms. They are found in plant juices and in milk. The type species is *L. mesenteroides.* [G. *leukos,* white, + *nostoc,* a genus of algae (a word coined by Paracelsus)]

L. mesenteroi′des, a species found in fermenting vegetables and other plant materials and in prepared meat products; it is an active slime (dextran) producer, the dextran commonly used as a plasma expander; it is the type species of the genus *L.*

leu·co pa·tent blue (loo′kō pat′ent) [C.I. 42051]. A sulfonated triphenylmethane dye reduced and decolorized with zinc and acetic acid to produce a stable solution; used to demonstrate hemoglobin peroxidase. SYN patent blue V.

leu·co·vo·rin (loo′kō-vōr-in). SYN folinic acid.

l. calcium, the calcium salt of leucovorin (folinic acid); used to counteract toxic effects of folic acid antagonists, for the treatment of megaloblastic anemias, and as an adjunct to cyanocobalamin in pernicious anemia. SYN calcium folinate.

Leudet, Théodor E., French physician, 1825–1887. SEE L. *tinnitus.*

leu·en·keph·a·lin (loo-en-kef′ă-lin). SEE enkephalins.

△**leuk-.** SEE leuko-.

leuk·a·ne·mia (loo-kă-nē′mē-ă). Obsolete term for erythroleukemia. [leukemia + anemia]

leuk·a·phe·re·sis (look′ă-fĕ-rē′sis). A procedure, analogous to plasmapheresis, in which leukocytes are removed from the withdrawn blood and the remainder of the blood is retransfused into the donor. [leuko- + G. *aphairesis,* a withdrawal]

leu·ke·mia (loo-kē′mē-ă). Progressive proliferation of abnormal leukocytes found in hemopoietic tissues, other organs, and usually in the blood in increased numbers. L. is classified by the dominant cell type, and by duration from onset to death. This occurs in *acute l.* within a few months in most cases, and is associated with acute symptoms including severe anemia, hemorrhages, and slight enlargement of lymph nodes or the spleen. The duration of *chronic l.* exceeds one year, with a gradual onset of symptoms of anemia or marked enlargement of spleen, liver, or lymph nodes. SYN leukocytic sarcoma. [leuko- + G. *haima,* blood]

acute lymphocytic leukemia (ALL), SEE lymphocytic l.

acute promyelocytic l., l. presenting as a severe bleeding disorder, with infiltration of the bone marrow by abnormal promyelocytes and myelocytes, a low plasma fibrinogen, and defective coagulation.

adult T-cell l. (ATL), SYN adult T-cell *lymphoma.*

aleukemic l., l. in which abnormal (or leukemic) cells are absent in the peripheral blood.

basophilic l., basophilocytic l., a form of granulocytic l. in which there are unusually great numbers of basophilic granulocytes in the tissues and circulating blood; in some instances, the immature and mature basophilic forms may represent from 40 to 80% of the total numbers of white blood cells. SYN mast cell l.

chronic granulocytic l., SYN chronic myelocytic l.

chronic myelocytic l., a heterogeneous group of myeloproliferative disorders that may evolve into acute l. in late stages (i.e., blast crisis.) SYN chronic granulocytic l., chronic myelogenous l., chronic myeloid l.

chronic myelogenous l. (CML), SYN chronic myelocytic l.

chronic myeloid l., SYN chronic myelocytic l.

l. cu′tis, yellow-brown, red, blue-red, or purple, sometimes nodular lesions associated with diffuse infiltration of leukemic cells in the skin; the involvement may be diffuse and generalized, i.e., so-called universal l. cutis, or it may be localized.

embryonal l., SYN stem cell l.

eosinophilic l., eosinophilocytic l., a form of granulocytic l. in which there are conspicuous numbers of eosinophilic granulocytes in the tissues and circulating blood, or in which such cells are predominant; in chronic disease of this type, the total white blood cell count may be as high as 200,000–250,000 per mm^3, with as many as 80 or 90% being eosinophils, chiefly adult forms.

granulocytic l., a form of l. characterized by an uncontrolled proliferation of myelopoietic cells in the bone marrow and in extramedullary sites, and the presence of large numbers of immature and mature granulocytic forms in various tissues (and organs) and in the circulating blood; the total count may range from 1000 (aleukemic variety) to several hundred thousand per cu mm. The predominant cell is usually of the neutrophilic series, but, in a few instances, eosinophilic or basophilic granulocytes, or even megakaryocytes, may represent the chief form; early in granulocytic l., the circulating blood may contain excessive numbers of all of the granulocytic forms. SYN leukemic myelosis (1), myelocytic l., myelogenic l., myelogenous l., myeloid l.

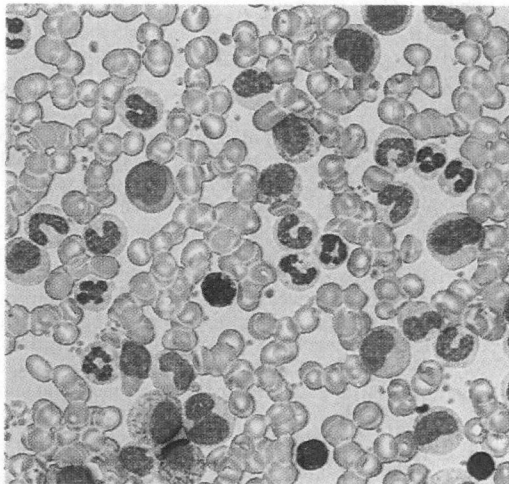

granulocytic leukemia (blood smear): high leukocyte count, with myeloblasts

hairy cell l., a rare, usually chronic disorder characterized by proliferation of hairy cells in reticuloendothelial organs and blood.

leukemic l., an obsolete redundant term sometimes used to em-

phasize the occurrence of abundant numbers of leukemic cells in the circulating blood; this classic form of l. is usually termed simply *leukemia.*

leukopenic l., a form of lymphocytic, granulocytic, or monocytic l. in which the total number of white blood cells in the circulating blood is in the normal range, or may be diminished to various levels that are significantly less than normal.

lymphatic l., SYN lymphocytic l.

lymphoblastic l., acute lymphocytic l. in which the abnormal cells are chiefly (or almost totally) blast forms of the lymphocytic series, or in which unusually large numbers of the immature forms occur in association with adult lymphocytes.

lymphocytic l., a variety of l. characterized by an uncontrolled proliferation and conspicuous enlargement of lymphoid tissue in various sites (e.g., lymph nodes, spleen, bone marrow, lungs), and the occurrence of increased numbers of cells of the lymphocytic series in the circulating blood and in various tissues and organs; in chronic disease, the cells are adult lymphocytes, whereas conspicuous numbers of lymphoblasts are observed in the more acute syndromes. SYN lymphatic l., lymphoid l.

lymphoid l., SYN lymphocytic l.

mast cell l., SYN basophilic l.

mature cell l., chronic granulocytic l.

megakaryocytic l., an unusual form of myelopoietic disease that is characterized by a seemingly uncontrolled proliferation of megakaryocytes in the bone marrow, and sometimes by the presence of a considerable number of megakaryocytes in the circulating blood. When bone marrow is examined at various intervals in some instances of chronic myelocytic l., the proliferation of megakaryocytes is more prominent than that of the granulocytes; at such times, the circulating blood may contain megakaryocytes or fragments of megakaryocytic nuclei and cytoplasm, or both, amounting to as much as 5 or 6% of the total number of leukocytes.

meningeal l., infiltration of the meninges by leukemic cells, a common occurrence in relapse following systemic administration of chemotherapeutic agents to leukemia patients.

micromyeloblastic l., a form of myelocytic l. in which relatively large proportions of micromyeloblasts are found in the circulating blood and in bone marrow and other tissues.

mixed l., mixed cell l., term infrequently used as a designation for granulocytic l., thereby emphasizing the occurrence of different types of cells in the myeloid series (i.e., neutrophilic, eosinophilic, and basophilic granulocytes), in contrast to the comparatively monotonous pattern observed in lymphocytic and monocytic l.

monocytic l., a form of l. characterized by large numbers of cells that can be definitely identified as monocytes, in addition to larger, apparently related cells formed from the uncontrolled proliferation of the reticuloendothelial tissue; l. in which these two types of cells seem to "overrun" the usual sites of the reticuloendothelial system, and occur in conspicuous numbers in the circulating blood, is frequently referred to as the Schilling type of monocytic l., or sometimes as true monocytic l. The disease runs an acute or subacute course in older persons, and is characterized by swelling of gums, oral ulceration, bleeding in skin or mucous membranes, secondary infection, and splenomegaly.

murine l., a leukemic disorder of mice caused by a number of different type C retroviruses.

myeloblastic l., a form of granulocytic l. in which there are large numbers of myeloblasts in various tissues (and organs) and in the circulating blood; the immature forms may amount to 30–60% (or even a greater proportion) of the increased total number of white blood cells. Used synonymously with acute granulocytic l. SYN leukemic myelosis (2).

myelocytic l., myelogenic l., myelogenous l., myeloid l., SYN granulocytic l.

myelomonocytic l., a variant of granulocytic l. with monocytosis in the peripheral blood. SYN Naegeli type of monocytic l.

Naegeli type of monocytic l., SYN myelomonocytic l.

natural killer cell l., a l. originating from cells of natural killer cell origin; often associated with the presence of monoclonal Epstein-Barr virus infecting tumor cells; usually indicates a leukemic subtype of poor prognosis.

le

neutrophilic l., an unusual form of chronic granulocytic l. in which the greatly increased number of leukocytes in the circulating blood are mature polymorphonuclear neutrophils, with virtually no young or immature granulocytes being observed.

plasma cell l., an unusual disease characterized by leukocytosis and other signs and symptoms that are suggestive of l., in association with diffuse infiltrations and aggregates of plasma cells in the spleen, liver, bone marrow, and lymph nodes, and the presence of considerable numbers of plasma cells in the circulating blood; the total number of leukocytes in the latter may range from normal levels to 80,000 or 90,000/mm^3, and 5–90% may be plasma cells; multiple myelomas are observed in some examples of plasma cell l., but discrete nodules are not formed in bone. Although there are other clinicopathologic differences in the two conditions, they may be phases of the same basic process.

polymorphocytic l., granulocytic l., especially any variety in which the predominant cells are mature, segmented granulocytes.

Rieder cell l., a special form of acute granulocytic l. in which the affected tissues and the circulating blood contain relatively large numbers of atypical myeloblasts (i.e., Rieder cells) that have the usual, faintly granular, immature type of cytoplasm, and a bizarre, comparatively mature nucleus with several wide and deep indentations (suggestive of lobulation).

Schilling type of monocytic l., SEE monocytic l.

splenic l., a form of l. in which there is an unusually great degree of enlargement of the spleen, as observed frequently in chronic granulocytic l.

stem cell l., a form of l. in which the abnormal cells are thought to be the precursors of lymphoblasts, myeloblasts, or monoblasts. SYN embryonal l.

subleukemic l., a form of l. in which abnormal cells are present in the peripheral blood, but the total leukocyte count is not elevated. SYN hypoleukemia, leukopenic myelosis, subleukemic myelosis, subleukemia.

leu·ke·mic (loo-kē'mik). Pertaining to, or having the characteristics of, any form of leukemia.

leu·ke·mid (loo-kem'id). Any nonspecific type of cutaneous lesion that is frequently associated with leukemia, but is not a localized accumulation of leukemic cells; e.g., petechiae, vesicles, wheals, bullae, hematomas, and the lesions of exfoliative dermatitis and herpes zoster. [leuko- + G. *haima*, blood, + *id* (1)]

leu·ke·mo·gen (loo-kē'mō-jen). Any substance or entity (e.g., benzene, ionizing radiation) considered to be a causal factor in the occurrence of leukemia.

leu·ke·mo·gen·e·sis (loo-kē-mō-jen'ĕ-sis). The causation (or induction), development, and progression of a leukemic disease. [leukemia + G. *genesis*, production]

leu·ke·mo·gen·ic (loo-kē-mō-jen'ik). Pertaining to the causation, induction, and development of leukemia; manifesting the ability to cause leukemia.

leu·ke·moid (loo-kē'moyd). Resembling leukemia in various signs and symptoms, especially with reference to changes in the circulating blood. SEE ALSO leukemoid reaction. [leukemia + G. *eidos*, resemblance]

leu·ke·moid re·ac·tion. A moderate, advanced, or sometimes extreme degree of leukocytosis in the circulating blood, similar to that occurring in various forms of leukemia, but not the result of leukemic disease; usually, there is a disproportionate increase in the number of forms (including immature stages) in one series of leukocytes, and various examples of myelocytic, lymphocytic, monocytic, or plasmocytic l. r. may be also indistinguishable from leukocytosis that is associated with certain forms of leukemia. L. r.'s are sometimes observed as a feature of: 1) infectious disease caused by certain bacteria and other biologic agents, e.g., tuberculosis, diphtheria, and chickenpox; 2) intoxication of various types, e.g., eclampsia, serious burns, and mustard gas poisoning; 3) malignant neoplasms, e.g., carcinoma of the colon, of the lung, of the kidney, or of other organs; 4) acute hemorrhage or hemolysis.

lymphocytic l. r., leukocytosis of varying degree, with adult lymphocytes and immature forms amounting to 40% (or more) of the total number of white blood cells in the circulating blood; may be

observed in association with pertussis, infectious mononucleosis, gonorrhea, chickenpox, and sarcoidosis.

monocytic l. r., leukocytosis of varying degree, e.g., 30,000–40,000/mm^3, with adult monocytes and immature forms amounting to 30% (or more) of the total number of white blood cells in the circulating blood; may be observed in association with tuberculosis, especially the first infection, miliary type.

myelocytic l. r., leukocytosis of at least moderate degree, e.g., 50,000 or more per mm^3, with a few immature forms, e.g., 1 or 2% myelocytes, but chiefly mature polymorphonuclear leukocytes in the circulating blood; may be observed in association with tuberculosis, chronic osteomyelitis, various types of empyema, malaria, pneumococcal pneumonia, meningococcal meningitis, Hodgkin disease, and metastases of carcinoma in the bone marrow.

plasmocytic l. r., the presence of unusual numbers of plasma cells, i.e., plasmocytosis, in the bone marrow; may be observed in association with sarcoidosis, rheumatoid arthritis, cirrhosis, Hodgkin disease, and certain of the so-called vascular collagen diseases.

leu·kin (loo'kin). A thermostable bactericidal substance extracted from leukocytes. SYN leucin. [*leuk*ocyte + -in]

leuko-, leuk-. White; white blood cells. For some words beginning thus, see leuc- and leuco-. [G. *leukos*, white]

leu·ko·ag·glu·ti·nin (loo'kō-ă-gloo'ti-nin). An antibody that agglutinates white blood cells.

leu·ko·bil·in (loo-kō-bil'in). SYN white *bile*. [leuko- + L. *bilis*, bile]

leu·ko·blast (loo'kō-blast). An immature granular leukocyte. SYN proleukocyte. [leuko- + G. *blastos*, germ]

leu·ko·blas·to·sis (loo'kō-blas-tō'sis). A general term for the abnormal proliferation of leukocytes, especially that occurring in myelocytic and lymphocytic leukemia.

leu·ko·chlo·ro·ma (loo'kō-klō-rō'mă). Obsolete term for myelocytomatosis. [leuko- + G. *chlōros*, green, + -*oma*, tumor]

leu·ko·ci·din (loo-kos'i-din, loo-kō-sī'din). A heat-labile substance that is elaborated by many strains of *Staphylococcus aureus*, *Streptococcus pyogenes*, and pneumococci and manifests a destructive action on leukocytes, with or without lysis of the cells. [leukocyte + L. *caedo*, to kill]

leu·ko·co·ria, leu·ko·ko·ria (loo-kō-kō'rē-ă, loo-kō-kō'rē-ă). Reflection from a white mass within the eye giving the appearance of a white pupil. SYN leukokoria, white pupillary *reflex*. [*leuko-* white, + G. *korē*, pupil]

leu·ko·cy·tac·tic (loo'kō-sī-tak'tik). SYN leukocytotactic.

leu·ko·cy·tal (loo-kō-sī'tăl). SYN leukocytic.

leu·ko·cy·tax·ia, leu·ko·cy·tax·is (loo'kō-sī-tak'sē-ă, -tak'sis). SYN leukocytotaxia.

leu·ko·cyte (loo'kō-sīt). A type of cell formed in the myelopoietic, lymphoid, and reticular portions of the reticuloendothelial system in various parts of the body, and normally present in those sites and in the circulating blood (rarely in other tissues). Under various abnormal conditions, the total numbers or proportions, or both, may be characteristically increased, decreased, or not altered, and they may be present in other tissues and organs. L.'s represent three lines of development from primitive elements: myeloid, lymphoid, and monocytic series. On the basis of features observed with various methods of staining with polychromatic dyes (e.g., Wright stain). cells of the myeloid series are frequently termed granular l.'s, or granulocytes; cells of the lymphoid and monocytic series also have granules in the cytoplasm but, owing to their tiny, inconspicuous size and different properties (frequently not clearly visualized with routine methods), lymphocytes and monocytes are sometimes termed nongranular or agranular l.'s. Granulocytes are commonly known as polymorphonuclear l.'s (also polynuclear or multinuclear l.'s), inasmuch as the mature nucleus is divided into two to five rounded or ovoid lobes that are connected with thin strands or small bands of chromatin; they consist of three distinct types: neutrophils, eosinophils, and basophils, named on the basis of the staining reactions of the cytoplasmic granules. Cells of the lymphocytic series occur as two, somewhat arbitrary, normal varieties: small and large lymphocytes; the former represent the ordinary forms and are conspicuously more numerous in the circulating blood and normal lymphoid tissue; the latter may be found in normal circulating blood, but are more easily observed in lymphoid tissue. The small lymphocytes have nuclei that are deeply or densely stained (the chromatin is coarse and bulky) and almost fill the cells, with only a slight rim of cytoplasm around the nuclei; the large lymphocytes have nuclei that are approximately the same size as, or only slightly larger than, those of the small forms, but there is a broader, easily visualized band of cytoplasm around the nuclei. Cells of the monocytic series are usually larger than the other l.'s, and are characterized by a relatively abundant, slightly opaque, pale blue or blue-gray cytoplasm that contains myriad extremely fine reddish-blue granules. Monocytes are usually indented, reniform, or shaped similarly to a horseshoe, but are sometimes rounded or ovoid; their nuclei are usually large and centrally placed and, even when eccentrically located, are completely surrounded by at least a small band of cytoplasm. SYN white blood cell. [leuko- + G. *kytos*, cell]

acidophilic l., SYN eosinophilic l.

agranular l., SYN nongranular l.

basophilic l., a polymorphonuclear l. characterized by many large, coarse, metachromatic granules (dark purple or blue-black when treated with Wright or similar stains) that usually fill the cytoplasm and may almost mask the nucleus; these l.'s are unique in that they usually do not occur in increased numbers as the result of acute infectious disease, and their phagocytic qualities are probably not significant; the granules, which contain heparin and histamine, may degranulate in response to hypersensitivity reactions and can be of significance in general inflammation. SYN basocyte, basophilocyte, mast l.

cystinotic l., a l. having an enhanced content of cystine, found in patients with disorders characterized by the storage of cystine; within the l., the cystine, largely in noncrystalline form, is associated with dense lysosomal particles.

endothelial l., obsolete term for a monocyte, a type of l. thought to be derived from reticuloendothelial tissue.

eosinophilic l., a polymorphonuclear l. characterized by many large or prominent, refractile, cytoplasmic granules that are fairly uniform in size and bright yellow-red or orange when treated with Wright or similar stains; the nuclei are usually larger than those of neutrophils, do not stain as deeply, and characteristically have two lobes (a third lobe is sometimes interposed on the connecting strand of chromatin); these l.'s are motile phagocytes with distinctive antiparasitic functions. SYN acidophilic l., eosinocyte, eosinophil, eosinophile, oxyphil (2), oxyphile, oxyphilic l.

filament polymorphonuclear l., any mature polymorphonuclear l., especially a neutrophilic l., in which the lobes of the nucleus are interconnected with a thin strand or filament of chromatin.

globular l., a type of wandering cell with a small, round nucleus found in the epithelium and lamina propria of the intestinal mucosa of many animals; its cytoplasm contains large eosinophilic globules or droplets.

granular l., any one of the polymorphonuclear l.'s, especially a neutrophilic l. SEE ALSO granulocyte, basophilic l., eosinophilic l.

hyaline l., obsolete term for a monocyte, and for a mononuclear macrophage in various lesions.

mast l., SYN basophilic l.

motile l., any l. that manifests active ameboid movement, especially a mature granulocytic l. (eosinophils are less motile than neutrophils or basophils); monocytes manifest a slow, but persistent, wavelike movement.

multinuclear l., SYN polymorphonuclear l.

neutrophilic l., a neutrophilic granulocyte, the most frequent of the polymorphonuclear l.'s, and also the most active phagocyte among the various types of white blood cells; when treated with Wright stain (or similar preparations), the fairly abundant cytoplasm is faintly pink, and numerous tiny, slightly refractile, relatively bright pink or violet-pink, diffusely scattered granules are recognizable in the cytoplasm; the deeply stained blue or purple-blue nucleus is sharply distinguished from the cytoplasm and is distinctly lobated, with thin strands of chromatin connecting the three to five lobes.

nonfilament polymorphonuclear l., a neutrophil, basophil, or eosinophil that is not completely matured, i.e., the lobes of the nuclei remain connected with bands of chromatin, in contrast to the thin strands observed in mature cells.

nongranular l., a general, nonspecific term frequently used with reference to lymphocytes, monocytes, and plasma cells; although the cytoplasm of a lymphocyte or monocyte contains tiny granules, it is "nongranular" in comparison with that of a neutrophil, basophil, or eosinophil. SEE ALSO leukocyte. SYN agranular l.

nonmotile l., a term sometimes used with reference to lymphocytes, monocytes, and plasma cells; although such forms actually have some degree of motility, they are "nonmotile" in comparison with the actively ameboid neutrophilic, basophilic, and eosinophilic l.'s.

oxyphilic l., SYN eosinophilic l.

polymorphonuclear l., polynuclear l., common term for granulocyte or granulocytic l.; the term includes basophilic, eosinophilic, and neutrophilic l.'s, but is usually used especially with reference to the neutrophilic l.'s. SYN multinuclear l.

segmented l., any mature polymorphonuclear l., especially a neutrophilic l.

transitional l., obsolete term for a monocyte.

Türk l., SYN Türk *cell.*

leu·ko·cy·the·mia (loo′kō-sī-thē′mē-ă). Obsolete term for leukemia. [leukocyte + G. *haima,* blood]

leu·ko·cyt·ic (loo-kō-sit′ik). Pertaining to or characterized by leukocytes. SYN leukocytal.

leu·ko·cy·to·blast (loo-kō-sī′tō-blast). A nonspecific term for any immature cell from which a leukocyte develops, including lymphoblast, myeloblast, and the like. [leukocyte + G. *blastos,* germ]

leu·ko·cy·toc·la·sis (loo′kō-sī-tok′lă-sis). Karyorrhexis of leukocytes. [leuko- + G. *kytos,* cell, + *klasia,* a breaking]

leu·ko·cy·to·gen·e·sis (loo′kō-sī-tō-jen′ĕ-sis). The formation and development of leukocytes. [leukocyte + G. *genesis,* production]

leu·ko·cy·toid (loo′kō-sī-toyd). Resembling a leukocyte. [leukocyte + G. *eidos,* resemblance]

leu·ko·cy·tol·y·sin (loo′kō-sī-tol′i-sin). Any substance (including lytic antibody) that causes dissolution of leukocytes. SYN leukolysin.

leu·ko·cy·tol·y·sis (loo′kō-sī-tol′i-sis). Dissolution or lysis of leukocytes. SYN leukolysis. [leukocyte + G. *lysis,* dissolution]

leu·ko·cy·to·lyt·ic (loo′kō-sī-tō-lit′ik). Pertaining to, causing, or manifesting leukocytolysis. SYN leukolytic.

leu·ko·cy·to·ma (loo′kō-sī-tō′mă). Obsolete term for a fairly well circumscribed, nodular, dense accumulation of leukocytes. [leukocyte + G. *-oma,* tumor]

leu·ko·cy·tom·e·ter (loo′kō-sī-tom′ĕ-ter). A standardized glass slide that is suitably ruled for counting the leukocytes in a measured volume of accurately diluted blood (or other specimens). [leukocyte + G. *metron,* measure]

leu·ko·cy·to·pe·nia (loo′kō-sī-tō-pē′nē-ă). SYN leukopenia.

leu·ko·cy·to·pla·nia (loo′kō-sī-tō-plā′nē-ă). Movement of leukocytes from the lumens of blood vessels, through serous membranes, or in the tissues. [leukocyte + G. *plane,* a wandering]

leu·ko·cy·to·poi·e·sis (loo′kō-sī-tō-poy-ē′sis). SYN leukopoiesis. [leukocyte + G. *poiēsis,* a making]

leu·ko·cy·to·sis (loo′kō-sī-tō′sis). An abnormally large number of leukocytes, as observed in acute infections, inflammation, hemorrhage, and other conditions. A white blood cell count of 10,000 or more per mm^3 usually indicates l. Most examples of l. represent a disproportionate increase in the number of cells in the neutrophilic series, and the term is frequently used synonymously with the designation neutrophilia. L. of 15,000–25,000/mm^3 is frequently observed in various pathologic conditions, and values as high as 40,000 are not unusual; occasionally, as in some examples of leukemoid reactions, white blood cell counts may range up to 100,000/mm^3. [leukocyte + G. *-osis,* condition]

absolute l., an actual increase in the total number of leukocytes in the circulating blood, as distinguished from a relative increase (such as that observed in dehydration).

le

agonal l., SYN terminal l.

basophilic l., the presence of an abnormally large number of basophilic granulocytes in the blood. SYN basocytosis.

digestive l., l. occurring normally after ingestion of food.

distribution l., an abnormally large proportion of one or more types of leukocytes.

emotional l., an abnormally high white blood cell count that is thought to be related only to an emotional disturbance.

eosinophilic l., a form of relative l. in which the greatest proportionate increase is in the eosinophils. SYN eosinophilia.

lymphocytic l., SYN lymphocytosis.

monocytic l., SYN monocytosis.

neutrophilic l., SYN neutrophilia.

l. of the newborn, an apparently "physiologic" l. usually observed in newborn infants, in whom the white blood cell counts are usually greater than 10,000/mm^3, and sometimes range to 45,000/mm^3, resulting chiefly from increased numbers of neutrophils (especially single and bilobed forms). On the third or fourth day of life, the count generally decreases rapidly, and then fluctuates for several days; beginning about the fourth week of life, a relative lymphocytosis is observed, and this normally continues for a few years.

physiologic l., any form of l. that is associated with apparently normal situations and that is not directly related to a pathologic condition; e.g., the temporary increase in the total number of white blood cells that may occur during a single day, or from day to day, as well as in the newborn period, during childhood, after strenuous exercise, during attacks of paroxysmal tachycardia, and in association with various other situations.

relative l., an increased proportion of one or more types of leukocytes in the circulating blood, without an actual increase in the total number of white blood cells.

terminal l., one that occurs in a person just prior to death, especially in one who has a "slow death." SYN agonal l.

leu·ko·cy·to·tac·tic (loo′kō-sī-tō-tak′tik). Pertaining to, characterized by, or causing leukocytotaxia. SYN leukocytactic, leukotactic.

leu·ko·cy·to·tax·ia (loo-kō-sī-tō-tak′sē-ă). **1.** The active ameboid movement of leukocytes, especially the neutrophilic granulocytes, either toward (**positive l.**) or away from (**negative l.**) certain microorganisms as well as various substances frequently formed in inflamed tissue. **2.** The property of attracting or repelling leukocytes. SYN leukocytaxia, leukocytaxis, leukotaxia, leukotaxis. [leukocyte + G. *taxis,* arrangement]

leu·ko·cy·to·tox·in (loo′kō-sī-tō-tok′sin). Any substance that causes degeneration and necrosis of leukocytes, including leukolysin and leukocidin. SYN leukotoxin. [leukocyte + G. *toxikon,* poison]

leu·ko·cy·tu·ria (loo′kō-sī-too′rē-ă). The presence of leukocytes in urine that is recently voided or collected by means of a catheter. [leukocyte + G. *ouron,* urine]

leu·ko·der·ma (loo-kō-der′mă). An absence of pigment, partial or total, in the skin. SYN hypomelanosis, leukopathia, leukopathy. [leuko- + G. *derma,* skin]

acquired l., SYN vitiligo.

l. acquisi′tum centrifu′gum, SYN halo *nevus.*

l. col′li, SYN syphilitic l.

syphilitic l., a fading of the roseola of secondary syphilis, leaving reticulated depigmented and hyperpigmented areas located chiefly on the sides of the neck. SYN l. colli, melanoleukoderma colli.

leu·ko·der·ma·tous (loo-kō-der′mă-tŭs). Relating to or resembling leukoderma.

leu·ko·don·tia (loo-kō-don′shē-ă). The condition of having white teeth. [leuko- + G. *odous,* tooth]

leu·ko·dys·tro·phia (loo-kō-dis-trō′fē-ă). SYN leukodystrophy.

l. cer′ebri progressi′va, SYN leukodystrophy.

leu·ko·dys·tro·phy (loo-kō-dis′trō-fē). Term for a group of white matter diseases, some familial, characterized by progressive cerebral deterioration usually in early life, and pathologically by primary absence or degeneration of the myelin of the central and peripheral nervous systems with glial reaction; probably related to a defect in lipid metabolism; most l.'s are autosomal recessive, several X-linked recessive, and a few autosomal dominant. SEE ALSO Canavan *disease.* SYN leukodystrophia cerebri progressiva, leukodystrophia, sclerosis of white matter. [leuko- + G. *dys,* bad, + *trophē,* nourishment]

adrenal l., sudanophilic leukodystrophy with bronzing of skin and adrenal atrophy. A metabolic disorder of young males, characterized by widespread myelin degeneration and associated adrenal insufficiency. The myelin degeneration is massive in various portions of the brain and sometimes the spinal cord, with the accumulation of degradation products of myelin in macrophages: sudanophilic demyelination; atrophy is present in the adrenal glands and testes, and markedly increased amounts of very long-chain fatty acid are present in both the brain and adrenal glands. Symptoms include bronzing of the skin, dysarthria, cortical blindness, bilateral hemiplegia, pseudobulbar paralysis, and progressive dementia. Probably sex-linked recessive inheritance.

globoid cell l. [MIM*245200], a metabolic disorder of infancy or early childhood characterized by spasticity, seizures, and rapidly progressive cerebral degeneration, massive loss of myelin, severe astrocytic gliosis, and infiltration of the white matter with characteristic multinucleate globoid cells; metabolically there is gross deficiency of lysosomal cerebrosidase (galactosylceramide β-galactosidase); autosomal recessive inheritance, caused by mutation in the gene encoding glycosylceramidase (GALC) on 14q. SYN diffuse infantile familial sclerosis, galactosylceramide lipoidosis, Krabbe disease.

metachromatic l. [MIM*250100], a metabolic disorder, with onset usually in the second year of life and death often before 5 years, with loss of myelin and accumulation of metachromatic lipids (galactosyl sulfatidates) in the white matter of the central and peripheral nervous systems leading to motor symptoms, paralysis, convulsions, and progressive cerebral deterioration;. Autosomal recessive inheritance [MIM*249900 and MIM*250100], caused by mutation in either the arylsulfatase A gene (ARSA) on 22q or the prosaposin gene (PSAP) on 10q. There is a dominant form occurring in adults [MIM*156310]. SYN arylsulfatase A deficiency, sulfatide lipidosis.

l. with diffuse Rosenthal fiber formation, a metabolic disorder whose onset can be in infancy, adolescence, or adulthood; characterized pathologically by widespread cerebral demyelination with astrocyte and primitive oligodendroglial cell proliferation; refractile Rosenthal fibers result from the degeneration of these proliferating cells; etiology unknown, but possibly due to a metabolic defect of astrocytes; sex-linked recessive disorder.

leu·ko·en·ceph·a·li·tis (loo′kō-en-sef-ă-lī′tis). Encephalitis restricted to the white matter.

acute epidemic l., a disease characterized by acute onset of fever, followed by convulsions, delirium, and coma, and associated with perivascular demyelination and hemorrhagic foci in the central nervous system. SYN acute primary hemorrhagic meningoencephalitis, Strümpell disease (2).

acute hemorrhagic l., SYN acute necrotizing hemorrhagic *encephalomyelitis.*

acute necrotizing hemorrhagic l., SYN acute necrotizing hemorrhagic *encephalomyelitis.*

sclerosing l., SYN subacute sclerosing *panencephalitis.*

subacute sclerosing l., SYN subacute sclerosing *panencephalitis.*

leu·ko·en·ceph·a·lop·a·thy (loo′kō-en-sef-ă-lop′ă-thē). White matter changes first described in children with leukemia, associated with radiation and chemotherapy injury, often associated with methotrexate; pathologically characterized by diffuse reactive astrocytosis with multiple areas of necrotic foci without inflammation. [leuko- + G. *enkephalos,* brain, + *pathos,* suffering]

progressive multifocal l. (PML), a rare, subacute, afebrile disease characterized by areas of demyelinization surrounded by markedly altered neuroglia, including inclusion bodies in glial cells; it occurs usually in individuals with AIDS, leukemia, lymphoma, or other debilitating diseases, or in those who have been receiving immunosuppressive treatment. Caused by JC virus, a human polyoma virus. SYN progressive subcortical encephalopathy.

leu·ko·e·ryth·ro·blas·to·sis (loo′kō-ĕ-rith′rō-blas-tō′sis). Any anemic condition resulting from space-occupying lesions in the bone marrow; the circulating blood contains immature cells of the granulocytic series and nucleated red blood cells, frequently in numbers that are disproportionately large in relation to the degree of anemia. SYN leukoerythroblastic anemia, myelophthisic anemia, myelopathic anemia.

leu·ko·ki·net·ic (loo′kō-ki-net′ik). Pertaining to leukokinetics. [leukocyte + G. *kinētikos*, of motion, fr. *kineō*, to move]

leu·ko·ki·net·ics (loo′kō-ki-net′iks). The study of the formation, circulation, and fate of leukocytes, usually by use of a radioactive tracer. [leukocyte + G. *kinetikos*, of or for putting in motion]

leu·ko·ko·ria (loo-kō-kō′rē-ă). SEE leukocoria.

leu·ko·krau·ro·sis (loo′kō-kraw-rō′sis). SYN kraurosis vulvae.

leu·kol·y·sin (loo-kol′i-sin). SYN leukocytolysin.

leu·kol·y·sis (loo-kol′i-sis). SYN leukocytolysis.

leu·ko·lyt·ic (loo-kō-lit′ik). SYN leukocytolytic.

leu·ko·ma (loo-kō′mă). A dense white opacity of the cornea. [G. whiteness, a white spot in the eye, fr. *leukos,* white]

    adherent l., a cicatrix of the cornea to which a portion of the iris is attached.

leu·ko·ma·tous (loo-kō′mă-tŭs). Pertaining to leukoma.

leu·ko·mye·li·tis (loo′kō-mī-e-lī′tis). An inflammatory process involving the white matter of the spinal cord.

    necrotizing hemorrhage l., the pathological substrate responsible for the clinical disorder of acute necrotizing *myelitis*.

leu·ko·my·e·lop·a·thy (loo′kō-mī′ĕ-lop′ă-thē). Any systemic disease involving the white matter or the conducting tracts of the spinal cord. [leuko- + G. *myelos,* marrow, + *pathos,* suffering]

leu·kon (loo′kon). The total mass of circulating leukocytes as well as the cells and leukopoietic cells from which it originates.

leu·ko·ne·cro·sis (loo′kō-ne-krō′sis). SYN white *gangrene*. [leuko- + G. *nekrōsis,* deadness]

leu·ko·nych·ia (loo-kō-nik′ē-ă). The occurrence of smooth-surfaced white spots or patches under the nails, of unknown cause; the decoloration may be total or in the form of lines (striate or transverse l.) or dots (punctate l.). [leuko- + G. *onyx (onych-),* nail]

leu·ko·path·ia, leu·kop·a·thy (loo-kō-path′ē-ă, loo-kop′ă-thē). SYN leukoderma. [leuko- + G. *pathos,* disease]

leu·ko·pe·de·sis (loo′kō-pē-dē′sis). The movement of white blood cells (especially polymorphonuclear leukocytes) through the walls of capillaries and into the tissues. [leuko- + G. *pēdēsis,* a leaping]

leu·ko·pe·nia (loo-kō-pē′nē-ă). The antithesis of leukocytosis; any situation in which the total number of leukocytes in the circulating blood is less than normal, the lower limit of which is generally regarded as 4000–5000/mm^3. SYN leukocytopenia. [leuko(cyte) + G. *penia,* poverty]

basophilic l., a decrease in the number of basophilic granulocytes in the circulating blood (difficult to evaluate, owing to the small and variable number normally present). SYN basocytopenia, basopenia.

eosinophilic l., a decrease in the number of eosinophilic granulocytes normally present in the circulating blood.

lymphocytic l., SYN lymphopenia.

monocytic l., SYN monocytopenia.

neutrophilic l., SYN neutropenia.

leu·ko·pe·nic (loo-kō-pē′nik). Pertaining to leukopenia.

leu·ko·pla·kia (loo-kō-plā′kē-ă). A white patch of oral or female genital mucous membrane that cannot be wiped off and cannot be diagnosed clinically as any specific disease entity; in current usage, a clinical term without histologic connotation. SYN smoker's patches. [leuko- + G. *plax,* plate]

□ **hairy l.,** a white lesion appearing on the tongue, occasionally on the buccal mucosa, of patients with AIDS; a manifestation of Epstein-Barr virus infection in an immunocompromised host; the lesion appears raised, with a corrugated, shaggy, or "hairy" surface due to keratin projections.

Oral hairy leukoplakia was first recognized in 1981 as a

marker of immunosuppression in male homosexuals with AIDS. The incidence in persons with AIDS is about 20%. Oral hairy leukoplakia consists of white vertical folds or ridges, generally along the lateral borders of the tongue, but sometimes on its lower surface or on the buccal mucosa. Unlike the lesions of candidiasis (thrush), the patches cannot be scraped off. The condition is ordinarily asymptomatic, causing neither pain nor alteration of taste. Histologic study shows parakeratosis and koilocytosis with little inflammation. The lesion occasionally progresses to squamous cell carcinoma. Treatment with topical podophyllin or systemic acyclovir usually induces prompt regression of lesions.

---

l. vul′vae, a clinical term for hyperkeratotic white patches of the vulvar epithelium; biopsy is necessary for specific diagnosis.

leu·ko·poi·e·sis (loo′kō-poy-ē′sis). Formation and development of the various types of white blood cells. SYN leukocytopoiesis. [leuko- + G. *poiēsis,* a making]

leu·ko·poi·et·ic (loo′kō-poy-et′ik). Pertaining to or characterized by leukopoiesis, as manifested by portions of the bone marrow and reticuloendothelial and lymphoid tissues, which form (respectively) the granulocytes, monocytes, and lymphocytes.

leu·ko·pro·te·ase (loo-kō-prō′tē-ās). An ill-defined proteolytic enzyme product of polynuclear leukocytes, formed in an area of inflammation, that causes liquefaction of dead tissue.

leu·ko·ri·bo·fla·vin (loo-kō-rī′bō-flā-vin). The colorless non-fluorescing dihydro compound formed by the reduction of riboflavin.

leu·kor·rha·gia (loo-kō-rā′jē-ă). SYN leukorrhea. [leuko- + G. *rhēgnymi,* to burst forth]

leu·kor·rhea (loo-kō-rē′ă). Discharge from the vagina of a white or yellowish viscid fluid containing mucus and pus cells. SYN leukorrhagia. [leuko- + G. *rhoia,* flow]

menstrual l., intermittent l. recurring at or just before each menstrual period.

leu·kor·rhe·al (loo-kō-rē′ăl). Relating to or characterized by leukorrhea.

leu·ko·tac·tic (loo-kō-tak′tik). SYN leukocytotactic.

leu·ko·tax·ia (loo-kō-tak′sē-ă). SYN leukocytotaxia.

leu·ko·tax·ine (loo-kō-tak′sēn). A cell-free nitrogenous material prepared from injured, acutely degenerating tissue and from inflammatory exudates.

leu·ko·tax·is (loo-kō-tak′sis). SYN leukocytotaxia.

leu·ko·tome (loo′kō-tōm). An instrument for performing leukotomy.

leu·kot·o·my (loo-kot′ō-mē). Incision into the white matter of the frontal lobe of the brain. [leuko- + G. *tomē,* a cutting]

prefrontal l., SYN prefrontal *lobotomy*.

transorbital l., SYN transorbital *lobotomy*.

leu·ko·tox·in (loo-kō-tok′sin). SYN leukocytotoxin.

leu·ko·trich·ia (loo-kō-trik′ē-ă). Whiteness of the hair. [leuko- + G. *thrix,* hair]

leu·ko·tri·enes (LT) (loo-kō-trī′ēnz). Products of eicosanoid metabolism (usually, arachidonic acid) with postulated physiologic activity such as mediators of inflammation and roles in allergic reactions; they differ from the related prostaglandins and thromboxanes by not having a central ring; so named because they were originally discovered in association with leukocytes and of three conjugated double bonds; letters A through F identify the first six metabolites isolated, with subscript numbers to indicate the number of double bonds (e.g., leukotriene C$_4$).

peptidyl l., l. having one or more amino acids present; e.g., LTC$_4$ is an *S*-substituted glutathione, LTD$_4$ is an *S*-substituted cysteinylglycine, LTE$_4$ is an *S*-substituted cysteine, and LTF$_4$ (also known as γ-glutamyl-LTE$_4$) is an *S*-substituted γ-glutamylcysteine.

Leu·ko·vi·rus (loo′kō-vī′rŭs). Obsolete term for a former genus composed of the RNA tumor viruses now included in the family Retroviridae.

LEU M1. The epitope for a monoclonal antibody generated to

LE

the human histiocytic cell line that localizes to neutrophils, adherent monocytes, and a subgroup of activated T cells.

leu·pep·tin (loo-pep′tin). One of a number of modified tripeptide protease inhibitors from *Streptomyces* species that inhibits cathepsin B, papain, trypsin, plasmin, and cathepsin D. The most commonly used leupeptin is *N*-acetylleucylleucylarginal.

leu·pro·lide ac·e·tate (loo′prō-līd). A synthetic nonapeptide analog of naturally occurring gonadotropin-releasing hormone; used in the palliative treatment of advanced prostatic cancer.

leu·ro·cris·tine (loo′rō-kris′tin). SYN vincristine sulfate.

Lev, Maurice, U.S. pathologist, 1908–1994. SEE L. *disease, syndrome.*

Levaditi, Constantin, Romanian bacteriologist in Paris, 1879–1928. SEE L. *stain.*

lev·al·lor·phan tar·trate (lev-ă-lōr′fan). The *N*-allyl analog of levorphanol, antagonistic to the actions of narcotic analgesics; used in the treatment of respiratory depression due to overdosage of narcotics.

lev·am·iso·le (lē-vam′ĭ-sōl). Formerly used as an anthelmintic; increases immune responses and is used adjunctively with antineoplastic agents to improve response and suppress recurrence.

lev·an (le′van). SYN fructosan (1).

lev·an·su·crase (lev-an-soo′krās). An enzyme catalyzing transfer of the fructose moiety of sucrose to polyfructose (a levan), releasing D-glucose.

lev·ar·te·re·nol (lev-ar-tēr′ĕ-nol). SYN norepinephrine.

l. bitartrate, SYN *norepinephrine* bitartrate.

le·va·tor (le-vā′ter, tōr) [TA]. **1.** A surgical instrument for prying up the depressed part in a fracture of the skull. **2.** One of several muscles whose action is to raise the part to which it inserts. [L. a lifter, fr. *levo,* pp. *-atus,* to lift, fr. *levis,* light]

LeVeen, Harry H., U.S. surgeon, *1914. SEE LeV. *shunt.*

lev·el (le′vel). **1.** Any rank, position, or status in a graded scale of values. **2.** A test for determining such rank or position.

acoustic reference l., the biological reference l. for sound measurements. When the term decibel is used to indicate the noise l., a reference quantity is implied; this reference value is usually expressed as a sound pressure of 20 micronewtons per square meter. The reference l. is referred to as 0 decibels, the baseline of the scale of noise l.'s; this baseline is considered the weakest sound that can be heard by a person with very good hearing in an extremely quiet location. Other equivalent reference l.'s still being used include 0.0002 microbar and 0.0002 dyne per square centimeter. SEE ALSO sound pressure l.

l. of aspiration, in clinical psychology, the degree or quality of performance (exhibited in a testing situation) which a person desires to attain or feels he or she can achieve.

background l., the concentration (usually low) at which a substance or agent is present or occurs at a particular time and place in the absence of a specific hazard under investigation; an example is the background level of ionizing radiation.

Clark l., the l. of invasion of primary malignant melanoma of the skin; limited to the epidermis, I; into the underlying papillary dermis, II; to the junction of the papillary and reticular dermis, III; into the reticular dermis, IV; into the subcutaneous fat, V. The prognosis is worse with each successive deeper l. of invasion.

hearing l., the measure of the status of hearing as read directly on the hearing loss scale of an audiometer; described in decibels as a deviation from a standard value for zero on the audiometer.

loudness discomfort l., the intensity at which sound, particularly speech, causes discomfort.

most comfortable l., the greatest sound intensity that is comfortable.

saturation sound pressure l. (SSPL), a measure of the maximum output of a hearing aid.

sensation l., the amount in decibels that a stimulus is above the hearing threshold.

sensory acuity l., a technique for determining air conduction thresholds without masking and with masking presented by bone conduction to the forehead; the change in thresholds indicates the conductive hearing loss.

sound pressure l. (SPL), a measure of sound energy relative to 0.0002 dynes/cm², expressed in decibels.

uncomfortable l., the intensity of sound that causes discomfort.

window l., the CT number setting in Hounsfield units of the midpoint of the window width, which is the gray scale of the image; a typical window l. for imaging the lungs is −500; for the abdomen, 0.

Leventhal, Michael L., U.S. obstetrician-gynecologist, 1901–1971. SEE Stein-L. *syndrome.*

le·ver (lev′er, lē′ver). An instrument used to lift or pry. [Fr. *lever,* to lift]

dental l., SYN elevator (2).

le·ver·age (lē′ver-ij). **1.** The actual lift or elevating direction of a lever or elevator. **2.** The mechanical advantage gained thereby.

Levey, S., 20th century U.S. statistician. SEE L.-Jennings *chart.*

Lévi, E. Leopold, French endocrinologist, 1868–1933. SEE dominantly inherited L. *disease;* Lorain-L. *dwarfism, infantilism, syndrome.*

Levin, Abraham, U.S. physician, 1880–1940. SEE L. *tube.*

Levin, Max, U.S. neurologist, *1901. SEE Kleine-L. *syndrome.*

Levine, Samuel A., U.S. cardiologist, 1891–1966. SEE Lown-Ganong-L. *syndrome.*

Le·vin·ea (lĕ-vin′ē-ă). A former genus of bacteria (of the family Enterobacteriaceae) whose species are now assigned to the genus *Citrobacter.* [Max *Levine,* U.S. bacteriologist, *1889]

L. amalona′tica, SYN *Citrobacter amalonatica.*

L. diversus, SYN *Citrobacter diversus.*

L. malona′tica, SYN *Citrobacter diversus.*

lev·i·ta·tion (lev-i-tā′shŭn). Support of the patient on a cushion of air. [L. *levitas,* lightness]

Le·vi·vir·i·dae (lĕ-vi-vir′i-dē). Provisional name for a family of small, nonenveloped, isometric bacterial viruses with genomes of single-stranded positive sense RNA (MW 1×10^6). Virions adsorb to the sides of bacterial pili, and crystalline arrays are formed in infected bacteria. The type species is enterobacteria phage M52. [L. *levis,* light (not heavy)]

levo-. Left, toward or on the left side. [L. *laevus*]

le·vo·bu·no·lol hy·dro·chlo·ride (lē-vō-bū′nō-lol). A β-adrenergic blocking agent used primarily as an eye drop in the treatment of chronic open-angle glaucoma and ocular hypertension.

le·vo·car·dia (lē-vō-kar′dē-ă). Situs inversus of the other viscera but with the heart normally situated on the left; congenital cardiac lesions are commonly associated. [levo- + G. *kardia,* heart]

le·vo·car·di·o·gram (lē-vō-kar′dē-ō-gram). That part of the electrocardiogram that is the effect of the left ventricle.

levo·car·ni·tine (lē′vō-kar′nĭ-tēn). Used as a supplement for carnitine deficiency.

le·vo·cli·na·tion (lē′vō-kli-nā′shŭn). SYN levotorsion (2). [levo- + L. *clino,* pp. *-atus,* to bend]

levocycleduction. SYN sinistrotorsion.

le·vo·cy·clo·duc·tion (lē′vō-sī-klō-dŭk′shŭn). levotorsion of one eye. [levo- + cyclo- + L. *duco,* pp. *ductus,* to lead]

le·vo·do·pa (lē-vō-dō′pă). The biologically active form of dopa; an antiparkinsonian agent that is converted to dopamine. SYN L-dopa.

le·vo·duc·tion (lē-vō-dŭk′shŭn). Turning of one eye to the left; abduction of left eye or adduction of right eye. [levo- + L. *duco,* pp. *ductus,* to lead]

le·vo·form (lē′vō-fōrm). Denoting the structure of a substance that rotates the plane of polarized light counterclockwise (left); that is, as viewed by the observer looking toward the light source.

le·vo·glu·cose (lē-vō-gloo′kōs). D-Fructose. SEE fructose.

le·vo·gram (lē′vō-gram). Electrocardiographic record in an experimental animal representing spread of impulse through the left ventricle alone.

le·vo·gy·rate, le·vo·gy·rous (lē-vō-jī′rāt, -jī′rŭs). SYN levorotatory. [levo- + L. *gyro,* to turn in a circle]

le·vo·nor·def·rin (lē′vō-nōr-def′rin). Used as a nasal decongestant and as a vasoconstrictor given with infiltration anesthetics.

le·vo·pha·ce·top·er·ane (lē′vō-fa-sĕ-top′er′ān). An antidepressant with anorexigenic properties.

le·vo·pho·bia (lev′ō-fō′bē-ă). Fear of objects to the left.

le·vo·pro·pox·y·phene nap·syl·ate (lē′vō-prō-pok′si-fēn). An antitussive.

le·vo·ro·ta·tion (lē-vō-rō-tā′shŭn). 1. A turning or twisting to the left; in particular, the counterclockwise twist given the plane of plane-polarized light by solutions of certain optically active substances. Cf. dextrorotation. 2. SYN sinistrotorsion. [levo- + L. *roto,* to turn]

le·vo·ro·ta·to·ry (lē-vō-rō′tă-tōr-ē). 1. Denoting levorotation, or certain crystals or solutions capable of causing it; as a chemical prefix, usually abbreviated *l-* or (−). Cf. dextrorotatory. 2. Describing any leftward or anticlockwise rotation. SYN levogyrate, levogyrous.

lev·or·pha·nol tar·trate (lev-ōrf′ă-nol). An analgesic similar in action to morphine.

le·vo·tor·sion (lē-vō-tōr′shŭn). 1. SYN sinistrotorsion. 2. Rotation of the upper pole of the cornea of one or both eyes to the left. SYN levoclination. [levo- + L. *torsio,* a twisting]

le·vo·ver·sion (lē′vō-ver′zhŭn). 1. Version toward the left. 2. Conjugate turning of both eyes to the left. [levo- + L. *verto,* pp. *versus,* to turn]

Levret, André, French obstetrician, 1703–1780. SEE L. *forceps;* Mauriceau-L. *maneuver.*

lev·u·lan (lev′ū-lan). SYN fructosan (1).

lev·u·lic ac·id (lev′ū-lik). SYN levulinic acid.

lev·u·lin (lev′ū-lin). SYN fructosan (1).

lev·u·li·nate (lev′ū-lin-āt). A salt or ester of levulinic acid.

lev·u·lin·ic ac·id (lev-ū-lin′ik). 4-Oxopentanoic acid; formed by the action of hot, strong acids on hexoses. SEE ALSO δ-aminolevulinic acid. SYN levulic acid.

lev·u·lo·san (lev′ū-lō-san). SYN fructosan (1).

lev·u·lose (lev′ū-lōs). D-Fructose. SEE fructose.

lev·u·lo·se·mia (lev′ū-lō-sē′mē-ă). SYN fructosemia.

lev·u·lo·su·ria (lev′ū-lō-soo′rē-ă). SYN fructosuria.

Lévy, Gabrielle, French neurologist, 1886–1935. SEE Roussy-L. *disease, syndrome.*

Lewandowski, Felix, German dermatologist, 1879–1921. SEE Jadassohn-L. *syndrome.*

Lewis, Ivor, Welsh surgeon who in 1946 reported to the Royal College of Surgeons a two-stage esophagectomy by laparotomy and right thoracotomy, performed today as one procedure. SEE Ivor L. *esophagectomy.*

Lewis, Gilbert N., U.S. chemist, 1875–1946. SEE ALSO L. *acid, base;* second *law* of thermodynamics.

Lewis Blood Group, Le Blood Group. See Blood Groups Appendix.

lew·is·ite (loo′i-sīt). A war gas. It is a vesicant, a lung irritant like mustard gas, a systemic poison entering the circulation through the lungs or skin, and a mitotic poison arresting mitosis in the metaphase; dimercaprol is the antidote. SYN β-chlorovinyldichloroarsine. [W. Lee *Lewis,* U.S. chemist, 1898–1943]

Lewy (Lewey), Frederic H., German neurologist in the U.S., 1885–1950. SEE L. *bodies,* under *body;* Lewy body *dementia;* diffuse Lewy body *disease.*

lex·i·cal (leks′ĭ-kal). Denoting the vocabulary of speech or language.

♻-**lexis, -lexy.** Suffixes that properly relate to speech, although often confused with -legia (L. *lego,* to read) and thus erroneously employed to relate to reading. [G. *lexis,* word, speech, from *legō,* to say]

Leyden, Ernst V. von, German physician, 1832–1910. SEE L. *ataxia, crystals,* under *crystal, neuritis;* L.-Möbius muscular *dystrophy.*

Leydig, Franz von, German anatomist, 1821–1908. SEE L. *cells,* under *cell;* Leydig cell *tumor;* Sertoli-Leydig cell *tumor.*

ley·dig·ar·che (lī′dig-ar-kē). Obsolete term for the beginning of gonadal function in the male, e.g., male puberty. [Leydig (see Leydig cells), + G. *archē,* beginning]

Lf, L_f. SEE dose.

LFA Abbreviation for left frontoanterior position; lymphocyte function associated *antigen.*

LFP Abbreviation for left frontoposterior position.

LFT Abbreviation for left frontotransverse position.

LGSIL Abbreviation for low-grade squamous intraepithelial *lesion.*

LH Abbreviation for luteinizing *hormone.*

Lhermitte, Jean, French neurologist, 1877–1959. SEE L. *sign.*

LH/FSH-RF Abbreviation for luteinizing hormone/follicle-stimulating hormone-releasing *factor.*

LH-RF Abbreviation for luteinizing hormone-releasing *factor.*

LH-RH Abbreviation for luteinizing hormone-releasing *hormone.*

Li, Frederick P., 20th century epidemiologist. SEE L.-Fraumeni cancer *syndrome.*

Li Symbol for lithium.

lib·er·a·tor (lib′er-ā-ter, -tōr). An agent that stimulates or activates a physiological chemical or an enzymatic action.
    histamine l.'s, substances that cause the release of histamine from mast cells or basophils.

li·ber·ins (lib′er-ins). SYN releasing *factors.* [L. *libero,* to free, + -in]

lib·er·o·mo·tor (lib′er-ō-mō′ter). Relating to voluntary movements. [L. *liber,* free, + *motor,* mover]

li·bid·i·ni·za·tion (li-bid′i-ni-zā′shŭn). SYN erotization.

li·bid·i·nous (li-bid′i-nŭs). Lascivious; invested with or arousing sexual desire or energy. [L. *libidinosus,* fr. libido (libidin-), pleasure, desire]

li·bi·do (li-bē′dō, -bī′dō). 1. Conscious or unconscious sexual desire. 2. Any passionate interest or form of life force. 3. In jungian psychology, synonymous with psychic *energy.* [L. lust]
    object l., l. invested in the object, in contradistinction to that invested in the ego.

Libman, Emanuel, U.S. physician, 1872–1946. SEE L.-Sacks *endocarditis, syndrome.*

Liborius, Paul, 19th century Russian bacteriologist. SEE L. *method.*

li·brary (lī′brār-ē). A collection of cloned fragments that represent the entire genome.
    cDNA l., a collection of copy (cDNA) fragments that have been made by reverse transcriptase from the mRNA of a particular cell, organ, or organism.
    genomic l., l. in which both introns and exons are represented; a l. prepared from genomic DNA.
    l. screening, the process of selection of a desired clone from the collection.

lice (līs). Plural of louse.

li·chen (lī′ken). A discrete flat papule or an aggregate of papules giving a patterned configuration resembling lichen growing on rocks. [G. *leichēn,* lichen; a lichenlike eruption]
    l. myxedemato′sus, a lichenoid eruption of papules on the upper body of mucinous edema due to deposit of glycosaminoglycans in the skin and fibroblast proliferation, in the absence of endocrine disease. Monoclonal gammopathy is often present. SEE ALSO scleromyxedema. SYN papular mucinosis.
    l. ni′tidus, minute asymptomatic whitish or pinkish papules; lesions, which are flat-topped, rarely may coexist with l. planus and may involve male genitalia.
    l. nu′chae, l. simplex of the neck, usually in women.
    l. obtu′sus, a form in which the papules are large and rounded instead of flattened.
    oral (erosive) l. planus, oral manifestations of l. planus characterized by white striae (Wickham striae) of the oral mucous membrane and sometimes associated with ulceration; patients may or may not exhibit a history of cutaneous l. planus.
    l. planopila′ris, a rare, patchy alopecia with follicular hyperkera-

li

tosis of the scalp and lymphocytic perifolliculitis with l. planus elsewhere.

l. pla′nus, eruption of flat-topped, shiny, violaceous papules on flexor surfaces, male genitalia, and buccal mucosa of unknown cause; may form linear groups; microscopically characterized by a band-like subepidermal lymphocytic infiltrate. Spontaneous resolution is common after months to years.

l. pla′nus annula′ris, a form in which the papules are grouped in ring figures.

l. pla′nus follicula′ris, l. planus of the hair follicles, usually of the scalp.

l. pla′nus hypertro′phicus, verrucoid or warty lesions occurring on legs and thighs in association with l. planus elsewhere. SYN l. planus verrucosus.

l. pla′nus verruco′sus, SYN l. planus hypertrophicus.

l. ru′ber monilifor′mis, a rare dermatosis consisting of small reddish papules arranged in narrow beaded bands and covering large areas of the body.

l. sclero′sus et atro′phicus, an eruption consisting of pruritic white atrophic papules and plaques that may be discrete or confluent and may contain a central depression or a black keratotic plug microscopically showing epidermal hyperkeratosis and atrophy, superficial dermal edema and homogenization, and mid-dermal inflammation; occurs most commonly in prepubertal and postmenopausal females; vulval involvement was formerly called kraurosis vulvae.

l. scrofuloso′rum, small asymptomatic l. papules on the trunk of children with tuberculosis; acid-fast bacilli are not seen in the dermal granulomas. SYN papular tuberculid.

l. sim′plex chronicus, a thickened area of itching skin resulting from rubbing and scratching.

l. spinulo′sus, eruption of conical papules, of unknown cause, which have an adherent scaly surface; may be related to l. planus.

l. stria′tus, a self-limited papular eruption occurring primarily in children (more commonly in females); the lesions are arranged in linear groups and usually occur on one extremity.

li·chen·i·fi·ca·tion (lī′ken-i-fi-kā′shŭn). Leathery induration and thickening of the skin with hyperkeratosis, caused by scratching, as in atopic or chronic contact dermatitis. [lichen + L. *facio,* to make]

li·chen·in (lī′ken-in). A variety of polysaccharide obtained from Iceland moss; used as a demulcent. SYN moss starch.

li·chen·oid (lī′kĕ-noyd). **1.** Resembling lichen. **2.** Accentuation of normal skin markings observed in cases of chronic eczema. **3.** Microscopically resembling lichen planus.

Lichtenstein, Louis, U.S. physician, 1906–1977. SEE Jaffe-L. *disease.*

lic·o·rice (lik′ŏ-ris). SYN glycyrrhiza.

lid. SYN eyelid. [A.S. *hlid*]

granular l.'s, SYN trachoma.

lower l., SYN inferior *eyelid.*

upper l., SYN superior *eyelid.*

Liddell, Edward G.T., English neurophysiologist, 1895–1981. SEE L.-Sherrington *reflex.*

li·do·caine hy·dro·chlo·ride (lī′dō-kān). A local anesthetic with antiarrhythmic and anticonvulsant properties.

li·do·fla·zine (lī-dō-flā′zēn). A coronary vasodilator.

lie (lī). Relationship of the long axis of the fetus to that of the mother.

longitudinal l., that relationship in which the long axis of the fetus is longitudinal and roughly parallel to the long axis of the mother; the presenting part may be either the head or the breech.

oblique l., that relationship in which the long axis of the fetus crosses the maternal axis at an angle other than a right angle.

transverse l., that relationship in which the long axis of the fetus is transverse or at right angles to that of the mother.

unstable l., oblique orientation of the fetus that is neither transverse nor longitudinal, but that converts to one or the other before or during labor.

Lieberkühn, Johann N., German anatomist, 1711–1756. SEE

crypts of L., under *crypt;* L. *follicles,* under *follicle, glands,* under *gland.*

lie·ber·kühn (lē′ber-koon). A concave reflector around the objective of a microscope, for the purpose of directing a concentrated beam of light on the material being examined. [J.N. *Lieberkühn*]

Liebermann, Leo von S., Hungarian physician, 1852–1926. SEE Burchard-L. *reaction;* L.-Burchard *test.*

Liebermeister, Carl von, German physician, 1833–1901. SEE L. *rule.*

Liebig, Baron Justus von, German chemist, 1803–1873. SEE L. *theory.*

Liebow (lē′-bō), Averill A., Austrian-U.S. pulmonary pathologist, 1911–1978. SEE usual interstitial *pneumonia* of Liebow.

lie de·tec·tor. SYN polygraph (2).

li·en (lī′en). ✭official alternate term for spleen. [L.]

l. accesso′rius, ✭official alternate term for accessory *spleen.*

l. mo′bilis, SYN floating *spleen.*

l. succenturia′tus, SYN accessory *spleen.*

△**lien-, lieno-.** The spleen; most terms beginning thus are obsolete or obsolescent. SEE spleno-. [L. *lien*]

li·e·nal (lī′ĕ-năl). SYN splenic.

li·en·cu·lus (lī-en′kū-lŭs). SYN accessory *spleen.* [Mod. L. dim. of L. *lien,* spleen]

li·e·nec·to·my (lī′ĕ-nek′tō-mē). Obsolete term for splenectomy.

li·e·no·med·ul·lary (lī′ĕ-nō-med′ū-lār-ē). SYN splenomyelogenous. [lieno- + G. *medulla,* marrow]

li·e·no·my·e·log·e·nous (lī′ĕ-nō-mī-ĕ-loj′ĕ-nŭs). SYN splenomyelogenous.

li·e·no·pan·cre·at·ic (lī′ĕ-nō-pan′krē-at′ik). SYN splenopancreatic.

li·e·no·re·nal (lī′ĕ-nō-rē′năl). SYN splenorenal. [lieno- + L. *ren,* kidney]

li·en·ter·ic (lī-en-ter′ik). Relating to, or marked by, lientery.

li·en·tery (lī′en-ter-ē). Passage of undigested food in the stools. [G. *leienteria,* fr. *leios,* smooth, + *enteron,* intestine]

li·en·un·cu·lus (lī′ĕ-nun′kū-lŭs). SYN accessory *spleen.* [Mod. L. dim. of L. *lien,* spleen]

Liesegang, Ralph E., German chemist, 1869–1947. SEE L. *rings,* under *ring.*

Lieutaud, Joseph, French anatomist and pathologist, 1703–1780. SEE L. *body, triangle, trigone, uvula.*

life (līf). **1.** Vitality, the essential condition of being alive; the state of existence characterized by such functions as metabolism, growth, reproduction, adaptation, and response to stimuli. **2.** Living organisms such as animals and plants. [A.S. *lif*]

half-l., SEE half-life.

postnatal l., that interval of l. after birth; in humans, usually divided into periods: neonatal, infancy, childhood, adolescence, and adulthood.

prenatal l., that interval of l. between conception and birth; in humans, usually divided into embryonic and fetal periods.

quality of l., a patient's general well-being, including mental status, stress level, sexual function, and self-perceived health status.

sexual l., in psychiatry and psychoanalysis, the specifically erotic or sexual interests, fantasies, inclinations, and conduct of the patient.

vegetative l., the simple metabolic and reproductive activity of humans or animals, apart from the exercise of conscious mental or psychic processes.

life e·vents. Occurrences in one's daily life, some of which act as stressors.

life·span. 1. The duration of life of an individual. **2.** The normal or average duration of life of members of a given species. SEE ALSO longevity.

life-style. The set of habits and customs that is influenced by the lifelong process of socialization, including social use of substances such as alcohol and tobacco, dietary habits, exercise, etc., all of which have important implications for health.

LIGAMENT

lig·a·ment (lig′ă-ment) [TA]. **1.** A band or sheet of fibrous tissue connecting two or more bones, cartilages, or other structures, or serving as support for fasciae or muscles. **2.** A fold of peritoneum supporting any of the abdominal viscera. **3.** Any structure resembling a l. though not performing the function of such. **4.** The cordlike remains of a fetal vessel or other structure that has lost its original lumen. SYN ligamentum [TA]. [L. *ligamentum*, a band, bandage]

accessory l.'s, l.'s about a joint that are in addition to the articular capsule. They may lie within (intracapsular ligaments) or on the outside (extracapsular ligaments) of the articular capsule.

accessory plantar l.'s, SYN plantar l.'s.

accessory volar l.'s, SYN palmar l.'s.

acromioclavicular l. [TA], a fibrous band extending from the acromion of the scapula to the clavicle. SYN ligamentum acromioclaviculare [TA].

alar l.'s, one of a pair of short stout bands that extends from the side of the dens of the axis to the tubercle on the medial aspect of the occipital condyle; SYN check l.'s of odontoid.

alveolodental l., SYN periodontium.

anococcygeal l., a musculofibrous band that passes between the anus and the coccyx. SYN anococcygeal body, ligamentum anococcygeum, raphe anococcygea, Symington anococcygeal body.

anterior costotransverse l., SYN superior costotransverse l.

anterior cruciate l. [TA], the l. that extends from the anterior intercondylar area of the tibia to the posterior part of the medial surface of the lateral condyle of the femur. SYN ligamentum cruciatum anterius.

anterior l. of fibular head [TA], a l. uniting the anterior part of the head of the fibula to the tibia. SYN ligamentum capitis fibulae anterius [TA].

anterior l. of Helmholtz, SEE anterior l. of malleus.

anterior longitudinal l. [TA], the wide fibrous band interconnecting the anterolateral surfaces of the vertebral bodies, blending with the outer lamellae of the intervertebral disks as it passes between vertebrae. SYN ligamentum longitudinale anterius [TA], lacertus medius.

anterior l. of malleus [TA], consists of two portions: Meckel band, passing from the base of the anterior process to the spine of the sphenoid through the petrotympanic fissure; and the anterior l. of Helmholtz, extending from the anterior aspect of the neck of the malleus to the anterior boundary of the tympanic notch. SYN ligamentum mallei anterius [TA].

anterior meniscofemoral l. [TA], the ligamentous band that passes anterior to the posterior cruciate l., extending between the posterior portion of the lateral meniscus and the upper end of the anterior cruciate l. SYN ligamentum meniscofemorale anterius [TA], Humphry l.

anterior sacrococcygeal l. [TA], the continuation of the anterior longitudinal l. uniting the sacrum and coccyx. SYN ligamentum sacrococcygeum anterius [TA], ventral sacrococcygeal l.

anterior sacroiliac l.'s [TA], the strong fibrous bands that reinforce the sacroiliac joint anteriorly. SYN ligamenta sacroiliaca anteriora [TA], ventral sacroiliac l.'s.

anterior sacrosciatic l., SYN sacrospinous l.

anterior sternoclavicular l. [TA], a fibrous band that reinforces the sternoclavicular anteriorly. SYN ligamentum sternoclaviculare anterius [TA].

anterior talofibular l. [TA], the band of fibers that extends from the lateral malleolus to the neck of the talus. SYN ligamentum talofibulare anterius [TA].

anterior talotibial l., SYN anterior tibiotalar *part* of medial ligament of ankle joint; SEE ALSO medial l. of ankle joint.

anterior tibiofibular l. [TA], the l. that binds the anterior aspect of the tibiofibular syndesmosis. SYN ligamentum tibiofibulare anterius [TA].

anterior tibiotalar l., SYN anterior tibiotalar *part* of medial ligament of ankle joint.

anular i. [TA], one of a number of l.'s encircling various parts; the principal anular l.'s are those of the stapes, radius, and trachea. SEE anular l. of radius, anular l. of stapes, anular l.'s of trachea. SYN ligamentum anulare [TA], orbicular l.

anular l. of radius [TA], the l. that encircles and holds the head of the radius in the radial notch of the ulna, forming the proximal radioulnar joint and enabling pronation/supination of forearm; receives the radial collateral l. of the elbow. SYN ligamentum anulare radii [TA], ligamentum orbiculare radii, orbicular l. of radius.

anular l. of stapes [TA], a ring of elastic fibers that attaches the base of the stapes to the margin of the fenestra vestibuli. SYN ligamentum anulare stapedis [TA].

anular l.'s of trachea [TA], the fibrous membranes that connect adjacent tracheal cartilages. SYN ligamenta anularia trachealia [TA], ligamenta trachealia.

apical l. of dens [TA], a l. that extends from the apex of the dens of the axis to the anterior margin of the foramen magnum; includes vestiges of notochord. SYN ligamentum apicis dentis.

Arantius l., SYN *ligamentum* venosum.

arcuate popliteal l. [TA], a broad fibrous band attached above to the lateral condyle of the femur and passing medially and downward, blending with the posterior part of the fibrous capsule of the knee joint, arching over the tendon of the popliteus muscle. SYN ligamentum popliteum arcuatum [TA], popliteal arch, posterior l. of knee.

arcuate pubic l., SYN inferior pubic l.

arterial l., SYN *ligamentum* arteriosum.

l.'s of auditory ossicles [TA], the l.'s connecting the ear bones with one another and with the walls of the tympanic cavity. SYN ligamenta ossiculorum auditus [TA], ligamenta ossiculorum auditorium☆.

l.'s of auricle [TA], the three l.'s that attach the auricle to the side of the head: anterior l. of auricle (*ligamentum* auriculare anterius), which extends from the root of the zygomatic process to the spine of the helix; posterior l. of auricle (*ligamentum* auriculare posterius), which extends from the mastoid process to the conchal eminence; superior l. of auricle (*ligamentum* auriculare superius), which extends from the superior margin of the osseous external acoustic meatus to the spine of the helix. SYN ligamenta auricularia [TA], auricular l.'s, Valsalva l.'s.

auricular l.'s, SYN l.'s of auricle.

axis l. of malleus, SYN Helmholtz axis l.

Bardinet l., the posterior band of the ulnar collateral l. of the elbow.

Barkow l.'s, the anterior and posterior portions of the fibrous capsule of the elbow joint.

Bellini l., a fasciculus from the ischiofemoral portion of greater articular fibrous capsule of the hip that extends to the greater trochanter.

Berry l.'s, SYN lateral thyrohyoid l.

Bertin l., SYN iliofemoral l.

Bichat l., the lower fasciculus of the posterior sacroiliac l.

bifurcate l. [TA], a strong, V-shaped dorsal tarsal l. on the dorsum of the foot that passes from the calcaneus distal to the tarsal sinus and attaches to cuboid and navicular bones; it is divided into the calcaneocuboid l. and the calcaneonavicular l. SYN ligamentum bifurcatum [TA], bifurcated l.

bifurcated l., SYN bifurcate l.

Bigelow l., SYN iliofemoral l.

Botallo l., SYN *ligamentum* arteriosum.

Bourgery l., SYN oblique popliteal l.

broad l. of the uterus [TA], the peritoneal fold passing from the lateral margin of the uterus to the wall of the pelvis on either side, and in so doing also ensheathing the ovaries and uterine tubes. SYN ligamentum latum uteri [TA].

Brodie l., SYN transverse humeral l.

Burns l., SYN superior *horn* of falciform margin of saphenous opening.

li

calcaneocuboid l. [TA], the lateral part of the bifurcate l. SYN ligamentum calcaneocuboideum [TA].

calcaneofibular l. [TA], the middle of the three fascicles that form the lateral l. of the ankle joint, reinforcing the lateral side of the ankle joint and resisting excessive inversion of the foot; the remaining two l.'s of the lateral l.'s are the anterior and posterior talofibular l.'s. SYN ligamentum calcaneofibulare [TA].

calcaneonavicular l. [TA], the medial part of the bifurcate ligament. SYN ligamentum calcaneonaviculare [TA].

calcaneotibial l., SYN tibiocalcaneal *part* of medial ligament of ankle joint; SEE ALSO medial l. of ankle joint.

Caldani l., SYN coracoclavicular l.

Campbell l., SYN suspensory l. of axilla.

Camper l., SYN perineal *membrane*.

capsular l. [TA], thickened portions of the fibrous membrane of an articular capsule. SYN ligamentum capsulare [TA].

cardinal l. [TA], a fibrous band attached to the uterine cervix and the vault of the lateral fornix of the vagina; continuous with the tissue ensheathing the pelvic vessels. SYN ligamentum cardinale [TA], transverse cervical l.★, cervical l. of uterus, ligamentum transversale cervicis, Mackenrodt l.

caroticoclinoid l., the l. that connects the anterior to the middle clinoid process of the sphenoid bone.

carpometacarpal l.'s (dorsal and palmar) [TA], the l.'s uniting the metacarpal and carpal bones. SYN ligamenta carpometacarpalia (dorsalia/palmaria) [TA].

caudal l., SYN *retinaculum* caudale.

ceratocricoid l. [TA], one of three ligaments (anterior, posterior, and lateral) reinforcing the capsule of the cricothyroid articulation on either side. SYN ligamentum ceratocricoideum [TA].

cervical l. of uterus, SYN cardinal l.

check l.'s of eyeball, medial and lateral, SYN check l.'s of medial and lateral rectus muscles.

check l.'s of medial and lateral rectus muscles [TA], expansions of the sheaths of the medial and lateral rectus muscles of the eyeball that are attached, respectively, to the lacrimal bone and to the orbital tubercle of the zygomatic bone; they serve to prevent overaction of these muscles. Terminologia Anatomica recognizes only the check l. of lateral rectus muscle. SYN check l.'s of eyeball, medial and lateral.

check l.'s of odontoid, SYN alar l.'s.

chondroxiphoid l., SYN costoxiphoid l.

ciliary l., SYN ciliary *muscle*.

Civinini l., SYN pterygospinous l.

Clado l., a mesenteric fold running from the broad l. on the right side to the appendix.

coccygeal l., ★official alternate term for dural *part* of filum terminale.

collateral l. [TA], one of a number of l.'s on either side of, and serving as a radius of movement of, a joint having a hingelike movement; they occur at the following joints: elbow, knee, wrist, and the metacarpo- or metatarsophalangeal, proximal interphalangeal, and distal interphalangeal joints of the hands and feet. SYN ligamentum collaterale [TA].

Colles l., SYN reflected inguinal l.

conoid l. [TA], the medial part of the coracoclavicular l. that attaches to the conoid tubercle of the clavicle. The conoid ligament and its partner coracoclavicular ligament, the trapezoid ligament, passively suspend the free upper limb from the strut formed by the clavicle. SYN ligamentum conoideum [TA].

Cooper l.'s, (1) SYN suspensory l.'s of breast; **(2)** SYN pectineal l; **(3)** SYN transverse l. of elbow.

coracoacromial l. [TA], the heavy arched fibrous band that passes between the coracoid process and the acromion above the shoulder joint; the osseofibrous arch thus formed prevents upward dislocation of the shoulder (glenohumeral) joint. SYN ligamentum coracoacromiale [TA].

coracoclavicular l. [TA], the strong compound l. that unites the clavicle to the coracoid process; it is subdivided into the conoid ligamentum and the trapezoid ligamentum. The free upper limb is passively suspended from the clavicular "strut" by the coracocla-

vicular l.; the l. also plays an important role in preventing dislocation of the acromioclavicular joint. SYN ligamentum coracoclaviculare [TA], Caldani l.

coracohumeral l. [TA], the l. that passes from the base of the coracoid process to the greater tubercle of the humerus. SYN ligamentum coracohumerale [TA].

corniculopharyngeal l., SYN cricopharyngeal l.

coronary l. of knee, portions of the articular capsule of the knee joint that connect the circumference of the menisci with the margins of the condyles of the tibia.

coronary l. of liver [TA], peritoneal reflections from the liver to the diaphragm at the margins of the bare area of the liver. SYN ligamentum coronarium hepatis [TA].

costoclavicular l. [TA], the l. that connects the first rib and the clavicle near its sternal end; limits elavation of shoulder (at sternoclavicular joint). SYN ligamentum costoclaviculare [TA], rhomboid l.

costocolic l., SYN phrenicocolic l.

costotransverse l. [TA], the l. that connects the dorsal aspect of the neck of a rib to the ventral aspect of the corresponding transverse process. SEE ALSO lateral costotransverse l., superior costotransverse l. SYN ligamentum costotransversarium [TA], ligamentum colli costae, middle costotransverse l.

costoxiphoid l. [TA], the l. that connects the xiphoid process to the seventh, and often to the sixth, costal cartilages. SYN ligamentum costoxiphoideum [TA], chondroxiphoid l.

cotyloid l., SYN acetabular *labrum*.

Cowper l., the part of the fascia lata which is anterior to and provides origin for fibers of the pectineus muscle.

cricoarytenoid l. [TA], the l. that passes downward from the posterior border of the arytenoid cartilage to the lamina of the cricoid cartilage. SYN ligamentum cricoarytenoideum posterius, posterior cricoarytenoid l.

cricopharyngeal l. [TA], an elastic band connecting the tip of the corniculate (Santorini) cartilage and the lamina of the cricoid cartilage and continuing into the pharyngeal mucosa covering the cricoid lamina. SYN ligamentum cricopharyngeum [TA], corniculopharyngeal l., cricosantorinian l., jugal l., ligamentum corniculopharyngeum, ligamentum jugale.

cricosantorinian l., SYN cricopharyngeal l.

cricotracheal l. [TA], a midline fibrous band connecting the cricoid cartilage with the first ring of the trachea. SYN ligamentum cricotracheale [TA], cricotracheal membrane.

crucial l., (1) SEE inferior extensor *retinaculum*, superior extensor *retinaculum*; **(2)** SYN cruciate l.'s of knee; **(3)** SYN cruciate l. of the atlas; **(4)** SYN cruciform *part* of fibrous digital sheath.

cruciate l. of the atlas [TA], the strong l. that lies posterior to the dens of the axis holding it against the anterior arch of the atlas; it consists primarily of the transverse l. of the atlas that forms the cross-bar of the cross and is most important functionally, and longitudinal bands of the cruciform l., forming the upright or vertical beams of the cross. SYN ligamentum cruciforme atlantis [TA], crucial l. (3), cruciform l. of atlas, ligamentum cruciatum atlantis.

▪ **cruciate l.'s of knee,** the two l.'s that pass from the intercondylar area of the tibia to the intercondylar fossa of the femur. SEE anterior cruciate l., posterior cruciate l; SEE ALSO anterior cruciate l., posterior cruciate l. SYN crucial l. (2), ligamenta cruciata genus.

cruciate l. of leg, SYN inferior extensor *retinaculum*.

cruciform l. of atlas, SYN cruciate l. of the atlas.

Cruveilhier l.'s, SYN plantar l.'s.

cuboideonavicular l.'s [TA], l. uniting the cuboid bone with the navicular bone. SEE dorsal cuboideonavicular l., plantar cuboideonavicular l.'s. SYN ligamenta cuboideonaviculare [TA].

cuneocuboid l.'s [TA], ligament uniting the lateral cuneiform bone with the cuboid bone. SEE dorsal cuneocuboid l., cuneocuboid interosseous l., plantar cuneocuboid l. SYN ligamentum cuneocuboideum [TA].

cuneocuboid interosseous l. [TA], the fibrous band that unites adjacent margins of the distal end of the lateral cuneiform and cuboid bones. SYN interosseous cuneocuboid l., ligamentum cuneocuboideum interosseum.

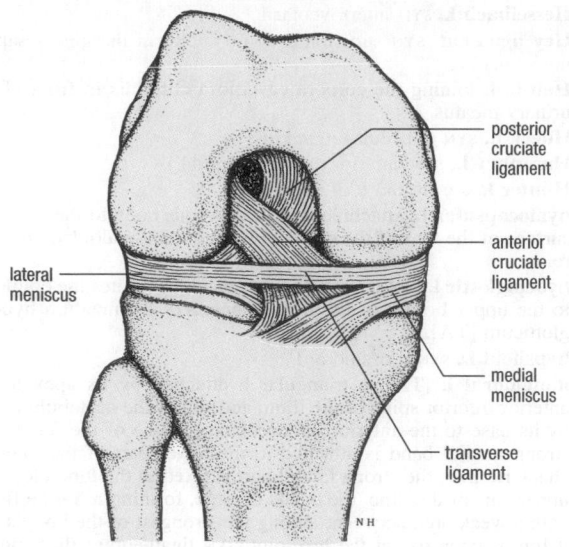

posterior
cruciate
ligament

anterior
cruciate
ligament

lateral
meniscus

medial
meniscus

transverse
ligament

N H

cruciate ligaments of knee

cuneometatarsal interosseous l.'s [TA], l.'s that pass from the cuneiform bones to the metatarsals, the one from the first cuneiform to the second metatarsal being the strongest. SYN ligamenta cuneometatarsalia interossea [TA], interosseous cuneometatarsal l.'s, Lisfranc l.'s.

cuneonavicular l.'s, l.'s uniting the medial cuneiform bone with the navicular. SEE ALSO dorsal cuneonavicular l.'s, plantar cuneonavicular l.'s.

cystoduodenal l., a peritoneal fold that sometimes passes from the gallbladder to the first part of the duodenum.

deep dorsal sacrococcygeal l., SYN deep posterior sacrococcygeal l.

deep posterior sacrococcygeal l., the continuation of the posterior longitudinal l. uniting the sacrum and coccyx. SYN deep dorsal sacrococcygeal l., ligamentum sacrococcygeum posterius profundum.

deep transverse metacarpal l. [TA], the l. that interconnects the palmar surface of the heads of the second to fifth metacarpals, being continuous with the palmar l.'s or palmar plates; it lies in the plane of the palmar interosseous fascia. SYN ligamentum metacarpale transversum profundum [TA], transverse metacarpal l.

deep transverse metatarsal l. [TA], the l. that interconnects the plantar surface of the heads of the metatarsals, being continuous with the plantar l.'s. SYN ligamentum metatarsale transversum profundum [TA], transverse metatarsal l.

deltoid l., ✩official alternate term for medial l. of ankle joint.

Denonvilliers l., SYN puboprostatic l.

dentate l. of spinal cord, rarely used variation on the spelling of denticulate l.

denticulate l. [TA], a serrated, shelflike extension of the spinal pia mater projecting in a frontal plane from either side of the cervical and thoracic spinal cord; its approximately 21 pointed processes fuse laterally with the arachnoid and dura mater midway between the exits of the roots of adjacent spinal nerves, with the highest process attaching immediately superior to foramen magnum. SYN ligamentum denticulatum [TA].

Denucé l., SYN quadrate l.

diaphragmatic l. of the mesonephros, the segment of the urogenital ridge that extends from the mesonephros to the diaphragm; becomes the suspensory l. of the ovary. SYN urogenital mesentery.

dorsal calcaneocuboid l., SEE bifurcate l.

dorsal carpal l., SYN extensor *retinaculum.*

dorsal carpometacarpal l.'s [TA], fibrous bands that connect the dorsal surfaces of the carpal and metacarpal bones. SYN ligamenta carpometacarpalia dorsalia [TA].

dorsal cuboideonavicular l. [TA], the dorsal tarsal l. that unites the dorsal surfaces of the cuboid and navicular bones of the tarsus. SYN ligamentum cuboideonaviculare dorsale [TA].

dorsal cuneocuboid l. [TA], one of the dorsal tarsal ligaments appearing as a fibrous band that unites the dorsal margins of the lateral cuneiform and cuboid bones. SYN ligamentum cuneocuboideum dorsale [TA].

dorsal cuneonavicular l.'s [TA], several l.'s connecting the dorsal surface of the navicular with the three cuneiform bones. SYN ligamenta cuneonavicularia dorsalia [TA].

dorsal intercuneiform l.'s [TA], the dorsal tarsal ligament extending between adjacent cuneiform bones.

dorsal metacarpal l.'s [TA], fibrous bands connecting the dorsal aspects of the bases of metacarpals two to five. SYN ligamenta metacarpalia dorsalia [TA].

dorsal metatarsal l.'s [TA], fibrous bands that connect the dorsal aspects of the bases of the metatarsals. SYN ligamenta metatarsalia dorsalia [TA].

dorsal radiocarpal l. [TA], the l. that extends from the distal end of the radius posteriorly to the proximal row of carpal bones. SYN ligamentum radiocarpale dorsale [TA].

dorsal sacroiliac l.'s, SYN posterior sacroiliac l.'s.

dorsal tarsal l.'s [TA], l.'s connecting dorsal aspects of the tarsal bones as a group; included in the group are the: talonavicular l. [TA] (ligamentum talonaviculare [TA]), bifurcate l. [TA] (ligamentum bifurcatum [TA]), and the following dorsal l.'s (ligamentum/a . . . dorsalia/e): intercuneiform [TA] (intercuneiformia [TA]), cuneocuboid [TA] (cuneocuboideum [TA]), cuboideonavicular [TA] (cuboideonaviculare [TA]), cuneonavicular [TA] (cuneonavicularia [TA]), and calcaneocuboid [TA] (calcaneocuboideum [TA]). SYN ligamenta tarsi dorsalia [TA].

dorsal tarsometatarsal l.'s [TA], strong, flat, longitudinal, and oblique bands reinforcing the dorsal aspects of the tarsometatarsal joints (joints between the metatarsals and the cuboid and cuneiform bones); the first metatarsal and medial cuneiform share an exclusive joint capsule, and the medial dorsal tarsometatarsal l.'s connect only those bones; the remaining metatarsals have attachments to multiple bones, with the ligaments reinforcing the dorsal aspect of their common joint capsule. SYN ligamenta tarsometatarsalia dorsalia [TA].

duodenorenal l., a fold of peritoneum occasionally passing from the termination of the hepatoduodenal l. to the front of the right kidney. SYN ligamentum duodenorenale.

l.'s of epididymis (inferior and superior), one of two folds (superior and inferior) of the tunica vaginalis between the epididymis and the testis. SYN ligamenta epididymidis (inferius et superius) [TA].

epihyal l., SYN stylohyoid l.

external collateral l. of wrist, SYN radial collateral l. of wrist joint.

extracapsular l.'s [TA], l.'s associated with a synovial joint but separate from and external to its articular capsule. SYN ligamenta extracapsularia [TA].

falciform l., SYN falciform *process* of sacrotuberous ligament.

falciform l. of liver [TA], a crescentic fold of peritoneum extending to the surface of the liver from the diaphragm and anterior abdominal wall; the round ligament lies in its free inferior border, derivative of embryonic ventral mesogastrium. SYN ligamentum falciforme hepatis [TA].

fallopian l., SYN inguinal l.

Ferrein l., SYN lateral l. of temporomandibular joint.

fibular collateral l. [TA], the cordlike l. that passes from the lateral epicondyle of the femur to the head of the fibula. SYN ligamentum collaterale fibulare [TA], lateral l. of knee, Winslow l.

fibular collateral l. of ankle, SYN lateral l. of ankle.

Flood l., a band of the coracohumeral ligament, attached to the lower part of the lesser tuberosity of the humerus.

fundiform l. of clitoris [TA], fibrous condensation of the subcutaneous tissue descending from the linea alba above the pubic symphysis to split and surround the root of the body of the clitoris, before fusing with the fascia of the clitoris. SYN ligamentum fundiforme clitoridis [TA].

fundiform l. of foot, SYN Retzius l.

fundiform l. of penis [TA], a band of elastic fibers of the superficial fascial layer that extends from the linea alba above the pubic symphysis splitting to surround the penis before attaching to the fascia of the penis. SYN ligamentum fundiforme penis [TA].

gastrocolic l. [TA], the major, apron-like portion of the greater omentum that extends between the stomach and the transverse colon. SYN ligamentum gastrocolicum [TA].

gastrodiaphragmatic l., SYN gastrophrenic l.

gastrolienal l., SYN gastrosplenic l.

gastrophrenic l. [TA], the portion of the greater omentum that extends from the greater curvature of the stomach to the inferior surface of the diaphragm. SYN ligamentum gastrophrenicum [TA], gastrodiaphragmatic l., phrenogastric l.

gastrosplenic l. [TA], the portion of the greater omentum that lies between the greater curvature of the stomach and the hilum of the spleen. SYN ligamentum gastrosplenicum [TA], ligamentum gastrolienale⁂, gastrolienal l., gastrosplenic omentum.

genital l., an embryonic mesenchymatous band providing support for the internal genitalia. SYN suspensory l. of gonad.

genitoinguinal l., in the fetus, a fold of the mesorchium containing the gubernaculum testis. SYN ligamentum genitoinguinale, plica gubernatrix.

Gerdy l., SYN suspensory l. of axilla.

Gillette suspensory l., SYN cricoesophageal *tendon.*

Gimbernat l., SYN lacunar l.

gingivodental l., SYN periodontium.

glenohumeral l.'s [TA], three fibrous bands (capsular ligaments) that reinforce the anterior part of the articular capsule of the shoulder joint; they are in continuity with the glenoid labrum at the supraglenoid tubercle of the scapula and blend with the fibrous capsule as it attaches to the anatomic neck of the humerus; they are conspicuous as folds or ridges on the internal aspect of the articular capsule. SYN ligamenta glenohumeralia [TA].

glenoid l., (1) SYN glenoid *labrum* of scapula; (2) SYN plantar l.'s.

glossoepiglottic l., an elastic ligamentous band passing from the base of the tongue to the epiglottis in the middle glossoepiglottic fold.

Günz l., a portion of the superficial layer of the obturator membrane.

hammock l., the part of the periodontium below the growing end of the root of the tooth.

l. of head of femur [TA], a flattened l. that passes from the fovea in the head of the femur to the borders of the acetabular notch (transverse acetabular l.); developmentally, an artery passes to the head of the femur with the l. which may or may not persist into adulthood; the l. does not contribute to the integrity of the joint or control movements there. SYN ligamentum capitis femoris [TA], ligamentum teres femoris, round l. of femur.

Helmholtz axis l., a l. forming the axis about which the malleus rotates; it consists of two portions extending from the anterior and the posterior border, respectively, of the tympanic notch to the malleus. SYN axis l. of malleus.

Hensing l., the left superior colic l.; a small serous horizontal or oblique fold sometimes found extending between the upper end of the descending colon and the abdominal wall. SEE phrenicocolic l.

hepatocolic l. [TA], an inconstant extension of the hepatoduodenal l. to the transverse colon. SYN ligamentum hepatocolicum [TA].

hepatoduodenal l. [TA], the portion of the lesser omentum that connects the liver and duodenum. SYN ligamentum hepatoduodenale [TA].

hepatoesophageal l. [TA], the part of the lesser omentum that extends between the liver and the abdominal part of the esophagus. SYN ligamentum hepatoesophageum [TA].

hepatogastric l. [TA], the part of the lesser omentum that extends between the liver and lesser curvature of the stomach. SYN ligamentum hepatogastricum [TA].

hepatorenal l. [TA], a prolongation of the coronary l. downward over the right kidney. SYN ligamentum hepatorenale [TA].

Hesselbach l., SYN interfoveolar l.

Hey ligament, SYN superior *horn* of falciform margin of saphenous opening.

Holl l., l. joining the corpora cavernosa clitoridis in front of the urinary meatus.

Hueck l., SYN trabecular *tissue* of sclera.

Humphry l., SYN anterior meniscofemoral l.

Hunter l., SYN round l. of uterus.

hyalocapsular l., attachment of the vitreous body to the posterior surface of the lens of the eye. SYN ligamentum hyaloideo-capsulare.

hyoepiglottic l. [TA], a short elastic band that unites the epiglottis to the upper border of the hyoid bone. SYN ligamentum hyoepiglotticum [TA].

hypsiloid l., SYN iliofemoral l.

iliofemoral l. [TA], a triangular l. attached by its apex to the anterior inferior spine of the ilium and rim of the acetabulum, and by its base to the anterior intertrochanteric line of the femur; the strong medial band is attached to the lower part of the intertrochanteric line; the strong lateral part is fixed to the tubercle at the upper part of this line; the bands diverge, forming a Y-like figure with a weak area between; among the strongest of the body's l.'s, it limits extension at the hip joint. SYN ligamentum iliofemorale [TA], Bertin l., Bigelow l., hypsiloid l., Y-shaped l.

iliolumbar l. [TA], the strong l. that connects the fourth and fifth lumbar vertebrae with the ilium, spanning the "notch" between the vertebral column and the wing of the ilium. SYN ligamentum iliolumbale [TA].

iliopectineal l., SYN iliopectineal *arch.*

iliotrochanteric l., the lateral strong band of the Y-shaped iliofemoral l.; it is attached below to the tubercle at the upper part of the intertrochanteric line.

inferior calcaneonavicular l., SYN plantar calcaneonavicular l.

inferior l. of epididymis [TA], the lower of the folds of the tunica vaginalis between the body of the epididymis and the testis. SYN ligamentum epididymidis inferius [TA].

inferior pubic l. [TA], the l. that arches across the inferior aspect of the pubic symphysis. SYN ligamentum pubicum inferius [TA], arcuate pubic l., ligamentum arcuatum pubis.

inferior transverse scapular l. [TA], an inconstant fibrous band that passes from the lateral border of the spine of the scapula to the posterior margin of the glenoid cavity. SYN ligamentum transversum scapulae inferius [TA], spinoglenoid l.

infundibulo-ovarian l., SYN ovarian *fimbria.*

infundibulopelvic l., SYN suspensory l. of ovary.

inguinal l. [TA], a fibrous band formed by the thickened inferior border of the aponeurosis of the external oblique that extends from the anterior superior spine of the ilium to the pubic tubercle, bridging muscular and vascular lacunae; forms the floor of the inguinal canal; gives origin to the lowermost fibers of internal oblique and transversus abdominis muscles. SEE ALSO *aponeurosis* of external oblique muscle. SYN ligamentum inguinale [TA], arcus inguinalis⁂, crural arch, fallopian arch, fallopian l., femoral arch, Poupart l.

inguinal l. of the kidney, the segment of the mesonephros extending to the inguinal region.

intercarpal l.'s [TA], three sets of short fibrous bands that bind together the two rows of carpal bones; according to their location they are named dorsal intercarpal l.'s (ligamenta intercarpalia dorsalia), interosseous intercarpal l.'s (ligamenta intercarpalia interossea), and palmar intercarpal l.'s (ligamenta intercarpalia palmaria). SYN ligamenta intercarpalia [TA].

interclavicular l. [TA], a strong l. that connects the two sternoclavicular joints across the upper border of the manubrium. SYN ligamentum interclaviculare [TA].

interclinoid l., a band of dura mater connecting the anterior and posterior clinoid processes of the sphenoid bone; may become ossified.

intercornual l., SYN lateral sacrococcygeal l.

intercostal l.'s, SYN intercostal *membranes,* under *membrane.*

intercuneiform l.'s [TA], fibrous bands that unite the cuneiform bones; they are arranged in three sets: dorsal intercuneiform l.'s (ligamenta intercuneiformia dorsalia), interosseous intercuneiform l.'s (ligamenta intercuneiformia interossea), and plantar intercuneiform l.'s (ligamenta intercuneiformia plantaria). SYN ligamenta intercuneiformia [TA].

interfoveolar l. [TA], fibrous or muscular strands that lie medial to the deep inguinal ring, extending from the lower border of the transversus muscle to the lacunar l. and pectineal fascia. SYN ligamentum interfoveolare [TA], Hesselbach l.

internal collateral l. of the wrist, SYN ulnar collateral l. of wrist joint.

interosseous cuneocuboid l., SYN cuneocuboid interosseous l.

interosseous cuneometatarsal l.'s, SYN cuneometatarsal interosseous l.'s.

interosseous metacarpal l.'s [TA], fibrous bands connecting the bases of metacarpals two to five; they extend between the dorsal and palmar metacarpal ligaments. SYN ligamenta metacarpalia interossea [TA].

interosseous metatarsal l.'s, SYN metatarsal interosseous l.'s.

interosseous sacroiliac l.'s [TA], short obliquely directed fibrous bands that pass between the sacrum and ilium in the narrow cleft behind the auricular surfaces of these bones. SYN ligamenta sacroiliaca interossea [TA].

interosseous talocalcaneal l., SYN talocalcaneal interosseous l.

interosseous tibiofibular l., the distal continuation of the interosseous membrane forming a strong l. that unites the distal end of the tibia and fibula; it lies deep to the posterior tibiofibular l. SYN transverse tibiofibular l.

interspinous l. [TA], bands of fibrous tissue that connect the spinous processes of adjacent vertebrae. SYN ligamentum interspinale [TA].

intertransverse l. [TA], one of the ligaments that connect the transverse processes of adjacent vertebrae. SYN ligamentum intertransversarium [TA].

intraarticular l. of costal head, SYN intraarticular l. of head of rib.

intraarticular l. of head of rib [TA], transverse fibers extending within the capsule from the ridge between the two facets on the head of the rib to the intervertebral disk. SYN intraarticular l. of costal head, ligamentum capitis costae intraarticulare.

intraarticular sternocostal l. [TA], a l. within the articular capsule between a costal cartilage and the sternum; especially well developed at second costal cartilage. SYN ligamentum sternocostale intraarticulare [TA].

intracapsular l.'s [TA], ligaments located within and separate from the articular capsule of a synovial joint. SYN ligamenta intracapsularia [TA].

ischiocapsular l., SYN ischiofemoral l.

ischiofemoral l. [TA], the thickened part of the capsule of the hip joint that passes from the ischium upward and laterally over the femoral neck; some of its fibers continue into the zona orbicularis. SYN ligamentum ischiofemorale [TA], ischiocapsular l., ligamentum ischiocapsulare.

jugal l., SYN cricopharyngeal l.

Krause l., SYN transverse perineal l.

laciniate l., SYN flexor *retinaculum* of lower limb.

lacunar l. [TA], a curved fibrous band that passes horizontally backward from the medial end of the inguinal l. to the pectineal line; it forms the medial boundary of the femoral ring. SEE ALSO *aponeurosis* of external oblique muscle. SYN ligamentum lacunare [TA], Gimbernat l.

Lannelongue l.'s, SYN sternopericardial l.'s.

lateral l. of ankle [TA], the calcaneofibular l., anterior talofibular l., and posterior talofibular l. together maintaining the integrity of the lateral aspect of the talocrural joint. SYN ligamentum collaterale laterale [TA], fibular collateral l. of ankle, lateral collateral l. of ankle.

lateral arcuate l. [TA], a thickening of the fascia of the quadratus lumborum muscle between the transverse process of the first lumbar vertebra and the twelfth rib on either side that gives attachment to a portion of the diaphragm (one of the Haller arches). SYN ligamentum arcuatum laterale [TA], arcus lumbocostalis lateralis, lateral lumbocostal arch.

lateral l. of bladder, condensations of fibroareolar tissue that pass one from each side of the bladder to blend with the pelvic fascia; smooth muscle is usually present in this tissue and is referred to as the rectovesicalis (musculus rectovesicalis). SYN ligamentum laterale vesicae [TA].

lateral collateral l. of ankle, SYN lateral l. of ankle.

lateral costotransverse l. [TA], the short quadrangular l., actually a thickening of the posterior aspect of the costotransverse joint, extending from the tip of the transverse process to the posterior surface of the neck of the rib. SYN ligamentum costotransversarium laterale [TA], ligamentum costotransversarium posterius, ligamentum tuberculi costae, posterior costotransverse l.

lateral l. of elbow, SYN radial collateral l. of elbow joint.

lateral l. of knee, SYN fibular collateral l.

lateral malleolar l., SEE anterior tibiofibular l., posterior tibiofibular l.

lateral l. of malleus [TA], a short fan-shaped l. converging from the posterior notch of the tympanic notch to the neck of the malleus. SYN ligamentum mallei laterale [TA].

lateral palpebral l. [TA], the band that attaches the tarsal plates to the orbital eminence of the zygomatic bone. SYN ligamentum palpebrale laterale [TA], ligamentum palpebrale externum, ligamentum tarsale externum.

lateral puboprostatic l., ✶official alternate term for puboprostatic l; SEE puboprostatic l.

lateral sacrococcygeal l. [TA], a l. that extends from the lateral inferior margin of the sacrum to the transverse process of the first coccygeal vertebra. SYN ligamentum sacrococcygeum laterale [TA], intercornual l.

lateral talocalcaneal l. [TA], a l. extending from the trochlea of the talus to the lateral surface of the calcaneus. SYN ligamentum talocalcaneum laterale [TA].

lateral temporomandibular l., SYN lateral l. of temporomandibular joint.

lateral l. of temporomandibular joint [TA], the capsular l. that passes obliquely down and backward across the lateral surface of the temporomandibular joint. SYN ligamentum laterale articulationis temporomandibularis [TA], Ferrein l., lateral temporomandibular l., ligamentum temporomandibulare, temporomandibular l.

lateral thyrohyoid l. [TA], thickened elastic bundle connecting the superior horn of the thyroid cartilage to the tip of the greater horn of the hyoid cartilage; forms the posterior border of the thyrohyoid membrane. SYN ligamentum thyrohyoideum laterale [TA], Berry l.'s, ligamentum hyothyroideum laterale.

lateral umbilical l., SYN *ligamentum* umbilicale laterale.

lateral l. of wrist, SYN radial collateral l. of wrist joint.

Lauth l., SYN transverse l. of the atlas.

l. of left superior vena cava, the obliterated left common cardinal vein that extends from the left brachiocephalic vein to the oblique vein of the left atrium.

left triangular l. of liver [TA], a triangular fold of fibrous connective tissue and peritoneum that extends from the left lobe of the liver to the diaphragm. SYN ligamentum triangulare sinistrum hepatis [TA].

l. of left vena cava [TA], the obliterated left common cardinal vein; it extends from the left brachiocephalic vein to the oblique vein of the left atrium. SYN ligamentum venae cavae sinistrae [TA].

lienophrenic l., SYN phrenicosplenic l.

lienorenal l., ✶official alternate term for splenorenal l.

Lisfranc l.'s, SYN cuneometatarsal interosseous l.'s.

Lockwood l., SYN suspensory l. of eyeball.

longitudinal l.'s, one of two extensive fibrous bands running the length of the vertebral column: the anterior longitudinal l. and the posterior longitudinal l. SEE ALSO anterior longitudinal l., posterior longitudinal l. SYN ligamenta longitudinalia.

long plantar l. [TA], a strong l. that extends from the calcaneus to the cuboid and lateral metatarsals on the plantar aspect of the

li

foot; part of the passive support system for maintaining the longitudinal arch of the foot. SYN ligamentum plantare longum [TA].

lumbocostal l. [TA], a strong band that unites the twelfth rib with the tips of the transverse processes of the first and second lumbar vertebrae. SYN ligamentum lumbocostale [TA].

Luschka l.'s, SYN sternopericardial l.'s.

Mackenrodt l., SYN cardinal l.

l.'s of malleus, SEE anterior l. of malleus, lateral l. of malleus, superior l. of malleus.

Mauchart l.'s, SEE alar l.'s.

Meckel l., SYN Meckel *band*.

medial l. of ankle joint [TA], compound l. consisting of four component l.'s which pass downward from the medial malleolus of the tibia to the tarsal bones: 1) tibionavicular l. (pars tibionavicularis [NA]), 2) tibiocalcaneal l. (pars tibiocalcanea [NA]), 3) anterior tibiotalar l. (pars tibiotalaris anterior [NA]), and 4) posterior tibiotalar l. (pars tibiotalaris posterior [NA]). SYN ligamentum collaterale mediale [TA], deltoid l.✶, ligamentum deltoideum✶, ligamentum mediale articulationis talocruralis, medial l. of talocrural joint, tibial collateral l. of ankle joint.

medial arcuate l. [TA], one of Haller arches; a tendinous thickening of the psoas fascia that extends from the body of the first lumbar vertebra to its transverse process on either side. A portion of the diaphragm arises from it. SYN ligamentum arcuatum mediale [TA], arcus lumbocostalis medialis, medial lumbocostal arch.

medial canthal l., SYN medial palpebral l.

medial collateral l. of elbow, SYN ulnar collateral l. of elbow joint.

medial l. of knee, SYN tibial collateral l.

medial palpebral l. [TA], the fibrous band that attaches the medial ends of the tarsal plates to the maxilla at the medial orbital margin. SYN ligamentum palpebrale mediale [TA], ligamentum tarsale internum, medial canthal l., tendo oculi, tendo palpebrarum.

medial puboprostatic l., ✶official alternate term for pubovesical l. (of male).

medial talocalcaneal l. [TA], a l. extending from the medial tuberosity of the posterior talar process and the sustentaculum tali. SYN ligamentum talocalcaneum mediale [TA].

medial l. of talocrural joint, SYN medial l. of ankle joint.

medial l. of temporomandibular joint [TA], the intracapsular bundle of fibers strengthening the medial part of the articular capsule of the temporomandibular joint; not as apparent as the lateral ligament. SYN ligamentum mediale articulationis temporomandibularis [TA].

medial umbilical l., SYN *cord* of umbilical artery.

medial l. of wrist, SYN ulnar collateral l. of wrist joint.

median arcuate l. [TA], a tendinous connection between the crura of the diaphragm that arches over the aorta, forming the anterosuperior margin of the aortic hiatus. SYN ligamentum arcuatum medianum [TA].

median cricothyroid l. [TA], the strong band that connects the cricoid and thyroid cartilages in the midline anteriorly; it is continuous posteriorly with the conus elasticus.

median thyrohyoid l. [TA], the central thickened portion of the thyrohyoid membrane. SYN ligamentum thyrohyoideum medianum [TA], ligamentum hyothyroideum medium.

median umbilical l. [TA], the remnant of the urachus, contained in the median umbilical fold; it persists as a midline fibrous cord between the apex of the bladder and the umbilicus. SYN ligamentum umbilicale medianum [TA], middle umbilical l., urachal l.

meniscofemoral l.'s [TA], one of two l.'s that extend from the posterior part of the lateral meniscus to the lateral surface of the medial meniscus: anterior meniscofemoral l. and posterior meniscofemoral l. SEE ALSO anterior meniscofemoral l., posterior meniscofemoral l. SYN ligamenta meniscofemoralia [TA].

metatarsal interosseous l.'s [TA], fibrous bands that connect the bases of the metatarsals; they extend between the dorsal and plantar metatarsal ligaments. SYN ligamenta metatarsalia interossea [TA], interosseous metatarsal l.'s.

middle costotransverse l., SYN costotransverse l.

middle umbilical l., SYN median umbilical l.

nuchal l., ✶official alternate term for *ligamentum* nuchae.

oblique l. of elbow joint, SYN oblique *cord* of interosseous membrane of forearm.

oblique popliteal l. [TA], reflected tendon of insertion of semimembranous muscle; a fibrous band that extends across the back of the knee from its separation from the direct tendon of insertion on the medial condyle of the tibia to the lateral condyle of the femur. SYN ligamentum popliteum obliquum [TA], Bourgery l.

occipitoaxial l.'s, l.'s connecting the axis with the occipital bone. SEE alar l.'s, apical l. of dens.

orbicular l., SYN anular l.

orbicular l. of radius, SYN anular l. of radius.

ovarian l., SYN l. of ovary.

l. of ovary [TA], a cordlike bundle of fibers passing to the side of the uterus from the lower end of the ovary, between the folds of the broad l. (mesovarium). SYN ligamentum ovarii proprium [TA], ligamentum uteroovaricum✶, ovarian l., proper l. of ovary.

palmar l.'s [TA], the fibrocartilaginous plates, one located on the anterior aspect of each metacarpophalangeal and interphalangeal joint of the hand, that are firmly attached to the bases of the phalanges and the heads of the next proximal bones; they are grooved to accommodate the long flexor tendons. SEE ALSO palmar l.'s of interphalangeal joints of hand, palmar l.'s of metacarpophalangeal joints. SYN ligamenta palmaria [TA], accessory volar l.'s.

palmar carpal l., SYN antebrachial flexor *retinaculum*.

palmar carpometacarpal l.'s [TA], fibrous bands that connect the palmar surfaces of the carpal and metacarpal bones. SYN ligamenta carpometacarpalia palmaria [TA].

palmar l.'s of interphalangeal joints of hand [TA], l.'s located on the anterior (palmar) aspect of the interphalangeal joints of the fingers, flanked by and connected to the collateral l.'s, forming the anterior portion of the joint capsule; lighter but similar in structure and function to the palmar l.'s of metacarpophalangeal joints. SEE ALSO palmar l.'s of metacarpophalangeal joints. SYN ligamenta palmaria articulationis interphalangeae manus [TA].

palmar metacarpal l.'s [TA], fibrous bands connecting the palmar aspects of the bases of metacarpals two to five. SYN ligamenta metacarpalia palmaria [TA].

palmar l.'s of metacarpophalangeal joints [TA], thick, dense, fibrocartilaginous ligaments located on the anterior (palmar) aspect of the metacarpophalangeal joints, flanked by and connected to the collateral ligaments, forming the anterior portion of the joint capsule; the ligaments are grooved longitudinally (relative to the digit) to accommodate the long flexor tendons of the digit; on each side of the groove they are attached to both the deep transverse metacarpal ligaments and fibrous sheaths of the fingers; they are firmly attached to the base of the proximal phalanges, deepening the "socket" of the phalangeal bases to accommodate the heads of the metacarpals, to which they are loosely attached, permitting free movement. SYN ligamenta palmaria articulationis metacarpophalangeae [TA], palmar plates.

palmar radiocarpal l. [TA], a strong l. that passes from the distal end of the radius to the proximal row of carpal bones on the anterior surface of the wrist joint. SYN ligamentum radiocarpale palmare [TA].

palmar ulnocarpal l. [TA], the fibrous band that passes from the ulnar styloid process to the carpal bones. SYN ligamentum ulnocarpale palmare [TA].

patellar l. [TA], a strong flattened fibrous band passing from the apex and adjoining margins of the patella to the tuberosity of the tibia; considered by some to be part of the tendon of the quadriceps femoris muscle, in which the patella is embedded as a sesamoid bone. SYN ligamentum patellae [TA].

pectinate l.'s of iridocorneal angle, SYN trabecular *tissue* of sclera.

pectinate l.'s of iris, SEE trabecular *tissue* of sclera.

pectineal l. [TA], a thick, strong fibrous band that passes laterally from the lacunar l. along the pectineal line of the pubis. This fibrous tissue on the bony surface allows the purchase of sutures in various procedures to repair inguinal herniae. SEE ALSO *aponeurosis* of external oblique muscle. SYN ligamentum pectineale [TA], Cooper l.'s (2).

peridental l., SYN periodontium.

periodontal l. [TA], SYN periodontium.

phrenicocolic l. [TA], a triangular fold of peritoneum attached to the left flexure of the colon and to the diaphragm, on which rests the inferior pole or extremity of the spleen. SYN ligamentum phrenicocolicum [TA], costocolic l.

phrenicolienal l., SYN phrenicosplenic l.

phrenicosplenic l. [TA], double fold of peritoneum (mesentery) extending between the diaphragm and spleen; this is a portion of the greater omentum, and distinctions between the phrenicosplenic ligament and adjacent ligaments, such as the gastrophrenic, gastrosplenic and splenorenal ligaments—all part of the same mesenteric sheet—are often nebulous. SYN ligamentum phrenicosplenicum [TA], lienophrenic l., ligamentum phrenicolienale, phrenicolienal l., phrenosplenic l., sustentaculum lienis.

phrenogastric l., SYN gastrophrenic l.

phrenosplenic l., SYN phrenicosplenic l.

pisohamate l. [TA], a strong fibrous band that extends from the pisiform bone to the hook of the hamate. SYN ligamentum pisohamatum [TA], pisounciform l., pisouncinate l.

pisometacarpal l. [TA], a strong fibrous band extending from the pisiform bone to the base of the fifth metacarpal bone; this l., together with the pisohamate l., forms the tendon of insertion of the flexor carpi ulnaris, in which the pisiform bone is like a sesamoid bone. SYN ligamentum pisometacarpeum [TA].

pisounciform l., SYN pisohamate l.

pisouncinate l., SYN pisohamate l.

plantar l.'s [TA], fibrocartilaginous plates located on the plantar aspect of each metatarsophalangeal and interphalangeal joint of the foot; the counterparts in the foot of the palmar l.'s in the hand. SEE ALSO plantar l.'s of interphalangeal joints of foot, plantar l.'s of metatarsophalangeal joints. SYN ligamenta plantaria [TA], accessory plantar l.'s, Cruveilhier l.'s, glenoid l. (2).

plantar calcaneocuboid l. [TA], a strong band that passes forward and medially from the plantar surface of the calcaneus to the cuboid bone, actually forming a part of the articular capsule of the calcaneocuboid joint; the shorter, deeper portion of the long plantar ligament. SYN ligamentum calcaneocuboideum plantare [TA].

plantar calcaneonavicular l. [TA], a dense fibroelastic l. that extends from the sustentaculum tali to the plantar surface of the navicular bone; it supports the head of the talus, actually forming part of the articular "socket" for the head of the talus. SYN ligamentum calcaneonaviculare plantare [TA], spring l.★, inferior calcaneonavicular l.

plantar cuboideonavicular l.'s [TA], the l.'s that unite the plantar surfaces of the cuboid and navicular bones of the tarsus. SYN ligamenta cuboideonavicularia plantaria [TA].

plantar cuneocuboid l. [TA], the fibrous band that unites the apex of the lateral cuneiform with the medial margin of the plantar suface of the cuboid. SYN ligamentum cuneocuboideum plantare [TA].

plantar cuneonavicular l.'s [TA], l.'s connecting the plantar surface of the navicular with the three cuneiform bones. SYN ligamenta cuneonavicularia plantaria [TA].

plantar l.'s of interphalangeal joints of foot [TA], l.'s located on the inferior (sole) aspect of the interphalangeal joints of the toes, flanked by and connected to the collateral ligaments, forming the plantar portion of the joint capsule; lighter but similar in structure and function to the palmar ligaments of metacarpophalangeal joints. SEE ALSO plantar l.'s of metatarsophalangeal joints. SYN ligamenta plantaria articulationis interphalangeae pedis [TA].

plantar l.'s of metatarsophalangeal joints [TA], thick, dense l.'s located on the inferior (sole) aspect of the metatarsophalangeal joints, flanked by and connected to the collateral l.'s, forming the plantar portion of the joint capsule; the l.'s are grooved longitudinally (relative to the digit) to accommodate the long flexor tendons of the digit; on each side of the groove they are attached to both the deep transverse metatarsal l.'s and fibrous sheaths of the toes; they are firmly attached to the base of the proximal phalanges, deepening the "socket" of the phalangeal bases to accommodate the heads of the metatarsals, to which they are loosely attached, permitting free movement. SYN ligamenta plantaria articulationis metatarsophalangeae [TA].

plantar metatarsal l.'s [TA], fibrous bands connecting the plantar aspects of the bases of the metatarsals. SYN ligamenta metatarsalia plantaria [TA].

plantar tarsal l.'s [TA], ligaments connecting plantar aspects of the tarsal bones as a group; included in the group are the: long plantar ligament [TA] (ligamentum plantare longum [TA]), and the following plantar ligaments (ligamentum/a . . . plantare/ia): calcaneocuboid [TA] (calcaneocuboideum [TA]), calcaneonavicular [TA] (calcaneonaviculare [TA]), cuneonavicular [TA] (cuneonavicularia [TA]), cuboideonavicular [TA] (cuboideonaviculare [TA]), intercuneiform [TA] (intercuneiformia [TA]), and cuneocuboid [TA] (cuneocuboideum [TA]). SYN ligamenta tarsi plantaria [TA].

plantar tarsometatarsal l.'s [TA], longitudinal and oblique bands reinforcing the plantar aspects of the tarsometatarsal joints (joints between the metatarsals and the cuboid and cuneiform bones); the medial bands are strongest; they become progressively weaker laterally. SYN ligamenta tarsometatarsalia plantaria [TA].

posterior costotransverse l., SYN lateral costotransverse l.

posterior cricoarytenoid l., SYN cricoarytenoid l.

posterior cruciate l. [TA], the strong fibrous cord that extends from the posterior intercondylar area of the tibia to the anterior part of the lateral surface of the medial condyle of the femur. SYN ligamentum cruciatum posterius [TA].

posterior l. of fibular head [TA], a l. uniting the posterior part of the head of the fibula to the tibia. SYN ligamentum capitis fibulae posterius [TA], posterior l. of head of fibula.

posterior l. of head of fibula, SYN posterior l. of fibular head.

posterior l. of incus [TA], ligamentous band extending from short crus of incus. SYN ligamentum incudis posterius [TA].

posterior l. of knee, SYN arcuate popliteal l.

posterior longitudinal l. [TA], the fibrous band interconnecting the posterior surfaces of the vertebral bodies; it narrows to pass between the pedicles and spreads out to blend with the outer lamellae of the posterior aspect of the anulus fibrosus of the intervertebral disks; forms the anterior wall of the vertebral canal. SYN ligamentum longitudinale posterius [TA].

posterior meniscofemoral l. [TA], the band that passes posterior to the posterior cruciate l. extending between the medial condyle of the femur and the posterior crus of the lateral meniscus. SYN ligamentum meniscofemorale posterius [TA], ligamentum cruciatum tertium genus, ligamentum menisci lateralis, Wrisberg l.

posterior occipitoaxial l., SYN tectorial *membrane* (of median atlantoaxial joint).

posterior sacroiliac l.'s [TA], the heavy fibrous bands that pass from the ilium to the sacrum posterior to the sacroiliac joint. SYN ligamenta sacroiliaca posteriora [TA], dorsal sacroiliac l.'s, ligamentum sacroiliacum posterius.

posterior sacrosciatic l., SYN sacrotuberous l.

posterior sternoclavicular l. [TA], a fibrous band that reinforces the sternoclavicular joint posteriorly. SYN ligamentum sternoclaviculare posterius [TA].

posterior talocalcaneal l. [TA], stout l. located immediately posterior to the lateral portion of the talocalcaneal interosseous l. and medial to the lateral talocalcaneal l. in the widest part of the tarsal sinus. SYN ligamentum talocalcaneum posterius [TA].

posterior talofibular l. [TA], the nearly horizontal fibrous band that extends from the posterior border of the talus to the malleolar fossa. SYN ligamentum talofibulare posterius [TA].

posterior talotibial l., SYN tibiotalar *part* of medial ligament of ankle joint; SEE ALSO medial l. of ankle joint.

posterior tibiofibular l. [TA], the fibrous band that horizontally crosses the posterior aspect of the tibiofibular syndesmosis, contributing the posterior "wall" of the "socket" which receives the trochlea of the talus. SYN ligamentum tibiofibulare posterius [TA].

posterior tibiotalar l., SYN tibiotalar *part* of medial ligament of ankle joint.

Poupart l., SYN inguinal l.

proper l. of ovary, SYN l. of ovary.

pterygomandibular l., SYN pterygomandibular *raphe*.

li

pterygospinal l., SYN pterygospinous l.

pterygospinous l. [TA], a membranous l. extending from the spine of the sphenoid to the upper part of the posterior border of the lateral plate of the sphenoid (lateral pterygoid plate). SYN ligamentum pterygospinale [TA], Civinini l., pterygospinal l.

pubocapsular l., SYN pubofemoral l.

pubofemoral l. [TA], a thickened part of the capsule of the hip joint that extends from the superior ramus of the pubis to the intertrochanteric line of the femur. SYN ligamentum pubofemorale [TA], ligamentum pubocapsulare, pubocapsular l.

puboprostatic l. [TA], the localized thickening of the superior fascia of the pelvic diaphragm anteriorly that anchors the prostate and neck of the bladder to the pubis on each side. It usually contains smooth muscle. SYN ligamentum puboprostaticum [TA], lateral puboprostatic l.☆, Denonvilliers l.

pubovesical l. (of female) [TA], in the female the fascial thickening comparable with the puboprostatic l. composed of medial and lateral pubovesical ligaments. SYN ligamentum pubovesicale (femininum) [TA].

pubovesical l. (of male) [TA], anteriormost portion of the tendinous arch of the pelvic fascia (a condensation of the superior fascia of the pelvic diaphragm) extending between the lower part of the pubic symphysis and the prostate and bladder; it forms the inferior boundary of the potential retropubic (prevesical) space. SYN ligamentum pubovesicale (masculinum) [TA], ligamentum mediale puboprostaticum☆, medial puboprostatic l.☆.

pulmonary l. [TA], two-layered fold formed as the pleura of the mediastinum is reflected onto the lung inferior to the root of the lung. SYN ligamentum pulmonale [TA], ligamentum latum pulmonis, Teutleben l.

quadrate l. [TA], fibers that pass from the distal margin of the radial notch of the ulna to the neck of the radius. SYN ligamentum quadratum [TA], Denucé l.

radial collateral l., SYN radial collateral l. of elbow joint.

radial collateral l. of elbow joint [TA], the l. that connects the lateral epicondyle of the humerus with the anular l. of the radius. SYN ligamentum collaterale radiale articulationis cubiti [TA], lateral l. of elbow, radial collateral l.

radial collateral l. of wrist joint [TA], the l. that extends distally from the styloid process of the radius to the carpal bones. SYN ligamentum collaterale carpi radiale articulationis radiocarpalis [TA], external collateral l. of wrist, lateral l. of wrist.

radiate l., SYN radiate l. of head of rib.

radiate carpal l. [TA], the ligament that extends from the capitate bone to the scaphoid, lunate, and triquetrum on the palmar side of the wrist. SYN ligamentum carpi radiatum [TA], radiate l. of wrist.

radiate l. of head of rib [TA], the radiate, stellate, or anterior costovertebral l. connecting the head of each rib to the bodies of the two vertebrae with which it articulates. SYN ligamentum capitis costae radiatum [TA], ligamentum radiatum, radiate l., stellate l.

radiate sternocostal l.'s [TA], fibers of the articular capsule that radiate from the costal cartilages to the anterior surface of the sternum. SYN ligamenta sternocostalia radiata [TA].

radiate l. of wrist, SYN radiate carpal l.

reflected inguinal l. [TA], slightly reinforced portion of the external oblique aponeurosis, formed by fibers derived from the medial portion of the inguinal ligament of one side that run medially and slightly superiorly, defining the inferior margin of the superficial inguinal ring; the fibers then pass on the deep aspect of the ipsilateral medial crus, crossing the linea alba and running within the contralateral aponeurosis to course parallel and superior to the contralateral inguinal ligament. SEE ALSO *aponeurosis* of external oblique muscle. SYN ligamentum reflexum [TA], Colles l., fascia triangularis abdominis, reflex l., triangular fascia.

reflex l., SYN reflected inguinal l.

Retzius l., the deep attachment of the inferior extensor retinaculum in the tarsal sinus, it acts as a sling for the extensor tendons of the toes. SYN fundiform l. of foot.

rhomboid l., SYN costoclavicular l.

right triangular l. of liver [TA], a triangular fold of peritoneum

that passes from the right lobe of the liver to the diaphragm; it is a formation of the coronary l., formed as the coronary l. makes an acute angle upon reaching its most lateral point on the right side as it surrounds the bare area of the liver. SYN ligamentum triangulare dextrum hepatis [TA].

ring l., SYN *zona* orbicularis (articulationis coxae).

round l. of elbow joint, SYN oblique *cord* of interosseous membrane of forearm.

round l. of femur, SYN l. of head of femur.

round l. of liver [TA], the remains of the umbilical vein running within the free edge of the falciform l. from umbilicus to the liver, where it continues within the fissure for the round l. to the origin of the left portal vein within the porta hepatis. SYN ligamentum teres hepatis [TA].

round l. of uterus [TA], a fibromuscular band that is attached to the uterus on either side in front of and below the opening of the uterine tube; it passes through the inguinal canal to the labium majus; corresponds to the spermatic cord of male in that it passes through the inguinal canal and gains similar coverings, but is not homologous, being a homolog of the gubernaculum testis. SYN ligamentum teres uteri [TA], Hunter l.

sacrodural l., a longitudinal bundle of fibrous filaments running from the midline of the inferior part of the dural sac to the posterior longitudinal ligament of the sacrum. SYN ligamentum sacrodurale.

sacrospinous l. [TA], the fibrous band that passes from the ischial spine to the sacrum and coccyx. SYN ligamentum sacrospinale [TA], anterior sacrosciatic l., ligamentum sacrospinosum.

sacrotuberous l. [TA], the l. that passes from the ischial tuberosity to the ilium, sacrum, and coccyx, transforming the sciatic notch to a large sciatic foramen, which is then further subdivided by the sacrospinous l. SYN ligamentum sacrotuberale [TA], ligamentum sacrotuberosum, posterior sacrosciatic l.

serous l., one of a number of peritoneal folds attaching certain of the viscera to the abdominal wall or to each other. SYN ligamentum serosum.

sheath l.'s, SEE fibrous *sheaths* of digits of hand, under *sheath*, fibrous digital *sheaths* of toes, under *sheath*, fibrous tendon *sheath*.

Simonart l.'s, SYN amnionic *band*.

skin l.'s [TA], one of the numerous small fibrous strands that extend through the superficial fascia attaching the deep surface of the dermis to the underlying deep fascia determining the mobility of the skin over the deep structures; these are particularly well developed over the breast where they are known as suspensory ligaments of the breast; they are also well-developed, but short, in the palms and soles. SYN retinaculum cutis [TA], retinaculum of skin.

Soemmerring l., small fibers attaching the lacrimal gland to the periorbita.

sphenomandibular l. [TA], the fibrous band that passes from the spine of the sphenoid bone to the lingula of the mandible; it is a primary passive support of the mandible serving as a "swinging axis", permitting depression and elevation around a transverse axis passing through the two lingulae, while at the same time permitting protraction and retraction. SYN ligamentum sphenomandibulare [TA].

spinoglenoid l., SYN inferior transverse scapular l.

spiral l. of cochlea, SYN spiral l. of cochlear duct.

spiral l. of cochlear duct [TA], the thickened periosteal lining of the bony cochlea forming the outer wall of the cochlear duct to which the basal lamina attaches. SYN ligamentum spirale ductus cochlearis [TA], crista spiralis, ligamentum spirale cochleae, spiral crest, spiral l. of cochlea.

splenorenal l. [TA], a peritoneal fold (portion of the greater omentum) that extends from the anterior aspect of the left kidney to the splenic hilum, conducting the splenic vessels from the posterior body wall to the spleen. SYN ligamentum splenorenale [TA], lienorenal l.☆, ligamentum lienorenale☆.

spring l., ☆official alternate term for plantar calcaneonavicular l.

Stanley cervical l.'s, fibers of the capsule of the hip joint reflected onto the neck of the femur.

stellate l., SYN radiate l. of head of rib.

sternoclavicular l.'s, l. uniting the clavicle to the manubrium of the sternum. SEE anterior sternoclavicular l., posterior sternoclavicular l. SYN ligamenta sternoclavicularia.

sternopericardial l.'s, fibrous bands that pass from the pericardium to the sternum. SYN ligamenta sternopericardiaca [TA], Lannelongue l.'s, Luschka l.'s.

stylohyoid l. [TA], a fibrous cord that passes from the tip of the styloid process to the lesser cornu of the hyoid bone; it is occasionally ossified. SYN ligamentum stylohyoideum [TA], epihyal l.

stylomandibular l. [TA], a condensation of the deep cervical fascia extending from the tip of the styloid process of the temporal bone to the posterior border of the angle of the jaw; blends with (is a thickening of) the parotid sheath. SYN ligamentum stylomandibulare [TA], stylomaxillary l.

stylomaxillary l., SYN stylomandibular l.

superficial dorsal sacrococcygeal l., SYN superficial posterior sacrococcygeal l.

superficial posterior sacrococcygeal l. [TA], the continuation of the supraspinal l. from the sacrum to the coccyx. SYN ligamentum sacrococcygeum posterius superficiale [TA], ligamentum sacrococcygeum dorsale superficiale*, superficial dorsal sacrococcygeal l.

superficial transverse metacarpal l. [TA], a thickening of the deep fascia in the most distal part of the (base) of the triangular palmar aponeurosis. SYN ligamentum metacarpale transversum superficiale [TA], Gerdy fibers, ligamentum natatorium.

superficial transverse metatarsal l. [TA], a thickening of the distal part (base) of the plantar aponeurosis, at the level of the heads of the metatarsal bones. SYN ligamentum metatarsale transversum superficiale [TA].

superior costotransverse l. [TA], the fibrous band that extends upward from the neck of a rib to the transverse process of the next higher vertebra. SYN ligamentum costotransversarium superius [TA], anterior costotransverse l., ligamentum costotransversarium anterius.

superior l. of epididymis [TA], the uppermost of the two folds of the tunica vaginalis between the head of the epididymis and the testis. SYN ligamentum epididymidis superius [TA].

superior l. of incus [TA], connects the body of the incus with the roof of the tympanic recess. SYN ligamentum incudis superius [TA].

superior l. of malleus [TA], a l. extending from the head of the malleus to the roof of the epitympanic recess. SYN ligamentum mallei superius [TA].

superior pubic l. [TA], fibers that pass transversely above the pubic symphysis. SYN ligamentum pubicum superius [TA].

superior transverse scapular l. [TA], the strong fibrous band that bridges the scapular notch creating a foramen that gives passage to the suprascapular nerve, while the suprascapular vessels pass over the l. superiorly. SYN ligamentum transversum scapulae superius [TA], suprascapular l.

suprascapular l., SYN superior transverse scapular l.

supraspinous l. [TA], the longitudinal fibrous band attached to the tips of the spinous processes of the vertebrae; in the cervical region it is altered to form the ligamentum nuchae. SYN ligamentum supraspinale [TA].

suspensory l. of axilla [TA], the continuation of the clavipectoral fascia downward to attach to the axillary fascia; it maintains the characteristic hollow of the armpit. SYN ligamentum suspensorium axillae [TA], Campbell l., Gerdy l.

suspensory l.'s of breast, well-developed retinacula cutis that extend from the fibrous stroma of the mammary gland to the overlying skin. SYN retinaculum cutis mammae*, suspensory retinaculum of breast*, Cooper l.'s (1), ligamenta suspensoria mammaria, suspensory l.'s of Cooper.

suspensory l. of clitoris [TA], a fibrous band at the deep fascial level that extends from the pubic symphysis to the deep fascia of the clitoris, anchoring the clitoris to the pubic symphysis. SYN ligamentum suspensorium clitoridis [TA].

suspensory l.'s of Cooper, SYN suspensory l.'s of breast.

suspensory l. of duodenum, *official alternate term for suspensory *muscle* of duodenum.

suspensory l. of esophagus, SYN cricoesophageal *tendon*.

suspensory l. of eyeball [TA], a thickening of the inferior part of the bulbar sheath that supports the eye within the orbit; it extends between the lateral and medial orbital margins and includes the medial and lateral check l.'s. SYN ligamentum suspensorium bulbi [TA], Lockwood l.

suspensory l. of gonad, SYN genital l.

suspensory l. of lens, SYN ciliary *zonule*.

suspensory l. of ovary [TA], a band of peritoneum that extends upward from the upper pole of the ovary; it contains the ovarian vessels and ovarian plexus of nerves. SYN ligamentum suspensorium ovarii [TA], Clado band, infundibulopelvic l.

suspensory l. of penis [TA], a fibrous band at the deep fascial layer that extends from the pubic symphysis to the deep fascia of the penis anchoring the roof of the penis. SYN ligamentum suspensorium penis [TA].

suspensory l. of testis, the cranial atrophic portion of the urogenital ridge attached to the cranial pole of the intraabdominal embryonic testis.

suspensory l. of thyroid gland [TA], one of several fibrous bands that pass from the sheath of the thyroid gland to the thyroid and cricoid cartilages. SYN ligamentum suspensorium glandulae thyroideae [TA].

sutural l., a delicate membrane binding the bones at the cranial sutures.

synovial l., one of the large synovial folds in a joint.

talocalcaneal l. [TA], any of three l.'s uniting the talus and calcaneus: talocalcaneal interosseous l., lateral talocalcaneal l., and medial talocalcaneal l. SYN ligamentum talocalcaneum [TA].

talocalcaneal interosseous l. [TA], a strong fibrous band occupying the tarsal sinus; one of three tarsal interosseous ligaments. SYN interosseous talocalcaneal l., ligamentum talocalcaneare interosseum.

talonavicular l. [TA], one of the dorsal tarsal ligaments, which occurs as a broad gap that passes from the dorsal side of the neck of the talus to the dorsal surface of the navicular bone. SYN ligamentum talonaviculare [TA].

tarsal l.'s [TA], the l.'s that interconnect the tarsal bones; they are grouped into three sets: dorsal tarsal l.'s, interosseous tarsal l.'s, and plantar tarsal l.'s, and are individually named according to their attachments. SYN ligamenta tarsi [TA].

tarsal interosseous l.'s [TA], deeper ligaments located between tarsal bones, connecting them together; group includes the talocalcaneal, cuneocuboid, and intercuneiform interosseous ligaments. SYN ligamenta tarsi interossea [TA].

tarsometatarsal l.'s [TA], the ligaments that unite tarsal and metatarsal bones; they are arranged in dorsal, plantar, and cuneometatarsal interosseous sets. SYN ligamenta tarsometatarsalia [TA].

temporomandibular l., SYN lateral l. of temporomandibular joint.

Teutleben l., SYN pulmonary l.

Thompson l., SYN iliopubic *tract*.

thyroepiglottic l. [TA], an elastic band that connects the petiole of the epiglottis to the interior of the thyroid cartilage near the superior thyroid notch. SYN ligamentum thyroepiglotticum [TA].

tibial collateral l. [TA], the broad fibrous band that passes from the medial epicondyle of the femur to the medial margin and medial surface of the tibia; the medial meniscus is attached to its deep surface; it is continuous with (is a thickening of) the fibrous capsule of the knee joint. SYN ligamentum collaterale tibiale [TA], medial l. of knee.

tibial collateral l. of ankle joint, SYN medial l. of ankle joint.

tibiocalcaneal l., SYN tibiocalcaneal *part* of medial ligament of ankle joint.

tibiofibular l., SEE anterior tibiofibular l., interosseous *membrane* of leg, posterior tibiofibular l. SEE ALSO tibiofibular *syndesmosis*.

tibionavicular l., SYN tibionavicular *part* of medial ligament of ankle joint.

transverse acetabular l. [TA], portion of the acetabular labrum

li

that passes across the acetabular notch. SYN ligamentum transversum acetabuli [TA], transverse l. of acetabulum.

transverse l. of acetabulum, SYN transverse acetabular l.

transverse atlantal l., SYN transverse l. of the atlas.

transverse l. of the atlas [TA], thick, strong, centrally flattened band spanning the vertebral foramen of the atlas as it extends from the medial aspect of one lateral mass to the other, passing dorsal to the dens with which it articulates; it forms the dorsal portion of the opening for the dens, tightly embracing its neck. It forms a part of the "cross-bar" of the cruciform l. of the atlas. SEE ALSO cruciate l. of the atlas. SYN ligamentum transversum atlantis [TA], Lauth l., transverse atlantal l.

transverse carpal l., SYN flexor *retinaculum*.

transverse cervical l., ✫official alternate term for cardinal l.

transverse crural l., SYN superior extensor *retinaculum*.

transverse l. of elbow, a bundle of fibers running from the olecranon to the coronoid process in association with the ulnar collateral l. SYN Cooper l.'s (3).

transverse genicular l., SYN transverse l. of knee.

transverse humeral l. [TA], a fibrous band running more or less obliquely from the greater to the lesser tuberosity of the humerus, bridging over the bicipital groove. SYN ligamentum transversum humeri [TA], Brodie l.

transverse l. of knee [TA], a transverse band that passes between the lateral and medial menisci in the anterior part of the knee joint. SYN ligamentum transversum genus [TA], transverse genicular l.

transverse l. of leg, SYN superior extensor *retinaculum*.

transverse metacarpal l., SYN deep transverse metacarpal l.

transverse metatarsal l., SYN deep transverse metatarsal l.

transverse l. of pelvis, SYN transverse perineal l.

transverse perineal l. [TA], the thickened anterior border of the perineal membrane. SYN ligamentum transversum perinei [TA], Krause l., ligamentum transversum pelvis, transverse l. of pelvis, transverse l. of perineum.

transverse l. of perineum, SYN transverse perineal l.

transverse tibiofibular l., SYN interosseous tibiofibular l.

trapezoid l. [TA], the lateral part of the coracoclavicular l. that attaches to the trapezoid line of the clavicle. SYN ligamentum trapezoideum [TA].

Treitz l., SYN suspensory *muscle* of duodenum.

triangular l., SYN perineal *membrane*.

triangular l.'s of liver, SEE right triangular l. of liver, left triangular l. of liver.

ulnar collateral l., SYN ulnar collateral l. of elbow joint.

ulnar collateral l. of elbow joint [TA], the triangular l. extending from the medial epicondyle of the humerus to the medial side of the coronoid process and olecranon of the ulna. SYN ligamentum collaterale ulnare articulationis cubiti [TA], medial collateral l. of elbow, ulnar collateral l.

ulnar collateral l. of wrist joint [TA], a l. that passes from the styloid process of the ulna to the pisiform and triquetrum. SYN internal collateral l. of the wrist, ligamentum collaterale carpi ulnare articulationis radiocarpalis, medial l. of wrist.

urachal l., SYN median umbilical l.

uterovesical l., a peritoneal fold extending from the uterus to the posterior portion of the bladder. SYN plica uterovesicalis, plica vesicouterina, uterovesical fold, vesicouterine l.

Valsalva l.'s, SYN l.'s of auricle.

venous l., SYN *ligamentum* venosum.

ventral sacrococcygeal l., SYN anterior sacrococcygeal l.

ventral sacroiliac l.'s, SYN anterior sacroiliac l.'s.

ventricular l., SYN vestibular l.

vertebropelvic l.'s, SEE iliolumbar l., sacrospinous l., sacrotuberous l.

vesicoumbilical l., one of the l.'s between the urinary bladder and the umbilicus. SEE median umbilical l., *cord* of umbilical artery.

vesicouterine l., SYN uterovesical l.

vestibular l. [TA], the inferior border of the quadrangular membrane that underlies the ventricular fold of the larynx. SYN ligamentum vestibulare [TA], ligamentum ventriculare, ventricular l.

vocal l. [TA], the band that extends on either side from the thyroid cartilage to the vocal process of the arytenoid cartilage; it is the thickened, free upper border of the conus elasticus of the larynx. SYN ligamentum vocale [TA].

volar carpal l., SYN flexor *retinaculum*.

Weitbrecht l., SYN oblique *cord* of interosseous membrane of forearm.

Winslow l., SYN fibular collateral l.

Wrisberg l., SYN posterior meniscofemoral l.

yellow l., SYN *ligamenta* flava, under *ligamentum*.

Y-shaped l., SYN iliofemoral l.

Zaglas l., a short thick fibrous band extending from the posterior superior spine of the ilium to the second transverse tubercle of the sacrum.

Zinn l., SYN common tendinous *ring* of extraocular muscles.

---

lig·a·men·ta (lig'ă-men'tă). Plural of ligamentum. [L.]

lig·a·men·to·pex·is, lig·a·men·to·pexy (lig'ă-men-tō-pek'sis, -pek'sē). Shortening of any ligament of the uterus. [ligament + G. *pēxis*, fixation]

lig·a·men·tous (lig'ă-men'tŭs). Relating to or of the form or structure of a ligament.

LIGAMENTUM

---

lig·a·men·tum, pl. **lig·a·men·ta** (lig'ă-men'tŭm, -men'tă) [TA]. SYN ligament. [L. a band, tie, fr. *ligo,* to bind]

l. acromioclavicula're [TA], SYN acromioclavicular *ligament*.

l. anococcy'geum, SYN anococcygeal *ligament*.

l. anula're [TA], SYN anular *ligament*.

l. anula're bul'bi, SYN trabecular *tissue* of sclera.

l. anula're digito'rum, SYN anular *part* of fibrous digital sheath of digits of hand and foot.

l. anula're ra'dii [TA], SYN anular *ligament* of radius.

l. anula're stape'dis [TA], SYN anular *ligament* of stapes.

ligamen'ta anula'ria trachea'lia [TA], SYN anular *ligaments* of trachea, under *ligament*.

l. ap'icis den'tis, SYN apical *ligament* of dens.

l. arcua'tum latera'le [TA], SYN lateral arcuate *ligament*.

l. arcua'tum media'le [TA], SYN medial arcuate *ligament*.

l. arcua'tum media'num [TA], SYN median arcuate *ligament*.

l. arcua'tum pu'bis, SYN inferior pubic *ligament*.

l. arterio'sum [TA], fibrous remnant of the ductus arteriosus extending between the aortic arch and the pulmonary trunk. SYN arterial ligament, Botallo ligament.

ligamen'ta auricula'ria [TA], SYN *ligaments* of auricle, under *ligament*.

l. bifurca'tum [TA], SYN bifurcate *ligament*.

l. calcaneocuboi'deum [TA], SYN calcaneocuboid *ligament*.

l. calcaneocuboi'deum planta're [TA], SYN plantar calcaneocuboid *ligament*.

l. calcaneofibula're [TA], SYN calcaneofibular *ligament*.

l. calcaneonavicula're [TA], SYN calcaneonavicular *ligament*.

l. calcaneonavicula're planta're [TA], SYN plantar calcaneonavicular *ligament*.

l. calcaneotibia'le, SYN tibiocalcaneal *part* of medial ligament of ankle joint; SEE ALSO medial *ligament* of ankle joint.

l. cap'itis cos'tae intraarticula're, SYN intraarticular *ligament* of head of rib.

l. cap'itis cos'tae radia'tum [TA], SYN radiate *ligament* of head of rib.

l. cap'itis fem'oris [TA], SYN *ligament* of head of femur.

l. cap'itis fib'ulae ante'rius [TA], SYN anterior *ligament* of fibular head.

l. cap′itis fib′ulae poste′rius [TA], SYN posterior *ligament* of fibular head.

ligamen′ta capitulo′rum transver′sa, SEE deep transverse metacarpal *ligament*, deep transverse metatarsal *ligament*.

l. capsula′re [TA], SYN capsular *ligament*.

l. cardinale [TA], SYN cardinal *ligament*.

l. car′pi dorsa′le, SYN extensor *retinaculum*.

l. car′pi radia′tum [TA], SYN radiate carpal *ligament*.

l. car′pi transver′sum, SYN flexor *retinaculum*.

l. car′pi vola′re, SYN flexor *retinaculum*.

ligamenta carpometacarpa′lia dorsa′lia [TA], SYN dorsal carpometacarpal *ligaments*, under *ligament*.

ligamen′ta carpometacarpa′lia (dorsalia/palmaria) [TA], SYN carpometacarpal *ligaments* (dorsal and palmar), under *ligament*.

ligamenta carpometacarpa′lia palma′ria [TA], SYN palmar carpometacarpal *ligaments*, under *ligament*.

l. cauda′le, SYN *retinaculum* caudale.

l. ceratocricoid′eum [TA], SYN ceratocricoid *ligament*.

l. collatera′le, pl. **ligamen′ta collatera′lia** [TA], SYN collateral *ligament*.

l. collatera′le car′pi radia′le articulationis radiocarpalis [TA], SYN radial collateral *ligament* of wrist joint.

l. collaterale carpi ulnare [TA],

l. collatera′le car′pi ulna′re articulationis radiocarpalis, SYN ulnar collateral *ligament* of wrist joint.

l. collatera′le fibula′re [TA], SYN fibular collateral *ligament*.

l. collaterale laterale [TA], SYN lateral *ligament* of ankle.

l. collaterale mediale [TA], SYN medial *ligament* of ankle joint.

l. collatera′le radia′le articulationis cubiti [TA], SYN radial collateral *ligament* of elbow joint.

l. collatera′le tibia′le [TA], SYN tibial collateral *ligament*.

l. collaterale ulnare articulationis cubiti [TA], SYN ulnar collateral *ligament* of elbow joint.

l. col′li cos′tae, SYN costotransverse *ligament*.

l. conoid′eum [TA], SYN conoid *ligament*.

l. coracoacromia′le [TA], SYN coracoacromial *ligament*.

l. coracoclavicula′re [TA], SYN coracoclavicular *ligament*.

l. coracohumera′le [TA], SYN coracohumeral *ligament*.

l. corniculopharyn′geum, SYN cricopharyngeal *ligament*.

l. corona′rium hep′atis [TA], SYN coronary *ligament* of liver.

l. costoclavicula′re [TA], SYN costoclavicular *ligament*.

l. costotransversa′rium [TA], SYN costotransverse *ligament*.

l. costotransversa′rium ante′rius, SYN superior costotransverse *ligament*.

l. costotransversa′rium latera′le [TA], SYN lateral costotransverse *ligament*.

l. costotransversa′rium poste′rius, SYN lateral costotransverse *ligament*.

l. costotransversa′rium supe′rius [TA], SYN superior costotransverse *ligament*.

l. costoxiphoi′deum [TA], SYN costoxiphoid *ligament*.

l. cotyloid′eum, SYN acetabular *labrum*.

l. cricoarytenoi′deum poste′rius, SYN cricoarytenoid *ligament*.

l. cricopharyn′geum [TA], SYN cricopharyngeal *ligament*.

l. cricotrachea′le [TA], SYN cricotracheal *ligament*.

ligamen′ta crucia′ta digito′rum, SYN cruciform *part* of fibrous digital sheath.

ligamen′ta crucia′ta ge′nus, SYN cruciate *ligaments* of knee, under *ligament*.

l. crucia′tum ante′rius, SYN anterior cruciate *ligament*.

l. crucia′tum atlan′tis, SYN cruciate *ligament* of the atlas.

l. crucia′tum cru′ris, SYN inferior extensor *retinaculum*.

l. crucia′tum poste′rius, SYN posterior cruciate *ligament*.

l. crucia′tum ter′tium ge′nus, SYN posterior meniscofemoral *ligament*.

l. crucifor′me atlan′tis, SYN cruciate *ligament* of the atlas.

ligamenta cuboideonaviculare [TA], SYN cuboideonavicular *ligaments*, under *ligament*.

l. cuboideonavicula′re dorsa′le [TA], SYN dorsal cuboideonavicular *ligament*.

ligamenta cuboideonavicula′ria planta′ria [TA], SYN plantar cuboideonavicular *ligaments*, under *ligament*.

l. cuneocuboideum [TA], SYN cuneocuboid *ligaments*, under *ligament*.

l. cuneocuboideum dorsa′le [TA], SYN dorsal cuneocuboid *ligament*.

l. cuneocuboideum interos′seum, SYN cuneocuboid interosseous *ligament*.

l. cuneocuboideum planta′re [TA], SYN plantar cuneocuboid *ligament*.

ligamen′ta cuneometatarsa′lia interos′sea [TA], SYN cuneometatarsal interosseous *ligaments*, under *ligament*.

ligamen′ta cuneonavicula′ria dorsa′lia [TA], SYN dorsal cuneonavicular *ligaments*, under *ligament*.

l. cuneonavicula′ria planta′ria [TA], SYN plantar cuneonavicular *ligaments*, under *ligament*.

l. deltoi′deum, ✫official alternate term for medial *ligament* of ankle joint.

l. denticula′tum [TA], SYN denticulate *ligament*.

l. duc′tus veno′si, SYN l. venosum.

l. duodenorena′le, SYN duodenorenal *ligament*.

ligamenta epididym′idis (inferius et superius) [TA], SYN *ligaments* of epididymis (inferior and superior), under *ligament*.

l. epididym′idis infe′rius [TA], SYN inferior *ligament* of epididymis.

l. epididym′idis supe′rius [TA], SYN superior *ligament* of epididymis.

ligamen′ta extracapsula′ria [TA], SYN extracapsular *ligaments*, under *ligament*.

l. falcifor′me, SYN falciform *process* of sacrotuberous ligament.

l. falcifor′me hep′atis [TA], SYN falciform *ligament* of liver.

ligamenta fla′va [TA], paired ligaments of yellow elastic fibrous tissue, which bind together the laminae of adjoining vertebrae, forming the dorsal wall of the vertebral canal between the vertebra or laminae; penetration of the ligamentum flavum with a trocar during epidural or spinal puncture produces a distinct feel ("pop"), letting the practitioner know that the tip of the trocar has entered the epidural space. SYN yellow ligament.

l. fundiforme clitoridis [TA], SYN fundiform *ligament* of clitoris.

l. fundifor′me pe′nis [TA], SYN fundiform *ligament* of penis.

l. gastrocol′icum [TA], SYN gastrocolic *ligament*.

l. gastroliena′le, ✫official alternate term for gastrosplenic *ligament*.

l. gastrophren′icum [TA], SYN gastrophrenic *ligament*.

l. gastrosple′nicum [TA], SYN gastrosplenic *ligament*.

l. genitoinguina′le, SYN genitoinguinal *ligament*.

ligamen′ta glenohumera′lia [TA], SYN glenohumeral *ligaments*, under *ligament*.

l. glenoida′le, SYN glenoid *labrum* of scapula.

l. hepatocol′icum [TA], SYN hepatocolic *ligament*.

l. hepatoduodena′le [TA], SYN hepatoduodenal *ligament*.

l. hepatoesopha′geum [TA], SYN hepatoesophageal *ligament*.

l. hepatogas′tricum [TA], SYN hepatogastric *ligament*.

l. hepatorena′le [TA], SYN hepatorenal *ligament*.

l. hyaloi′deo-capsula′re, SYN hyalocapsular *ligament*.

l. hyoepiglot′ticum [TA], SYN hyoepiglottic *ligament*.

l. hyothyroi′deum latera′le, SYN lateral thyrohyoid *ligament*.

l. hyothyroi′deum me′dium, SYN median thyrohyoid *ligament*.

l. iliofemora′le [TA], SYN iliofemoral *ligament*.

l. iliolumba′le [TA], SYN iliolumbar *ligament*.

l. iliopectinea′le, SYN iliopectineal *arch*.

l. incu′dis poste′rius [TA], SYN posterior *ligament* of incus.

l. incu′dis supe′rius [TA], SYN superior *ligament* of incus.

l. inguina′le [TA], SYN inguinal *ligament*.

ligamen′ta intercarpa′lia [TA], SYN intercarpal *ligaments*, under *ligament*.

li

l. intercarpalia dorsalia, dorsal intercarpal ligament. SEE intercarpal *ligaments,* under *ligament.*

l. intercarpalia interossea, interosseous intercarpal ligament. SEE intercarpal *ligaments,* under *ligament.*

l. intercarpalia palmaria, palmar intercarpal ligament. SEE intercarpal *ligaments,* under *ligament.*

l. interclavicula're [TA], SYN interclavicular *ligament.*

ligamen'ta intercosta'lia, SYN intercostal *membranes,* under *membrane.*

ligamen'ta intercuneifor'mia [TA], SYN intercuneiform *ligaments,* under *ligament.*

ligamenta intercuneiformia dorsalia, dorsal intercuneiform ligament. SEE intercuneiform *ligaments,* under *ligament.*

ligamenta intercuneiformia interossea, interosseous intercuneiform ligaments. SEE intercuneiform *ligaments,* under *ligament.*

ligamenta intercuneiformia plantaria, plantar intercuneiform ligaments. SEE intercuneiform *ligaments,* under *ligament.*

l. interfoveola're [TA], SYN interfoveolar *ligament.*

l. interspina'le [TA], SYN interspinous *ligament.*

l. intertransversa'rium [TA], SYN intertransverse *ligament.*

ligamen'ta intracapsula'ria [TA], SYN intracapsular *ligaments,* under *ligament.*

l. ischiocapsula're, SYN ischiofemoral *ligament.*

l. ischiofemora'le [TA], SYN ischiofemoral *ligament.*

l. juga'le, SYN cricopharyngeal *ligament.*

l. lacinia'tum, SYN flexor *retinaculum* of lower limb.

l. lacuna're [TA], SYN lacunar *ligament.*

l. latera'le articulatio'nis temporomandibula'ris [TA], SYN lateral *ligament* of temporomandibular joint.

l. laterale vesicae [TA], SYN lateral *ligament* of bladder.

l. la'tum pulmo'nis, SYN pulmonary *ligament.*

l. la'tum u'teri [TA], SYN broad *ligament* of the uterus.

l. lienorena'le, ⋆official alternate term for splenorenal *ligament.*

l. longitudina'le ante'rius [TA], SYN anterior longitudinal *ligament.*

l. longitudina'le poste'rius [TA], SYN posterior longitudinal *ligament.*

ligamenta longitudina'lia, SYN longitudinal *ligaments,* under *ligament.*

l. lumbocosta'le [TA], SYN lumbocostal *ligament.*

l. mal'lei ante'rius [TA], SYN anterior *ligament* of malleus.

l. mal'lei latera'le [TA], SYN lateral *ligament* of malleus.

l. mal'lei supe'rius [TA], SYN superior *ligament* of malleus.

l. malle'oli latera'lis, SEE anterior tibiofibular *ligament,* posterior tibiofibular *ligament.*

l. media'le, SYN anterior tibiotalar *part* of medial ligament of ankle joint.

l. media'le articulatio'nis talocrura'lis, SYN medial *ligament* of ankle joint.

l. media'le articulatio'nis temporomandibula'ris [TA], SYN medial *ligament* of temporomandibular joint.

l. mediale puboprostaticum, ⋆official alternate term for pubovesical *ligament* (of male).

l. menis'ci latera'lis, SYN posterior meniscofemoral *ligament.*

ligamen'ta meniscofemora'lia [TA], SYN meniscofemoral *ligaments,* under *ligament.*

l. meniscofemora'le ante'rius [TA], SYN anterior meniscofemoral *ligament.*

l. meniscofemora'le poste'rius [TA], SYN posterior meniscofemoral *ligament.*

l. metacarpa'le transver'sum profun'dum [TA], SYN deep transverse metacarpal *ligament.*

l. metacarpa'le transver'sum superficia'le [TA], SYN superficial transverse metacarpal *ligament.*

ligamen'ta metacarpa'lia dorsa'lia [TA], SYN dorsal metacarpal *ligaments,* under *ligament.*

ligamen'ta metacarpa'lia interos'sea [TA], SYN interosseous metacarpal *ligaments,* under *ligament.*

ligamen'ta metacarpa'lia palma'ria [TA], SYN palmar metacarpal *ligaments,* under *ligament.*

l. metatarsa'le transver'sum profun'dum [TA], SYN deep transverse metatarsal *ligament.*

l. metatarsa'le transver'sum superficia'le [TA], SYN superficial transverse metatarsal *ligament.*

ligamen'ta metatarsa'lia dorsa'lia [TA], SYN dorsal metatarsal *ligaments,* under *ligament.*

ligamen'ta metatarsa'lia interos'sea [TA], SYN metatarsal interosseous *ligaments,* under *ligament.*

ligamen'ta metatarsa'lia planta'ria [TA], SYN plantar metatarsal *ligaments,* under *ligament.*

l. natato'rium, SYN superficial transverse metacarpal *ligament.*

ligamen'ta navicularicuneifor'mia, SEE dorsal cuneonavicular *ligaments,* under *ligament,* plantar cuneonavicular *ligaments,* under *ligament.*

l. nu'chae [TA], a sagittal ligamentous band at the back of the neck, formed of thickened supraspinous ligaments; it extends from the external occipital protuberance to the posterior border of the foramen magnum cranially and to the seventh cervical spinous process caudally. SYN nuchal ligament⋆, apparatus ligamentosus colli.

l. orbicula're ra'dii, SYN anular *ligament* of radius.

ligamenta ossiculorum auditorium, ⋆official alternate term for *ligaments* of auditory ossicles, under *ligament.*

ligamen'ta ossiculo'rum audi'tus [TA], SYN *ligaments* of auditory ossicles, under *ligament.*

l. ova'rii pro'prium [TA], SYN *ligament* of ovary.

ligamen'ta palma'ria [TA], SYN palmar *ligaments,* under *ligament.*

ligamenta palmaria articulationis interphalangeae manus [TA], SYN palmar *ligaments* of interphalangeal joints of hand, under *ligament.*

ligamenta palmaria articulationis metacarpophalangeae [TA], SYN palmar *ligaments* of metacarpophalangeal joints, under *ligament.*

l. palpebra'le exter'num, SYN lateral palpebral *ligament.*

l. palpebra'le latera'le [TA], SYN lateral palpebral *ligament.*

l. palpebra'le media'le [TA], SYN medial palpebral *ligament.*

l. patel'lae [TA], SYN patellar *ligament.*

l. pectina'tum, pectinate ligaments of iridocorneal angle. SEE trabecular *tissue* of sclera.

l. pectina'tum an'guli iridocornea'lis, pectinate ligaments of iridocorneal angle. SEE trabecular *tissue* of sclera.

l. pectina'tum ir'idis, pectinate ligaments of iridocorneal angle. SEE trabecular *tissue* of sclera.

l. pectinea'le [TA], SYN pectineal *ligament.*

l. phrenicocol'icum [TA], SYN phrenicocolic *ligament.*

l. phrenicolienale, SYN phrenicosplenic *ligament.*

l. phrenicosplenicum [TA], SYN phrenicosplenic *ligament.*

l. pisohama'tum [TA], SYN pisohamate *ligament.*

l. pisometacarp'eum [TA], SYN pisometacarpal *ligament.*

l. planta're lon'gum [TA], SYN long plantar *ligament.*

ligamen'ta planta'ria [TA], SYN plantar *ligaments,* under *ligament.*

ligamenta plantaria articulationis interphalangeae pedis [TA], SYN plantar *ligaments* of interphalangeal joints of foot, under *ligament.*

ligamenta plantaria articulationis metatarsophalangeae [TA], SYN plantar *ligaments* of metatarsophalangeal joints, under *ligament.*

l. poplit'eum arcua'tum [TA], SYN arcuate popliteal *ligament.*

l. poplit'eum obli'quum [TA], SYN oblique popliteal *ligament.*

l. pterygospina'le [TA], SYN pterygospinous *ligament.*

l. pubicum inferius [TA], SYN inferior pubic *ligament.*

l. pu'bicum supe'rius [TA], SYN superior pubic *ligament.*

l. pubocapsula're, SYN pubofemoral *ligament.*

l. pubofemora'le [TA], SYN pubofemoral *ligament.*

l. puboprostat'icum [TA], SYN puboprostatic *ligament.*

l. puboprostat'icum latera'le, SEE puboprostatic *ligament.*

l. puboprostat′icum media′le, SEE puboprostatic *ligament*.

l. pubovesica′le (femininum) [TA], SYN pubovesical *ligament* (of female).

i. pubovesicale (masculinum) [TA], SYN pubovesical *ligament* (of male).

l. pulmona′le [TA], SYN pulmonary *ligament*.

l. quadra′tum [TA], SYN quadrate *ligament*.

l. radia′tum, SYN radiate *ligament* of head of rib.

l. radiocarpa′le dorsa′le [TA], SYN dorsal radiocarpal *ligament*.

l. radiocarpa′le palma′re [TA], SYN palmar radiocarpal *ligament*.

l. reflex′um [TA], SYN reflected inguinal *ligament*.

l. sacrococcyg′eum ante′rius [TA], SYN anterior sacrococcygeal *ligament*.

l. sacrococcygeum dorsale superficiale, ⭐official alternate term for superficial posterior sacrococcygeal *ligament*.

l. sacrococcyg′eum latera′le [TA], SYN lateral sacrococcygeal *ligament*.

l. sacrococcyg′eum poste′rius profun′dum, SYN deep posterior sacrococcygeal *ligament*.

l. sacrococcyg′eum poste′rius superficia′le [TA], SYN superficial posterior sacrococcygeal *ligament*.

l. sacrodura′le, SYN sacrodural *ligament*.

ligamen′ta sacroili′aca anterio′ra [TA], SYN anterior sacroiliac *ligaments*, under *ligament*.

ligamen′ta sacroili′aca interos′sea [TA], SYN interosseous sacroiliac *ligaments*, under *ligament*.

ligamen′ta sacroil′iaca posterio′ra [TA], SYN posterior sacroiliac *ligaments*, under *ligament*.

l. sacroili′acum poste′rius, SYN posterior sacroiliac *ligaments*, under *ligament*.

l. sacrospina′le [TA], SYN sacrospinous *ligament*.

l. sacrospino′sum, SYN sacrospinous *ligament*.

l. sacrotubera′le [TA], SYN sacrotuberous *ligament*.

l. sacrotubero′sum, SYN sacrotuberous *ligament*.

l. sero′sum, SYN serous *ligament*.

l. sphenomandibula′re [TA], SYN sphenomandibular *ligament*.

l. spira′le coch′leae, SYN spiral *ligament* of cochlear duct, spiral *ligament* of cochlear duct.

l. spirale ductus cochlearis [TA], SYN spiral *ligament* of cochlear duct.

l. splenorena′le [TA], SYN splenorenal *ligament*.

ligamenta sternoclavicularia, SYN sternoclavicular *ligaments*, under *ligament*.

l. sternoclavicula′re ante′rius [TA], SYN anterior sternoclavicular *ligament*.

l. sternoclavicula′re poste′rius [TA], SYN posterior sternoclavicular *ligament*.

l. sternocosta′le intraarticula′re [TA], SYN intraarticular sternocostal *ligament*.

ligamen′ta sternocosta′lia radia′ta [TA], SYN radiate sternocostal *ligaments*, under *ligament*.

ligamen′ta sternoper′icardi′aca [TA], SYN sternopericardial *ligaments*, under *ligament*.

l. stylohyoi′deum [TA], SYN stylohyoid *ligament*.

l. stylomandibula′re [TA], SYN stylomandibular *ligament*.

l. supraspina′le [TA], SYN supraspinous *ligament*.

ligamen′ta suspenso′ria mammaria, SYN suspensory *ligaments* of breast, under *ligament*.

l. suspensorium axillae [TA], SYN suspensory *ligament* of axilla.

l. suspensorium bulbi [TA], SYN suspensory *ligament* of eyeball.

l. suspenso′rium clitor′idis [TA], SYN suspensory *ligament* of clitoris.

l. suspensorium duodeni, ⭐official alternate term for suspensory *muscle* of duodenum.

l. suspensorium glandulae thyroideae [TA], SYN suspensory *ligament* of thyroid gland.

l. suspenso′rium ova′rii [TA], SYN suspensory *ligament* of ovary.

l. suspenso′rium pe′nis [TA], SYN suspensory *ligament* of penis.

l. talocalcaneum [TA], SYN talocalcaneal *ligament*.

l. talocalcanea′re interos′seum, SYN talocalcaneal interosseous *ligament*.

l. talocalcaneum latera′le [TA], SYN lateral talocalcaneal *ligament*.

l. talocalcaneum media′le [TA], SYN medial talocalcaneal *ligament*.

l. talocalcaneum posterius [TA], SYN posterior talocalcaneal *ligament*.

l. talofibula′re ante′rius [TA], SYN anterior talofibular *ligament*.

l. talofibula′re poste′rius [TA], SYN posterior talofibular *ligament*.

l. talonavicula′re [TA], SYN talonavicular *ligament*.

l. talotibia′le ante′rius, SYN anterior tibiotalar *part* of medial ligament of ankle joint; SEE ALSO medial *ligament* of ankle joint.

l. talotibia′le poste′rius, SYN tibiotalar *part* of medial ligament of ankle joint; SEE ALSO medial *ligament* of ankle joint.

l. tarsa′le exter′num, SYN lateral palpebral *ligament*.

l. tarsa′le inter′num, SYN medial palpebral *ligament*.

ligamen′ta tar′si [TA], SYN tarsal *ligaments*, under *ligament*.

ligamenta tarsi dorsalia [TA], SYN dorsal tarsal *ligaments*, under *ligament*.

ligamenta tarsi interossea [TA], SYN tarsal interosseous *ligaments*, under *ligament*.

ligamenta tarsi plantaria [TA], SYN plantar tarsal *ligaments*, under *ligament*.

ligamen′ta tarsometatarsa′lia [TA], SYN tarsometatarsal *ligaments*, under *ligament*.

ligamenta tarsometatarsalia dorsalia [TA], SYN dorsal tarsometatarsal *ligaments*, under *ligament*.

ligamenta tarsometatarsalia plantaria [TA], SYN plantar tarsometatarsal *ligaments*, under *ligament*.

l. temporomandibula′re, SYN lateral *ligament* of temporomandibular joint.

l. te′res fem′oris, SYN *ligament* of head of femur.

l. te′res hep′atis [TA], SYN round *ligament* of liver.

l. te′res u′teri [TA], SYN round *ligament* of uterus.

l. tes′tis, the caudal portion of the embryonic urogenital ridge; the upper third of the gubernaculum testis.

l. thyroepiglot′ticum [TA], SYN thyroepiglottic *ligament*.

l. thyrohyoi′deum latera′le [TA], SYN lateral thyrohyoid *ligament*.

l. thyrohyoi′deum media′num [TA], SYN median thyrohyoid *ligament*.

l. tibiofibula′re ante′rius [TA], SYN anterior tibiofibular *ligament*.

l. tibiofibula′re me′dium, SYN interosseous *membrane* of leg.

l. tibiofibula′re poste′rius [TA], SYN posterior tibiofibular *ligament*.

l. tibionavicula′re, SYN tibionavicular *part* of medial ligament of ankle joint.

ligamen′ta trachea′lia, SYN anular *ligaments* of trachea, under *ligament*.

l. transversa′le cervicis, SYN cardinal *ligament*.

l. transver′sum acetab′uli [TA], SYN transverse acetabular *ligament*.

l. transver′sum atlan′tis [TA], SYN transverse *ligament* of the atlas.

l. transver′sum cru′ris, SYN superior extensor *retinaculum*.

l. transver′sum ge′nus [TA], SYN transverse *ligament* of knee.

l. transversum humeri [TA], SYN transverse humeral *ligament*.

l. transver′sum pel′vis [TA], SYN transverse perineal *ligament*.

l. transver′sum perine′i [TA], SYN transverse perineal *ligament*.

l. transver′sum scap′ulae infe′rius [TA], SYN inferior transverse scapular *ligament*.

l. transver′sum scap′ulae supe′rius [TA], SYN superior transverse scapular *ligament*.

l. trapezoi′deum [TA], SYN trapezoid *ligament*.

l. triangula′re, SYN perineal *membrane*.

li

l. triangula're dex'trum hepatis [TA], SYN right triangular *ligament* of liver.

l. triangula're sinis'trum hepatis [TA], SYN left triangular *ligament* of liver.

l. tuber'culi cos'tae, SYN lateral costotransverse *ligament*.

l. ulnocarpa'le palma're [TA], SYN palmar ulnocarpal *ligament*.

l. umbilica'le latera'le, an old name for l. umbilicale mediale. SYN lateral umbilical ligament.

l. umbilica'le media'le, SYN *cord* of umbilical artery.

l. umbilica'le media'num [TA], SYN median umbilical *ligament*.

l. uteroovaricum, ⨯official alternate term for *ligament* of ovary.

l. ve'nae ca'vae sinis'trae [TA], SYN *ligament* of left vena cava.

l. veno'sum [TA], a thin fibrous cord, lying in the fissure of the ligamentum venosum, the remains of the ductus venosus of the fetus. SYN Arantius ligament, l. ductus venosi, venous ligament.

l. ventricula're, SYN vestibular *ligament*.

l. vestibula're [TA], SYN vestibular *ligament*.

l. voca'le [TA], SYN vocal *ligament*.

---

lig·and (lig'and, lī'gand). **1.** Any individual atom, group, or molecule attached to a central metal ion by multiple coordinate bonds; e.g., the porphyrin portion of heme, the corrin nucleus of the B$_{12}$ vitamins. **2.** An organic molecule attached to a tracer element, e.g., a radioisotope. **3.** A molecule that binds to a macromolecule, e.g., a l. binding to a receptor. **4.** The analyte in competitive binding assays, such as radioimmunoassay. **5.** An atom or group covalently attached to a specified carbon atom in an organic molecule. [L. *ligo,* to bind]

addressin l.'s, l.'s on cells for specific homing receptors on lymphocytes.

Fas l., a molecule on the surface of cytotoxic T cells that binds to its receptor, Fas, on the surface of other cells, initiating apoptosis in the target cell.

lig·and·in (lī-gan'din). SYN *glutathione S*-transferase.

li·gase (lī'gās). Generic term for enzymes (EC class 6) catalyzing the joining of two molecules coupled with the breakdown of a pyrophosphate bond in ATP or a similar compound. SEE ALSO synthetase.

li·gate (lī'gāt). To apply a ligature. [L. *ligo,* pp. *-atus,* to bind]

li·ga·tion (lī-gā'shŭn). **1.** Application of a ligature. **2.** The act of binding or annealing. [L. *ligatio,* fr. *ligo,* to bind]

blunt-end l., a reaction that joins two DNA duplexes directly at their blunt ends.

enzyme-catalyzed l., an enzyme-mediated joining of phosphodiester linkage of two stretches of DNA or RNA, or of peptide linkage of two polypeptides.

pole l., a l. at the root of an organ to shut off or diminish blood supply.

surgical l., in dentistry, the surgical exposure of an unerupted tooth so that a metal ligature can be placed around its cervix and fastened to an orthodontic appliance to facilitate eruption.

tooth l., the binding together of teeth with wire for stabilization and immobilization following traumatic injury or orthognathic surgery, or during periodontal therapy.

tubal l., interruption of the continuity of the oviducts by cutting, cautery, or by a plastic or metal device to prevent future conception.

li·ga·tor (lī'gā-ter, -tōr). An instrument used in the ligation of vessels in deep and nearly inaccessible parts.

lig·a·ture (lig'ă-choor). **1.** A thread, wire, fillet, or the like, tied tightly around a blood vessel, the pedicle of a tumor, or other structure to constrict it. **2.** In orthodontics, a wire or other material used to secure an orthodontic attachment or tooth to an archwire. [L. *ligatura,* a band or tie, fr. *ligo,* to tie]

elastic l., (1) a rubber l. that slowly constricts; **(2)** in orthodontics, a stretchable threadlike material that may be tied from a tooth to an archwire or from tooth to tooth to gain movement of these units.

intravascular l., balloon occlusion of the feeding vessels of a cerebral arteriovenous malformation.

nonabsorbable l., a permanent l. of inert material, such as silk, wire, or synthetic fiber, that does not undergo dissolution in human tissues.

occluding l., a l. to shut off completely the distal blood supply.

provisional l., a l. applied to an artery in continuity at the beginning of an operation to prevent hemorrhage, but removed when the operation is completed.

soluble l., a temporary l. of material that can be absorbed by human tissues.

Stannius l., a l. placed either around the junction between the sinus venosus and atrium of the frog or turtle heart (first Stannius l.) or around the atrioventricular junction (second Stannius l.); demonstrates that the cardiac impulse is conducted from sinus venosus to atria to ventricle, but that successive chambers possess automaticity since each may continue to beat, but the atria now have a slower rate than the sinus venosus, and the ventricle either does not contract or beats at a slower rate than the atria.

suboccluding l., a l. to diminish blood supply and encourage collateral circulation.

suture l., a l. applied by passing a needle with attached thread through or around a structure to more firmly secure the l.

light (līt). That portion of electromagnetic radiation (between 390 and 770 nm) to which the retina is sensitive (wavelength range of 380–780 nm). SEE ALSO lamp. [A.S. *leōht*]

cold l., (1) SYN bioluminescence (1); **(2)** fluorescent l. as opposed to incandescent l.

infrared l., SEE infrared.

invisible l., historic term for x-rays.

minimum l., SEE visual *threshold.*

polarized l., l. in which, as a result of reflection or transmission through certain media, the vibrations are all in one plane, transverse to the ray, instead of in all planes.

reflected l., l. directed backward from a mirror.

refracted l., bent rays of l. changed in passage from one transparent medium to another of unequal density. SEE ALSO refraction.

transmitted l., l. passed through a transparent medium.

Wood l., ultraviolet l. produced by Wood lamp.

light·en·ing (līt'en-ing). Sensation of decreased abdominal distention during the later weeks of pregnancy following the descent of the fetal head into the pelvic inlet.

light green SF yel·low·ish [C.I. 42095]. An acid arylmethane dye, used as a cytoplasmic stain in plant and animal histology; fades badly in bright light.

lig·ne·ous (lig'nē-us). Woody; having a woody feeling. [L. *ligneus,* wooden, fr. *lignum,* wood]

lig·nin (lig'nin). A random polymer of coniferyl alcohol accompanying cellulose and present in vegetable fiber and wood cells; a source of vanillin (by oxidation of l.); l. composition varies with plant species. It is one of the most abundant biopolymers in nature. [L. *lignum,* wood]

lig·no·cer·ic ac·id (lig-nō-sār'ik, -sēr'ik). An acid present in one type of sphingolipid and in small amounts in triacylglycerols. SYN *n*-tetracosanoic acid.

like·li·hood. A statement of the chance that an unknown quantity in reality has a particular value based on the readiness with which it would account for a given set of data; in this way the merits of various competing interpretations may be compared.

Likert, Rensis, U.S. social psychologist, *1903. SEE Likert *scale.*

Lillie, Ralph D., U.S. pathologist, 1896–1979. SEE Glenner-L. *stain* for pituitary. See entries under stain.

Lilly, John C., U.S. physiologist, *1915. SEE Silverman-L. *pneumotachograph.*

limb (lim) [TA]. **1.** An extremity; a member; an arm or leg. SYN member. **2.** A segment of any jointed structure. SEE ALSO leg, crus. [A.S. *lim*]

ampullary membranous l.'s of semicircular ducts [TA], the dilated ends of the three semicircular ducts, each of which contains a specialized thickening of the epithelium known as the ampullary crest. SYN crura membranacea ampullaria ductuum semicircularium [TA], ampullary crura of semicircular ducts.

anacrotic l., the ascending l. of an arterial pulse tracing.

anterior l. of internal capsule [TA], the portion of the internal capsule between the head of the caudate nucleus and the putamen; it lies anterior to the genu of the internal capsule. SYN crus anterius capsulae internae [TA].

anterior l. of stapes [TA], the anterior of the two delicate curving limbs of the stapes that pass from the head of the bone to the base or footplate. SYN crus anterius stapedis [TA], anterior crus of stapes.

l.'s of bony semicircular canals, SYN bony l.'s of semicircular canals.

bony l.'s of semicircular canals [TA], the extremities of the bony semicircular canals in which the corresponding membranous l.'s of the semicircular ducts are located; they are the common bony l.'s (crus osseum commune), simple bony l.'s (crus osseum simplex), and ampullary bony l.'s (crus ossea ampullaria). SYN crura of bony semicircular canals, crura ossea canalium semicircularium, l.'s of bony semicircular canals.

common membranous l. of membranous semicircular ducts, SYN common membranous l. of semicircular ducts.

common membranous l. of semicircular ducts [TA], the united, nonampullary ends of the superior and posterior semicircular ducts. SYN crus membranaceum commune ductuum semicircularium [TA], common crus of semicircular ducts, common membranous l. of membranous semicircular ducts.

l. of helix, SYN crus of helix.

inferior l., SYN lower l.

inferior l. of ansa cervicalis, *official alternate term for inferior root of ansa cervicalis.

lateral l., SYN lateral crus.

long l. of incus [TA], the process of the incus that articulates with the stapes. SYN crus longum incudis [TA], long crus of incus.

▣lower l. [TA], the hip, thigh, leg, ankle, and foot. SYN inferior member [TA], membrum inferius [TA], inferior l., lower extremity, pelvic l.

medial l., SYN medial crus.

pelvic l., SYN lower l.

phantom l., SYN phantom limb pain.

posterior l. of internal capsule [TA], that subdivision of the internal capsule caudal to the genu and located between the thalamus and lentiform nucleus. SYN crus posterius capsulae internae [TA].

posterior l. of stapes [TA], the posterior of the two delicate limbs of the stapes that connect the head and base or footplate of the bone. SYN crus posterius stapedis [TA], posterior crus of stapes.

retrolenticular l. of internal capsule, *official alternate term for retrolentiform l. of internal capsule.

retrolentiform l. of internal capsule [TA], the portion of the internal capsule located caudal to the posterior limb of the internal capsule and the lenticular (lentiform) nucleus. SEE ALSO retrolenticular part of internal capsule. SYN pars retrolentiformis cruris posterior [TA], retrolenticular l. of internal capsule*.

short l. of incus [TA], the short crus of incus; the process of the incus that fits into a depression (fossa incudis) in the epitympanic recess. SYN crus breve incudis [TA], short crus of incus.

simple membranous l. of semicircular duct [TA], the non-ampullary end of the lateral semicircular duct that opens independently into the utricle. SYN crus membranaceum simplex ductus semicircularis [TA], simple crus of semicircular duct.

sublenticular l. of internal capsule, *official alternate term for sublentiform l. of internal capsule.

sublentiform l. of internal capsule [TA], the portion of the internal capsule located ventral to caudal portions of the lenticular nucleus. SEE ALSO sublenticular part of internal capsule. SYN pars sublentiformis cruris posterioris [TA], sublenticular l. of internal capsule*.

superior l., SYN upper l.

superior l. of ansa cervicalis, *official alternate term for superior root of ansa cervicalis.

thoracic l., SYN upper l.

▣upper l. [TA], the shoulder, arm, forearm, wrist, and hand. SYN

membrum superius [TA], superior member [TA], superior l., thoracic l., upper extremity.

lim·bic (lim′bik). **1.** Relating to a limbus. **2.** Relating to the limbic *system.*

lim·bus, pl. **lim·bi** (lim′bŭs, lim′bī). The edge, border, or fringe of a part. [L. a border]

l. acetab′uli [TA], SYN acetabular *margin.*

l. alveola′ris, (1) SYN alveolar *arch* of mandible; **(2)** SYN alveolar *arch* of maxilla.

l. anterior palpebrae [TA], SYN anterior palpebral *margin.*

l. of cornea, SYN corneal l.

l. cor′neae, SYN corneal l.

corneal l. [TA], the margin of the cornea overlapped by the sclera. SYN corneal margin, corneoscleral junction, l. corneae, l. of cornea, sclerocorneal junction.

l. fos′sae ova′lis [TA], a muscular ring surrounding the fossa ovalis in the wall of the right atrium of the heart. SYN anulus ovalis, margin of fossa ovalis, Vieussens anulus, Vieussens isthmus, Vieussens l., Vieussens ring.

l. lam′inae spira′lis os′seae [TA], SYN l. of osseous spiral lamina.

l. membra′nae tym′pani, SYN l. of tympanic membrane.

l. of osseous spiral lamina [TA], the border of the spiral lamina; the thickened periosteum covering the upper plate of the bony spiral lamina of the cochlea. SYN l. laminae spiralis osseae [TA].

lim′bi palpebra′les [TA], SYN palpebral *margins,* under *margin.*

l. penicilla′tus, SYN brush *border.*

l. posterior palpebrae [TA],

l. sphenoidalis [TA], SYN l. of sphenoid (bone).

l. of sphenoid (bone) [TA], variably prominent ridge on the body of the sphenoid (bone) forming the posterior border of the jugum sphenoidale and the anterior border of the prechiasmatic sulcus. SYN l. sphenoidalis [TA].

l. stria′tus, SYN striated *border.*

l. of tympanic membrane, margin of the tympanic membrane attaching to the tympanic sulcus. SYN l. membranae tympani.

Vieussens l., SYN l. fossae ovalis.

lime (līm). **1.** CaO; an alkaline earth oxide occurring in grayish white masses (quicklime); on exposure to the atmosphere it becomes converted into calcium hydrate and calcium carbonate (air-slaked l.); direct addition of water to calcium oxide produces calcium hydrate (slaked l.). SYN calcium oxide, calx (1). **2.** Fruit of the l. tree, *Citrus medica* (family Rutaceae), which is a source of ascorbic acid and acts as an antiscorbutic agent. [O.E. *līm,* birdlime]

air-slaked l., SEE lime (1).

chlorinated l., a mixture of varying proportions of complexes of chlorine with calcium oxide and calcium hydroxide. Contains 24–37% available chlorine. Decomposes in moist conditions to liberate chlorine. Strong irritant due to chlorine vapors. Used for disinfecting drinking water, sewage etc.; in the bleaching of wood pulp, linen, cotton, straw, oils, soaps, and laundry; as an oxidizer; in destroying caterpillars; and as a decontaminant for mustard gas and similar substances. SYN bleaching powder.

slaked l., SEE lime (1).

sulfurated l., SYN crude *calcium* sulfide.

li·men, pl. **li·mi·na** (lī′men, lim′i-nă) [TA]. **1.** Entrance; the external opening of a canal or space, such as l. insulae [TA]. **2.** SYN threshold. [L.]

difference l., a barely noticeable change in the intensity or frequency of a stimulus.

l. in′sulae [TA], the band of transition between the anterior portion of the gray matter of the insula and the anterior perforated substance; it is formed by a narrow strip of olfactory cortex along the lateral side of the lateral olfactory stria. SYN threshold of island of Reil.

l. na′si [TA], a ridge marking the boundary between the nasal cavity proper and the vestibule. SYN threshold of nose.

lim·er·ence (lim′er-ens). Emotional excitement of being in love.

limes (L) (lī′mēz). A boundary, limit, or threshold. SEE ALSO L *doses,* under *dose.* [L.]

li

lim·i·nal (lim′i-năl). **1.** Pertaining to a threshold. **2.** Pertaining to a stimulus just strong enough to excite a tissue, e.g., nerve or muscle. [L. *limen* (*limin-*), a threshold]

lim·i·nom·e·ter (lim-i-nom′ĕ-ter). An instrument for measuring the strength of a stimulus which is barely sufficient to produce a reflex response. [L. *limen*, threshold, + G. *metron*, measure]

lim·it. A boundary or end. [L. *limes*, boundary]

critical l., the upper or lower boundary of a laboratory test result that indicates a life-threatening value.

elastic l., the greatest stress to which a material may be subjected and still be capable of returning to its original dimensions when the forces are released.

Hayflick l., the l. of human cell division in subcultures; such cells typically divide only about 50 times before dying out.

permissible exposure l., an occupational health standard to safeguard workers against dangerous contaminants in the workplace.

proportional l., the greatest stress that a material is capable of sustaining without any deviation from proportionality of stress to strain (Hooke law).

quantum l., the shortest wavelength found in an x-ray spectrum.

short-term exposure l. (STEL), the maximum concentration of a chemical to which workers may be exposed continuously for up to 15 minutes without danger to health or work efficiency and safety.

tolerance l.'s, specified performance l.'s for allowable error for a test; the l.'s selected should depend on both the effect of the error on the clinical significance of a test and on what is technically achievable.

Lim·na·tis ni·lot·i·ca (lim-nā′tis nī-lot′i-kă). The horse leech; a species of land-leech of southern Europe and northern Africa which may infest the nostrils or gullet and, attaching itself to the mucous membrane, may cause hemorrhages and anemia in horses and other animals drinking leech-infested water. [G. *limnē*, pool]

lim·ne·mia (lim-nē′mē-ă). SYN chronic *malaria*. [G. *limnē*, marsh, + *haima*, blood]

lim·ne·mic (lim-nē′mik). Suffering from chronic malaria.

lim·nol·o·gy (lim-nol′ō-jē). Study of the physical, chemical, meteorologic, and biologic conditions in fresh water; a branch of ecology. [G. *limnē*, pool, + *logos*, study]

li·mon, gen. **li·mo·nis** (lī′mon, li-mō′nis). SYN lemon. [L.]

li·moph·thi·sis (lī-mof′thī-sis). Rarely used term for emaciation from lack of sufficient nourishment. [G. *limos*, hunger, + *phthisis*, wasting]

limp. A lame walk with a yielding step; asymmetrical gait. SEE ALSO claudication.

LINAC Acronym of linear *accelerator*.

lin·co·my·cin (lin-kō-mī′sin). An antibacterial substance, composed of substituted pyrrolidine and octapyranose moities, produced by *Streptomyces lincolnensis;* active against Gram-positive organisms; used medicinally as l. hydrochloride.

linc·ture, linc·tus (link′choor, link′tŭs). An electuary or a confection; originally a medicinal preparation taken by licking. [L. *lingo*, pp. *linctus*, to lick]

lin·dane (lin′dān). Used as a scabicide, pediculicide, and insecticide (10 times more toxic for houseflies than DDT).

Lindau, Arvid, Swedish pathologist, 1892–1958. SEE L. *disease, tumor;* von Hippel-L. *syndrome.*

Lindbergh, Charles A., U.S. aviator, 1902–1974. SEE Carrel-L. *pump.*

Lindner, Karl D., Austrian ophthalmologist, 1883–1961. SEE L. *bodies,* under *body.*

Lindqvist, Johan Torsten, Swedish physician, *1906. SEE Fahraeus-L. *effect.*

LINE

line (līn) [TA]. **1.** A mark, strip, or streak. In anatomy, a long, narrow mark, strip, or streak distinguished from the adjacent tissues by color, texture, or elevation. SEE ALSO linea. **2.** A unit of measurement used by histologists in the 19th century; it varied in different countries from $\frac{1}{10}$–$\frac{1}{12}$ of an English inch. **3.** A laboratory derivative of a stock of organisms maintained under defined physical conditions. **4.** A section of tubing supplying fluid or conducting impulses for monitoring equipment; e.g., intravenous l., arterial l. SYN linea [TA]. [L. *linea,* a linen thread, a string, line, fr. *linum,* flax]

absorption l.'s, the dark l.'s in the solar spectrum due to absorption by the solar and the earth's atmosphere; the phenomenon occurs because rays passing from an incandescent body through a colder medium are absorbed by elements in that medium.

accretion l.'s, l.'s seen in microscopic sections of the enamel, marking successive layers of added material.

alveolonasal l., a l. connecting the alveolar point and the nasion.

Amberg lateral sinus l., a l. dividing the angle formed by the anterior edge of the mastoid process and the temporal l.

anocutaneous l. [TA], inferior border of the anal pecten where the stratified squamous epithelium changes from the hairless anoderm to typical (hairy) skin; commonly coincides with the inferior border of the internal anal sphincter. SYN linea anorectalis [TA].

anterior axillary l. [TA], a vertical line extending inferiorly from the anterior axillary fold. SYN linea axillaris anterior [TA], linea preaxillaris, preaxillary l.

anterior junction l., radiographic projection of the mediastinal tissue septum between the upper lobes behind the sternum.

anterior median l. [TA], the line of intersection of the midsagittal plane with the anterior surface of the body. SYN linea mediana anterior [TA].

arcuate l. [TA], an arching or bow-shaped l. SEE arcuate l. of ilium, arcuate l. of rectus sheath. SYN linea arcuata [TA].

arcuate l. of ilium [TA], the iliac portion of the linea terminalis of the bony pelvis. SYN linea arcuata ossis ilii [TA].

arcuate l. of rectus sheath [TA], a crescentic line, not always clearly defined, which marks the lower limit of the posterior layer of the sheath of the rectus abdominis muscle. SYN linea arcuata vaginae musculi recti abdominis [TA], Douglas l., linea semicircularis, semicircular l.

arterial l., an intraarterial catheter.

axillary l., SEE anterior axillary l., midaxillary l., posterior axillary l.

Baillarger l.'s, two laminae of white fibers that course parallel to the surface of the cerebral cortex and are visible as the stria of the internal pyramidal layer [TA] in cortical layer V (outer l.) and the stria of the internal granular layer [TA] in cortical layer IV (inner l.) that appear in myelin stained sections cut perpendicular to the surface; the l. of Gennari in the calcarine cortex represents the outer of these lines. SYN stria laminae granularis internae [TA], stria laminae pyramidalis internae [TA], Baillarger bands.

base l., SEE orbitomeatal *plane* (1).

basinasal l., a l. connecting the basion and the nasion. SYN nasobasilar l.

Beau l.'s, transverse grooves on the fingernails following severe febrile disease, malnutrition, trauma, myocardial infarction, etc.

l. of Bechterew, SYN *band* of Kaes-Bechterew.

bismuth l., a black zone on the free marginal gingiva, often the first sign of poisoning from prolonged parenteral administration of bismuth.

black l., SYN *linea* nigra.

l.'s of Blaschko, a pattern of distribution of skin lesions or pigmentary anomalies; linear on the extremities, S-shaped curves on the abdomen, and V-shaped on the back, thought to result from genetic mosaicism (q.v.) and the interplay of transverse clonal proliferation and longitudinal growth and flexion of the embryo.

blue l., a bluish l. along the free border of the gingiva, occurring in chronic heavy metal poisoning.

Brödel bloodless l., l. running somewhat posterior to the lateral convex border of the kidney between anterior and posterior renal segments demarcating the areas of distribution of the anterior and posterior branches of the renal artery; it is in fact only relatively avascular.

Burton l., a bluish l. on the free border of the gingiva, occurring in lead poisoning.

calcification l.'s of Retzius, incremental l.'s of rhythmic deposition of successive layers of enamel matrix during development. SYN l.'s of Retzius.

Camper l., the l. running from the inferior border of the ala of the nose to the superior border of the tragus of the ear.

cell l., (1) in tissue culture, the cells growing in the first or later subculture from a primary culture. SEE ALSO established cell l; (2) a clone of cultured cells derived from an identified parental cell type.

cement l., the refractile boundary of an osteon or interstitial lamellar system in compact bone.

cervical l., a continuous anatomical irregular curved l. marking the cervical end of the crown of a tooth and the cementoenamel junction.

Chamberlain l., a l. drawn from the posterior margin of the hard palate to the dorsum of the foramen magnum; in basilar impression, the odontoid process rises above this l.

Chaussier l., the anteroposterior l. of the corpus callosum as appearing on median section of the brain.

choroid l. [TA], SYN *tenia* choroidea.

Clapton l., a greenish discoloration of the marginal gingiva in cases of chronic copper poisoning.

cleavage l.'s, SYN tension l.'s.

Conradi l., a l. extending from the base of the ensiform cartilage to the apex beat of the heart, corresponding approximately to the lower edge of the cardiac area.

contour l.'s of Owen, SYN Owen l.'s.

Correra l., SYN pleural l.'s.

costal l. of pleural reflection, surface projection of the sharp l. along which the costal part of the parietal pleura becomes continuous with the diaphragmatic part inferiorly; this l. intersects midclavicular l. at the level of the 8th rib, the midaxillary l. at the level of the 10th rib, and the paravertebral l. at the level of the 12th rib; thoracentesis is performed one rib level higher in these l.'s.

costoclavicular l., SYN parasternal l.

costophrenic septal l.'s, SYN Kerley B l.'s.

Crampton l., a l. from the apex of the cartilage of the last rib downward and forward nearly to the crest of the ilium, then forward parallel with it to a little below the anterior superior spine; a guide to the common iliac artery.

Daubenton l., the l. passing between the opisthion and the basion. SEE ALSO Daubenton *angle*, Daubenton *plane*.

l. of demarcation, a zone of inflammatory reaction separating a gangrenous area from healthy tissue.

demarcation l. of retina, junction of avascular and vascular retina in retinopathy of prematurity; line marking the limits of an old retinal detachment.

Dennie l., SYN Dennie-Morgan *fold*.

dentate l., SYN pectinate l.

developmental l.'s, SYN developmental *grooves*, under *groove*.

Douglas l., SYN arcuate l. of rectus sheath.

Eberth l.'s, l.'s appearing between the cells of the myocardium when stained with silver nitrate.

Egger l., seldom-used term for the circular l. of adhesion between the vitreous and posterior lens.

Ehrlich-Türk l., seldom-used term for the vertical, thin deposition of material on the posterior surface of the cornea in uveitis.

epiphysial l. [TA], the line of junction of the epiphysis and diaphysis of a long bone where growth in length occurs. SYN linea epiphysialis [TA], synchondrosis epiphyseos.

established cell l., cells that demonstrate the potential for indefinite subculture in vitro.

Farre l., a whitish l. marking the insertion of the mesovarium at the hilum of the ovary.

Feiss l., a l. running from the medial malleolus to the plantar aspect of the first metatarsophalangeal joint.

Ferry l., an iron l. occurring in the corneal epithelium anterior to a filtering *bleb*.

l. of fixation, a l. joining the object (or point of fixation) with the fovea.

Fleischner l.'s, coarse linear shadows on a chest radiograph, indicating bands of subsegmental atelectasis.

Fraunhofer l.'s, a number of the most prominent of the absorption l.'s of the solar spectrum.

fulcrum l., an imaginary l. around which a removable partial denture tends to rotate. SYN rotational axis.

l. of Gennari, a prominent white line appearing in perpendicular sections of the visual cortex (Brodmann area 17) at about midthickness of the cortical gray matter, corresponding to the particularly well-developed outer line of Baillarger of that cortical area, and composed largely of tangentially disposed intracortical association fibers. SYN occipital stripe [TA], stria occipitalis [TA], occipital l.☆, Gennari band, Gennari stria, stripe of Gennari.

germ l., a collection of haploid cells derived from the specialized cells of the primitive gonad.

gluteal l.'s [TA], one of three rough curved lines on the outer surface of the ala of the ilium: anterior gluteal l., inferior gluteal l., and posterior gluteal l.; the two areas bounded by these give attachment to the gluteus minimus muscle below and gluteus medius above. SYN lineae gluteae [TA].

Granger l., on lateral skull radiographs, the l. produced by the groove of the optic chiasm or *sulcus* prechiasmaticus.

growth arrest l.'s, dense l.'s parallel to the growth plates of long bones on radiographs, representing temporary slowing or cessation of longitudinal growth. SYN Harris l.'s.

Gubler l., the level of the superficial origin of the trigeminus on the pons, a lesion below which causes Gubler paralysis.

gum l., the position of the margin of the gingiva in relation to the teeth in the dental arch.

Haller l., SYN *linea* splendens.

Hampton l., a thin radiolucent band across the neck of a contrast-filled benign gastric ulcer, indicating mucosal edema. Cf. Carman *sign*.

Harris l.'s, SYN growth arrest l.'s.

Head l.'s, bands of cutaneous hyperesthesia associated with acute or chronic inflammation of the viscera. SYN Head zones, tender l.'s, tender zones.

Hensen l., SYN H *band*.

highest nuchal l. [TA], a line above and parallel to the superior nuchal line on the external surface of the occipital bone; it gives attachment to the epicranial aponeurosis and occipitalis muscle. SYN linea nuchae suprema [TA].

high lip l., the greatest height to which the lip is raised in normal function or during the act of smiling broadly.

Hilton white l., SYN white l. of anal canal.

His l., a l. extending from the tip of the anterior nasal spine (acanthion) to the hindmost point on the posterior margin of the foramen magnum (opisthion), dividing the face into an upper and a lower, or dental part.

Holden l., the crease or furrow of the skin of the groin caused by flexion of the thigh.

Hudson-Stähli l., a brown, horizontal l. across the lower third of the cornea, occasionally seen in the aged and also in association with corneal opacities.

Hunter l., SYN *linea* alba.

Hunter-Schreger l.'s, SYN Hunter-Schreger *bands*, under *band*.

iliopectineal l., SYN *linea* terminalis of pelvis.

imbrication l.'s of von Ebner, incremental l.'s in the dentin of the tooth that reflect variations in mineralization during dentin formation; the distance between the l.'s corresponds to the daily rate of dentin formation. SYN incremental l.'s of von Ebner.

li

Head lines		
organ	**dermatomic area**	**side of body**
heart	C3–4–T1–5	right front
thoracic aorta	C3–4–T1–7	both sides
ribs	T2–12	ipsilateral
lungs	C3–4	ipsilateral
esophagus	T1–8	both sides
stomach	T (5) 6–9	left
liver and gallbladder	T (5) 6–9 (10)	right
pancreas	T6–9	left front
duodenum	T6–10	right
jejunum	T8–11	left
ileum	T9–11	both sides
cecum, proximal colon	T9–10–L1	right
distant colon	T9–L1	left
rectum	T9–L1	left
kidney and ureter	T9–L1 (2)	ipsilateral
uterus and ovaries	T12–L1	ipsilateral
peritoneum	T5–12	both sides
spleen	T6–10	left

C = cervical segments, T = thoracic segments, L = lumbar segments

incremental l.'s, (1) in the enamel, calcification l.'s of Retzius; **(2)** in the dentin, imbrication or incremental l.'s of von Ebner, and Owen l.'s.

incremental l.'s of von Ebner, SYN imbrication l.'s of von Ebner.

inferior nuchal l. [TA], a ridge that extends laterally from the external occipital crest toward the jugular process of the occipital bone. SYN linea nuchae inferior [TA].

inferior temporal l. of parietal bone [TA], the lower of two curved lines on the parietal bone; it marks the outer limit of attachment of the temporalis muscle. SYN linea temporalis inferior ossis parietalis [TA], temporal ridge.

infracostal l., SYN subcostal *plane*.

intercondylar l. of femur [TA], a faint transverse ridge separating the floor of the intercondylar fossa from the popliteal surface of the femur; it affords attachment to the posterior portion of the articular capsule of the knee. SYN linea intercondylaris femoris [TA].

intermediate l. of iliac crest, SYN intermediate *zone* of iliac crest.

interspinal l., l. passing through both anterior superior iliac spines indicating the interspinal *plane*. SYN linea interspinalis.

intertrochanteric l. [TA], a rough line that separates the neck and shaft of the femur anteriorly; it passes downward and medially from the greater trochanter to the lesser trochanter and continues into the medial lip of the linea aspera. SYN linea intertrochanterica [TA], linea spiralis, spiral l.

intertubercular l., horizontal l. passing through tubercles of both iliac crests, indicating the intertubercular *plane*. SYN linea intertubercularis.

iron l., deposition of l. in the corneal epithelium.

isoelectric l., the baseline of the electrocardiogram, recorded in the TP interval during rhythms with P waves.

l. of Kaes, SYN *band* of Kaes-Bechterew.

Kerley A l.'s, images of deep interlobular septa; longer, thicker, and more central than Kerley B l.'s; usually in upper lobes.

Kerley B l.'s, fine peripheral septal l.'s. SYN costophrenic septal l.'s.

Kerley C l.'s, a nonspecific fine reticular pattern on chest radiographs.

Kilian l., a transverse l. marking the promontory of the pelvis.

Langer l.'s, SYN tension l.'s.

Lanz l., SYN interspinous *plane*.

lead l., deposits of lead sulfide in the gingiva in areas of chronic inflammation.

Looser l.'s, radiolucent bands in the cortex of a bone; usually indicates osteomalacia. SYN Looser zones.

low lip l., (1) the lowest position of the lower lip during the act of smiling or voluntary retraction; **(2)** the lowest position of the upper lip at rest.

M l., a fine l. in the center of the A band of the sarcomere of striated muscle myofibrils. SYN M band, mesophragma.

Mach l., the apparent l. of contrasting density bordering a soft tissue shadow on a radiograph; it is an optical illusion constructed by the observer's retina.

mammary l., a transverse l. drawn between the two nipples.

mammillary l. [TA], a vertical line passing through the nipple on either side. SYN linea mammillaris [TA], nipple l.

McKee l., a l. drawn from the tip of the cartilage of the eleventh rib to a point 3.5 cm medial to the anterior superior spine, then curved downward, forward, and inward to just above the deep inguinal ring; a guide to the common iliac artery.

median l., SEE anterior median l., posterior median l.

Mees l.'s, horizontal white bands of the nails seen in chronic arsenical poisoning, and occasionally in leprosy. SYN Mees stripes.

mercurial l., a bluish brown pigmentation seen at the gingival margin and associated with mercury poisoning (mercurial stomatitis).

Meyer l., a l. through the axis of the big toe and passing the midpoint of the heel in a normal foot.

midaxillary l. [TA], a vertical line intersecting a point midway between the anterior and posterior axillary folds or lines. SYN linea axillaris media [TA], linea medio-axillaris, middle axillary l.

midclavicular l. [TA], a vertical line passing through the midpoint of the clavicle. SYN linea medioclavicularis [TA].

middle axillary l., SYN midaxillary l.

milk l., SYN mammary *ridge*.

Monro l., SYN Monro-Richter l.

Monro-Richter l., a l. passing from the umbilicus to the anterior superior iliac spine. McBurney point occurs on this line. SYN Monro l., Richter-Monro l.

Muehrcke l.'s, white l.'s, parallel with the lunula and separated from each other by normal pink areas; associated with hypoalbuminemia; the l.'s do not move outward with nail growth, but disappear when the serum albumin returns to normal.

mylohyoid l. [TA], a ridge on the inner surface of the mandible running from a point inferior to the mental spine upward and backward to the ramus behind the last molar tooth; it gives attachment to the mylohyoid muscle and the lowermost part of the superior constrictor of the pharynx. SYN linea mylohyoidea [TA], mylohyoid ridge.

nasobasilar l., SYN basinasal l.

Nélaton l., a l. drawn from the anterior superior iliac spine to the tuberosity of the ischium; normally the greater trochanter lies in this l., but in cases of iliac dislocation of the hip or fracture of the neck of the femur the trochanter is felt above the l. SYN Roser-Nélaton l.

neonatal l., in deciduous teeth, a l. of demarcation between prenatal and postnatal enamel. SYN neonatal ring.

nipple l., SYN mammillary l.

Obersteiner-Redlich l., SYN Obersteiner-Redlich *zone*.

oblique l. [TA], a diagonal, sloping or slanting l.; a l. which is neither parallel nor perpendicular, neither horizontal nor vertical. SEE oblique l. of mandible, oblique l. of thyroid cartilage. SYN linea obliqua [TA].

oblique l. of mandible [TA], the l. on the external surface of the mandible that extends from the mental tubercle to the ramus and separates the alveolar and basilar parts of the bone. SYN linea obliqua mandibulae [TA], external oblique ridge.

oblique l. of thyroid cartilage [TA], a ridge on the outer surface of the thyroid cartilage that gives attachment to the sternothyroid and thyrohyoid muscles. SYN linea obliqua cartilaginis thyroideae [TA].

occipital l., *official alternate term for l. of Gennari.

l. of occlusion, the alignment of the occluding surfaces of the teeth in the horizontal plane. SEE ALSO occlusal *plane*.

Ogston l., a l. drawn from the adductor tubercle of the femur to the intercondylar notch; a guide to resection of the medial condyle for knock-knee.

Ohngren l., a theoretical plane passing between the medial canthus of the eye and the angle of the mandible; used as an arbitrary dividing l. in classifying localized tumors of the maxillary sinus; tumors above the l. invade vital structures early and have a poorer prognosis, whereas those below the l. have a more favorable prognosis.

orbitomeatal l., SEE orbitomeatal *plane*.

Owen l.'s, accentuated incremental l.'s in the dentin thought to be due to disturbances in the mineralization process. SYN contour l.'s of Owen.

paraspinal l., radiographic image of the interface between the lung and paravertebral soft tissues.

parasternal l. [TA], a vertical line equidistant from the sternal and midclavicular lines. SYN linea parasternalis [TA], costoclavicular l.

paravertebral l. [TA], a vertical line corresponding to the tips of the transverse processes of the vertebrae. SYN linea paravertebralis [TA].

Paris l., a unit of microscopic measurement as used in Kölliker's *Mikroskopische Anatomie;* it was equal to 0.0888138 of an inch.

Paton l.'s, SYN striae retinae, under *stria*.

pectinate l. [TA], the l. between the simple columnar epithelium of the rectum and the stratified epithelium of the anal canal, usually defined as being at the level of the anal valves at the bases of the anal columns. SYN linea pectinata canalis analis [TA], dentate l.

pectineal l. of femur [TA], a ridge running down the posterior surface of the shaft of the femur from the lesser trochanter to which the pectineus muscle attaches; continuous superiorly with intertrochanteric line and inferiorly with the medial lip of the linea aspera. SYN linea pectinea femoris [TA].

pectineal l. of pubis, SYN *pecten* pubis.

PICC l., acronym for *p*eripherally *i*nserted *c*entral *c*atheter; a long-term central venous catheter, inserted peripherally.

pleural l.'s, on a chest radiograph, the shadow of the soft tissues between the aerated lung and the bones of the thorax. SYN Correra l., pleural stripe.

l.'s of pleural reflection, lines, usually projected onto the surface of the thoracic wall, indicating the abrupt change in direction of the parietal pleura as it passes from one wall of the pulmonary cavity to another. SEE ALSO vertebral l. of pleural reflection.

pleuroesophageal l., on a frontal chest radiograph, the image of the interface between the right lung and esophagus, the boundary of the azygoesophageal recess.

Poirier l., a l. extending from the nasion to the lambda.

popliteal l., SYN soleal l.

postaxillary l., SYN posterior axillary l.

posterior axillary l. [TA], a vertical line extending inferiorly from the posterior axillary fold. SYN linea axillaris posterior [TA], linea postaxillaris, postaxillary l.

posterior junction l., radiographic image of the mediastinal septum between the upper lobes behind the esophagus, above the aortic arch.

posterior median l. [TA], the line of intersection of the midsagittal plane with the posterior surface of the body. SYN linea mediana posterior [TA].

Poupart l., a vertical l. passing through the center of the inguinal ligament on either side; it marks off the hypochondriac, lumbar, and iliac from the epigastric, umbilical, and hypogastric regions, respectively.

preaxillary l., SYN anterior axillary l.

Reid base l., a l. drawn from the inferior margin of the orbit to the auricular point (center of the orifice of the external acoustic meatus) and extending backward to the center of the occipital bone. Used as the zero plane in computed tomography.

retentive fulcrum l., (1) an imaginary l. connecting the retentive points of clasp arms on retaining teeth adjacent to mucosa-borne denture bases; (2) an imaginary l. connecting the retentive points of clasp arms, around which l. the denture tends to rotate when subjected to forces such as the pull of sticky foods.

l.'s of Retzius, SYN calcification l.'s of Retzius.

Richter-Monro l., SYN Monro-Richter l.

Roser-Nélaton l., SYN Nélaton l.

rough l., SYN *linea* aspera.

sagittal l., any l. parallel to the midline, indicating (occurring within) a sagittal *plane*.

Salter incremental l.'s, transverse l.'s sometimes seen in dentin, due to improper calcification.

S-BP l., a l. connecting the sella with the Bolton point; it indicates the posterior portion of the cranial base in cephalometrics.

scapular l. [TA], a vertical line passing through the inferior angle of the scapula. SYN linea scapularis [TA].

Schreger l.'s, SYN Hunter-Schreger *bands*, under *band*.

semicircular l., SYN arcuate l. of rectus sheath.

semicircular l. of Douglas, a crescent-shaped l. that defines the end of the posterior fascial sheath of the rectus abdominis muscle.

semilunar l., SYN *linea* semilunaris.

septal l.'s, radiographic images of thickened interlobular septa, most often along the lateral border of lung, extending to pleura; Kerley A and B l.'s; usually caused by septal edema and fibrosis, also carcinomatosis.

Sergent white l., SYN white l. (2).

Shenton l., a curved l. formed by the top of the obturator foramen and the inner side of the neck of the femur, seen on an anteroposterior frontal radiograph of a normal hip joint; it is disturbed in lesions of the joint such as dislocation or fracture.

S-N l., a l. connecting a point (S) representing the center of the sella turcica with the frontonasal junction (N); it denotes the anterior portion of the cranial base in cephalometrics.

soleal l. [TA], a ridge that extends obliquely downward and medially across the back of the tibia from the fibular articular facet; it gives origin to the soleus muscle. SYN linea musculi solei [TA], l. for soleus muscle, linea poplitea, popliteal l.

l. for soleus muscle, SYN soleal l.

Spigelius l., SYN *linea* semilunaris.

spiral l., SYN intertrochanteric l.

stabilizing fulcrum l., an imaginary l. connecting occlusal rests, around which l. the denture tends to rotate under masticatory force.

sternal l. [TA], a vertical line corresponding to the lateral margin of the sternum. SYN linea sternalis [TA].

sternal l. of pleural reflection, surface projection of the sharp l. along which the costal part of the parietal pleura becomes continuous with the mediastinal part anteriorly; the right and left sternal l.'s of pleural reflection are parallel to the median plane, posterior to the sternum, at the level of costal cartilages 2–4; at the level of the costal cartilage 4, the left l. turns laterally to parallel the left margin of the sternum, creating a "notch" that is shallower than the cardiac notch of the left lung and an area where the pericardial sac contacts the anterior thoracic wall without intervening pleura sac—significant for pericardiocentesis.

Stocker l., a fine l. of pigment in the corneal epithelium near the head of a pterygium.

subcostal l., a transverse l. transecting the inferiormost border of the thoracic cage, indicating the subcostal *plane*. SEE ALSO subcostal *plane*. SYN linea subcostalis.

superior nuchal l. [TA], the ridge that extends laterally from the external occipital protuberance toward the lateral angle of the occipital bone; it gives attachment to the trapezius, sternocleidomastoid, and splenius capitis muscles. SYN linea nuchae superior [TA].

superior temporal l. of parietal bone [TA], the upper of two curved lines on the parietal bone; the temporal fascia is attached to it. SYN linea temporalis superior ossis parietalis [TA], temporal ridge.

supracrestal l., a transverse l. transecting the high point of both

li

iliac crests, indicating the supracristal *plane*. SEE ALSO supracristal *plane*. SYN linea supracristalis.

survey l., (1) a l. scribed on an abutment tooth of a dental cast by means of a dental surveyor indicating the height of contour of the tooth according to a specific path of insertion; **(2)** a l. which serves as a guide in the proper location of various parts of a clasp assembly for a removable partial denture. SYN clasp guideline, Cummer guideline.

Sydney l., SYN Sydney *crease*.

sylvian l., the l. of the posterior limb of the lateral sulcus (sylvian fissure) of the cerebral cortex.

temporal l., SEE inferior temporal l. of parietal bone, superior temporal l. of parietal bone.

temporal l. of frontal bone [TA], anterior continuation of the inferior temporal line of the temporal bone onto the lateral aspect of the external surface of the frontal bone, demarcating the temporal surface of the bone. SYN linea temporalis ossis frontalis [TA].

tender l.'s, SYN Head l.'s.

tension l.'s [TA], lines that can be extrapolated by connecting linear openings made when a round pin is driven into the skin of a cadaver, resulting from the principal axis of orientation of the subcutaneous connective tissue (collagen) fibers of the dermis; they vary in direction with the region of the body surface. SYN lineae distractionis [TA], cleavage l.'s, Langer l.'s.

terminal l., SYN *linea* terminalis of pelvis.

Topinard l., a l. running between the glabella and the mental point.

tram l.'s, the images of bronchial walls on a plain chest radiograph. When seen distally, indicative of bronchiectasis or chronic bronchitis; usually thickened; colloq., British. SYN radiographic parallel line shadow.

trapezoid l. [TA], the area on the inferior surface of the clavicle near its lateral extremity on which the trapezoid ligament attaches. SYN linea trapezoidea [TA], trapezoid ridge.

Ullmann l., the l. of displacement in spondylolisthesis.

vertebral l. of pleural reflection, approximation of the more gradual reflection of the costal part of the parietal pleura onto the mediastinum posteriorly.

Vesling l., SYN *raphe* of scrotum.

vibrating l., the imaginary l. across the posterior part of the palate, marking the division between the movable and immovable tissues.

l. of vision, SYN visual *axis*.

Wegner l., a narrow, whitish, slightly curved l. representing an area of preliminary calcification at the junction of the epiphysis and diaphysis of a long bone, related to syphilitic epiphysitis.

white l., (1) SYN *linea* alba; **(2)** a pale streak appearing within 30 to 60 seconds after stroking the skin with a fingernail, and lasting for several minutes; regarded as a sign of diminished arterial tension. SYN Sergent white l.

white l. of anal canal, a bluish pink, narrow, wavy zone in the mucosa of the anal canal below the pectinate l. at the level of the interval between the subcutaneous part of the external sphincter and the lower border of the internal sphincter, said to be palpable. SYN Hilton white l.

white l. of Toldt, (1) lateral reflection of posterior parietal pleura of abdomen over the mesentery of the ascending and descending colon. **(2)** junction of parietal peritoneum with Denonvilliers fascia.

Z l., a cross-striation bisecting the I band of striated muscle myofibrils and serving as the anchoring point of actin filaments at either end of the sarcomere. SYN intermediate disk, Z band, Z disk.

l.'s of Zahn, riblike markings seen by the naked eye on the surface of antemortem thrombi; they consist of a branching framework of platelets and fibrin separating the coagulated blood cells. SYN striae of Zahn.

Zöllner l.'s, figures devised to show the possibility of optical illusions; a common one consists of two parallel l.'s which are met by numerous short lines obliquely placed; the parallel lines then seeming to converge or diverge.

LINEA

lin·ea, gen. and pl. **lin·e·ae** (lin′ē-ă, -ē-ē) [TA]. SYN line. [L.]

l. al′ba [TA], a fibrous band running vertically the entire length of the midline of the anterior abdominal wall, receiving the attachments of the oblique and transverse abdominal muscles. SYN Hunter line, white line (1).

l. anorectalis [TA], SYN anocutaneous *line*.

l. arcua′ta [TA], SYN arcuate *line*.

l. arcua′ta os′sis il′ii [TA], SYN arcuate *line* of ilium.

l. arcua′ta vagi′nae mus′culi rec′ti abdom′inis [TA], SYN arcuate *line* of rectus sheath; SEE ALSO rectus *sheath*, posterior *layer* of rectus sheath.

l. as′pera [TA], a rough ridge with two pronounced lips running down the posterior surface of the shaft of the femur; the lateral lip of the linea aspera is a continuation of the gluteal tuberosity, the medial lip of the intertrochanteric line; it affords attachment to the vastus medialis, adductor longus, adductor magnus, adductor brevis, the short head of the biceps, and the vastus lateralis muscles as well as to the intermuscular septa of the thigh. SYN rough line.

lin′eae atroph′icae, SYN *striae* cutis distensae, under *stria*.

l. axilla′ris ante′rior [TA], SYN anterior axillary *line*.

l. axilla′ris me′dia [TA], SYN midaxillary *line*.

l. axilla′ris poste′rior [TA], SYN posterior axillary *line*.

l. cor′neae seni′lis, SYN *arcus* senilis.

lineae distractionis [TA], SYN tension *lines*, under *line*.

l. epiphysia′lis [TA], SYN epiphysial *line*.

l. glu′tea ante′rior, anterior gluteal line. SEE gluteal *lines*, under *line*.

lineae glu′teae [TA], SYN gluteal *lines*, under *line*.

l. glutea inferior, inferior gluteal line. SEE gluteal *lines*, under *line*.

l. glutea posterior, posterior gluteal line. SEE gluteal *lines*, under *line*.

l. intercondyla′ris fem′oris [TA], SYN intercondylar *line* of femur.

l. interme′dia cris′tae ili′acae [TA], SYN intermediate *zone* of iliac crest.

l. interspina′lis, SYN interspinal *line*; SEE ALSO interspinous *plane*.

l. intertrochanter′ica [TA], SYN intertrochanteric *line*.

l. intertubercula′ris, SYN intertubercular *line*; SEE ALSO intertubercular *plane*.

l. mammilla′ris [TA], SYN mammillary *line*.

l. media′na ante′rior [TA], SYN anterior median *line*.

l. media′na poste′rior [TA], SYN posterior median *line*.

l. medio-axilla′ris, SYN midaxillary *line*, midaxillary *line*.

l. medioclavicula′ris [TA], SYN midclavicular *line*.

l. mus′culi sol′ei [TA], SYN soleal *line*.

l. mylohyoi′dea [TA], SYN mylohyoid *line*.

l. ni′gra, the l. alba in pregnancy, which then becomes pigmented. SYN black line.

l. nu′chae infe′rior [TA], SYN inferior nuchal *line*.

l. nu′chae media′na, SYN external occipital *crest*.

l. nu′chae supe′rior [TA], SYN superior nuchal *line*.

l. nu′chae supre′ma [TA], SYN highest nuchal *line*.

l. obli′qua [TA], SYN oblique *line*.

l. obliqua cartilag′inis thyroi′deae [TA], SYN oblique *line* of thyroid cartilage.

l. obliqua mandib′ulae [TA], SYN oblique *line* of mandible.

l. parasterna′lis [TA], SYN parasternal *line*.

l. paravertebra′lis [TA], SYN paravertebral *line.*

l. pectinata canalis analis [TA], SYN pectinate *line.*

l. pecti′nea femoris [TA], SYN pectineal *line* of femur.

l. poplit′ea, SYN soleal *line.*

l. postaxilla′ris, SYN posterior axillary *line,* posterior axillary *line.*

l. preaxilla′ris, SYN anterior axillary *line,* anterior axillary *line.*

l. scapula′ris [TA], SYN scapular *line.*

l. semicircula′ris, SYN arcuate *line* of rectus sheath.

l. semiluna′ris [TA], the slight groove in the external abdominal wall parallel to the lateral edge of the rectus sheath. SYN semilunar line, Spigelius line.

l. spira′lis, SYN intertrochanteric *line.*

l. splen′dens, a thickened band of pia mater along the midline of the anterior surface of the spinal cord. SYN Haller line.

l. sterna′lis [TA], SYN sternal *line.*

l. subcosta′lis, SYN subcostal *line;* SEE ALSO subcostal *plane.*

l. supracrista′lis, SYN supracrestal *line;* SEE ALSO supracrestal *plane.*

l. tempora′lis infe′rior ossis parietalis [TA], SYN inferior temporal *line* of parietal bone.

l. temporalis ossis frontalis [TA], SYN temporal *line* of frontal bone.

l. tempora′lis supe′rior ossis parietalis [TA], SYN superior temporal *line* of parietal bone.

l. termina′lis of pelvis [TA], an oblique ridge on the inner surface of the ilium and continued on the pubis, which forms the lower boundary of the iliac fossa; it separates the true from the false pelvis. SYN l. terminalis pelvis [TA], iliopectineal line, terminal line.

l. terminalis pelvis [TA], SYN l. terminalis of pelvis.

lineae transver′sae ossis sacri [TA], SYN transverse *ridges* of sacrum, under *ridge.*

l. trapezoi′dea [TA], SYN trapezoid *line.*

---

lin·e·age (lĭn′aj, lĭn′ē-āj). Descent in a line from a common progenitor or source. [O. Fr. *ligne,* line of descent]

lin·e·ar (lĭn′ē-ăr). Pertaining to or resembling a line.

linearity (lin-ē-ar′ĭ-tē). A relationship between two quantities whereby a change in one causes a directly proportional change in the other. [L. *linearis,* linear, fr. *linea,* line]

line·breed·ing. Practice of successive inbreeding of closely related individuals with the object of concentrating desirable or scientifically interesting genetic characteristics of some individual or group.

li·ner (lī′ner). A layer of protective material.

asbestos l., a layer of asbestos used to line a dental casting ring so that during the heating and expansion of the investment the compression of the l. will free the investment from the restraint of the ring.

cavity l., SYN varnish (dental).

LINES Abbreviation for long interspersed *elements,* under *element.*

Lineweaver, Hans, U.S. physical chemist, *1907. SEE L.-Burk *equation, plot.*

Ling, Per Henrik, Swedish hygienist, 1776–1839. SEE L. *method.*

Lin·gel·sheim·ia (lin′jels-hii′mē-ă). SYN *Acinetobacter.* [W. von Lingelsheim]

L. anitra′ta, SYN *Acinetobacter calcoaceticus.*

lin·gua, gen. and pl. **lin·guae** (ling′gwă, ling′gwē). 1. SYN tongue (1). 2. SYN tongue (2). [L. tongue]

l. cerebel′li, SYN *lingula* of cerebellum.

l. fissura′ta, SYN fissured *tongue.*

l. frena′ta, a tongue with a very short frenum constituting tongue-tie.

l. geograph′ica,

l. ni′gra, SYN black *tongue.*

l. plica′ta, SYN fissured *tongue.*

lin·gual (ling′gwăl). 1. Relating to the tongue or any tonguelike part. SYN glossal. 2. Next to or toward the tongue.

Lin·guat·u·la (ling-gwat′ū-lă). A genus of endoparasitic blood-sucking arthropods (family Linguatulidae, class Pentastomida), commonly known as tongue worms; once thought to be degenerate Acarina, but now generally considered to be a small but distinctive early offshoot of the Arthropoda. Adult worms are found in lungs or air passages of various hosts (e.g., reptiles, birds, carnivores); young worms are found in a great variety of hosts, including humans, but chiefly in animals that serve as prey. [L. *linguatu,* tongued, + -*ula,* dim. suffix]

L. rhina′ria, SYN *L. serrata.*

L. serra′ta, a species most common in Europe, but also found in the United States, South America, and probably elsewhere; the adult is a whitish, soft, flattened, annulated worm equipped with hooks by which it attaches itself to the nasal mucosa of dogs and other canids; the larvae develop in the liver and lymph nodes of rodents, swine, cattle, and sometimes humans and other primates. SYN *L. rhinaria.*

lin·guat·u·li·a·sis (ling-gwat-ū-lī′ă-sis). Infection with *Linguatula.* SEE ALSO halzoun.

Lin·gua·tu·li·dae (ling-gwat′ū-li-dē). One of the families of Pentastomida of medical interest, the other being the Porocephalidae. L. have flattened bodies; adults inhabit the nasal cavities of various carnivores, such as the dog and cat, and larval forms are found in tissues of rodents, herbivores, and other animals; both larvae and adults have been reported from humans.

lin·gui·form (ling′gwi-fōrm). Tongue-shaped.

lin·gu·la, pl. **lin·gu·lae** (ling′gū-lă, -lē) [TA]. 1. A term applied to several tongue-shaped processes. 2. When not qualified, the l. of cerebellum. [L. dim. of *lingua,* tongue]

l. cerebel′li [TA], SYN l. of cerebellum.

l. of cerebellum [TA], a tongue-shaped sequence of flattened cerebellar folia forming the anterior (or superior) extreme of the cerebellar vermis, extending forward on the surface of the superior medullary velum between the two emerging superior cerebellar peduncles. SYN l. cerebelli [TA], alae lingulae cerebelli, lingua cerebelli, tongue of cerebellum.

l. of left lung [TA], an inferomedial projection from the anterior aspect of the upper lobe of the left lung which bounds the cardiac notch inferiorly. SYN l. pulmonis sinistri [TA].

l. of mandible [TA], a pointed tongue of bone overlapping the mandibular foramen, giving attachment to the sphenomandibular ligament. SYN l. mandibulae [TA], mandibular tongue, Spix spine.

l. mandib′ulae [TA], SYN l. of mandible.

l. pulmo′nis sinis′tri [TA], SYN l. of left lung.

sphenoidal l. [TA], a slender process projecting posteriorly between the body and greater wing of the sphenoid bone, on either side, forming the lateral margin of the carotid groove. In the dry skull, it projects into the foramen lacerum. SYN l. sphenoidalis [TA].

l. sphenoida′lis [TA], SYN sphenoidal l.

lin·gu·lar (ling′gū-lăr). Pertaining to any lingula.

lin·gu·lec·to·my (ling′gū-lek′tō-mē). Excision of the lingular portion of the left upper lobe of the lung.

linguo-. The tongue. [L. *lingua*]

lin·guo·cli·na·tion (ling′gwō-kli-nā′shŭn). Axial inclination of a tooth when the crown is inclined toward the tongue more than is normal.

lin·guo·clu·sion (ling-gwō-kloo′zhŭn). Displacement of a tooth toward the interior of the dental arch, or toward the tongue. SEE ALSO lingual *occlusion* (2). SYN lingual occlusion (1).

lin·guo·dis·tal (ling-gwō-dis′tăl). Relating to the lingual and distal part of the tooth, e.g., the l. cusp. SEE ALSO distolingual.

lin·guo·gin·gi·val (ling-gwō-jin′ji-văl). 1. Relating to the gingival third of the lingual surface of a tooth. 2. Relating to the angle or point of junction of the lingual border and gingival line on the distal or mesial surface of an incisor tooth.

lin·guo·oc·clu·sal (ling′gwō-ŏ-kloo′săl). Relating to the line of junction of the lingual and occlusal surfaces of a tooth.

lin·guo·pap·il·li·tis (ling′gwō-pap′i-lī′tis). Small painful ulcers involving the papillae on the tongue margins.

lin·guo·plate (ling′gwō-plāt). A partial denture major connector formed as a lingual bar extended to cover the cingula of the lower anterior teeth. SYN lingual plate.

lin·guo·ver·sion (ling′gwō-ver-zhŭn). Malposition of a tooth lingual to the normal position.

lin·i·ment (lin′i-ment). A liquid preparation for external application or application to the gums; they may be clear dispersions, suspensions, or emulsions, and are frequently applied by friction to the skin; used as counterirritants, rubefacients, anodynes, or cleansing agents. [L., fr. *lino,* to smear]

li·nin (lī′nin). 1. A bitter glycoside obtained from *Linum catharticum* (family Linaceae). 2. A protein in linseed. 3. Obsolete term for the threadlike, nonstaining (achromatic) substance of the cell nucleus, on which chromatin granules were thought to be suspended. [L. *linum,* fr. G. *linon,* flax]

lin·ing (līn′ing). A coating applied to the pulpal wall(s) of a restorative dental preparation to protect the pulp from thermal or chemical irritation; usually a vehicle containing a varnish, resin, and/or calcium hydroxide.

li·ni·tis (li-nī′tis, lī-nī′tis). Inflammation of cellular tissue, specifically of the perivascular tissue of the stomach. [G. *linon,* flax, linen cloth, + *-itis,* inflammation]

l. plas′ti·ca, originally believed to be an inflammatory condition, but now recognized to be due to infiltrating scirrhous carcinoma causing extensive thickening of the wall of the stomach; often called leather-bottle stomach.

link. A connection; bond.

tip l.'s, connections between the stereocilia of auditory and vestibular hair cells.

link·age (lingk′ij). 1. A chemical covalent bond. 2. The relationship between syntenic loci sufficiently close that the respective alleles are not inherited independently by the offspring; a characteristic of loci, not genes.

genetic l., SEE linkage (2).

medical record l., the assemblage of lifetime or long-term individual medical histories from vital and medical data derived from multiple sources.

record l., a method of assembling the information contained in two or more sets of medical records, or a set of medical records and vital records such as birth or death certificates, and a procedure to ensure that each individual's records are counted only once; facilitated by a unique numbering system such as the Hogben number or soundex code to identify individuals with precision.

sex l., inheritance of a trait or a sex chromosome or gonosome. A man receives all his sex-linked genes from his mother and transmits them all to his daughters but not to his sons; a recessive sex-linked character is much more likely to be expressed in the male. SEE ALSO sex *chromosomes,* under *chromosome.*

linked. Said of two genetic loci that exhibit genetic linkage.

link·er. A fragment of synthetic DNA containing a restriction site that may be used for splicing genes.

link·er scan·ning. A type of deletion mutagenesis where the distance and/or reading frame between potentially important regions is maintained by replacement with a synthetic oligonucleotide of known sequence.

Linné, Carl von, Swedish botanist and physician, 1707-1778. SEE linnaean *system* of nomenclature.

Li·nog·na·thus (li-nog′nă-thŭs). A genus of sucking lice (order Anoplura, family Linognathidae) that includes the species *L. africanus,* the African blue louse of sheep and goats; *L. ovillus,* the sheep body louse; *L. pedalis,* the foot louse of sheep; *L. setosus,* the sucking louse of the dog and other canids; *L. stenopsis,* the sucking louse of goats; and *L. vituli,* the "long-nosed" sucking louse, ox louse, or blue louse of cattle. [G. *linon,* flax, thread, + *gnathos,* jaw]

li·no·le·ate (li-nō′lē-āt). Salt of linoleic acid.

lin·o·le·ic ac·id (lin-ō-lē′ik). 9,12-Octadecadienoic acid; a doubly unsaturated fatty acid, occurring widely in plant glycerides, that is essential in nutrition in mammals. SYN linolic acid. [L. *linum,* flax, + *oleum,* oil]

lin·o·len·ic ac·id (lin-ō-len′ik). 9,12,15-Octadecatrienoic acid

(also referred to as α-l); an unsaturated fatty acid that is essential in the nutrition of mammals. γ-L. a. is 6,9,12-octadecatrienoic acid.

linolic acid. SYN linoleic acid.

lin·seed (lin′sēd). The dried ripe seed of *Linum usitatissimum* (family Linaceae), flax, the fiber of which is used in the manufacture of linen; an infusion was used as a demulcent in catarrhal affections of the respiratory and urogenital tracts, and the ground seeds are used in making poultices. SYN flaxseed. [G. *linon,* flax]

l. oil, a fatty oil expressed from the ripe seeds of *Linum usitatissimum;* used in the preparation of lime liniment. SYN flaxseed oil.

lint. A soft, absorbent material rarely used in surgical dressings, usually in the form of a thick, loosely woven material (sheet or patent l.). [O.E. *lin,* flax]

△**lio-.** SEE leio-.

LIP Acronym for lymphocytic interstitial pneumonia or lymphoid interstitial pneumonia. SEE lymphocytic interstitial *pneumonia.*

lip [TA]. 1. One of the two muscular folds with an outer membrane having a stratified squamous cell epithelial surface layer that bound the mouth anteriorly. 2. Any liplike structure bounding a cavity or groove. SEE ALSO labium, labrum. SYN labium (1) [TA]. [A.S. *lippa*]

acetabular l., SYN acetabular *labrum.*

anterior l. of external os of uterus [TA], the portion of the vaginal part of the uterine cervix that bounds the ostium anteriorly intervening between the ostium and the anterior vaginal fornix. It is slightly shorter than the posterior lip. SYN labium anterius ostii uteri [TA], anterior l. of uterine os.

anterior l. of uterine os, SYN anterior l. of external os of uterus.

articular l., SYN labrum (3).

cleft l., a congenital facial abnormality of the l. (usually of the upper l.) resulting from failure of union of the medial and lateral nasal prominences and maxillary process; frequently but not necessarily associated with cleft alveolus and cleft palate. In many families and in various forms [MIM*119300, *119500, *119530, *119540, and *119550] there seems to be autosomal dominant inheritance; likewise for X-linked inheritance [MIM*303400]. But generally, as with the supposed autosomal recessive forms, the genetics is more confusing and may represent a variable feature of a syndrome. SYN harelip.

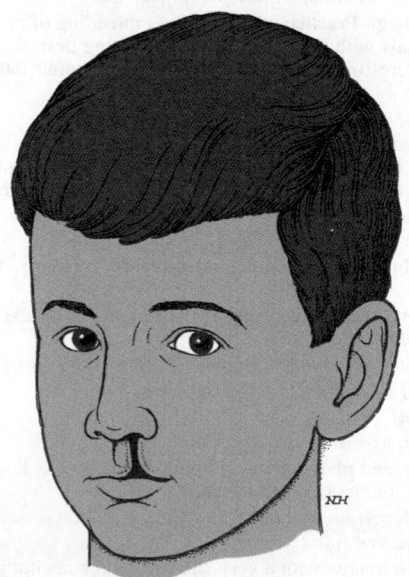

cleft lip

double l., congenital or acquired excess tissue on the inner mucosal aspect of the l.; may be a manifestation of Ascher syndrome.

external l. of iliac crest, SYN outer l. of iliac crest.

glenoidal l., SYN glenoid *labrum* of scapula.

Hapsburg l., SEE Hapsburg *jaw.*

inner l. of iliac crest [TA], the roughened inner margin of the crest that gives attachment to parts of the transversus abdominis, quadratus lumborum, and erector spinae muscles. SYN labium internum cristae iliacae [TA], internal l. of iliac crest.

internal l. of iliac crest, SYN inner l. of iliac crest.

large pudendal l., SYN *labium* majus.

lateral l. of linea aspera [TA], the lateral margin of the linea aspera of the femur that gives attachment to the lateral intermuscular septum and the short head of the biceps femoris muscles. SYN labium laterale lineae asperae [TA].

lower l. [TA], the muscular fold bounding the opening of the mouth inferiorly. SYN labium inferius oris [TA].

medial l. of linea aspera [TA], the medial margin of the linea aspera of the femur that provides attachment for part of the vastus medialis muscle. SYN labium mediale lineae asperae [TA].

l.'s of mouth [TA], fleshy folds with skin externally and oral mucosa internally that surround the oval fissure and form the anterior walls of the oral vestibule; with the enclosed orbicularis oris and various dilator muscles, the lips constitute the cranial sphincter of the alimentary tract. SYN labia oris [TA].

outer l. of iliac crest [TA], the roughened outer margin of the crest that gives attachment to the external oblique and latissimus dorsi muscles above and to the fascia lata and the tensor fasciae latae muscle below. SYN labium externum cristae iliacae [TA], external l. of iliac crest.

posterior l. of external os of uterus [TA], the portion of the uterine cervix that bounds the ostium posteriorly. It is slightly longer than the anterior lip, intervening between the cervical canal and the posterior fornix of the vagina. SYN labium posterius ostii uteri [TA].

rhombic l., the thickened alar plate of the embryonic rhombencephalon.

small pudendal l., SYN *labium* minus.

tympanic l. of limbus of spiral lamina, SYN tympanic l. of spiral limbus.

tympanic l. of spiral limbus [TA], the lower, long periosteal extension of the limbus laminae spiralis osseae that rests on the basilar lamina of the spiral organ (of Corti). SYN labium limbi tympanicum limbi spiralis ossei [TA], labium limbi tympanicum laminae spiralis ossei, tympanic labium of limbus of spiral lamina, tympanic l. of limbus of spiral lamina.

upper l. [TA], the muscular fold forming the superior border of the mouth. SYN labium superius oris [TA].

vestibular l. of limbus of spiral lamina, SYN vestibular l. of spiral limbus.

vestibular l. of spiral limbus [TA], the upper, short periosteal extension of the limbus laminae spiralis osseae which provides the central attachment for the tectorial membrane. SYN labium limbi vestibulare limbi spiralis ossei [TA], labium limbi vestibulare laminae spiralis ossei, lamina dentata, vestibular labium of limbus of spiral lamina, vestibular l. of limbus of spiral lamina.

△**lip-.** SEE lipo-.

li·pan·cre·a·tin (li-pan′krē-ă-tin, -krē′ă-tin). SYN pancrelipase.

lip·a·ro·cele (lip′ă-rō-sēl). An omental hernia. [G. *liparos,* fatty, + *kēlē,* tumor, hernia]

li·pase (lip′ās). 1. In general, any fat-splitting or lipolytic enzyme; a carboxylesterase; e.g., triacylglycerol lipase, phospholipase A_2, lipoprotein lipase. 2. SYN *triacylglycerol* lipase.

lip·ec·to·my (lip-ek′tō-mē). Surgical removal of fatty tissue, as in cases of adiposity. [lipo- + G. *ektomē,* excision]

lip·e·de·ma (lip′e-dē′mă). Chronic swelling, usually of the lower extremities, particularly in middle-aged women, caused by the widespread even distribution of subcutaneous fat and fluid. [lipo- + G. *oidēma,* swelling]

li·pe·mia (lip-ē′mē-ă). The presence of an abnormally high concentration of lipids in the circulating blood. SYN hyperlipidemia, hyperlipoidemia, lipidemia, lipoidemia. [lipid + G. *haima,* blood]

alimentary l., relatively transient l. occurring after the ingestion of foods with a large content of fat. SYN postprandial l.

diabetic l., development of lactescent plasma upon ingestion of dietary lipids; a rare manifestation of uncontrolled diabetes mellitus caused by defective metabolism of dietary lipids and abolished by the administration of insulin.

postprandial l., SYN alimentary l.

l. retina′lis, a creamy appearance of the retinal blood vessels that occurs when the lipids of the blood exceed 5%.

li·pe·mic (li-pē′mik). Relating to lipemia.

lip·id (lip′id). "Fat-soluble," an operational term describing a solubility characteristic, not a chemical substance, i.e., denoting substances extracted from animal or vegetable cells by nonpolar solvents; included in the heterogeneous collection of materials thus extractable are fatty acids, glycerides and glyceryl ethers, phospholipids, sphingolipids, long-chain alcohols and waxes, terpenes, steroids, and "fat-soluble" vitamins such as A, D, and E. [G. *lipos,* fat]

l. A, the glycolipid component of lipopolysaccharide responsible for its endotoxic activity.

anisotropic l., a l. in the form of doubly refractive droplets.

anular l., the layer(s) of l. bound to and/or surrounding an integral membrane protein.

brain l., impure cephalin possessing marked hemostatic action when locally applied.

compound l.'s, l. that can be hydrolyzed under alkali conditions to generate smaller constituents.

isotropic l., a l. occurring in the form of singly refractive droplets.

simple l.'s, SYN homolipids.

lip·i·de·mia (lip′i-dē′mē-ă). SYN lipemia.

lip·i·do·ly·tic (lip′ĭ-dō-lit′ik). Causing breakdown of lipid. [lipid + G. *lysis,* loosening]

lip·i·do·sis, pl. **lip·i·do·ses** (lip-i-dō′sis, -sēz). Hereditary abnormality of lipid metabolism that results in abnormal amounts of lipid deposition; classification is typically based on the responsible enzymatic deficiency and type of lipid involved. Such enzymatic activity takes place in the lysosomes, and the abnormal products appear as lysosomal storage diseases. Sphingolipidoses make up the largest portion of recognized lipidoses, including abnormal metabolism of gangliosides, ceramides, and cerebrosides. [lipid + G. *-ōsis,* condition]

ceramide lactoside l., an inherited disorder associated with an accumulation of ceramide lactoside due to a deficiency of ceramide lactosidase; results in progressive brain damage with liver and spleen enlargement.

cerebral l., SYN cerebral *sphingolipidosis.*

cerebroside l., SYN Gaucher *disease.*

ganglioside l., SYN gangliosidosis.

glycolipid l., SYN Fabry *disease.*

sphingomyelin l., SYN Niemann-Pick *disease.*

sulfatide l., SYN metachromatic *leukodystrophy.*

Lipmann, Fritz A., German-U.S. biochemist in the U.S. and Nobel laureate, 1899–1986. SEE Warburg-L.-Dickens-Horecker *shunt.*

△**lipo-, lip-.** Fatty, lipid. [G. *lipos,* fat]

lip·o·am·ide (lip-ō-am′īd, -am′id). SEE lipoic acid.

lip·o·am·ide de·hy·dro·gen·ase. SYN dihydrolipoamide dehydrogenase.

lip·o·am·ide di·sul·fide. Oxidized lipoic acid in amide combination with the ε-amino group of an L-lysyl residue of pyruvic acid dehydrogenase.

lip·o·am·ide re·duc·tase (NADH). SYN dihydrolipoamide dehydrogenase.

lip·o·ar·thri·tis (lip′ō-ar-thrī′tis). Inflammation of the periarticular fatty tissues of the knee. [lipo- + arthritis]

lip·o·ate (lip′ō-āt). A salt or ester of lipoic acid.

lip·o·ate ace·tyl·trans·fer·ase. SYN dihydrolipoamide S-acetyltransferase.

lip·o·a·tro·phia (lip′ō-ă-trō′fē-ă). SYN lipoatrophy.

l. annula′ris, a rare condition of unknown cause characterized by localized panatrophy, a depressed area encircling the arm with sclerosis and atrophy of fat.

li

l. circumscrip′ta, localized fat atrophy.

lip·o·at·ro·phy (lip-ō-at′rō-fē). Loss of subcutaneous fat, which may be total, congenital, and associated with hepatomegaly, excessive bone growth, and insulin-resistant diabetes. SYN Lawrence-Seip syndrome, lipoatrophia, lipoatrophic diabetes. [G. *lipos,* fat, + *a-,* priv. + *trophē,* nourishment]

insulin l., SYN insulin *lipodystrophy.*

partial l., SYN progressive *lipodystrophy.*

lip·o·blast (lip′ō-blast). An embryonic fat cell. [lipo- + G. *blastos,* germ]

lip·o·blas·to·ma (lip′ō-blas-tō′mă). A benign subcutaneous tumor composed of embryonal fat cells separated into distinct lobules, occurring usually in infants.

lip·o·blas·to·ma·to·sis (lip′ō-blas-tō-mă-tō′sis). A diffuse form of lipoblastoma that infiltrates locally but does not metastasize.

lip·o·car·di·ac (lip′ō-kar′dē-ak). **1.** Relating to fatty heart. **2.** Denoting a person suffering from fatty degeneration of the heart. [lipo- + G. *kardia,* heart]

lip·o·cat·a·bol·ic (lip′ō-kat-ă-bol′ik). Relating to the breakdown (catabolism) of fat.

lip·o·cer·a·tous (lip-ō-ser′ă-tŭs). SYN adipoceratous.

lip·o·cere (lip′ō-sēr). SYN adipocere. [lipo- + L. *cera,* wax]

lip·o·chon·dria (lip′ō-kon′drē-ă). Temporary storage vacuoles of lipids found in the Golgi apparatus. SEE ALSO phytosterolemia. [lipo- + mitochondria]

lip·o·chon·dro·dys·tro·phy (lip′ō-kon-drō-dis′trō-fē). SYN Hurler *syndrome.*

lip·o·chrome (lip′ō-krōm). **1.** A pigmented lipid, e.g., lutein, carotene. SYN chromolipid. **2.** A term sometimes used to designate the wear-and-tear pigments, e.g., lipofuscin, hemofuscin, ceroid. More precisely, l.'s are yellow pigments that seem to be identical to carotene and xanthophyll and are frequently found in the serum, skin, adrenal cortex, corpus luteum, and arteriosclerotic plaques, as well as in the liver, spleen, and adipose tissue; l.'s do not stain with the ordinary dyes for fat. **3.** The pigment produced by certain bacteria. [lipo- + G. *chroma,* color]

li·poc·la·sis (li-pok′lă-sis). SYN lipolysis. [lipo- + G. *klasis,* a breaking]

lip·o·clas·tic (lip-ō-klas′tik). SYN lipolytic.

lip·o·crit (lip′ō-krit). An apparatus and procedure for separating and volumetrically analyzing the amount of lipid in blood or other body fluid. [lipo- + G. *krinō,* to separate]

lip·o·cyte (lip′ō-sīt). SYN fat-storing *cell.* [lipo- + G. *kytos,* cell]

lip·o·der·moid (lip-ō-der′moyd). Congenital, yellowish-white, fatty, benign tumor located subconjunctivally. [lipo- + dermoid]

lip·o·di·er·e·sis (lip′ō-dī-er′ĕ-sis). SYN lipolysis. [lipo- + G. *diairesis,* division]

lip·o·dys·tro·phia (lip′ō-dis-trō′fē-ă). SYN lipodystrophy.

l. progessi′va supe′rior, SYN progressive *lipodystrophy.*

lip·o·dys·tro·phy (lip-ō-dis′trō-fē). Defective metabolism of fat. SYN lipodystrophia. [lipo- + G. *dys-,* bad, difficult, + *trophē,* nourishment]

congenital total l. [MIM*269700], characterized by almost complete lack of subcutaneous fat, accelerated rate of growth and skeletal development during the first 3–4 years of life, muscular hypertrophy, cardiac enlargement, hepatosplenomegaly, acanthosis nigricans, hypertrichosis, renal enlargement, hypertriglyceridemia, and hypermetabolism; autosomal recessive inheritance. SYN Berardinelli syndrome, Seip syndrome.

familial partial l. [MIM*151660], characterized by symmetric lipoatrophy of the trunk and limbs but the face is spared; with full rounded face, xanthomata, acanthosis nigricans, and insulin-resistant hyperglycemia; there is accumulation of fat around the neck and shoulders and genitalia. SYN Kobberling-Dunnigan syndrome.

insulin l., dystrophic atrophy of subcutaneous tissues in diabetics at the site of frequent injections of insulin. SYN insulin lipoatrophy.

membranous l., a rare metabolic disease in which bone marrow fat cells are transformed into thick convoluted PAS-staining membranes enclosing weakly osmophilic material; leads to pro-

gressive cystic resorption of limb bones and dementia with sudanophilic leukodystrophy.

progressive l., a condition characterized by a complete loss of the subcutaneous fat of the upper part of the torso, the arms, neck, and face, sometimes with an increase of fat in the tissues about and below the pelvis. SYN Barraquer disease, lipodystrophia progessiva superior, partial lipoatrophy, Simons disease.

lip·o·e·de·ma (lip′ō-e-dē′mă). Edema of subcutaneous fat, causing painful swellings, especially of the legs in women. SYN cellulite (2).

lip·o·fec·tin (lĭp′ō-fek′tin). A mixture predominantly of phospholipids used for aiding in the transfer of DNA into cells.

lip·o·fec·tion (lĭp′ō-fek′shŭn). The process of injecting a lipid-complexed or contained DNA into eucaryotic cells. [lipo- + trans-*fection*]

li·pof·er·ous (lip-of′er-ŭs). Transporting fat. [lipo- + L. *fero,* to carry]

lip·o·fi·bro·ma (lip′ō-fī-brō′mă). A benign neoplasm of fibrous connective tissue, with conspicuous numbers of adipose cells.

lip·o·fus·cin (lip-ō-fūs′in). Brown pigment granules representing lipid-containing residues of lysosomal digestion and considered one of the aging or "wear and tear" pigments; found in liver, kidney, heart muscle, adrenal, and ganglion cells.

lip·o·fus·ci·no·sis (lip′ō-fūs-i-nō′sis). Abnormal storage of any one of a group of fatty pigments.

ceroid l., SYN Batten *disease.*

neuronal ceroid l., a group of diseases characterized by accumulation of abnormal pigments in tissue (previously classified as cerebral sphingolipidoses). Major subtypes include chronic juvenile form (Batten disease), slowly progressive behavior and visual symptoms, autosomal recessive inheritance; acute, late infantile form (Bielschowsky disease); autosomal recessive inheritance; chronic adult form (Kufs disease), variable inheritance; acute infantile form (Santavuori-Haltia disease), fulminating motor and mental deterioration often associated with myoclonic seizures. Minor forms have also been described.

lip·o·gen·e·sis (lip-ō-jen′ĕ-sis). The production of fat, either fatty degeneration or fatty infiltration; also applied to the normal deposition of fat or to the conversion of carbohydrate or protein to fat. SYN adipogenesis. [lipo- + G. *genesis,* production]

lip·o·gen·ic (lip-ō-jen′ik). Relating to lipogenesis. SYN adipogenic, adipogenous, lipogenous.

li·pog·e·nous (li-poj′ĕ-nŭs). SYN lipogenic.

lip·o·gran·u·lo·ma (lip′ō-gran-ū-lō′mă). A nodule or focus of granulomatous inflammation (usually of the foreign-body type) in association with lipid material deposited in tissues, e.g., after the injection of certain oils. SEE ALSO paraffinoma. SYN eleoma, oil tumor, oleogranuloma, oleoma.

lip·o·gran·u·lo·ma·to·sis (lip′ō-gran′ū-lō-mă-tō′sis). **1.** Presence of lipogranulomas. **2.** Local inflammatory reaction to necrosis of adipose tissue.

disseminated l., a form of mucolipodosis, developing soon after birth because of deficiency of ceramidase; characterized by swollen joints, subcutaneous nodules, lymphadenopathy, and accumulation in lysosomes of affected cells of PAS-positive lipid consisting of ceramide. SYN Farber disease, Farber syndrome.

lip·o·he·mia (lip-ō-hē′mē-ă). Obsolete term for lipemia.

li·po·ic ac·id (li-pō′ik). Functions as the amide (lipoamide) in the disulfide (–S–S–) form in the transfer of "active aldehyde" (acetyl), the two-carbon fragment resulting from decarboxylation of pyruvate from α-hydroxyethylthiamin pyrophosphate to acetyl-CoA, itself being reduced to the dithiol form (i.e., dihydrolipoic acid) in the process; present in yeast and liver extracts, and may be useful in the treatment of mushroom poisoning. L. a. is also an essential component of other α-keto acid dehydrogenase complexes. SYN acetate replacement factor, ovoprotogen, protogen, protogen A, pyruvate oxidation factor, thioctic acid.

lip·oid (lip′oyd). **1.** Resembling fat. **2.** Former term for lipid. SYN adipoid. [lipo- + G. *eidos,* appearance]

lip·oi·de·mia (lip-oy-dē′mē-ă). SYN lipemia.

lip·oi·do·sis (lip-oy-do'sis). Presence of anisotropic lipoids in the cells.

cerebroside l. (ser-ē'brō-sīd), a group of lysosomal storage diseases characterized by accumulation of lipid in cells of affected tissue and commonly accompanied by a manifest derangement of central nervous system development; e.g., Gaucher *disease* and Krabbe *disease*.

l. cor'neae, SYN *arcus* senilis.

l. cu'tis et muco'sae, SYN lipoid *proteinosis*.

galactosylceramide l., SYN globoid cell *leukodystrophy*.

lip·o·in·jec·tion (lip-ō-in-jek'shun). Augmentation of tissue with fat cells after atrophy, as in vocal cord paralysis or scarring.

lip·o·lip·oi·do·sis (lip'ō-lip-oy-dō'sis). Fatty infiltration, both neutral fats and anisotropic lipoids being present in the cells. SEE ALSO liposis (2).

li·pol·y·sis (li-pol'i-sis). The splitting up (hydrolysis), or chemical decomposition, of fat. SYN lipoclasis, lipodieresis. [lipo- + G. *lysis*, dissolution]

lip·o·lyt·ic (lip-ō-lit'ik). Relating to or causing lipolysis. SYN lipoclastic.

li·po·ma (li-pō'mă). A benign neoplasm of adipose tissue, composed of mature fat cells. SYN adipose tumor. [lipo- + G. *-oma*, tumor]

l. annula're col'li, an encircling growth of l. (or coalescent l.'s) in the neck, resulting in a collar-like enlargement. SEE ALSO Madelung *neck*.

l. arbores'cens, an irregularly shaped l. involving the synovial membrane of a joint, resulting in fingerlike or treelike hyperplastic folds in the villi.

atypical l., l., occurring primarily in older men on the posterior neck, shoulders, and back, which is benign but microscopically atypical, containing giant cells with multiple overlapping nuclei forming a circle. SYN pleomorphic l.

l. capsula're, a well-circumscribed mass resulting from a greatly increased amount of adipose tissue adjacent to the breast.

l. caverno'sum, SYN angiolipoma.

l. fibro'sum, SYN fibrolipoma.

l. myxomatodes, SYN myxolipoma.

l. ossif'icans, a l. in which metaplasia occurs and small foci of bone are formed.

l. petri'ficans, a l. in which degeneration and necrosis results in a considerable amount of dystrophic calcification.

pleomorphic l., SYN atypical l.

spindle cell l., a microscopically distinctive benign form of l. in which adipose tissue is infiltrated by fibroblasts and collagen; usually found in the shoulder or neck of elderly men.

telangiectatic l., SYN angiolipoma.

li·po·ma·toid (li-pō'mă-toyd). Resembling a lipoma, frequently said of accumulations of adipose tissue that is not thought to be neoplastic.

lip·o·ma·to·sis (lip'ō-mă-tō'sis). SYN adiposis.

encephalocraniocutaneous l., a rare syndrome of multiple fibrolipomas or angiofibromas of the face, scalp, and neck present at birth, sometimes with symptomatic intracranial lipomas.

mediastinal l., increased mediastinal fat caused by taking steroids.

multiple symmetric l., accumulation and progressive enlargement of collections of adipose tissue in the subcutaneous tissue of the head, neck, upper trunk, and upper portions of the upper extremities; seen primarily in adult males and of unknown cause. SYN Launois-Bensaude syndrome, Madelung disease, symmetric adenolipomatosis.

l. neurot'ica, SYN *adiposis* dolorosa.

li·po·ma·tous (li-pō'mă-tŭs). Pertaining to or manifesting the features of lipoma, or characterized by the presence of a lipoma (or lipomas).

lip·o·me·nin·go·cele (lip'ō-mě-ning'gō-sēl). An intraspinal cauda equinal lipoma associated with a spina bifida. [lipo- + G. *mēninx*, membrane, + *kēlē*, tumor]

lip·o·mu·co·pol·y·sac·cha·ri·do·sis (lip'ō-mū"ko-pol-ē-sak'ă-ri-dō'sis). SYN *mucolipidosis* I.

lip·o·nu·cle·o·pro·teins (lip'ō-noo'klē-ō-prō'tēnz). Associations or complexes containing lipids, nucleic acids, and proteins.

Lip·o·nys·sus (lip-ō-nis'ŭs). Former name for *Ornithonyssus*. [lipo- + G. *nyssō*, to prick]

lip·o·pe·nia (lip-ō-pē'nē-ă). An abnormally small amount, or a deficiency, of lipids in the body. [lipo- + G. *penia*, poverty]

lip·o·pe·nic (lip-ō-pē'nik). **1.** Relating to or characterized by lipopenia. **2.** An agent or drug that produces a reduction in the concentration of lipids in the blood.

lip·o·pep·tid, lip·o·pep·tide (lip-ō-pep'tid, lip-ō-pep'tīd). A compound or complex of lipid and amino acids.

lip·o·phage (lip'ō-fāj). A cell that ingests fat. [G. *lipos*, fat, + *phagō*, to eat]

lip·o·phag·ic (lip-ō-fā'jik). Relating to lipophagy.

lip·oph·a·gy (lip-of'ă-jē). Ingestion of fat by a lipophage. [lipo- + G. *phagō*, to eat]

lip·o·phan·er·o·sis (lip'ō-fan-er-ō'sis). A change in certain cells whereby previously invisible fat becomes demonstrable as small sudanophilic droplets. SEE fatty *degeneration*. [lipo- + G. *phaneros*, visible, + *-osis*, condition]

lip·o·phil (lip'ō-fil). A substance with lipophilic (hydrophobic) properties. [lipo- + G. *philos*, fond of]

lip·o·phil·ic (lip-ō-fil'ik). Capable of dissolving, of being dissolved in, or of absorbing lipids.

lip·o·phos·pho·di·es·ter·ase I (lip'ō-fos'-fō-dī-es'ter-ās). SYN *phospholipase* C.

lip·o·phos·pho·di·es·ter·ase II. SYN *phospholipase* D.

lip·o·pol·y·sac·cha·ride (LPS) (lip'ō-pol'ē-sak'ă-rīd). **1.** A compound or complex of lipid and carbohydrate. **2.** The l. (endotoxin) released from the cell walls of Gram-negative organisms that produces septic shock.

🔲 **lip·o·pro·tein** (lip-ō-prō'tēn, lī-pō-). Any complex or compound containing both lipid and protein. L.'s are important constituents of biological membranes and of myelin. Conjugation with protein facilitates transport of lipids, which are hydrophobic, in the aqueous medium of the plasma. Plasma l.'s can be separated by ultracentrifugation, electrophoresis, or immunoelectrophoresis; they migrate electrophoretically with α- and β-globulins, but are usually classified according to their densities (flotation constants). The principal classes by density are chylomicrons, which transport dietary cholesterol and triglycerides from the intestine to the liver and other tissues; very low density l.'s (VLDL), which transport triglycerides from intestine and liver to muscle and adipose tissue; low density l.'s (LDL), which transport cholesterol to tissues other than the liver; and high density l.'s (HDL), which transport cholesterol to the liver for excretion in bile. The properties of these and other plasma l.'s are set forth in the accompanying table. The protein moiety of a l. is called an apolipoprotein (or apoprotein). Besides rendering lipids soluble, some apolipoproteins perform biochemical functions such as enzyme activation. The apolipoproteins of plasma l.'s are synthesized by the liver and intestinal mucosal cells and vary in molecular weight from 7000 to 500,000. Protein makes up more than 50% of some HDLs but only 1% of chylomicrons. As the proportion of lipid in a l. increases, its density decreases. A plasma l. particle is typically spherical, with a hydrophobic core of triacylglycerol, cholesteryl esters, and apolar amino acid residues surrounded by hydrophilic protein structures and phospholipids.

> The concentrations of certain serum lipoproteins correlate closely with the risk of atherosclerosis. An HDL cholesterol level below 35 mg/dL (0.90 mmol/L), an LDL cholesterol level above 160 mg/dL (4.15 mmol/L), and a fasting triglyceride level above 250 mg/dL are all independent risk factors for coronary artery disease. Although dietary factors are important in some persons, basal levels of lipoprotein, cholesterol, and triglycerides depend chiefly on heredity. Several phenotypes of familial hyperlipoproteinemia associated with risk of premature cardiovascular disease and death have been identified. SEE hyperlipopro-

li

teinemia. Medical management of patients with coronary artery disease (myocardial infarction, angina pectoris, history of coronary artery bypass graft or coronary angioplasty) and other atherosclerotic disorders (peripheral arterial disease, abdominal aortic aneurysm, carotid artery disease) includes detection and correction of hypercholesterolemia and hyperlipoproteinemia. Reducing elevated LDL cholesterol diminishes the risk of coronary artery disease; besides halting the progression of atherosclerosis, it may even shrink established atherosclerotic lesions. Of persons with elevated LDL cholesterol, 75% can achieve normal levels with diet, weight reduction, and exercise; the remainder need drug treatment. Factors besides familial hyperlipoproteinemias that can elevate LDL cholesterol include diabetes mellitus, hypothyroidism, nephrotic syndrome, obstructive liver disease, and drugs (progestogens, anabolic steroids, corticosteroids, thiazide diuretics). Dietary saturated fat raises LDL cholesterol more than any other dietary component, cholesterol itself not excepted.

l. (a), a l. consisting of an LDL particle to which a large glycoprotein, apolipoprotein (a), is covalently bonded. Elevation of the concentration in serum has been identified as a risk factor for coronary artery disease.

Elevation of plasma lipoprotein (a) above 30 mg/dL is a strong independent risk factor for coronary artery disease and possibly for stroke. A unique feature of lipoprotein (a) is the structural similarity of its nonlipid moiety, apolipoprotein (a), to plasminogen. This similarity allows it to bind to endothelium and to proteins of cellular membranes. It inhibits fibrinolysis by competing for plasminogen binding sites and also favors lipid deposition and stimulates smooth muscle cell proliferation. Niacin and estrogen lower Lp(a), but HMG-CoA reductase inhibitors, fibrates, and bile acid sequestrants do not.

α_1-**l.,** A lipoprotein fraction of relatively low molecular weight, high density, rich in phospholipids, and found in the α_1-globulin fraction of human plasma.

β_1-**l.,** A lipoprotein fraction of relatively high molecular weight, low density, rich in cholesterol, and found in the β-globulin fraction of human plasma.

intermediate density l. (IDL), class of l.'s formed in degradation of very low density l.'s; about half are cleared quickly from the plasma into the liver by receptor-mediated endocytosis; the other half are degraded into low density lipoproteins.

l. Lp(a), a l. composed of an LDL particle combined with an additional protein, Lp(a) specific protein; elevated levels have been identified as a risk factor for coronary artery disease; elevations may be treated with niacin.

malondialdehyde-modified low-density l., IDL molecule with aldehyde-substituted lysine residue(s) in the apoprotein moiety, resulting from oxidative reaction accompanying prostaglandin synthesis and platelet aggregation.

l.-X, An abnormal low-density lipoprotein found in patients with obstructive jaundice.

lip·o·pro·tein li·pase. An enzyme that hydrolyzes one fatty acid from a triacylglycerol; its activity is enhanced by heparin and inactivated by heparinase. It is activated by apolipoprotein C-II; a deficiency of l. l. is associated with familial hyperlipoproteinemia type I. SEE ALSO familial lipoprotein lipase *inhibitor,* clearing *factors,* under *factor.* SYN diacylglycerol lipase, diglyceride lipase.

lip·o·sar·co·ma (lip'ō-sar-kō'mă). A malignant neoplasm of adults that occurs especially in the retroperitoneal tissues and the thigh, usually deep in the intermuscular or periarticular planes; histologically, l. is a large tumor that may be composed of well-differentiated fat cells or may be dedifferentiated, either myxoid, round-celled, or pleomorphic, usually in association with a rich network of capillaries; recurrences are common, and dedifferentiated l. metastasizes to the lungs or serosal surfaces. [lipo- + *sarx,* flesh, + -*oma,* tumor]

li·po·sis (li-pō'sis). **1.** SYN adiposis. **2.** Fatty infiltration, neutral fats being present in the cells. SEE ALSO lipolipoidosis. [lipo- + G. -*osis,* condition]

li·pos·i·tol (lip-os'i-tol). SYN inositol.

lip·o·sol·u·ble (lip-ō-sol'ū-bl). Fat-soluble.

lip·o·some (lip'ō-sōm). **1.** A spherical particle of lipid substance suspended in an aqueous medium within a tissue. **2.** Any small, roughly spherical artificial vesicle consisting of a lipid bilayer enclosing some of the suspending medium. [lipo- + G. *sōma,* body]

lip·o·suc·tion (lip'ō-sŭk-shun). Method of removing unwanted subcutaneous fat using percutaneously placed suction tubes.

tumescent l., l. performed after subcutaneous infusion of lidocaine solution and the use of microcannulae.

wet-technique l., l. performed after subcutaneous infusion of dilute epinephrine solution.

lip·o·suc·tion·ing (lip'ō-sŭk'shŭn-ing). Removal of fat by high vacuum pressure; used in body contouring.

lip·o·thi·am·ide py·ro·phos·phate (lip-ō-thī'am-īd). Name once given to the coenzymes of the multienzyme complex catalyzing the formation of acetyl-CoA from pyruvate and involving lipoamide and thiamin pyrophosphate, on the assumption that they were a single compound. SEE lipoic acid.

lip·o·tro·phic (lip-ō-trof'ik). Relating to lipotrophy.

li·pot·ro·phy (li-pot'rō-fē). An increase of fat in the body. [lipo- + G. *trophē,* nourishment]

lip·o·tro·pic (lip-ō-trop'ik). **1.** Pertaining to substances preventing or correcting excessive fat deposits in liver such as occurs in choline deficiency. **2.** Relating to lipotropy.

lip·o·tro·pin (li-pō-trō'pin). A pituitary hormone mobilizing fat from adipose tissue. β-L. is a single-chain peptide of 91 amino acyl residues that contains the sequences of endorphins, metenkephalin, and β-melanotropin; γ-l. is shorter and is identical in sequence to the N-terminal 58 residues of β-lipotropin; both contain sequences common to ACTH and β-melanotropin. SYN lipid-mobilizing hormone, lipotropic hormone, lipotropic pituitary hormone.

plasma lipoproteins						
class	density (g/ml)	diameter (nm)	apolipoproteins	protein (%)	triglyceride (%)	cholesterol (free and esterified) (%)
chylomicrons	<0.95	90–1000	A-1, A-2, B-48, C-2, C-3, E	1–2	88	4
very-low-density lipoproteins (VLDL)	0.95–1.006	30–90	B-100, C-1, C-2, C-3, E	7–10	56	23
intermediate-density lipoproteins (IDL)	1.006–1.019	25–30	B-100	11	43	29
low-density lipoproteins (LDL)	1.019–1.063	20–25	B-100	21	58	13
high-density lipoproteins (HDL)						
HDL₂	1.063–1.125	10–20	A-1, A-2, A-4, C-1, C-2, C-3, D	33	41	16
HDL₃	1.125–1.210	7.5–10		57	35	13

li·pot·ro·py (li-pot′rō-pē). **1.** Affinity of basic dyes for fatty tissue. **2.** Prevention of accumulation of fat in the liver. **3.** Affinity of nonpolar substances for each other. [lipo- + G. *tropē,* turning]

lip·o·vac·cine (lip′ō-vak-sēn). A vaccine suspended in vegetable oil as a solvent. SEE adjuvant *vaccine.*

lip·o·vi·tel·lin (lip′ō-vi-tel′in). SYN vitellin.

li·pox·e·nous (li-pok′sĕ-nŭs). Pertaining to lipoxeny.

li·pox·e·ny (li-pok′sĕ-nē, lī-). Desertion of the host by a parasite when the development of the latter is complete. [G. *leipō,* to leave, + *xenos,* host]

li·pox·i·dase (li-poks′i-dās). SYN lipoxygenase.

li·pox·y·ge·nase (li-poks′ē-jĕ-nās). A class of enzymes that catalyzes the oxidation of unsaturated fatty acids with O_2 to yield hydroperoxides of the fatty acids; 5-l. catalyzes the first step in leukotriene biosynthesis, acting on arachidonate. SYN carotene oxidase, lipoxidase.

lip·o·yl (lip′ō-il). The acyl radical of lipoic acid.

lip·o·yl de·hy·dro·gen·ase. SYN dihydrolipoamide dehydrogenase.

lip·ping (lip′ing). The formation of a liplike structure, as at the articular end of a bone in osteoarthritis.

lip·pi·tude, lip·pi·tu·do (lip′i-tood, lip-i-too′dō). SYN blear *eye.* [L., fr. *lippus,* blear-eyed]

Lipschütz, Benjamin, Austrian physician, 1878–1931. SEE L. *cell.*

li·pu·ria (li-poo′rē-ă). Presence of lipids in the urine. SYN adiposuria. [lipo- + G. *ouron,* urine]

li·pur·ic (li-poo′rik). Pertaining to lipuria.

liq·ue·fa·cient (lik′we-fā′shent). **1.** Making liquid; causing a solid to become liquid. **2.** Denoting a resolvant supposed to cause the resolution of a solid tumor by liquefying its contents. [L. *liquefacio,* pres. p. *-faciens,* to make fluid, fr. *liqueo,* to be liquid]

liq·ue·fac·tion (lik-wĕ-fak′shŭn). The act of becoming liquid; change from a solid to a liquid form. [see liquefacient]

liq·ue·fac·tive (lik-wĕ-fak′tiv). Relating to liquefaction.

li·queur (li-ker′). A cordial; a spirit containing sugar and aromatics. [Fr.]

liq·uid (l) (lik′wid). **1.** An inelastic substance, like water, that is neither solid nor gaseous and in which the molecules are relatively free to move with respect to each other yet still are restricted by intermolecular forces. **2.** Flowing like water. [L. *liquidus*]

Cotunnius l., SYN perilymph.

li·quor, gen. **li·quor·is,** pl. **li·quo·res** (lik′er, -wōr-is, -wō′rēs) [TA]. **1.** Any liquid or fluid. **2.** A term used for certain body fluids. **3.** The pharmacopoeial term for any aqueous solution (not a decoction or infusion) of a nonvolatile substance and for aqueous solutions of gases. SEE ALSO solution. [L.]

l. am′nii, SYN amnionic *fluid.*

l. cerebrospina′lis [TA], SYN cerebrospinal *fluid.*

l. cotun′nii, SYN perilymph.

l. enter′icus, intestinal secretions.

l. follic′uli, the fluid within the antrum of the ovarian follicle.

malt l., a beverage brewed from malt, such as beer or ale.

Morgagni l., a fluid found postmortem between the epithelium and the fibers of the lens, resulting from the liquefaction of a semifluid material existing there during life. SYN Morgagni humor.

mother l., the saturated solution remaining after a crystallization or precipitation.

Scarpa l., SYN endolymph.

spirituous l., a strong alcoholic l. obtained by distillation, such as whiskey.

vinous l., SYN wine (1).

li·quo·rice (lik′ō-ris). SYN glycyrrhiza.

li·quor·rhea (lik-ō-rē′ă). The flow of liquid. [L. *liquor,* fluid, + G. *rhoia,* flow]

Lisch, Karl, Austrian ophthalmologist, *1907. SEE L. *nodule.*

Lisfranc (de St. Martin), Jacques, French surgeon, 1790–1847.

SEE L. *amputation, joints,* under *joint, ligaments,* under *ligament, operation;* scalene *tubercle* of L.

lis·in·o·pril (līs-in′ō-pril). An angiotensin-converting enzyme inhibitor used in the treatment of hypertension.

Lison, Lucien, Belgian scientist, *1907. SEE L.-Dunn *stain.*

lisp·ing. Mispronunciation of the sibilants *s* and *z*. SYN parasigmatism, sigmatism.

lis·sa·mine rho·da·mine B 200 (lis′să-mēn rō′dă-mēn). SYN sulforhodamine B.

Lissauer, Heinrich, German neurologist, 1861–1891. SEE L. *bundle, column, fasciculus, tract,* marginal *zone; column* of Spitzka-L.

lis·sen·ce·pha·lia (lis′en-sĕ-fā′lē-ă). SYN agyria. [G. *lissos,* smooth, + *enkephalos,* brain]

lis·sen·ce·phal·ic (lis′en-sĕ-fal′ik). Pertaining to, or characterized by, lissencephalia.

lis·sen·ceph·a·ly (lis-en-sef′ă-lē). SYN agyria. [G. *lissos,* smooth, + *enkephalos,* brain]

lis·sive (lis′iv). Having the property of relieving muscle spasm without causing flaccidity. [G. *lissos,* smooth]

lis·so·sphinc·ter (lis′ō-sfingk′ter). A sphincter of smooth musculature. SYN smooth muscular sphincter. [G. *lissos,* smooth, + sphincter]

lis·so·trich·ic, lis·sot·ri·chous (lis-ō-trik′ik, -trik′ŭs). Having straight hair. [G. *lissos,* smooth, + *thrix (trich-),* hair]

Lister, Joseph (Lord Lister), English surgeon, 1827–1912. SEE *Listerella; Listeria;* listerism; L. *dressing, method, tubercle.*

Lis·ter·el·la (lis′ter-el′ă). In bacteriology, a rejected generic name sometimes cited as a synonym of *Listeria.* The type species is *L. hepatolytica.* [Joseph *Lister*]

Lis·te·ria (lis-tēr-ē-ă). A genus of aerobic to microaerophilic, motile, peritrichous bacteria containing small, coccoid, Gram-positive rods; these organisms tend to produce chains of 3–5 cells and, in the rough state, elongated and filamentous forms. Cells 18–24 hours old may show a palisade arrangement with a few V or Y forms; the bacteria produce acid but no gas from glucose and are found in the feces of humans and other animals, on vegetation, and in silage and are parasitic on poikilothermic and warm-blooded animals, including humans. The type species is *L. monocytogenes.* [Joseph *Lister*]

L. denitri′ficans, a bacterial species reclassified as *Jonesia denitrificans.*

L. gra′yi, a bacterial species found in the feces of chinchillas.

L. monocytog′enes, a bacterial species causing meningitis, encephalitis, septicemia, endocarditis, abortion, abscesses, and local purulent lesions; it is often fatal; it is found in healthy ferrets, insects, and the feces of chinchillas, ruminants, and humans, as well as in sewage, decaying vegetation, silage, soil, and fertilizer. Sometimes involved in infections in immunocompromised hosts. A causative agent of perinatal infections, neonatal sepsis and septicemia. Also recently linked to food-borne diseases especially associated with meat and dairy products.

lis·te·ri·o·sis (lis-tēr′ē-ō′sis). A sporadic disease of animals and humans, particularly those who are immunocompromised or pregnant, caused by the bacterium, *Listeria monocytogenes.* The infection in sheep and cattle frequently involves the central nervous system, causing various neurologic signs; in monogastric animals and fowl, the chief manifestations are septicemia and necrosis of the liver. Meningitis, bacteremia, and focal metastatic disease are associated with listeriosis. SYN listeria meningitis. [fr. organism *Listeria*]

lis·ter·ism (lis′ter-izm). SYN Lister *method.*

Listing, Johann B., German physiologist, 1808–1882. SEE L. reduced *eye, law.*

Liston, Robert, English surgeon, 1794–1847. SEE L. *knives,* under *knife, shears.*

li·sur·ide (lī′soor-īd). A soluble ergot derivative with endocrine effects similar to those of bromocriptine; a serotonin inhibitor.

li·ter (L, l) (lē′ter). A measure of capacity of 1000 cubic centimeters or 1 cubic decimeter; equivalent to 1.056688 quarts (U.S., liquid). [Fr., fr. G. *litra,* a pound]

li

literature.

gray l., reports containing data, e.g., on health and disease in a population, that are unpublished or have limited distribution. Examples include local health department reports and masters' and doctoral dissertations lodged in university libraries.

⚠**lith-.** SEE litho-.

lith·a·gogue (lith'ă-gog). Causing the dislodgment or expulsion of calculi, especially urinary calculi. [litho- + G. *agōgos*, drawing forth]

lith·arge (lith'arj). SYN *lead* monoxide. [litho- + G. *argyros*, silver]

li·thec·to·my (li-thek'tō-mē). SYN lithotomy. [litho- + G. *ektomē*, excision]

li·thi·a·sis (li-thī'ă-sis). Formation of calculi of any kind, especially of biliary or urinary calculi. [litho- + G. *-iasis*, condition]

l. conjuncti'vae, hard nodules caused by deposition of calcareous material in areas of cellular degeneration in Henle glands.

2,8-dihydroxyadenine l., formation of calculi of 2,8-dihydroxyadenine due to a deficiency or reduced activity of adenine phosphoribosyltransferase.

pancreatic l., the formation of stones in the pancreas, usually associated with chronic inflammation and obstruction of the pancreatic ducts.

lith·ic ac·id (lith'ik). SYN uric acid.

lith·i·um (Li) (lith'ē-ŭm). An element of the alkali metal group, atomic no. 3, atomic wt. 6.941. Many of its salts have clinical applications. [Mod. L. fr. G. *lithos*, a stone]

l. bromide, LiBr; a white deliquescent powder, used as a sedative and hypnotic.

l. carbonate, an antirheumatic and antilithic agent, also used in the treatment and prophylaxis of depressive, hypomanic, and manic phases of bipolar affective disorders.

l. citrate, a diuretic and antirheumatic, also used in the treatment of manic psychosis.

effervescent l. citrate, a preparation containing l. citrate, sodium bicarbonate, tartaric acid, and citric acid; same use as potassium or sodium citrate.

l. tungstate, used in electron microscopy as a negative stain.

⚠**litho-, lith-.** A stone, calculus, calcification. [G. *lithos*]

Lith·o·bi·us (li-thō'bē-ŭs). A genus of centipedes characterized by 15 pairs of legs. Species common in the U.S. include *L. multidentatus* and *L. forficatus*. [litho- + G. *bios*, life]

lith·o·cho·lic ac·id (lith-ō-kō'lik). One of the acids isolated from human bile as well as from that of cows, rabbits, sheep, and goats.

lith·o·clast (lith'ō-klast). SYN lithotrite. [litho- + G. *klastos*, broken]

lith·o·gen·e·sis, li·thog·e·ny (lith-ō-jen'ě-sis, lith-oj'ě-nē). Formation of calculi. [litho- + G. *genesis*, production]

lith·o·gen·ic (lith-ō-jen'ik). Promoting the formation of calculi.

lith·og·e·nous (lith-oj'ě-nŭs). Calculus-forming.

lith·oid (lith'oyd). Resembling a calculus or stone. [litho- + G. *eidos*, resemblance]

lith·o·kel·y·pho·pe·di·on, lith·o·kel·y·pho·pe·di·um (lith-ō-kel'ě-fō-pē'dē-on, -ŭm). A lithopedion in which the fetal parts in contact with the surrounding membranes, as well as the membranes, are calcified. [litho- + G. *kelyphos*, husk, shell, + *paidion*, child]

lith·o·kel·y·phos (lith-ō-kel'ě-fos). A type of lithopedion in which the fetal membranes alone undergo calcification. [litho- + G. *kelyphos*, rind, shell]

lith·o·labe (lith'ō-lāb). Obsolete instrument for holding a bladder calculus during its removal. [litho- + G. *lambanō*, *labein*, to grasp]

li·thol·a·paxy (li-thol'ă-pak-sē). The technique of crushing a stone in the bladder and washing out the fragments through a catheter. [litho- + G. *lapaxis*, an emptying out]

li·thol·y·sis (li-thol'i-sis). The dissolution of urinary calculi. [litho- + G. *lysis*, dissolution]

lith·o·lyte (lith'ō-līt). An instrument for injecting calculary solvents.

lith·o·lyt·ic (li-thō-lit'ik). **1.** Tending to dissolve calculi. **2.** An agent having such properties. [litho- + G. *lysis*, dissolution]

lith·o·myl (lith'ō-mil). An instrument for pulverizing a stone in the bladder. [litho- + G. *mylē*, mill]

lith·o·ne·phri·tis (lith'ō-ne-frī'tis). Interstitial nephritis associated with calculus formation.

lith·o·pe·di·on, lith·o·pe·di·um (lith-ō-pē'dē-on, -ŭm). A retained fetus, usually extrauterine, that has become calcified. [litho- + G. *paidion*, small child]

lith·o·tome (lith'ō-tōm). A knife used in lithotomy.

li·thot·o·mist (li-thot'ō-mist). A person skilled in lithotomy.

li·thot·o·my (li-thot'ō-mē). Cutting for stone; a cutting operation for the removal of a calculus, especially a vesical calculus. SYN lithectomy. [litho- + G. *tomē*, incision]

high l., SYN suprapubic l.

lateral l., l. in which the perineum is incised to one side of the median line.

marian l., SYN median l. [L. *mas* (*mar*-), male]

median l., l. in which the perineal incision is made in the median raphe. SYN marian l.

perineal l., l. in which the bladder is approached by an incision in the perineum.

prerectal l., l. by an incision in the midline of the perineum anterior to anus.

suprapubic l., l. in which the bladder is entered by an incision immediately above the symphysis pubis. SYN high l.

vaginal l., l. in which the bladder or ureter is entered through an incision in the vagina.

vesical l., SYN cystolithotomy.

lith·o·tre·sis (lith-ō-trē'sis). The boring of holes in a calculus to facilitate its crushing. [litho- + G. *trēsis*, a boring]

lith·o·trip·sy (lith'ō-trip-sē). The crushing of a stone in the renal pelvis, ureter, or bladder, by mechanical force or focused sound energy. SYN lithotrity. [litho- + G. *tripsis*, a rubbing]

electrohydraulic shock wave l. (ESWL), destruction of calculi (urinary tract or other) by fragmentation using shock waves sent transcutaneously via ultrasound transducers.

📖**extracorporeal shock wave l. (ESWL)** (lith'ō-trip'sē), breaking up of renal or ureteral calculi by focused sound energy.

shock wave l., a method of fragmenting calculi.

ultrasonic l., the demolition of calculi by high frequency sound waves.

lith·o·trip·tic (lith-ō-trip'tik). **1.** Relating to lithotripsy. **2.** An agent that effects the dissolution of a calculus.

lith·o·trip·tor (lith-ō-trip'tŏr). A device used to crush or fragment a calculus in lithotripsy.

lith·o·trip·tos·co·py (lith'ō-trip-tos'kŏ-pē). Crushing of a stone in the bladder under direct vision by use of a lithotriptoscope. [litho- + G. *tribō*, to rub, crush, + *skopeō*, to view]

lith·o·trite (lith'ō-trīt). A mechanical instrument used to crush a urinary calculus in lithotripsy. SYN lithoclast. [litho- + L. *tero*, pp. *tritus*, to rub]

li·thot·ri·ty (li-thot'ri-tē). SYN lithotripsy.

lith·o·troph (lith'ō-trof). An organism whose carbon needs are satisfied by carbon dioxide. Cf. chemoautotroph.

lith·u·re·sis (lith'ū-rē'sis). The passage of gravel in the urine. [litho- + G. *ourēsis*, urination]

li·thu·ria (li-thoo'rē-ă). Excretion of uric acid or urates in large amount in the urine. [lithic (acid) + G. *ouron*, urine]

lit·mus (lit'mŭs) [old C.I. 1242]. A blue coloring matter obtained from *Roccella tinctoria* and other species of lichens, the principal component of which is azolitmin; used as an indicator (reddened by acids and turned blue again by alkalies). [a corruption of *lacmus*, fr. Dutch *lakmoes*]

lit·ter (lit'er). **1.** A stretcher or portable couch for moving the sick or injured. **2.** A group of animals of the same parents, born at the same time. SYN brood (1). [Fr. *litière*; fr. *lit*, bed]

Little, James, U.S. surgeon, 1836–1885. SEE L. *area.*

Little, William J., English surgeon, 1810–1894. SEE L. *disease.*

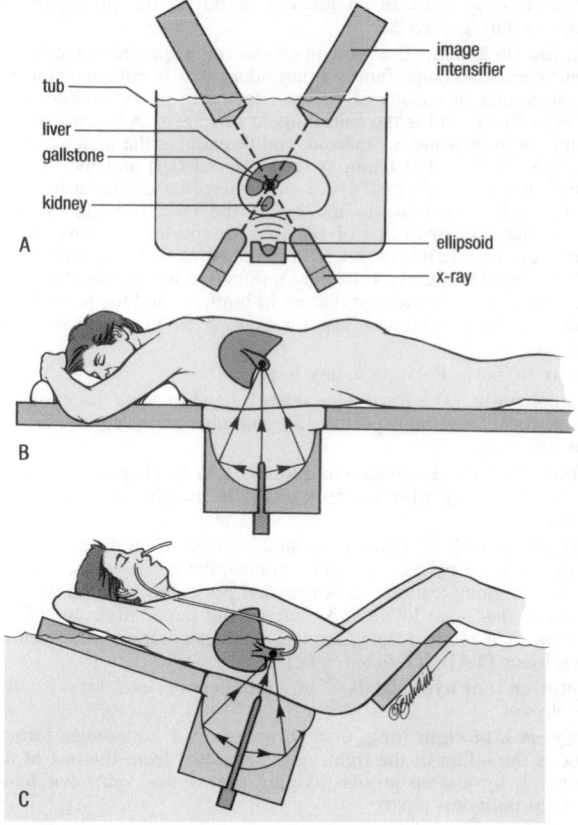

A

B

C

extracorporeal shock wave lithotripsy: (A) gallbladder stone is localized by imaging; shock waves are generated in ellipsoid reflector and transmitted through water to stone; (B) positioning of patient for treatment of stones located in gallbladder; fluid-filled bag is recessed in table and transmits shock wave from generator to patient's skin; (C) positioning of patient for treatment of stones located in common bile duct; the patient is partially submerged in a water bath; nasobiliary tube is used to introduce contrast material to permit visualization and localization of stone and to decompress biliary tree

Labels on figure A: image intensifier, tub, liver, gallstone, kidney, ellipsoid, x-ray

---

Littré, Alexis, French anatomist, 1658–1726. SEE L. *glands,* under *gland, hernia.*

Litzmann, Karl K.T., German gynecologist, 1815–1890. SEE L. *obliquity.*

live·birth, live birth (līv′berth). The birth of an infant who shows evidence of life after birth. SEE ALSO liveborn *infant.*

li·ve·do (li-vē′dō). A bluish discoloration of the skin, either in limited patches or general. [L. lividness, fr. *liveo,* to be black and blue]

postmortem l., a purple coloration of dependent parts, except in areas of contact pressure, appearing within one half to two hours after death, as a result of gravitational movement of blood within the vessels. SYN postmortem hypostasis, postmortem lividity, postmortem suggillation.

l. reticula′ris, a persistent purplish network-patterned discoloration of the skin caused by dilation of capillaries and venules due to stasis or changes in underlying blood vessels including hyalinization; rarely appears as a developmental defect. SYN dermatopathia pigmentosa reticularis.

l. reticula′ris idiopath′ica, an extensive and permanent form of l. reticularis; in rare instances associated with central arterial disease.

l. reticula′ris symptomat′ica, a discoloration or mottling of the skin due to some demonstrable cause, such as seen in erythema ab igne, and in certain tuberculids. SEE ALSO *cutis* marmorata.

l. telangiectat′ica, a permanent mottling of the skin due to an anomaly, probably congenital, of the cutaneous capillaries; a form of l. reticularis.

liv·e·doid (liv′ĕ-doyd). Pertaining to or resembling livedo.

▣ **liv·er** (liv′er) [TA]. The largest gland of the body, lying beneath the diaphragm in the right hypochondrium and upper part of the epigastric region; it is of irregular shape and weighs from 1–2 kg, or about ¹⁄₄₀ the weight of the body. As an exocrine gland it secretes bile; it initially receives most absorbed nutrients via the portal vein; it detoxifies and is also of great importance in fat, carbohydrate, and protein metabolism and stores glycogen. SYN hepar [TA]. [A.S. *lifer*]

cardiac l., SYN cardiac *cirrhosis.*

desiccated l., a dried undefatted powder prepared from mammalian l.'s used as human food; contains riboflavin, nicotinic acid, and choline; used in the treatment of macrocytic anemias and as a nutritional supplement.

fatty l., yellow discoloration of the l. due to fatty degeneration of l. parenchymal cells. SYN hepatic steatosis.

hobnail l., in Laënnec cirrhosis, the contraction of scar tissue and hepatic cellular regeneration which causes a nodular appearance of the l.'s surface.

lardaceous l., SYN waxy l.

left l. [TA], portion of the liver receiving blood from the left branches of the hepatic artery and portal vein, and from which bile is drained via the left hepatic duct; the plane of the middle hepatic vein (demarcated externally on the visceral surface by the fossae for the gallbladder and inferior vena cava and on the diaphragmatic surface by a line extrapolated from the gallbladder to the terminal inferior vena cava) separates left from right liver. SYN pars hepatis sinistra [TA], left part of liver☆.

nutmeg l., chronic passive congestion of the l., causing accentuation of the lobular pattern with red central and yellow or tan periportal zones.

pigmented l., a l. that contains pigment, such as occurs in Dubin-Johnson *syndrome,* hemochromatosis, long-standing malaria.

polycystic l., gradual cystic dilation of intralobular bile ducts (Meyenburg complexes) that fail to involute in embryologic development of the l.; frequently associated with bilateral congenital polycystic kidneys and occasionally with cystic involvement of the pancreas, lungs, and other organs. SYN polycystic liver disease.

posterior l., ☆official alternate term for posterior hepatic *segment* I.

right l. [TA], portion of the l. receiving blood from the right branches of the hepatic artery and portal vein, and from which bile is drained via the right hepatic duct; the plane of the middle hepatic vein (demarcated externally on the visceral surface by the fossae for the gallbladder and inferior vena cava and on the diaphragmatic surface by a line extrapolated from the gallbladder to the terminal inferior vena cava) separates right from left liver. SYN pars hepatis dextra [TA], right part of liver☆.

wandering l., SYN hepatoptosis.

waxy l., amyloid degeneration of the l. SYN lardaceous l.

liv·e·tin (liv′ĕ-tin). Any of the three major water-soluble proteins in egg yolk: α-**livetin,** serum albumin; β-**livetin,** α-glycoprotein; γ-**livetin,** serum γ-globulin.

liv·id. Having a black and blue or a leaden or ashy gray color, as in discoloration from a contusion, congestion, or cyanosis. [L. *lividus,* being black and blue]

li·vid·i·ty (li-vid′i-tē). The state of being livid.

postmortem l., SYN postmortem *livedo.*

li·vor (lī′vōr). The livid discoloration of the skin on the dependent parts of a corpse. [L. a black and blue spot]

lix·iv·i·um (lik-siv′ē-ŭm). SYN lye. [L. ntr. of *lixivius,* made into lye]

LLAT Abbreviation for *lysolecithin*-lecithin acyltransferase.

LLETZ. Abbreviation for large loop excision of transformation zone of the cervix of the uterus.

LLL Abbreviation for left lower lobe (of lung).

Lloyd, John Uri, U.S. pharmacist, 1849–1936. Noted for investi-

Ll

gational work in plant chemistry and phytochemistry as applied to medicines, alkaloids, and glucosides.

Lloyd re·a·gent. See under reagent.

LLQ Abbreviation for left lower quadrant (of abdomen).

LM Abbreviation for licentiate in midwifery.

lm Abbreviation for lumen (2).

LMA Abbreviation for left mentoanterior position.

LMP 1. Abbreviation for left mentoposterior position; last menstrual period; latent membrane *protein*; low molecular weight *proteins*, under *protein*. **2.** Gene product of Epstein-Barr virus (latent membrane protein).

LMT Abbreviation for left mentotransverse position.

L-α-nar·co·tine. SYN noscapine.

LNPF Abbreviation for lymph node permeability *factor*.

Lo, L₀. SEE Lo *dose*.

LOA Abbreviation for left occipitoanterior position.

load (lōd). **1.** A departure from normal body content, as of water, salt, or heat; positive l.'s are quantities in excess of the normal; negative l.'s are quantities in deficit. **2.** The quantity of a measurable entity borne by an object or organism. [M.E. *lode*, fr. A.S. lād,]

electronic pacemaker l., the impedance to the output, the standard l. being 500 ohms resistance ± 1%.

genetic l., the aggregate of more or less harmful genes that are carried, mostly hidden, in the genome that may be transmitted to descendants and cause morbidity and disease; in classical genetic dynamics, genetic l. may be seen as undischarged genetic debts that result from previous mutations, each of which is supposed to exact an average number of lethal equivalents dependent only on the pattern of inheritance, regardless of how mild or severe the phenotype may be.

viral l., the plasma level of viral RNA, as determined by various techniques including target amplification assay by reverse transcriptase polymerase chain reaction and branched DNA technology with signal amplification. Because levels of detection vary with method, results of testing by different methods are not comparable.

> Serial measurement of HIV viral load has become a standard procedure in monitoring the course of AIDS. Reported as the number of copies of viral RNA per mL of plasma, assessment of viral load provides important information about the number of lymphoid cells actively infected with HIV. This laboratory procedure has supplanted the CD4 count as an indicator of prognosis of persons infected with HIV, in determining when to start antiretroviral therapy, and in measuring the response to therapy. Because the CD4 count is regarded as superior in determining the level of immune compromise and the risk of opportunistic infection, both tests are currently used. Antiretroviral therapy is started when plasma HIV RNA concentration exceeds 5000 copies/mL. When, as a result of treatment, the number of copies of viral RNA falls below the level that can be detected by standard methods, replication of HIV is considered to have been suppressed. In no case, however, has AIDS been cured, nor has viral proliferation remained arrested after cessation of antiretroviral therapy.

load·ing (lōd'ing). Administration of a substance for the purpose of testing metabolic function.

carbohydrate l., a procedure, popular with long-distance runners and other athletes, of filling muscles with a large glycogen pool prior to an athletic event; often, the athlete consumes very few carbohydrates for three days, followed by a largely carbohydrate diet for the last three days before the event.

salt l., the administration of 2 g of sodium chloride (with a regular diet) 3 times a day for 4 days; a diagnostic test in primary aldosteronism, in which the salt l. produces a typical plasma electrolyte and hormonal pattern.

soda l., a procedure adopted by a number of athletes of ingesting

sodium bicarbonate in an attempt to buffer the production of protons during exercise.

Loa loa (lō'ă lō'ă). The African eye worm, a species of the family Onchocercidae (superfamily Filarioidea) that is indigenous to the western part of equatorial Africa, especially in the region of the Congo River, and is the causal agent of loiasis. Adult worms are white or gray-white, cylindroid, and threadlike, the males averaging 25–35 by 0.3–0.4 mm (with a curved tail) and the females ranging from 50–60 by 0.4–0.6 mm; microfilariae are ensheathed, with nuclei extending to the tip of the tail. The life cycle is somewhat similar to that of *Wuchereria* species; humans are the only known definitive host, and parasites are transmitted by *Chrysops* flies (family Tabanidae); infective larvae from the latter require 3 years or more to mature in humans, and the adult forms may persist in a human host for as long as 17 years. SEE ALSO loiasis.

lo·bar (lō'bar). Relating to any lobe.

l. nephronia, (**1**) a focal renal mass related to acute infection. (**2**) acute focal bacterial nephritis. (**3**) renal phlegmon (not an abscess; no free pus).

lo·bate (lō'bāt). **1.** Divided into lobes. **2.** Lobe-shaped; denoting a bacterial colony with a deeply undulate margin. SYN lobose, lobous.

lobe (lōb) [TA]. **1.** One of the subdivisions of an organ or other part, bounded by fissures, sulci, connective tissue septa, or other structural demarcations. **2.** A rounded projecting part, as the l. of the ear. SEE ALSO lobule. **3.** One of the larger divisions of the crown of a tooth, formed from a distinct point of calcification. SYN lobus [TA]. [G. *lobos*, lobe]

anterior l. of hypophysis, ☆official alternate term for adenohypophysis.

az'ygos l. of right lung, a small accessory l. sometimes formed above the hilum of the right lung; separated from the rest of the upper l. by a deep groove lodging the azygos vein. SYN lobus azygos pulmonis dextri.

caudate l., ☆official alternate term for posterior hepatic *segment* l.

cerebral l.'s, SYN lobi cerebri, under *lobus*.

cuneiform l., SYN biventer *lobule*.

ear l., SYN *lobule* of auricle.

falciform l., SYN cingulate *gyrus*.

flocculonodular l. [TA], the small posterior and inferior subdivision of the cerebellar cortex that borders the line of attachment of the choroid roof of the rhomboid fossa, and consists of the left and right flocculus together with the unpaired nodulus (the most posterior of the folia composing the vermis cerebelli). Its major afferent connections come from the vestibular nuclei and directly from the vestibular nerve; it projects largely to the vestibular nuclei, directly and by way of the fastigial nucleus. SYN lobus flocculonodularis [TA].

frontal l. [TA], SYN frontal l. of cerebrum.

frontal l. of cerebrum [TA], the portion of each cerebral hemisphere anterior to the central sulcus. SYN frontal l. [TA], lobus frontalis [TA].

glandular l. of hypophysis, SYN adenohypophysis.

Home l., the enlarged middle l. of the prostate gland.

inferior l. of (left / right) lung, it is located below and behind the oblique fissure and contains five bronchopulmonary segments: superior (S VI), medial basal (S VII), anterior basal (S VIII), lateral basal (S IX), and posterior basal (S X). SYN lobus inferior pulmonis dextri et sinistri [TA], lower l. of lung ☆.

insular l., ☆official alternate term for *lobus* insula.

kidney l.'s [TA], one of the subdivisions of the kidney, consisting of a renal pyramid and the cortical tissue associated with it. SYN lobus renalis [TA], renal l.

left l. [TA], the left subdivision of several glands, e.g., prostate, thyroid, thymus. SYN lobus sinister [TA].

left l. of liver [TA], it is separated from the much larger right lobe anterior and superior to the falciform and coronary ligaments, and from the quadrate and caudate lobes by the fissure for the ligamentum teres and the fissure for the ligamentum venosum. The lobes of the liver are not functional units, being defined by external structures; the distribution of the portal vein, hepatic artery, and bile ducts does not correspond to the gross lobar divisions of the liver. SYN lobus hepatis sinister [TA], divisio lateralis sinistra⋆, lateral division of left liver⋆.

limbic l. [TA], as originally defined by P. Broca: the nearly closed ring of the brain structures surrounding the hilus, or margin, of the cerebral hemisphere of mammals; it is composed of the fornicate gyrus (cingulate gyrus, fasciolar gyrus, parahippocampal gyrus, and uncus), and the hippocampus. SEE limbic *system*. SYN lobus limbicus [TA].

lingual l., SYN *cingulum* of tooth.

lower l. of lung, ⋆official alternate term for inferior l. of (left / right) lung.

l.'s of mammary gland [TA], the 15–20 separate portions of the mammary gland that radiate from the central area deep to the nipplelike wheel spokes and make up the body of the mammary gland; each is drained by a single lactiferous duct. SYN lobi glandulae mammariae [TA].

middle l. of prostate [TA], the portion of the prostate lying between the urethra and the ejaculatory ducts; indistinct unless hypertrophied. SYN lobus medius prostatae [TA], Morgagni caruncle.

middle l. of right lung [TA], it is located anteriorly between the horizontal and oblique fissures and includes lateral (S IV) and medial (S V) bronchopulmonary segments. SYN lobus medius pulmonis dextri [TA].

nervous l., SYN neurohypophysis.

neural l. of hypophysis, the bulbous part of the neurohypophysis attached to the hypothalamus by the infundibulum. It is composed of pituicytes, blood vessels, and terminals of nerve fibers from the supraoptic and paraventricular nuclei.

occipital l. [TA], SYN occipital l. of cerebrum.

occipital l. of cerebrum [TA], the posterior, somewhat pyramid-shaped part of each cerebral hemisphere, demarcated by no distinct surface markings on the lateral convexity of the hemisphere from the parietal and temporal lobes, but sharply delineated from the parietal lobe by the parieto-occipital sulcus on the medial surface. SYN lobus occipitalis [TA], occipital l. [TA].

parietal l. [TA], SYN parietal l. of cerebrum.

parietal l. of cerebrum [TA], the middle portion of each cerebral hemisphere, separated from the frontal lobe by the central sulcus, from the temporal lobe by the lateral sulcus in front and an imaginary line projected posteriorly, and from the occipital lobe only partially by the parieto-occipital sulcus on its medial aspect. SYN lobus parietalis [TA], parietal l. [TA].

placental l.'s, cotyledons of the human placenta, viewed on the maternal surface as irregularly shaped elevations or l.'s.

polyalveolar l., a type of congenital anomaly where a severalfold increase in the total alveolar number leads to congenital lobar emphysema.

posterior l. of hypophysis, SYN neurohypophysis.

l. of prostate [TA], one of the lateral lobes (right or left) or the middle lobe or isthmus of the prostate; in the adult the lobes are ill-defined. SYN lobus prostatae [TA].

pyramidal l. of thyroid gland [TA], an inconstant narrow lobe of the thyroid gland that arises from the upper border of the isthmus and extends upward, sometimes as far as the hyoid bone; it marks the point of continuity with the thyroglossal duct. SYN lobus pyramidalis glandulae thyroideae [TA], Lallouette pyramid, Morgagni appendix, pyramid of thyroid.

quadrate l., (1) a lobe on the inferior surface of the liver located between the fossa for the gallbladder and the fissure for the ligamentum teres; (2) SYN quadrangular *lobule*; (3) SYN precuneus.

renal l., SYN kidney l.'s.

Riedel l., an occasional tonguelike process extending downward from the right l. of the liver lateral to the gallbladder; a similar process may, though rarely, extend from the left lobe. SYN lobus appendicularis, lobus linguiformis.

right l. [TA], the right subdivision of several glands, e.g., prostate, thyroid, thymus. SYN lobus dexter [TA].

right l. of liver [TA], the largest lobe of the liver, separated from

the left lobe anteriorly and superiorly by the falciform and coronary ligaments and from the caudate and quadrate lobes by the sulcus for the vena cava and the fossa for the gallbladder. SYN lobus hepatis dexter [TA].

Spigelius l., SYN posterior hepatic *segment* I.

superior l. of (right/left) lung, the lobe of the right lung that lies above the oblique and horizontal fissures and includes the apical (S I), posterior (S II), and anterior (S III) bronchopulmonary segments; in the left lung, the lobe lies above the oblique fissure and contains the apicoposterior (S I + II), anterior (S III), superior lingular (S IV), and inferior lingular (S V) segments. SYN lobus superior pulmonis (dextri et sinistri) [TA], upper l. of lung⋆.

supplemental l., in dental anatomy, an extra l.; one that is not included in the typical formation of a tooth.

temporal l. [TA], a long l., the lowest of the major subdivisions of the cortical mantle, forming the posterior two-thirds of the ventral surface of the cerebral hemisphere, separated from the frontal and parietal l.'s above it by the lateral sulcus arbitrarily delineated by an imaginary plane from the occipital l. with which it is continuous posteriorly. The temporal l. has a heterogeneous composition: in addition to a large neocortical component consisting of the superior, middle, and inferior temporal gyri and the lateral and medial occipitotemporal gyri, it includes the largely juxtallocortical parahippocampal gyrus with its paleocortical (olfactory) uncus and, beneath the latter, the amygdala. SYN lobus temporalis [TA], temporal cortex.

l.'s of thyroid gland [TA], the two major divisions of the gland lying on the right and left side of the trachea and connected by the isthmus. A smaller pyramidal lobe is frequently present as an upward extension from the isthmus. SYN lobi glandulae thyroideae [TA].

upper l. of lung, ⋆official alternate term for superior l. of (right/left) lung.

lo·bec·to·my (lō-bek'tō-mē). Excision of a lobe of any organ or gland. [G. *lobos,* lobe, + *ektomē,* excision]

lo·be·lia (lō-bē'lē-ă). **1.** The dried leaves and tops of *Lobelia inflata* (family Lobeliaceae); it contains several alkaloids: lobeline, lobelamine, lobelanidine, lobelanine, norlobelanine, norlobelanidine, and isolobelanine. The fluid extract and the tincture have been used as an expectorant in asthma and chronic bronchitis. **2.** One of a class of alkaloids isolated from l. (1). **3.** Any plant of the genus *Lobelia.* SYN asthma-weed (1), wild tobacco.

lo·be·line, lo·be·lin (lō'bĕ-lēn, lob'ĕ-lēn, -lin). A piperidylacetophenone; an alkaloid of lobelia with the same actions as nicotine, but with less potency.

l. sulfate, a form of l. occurring in yellow friable masses, soluble in water; used in whooping cough and asthma; it has been suggested as a smoking deterrent.

lo·bi (lō'bī). Plural of lobus. [L.]

lo·bi·tis (lō-bī'tis). Inflammation of a lobe.

Lobo, Jorge, Brazilian physician, 1900–1979. SEE L. *disease.*

Lo·boa lo·boi (lō-bō'ă lō-bō'ē). A species of fungus causing lobomycosis. The organism has not been grown in culture.

lo·bo·my·co·sis (lō-bō-mī-kō'sis). A chronic localized mycosis of the skin reported from South America resulting in granulomatous nodules or keloids that contain budding, thick-walled cells about 9 μm in diameter, i.e., the tissue form of *Loboa loboi,* the causative fungus, which has not been cultured. Also occurs in dolphins. SYN Lobo disease.

lo·bo·po·di·um, pl. **lo·bo·po·dia** (lō'bō-pō'dē-ŭm, -dē-ă). A thick lobose pseudopodium. [G. *lobos,* lobe, + *pous,* foot]

lo·bose, lo·bous (lō'bōs, lō'bŭs). SYN lobate.

lo·bot·o·my (lō-bot'ō-mē). **1.** Incision into a lobe. **2.** Division of one or more nerve tracts in a lobe of the cerebrum. [G. *lobos,* lobe, + *tomē,* a cutting]

prefrontal l., division of one or more nerve tracts in the prefrontal area of the brain for surgical treatment of pain and emotional disorder. SYN prefrontal leukotomy.

transorbital l., l. by an approach through the roof of the orbit, behind the frontal sinus. SYN transorbital leukotomy.

lo

Lobry de Bruyn, Cornelius A., Dutch chemist, 1857–1904. SEE L. de B.-van Ekenstein *transformation*.

Lobstein, Johann F.D., German pathologist, 1777–1840. SEE L. *ganglion*.

lob·u·lar (lob′ū-lăr). Relating to a lobule.

lob·u·late, lob·u·lat·ed (lob′ū-lāt, -ed). Divided into lobules.

lob·ule (lob′ūl) [TA]. A small lobe or subdivision of a lobe. SYN lobulus [TA].

ala central l. [TA], SYN *wing* of central lobule. SYN pars inferior alae lobuli centralis [TA], pars superior ali lobuli centralis [TA].

ansiform l., comprises the greater part of the hemisphere of the cerebellum; its superior and inferior surfaces are separated by the horizontal fissure into major parts known as crus I (superior semilunar lobule) and crus II (inferior semilunar lobule).

anterior lunate l., SYN superior semilunar l.

l. of auricle [TA], the lowest part of the auricle; it consists of fat and fibrous tissue not reinforced by the auricular cartilage; it is often utilized as a site to obtain a small sample of blood using a lancet. SYN lobulus auriculae [TA], ear lobe.

biventer l. [TA], a l. on the undersurface of each cerebellar hemisphere, divided by a curved sulcus into a lateral and medial portion; it corresponds to the pyramid of the vermis. SYN lobulus biventer [TA], biventral l., cuneiform lobe, lobulus biventralis, lobulus cuneiformis.

biventral l., SYN biventer l.

central l. [TA], SYN central l. of cerebellum.

central l. of cerebellum, a division of the superior vermis of the cerebellum between the lingula and the culmen consisting of lobules II and III. SYN central l. [TA], lobulus centralis corporis cerebelli [TA].

conical l.'s of epididymis, ☆official alternate term for l.'s of epididymis.

cortical l.'s of kidney, one of the subdivisions of the kidney, consisting of a medullary ray and that portion of the convoluted part (renal corpuscles and convoluted tubules) associated with its collecting duct. SYN lobulus corticalis renalis, renal cortical l., renculus (1), reniculus (1), renunculus (1).

crescentic l.'s of the cerebellum, archaic term for *lobulus* semilunaris inferior and *lobulus* semilunaris superior.

l.'s of epididymis [TA], the coiled portion of the efferent ductules that constitute the head of the epididymis; these join the ductus epididymidis. SYN lobuli epididymidis [TA], coni epididymidis☆, conical l.'s of epididymis☆, coni vasculosi, Haller cones, vascular cones.

gracile l. [TA], the anterior portion of the posteroinferior lobule of the cerebellum, the posterior portion being the semilunar l. inferior; the two are continuous with the tuber of the vermis. SYN lobulus paramedianus [TA], lobulus gracilis☆, paramedian l.☆, slender l.

hepatic l., SYN l.'s of liver.

inferior parietal l. [TA], the area of the parietal lobe of the cerebrum lying below the interparietal sulcus; it contains the angular and the supramarginal gyri. SYN lobulus parietalis inferior [TA], inferior parietal gyrus.

inferior semilunar l. [TA], the part of the superior surface of the cerebellar hemisphere lying behind the horizontal fissure. SYN lobulus semilunaris inferior [TA], crus II, posterior lunate l.

l.'s of liver [TA], the conceptual polygonal histologic unit of the liver consisting of masses of liver cells arranged around a central vein, a terminal branch of one of the hepatic veins; at the periphery are located preterminal and terminal branches of the portal vein, hepatic artery, and bile duct; hepatic lobules have anatomic reality in pig liver or pathologically in humans, when fibrous septa are present. SYN lobulus hepatis [TA], hepatic l.

l.'s of mammary gland [TA], subdivisions of the lobes of the mammary gland. SYN lobuli glandulae mammariae [TA].

paracentral l. [TA], a division of the medial aspect of the cerebral cortex, lying above the cingulate sulcus and bounded by the paracentral sulcus in front and the marginal part of the cingulate sulcus behind; this l. is formed by the anterior paracentral gyrus

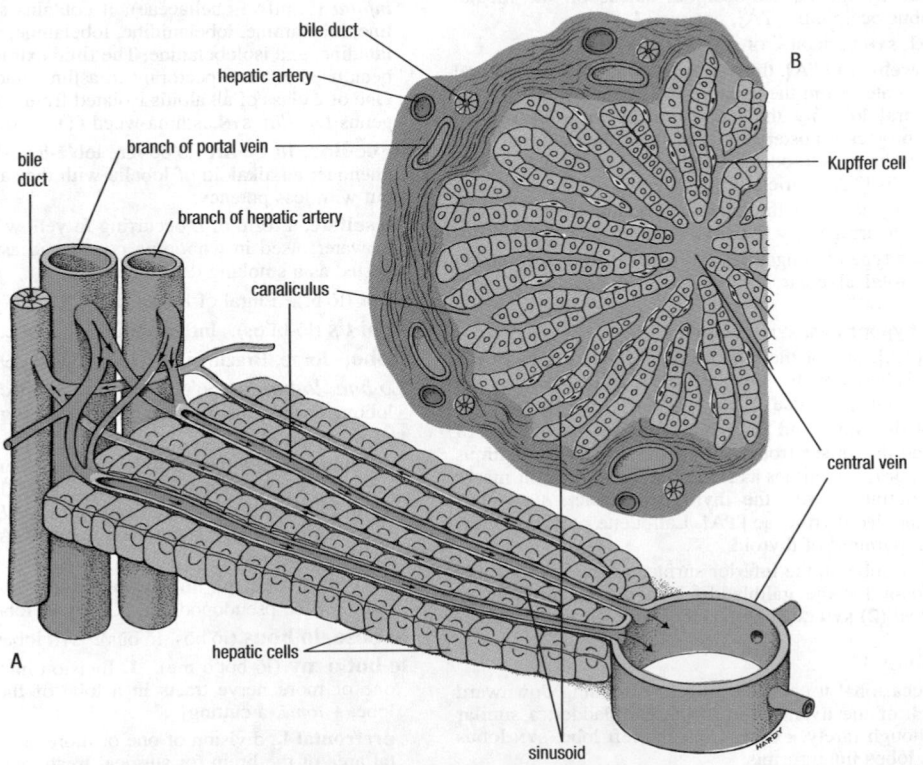

liver lobule and sinusoids: (A) schematic diagram of section of liver lobule, (B) cross section of a liver lobule

and the posterior paracentral gyrus. SYN lobulus paracentralis [TA].

paramedian l., ⋆official alternate term for gracile l.

portal l. of liver, a conceptual unit of the liver, emphasizing its exocrine function in bile secretion, which comprises a roughly triangular shaped cross-sectional area with a portal canal at its center and three or more venae centrales hepatis at its periphery.

posterior lunate l., SYN inferior semilunar l.

primary pulmonary l., SYN pulmonary *acinus*.

quadrangular l., the main portion of the superior part of each hemisphere of the cerebellum, corresponding in current terminology to the anterior quadrangular lobule; the hemisphere portions of the culmen (lobules IV and V) of the vermis consist of an anterior part (lobule HIV) and a posterior part (lobule HV); located between the preculminate and primary fissures. SYN lobulus quadrangularis, lobulus quadratus (1), lobus quadratus, quadrate lobe (2), quadrate l. (1).

quadrate l., (1) SYN quadrangular l; **(2)** SYN precuneus.

renal cortical l., SYN cortical l.'s of kidney.

respiratory l., SYN pulmonary *acinus*.

secondary pulmonary l., a pyramidal mass of lung tissue whose sides are bounded by the incomplete interlobular connective tissue septa and whose base, which is 1 to 2 cm in diameter, usually faces the pleural surface of the lung; l.'s that occupy a more central position in the lung are not well defined and are considered to consist of three to five pulmonary acini with proximate terminal bronchioles.

simple l. [TA], the smaller anterior part of the posterior lobe of the cerebellum, demarcated by the primary fissure from the anterior lobe rostrally and by the posterior superior fissure from the large ansiform lobule caudally. SYN lobulus simplex [TA].

slender l., SYN gracile l.

superior parietal l. [TA], the area of the convex surface of the parietal lobe of the cerebrum lying between the longitudinal fissure and the interparietal sulcus caudal to the postcentral gyrus; it is continuous with the precuneus on the medial aspect of the hemisphere. SYN lobulus parietalis superior [TA], superior parietal gyrus.

superior semilunar l. [TA], the part of the superior surface of the cerebellar hemisphere lying between the horizontal and ansoparamedian fissures and adjoining the folium and parts of the tuber of the vermis. SYN lobulus semilunaris superior [TA], anterior lunate l., crus I.

l.'s of testis [TA], the subdivisions of the parenchyma of the testis formed by delicate fibrous septa that pass inward from the tunica albuginea to converge at the mediastinum testis. SYN lobuli testis [TA].

l.'s of thymus [TA], areas of thymic tissue 0.5 to 2 mm in diameter with a cortex and medulla. SYN lobuli thymi [TA].

l.'s of thyroid gland [TA], the subdivisions of the lobe of the thyroid gland, consisting of incompletely separated, irregular groups of thyroid follicles (20–40 in number) bound together by delicate connective tissue. SYN lobuli glandulae thyroideae [TA].

lob·u·let, lob·u·lette (lob′ū-let′). A very small lobule or one of the smaller subdivisions of a lobule.

lob·u·lus, gen. and pl. **lob·u·li** (lob′ū-lŭs, -ū-lī) [TA]. SYN lobule. [Mod. L. dim. of *lobus*, lobe]

l. auric′ulae [TA], SYN *lobule* of auricle.

l. biven′ter [TA], SYN biventer *lobule*.

l. biventra′lis, SYN biventer *lobule*.

l. centra′lis corporis cerebel′li [TA], SYN central *lobule* of cerebellum.

l. cli′vi, SYN declive.

l. cortica′lis rena′lis, SYN cortical *lobules* of kidney, under *lobule*.

l. cul′minis, SYN culmen.

l. cune′iform′is, SYN biventer *lobule*.

lob′uli epididym′idis [TA], SYN *lobules* of epididymis, under *lobule*.

l. fo′lii, the part of the superior vermis of the cerebellum lying immediately behind the posterior superior fissure and caudal to the l. clivi.

l. fusifor′mis, SYN fusiform *gyrus*.

lob′uli glan′dulae mamma′riae [TA], SYN *lobules* of mammary gland, under *lobule*.

lob′uli glan′dulae thyroi′deae [TA], SYN *lobules* of thyroid gland, under *lobule*.

l. grac′ilis, ⋆official alternate term for gracile *lobule*.

l. hep′atis [TA], SYN *lobules* of liver, under *lobule*.

l. paracentra′lis [TA], SYN paracentral *lobule*.

l. paramedianus [TA], SYN gracile *lobule*.

l. parieta′lis infe′rior [TA], SYN inferior parietal *lobule*.

l. parieta′lis supe′rior [TA], SYN superior parietal *lobule*.

l. quadrangula′ris, SYN quadrangular *lobule*.

l. quadra′tus, (1) SYN quadrangular *lobule*; **(2)** SYN precuneus.

l. semiluna′ris infe′rior [TA], SYN inferior semilunar *lobule*.

l. semiluna′ris supe′rior [TA], SYN superior semilunar *lobule*.

l. sim′plex [TA], SYN simple *lobule*.

lob′uli tes′tis [TA], SYN *lobules* of testis, under *lobule*.

lobuli thy′mi [TA], SYN *lobules* of thymus, under *lobule*.

lo·bus, gen. and pl. **lo·bi** (lō′bŭs, lō′bī) [TA]. SYN lobe. [LL. fr. G. *lobos*]

l. ante′rior hypophys′eos [TA], SYN adenohypophysis.

l. appendicula′ris, SYN Riedel *lobe*.

l. azygos pulmonis dextri, SYN azygos *lobe* of right lung.

l. cauda′tus, ⋆official alternate term for posterior hepatic *segment* I.

lobi cer′ebri [TA], the major divisions of the cerebral hemisphere; they include the frontal, parietal, temporal, and occipital lobes, named for the overlying bones of the skull, and the limbic lobe. The insula may also be regarded as a lobe (lobus insularis [TA]) because it is separated from the frontal, parietal, and temporal opercula by the circular sulcus of the insula [TA]. SYN cerebral lobes.

l. cli′vi, obsolete term for the clivus monticuli and the posterior crescentic lobules of the cerebellum, considered as one lobe.

l. dex′ter [TA], SYN right *lobe*.

l. falcifor′mis, SYN cingulate *gyrus*.

l. flocculonodularis [TA], SYN flocculonodular *lobe*.

l. fronta′lis [TA], SYN frontal *lobe* of cerebrum.

lo′bi glan′dulae mamma′riae [TA], SYN *lobes* of mammary gland, under *lobe*.

lo′bi glan′dulae thyroi′deae [TA], SYN *lobes* of thyroid gland, under *lobe*.

l. glandula′ris hypophys′eos, SYN adenohypophysis.

l. hep′atis dex′ter [TA], SYN right *lobe* of liver.

l. hep′atis sinis′ter [TA], SYN left *lobe* of liver.

l. inferior pulmonis dextri et sinistri [TA], SYN inferior *lobe* of (left / right) lung.

l. insula [TA], the area of cerebral cortex located internal to the lateral sulcus and separated from the adjacent frontal, parietal and temporal opercula by the circular sulcus of the insula; composed of short and long gyri separated by the central sulcus of the insula. SEE ALSO insula. SYN insular lobe⋆, l. insularis⋆, insular part, pars insularis.

l. insularis, ⋆official alternate term for l. insula.

l. limbicus [TA], SYN limbic *lobe*.

l. linguifor′mis, SYN Riedel *lobe*.

l. me′dius pro′statae [TA], SYN middle *lobe* of prostate.

l. me′dius pulmo′nis dex′tri [TA], SYN middle *lobe* of right lung.

l. nervo′sus [TA], SYN neurohypophysis.

l. occipita′lis [TA], SYN occipital *lobe* of cerebrum.

l. parieta′lis [TA], SYN parietal *lobe* of cerebrum.

l. poste′rior hypophys′eos, ⋆official alternate term for neurohypophysis; SEE ALSO pituitary *gland*.

l. pro′statae [TA], SYN *lobe* of prostate.

l. pyramida′lis glan′dulae thyroi′deae [TA], SYN pyramidal *lobe* of thyroid gland.

l. quadra′tus, SYN quadrangular *lobule*.

l. rena′lis [TA], SYN kidney *lobes*, under *lobe*.

l. sinis′ter [TA], SYN left *lobe*.

lo

l. supe′rior pulmo′nis (dextri et sinistri) [TA], SYN superior *lobe* of (right/left) lung.

l. tempora′lis [TA], SYN temporal *lobe.*

LOCA Abbreviation for low osmolar contrast *agent.*

lo·cal (lō′kăl). Having reference or confined to a limited part; not general or systemic. [L. *localis,* fr. *locus,* place]

lo·cal·i·za·tion (lō′kăl-i-zā′shŭn). **1.** Limitation to a definite area. **2.** The reference of a sensation to its point of origin. **3.** The determination of the location of a morbid process.

auditory l., in sensory psychology, the naming or pointing to directions from which sounds emanate.

cerebral l., (1) the mapping of the cerebral cortex into areas and the correlation of the various areas with cerebral function. **(2)** determination of the site of a brain lesion on the basis of the signs and symptoms manifested by the patient or by neuroimaging.

germinal l., SYN fate *map.*

radiotherapy l., planning the size and alignment of radiation beams to encompass the neoplasm to be treated.

spatial l., the reference of a visual sensation to a definite locality in space.

stereotaxic l., l. of intracerebral nuclei by coordinates with reference to anatomic landmarks in the brain.

lo·cal·ized (lō′kăl-īzd). Restricted or limited to a definite part.

lo·cant (lō′kant). A number or letter preceding a substituent name in the name of a complex chemical that specifies the position (location) of the substituent on the parent molecule; e.g., 5 in 5-methyluridine, *S* in *S*-adenosylmethionine.

lo·ca·tor (lō′kā-ter, tōr). An instrument or apparatus for finding the position of a foreign object in tissue.

🖻 **lo·chia** (lō′kē-ă). Discharges from the vagina of mucus, blood, and tissue debris, following childbirth. [G. neut. pl. of *lochios,* relating to childbirth, fr. *lochos,* childbirth]

lochia		
name (color)	**composition**	**times (varies for individuals)**
lochia rubra (red)	mainly blood, tissue debris, decidua (occasionally vernix caseosa, lanugo, meconium)	1st–3rd day (first week)
lochia fusca (brownish)	increasing hemolysis, less blood; serous secretion (lymph, leukocytes)	3rd–7th day (second week)
lochia serosa (serous)	leukocytes, decidual cells, cervical mucus	7th–14th day
lochia flava (yellowish)	mainly leukocytes, bacteria, detritus (so-called physiologic endometritis)	2nd–3rd week
lochia alba (grayish)	decline of weekly flow; endometrial epithelializing; clear mucous secretion of uterine glands	3rd (4th) week

l. al′ba, the last discharge no longer tinged with blood.

l. ru′bra, the initial discharge stained with blood.

l. sanguinolen′ta, thick, dark red vaginal discharge seen a few days after delivery.

l. sero′sa, a thin and watery l.

lo·chi·al (lō′kē-ăl). Relating to the lochia.

lo·chi·o·me·tra (lō-kē-ō-mē′tră). Distention of the uterus with retained lochia. [G. *mētra,* womb]

lo·chi·or·rha·gia (lō-kē-ō-rā′jē-ă). SYN lochiorrhea. [lochia + G. *rhēgnymi,* to burst forth]

lo·chi·or·rhea (lō-kē-ō-rē′ă). Profuse flow of the lochia. SYN lochiorrhagia. [lochia + G. *rhoia,* a flow]

lo·ci (lō′sī). Plural of locus.

lock (lok). A device for holding or closing.

English l., articulation of the blades of obstetrical forceps consist-

ing of a socket on the shank at the junction with the handle in a similar socket on the other shank; used in Simpson forceps.

sliding l., a slot on one shank of obstetrical forceps (as in Kjelland forceps) that allows the shanks to move forward and backward independently.

Locke, Frank S., British physiologist, 1871–1949. SEE Cabot-L. *murmur;* L. *solutions,* under *solution;* L.-Ringer *solution.*

lock·jaw (lok′jaw). SYN trismus.

Lockwood, Charles B., English anatomist and surgeon, 1858–1914. SEE L. *ligament.*

LOCM Abbreviation for low osmolar contrast *medium.*

lo·co·mo·tive (lō-kō-mō′tiv). SYN locomotor.

lo·co·mo·tor (lō-kō-mō′ter). Relating to locomotion, or movement from one place to another. SYN locomotive, locomotory. [L. *locus,* place, + L. *moveo,* pp. *motus,* to move]

lo·co·mo·to·ri·al (lō-kō-mō-tō′rē-ăl). Relating to the locomotorium.

lo·co·mo·to·ri·um (lō′kō-mō-tō′rē-ŭm). The locomotor apparatus of the body. [L. *locus,* place, + *motorius,* moving]

lo·co·mo·to·ry (lō-kō-mō′tō-rē). SYN locomotor.

loc·u·lar (lok′ū-lăr). Relating to a loculus.

loc·u·late (lok′ū-lāt). Containing numerous loculi.

loc·u·la·tion (lok-ū-lā′shŭn). **1.** A loculate region in an organ or tissue, or a loculate structure formed between surfaces of organs, mucous or serous membranes, and so on. **2.** The process that results in the formation of a loculus or loculi.

loc·u·lus, pl. **loc·u·li** (lok′ū-lŭs, -lī). A small cavity or chamber. [L. dim. of *locus,* place]

lo·cum ten·ant (lō′kum tĕn′ent). A temporary substitution of one physician by another. SYN locum tenens. [partial anglicization of *locum tenens*]

lo·cum ten·ens (lō′kum tĕn′ens). SYN locum tenant. [L. one holding a place]

lo·cus, pl. **lo·ci** (lō′kŭs, lō′sī). **1.** A place; usually, a specific site. **2.** The position that a gene occupies on a chromosome. **3.** The position of a point, as defined by the coordinates on a graph. [L.]

l. caeru′leus [TA], a shallow depression, of a blue color in the fresh brain, lying laterally in the most rostral portion of the rhomboidal fossa near the cerebral aqueduct; it lies near the lateral wall of the fourth ventricle and consists of about 20,000 melanin-pigmented neuronal cell bodies whose norepinephrine-containing axons have a remarkably wide distribution in the cerebellum as well as in the hypothalamus and cerebral cortex. SYN l. cinereus, l. ferrugineus, substantia ferruginea.

l. cine′reus, SYN l. caeruleus.

cis-acting **l.,** a section of DNA that affects the activity of DNA sequences on that same molecule of DNA.

complex l., a set of closely linked genetic loci with a common function, as in the major histocompatibility complex l.

l. of control, a theoretical construct designed to assess a person's perceived control over his/her own behavior; classified as *internal* if the person feels in control of events, *external* if others are perceived to have that control.

l. ferrugin′eus, SYN l. caeruleus.

genetic l., the set of homologous parts of a pair of chromosomes that may be occupied by allelic genes. The l. thus comprises a pair of locations (except in the X chromosome in males). The concept of a l. is somewhat idealized, not taking into account accidents that may occur in meiosis such as duplication of loci as a result of unequal crossing-over, translocations, inversions, etc.

marker l., a l. on a chromosome or in a stretch of DNA that can be identified (e.g., a restriction fragment length polymorphism) and can serve in linkage analysis and in the isolation of a disease gene. SEE ALSO linkage *marker.*

l. ni′ger, SYN *substantia* nigra.

l. perfora′tus anti′cus, SYN anterior perforated *substance.*

l. perfora′tus posti′cus, SYN posterior perforated *substance.*

sex-linked l., any l. that in normal karyotypes is borne on a heterosome; commonly but incorrectly applied to an X-linked l.

X-linked l., any l. that in normal karyotypes is borne on the X chromosome.

Y-linked l., any (haploid) l. that in normal karyotypes is borne on the Y chromosome. The known content is so far small.

lod score (lod skōr). A number used in genetic linkage studies; logarithm (decadic) of the odds in favor of genetic linkage. [*logarithm* + *odds*]

Loeb, Leo, U.S. pathologist, 1869–1959. SEE L. *deciduoma.*

Loeffler, Friedrich A.J., German bacteriologist and surgeon, 1852–1915. SEE L. *bacillus,* blood culture *medium, stain,* caustic *stain, methylene blue;* Klebs-L. *bacillus;* Loeffler *syndrome* I; Loeffler *syndrome* II.

Loevit, Moritz, Austrian pathologist, 1851–1918. SEE L. *cell.*

Loewenthal, Wilhelm, German physician, 1850–1894. SEE L. *bundle, reaction, tract.*

lo·fen·ta·nil (lō-fen′tă-nil). A potent, long-lasting narcotic and analgesic that is chemically related to fentanyl.

Löffler, Wilhelm, Swiss physician, 1887–1972. SEE L. *disease, endocarditis,* parietal fibroplastic *endocarditis, syndrome.*

⌂**log-.** SEE logo-.

Logan, William H.G., early 20th century U.S. plastic surgeon. SEE L. *bow.*

log·a·rithm (lŏg′ar-ridhm). If a number, *x*, is expressed as a power of another number, *y*, i.e., if $x = y^n$, then n is said to be the logarithm of *x* to base *y*. Common logarithms are to the base 10; natural or Napierian logarithms are to the base e, a mathematical constant. [G. *logos,* word, ratio, + *arithmos,* number]

log·e·tro·nog·ra·phy (log-ĕ-tron-og′ră-fē). A method of photographic printing in which fine details are emphasized by electronic enhancement of their contrast; formerly used for reproducing radiographic images.

⌂**-logia.** **1.** The study of the subject noted in the body of the word, or a treatise on the same; the Eng. equivalent is -logy, or, with a connecting vowel, -ology. [G. *logos,* discourse, treatise] **2.** Collecting or picking. [G. *legō,* to collect]

lo·git (lŏg′it). The logarithm of the ratio of frequencies of two different categorical and mutually exclusive outcomes such as healthy and sick.

⌂**logo-, log-.** Speech, words. [G. *logos,* word, discourse]

log·o·pe·dia (log-ō-pē′dē-ă). SYN logopedics.

log·o·pe·dics (log′ō-pē′diks). A branch of science concerned with the physiology and pathology of the organs of speech and with the correction of speech defects. SYN logopedia. [logo- + G. *pais* (*paid-*), child]

log·or·rhea (log-ō-rē′ă). Rarely used term for abnormal or pathologic talkativeness or garrulousness. [logo- + G. *rhoia,* a flow]

log·o·spasm (log′ō-spazm). **1.** SYN stuttering. **2.** SYN explosive *speech.* [logo- + G. *spasmos,* spasm]

log·o·ther·a·py (log′ō-thār′ă-pē). A form of psychotherapy which places special emphasis on the patient's spiritual life and on the physician as "medical minister." [logo- + G. *therapeia,* cure]

⌂**-logy.** SEE -logia. [G. *logos,* treatise, discourse]

Lohlein-Baehr le·sion. See under lesion.

lo·i·a·sis (lō-ī′ă-sis). A chronic disease caused by the filarial nematode *Loa loa,* with symptoms and signs first occurring approximately 3–4 years after a bite by an infected tabanid fly. When the infective larvae mature, the adult worms move about in an irregular course through the connective tissue of the body (as rapidly as 1 cm per minute), frequently becoming visible beneath the skin and mucous membranes; e.g., in the back, scalp, chest, inner surface of the lip, and especially on the conjunctiva. The worms provoke hyperemia and exudation of fluid, often a host response to the worm products, a Calabar or fugitive swelling which causes no serious damage and subsides as the parasites move on; the patient is annoyed by the "creeping" in the tissues and intense itching, as well as occasional pain, especially when the swelling is in the region of tendons and joints. Most patients have an eosinophilia of 10–30 or 40% in the circulating blood. SYN Calabar swelling, fugitive swelling.

loin (loyn). The part of the side and back between the ribs and the pelvis. SYN lumbus. [Fr. *longe;* E. *lumbus*]

Lok, SEE Luer-Lok *syringe.*

lo·li·ism (lō′li-izm). Poisoning by the seeds of a grass, *Lolium temulentum* (in the form of flour made into bread), characterized by giddiness, tremor, green vision, dilated pupils, prostration, and sometimes vomiting. [L. *lolium,* darnel, tares]

Lombard, Etienne, French physician, 1868–1920. SEE L. voice-reflex *test.*

lo·mus·tine (lō-mŭs′tēn). An antineoplastic agent. SYN CCNU.

Long, John H., U.S. physician, 1856–1927. SEE L. *coefficient, formula.*

long-chain ac·yl-CoA de·hy·dro·gen·ase. SEE *acyl-CoA* dehydrogenase (NADPH).

long-chain fat·ty ac·id-CoA li·gase. Fatty acid thiokinase (long-chain), a ligase forming acyl-CoA, AMP, and pyrophosphate from long-chain fatty acids, ATP, and coenzyme A. SYN acyl-activating enzyme (1), dodecanoyl-CoA synthetase.

lon·gev·i·ty (lon-jev′i-tē). Duration of a particular life beyond the norm for the species. SEE ALSO lifespan. SYN macrobiosis.

lon·gi·tu·di·nal (lon′ji-too′di-năl) [TA]. **1.** Running lengthwise; in the direction of the long axis of the body or any of its parts. SYN longitudinalis [TA]. **2.** Studied over a period of time, diachronic; contrast with cross-sectional or synchronic, which give equivalent results only under certain strict conditions of stability and equilibrium. Strict attention to these conditions is of the greatest importance in the study of survivorship either in demographics or in cell economy (such as the survival pattern of the erythrocytes and platelets). [L. *longitudo,* length]

lon·gi·tu·di·na·lis (lon′ji-too′di-nā′lis) [TA]. SYN longitudinal (1).

lon·gi·type (lon′ji-tūp). SYN ectomorph.

Longmire, William P., Jr., U.S. surgeon, 1913–1977. SEE L. *operation.*

Looney, Joseph M., U.S. biochemist, *1896. SEE Folin-Looney *test.*

loop (loop). **1.** A sharp curve or complete bend in a vessel, cord, or other cylindrical body, forming an oval or circular ring. SEE ALSO ansa. **2.** A wire (usually of platinum or nichrome) fixed into a handle at one end and bent into a circle at the other, rendered sterile by flaming, and used to transfer microorganisms. [M.E. *loupe*]

Biebl l., a continuous l. of small intestine brought through the abdominal wall to a subcutaneous location, for observation of motility.

bulboventricular l., the portion of the early-somite embryonic cardiac tube that evolves into the ventricle and bulbus cordis. SYN ventricular l.

capillary l., small blood vessel in the dermal papillae.

cervical l., SYN ansa *cervicalis.*

cruciform l.'s, a secondary structure of DNA formed by the hydrogen bonding of self-complementary regions.

D l., a structure in replicating circular DNA. SYN displacement l.

displacement l., SYN D l.

gamma l., the reflex arc consisting of small anterior horn cells and neuroma, their small fibers projecting to the intrafusal bundle producing its contraction, which initiates the afferent impulses that pass through the posterior root to the anterior horn cells, inducing a stretch reflex. SYN gamma motor neurons, gamma motor system, Granit l.

Gerdy interatrial l., a muscular fasciculus in the interatrial septum of the heart, passing backward from the atrioventricular groove.

Granit l., SYN gamma l.

hairpin l.'s, single-stranded DNA and RNA can fold back on itself under the proper conditions forming irregular double-helical l.'s.

Henle l., SYN nephronic l.

l. of hypoglossal nerve, SYN ansa *cervicalis.*

Hyrtl l., a communicating l. between the right and left hypoglos-

lo

sal nerves, lying between the geniohyoid and genioglossus muscles or in the substance of the geniohyoid; it is found in about one in ten persons. SYN Hyrtl anastomosis.

lenticular l., the pallidal efferent fibers curving around the medial border of the internal capsule. SYN ansa lenticularis [TA], lenticular ansa.

memory l., an electronic device for retrieving data that had been stored and/or displayed upon the oscilloscope at an earlier time; used for reviewing electrical events immediately preceding a specific disturbance.

Meyer-Archambault l., the fibers of the visual radiation that loop around the tip of the temporal horn.

nephronic l., the U-shaped part of the nephron extending from the proximal to the distal convoluted tubules, consisting of descending and ascending limbs, located in the medulla renalis and medullary ray. SYN Henle ansa, Henle l.

peduncular l., SYN *ansa* peduncularis.

l.'s of spinal nerves, loops of the spinal nerves, connecting ventral primary rami of the spinal nerves. SYN ansae nervorum spinalium.

subclavian l., SYN *ansa* subclavia.

vector l., a smooth or irregular, usually elliptical, curve representing the average direction and magnitude of the heart's action from moment to moment throughout the cardiac cycle. SEE ALSO vector (2), vectorcardiogram.

ventricular l., SYN bulboventricular l.

Vieussens l., SYN *ansa* subclavia.

loos·en·ing of as·so·ci·a·tion. A manifestation of a severe thought disorder characterized by the lack of an obvious connection between one thought or phrase and the next, or with the response to a question.

Looser, Emil, Swiss physician, 1877–1936. SEE L. *zones,* under *zone.*

LOP Abbreviation for left occipitoposterior position.

lop-ear (lop'ēr). Congenital abnormality of the external ear, with poor development of helix and anthelix. SYN bat ear.

lo·per·am·ide hy·dro·chlo·ride (lō-per'ă-mīd). An antiperistaltic agent used to treat diarrhea.

loph·o·dont (lof'ŏ-dont). Having the crowns of the molar teeth formed in transverse or longitudinal crests or ridges, in contrast to bunodont. [G. *lophos,* ridge, + *odous,* tooth]

Lo·phoph·o·ra wil·liam·sii (lō-fof'ŏ-ră wil-yăm'sē-ī). The botanical origin of peyote (mescal button); it contains over a dozen alkaloids, of which mescaline is the most important; others are pellotine, anhalomine, anhalonidine, anhalamine, anhalinine, anhalidine, and lophophorine.

lo·phot·ri·chate (lō-fot'ri-kāt). SYN lophotrichous.

lo·phot·ri·chous (lō-fot'ri-kŭs). Referring to a bacterial cell with two or more flagella at one or both poles. SYN lophotrichate. [G. *lophos,* crest, + *thrix,* hair]

lo·pre·mone (lō'pre-mōn). Former name for protirelin.

Lorain, Paul, French physician, 1827–1875. SEE L. *disease;* L.-Lévi *dwarfism, infantilism, syndrome.*

lor·a·ze·pam (lō-ră'ză-pam). An antianxiety drug of the benzodiazepine group.

lor·cai·nide (lor-kă-nīd). An antiarrhythmic agent used for the treatment of ventricular arrhythmias; much like a cardiac depressant (antiarrhythmic).

lor·do·sco·li·o·sis (lor'dō-skō-lē-ō'sis). Combined backward and lateral curvature of the spine. [G. *lordos,* bent back, + *skoliōsis,* crookedness, fr. *skolios,* bent, aslant]

lor·do·sis (lor-dō'sis) [TA]. An anteriorly convex curvature of the vertebral column; the normal lordoses of the cervical and lumbar regions are secondary curvatures of the vertebral column, acquired postnatally. SYN hollow back, saddle back. [G. *lordōsis,* a bending backward]

cervical l. [TA], the normal, anteriorly convex curvature of the cervical segment of the vertebral column; cervical lordosis is a secondary curvature of the vertebral column, acquired postnatally as the infant lifts its head. SYN l. cervicis [TA], l. colli[*].

l. cervicis [TA], SYN cervical l.

l. colli, [*]official alternate term for cervical l.

l. lumbalis [TA], SYN lumbar l.

lumbar l. [TA], the normal, anteriorly convex curvature of the lumbar segment of the vertebral column; lumbar l. is a secondary curvature of the vertebral column, acquired postnatally as the upright posture is assumed when one learns to walk. SYN l. lumbalis [TA], lumbar flexure.

lor·dot·ic (lōr-dot'ik). Pertaining to or marked by lordosis.

Lorenz, Adolf, Austrian surgeon, 1854–1946. SEE L. *sign.*

Loschmidt, Joseph (Johann), Czech chemist and physicist, 1821–1895. SEE L. *number.*

LOT Abbreviation for left occipitotransverse position.

lo·tion (lō'shŭn). A class of pharmacopeial preparations that are liquid suspensions or dispersions intended for external application; some consist of finely powdered, insoluble solids held in more or less permanent suspension by suspending agents or surface-active agents, or both; others are oil-in-water emulsions stabilized by surface-active agents. [L. *lotio,* a washing, fr. *lavo,* to wash]

Louis, Pierre C.A., French physician, 1787–1872. SEE L. *angle, law.*

Louis-Bar, Denise, mid-20th century French physician. SEE Louis-Bar *syndrome.*

loupe (loop). A magnifying lens. [Fr.]

binocular l., a magnifying device, attached to spectacles or a headband, worn as a visual aid when performing operations on small structures.

louse, pl. **lice** (lows, līs). Common name for members of the ectoparasitic insect orders Anoplura (sucking lice) and Mallophaga (biting lice). Important species are *Felicola subrostrata* (cat l.), *Goniocotes gallinae* (fluff l.), *Goniodes dissimilis* (brown chicken l.), *Haemodipsus ventricosus* (rabbit l.), *Lipeurus caponis* (wing l.), *Menacanthus stramineus* (chicken body l.), *Pthirus pubis* (crab or pubic l.), and *Polyplax serratus* (mouse l.). [A.S. *lūs*]

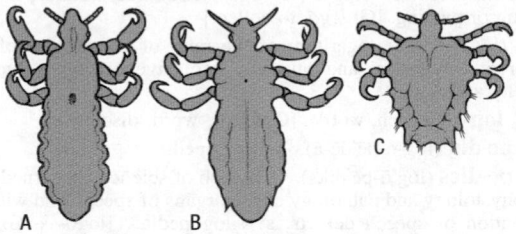

common lice of humans: (A) head louse (*Pediculus humanus capitis*), (B) body louse (*Pediculus humanus humanus*), (C) pubic louse (*Pthirus pubis*)

biting l., chewing l., feather l., ectoparasites (order Mallophaga) chiefly found on birds, where they feed on feathers, hair, epidermal debris, and (less commonly) on blood; they possess nipperlike, heavily sclerotized mandibles and a characteristic broad head; many species are host-specific.

sea l., the very small larvae of the thimble jellyfish (*Linuche unguiculata*).

sucking l., blood-sucking mammalian ectoparasites (order Anoplura), characterized by a narrow head with piercing and sucking mouthparts that lie in a sac concealed in the head.

lousy (low'sē). SYN pediculous.

lo·va·stat·in (lō-vă-stat'in). A cholesterol-lowering agent, isolated from a strain of *Aspergillus terreus,* that reduces both normal and elevated serum cholesterol. SYN mevinolin.

Lovén, Otto C., Swedish physician, 1835–1904. SEE L. *reflex.*

Lovibond, J.L., 20th century English dermatologist. SEE Lovibond *angle,* Lovibond profile *sign.*

Lowe, Charles U., U.S. pediatrician, *1921. SEE L. *syndrome;* L.-Terrey-MacLachlan *syndrome.*

Löwenberg, Benjamin B., French laryngologist, 1836–1905. SEE L. *canal, forceps, scala.*

Lower, SYN inferior. SEE L. *ring, tubercle.*

Lown, Bernard, U.S. cardiologist, *1921. SEE L.-Ganong-Levine *syndrome.*

Lowry, Oliver H., U.S. biochemist, *1910. SEE L.-Folin *assay;* Lowry protein *assay.*

Lowry, R. Brian, 20th century Irish medical geneticist in Canada. SEE Coffin-L. *syndrome.*

Lowsley, Oswald S., U.S. urologist, 1884–1955. SEE L. *tractor.*

lox·a·pine (lok′să-pēn). 2-Chloro-11-(4-methyl-1-piperazinyl)-dibenz[*b,f*][1,4]-oxazepine; a neuroleptic antipsychotic agent used as the succinate and hydrochloride salts.

Lox·os·ce·les (lok-sos′ĕ-lēz). A genus of venomous spiders, the brown spiders, marked by a fiddle-shaped pattern on the cephalothorax, and found chiefly in South America. They inflict a highly ulcerative, spreading dermal lesion at the site of the bite (loxoscelism). Important species include *L. laeta,* the Chilean brown recluse spider; *L. reclusus,* the brown recluse spider of North America; and *L. rufipes,* the Peruvian brown spider. [G. *loxos,* oblique, + *skelos,* leg]

lox·os·ce·lism (lok-sos′ĕ-lizm). A clinical illness produced by the brown recluse spider, *Loxosceles reclusus,* of North America; characterized by gangrenous slough at the site of the bite, nausea, malaise, fever, hemolysis, and thrombocytopenia.

Lox·o·tre·ma ova·tum (lok-sō-trē′mă ō-vā′tŭm). Former name for *Metagonimus yokogawai.* [G. *loxos,* slanting, + *trēma,* a hole; L. *ovatus,* egg-shaped]

loz·enge (loz′enj). SYN troche. [Fr. *losange,* fr. *lozangé,* rhombic]

LPH Abbreviation for lipotropic *hormone.*

L.P.N. Abbreviation for licensed practical *nurse.*

LPO Abbreviation for left posterior oblique, a radiographic projection.

LPS Abbreviation for lipopolysaccharide.

Lr Symbol for lawrencium.

Lr, L$_r$ SEE Lr *dose.*

L.R.C.P. Abbreviation for Licentiate of the Royal College of Physicians (of England).

L.R.C.P.(E) Abbreviation for Licentiate of the Royal College of Physicians (Edinburgh).

L.R.C.P.(I) Abbreviation for Licentiate of the Royal College of Physicians (Ireland).

L.R.C.S. Abbreviation for Licentiate of the Royal College of Surgeons (of England).

L.R.C.S.(E) Abbreviation for Licentiate of the Royal College of Surgeons (Edinburgh).

L.R.C.S.(I) Abbreviation for Licentiate of the Royal College of Surgeons (Ireland).

LRF Abbreviation for luteinizing hormone-releasing *factor.*

L.R.F.P.S. Abbreviation for Licentiate of the Royal Faculty of Physicians and Surgeons, a Scottish institution.

LRH Abbreviation for luteinizing hormone-releasing *hormone.*

LSA Abbreviation for left sacroanterior position.

LSD Abbreviation for *lysergic acid* diethylamide.

LSF Abbreviation for line spread *function.*

LSIL Abbreviation for low-grade squamous intraepithelial *lesion.*

LSP Abbreviation for left sacroposterior position.

LST Abbreviation for left sacrotransverse position.

LT Abbreviation for leukotrienes, usually followed by another letter with a subscript number; e.g., LTA$_4$, LTC$_4$.

LTM Abbreviation for long-term *memory.*

LTP Abbreviation for laser *trabeculoplasty.*

LTR Abbreviation for long terminal repeat *sequences,* under *sequence.*

Lu Symbol for lutetium.

Lubarsch, Otto, German pathologist, 1860–1933. SEE L. *crystals,* under *crystal.*

Luc, Henri, French laryngologist, 1855–1925. SEE L. *operation;* Caldwell-L. *operation;* Ogston-L. *operation.*

lu·can·thone hy·dro·chlo·ride (loo-kan′thŏn). Used in the treatment of urinary schistosomiasis (*Schistosoma haematobium*) and intestinal schistosomiasis (*S. mansoni*).

Lucas, Richard C., English anatomist and surgeon, 1846–1915. SEE L. *groove.*

lu·cen·so·my·cin (loo-sen-sō-mī′sin). An antibiotic isolated from cultures of *Streptomyces lucensis;* an antifungal agent. SYN lucimycin.

lu·cent (loo′sent). Bright; clear; translucent. [L. *luceo,* to shine]

lu·cid (loo′sid). Clear, not obscured or confused, as in a l. moment or l. spoken expression. [L. *lucidus,* clear]

lu·cid·i·fi·ca·tion (loo-sid′i-fi-kā′shŭn). SYN clarification. [L. *lucidus,* clear, + *facio,* to make]

lu·cid·i·ty (loo-sid′i-tē). The quality or state of being lucid.

lu·cif·er·as·es (loo-sif′er-ās-ĕz). Enzymes present in certain luminous organisms that act to bring about the oxidation of luciferins; energy produced in the process is liberated as bioluminescence; such enzymes can be used to detect very low concentrations of metabolites.

lu·cif·er·ins (loo-sif′er-inz). Chemical substances present in certain luminous organisms that, when acted upon by luciferases, produce bioluminescence. [L. *lux,* light + *fero.* to bear]

lu·cif·u·gal (loo-sif′ū-găl). Avoiding light. [L. *lux,* light, + *fugio,* to flee from]

Lu·cil·ia (loo-sil′ē-ă). A genus of scavenging blowflies (family Calliphoridae), commonly called bluebottle or greenbottle flies, whose larvae feed on carrion or excrement; they occasionally cause wound infestation or myiasis.

L. cae′sar, a species whose larvae formerly were used in the treatment of septic wounds. SEE ALSO *Phormia regina.*

L. illus′tris, a metallic blue-green blowfly widely distributed in North America; the eggs are deposited chiefly on animal carcasses.

L. serica′ta, SYN *Phaenicia sericata.*

lu·ci·my·cin (loo-si-mī′sin). SYN lucensomycin.

Lucio, R., Mexican physician, 1819–1866. SEE L. *leprosy;* Lucio leprosy *phenomenon.*

lu·cip·e·tal (loo-sip′i-tăl). Seeking light. [L. *lux,* light, + *peto,* to seek]

Lucké, Balduin, U.S. pathologist, 1889–1954. SEE L. *virus.*

Lücke, George A., German surgeon, 1829–1894. SEE L. *test.*

lüc·ken·schä·del (luk-en-shā′dl). Craniolacunia with meningocele or encephalocele. [Ger. *Lücke,* gap + *Schädel,* skull]

Ludwig, Daniel, German anatomist, 1625–1680. SEE L. *angle.*

Ludwig, Karl F.W., German anatomist and physiologist, 1816–1895. SEE depressor *nerve* of L.; L. *ganglion, labyrinth, nerve, stromuhr.*

Ludwig, Kurt, German anatomist, *1922. SEE Klinger-L. acid-thionin *stain* for sex chromatin.

Ludwig, Wilhelm Friedrich von, German surgeon, 1790–1865. SEE L. *angina.*

Luebering, J. SEE Rapoport-Luebering *shunt.*

Luer, German instrument maker, †1883. SEE L. *syringe;* L.-Lok *syringe.*

lu·es (loo′ēz). A plague or pestilence; specifically, syphilis. [L. pestilence]

l. vene′rea, SYN syphilis.

lu·et·ic (loo-et′ik). SYN syphilitic.

Luft, John H., U.S. histologist, *1927. SEE L. potassium permanganate *fixative.*

Luft, Rolf, Swedish endocrinologist, *1914. SEE L. *disease.*

Lugol, Jean G.A., French physician, 1786–1851. SEE Lugol iodine *solution.*

Lukes, L.J., 20th century U.S. pathologist. SEE L.-Collins *classification.*

Lukes-Collins clas·si·fi·ca·tion. See under classification.

LUL Abbreviation for left upper lobe (of lung).

lu·lib·er·in (loo-lib′er-in). A decapeptide hormone from the hypothalamus that stimulates the anterior pituitary to release both follicle-stimulating hormone and luteinizing hormone; gonadotropin-releasing hormone. SYN luteinizing hormone-releasing hormone. [*luteinizing hormone* + L. *libero*, to free, + *-in*]

lum·ba·go (lŭm-bā′gō). Pain in mid and lower back; a descriptive term not specifying cause. [L. fr. *lumbus*, loin]

ischemic l., an ischemic form of backache characterized by a painful cramp of the muscles in the lumbar region incited by the exertion of walking or standing and promptly relieved by rest.

lum·bar (lŭm′bar). Relating to the loins, or the part of the back and sides between the ribs and the pelvis. [L. *lumbus*, a loin]

lum·bar·i·za·tion (lŭm′bar-i-zā′shŭn). A congenital anomaly of the lumbosacral junction characterized by development of the first sacral vertebra as a lumbar vertebra, resulting in six lumbar vertebrae instead of five.

lum·bi (lŭm′bī). Plural of lumbus. [L.]

lum·bo·ab·dom·i·nal (lŭm′bō-ab-dom′i-năl). Relating to the sides and front of the abdomen.

lum·bo·cos·tal (lŭm′bō-kos′tăl). 1. Relating to the lumbar and the hypochondriac regions. 2. Relating to the lumbar vertebrae and the ribs; denoting a ligament connecting the first lumbar vertebra with the neck of the twelfth rib. [L. *lumbus*, loin, + *costa*, rib]

lum·bo·il·i·ac (lŭm-bō-il′ē-ak). SYN lumboinguinal.

lum·bo·in·gui·nal (lŭm′bō-ing′gwi-năl). Relating to the lumbar and the inguinal regions. SYN lumboiliac. [L. *lumbus*, loin, + *inguen* (*inguin-*), groin]

lum·bo·ova·ri·an (lŭm-bō-ō-vā′rē-an). Relating to the ovary and the lumbar regions.

lum·bo·sa·cral (lŭm′bō-sā′krăl). Relating to the lumbar vertebrae and the sacrum. SYN sacrolumbar.

lum·bri·cal (lŭm′bri-kăl). SYN lumbricoid (1). [L. *lumbricus*, earthworm]

lum·bri·ca·lis. SEE lumbricals (lumbrical *muscles*) of hand, under *muscle*, lumbricals (lumbrical *muscles*) of foot, under *muscle*.

lum·bri·ci·dal (lŭm-bri-sī′dăl). Destructive to lumbricoid (intestinal) worms.

lum·bri·cide (lŭm′bri-sīd). An agent that kills lumbricoid (intestinal) worms. [L. *lumbricus*, worm, + *caedo*, to kill]

lum·bri·coid (lŭm′bri-koyd). 1. Denoting or resembling a roundworm, especially *Ascaris lumbricoides*. SYN lumbrical, lumbricus (1). SEE ALSO scolecoid (2), vermiform. 2. Obsolete common name for *Ascaris lumbricoides*. [L. *lumbricus*, earthworm, + G. *eidos*, resemblance]

lum·bri·co·sis (lŭm′bri-kō′sis). Infection with round intestinal worms.

lum·bri·cus (lŭm′bri-kŭs). 1. SYN lumbricoid (1). 2. Obsolete name for *Ascaris lumbricoides*. [L. earthworm]

lum·bus, gen. and pl. **lum·bi** (lŭm′bŭs, -bī). SYN loin. [L.]

lu·men, pl. **lu·mi·na**, **lu·mens** (loo′men, -min-ă, -menz). 1. The space in the interior of a tubular structure, such as an artery or the intestine. 2 (lm). The unit of luminous flux; the luminous flux emitted in a unit solid angle of 1 steradian by a uniform point source of light having a luminous intensity of 1 candela. 3. The volume enclosed within the membranes of a mitochondrion or of the endoplasmic reticulum. 4. The bore of a catheter or hollow needle. [L. light, window]

false l., in a dissecting aneurysm, the abnormal channel within the wall of the involved artery.

residual l., SYN residual *cleft*.

true l., in a dissecting aneurysm, the channel representing the actual intima-lined artery.

lu·mi·chrome (loo′mi-krōm). 7,8-Dimethylalloxazine; riboflavin minus its ribityl side chain; produced by ultraviolet irradiation of riboflavin in acid solution.

lu·mi·fla·vin (loo′mi-flā-vin). 7,8,10-Trimethylisoalloxazine; a yellow photoderivative of riboflavin, bearing a methyl group in place of the ribityl; produced by ultraviolet irradiation of riboflavin in alkaline solution.

lu·mi·na (loo′mi-nă). Plural of lumen. [L.]

lu·mi·nal (loo′mi-năl) [TA]. Relating to the lumen of a blood vessel or other tubular structure. SYN luminalis [TA].

luminalis [TA]. SYN luminal.

lu·mi·nance (loo′mi-năns). The brightness of an object, expressed as the luminous flux per unit solid angle per unit projected area, measured in lamberts or in candelas per square meter. [L. *lumino*, to light up, fr. *lumen*, light]

lu·mi·nes·cence (loo-mi-nes′ens). Emission of light from a body as a result of a chemical reaction. SEE bioluminescence. [L. *lumen*, light]

lu·mi·nif·er·ous (loo-mi-nif′er-ŭs). Producing or conveying light. [L. *lumen*, light, + *fero*, to carry]

lu·mi·no·phore (loo′mi-nō-fōr). An atom or atomic grouping in an organic compound that increases its ability to emit light. [L. *lumen*, light, + G. *phoros*, bearing]

lu·mi·nous (loo′mi-nŭs). Emitting light, with or without accompanying heat. [L. *lumen*, light]

lu·mi·rho·dop·sin (loo′mi-rō-dop′sin). An intermediate between rhodopsin and all-*trans*-retinal plus opsin during bleaching of rhodopsin by light; formed from bathorhodopsin and converted to metarhodopsin I with a half-life of about 20 μs. [L. *lumen*, light, + G. *rhodon*, rose, + *opsis*, vision]

lum·is·ter·ol (loom-ē-stēr′ol). 1. A by-product in ergocalciferol biosynthesis. 2. A phosphorylated derivative of ribulose that is an intermediate in the pentose monophosphate shunt.

lump·ec·to·my (lŭm-pek′tō-mē). Removal of either a benign or malignant lesion from the breast with preservation of essential anatomy of the breast; tylectomy involving breast tissue. [lump + G. *ektomē*, excision]

Luna, Lee G., 20th century U.S. medical technologist. SEE L.-Ishak *stain*.

lu·na·cy (loo′nă-sē). 1. An obsolete term for a form of insanity characterized by alternating lucid and insane periods, believed to be influenced by phases of the moon. 2. Any form of insanity. 3. Insanity as defined variously by law. [L. *luna*, moon]

lu·nar (loo′ner). 1. Relating to the moon or to a month. 2. Resembling the moon in shape, especially a half moon. SYN lunate (1) [TA], semilunar. SEE ALSO crescentic. 3. Relating to silver (the moon was the symbol of silver in alchemy). [L. *luna*, moon]

lunar caustic. SYN toughened *silver* nitrate.

lu·na·re (loo-nā′rē). SYN lunate (*bone*).

lu·nate (loo′nāt) [TA]. 1. SYN lunar (2). 2. Relating to the lunate bone.

lu·na·tic (loo′nă-tik). Obsolete term for a mentally ill person. [see lunacy]

lu·na·to·ma·la·cia (loo-nā′tō-mă-lā′shē-ă). SYN Kienböck *disease*.

lung (lŭng) [TA]. One of a pair of viscera occupying the pulmonary cavities of the thorax, the organs of respiration in which aeration of the blood takes place. In humans, the right l. is slightly larger than the left and is divided into three lobes (an upper, a middle, and a lower or basal), while the left has but two lobes (an upper and a lower or basal). Each l. is irregularly conical in shape, presenting a blunt upper extremity (the apex), a concave base following the curve of the diaphragm, an outer convex surface (costal surface), a generally concave inner or medial surface (mediastinal surface), a thin and sharp anterior border, and a rounded posterior border. SYN pulmo [TA]. [A.S. *lungen*]

air-conditioner l., an extrinsic allergic alveolitis caused by forced air contaminated by thermophilic actinomycetes and other organisms.

bird-breeder's l., **bird-fancier's l.**, extrinsic allergic alveolitis caused by inhalation of particulate avian emanations; sometimes specified by avian species, e.g., pigeon-breeder's l., budgerigar-breeder's l. SYN bird-breeder's disease.

black l., a form of pneumoconiosis, common in coal miners, characterized by deposits of carbon particles in the l. SYN miner's l. (2).

brown l., obstructive airway disease with asthma produced by exposure to cotton dust, flax, or hemp. SEE ALSO byssinosis.

butterfly l., hemorrhagic markings appearing on an animal's l. after inoculation with *Leptospira interrogans* (*L. icterohaemorrhagiae*).

cardiac l., disturbance in pulmonary anatomy and physiology secondary to valvular disease of the heart or to other disturbances of circulation incident to cardiac disease.

cheese worker's l., extrinsic allergic alveolitis caused by inhalation of spores of *Penicillium casei* from moldy cheese.

collier l., SYN anthracosis.

cystic l., SYN honeycomb l.

endstage l., severe diffuse interstitial fibrosis and honeycombing.

farmer's l., a hypersensitivity pneumonitis characterized by fever and dyspnea, caused by inhalation of organic dust from moldy

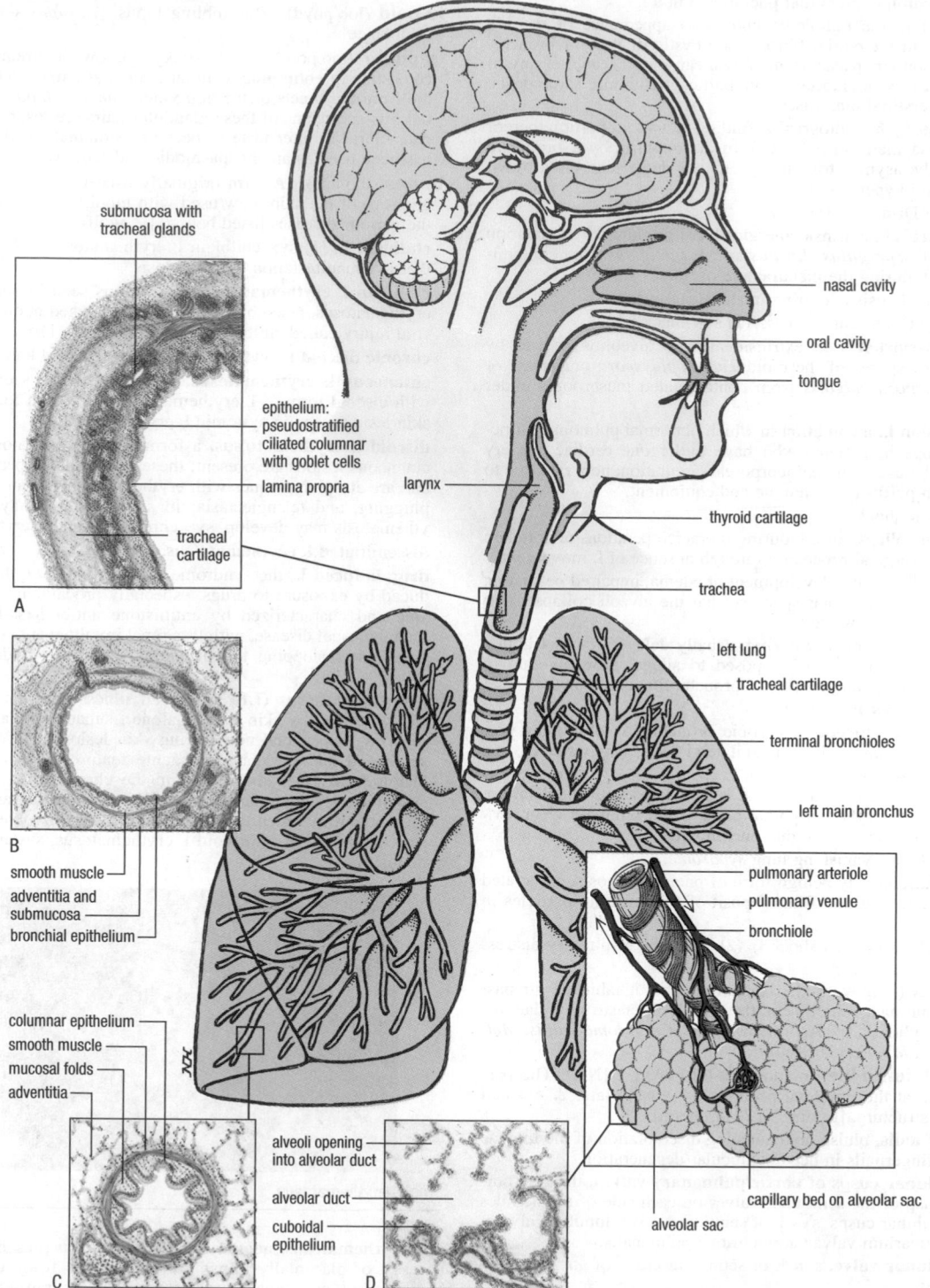

submucosa with tracheal glands

epithelium: pseudostratified ciliated columnar with goblet cells

lamina propria

tracheal cartilage

A

smooth muscle
adventitia and submucosa
bronchial epithelium

B

columnar epithelium
smooth muscle
mucosal folds
adventitia

alveoli opening into alveolar duct

alveolar duct

cuboidal epithelium

C   D

nasal cavity

oral cavity

tongue

larynx

thyroid cartilage

trachea

left lung

tracheal cartilage

terminal bronchioles

left main bronchus

pulmonary arteriole
pulmonary venule
bronchiole

capillary bed on alveolar sac

alveolar sac

lungs and respiratory anatomy: (A) trachea (panoramic, transverse section); (B) intrapulmonary bronchus; (C) terminal bronchiole; (D) respiratory bronchiole with alveoli

lu

hay containing spores of thermophilic actinomycetes such as *Micromonospora vulgaris*, *M. faeni*, and *Thermopolyspora polyspora*, which thrive in the elevated temperatures of hay lofts and silos; repeated exposure may result in alveolar sensitization and, ultimately, granulomatous lung disease with severe disability. SYN thresher's l.

fibroid l., chronic interstitial pneumonia in a l.

honeycomb l., the radiologic and gross appearance of the l.'s resulting from interstitial fibrosis and cystic dilation of bronchioles and distal air spaces; of unknown cause or a sequel of any of several diseases, including eosinophilic granuloma, sarcoidosis, and any interstitial lung disease. SYN cystic l.

hyperlucent l., the radiographic finding that a l. or portion thereof is less dense than normal, as from air trapping by a bronchial foreign body, asymmetric emphysema, or decreasing blood flow. SEE unilateral hyperlucent l.

iron l., SYN Drinker *respirator.*

malt-worker's l., extrinsic allergic alveolitis caused by inhalation of spores of *Aspergillus clavatus* and *A. fumigatus* from contaminated barley during the manufacture of beer.

mason's l., silicosis occurring in stone masons.

miner's l., (1) SYN anthracosis; **(2)** SYN black l.

mushroom-worker's l., extrinsic allergic alveolitis caused by inhalation of spores of the mold *Thermopolyspora polyspora* or *Micromonospora vulgaris* from contaminated mushrooms under cultivation.

postperfusion l., a condition in which abnormal pulmonary function develops in patients who have undergone cardiac surgery involving the use of an extracorporeal circulation; now rare due to advances in perfusion technique and equipment.

pump l., SYN shock l.

quiet l., the collapse of a l. during thoracic operations undertaken to facilitate surgical procedure through absence of l. movement.

shock l., in shock, the development of edema, impaired perfusion, and reduction in alveolar space so that the alveoli collapse. SYN pump l., wet l. (1), white l.

silo-filler's l., pulmonary *edema*, usually delayed for 1–4 hours, occurring in an individual exposed to silage, probably due to nitrogen dioxide; can progress to bronchiolitis obliterans.

thresher's l., SYN farmer's l.

unilateral hyperlucent l., chronic bronchiolitis obliterans predominating on one side. SEE unilateral lobar *emphysema;* SEE ALSO Swyer-James *syndrome* (2).

uremic l., perihilar edema of the l. associated with renal failure and hypertension; the peripheral parts of the l. remain clear. SYN uremic pneumonia (1), uremic pneumonitis.

vanishing l., SEE vanishing lung *syndrome.*

welder's l., relatively benign form of pneumoconiosis, associated with welding, resulting from deposit of fine metallic particles in the l.

wet l., white l., (1) SYN shock l; **(2)** SYN adult respiratory distress *syndrome.*

lung·worms (lŭng'wermz). Nematodes that inhabit the air passages of animals, chiefly in the family Metastrongylidae (or Protostrongylidae). SEE *Aelurostrongylus, Crenosoma vulpis, Metastrongylus, Muellerius capillaris.*

lu·nu·la, pl. **lu·nu·lae** (loo'noo-lă, -lē) [TA]. **1** [NA]. The pale arched area at the proximal portion of the nail plate. **2.** A small semilunar structure. [L. dim. of *luna,* moon]

azure l. of nails, bluish nonblanching discoloration of the lunulae of all the fingernails in hepatolenticular degeneration.

l. of semilunar cusps of aortic/pulmonary valves, the free border of a cusp of the semilunar valves on each side of the nodules of the semilunar cusps. SYN l. of semilunar valve, lunulae valvularum semilunarium valvae aortae/trunci pulmonalis.

l. of semilunar valve, SYN l. of semilunar cusps of aortic/pulmonary valves.

l. unguis, SYN *lunule* of nail.

lunulae valvularum semilunarium valvae aortae/trunci pulmonalis, SYN l. of semilunar cusps of aortic/pulmonary valves.

lunule. 1 [TA]. SYN l. of nail. **2.** A small semilunar structure.

l. of nail, the pale arched area at the proximal portion of the nail plate. SYN arcus unguium, half-moon, lunula unguis, lunule (1), selene unguium.

lu·pin·i·dine (loo-pin'i-dēn). SYN sparteine.

lu·pi·no·sis (loo-pi-nō'sis). SYN lathyrism. [L. *lupinus,* lupine, fr. *lupus,* wolf]

lu·poid (loo'poyd). Resembling lupus. [L. *lupus* + G. *eidos,* resemblance]

lu·pu·lin (loo'poo-lin). A sticky, yellowish, granular material consisting of entire multicellular glandular hairs (trichomes) from the fruit and bracts of the hop vine, *Humulus lupulus;* the essential oils and resins of these glandular hairs are responsible for the characteristic bitter taste of beer or medicinals made from hops; has been used as an antispasmodic and sedative. SYN humulin.

lu·pus (loo'pŭs). A term originally used to depict erosion (as if gnawed) of the skin, now used with modifying terms designating the various diseases listed below. [L. wolf]

chilblain l., (1) SYN chilblain l. erythematosus; **(2)** lupus pernio that is a manifestation of sarcoidosis.

chilblain l. erythematosus, skin lesions seen in patients with l. erythematosus, resembling the small, hardened nodular areas of a cold injury called chilblains. SYN chilblain l. (1).

chronic discoid l. erythemato'sus, SYN discoid l. erythematosus.

cutaneous l. erythematosus, (1) skin disease seen in patients with discoid form of l. erythematosus; **(2)** a term for a variety of skin lesions seen in systemic l. erythematosus.

discoid l. erythemato'sus, a form of l. erythematosus in which cutaneous lesions are present; these commonly appear on the face and are atrophic plaques with erythema, hyperkeratosis, follicular plugging, and telangiectasia; in some instances systemic l. erythematosis may develop. SYN chronic discoid l. erythematosus.

disseminated l. erythemato'sus, SYN systemic l. erythematosus.

drug-induced l., the syndrome of systemic l. erythematosus induced by exposure to drugs, especially procainamide or hydralazine and characterized by antihistone antibodies. More benign than the usual disease, with less renal involvement. The syndrome clears after stopping the offending drug. SYN hydralazine syndrome.

l. erythemato'sus (LE, L.E.), an illness that may be chronic (characterized by skin lesions alone), subacute (characterized by recurring superficial nonscarring skin lesions that are more disseminated and present more acute features both clinically and histologically than those seen in the chronic discoid phase), or systemic or disseminated (in which antinuclear antibodies are present and in which there is almost always involvement of vital structures). SEE ALSO discoid l. erythematosus, systemic l. erythematosus.

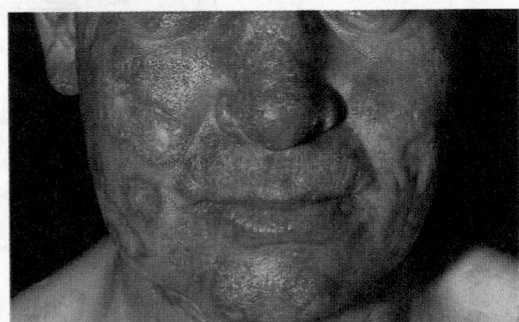

lupus erythematosus

l. erythematosus, neonatal, l. erythematosus present at birth as a result of placentally transmitted antibodies from a mother with systemic l. erythematosus; characterized by transient hematopoietic and cutaneous lesions and permanent cardiac abnormalities.

l. erythemato'sus profun'dus, a subcutaneous panniculitis with marked lymphocyte infiltration of fat lobules giving rise to deep-seated, firm, rubbery nodules that sometimes become ulcerated, usually of the face; may occur in systemic and localized l. erythematosus. SYN l. profundus.

l. livedo, persistent cyanotic lesions on the extremities, associated with the cutaneous manifestations of Raynaud disease.

l. milia′ris dissemina′tus facie′i, a milletlike papular eruption of the face associated with a (histopathologically) tuberculoid perifollicular infiltration but probably related to rosacea rather than tuberculous infection.

neonatal l., l. erythematosus occurring in newborn children of mothers who had lupus during pregnancy; anti-SSA antibodies usually should be screened for; 50% have anti-nuclear antibodies. A variety of skin lesions are seen, which can resolve or leave scarring; the syndrome usually resolves; however, cardiac manifestations can be fatal. Some children develop systemic lupus later in life.

l. per′nio, chronic indurated purple granulomatous skin of sarcoidosis lesion, clinically resembling frostbite, involving ears, cheeks, nose, lips, and forehead; usually with intrathoracic sarcoidosis.

l. profundus (prō-fŭn′dŭs), SYN l. erythematosus profundus. [L. deep]

l. serpigino′sus, a cutaneous tuberculous lesion that spreads peripherally, healing centrally with scar formation.

systemic l. erythemato′sus (SLE), an inflammatory connective tissue disease with variable features, frequently including fever, weakness and fatigability, joint pains or arthritis resembling rheumatoid arthritis, diffuse erythematous skin lesions on the face, neck, or upper extremities, with liquefaction degeneration of the basal layer and epidermal atrophy, lymphadenopathy, pleurisy or pericarditis, glomerular lesions, anemia, hyperglobulinemia, and a positive LE cell test, with serum antibodies to nuclear protein and sometimes to double-stranded DNA and other substances. SYN disseminated l. erythematosus.

l. vulga′ris, cutaneous tuberculosis with characteristic nodular lesions on the face, particularly about the nose and ears.

LUQ Abbreviation for left upper quadrant (of abdomen).

lu·ra (loo′ră). The contracted termination of the infundibulum of the brain. [L. the mouth of a bottle]

lu·ral (loo′răl). Pertaining to the lura.

Luschka, Hubert, German anatomist, 1820–1875. SEE L. *bursa, cartilage, ducts,* under *duct, gland,* cystic *glands,* under *gland, joints,* under *joint, ligaments,* under *ligament, sinus, tonsil; foramen* of L.

Luse, Sarah A., U.S. physician, 1918–1970. SEE L. *bodies,* under *body.*

lus·i·tropic (loos-ē-trō′pik). Relating to lusitropy.

lus·it·ropy (loos-it′trō-pē). Relaxation functions of cardiac muscle and chambers.

lute (loot). To seal or fasten with wax or cement. [L. *lutum,* mud]

lu·te·al (loo′tē-ăl). Relating to the corpus luteum; l. cells, l. hormone, etc. SYN luteus. [L. *luteus,* saffron-yellow]

lu·te·ci·um (loo-tē′sē-ŭm). SYN lutetium.

lu·te·in (loo′tē-in). **1.** The yellow pigment in the corpus luteum, in the yolk of eggs, or any lipochrome. **2.** SYN xanthophyll. **3.** The dried powdered corpora lutea of the hog, formerly used as a progesterone source. [L. *luteus,* saffron-yellow]

lu·te·in·i·za·tion (loo′tē-in-i-zā′shŭn). Transformation of the mature ovarian follicle and its theca interna into a corpus luteum after ovulation; formation of luteal tissue, which appears yellow in some species.

lu·te·i·nize (loo′tē-ĭ-nīz). To form luteal tissue.

lu·te·i·no·ma (loo′tē-i-nō′mă). SYN luteoma.

Lutembacher, René, French cardiologist, 1887–1916. SEE L. *syndrome.*

lu·te·o·gen·ic (loo′tē-ō-jen′ik). Luteinizing; inducing the production or growth of corpora lutea.

lu·te·o·hor·mone (loo′tē-ō-hōr′mōn). SYN progesterone.

lu·te·ol, lu·te·ole (loo′tē-ol, -ōl). SYN xanthophyll.

lu·te·o·lin (loo-tē-ō′lin). The aglycon of galuteolin and cynaroside. SYN cyanidenon.

lu·te·ol·y·sin (loo-tē-ol′i-sin). Any agent, natural or compounded, that destroys the function of the corpus luteum. [L. *luteus,* saffron-yellow, + G. *lysis,* dissolution]

lu·te·ol·y·sis (loo-tē-ol′i-sis). Degeneration or destruction of ovarian luteinized tissue.

lu·te·o·lyt·ic (loo-tē-ō-lit′ik). Promoting or characteristic of luteolysis.

lu·te·o·ma (loo-tē-ō′mă). An ovarian tumor of granulosa or thecalutein cell origin, producing progesterone effects on the uterine mucosa. SYN luteinoma.

pregnancy l., a benign lutein cell tumor of the ovary.

lu·te·o·tro·pic, lu·te·o·tro·phic (loo′tē-ō-trop′ik, -trof′ik). Having a stimulating action on the development and function of the corpus luteum.

lu·te·ti·um (Lu) (loo-tē′shē-ŭm). A rare earth element; atomic no. 71, atomic wt. 174.967. SYN lutecium. [L. *Lutetia,* Paris]

lu·te·us (loo-tē′ŭs). SYN luteal. [L.]

Lu·ther·an Blood Group, Lu Blood Group. See Blood Groups Appendix.

lu·tro·pin (loo′trō-pin). One of two glycoprotein hormones that stimulate the final ripening of the follicles and the secretion of progesterone by them, their rupture to release the egg, and the conversion of the ruptured follicle into the corpus luteum. SYN interstitial cell-stimulating hormone, luteinizing hormone, luteinizing principle.

lu·tu·trin (loo′too-trin). A water-soluble protein-like fraction extracted from the corpus luteum of sows' ovaries, resembling relaxin; it causes uterine relaxation and is used in dysmenorrhea.

Lutz, Alfredo, Brazilian physician, 1855–1940. SEE L.-Splendore-Almeida *disease.*

Lutz·o·my·ia (loot-zō-mī′ă). A genus of New World sandflies or bloodsucking midges (family Psychodidae) that serve as vectors of leishmaniasis and Oroyo fever; formerly combined with the Old World sandfly genus *Phlebotomus.*

L. flaviscutella′ta, a sandfly species that is a vector of *Leishmania mexicana,* the agent of chiclero ulcer. SYN *Phlebotomus flaviscutellatus.*

L. interme′dius, one of a group of sandfly species that are vectors of *Leishmania braziliensis,* the agent of espundia.

L. longipal′pis, SYN *Phlebotomus longipalpis.*

L. peruen′sis, a sandfly species that is a vector of *Leishmania peruviana,* the agent of uta.

lux (lx) (lŭks). A unit of light or illumination; the reception of a luminous flux of 1 lumen per square meter of surface. SYN candlemeter, meter-candle. [L. light]

lux·a·tio (lŭk-sā′shē-ō). SEE luxation. [L. *luxo,* pp. *-atus,* to dislocate]

l. erec′ta, subglenoid dislocation of the head of the humerus in which the arm is raised and abducted and cannot be lowered.

l. perinea′lis, a condition in which the head of the femur is dislocated to the perineum.

lux·a·tion (lŭk-sā′shŭn). **1.** SYN dislocation. **2.** In dentistry, the dislocation or displacement of the condyle in the temporomandibular fossa, or of a tooth from the alveolus. [L. *luxatio*]

Malgaigne l., SYN nursemaid's *elbow.*

Lux·ol fast blue. Name for a group of closely related copper phthalocyanin dyes used as stains (with PAS, PTAH, hematoxylin, silver nitrate, etc.) for myelin in nerve fibers.

lux·us (lŭks′ŭs). Excess of any sort. [L. extravagance, luxury]

Luys, Jules Bernard, French physician, 1828–1897. SEE L. *body;* centre médian de L.; *corpus* luysi; *nucleus* of L.

LVET Abbreviation for left ventricular ejection *time.*

L.V.N. Abbreviation for licensed vocational *nurse.*

Lw Former symbol for lawrencium.

lx Abbreviation for lux.

ly·ase (lī′ās). Class name for those enzymes removing groups nonhydrolytically (EC class 4); prefixes such as "hydro-" and "ammonia-" are used to indicate the type of reaction. Trivial names for lyases include synthases, decarboxylases, aldolases, dehydratases. Cf. synthase, synthetase.

ly

ly·can·thro·py (lī-kan′thrō-pē). The morbid delusion that one is a wolf, possibly a mental atavism of the werewolf superstition. [G. *lykos,* wolf, + *anthrōpos,* man]

ly·coc·to·nine (lī-kok′tō-nēn). An alkaloid, $C_{25}H_{41}NO_7$, obtained from *Aconitum lycoctonum,* an exceedingly poisonous species of aconite; it also occurs in other species of *Aconitum* and *Delphinium.*

ly·co·pene (lī′kō-pēn). Ψ,Ψ-Carotene; the characteristic red pigment of the tomato that may be considered chemically as the parent substance from which all natural carotenoid pigments are derived; an unsaturated hydrocarbon made up of eight isoprene units, two of them hydrogenated, with 11 conjugated double bonds.

ly·co·pe·ne·mia (lī′kō-pě-nē′mē-ă). A condition in which there is a high concentration of lycopene in the blood, producing carotenoidlike yellowish pigmentation of the skin; found in people who consume excessive amounts of tomatoes or tomato juice, or lycopene-containing fruits and berries. [lycopene + G. *haima,* blood]

Ly·co·per·don (līkō-per′don). A genus of fungi (family Lycoperdaceae), some species of which have been used medicinally, e.g., in folk medicine, by nasal inhalation to treat epistaxis. The spores of *L. bovista* (*L. gemmatum, L. caelatum*) and of *L. pyriforme* may rarely produce lycoperdonosis. SYN puffball. [G. *lykos,* wolf, + *perdomai,* to break wind]

ly·co·per·do·no·sis (lī′kō-per-don-ō′sis). A persisting pneumonitis following inhalation of spores of the puffballs *Lycoperdon pyriforme* and *L. bovista.*

ly·coph·o·ra (lī-kof′ō-ră). The 10-hooked larva of primitive tapeworms of the subclass Cestodaria.

ly·co·po·di·um (lī-kō-pō′dē-ŭm). The spores of *Lycopodium clavatum* (family Lycopodiaceae) and other species of *L.;* a yellow, tasteless, and odorless powder; was used as a dusting powder and in pharmacy to prevent the agglutination of pills in a box. SYN club moss, vegetable sulfur. [G. *lykos,* wolf, + *pous,* foot]

lye (lī). The liquid obtained by leaching wood ashes. SEE *potassium* hydroxide, *sodium* hydroxide. SYN lixivium. [A.S. *leáh*]

Lyell, Aian. SEE L. *disease, syndrome.*

Lym·naea (lim-nē′ă). A genus of snails, species of which are invertebrate hosts for the liver or sheep liver fluke, *Fasciola hepatica,* and other trematodes. [G. *limnē,* marsh]

lymph (limf) [TA]. A clear, transparent, sometimes faintly yellow and slightly opalescent fluid that is collected from the tissues throughout the body, flows in the lymphatic vessels (through the l. nodes), and is eventually added to the venous blood circulation. L. consists of a clear liquid portion, varying numbers of white blood cells (chiefly lymphocytes), and a few red blood cells. SYN lympha [TA]. [L. *lympha,* clear spring water]

aplastic l., l. containing a relatively large number of leukocytes, but comparatively little fibrinogen; such l. does not form a good clot and manifests only a slight tendency to become organized. SYN corpuscular l.

blood l., l. exuded from the blood vessels and not derived from the fluid in the tissue spaces.

corpuscular l., SYN aplastic l.

croupous l., a form of inflammatory l. with an unusually large content of fibrinogen; as a result of the fibrin that is formed in relatively dense mats, a pseudomembrane is likely to be produced.

dental l., SYN dentinal *fluid.*

euplastic l., l. that contains relatively few leukocytes, but a comparatively high concentration of fibrinogen; such l. clots fairly well and tends to become organized with fibrous tissue.

fibrinous l., a euplastic or croupous l.

inflammatory l., a faintly yellow, usually coagulable fluid (i.e., euplastic l.) that collects on the surface of an acutely inflamed membrane or cutaneous wound.

intercellular l., the fluid in the potential spaces between cells in the various organs and tissues.

intravascular l., l. within the lymphatic vessels, in contrast to intercellular l. and l. that has exuded from the vessels.

plastic l., inflammatory l. that has a tendency to become organized.

tissue l., true l., i.e., l. derived chiefly from fluid in tissue spaces (in contrast to blood l.).

vaccine l., vaccinia l., that collected from the vesicles of vaccinia infection, and used for active immunization against smallpox.

△**lymph-.** SEE lympho-.

lym·pha (lim′fă) [TA]. SYN lymph. [L.]

lym·pha·den (limf′ă-den). SYN lymph node. [lymph- + G. *adēn,* gland]

△**lymphaden-.** SEE lymphadeno-.

lym·phad·e·nec·to·my (lim-fad-ě-nek′tō-mē). Excision of lymph nodes. [lymphadeno- + G. *ektomē,* excision]

lym·phad·e·ni·tis (lim′-fad′ě-nī′tis). Inflammation of a lymph node or lymph nodes. [lymphadeno- + G. *-itis,* inflammation]

dermatopathic l., SYN dermatopathic *lymphadenopathy.*

mesenteric l., SYN mesenteric *adenitis.*

paratuberculous l., old term for chronic inflammation of certain lymph nodes, not specifically tuberculous (i.e., tubercle bacilli are not demonstrable), but associated with proved tuberculous inflammation in another part or organ of the body.

regional l., inflammation of a group of lymph nodes receiving drainage from a site of infection.

regional granulomatous l., SYN catscratch *disease.*

tuberculosis l., SYN tuberculous l.

tuberculous l., l. resulting from infection by *Mycobacterium tuberculosis;* tuberculosis of the lymph nodes. SYN tuberculosis l.

△**lymphadeno-, lymphaden-.** The lymph nodes. [L. *lympha,* spring water, + G. *adēn,* gland]

▣**lym·phad·e·nog·ra·phy** (lim-fad′ě-nog′ră-fē). Radiographic visualization of lymph nodes after injection of a contrast medium; lymphography. [lymphadeno- + G. *graphō,* to write]

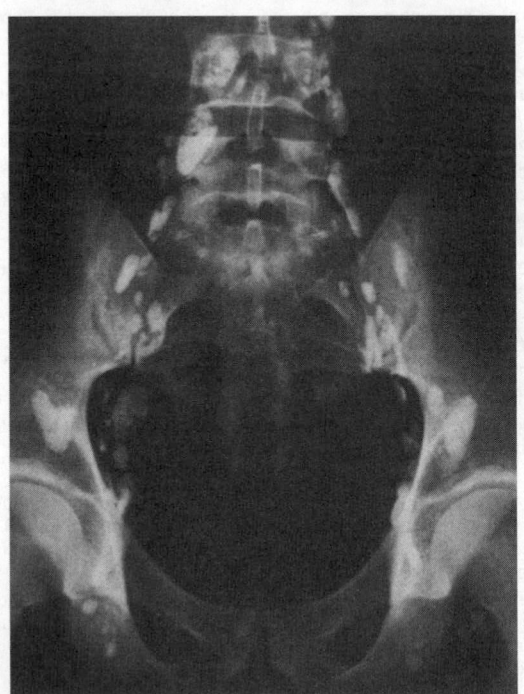

lymphadenography: storage phase

lym·phad·e·noid (lim-fad′ě-noyd). Relating to, or resembling, or derived from a lymph node. [lymphadeno- + G. *eidos,* resemblance]

lym·phad·e·no·ma (lim-fad′ě-nō′mă). Obsolete term for: **1.** An enlarged lymph node. **2.** SYN Hodgkin *disease.* [lymphadeno- + G. *-ōma,* tumor]

lym·phad·e·nop·a·thy (lim-fad-ě-nop′ă-thē). Any disease process affecting a lymph node or lymph nodes. [lymphadeno- + G. *pathos,* suffering]

angioimmunoblastic l. with dysproteinemia (AILD), a lymphoproliferative disorder characterized by generalized l., hepatosplenomegaly, fever, sweats, weight loss, skin lesions, and pruritus with hypergammaglobulinemia; occurs primarily in older adults, often with fatal outcome. Proliferation of B cells, deficiency of T cells have been demonstrated. SYN immunoblastic l.

bulky l., SYN bulky *disease.*

dermatopathic l., enlargement of lymph nodes, with proliferation of pale-staining interdigitating reticulum cells and macrophages containing fat and melanin; secondary to various forms of dermatitis. SYN dermatopathic lymphadenitis.

immunoblastic l., SYN angioimmunoblastic l. with dysproteinemia.

persistent generalized l., a syndrome characterized by reactive hyperplasia of lymph nodes (of at least one month's duration and at two different body sites, not including the inguinal area) in patients infected with the human immunodeficiency virus. The lymph node lesions progress from benign reactive hyperplasia through a stage of mixed follicular hyperplasia, to follicular involution with lymphocyte depletion. Many go on to a malignant non-Hodgkin lymphoma.

lym·phad·e·no·sis (lim-fad'ĕ-nō'sis). The basic underlying proliferative process that results in enlargement of lymph nodes, as in lymphocytic leukemia and certain inflammations. [lymphadeno- + G. *-osis,* condition]

benign l., SYN infectious *mononucleosis.*

lym·phad·e·no·va·rix (lim-fad'ĕ-nō-vā'riks). Varicose deformity of a lymph node associated with lymphangiectasis. [lymphadeno- + L. *varix*]

lym·pha·gogue (limf'ă-gog). An agent that increases the formation and flow of lymph. [lymph + G. *agōgos,* drawing forth]

lym·phan·ge·i·tis (lim-fan'jē-ī'tis). SYN lymphangitis.

△**lymphangi-.** SEE lymphangio-.

lym·phan·gi·al (lim-fan'jē-ăl). Relating to a lymphatic vessel.

lym·phan·gi·ec·ta·sis, lym·phan·gi·ec·ta·sia (lim-fan'jē-ek'tă-sis, -ek-tā'zē-a). Dilation of the lymphatic vessels, the basic process that may result in the formation of a lymphangioma. SYN lymphectasia, telangiectasia lymphatica. [lymphangio- + G. *ektasis,* a stretching]

cavernous l., SYN lymphangioma cavernosum.

cystic l., SYN lymphangioma cysticum.

intestinal l. [MIM*152800], familial l. with intestinal loss of lymph causing lymphocytopenia and hypogammaglobulinemia.

simple l., SYN lymphangioma simplex.

lym·phan·gi·ec·tat·ic (lim-fan'jē-ek-tat'ik). Relating to or characterized by lymphangiectasis.

lym·phan·gi·ec·to·my (lim-fan'jē-ek'tō-mē). Excision of a lymph channel. [lymphangio- + G. *ektomē,* excision]

lym·phan·gi·i·tis (lim-fan'jē-ī'tis). SYN lymphangitis.

△**lymphangio-, lymphangi-.** The lymphatic vessels. [L. *lympha,* spring water, + G. *angeion,* vessel]

lym·phan·gi·o·en·do·the·li·o·ma (lim-fan'jē-ō-en'dō-thē-lē-ō'mă). Old term for combined lymphatico-venous malformation. [lymphangio- + endothelium + *-oma,* tumor]

lym·phan·gi·og·ra·phy (lim-fan'jē-og'ră-fē). Radiographic demonstration of lymphatics and lymph nodes following the injection of a contrast medium; lymphography. [lymphangio- + G. *graphō,* to write]

lymphangioleiomyomatosis. A rare disorder of unknown etiology seen in women of reproductive age and in patients of either sex with tuberous sclerosis. Pulmonary complications are due to hamartomatous proliferation of smooth muscle cells preferentially along bronchovascular structures resulting in obliteration of the airways and consecutive development of cysts in the lungs. Usually progressive, leading to death from respiratory failure. Treatment by lung transplantation has been successful. SYN lymphangiomyomatosis.

lym·phan·gi·ol·o·gy (lim-fan-jē-ol'ō-jē). The branch of medical

science concerned with the lymphatic vessels. SYN lymphology. [lymphangio- + G. *logos,* study]

lym·phan·gi·o·ma (lim-fan'jē-ō'mă). Old term for a mass of anomalous lymphatic vessels or channels that vary in size, are usually greatly dilated, and are lined with normal endothelial cells; lymphoid tissue is usually present in the peripheral portions of the lesions, which are present at birth, or shortly thereafter, and probably represent maldevelopment of lymphatic vessels (rather than true neoplasms); they occur most frequently in the neck and axilla, but may also develop in the arm, mesentery, retroperitoneum, and other sites. [lymphangio- + G. *-oma,* tumor]

l. caverno'sum, a condition of conspicuous dilation of lymphatic vessels in a fairly circumscribed region, frequently with the formation of cavities or "lakes" filled with lymph. SYN cavernous lymphangiectasis.

l. circumscrip'tum, a congenital nevoid lesion consisting of a circumscribed group of tense lymph vesicles.

l. cys'ticum, a condition characterized by a fairly well circumscribed group of several or numerous cystlike, dilated vessels or spaces lined with endothelium and filled with lymph. SYN cystic lymphangiectasis.

l. sim'plex, a circumscribed region or focus of several to numerous lymphatic vessels that are moderately dilated. SYN simple lymphangiectasis.

l. tubero'sum mul'tiplex, a cutaneous lesion characterized by multiple, slightly red, cystlike nodules (located chiefly on the trunk), resulting from fairly large lymphatic vessels and spaces, and groups of proliferating endothelial cells; the lesion has some gross resemblance to spiradenoma, except for the characteristic location.

l. xanthelasmoid'eum, a capillary l. with colloid degeneration of the elastic tissues of the skin, characterized by yellow-brown or gray-brown plaques that may be only slightly raised above the surface of the skin.

lym·phan·gi·o·ma·tous (lim-fan'jē-ō'mă-tŭs). Pertaining to, characterized by, or containing lymphangioma.

lymph·an·gi·o·my·o·ma·to·sis (lim-fan'gē-ō-mī'ō-ma-tō'sis). SYN lymphangioleiomyomatosis. [lymphangio- + myoma + *-osis,* condition]

lym·phan·gi·on (lim-fan'jē-on). A lymphatic vessel. SEE lymph *vessels,* under *vessel.* [L. *lympha,* lymph, + G. *angeion,* vessel]

lym·phan·gi·o·phle·bi·tis (lim-fan'jē-ō-flē-bī'tis). Inflammation of the lymphatic vessels and veins.

lym·phan·gi·o·plas·ty (lim-fan'jē-ō-plas-tē). Surgical alteration of lymphatic vessels. [lymphangio- + G. *plastos,* formed]

lym·phan·gi·o·sar·co·ma (lim-fan'jē-ō-sar-kō'mă). A malignant neoplasm derived from vascular tissue, i.e., an angiosarcoma, in which the neoplastic cells originate from the endothelial cells of lymphatic vessels, usually developing in the arm several years after radical mastectomy.

lym·phan·gi·ot·o·my (lim-fan'jē-ot'ō-mē). Incision of lymphatic vessels. [lymphangio- + G. *tomē,* incision]

lym·phan·gi·tis (lim-fan-jī'tis). Inflammation of the lymphatic vessels. SYN lymphangeitis, lymphangiitis. [lymphangio- + G. *-itis,* inflammation]

l. carcinomato'sa, extensive lymphatic permeation by tumor cells, with surrounding fibrosis, producing visible or palpable cords, especially in pleura or skin overlying a carcinoma.

lym·pha·phe·re·sis (lim'fă-fĕ-rē'sis). SYN lymphocytapheresis.

lym·phat·ic (lim-fat'ik). **1.** Pertaining to lymph. **2.** A vascular channel that transports lymph. **3.** Sometimes used to pertain to a sluggish or phlegmatic characteristic. SYN vas lymphaticum. [L. *lymphaticus,* frenzied; Mod. L. use, of or for lymph]

afferent l., a l. vessel entering, or bringing lymph to, a node. SYN afferent vessel (3), vas lymphaticum afferens.

efferent l., SYN *vas efferens* (1).

lym·phat·i·cos·to·my (lim-fat-i-kos'tō-mē). Making an opening into a lymphatic duct. [lymphatic + G. *stoma,* mouth]

lymph·at·ics (lim-fat'iks). SYN lymph *vessels,* under *vessel.*

lym·pha·ti·tis (lim-fă-tī'tis). Obsolete term for inflammation of the lymphatic vessels or lymph nodes. [lymphatic + G. -*itis*, inflammation]

lym·pha·tol·o·gy (lim-fă-tol′ō-jē). The study of the lymphatic system. [lymphatic + G. *logos*, study]

lym·pha·tol·y·sis (lim′fă-tol′i-sis). Obsolete term for destruction of the lymphatic vessels or lymphoid tissue, or both. [lymphatic + G. *lysis*, dissolution]

lym·pha·to·lyt·ic (lim′fă-tō-lit′ik). Pertaining to or characterized by lymphatolysis.

lym·phec·ta·sia (lim-fek-tā′zē-ă). SYN lymphangiectasis. [lymph + G. *ektasis*, a stretching]

lymph·e·de·ma (limf′e-dē′mă). Swelling (especially in subcutaneous tissues) as a result of obstruction of lymphatic vessels or lymph nodes and the accumulation of large amounts of lymph in the affected region. SEE ALSO elephantiasis. [lymph + G. *oidēma*, a swelling]

congenital l., SEE hereditary l.

hereditary l., permanent pitting edema usually confined to the legs; two types, congenital (Milroy disease [MIM*153100], caused by mutation in the FMS-like tyrosine kinase 4 gene (FLT4) on 5q, or with onset at about the age of puberty (Meige disease [MIM*153200]); autosomal dominant inheritance.

l. prae′cox, SYN primary l.

primary l., a form of l. observed chiefly in young women and girls, characterized by diffuse swelling of the lower extremities. SYN l. praecox.

lym·phe·mia (lim-fē′mē-ă). The presence of unusually large numbers of lymphocytes or their precursors, or both, in the circulating blood. [lymph(ocyte) + G. *haima*, blood]

lym·phi·za·tion (lim-fi-zā′shŭn). The formation of lymph.

LYMPH NODE

lymph node [TA]. One of numerous round, oval, or bean-shaped bodies located along the course of lymphatic vessels, varying greatly in size (1–25 mm in diameter) and usually presenting a depressed area, the hilum, on one side through which blood vessels enter and efferent lymphatic vessels emerge. The structure consists of a fibrous capsule and internal trabeculae supporting lymphoid tissue and lymph sinuses; lymphoid tissue is arranged in nodules in the cortex and cords in the medulla of a node, with afferent vessels entering at many points of the periphery. SYN nodus lymphoideus [TA], lymphonodus☆, nodus lymphaticus☆, lymph gland, lymphaden, lymphoglandula.

abdominal l. n.'s [TA], the parietal and visceral l. n.'s of the abdomen, collectively. SYN nodi lymphoidei abdominis [TA].

l. n.'s of abdominal organs, SYN visceral l. n.'s of abdomen.

accessory l. n.'s [TA], the nodes of the lateral deep cervical group that are located along the accessory nerve; their efferent vessels pass to the supraclavicular l. n.'s. SYN nodi lymphoidei accessorii [TA], accessory nerve l. n.'s, companion l. n.'s of accessory nerve, nodi lymphatici comitantes nervi accessorii.

accessory nerve l. n.'s, SYN accessory l. n.'s.

anorectal l. n.'s, SYN pararectal l. n.'s.

anterior axillary l. n.'s, ☆official alternate term for pectoral axillary l. n.'s.

l. n. of anterior border of omental foramen [TA], one of the hepatic nodes located adjacent to the omental foramen. SYN nodus lymphoideus foraminalis [TA], foraminal l. n., foraminal node.

anterior cervical l. n.'s [TA], the group of l. n.'s located in the anterior region of the neck, divided into superficial and deep groups. SYN nodi lymphoidei cervicales anteriores [TA].

anterior deep cervical l. n.'s, SYN deep anterior cervical l. n.'s.

anterior jugular l. n.'s, SYN anterior superficial cervical l. n.'s.

anterior mediastinal l. n.'s, SYN brachiocephalic l. n.

anterior superficial cervical l. n.'s [TA], the l. n.'s in the subcutaneous tissue of the anterior region of the neck. SYN nodi lym-

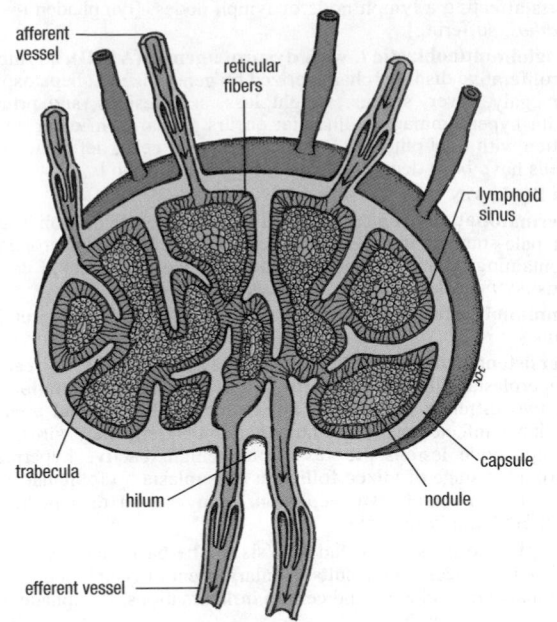

lymph node

phoidei cervicales anteriores superficiales [TA], anterior jugular l. n.'s, nodi lymphoidei jugulares anteriores.

anterior tibial l. n. [TA], a small inconstant l. n. in front of the interosseous membrane along the upper part of the anterior tibial vessels. SYN nodus tibialis anterior [TA], anterior tibial node.

apical axillary l. n.'s [TA], the group of l. n.'s located at the apex of the axillary fossa that receive lymphatic drainage from other groups of axillary l. n.'s and then drain in turn into the subclavian lymphatic trunk. SYN nodi lymphoidei axillares apicales [TA].

appendicular l. n.'s [TA], visceral nodes along the appendicular vessels in the mesoappendix; they receive afferent vessels from the vermiform appendix and send efferent vessels to the ileocolic l. n.'s. SYN nodi lymphoidei appendiculares [TA].

l. n. of arch of azygos vein [TA], a visceral l. n. of the right brachiocephalic group located adjacent to the arch of the azygos vein. SYN nodus lymphoideus arcus venae azygos [TA], l. n. of azygos arch, nodus lymphoideus arcus venae azygos.

l. n.'s around cardia of stomach [TA], a group of lymph nodes surrounding the cardia of the stomach. SYN anulus lymphaticus cardiae [TA], cardiac lymphatic ring, lymphatic ring of cardiac part of stomach.

axillary l. n.'s [TA], numerous nodes around the axillary veins that receive the lymphatic drainage from the upper limb, scapular region and pectoral region (including mammary gland); they drain into the subclavian trunk. SYN nodi lymphoidei axillares [TA], axillary glands.

l. n. of azygos arch, SYN l. n. of arch of azygos vein.

bifurcation l. n.'s, SYN inferior tracheobronchial l. n.'s.

brachial l. n.'s, SYN humeral axillary l. n.'s.

brachiocephalic l. n., located in the superior mediastinum in relation to the great vessels, these nodes receive lymph from the thymus, pericardium, and right side of the heart; their efferent vessels join those of the tracheal nodes to form the bronchomediastinal trunks. SYN nodi lymphoidei brachiocephalici [TA], anterior mediastinal l. n.'s, nodi lymphoidei mediastinales anteriores.

bronchopulmonary l. n.'s [TA], l. n.'s in the hilum of the lung that receive lymph from the pulmonary l. n.'s, and drain to the tracheobronchial nodes. SYN nodi lymphoidei bronchopulmonales [TA], hilar l. n.'s.

buccal l. n., one of the chain of facial l. n.'s located superficial to the buccinator muscle. SYN nodus lymphoideus buccinatorius [TA], buccinator node, buccal node, nodus buccinatorius.

carinal l. n.'s, SYN inferior tracheobronchial l. n.'s.

celiac l. n.'s [TA], visceral nodes located along the celiac trunk that drain lymph from the stomach, duodenum, pancreas, spleen, and biliary tract and drain to the cisterna chyli via the right and left intestinal lymphatic trunks. SYN nodi lymphoidei coeliaci [TA].

central axillary l. n.'s [TA], nodes located around the midportion of the axillary vein; they receive afferent vessels from the humeral (lateral), pectoral (anterior), and subscapular (posterior) groups of axillary nodes and send efferent vessels to the apical group of axillary l. n.'s; SYN nodi lymphoidei axillares centrales [TA].

central mesenteric l. n.'s, SYN central superior mesenteric l. n.'s; SEE ALSO mesenteric l. n.'s.

central superior mesenteric l. n.'s [TA], the mesenteric l. n.'s located along the intestinal (jejunal and ileal) branches of the superior mesenteric artery. SYN nodi lymphoidei superiores centrales [TA], central mesenteric l. n.'s, middle group of mesenteric l. n.'s.

colic l. n.'s, SYN nodi lymphatici colici. SEE left colic l. n.'s, middle colic l. n.'s, right colic l. n.'s.

common iliac l. n.'s [TA], parietal nodes located in association with the common iliac vein; they are subdivided into five groups: intermediate common iliac l. n.'s, between the common iliac artery and vein; lateral common iliac l. n.'s lateral to the vein; medial common iliac l. n.'s, medial to the vein; promontorial common iliac l. n.'s at the sacral promontory; and subaortic common iliac l. n.'s, at the bifurcation of the aorta; they all receive afferent vessels from the external and internal iliac nodes and send efferent vessels to the lumbar nodes. SYN nodi lymphoidei iliaci communes [TA].

companion l. n.'s of accessory nerve, SYN accessory l. n.'s.

cubital l. n.'s [TA], two groups of nodes, superficial and deep, lying along the basilic vein above the medial epicondyle; they receive afferents from the ulnar side of the forearm and hand, and send efferents to the brachial nodes. SYN nodi lymphoidei cubitales [TA], l. n.'s of elbow.

cystic l. n. [TA], a visceral l. n. at the neck of the gallbladder draining lymph into the hepatic nodes. SYN nodus lymphoideus cysticus [TA], cystic node.

deep anterior cervical l. n.'s [TA], the l. n.'s near the larynx, trachea, and thyroid gland. SYN anterior deep cervical l. n.'s, nodi lymphoidei cervicales anteriores profundi.

deep inguinal l. n.'s [TA], several small inconstant nodes (proximal, intermediate, and distal) deep to the fascia lata and medial to the femoral vein; they receive lymph from the deep structures of the lower limb, from the glans penis and from superficial inguinal nodes; efferents pass to the external iliac nodes. SYN nodi lymphoidei inguinales profundi.

deep lateral cervical l. n.'s [TA], the l. n.'s located in the posterior triangle of the neck deep to the investing layer of cervical fascia; they empty into the jugular trunk on the right or left side; the group is subdivided into four smaller chains: superior deep cervical nodes, inferior deep cervical nodes, accessory nodes, and supraclavicular nodes. SYN nodi lymphoidei cervicales laterales profundi [TA].

deep parotid l. n.'s [TA], the group of l. n.'s associated with the parotid gland lying deep to the parotid masseteric fascia. SYN nodi lymphoidei parotidei profundi [TA].

l. n.'s of elbow, SYN cubital l. n.'s.

external iliac l. n.'s [TA], parietal nodes located in association with the external iliac vein; they are subdivided into three groups: intermediate external iliac l. n.'s, between the vein and the external iliac artery; lateral external iliac l. n.'s, and medial external iliac l. n.'s, medial to the vein; they all receive afferent vessels from the inguinal nodes, lower abdominal wall, and pelvic viscera, and send efferent vessels to the common iliac nodes. SYN nodi lymphoidei iliaci externi [TA].

facial l. n.'s [TA], a chain of l. n.'s lying along the facial vein that receive afferent vessels from the eyelids, nose, cheek, lip, and gums, and send efferent vessels to the submandibular nodes. SYN nodi lymphoidei faciales [TA].

fibular l. n., a small inconstant l. n. located along the course of the fibular vein (venae comitantes). SYN nodus lymphoideus fibularis [TA], fibular node, peroneal l. n.

foraminal l. n., SYN l. n. of anterior border of omental foramen.

gastroduodenal l. n.'s, SYN pyloric l. n.'s.

gluteal l. n.'s [TA], parietal nodes of the internal iliac nodes; they are subdivided into two groups: interior gluteal nodes, located along the inferior gluteal vein; superior gluteal nodes located along the superior gluteal vein. SYN nodi lymphoidei gluteales [TA].

l. n.'s of head and neck [TA], l. n.'s located in and draining the head and neck regions, ultimately draining via the jugular lymphatic trunks. SYN nodi lymphoidei capitis et colli [TA].

hepatic l. n.'s [TA], visceral nodes located along the hepatic artery as far as the porta hepatis; they drain the liver, gallbladder, stomach, duodenum, and pancreas, and send efferents to the celiac nodes. SYN nodi lymphoidei hepatici [TA].

hilar l. n.'s, SYN bronchopulmonary l. n.'s.

humeral axillary l. n.'s [TA], l. n.'s along the brachial vein that receive lymph drainage from most of the free upper limb and send efferent vessels to the central axillary l. n.'s. SYN nodi lymphoidei axillares humerales [TA], lateral axillary l. n.'s*, nodi lymphoidei axillares laterales*, brachial l. n.'s, nodi lymphoidei brachiales.

ileocolic l. n.'s [TA], visceral nodes located along the ileocolic artery that drain lymph from the ascending colon to the superior mesenteric nodes. SYN nodi lymphoidei ileocolici [TA].

inferior epigastric l. n.'s [TA], three or four parietal nodes placed along the inferior epigastric vessels; they receive afferents from the lower abdominal wall and empty into the external iliac nodes. SYN nodi lymphoidei epigastrici inferiores [TA].

inferior mesenteric l. n.'s [TA], visceral nodes located along the inferior mesenteric artery and its branches that drain the upper part of the rectum, the sigmoid colon, and descending colon. SYN nodi lymphoidei mesenterici inferiores [TA].

inferior phrenic l. n.'s [TA], small l. n.'s associated with the inferior phrenic vessels. SYN nodi lymphoidei phrenici inferiores [TA].

inferior tracheobronchial l. n.'s [TA], several large l. n.'s inferior to the tracheal bifurcation; they receive afferents from the bronchopulmonary nodes and the heart, and send efferents to the superior tracheobronchial and tracheal nodes. SYN bifurcation l. n.'s, carinal l. n.'s, nodi lymphoidei tracheobronchiales inferiores.

infraauricular deep parotid l. n.'s [TA], small l. n.'s located deep to the parotid fascia and below the ear. SYN infraauricular subfascial parotid l. n.'s, nodi lymphoidei parotidei profundi infra-auriculares.

infraauricular subfascial parotid l. n.'s, SYN infraauricular deep parotid l. n.'s.

intercostal l. n.'s [TA], one or two small nodes located posteriorly in each intercostal space; they receive lymph from the parietal pleura, intercostal space, and posterior body wall; the nodes in the upper spaces empty into the thoracic duct; the nodes in the lower spaces form a descending intercostal trunk that opens into the cisterna chyli. SYN nodi lymphoidei intercostales [TA].

interiliac l. n.'s [TA], several l. n.'s located between the external and internal iliac arteries and the obturator artery; these nodes are considered by some to be part of the medial external iliac nodes. SYN nodi lymphoidei interiliaci [TA].

intermediate lacunar l. n. [TA], an inconstant l. n. of the external iliac nodes frequently occurring between the external iliac artery and vein at the vascular space of the subinguinal compartment. SYN nodus lymphoideus lacunaris intermedius [TA], intermediate lacunar node.

intermediate lumbar l. n.'s [TA], the chain of lymph nodes located between the aorta and the inferior vena cava. SYN nodi lymphoidei lumbales intermedii [TA], lumbar l. n.'s.

internal iliac l. n.'s [TA], nodes that lie along the internal iliac artery and its branches; they receive lymph from the pelvic viscera, the gluteal region, and the deep parts of the perineum, and send efferent vessels to the common iliac nodes. SYN nodi lymphoidei iliaci interni [TA].

ly

interpectoral l. n.'s [TA], small l. n.'s located between the pectoralis major and minor muscles; they receive lymph from the muscles and the mammary gland, and deliver lymph to the axillary lymphatic plexus. SYN nodi lymphoidei interpectorales [TA].

intraglandular deep parotid l. n.'s [TA], small l. n.'s of the deep parotid group lying within the parotid gland. SYN nodi lymphoidei parotidei intraglandulares [TA], intraglandular parotid l. n.'s.

intraglandular parotid l. n.'s, SYN intraglandular deep parotid l. n.'s.

intrapulmonary l. n.'s [TA], small nodes that occur along the bronchi within the parenchyma of the lung; they receive the drainage from localized areas of the lung and send efferents to bronchopulmonary nodes. SYN nodi lymphoidei intrapulmonales [TA], nodi lymphoidei pulmonales, pulmonary l. n.'s.

jugulodigastric l. n. [TA], a prominent l. n. in the deep lateral cervical group lying below the digastric muscle and anterior to the internal jugular vein; it receives lymphatic drainage from the pharynx, palatine tonsil, and tongue. SYN nodus lymphoideus jugulodigastricus [TA], jugulodigastric node, subdigastric node.

juguloomohyoid l. n. [TA], a l. n. of the lateral deep cervical group that lies above the intermediate tendon of the omohyoid muscle and anterior to the internal jugular vein; it receives lymphatic drainage from the submental, submandibular, and deep anterior cervical nodes; its efferent vessels go to other deep lateral cervical nodes. SYN nodus lymphoideus juguloomohyoideus [TA], juguloomohyoid node.

juxtaesophageal l. n.'s [TA], several nodes located along either side of the esophagus; they receive lymph from both the esophagus and the lungs. SYN nodi lymphoidei juxtaesophageales [TA], nodi lymphoidei juxtaesophageales pulmonales.

juxta-intestinal mesenteric l. n.'s [TA], the mesenteric l. n.'s located in immediate proximity to the jejunum or ileum. SYN nodi lymphoidei juxtaintestinales [TA].

lateral axillary l. n.'s, ✕official alternate term for humeral axillary l. n.'s.

lateral jugular l. n.'s, deep nodes of the lateral cervical nodes lying lateral to the internal jugular vein; they usually empty into the jugular trunk. SYN nodi lymphoidei jugulares laterales.

lateral lacunar l. n. [TA], a l. n. of the external iliac group located lateral to the external iliac artery at the vascular space of the subinguinal compartment. SYN nodus lymphoideus lacunaris lateralis [TA], lateral lacunar node.

lateral pericardial l. n.'s [TA], small l. n.'s located along the pericardiacophrenic vessels, they drain the pericardium. SYN nodi lymphoidei pericardiales laterales [TA].

left colic l. n.'s [TA], small nodes along the left colic artery and its branches that drain the left flexure and upper part of the descending colon; efferent vessels pass to the inferior mesenteric nodes. SYN nodi lymphoidei colici sinistri [TA].

left gastric l. n.'s [TA], nodes located along the left gastric artery and its branches; they are divided into paracardial, upper and lower groups. SYN nodi lymphoidei gastrici sinistri [TA], superior gastric l. n.'s.

left gastroepiploic l. n.'s, SYN left gastroomental l. n.'s.

left gastroomental l. n.'s [TA], nodes located in the greater omentum along the left gastroepiploic artery that drain part of the greater curvature of the stomach and greater omentum. SYN nodi lymphoidei gastroomentales sinistri [TA], left gastroepiploic l. n.'s.

left lumbar l. n.'s [TA], the chain of l. n.'s associated with the aorta in the abdomen; it is divided into three groups: lateral aortic l. n.'s on the left of the aorta; pre-aortic l. n.'s in front of the aorta; post-aortic l. n.'s, behind the aorta. SYN nodi lymphoidei lumbales sinistri [TA], lumbar l. n.'s.

l. n. of ligamentum arteriosum [TA], an inconstant l. n. of the anterior mediastinal group located adjacent to the ligamentum arteriosum. SYN nodus lymphoideus ligamenti arteriosi [TA], node of ligamentum arteriosum.

lingual l. n.'s [TA], l. n. along the lingual vein receiving drainage from the tongue (except tip); drain to submandibular l. n.'s. SYN nodi lymphoidei linguales [TA].

l. n.'s of lower limb [TA], the l. n.'s located in and draining the lower limb as a group; includes inguinal, popliteal, tibial, and fibular nodes. SYN nodi lymphoidei membri inferioris [TA].

lumbar l. n.'s, SYN right lumbar l. n.'s, intermediate lumbar l. n.'s, left lumbar l. n.'s.

malar l. n. [TA], one of the facial l. n.'s located near the zygomatic minor muscle. SYN nodus lymphoideus malaris [TA], malar node.

mandibular l. n. [TA], one of the facial l. n.'s located by the facial artery near the point it crosses the mandible. SYN nodus lymphoideus mandibularis [TA], mandibular nodes.

mastoid l. n.'s [TA], two or three nodes in the region of the mastoid process; they receive afferent lymphatic vessels from the scalp and auricle and send efferent vessels to the superior deep cervical nodes. SYN nodi lymphoidei mastoidei [TA], retroauricular l. n.'s.

medial lacunar l. n. [TA], a l. n. of the external iliac group located medial to the external iliac vein at the vascular space of the subinguinal compartment. SYN nodus lymphoideus lacunaris medialis [TA], medial lacunar node.

mesenteric l. n.'s [TA], nodes located in the mesentery; they are of three classes: ileocolic l. n.'s, juxtaintestinal mesenteric l. n.'s, and the central superior group of mesenteric l. n.'s. SYN nodi lymphoidei mesenterici [TA].

mesocolic l. n.'s [TA], nodes located in the mesocolon; they are of two classes: paracolic l. n.'s, located in immediate proximity to the colon; colic l. n.'s located along the arteries supplying the colon. SYN nodi lymphoidei mesocolici [TA], nodi lymphoidei paracolici.

middle colic l. n.'s [TA], nodes along the middle colic artery and its branches that drain the right colic flexure and most of the transverse colon. SYN nodi lymphoidei colici medii [TA].

middle group of mesenteric l. n.'s, SYN central superior mesenteric l. n.'s.

middle rectal l. n., a l. n. along the middle rectal artery that receives afferents from the pararectal nodes and sends efferents to the internal iliac nodes. SYN middle rectal node, nodus lymphoideus rectalis medius.

nasolabial l. n. [TA], one of the facial l. n.'s located near the junction of the superior labial and facial arteries. SYN nodus lymphoideus nasolabialis [TA], nasolabial node.

obturator l. n.'s [TA], nodes of the internal iliac group located along the obturator artery. SYN nodi lymphoidei obturatorii [TA].

occipital l. n.'s [TA], one or two small nodes along the occipital vessels close to the trapezius muscle that receive afferents from the posterior scalp and drain into the superior deep lateral cervical nodes; these are the most posterior nodes of the pericervical collar of lymph nodes of the head and neck, which receive the drainage from the head. SYN nodi lymphoidei occipitales [TA].

pancreatic l. n.'s [TA], nodes draining the body and tail of the pancreas; they are subdivided into two groups: inferior pancreatic l. n.'s [TA] (nodi lymphoidei pancreatici inferiores [TA]), located along the inferior pancreatic artery; superior pancreatic l. n.'s [TA] (nodi lymphoidei pancreatici superiores [TA]), located along the splenic artery near the origin of its pancreatic branches. SYN nodi lymphoidei pancreatici [TA].

pancreaticoduodenal l. n.'s [TA], nodes along the superior and inferior pancreaticoduodenal arteries. SYN nodi lymphoidei pancreaticoduodenales [TA].

pancreaticosplenic l. n.'s, l. n.'s of the pancreatic tail and spleen, receiving afferents from both organs plus the greater curvature of the stomach; they drain to the celiac l. n.'s. SYN nodi lymphoidei pancreaticosplenales [TA], nodi lymphoidei pancreaticolienales.

paramammary l. n.'s [TA], several l. n.'s on the lateral side of the mammary gland that receive afferents from the mammary gland and send efferents to the axillary pectoral group of l. n.'s. The paramammary l. n.'s are commonly considered as part of the pectoral axillary nodes. SYN nodi lymphoidei paramammarii [TA].

pararectal l. n.'s [TA], nodes located on either side of the rectum; they send efferents to the middle and superior rectal nodes. SYN nodi lymphoidei pararectales [TA], anorectal l. n.'s, nodi lymphoidei anorectales.

parasternal l. n.'s [TA], a number of small nodes that lie along the course of the internal thoracic vessels; lymph enters these nodes from the anterior intercostal spaces, pericardium, diaphragm, liver and medial mammary gland; the efferent vessels pass upward to join the bronchomediastinal trunk of the same side. SYN nodi lymphoidei parasternales [TA].

paratracheal l. n. [TA], nodes along the sides of the trachea in the neck and in the posterior mediastinum; receive drainage of superior (and inferior) tracheobranchial nodes, trachea, and esophagus; drain to bronchomediastinal lymphatic trunk(s), thoracic duct. SYN nodi lymphoidei paratracheales [TA], tracheal l. n.'s.

parauterine l. n.'s [TA], nodes on either side of the uterus draining lymph to the internal iliac nodes and to the lumbar nodes via lymphatic vessels following the ovarian arteries. SYN nodi lymphoidei parauterini [TA].

paravaginal l. n.'s [TA], l. n.'s in association with the vagina; they drain to the internal iliac nodes. SYN nodi lymphoidei paravaginales [TA].

paravesical l. n.'s, the l. n.'s located around the urinary bladder and, in the male, the prostate; there are three groups: prevesicular l. n.'s, in front of the bladder; lateral vesical l. n.'s, on the right and left sides; postvesicular l. n.'s behind the bladder.

parietal l. n.'s [TA], the l. n.'s draining the walls of the abdomen or of the pelvis (as opposed to the visceral nodes draining the abdominopelvic viscera). SYN nodi lymphoidei parietales [TA], parietal nodes.

pectoral axillary l. n.'s [TA], l. n.'s located along the lateral thoracic vein; they receive the drainage of the pectoral region, including most of the drainage of the breast. SYN nodi lymphoidei axillares pectorales [TA], anterior axillary l. n.'s★, nodi lymphoidei axillares anteriores.

pelvic l. n.'s [TA], the parietal and visceral l. n.'s of the pelvis, collectively. SYN nodi lymphoidei pelvis [TA].

peroneal l. n., SYN fibular l. n.

popliteal l. n.'s [TA], two groups of nodes located in the popliteal fossa: the superficial popliteal l. n.'s, located around the termination of the small saphenous vein, that drain the skin of the back of the leg and lateral side of the foot; and the deep popliteal l. n.'s, located around the popliteal vessels, that drain the superficial group, the deep structures of the leg, and the knee joint. SYN nodi lymphoidei popliteales [TA].

posterior axillary l. n.'s, ★official alternate term for subscapular axillary l. n.'s.

posterior mediastinal l. n.'s, SYN prevertebral l. n.'s.

posterior tibial l. n. [TA], a small inconstant l. n. located along the course of the posterior tibial artery. SYN nodus lymphoideus tibialis posterior [TA], posterior tibial node.

preauricular deep parotid l. n.'s [TA], small l. n.'s located deep to the parotid fascia and in front of the ear. SYN nodi lymphoidei parotidei profundi preauriculares [TA].

prececal l. n.'s [TA], nodes located in front of the cecum draining lymph to the ileocolic nodes. SYN nodi lymphoidei precaecales [TA].

prelaryngeal l. n.'s [TA], l. n.'s of the deep anterior cervical group that lie in front of the larynx; they drain into the lateral deep lateral cervical nodes. SYN nodi lymphoidei prelaryngeales [TA].

prepericardial l. n.'s [TA], several small l. n.'s located between the pericardium and the sternum, in the anterior mediastinum. SYN nodi lymphoidei prepericardiaci [TA].

pretracheal l. n.'s [TA], l. n.'s of the deep anterior cervical group that lie in front of the trachea; they drain into the deep lateral cervical group or into the parasternal nodes. SYN nodi lymphoidei pretracheales [TA].

prevertebral l. n.'s [TA], nodes located along the thoracic aorta; they receive vessels from the esophagus, diaphragm, liver, and pericardium and send efferents to the thoracic duct and bronchomediastinal lymphatic trunk(s). SYN nodi lymphoidei prevertebrales★, nodi lymphoidei mediastinales posteriores, posterior mediastinal l. n.'s.

proximal deep inguinal l. n. [TA], one of the deep inguinal l. n.'s located in or adjacent to the femoral canal; sometimes mistaken for a femoral hernia when enlarged. SYN nodus lymphoideus proximalis profundus [TA], node of Cloquet, Rosenmüller gland, Rosenmüller node.

pulmonary l. n.'s, SYN intrapulmonary l. n.'s.

pyloric l. n.'s [TA], group of lymph nodes surrounding the pylorus, draining lymph into the right gastric or the right gastroomental l. n.'s; it is divided into three smaller groups: suprapyloric nodes, superior to the pylorus; subpyloric nodes, inferior to the pylorus; and retropyloric nodes, posterior to the pylorus. SYN gastroduodenal l. n.'s, nodi lymphoidei pylorici.

retroauricular l. n.'s, SYN mastoid l. n.'s.

retrocecal l. n.'s [TA], nodes located behind the cecum draining lymph into the ileocolic nodes. SYN nodi lymphoidei retrocecales [TA].

retropharyngeal l. n.'s [TA], the three groups of l. n.'s, one median and two lateral, located between the pharynx and the prevertebral layer of cervical fascia; they receive lymph from the nasopharynx, the auditory tube, and the atlanto-occipital and atlantoaxial joints. SYN nodi lymphoidei retropharyngeales [TA].

retropyloric l. n.'s [TA], a group of l. n.'s located behind the pylorus. SYN nodi lymphoidei retropylorici [TA], retropyloric nodes.

right colic l. n.'s [TA], nodes located along the right colic artery that drain the upper part of the ascending colon. SYN nodi lymphoidei colici dextri [TA].

right gastric l. n.'s [TA], small nodes along the course of the right gastric artery that drain part of the lesser curvature of the stomach. SYN nodi lymphoidei gastrici dextri [TA].

right gastroepiploic l. n.'s, SYN right gastroomental l. n.'s.

right gastroomental l. n.'s [TA], nodes located in the greater omentum along the right gastroepiploic artery that drain part of the greater curvature of the stomach and the greater omentum. SYN nodi lymphoidei gastroomentales dextri [TA], right gastroepiploic l. n.'s.

right lumbar l. n.'s [TA], the chain of nodes associated with the inferior vena cava; it is divided into three groups: lateral caval nodes, on the right of the inferior vena cava; precaval nodes, anterior to the inferior vena cava; postcaval nodes, posterior to the inferior vena cava. SYN nodi lymphoidei lumbales dextri [TA], lumbar l. n.'s.

sacral l. n.'s [TA], nodes in the concavity of the sacrum that drain the rectum and posterior pelvic wall. SYN nodi lymphoidei sacrales [TA].

sentinel l. n., the first l. n. to receive lymphatic drainage from a malignant tumor; the sentinel node is identified as the first to take up a radionuclide or dye injected into the tumor; increasingly used in operations for melanoma and breast cancer; if the sentinel node is free of metastasis, more distal nodes are also free. SEE ALSO signal l. n. SYN sentinel node.

sigmoid l. n.'s [TA], nodes of the inferior mesenteric group, located along the sigmoid arteries. SYN nodi lymphoidei sigmoidei [TA].

signal l. n., a firm supraclavicular l. n., especially on the left side, sufficiently enlarged that it is palpable from the cutaneous surface; such a l. n. is so termed because it may be the first recognized presumptive evidence of a malignant neoplasm in one of the viscera. A signal l. n. that is known to contain a metastasis from a malignant neoplasm is sometimes designated by an old eponym, Troisier *ganglion*. SEE ALSO sentinel l. n. SYN jugular gland, Virchow node.

splenic l. n.'s [TA], nodes near the hilum of the spleen; they receive afferents from the spleen and stomach, and send efferents to the pancreatic-postsplenic and celiac nodes. SYN nodi lymphoidei splenici [TA], nodi lymphoidei lienales★.

subaortic l. n.'s [TA], nodes of the common iliac group located at the bifurcation of the aorta. SYN nodi lymphoidei subaortici [TA].

submandibular l. n.'s [TA], four or five nodes that lie in relationship to the mandible and the submandibular gland; they receive vessels from the face below the eye and from the tongue and drain into the superior deep cervical nodes, particularly the jugulodigastric node; these nodes are part of the pericervical col-

ly

lar of lymph nodes that initially receive drainage from the head. SYN nodi lymphoidei submandibulares [TA].

submental l. n.'s [TA], small nodes that lie superficial to the mylohyoid muscle; they receive afferents from the lower lip, chin, and the tip of the tongue, and send efferents to the deep lateral cervical nodes; these nodes are part of the pericervical collar of lymph nodes that initially receives drainage from the head. SYN nodi lymphoidei submentales [TA].

subpyloric l. n.'s [TA], a group of pyloric nodes located below the pylorus. SYN nodi lymphoidei subpylorici [TA], subpyloric node.

subscapular axillary l. n.'s [TA], l. n.'s of the axillary region located along the subscapular vein and its tributaries; they receive afferent vessels from the dorsal surface of the thorax and scapular region and send efferent vessels to the central group of l. n.'s. SYN nodi lymphoidei axillares subscapulares [TA], nodi lymphoidei axillares posteriores⋆, posterior axillary l. n.'s⋆.

superficial inguinal l. n.'s [TA], a group of 12–20 nodes that lie in the subcutaneous tissue below the inguinal ligament and along the terminal part of the great saphenous vein; they drain the skin and subcutaneous tissue of the lower abdominal wall, perineum, buttock, external genitalia, and lower limb; they are subdivided into three groups: inferior (vertical) group of superficial inguinal l. n.'s, located inferior to the saphenous opening, receiving drainage of the lower limb; superolateral (lateral horizontal) superficial inguinal l. n.'s located lateral to the saphenous opening, receiving drainage of lateral buttock and lower anterior abdominal wall; and superomedial (medial horizontal) superficial inguinal l. n.'s, located medial to the saphenous opening, receiving drainage of the perineum and external genitalia. SYN nodi lymphoidei inguinales superficiales [TA].

superficial lateral cervical l. n.'s [TA], 1–4 nodes lying along the external jugular vein; they drain the skin and superficial structures over the region of the sternocleidomastoid muscle and send efferent vessels to the deep lateral cervical l. n.'s. SYN nodi lymphoidei cervicales laterales superficiales [TA].

superficial parotid l. n.'s [TA], several small l. n.'s located in the subcutaneous tissue in the parotid region. SYN nodi lymphoidei parotidei superficiales [TA].

superior gastric l. n.'s, SYN left gastric l. n.'s.

superior mesenteric l. n.'s [TA], the numerous nodes located in the mesentery along the superior mesenteric artery; they receive lymph from the central mesenteric l. n.'s and drain into the intestinal lymph trunk. SYN nodi lymphoidei mesenterici superiores [TA], nodi lymphoidei centrales.

superior phrenic l. n.'s [TA], three groups of small nodes, anterior, middle, and posterior, on the upper surface of the diaphragm; they receive afferents from the liver, diaphragm, and intercostal spaces and send efferents to parasternal and posterior mediastinal nodes. SYN nodi lymphoidei phrenici superiores [TA].

superior rectal l. n.'s [TA], nodes of the inferior mesenteric group, located along the superior rectal artery. SYN nodi lymphoidei rectales superiores [TA].

superior tracheobronchial l. n.'s [TA], several large lymph nodes of the posterior mediastinum located superior to the bronchi at their union with the trachea; receives lymph from inferior tracheobronchial lymph nodes and bronchopulmonary nodes; drain to paratracheal nodes. SYN nodi lymphoidei tracheobronchiales superiores [TA].

supraclavicular l. n.'s [TA], the portion of the inferior deep lateral cervical nodes located between the inferior belly of the omohyoid muscle and the clavicle; afferent vessels come from adjacent regions including the mediastinum; efferent vessels terminate in the subclavian trunk. SYN nodi lymphoidei supraclaviculares [TA].

suprapyloric l. n. [TA], a l. n. located above the pylorus. SYN nodus lymphoideus suprapyloricus [TA], suprapyloric node.

thoracic l. n.'s [TA], the parietal and visceral l. n.'s of the thorax, collectively. SYN nodi lymphoidei thoracis [TA].

thyroid l. n.'s [TA], nodes of the deep anterior cervical group located around the thyroid gland; they drain into the deep lateral cervical group. SYN nodi lymphoidei thyroidei [TA].

tracheal l. n.'s, SYN paratracheal l. n.

l. n.'s of upper limb [TA], lymph nodes located in and draining the upper limb, ultimately drained by the subclavian lymphatic trunk; included are the axillary, interpectoral, deltopectoral (infraclavicular), brachial, and cubital nodes. SYN nodi lymphoidei membri superioris [TA].

visceral l. n.'s [TA], the l. n.'s draining the viscera of the abdomen or of the pelvis as opposed to the parietal nodes draining the body walls. SYN nodi lymphoidei viscerales [TA], visceral nodes.

visceral l. n.'s of abdomen [TA], the numerous l. n.'s receiving lymph from abdominal organs located in association with the visceral branches of the aorta. SYN nodi lymphoidei abdominis viscerales [TA], l. n.'s of abdominal organs.

⌂**lympho-, lymph-.** Lymph. [L. *lympha,* spring water]

lym·pho·blast (lim′fō-blast). A young immature cell that matures into a lymphocyte and is characterized by more abundant cytoplasm than in a lymphocyte, a nucleus in which the chromatin is finer than in a lymphocyte (but coarser than in a myeloblast), and one or two rather prominent nucleoli. SYN lymphocytoblast. [lympho- + G. *blastos,* germ]

lym·pho·blas·tic (lim-fō-blas′tik). Pertaining to the production of lymphocytes.

lym·pho·blas·to·ma (lim-fō-blas-tō′mă). SYN lymphoblastic *lymphoma.* [lymphoblast + G. *-oma,* tumor]

giant follicular l., SYN nodular *lymphoma.*

lym·pho·blas·to·sis (lim′fō-blas-tō′sis). The presence of lymphoblasts in the peripheral blood; sometimes used as a synonym for acute lymphocytic leukemia. [lymphoblast + G. *-osis,* condition]

lym·pho·cele (lim′fō-sēl). A cystic mass that contains lymph, usually from diseased or injured lymphatic channels. SYN lymphocyst. [lympho- + G. *kēlē,* tumor]

lym·pho·cer·as·tism (lim-fō-ser′as-tizm). Obsolete term for the process of formation of cells in the lymphocytic series. [lympho- + G. *kerastos,* mixed, mingled]

lym·pho·ci·ne·sis, lym·pho·ci·ne·sia (lim′fō-si-nē′sis, nē-zē-ă). SYN lymphokinesis.

lym·pho·cyst (lim′fō-sist). SYN lymphocele. [lympho- + G. *kystis,* bladder]

lym·pho·cy·ta·phe·re·sis (lim′fō-sīt-ăf-ĕ-rē′sis). Separation and removal of lymphocytes from the withdrawn blood, with the remainder of the blood retransfused into the donor. SYN lymphapheresis. [lymphocyte + G. *aphairesis,* a withdrawal]

▊**lym·pho·cyte** (lim′fō-sīt). A white blood cell formed in lymphatic tissue throughout the body (e.g., lymph nodes, spleen, thymus, tonsils, Peyer patches, and sometimes in bone marrow) and in normal adults making up approximately 22–28% of the total number of leukocytes in the circulating blood. L.'s are generally small (7–8 μm), but larger forms are frequent (10–20 μm); with Wright (or a similar) stain, the nucleus is deeply colored (purple-blue), and is composed of dense aggregates of chromatin within a sharply defined nuclear membrane; the nucleus is usually round, but may be slightly indented, and is eccentrically situated within a relatively small amount of light blue cytoplasm that ordinarily contains no granules; especially in larger forms, the cytoplasm may be fairly abundant and include several bright red-violet fine granules; in contrast to granules of the myeloid series of cells, those in l.'s do not yield a positive oxidase or peroxidase reaction. L.'s are divided into 2 principal groups, termed T and B cells, based on their surface molecules as well as function. Natural killer cells, which are large granular l.'s, represent a small percentage of the l. population. SYN lymph cell, lympholeukocyte. [lympho- + G. *kytos,* call]

B l., an immunologically important l. that is not thymus-dependent, is of short life, and resembles the bursa-derived l. of birds in that it is responsible for the production of immunoglobulins, i.e., it is the precursor of the plasma cell and expresses immunoglobulins on its surface but does not release them. It does not play a direct role in cell-mediated immunity. SEE ALSO T l. SYN B cell (2).

pre-B l., an early B-lymphoid type cell that is recognized by

lymphocytes

	T- lymphocytes	B-lymphocytes
place of formation	marrow (from undifferentiated stem cells)	
regulating organ or place of differentiation	thymus	lymphoid tissue of intestine (Peyer's patches); in birds, bursa of Fabricius
function	cell-transmitted immunity	humoral immunity
cell function forms	T-memory, killer, helper, suppressor cells	B-memory, antibody-producing cells (plasma cells)
interactions	see "immunity" (and diagram s.v.)	
surface characteristics of cell membrane	surface structures, distinguished by monoclonal antibodies (see "marker")	
	T-cell (antigen) receptor	receptor for complement factor C3
	receptor for sheep erythrocyte (sheep red blood cell); shown by rosette test	receptor for mouse erythrocyte
transformation (blastogenesis, mitosis) stimulants	antigens (e.g., transplantation or tissue, bacterial antigen), mitogens (e.g., phytohemagglutinin [PHA], concanavalin A [con A])	antigens (indirect), interleukin II, pokeweed mitogen (PWM)
soluble products of activated lymphocytes	lymphokines	immunoglobulins (antibodies)
defects	see "immunodeficiency"	
malignant proliferation	see "lymphoma" (diagram), lymphatic leukemia	

immunofluorescence as a μ-positive, L-chain-negative bone marrow cell.

Rieder l., an abnormal form of l. that has a greatly indented (or lobed), slightly twisted nucleus; such cells are usually observed in certain examples of chronic lymphocytic leukemia.

T l., a thymocyte-derived l. of immunologic importance that is long-lived (months to years) and is responsible for cell-mediated immunity. T l.'s form rosettes with sheep erythrocytes and, in the presence of transforming agents (mitogens), differentiate and divide. These cells have characteristic CD3 surface markers and may be further divided into subsets according to function, such as helper, cytotoxic, etc. SEE ALSO B l. SYN T cell.

transformed l., SEE lymphocyte *transformation.*

tumor-infiltrating l.'s (TIL, TILS) (lim'fō-sītz), l.'s collected from the site of a tumor and exposed to IL-2 in vitro to expand the population. When these cells are injected back into the tumor-bearing host, they will specifically kill the tumor from which they originated.

lym·pho·cy·the·mia (lim'fō-sī-the'mē-ă). SYN lymphocytosis.

lym·pho·cyt·ic (lim-fō-sit'ik). Pertaining to or characterized by lymphocytes.

lym·pho·cy·to·blast (lim-fō-sī'tō-blast). SYN lymphoblast. [lymphocyte + G. *blastos,* germ]

lym·pho·cy·to·ma (lim'fō-sī-tō'mă). A circumscribed nodule or mass of mature lymphocytes, grossly resembling a neoplasm. [lymphocyte + G. *-oma,* tumor]

benign l. cutis, a soft red to violaceous skin nodule often involv-

ing the head, caused by dense infiltration of the dermis by lymphocytes and histiocytes, often forming lymphoid follicles, separated from the epidermis by a narrow noninfiltrating layer. SYN cutaneous pseudolymphoma, Spiegler-Fendt sarcoid.

lym·pho·cy·to·pe·nia (lim'fō-sī-tō-pē'nē-ă). SYN lymphopenia.

lym·pho·cy·to·poi·e·sis (lim'fō-sī-tō-poy-ē'sis). The formation of lymphocytes. [lymphocyte + G. *poiēsis,* a making]

lym·pho·cy·to·sis (lim'fō-sī-tō'sis). A form of actual or relative leukocytosis in which there is an increase in the number of lymphocytes. SYN lymphocythemia, lymphocytic leukocytosis.

lym·pho·der·ma (lim'fō-der'mă). A condition resulting from any disease of the cutaneous lymphatic vessels. [lympho- + G. *derma,* skin]

lym·pho·duct (lim'fō-dŭkt). A lymphatic vessel. SEE lymph *vessels,* under *vessel.* [lympho- + L. *ductus,* a leading]

lym·pho·gen·e·sis (lim-fō-gen'ĕ-sis). Lymph production. [lympho- + G. *genesis,* production]

lym·pho·gen·ic (lim-fō-jen'ik). SYN lymphogenous (1).

lym·phog·e·nous (lim-foj'ĕ-nŭs). 1. Originating from lymph or the lymphatic system. SYN lymphogenic. 2. Producing lymph.

lym·pho·glan·du·la (lim-fō-glan'doo-lă). SYN lymph node.

lym·pho·gran·u·lo·ma (lim'fō-gran-ū-lō'mă). Old nonspecific term used with reference to a few basically dissimilar diseases in which the pathologic processes result in granulomas or granulomalike lesions, especially in various groups of lymph nodes (which then become conspicuously enlarged).

l. benig'num, old term for sarcoidosis.

l. ingina'le, SYN venereal l.

l. malig'num, old term for Hodgkin disease.

Schaumann l., old eponym for sarcoidosis.

venereal l., l. vene'reum, a venereal infection usually caused by *Chlamydia trachomatis,* and characterized by a transient genital ulcer and inguinal adenopathy in the male; in the female, perirectal lymph nodes are involved and rectal stricture is a common occurrence. SYN Favre-Durand-Nicholas disease, l. inguinale, Nicolas-Favre disease, tropical bubo.

lym·pho·gran·u·lo·ma·to·sis (lim-fō-gran'ū-lō-mă-tō'sis). Any condition characterized by the occurrence of multiple and widely distributed lymphogranulomas.

lym·phog·ra·phy (lim-fog'ră-fē). Visualization of lymphatics (lymphangiography) and lymph nodes (lymphadenography) by radiography following the intralymphatic injection of a contrast medium, usually an iodized oil. [lympho- + *graphō,* to write]

lym·pho·his·ti·o·cy·to·sis (lim'fō-his'tē-ō-sī-tō'sis). Proliferation or infiltration of lymphocytes and histiocytes.

familial erythrophagocytic l. (FEL), SYN familial hemophagocytic l.

familial hemophagocytic l. (FMLH), an extremely rare, usually fatal disease of childhood characterized by multiorgan infiltration with activated macrophages and lymphocytes. The disease is often familial and appears to be inherited as an autosomal recessive trait. SYN familial erythrophagocytic l.

lym·phoid (lim'foyd). Resembling lymph or lymphatic tissue, or pertaining to the lymphatic system. [lympho- + G. *eidos,* appearance]

lym·phoi·dec·to·my (lim-foy-dek'tō-mē). Excision of lymphoid tissue. [lymphoid + G. *ektomē,* excision]

lym·phoi·do·cyte (lim-foy'dō-sīt). A primitive mesenchymal cell believed to be capable of differentiating into all types of lymphoid cells, including lymphocytes, littoral cells, and reticular cells of lymph nodes.

lym·pho·kine (lim'fō-kīnz). Hormonelike peptide, released by activated lymphocytes, that mediates immune response; a cytokine obtained from lymphocytes. [*lympho*cyte + G. *kineō,* to set in motion]

lym·pho·ki·ne·sis (lim'fō-ki-nē'sis). 1. Circulation of lymph in the lymphatic vessels and through the lymph nodes. 2. Movement of endolymph in the semicircular canals of the inner ear. SYN lymphocinesis, lymphocinesia. [lympho- + G. *kinēsis,* movement]

ly

lym·pho·leu·ko·cyte (lim′fō-loo′kō-sīt). SYN lymphocyte.

lym·phol·o·gy (lim-fol′ō-jē). SYN lymphangiology. [lympho- + G. *logos,* study]

⬛lym·pho·ma (lim-fō′mă). Any neoplasm of lymphoid tissue; in general use, synonymous with malignant l. [lympho- + G. *-oma,* tumor]

adult T-cell l. (ATL), an acute or subacute disease associated with a human T-cell virus, with lymphadenopathy, hepatospleno-megaly, skin lesions, peripheral blood involvement, and hypercalcemia. SYN adult T-cell leukemia.

anaplastic large cell l., a form of lymphoma characterized by anaplasia of cells, sinusoidal growth, and immunoreactivity with CD30 (Ki-1 or Ber-H2). SYN Ki-1+ l.

benign l. of the rectum, obsolete term for a rectal polyp composed of lymphoid tissue with follicle formation, covered by mucosa.

⬛Burkitt l., a form of malignant l. reported in African children, frequently involving the jaw and abdominal lymph nodes. Geographic distribution of Burkitt l. suggests that it is found in areas with endemic malaria. It is primarily a B-cell neoplasm and is believed to be caused by Epstein-Barr virus, a member of the family Herpesviridae, which can be isolated from tumor cells in culture; occasional cases of l. with similar features have been reported in the United States.

chronic lymphocytic l., a type of low-grade non-Hodgkin l. characterized by lymphocytosis, lymphadenoathy, and, in late stages, hepatosplenomegaly; may evolve into chronic lymphocytic leukemia over the course of several years.

diffuse small cleaved cell l., diffuse poorly differentiated lymphocytic l.; follicular center cell l. that lacks a follicular pattern; malignancy is of intermediate grade.

extranodal marginal zone l., SYN MALToma.

follicular l., SYN nodular l.

follicular predominantly large cell l., a B-cell l. of intermediate malignancy.

follicular predominantly small cleaved cell l., SYN poorly differentiated lymphocytic l.

histiocytic l., a malignant tumor of reticular tissue composed predominantly of neoplastic histiocytes. SEE ALSO large cell l.

Hodgkin l., SYN Hodgkin *disease.*

immunoblastic l., a monomorphous proliferation of immuno-

comparison of working formulation (WF) and Revised European-American Lymphoma (REAL) classification			
WF category *	**frequency** † **(%)**	**REAL classification‡**	
		B-cell neoplasms	**T-cell neoplasms**
A. small lymphocytic consistent with CLL	4	B-cell CLL/SLL/PLL marginal zone/MALT mantle cell	T-cell CLL/PLL LGL
plasmacytoid		lymphoplasmacytoid	
B. follicular, predominantly small cleaved cell	26	follicle center, follicular, grade I mantle zone marginal zone	
C. follicular, mixed small cleaved and large cell	9	follicle center, follicular, grade II marginal zone/MALT	
D. follicular, large cell	4	follicle center, follicular, grade III	
E. diffuse, small cleaved cell	8	mantle cell follicle center, diffuse small cell marginal zone/MALT	T-cell CLL/PLL LGL peripheral T-cell, unspecified ATL/L angioimmunoblastic angiocentric
F. diffuse, mixed small and large cell	7	large B-cell lymphoma (rich in T-cells) follicle center, diffuse small cell lymphoplasmacytoid marginal zone/MALT mantle cell	peripheral T-cell, unspecified ATL/L angioimmunoblastic angiocentric
G. diffuse, large cell	22	diffuse large B-cell lymphoma	peripheral T-cell, unspecified ATL/L angioimmunoblastic angiocentric
H. large cell immunoblastic	9	diffuse large B-cell lymphoma	peripheral T-cell, unspecified ATL/L angioimmunoblastic angiocentric anaplastic large-cell
I. lymphoblastic	5	precursor B-lymphoblastic	precursor T-lymphoblastic
J. small noncleaved cell Burkitt non-Burkitt	6	Burkitt high-grade B-cell, Burkitt-like	peripheral T-cell, unspecified

* categories A–C = low grade (survival 5–10 or more years untreated); D–G = intermediate grade (survival 2–5 years untreated); H–J = high grade (survival 0.5–2.0 years untreated); categories D–H are also called aggressive lymphomas

† ATL/L, adult T-cell lymphoma/leukemia; CLI, chronic lymphocytic leukemia; LGL, large granular lymphocyte leukemia; MALT, mucosa-associated lymphoid tissue; PLL, prolymphocytic leukemia; SLL, small lymphocytic lymphoma

‡ lymphoma

blasts involving the lymph nodes; it may develop in some patients with angioimmunoblastic lymphadenopathy.

Ki-1+ l., SYN anaplastic large cell l.

large cell l., l. composed of large mononuclear cells of undetermined type. Many l.'s formerly classified as histiocytic have in recent years been shown to consist of large lymphocytes.

Lennert l., malignant l. with a high proportion of diffusely scattered epithelioid cells, tonsillar involvement, and an unpredictable course.

lymphoblastic l., a diffuse l. in children, with supradiaphragmatic distribution and T lymphocytes having convoluted nuclei; many patients develop acute lymphoblastic leukemia. SYN lymphoblastoma.

malignant l., general term for ordinarily malignant neoplasms of lymphoid and reticuloendothelial tissues which present as apparently circumscribed solid tumors composed of cells that appear primitive or resemble lymphocytes, plasma cells, or histiocytes. L.'s appear most frequently in lymph nodes, spleen, or other normal sites of lymphoreticular cells; when disseminated, L.'s, especially of the lymphocytic type, may invade the peripheral blood and manifest as leukemia. L.'s are classified by cell type, degrees of differentiation, and nodular or diffuse pattern; Hodgkin disease and Burkitt l. are special forms.

mantle cell l., a clinically and biologically distinct B-cell neoplasm with a recurring acquired genetic abnormality, the t(11;14) translocation, and a heterogeneous histologic appearance that may lead to confusion with reactive or other neoplastic lymphoproliferative disorders.

marginal zone l., a heterogeneous group of neoplasms originating from the B-cell–rich zones of the lymph nodes, spleen, or extranodal lymphoid tissue. Those tumors originating from mucosa-associated lymphoid tissue (MALT), most often in the stomach, intestines, salivary glands, and lungs, are called MALTomas.

Mediterranean l., SYN immunoproliferative small intestinal *disease.*

nodular l., malignant l. arising from lymphoid follicular B cells which may be small or large, growing in a nodular pattern. SYN follicular l., giant follicular lymphoblastoma.

nodular histiocytic l., SYN poorly differentiated lymphocytic l.

non-Hodgkin l. (NHL), a l. other than Hodgkin disease, classified by Rappaport into a nodular or diffuse tumor pattern and by cell type; a working or international formulation separates such l.'s into low, intermediate, and high grade malignancy and into cytologic subtypes reflecting follicular center cell or other origin.

peripheral T-cell l., unspecified, a heterogeneous group of T-cell neoplasms expressing typical T-cell markers such as CD2, CD3, CD5, and either T-cell α/β or γ/δ receptors.

poorly differentiated lymphocytic l., a B-cell l. with nodular or diffuse lymph node or bone marrow involvement by large lymphoid cells. SYN follicular predominantly small cleaved cell l., nodular histiocytic l.

small lymphocytic l., SYN well-differentiated lymphocytic l.

T-cell–rich, B-cell l., a B-cell l. in which more than 90% of the cells are of T-cell origin, masking the large cells that form the neoplastic B-cell component. SEE ALSO adult T-cell l.

well-differentiated lymphocytic l., essentially the same disease as chronic lymphocytic leukemia, except that lymphocytes are not increased in the peripheral blood; lymph nodes are enlarged and other lymphoid tissue or bone marrow is infiltrated by small lymphocytes. SYN small lymphocytic l.

lym·pho·ma·toid (lim-fō′mă-toyd). Resembling a lymphoma.

lym·pho·ma·to·sis (lim′fō-mă-to′sis). Any condition characterized by the occurrence of multiple, widely distributed sites of involvement with lymphoma.

lym·pho·ma·tous (lim-fō′mă-tŭs). Pertaining to or characterized by lymphoma.

lym·pho·no·dus. ☆official alternate term for lymph node.

lym·pho·path·i·a (lim-fō-path′ē-ă). SYN lymphopathy.

lym·phop·a·thy (lim-fop′ă-thē). Any disease of the lymphatic vessels or lymph nodes. SYN lymphopathia. [lympho- + G. *pathos,* suffering]

lym·pho·pe·nia (lim-fō-pē′nē-ă). A reduction, relative or absolute, in the number of lymphocytes in the circulating blood. SYN lymphocytic leukopenia, lymphocytopenia. [lympho- + G. *penia,* poverty]

lym·pho·plas·ma·phe·re·sis (lim′fō-plaz′mă-fĕ-rē′sis). Separation and removal of lymphocytes and plasma from the withdrawn blood, with the remainder of the blood retransfused into the donor. [lymphocyte + plasma + G. *aphairesis,* a withdrawal]

lym·pho·poi·e·sis (lim-fō-poy-ē′sis). The formation of lymphatic tissue. [lympho- + G. *poiēsis,* a making]

lym·pho·poi·et·ic (lim-fō-poy-et′ik). Pertaining to or characterized by lymphopoiesis.

lym·pho·re·tic·u·lo·sis (lim′fō-rĕ-tik-ū-lō′sis). Proliferation of the reticuloendothelial cells (macrophages) of the lymph nodes.

benign inoculation l., SYN catscratch *disease.*

lym·phor·rha·gia (lim-fō-rā′jē-ă). SYN lymphorrhea. [lympho- + G. *rhēgnymi,* to burst forth]

lym·phor·rhea (lim-fō-rē′ă). An escape of lymph onto the surface of the skin from ruptured, torn, or cut lymphatic vessels. SYN lymphorrhagia. [lympho- + G. *rhoia,* a flow]

lym·phor·rhoid (lim′fō-royd). A dilation of a lymph channel, resembling a hemorrhoid. [lymph + -*rrhoid,* tending to leak, on the analogy of *hemorrhoid*]

lym·pho·scin·tig·ra·phy (lim′fō-sin-tig′ră-fē). Scintillation scanning of lymphatics or lymph nodes following intralymphatic or subcutaneous injection of a radionuclide.

lym·pho·sis (lim-fō′sis). Obsolete term for lymphocytic *leukemia.*

lym·phos·ta·sis (lim-fos′tă-sis). Obstruction of the normal flow of lymph. [lympho- + G. *stasis,* a standing still]

lym·pho·tax·is (lim-fō-tak′sis). The exertion of an effect that attracts or repels lymphocytes. [lympho- + G. *taxis,* orderly arrangement]

lym·pho·tox·ic·i·ty (lim′fō-tok-sis′i-tē). Toxicity to lymphocytes.

lym·pho·tox·in (lim′fō-tok-sin). A lymphokine from T lymphocytes that lyses or damages many cell types.

lym·phot·ro·phy (lim-fot′rō-fē). Nourishment of the tissues by lymph in parts devoid of blood vessels. [lympho- + G. *trophē,* nourishment]

lym·phu·ria (lim-foo′rē-ă). Discharge of lymph in the urine. [lympho- + G. *ouron,* urine]

Lynch, Henry T., 20th century U.S. oncologist. SEE L. *syndrome.*

lyn·es·tre·nol (lin-es′tren-ol). A progestational agent, used with mestranol as an oral contraceptive. SYN ethinylestrenol.

△lyo-. Dissolution. SEE ALSO lyso-. [G. *lyō,* to loosen, dissolve]

ly·o·en·zyme (lī-ō-en′zīm). **1.** Any enzyme existing in the cell in soluble form. **2.** A soluble enzyme.

ly·ol·y·sis (lī-ol′i-sis). Rarely used term for solvolysis.

Lyon, B. B. Vincent, U.S. physician, 1880–1953. SEE Meltzer-L. *test.*

Lyon, Mary F., English cytogeneticist, *1925. SEE L. *hypothesis;* lyonization.

ly·on·i·za·tion (lī′on-i-zā′shŭn). The normal phenomenon that wherever there are two or more haploid sets of X-linked genes in each cell all but one of the genes are inactivated apparently at random and have no phenotypic expression. L. is usual but not invariable for all loci. Its randomness explains the more variable espressivity of X-linked traits in women than in men. L. occurs in men with the Klinefelter (XXY) karyotype. SEE ALSO gene dosage *compensation.* SYN Lyon hypothesis, X-inactivation. [M. *Lyon*]

ly·o·phil, ly·o·phile (lī′ō-fil, -fīl). A substance that is lyophilic.

ly·o·phil·ic (lī-ō-fil′ik). **1.** In colloid chemistry, denoting a dispersed phase having a pronounced affinity for the dispersion medium; when the dispersed phase is l., the colloid is usually a reversible one. **2.** Denoting a preference for the solvent. SYN lyotropic. [lyo- + G. *phileō,* to love]

ly·oph·i·li·za·tion (lī-of′i-li-zā′shŭn). **1.** The process of isolating a solid substance from solution by freezing the solution and evaporating the ice under vacuum. **2.** The process of imparting lyophilic properties to a substance. SYN freeze-drying.

ly

ly·o·phobe (lī'ō-fōb). A substance that is lyophobic.

ly·o·pho·bic (lī-ō-fo'bik). **1.** In colloid chemistry, denoting a dispersed phase having but slight affinity for the dispersion medium; when the dispersed phase is l., the colloid is usually an irreversible one. **2.** Denoting a lack of preference or rejection of the solvent. [lyo- + G. *phobos*, fear]

ly·o·sorp·tion (lī-ō-sōrp'shŭn). Adsorption of a liquid on a solid surface.

ly·o·tro·pic (lī-ō-trop'ik). SYN lyophilic. [lyo- + G. *tropē*, a turning]

ly·pres·sin (lī'pres-in). Vasopressin-containing lysine in position 8; an antidiuretic and vasopressor hormone. SYN 8-lysine vasopressin.

ly·ra (lī'rǎ). A lyre-shaped structure. [L. and G. lyre]

   l. davidis, lyre of David, obsolete terms for *commissura* fornicis.

   l. uteri'na, SYN palmate *folds* of cervical canal, under *fold.*

Lys Symbol for lysine or lysyl.

△**lys-.** SEE lyso-.

ly·sate (lī'sāt). Material produced by the destructive process of lysis.

lyse (līz). To break up, to disintegrate, to effect lysis. SYN lyze.

ly·se·mia (lī-sē'mē-ǎ). Disintegration or dissolution of red blood cells and the occurrence of hemoglobin in the circulating plasma and in the urine. [lyso- + G. *haima*, blood]

ly·serg·am·ide (lī-serj'ǎ-mīd). SYN *lysergic* amide.

ly·ser·gic ac·id (lī-ser'jik). The D-isomer is a cleavage product of alkaline hydrolysis of ergot alkaloids; occurs as shiny crystals, slightly soluble in water; a psychotomimetic.

   l. a. amide, a psychotomimetic agent present in *Rivea corymbosa* and *Ipomoea tricolor;* possesses less hallucinogenic potency than does l. a. diethylamide. SYN ergine, lysergamide.

   l. a. diethylamide (LSD), peripherally, a serotonin antagonist; 1 to 2 µg per kg induces hallucinatory states of a visual rather than auditory nature; its use may precipitate psychoses; it has been occasionally used in the treatment of chronic alcoholism and psychotic disorders. SYN lysergide.

   l. a. monoethylamide, a psychotomimetic agent present in *Rivea corymbosa* and *Ipomoea tricolor;* possesses less hallucinatory potency than does l. a. diethylamide.

ly·ser·gide (lī-ser'jīd). SYN *lysergic acid* diethylamide.

ly·ser·gol (lī-sŭr-jol). A semisynthetic ergot alkaloid.

ly·sin (lī'sin). **1.** A specific complement-fixing antibody that acts destructively on cells and tissues; the various types are designated in accordance with the form of antigen that stimulates the production of the l., e.g., hemolysin, bacteriolysin. **2.** Any substance that causes lysis.

ly·sine (K, Lys) (lī'sēn). 2,6-Diaminohexanoic acid; the L-isomer is a nutritionally essential α-amino acid of mammals found in many proteins; distinguished by an ε-amino group.

   l. decarboxylase, an enzyme that catalyzes the decarboxylation of L-l., with the production of cadaverine and CO_2.

ly·si·ne·mia (lī-si-nē'mē-ǎ). SEE hyperlysinemia.

8-ly·sine va·so·pres·sin. SYN lypressin.

ly·sin·i·um (lī-sin'ē-um). The cation form of lysine, either lysinium (+1) or lysinium (+2).

ly·sin·o·gen (lī-sin'ō-jen). An antigen that stimulates the formation of a specific lysin.

ly·si·no·gen·ic (lī'si-nō-jen'ik). Having the property of a lysinogen.

ly·sin·u·ria (lī-si-noo'rē-ǎ). The presence of lysine in the urine.

ly·sis (lī'sis). **1.** Destruction of red blood cells, bacteria, and other structures by a specific lysin, usually referred to by the structure destroyed (e.g., hemolysis, bacteriolysis, nephrolysis); may be due to a direct toxin or an immune mechanism, such as antibody reacting with antigen on the surface of a target cell, usually by binding and activation of a series of proteins in the blood with enzymatic activity (complement system). **2.** Gradual subsidence of the symptoms of an acute disease, a form of the recovery process, as distinguished from crisis. [G. dissolution or loosening]

   bystander l., complement-mediated l. of nearby cells in the vicinity of a complement activation site.

△**lyso-, lys-.** Lysis, dissolution. SEE ALSO lyo-. [G. *lysis*, a loosening]

ly·so·ceph·a·lin (lī-sō-sef'ǎ-lin). A lysophosphatidic acid esterified with serine or ethanolamine, i.e., a lysophosphatidylserine or -ethanolamine; analogous to lysolecithin.

ly·so·gen (lī'sō-jen). **1.** That which is capable of inducing lysis. **2.** A bacterium in the state of lysogeny. **3.** Any antigen that stimulates lysin production. [lysin + G. *-gen,* producing]

ly·so·gen·e·sis (lī-sō-jen'ĕ-sis). The production of lysins.

ly·so·gen·ic (lī-sō-jen'ik). **1.** Causing or having the power to cause lysis, as the action of certain antibodies and chemical substances. **2.** Pertaining to bacteria in the state of lysogeny.

ly·so·ge·nic·i·ty (lī'sō-jĕ-nis'i-tē). The property of being lysogenic.

ly·so·ge·ni·za·tion (lī'sō-jĕ-ni-zā'shŭn, lī-soj'ĕ-ni-zā'shŭn). The process by which a bacterium becomes lysogenic.

ly·sog·e·ny (lī-soj'ĕ-nē). The phenomenon by which a bacterium is infected by a temperate bacteriophage whose DNA is integrated into the bacterial genome and replicates along with the bacterial DNA but remains latent or unexpressed; triggering of the lytic cycle may occur spontaneously or by certain agents and will result in the production of bacteriophage and lysis of the bacterial cell.

ly·so·ki·nase (lī-sō-kī'nās). Term for activator agents (e.g., streptokinase, urokinase, staphylokinase) that produce plasmin by indirect or multiple-stage action on plasminogen.

ly·so·lec·i·thin (lī-sō-les'i-thin). A lysophosphatidylcholine; capable of lysing erythrocytes.

   l.-lecithin acyltransferase (LLAT), an enzyme that catalyzes the reversible reaction of l. and another phospholipid (e.g., phosphatidylethanolamine) to form lecithin and lysophosphatidylethanolamine; a major route in the restructuring of lecithin.

ly·so·lec·i·thin·ase (lī-sō-les'i-thin-ās). SYN *lysophospholipase.*

ly·so·phos·pha·tid·ic ac·id (lī'sō-fos'fǎ-tid'ik). A phosphatidic acid in which only one of the two hydroxyl groups of the glycerophosphate is esterified; most commonly, when carbon-1 of the glycerol moiety is esterified (e.g., 1-acylglycerol-3-phosphate).

   l. a. acyltransferase, 1-acylglycerol-3-phosphate acyltransferase, 1-acylglycerol-3-phosphate acyltransferase.

ly·so·phos·pha·ti·dyl·cho·line (lī'sō-fos'fǎ-tī'dil-kō'lēn). A phosphatidylcholine in which a fatty acid has been removed from the C2 position of the glycerol group.

ly·so·phos·pha·ti·dyl·ser·ine (lī'sō-fos'fǎ-tī'dil-ser'ēn). Phosphatidylserine from which one fatty acid residue has been removed from the glycerol moiety, typically at carbon-2. Cf. lysophosphatidic acid.

ly·so·phos·pho·li·pase (lī'sō-fos'fō-lip'ās). A hydrolase removing the single acyl group from a lysolecithin, producing glycerophosphocholine and the free fatty acid anion. SYN lecithinase B, lysolecithinase, phospholipase B (1).

ly·so·some (lī'sō-sōm). A cytoplasmic membrane-bound vesicle measuring 5-8 nm (primary l.) and containing a wide variety of glycoprotein hydrolytic enzymes active at an acid pH; serves to digest exogenous material, such as bacteria, as well as effete organelles of the cells. [lyso- + G. *soma*, body]

   definitive l.'s, SYN secondary l.'s.

   primary l.'s, l.'s produced at the Golgi apparatus where hydrolytic enzymes are incorporated; they fuse with phagosomes or pinosomes to become secondary l.'s.

   secondary l.'s, l.'s in which lysis takes place, owing to the activity of hydrolytic enzymes; they are believed to eventually become residual bodies. SYN definitive l.'s, digestive vacuole.

ly·so·staph·in (lī-sō-staf'in). A peptidase enzyme produced by certain strains of staphylococcus microorganisms with antibacterial activity against staphylococci.

ly·so·type (li'so-typ). A type within a bacterial species determined by its reaction to specific phages. [lyso + type]

ly·so·zyme (lī'sō-zīm). An enzyme hydrolyzing 1,4-β links between *N*-acetylmuramic acid and *N*-acetyl-D-glucosamine, and thus destructive to cell walls of certain bacteria; present in tears and some other body fluids, in egg white, and in some plant tissues; used in the prevention of caries and in the treatment of infant formulas. SYN mucopeptide glycohydrolase, muramidase.

Lys·sa·vi·rus (lis′ă-vī-rŭs). A genus of viruses (family Rhabdoviridae) that includes the rabies virus group.

Australian bat L., a species that has caused a fatal rabieslike disease in a woman in Australia.

European bat L., two species (1 & 2) causing rabieslike diseases in humans in Europe; transmitted by bite of insectivorous bats.

ly·syl (K) (lī′sil). The univalent radical of lysine.

l. hydroxylase, an enzyme that acts on specific lysyl residues in certain proteins (e.g., collagens) with α-ketoglutarate and O_2 to produce δ-hydroxylysyl residues, succinate, and CO_2; this enzyme, which requires Fe^{2+} and ascorbate, is deficient in Ehlers-Danlos syndrome type VI. SYN l. 2-oxoglutarate dioxygenase.

l. oxidase, an enzyme, which requires Cu^{2+} and O_2, that oxidizes certain lysyl residues in collagen to allysyl residues and hydroxylysyl residues to hydroxyallysyl residues; this is a required step for the cross-linking (via aldol condensations and Amadori rearrangements) of collagen strands; a lower activity of this enzyme is associated with occipital horn syndrome.

l. 2-oxoglutarate dioxygenase, SYN l. hydroxylase.

ly·syl-brad·y·ki·nin (lī′sil-brad-ē-kī′nin). SYN kallidin.

Lyth·o·glyph·op·sis (lith-ō-glif-op′-sis). A genus of amphibious freshwater operculate snails of the family Hydrobiidae (subfamily Hydrobiinae; subclass Prosobranchiata). In the Mekong River delta, *Lythoglyphopsis aperta* serves as an intermediate host of the blood fluke, *Schistosoma mekongi.*

lyt·ic (lit′ik). Pertaining to lysis; used colloq. as an abbreviation for osteolytic.

lyx·i·tol (lik′si-tol). A pentitol (reduced lyxose) occurring in lyxoflavin.

lyx·o·fla·vin (lik-sō-flā′vin). A compound similar to riboflavin except that D-lyxitol is present in place of the D-ribitol group; present in small quantity in cardiac muscle.

lyx·ose (lik′sōs). An aldopentose; D-l. is epimeric with both D-arabinose and D-xylose; L-l. is epimeric with D-ribose.

lyx·u·lose (liks′ū-lōs). The 2-keto derivative of lyxose.

lyze (līz). SYN lyse.

ly

μ **1.** The 12th letter of the Greek alphabet, mu. **2.** Symbol for micro- (2); micron; dynamic *viscosity*; magnetic or electric dipole moment of a molecule; chemical *potential*; denotes the position of a substituent located on the 12th atom from the carboxyl or other functional group.

μ$_N$ Symbol for nuclear *magneton*.

μ$_B$ 1. Symbol for Bohr *magneton*.

μμ micromicro-; micromicron.

μμg Symbol for micromicrogram.

μΩ Symbol for microhm.

μC Symbol for microcoulomb.

μCi Symbol for microcurie.

μg Symbol for microgram.

μl, μL Symbol for microliter.

μm Symbol for micrometer.

μmol Symbol for micromole.

μmol/L Symbol for micromolar.

μV Symbol for microvolt.

M 1. Symbol for mega- (2); morgan; molarity (moles per liter, also written *M* or M); myopia or myopic; methionine; 6-mercaptopurine ribonucleoside in a nucleic acid; L. *misce*, mix; metal. **2.** Symbol for a blood factor. See entries under MNSs blood group, Blood Groups Appendix.

M. Abbreviation for L. *misce*, mix.

M Symbol for molarity.

M_r Symbol for molecular weight *ratio* or relative molecular *mass*.

m Symbol for meter; milli-; minim; mass; magnetic dipole moment; molality.

mμ Symbol for millimicron.

M Symbol for moles per liter (also written M or *M*).

△m- Abbreviation for meta- (2).

MA Abbreviation for mental *age*; mentoanterior *position*.

ma, mA Abbreviation for milliampere.

MAA Abbreviation for macroaggregated *albumin*.

MAB Abbreviation for monoclonal *antibody*.

MAC 1. Abbreviation for minimal anesthetic *concentration*; minimal alveolar *concentration*; membrane attack *complex*. **2.** Abbreviation for *Mycobacterium avium complex*. SEE *Mycobacterium avium-intracellulare complex*.

△Mac-. For proper names beginning thus, see also Mc-.

Ma·ca·ca (mă-kah′kă). A large genus of Old World monkeys (family Cercopithecidae) that includes the macaque and rhesus monkeys, and the Barbary apes. *M. mulatta*, the rhesus monkey, is used as a research animal. [Pg. *macaco*, monkey]

ma·caque (mă-kahk′). SEE *Macaca*. [Fr.]

MacConkey, Alfred T., British bacteriologist, 1861–1931. SEE MacConkey *agar*.

Mace, MACE Acronym for *m*ethyl*c*hloroform 2-chlor*ace*tophenone (the classical lacrimator) in a light petroleum dispersant and a pressurized propellant.

mac·er·ate (mas′er-āt). To soften by steeping or soaking. [see maceration]

mac·er·a·tion (mas-er-ā′shŭn). **1.** Softening by the action of a liquid. **2.** Softening of tissues after death by nonputrefactive (sterile) autolysis; seen especially in the stillborn, with detachment of the epidermis. [L. *macero*, pp. *-atus*, to soften by soaking]

Macewen, Sir William, Scottish surgeon, 1848–1924. SEE M. *sign, symptom, triangle*.

Mach, Ernst, Austrian scientist, 1838–1916. SEE M. *band, number*.

ma·chine (mă-shēn′). Any mechanical apparatus or device. [L. *machina*, contrivance]

anesthesia m., equipment used for inhalation anesthesia, including flowmeters, vaporizers, and sources of compressed gases, but not including the anesthetic circuit or mechanisms for elimination of carbon dioxide.

∎heart-lung m., a device incorporating a blood pump (artificial heart) and a blood oxygenator (artificial lung) to provide extracorporeal circulation and oxygenation of the blood during cardiac surgery.

panoramic rotating m., an x-ray machine using a reciprocating motion of the tube and extraoral film to produce a radiograph of all the teeth and surrounding structures. SEE ALSO tomography.

Mackay, Ralph Stuart, U.S. physicist, *1924. SEE M.-Marg *tonometer*.

Mackenrodt, Alwin K., German gynecologist, 1859–1925. SEE M. *ligament*.

Mackenzie, Sir James, Scottish physician practicing in London, 1853–1925. SEE M. *polygraph*.

Mackenzie, Richard J., Scottish surgeon, 1821–1854. SEE M. *amputation*.

MacLachlan, Elsie A., 20th century researcher. SEE Lowe-Terrey-MacL. *syndrome*.

Macleod, William Mathieson, British physician, 1911–1977. SEE M. *syndrome;* Swyer-James-MacLeod *syndrome*.

Macleod, Roderick, Scottish physician, 1795–1852. SEE M. *rheumatism*.

ma·clur·in (mă-kloor′in) [C.I. 75240]. A natural dye associated with morin and derived from fustic; used to dye fabrics with various metal mordants. It turns deep green on addition of ferric chloride.

MacNeal, Ward J., U.S. bacteriologist, 1881–1946. SEE M. tetrachrome blood *stain;* Novy and M. blood *agar*.

△macr-. SEE macro-.

Mac·ra·can·tho·rhyn·chus (mak′ră-kan-thō-ring′kŭs). A genus of giant thorny-headed worms (class Acanthocephala). [macro- + G. *akantha*, thorn, + *rhynchos*, snout]

M. hirudina′ceus, the giant thorny-headed worm of the pig, approximately the size of the giant roundworm (*Ascaris*); it inhabits the intestinal tract where nodules develop at the site of penetration of the spiny proboscis of each worm; it has occasionally been reported in man; transmission is by ingestion of infected insects, frequently dung beetles or cockroaches that have fed on feces of infected pigs containing viable eggs and have developed the cystacanth stage infective to the vertebrate host, including humans.

mac·ren·ceph·a·ly, mac·ren·ce·pha·lia (mak′ren-sef′ă-lē, -sĕ-fā′lē-ă). Hypertrophy of the brain; the condition of having a large brain. [macro- + G. *enkephalos*, brain]

△macro-, macr-. Large, long. SEE ALSO mega-, megalo-. [G. *makros*]

mac·ro·ad·e·no·ma (mak′rō-ad-ĕ-nō′mă). A pituitary adenoma larger than 10 mm in diameter.

mac·ro·am·y·lase (mak-rō-am′i-lās). Descriptive term applied to a form of serum amylase in which the enzyme is present as a complex joined to a globulin; the molecular weight of the enzyme alone is 50,000, whereas that of the complex probably exceeds 160,000; hence, renal excretion of the complex is not appreciable.

mac·ro·am·y·la·se·mia (mak′rō-am′i-lā-sē′mē-ă). A form of hyperamylasemia, in which a portion of serum amylase exists as macroamylase. [macroamylase + G. *haima*, blood]

mac·ro·bac·te·ri·um (mak′rō-bak-tēr′ē-ŭm). SYN megabacterium.

△ **Combining Forms**	☆ **Official alternate Terminologia Anatomica term**
∎ **Indicates term is illustrated, see Illustration Index**	
	[MIM] Mendelian Inheritance in Man
SYN **Synonym**	
Cf. **Compare**	C.I. **Colour Index**
[NA] Nomina Anatomica	
[TA] Terminologia Anatomica	**High Profile Term**

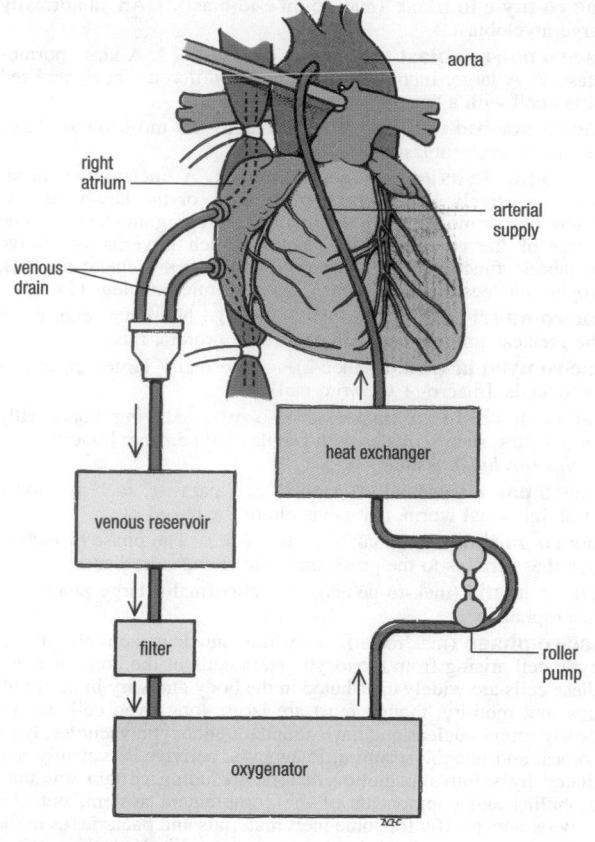

heart-lung machine

mac·ro·bi·o·sis (mak′rō-bī-ō′sis). SYN longevity. [macro- + G. *bios*, life]

mac·ro·bi·ote (mak-rō-bī′ōt). An organism that is long-lived. [macro- + G. *bios*, life]

mac·ro·bi·ot·ic (mak′rō-bī-ot′ik). **1.** Long lived. **2.** Tending to prolong life.

mac·ro·bi·ot·ics (mak′rō-bī-ot′iks). The study of the prolongation of life.

mac·ro·blast (mak′rō-blast). A large erythroblast. [macro- + G. *blastos*, germ]

mac·ro·ble·pha·ron (mak′rō-blef′ar-on). An abnormally large eyelid. [macro- + G. *blepharon*, eyelid]

mac·ro·bra·chia (mak-rō-brā′kē-ă). Condition of having abnormally thick or long arms. [macro- + G. *brachión*, arm]

mac·ro·car·dia (mak-rō-kar′dē-ă). SYN cardiomegaly.

mac·ro·ce·phal·ic, mac·ro·ceph·a·lous (mak′rō-se-fal′ik, -sef′ă-lŭs). SYN megacephalic. [macro- + G. *kephalē*, head]

mac·ro·ceph·a·ly, mac·ro·ce·pha·lia (mak-rō-sef′ă-lē, -sĕ-fā′lē-ă). SYN megacephaly. [macro- + G. *kephalē*, head]

mac·ro·chei·lia, mac·ro·chi·lia (mak-rō-kī′lē-ă). **1.** Abnormally enlarged lips. SYN macrolabia. **2.** Cavernous lymphangioma of the lip, a condition of permanent swelling of the lip resulting from the presence of greatly distended lymphatic spaces. [macro- + G. *cheilos*, lip]

mac·ro·chei·ria, mac·ro·chi·ria (mak-rō-kī′rē-ă). A condition characterized by abnormally large hands. SYN cheiromegaly, chiromegaly, megalocheiria, megalochiria. [macro- + G. *cheir*, hand]

mac·ro·chem·is·try (mak-rō-kem′is-trē). The use of chemical procedures, the reactions of which (color change, effervescence, etc.) are visible to the unaided eye. Cf. microchemistry.

mac·ro·chy·lo·mi·cron (mak′rō-kī-lō-mī′kron). An unusually large chylomicron.

mac·ro·cne·mia (mak-rō-nē′mē-ă). A condition characterized by enlargement of the legs below the knee. [macro- + G. *knēmē*, leg]

mac·ro·coc·cus (mak′rō-kok′ŭs). SYN megacoccus.

mac·ro·co·lon (mak′rō-kō′lon). A sigmoid colon of unusual length; a variety of megacolon.

mac·ro·co·nid·i·um, pl. **mac·ro·co·nid·ia** (mak′rō-kō-nid′ē-ŭm, -ă). **1.** A conidium, or exospore, of large size. **2.** In fungi, the larger of two distinctively different-sized types of conidia in a single species, thick- or thin-walled and composed of 2 to 10 cells; characteristic of most dermatophytes and some other genera e.g., *Histoplasma, Fusarium.* [macro- + Mod. L. dim. fr. G. *konis,* dust]

mac·ro·cor·nea (mak-rō-kōr′nē-ă). An abnormally large cornea.

mac·ro·cra·ni·um (mak-rō-krā′nē-ŭm). An enlarged skull, especially the bones containing the brain, as seen in hydrocephalus; the face appears relatively small in comparison.

mac·ro·cry·o·glob·u·lin (mak-rō-krī-ō-glob′ū-lin). A macroglobulin that has the properties of a cryoglobulin.

mac·ro·cry·o·glob·u·li·ne·mia (mak-rō-krī-ō-glob′ū-lin-ē′mē-ă). The presence of cold-precipitating macroglobulins in the peripheral blood; such macrocryoglobulins are often called cold hemagglutinins.

mac·ro·cyst (mak′rō-sist). A cyst of macroscopic proportions.

mac·ro·cyte (mak′rō-sīt). A large erythrocyte, such as those observed in pernicious anemia. SYN macroerythrocyte. [macro- + G. *kytos,* a hollow (cell)]

mac·ro·cy·the·mia (mak′rō-sī-thē′mē-ă). The occurrence of unusually large numbers of macrocytes in the circulating blood. SYN macrocytosis, megalocythemia, megalocytosis. [macrocyte + G. *haima,* blood]

   hyperchromatic m., an inexact term frequently used for macrocytes that contain an unusually large amount of hemoglobin, but are actually normochromic; although the total mass of hemoglobin is greater than normal (owing to the large cells), the percentage of hemoglobin in the cells is not greater than normal.

mac·ro·cy·to·sis (mak′rō-sī-tō′sis). SYN macrocythemia. [macrocyte + G. *-osis,* condition]

mac·ro·dac·tyl·ia, mac·ro·dac·tyl·ism, mac·ro·dac·ty·ly (mak-rō-dak-til′ē-ă, -dak′til-izm, dak′ti-lē). SYN megadactyly.

mac·ro·dont (mak′rō-dont). **1.** A tooth of abnormally large and frequently distorted proportions; the condition may be localized or generalized. **2.** Denoting a skull with a dental index above 44. SYN megadont, megalodont. [macro- + G. *odous (odont-),* tooth]

mac·ro·don·tia, mac·ro·don·tism (mak-rō-don′shē-ă, -don′tizm). The state of having abnormally large teeth. SYN megadontism, megalodontia.

mac·ro·dys·tro·phia li·po·ma·to·sa (mak′rō-dis-trō′fē-ă lip-ō-mă-tō′să). A rare nonfamilial disease characterized by enlargement of the fingers by lipomas, with painful degenerative arthropathy of the metacarpophalangeal and interphalangeal joints.

mac·ro·ele·ments (mak′rō-el′ĕ-ments). Inorganic nutrients needed in relatively high daily amounts (i.e., more than 100 mg per day) e.g., calcium, phosphorus, sodium, etc. SYN macrominerals.

mac·ro·en·ceph·a·lon (mak′rō-en-sef′ă-lon). SYN megaloencephalon. [macro- + G. *enkephalos,* brain]

mac·ro·e·ryth·ro·blast (mak′rō-ĕ-rith′rō-blast). A large erythroblast. SYN macronormochromoblast.

mac·ro·e·ryth·ro·cyte (mak′rō-ĕ-rith′rō-sīt). SYN macrocyte.

mac·ro·es·the·sia (mak′rō-es-thē′zē-ă). A subjective sensation that all objects are larger than they are. [macro- + G. *aisthēsis,* sensation]

mac·ro·ga·mete (mak-rō-gam′ēt). The female element in anisogamy; it is the larger of the two sex cells, with more reserve material, and usually nonmotile. SYN megagamete. [macro- + G. *gametē,* wife]

mac·ro·ga·me·to·cyte (mak′rō-gă-mē′tō-sīt). The female gametocyte or mother cell producing the female or macrogamete

ma

among fungi or protozoa that undergo anisogamy. SYN macrogamont.

mac·ro·gam·ont (mak-rō-gam′ont). SYN macrogametocyte.

ma·crog·a·my (mă-krog′ă-mē). Conjugation of two adult cells or gametes. [macro- + G. *gamos*, marriage]

mac·ro·gas·tria (mak-rō-gas′trē-ă). SYN megalogastria.

mac·ro·gen·i·to·so·mia (mak′rō-jen′i-tō-sō′mē-ă). Excessive bodily and genital development. [macro- + L. *genitalis*, genital, + G. *sōma*, body]

m. prae′cox, a disorder in which gonadal maturation (puberty) and the adolescent growth spurt in bodily height occur in the first decade of life; often associated with a pineal tumor or lesions in hypothalamic areas known to regulate gonadotrophin secretion. SYN Pellizzi syndrome.

m. prae′cox su′prarena′lis, precocious somatic growth and isosexual maturation of secondary sexual characteristics, resulting from an adrenocortical tumor.

ma·crog·lia (ma-krog′lē-ă). SYN astrocyte. [macro- + G. *glia*, glue]

mac·ro·glob·u·lin·e·mia (mak′rō-glob′ū-li-nē′mē-ă). The presence of increased levels of macroglobulins in the circulating blood.

Waldenström m., m. occurring in elderly persons, characterized by proliferation of cells resembling lymphocytes or plasma cells in the bone marrow, anemia, increased sedimentation rate, and hyperglobulinemia with a narrow peak in γ-globulin or β$_2$-globulin at about 19 S units. The spleen, liver, or lymph nodes are often enlarged and there is frequently purpura or mucosal bleeding. SYN hyperglobulinemic purpura, Waldenström purpura, Waldenström syndrome.

mac·ro·glob·u·lins (mak-rō-glob′ū-lins). Plasma globulins of unusually large molecular weight, e.g., as much as 1,000,000; α$_2$-macroglobulin inhibits thrombin and other proteases.

mac·ro·glos·sia (mak-rō-glos′ē-ă). Enlargement of the tongue, either developmental in origin or secondary to a neoplasm or vascular hamartoma. SYN megaloglossia. [macro- + G. *glōssa*, tongue]

mac·ro·gna·thia (mak-rō-nā′thē-ă). Enlargement or elongation of the jaw. SYN megagnathia. [macro- + G. *gnathos*, jaw]

ma·crog·ra·phy (mă-krog′ră-fē). Rarely used term for writing with very large letters. SYN megalographia. [macro- + G. *graphō*, to write]

mac·ro·gy·ria (mak-rō-jī′rē-ă). SYN pachygyria. [macro- + G. *gyros*, circle (gyrus)]

mac·ro·la·bia (mak′rō-lā′bē-ă). SYN macrocheilia (1). [macro- + L. *labium*, lip]

mac·ro·leu·ko·blast (mak-rō-loo′kō-blast). An unusually large leukoblast.

mac·ro·lide (mak′rō-līd). A natural lactone, whose ring is large, usually of 14–20 atoms; several antibiotics, including erythromycin, are macrolides. They inhibit protein biosynthesis.

mac·ro·lides (mak′rō-līdz). A class of antibiotics discovered in streptomycetes, characterized by molecules made up of large-ring lactones; e.g., erythromycin; many inhibit protein biosynthesis.

mac·ro·mas·tia, mac·ro·ma·zia (mak-rō-mas′tē-a, -mā′zē-ă). Abnormally large breasts. SEE ALSO hypermastia (2). [macro- + G. *mastos*, breast]

mac·ro·mel·a·no·some (mak-rō-mel′ă-nō-sōm). SYN giant *melanosome*.

mac·ro·me·lia (mak-rō-mē′lē-ă). Abnormal size of one or more of the limbs. SYN megalomelia. [macro- + G. *melos*, limb]

mac·ro·mere. A blastomere of large size, as in amphibians. [macro- + G. *meros*, part]

mac·ro·mer·o·zo·ite (mak′rō-mer-ō-zō′īt). A large merozoite. SYN megamerozoite. [macro- + G. *meros*, part, + *zōon*, animal]

mac·ro·min·er·als (mak-rō-min-er-alz). SYN macroelements.

mac·ro·mol·e·cule (mak-rō-mol′ĕ-kūl). A molecule of colloidal size; e.g., proteins, polynucleic acids, polysaccharides.

mac·ro·mon·o·cyte (mak-rō-mon′ō-sīt). An unusually large monocyte.

mac·ro·my·e·lo·blast (mak-rō-mī′ĕ-lō-blast). An abnormally large myeloblast.

mac·ro·nor·mo·blast (mak-rō-nōr′mō-blast). **1.** A large normoblast. **2.** A large, incompletely hemoglobiniferous, nucleated red blood cell with a "cart-wheel" nucleus.

mac·ro·nor·mo·chro·mo·blast (mak′rō-nōr-mō-krō′mō-blast). SYN macroerythroblast.

mac·ro·nu·cle·us (mak-rō-noo′klē-ŭs). **1.** A nucleus that occupies a relatively large portion of the cell, or the larger nucleus where two or more are present in a cell. SYN meganucleus. **2.** The larger of the two nuclei in ciliates, which governs vegetative metabolic functions and not reproduction. SYN somatic nucleus, trophic nucleus, trophonucleus. SEE ALSO micronucleus (2).

mac·ro·nu·tri·ents (mak-rō-noo′trē-ents). Nutrients required in the greatest amount; e.g., carbohydrates, protein, fats.

mac·ro·nych·ia (mak-rō-nik′ē-ă). Abnormally large fingernails or toenails. [macro- + G. *onyx*, nail]

mac·ro·or·chid·ism (mak-rō-ōr′kǐ-dizm). Having abnormally large testes; seen in males with fragile X syndrome. [macro- + G. *orchis* (*orchid-*), testicle]

mac·ro·par·a·site (mak-rō-par′ă-sīt). A parasite, such as a louse or an intestinal worm, that is visible to the naked eye.

mac·ro·pa·thol·o·gy (mak′rō-pa-thol′ŏ-jē). The phase of pathology that pertains to the gross anatomic changes in disease.

mac·ro·pe·nis (mak-rō-pē′nis). An abnormally large penis. SYN macrophallus.

mac·ro·phage (mak′rō-fāj). Any mononuclear, actively phagocytic cell arising from monocytic stem cells in the bone marrow; these cells are widely distributed in the body and vary in morphology and motility, though most are large, long-lived cells with a nearly round nucleus and have abundant endocytic vacuoles, lysosomes, and phagolysosomes. Phagocytic activity is typically mediated by serum recognition factors, including certain immunoglobulins and components of the complement system, but also may be nonspecific for some inert materials and bacteria, as in the case of alveolar m.'s; m.'s also are involved in both the production of antibodies and in cell-mediated immune responses, participate in presenting antigens to lymphocytes, and secrete a variety of immunoregulatory molecules. SYN macrophagocyte, rhagiocrine cell. [macro- + G. *phagō*, to eat]

activated m., a mature m., in an active metabolic state, that is cytotoxic to tumor/target cells, usually following exposure to certain cytokines. SYN armed m.

alveolar m., a vigorously phagocytic m. on the epithelial surface of lung alveoli where it ingests inhaled particulate matter. SYN coniophage, dust cell.

armed m., SYN activated m.

fixed m., a relatively immotile m. found in connective tissue, lymph nodes, spleen, and bone marrow. SYN resting wandering cell.

free m., an actively motile m. typically found in sites of inflammation.

Hansemann m., obsolete term for large histiocytes with abundant cytoplasm that may contain Michaelis-Gutmann bodies and one or several nuclei; described in lesions of malacoplakia.

inflammatory m., a m. found at sites of inflammation.

tangible body m., a m. that specializes in phagocytosis of lymphoid cells.

mac·ro·phag·o·cyte (mak-rō-fag′ō-sīt). SYN macrophage.

mac·ro·phal·lus (mak-rō-fal′lŭs). SYN macropenis. [macro- + G. *phallos*, penis]

mac·roph·thal·mia (mak-rof-thal′mē-ă). SYN megalophthalmos. [macro- + G. *ophthalmos*, eye]

mac·ro·po·dia (mak-rō-pō′dē-ă). Abnormally large feet. SYN megalopodia, pes gigas. [macro- + G. *pous*, foot]

mac·ro·pol·y·cyte (mak-rō-pol′ē-sīt). An unusually large polymorphonuclear neutrophilic leukocyte that contains a multisegmented nucleus (e.g., 8, 10, or more lobes); the arrangement of chromatin is less compact than in the normal neutrophil, and the cytoplasmic granules tend to be larger and more acidophilic. Such changes frequently precede significant alterations in the red blood cells, e.g., as in pernicious anemia and certain other forms of anemia. [macro- + G. *polys,* many, + *kytos,* cell]

mac·ro·pro·my·e·lo·cyte (mak′rō-prō-mī′ĕ-lō-sīt). An unusually large promyelocyte.

mac·ro·pro·so·pia (mak′rō-prō-sō′pē-ă). A condition in which the face is too large in proportion to the size of the cranial vault. SYN megaprosopia. [macro- + G. *prosōpon,* face]

mac·ro·pro·so·pous (mak-rō-prō′sō-pŭs, -prō-sō′pŭs). Relating to or exhibiting macroprosopia. SYN megaprosopous.

ma·crop·sia (mă-krop′sē-ă). Perception of objects as larger than they are. [macro- + G. *opsis,* vision]

mac·ro·rhin·ia (mak-rō-rin′ē-ă). Excessive size of the nose, either congenital or pathologic. [macro- + G. *rhis* (*rhin-*), nose]

mac·ro·sce·lia (mak-rō-sē′lē-ă). Abnormally increased length or thickness of the legs. [macro- + G. *skelos,* leg]

mac·ro·scop·ic (mak-rō-skop′ik). **1.** Of a size visible with the naked eye or without the use of a microscope. **2.** Relating to macroscopy.

ma·cros·co·py (mă-kros′kŏ-pē). Examination of objects with the naked eye. [macro- + G. *skopeō,* to view]

mac·ro·sig·moid (mak-rō-sig′moyd). Enlargement or dilation of the sigmoid colon. SYN megasigmoid.

ma·cro·sis (mă-krō′sis). Increase in length or volume. [G.]

mac·ros·mat·ic (mak′roz-mat′ik). Denoting an abnormally keen olfactory sense. [macro- + G. *osmē,* smell]

mac·ro·so·mia (mak-rō-sō′mē-ă). Abnormally large size of the body. SYN megasomia. [macro- + G. *sōma,* body]

mac·ro·splanch·nic (mak-rō-splangk′nik). SYN megalosplanchnic.

mac·ro·spore (mak′rō-spōr). The larger of two spore types of certain protozoans or fungi. SYN megalospore, megaspore. [macro- + G. *sporos,* seed]

mac·ro·ster·e·og·no·sis (mak′rō-ster-ē-og-nō′sis). An error of perception in which objects appear larger than they are. [macro- + G. *stereos,* solid, + *gnōsis,* recognition]

mac·ro·sto·mia (mak-rō-stō′mē-ă). Abnormally large size of the mouth resulting from failure of fusion between the maxillary and mandibular processes of the embryonic face. [macro- + G. *stoma,* mouth]

mac·ro·tia (mak-rō′shē-ă). Congenital excessive enlargement of the auricle or pinna. [macro- + G. *ous,* ear]

mac·ro·tome (mak′rō-tōm). An instrument for making gross anatomic sections. [macro- + G. *tomē,* cutting]

mac·u·la, pl. **mac·u·lae** (mak′ū-lă, -ū-lē). **1** [TA]. A circumscribed flat area, up to 1.0 cm in diameter, perceptibly different in color from the surrounding tissue. **2.** A small, discolored patch or spot on the skin, neither elevated above nor depressed below the skin's surface. SEE ALSO spot. **3.** The neuroepithelial sensory receptors of the utricle and saccule of the vestibular labyrinth collectively. SYN maculae utriculosaccularis [TA]. SEE ALSO *neuroepithelium* of macula. SYN macule, spot (1). [L. a spot]

mac′ulae acus′ticae, SEE m. of saccule, m. of utricle.

m. adher′ens, SYN desmosome.

m. al′bida, pl. **mac′ulae al′bidae,** gray-white or white, rounded or irregularly shaped, slightly opaque patches or spots that are sometimes observed postmortem in the epicardium, especially in middle-aged or older persons; they result from fibrous thickening, and sometimes hyalinization, of the epicardium; similar lesions may also occur in the visceral layer of the peritoneum. SYN m. lactea, m. tendinea, tache blanche, tache laiteuse (2), tendinous spot, white spot.

m. atroph′ica, an atrophic glistening white spot on the skin.

m. ceru′lea, a bluish stain on the skin caused by the bites of fleas or lice, especially pediculosis pubis. SYN blue spot (1).

m. commu′nicans, SYN gap *junction.*

m. commu′nis, the thickened area in the medial wall of the auditory vesicle that later subdivides to form the maculae of the sacculus and utriculus as well as the cristae of the ampullae of the semicircular ducts.

m. cor′neae, a moderately dense opacity of the cornea. SYN corneal spot.

m. cribro′sa, pi. **mac′ulae cribro′sae** [TA], one of three areas on the wall of the vestibule of the labyrinth, marked by numerous foramina giving passage to nerve filaments supplying portions of the membranous labyrinth; **m. cribrosa inferior** [TA], located in the posterior bony ampulla for passage of posterior ampullary nerve fibers; **m. cribrosa media** [TA], area near the base of the cochlea through which the saccular nerve fibers pass; **m. cribrosa superior** [TA], perforated area above the elliptical recess for passage of the utriculoampullary nerve fibers; m. cribrosa quarta, a name sometimes applied to the opening for the cochlear nerve.

m. cribrosa quarta, a name sometimes applied to the opening for the cochlear nerve.

m. den′sa, a closely packed group of densely staining cells in the distal tubular epithelium of a nephron, in direct apposition to the juxtaglomerular cells; they may function as either chemoreceptors or as baroreceptors feeding information to the juxtaglomerular cells.

false m., an extrafoveal point of fixation.

m. fla′va, a yellowish spot at the anterior extremity of the rima glottidis where the two vocal folds join.

m. gonorrho′ica, a spot of red brighter than the surrounding membrane, at the congested orifice of the duct of Bartholin gland, sometimes seen in gonorrhea.

honeycomb m., edema of the macular region of the retina.

m. lac′tea, SYN m. albida.

m. lu′tea [TA], SYN m. of retina.

m. pellu′cida, SYN follicular *stigma.*

m. of retina [TA], an oval area of the sensory retina, 3 by 5 mm, temporal to the optic disk corresponding to the posterior pole of the eye; at its center is the central fovea, which contains only retinal cones. SYN m. lutea [TA], area centralis, m. retinae, macular area, punctum luteum, Soemmerring spot, yellow spot.

m. ret′inae, SYN m. of retina.

m. of saccule [TA], the oval neuroepithelial sensory receptor in the anterior wall of the saccule; hair cells of the neuroepithelium support the statoconial membrane and have terminal arborizations of vestibular nerve fibers around their bodies. SYN m. sacculi [TA], saccular spot.

m. sac′culi [TA], SYN m. of saccule.

m. tendin′ea, SYN m. albida.

m. of utricle [TA], the neuroepithelial sensory receptor in the inferolateral wall of the utricle; hair cells of the neuroepithelium support the statoconial membrane and have terminal arborizations of vestibular nerve fibers around their bodies; sensitive to linear acceleration in the longitudinal axis of the body and to gravitational influences. SYN m. utriculi [TA], utricular spot.

m. utric′uli [TA], SYN m. of utricle.

maculae utriculosaccularis [TA], SYN macula (3).

mac·u·lar, mac·u·late (mak′ū-lăr, -lāt). **1.** Relating to or marked by macules. **2.** Denoting the central retina, especially the macula retinae.

mac·ule (mak′ūl). SYN macula. [L. *macula,* spot]

ash-leaf m., a hypopigmented, often ash leaf-shaped macule that is present at birth in many patients with tuberous sclerosis.

mac·u·lo·ce·re·bral (mak′ū-lō-ser′ĕ-brăl). Relating to the macula lutea and the brain; denoting a type of nervous disease marked by degenerative lesions in both the retina and the brain.

mac·u·lo·er·y·the·ma·tous (mak′ū-lō-er-i-thē′mă-tŭs). Denoting lesions that are erythematous and macular, covering wide areas.

mac·u·lo·pap·ule (mak′ū-lō-pap′ūl). A lesion with a flat base surrounding a papule in the center.

mac·u·lop·a·thy (mak-ū-lop′ă-thē). Any pathological condition of the macula lutea. SYN macular retinopathy.

bull's-eye m., an ocular condition in which edema or degeneration of the sensory retina at the posterior pole of the eye causes alternating areas of light and dark, as in a target; seen in toxic, inflammatory, and hereditary conditions.

cystoid m., cystic degeneration of the central retina that may

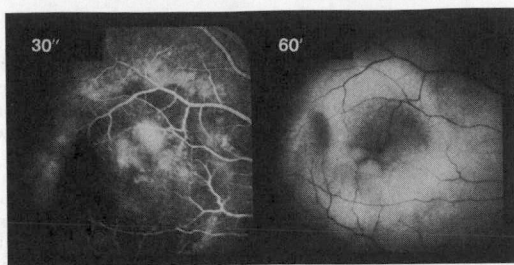

bull's-eye maculopathy: fluorescein angiogram showing macular degeneration of the right eye

occur after cataract extraction, in senile macular degeneration, and in other retinal abnormalities.

familial pseudoinflammatory m., familial macular degeneration resembling inflammatory changes.

nicotinic acid m., m. observed in persons taking 3000 mg or more of nicotinic acid daily; normal vision returns after this medication is discontinued.

solar m., damage to the fovea centralis of the retina and the adjacent choroid due to the thermal action of infrared rays, consequent to sungazing or watching a solar eclipse without sufficient eye protection. SEE ALSO photoretinopathy. SYN eclipse blindness, solar blindness.

mad. A non-medical, pejorative term for: **1.** Rabid. **2.** Mentally ill; insane. [A.S. *gemād*]

mad·a·ro·sis (mad-ă-rō′sis). **1.** SYN milphosis. **2.** SYN *alopecia adnata.* [G. a falling off of the eyelashes, fr. *madaō,* to fall off (of hair)]

mad·der (mad′er). **1.** The dried and powdered root of *Rubia tinctorum* (family Rubiaceae); it contains several glycosides that upon fermentation give the red dyes alizarin and purpurin. When m. (or alizarin) is fed to young animals, the calcium in newly deposited bone salt, hydroxyapatite, is stained red. **2.** Any dye obtained from plants of the madder family (Rubiaceae). SYN turkey red. [A.S. *maedere*]

Maddox, Ernest E., English ophthalmologist, 1860–1933. SEE M. *rod.*

Madelung, Otto W., German surgeon, 1846–1926. SEE M. *deformity, disease, neck.*

Madlener, Max, German surgeon, 1868–1951. SEE M. *operation.*

mad·ness (mad′nes). The state of being mad.

Madsen, Thorvald J.M., 1870–1957. SEE Arrhenius-M. *theory.*

Mad·u·rel·la (mad′ū-rel′ă). A genus of fungi including a number of species, such as *M. grisea* and *M. mycetomi,* that cause mycetoma. [*Madura,* India]

ma·du·ro·my·co·sis (mad′ū-rō-mī-kō′sis). SYN mycetoma. [*Madura,* India, + mycosis]

MAF Abbreviation for macrophage-activating *factor.*

ma·fe·nide (mā′fe-nīd). A topical antibacterial agent active against anaerobic pathogens. M. acetate is the preferred salt for ointment; m. hydrochloride is the preferred salt for solution. SYN 4-homosulfanilamide.

Maffucci, Angelo, Italian physician and anatomic pathologist, 1847–1903. SEE M. *syndrome.*

mag·al·drate (mag′al-drāt). A chemical combination of aluminum hydroxide and magnesium hydroxide, used as an antacid.

Magendie, François, French physiologist, 1783–1855. SEE *foramen* of M.; Bell-M. *law;* M. *law, spaces,* under *space;* M.-Hertwig *sign, syndrome.*

ma·gen·stras·se (mag′en-stras′e). SYN gastric *canal.* [Ger. *Magen,* stomach, + *Strasse,* road]

mag·got (mag′ot). A fly larva or grub.

cheese m., SYN *Philopia casei.*

surgical m., a sterilized botfly maggot used in an obsolete therapy of wound debridement and removal of necrotic tissues.

Magill, Sir Ivan Whiteside, British anesthesiologist, 1888–1975. SEE M. *forceps.*

mag·is·tral (maj′is-trăl). Denoting a preparation compounded according to a physician's prescription, in contrast to officinal (derived from a pharmacist's stock). [L. *magister,* master]

mag·ma (mag′mă). **1.** A soft mass left after extraction of the active principles. **2.** A salve or thick paste. [G. a soft mass or salve, fr. *massō,* to knead]

m. reticula′re, delicate noncellular strands running between the yolk sac and the outer wall of the blastocyst which is the early chorionic sac.

Magnan, Valentin J.J., Paris psychiatrist, 1835–1916. SEE M. *trombone movement, sign.*

mag·ne·sia (mag-nē′zhŭh). SYN *magnesium* oxide. [see magnesium]

calcined m., SYN *magnesium* oxide.

m. magma, SYN *milk* of magnesia.

mag·ne·si·um (Mg) (mag-nē′zē-ŭm). An alkaline earth element, atomic no. 12, atomic wt. 24.3050, that oxidizes to magnesia; a bioelement, many salts have clinical applications. [Mod. L. fr. G. *Magnēsia,* a region in Thessaly]

m. aluminum silicate, an antacid. SYN aluminum magnesium silicate.

m. bacteriopheophytinate, SEE bacteriochlorophyll.

m. benzoate, has been used in gout and rheumatoid arthritis.

m. carbonate, used in gastric and intestinal acidity and as a laxative.

m. chloride, has been used as a laxative.

m. citrate, a laxative; usually administered as an effervescent flavored beverage.

effervescent m. citrate, m. carbonate, citric acid, sodium bicarbonate, and sugar, moistened with alcohol, passed through a sieve, and dried to a coarse granular powder; used as a laxative.

effervescent m. sulfate, effervescent Epsom salt; m. sulfate, sodium bicarbonate, tartaric acid, and citric acid, moistened, passed through a sieve, and dried to a coarse granular powder; a purgative.

m. hydroxide, an antacid and laxative.

m. lactate, a laxative.

m. oxide, used as an antacid and laxative. SYN calcined magnesia, magnesia.

m. peroxide, decomposes in water to hydrogen peroxide; used as an ingredient in dentifrices and in antiseptic dusting powder.

m. phytinates, chlorophyll *a* and *b.* See entries under chlorophyll.

m. salicylate, a sodium-free salicylate derivative with anti-inflammatory, analgesic, and antipyretic actions; used for relief of mild to moderate pain.

m. stearate, a compound of m. with variable proportions of stearic and palmitic acids; used in the preparation of tablets, as a lubricant, and as an ingredient in some baby powders.

m. sulfate, active ingredient of most natural laxative waters; used as a promptly acting cathartic in certain poisonings, in the treatment of increased intracranial pressure and edema, as an anticonvulsant in eclampsia (when administered intravenously), and as an anti-inflammatory (when applied locally). SYN Epsom salts.

tribasic m. phosphate, tertiary m. phosphate, it is used as an antacid but it does not produce systemic alkalization; 1 g is equivalent in neutralizing power to about 0.46 g of sodium bicarbonate.

m. trisilicate, a compound of m. oxide and silicon dioxide with varying proportions of water; occurs in nature as meerschaum, pararepiolite, and repiolite; a gastric antacid.

mag·net. **1.** A body that has the property of attracting particles of iron, cobalt, nickel, or any of various metallic alloys and that when freely suspended tends to assume a definite direction between the magnetic poles of the earth (magnetic polarity). **2.** A bar or horseshoe-shaped piece of iron or steel that has been made magnetic by contact with another m. or, as in an electromagnet, by passage of electric current around a metallic (iron) core. **3.** An electromagnet built in a cylindrical configuration to accommodate a patient in its core, for magnetic resonance imaging. [G. *magnēs*]

superconducting m., a m. whose coils are cooled, usually with liquid helium, to a temperature at which the metal becomes superconducting, effectively removing all electrical resistance.

mag·net·ic. 1. Relating to or characteristic of a magnet. **2.** Possessing magnetism.

mag·ne·tism (mag′nĕ-tizm). The property of mutual attraction or repulsion possessed by magnets.

animal m., a psychic force akin to the property of mutual attraction or repulsion possessed by metal magnets and once believed to be the principal factor in hypnosis, which thus was called animal m. SEE hypnosis, mesmerism.

mag·ne·to·car·di·og·ra·phy (mag′nĕ-tō-kar-dē-og′ră-fē). Measurement of the magnetic field of the heart, produced by the same ionic currents that generate the electrocardiogram, and showing characteristic P, QRS, T, and U waves.

mag·ne·to·en·ceph·a·lo·gram (MEG) (mag-nē′tō-en-sef′ă-lō-gram). A Gauss-time record of the magnetic field of the brain.

mag·ne·to·en·ceph·a·log·ra·phy (mag-nē′tō-en-sef-ă-log′ră-fē). The process of recording the brain's magnetic field.

mag·ne·tom·e·ter (mag-nĕ-tom′ĕ-ter). An instrument for detecting and measuring the magnetic field.

mag·ne·ton (mag′nĕ-ton). A unit of measurement of the magnetic moment of a particle (e.g., atom or subatomic particle).

Bohr m. (μ_B), a constant in the equation relating the difference in energies between parallel and antiparallel spin alignments of electrons in a magnetic field; the net magnetic moment of one unpaired electron; used in electron spin resonance spectrometry for detection and estimation of free radicals; the smallest unit of magnetic moment (approximately 9.274×10^{-24} J T^{-1}). SYN electron m.

electron m., SYN Bohr m.

nuclear m. (μ_N), a constant in the equation relating the difference in energies between parallel and antiparallel spin alignments of atomic nuclei in a magnetic field; used in nuclear magnetic resonance spectrometry; 5.05×10^{-27} J T^{-1}.

mag·ne·to·ther·a·py (mag-nē′tō-thār′ă-pē). Attempted treatment of disease by application of magnets or induced magnetic fields.

mag·ni·fi·ca·tion (mag′ni-fi-kā′shŭn). **1.** The seeming increase in size of an object viewed under the microscope; when noted, this increased size is expressed by a figure preceded by ×, indicating the number of times its diameter is enlarged. **2.** The increased amplitude of a tracing, as of a muscular contraction, caused by the use of a lever with a long writing arm, i.e., one in which the fulcrum is placed nearer to the muscle than to the writing point. [L. *magnifico,* pp. *-atus,* to magnify]

mag·ni·tude (mag′ni-tood). Size or extent.

average pulse m., the amplitude of pulse averaged throughout its duration; identical with peak amplitude for a square wave or pulse without droop.

peak m., the greatest amplitude.

mag·no·cel·lu·lar (mag′nō-sel′ū-lăr). Composed of cells of large size. [L. *magnus,* large, + cellular]

mag·num (mag′nŭm). SYN capitate (1). [L. *magnus,* large]

Magnus, Rudolph, German physiologist, 1873–1927. SEE M. sign.

mag·nus (mag′nŭs). Large; great; denoting a structure of large size. [L.]

Mahaim, Ivan, 20th century cardiologist, 1897–1965. SEE M. *fibers,* under *fiber.*

Ma-huang (mah-hwahng). Name for *Ephedra equisetina.* [Chinese]

MAI Abbreviation for *Mycobacterium avium-intracellulare.* SEE ALSO *Mycobacterium avium-intracellulare complex.*

maidenhair tree. SYN *Ginkgo biloba.*

maid·en·head (mā′den-hed). Obsolete term for the intact hymen of a virgin.

mai·dism (mā′dizm). SYN pellagra. [*Zea mays,* maize]

Maier, Rudolf, German physician, 1824–1888. SEE M. *sinus.*

maim (mām). To disable or cripple by an injury.

main (man). SYN hand. [Fr.]

m. succulente, SYN Marinesco succulent *hand.*

main·frame (mān′frām). A large digital computer, such as would be used in a hospital for information management. Cf. mini.

main·stream·ing (mān′strēm-ing). Providing the least restrictive environment (socially, physically, and educationally) for chronically disabled individuals by introducing them into the natural environment rather than segregating them into homogeneous groups living in sheltered environments under constant supervision.

main·tain·er (mān-tā′ner). A device utilized to hold or keep teeth in a given position.

space m., an orthodontic appliance used to prevent the loss of space or the shifting of teeth following extraction or premature loss of teeth. SYN space retainer.

main·te·nance (mān′ten-ans). **1.** A therapeutic regimen intended to preserve benefit. Cf. compliance (2), adherence (2). **2.** The extent to which the patient continues good heath practices without supervision, incorporating them into a general life-style. Cf. compliance. [M.E., fr O.Fr., fr. Mediev. L. *manuteneo,* to hold in the hand]

maise oil (māz). SYN corn oil.

Maissiat, Jacques H., French anatomist, 1805–1878. SEE M. *band.*

Majocchi, Domenico, Italian dermatologist, 1849–1929. SEE M. *granulomas,* under *granuloma.*

ma·jor (mā′jŏr). Larger or greater in size of two similar structures. [L. comparative of *magnus,* great]

Makeham, William Matthew, English actuary, †1892. SEE M. *hypothesis.*

mal (mahl) A disease or disorder. [Fr. fr. L. *malum,* an evil]

m. de la rosa, m. rosso, SYN pellagra.

m. del pinto, SYN pinta.

m. de Meleda, endemic symmetrical keratoderma of the extremities occurring on the island of Meleda off the coast of Dalmatia, in Eastern Europe.

m. de mer, SYN seasickness.

grand m. (grahn), SYN generalized tonic-clonic *seizure.*

m. morado (mal mō-rä′ďo), purplish skin discoloration seen in acute attacks of onchodermatitis caused by *Onchocerca volvulus* in Central America. [Sp. *mal,* disease, + *morado,* purple]

petit m. (pĕ-tē′), SEE petit mal *seizure.* [Fr. small]

mal-. Ill, bad; opposite of eu-. Cf. dys-, caco-. [L. *malus,* bad]

ma·la (mā′lă). **1.** SYN cheek. **2.** SYN zygomatic *bone.* [L. cheek bone]

mal·ab·sorp·tion (mal-ab-sōrp′shŭn). Imperfect, inadequate, or otherwise disordered gastrointestinal absorption.

congenital selective glucose and galactose m., an inherited disorder in which D-glucose and D-galactose accumulate in the intestinal lumen and exert an osmotic effect; leads to abdominal fullness, abdominal pain, and diarrhea.

enterocyte cobalamin m., an inherited disorder of impaired transintestinal transport of cobalamin; symptoms are similar to a vitamin B$_{12}$ deficiency.

fructose m., an inborn error in metabolism in which oral D-fructose is incompletely absorbed; results in abdominal symptoms and diarrhea.

hereditary folate m., an inherited disorder in which there is defective transport of folates in intestine and choroid plexus, results in megaloblastic anemia and neurologic abnormalities.

Malacarne, Michele V.G., Italian surgeon, 1744–1816. SEE M. *pyramid, space.*

mal·a·chite green (mal′ă-kīt) [C.I. 42000]. A dye that has been used as a wound antiseptic, as a treatment of mycotic skin infections, and in biologic staining of tissues and bacteria. [G. *malachē,* a mallow]

ma·la·cia (mă-lā′shē-ă). A softening or loss of consistency and contiguity in any of the organs or tissues. Also used as a combining form in the suffix position. SYN mollities (2). SYN malacosis. [G. *malakia,* a softness]

ma·la·cic (mă-lā′sik). SYN malacotic.

maldigestion or malabsorption

Intraluminal Stage

defect at secretory (pancreatic) stage
    absence of trypsin, lipase, or colipase (inherited)
    cystic fibrosis*
    pancreatectomy
    chronic pancreatitis
    carcinoma of the pancreas*
    defective stimulation due to intestinal disease or gastric surgery
    obstruction of pancreatic duct
    Zollinger-Ellison syndrome
    malnutrition

defect at biliary stage
    parenchymal liver disease*
    biliary obstruction*
    terminal ileal disease*
    resection of terminal ileum*
    administration of cholestyramine
    bacterial action as a result of stasis or bacterial overgrowth

Small Intestinal Stage

defect at surface stage
    enterokinase deficiency (inherited)
    disaccharidase deficiencies (inherited and acquired)

defect at cellular and delivery stage
    amino acid transport defects
    primary vitamin B_{12} malabsorption
    massive resection
    radiation enteritis
    intestinal ischemia
    celiac sprue
    tropical sprue*
    ulcerative colitis
    regional enteritis
    Whipple's disease
    primary intestinal lymphoma
    hypogammaglobulinemia
    food allergy
    amyloidosis
    parasitized states

Multiple Stage Defects

    postgastrectomy
    diabetes mellitus
    endocrinopathies
    collagen disease
    administration of neomycin

* most common diseases

---

malaco-. Soft, softening. [G. *malakos*, soft; *malakia*, a softness]

mal·a·co·pla·kia, mal·a·ko·pla·kia (mal'ă-kō-plā'kē-ă, mal'ă-kō-plā'kē-a). Rare lesion in the mucosa of the urinary bladder and other organs, more frequent in women, characterized by numerous mottled yellow and gray soft plaques and nodules that consist of numerous macrophages and calcospherites (Michaelis-Guttmann bodies) that may form around intracellular bacteria, usually *Escherichia coli.* [malaco- + G. *plax*, plate, plaque]

mal·a·co·sis (mal'ă-kō'sis). SYN malacia.

mal·a·cot·ic (mal'ă-kot'ik). Pertaining to or characterized by malacia. SYN malacic.

ma·lac·tic (mă-lak'tik). SYN emollient. [G. *malaktikos*, softening]

ma·la·die (mal'ă-dē'). SYN malady. [Fr.]

  m. de Roger, SYN Roger *disease*. [Fr.]

  m. des jambes (mal'ă-dē' dĕ zhamb'), ill-defined disease seen among rice-growers in Louisiana.

mal·ad·just·ment (mal-ad-jŭst'ment). In the mental health professions, an inability to cope with the problems and challenges of everyday living. [mal- + *adjust*, fr. O.Fr. *adjuster*, fr. L.L. *adjuxto*, to put close to, + -ment]

  social m., m. without manifest psychiatric disorder, as that occasioned by an inability to cope with social situations.

mal·a·dy (mal'ă-dē). A disease or illness. SYN maladie. [Fr. *maladie*, illness]

ma·lag·ma (mă-lag'mă). A cataplasm or emollient. [G. a poultice]

mal·aise (mă-lāz'). A feeling of general discomfort or uneasiness, an "out-of-sorts" feeling, often the first indication of an infection or other disease. [Fr. discomfort]

mal·a·lign·ment (mal-ă-līn'ment). Displacement of a tooth or teeth from a normal position in the dental arch.

ma·lar (mā'lăr). Relating to the mala, the cheek or cheek bones.

MALARIA

ma·lar·ia (mă-lār'ē-ă). A disease caused by the presence of the sporozoan *Plasmodium* in human or other vertebrate red blood cells, usually transmitted to humans by the bite of an infected female mosquito of the genus *Anopheles* that previously sucked the blood from a person with m. Human infection begins with the exoerythrocytic cycle in liver parenchyma cells, followed by a series of erythrocytic schizogenous cycles repeated at regular intervals; production of gametocytes in other red cells provides future gametes for another mosquito infection; characterized by episodic severe chills and high fever, prostration, occasionally fatal termination. SEE tropical *diseases*, under *disease.* SEE ALSO *Plasmodium.* SYN jungle fever, marsh fever, paludal fever. [It. *malo* (fem. *mala*), bad, + *aria*, air, referring to the old theory of the miasmatic origin of the disease]

  acute m., a form of m. that may be intermittent or remittent, consisting of a chill accompanied and followed by fever with its attendant general symptoms and terminating in a sweating stage; the paroxysms, caused by release of merozoites from infected cells, typically recur every 48 hours in tertian (vivax or ovale) m., every 72 hours in quartan (malariae) m., and at indefinite but frequent intervals, usually about 48 hours, in malignant tertian (falciparum) m., but in many cases the periodicity is not well established.

  airport m., m. inadvertently imported by transport of an infected anopheline mosquito on an airplane.

  algid m., a form of falciparum m. chiefly involving the gut and other abdominal viscera; gastric algid m. is characterized by persistent vomiting; dysenteric algid m. is characterized by bloody diarrheic stools in which enormous numbers of infected red blood cells are found.

  autochthonous m., disease acquired by mosquito transmission in an area where m. regularly occurs.

  benign tertian m., SYN vivax m.

  bilious remittent m., a form of falciparum m. characterized by bilious vomiting, bilious diarrhea, etc.

  cerebral m., a form of falciparum m. characterized by cerebral involvement, with extreme hyperthermia and headache, and a case fatality rate of about 50%.

  chronic m., m. that develops after frequently repeated attacks of one of the acute forms, usually falciparum m.; it is characterized by profound anemia, enlargement of the spleen, emaciation, mental depression, sallow complexion, edema of ankles, feeble digestion, and muscular weakness. SYN limnemia, malarial cachexia.

  m. comato'sa, falciparum m. complicated by coma.

  double tertian m., SEE quotidian m.

  dysenteric algid m., SEE algid m.

  falciparum m., m. caused by *Plasmodium falciparum* and characterized by malarial paroxysms of severe form that typically occur every 48 hours with acute cerebral, renal, or gastrointestinal manifestations in severe cases, chiefly caused by the large number of red blood cells affected and the tendency for infected red cells to become sticky and clump, thus blocking capillaries. SEE ALSO malarial *knobs,* under *knob.* SYN aestivoautumnal fever, falciparum fever, malignant tertian fever, malignant tertian m., pernicious m.

gastric algid m., SEE algid m.

induced m., m. acquired by artificial means, e.g., via blood transfusion, common syringes, or malariotherapy.

intermittent m., a malarial fever, usually of the tertian or quartan type, in which there is complete apyrexia, with absence of the other symptoms, in the intervals between the paroxysms.

malariae m., a malarial fever with paroxysms that typically recur every 72 hours or every fourth day, reckoning the day of the paroxysm as the first; due to the schizogony and release of merozoites from infected cells, with invasion of new red blood corpuscles by *Plasmodium malariae.* SYN quartan fever, quartan m.

malignant tertian m., SYN falciparum m.

monkey m., SYN simian m.

nonan m., a malarial fever with paroxysms that occur every ninth day, i.e., every eighth day following the preceding paroxysm, the day of each paroxysm being included in the computation.

ovale m., ovale tertian m., m. caused by *Plasmodium ovale.*

pernicious m., SYN falciparum m.

quartan m., SYN malariae m.

quotidian m., m. in which the paroxysms occur daily; usually a double tertian m., in which there is an infection by two distinct groups of *Plasmodium vivax* parasites sporulating alternately every 48 hours, but also may be an infection by the pernicious form of malarial parasite, *P. falciparum,* combined with *P. vivax,* or infection by two distinct *P. falciparum* generations, which mature on different days; also may develop from infection with *P. knowlesi.* SYN quotidian fever.

relapsing m., renewal of clinical activity at some interval after the primary attack.

remittent m., a malarial fever, usually of the severe falciparum type, in which the temperature falls but not to the normal level during the interval between two pronounced paroxysms.

simian m., plasmodial infection of monkeys and apes, as with human m., transmitted chiefly by anopheline mosquitoes; a number of *Plasmodium* species are responsible, with Southeast Asia and Africa being the apparent centers of evolution; among the 20 plasmodial agents described from nonhuman primates, some resemble and induce a malarial infection similar to those caused by the four species of *Plasmodium* from humans, from which the agents of human m. appear to be derived. SYN monkey m.

tertian m., SYN vivax m.

therapeutic m., intentionally induced m., formerly used against neurosyphilis and certain other paralytic diseases. SYN malariotherapy.

vivax m., a malarial fever with paroxysms that typically recur every 48 hours or every other day (every third day, reckoning the day of the paroxysm as the first); the fever is induced by release of merozoites and their invasion of new red blood corpuscles. SYN benign tertian fever, benign tertian m., tertian fever, tertian m., vivax fever.

ma·lar·i·al (mă-lār′ē-ăl). Pertaining to or affected with malaria.

ma·lar·i·ol·o·gy (mă-lār-ē-ol′ō-jē). A study of malaria in all aspects, with particular reference to epidemiology and control.

ma·lar·i·o·ther·a·py (ma-lar-ē-ō-ther′a-pē). SYN therapeutic *malaria.*

ma·lar·i·ous (mă-lār′ē-ŭs). Relating to or characterized by the prevalence of malaria.

Malassez, Louis C., French physiologist, 1842–1910. SEE *Malassezia;* M. epithelial *rests,* under *rest.*

Ma·las·sez·ia (mal-ă-sā′zē-ă). A genus of fungi (family Cryptococcaceae) of low pathogenicity that lack the ability to synthesize medium-chain and long-chain fatty acids and require an exogenous supply of these lipids for growth as can be found in the skin. [L. C. *Malassez*]

M. fur′fur, a fungus species that is normal skin flora but can cause tinea versicolor, folliculitis, or fungemia in patients receiving intravenous lipids. SYN *Pityrosporum orbiculare, Pityrosporum ovale.*

M. ova′lis, a species of yeast found in superficial epidermal scales and hair follicles on oily skin, of borderline pathogenicity; may cause seborrheic dermatitis associated with immune deficiency.

M. pachydermatis, a fungus occasionally isolated from skin lesions of humans and animals; a rare cause of fungemia in patients receiving intravenous lipids.

mal·as·sim·i·la·tion (mal′ă-sim-i-lā′shŭn). Rarely used term for incomplete or faulty assimilation; malabsorption.

ma·late (mal′āt). A salt or ester of malic acid.

m. dehydrogenase, an enzyme that catalyzes, through NAD^+ or $NADP^+$, the dehydrogenation of malate to oxaloacetate or its decarboxylation to pyruvate and CO_2. At least six m. dehydrogenases are known, distinguished by their products, use of NAD^+ or $NADP^+$, and specificity of substrate (one acts on D-m., the rest act on L-m.); one is an enzyme in the tricarboxylic acid cycle. SYN malic acid dehydrogenase, malic dehydrogenase, malic enzyme, pyruvic-malic carboxylase.

m. synthase, an enzyme catalyzing the reversible condensation of acetyl-CoA with glyoxylate and water to form L-malate and coenzyme A; an enzyme in the glyoxylate cycle. SYN glyoxylate transacetylase, malate-condensing enzyme.

mal·a·thi·on (mal-ă-thī′on, mă-lā′thi-on). An organophosphorous compound used as an insecticide and veterinary ectoparasiticide; considered to be less toxic than parathion.

mal·ax·a·tion (mal′ak-sā′shŭn). **1.** Formation of ingredients into a mass for pills and plasters. **2.** A kneading process in massage. [L. *malaxo,* pp. *-atus,* to soften]

mal·di·ges·tion (mal-dī-jes′chŭn). Imperfect digestion.

Mal·do·na·do-San Jo·se stain. See under stain.

male (māl). **1.** In zoology, denoting the sex to which those belong that produce spermatozoa; an individual of that sex. **2.** SYN masculine. [L. *masculus,* fr. *mas,* male]

genetic human m., **(1)** an individual with a karyotype containing a Y chromosome; **(2)** an individual whose cell nuclei do not contain Barr sex chromatin bodies, which are normally present in females. Patients with ambiguous sexual development and those with Turner syndrome are classed as genetic m.'s or genetic females according to the absence or presence of Barr bodies even though their sex chromosome complement may suggest otherwise.

XX m., a clear male phenotype in the presence of a 46,XX karyotype; presumably the vital parts of the Y chromosome are located elsewhere in the genome as a result of translocation at least in some of these persons.

XXY m., SEE Klinefelter *syndrome.*

XYY m., SEE XYY *syndrome.*

Malecot, Achille-Etienne, French surgeon, *1852. SEE M. *catheter.*

ma·le·ic ac·id (mă-lē′ik). Butenedioic acid; the *cis* isomer of fumaric acid; used for preparing maleate salts of antihistaminics and similar drugs. SYN toxilic acid.

mal·e·mis·sion (mal-ē-mish′ŭn). Failure to eject semen from the penis at orgasm. [mal- + L. *e-mitto,* pp. *missus,* to send out]

mal·e·rup·tion (mal-ē-rŭp′shŭn). Faulty eruption of teeth.

ma·ley·lac·e·to·ac·e·tate (mal′a-il-as′e-tō-as′e-tāt). An intermediate in L-phenylalanine and L-tyrosine catabolism; accumulates in certain inherited disorders of tyrosine metabolism.

m. *cis,trans*-isomerase, an enzyme that catalyzes the reversible conversion of m. to 4-fumarylacetoacetate; an enzyme that participates in L-tyrosine catabolism; a deficiency of this enzyme is associated with tyrosinemia type IB.

mal·for·ma·tion (mal-fōr-mā′shŭn). Failure of proper or normal development; more specifically, a primary structural defect that results from a localized error of morphogenesis; e.g., cleft lip. Cf. deformation.

Arnold-Chiari m., malformed posterior fossa structures associated with caudad traction and displacement of the rhombencephalon as caused by tethering of the spinal cord; may or may not be accompanied by spina bifida and associated anomalies such as

ma

meningomyelocele; this m. is usually multifactorial in inheritance; very weak evidence of autosomal recessive inheritance [MIM*207950]. syn Arnold-Chiari deformity, Arnold-Chiari syndrome, cerebellomedullary malformation syndrome.

cystic adenomatoid m., a rare developmental lung-bud abnormality which results in stillbirth, acute progressive respiratory disease of newborns, or protracted childhood pneumonias; this m. combines features of a hamartoma, dysplastic growth, and tumorous growth. Three types have been described, based chiefly on cyst diameters: Type I: up to 10 cm; Type II: less than 1.2 cm; Type III: less than 0.5 cm.

mermaid m., syn sirenomelia.

Michel m., hypoplasia of the petrous pyramid and aplasia of the inner ear.

venous m., syn venous *angioma*.

mal·func·tion (mal-fŭnk′shŭn). Disordered, inadequate, or abnormal function.

Malgaigne, Joseph F., French surgeon, 1806–1865. see M. *amputation, fossa, hernia, luxation, triangle.*

Malherbe, Albert, 1845–1915. see M. calcifying *epithelioma.*

mal·ic ac·id (mal′ik, mā′lik). Hydroxysuccinic acid; an acid found in apples and various other tart fruits; an intermediate in the tricarboxylic acid cycle, the glyoxylate cycle, and in a shuttle system. syn monohydroxysuccinic acid.

mal·ic ac·id de·hy·dro·gen·ase. syn *malate* dehydrogenase.

mal·ic de·hy·dro·gen·ase. syn *malate* dehydrogenase.

ma·lig·nan·cy (mă-lig′nan-sē). The property or condition of being malignant.

ma·lig·nant (mă-lig′nănt). **1.** Resistant to treatment; occurring in severe form, and frequently fatal; tending to become worse and leading to an ingravescent course. **2.** In reference to a neoplasm, having the property of locally invasive and destructive growth and metastasis. [L. *maligno,* pres. p. *-ans* (*ant-*), to do anything maliciously]

ma·lin·ger (mă-ling′ger). To engage in malingering.

ma·lin·ger·er (mă-ling′ger-er). One who engages in malingering.

ma·lin·ger·ing (mă-ling′ger-ing). Feigning illness or disability to escape work, excite sympathy, or gain compensation. [Fr. *malingre,* poor, weakly]

mal·in·ter·dig·i·ta·tion (mal′in-ter-dij′i-tā′shŭn). Faulty intercuspation of teeth.

Mall, Franklin Paine, U.S. anatomist and embryologist, 1862–1917. see M. *formula, ridges,* under *ridge;* periportal *space* of M.

mal·le·a·ble (mal′ē-ă-bl). Capable of being shaped by being beaten or by pressure; a property of certain metals such as gold and silver. [L. *malleus,* a hammer]

mal·le·brin (mal′e-brin). syn *aluminum* chlorate nonahydrate.

mal·le·o·in·cu·dal (mal′ē-ō-ing′koo-dăl). Relating to the malleus and the incus in the tympanum.

mal·le·o·lar (mă-lē′ō-lăr). Relating to one or both malleoli.

mal·le·o·lus, pl. **mal·le·o·li** (ma-lē′ō-lŭs, -lī) [TA]. A rounded bony prominence such as those on either side of the ankle joint. [L. dim. of *malleus,* hammer]

external m., syn lateral m.

inner m., syn medial m.

internal m., syn medial m.

lateral m. [TA], the process at the lateral side of the lower end of the fibula, forming the projection of the lateral part of the ankle; the lateral malleolus extends farther inferiorly than the medial malleolus. syn m. lateralis [TA], external m., extramalleolus, outer m.

m. latera′lis [TA], syn lateral m.

medial m. [TA], the process at the medial side of the lower end of the tibia, forming the projection of the medial side of the ankle; the medial m. lies superior to the level of the lateral malleolus. syn m. medialis [TA], inner m., internal m.

m. media′lis [TA], syn medial m.

outer m., syn lateral m.

mal·le·ot·o·my (mal′ē-ot′ō-mē). Division of the malleus. [malleus + G. *tomē,* incision]

mal·le·us, gen. and pl. **mal·lei** (mal′ē-ŭs, mal′ē-ī) [TA]. The largest of the three auditory ossicles, resembling a club rather than a hammer; it is regarded as having a head, below which is the neck, and from this diverge the handle or manubrium, and the slender, anterior process; from the base of the manubrium the short lateral process arises. The manubrium and lateral process are firmly attached to the tympanic membrane, and the head articulates with a saddle-shaped surface on the body of the incus. syn hammer. [L. a hammer]

Mal·loph·a·ga (mă-lof′ă-gă). An order of biting lice that cause irritation by feeding on hair, feathers, and skin, and on blood and exudates when present; most species are found on birds, but some are found on common domestic animals. The genera *Menacanthus* and *Menopon* (family Menoponidae) attack domestic fowl, as do *Columbicola, Chelopistes, Lipeurus,* and other genera of the family Philopteridae, while *Bovicola, Felicola,* and *Trichodectes* (family Trichodectidae) infest domestic mammals. [G. *mallos,* wool, + *phagein,* to eat]

Mallory, Frank B., U.S. pathologist, 1862–1941. see M. *bodies,* under *body;* picro-M. trichrome *stain.* See entries under stain.

Mallory, G. Kenneth, U.S. pathologist, *1926. see M.-Weiss *lesion, syndrome, tear.*

mal·nu·tri·tion (mal-noo-trish′ŭn). Faulty nutrition resulting from malabsorption, poor diet, or overeating.

malignant m., syn kwashiorkor.

protein m., undernutrition resulting from inadequate intake of protein; characteristic manifestations include nutritional *edema,* kwashiorkor.

mal·oc·clu·sion (mal-ō-kloo′zhŭn). **1.** Any deviation from a physiologically acceptable contact of opposing dentitions. **2.** Any deviation from a normal occlusion.

mal·on·ate (măl′on-āt). The salt or ester of malonic acid.

mal·on·ate sem·i·al·de·hyde. The transaminated product of β-alanine; elevated in hyper-β-alaninemia.

Maloney bou·gies. See under bougie.

ma·lo·nic ac·id (mă-lō′nik, -lon′ik). A dicarboxylic acid of importance in intermediary metabolism; an inhibitor of succinate dehydrogenase. syn propanedioic acid.

mal·o·nyl (mal′ō-nil). The divalent moiety derived from malonic acid.

m. transacylase, syn ACP-malonyltransferase.

mal·o·nyl-CoA. The condensation product of malonic acid and coenzyme A, an intermediate in fatty acid biosynthesis. syn malonylcoenzyme A.

mal·o·nyl·co·en·zyme A (mal′ō-nil-kō-en′zīm). syn malonyl-CoA.

mal·o·nyl·u·rea (mal′ō-nil-ū-rē′ă). syn barbituric acid.

Malpighi, Marcello, Italian anatomist, histologist, and embryologist, 1628–1694. see malpighian *bodies,* under *body;* malpighian *capsule;* malpighian *cell;* malpighian *corpuscles,* under *corpuscle;* malpighian *glands,* under *gland;* malpighian *glomerulus;* malpighian *layer;* malpighian *nodules,* under *nodule;* malpighian *pyramid;* malpighian *rete;* malpighian *stigmas,* under *stigma;* malpighian *stratum;* malpighian *tubules,* under *tubule;* malpighian *tuft;* malpighian *vesicles,* under *vesicle.*

mal·pi·ghi·an (mahl-pig′ē-an). Described by or attributed to Marcello Malpighi.

mal·po·si·tion (mal-pō-zish′ŭn). syn dystopia.

mal·prac·tice (mal-prak′tis). Mistreatment of a patient through ignorance, carelessness, neglect, or criminal intent.

mal·pre·sen·ta·tion (mal′prē-sen-tā′shŭn). Faulty presentation of the fetus; presentation of any part other than the occiput.

mal·ro·ta·tion (mal-rō-tā′shŭn). Failure during embryonic development of normal rotation of all or part of an organ or system such as gut tube or kidney.

MALT Abbreviation for mucosa-associated lymphoid *tissue.*

malt (mawlt). The seed of barley or other grain, artificially germinated and dried, containing dextrin, maltose, small amounts of glucose, and amylolytic enzymes. Used in the form of an extract as a digestive and flavoring agent. [A.S. *mealt*]

malt·ase (mawl-tās). SEE α-D-glucosidase.

acid m., SYN exo-1,4-α-D-glucosidase.

mal·to·bi·ose (mawl-tō-bī′ōs). SYN maltose.

MALToma. B-cell lymphoma of mucosa-associated lymphoid tissue. SYN extranodal marginal zone lymphoma.

mal·tose (mawl-tōs). A disaccharide formed in the hydrolysis of starch and consisting of two D-glucose residues bound by a 1,4-α-glycoside link. SYN malt sugar, maltobiose.

mal·to·tet·rose (mawl-tō-tet′rōs). A saccharide composed of four D-glucose units in the α-1,4 linkage.

ma·lum (mā′lŭm). A disease. [L. an evil]

m. artic′ulorum seni′lis, arthritis in the aged.

m. per′forans pe′dis, perforating ulcer of the foot occurring in certain neuropathies.

m. vene′reum, SYN syphilis.

mal·un·ion (mal-ūn′yŭn). M. of the ends of a broken bone resulting in a deformity or a crooked limb; frequently used interchangeably with faulty m. SYN vicious union.

ma·man·pi·an (mă-mon-pē-on′). Formerly used term for mother *yaw.* [Fr. *maman,* mother + *pian,* yaw]

mam·e·lon (mam′ĕ-lon). One of the rounded prominences, three in number, on the cutting edge of an incisor tooth when it first pierces the gum. [Fr. nipple]

mam·e·lon·at·ed (mam′ĕ-lon-āt-ed). Having rounded, teatlike elevations; nodulated. [Fr. *mamelon,* nipple]

mam·e·lo·na·tion (mam′ĕ-lŏ-nā′shŭn). The formation of rounded projections or nodules on bony and other structures.

△**mamil-, mamilli-.** The mamillae. SEE ALSO mammil-. Cf. thelo-. [L. *mamilla,* nipple]

mam·ma, gen. and pl. **mam·mae** (mam′ă, mam′ē) [TA]. SYN breast. SEE ALSO mammary *gland.* [L.]

m. accesso′ria [TA], SYN accessory *breast.*

m. errat′ica, a supernumerary breast aberrantly located, i.e., in some part other than the milk line.

m. masculi′na [TA], SYN male *breast.*

supernumerary m., SYN accessory *breast.*

m. viri′lis, SYN male *breast.*

mam·mal (mam′ăl). An animal of the class Mammalia.

mam·mal·gia (mă-mal′jē-ă). SYN mastodynia. [L. *mamma,* breast, + G. *algos,* pain]

Mam·ma·lia (mă-mā′lē-ă). The highest class of living organisms; it includes all the vertebrate animals (monotremes, marsupials, and placentals) that suckle their young, possess hair, and (except for the egg-laying monotremes) bring forth living young rather than eggs. [L. *mamma,* breast]

mam·ma·plas·ty (mam′ă-plas-tē). Plastic surgery of the breast to alter its shape, size, or position, or all of these. SYN mammoplasty, mastoplasty. [L. *mamma,* breast, + G. *plastos,* formed]

augmentation m., plastic surgery to enlarge the breast, often by insertion of an implant.

reconstructive m., making a simulated breast by plastic surgery, to replace a breast that has been removed.

reduction m., plastic surgery of the breast to reduce its size and (frequently) to improve its shape and position.

mam·ma·ry (mam′ă-rē). Relating to the breasts.

mam·mec·to·my (ma-mek′tō-mē). SYN mastectomy. [L. *mamma,* breast, + *ektomē,* excision]

mam·mi·form (mam′i-fōrm). Resembling a breast; breast-shaped. SYN mammose (1). [L. *mamma,* breast, + *forma,* form]

△**mammil-, mammilli-.** The mamillae. SEE ALSO mamil-. Cf. thelo-. [L. *mammilla (mamilla),* nipple]

mam·mil·la, pl. **mam·mil·lae** (mă-mil′ă, mă-mil′ē). **1.** A small rounded elevation resembling the female breast. **2.** SYN nipple. [L. nipple]

mam·mil·la·plas·ty (ma-mil′ă-plas-tē). Plastic surgery of the nipple and areola. [L. *mammilla,* nipple, + G. *plastos,* formed]

mam·mil·la·re (mam-i-lā′rē) [TA]. SYN mammillary. [L.]

mamm·il·lar·ia. SEE mammillary *body.*

mam·mil·lary (mam′i-lār-ē) [TA]. Relating to or shaped like a nipple. SYN mammillare [TA].

mam·mil·late (mam′i-lāt). Studded with nipple-like projections.

mam·mil·la·tion (mam-i-lā′shŭn). **1.** A nipple-like projection. **2.** The condition of being mamillated.

mam·mil·li·form (mă-mil′i-fōrm). Nipple-shaped. [L. *mamilla,* nipple, + *forma,* form]

mam·mil·li·tis (mam-i-lī′tis). Inflammation of the nipple. [L., *mamilla,* nipple, + G. *-itis,* inflammation]

△**mammo-.** The breasts. Cf. masto-. [L. *mamma,* breast]

🔲**mam·mo·gram** (mam′ō-gram). The record produced by mammography.

🔲**mam·mog·ra·phy** (ma-mog′ră-fē). Radiologic examination of the female breast with equipment and techniques designed to screen for cancer. [mammo- + G. *graphō,* to write]

Mammography can detect carcinoma of the breast sometimes as early as 2 years before it becomes palpable and in many cases before lymph node metastasis has occurred. Mammographic findings that strongly suggest carcinoma are microcalcifications and ill-defined densities within breast tissue. These findings are not specific, however, and the cumulative probability of a woman's having a false-positive mammogram during 10 years of annual examinations approaches 50%. Scintimammography after intravenous injection of Tc-99m sestamibi may be used to follow up an equivocal mammogram. Positron emission tomography (PET) has shown promise in discriminating between benign and malignant breast masses as well as in detecting axillary lymph node metastases in patients with newly diagnosed breast cancer and distant metastases in patients with advanced or recurrent breast carcinoma. Because of the high cost of this procedure, its use is currently limited to high-risk subjects and those with dense breasts. The value of mammography in the early detection of breast cancer is well established for women of average risk aged 50–69 years. For this group, annual mammography reduces breast cancer mortality by 30–40%. Analysis of numerous clinical studies has revealed that mammograms may not save lives for healthy women under 50 (only 17% of all breast cancers occur in women under 40). The higher density of breast tissue in younger women limits the ability of radiography to identify tumors in women aged 40–50, for whom ultrasonography is preferred in evaluation of palpable breast lesions. Research has suggested that for a small fraction of women, exposure to radiation during mammography may actually trigger breast cancer. The American Cancer Society, the National Cancer Institute, and the American College of Radiology recommend a baseline mammogram for all women by age 40 and annual mammograms after age 50. Mammograms should begin at age 25 for women who are at special risk because of family history. Because some 10% of breast cancers that can be felt on examination are missed by mammography, annual examination of the breasts by a physician is also recommended. Surveillance by the Food and Drug Administration has shown an improvement in the sensitivity of mammograms during the past 5 years, largely because of improvements in screen and film systems. A digital scanning technique approved in 1998 further enhances the detection of microcalcifications and spiculated masses on mammography. However, mammography remains a screening procedure, and diagnosis of breast lesions depends on physical examination and biopsy findings. Federal law requires all facilities in the U.S. that perform mammography to provide each examinee with a report of the results in clear, simple language within 30 days after the examination, besides a detailed report to the physician who ordered the examination. See Also carcinoma of the breast.

Mam·mo·mon·o·ga·mus (mam′ō-mon-og′ă-mus). Genus of syngamid trematode (family Syngamidae) found in the respiratory system of ruminants and occasionally reported in humans; worms usually joined together in a Y-shaped formation.

M. laryngeus, nematode found in upper respiratory tract of some mammals; approximately 100 human cases, most from Caribbean islands; worm is red to reddish-brown; copulating male and female present a Y shape; life cycle not known.

mam·mo·plas·ty (mam′ō-plas-tē). SYN mammaplasty. [mammo- + G. *plastos,* formed]

mam·mose (mam′mōs). **1.** SYN mammiform. **2.** Having large breasts.

mam·mo·so·ma·to·troph (mam′ō-sō-mat′ō-trof). A cell of the adenohypophysis that produces prolactin and somatotropin.

mam·mot·o·my (ma-mot′ō-mē). SYN mastotomy. [mammo- + G. *tomē,* incision]

mam·mo·troph (mam′ō-trof). An acidophilic cell of the adenohypophysis that produces prolactin. SYN prolactin cell.

mam·mo·tro·pic, mam·mo·tro·phic (mam-ō-trop′ik, -trof′ik). Having a stimulating effect upon the development, growth, or function of the mammary glands. [mammo- + G. *tropos,* a turning]

mam·mo·tro·pin, mam·mo·tro·phin (mam-ō-trō′pin, -trō′fin). Obsolete term for prolactin.

Man Symbol for mannose and mannosyl.

management.

> **case m.,** a process whereby covered persons with specific health care needs are identified and an efficient treatment plan formulated and implemented to produce the most cost-effective outcomes.

> **component m.,** the approach to health care cost containment that involves trying to control individual components such as drug, hospitalization, or laboratory testing costs. SEE ALSO managed *care.*

man·chette (man-shet′). A conical array of microtubules that invests the nucleus of a spermatid; believed to play a role in shaping the nucleus during spermatogenesis. [Fr. cuff, dim. of *manche,* sleeve, fr. L. *manicae;* fr. *manus,* hand]

man·del·ate (man′de-lāt). A salt or ester of mandelic acid.

man·del·ic ac·id (man-del′ik). A urinary antibacterial agent (both bactericidal and bacteriostatic). SYN hydroxytoluic acid, phenylglycolic acid. [Ger. *Mandel,* almond]

Mandelin re·a·gent. See under reagent.

man·de·lyt·ro·pine (man-de-lit′rō-pēn). SYN homatropine.

■man·di·ble (man′di-bl) [TA]. A U-shaped bone (in superior view), forming the lower jaw, articulating by its upturned extremities with the temporal bone on either side. SYN mandibula [TA], jaw bone, lower jaw, mandibulum, submaxilla.

man·dib·u·la, pl. **man·dib·u·lae** (man-dib′ū-lă, -lē) [TA]. SYN mandible. [L. a jaw, fr. *mando,* pp. *mansus,* to chew]

man·dib·u·lar (man-dib′ū-lăr). Relating to the lower jaw. SYN inframaxillary, submaxillary (1).

man·dib·u·lec·to·my (man-dib-ū-lek′tō-mē). Resection of the lower jaw. [mandibula + G. *ektomē,* excision]

man·dib·u·lo·fa·cial (man-dib′ū-lō-fā′shăl). Relating to the mandible and the face.

man·dib·u·lo·oc·u·lo·fa·cial (man-dib′ū-lō-ok′ū-lō-fā′shăl). Relating to the mandible and the orbital part of the face.

man·dib·u·lo·pha·ryn·ge·al (man-dib′ū-lō-fa-rin′jē-ăl). Relating to the mandible and the pharynx; denoting the region between the pharynx and the ramus of the mandible, in which are found the internal carotid artery, the internal jugular vein, and the vagus, glossopharyngeal, accessory, and hypoglossal nerves.

man·dib·u·lum (man-dib′ū-lŭm). SYN mandible.

man·drag·o·ra (man-drag′ō-ră). The European mandrake, *Mandragora officinalis,* or *Atropa mandragora* (family Solanaceae), the mandrake of the Bible; its properties are similar to those of stramonium, hyoscyamus, and belladonna. [G. *mandragoras*]

man·drake (man′drāk). **1.** SEE mandragora. **2.** SEE podophyllum. [thr. L., fr. G. *mandragoras*]

> **wild m.,** SYN podophyllum *resin.*

man·drel, man·dril. **1.** The shaft or spindle to which a tool is

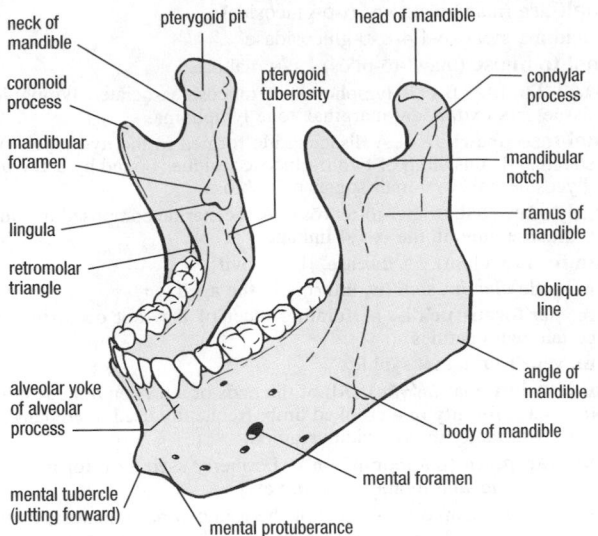

attached and by means of which it is rotated. **2.** SYN mandrin. **3.** In dentistry, an instrument used in a handpiece to hold a disk, stone, or cup used for grinding, smoothing, or finishing. [G. *mandra,* a stable; the bed in which a ring's stone is set]

man·drill. Common name for a species of monkey of the genus *Cynocephalus,* with a short tail and doglike head.

man·drin. A stiff wire or stylet inserted in the lumen of a soft catheter to give it shape and firmness while passing through a hollow tubular structure. SYN mandrel (2), mandril. [Fr. *mandrin,* mandrel]

ma·neu·ver (mă-noo′ver). A planned movement or procedure. [Fr. *manoeuvre,* fr. L. *manu operari,* to work by hand]

> **Adson m.,** SYN Adson *test.*

> **Barlow m.,** test for hip instability, with dislocation occurring with flexion, adduction, and posterior force. SYN Barlow test.

> **Bill m.,** forceps rotation of the fetal head at mid-pelvis before extraction of the head.

> **Bracht m.,** delivery of a fetus in breech position by extension of the legs and trunk of the fetus over the symphysis pubis and abdomen of the mother; the fetal head is born spontaneously as the legs and trunk are lifted above the maternal pelvis, and as the body of the infant is extended by the operator.

> **Buzzard m.,** testing the patellar reflex while the sitting patient makes firm pressure on the floor with the toes.

> **Credé m.'s,** SYN Credé *methods,* under *method.*

> **Dix-Hallpike m.,** test for eliciting paroxysmal vertigo and nystagmus in which the patient is brought from the sitting to the supine position with the head hanging over the examining table and turned to the right or left; vertigo and nystagmus are elicited when the head is rotated toward the affected ear.

> **Ejrup m.,** demonstration of collateral circulation by reduction in the prominence of activity of the greater arteries and reduced pulse volume following muscular activity.

> **Hampton m.,** rolling a supine patient to the right and then left side to obtain an air contrast radiograph of the contrast-coated antrum and duodenum in gastrointestinal fluoroscopy.

> **■Heimlich m.,** an action designed to expel an obstructing bolus of food from the throat by placing a fist on the abdomen between the navel and the costal margin, grasping the fist from behind with the other hand, and forcefully thrusting it inward and upward so as to force the diaphragm upward, forcing air up the trachea to dislodge the obstruction.

> **Hillis-Müller m.,** manual pressure on the term fundus while a finger in the vagina determines the descent of the head into the pelvis.

Figure labels (mandible diagram): neck of mandible · pterygoid pit · head of mandible · coronoid process · pterygoid tuberosity · condylar process · mandibular foramen · mandibular notch · lingula · ramus of mandible · retromolar triangle · oblique line · alveolar yoke of alveolar process · angle of mandible · body of mandible · mental foramen · mental tubercle (jutting forward) · mental protuberance

mandible: left-front view

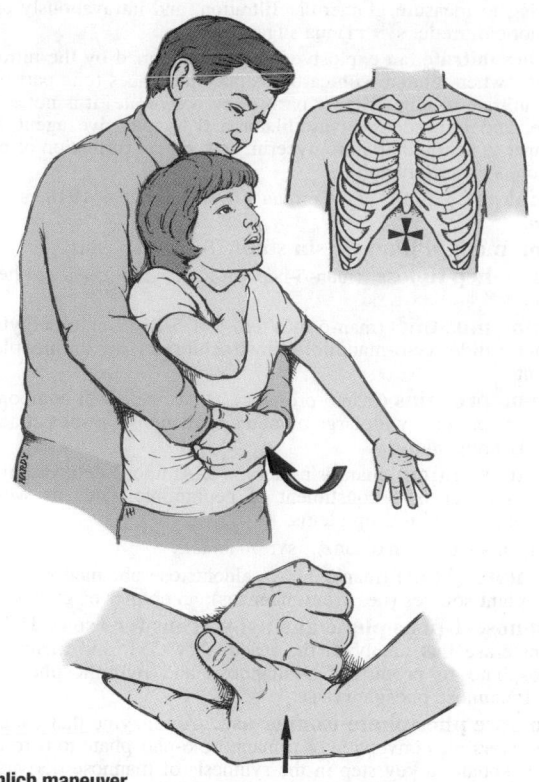

Heimlich maneuver

Hueter m., pressing the patient's tongue downward and forward with the left forefinger in passing a stomach tube.

Jendrassik m., a method of emphasizing the patellar reflex: the subject hooks the hands together by the flexed fingers and pulls against them with all possible strength.

LeCompte m., a repair of double outlet right ventricle with pulmonary stenosis and other abnormalities of ventricular arterial connection and ventricular septal defect in which the LV is connected to the aorta and the RV to the pulmonary artery using a technique that does not require an extracardiac conduit. SYN Le-Compte operation.

Leopold m.'s, four m.'s employed to determine fetal position: 1) determination of what is in the fundus; 2) evaluation of the fetal back and extremities; 3) palpation of the presenting part above the symphysis; 4) determination of the direction and degree of flexion of the head.

load-and-shift m., a test of shoulder instability in which the humeral head is pushed against the glenoid and moved anteriorly and posteriorly.

Mauriceau m., a method of assisted breech delivery in which the infant's body is astraddle the right forearm, and the middle finger of the right hand is in the fetal mouth to maintain flexion while traction is made upon the shoulders by the other hand. SYN Mauriceau-Levret m.

Mauriceau-Levret m., SYN Mauriceau m.

McDonald m., measurement of uterus from the upper border of the symphysis to a line tangential to the fundus over the abdomen with a tape to determine the height of the uterus; each centimeter approximately corresponds to the gestational age in weeks from 20–34 weeks' gestation.

McRoberts m., m. to reduce a fetal shoulder dystocia by flexion of the maternal hips.

Müller m., after a forced expiration, an attempt at inspiration is made with closed mouth and nose or closed glottis, whereby the negative pressure in the chest and lungs is made very subatmospheric; the reverse of Valsalva m.

Ortolani m., a m. for reduction of hip dislocation, using thigh flexion and abduction with anterior movement of the femoral head; reduction is accompanied by palpable reseating of the femoral head in the acetabulum. SYN Ortolani test.

Phalen m., m. in which the wrist is maintained in volar flexion; paresthesia occurring in the distribution of the median nerve within 60 sec may be indicative of carpal tunnel syndrome.

Pinard m., in management of a frank breech presentation, pressure on the popliteal space is made by the index finger while the other three fingers flex the leg while sliding it along the other thigh as the foot of the flexed leg is brought down and out.

Ritgen m., delivery of a child's head by pressure on the perineum while controlling the speed of delivery by pressure with the other hand on the head.

Scanzoni m., forceps rotation and traction in a spiral course, with reapplication of forceps for delivery.

Sellick m., pressure applied to the cricoid cartilage, to prevent regurgitation during tracheal intubation in the anesthetized patient.

Valsalva m., any forced expiratory effort ("strain") against a closed airway, whether at the nose and mouth or at the glottis, the reverse of Müller m.; because high intrathoracic pressure impedes venous return to the right atrium, this m. is used to study cardiovascular effects of raised peripheral venous pressure and decreased cardiac filling and cardiac output, as well as post-strain responses.

Wigand m., an assisted breech delivery with pressure above the symphysis while the fetus lies astraddle the operator's other arm.

Zavanelli m., SYN cephalic *replacement.*

man·ga·nese (Mn) (mang′gǎ-nēz). A metallic element resembling and often associated, particularly in ores, with iron; atomic no. 25, atomic wt. 54.94; manganous salts are sometimes used in medicine. SYN manganum. [Mod. L. *manganesium, manganum,* an altered form of *magnesium*]

man·gan·ic (mang-gan′ik). Denoting the trivalent cation of manganese, Mn^{3+}.

man·ga·nous (mang′gǎ-nŭs). Denoting the divalent cation of manganese, Mn^{2+}.

man·ga·num (man′gǎ-nŭm). SYN manganese. [L.]

mange (mānj). A cutaneous disease of domestic and wild animals caused by any one of several genera of skin-burrowing mites; in humans, mite infestations are usually referred to as scabies. [Fr. *manger,* to eat]

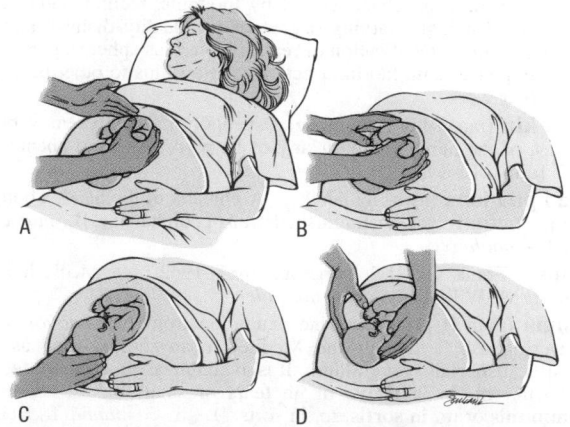

Leopold maneuvers: (A) first maneuver, palpate superior surface of fundus, (B) second maneuver, palpate sides of uterus to determine which direction fetal back is facing, (C) third maneuver, palpate to discover what is at inlet of pelvis, (D) fourth maneuver, assuming fetus has been found to be in a cephalic presentation, fetal attitude should then be determined (degree of flexion)

demodectic m., an infestation of the hair follicles and sebaceous glands with mites of the genus *Demodex;* they occur in humans and a number of domesticated animals; although asymptomatic in

ma

most species, these mites can cause severe and extensive dermatitis ("red mange") in dogs. SEE *Demodex*.

sarcoptic m., a cutaneous disease of animals caused by mites of the genus *Sarcoptes* including *Sarcoptes scabiei*.

Manhold, John H., U.S. dentist, *1919 SEE Volpe-M. *Index*.

ma·nia (mā'nē-ă). An emotional disorder characterized by euphoria or irritability, increased psychomotor activity, rapid speech, flight of ideas, decreased need for sleep, distractibility, grandiosity, and poor judgment; usually occurs in bipolar disorder. SEE manic-depressive, manic *excitement*. [G. frenzy]

acute m., SYN manic *excitement*.

△**-mania.** An abnormal love for, or morbid impulse toward, some specific object, place, or action. [G. frenzy]

ma·ni·ac (mā'nē-ak). **1.** Obsolete term for a mentally ill or disturbed person. **2.** One suffering from mania.

ma·ni·a·cal (mă-nī'ă-kăl). Relating to or characterized by mania. SEE amok. SYN manic.

man·ic (man'ik, mā'nik). SYN maniacal.

man·ic-de·pres·sive. 1. Pertaining to a manic-depressive psychosis (bipolar *disorder*). **2.** One suffering from such a disorder.

manicky (man'i-kē). Behavior characteristic of the manic phase of bipolar disorder.

man·i·fes·ta·tion (man'i-fes-tā'shŭn). The display or disclosure of characteristic signs or symptoms of an illness. [L. *manifestus*, caught in the act]

behavioral m., a m. characterized by defects in personality structure and attendant behavior with minimal anxiety and little or no sense of distress, indicative of a psychiatric disorder; occasionally encephalitis or head injury will produce the clinical picture which is properly diagnosed as chronic brain disorder with behavioral m.'s.

neurotic m., a m. characterized by such defenses as conversion, dissociation, displacement, phobia formation, or repetitive thoughts and acts being utilized to handle anxiety; in contrast to psychotic m.'s, gross distortion or falsification of reality is not exhibited, and gross disintegration of the personality is not usually observed.

psychophysiologic m., a m. characterized by the visceral expression of affect, the symptoms due to a chronic and exaggerated state of the physiologic expression of emotion with the feeling repressed; such m.'s are commonly characteristic of psychosomatic disorders.

psychotic m., a m. characterized by thoughts, feelings, and behavior evidencing a varying degree of personality disintegration and distortion or falsification of reality in various spheres; persons exhibiting such a m. fail in effective relationships to other people or to their work.

man·i·kin (man'i-kin). A model, especially one with removable pieces, of the human body or any of its parts. SEE ALSO phantom (2). [dim. of *man*]

man·i·pha·lanx (man'i-fā'langks). A phalanx of the hand; a bony segment of a finger; distinguished from pediphalanx. [L. *manus*, hand, + *phalanx*]

Mann, Frank C., U.S. surgeon, 1887–1962. SEE M.-Bollman *fistula;* M.-Williamson *operation, ulcer.*

man·na (man'ă). A saccharine exudation from *Fraxinus ornus*, flowering ash, a tree of the Mediterranean shores, used as a laxative, especially for children. It is available as **m. cannellata,** a flake m.; **m. in lacrimis,** m. in tears or small flakes; and **m. communis** or **m. in sortis,** m. in sorts. [L., fr. G. *manna,* fr. Heb. *mān*]

man·nans (man'anz). **1.** Polysaccharides of mannose, found in various legumes and in the ivory nut. **2.** Polysaccharides in which mannose is the monosaccharide present in highest proportion. SYN mannosans.

man·ner·ism (man'er-izm). A peculiar or unusual characteristic mode of movement, action, or speech.

man·nite (man'īt). SYN mannitol.

man·ni·tol (man'i-tol). The hexahydric alcohol, widespread in plants, derived by reduction of fructose; used in renal function testing to measure glomerular filtration, and intravenously as an osmotic diuretic. SYN manna sugar, mannite.

m. hexanitrate, an explosive compound formed by the nitration of m.; when diluted with carbohydrate substances (one part of m. hexanitrate to nine or more parts of carbohydrate) it is not explosive, and is used as a vasodilator and hypotensive agent; it is slower in action than nitroglycerin; acts via the formation of nitric oxide. SYN nitromannitol.

Mannkopf, Emil W., German physician, 1836–1918. SEE M. *sign*.

Mann meth·yl blue-e·o·sin stain. See under stain.

man·no·hep·tu·lose (man-ō-hep'too-lōs). SEE D-*manno*-heptulose.

man·no·mus·tine (man-ō-mŭs'tēn). 1-6-Bis(2-chloroethylamino)-1,6-dideoxy-D-mannitol dihydrochloride; an antineoplastic agent.

man·no·pro·teins (man'ō-prō-tēnz). Yeast cell wall components that are proteins with large numbers of mannose groups attached; highly antigenic.

man·no·sa·mine (man-ōs'a-mēn). 2-Amino-2-deoxymannose; the D-isomer is a constituent of neuraminic acids as well as mucolipids and mucoproteins.

man·no·sans (man'o-sanz). SYN mannans.

man·nose (Man) (man'ōs). An aldohexose obtained from various plant sources (i.e., from mannans); an epimer of glucose.

man·nose-1-phos·phate gua·nyl·yl·trans·fer·ase (GDP). A transferase that catalyzes the reaction of GTP and mannose 1-phosphate to produce GDPmannose and pyrophosphate. SYN GDPmannose phosphorylase.

man·nose·phos·phate isom·er·ase. An enzyme that catalyzes the reversible conversion of D-mannose 6-phosphate to D-fructose 6-phosphate; a key step in the synthesis of mannose derivatives, as well as the entry of mannose into the central pathways of carbohydrate metabolism.

man·no·si·dases (man-ō'si-dās'es). A group of enzymes that catalyze the hydrolysis of terminal, non-reducing D-mannose residues of mannosides (particularly in glycoproteins and glycolipids); α-m. act on α-D-mannosides while β-m. act on β-D-mannosides; a deficiency of α-m. is associated with mannosidosis.

man·no·side (man'ō-sīd). A glycoside of mannose.

man·no·si·do·sis (man'ō-si-dō'sis) [MIM*248500]. Congenital deficiency of α-mannosidase; associated with coarse facial features, enlarged tongue, mental retardation, kyphosis, radiographic skeletal abnormalities, and vacuolated lymphocytes, with accumulation of mannose in tissues; autosomal recessive inheritance, caused by mutation in the alpha-mannosidase gene (MANB) on chromosome 19p.

man·nu·ron·ic ac·id (man-ū-ron'ik). Uronic acid derived from the oxidation of mannose; a component of alginic acid.

man-of-war.

Portuguese m., SYN *Physalia physalis.*

ma·nom·e·ter (mă-nom'ě-ter). An instrument for indicating the pressure of any fluid or the difference in pressure between two fluids, whether gas or liquid. [G. *manos*, thin, scanty, + *metron*, measure]

aneroid m., a m. in which the pressure is indicated by a revolving pointer moved by a diaphragm or Bourdon tube exposed to the pressure. SYN dial m.

dial m., SYN aneroid m.

differential m., any device that indicates the difference in pressure between two fluids, regardless of any changes in their absolute pressures.

mercurial m., an m. in which the varying pressures are shown by differences of elevation in a column of mercury.

man·o·met·ric (man-ō-met'rik). Relating to a manometer.

ma·nom·e·try (mă-nom'ě-trē). Measurement of the pressure of gases or fluids by means of a manometer. SYN manoscopy. [see manometer]

esophageal m., measurement of intra-esophageal pressures at one or more sites by intraluminal pressure-sensitive instruments.

ma·nos·co·py (mă-nos′kŏ-pē). SYN manometry.

man. pr. Abbreviation for L. *mane primo*, early morning, first thing in the morning.

Manson, Sir Patrick, English authority on tropical medicine, 1844–1922. SEE *Mansonella; Mansonia;* M. *disease, schistosomiasis; Schistosoma mansoni; schistosomiasis* mansoni; M. eye worm.

Man·son·el·la (man-sō-nel′ă). A genus of filaria, widely distributed in tropical Africa and South America, that infects the peritoneal cavity, serous surfaces, or skin of humans and other primates with unsheathed microfilariae. The important human parasites *M. perstans* and *M. streptocerca* formerly were placed in the genera *Dipetalonema, Acanthocheilonema,* and *Tetrapetalonema.*

M. demarqua′yi, SYN *M. ozzardi.*

M. ozzar′di, a filarial parasite occurring in Yucatan, Panama, Colombia, northern Argentina, Guyana, French Guiana, and the islands of St. Vincent and Dominica, causing mansonelliasis; the microfilariae are not ensheathed, and there are no nuclei in the pointed tail; the life cycle is similar to that of *Wuchereria bancrofti;* humans are the only known definitive host, and the intermediate hosts are biting midges, *Culicoides furens* and possibly *C. paraensis.* SYN *M. demarquayi, M. tucumana.*

M. per′stans, the "persistent filaria," a species widely prevalent in tropical Africa and northern South America where it infects human peritoneal and other body cavities, but is non- or mildly pathogenic; characteristic subperiodic microfilariae occur in peripheral blood. It is transmitted in Africa by the biting midges *Culicoides austeni* and *C. grahami.*

M. streptocer′ca, a filarial species in humans that produces nonperiodic sheathless microfilariae found in the circulating blood; may cause a lichenoid condition or edema of the skin; commonly found in the corium of the skin of west African residents and transmitted by the biting midge, *Culicoides grahami.*

M. tucuma′na, SYN *M. ozzardi.*

man·so·nel·li·a·sis (man′sō-nel-ī′ă-sis). Infection with a species of *Mansonella,* transmitted to humans by biting midges of the genus *Culicoides;* adult worms live in the serous cavities, especially the peritoneal cavity, in mesenteric and perivisceral adipose tissue, and in the skin.

man·son·el·lo·sis (man-sō-nel′lō-sis). Infection with the filarial parasite *Mansonella ozzardi.*

Man·so·ni·a (man-sō′nē-ă). A genus of brown or black medium-sized mosquitoes (tribe Culicini), often having banded abdomen and legs; larvae and pupae have modified breathing tubes enabling them to pierce aquatic plants to obtain air. M. mosquitoes are distributed worldwide and, in tropical areas, are important vectors of *Brugia malayi;* in some areas they also transmit *Wuchereria bancrofti.* [P. *Manson*]

Man·so·noi·des (man-sō-noy′dēz). A subgenus of *Mansonia.*

Mantel, Nathan, U.S. biostatistician, *1927. SEE Mantel-Haenszel *test.*

man·tle (man′tl). **1.** A covering layer. **2.** SYN cerebral *cortex.*

brain m., SYN cerebral *cortex.*

myoepicardial m., the dorsal wall of the primitive pericardium which, in the early somite embryo, becomes both the epicardium and the myocardium.

Mantoux, Charles, French physician, 1877–1947. SEE M. *pit, test.*

man·u·al Eng·lish. A means of communicating in English with a person with profound hearing impairment by a combination of signs, finger spelling, and gestures.

ma·nu·bri·um, pl. **ma·nu·bria** (mă-noo′brē-ŭm, -ă) [TA]. The portion of the sternum or of the malleus that represents the handle of a sword or hammer. [L. handle]

m. mal′lei, SYN m. of malleus.

m. of malleus, the handle of the malleus; the portion that extends downward, inward, and backward from the neck of the malleus; it is embedded throughout its length in the tympanic membrane. SYN m. mallei.

m. ster′ni [TA], SYN m. of sternum.

m. of sternum [TA], the upper segment of the sternum, a flat-

tened, roughly triangular bone, occasionally fused with the body of the sternum, forming with it a slight angle, the sternal angle. SYN m. sterni [TA], episternum, presternum.

man·u·dy·na·mom·e·ter (man′ū-dī-nă-mom′ĕ-ter). In dentistry, a device for measuring the force exerted by the thrust of an instrument. [L. *manus,* hand, + G. *dynamis,* force, + *metron,* measure]

ma·nus, gen. and pl. **ma·nus** (mā′nŭs) [TA]. SYN hand. [L.]

MAO Abbreviation for monoamine oxidase.

MAOI Abbreviation for monoamine oxidase *inhibitor.*

map. A representation of a region or structure; e.g., of a stretch of DNA.

choroplethic m., a method of mapping to display quantitative information such as death rates in defined jurisdictions (states, counties, etc.) by color coding or shading. [G. *chōros,* district, + *plēthos,* multitude, + -ic]

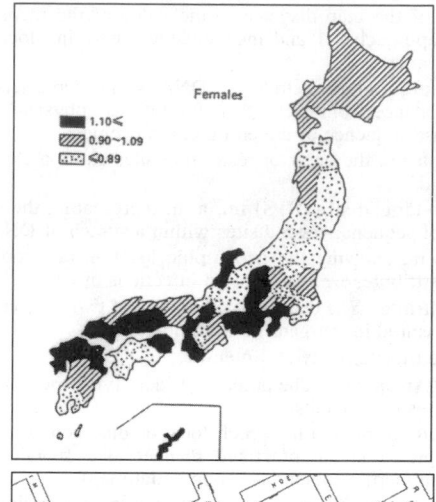

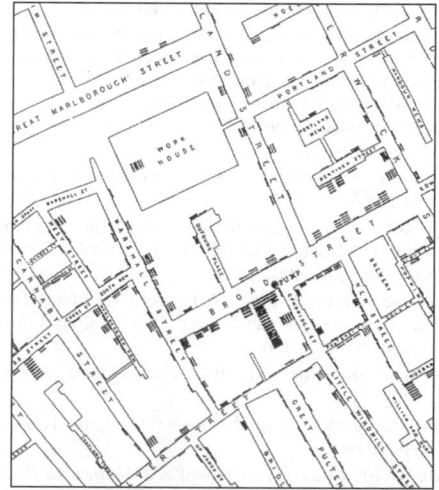

choroplethic and spot maps: choroplethic map (top) shows regional differences of hip fracture incidence in Japan; spot map (bottom), part of John Snow's map of Soho, London, showing the distribution of cholera cases in dwellings near the Broad Street pump in 1849

chromosome m., a systematic, semiabstract representation of the physical position of loci on a karyotype. Cf. genetic m.

conformational m., SYN Ramachandran *plot.*

contig m., a physical m. of a chromosome or stretch of DNA constructed from sets of overlapping clones (contigs).

cytogenetic m., a m. in which the classical bonding pattern of a chromosome is shown.

ma

map 1064 **margin**

fate m., determination in very young embryos of the cellular origin of specific organs or structures. SYN germinal localization.

genetic m., an abstract representation of the ordered array of genetic loci such that the interval between entries has algebraic signs and magnitude proportional to the expected number of crossings over between them and distances are algebraically additive; e.g., on a m. the combined distance between locus A and locus C is the algebraic sum of the two distances between loci A and B, and B and C.

isodemographic m., diagrammatic method of displaying countries or administrative jurisdictions within a country in two-dimensional m.'s with each area directly proportional to the population density of the country or jurisdiction. [iso- + G. *dēmos*, people, + *graphō*, to write + -ic]

linkage m., an abstract mathematical representation of genetic loci that conserves order of loci which are spaced in such a way that the distances are algebraically additive; conventionally, a map is scaled so that as distances between loci become smaller the ratio of the map distance to the value of the recombination fraction approaches 1 and independently assorting loci are infinitely far apart.

physical m., a m. of a stretch of DNA with ordered landmarks a known distance from each other; the ultimate physical m. would be the base sequence of the entire chromosome.

restriction m., the order of restriction sites along a chromosome or plasmid.

sequence-tagged site (STS) m., a m. representing the order and spacing of sequence-tagged sites within a stretch of DNA.

spot m., m. showing the geographic location of people with a specific attribute, e.g., cases of an infectious disease.

map dis·tance. The degree of separation of two loci on a linkage map, measured in morgans or centimorgans.

map·pine (map'ēn). SYN bufotenine.

map·ping (map'ing). The process of identifying the relative position of sites or elements.

cardiac m., a method by which local cardiac potentials are spatially depicted in an integrated manner as a function of time (isochrone map) or potential (isopotential map).

chromosome m., the process of determining the position of loci on specific chromosomes and constructing a diagram of each chromosome showing the relative positions of loci; techniques include family studies with linkage analysis, somatic cell hybridization, and chromosome deletion mapping.

gene m., SEE genetic *map*.

S1 nuclease m., a method for locating the 5' end of a transcript in a mixture of RNA.

map·ping func·tion. In linkage analysis, a formula that converts the recombination fraction (which is on the probability scale) into map distance (in morgans).

ma·pro·ti·line (ma-prō'ti-lēn). A tricyclic antidepressant used in the treatment of various depressive illnesses, and for relief of anxiety associated with depression.

MAPs Abbreviation for microtubule-associated *proteins*, under *protein*.

Marañón, Gregorio, Spanish endocrinologist, 1887–1960. SEE M. *sign;* syndrome.

ma·ran·tic (mă-ran'tik). SYN marasmic. [G. *marantikos*, wasting]

ma·ras·mic (mă-raz'mik). Relating to or suffering from marasmus. SYN marantic.

ma·ras·moid (mă-raz'moyd). Resembling marasmus. [G. *marasmos*, withering, + *eidos*, resemblance]

ma·ras·mus (mă-raz'mŭs). Cachexia, especially in young children, primarily due to prolonged dietary deficiency of protein and calories. SYN marantic atrophy, Parrot disease (2), pedatrophia, pedatrophy. [G. *marasmos*, withering]

nutritional m., extreme weakness and wasting secondary to malnutrition.

marc (mark). The residue remaining after percolation of a drug. [Fr. fr. *marcher*, to trample]

Marcacci, Arturo, Italian physiologist, 1854–1915. SEE M. *muscle.*

Marchand, Felix J., German pathologist, 1846–1928. SEE M. *adrenals,* under *adrenal, rest,* wandering *cell.*

Marchant, Gérard T.J., French surgeon, 1850–1903. SEE M. *zone.*

Marchesani, Oswald, 1900–1952. SEE Weill-M. *syndrome.*

Marchetti, Andrew A., U.S. obstetrician and gynecologist, 1901–1970. SEE Marshall-M. *test;* Marshall-M.-Krantz *operation.*

Marchi, Vittorio, Italian physician, 1851–1908. SEE M. *fixative, reaction, stain, tract.*

Marchiafava, Ettore, Italian pathologist, 1847–1935. SEE M.-Bignami *disease;* M.-Micheli *anemia, syndrome.*

mar·cid (mar'sid). Emaciating; wasting away. [L. *marcidus;* fr. *marceo,* to wither]

Marcille, Maurice, 1871–1941. SEE M. *triangle.*

mar·cor (mar'kōr). Obsolete term for marasmus. [L. fr. *marceo,* to wither]

Marcus Gunn, Robert. SEE Gunn.

Marek, Josef, Hungarian veterinarian and pathologist, 1868–1952. SEE M. disease *virus.*

marenostrin. SYN pyrin.

Marey, Étienne Jules, French physiologist, 1830–1904. SEE M. *law.*

Marfan, Antoine Bernard-Jean, French pediatrician, 1858–1942. SEE M. *disease, law, syndrome.*

mar·fan·oid (mar'fan-oyd). A term used of those whose phenotype bears a superficial resemblence to that of Marfan syndrome.

Marg, Elwin, U.S. physicist, *1918. SEE Mackay-M. *tonometer.*

Mar·gar·o·pus (mar-gar'ō-pŭs). A genus of ixodid ticks closely resembling *Boophilus,* but not having festoons or ornamentations; they are characterized by greatly enlarged posterior legs and a prolonged median plate. [G. *margaros,* pearl oyster, + *pous,* foot]

M. winthe'mi, the one-host South American winter horse tick; it also sometimes attacks cattle and sheep.

mar·gin (mar'jin) [TA]. A boundary, edge, or border, as of a surface or structure. SEE ALSO border, edge. SYN margo [TA]. [L. *margo,* border, edge]

acetabular m. [TA], the rim of bone around the acetabulum to which is attached the labrum acetabulare. SYN limbus acetabuli [TA], m. of acetabulum [TA], margo acetabularis ☆.

m. of acetabulum [TA], SYN acetabular m.

anterior m., SYN anterior *border.*

anterior palpebral m. [TA], the anterior edge of the free margin of each eyelid, along close to which the eyelashes are embedded. SYN limbus anterior palpebrae [TA], anterior border of eyelids.

articular m., SYN glenoid *labrum* of scapula.

cavity m., the periphery of a filling, the line of junction between a restoration and the external surface of a tooth.

cervical m., (1) SYN gingival m; (2) termination of a restoration in the gingival area.

cervical m. of tooth, SYN *neck* of tooth.

ciliary m. of iris [TA], the peripheral border of the iris attached to the ciliary body. SYN margo ciliaris iridis [TA], ciliary border of iris.

corneal m., SYN corneal *limbus.*

costal m. [TA], that portion of the inferior aperture of the thorax formed by the articulated cartilages of the seventh to tenth (false) ribs. SYN arcus costalis [TA], costal arch ☆, arcus costarum.

m.'s of eyelids, SYN palpebral m.'s.

falciform m. of saphenous opening [TA], the sharply curved, free margin of the saphenous opening in the fascia lata; medially, it ends in a superior and an inferior horn. SYN margo falciformis hiatus sapheni [TA], margo arcuatus hiatus sapheni ☆.

fibular m. of foot, SYN lateral *border* of foot.

m. of fossa ovalis, SYN *limbus* fossae ovalis.

free m., SYN free *border.*

free m. of eyelids, the unattached inferior edge of the upper lid and superior edge of the lower lid, where the anterior (cutaneous) surface of the eyelid meets the posterior (conjunctival) surface of the eyelid. The free m.'s of the eyelids bound the rima palpebrarum, and each free m. has an anterior and posterior m. SEE ALSO palpebral m.'s.

frontal m., SYN frontal *border.*

frontal m. of sphenoid [TA], the margin of the greater wing of the sphenoid bon that articulates with the frontal bone. SYN margo frontalis ossis sphenoidalis [TA], frontal border of sphenoid bone.

gingival m., (1) the most coronal portion of the gingiva surrounding the tooth; **(2)** the edge of the free gingiva. SYN cervical m. (1), gingival crest.

incisal m. [TA], the part of an anterior tooth farthest from the apex of the root. SYN margo incisalis [TA], cutting edge (2), incisal edge, incisal surface, shearing edge.

inferior m., SYN inferior *border.*

inferolateral m., SYN inferolateral m. of cerebral hemisphere.

inferolateral m. of cerebral hemisphere [TA], the irregular, discontinuous margin of the cerebral hemisphere at the junction of the inferior and superolateral surfaces. SYN margo inferolateralis [TA], inferolateral m., margo inferior cerebri.

inferomedial m. of cerebral hemisphere [TA], the irregular border of the cerebral hemisphere at the junction of the inferior and medial surfaces. SYN margo inferomedialis hemispherii cerebri [TA], margo medialis cerebri.

infraorbital m., the inferior half of the orbital rim, or the lower border of the orbital opening, formed by the maxilla medially and the zygomatic bone laterally. SEE orbital m. SYN margo infraorbitalis.

interosseous m., SYN interosseous *border.*

lacrimal m. of maxilla [TA], the margin of the nasal surface of the maxilla that articulates with the lacrimal bone. SYN margo lacrimalis maxillae [TA], lacrimal border of maxilla.

lambdoid m. of occipital bone, SYN lambdoid *border* of occipital bone.

lateral m., SYN lateral *border.*

mastoid m. of occipital bone, SYN mastoid *border* of occipital bone.

medial m., SYN medial *border.*

mesovarian m. of ovary, SYN mesovarian *border* of ovary.

nasal m. of frontal bone [TA], the border of the frontal bone that articulates with the nasal bones. SYN margo nasalis ossis frontalis [TA], nasal border of frontal bone.

occipital m., SYN occipital *border.*

occipital m. of temporal bone [TA], that part of the temporal bone that articulates with the occipital squama. SYN margo occipitalis ossis temporalis [TA], occipital border of temporal bone.

m. of orbit, SYN orbital m.

orbital m. [TA], the mostly sharp edge of the orbital opening which is the peripheral border of the base of the pyramid-shaped orbit. The superior half of the orbital m. is the supraorbital margin; the inferior half is the infraorbital margin. The frontal, maxillary, and zygomatic bones contribute to the orbital m., which is generally strong to protect the orbital contents. Weak, potential fracture sites of the m. coincide with the sutures between the participating bones. SYN margo orbitalis [TA], m. of orbit, orbital rim.

orbital m. of eyelids, the outer or peripheral attached borders of the upper and lower eyelids; the "root" of the eyelids, along which it is attached to the orbital rim.

palpebral m.'s [TA], the anterior and posterior edges of the free margin of the upper and lower eyelids. SEE ALSO anterior palpebral m., posterior palpebral m. SYN limbi palpebrales [TA], margo palpebrae [TA], borders of eyelids, m.'s of eyelids.

parietal m., SYN parietal *border.*

parietal m. of frontal bone [TA], the margin of the frontal bone that articulates with the parietal bone. SYN margo parietalis ossis frontalis [TA], parietal border of frontal bone.

parietal m. of greater wing of sphenoid [TA], the margin of the greater wing of the sphenoid that articulates with the parietal bone. SYN margo parietalis alaris majoris ossis sphenoidalis [TA], margo parietalis ossis sphenoidalis, parietal border of sphenoid bone.

posterior palpebral m. [TA], the posterior edge of the free mar-

gin of each eyelid, which is also the border of the conjunctiva. SYN posterior border of eyelids.

psoas m., in abdominal radiography, the appearance of the fat stripe delineating the lateral margin of the psoas muscle shadow; shows a normal retroperitoneum when visible.

pupillary m. of iris [TA], the inner border of the iris that forms the edge of the pupil. SYN margo pupillaris iridis [TA], pupillary border of iris.

right m. of heart, SYN right *border* of heart.

m. of safety, the range between the minimal therapeutic dose and the minimal toxic dose of a drug.

sphenoidal m. of temporal bone [TA], the part of the border of the squamous part of the temporal bone that articulates with the greater wing of the sphenoid. SYN margo sphenoidalis ossis temporalis [TA], sphenoidal border of temporal bone.

squamosal m.,

squamosal m. of greater wing of sphenoid [TA], the margin of the greater wing of the sphenoid bone that articulates with the squamous part of the temporal bone. SYN margo squamosus alaris majoris ossis sphenoidalis [TA], margo squamosus ossis sphenoidalis, squamous border of sphenoid bone.

squamous m., SYN squamosal *border.*

superior m. of cerebral hemisphere [TA], the curved margin of the cerebral hemisphere at the junction of the superolateral and medial surfaces. SYN margo superior hemispherii cerebri [TA], margo superomedialis, superomedial m.

superomedial m., SYN superior m. of cerebral hemisphere.

supraorbital m. [TA], the superior half of the orbital rim, which constitutes the curved superior border of the orbital opening, formed by the frontal bone. SEE orbital m. SYN margo supraorbitalis [TA], supraorbital arch, supraorbital ridge.

m. of tongue [TA], the lateral border that separates the dorsum from the inferior surface of the tongue on each side, the two borders meeting anteriorly at the apex. SYN margo linguae [TA].

ulnar m. of forearm, SYN ulnar *border* of forearm.

zygomatic m. of greater wing of sphenoid bone, the border of the greater wing of the sphenoid that articulates with the zygomatic bone. SYN margo zygomaticus alaris majoris ossis sphenoidalis [TA], margo zygomaticus alae majoris, zygomatic border of greater wing of sphenoid bone.

mar·gi·nal (mar′ji-năl). Relating to a margin.

Mar·gi·nal Line Cal·cu·lus In·dex (MLC). An index which scores supragingival calculus found in cervical areas paralleling marginal gingiva.

mar·gin·a·tion (mar′ji-nā′shŭn). A phenomenon that occurs during the relatively early phases of inflammation; as a result of dilation of capillaries and slowing of the bloodstream, leukocytes tend to occupy the periphery of the cross-sectional lumen and adhere to the endothelial cells that line the vessels.

m. of placenta, SEE *placenta* marginata.

mar·gi·nes (mar′ji-nēz). Plural of margo. [L.]

mar·go, gen. **mar·gi·nis,** pl. **mar·gi·nes** (mar′gō, mar′ji-nis, -nēz) [TA]. SYN margin, border. [L.]

m. acetabularis, ☆official alternate term for acetabular *margin.*

m. anterior [TA], SYN anterior *border.*

m. anterior corporis pancreatis [TA], SYN anterior *border* of body of pancreas.

m. anterior fibulae [TA], SYN anterior *border* of fibula.

m. anterior pancreatis, SYN anterior *border* of body of pancreas.

m. anterior pulmonis [TA], SYN anterior *border* of lung.

m. anterior radii [TA], SYN anterior *border* of radius.

m. anterior testis [TA], SYN anterior *border* of testis.

m. anterior tibiae [TA], SYN anterior *border* of tibia.

m. anterior ulnae [TA], SYN anterior *border* of ulna.

m. arcuatus hiatus sapheni, ☆official alternate term for falciform *margin* of saphenous opening.

m. cilia′ris i′ridis [TA], SYN ciliary *margin* of iris.

m. dex′ter cor′dis [TA], SYN right *border* of heart.

m. falcifor′mis hiatus sapheni [TA], SYN falciform *margin* of saphenous opening.

ma

m. fibula′ris pedis, ☆official alternate term for lateral *border* of foot.

m. frontalis [TA], SYN frontal *border*.

m. frontalis ossis parietalis [TA], SYN frontal *border* of parietal bone.

m. frontalis ossis sphenoidalis [TA], SYN frontal *margin* of sphenoid.

m. incisa′lis [TA], SYN incisal *margin*.

m. inferior [TA], SYN inferior *border*.

m. inferior cer′ebri, SYN inferolateral *margin* of cerebral hemisphere.

m. inferior corporis pancreatis [TA], SYN inferior *border* of body of pancreas.

m. inferior corporis splenis, SYN inferior *border* of body of pancreas.

m. inferior hep′atis [TA], SYN inferior *border* of liver.

m. inferior pancrea′tis, SYN inferior *border* of body of pancreas.

m. inferior pulmo′nis [TA], SYN inferior *border* of lung.

m. inferior splenis [TA], SYN inferior *border* of spleen.

m. inferolatera′lis [TA], SYN inferolateral *margin* of cerebral hemisphere.

m. inferomedia′lis hemispherii cerebri [TA], SYN inferomedial *margin* of cerebral hemisphere.

m. infraorbita′lis, SYN infraorbital *margin*.

m. interosseus [TA], SYN interosseous *border*.

m. interos′seus fib′ulae [TA], SYN interosseous *border* of fibula.

m. interos′seus ra′dii [TA], SYN interosseous *border* of radius.

m. interos′seus tib′iae [TA], SYN interosseous *border* of tibia.

m. interos′seus ul′nae [TA], SYN interosseous *border* of ulna.

m. lacrima′lis maxillae [TA], SYN lacrimal *margin* of maxilla.

m. lambdoideus ossis occipitalis [TA], SYN lambdoid *border* of occipital bone.

m. lambdoid′eus squa′mae occipita′lis, SYN lambdoid *border* of occipital bone.

m. lateralis [TA], SYN lateral *border*.

m. latera′lis antebra′chii, ☆official alternate term for radial *border* of forearm.

m. latera′lis humer′i [TA], SYN lateral *border* of humerus.

m. latera′lis pe′dis [TA], SYN lateral *border* of foot.

m. latera′lis re′nis [TA], SYN lateral *border* of kidney.

m. latera′lis scap′ulae [TA], SYN lateral *border* of scapula.

m. latera′lis un′guis [TA], SYN lateral *border* of nail.

m. liber [TA], SYN free *border*.

m. li′ber ova′rii [TA], SYN free *border* of ovary.

m. li′ber un′guis [TA], SYN free *border* of nail.

m. lin′guae [TA], SYN *margin* of tongue.

m. mastoideus ossis occipitalis [TA], SYN mastoid *border* of occipital bone.

m. mastoi′deus squa′mae occipita′lis, SYN mastoid *border* of occipital bone.

m. media′lis [TA], SYN medial *border*.

m. media′lis antebra′chii, ☆official alternate term for ulnar *border* of forearm.

m. media′lis cer′ebri, SYN inferomedial *margin* of cerebral hemisphere.

m. media′lis glan′dulae suprarena′lis [TA], SYN medial *border* of suprarenal gland.

m. media′lis humer′i [TA], SYN medial *border* of humerus.

m. media′lis pe′dis [TA], SYN medial *border* of foot.

m. media′lis re′nis [TA], SYN medial *border* of kidney.

m. media′lis scap′ulae [TA], SYN medial *border* of scapula.

m. media′lis tib′iae [TA], SYN medial *border* of tibia.

m. mesova′ricus ovarii, SYN mesovarian *border* of ovary.

m. nasa′lis os′sis fronta′lis [TA], SYN nasal *margin* of frontal bone.

m. occipita′lis [TA], SYN occipital *border*.

m. occipita′lis os′sis parieta′lis [TA], SYN occipital *border* of parietal bone.

m. occipita′lis os′sis tempora′lis [TA], SYN occipital *margin* of temporal bone.

m. occul′tus un′guis [TA], SYN hidden *border* of nail.

m. orbitalis [TA], SYN orbital *margin*.

m. pal′pebrae [TA], SYN palpebral *margins*, under *margin*.

m. parieta′lis [TA], SYN parietal *border*.

m. parietalis alaris majoris ossis sphenoidalis [TA], SYN parietal *margin* of greater wing of sphenoid.

m. parieta′lis os′sis fronta′lis [TA], SYN parietal *margin* of frontal bone.

m. parieta′lis os′sis sphenoida′lis, SYN parietal *margin* of greater wing of sphenoid.

m. parieta′lis os′sis tempora′lis, SYN parietal *border* of squamous part of temporal bone.

m. parietalis partis squamosae ossis temporalis [TA], SYN parietal *border* of squamous part of temporal bone.

m. poste′rior fib′ulae [TA], SYN posterior *border* of fibula.

m. poste′rior par′tis petro′sae os′sis tempora′lis [TA], SYN posterior *border* of petrous part of temporal bone.

m. poste′rior ra′dii [TA], SYN posterior *border* of radius.

m. poste′rior tes′tis [TA], SYN posterior *border* of testis.

m. poste′rior ul′nae [TA], SYN posterior *border* of ulna.

m. pupilla′ris ir′idis [TA], SYN pupillary *margin* of iris.

m. radia′lis antebra′chii [TA], SYN radial *border* of forearm.

m. sagitta′lis os′sis parieta′lis [TA], SYN sagittal *border* of parietal bone.

m. sphenoida′lis os′sis tempora′lis [TA], SYN sphenoidal *margin* of temporal bone.

m. squamo′sus [TA], SYN squamosal *border*.

m. squamosus alaris majoris ossis sphenoidalis [TA], SYN squamosal *margin* of greater wing of sphenoid.

m. squamo′sus os′sis parieta′lis [TA], SYN squamosal *border* of parietal bone.

m. squamo′sus os′sis sphenoida′lis, SYN squamosal *margin* of greater wing of sphenoid.

m. superior corporis pancreatis [TA], SYN superior *border* of body of pancreas.

m. supe′rior glan′dulae suprarena′lis [TA], SYN superior *border* of suprarenal gland.

m. supe′rior hemispherii cer′ebri [TA], SYN superior *margin* of cerebral hemisphere.

m. supe′rior pancrea′tis, SYN superior *border* of body of pancreas.

m. superior par′tis petro′sae os′sis tempora′lis [TA], SYN superior *border* of petrous part of temporal bone.

m. supe′rior scap′ulae [TA], SYN superior *border* of scapula.

m. supe′rior splenis [TA], SYN superior *border* of spleen.

m. superomedia′lis, SYN superior *margin* of cerebral hemisphere.

m. supraorbita′lis [TA], SYN supraorbital *margin*.

m. tibia′lis pe′dis, ☆official alternate term for medial *border* of foot.

m. ulna′ris antebra′chii [TA], SYN ulnar *border* of forearm.

m. u′teri [TA], SYN *border* of uterus.

m. zygomat′icus a′lae majo′ris, SYN zygomatic *margin* of greater wing of sphenoid bone.

m. zygomaticus alaris majoris ossis sphenoidalis [TA], SYN zygomatic *margin* of greater wing of sphenoid bone.

Marie, Pierre, French neurologist, 1853–1940. SEE M. *ataxia;* Charcot-M.-Tooth *disease;* Bamberger-M. *disease, syndrome;* M.-Strümpell *disease;* Strümpell-M. *disease;* Brissaud-M. *syndrome;* Foix-Cavany-Marie *syndrome*.

mar·i·hua·na (mar-i-wah′nă). Popular name for the dried flowering leaves of *Cannabis sativa*, which are smoked as cigarettes, "joints," or "reefers." In the U.S. m. includes any part of, or any extracts from, the female plant. Alternative spellings are mariguana, marijuana. SEE ALSO cannabis. [fr. Sp. *Maria-Juana,* Mary-Jane]

Marinesco, Georges, Roumanian neurologist, 1863–1938. SEE M. succulent *hand;* M.-Garland *syndrome;* Marinesco-Sjögren *syndrome*.

mar·i·no·bu·fo·tox·in (mar′i-nō-boo′fō-toks-in). A poison produced by the parotid gland of *Bufo marinus* (family Bufonidae), a large toad native to Central and South America; used in tropical countries for insect control.

Marion, Georges, French urologist, 1869–1932. SEE M. *disease.*

Mariotte, Edmé, French physicist, 1620–1684. SEE M. *bottle, experiment, law,* blind *spot.*

mar·i·po·sia (măr-i-pō′zē-ă). Thallasoposia; rarely used term for abnormal consumption of sea water as a result of psychogenic factors. SYN thalassoposia. [L. *mare,* the sea, + G. *posis,* drinking]

Marjolin, Jean N., French physician, 1780–1850. SEE M. *ulcer.*

mar·jo·ram (mar′jō-ram). Sweet, leaf, or garden m. whose leaves, with and without a small portion of the flowering tops of *Majorana hortensis* (*Origanum majorana*) (family Labiatae), are used as seasoning and medicinally as a stimulant, carminative, and emmenagogue.

mark. 1. Any spot, line, or other figure on the cutaneous or mucocutaneous surface, visible through difference in color, elevation, or other peculiarity. [A.S. *mearc*]

alignment m., m.'s made in tracings while the kymograph or other recording apparatus is at rest in order to indicate the time relations between two tracings inscribed one above the other, e.g., jugular and radial pulses.

stretch m.'s, SYN *striae* cutis distensae, under *stria.*

mark·er. 1. A device used to make a mark or to indicate measurement. 2. A characteristic or factor by which a cell or molecule can be recognized or identified. 3. A locus containing two or more alleles that, being harmless, are common and therefore yield high frequencies of heterozygotes which facilitate linkage *analysis.*

allotypic m., SYN allotype.

cell m., an identifying characteristic of a cell; e.g., formation of rosettes with sheep erythrocytes as a m. of T lymphocytes, or the presence of surface immunoglobulin as a m. of B lymphocytes.

cell surface m., a surface protein, glycoprotein, or group of proteins that distinguish a cell or subset of cells from another defined subset of cells.

genetic m., SYN genetic *determinant.*

linkage m., a locus at which there is a high probability of heterozygotes (indispensible state for linkage analysis), but in itself perhaps of no clinical interest. SEE ALSO marker *locus.*

oncofetal m., a tumor m. produced by tumor tissue and by fetal tissue of the same type as the tumor, but not by normal adult tissue from which the tumor arises.

polymorphic genetic m., inherited characteristic that occurs within a given population as two or more traits.

time m., an instrument that marks the time, usually in seconds or fractions of seconds, on a kymograph record in physiologic experiments.

tumor m., a substance, released into the circulation by tumor tissue, whose detection in the serum indicates the presence of tumor.

type of tumor	marker
testicular carcinoma, choriocarcinoma	β-subunit of human choriogonadotropin (β-HCG) and α-1-fetoprotein (AFP)
multiple myeloma	immunoglobulins, Bence Jones protein
neuroblastoma, pheochromocytoma	catecholamines, vanillylmandelic acid, metanephrines
carcinoid, primary liver-cell carcinoma	5-hydroxyindoleacetic acid α-1-fetoprotein
medullary thyroid gland carcinoma	calcitonin
malignant lymphoma, leukemia	surface antigens

tumor markers used in primary diagnoses

Markov, Andrei, Russian mathematician, 1865–1922. SEE Markov *process.*

Marme re·a·gent. See under reagent.

mar·mo·rat·ed (mar′mō-rā-ted). Denoting a condition in which the appearance of the skin is streaked like marble. SEE ALSO *cutis* marmorata. [L. *marmoratus,* marbled]

mar·mot (mar′mot). A woodchuck or groundhog; a hibernating rodent that may serve as reservoir host of plague bacillus in North America. [Fr. *marmotte*]

Maroteaux, Pierre, French medical geneticist, *1926. SEE M.-Lamy *syndrome.*

Marquis re·a·gent. See under reagent.

mar·row (mar′ō) [TA]. 1. A highly cellular hematopoietic connective tissue filling the medullary cavities and spongy epiphyses of bones; it becomes predominantly fatty with age, particularly in the long bones of the limbs. 2. Any soft gelatinous or fatty material resembling the m. of bone. SEE ALSO medulla. [A.S. *mearh*]

bone m. [TA], the soft, pulpy tissue filling the medullary cavities of bones, having a stroma of reticular fibers and cells; it differs in consistency by age and location. SEE ALSO gelatinous bone m., red bone m., yellow bone m. SYN medulla ossium [TA].

gelatinous bone m. [TA], degenerated marrow of cranial bones in old age.

red bone m. [TA], bone marrow in which the stroma primarily contain the developmental stages of erythrocytes, leukocytes, and megakaryocytes; it is present throughout the skeleton during fetal life and at birth. After the fifth postnatal year, it is gradually replaced in the long bones by yellow marrow. SYN medulla ossium rubra [TA].

spinal m., SYN spinal *cord.*

yellow bone m. [TA], bone m. in which the stroma of the reticular network are largely filled primarily with fat; it replaces red marrow in the long bones after the fifth year of life. SYN medulla ossium flava [TA].

Marshall, Don, U.S. ophthalmologist, *1905. SEE M. *syndrome.*

Marshall, Eli K., U.S. pharmacologist, 1889–1966. SEE M. *method.*

Marshall, John, English anatomist, 1818–1891. SEE M. vestigial *fold,* oblique *vein.*

Marshall, Victor F., U.S. urologist, *1913. SEE M. *test;* M.-Marchetti *test;* M.-Marchetti-Krantz *operation.*

Mar·shal·la·gia mar·shalli (mar-sha-lā′jē-ă mar-shal′ī). One of the medium stomach worms of the nematode family Trichostrongylidae, found in the abomasum of sheep, goats, camels, and various wild ruminants.

marsh·mal·low root (marsh′mal-ō). SYN althea.

mar·su·pi·al (mar-soo′pē-ăl). 1. A member of the order Marsupalia, which includes such mammals as kangaroos, wombats, bandicoots, and opossums, the female of which has an abdominal pouch for carrying the young. 2. Of or pertaining to marsupials. [L. *marsupium,* a pouch]

mar·su·pi·al·i·za·tion (mar-soo′pē-ăl-i-zā′shŭn). Exteriorization of a cyst or other such enclosed cavity by resecting the anterior wall and suturing the cut edges of the remaining wall to adjacent edges of the skin, thereby creating a pouch. [L. *marsupium,* pouch]

mar·su·pi·um (mar-soo′pē-ŭm). 1. SYN scrotum. 2. A pouch or sac; e.g., in marsupials. [L. pouch]

Martegiani, J., 19th century Italian anatomist. SEE M. *area, funnel.*

Martin, August E., German gynecologist, 1847–1933. SEE M. *tube;* M.-Gruber *anastomosis.*

Martin, Henry A., U.S. surgeon, 1824–1884. SEE M. *bandage, disease.*

Martin, J.E. SEE Thayer-M. *medium.*

Martinotti, Giovanni, Italian physician, 1857–1928. SEE M. *cell.*

mar·ti·us yel·low (marsh′ē-ŭs) [C.I. 10315]. An acid dye used as a stain in plant and animal histology, and as a light filter for photomicrography. [Karl A. *Martius,* Ger. chemist, *1920]

ma

Martorell, Fernando Otzet, Spanish cardiologist, 1906–1984. SEE M. *syndrome.*

Mar·y·land co·ma scale. SEE coma *scale.*

mas·cha·le (mas′kăl-ē). SYN axilla. [G.]

mas·chal·y·per·i·dro·sis (mas′kăl-i-per-i-drō′sis). Excessive sweating in the axillae. [G. *maschalē,* axilla, + *hyper,* over, + *hidrōs,* sweat]

mas·cu·line (mas′kū-lin). Relating to or marked by the characteristics of the male sex or gender. SYN male (2), masculinus. [L. *masculus,* male, fr. *mas,* male]

mas·cu·line pro·test. Adler term to describe the movement of individuals from passive to active roles in a desire to escape from the feminine role.

mas·cu·lin·i·ty (mas-kū-lin′i-tē). The qualities and characteristics of a male.

mas·cu·lin·i·za·tion (mas′kū-lin-i-zā′shŭn). The condition marked by the attainment of male characteristics, such as facial hair, either physiologically as part of male maturation, or pathologically by individuals of either sex. [L. *masculus,* male]

mas·cu·li·nize (mas′kū-li-nīz). To confer the qualities or characteristics peculiar to the male.

mas·cu·li·nus (mas-kū-lī′nŭs). SYN masculine, masculine. [L.]

Masini, Giulio, Italian physician, 1874–1937.

mask (mask). **1.** Any of a variety of disease states producing alteration or discoloration of the skin of the face. **2.** The expressionless appearance seen in certain diseases; e.g., Parkinson facies. **3.** A facial bandage. **4.** A shield designed to cover the mouth and nose for maintenance of antiseptic conditions. **5.** A device designed to cover the mouth and nose for administration of inhalation anesthetics, oxygen, or other gases.

ecchymotic m., a dusky discoloration of the head and neck occurring when the trunk has been subjected to sudden and extreme compression, as in traumatic asphyxia.

Hutchinson m., the sensation experienced in tabetic neurosyphilis as if the face were covered with a m. or with cobwebs.

laryngeal m., a tubular oropharyngeal airway with an inflatable rim at the distal end that when inflated creates an airtight seal immediately above the larynx.

nonrebreathing m., a m. fitted with both an inhalation valve and an exhalation valve so that all exhaled gas is vented to the external atmosphere and inhaled gas comes only from a reservoir connected to the m.

tropical m., SYN *chloasma* bronzinum.

masked (maskt). Concealed.

mask·ing. 1. The use of noise of any kind to interfere with the audibility of another sound. For any given intensity, low-pitched tones have a greater m. effect than those of a high pitch. **2.** In audiology, the use of a noise applied to one ear while testing the hearing of the other ear. **3.** The hiding of smaller rhythms in the brain wave record by larger and slower ones whose wave form they distort. **4.** In dentistry, an opaque covering used to camouflage the metal parts of a prosthesis. **5.** In radiography, superimposition of an altered positive image on the original negative to produce an enhanced copy photographically. SEE subtraction.

unsharp m., in radiography, superimposing a blurred negative of a radiograph to cancel large density differences, leaving fine detail more visible.

Maslow, Abraham H., U. S. psychologist, 1908–1970. SEE M. *hierarchy.*

mas·och·ism (mas′ō-kizm, maz′ō-). **1.** Passive algolagnia; a form of perversion, often sexual in nature, in which a person experiences pleasure in being abused, humiliated, or maltreated. Cf. sadism. **2.** A general orientation in life that personal suffering relieves guilt and leads to a reward. [Leopold von Sacher-*Masoch,* Austrian novelist, 1836–1895]

mas·och·ist (mas′ō-kist). The passive party in the practice of masochism.

Mason, Edward E., U.S. surgeon, *1920.

MASS Acronym for *m*itral valve prolapse, *a*ortic anomalies, *s*keletal changes, and *s*kin changes. SEE MASS *syndrome.*

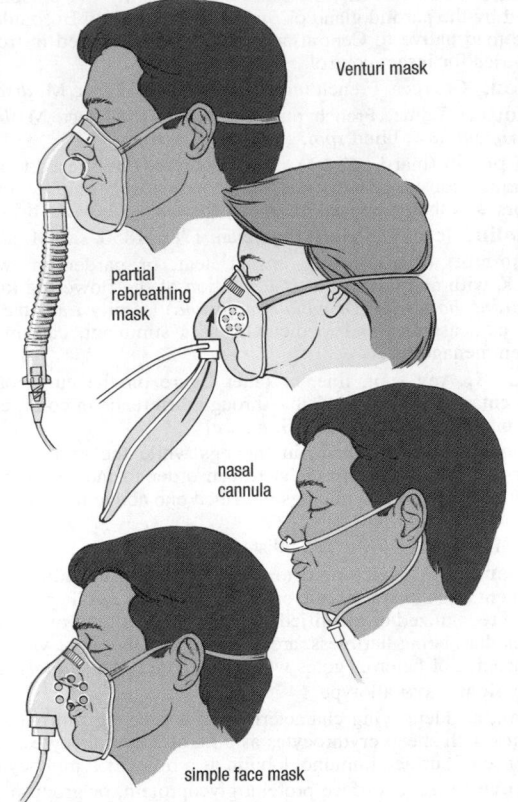

Venturi mask

partial rebreathing mask

nasal cannula

simple face mask

oxygen masks

mass (m). **1.** A lump or aggregation of coherent material. SYN massa [TA]. **2.** In pharmacy, a soft solid preparation containing an active medicinal agent, of such consistency that it can be divided into small pieces and rolled into pills. **3.** One of the seven fundamental quantities in the SI system; its unit is the kilogram, defined as the m. of the international prototype of the kilogram, which is made of platinum-iridium and kept at the International Bureau of Weights and Measures. **4.** The quantity of matter in a body or substance. [L. *massa,* a doughlike mass]

apperceptive m., the already existing knowledge base in a similar or related area with which the new perceptual material is articulated.

filar m., SYN reticular *substance* (1).

injection m., colored solutions or suspensions injected into the vascular system to render vessels and their walls prominent; useful for gross preparations and for study under low magnification after clearing; most fluids contain warm gelatin and the coloring materials are carmine, Berlin blue, or carbon.

inner cell m., the cells at the embryonic pole of the blastocyst concerned with formation of the body of the embryo *per se.* SYN embryoblast.

intermediate m., SYN interthalamic *adhesion.*

lateral m. of atlas [TA], the thick weight-bearing lateral part of the atlas on each side that articulates above with the occipital condyle and below with the axis. SYN massa lateralis atlantis [TA].

lateral m. of ethmoid bone, SYN ethmoidal *labyrinth.*

molar m., SEE molecular *weight.*

molecular m., SYN molecular *weight.*

pilular m., the mixture of drug(s), excipients, diluents and binders with a suitable amount of liquid to form a plastic mass which can be rolled into a long rod and cut into the appropriate number of units for pills to be rolled from. SYN pill mass.

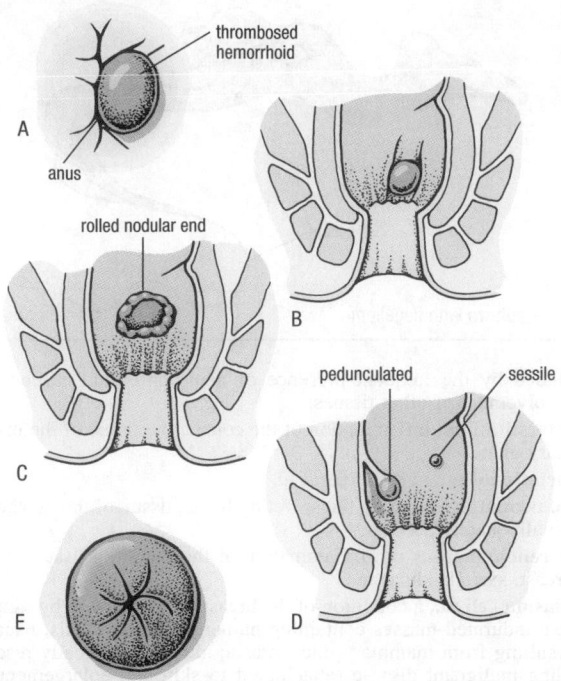

anal and rectal masses: (A) external hemorrhoid, (B) internal hemorrhoid, (C) rectal tumor, (D) rectal polyps, (E) rectal prolapse

relative molecular m. (*M*$_r$), SYN molecular *weight*.

sclerotic cemental m., benign fibro-osseous jaw lesions of unknown etiology, occurring predominantly in middle-aged black females, which present as large painless radiopaque masses usually involving several quadrants of the jaw. SYN florid osseous dysplasia, cemental dysplasia.

tubular excretory m., the m. of functioning excretory tubules of the kidney determined from the excretion of measurable compounds processed in the kidney primarily by tubular secretion.

mas·sa, gen. and pl. **mas·sae** (mas'să, mas'sē) [TA]. SYN mass (1). [L.]

m. interme′dia, ☆official alternate term for interthalamic *adhesion.*

m. latera′lis atlan′tis [TA], SYN lateral *mass* of atlas.

mas·sage (mă-sahzh′). A method of manipulation of the body or portion thereof by rubbing, pinching, kneading, tapping, etc. SYN tripsis (2). [Fr. from G. *massō,* to knead]

cardiac m., SYN heart m.

closed chest m., rhythmic compression of the heart between sternum and spine by depressing the lower sternum backward with the heels of the hands, the patient lying supine. SYN external cardiac m.

external cardiac m., SYN closed chest m.

gingival m., mechanical stimulation of the gingiva by rubbing or pressure.

heart m., rhythmic m. of the heart either in an open chest or through the chest wall to renew failed circulation during cardiac resuscitation. SYN cardiac m.

open chest m., rhythmic manual compression of the ventricles of the heart with the hand inside the thoracic cavity.

prostatic m., (1) manual expression of prostatic secretions by digital rectal technique; **(2)** the emptying of prostatic acini and ducts by repeated downward compression maneuvers, for treatment of various congestive and inflammatory prostatic conditions.

vibratory m., very rapid tapping of the surface effected by means of an instrument, usually with an elastic tip. SYN seismotherapy, sismotherapy, vibrotherapeutics.

Masselon, Julián, French physician, 1844–1917. SEE M. *spectacles.*

mas·se·ter. SEE masseter (*muscle*).

mas·seur (mă-ser′). **1.** A man who massages. **2.** An instrument used in mechanical massage. [Fr. see *massage*]

mas·seuse (mă-sooz′). A woman who massages.

mas·si·cot (mas′i-kot). SYN *lead* monoxide.

Masson, Pierre, Canadian pathologist, 1880–1959. SEE M.-Fontana ammoniac silver *stain.* See entries under stain.

mas·so·ther·a·py (mas-ō-thār′ă-pē). The therapeutic use of massage. [G. *massō,* to knead, + *therapeia,* treatment]

MAST Abbreviation for military antishock trousers.

△**mast-.** SEE masto-.

mast·ad·e·ni·tis (mast′ad-ĕ-nī′tis). SYN mastitis. [masto- + G. *adēn,* gland, + *-itis,* inflammation]

mast·ad·e·no·ma (mast′ad-ĕ-nō′mă). An adenoma of the breast. [masto- + G. *adēn,* gland, + *-ōma,* tumor]

Mast·ad·e·no·vi·rus (mast-ad′ĕ-nō-vī′rŭs). A genus of the family Adenoviridae, including adenoviruses that infect mammals, with over 40 antigenic types (species) being infective for humans. They cause respiratory infections in children, epidemic acute respiratory disease in military recruits, acute follicular conjunctivitis in adults, epidemic keratoconjunctivitis and gastroenteritis; many infections are inapparent. [G. *mastos,* breast, hence mammal, + adenovirus]

mas·tal·gia (mas-tal′jē-ă). SYN mastodynia. [masto- + G. *algos,* pain]

mas·tat·ro·phy, mas·ta·tro·phia (mas-tat′rō-fē, mast-ă-trō′fē-ă). Atrophy or wasting of the breasts. [masto- + atrophy]

mas·tauxe (mas-tawk′sē). Hypertrophy of the breast. [masto- + G. *auxē,* increase]

mas·tec·to·my (mas-tek′tō-mē). Excision of the breast. SYN mammectomy. [masto- + G. *ektomē,* excision]

extended radical m., excision of the entire breast including the nipple, areola, and overlying skin, as well as the pectoral muscles and the lymphatic-bearing tissues of the axilla and chest wall and internal mammary chain of lymph nodes.

modified radical m., excision of the entire breast including the nipple, areola, and overlying skin, as well as the lymphatic-bearing tissue in the axilla with preservation of the pectoral muscles.

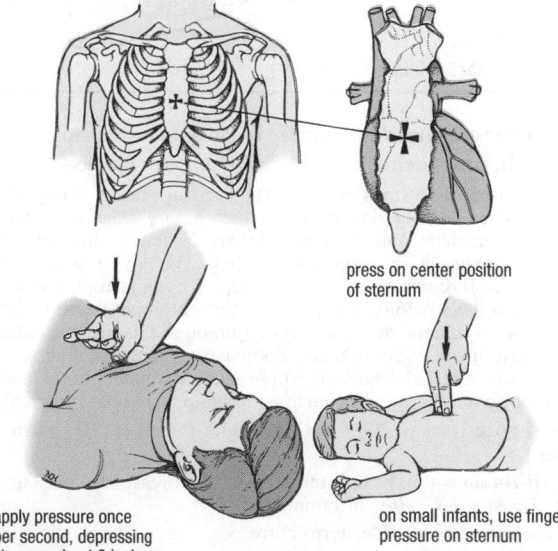

apply pressure once per second, depressing sternum about 2 inches

press on center position of sternum

on small infants, use finger pressure on sternum

closed chest massage

radical m., excision of the entire breast including the nipple, areola, and overlying skin, as well as the pectoral muscles, lym-

ma

phatic-bearing tissue in the axilla, and various other neighboring tissues. SYN Halsted operation (2).

simple m., excision of the breast including the nipple, areola, and some of the overlying skin. SYN total m.

subcutaneous m., excision of the breast tissues, but sparing the skin, nipple, and areola; usually followed by implantation of a prosthesis.

total m., SYN simple m.

Master, Arthur M., U.S. physician, 1895–1973. SEE M. *test*, two-step exercise *test*.

Masters, William H., U.S. gynecologist, *1915. SEE Allen-M. *syndrome*.

mas·tic (mas′tik). A resinous exudate from *Pistacia lentiscus* (family Anacardiaceae), a small tree of the Mediterranean shores; used in chewing gum, as an enteric coating, and as a temporary filling material in dentistry. SYN mastich, mastiche. [G. *mastichē,* the resin of the mastich tree]

mas·ti·cate (mas′ti-kāt). To chew; to perform mastication.

mas·ti·ca·tion (mas-ti-kā′shŭn). The process of chewing food in preparation for deglutition and digestion; the act of grinding or comminuting with the teeth. [L. *mastico,* pp. *-atus,* to chew]

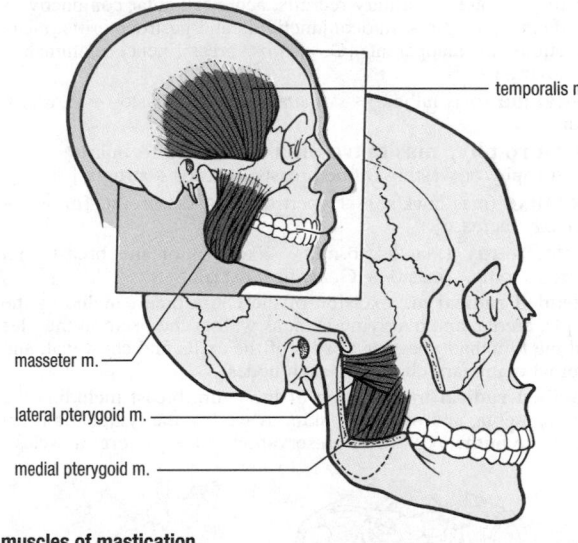

muscles of mastication

temporalis m.

masseter m.

lateral pterygoid m.

medial pterygoid m.

mas·ti·ca·to·ry (mas′ti-kă-tō-rē). Relating to mastication.

mas·tich, mas·ti·che (mas′tik, mas′ti-kē). SYN mastic.

Mas·ti·goph·o·ra (mas′ti-gof′ŏ-ră). The flagellates, a subphylum of Protozoa having one or more locomotory flagella, a single vesicular nucleus, and symmetric binary fission; sexual reproduction is unknown in many groups (e.g., *Volvox, Trypanosoma, Euglena*). It consists of two classes: Phytomastigophorea (to which *Euglena* belongs), which contains chlorophyll and is therefore photosynthetic and holophytic (although this has secondarily been lost in some groups), and Zoomastigophorea (including *Trypanosoma* and *Leishmania*), which lacks chromatophores and is heterotrophic. [G. *mastix (mastig-),* a whip, + *phoros,* bearing]

mas·ti·gote (mas′ti-gōt). An individual flagellate. [G. *mastix,* a whip]

mas·ti·tis (mas-tī′tis). Inflammation of the breast. SYN mastadenitis. [masto- + G. *-itis,* inflammation]

chronic cystic m., older term corresponding to fibrocystic *condition* of the breast.

gargantuan m., obsolete term for chronic inflammation of the breast with great enlargement of the gland.

glandular m., SYN parenchymatous m.

granulomatous m., a rare granulomatous inflammation of lobular breast tissue, with multinucleated giant cells; sarcoidosis is ex-

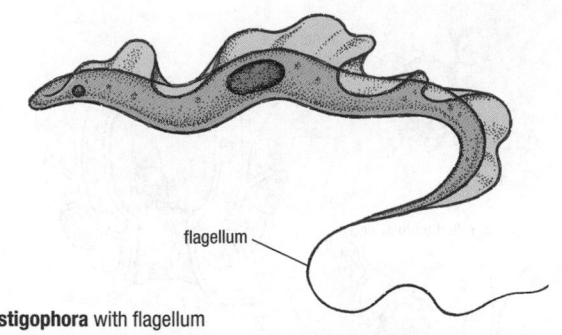

Mastigophora with flagellum

flagellum

cluded by the frequent presence of neutrophils and absence of involvement of other tissues.

interstitial m., inflammation of the connective tissue of the mammary gland.

lactational m., SYN puerperal m.

m. neonator′um, m. in the secreting breast tissue of the newborn, usually staphylococcal.

parenchymatous m., inflammation of the secreting tissue of the breast. SYN glandular m.

plasma cell m., a condition of the breasts characterized by tumor-like indurated masses containing numerous plasma cells, usually resulting from mammary duct ectasia; although clinically resembling malignant disease (attachment to skin and enlargement of axillary lymph nodes), it is not neoplastic.

puerperal m., m., usually suppurative, occurring in the later part of the puerperium. SYN lactational m.

retromammary m., SYN submammary m.

stagnation m., painful distention of the breast occurring during the latter days of pregnancy and the first days of lactation.

submammary m., inflammation of the tissues lying deep to the mammary gland. SYN retromammary m.

suppurative m., inflammation of the breast due to infection with pyogenic bacteria.

masto-, mast-. The breast; the mastoid. Cf. mammo-, mazo-. [G. *mastos*]

mas·toc·cip·i·tal (mast′ok-sip′-i-tăl). SYN masto-occipital.

mas·to·cyte (mas′tō-sīt). SYN mast *cell*.

mas·to·cy·to·gen·e·sis (mas′tō-sī′tō-jen′ĕ-sis). Formation and development of mast cells. [mastocyte + G. *genesis* production]

mas·to·cy·to·ma (mas′tō-sī-tō′mă). A fairly well-circumscribed accumulation or nodular focus of mast cells, grossly resembling a neoplasm. [mastocyte + G. *-oma,* tumor]

mas·to·cy·to·sis (mas′tō-sī-tō′sis). Abnormal proliferation of mast cells in a variety of tissues; may be systemic, involving a variety of organs, or cutaneous (urticaria pigmentosa). [mastocyte + G. *-osis,* condition]

diffuse m., infiltration of many organ systems by mast cells with varied clinical manifestations that can include fever, weight loss, flushing, bronchospasm, rhinorrhea, palpitations, dyspnea, diarrhea, gastrointestinal bleeding, and hypotension. SYN systemic m.

diffuse cutaneous m., a benign process consisting of focal cutaneous infiltrates composed of mast cells; lesions are flat or slightly elevated, form wheals and itch when stroked; bone lesions may occur.

systemic m., SYN diffuse m.

mas·to·dyn·ia (mas-tō-din′ē-ă). Pain in the breast. SEE ALSO mammary *neuralgia*. SYN mammalgia, mastalgia. [masto- + G. *odynē,* pain]

mas·toid (mas′toyd). **1.** Resembling a mamma; breast-shaped. **2.** Relating to the m. process, antrum, cells, etc. SYN mastoidal. [masto- + G. *eidos,* resemblance]

mas·toi·dal (mas-toy′dăl). SYN mastoid (2).

mas·toi·da·le (mas-toy-dā′lē). The lowest point on the contour of the mastoid process.

mas·toid·ec·to·my (mas′toy-dek′tō-mē). A group of operations on the mastoid process of the temporal bone and middle ear to drain, expose, or remove an infectious, inflammatory, or neoplastic lesion. [mastoid (process) + G. *ektomē,* excision]

complete m., an operation to exenterate the air cell system from the mastoid process of the temporal bone for the drainage of the suppuration in acute mastoiditis. SYN simple m.

modified radical m., an operation for the management of cholesteatoma that lies lateral to the remnant of the tympanic membrane and middle-ear ossicles; involves exenteration of the remaining air cells of the mastoid process and removal of the posterior and superior walls of the external auditory canal to open the mastoid and attic of the middle ear to the outside and preserve hearing.

radical m., an operation for the management of extensive cholesteatoma; involves exenteration of the remaining mastoid air cells and removal of the posterior and superior walls of the external auditory canal and the remnants of the tympanic membrane and middle-ear ossicles to exteriorize the mastoid cavity and middle ear through the external auditory canal. SYN tympanomastoidectomy.

simple m., SYN complete m.

mas·toid·i·tis (mas-toy-dī′tis). Inflammation of any part of the mastoid process. SYN mastoid empyema.

sclerosing m., a chronic m. in which the trabeculae are greatly thickened, tending to obliterate the cells.

mas·ton·cus (mas-tong′kŭs). A tumor or swelling of the breasts. [masto- + G. *onkos,* mass]

mas·to-oc·cip·i·tal (mas′tō-ok-sip′i-tăl). Relating to the mastoid portion of the temporal bone and to the occipital bone, denoting the suture uniting them. SYN mastoccipital.

mas·to·pa·ri·e·tal (mas′tō-pa-rī′ĕ-tăl). Relating to the mastoid portion of the temporal bone and to the parietal bone, denoting the suture uniting them.

mas·top·a·thy (mas-top′ă-thē). Any disease of the breasts. [masto- + G. *pathos,* suffering]

mas·to·pexy (mas′tō-pek-sē). Plastic surgery to elevate a ptotic breast in normal position, often with some improvement in shape. [masto- + G. *pēxis,* fixation]

mas·to·pla·sia (mas-tō-plā′zē-ă). Enlargement of the breast. [masto- + G. *plasis,* a molding]

mas·to·plas·ty (mas′tō-plas-tē). SYN mammaplasty. [masto- + G. *plastos,* formed]

mas·top·to·sis (mas-top-tō′sis). Ptosis or sagging of the breast. [masto- + G. *ptōsis,* a falling]

mas·tor·rha·gia (mas-tō-rā′jē-ă). Hemorrhage from a breast. [masto- + G. *rhēgnymi,* to burst forth]

mas·to·squa·mous (mas′tō-skwā′mŭs). Relating to the mastoid and the squamous portions of the temporal bone.

mas·to·syr·inx (mas′tō-sir′ingks). A fistula of the mammary gland. [masto- + G. *syrinx,* tube]

mas·tot·o·my (mas-tot′ō-mē). Incision of the breast. SYN mammotomy. [masto- + G. *tomē,* incision]

mas·tur·bate (mas′ter-bāt). To practice masturbation. [L. *masturbari,* pp. *masturbatus*]

mas·tur·ba·tion (mas′ter-bā′shung). Self-stimulation of the genitals for erotic pleasure, often resulting in orgasm.

MAT Abbreviation for multifocal atrial *tachycardia.*

Matas, Rudolph, U.S. surgeon, 1860–1957.

match·ing. The process of making a study group and a comparison group in an epidemiological study comparable with respect to extraneous or confounding factors such as age, sex, weight.

impedance m., the force delivered through the mechanical advantages of the tympanic ossicles and the area ratio of the tympanic membrane to the oval window to overcome the acoustic impedance between the ambient air and the fluid in the inner ear.

maté (mah-tā′). The dried leaves of *Ilex paraguayensis* and other species of *Ilex* (family Aquifoliaceae), shrubs growing in Paraguay and Brazil, which contain caffeine and tannin; used in South American countries as a beverage and medicinally as a diuretic and diaphoretic, and for the relief of headache. SYN Paraguay tea. [Sp. *maté,* a vessel in which the leaves are prepared]

mat·er (ma′ter). The "sheltering" coverings of the central nervous system. SEE *arachnoid* mater, dura mater, pia mater. [L. mother]

arachnoidea mater cranialis [TA], SYN cranial *arachnoid* mater.

arachnoidea mater encephali, ☆official alternate term for cranial *arachnoid* mater.

cranial pia mater [TA], the pia mater found specifically around the brain; contiguous with the arachnoid mater via the arachnoid trabeculae. SEE ALSO pia mater. SYN pia mater encephali☆.

pia mater encephali, ☆official alternate term for cranial pia mater.

pia mater spinalis [TA], SYN spinal pia mater; SEE ALSO pia mater.

spinal arachnoid mater [TA], SEE spinal *arachnoid* mater; SEE ALSO *arachnoid* mater.

spinal pia mater [TA], the pia mater found specifically around the spinal cord; includes specializations such as the denticulate ligaments. SEE ALSO pia mater. SYN pia mater spinalis [TA].

ma·te·ria (mă-tē′rē-ă). Substance or matter. [L. substance]

m. al′ba, accumulation or aggregation of microorganisms, desquamated epithelial cells, blood cells and food debris loosely adherent to surfaces of plaques, teeth, gingiva or dental appliances. [L. white matter]

m. med′ica, **(1)** that aspect of medical science concerned with the origin and preparation of drugs, their doses, and their mode of administration; **(2)** any agent used therapeutically. SEE ALSO pharmacognosy, pharmacology. [L. medical matter]

ma·te·ri·al (mă-tēr′ē-ăl). That of which something is made or composed; the constituent element of a substance. [L. *materialis,* fr. *materia,* substance]

base m., any substance from which a denture base may be made, such as shellac, acrylic resin, vulcanite, polystyrene, metal, etc.

by-product m., radioactive material produced by nuclear fission or by neutron irradiation in a nuclear reactor or similar device.

certified reference m. (CRM), a reference m. documented by or traceable to a certificate or publication from a reputable source and that states the values of the properties concerned.

contrast m., SYN contrast *medium.*

cross-reacting m. (CRM), a substance sufficiently different from a reference substance (R) to have a perceptibly different function from R, but similar enough to react with anti-R antibodies.

dental m., any m. used in dentistry.

genetic m., the carrier of hereditary information; in higher organisms it is duplex DNA.

impression m., any substance or combination of substances used for making a negative reproduction or impression.

plastic restoration m., in dentistry, any m. that may be shaped directly to the tooth cavity, such as amalgam, cement, or resin.

restorative dental m.'s, m.'s used to replace oral tissues in dentistry; e.g., amalgam, gold alloys, cements, porcelain, plastics, and denture m.'s.

ma·te·ri·es mor·bi (mă-tē′rē-ēz mōr′bī). The substance acting as the immediate cause of a disease. [L. the matter of disease]

ma·ter·nal (mă-ter′năl). Relating to or derived from the mother. [L. *maternus,* fr. *mater,* mother]

ma·ter·ni·ty (mă-ter′ni-tē). Motherhood. [see maternal]

mat·ing (māt′ing). The pairing of male and female for the purpose of reproduction.

assortative m., selection of a mate with preference for (or aversion to) a particular genotype, i.e., nonrandom m. SYN nonrandom m.

cross m., SEE cross.

nonrandom m., SYN assortative m.

random m., a practice of m. in which any egg has an equal opportunity of being fertilized by any sperm; thus the chance of one genotype at a particular locus combining with another genotype at that locus is random. SYN panmixis.

mat·rass (mat′răs). A long-necked glass vessel used for heating dry substances in chemical manipulations. [Fr. *matras*]

mat·ri·cal (mat'ri-kăl). Relating to any matrix. SYN matricial.

mat·ri·ca·ria (mat-ri-kā'rē-ă). The flowers of *Matricaria chamomilla* (family Compositae); used internally as a tonic and externally as a counterirritant. SEE ALSO chamomile. [L. *matrix,* womb]

ma·tri·ces (mā'tri-sēz, mat'rĭ-sēz). Plural of matrix. [L.]

ma·tri·cial (mă-trish'ăl). SYN matrical.

mat·ri·cide (mat'ri-sīd). 1. The killing of one's mother. Cf. patricide. 2. One who commits such an act. [L. *mater,* mother, + *caedo,* to kill]

mat·ri·lin·e·al (mat-ri-lin'ē-ăl). Denoting descent through the female line. [L. *mater,* mother, + *linea,* line]

ma·trix, pl. **ma·tri·ces** (mā'triks, mat'riks; mā'tri-sēz, mat'ri-sēz). 1 [NA]. The formative portion of a tooth or a nail. 2. The intercellular substance of a tissue. 3. A surrounding substance within which something is contained or embedded, e.g., the fatty tissue in which blood vessels or lymph nodes lie; provides a matrix for these embedded structures. 4. A mold in which anything is cast or swaged; a counterdie; a specially shaped instrument, plastic material, or metal strip used for holding and shaping the material used in filling a tooth cavity. 5. A rectangular array of numbers or symbol quantities that simplify the execution of linear operations of tedious complexity, e.g., the ITO method; the theory of matrices is widely used in solving simultaneous equations and in population genetics. [L. womb; female breeding animal]

amalgam m., a device used during placement of the amalgam mass within a compound cavity preparation, facilitating proper condensation and contour thereof by providing a confining wall.

bone m., the intercellular substance of bone tissue consisting of collagen fibers, ground substance, and inorganic bone salts.

cartilage m., the intercellular substance of cartilage consisting of fibers and ground substance.

cell m., SYN cytoplasmic m.

cytoplasmic m., a fluid cytoplasmic substance filling the interstices of the cytoskeleton. SYN cell m., cytomatrix.

external m., the substance occupying the space between the inner and outer membrane of any organelle (e.g., mitochondria) with a double membrane.

identity m., a square m. in which the quantities on the diagonal from top left to bottom right are all equal to 1 and all the other entries are 0.

mitochondrial m., SYN m. mitochondrialis.

m. mitochondria'lis, the substance occupying the space enclosed by the inner membrane of a mitochondrion; it contains enzymes, filaments of DNA, ribosomes, granules, and inclusions of protein crystals, glycogen, and lipid. SYN mitochondrial m.

nail m. [TA], the area of the corium on which the nail rests; it is extremely sensitive and presents numerous longitudinal ridges on its surface. According to some anatomists, the nail bed is the portion covered by the body of the nail, the nail bed being only the part on which the root of the nail rests. SYN m. unguis [TA], keratogenous membrane, nail bed, onychostroma.

nuclear m., the network of protein fibers both around the outside of the nucleus as well as inside the nucleus.

square m., a m. in which the numbers of rows and columns are equal.

territorial m., SYN cartilage *capsule.*

m. un'guis [TA], SYN nail m.

mat·ter. SYN substance. SEE ALSO substance. [L. *materies,* substance]

gray m. [TA], those regions of the brain and spinal cord which are made up primarily of the cell bodies and dendrites of nerve cells rather than myelinated axons. SYN gray substance [TA], substantia grisea [TA], substantia cinerea.

pontine gray m., SYN pontine *nuclei,* under *nucleus.*

white m. [TA], those regions of the brain and spinal cord that are largely or entirely composed of nerve fibers and contain few or no neuronal cell bodies or dendrites. SYN alba, substantia alba, white substance.

mat·u·rate (mat'ū-rāt). To suppurate. [L. *maturo,* pp. -*atus,* to make ripe, fr. *maturus,* ripe]

mat·u·ra·tion (mat-ū-rā'shŭn). 1. Achievement of full development or growth. 2. Developmental changes that lead to maturity. 3. Processing of a macromolecule; e.g., posttranscriptional modification of RNA or posttranslational modification of proteins. 4. The overall process leading to the incorporation of a viral genome into a capsid and the development of a complete virion. [L. *maturatio,* a ripening, fr. *maturus,* ripe]

ma·ture (mă-choor', -toor). 1. Ripe; fully developed. 2. To ripen; to become fully developed. [L. *maturus,* ripe]

ma·tu·ri·ty (mă-choor'i-tē). A state of full development or completed growth.

Mauchart (Mauchard), Burkhard D., German anatomist, 1696–1751. SEE M. *ligaments,* under *ligament.*

Maurer, Georg, German physician in Sumatra, *1909. SEE M. *clefts,* under *cleft,* *dots,* under *dot.*

Mauriac, Pierre, French physician, *1882. SEE M. *syndrome.*

Mauriceau, François, French obstetrician, 1637–1709. SEE M. *maneuver;* M.-Levret *maneuver.*

Mauthner, Ludwig, Austrian ophthalmologist, 1840–1894. SEE M. *sheath.*

max·il·la, gen. and pl. **max·il·lae** (mak-sil'ă, mak-sil'ē) [TA]. An irregularly shaped pneumatized bone, supporting the superior teeth and taking part in the formation of the orbit, hard palate, and nasal cavity and containing the maxillary sinus. SYN upper jaw bone, upper jaw. [L. jawbone]

max·il·lary (mak'si-lār-ē). Relating to the maxilla, or upper jaw.

max·il·lec·to·my (mak-sil-ek'tō-mē). Resection of the maxilla. [maxilla + G. *ektomē,* excision]

max·il·li·tis (mak'si-lī'tis). Inflammation of the maxilla.

max·il·lo·den·tal (mak-sil'ō-den'tăl). Relating to the upper jaw and its associated teeth.

max·il·lo·fa·cial (mak-sil'ō-fā'shăl). Pertaining to the jaws and face, particularly with reference to specialized surgery of this region.

max·il·lo·ju·gal (mak-sil'ō-joo'găl). Relating to the maxilla and the zygomatic bone.

max·il·lo·man·dib·u·lar (mak-sil'ō-man-dib'ū-lăr). Relating to the upper and lower jaws.

max·il·lo·pal·a·tine (mak-sil'ō-pal'ă-tīn). Relating to the maxilla and the palatine bone.

max·il·lot·o·my (mak-si-lot'ō-mē). Surgical sectioning of the maxilla to allow movement of all or a part of the maxilla into the desired portion. [maxilla + G. *tomē,* incision]

max·il·lo·tur·bi·nal (mak-sil'lō-ter'bi-năl). Relating to the inferior nasal concha.

Maximow, Alexander A., Russian physician in U.S., 1874–1928. SEE M. *stain* for bone marrow.

max·i·mum (mak'si-mŭm). The greatest amount, value, or degree attained or attainable. [L. neuter of *maximus,* greatest]

glucose transport m., the maximal rate of reabsorption of glucose from the glomerular filtrate; it amounts to approximately 320 mg/min in humans.

transport m. (Tm), the maximal rate of secretion or reabsorption of a substance by the renal tubules. SYN tubular m.

tubular m. (Tm), SYN transport m.

May, Richard, German physician. SEE M.-Hegglin *anomaly.*

May ap·ple. SYN podophyllum.

Mayer, Paul, German histologist, 1848–1923. SEE M. hemalum *stain,* mucicarmine *stain,* muchematein *stain.*

Mayer, Karl, W., German gynecologist, 1795–1868. SEE M. *pessary;* M.-Rokitansky-Küster-Hauser *syndrome.*

Mayer, Karl, Austrian neurologist, 1862–1932. SEE M. *reflex.*

May-Grünwald stain. See under stain.

may·id·ism (mā'id-izm). SYN pellagra. [*Zea mays,* maize]

Mayo, Charles H., U.S. surgeon, 1865–1939. SEE M. *bunionectomy.*

Mayo, William J., U.S. surgeon, 1861–1939. SEE M. *operation,* *vein.*

Mayo-Robson, Sir Arthur W., British surgeon, 1853–1933. SEE Mayo-Robson *point;* Mayo-Robson *position.*

Mayou, Marmaduke Stephen, British ophthalmologist, 1876–1934. SEE Batten-M. *disease.*

ma·za·mor·ra (maz-ă-mōr′ă). Name given in Puerto Rico to a dermatitis caused by penetration of the skin by hookworm larvae.

maze (māz). A labyrinth; frequently used to study higher functions of the nervous system in rats. [M.E. *masen,* to confuse]

ma·zin·dol (mā′zin-dol). An isoindole anorexiant that is distinctive in not having the phenethylamine chain common to sympathomimetic amines.

mazo-. The breast. SEE ALSO masto-. [G. *mazos*]

Mazzoni, Vittorio, Italian physician, 1880–1940. SEE M. *corpuscle;* Golgi-M. *corpuscle.*

Mazzotti, Luigi, Mexican physician specializing in tropical medicine in mid-20th century. SEE Mazzotti *reaction,* Mazzotti *test.*

Mb, MbCO, MbO₂ myoglobin and its combinations with CO and O₂ (oxymyoglobin), respectively.

MBC Abbreviation for maximum breathing *capacity.*

M.C. Abbreviation for *Magister Chirurgiae,* Master of Surgery; Medical Corps.

mc Former abbreviation for millicurie.

MCAD Abbreviation for medium-chain acyl-CoA dehydrogenase.

McArdle, Brian, 20th century British neurologist. SEE McA. *disease;* McA.-Schmid-Pearson *disease;* McA. *syndrome.*

McBurney, Charles, U.S. surgeon, 1845–1913. SEE McB. *incision, point, sign.*

McCall, M.L., 20th century U.S. gynecologist. SEE M. culdoplasty *procedure.*

McCarthy, Daniel J., U.S. neurologist, 1874–1958. SEE McC. *reflexes,* under *reflex.*

McClintock, Barbara, 1902–1992, 1993 Nobel Prize winner for her work in the genetics of corn.

McCrea, Lowrain E., U.S. urologist, *1896. SEE McC. *sound.*

McCune, Donovan James, U.S. pediatrician, 1902–1976. SEE M.-Albright *syndrome.*

McDonald, Ellice, U.S. gynecologist, 1876–1955. SEE McD. *maneuver.*

McGoon, Dwight C., U.S. surgeon, *1925. SEE McG. *technique.*

MCH Abbreviation for mean corpuscular *hemoglobin.*

M.Ch. Abbreviation for *Magister Chirurgiae,* Master of Surgery.

MCHC Abbreviation for mean corpuscular hemoglobin *concentration.*

mCi Abbreviation for millicurie.

McKee, George Kenneth, British orthopedic surgeon, *1930. SEE McK. *line.*

McKusick, Victor Almon, U.S. physician, *1921. SEE McKusick metaphyseal *dysplasia.*

McLean, Malcolm, U.S. obstetrician, 1848–1924. SEE Tucker-McL. *forceps.*

MCMI Abbreviation for Millon clinical multiaxial *inventory.*

McMurray, Thomas P., British surgeon, 1887–1949. SEE McM. *test.*

m-cone. Middle wavelength sensitive cone (green cone).

MCP-1 Abbreviation for monocyte chemoattractant *protein*-1.

McPhail, M.K., Canadian physiologist, *1907. SEE McP. *test.*

MCR Abbreviation for steroid metabolic clearance *rate.*

McReynolds, John O., U.S. ophthalmologist, 1865–1942.

M-CSF Abbreviation for macrophage colony-stimulating *factor.*

MCV Abbreviation for mean corpuscular *volume.*

McVay, Chester B., U.S. surgeon, *1911. SEE McV. *operation.*

MD Abbreviation for methyldichloroarsine.

M.D. Abbreviation of *Medicinae Doctor,* Doctor of Medicine.

Md Symbol for mendelevium.

MDF Abbreviation for myocardial depressant *factor.*

m. dict. Abbreviation for [L] *more dicto,* as directed.

MDMA A centrally active phenethylamine derivative related to amphetamine and methamphetamine, with central nervous system excitant and hallucinogenic properties. SYN 3,4-methylenedioxymethamphetamine.

MDNCF Abbreviation for monocyte-derived neutrophil chemotactic *factor.*

M'Dowel, Benjamin G., Irish anatomist, 1829–1885. SEE *frenulum* of M.

M.D.S. Abbreviation of Master of Dental Surgery.

Me Symbol for methyl.

Meadows, William Robert, U.S. cardiologist, *1919. SEE M. *syndrome.*

meal (mēl). **1.** The food consumed at regular intervals or at a specified time. **2.** Ground flour from a grain.

Boyden m., a m. consisting of three or four egg yolks, beaten up in milk and seasoned with sugar, port wine, etc., used to test the evacuation time of the gallbladder; two-thirds to three-quarters of the contents will be normally evacuated within 40 minutes.

Lundh m., a meal of skimmed milk powder mixed with corn oil and dextrose used to assess pancreatic function.

test m., (1) toast and tea, or crackers and tea, or gruel or other bland food, given to stimulate gastric secretion before withdrawing gastric contents for analysis; (2) administration of food containing a substance thought to be responsible for symptoms, such as an allergic reaction.

mean (mēn). A statistical measurement of central tendency or average of a set of values, usually assumed to be the arithmetic m. unless otherwise specified. [M.E., *mene* fr. O.Fr., fr. L. *medianus,* in the middle]

arithmetic m., the m. calculated by adding a set of values and then dividing the sum by the number of values.

geometric m., the m. calculated as the antilogarithm of the arithmetic mean of the logarithms of the individual values; it can also be calculated as the *n*th root of the product of *n* values.

harmonic m., the m. calculated as the number of values being averaged, divided by the sum of their reciprocals.

regression of the m., if, for a symmetrical population with a single mode, a measurement, selected because it is extreme, is repeated, on average the second reading will be closer to the m. than the first.

standard error of the m. (SEM), a statistical index of the probability that a given sample m. is representative of the m. of the population from which the sample was drawn.

mea·sle (mē′zl). **1.** The larva (*Cysticercus cellulosae*) of *Taenia solium,* the pork tapeworm; *C. cellulosae* is less frequently used to designate cysticerci of *T. solium.* **2.** The larva (*Cysticercus bovis*) of *Taenia saginata,* the beef tapeworm; the term *C. bovis* is less frequently used to designate cysticerci of *T. bovis.*

mea·sles (mē′zlz). **1.** An acute exanthematous disease, caused by m. virus (genus Morbillivirus), a member of the family Paramyxoviridae, and marked by fever and other constitutional disturbances, a catarrhal inflammation of the respiratory mucous membranes, and a generalized maculopapular eruption of a dusky red color; the eruption occurs early on the buccal mucous membrane in the form of Koplik spots, a manifestation utilized in early diagnosis; average incubation period is from 10–12 days. Recovery is usually rapid but respiratory complications and otitis media caused by secondary bacterial infections are common. Encephalitis occurs rarely. Subacute sclerosing parencephalitis may occur later and is associated with chronic infection. SYN morbilli. **2.** A disease of swine caused by the presence of *Cysticercus cellulosae,* the measle or larva of *Taenia solium,* the pork tapeworm. **3.** A disease of cattle caused by the presence of *Cysticercus bovis,* the measle or larva of *Taenia saginata,* the beef tapeworm of humans. [D. *maselen*]

atypical m., sometimes severe, unusual clinical manifestation of natural m. virus infection in persons with waning vaccination immunity, particularly in those who had received formaldehyde-inactivated vaccine; an accelerated allergic reaction apparently resulting from an anamnestic antibody response, characterized by high fever, absence of Koplik spots, a shortened prodromal period, atypical rash, and pneumonia.

me

black m., (1) SYN hemorrhagic m; (2) SYN Rocky Mountain spotted *fever*.

German m., SYN rubella.

hemorrhagic m., a severe form in which the eruption is dark in color due to effusion of blood into affected areas of the skin. SYN black m. (1).

three-day m., SYN rubella.

tropical m., a disease of uncertain character, somewhat resembling rubella, occurring in southern China.

mea·sly (mēz'lē). Pertaining to pork or beef infected with the cysticerci of the tapeworms *Taenia solium* or *Taenia saginata*, respectively.

mea·sure (mezh'er). **1.** To determine the magnitude or quantity of a substance by comparing it to some accepted standard or by calculation. **2.** A specified magnitude of a physical quantity. **3.** A graduated instrument used to measure an object or substance. [O.F. *mesure*, fr. L. *mensura*, fr. *metior*, to measure]

Geneva lens m., a device for measuring the radii of the curvature of a spectacle lens. SYN lens clock. [*Geneva*, Switzerland]

mea·sure·ment (mezh'ŭr-ment). Determination of a dimension or quantity.

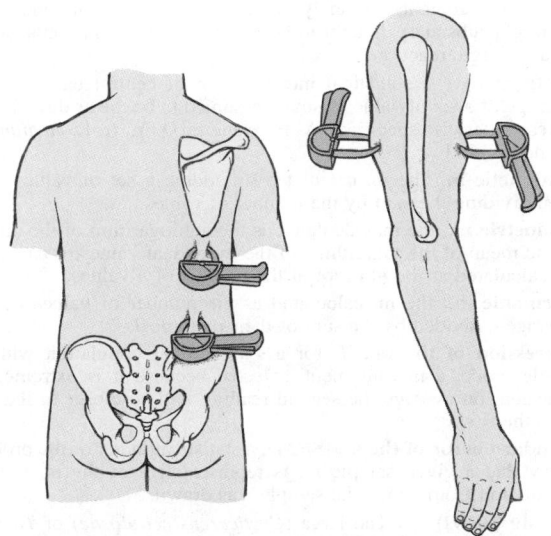

skinfold measurement: with calipers at standard sites provides an accurate estimate of subcutaneous fat

---

end-point m., analytical m. at the end of a chemical reaction, as opposed to making the m. while the reaction proceeds.

kinetic m., continuous or frequent monitoring of the readings during a chemical reaction to determine its rate.

nasion-pogonion m., SYN facial *plane*.

mea·sures of cen·tral ten·den·cy. General term for several characteristics of the distribution of a set of measurements or values around a value or values at or near the middle of the set; the principal measures of central tendency are mean, median, and mode.

me·a·tal (mē-ā'tăl). Relating to a meatus.

meato-. Meatus. [L. *meatus*, passage]

me·a·tom·e·ter (mē-ă-tom'ĕ-ter). An instrument for measuring the size of a meatus, especially the meatus of the urethra. [meato- + G. *metron*, measure]

me·a·to·plas·ty (mē'ă-tō-plas-tē). Enlargement or other surgical reconfiguring of a meatus or canal, e.g., the external auditory meatus or the urethral meatus.

me·a·tor·rha·phy (mē-ă-tōr'ă-fē). Closing by suture of the wound made by performing a meatomy. [meato- + G. *rhaphē*, suture]

me·at·o·scope (mē-at'ō-skōp). A form of speculum for examining a meatus, especially the meatus of the urethra. [meato- + G. *skopeō*, to view]

me·a·tos·co·py (mē-ă-tos'kŏ-pē). Inspection, usually instrumental, of any meatus, especially of the meatus of the urethra. [meato- + G. *skopeō*, to view]

me·at·o·tome (mē-at'ō-tōm). A knife with short cutting edge for use in meatotomy.

me·a·tot·o·my (mē-ă-tot'ō-mē). An incision made to enlarge a meatus, e.g., of the urethra or ureter. [meato- + G. *tomē*, incision]

me·a·tus, pl. **me·a·tus** (mē-ā'tŭs) [TA]. A passage or channel, especially the external opening of a canal. SYN external opening. [L. a going, a passage, fr. *meo*, pp. *meatus*, to go, pass]

acoustic m., SYN external acoustic m.

m. acus'ticus exter'nus [TA], SYN external acoustic m.

m. acus'ticus inter'nus [TA], SYN internal acoustic m.

external acoustic m. [TA], the passage leading inward through the tympanic portion of the temporal bone, from the auricle to the tympanic membrane; it consists of a bony (inner) portion and a fibrocartilaginous (outer) portion, the cartilaginous external acoustic meatus. SYN m. acusticus externus [TA], acoustic m., antrum auris, auditory canal, ear canal, external auditory m.

external auditory m., SYN external acoustic m.

external urinary m., ☆official alternate term for external urethral *orifice*.

fish-mouth m., a red and swollen condition of the orifice of the urethra (urinary m.) in gonorrhea.

internal acoustic m. [TA], a canal beginning at the opening of the internal acoustic meatus in the posterior cranial fossa, passing laterally through the petrous portion of the temporal bone to end at the fundus, where a thin plate of bone separates it from the vestibule; it gives passage to the facial and vestibulocochlear nerves together with the labyrinthine artery and veins. SYN m. acusticus internus [TA], internal auditory m.

internal auditory m., SYN internal acoustic m.

nasal m. [TA], any of four passages in the nasal cavity formed by the projection of the conchae: inferior nasal m. [TA] (meatus nasi inferior [TA]), lies below the inferior concha; middle nasal m. [TA] (meatus nasi medius [TA]), lies between the middle and inferior conchae; superior nasal m. [TA] (meatus nasi superior [TA]), lies between the superior and middle conchae; common nasal m. [TA] (meatus nasi communis [TA]) is the part of the nasal cavity between the conchae and the nasal septum. SYN m. nasi [TA].

m. na'si [TA], SYN nasal m.

nasopharyngeal m. [TA], the posterior part of the nasal cavity from the posterior limits of the conchae to the choanae. SYN m. nasopharyngeus [TA], nasopharyngeal passage.

m. nasopharyn'geus [TA], SYN nasopharyngeal m.

ureteral m., SYN ureteric *orifice*.

m. urina'rius, SYN external urethral *orifice*.

me·ban·a·zine (mē-ban'ă-zēn). An antidepressant with inhibitory effect on monoamine oxidase.

me·ben·da·zole (mē-ben'dă-zōl). An effective broad-spectrum nematicidal agent against intestinal nematodes such as pinworm, hookworm, whipworm, and *Ascaris*.

me·bev·er·ine hy·dro·chlo·ride (mĕ-bev'er-ēn). An intestinal antispasmodic.

me·bro·phen·hy·dra·mine (mĕ-brō-fen-hī'dră-mēn). An H₁ antihistaminic.

me·but·a·mate (mĕ-bū'tă-māt). Chemically, it differs only slightly from meprobamate, and possesses similar CNS-depressant properties.

mec·a·myl·a·mine hy·dro·chlo·ride (mek'ă-mil'ă-mēn). A secondary amine that blocks transmission of impulses at autonomic ganglia (similar to but more effective than hexamethonium); used in the management of severe hypertension.

me·chan·i·cal (mĕ-kan'i-kăl). **1.** Performed by means of some apparatus, not manually. **2.** Explaining phenomena in terms of mechanics. **3.** Automatic. [G. *mechanikos*, relating to a machine, fr. *mēchanē*, a contrivance, machine]

me·chan·i·co·re·cep·tor (mĕ-kan′i-kō-rē-sep′ter, tōr). SYN mechanoreceptor.

me·chan·ics (mĕ-kan′iks). The science of the action of forces in promoting motion or equilibrium. [see mechanical]

body m., the study of the action of muscles in producing motion or posture of the body.

mech·a·nism (mek′ă-nizm). **1.** An arrangement or grouping of the parts of anything that has a definite action. **2.** The means by which an effect is obtained. **3.** The chain of events in a particular process. **4.** The detailed description of a reaction pathway. [G. *mēchanē*, a contrivance]

association m., the cerebral m. whereby the memory of past sensations may be compared or associated with present ones.

countercurrent m., a system in the renal medulla that facilitates concentration of the urine as it passes through the renal tubules. SEE countercurrent exchanger, countercurrent multiplier.

defense m., **(1)** a psychological means of coping with conflict or anxiety, e.g., conversion, denial, dissociation, rationalization, repression, sublimation; **(2)** the psychic structure underlying a coping strategy; **(3)** immunologic m. vs. non-specific defense m.

double displacement m., SYN ping-pong m.

Douglas m., m. of spontaneous evolution in transverse lie; extreme lateral flexion of the vertebral column with birth of the lateral aspect of thorax before the buttocks.

Duncan m., passage of the placenta from the uterus with the rough side foremost.

gating m., **(1)** occurrence of the maximum refractory period among cardiac conducting cells approximately 2 mm proximal to the terminal Purkinje fibers in the ventricular muscle, beyond which the refractory period is shortened through a sequence of Purkinje cells, transitional cells, and muscular cells; gating m. may be a cause of ventricular aberration, bidirectional tachycardia, and concealed extrasystoles; **(2)** a m. by which painful impulses may be blocked from entering the spinal cord. Cf. gate-control *theory*.

immunologic m., the groups of cells (chiefly lymphocytes and cells of the reticuloendothelial system) that function in establishing active acquired immunity (induced sensitivity, allergy).

ordered m., a scheme for substrate binding and product release for multisubstrate enzymes; for a two-substrate two-product enzyme with an ordered m., one particular substrate has to first bind to the enzyme, followed by the other substrate; chemistry then occurs, and products are formed and are released from the enzyme in a distinct order. More complex ordered schemes exist for enzymes having more than two substrates. Some of the dehydrogenases have such a m. SYN ordered.

ordered on-random off m., a scheme for substrate binding and product release for multisubstrate enzymes; for a two-substrate two-product enzyme with this m., the reactants have to bind to the enzyme in a distinct order; however, once the products are formed they may dissociate from the enzyme in either order. It has been suggested that pyruvate kinase has such a mechanism. The random on-ordered off m. is simply the reverse of this m.

ping-pong m., a special multisubstrate reaction in which, for a two-substrate, two-product (i.e., bi-bi) system, an enzyme reacts with one substrate to form a product and a modified enzyme, the latter then reacting with a second substrate to form a second, final product, and regenerating the original enzyme. An example of such a m. is found in the aminotransferases. More complex ping-pong m.'s exist for enzymes having more than two substrates. SYN double displacement m.

pressoreceptive m., the pressoreceptor system, especially of the carotid sinuses and aortic arch.

proprioceptive m., the m. of sense of position and movement, by which muscular movements can be adjusted to a great degree of accuracy and equilibrium maintained.

random m., a scheme for substrate binding and product release for a multisubstrate enzyme; for a two-substrate two-product enzyme with this m., either substrate can bind first and, after the reaction has taken place, either product can be the first to dissociate from the enzyme. Brain hexokinase has a random m. More

complex random m.'s exist for enzymes having more than two substrates.

re-entrant m., the probable basis of most arrhythmias, requiring at least three criteria in the heart: 1. a loop circuit, 2. unidirectional block, 3. slowed conduction. Impulses enter the loop circuit and divide in both directions (blocked in one direction only), negotiate the loop circuit to the area of block where the slowed conduction has allowed the impulse to arrive at a time when the tissue proximal to the unidirectional block has recovered and will permit its passage in the opposite direction.

Schultze m., expulsion of the placenta with the fetal surface foremost.

mech·a·no·car·di·og·ra·phy (mek′ă-nō-kar-dē-og′ră-fē). Use of graphic tracings reflecting the mechanical effects of the heartbeat, such as the carotid pulse tracing or apexcardiogram; phonocardiography is also usually considered a form of m.

mech·a·no·cyte (mek′ă-nō-sīt). An in vitro tissue culture fibroblast.

mech·a·no·pho·bia (mek′ă-nō-fō′bē-ă). Morbid fear of machinery. [G. *mēchanē*, machine, + *phobos*, fear]

mech·a·no·re·cep·tor (mek′ă-nō-rē-sep′tŏr). A receptor which responds to mechanical pressure or distortion; e.g., receptors in the carotid sinuses, touch receptors in the skin. SYN mechanicoreceptor.

mech·a·no·re·flex (mek′ă-nō-rē′fleks). A reflex triggered by stimulation of a mechanoreceptor.

mech·a·no·ther·a·py (mek′ă-nō-thār′ă-pē). Treatment of disease by means of apparatus or mechanical appliances of any kind. [G. *mēchanē*, machine, + *therapeia*, treatment]

mèche (māsh). A strip of gauze or other material used as a tent or drain. [Fr. wick]

mech·lor·eth·a·mine hy·dro·chlo·ride (mek′lōr-eth′ă-mēn). It is cytotoxic for all cells, but with a special affinity for bone marrow, lymphatic tissues, and rapidly proliferating cells of certain neoplasms. Used for the palliative treatment of Hodgkin disease, lymphosarcoma, and certain chronic leukemias. SYN mustine hydrochloride.

me·cism (mē′sizm). Abnormal elongation of the body or one or more of its parts. [G. *mēkos*, length, *-ismos*, condition]

Me·cis·to·cir·rus (mē-sis-tō-sir′ŭs). A monotypic genus of trichostrongylid nematodes (subfamily Mecistocirrinae), with the single species, *M. digitatus;* it is not grossly distinguished from *Haemonchus contortus* and has about the same effect on the host. *M.* is distributed chiefly in Asia in cattle, sheep, buffalo, bison, the stomach of pigs, and occasionally in humans. [G. *mēkistos*, very long, + L. *cirrus*, curl, the protruding male organ of a nematode]

Meckel, Johann F., the elder, German anatomist and obstetrician, 1714–1774. SEE M. *band, cavity, ganglion, ligament, space.*

Meckel, Johann F., the younger, German comparative anatomist and embryologist, 1781–1833. SEE M. *scan, syndrome, cartilage, diverticulum, plane;* M.-Gruber *syndrome.*

Mecke re·a·gent. See under reagent.

me·clas·tine (mĕ-klas′tēn). SYN clemastine.

mec·li·zine hy·dro·chlo·ride (mek′li-zēn). An H_1 antihistaminic useful in the prevention and relief of motion sickness and symptoms caused by vestibular disorders. SYN meclozine hydrochloride.

mec·lo·fen·a·mate so·di·um (mek-lō-fen′ă-māt). A nonsteroidal anti-inflammatory agent with analgesic and antipyretic actions.

mec·lo·fen·a·mic ac·id (mĕ-klō-fen-am′ik). An NSAID used for inflammatory conditions and dysmenorrhea; also antipyretic.

mec·lo·fen·ox·ate (mek′lō-fen-ok′sāt). An analeptic.

mec·lo·zine hy·dro·chlo·ride (mek′lō-zēn). SYN meclizine hydrochloride.

me·com·e·ter (mē-kom′ĕ-ter). An instrument, such as calipers with a scale attachment, for measurement of newborn infants. [G. *mēkos*, length, + *metron*, measure]

mec·o·nate (mek′ŏ-nāt). A salt or ester of meconic acid. [G. *mēkōn*, poppy]

me

me·con·ic ac·id (me-kon'ik). Obtained from opium; it forms soluble salts (meconates) with many of the alkaloids of opium.

mec·o·nin (mek'ŏ-nin). $C_{10}H_{10}O_4$; the lactone of meconic acid, found also in *Hydrastis canadensis;* a hypnotic. SYN opianyl.

me·co·ni·or·rhea (mē-kō'nē-ō-rē'ă). Passage, by the newborn infant, of an abnormally large amount of meconium. [meconium + G. *rhoia,* flow]

me·co·ni·um (mē-kō'nē-ŭm). **1.** The first intestinal discharges of the newborn infant, greenish in color and consisting of epithelial cells, mucus, and bile. **2.** SYN opium. [L., fr. G. *mēkōnion,* dim. of *mēkōn,* poppy]

me·daz·e·pam hy·dro·chlo·ride (mĕ-daz'ĕ-pam). An antianxiety agent.

med·fal·an (med'fal-an). SYN medphalan.

me·dia (mē'dē-ă). **1.** SYN *tunica* media. **2.** Plural of medium. [L. fem. of *medius,* middle]

me·di·ad (mē'dē-ad). Toward the middle line.

🔲 **me·di·al** (mē'dē-ăl) [TA]. Relating to the middle or center; nearer to the median or midsagittal plane. SYN medialis [TA]. [L. *medialis,* middle]

me·di·a·lec·i·thal (mē'dē-ă-les'i-thăl). Denoting an egg with a moderate amount of yolk, as in amphibians. [L. *medialis,* medial, + G. *lekithos,* egg yolk]

me·di·a·lis (mē-dē-ā'lis) [TA]. SYN medial, medial. [L.]

med·i·al·i·za·tion (mēd-ē-al-ĭ-zā'shun). An operation to move a part toward the midline, such as the arytenoid cartilage or vocal cord in vocal cord paralysis.

me·di·an (mē'dē-an). **1.** Central; middle; lying in the midline. SYN medianus. **2.** The middle value in a set of measurements; like the mean, a measure of central tendency. [L. *medianus,* middle]

me·di·a·nus (mē-dē-ā'nŭs). SYN median (1). [L.]

me·di·as·ti·nal (mē'dē-as-tī'năl). Relating to the mediastinum.

me·di·as·ti·ni·tis (mē'dē-as-ti-nī'tis). Inflammation of the cellular tissue of the mediastinum.

fibrosing m., SYN mediastinal *fibrosis.*

fibrous m., scarring of mediastinal structures of unknown origin or due to infection.

idiopathic fibrous m., SYN mediastinal *fibrosis.*

me·di·as·ti·nog·ra·phy (mē'dē-as-ti-nog'ră-fē). Radiography of the mediastinum. [mediastinum + G. *graphō,* to write]

gaseous m., radiography of the mediastinum after injection of air (artificial pneumomediastinum), an obsolete procedure.

me·di·as·tin·o·per·i·car·di·tis (me'dē-as'tin-ō-per'i-kar-dī'tis). Inflammation of the pericardium and of the surrounding mediastinal cellular tissue.

me·di·as·tin·o·scope (mē-dē-as'tin'-ō-skōp). An endoscope for inspection of the mediastinum through a suprasternal incision.

me·di·as·ti·nos·co·py (mē'dē-as-ti-nos'kŏ-pē). Endoscopic examination of the mediastinum through a suprasternal incision, usually for biopsy of paratracheal lymph nodes. [mediastinum + G. *skopeō,* to view]

anterior m., modification of the Chamberlain *procedure* in which a mediastinoscope is used for exploration of the anterior mediastinum and subaortic regions.

extended m., cervical m. in which, in addition to the standard pre- and paratracheal exploration, the mediastinoscope is passed anterior to the innominate artery and aortic arch to provide access to the subaortic (aortopulmonary window) and anterior mediastinal lymph nodes; an alternative to the Chamberlain *procedure.*

me·di·as·ti·not·o·my (mē'dē-as-ti-not'ō-mē). Incision into the mediastinum. [mediastinum + G. *tomē,* incision]

anterior m., SYN Chamberlain *procedure.*

me·di·as·ti·num (me'dē-as-tī'nŭm). **1.** A septum between two parts of an organ or a cavity. **2** [TA]. The median partition of the thoracic cavity, covered by the mediastinal part of the parietal pleura and containing all the thoracic viscera and structures except the lungs. It is divided arbitrarily into two major divisions: a superior mediastinum [TA] (mediastinum superus [TA]), which lies directly superior to a horizontal plane intersecting the sternal angle and approximately the T4–5 intervertebral disk, and an

inferior mediastinum [TA] (mediastinum inferius [TA]) inferior to that plane; the latter is, in turn, subdivided in 3 parts: a middle mediastinum [TA] (mediastinum medium [TA]), which is coterminus with the pericardial sac containing the heart, a nearly potential anterior mediastinum [TA] (mediastinum anterius [TA]) lying in front, and a posterior mediastinum [TA] (mediastinum posterius [TA]) behind, containing the esophagus, descending aorta, and thoracic duct. SYN interpleural space, interpulmonary septum, mediastinal space, septum mediastinale. [Mod. L. a middle septum, fr. Mediev. L. *mediastinus,* medial, fr. L. *mediastinus,* a lower servant, fr. *medius,* middle]

anterior m. [TA], the narrow nearly potential space region between the pericardium posteriorly and the sternum anteriorly containing the thymus or its remnants, some lymph nodes and vessels and branches of the internal thoracic artery. SYN m. anterius [TA].

m. ante'rius [TA], SYN anterior m.

inferior m. [TA], the region below a horizontal plane transecting approximately the T4–5 intervertebral disk posteriorly and the sternal angle anteriorly, demarcating the inferior limit of the superior mediastinum. It is subdivided into three regions: middle, anterior, and posterior. SYN m. inferius [TA].

m. infe'rius [TA], SYN inferior m.

m. me'dium [TA], SYN middle m.

middle m. [TA], the large central portion of the inferior m., which includes the pericardium and the contained heart, as well as the phrenic nerves and cardiacophrenic vessels. SYN m. medium [TA].

posterior m. [TA], lies between the pericardium anteriorly and the vertebral column posteriorly and below the level of the plane that intersects the sternal angle and the T4–5 intervertebral disk. It contains the descending aorta, thoracic duct, esophagus, azygos veins, and vagus nerves. SYN m. posterius [TA], postmediastinum.

m. poste'rius [TA], SYN posterior m.

superior m. [TA], part of the mediastinum lying superior to the horizontal plane intersecting the sternal angle and approximately the T4–5 intervertebral disc (i.e., above the pericardium); it contains the arch of the aorta and the vessels arising from it, the brachiocephalic veins, and upper portion of the superior vena cava, the trachea, the esophagus, the thoracic duct, the thymus, and the phrenic, vagus, cardiac, and left recurrent laryngeal nerves. SYN m. superius [TA].

m. supe'rius [TA], SYN superior m.

m. tes'tis [TA], SYN m. of testis.

m. of testis [TA], a mass of fibrous tissue continuous with the tunica albuginea, projecting into the testis from its posterior border; testicular septa radiate as continuations surrounding the testicular lobules. SYN m. testis [TA], corpus highmori, corpus highmorianum, Highmore body, septum of testis.

me·di·ate. 1 (mē'dē-it). Situated between; intermediate. **2** (mē'dē-āt). To effect something by means of an intermediary substance, as in complement-mediated phagocytosis. [L. *mediatus,* fr. *medio,* pp. *-atus,* to divide in the middle]

me·di·a·tion (mē-dē-ā'shŭn). The action of an intermediary substance (mediator).

me·di·a·tor (mē'dē-ā-ter, -tōr). An intermediary substance or thing.

pharmacologic m.'s of anaphylaxis, substances released from mast (and other) cells by the reaction of antigen and specific homocytotropic antibody on their surfaces; they include histamine, slow-reacting substance of anaphylaxis (SRS-A), bradykinin, and (in some species of animals) serotonin.

med·i·ca·ble (med'i-kă-bl). Treatable, with hope of a cure.

med·i·cal (med'i-kăl). **1.** Relating to medicine or the practice of medicine. SYN medicinal (2). **2.** SYN medicinal (1). [L. *medicalis,* fr *medicus,* physician]

med·i·cal corps. The subdivision of a military organization, such as the U.S. Army, devoted to medical care of the troops.

med·i·cal tran·scrip·tion·ist. An individual who performs machine transcription of physician-dictated medical reports concerning a patient's health care, which become part of the patient's permanent medical record; a certified m. t. (CMT) has satisfied the requirements for certification by the American Association for Medical Transcription.

me·dic·a·ment (me-dik′ă-ment, med′i-kă-ment). A medicine, medicinal application, or remedy. [L. *medicamentum*, medicine]

med·i·ca·men·to·sus (med′i-kă-men-tō′sŭs). Relating to a drug; denoting a drug eruption. [L.]

med·i·cate (med′i-kāt). **1.** To treat disease by the giving of drugs. **2.** To impregnate with a medicinal substance. [L. *medico*, pp. *-atus*, to heal]

med·i·cat·ed (med′i-kāt-ed). Impregnated with a medicinal substance.

med·i·ca·tion (med-i-kā′shŭn). **1.** The act of medicating. **2.** A medicinal substance, or medicament.

ionic m., SYN iontophoresis.

maintenance medication, m. taken to stabilize an illness or symptoms of illness.

preanesthetic m., drugs administered prior to an anesthetic to decrease anxiety and to obtain a smoother induction of, maintenance of, and emergence from anesthesia.

sublingual m., a drug dosage form intended to be used by placement under the tongue; the drug (e.g., nitroglycerin) is absorbed from the mucosal tissues and bypasses the gastrointestinal tract, where it may be partially or totally degraded.

med·i·ca·tor (med′i-kā-ter, -tōr). **1.** An instrument for use in making therapeutic applications to the deeper parts of the body. **2.** One who gives medicaments for the relief of disease; sometimes applied in derision to one who prescribes drugs excessively for minor ailments.

me·di·ce·phal·ic (mē′dē-se-fal′ik). Median cephalic, denoting the communicating vessel between the median and the cephalic veins of the forearm.

me·dic·i·nal (mĕ-dis′i-năl). **1.** Relating to medicine having curative properties. SYN medical (2). **2.** SYN medical (1).

me·dic·i·nal scar·let red. SYN scarlet red.

med·i·cine (med′i-sin). **1.** A drug. **2.** The art of preventing or curing disease; the science concerned with disease in all its relations. **3.** The study and treatment of general diseases or those affecting the internal parts of the body, especially those not usually requiring surgical intervention. [L. *medicina*, fr. *medicus*, physician (see medicus)]

adolescent m., the branch of medicine concerned with the treatment of youth in the approximate age range of 13 to 21 years. SYN hebiatrics.

aerospace m., a branch of m. combining the areas of concern of both aviation and space m.

alternative m., a term referring to a heterogeneous group of hygienic, diagnostic, and therapeutic philosophies and practices whose theoretical bases and techniques diverge from those of modern scientific m. Some of these differ from traditional m. only in preferring natural hygienic and therapeutic methods to drug treatment and surgery; some are supernatural, magical, or cultist, with roots in ancient or modern philosophical or religious systems; some are based on naive, false, or inconsistent notions of anatomy, physiology, psychology, pathology, and pharmacology; and some are fraudulent schemes designed to exploit unsophisticated health care consumers and those whose perceived health needs have not been met by scientific m. Alternative health practices have been imported into some parts of the U.S. by migrant populations, particularly Asians and Hispanics. Many branches of alternative m. have in common a holistic view of human health, emphasizing integration of body, mind, and spirit. All have failed to gain acceptance as part of mainstream m. because they lack both a plausible scientific basis and evidence of efficacy. SYN complementary m., holistic m. (2).

> Americans make more visits annually to alternative medicine (AM) practitioners than to primary care physicians, and the total cost of AM in this country exceeds $21 billion a year. Three-fifths of adults queried have made use of AM within the past year, but only 5% rely on it exclusively. AM appeals particularly to people of advanced education, those who believe strongly in the role of the mind in health and disease, and those with an interest in esoteric forms of spirituality and personal growth psychology. Users of AM tend to be in poorer general health than others and to have certain chronic conditions (including anxiety, depression, headache, and backache), but dissatisfaction with conventional medicine appears to be less important in their choice than a preference for a healing system that is congruent with their personal beliefs and values. Practitioners of some forms of AM are overtly hostile to traditional medicine and habitually impugn the competence and integrity of legitimate health practitioners. On the other hand, alternative methods such as acupuncture and hypnosis are employed by some physicians, particularly those espousing a holistic view of medical practice. Some insurance plans provide coverage for certain alternative therapies, such as acupuncture, biofeedback, and massage therapy. Although the use of AM may benefit some people by providing hope and needed emotional support, exerting placebo effects, or relieving symptoms through mechanisms not yet understood, it prevents many from receiving appropriate diagnosis and treatment. Moreover, alternative therapies can interact adversely with more orthodox forms of treatment, and some are inherently dangerous to health. In 1992, the U.S. Congress established the Office of Alternative Medicine (OAM) within the Office of the Director, National Institutes of Health to facilitate the full scientific evaluation of alternative therapies, to establish a clearinghouse for the exchange of information, and to support research training in topics related to AM that are not typically included in the training curriculum of mainstream health professionals. In 1998 OAM was renamed the National Center for Complementary and Alternative Medicine (NCCAM) and accorded a $50 million annual budget. Philosophies or methods of alternative diagnosis or treatment that are popular in the U.S. include acupressure, acupuncture, aromatherapy, biofeedback, chelation therapy, chiropractic, Christian Science, herbal medicine, homeopathy, hydrotherapy, hypnotherapy, iridology, macrobiotics, massage therapy, meditation, megavitamin therapy, moxibustion, naturopathy, osteopathy, relaxation techniques, rolfing, shiatsu, tai chi, and yoga.

aviation m., the study and practice of m. as it applies to physiologic problems peculiar to aviation. SYN aeromedicine.

behavioral m., an interdisciplinary field concerned with the development and integration of behavioral and biomedical science knowledge and techniques relevant to health and illness, and to its application to prevention, diagnosis, treatment, and rehabilitation.

clinical m., the study and practice of m. in relation to the care of patients; the art of m. as distinguished from laboratory science.

community m., the study of health and disease in a defined community; the practice of m. in such a setting.

comparative m., a field of study concentrating on similarities and differences between veterinary m. and human m.

complementary m., SYN alternative m.

defensive m., diagnostic or therapeutic measures conducted primarily as a safeguard against possible subsequent malpractice liability.

desmoteric m., the branch of medical practice that deals with health problems occurring among prison inmates. [G. *desmōtērion*, prison, fr. *deo*, to bind, + -ic]

electrodiagnostic m., the specific area of medical practice in which specially trained physicians use information from the clinical history and physical examination, along with the scientific method of recording and analyzing biologic electrical potentials, to diagnose and treat neuromuscular disorders.

evidence-based m., the process of applying relevant information derived from peer-reviewed medical literature to address a specific clinical problem; the application of simple rules of science and common sense to determine the validity of the information; and the application of the information to the clinical problem. SEE

me

ALSO Cochrane *collaboration*, clinical practice *guidelines*, under *guideline*.

experimental m., the scientific investigation of medical problems by experimentation upon animals or by clinical research.

family m., the medical specialty concerned with providing continuous, comprehensive care to all age groups, from first patient contact to terminal care, with special emphasis on care of the family as a unit.

folk m., treatment of ailments outside of organized medicine by remedies and simple measures based upon experience and knowledge handed on from generation to generation.

forensic m., (1) the relation and application of medical facts to legal matters; (2) the law in its bearing on the practice of medicine. SYN legal m., medical jurisprudence.

geriatric m., a specialty of m. that is concerned with the disease and health problems of older people, usually those over 65 years of age. Considered a subspecialty of internal medicine.

holistic m., (1) an approach to medical care that emphasizes the study of all aspects of a person's health, especially that a person should be considered as a unit, including psychological as well as social and economic influences on health status. (2) SYN alternative m.

hyperbaric m., the medicinal use of high barometric pressure, usually in specially constructed chambers, to increase oxygen content of blood and tissues.

internal m. (IM), the branch of m. concerned with nonsurgical diseases in adults, but not including diseases limited to the skin or to the nervous system.

legal m., SYN forensic m.

maternal-fetal m., a subspecialty of obstetrics/gynecology devoted to the study of the obstetrical, medical, and surgical complications of pregnancy. SYN fetology.

military m., the practice of m. as applied to the special circumstances associated with military life.

neonatal m., SYN neonatology.

nuclear m., the clinical discipline concerned with the diagnostic and therapeutic uses of radionuclides, including sealed radiation sources.

osteopathic m., SYN osteopathy (2).

patent m., a m., usually originally patented, advertised to the public.

perinatal m., SYN perinatology.

physical m., the study and treatment of disease mainly by mechanical and other physical methods. SYN physiatry.

podiatric m., SYN podiatry.

preventive m., the branch of medical science concerned with the prevention of disease and with promotion of physical and mental health, through study of the etiology and epidemiology of disease processes.

proprietary m., a medicinal compound the formula and mode of manufacture of which are the property of the maker.

psychosomatic m., the study and treatment of diseases, disorders, or abnormal states in which psychological processes resulting in physiological reactions are believed to play a prominent role.

quack m., a compound advertised falsely as curative of a certain disease or diseases. Cf. nostrum.

social m., a specialized field of medical knowledge concentrating on the social, cultural and economic impact of medical phenomena.

socialized m., the organization and control of medical practice by a government agency, the practitioners being employed by the organization from which they receive standardized compensation for their services, and to which the public contributes usually in the form of taxation rather than fee-for-service.

space m., the field of m. concerned with physiologic diseases or disturbances resulting from the unique conditions of space travel.

sports m., a field of m. that uses a holistic, comprehensive, and multidisciplinary approach to health care for those engaged in a sporting or recreational activity.

tropical m., the branch of m. concerned with diseases, mainly of parasitic origin, in areas having a tropical climate.

veterinary m., the field concerned with the diseases and health of all animal species other than humans.

△**medico-.** Medical. Cf. iatro-. [L. *medicus,* physician]

med·i·co·bi·o·log·ic, med·i·co·bi·o·log·i·cal (med'i-kō-bī-ō-loj' ik, -loj'i-kăl). Pertaining to the biologic aspects of medicine.

med·i·co·chi·rur·gi·cal (med'i-kō-kī-rŭr'ji-kăl). Relating to both medicine and surgery, or to both physicians and surgeons. [medico- G. *cheirourgia,* surgery]

med·i·co·le·gal (med'i-kō-lē'găl). Relating to both medicine and the law. SEE ALSO forensic *medicine.* [medico- + L. *legalis,* legal]

med·i·co·me·chan·i·cal (med'i-kō-mě-kan'i-kăl). Relating to both medicinal and mechanical measures in therapeutics.

med·i·co·phys·i·cal (med'i-kō-fiz'i-kăl). Relating to disease and the condition of the body in general; e.g., a m. examination, in which a person is examined in order to determine the presence or absence of disease as well as to note the general physical condition.

med·i·co·psy·chol·o·gy (med'i-kō-sī-kol'ō-jē). Psychology in its relation to medicine. SEE medical *psychology,* health *psychology.*

△**medio-, medi-.** Middle, median. [L. *medius*]

me·di·o·car·pal (mē'dē-ō-kar'păl). SYN midcarpal.

me·di·oc·cip·i·tal (mē'dē-ok-sip'i-tăl). SYN midoccipital.

me·di·o·dens (mē'dē-ō-dens). A supernumerary tooth located between the two maxillary central incisors. [medio- + L. *dens,* tooth]

me·di·o·dor·sal (mē'dē-ō-dōr'săl). Relating to the median plane and the dorsal plane.

me·di·o·lat·er·al (mē'dē-ō-lat'er-ăl). Relating to the median plane and a side.

me·di·o·ne·cro·sis (mē'dē-ō-ne-krō'sis). Necrosis of a tunica media.

m. of the aorta, SYN cystic medial *necrosis.*

m. aor'tae idiopath'ica cys'tica, SYN cystic medial *necrosis.*

me·di·o·tar·sal (mē'dē-ō-tar'săl). SYN midtarsal.

me·di·o·tru·sion (mē'dē-ō-troo'zhŭn). A thrusting of the mandibular condyle toward the midline during movement of the mandible. [medio- + L. *trudo,* pp. *trusus,* to thrust]

me·di·o·type (mē'dē-ō-tīp). SYN mesomorph.

me·di·sect (mē'di-sekt). To incise in the median line. [L. *medius,* middle, + *seco,* pp. *sectus,* to cut]

me·di·um, pl. **me·dia** (mē'dē-ŭm, -ă). **1.** A means; that through which an action is performed. **2.** A substance through which impulses or impressions are transmitted. **3.** SYN culture m. **4.** The liquid holding a substance in solution or suspension. **5.** Any of the substances in which a chromatographic or electrophoretic separation is effected. [L. neuter of *medius,* middle]

Acanthamoeba **m.,** nonnutrient agar plates with an *E. coli* overlay used to detect the presence of *Acanthamoeba* or *Naegleria* from tissue or soil samples.

Balamuth aqueous egg yolk infusion m., used to detect the presence of intestinal amebae, primarily *Entamoeba histolytica.*

Boeck and Drbohlav Locke-egg-serum m., m. of whole eggs, human serum, and rice powder used to detect the presence of intestinal amebae, primarily *Entamoeba histolytica.*

clearing m., a m. used in histology for making specimens translucent or transparent.

complete m., a m. for an in vitro culture that contains the supplemental nutrients as well as the basic nutrients to support fastidious or mutant growth requirements.

contrast m., any internally administered substance that has a different opacity from soft tissue on radiography or computed tomography; includes barium, used to opacify parts of the gastrointestinal tract; water-soluble iodinated compounds, used to opacify blood vessels or the genitourinary tract; may refer to air occurring naturally or introduced into the body; also, paramagnetic substances used in magnetic resonance imaging. SYN contrast agent, contrast material.

culture m., a substance, either solid or liquid, used for the cultivation, isolation, identification, or storage of microorganisms. SYN growth m., medium (3), nutrient m.

Czapek-Dox m., SYN Czapek solution *agar.*

Diamond TYM m., m. of trypticase, yeast extract, maltose, and serum used to detect the presence of *Trichomonas vaginalis.*

dispersion m., SYN external *phase.*

Dorset culture egg m., a m. for cultivating *Mycobacterium tuberculosis;* it consists of the whites and yolks of four fresh eggs and a solution of sodium chloride.

Eagle basal m., a solution of various salts containing 13 naturally occurring amino acids, several vitamins, two antibiotics, and phenol red; used as a tissue culture medium.

Eagle minimum essential m. (MEM), a tissue culture m. similar to Eagle basal medium but with different amounts and a few exclusions (e.g., antibiotics and phenol red).

Endo m., SYN Endo *agar.*

external m., SYN external *phase.*

growth m., SYN culture m.

high osmolar contrast m. (HOCM), SYN high osmolar contrast *agent.*

Lash casein hydrolysate-serum m., used to detect the presence of *Trichomonas vaginalis.*

Loeffler blood culture m., a culture m. consisting of beef blood serum, sheep blood serum, and beef bouillon containing peptone, glucose, and sodium chloride; used for the isolation of *Corynebacterium diphtheriae.*

Lowenstein-Jensen m., SYN Lowenstein-Jensen culture m.

Lowenstein-Jensen culture m., primary mycobacterial recovery media composed of fresh whole eggs, defined salts, glycerol, potato flour, and malachite green (as an inhibitory agent). SYN Lowenstein-Jensen m.

low osmolar contrast m. (LOCM), SYN low osmolar contrast *agent.*

McCarey-Kaufmann media, a culture solution used for storage of enucleated eyes for corneal *transplantation.*

motility test m., a culture m. with a concentration of agar that produces a less solid consistency than usual and allows motile organisms to grow away from the line of inoculation; used to differentiate species of bacteria.

mounting m., a substance, usually resinous, used for mounting a cover glass on histologic suspensions.

Mueller-Hinton m., an agar-based m. composed of beef infusion, casamino acids, and starch; the recommended medium for antibacterial susceptibility tests for most common aerobic and facultatively anaerobic bacteria.

NNN m., agar slant overlaid with defibrinated rabbit blood used to detect the presence of leishmania or *Trypanosoma cruzi.*

nutrient m., SYN culture m.

passive m., a m. that produces no change in the specimens placed in it.

selective m., a culture m. containing ingredients that inhibit growth of contaminants or microorganisms other than that desired.

separating m., (1) any coating which serves to prevent one surface from adhering to another; **(2)** in dentistry, a material usually applied to a cast to facilitate separation from the resin denture base after curing; a coating on impressions to facilitate removal of the cast.

Simmons citrate m., a diagnostic m. used in the differentiation of species of Enterobacteriaceae, based on their ability to utilize sodium citrate as the sole source of carbon.

support m., the material in which separation takes place, as in separation of components in electrophoresis.

Thayer-Martin m., SYN Thayer-Martin *agar.*

transport m., a m. for transporting clinical specimens to the laboratory for examination.

TY1-S-33 m., m. of biosate peptone, dextrose, vitamins, and bovine serum used to detect the presence of *Entamoeba histolytica.*

TYSGM-9 m., m. of gastric mucin, nutrient broth, bovine serum, and rice starch used to detect the presence of *Entamoeba histolytica.*

me·di·um-chain ac·yl-CoA de·hy·dro·gen·ase (MCAD). SEE *acyl-CoA* dehydrogenase (NADPH).

me·di·us (mē′dē-ŭs). SYN middle. [L.]

MEDLARS Abbreviation for Medical Literature Analysis and Retrieval System, a computerized index system of the U.S. National Library of Medicine.

MEDLINE. [MEDLARS-on-line] A computer-based telephone and internet linkage to MEDLARS for rapid provision of medical bibliographies.

med·pha·lan (med′fă-lan). An antineoplastic agent. SYN medfalan.

med·ro·ges·tone (med-rō-jes′tōn). An oral progestin.

me·drox·y·pro·ges·ter·one ac·e·tate (med-rok′sē-prō-jes′ter-ōn). A progestational agent that is active orally as well as parenterally, and more potent than progesterone; used to control uterine bleeding and, in combination with ethynyl estradiol, as an oral contraceptive.

med·ryl·a·mine (med-ril′ă-mēn). An H₁ antihistaminic.

med·ry·sone (med′ri-sōn). A glucocorticoid used topically as an anti-inflammatory agent, usually on the eye.

me·dul·la, pl. **me·dul·lae** (me-dool′ă, me-dool′ē) [TA]. Any soft marrow-like structure, especially in the center of a part. SEE ALSO m. oblongata. SYN substantia medullaris (1). [L. marrow, fr. *medius,* middle]

m. of adrenal gland, ✩official alternate term for m. of suprarenal gland.

m. glan′dulae suprarena′lis [TA], SYN m. of suprarenal gland.

m. of hair shaft, the central axis of some hairs, containing a column of large vacuolated and keratinized cells; the medullary portion is surrounded by the cortex.

m. of kidney, SYN renal m.

m. of lymph node [TA], the central portion of a node consisting of cordlike masses of lymphocytes, plasma cells, and macrophages in a stroma of reticular fibers separated by lymph sinuses; it reaches the surface of the node at the hilum. SYN m. nodi lymphoidei [TA].

m. no′di lymphoidei [TA], SYN m. of lymph node.

m. oblonga′ta [TA], the most caudal subdivision of the brainstem, immediately continuous with the spinal cord, extending from the lower border of the decussation of the pyramid to the pons; its ventral surface resembles that of the spinal cord except for the bilateral prominence of the inferior olive; the dorsal surface of its upper half forms part of the floor of the fourth ventricle. Motor nuclei of the m. oblongata include the hypoglossal nucleus, the dorsal motor nucleus, inferior salivatory nucleus, and the nucleus ambiguus; sensory nuclei include the nuclei of the posterior column (gracile and cuneate), the cochlear and vestibular nuclei, the mid and caudal portions of the spinal trigeminal nucleus, and the nucleus of the solitary tract. SEE ALSO medulla. SYN myelencephalon [TA], oblongata.

m. os′sium [TA], SYN bone *marrow.*

m. os′sium fla′va [TA], SYN yellow bone *marrow.*

m. os′sium ru′bra [TA], SYN red bone *marrow.*

renal m. [TA], the inner, darker portion of the kidney parenchyma consisting of the renal pyramids. SYN m. renalis [TA], m. of kidney.

m. rena′lis [TA], SYN renal m.

m. spina′lis [TA], SYN spinal *cord.*

suprarenal m., SYN m. of suprarenal gland.

m. of suprarenal gland [TA], it is composed principally of anastomosing cords of cells in the core of the gland; the cells display a chromaffin reaction because of the presence of epinephrine and norepinephrine in their granules. SYN m. glandulae suprarenalis [TA], m. of adrenal gland✩, suprarenal m.

me·dul·lar (med-ool′ăr). SYN medullary.

med·ul·lary (med′ul-er-ē, med′oo-lār-ē). Relating to the medulla or marrow. SYN medullar.

med·ul·lat·ed (med′ŭ-lā-ted, med′oo-). **1.** Having a medulla or medullary substance. **2.** SYN myelinated.

me

med·ul·la·tion (med'ŭ-lā'shŭn, med'oo-). **1.** Acquiring, or the act of formation of, marrow or medulla. **2.** SYN myelination.

med·ul·lec·to·my (med-oo-lek'tō-mē, med-ū-). Excision of any medullary substance. [medulla + G. *ektomē*, excision]

med·ul·li·za·tion (med'ŭ-li-zā'shŭn, med'ū-). Enlargement of the medullary spaces in the treatment of various skeletal disorders.

△**medullo-.** Medulla. Cf. myel-. [L. *medulla*]

me·dul·lo·ar·thri·tis (med-ŭ-lō-ar-thrī'tis). Inflammation of the cancellous articular extremity of a long bone.

🖬**me·dul·lo·blas·to·ma** (med'ŭ-lō-blas-tō'mă). A tumor consisting of neoplastic cells that resemble the undifferentiated cells of the primitive medullary tube; m.'s are usually located in the vermis of the cerebellum, and may be implanted discretely or coalescently on the surfaces of the cerebellum, brainstem, and spinal cord; they comprise approximately 3% of all intracranial neoplasms, and occur most frequently in children; the neoplastic cells are compactly arranged, rounded or ovoid, with hyperchromatic nuclei and relatively scant cytoplasm, and lie in small and poorly defined groups, or, occasionally, in a pseudorosette pattern (Homer-Wright rosette). A type of primitive neuroectodermal tumor.

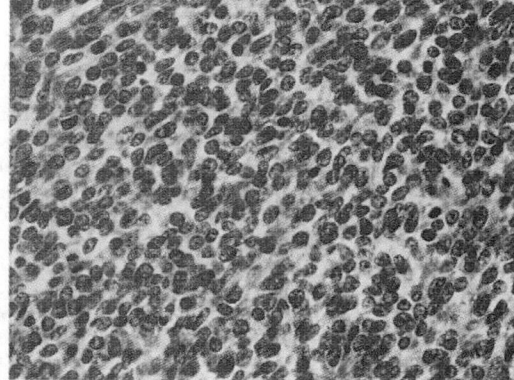

medulloblastoma: note diffuse proliferation of undifferentiated cells

desmoplastic m., subtype of m. with a biphasic pattern of compact sheets of undifferentiated cells alternating with islands of more loosely cohesive cells, generally occurs in adolescence and young adults and has a better prognosis than the usual m.

melanotic m., a rare variant of m. in which melanin-pigmented cells are present.

me·dul·lo·cell (med'ŭ-lō-sel, med'oo-). SYN myelocyte (2).

me·dul·lo·ep·i·the·li·o·ma (me'dŭ-lō-ep'ĭ-thē-lē-ō'mă). A rare, primitive, rapidly growing intracranial neoplasm thought to originate from the cells of the embryonic medullary canal and hence included with ependymoblastomas by some neuropathologists; ganglion cells and astrocyte maturation have also been reported. Tumors that occur in the ciliary body are referred to as embryonal m.'s. [medullo- + epithelium + -*oma*, tumor]

adult m., SYN malignant ciliary *epithelioma*.

embryonal m., an epitheliomatous tumor of the nonpigmented layer of the ciliary epithelium. SYN embryonal tumor of ciliary body.

me·dul·lo·my·o·blas·to·ma (med'ŭ-lō-mī'ō-blas-tō'mă). A rare histologic variant of medulloblastoma with scattered smooth and striated muscle cells incorporated into the neoplasm.

Meeh, K., 19th century German physiologist. SEE M. *formula;* M.-Dubois *formula.*

Mees, R.A., 20th century Dutch physician. SEE M. *lines,* under *line, stripes,* under *stripe.*

Meesman, A., German ophthalmologist, 1888–1969. SEE M. *dystrophy.*

mef·e·nam·ic ac·id (me-fĕ-nam'ik). An aspirinlike analgesic with antiinflammatory properties.

me·fen·o·rex hy·dro·chlo·ride (me-fen'ŏ-reks). A sympathomimetic drug with anorexic activity.

me·fex·a·mide (mĕ-fek'ă-mīd). An antidepressant.

mef·lo·quine (mef'lō-kwin). An antimalarial resembling quinine and chloroquine.

MEG Abbreviation for magnetoencephalogram.

△**mega-. 1.** Combining form meaning large, oversize; opposite of micro-. SEE ALSO macro-, megalo-. **2 (M).** Prefix used in the SI and metric system to signify multiples of one million (10^6). [G. *megas,* big]

meg·a·bac·te·ri·um (meg'ă-bak-tēr'ē-ŭm). A bacterium of unusually large size. SYN macrobacterium.

meg·a·ca·ly·co·sis (meg'ă-kal-ĭ-kō-sis). **1.** Congenital, nonobstructive enlargement of renal calices. **2.** Excessively large number of calices. [mega- + G. *kalyx,* cup of a flower, + -*osis,* condition]

meg·a·car·dia (meg-ă-kar'dē-ă). SYN cardiomegaly.

meg·a·car·y·o·blast (meg-ă-kar'ē-ō-blast). SYN megakaryoblast.

meg·a·car·y·o·cyte (meg-ă-kar'ē-ō-sīt). SYN megakaryocyte.

meg·a·ce·pha·lia (meg-ă-se-fā'lē-ă). SYN megacephaly.

meg·a·ce·phal·ic (meg'ă-se-fal'ik). Relating to or characterized by megacephaly. SYN macrocephalic, macrocephalous, megacephalous.

meg·a·ceph·a·lous (meg-ă-sef'ă-lŭs). SYN megacephalic.

meg·a·ceph·a·ly (meg-ă-sef'ă-lē). A condition, either congenital or acquired, in which the head is abnormally large; usually applied to an adult skull with a capacity of over 1450 ml. SYN leontiasis ossea, macrocephaly, macrocephalia, megacephalia, megalocephaly, megalocephalia, Virchow disease. [mega- + G. *kephalē,* head]

meg·a·cins (meg'ă-sinz). Antibacterial proteins produced by strains of *Bacillus megaterium.*

meg·a·coc·cus, pl. **meg·a·coc·ci** (meg'ă-kok'ŭs, -kok'sī). A coccus of unusually large size. SYN macrococcus.

meg·a·co·lon (meg'ă-kō'lon). A condition of extreme dilation of the colon. SYN giant colon.

acquired m., m. occurring on the basis of an acquired disease; occurs in inflammatory bowel disease (toxic m.) and Chagas *disease* (South American *trypanosomiasis*).

congenital m., m. congen'itum, congenital dilation and hypertrophy of the colon due to absence (aganglionosis) or marked reduction (hypoganglionosis) in the number of ganglion cells of the myenteric plexus of the rectum and a varying but continuous length of gut above the rectum; also seen in dogs. SYN Hirschsprung disease.

idiopathic m., an acquired m., found in children and adults, without distal obstruction or absence of ganglion cells; the muscle of the dilated colon is thin.

toxic m., acute nonobstructive dilation of the colon, seen in fulminating ulcerative colitis and Crohn disease.

meg·a·cy·cle (meg'ă-sī-kl). One million cycles per second.

meg·a·cys·tis (meg'ă-sis-tis). Pathologically large bladder in children. SYN megalocystis. [mega- + *kystis,* bladder]

meg·a·dac·ty·ly, meg·a·dac·tyl·ia, meg·a·dac·tyl·ism (meg-ă-dak'ti-lē, -dak-til'ē-ă -dak'til-izm). Condition characterized by enlargement of one or more digits (fingers or toes). SYN dactylomegaly, macrodactylia, macrodactylism, macrodactyly, megalodactylia, megalodactylism, megalodactyly. [mega- + G. *daktylos,* digit]

meg·a·dol·i·cho·co·lon (meg'ă-dol'i-kō-kō'lon). Excessive length and dilation of the colon. [mega- + G. *dolichos,* long, + *kōlon,* colon]

meg·a·dont (meg'ă-dont). SYN macrodont. [mega- + G. *odous (odont-),* tooth]

meg·a·don·tism (meg-ă-don'tizm). SYN macrodontia.

meg·a·dyne (meg'ă-dīn). One million dynes.

meg·a·e·soph·a·gus (meg'ă-ē-sof'ă-gŭs, meg'ă-e-sof'). Great enlargement of the lower portion of the esophagus, as seen in patients with achalasia and Chagas disease.

meg·a·ga·mete (meg-ă-gam'ēt). SYN macrogamete.

meg·a·gna·thia (meg-ă-nā'thē-ă). SYN macrognathia.

meg·a·hertz (MHz) (meg′ă-hertz). One million hertz.

▣**meg·a·kar·y·o·blast** (meg-ă-kar′ē-ō-blast). The precursor of a megakaryocyte. SYN megacaryoblast.

meg·a·kar·y·o·cyte (meg-ă-kar′ē-ō-sīt). A large cell (as much as 100 μm in diameter) with a polyploid nucleus that is usually multilobed; m.'s are normally present in bone marrow, not in the circulating blood, and give rise to blood platelets. SYN megacaryocyte, megalokaryocyte, thromboblast. [mega- + G. *karyon*, nut (nucleus), + *kytos*, hollow vessel (cell)]

△**megal-.** SEE megalo-.

meg·a·lec·i·thal (meg-ă-les′i-thăl). Denoting an egg rich in yolk, as in bony fishes, reptiles, and birds. [mega- + G. *lekithos*, yolk]

meg·al·gia (meg-al′jē-ă). Very severe pain. [mega- + G. *algos*, pain]

△**megalo-, megal-.** Large; opposite of micro-. SEE ALSO macro-, mega-. [G. *megas* (*megal-*)]

meg·a·lo·blast (meg′ă-lō-blast). A large, nucleated, embryonic type of cell that is a precursor of erythrocytes in an abnormal erythropoietic process observed in pernicious anemia; a m.'s four stages of development are as follows: 1) promegaloblast, 2) basophilic m., 3) polychromatic m., 4) orthochromatic m. SEE ALSO erythroblast. [megalo- + G. *blastos*, + germ, sprout]

meg·a·lo·car·dia (meg′ă-lō-kar′dē-ă). SYN cardiomegaly. [megalo- + G. *kardia*, heart]

meg·a·lo·ceph·a·ly, meg·a·lo·ce·pha·lia (meg′ă-lō-sef′ă-lē, -sĕ-fā′lē-ă). SYN megacephaly.

meg·a·lo·chei·ria, meg·a·lo·chi·ria (meg′ă-lō-kī′rē-ă). SYN macrocheiria. [megalo- + G. *cheir*, hand]

meg·a·lo·cor·nea (meg′ă-lō-kōr′nē-ă). SYN keratoglobus.

meg·a·lo·cys·tis (meg′ă-lō-sis′tis). SYN megacystis. [megalo- + G. *kystis*, bladder]

meg·a·lo·cyte (meg′ă-lō-sīt). A large (10–20 μm) nonnucleated red blood cell. [megalo- + G. *kytos*, cell]

meg·a·lo·cy·the·mia (meg′ă-lō-sī-thē′mē-ă). SYN macrocythemia.

meg·a·lo·cy·to·sis (meg′ă-lō-sī-tō′sis). SYN macrocythemia.

meg·a·lo·dac·tyl·ia, meg·a·lo·dac·tyl·ism, meg·a·lo·dac·ty·-ly (meg′ă-lō-dak-til′ē-ă, -dak′til-izm, -dak′ti-lē). SYN megadactyly.

meg·a·lo·dont (meg′ă-lō-dont). SYN macrodont.

meg·a·lo·don·tia (meg′ă-lō-don′shē-ă). SYN macrodontia.

meg·a·lo·en·ce·phal·ic (meg′ă-lō-en′sĕ-fal′ik). Denoting an abnormally large brain.

meg·a·lo·en·ceph·a·lon (meg′ă-lō-en-sef′ă-lon). An abnormally large brain. SYN macroencephalon. [megalo- + G. *enkephalos*, brain]

meg·a·lo·en·ceph·a·ly (meg′ă-lō-en-sef′ă-lē). Abnormal largeness of the brain. [megalo- + G. *enkephalon*, brain]

meg·a·lo·en·ter·on (meg′ă-lō-en′ter-on). Abnormal largeness of the intestine. SYN enteromegaly, enteromegalia. [megalo- + G. *enteron*, intestine]

meg·a·lo·gas·tria (meg′ă-lō-gas′trē-ă). Abnormally large size of the stomach. SYN macrogastria. [megalo- + G. *gastēr*, stomach]

meg·a·lo·glos·sia (meg′ă-lō-glos′sē-ă). SYN macroglossia. [megalo- + G. *glōssa*, tongue]

meg·a·lo·graph·ia (meg′ă-lō-graf′ē-ă). SYN macrography.

meg·a·lo·kar·y·o·cyte (meg′ă-lō-kar′ē-ō-sīt). SYN megakaryocyte.

meg·a·lo·ma·nia (meg′ă-lō-mā′nē-ă). **1.** A type of delusion in which the individual considers himself or herself possessed of greatness. He/she believes him/herself to be Christ, God, Napoleon, etc., or everyone and everything, including a lawyer, physician, clergyman, merchant, prince, ace athlete in all divisions of sport, etc. **2.** Morbid verbalized overevaluation of oneself or of some aspect of oneself. [megalo- + G. *mania*, frenzy]

meg·a·lo·ma·ni·ac (meg′ă-lō-mā′nē-ak). A person exhibiting megalomania.

meg·a·lo·me·lia (meg′ă-lō-mē′lē-ă). SYN macromelia.

meg·a·loph·thal·mos (meg′ă-lof-thal′mŭs). Congenital large globe. SYN macrophthalmia, megophthalmus. [megalo- + G. *ophthalmos*, eye]

anterior m., SYN keratoglobus.

meg·a·lo·po·dia (meg′ă-lō-pō′dē-ă). SYN macropodia. [megalo- + G. *pous*, foot]

meg·a·lo·splanch·nic (meg′ă-lō-splangk′nik). Having abnormally large viscera. SYN macrosplanchnic. [megalo- + G. *splanchnon*, viscus]

meg·a·lo·sple·nia (meg′ă-lō-splē′nē-ă). SYN splenomegaly.

meg·a·lo·spore (meg′ă-lō-spōr). SYN macrospore.

meg·a·lo·syn·dac·ty·ly, meg·a·lo·syn·dac·tyl·ia (meg′ă-lō-sin-dak′ti-lē, -dak-til′ē-ă). Condition of webbed or fused fingers or toes of large size. [megalo- + G. *syn*, together, + *daktylos*, finger]

meg·a·lo·u·re·ter (meg′ă-lō-ū-rē′ter). SYN ureterectasia. SYN megaureter.

meg·a·lo·u·re·thra (meg′ă-lō-ū-rē′thră). Congenital dilation of the urethra.

△**-megaly.** Large. [G. *megas* (*megal-*)]

meg·a·mer·o·zo·ite (meg′ă-mer-ō-zō′ĭt). SYN macromerozoite.

meg·a·nu·cle·us (meg-ă-noo′klē-ŭs). SYN macronucleus (1).

megapoietin (meg′ă-poy′ĕ-tin). SYN thrombopoietin. [mega- + G. *poiētēs*, maker, + -in]

meg·a·pro·so·pia (meg′ă-prō-sō′pē-ă). SYN macroprosopia. [mega- + G. *prosōpon*, face]

meg·a·pros·o·pous (meg-ă-pros′ō-pŭs). SYN macroprosopous.

meg·a·rec·tum (meg-ă-rek′tŭm). Extreme dilation of the rectum.

meg·a·seme (meg′ă-sēm). Denoting an orbital aperture with an index above 89. [mega- + G. *sēma*, sign]

meg·a·sig·moid (meg-ă-sig′moyd). SYN macrosigmoid.

meg·a·so·mia (meg-ă-sō′mē-ă). SYN macrosomia.

meg·a·spore (meg′ă-spōr). SYN macrospore.

meg·a·throm·bo·cyte (meg-ă-throm′bō-sīt). A large blood platelet, especially a young one recently released from the bone marrow. [mega- + G. *thrombos*, clot, + *kytos*, cell]

meg·a·u·re·ter (meg′ă-ū-rē′ter). SYN megaloureter.

primary m., independent ureteral dilation; may be nonobstructive or related to congenital distal ureteral obstruction.

secondary m., hydroureter secondary to vesicoureteral reflux or distal obstruction.

meg·a·volt (meg′ă-vōlt). One million volts.

meg·a·volt·age (meg′ă-vol′tij). In radiation therapy, a term for voltage above one million volts.

me·ges·trol ac·e·tate (me-jes′trōl). A synthetic progestin with progestational effects similar to those of progesterone; current uses include palliation in breast cancer and as an appetite stimulant in advanced malignancy.

meg·lit·in·ides (meg-lit′in-īdz). A class of oral glucose-lowering drugs that act by closing ATP-dependent potassium channels in pancreatic beta cells, thus causing calcium channel opening and subsequent insulin release.

meg·lu·mine (meg′loo-mēn). USAN-approved contraction for *N*-methylglucamine.

m. acetrizoate, a radiographic contrast medium. SEE acetrizoate sodium.

m. diatrizoate, a water-soluble organic iodine compound formerly used for excretory urography, for contrast visualization of the cardiovascular system, and orally for opacification of the gastrointestinal tract. SYN methylglucamine diatrizoate.

m. iothalamate, *N*-methylglucamine salt of iothalamic acid (60% solution); a diagnostic radiopaque medium for intravascular use in angiography and urography.

meg·ohm (meg′ōm). One million ohms.

meg·oph·thal·mus (meg-of-thal′mŭs). SYN megalophthalmos.

meg·ox·y·cyte (meg-oks′ē-sīt). SYN megoxyphil.

meg·ox·y·phil, meg·ox·y·phile (meg-oks′ē-fil, fīl). An eosinophilic leukocyte containing coarse granules. SYN megoxycyte. [mega- + G. *oxys*, acid, + *phileō*, to like]

me·grim (mē′grim). Obsolete term for migraine.

me

Meibom (Meibomius), Hendrik (Heinrich), German anatomist, 1638–1700. SEE meibomian *cyst*, meibomian *glands*, under *gland*, meibomian *sty*.

mei·bo·mi·an (mī-bō'mē-an). Attributed to or described by Meibom.

mei·bo·mi·tis, mei·bo·mi·a·ni·tis (mī'bō-mī'tis, mī-bō'mē-ă-nī'tis). Inflammation of the meibomian glands.

Meier, Georg, German serologist, *1875. SEE Porges-M. *test*.

Meige, Henri, French physician, 1866–1940. SEE M. *disease*.

Meigs, Joe V., U.S. gynecologist, 1892–1963. SEE M. *syndrome*.

Meinicke, Ernst, German physician, 1878–1945. SEE M. *test*.

△**meio-.** For words beginning thus and not found here, see mio-.

🔲**mei·o·sis** (mī-ō'sis). A special process of cell division comprising two nuclear divisions in rapid succession that result in four gametocytes, each containing half the number of chromosomes found in somatic cells. SYN meiotic division. [G. *meiōsis*, a lessening]

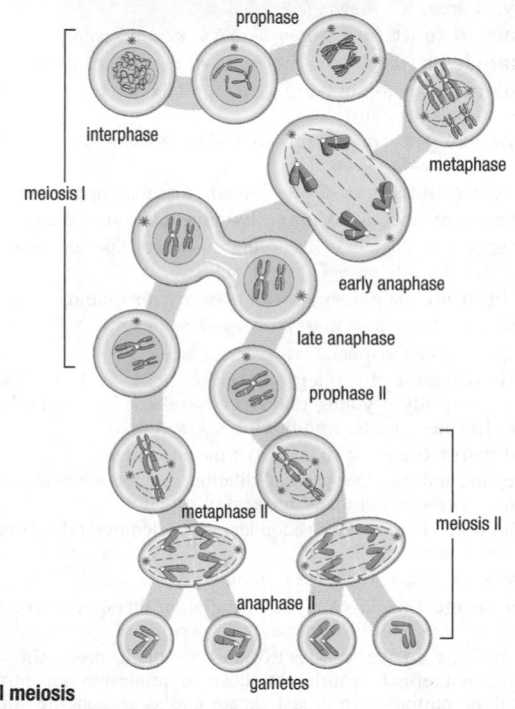

prophase
interphase
meiosis I
metaphase
early anaphase
late anaphase
prophase II
metaphase II
meiosis II
anaphase II
gametes
cell meiosis

mei·ot·ic (mī-ot'ik). Pertaining to meiosis.

Meissel. SEE Wachstein-Meissel *stain* for calcium-magnesium-ATPase.

Meissner, Georg, German histologist, 1829–1905. SEE M. *corpuscle, plexus*.

mel. **1.** SYN honey. **2.** Unit of pitch; a pitch of 1000 mels results from a simple tone of frequency 1000 Hz at 40 dB above the normal threshold of audibility.

△**mel-, melo-.** **1.** Limb. [G. *melos*] **2.** A cheek. [G. *mēlon*] **3.** Honey, sugar. SEE ALSO meli-. [L. *mel, mellis,* G. *meli, melitos*] **4.** Sheep. [G. *mēlon*]

me·lag·ra (mě-lag'ră). Rheumatic or myalgic pains in the arms or legs. [G. *melos,* limb, + *agra,* seizure]

me·lal·gia (mě-lal'jē-ă). Pain in a limb; specifically, burning pain in the feet extending up the leg and even to the thigh. [G. *melos,* a limb, + *algos,* pain]

mel·a·mine form·al·de·hyde (mel'ă-mēn). SYN melamine *resin*.

△**melan-, melano-.** Black, extreme darkness of hue. [G. *melas*]

mel·an·cho·lia (mel-an-kō'lē-ă). **1.** A severe form of depression marked by anhedonia, insomnia, psychomotor changes, and guilt. **2.** A symptom occurring in other conditions, marked by depres-

sion of spirits and by a sluggish and painful process of thought. SYN melancholy. [melan- + G. *cholē,* bile. See humoral *doctrine*]

hypochondriacal m., m. with many associated physical complaints, often with little basis in fact.

involutional m., a depressive disorder of middle life, commonly associated with the climacteric.

mel·an·chol·ic (mel-an-kol'ik). **1.** Relating to or characteristic of melancholia. **2.** Formerly, denoting a temperament characterized by irritability and a pessimistic outlook. **3.** A person who is exhibiting melancholia.

mel·an·choly (mel'an-kol-ē). SYN melancholia.

mel·a·ne·mia (mel-ă-nē'mē-ă). The presence of dark brown, almost black, or black granules of insoluble pigment (melanin) in the circulating blood. [melan- + G. *haima,* blood]

mel·a·nif·er·ous (mel-ă-nif'er-ŭs). Containing melanin or other black pigment. [melan- (melanin) + L. *ferro,* to carry]

mel·a·nin (mel'ă-nin). Any of the dark brown to black polymers of indole-5,6-quinone and/or 5,6-dihydroxyindole 2-carboxylic acid that normally occur in the skin, hair, pigmented coat of the retina, and inconstantly in the medulla and zona reticularis of the adrenal gland. M. may be formed in vitro or biologically by oxidation of L-tyrosine or L-tryptophan, the usual mechanism being the enzymatic oxidation of L-tyrosine to 3,4-dihydroxy-L-phenylalanine (dopa) and dopaquinone by monophenol monooxygenase, and the further oxidation (probably spontaneous) of this intermediate to m. Cf. eumelanin, pheomelanin. SYN melanotic pigment. [G. *melas (melan-),* black]

artificial m., factitious m., SYN melanoid.

mel·a·nism (mel'ă-nizm). Unusually marked, diffuse, melanin pigmentation of body hair and skin (usually not affecting the iris). SEE ALSO melanosis.

△**melano-.** SEE melan-.

mel·a·no·ac·an·tho·ma (mel'ă-nō-ak-an-thō'mă). A seborrheic keratosis with melanin pigmentation associated with proliferation of intraepidermal melanocytes. [melano- + G. *akantha,* thorn, + suffix -*ōma,* tumor]

mel·a·no·am·e·lo·blas·to·ma (mel'ă-nō-am'ě-lō-blas-tō'mă). SYN melanotic neuroectodermal *tumor* of infancy. [melano- + ameloblastoma]

mel·a·no·blast (mel'ă-nō-blast). A cell derived from the neural crest; it migrates to various parts of the body early in embryonic life, and then becomes a mature melanocyte capable of forming melanin. [melano- + G. *blastos,* germ, sprout]

mel·a·no·cyte (mel'ă-nō-sīt). A pigment-producing cell located in the basal layer of the epidermis with branching processes by means of which melanosomes are transferred to epidermal cells, resulting in pigmentation of the epidermis. SYN melanodendrocyte, pigment cell of skin. [melano- + G. *kytos,* cell]

mel·a·no·cy·to·ma (mel'ă-nō-sī-tō'mă). **1.** A pigmented tumor of the uveal stroma. **2.** Usually benign melanoma of the optic disk, appearing in markedly pigmented individuals as a small deeply pigmented tumor at the edge of the disk, sometimes extending into the retina and choroid; malignant metaplasia is rare. [megalo- + cyto- + G. -*oma;* tumor]

mel·a·no·den·dro·cyte (mel'ă-nō-den'drō-sīt). SYN melanocyte. [melano- + G. *dendron,* tree, + *kytos,* a hollow (cell)]

mel·a·no·der·ma (mel'ă-nō-der'mă). **1.** An abnormal darkening of the skin by deposition of excess melanin. **2.** Hyperpigmentation of the skin by melanin or deposition of dark substances such as silver, iron, and drug derivatives. [melano- + G. *derma,* skin]

m. cachectico'rum, m. of the cachectic, occurring in certain chronic diseases, such as malaria and tuberculosis.

parasitic m., excoriations and m. caused by scratching the bites of the body louse, *Pediculus corporis.* SYN vagabond's disease, vagrant's disease.

racial m., the normally dark skin of members of some nonwhite races.

senile m., cutaneous pigmentation occurring in the aged. SYN melasma universale.

mel·a·no·der·ma·ti·tis (mel'ă-nō-der-mă-tī'tis). Excessive deposit of melanin in an area of dermatitis.

me·la·no·gen (mĕ-lan′ō-jen, mel′ă-nō-jen). A colorless substance that may be converted into melanin; e.g., some patients with widespread metastases of melanoma excrete m. in their urine, and melanin is formed when the urine is exposed to air (i.e., oxidized) for a few hours. [melanin + G. *-gen,* producing]

mel·a·no·ge·ne·mia (mel′ă-nō-jĕ-nē′mē-ă). The presence of melanin precursors in the blood; may occur in malignant melanoma with metastasis. [melanogen + G. *haima,* blood]

mel·a·no·gen·e·sis (mel′ă-nō-jen′ĕ-sis). Formation of melanin. [melanin + G. *genesis,* production]

mel·a·no·glos·sia (mel′ă-nō-glos′ē-ă). SYN black *tongue.* [melano- + G. *glōssa,* tongue]

mel·a·noid (mel′ă-noyd). A dark pigment, resembling melanin, formed from glucosamines in chitin. SYN artificial melanin, factitious melanin.

mel·a·no·ker·a·to·sis (mel′ă-nō-ker-ă-tō′sis). Migration of conjunctival melanoblasts into the cornea. [melano- + kerato- + G. *-osis,* condition]

mel·a·no·leu·ko·der·ma (mel′ă-nō-loo-kō-der′mă). Marbled, or marmorated, skin. [melano- + G. *leukos,* white, + *derma,* skin]
m. col′li, SYN syphilitic *leukoderma.*

mel·an·o·li·ber·in (mel′ă-nō-lib′er-in). A hexapeptide similar to oxytocin; it stimulates the release of melanotropin. SYN melanotropin-releasing factor, melanotropin-releasing hormone. [melanotropin + L. *libero,* to free, + -in]

mel·a·no·ma (mel′ă-nō′mă). A malignant neoplasm, derived from cells that are capable of forming melanin, arising most commonly in the skin of any part of the body, or in the eye, and, rarely, in the mucous membranes of the genitalia, anus, oral cavity, or other sites; occurs mostly in adults and may originate *de novo* or from a pigmented nevus or lentigo maligna. In the early phases, the cutaneous form is characterized by proliferation of cells at the dermal-epidermal junction which soon invade adjacent tissues. The cells vary in amount and pigmentation of cytoplasm; the nuclei are relatively large and frequently bizarre in shape, with prominent acidophilic nucleoli; and mitotic figures tend to be numerous. Prognosis correlates with the depth of skin invasion. M.'s frequently metastasize widely; regional lymph nodes, skin, liver, lungs, and brain are likely to be involved. Intense, intermittent sun exposure, especially of fair-skinned children, increases the risk of m. later in life. SYN malignant m. [melano- + G. *-ōma,* tumor]

acral lentiginous m., a form of malignant lentigo m. that occurs in palms, soles, and subungual areas.

amelanotic m., an anaplastic m. consisting of cells derived from melanocytes but not forming melanin.

benign juvenile m., SYN Spitz *nevus.*

Cloudman m., a transplantable m. that arose spontaneously in a mouse of DBA strain, and which grows and metastasizes in mice of related strains.

desmoplastic malignant m. (dez-mō-plas-mik), a m. with marked fibrosis surrounding atypical spindle-shaped melanocytes in the dermis, tending to invade widely around small nerves.

Harding-Passey m., a melanin-forming tumor that arose spontaneously in a non-inbred mouse, and that is transplantable to mice of many strains but does not ordinarily metastasize.

◨**malignant m.,** SYN melanoma.

malignant lentigo m., a m. arising (in unusual cases) from a malignant lentigo.

malignant m. in situ, a m. limited to the epidermis and composed of nests of atypical melanocytes and scattered single cells extending into the upper epidermis; local excision is curative although the lesion, if untreated, may soon invade the dermis. Malignant lentigo may be considered a slowly progressive type of malignant m. in situ.

minimal deviation m., a malignant m. showing less cytologic atypia than is usual in m. cells that nevertheless demonstrate asymmetric expansile invasion of the dermis, or metastasis.

◨**nodular m.,** primary cutaneous m. that presents as rapidly growing smoothly spheroid or ulcerated nodules in which tumor cells microscopically invade the dermis beneath all of the lateral epidermal margins of involvement.

subungual m., a m. beginning in the skin at the border of or beneath the nail, usually of acral lentiginous type (q.v.).

superficial spreading m., primary cutaneous m. characterized by intraepidermal growth extending laterally beyond the site of dermal invasion.

mel·a·no·ma·to·sis (mel′ă-nō-mă-tō′sis). A condition characterized by numerous, widespread lesions of melanoma. [melanoma + G. *-osis,* condition]

mel·a·no·nych·ia (mel′ă-nō-nik′ē-ă). Black pigmentation of the nails. [melano- + G. *onyx* (*onych-*), nail]

mel·a·nop·a·thy (mel′ă-nop′ă-thē). Any disease marked by abnormal pigmentation of the skin. [melano- + G. *pathos,* suffering]

mel·a·no·phage (mel′ă-nō-fāj, mĕ-lan′ō-fāj). A histiocyte that has phagocytized melanin. [melano- + G. *phagein,* to eat]

mel·a·no·phore (mel′ă-nō-fōr, mĕ-lan′ō-fōr). A dermal pigment cell that does not secrete its pigment granules but participates in rapid color changes by intracellular aggregation and dispersal of melanosomes; it is well developed in fish, amphibians, and reptiles, but absent in humans. [melano- + G. *phoros,* bearing]

mel·a·no·pla·kia (mel′ă-nō-plā′kē-ă). The occurrence of pigmented patches on the tongue and buccal mucous membrane. [melano- + G. *plax,* plate, plaque]

mel·a·no·pro·tein (mel′ă-nō-prō′tēn). A protein complex containing melanin.

mel·a·nor·rha·gia (mel′ă-nō-rā′jē-ă). SYN melena. [melano- + G. *rhēgnymi,* to burst forth]

mel·a·nor·rhea (mel′ă-nō-rē′ă). SYN melena. [melano- + G. *rhoia,* a flow]

mel·a·no·sis (mel-ă-nō′sis). Abnormal dark brown or brown-black pigmentation of various tissues or organs, as the result of melanin or, in some situations, other substances that resemble melanin to varying degrees; e.g., m. of the skin may occur in widespread metastatic melanoma, sunburn, during pregnancy, and as a result of chronic infections. [melano- + G. *-osis,* condition]
m. co′li, m. of the large intestinal mucosa due to accumulation of pigment of uncertain composition within macrophages in the lamina propria.

neurocutaneous m., cutaneous giant pigmented nevi associated with m. of the leptomeninges; malignant melanomas may develop in the skin or meninges.

oculodermal m., pigmentation of the sclera and skin around the eye, usually unilateral; seen especially in women of Asian descent. SYN Ota nevus.

pustular m., a transient, benign, pustular rash of unknown etiology seen in neonates; leaves a hyperpigmented base when the pustule resolves.

Riehl m., a brown pigmentary condition of the exposed portions of the skin of the neck and face with melanin pigment in dermal macrophages, thought to result from photodermatitis due to materials, such as cosmetic ingredients, or oils encountered in various occupations.

mel·a·no·some (mel′ă-nō-sōm). The generally oval pigment granule (0.2 by 0.6 μm) produced by melanocytes. SYN eumelanosome. [melano- + G. *sōma,* body]

giant m., a large spherical m. (1 to 6 μ in diameter) formed in the cytoplasm of melanocytes in café-au-lait spots and other melanocytic disorders. SYN macromelanosome.

mel·an·o·sta·tin. Inhibits synthesis and release of melanotropin; neuropeptide Y. SYN melanotropin release-inhibiting hormone. [melanotropin + G. *states,* stationary, + -in]

mel·a·not·ic (mel′ă-not′ik). **1.** Pertaining to the presence, normal or pathologic, of melanin. **2.** Relating to or characterized by melanosis.

mel·a·no·ton·in (mel′ă-nō-tō-nin). SEE melatonin.

mel·a·not·ri·chous (mel-ă-not′ri-kŭs). Having black hair. [melano- + G. *thrix* (*trich-*), hair]

mel·a·no·troph (mel′ă-nō-trōf). A cell of the intermediate lobe of the hypophysis that produces melanotropin. [melano- + G. *trophē,* nourishment]

mel·a·no·tro·phin (mel′ă-nō-trō′fin). SYN melanotropin. [melano- + G. *trophē,* nourishment, + -in]

me

mel·a·no·tro·pin (mel'ă-nō-trō'pin). A polypeptide hormone secreted by the intermediate lobe of the hypophysis in humans (in neurohypophysis in certain other species) which causes dispersion of melanin by melanophores, resulting in darkening of the skin, presumably by promoting melanin synthesis; this effect is readily demonstated in some lower vertebrates, such as frogs and fish; α-m. is an *N*-acetylated peptide with 13 amino acids; β-m. has 22 amino acids. SYN intermedin, melanocyte-stimulating hormone, melanophore-expanding principle, melanotrophin.

mel·a·nu·ria (mel-ă-noo'rē-ă). The excretion of urine of a dark color, resulting from the presence of melanin or other pigments or from the action of phenol, creosote, resorcin, and other coal tar derivatives. [melano- + G. *ouron,* urine]

mel·a·nu·ric (mel-ă-noo'rik). Pertaining to or characterized by melanuria.

mel·ar·so·prol (me-lar'sō-prol). Used in the treatment of the meningoencephalitic stages of trypanosomiasis; may produce a fatal reactive encephalopathy.

MELAS An acronym for mitochondrial myopathy, encephalopathy, lactacidosis, and stroke; an inherited disorder of the respiratory chain, either a deficiency of NADH:ubiquinone oxidoreductase (complex I of the chain) or of cytochrome *c* oxidase.

MELAS Acronym for *m*itochondrial myopathy, *e*ncephalopathy, *l*actic *a*cidosis, and *s*trokelike episodes. One of the mitochondrial disorders, this condition is usually hereditary, with a mutation at the mitochondrial genome at locus 3243.

me·las·ma (mě-laz'mă). A patchy pigmentation of sun-exposed skin, seen most commonly in pregnancy. SEE ALSO chloasma. [G. a black color, a black spot]

    m. gravida'rum, chloasma occurring in pregnancy.

    m. universa'le, SYN senile *melanoderma.*

mel·a·ton·in (mel-ă-tōn'in). *N* -Acetyl-5-methoxytryptamine; a substance formed by the mammalian pineal gland, which appears to depress gonadal function in mammals and causes contraction of amphibian melanophores; a precursor is serotonin; m. is rapidly metabolized and is taken up by all tissues; it is involved in circadian rhythms. [melanophore + G. *tonos,* contraction, + -in]

> Melatonin secretion is linked to both the sleep-wakefulness and light-dark cycles. Ocular perception that ambient light is dimming has been shown to trigger, via neural pathways involving the hypothalamus, increased secretion of melatonin by the pineal gland. Serum levels increase 10-fold just before sleep and peak around midnight. Twenty-four-hour secretion is higher in winter than in summer. The decline of melatonin secretion with age has been blamed for the tendency to insomnia in the elderly. Because melatonin acts as an antioxidant in counteracting free radicals, it has been promoted as a means of delaying aging and preventing cancer, heart disease, and Alzheimer dementia. It has also been proposed as an antidepressant because serotonin (5-hydroxytryptamine), whose metabolism is known to be disordered in clinical depression, is a chemical precursor of melatonin. Adequately controlled, large-scale studies of the efficacy, safety, and optimum dosage of melatonin are lacking. There is experimental evidence that long-term administration can reset the circadian pacemaker. Anecdotal reports suggest that shorter courses can hasten recovery from jet lag and facilitate adaptation to night-shift work. In one controlled study of 15 emergency physicians, melatonin did not improve sleep when subjects returned to a normal sleep pattern after working night shifts. The direct soporific effect of melatonin varies widely from person to person. Limited studies suggest that it may increase the duration of restful nighttime sleep in the elderly. High doses of melatonin result in prolonged elevation of serum melatonin level and increased production of prolactin by the pituitary gland. Unlike most hormones, melatonin is readily absorbed from the digestive tract and is a component of some foods. Hence therapeutic formulations are not subject to federal drug regulations or purity standards. Testing of commercially available preparations of melatonin has indicated

both variation in potency and the presence of possibly harmful contaminants.

Melchior. J.C., Danish physician. SEE Dyggve-Melchior-Clausen *syndrome.*

me·le·na (me-lē'nă). Passage of dark-colored, tarry stools, due to the presence of blood altered by the intestinal juices. Cf. hematochezia. SYN melanorrhagia, melanorrhea. [G. *melaina,* fem. of *melas,* black]

    m. neonato'rum, m. of the newborn; m. occurring in young infants.

    m. spu'ria, passage in the stool of blood that has been swallowed, especially that swallowed by nurslings from a fissured nipple.

    m. ve'ra, true m. as distinguished from m. spuria.

mel·e·nem·e·sis (mel-ě-nem'ě-sis). Vomiting of dark-colored or blackish material. SEE ALSO black *vomit.* [G. *melas,* black, + *emesis,* vomiting]

Meleney, Frank L., U.S. surgeon, 1889–1963. SEE M. *gangrene, ulcer.*

mel·en·ges·trol ac·e·tate (mel-en-jes'trōl). A progestational agent.

mel·e·tin (mel'ě-tin). SYN quercetin.

⌂meli-. Honey, sugar. SEE ALSO mel- (3). [G. *meli*]

mel·i·bi·ase (mel-i-bī'ās). SYN α-D-galactosidase.

mel·i·bi·ose (mel-i-bī'ōs). A disaccharide formed by the hydrolysis of raffinose by β-fructofuranosidase; also present in plant juices.

mel·i·ce·ra, mel·i·ce·ris (mel-i-sē'ră, mel-i-sē'ris). A hygroma or other type of cyst that contains a relatively thick, tenacious, semifluid material. [G. *meli- kēris,* a tumor, fr. *melikēron,* honeycomb, fr. *meli,* honey, + *kēros,* wax]

mel·i·oi·do·sis (mel'ē-oy-dō'sis). An infectious disease of rodents in India and Southeast Asia that is caused by *Pseudomonas pseudomallei* and is communicable to humans. The characteristic lesion is a small caseous nodule, found generally throughout the body, which breaks down into an abscess; symptoms vary according to the tracts or organs involved. SYN pseudoglanders, Whitmore disease. [G. *mēlis,* a distemper of asses, + *eidos,* resemblance, + *-osis,* condition]

me·lis·sa (me-lis'ă). The leaves from the tops of *Melissa officinalis* (family Labiatae), a plant of southern Europe; a diaphoretic. SYN sweet balm. [G. a bee]

me·lis·sic ac·id (me-lis'ik). A long-chain saturated fatty acid found in waxes. [G. *melissa,* bee + -ic]

me·lis·so·pho·bia (mě-lis'ō-fō'bē-ă). SYN apiphobia. [G. *melissa,* bee, + *phobos,* fear]

me·li·tis (mē-lī'tis). Inflammation of the cheek. [G. *mēlon,* cheek, + *-itis,* inflammation]

mel·i·tose (mel'i-tōs). SYN raffinose.

mel·i·tra·cen hy·dro·chlo·ride (mel-i-trā'sen). An antidepressant.

mel·i·tri·ose (mel-i-trī'ōs). SYN raffinose.

mel·it·tin (mel'i-tin). The principal component in bee venom; m. is a peptide amide containing 26 amino acids and is a hemolysin. [G. *melitta,* bee, + -in]

Melkersson, Ernst G., Swedish physician, 1898–1932. SEE M.-Rosenthal *syndrome.*

mel·li·tum, gen. **mel·li·ti,** pl. **mel·li·ta** (me-lī'tŭm, -tī, tă). A pharmaceutical preparation with honey as an excipient. [L. neut. of *mellitus,* honeyed]

Melnick, John C., U.S. radiologist, *1928. SEE Melnick-Needles *osteodysplasty;* M.-Needles *syndrome.*

⌂melo-. SEE mel-.

mel·o·did·y·mus (mel'ō-did'ĭ-mus). A fetus with a supernumerary limb. [melo- + G. *didymos,* twin]

mel·o·ma·nia (mel-ō-mā'nē-ă). An abnormal fascination with or devotion to music. [L. *melos,* song + *mania,* frenzy]

mel·o·me·lia (mel-ō-mē'lē-ă). A malformation in which the fetus has one or more rudimentary limbs in addition to the normal limbs. Cf. micromelia. [G. *melos,* limb]

mel·o·plas·ty (mel′ō-plas-tē). Old term for plastic surgery of the cheek; also for "facelift". [melo- + G. *plastos,* formed]

mel·o·rhe·os·to·sis (mel′ō-rē-os-tō′sis). Rheostosis confined to the long bones. [G. *melos,* limb, + *rheos,* stream, + *osteon,* bone, + *-ōsis*]

me·los·chi·sis (me-los′ki-sis). Congenital cleft in the face. [G. *mēlon,* cheek, + *schisis,* a cleaving]

me·lo·tia (me-lō′shē-ă). Congenital displacement of the auricle onto the cheek. [G. *mēlon,* cheek, + *ous,* ear]

mel·pha·lan (mel′fă-lan). L-Phenylalanine mustard; L-sarcolysine; L-3-[*p*-[*bis*(2-chloroethyl)amino]phenyl]alanine; a phenylalanine derivative of nitrogen mustard; an alkalylating antineoplastic agent.

melt. Denature, used to describe RNA polymerase action in decoupling DNA base pairs.

Meltzer, Samuel J., U.S. physiologist, 1851–1920. SEE M. *law;* M.-Lyon *test.*

MEM Abbreviation for Eagle minimum essential *medium.*

mem·ber. SYN limb (1). [L. *membrum*]

   inferior m. [TA], SYN lower *limb.*

   superior m. [TA], SYN upper *limb.*

   virile m., obsolete term for penis.

mem·bra (mem′bră). Plural of membrum. [L.]

MEMBRANA

---

mem·bra·na, gen. and pl. **mem·bra·nae** (mem-brā′nă, -brā′nē) [TA]. SYN membrane (1). [L.]

   m. abdom′inis, SYN peritoneum.

   m. adamanti′na, SYN enamel *cuticle.*

   m. adventi′tia, (1) SYN adventitia; **(2)** SYN *decidua* capsularis.

   m. atlan′to-occipita′lis ante′rior [TA], SYN anterior atlanto-occipital *membrane.*

   m. atlan′to-occipita′lis poste′rior [TA], SYN posterior atlanto-occipital *membrane.*

   m. basa′lis duc′tus semicircula′ris, SYN basal *membrane* of semicircular duct.

   m. basila′ris, SYN basal *lamina* of cochlear duct.

   m. capsula′ris, the hyaloid vascular network around the posterior pole of the lens in the embryo.

   m. capsulopupilla′ris, the lateral portion of the vascular tunic of the lens of the eye in the embryo.

   m. carno′sa, SYN dartos *fascia.*

   m. cer′ebri, any one of the cerebral meninges.

   m. choriocapilla′ris, SYN capillary *lamina* of choroid.

   m. cor′dis, SYN pericardium.

   m. cricothyroi′dea, SYN cricothyroid *membrane.*

   m. decid′ua, SYN deciduous *membrane.*

   m. e′boris, the lining membrane of the pulp cavity of a tooth, consisting of the odontoblastic layer. SYN ivory membrane.

   m. fibroelas′tica laryn′gis [TA], SYN fibroelastic *membrane* of larynx.

   m. fibro′sa capsulae articularis [TA], SYN fibrous *layer* of joint capsule.

   m. flac′cida, SYN flaccid *part* of tympanic membrane.

   m. fus′ca, SYN suprachoroid *lamina* of sclera.

   m. germinati′va, SYN blastoderm.

   m. granulo′sa, SYN *stratum* granulosum folliculi ovarici vesiculosi.

   m. hyaloi′dea, SYN posterior limiting *lamina* of cornea.

   m. hyothyroi′dea, SYN thyrohyoid *membrane.*

   membran′ae intercosta′les [TA], SYN intercostal *membranes,* under *membrane.*

   m. intercosta′lis exter′na [TA], SYN external intercostal *membrane.*

   m. intercosta′lis inter′na [TA], SYN internal intercostal *membrane.*

   m. interos′sea antebra′chii [TA], SYN interosseous *membrane* of forearm.

   m. interos′sea cru′ris [TA], SYN interosseous *membrane* of leg.

   m. lim′itans, (1) SYN limiting *membrane* of retina; **(2)** limiting membrane separating the neural parenchyma from the pia and blood vessels.

   m. lim′itans gli′ae, SYN glial limiting *membrane.*

   m. muco′sa, SYN mucosa.

   m. nic′titans, SYN *plica* semilunaris of conjunctiva (2).

   m. obturato′ria [TA], SYN obturator *membrane.*

   m. perine′i [TA], SYN perineal *membrane.*

   m. pituito′sa, SYN *mucosa* of nose.

   m. preformati′va, the thickened m. formed by fusion of Korff fibers and the basement membrane of the ameloblasts in a developing tooth.

   m. pro′pria duc′tus semicircula′ris, SYN proper *membrane* of semicircular duct.

   m. propria of semicircular duct, SYN proper *membrane* of semicircular duct.

   m. pupilla′ris, SYN pupillary *membrane.*

   m. quadrangula′ris [TA], SYN quadrangular *membrane.*

   m. reticula′ris organi spiralis [TA], SYN reticular *membrane* of spinal organ.

   m. sero′sa, (1) SYN serosa, chorion; **(2)** SYN serosa (2).

   m. seroti′na, obsolete synonym of *decidua* basalis.

   m. spira′lis, ⭐official alternate term for tympanic *surface* of cochlear duct.

   m. stape′dis [TA], SYN stapedial *membrane.*

   m. statoconio′rum [TA], SYN otolithic *membrane.*

   m. ster′ni [TA], SYN sternal *membrane.*

   m. stria′ta, SYN *zona* striata.

   m. succin′gens, SYN pleura. [L. *succingere,* to surround]

   m. suprapleura′lis [TA], SYN suprapleural *membrane.*

   m. synovia′lis [TA], SYN synovial *membrane.*

   m. tecto′ria (articulationis atlantoaxialis medianae) [TA], SYN tectorial *membrane* (of median atlantoaxial joint).

   m. tecto′ria duc′tus cochlea′ris [TA], SYN tectorial *membrane* of cochlear duct.

   m. ten′sa, SYN tense *part* of the tympanic membrane.

   m. thyrohyoi′dea [TA], SYN thyrohyoid *membrane.*

   m. tym′pani [TA], SYN tympanic *membrane.*

   m. tym′pani secunda′ria [TA], SYN secondary tympanic *membrane.*

   m. versic′olor, SYN tapetum (2).

   m. vestibula′ris ductus cochlearis, ⭐official alternate term for vestibular *surface* of cochlear duct.

   m. vi′brans, SYN tense *part* of the tympanic membrane.

   m. vitelli′na, (1) the membrane enveloping the yolk; specifically, the thickened cell membrane of large-yolked ova; SYN ovular membrane, vitelline membrane. **(2)** sometimes used to designate the zona pellucida of a mammalian ovum. SYN yolk membrane.

   m. vit′rea, SYN posterior limiting *lamina* of cornea.

---

mem·bra·na·ceous (mem-bră-nā′shŭs). SYN membranous.

mem·bra·nate (mem′bră-nāt). Of the nature of a membrane.

MEMBRANE

---

mem·brane (mem′brān). **1.** A thin sheet or layer of pliable tissue, serving as a covering or envelope of a part, as the lining of a cavity, as a partition or septum, or to connect two structures. SYN membrana [TA]. **2.** SYN biomembrane. [L. *membrana,* a skin or membrane that covers parts of the body, fr. *membrum,* a member]

me

adamantine m., SYN enamel *cuticle*.

allantoid m., SYN allantois.

alveolocapillary m., the pulmonary diffusion barrier.

alveolodental m., SYN periodontium.

anal m., the dorsal portion of the embryonic cloacal m. after its division by the urorectal septum.

anterior atlanto-occipital m. [TA], the fibrous layer that extends from the anterior arch of the atlas to the anterior margin of the foramen magnum of the occipital bone. SYN membrana atlanto-occipitalis anterior [TA].

arachnoid m., SYN *arachnoid* mater.

atlanto-occipital m., SEE anterior atlanto-occipital m., posterior atlanto-occipital m.

Barkan m., a theoretical tissue covering the trabecular *meshwork*; thought to obstruct aqueous *humor* outflow and be responsible for congenital glaucoma.

basal m. of semicircular duct, the basal m. underlying the epithelium of the semicircular duct. SYN basal lamina of semicircular duct, membrana basalis ductus semicircularis.

basement m., an amorphous extracellular layer closely applied to the basal surface of epithelium and also investing muscle cells, fat cells, and Schwann cells; thought to be a selective filter and to serve both structural and morphogenetic functions. It is composed of three successive layers (lamina lucida, lamina densa, and lamina fibroreticularis), a matrix of collagen (of which type IV is unique to this membrane), and several glycoproteins. SYN basement lamina, basilemma.

basilar m. of cochlear duct, SYN basal *lamina* of cochlear duct.

Bichat m., the inner elastic m. of arteries.

Bogros serous m., a m. of the episcleral space (of Tenon).

Bowman m., SYN anterior limiting *layer* of cornea.

Bruch m., SYN *lamina* basalis choroideae.

Brunn m., the epithelium of the olfactory region of the nose.

bucconasal m., a thin, transient epithelial sheet separating the primitive nasal cavity from the stomodeum in the 7-week-old human embryo. SYN oronasal m.

buccopharyngeal m., a bilaminar (ectoderm and endoderm) m. derived from the prochordal plate; after the embryonic head fold has evolved it lies at the caudal limit of the stomodeum. SYN oral m., oropharyngeal m.

cell m., the protoplasmic boundary of all cells that controls permeability and may serve other functions through surface specializations; e.g., active ion transport absorption by formation of pinocytotic vesicles; receptor-mediated antigen recognition, etc.; its fine structure is trilaminar and consists of the electron-dense lamina externa and lamina interna with an electron-lucent lamina intermedia. SYN cytolemma, cytomembrane, plasma m., plasmalemma, plasmolemma, Wachendorf m. (2).

chorioallantoic m., extraembryonic m. formed by fusion of chorion and allantois.

choroid m. [TA], SYN *tela* choroidea.

cloacal m., a transitory m. in the caudal area of the embryo, separating the proctodeum from the cloaca; it is divided into anal and genitourinary m.'s that break down during the 8th to 9th week of human development to establish the external opening for the alimentary and genitourinary tracts.

closing m.'s, thin sheets, composed of ectoderm externally and endoderm internally, which separate the pharyngeal pouches from the overlying branchial clefts in the early embryo. SYN pharyngeal m.'s.

Corti m., SYN tectorial m. of cochlear duct.

cricothyroid m., one of the bilateral m.'s extending between the arch of the cricoid cartilage and the inferior edge of the thyroid lamina on each side of the midline, which is occupied by the thicker median cricothyroid ligament. SEE ALSO *conus* elasticus, median cricothyroid *ligament*. SYN membrana cricothyroidea.

cricotracheal m., SYN cricotracheal *ligament*.

cricovocal m., ✶official alternate term for *conus* elasticus.

croupous m., SYN false m.

deciduous m., the mucous m. of the pregnant uterus that has already undergone certain changes, under the influence of the ovulation cycle, to fit it for the implantation and nutrition of the ovum; so called because the m. is cast off after labor. SYN caduca, decidua, Hunter m., membrana decidua.

Descemet m., SYN posterior limiting *lamina* of cornea.

diphtheritic m., the false m. forming on the mucous surfaces in diphtheria.

double m., two biomembrane layers, with an intermembranal space, surrounding certain organelles (e.g., mitochondria) or structures.

drum m., SYN tympanic m.

Duddell m., SYN posterior limiting *lamina* of cornea.

dysmenorrheal m., a m., resembling the decidua, cast off in cases of membranous dysmenorrhea.

egg m., the investing envelope of the ovum; a **primary egg m.** is produced from ovarian cytoplasm (e.g., a vitelline m.); a **secondary egg m.** is the product of the ovarian follicle (e.g., the zona pellucida); a **tertiary egg m.** is secreted by the lining of the oviduct (e.g., a shell).

elastic m., a m. formed of elastic connective tissue, present as fenestrated lamellae in the coats of the arteries and elsewhere.

embryonic m., SYN fetal m.

enamel m., the internal layer of the enamel organ formed by the enamel cells.

epipapillary m., (1) a congenital m. covering the optic disk; (2) the glial remnants of Bergmeister *papilla*.

epiretinal m., a m., usually acquired, covering a portion of the retina and composed of fibrous tissue from metaplasia of retinal pigment epithelial cells or glia.

exocelomic m., a layer of cells delaminated from the inner surface of the blastocystic cytotrophoblast and from the envelope of the primary yolk sac during the second week of embryonic life. SYN Heuser m.

external intercostal m. [TA], the m. that replaces the external intercostal muscle anteriorly, between costal cartilages. SYN membrana intercostalis externa [TA].

extraembryonic m., SYN fetal m.

false m., a thick, tough fibrinous exudate or slough on the surface of a mucous m. or the skin, as seen in diphtheria. SYN croupous m., pseudomembrane.

fenestrated m., an elastic m., as in elastic laminae of arteries.

fertilization m., a viscous m. formed on the inner surface of the vitelline m. from the cytoplasm of the egg cell after entry of the sperm, preventing the entry of additional sperm.

fetal m., a structure or tissue that develops from the fertilized ovum but does not form part of the embryo proper. SYN embryonic m., extraembryonic m.

fibroelastic m. of larynx [TA], a layer of fibrous and elastic fibers, taking the place of the submucosa in the larynx. It is divided by the laryngeal ventricle into two parts: the quadrangular m. superiorly and the conus elasticus inferiorly. SYN membrana fibroelastica laryngis [TA].

fibrous m. of joint capsule, ✶official alternate term for fibrous *layer* of joint capsule.

Fielding m., SYN tapetum (2).

flaccid m., SYN flaccid *part* of tympanic membrane.

germ m., germinal m., SYN blastoderm.

glassy m., (1) the basement m. present between the stratum granulosum and the theca interna of a vesicular ovarian follicle; it becomes very prominent in large atretic follicles; (2) the basement m. and associated connective tissue of the hair follicle. SYN hyaline m. (2).

glial limiting m., a dense, resilient m. forming the true capsule of the brain and spinal cord, composed of the processes of astrocytes (macroglia cells) and covered throughout by the pia mater, which firmly adheres to it; the two m.'s are collectively called the pial-glial m. SYN membrana limitans gliae.

Henle m., SYN *lamina* basalis choroideae.

Henle fenestrated elastic m., SYN elastic *laminae* of arteries, under *lamina*.

Heuser m., SYN exocelomic m.

Hunter m., SYN deciduous m.

Huxley m., SYN Huxley *layer*.

hyaline m., (1) the thin, clear basement m. beneath certain epithelia; (2) SYN glassy m. (2).

hyaloid m., SYN posterior limiting *lamina* of cornea.

hyoglossal m., posterior widening of the lingual septum connecting the root of the tongue to the hyoid bone; the inferior fibers of the genioglossus are attached to it and by this means to the upper anterior body of the hyoid bone near the midline.

inner m., the smaller of a double m.

intercostal m.'s [TA], the membranous portion of the intercostal muscle layers between ribs. SYN membranae intercostales [TA], intercostal ligaments, ligamenta intercostalia.

internal intercostal m. [TA], the m. that replaces the internal intercostal muscle posteriorly, medial to the angles of the ribs. SYN membrana intercostalis interna [TA].

interosseous m. of forearm [TA], the dense m. that connects the interosseous margins of the radius and ulna, forming the radioulnar syndesmosis, and with those bones separating the flexor and extensor compartments of the forearm. SYN membrana interossea antebrachii [TA].

interosseous m. of leg [TA], the dense fibrous layer that connects the interosseous margins of the tibia and fibula, forming the upper portion of the tibiofibular syndesmosis and, with the bones and intermuscular septa, creating anterior and posterior comparments of the leg. SYN membrana interossea cruris [TA], ligamentum tibiofibulare medium.

ivory m., SYN *membrana eboris*.

Jackson m., a thin vascular m. or veillike adhesion, covering the anterior surface of the ascending colon from the cecum to the right flexure; it may cause obstruction by kinking of the bowel. SYN Jackson veil.

keratogenous m., SYN nail *matrix*.

limiting m. of retina, one of two layers of the retina: **internal limiting m.,** formed by the expanded inner ends of Müller fibers; **outer limiting m.,** not a m. but a row of junctional complexes. SYN membrana limitans (1).

medullary m., SYN endosteum.

mitochondrial m., the double biomembrane surrounding the mitochondrion.

mucous m.'s, ✕official alternate term for mucosa.

mucous m. of bronchus, ✕official alternate term for *mucosa* of bronchi.

mucous m. of ductus deferens, ✕official alternate term for *mucosa* of ductus deferens.

mucous m. of esophagus, ✕official alternate term for *mucosa* of esophagus.

mucous m. of female urethra, ✕official alternate term for *mucosa* of female urethra.

mucous m. of gallbladder, ✕official alternate term for *mucosa* of gallbladder.

mucous m. of large intestine, ✕official alternate term for *mucosa* of large intestine.

mucous m. of larynx, ✕official alternate term for *mucosa* of larynx.

mucous m. of male urethra, SYN *mucosa* of male urethra.

mucous m. of nose, ✕official alternate term for *mucosa* of nose.

mucous m. of pharyngotympanic auditory tube, ✕official alternate term for *mucosa* of pharyngotympanic (auditory) tube.

mucous m. of pharynx, SYN *mucosa* of pharynx.

mucous m. of small intestine, ✕official alternate term for *mucosa* of small intestine.

mucous m. of stomach, ✕official alternate term for *mucosa* of stomach.

mucous m. of tongue, ✕official alternate term for *mucosa* of tongue.

mucous m. of trachea, ✕official alternate term for *mucosa* of trachea.

mucous m. of tympanic cavity, ✕official alternate term for *mucosa* of tympanic cavity.

mucous m. of ureter, ✕official alternate term for *mucosa* of ureter.

mucous m. of urinary bladder, ✕official alternate term for *mucosa* of (urinary) bladder.

mucous m. of uterine tube, ✕official alternate term for *mucosa* of uterine tube.

mucous m. of vagina, ✕official alternate term for *mucosa* of vagina.

Nasmyth m., SYN enamel *cuticle*.

nictitating m., SYN *plica* semilunaris of conjunctiva (2).

Nitabuch m., a layer of fibrin between the boundary zone of compact endometrium and the cytotrophoblastic shell in the placenta. SYN Nitabuch layer, Nitabuch stria.

nuclear m., SYN nuclear *envelope*.

obturator m. [TA], the thin m. of strong interlacing fibers filling the obturator foramen and with the surrounding bone, giving origin to the obturator externus and internus muscles. SYN membrana obturatoria [TA].

olfactory m., SYN olfactory *region* of nose.

oral m., SYN buccopharyngeal m.

oronasal m., SYN bucconasal m.

oropharyngeal m., SYN buccopharyngeal m.

otolithic m., a gelatinous m. supported by the hairs of the hair cells of the maculae of the saccule and utriculus of the inner ear; adhering to the surface are numerous crystalline particles called otoliths (statoconia). SYN membrana statoconiorum [TA], statoconial m.

outer m., the larger of the two m.'s of a double m.

ovular m., SYN *membrana* vitellina (1).

Payr m., a fold of peritoneum that crosses over the left flexure of the colon.

pericardiopleural m., SYN pleuropericardial *fold*.

peridental m., SYN periodontium.

perineal m. [TA], the layer of fascia extending between the ischiopubic rami inferior to the sphincter urethrae and the deep transverse perineal muscles. SYN membrana perinei [TA], Camper ligament, ligamentum triangulare, triangular ligament.

periodontal m., ✕official alternate term for periodontium.

periorbital m., SYN periorbita.

pharyngeal m.'s, SYN closing m.'s.

pial-glial m., the dual outer lining of the brain and spinal cord, composed of the glial limiting m. and the pia mater.

pituitary m., SYN *mucosa* of nose.

placental m., the semipermeable layer of fetal tissue separating the maternal from the fetal blood in the placenta; composed of: 1) endothelium of the fetal vessels in the chorionic villi, 2) stromata of the villi, 3) cytotrophoblast (negligible after the fifth month of gestation), and 4) syncytial trophoblast covering the villi; the placental m. acts as a selective m. regulating passage of substances from the maternal to the fetal blood. SYN placental barrier.

plasma m., SYN cell m.

pleuropericardial m., SYN pleuropericardial *fold*.

pleuroperitoneal m., SYN pleuroperitoneal *fold*.

posterior atlanto-occipital m. [TA], the fibrous membrane that attaches between the posterior arch of the atlas and the posterior margin of the foramen magnum. SYN membrana atlanto-occipitalis posterior [TA].

postsynaptic m., that part of the plasma m. of a neuron or muscle fiber with which an axon terminal forms a synaptic junction; in many instances, at least part of such a small postsynaptic m. patch shows characteristic morphological modifications such as greater thickness and higher electron density, believed to correspond to the transmitter-sensitive receptor site of such synapses.

presynaptic m., that part of the plasma m. of an axon terminal that faces the plasma m. of the neuron or muscle fiber with which the axon terminal establishes a synaptic junction; many synaptic junctions exhibit structural presynaptic characteristics, such as conical, electron-dense internal protrusions, that distinguish it from the remainder of the axon's plasma m. SEE ALSO synapse.

primary egg m., SEE egg m.

proligerous m., SYN *cumulus* oöphorus.

proper m. of semicircular duct [TA], the meshwork of connective tissue fibers between the semicircular duct and the bony

me

semicircular canal; it forms a delicate meshwork within the otherwise perilymph-filled perilymphatic space. SYN membrana propria ductus semicircularis, membrana propria of semicircular duct.

prophylactic m., SYN pyogenic m.

pupillary m., remnants of the central portion of the anterior layer of the iris stroma (the iridopupillary lamina) which occludes the pupil in fetal life, and normally atrophies about the seventh month of gestation. Persistent strands usually stretch across the pupil from one iris collarette to the other, without touching the pupillary margin. Failure to regress is a rare cause of congenital blindness. SYN membrana pupillaris, Wachendorf m. (1).

pyogenic m., a layer of pus cells lining an abscess cavity which have not yet autolyzed. SYN prophylactic m.

quadrangular m. [TA], portion of the fibroelastic membrane of the larynx that lies superior to the laryngeal ventricle; its slightly thickened inferior edge, the vestibular ligament, unlerlies the vestibular fold of the larynx; it attaches anteriorly to the epiglottis and posteriorly to the lateral margin of the arytenoid and corniculate cartilages; its upper portion underlies the mucosa of the aryepiglottic fold, which separates the laryngeal vestibule from the piriform fossa of the laryngopharynx. SYN membrana quadrangularis [TA], Tourtual m.

Reissner m., SYN vestibular *surface* of cochlear duct.

reticular m. of spinal organ, the m. formed by cuticular plates of the cells of the spiral organ of Corti; it appears netlike when viewed from above. SYN membrana reticularis organi spiralis [TA].

Rivinus m., SYN flaccid *part* of tympanic membrane.

round window m., SYN secondary tympanic m.

Ruysch m., SYN capillary *lamina* of choroid.

Scarpa m., SYN secondary tympanic m.

schneiderian m., SYN *mucosa* of nose.

Schultze m., SYN olfactory *region* of nasal mucosa.

secondary egg m., SEE egg m.

secondary tympanic m. [TA], the m. closing the round window (fenestra cochleae). SYN membrana tympani secundaria [TA], round window m., Scarpa m.

semipermeable m., a m. that is relatively permeable to the solvent but relatively impermeable to all or at least some of the solutes in either or both of the solutions separated by the m.

serous m., SYN serosa.

Shrapnell m., SYN flaccid *part* of tympanic membrane.

spiral m., ⁎official alternate term for tympanic *surface* of cochlear duct.

stapedial m. [TA], the delicate mucosal layer that bridges the space between the crura and base of the stapes. SYN membrana stapedis [TA].

statoconial m., SYN otolithic m.

sternal m. [TA], interlacing fibers from the anterior costosternal ligaments covering the anterior surface of the sternum. SYN membrana sterni [TA].

striated m., SYN *zona* striata.

suprapleural m. [TA], the thickened portion of endothoracic fascia extending over the cupola of the pleura and reinforcing it; it attaches to the inner border of the first rib and to the transverse process of the seventh cervical vertebra. SYN membrana suprapleuralis [TA], Sibson aponeurosis, Sibson fascia.

synovial m. [TA], the connective tissue m. that lines the cavity of a synovial joint and produces the synovial fluid; it lines all internal surfaces of the cavity except for the articular cartilage of the bones. SYN membrana synovialis [TA], stratum synoviale, synovium.

tectorial m. of cochlear duct [TA], a gelatinous m. that overlies the spiral organ (Corti) in the inner ear. SYN membrana tectoria ductus cochlearis [TA], Corti m., tectorium (2).

tectorial m. (of median atlantoaxial joint) [TA], the upward continuation of the anterior part of the posterior longitudinal ligament attached to (spanning between) the upper surface of the basilar portion of the occipital bone and the bodies of the second and third cervical vertebrae; it forms a "roof" over the median atlantoaxial joint. SYN membrana tectoria (articulationis atlantoax-

ialis medianae) [TA], apparatus ligamentosus weitbrechti, posterior occipitoaxial ligament.

tertiary egg m., SEE egg m.

thyrohyoid m. [TA], a thin, fibrous, membranous sheet filling the gap between the hyoid bone and the thyroid cartilage. SYN membrana thyrohyoidea [TA], membrana hyothyroidea.

Toldt m., the anterior layer of the renal fascia.

Tourtual m., SYN quadrangular m.

▌**tympanic m.** [TA], a thin tense m. forming the greater part of the lateral wall of the tympanic cavity and separating it from the external acoustic meatus; it constitutes the boundary between the external and middle ear; it is a trilaminar membrane covered with skin on its external surface, mucosa in its internal surface, is covered on both surfaces with epithelium, and, in the tense part, has an intermediate layer of outer radial and inner circular collagen fibers. SYN membrana tympani [TA], drum m., drum, drumhead, m. of tympanum, myringa, myrinx.

m. of tympanum, SYN tympanic m.

undulating m., undulatory m., a locomotory organelle of certain flagellate (trypanosome and trichomonad) parasites, consisting of a finlike extension of the limiting m. with the flagellar sheath; wavelike rippling of the undulating m. produces a characteristic movement.

unit m., the trilaminar structure of the plasmalemma and other intercellular m.'s, when seen in cross-section with the electron microscope, composed of two electron-dense laminae approximately 20 Å thick separated by a less dense lamina 35 Å thick.

urogenital m., the ventral portion of the embryonic cloacal m. after its division by the urorectal septum.

urorectal m., in the embryo, urorectal septum separating the cloaca into urogenital sinus and rectum. SYN urorectal fold.

uteroepichorial m., rarely used term for *decidua* parietalis.

vaginal synovial m., SYN synovial tendon *sheath*.

vestibular m., ⁎official alternate term for vestibular *surface* of cochlear duct.

virginal m., obsolete term for hymen.

vitelline m., SYN *membrana* vitellina (1).

vitreous m., (1) SYN posterior limiting *lamina* of cornea; **(2)** a condensation of fine collagen fibers in places in the cortex of the vitreous body; formerly thought to form a m. or capsule at its periphery; **(3)** SYN *lamina* basalis choroideae.

Wachendorf m., (1) SYN pupillary m; **(2)** SYN cell m.

yolk m., SYN *membrana* vitellina.

Zinn m., the anterior layer of the iris.

---

mem·bra·nec·to·my (mem-bră-nek′tō-mē). Removal of the membranes of a subdural hematoma. [membrane + G. *ektomē*, excision]

mem·bra·nelle (mem-bră-nel′). A minute membrane formed of fused cilia, found in certain ciliate protozoa.

mem·bra·ni·form (mem-brā′ni-fōrm). Of the appearance or character of a membrane. SYN membranoid.

mem·bra·no·car·ti·lag·i·nous (mem′bră-nō-kar-ti-laj′i-nŭs). **1.** Partly membranous and partly cartilaginous. **2.** Derived from both a mesenchymal membrane and cartilage; denoting certain bones.

mem·bra·noid (mem′bră-noyd). SYN membraniform.

mem·bra·nous (mem′bră-nŭs). Relating to or of the form of a membrane. SYN hymenoid (1), membranaceous.

mem·brum, pl. **mem·bra** (mem′brŭm, mem′bră). A limb; a member. [L. member]

m. infe′rius [TA], SYN lower *limb*.

m. mulieb′re, obsolete term for clitoris.

m. supe′rius [TA], SYN upper *limb*.

m. vir′ile, SYN penis.

mem·o·ry (mem′ŏ-rē). **1.** General term for the recollection of that which was once experienced or learned. **2.** The mental information processing system that receives (registers), modifies, stores, and retrieves informational stimuli; composed of three stages: encoding, storage, and retrieval. [L. *memoria*]

affect m., the emotional element recurring whenever a significant experience is recalled.

anterograde m., m. for that which occurred after an event such as a brain injury.

long-term m. (LTM), that phase of the m. process considered the permanent storehouse of information which has been registered, encoded, passed into the short-term m., coded, rehearsed, and finally transferred and stored for future retrieval; material and information retained in LTM underlies cognitive abilities.

remote m., m. for events of long ago as opposed to recent events.

retrograde m., m. for that which occurred before an event such as a brain injury.

screen m., in psychoanalysis, a consciously tolerable m. that unwittingly serves as a cover for another associated m. which would be emotionally painful if recalled.

selective m., reception or retrieval of only some of the events in an experience.

senile m., m. that is good for remote events, often in contrast to current events; characteristically seen in aged or demented persons.

short-term m. (STM), that phase of the m. process in which stimuli that have been recognized and registered are stored briefly; decay occurs rapidly, sometimes within seconds, but may be held indefinitely by using rehearsal as a holding process by which to recycle material over and over through STM. SYN temporary m.

subconscious m., information not immediately available for recall.

temporary m., SYN short-term m.

MEN Abbreviation for multiple endocrine *neoplasia.*

MEN1 Abbreviation for multiple endocrine *neoplasia,* type 1.

MEN2A Abbreviation for multiple endocrine *neoplasia,* type 2A.

men·ac·me (me-nak′mē). The period of menstrual activity in a woman's life. [G. *mēn,* month, + *akmē,* prime]

men·a·di·ol di·ac·e·tate (men-ă-dī′ol). Menadiol acetylated at both hydroxyl groups; a prothrombogenic vitamin. SYN acetomenaphthone, vitamin K_4.

men·a·di·ol so·di·um di·phos·phate. A dihydro derivative of menadione, with similar vitamin K activity.

men·a·di·one (men-ă-dī′ōn). The root of compounds that are 3-multiprenyl derivatives of m. and known as the menaquinones or vitamins K_2. SYN menaphthone, vitamin K_3.

m. reductase, SYN *NADPH* dehydrogenase (quinone).

m. sodium bisulfite, it possesses the same action and is used for the same purposes as m. or vitamin K; it differs, however, from m. in being water-soluble.

men·aph·thone (men-ă-naf′thōn). SYN menadione.

men·a·quin·one (MK, MQ) (men′ă-kwin′ōn, -kwī′nōn). The class name for a series of 2-methyl-3-all-*trans*-polyprenyl)-1,4-naphthoquinones (vitamins K_2).

men·a·quin·one-6 (MK-6). Hexaprenylmenaquinone; prenylmenaquinone-6; isolated from putrified fish meal; potency is about 60% of that of phylloquinone (vitamin K_1). SYN farnoquinone, vitamin K_2, vitamin $K_2(30)$.

men·a·quin·one-7 (MK-7). Menaquinone-6 with a 3-heptaprenyl side chain. SYN vitamin $K_2(35)$.

men·ar·che (me-nar′kē). Establishment of the menstrual function; the time of the first menstrual period. [G. *mēn,* month, + *archē,* beginning]

men·ar·che·al, men·ar·chi·al (me-nar′kē-ăl). Pertaining to the menarche.

Mendel, Gregor J., Austrian geneticist, 1822–1884. SEE mendelian *character;* mendelian *inheritance;* mendelian *ratio;* M. first *law,* second *law.*

Mendel, Kurt, German neurologist, 1874–1946. SEE M. instep *reflex;* Bechterew-M. *reflex.*

Mendeléeff (Mendeleev), Dimitri (Dmitri) I., Russian chemist, 1834–1907. SEE mendelevium; M. *law.*

men·de·le·vi·um (Md) (men-dě-lē′vē-ŭm). An element, atomic no. 101, atomic wt. 258.1, prepared in 1955 by bombardment of einsteinium with alpha particles. [*D. Mendeléeff*]

men·de·li·an (men-dē′lē-ăn). Attributed to or described by Gregor Mendel; usually referring to the behavior and the mechanism of the genetic transmission of single-locus traits.

***Men·de·li·an In·her·i·tance in Man* (MIM).** A standard, comprehensive, regularly updated reference source for traits in humans that have been shown to be mendelian or that are thought on reasonable grounds to be so. Each entry has a six-digit catalog number. Those securely established (by molecular biology or by extensive clinical studies) are marked with an asterisk.

men·del·ism (men′del-izm). The hereditary principles of single gene traits derived from Mendel laws.

men·del·iz·ing (men′del-īz-ing). Denoting a pattern of inheritance of a trait that corresponds phenotypically to the segregation of known or putative genes at one genetic locus.

Mendelson, Curtis L., U.S. physician, *1913.

Ménétrier, Pierre E., French physician, 1859–1935. SEE M. *disease, syndrome.*

Menge, Karl, German gynecologist, 1864–1945. SEE M. *pessary.*

Ménière, Prosper, French physician, 1799–1862. SEE M. *disease, syndrome.*

mening-. SEE meningo-.

me·nin·ge·al (mě-nin′jē-ăl, men′in-jē′ăl). Relating to the meninges.

me·nin·ge·o·cor·ti·cal (mě-nin′jē-ō-kōr′ti-kăl). SYN meningocortical.

me·nin·ge·or·rha·phy (mě-nin′jē-ōr′ă-fē). Suture of the cranial or spinal meninges or of any membrane. [G. *mēninx (mēning-),* membrane, + *rhaphē,* suture]

me·nin·ges (mě-nin′jēz) [TA]. Plural of meninx.

me·nin·gi·o·an·gi·o·ma·to·sis (mě-nin′jē-ō-an′jē-ō-mă-tō-sis). Proliferation of vessels and meningothelial cells, associated with epilepsy and neurofibromatosis.

me·nin·gi·o·ma (mě-nin′jē-ō′mă). A benign, encapsulated neoplasm of arachnoidal origin, occurring most frequently in adults; most frequent form consists of elongated, fusiform cells in whorls and pseudolobules with psammoma bodies frequently present; m.'s tend to occur along the superior sagittal sinus, along the sphenoid ridge, or in the vicinity of the optic chiasm; in addition to meningothelial m., fibrous, transitional, metaplastic, psammomatous, secretory, clear cell, papillary, chordoid, and lymphoplasmocytic varieties are recognized. [mening- + G. -*oma,* tumor]

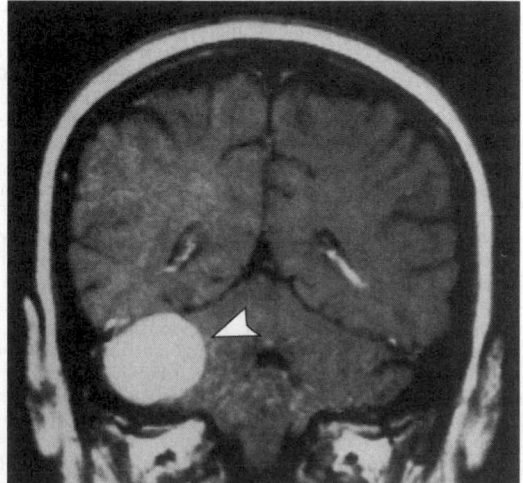

meningioma: meningioma in the right cerebellopontine angle (MRI, after injection of contrast medium)

cutaneous m., a lesion in the skin and subcutis composed of meningeal cells; occurs as a developmental lesion in children or as an extension of an intracranial m. in adults.

malignant m., m. that either invades brain parenchyma or metastasizes.

psammomatous m., a firm cellular neoplasm derived from fibrous tissue of the meninges, choroid plexus, and certain other structures associated with the brain, characterized by the formation of multiple, discrete, concentrically laminated, calcareous bodies (psammoma bodies); most of these neoplasms are histologically benign, but may lead to severe symptoms as a result of compressing the brain. SYN sand tumor, Virchow psammoma.

me·nin·gi·o·ma·to·sis (mĕ-nin'jē-ō-mă-tō'sis). The presence of multiple meningiomas, sometimes seen in von Recklinghausen disease.

me·nin·gism (men'in-jizm, mĕ-nin'jizm). A condition in which the symptoms simulate a meningitis, but in which no actual inflammation of these membranes is present. SYN pseudomeningitis.

men·in·git·ic (men'in-jit'ik). Relating to or characterized by meningitis.

men·in·gi·tis, pl. **men·in·git·i·des** (men-in-jī'tis, -jit'i-dēz; -jit'i-dēz). Inflammation of the membranes of the brain or spinal cord. SEE ALSO arachnoiditis, leptomeningitis. SYN cerebrospinal m. [mening- + G. *itis,* inflammation]

basilar m., m. at the base of the brain, due usually to tuberculosis, syphilis, or any low-grade chronic granulomatous process; may result in an internal hydrocephalus.

cerebrospinal m., SYN meningitis.

eosinophilic m., SYN angiostrongylosis.

epidemic cerebrospinal m., SYN meningococcal m.

epidural m., SYN *pachymeningitis* externa.

external m., SYN *pachymeningitis* externa.

internal m., SYN *pachymeningitis* interna.

listeria m., SYN listeriosis.

meningococcal m., an acute infectious disease of children and young adults, caused by *Neisseria meningitidis* characterized by fever, headache, photophobia, vomiting, nuchal rigidity, seizures, coma, and a purpuric eruption; even in the absence of m., meningococcemia can induce toxic phenomena such as vasculitis, disseminated intravascular coagulation, shock, and Waterhouse-Friderichsen syndrome due to adrenal hemorrhage; late complications include paralysis, mental retardation, and gangrene of extremities. SYN cerebrospinal fever, epidemic cerebrospinal m.

Approximately 2500 cases of invasive meningococcal disease occur annually in the U.S., with a case fatality rate of 10–15%. The incidence of endemic meningococcal disease peaks between late winter and early spring. Attack rates and case fatality rates are highest among children aged 6–12 months. Household exposure to tobacco smoke is a risk factor for meningococcal disease in children. Organisms are spread from person to person by direct contact and in saliva and respiratory secretions. The epidemiology of meningococcal disease is poorly understood. The nasopharyngeal carriage rate in the general population is 5–10%. This asymptomatic carrier state can persist for months or years and may confer protection against invasive disease. During epidemics of meningococcal meningitis, the carrier rate can approach 95%, yet fewer than 1% may develop the disease. Diagnosis is established by the finding of meningococci in cerebrospinal fluid or blood. Because meningococcemia can progress fulminantly to an irreversible stage, intravenous penicillin G, ampicillin, or chloramphenicol is begun as soon as the diagnosis is suspected, usually before laboratory confirmation. Intensive support of vital functions is crucial during the acute phase. Close contacts of known cases are treated prophylactically with rifampin or ciprofloxacin; mass prophylaxis may be appropriate in a confirmed institutional outbreak. A quadrivalent vaccine has been effective in preventing meningococcal disease due to serogroups A, C, W-135, and Y. Shortcomings of the vaccine are that it does not protect against serogroup B, which causes 30–40% of meningo-

coccal disease in the U.S.; does not interrupt the carrier state; does not induce immunity quickly enough to protect a person already infected; and protects for only 4–5 years. Routine immunization is recommended only for military recruits, travelers to endemic areas, and others known to be at long-term high risk. A major objection to infant vaccination has been the poor induction of immunity in this age group to serogroup C, which causes 45% of meningitis in the U.S. Use of a meningococcal C vaccine conjugated to protein has yielded high initial titers of anticapsular and bactericidal antibody in infants and toddlers, as well as more prolonged protection and better response to booster doses.

Mollaret m., a recurrent aseptic m.; febrile illness accompanied by headaches, malaise, meningeal signs, and cerebrospinal fluid monocytes.

neoplastic m., infiltration of subarachnoid space by neoplastic cells, typically medulloblastoma or metastatic carcinoma. SYN neoplastic arachnoiditis.

occlusive m., leptomeningitis causing occlusion of the spinal fluid pathways.

otitic m., infection of the meninges secondary to otitis media or mastoiditis.

serous m., acute m. with secondary external hydrocephalus.

tuberculous m., inflammation of the cerebral leptomeninges marked by the presence of granulomatous inflammation; it is usually confined to the base of the brain (basilar m., internal hydrocephalus) and is accompanied in children by an accumulation of spinal fluid in the ventricles (acute hydrocephalus). SYN cerebral tuberculosis (1).

⌂**meningo-, mening-.** The meninges. [G. *mēninx,* membrane]

ℹ**me·nin·go·cele** (mĕ-ning'gō-sēl). Protrusion of the membranes of the brain or spinal cord through a defect in the skull or spinal column. [meningo- + G. *kēlē,* tumor]

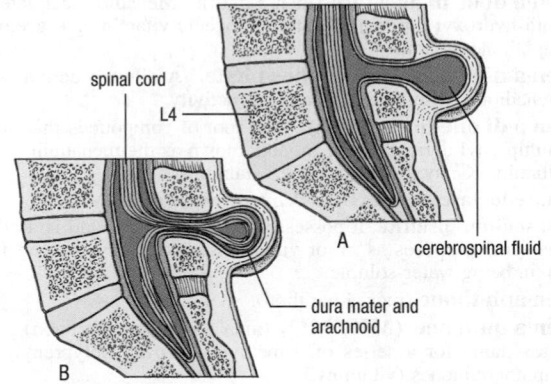

spinal cord
L4
A
cerebrospinal fluid
dura mater and arachnoid
B

meningocele (A) and **meningomyelocele:** occurring between L4 and L5 vertebrae

spurious m., an extracranial or extraspinal accumulation of cerebrospinal fluid, due to meningeal tear. SYN traumatic m.

traumatic m., SYN spurious m.

me·nin·go·coc·ce·mia (mĕ-ning'gō-kok-sē'mē-ă). Presence of meningococci (*N. meningitidis*) in the circulating blood.

acute fulminating m., rapidly moving systemic infection with *Neisseria meningitidis,* usually without meningitis, characterized by rash, usually petechial or purpuric, high fever, and hypotension. May lead to death within hours.

me·nin·go·coc·cus, pl. **me·nin·go·coc·ci** (mĕ-ning'gō-kok'ŭs, -kok'sī). SYN *Neisseria meningitidis.* [meningo- + G. *kokkos,* berry]

me·nin·go·cor·ti·cal (mĕ-ning'gō-kōr'ti-kăl). Relating to the meninges and the cortex of the brain. SYN meningeocortical.

me·nin·go·cyte (mĕ-ning'gō-sīt). A mesenchymal epithelial cell of the subarachnoid space; it may become a macrophage. [meningo- + G. *kytos*, cell]

me·nin·go·en·ceph·a·li·tis (mě-ning'gō-en-sef'ăl-ī'tis). An inflammation of the brain and its membranes. SYN cerebromeningitis, encephalomeningitis. [meningo- + G. *enkephalos*, brain, + *-itis*, inflammation]

acute primary hemorrhagic m., SYN acute epidemic *leukoencephalitis.*

biundulant m., SYN tick-borne *encephalitis* (Central European subtype).

chronic progressive syphilitic m., SYN paretic *neurosyphilis.*

eosinophilic m., a disease caused by infection with the rat lungworm, *Angiostrongylus cantonensis,* whose larvae, ingested with infected slugs or land snails (or some unidentified transport host), migrate from intestine to the meninges of the brain where the disease is produced; it is usually mild, of short duration, and characterized by fever, eosinophilia, and white blood cells (rarely nematode larvae) in the spinal fluid.

herpetic m., a severe form of m. caused by herpesvirus type 1 and associated with a high mortality rate.

mumps m., a usually benign nervous system infection arising during the active phase of clinical mumps parotiditis.

primary amebic m., an invasive, rapidly fatal cerebral infection by soil amebae, chiefly *Naegleria fowleri,* found in humans and other primates and experimentally in rodents; the disease is characterized by a high fever, neck rigidity, and symptoms associated with upper respiratory infection such as cough and nausea; although organisms have been cultured from various organs, the brain is the primary focus, especially the olfactory lobes and cerebral cortex, which are first attacked by the amebae that enter from nasal mucosa through the cribriform plate; death usually occurs two to three days after onset of symptoms.

syphilitic m., a secondary or tertiary stage manifestation of syphilis; rarely fatal.

me·nin·go·en·ceph·a·lo·cele (mě-ning'gō-en-sef'ă-lō-sēl). A protrusion of the meninges and brain through a congenital defect in the cranium, usually in the frontal or occipital region. SYN encephalomeningocele. [meningo- + G. *enkephalos*, brain, + *kēlē*, hernia]

me·nin·go·en·ceph·a·lo·my·e·li·tis (mě-ning'gō-en-sef'ă-lō-mī-ě-lī'tis). Inflammation of the brain and spinal cord together with their membranes. [meningo + G. *enkephalos*, brain, + *myelos*, marrow, + *-itis*, inflammation]

me·nin·go·en·ceph·a·lop·a·thy (mě-ning'gō-en-sef-ă-lop'ă-thē). Disorder affecting the meninges and the brain. SYN encephalomeningopathy. [meningo- + G. *enkephalos*, brain, + *pathos*, suffering]

me·nin·go·my·e·li·tis (mě-ning'gō-mī'ě-lī'tis). Inflammation of the spinal cord and of its enveloping arachnoid and pia mater, and less commonly also of the dura mater. [meningo- + G. *myelos*, marrow, + *-itis*, inflammation]

me·nin·go·my·e·lo·cele (mě-ning-gō-mī'ě-lō-sēl). Protrusion of the spinal cord and its membranes through a defect in the vertebral column. SYN myelocystomeningocele, myelomeningocele. [meningo- + G. *myelos*, marrow, + *kēlē*, tumor]

me·nin·go-os·te·o·phle·bi·tis (mě-ning'gō'os-tē-ō-flě-bī'tis). Inflammation of the veins of the periosteum.

me·nin·go·ra·dic·u·lar (mě-ning'gō-ra-dik'ū-lăr). Relating to the meninges covering cranial or spinal nerve roots. [meningo- + L. *radix*, root]

me·nin·go·ra·dic·u·li·tis (mě-ning'gō-ra-dik-ū-lī'tis). Inflammation of the meninges and roots of the nerves.

me·nin·gor·rha·chid·i·an (mě-ning'gō-ra-kid'ē-an). Relating to the spinal cord and its membranes. [meningo- + G. *rhachis*, spine]

me·nin·gor·rha·gia (mě-ning'gō-rā'jē-ă). Hemorrhage into or beneath the cerebral or spinal meninges. [meningo- + G. *rhēgnymi*, to burst forth]

men·in·go·sis (men'ing-gō'sis). Membranous union of bones, as in the skull of the newborn. [meningo- + G. *-ōsis*, condition]

me·nin·go·vas·cu·lar (mě-ning'gō-vas'kū-lăr). Concerning the blood vessels in the meninges; or the meninges and blood vessels.

men·in·gu·ria (men-ing-goo'rē-ă). The passage of membraniform shreds in the urine. [meningo- + G. *ouron*, urine]

⊞**me·ninx,** gen. **me·nin·gis,** pl. **me·nin·ges** (mē'ninks, -jēz; men'ingks; mě-nin'jes) [TA]. Any membrane; specifically, one of the membranous coverings of the brain and spinal cord. SEE ALSO *arachnoid* mater, dura mater, pia mater, leptomeninx. [Mod. L. fr. G. *mēninx*, membrane]

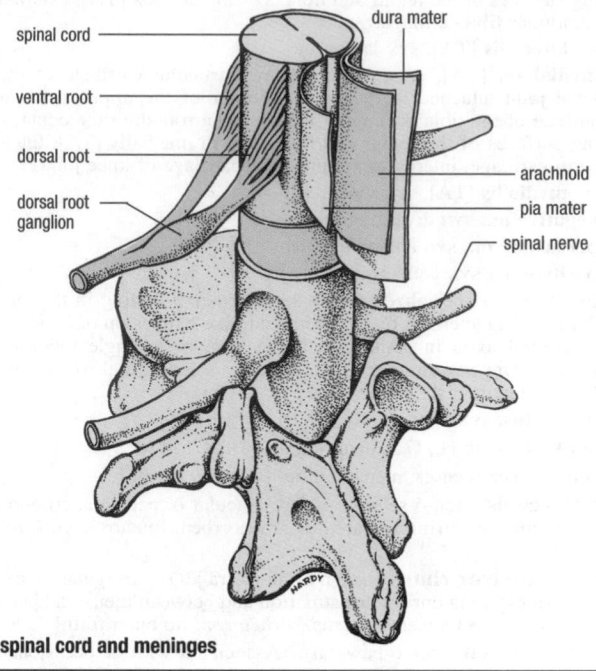

spinal cord and meninges

m. fibro'sa, rarely used term for dura mater.

m. primiti'va, SYN primitive m.

primitive m., the embryonic loose mesenchymatous tissue surrounding the brain and spinal cord; from it the three definite meninges (arachnoid mater, dura mater, and pia mater) are derived. SYN m. primitiva.

m. ten'uis, SYN leptomeninx.

vascular m., rarely used term for pia mater. SYN m. vasculosa.

m. vasculo'sa, SYN vascular m.

men·is·cec·to·my (men'i-sek'tō-mē). Excision of a meniscus, usually from the knee joint. [G. *mēniskos*, crescent (meniscus) + *ektomē*, excision]

me·nis·ci (mě-nis'sī). Plural of meniscus.

men·is·ci·tis (men'i-sī'tis). Inflammation of a fibrocartilaginous meniscus. [G. *mēniskos*, crescent (meniscus), + *-itis*, inflammation]

me·nis·co·cyte (mě-nis'kō-sīt). SYN sickle *cell.* [G. *mēniskos*, a crescent, + *kytos*, a hollow (cell)]

me·nis·co·pexy (mě-nis'kō-pek-sē). Surgical procedure anchoring the medial meniscus to its former attachment. SYN meniscorrhaphy. [menisco- + G. *pēxis*, fixation]

men·is·cor·rha·phy (men-is-kōr'ă-fē). SYN meniscopexy. [menisco- + G. *rhaphē*, suture]

me·nis·co·tome (mě-nis'kō-tōm). An instrument used in the removal of a meniscus. [G. *mēniskos*, crescent (meniscus) + *tomē*, incision]

⊞**me·nis·cus,** pl. **me·nis·ci** (mě-nis'kŭs, mě-nis'sī). **1.** SYN meniscus *lens.* **2** [TA]. A crescent-shaped intraarticular fibrocartilage found in certain joints. **3.** A crescent-shaped fibrocartilaginous structure of the knee, the acromio- and sternoclavicular and the temporomandibular joints. [G. *mēniskos*, crescent]

articular m., SYN meniscus *lens.*

m. articula'ris, SYN meniscus *lens.*

me

converging m., a convexoconcave lens in which the power of the convexity exceeds that of the concavity. SYN positive m.

diverging m., a convexoconcave lens in which the power of the concavity exceeds that of the convexity. SYN negative m.

lateral m. [TA], crescent-shaped intraarticular cartilage of the knee joint attached to the lateral border of the upper articular surface of the tibia, occupying the space surrounding the contacting surfaces of the femur and tibia. SYN m. lateralis [TA], external semilunar fibrocartilage.

m. latera'lis [TA], SYN lateral m.

medial m. [TA], crescent-shaped intraarticular cartilage of the knee joint attached to the medial border of the upper articular surface of the tibia occupying the space surrounding the contacting surfaces of the femur and tibia. SYN m. medialis [TA], falciform cartilage, internal semilunar fibrocartilage of knee joint.

m. media'lis [TA], SYN medial m.

negative m., SYN diverging m.

periscopic m., SYN aplanatic *lens.*

positive m., SYN converging m.

tactile m., a specialized tactile sensory nerve ending in the epidermis, characterized by a terminal cuplike expansion of an intraepidermal axon in contact with the base of a single modified keratinocyte. SYN m. tactus, Merkel corpuscle, Merkel tactile cell, Merkel tactile disk, tactile disk.

m. tac'tus, SYN tactile m.

Menkes, John H., U.S. neurologist, *1928. SEE M. *syndrome.*

⌂**meno-.** The menses, menstruation. [G. *mēn,* month]

men·o·ce·lis (men-ō-sē'lis). A dark macular or petechial eruption sometimes occurring in cases of amenorrhea. [meno- + G. *kēlis,* spot]

men·o·me·tror·rha·gia (men'ō-mē-trō-rā'jē-ă). Irregular or excessive bleeding during menstruation and between menstrual periods. [meno- + G. *mētra,* uterus, + *rhēgnymi,* to burst forth]

men·o·pau·sal (men'ō-paw-zăl). Associated with or occasioned by the menopause.

men·o·pause (men'ō-pawz). Permanent cessation of the menses; termination of the menstrual life. [meno- + G. *pausis,* cessation]

premature m., failure of cyclic ovarian function before age 40. SYN premature ovarian failure.

men·o·pha·nia (men-ō-fā'nē-ă). First sign of the menses at puberty. [meno- + G. *phainō,* to show]

Men·o·pon (men'ō-pon). A genus of biting lice (family Menoponidae, order Mallophaga) found on birds; it includes important pests that infect domestic fowl, such as *M. gallinae (M. pallidum),* the shaft louse of poultry, a light yellow louse about 1.7 to 2.0 mm long, found on barnyard fowl, ducks, and pigeons.

men·or·rha·gia (men-ō-rā'jē-ă). SYN hypermenorrhea. [meno- + G. *rhēgnymi,* to burst forth]

men·or·rhal·gia (men-ō-ral'jē-ă). SYN dysmenorrhea. [meno- + G. *algos,* pain]

men·o·tro·pins (men-ō-trō'pinz). Extract of postmenopausal urine containing primarily the follicle-stimulating hormone. SEE ALSO human menopausal *gonadotropin,* urofollitropin.

men·o·u·ria (men-ō-ū'rē-ă). Menstruation occurring through the urinary bladder as a result of vesicouterine fistula. [meno- + G. *ouron,* urine, + *-ia,* condition]

men·o·xe·nia (men-ō-zē'nē-ă, men'ok-sē'nē-ă). Any abnormality of menstruation. [meno- + G. *xenos,* strange]

men·ses (men'sēz). A periodic physiologic hemorrhage, occurring at approximately 4-week intervals, and having its source from the uterine mucous membrane; usually the bleeding is preceded by ovulation and predecidual changes in the endometrium. SEE ALSO menstrual *cycle.* SYN menstrual period. [L. pl. of *mensis,* month]

men·stru·al (men'stroo-ăl). Relating to the menses. [L. *menstrualis*]

men·stru·ant (men'stroo-ant). Menstruating.

men·stru·ate (men'stroo-āt). To undergo menstruation. [L. *menstruo,* pp. *-atus,* to be menstruant]

▣**men·stru·a·tion** (men-stroo-ā'shŭn). Cyclic endometrial shedding and discharge of a bloody fluid from the uterus during the menstrual cycle. [see menstruate]

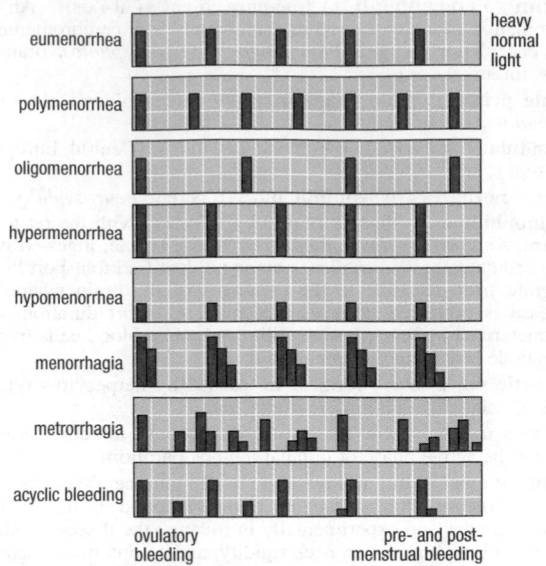

menstruation: abnormalities as shown in Kaltenbach chart

anovular m., menstrual bleeding without recent ovulation; also occurs in subhuman primates. SYN anovulational m., nonovulational m.

anovulational m., SYN anovular m.

nonovulational m., SYN anovular m.

retained m., SYN hematocolpos.

retrograde m., a flow of menstrual blood back through the fallopian tubes; it sometimes carries with it endometrial cells.

supplementary m., bleeding from the navel or urinary tract due to endometriosis occurring at the time of m.

suppressed m., nonappearance of menstrual bleeding from whatever cause.

vicarious m., bleeding from any surface other than the mucous membrane of the uterine cavity, occurring periodically at the time when the normal m. should take place.

men·stru·um, pl. **men·strua** (men'stroo-ŭm, -stroo-ă). Old term for solvent. [Mediev. L. menstrual fluid, thought to possess certain solvent properties, ntr. of L. *menstruus,* monthly]

men·su·al (men'soo-ăl, -shoo-ăl). Monthly. [L. *mensis,* month]

men·su·ra·tion (men-soo-rā'shŭn). The act or process of measuring. [L. *mensuratio,* fr. *mensuro,* to measure]

men·tal. **1.** Relating to the mind. [L. *mens (ment-),* mind] **2.** Relating to the chin. SYN genial, genian. [L. *mentum,* chin]

men·ta·lis (men-tā'lis). SEE mentalis *(muscle).* [L.]

men·tal·i·ty (men-tal'i-tē). The functional attributes of the mind; mental activity.

men·ta·tion (men-tā'shŭn). The process of reasoning and thinking.

Menten, Maud L., Canadian pathologist in U.S., 1879–1960. SEE Michaelis-M. *constant, hypothesis.*

Men·tha (men'thă). A genus of plants of the family Labiatae. *M. piperita* is peppermint; *M. pulegium,* pennyroyal; *M. viridis,* spearmint. SYN mint. [L.]

men·thane (men'thān). The monocyclic terpene parent of alcohols such as menthol and terpin.

men·thol. An alcohol obtained from peppermint oil or other mint oils, or prepared synthetically; used as an antipruritic and topical anesthetic, in nasal sprays, cough drops, and inhalers, and as a flavoring agent. SYN peppermint camphor.

camphorated m., a liquid obtained by triturating equal parts of camphor and m.; was used locally as a counterirritant and (diluted) as a spray in rhinitis and pharyngitis.

men·thyl sa·lic·y·late. Used as a sunscreen to filter out ultraviolet light in preparations to protect the skin from sunburn.

men·to·ia·bi·a·lis (men′tō-lā-bē-ā′lis). The mentalis and depressor labii inferioris considered as one muscle. [L.]

men·ton. In cephalometrics, the lowermost point in the symphysial shadow as seen on a lateral jaw projection. [L. *mentum,* chin]

men·to·plas·ty (men′tō-plas-tē). Plastic surgery of the chin, whereby its shape or size is altered. [L. *mentum,* chin, + G. *plastos,* formed]

men·tum, gen. **men·ti** (men′tŭm, -tī) [TA]. SYN chin. [L.]

men·yan·thes (men-yan′thēz). SYN buckbean.

mep·a·crine hy·dro·chlo·ride (mep′ă-krēn). SYN quinacrine hydrochloride.

mep·a·zine ac·e·tate (mep′ă-zēne). A phenothiazine derivative with actions and uses similar to those of chlorpromazine. Also available as m. a. hydrochloride.

me·pen·zo·late bro·mide (me-pen′zō-lāt). An anticholinergic drug.

me·per·i·dine hy·dro·chlo·ride (me-per′i-dēn). A widely used narcotic analgesic. SYN pethidine.

me·phen·e·sin (me-fen′ĕ-sin). A centrally acting skeletal muscle relaxant; also available as m. carbamate.

me·phen·ter·mine (me-fen′ter-mēn). A sympathomimetic amine.

m. sulfate, used topically as a nasal decongestant and systemically for its pressor effects in acute hypotensive states.

me·phen·y·to·in (mĕ-fen′i-tō-in). An anticonvulsant used when safer agents prove inadequate; used in drug metabolism studies.

me·phit·ic (me-fit′ik). Foul, poisonous, or noxious. [L. *mephitis,* a noxious exhalation]

meph·o·bar·bi·tal (mef-ō-bar′bi-tawl). Used as a sedative and long-acting hypnotic, and as an anticonvulsant in the management of epilepsy; converted to phenobarbital in the body.

me·piv·a·caine hy·dro·chlo·ride (me-piv′ă-kān). A local anesthetic agent.

me·pro·ba·mate (me-prō′bă-māt). A skeletal muscle relaxant with action similar to that produced by mephenesin but of longer duration; used in the management of certain disorders associated with abnormal motor activity, as a mild hypnotic, and as an antianxiety agent.

mep·ta·zi·nol (mep-tāz′ĭ-nol). A narcotic analgesic mixed agonist/antagonist (like pentazocine) which is about one-tenth as potent as morphine in producing analgesia. Though its abuse potential is less than that of pure agonists, the drug can precipitate an abstinence syndrome in persons dependent on opioids.

me·pyr·a·mine ma·le·ate (me-pir′ă-mēn). SYN pyrilamine maleate.

me·pyr·a·pone (me-pir′ă-pōn). SYN metyrapone.

mEq, meq Abbreviation for milliequivalent.

♻**-mer.** **1.** Chemical suffix attached to a prefix such as mono-, di-, poly-, tri-, etc., to indicate the smallest unit of a repeating structure; e.g., polymer. **2.** Suffix denoting a member of a particular group; e.g., isomer, enantiomer.

me·ral·gia (me-ral′jē-ă). Pain in the thigh; specifically, m. paresthetica. [G. *mēros,* thigh, + *algos,* pain]

m. paresthet′ica, burning pain, tingling, pruritus, or formication along the lateral aspect of the thigh in the distribution of the lateral femoral cutaneous nerve due to entrapment of that nerve; affected skin area often is hyperesthetic. SYN Bernhardt disease, Bernhardt-Roth syndrome.

mer·al·lu·ride (mer-al′ū-rīd). A mercurial diuretic.

mer·bro·min (mer-brō′min). The disodium salt of 2,7-dibromo-4-hydroxymercurifluorescein; an organic mercurial antiseptic compound that also has staining properties similar to those of eosin and phloxine, with strong affinity for cytoplasmic structures; also used histochemically to stain protein-bound sulfhydryl and disulfide groups for bright-field and fluorescence microscopy. SYN mercurochrome.

mer·cap·tal (mer-kap′tăl). A substance derived from an aldehyde by the replacement of the bivalent oxygen by two thioalkyl (–SR) groups.

mer·cap·tan (mer-kap′tan). **1.** A class of substances in which the oxygen of an alcohol has been replaced by sulfur (e.g., cysteine). SYN thioalcohol. SEE thiol. **2.** In dentistry, a class of elastic impression compounds sometimes referred to as rubber base materials.

methyl m., formed in the intestines by bacterial action on sulfur-containing proteins and appears in urine after ingestion of asparagus (contributing to the characteristic odor); also used in the manufacture of various organic sulfur-containing pesticides and fungicides.

♻**mercapto-.** Prefix indicating the presence of a thiol group, –SH.

mer·cap·to·a·ce·tic ac·id (mer-kap′tō-ă-sē′tik). SYN thioglycolic acid.

mer·cap·to·eth·a·nol (mer-kap′tō-eth′ă-nol). A commonly used reducing agent.

β-mercaptoethanol. SYN 2-mercaptoethanol.

2-mer·cap·to·eth·a·nol (mer-kap′tō-eth-ăn-ol). A reagent used to reduce disulfide bonds, particularly in proteins, and to prevent their formation. SYN β-mercaptoethanol.

mer·cap·tol (mer-kap′tol). A substance derived from a ketone by the replacement of the bivalent oxygen by two thioalkyl (–SR) groups.

3-mer·cap·to·lac·tate (mer-kap′tō-lak-tāt). A product of cysteine catabolism; formed by the action of lactate dehydrogenase on 3-mercaptopyruvate that was, in turn, formed by transamination of cysteine; present in normal human urine as a mixed disulfide with cysteine; elevated in the urine in individuals with mercapto-lactate-cysteine disulfiduria.

mer·cap·to·lac·tate-cys·te·ine di·sul·fid·u·ria. Elevated levels of the mixed disulfide of 3-mercaptolactate and cysteine in the urine.

mer·cap·tom·er·in so·di·um (mer-kap-tom′ĕ-rin, mer-kap-tō-mer′in). A mercurial diuretic.

6-mer·cap·to·pu·rine (Shy) (mer-kap-tō-poor′ēn). An analogue of hypoxanthine and of adenine; an antineoplastic agent.

3-mer·cap·to·py·ru·vate (mer-kap′tō-pī-roo-vāt). The transaminated product of cysteine; formed in cysteine catabolism; elevated in individuals with a deficiency of 3-m. sulfurtransferase.

3-m. sulfurtransferase, an enzyme that is a part of the cysteine catabolic pathway; it catalyzes the conversion of 3-m. to pyruvate and H₂S; a deficiency of this enzyme will result in elevated urine concentrations of 3-m. as well as of 3-mercaptolactate, both in the form of disulfides with cysteine.

mer·cap·tu·ric ac·id (mer-kap-tūr′ik). A condensation product of L-cysteine with aromatic compounds, such as bromobenzene, and usually acetylated; formed biologically via glutathione in the liver and excreted in the urine; an *S*-substituted *N*-acetylated L-cysteine. Cf. mercapturic acid *pathway*.

Mercier, Louis A., French urologist, 1811–1882. SEE M. *bar, sound, valve;* median *bar* of M.

mer·co·cre·sols (mer-kō-krē′solz). A mixture consisting of equal parts by weight of *sec*-amyltricresol and *o*-hydroxy-phenylmercuric chloride; it possesses fungicidal, germicidal, and bacteriostatic action.

mer·cu·ma·til·in (mer′kū-mă-til′in, -mat′i-lin). A mercurial diuretic; also available as m. sodium.

mer·cu·ra·mide (mer-koo′ră-mīd). SYN mersalyl.

mer·cu·ri·al (mer-kū′rē-ăl). **1.** Relating to mercury. **2.** Any salt of mercury used medicinally. **3.** Having the characteristic of rapid, changing moods.

mer·cu·ri·a·len·tis (mer-kū′rē-ă-len′tis). A brown discoloration of the anterior capsule of the lens caused by mercury; early sign of mercurial poisoning.

mer·cu·ri·a·lism (mer-kū′rē-ă-lizm). SYN mercury *poisoning.*

***p*-mer·cur·i·ben·zo·ate** (mer-kūr-i-ben′zō-āt). A commonly used enzyme inhibitor because of its reaction with sulfhydryl groups; usually *p*-chloromercuribenzoate or *p*-hydroxymercuribenzoate is used.

me

mer·cu·ric (mer-kū′rik). Denoting a salt of mercury in which the ion of the metal is bivalent, as in corrosive sublimate, mercuric chloride, $HgCl_2$; the mercurous chloride is calomel, HgCl.

mer·cu·ric chlo·ride. A topical antiseptic and disinfectant for inanimate objects. SYN corrosive sublimate, mercury bichloride, mercury perchloride, corrosive mercury chloride.
  ammoniated m. c., SYN ammoniated *mercury.*

mer·cu·ric io·dide, red. Has been used as an antiseptic and as a disinfectant for inanimate objects. SYN mercury biniodide, mercury deutoiodide.

mer·cu·ric ole·ate. An ointment-like preparation used in parasitic skin diseases.

mer·cu·ric ox·ide, red. The red precipitate of HgO; it has been used externally as an antiseptic in chronic skin diseases and fungus infections. SYN red precipitate.

mer·cu·ric ox·ide, yel·low. The yellow precipitate of HgO; used externally as an antiseptic in the treatment of inflammatory conditions of the eyelids and the conjunctivae. SYN yellow precipitate.

mer·cu·ric sa·lic·y·late. A powder used externally in the treatment of parasitic and fungus skin diseases. SYN mercury subsalicylate.

mer·cu·ro·chrome (mer-kur′ō-krōm). SYN merbromin.

mer·cu·ro·phen (mer-kū′-rō-fen). A local antiseptic.

mer·cu·ro·phyl·line so·di·um (mer-kūr-of′i-lēn). The sodium salt of β-methoxy-γ-hydroxymercuripropylamide of trimethylcyclopentanedicarboxylic acid, and theophylline; a mercurial diuretic.

mer·cu·rous (mer-kū′rŭs, mer′kū-rŭs). Denoting a salt of mercury in which the ion of the metal is univalent, as in calomel, mercurous chloride, HgCl; the mercuric chloride is corrosive sublimate, $HgCl_2$.

mer·cu·rous chlo·ride. SYN calomel.

mer·cu·rous io·dide. Used externally as an ointment in eye diseases. SYN mercury protoiodide, yellow mercury iodide.

mer·cu·ry (Hg) (mer′kū-rē). A dense liquid metallic element, atomic no. 80, atomic wt. 200.59; used in thermometers, barometers, manometers, and other scientific instruments; some salts and organic mercurials are used medicinally; care must be followed with its handling; [197]Hg (half-life of 2.672 days) and [203]Hg (half-life of 46.61 days) have been used in brain and renal scanning. SYN hydrargyrum, quicksilver. [L. *Mercurius,* Mercury, the god of trade, messenger of the gods; in Mediev. L., quicksilver, mercury]
  ammoniated m., used in ointment for the treatment of skin diseases. SYN ammoniated mercuric chloride, white mercuric precipitate.
  m. bichloride, m. perchloride, corrosive m. chloride, SYN mercuric chloride.
  m. biniodide, SYN mercuric iodide, red.
  m. deutoiodide, SYN mercuric iodide, red.
  m. protoiodide, SYN mercurous iodide.
  m. subsalicylate, SYN mercuric salicylate.
  yellow m. iodide, SYN mercurous iodide.

⌂**mere-, mero-.** Part; also indicating one of a series of similar parts. SEE ALSO -mer. [G. *mēros,* share]

Merendino, K. Alvin, U.S. surgeon, 1914–1985. SEE M. *technique.*

mer·e·prine (mer′ĕ-prēn). SYN doxylamine succinate.

Meretoja, J., Finnish physician. SEE Meretoja *syndrome.*

me·rid·i·an (mĕ-rid′-ē-an). **1** [TA]. A line encircling a globular body at right angles to its equator and touching both poles, or the half of such a circle extending from pole to pole. SYN meridianus [TA]. **2.** In acupuncture, the lines connecting different anatomical sites. [L. *meridianus,* pertaining to midday, on the south side, southern]
  m. of cornea, any line bisecting the cornea through its apex.
  m.'s of eyeball [TA], lines surrounding the surface of the eyeball passing through both anterior and posterior poles. SYN meridiani bulbi oculi [TA].

me·rid·i·ani (mĕ-rid-ē-ā′nī). Plural of meridianus.

me·rid·i·a·nus, pl. **me·rid·i·ani** (mĕ-rid′ē-ā′nŭs, -nī) [TA]. SYN meridian (1). [L.]
  meridiani bul′bi oc′uli [TA], SYN *meridians* of eyeball, under *meridian.*

me·rid·i·o·nal (mĕ-rid′ē-ŏ-năl). Relating to a meridian.

mer·i·spore (mer′i-spōr). A secondary spore, one resulting from the segmentation of another (compound or septate) spore. [G. *meros,* a part, + *sporos,* seed]

mer·i·ste·mat·ic (mer′is-tĕ-mat′ik). Pertaining (in fungi) to an area (meristem) of the hyphae or of other specialized structures from which new growth occurs. [G. *merizein,* to divide]

me·ris·tic (mĕ-ris′tik). Symmetrical; that which can be divided evenly; denoting bilateral or longitudinal symmetry in the arrangement of parts in one organism. [G. *meristikos,* suitable for dividing]

Merkel, Friedrich S., German anatomist and physiologist, 1845–1919. SEE M. cell *tumor, corpuscle,* tactile *cell,* tactile *disk.*

Merkel, Karl L., German anatomist and laryngologist, 1812–1876. SEE M. *filtrum* ventriculi, *fossa, muscle.*

Mer·mis (mer′mis). Genus of long, opaque nematodes; larval stages passed in the hemocylic cavity of insects, particularly grasshoppers, while adults are free-living in the soil. Accidental ingestion by humans causes infection.
  M. nigrescens, nematode species found in soil that deposits eggs on above-ground plants; normal host grasshoppers; has been recovered from alimentary and urogenital tracts of humans but infections are rare.

⌂**mero-.** SEE mere-.

mer·o·a·cra·nia (mer′ō-ă-krā′nē-ă). Congenital lack of a part of the cranium other than the occipital bone. [mero- + G. *a-* priv. + *kranion,* skull]

mer·o·an·en·ceph·a·ly (mer′ō-an-en-sef′ă-lē). A type of anencephaly in which the brain and cranium are present in rudimentary form. [mero- + G. *an-* priv. + *enkephalos,* brain]

mer·o·crine (mer′ō-krin, -krīn, -krēn). SEE merocrine *gland.* [mero- + G. *krinō,* to separate]

mer·o·di·a·stol·ic (mer′ō-dī-ă-stol′ik). Partially diastolic; relating to a part of the diastole of the heart. [mero- + diastole]

mer·o·gas·tru·la (mer′ō-gas′troo-lă). The gastrula of a meroblastic ovum.

mer·o·gen·e·sis (mer-ō-jen′ĕ-sis). **1.** Reproduction by segmentation. **2.** Cleavage of an ovum. [mero- + G. *genesis,* origin]

mer·o·ge·net·ic, mer·o·gen·ic (mer-ō-jĕ-net′ik, -ō-jen′ik). Relating to merogenesis.

me·rog·o·ny (mĕ-rog′ō-nē). **1.** The incomplete development of an ovum that has been disorganized. **2.** A form of asexual schizogony, typical of sporozoan protozoa, in which the nucleus divides several times before the cytoplasm divides; the schizont divides to form merozoites in this asexual phase of the life cycle. [mero- + G. *gonē,* generation]

mer·o·me·lia (mer-ō-mē′lē-ă). Partial absence of a free limb (exclusive of girdle); e.g., hemimelia, phocomelia. [mero- + G. *melos,* a limb]

mer·o·mi·cro·so·mia (mer′ō-mī′krō-sō′mē-ă). Abnormal smallness of some portion of the body; local dwarfism. [mero- + G. *mikros,* small, + *sōma,* body]

mer·o·my·o·sin (mer-ō-mī′ō-sin). A subunit of the tryptic digestion of myosin; two types are produced, H-m. and L-m.
  H-m., heavy-m., one of the relatively heavy products (mol. wt. about 350,000) of the action of trypsin on myosin; it carries the ATPase activity of myosin.
  L-m., light-m., the relatively low molecular weight product (mol. wt. about 120,000) of the tryptic digestion of myosin.

mer·ont (mer′ont). A stage in the life cycle of sporozoans in which multiple asexual fission (schizogony) occurs, resulting in production of merozoites. SEE ALSO schizont.

mer·o·ra·chis·chi·sis, mer·or·rha·chis·chi·sis (mer′ō-ră-kis′ki-sis). Fissure of a portion of the spinal cord. SYN rachischisis partialis. [mero- + G. *rhachis,* spine, + *schisis,* fissure]

me·ros·mia (me-roz'mē-ă). A condition in which the perception of certain odors is wanting; analogous to color blindness. [mero- + G. *osmē*, smell]

mer·o·spor·an·gi·um (mer'ō-spōr-ran'-jē-ŭm). A cylindrical small sporangium containing few spores and found in certain Zygomycetes. [G. *meros*, part, + sporangium]

mer·o·sys·tol·ic (mer'ō-sis-tol'ik). Partially systolic; relating to a portion of the systole of the heart. [mero- + systole]

me·rot·o·my (me-rot'ō-mē). The procedure of cutting into parts, as the cutting of a cell into separate parts to study their capacity for survival and development. [mero- + G. *tomē*, incision]

mer·o·zo·ite (mer-ō-zō'īt). The motile infective stage of sporozoan protozoa that results from schizogony or a similar type of asexual reproduction; e.g., endodyogeny or endopolygeny. M.'s form at the surface of schizonts, blastophores, or invaginations into schizonts, and are responsible for the vast reproductive powers of sporozoan parasites; this is seen in human malaria, where the cyclic production of m.'s produces the typical fever and chill syndrome. SYN endodyocyte (2). [mero- + G. *zōon*, animal]

me·ro·zy·gote (mē-rō-zī'gōt). In microbial genetics, an organism that, in addition to its own original genome (endogenote), contains a fragment (exogenote) of a genome from another organism; the relatively small size of the exogenote permits a diploid condition for only a limited region of the endogenote. [mero- + G. *zygōtos*, yoked]

mer·pha·lan (mer'fă-lan). The racemic mixture of melphalan and medphalan; an antineoplastic agent. SYN sarcolysine.

MERRF Acronym for *myoclonic epilepsy with ragged red fiber myopathy*. One of the mitochondrial disorders, this condition is caused by a point mutation of the mitochondria genome locus 8344, where transfer RNA is coded.

Merrifield, R. Bruce, U.S. biochemist and Nobel laureate, *1921. SEE M. *synthesis*.

Merrifield knife. See under knife.

Merritt, Katharine K., U.S. pediatrician, *1886. SEE Kasabach-M. *syndrome*.

mer·sa·lyl (mer'să-lil). Sodium salt of (3-hydroxymercuric-2-methoxypropyl)salicylamide-*O*-acetic acid; a mercurial diuretic. SYN mercuramide.

  m. acid, a mixture of *o*-carboxymethylsalicyl-(3-hydroxymercuric-2-methoxypropyl)amide and its anhydrides; same use as m.

  m. theophylline, m. plus theophylline added to inhibit decomposition of m.

Méry, Jean, French anatomist, 1645–1722. SEE M. *gland*.

Merzbacher, Ludwig, German physician in Argentina, 1875–1942. SEE M.-Pelizaeus *disease;* Pelizaeus-M. *disease*.

⚠ **mes-.** SEE meso-.

me·sad (mē'zad, mē'sad). Passing or extending toward the median plane of the body or of a part. SYN mesiad. [G. *mesos*, middle, + L. *ad*, to]

me·sal (mē'zăl, mē'săl). Rarely used term referring to the median plane of the body or a part. [G. *mesos*, middle]

mes·a·me·boid (mez-ă-mē'boyd). Minot's term for a primitive, "wandering" cell derived from mesoderm, probably a hemocytoblast. [mes- + G. *amoibē*, change (ameba), + *eidos*, resemblance]

mes·an·gi·al (mes-an'jē-ăl). Referring to the mesangium.

mes·an·gi·um (mes-an'jē-ŭm). A central part of the renal glomerulus between capillaries; mesangial cells are phagocytic and for the most part separated from capillary lumina by endothelial cells. [mes- + G. *angeion*, vessel]

  extraglomerular m., mesangial cells that fill the triangular space between the macula densa and the afferent and efferent arterioles of the juxtaglomerular apparatus. SYN polkissen of Zimmermann.

mes·a·or·ti·tis (mes-ā-ōr-tī'tis). Inflammation of the middle or muscular coat of the aorta. [mes- + aortitis]

mes·a·re·ic, mes·a·ra·ic (mes-ă-rā'ik). SYN mesenteric. [G. *mesaraion*, mesentery, fr. *mesos*, middle, + *araia*, flank, belly]

mes·ar·ter·i·tis (mes-ar-ter-ī'tis). Inflammation of the middle (muscular) coat of an artery. [mes- + arteritis]

me·sat·i·ce·phal·ic (mĕ-sat'i-se-fal'ik). SYN mesocephalic. [G. *mesatos*, midmost, + *kephalē*, head]

me·sat·i·pel·lic, me·sat·i·pel·vic (mĕ-sat'i-pel'ik, -pel'vik). Denoting an individual with a pelvic index between 90 and 95; the superior strait has a round appearance, with the transverse diameter longer than the anteroposterior by 1 cm or less. [G. *mesatos*, midmost, + *pellis*, a bowl (pelvis)]

mes·ax·on (mez-ak'son, mes-). The plasma membrane of the neurolemma that is folded in to surround a nerve axon. In electron micrographs this double layer resembles a mesentery in appearance.

mes·cal but·tons (mes'kal). The dried slices of the cactus *Lophophora williamsii* containing mescaline and related alkaloids.

mes·ca·line (mes'kă-lēn). The most active alkaloid present in the buttons of the mescal cactus, *Lophophora williamsii*. M. produces psychotomimetic effects similar to those produced by LSD: alteration in mood, changes in perception, reveries, visual hallucinations, delusions, depersonalization, mydriasis, hippus, and increases in body temperature and blood pressure; psychic dependence, tolerance, and cross tolerance to LSD and psilocybin develop; the principal component of peyote.

mes·ec·to·derm (mez-ek'tō-derm). 1. Cells in the area around the dorsal lip of the blastopore where mesoderm and ectoderm undergo a process of separation. 2. That part of the mesenchyme derived from ectoderm, especially from the neural crest in the cephalic region in very young embryos. SYN ectomesenchyme. [mes- + ectoderm]

mes·en·ce·phal·ic (mez-en'se-fal'ik). Relating to the mesencephalon.

mes·en·ceph·a·li·tis (mez'en-sef'ă-lī'tis). Inflammation of the midbrain (mesencephalon).

mes·en·ceph·a·lon (mez-en-sef'ă-lon) [TA]. That part of the brainstem developing from the middle of the three primary cerebral vesicles of the embryo (the caudal of these being the rhombencephalon or hindbrain, the rostral the prosencephalon or forebrain). In the adult, the m. is characterized by the unique conformation of its roof plate, the lamina tecti (tectal plate [TA] or quadrigeminal plate [TAalt]. composed of the bilaterally paired superior and inferior colliculus, and by the massive paired prominence of the crus cerebri at its ventral surface. On transverse section, its patent central canal, the cerebral aqueduct, is surrounded by a prominent ring of gray matter poor in myelinated fibers; the periaqueductal gray is ventrally and laterally adjoined by the myelin-rich mesencephalic tegmentum, and covered dorsally by the mesencephalic tectal plate. Prominent cell groups of the m. include the motor nuclei of the trochlear and oculomotor nerves, the red nucleus, and the substantia nigra. SYN midbrain vesicle☆, midbrain☆. [mes- + G. *enkephalos*, brain]

mes·en·ceph·a·lot·o·my (mez'en-sef'ă-lot'ō-mē). 1. The sectioning of any structure in the midbrain, especially of the spinothalamic tracts for the relief of intractable pain or the cerebral peduncle for dyskinesias. 2. A mesencephalic spinothalamic tractotomy. [mesencephalon + G. *tomē*, incision]

me·sen·chy·ma (mĕ-seng'ki-mă, mĕ-zeng'). SYN mesenchyme.

me·sen·chy·mal (mĕ-seng'ki-măl, mez-eng-kī'măl). Relating to the mesenchyme.

mes·en·chyme (mez'en-kīm). 1. An aggregation of mesenchymal or fibroblastlike cells. 2. Primordial embryonic connective tissue consisting of mesenchymal cells, usually stellate in form, supported in interlaminar jelly. SYN mesenchyma. [mes- + G. *enkyma*, infusion]

  interzonal m., an area of avascular m. between adjacent skeletal elements in the embryo; it denotes the region of future joints.

  synovial m., vascular m. surrounding the interzonal m.; it develops into the synovial membrane of a joint.

mes·en·chy·mo·ma (mez'en-kī-mō'mă). Rarely used term for a neoplasm in which there is a mixture of mesenchymal derivatives, other than fibrous tissue. A **benign m.** may contain foci of vascular, muscular, adipose, osteoid, osseous, and cartilaginous tissue; such neoplasms are sometimes classed under a compounded name, e.g., angioleiomyolipoma, and the like, but the broader term may be preferred. A **malignant m.** may also occur as a

me

similar mixture of two or more types of mesenchymal cells that are malignant (other than fibrous tissue cells).

mes·en·ter·ic (mez-en-ter′ik). Relating to the mesentery. SYN mesareic, mesaraic.

mes·en·ter·i·o·lum (mez-en-ter-ē′ō-lŭm). A small mesentery, as one of an intestinal diverticulum. SYN mesoenteriolum. [Mod. L. dim. of *mesenterium,* mesentery]

m. proces′sus vermifor′mis, SYN mesoappendix.

mes·en·ter·i·o·pexy (mes′en-ter-ē-ō-pek′sē). Fixation or attachment of a torn or incised mesentery. SYN mesopexy. [mesentery + G. *pēxis,* fixation]

mes·en·ter·i·or·rha·phy (mez′en-ter-ē-ōr′ă-fē). Suture of the mesentery. SYN mesorrhaphy. [mesentery + G. *rhaphē,* suture]

mes·en·ter·i·pli·ca·tion (mez′en-ter-i-pli-kā′shŭn). Reducing redundancy of a mesentery by making one or more tucks in it. [mesentery + L. *plico,* pp. *-atus,* to fold]

mes·en·ter·i·tis (mez′en-ter-ī′tis). Inflammation of the mesentery.

mes·en·te·ri·um (mez′en-ter′ē-ŭm) [TA]. SYN mesentery, mesentery. [Mod. L.]

m. dorsa′le commu′ne, SYN mesentery (2).

mes·en·ter·on (mez-en′ter-on). The midportion of the insect alimentary canal and site of digestion; the m. may possess anterior finger-like projections, the gastric ceca, and a tubular anterior midgut, followed posteriorly by the saccular ventriculus, or stomach. [mes- + G. *enteron,* intestine]

mes·en·tery (mes′en-ter-ē) [TA]. **1.** A double layer of peritoneum attached to the abdominal wall and enclosing in its fold a portion or all of one of the abdominal viscera, conveying to it its vessels and nerves. **2.** The fan-shaped fold of peritoneum suspending the greater part of the small intestines (jejunum and ileum) and attaching it to the posterior abdominal wall at the root of the m. (radix mesenterii). SYN mesenterium dorsale commune, mesostenium. SYN mesenterium [TA]. [Mod. L. *mesenterium,* fr. G. *mesenterion,* fr. G. *mesos,* middle, + *enteron,* intestine]

m. of appendix, SYN mesoappendix.

m. of cecum, SYN mesocecum.

m. of lung, SYN mesopneumonium.

m. of sigmoid colon, SEE mesocolon.

m. of transverse colon, SEE mesocolon.

urogenital m., SYN diaphragmatic *ligament* of the mesonephros.

mesh·work. SEE network.

trabecular m., SYN trabecular *tissue* of sclera.

me·si·ad (mē′zē-ad, mes′ē-ad). SYN mesad.

me·si·al (mē′zē-ăl, mes′ē-ăl) [TA]. SYN proximal. [G. *mesos,* middle]

△**mesio-.** Mesial (especially in dentistry). [G. *mesos,* middle]

me·si·o·buc·cal (mē′zē-ō-bŭk′ăl). Relating to the mesial and buccal surfaces of a tooth; denoting especially the angle formed by the junction of these two surfaces.

me·si·o·buc·co-oc·clu·sal (mē′zē-ō-bŭk′ō-ŏ-kloo′săl). Relating to the angle formed by the junction of the mesial, buccal, and occlusal surfaces of a bicuspid or molar tooth.

me·si·o·buc·co·pul·pal (mē′zē-ō-bŭk′ō-pŭl′păl). Relating to the angle denoting the junction of mesial, buccal and pulpal surfaces in a tooth cavity preparation.

me·si·o·cer·vi·cal (mē′zē-ō-ser′vi-kăl). **1.** Relating to the line angle of a cavity preparation at the junction of the mesial and cervical walls. **2.** Pertaining to the area of a tooth at the junction of the mesial surface and the cervical region.

me·si·o·clu·sion (mē′zē-ō-kloo′zhŭn). A malocclusion in which the mandibular arch articulates with the maxillary arch in a position mesial to normal; in Angle classification, a Class III malocclusion. SYN mesial occlusion (2).

me·si·o·dens (mē′zē-ō-denz). A supernumerary tooth located in the midline of the anterior maxillae, between the maxillary central incisor teeth. [mesio- + L. *dens,* tooth]

me·si·o·dis·tal (mē′zē-ō-dis′tăl). Denoting the plane or diameter of a tooth cutting its mesial and distal surfaces.

me·si·o·dis·toc·clu·sal (MOD) (mē′zē-ō-dist′ō-kloo′săl, -zăl). Denoting three-surface cavity or cavity preparation or restoration (class 2, Black classification) in the premolars (bicuspids) and molars.

me·si·o·gin·gi·val (mē′zē-ō-jin′ji-văl). Relating to the angle formed by the junction of the mesial surface with the gingival line of a tooth.

me·si·o·gnath·ic (mē′zē-ō-nath′ik). Denoting malposition of one or both jaws forward from their normal position.

me·si·o·in·ci·sal (mē′zē-ō-in-sī′săl, -zăl). Relating to the mesial and incisal surfaces of a tooth; denoting the angle formed by their junction.

me·si·o·la·bi·al (mē′zē-ō-lā′bē-ăl). Relating to the mesial and labial surfaces of a tooth; denoting especially the angle formed by their junction.

me·si·o·lin·gual (mē′zē-ō-ling′gwăl). Relating to the mesial and lingual surfaces of a tooth; denoting especially the angle formed by their junction.

me·si·o·lin·guo-oc·clu·sal (mē′zē-ō-ling′gwō-ŏ-kloo′săl, -zăl). Denoting the angle formed by the junction of the mesial, lingual, and occlusal surfaces of a bicuspid or molar tooth.

me·si·o·lin·guo·pul·pal (mē′zē-ō-ling′gwō-pŭl′păl). Relating to the angle denoting the junction of the mesial, lingual, and pulpal surfaces in a tooth cavity preparation.

me·sio-oc·clu·sal (mē′zē-ō-ō-kloo′săl, -zăl). Denoting the angle formed by the junction of the mesial and occlusal surfaces of a bicuspid or molar tooth.

me·sio-oc·clu·sion (mē′zē-ō-ō-kloo′zhŭn). SYN mesial *occlusion* (1).

me·si·o·place·ment (mē′zē-ō-plās′ment). SYN mesioversion.

me·si·o·pul·pal (mē′zē-ō-pŭl′păl). Pertaining to the inner wall or floor of a cavity preparation on the mesial side of a tooth.

me·si·o·ver·sion (mē′zē-ō-ver-zhŭn). Malposition of a tooth mesial to normal, in an anterior direction following the curvature of the dental arch. SYN mesial displacement, mesioplacement.

Mesmer, F. A., Austrian physician, 1733–1815. SEE mesmerism.

mes·mer·ism (mes′mer-izm). A system of therapeutics from which were developed hypnotism and therapeutic suggestion. [F.A. *Mesmer,* Austrian physician, 1734–1815]

mes·mer·ize (mes′mer-īz). Obsolete term for hypnotize. [see mesmerism]

△**meso-, mes-.** **1.** Middle, mean, intermediacy. **2.** A mesentery, mesentery-like structure. **3.** A prefix denoting a compound, containing more than one chiral center, having an internal plane of symmetry; such compounds do not exhibit optical activity (e.g., *meso*-cystine). [G. *mesos*]

mes·o·ap·pen·dix (mez′ō-ă-pen′diks) [TA]. The short mesentery of the appendix lying behind the terminal ileum, in which the appendicular artery courses. SYN mesenteriolum processus vermiformis, mesentery of appendix.

mes·o·ar·i·um (mez-ō-ār′ē-ŭm). SYN mesovarium.

mes·o·bi·lane (mez-ō-bī′lān). A reduced mesobilirubin with no double bonds between the pyrrole rings and, consequently, colorless. SEE ALSO bilirubinoids. SYN mesobilirubinogen, urobilinogen IXα.

mes·o·bi·lene, mesobilene- (mez-ō-bī′lēn). A bilirubinoid. SEE urobilin. SYN urobilin IXα.

mes·o·bil·i·ru·bin (mez′ō-bil-i-roo′bin). A compound differing from bilirubin only in that the vinyl groups of bilirubin are reduced to ethyl groups. SEE ALSO bilirubinoids.

mes·o·bil·i·ru·bin·o·gen (mez′ō-bil-i-roo-bin′ō-jen). SYN mesobilane.

mes·o·bil·i·vi·o·lin (mez′ō-bil-i-vī-ō′lin). A bilirubinoid.

mes·o·blast (mez′ō-blast). SYN mesoderm. [meso- + G. *blastos,* germ]

mes·o·blas·te·ma (mez′ō-blas-tē′mă). All the cells collectively which constitute the early undifferentiated mesoderm. [meso- + G. *blastēma,* a sprout]

mes·o·blas·tem·ic (mez′ō-blas-tē′mik). Relating to or derived from the mesoblastema.

mes·o·blas·tic (mez′ō-blas′tik). Relating to or derived from the mesoderm.

mes·o·car·dia (mez′ō-kar′dē-ă). **1.** Atypical position of the heart in a central position in the chest, as in early embryonic life. **2.** Plural of mesocardium. [meso- + G. *kardia*, heart]

mes·o·car·di·um, pl. **mes·o·car·dia** (mez-ō-kar′dē-ŭm). The double layer of splanchnic mesoderm supporting the embryonic heart in the pericardial cavity. It disappears before birth. [meso- + G. *kardia*, heart]

dorsal m., the part of the m. dorsal to the embryonic heart; it breaks down to form the transverse sinus of the pericardium.

ventral m., the part of the m. ventral to the embryonic cardiac tube; transitory in all vertebrates; in the higher mammals, it breaks through as soon as its component layers of epicardium make contact with each other.

mes·o·car·pal (mez′ō-kar′păl). SYN midcarpal.

mes·o·ce·cal (mez′ō-sē′kăl). Relating to the mesocecum.

mes·o·ce·cum (mez′ō-sē′kŭm). Part of the mesocolon, supporting the cecum, that occasionally persists when the ascending colon becomes retroperitoneal during fetal life. SYN mesentery of cecum. [meso- + cecum]

mes·o·ce·phal·ic (mez′ō-se-fal′ik). Having a head of medium length; denoting a skull with a cephalic index between 75 and 80 and with a capacity of 1350 to 1450 ml, or an individual with such a skull. SYN mesaticephalic, mesocephalous, normocephalic. [meso- + G. *kephalē*, head]

mes·o·ceph·a·lous (mez′ō-sef′ă-lŭs). SYN mesocephalic.

Mes·o·ces·toi·des (mez-ō-ses-toy′dēz). Tapeworm genus found in carnivorous mammals, such as foxes; mites probably intermediate hosts; few human cases identified in Japan, the United States, and China.

mes·o·col·ic (mez′ō-kol′ik). Relating to the mesocolon.

mes·o·co·lon (mez′ō-kō′lon) [TA]. The fold of peritoneum attaching the colon to the posterior abdominal wall; ascending m. [TA] (m. ascendens [TA]), transverse m. [TA] (m. transversum [TA]), descending m. [TA] (m. descendens [TA]), and sigmoid m. [TA] (m. sigmoideum [TA]) correspond to the respective divisions of the colon; the ascending and descending portions are usually fused to the peritoneum of the posterior abdominal wall, but can be mobilized. [meso- + *kolon*, colon]

mes·o·co·lo·pexy (mez′ō-kō′lō-pek-sē). An operation for shortening the mesocolon, for correction of undue mobility and ptosis. SYN mesocoloplication. [meso- + G. *kolon*, colon, + *pēxis*, fixation]

mes·o·co·lo·pli·ca·tion (mes′ō-kō′lō-pli-kā′shŭn). SYN mesocolopexy. [meso- + G. *kolon*, colon, + L. *plico*, pp. *-atus*, to fold]

mes·o·cord (mez′ō-kōrd). A fold of amnion that sometimes binds a segment of the umbilical cord to the placenta.

mes·o·cu·ne·i·form (mez-ō-koo′nē-i-fōrm). SYN intermediate cuneiform (*bone*).

mes·o·derm (mez′ō-derm). The middle of the three primary germ layers of the embryo (the others being ectoderm and endoderm); m. is the origin of connective tissues, myoblasts, blood, the cardiovascular and lymphatic systems, most of the urogenital system, and the lining of the pericardial, pleural, and peritoneal cavities. SYN mesoblast. [meso- + G. *derma*, skin]

branchial m., m. surrounding the primitive stomodeum and pharynx; it contributes to the pharyngeal arches.

extraembryonic m., extraembryonic cells which, though derived from the zygote, are not part of the embryo proper and contribute to the fetal membranes (e.g., amnion). SYN primary m.

gastral m., m. in lower vertebrates formed by constriction from the roof of the archenteron or yolk sac.

intermediate m., a continuous band of m. between the segmented paraxial m. medially and the lateral plate m. laterally; from it develops the nephrogenic cord.

intraembryonic m., m. derived from the primitive streak and lying between the ectoderm and endoderm. SYN secondary m.

lateral m., SYN lateral plate m.

lateral plate m., the peripheral portion of intraembryonic m. that is continuous with the extraembryonic m. beyond the margins of the embryonic disk; it forms the somatic and splanchnic m. between which develops the intraembryonic celom. SYN lateral m.

paraxial m., the m. lying at either side of the midline embryonic notochord; on segmentation, it forms the paired somites.

primary m., SYN extraembryonic m.

prostomial m., m. that arises in lower vertebrates by continued proliferation at the lateral lips of the blastopore.

secondary m., SYN intraembryonic m.

somatic m., the m. adjacent to the ectoderm in the early embryo, after formation of the intraembryonic celom; the limbs and body wall are derived, in part, from it.

somitic m., m. derived from cells situated in or derived from somites.

splanchnic m., the layer of lateral plate m. adjacent to the endoderm.

visceral m., the splanchnic m. or the branchial m.

mes·o·der·mal (mez-ō-der′mal). Pertaining to the mesoderm.

mes·o·der·mic (mez-ō-der′mik). Relating to the mesoderm.

mes·o·di·a·stol·ic (mez-ō-dī-ă-stol′ik). Middiastolic.

mes·o·dont (mez′ō-dont). Having teeth of medium size; denoting a skull with a dental index between 42 and 43.9. [meso- + G. *odous*, tooth]

mes·o·du·o·de·nal (mez′ō-doo-ō-dē′năl). Relating to the mesoduodenum.

mes·o·du·o·de·num (mez′ō-doo′ō-dē′nŭm, -doo-od′ĕ-nŭm). The mesentery of the duodenum.

mes·o·en·te·ri·o·lum (mes′ō-en-ter-ē′ō-lŭm). SYN mesenteriolum.

mes·o·ep·i·did·y·mis (mez-ō-ep-i-did′i-mis). An occasional fold of the tunica vaginalis binding the epididymis to the testis. [meso- + epididymis]

mes·o·gas·ter (mez-ō-gas′ter). SYN mesogastrium.

mes·o·gas·tric (mez-ō-gas′trik). Relating to the mesogastrium.

mes·o·gas·tri·um (mez-ō-gas′trē-ŭm). In the embryo, the mesentery of the dilated portion of the enteric canal that is the future stomach; it gives rise to the greater omentum and consequently is involved in the formation of the omental bursa. The spleen and body of the pancreas develop within it, and thus the splenorenal and gastrosplenic ligaments are derivatives of the (dorsal) mesogastrium. SYN dorsal m., mesogaster. [meso- + G. *gastēr* stomach]

dorsal m., SYN mesogastrium.

ventral m., the primitive midline mesentery extending between future stomach and proximal duodenum and the anterior abdominal wall superior to the umbilicus (umbilical vein). The liver develops within it, and consequently the lesser omentum, coronary and falciform ligaments are derivatives of it. The umbilical vein runs in its caudal free edge, becoming the postnatal round ligament of the liver.

mes·o·gen·ic (mez-ō-jen′ik). Denoting the virulence of a virus capable of inducing lethal infection in embryonic hosts, after a short incubation period, and an inapparent infection in immature and adult hosts; used in characterizing Newcastle disease virus, particularly strains used in parenteral vaccination of chickens. [meso- + G. *-gen*, producing]

me·sog·li·a (me-sog′lē-ă). Neuroglial cells of mesodermal origin. SEE ALSO microglia. SYN mesoglial cells. [meso- + G. *glia*, glue]

mes·o·glu·te·al (mez′ō-gloo′tē-ăl). Relating to the musculus gluteus medius.

mes·o·glu·te·us (mez′ō-gloo-tē′ŭs). SYN gluteus medius (*muscle*).

mes·o·gnath·ic (mez-ō-nath′ik, -og-nath′ik). **1.** Relating to the mesognathion. **2.** SYN mesognathous.

mes·o·gna·thi·on (mez′ō-nā′thē-on, -og-nā′thē-on, nath′ē-on). The lateral segment of the premaxillary or incisive bone external to the endognathion. [meso- + G. *gnathos*, jaw]

me·sog·na·thous (me-zog′nă-thŭs). Having a face with slightly projecting jaw, one with a gnathic index from 98 to 103. SYN mesognathic (2).

mes·o·il·e·um (mez-ō-il′ē-ŭm). The mesentery of the ileum.

mes·o·je·ju·num (mez'ō-je-joo'nŭm). The mesentery of the jejunum.

me·sol·o·bus (me-sol'ŏ-bŭs). Obsolete term for *corpus* callosum. [meso- + L. *lobus*, lobe]

mes·o·lym·pho·cyte (mez-ō-lim'fō-sīt). A mononuclear leukocyte of medium size, probably a lymphocyte, with a deeply staining nucleus of large size but relatively smaller than that in most lymphocytes. [meso- + lymphocyte]

mes·o·me·lia (mez-ō-mē'lē-ă). The condition of having abnormally short forearms and lower legs. [meso- + G. *melos*, limb]

mes·o·mel·ic (mez-ō-mē'lik). Pertaining to the middle segment of a limb.

mes·o·mere (mez'ō-mēr). **1.** A blastomere of a size intermediate between a macromere and a micromere. **2.** The zone between an epimere and a hypomere. [meso- + G. *meros*, part]

mes·o·mer·ic (mez-ō-mer'ik). Pertaining to mesomerism.

me·som·er·ism (mĕ-som'er-izm). Displacement or delocalization of electrons within a molecule in such a way as to create fractional charges on different parts of the molecule; resonance.

mes·o·me·tri·um (mez'ō-mē'trē-ŭm). The broad ligament of the uterus, below the mesosalpinx. [meso- + G. *mētra*, uterus]

mes·o·morph (mez'ō-mōrf). A constitutional body type or build (biotype or somatotype) in which tissues that originate from the mesoderm prevail; from the morphological standpoint, there is a balance between trunk and limbs. SEE ALSO hypermorph, hypomorph, ectomorph, endomorph. SYN mediotype. [meso- + G. *morphē*, form]

mes·o·mor·phic (mez-ō-mōrf'ik). Relating to mesomorphs.

me·son (mez'on, mē'zon, mes'on). An elementary particle having a rest mass intermediate in value between the mass of an electron and that of a proton. [G. neuter of *mesos*, middle]

mes·o·neph·ric (mez-ō-nef'rik). Relating to the mesonephros.

mes·o·neph·roi (mez-ō-nef'roy). Plural of mesonephros.

mes·o·ne·phro·ma (mez'ō-ne-frō'mă). Obsolete term for a relatively rare malignant neoplasm of the ovary and corpus uteri, thought to originate in mesonephric structures that become misplaced in ovarian tissue during embryonic development; characterized by a tubular pattern, with focal proliferation of epithelial cells with clear cytoplasm or of the hob-nail type; so-called glomeruloid structures are reported, i.e., small convolutions or tufts of tiny tubate formations with capillaries extending into the spaces. SYN clear cell carcinoma, mesonephric adenocarcinoma, mesonephroid tumor, wolffian duct carcinoma. [mesonephros + -*oma*, tumor]

mes·o·neph·ros, pl. **mes·o·neph·roi** (mez'ō-nef'ros, -roy). One of three excretory organs appearing in the evolution of vertebrates; in life forms with a metanephros, the m. is located between the regressing pronephros and the metanephros, cephalic to the latter. In young mammalian embryos, the m. is well developed and briefly functional until establishment of the metanephros, the definitive kidney; in older embryos, the m. undergoes regression as an excretory organ, but its duct system is retained in the male as the epididymis and ductus deferens. SYN middle kidney, wolffian body. [meso- + G. *nephros*, kidney]

mes·o·neu·ri·tis (mez'ō-noo-rī'tis). Inflammation of a nerve or of its connective tissue without involvement of its sheath.

nodular m., inflammation of the connective tissue beneath the nerve sheath, with the formation of circumscribed fibrous thickenings.

meso-on·to·morph (mez-ō-on'tō-mōrf). A broad, stocky individual. [meso- + G. *ōn*, being, + *morphē*, form]

mes·o·pexy (mez'ō-pek-sē). SYN mesenteriopexy.

mes·o·phil, mes·o·phile (mez'ō-fil, -fīl). A microorganism with an optimum temperature between 25°C and 40°C, but growing within the limits of 10°C and 45°C. [meso- + G. *philos*, fond]

mes·o·phil·ic (mez'ō-fil'ik). Pertaining to a mesophil.

mes·o·phle·bi·tis (mez'ō-flĕ-bī'tis). Inflammation of the middle coat of a vein. [meso- + phlebitis]

mes·o·phrag·ma (mez-ō-frag'mă). SYN M *line*. [meso- + G. *phragma*, a fence]

me·soph·ry·on (mez-of'ri-on). SYN glabella (2). [meso- + Gr. *ophrys*, eyebrow]

me·sop·ic (me-zō'pik). Pertaining to illumination between the photopic and scotopic ranges. [meso- + G. *opsis*, vision]

mes·o·pneu·mo·ni·um (mez'ō-noo-mō'nē-um). The reflection of pleura surrounding the root of the lung (including the pulmonary ligament inferiorly) as parietal pleura becomes continuous with the visceral pleura of the lung. SYN mesentery of lung, pleural isthmus.

mes·o·por·phy·rins (mez-ō-pōr'fi-rinz). Porphyrin compounds resembling the protoporphyrins except that the vinyl side chains of the latter are reduced to ethyl side chains; e.g., mesobilane.

mes·o·proc·ton. SYN rectosacral *fascia*.

mes·o·pro·sop·ic (mez'ō-prō-sop'ik). Having a face of moderate width, i.e., with a facial index of about 90. [meso- + G. *prosōpon*, face]

mes·o·pul·mon·um (mez-ō-pŭl'mon-ŭm). The mesentery of the embryonic lung. [meso- + L. *pulmo*, lung]

me·sor·chi·al (mez-ōr'kē-ăl). Relating to the mesorchium.

me·sor·chi·um (mez-ōr'kē-ŭm). **1.** In the fetus, a fold of tunica vaginalis testis supporting the mesonephros and the developing testis. **2.** In the adult, a fold of tunica vaginalis testis between the testis and epididymis. [meso- + G. *orchis*, testis]

mes·o·rec·tum (mez'ō-rek'tŭm). The peritoneal investment of the rectum, covering the upper part only.

mes·o·rid·a·zine be·syl·ate (mez-ō-rid'ă-zēn). A biotransformation product of thioridazine; an antipsychotic.

mes·or·rha·phy (mez-ōr'ă-fē). SYN mesenteriorrhaphy.

mes·or·rhine (mez'ō-rin). Having a nose of moderate width. Denoting a skull with a nasal index from 47 to 51 (Frankfort agreement) or 48 to 53 (Broca). [meso- + G. *rhis* (rhin-), nose]

mes·o·sal·pinx (mez'ō-sal'pinks) [TA]. The part of the broad ligament investing the uterine (fallopian) tube. [meso- + G. *salpinx*, trumpet]

mes·o·scope (mez'ō-skōp). An instrument for viewing objects that are larger than microscopic but cannot be seen distinctly with the naked eye. [meso- + G. *skopeō*, to view]

mes·o·seme (mez'ō-sēm). Denoting an orbital aperture with an index between 84 and 89; characteristic of the white race. [meso- + G. *sēma*, sign]

mes·o·sig·moid (mez'ō-sig'moyd). Sigmoid mesocolon. SEE mesocolon.

mes·o·sig·moid·i·tis (mes'ō-sig-moy-dī'tis). Inflammation of the mesosigmoid.

mes·o·sig·moid·o·pexy (mez-ō-sig-moy'dō-pek-sē). Surgical fixation of the mesosigmoid.

mes·o·so·ma·tous (mez'ō-so'mă-tŭs). Denoting a person of medium height.

mes·o·some (mes'ōsom). A convoluted membranous body formed by involution of the plasma membranes of certain bacteria; it functions in cellular respiration and septum formation. [meso + G. *soma*, body]

mes·o·so·mia (mez'ō-sō'mē-ă). Medium height. [meso- + G. *sōma*, body]

mes·o·ste·ni·um (mez'ō-stē'nē-ŭm). SYN mesentery (2).

mes·o·ster·num (mez'ō-ster'nŭm). SYN *body* of sternum. [meso- + G. *sternon*, chest]

mes·o·sys·tol·ic (mez'ō-sis-tol'ik). Midsystolic.

mes·o·tar·sal (mez'ō-tar'săl). SYN midtarsal.

mes·o·ten·di·ne·um (mez'ō-ten-din'ē-ŭm) [TA]. SYN mesotendon.

mes·o·ten·don (mez'ō-ten'don) [TA]. The synovial layers that pass from a tendon to the wall of a tendon sheath in certain places where tendons lie within osteofibrous canals. In most instances, the m. degenerates, leaving only the vinculae. SYN mesotendineum [TA].

mes·o·the·lia (mez-ō-thē'lē-ă). Plural of mesothelium.

mes·o·the·li·al (mez-ō-thē'lē-ăl). Relating to the mesothelium.

🔲**mes·o·the·li·o·ma** (mez'ō-thē-lē-ō'mă). A rare neoplasm derived from the lining cells of the pleura and peritoneum which grows as a thick sheet covering the viscera, and is composed of spindle cells or fibrous tissue which may enclose glandlike spaces lined by cuboidal cells. [mesothelium + G. -oma, tumor]

benign m., SYN solitary fibrous *tumor.*

benign m. of genital tract, SYN adenomatoid *tumor.*

mes·o·the·li·um, pl. **mes·o·the·lia** (mez-ō-thē′lē-ŭm, -lē-ă). A single layer of flattened cells forming an epithelium that lines serous cavities; e.g., peritoneum, pleura, pericardium. [meso- + epithelium]

mes·o·tho·ri·um (mez′ō-thōr′ē-ŭm). The first two disintegration products of thorium; mesothorium 1 is ^{228}Ra, a beta emitter with a half-life of 6.7 years, decaying into mesothorium 2, which is ^{228}Ac, a beta emitter with a half-life of 6.13 hr, which disintegrates to radiothorium (^{228}Th).

mes·o·tro·pic (mez′ō-trop′ik). Turned toward the median plane. [meso- + G. *tropē,* a turning]

mes·o·tym·pan·um (mez-ō-tim′pan-um). The portion of the middle ear medial to the tympanic membrane.

mes·o·u·ran·ic (mes′ō-ū-ran′ik). Having a palatal index between 110 and 115. SYN mesuranic. [meso- + G. *ouranos,* palate]

mes·o·va·ri·um, pl. **mes·o·va·ria** (mez′ō-vā′rē-ŭm, -ă) [TA]. Portion of the broad ligament of the uterus that reflects onto and suspends the ovary. SYN mesoarium. [meso- + L. *ovarium,* ovary]

Mes·o·zoa (mez-ō-zō′ă). A small phylum of about 50 species of parasites of marine invertebrates with complex life cycles. M. are classified with the Metazoa, but they are regarded by some observers as intermediate between unicellular and multicellular animals; others consider them a degenerate group of flatworms. M. are divided into two very distinct orders, the Orthonectida and Dicyemida; the latter are nephridial parasites of squids, octopods, and cuttlefish. [meso- + G. *zōon,* animal]

mes·sen·ger (mes′en-jer). **1.** That which carries a message. **2.** Having message-carrying properties.

first m., a hormone that binds to a receptor on the surface cell and, in so doing, communicates with intracellular metabolic processes.

second m., an intermediary molecule that is generated as a consequence of hormone-receptor interaction; e.g., see adenosine 3′,5′-cyclic monophosphate, guanosine 3′,5′-cyclic monophosphate, calcium, inositide.

mes·sen·ger RNA (mRNA). See under ribonucleic acid.

mes·tan·o·lone (mes-tan′ŏ-lōn). An androgenic steroid with anabolic properties.

mes·tene·di·ol (mes-tēn′dī-ol). SYN methandriol.

mes·tra·nol (mes′tră-nōl). The 3-methyl ether of ethynyl estradiol; an estrogen used in many oral contraceptive preparations.

me·sul·phen (mĕ-sŭl′fen). A topical scabicide with antipruritic properties.

me·su·ran·ic (mez′ū-ran′ik). SYN mesouranic.

MET Abbreviation for metabolic *equivalent.*

Met Symbol for methionine or methionyl.

♻**meta-.** In medicine and biology, a prefix denoting the concept of after, subsequent to, behind, or hindmost. Cf. post-. [G. after, between, over]

♻**meta-.** **1.** In chemistry, an italicized prefix denoting joint, action sharing. **2** (*m-*). In chemistry, an italicized prefix denoting a compound formed by two substitutions in the benzene ring separated by one carbon atom, i.e., linked to the first and third, second and fourth, etc., carbon atoms of the ring. For terms beginning with *meta-,* or *m-,* see the specific name. [G. after, between, over]

met·a·anal·y·sis (met′ă-ă-nal′i-sis). The process of using statistical methods to combine the results of different studies; systematic, organized, and structured evaluation of a problem using information, commonly in the form of statistical tables, from a number of different studies of a problem.

me·tab·a·sis (mĕ-tab′ă-sis). Rarely used term for a change of any kind in symptoms or course of a disease. [G. a passing over, change, fr. *metabainō,* to pass over]

met·a·bi·o·sis (met′ă-bī-ō′sis). Dependence of one organism on

another for its existence. SEE ALSO commensalism, mutualism, parasitism. [meta- + G. *biōsis,* way of life]

met·a·bol·ic (met-ă-bol′ik). Relating to metabolism.

met·a·bo·lim·e·ter (met′ă-bŏ-lim′ĕ-ter). A modified calorimeter for measuring the rate of basal metabolism.

me·tab·o·lin (mĕ-tab′ō-lin). SYN metabolite.

me·tab·o·lism (mĕ-tab′ō-lizm). **1.** The sum of the chemical and physical changes occurring in tissue, consisting of anabolism, those reactions that convert small molecules into large, and catabolism, those reactions that convert large molecules into small, including both endogenous large molecules as well as biodegradation of xenobiotics. **2.** Often incorrectly used as a synonym for either anabolism or catabolism. [G. *metabolē,* change]

basal m., oxygen utilization of an individual during minimal physiologic activity while awake; an obsolete test determined by measuring oxygen consumption of a fasting subject at complete bodily and mental rest and a room temperature of 20°C. SYN basal metabolic rate.

carbohydrate m., oxidation, breakdown, and synthesis of carbohydrates in the tissues.

electrolyte m., the chemical changes that various essential minerals (e.g., sodium, potassium, calcium, magnesium) undergo in the tissues.

energy m., those metabolic reactions whose role is to release or to provide energy.

fat m., oxidation, decomposition, and synthesis of fats in the tissues.

first-pass m., the intestinal and hepatic degradation or alteration of a drug or substance taken by mouth, after absorption, removing some of the active substance from the blood before it enters the general circulation. SYN first-pass effect.

inborn error of m., a genetic biochemical disorder of a specific enzyme that forms a metabolic block, e.g., phenylketonuria.

intermediary m., the sum of all metabolic reactions between uptake of foodstuffs and formation of excretory products.

oxidative m., SYN ventilation (2).

primary m., metabolic processes central to most cells; e.g., biosynthesis of macromolecules, energy production, turnover, etc.

protein m., decomposition and synthesis of protein in the tissues. SYN proteometabolism.

respiratory m., the exchange of respiratory gases in the lungs, oxidation of foodstuffs in the tissues, and production of carbon dioxide and water.

secondary m., metabolic processes in which substances (such as pigments, alkaloids, terpenes, etc.) are only synthesized in certain types of tissues or cells or are only synthesized under certain conditions.

me·tab·o·lite (mĕ-tab′ō-līt). Any product or substrate (foodstuff, intermediate, waste product) of metabolism, especially of catabolism. SYN metabolin.

primary m., a m. synthesized in a step in primary metabolism.

secondary m., a m. synthesized in a step in secondary metabolism.

me·tab·o·lize (mĕ-tab′ō-līz). To undergo the chemical changes of metabolism.

met·a·car·pal (met′ă-kar′păl). **1.** Relating to the metacarpus. **2.** Any one of the metacarpal bones. SEE metacarpal (*bones*) [I–V], under *bone.*

met·a·car·pec·to·my (met′ă-kar-pek′tō-mē). Excision of one or all of the metacarpals. [metacarpus + G. *ektomē,* excision]

met·a·car·po·pha·lan·ge·al (met′ă-kar′pō-fă-lan′jē-ăl). Relating to the metacarpus and the phalanges; denoting the articulations between them.

met·a·car·pus, pl. **met·a·car·pi** (met′ă-kar′pŭs, -kar′pī). The five bones of the hand between the carpus and the phalanges. [meta- + G. *karpos,* wrist]

met·a·cen·tric (met-ă-sen′trik). Having the centromere about equidistant from the extremities, said of a chromosome. [meta- + G. *kentron,* circle]

met·a·cer·ca·ria, pl. **met·a·cer·ca·ri·ae** (met′ă-ser-kar′ē-ă, -ē). The post-cercarial encysted stage in the life history of a fluke,

me

prior to transfer to the definitive host. Some cercariae attach themselves to grass or other vegetation, form m., and later are ingested by herbivores, as in *Fasciola* and similar forms; others encyst in muscles of fish, as in *Clonorchis*, or in crayfish, as in *Paragonimus*. [meta- + G. *kerkos*, tail]

met·a·ces·tode (met-ă-ses′tōd). The larval stages of a tapeworm, including the metamorphosis of the oncosphere to the first evidence of sexuality in the adult worm, differentiation of the scolex, and beginning of proglottid formation; it includes the procercoid and plerocercoid stages of pseudophyllid cestodes, and the cysticercus, cysticercoid, coenurus, and hydatid stages of cyclophyllidean cestodes.

met·a·chlo·ral (met-ă-klō′răl). SYN *m*-chloral.

met·a·chro·ma·sia (met′ă-krō-mā′zē-ă). **1.** The condition in which a cell or tissue component takes on a color different from the dye solution with which it is stained. SYN metachromatism (2). **2.** A change in the characteristic color of certain basic thiazine dyes, such as toluidine blue, when the dye molecules are bound in proximate array to tissue polyanionic polymers, such as glycosaminoglycans. [meta- + G. *chrōma*, color]

met·a·chro·mat·ic (met′ă-krō-mat′ik). Denoting cells or dyes that exhibit metachromasia. SYN metachromophil, metachromophile.

met·a·chro·ma·tism (met-ă-krō′mă-tizm). **1.** Any color change, whether natural or produced by basic aniline dyes. **2.** SYN metachromasia (1). [meta- + G. *chrōma*, color]

met·a·chrom·ing (met′ă-krō′ming). The process of mixing a metal mordant with a dye before applying the dye to a tissue or fabric.

met·a·chro·mo·phil, met·a·chro·mo·phile (met-ă-krō′mō-fil, -fīl). SYN metachromatic. [meta- + G. *chrōma*, color, + *philos*, fond]

me·tach·ro·nous (mĕ-tak′rō-nŭs). Not synchronous; multiple separate occurrences, such as multiple primary cancers developing at intervals. [meta- + G. *chronos*, time]

met·a·chro·sis (met-ă-krō′sis). A change of color, such as occurs in certain animals, e.g., the chameleon, by expansion and contraction of chromatophores. [meta- + G. *chrōsis*, a coloring]

met·a·cone (met′ă-kōn). The distobuccal cusp of an upper molar tooth. [meta- + G. *kōnos*, cone]

met·a·co·nid (met-ă-kon′id, -kō′nid). The mesolingual cusp of a lower molar tooth.

met·a·con·trast (met-ă-kon′trast). Inhibition of the brightness of illumination when an adjacent visual field is illuminated.

met·a·con·ule (met-ă-kon′ūl). The distal intermediate cusp of an upper molar tooth. [meta- + G. *kōnos*, a cone]

met·a·cre·sol (met-ă-krē′sol). SYN *m*-cresol.

met·a·cryp·to·zo·ite (met′ă-krip-tō-zō′īt). The exoerythrocytic stage that develops from merozoites formed by the first, or cryptozoite, generation; the cryptozoite and metacryptozoite generations comprise the primary exoerythrocytic stages of malaria development (prepatent period) prior to infection of red blood cells. [meta- + G. *kryptos*, hidden, + *zōon*, animal]

met·a·dys·en·tery (met-ă-dis′en-tār-ē). Old term for bacillary *dysentery*.

Met·a·gon·i·mus (met-ă-gon′i-mŭs). A genus of flukes (superfamily Heterophyundea) that encyst on fish and infect various fish-eating animals, including humans. *M. yokogawai*, an intestinal fluke widely distributed in the Far East and the Balkans and one of the smallest (1–2.5 mm) flukes infecting humans, is passed from *Semisulcospira* snails to cyprinoid fish and then to humans and other fish-eating mammals and birds. [meta- + G. *gonimos*, productive]

met·a·ic·ter·ic (met-ă-ik′ter-ik). Occurring as a sequel of jaundice. [meta- + G. *ikterikos*, jaundiced]

met·a·in·fec·tive (met′ă-in-fek′tiv). Occurring subsequent to an infection; denoting specifically a febrile condition sometimes observed during convalescence from an infectious disease.

met·a·ki·ne·sis, met·a·ki·ne·sia (met′ă-ki-nē′sis, -ki-nē′sē-ă). Moving apart; the separation of the two chromatids of each chro-

mosome and their movement to opposite poles in the anaphase of mitosis. [meta- + G. *kinēsis*, movement]

met·al (M) (met′ăl). One of the electropositive elements, either amphoteric or basic, usually characterized by properties such as luster, malleability, ductility, the ability to conduct electricity, and the tendency to lose rather than gain electrons in chemicals. [L. *metallum*, a mine, a mineral, fr. G. *metallon*, a mine, pit]

> **alkali m.,** an alkali of the family Li, Na, K, Rb, Cs, and Fr, all of which have highly ionized hydroxides. SYN alkali (3).
>
> **alkali earth m.,** SEE alkaline earth *elements*, under *element*.
>
> **Babbitt m.,** an alloy of antimony, copper, and tin; used occasionally in dentistry.
>
> **base m., basic m.,** a m. that is readily oxidized; e.g., iron, copper.
>
> **colloidal m.,** a colloidal solution of a m. obtained by passing electric sparks between terminals of the m. in distilled water. SYN electrosol.
>
> **d'Arcet m.,** an alloy of lead, bismuth, and tin; used in dentistry.
>
> **fusible m.,** a m. with a low melting point.
>
> **heavy m.,** a m. with a high specific gravity, typically larger than 5; e.g., Fe, Co, Cu, Mn, Mo, Zn, V.
>
> **light m.,** a m. with a specific gravity of less than 4.
>
> **noble m.,** a m. that cannot be oxidized by heat alone, nor readily dissolved by acid; e.g., gold, platinum. SYN noble element.
>
> **rare earth m.,** SEE lanthanides.
>
> **respiratory m.,** a m. present in certain respiratory pigments; e.g., iron, manganese, copper, vanadium.

met·al·de·hyde (met-al′dĕ-hīd). A polymer of acetaldehyde. [meta- + aldehyde]

me·tal·lic (mĕ-tal′ik). Relating to, composed of, or resembling metal.

metallo-. Metal, metallic. [see metal]

me·tal·lo·cy·a·nide (mĕ-tal-ō-sī′ă-nīd). A compound of cyanogen with a metal forming an ionic radical that combines with a basic element to form a salt; e.g., potassium ferricyanide, $K_3Fe(CN)_6$.

me·tal·lo·en·zyme (mĕ-tal-ō-en′zīm). An enzyme containing a metal (ion) as an integral part of its active structure; e.g., cytochromes (Fe, Cu), aldehyde oxidase (Mo), catechol oxidase (Cu), carbonic anhydrase (Zn).

me·tal·lo·fla·vo·de·hy·drog·e·nase (mĕ-tal′ō-flā′vō-dē-hī′drō-jen-ās). A type of oxidizing enzyme, containing one of the flavin nucleotides as coenzyme, plus a metal ion that is also necessary to the action; the metal may be Fe (as in succinate dehydrogenase), Cu (as in urate oxidase), or Mo (as in xanthine oxidase).

me·tal·lo·fla·vo·en·zyme (mĕ-tal′ō-flā-vō-en′zīm). An enzyme that contains one of the flavin nucleotides and at least one metal ion as a required part of its active structure.

me·tal·lo·fla·vo·pro·tein (mĕ-tal′ō-flā′vō-prō-tēn). A protein containing a flavin entity and at least one metal ion.

met·al·loid (met′ă-loyd). Resembling a metal in at least one amphoteric form; e.g., silicon and germanium as semiconductors. [metal + G. *eidos*, resemblance]

me·tal·lo·phil·ia (mĕ-tal′ō-fil′ē-ă). Affinity for metal salts; e.g., the affinity of the cytoplasm of cells of the reticuloendothelial system for silver carbonate stain and salts of gold and iron. [metallo- + G. *philos*, fond]

me·tal·lo·pho·bia (mĕ-tal-ō-fō′bē-ă). Morbid fear of metal objects. [G. *metallon*, metal, + *phobos*, fear]

me·tal·lo·por·phy·rin (mĕ-tal-ō-pōr′fi-rin). A combination of a porphyrin with a metal, e.g., Fe (heme), Mg (as in chlorophyll), Cu (in hemocyanin), Zn.

me·tal·lo·pro·tein (mĕ-tal-ō-prō′tēn). A protein with a tightly bound metal ion or ions; e.g., hemoglobin.

metalloproteinase (met′a-lō-prō′tēn-āz). A family of protein-hydrolyzing endopeptidases that contain zinc ions as part of the active structure.

> **matrix m.,** a subfamily of endopeptidases that hydrolyze extracellular proteins, especially collagens and elastin. By regulating the integrity and composition of the extracellular matrix, these enzymes play a pivotal role in the control of signals elicited by

matrix molecules that regulate cell proliferation, differentiation, and death.

me·tal·lo·thi·o·nein (mĕ-tal-ō-thī′ō-nēn). Any of a group of small proteins, rich in cysteinyl residues, that is synthesized in the liver and kidney in response to the presence of divalent ions (zinc, mercury, cadmium, copper, etc.) and that binds these ions tightly; of importance in ion transport and detoxification; the apoprotein is thionein.

met·a·lu·et·ic (met′ă-loo-et′ik). **1.** SYN metasyphilitic (1). **2.** SYN metasyphilitic (2). **3.** SYN parasyphilitic. [meta- + L. *lues,* pestilence]

met·a·mer (met′ă-mer). **1.** An entity that is similar to, but ultimately differentiable from, another entity. **2.** Structural isomer. [meta- + -mer]

met·a·mere (met′ă-mēr). One of a series of homologous segments in the body. SEE ALSO somite. [meta- + G. *meros,* part]

met·a·mer·ic (met-ă-mer′ik). **1.** Relating to or showing metamerism, or occurring in a metamere. **2.** Referring to a metamer.

me·tam·er·ism (me-tam′er-izm). **1.** A type of anatomic structure exhibiting serially homologous metameres; in primitive forms, such as the annelids, the metameres are almost alike in structure; in vertebrates, specialization in the cephalic region masks the underlying m., which is still clearly evident in serially repeated vertebrae, ribs, intercostal muscles, and spinal nerves, and in young vertebrate embryos. **2.** In chemistry, rarely used synonym for structural isomerism.

met·a·mor·phop·sia (met′ă-mōr-fop′sē-ă). Distortion of visual images. [meta- + G. *morphē,* shape, + *opsis,* vision]

met·a·mor·pho·sis (met-ă-mōr′fŏ-sis, -mōr-fō′sis). **1.** A change in form, structure, or function. **2.** Transition from one developmental stage to another. SYN allaxis, transformation (1). [G. *metamorphosos,* transformation fr. *meta,* beyond, over, + *morphē,* form]

complete m., insect development from egg, through successive larval instars, pupa, and adult; the latter is distinct from the first two forms of the insect, permitting specialization of feeding (larval) and reproductive-flying functions (adult); characteristic of the higher insect orders, such as Coleoptera (beetles), Hymenoptera (bees, wasps, ants), Diptera (two-winged flies), and Siphonaptera (fleas). SYN holometabolous m.

fatty m., the appearance of microscopically visible droplets of fat in the cytoplasm of cells. SEE ALSO fatty *degeneration.* SYN fatty change.

heterometabolous m., SYN incomplete m.

holometabolous m., SYN complete m.

incomplete m., the development of a nymph into the imago which in many respects resembles the former; characteristic of more primitive insect orders, such as Heteroptera (true bugs), Orthoptera (locusts, grasshoppers), and Blatterria (roaches). SYN heterometabolous m.

retrograde m., SYN degeneration (3); **(1)** SYN cataplasia.

met·a·mor·phot·ic (met′ă-mōr-fot′ik). Relating to or marked by metamorphosis.

met·a·my·el·o·cyte (met-ă-mī′el-ō-sīt). A transitional form of myelocyte with nuclear construction that is intermediate between the mature myelocyte (myelocyte C of Sabin) and the two-lobed granular leukocyte. SYN juvenile cell. [meta- + G. *myelos,* marrow, + *kytos,* cell]

met·a·neph·ric (met-ă-nef′rik). Of or pertaining to the metanephron.

met·a·neph·rine (met-ă-nef′rin). A catabolite of epinephrine found, together with normetanephrine, in the urine and in some tissues, resulting from the action of catechol-*O*-methyltransferase on epinephrine; has no sympathomimetic actions.

met·a·neph·ro·gen·ic, met·a·ne·phrog·e·nous (met′ă-nef-rō-jen′ik, -nĕ-froj′ĕ-nŭs). Applied to the more caudal part of the intermediate mesoderm which, under the inductive action of the metanephric diverticulum, has the potency to form metanephric tubules. [meta- + G. *nephros,* kidney, + *-gen,* producing]

met·a·neph·ros, pl. **met·a·neph·roi** (met-ă-nef′ros, -roy). The most caudally located of the three excretory organs appearing in

the evolution of the vertebrates (the others being the pronephros and the mesonephros); in mammalian embryos, the m. develops caudal to the mesonephros during its regression, becoming the permanent kidney. SYN hind kidney. [meta- + G. *nephros,* kidney]

met·a·neu·tro·phil, met·a·neu·tro·phile (met-ă-noo′trō-fil, -fīl). Not staining normally with neutral dyes. [meta- + L. *neuter,* neither, + G. *philos,* fond]

met·a·nil yel·low (mĕt′ă-nil) [C.I. 13065]. A monoazo acid dye, $C_{18}H_{14}N_3O_3SNa$, used as a cytoplasmic and connective tissue stain.

metaperiodic acid. SYN periodic acid (1).

met·a·phase (met′ă-fās). The stage of mitosis or meiosis in which the chromosomes become aligned on the equatorial plate of the cell separating the centromeres. In mitosis and in the second meiotic division, the centromeres of each chromosome divide and the two daughter centromeres are directed toward opposite poles of the cell; in the first division of meiosis, the centromeres do not divide but the centromeres of each pair of homologous chromosomes become directed toward opposite poles. [meta- + G. *phasis,* an appearance]

met·a·phos·phor·ic ac·id (met′ă-fos-fōr′ik). SYN glacial *phosphoric acid.*

met·a·phy·si·al, met·a·phy·se·al (met-ă-fiz′ē-ăl). Relating to a metaphysis.

me·taph·y·sis, pl. **me·taph·y·ses** (mĕ-taf′i-sis, -sēz) [TA]. A conical section of bone between the epiphysis and diaphysis of long bones. [meta- + G. *physis,* growth]

me·taph·y·si·tis (mĕ-taf′i-sī′tis). Inflammation of the metaphysis.

met·a·pla·sia (met-ă-plā′zē-ă). Abnormal transformation of an adult, fully differentiated tissue of one kind into a differentiated tissue of another kind; an acquired condition, in contrast to heteroplasia. SYN metaplasis (2). [G. *metaplasis,* transformation]

agnogenic myeloid m., SYN primary myeloid m.

apocrine m., alteration of acinar epithelium of breast tissue to resemble apocrine sweat glands; seen commonly in fibrocystic disease of the breasts.

autoparenchymatous m., m. occurring in the parenchymal cells proper to the tissue.

Barrett m., SYN Barrett *syndrome.*

coelomic m., potential of coelomic epithelium to differentiate into several different histologic cell types.

intestinal m., the transformation of mucosa, particularly in the stomach, into glandular mucosa resembling that of the intestines, although usually lacking villi.

myeloid m., a syndrome characterized by anemia, enlargement of the spleen, nucleated red blood cells and immature granulocytes in the circulating blood, and conspicuous foci of extramedullary hemopoiesis in the spleen and liver; may develop in the course of polycythemia rubra vera; there is a high incidence of development of myeloid leukemia.

primary myeloid m., myeloid m. occurring as the primary condition, often in association with myelofibrosis. SYN agnogenic myeloid m.

secondary myeloid m., myeloid m. occurring in individuals with another disease. SYN symptomatic myeloid m.

squamous m., the transformation of glandular or mucosal epithelium into stratified squamous epithelium. SYN epidermalization.

squamous m. of amnion, SYN *amnion* nodosum.

symptomatic myeloid m., SYN secondary myeloid m.

me·tap·la·sis (mĕ-tap′lă-sis). **1.** The stage of completed growth or development of the individual. **2.** SYN metaplasia. [G. a transformation]

met·a·plas·tic (met-ă-plas′tik). Pertaining to metaplasia or metaplasis.

met·a·plex·us (met′ă-plek′sŭs). The choroid plexus in the fourth ventricle of the brain. [meta- + L. *plexus,* an interweaving]

met·a·poph·y·sis (met′ă-pof′i-sis). SYN mammillary *process* of lumbar vertebra. [meta- + G. *apophysis,* a process]

met·a·pore (met′ă-pōr). Rarely used term for *apertura* mediana ventriculi quarti. [meta- + G. *poros,* pore]

met·a·pro·tein (met-ă-prō′tēn). Nondescript term for a derived

me

protein obtained by the action of acids or alkalies, soluble in weak acids or alkalies but insoluble in neutral solutions; e.g., albuminate.

met·a·pro·ter·e·nol sul·fate (met′ă-prō-ter′ĕ-nol). A sympathomimetic bronchodilator used for the treatment of bronchospasm in asthma and chronic obstructive lung disease. It has relatively greater effect on β_2-adrenergic receptors than β_1, conferring some selectivity in relaxing bronchiolar smooth muscle as compared with cardiac stimulation. SYN orciprenaline sulfate.

met·a·psy·chol·o·gy (met′ă-sī-kol′ō-jē). 1. A systematic attempt to discern and describe what lies beyond the empirical facts and laws of psychology, such as the relations between body and mind, or concerning the place of the mind in the universe. 2. In psychoanalysis, or psychoanalytic m., psychology concerning the fundamental assumptions of the freudian theory of the mind, which entail five points of view: 1) dynamic, concerning psychologic forces; 2) economic, concerning psychologic energy; 3) structural, concerning psychologic configurations; 4) genetic, concerning psychologic origins; 5) adaptive, concerning psychologic relations with the environment. [G. *meta,* beyond, transcending, + psychology]

met·a·py·ret·ic (met′ă-pī-ret′ik). SYN postfebrile. [meta- + G. *pyretos,* fever]

met·a·py·ro·cat·e·chase (met′ă-pī-rō-kat′ĕ-kās). SYN catechol 2,3-dioxygenase.

met·a·ram·i·nol bi·tar·trate (met-ă-ram′i-nol). A potent sympathomimetic amine used for the elevation and maintenance of blood pressure in acute hypotensive states and topically as a nasal decongestant.

met·a·rho·dop·sin (met-ă-rō-dop′sin). A light-activated form of rhodopsin; m. I is formed from lumirhodopsin and is converted to m. II; m. II is the form of rhodopsin that releases all-*trans*-retinal.

met·ar·te·ri·ole (met′ar-tēr′ē-ōl). One of the small peripheral blood vessels between the arterioles and the true capillaries that contain scattered groups of smooth muscle fibers in their walls. [meta- + arteriole]

met·a·ru·bri·cyte (met-ă-roo′bri-sīt). Orthochromatic normoblast. SEE normoblast.

pernicious anemia type m., orthochromatic megaloblast. SEE megaloblast.

met·a·sta·ble (met′ă-stā-bl). 1. Of uncertain stability; in a condition to pass into another phase when slightly disturbed; e.g., water, when cooled below the freezing point may remain liquid but will at once congeal if a piece of ice is added. 2. Denoting the excited condition of the nucleus of a radionuclide isomer that reaches a lower energy state by the process of isomeric transition decay without changing its atomic number or weight; e.g., $^{99m}_{43}$Tc → $^{99}_{43}$Tc + γ. [meta- + L. *stabilis,* stable]

▣**me·tas·ta·sis,** pl. **me·tas·ta·ses** (mĕ-tas′tă-sis, -sēz). 1. The shifting of a disease or its local manifestations, from one part of the body to another, as in mumps when the symptoms referable to the parotid gland subside and the testis becomes affected. 2. The spread of a disease process from one part of the body to another, as in the appearance of neoplasms in parts of the body remote from the site of the primary tumor; results from dissemination of tumor cells by the lymphatics or blood vessels or by direct extension through serous cavities or subarachnoid or other spaces. 3. Transportation of bacteria from one part of the body to another, through the bloodstream (hematogenous m.) or through lymph channels (lymphogenous m.). SYN secondaries (1). [G. a removing, fr. *meta,* in the midst of, + *stasis,* a placing]

biochemical m., the transportation and induction of abnormal immunochemical specificities in apparently normal organs.

calcareous m., the deposit of calcareous material in remote tissues in the event of extensive resorption of osseous tissue in caries, malignant neoplasms, and so on.

hematogenous m., SEE metastasis.

in-transit m., in melanoma, a metastatic deposit occurring in the lymphatic pathway between the primary tumor and its draining lymph nodes.

lymphogenous m., SEE metastasis.

pulsating metastases, metastases to bone, usually from hyperne-

phromas, but occasionally from thyroid tumors; considerablee vascularity may have expansile pulsation and a continuous bruit.

satellite m., m. within the immediate vicinity of a primary malignant neoplasm; e.g., skin adjacent to a melanoma.

me·tas·ta·size (mĕ-tas′tă-sīz). To pass into or invade by metastasis.

met·a·stat·ic (met-ă-stat′ik). Relating to metastasis.

met·a·ster·num (met′ă-ster′nŭm). SYN xiphoid *process.*

met·a·stron·gyle (met-ă-stron′jīl). Common name for members of the genus *Metastrongylus* or of the family Metastrongylidae.

Met·a·stron·gy·lus (met-ă-stron′ji-lŭs). A genus of nematode lungworms (family Metastrongylidae), the only genus in its subfamily (Metastrongylinae). The four known species are found only in pigs; transmission is by earthworm intermediate hosts. [meta- + G. *strongylos,* round]

met·a·syph·i·lis (met-ă-sif′i-lis). 1. The constitutional state due to congenital syphilis without local lesions. 2. SYN parasyphilis.

met·a·syph·i·lit·ic (met′ă-sif-i-lit′ik). 1. Relating to metasyphilis. SYN metaluetic (1). 2. Following or occurring as a sequel of syphilis. SYN metaluetic (2). 3. SYN parasyphilitic.

met·a·tar·sal (met′ă-tar′săl). 1. Relating to the metatarsus or to one of the metatarsal bones. SEE metatarsal (*bones*) [I–V], under *bone.* 2. Any one of the metatarsal bones.

met·a·tar·sal·gia (met′ă-tar-sal′jē-ă). Pain in the forefoot in the region of the heads of the metatarsals. [meta- + G. *algos,* pain]

Morton m., SYN Morton *neuralgia.*

met·a·tar·sec·to·my (met′ă-tar-sek′tō-mē). Excision of the metatarsus. [metarsus + G. *ektomē,* excision]

met·a·tar·so·pha·lan·ge·al (met′ă-tar′sō-fă-lan′jē-ăl). Relating to the metatarsal bones and the phalanges; denoting the articulations between them.

met·a·tar·sus, pl. **me·ta·tar·si** (met′ă-tar′sŭs, -sī). The distal portion of the foot between the instep and the toes, having as its skeleton the five long bones (metatarsal bones) articulating proximally with the cuboid and cuneiform bones and distally with the phalanges. [meta- + G. *tarsos,* tarsus]

m. adductova′rus, fixed deformity of the foot in which both adductus and varus vectors contribute to the resultant foot posture.

m. adduc′tus, a fixed deformity of the foot in which the forepart of the foot is angled away from the main longitudinal axis of the foot toward the midline; usually congenital in origin. SYN intoe.

m. atav′icus, abnormal shortness of the first metatarsal bone as compared with the second.

m. la′tus, deformity caused by sinking down of the transverse arch of the foot. SYN talipes transversoplanus.

m. va′rus, fixed deformity of the foot in which the forepart of the foot is rotated on the long axis of the foot, so that the plantar surface faces the midline of the body.

met·a·thal·a·mus (met′ă-thal′ă-mŭs) [TA]. The caudoventral part of the thalamus, consisting of the medial and lateral geniculate bodies. [meta- + G. *thalamos,* thalamus]

me·tath·e·sis (me-tath′ĕ-sis). 1. Transfer of a pathologic product (e.g., a calculus) from one place to another where it causes less inconvenience or injury, when it is not possible or expedient to remove it from the body. 2. In chemistry, a double decomposition, wherein a compound, A-B, reacts with another compound, C-D, to yield A-C + B-D, or A-D + B-C. [meta- + G. *thesis,* a placing]

met·a·troph (met′ă-trof). An organism that requires complex organic sources of carbon and nitrogen for growth.

met·a·tro·phic (met-ă-trof′ik). Denoting the ability to undertake anabolism or to obtain nourishment from varied sources, i.e., both nitrogenous and carbonaceous organic matter. [meta- + G. *trophē,* nourishment]

met·a·tro·pic (met-ă-trop′ik). Denoting a reversion to a previous state. [meta- + G. *tropē,* a turning]

met·a·typ·i·cal (met-ă-tip′i-kăl). Pertaining to tissue that is formed of elements identical to those occurring in that site under normal conditions, but the various elements are not arranged in the usual normal pattern.

me·tax·a·lone (mĕ-tak'să-lōn). A centrally acting skeletal muscle relaxant.

Met·a·zoa (met-ă-zō'ă). A subkingdom of the kingdom Animalia, including all multicellular animal organisms in which the cells are differentiated and form tissues; distinguished from the subkingdom Protozoa, or unicellular animal organisms. [meta- + G. *zōon,* animal]

met·a·zo·o·no·sis (met'ă-zō-ō-nō'sis). A zoonosis that requires both a vertebrate and an invertebrate host for completion of its life cycle; e.g., the arbovirus infections of humans and other vertebrates. [meta- + G. *zōon,* animal, + *nosos,* disease]

Metchnikoff, Elie, Russian biologist in Paris and Nobel laureate, 1845–1916. SEE M. *theory.*

met·en·ce·phal·ic (met'en-se-fal'ik). Relating to the metencephalon.

met·en·ceph·a·lon (met'en-sef'ă-lon) [TA]. The anterior of the two major subdivisions of the rhombencephalon (the posterior being the myelencephalon or medulla oblongata), composed of the pons and the cerebellum. [meta- + G. *enkephalos,* brain]

Metenier sign. See under sign.

met·en·keph·a·lin (met-en-kef'ă-lin). SEE enkephalins.

me·te·or·ism (mē'tē-ŏ-rizm). SYN tympanites. [G. *meteōrismos,* a lifting up]

me·te·or·op·a·thy (mē'tē-ōr-op'ă-thē). Rarely used term for ill health due to climatic conditions. [G. *meteōra,* things high in the air, + *pathos,* suffering]

me·te·or·o·tro·pic (mē'tē-ōr-ō-trop'ik). Denoting diseases affected in their incidence by the weather. [G. *meteōra,* things high in the air, + G. *tropos,* a turning]

me·ter (m) (mē'ter). **1.** The fundamental unit of length in the SI and metric systems, equivalent to 39.37007874 inches. Defined to be the length of the path traveled by light in a vacuum in $1/299792458$ sec. **2.** A device for measuring the quantity of that which passes through it. [Fr. *metre;* G. *metron,* measure]

potential acuity m. (PAM), instrument used to project an image such as Snellen *test types* through a cataractous lens onto the retina in order to predict likely visual function if the cataract were removed.

rate m., a device that continuously displays the magnitude of events averaged over varying time intervals.

ventilation m., a m. used to measure tidal and minute ventilatory volumes.

Venturi m., a device for measuring flow of a fluid in terms of the drop in pressure when the fluid flows into the constriction of a Venturi tube.

me·ter-can·dle (mē'ter-kan'dl). SYN lux.

met·er·ga·sia (met-er-gā'zē-ă). Change of function. [G. *meta,* denoting change, + *ergasia,* work]

me·ter·go·line (mē'ter-gō-lēn). An ergot derivative with a pharmacological profile similar to methysergide; a nonselective blocker of serotonin receptors. Used as an analgesic in migraine headache. SYN methergoline.

met·es·trus, met·es·trum (met-es'trŭs, -trŭm). The period between estrus and diestrus in the estrous cycle. [meta- + estrus]

met·for·min (met-fōr'min). An oral hypoglycemic agent.

meth-, metho-. Chemical prefixes usually denoting a methyl, methoxy group.

meth·a·cho·line chlo·ride (meth'ă-kō-lēn). A derivative of acetylcholine; a parasympatomimetic agent used as a bronchoconstrictor in testing for bronchial hyperreactivity.

meth·a·cryl·ic ac·id (meth'ă-kril'ik). Occurs in oil from Roman camomile; used in the manufacture of methacrylate resins and plastics. SYN methylacrylic acid.

meth·a·cy·cline hy·dro·chlo·ride (meth-ă-sī'klēn). An antimicrobial agent.

meth·a·done hy·dro·chlo·ride (meth'ă-dōn). A synthetic narcotic drug; an orally effective analgesic similar in action to morphine but with slightly greater potency and longer duration. It produces psychic and physical dependence as with morphine, but withdrawal symptoms are somewhat milder; used as a replace-

ment (oral route) for morphine and heroin; also used during withdrawal treatment in morphine and heroin addiction.

meth·al·len·es·tril (meth'ă-len-es'tril). An orally effective, nonsteroid estrogenic compound.

meth·am·phet·a·mine hy·dro·chlo·ride (meth-am-fet'ă-mēn). A sympathomimetic agent that exerts greater stimulating effects upon the central nervous system than does amphetamine (hence street name, "speed"); widely used by drug abusers via the oral and intravenous ("mainlining") routes; strong psychic dependence may develop. When converted to the freebase (methamphetamine) it can be smoked like crack cocaine and is referred to as "ICE". SYN methylamphetamine hydrochloride.

meth·am·py·rone (meth-am-pī'rōn). SYN dipyrone.

meth·an·di·e·none (meth-an-dī'ĕ-nōn). SYN methandrostenolone.

meth·an·dri·ol (meth-an'drē-ol). The methyl derivative of androstenediol, with similar actions and uses. SYN mestenediol.

meth·an·dro·sten·o·lone (meth-an-drō-sten'ō-lōn). An orally effective anabolic steroid that may promote nitrogen retention when combined with an adequate diet; in addition, it can exert typically androgenic effects. SYN methandienone.

meth·ane (meth'ān). CH_4; an odorless gas produced by the decomposition of organic matter; explosive when mixed with 7 or 8 volumes of air, constituting then the firedamp in coal mines. SYN marsh gas.

Meth·a·no·bac·te·ri·a·ce·ae (meth'ă-nō-bak-tēr-ē-ā'sē-ē). Archaea bacteria containing Gram-negative and Gram-positive, motile or nonmotile, strictly anaerobic rods and cocci, which obtain energy either by the reduction of carbon dioxide to form methane or by the fermentation of compounds such as acetate and methanol with the production of methane and carbon dioxide; they are found in anaerobic habitats such as sediments of natural waters, soil, anaerobic sewage digestors, and the gastrointestinal tract of animals.

meth·a·no·gen (meth-an'ō-jen). Any methane-producing bacterium of the family Methanobacteriaceae.

meth·a·nol (meth'ă-nol). SYN methyl *alcohol.*

meth·an·the·line bro·mide (meth-an'thĕ-lēn). An anticholinergic drug.

meth·a·pyr·i·lene (meth-ă-pir'i-lēn). An H_1 tihistamine. M. fumarate is administered topically on the skin; m. hydrochloride is the preferred salt for oral or parenteral use.

meth·a·qua·lone (meth-ă-kwā'lōn). A sedative and hypnotic, also a drug of abuse; available as the hydrochloride.

meth·ar·bi·tal (meth-ar'bi-tahl). An *N*-methylated derivative of barbital with anticonvulsant properties similar to those of phenobarbital; converted to barbital in the body.

meth·ar·gen (meth'ar-jen). A topical antiseptic agent.

meth·a·zo·la·mide (meth-ă-zol'ă-mīd). A carbonic anhydrase inhibitor with uses similar to those of acetazolamide.

metHb Abbreviation for methemoglobin.

meth·dil·a·zine hy·dro·chlo·ride (meth-dil'ă-zēn). A phenothiazine compound with antihistaminic activity; used in the treatment of various dermatoses to relieve pruritus.

met·hem·al·bu·min (met'hĕm-al-boo'min, -hem-al'boo-min). An abnormal compound formed in the blood as a result of heme combining with plasma albumin.

met·hem·al·bu·mi·ne·mia (met'hĕm-al-boo-min-ē'mē-ă). The presence of methemalbumin in the circulating blood, indicative of intravascular hemolysis with rapid hemoglobin breakdown; found in some patients with blackwater fever or paroxysmal nocturnal hemoglobinuria; described as a means of differentiating severe (hemorrhagic) from mild (edematous) pancreatitis, and also has been described in other acute conditions such as strangulation obstruction of intestine and mesenteric artery occlusion.

met·he·mo·glo·bin (metHb) (met-hē-mō-glō'bin). A transformation product of oxyhemoglobin because of the oxidation of the normal Fe^{2+} to Fe^{3+}, thus converting ferroprotoporphyrin to ferriprotoporphyrin; it contains water in firm union with ferric iron, thus being chemically different from oxyhemoglobin and useless for respiration; found in sanguineous effusions and in the circulat-

me

ing blood after poisoning with acetanilid, potassium chlorate, and other substances. SYN ferrihemoglobin.

m. reductase, a flavoenzyme catalyzing the reduction of m. to hemoglobin in the red blood cell.

met·he·mo·glo·bi·ne·mia (met-hē'mō-glō-bi-nē'mē-ă, meth'ĕ-mō-). The presence of methemoglobin in the circulating blood; when severe, there is inadequate oxygenation of the tissues. Methemoglobin causes the blood to have a brownish color, which may be mistaken for cyanosis. [methemoglobin + G. *haima*, blood]

acquired m., m. caused by various chemical agents, such as nitrites or topical anesthetics. SYN enterogenous m., secondary m.

congenital m., (1) m. due to formation of any one of a group of abnormal α chain [MIM*141800] or β chain [MIM*141900] hemoglobins collectively known as hemoglobin M. Slate-gray cyanosis occurs in early infancy, without pulmonary or cardiac disease, and is resistant to ascorbic acid or methylene blue therapy; autosomal dominant inheritance; (2) m. due to deficiency of cytochrome b_5 reductase [MIM*250790] or methemoglobin reductase [MIM*250700], the enzyme responsible for reduction of intraerythrocyte methemoglobin; cyanosis is improved by ascorbic acid or methylene blue; autosomal recessive inheritance; SYN hereditary m., hereditary methemoglobinemic cyanosis, primary m.

enterogenous m., SYN acquired m.

hereditary m., SYN congenital m.

primary m., SYN congenital m.

secondary m., SYN acquired m.

met·he·mo·glo·bi·nu·ria (met-hē'mō-glō-bi-noo'rē-ă, meth'ĕ-mō-). The presence of methemoglobin in the urine. [methemoglobin + G. *ouron*, urine]

meth·en·a·mine (me-then'ă-mēn). A condensation product obtained by the action of ammonia upon formaldehyde; in an acid urine, it decomposes to yield formaldehyde, a urinary antiseptic. SYN hexamine.

m. hippurate, a urinary antiseptic.

m. mandelate, a urinary antiseptic.

m. salicylate, a uric acid solvent and urinary antiseptic.

meth·en·a·mine-sil·ver. A hexamethylenetetramine-silver complex prepared by adding silver nitrate to methenamine; a white precipitate appears in the solution which dissolves upon shaking and is stable under refrigeration; used in various histological and histochemical staining methods. SEE ALSO Gomori methenamine-silver *stain*, under *stain*.

meth·ene (meth'ēn). The moiety =CH–.

N^5,N^{10}-**meth·e·nyl·tet·ra·hy·dro·fol·ic ac·id.** SYN anhydroleucovorin.

N^5,N^{10}-**meth·e·nyl·tet·ra·hy·dro·fo·late.** A one-carbon derivative of tetrahydrofolate; used in purine biosynthesis.

meth·er·go·line. SYN metergoline.

meth·i·cil·lin so·di·um (meth-i-sil'in). A semisynthetic penicillin salt for parenteral administration; restriction of its use to infections caused by penicillin G-resistant staphylococci is recommended; it is less effective than penicillin G in infections caused by hemolytic streptococci, pneumococci, gonococci, and penicillin G-sensitive staphylococci. SYN sodium methicillin.

meth·im·a·zole (me-thim'ă-zōl). An antithyroid drug similar in action to propylthiouracil.

me·thi·o·dal so·di·um (meth-ī'ō-dăl). An iodine-containing radiopaque medium, CH_2ISO_3Na or sodium methanesulfonate, formerly used for examination of the urinary tract.

me·thi·o·nine (Met, M) (me-thī'ō-nēn). 2-Amino-4-(methylthio)butyric acid; the L-isomer is a nutritionally essential amino acid and the most important natural source of "active methyl" groups in the body, hence usually involved in methylations in vivo; the DL-form is used as an adjunct in the treatment of liver diseases.

active m., SYN S-adenosyl-L-methionine.

m. adenosyltransferase, an enzyme catalyzing the condensation of L-methionine and ATP, forming S-adenosyl-L-methionine, orthophosphate, and pyrophosphate; a deficiency of the hepatic enzyme will result in hypermethionemia. SYN methionine-activating enzyme.

m. sulfoxime, a toxic derivative of m. formed when proteins containing it are treated with nitrogen chloride to give –SO(NH)-CH₃ in place of –SCH₃.

m. synthase, tetrahydropteroylglutamate methyltransferase; methionine-homocysteine methyltransferase; an enzyme that catalyzes the reaction of N^5-methyltetrahydrofolate with L-homocysteine to form tetrahydrofolate and L-methionine; a cobalamin-requiring enzyme; a deficiency of this enzyme results in an accumulation of L-homocysteine and neurological abnormalities. SYN tetrahydrofolate methyltransferase.

me·this·a·zone (mĕ-this'ă-zōn). An antiviral agent.

meth·i·tu·ral (me-thi't-oo-ral). An intravenous thiobarbiturate resembling thiopental and used for the induction of anesthesia; exerts a brief effect due to rapid redistribution in the body after a single injection.

me·thix·ene hy·dro·chlo·ride (me-thik'sēn). An anticholinergic agent.

△**metho-.** SEE meth-.

meth·o·car·ba·mol (meth-ō-kar'bă-mol). A centrally acting skeletal muscle relaxant, chemically related to mephenesin carbamate; it is slower in onset of action but of longer duration, and may be administered intravenously, intramuscularly, or orally.

METHOD

meth·od (meth'ŏd). The mode or manner or orderly sequence of events of a process or procedure. SEE ALSO fixative, operation, procedure, stain, technique. [G. *methodos;* fr. *meta,* after, + *hodos,* way]

Abell-Kendall m., a standard reference m. for estimation of total serum cholesterol involving saponification of cholesterol ester by hydroxide, extraction with petroleum ether, and color development with acetic anhydride-sulfuric acid; the m. avoids interference by bilirubin, protein, and hemoglobin.

activated sludge m., a m. of sewage disposal in which the sewage is treated with 15% bacterially active, liquid sludge, which is produced by repeated vigorous aeration of fresh sewage to form floccules or sediment; when this flocculation process is complete, the resulting activated sludge contains large numbers of bacteria, together with yeasts, molds, and protozoa, which actively effect the oxidation of organic compounds; this mixture is piped to a sedimentation tank, the effluent from which is completely treated sewage.

Altmann-Gersh m., the m. of rapidly freezing a tissue and dehydrating it in a vacuum.

Anel m., ligation of an artery immediately above (on the proximal side of) an aneurysm.

Antyllus m., ligation of the artery above and below an aneurysm, followed by incision into and emptying of the sac.

aristotelian m., a m. of study that stresses the relation between a general category and a particular object.

Ashby m., a differential agglutination m. for estimating erythrocyte life span; compatible blood possessing a group factor that the recipient lacks is transferred to the recipient; after the transfusion, sera with potent agglutinins for the recipient's red cells are added to samples of the recipient's blood, and the unagglutinated red cells are counted; using this technique the red cell life span in normal persons is found to be 110–120 days.

auxanographic m., a m. for the study of bacterial enzymes in which agar is mixed with the material (e.g., starch or milk) which is to serve as an indicator of the enzyme action and is inoculated and plated; if the bacteria produce enzymes digesting the admixed material, there will be a zone of clearing in the medium about each colony. SYN diffusion m.

Barraquer m., SYN zonulolysis.

Beck m., a permanent opening into the stomach made from its greater curvature.

Bier m., (1) SYN intravenous regional *anesthesia*; **(2)** treatment of various surgical conditions by reactive hyperemia.

Billings m., a contraceptive m. that involves periods of abstinence determined by changes in cervical mucus.

Born m. of wax plate reconstruction, the making of three-dimensional models of structures from serial sections; it depends on the building up of a series of wax plates, cut out to scaled enlargements of the individual sections involved in the region to be reconstructed.

Brasdor m., treatment of aneurysm by ligation of the artery immediately below (on the distal side of) the tumor.

Callahan m., SYN chloropercha m.

capture-recapture m., originally, a technique developed by biologists to track wild animal populations; now adapted for epidemiological studies of elusive human populations (e.g., prostitutes, teen runaways, IV drug users).

Charters m., a method of toothbrushing utilizing a restricted circular motion with the bristles inclined coronally at a 45 degree angle.

Chayes m., a m. of replacing lost teeth utilizing a mechanical device for the fixation and stabilization of the dental prosthesis which allows "movement in function" of the abutment teeth.

chloropercha m., a m. of filling the root canals of teeth by dissolving gutta-percha cones in a chloroform-rosin medium within the root canal. SYN Callahan m., Johnson m.

closed circuit m., a m. for measuring oxygen consumption in which the subject rebreathes an initial quantity of oxygen through a carbon dioxide absorber and the decrease in the volume of oxygen being rebreathed is noted.

Cobb m., a technique used in scoliosis to determine the degree of curvature of the spine; the measurement is made by drawing a perpendicular to a line drawn across the superior endplate of the upper-end (most tilted) vertebra and the inferior endplate of the lower-end vertebra; the angle formed by the intersection of the two perpendicular lines is the Cobb angle, which is the measure of the magnitude of the curve.

combined m.'s, varying combinations of the oral auditory m. and the manual visual m. of education of deaf children. SEE ALSO oral auditory m., manual visual m., total *communication*.

confrontation m., a m. of perimetry; the examiner compares the patient's visual fields with the examiner's own by facing the patient who has one eye covered and the other fixed upon the corresponding (confronting) eye of the examiner. The examiner then holds a finger midway between them and moves it slowly in different directions until the patient fails to see it. In each instance the finger is moved again toward the original position until the patient can just see it.

cooled-knife m., the cutting of frozen sections with a knife cooled to a few degrees below the freezing point.

copper sulfate m., a m. for the determination of specific gravity of blood or plasma in which the blood or plasma is delivered by drops into solutions of copper sulfate graded in specific gravity by increments of 0.004, each of the bottles of solution being within the expected range of the blood or plasma sample; the specific gravity of the copper sulfate solution in which the drop of blood or plasma remains suspended indefinitely indicates the specific gravity of the sample.

correlational m., a statistical m., most often used in clinical and other applied areas of psychology, to study the relationship which exists between one characteristic and another in an individual.

Credé m.'s, (1) instillation of one drop of a 2% solution of silver nitrate into each eye of the newborn infant, to prevent ophthalmia neonatorum; **(2)** resting the hand on the fundus uteri from the moment of the expulsion of the fetus, and gently rubbing in case of hemorrhage or failing contraction; then, when the afterbirth is loosened it is expelled by firm compression or squeezing of the fundus by the hand; **(3)** use of manual pressure on a bladder, particularly a paralyzed bladder, to express urine. SYN Credé maneuvers.

cross-sectional m., in developmental psychology, the study of the life span involving comparison of groups of individuals at different age levels. Cf. longitudinal m.

Deaver m., a m. of motor reeducation.

definitive m., an analytical procedure for the measurement of a specified analyte in a specified material which is known to give essentially the true value for the concentration of the analyte.

Dick m., SYN Dick *test*.

diffusion m., SYN auxanographic m.

direct m. for making inlays, in dentistry, an inlay technique in which the wax pattern is made directly in the prepared cavity in the tooth. SYN direct technique.

disk sensitivity m., a procedure for testing the relative effectiveness of various antibiotics; small disks of paper (or other suitable material) are impregnated with known, appropriate amounts of antibiotic, and then placed on the surface of semisolid medium that has been previously inoculated with the organism being tested; after suitable periods of incubation at 37°C, the lack of growth in zones about the various disks indicates the relative effectiveness of the antibiotic.

double antibody m., SYN double antibody *precipitation*.

Edman m., SEE phenylisothiocyanate.

Eggleston m., obsolete term for rapid digitalization by means of large doses of digitalis leaf or tincture frequently repeated.

Eicken m., facilitation of hypopharyngoscopy by means of forward traction on the cricoid cartilage by a laryngeal probe.

encu m., a means of simplifying the calculation of risk in genetic counseling for autosomal dominant traits by converting all pertinent evidence into encu units.

ensu m., a means of simplifying the calculation of risk in genetic counseling for X-linked traits by converting all pertinent evidence into ensu units.

experimental m., in experimental psychology, control of environmental, physiological, or attitudinal factors to observe dependent changes in aspects of experience and behavior.

Fick m., in 1870 A. Fick proposed that cardiac output can be calculated as the quotient of total body oxygen consumption divided by the difference in oxygen content of arterial blood and mixed venous blood. In the direct Fick m. all variables are measured. The indirect Fick m. employs a variety of means to avoid measuring mixed venous oxygen content. By extension, the Fick m. may be used to measure cardiac output or organ blood flow with any indicator substance for which the rate of uptake or consumption, and the arterial and mixed venous concentrations, can be measured, provided the indicator does not enter or leave the system by any route not being measured. SYN Fick principle.

flash m., sterilization of milk by raising it rapidly to a temperature of 178°F, holding it there for a short time, and reducing it rapidly to 40°F.

flotation m., any of several procedures for concentrating helminth eggs for more reliable results when eggs are difficult to find in direct examination; the flotation m.'s depend on flotation of helminth eggs on the surface of a liquid of sufficiently high specific gravity, approximately 1.180; 1 part feces mixed in about 10 parts saturated saline will float most protozoan cysts and nonoperculated helminth eggs. SEE ALSO zinc sulfate flotation centrifugation m.

Gärtner m., a m. of measuring venous pressure, based upon Gärtner vein phenomenon; with the patient sitting erect, a vein is selected on the back of the hand that is held dependent, well below the level of the right atrium, and then is raised slowly; when the vein is observed to collapse, the distance between its level and that of the atrium is measured with a millimeter rule; this distance gives the venous pressure in millimeters of blood; thus the vein itself is used as a manometer communicating with the right atrium; highly inaccurate, especially in elderly subjects.

Gerota m., injection of the lymphatics with a dye that is soluble in chloroform or ether but not in water; alkannin, red sulfide of mercury, and Prussian blue are said to be suitable for this purpose.

glucose oxidase m., a highly specific m. for measurement of glucose in serum or plasma by reaction with glucose oxidase, in which gluconic acid and hydrogen peroxide are formed.

Gruber m., a modification of the Politzer m. in which the patient

me

does not swallow, but says "hoc" at the instant of compression of the bag.

Hamilton-Stewart m., formula to calculate cardiac output after intravenous indicator dye injection; blood flow in liters per minute is given by dividing the amount of injectant in milligrams by the product of the average dye concentration in the initial curve of the dye concentration sampled at a given point in the circulation and multiplied by the dose of dye (in milligrams) to write the curve from appearance to disappearance (in the absence of any recirculation). SYN Hamilton-Stewart formula, indicator dilution m., Stewart-Hamilton m.

Hammerschlag m., a hydrometric m. of determining the specific gravity of the blood by allowing a drop of blood to fall into each of a series of tubes containing mixtures of chloroform and benzene of known graded specific gravities; the specific gravity of that mixture in which the drop remains exactly suspended, neither rising nor falling, corresponds to the specific gravity of the blood sample.

hexokinase m., the most specific m. for measuring glucose in serum or plasma, wherein hexokinase plus ATP transforms glucose to glucose 6-phosphate plus ADP; glucose 6-phosphate is then reacted with NADP and glucose 6-phosphate dehydrogenase to form NADP which is measured spectrophotometrically.

Hilton m., division of the nerves supplying a part, for the relief of pain in ulcers.

Hirschberg m., a m. of measuring the amount of deviation of a strabismic eye, by observing the reflection of a light fixated by the straight eye on the cornea of the deviating eye.

Hung method, SYN Wilson m.

immunofluorescence m., any m. in which a fluorescent-labeled antibody is used to detect the presence or determine the location of the corresponding antigen.

impedance m., a m. for localizing brain structures by measuring impedance of electric current.

indicator dilution m., SYN Hamilton-Stewart m.

indirect m. for making inlays, a method whereby the inlay is constructed entirely on a model made from an impression of the prepared tooth or teeth in the mouth. SYN indirect technique.

indophenol m., a m. of determining quantitatively the amount of vitamin C in plant and animal tissue based on the rapid reduction of a standardized indophenol solution to a colorless compound by vitamin C in acid solution.

introspective m., in functionalism, the systematic study of mental phenomena by contemplating the processes in one's own conscious experiences.

ITO m., a concise matrix m. for computing the distribution of genotypes of relatives that at one locus may share no genes in common, one, or both.

Johnson m., SYN chloropercha m.

Keating-Hart m., fulguration in the treatment of external cancer or of the field of operation after the removal of a malignant growth.

Kety-Schmidt m., a m. for measuring organ blood flow first applied to the brain in 1944 by C. F. Schmidt and S. S. Kety. A chemically inert indicator gas is equilibrated with the tissue of the organ of interest and the rate of disappearance from the organ is measured. Blood flow is calculated on the assumption that the tissue and venous blood concentrations of the indicator gas are in diffusion equilibrium at all blood flow rates and that the rate of disappearance of the indicator from the tissue is a function of how much is in the tissue at any time, i.e., it is assumed to be an exponential disappearance.

Kjeldahl m., SEE macro-Kjeldahl m., micro-Kjeldahl m.

Lamaze m., a technique of psychoprophylactic preparation for childbirth, designed to minimize the pain of labor.

Langendorff m., perfusion of the isolated mammalian heart by carrying fluid under pressure into the sectioned aorta, and thus into the coronary system.

Lee-White m., a m. for determining coagulation time of venous blood in tubes of standard bore at body temperature.

Liborius m., a m. for culturing anaerobic bacteria; a stab culture is made in the appropriate agar medium, then more of the same medium is liquefied and poured into the test tube on top of the stab culture, effectually sealing it from the air.

Ling m., gymnastic exercises (as in Swedish movements) without the use of apparatus.

Lister m., antiseptic surgery, as first advocated by Lister in 1867; his operations were performed under a cloud of diluted carbolic acid spray, the instruments were dipped in a carbolic solution before use, and the wound was dressed with a thick layer of carbolized gauze; from this was developed the present practice of aseptic surgery. SYN listerism.

lod m., a method of linkage analysis using an examination of the common logarithm of the ratio of the likelihood for a particular value of the recombination fraction to that if the recombination fraction is 0.5 (i.e., no linkage); thus, a lod score of 3 at a recombination fraction of 0.2 means that the data are 1000 times more readily explained by supposing a recombination fraction of 0.2 than by supposing the loci are unlinked and the recombination fraction is 0.5. [logarithm of the odds]

longitudinal m., in developmental psychology, the study of the life span of one individual involving comparisons of different age levels. Cf. cross-sectional m.

macro-Kjeldahl m., a procedure for analyzing the content of nitrogenous compounds in urine, serum, or other specimens, usually to determine relatively large amounts of nitrogen (e.g., 20–100 mg); the specimen is treated with a digestion mixture (copper sulfate and sulfuric acid), heated thoroughly, and made alkaline with a solution of sodium hydroxide; ammonia is then distilled from the mixture, trapped in a boric acid-indicator solution, and titrated with standard hydrochloric or sulfuric acid.

manual visual m., an approach to the education of deaf children that emphasizes the role of vision in communication and the early and consistent use of ASL or other national sign languages. SEE ALSO oral auditory m., combined m.'s, total *communication*.

Marshall m., a quantitative procedure for estimating free and conjugated sulfanilamide in body fluids.

micro-Astrup m., an interpolation technique for acid-base measurement, based on pH and the use of the Siggaard-Andersen nomogram to determine the base deficit as an expression of metabolic acidosis and the arterial P_{CO_2} as an expression of respiratory acidosis or alkalosis.

micro-Kjeldahl m., a modification of the macro-Kjeldahl m. designed for the analysis of nitrogenous compounds in relatively small quantities, e.g., specimens in which the total content of nitrogen is in the range of 1 to a few milligrams.

microsphere m., a m. for measuring organ blood flow by indicator dilution, but more importantly, a m. for measuring the distribution of cardiac output or the intraorgan distribution of blood flow. To measure distribution of flow, neutrally buoyant, chemically inert microspheres that have an indicator property (e.g., radioactivity) are injected into a cardiac chamber or arterial blood. They are presumed to distribute in proportion to the distribution of arterial blood flow. Injected sphere size is selected to be large enough to embolize the vessels of interest. Injected quantity is selected to be large enough to provide statistically meaningful samples and small enough not to alter the organ blood flow under investigation. Organ samples are taken to quantify the distribution of the microspheres and hence the flow. SEE Fick m., Stewart-Hamilton m.

Moore m., treatment of aneurysm by the introduction of silver or zinc wire into the sac to induce fibrin deposition.

Needles split cast m., SYN split cast m.

Nikiforoff m., the fixing of blood films by immersion for 5 to 15 minutes in absolute alcohol, a mixture of equal parts of alcohol and ether, or pure ether.

Ochsner m., an obsolete treatment for appendicitis (by peristaltic rest), when surgery is not advisable.

open circuit m., a m. for measuring oxygen consumption and carbon dioxide production by collecting the expired gas over a known period of time and measuring its volume and composition.

oral auditory m., an approach to the education of deaf children that emphasizes early auditory training, speech and speech reading, and early and consistent use of high quality amplification for residual hearing. SEE ALSO manual visual m., combined m.'s, total *communication*.

Orsi-Grocco m., palpatory percussion of the heart.

Ouchterlony method, SYN Ouchterlony *test*.

Pachon m., cardiography carried out with the patient lying on the left side.

paracelsian m., the treatment of disease using chemical agents only.

parallax m., localization of a foreign body by observing the direction of its motion on a fluoroscopic screen while moving the x-ray tube or the screen.

Pavlov m., the m. of studying conditioned reflex activity by the observation of a motor indicator, such as the salivary or electroencephalographic response.

Politzer m., inflation of the eustachian tube and tympanum by forcing air into the nasal cavity at the instant the patient swallows.

Porges m., a m. of destroying the capsule of bacteria by heating with N/4 hydrochloric acid and neutralizing with NaOH.

Purmann m., treatment of aneurysm by extirpation of the sac.

Quick m., SYN prothrombin *test*.

reference m., an analytical procedure sufficiently free of random or systematic error to make it useful for validating proposed new analytical procedures for the same analyte.

Rehfuss m., m. of fractional measurement of gastric activity: a fine tube with fenestrated metal tip is passed into the stomach after a test meal, and small quantities (6 or 8 ml) of the stomach contents are removed at 15-min intervals and examined.

rhythm m., a natural contraceptive m. that spaces human sexual intercourse to avoid the fertile period of the menstrual cycle. SYN rhythm (2).

Rideal-Walker m., SEE Rideal-Walker *coefficient*.

Roux m., division of the mandible in the median line, to facilitate the operation of ablation of the tongue.

Sanger m., the m. for the sequencing of DNA employing an enzyme that can polymerase DNA and labeled nucleotides.

Scarpa m., cure of aneurysm by ligation of the artery at some distance above the sac.

Schäfer m., an obsolete m. of resuscitation in cases of drowning or asphyxia; the patient is laid face downward and natural breathing is imitated by gentle intermittent pressure over the lower part of the thorax at the rate of about 15 times a minute.

Schede m., filling of the defect in bone, after removal of a sequestrum or scraping away carious material, by allowing the cavity to fill with blood which may become organized (Schede clot).

Schick m., SYN Schick *test*.

Schmidt-Thannhauser m., a m. for fractionation of nucleic acid, based upon the fact that RNA but not DNA is hydrolyzed to nucleotides by alkali; RNA can be hydrolyzed in about 2 h in 0.75 N NaOH, but 18 h and 0.3 N NaOH usually are used.

Schweninger m., a method suggested to reduce obesity by restricting intake of fluid.

Shaffer-Hartmann m., an obsolete m. for the quantitative determination of glucose in biological fluids, based on the reduction of copper by the reducing group of the sugar.

Somogyi m., SEE Somogyi *unit*.

split cast m., (1) a procedure for placing indexed casts on an articulator to facilitate their removal and replacement on the instrument; **(2)** the procedure of checking the ability of an articulator to receive or be adjusted to a maxillomandibular relation record. SYN Needles split cast m.

Stas-Otto m., a m. of extraction of alkaloids from plants and animal bodies: the substance is digested in alcohol and tartaric acid, the fatty and resinous matters are precipitated with water, the fluid is made alkaline, and the alkaloids are extracted with ether or chloroform.

Stewart-Hamilton m., SYN Hamilton-Stewart m.

Thane m., a m. for indicating the position of the central sulcus (Rolando fissure) of the brain; the upper end of the sulcus corresponds to the midpoint of a line drawn from the glabella to the inion.

Theden m., treatment of aneurysms or of large sanguineous effusions by compression of the entire limb with a roller bandage.

Thezac-Porsmeur m., heat treatment of infected wounds by focusing of sun's rays on suppurating area by means of a lens mounted in a cylinder of canvas.

thiochrome m., a m. for the determination of thiamin based upon the production of thiochrome when the vitamin is oxidized by alkaline ferricyanide to yield the fluorescent compound, thiochrome.

twin m., a general means of genetic analysis that capitalizes on the fact that while twins have the same age and the same intrauterine environment, identical (monozygotic) twins have the same genotype but dizygotic twins are no more alike than sibs and may be of different sex.

ultropaque m., a rapid m. for examining thick (1–3 mm) sections of fresh tissue with the ultramicroscope, making use of an objective built in an illuminator so that the light is reflected down upon the tissue.

u-score m., an older, simpler, but somewhat less efficient method of linkage analysis than that by maximum likelihood estimation.

Wardrop m., treatment of aneurysm by ligation of the artery at some distance beyond the sac, leaving one or more branches of the artery between the sac and the ligature.

Westergren m., a procedure for estimating the sedimentation rate of red blood cells in fluid blood by mixing venous blood with an aqueous solution of sodium citrate and allowing it to stand in an upright standard pipette (200 mm long) filled to the zero mark; the fall of the red blood cells, in millimeters, is then observed in 1 hr; the normal rate for men is 0–15 mm (average, 4 mm), and for women 0–20 mm (average, 5 mm).

Wheeler m., a surgical procedure for correction of cicatricial ectropion.

Wilson m., a simple saline flotation m. for concentrating helminth eggs in the feces. SEE flotation m. SYN Hung method.

zinc sulfate flotation centrifugation m., a flotation m. in which the fecal specimen is suspended in tap water, strained through wet gauze, centrifuged, resuspended in tap water, washed and recentrifuged several times, and then suspended in 33% solution of zinc sulfate and centrifuged at top speed for 45–60 sec; a bacteriologic loop may be used to pick up the surface layer, which contains protozoan cysts and helminth eggs.

---

meth·od·ism (meth′ŏd-izm). SYN solidism.

meth·o·dol·o·gy (meth′u-dol-ō-jē). The scientific study or logical analysis of methods.

meth·o·hex·i·tal so·di·um (meth-ō-heks′i-tawl). An ultra-short-acting barbiturate used intravenously for induction and for general anesthesia of short duration.

meth·o·phen·a·zine (me-thō-fen′ă-zēn). An antipsychotic.

meth·o·pho·line (me-thō-fō′lēn). An analgesic.

meth·op·ter·in (meth-op′ter-in). A folic acid antagonist.

meth·or·phi·nan (meth-ōr′fi-nan). SEE dextromethorphan hydrobromide, levorphanol tartrate.

meth·o·ser·pi·dine (meth-ō-ser′pi-dēn). An antihypertensive agent similar in its actions to reserpine.

meth·o·trex·ate (meth-ō-trek′sāt). A folic acid antagonist used as an antineoplastic agent; used to treat psoriasis and rheumatoid arthritis. SYN amethopterin.

meth·o·tri·mep·ra·zine (meth′ō-trī-mep′ră-zēn). A phenothiazine analgesic.

me·thox·a·mine hy·dro·chlo·ride (me-thok′să-mēn). A sympathomimetic amine.

me·thox·sa·len (me-thok′să-len). A methoxypsoralen derivative that increases melanin production in the skin when exposed to ultraviolet light; used orally and topically in the treatment of idiopathic vitiligo, and also as a suntan accelerator and sun protectant.

△**methoxy-.** Chemical prefix denoting substitution of a methoxyl group.

me

4-me·thox·y·ben·zo·ic ac·id (meth-ok′sē-ben-zō′ik). SYN anisic acid.

me·thox·y·chlor (mĕ-thok′sē-klōr). An insecticide resembling DDT; ectoparasiticide.

me·thox·y·flu·rane (me-thok-sē-floor′ān). A potent inhalation anesthetic no longer in use because of high-output renal failure caused by increased plasma concentrations of inorganic fluoride, a metabolic breakdown product of m.

3-me·thox·y-4-hy·drox·y·man·del·ic ac·id. SEE vanillylmandelic acid.

5-me·thox·y·in·dole-3-ac·e·tate (meth-oks′ē-in-dōl). An intermediate of tryptophan and serotonin degradation; excreted as conjugates.

me·thox·yl (me-thok′sil). The group, –OCH₃.

me·thox·y·phen·a·mine hy·dro·chlo·ride (me-thok-sē-fen′ă-mēn). A sympathomimetic amine.

5-me·thox·y·trypt·a·mine (meth-oks′ē-trip-ta-mēn). An intermediate in the degradation of L-tryptophan and serotonin.

meth·sco·pol·a·mine bro·mide (meth-skō-pol′ă-mēn). A parasympatholytic drug similar to atropine; the methyl nitrate has the same action and uses.

meth·sux·i·mide (meth-sŭk′si-mīd). An antiepileptic effective against petit mal and psychomotor epilepsy; similar to ethosuximide.

meth·y·clo·thi·a·zide (meth′i-klō-thī′ă-zīd). An orally effective diuretic and antihypertensive agent of the thiazide group.

meth·yl (Me) (meth′il). The moiety, –CH₃. [G. *methy,* wine, + *hylē,* wood]

active m., a m. group attached to a quaternary ammonium ion or a tertiary sulfonium ion that can take part in transmethylation reactions; e.g., m. groups in choline and in *S*-adenosyl-L-methionine, which are thus m. donors.

m. aldehyde, SYN formaldehyde.

angular m., a m. group attached to carbon 10 (between rings A and B) or to carbon 13 (between rings C and D) of the steroid nucleus.

m. chloride, SYN chloromethane.

m. cysteine hydrochloride, the methyl ester of cysteine hydrochloride; a mucolytic agent.

m. hydroxybenzoate, SYN methylparaben.

m. isobutyl ketone, in high concentrations it has narcotic action; in relatively low concentrations it may be irritating to the eyes and mucous membranes.

m. methacrylate, a thermoplastic material used for denture bases and as an embedding material for electron microscopy.

m. nicotinate, nicotinic acid methyl ester, used as rubefacient.

2-meth·yl·a·ce·to·a·ce·tyl-CoA thi·o·lase. An enzyme that is part of the L-isoleucine degradation pathway; it catalyzes the conversion of 2-methylacetoacetyl-CoA to acetyl-CoA and propionyl-CoA. A deficiency of this enzyme leads to an accumulation of 2-methylacetoacetyl-CoA, causing episodes of severe metabolic acidosis and ketosis.

meth·yl·a·cryl·ic ac·id (meth′il-ă-kril′ik). SYN methacrylic acid.

meth·yl·am·phet·a·mine hy·dro·chlo·ride (meth′il-am-fet′ă-mēn). SYN methamphetamine hydrochloride.

***N*-methyl D-aspartic acid.** SYN NMDA.

meth·yl·ate (meth′i-lāt). **1.** To mix with methanol. **2.** To introduce a methyl group. **3.** A compound in which a metal ion methyl replaces the alcoholic hydrogen of alcohol.

meth·yl·a·tion (meth-i-lā′shŭn). Addition of methyl groups; in histochemistry, used to esterify carboxyl groups and remove sulfate groups by treating tissue sections with hot methanol in the presence of hydrochloric acid; the net effect being to reduce tissue basophilia and abolish metachromasia.

restriction m., the enzymatic addition of methyl groups to selected adenine and cytosine residues to protect from hydrolysis by certain restriction enzymes.

meth·yl·at·ro·pine bro·mide (meth-il-at′rō-pēn, -pin). A quaternary derivative of atropine that is less lipid soluble and hence produces fewer central nervous system actions; a cycloplegic. SYN atropine methylbromide.

meth·yl·ben·zene (meth-il-ben′zēn). SYN toluene.

meth·yl·ben·ze·tho·ni·um chlo·ride (meth′il-ben-zĕ-thō′nē-ŭm). A quaternary ammonium compound having a surface action like that of other cationic detergents; generally germicidal and bacteriostatic; used to rinse infant diapers and bed linen in the prevention of ammonia dermatitis.

meth·yl blue [C.I. 42780]. A sulfonated triphenylrosaniline dye used as a stain for cytoplasm, collagen, and Negri bodies, and as an antiseptic.

meth·yl bro·mide. Used in ionization chambers; for degreasing wool; extracting oils from nuts, seeds, flowers; used as an insect fumigant for mills, warehouses, vaults, ships, freight cars; also as a soil fumigant.

***N*-meth·yl·car·no·sine** (meth-il-kar′nō-sēn). SYN anserine (2).

meth·yl-CCNU. A nitrosourea antineoplastic agent resembling carmustine (BCNU) and lomustine (CCNU). SYN semustine.

meth·yl·cel·lu·lose (meth-il-sel′ū-lōs). A methyl ester of cellulose that forms a colorless viscous liquid when dissolved in water, alcohol, or ether; used to increase bulk of the intestinal contents, to relieve constipation, or of the gastric contents, to reduce appetite in obesity; also used dissolved in water as a spray to cover burned areas and as a suspending agent in pharmaceuticals and foods.

meth·yl·chlo·ro·form (meth-il-chlōr′ō-fōrm). SYN trichloroethane.

3-meth·yl·chol·an·threne, 20-meth·yl·chol·an·threne (meth′il-kōl-an′thrēn). A highly carcinogenic hydrocarbon that can be formed chemically from deoxycholic or cholic acids, or from cholesterol; it induces the synthesis of cytochrome P-450 mRNA; the choice between 3- or 20- for the methyl group depends upon whether hydrocarbon (inner) or steroid (outer) numbering is chosen; in the latter case, the formal relationship to the cholic acids and cholesterol is clear.

meth·yl·cit·rate (meth-il-sit′trāt). A minor metabolite that accumulates in individuals with propionic acidemia.

meth·yl·co·bal·a·min (meth-il-kō-bal′a-mēn). SYN *vitamin* B₁₂.

3-meth·yl·cro·ton·yl-CoA (meth-il-krō′ton-il). An intermediate in the degradation of L-leucine; accumulates in a deficiency of 3-methylcrotonyl-CoA carboxylase.

3-methylcrotonyl-CoA carboxylase, a biotin-dependent enzyme in the pathway of L-leucine degradation that catalyzes the reaction of 3-methylcrotonyl-CoA with CO_2, ATP, and water to form ADP, orthophosphate, and 3-methylcrotonyl-CoA; a deficiency of this enzyme causes episodes of severe metabolic acidosis.

5-meth·yl·cy·to·sine (meth′il-sī′tō-sēn). A minor base that is present in both bacterial and human DNA.

meth·yl·di·chlo·ro·ar·sine (MD) (meth′il-dī-klōr-ō-ar′sēn). A vesicant; irritating to the respiratory tract and will produce lung injury and eye injury; has been used in certain military operations.

meth·yl·do·pa (meth-il-dō′pă). An antihypertensive agent, also used as the ethyl ester hydrochloride, with the same action and uses. SYN alpha methyl dopa.

meth·yl·ene (meth′i-lēn). The moiety, –CH₂–.

meth·yl·ene az·ure. SYN *azure* I.

meth·yl·ene blue [C.I. 52015]. A basic dye easily oxidized to azure, with dye mixtures; used in histology and microbiology, to stain intestinal protozoa in wet mount preparations, to track RNA and RNase in electrophoresis, and as an antidote for methemoglobinemia; its redox indicator properties are useful in milk bacteriology.

Kühne m. b., m. b. in absolute alcohol and phenol solution.

Loeffler m. b., a stain for diphtheria organisms that contains m. b. in dilute ethanol plus a slight amount of potassium hydroxide; dye solution gives best results when aged to a polychrome state.

new m. b. [C.I. 52030], a basic thiazin dye used for supravital staining of reticulocytes in blood smears.

polychrome m. b., an alkaline solution of m. b. that undergoes progressive oxidative demethylation with aging (ripening) to produce a mixture of m. b., azures, and methylene violet; boiling with sodium carbonate or other oxidizing agents accomplishes this result quickly, although it is not as highly regarded.

meth·yl·ene chlo·ride. Mobile liquid with a pungent odor; harmful vapor. Organic solvent used for cellulose acetate plastic; degreasing and cleaning fluids; and in food processing. Pharmaceutical aid (solvent).

3,4-meth·yl·ene·di·oxy·meth·am·phet·a·mine. SYN MDMA.

meth·yl·ene·suc·cin·ic ac·id (meth′il-ēn-sŭk′sin-ik). SYN itaconic acid.

N^5,N^{10}-meth·yl·ene·tet·ra·hy·dro·fo·late re·duc·tase. An enzyme that converts N^5,N^{10}-methylenetetrahydrofolate to N^5,N^{10}-methenyltetrahydrofolate using NADP$^+$; a deficiency of this enzyme results in an accumulation of L-homocysteine and severe neurological disturbances.

meth·yl·ene white. SYN leucomethylene blue.

meth·yl·en·o·phil, meth·yl·en·o·phile (meth-i-lēn′ō-fil, -fīl). Staining readily with methylene blue; denoting certain cells and histologic structures. SYN methylenophilic, methylenophilous. [methylene + G. *philos*, fond]

meth·yl·en·o·phil·ic, meth·yl·e·noph·i·lous (meth′i-lē-nō-fil′ik, meth′il-ĕ-nof′i-lŭs). SYN methylenophil.

meth·yl·er·go·met·rine ma·le·ate (meth′il-er-gō-met′rēn). SYN methylergonovine maleate.

meth·yl·er·go·no·vine ma·le·ate (meth′il-er-gō-nō′vēn). A partially synthesized derivative of lysergic acid with oxytocic action, used to prevent or treat postpartum uterine atony and hemorrhage. SYN methylergometrine maleate.

meth·yl·glu·ca·mine (meth-il-gloo′kă-mēn). Cation commonly used in water-soluble iodinated radiographic contrast media. SYN N-methylglucamine.

m. diatrizoate, SYN *meglumine* diatrizoate.

N-meth·yl·glu·ca·mine. SYN methylglucamine.

3-meth·yl·glu·ta·con·ic ac·i·du·ria (meth-il-gloo-ta-kon′ik). Elevated levels of 3-methylglutaconic acid in the urine. An inherited disorder whose mild form is a result of a deficiency of 3-methylglutaconyl-CoA hydratase, leading to delayed speech development.

3-meth·yl·glu·ta·con·yl-CoA hy·dra·tase. An enzyme that catalyzes the reaction of *trans*-3-methylglutaconyl-CoA and water to form 3-hydroxy-3-methylglutaconyl-CoA; this enzyme participates in the pathway for L-leucine degradation; a deficiency of this enzyme will result in 3-methylglutaconic aciduria.

meth·yl·gly·ox·al (meth′il-glī-ok′săl). Pyruvaldehyde; the aldehyde of pyruvic acid; an intermediate of carbohydrate metabolism in certain organisms. SYN pyruvic aldehyde.

m. bis(guanylhydrazone), an antineoplastic agent.

meth·yl·gly·ox·a·lase (meth′il-glī-oks′ă-lās). SYN lactoylglutathione lyase.

meth·yl green [C.I. 42585]. A basic triphenylmethane dye used as a chromatin stain and, in combination with pyronin, for differential staining of RNA (red) and DNA (green); also used as a tracking dye for DNA in electrophoresis.

meth·yl·hex·ane·a·mine (meth′il-hek-sān′ă-mēn, -min). A volatile sympathetic amine base, used as an inhalant nasal decongestant.

N-meth·yl·his·tid·ine (meth′il-his′ti-dēn). A methylated derivative of histidine found in actin; in the breakdown of actin and myosin, N-methylhistidine is released into the urine; urinary output of N-methylhistidine is a reliable index of the rate of myofibrillar protein breakdown in musculature.

meth·yl·ki·nase (meth′il-kī′nās). SYN methyltransferase.

meth·yl·mal·o·nate sem·i·al·de·hyde (meth′il-mă-lon-āt). An intermediate in L-valine catabolism; elevated in certain inborn disorders.

meth·yl·ma·lon·ic ac·id (meth′il-mă-lon′ik). 2-Methylpropanedioic acid, an important intermediate in fatty acid metabolism; seen in elevated levels in cases of vitamin B$_{12}$ deficiency. Note that methylmalonate is not methyl malonate, which is the dimethyl ester of malonate. SYN isosuccinic acid.

meth·yl·ma·lon·ic ac·i·de·mia. SYN ketotic *hyperglycinemia*.

meth·yl·ma·lon·ic ac·i·du·ria. Excretion of excessive amounts of methylmalonic acid in urine owing to deficient activity of methylmalonyl-CoA mutase or deficient cobalamin reductase. Two types occur: 1) an inborn error of metabolism resulting in severe ketoacidosis shortly after birth, with long-chain urinary ketones; autosomal recessive inheritance, caused by mutations in the methylmalonyl-CoA mutase gene (MCM) on chromosome 6p [MIM*251000]; 2) acquired, a type due to vitamin B$_{12}$ deficiency [MIM*251110] due to defective synthesis of adenosylcobalamin.

meth·yl·mal·o·nyl-CoA. An intermediate in the degradation of several metabolites (e.g., valine, methionine, odd-chain fatty acids, threonine); elevated in cases of pernicious anemia.

m.-CoA epimerase, an enzyme that catalyzes the interconversion of D-m.-CoA and L-m.-CoA.

m.-CoA mutase, an enzyme that catalyzes a reversible interconversion of L-methylmalonyl-CoA and succinyl-CoA; a cobalamin-dependent enzyme; deficiency of this enzyme will result in methylmalonic acidemia.

meth·yl·mer·cu·ry. SYN dimethylmercury.

meth·yl·mor·phine (meth-il-mōr′fēn). SYN codeine.

meth·yl·ol (meth′i-lol). Hydroxymethyl; the moiety, –CH$_2$OH.

meth·yl or·ange. A weakly acid dye used as a pH indicator (red at 3.2, yellow at 4.4). SYN helianthine.

meth·y·lose (meth′i-lōs). A sugar in which the carbon atom farthest from the carbonyl group is a methyl (CH$_3$).

meth·yl·par·a·ben (meth-il-par′ă-ben). An antifungal preservative. SYN methyl hydroxybenzoate.

meth·yl·pen·tose (meth-il-pen′tōs). A hexose (a 6-deoxyhexose) in which carbon-6 is part of a methyl group; e.g., rhamnose, fucose.

meth·yl·phen·i·date hy·dro·chlo·ride (meth-il-fen′i-dāt). A central nervous system stimulant used to produce mild cortical stimulation in various types of depressions; commonly used in the treatment of hyperkinetic or hyperactive (attention deficit disorder) children.

meth·yl·pred·nis·o·lone (meth′il-pred-nis′ŏ-lōn). An anti-inflammatory glucocorticoid.

m. acetate, has the same actions and uses as m.; aqueous suspensions are suitable for intrasynovial and soft tissue injection.

sodium m. succinate, it has the same metabolic and anti-inflammatory actions as the parent compound, m.; because of its solubility it can be administered in small volumes.

meth·yl red. A weakly acid dye used as a pH indicator (red at 4.8, yellow at 6.0); easily reduced with loss of color, and pH readings must be made rapidly.

5-meth·yl·res·or·cin·ol (meth′il-rē-sōr′sin-ol). SYN orcinol.

meth·yl·ros·an·i·line chlo·ride (meth′il-rō-zan′i-lēn, -lin). SYN crystal violet.

meth·yl sa·lic·y·late. The methyl ester of salicylic acid, produced synthetically or distilled from *Gaultheria procumbens* (family Ericaceae) or from *Betula lenta* (family Betulaceae); used externally and internally for the treatment of various forms of rheumatism. SYN checkerberry oil, gaultheria oil, sweet birch oil, wintergreen oil.

methyl-*tert*-butyl ether (MTBE). Used to dissolve gallbladder stones.

meth·yl·tes·tos·ter·one (meth′il-tes-tos′ter-ōn). A methyl derivative of testosterone, with the same actions and uses, except that it is active when given orally or sublingually. Used in the treatment of hypogenitalism. SYN 17α-methyltestosterone.

17α-meth·yl·tes·tos·ter·one. SYN methyltestosterone.

N^5-meth·yl·tet·ra·hy·dro·fo·late (meth-il-tet′ra-hī-drō-fōl-āt). An active one-carbon derivative of tetrahydrofolate that participates in the S-methylation of L-homocysteine.

N^5-m.:homocysteine methyltransferase, SEE *methionine* synthase.

meth·yl·thi·o·a·den·o·sine (meth′il-thī′ō-ă-den′ō-sēn). Adenosine carrying an –SCH$_3$ group in place of OH at position 5′; the –SCH$_3$ group is transferred to α-aminobutyric acid to form L-methionine in some bacteria. M. is formed from S-adenosyl-L-

me

methionine in the course of spermidine synthesis by loss of the alanine moiety. SYN thiomethyladenosine.

meth·yl·thi·o·u·ra·cil (meth′il-thī-ō-ū′ră-sil). An antithyroid compound with the same action as propylthiouracil, but with a smaller dose required.

meth·yl·to·col (meth-il-tō′kol). A methylated tocol; e.g., tocotrienol, the tocopherols.

meth·yl·trans·fer·ase (meth-il-trans′fer-ās). Any enzyme transferring methyl groups from one compound to another. SYN demethylase, methylkinase, transmethylase.

meth·yl vi·o·let [C.I. 42535]. Mixtures of tetra-, penta-, or pararosanilin which vary in shade of violet depending on the extent of methylation (designated R for reddish shades, B for bluish shades); the hexamethyl compound is known as crystal violet, the pentamenthyl compound is methyl violet 6B. As stains, m. v. has many bacteriological, histological, and cytological applications.

meth·yl·xan·thines (meth′il-zan′thinz). A chemical group of drugs derived from xanthine (a purine derivative); members of the group include theophylline, caffeine, and theobromine.

meth·yl yel·low. SYN butter yellow.

meth·y·pry·lon, meth·y·pry·lone (meth-i-prī′lon, -lōn). A sedative and hypnotic.

meth·y·ser·gide ma·le·ate (meth-i-ser′jīd). A serotonin antagonist, weakly adrenolytic, chemically related to methylergonovine; used in the prophylactic treatment of vascular headache (migraine); untoward effects are common.

me·thys·ti·cum (mĕ-this′ti-kŭm). The root of *Piper methysticum* (family Piperaceae), a plant of the Pacific islands, used by the natives as an intoxicant. It has been used in diarrhea and in inflammatory affection of the urogenital tract. SYN kava (1).

metMb Abbreviation for metmyoglobin.

met·my·o·glo·bin (metMb) (met′mī-ō-glō′bin). Myoglobin in which the ferrous ion of the heme prosthetic group is oxidized to ferric ion; ferrimyoglobin.

met·o·clo·pra·mide hy·dro·chlo·ride (met′ō-klō-pram′īd). An antiemetic agent.

met·o·cur·ine io·dide (met-ō-kūr′ēn). A nondepolarizing neuromuscular blocking agent used to provide relaxation during surgical operations. SYN dimethyl *d*-tubocurarine, dimethyl tubocurarine iodide.

me·tol·a·zone (me-tol′ă-zōn). A diuretic with antihypertensive activity.

me·top·a·gus (mĕ-top′ă-gŭs). Conjoined twins united at the forehead. SEE conjoined *twins*, under *twin*. [G. *metōpon*, forehead, + *pagos*, something fixed]

me·top·ic (me-tō′pik, me-top′ik). Relating to the forehead or anterior portion of the cranium. [G. *metōpon*, forehead]

me·to·pi·on (mĕ-tō′pē-on). A craniometric point midway between the frontal eminences. SYN metopic point. [G. *metōpon*, forehead]

met·o·pism (met′ō-pizm). Persistence of the frontal suture in the adult. [G. *metōpon*, forehead]

met·o·po·plas·ty (met′ŏ-pō-plas-tē, me-top′ō-plas-tē). Plastic surgery of the skin or bone of the forehead. [G. *metōpon*, forehead, + *plastos*, formed]

met·o·pos·co·py (met′ŏ-pos′kŏ-pē). The study of physiognomy. [G. *metōpon*, forehead, + *skopeō*, to view]

me·to·pro·lol tar·trate (me-tō′prō-lol). A β-adrenergic blocking agent used in the treatment of hypertension; exhibits some cardioselectivity.

Met·or·chis (met-ōr′kis). A genus of opisthorchid fish-borne flukes parasitic in the gallbladder of fish-eating mammals and birds, common in north temperate regions. *M. conjunctus* is a species that occurs in dogs and cats, and occasionally in humans, in North America. [G. *meta*, behind, + *orchis*, testicle]

me·tox·e·nous (me-tok′sĕ-nŭs). SYN heterecious. [G. *meta*, beyond, + *xenos*, host]

me·tox·e·ny (me-tok′sĕ-nē). 1. SYN heterecism. 2. Change of host by a parasite. [G. *meta*, beyond, + *xenos*, host]

⌂**metr-, metra-, metro-.** The uterus. SEE ALSO hystero- (1), utero-. [G. *mētra*]

me·tra (mē′tră). SYN uterus. [G. uterus]

me·tra·to·nia (mē-tră-tō′nē-ă). SYN postpartum *atony*. [metra- + G. *a-* priv. + *tonos*, tension]

me·tria (mē′trē-ă). Pelvic cellulitis or other inflammatory affection in the puerperal period. [G. *mētra*, uterus]

met·ric (met′rik). Quantitative; relating to measurement. SEE metric *system*. [G. *metrikos*, fr. *metron*, measure]

me·tri·fo·nate (me-trī′fō-nāt). SYN trichlorfon.

met·ri·o·ce·phal·ic (met′rē-ō-se-fal′ik). Having a head well proportioned to height; denoting a skull with an index between 72 and 77. SEE ALSO orthocephalic. [G. *metrios*, moderate, fr. *metron*, measure, + *kephalē*, head]

me·tri·tis (mē-trī′tis). Inflammation of the uterus. [G. *mētra*, uterus, + *-itis*, inflammation]

me·triz·a·mide (me-triz′ă-mīd). SYN metrizoate sodium.

met·ri·zo·ate so·di·um (met-ri-zō′āt). A diagnostic radiopaque medium. SYN metrizamide.

⌂**metro-.** SEE metr-. [G. *mētra*, uterus]

me·tro·cyte (mē′trō-sīt). SYN mother *cell*. [G. *mētēr*, mother, + *kytos*, a hollow (cell)]

me·tro·dy·na·mom·e·ter (mē-trō-dī′nă-mom′ĕ-ter). Instrument for measuring the force of uterine contractions. [metro- + G. *dynamis*, power, + *metron*, measure]

me·tro·dyn·ia (mē-trō-dī′nē-ă). SYN hysteralgia. [metro- + G. *odynē*, pain]

me·tro·lym·phan·gi·tis (mē′trō-lim-fan-jī′tis). Inflammation of the uterine lymphatics. [metro- + lymphangitis]

met·ro·ni·da·zole (met-rō-ni′dă-zōl). An orally effective trichomonicide used in the treatment of infections caused by *Trichomonas vaginalis* and *Entamoeba histolytica* and Gram-negative anaerobic bacteria. Can produce a disulfiram reaction when combined with alcohol.

me·tron·o·scope (mĕ-tron′ō-skōp). A tachistoscopic apparatus that exposes for timed intervals short selections of printed matter for reading; used in testing and developing reading speed. [G. *metron*, measure, + *skopeō*, to view]

me·tro·path·ia (mē-trō-path′ē-ă). SYN metropathy. [L.]
 m. hemorrhag′ica, abnormal, excessive, often continuous uterine bleeding due to persistence and exaggeration of the follicular phase of the menstrual cycle; the endometrium is the seat of glandular hyperplasia with cyst formation. SEE Swiss cheese *endometrium.*

me·tro·path·ic (mē-trō-path′ik). Relating to or caused by uterine disease.

me·trop·a·thy (mē-trop′ă-thē). Any disease of the uterus, especially of the myometrium. SYN metropathia. [metro- + G. *pathos*, suffering]

me·tro·per·i·to·ni·tis (mē′trō-per-i-tō-nī′tis). SYN perimetritis. [metro- + peritonitis]

me·tro·phle·bi·tis (mē′trō-flĕ-bī′tis). Inflammation of the uterine veins usually following childbirth. [metro- + G. *phleps*, vein, + *-itis*, inflammation]

met·ro·plas·ty (met′trō-plas-tē, mē′trō-). SYN uteroplasty.

me·tror·rha·gia (mē-trō-rā′jē-ă). Any irregular, acyclic bleeding from the uterus between periods. [metro- + G. *rhēgnymi*, to burst forth]

me·tror·rhea (mē-trō-rē′ă). Discharge of mucus or pus from the uterus. [metro- + G. *rhoia*, a flow]

me·tro·sal·pin·gi·tis (mē′trō-sal-pin-jī′tis). Inflammation of the uterus and of one or both fallopian tubes. [metro- + G. *salpinx*, trumpet (oviduct), + *-itis*, inflammation]

me·tro·stax·is (mē-trō-stak′sis). Small but continuous hemorrhage of the uterine mucous membrane. [metro- + G. *staxis*, a dripping]

me·tro·ste·no·sis (mē′trō-ste-nō′sis). A narrowing of the uterine cavity. [metro- + G. *stenōsis*, a narrowing]

me·trot·o·my (mē-trot′ō-mē). SYN hysterotomy. [metro- + G. *tomē,* incision]

me·tyr·a·pone (mĕ-tir′ă-pōn). An inhibitor of adrenocortical steroid C-11 β-hydroxylation, administered orally or intravenously to determine the ability of the pituitary gland to increase its secretion of corticotropin; because 11-deoxycorticosteroids, as a consequence of m. administration, only weakly inhibit pituitary corticotropin secretion, the normal pituitary gland will appreciably increase its output of this hormone. SYN mepyrapone.

me·ty·ro·sine (mĕ-tī′rō-sin, -sēn). An inhibitor of tyrosine hydroxylase and therefore a powerful inhibitor of catecholamine synthesis; used for controlling the manifestations of pheochromocytoma, in preoperative preparation, or in instances where surgical resection is contraindicated or incomplete.

Mev Symbol for 1 million electron-volts.

mev·a·lo·nate (mev-ă-lon′at). The salt or ester of mevalonic acid.
m. kinase, an enzyme that catalyzes the reaction of m. and ATP to form ADP and m. 5-phosphate; this enzyme participates in the pathway for steroid synthesis; a deficiency of this enzyme will lead to mevalonic aciduria and lack of development.

mev·a·lon·ic ac·id (mev-ă-lon′ik). Precursor of squalene, steroids, terpenes, and dolichol.

mev·a·lon·ic ac·i·du·ria. Elevated levels of mevalonic acid in the urine; associated with a deficiency of mevalonate kinase.

mev·a·sta·tin (mev′ă-stat-in). Fungal metabolite which is a potent inhibitor of HMG-CoA reductase, the rate-controlling enzyme in cholesterol biosynthesis. The drug, similar to lovastatin, pravastatin and simvastatin, is used in the treatment of hyperlipidemia.

me·vin·o·lin (me-vin′ō-lin). SYN lovastatin.

mex·e·none (mek′sĕ-nōn). A sun-screening agent.

mex·il·e·tine (meks-il′ĕ-tēn). A cardiac antiarrhythmic drug used to treat ventricular arrhythmias; resembles lidocaine in its actions but is orally effective.

mex·il·e·tine hy·dro·chlo·ride (meks-il′ĕ-tēn). An orally active antiarrhythmic agent used to suppress symptomatic ventricular arrhythmias; resembles lidocaine in its actions but is orally effective.

Meyenburg, H. von, Swiss pathologist, *1877. SEE M. *complex, disease;* M.-Altherr-Uehlinger *syndrome.*

Meyer, Adolf, U.S. psychiatrist, 1866–1950. SEE M.-Archambault *loop.*

Meyer, Edmund V., German laryngologist, 1864–1931. SEE M. *cartilages,* under *cartilage.*

Meyer, Georg H., Swiss anatomist, 1815–1892. SEE M. *line, sinus.*

Meyer, Hans H., German pharmacologist, 1853–1939. SEE M.-Overton *rule, theory* of narcosis.

Meyer, Willy, U.S. surgeon, 1858–1932. SEE M. *reagent.*

Meyer-Betz, Friedrich, 20th century German physician. SEE Meyer-Betz *disease;* Meyer-Betz *syndrome.*

Meyerhof, Otto F., German-U.S. biochemist and Nobel laureate, 1884–1951. SEE Embden-M. *pathway;* Embden-M.-Parnas *pathway;* M. oxidation *quotient.*

Meyer-Schwickerath, Gerhard Rudolph Edmund, German ophthalmologist, *1920.

Meynert, Theodor H., Vienna neurologist, 1833–1892. SEE retroflex *bundle* of Meynert; M. *cells,* under *cell, commissure, decussation; fasciculus* of Meynert; M. *layer.*

mez·lo·cil·lin so·di·um (mez-lō-sil′in). $C_{21}H_{24}NaN_5O_8S_2$; an extended spectrum penicillin antibiotic used intravenously and intramuscularly.

Mg Symbol for magnesium.

mg Symbol for milligram.

MGP Abbreviation for matrix Gla *protein.*

MGUS Abbreviation for monoclonal *gammopathy* of unknown significance.

MHC Abbreviation for major histocompatibility *complex,* minor histocompatibility *complex.*

mho (mō). SYN siemens. [*ohm* reversed]

MHz Symbol for megahertz.

MI Abbreviation for myocardial *infarction.*

mi·an·ser·in hy·dro·chlo·ride (mē-an′ser-in). An H_1 antihistaminic with antiserotonin activity.

mibefradil (mib-ef′ra-dil). A tetralol derivative in a new class of calcium antagonists that block at T-type channels; used to treat mild to moderate hypertension and angina pectoris.

Mibelli, Vittorio, Italian dermatologist, 1860–1910. SEE M. *angiokeratomas,* under *angiokeratoma, disease.*

MIC Abbreviation for minimal inhibitory *concentration.*

mi·ca·to·sis (mī′kă-tō-sis). Pneumoconiosis due to inhalation of mica particles.

mi·cel·lar (mī-sel′er, mi-). Having the properties of an assemblage of micelles, i.e., of a gel.

mi·celle (mi-sel′, mī-sel′). 1. Nägeli term for elongated sub(light)-microscopic particles, detected in hydrogels, of supramolecular character and crystalline structure; now defined as one of two classes of colloidal particle: those consisting of many molecules, the other class being single macromolecules light- or submicroscopic in size. A m. is thus a structural unit of the disperse phase in a gel, a unit whose repetition in three dimensions constitutes the micellar structure of the gel; it does not denote the individual particles in free suspension or solution, or the unit structure of a crystal. 2. Any water-soluble aggregate, spontaneously and reversibly, formed from amphiphile molecules. 3. A hypothetical ordered region in a natural fiber such as cellulose. [L. *micella,* small morsel, dim. of *mica,* morsel, grain]

Michaelis, Leonor, German-U.S. chemist, 1875–1949. SEE M.-Gutmann *body;* M. *constant;* M.-Menten *constant, equation, hypothesis.*

Michel, Gaston, French surgeon, 1874–1937. SEE Michel *spur.*

Michel, M., 19th century French physician. SEE M. *malformation.*

Micheli, Ferdinando, Italian physician, 1872–1936. SEE Marchiafava-M. *anemia, syndrome.*

mi·con·a·zole ni·trate (mī-kon′ă-zōl). An antifungal agent.

⌂**micr-.** SEE micro-.

mi·cren·ce·pha·lia (mī′kren-se-fā′lē-ă). SYN micrencephaly.

mi·cren·ceph·a·lous (mī-kren-sef′ă-lŭs). Having a small brain.

mi·cren·ceph·a·ly (mī-kren-sef′ă-lē). Abnormal smallness of the brain. SYN micrencephalia, microencephaly. [micro- + G. *enkephalos,* brain]

⌂**micro-, micr-.** 1. Prefixes denoting smallness. 2 (μ). Prefix used in the SI and metric system to signify submultiples of one-millionth (10^{-6}) of such unit. 3. In chemistry, prefix to terms denoting chemical examination, methods, etc. that utilize minimal quantities of the substance to be examined; e.g., a drop or two in place of 1 or more mL. 4. Combining forms meaning microscopic; opposite of macro-, megalo-. [G. *mikros,* small]

mi·cro·ab·scess (mī′krō-ab′ses). A very small circumscribed collection of leukocytes in solid tissues.
Munro m., a microscopic collection of polymorphonuclear leukocytes found in the stratum corneum in psoriasis. SYN Munro abscess.
Pautrier m., a microscopic lesion in the epidermis, seen in mycosis fungoides; it is composed of the same type of atypical mononuclear cells as those that form the infiltrate in the corium. SYN Pautrier abscess.

mi·cro·ad·e·no·ma (mī′krō-ad-ĕ-nō′mă). A pituitary adenoma less than 10 mm in diameter.

mi·cro·ae·ro·bi·on (mī′krō-ā-rō′bĭ-on). A microaerophilic microorganism.

mi·cro·aer·o·phil, mi·cro·aer·o·phile (mī-krō-ār′ō-fil, -fīl). 1. An aerobic bacterium that requires oxygen, but less than is present in the air, and grows best under modified atmospheric conditions. 2. Relating to such an organism. SYN microaerophilic, microaerophilous. [micro- + G. *aēr,* air, + *philos,* fond]

mi·cro·aer·o·phil·ic (mī′krō-ār-ō-fil′ik). SYN microaerophil (2).

mi·cro·aer·oph·i·lous (mī′krō-ār-ōf′i-lŭs). SYN microaerophil (2).

mi

mi·cro·aer·o·sol (mī-krō-ār′ō-sol). A suspension in air of particles that are submicronic or, more frequently, from 1–10; μm in diameter.

microalbuminuria (mī′krō-al-boo-min-ū′rē-ă). A slight increase in urinary albumin excretion that can be detected using immunoassays but not using conventional urine protein measurements; an early marker for renal disease in patients with diabetes. [micro- + albuminuria]

mi·cro·a·nal·y·sis (mī′krō-ă-nal′i-sis). Analytic techniques involving unusually small samples.

mi·cro·a·nas·to·mo·sis (mī′krō-ă-nas-tō-mō′sis). Anastomosis of minute structures performed under an operating microscope.

mi·cro·a·nat·o·mist (mī′krō-ă-nat′ō-mist). SYN histologist.

mi·cro·a·nat·o·my (mī′krō-ă-nat′ŏ-mē). SYN histology.

mi·cro·an·eu·rysm (mī′krō-an′ū-rizm). Focal dilation of retinal capillaries occurring in diabetes mellitus, retinal vein obstruction, and absolute glaucoma, or of arteriolocapillary junctions in many organs in thrombotic thrombocytopenic purpura.

mi·cro·an·gi·og·ra·phy (mī′krō-an-jē-og′ră-fē). Radiography of the finer vessels of an organ after the injection of a contrast medium and enlargement of the resulting radiograph. SYN microarteriography. [micro- + angiography]

mi·cro·an·gi·op·a·thy (mī′krō-an-jē-op′ă-thē). SYN capillaropathy.

    thrombotic m., thrombosis within small blood vessels, as in thrombotic thrombocytopenic purpura.

mi·cro·an·gi·os·co·py (mī′krō-an-jē-os′kŏ-pē). SYN capillarioscopy.

mi·cro·ar·te·ri·og·ra·phy (mī′krō-ar-tēr-ē-og′ră-fē). SYN microangiography.

microatelectasis. SYN adhesive *atelectasis.*

mi·cro·bal·ance (mī′krō-bal-ans). A balance designed for use in weighing unusually small samples of materials.

mi·crobe (mī′krōb). Any very minute organism. As originated, the word was intended as a collective term for the large variety of microorganisms then known in the 19th century; modern usage has retained the original collective meaning but expanded it to include both microscopic and ultramicroscopic organisms (spirochetes, bacteria, rickettsiae, and viruses). These organisms are considered to form a biologically distinctive group, in that the genetic material is not surrounded by a nuclear membrane, and mitosis does not occur during replication. [Fr., fr. G. *mikros,* small, + *bios,* life]

mi·cro·bi·al (mī-krō′bē-ăl). Relating to a microbe or to microbes. SYN microbic, microbiotic (2).

mi·cro·bi·al as·so·ci·ates (mī-krō′bē-ăl ă-sō′shē-ăts). SYN flora (2).

mi·cro·bic (mī-krō′bik). SYN microbial.

mi·cro·bi·ci·dal (mī-krō′bi-sī′dăl). Destructive to microbes. SYN microbicide (1).

mi·cro·bi·cide (mī-krō′bi-sīd). **1.** SYN microbicidal. **2.** An agent destructive to microbes; a germicide; an antiseptic. [microbe + L. *caedo,* to kill]

mi·cro·bi·o·log·ic (mī′krō-bī-ō-loj′ik). Relating to microbiology.

mi·cro·bi·ol·o·gist (mī′krō-bī-ol′ō-jist). One who specializes in the science of microbiology.

mi·cro·bi·ol·o·gy (mī′krō-bī-ol′ō-jē). The science concerned with microorganisms, including fungi, protozoa, bacteria, and viruses. [Fr. *microbiologie*]

mi·cro·bi·ot·ic (mī′krō-bī-ot′ik). **1.** Short-lived. **2.** SYN microbial.

mi·cro·bism (mī′krō-bizm). Infection with microbes.

    latent m., the presence of pathogenic microorganisms in the body that elicit no symptoms; the condition of a pathogen carrier.

mi·cro·blast (mī′krō-blast). A small, nucleated, red blood cell. [micro- + G. *blastos,* sprout, germ]

mi·cro·ble·pha·ria (mī′krō-ble-far′ē-ă). SYN microblepharon.

mi·cro·bleph·a·rism (-blef′ăr-izm). SYN microblepharon.

mi·cro·bleph·a·ron (-blef′ă-ron). Eyelids with abnormal vertical shortness. SYN microblepharia, microblepharism. [micro + G. *blepharon,* eyelid + -*ia,* condition]

mi·cro·body (mī′krō-bod-ē). A cytoplasmic organelle, bounded by a single membrane and containing oxidative enzymes. M.'s include peroxisomes and glyoxysomes.

mi·cro·bra·chia (mī-krō-brā′kē-ă). Abnormal smallness of the arms. [micro- + G. *brachiōn,* arm]

mi·cro·bren·ner (mī-krō-bren′er). An electric cautery with needle point. [micro- + Ger. *Brenner,* burner]

mi·cro·cal·ci·fi·ca·tions (mī′krō-kal-si-fi-kā′shuns). Calcifications less than 1 mm in diameter as seen on mammography; often associated with malignant lesions. [micro- + calcification]

mi·cro·car·dia (mī-krō-kar′dē-ă). Abnormal smallness of the heart. [micro- + G. *kardia,* heart]

mi·cro·cen·trum (mī-krō-sen′trŭm). SYN cytocentrum. [micro- + G. *kentron,* center]

mi·cro·ce·pha·lia (mī-krō-se-fā′lē-ă). SYN microcephaly.

mi·cro·ce·phal·ic (mī′krō-sĕ-fal′ik). Having a small head. SYN microcephalous, nanocephalous, nanocephalic.

mi·cro·ceph·a·lism (mī-krō-sef′ă-lizm). SYN microcephaly.

mi·cro·ceph·a·lous (mī-krō-sef′ă-lŭs). SYN microcephalic.

mi·cro·ceph·a·ly (mī-krō-sef′ă-lē). Abnormal smallness of the head; applied to a skull with a capacity below 1350 ml. Usually associated with mental retardation. SYN microcephalia, microcephalism, nanocephalia, nanocephaly. [micro- + G. *kephalē,* head]

    encephaloclastic m., complex growth disturbances in the brain as a result of regressive changes in fetal life.

    schizencephalic m., dysgenic process resulting in focal cerebral defects.

mi·cro·chei·lia, mi·cro·chi·lia (mī-krō-kī′lē-ă). Smallness of the lips. [micro- + G. *cheilos,* lip]

mi·cro·chei·ria, mi·cro·chi·ria (mī-krō-kī′rē-ă). Smallness of the hands. [micro- + G. *cheir,* hand]

mi·cro·chem·is·try (mī-krō-kem′is-trē). The use of chemical procedures involving minute quantities or reactions not visible to the unaided eye. Cf. macrochemistry.

micro·chim·er·ism (mī-krō-kim′er-izm). The presence of donor cells in a graft recipient, or of fetal cells remaining in maternal circulation, which can be detected by molecular methods but not by flow cytometry.

mi·cro·cide (mī′krō-sīd). SYN *glucose* oxidase.

mi·cro·cin·e·ma·tog·ra·phy (mī′kro-sin-ĕ-mă-tog′ră-fē). The application of moving pictures taken through magnifying lenses to the study of an organ or system in motion; e.g., the circulation in living embryos. [micro- + G. *kinēma,* movement, + *graphō,* to write]

mi·cro·cir·cu·la·tion (mī′krō-sir-kū-lā′shŭn). Passage of blood in the smallest vessels, namely arterioles, capillaries, and venules.

Mi·cro·coc·ca·ce·ae (mī′krō-kok-ā′sē-ē). A family of bacteria (order Eubacteriales) containing Gram-positive spherical cells which occur singly or in pairs, tetrads, packets, irregular masses, or even chains. Rarely are these organisms motile. Free-living, saprophytic, parasitic, and pathogenic species occur. The type genus is *Micrococcus.*

mi·cro·coc·ci (mī′krō-kok′sī). Plural of micrococcus.

Mi·cro·coc·cus (mī′krō-kok-ŭs). A genus of bacteria (family Micrococcaceae) containing Gram-positive, spherical cells that occur in irregular masses. Some species are motile or produce motile mutants. These organisms are saprophytic, facultatively parasitic, or parasitic but are not truly pathogenic. The type species is *M. luteus.* It is the type genus of the family Micrococcaceae. [micro- + G. *kokkos,* berry]

    M. conglomera′tus, a bacterial species found in infections, milk, dairy products, dairy utensils, and water.

    M. lu′teus, a saprophytic species found in milk and dairy products and on dust particles, it has caused meningitis in humans; it is the type species of the genus *M.*

    M. var′ians, former name for *Kocuria varians.*

mi·cro·coc·cus, pl. **mi·cro·coc·ci** (mī′krō-kok′ŭs, -kok′sī). A vernacular term used to refer to any member of the genus *Micro-coccus*.

mi·cro·co·li·tis (mī′krō-kō-lī′tis). Colitis that is not seen by endoscopy, but in which microscopic examination of biopsies shows nonspecific mucosal inflammation.

mi·cro·co·lon (mī′krō-kō-lon). A small-caliber unused colon, seen in the neonate on radiographic contrast enema; usually a consequence of intestinal atresia or meconium ileus.

mi·cro·col·o·ny (mī′krō-kol-ō-nē). A colony of bacteria visible only under a low power microscope.

mi·cro·co·nid·i·um, pl. **mi·cro·co·nid·ia** (mī′krō-kō-nid′ē-ŭm, -ă). In fungi, the smaller of two distinctively different-sized types of conidia in a single species, usually single-celled and spherical, ovoid, pyriform, or clavate.

mi·cro·co·ria (mī-krō-kō′rē-ă). A congenitally small pupil with an inability to dilate. [micro- + G. *korē*, pupil]

mi·cro·cor·nea (mī′krō-kōr′nē-ă). An abnormally small cornea.

mi·cro·cou·lomb (μC) (mī-krō-koo′lom). One-millionth of a coulomb.

mi·cro·crys·tal·line (mī′krō-krys′tă-lin). Occurring in minute crystals.

mi·cro·cu·rie (μCi) (mī′krō-kū′rē). One-millionth of a curie; a quantity of any radionuclide with 3.7×10^4 disintegrations per second.

mi·cro·cyst (mī′krō-sist). A tiny cyst, frequently of such dimensions that a magnifying lens or microscope is required for observation.

mi·cro·cyte (mī′krō-sīt). A small (5 μm or less) nonnucleated red blood cell. SYN microerythrocyte. [micro- + G. *kytos*, cell]

mi·cro·cy·the·mia (mī′krō-sī-thē′mē-ă). The presence of many microcytes in the circulating blood. SYN microcytosis. [microcyte + G. *haima*, blood]

▮ **mi·cro·cy·to·sis** (mī′krō-sī-tō′sis). SYN microcythemia. [microcyte + G. *-osis*, condition]

mi·cro·dac·tyl·ia (mī′krō-dak-til′ē-ă). SYN microdactyly.

mi·cro·dac·ty·lous (mī-krō-dak′ti-lŭs). Relating to or characterized by microdactyly.

mi·cro·dac·ty·ly (mī-krō-dak′ti-lē). Smallness or shortness of the fingers or toes. SYN microdactylia. [micro- + G. *dactylos*, finger, toe]

microdialysis. A method of studying extracellular fluid composition and response to exogenous agents, utilizing a tiny tubular probe with a dialysis membrane and fluid flow rates of 1–3 μL/min, inserted into tissues.

mi·cro·dis·sec·tion (mī′krō-di-sek′shŭn). Dissection of tissues under a microscope or magnifying glass, usually done by teasing the tissues apart by means of needles.

mi·cro·dont (mī′krō-dont). Having small teeth; denoting a skull with a dental index below 41.9. [micro- + G. *odous (odont-)*, tooth]

mi·cro·don·tia, mi·cro·don·tism (mī-krō-don′shē-ă, -don′tizm). A condition in which a single tooth, or pairs of teeth, or the whole dentition, may be disproportionately small. [micro- + G. *odous*, tooth]

mi·cro·dose (mī′krō-dōs). A very small dose.

mi·cro·drep·a·no·cy·to·sis (mī′krō-drep′ă-nō-sī-tō′sis). A chronic hemolytic anemia resulting from interaction of the genes for sickle cell anemia and thalassemia. [microcytosis + drepanocytosis]

mi·cro·dys·ge·ne·sia (mī′krō-dis-ge-nē′sē-ă). Increase in partially distopic neurons in the stratum zonale, white matter, hippocampus and cerebellar cortex, producing an indistinct border between cortex and subcortical white matter and a columnar arrangement of cortical neurons; seen in patients with primary generalized epilepsy. [micro- + dys- + G. *genesis*, production]

mi·cro·e·lec·trode (mī′krō-ē-lek′trōd). An electrode of very fine caliber consisting usually of a fine wire or a glass tube of capillary diameter (10 μm to 1 mm) drawn to a fine point and filled with saline or a metal such as gallium or indium (while melted);

used in physiologic experiments to stimulate or to record action currents of extracellular or intracellular origin.

microelements (mī′krō-el′ĕ-ments). SYN trace *elements*, under *element*.

mi·cro·en·ceph·a·ly (mī′krō-en-sef′ă-lē). SYN micrencephaly.

mi·cro·e·ryth·ro·cyte (mī′krō-ĕ-rith′rō-sīt). SYN microcyte.

mi·cro·ev·o·lu·tion (mī′krō-ev-ŏ-loo′shŭn). The evolution of bacteria and other microorganisms through mutations.

mi·cro·fi·bril (mi-kro-fi′bril). A very small fibril having an average diameter of 13 nm; it may be a bundle of still smaller elements, the microfilaments.

mi·cro·fil·a·ment (mī-krō-fil′ă-ment). The finest filamentous element of the cytoskeleton, having a diameter of about 5 nm and consisting primarily of actin. SEE ALSO actin *filament*.

mi·cro·fil·a·re·mia (mī′krō-fil-ă-rē′mē-ă). Infection of the blood with microfilariae. M. caused by *Wuchereria bancrofti* is characterized by sharp nocturnal periodicity, apparently tied to the nocturnal habits of the vector mosquitoes; in geographic areas where mosquitoes are not strictly night-biters (as in parts of Polynesia), the microfilarial periodicity is modified or absent. SEE ALSO periodic *filariasis*.

mi·cro·fi·lar·ia, pl. **mi·cro·fi·lar·i·ae** (mī′krō-fi-lar′ē-ă, -ē). Term for embryos of filarial nematodes in the family Onchocercidae. In the past this term has been used as a generic designation (e.g., *Microfilaria bancrofti*, *M. malaya*). SEE *Filaria*.

mi·cro·film (mī′krō-film). **1.** A photographic film bearing greatly reduced images of printed records. **2.** To record on microfilm.

mi·cro·flo·ra (mī′krō-flō-rā). The bacteria and fungi that inhabit an area.

mi·cro·ga·mete (mī-krō-gam′ēt). The male element in anisogamy, or conjugation of cells of unequal size; it is the smaller of the two cells and actively motile. [micro- + G. *gametēs*, husband]

mi·cro·ga·me·to·cyte (mī-krō-gam′ĕ-tō-sīt). The mother cell producing the microgametes, or male elements of sexual reproduction in sporozoan protozoans and fungi. SYN microgamont.

mi·cro·gam·ont (mī-krō-gam′ont). SYN microgametocyte.

mi·crog·a·my (mī-krog′ă-mē). Conjugation between two young cells, the recent product of sporulation or some other form of reproduction. [micro- + G. *gamos*, marriage]

mi·cro·gas·tria (mī-krō-gas′trē-ă). Smallness of the stomach. [micro- + G. *gastēr*, stomach]

mi·cro·gen·ia (mī-krō-jēn′ē-ă). Abnormal smallness of the chin resulting from the underdevelopment of the mental symphysis. [micro- + G. *geneion*, chin]

mi·cro·gen·i·tal·ism (mī-krō-jen′i-tal-izm). Abnormal smallness of the external genital organs.

mi·crog·lia (mī-krog′lē-ă). Small neuroglial cells, possibly of mesodermal origin, which may become phagocytic, in areas of neural damage or inflammation. SYN Hortega cells, microglia cells, microglial cells. [micro- + G. *glia*, glue]

mi·crog·li·a·cyte (mī-krōg′lē-ă-sīt). A cell, especially an embryonic cell, of the microglia. [micro- + G. *glia*, glue, + *kytos*, cell]

mi·crog·li·o·ma (mī-krog′lē-ō′mă). Obsolete term for an intracranial neoplasm of microglial cell origin that is structurally similar to lymphoma. [microglia + G. *-oma*, tumor]

mi·cro·gli·o·ma·to·sis (mī′krō-glē-ō-mă-tō′sis). Obsolete term for a condition characterized by the presence of multiple microgliomas.

mi·crog·li·o·sis (mī-krog′lē-ō′sis). Presence of microglia in nervous tissue secondary to injury. [microglia + G. *-osis*, condition]

mi·cro·glob·u·lin (mī-krō-glob′oo-lin). **1.** Any serum or urinary globulin of molecular mass below about 40 kd, including especially Bence Jones *proteins*, under *protein*. **2.** On occasions, a term used to refer to 7S immunoglobins (e.g., IgG).

β-m., a polypeptide of 11,600 Da that forms the light chain of class 1 major histocompatibility antigens and can therefore be detected on all cells bearing these antigens. Free β-m. is found in the blood and urine of patients with certain diseases, including Wilson *disease*, cadmium poisoning, and renal tubular *acidosis*.

β₂-m., the light chain of the histocompatibility class I molecule.

mi

This chain is invariant within a given species; found in elevated levels in individuals with Wilson disease and in alcohol-induced liver cirrhosis.

mi·cro·glos·sia (mī-krō-glos′ē-ă). Smallness of the tongue. [micro- + G. *glōssa,* tongue]

mi·cro·gna·thia (mī-krō-nā′thē-ă, mī-krog-nath′ē-ă). Abnormal smallness of the jaws, especially of the mandible. [micro- + G. *gnathos,* jaw]

m. with peromelia, hypoplasia of the mandible with malformed and missing teeth, birdlike face, and severe deformities of the hands and forearms and sometimes of feet and legs. SYN Hanhart syndrome.

mi·cro·gram (μg, γ) (mī′krō-gram). One-millionth of a gram.

mi·cro·graph (mī′krō-graf). **1.** An instrument that magnifies the microscopic movements of a diaphragm by means of light interference and records them on a moving photographic film; may be used for recording various pulse curves, sound waves, and any forms of motion that may be communicated through the air to a diaphragm. **2.** SYN photomicrograph. [micro- + G. *graphō,* to write]

electron m., the image produced by the electron beam of an electron microscope, recorded on an electron-sensitive plate or film.

light m., a photograph produced by means of a light microscope.

mi·crog·ra·phy (mī-krog′ră-fē). **1.** Writing with very minute letters, sometimes observed in psychoses and in paralysis agitans. **2.** A description of objects seen with a microscope. **3.** SYN photomicrography. [micro- + G. *graphō,* to write]

mi·cro·gy·ria (mī-krō-jī′rē-ă). Abnormal narrowness of the cerebral convolutions. [micro- + G. *gyros,* convolution]

mi·cro·he·pat·ia (mī-krō-he-pat′ē-ă). Abnormal smallness of the liver. [micro- + G. *hepar (hepat-),* liver]

mi·cro·het·er·o·gene·i·ty (mī′krō-het′er-ō-jĕ-nē′i-tē;nĕ′i-tē). Slight differences in structure between essentially identical molecules; e.g., in the saccharide portion of a glycoprotein.

mi·crohm (μΩ) (mī′krōm). One-millionth of an ohm. SYN microohm.

mi·cro·in·cin·er·a·tion (mī′krō-in-sin′ĕ-rā′shŭn). Combustion, in a furnace, of organic constituents in a tissue section so that the remaining mineral ash can be examined microscopically. SYN spodography.

mi·cro·in·cis·ion (mī-krō-in-sizh′ŭn). An incision made with the aid of a microscope.

mi·cro·in·jec·tor (mī′krō-in-jek-tor). An instrument for infusion of very small amounts of fluids or drugs into animals or humans.

mi·cro·in·va·sion (mī′krō-in-vā′zhŭn). Invasion of tissue immediately adjacent to a carcinoma in situ, the earliest stage of malignant neoplastic invasion.

mi·cro·kat·al (mī′krō-kat′ăl). One-millionth of a katal.

mi·cro·ky·mat·o·ther·a·py (mī′krō-kī-mat′ō-thār′ă-pē). Treatment with high frequency radiations of 3,000,000,000 Hz (3000 MHz), at a wavelength of 10 cm. SYN microwave therapy. [micro- + G. *kyma,* a wave, + *therapeia,* treatment]

mi·cro·leu·ko·blast (mī-krō-loo′kō-blast). SYN micromyeloblast.

mi·cro·li·ter (μl, μL) (mī′krō-lē-ter). One-millionth of a liter.

mi·cro·lith (mī′krō-lith). A minute calculus, usually multiple, sometimes constituting a coarse sand called gravel. [micro- + G. *lithos,* stone]

mi·cro·li·thi·a·sis (mī-krō-li-thī′ă-sis). The formation, presence, or discharge of minute concretions, or gravel, e.g., testicular microlithiasis.

pulmonary alveolar m., microscopic granules of calcium or bone disseminated throughout the lungs.

mi·crol·o·gy (mī-krol′ō-jē). The science concerned with microscopic objects, of which histology is a branch. [micro- + G. *logos,* study]

mi·cro·ma·nip·u·la·tion (mī′krō-mă-nip′ū-lā′shŭn). Dissection, teasing, stimulation, etc., under the microscope, of minute structures; e.g., tissue cells or unicellular organisms.

mi·cro·ma·nip·u·la·tor (mī′krō-mă-nip′ū-lā′ter, -tōr). An instru-

ment used in micromanipulation, whereby microdissection, microinjection, and other maneuvers are performed, usually with the aid of a microscope.

mi·cro·ma·zia (mī-krō-mā′zē-ă). Condition in which the breasts are rudimentary and functionless. [micro- + G. *mazos,* breast]

mi·cro·me·lia (mī-krō-mē′lē-ă). Condition of having disproportionately short or small limbs. SEE ALSO achondroplasia. SYN nanomelia. [micro- + G. *melos,* limb]

mi·cro·mere (mī′krō-mēr). A blastomere of small size; for example, one of the blastomeres at the animal pole of an amphibian egg. [micro- + G. *meros,* a part]

mi·cro·mer·o·zo·ite (mī′krō-mer-ō-zō′īt). A small merozoite.

mi·cro·me·tas·ta·sis (mī′krō-mĕ-tas′tă-sis). A stage of metastasis when the secondary tumors are too small to be clinically detected, as in micrometastatic disease.

mi·cro·met·a·stat·ic (mī′krō-met-ă-stat′ik). Denoting or characterized by micrometastasis, as in m. disease.

mi·crom·e·ter (μm) (mī-krom′ĕ-ter). **1.** One-millionth of a meter; formerly called micron. **2.** A device for measuring various types of objects in an accurate and precise manner; in medicine and biology, the term is usually used with reference to a glass slide or lens that is accurately marked for measuring microscopic forms. [micro- + G. *metron,* measure]

caliper m., a gauge with a calibrated m. screw for the measurement of thin objects such as microscope cover glasses and slides.

filar m., an ocular micrometer with a line moved by a ruled drum such that a movement of the line of 5 μm or less may be made in relation to fixed parallel lines.

ocular m., a glass disk that fits in a microscope eyepiece and that has a ruled scale; when calibrated with a slide m., direct measurements of a microscopic object can be made.

slide m., a scale made on a microscope slide with lines ruled in divisions, usually, of 0.01 mm; typically used to calibrate an ocular m.

mi·crom·e·try (mī-krom′ĕ-trē). Measurement of objects with some type of micrometer and a microscope.

△**micromicro-** (μμ). Prefix formerly used to signify one-trillionth (10^{-12}); now pico-.

mi·cro·mi·cro·gram (μμg) (mī′krō-mī′krō-gram). Former term for picogram.

mi·cro·mi·cron (μμ) (mī-krō-mī′kron). Former term for picometer.

mi·cro·min·er·als (mī-krō-min′er-ălz). SYN trace *elements,* under *element.*

mi·cro·mo·lar (μmol/L) (mī-krō-mō′lar). Denoting a concentration of 10^{-6} mol/L.

mi·cro·mole (μmol) (mī′krō-mōl). One-millionth of a mole.

mi·cro·mo·to·scope (mī′krō-mō′tō-skōp). A cinematoscope for representing the movements of amebas and other motile microscopic objects. [micro- + L. *motus,* motion, + G. *skopeō,* to view]

mi·cro·my·e·lia (mī′krō-mī-ē′lē-ă). Abnormal smallness or shortness of the spinal cord. [micro- + G. *myelos,* marrow]

mi·cro·my·el·o·blast (mī-krō-mī′el-ō-blast). A small myeloblast, often the predominating cell in myeloblastic leukemia. SYN microleukoblast.

mi·cron (μ) (mī′kron). Former term for micrometer.

mi·cro·nee·dle (mī′krō-nē′dl). A small glass needle used in micrurgical manipulation.

mi·cro·neme (mī′krō-nēm). A small, osmiophilic, cordlike twisted organelle found in the anterior region of many sporozoans; one of the characteristics that helps to define the subphylum Apicomplexa. SYN sarconeme. [micro- + G. *nēma,* thread]

mi·cron·ic (mī-kron′ik). Of the size of 1 micron (micrometer).

mi·cro·nod·u·lar (mī′krō-nod′ū-lăr). Characterized by the presence of minute nodules; denoting a somewhat coarser appearance than that of a granular tissue or substance. [G. *mikros,* small]

mi·cro·nu·cle·us (mī-krō-noo′klē-ŭs). **1.** A small nucleus in a large cell, or the smaller nuclei in cells that have two or more such structures. **2.** The smaller of the two nuclei in ciliates dividing mitotically and bearing specific inheritable material. SYN gametic nucleus, germ nucleus, gonad nucleus, karyogonad, reproductive nucleus. SEE ALSO macronucleus (2).

mi·cro·nu·tri·ents (mī-krō-noo′trē-ents). Essential food factors required in only small quantities by the body; e.g., vitamins, trace minerals. SYN trace nutrient.

mi·cro·nych·ia (mī-krō-nik′ē-ă). Abnormal smallness of nails. [micro- + G. *onyx*, nail]

mi·cro·nys·tag·mus (mī′krō-nis-tag′mŭs). Nystagmus of so small an amplitude that it is not detected by the usual clinical tests. SYN minimal amplitude nystagmus. [micro- + G. *nystagmos*, a nodding]

mi·cro·ohm (mī′krō-ōm). SYN microhm.

mi·cro·or·gan·ism (mī′krō-ōr′gan-izm). A microscopic organism (plant or animal).

mi·cro·par·a·site (mī-krō-par′ă-sīt). A parasitic microorganism.

mi·cro·pa·thol·o·gy (mī′krō-pa-thol′ō-jē). Obsolete term for the microscopic study of disease changes. [micro- + G. *pathos*, suffering, + *logos*, study]

mi·cro·pe·nis (mī-krō-pē′nis). Abnormally small penis. SYN microphallus.

mi·cro·phage (mī′krō-fāj). A polymorphonuclear leukocyte that is phagocytic. SEE ALSO phagocyte. SYN microphagocyte. [micro- + phag(ocyte)]

mi·cro·phag·o·cyte (mī-krō-fāj′ō-sīt). SYN microphage.

mi·cro·phal·lus (mī-krō-fal′ŭs). SYN micropenis.

mi·cro·pho·bia (mī-krō-fō′bē-ă). Fear of minute objects, microorganisms, germs, etc. [micro- + G. *phobos*, fear]

mi·cro·phone (mī′krō-fōn). An instrument for converting sounds to electrical impulses. [micro- + G. *phōnē*, sound]

mi·cro·pho·nia, mi·croph·o·ny (mī-krō-fō′nē-ă, mī-krof′ŏ-nē). SYN hypophonia. [micro- + G. *phōnē*, voice]

mi·cro·pho·no·scope (mī-krō-fō′nō-skōp). A stethoscope with a diaphragm attachment for magnifying the sound.

mi·cro·pho·to·graph (mī-krō-fō′tō-graf). A minute photograph of any object, as distinguished from a photomicrograph.

mi·croph·thal·mia (mī′krof-thal′mē-ă). SYN microphthalmos.

colobomatous m., a congenital defect occurring along an embryonic fissure in a small eye, sometimes associated with cysts.

mi·croph·thal·mos (-thal′mos). Abnormal smallness of the eye. SYN microphthalmia, nanophthalmia, nanophthalmos. [micro + G. *ophthalmos*, eye]

mi·cro·pi·pette, mi·cro·pi·pet (mī′krō-pi-pet′, -pī-pet′). A pipette designed for the measurement of very small volumes.

mi·cro·pla·nia (mī-krō-plā′nē-ă). Decreased horizontal diameter of erythrocytes. [micro- + L. *planus*, flat]

mi·cro·pla·sia (mī-krō-plā′zē-ă). Stunted growth, as in dwarfism. [micro- + G. *plasis*, a shaping, forming]

mi·cro·pleth·ys·mog·ra·phy (mī′krō-pleth-iz-mog′ră-fē). The technique of measuring minute changes in the volume of a part as a result of blood flow into or out of it.

mi·cro·po·dia (mī-krō-pō′dē-ă). Abnormal smallness of the feet. [micro- + G. *pous*, foot]

mi·cro·pore (mī′krō-pōr). An organelle formed by the pellicle of all stages of sporozoan protozoa of the subphylum Apicomplexa and also found in developmental stages that may lack the inner pellicle layer; it is composed of two concentric rings (in transverse section), the inner of which corresponds with an invagination of the outer pellicle membrane. M.'s thus far observed seem to serve as feeding organelles; their role in nonfeeding developmental forms is unknown. [micro- + G. *poros*, pore]

mi·cro·pro·my·el·o·cyte (mī′krō-prō-mī′el-ō-sīt). A cell derived from a promyelocyte.

mi·cro·pro·so·pia (mī′krō-prō-sō′pē-ă). A condition characterized by an abnormally small or imperfectly developed face. [micro- + G. *prosōpon*, face]

mi·crop·sia (mī-krop′sē-ă). Perception of objects as smaller than they are. [micro- + G. *opsis*, sight]

mi·cro·punc·ture (mī′krō-pŭnk-choor). A small puncture made with the aid of a microscope.

mi·cro·pyle (mī′krō-pīl). **1.** Minute opening believed to exist in the investing membrane of certain ova as a point of entrance for the spermatozoon. **2.** Former name for micropore. [micro- + G. *pylē*, gate]

mi·cro·ra·di·og·ra·phy (mī′krō-rā-dē-og′ră-fē). Making radiographs of histologic sections of tissue for enlargement. SEE ALSO historadiography.

mi·cro·re·frac·tom·e·ter (mī′krō-rē-frak-tom′ě-ter). A refractometer used in the study of blood cells.

mi·cro·res·pi·rom·e·ter (mī′krō-res-pi-rom′ě-ter). An apparatus for measuring the utilization of oxygen by small particles of isolated tissues or cells or particles of cells.

mi·cro·sac·cades (mī′krō-să-kādz′). Minute to-and-fro movements of the eyes. [micro- + Fr. *saccade*, sudden check (of a horse)]

mi·cro·scin·tig·ra·phy (mī′krō-sin-tig′ră-fē). Imaging of small anatomic structures by use of a radionuclide in conjunction with a special collimator which "magnifies" the image; for example, the use of technetium-99m in conjunction with a pinhole collimator to image the lacrimal drainage. [micro- + scintigraphy]

mi·cro·scope (mī′krō-skōp). An instrument that gives an enlarged image of an object or substance that is minute or not visible with the naked eye; usually the term denotes a compound m.; for low magnifications, the term simple m., or magnifying glass, is used. [micro- + G. *skopeō*, to view]

binocular m., a m. having two eyepieces; it may be a compound m. or a stereoscopic m.

color-contrast m., a type of m. in which the condenser stop is of one color and the annulus is a complement of it so that unstained objects are observed in one color on a field of the other.

comparator m., a device constructed with one or more m.'s having micrometer eyepieces used to measure dimensional changes during setting or temperature changes.

compound m., a m. having two or more magnifying lenses.

confocal m., a m. that allows the observer to visualize objects in a single plane of focus, thereby creating a sharper image (usually the objects are fluorescent molecules); a refinement of this m. uses optical sectioning and a computer to record serial sections. This permits three-dimensional reconstruction.

dark-field m., a m. that has a special condenser and objective with a diaphragm or stop that scatters light from the object observed, with the result that the object appears bright on a dark background.

electron m., a visual and photographic m. in which electron beams with wavelengths thousands of times shorter than visible light are utilized in place of light, thereby allowing much greater resolution and magnification; in this technique, the electrons are transmitted through a very thin section of an embedded and dehydrated specimen maintained in a vacuum.

fluorescence m., SEE fluorescence *microscopy*.

flying spot m., a m. in which a moving spot of light is imaged in the object plane, the energy transmitted by the specimen being detected with a photoelectric cell; the light source may be a cathode ray tube, a scanning disk or drum, or an oscillating mirror.

infrared m., a m. that is equipped with infrared transmitting optics and that measures the infrared absorption of minute samples with the aid of photoelectric cells; images may be observed with image converters or television.

interference m., a specially constructed m. in which the entering light is split into two beams which pass through the specimen and are recombined in the image plane where the interference effects make the transparent (invisible) refractile object details become visible as intensity differences; permits measurements of light retardation, index of refraction, and thickness and mass of specimen; it is useful in the examination of living or unstained cells.

laser m., a m. in which a laser beam is focused on a microscopic field, causing it to vaporize; the emitted radiation is analyzed by means of a microspectrophotometer; at a low intensity the laser is employed as the light source in an interference m.

light m., a class of m. that forms a magnified image using visible light.

mi

opaque m., SYN epimicroscope.

operating m., SYN surgical m.

phase m., phase-contrast m., a specially constructed m. that has a special condenser and objective containing a phase-shifting ring whereby small differences in index of refraction are made visible as intensity or contrast differences in the image; particularly useful for examining structural details in transparent specimens such as living or unstained cells and tissues.

polarizing m., a m. equipped with a polarizing filter below and above the specimen which forms an image by the influence of specimen birefringence on polarized light; the polarizing direction of the two filters is typically adjustable which, together with a graduated rotating stage, permits measurement of the angular value of different refractive indices in either biological or chemical specimens.

Rheinberg m., a modified form of dark-field m. in which the central opaque stop in the condenser is replaced by a colored filter, producing a background of contrasting color against which the specimen is illuminated.

scanning electron m., a m. in which the object in a vacuum is scanned in a raster pattern by a slender electron beam, generating reflected and secondary electrons from the specimen surface that are used to modulate the image on a synchronously scanned cathode ray tube; with this method a three-dimensional image is obtained, with both high resolution and great depth of focus.

simple m., single m., a m. that has a single magnifying lens.

stereoscopic m., a m. having double eyepieces and objectives and thus independent light paths, giving a three-dimensional image.

stroboscopic m., a m. that has a light source that flashes at a constant rate so that an analysis of the motility of an object may be made; it may be used for high speed or low speed (time-lapse) cinephotomicrography.

surgical m., a binocular m. used to obtain good visualization of fine structures in the operating field; in the standing type of m., a motorized zoom lens system operated by hand or foot controls provides an adjustable working distance; in headborne models, interchangeable oculars provide the magnification needed. SYN operating m.

television m., a m. in which the image is observed by a television camera that produces a television display; it is used for quantitative studies, display to a large audience, or examinations in ultraviolet and infrared regions of the spectrum.

ultra-m., SEE ultramicroscope.

ultrasonic m., a m. that has lenses designed to use acoustic energy so that the ultrasonic wavelengths may be utilized; by means of transducers, the information is translated to a form that may be visualized or recorded.

ultraviolet m., a m. having optics of quartz and fluorite that allow transmission of light waves shorter than those of the visible spectrum, i.e., below 400 nm; the image is made visible by photography, fluorescence of special glasses, or television; in a scanning instrument the receptor is a multiplier phototube.

x-ray m., a m. in which images are obtained by using x-rays as an energy source that are recorded on a very fine-grained film, or the image is enlarged by projection; if film is used, it may be examined with the light m. at fairly high magnifications.

mi·cro·scop·ic, mi·cro·scop·i·cal (mī-krō-skop'ik, -i-kăl). **1.** Of minute size; visible only with the aid of the microscope. **2.** Relating to a microscope.

mi·cros·co·py (mī-kros'kŏ-pē). Investigation of minute objects by means of a microscope. SEE ALSO microscope.

electron m., examination of minute objects by use of an electron microscope.

epiluminescence m., low-power m. (×50–×100), commonly a television *microscope* applied to a glass slide covering mineral oil on the surface of a skin lesion, e.g., to determine malignancy in pigmented lesions. SYN surface m.

fluorescence m., a procedure based on the fact that fluorescent materials emit visible light when they are irradiated with ultraviolet or violet-blue visible rays; some materials manifest this property naturally, whereas others may be treated with fluorescent solutions (somewhat analogous to staining); when the absorption

of the specimen is in the relatively long ultraviolet range, a filter that transmits these radiations is used, and a yellow filter is placed on or in the ocular; the background field is then dark, and any yellow or red fluorescence becomes visible.

immersion m., SEE immersion.

immune electron m., electron m. of biological specimens to which specific antibody has been bound.

immunofluorescence m., SEE immunofluorescence.

Nomarski interference m., SEE Nomarski *optics*.

surface m., SYN epiluminescence m.

time-lapse m., m. in which the same object (e.g., a cell) is photographed at regular time intervals over several hours.

mi·cro·seme (mī'krō-sēm). Denoting a skull with an orbital index below 84. [micro- + G. *sēma*, sign]

mi·cro·sides (mī'krō-sīdz). Fatty acid esters of trehalose and mannose isolated from diphtheria bacilli.

mi·cros·mat·ic (mī'kroz-mat'ik). Having a weakly developed sense of smell. [micro- + G. *osmē*, sense of smell]

mi·cro·some (mī'krō-sōm). One of the small spherical vesicles derived from the endoplasmic reticulum after disruption of cells and ultracentrifugation. [micro- + G. *sōma*, body]

mi·cro·so·mia (mī-krō-sō'mē-ă). Abnormal smallness of body, as in dwarfism or as in a fetus. SYN nanocormia. [micro- + G. *sōma*, body]

mi·cro·spec·tro·pho·tom·e·try (mī'krō-spek-trō-fō-tom'ĕ-trē). A technique for characterizing and quantitating nucleoproteins in single cells or cell organelles by their natural absorption spectra (ultraviolet) or after binding stoichiometrically in selective cytochemical staining reactions, as in the Feulgen stain for DNA. SEE ALSO cytophotometry.

mi·cro·spec·tro·scope (mī-krō-spek'trō-skōp). An instrument for observing the optical spectrum of microscopic objects.

micro·sphere (mī'krō-sfēr). Tiny globules of radiolabeled material such as macroaggregated albumin, about 15 microns in size.

mi·cro·sphe·ro·cy·to·sis (mī'krō-sfēr'ō-sī-tō'sis). SYN spherocytosis.

mi·cro·sphyg·my (mī'krō-sfig'mē). Smallness of the pulse. SYN microsphyxia. [micro- + G. *sphygmos*, pulse]

mi·cro·sphyx·ia (mī-krō-sfik'sē-ă). SYN microsphygmy. [micro- + G. *sphyxis*, pulse]

mi·cro·splanch·nic (mī-krō-splangk'nik). Referring to smallness of the abdominal viscera. [micro- + G. *splanchna*, viscera]

mi·cro·sple·nia (mī-krō-sple'nē-ă). Abnormal smallness of the spleen.

Mi·cro·spo·ra (mī-krō-spōr'ă). A protozoan phylum that includes the genus *Nosema* and *Encephalitozoon*, and is characterized by the presence of unicellular spores with an imperforate wall and an extrusion apparatus having a polar tube and a polar cap; mitochondria are absent. They are intracellular parasites of invertebrates and lower vertebrates, with rare examples in higher vertebrates. SYN Cnidospora. [micro- + G. *sporos*, seed]

Mi·cro·spo·ra·si·da (mī'krō-spōr-as'i-dă). SYN Microsporida.

Mi·cro·spo·rida (mī-krō-spō'ri-dă). An order of the protozoan class Microsporea and phylum Microspora, characterized by minute spores with a single long, coiled, tubular filament enclosing the infective cell or sporoplasm. They are typically parasites of invertebrates and lower vertebrates, although fish and higher vertebrates (including man) have been infected. The order includes genera such as *Encephalitozoon* and *Nosema*. SYN Cnidosporidia, Microsporasida.

mi·cro·spor·id·ia (mī'krō-spōr-id'ē-ă). Common name for members of the protozoan phylum Microspora. It includes some 80 genera parasitizing all classes of vertebrates and many invertebrates, especially the insects. Several genera, such as *Encephalitozoon*, *Enterocytozoon*, *Nosema*, *Vittaforma*, *Pleistophora*, and *Trachipleistophora* have been implicated in the infection of immunocompromised humans.

mi·cro·spo·rid·i·a·sis (mī'krō-spō-ri-dī'a-sis). SEE microsporidiosis.

mi·cro·spo·rid·i·o·sis, mi·cro·spo·rid·i·a·sis (mī-krō-spō-rid-ē-ō'sis, mī'krō-spō-ri-dī'a-sis). Infection with a member of the phylum Microspora, the microsporidians.

Mi·cros·po·rum (mī-kros'pŏ-rŭm, mī-krō-spō'rŭm). A genus of pathogenic fungi causing dermatophytosis. In appropriate culture media, characteristic macroconidia are seen; microconidia are rare in most species. [micro- + G. *sporos,* seed]

M. audoui'nii, an anthrophilic fungal species of fungi that has caused epidemic tinea capitis in children.

M. ca'nis, the principal cause of ringworm in dogs and cats and a zoophilic fungal species of fungi causing sporadic dermatophytosis in humans, especially tinea capitis in children with cats and dogs.

M. canis, var. distor'tum, a zoophilic fungal species that causes dermatophytosis in humans and animals; seen among laboratory animal handlers.

M. ferrugin'eum, an anthropophilic fungal species that causes dermatophytosis, primarily in Japan and the Far East.

M. ful'vum, a geophilic fungal species that causes dermatophytosis in humans and is a member of the *M. gypseum* complex whose ascomyceous state elevates it to the rank of a specific species.

M. galli'nae, a fungal species that causes dermatophytosis in fowl and, occasionally, in humans; due to its broadly clavate macroconidia, it was erroneously classified as a species of *Trichophyton.*

M. gyp'seum, a cause of ringworm in dogs and horses and occasionally other animal species; a geophilic complex of fungal species causing sporadic dermatophytosis in humans.

M. na'num, a geophilic fungal species that is the principal cause of ringworm in pigs; rarely causes dermatophytosis in humans.

M. persic'olor, a geophilic fungal species that causes dermatophytosis in voles, field voles, and, occasionally, humans; its ascomycetous state is *Nannizzia persicolor.*

M. vanbreusegh'emi, a zoophilic fungal species that causes dermatophytosis in dogs and squirrels, and occasionally in humans.

mi·cro·steth·o·phone (mī-krō-steth'ō-fōn). SYN microstethoscope. [micro- + G. *stēthos,* chest, + *phōnē,* sound]

mi·cro·steth·o·scope (mī-krō-steth'ō-skōp). A very small stethoscope that amplifies the sounds heard. SYN microstethophone.

mi·cro·sto·mia (mī-krō-stō'mē-ă). Smallness of the oral aperture. [micro- + G. *stoma,* mouth]

mi·cro·sur·gery (mī-krō-ser'jer-ē). Surgical procedures performed under the magnification of a surgical microscope.

mi·cro·su·ture (mī-krō-soo'choor). Tiny caliber suture material, often 9-0 or 10-0, with an attached needle of corresponding size, for use in microsurgery.

mi·cro·sy·ringe (mī'krō-si-rinj'). A hypodermic syringe that has a micrometer screw attached to the piston, whereby accurately measured minute quantities of fluid may be injected.

mi·cro·the·lia (mī-krō-thē'lē-ă). Smallness of the nipples. [micro- + G. *thēlē,* nipple]

mi·cro·tia (mī-krō'shē-ă). Smallness of the auricle of the ear with a blind or absent external auditory meatus. [micro- + G. *ous,* ear]

Mi·cro·ti·nae (mī-krot'in-ē). The rodent subfamily comprising voles or lemmings.

mi·cro·tine (mī'krō-tēn). Relating to voles or lemmings.

mi·cro·tome (mī'krō-tōm). An instrument for making sections of biological tissue for examination under the microscope. SEE ALSO ultramicrotome. SYN histotome.

mi·crot·o·my (mī-krot'ō-mē). The making of thin sections of tissues for examination under the microscope. SYN histotomy. [micro- + G. *tomē,* incision]

mi·cro·to·nom·e·ter (mī'krō-tō-nom'ĕ-ter). A small tonometer invented by Krogh, originally intended for animals but later adapted to humans, for determining the tensions of oxygen and carbon dioxide in arterial blood; it provides the means of bringing a small bubble of air into gaseous equilibrium with a sample of blood obtained by arterial puncture. [micro- + G. *tonos,* tone, + *metron,* measure]

Mi·cro·trom·bid·i·um (mī'krō-trom-bid'ē-ŭm). A genus of chigger or harvest mites that cause severe itching from the presence of the larval stage (chigger) in the skin. [micro- + Mod. L. *trombidium,* a timid one]

mi·cro·tro·pia (mī-krō-trō'pē-ă). Strabismus of less than four degrees, associated with amblyopia, eccentric fixation, or anomalous retinal correspondence. [micro- + G. *tropē,* a turn, turning]

mi·cro·tu·bule (mī-krō-too'būl). A hollow, cylindrical cytoplasmic element, 20–27 nm in diameter and of variable length, that occurs widely in the cytoskeleton, cilia, and flagella of cells; m.'s play a role in the maintenance of cell shape and increase in number during mitosis and meiosis, where they are related to movement of the chromosomes by the nuclear spindle.

subpellicular m., a m. lying beneath the unit membrane (pellicle) of many protozoans, often as a palisade of longitudinally arranged fibrils connected by fine lateral bridges that support the external cell form; in certain sporozoan stages a fixed number of m.'s are found, extending longitudinally from the polar ring. SYN subpellicular fibril.

mi·cro·ves·i·cle (mī-krō-ves'i-kl). A fluid-filled space formed within the epidermis that is too small to be recognized as a blister.

mi·cro·vil·lus, pl. **mi·cro·vil·li** (mī-krō-vil'ŭs, -vil'ī). One of the minute projections of cell membranes greatly increasing surface area; microvilli form the striated or brush borders of certain cells.

Mi·cro·vir·i·dae (mī-krō-vir'i-dē). A family of small, spherical, bacterial viruses with a genome of single-stranded DNA (MW 1.7 × 10⁶).

mi·cro·volt (μV) (mī'krō-vōlt). One-millionth of a volt.

mi·cro·waves (mī'krō-wāvz). That portion of the radio wave spectrum of shortest wavelength, including the region with wavelengths of 1 mm to 30 cm (1000–300,000 megacycles per second). SYN microelectric waves.

mi·cro·weld·ing (mī-krō-weld'ing). A method of fastening or joining stainless steel sutures or such sutures to needles.

mi·crox·y·phil (mī-krok'si-fil). A multinuclear oxyphil leukocyte. [micro- + G. *oxys,* acid, + *philos,* fond]

mi·cro·zo·on (mī-krō-zō'on). A microscopic form of the animal kingdom; a protozoon. [micro- + G. *zōon,* animal]

mi·crur·gi·cal (mī-krer'ji-kăl). Relating to procedures performed on minute structures under a microscope. [micro- + G. *ergon,* work]

mic·tion (mik'shŭn). SYN urination.

mic·tu·rate (mik'choo-rāt). SYN urinate. [see micturition]

mic·tu·ri·tion (mik-choo-rish'ŭn). **1.** SYN urination. **2.** The desire to urinate. **3.** Frequency of urination. [L. *micturio,* to desire to make water]

MID Abbreviation for minimal infecting *dose.*

mid-. Middle. [A.S. *mid, midd*]

mi·daz·o·lam hy·dro·chlo·ride. A short-acting injectable benzodiazepine central nervous system depressant used for preoperative sedation.

mid·body (mid'bod'ē). A dense stalk of residual interzonal spindle fibers (microtubules) and actin-containing filaments that is formed during anaphase of mitosis and connects daughter cells during telophase; m.'s are frequently observed between spermatids. SYN intermediate body of Flemming.

mid·brain (mid'brān). ✱official alternate term for mesencephalon.

mid·car·pal (mid'kar-păl). **1.** Relating to the central part of the carpus. **2.** Denoting the articulation between the two rows of carpal bones. SYN carpocarpal. SYN mediocarpal, mesocarpal.

mid·dle (mid'el). Denoting an anatomical structure that is between two other similar structures or that is midway in position. SYN medius.

midge (midj). The smallest of the biting flies, in the genus *Culicoides;* swarms may attack humans and other animals; vectors of filarial infections. [O.E. *mycg*]

mid·grac·ile (mid-gras'il). Denoting an occasional fissure dividing the gracile lobe of the cerebellum into two parts.

mid·gut (mid'gŭt). **1.** The central portion of the digestive tube; the distal duodenum, small intestine, and proximal colon. **2.** The portion of the embryonic gut tract between the foregut and the hindgut which originally is open to the yolk sac.

mid·men·stru·al (mid′men′stroo-ăl). Denoting the several days midway in time between two menstrual periods.

mid·oc·cip·i·tal (mid′ok-sip′i-tăl). Relating to the central portion of the occiput. SYN medioccipital.

mid·pain (mid′pān). SYN intermenstrual *pain* (1).

mid·plane (mid′plān). SYN pelvic *plane* of least dimensions.

mid·riff (mid′rif). SYN diaphragm (1). [A.S. *mid,* middle, + *hrif,* belly]

mid·sec·tion (mid′sek-shŭn). A cut or section through the middle of an organ.

mid·ster·num (mid′ster′nŭm). SYN *body* of sternum.

mid·tar·sal (mid′tar′săl). Relating to the middle of the tarsus. SYN mediotarsal, mesotarsal.

mid·wife (mid′wīf). A person qualified to practice midwifery, having specialized training in obstetrics and child care. [A.S. *mid,* with, + *wif,* wife]

mid·wife·ry (mid′wīf′rē, mid-wif′ĕ-rē). Independent care of essentially normal, healthy women and infants by a midwife, antepartally, intrapartally, postpartally, and/or obstetrically in a hospital, birth center, or home setting, and including normal delivery of the infant, with medical consultation, collaborative management, and referral of cases in which abnormalities develop; strong emphasis is placed on educational preparation of parents for childbearing and childrearing, with an orientation toward childbirth as a normal physiological process requiring minimal intervention.

Miescher, Johann F., Swiss pathologist, 1811–1887. SEE M. *elastoma, granuloma, tubes,* under *tube.*

MIF Abbreviation for migration-inhibitory *factor.*

mife·pris·tone (mif′pris-tōn). Synthetic chemical compound with antiprogesterone properties used for early pregnancy termination; the substance binds with glucocorticoid receptors resulting in increased adrenal gland secretion. SYN RU-486.

mi·graine (mī′grān, mi-grān′). A symptom complex occurring periodically and characterized by pain in the head (usually unilateral), vertigo, nausea and vomiting, photophobia, and scintillating appearances of light. Classified as classic m., common m., cluster headache, hemiplegic m., ophthalmoplegic m., and ophthalmic m. SYN bilious headache, blind headache, hemicrania (1), sick headache, vascular headache. [through O. Fr., fr. G. *hēmi- krania,* pain on one side of the head, fr. *hēmi-,* half, + *kranion,* skull]

abdominal m., (1) m. in children accompanied by paroxysmal abdominal pain. This must be distinguished from similar symptoms requiring surgical attention. **(2)** a disorder that causes intermittent abdominal pain and is believed to be related to m.; abdominal m. has some of the features of m., e.g., there may be a strong family history of migraine headaches, and the condition may be relieved by sleep; however, a headache may not be present. The diagnosis depends on excluding other causes of abdominal pain.

acephalgic m., a classic m. episode in which the teichopsia is not followed by a headache. SYN m. without headache.

basilar m., a m. accompanied by transient brainstem signs (vertigo, tinnitus, perioral numbness, diplopia, etc.) thought to be due to vasospastic narrowing of the basilar artery.

classic m., a form of hemicrania m. preceded by a scintillating scotoma (teichopsia).

common m., a form of m. headache without the visual prodrome, that is not limited on one side of the head but nevertheless is recognizable as m. because of the stereotyped course; the tendency to nausea, photophobia, and phonophobia; and the relief produced by sleep.

complicated m., a m. attack during which an infarction of tissue takes place.

fulgurating m., m. characterized by its abrupt commencement and the severity of the episode.

Harris m., SYN periodic migrainous *neuralgia.*

hemiplegic m., a form associated with transient hemiplegia.

ocular m., a form of m. with transient monocular vision loss, typically in young adults, that may or may not be associated with headache around the eye. SYN retinal m.

ophthalmoplegic m., a form of m. associated with paralysis of the extraocular muscles.

retinal m., SYN ocular m.

m. without headache, SYN acephalgic m.

mi·gra·tion (mī-grā′shŭn). **1.** Passing from one part to another, said of certain morbid processes or symptoms. **2.** SYN diapedesis. **3.** Movement of a tooth or teeth out of normal position. **4.** Movement of molecules during electrophoresis, centrifugation, or diffusion. [L. *migro,* pp. *-atus,* to move from place to place]

branch m., a process in which the cross connection around the position where two DNA helices are joined moves along the strands.

epithelial m., apical shift of epithelial attachment, exposing more of the tooth crown.

m. of ovum, the transperitoneal passage of an ovum from the ovarian follicle into the uterine tube.

MIH Abbreviation for melanotropin release-inhibiting *hormone.*

Mikity, Victor G., U.S. radiologist, *1919. SEE Wilson-M. *syndrome.*

Mikulicz, Johannes von-Radecki, Polish surgeon in Germany, 1850–1905. SEE M. *aphthae,* under *aphtha, cells,* under *cell, clamp, disease, drain, operation, syndrome;* M.-Vladimiroff *amputation;* Vladimiroff-M. *amputation;* Heineke-Mikulicz *pyloroplasty.*

Miles, William E., British surgeon, 1869–1947. SEE M. *operation.*

mil·ia (mil′ē-ă). Plural of milium.

mil·i·a·ria (mil-ē-ā′rē-ă). An eruption of minute vesicles and papules due to retention of fluid at the orifices of sweat glands. SYN miliary fever (2). [L. *miliarius,* relating to millet, fr. *milium,* millet]

m. al′ba, m. with vesicles containing a milky fluid.

apocrine m., SYN Fox-Fordyce *disease.*

m. crystalli′na, a noninflammatory form of m. in which the fragile subcorneal vesicles, about 100 mm in diameter, are filled with clear fluid. SYN crystal rash, sudamina (2).

m. profun′da, pale firm papules, most commonly on the trunk; m. profunda is asymptomatic and results from severe damage to the sweat ducts after repeated episodes of m. rubra. Heat stress may cause collapse because of the high proportion of nonfunctional sweat glands.

m. ru′bra, an eruption of pruritic macules with small central vesicles at the orifices of sweat glands, accompanied by redness and inflammatory reaction of the skin. SYN heat rash, prickly heat, summer rash, wildfire rash.

mil·i·a·ry (mil′ē-ā-rē, mil′yă-rē). **1.** Resembling a millet seed in size (about 2 mm). **2.** Marked by the presence of nodules of millet seed size on any surface. [see miliaria]

mil·ieu (mēl-ū′). **1.** Surroundings; environment. **2.** In psychiatry, the social setting of the mental patient, e.g., the family setting or a hospital unit. [Fr. *mi,* fr. L. *medius,* middle, + *lieu,* fr. L. *locus,* place]

m. intérieur, m. inter′ne, the internal environment; the fluids bathing the tissue cells of multicellular animals.

mil·i·tar·y an·ti·shock trou·sers (MAST). SYN pneumatic antishock *garment.*

mil·i·um, pl. **mil·ia** (mil′ē-ŭm, -ē-ă). A tiny subepidermal keratinous cyst, usually multiple and therefore commonly referred to in the plural. M. may be primary (developmental), occurring predominantly on the face in infants and adults, or retention cysts secondary to causes of scarring or subepidermal blisters involving adnexal epithelium. SYN whitehead (1). [L. millet]

milk. 1. A white liquid, containing proteins, sugar, and lipids, secreted by the mammary glands, and designed for the nourishment of the young. SYN lac (1). **2.** Any whitish milky fluid; e.g., the juice of the coconut or a suspension of various metallic oxides. **3.** A pharmacopeial preparation that is a suspension of insoluble drugs in a water medium; distinguished from gels mainly in that the suspended particles of m. are larger. **4.** SYN strip (1). [A.S. *meolc*]

acidophilus m., m. inoculated with a culture of *Bacillus acidophilus.*

m. of bismuth, a suspension of bismuth hydroxide and bismuth subcarbonate in water; used in gastrointestinal disorders as a protective agent.

buddeized m., SEE Budde *process.*

certified m., cow's m. that does not have more than the maximal permissible limit of 10,000 bacteria per ml at any time prior to delivery to the consumer, and that must be cooled to 10°C or less and maintained at that temperature until delivery.

certified pasteurized m., cow's m. in which the maximum permissible limit for bacteria should not be more than 10,000 bacteria per ml before pasteurization and not more than 500 bacteria per ml after pasteurization; it must be cooled to 7.2°C or less and maintained at that temperature until delivery.

condensed m., a thick liquid prepared by the partial evaporation of cow's m., with or without the addition of sugar.

fortified m., m. to which some essential nutrient, usually vitamin D, has been added.

fortified vitamin D m., m. produced through direct addition of vitamin D; standardized at 400 USP units per quart.

irradiated vitamin D m., cow's m. exposed in a thin film to ultraviolet light and standardized to contain 400 USP units of vitamin D per quart.

lactobacillary m., m. inoculated with a culture of *Bacillus acidophilus, B. bulgaricus,* or other lactic acid-forming microorganism.

m. of magnesia, mixture of magnesium hydroxide; an aqueous solution of magnesium hydroxide, used as an antacid and laxative. SYN magnesia magma.

metabolized vitamin D m., m. produced by feeding irradiated yeast to cows; standardized to contain not less than 400 USP units per quart.

modified m., cow's m. altered, by increasing the fat and reducing the amount of protein, to resemble human m. in composition.

perhydrase m., m. treated by the addition of hydrogen peroxide. SEE Budde *process.*

skim m., skimmed m., the aqueous (noncream) part of m. from which casein is isolated.

m. of sulfur, SYN precipitated *sulfur.*

vitamin D m., cow's m. to which vitamin D has been added, to contain 400 USP units of vitamin D per quart.

witch's m., a secretion of colostrum-like m. sometimes occurring in the glands of newborn infants of either sex 3 to 4 days after birth and lasting a week or two; due to endocrine stimulation from the mother before birth.

Milkman, Louis A., U.S. roentgenologist, 1895–1951. SEE M. *syndrome.*

milk·pox (milk'poks). SYN alastrim.

Millard, Auguste L.J., French physician, 1830–1915. SEE M.-Gubler *syndrome.*

Miller, Willoughby D., U.S. dentist, 1853–1907. SEE M. chemicoparasitic *theory.*

Miller, Thomas Grier, U.S. physician, *1886. SEE M.-Abbott *tube.*

mil·let seed (mil'et). The seed of a grass, formerly used as a rough designation of size of about 2 mm in diameter.

⌂**milli- (m).** Prefix used in the SI and metric system to signify submultiples of one-thousandth (10^{-3}). [L. *mille,* one thousand]

mil·li·am·pere (ma, mA) (mil'ē-am'pēr). One thousandth of an ampere.

mil·li·bar (mil'i-bar). One-thousandth of a bar; 100 newtons/sq

m; 0.75006 mm Hg; standard atmospheric pressure is 1013 millibars.

mil·li·cu·rie (mc, mCi) (mil'i-kū'rē). A unit of radioactivity equivalent to 3.7×10^7 disintegrations per second.

mil·li·e·quiv·a·lent (mEq, meq) (mil'i-ē-kwiv'ă-lent). One-thousandth equivalent; 10^{-3} mol divided by valence.

mil·li·gram (mg) (mil'i-gram). One-thousandth of a gram.

mil·li·lam·bert (mil-i-lam'bert). One thousandth of a lambert; a unit of brightness equal to 0.929 lumen per square foot (roughly, 1 equivalent footcandle).

mil·li·li·ter (mil'i-lē-ter). One-thousandth of a liter.

mil·li·me·ter (mm) (mil'i-mē-ter). One-thousandth of a meter.

⌂**millimicro-.** Prefix formerly used to signify submultiples of one-billionth (10^{-9}); now nano-.

mil·li·mi·cron (mμ) (mil'i-mī-kron). Former term for nanometer.

mil·li·mole (mmol) (mil'i-mōl). One-thousandth of a gram-molecule.

mil·ling-in (mil'ing-in). Refining the occlusion of teeth by the use of abrasives between their occluding surfaces while the dentures are rubbed together in the mouth or on the articulator.

mil·li·os·mole (mil'i-oz-mōl). One-thousandth of an osmole.

mil·li·pede (mil'i-pēd). A venomous nonpredaceous arthropod of the order Diplopoda, characterized by two pairs of legs per leg-bearing segment. The venom is purely defensive, oozed or squirted from pores along the body, producing irritation to the skin or severe inflammation if it reaches the eyes. [milli- + L. *pes, pedis,* foot]

mil·li·sec·ond (ms, msec) (mil'i-sek'ŏnd). One-thousandth of a second.

mil·li·volt (mV) (mil'i-vōlt). One thousandth of a volt.

Millon, Auguste N.E., French chemist, 1812–1867. SEE M. *reaction, reagent;* M.-Nasse *test.*

mil·pho·sis (mil-fō'sis). Loss of eyelashes. SYN madarosis (1). [G. *milphōsis*]

mil·ri·none (mil'ri-nōn). A xanthine oxidase inhibitor which increases the force of contraction of the heart; used in congestive heart failure; resembles amrinone; cardiotonic.

Milroy, William F., U.S. physician, 1855–1942. SEE M. *disease.*

MIM Abbreviation for *Mendelian Inheritance in Man.*

mi·me·sis (mi-mē'sis, mī-). **1.** Hysterical simulation of organic disease. **2.** The symptomatic imitation of one organic disease by another. [G. *mimēsis,* imitation, fr. *mimeomai,* to mimic]

mi·met·ic (mi-met'ik, mī-). Relating to mimesis. [G. *mimētikos,* imitative]

mim·ic (mim'ik). To imitate or simulate. [G. *mimikos,* imitating, fr. *mimos,* a mimic]

mim·ma·tion (mi-mā'shŭn). A form of stammering in which the m-sound is given to various letters. [Ar. *mim,* the letter m]

min. Abbreviation for minute.

mind. 1. The organ or seat of consciousness and higher functions of the human brain, such as cognition, reasoning, willing, and emotion. **2.** The organized totality of all mental processes and psychic activities, with emphasis on the relatedness of the phenomena. [A.S. *gemynd*]

prelogical m., SYN prelogical *thinking.*

subconscious m., SYN subliminal *self.*

mind-read·ing. SYN telepathy.

min·er·al (min'er-ăl). Any homogeneous inorganic material usu-

milk														
	specific gravity	protein %	fat %	carbohydrate (lactose) %	ash %	joule/ 100 ml	mineral content, mg %							
							Na	K	Ca	Mg	Fe	Cl	P	citric acid
human milk	1.030	1.1–1.5	2.5–4.8	6–7.1	0.20	293	14	53	30	4	0.15	30	15	120
cow milk	1.031	3.1–4.0	3.5–4.8	4–4.8	0.75	285	45	160	126	12	0.18	126	98	250
goat milk	1.031	3.7–4.0	4.0–4.8	4–4.8	0.80	293	79	145	128	12	0.21	128	100	150

mi

ally found in the earth's crust. [L. *mineralis,* pertaining to mines, fr. *mino,* to mine]

min·er·al·i·za·tion (mĭn′er-al-i-zā′shŭn). The introduction of minerals into a structure, as in the normal mineralization of bones and teeth or the pathologic mineralization of tissues, i.e., dystrophic or metastatic calcification.

min·er·al·o·coid (min-er-al′ō-koyd). SYN mineralocorticoid.

min·er·al·o·cor·ti·coid (min′er-al-ō-kōr′ti-koyd). One of the steroids of the adrenal cortex that influences water and electrolyte (particularly sodium and potassium ions) metabolism and balance. SYN mineralocoid.

min·er·al oil. A mixture of liquid hydrocarbons obtained from petroleum, used as a vehicle in pharmaceutical preparations; occasionally used as an intestinal lubricant; can interfere with absorption of fat-soluble vitamins. SYN heavy liquid petrolatum, liquid paraffin, liquid petroleum.

min·er·al·o·tro·pic (min-er-al′ō-trō′pik). Concerning the action of or relating to mineralocorticoids.

mini (mi′nē). A moderate-sized computer that can serve many users in a department, or one dedicated to a complex computational function such as computed tomography or magnetic resonance imaging; smaller and slower than a mainframe, more complex and powerful than a personal computer. [It. *miniatura,* decoration of manuscripts, fr. L. *minium,* red lead]

min·i·lap·a·rot·o·my (min′ē-lap-ă-rot′ō-mē). Technique for sterilization by surgical ligation of the fallopian tubes, performed through a small suprapubic or infraumbilical incision.

min·im (m). **1.** A fluid measure, ¹⁄₆₀ of a fluidrachm; in the case of water about one drop. **2.** Smallest; least; the smallest of several similar structures. [L. *minimus,* least]

min·i·mum (min-i-mum). The smallest amount or lowest limit. [L. smallest, least]

min·i·my·o·sin (min-ē-mī′ō-sin). A protein similar to myosin in having a globular actin-binding domain and a short tail that can bind to membranes but lacking a long α-helical tail; believed to have a role in filopodium extension in the growth cone of neurons.

minithoracotomy. See under thoracotomy.

min·o·cy·cline (min-ō-sī′klēn). A substituted naphthacene-carboxamide; an antibacterial drug related to tetracycline.

mi·nor (mī′ner). Smaller; lesser; denoting the smaller of two similar structures. [L.]

mi·nox·i·dil (mi-nok′si-dil). An antihypertensive agent used for treatment of premature hair loss; sometimes used topically on the scalp to increase hair growth.

mint. SYN Mentha. [G. *mintha*]

⌂**mio-.** Less. [G. *meiōn*]

mi·o·did·y·mus, mi·od·y·mus (mī-ō-did′i-mŭs, mī-od′i-mŭs). Unequal conjoined twins with the head of the smaller twin joined to the occipital region of the head of the larger twin. SEE conjoined *twins,* under *twin.* [mio- + G. *didymos,* twin]

mi·o·lec·i·thal (mī-ō-les′i-thal). Denoting an egg with little yolk which is uniformly dispersed throughout the egg. [mio- + G. *lekithos,* egg yolk]

mi·o·pra·gia (mī-ō-prā′jē-ă). Diminished functional activity in a part. [mio- + G. *prassō,* to do]

mi·o·pus (mī-ō′pŭs). Unequal conjoined twins with heads united in such a manner that one face is rudimentary. SEE conjoined *twins,* under *twin.* [mio- + *ōps,* eye]

mi·o·sis (mī-ō′sis). **1.** Contraction of the pupil. **2.** Incorrect alternative spelling for meiosis. [G. *meiōsis,* a lessening]

paralytic m., m. due to paralysis of the dilator muscle of the pupil.

spastic m., m. due to spasmodic contraction of the sphincter muscle of the pupil.

mi·ot·ic (mī-ot′ik). **1.** Relating to or characterized by constriction of the pupil. **2.** An agent that causes the pupil to constrict so that the pupils are small.

MIP Abbreviation for maximum intensity *projection.*

MIP Abbreviation for macrophage inflammatory *protein.*

mi·ra·cid·i·um, pl. **mi·ra·cid·ia** (mī-ră-sid′ē-ŭm, -ă). The ciliated first-stage larva of a trematode that emerges from the egg and must penetrate into the tissues of an appropriate intermediate host snail if it is to continue its life cycle; followed by development into a mother sporocyst and by production of a number of offspring of successive larval generations. SEE ALSO sporocyst (1). [G. *meirakidion,* boy]

Mirchamp sign. See under sign.

mire (mēr). One of the test objects in the ophthalmometer; its image (also called a m.), mirrored on the corneal surface, is measured to determine the radii of curvature of the cornea. [L. *miror,* pp. *-atus,* to wonder at]

mi·rex (mī′reks). Benzene derivative used as insecticide and fire retardant for plastics, rubber, paint, paper, electrical goods; likely carcinogen.

Mirizzi, P.L., 20th century Argentinian physician. SEE M. *syndrome.*

mir·ror (mir′ŏr). A polished surface reflecting the rays of light reflected from objects in front of it. [Fr. *miroir,* fr. L. *miror,* to wonder at]

concave m., a spherical reflecting surface that constitutes a segment of the interior of a sphere.

convex m., a spherical reflecting surface that constitutes a segment of the exterior of a sphere.

head m., a circular concave m. attached to a head band, used to project a beam of light into a cavity, such as the nose or larynx, for purposes of examination and permitting binocular vision.

mouth m., a small m. on a handle used to facilitate visualization in the examination of the teeth.

van Helmont m., obsolete term for central *tendon* of diaphragm.

mir·ror-writ·ing (mir′ŏr-rīt-ing). Writing backward, from right to left, the letters appearing like ordinary writing seen in a mirror. SYN retrography.

mir·yach·it (mir-yach′it). A nervous affection observed in Siberia. SEE jumping *disease.*

MIS Abbreviation for müllerian inhibiting *substance.*

mis·an·dry (mis′an-drē). Aversion to or hatred of men. [G. *miseō,* to hate, + *anēr, andros,* male]

mis·an·thro·py (mis-an′thrō-pē). Aversion to and hatred of human beings. [G. *miseō,* to hate, + *anthrōpos,* man]

mis·car·riage (mis-kar′ij). Spontaneous expulsion of the products of pregnancy before the middle of the second trimester. SYN spontaneous abortion.

mis·car·ry (mis-kar′ē). To have a miscarriage.

mis·ce·ge·na·tion (mis′e-jĕ-nā′shŭn). Marriage or interbreeding of individuals of different races. [L. *misceo,* to mix, + *genus,* descent, race]

mis·ci·ble (mis′i-bl). Capable of being mixed and remaining so after the mixing process ceases. [L. *misceo,* to mix]

mis·di·ag·no·sis (mis′dī-ag-nō′sis). A wrong or mistaken diagnosis.

mi·sog·a·my (mi-sog′ă-mē). Aversion to marriage. [G. *miseō,* to hate, + *gamos,* marriage]

mi·sog·y·ny (mi-soj′i-nē). Aversion to or hatred of women. [G. *miseō,* to hate, + *gynē,* woman]

mis·o·pe·dia, mis·op·e·dy (mis-ō-pē′dē-ă, -op′ĕ-dē). Aversion to or hatred of children. [G. *miseō,* to hate, + *pais* (*paid-*), child]

mi·so·pros·tol (mī-sō-prost′ol). A prostaglandin analog used in the treatment of ulcer disease; particularly useful in persons taking nonsteroidal anti-inflammatory drugs; antiulcerative.

mis·sense (mis′ens). As used in genetics, a mutation that causes a sequence such that there is a substitution of one amino acid residue for another.

m. suppression, a mutation in tRNA that allows for incorporation of an amino acid residue that allows for full function of the gene product.

mis·tle·toe (mis′l-tō). SYN viscum (1).

MIT Abbreviation for monoiodotyrosine.

Mitchell. SEE Weir Mitchell.

mite (mīt). A minute arthropod of the order Acarina, a vast assemblage of parasitic and (primarily) free-living organisms. Most are still undescribed, and only a relatively small number are of medical or veterinary importance as vectors or intermediate hosts of pathogenic agents, by directly causing dermatitis or tissue damage, or by causing blood or tissue fluid loss. The six-legged larvae of trombiculid m.'s, the chigger m.'s (*Trombicula*), are parasitic of humans and many mammals and birds, and are important as vectors of scrub typhus (tsutsugamushi disease) and other rickettsial agents. Some other important m.'s are *Acarus hordei* (barley m.), *Demodex folliculorum* (follicular or mange m.), *Dermanyssus gallinae* (red hen m.), *Ornithonyssus bacoti* (tropical rat m.), *m. bursa* (tropical fowl m.), *m. sylviarum* (northern fowl m.), *Pyemotes tritici* (straw or grain itch m.), and *Sarcoptes scabiei* (itch m.). [A.S.]

mith·ra·my·cin (mith-ră-mī′sin). An antibiotic produced by *Streptomyces argillaceus* and *S. tanashiensis;* possesses antineoplastic activity. SYN aureolic acid, mitramycin.

mith·ri·da·tism (mith′ri-dā′tizm, mith-rid′ă-tizm). Immunity against the action of a poison produced by small and gradually increasing doses of the same. [*Mithridates,* King of Pontus (132–63 B.C.), supposedly an unsuccessful suicide (by poison) because of repeated small doses taken to become invulnerable to assassination by poison]

mi·ti·ci·dal (mī-ti-sī′dăl). Destructive to mites.

mi·ti·cide (mī′ti-sīd). An agent destructive to mites. [mite + L. *caedo,* to kill]

mit·i·gate (mit′i-gāt). SYN palliate. [L. *mitigo,* pp. *-atus,* to make mild or gentle, fr. *mitis,* mild, + *ago,* to do, make]

mi·tis (mī′tis). Mild. [L.]

mi·to·chon·dria (-ă). Plural of mitochondrion.

mi·to·chon·dri·al (mī-tō-kon′drē-ăl). Relating to mitochondria.

mi·to·chon·dri·on, pl. **mi·to·chon·dria** (mī-tō-kon′drē-on, -ă). An organelle of the cell cytoplasm consisting of two sets of membranes, a smooth continuous outer coat and an inner membrane arranged in tubules or more often in folds that form platelike double membranes called cristae; mitochondria are the principal energy source of the cell and contain the cytochrome enzymes of terminal electron transport and the enzymes of the citric acid cycle, fatty acid oxidation, and oxidative phosphorylation. SYN Altmann granule (2). [G. *mitos,* thread, + *chondros,* granule, grits]

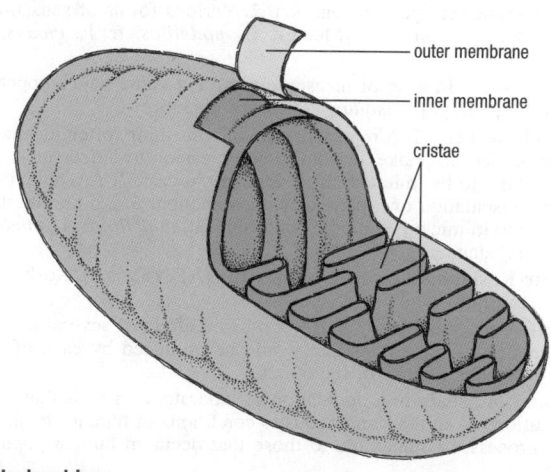

— outer membrane
— inner membrane
— cristae

mitochondrion

m. of hemoflagellates, the "mother m.," from which smaller mitochondria appear to arise.

mi·to·gen (mī′tō-jen). A substance frequently derived from plants that stimulates mitosis and lymphocyte transformation; includes not only lectins such as phytohemagglutinins and concanavalin A, but also substances from streptococci (associated with streptolysin S) and from strains of α-toxin-producing staphylococci. SYN transforming agent (1). [mitosis + G. *-gen,* producing]

pokeweed m. (PWM), a m. (lectin) from *Phytolacca americana* (pokeweed) which stimulates chiefly B lymphocytes.

mi·to·gen·e·sis (mī-tō-jen′ĕ-sis). The process of induction of mitosis in or transformation of a cell. [mitosis + G. *genesis,* origin]

mi·to·ge·net·ic (mī′tō-jĕ-net′ik). Pertaining to the factor or factors promoting cell mitosis.

mi·to·gen·ic (mī-tō-jen′ik). Causing mitosis or transformation.

mi·to·my·cin (mī-tō-mī′sin). Antibiotic produced by *Streptomyces caespitosus,* variants of which are designated m. A, m. B, etc.; m. C is an antineoplastic agent and a bacteriocide; inhibits DNA synthesis.

mi·to·plast (mī′tō-plast). A mitochondrion without its outer membrane.

mi·to·sis, pl. **mi·to·ses** (mī-tō′sis, -sēz). The usual process of somatic reproduction of cells consisting of a sequence of modifications of the nucleus (prophase, prometaphase, metaphase, anaphase, telophase) that result in the formation of two daughter cells with exactly the same chromosome and nuclear DNA content as that of the original cell. SEE ALSO cell *cycle.* SYN indirect nuclear division, mitotic division. [G. *mitos,* thread]

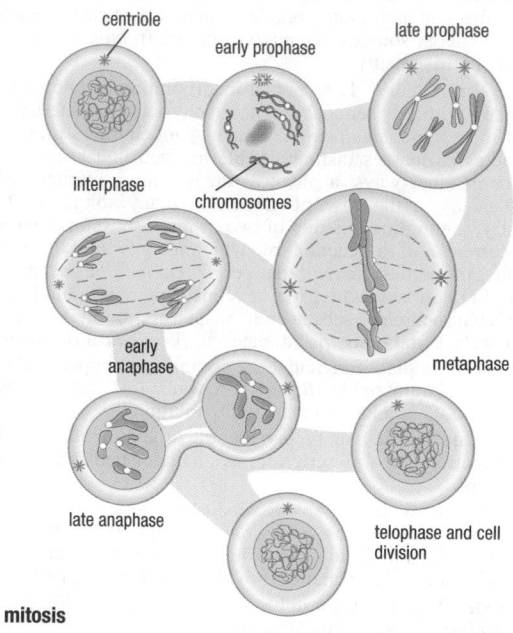

centriole
early prophase
late prophase
interphase
chromosomes
early anaphase
metaphase
late anaphase
telophase and cell division

cell mitosis

heterotype m., a variety of m. in which the halved chromosomes are united at their ends forming ringlike figures. Occurs in the first division of meiosis.

multipolar m., a pathologic form in which the spindle has three or more poles, resulting in the formation of a corresponding number of nuclei.

somatic m., the ordinary process of m. as it occurs in the somatic or body cells, characterized by the formation of the prescribed number of chromosomes, appropriate for the species (in humans the number is 46).

mi·to·tane (mī′tō-tān). An antineoplastic agent.

mi·tot·ic (mī-tot′ik). Relating to or marked by mitosis.

mi·to·xan·trone hy·dro·chlo·ride (mī-tō-zan′trōn). A synthetic anti-neoplastic used intravenously in the initial therapy for acute nonlymphocytic leukemia in adults.

mi·tral (mī′trăl). **1.** Relating to the mitral or bicuspid valve. **2.** Shaped like a bishop's miter; denoting a structure resembling the shape of a headband or turban. [L. *mitra,* a coif or turban]

mi·tral·i·za·tion (mī′tră-li-zā′shŭn). Straightening of the left heart border on a chest radiograph due to prominence of the left atrial appendage or the pulmonary outflow tract; an unreliable indication of mitral valve disease.

mi

mit·ra·my·cin (mit-ră-mī′sin). SYN mithramycin.

Mitrofanoff, Paul, French pediatric surgeon, *1934. SEE Mitrofanoff *principle*.

Mitsuda, Kensuke, Japanese physician, 1876–1964. SEE M. *antigen, reaction*.

Mitsuo, Gentaro, Japanese ophthalmologist, 1876–1913. SEE M. *phenomenon*.

mit·tel·schmerz (mit′el-schmărts). Abdominal pain occurring at the time of ovulation, resulting from irritation of the peritoneum by bleeding from the ovulation site. SYN intermenstrual pain (2), middle pain. [Ger. Mittelschmerz, middle + pain]

mi·vac·ur·i·um (mī′vă-kŭr′ē-ŭm). A neuromuscular blocking agent resembling *d*-tubocurarine, but having a shorter duration of action.

mix·ing (mik′sing). The mingling or blending of particles or components, especially of different kinds.

phenotypic m., a nongenetic interaction in which virus particles released from a cell that is infected with two different viruses have components from both the infecting agents, but with a genome from one of them.

mix·o·tro·phy (miks-o′trō-fē). The property of certain microorganisms that can assimilate organic compounds as carbon sources but not as energy sources. [G. *mixis*, mixture, fr. *mignumi*, to mix, + *trophē*, nourishment]

mix·ture (miks′chŭr). 1. A mutual incorporation of two or more substances, without chemical union, the physical characteristics of each of the components being retained. A **mechanical m.** is a m. of particles or masses distinguishable as such under the microscope or in other ways; a **physical m.** is a more intimate m. of molecules, as in the case of gases and many solutions. 2. In chemistry, a mingling together of two or more substances without the occurrence of a reaction by which they would lose their individual properties, i.e., without permanent gain or loss of electrons. 3. In pharmacy, a preparation, consisting of a liquid holding an insoluble medicinal substance in suspension by means of acacia, sugar, or some other viscid material. [L. *mixtura* or *mistura*]

Bordeaux m., a plant fungicidal m., comprising copper sulfate (5 parts) and calcium oxide (5 parts) in water (400 parts) freshly mixed; the CaO is added to the CuSO₄ solution.

extemporaneous m., a m. prepared at the time ordered, according to the directions of a prescription, as distinguished from a stock preparation.

Seidlitz m., a m. of 3 parts Rochelle salt and 1 part sodium bicarbonate. Ten grams of the m. are employed with 2.17 g tartaric acid for one Seidlitz powder. The powder, which effervesces when placed in water, was widely used as a cathartic.

Miyagawa, Yoneji, Japanese bacteriologist, 1885–1959. SEE *Miyagawanella*; M. *bodies*, under *body*.

Mi·ya·ga·wa·nel·la (mē′yă-gah′wă-nel′ă). Formerly considered a genus of Chlamydiaceae, but now synonymous with *Chlamydia*. [Y. *Miyagawa*]

MK Abbreviation for menaquinone.

MK-6 Abbreviation for menaquinone-6.

MK-7 Abbreviation for menaquinone-7.

MLC Abbreviation for Marginal Line Calculus Index.

MLD, mld Abbreviation for minimal lethal *dose*.

mlRNA Abbreviation for messengerlike RNA.

mM, mM Abbreviation for millimolar.

mm Abbreviation for millimeter.

MMMT Abbreviation for malignant mixed müllerian *tumor* or malignant mixed mesodermal tumor.

M-mode. A diagnostic ultrasound presentation of the temporal changes in echoes in which the depth of echo-producing interfaces is displayed along one axis with time (T) along the second axis; motion (M) of the interfaces toward and away from the transducer is displayed. SYN TM-mode.

mmol Abbreviation for millimole.

MMPI Abbreviation for Minnesota Multiphasic Personality Inventory *test*.

MMR Abbreviation for measles, mumps, and rubella *vaccine*.

Mn Symbol for manganese.

M′Naghten, Daniel, British criminal, tried in March, 1843. SEE M. *rule*.

MND Abbreviation for motor neuron *disease*.

mne·me (nē′mē). The enduring quality in the mind that accounts for the facts of memory; the engram of a specific experience. [G. *mnēmē*, memory]

mne·men·ic, mne·mic (nē-men′ik, nē′mik). Relating to memory.

mne·mism (nē′mizm). SYN mnemic *hypothesis*. [G. *mnēmē*, memory]

mne·mon·ic (nē-mon′ik). SYN anamnestic (1).

mne·mon·ics (nē-mon′iks). The art of improving the memory; a system for aiding the memory. [G. *mnēmonikos*, mnemonic, pertaining to memory]

MNSs blood group. See Blood Groups appendix.

M.O. Abbreviation for Medical Officer.

Mo Symbol for molybdenum.

⁹⁹Mo. Abbreviation for molybdenum-99.

MoAb Abbreviation for monoclonal *antibody*.

mo·bi·li·za·tion (mō′bi-li-zā′shŭn). 1. Making movable; restoring the power of motion in a joint. 2. The act or the result of the act of mobilizing; exciting a hitherto quiescent process into physiologic activity. SEE ALSO mobilize. 3. The process by which a conjugative plastid brings about the transfer from one cell to another of DNA.

stapes m., an operation to remobilize the footplate of the stapes to relieve conductive hearing impairment caused by its immobilization through otosclerosis or other middle ear disease.

mo·bi·lize (mō′bi-līz). 1. To liberate material stored in the body; more specifically, to move a substance from tissue stores into the bloodstream. 2. To excite quiescent material to physiologic activity. [Fr. *mobiliser*, to liberate, make ready, fr. L. *mobilis*, movable]

Mobitz, Woldemar, German cardiologist, *1889. SEE M. types of atrioventricular *block*.

Möbius, Paul J., German physician, 1853–1907. SEE M. *sign, syndrome*; Leyden-M. muscular *dystrophy*.

MOD Abbreviation for mesiodistocclusal.

mo·dal·i·ty (mō-dal′i-tē). 1. A form of application or employment of a therapeutic agent or regimen. 2. Various forms of sensation, e.g., touch, vision, etc.. [Mediev. L. *modalitas*, fr. L. *modus*, a mode]

mode (mōd). In a set of measurements, that value which appears most frequently. [L. *modus*, a measure, quantity]

mod·el (mod′ĕl). 1. A representation of something, often idealized or modified to make it conceptually easier to understand. 2. Something to be imitated. 3. In dentistry, a cast. 4. A mathematical representation of a particular phenomenon. 5. An animal that is used to mimic a pathologic condition. [It. *midello*, fr. L. *modus*, measure, standard]

Adair-Koshland-Némethy-Filmer m. (AKNF), SYN Koshland-Némethy-Filmer m.

additive m., a m. in which the combined effect of several factors is the sum of the effects that would be produced by each of the factors in the absence of the others.

animal m., study in a population of laboratory animals that uses conditions of animals analogous to conditions of humans to simulate processes comparable to those that occur in human populations.

Armitage-Doll m., a m. of carcinogenesis with the premise that the main variable determining change in risk is not age but time.

Bingham m., a m. representing the flow behavior of a Bingham plastic, in the idealized case.

biomedical m., a conceptual m. of illness that excludes psychological and social factors and includes only biological factors in an attempt to understand a person's medical illness or disorder.

biopsychosocial m., a conceptual m. that assumes that psychological and social factors must also be included along with the biological in understanding a person's medical illness or disorder.

cloverleaf m., a m. for the structure of tRNA; so named because the structure roughly resembles a cloverleaf.

computer m., a mathematical representation of the functioning of a system, presented in the form of a computer program. SYN computer simulation.

concerted m., SYN Monod-Wyman-Changeux m.

cooperativity m., a m. used to explain the property of cooperativity observed in certain enzymes; e.g., allosterism or hysteresis.

fluid mosaic m., a m. for the structure of a biomembrane, with lateral diffusibility of constituents and little, if any, flip-flop motion.

genetic m., a formalized conjecture about the behavior of a heritable structure in which the component terms are intended to have literal interpretation as standard structures of empirical genetics.

induced fit m., (1) a m. to suggest a mode of action of enzymes in which the substrate binds to the active site of the protein, causing a conformational change in the protein; **(2)** SYN Koshland-Némethy-Filmer m.

Koshland-Némethy-Filmer m. (KNF model), a m. to explain the allosteric form of cooperativity; in this m., in the absence of ligands, the protein exists in only one conformation; upon binding, the ligand induces a conformational change that may be transmitted to other subunits. SYN Adair-Koshland-Némethy-Filmer m., induced fit m. (2).

lock-and-key m., a m. used to suggest the mode of operation of an enzyme in which the substrate fits into the active site of the protein like a key into a lock.

logistic m., a statistical m.; in epidemiology, a m. of risk as a function of exposure to a risk factor.

mathematical m., representation of a system, process, or relationship in mathematical form, using equations to simulate the behavior of the system or process under study.

medical m., a set of assumptions that views behavioral abnormalities in the same framework as physical disease or abnormalities.

Monod-Wyman-Changeux m. (MWC m.), a m. used to explain the allosteric form of cooperativity; in this m., an oligomeric protein can exist in two conformational states in the absence of the ligand; these states are in equilibrium and the one that is predominant has a lower affinity for the ligand (which binds to the protein in a rapid equilibrium fashion). SYN concerted m.

multiplicative m., a m. in which the joint effect of two or more causes is the product of their effects if they were acting alone.

multistage m., a mathematical m., mainly for carcinogenesis, based on the theory that a specific carcinogen may affect one among a number of stages in the development of cancer.

MWC m., abbreviation for Monod-Wyman-Changeux m.

pathologic m., an animal or animal stock that by inheritance or by artificial manipulation develops a disorder similar to some disease of interest and hence directly or by analogy furnishes evidence of its pathogenesis and may be used as a m. for the study of preventive or therapeutic measures.

Reed-Frost m., mathematical m. of infectious disease transmission and herd immunity. The m. gives the number of new cases of an infection that can be expected in a specified time in a closed, freely mixing population of immune and susceptible individuals, with varying assumptions about frequency of contact.

Sartwell incubation m., mathematical m. based on empirical observations, showing that incubation periods for communicable diseases have a log-normal distribution; m. holds true for certain kinds of cancers that have well-defined external causes.

statistical m., a formal representation for a class of processes that allows a means of analyzing results from experimental studies, such as the Poisson m. or the general linear m.; it need not propose a process literally interpretable in the context of the individual case.

mod·el·ing (mod'ĕl-ing). **1.** In learning theory, the acquiring and learning of a new skill by observing and imitating that behavior being performed by another individual. **2.** In behavior modification, a treatment procedure whereby the therapist or another significant person presents (models) the target behavior that the learner is to imitate and make part of repertoire. **3.** A continuous process by which a bone is altered in size and shape during its growth by resorption and formation of bone at different sites and rates. **4.** A process by which a representation of an entity is formed.

mod·i·fi·ca·tion (mod'i-fi-kā'shŭn). **1.** A nonhereditary change in an organism; e.g., one that is acquired from its own activity or environment. **2.** A chemical or structural alteration in a molecule.

behavior m., the systematic use of principles of conditioning and learning, especially operant or instrumental conditioning, to teach certain skills or to extinguish undesirable behaviors, attitudes, or phobias.

chemical m., alteration in the structure of a molecule, typically a macromolecule such as a protein, by chemical means; often, the covalent addition by some reagent.

covalent m., alteration in the structure of a macromolecule by enzymatic means, resulting in a change in the properties of that macromolecule; frequently, this type of m. is physiologically relevant.

mod·i·fi·er (mod'ĭ-fī-er). That which alters or limits.

biologic response modifier, agent that modifies host responses to neoplasms by enhancing immune systems or reconstituting impaired immune mechanisms.

mo·di·o·lus, pl. **mo·di·o·li** (mō-dī'ō-lŭs, -ō-lī) **1** [tA]. The central cone-shaped core of spongy bone about which turns the spiral canal of the modiolus. **2.** SYN m. of angle of mouth. [L., the nave of a wheel]

m. of angle of mouth [TA], a point near the corner of the mouth where several muscles of facial expression converge. SYN m. anguli oris [TA], columella cochleae, m. labii, modiolus (2).

m. anguli oris [TA], SYN m. of angle of mouth.

m. la'bii, SYN m. of angle of mouth.

mod·u·la·tion (mod-ū-lā'shŭn). **1.** The functional and morphologic fluctuation of cells in response to changing environmental conditions. **2.** Systematic variation in a characteristic (e.g., frequency, amplitude) of a sustained oscillation to code additional information. **3.** A change in the kinetics of an enzyme or metabolic pathway. **4.** The regulation of the rate of translation of mRNA by a modulating codon. [L. *modulor,* to measure off properly]

biochemical m., term describing the m. (either enhancement of activity or reduction of toxicity) of a chemotherapeutic agent by another agent, which may or may not have antineoplastic activity of its own.

mod·u·la·tor. That which regulates or adjusts.

selective estrogen receptor modulator (SERM), pharmaceutical agent with selective estrogen receptor affinity; current preparations have a primary effect on bone and cardiovascular tissues and less effect on endometrial, genital, and breast tissues.

mo·du·lus (moj'ū-lŭs, mod'ū-). A coefficient expressing the magnitude of a physical property by a numerical value. [L. dim. of *modus,* a measure, quantity]

bulk m., SYN m. of volume elasticity.

m. of elasticity, a coefficient expressing the ratio between stress per unit area acting to deform a body and the amount of deformation that results from it.

m. of volume elasticity, a coefficient expressing the ratio between pressure acting to change the volume of a substance and the amount of change that results from it. SYN bulk m.

Young m., a type of m. of elasticity which specifies the force applied to a body in one direction, per unit cross-sectional area of the body perpendicular to that direction, divided by the fractional change in length of the body in that direction.

Moeller, Julius O.L., German surgeon, 1819–1887. SEE M. *glossitis.*

Moeller, Alfred, German bacteriologist, *1868. SEE M. grass *bacillus.*

mo·fe·bu·ta·zone (mof-ĕ-būtă-zōn). An anti-inflammatory agent used for the treatment of arthritis.

mog·i·ar·thria (moj-i-ar'thrē-ă). Speech defect due to muscular incoordination. [G. *mogis,* with difficulty, + *arthroō,* to articulate]

mog·i·la·lia (moj-i-lā'lē-ă). Stuttering, stammering, or any speech defect. SYN molilalia. [G. *mogis,* with difficulty, + *lalia,* speech]

mog·i·pho·nia (moj-i-fō'nē-ă). Laryngeal spasm occurring in

mo

public speakers as a result of overuse of the voice. [G. *mogis*, with difficulty, + *phōnē*, voice]

Mohrenheim, Joseph J. Freiherr von, Austrian-Russian surgeon, 1755–1799. SEE M. *fossa, space.*

Mohs, Frederic E., U.S. surgeon, *1910, who as a medical student devised a system of microscopicaly controlled removal of skin tumors. SEE M. fresh tissue chemosurgery *technique, chemosurgery.*

Mohs, Friedrich, German mineralogist, 1773–1839. SEE M. *scale.*

moi·e·ty (moy′i-tē). **1.** Originally, a half; now, loosely, a portion of something. **2.** Functional group. [M.E. *moite,* a half]

mol Abbreviation for mole (4).

mo·lal (mō′lăl). Denoting 1 mol of solute dissolved in 1000 g of solvent; such solutions provide a definite ratio of solute to solvent molecules. Cf. molar (4).

mo·lal·i·ty (m) (mō-lal′i-tē). Moles of solute per kilogram of solvent; the molarity is equal to mρ/(1 + mM), where m is the molality, ρ is the density of the solution, and M is the molar mass of the solute. Cf. molarity.

mo·lar (mō′lăr). **1.** Denoting a grinding, abrading, or wearing away. [L. *molaris,* relating to a mill, millstone] **2.** SYN molar *tooth.* **3.** Massive; relating to a mass; not molecular. [L. *moles,* mass] **4.** Denoting a concentration of 1 gram-molecular weight (1 mol) of solute per liter of solution, the common unit of concentration in chemistry. Cf. molal. **5.** Denoting specific quantity, e.g., m. volume (volume of 1 mol).

first m., first permanent m., sixth permanent tooth or fourth deciduous tooth in the maxilla and mandible on either side of the midsagittal plane of the head following the arch form.

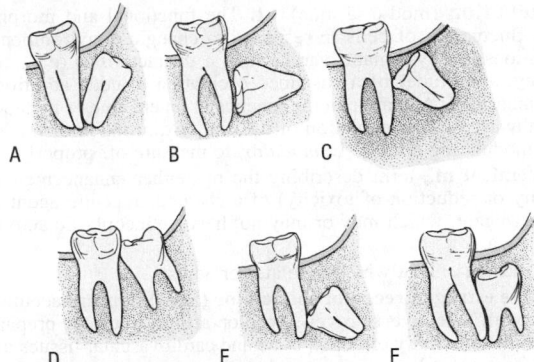

impacted mandibular third molar: (A) distoangular; (B) horizontal; (C) mesioangular; (D) high level; (E) low level; (F) vertical

Moon m.'s, small dome-shaped first m. teeth occurring in congenital syphilis.

mulberry m., a m. tooth with alternating nonanatomical depressions and rounded enamel nodules on its crown surface, usually associated with congenital syphilis.

second m., seventh permanent or fifth deciduous tooth in the maxilla and mandible on either side of the midsagittal plane of the head following the arch form.

sixth-year m., the first permanent m. tooth.

third m., SYN third-year molar *tooth.*

twelfth-year m., the second permanent m. tooth.

mo·lar·i·form (mō-lar′i-fōrm). Having the form of a molar tooth. [molar (tooth) + L. *forma,* form]

mo·lar·i·ty (M, M) (mō-lar′i-tē). Moles per liter of solution (mol/L). Cf. molality.

mold (mōld). **1.** A filamentous fungus, generally a circular colony that may be cottony, wooly, etc., or glabrous, but with filaments not organized into large fruiting bodies, such as mushrooms. **2.** A shaped receptacle into which wax is pressed or fluid plaster is poured in making a cast. **3.** To shape a mass of plastic material according to a definite pattern. **4.** To change in shape; denoting

especially the adaptation of the fetal head to the pelvic canal. **5.** The term used to specify the shape of an artificial tooth (or teeth). SYN mould.

pink bread m., SYN *Neurospora.*

mold·ing (mōld′ing). Shaping by means of a mold.

border m., the shaping of an impression material by the manipulation or action of the tissues adjacent to the borders of an impression. SYN muscle-trimming, tissue m., tissue-trimming.

compression m., (1) the act of pressing or squeezing together to form a shape in a mold; (2) the adaptation of a plastic material to the negative form of a split mold by pressure. SEE ALSO injection m.

injection m., the adaptation of a plastic material to the negative form of a closed mold by forcing the material into the mold through appropriate gateways. SEE ALSO compression m. (2).

tissue m., SYN border m.

mole (mōl). **1.** SYN nevus (2). **2.** SYN *nevus* pigmentosus. [A.S. *māēl* (L. *macula*), a spot] **3.** An intrauterine mass formed by the degeneration of the partly developed products of conception. [L. *moles,* mass] **4 (mol).** In the SI system, the unit of amount of substance, defined as that amount of a substance containing as many "elementary entities" as there are atoms in 0.0120 kg of carbon-12; "elementary entities" may be atoms, molecules, ions, or any describable entity or defined mixture of entities and must be specified when this term is used; in practical terms, the mole is 6.0221367×10^{23} "elementary entities." SEE ALSO Avogadro *number.*

carneous m., SYN fleshy m.

cystic m., SYN hydatidiform m.

fleshy m., a uterine mass occurring after fetal death and consisting of blood clots, fetal membranes, and placenta. SYN carneous m.

hairy m., SYN *nevus* pilosus.

hydatidiform m., hydatid m. [MIM*231090], a vesicular or polycystic mass resulting from the proliferation of the trophoblast, with hydropic degeneration and avascularity of the chorionic villi; the abnormal tissue typically results from expression of paternally derived chromosomes and a loss of maternal chromosomes. SYN cystic m., gestational trophoblastic disease.

invasive m., SYN *chorioadenoma* destruens.

mo·lec·u·lar (mō-lek′ū-lăr). Relating to molecules.

mo·lec·u·lar·i·ty (mō-lek′ū-lār′i-tē). The number of reactants in an elementary reaction. For example, a reaction involving one reactant is unimolecular; reactions involving two compounds are bimolecular. Molecularity and order are not synonymous. Cf. order (2).

mol·e·cule (mol′ě-kūl). The smallest possible quantity of a di-, tri-, or polyatomic substance that retains the chemical properties of the substance. [Mod. L. *molecula,* dim. of L. *moles,* mass]

accessory m.'s, cell surface adhesion m.'s on T cells that are involved in binding of one cell to another cell activation, and in signal transduction, e.g., CD4.

adhesion m.'s, m.'s that are involved in T helper-accessory cell, T helper-B cell, and T cytotoxic-target cell interactions; extracellular matrix proteins that attract leukocytes from the circulation.

cell adhesion m. (CAM), proteins that hold cells together, e.g., uvomorulin, and hold them to their substrates, e.g., laminin.

chimeric m., a m. (usually a biopolymer) containing sequences derived from two different genes; specifically, from two different species. Cf. chimera.

class I m., a major histocompatibility complex antigen made up of two noncovalently bonded polypeptide chains, one glycosylated, heavy, and variable with antigen specificity; the other chain is β_2-microglobulin.

class II m., a major histocompatibility complex membrane-piercing antigen made up of two noncovalently bonded polypeptide chains designated α and β.

costimulatory m., membrane-bound or secreted product of accessory cells that is required for signal transduction.

endothelial-leukocyte adhesion m. (E-LAM), a glycoprotein on the surface of endothelial cells that is involved in blood leukocyte attachment to vessel walls as well as emigration from the vessels into the tissues.

gram-molecule, the amount of a substance with a mass in grams equal to its molecular weight; e.g., a m. of hydrogen weighs 2.016 g, that of water 18.015 g.

intercellular adhesion m.-1 (ICAM-1), a glycoprotein that is expressed on a variety of cells. It is the ligand for LFA-1 as well as the receptor for the rhinoviruses.

lectin pathway m., the binding of mannose-binding protein to bacterial carbohydrates resulting in activation of the complement pathway.

mol·i·la·lia (mol′i-lā′lē-ă). SYN mogilalia. [G. *molis,* with difficulty (a later form of *mogis*), + *lalia,* talking]

mo·lim·i·na (-lim′i-nă).

menstrual m., SYN premenstrual *syndrome.*

mo·lin·done hy·dro·chlo·ride (mō-lin′dōn). An antipsychotic.

Molisch, Hans, Austrian chemist, 1856–1937. SEE M. *test.*

Moll, Jacob A., Dutch oculist, 1832–1914. SEE M. *glands,* under *gland.*

mol·li·ti·es (mō-lish′i-ēz). **1.** Characterized by a soft consistency. **2.** SYN malacia. [L. *mollis,* soft]

mol·lusc (mol′ŭsk). SYN mollusk.

Mol·lus·ca (mo-lŭs′kă). A phylum of the subkingdom Metazoa with soft, unsegmented bodies, consisting of an anterior head, a dorsal visceral mass and a ventral foot. Most forms are enclosed in a protective calcareous shell. M. includes the classes Gastropoda (snails, whelks, slugs), Pelecypoda (oysters, clams, mussels), Cephalopoda (squids, octopuses), Amphineura (chitons), Scaphopoda (tooth shells), and the class of primitive metameric mollusks, Monoplacophora. [L. *mollusca,* a nut with a thin shell, fr. *mollis,* soft]

Mol·lusc·i·pox·vi·rus (mol′lusk-′e-poks-vī-rus). A genus in the family Poxviridae; causes localized wartlike skin lesions. SYN molluscum contagiosum.

mol·lus·cum (mo-lŭs′kŭm). A disease marked by the occurrence of soft rounded tumors of the skin. [L. *molluscus,* soft]

⧉ m. contagio′sum, SYN Molluscipoxvirus.

mol·lusk (mol′ŭsk). Common name for members of the phylum Mollusca, although usually restricted to the gastropods and bivalves. SYN mollusc.

Moloney, Paul J., Canadian physician, 1870–1939. SEE M. *test.*

Moloney, John B., 20th century U.S. oncologist. SEE M. *virus.*

Moloy, Howard C., U.S. obstetrician, 1903–1953. SEE Caldwell-M. *classification.*

molt (mōlt). To cast off feathers, hair, or cuticle; to undergo ecdysis. SEE ALSO desquamate. SYN moult. [L. *muto,* to change]

mol wt Abbreviation for molecular *weight.*

mo·lyb·date (mō-lib′dāt). A salt of molybdic acid.

mo·lyb·den·ic, mo·lyb·de·nous (mō-lib′den-ik, -den-ŭs). Relating to molybdenum.

mo·lyb·de·num (Mo) (mō-lib′dĕ-nŭm). A silvery white metallic element, atomic no. 42, atomic wt. 95.94; a bioelement found in a number of proteins (e.g., xanthine oxidase). SEE molybdenum target *tube.* [G. *molybdaina,* a piece of lead; a metal, prob. galena, fr. *molybdos,* lead]

mo·lyb·de·num-99 (⁹⁹Mo). A reactor-produced radioisotope of molybdenum with a half-life of 2.7476 days, used in radionuclide generators for the production of technetium-99m.

adhesion molecules involved in leukocyte migration

molecule	structure	location	ligand(s)	function
P-selectin	selectin	endothelium neutrophils platelets	sLeX = sialyl Lewis X (carbohydrate)	acute inflammation neutrophil adhesion hemostasis
E-selectin	selectin	endothelium	sialyl Lewis X (eg. CD15)	leucocyte slowing
L-selectin	selectin	lymphocytes neutrophils	sialyl Lewis X	HEV binding slowing
ICAM-1	Ig family	endothelium (inducible)	LFA-1 CR3, CR4	adhesion and migration
ICAM-2	Ig family	endothelium	LFA-1	adhesion and migration
VCAM-1	Ig family	endothelium (inducible)	VLA-4 LPAM	adhesion
MAdCAM-1	Ig family sialylated	lymphoid endothelium	LPAM L-selectin	lymphocyte homing
PECAM	Ig family	endothelium lymphocytes	PECAM ?	adhesion activation migration guidance
LFA-1	$\alpha_L\beta_2$ integrin	leukocytes	ICAM-1, ICAM-2 CR3	migration
CR3	$\alpha_M\beta_2$ integrin	phagocytes	ICAM-1, ICAM-2 C3bi fibronectin	migration immune complex uptake
CR4	$\alpha_X\beta_2$ integrin	phagocytes	ICAM-1 ICAM-2 C3bi	adhesion immune complex uptake
VLA-4	$\alpha_4\beta_1$ integrin	lymphocytes	VCAM-1 LPAM fibronectin	adhesion at inflammatory sites and HEVs
LPAM	$\alpha_4\beta_7$ integrin	lymphocytes	MAdCAM-1	migration to lymphoid tissue
GlyCAM-1	sialoglycoprotein (soluble)	high endothelial venules	L-selectin	control of adhesion
PSGL-1	sialoglycoprotein	neutrophils	P-selectin	slowing in acute inflammation
CLA	glycoprotein	lymphocytes	E-selectin	lymphocyte migration to skin

mo

mo·lyb·dic (mō-lib′dik). Denoting molybdenum in the 6+ state, as in MoO₃.

mo·lyb·dic ac·id. $MoO_3 \cdot H_2O$; a yellowish crystalline acid, forming molybdates; used in the determination of phosphorus or phosphate.

mo·lyb·do·en·zymes (mō-lib′dō-en′zīmz). Enzymes that require a molybdenum ion as a component (e.g., xanthine oxidase).

mo·lyb·do·fla·vo·pro·teins (mō-lib′dō-flā′vō-prō′tēnz). Proteins that require a molybdenum ion and a flavin nucleotide as a part of its naturally occurring structure (e.g., aldehyde dehydrogenase).

mo·lyb·dop·ter·in (mō-lib-op′ter-in). A pterin derivative that complexes with molybdenum to form the molybdenum cofactor required by several enzymes.

mo·lyb·dous (mō-lib′dŭs). Denoting molybdenum in the 4+ state, as in MoO₂.

mo·lys·mo·pho·bia (mō-liz-mō-fō′bē-ă). Morbid fear of infection. [G. *molysma*, filth, infection, + *phobos*, fear]

mo·ment (mō′ment). The product of a quantity times a distance. [L. *momentum* (for *movimentum*), motion, moment, fr. *moveo*, to move]

dipole m., the product of one of the two charges of a dipole and the distance that separates them; an important measure of the degree of polarity of many biomolecules.

mom·ism (mom′izm). A term relating to excessive or overbearing mothering, especially as attributed to American cultural stereotypes.

△**mon-.** SEE mono-.

mo·nad (mō′nad, mon′ad). **1.** A univalent element or radical. **2.** A unicellular organism. **3.** In meiosis, the single chromosome derived from a tetrad after the first and second maturation divisions. [G. *monas*, the number one, unity]

Monakow, Constantin von, Swiss histologist, 1853–1930. SEE M. *bundle, nucleus, syndrome, tract.*

mon·am·ide (mon-am′id). SYN monoamide.

mon·am·ine (mon-am′in). SYN monoamine.

mon·am·i·nu·ria (mon′am-i-noo′rē-ă). SYN monoaminuria.

mon·an·gle (mon′ang-gl). Having only one angle, denoting a dental instrument that has only one angle between the handle or shaft and the working portion (blade or nib).

mon·ar·da (mon-ar′dă). The leaves of *Monarda punctata* (family Labiatae), American horsemint, a labiate plant of the U.S. east of the Mississippi; the main commercial source of natural thymol; used as a carminative in colic.

mon·ar·thric (mon-ar′thrik). SYN monarticular.

mon·ar·thri·tis (mon-ar-thrī′tis). Arthritis of a single joint.

mon·ar·tic·u·lar (mon-ar-tik′ū-lăr). Relating to a single joint. SYN monarthric, uniarticular.

mon·as·ter (mon-as′ter). The single star figure at the end of prophase in mitosis. SYN mother star. [mono- + G. *astēr*, star]

mon·a·tom·ic (mon-ă-tom′ik). **1.** Relating to or containing a single atom. **2.** SYN monovalent (1).

mon·au·ral (mon-aw′răl). Pertaining to one ear. [mono- + L. *auris*, ear]

mon·ax·on·ic (mon-aks-on′ik). **1.** Having but one axis, being therefore elongated and slender. **2.** Having one axon. [mono- + G. *axōn*, axle]

Mönckeberg, Johann G., German pathologist, 1877–1925. SEE M. *arteriosclerosis, calcification, degeneration, sclerosis.*

Mondini. C., Italian physician, 1729–1803. SEE Mondini *hearing impairment*, Mondini *dysplasia*.

Mondonesi, Filippo, Italian physician. SEE M. *reflex.*

Mondor, Henri, French surgeon, 1885–1962. SEE M. *disease.*

△**-mone.** A termination denoting a hormone or hormonelike substance. [Fr. hormone]

Mo·ne·ra (mō-nē′ră). The prokaryotes, a kingdom of primitive microbial organisms characterized by having no defined nucleus or chromosomes; DNA that is not membrane-bound; and absence of centrioles, mitotic spindle, microtubules, and mitochondria;

division of the ill-defined nuclear zone (nucleoid) is by separation of two masses attached to parts of the cell membrane, then growing apart (a form of amitosis). M. includes the blue-green algae and bacteria; viruses, which lack a true cell, may have originated as "escaped nucleic acids" or "wild genes" from eukaryotic cells and are not included. [pl. of Mod. L. *moneron*, fr. G. *monērēs*, solitary]

mo·ne·ran (mō-nē′ran). A member of the prokaryote kingdom Monera.

mon·es·trous (mon-es′trŭs). Having but one estrous cycle in a mating season.

Monge Medrano, Carlos, Peruvian professor of medicine and high altitude specialist, 1884–1970. SEE Monge *disease.*

mon·go·li·an (mon-gō′lē-ăn). **1.** Relating to a member of the Mongolian race. **2.** *Obsolete.* Relating to Down syndrome (because of the Asian-appearing facies).

mo·nil·e·thrix (mō-nil′ĕ-thriks). An autosomal dominant trichodystrophy in which brittle hairs show a series of constrictions, usually without a medulla. SYN beaded hair, moniliform hair. [L. *monile*, necklace, + G. *thrix*, hair]

Mo·nil·i·a (mo-nil′ē-ă). Generic term for a group of fungi that are commonly known as fruit molds; the sexual state is *Neurospora*. A few closely related pathogenic organisms formerly classified in this genus are now properly termed *Candida*. [L. *monile*, necklace]

Mo·nil·i·a·ce·ae (mō-nil-ē-ā′sē-ē). A family of Fungi Imperfecti (order Moniliales) which includes *Sporothrix schenckii*, the causative agent of sporotrichosis.

mo·nil·i·al (mō-nil′ē-ăl). Precisely, pertaining to the *Monilia*, but, in medicine, frequently used incorrectly with reference to the genus *Candida*.

mon·i·li·a·sis (mō-ni-lī′ă-sis). SYN candidiasis.

mo·nil·i·form (mō-nil′i-fōrm). Shaped like a string of beads or beaded necklace. [L. *monile*, necklace, + *forma*, appearance]

Mo·nil·i·for·mis (mō-nil-i-fōr′mis). A genus of the class (or phylum) Acanthocephala, the thorny-headed worms. *M. dubius*, the common spiny-headed worm of house rats, is transmitted by infected cockroaches, *Periplaneta americana*; a few infections in humans have been reported. *M. moniliformis* is a species normally found in rodents and is a rare parasite of humans. [L. *monile*, necklace, + *forma*, appearance]

mon·ism (mō′nizm). A metaphysical system in which all of reality is conceived as a unified whole. [G. *monos*, single]

mo·nis·tic (mo-nis′tik). Pertaining to monism.

mon·i·tor (mon′i-ter, -tōr). A device that displays and/or records specified data for a given series of events, operations, or circumstances. [L., one who warns, fr. *moneo*, pp. *monitum*, to warn]

cardiac m., an electronic m. which, when connected to the patient, signals each heart beat with a flashing light, an electrocardiographic curve, an audible signal, or all three.

▣**electronic fetal m.,** an instrument for continuous monitoring of the fetal heart before or during labor.

Holter m., a technique for long-term, continuous usually ambulatory, recording of electrocardiographic signals on magnetic tape for scanning and selection of significant but fleeting changes that might otherwise escape notice.

home m., a m. for heart and respiratory rate, usually used for infants believed to be at risk for sudden infant death syndrome or apnea.

mon·i·tor·ing. **1.** Performance and analysis of routine measurements aimed at detecting a change in the environment or health status of a population. **2.** Ongoing measurement of performance of a health service. **3.** Continuous oversight of implementation of an activity.

mon·key-paw (mong′kē-paw). SYN ape *hand.*

mon·key·pox (mŏng′kē-poks). A disease of monkeys and, rarely, of humans caused by the monkeypox virus, a member of the family Poxviridae; the human disease is serious and clinically resembles smallpox.

monks·hood (monks′hud). SEE aconite.

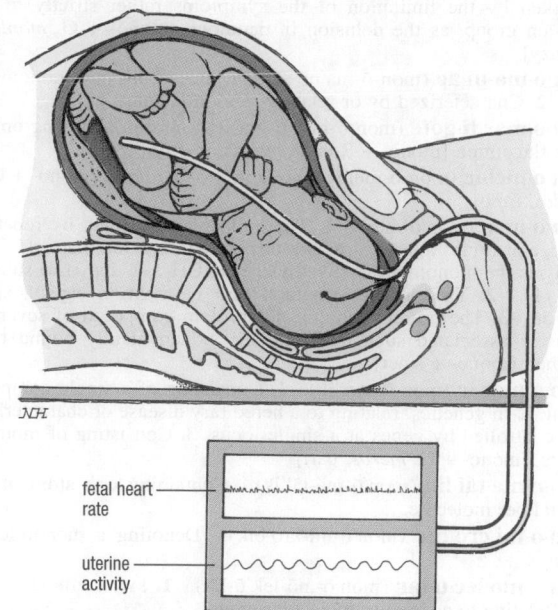

fetal heart rate

uterine activity

electronic fetal monitoring

⌂**mono-, mon-.** The participation or involvement of a single element or part. Cf. uni-. [G. *monos*, single]

mon·o·ac·yl·glyc·er·ol (mon-ō-ās-il-gli′ser-ol). Glycerol with an acyl moiety esterified to position 1 (i.e., 1-m.) or position 2 (i.e., 2-m.); an intermediate in the degradation and synthesis of lipids; 2 m.'s are a major end product of triacylglycerol degradation. SYN monoglyceride.

m. acyltransferase, an intestinal enzyme that catalyzes the reaction of 2-m. and acyl-CoA to form coenzyme A and 1,2-diacylglycerol.

m. lipase, an enzyme that catalyzes the hydrolysis of m. to produce a fatty acid anion and glycerol; a part of lipid degradation.

mon·o·a·me·lia (mon-ō-ă-mē′lē-ă). Absence of one limb.

mon·o·am·ide (mon-ō-am′īd, -id). A molecule containing one amide group. SYN monamide.

mon·o·am·ine (mon-ō-am′īn, -in). A molecule containing one amine group. SYN monamine.

mon·o·am·ine ox·i·dase (MAO). SYN *amine* oxidase (flavin-containing).

mon·o·am·i·ner·gic (mon′ō-am-i-ner′jik). Referring to nerve cells or fibers that transmit nervous impulses by the medium of a catecholamine or indolamine. [monoamine + G. *ergon*, work]

mon·o·am·i·nu·ria (mon′ō-am-i-noo′rē-ă). The excretion of any monoamine in the urine. SYN monaminuria.

mon·o·am·ni·ot·ic (mon′ō-am-nē-ot′ik). Denoting two or more progeny of a multiple pregnancy that have shared a common amniotic sac.

mon·o·as·so·ci·at·ed (mon′ō-ă-sō′shē-ā-tĕd). Denoting a germ-free organism that becomes colonized by a single microbial species.

mon·o·aux·o·troph (mon-ō-auks′ō-troph). A mutant microorganism that requires a particular nutrient that is not required by the wild-type organism. Cf. auxotroph, polyauxotroph.

mon·o·bac·tam (mon-ō-bak′tam). A class of antibiotic that has a monocyclic β-lactam nucleus and is structurally different from other β-lactams; e.g., aztreonam.

mon·o·ba·sic (mon-ō-bā′sik). Denoting an acid with only one replaceable hydrogen atom, or only one replaced hydrogen atom.

mon·o·ben·zone (mon-ō-ben′zōn). A melanin-pigment inhibiting agent; used topically for the treatment of hyperpigmentation caused by formation of melanin.

mon·o·blast (mon′ō-blast). An immature cell that develops into a monocyte. [mono- + G. *blastos*, germ]

mon·o·bra·chi·us (mon-ō-brā′kē-ŭs). The condition of being one-armed. [mono- + G. *brachiōn*, arm]

mon·o·bro·mat·ed, mon·o·bro·mi·nat·ed (mon-ō-brō′māt-ed, -brō′min-āt-ed). Denoting a chemical compound with one atom of bromine per molecule.

mon·o·car·di·an (mon-ō-kar′dē-an). Having a heart with a single atrium and ventricle.

mon·o·ceph·a·lus (mon-ō-sef′ă-lŭs). SYN syncephalus.

mon·o·chlor·phen·am·ide (mon′ō-klōr-fen′ă-mīd). SYN clofenamide.

mon·o·cho·ri·al (mon-ō-kō-rē′ăl). SYN monochorionic.

mon·o·cho·ri·on·ic (mon′ō-kōr-ē-on′ik). Relating to or having a single chorion; denoting monovular twins. SYN monochorial.

mon·o·chro·ic (mon-ō-krō′ik). SYN monochromatic.

mon·o·chro·ma·sia (mon′ō-krō-mā′zē-ă). SYN achromatopsia.

mon·o·chro·ma·sy (mon-ō-krō′mă-sē). SYN achromatopsia.

mon·o·chro·mat·ic (mon′ō-krō-mat′ik). **1.** Having but one color. **2.** Indicating a light of a single wavelength. **3.** Relating to or characterized by monochromatism. SYN monochroic, monochromic.

mon·o·chro·ma·tism (mon-ō-krō′mă-tizm). **1.** The state of having or exhibiting only one color. **2.** SYN achromatopsia. [mono- + G. *chrōma*, color]

blue cone m., SEE incomplete *achromatopsia*.

pi cone m., SEE incomplete *achromatopsia*.

rod m., SYN complete *achromatopsia*.

mon·o·chro·mat·o·phil, mon·o·chro·mat·o·phile (mon′ō-krō-mat′ō-fil, -fīl). **1.** Taking only one stain. **2.** A cell or any histologic element staining with only one kind of dye. SYN monochromophil, monochromophile. [mono- + G. *chrōma*, color, + *philos*, fond]

mon·o·chro·ma·tor (mon-ō-krō′mā-ter, -tōr). A prism or diffraction grating used in spectrophotometry to isolate a narrow spectral range.

mon·o·chro·mic (mon-ō-krō′mik). SYN monochromatic.

mon·o·chro·mo·phil, mon·o·chro·mo·phile (mon-ō-krō′mō-fil, -fīl). SYN monochromatophil.

mon·o·cis·tron·ic (mon-ō-sis-tron′ik). Referring to fully processed mRNA that codes for a single protein.

mon·o·cle (mon′ŏ-kl). A lens used for one eye, usually in the correction of presbyopia.

mon·o·clin·ic (mon-ō-klin′ik). Relating to crystals with a single oblique inclination. [mono- + G. *klinō*, to incline]

mon·o·clo·nal (mon-ō-klō′năl). In immunochemistry, pertaining to a protein from a single clone of cells, all molecules of which are the same; e.g., in the case of Bence Jones protein, the chains are all κ or λ.

mon·o·cra·ni·us (mon-ō-krā′nē-ŭs). SYN syncephalus. [mono- + G. *kranion*, cranium]

mon·o·crot·ic (mon′ō-krot′ik). Denoting a pulse the curve of which presents no notch or subsidiary wave in its descending line. [mono- + G. *krotos*, a beat]

mon·oc·ro·tism (mon-ok′rō-tizm). The state in which the pulse is monocrotic. [mono- + G. *krotos*, a beat]

mo·noc·u·lar (mon-ok′ū-lăr). Relating to, affecting, or visible by one eye only. [mono- + L. *oculus*, eye]

mo·noc·u·lus (mon-ok′ū-lŭs). **1.** SYN cyclops. **2.** A bandage applied to one eye only. [L. a one-eyed man, a hybrid word fr. G. *monos*, single, + L. *oculus*, eye]

▣**mon·o·cyte** (mon′ō-sīt). A relatively large mononuclear leukocyte (16–22 μm in diameter), that normally constitutes 3–7% of the leukocytes of the circulating blood, and is normally found in lymph nodes, spleen, bone marrow, and loose connective tissue. When treated with the usual dyes, m.'s manifest an abundant pale blue or blue-gray cytoplasm that contains numerous, fine, dust-like, red-blue granules; vacuoles are frequently present; the nucleus is usually indented, or slightly folded, and has a stringy chromatin structure that seems more condensed where the delicate

mo

strands are in contact. SEE ALSO monocytoid *cell*, endothelial *leukocyte*. [mono- + G. *kytos,* cell]

mon·o·cy·to·pe·nia (mon'ō-sī-tō-pē'nē-ă). Diminution in the number of monocytes in the circulating blood. SYN monocytic leukopenia, monopenia. [mono- + G. *kytos,* cell, + *penia,* poverty]

mon·o·cy·to·sis (mon'ō-sī-tō'sis). An abnormal increase in the number of monocytes in the circulating blood. SYN monocytic leukocytosis.

Monod, Jacques L., French biochemist and Nobel laureate, 1910–1976. SEE Monod-Wyman-Changeux *model.*

mon·o·dac·ty·ly, mon·o·dac·tyl·ism (mon-ō-dak'ti-lē, -dak'-tilizm). The presence of a single finger on the hand, or a single toe on the foot. [mono- + G. *daktylos,* digit]

mon·o·dis·perse (mon'ō-dis-pers). Of relatively uniform size; said of aerosol suspensions with size variation of less than ±20%.

mon·o·eth·a·nol·a·mine (mon'ō-eth-ă-nol'ă-mēn). A surfactant; the oleate is used as a sclerosing agent in the treatment of varicose veins.

mon·o·ga·met·ic (mon'ō-gă-met'ik). SYN homogametic.

mo·nog·a·my (mon-og'ă-mē). The marriage or mating system in which each partner has but one mate. [mono- + G. *gamos,* marriage]

mon·o·gen·e·sis (mon-ō-jen'ĕ-sis). **1.** The production of similar organisms in each generation. **2.** The production of young by one parent only, as in nonsexual generation and parthenogenesis. **3.** The process of parasitizing a single host, in which the life cycle of the parasite is passed; e.g., *Boophilus annulatus,* the one-host cattle tick, or certain trematodes of the order Monogenea. [mono- + G. *genesis,* origin, production]

mon·o·ge·net·ic (mon'ō-jĕ-net'ik). Relating to monogenesis. SYN monoxenous.

mon·o·gen·ic (mon-ō-jen'ik). Relating to a hereditary disease or syndrome, or to an inherited characteristic, controlled by alleles at a single genetic locus.

mo·nog·e·nous (mŏ-noj'ĕ-nŭs). Asexually produced, as by fission, gemmation, or sporulation.

mon·o·ger·mi·nal (mon-ō-jer'mi-năl). SYN unigerminal.

mon·o·glyc·er·ide (mon-ō-gli'ser-īd). SYN monoacylglycerol.

mon·o·graph (mon'ō-graf). A treatise on a particular subject or specific aspect of a subject. [mono- + G. *graphē,* a writing]

mon·o·hy·drat·ed (mon-ō-hī'drā-ted). Containing or united with a single molecule of water per molecule of substance.

mon·o·hy·dric (mon-ō-hī'drik). Having but one hydrogen atom in the molecule.

mon·o·hy·drox·y·succinic ac·id (mon-ō-hī-droks'ē-suk-sin'ik). SYN malic acid.

mon·o·i·de·ism (mon'ō-ī-dē'izm). A marked preoccupation with one idea or subject; a slight degree of monomania. [mono- + G. *idea,* form, idea]

mon·o·in·fec·tion (mon'ō-in-fek'shoon). Simple infection with a single variety of microorganism.

mon·o·i·o·do·ty·ro·sine (MIT) (mon'ō-ī-ō'dō-tī-rō-sēn). An intermediate in thyroid hormone synthesis.

mon·o·i·so·ni·tro·so·ac·e·tone (mon'ō-ī'sō-nī-trō'sō-as'ĕ-tōn). SYN isonitrosoacetone.

mon·o·kine (mon'ō-kīn). Cytokines secreted by both monocytes and macrophages. These substances influence the activity of other cells. SEE cytokine. [monocyte + G. *kineō,* to set in motion]

mon·o·lay·ers (mon-ō-lā'erz). **1.** Films, one molecule thick, formed on water by certain substances, such as proteins and fatty acids, characterized by molecules containing some atom groupings that are soluble in water and other atom groupings that are insoluble in water. **2.** A confluent sheet of cells, one cell deep, growing on a surface in a cell culture.

mon·o·loc·u·lar (mon-ō-lok'ū-lăr). Having one cavity or chamber. SYN unicameral, unicamerate. [mono- + L. *loculus,* a small place]

mon·o·ma·nia (mon-ō-mā'nē-ă). An obsession or abnormally extreme enthusiasm for a single idea or subject; a psychosis

marked by the limitation of the symptoms rather strictly to a certain group, as the delusion in paranoia. [mono- + G. *mania,* frenzy]

mon·o·ma·ni·ac (mon-ō-mā'nē-ak). **1.** One exhibiting monomania. **2.** Characterized by or relating to monomania.

mon·o·mas·ti·gote (mon-ō-mas'ti-gōt). A mastigote having only one flagellum. [mono- + Roman *mastix, a whip*]

mon·o·mel·ic (mon-ō-mel'ik). Relating to one limb. [mono- + G. *melos,* limb]

mon·o·mer (mon'ō-mer). **1.** The molecular unit that, by repetition, constitutes a large structure or polymer; e.g., ethylene, $H_2C=CH_2$, is the monomer of polyethylene, $H(CH_2)_nH$. SEE ALSO subunit (1). **2.** The protein structural unit of a virion capsid. SEE virion. **3.** The protein subunit of a protein composed of several loosely associated such units, usually noncovalently bound together. [mono- + -mer]

mon·o·mer·ic (mon-ō-mer'ik). **1.** Consisting of a single component. **2.** In genetics, relating to a hereditary disease or characteristic controlled by genes at a single locus. **3.** Consisting of monomers. [mono- + G. *meros,* part]

mon·o·me·tal·lic (mon'ō-mĕ-tal'ik). Containing one atom of a metal per molecule.

mon·o·mi·cro·bic (mon'ō-mī-krō'bik). Denoting a monoinfection.

mon·o·mo·lec·u·lar (mon'ō-mō-lek'ū-lăr). **1.** SYN unimolecular. **2.** Relating to a singular molecular entity.

mon·o·mor·phic (mon-ō-mōr'fik). Of one shape; unchangeable in shape. [mono- + G. *morphē,* shape]

mon·om·pha·lus (mon-om'fă-lŭs). SYN omphalopagus. [mono- + G. *omphalos,* umbilicus]

mon·o·my·o·ple·gia (mon'ō-mī'ō-plē'jē-ă). Paralysis limited to one muscle. [mono- + G. *mys,* muscle, + *plēgē,* a stroke]

mon·o·my·o·si·tis (mon'ō-mī-ō-sī'tis). Inflammation of a single muscle.

mon·o·neme (mon'ō-nēm). An unpaired helix of nucleic acid, as occurs in a chromatid.

mon·o·neu·ral, mon·o·neu·ric (mon'ō-noo'răl, -noo'rik). **1.** Having only one neuron. **2.** Supplied by a single nerve.

mononeuritis multiplex. SYN *mononeuropathy* multiplex.

mon·o·neu·rop·a·thy (mon'ō-noo-rop'ă-thē). Disorder involving a single nerve.

  m. mul'tiplex, nontraumatic involvement of two or more portions of the peripheral nervous system (e.g., roots, plexus elements, nerve trunks), usually sequentially and in different areas of the body; most often the result of vasculitides. SYN mononeuritis multiplex.

mon·o·nu·cle·ar (mon-ō-noo'klē-ăr). Having only one nucleus; used especially in reference to blood cells.

mon·o·nu·cle·o·sis (mon'ō-noo-klē-ō'sis). Presence of abnormally large numbers of mononuclear leukocytes in the circulating blood, especially with reference to forms that are not normal.

🔲**infectious m.,** an acute febrile illness of young adults caused by the Epstein-Barr virus, a member of the Herpesviridae family; frequently spread by saliva transfer; characterized by fever, sore throat, enlargement of lymph nodes and spleen, and leukopenia that changes to lymphocytosis during the second week; the circulating blood usually contains abnormal, large T lymphocytes that resemble monocytes even though B cells are infected, and there is heterophil antibody that may be completely adsorbed on beef erythrocytes, but not on guinea pig kidney antigen. Collections of the characteristic abnormal lymphocytes may be present not only in the lymph nodes and spleen, but in various other sites, such as the meninges, brain, and myocardium. SYN benign lymphadenosis, glandular fever.

mon·o·nu·cle·o·tide (mon-ō-noo'klē-ō-tīd). SYN nucleotide.

mon·o·oc·tan·o·in (mon'ō-ok'-ta'nō'in). A semisynthetic esterified glycerol used as a solubilizing agent for radiolucent gallstones retained in the biliary tract following cholecystectomy.

mon·o·ox·y·ge·na·ses (mon-ō-ok'si-jĕ-nā-sez). Oxidoreductases that induce the incorporation of one atom of oxygen from O_2 into the substance being oxidized.

mon·o·pa·re·sis (mon′o-pa-rē′sis, -par′ĕ-sis). Paresis affecting a single extremity or part of an extremity.

mon·o·par·es·the·sia (mon′ō-par-es-thē′zē-ă). Paresthesia affecting a single region only.

mon·o·path·ic (mon-ō-path′ik). Relating to a monopathy.

mo·nop·a·thy (mon-op′ă-thē). **1.** A single uncomplicated disease. **2.** A local disease affecting only one organ or part. [mono- + G. *pathos*, suffering]

mon·o·pe·nia (mon-ō-pē′nē-ă). SYN monocytopenia.

mo·noph·a·gism (mŏ-nof′ă-jizm). Habitual eating of but one kind of food or but one meal a day when the latter is clearly an aberration. [mono- + G. *phagō*, to eat]

mon·o·pha·sia (mon-ō-fā′zē-ă). Inability to speak other than a single word or sentence. [mono- + G. *phasis*, speech]

mon·o·pha·sic (mon-ō-fā′zik). **1.** Marked by monophasia. **2.** Occurring in or characterized by only one phase or stage. **3.** Fluctuating from the baseline in one direction only.

mon·o·phe·nol mon·o·ox·y·gen·ase (mon-ō-fē′nol). **1.** A copper-containing oxidoreductase that catalyzes the oxidation of *o*-diphenols to *o*-quinones by O_2, with the incorporation of one of the two oxygen atoms in the product; it also catalyzes the oxidation of monophenols, such as L-tyrosine, to dihydroxy-L-phenylalanine (dopa), a precursor of melanin and epinephrine (catecholamines), and can act as a catechol oxidase; a deficiency of this enzyme is observed in a number of forms of albinism. SYN cresolase, monophenol oxidase, tyrosinase. **2.** SYN laccase.

mon·o·phe·nol ox·i·dase. SYN monophenol monooxygenase (1).

mon·o·pho·bia (mon-ō-fō′bē-ă). Morbid fear of solitude or of being left alone. [mono- + G. *phobos*, fear]

mon·oph·thal·mos (mon-of-thal′mos). Failure of outgrowth of a primary optic vesicle with absence of ocular tissues; the remaining eye is often maldeveloped. [mono- + G. *ophthalmos*, eye]

mon·oph·thal·mus (mon′of-thal′mŭs). SYN cyclops. [mono- + G. *ophthalmos*, eye]

mon·o·phy·let·ic (mon′ō-fī-let′ik). **1.** Having a single cell type of origin; derived from one line of descent, in contrast to polyphyletic. **2.** In hematology, relating to monophyletism. [mono- + G. *phylē*, tribe]

mon·o·phy·le·tism (mon-ō-fī′lĕ-tizm). In hematology, the theory that all the blood cells are derived from one common stem cell or histioblast. SYN monophyletic theory. [mono- + G. *phylē*, tribe]

mon·o·phy·o·dont (mon-ō-fī′ō-dont). Having one set of teeth only; without deciduous dentition. [mono- + G. *phyō*, to grow, + *odous* (*odont*-), tooth]

mon·o·plas·mat·ic (mon′ō-plas-mat′ik). Formed of but one tissue. [mono- + G. *plasma*, thing formed]

mon·o·plast (mon′ō-plast). A unicellular organism that retains the same structure or form throughout its existence. [mono- + G. *plastos*, formed]

mon·o·plas·tic (mon-ō-plas′tik). Undergoing no change in structure; relating to a monoplast.

mon·o·ple·gia (mon-ō-plē′jē-ă). Paralysis of one limb. [mono- + G. *plēgē*, a stroke]

m. masticato′ria, unilateral paralysis of the muscles of mastication (masseter, temporal, pterygoid).

mon·o·ploid (mon′ō-ployd). SYN haploid. [mono- + G. *ploides*, in form]

mon·o·po·dia (mon-ō-pō′dē-ă). Malformation in which only one foot is externally recognizable. [mono- + G. *pous*, foot]

mon·ops (mon′ops). SYN cyclops. [mono- + G. *ōps*, eye]

mon·o·pty·chi·al (mon-ō-tī′kē-ăl). Arranged in a single but folded layer, as the cells in the epithelium of the gallbladder or certain glands. [mono- + G. *ptychē*, fold]

mon·or·chia (mon-ōr′kē-ă). SYN monorchism.

mon·or·chid·ic, mon·or·chid (mon-ōr-kid′ik, mon-ōr′kid). **1.** Having only one testis. **2.** Having apparently only one testis, the other being undescended.

mon·or·chid·ism (mon-ōr′ki-dizm). SYN monorchism.

mon·or·chism (mon′ōr-kizm). A condition in which only one testis is apparent, the other being absent or undescended. SYN monorchia, monorchidism. [mono- + G. *orchis*, testis]

mon·o·rec·i·dive (mon-o-res′i-dēv). Denoting a late or tertiary manifestation of syphilis which takes the form of an ulcerated papule located at the site of the original chancre. [mono- + L. *recidivus*, relapsing]

mon·o·rhin·ic (mon-ō-rin′ik). Single-nosed; used to characterize conjoined twins in which only a single nose cavity is evident. [mono- + G. *rhis* (*rhin*-), nose]

mon·o·sac·cha·ride (mon-ō-sak′ă-rīd). A carbohydrate that cannot form any simpler sugar by simple hydrolysis; e.g., pentoses, hexoses. SYN monose.

mon·o·scel·ous (mon-ō-sel′ŭs, -skel′ŭs). Having only one leg. [mono- + G. *skelos*, leg]

mon·o·sce·nism (mon-ō-sē′nizm). Morbid concentration on some past experience. [mono- + G. *skēnē*, tent (stage drop)]

mon·ose (mon′ōs). SYN monosaccharide.

mon·o·so·di·um glu·ta·mate (MSG) (mon-ō-sō′dē-ŭm gloo′tă-māt). The monosodium salt of the naturally occurring L form of glutamic acid; used as a flavor enhancer that is a cause or contributing factor to "Chinese restaurant" syndrome; also used intravenously as an adjunct in treatment of encephalopathies associated with hepatic disease.

mon·o·some (mon′ō-sōm). **1.** SYN accessory *chromosome*. **2.** Obsolete term for ribosome. **3.** A structure consisting of a single ribosome bound to a molecule of mRNA. [mono- + chromosome]

mon·o·so·mia (mon-ō-sō′mē-ă). In conjoined twins, a condition in which there are two heads and a single trunk. SEE conjoined *twins*, under *twin*. [mono- + G. *sōma*, body]

mon·o·so·mic (mon-ō-sō′mik). Relating to monosomy.

mon·o·so·mous (mon-ō-sō′mŭs). Characterized by or pertaining to monosomia.

mon·o·so·my (mon′ō-sō-mē). Absence of one chromosome of a pair of homologous chromosomes. SEE ALSO chromosomal *deletion*. [see monosome]

mon·o·sper·my (mon′ō-sper-mē). Fertilization by the entrance of only one spermatozoon into the egg. [mono- + G. *sperma*, seed]

Mon·o·spo·ri·um ap·i·o·sper·mum (mon-ō-spō′rē-ŭm ap′ē-ō-sper′mŭm). Former name for *Scedosporium apiospermum*. Telemorph is *Pseudallescheria boydii*.

Mo·nos·to·ma (mō-nos′tō-mă, mon-ō-stō′mă). Archaic name for a genus of trematodes, based on the presence of a single sucker. [mono- + G. *stoma*, mouth]

mon·o·stome (mon′ō-stōm). Common name for digenetic trematodes that possess a single sucker, oral or ventral, rather than both. SEE ALSO *Monostoma*. [mono- + G. *stoma*, mouth]

mon·o·stot·ic (mon-os-tot′ik). Involving only one bone. [mono- + G. *osteon*, bone]

mon·o·stra·tal (mon-ō-strā′tăl). Composed of a single layer. [mono- + L. *stratum*, layer]

mon·o·sub·sti·tut·ed (mon-ō-sŭb′sti-too-tĕd). In chemistry, denoting an element or radical, only one atom or unit of which is found in each molecule of a substitution compound.

mon·o·symp·to·mat·ic (mon′ō-simp-tō-mat′ik). Denoting a disease or morbid condition manifested by only one marked symptom.

mon·o·sy·nap·tic (mon′ō-si-nap′tik). Referring to direct neural connections (those not involving an internuncial neuron); e.g., the direct connection between primary sensory nerve cells and motor neurons characterizing the monosynaptic reflex arc.

mon·o·syph·i·lide (mon-o-sif′i-lid). Marked by the occurrence of a single syphilitic lesion.

mon·o·ter·penes (mon-ō-ter′pēnz). Hydrocarbons or their derivatives formed by the condensation of two isoprene units, and therefore containing 10 carbon atoms; e.g., camphor; often containing a cyclic structure.

mon·o·ther·mia (mon-ō-ther′mē-ă). Evenness of bodily temperature; absence of an evening rise in body temperature. [mono- + G. *thermē*, heat]

mo

mon·o·thi·o·glyc·er·ol (mon'ō-thī-ō-glis'er-ol). Used to promote wound healing. SYN thioglycerol.

mo·not·o·cous (mŏ-not'ō-kŭs). Producing a single offspring at a birth. [mono- + G. *tokos,* birth]

Mon·o·tre·ma·ta (mon-ō-trē'mă-tă). An order of egg-laying mammals that have a cloaca or common chamber that receives digestive, urinary, and reproductive products; only Australia has such forms, the duck-billed platypus (*Ornithorhynchus*) and the echidna (*Tachyglossus*). [mono- + G. *trēma,* a hole]

mon·o·treme (mon'ō-trēm). A member of the order Monotremata.

mo·not·ri·chate (mŏ-not'ri-kāt). SYN monotrichous.

mo·not·ri·chous (mŏ-not'ri-kŭs). Denoting a microorganism possessing a single flagellum or cilium. SYN monotrichate, uniflagellate.

mon·o·va·lence, mon·o·va·len·cy (mon-ō-vā'lens, -vā'len-sē). A combining power (valence) equal to that of a hydrogen atom. SYN univalence, univalency.

mon·o·va·lent (mon-ō-vā'lent). **1.** Having the combining power (valence) of a hydrogen atom. SYN monatomic (2), univalent. **2.** Pertaining to a monovalent (specific) antiserum to a single antigen or organism.

mon·ox·e·nous (mon-oks'ē-nŭs). SYN monogenetic. [mono- + G. *xenos,* stranger]

mon·ox·ide (mon-ok'sīd). Any oxide having only one atom of oxygen; e.g., CO.

mon·o·zo·ic (mon-ō-zō'ik). Unisegmented, as in cestodarian tapeworms. SEE polyzoic.

mon·o·zy·got·ic, mon·o·zy·gous (mon-ō-zī-got'ik, -zī'gŭs). SYN unigerminal. SEE monozygotic *twins,* under *twin.* [mono- + G. *zygōtos,* yoked]

Monro, Alexander Sr., Scottish anatomist and surgeon, 1697–1767. SEE *bursa* of M.

Monro, Alexander, Jr., Scottish anatomist, 1733–1817. SEE M. *doctrine, foramen, line, sulcus;* M.-Kellie *doctrine;* M.-Richter *line;* Richter-M. *line.*

mons, gen. **mon·tis,** pl. **mon·tes** (monz, mon'tis, mon'tēz) [TA]. An anatomical prominence or slight elevation above the general level of the surface. [L. a mountain]

m. pu'bis [TA], the prominence caused by a pad of fatty tissue over the symphysis pubis in the female. SYN pubes (2) [TA], m. veneris, pubic bone.

m. ure'teris, a pinkish prominence on the wall of the bladder marking each ureteral orifice.

m. ven'eris, SYN m. pubis. [L. *Venus*]

Monson, George S., U.S. dentist, 1869–1933. SEE M. *curve;* anti-M. *curve.*

mon·ster. Outmoded term for a malformed embryo, fetus, or individual. See entries beginning with terato-. SEE teras. [L. *monstrum,* an evil omen, a prodigy, a wonder]

mon·tan·ic ac·id (mon-tan'ik). SYN octacosanoic acid. [montan (wax)]

Monteggia, Giovanni B., Italian surgeon, 1762–1815. SEE M. *fracture.*

montelukast sodium (mon-te-loo'kast). A competitive and selective Cys-LT$_1$-receptor antagonist that acts as a blocker of leukotrienes, which are potent endogenous bronchoconstrictors. A prophylactic; not useful to treat an ongoing attack of asthma.

Montgomery, William F., Irish obstetrician, 1797–1859. SEE M. *follicles,* under *follicle, glands,* under *gland, tubercles,* under *tubercle.*

mon·tic·u·lus, pl. **mon·tic·u·li** (mon-tik'ū-lŭs, -lī). **1.** Any slight rounded projection above a surface. **2.** The central portion of the superior vermis forming a projection on the surface of the cerebellum; its anterior and most prominent portion is called the culmen, its posterior sloping portion, the declive. [L. dim. of *mons,* mountain]

palmar monticuli, three small elevations in the distal palm corresponding to the window-like deficiencies in the distal palmar

aponeurosis between the four longitudinal bundles and proximal to the superficial transverse metacarpal ligament.

mood (mood). The pervasive feeling, tone, and internal emotional state of an individual which, when impaired, can markedly influence virtually all aspects of a person's behavior or his or her perception of external events.

mood swing. Oscillation of a person's emotional feeling tone between periods of euphoria and depression.

Moon, Henry, English surgeon, 1845–1892. SEE M. *molars,* under *molar.*

Moon, Robert C., U.S. ophthalmologist, 1844–1914. SEE Laurence-M. *syndrome.*

Moore, Robert Foster, British ophthalmologist, 1878–1963. SEE M. lightning *streaks,* under *streak.*

Moore, Charles H., English surgeon, 1821–1870. SEE M. *method.*

Mooren, Albert, German ophthalmologist, 1828–1899. SEE M. *ulcer.*

Mooser, Hermann, Swiss pathologist in Mexico, 1891–1971. SEE M. *bodies,* under *body.*

MOPP Acronym for *m*echlorethamine, *o*ncovin (vincristine), *p*rocarbazine, and *p*rednisone, a chemotherapy regimen used in the treatment of Hodgkin disease.

Morand, Sauveur F., French surgeon, 1697–1773. SEE M. *foot, spur.*

Morax, Victor, French ophthalmologist, 1866–1935. SEE *Moraxella.*

Mor·ax·el·la (mōr'ak-sel'ă). A genus of obligately aerobic nonmotile bacteria (family Neisseriaceae) containing Gram-negative coccoids or short rods that usually occur in pairs. They do not produce acid from carbohydrates, are oxidase positive and penicillin-susceptible, and infect the mucous membranes of humans and other mammals. The type species is *M. lacunata.* [V. *Morax*]

M. anatipes'tifer, a bacterial species causing a respiratory disease in ducklings.

M. catarrha'lis, a bacterial species that causes upper respiratory tract infections, particularly in immunocompromised hosts; the type species of the genus M. SYN *Branhamella catarrhalis.*

M. kingae, SYN *Kingella kingae.*

M. lacuna'ta, a bacterial species causing conjunctivitis in humans; it is the type species of the genus *M.*

M. nonliquefa'ciens, a bacterial species found in the respiratory tract of humans, especially in the nose; usually not pathogenic, but occasionally causes sinusitis.

M. osloen'sis, a bacterial species found in the genitourinary tract, blood, spinal and chest fluids, and nose; rarely found in the respiratory tract; usually not pathogenic, although some strains have been isolated from serious pathologic conditions in humans.

M. phenylpyru'vica, a bacterial species of unknown pathogenicity found in the genitourinary tract, blood, cerebrospinal fluid, and in pus from various lesions.

mor·bid (mōr'bid). **1.** Diseased or pathologic. **2.** In psychology, abnormal or deviant. [L. *morbidus,* ill, fr. *morbus,* disease]

mor·bid·i·ty (mōr-bid'i-tē). **1.** A diseased state. **2.** The ratio of sick to well in a community. SYN morbility. SEE ALSO morbidity *rate.* **3.** The frequency of the appearance of complications following a surgical procedure or other treatment.

maternal m., medical complications in a woman caused by pregnancy, labor, or delivery.

puerperal m., illness arising during the first 10 days of the postpartum period, i.e., a temperature of 38°C (100.4°F) or more on any two days of the first 10, excluding the first 24 hours.

mor·bif·ic (mōr-bif'ik). SYN pathogenic. [L. *morbus,* disease, + *facio,* to make]

mor·big·e·nous (mor-bij'ē-nŭs). SYN pathogenic. [L. *morbus,* disease, + G. *-gen,* producing]

mor·bil·i·ty (mōr-bil'i-tē). SYN morbidity (2).

mor·bil·li (mōr-bil'ī). SYN measles (1). [Mediev. L. *morbillus,* dim. of L. *morbus,* disease]

mor·bil·li·form (mōr-bil'i-fōrm). Resembling measles (1). [see morbilli]

Mor·bil·li·vi·rus (mōr-bil′i-vī′rŭs). A genus in the family Paramyxoviridae, including measles, canine distemper, and bovine rinderpest viruses.

equine M., a species causing a fatal respiratory disease in horses and humans in Australia, with encephalitis also seen in some human cases. SYN Hendra virus.

mor·bi·lous (mōr-bil′ŭs). Relating to measles (1). [see morbilli]

mor·bus (mōr′bŭs). SYN disease (1). [L. disease]

mor·bus Ad·di·so·nii (mōr′bus ad′ĭ-son-ē). SYN chronic adreno-cortical *insufficiency.*

mor·cel (mōr-sel′). To remove piecemeal. [Fr. *morceler,* to subdivide]

mor·cel·la·tion (mōr-se-lā′shŭn). Division into and removal of small pieces, as of a tumor. SYN morcellement. [Fr. *morceler,* to subdivide]

mor·celle·ment (mōr-sel-maw′). SYN morcellation. [Fr.]

mor·dant (mōr′dant). **1.** A substance capable of combining with a dye and the material to be dyed, thereby increasing the affinity or binding of the dye; e.g., a m. commonly used to promote staining with hematoxylin is alum. **2.** To treat with a m. [L. *mordeo,* to bite]

mor. dict. Abbreviation for L. *more dicto,* as directed.

Morel, Benedict A., French psychiatrist, 1809–1873. SEE M. *ear;* Stewart-M. *syndrome.*

Mo·re·ra·stron·gy·lus cos·tar·i·cen·sis (mōr′er-ă-stron′ji-lŭs kos′tar-i-sen′sis). SYN *Angiostrongylus costaricensis.*

mo·res (mo′rāz). A concept used in the behavioral and social sciences to refer to centrally important and accepted folkways, and cultural norms which embody the fundamental moral views of a group. [L. pl. of *mos,* custom]

Morgagni, Giovanni B., Italian anatomist and pathologist, 1682–1771. SEE morgagnian *cyst;* M. *appendix, cartilage, caruncle, cataract, columns,* under *column, concha, crypts,* under *crypt, disease, foramen;* Morgagni foramen *hernia;* M. *fossa, fovea, frenum, globules,* under *globule, humor, hydatid, lacuna, liquor, nodule, prolapse, retinaculum, sinus, spheres,* under *sphere, syndrome, tubercle, valves,* under *valve, ventricle;* M.-Adams-Stokes *syndrome; frenulum* of M.

Morgan, Harry de R., British physician, 1863–1931. SEE M. *bacillus.*

mor·gan (M) (mōr′găn). The standard unit of genetic distance on the genetic map: the distance between two loci such that on average one crossing over will occur per meiosis; for working purposes, the centimorgan (0.01 M) is used. [T.H. *Morgan,* U.S. geneticist, 1866–1945]

Mor·gan·el·la (mōr′gan-el′-ah). A genus (family Enterobacteriaceae) of Gram-negative, facultatively anaerobic, chemoorganotrophic, straight rods that are motile by peritrichous flagella; found in feces of human beings, other animals, and reptiles; can cause opportunistic infections of the blood, respiratory tract, wounds, and urinary tract.

M. morganii, type species of the genus M. SYN Morgan bacillus.

morgue (mōrg). **1.** A building or room in a hospital or other facility where the dead are kept pending autopsy, burial, or cremation. **2.** A building where unidentified dead are kept pending identification before burial. SYN mortuary (2). [Fr.]

Mori, O., 20th century Japanese pathologist. SEE Harada-M. filter paper strip *culture.*

mo·ria (mōr′ē-ă). **1.** Rarely used term denoting foolishness or dullness of comprehension. SYN hebetude. **2.** Rarely used term for a mental state marked by frivolity, joviality, an inveterate tendency to jest, and inability to take anything seriously. [G. *mōria,* folly, fr. *mōros,* stupid, dull]

mor·i·bund (mōr′i-bŭnd). Dying; at the point of death. [L. *moribundus,* dying, fr. *morior,* to die]

mo·rin (mōr′in) [C.I. 75660]. A natural yellow dye obtained from fustic and other members of the mulberry family and often associated with the dye maclurin; used as a fluorochrome for detection of metals, particularly aluminum. Fluorescent morinates are also formed with beryllium, gallium, indium, scandium, thorium, titanium, and zirconium.

Morison, James R., British surgeon, 1853–1939. SEE M. *pouch.*

Mörner, Karl A.H., Swedish chemist, 1855–1917. SEE M. *test.*

morn·ing glo·ry (mōr′ning glō′rē). **1.** SYN *Ipomoea rubrocoerulea* var. *praecox.* **2.** SYN *Rivea corymbosa.*

morn·ing glo·ry seeds. The seeds of morning glories, *Rivea corymbosa,* have been used for mind-altering purposes; hallucinogenic; intoxicant.

Moro, Ernst, German physician, 1874–1951. SEE M. *reflex.*

mo·ron (mōr′on). An obsolete term for a subclass of mental retardation or the individual classified therein. [G. *mōros,* stupid]

mo·rox·y·dine (mŏ-rok′si-dēn). An antiviral agent.

morph-. SEE morpho-.

mor·phea (mōr-fē′ă). Cutaneous lesion(s) characterized by indurated, slightly depressed plaques of thickened dermal fibrous tissue of a whitish or yellowish-white color surrounded by a pinkish or purplish halo. Lesions occur at any age, without systemic involvement, and usually resolve after a few years. SYN localized scleroderma. [G. *morphē,* form, figure]

m. gutta′ta, a form of m. with small discrete, white, waxy, indurated lesions. SYN white spot disease.

m. linea′ris, SYN linear *scleroderma.*

mor·pheme (mōr′fēm). The smallest linguistic unit with a meaning. [G. *morphē,* form + *-eme,* from *phoneme,* G. *phēmē,* utterance]

mor·phine (mōr′fēn, mōr-fēn′). The major phenanthrene alkaloid of opium, which contains 9–14% of anhydrous m. It produces a combination of depression and excitation in the central nervous system and some peripheral tissues; predominance of either central stimulation or depression depends upon the species and dose; repeated administration leads to the development of tolerance, physical dependence, and (if abused) psychic dependence. Used as an analgesic, sedative, and anxiolytic. [L. *Morpheus,* god of dreams or of sleep]

m. hydrochloride, white acicular or cubical crystals of bitter taste, soluble in about 25 parts of water.

m. sulfate (MS), m. used for formulation of tablets as well as solutions for parenteral, epidural, or intrathecal injection to relieve pain.

morpho-, morph-. Form, shape, structure. [G. *morphē*]

mor·pho·gen·e·sis (mōr-fō-jen′ĕ-sis). **1.** Differentiation of cells and tissues in the early embryo that establishes the form and structure of the various organs and parts of the body. **2.** The ability of a molecule or group of molecules (particularly macromolecules) to assume a certain shape. [morpho- + G. *genesis,* production]

mor·pho·ge·net·ic (mōr′fō-jĕ-net′ik). Relating to morphogenesis.

mor·pho·log·ic (mōr-fō-loj′ik). Relating to morphology.

mor·phol·o·gy (mōr-fol′ō-jē). The science concerned with the configuration or the structure of animals and plants. [morpho- + G. *logos,* study]

mor·pho·met·ric (mōr′fō-met′rik). Pertaining to morphometry.

mor·phom·e·try (mōr-fom′ĕ-trē). The measurement of the form of organisms or their parts. [morpho- + G. *metron,* measure]

mor·phon (mōr′fon). Any one of the individual structures entering into the formation of an organism; a morphologic element, such as a cell. [G. *morphē,* form]

mor·pho·phys·i·ol·o·gy (mōr-fō-fiz-ē-ol′ō-jē). SYN functional *anatomy.*

mor·pho·sis (mōr-fō′sis). Mode of development of a part. [G. formation, act of forming]

mor·pho·syn·the·sis (mōr-fō-sin′thĕ-sis). An awareness of space and of body schema represented in the parietal lobes of the cerebral cortex. [morpho- + synthesis]

mor·pho·type (mōr′fō-tīp). An infrasubspecific group of bacterial strains distinguishable from other strains of the same species on the basis of morphologic characters which may or may not be associated with a change in serologic state. [morpho- + G. *typos,* stamp, model]

mo

Morquio, Louis, Uruguayan physician, 1867–1935. SEE M. *disease, syndrome;* M.-Ullrich *disease;* Brailsford-Morquio *disease.*

mor·rhu·ate so·di·um (mōr′roo-āt). The sodium salts of the fatty acids of cod liver oil; a sclerosing agent used in the treatment of varicose veins, mixed with a local anesthetic. [fr. *Gadus morrhua,* cod]

Morrison, Ashton B., Irish pathologist in the U.S., *1922. SEE Verner-M. *syndrome.*

mors, gen. **mor·tis** (mōrz, mōr′tis). SYN death. [L.]

m. thy′mica, obsolete term for sudden death in young children, usually the result of infection; formerly erroneously attributed to an enlarged thymus. SEE ALSO sudden infant death *syndrome.*

mor·si·ca·tio (mor-sik′ă-tē-ō). Habitual nibbling of the lips (labiorum), tongue (linguae), or buccal mucosa (buccarum); often produces a shaggy white lesion. [L. biting, fr. *mordeo,* to bite]

morsicatio buccarum, white elevations of buccal mucosa caused by the pressure of molar teeth. [L. chewing of the cheeks]

mor. sol. Abbreviation for L. *more solito,* as usual, as customary.

mor·su·lus (mōr′soo-lŭs). SYN troche. [Mod. L. dim. of L. *morsus,* a bite]

mor·tal (mōr′tăl). **1.** Pertaining to or causing death. **2.** Destined to die. [L. *mortalis,* fr. *mors,* death]

mor·tal·i·ty (mōr-tal′i-tē). **1.** The state of being mortal. **2.** SYN death rate. **3.** A fatal outcome. [L. *mortalitas,* fr. *mors* (*mort-*), death]

perinatal m. (per′ē-nā-tal), m. around the time of birth, conventionally limited to the period from 28 weeks' gestation to 1 week postnatal.

mor·tar (mōr′tăr). A vessel with rounded interior in which crude drugs and other substances are crushed or bruised by means of a pestle. [L. *mortarium*]

Mor·ti·er·el·la (mōr′tē-ĕ-rel′ă). A genus of saprophytic fungi (class Zygomycetes, family Mucoraceae) commonly found in nature; pathogenicity doubtful.

mor·ti·fi·ca·tion (mōr′ti-fi-kā′shŭn). SYN gangrene (1). [L. *mors* (*mort-*), death, + *facio,* to make]

mor·tise (mōr′tēs). The seating for the talus formed by the union of the distal fibula and the tibia at the ankle joint. [M.E., fr. O.Fr., fr. Ar. *murtazz,* fastened]

Morton, Dudley J., U.S. orthopedist, 1884–1960. SEE M. *syndrome.*

Morton, Samuel G., U.S. physician, 1799–1851. SEE M. *plane.*

Morton, Thomas G., U.S. physician, 1835–1903. SEE M. *neuralgia;* Morton *metatarsalgia.*

mor·tu·ary (mōr′tū-ār-ē). **1.** Relating to death or to burial. **2.** SYN morgue. [L. *mortuus,* dead, part. adj. fr. *morior,* pp. *mortuus,* to die]

mor·u·la (mōr′oo-lă, mōr′ū-). The solid mass of blastomeres resulting from the early cleavage divisions of the zygote. In ova with little yolk, the m. is a spheroidal mass of cells; in forms with considerable yolk, the configuration of the m. stage is greatly modified. [Mod. L. dim. of L. *morus,* mulberry]

mor·u·la·tion (mōr-oo-lā′shŭn, mōr-ū-). Formation of the morula.

mor·u·loid (mōr′oo-loyd, mōr′ū-). **1.** Resembling a morula. **2.** Shaped like a mulberry.

Morvan, Augustin, French physician, 1819–1897. SEE M. *chorea, disease.*

mo·sa·ic (mō-zā′ik). **1.** Inlaid; resembling inlaid work. **2.** The juxtaposition in an organism of genetically different tissues; it may occur normally (as in lyonization, *q.v.*), or pathologically, as an occasional phenomenon. From somatic mutation (gene mosaicism), an anomaly of chromosome division resulting in two or more types of cells containing different numbers of chromosomes (chromosome mosaicism), or chimerism (cellular mosaicism). [Mod. L. *mosaicus, musaicus,* pertaining to the Muses, artistic]

mo·sa·i·cism (mō-zā′i-sizm). Condition of being mosaic (2).

cellular m., a chimerism in which a tissue contains cells from different zygotes; e.g., in humans, involving erythrocytes.

chromosome m., SEE mosaic (2).

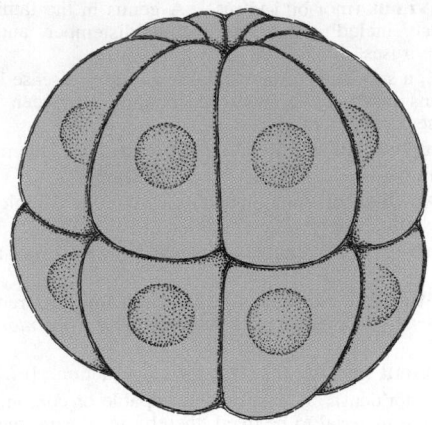
morula

gene m., SEE mosaic (2).

germinal m., gonadal m., a state in which some of the germ cells of the gonad are of a form not present in either parent, because of mutation in an intermediate progenitor of these cells.

Moschcowitz, Eli, U.S. physician, 1879–1964. SEE Moschcowitz *test.*

mos·chus (mos′kŭs). Musk. [G. *moschos,* musk]

Mosenthal, Herman Otto, American physician, 1878–1954. SEE Mosenthal *test.*

Mosler, Karl F., German physician, 1831–1911. SEE M. *diabetes, sign.*

mos·qui·to, pl. **mos·qui·toes** (mŭs-kē′tō, -tōs). A blood-sucking dipterous insect of the family Culicidae. *Aedes, Anopheles, Culex, Mansonia,* and *Stegomyia* are the genera containing most of the species involved in the transmission of protozoan and other disease-producing parasites. [Sp. dim. of *mosca,* fly, fr. L. *musca,* a fly]

Moss, Gerald, U.S. physician, 1931–1973. SEE M. *tube.*

Moss, Melvin L., U.S. oral pathologist, *1923. SEE Gorlin-Chaudhry-M. *syndrome.*

moss. **1.** Any low growing, delicate cryptogamous plant of the class Musci. **2.** Popularly, any one of a number of lichens and seaweeds. [A.S. *meōs*]

Ceylon m., a red seaweed; a source of agar.

club m., SYN lycopodium.

Iceland m., SYN cetraria.

Irish m., SYN chondrus (2).

muskeag m., SYN sphagnum m.

pearl m., SYN chondrus (2).

peat m., SYN sphagnum m.

sphagnum m., a highly absorbent m. used as a substitute for absorbent cotton or gauze in surgical dressing and sanitary napkins. SYN muskeag m., peat m.

Mosso, Angelo, Italian physiologist, 1846–1910. SEE M. *ergograph, sphygmomanometer.*

Motais, Ernst, French ophthalmologist, 1845–1913. SEE M. *operation.*

mote (mōt). A small particle; a speck. [A.S. *mot*]

blood m.'s, SYN hemoconia.

moth·er (mŭth′er). **1.** The female parent. **2.** Any cell or other structure from which other similar bodies are formed. [A.S. *mōdor*]

surrogate m., a woman who has been contracted with to carry a pregnancy for another woman or couple.

mo·tile (mō′til). **1.** Having the power of spontaneous movement. **2.** Denoting the type of mental imagery in which one learns and recalls most readily that which has been felt, i.e., having a kinesthetic representational system. Cf. audile. **3.** A person having such mental imagery. [see motion]

mo·til·in (mō-til′in). A 22-amino acid polypeptide occurring in duodenal mucosa as a controller of normal gastrointestinal motor activity; in minute (ng) doses it induces powerful motor activity increases in the fundic gland area and antral pouches of the stomach, with an increase in pepsin output from the former. [motility + -in]

mo·til·i·ty (mō-til′i-tē). The power of spontaneous movement.

mo·tion (mō′shŭn). **1.** A change of place or position. Cf. movement (1). **2.** SYN defecation. **3.** SYN stool. [L. *motio,* movement, fr. *moveo,* pp. *motus,* to move]

brownian m., SYN brownian *movement.* [R. Brown, British botanist, 1773–1858]

continuous passive m. (CPM), a technique in which a joint, usually the knee, is moved constantly through a variable range of motion to prevent stiffness and to increase the range of motion; most often accomplished using a motorized device specifically designed for this purpose.

mo·ti·va·tion (mō-ti-vā′shŭn). In psychology, the aggregate of all the individual motives, needs, and drives operative in an individual at any given moment which influence will and cause behavior. [ML. *motivus,* moving]

extrinsic m., the search for satisfaction, or to avoid dissatisfaction, through nontask aspects of the environment such as seeking comfort, safety, and security from others or through the efforts of others.

intrinsic m., derivation of personal satisfaction through self-initiated achievement and behavior.

personal m., an individual's predispositions and expectations that give meaning and direction to personality functioning.

mo·tive (mō′tiv). **1.** An acquired predisposition, need, or specific state of tension within an individual which arouses, maintains, and directs behavior toward a goal. SYN learned drive. **2.** The reason attributed to or given by an individual for a behavioral act. Cf. instinct. [L. *moveo,* to move, to set in motion]

achievement m., an acquired, chronic need to succeed in the face of recognizable obstacles; its strength is usually diagnosed from recurring themes in stories told by the individual while taking a thematic apperception test or from other assessment instruments used by clinical psychologists.

mastery m., an acquired need to be assertive, to stand out in a crowd, to be dominant.

mo·to·fa·cient (mō-tō-fā′shent). Causing motion; denoting the second phase of muscular activity in which actual movement is produced. [L. *motus,* motion, + *facio,* to make]

mo·to·neu·ron (mō′tō-noo′ron). SYN motor *neuron.*

mo·tor (mō′ter). **1.** In anatomy and physiology, denoting those neural structures which by the impulses generated and transmitted by them cause muscle fibers or pigment cells to contract, or glands to secrete. SEE ALSO motor *cortex,* motor *endplate,* motor *neuron.* **2.** In psychology, denoting the organism's overt reaction to a stimulus (motor response). [L. a mover, fr. *moveo,* to move]

m. oc′uli, SYN oculomotor *nerve* [CN III].

plastic m., an artificial point of attachment on an amputation stump to which is fastened the cord or extensor by which movement is transmitted to an artificial limb; used in cinematization.

mo·tor·i·al (mō-tōr′ē-ăl). Relating to motion, to a motor nerve or the motor nucleus.

mo·tor·me·ter (mō′ter-mē′ter). A device for determining the amount, force, and rapidity of movement.

MOTT Term used to describe mycobacteria other than *Mycobacterium tuberculosis, M. bovis,* and *M. africanum,* (*M. tuberculosis*-complex).

mot·tle (mot′tl). Fine inhomogeneity of an area of generally uniform opacity on a photograph or radiograph; noise. [fr. *motley,* fr. M.E. *mot,* speck]

quantum m., m. caused by the statistical fluctuation of the number of photons absorbed by the intensifying screens to form the light image on the film; faster screens produce more quantum m.

mot·tling (mot′ling). An area of skin composed of macular lesions of varying shades or colors. [E. *motley,* variegated in color]

Motulsky dye re·duc·tion test. See under test.

mou·lage (moo-lazh′). A reproduction in wax of a skin lesion, tumor, or other pathologic state. [F. a molding]

mould (mōld). SYN mold.

moult (mōlt). SYN molt.

mound·ing (mownd′ing). SYN myoedema.

Mounier-Kuhn, Pierre, French physician, *1901. SEE Mounier-Kuhn *syndrome.*

mount (mownt). **1.** To prepare for microscopic examination. **2.** To climb on for purposes of copulation. **3.** To organize and present, as a fever, an immunologic response, etc.

mount·ing (mownt′ing). In dentistry, the laboratory procedure of attaching the maxillary and/or mandibular cast to an articulator.

split cast m., (1) a cast with key grooves on its base, mounted on an articulator for the purpose of easy removal and accurate replacement; split remounting metal plates may be used instead of grooves in casts; (2) a means for testing the accuracy of articulator adjustment.

mourn (mōrn). To express grief or sorrow as a result of loss. In psychoanalysis, mourning is the frequently unexpressed process of responding to loss of a cathected object which, in contrast to melancholia, usually does not involve loss of self-esteem. [O.E. *murnan*]

mouse (mows). A small rodent belonging to the genus *Mus.*

joint m.'s, Small fibrous, cartilaginous, or bony loose bodies in the synovial cavity of a joint.

---

knockout m., a m. from whose genome a single gene has been artificially deleted.

Experimental animals lacking specific genes have become valuable research tools in many branches of medicine, including genetics, physiology, pharmacology, immunology, cell biology, and oncology. A transgenic animal is one into whose genome a foreign gene, constructed by recombinant DNA technology, has been deliberately inserted. Placement of the inserted gene at a specific locus in the genome is made possible by incorporating it in a vector in which it is flanked by DNA sequences unique to the target site. The artificial genetic material is introduced into an embryo, which then develops into a chimera whose tissues contain both normal cells and cells containing the transgene. Matings among such animals yield some offspring that are homozygous for the transgene. If the inserted gene is a nonfunctional (null) allele, it deletes or "knocks out" the normal, wild allele. Not only is the deleted gene not expressed, but the offspring of matings among homozygous individuals constitute a pure strain, all of whose members lack the gene. Although theoretically any animal could be subjected to the knockout technique, mice have been used almost exclusively. Mice are small and easily maintained, and they reproduce rapidly and have a short life span. In addition, mouse and human genomes are strikingly similar, with about 75% correspondence of genes. The fact that knockout mice lacking a wide variety of genes are often phenotypically normal indicates that the mouse genome, like that of human beings, often has sufficient redundancy to compensate for a single missing pair of alleles. Knockout mice lacking the p53 tumor suppressor gene are used in studies of carcinogenesis, while those lacking the gene for the LDL receptor constitute an animal model of human familial hypercholesterolemia. Knockout mice have proved valuable in revealing the functions of genes for which mutant strains were not previously available.

---

multimammate m., an African rodent, *Praomys natalensis,* widely used in cancer research.

New Zealand mice, inbred strains of mice, either black (NZB) or white (NZW), unique among strains used in experimental immunology because of their proclivity to spontaneous immunologic abnormalities and disorders including systemic lupus erythematosus similar to that found in humans.

mo

nude m., a hairless mutant m. with thymic hypoplasia, lacking T cells.

transgenic m.'s (tranz′jen-ik), Mice that have a piece of foreign DNA integrated into their genome.

mouth (mowth). **1.** SYN oral *cavity.* **2.** The opening, usually the external opening, of a cavity or canal. SEE os (2), ostium, orifice, stoma (2). [A.S. *mūth*]

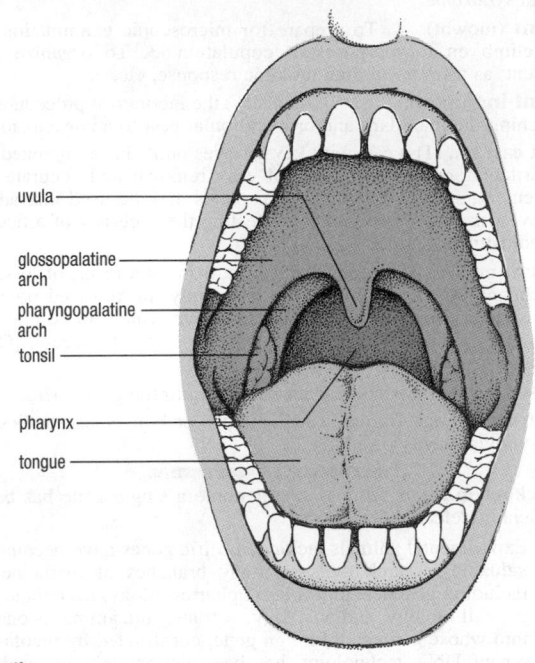

uvula

glossopalatine arch

pharyngopalatine arch

tonsil

pharynx

tongue

mouth

carp m., a m. like that of the carp, with downturning of the corners; observed in Cornelia de Lange syndrome and Silver-Russell dwarfism.

denture sore m., mucosal erythema underlying a denture base, usually representing inflammation caused by ill-fitting dentures, poor oral hygiene, or *Candida albicans.*

scabby m., SYN orf.

sore m., SEE soremouth.

tapir m., protrusion of the lips due to weakness of the orbicularis oris muscles; seen with some dystrophies. SYN bouche de tapir.

trench m., SYN necrotizing ulcerative *gingivitis.*

m. of the womb, SYN external *os* of uterus.

mouth guard. A pliable plastic device, adapted to cover the maxillary teeth, which is worn to reduce potential injury to oral structures during participation in contact sports.

mouth stick. A prosthesis which is held by the teeth and utilized by handicapped persons to perform such actions as typing, painting, and lifting small objects.

mouth·wash. A medicated liquid used for cleaning the mouth and treating diseased states of its mucous membranes. SYN collutorium, collutory.

move·ment (moov′ment). **1.** The act of motion; said of the entire body or of one or more of its members or parts. **2.** SYN stool. **3.** SYN defecation. [L. *moveo,* pp. *motus,* to move]

active m., (1) m. effected by the organism itself, unaided by external influences. (2) in physical therapy, a m. that is effected entirely by the patient's muscles, often with the guidance of the therapist.

adversive m., a rotation of the eyes, head, or trunk about the long axis of the body.

after-m., SEE aftermovement.

ameboid m., the form of m. characteristic of the protoplasm of leukocytes, amebae, and other unicellular organisms; it involves the massing of the protoplasm at a point where surface pressure is least and its extrusion in the form of a pseudopod; the protoplasm may return to the body of the cell, resulting in the retraction of the pseudopod, or the entire mass may flow into the latter and thereby result in locomotion of the cell. SYN streaming m.

assistive m., in physical therapy, a m. which is effected with the graduated assistance of the therapist.

associated m.'s, normal involuntary limb m.'s that accompany voluntary movement, e.g., arm swing with walking.

Bennett m., the bodily lateral m. or lateral shift of the mandible during a laterotrusive m.

border m.'s, any extreme compass of mandibular m. limited by bone, ligaments, or soft tissues; usually applied to horizontal mandibular m.'s.

border tissue m.'s, the action of the muscles and other tissues adjacent to the borders of a denture.

bowel m., defecation.

brownian m., erratic, nondirectional, zigzag m. observed by ultramicroscope in certain colloidal solutions and by microscope in suspensions of light particulate matter that results from the jostling or bumping of the larger particles by the molecules in the suspending medium which are regarded as being in continuous motion. SYN brownian motion, brownian-Zsigmondy m., molecular m., pedesis.

brownian-Zsigmondy m., SYN brownian m.

cardinal ocular m.'s, eye rotations to the right and left, upward to the right and left, and downward to the right and left, to diagnose positions of gaze.

choreic m., an involuntary spasmodic twitching or jerking in groups of muscles not associated in the production of definite purposeful m.'s.

ciliary m., the rhythmic, sweeping m. of epithelial cell cilia, of ciliate protozoans, or the sculling m. of flagella, effected possibly by the alternate contraction and relaxation of contractile threads (myoids) on one side of the cilium or flagellum.

circus m., a contraction or excitation wave traveling continuously in circular fashion around a ring of muscle or through the wall of the heart. SYN circus rhythm.

cogwheel ocular m.'s, loose, jerky ocular rotations replacing smooth following rotations.

conjugate m. of eyes, rotation of the two eyes in the same direction. SEE ALSO version (4).

decomposition of m., a manifestation of cerebellar disease in which a muscular movement is not carried out smoothly but in a series of component motions.

disconjugate m. of eyes, rotation of the two eyes in opposite directions, as in convergence or divergence.

drift m.'s, SYN drifts.

fetal m., the m. characteristic of the fetus *in utero;* usually commences between the sixteenth and eighteenth weeks of pregnancy. SEE ALSO quickening.

fixational ocular m., rotation of the eyes during voluntary fixation on an object; tremors, flicks, and drifts occur.

flick m.'s, SYN flicks.

free mandibular m.'s, (1) any mandibular m.'s made without tooth interference; **(2)** any uninhibited m.'s of the mandible.

functional mandibular m.'s, all natural, proper, or characteristic m.'s of the mandible made during speech, mastication, yawning, swallowing, and other associated m.'s.

fusional m., a reflex m. that tends to move the visual axes to the object of fixation so that stereoscopic vision is possible.

hinge m., an opening or closing m. of the mandible on the hinge axis.

intermediary m.'s, in dentistry, all m.'s between the extremes of mandibular excursions.

lateral m., in dentistry, m. of the mandible to the side.

Magnan trombone m., an involuntary forward and back m. of the tongue when it is drawn out of the mouth; may be seen in several basal ganglia disorders.

mandibular m., (1) m.'s of the lower jaw; **(2)** all changes in position of which the mandible is capable.

mass m., SYN mass *peristalsis*.

molecular m., SYN brownian m.

morphogenetic m., the streaming of cells in the early embryo to form tissues or organs.

muscular m., m. caused by the contraction of the myofibrils of the muscle cells.

neurobiotactic m., the streaming of nerve cells toward the area from which they receive the most stimuli.

non-rapid eye m. (NREM), slow oscillation of the eyes during sleep.

opening m., in dentistry, m. of the mandible executed during jaw separation.

paradoxical m. of eyelids, spontaneous, involuntary elevation or lowering of the eyelids, associated with m. of extraocular muscles or muscles of mastication (external pterygoids). SEE jaw winking.

paradoxical vocal cord m., adduction of the vocal cords on inspiration, resulting in stridor and airway obstruction.

passive m., (1) m. imparted to an organism or any of its parts by external agency. **(2)** in physical therapy, a m. that is effected entirely by the therapist without the assistance of the patient's muscles.

pendular m., a to-and-fro m. of the intestine, without any propelling or peristaltic action, whereby the contents are churned and thoroughly mixed with the intestinal ferments.

protoplasmic m., m. produced by the inherent power of contraction and relaxation of protoplasm; such m.'s are of three kinds: muscular, streaming, and ciliary.

rapid eye m.'s (REM), symmetrical quick scanning m.'s of the eyes occurring many times during sleep in clusters for 5 to 60 minutes; associated with dreaming.

reflex m., an involuntary m. resulting from a sensory stimulus.

resistive m., in physical therapy, a m. made by the patient against the efforts of the therapist, or one forced by the operator against the resistance of the patient.

saccadic m., (1) a quick rotation of the eyes from one fixation point to another as in reading; **(2)** the rapid correction m. of a jerky nystagmus, as in labyrinthine and optokinetic nystagmus.

streaming m., SYN ameboid m.

Swedish m.'s, a form of kinesitherapy in which certain systematized m.'s of the body and limbs are regulated by resistance made by an attendant. SYN Swedish gymnastics.

translatory m., the motion of the body at any instant when all points within the body are moving at the same velocity and in the same direction.

vermicular m., SYN peristalsis.

moxa (mok'să). A cone or cylinder of cotton wool or other combustible material, placed on the skin and ignited in order to produce counterirritation. SEE ALSO moxibustion. [Jap. *moe kusa,* burning herb]

mox·a·lac·tam (moks-a-lak'tam). A third-generation cephalosporin with a broad spectrum of antibacterial action; causes bleeding disorders, which limit its use.

mox·i·bus·tion (mok-sĭ-bŭs'chŭn). Burning of herbal agents, such as moxa, on the skin as a counterirritant in the treatment of disease; a component of traditional Chinese and Japanese medicine.

mox·i·sy·lyte (mok-sĭ'si-līt). Used as an α-adrenergic blocking agent for treatment of peripheral vascular disease. SYN thymoxamine.

MP Abbreviation for mentoposterior *position*.

m.p. 1. Abbreviation for melting *point*. **2.** Abbreviation for [L] *modo praescripto,* in the manner prescribed.

MPD Abbreviation for maximum permissible *dose*.

MPR Abbreviation for mannose-6-phosphate *receptors,* under *receptor.*

MPS Abbreviation for mononuclear phagocyte *system*.

MPTP Piperidine derivative which causes irreversible symptoms of parkinsonism in humans and monkeys. A by-product of illicitly manufactured meperidine that caused numerous cases of parkinsonism. Used as an experimental tool in research on parkinsonism.

MQ Former abbreviation for menaquinone; now MK.

MRA Abbreviation for MR *angiography*.

M.R.C.P. Abbreviation for Member of the Royal College of Physicians (of England).

M.R.C.P.(E) Abbreviation for Member of the Royal College of Physicians (Edinburgh).

M.R.C.P.(I) Abbreviation for Member of the Royal College of Physicians (Ireland).

M.R.C.S. Abbreviation for Member of the Royal College of Surgeons (England).

M.R.C.S.(E) Abbreviation for Member of the Royal College of Surgeons (Edinburgh).

M.R.C.S.(I) Abbreviation for Member of the Royal College of Surgeons (Ireland).

MRD, mrd Abbreviation for minimal reacting *dose*.

MRF Abbreviation for melanotropin-releasing *factor*.

MRH Abbreviation for melanotropin-releasing *hormone*.

MRI Abbreviation for magnetic resonance *imaging*.

mRNA Abbreviation for messenger RNA. See entries under ribonucleic acid.

MS Abbreviation for multiple *sclerosis; morphine* sulfate; mitral *stenosis*; and myasthenic *syndrome* (Lambert-Eaton syndrome).

ms Abbreviation for millisecond.

M.S.D. Abbreviation for Master of Science in Dentistry.

msec Abbreviation for millisecond.

MSG Abbreviation for monosodium glutamate.

MSH Abbreviation for melanocyte-stimulating *hormone*.

MTBE Abbreviation for methyl-*tert*-butyl ether.

MTF Abbreviation for modulation transfer *function*.

m.u. Abbreviation for mouse *unit*.

mu (mū). Twelfth letter of the Greek alphabet, μ.

mu·case (mū'kās). SYN mucinase.

Much, Hans C.R., German physician, 1880–1932. SEE M. *bacillus*.

Mucha, Victor, Austrian dermatologist, 1877–1919. SEE M.-Habermann *disease*.

muci-. Mucous, mucin. SEE ALSO muco-, myxo-. [L. *mucus*]

mu·ci·car·mine (mū-si-kar'mīn). A red stain containing aluminum chloride and carmine; used to detect epithelial mucins and mucin-secreting adenocarcinomas; also used to demonstrate the capsule of *Cryptococcus neoformans* and other fungi.

mu·cid (mū'sid). SYN muciparous.

mu·cif·er·ous (mū-sif'er-ŭs). SYN muciparous.

mu·ci·fi·ca·tion (mū'si-fi-kā'shŭn). A change produced in the vaginal mucosa of spayed experimental animals following stimulation with estrogen; characterized by the formation of tall columnar cells secreting mucus. [L. *mucus* + *facio,* to make]

mu·ci·form (mū'si-fōrm). Resembling mucus. SYN blennoid, mucoid (2).

mu·cig·e·nous (mū-sij'ĕ-nŭs). SYN muciparous.

mu·ci·he·ma·te·in (mū-si-hē'mă-tē-in). A violet-blue staining fluid containing aluminum chloride and hematein; used to detect connective tissue mucins.

mu·ci·lage (mū'si-lij). A pharmacopeial preparation consisting of a solution in water of the mucilaginous principles of vegetable substances; used as a soothing application to the mucous membranes and in the preparation of official and extemporaneous mixtures. [L. *mucilago*]

mu·ci·lag·i·nous (mū-sĭ-laj'i-nŭs). **1.** Resembling mucilage; i.e., adhesive, viscid, sticky. **2.** SYN muciparous.

mu·cin (mū'sin). A secretion containing carbohydrate-rich glycoproteins such as that from the goblet cells of the intestine, the submaxillary glands, and other mucous glandular cells; it is also present in the ground substance of connective tissue, especially mucous connective tissue, is soluble in alkaline water, and is precipitated by acetic acid; m.'s act as lubricants and protectants of the linings of body cavities.

gastric m., a white or yellowish powder which forms a viscous

mu

opalescent fluid with water, prepared from mucosa of hog's stomach by pepsin-hydrochloric acid digestion and precipitation of the supernatant fluid with 60% alcohol; used in peptic ulcer for its protective and lubricating action.

mu·cin·ase (mū′si-nās). A term specifically applied to hyaluronate lyase, hyaluronoglucosaminidase, and hyaluronoglucuronidase (hyaluronidases), but more loosely to any enzyme that hydrolyzes mucopolysaccharide substances (mucins). SYN mucase, mucopolysaccharidase.

mu·ci·ne·mia (mū-si-nē′mē-ă). The presence of mucin in the circulating blood. SYN myxemia. [mucin + G. *haima,* blood]

mu·cin·o·gen (mū′sin-ō-jen). A glycoprotein that forms mucin through the imbibition of water. [mucin + G. *-gen,* producing]

mu·ci·noid (mū′si-noyd). **1.** SYN mucoid (1). **2.** Resembling mucin.

mu·ci·no·lyt·ic (mū′si-nō-lit′ik). Capable of bringing about the hydrolysis of mucin, as by a mucinase.

mu·ci·no·sis (mū-si-nō′sis). A condition in which mucin is present in the skin in excessive amounts, or in abnormal distribution; classified as: **metabolic m.**, diffuse or pretibial myxedema, lichen myxedematosus, gargoylism; **secondary m.**, degeneration in tumors; **localized m.**, follicular, papular, plaquelike, focal, and myxoid or synovial cyst. [mucin + G. *-osis,* condition]

cutaneous focal m., flesh-colored papules of the skin, composed of homogenous mucinous material with scattered fibroblasts.

follicular m., a relatively uncommon benign eruption of discrete erythematous lesions progressing to alopecia on the face or scalp, usually in young people, in which there are cystic mucinous changes in the epithelium of hair follicles in the involved area; may also develop in mycosis fungoides.

oral focal m., an area of myxomatous connective tissue; the mucosal counterpart of cutaneous focal m.

papular m., SYN *lichen* myxedematosus.

reticular erythematous m. (REM), SYN REM *syndrome.*

mu·ci·nous (mū′si-nŭs). Relating to or containing mucin. SYN mucoid (3).

mu·ci·nu·ria (mū-si-nū′rē-ă). The presence of mucin in the urine. [mucin + G. *ouron,* urine]

mu·cip·a·rous (mū-sip′ă-rŭs). Producing or secreting mucus. SYN blennogenic, blennogenous, mucid, muciferous, mucigenous, mucilaginous (2). [mucin + L. *pario,* to bring forth, bear]

mu·ci·tis (mū-sī′tis). Inflammation of a mucous membrane.

Muckle, T.J., 20th century Canadian pediatrician. SEE M.-Wells *syndrome.*

muco-. Mucus, mucous (mucous membrane). SEE ALSO muci-, myxo-. [L. *mucus*]

mu·co·cele (mū′kō-sēl). **1.** SYN mucous *cyst.* **2.** A retention cyst of the salivary gland, lacrimal sac, paranasal sinuses, appendix, gallbladder, or other site. [muco- + G. *kēlē,* tumor, hernia]

mu·co·cil·i·ary (mū-kō-sil′ē-ă-rē). Related to the interaction of mucus and ciliated epithelium.

mu·coc·la·sis (mū-kok′lă-sis). Obsolete term for denudation of any mucous surface. [muco- + G. *klasis,* a breaking off]

mu·co·co·li·tis (mū′kō-kō-lī′tis). SYN mucous *colitis.*

mu·co·col·pos (mū-kō-kol′pos). Presence of mucus in the vagina. [muco- + G. *kolpos,* vagina]

mu·co·cu·ta·ne·ous (mū′kō-kū-tā′nē-ŭs). Relating to mucous membrane and skin; denoting the line of junction of the two at the nasal, oral, vaginal, and anal orifices. SYN cutaneomucosal.

mu·co·en·ter·i·tis (mū′kō-en-ter-ī′tis). **1.** Inflammation of the intestinal mucous membrane. **2.** SYN mucomembranous *enteritis.*

mu·co·ep·i·der·moid (mū′kō-ep-i-der′moyd). Denoting a mixture of mucus-secreting and epithelial cells, as in m. carcinoma.

mu·co·glob·u·lin (mū-kō-glob′ū-lin). A glycoprotein or mucoprotein in which the protein component is a globulin.

mu·coid (mū′koyd). **1.** General term for a mucin, mucoprotein, or glycoprotein. SYN mucinoid (1). **2.** SYN muciform. **3.** SYN mucinous. [mucus + G. *eidos,* appearance]

mu·co·lip·i·do·sis, pl. **mu·co·lip·i·do·ses** (mū′kō-lip-i-dō′sis, -sēz). Any of a group of lysosomal storage diseases in which

symptoms of visceral and mesenchymal mucopolysaccharide, glycoprotein, oligosaccharide, or glycolipid storage are present; clinically, they bear a superficial resemblance to the mucopolysaccharidoses; autosomal recessive inheritance. [muco- + lipid + *-osis,* condition]

m. I [MIM*256550], m. somewhat like a mild form of Hurler *syndrome* with coarse facial features, macular cherry red spots, myoclonus epilepsy, mild dysostosis multiplex, and moderate mental retardation due to neuraminidase deficiency; autosomal recessive inheritance caused by mutation in the neuraminidase gene (NEU) on 6p. SYN lipomucopolysaccharidosis.

m. II [MIM*252500], a metabolic disorder with onset in early childhood characterized by clinical and radiographic findings similar to those in Hurler *syndrome* including gum hypertrophy, thoracic dysplasia, congenital hip dislocation, and mental retardation; vacuolated lymphocytes and unusual inclusion bodies in cultured fibroblasts (I-cells) are found; lysosomal enzymes are increased in serum, spinal fluid, and urine; urinary mucopolysaccharides are normal; associated with a deficiency of *N*-acetylglucosaminyl-1-phosphotransferase; autosomal recessive inheritance. SYN I-cell disease, inclusion cell disease.

m. III [MIM*252600], m. with mild Hurlerlike symptoms, restricted joint mobility, short stature, mild mental retardation, and dysplastic skeletal changes, especially of the hip; aortic and mitral valve disease are often present; associated with a deficiency of *N*-acetyl-α-glucosaminidase or other enzyme deficiencies such as lysosomal enzyme *N*-acetylglucosaminyl-1-phosphotransferase in mutant fibroblasts lacks the ability to recognize lysosomal enzymes and specific substrates for phosphorylation; autosomal recessive inheritance. SYN pseudo-Hurler polydystrophy, pseudopolydystrophy.

m. IV [MIM*252650], psychomotor retardation with cloudy corneas and retinal degeneration, with inclusion cells in cultured fibroblasts; the pathogenesis is uncertain; autosomal recessive inheritance.

mu·col·y·sis (mū-kol′i-sis). The solution, digestion, or liquefaction of mucus. [muco- + G. *lysis,* dissolution]

mu·co·lyt·ic (mū-kō-lit′ik). Capable of dissolving, digesting, or liquefying mucus.

mu·co·mem·bra·nous (mū′kō-mem′bră-nŭs). Relating to a mucous membrane.

mu·co·pep·tide (mū-kō-pep′tīd). **1.** A peptide found in combination with polysaccharides containing muramic or sialic acids. **2.** SYN peptidoglycan.

m. glycohydrolase, SYN lysozyme.

mu·co·per·i·os·te·al (mū′kō-per-ē-os′tē-ăl). Relating to mucoperiosteum.

mu·co·per·i·os·te·um (mū′kō-per-ē-os′tē-ŭm). Mucous membrane and periosteum so intimately united as to form practically a single membrane, as that covering the hard palate.

mu·co·pol·y·sac·cha·ri·dase (mū′kō-pol-ē-sak′ă-ri-dās). SYN mucinase, β-*d*-glucuronidase *deficiency.*

mu·co·pol·y·sac·cha·ride (mū′kō-pol-ē-sak′ă-rīd). General term for a protein-polysaccharide complex obtained from proteoglycans and containing as much as 95% polysaccharide; m.'s include the blood group substances. A more modern term is glycosaminoglycan, as all of the known six classes contain major amounts of D-glucosamine and D-galactosamine.

mu·co·pol·y·sac·cha·ri·do·sis, pl. **mu·co·pol·y·sac·cha·ri·do·ses** (mū′kō-pol-ē-sak′ă-ri-dō′sis, -sēz). Any of a group of lysosomal storage diseases that have in common a disorder in metabolism of mucopolysaccharides, as evidenced by excretion of various mucopolysaccharides in urine and infiltration of these substances into connective tissue, with resulting various defects of bone, cartilage, connective tissue, and other organs.

type IH m., SYN Hurler *syndrome.*

type I H/S m., SYN Hurler-Scheie *syndrome.*

type II m., SYN Hunter *syndrome.*

type III m., SYN Sanfilippo *syndrome.*

type IS m., SYN Scheie *syndrome.*

type IVA, B m., SYN Morquio *syndrome.*

type V m., former designation for Scheie *syndrome.*

type VI m., SYN Maroteaux-Lamy *syndrome.*

type VII m., (1) SYN Sly *syndrome*; (2) SYN Di Ferrante *syndrome.*

mu·co·poi·y·sac·cha·ri·du·ria (mū′kō-pol-ē-sak′ă-ri-doo′rē-ă). The excretion of mucopolysaccharides in the urine.

mu·co·pro·tein (mū-kō-prō′tēn). General term for a protein-polysaccharide complex, usually implying that the protein component is the major part of the complex, in contradistinction to mucopolysaccharide; m.'s include the α₁- and α₂-globulins of serum (and others). Sometimes called glycoproteins, although this term usually refers to those m.'s containing less than 4% carbohydrate.

Tamm-Horsfall m., the matrix of urinary casts derived from the secretion of renal tubular cells.

mu·co·pu·ru·lent (mū-kō-poo′roo-lent). Pertaining to an exudate that is chiefly purulent (pus), but containing relatively conspicuous proportions of mucous material. SYN puromucous.

mu·co·pus (mū′kō-pŭs). A mucopurulent discharge; a mixture of mucous material and pus. SYN mycopus.

Mu·cor (mū′kōr). A genus of fungi (class Zygomycetes, family Mucoraceae), most species of which are saprobic; several are pathogenic and may cause zygomycosis in humans.

Mu·co·ra·ce·ae (mū′kōr-a′sē-ē). A family of fungi (class Zygomycetes) comprising terrestrial, aquatic, and sometimes parasitic organisms; includes the genera *Mucor*, *Absidia*, *Rhizopus*, *Rhizomucor*, *Apophysomyces*, and *Mortierella*. Although the various species of the genera are ordinarily saprobic, free-living forms, some of them cause mucormycosis in humans. [L. *mucor*, mold]

Mucorales (moo-kor-al′ez). An order of the fungal class Zygomycetes that contains all the species causing mucormycosis in humans. The genera include *Cunninghamella*, *Rhizopus*, *Absidia*, *Rhlizomucor*, *Mucor*, *Apophysomyces*, *Saksenaea*, *Syncepthalastrum*, and *Cokeromyces*. *Mortierella* species are included but are of doubtful pathogenicity for humans.

mu·cor·my·co·sis (mū′kōr-mī-kō′sis). Infection with fungi of the order Mucorales; to be distinguished from zygomycosis, a broader term that includes infections caused by fungi of the order Entomophthorales.

mu·co·sa (mū-kō′să) [TA]. A mucous tissue lining various tubular structures, consisting of epithelium, lamina, propria, and, in the digestive tract, a layer of smooth muscle (muscularis mucosae). SYN tunica mucosa [TA], mucous membranes✶, membrana mucosa, mucosal tunics, mucous tunics. [L. fem. of *mucosus*, mucous]

alveolar m., the mucous membrane apical to the attached gingiva.

m. of bronchi [TA], the inner coat of a bronchus. SYN tunica mucosa bronchi [TA], mucous membrane of bronchus✶, bronchial m.

bronchial m., SYN m. of bronchi.

m. of colon, the lining coat of the colon. SYN tunica mucosa coli.

m. of ductus deferens [TA], the inner layer of the ductus deferens. SYN tunica mucosa ductus deferentis [TA], mucous membrane of ductus deferens✶.

esophageal m., SYN m. of esophagus.

m. of esophagus [TA], the inner coat of the esophagus. SYN tunica mucosa esophagi [TA], mucous membrane of esophagus✶, esophageal m.

m. of female urethra [TA], the inner mucosal layer of the female urethra. SYN tunica mucosa urethrae femininae [TA], mucous membrane of female urethra✶.

m. of gallbladder [TA], the inner coat of the gallbladder. SYN tunica mucosa vesicae biliaris [TA], mucous membrane of gallbladder✶, tunica mucosa vesicae felleae✶.

gastric m., SYN m. of stomach.

gingival m., that portion of the oral mucous membrane that covers and is attached to the necks of the teeth and the alveolar process of the jaws; it is demarcated from lining m. on the facial aspect by a clearly defined line which marks the mucogingival junction, and, in contrast to the lining m., is keratinized and

lighter in color; on the palatal surface, the gingiva blends imperceptibly with the palatal m.

m. of large intestine [TA], the mucosal lining (epithelium, lamina propria, and muscularis mucosae) of the wall of all the parts of the large intestine (cecum, colon, rectum, and anal canal) collectively. SYN tunica mucosa intestini crassi [TA], mucous membrane of large intestine✶.

laryngeal m., SYN m. of larynx.

m. of larynx [TA], the mucous coat of the larynx. SYN tunica mucosa laryngis [TA], mucous membrane of larynx✶, laryngeal m.

lingual m., SYN m. of tongue.

m. of male urethra [TA], innermost layer of urethra including an epithelium typical of the urinary tract (a transitional epithelium or urothelium) proximal to the openings of the ejaculatory ducts and typical of the genital tract (a stratified columnar epithelium) distally that continues through the intermediate and most of the spongy urethra, changing again to a stratified squamous epithelium in the region of the navicular fossa; many recesses occur in the mucosa of the spongy portion that continue into tubular, branching mucous glands. SYN tunica urethrae masculinae [TA], mucous membrane of male urethra.

m. of mouth [TA], the mucous membrane of the oral cavity, including the gingiva. SYN oral m. [TA], tunica mucosa oris [TA].

nasal m., SYN m. of nose.

m. of nose [TA], the lining of the nasal cavity, it is continuous with the skin in the vestibule of the nose and with the mucosa of the nasopharynx, the paranasal sinuses, and the nasolacrimal duct and contains goblet cells; it is subdivided into the olfactory region and respiratory region. SYN tunica mucosa nasi [TA], mucous membrane of nose✶, membrana pituitosa, nasal m., pituitary membrane, schneiderian membrane.

olfactory m., SYN olfactory *region* of mucosa of nose.

oral m. [TA], SYN m. of mouth.

pharyngeal m., SYN m. of pharynx.

m. of pharyngotympanic (auditory) tube [TA], the lining coat of the auditory tube. SYN tunica mucosa tubae auditivae [TA], mucous membrane of pharyngotympanic auditory tube✶, tunica mucosa tubae auditoriae.

m. of pharynx [TA], the mucous coat of the pharynx. SYN tunica mucosa pharyngis [TA], mucous membrane of pharynx, pharyngeal m.

m. of renal pelvis [TA], innermost of three layers of the wall of the renal pelvis, identical in structure to that of the ureter, that is, consisting of a transitional epithelium (urothelium) and an underlying lamina propria. SYN tunica mucosa pelvis renalis [TA].

respiratory m., pseudostratified ciliated columnar epithelium with goblet cells and a lamina propria containing, in addition to connective tissue, numerous seromucous glands and in some regions many thin-walled veins that line the airways; it includes the respiratory region of the nasal mucosa [TA] (pars respiratoria tunicae mucosae nasi [TA]), m. of the trachea [TA] (tunica mucosa tracheae [TA]), and m. of bronchi [TA] (tunica mucosa bronchi [TA]). SEE respiratory *region* of mucosa of nasal cavity.

m. of seminal gland [TA], the mucous membrane lining the seminal gland (vesicle). SYN tunica mucosa vesiculae seminalis✶, m. of seminal vesicle.

m. of seminal vesicle, SYN m. of seminal gland.

m. of small intestine [TA], the mucous coat of the small intestine. SYN tunica mucosa intestini tenuis [TA], mucous membrane of small intestine✶.

m. of stomach [TA], the mucous layer of the stomach. SYN tunica mucosa gastrica [TA], mucous membrane of stomach✶, gastric m.

m. of tongue [TA], the mucosa forming the surface of the tongue; that of the dorsum of the tongue appears velvety due to the presence of vast numbers of papillae; that of the inferior surface is smooth and thinner. SYN tunica mucosa linguae [TA], mucous membrane of tongue✶, lingual m.

m. of trachea [TA], the inner mucous layer of the trachea. SYN tunica mucosa tracheae [TA], mucous membrane of trachea✶, tracheal m.

mu

tracheal m., SYN m. of trachea.

m. of tympanic cavity [TA], the mucosal lining of the tympanic cavity and the structures in it. SYN tunica mucosa cavitatis tympani [TA], mucous membrane of tympanic cavity✳.

m. of ureter [TA], the inner mucosal layer of the ureter. SYN tunica mucosa ureteris [TA], mucous membrane of ureter✳.

m. of urethra [TA], SEE m. of female urethra, m. of male urethra.

m. of (urinary) bladder [TA], the inner coat of the urinary bladder. SYN tunica mucosa vesicae urinariae [TA], mucous membrane of urinary bladder✳.

m. of uterine tube [TA], the inner mucosal layer of the uterine tube. SYN tunica mucosa tubae uterinae [TA], mucous membrane of uterine tube✳.

m. of vagina [TA], the mucosal layer of the vagina. SYN tunica mucosa vaginae [TA], mucous membrane of vagina✳, vaginal m.

vaginal m., SYN m. of vagina.

mu·co·sal (mū-kō'săl). Relating to the mucosa or mucous membrane.

mu·co·san·guin·e·ous, mu·co·san·guin·o·lent (mū'kō-sang-gwin'ē-ŭs, -ŏ-lent). Pertaining to an exudate or other fluid material that has a relatively high content of blood and mucus. [muco- + L. *sanguis,* blood]

mu·co·sec·to·my (mū-kō-sek'tō-me). Excision of the mucosa, usually of the rectum prior to ileoanal anastomosis. [mucosa + G. *ektomē,* excision]

mu·co·se·rous (mū-kō-sē'rŭs). Pertaining to an exudate or secretion that consists of both mucus and serum or a watery component.

mu·co·stat·ic (mū-kō-stat'ik). **1.** Denoting the normal relaxed condition of mucosal tissues covering the jaws. **2.** Arresting the secretion of mucus. [muco- + G. *stasis,* a standing]

mu·cous (mū'kŭs). Relating to mucus or a m. membrane. [L. *mucosus,* mucous, fr. *mucus*]

mu·co·vis·ci·do·sis (mū'kō-vis-i-dō'sis). SYN cystic *fibrosis.* [myco- + G. *toxikon,* poison, + -osis, condition]

mu·cro, pl. **mu·cron·es** (mū'krō, mū-krō'nēz). A term applied to the pointed extremity of a structure. [L. point, sword]

m. cor'dis, obsolete term for *apex* of heart.

m. ster'ni, SYN xiphoid *process.*

mu·cron (mū'kron). Attachment organelle of aseptate gregarines, similar to an epimerite; the latter is set off from the rest of the gregarine body by a septum.

mu·cro·nate (mū'krō-nāt). SYN xiphoid. [L. *mucronatus,* pointed]

mu·cus (mū'kŭs). The clear viscid secretion of the mucous membranes, consisting of mucin, epithelial cells, leukocytes, and various inorganic salts dissolved in water. [L.]

glairy m., SYN pituita.

Muehrcke, Robert C., 20th century U.S. nephrologist. SEE Muehrcke *bands,* under *band;* M. *lines,* under *line;* Muehrcke *sign.*

Mueller. U.S. manufacturer of surgical instruments. SEE Mueller electronic *tonometer.*

Muel·le·ri·us cap·il·la·ris (mū-ler'ē-ŭs kap-il-lā'ris). One of the most common species of hair lungworms (subfamily Protostrongylinae) of sheep, goats, and deer. It is smaller than *Dictyocaulus,* inhabits the smaller bronchi and lung parenchyma, and is relatively nonpathogenic to its host.

MUGA Acronym for multiple-gated acquisition *scan.*

Muir, Edward G., British surgeon, 1906–1973. SEE M.-Torre *syndrome.*

Mules, Philip H., English ophthalmologist, 1843–1905. SEE M. *operation.*

mu·li·e·bria (moo'lē-ē'brē-ă). The female genital organs. [L. neut pl. of *muliebris,* relating to *mulier,* a woman]

Müller, Friedrich von, German physician, 1858–1941. SEE M. *sign.*

Müller, Heinrich, German anatomist, 1820–1864. SEE M. radial *cells,* under *cell, fibers,* under *fiber, muscle, trigone.*

Müller, Hermann F., German histologist, 1866–1898. SEE formol-M. *fixative;* M. *fixative.*

Müller, Johannes P., German anatomist, physiologist, and pathologist, 1801–1858. SEE M. *capsule, duct, law, maneuver, tubercle;* müllerian *agenesis.*

Müller, Leopold, Czechoslovakian ophthalmologist, 1862–1936.

Müller, Peter, German obstetrician, 1836–1922. SEE Hillis-M. *maneuver.*

Müller, Walther, 20th century German physicist. SEE Geiger-M. *counter, tube.*

mül·le·ri·an (mū-ler'ē-an). Attributed to or described by Johannes Müller.

mul·ling (mŭl'ing). In dentistry, the final step of mixing dental amalgam, when the triturated mass is kneaded to complete the amalgamation.

mult·ang·u·lar (mŭl-tang'gū-lăr). Having many angles.

multi-. Many. SEE ALSO pluri-. Cf. poly-. [L. *multus,* much]

mul·ti·ar·tic·u·lar (mŭl'tē-ar-tik'ū-lăr). Relating to or involving many joints. SYN polyarthric, polyarticular. [multi- + L. *articulus,* joint]

mul·ti·bac·il·lary (mŭl-tē-bas'i-lār-ē). Made up of, or denoting the presence of, many bacilli.

mul·ti·cap·su·lar (mŭl-tē-kap'soo-lăr). Having numerous capsules.

mul·ti·cel·lu·lar (mŭl-tē-sel'ū-lăr). Composed of many cells.

Mul·ti·ceps (mŭl'ti-seps). A genus of taeniid tapeworms in which the larval forms in herbivores occur in the form of a coenurus (multiple scoleces invaginated within a single cyst). [multi- + L. *caput,* head]

M. mul'ticeps, a species the mature form of which occurs in the intestines of dogs; the coenurus develops in the brains of herbivorous animals, especially sheep; the cyst is often called *Coenurus cerebralis.*

M. seria'lis, a species the mature form of which is found in the intestine of dogs; the coenurus is found in the subcutaneous tissues of rabbits.

mul·ti·col·lin·e·ar·i·ty (mŭl'tē-kol'in-ē-ar'i-tē). In multiple regression analysis, a situation in which at least some independent variables in a set are highly correlated with each other. [multi- + L. *col-lineo,* to line up together]

mul·ti·CSF Abbreviation for multicolony-stimulating *factor.*

mul·ti·cus·pid (mŭl-tē-kŭs'pid). SYN multicuspidate (2).

mul·ti·cus·pi·date (mŭl-tē-kŭs'pi-dāt). **1.** Having more than two cusps. **2.** A molar tooth with three or more cusps or projections on the crown. SYN multicuspid.

mul·ti·en·zyme (mŭl'tī-en'zīm, mŭl'tē-). Referring to several enzymes; e.g., multienzyme complex.

mul·ti·fe·ta·tion (mŭl-tē-fe-tā'shŭn). SYN superfetation.

mul·ti·fid (mŭl'tē-fid). Divided into many clefts or segments. SYN multifidus (1). [L. *multifidus,* fr. *multus,* much, + *findo,* to cleave]

mul·tif·i·dus (mŭl-tif'i-dŭs). **1.** SYN multifid. **2.** SEE multifidus (*muscle*). [L.]

mul·ti·fo·cal (mŭl-tē-fō'kăl). Relating to or arising from many foci.

mul·ti·form (mŭl'ti-fōrm). SYN polymorphic.

mul·ti·glan·du·lar (mŭl-tē-glan'dū-lăr). SYN pluriglandular.

mul·ti·grav·i·da (mŭl-tē-grav'i-dă). A pregnant woman who has been pregnant one or more times previously. [multi- + L. *gravida,* pregnant]

mul·ti·in·fec·tion (mŭl'tē-in-fek'shŭn). Mixed infection with two or more varieties of microorganisms developing simultaneously.

mul·ti·lo·bar, mul·ti·lo·bate, mul·ti·lobed (mŭl-tē-lō'bar, -lō'bāt, -lōbd'). Having several lobes.

mul·ti·lob·u·lar (mŭl-tē-lob'ū-lăr). Having many lobules.

mul·ti·lo·cal (mŭl-tē-lō'kăl). Denoting traits with an etiology comprising effects of multiple genetic loci operating together and simultaneously. Cf. galtonian.

mul·ti·loc·u·lar (mŭl-tē-lok'ū-lăr). Many-celled; having many compartments or loculi. SYN plurilocular.

mul·ti·mam·mae (mŭl-tē-mam′ē). SYN polymastia. [multi- + L. *mamma,* breast]

mul·ti·no·dal (mŭl-tē-nō′dăl). Having many nodes.

mul·ti·nod·u·lar, mul·ti·nod·u·late (mŭl-tē-nod′ū-lăr, -ū-lāt). Having many nodules.

mul·ti·nu·cle·ar, mul·ti·nu·cle·ate (mŭl-tē-noo′klē-ăr, -āt). Having two or more nuclei. SYN plurinuclear, polynuclear, polynucleate.

mul·ti·nu·cle·o·sis (mool′tē-nook-lē-ō′sis). SYN polynucleosis.

mul·tip·a·ra (mŭl-tip′ă-ră). A woman who has given birth at least two times to an infant, liveborn or not, weighing 500 g or more, or having an estimated length of gestation of at least 20 weeks. [multi- + L. *pario,* to bring forth, to bear]
grand m., a m. who has given birth five or more times.

mul·ti·par·i·ty (mŭl-tē-păr′i-tē). Condition of being a multipara.

mul·tip·a·rous (mŭl-tip′ă-rŭs). Relating to a multipara.

mul·ti·par·tial (mŭl′tē-par′shăl). Polyvalent, with respect to an antiserum.

mul·ti·ple (mŭl′ti-pl). Manifold; repeated several times; occurring in several parts at the same time, as m. arthritis, m. neuritis. [L. *multiplex,* fr. *multus,* many, + *plico,* pp. *-atus,* to fold]

mul·ti·po·lar (mŭl-tē-pō′lăr). Having more than two poles; denoting a nerve cell in which the branches project from several points.

mul·ti·root·ed (mŭl-tē-root′ed). Having more than two roots.

mul·ti·ro·ta·tion (mŭl′tē-rō-tā′shŭn). SYN mutarotation.

mul·ti·sub·strate (mŭl-tī-sub′stāt, mŭl-tē′-). Referring to an enzyme, receptor, or acceptor protein, which requires two or more substrates.

mul·ti·sy·nap·tic (mŭl′tē-si-nap′tik). SYN polysynaptic.

mul·ti·va·lence, mul·ti·va·len·cy (mŭl-tē-vā′lens, -vā′len-sē). The state of being multivalent.

mul·ti·va·lent (mŭl-tē-vā′lent). **1.** In chemistry, having a combining power (valence) of more than one hydrogen atom. **2.** Efficacious in more than one direction. **3.** An antiserum specific for more than one antigen or organism. **4.** Antigen or antibody with a combining power greater than two. SYN polyvalent (1).

mum·mi·fi·ca·tion (mŭm′i-fi-kā′shŭn). **1.** SYN dry *gangrene.* **2.** Shrivelling of a dead, retained fetus. **3.** In dentistry, treatment of inflamed dental pulp with fixative drugs (usually formaldehyde derivatives) in order to retain teeth so treated for relatively short periods; generally acceptable only for primary (deciduous) teeth. [mummy + L. *facio,* to make]

mumps (mŭmps). An acute infectious and contagious disease caused by a mumps virus of the genus Rubulavirus and characterized by fever, inflammation and swelling of the parotid gland, sometimes of other salivary glands, and occasionally by inflammation of the testis, ovary, pancreas, or meninges. SYN epidemic parotiditis. [dialectic Eng. *mump,* a lump or bump]
metastatic m., m. complicated by involvement of organs other than parotid glands, such as the testis, breast, or pancreas.

mumpvirus. SYN Rubulavirus.

Münchhausen, Baron Karl F.H. von, German nobleman, soldier, and raconteur, 1720–1797. SEE Munchausen *syndrome;* Munchausen *syndrome* by proxy.

Munro, William J., Australian dermatologist, 1863–1908. SEE M. *abscess, microabscess.*

Munro, John C., U.S. surgeon, 1858–1910. SEE M. *point.*

Munsell, Albert H., U.S. artist, 1858–1918. SEE Farnsworth-M. color *test.*

Munsell, Hazel E., U.S. chemist, *1891. SEE Sherman-M. *unit.*

Munson, Edward Sterling, U.S. ophthalmologist, *1933. SEE Munson *sign.*

Münzer, Egmont, Austrian physician, 1865–1924. SEE *tract* of M. and Wiener.

Mur Abbreviation for muramic acid.

mu·ral (mū′răl). Relating to the wall of any cavity. [L. *muralis;* fr. *murus,* wall]

mu·ram·ic ac·id (Mur) (mū-ram′ik). 2-Amino-3-*O*-(1-carboxy-

ethyl)-2-deoxy-D-glucose; D-glucosamine and lactate in ether linkage between the 3 and 2 positions, respectively; a constituent of the mureins in bacterial cell walls.

mu·ram·i·dase (mū-ram′i-dās). SYN lysozyme.

mu·reins (mūr′ēnz). Peptidoglycans composing the sacculus or cell casing of bacteria, consisting of linear polysaccharides of alternating *N*-acetyl-D-glucosamine and *N*-acetylmuramic acid units, to the lactate side chains of which are linked oligopeptides; independent chains are cross-linked in three dimensions via the peptides or the 6-OH groups (the latter may be linked via phosphate to a teichoic acid). [L. *murus,* wall]

Muret, Paul-Louis, French physician, *1878. SEE Quénu-M. *sign.*

mu·rex·ide (mū-rek′sīd, -sid). The ammonium salt of purpuric acid, formerly used as a dye but superseded by the aniline colors.

mu·ri·ate (mū′rē-āt). Former term for chloride. [L. *muria,* brine]

mu·ri·at·ic (mū-rē-at′ik). Relating to brine. [L. *muriaticus,* pickled in brine, fr. *muria,* brine]

mu·ri·at·ic ac·id. SYN hydrochloric acid.

Mu·ri·dae (mū′ri-dē). The largest family of Rodentia and of mammals, embracing the Old World mice and rats. [L. *mus* (*mur-*), a mouse]

mu·ri·form (mūr′i-fōrm). Multicellular with cross and longitudinal septa; denoting an aggregation of cells fitting together like stones in a stone wall. [L. *murus,* wall, + -form]

mu·rine (mū′rīn, -rin, -rēn). Relating to animals of the family Muridae. [L. *murinus,* relating to mice, fr. *mus* (*mur-*), a mouse]

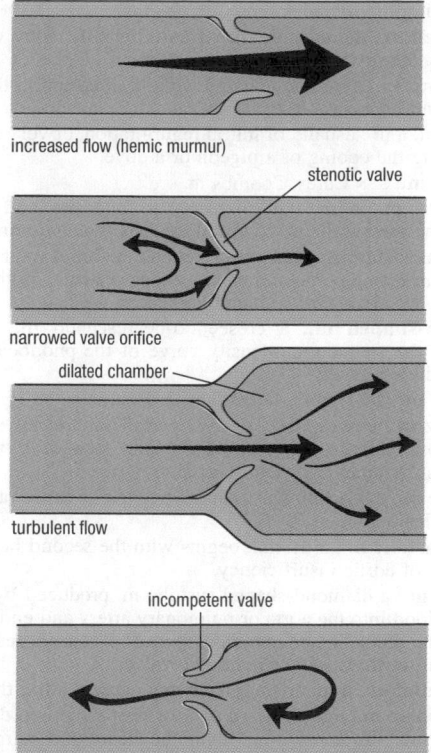

increased flow (hemic murmur)

stenotic valve

narrowed valve orifice

dilated chamber

turbulent flow

incompetent valve

backward flow (regurgitation)

origin of cardiac murmurs

mur·mur (mer′mer). **1.** A soft sound, like that made by a somewhat forcible expiration with the mouth open, heard on auscultation of the heart, lungs, or blood vessels. SYN susurrus. **2.** An other-than-soft sound, which may be loud, harsh, frictional, etc.; e.g., organic cardiac m.'s may be soft or loud and harsh; pericardial m.'s usually are frictional and are more properly described as "rubs" rather than m.'s. [L.]

accidental m., an evanescent cardiac m. not due to valvular lesion.

anemic m., a nonvalvular m. heard on auscultation of the heart and large blood vessels in cases of profound anemia associated mainly with turbulent blood flow due to decreased blood viscosity.

aneurysmal m., a systolic or systolic-diastolic m. heard over some cardiac aneurysms.

aortic m., a m. produced at the aortic orifice, either obstructive or regurgitant.

arterial m., a m. heard on auscultating an artery.

atriosystolic m., SYN presystolic m.

Austin Flint m., SYN Austin Flint *phenomenon*, Flint m.

bellows m., a blowing m.

brain m., sounds produced by intracranial aneurysms or arterial venous aneurysms in congenital dysplastic angiomatosis.

Cabot-Locke m., an early diastolic m., like that of aortic insufficiency, heard best at the left lower sternal border in severe anemia.

cardiac m., a m. produced within the heart, at one of its valvular orifices or across ventricular septal defects.

cardiopulmonary m., an innocent extracardiac m., synchronous with the heart's beat but disappearing when the breath is held, believed due to movement of air in a segment of lung compressed by the contracting heart. SYN cardiorespiratory m.

cardiorespiratory m., SYN cardiopulmonary m.

Carey Coombs m., a blubbering apical middiastolic m. occurring in the acute stage of rheumatic mitral valvulitis and disappearing as the valvulitis subsides. SYN Coombs m.

Cole-Cecil m., the diastolic m. of aortic insufficiency when well or predominantly heard in the left axilla.

continuous m., a m. that is heard without interruption throughout systole and into diastole.

cooing m., a m., usually of mitral regurgitation, of very high pitch resembling the cooing of a pigeon or a dove.

Coombs m., SYN Carey Coombs m.

crescendo m., a m. that increases in intensity and suddenly ceases; the presystolic m. of mitral stenosis is a common example.

Cruveilhier-Baumgarten m., a venous m. heard over collateral veins, connecting portal and caval venous systems, on the abdominal wall. SEE ALSO Cruveilhier-Baumgarten *sign*.

diamond-shaped m., a crescendo-decrescendo m., from the shape of the frequency intensity curve of the phonocardiogram, often audible as such.

diastolic m. (DM), a m. heard during diastole.

Duroziez m., a two-phase m. over peripheral arteries, especially the femoral artery, due to rapid ebb and flow of blood during aortic insufficiency. SYN Duroziez sign.

dynamic m., a heart m. due to anemia or to any cause other than a valvular lesion.

early diastolic m., a m. that begins with the second heart sound, as the m. of aortic insufficiency.

ejection m., a diamond-shaped systolic m. produced by the ejection of blood into the aorta or pulmonary artery and ending by the time of the second heart sound component produced, respectively, by closing of the aortic or pulmonic valve.

endocardial m., a m. arising, from any cause, within the heart.

extracardiac m., a bruit heard over or near the precordium originating from structures other than the heart; the term includes pericardial friction rubs and cardiopulmonary m.'s.

Flint m., a diastolic m., similar to that of mitral stenosis, heard best at the cardiac apex in some cases of free aortic insufficiency; it is thought to be caused by the turbulent regurgitating stream from the aorta mixing into the stream simultaneously entering from the left atrium through the mitral valve, causing posterior movement of the anterior leaflet of the mitral valve with transient acceleration of blood flow through the mitral valve. SYN Austin Flint m.

Fräntzel m., m. of mitral stenosis when louder at its beginning and end than in its midportion.

friction m., SYN friction *sound*.

functional m., a cardiac m. not associated with a significant heart lesion. SYN innocent m., inorganic m.

Gibson m., the typical continuous "machinerylike" m. of patent ductus arteriosus.

Graham Steell m., an early diastolic m. of pulmonic insufficiency secondary to pulmonary hypertension, as in mitral stenosis and various congenital defects associated with pulmonary hypertension. SYN Steell m.

Hamman m., a crunching precordial sound synchronous with the heart beat; heard in mediastinal emphysema; also known as Hamman crunch.

hemic m., a cardiac or vascular m. heard in anemic persons who have no valvular lesion, probably due to the increased blood velocity and turbulence that characterizes anemia.

Hodgkin-Key m., a musical diastolic m. associated with retroversion of an aortic cusp; often very loud.

holosystolic m., SYN pansystolic m.

hourglass m., one in which there are two areas of maximum loudness decreasing to a point midway between the two.

innocent m., SYN functional m.

inorganic m., SYN functional m.

late apical systolic m., a m. previously considered benign, or even extracardiac, with a possible relationship to pericardial disease; it often represents mitral insufficiency, often localized and of moderate severity but with propensity for developing bacterial endocarditis, and is frequently associated with systolic click and mitral prolapse (Barlow syndrome; a balloon or billowing mitral valve leaflet) often producing a click, murmur, or both, as it prolapses during systole into the left atrium.

late diastolic m., SYN presystolic m.

machinery m., the long "continuous" rumbling m. of patent ductus arteriosus.

middiastolic m., a m. beginning after the A-V valves have opened in diastole, i.e., an appreciable time after the second heart sound, as the m. of mitral stenosis.

mill wheel m., churning cardiac m. produced by air embolism to the heart; also heard in pneumohydropericardium. SYN water wheel m.

mitral m., a m. produced at the mitral valve, either obstructive or regurgitant.

musical m., a cardiac or vascular m. having a high-pitched musical character.

nun's m., SYN venous *hum*.

obstructive m., a m. caused by narrowing of one of the valvular orifices.

organic m., a m. caused by an organic lesion.

pansystolic m., a m. occupying the entire systolic interval, from first to second heart sounds. SYN holosystolic m.

pericardial m., a friction sound, synchronous with the heart movements, heard in certain cases of pericarditis.

pleuropericardial m., a pleural friction sound over the pericardial region, synchronous with the heart's action, and simulating a pericardial m. (rub).

presystolic m., a m. heard at the end of ventricular diastole (during atrial systole if in sinus rhythm), usually due to obstruction at one of the atrioventricular orifices. SYN atriosystolic m., late diastolic m.

pulmonary m., pulmonic m., a m. produced at the pulmonary orifice of the heart, either obstructive or regurgitant.

regurgitant m., a m. due to leakage or backward flow at one of the valvular orifices of the heart.

respiratory m., SYN vesicular *respiration*.

Roger m., a loud pansystolic m. maximal at the left sternal border, caused by a small ventricular septal defect. SYN bruit de Roger, Roger bruit.

sea gull m., a m. imitating the cooing sound of a seagull nearly always due to aortic stenosis or mitral regurgitation.

seesaw m., SYN to-and-fro m.

Steell m., SYN Graham Steell m.

stenosal m., an arterial m. due to narrowing of the vessel from pressure or organic change.

Still m., an innocent musical m. resembling the noise produced by a twanging string; almost exclusively in young children, of uncertain origin and ultimately disappearing.

systolic m., a m. heard during ventricular systole.

to-and-fro m., m. heard in both systole and diastole of the heart, as in aortic stenosis and insufficiency. SYN seesaw m.

tricuspid m., a m. produced at the tricuspid orifice, either obstructive or regurgitant.

vascular m., a m. originating in a blood vessel.

venous m., a m. heard over a vein.

vesicular m., SYN vesicular *respiration.*

water wheel m., SYN mill wheel m.

mu·ro·mo·nab-CD3 (mū-rō-mō′nab). A murine monoclonal antibody to the T3 (CD3) antigen of human T lymphocytes, used as an immunosuppressant in the treatment of acute allograft rejection following renal transplantation.

Murphy, John B., U.S. surgeon, 1857–1916. SEE M. *drip, button, percussion.*

Mus (mŭs). A genus of the family Muridae that includes about 16 species of mice; domesticated strains are numerous and genetically well defined, the most popular being the albino and piebald strains. [L. *mus* (*mur*-), a mouse]

Mus·ca (mŭs′kă). A genus of flies (family Muscidae, order Diptera) that includes the common housefly, *M. domestica,* a species universally associated with humans, particularly under unsanitary conditions; it breeds in filth and organic waste, and is involved in the mechanical transfer of numerous pathogens. [L. fly]

mus·cae vol·i·tan·tes (mŭs′sē, mŭs′kē vol-i-tan′tēs). Floaters; appearance of moving spots before the eyes, arising from remnants of the embryologic hyaloid vascular system in the vitreous humor. [L. pl. of *musca,* fly; pres. ppl. of *volito,* to fly to and fro]

mus·ca·rine (mŭs′kă-rēn, -rin). A toxin with neurologic effects, first isolated from *Amanita muscaria* (fly agaric) and also present in some species of *Hebeloma* and *Inocybe.* The quaternary trimethylammonium salt of 2-methyl-3-hydroxy-5-(aminomethyl)-tetrahydrofuran, it is a cholinergic substance whose pharmacologic effects resemble those of acetylcholine and postganglionic parasympathetic stimulation (cardiac inhibition, vasodilation, salivation, lacrimation, bronchoconstriction, gastrointestinal stimulation).

mus·ca·rin·ic (mŭs-kă-rin′ik). **1.** Having a muscarinelike action, i.e., producing effects that resemble postganglionic parasympathetic stimulation. **2.** An agent that stimulates the postganglionic parasympathetic receptor. SEE ALSO muscarine, nicotinic.

mus·ca·rin·ism (mŭs′kă-rin-izm). SYN mycetism.

Mus·ci (mŭs′sī). The class of plants that includes the mosses. [L. pl. of *muscus,* moss]

mus·ci·cide (mŭs′i-sīd). An agent destructive to flies. [L. *musca,* fly, + *caedo,* to kill]

Mus·ci·dae (mŭs′i-dē). The family of flies (order Diptera) that includes the houseflies (*Musca*) and stable flies (*Stomoxys*). [L. *musca,* fly]

mus·ci·mol (mus′ĭ-mol). An alkaloid extracted from the poison mushroom *Amanita muscaria;* selectively stimulates receptors for γ-aminobutyric acid (GABA) and is used as a molecular probe to study GABA receptors; a potent CNS depressant, m. inhibits motor function and can lead to psychosis.

MUSCLE

[1] **mus·cle** (mŭs′ĕl) [TA]. A primary tissue, consisting predominantly of highly specialized contractile cells, which may be classified as skeletal m., cardiac m., or smooth m.; microscopically, the latter is lacking in transverse striations characteristic of the other two types; one of the contractile organs of the body by which movements of the various organs and parts are effected; typical m. is a mass of m. fibers (venter or belly), attached at each

extremity, by means of a tendon, to a bone or other structure; the more proximal or more fixed attachment is called the *origin,* the more distal or more movable attachment is the *insertion;* the narrowing part of the belly that is attached to the tendon of origin is called the caput or head. For gross anatomic description, see musculus. SYN musculus [TA]. [L. *musculus*]

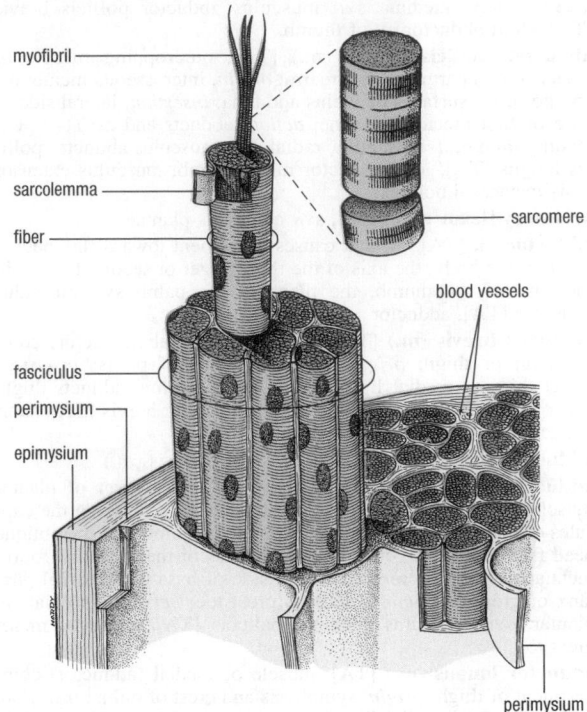

skeletal muscle: diagram of the connective tissue components; the relationships between a muscle bundle (fasciculus), a single muscle cell (fiber), and a myofibril also are indicated

m.'s of abdomen [TA], m.'s forming the wall of the abdomen including rectus abdominis, external and internal oblique m.'s, transversus abdominis, and quadratus abdominis. SYN musculi abdominis.

abdominal external oblique (m.), SYN external oblique (m.).

abdominal internal oblique m., SYN internal oblique (m.).

abductor (m.) [TA], m. that causes movement away from the median plane of body, axis of middle finger, or axis of second toe, or in the case of the thumb, anterior to the plane of the palm. SYN musculus abductor [TA], abductor.

abductor digiti minimi (m.) of foot [TA], muscle of first layer of plantar muscles; *origin,* lateral and medial processes of calcaneal tuberosity; *insertion,* lateral side of proximal phalanx of fifth toe; *action,* abducts and flexes little toe; *nerve supply,* lateral plantar nerve. SYN musculus abductor digiti minimi pedis [TA], abductor m. of little toe, musculus abductor digiti quinti (2).

abductor digiti minimi (m.) of hand [TA], superficial hypothenar muscle of palm; *origin,* pisiform bone and pisohamate ligament; *insertion,* medial side of base of proximal phalanx of the little finger; *action,* abducts and flexes little finger; *nerve supply,* deep branch of ulnar. SYN musculus abductor digiti minimi manus [TA], abductor m. of little finger, musculus abductor digiti quinti (1).

abductor m. of great toe, SYN abductor hallucis (m.).

abductor hallucis (m.) [TA], muscle of third layer of plantar muscles; *origin,* medial process of calcaneal tuberosity, flexor retinaculum, and plantar aponeurosis; *insertion,* medial side of proximal phalanx of great toe; *action,* abducts great toe; *nerve supply,* medial plantar. SYN musculus abductor hallucis [TA], abductor m. of great toe.

mu

abductor m. of little finger, SYN abductor digiti minimi (m.) of hand.

abductor m. of little toe, SYN abductor digiti minimi (m.) of foot.

abductor pollicis brevis (m.) [TA], superficial thenar muscle *origin*, tubercle of trapezium and flexor retinaculum; *insertion*, lateral side of proximal phalanx of thumb; *action*, abducts thumb; *nerve supply*, median. SYN musculus abductor pollicis brevis [TA], short abductor m. of thumb.

abductor pollicis longus (m.) [TA], outcropping muscle of posterior compartment of forearm; *origin*, interosseous membrane and posterior surfaces of radius and ulna; *insertion*, lateral side of base of first metacarpal bone; *action*, abducts and assists in extending thumb; *nerve supply*, radial. SYN musculus abductor pollicis longus [TA], long abductor m. of thumb, musculus extensor ossis metacarpi pollicis.

accessory flexor m. of foot, SYN quadratus plantae (m.).

adductor m. [TA], m. that causes movement toward the median plane of the body, the axis of the third finger or second toe, or, in the case of the thumb, the plane of the palm. SYN musculus adductor [TA], adductor.

adductor brevis (m.) [TA], muscle of medial (adductor) compartment of thigh; *origin*, superior ramus of pubis; *insertion*, upper third of medial lip of linea aspera; *action*, adducts thigh; *nerve supply*, obturator. SYN musculus adductor brevis [TA], short adductor m.

adductor m. of great toe, SYN adductor hallucis (m.).

adductor hallucis (m.) [TA], muscle of third layer of plantar muscles; *origin*, by two heads, the transverse head from the capsules of the lateral four metatarsophalangeal joints and the oblique head from the lateral cuneiform and bases of the third and fourth metatarsal bones; *insertion*, lateral side of base of proximal phalanx of great toe; *action*, adducts great toe; *nerve supply*, lateral plantar. SYN musculus adductor hallucis [TA], adductor m. of great toe.

adductor longus (m.) [TA], muscle of medial (adductor) compartment of thigh; *origin*, symphysis and crest of pubis; *insertion*, middle third of medial lip of linea aspera; *action*, adducts thigh; *nerve supply*, obturator. SYN musculus adductor longus [TA], long adductor m.

adductor magnus (m.) [TA], muscle of medial (adductor) compartment of thigh; *origin*, ischial tuberosity and ischiopubic ramus; *insertion*, linea aspera and adductor tubercle of femur; *action*, adducts and extends thigh; *nerve supply*, obturator and sciatic. SYN musculus adductor magnus [TA], great adductor m.

adductor minimus (m.) [TA], a small flat m. of the medial (adductor) compartment of thigh constituting the upper portion of the adductor magnus, *insertion*, the space above linea aspera. SYN musculus adductor minimus [TA].

adductor pollicis (m.) [TA], intrinsic muscle of palm; *origin*, by two heads, the transverse head from the shaft of the third metacarpal and the oblique head from the front of the base of the second metacarpal, the trapezoid and capitate bones; *insertion*, medial side of base of proximal phalanx of thumb; *action*, adducts thumb; *nerve supply*, ulnar. SYN musculus adductor pollicis [TA], adductor m. of thumb.

adductor m. of thumb, SYN adductor pollicis (m.).

Albinus m., (1) SYN risorius (m.); **(2)** SYN scalenus minimus (m.).

m.'s of anal triangle [TA], voluntary m.'s of region posterior to perineal body and transverse perineal m.'s and anterior to the inferior margins of gluteus maximus m.'s; includes levator ani (including puborectalis), and all portions of the external anal sphincter. SYN musculi regionis analis [TA].

anconeus m. [TA], *origin*, back of lateral condyle of humerus; *insertion*, olecranon process and posterior surface of ulna; *action*, extends forearm and abducts ulna in pronation of wrist; *nerve supply*, radial. SYN musculus anconeus [TA], anconeus.

anorectoperineal m.'s [TA], smooth m. fibers that pass forward from the longitudinal m. layer of the rectum to the membranous urethra in the male. SYN musculi anorectoperineales [TA], musculi rectourethrales✗, rectourethral m.'s✗.

antagonistic m.'s, two or more m.'s that produce opposite movements (function), the contraction of one having the potential, in theory, to "neutralize" that of the other; however, in so doing, they are frequently acting as synergists in fixing the moving part.

anterior auricular m., SYN auricularis anterior (m.).

anterior cervical intertransversarii (m.'s) [TA], deep muscle of back; *origin*, anterior tubercles of cervical transverse processes; *insertion*, anterior tubercle of next superior transverse process; *action*, abducts cervical vertebrae; *nerve supply*, ventral branch of cervical nerves. SYN musculi intertransversarii anteriores cervicis [TA], anterior cervical intertransverse m.'s.

anterior cervical intertransverse m.'s, SYN anterior cervical intertransversarii (m.'s).

anterior rectus m. of head, SYN rectus capitis anterior (m.).

anterior scalene m., ✗official alternate term for scalenus anterior (m.).

anterior serratus m., SYN serratus anterior (m.).

anterior tibial m., SYN tibialis anterior (m.).

antigravity m.'s, the m.'s that maintain the posture characteristic of a given animal species. In most mammals they are the extensor m.'s.

antitragicus (m.) [TA], a band of transverse muscular fibers on the outer surface of the antitragus, arising from the border of the intertragic notch and inserted into the antihelix and tail of the helix. SYN musculus antitragicus [TA], m. of antitragus.

m. of antitragus, SYN antitragicus (m.).

appendicular m., one of the skeletal m.'s of the limbs.

arrector m. of hair [TA], bundles of smooth m. fibers, attached to the deep part of the hair follicles, passing outward alongside the sebaceous glands to the papillary layer of the dermis; they act to pull the hairs erect, causing "goose bumps" or "goose flesh" (cutis anserina) in humans but increasing depth (efficiency) of fur/hair coats of most animals. SYN musculus arrector pili [TA], arrector pili m.'s, erector m. of hair.

arrector pili m.'s, SYN arrector m. of hair.

articular m., a m. that inserts directly onto the capsule of a joint, acting to retract the capsule in certain movements. SYN musculus articularis.

articular m. of elbow, SYN articularis cubiti (m.).

articularis cubiti (m.) [TA], the name applied to a small slip of the medial head of the triceps that inserts into the capsule of the elbow joint. SYN musculus articularis cubiti [TA], articular m. of elbow, subanconeus m.

articularis genus (m.) [TA], deep, distal portion of vastus intermedius m.; *origin*, lower fourth of anterior surface of shaft of femur; *insertion*, suprapatellar bursa of knee joint; *action*, retracts suprapatellar bursa, during extension of knee; *nerve supply*, femoral. SYN musculus articularis genus [TA], articular m. of knee, Dupré m., subcrural m., subcruralis, subcrureus, subquadricipital m.

articular m. of knee, SYN articularis genus (m.).

aryepiglottic m., SYN aryepiglottic *part* of oblique arytenoid muscle.

m.'s of auditory ossicles [TA], the m. stapedius and m. tensor tympani. SYN musculi ossiculorum auditus [TA], musculi ossiculorum auditoriorum✗.

auricular m.'s [TA], small muscles associated with the auricle, having little function in humans. SYN musculi auriculares [TA].

auricularis anterior (m.) [TA], *origin*, epicranial aponeurosis, *insertion*, cartilage of auricle; *action*, draws pinna of ear upward and forward; *nerve supply*, facial. Considered by some to be the anterior part of the temporoparietalis m. SYN anterior auricular m., musculus attrahens aurem, musculus attrahens auriculam, musculus auricularis anterior, zygomaticoauricularis.

auricularis posterior (m.) [TA], facial muscle of external ear; *origin*, mastoid process; *insertion*, posterior portion of root of auricle; *action*, draws back the pinna; *nerve supply*, facial. SYN musculus auricularis posterior [TA], musculus retrahens aurem, musculus retrahens auriculam, posterior auricular (m.).

auricularis superior (m.) [TA], facial muscle associated with external ear; *origin*, galea aponeurotica; *insertion*, cartilage of auricle; *action*, draws pinna of ear upward and backward; *nerve supply*, facial. Considered by some to be the posterior part of the temporoparietal muscle. SYN musculus auricularis superior [TA], attollens aurem, attollens auriculam, musculus attollens aurem, musculus attollens auriculam, superior auricular m.

axial m., one of the skeletal m.'s of the trunk or head.

axillary arch m., SYN pectorodorsalis m.

m.'s of back [TA], the m.'s of the back in general, including the thoracoappendicular m.'s attaching the shoulder girdle to the trunk posteriorly, the posterior serratus m.'s, and the erector spinae and transversospinalis m.'s. SYN musculi dorsi [TA], dorsal m.'s.

m.'s of back proper [TA], m.'s of the back innervated by the dorsal primary rami of spinal nerves; includes erector spinae, transversospinalis, interspinales, and anterior and lateral intertransversii m.'s; excludes the superficial back m.'s which are appendicular and are innervated by ventral rami, and the trapezius, innervated by the spinal accessory nerve. SYN musculi dorsi proprii [TA], deep m.'s of back, true m.'s of back.

Bell m., a band of muscular fibers, forming a slight fold in the wall of the bladder, running from the uvula to the opening of the ureter on either side, bounding the trigonum.

biceps m. of arm, SYN biceps brachii (m.).

biceps brachii (m.) [TA], superficial muscle of anterior (flexor) compartment of arm; *origin,* long head from supraglenoidal tubercle of scapula, short head from coracoid process; *insertion,* tuberosity of radius; *action,* flexes elbow and supinates forearm (it is the primary supinator of the forearm); *nerve supply,* musculocutaneous. SYN musculus biceps brachii [TA], biceps m. of arm.

biceps femoris (m.) [TA], hamstring muscle of posterior compartment of thigh; *origin,* long head (caput longum) from tuberosity of ischium, short head (caput breve) from lower half of lateral lip of linea aspera; *insertion,* head of fibula; *action,* flexes knee and rotates the flexed leg laterally; *nerve supply,* long head, tibial, short head, fibular. SYN musculus biceps femoris [TA], biceps m. of thigh, musculus biceps flexor cruris.

biceps m. of thigh, SYN biceps femoris (m.).

bipennate m., SYN pennate m.

Bochdalek m., SYN *musculus* triticeoglossus.

Bowman m., SYN ciliary m.

brachial m., SYN brachialis (m.).

brachialis (m.) [TA], deep muscle of anterior (flexor) compartment of arm; *origin,* lower two-thirds of anterior surface of humerus; *insertion,* coronoid process of ulna; *action,* flexes elbow; *nerve supply,* musculocutaneous, usually with a minor contribution from the radial. SYN musculus brachialis [TA], brachial m.

brachioradial m., SYN brachioradialis (m.).

brachioradialis (m.) [TA], muscle of posterior (extensor) compartment of forearm; *origin,* lateral supracondylar ridge of humerus; *insertion,* anterior aspect of base of styloid process of radius; *action,* flexes elbow and assists in returning the pronated or supinated limb to the neutral position; *nerve supply,* (common) radial. SYN musculus brachioradialis [TA], brachioradial m.

branchiomeric m.'s, the m.'s associated with the branchial arches; they provide a large portion of the musculature for the face and neck; the myoblasts for these m.'s originate from paroxial mesoderm, while the neural crest provides their connective tissue.

Braune m., SYN puborectalis (m.).

broadest m. of back, SYN latissimus dorsi (m.).

bronchoesophageal m., SYN bronchoesophageus (m.).

bronchoesophageus (m.) [TA], muscular fascicles, arising from the wall of the left bronchus, which reinforce the musculature of the esophagus. SYN musculus bronchoesophageus [TA], bronchoesophageal m.

Brücke m., the part of the ciliary m. formed by the meridional fibers. SYN Crampton m.

buccinator (m.) [TA], facial muscle of cheek; *origin,* posterior portion of alveolar portion of maxilla and mandible and pterygomandibular raphe; *insertion,* angle of mouth; also become interspersed with more horizontal portions of the orbicularis oris; *action,* flattens cheek, retracts angle of mouth; plays an important role in mastication, working with tongue and orbicularis oris muscle to keep food between teeth; when it is paralyzed, as in Bell palsy, food accumulates in the oral vestibule; *nerve supply,* facial. SYN musculus buccinator [TA], cheek m.

bulbocavernosus m., SYN bulbospongiosus (m.).

bulbospongiosus (m.) [TA], perineal muscle; in the male: *origin,* the perineal membrane fascia on the dorsum of the bulb of the penis; *insertion,* central tendon of the perineum and the median raphe on the free surface of the bulb; *action,* voluntarily constricts bulbous urethra when attempting to expel last drops following urination, or spasmodically with, and following, ejaculation to expel semen. In the female: *origin,* the dorsum of the clitoris, the corpus cavernosum, and the perineal membrane; *insertion,* central tendon of the perineum; *action,* acts as a weak sphincter of the vagina; when developed, is a part of "cross-member musculature" of pelvic floor that resists prolapse of pelvic viscera; surrounds and compresses greater vestibular gland, especially during erection of bulb of vestibule, expressing secretion. *Nerve supply,* pudendal (deep perineal branch). SYN musculus bulbospongiosus [TA], bulbocavernosus m., musculus bulbocavernosus, musculus ejaculator seminis, musculus sphincter vaginae, sphincter vaginae.

cardiac m., the involuntary m. comprising the myocardium and walls of the pulmonary veins and superior vena cava, consisting of anastomosing transversely striated m. fibers formed of cells united at intercalated disks; the one or two nuclei of each cell are centrally located and the longitudinally arranged myofibrils have considerable sarcoplasm around them; connective tissue is limited to reticular and fine collagenous fibers; contraction is rhythmic and intrinsically stimulated. SYN m. of heart.

Casser perforated m., SYN coracobrachialis m.

ceratocricoid (m.) [TA], an inconstant fasciculus from the posterior cricoarytenoid m. inserted into the inferior horn of the thyroid cartilage. SYN musculus ceratocricoideus [TA], Merkel m.

ceratoglossus (m.) [TA], main, posterior part of hyoglossus m. (vs. chondroglossus) arising from the greater horn of the hyoid bone. SYN musculus ceratoglossus [TA].

cervical iliocostal m., SYN iliocostalis cervicis (m.).

cervical interspinal m., SYN interspinales cervicis (m.'s).

cervical interspinales m.'s, SYN interspinales cervicis (m.'s).

cervical longissimus m., SYN longissimus cervicis (m.).

cervical rotator m.'s, SYN rotatores cervicis (m.'s).

cheek m., SYN buccinator (m.).

chin m., SYN mentalis (m.).

chondroglossus m. [TA], lesser part of hyoglossus, arising as fibers from lesser horn of hyoid bone, which are separated from the main part of the hyoglossus (the ceratoglossus) by slips of genioglossus muscle. SYN musculus chondroglossus.

ciliary m. [TA], the intrinsic smooth m. of the ciliary body of eyeball; it consists of circular fibers [TA] (fibrae circulares [TA]), radial fibers [TA] (fibrae radialis [TA]), meridional fibers [TA] (fibrae meridoneales [TA]), and longitudinal fibers [TA] (fibrae longitudinales [TA]); *action,* in contracting, its diameter is reduced (like a sphincter's), reducing tensile (stretching) forces on lens, allowing the lens to thicken for near vision (accommodation). SYN musculus ciliaris [TA], Bowman m., ciliary ligament.

coccygeal m., SYN coccygeus m.

coccygeus m. [TA], striated pelvic muscle associated with the deep (pelvic) aspect of the sacrospinous ligament, forming part of the pelvic diaphragm; *origin,* spine of ischium and sacrospinous ligament; *insertion,* sides of lower part of sacrum and upper part of coccyx; *action,* with the sacrospinous ligament assists in support of pelvic floor, theoretically increasingly so when intraabdominal pressures increase; *nerve supply,* third and fourth sacral. SYN musculus coccygeus [TA], coccygeal m., ischiococcygeus, musculus ischiococcygeus.

m.'s of coccyx, the m.'s of the coccyx considered as a group, including the musculus coccygeus and the inconstant ventral and dorsal sacrococcygeal m.'s. SYN musculi coccygei.

Coiter m., SYN corrugator supercilii (m.).

compressor urethra (m.) [TA], part of the external urethral sphincter complex of m. consisting of a slender muscular band spanning between the more posterior aspects of the ischiopubic rami but looping anterior to the urethra so that its contraction pulls posteriorly on the urethra,, compressing its anterior wall against the posterior wall, closing the urethra like a gentle kink in a hose; Terminologia Anatomica lists this m. only for the female,

mu

but a similar structure has been described for the male. SYN musculus compressor urethrae [TA].

coracobrachial m., SYN coracobrachialis m.

coracobrachialis m. [TA], muscle of anterior (flexor) compartment of arm; *origin*, coracoid process of scapula; *insertion*, middle of medial border of humerus; *action*, adducts and flexes the arm; acts as a shunt muscle in resisting downward dislocation of shoulder joint; *nerve supply*, musculocutaneous. SYN musculus coracobrachialis [TA], Casser perforated m., coracobrachial m.

corrugator m., SYN corrugator supercilii (m.).

corrugator cutis m. of anus, muscle of anal triangle with muscle fibers radiating from the superficial portion of the external sphincter to the deep aspect of the perianal skin, said to cause puckering of that skin, which contributes to the air/water-tight "seal" of the anal canal. SYN musculus corrugator cutis ani.

corrugator supercilii (m.) [TA], facial muscle of forehead; *origin*, from orbital portion of m. orbicularis oculi and nasal prominence; *insertion*, skin of eyebrow; *action*, draws medial end of eyebrow downward and wrinkles forehead vertically, conveying expression of deep thought, worry, or concern; *nerve supply*, facial. SYN musculus corrugator supercilii [TA], Coiter m., corrugator m., wrinkler m. of eyebrow.

cowl m., SYN trapezius (m.).

Crampton m., SYN Brücke m.

cremaster m. [TA], *origin*, continuation of fibers from inferiormost internal oblique m. and slips arising from the inguinal ligament; *insertion*, becomes interspersed within cremasteric fascia of spermatic cord and intermediate covering of testis; in the female, the round ligament of the uterus; *action*, elevate testicle; *nerve supply*, genital branch of genitofemoral. SYN musculus cremaster [TA], Riolan m. (2).

cricopharyngeus m., ✭official alternate term for cricopharyngeal *part* of inferior constrictor (muscle) of pharynx.

cricothyroid m. [TA], intrinsic laryngeal muscle; *origin*, anterior surface of arch of cricoid; *insertion*, the anterior or straight part passes upward to ala of thyroid; the posterior or oblique part passes more outward to inferior horn of thyroid; *action*, acts at cricothyroid joint, pulling anterior aspects of thyroid and cricoid cartilages together, rotating the superior portion of the cricoid lamina and arytenoid cartilages posteriorly, causing vocal folds to tense, increasing the pitch of voice tone; the antagonist of this movement is the thyroarytenoid muscle; *nerve supply*, external laryngeal branch of superior laryngeal nerve (from vagus). SYN musculus cricothyroideus [TA].

cruciate m., a general type of m. in which the m.'s or bundles of m. fibers cross in an X-shaped configuration; e.g., the oblique arytenoid m.'s. SYN musculus cruciatus.

cutaneous m. [TA], a m. that lies in the subcutaneous tissue and attaches to the skin; it may or may not have a bony attachment. The m.'s of expression are the chief examples of cutaneous m.'s in the human. SYN musculus cutaneus [TA].

dartos m., smooth muscle fibers interspersed within the dartos fascia (superficial fascia of scrotum), causing contraction of the scrotum, as when experiencing a cool environmental temperature. SEE ALSO dartos *fascia*.

deep m.'s of back, SYN m.'s of back proper.

deep flexor (m.) of fingers, SYN flexor digitorum profundus (m.).

deep transverse perineal m. [TA], *origin*, ramus of ischium; *insertion*, with its fellow in the perineal body; *action*, with superficial transverse perineal m. in forming the transverse element of cross-member (the sagittal element being formed by bulbospongiosus and external anal sphincter muscles) that provides support of the perineum and the pelvic diaphragm above it during increased abdominopelvic pressure; in males, it adds support to the bulb of the penis; *nerve supply*, pudendal (dorsal nerve of penis/clitoris). SYN musculus transversus perinei profundus [TA], deep transverse m. of perineum.

deep transverse m. of perineum, SYN deep transverse perineal m.

deltoid (m.) [TA], intrinsic (scapulohumeral) m. of shoulder joint; *origin*, lateral third of anterior border of clavicle, lateral and posterior border of acromion process, lower border of spine of scapula; *insertion*, lateral side of shaft of humerus (deltoid tuber-

osity) a little above its middle; *action*, its anterior, middle, and posterior portions act independently to produce abduction, flexion, extension, and rotation of the humerus at the shoulder joint; *nerve supply*, axillary (fifth and sixth cervical spinal cord segments via the brachial plexus). SYN musculus deltoideus [TA].

depressor anguli oris (m.) [TA], facial muscle of mouth; *origin*, anterolateral base of mandible anteriorly; *insertion*, blends with other m.'s in lower lip near angle of mouth; *action*, pulls down corners of mouth; *nerve supply*, facial. SYN musculus depressor anguli oris [TA], musculus triangularis (2) [TA], triangular m. (2) [TA], musculus triangularis labii inferioris.

depressor m. of epiglottis, SYN thyroepiglottic *part* of thyroarytenoid (muscle).

depressor m. of eyebrow, SYN depressor supercilii (m.).

depressor labii inferioris (m.) [TA], facial muscle of mouth; *origin*, anterior portion of base of mandible; *insertion*, interdigitates with fibers of orbicularis oris m. to reach skin of lower lip; *action*, depresses lower lip; *nerve supply*, facial. SYN musculus depressor labii inferioris [TA], depressor m. of lower lip, musculus quadratus labii inferioris, musculus quadratus menti.

depressor m. of lower lip, SYN depressor labii inferioris (m.).

depressor septi nasi (m.) [TA], facial muscle of nose; a vertical fasciculus from the maxilla superior to the central incisor passing upward along the median line of the upper lip to insert into the mobile part of the nasal septum; *action*, works with alar (dilator) part of the nasalis muscle to widen the nares during deep inspiration; depresses septum; *nerve supply*, buccal branch of facial. SYN musculus depressor septi [TA], depressor (m.) of septum.

depressor (m.) of septum, SYN depressor septi nasi (m.).

depressor supercilii (m.) [TA], facial muscle arising from nasal part of frontal bone, medial to the corrugator supercili and inserting into the skin underlying the middle of the eyebrow; *action*, depresses eyebrow; *nerve supply*, facial. SYN musculus depressor supercilii [TA], depressor m. of eyebrow.

detrusor (m.) [TA], the muscular coat of the urinary bladder, which, along with gravity and increased intraabdominal pressure, facilitates emptying of bladder during urination by its contraction. SYN musculus detrusor urinae [TA].

digastric (m.) [TA], **(1)** one of the suprahyoid group of m.'s consisting of two bellies united by a central tendon that passes through a fascial loop connected to the body of the hyoid bone; *origin*, by posterior belly from the digastric groove medial to the mastoid process; *insertion*, by anterior belly into lower border of mandible near midline; *action*, elevates the hyoid when mandible is fixed; depresses the mandible when hyoid is fixed; *nerve supply*, posterior belly from facial, anterior belly by nerve to the mylohyoid from the mandibular division of trigeminal; SYN musculus biventer [TA], musculus digastricus [TA], two-bellied m. [TA], biventer mandibulae, musculus biventer mandibulae. **(2)** a m. with two fleshy bellies separated by a fibrous insertion;

dilator m. [TA], a m. that opens an orifice or dilates the lumen of an organ; it is the dilating or opening component of a pylorus (the other component is the sphincter m.). SYN musculus dilatator [TA], musculus dilator.

dilator (m.) of ileocecal sphincter, the longitudinal muscular fibers that open the ileal orifice at the level of the cecocolic junction. SYN musculus dilator pylori ilealis.

dilator pupillae m. [TA], intrinsic "muscle" of eyeball; radially disposed layer of muscular processes of the myoepithelial cells that form the epithelium of the posterior surface of the iris, which extends from the pupillary to the ciliary margin; sympathetic stimulation causes contraction, which slowly dilates the pupil to allow more light to reach the retina. SYN musculus dilator pupillae [TA], dilator iridis, dilator of pupil, musculus dilator iridis.

dilator (m.) of pylorus, the longitudinal muscular fibers that open the gastroduodenal junction. SYN musculus dilator pylori gastroduodenalis.

dorsal m.'s, SYN m.'s of back.

dorsal interossei (interosseous m.'s) of foot [TA], four intrinsic muscles of the fourth layer of plantar muscles; *origin*, from sides of adjacent metatarsal bones; *insertion*, first into medial, second into lateral side of proximal phalanx of second toe, third and fourth into lateral side of proximal phalanx of third and fourth toes; *action*, abduct toes 2–4 from an axis through the second toe; *nerve supply*, lateral plantar. SYN musculi interossei dorsalis pedis [TA].

dorsal interossei (interosseous m.'s) of hand [TA], four intrinsic muscles of the hand; *origin*, sides of adjacent metacarpal bones; *insertion*, proximal phalanges and extensor expansion, first on radial side of index, second on radial side of middle finger, third on ulnar side of middle finger, fourth on ulnar side of ring finger; *action*, abduct fingers 2–4 from the axis of the middle finger, *nerve supply*, ulnar. SYN musculi interossei dorsalis manus [TA].

dorsal sacrococcygeal m., SYN dorsal sacrococcygeus m.

dorsal sacrococcygeus m., an inconstant and poorly developed muscle on the dorsal surfaces of the sacrum and coccyx, the remains of a portion of the tail musculature of lower animals. SYN dorsal sacrococcygeal m., musculus extensor coccygis, musculus sacrococcygeus dorsalis, musculus sacrococcygeus posterior.

Dupré m., SYN articularis genus (m.).

Duverney m., SYN lacrimal *part* of orbicularis oculi muscle; SEE orbicularis oculi (m.).

elevator m. of anus, SYN levator ani (m.).

elevator (m.) of prostate, SYN puboprostaticus (m.).

elevator m. of rib, SYN levatores costarum (m.'s).

elevator (m.) of scapula, SYN levator scapulae (m.).

(elevator) m. of soft palate, SYN levator veli palatini (m.).

elevator (m.) of thyroid gland, SYN levator (m.) of thyroid gland.

elevator (m.) of upper eyelid, SYN levator palpebrae superioris (m.).

elevator m. of upper lip, SYN levator labii superioris (m.).

elevator m. of upper lip and wing of nose, SYN levator labii superioris alaeque nasi (m.).

epicranial m., SYN epicranius (m.).

epicranius (m.) [TA], compound facial (scalp) muscle composed of the epicranial aponeurosis and the m.'s inserting into it, i.e., the occipitofrontalis m. and temporoparietalis m. SYN musculus epicranius [TA], epicranial m., scalp m.

erector m. of hair, SYN arrector m. of hair.

erector spinae (m.'s) [TA], proper muscles of back; *origin*, from sacrum, ilium, and spines of lumbar vertebrae; it divides into three columns, iliocostalis m., longissimus m., and spinalis m., which insert into ribs and vertebrae with additional muscle slips joining the columns at successively higher levels; *action*, extends and laterally flexes vertebral column; *nerve supply*, dorsal primary rami of spinal nerves. SYN musculus erector spinae [TA], erector m. of spine, musculus sacrospinalis.

erector m. of spine, SYN erector spinae (m.'s).

extensor m. [TA], m. producing extension, i.e., a movement that produces straightening, or an increase in the angle of a joint. SYN musculus extensor [TA].

extensor carpi radialis brevis (m.) [TA], muscle of posterior compartment of forearm; *origin*, lateral epicondyle of humerus; *insertion*, base of third metacarpal bone; *action*, extends and abducts hand at wrist joint; *nerve supply*, deep radial. SYN musculus extensor carpi radialis brevis [TA], short radial extensor m. of wrist.

extensor carpi radialis longus (m.) [TA], muscle of posterior (extensor) compartment of forearm; *origin*, lateral supracondylar ridge of humerus; *insertion*, posterior aspect of base of second metacarpal bone; *action*, extends and abducts hand at wrist joint; *nerve supply*, radial. SYN musculus extensor carpi radialis longus [TA], long radial extensor m. of wrist.

extensor carpi ulnaris (m.) [TA], muscle of posterior (extensor) compartment of forearm; *origin*, lateral epicondyle of humerus (humeral head) and oblique line and posterior border of ulna (ulnar head); *insertion*, base of fifth metacarpal bone; *action*, extends and adducts hand at wrist joint; *nerve supply*, radial (posterior interosseous). SYN musculus extensor carpi ulnaris [TA], ulnar extensor (m.) of wrist.

extensor digiti minimi (m.) [TA], muscle of posterior (extensor) compartment of forearm; *origin*, lateral epicondyle of humerus; *insertion*, dorsum of proximal, middle, and distal phalanges of little finger; *action*, extends little finger; *nerve supply*, radial

(posterior interosseous). SYN musculus extensor digiti minimi [TA], extensor (m.) of little finger, musculus extensor digiti quinti proprius, musculus extensor minimi digiti.

extensor digitorum m. [TA], muscle of posterior (extensor) compartment of forearm; *origin*, lateral epicondyle of humerus; *insertion*, by four tendons into the base of the proximal and middle and base of the distal phalanges; *action*, extends fingers, especially at metacarpophalangeal joint; *nerve supply*, radial (posterior interosseous). SYN musculus extensor digitorum [TA], extensor (m.) of fingers, musculus extensor digitorum communis.

extensor digitorum brevis (m.) [TA], intrinsic muscle of dorsum of foot; *origin*, dorsal surface of calcaneus; *insertion*, by four tendons fusing with those of the extensor digitorum longus, and by a slip attached independently to the base of the proximal phalanx of the great toe; *action*, extends four lateral toes (II–V); *nerve supply*, deep fibular. SYN musculus extensor digitorum brevis [TA], musculus extensor brevis digitorum, short extensor (m.) of toes.

extensor digitorum brevis (m.) of hand, a short extensor muscle of the fingers of rare occurrence, and comparable to the short extensor of the toes. SYN musculus extensor digitorum brevis manus, Pozzi m.

extensor digitorum longus (m.) [TA], muscle of anterior (extensor/dorsiflexor) compartment of leg; *origin*, lateral condyle of tibia, upper two-thirds of anterior margin of fibula; *insertion*, by four tendons to the dorsal surfaces of the bases of the proximal, middle, and distal phalanges of the second to fifth toes; *action*, extends the four lateral toes; *nerve supply*, deep fibular. SYN musculus extensor digitorum longus [TA], long extensor (m.) of toes, musculus extensor longus digitorum.

extensor (m.) of fingers, SYN extensor digitorum m.

extensor hallucis brevis (m.) [TA], intrinsic muscle of dorsum of foot considered by some anatomists as the medial belly of extensor digitorum brevis muscle; *origin,* dorsal calcaneus; *insertion,* via a stout aspect of the base of the proximal phalanx of the great toe; *action,* extends great toe; *nerve supply,* deep fibular. of which is inserted into the base of the proximal phalanx of the great toe. SYN musculus extensor hallucis brevis [TA], short extensor (m.) of great toe.

extensor hallucis longus (m.) [TA], muscle of anterior (extensor/dorsiflexor) compartment of leg; *origin*, anterior surface of fibula and interosseous membrane; *insertion*, dorsal aspect of base of distal phalanx of great toe; *action*, extends the great toe; *nerve supply*, deep fibular. SYN musculus extensor hallucis longus [TA], long extensor (m.) of great toe.

extensor indicis (m.) [TA], muscle of posterior (extensor) compartment of forearm; *origin*, dorsal surface of distal ulna and adjacent interosseous membrane; *insertion*, extensor expansion of index finger; *action*, independently extends the index finger and assists in extending hand at wrist joint; *nerve supply*, radial (posterior interosseous). SYN musculus extensor indicis [TA], index extensor (m.), musculus extensor indicis proprius.

extensor (m.) of little finger, SYN extensor digiti minimi (m.).

extensor pollicis brevis (m.) [TA], muscle of posterior (extensor) compartment of forearm; *origin*, dorsal surface of distal radius and adjacent interosseous membrane; *insertion*, posterior aspect of base of proximal phalanx of thumb; *action*, extends and abducts the thumb at metacarpophalangeal joint; *nerve supply*, radial joint (posterior interosseous). SYN musculus extensor pollicis brevis [TA], musculus extensor brevis pollicis, short extensor (m.) of thumb.

extensor pollicis longus (m.) [TA], muscle of posterior (extensor) compartment of forearm; *origin*, posterior surface of middle of shaft of ulna; *insertion*, dorsal aspect of base of distal phalanx of thumb; *action*, extends distal phalanx of thumb; *nerve supply*, radial (posterior interosseous). SYN musculus extensor pollicis longus [TA], long extensor (m.) of thumb, musculus extensor longus pollicis.

external intercostal (m.) [TA], flat muscle of thorax arising from lower border of one rib and pass obliquely downward and forward to be inserted into the upper border of rib below; *action*, contract during inspiration to elevate ribs; also to maintain tension in the

mu

intercostal spaces to resist inward movement during inspiration; *nerve supply*, intercostal. SYN musculus intercostales externi [TA].

external oblique (m.) [TA], flat muscle of abdomen; *origin*, external surfaces of fifth to twelfth ribs; *insertion*, anterior half of lateral lip of iliac crest and inguinal ligament inferiorly, and continuing medially as part of the anterior layer of the rectus sheath; *action*, supports and compresses abdominal viscera; flexes and rotates trunk; *nerve supply*, thoracoabdominal nerves. SYN musculus obliquus externus abdominis [TA], abdominal external oblique (m.).

external obturator m., SYN obturator externus (m.).

external pterygoid m., SYN lateral pterygoid (m.).

external m. m. of anus, SYN external anal *sphincter*.

extraocular m.'s [TA], the m.'s within the orbit but outside of eyeball, including the four rectus muscles (superior, inferior, medial and lateral); two oblique muscles (superior and inferior), and the levator of the superior eyelid (levator palpebrae superioris). SYN musculi externi bulbi oculi [TA], extrinsic m.'s of eyeball⋆, m.'s of eyeball, musculi bulbi, ocular m.'s.

extrinsic m.'s, m.'s arising outside of, but which act upon, the structure under consideration. For example, the m.'s operating the hand but having fleshy bellies located in the forearm.

extrinsic m.'s of eyeball, ⋆official alternate term for extraocular m.'s.

m.'s of eyeball, SYN extraocular m.'s.

facial m.'s [TA], the numerous m.'s supplied by the facial nerve that are attached to and move the skin of the face. Terminologia Anatomica includes the buccinator m. in this group because of its innervation and embryonic origin, even though it functions primarily in mastication. SYN mimetic m.'s, m.'s of facial expression, musculi faciei.

m.'s of facial expression, SYN facial m.'s.

femoral m., SYN vastus intermedius (m.).

fibularis brevis (m.) [TA], *origin*, lower two-thirds of lateral surface of fibula; *insertion*, base of fifth metatarsal bone; *action*, everts foot; *nerve supply*, superficial peroneal. SYN musculus fibularis brevis [TA], musculus peroneus brevis⋆, peroneus brevis (m.)⋆, short fibular m., short peroneal m.

fibularis longus (m.) [TA], *origin*, upper two-thirds of outer surface of fibula and lateral condyle of tibia; *insertion*, by tendon passing behind lateral malleolus and across sole of foot to medial cuneiform and base of first metatarsal; *action*, plantar flexes and everts foot; *nerve supply*, superficial peroneal. SYN musculus fibularis longus [TA], musculus peroneus longus⋆, peroneus longus (m.)⋆, long fibular m., long peroneal m.

fibularis tertius (m.) [TA], *origin*, in common with m. extensor digitorum longus; *insertion*, dorsum of base of fifth metatarsal bone; *nerve supply*, deep branch of peroneal; *action*, assists in dorsiflexion and eversion of foot. SYN musculus fibularis tertius [TA], musculus peroneus tertius⋆, peroneus tertius (m.)⋆, third peroneal m.

fixator m., a m. that acts as a stabilizer of one part of the body during movement of another part.

flat m. [TA], broad, relatively thin, sheetlike muscle, e.g., muscles of the anterolateral abdominal wall (external and internal oblique, transversus abdominis). SYN musculus plana [TA].

flexor m. [TA], muscle producing flexion, i.e., a movement that bends or decreases the angle of joints. SYN musculus flexor [TA].

flexor accessorius (m.), ⋆official alternate term for quadratus plantae (m.).

flexor carpi radialis (m.) [TA], muscle of the anterior (flexor) compartment of forearm; *origin*, common flexor origin of medial condyle of humerus; *insertion*, anterior surface of the base of the second and most often sending a slip to that of the third metacarpal bone; *action*, flexes and abducts wrist; *nerve supply*, median; its tendon travels in its own canal roofed by a layer of the transverse carpal ligament. SYN musculus flexor carpi radialis [TA], radial flexor (m.) of wrist.

flexor carpi ulnaris (m.) [TA], muscle of anterior (flexor) compartment of forearm; *origin*, via a humeral head from the medial condyle of humerus and an ulnar head from the olecranon and upper three-fifths of posterior border of ulna; *insertion*, pisiform bone, but is continued to the fifth metacarpal bone via the pisometacarpal ligament; *action*, flexes and adducts the hand at the wrist joint ulnarward; *nerve supply*, ulnar. SYN musculus flexor carpi ulnaris [TA], ulnar flexor (m.) of wrist.

flexor digiti minimi brevis (m.) of foot [TA], muscle of third layer of plantar muscles; *origin*, base of metatarsal bone of the little toe and sheath of fibularis longus muscle; *insertion*, lateral surface of base of proximal phalanx of little toe; *action*, flexes the little toe at the metacarpophalangeal joint; *nerve supply*, lateral plantar. SYN musculus flexor digiti minimi brevis pedis [TA], short flexor (m.) of little toe.

flexor digiti minimi brevis (m.) of hand [TA], hypothenar muscle of palm; *origin*, hook of hamate bone; *insertion*, medial side of proximal phalanx of little finger; *action*, flexes little finger at the metacarpophalangeal joint; *nerve supply*, deep branch of ulnar. SYN musculus flexor digiti minimi brevis manus [TA], short flexor (m.) of little finger.

flexor digitorum brevis (m.) [TA], muscle of first layer of lantar muscles; *origin*, medial tubercle of calcaneus and plantar aponeurosis; *insertion*, middle phalanges of four lateral toes by tendons perforated by those of the flexor digitorum longus; *action*, flexes lateral four toes; *nerve supply*, medial plantar. SYN musculus flexor digitorum brevis [TA], musculus flexor brevis digitorum, short flexor (m.) of toes.

flexor digitorum longus (m.) [TA], muscle of deep posterior or flexor (plantar flexor) compartment of leg; *origin*, middle third of posterior surface of tibia; *insertion*, by four tendons, perforating those of the flexor brevis, into bases of distal phalanges of four lateral toes; *action*, flexes second to fifth toes; *nerve supply*, tibial nerve. SYN musculus flexor digitorum longus [TA], long flexor (m.) of toes, musculus flexor longus digitorum.

flexor digitorum profundus (m.) [TA], muscle of deep layer of anterior (flexor) compartment of forearm; *origin*, anterior surface of proximal third of ulna; *insertion*, by four tendons, piercing those of the flexor digitorum superficialis, into anterior aspect of the base of distal phalanx of each finger; *action*, flexes distal interphalangeal joint of fingers; *nerve supply*, ulnar and median (anterior interosseous muscle). SYN musculus flexor digitorum profundus [TA], deep flexor (m.) of fingers, musculus flexor profundus.

flexor digitorum superficialis (m.) [TA], intermediate muscle of anterior (flexor) compartment of forearm; *origin*, via a humeroulnar head from the medial epicondyle of the humerus, the medial border of the coronoid process, and a tendinous arch between these points, and a radial head from the oblique line and middle

movements of the eyes and muscles employed				
sideways motion (ab- and adduction)	**vertical motion**	**oblique motion**		**rolling motion**
dextroversion	**elevation (lifting)**	**dextroelevation**	**levoelevation**	**extorsion (outward rolling)**
right eye: lateral rectus	superior rectus	right eye: superior rectus	left eye: superior rectus	inferior rectus
left eye: medial rectus	inferior oblique	left eye: inferior oblique	right eye: inferior oblique	inferior oblique
levoversion	**depression (lowering)**	**dextrodepression**	**levodepression**	**intorsion (inward rolling)**
right eye: medial rectus	inferior rectus	right eye: inferior rectus	left eye: inferior rectus	superior rectus
left eye: lateral rectus	inferior oblique	left eye: superior oblique	right eye: superior oblique	superior oblique

third of the lateral border of the radius; *insertion*, by four split tendons, passing to either side of the flexor digitorum profundus tendons, into sides of middle phalanx of each finger; *action*, flexes proximal interphalangeal joint of the fingers; *nerve supply*, median. SYN musculus flexor digitorum superficialis [TA], musculus flexor digitorum sublimis, musculus flexor sublimis, superficial flexor (m.) of fingers.

flexor hallucis brevis (m.) [TA], thenar muscle of palm; *origin*, medial surface of cuboid and middle and lateral cuneiform bones; *insertion*, by two tendons, embracing that of the flexor longus hallucis, into the sides of the base of the proximal phalanx of the great toe; *action*, flexes great toe; *nerve supply*, medial and lateral plantar. SYN musculus flexor hallucis brevis [TA], musculus flexor brevis hallucis, short flexor (m.) of great toe.

flexor hallucis longus (m.) [TA], muscle of deep posterior (plantar flexor) compartment of leg; *origin*, lower two-thirds of posterior surface of fibula; *insertion*, base of distal phalanx of great toe; *action*, flexes great toe; *nerve supply*, medial plantar. SYN musculus flexor hallucis longus [TA], long flexor (m.) of great toe, musculus flexor longus hallucis.

flexor pollicis brevis (m.) [TA], thenar muscle of palm; *origin*, superficial portion from flexor retinaculum of wrist, deep portion from ulnar side of first metacarpal bone; *insertion*, palmar aspect of base of proximal phalanx of thumb; *action*, flexes proximal phalanx of thumb; *nerve supply*, median (superficial head) and deep branch of ulnar (deep head). Some authors consider the deep head to be the first in a series of four palmar interossei muscles of the hand. SYN musculus flexor pollicis brevis [TA], short flexor (m.) of thumb.

flexor pollicis longus (m.) [TA], muscle of deep layer of anterior (flexor) compartment of forearm; *origin*, anterior surface of middle third of radius; *insertion*, palmar aspect of distal phalanx of thumb; *action*, flexes thumb at interphalangeal joint; *nerve supply*, median (anterior interosseous). SYN musculus flexor pollicis longus [TA], long flexor m. of thumb, musculus flexor longus pollicis.

four-headed m. [TA], having four heads; denoting a muscle of the thigh, m. femoris muscle, and—uncommonly—one of the calf, m. surae muscle, or the combined gastrocnemius (with two heads), soleus, and plantaris, more commonly called triceps surae muscle, the plantaris being counted as a separate muscle. SYN quadriceps.

frontalis m., SYN frontal *belly* of occipitofrontalis muscle.

fusiform m. [TA], one that has a fleshy belly, tapering at either extremity. SYN musculus fusiformis [TA], spindle-shaped m.

Gantzer m., an accessory m. extending from the superficial flexor of the digits to the deep flexor of the digits.

gastrocnemius (m.) [TA], superficial muscle of posterior (plantar flexor) compartment of leg; *origin*, by two heads (lateral and medial) from the lateral and medial condyles of the femur; *insertion*, with soleus by tendo calcaneus into lower half of posterior surface of calcaneus; *action*, plantar flexion of foot; *nerve supply*, tibial. SYN musculus gastrocnemius [TA], gastrocnemius.

Gavard m., oblique fibers in the muscular coat of the stomach.

genioglossal m., SYN genioglossus (m.).

genioglossus (m.) [TA], one of the paired lingual m.'s; *origin*, mental spine of the mandible; *insertion*, lingual fascia beneath the mucous membrane and epiglottis; *action*, depresses and protrudes the tongue; *nerve supply*, hypoglossal. SYN musculus genioglossus [TA], genioglossal m., genioglossus, musculus geniohyoglossus.

geniohyoid (m.) [TA], one of the suprahyoid muscles of the neck; *origin*, mental spine of mandible; *insertion*, body of hyoid bone; *action*, draws hyoid forward, or depresses jaw when hyoid is fixed; *nerve supply*, fibers from ventral primary rami of first and second cervical spinal nerves conveyed by the hypoglossal nerve. SYN musculus geniohyoideus [TA], geniohyoid, geniohyoideus.

gluteus maximus (m.) [TA], superficial muscle of buttock; *origin*, ilium behind posterior gluteal line, posterior surface of sacrum and coccyx, and sacrotuberous ligament; *insertion*, iliotibial band of fascia lata (superficial three-quarters) and gluteal ridge (deep inferior one-quarter) of femur; *action*, extends thigh, especially from the flexed position, as in climbing stairs or rising from

a sitting position; *nerve supply*, inferior gluteal. SYN musculus gluteus maximus [TA].

gluteus medius (m.) [TA], intermediate muscle of buttock; *origin*, ilium between anterior and posterior gluteal lines; *insertion*, lateral surface of greater trochanter; *action*, abducts and medially rotates thigh; *nerve supply*, superior gluteal. SYN musculus gluteus medius [TA], mesogluteus.

gluteus minimus (m.) [TA], deep muscle of buttock; *origin*, ilium between anterior and inferior gluteal lines; *insertion*, greater trochanter of femur; *action*, abducts and medially rotates thigh; *nerve supply*, superior gluteal. SYN musculus gluteus minimus [TA].

gracilis (m.) [TA], muscle of medial compartment of thigh; *origin*, ramus of pubis near symphysis; *insertion*, shaft of tibia below medial tuberosity (see *pes* anserinus); *action*, adducts thigh, flexes knee, rotates leg medially; *nerve supply*, obturator. SYN musculus gracilis [TA], gracilis (2).

great adductor m., SYN adductor magnus (m.).

greater pectoral m., SYN pectoralis major (m.).

greater posterior rectus m. of head, SYN rectus capitis posterior major (m.).

greater psoas m., SYN psoas major (m.).

greater rhomboid m., SYN rhomboid major (m.).

greater zygomatic m., SYN zygomaticus major (m.).

Guthrie m., SYN external urethral *sphincter*.

hamstring m.'s, the m.'s at the back of the thigh, comprising the long head of biceps, the semitendinosus, and the semimembranosus m.'s; hamstring m.'s arise from ischial tuberosity, act across both hip and knee joints, and are innervated by the tibial nerve.

m.'s of head [TA], the m.'s of expression, of mastication, and the suboccipital m.'s in general. SYN musculi capitis [TA].

m. of heart, SYN cardiac m.

helicis major (m.) [TA], auricular muscle occurring as a narrow band of muscular fibers on the anterior border of the helix of the auricle, arising from the spine and inserted at the point where the helix becomes transverse. SYN musculus helicis major [TA], large m. of helix.

helicis minor (m.) [TA], auricular muscle occurring as a band of oblique fibers covering the crus of the helix of the auricle. SYN musculus helicis minor [TA], smaller m. of helix.

Horner m., SYN lacrimal *part* of orbicularis oculi muscle; SEE orbicularis oculi (m.).

Houston m., SYN *compressor* venae dorsalis penis.

hyoglossal m., SYN hyoglossus (m.).

hyoglossus (m.) [TA], muscle of tongue; *origin*, body and greater horn of hyoid bone; *insertion*, side of the tongue; *action*, retracts and pulls down side of tongue; *nerve supply*, motor by hyoglossal, sensory by lingual. SYN musculus hyoglossus [TA], hyoglossal m., hyoglossus.

iliac m., SYN iliacus (m.).

iliacus (m.) [TA], *origin*, iliac fossa; *insertion*, via a common tendon with psoas major into anterior surface of lesser trochanter of the femur, and capsule of hip joint; *action*, flexes thigh and rotates it medially; *nerve supply*, lumbar plexus. SYN musculus iliacus [TA], iliac m.

iliacus minor (m.), the fibers of the iliacus arising from the anterior inferior iliac spine and inserted into the iliofemoral ligament, sometimes distinctly separate from the rest of the muscle. SYN musculus iliacus minor, musculus iliocapsularis.

iliococcygeal m., SYN iliococcygeus (m.).

iliococcygeus (m.) [TA], the posterior part of the levator ani; *origin*, tendinous arch of the levator ani muscle (obturator fascia); *insertion*, anococcygeal ligament and coccyx; *action*, resistance to increase intrapelvic pressure, postdefecatory elevation of anal canal. SYN musculus iliococcygeus [TA], iliococcygeal m.

iliocostal m., SYN iliocostalis (m.).

iliocostalis (m.) [TA], the lateral division of the erector spinae, having three subdivisions: iliocostalis lumborum m., iliocostalis thoracis m., and iliocostalis cervicis m. SYN musculus iliocostalis [TA], iliocostal m.

iliocostalis cervicis (m.) [TA], deep back (erector spinae) muscle;

mu

origin, angles of upper six ribs; *insertion*, transverse processes of middle cervical vertebrae; *action*, extends, abducts, and rotates cervical vertebrae; *nerve supply*, dorsal branches of upper thoracic nerves. SYN musculus iliocostalis cervicis [TA], cervical iliocostal m., cervicalis ascendens (1), musculus cervicalis ascendens.

iliocostalis lumborum (m.) [TA], deep back (erector spinae) muscle; *origin*, posterior aspect of sacrum and thoracolumbar fascia; *insertion*, the angles of lower six ribs; *action*, extends, abducts, and rotates lumbar vertebrae; *nerve supply*, dorsal branches of thoracic and lumbar nerves. SYN musculus iliocostalis lumborum [TA], lumbar iliocostal m., musculus sacrolumbalis.

iliocostalis thoracis (m.) [TA], deep back (erector spinae) muscle; *origin*, medial side of angles of lower six ribs; *insertion*, angles of upper six ribs; *action*, extends, abducts, and rotates thoracic vertebrae; *nerve supply*, dorsal branches of thoracic nerves. SYN musculus iliocostalis thoracis [TA], musculus iliocostalis dorsi.

iliopsoas (m.) [TA], a compound muscle, consisting of the iliacus m. and psoas major m. inserting via a common tendon into the anterior surface of the lesser trochanter of the femur. SYN musculus iliopsoas [TA].

index extensor (m.), SYN extensor indicis (m.).

inferior constrictor (m.) of pharynx [TA], lowest part of outer "circular" muscle layer of pharynx; *origin*, outer surfaces of thyroid (thyropharyngeal part [TA]) and cricoid (cricopharyngeal part [TA], musculus cricopharyngeus [TA]; superior or upper esophageal sphincter m.) cartilages; *insertion*, pharyngeal raphe in the posterior portion of wall of pharynx; *action*, narrows lower part of pharynx in swallowing, the cricopharyngeal part has a sphincteric function for the esophagus, allowing some voluntary control of eructation and reflux; *nerve supply*, pharyngeal plexus (cranial root of accessory nerve via the vagus) and rami of the external and recurrent laryngeal nerves. SYN musculus constrictor pharyngis inferior [TA], laryngopharyngeus, musculus laryngopharyngeus, superior esophageal sphincter.

inferior gemellus (m.) [TA], deep muscle of gluteal region; *origin*, tuberosity of ischium; *insertion*, tendon of m. obturator internus; *action*, rotates thigh laterally; *nerve supply*, sacral plexus. SYN musculus gemellus inferior [TA], gemellus.

inferior lingual m., SYN inferior longitudinal m. of tongue.

inferior longitudinal m. of tongue [TA], an intrinsic m. of the tongue, cylindrical in shape, occupying the underpart on either side; *action*, shortens the lower part of the tongue; *nerve supply*, motor by hypoglossal, sensory by lingual. SYN musculus longitudinalis inferior linguae [TA], inferior lingual m.

inferior oblique (m.) [TA], extraocular muscle in orbit; *origin*, orbital plate of maxilla lateral to the lacrimal groove; *insertion*, sclera between the superior and lateral recti; *action*, primary, extorsion; secondary, elevation and abduction; *nerve supply*, oculomotor (inferior branch). SYN musculus obliquus inferior [TA].

inferior oblique m. of head, SYN obliquus capitis inferior (m.).

inferior posterior serratus m., SYN serratus posterior inferior (m.).

inferior rectus (m.) [TA], extraocular muscle in orbit; *origin*, inferior part of the common tendinous ring; *insertion*, inferior part of sclera of the eye; *action*, primary, depression; secondary, adduction and extorsion; *nerve supply*, oculomotor (inferior branch). SYN musculus rectus inferior [TA].

inferior tarsal m. [TA], poorly developed smooth m. in the lower eyelid that acts to widen the palpebral fissure. SYN musculus tarsalis inferior [TA].

infrahyoid m.'s [TA], the small, flat m.'s inferior to the hyoid bone including the sternohyoid, omohyoid, sternothyroid, thyrohyoid, and levator m. of the thyroid gland. SYN musculi infrahyoidei [TA], strap m.'s.

infraspinatus (m.) [TA], intrinsic (scapulohumeral) muscle of shoulder joint, the tendon of which contributes to the formation of the rotator cuff; *origin*, infraspinous fossa of scapula; *insertion*, middle facet of greater tubercle of humerus; *action*, extends arm and rotates it laterally; its tonic contraction helps to hold the head of the humerus in the shallow glenoid fossa; *nerve supply*, suprascapular (from fifth to sixth cervical spinal nerves). SYN musculus infraspinatus [TA].

innermost intercostal (m.) [TA], flat muscle of thorax that occurs as a layer parallel to and essentially part of the internal intercostal m. but separated from it by the intercostal vessels and nerves. See also entries under internal intercostal muscle for attachment, action and nerve supply. SYN musculus intercostalis intimus [TA].

intermediate great m., SYN vastus intermedius (m.).

intermediate vastus (m.), SYN vastus intermedius (m.).

internal intercostal (m.) [TA], flat muscle of thorax arising from lower border of rib and passes obliquely downward and backward to be inserted into upper border of rib below; *action*, contract during expiration, also maintain tension in the intercostal spaces to resist mediolateral movement; *nerve supply*, intercostal. SYN musculus intercostalis internus [TA].

internal oblique (m.) [TA], flat muscle of anterolateral abdominal wall; *origin*, iliac fascia deep to lateral part of inguinal ligament, anterior half of crest of ilium, and lumbar fascia; *insertion*, tenth to twelfth ribs, with aponeurosis contributing to the sheath of rectus; some of the fibers from inguinal ligament terminate in the conjoint tendon; *action*, diminishes capacity of abdomen, flexes lumbar vertebral column (bends thorax forward); *nerve supply*, lower thoracic. SYN musculus obliquus internus abdominis [TA], abdominal internal oblique m.

internal obturator m., SYN obturator internus (m.).

internal pterygoid m., SYN medial pterygoid (m.).

internal m. m. of anus, SYN internal anal *sphincter*.

interosseous m.'s [TA], m.'s which arise from and run between the long (metacarpal and metatarsal) bones of the hand and foot, extending to and producing movement of the digits. SEE ALSO dorsal interossei (interosseous m.'s) of foot, dorsal interossei (interosseous m.'s) of hand, palmar interossei (interosseous m.'s), plantar interossei (interosseous m.'s). SYN musculi interossei [TA].

interspinal m.'s, SYN interspinales (m.'s).

interspinales (m.'s) [TA], the paired m.'s between spinous processes of adjacent vertebrae; subdivided into cervical, thoracic, and lumbar m.'s. SYN musculi interspinales [TA], interspinal m.'s.

interspinales cervicis (m.'s) [TA], continuation of deep back muscle into neck; *origin*, tubercle of spinous process of cervical vertebra; *insertion*, tubercle of spinous process of next superior vertebra; *action*, extends the neck; *nerve supply*, dorsal rami of cervical nerves. SYN cervical interspinal m., cervical interspinales m.'s, musculus interspinalis cervicis.

interspinales lumborum (m.'s) [TA], deep muscle of lower back; *origin*, superior margin of lumbar spinous process; *insertion*, inferior margin of next superior spinous process; *action*, extends lumbar vertebrae; *nerve supply*, dorsal primary rami of lumbar spinal nerves. SYN musculus interspinalis lumborum [TA], lumbar interspinal m.

interspinales thoracis (m.'s) [TA], often poorly developed or absent deep muscles of back spanning between spinous process of thoracic vertebrae; *action*, extends thoracic vertebrae; *nerve supply*, dorsal primary rami of thoracic nerves. SYN musculus interspinalis thoracis [TA], thoracic interspinal m., thoracic interspinales m.'s.

intertransversarii (m.'s) [TA], the paired m.'s between transverse processes of adjacent vertebrae; there are anterior and posterior m.'s in the cervical region; lateral and medial m.'s in the lumbar region; and single m.'s in the thoracic region. SYN musculi intertransversarii [TA], intertransverse m.'s.

intertransverse m.'s, SYN intertransversarii (m.'s).

intrinsic m.'s, m.'s fully contained (origin, belly, and insertion) within the structure under consideration. For example, the interossei and lumbrical m.'s are intrinsic m.'s of the hand.

intrinsic m.'s of foot, m.'s fully contained (origin, belly, insertion) in the foot and toes. These m.'s are arranged in four layers and all are innervated by the plantar branches of the tibial nerve. Although they may be capable of producing the actions described under their individual entries, as a group the primary function of the intrinsic m.'s of the foot is to provide dynamic support of the longitudinal arch of the foot, resisting the forces which act momentarily to spread the arch during walking and running.

involuntary m.'s, m.'s not ordinarily under control of the will; except in the case of the heart, they are composed of smooth (nonstriated) muscle fibers, innervated by the autonomic nervous system.

ischiocavernous (m.) [TA], muscle of urogenital triangle; *origin*, ramus of ischium; *insertion*, corpus cavernosum penis (or clitoridis); *action*, compresses the crus of the penis (or clitoris) forcing blood in its sinuses into the distal part of the corpus cavernosum and diminishing egress of venous blood; *nerve supply*, pudendal (perineal). SYN musculus ischiocavernosus [TA], musculus erector clitoridis, musculus erector penis.

Jung m., SYN pyramidal m. of auricle.

Kohlrausch m., the longitudinal m.'s of the rectal wall.

Landström m., microscopic m. fibers in the fascia behind and about the eyeball, attached anteriorly to the lids and anterior orbital fascia; its action is to draw the eyeball forward and the lids backward, resisting the pull of the four orbital m.'s.

Langer m., SYN pectorodorsalis m.

large m. of helix, SYN helicis major (m.).

m.'s of larynx [TA], the intrinsic m.'s that regulate the length, position, and tension of the vocal cords and serve as sphincters and dilators of the airway, adjusting the size of the openings between the aryepiglottic folds, the ventricular folds and the vocal folds. SYN musculi laryngis [TA].

lateral cricoarytenoid (m.) [TA], an intrinsic muscle of larynx; *origin*, upper margin of arch of cricoid cartilage; *insertion*, muscular process of arytenoid; *action*, adducts vocal folds (narrows rima glottidis); *nerve supply*, recurrent laryngeal. SYN musculus cricoarytenoideus lateralis [TA].

lateral great m., SYN vastus lateralis (m.).

lateral lumbar intertransversarii (m.'s) [TA], deep muscle of lower back; *origin*, transverse processes of lumbar vertebrae; *insertion*, next superior transverse process; *action*, abducts lumbar vertebrae; *nerve supply*, ventral branches of lumbar nerves. SYN musculi intertransversarii laterales lumborum [TA], lateral lumbar intertransverse m.'s.

lateral lumbar intertransverse m.'s, SYN lateral lumbar intertransversarii (m.'s).

lateral posterior cervical intertransversarii m.'s [TA], SEE posterior cervical intertransversarii (m.'s).

lateral pterygoid (m.) [TA], masticatory muscle of infratemporal fossa; *origin*, inferior head from lateral lamina of pterygoid process; superior head from infratemporal crest and adjacent greater wing of the sphenoid; *insertion*, into pterygoid fovea of mandible and articular disk and capsule of temporomandibular joint; *action*, protrudes lower jaw to enable opening of mouth; unilateral contraction deviates chin laterally, enabling grinding motion for chewing; *nerve supply*, nerve to lateral pterygoid from mandibular division of trigeminal. SYN musculus pterygoideus lateralis [TA], external pterygoid m., musculus pterygoideus externus.

lateral rectus (m.) [TA], extraocular muscle in orbit; *origin*, lateral part of the common tendinous ring that bridges superior orbital fissure; *insertion*, lateral part of sclera of eye; *action*, abduction; *nerve supply*, abducens. SYN musculus rectus lateralis [TA], abducens oculi, musculus rectus externus.

lateral rectus m. of the head, SYN rectus capitis lateralis (m.).

lateral vastus (m.), SYN vastus lateralis (m.).

latissimus dorsi (m.) [TA], thoracoappendicular muscle (superficial muscle of back); *origin*, spinous processes of lower five or six thoracic and the lumbar vertebrae, median ridge of sacrum, and outer lip of iliac crest; *insertion*, with teres major into posterior lip of bicipital groove of humerus; *action*, adducts arm, rotates it medially, and extends it; *nerve supply*, thoracodorsal. SYN musculus latissimus dorsi [TA], broadest m. of back.

lesser rhomboid m., SYN rhomboid minor (m.).

lesser zygomatic m., SYN zygomaticus minor (m.).

levator anguli oris (m.) [TA], facial muscle of upper lip; *origin*, canine fossa of maxilla; *insertion*, orbicularis oris and skin at angle of mouth; *action*, raises angle of mouth; *nerve supply*, facial. SYN musculus levator anguli oris [TA], musculus caninus, musculus triangularis labii superioris.

levator ani (m.) [TA], compound muscle of pelvis; formed by pubococcygeus and iliococcygeus m.'s; *origin*, posterior body of pubis, tendinous arch of the levator ani (obturator fascia), and spine of ischium; *insertion*, anococcygeal ligament, sides of the lower part of the sacrum and of coccyx; *action*, resists prolapsing forces and draws the anus upward following defecation; supports the pelvic viscera; *nerve supply*, nerve to levator ani (fourth sacral spinal nerve). SYN musculus levator ani [TA], elevator m. of anus.

levatores costarum longi (m.'s) [TA], vertebrothoracic (costovertebral) muscles; *insertion*, the second rib below their origin; *action*, raise ribs; *nerve supply*, intercostal. SYN musculi levatores costarum longi [TA], long levatores costarum (m.'s).

levatores costarum (m.'s) [TA], muscle of thorax; *origin*, tips of transverse processes of C7 and T1–T11 vertebrae; *insertion*, ribs, between tubercle and angle; *action*, elevate ribs for deep inspiration; *nerve*, dorsal rami of C8–T11 spinal nerves. SEE levatores costarum longi (m.'s), levatores costarum breves (m.'s). SYN musculi levatores costarum [TA], elevator m. of rib, musculus levator costae.

levatores costarum breves (m.'s) [TA], *origin*, the transverse processes of last cervical and eleven thoracic vertebrae; *insertion* ribs immediately below, between angle and tubercle. SYN musculi levatores costarum breves [TA], short levatores costarum (m.'s).

levator labii superioris (m.) [TA], facial muscle of upper lip; *origin*, maxilla below infraorbital foramen; *insertion*, interspersed with orbicularis oris to reach skin of upper lip; *action*, elevates upper lip; *nerve supply*, facial. SYN musculus levator labii superioris [TA], caput infraorbitale quadrati labii superioris, elevator m. of upper lip.

levator labii superioris alaeque nasi (m.) [TA], facial muscle of upper lip and nose; *origin*, root of nasal process of maxilla; *insertion*, wing of nose and orbicularis oris m. of upper lip; *action*, elevates upper lip and wing of nose; *nerve supply*, facial. SYN musculus levator labii superioris alaeque nasi [TA], caput angulare quadrati labii superioris, elevator m. of upper lip and wing of nose.

levator palati (m.), SYN levator veli palatini (m.).

levator palpebrae superioris (m.) [TA], extraocular muscle in orbit; *origin*, orbital surface of the lesser wing of the sphenoid, above and anterior to the optic canal; *insertion*, skin of eyelid, tarsal plate, and orbital walls, by medial and lateral expansions of the aponeurosis of insertion; *action*, raises the upper eyelid; *nerve supply*, oculomotor. SYN musculus levator palpebrae superioris [TA], elevator (m.) of upper eyelid, musculus orbitopalpebralis, palpebralis.

levator prostatae (m.), ✱ official alternate term for puboprostaticus (m.).

levator scapulae (m.) [TA], extrinsic muscle of the shoulder; *origin*, from posterior tubercles of transverse processes of four upper cervical vertebrae; *insertion*, into superior angle of scapula; *action*, raises the scapula; *nerve supply*, dorsal scapular nerve. SYN musculus levator scapulae [TA], elevator (m.) of scapula, musculus levator anguli scapulae.

levator (m.) of thyroid gland [TA], a fasciculus occasionally passing from the thyrohyoid m. to the isthmus of the thyroid gland. SYN musculus levator glandulae thyroideae [TA], elevator (m.) of thyroid gland, Soemmerring m.

levator veli palatini (m.) [TA], muscle of soft palate; *origin*, apex of petrous portion of temporal bone and lower part of cartilaginous pharyngotympanic (auditory) tube; *insertion*, aponeurosis of soft palate; *action*, raises soft palate; through the expansion of its fleshy belly during contraction, it helps to "push" open the auditory tube for equilibration of pressure; *nerve supply*, pharyngeal plexus (cranial root of accessory nerve). SYN musculus levator veli palatini [TA], (elevator) m. of soft palate, levator palati (m.), musculus levator palati, musculus petrostaphylinus.

lingual m.'s, SYN m.'s of tongue.

long abductor m. of thumb, SYN abductor pollicis longus (m.).

long adductor m., SYN adductor longus (m.).

long extensor (m.) of great toe, SYN extensor hallucis longus (m.).

long extensor (m.) of thumb, SYN extensor pollicis longus (m.).

long extensor (m.) of toes, SYN extensor digitorum longus (m.).

long fibular m., SYN fibularis longus (m.).

mu

long flexor (m.) of great toe, SYN flexor hallucis longus (m.).

long flexor m. of thumb, SYN flexor pollicis longus (m.).

long flexor (m.) of toes, SYN flexor digitorum longus (m.).

long m. of head, SYN longus capitis (m.).

longissimus (m.) [TA], the intermediate division of the erector spinae m. having three subdivisions: longissimus capitis m., longissimus cervicis m., and longissimus thoracis m. SYN musculus longissimus [TA].

longissimus capitis (m.) [TA], intermediate erector spinae muscle in neck; *origin*, from transverse processes of upper thoracic and transverse and articular processes of lower and middle cervical vertebrae; *insertion*, into mastoid process; *action*, keeps head erect, draws it backward or to one side; *nerve supply*, dorsal primary rami of cervical spinal nerves. SYN musculus longissimus capitis [TA], musculus complexus minor, musculus trachelomastoideus, musculus transversalis capitis.

longissimus cervicis (m.) [TA], intermediate erector spinae muscle in neck; *origin*, transverse processes of upper thoracic vertebrae; *insertion*, transverse processes of middle and upper cervical vertebrae; *action*, extends cervical vertebrae; *nerve supply*, dorsal primary rami of lower cervical and upper thoracic spinal nerves. SYN musculus longissimus cervicis [TA], cervical longissimus m., musculus transversalis cervicis, musculus transversalis colli.

longissimus thoracis (m.) [TA], intermediate erector spinae muscle of back; *origin*, with iliocostalis and from transverse processes of lower thoracic vertebrae; *insertion*, by lateral slips into most or all of the ribs between angles and tubercles and into tips of transverse processes of upper lumbar vertebrae, and by medial slips into accessory processes of upper lumbar and transverse processes of thoracic vertebrae; *action*, extends vertebral column; *nerve supply*, dorsal primary rami of thoracic and lumbar spinal nerves. SYN musculus longissimus thoracis [TA], musculus longissimus dorsi, thoracic longissimus m.

long levatores costarum (m.'s), SYN levatores costarum longi (m.'s).

long m. of neck, SYN longus colli (m.).

long palmar m., SYN palmaris longus (m.).

long peroneal m., SYN fibularis longus (m.).

long radial extensor m. of wrist, SYN extensor carpi radialis longus (m.).

longus capitis (m.) [TA], prevertebral muscle of neck; *origin*, anterior tubercles of transverse processes of third to sixth cervical vertebrae; *insertion*, basilar process of occipital bone; *action*, twists or flexes neck anteriorly; *nerve supply*, cervical plexus. SYN musculus longus capitis [TA], long m. of head, musculus rectus capitis anticus major.

longus colli (m.) [TA], prevertebral muscle of neck; medial part: *origin*, the bodies of the third thoracic to the fifth cervical vertebrae; *insertion*, the bodies of the second to fourth cervical vertebrae; superolateral part: *origin*, the anterior tubercles of the transverse processes of the third to fifth cervical vertebrae; *insertion*, the anterior tubercle of the atlas; inferolateral part: *origin*, the bodies of the first to third thoracic vertebrae; *insertion*, the anterior tubercles of the transverse processes of the fifth and sixth cervical vertebrae; *action*, for all three parts, twist neck and flex neck anteriorly; *nerve supply*, for all three parts, ventral primary rami of cervical spinal nerves (cervical plexus). SYN musculus longus colli [TA], long m. of neck.

lumbar iliocostal m., SYN iliocostalis lumborum (m.).

lumbar interspinal m., SYN interspinales lumborum (m.'s).

lumbar quadrate m., SYN quadratus lumborum (m.).

lumbar rotator m.'s, SYN rotatores lumborum (m.'s).

lumbricals (lumbrical m.'s) of foot [TA], four intrinsic m.'s of second layer of plantar muscles; *origin*, first: from tibial side of tendon to second toe of flexor digitorum longus; second, third, and fourth: from adjacent sides of all four tendons of this m.; *insertion*, tibial side of extensor tendon on dorsum of each of the four lateral toes; *action*, flex the proximal and extend the middle and distal phalanges; *nerve supply*, lateral (second to fourth lumbricals) and medial (first lumbrical) plantar. SYN musculus lumbricalis pedis [TA].

lumbricals (lumbrical m.'s) of hand [TA], four intrinsic mus-

cles of the palm; *origin*, the two lateral: from the radial side of the tendons of the flexor digitorum profundus going to the index and middle fingers; the two medial: from the adjacent sides of the second and third, and third and fourth tendons; *insertion*, radial side of extensor tendon on dorsum of each of the four fingers; *action*, flexes metacarpophalangeal joint and extends the proximal and distal interphalangeal joint; *nerve supply*, the two radial m.'s by the median, the two ulnar m.'s by the ulnar. SYN musculus lumbricalis manus [TA].

Marcacci m., a sheet of smooth m. fibers underlying the areola and nipple of the mammary gland.

masseter (m.) [TA], masticatory muscle of posterior cheek; *origin*, superficial part: inferior border of the anterior two-thirds of the zygomatic arch; deep part: inferior border and medial surface of the zygomatic arch; *insertion*, lateral surface of ramus and coronoid process of the mandible; *action*, elevates mandible (closes jaw); *nerve supply*, masseteric branch of mandibular division of trigeminal. SYN musculus masseter [TA].

m.'s of mastication, SYN masticatory m.'s.

masticatory m.'s [TA], m.'s derived from the first (mandibular) arch used in chewing; all receive innervation from the motor root of the trigeminal nerve via its mandibular division; includes masseter m., temporalis m., lateral pterygoid m., and medial pterygoid m. SYN m.'s of mastication.

medial great m., SYN vastus medialis (m.).

medial lumbar intertransversarii (m.'s) [TA], part of deep muscles of back; *origin*, accessory and mammillary processes of lumbar vertebrae; *insertion*, corresponding processes of next superior vertebra; *action*, abducts lumbar vertebrae; *nerve supply*, dorsal primary rami of lumbar spinal nerves. SYN musculi intertransversarii mediales lumborum [TA], medial lumbar intertransverse m.'s.

medial lumbar intertransverse m.'s, SYN medial lumbar intertransversarii (m.'s).

medial posterior cervical intertransversarii (m.'s, SEE posterior cervical intertransversarii (m.'s).

medial pterygoid (m.) [TA], masticatory muscle of infratemporal fossa; *origin*, pterygoid fossa of sphenoid and tuberosity of maxilla; *insertion*, medial surface of mandible between angle and mylohyoid groove; *action*, elevates mandible closing jaw; *nerve supply*, nerve to medial pterygoid from mandibular division of trigeminal. SYN musculus pterygoideus medialis [TA], internal pterygoid m., musculus pterygoideus internus.

medial rectus (m.) [TA], extraocular muscle in orbit; *origin*, medial part of the anulus tendineus communis; *insertion*, medial part of sclera of the eye; *action*, adduction; *nerve supply*, oculomotor. SYN musculus rectus medialis [TA], musculus rectus internus.

medial vastus (m.), SYN vastus medialis (m.).

mentalis (m.) [TA], facial muscle of chin; *origin*, incisor fossa of mandible; *insertion*, skin of chin; *action*, raises and wrinkles skin of chin, thus elevating the lower lip; *nerve supply*, facial. SYN musculus mentalis [TA], chin m., musculus levator labii inferioris.

Merkel m., SYN ceratocricoid (m.).

middle constrictor (m.) of pharynx [TA], intermediate part of outer "circular" muscle layer of pharynx; *origin*, stylohyoid ligament, lesser cornu of the hyoid bone (chondropharyngeal part [TA]) and greater cornu of the hyoid bone (ceratopharyngeal part [TA]); *insertion*, pharyngeal raphe in the posterior wall of the pharynx; *action*, narrows pharynx in the act of swallowing; *nerve supply*, pharyngeal plexus. SYN musculus constrictor pharyngis medius [TA].

middle scalene m., ✱official alternate term for scalenus medius (m.).

mimetic m.'s, SYN facial m.'s.

Müller m., (1) SYN orbitalis (m.); (2) SYN circular *fibers*, under *fiber*; (3) SYN superior tarsal m.

multifidus (m.) [TA], intermediate layer of deepest (transversospinales) muscles of back; *origin*, from the sacrum, sacroiliac ligament, mamillary processes of the lumbar vertebrae, transverse processes of thoracic vertebrae, and articular processes of last four cervical vertebrae; *insertion*, into the spinous processes of all the vertebrae up to and including the axis; *action*, rotates vertebral column; *nerve supply*, dorsal primary rami of spinal nerves. SYN musculus multifidus [TA], musculus multifidus spinae.

multipennate m. [TA], a m. with several central tendons toward which the m. fibers converge like the barbs of feathers. SYN musculus multipennatus [TA].

mylohyoid (m.) [TA], muscle of floor of mouth; *origin*, mylohyoid line of mandible; *insertion*, upper border of hyoid bone and raphe separating m. from its fellow; *action*, elevates floor of mouth and the tongue, depresses jaw when hyoid is fixed; *nerve supply*, nerve to mylohyoid from mandibular division of trigeminal. SYN musculus mylohyoideus [TA], diaphragm of mouth, diaphragma oris, mylohyoideus.

nasal m., SYN nasalis (m.).

nasalis (m.) [TA], facial muscle of nose; compound m. consisting of: a transverse part [TA] (pars transversa [TA], musculus compressor naris) arising from the maxilla above the root of the canine tooth on each side and forming an aponeurosis across the bridge of the nose; and an alar part [TA] (pars alaris [TA], musculus dilator naris) arising from the maxilla above the lateral incisor and attaching to the wing of the nose; the alar part dilates the nostril; *nerve supply*, facial. SYN musculus nasalis [TA], nasal m.

m.'s of neck [TA], the anterolateral m.'s of the neck including the platysma, sternocleidomastoid, suprahyoid m.'s, infrahyoid m.'s, longus colli and scalene m.'s. SYN musculi colli [TA], musculi cervicis ✫.

m. of notch of helix, SYN m. of terminal notch.

oblique arytenoid m. [TA], intrinsic laryngeal muscle; *origin*, muscular process of arytenoid cartilage; *insertion*, summit of arytenoid cartilage of opposite side and continuing as the aryepiglottic muscle in the aryepiglottic fold to the epiglottis; *action*, narrows or closes the interarytenoid portion of the rima glottidis; *nerve supply*, recurrent laryngeal. SYN musculus arytenoideus obliquus [TA], arytenoideus.

oblique m. of auricle [TA], a thin band of oblique muscular fibers extending from the upper part of the eminence of the concha to the convexity of the helix, running across the groove corresponding to the inferior crus of the anthelix. SYN musculus obliquus auriculae [TA], oblique auricular m., Tod m.

oblique auricular m., SYN oblique m. of auricle.

obliquus capitis inferior (m.) [TA], suboccipital muscle that, despite its name, has no attachment to the cranium; *origin*, spinous process of axis; *insertion*, transverse process of the atlas; *action*, rotates head; *origin*, spinous process of axis; *insertion*, transverse process of the atlas; *nerve supply*, suboccipital. SEE ALSO suboccipital m.'s. SYN musculus obliquus capitis inferior [TA], inferior oblique m. of head.

obliquus capitis superior (m.) [TA], suboccipital muscle; *origin*, transverse process of atlas; *insertion*, lateral third of inferior nuchal line; *action*, rotates head; *nerve supply*, suboccipital. SEE ALSO suboccipital m.'s. SYN musculus obliquus capitis superior [TA], superior oblique m. of head.

obturator externus (m.) [TA], muscle of medial (adductor) compartment of thigh; *origin*, lower half of margin of obturator foramen and adjacent part of external surface of obturator membrane; *insertion*, trochanteric fossa of greater trochanter; *action*, rotates thigh laterally; *nerve supply*, obturator. SYN musculus obturator externus [TA], external obturator m.

obturator internus (m.) [TA], intrapelvic muscle extending into gluteal region; *origin*, pelvic surface of obturator membrane and margin of obturator foramen; *insertion*, passes out of pelvis through lesser sciatic foramen, in so doing, making a 90° turn to insert into the medial surface of greater trochanter; *action*, rotates thigh laterally; *nerve supply*, nerve to obturator internus (sacral plexus). SYN musculus obturator internus [TA], internal obturator m.

occipitalis m., SYN occipital *belly* of occipitofrontalis muscle.

occipitofrontal m., SYN occipitofrontalis (m.).

occipitofrontalis (m.) [TA], compound facial muscle part of epicranius muscle; the occipital belly (occipitalis m.) arises from the occipital bone and inserts into the galea aponeurotica; the frontal belly (frontalis m.) arises from the galea and inserts into the skin of the eyebrow and nose; *action*, to move the scalp; *nerve supply*, facial. SYN musculus occipitofrontalis [TA], occipitofrontal m.

ocular m.'s, SYN extraocular m.'s.

Oehl m.'s, strands of m. fibers in the chordae tendineae of the left atrioventricular valve.

omohyoid (m.) [TA], infrahyoid muscle; formed of two bellies attached to intermediate tendon; *origin*, by inferior belly from upper border of scapula between superior angle and notch; *insertion*, by superior belly into hyoid bone; *action*, depresses hyoid; *nerve supply*, upper cervical spinal nerves through ansa cervicalis. SYN musculus omohyoideus [TA], omohyoid.

opponens m. [TA], m. that facilitates the opposing of pad of distal phalanx of thumb to the pads of other fingers, especially that of the little finger. SYN musculus opponens [TA].

opponens digiti minimi (m.) [TA], hypothenar muscle of palm; *origin*, hamulus of the hamate bone and transverse carpal ligament; *insertion*, shaft of fifth metacarpal; *action*, "cups" palm, drawing ulnar side of hand toward center of palm; *nerve supply*, ulnar. SYN musculus opponens digiti minimi [TA], musculus opponens digiti quinti, musculus opponens minimi digiti, opposer (m.) of little finger.

opponens pollicis (m.) [TA], thenar muscle of palm; *origin*, ridge of trapezium and transverse carpal ligament (flexor retinaculum); *insertion*, anterior surface of the full length of the shaft of the first metacarpal bone; *action*, acts at carpometacarpal joint to "cup" palm, enabling one to oppose thumb to other fingers; *nerve supply*, median. SYN musculus opponens pollicis [TA], opposer (m.) of thumb.

opposer (m.) of little finger, SYN opponens digiti minimi (m.).

opposer (m.) of thumb, SYN opponens pollicis (m.).

orbicular m. [TA], a sphincterlike sheet of m. that encircles an orifice such as the mouth or the palpebral fissures. SYN musculus orbicularis [TA], orbicularis m., orbicularis (2).

orbicular m. of eye, SYN orbicularis oculi (m.).

orbicularis m., SYN orbicular m.

orbicularis oculi (m.) [TA], facial muscle of eyelids; consists of three portions: orbital part, or external portion, which arises from frontal process of maxilla and nasal process of frontal bone, encircles aperture of orbit, and is inserted near origin; palpebral part, or internal portion, which arises from medial palpebral ligament, passes through each eyelid, and is inserted into lateral palpebral raphe; lacrimal part (tensor tarsi muscle, Duverney or Horner muscle) arises from posterior lacrimal crest and passes across lacrimal sac to join palpebral portion; *action*, closes eye, wrinkles forehead vertically; *nerve supply*, zygomatic and temporal branches of facial. SYN musculus orbicularis oculi [TA], musculus orbicularis palpebrarum, orbicular m. of eye, sphincter oculi.

orbicularis oris (m.) [TA], facial muscle of mouth; *origin*, by nasolabial band from septum of the nose, by superior incisive bundle from incisor fossa of maxilla, by inferior incisive bundle from lower jaw each side of symphysis; *insertion*, fibers surround mouth between skin and mucous membrane of lips and cheeks, and are blended with other m.'s; *action*, closes lips; *nerve supply*, facial. SYN musculus orbicularis oris [TA], musculus sphincter oris, orbicular m. of mouth, sphincter oris.

orbicular m. of mouth, SYN orbicularis oris (m.).

orbital m., SYN orbitalis (m.).

orbitalis (m.) [TA], a rudimentary nonstriated m., crossing the infraorbital groove and sphenomaxillary fissure, intimately united with the periosteum of the orbit. SYN musculus orbitalis [TA], Müller m. (1), orbital m.

palatoglossus (m.) [TA], palatine muscle that forms anterior pillar of tonsillar fossa; *origin*, oral surface of soft palate; *insertion*, side of tongue; *action*, raises back of tongue and narrows fauces; *nerve supply*, pharyngeal plexus (cranial root of accessory nerve). SYN musculus palatoglossus [TA], glossopalatinus, musculus glossopalatinus, palatoglossus.

palatopharyngeal (m.), SYN palatopharyngeus (m.).

palatopharyngeus (m.) [TA], *origin*, soft palate; forms the posterior pillar of the fauces or tonsillar fossa; *insertion*, posterior border of thyroid cartilage and aponeurosis of pharynx as it be-

mu

comes part of the inner longitudinal muscle layer of the pharynx; *action*, narrows fauces, depresses soft palate, elevates pharynx and larynx; *nerve supply*, pharyngeal plexus (cranial root of accessory nerve). SYN musculus palatopharyngeus [TA], musculus pharyngopalatinus, palatopharyngeal (m.), palatopharyngeus, pharyngopalatinus, pharyngostaphylinus.

palatouvularis m., SYN m. of uvula.

palmar interossei (interosseous m.'s) [TA], three intrinsic m.'s in the hand; *origin*, first: ulnar side of second metacarpal; second and third: radial sides of fourth and fifth metacarpals; *insertion*, first: into ulnar side of index; second and third: into radial sides of ring and little fingers; *action*, adducts fingers toward axis of middle finger; *nerve supply*, ulnar. SEE ALSO flexor pollicis brevis (m.). SYN musculus interosseus palmaris [TA], musculus interosseus volaris.

palmaris brevis (m.) [TA], cutaneous muscle of hand; *origin*, ulnar side of central portion of the palmar aponeurosis; *insertion*, skin of ulnar side of hand; *action*, wrinkles skin on medial side of palm; *nerve supply*, ulnar. SYN musculus palmaris brevis [TA], short palmar m.

palmaris longus (m.) [TA], muscle of superficial layer of anterior (flexor) compartment of forearm; *origin*, medial epicondyle of humerus; *insertion*, flexor retinaculum of wrist and palmar fascia; *action*, tenses palmar fascia and flexes the hand and forearm; is absent about 20% of the time; when tensed, its tendon stands out sharply at the wrist and overlies the median nerve; *nerve supply*, median. SYN musculus palmaris longus [TA], long palmar m.

panniculus carnosus m., (1) a sheet of m., lying beneath the skin, by which the skin can be made to shiver; it is especially well developed in the horse; (2) in humans, platysma.

papillary m. [TA], one of the group of myocardial bundles which terminate in the chordae tendineae that attach to the cusps of the atrioventricular valves; each ventricle has an anterior and a posterior papillary muscle; the right ventricle sometimes has a septal papillary muscle. SYN musculus papillaris [TA].

pectinate m.'s [TA], prominent ridges of atrial myocardium located on the inner surface of much of the right atrium and both auricles. SYN musculi pectinati [TA], pectinate fibers.

pectineal m., SYN pectineus (m.).

pectineus (m.) [TA], *origin*, crest of pubis; *insertion*, pectineal line of femur; *action*, adducts thigh and assists in flexion; *nerve supply*, obturator and femoral. SYN musculus pectineus [TA], pectineal m.

pectoralis major (m.) [TA], superficial thoracoappendicular muscle of chest; *origin*, clavicular part [TA] (pars clavicularis [TA]), medial half of clavicle; sternocostal part [TA] (pars sternocostalis [TA]), anterior surface of manubrium and body of sternum and cartilages of first to sixth ribs; abdominal part [TA] (pars abdominalis [TA]), aponeurosis of external oblique; *insertion*, crest of greater tubercle of humerus; *action*, adducts and medially rotates arm; *nerve supply*, anterior thoracic. SYN musculus pectoralis major [TA], greater pectoral m.

pectoralis minor (m.) [TA], deep thoracoappendicular muscle of chest; *origin*, third to fifth ribs at the costochondral articulations; *insertion*, tip of coracoid process of scapula; *action*, draws down scapula or raises ribs; *nerve supply*, medial pectoral nerve. SYN musculus pectoralis minor [TA], smaller pectoral m.

pectorodorsal m., SYN pectorodorsalis m.

pectorodorsalis m., an anomalous m. or tendinus slip that passes across the axilla from the pectoralis major to insert with the latissimus dorsi onto the humerus. Though to be a vestige of the panniculus carnosus muscle of lower mammals. SYN axillary arch m., axillary arch, Langer arch, Langer m., pectorodorsal m.

pennate m., a muscle with a central tendon toward which the fibers converge on either side like the barbs of a feather. SYN musculus pennatus [TA], bipennate m., musculus bipennatus. SEE semipennate m.

perineal m.'s [TA], the muscles located in the perineal region; these are the external anal sphincter, the superficial transverse perineal m., ischiocavernosus m., bulbospongiosus m., deep transverse perineal m., and sphincter urethrae m. SYN musculi perinei [TA].

peroneus brevis (m.), ☆official alternate term for fibularis brevis (m.).

peroneus longus (m.), ☆official alternate term for fibularis longus (m.).

peroneus tertius (m.), ☆official alternate term for fibularis tertius (m.).

piriform m., SYN piriformis (m.).

piriformis (m.) [TA], muscle extending from pelvis into gluteal region; *origin*, margins of pelvic sacral foramina and greater sciatic notch of ilium; *insertion*, upper border of greater trochanter; *action*, rotates thigh laterally; *nerve supply*, nerve to piriformis (sciatic plexus). SYN musculus piriformis [TA], musculus pyriformis, piriform m.

plantar m., SYN plantaris (m.).

plantar interossei (interosseous m.'s), three intrinsic m.'s of foot; *origin*, the medial side of the third, fourth, and fifth metatarsal bones; *insertion*, corresponding side of proximal phalanx of the same toes; *action*, adducts three lateral toes; *nerve supply*, lateral plantar. SYN musculi interossei plantaris [TA].

plantaris (m.) [TA], small muscle of superficial posterior (plantar flexor) compartment of leg; *origin*, lateral supracondylar ridge; *insertion*, medial margin of tendo achillis and deep fascia of ankle; *action*, traditionally described as plantar flexion of foot; many investigators now believe the plantaris muscle to be primarily a proprioceptive organ; *nerve supply*, tibial nerve. SYN musculus plantaris [TA], musculus tibialis gracilis, plantar m.

plantar quadrate m., SYN quadratus plantae (m.).

platysma (m.) [TA], facial muscle in neck region; *origin*, subcutaneous layer and fascia covering pectoralis major and deltoid at level of first or second rib; *insertion*, lower border of mandible, risorius and platysma of opposite side; *action*, depresses lower lip, forms ridges in skin of neck and upper chest when jaws are "clenched", denoting stress, anger; *nerve supply*, cervical branch of facial. SYN platysma [TA], musculus platysma myoides, musculus platysma, musculus subcutaneus colli, musculus tetragonus.

pleuroesophageal (m.), SYN pleuroesophageus (m.).

pleuroesophageus (m.) [TA], muscular fasciculi, arising from the mediastinal pleura, which reinforce musculature of esophagus. SYN musculus pleuroesophageus [TA], pleuroesophageal (m.).

popliteal m., SYN popliteus (m.).

popliteus (m.) [TA], muscle forming floor of popliteal fossa; *origin*, lateral condyle of femur; *insertion*, posterior surface of tibia above oblique line; *action*, from the fully extended and "locked" position, rotates the femur medially, on the fixed (planted) tibial plateau about 5°, "unlocking" the knee to enable flexion to occur; *nerve supply*, tibial. SYN musculus popliteus [TA], popliteal m., popliteus (3).

posterior auricular (m.), SYN auricularis posterior (m.).

posterior cervical intertransversarii (m.'s) [TA], *origin*, lateral muscles: posterior tubercle of cervical transverse process; medial muscles: transverse process; *insertion*, corresponding parts of next superior transverse process; *action*, abducts cervical vertebrae; *nerve supply*, lateral part: ventral primary rami of cervical spinal nerves; medial part: dorsal primary rami of cervical spinal nerves. SYN musculi intertransversarii posteriores cervicis [TA], posterior cervical intertransverse m.'s.

posterior cervical intertransverse m.'s, SYN posterior cervical intertransversarii (m.'s).

posterior cricoarytenoid (m.) [TA], intrinsic muscle of larynx; *origin*, depression on posterior surface of lamina of cricoid; *insertion*, muscular process of arytenoid; *action*, abducts vocal folds, widening rima glottidis as for taking a deep breath; *nerve supply*, recurrent laryngeal. SYN musculus cricoarytenoideus posterior [TA].

posterior scalene m., ☆official alternate term for scalenus posterior (m.).

posterior tibial m., SYN tibialis posterior (m.).

Pozzi m., SYN extensor digitorum brevis (m.) of hand.

procerus (m.) [TA], facial muscle of central forehead; *insertion*, into frontalis; *action*, assists frontalis; *origin*, from membrane covering bridge of nose; *nerve supply*, branch of facial. SYN musculus procerus [TA], musculus pyramidalis nasi, procerus.

pronator (m.) [TA], m. that twists forearm about a longitudinal axis from the supinated or neutral position toward one in which the dorsum of the hand is directed anteriorly from the anatomical position. SYN musculus pronator [TA].

pronator quadratus (m.) [TA], muscle of deep layer of anterior (flexor) compartment of forearm; *origin*, distal fourth of anterior surface of ulna; *insertion*, distal fourth of anterior surface of radius; *action*, pronates forearm; *nerve supply*, anterior interosseous. SYN musculus pronator quadratus [TA], quadrate pronator m.

pronator teres (m.) [TA], muscle of superficial layer of anterior compartment of forearm; *origin*, superficial (humeral) head from the common flexor origin on the medial epicondyle of the humerus, deep (ulnar) head from the medial side of the coronoid process of the ulna; *insertion*, middle of the lateral surface of the radius; *action*, pronates forearm; *nerve supply*, median. SYN musculus pronator teres [TA], musculus pronator radii teres, round pronator m.

psoas major (m.) [TA], groin muscle; *origin*, bodies of vertebrae and intervertebral disks from the twelfth thoracic to the fifth lumbar, and transverse processes of the lumbar vertebrae; *insertion*, forms a common insertion with iliacus m.'s into lesser trochanter of femur; *action*, primary flexor of hip joint; *nerve supply*, lumbar plexus (ventral rami of first, second and usually third lumbar spinal nerves). SYN musculus psoas major [TA], greater psoas m.

psoas minor (m.) [TA], an inconstant m., absent in about 40%; *origin*, bodies of twelfth thoracic and first lumbar vertebrae and disk between them; *insertion*, iliopubic eminence via iliopectineal arch (iliac fascia); *action*, assists in flexion of lumbar spine; *nerve supply*, lumbar plexus. SYN musculus psoas minor [TA], smaller psoas (m.).

puboanalis (m.) [TA], part of pubococcygeus m., the fibers of which insert onto the external surface of the anal canal. SYN musculus puboanalis [TA].

pubococcygeal m., SYN pubococcygeus (m.).

pubococcygeus (m.) [TA], anterior part of the levator ani, arising from the pelvic surface of the body of the pubis and adjacent tendinous arch of obturator fascia, attaching to the coccyx. SYN musculus pubococcygeus [TA], pubococcygeal m.

puboperinealis (m.) [TA], part of pubococcygeus m., the fibers of which insert into the perineal body. SYN musculus puboperinealis [TA].

puboprostatic (m.), SYN puboprostaticus (m.).

puboprostaticus (m.) [TA], smooth m. fibers within the puboprostatic ligament. SYN musculus puboprostaticus [TA], levator prostatae (m.).⭐, musculus levator prostatae⭐, elevator (m.) of prostate, puboprostatic (m.).

puborectal m., SYN puborectalis (m.).

puborectalis (m.) [TA], the medial part of the pubococcygeus m. (levator ani) that passes from the body of the pubis around the posterior aspect of the anus to form a muscular sling at the level of the anorectal junction; it contracts to increase the anorectal (perineal) flexure during a peristalsis to maintain fecal continence and relaxes to allow defecation. SYN musculus puborectalis [TA], Braune m., puborectal m.

pubovaginal m., SYN pubovaginalis (m.).

pubovaginalis (m.) [TA], in the female, the most medial fibers of the pubococcygeus m. (levator ani) that extend from the pubis into the lateral walls of the vagina. SYN musculus pubovaginalis [TA], pubovaginal m.

pubovesical m., SYN pubovesicalis (m.).

pubovesicalis (m.) [TA], smooth m. fibers within the pubovesical ligament in the female. SYN musculus pubovesicalis [TA], pubovesical m.

pyramidal m., SYN pyramidalis (m.).

pyramidal m. of auricle [TA], an occasional prolongation of the fibers of the tragicus to the spine of the helix. SYN musculus pyramidalis auriculae [TA], Jung m., pyramidal auricular m.

pyramidal auricular m., SYN pyramidal m. of auricle.

pyramidalis (m.) [TA], muscle of inferior abdomen; *origin*, crest of pubis; *insertion*, lower portion of linea alba; *action*, makes linea alba tense; *nerve supply*, subcostal. SYN musculus pyramidalis [TA], pyramidal m.

quadrate m. [TA], a m. that is approximately square or four-sided. SYN musculus quadratus [TA], quadratus m.

quadrate m. of loins, SYN quadratus lumborum (m.).

quadrate pronator m., SYN pronator quadratus (m.).

quadrate m. of sole, SYN quadratus plantae (m.).

quadrate m. of thigh, SYN quadratus femoris (m.).

quadrate m. of upper lip, SYN *musculus* quadratus labii superioris.

quadratus m., SYN quadrate m.

quadratus fem'oris (m.) [TA], deep muscle of inferior gluteal (buttock) region; *insertion*, intertrochanteric ridge; *origin*, lateral border of tuberosity of ischium; *action*, rotates thigh laterally; *nerve supply*, nerve to quadratus femoris (sacral plexus). SYN musculus quadratus femoris [TA], quadrate m. of thigh.

quadratus lumborum (m.) [TA], flat muscle of posterior abdominal wall; *origin*, iliac crest, iliolumbar ligament, and transverse processes of lower lumbar vertebrae; *insertion*, twelfth rib and transverse processes of upper lumbar vertebrae; *action*, abducts trunk; *nerve supply*, ventral primary rami of upper lumbar spinal nerves. SYN musculus quadratus lumborum [TA], lumbar quadrate m., quadrate m. of loins.

quadratus plantae (m.) [TA], muscle of second layer of plantar muscles; *origin*, by two heads from the lateral and medial borders of the inferior surface of the calcaneus; *insertion*, tendons of flexor digitorum longus; *action*, assists long flexor; *nerve supply*, lateral plantar. SYN musculus quadratus plantae [TA], flexor accessorius (m.).⭐, musculus flexor accessorius⭐, accessory flexor m. of foot, caro quadrata sylvii, musculus pronator pedis, plantar quadrate m., quadrate m. of sole.

quadriceps fem'oris (m.) [TA], anterior thigh muscles; *origin*, by four heads: rectus femoris, vastus lateralis, vastus intermedius, and vastus medialis; *insertion*, patella, and thence by patellar ligament to tibial tuberosity; *action*, extends leg; flexes thigh by action of rectus femoris; *nerve supply*, femoral. SYN musculus quadriceps femoris [TA], musculus quadriceps [TA], musculus quadriceps extensor femoris, quadriceps m. of thigh.

quadriceps m. of thigh, SYN quadriceps femoris (m.).

radial flexor (m.) of wrist, SYN flexor carpi radialis (m.).

rectococcygeal m., SYN rectococcygeus (m.).

rectococcygeus (m.) [TA], a band of smooth m. fibers passing from the posterior surface of the rectum to the anterior surface of second or third coccygeal segment. SYN musculus rectococcygeus [TA], rectococcygeal m.

rectourethral m.'s, ⭐official alternate term for anorectoperineal m.'s.

rectouterine m., SYN rectouterinus (m.).

rectouterinus (m.) [TA], a band of fibrous tissue and smooth muscle fibers passing between the cervix of the uterus and the rectum in the rectouterine fold, on either side. SYN musculus rectouterinus [TA], rectouterine m.

rectovesical m., SYN rectovesicalis (m.).

rectovesicalis (m.) [TA], smooth m. fibers in the sacrogenital fold in the male; they correspond to rectouterinus m. of female. SYN musculus rectovesicalis [TA], rectovesical m.

rectus m. of abdomen, SYN rectus abdominis (m.).

rectus abdominis (m.) [TA], m. of ventral abdominal wall, flanking the linea alba, and characterized by tendinous intersections separating its length into multiple bellies; *origin*, crest and symphysis of the pubis; *insertion*, xiphoid process and fifth to seventh costal cartilages; *action*, flexes lumbar vertebral column, draws thorax downward toward pubis; *nerve supply*, thoracoabdominal nerves. SYN musculus rectus abdominis [TA], rectus m. of abdomen.

rectus capitis anterior (m.) [TA], suboccipital (prevertebral) muscle; *origin*, transverse process and lateral mass of atlas; *insertion*, basilar process of occipital bone; *action*, turns and inclines head forward; *nerve supply*, ventral primary ramus of first and second cervical spinal nerve. SYN musculus rectus capitis anterior [TA], anterior rectus m. of head, musculus rectus capitis anticus minor.

mu

rectus capitis lateralis (m.) [TA], suboccipital (prevertebral) muscle of upper neck; *origin*, transverse process of atlas; *insertion*, jugular process of occipital bone; *action*, inclines head to one side; *nerve supply*, ventral primary ramus of first cervical spinal nerve. SYN musculus rectus capitis lateralis [TA], lateral rectus m. of the head.

rectus capitis posterior major (m.) [TA], muscle of suboccipital triangle; *origin*, spinous process of axis; *insertion*, middle of inferior nuchal line of occipital bone; *action*, rotates and draws head backward; *nerve supply*, dorsal branch of first cervical (suboccipital). SEE ALSO suboccipital m.'s. SYN musculus rectus capitis posterior major [TA], greater posterior rectus m. of head, musculus rectus capitis posticus major.

rectus capitis posterior minor (m.) [TA], muscle of suboccipital triangle; *origin*, from posterior tubercle of atlas; *insertion*, medial third of inferior nuchal line of occipital bone; *action*, rotates head and draws it backward; *nerve supply*, dorsal branch of first cervical (suboccipital). SEE ALSO suboccipital m.'s. SYN musculus rectus capitis posterior minor [TA], musculus rectus capitis posticus minor, smaller posterior rectus m. of head.

rectus femoris (m.) [TA], anterior (superficial) middle head of quadriceps femoris; *origin*, anterior inferior spine of ilium and upper margin of acetabulum; *insertion*, via common tendon of quadriceps femoris into patella, and via patellar ligament to tibial tuberosity. SYN musculus rectus femoris [TA], rectus m. of thigh.

rectus m. of thigh, SYN rectus femoris (m.).

red m., slow-twitch m. in which small dark "red" m. fibers predominate; myoglobin is abundant and great numbers of mitochondria occur, characterized by slow, sustained (tonic) contraction. Contrast with white m.

Reisseisen m.'s, microscopic smooth m. fibers in the smallest bronchial tubes.

rhomboid major (m.) [TA], thoracoappendicular muscle; *origin*, spinous processes and corresponding supraspinous ligaments of first four thoracic vertebrae; *insertion*, medial border of scapula below spine; *action*, draws scapula toward vertebral column; *nerve supply*, dorsal of scapula nerve. SYN musculus rhomboideus major [TA], greater rhomboid m.

rhomboid minor (m.) [TA], thoracoappendicular muscle; *origin*, spinous processes of sixth and seventh cervical vertebrae; *insertion*, medial margin of scapula above spine; *action*, draws scapula toward vertebral column and slightly upward; *nerve supply*, dorsal nerve of scapula. SYN musculus rhomboideus minor [TA], lesser rhomboid m.

rider's m.'s, the adductor m.'s of the thigh, which come into play especially in horseback riding.

Riolan m., (1) marginal fibers of the palpebral part of the orbicularis oculi (m.); **(2)** SYN cremaster m.

risorius (m.) [TA], facial muscle of mouth; *origin*, from platysma and fascia of masseter; *insertion*, orbicularis oris and skin at corner of mouth; *action*, draws angle of mouth laterally, lenghthening rima oris; *nerve supply*, facial. SYN musculus risorius [TA], Albinus m. (1), Santorini m.

rotator m., (1) one of the rotatores (m.'s); **(2)** m. that produces a rotation, alone or in concert with other rotators, around an axis, e.g., rotator m.'s of vertebral column. SYN musculus rotator [TA], rotator.

rotatores (m.'s) [TA], deepest of the three layers of transversospinalis m.'s, chiefly developed in the thoracic region; they arise from the transverse process of one vertebra and are inserted into the root of the spinous process of the next two or three vertebrae above; *action*, traditionally described as a column, it is more likely that these m.'s, provided with a very high density of m. spindles, are organs of proprioception; *nerve supply*, dorsal primary rami of the spinal nerves. SYN musculi rotatores [TA].

rotatores cervicis (m.'s) [TA], the rotator m.'s attached to the cervical vertebrae. SYN musculi rotatores cervicis [TA], cervical rotator m.'s.

rotatores lumborum (m.'s) [TA], the rotator m.'s of the lumbar vertebrae. SYN musculi rotatores lumborum [TA], lumbar rotator m.'s.

rotatores thoracis (m.'s) [TA], the rotators of the thoracic vertebrae. SYN musculi rotatores thoracis [TA], thoracic rotator m.'s.

Rouget m., SYN circular *fibers*, under *fiber*.

round pronator m., SYN pronator teres (m.).

Ruysch m., the muscular tissue of the fundus of the uterus.

salpingopharyngeal m., SYN salpingopharyngeus (m.).

salpingopharyngeus (m.) [TA], *origin*, medial lamina of cartilaginous part of auditory tube; *insertion*, longitudinal muscular layer of pharynx in association with m. palatopharyngeus; *action*, assists in elevating pharynx and, according to some, assists in opening the auditory tube during swallowing; *nerve supply*, pharyngeal plexus. SYN musculus salpingopharyngeus [TA], salpingopharyngeal m.

Santorini m., SYN risorius (m.).

sartorius (m.) [TA], superficial anterior thigh muscle; *origin*, anterior superior spine of ilium; *insertion*, medial border of tuberosity of tibia; *action*, flexes thigh and leg, rotates leg medially and thigh laterally; *nerve supply*, femoral. SYN musculus sartorius [TA], tailor's m.

scalenus anterior (m.) [TA], lateral muscle of inferior half of neck; *origin*, anterior tubercles of transverse processes of third to sixth cervical vertebrae; *insertion*, scalene tubercle of first rib; *action*, raises first rib; *nerve supply*, cervical plexus. SYN musculus scalenus anterior [TA], anterior scalene m.✩, musculus scalenus anticus.

scalenus medius (m.) [TA], lateal muscle of inferior half of neck; *origin*, costotransverse lamellae of transverse processes of second to sixth cervical vertebrae; *insertion*, first rib posterior to subclavian artery; *action*, raises first rib; *nerve supply*, cervical plexus. SYN musculus scalenus medius [TA], middle scalene m.✩.

scalenus minimus (m.) [TA], an occasional independent muscular fasciculus between the scalenus anterior and medius, and having the same action and innervation. SYN musculus scalenus minimus [TA], Albinus m. (2), Sibson m., smallest scalene m.

scalenus posterior (m.) [TA], lateal muscle of inferior half of neck; *origin*, posterior tubercles of transverse processes of fourth to sixth cervical vertebrae; *insertion*, lateral surface of second rib; *action*, elevates second rib; *nerve supply*, cervical and brachial plexuses. SYN musculus scalenus posterior [TA], posterior scalene m.✩, musculus scalenus posticus.

scalp m., SYN epicranius (m.).

scapulohumeral m.'s [TA], intrinsic m.'s of the shoulder joint originating on the scapula and inserting into and acting upon the humerus, producing motion of the glenohumeral joint; includes supraspinatus, infraspinatus, teres minor and major, and subscapularis. SYN musculi scapulohumerales [TA].

Sebileau m., deep fibers of the dartos tunic which pass into the scrotal septum.

second tibial m., SYN *musculus* tibialis secundus.

semimembranosus (m.) [TA], deep hamstring muscle of posterior (flexor) compartment of thigh; *origin*, tuberosity of ischium; *insertion*, medial condyle of tibia and by membrane to tibial collateral ligament of knee joint, popliteal fascia, and via its reflected tendon of insertion (oblique popiteal ligament) lateral condyle of femur; *action*, flexes knee and rotates leg medially when knee is flexed; and contributes to the stability of extended knee by making capsule of knee joint tense; *nerve supply*, tibial. SYN musculus semimembranosus [TA].

semipennate m. [TA], a muscle with a lateral tendon to which the fibers are attached obliquely, like one half of a feather. SYN musculus semipennatus [TA], musculus unipennatus✩, unipennate m.✩.

semispinal m., SYN semispinalis m.

semispinal m. of head, SYN semispinalis capitis (m.).

semispinalis m. [TA], the most superficial layer of the three layers of the transversospinal m.; comprised of semispinalis capitis, semispinalis cervicis, and semispinalis thoracis m.'s. SYN musculus semispinalis [TA], semispinal m.

semispinalis capitis (m.) [TA], *origin*, transverse processes of five or six upper thoracic and articular processes of four lower cervical vertebrae; *insertion*, occipital bone between superior and inferior nuchal lines; *action*, rotates head and draws it backward; *nerve supply*, dorsal primary rami of cervical spinal nerves. SYN musculus semispinalis capitis [TA], musculus complexus, semispinal m. of head.

semispinalis cervicis (m.) [TA], continuous with m. semispinalis thoracis; *origin*, transverse processes of second to fifth thoracic vertebrae; *insertion*, spinous processes of axis and third to fifth cervical vertebrae; *action*, extends cervical spine; *nerve supply*, dorsal primary rami of cervical and thoracic spinal nerves. SYN musculus semispinalis cervicis [TA], musculus semispinalis colli✕, semispinal m. of neck.

semispinalis thoracis (m.) [TA], *origin*, transverse processes of fifth to eleventh thoracic vertebrae; *insertion*, spinous processes of first four thoracic and fifth and seventh cervical vertebrae; *action*, extends vertebral column; *nerve supply*, dorsal primary rami of cervical and thoracic spinal nerves. SYN musculus semispinalis thoracis [TA], musculus semispinalis dorsi, semispinal m. of thorax.

semispinal m. of neck, SYN semispinalis cervicis (m.).

semispinal m. of thorax, SYN semispinalis thoracis (m.).

semitendinosus (m.) [TA], superficial medial hamstring muscle of posterior (flexor) compartment of thigh; *origin*, ischial tuberosity; *insertion*, medial surface of the upper fourth of shaft of tibia; *action*, extends thigh, flexes leg and rotates it medially; *nerve supply*, tibial. SYN musculus semitendinosus [TA].

serratus anterior (m.) [TA], thoracoappendicular (scapulothoracic) muscle; *origin*, from center of lateral aspect of first eight to nine ribs; *insertion*, superior and inferior angles and intervening medial margin of scapula; *action*, rotates scapula and pulls it forward, elevates ribs; *nerve supply*, long thoracic from brachial plexus. SYN musculus serratus anterior [TA], anterior serratus m., costoscapularis, musculus serratus magnus.

serratus posterior inferior (m.) [TA], lower intermediate muscle of back; *origin*, with latissimus dorsi, from spinous processes of two lower thoracic and two upper lumbar vertebrae; *insertion*, into lower borders of last four ribs; *action*, draws lower ribs backward and downward; *nerve supply*, ninth to twelfth intercostal. SYN musculus serratus posterior inferior [TA], inferior posterior serratus m.

serratus posterior superior (m.) [TA], upper intermediate muscle of back; *origin*, from spinous processes of two lower cervical and two upper thoracic vertebrae; *insertion*, into lateral side of angles of second to fifth ribs; *nerve supply*, first to fourth intercostals. SYN musculus serratus posterior superior [TA], superior posterior serratus m.

shawl m., obsolete term for trapezius (m.).

short abductor m. of thumb, SYN abductor pollicis brevis (m.).

short adductor m., SYN adductor brevis (m.).

short extensor (m.) of great toe, SYN extensor hallucis brevis (m.).

short extensor (m.) of thumb, SYN extensor pollicis brevis (m.).

short extensor (m.) of toes, SYN extensor digitorum brevis (m.).

short fibular m., SYN fibularis brevis (m.).

short flexor (m.) of great toe, SYN flexor hallucis brevis (m.).

short flexor (m.) of little finger, SYN flexor digiti minimi brevis (m.) of hand.

short flexor (m.) of little toe, SYN flexor digiti minimi brevis (m.) of foot.

short flexor (m.) of thumb, SYN flexor pollicis brevis (m.).

short flexor (m.) of toes, SYN flexor digitorum brevis (m.).

short levatores costarum (m.'s), SYN levatores costarum breves (m.'s).

short palmar m., SYN palmaris brevis (m.).

short peroneal m., SYN fibularis brevis (m.).

short radial extensor m. of wrist, SYN extensor carpi radialis brevis (m.).

shunt m. [TA], m. that, rather than producing observable motion, contracts to resist dislocating forces occurring at joints, e.g., the coracobrachialis, short head of biceps, and long head of triceps all contract to resist downward dislocating forces at the shoulder joint, as when toting luggage.

Sibson m., SYN scalenus minimus (m.).

skeletal m., grossly, a collection of striated m. fibers connected at either or both extremities with the bony framework of the body; it may be an appendicular or an axial m.; histologically, a m. consisting of elongated, multinucleated, transversely striated skeletal m. fibers together with connective tissues, blood vessels, and nerves; individual m. fibers are surrounded by fine reticular and collagen fibers (endomysium); bundles (fascicles) of m. fibers are surrounded by irregular connective tissue (perimysium); the entire m. is surrounded, except at the m. tendon junction, by a dense connective tissue (epimysium). SYN musculus skeleti.

smaller m. of helix, SYN helicis minor (m.).

smaller pectoral m., SYN pectoralis minor (m.).

smaller posterior rectus m. of head, SYN rectus capitis posterior minor (m.).

smaller psoas (m.), SYN psoas minor (m.).

smallest scalene m., SYN scalenus minimus (m.).

smooth m., one of the m. fibers of the internal organs, blood vessels, hair follicles, etc.; contractile elements are elongated, usually spindle-shaped cells with centrally located nuclei and a length from 20 to 200 μm, or even longer in the pregnant uterus; although transverse striations are lacking, both thick and thin myofibrils occur; smooth m. fibers are bound together into sheets or bundles by reticular fibers, and frequently elastic fiber nets are also abundant. SEE ALSO involuntary m.'s. SYN unstriated m., unstriped m., visceral m.

Soemmerring m., SYN levator (m.) of thyroid gland.

soleus (m.) [TA], muscle of superficial posterior (plantar flexor) compartment of leg; *origin*, posterior surface of head and upper third of shaft of fibula, oblique line and middle third of medial margin of tibia, and a tendinous arch passing between tibia and fibula over the popliteal vessels; *insertion*, with gastrocnemius by tendo calcaneus (achillis) into tuberosity of calcaneus; *action*, plantar flexion of foot; *nerve supply*, tibial. SYN musculus soleus [TA].

sphincter m. [TA], SYN sphincter.

m. m. of common bile duct, SYN *sphincter* of (common) bile duct.

sphincter m. of pancreatic duct, SYN *sphincter* of pancreatic duct.

sphincter m. of pupil, SYN *sphincter* pupillae.

sphincter m. of pylorus, SYN pyloric *sphincter*.

sphincter m. of urethra, SYN external urethral *sphincter*.

sphincter m. of urinary bladder, SYN internal urethral *sphincter*.

spinal m., SYN spinalis (m.).

spinal m. of head, SYN spinalis capitis (m.).

spinalis (m.) [TA], the medial component of the erector spinae muscle; it is comprised of the spinalis capitis, spinalis cervicis, and spinalis thoracis muscles. SYN musculus spinalis [TA], spinal m.

spinalis capitis (m.) [TA], an inconstant extension of spinalis cervicis to the occipital bone, sometimes fusing with semispinalis capitis. SYN musculus spinalis capitis [TA], biventer cervicis, spinal m. of head.

spinalis cervicis (m.) [TA], an inconstant or rudimentary muscle; *origin*, spinous processes of sixth and seventh cervical vertebrae; *insertion*, spinous processes of axis and third cervical vertebra; *action*, extends cervical spine; *nerve supply*, dorsal primary rami of cervical. SYN musculus spinalis cervicis [TA], musculus spinalis colli, spinal m. of neck.

spinalis thoracis (m.) [TA], *origin*, spinous processes of upper lumbar and two lower thoracic vertebrae; *insertion*, spinous processes of middle and upper thoracic vertebrae; *action*, supports and extends vertebral column; *nerve supply*, dorsal primary rami of thoracic and upper lumbar. SYN musculus spinalis thoracis [TA], musculus spinalis dorsi, spinal m. of thorax.

spinal m. of neck, SYN spinalis cervicis (m.).

spinal m. of thorax, SYN spinalis thoracis (m.).

spindle-shaped m., SYN fusiform m.

splenius (m.'s) [TA], SYN musculi splenii [TA].

splenius capitis (m.) [TA], flat superficial muscle of the posterior neck, distinguished from the splenius cervicis primarily by its insertion onto the cranium; *origin*, from ligamentum nuchae of last four cervical vertebrae and supraspinous ligament of first and

mu

second thoracic vertebrae; *insertion*, lateral half of superior nuchal line and mastoid process; *action*, rotates head and extends neck; *nerve supply*, dorsal primary rami of second to sixth cervical spinal nerves. SYN musculus splenius capitis [TA], splenius m. of head.

splenius cervicis (m.) [TA], flat superficial muscle of the posterior neck, distinguished from the splenius capitis primarily by its insertion onto the cervical vertebrae; *origin*, from supraspinous ligament and spinous processes of third to fifth thoracic vertebrae; *insertion*, posterior tubercles of transverse processes of first and second (sometimes third) cervical vertebrae; *action*, rotates and extends neck; *nerve supply*, dorsal primary rami of fourth to eighth cervical spinal nerves. SYN musculus splenius cervicis [TA], musculus splenius colli, splenius m. of neck.

splenius m. of head, SYN splenius capitis (m.).

splenius m. of neck, SYN splenius cervicis (m.).

stapedius (m.) [TA], one of the muscles of the auditory ossicles; *origin*, internal walls of pyramidal eminence in tympanic cavity; *insertion*, neck of the stapes; *action*, dampens vibration of stapes by drawing head of stapes backward as a result of a protective reflex stimulated by loud noise; *nerve supply*, facial. SYN musculus stapedius [TA], stapedius.

sternal m., SYN sternalis (m.).

sternalis (m.) [TA], an inconstant muscle, running parallel to the sternum across the costosternal origin of the pectoralis major, and usually connected with the sternocleidomastoid and rectus abdominis muscles due to their common development source. SYN musculus sternalis [TA], musculus rectus thoracis, sternal m.

sternochondroscapular m., an occasional muscle arising from the manubrium of the sternum and first costal cartilage and passing lateralward and backward to be inserted into the upper border of the scapula. SYN musculus sternochondroscapularis.

sternoclavicular m., an occasional m. a slip from the subclavius muscle, passing from the upper part of the sternum to the clavicle beneath the pectoralis major m. SYN musculus sternoclavicularis.

sternocleidomastoid (m.) (SCM) [TA], superficial muscle of the anterolateral neck; *origin*, by two heads from anterior surface of manubrium of the sternum and sternal end of clavicle; *insertion*, mastoid process and lateral half of superior nuchal line; *action*, turns head obliquely to opposite side; when acting together, flex the neck and extend the head; *nerve supply*, motor by accessory, sensory by cervical plexus. SYN musculus sternocleidomastoideus [TA], sternomastoid m.

sternocostalis m., SYN transversus thoracis (m.).

sternohyoid (m.) [TA], infrahyoid (strap) muscle of anterior neck; *origin*, posterior surface of manubrium sterni and first costal cartilage; *insertion*, body of hyoid bone; *action*, depresses hyoid bone; *nerve supply*, upper cervical via spinal nerves(ansa cervicalis). SYN musculus sternohyoideus [TA].

sternomastoid m., SYN sternocleidomastoid (m.).

sternothyroid (m.) [TA], infrahyoid (strap) muscle of anterior neck; *origin*, posterior surface of manubrium of sternum and first or second costal cartilage; *insertion*, oblique line of thyroid cartilage; *action*, depresses larynx; *nerve supply*, upper cervical via spinal nerves (ansa cervicalis). SYN musculus sternothyroideus [TA].

straight m. [TA], member(s) of a group of m.'s that proceed either in a more direct or more nearly vertical or horizontal direction than other muscles of the group, e.g., rectus m.'s of extraocular or suboccipital m.'s. SYN musculus rectus [TA].

strap m.'s, SYN infrahyoid m.'s.

striated m., skeletal or voluntary m. in which cross striations occur in the fibers as a result of regular overlapping of thick and thin myofilaments; contrast with smooth muscle. Although cardiac muscle (which is not voluntary muscle) is also striated in appearance, the term "striated muscle" is commonly used as a synonym for voluntary, skeletal muscle.

styloauricular (m.), an occasional small m. extending from the root of the styloid process to the cartilage of the meatus of the ear. SYN musculus styloauricularis.

styloglossus (m.) [TA], extrinsic muscle of tongue; *action*, retracts tongue; *origin*, lower end of styloid process; *insertion*, side and undersurface of tongue; *nerve supply*, hypoglossal. SYN musculus styloglossus [TA].

stylohyoid (m.) [TA], *origin*, styloid process of temporal bone; *insertion*, hyoid bone by two slips on either side of intermediate tendon of digastric; *action*, elevates hyoid bone; *nerve supply*, facial. SYN musculus stylohyoideus [TA].

stylopharyngeal m., SYN stylopharyngeus (m.).

stylopharyngeus (m.) [TA], *origin*, root of styloid process; *insertion*, thyroid cartilage and wall of pharynx (becomes part of the longitudinal coat): *action*, elevates pharynx and larynx; *nerve supply*, glossopharyngeal. SYN musculus stylopharyngeus [TA], stylopharyngeal m.

subanconeus m., SYN articularis cubiti (m.).

subclavian m., SYN subclavius (m.).

subclavius (m.) [TA], thoracoappendicular muscle; *origin*, first costal cartilage; *insertion*, inferior surface of acromial end of clavicle; *action*, fixes clavicle or elevates first rib; *nerve supply*, subclavian from brachial plexus. SYN musculus subclavius [TA], subclavian m.

subcostal m. [TA], one of a number of inconstant muscles of the posterolateral thoracic wall having the same direction as the internal intercostal muscles but extending across (deep to) one or more ribs. SYN musculus subcostalis [TA], musculus infracostalis.

subcrural m., SYN articularis genus (m.).

suboccipital m.'s [TA], a group of muscles located immediately below the occipital bone; they are: rectus capitis anterior muscle, rectus capitis posterior major and minor muscles, rectus capitis lateralis m., obliquus capitis superior and inferior muscles; innervated by suboccipital nerve; although actions are described, it is held by many authorities that these muscles act primarily as organs of proprioception. SYN musculi suboccipitales [TA].

subquadricipital m., SYN articularis genus (m.).

subscapular m., SYN subscapularis (m.).

subscapularis (m.) [TA], intrinsic (scapulohumeral) muscle of shoulder joint, the tendon of which contributes to the formation of the rotator cuff; *origin*, subscapular fossa; *insertion*, lesser tuberosity of humerus; *action*, rotates arm medially; its tonic contraction helps to hold the head of the humerus in the shallow glenoid fossa; *nerve supply*, upper and lower subscapular from posterior cord of brachial plexus (fifth and sixth cervical spinal nerves). SYN musculus subscapularis [TA], subscapular m.

superficial back m.'s, m.'s originating from the vertebral column and having their fleshy bellies located in the back, but inserting onto the appendicular skeleton of the upper limb or the ribs. They are not innervated by dorsal primary rami of spinal nerves, as are the deep or true m.'s of the back; includes the trapezius m. (innervated by spinal accessory nerve) and latissimus dorsi, rhomboids, levator scapulae, and thoracic m.'s (innervated by ventral primary rami of spinal nerves, or derivatives thereof).

superficial flexor (m.) of fingers, SYN flexor digitorum superficialis (m.).

superficial lingual m., SYN superior longitudinal m. of tongue.

superficial transverse perineal m. [TA], an inconstant muscle of the urogenital triangle; *origin*, ramus of ischium; *insertion*, central tendon of perineum acting with other perineal muscles of resist increased intrapelvic pressure; *action*, draws back and fixes the central tendon of the perineum; *nerve supply*, pudendal (perineal). SYN musculus transversus perinei superficialis [TA], superficial transverse m. of perineum, Theile m.

superficial transverse m. of perineum, SYN superficial transverse perineal m.

superior auricular m., SYN auricularis superior (m.).

superior gemellus (m.) [TA], deep muscle of gluteal region; *origin*, ischial spine and margin of lesser sciatic notch; *insertion*, tendon of m. obturator internus; *action*, rotates thigh laterally; *nerve supply*, sacral plexus. SYN musculus gemellus superior [TA], gemellus.

superior longitudinal m. of tongue [TA], an intrinsic muscle of the tongue, running from base to tip on the dorsum just beneath the mucous membrane; *action*, shortens the upper part of the tongue; *nerve supply*, motor by hypoglossal, sensory by lingual.

SYN musculus longitudinalis superior linguae [TA], superficial lingual m.

superior oblique (m.) [TA], extraocular muscle in orbit; *origin*, above the medial margin of the optic canal; *insertion*, by a tendon passing through the trochlea, or pulley, and then reflected backward, downward, and laterally to the sclera between the superior and lateral recti; *action*, primary, intorsion; secondary, depression and abduction; *nerve supply*, trochlear nerve. SYN musculus obliquus superior [TA].

superior oblique m. of head, SYN obliquus capitis superior (m.).

superior pharyngeal constrictor (m.) [TA], uppermost component of the outer "circular" muscle layer of pharynx; *origin*, medial pterygoid plate (pterygopharyngeal part [TA]), pterygomandibular raphe (buccopharyngeal part [TA]), mylohyoid line of mandible (mylopharyngeal part [TA]), and the mucous membrane of the floor of the mouth and the side of the tongue (glossopharyngeal part [TA]); *insertion*, pharyngeal raphe in the posterior wall of the pharynx; *action*, narrows pharynx; helps to seal nasopharynx off from oropharynx and contracts in a peristaltic manner during swallowing; *nerve supply*, pharyngeal plexus. SYN musculus constrictor pharyngis superior [TA], musculus cephalopharyngeus.

superior posterior serratus m., SYN serratus posterior superior (m.).

superior rectus (m.) [TA], extraocular muscle in orbit; *origin*, superior part of common tendinous ring; *insertion*, superior part of sclera of the eye; *action*, primary, elevation; secondary, adduction and intorsion; *nerve supply*, oculomotor. SYN musculus rectus superior [TA], attollens oculi.

superior tarsal m. [TA], a well-defined layer of smooth muscle that extends from the aponeurosis of the m. levator palpebrae superioris to the superior tarsus; it is innervated by sympathetic nerves and acts to hold the upper lid in an elevated position; its paralysis in Horner syndrome result in ptosis. SYN musculus tarsalis superior [TA], Müller m. (3).

supinator (m.) [TA], (1) muscle of deep layer of proximal part of posterior compartment of forearm; *origin*, lateral epicondyle of humerus radial collateral and anular ligaments, and supinator ridge of ulna; *insertion*, anterior and lateral surface of radius; *action*, supinates the forearm; *nerve supply*, radial (posterior interosseous). (2) a m. that supinates, i.e., twists the forearm about a longitudinal axis from the pronated or neutral position toward one in which the palms face anteriorly (in the anatomic position). SYN musculus supinator [TA], supinator [TA], musculus supinator radii brevis.

supraclavicular m., an anomalous muscular slip running from the upper edge of the manubrium of the sternum lateralward to about the middle of the upper surface of the clavicle. SYN musculus supraclavicularis.

suprahyoid m.'s [TA], the group of muscles attached to the upper part of the hyoid bone including the digastric, stylohyoid, mylohyoid, and geniohyoid muscles. SYN musculi suprahyoidei [TA].

supraspinalis (m.), one of a number of muscular bands passing between the tips of the spinous processes of the cervical vertebrae. SYN musculus supraspinalis.

supraspinatus (m.) [TA], intrinsic (scapulohumeral) muscle of shoulder joint, the tendon of which contributes to the rotator cuff; *origin*, supraspinous fossa of scapula; *insertion*, greater tuberosity of humerus; *action*, initiates abduction of arm; its tonic contraction helps to hold the head of the humerus in the shallow glenoid fossa; *nerve supply*, suprascapular from fifth and sixth cervical. SYN musculus supraspinatus [TA], supraspinous m.

supraspinous m., SYN supraspinatus (m.).

suspensory m. of duodenum [TA], a broad flat band of smooth muscle and fibrous tissue attached to the right crus of the diaphragm and to the duodenum at its junction with the jejunum. SYN musculus suspensorius duodeni [TA], ligamentum suspensorium duodeni☆, suspensory ligament of duodenum☆, Treitz ligament, Treitz m.

synergistic m.'s, m.'s having a similar and mutually helpful function or action.

tailor's m., SYN sartorius (m.).

temporal m., SYN temporalis (m.).

temporalis (m.) [TA], superiormost masticatory muscle; *origin*, temporal fossa; *insertion*, coronoid process of mandible and anterior border of ramus; *action* elevates mandible (closes jaw); its posterior, nearly horizontally-oriented fibers are the primary retractors of the protruded mandible. *nerve supply*, deep temporal branches of mandibular division of trigeminal. SYN musculus temporalis [TA], temporal m., temporalis.

temporoparietal m., SYN temporoparietalis (m.).

temporoparietalis (m.) [TA], the part of epicranius m. that arises from the lateral part of the epicranial aponeurosis and inserts in the cartilage of the auricle. SYN musculus temporoparietalis [TA], temporoparietal m.

tensor fasciae latae (m.) [TA], anterior muscle of gluteal region (abductor compartment of thigh); *origin*, anterior superior spine and adjacent lateral surface of the ilium; *insertion*, iliotibial band of fascia lata; *action*, tenses fascia lata; flexes, abducts and medially rotates thigh; *nerve supply*, superior gluteal. SYN musculus tensor fasciae latae [TA], tensor (m.) of fascia lata☆, musculus tensor fasciae femoris.

tensor (m.) of fascia lata, ☆official alternate term for tensor fasciae latae (m.).

tensor (m.) of soft palate, SYN tensor veli palati (m.).

tensor tarsi m., lacrimal part of orbicularis oculi muscle. SEE orbicularis oculi (m.).

tensor tympani (m.) [TA], muscle of auditory ossicles; *origin*, the cartilaginous part of the pharyngotympanic (auditory) tube and the walls of its hemicanal just above the bony portion of the pharyngotympanic tube; *insertion*, handle of malleus; *action*, draws the handle of the malleus medially tensing the tympanic membrane to protect it from excessive vibration by loud sounds. *nerve supply*, branches of trigeminal through the otic ganglion. SYN musculus tensor tympani [TA], tensor (m.) of tympanic membrane, Toynbee m.

tensor (m.) of tympanic membrane, SYN tensor tympani (m.).

tensor veli palati (m.) [TA], muscle that tenses the soft palate so that the tongue may compress the food bolus against it during swallowing, forcing the mass into the oropharynx; *origin*, scaphoid fossa of sphenoid, cartilaginous and membranous part of pharyngotympanic (auditory) tube and spine of sphenoid; *insertion*, posterior border of hard palate and aponeurosis of soft palate; *action*, tenses the soft palate for swallowing; contributes to opening of auditory tube to enable equilibration of pressure; *nerve supply*, branches of trigeminal nerve through the otic ganglion. SYN musculus tensor veli palatini [TA], musculus palatosalpingeus, tensor (m.) of soft palate.

teres major (m.) [TA], intrinsic (scapulohumeral) muscle of shoulder joint; *origin*, inferior angle and lower third of border of scapula; *insertion*, medial border of intertubercular groove of humerus; *action*, adducts and extends arm and rotates it medially; *nerve supply*, lower subscapular from posterior cord of brachial plexus (fifth and sixth cervical spinal nerves). SYN musculus teres major [TA].

teres minor (m.) [TA], intrinsic (scapulohumeral) muscle of shoulder joint, the tendon of which contributes to formation of the rotator cuff; *origin*, upper two-thirds of the lateral border of scapula; *insertion*, lower facet of greater tuberosity of humerus; *action*, adducts arm and rotates it laterally; its tonic contraction helps to hold the head of the humerus in the shallow glenoid fossa; *nerve supply*, axillary (fifth and sixth cervical spinal nerves). SYN musculus teres minor [TA].

m. of terminal notch [TA], an occasional m. on the cranial surface of the auricle spanning the antitragohelicine fissure. SYN musculus incisurae helicis [TA], m. of notch of helix, musculus intertragicus.

Theile m., SYN superficial transverse perineal m.

third peroneal m., SYN fibularis tertius (m.).

thoracic interspinal m., SYN interspinales thoracis (m.'s).

thoracic interspinales m.'s, SYN interspinales thoracis (m.'s).

thoracic intertransversarii (m.'s) [TA], deep muscles of upper back; *origin*, transverse processes of thoracic vertebrae; *insertion*, next superior transverse process; *action*, abducts thoracic verte-

mu

brae; *nerve supply*, dorsal primary rami of thoracic nerves. SYN musculi intertransversarii thoracis [TA], thoracic intertransverse m.'s.

thoracic intertransverse m.'s, SYN thoracic intertransversarii (m.'s).

thoracic longissimus m., SYN longissimus thoracis (m.).

thoracic rotator m.'s, SYN rotatores thoracis (m.'s).

thoracoappendicular m.'s [TA], extrinsic m.'s of the upper limb, having an origin from the axial skeleton of the trunk (ribs and spinous processes of cervicothoracic vertebrae) and inserting into the appendicular skeleton of the upper limb. SYN musculi thoracoappendiculares [TA].

m.'s of thorax [TA], the muscles attaching to the rib cage including the pectoral muscles, serratus anterior, subclavius, levator muscles, intercostal muscles, transverse thoracic muscle, subcostal muscles, and diaphragm. SYN musculi thoracis [TA].

three-headed m. [TA], complex m. in which three separate heads of origin converge to insert via a common tendon, e.g., triceps brachii, triceps coxae, or triceps surae. SYN musculus triceps [TA], triceps (m.) [TA]. [L. fr. *tri-*, three, + *caput*, head]

thyroarytenoid (m.) [TA], intrinsic muscle of larynx; *origin*, inner surface of thyroid cartilage; *insertion*, muscular process and outer surface of arytenoid; *action*, decreases tension on (relaxes) vocal cords lowering the pitch of the voice tone; it is antagonistic to the cricothyroid muscle in this action; *nerve supply*, recurrent laryngeal. SYN musculus thyroarytenoideus [TA], musculus thyroarytenoideus externus.

thyroepiglottic m., thyroepiglottidean m., SYN thyroepiglottic *part* of thyroarytenoid (muscle).

thyrohyoid (m.) [TA], infrahyoid (strap) muscle of anterior neck that appears to be a continuation of the sternothyroid; *origin*, oblique line of thyroid cartilage; *insertion*, body of hyoid bone; *action*, approximates hyoid bone to the larynx; *nerve supply*, upper cervical spinal nerves carried by hypoglossal. SYN musculus thyrohyoideus [TA].

tibialis anterior (m.) [TA], medial muscle of anterior (dorsiflexor) compartment of leg; *origin*, upper two-thirds of lateral surface of tibia, interosseous membrane, and overlying crural fascia; *insertion*, medial cuneiform and base of first metatarsal; *action*, dorsiflexion and inversion of foot; provides dynamic support of longitudinal and transverse arches of foot; *nerve supply*, deep peroneal. SYN musculus tibialis anterior [TA], anterior tibial m., musculus tibialis anticus.

tibialis posterior (m.) [TA], most anterior (deepest) muscle of deep posterior (plantar flexor) compartment of leg; *origin*, soleal line and posterior surface of tibia, the head and shaft of the fibula between the medial crest and interosseous border, and the posterior surface of interosseous membrane; *insertion*, navicular, three cuneiform, cuboid, and second, third, and fourth metatarsal bones; *action*, plantar flexion and inversion of foot; *nerve supply*, tibial. SYN musculus tibialis posterior [TA], musculus tibialis posticus, posterior tibial m.

Tod m., SYN oblique m. of auricle.

m.'s of tongue [TA], the extrinsic m.'s include the genioglossus, hyoglossus, chondroglossus, and styloglossus m.'s; the intrinsic muscles are the vertical, transverse, and the superior and inferior longitudinal; all are innervated by the hypoglssal nerve. SYN musculi linguae [TA], lingual m.'s.

Toynbee m., SYN tensor tympani (m.).

trachealis (m.) [TA], the band of mostly transversely disposed smooth muscular fibers in the fibrous membrane connecting posteriorly the ends of the tracheal rings; *action,* reduces caliber of trachea. SYN musculus trachealis [TA].

tracheloclavicular m., an anomalous muscle occasionally arising from the cervical vertebrae and inserted into the lateral end of the clavicle. SYN musculus tracheloclavicularis.

tragicus (m.) [TA], one of the auricular muscles occurring as a band of vertical muscular fibers on the outer surface of the tragus of the auricle. SYN musculus tragicus [TA], m. of tragus, Valsalva m.

m. of tragus, SYN tragicus (m.).

transverse m. of abdomen, SYN transversus abdominis (m.).

transverse arytenoid (m.) [TA], intrinsic muscle of larynx; a band of muscular fibers passing between the two arytenoid cartilages posteriorly; *action*, narrows the intercartilaginous portion of the rima glottidis; *nerve supply*, recurrent laryngeal. SYN musculus arytenoideus transversus [TA], arytenoideus.

transverse m. of auricle, a band of sparse muscular fibers on the cranial surface of the auricle, extending from the eminence of the concha to the eminence of the scapha. SYN musculus transversus auriculae [TA], transverse auricular m. ✫.

transverse auricular m., ✫official alternate term for transverse m. of auricle.

transverse m. of chin, SYN transversus menti (m.).

transverse m. of nape, SYN transversus nuchae (m.).

transverse m. of thorax, SYN transversus thoracis (m.).

transverse m. of tongue [TA], an intrinsic muscle of the tongue, the fibers of which arise from the septum and radiate to the dorsum and sides; *action*, decreases lateral dimension of the tongue; *nerve supply*, hypoglossal for motor, lingual for sensory. SYN musculus transversus linguae [TA].

transversospinal m., SYN transversospinales (m.'s).

transversospinales (m.'s) [TA], the group of deep back muscles that originate from transverse processes of vertebrae and pass to spinous processes of higher vertebrae; they act as rotators and include the semispinalis (capitis, cervicis, thoracis), multifidus, and rotatores (cervicis, thoracis, lumborum) muscles. All are innervated by dorsal primary rami of spinal nerves. SYN musculi transversospinales [TA], transversospinal m., transversospinales.

transversus abdominis (m.) [TA], deepest layer of flat muscles of the anterolateral abdominal wall; *origin*, seventh to twelfth costal cartilages, lumbar fascia, iliac crest, and inguinal ligament; *insertion*, xiphoid cartilage and linea alba and, through the conjoint tendon, pubic tubercle and pecten; *action*, compresses abdominal contents; rotates and flexes trunk; *nerve supply*, lower thoracic. SYN musculus transversus abdominis [TA], musculus transversalis abdominis, transverse m. of abdomen.

transversus menti (m.) [TA], facial muscle of chin formed as inconstant fibers of the depressor anguli oris m. continue into the neck and cross to the opposite side inferior to the chin. SYN musculus transversus menti [TA], transverse m. of chin.

transversus nuchae (m.) [TA], an occasional muscle passing between the tendons of the trapezius and sternocleidomastoid, possibly a fasciculus of the posterior auricular muscle. SYN musculus transversus nuchae [TA], transverse m. of nape.

transversus thoracis (m.) [TA], internal muscle of thorax; *origin*, dorsal surface of xiphoid process and lower portion of dorsal surface of body of sternum; *insertion*, second to sixth costal cartilages; *action*, contributes to depression of ribs, narrowing chest; *nerve supply*, intercostal. SYN musculus transversus thoracis [TA], musculus triangularis sterni, sternocostalis m., transverse m. of thorax.

trapezius (m.) [TA], extrinsic (thoracoappendicular) muscle of shoulder; *origin*, medial third of superior nuchal line, external occipital protuberance, ligamentum nuchae, spinous processes of seventh cervical and the thoracic vertebrae and corresponding supraspinous ligaments; *insertion*, lateral third of posterior surface of clavicle, anterior side of acromion, and upper and medial border of the spine of the scapula; *action*, when scapulae are fixed, portions of muscle can act independently: cervical portion elevates scapula, thoracic portion contributes to depression of scapula; upper and lowermost portions act simultaneously to rotate glenoid fossa superiorly; when the entire muscle and especially middle part contracts, the scapulae retract; draws head to one side or backward; *nerve supply*, motor by accessory, sensory by cervical plexus. SYN musculus trapezius [TA], cowl m., trapezius.

Treitz m., SYN suspensory m. of duodenum.

triangular m. [TA], **(1)** a three-sided muscle; SYN musculus triangularis (1) [TA]. **(2)** SYN depressor anguli oris (m.).

triceps (m.) [TA], SYN three-headed m.

triceps m. of arm, SYN triceps brachii (m.).

triceps brachii (m.) [TA], three-headed muscle of posterior (extensor) compartment of arm; *origin*, long or scapular head: lateral border of scapula below glenoid fossa, lateral head: lateral and posterior surface of humerus below greater tubercle, medial head: posterior surface of humerus below radial groove; *insertion*, olecranon of ulna; *action*, extends elbow; *nerve supply*, radial. SYN musculus triceps brachii [TA], triceps m. of arm.

triceps (m.) of calf, SYN triceps surae (m.).

triceps coxae (m.), the obturator internus and superior and inferior gemellus m.'s considered as one muscle, inserting via a single common tendon into the greater trochanter of the femur. SYN musculus triceps coxae, triceps (m.) of hip.

triceps (m.) of hip, SYN triceps coxae (m.).

triceps surae (m.) [TA], the two bellies of the gastrocnemius and soleus considered as one muscle inserting via the calcaneal tendon into the calcaneal tuberosity. SYN musculus triceps surae [TA], triceps (m.) of calf.

true m.'s of back, SYN m.'s of back proper.

two-bellied m. [TA], SYN digastric (m.) (1).

two-headed m. [TA], a muscle with two origins or heads. Commonly used to refer to the biceps brachii (m.).

ulnar extensor (m.) of wrist, SYN extensor carpi ulnaris (m.).

ulnar flexor (m.) of wrist, SYN flexor carpi ulnaris (m.).

unipennate m., ☆official alternate term for semipennate m.

unstriated m., unstriped m., SYN smooth m.

m.'s of urogenital triangle [TA], m.'s located between ischiopubic rami and anterior to a line connecting ischial tuberosities, includes bulbospongiosus, ischiocavernosus, and transverse perineal m.'s and the external urethral sphincter. SYN musculi regionis urogenitalis [TA].

m. of uvula [TA], intrinsic muscle of soft palate; *origin*, posterior nasal spine; *insertion*, forms chief bulk of the uvula; *action*, raises the uvula; *nerve supply*, pharyngeal plexus. SYN musculus uvulae [TA], musculus azygos uvulae, palatouvularis m., uvular m., uvularis.

uvular m., SYN m. of uvula.

Valsalva m., SYN tragicus (m.).

vastus intermedius (m.) [TA], central deep head of quadriceps muscle of anterior (extensor) compartment of thigh; *origin*, upper three-fourths of anterior surface of shaft of femur; *insertion*, tibial tuberosity by way of common tendon of quadriceps femoris and patellar ligament; *action*, extends leg; *nerve supply*, femoral. SYN musculus vastus intermedius [TA], crureus, femoral m., intermediate great m., intermediate vastus (m.).

vastus lateralis (m.) [TA], lateral head of quadriceps muscle of anterior (extensor) compartment of thigh; *origin*, lateral lip of linea aspera as far as great trochanter; *insertion*, tibial tuberosity by way of common tendon of quadriceps femoris and patellar ligament; *action*, extends leg; *nerve supply*, femoral. SYN musculus vastus lateralis [TA], lateral great m., lateral vastus (m.), musculus vastus externus.

vastus medialis (m.) [TA], medial head of quadriceps muscle of anterior (extensor) compartment of thigh; *origin*, medial lip of linea aspera; *insertion*, tibial tuberosity by way of common tendon of quadriceps femoris and ligamentum patellae; *action*, extends leg; *nerve supply*, femoral. SYN musculus vastus medialis [TA], medial great m., medial vastus (m.), musculus vastus internus.

ventral sacrococcygeal m., SYN ventral sacrococcygeus (m.).

ventral sacrococcygeus (m.), an inconstant muscle on the pelvic surfaces of the sacrum and coccyx, the remains of a portion of the tail musculature of lower animals. SYN musculus sacrococcygeus anterior, musculus sacrococcygeus ventralis, ventral sacrococcygeal m.

vertical m. of tongue [TA], an intrinsic muscle of the tongue, consisting of fibers that pass from the aponeurosis of the dorsum to the aponeurosis of the inferior surface; *action*, decreases the superior to inferior dimension of (flattens) the tongue; *nerve supply*, hypoglossal for motor, lingual for sensory. SYN musculus verticalis linguae [TA].

vestigial m., an imperfect structure in humans corresponding to a functioning m. in the lower animals.

visceral m., SYN smooth m.

vocal m., SYN vocalis (m.).

vocalis (m.) [TA], intrinsic muscle of the larynx formed by a number of the most medial and finer fibers of the thyroaryteroid m. attached directly to the outer side of the vocal ligament; *origin*, depression between the two laminae of thyroid cartilage; *insertion*, portions of vocal ligament and vocal process of arytenoid; *action*, shortens and relaxes portions of vocal cords; *nerve supply*, recurrent laryngeal. SYN musculus vocalis [TA], musculus thyroarytenoideus internus, vocal m.

voluntary m., one whose action is under the control of the will; all the striated m.'s, except the heart, are voluntary m.'s.

white m., a rapid or fast-twitch m. in which pale large "white" fibers predominate; mitochondria and myoglobin are relatively sparse compared with red m.; involved in phasic contraction.

Wilson m., (1) SYN external urethral *sphincter*; (2) certain fibers of the levator ani.

wrinkler m. of eyebrow, SYN corrugator supercilii (m.).

zygomaticus major (m.) [TA], facial muscle of anterior cheek extending to upper lip; *origin*, zygomatic bone anterior to temporozygomatic suture; *insertion*, muscles at angle of mouth; *action*, draws upper lip upward and laterally; *nerve supply*, facial. SYN musculus zygomaticus major [TA], greater zygomatic m., musculus zygomaticus.

zygomaticus minor (m.) [TA], facial muscle of anterior cheek extending to upper lip; *origin*, zygomatic bone posterior to zygomaticomaxillary suture; *insertion*, orbicularis oris of upper lip; *action*, draws upper lip upward and outward; *nerve supply*, facial. SYN musculus zygomaticus minor [TA], caput zygomaticum quadrati labii superioris, lesser zygomatic m.

mus·cle-bound (mŭs'ĕl-bownd). Denoting a condition in which individual muscles are overdeveloped but dyssynergic in concerted action.

mus·cle-trim·ming. SYN border *molding*.

mus·cone (mŭs'kōn). Muskone.

mus·cu·la·mine (mŭs'kūl-ă-mēn). SYN spermine.

mus·cu·lar (mŭs'kū-lăr). **1.** Relating to a muscle or the muscles. **2.** Having well developed musculature.

mus·cu·la·ris (mŭs-kū-lā'ris). The muscular coat of a hollow organ or tubular structure. [Mod. L. muscular]

m. muco'sae, the thin layer of smooth muscle found in most parts of the digestive tube located outside the m. propria mucosae and adjacent to the tela submucosa. SYN lamina muscularis mucosae, muscular layer of mucosa.

mus·cu·lar·i·ty (mŭs'kū-lar'i-tē). The state or condition of having well developed muscles.

🔊 **mus·cu·la·ture** (mŭs'kū-lă-choor). The arrangement of the muscles in a part or in the body as a whole.

mus·cu·lo·ap·o·neu·rot·ic (mŭs'kū-lō-ap'ō-noo-rot'ik). Relating to muscular tissue and an aponeurosis of origin or insertion.

mus·cu·lo·cu·ta·ne·ous (mŭs'kū-lō-kū-tā'nē-ŭs). Relating to both muscle and skin. SYN myocutaneous, myodermal.

mus·cu·lo·mem·bra·nous (mŭs'kū-lō-mem'bră-nŭs). Relating to both muscular tissue and membrane; denoting certain muscles, such as the occipitofrontalis, that are largely membranous.

mus·cu·lo·phren·ic (mŭs'kū-lō-fren'ik). Relating to the muscular portion of the diaphragm; denoting an artery supplying this part.

mus·cu·lo·skel·e·tal (mŭs'kū-lō-skel'ĕ-tăl). Relating to muscles and to the skeleton, as, for example, the m. system.

mus·cu·lo·spi·ral (mŭs'kū-lō-spī'răl). Denoting the musculospiral nerve. SEE radial *nerve*.

mus·cu·lo·ten·di·nous (mŭs'kū-lō-ten'di-nŭs). Relating to both muscular and tendinous tissues.

mus·cu·lo·tro·pic (mŭs'kū-lō-trop'ik). Affecting, acting upon, or attracted to muscular tissue.

mu

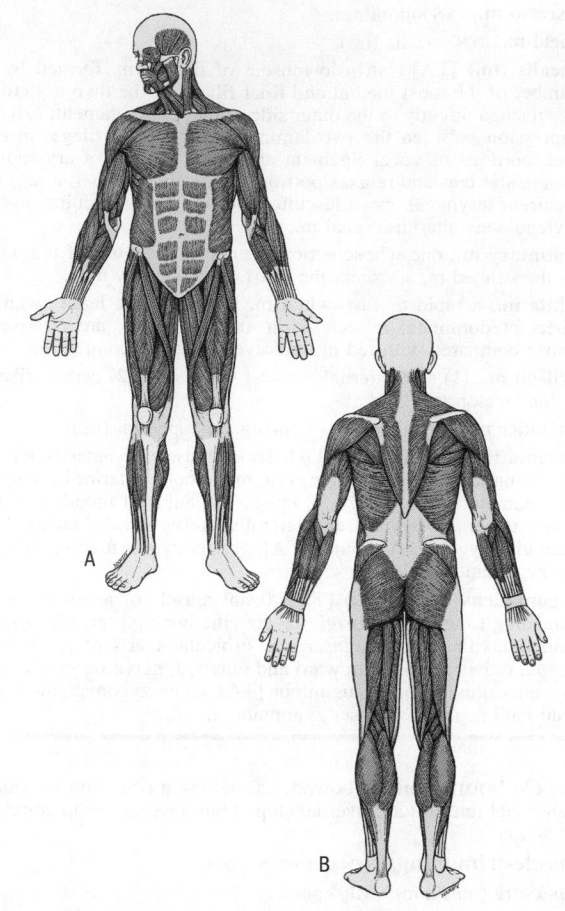

musculature: (A) anterior view, (B) posterior view

MUSCULUS

mus·cu·lus, gen. and pl. **mus·cu·li** (mŭs′kū-lŭs, -kū-lī) [TA]. SYN muscle. For histologic description, see muscle. [L. a little mouse, a muscle, fr. *mus* (*mur*-), a mouse]

mus′culi abdom′inis, SYN *muscles* of abdomen, under *muscle*.

m. abductor [TA], SYN abductor (*muscle*).

m. abduc′tor dig′iti min′imi ma′nus [TA], SYN abductor digiti minimi (*muscle*) of hand.

m. abduc′tor dig′iti min′imi pe′dis [TA], SYN abductor digiti minimi (*muscle*) of foot.

m. abduc′tor dig′iti quin′ti, (1) SYN abductor digiti minimi (*muscle*) of hand; **(2)** SYN abductor digiti minimi (*muscle*) of foot.

m. abduc′tor hal′lucis [TA], SYN abductor hallucis (*muscle*).

m. abduc′tor pol′licis bre′vis [TA], SYN abductor pollicis brevis (*muscle*).

m. abduc′tor pol′licis lon′gus [TA], SYN abductor pollicis longus (*muscle*).

m. adductor [TA], SYN adductor *muscle*.

m. adduc′tor bre′vis [TA], SYN adductor brevis (*muscle*).

m. adduc′tor hal′lucis [TA], SYN adductor hallucis (*muscle*).

m. adduc′tor lon′gus [TA], SYN adductor longus (*muscle*).

m. adduc′tor mag′nus [TA], SYN adductor magnus (*muscle*).

m. adduc′tor min′imus [TA], SYN adductor minimus (*muscle*).

m. adduc′tor pol′licis [TA], SYN adductor pollicis (*muscle*).

m. anco′neus [TA], SYN anconeus *muscle*.

musculi anorectoperineales [TA], SYN anorectoperineal *muscles*, under *muscle*.

m. antitrag′icus [TA], SYN antitragicus (*muscle*).

m. arrector pili [TA], SYN arrector *muscle* of hair.

m. articula′ris, SYN articular *muscle*.

m. articula′ris cu′biti [TA], SYN articularis cubiti (*muscle*).

m. articula′ris ge′nus [TA], SYN articularis genus (*muscle*).

m. aryepiglot′ticus, SYN aryepiglottic *part* of oblique arytenoid muscle.

m. arytenoi′deus obli′quus [TA], SYN oblique arytenoid *muscle*.

m. arytenoi′deus transver′sus [TA], SYN transverse arytenoid (*muscle*).

m. aryvoca′lis, a number of the deeper fibers of the vocalis muscle attached directly to the outer side of the true vocal cord.

m. attol′lens au′rem, m. attol′lens auric′ulam, SYN auricularis superior (*muscle*).

m. a′ttrahens au′rem, m. a′ttrahens auric′ulam, SYN auricularis anterior (*muscle*).

musculi auriculares [TA], SYN auricular *muscles*, under *muscle*.

m. auricula′ris ante′rior, SYN auricularis anterior (*muscle*).

m. auricula′ris poste′rior [TA], SYN auricularis posterior (*muscle*).

m. auricula′ris supe′rior [TA], SYN auricularis superior (*muscle*).

m. az′ygos u′vulae, SYN *muscle* of uvula.

m. bi′ceps bra′chii [TA], SYN biceps brachii (*muscle*).

m. bi′ceps fem′oris [TA], SYN biceps femoris (*muscle*).

m. bi′ceps flex′or cru′ris, SYN biceps femoris (*muscle*).

m. bipenna′tus, SYN pennate *muscle*.

m. biventer [TA], SYN digastric (*muscle*) (1).

m. biven′ter mandib′ulae, SYN digastric (*muscle*) (1).

m. brachia′lis [TA], SYN brachialis (*muscle*).

m. brachioradia′lis [TA], SYN brachioradialis (*muscle*).

m. bronchoesopha′geus [TA], SYN bronchoesophageus (*muscle*).

m. buccina′tor [TA], SYN buccinator (*muscle*).

m. buccopharyn′geus, SEE superior pharyngeal constrictor (*muscle*).

mus′culi bul′bi, SYN extraocular *muscles*, under *muscle*.

m. bulbocaverno′sus, SYN bulbospongiosus (*muscle*).

m. bulbospongio′sus [TA], SYN bulbospongiosus (*muscle*).

m. cani′nus, SYN levator anguli oris (*muscle*).

mus′culi cap′itis [TA], SYN *muscles* of head, under *muscle*.

m. cephalopharyn′geus, SYN superior pharyngeal constrictor (*muscle*).

m. ceratocricoi′deus [TA], SYN ceratocricoid (*muscle*).

m. ceratoglossus [TA], SYN ceratoglossus (*muscle*).

m. ceratopharyn′geus, SEE middle constrictor (*muscle*) of pharynx.

m. cervica′lis ascen′dens, SYN iliocostalis cervicis (*muscle*).

musculi cervicis, ☆official alternate term for *muscles* of neck, under *muscle*.

m. chondroglos′sus, SYN chondroglossus *muscle*.

m. chondropharyn′geus, SEE middle constrictor (*muscle*) of pharynx.

m. cilia′ris [TA], SYN ciliary *muscle*.

m. cleidoepitrochlea′ris, the anterior portion of the deltoid, arising from the clavicle.

m. cleidomastoi′deus, the portion of the sternocleidomastoid muscle passing between the clavicle and the mastoid process.

m. cleido-occipita′lis, the portion of the sternocleidomastoid muscle between the clavicle and the superior nuchal line.

mus′culi coccyg′ei, SYN *muscles* of coccyx, under *muscle*.

m. coccyg′eus [TA], SYN coccygeus *muscle*.

mus′culi col′li [TA], SYN *muscles* of neck, under *muscle*.

m. complex′us, SYN semispinalis capitis (*muscle*).

m. complex′us mi′nor, SYN longissimus capitis (*muscle*).

m. compres′sor na′ris, SEE nasalis (*muscle*).

m. compressor urethrae [TA], SYN compressor urethra (*muscle*).

m. constric′tor pharyn′gis infe′rior [TA], SYN inferior constrictor (*muscle*) of pharynx.

m. constric′tor pharyn′gis me′dius [TA], SYN middle constrictor (*muscle*) of pharynx.

m. constric′tor pharyn′gis supe′rior [TA], SYN superior pharyngeal constrictor (*muscle*).

m. constric′tor ure′thrae, SYN external urethral *sphincter*.

m. coracobrachia′lis [TA], SYN coracobrachialis *muscle*.

m. corruga′tor cu′tis a′ni, SYN corrugator cutis *muscle* of anus.

m. corruga′tor supercil′ii [TA], SYN corrugator supercilii (*muscle*).

m. cremas′ter [TA], SYN cremaster *muscle*.

m. cricoarytenoi′deus latera′lis [TA], SYN lateral cricoarytenoid (*muscle*).

m. cricoarytenoi′deus poste′rior [TA], SYN posterior cricoarytenoid (*muscle*).

m. cricopharyn′geus, SEE inferior constrictor (*muscle*) of pharynx.

m. cricothyroi′deus [TA], SYN cricothyroid *muscle*.

m. crucia′tus, SYN cruciate *muscle*.

m. cuta′neus [TA], SYN cutaneous *muscle*.

m. deltoi′deus [TA], SYN deltoid (*muscle*).

m. depres′sor an′guli o′ris [TA], SYN depressor anguli oris (*muscle*).

m. depres′sor la′bii inferio′ris [TA], SYN depressor labii inferioris (*muscle*).

m. depres′sor sep′ti [TA], SYN depressor septi nasi (*muscle*).

m. depres′sor supercil′ii [TA], SYN depressor supercilii (*muscle*).

m. detru′sor uri′nae [TA], SYN detrusor (*muscle*).

m. diaphrag′ma, SEE diaphragm.

m. digas′tricus [TA], SYN digastric (*muscle*) (1).

m. dilata′tor [TA], SYN dilator *muscle*.

m. dila′tor, SYN dilator *muscle*.

m. dila′tor i′ridis, SYN dilator pupillae *muscle*.

m. dila′tor na′ris, SEE nasalis (*muscle*).

m. dila′tor pupil′lae [TA], SYN dilator pupillae *muscle*.

m. dila′tor pylo′ri gastroduodena′lis, SYN dilator (*muscle*) of pylorus.

m. dila′tor pylo′ri ilea′lis, SYN dilator (*muscle*) of ileocecal sphincter.

m. dila′tor tu′bae, that portion of m. tensor veli palatini that attaches to the mucous membrane of the auditory tube; formerly described as a separate muscle.

mus′culi dor′si [TA], SYN *muscles* of back, under *muscle*.

musculi dorsi proprii [TA], SYN *muscles* of back proper, under *muscle*.

m. ejacula′tor sem′inis, SYN bulbospongiosus (*muscle*).

m. epicra′nius [TA], SYN epicranius (*muscle*).

m. epitrochleoanco′neus, an occasional muscle *origin*, from the back of the medial condyle of the humerus, and *insertion* into the medial side of the olecranon process.

m. erec′tor clitor′idis, SYN ischiocavernous (*muscle*).

m. erec′tor pe′nis, SYN ischiocavernous (*muscle*).

m. erec′tor spi′nae [TA], SYN erector spinae (*muscles*), under *muscle*.

m. extensor [TA], SYN extensor *muscle*.

m. exten′sor bre′vis digito′rum, SYN extensor digitorum brevis (*muscle*).

m. exten′sor bre′vis pol′licis, SYN extensor pollicis brevis (*muscle*).

m. exten′sor car′pi radia′lis bre′vis [TA], SYN extensor carpi radialis brevis (*muscle*).

m. exten′sor car′pi radia′lis lon′gus [TA], SYN extensor carpi radialis longus (*muscle*).

m. exten′sor car′pi ulna′ris [TA], SYN extensor carpi ulnaris (*muscle*).

m. exten′sor coccyg′is, SYN dorsal sacrococcygeus *muscle*.

m. exten′sor dig′iti min′imi [TA], SYN extensor digiti minimi (*muscle*).

m. exten′sor dig′iti quin′ti pro′prius, SYN extensor digiti minimi (*muscle*).

m. exten′sor digito′rum [TA], SYN extensor digitorum *muscle*.

m. exten′sor digito′rum bre′vis [TA], SYN extensor digitorum brevis (*muscle*).

m. exten′sor digito′rum bre′vis ma′nus, SYN extensor digitorum brevis (*muscle*) of hand.

m. exten′sor digito′rum commu′nis, SYN extensor digitorum *muscle*.

m. exten′sor digito′rum lon′gus [TA], SYN extensor digitorum longus (*muscle*).

m. exten′sor hal′lucis bre′vis [TA], SYN extensor hallucis brevis (*muscle*).

m. exten′sor hal′lucis lon′gus [TA], SYN extensor hallucis longus (*muscle*).

m. exten′sor in′dicis [TA], SYN extensor indicis (*muscle*).

m. exten′sor in′dicis pro′prius, SYN extensor indicis (*muscle*).

m. exten′sor lon′gus digito′rum, SYN extensor digitorum longus (*muscle*).

m. exten′sor lon′gus pol′licis, SYN extensor pollicis longus (*muscle*).

m. exten′sor min′imi dig′iti, SYN extensor digiti minimi (*muscle*).

m. exten′sor os′sis metacar′pi pol′licis, SYN abductor pollicis longus (*muscle*).

m. exten′sor pol′licis bre′vis [TA], SYN extensor pollicis brevis (*muscle*).

m. exten′sor pol′licis lon′gus [TA], SYN extensor pollicis longus (*muscle*).

musculi externi bulbi oculi [TA], SYN extraocular *muscles*, under *muscle*.

mus′culi faciei, SYN facial *muscles*, under *muscle*.

m. fibula′ris brev′is [TA], SYN fibularis brevis (*muscle*).

m. fibula′ris long′us [TA], SYN fibularis longus (*muscle*).

m. fibula′ris ter′tius [TA], SYN fibularis tertius (*muscle*).

m. flexor [TA], SYN flexor *muscle*.

m. flex′or accesso′rius, ✩official alternate term for quadratus plantae (*muscle*).

m. flex′or bre′vis digito′rum, SYN flexor digitorum brevis (*muscle*).

m. flex′or bre′vis hal′lucis, SYN flexor hallucis brevis (*muscle*).

m. flex′or car′pi radia′lis [TA], SYN flexor carpi radialis (*muscle*).

m. flex′or car′pi ulna′ris [TA], SYN flexor carpi ulnaris (*muscle*).

m. flex′or dig′iti min′imi brev′is ma′nus [TA], SYN flexor digiti minimi brevis (*muscle*) of hand.

m. flex′or dig′iti min′imi brev′is pe′dis [TA], SYN flexor digiti minimi brevis (*muscle*) of foot.

m. flex′or digito′rum bre′vis [TA], SYN flexor digitorum brevis (*muscle*).

m. flex′or digito′rum lon′gus [TA], SYN flexor digitorum longus (*muscle*).

m. flex′or digito′rum profun′dus [TA], SYN flexor digitorum profundus (*muscle*).

m. flex′or digito′rum subli′mis, SYN flexor digitorum superficialis (*muscle*).

m. flex′or digito′rum superficia′lis [TA], SYN flexor digitorum superficialis (*muscle*).

m. flex′or hal′lucis bre′vis [TA], SYN flexor hallucis brevis (*muscle*).

m. flex′or hal′lucis lon′gus [TA], SYN flexor hallucis longus (*muscle*).

m. flex′or lon′gus digito′rum, SYN flexor digitorum longus (*muscle*).

m. flex′or lon′gus hal′lucis, SYN flexor hallucis longus (*muscle*).

m. flex′or lon′gus pol′licis, SYN flexor pollicis longus (*muscle*).

m. flex′or pol′licis bre′vis [TA], SYN flexor pollicis brevis (*muscle*).

mu

m. **flex'or pol'licis lon'gus** [TA], SYN flexor pollicis longus (*muscle*).

m. **flex'or profun'dus,** SYN flexor digitorum profundus (*muscle*).

m. **flex'or subli'mis,** SYN flexor digitorum superficialis (*muscle*).

m. **fronta'lis,** SEE occipitofrontalis (*muscle*).

m. **fusifor'mis** [TA], SYN fusiform *muscle*.

m. **gastrocne'mius** [TA], SYN gastrocnemius (*muscle*).

m. **gemel'lus infe'rior** [TA], SYN inferior gemellus (*muscle*).

m. **gemel'lus supe'rior** [TA], SYN superior gemellus (*muscle*).

m. **genioglos'sus** [TA], SYN genioglossus (*muscle*).

m. **geniohyoglos'sus,** SYN genioglossus (*muscle*).

m. **geniohyoi'deus** [TA], SYN geniohyoid (*muscle*).

m. **glossopalati'nus,** SYN palatoglossus (*muscle*).

m. **glossopharyn'geus,** SEE superior pharyngeal constrictor (*muscle*).

m. **glu'teus max'imus** [TA], SYN gluteus maximus (*muscle*).

m. **glu'teus me'dius** [TA], SYN gluteus medius (*muscle*).

m. **glu'teus min'imus** [TA], SYN gluteus minimus (*muscle*).

m. **grac'ilis** [TA], SYN gracilis (*muscle*).

m. **hel'icis ma'jor** [TA], SYN helicis major (*muscle*).

m. **hel'icis mi'nor** [TA], SYN helicis minor (*muscle*).

m. **hyoglos'sus** [TA], SYN hyoglossus (*muscle*).

m. **hypopharyn'geus,** SEE middle constrictor (*muscle*) of pharynx.

m. **ili'acus** [TA], SYN iliacus (*muscle*).

m. **ili'acus mi'nor,** SYN iliacus minor (*muscle*).

m. **iliocapsula'ris,** SYN iliacus minor (*muscle*).

m. **il'iococcyg'eus** [TA], SYN iliococcygeus (*muscle*).

m. **iliocosta'lis** [TA], SYN iliocostalis (*muscle*).

m. **iliocosta'lis cer'vicis** [TA], SYN iliocostalis cervicis (*muscle*).

m. **iliocosta'lis dor'si,** SYN iliocostalis thoracis (*muscle*).

m. **iliocosta'lis lumbo'rum** [TA], SYN iliocostalis lumborum (*muscle*).

m. **iliocosta'lis thora'cis** [TA], SYN iliocostalis thoracis (*muscle*).

m. **iliopso'as** [TA], SYN iliopsoas (*muscle*).

m. **incisi'vus la'bii inferior'is,** inferior incisive bundle of origin of orbicularis oris m.

m. **incisi'vus la'bii superior'is,** superior incisive bundle of origin of orbicularis oris m.

m. **incisu'rae hel'icis** [TA], SYN *muscle* of terminal notch.

m. **infracosta'lis,** pl. **musculi infracosta'les,** SYN subcostal *muscle*.

mus'culi infrahyoi'dei [TA], SYN infrahyoid *muscles*, under *muscle*.

m. **infraspina'tus** [TA], SYN infraspinatus (*muscle*).

m. **intercosta'les exter'ni,** pl. **mus'culi intercosta'les exter'ni** [TA], SYN external intercostal (*muscle*).

m. **intercosta'lis inter'nus,** pl. **mus'culi intercosta'les inter'ni** [TA], SYN internal intercostal (*muscle*).

m. **intercosta'lis in'timus,** pl. **mus'culi intercosta'les in'timi** [TA], SYN innermost intercostal (*muscle*).

musculi interos'sei [TA], SYN interosseous *muscles*, under *muscle*.

musculi interos'sei dorsa'lis ma'nus, pl. **mus'culi interos'sei dorsa'les ma'nus,** [TA], SYN dorsal interossei (interosseous *muscles*) of hand, under *muscle*.

musculi interos'sei dorsa'lis pe'dis, pl. **mus'culi interos'sei dorsa'les pe'dis,** [TA], SYN dorsal interossei (interosseous *muscles*) of foot, under *muscle*.

musculi interos'seus planta'ris [TA], SYN plantar interossei (interosseous *muscles*), under *muscle*.

m. **interos'seus palma'ris,** pl. **mus'culi interos'sei palma'res** [TA], SYN palmar interossei (interosseous *muscles*), under *muscle*.

m. **interos'seus vola'ris,** SYN palmar interossei (interosseous *muscles*), under *muscle*.

mus'culi interspina'les [TA], SYN interspinales (*muscles*), under *muscle*.

m. **interspina'lis cer'vicis,** SYN interspinales cervicis (*muscles*), under *muscle*.

m. **interspina'lis lumbo'rum** [TA], SYN interspinales lumborum (*muscles*), under *muscle*.

m. **interspina'lis thora'cis** [TA], SYN interspinales thoracis (*muscles*), under *muscle*.

m. **intertra'gicus,** SYN *muscle* of terminal notch.

mus'culi intertransversa'rii [TA], SYN intertransversarii (*muscles*), under *muscle*.

mus'culi intertransversa'rii anterio'res cer'vicis [TA], SYN anterior cervical intertransversarii (*muscles*), under *muscle*.

mus'culi intertransversa'rii latera'les lumbo'rum [TA], SYN lateral lumbar intertransversarii (*muscles*), under *muscle*.

mus'culi intertransversa'rii media'les lumbo'rum [TA], SYN medial lumbar intertransversarii (*muscles*), under *muscle*.

mus'culi intertransversa'rii posterio'res cer'vicis [TA], SYN posterior cervical intertransversarii (*muscles*), under *muscle*.

mus'culi intertransversa'rii thora'cis [TA], SYN thoracic intertransversarii (*muscles*), under *muscle*.

m. **ischiocaverno'sus** [TA], SYN ischiocavernous (*muscle*).

m. **ischiococcyg'eus,** SYN coccygeus *muscle*.

m. **keratopharyn'geus,** SEE middle constrictor (*muscle*) of pharynx.

mus'culi laryn'gis [TA], SYN *muscles* of larynx, under *muscle*.

m. **laryngopharyn'geus,** SYN inferior constrictor (*muscle*) of pharynx.

m. **latis'simus dor'si** [TA], SYN latissimus dorsi (*muscle*).

m. **leva'tor a'lae na'si,** portion of m. levator labii superioris alaeque nasi muscle inserting into wing of nose.

m. **leva'tor an'guli o'ris** [TA], SYN levator anguli oris (*muscle*).

m. **leva'tor an'guli scap'ulae,** SYN levator scapulae (*muscle*).

m. **leva'tor a'ni** [TA], SYN levator ani (*muscle*).

m. **leva'tor cos'tae,** pl. **mus'culi levato'res costa'rum,** SYN levatores costarum (*muscles*), under *muscle*.

mus'culi levato'res costa'rum [TA], SYN levatores costarum (*muscles*), under *muscle*.

musculi levatores costa'rum breves [TA], SYN levatores costarum breves (*muscles*), under *muscle*.

musculi levatores costa'rum longi [TA], SYN levatores costarum longi (*muscles*), under *muscle*.

m. **leva'tor glan'dulae thyroi'deae** [TA], SYN levator (*muscle*) of thyroid gland.

m. **leva'tor la'bii inferio'ris,** SYN mentalis (*muscle*).

m. **leva'tor la'bii superio'ris** [TA], SYN levator labii superioris (*muscle*).

m. **leva'tor la'bii superio'ris alae'que na'si** [TA], SYN levator labii superioris alaeque nasi (*muscle*).

m. **leva'tor pala'ti,** SYN levator veli palatini (*muscle*).

m. **leva'tor pal'pebrae superio'ris** [TA], SYN levator palpebrae superioris (*muscle*).

m. **leva'tor pro'statae,** ⋆official alternate term for puboprostaticus (*muscle*).

m. **leva'tor scap'ulae** [TA], SYN levator scapulae (*muscle*).

m. **leva'tor ve'li palati'ni** [TA], SYN levator veli palatini (*muscle*).

mus'culi lin'guae [TA], SYN *muscles* of tongue, under *muscle*.

m. **longis'simus** [TA], SYN longissimus (*muscle*).

m. **longis'simus cap'itis** [TA], SYN longissimus capitis (*muscle*).

m. **longis'simus cer'vicis** [TA], SYN longissimus cervicis (*muscle*).

m. **longis'simus dor'si,** SYN longissimus thoracis (*muscle*).

m. **longis'simus thora'cis** [TA], SYN longissimus thoracis (*muscle*).

m. **longitudina'lis infe'rior linguae** [TA], SYN inferior longitudinal *muscle* of tongue.

m. **longitudina'lis supe'rior linguae** [TA], SYN superior longitudinal *muscle* of tongue.

m. **lon'gus cap'itis** [TA], SYN longus capitis (*muscle*).

m. **lon'gus col'li** [TA], SYN longus colli (*muscle*).

m. **lumbrica'lis ma'nus,** pl. **mus'culi lumbrica'les ma'nus** [TA], SYN lumbricals (lumbrical *muscles*) of hand, under *muscle*.

m. lumbrica′lis pe′dis, pl. **mus′culi lumbrica′les pe′dis** [TA], SYN lumbricals (lumbrical *muscles*) of foot, under *muscle*.

m. masse′ter [TA], SYN masseter (*muscle*).

m. menta′lis [TA], SYN mentalis (*muscle*).

m. multif′idus [TA], SYN multifidus (*muscle*).

m. multif′idus spi′nae, SYN multifidus (*muscle*).

m. multipenna′tus [TA], SYN multipennate *muscle*.

m. mylohyoi′deus [TA], SYN mylohyoid (*muscle*).

m. mylopharyn′geus, SEE superior pharyngeal constrictor (*muscle*).

m. nasa′lis [TA], SYN nasalis (*muscle*).

m. obli′quus auric′ulae [TA], SYN oblique *muscle* of auricle.

m. obli′quus cap′itis infe′rior [TA], SYN obliquus capitis inferior (*muscle*).

m. obli′quus cap′itis supe′rior [TA], SYN obliquus capitis superior (*muscle*).

m. obli′quus exter′nus abdom′inis [TA], SYN external oblique (*muscle*).

m. obli′quus infe′rior [TA], SYN inferior oblique (*muscle*).

m. obli′quus inter′nus abdom′inis [TA], SYN internal oblique (*muscle*).

m. obli′quus supe′rior [TA], SYN superior oblique (*muscle*).

m. obtura′tor exter′nus [TA], SYN obturator externus (*muscle*).

m. obtura′tor inter′nus [TA], SYN obturator internus (*muscle*).

m. occipita′lis, SEE occipitofrontalis (*muscle*).

m. occipitofronta′lis [TA], SYN occipitofrontalis (*muscle*).

m. omohyoi′deus [TA], SYN omohyoid (*muscle*).

m. oppo′nens [TA], SYN opponens *muscle*.

m. oppo′nens dig′iti min′imi [TA], SYN opponens digiti minimi (*muscle*).

m. oppo′nens dig′iti quin′ti, SYN opponens digiti minimi (*muscle*).

m. oppo′nens min′imi dig′iti, SYN opponens digiti minimi (*muscle*).

m. oppo′nens pol′licis [TA], SYN opponens pollicis (*muscle*).

m. orbicula′ris [TA], SYN orbicular *muscle*.

m. orbicula′ris oc′uli [TA], SYN orbicularis oculi (*muscle*).

m. orbicula′ris o′ris [TA], SYN orbicularis oris (*muscle*).

m. orbicula′ris palpebra′rum, SYN orbicularis oculi (*muscle*).

m. orbita′lis [TA], SYN orbitalis (*muscle*).

m. orbitopalpebra′lis, SYN levator palpebrae superioris (*muscle*).

musculi ossiculorum auditoriorum, ☆official alternate term for *muscles* of auditory ossicles, under *muscle*.

mus′culi ossiculo′rum audi′tus [TA], SYN *muscles* of auditory ossicles, under *muscle*.

m. palatoglos′sus [TA], SYN palatoglossus (*muscle*).

m. palatopharyn′geus [TA], SYN palatopharyngeus (*muscle*).

m. palatosalpin′geus, SYN tensor veli palati (*muscle*).

m. palatostaphyli′nus, a bundle of muscular fibers from the tensor veli palatini joining the m. uvulae.

m. palma′ris bre′vis [TA], SYN palmaris brevis (*muscle*).

m. palma′ris lon′gus [TA], SYN palmaris longus (*muscle*).

m. papilla′ris [TA], SYN papillary *muscle*.

mus′culi pectina′ti [TA], SYN pectinate *muscles*, under *muscle*.

m. pectin′eus [TA], SYN pectineus (*muscle*).

m. pectora′lis ma′jor [TA], SYN pectoralis major (*muscle*).

m. pectora′lis mi′nor [TA], SYN pectoralis minor (*muscle*).

m. pennatus [TA], SYN pennate *muscle*.

mus′culi perine′i [TA], SYN perineal *muscles*, under *muscle*.

m. peroneocalca′neus, an occasional muscle arising from the shaft of the fibula and inserted into the calcaneus.

m. perone′us bre′vis, ☆official alternate term for fibularis brevis (*muscle*).

m. perone′us lon′gus, ☆official alternate term for fibularis longus (*muscle*).

m. perone′us ter′tius, ☆official alternate term for fibularis tertius (*muscle*).

m. petropharyn′geus, an occasional accessory levator muscle of the pharynx, arising from the undersurface of the petrous portion of the temporal bone and inserted into the pharynx.

m. petrostaphyli′nus, SYN levator veli palatini (*muscle*).

m. pharyngopalati′nus, SYN palatopharyngeus (*muscle*).

m. pirifor′mis [TA], SYN piriformis (*muscle*).

m. plana [TA], SYN flat *muscle*.

m. planta′ris [TA], SYN plantaris (*muscle*).

m. platys′ma, SYN platysma (*muscle*).

m. platys′ma myoi′des, SYN platysma (*muscle*).

m. pleuroesopha′geus [TA], SYN pleuroesophageus (*muscle*).

m. poplit′eus [TA], SYN popliteus (*muscle*).

m. proce′rus [TA], SYN procerus (*muscle*).

m. prona′tor [TA], SYN pronator (*muscle*).

m. prona′tor pe′dis, SYN quadratus plantae (*muscle*).

m. prona′tor quadra′tus [TA], SYN pronator quadratus (*muscle*).

m. prona′tor ra′dii te′res, SYN pronator teres (*muscle*).

m. prona′tor te′res [TA], SYN pronator teres (*muscle*).

m. prostat′icus, SYN muscular *substance* of prostate.

m. pso′as ma′jor [TA], SYN psoas major (*muscle*).

m. pso′as mi′nor [TA], SYN psoas minor (*muscle*).

m. pterygoi′deus exter′nus, SYN lateral pterygoid (*muscle*).

m. pterygoi′deus inter′nus, SYN medial pterygoid (*muscle*).

m. pterygoi′deus latera′lis [TA], SYN lateral pterygoid (*muscle*).

m. pterygoi′deus media′lis [TA], SYN medial pterygoid (*muscle*).

m. pterygopharyn′geus, SEE superior pharyngeal constrictor (*muscle*).

m. pterygospino′sus, a muscular slip, occasionally present, passing between the spine of the sphenoid bone and the posterior margin of the lateral pterygoid plate.

m. puboanalis [TA], SYN puboanalis (*muscle*).

m. pubococcyg′eus [TA], SYN pubococcygeus (*muscle*).

m. puboperinealis [TA], SYN puboperinealis (*muscle*).

m. puboprostat′icus [TA], SYN puboprostaticus (*muscle*).

m. puborecta′lis [TA], SYN puborectalis (*muscle*).

m. pubovagina′lis [TA], SYN pubovaginalis (*muscle*).

m. pubovesica′lis [TA], SYN pubovesicalis (*muscle*).

m. pyramida′lis [TA], SYN pyramidalis (*muscle*).

m. pyramida′lis auric′ulae [TA], SYN pyramidal *muscle* of auricle.

m. pyramida′lis na′si, SYN procerus (*muscle*).

m. pyrifor′mis, SYN piriformis (*muscle*).

m. quadra′tus [TA], SYN quadrate *muscle*.

m. quadra′tus fem′oris [TA], SYN quadratus femoris (*muscle*).

m. quadra′tus la′bii inferio′ris, SYN depressor labii inferioris (*muscle*).

m. quadra′tus la′bii superior′is, composed of three heads usually described as three separate muscles; they are the caput angulare or levator labii superioris alaeque nasi muscle; caput infraorbitale or levator labii superioris muscle; caput zygomaticum or zygomaticus minor muscle. SYN quadrate muscle of upper lip.

m. quadra′tus lumbo′rum [TA], SYN quadratus lumborum (*muscle*).

m. quadra′tus men′ti, SYN depressor labii inferioris (*muscle*).

m. quadra′tus plan′tae [TA], SYN quadratus plantae (*muscle*).

m. quadriceps [TA], SYN quadriceps femoris (*muscle*).

m. quad′riceps exten′sor fem′oris, SYN quadriceps femoris (*muscle*).

m. quad′riceps fem′oris [TA], SYN quadriceps femoris (*muscle*).

m. rectococcyg′eus [TA], SYN rectococcygeus (*muscle*).

musculi rectourethra′les, ☆official alternate term for anorectoperineal *muscles*, under *muscle*.

m. rectouteri′nus [TA], SYN rectouterinus (*muscle*).

m. rectovesica′lis [TA], SYN rectovesicalis (*muscle*).

m. rectus [TA], SYN straight *muscle*.

m. rec′tus abdom′inis [TA], SYN rectus abdominis (*muscle*).

m. rec′tus cap′itis ante′rior [TA], SYN rectus capitis anterior (*muscle*).

m. rec′tus cap′itis anti′cus ma′jor, SYN longus capitis (*muscle*).

mu

m. rec'tus cap'itis anti'cus mi'nor, SYN rectus capitis anterior (*muscle*).

m. rec'tus cap'itis latera'lis [TA], SYN rectus capitis lateralis (*muscle*).

m. rec'tus cap'itis poste'rior ma'jor [TA], SYN rectus capitis posterior major (*muscle*).

m. rec'tus cap'itis poste'rior mi'nor [TA], SYN rectus capitis posterior minor (*muscle*).

m. rec'tus cap'itis posti'cus ma'jor, SYN rectus capitis posterior major (*muscle*).

m. rec'tus cap'itis posti'cus mi'nor, SYN rectus capitis posterior minor (*muscle*).

m. rec'tus exter'nus, SYN lateral rectus (*muscle*).

m. rec'tus fem'oris [TA], SYN rectus femoris (*muscle*).

m. rec'tus infe'rior [TA], SYN inferior rectus (*muscle*).

m. rec'tus inter'nus, SYN medial rectus (*muscle*).

m. rec'tus latera'lis [TA], SYN lateral rectus (*muscle*).

m. rec'tus media'lis [TA], SYN medial rectus (*muscle*).

m. rec'tus supe'rior [TA], SYN superior rectus (*muscle*).

m. rec'tus thora'cis, SYN sternalis (*muscle*).

musculi regionis analis [TA], SYN *muscles* of anal triangle, under *muscle*.

musculi regionis urogenitalis [TA], SYN *muscles* of urogenital triangle, under *muscle*.

m. ret'rahens au'rem, m. ret'rahens auric'ulam, SYN auricularis posterior (*muscle*).

m. rhomboatloi'deus, an occasional muscle arising with the rhomboids from the cervical and thoracic vertebrae and inserted into the atlas.

m. rhomboi'deus ma'jor [TA], SYN rhomboid major (*muscle*).

m. rhomboi'deus mi'nor [TA], SYN rhomboid minor (*muscle*).

m. riso'rius [TA], SYN risorius (*muscle*).

m. rotator [TA], SYN rotator *muscle*.

mus'culi rotato'res [TA], SYN rotatores (*muscles*), under *muscle*.

mus'culi rotato'res cer'vicis [TA], SYN rotatores cervicis (*muscles*), under *muscle*.

mus'culi rotato'res lumbo'rum [TA], SYN rotatores lumborum (*muscles*), under *muscle*.

mus'culi rotato'res thora'cis [TA], SYN rotatores thoracis (*muscles*), under *muscle*.

m. sacrococcyg'eus ante'rior, SYN ventral sacrococcygeus (*muscle*).

m. sacrococcyg'eus dorsa'lis, SYN dorsal sacrococcygeus *muscle*.

m. sacrococcyg'eus poste'rior, SYN dorsal sacrococcygeus *muscle*.

m. sacrococcyg'eus ventra'lis, SYN ventral sacrococcygeus (*muscle*).

m. sacrolumba'lis, SYN iliocostalis lumborum (*muscle*).

m. sacrospina'lis, SYN erector spinae (*muscles*), under *muscle*.

m. salpingopharyn'geus [TA], SYN salpingopharyngeus (*muscle*).

m. sarto'rius [TA], SYN sartorius (*muscle*).

m. scale'nus ante'rior [TA], SYN scalenus anterior (*muscle*).

m. scale'nus anti'cus, SYN scalenus anterior (*muscle*).

m. scale'nus me'dius [TA], SYN scalenus medius (*muscle*).

m. scale'nus min'imus [TA], SYN scalenus minimus (*muscle*).

m. scale'nus poste'rior [TA], SYN scalenus posterior (*muscle*).

m. scale'nus posti'cus, SYN scalenus posterior (*muscle*).

musculi scapulohumerales [TA], SYN scapulohumeral *muscles*, under *muscle*.

m. semimembrano'sus [TA], SYN semimembranosus (*muscle*).

m. semipennatus [TA], SYN semipennate *muscle*.

m. semispina'lis [TA], SYN semispinalis *muscle*.

m. semispina'lis cap'itis [TA], SYN semispinalis capitis (*muscle*).

m. semispina'lis cer'vicis [TA], SYN semispinalis cervicis (*muscle*).

m. semispina'lis col'li, ✩official alternate term for semispinalis cervicis (*muscle*).

m. semispina'lis dor'si, SYN semispinalis thoracis (*muscle*).

m. semispina'lis thora'cis [TA], SYN semispinalis thoracis (*muscle*).

m. semitendino'sus [TA], SYN semitendinosus (*muscle*).

m. serra'tus ante'rior [TA], SYN serratus anterior (*muscle*).

m. serra'tus mag'nus, SYN serratus anterior (*muscle*).

m. serra'tus poste'rior infe'rior [TA], SYN serratus posterior inferior (*muscle*).

m. serra'tus poste'rior supe'rior [TA], SYN serratus posterior superior (*muscle*).

m. skel'eti, SYN skeletal *muscle*.

m. sol'eus [TA], SYN soleus (*muscle*).

m. sphinc'ter [TA], SYN sphincter.

m. sphinc'ter ampullae biliaropancrea'ticae, ✩official alternate term for *sphincter* of hepatopancreatic ampulla.

m. sphinc'ter ampullae, ✩official alternate term for *sphincter* of hepatopancreatic ampulla.

m. sphinc'ter ampullae hepatopancrea'ticae [TA], SYN *sphincter* of hepatopancreatic ampulla.

m. sphinc'ter a'ni exter'nus [TA], SYN external anal *sphincter*.

m. sphinc'ter a'ni inter'nus [TA], SYN internal anal *sphincter*.

m. sphinc'ter ductus biliaris, ✩official alternate term for *sphincter* of (common) bile duct.

m. sphinc'ter duc'tus chole'dochi [TA], SYN *sphincter* of (common) bile duct.

m. sphinc'ter duc'tus pancrea'tici, SYN *sphincter* of pancreatic duct.

m. sphinc'ter o'ris, SYN orbicularis oris (*muscle*).

m. sphinc'ter palatopharyn'geus, ✩official alternate term for posterior *fascicle* of palatopharyngeus muscle.

m. sphinc'ter pupil'lae [TA], SYN *sphincter* pupillae.

m. sphinc'ter pylo'ri [TA], SYN pyloric *sphincter*.

m. sphinc'ter ure'thrae externus, SYN external urethral *sphincter*.

m. sphinc'ter urethrae externus femininae [TA], SYN external urethral *sphincter* of female.

m. sphinc'ter urethrae externus masculinae [TA], SYN external urethral *sphincter* of male.

m. sphinc'ter urethrae internus, ✩official alternate term for internal urethral *sphincter*.

m. sphinc'ter urethrovaginalis [TA], SYN urethrovaginal *sphincter*.

m. sphinc'ter vagi'nae, SYN bulbospongiosus (*muscle*).

m. sphinc'ter vesi'cae, SYN internal urethral *sphincter*.

m. spina'lis [TA], SYN spinalis (*muscle*).

m. spina'lis cap'itis [TA], SYN spinalis capitis (*muscle*).

m. spina'lis cer'vicis [TA], SYN spinalis cervicis (*muscle*).

m. spina'lis col'li, SYN spinalis cervicis (*muscle*).

m. spina'lis dor'si, SYN spinalis thoracis (*muscle*).

m. spina'lis thora'cis [TA], SYN spinalis thoracis (*muscle*).

musculi splenii [TA], SYN splenius (*muscles*), under *muscle*.

m. sple'nius cap'itis [TA], SYN splenius capitis (*muscle*).

m. sple'nius cer'vicis [TA], SYN splenius cervicis (*muscle*).

m. sple'nius col'li, SYN splenius cervicis (*muscle*).

m. stape'dius [TA], SYN stapedius (*muscle*).

m. sterna'lis [TA], SYN sternalis (*muscle*).

m. sternochondroscapula'ris, SYN sternochondroscapular *muscle*.

m. sternoclavicula'ris, SYN sternoclavicular *muscle*.

m. sternocleidomastoi'deus [TA], SYN sternocleidomastoid (*muscle*).

m. sternofascia'lis, an occasional muscular slip arising from the manubrium of the sternum and inserted into the fascia of the neck.

m. sternohyoi'deus [TA], SYN sternohyoid (*muscle*).

m. sternothyroi'deus [TA], SYN sternothyroid (*muscle*).

m. styloauricula'ris, SYN styloauricular (*muscle*).

m. styloglos'sus [TA], SYN styloglossus (*muscle*).

m. stylohyoi'deus [TA], SYN stylohyoid (*muscle*).

m. stylolaryn'geus, that part of the stylopharyngeus which is inserted into the thyroid cartilage.

m. **stylopharyn′geus** [TA], SYN stylopharyngeus (*muscle*).

m. **subcla′vius** [TA], SYN subclavius (*muscle*).

m. **subcosta′lis**, pl. **mus′culi subcosta′les** [TA], SYN subcostal *muscle*.

m. **subcuta′neus col′li**, SYN platysma (*muscle*).

mus′culi suboccipita′les [TA], SYN suboccipital *muscles*, under *muscle*.

m. **subscapula′ris** [TA], SYN subscapularis (*muscle*).

m. **supina′tor** [TA], SYN supinator (*muscle*).

m. **supina′tor lon′gus**, obsolete and inaccurate term for brachioradialis (*muscle*).

m. **supina′tor ra′dii brev′is**, SYN supinator (*muscle*).

m. **supraclavicula′ris**, SYN supraclavicular *muscle*.

mus′culi suprahyoi′dei [TA], SYN suprahyoid *muscles*, under *muscle*.

m. **supraspina′lis**, SYN supraspinalis (*muscle*).

m. **supraspina′tus** [TA], SYN supraspinatus (*muscle*).

m. **suspenso′rius duode′ni** [TA], SYN suspensory *muscle* of duodenum.

m. **tarsa′lis infe′rior** [TA], SYN inferior tarsal *muscle*.

m. **tarsa′lis supe′rior** [TA], SYN superior tarsal *muscle*.

m. **tempora′lis** [TA], SYN temporalis (*muscle*).

m. **temporoparieta′lis** [TA], SYN temporoparietalis (*muscle*); SEE ALSO auricularis anterior (*muscle*), auricularis superior (*muscle*).

m. **ten′sor fas′ciae fem′oris**, SYN tensor fasciae latae (*muscle*).

m. **ten′sor fas′ciae la′tae** [TA], SYN tensor fasciae latae (*muscle*).

m. **ten′sor tar′si**, SYN lacrimal *part* of orbicularis oculi muscle; SEE orbicularis oculi (*muscle*).

m. **ten′sor tym′pani** [TA], SYN tensor tympani (*muscle*).

m. **ten′sor ve′li palati′ni** [TA], SYN tensor veli palati (*muscle*).

m. **te′res ma′jor** [TA], SYN teres major (*muscle*).

m. **te′res mi′nor** [TA], SYN teres minor (*muscle*).

m. **tetrago′nus**, SYN platysma (*muscle*).

mus′culi thora′cis [TA], SYN *muscles* of thorax, under *muscle*.

musculi thoracoappendiculares [TA], SYN thoracoappendicular *muscles*, under *muscle*.

m. **thyroarytenoi′deus** [TA], SYN thyroarytenoid (*muscle*).

m. **thyroarytenoi′deus exter′nus**, SYN thyroarytenoid (*muscle*).

m. **thyroarytenoi′deus inter′nus**, SYN vocalis (*muscle*).

m. **thyroepiglot′ticus**, SYN thyroepiglottic *part* of thyroarytenoid (*muscle*).

m. **thyrohyoi′deus** [TA], SYN thyrohyoid (*muscle*).

m. **thyropharyn′geus**, SEE inferior constrictor (*muscle*) of pharynx.

m. **tibia′lis ante′rior** [TA], SYN tibialis anterior (*muscle*).

m. **tibia′lis anti′cus**, SYN tibialis anterior (*muscle*).

m. **tibia′lis gra′cilis**, SYN plantaris (*muscle*).

m. **tibia′lis poste′rior** [TA], SYN tibialis posterior (*muscle*).

m. **tibia′lis posti′cus**, SYN tibialis posterior (*muscle*).

m. **tibia′lis secun′dus**, an inconstant muscle, of small size, arising from the back of the tibia and inserted into the articular capsule of the ankle joint. SYN second tibial muscle.

m. **tibiofascia′lis ante′rior, m. tibiofascia′lis anti′cus**, separate fibers of the tibialis anterior inserted into the fascia of the dorsum of the foot.

m. **trachea′lis** [TA], SYN trachealis (*muscle*).

m. **tracheloclavicula′ris**, SYN tracheloclavicular *muscle*.

m. **trachelomastoi′deus**, SYN longissimus capitis (*muscle*).

m. **tra′gicus** [TA], SYN tragicus (*muscle*).

m. **transversa′lis abdom′inis**, SYN transversus abdominis (*muscle*).

m. **transversa′lis cap′itis**, SYN longissimus capitis (*muscle*).

m. **transversa′lis cer′vicis, m. transversa′lis col′li**, SYN longissimus cervicis (*muscle*).

m. **transversa′lis na′si**, SEE nasalis (*muscle*).

musculi transversospina′les [TA], SYN transversospinales (*muscles*), under *muscle*.

m. **transver′sus abdom′inis** [TA], SYN transversus abdominis (*muscle*).

m. **transver′sus auric′ulae** [TA], SYN transverse *muscle* of auricle.

m. **transver′sus lin′guae** [TA], SYN transverse *muscle* of tongue.

m. **transver′sus men′ti** [TA], SYN transversus menti (*muscle*).

m. **transver′sus nu′chae** [TA], SYN transversus nuchae (*muscle*).

m. **transver′sus perine′i profun′dus** [TA], SYN deep transverse perineal *muscle*.

m. **transver′sus perine′i superficia′lis** [TA], SYN superficial transverse perineal *muscle*.

m. **transver′sus thora′cis** [TA], SYN transversus thoracis (*muscle*).

m. **trape′zius** [TA], SYN trapezius (*muscle*).

m. **triangula′ris** [TA], **(1)** [NA], SYN triangular *muscle* (1); **(2)** SYN depressor anguli oris (*muscle*).

m. **triangula′ris la′bii inferior′is**, SYN depressor anguli oris (*muscle*).

m. **triangula′ris la′bii superior′is**, SYN levator anguli oris (*muscle*).

m. **triangula′ris ster′ni**, SYN transversus thoracis (*muscle*).

m. **tri′ceps** [TA], SYN three-headed *muscle*.

m. **tri′ceps bra′chii** [TA], SYN triceps brachii (*muscle*).

m. **tri′ceps cox′ae**, SYN triceps coxae (*muscle*).

m. **tri′ceps su′rae** [TA], SYN triceps surae (*muscle*).

m. **triticeoglos′sus**, an occasional thin band of muscular fibers passing between the root of the tongue and the triticeal cartilage. SYN Bochdalek muscle.

m. **unipenna′tus**, ✳official alternate term for semipennate *muscle*.

m. **u′vulae** [TA], SYN *muscle* of uvula.

m. **vas′tus exter′nus**, SYN vastus lateralis (*muscle*).

m. **vas′tus interme′dius** [TA], SYN vastus intermedius (*muscle*).

m. **vas′tus inter′nus**, SYN vastus medialis (*muscle*).

m. **vas′tus latera′lis** [TA], SYN vastus lateralis (*muscle*).

m. **vas′tus media′lis** [TA], SYN vastus medialis (*muscle*).

m. **ventricula′ris**, fibers of the thyroarytenoid which pass into the vestibular fold (false vocal cord).

m. **vertica′lis lin′guae** [TA], SYN vertical *muscle* of tongue.

m. **voca′lis** [TA], SYN vocalis (*muscle*).

m. **zygomat′icus**, SYN zygomaticus major (*muscle*).

m. **zygomat′icus ma′jor** [TA], SYN zygomaticus major (*muscle*).

m. **zygomat′icus mi′nor** [TA], SYN zygomaticus minor (*muscle*).

---

mush·bite (mŭsh′bīt). A maxillomandibular record made by introducing a mass of soft wax into the patient's mouth and instructing the patient to bite into it to the desired degree; not a generally accepted procedure.

mu·si·co·ther·a·py (mū′sik-ō-thār′ă-pē). An adjunctive treatment of mental disorders by means of music.

Musset, L.C. Alfred de, French poet, 1810–1857; person in whom Musset *sign* was studied. SEE M. *sign.*

mus·si·ta·tion (mŭs-i-tā′shŭn). Movements of the lips as if speaking, but without sound; observed in delirium, semicoma, and severe Parkinson disease. [L. *mussito,* to murmur constantly, fr. *musso,* pp. -*atus,* to mutter]

Mussy. SEE Guéneau de Mussy.

must (mŭst). Unfermented juice of the grape or other fruits. [L. *mustum,* new wine, ntr. of *mustus,* fresh]

Mustard, William T., Canadian thoracic surgeon, 1914–1987. SEE M. *operation, procedure.*

mus·tard (mŭs′tard). **1.** The dried ripe seeds of *Brassica alba* (white m.) and *B. nigra* (black m.) (family Cruciferae). **2.** SYN mustard *gas.* [O.Fr. *moustarde,* fr. L. *mustum,* must]

black m., the dried ripe seed of *Brassica nigra* or of *B. juncea;* it is the source of allyl isothiocyanate; it contains sinigrin (potassium myronate); myrosin; sinapine sulfocyanate; erucic, behenic, and synapolic acids; and fixed oil; a prompt emetic, a rubefacient, and a condiment.

m. chlorohydrin, SYN hemisulfur m.

mu

hemisulfur m., an antineoplastic agent. SYN m. chlorohydrin, semisulfur m.

nitrogen m.'s (HN2), compounds of the general formula R—N(CH₂CH₂C1) the prototype is HN-2 nitrogen m., mechlorethamine, in which R is CH₃. Some have been used therapeutically for their destructive action upon lymphoid tissue in lymphosarcoma, leukemia, Hodgkin disease, and certain other cancers; most are blister agents. SEE ALSO mechlorethamine hydrochloride.

semisulfur m., SYN hemisulfur m.

sulfur m., SYN mustard *gas.*

uracil m., SEE *uracil* mustard.

white m., the ripe seeds of *Brassica (Sinapis) alba;* less pungent than black m., but with the same constituents and uses.

mus·tard oil. Term applied to any of the organic isothiocyanates in general, but more specifically to allyl isothiocyanate; such oils are metabolically convertible to thiocyanates and may thus lead to goiter.

expressed m. o., the fixed oil expressed from the seeds of *Brassica alba* and *B. nigra;* it contains the glycerides of oleic, arachidic, and other fatty acids; used as salad oil and in the manufacture of oleomargarine.

volatile m. o., SYN *allyl* isothiocyanate.

mus·tine hy·dro·chlo·ride (mŭs′tēn). SYN mechlorethamine hydrochloride.

mu·ta·cism (mū′tă-sizm). SYN mytacism.

mu·ta·gen (mū′tă-jen). Any agent that promotes a mutation or causes an increase in the rate of mutational events, e.g., radioactive substances, x-rays, or certain chemicals. [L. *muto,* to change, + G. *-gen,* producing]

frame-shift m., a m., such as an acridine derivative, that causes a reading-frame-shift mutation; codons (base triplets) are read out of phase and different amino acids are utilized.

mu·ta·gen·e·sis (mū-tă-jen′ĕ-sis). **1.** Production of a mutation. **2.** Production of genetic alteration through use of chemicals or radiation.

cassette m., the production of mutants within a region (often bounded by unique restriction sites) by the use of synthetic oligonucleotides that fill the gap with mutants designed into the synthetic genetic material.

insertional m., mutation caused by insertion of new genetic material into a normal gene, particularly of retroviruses into chromosomal DNA.

site-directed m., the controlled alterations of selected regions of a DNA molecule.

mu·ta·gen·ic (mū-tă-jen′ik). Promoting mutation.

mu·tant (myu′tant). **1.** A phenotype in which a mutation is manifested. **2.** A gene that is rare and usually harmful, in contrast to a wild-type gene, not necessarily generated recently.

active m., a m. with overt phenotypic expression.

amber m., a m. with a mutation resulting in a UAG codon.

auxotrophic m., m. with a nutritional requirement not present in the wild-type organism. SYN defective organism, deficiency m.

cold-sensitive m., a m. that is defective at low temperature but functional at normal temperature. Cf. temperature-sensitive m.

conditional-lethal m., SYN conditionally lethal m.

conditionally lethal m., a viral m. that can replicate under some (permissive) conditions but not under other (restrictive or nonpermissive) conditions, the parent (wild-type) strain being able to replicate under both conditions. SEE suppressor-sensitive m., temperature-sensitive m. SYN conditional-lethal m.

deficiency m., SYN auxotrophic m.

inactive m., a m. that is not phenotypically manifest. SYN silent m.

petite m., a m. with a mutation that caused the microorganism to grow very slowly or to form small colonies. [Fr. small]

quick-stop m., a bacterial m. that ceases replication immediately when the temperature reaches a certain level. Cf. temperature-sensitive m.

silent m., SYN inactive m.

suppressor-sensitive m., a conditionally lethal, host range, bacteriophage m. that produces nonsense codons and can replicate only

in a host bacterium able to translate the nonsense codon; the mutation's effects are lethal (i.e., prevent replication of the virus) in a bacterium without such a suppressor mechanism.

temperature-sensitive m., a viral m. that is able to replicate at one portion of a temperature range but not at another, the parent (wild-type) strain being able to replicate over the whole temperature range; usually a product is not made at the elevated temperature. Cf. cold-sensitive m., quick-stop m.

uninducible m., a m. that cannot be induced.

virulent phage m., a m. of a phage that is unable to establish lysogeny.

mu·ta·ro·tase (mū′tă-rō-tās). SYN aldose 1-epimerase.

mu·ta·ro·ta·tion (mū′tă-rō-tā′shŭn). The process of changing specific rotation at a given wavelength; e.g., a solution of α-D-glucose recrystallized from its solution in acetic acid and freshly dissolved in water gives a rotation of $[\alpha]_D^{20} = +112.2°$, but when recrystallized from a boiling aqueous solution (as the β-form) it shows an initial rotation of $[\alpha]_D^{20} = +18.7°$; either solution upon standing slowly changes its specific rotation to a value of $[\alpha]_D^{20} = +52.7°$, indicating a mixture of the two forms of D-glucose. SYN birotation, multirotation.

mu·tase (mū′tās). Any enzyme that catalyzes the apparent migration of groups within one molecule, e.g., phosphoglycerate phosphomutase; sometimes the transfer is from one molecule to another, e.g., phosphoglucomutase, phosphoglyceromutase (both phosphotransferases).

mu·ta·tion (mū-tā′shŭn). **1.** A change in the chemistry of a gene that is perpetuated in subsequent divisions of the cell in which it occurs; a change in the sequence of base pairs in the chromosomal molecule. **2.** De Vries term for the sudden production of a species, as distinguished from variation. [L. *muto,* pp. *-atus,* to change]

addition m., SYN reading-frame-shift m.

addition-deletion m., SYN reading-frame-shift m.

amber m., a m. that results in the formation of the codon UAG, which results in the premature termination of a polypeptide chain. Cf. suppressor m.

back m., reversion of a gene to an ancestral form due to further m. to the original codon or one coding for the same amino acid. SYN reverse m.

deletion m., SYN reading-frame-shift m.

frame-shift m., SYN reading-frame-shift m.

induced m., a m. caused by exposure to a mutagen.

lethal m., a mutant trait that leads to a phenotype incompatible with effective reproduction.

missense m., a m. in which a base change or substitution results in a codon that causes insertion of a different amino acid into the growing polypeptide chain, giving rise to an altered protein. [missense by analogy with non-sense]

natural m., SYN spontaneous m.

neutral m., a m. with a negligible impact on genetic fitness.

new m., redundant term for a heritable trait present in the offspring but in neither parent, i.e., not a pre-existing mutant form inherited.

nonsense m., SYN suppressor m.

ochre m., a m. yielding the termination codon UAA, resulting in premature termination of a polypeptide chain. Cf. suppressor m.

opal m., SYN umber m.

point m., a m. that involves a single nucleotide; it may consist of loss of a nucleotide, substitution of one nucleotide for another, or the insertion of an additional nucleotide.

reading-frame-shift m., a m. that results from insertion or deletion of a single nucleotide into, or from, the normal DNA sequence; since the genetic code is read three nucleotides at a time, all nucleotide triplets distal to the mutation will be one step out of phase and misread, and hence translated as different amino acids. SYN addition m., addition-deletion m., deletion m., frame-shift m.

reverse m., SYN back m.

silent m., the form of a genetic trait distinguishable at the genotypic level but not at the level of arbitrary phenotype (e.g., clinical, immunological, or electrophoretic).

site specific m., an alteration of the structure of a gene at a specific sequence, usually referring to experimentally produced changes in gene sequence.

somatic m., a m. occurring in the general body cells (as opposed to the germ cells) and hence not transmitted to progeny.

spontaneous m., a m. that arises naturally and not as a result of exposure to mutagens. SYN natural m.

suppressor m., (1) a second m. that alters the anticodon in a tRNA so that it can recognize a nonsense (stop) codon, thus suppressing termination of the amino acid chain. Cf. amber m., ochre m., umber m; **(2)** genetic changes such that the effect of a m. in one place can be masked by a second m. in another location. There are two types: intergenic suppression (occurring in a different gene) and intragenic suppression (occurring in the same gene but at a different site). SYN nonsense m.

transition m., a point m. involving substitution of one base-pair for another, i.e., replacement of one purine for another and of one pyrimidine for another pyrimidine without change in the purine-pyrimidine orientation.

transversion m., a point m. involving base substitution in which the orientation of purine and pyrimidine is reversed, in contradistinction to transition m.

umber m., a m. yielding the termination codon UGA, resulting in premature termination of a polypeptide chain. Cf. suppressor m. SYN opal m.

up promoter m., a m. that increases the frequency of initiation of transcription.

mute (mūt). **1.** Unable or unwilling to speak. **2.** A person who has not the faculty of speech. [L. *mutus*]

mu·tein (mū′tēn). A term used for a protein arising as a result of a mutation. [*mut*ation + prot*ein*]

mu·ti·la·tion (mū-ti-lā′shŭn). Disfigurement or injury by removal or destruction of any conspicuous or essential part of the body. [L. *mutilatio,* fr. *mutilo,* pp. *-atus,* to maim]

mut·ism (mū′tizm). **1.** The state of being silent. **2.** Organic or functional absence of the faculty of speech. [L. *mutus,* mute]

akinetic m., subacute or chronic state of altered consciousness, in which the patient appears alert intermittently, but is not responsive, although his/her descending motor pathways appear intact; due to lesions of various cerebral structures. SYN coma vigil.

elective m., m. due to psychogenic causes. SYN voluntary m.

voluntary m., SYN elective m.

mu·ton (mū′ton). In genetics, the smallest unit of a chromosome in which alteration can be effective in causing a mutation (a single nucleotide change). [*mut*ation + *-on*]

mu·tu·al·ism (mū′tū-ăl-izm). Symbiotic relationship in which both species derive benefit. Cf. commensalism, metabiosis, parasitism.

mu·tu·al·ist (mū′tū-ăl-ist). SYN symbion. [L. *mutuus,* in return, mutual]

Mv Obsolete abbreviation for mendelevium.

mV Abbreviation for millivolt.

MVV Abbreviation for maximum voluntary *ventilation.*

MW Abbreviation for molecular *weight.*

my·al·gia (mī-al′jē-ă). Muscular pain. SYN myodynia. [G. *mys,* muscle, + *algos,* pain]

epidemic m., SYN epidemic *pleurodynia.*

m. ther′mica, SYN heat *cramps,* under *cramp.*

my·as·the·nia (mī-as-thē′nē-ă). Muscular weakness. [G. *mys,* muscle, + *astheneia,* weakness]

m. angioscler ot′ica, SYN intermittent *claudication.*

m. gravis, a disorder of neuromuscular transmission marked by fluctuating weakness and fatigue of certain voluntary muscles, including those innervated by brainstem motor nuclei; caused by a marked reduction in the number of acetylcholine receptors in the postsynaptic membrane of the neuromuscular junction, resulting from an autoimmune mechanism. SYN Goldflam disease.

my·as·then·ic (mī′as-then′ik). Relating to myasthenia.

my·a·to·nia, my·at·o·ny (mī-ă-tō′nē-ă, mī-at′ō-nē). Abnormal extensibility of a muscle. [G. *mys,* muscle, + *a* priv. + *tonos,* tone]

m. congen′ita, SYN *amyotonia* congenita.

my·at·ro·phy (mī-at′rō-fē). SYN muscular *atrophy.*

my·ce·lia (mī-sē′lē-ă). Plural of mycelium.

my·ce·li·an (mī-sē′lē-an). Pertaining to a mycelium.

my·ce·li·oid (mī-sē′lē-oyd). Resembling a mycelium. [mycelium + G. *eidos,* resemblance]

my·ce·li·um, pl. **my·ce·lia** (mī-sē′lē-ŭm, -ă). The mass of hyphae making up a colony of fungi. [G. *mykēs,* fungus, + *hēlos,* nail, wart, excrescence on animal or plant]

aerial m., the portion of m. that grows upward or outward from the surface of the substrate, and from which propagative spores develop in or on characteristic structures that are distinctive for various generic groups.

nonseptate m., one in which there are no septa, or "cross-walls," in the hyphae; inasmuch as the latter are not divided into numerous individual cells, the multinucleated protoplasm may flow throughout the tubelike structures.

septate m., one in which septa, or "cross-walls," divide the hyphae into numerous uninucleated or multinucleated cells.

△**mycet-, myceto-.** Fungus. SEE ALSO myco-. [G. *mykēs,* fungus]

my·cete (mī′sēt). A fungus. [G. *mykēs,* fungus]

my·ce·tism, my·ce·tis·′mus (mī′sē-tizm, -tiz′mŭs). Poisoning by certain species of mushrooms. SYN muscarinism. [G. *mykēs,* fungus]

m. cerebra′lis, a condition characterized by transient hallucinogenic symptoms following ingestion of mushrooms such as *Psilocybe* and *Panaeolus.*

m. cholifor′mis, a severe and occasionally fatal illness due to the consumption of *Amanita phalloides* and other poisonous mushroom species.

m. gastrointestina′lis, a relatively mild type of mushroom poisoning characterized by nausea, vomiting, and diarrhea and caused by eating certain species of *Boletus, Lactarius, Entoloma,* and *Lepiota.*

m. nervo′sa, mushroom poisoning that involves the parasympathetic nervous system and causes gastrointestinal distress, after consumption of species such as *Amanita, Inocybe,* and *Clitocybe.*

m. sanguina′reus, a transient hemoglobinuria and jaundice caused by eating the mushroom *Helvella esculenta,* either raw or cooked.

my·ce·to·ge·net·ic, my·ce·to·gen·ic (mī-sē′tō-jĕ-net′ik, mī′sē-tō-; -jen′ik). Caused by fungi. SYN mycetogenous. [G. *mykēs,* fungus, + *gennētos,* begotten]

my·ce·tog·e·nous (mī-sē-toj′ĕ-nŭs). SYN mycetogenetic.

my·ce·to·ma (mī-sē-tō′mă). A chronic infection involving the subcutaneous tissue, skin, and contiguous bone; characterized by the formation of localized lesions with tumefactions and multiple draining sinuses. The exudate contains granules that may be yellow, white, red, brown, or black, depending upon the causative agent. M. is caused by two principal groups of microorganisms: 1) actinomycetoma is caused by actinomycetes, including species of *Streptomyces, Actinomadurae,* and *Nocardia,* 2) eumycetoma is caused by true fungi, including species of *Madurella, Exophiala, Pseudallescheria, Curvularia, Neotestudina, Pyrenochaeta, Aspergillus, Leptosphaeria, Plemodomus, Polycytella, Fusarium, Phialophora, Corynespora, Cylindrocarpon, Pseudochaetosphaeronema, Bipolaris,* and *Acremonium.* SYN Madura boil, Madura foot, maduromycosis.

△**myco-.** Fungus. SEE ALSO mycet-. [G. *mykēs,* fungus]

my·co·bac·te·ria (mī′kō-bak-tē′rē-ă). Organisms belonging to the genus *Mycobacterium.*

atypical m., species of mycobacteria other than *M. tuberculosis* or *M. bovis* that can cause disease in immunocompromised humans; being replaced by the designation of MOTT (Mycobacteria Other Than Tuberculosis).

Runyon group I m., m. that produce a bright yellow color when grown in the presence of light. Organisms placed in this group include *Mycobacterium kansasii.* SYN photochromogens.

Runyon group II m., m. that produce a yellow pigment even when grown in the dark; when grown in the light, the pigment is orange. These organisms behave as saprophytes do in humans and are usually nonpathogenic to laboratory animals. SYN scotochromogens.

Runyon group III m., m. that are either colorless or that slowly produce a light yellow pigment when grown in the presence of light. Organisms placed in this group include *Mycobacterium avium* and *M. intracellulare*. SYN nonchromogens.

Runyon group IV m., m. that grow rapidly and that do not produce pigment. Organisms placed in this group belong to such species as *Mycobacterium ulcerans* and *M. marinum*.

My·co·bac·te·ri·a·ce·ae (mī′kō-bak-tēr-ē-ā′sē-ē). A family of aerobic bacteria (order Actinomycetales) containing Gram-positive, spherical to rod-shaped cells. Branching does not occur under ordinary cultural conditions. They are usually acid-fast. They occur in soil and dairy products and as parasites on humans and other animals. The type genus is *Mycobacterium*.

my·co·bac·te·ri·o·sis (mī′kō-bak-tēr′ē-ō′sis). Infection with mycobacteria.

My·co·bac·te·ri·um (mī′kō-bak-tēr′ē-ŭm). A genus of aerobic, nonmotile bacteria (family Mycobacteriaceae) containing Gram-positive, acid-fast, slender, straight or slightly curved rods; slender filaments occasionally occur, but branched forms rarely are produced. Parasitic and saprophytic species occur. A number of species are associated with infections in immunocompromised people, especially those with AIDS. The type species is *M. tuberculosis*. It is the type genus of the family Mycobacteriaceae. [myco- + bacterium]

M. absces′sus, SYN *M. chelonae* subsp. *abscessus.*

M. a′vium, a bacterial species causing tuberculosis in fowl and other birds. Causes opportunistic infections in humans.

M. avium-intracellulare complex, an opportunistic agent of infection, particularly in people with AIDS. Difficult to treat because *M. avium-intracellulare* is resistant to many antibiotics. The organism may also cause chronic lower respiratory tract infections in patients who are not severely immunocompromised, especially those with underlying abnormal lung parenchyma.

M. bo′vis, a bacterial species that is the primary cause of tuberculosis in cattle; transmissible to humans and other animals, causing tuberculosis. SYN tubercle bacillus (2).

M. chelo′nae, rapid-growing mycobacterium (Runyon group IV) that cause sporadic infection in any tissue or organ system in humans following cardiothoracic surgery, peritoneal- and hemodialysis, augmentation mammaplasty, arthroplasty, and immunocompromised patients.

M. chelo′nae subsp. *absces′sus,* a bacterial species originally found in a traumatic infection of the knee. SYN *M. abscessus.*

M. fortui′tum, a saprophytic bacterial species found in soil and in infections of humans, cattle, and cold-blooded animals. Causes skin abscesses.

M. intracellula′re, a bacterial species found in lung lesions and sputum of humans; may cause bone and tendon-sheath lesions in rabbits; some strains are pathogenic for mice. Recently linked to opportunistic infections in humans. SYN Battey bacillus.

M. kansas′ii, a bacterial species causing a tuberculosislike pulmonary disease; found to cause rare infections (and usually lesions) in spinal fluid, spleen, liver, pancreas, testes, hip joint, knee joint, finger, wrist, and lymph nodes.

M. lep′rae, a bacterial species that causes Hansen disease (leprosy); an obligatory intracellular mycobacterium that has not been propagated in the laboratory, but that will survive in the 9-banded armadillo (*Dasypus novemcinctus*). SYN Hansen bacillus, leprosy bacillus.

M. maria′num, former name for *M. scrofulaceum.*

M. mari′num, a bacterial species causing spontaneous tuberculosis in salt water fish; it also occurs in other cold-blooded animals, in some aquaria and swimming pools in which it may cause human cutaneous infection (see swimming pool *granuloma*), irrigation canals and ditches, and ocean beaches.

M. micro′ti, a bacterial species causing generalized tuberculosis in voles; transmissible to guinea pigs, rabbits, and calves, causing localized infections.

M. paratuberculo′sis, a bacterial species causing Johne disease, a chronic enteritis in cattle.

M. phle′i, a bacterial species found in soil and dust and on plants. SYN Moeller grass bacillus.

M. scrofula′ceum, a bacterial species frequently associated with cervical adenitis in children.

M. smeg′matis, a saprophytic bacterial species of bacteria found in smegma from the genitalia of humans and many of the lower animals; it is also found in soil, dust, and water.

🄸*M. tuberculo′sis,* a bacterial species that causes tuberculosis in humans; it is the type species of the genus *M.* SYN Koch bacillus, tubercle bacillus (1).

M. ul′cerans, a bacterial species causing Buruli ulcers in humans; transmissible from soil, usually after an injury, and possibly by an insect vector.

M. vaccae, a rapidly growing scotochromogenic, nonpathogenic species that is distributed widely in nature.

M. xen′opi, a bacterial species found in a skin lesion of a cold-blooded animal, *Xenopus laevis;* a rare cause of nosocomial human pulmonary tuberculosis.

my·co·bac·tin (mī′kō-bak′tin). A complex lipid factor reported to be required for the growth of *Mycobacterium tuberculosis* in human plasma; appears to be identical with the lipid factor extracted from *M. phlei* and essential for the growth of *M. johnei.*

my·co·cide (mī′kō-sīd). SYN fungicide. [myco- + L. *caedo,* to kill]

my·co·der·ma·ti·tis (mī′kō-der-mă-tī′tis). An obsolete term to designate an eruption of mycotic (fungus, yeast, mold) origin.

my·co·gas·tri·tis (mī′kō-gas-trī′tis). Inflammation of the stomach due to the presence of a fungus. [myco- + G. *gastēr,* stomach, + -*itis,* inflammation]

my·col·ic ac·ids (mī-kol′ik). Long-chain cyclopropanecarboxylic acids (C_{19}–C_{21}), further substituted by long-chain (C_{24}–C_{30}) alkanes containing free hydroxyl groups, found in certain bacteria; these waxy substances appear to be responsible for the acid-fastness of the bacteria that contain them. SYN mykol.

my·col·o·gist (mī-kol′ŏ-jist). A person specializing in mycology.

my·col·o·gy (mī-kol′ō-jē). The study of fungi: their classification, edibility, cultivation, and biology. [myco- + G. *logos,* study]

medical m., the study of fungi that produce disease in humans and other animals, and of the diseases they produce, their ecology, and their epidemiology.

my·co·phage (mī′kō-fāj). A virus, the host of which is a fungus, in contradistinction to a bacteriophage, the host of which is a bacterium. SEE ALSO mycovirus. [myco- + G. *phagō,* to eat]

My·co·plas·ma (mī′kō-plaz′mă). A genus of aerobic to facultatively anaerobic bacteria (family Mycoplasmataceae) containing Gram-negative cells that do not possess a true cell wall but are bounded by a three-layered membrane; they do not revert to bacteria containing cell walls or cell wall fragments. The minimal reproductive units of these organisms are 0.2–0.3 μm in diameter. The cells are pleomorphic, and in liquid media appear as coccoid bodies, rings, or filaments. Colonies of most species consist of a central core, growing down into the medium, surrounded by superficial peripheral growth. They require sterol for growth. They also require enrichment with serum or ascitic fluid. These organisms are found in humans and other animals and can be pathogenic. The type species is *M. mycoides.* SYN Asterococcus. [myco- + G. *plasma,* something formed (plasm)]

M. bucca′le, a species which is an infrequent parasitic inhabitant of the human oropharynx; it is the predominant mycoplasma in the oropharynx of nonhuman primates.

M. fau′cium, a bacterial species that is a rare member of the normal flora of the human oropharynx; it is occasionally found in the oropharynx of nonhuman primates.

M. fermen′tans, a bacterial species found in ulcerative genital lesions associated with fusiform bacteria and spirilla and also on the apparently normal genital mucosa of humans.

M. genita′lium, a bacterial species that may be a causative agent of urethritis; cross-reacts immunologically with *M. pneumoniae;* can cause serious infections involving the respiratory tract, heart, bloodstream, central nervous system, and prosthetic valves and joints.

M. hom′inis, a bacterial species that is the causative agent of pelvic inflammatory disease and other genitourinary tract infections; can also cause chorioamnionitis and postpartum fever; can be an oropharyngeal commensal and has caused nosocomial wound infections.

M. laidla′wii, SYN *Acholeplasma laidlawii.*

M. ora′le, a bacterial species of *M.* associated with the buccal and pharyngeal cavities of humans and animals.

M. pharyn′gis, a bacterial species occurring as a commensal in the human oropharynx.

M. pneumo′niae, a bacterial species causing otitis and upper and lower respiratory tract disease including primary atypical pneumonia in human beings. SYN Eaton agent.

M. saliva′rium, a bacterial species found in the human pharynx.

my·co·plas·ma, pl. **my·co·plas·ma·ta** (mī′kō-plaz′mă, -plaz′mah-tă). A vernacular term used only to refer to any member of the genus *Mycoplasma.*

My·co·plas·ma·ta·les (mī′kō-plaz′mă-tā′lēz). An order of Gram-negative bacteria containing cells which are bounded by a three-layered membrane but which do not possess a true cell wall. The minimal reproductive units are 0.2 to 0.3 μm in diameter. Pathogenic and saprophytic species occur. These organisms reproduce through the breaking up of branched filaments into coccoid, filterable elementary bodies. The order includes the so-called pleuropneumonia-like *organisms*, under *organism* (PPLO).

my·co·pus (mī′kō-pŭs). SYN mucopus.

my·cose (mī′kōs). SYN trehalose.

my·co·sis, pl. **my·co·ses** (mī-kō′sis, -sēz). Any disease caused by a fungus (filamentous or yeast). [myco- + G. *-osis*, condition]

m. framboesioi′des, SYN yaws.

⚠**m. fungoi′des,** a chronic progressive lymphoma arising in the skin that initially simulates eczema or other inflammatory dermatoses; the appearance of plaques is associated with acanthosis and bandlike infiltration of the upper dermis by a pleomorphic infiltrate including helper T lymphocytes with large, convoluted nuclei that also collect in clear spaces in the lower epidermis (Pautrier microabscesses); in advanced cases, ulcerated tumors and infiltration of lymph nodes may occur.

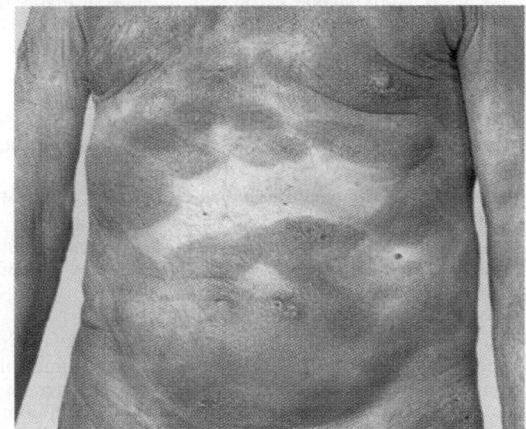

mycosis fungoides

m. intestina′lis, gastroenteric form of anthrax, the symptoms of which are those of gastroenteritis followed by toxemia and general depression.

my·co·stat·ic (mī-kō-stat′ik). SYN fungistatic.

my·cos·ter·ols (mī-kos′ter-olz). Sterols obtained from fungi.

my·cot·ic (mī-kot′ik). Relating to or caused by a fungus.

my·co·tox·i·co·sis (mī′kō-tok-si-kō′sis). Poisoning due to the ingestion of preformed substances produced by the action of certain fungi on particular foodstuffs or ingestion of the fungi themselves; e.g., ergotism. [myco- + G. *toxikon*, poison, + *-osis*, condition]

my·co·tox·in (mī′kō-tok-sinz). Toxic compound produced by cer-

tain fungi; some are used for medicinal purposes; e.g., muscarine, psilocybin.

my·co·vi·rus (mī′kō-vī-rŭs). A virus that infects fungi.

my·da·le·ine (mī-dā′lē-ēn). A poisonous ptomaine formed in putrefying liver and other viscera; it acts specifically upon the heart, causing arrest of its action in diastole. [G. *mydaleos*, moldy, fr. *mydos*, dampness]

my·da·tox·in (mī-dă-tok′sin). A ptomaine from putrefying viscera and flesh. [G. *mydos*, dampness, decay, + *toxikon*, poison]

my·dri·a·sis (mi-drī′ă-sis). Dilation of the pupil. [G.]

  alternating m., m. alternately affecting each eye.

  amaurotic m., a moderate widening of both pupils resulting from impaired visual input from one or both eyes.

  paralytic m., pupillary dilation due to paralysis of the sphincter muscle of the pupil induced by anticholinergic drugs given topically or systemically, or resulting from lesions of the oculomotor nucleus or nerve, contusion of the eyeball, or glaucoma.

  spastic m., pupillary dilation due to contraction of the dilator muscle of the pupil induced by adrenergic drugs or by stimulation of the sympathetic pathway.

myd·ri·at·ic (mi-drē-at′ik). **1.** Causing mydriasis or dilation of the pupil. **2.** An agent that dilates the pupil.

my·ec·to·my (mī-ek′tō-mē). Excision of a portion of a muscle. [G. *mys*, muscle, + *ektomē*, excision]

my·ec·to·py, my·ec·to·pia (mī-ek′tō-pē, mī-ek-tō′pē-ă). Rarely used term for dislocation of a muscle. [G. *mys*, muscle, + *ektopos*, out of place]

♻**myel-, myelo-. 1.** The bone marrow. **2.** The spinal cord and medulla oblongata. Cf. medullo-. **3.** The myelin sheath of nerve fibers. [G. *myelos*, medulla, marrow]

my·el·ap·o·plexy (mī′el-ap′ō-plek′sē). SYN hematomyelia. [myel- + G. *apoplēxia*, apoplexy]

my·el·a·te·lia (mī′el-ă-tē′lē-ă). Developmental defect of the spinal cord. [myel- + G. *ateleia*, incompleteness]

my·el·auxe (mī-el-awk′sē). Hypertrophy of the spinal cord. [myel- + G. *auxē*, increase]

my·e·le·mia (mī-ĕ-lē′mē-ă). Rarely used term for myelocytosis. [myel- + G. *haima*, blood]

my·el·en·ceph·a·lon (mī′el-en-sef′ă-lon) [TA]. SYN *medulla* oblongata. [myel- + G. *enkephalos*, brain]

my·el·ic (mī-el′ik). Relating to (1) the spinal cord, or (2) bone marrow.

my·e·lin (mī′ĕ-lin). **1.** The lipoproteinaceous material, composed of regularly alternating membranes of lipid lamellae (cholesterol, phospholipids, sphingolipids, phosphatidates) and protein, of the myelin sheath. **2.** Droplets of lipid formed during autolysis and postmortem decomposition.

my·e·li·nat·ed (mī′ĕ-li-nāt-ed). Having a myelin sheath. SYN medullated (2).

my·e·li·na·tion (mī′ĕ-li-nā′shŭn). The acquisition, development, or formation of a myelin sheath around a nerve fiber. SYN medullation (2), myelinization, myelinogenesis.

my·e·lin·ic (mī′ĕ-lin′ik). Relating to myelin.

my·e·lin·i·za·tion (mī′ĕ-li-nī-zā′shŭn). SYN myelination.

my·e·li·noc·la·sis (mī′ĕ-li-nok′lă-sis). Destruction of myelin. SEE ALSO demyelination, dysmyelination. [myelin + G. *klasis*, a breaking]

my·e·lin·o·gen·e·sis (mī′ĕ-lin-ō-jen′ĕ-sis). SYN myelination. [myelin + G. *genesis*, production]

my·e·li·nol·y·sis (mī′ĕ-li-nol′i-sis). Dissolution of the myelin sheaths of nerve fibers. [myelin + G. *lysis*, dissolution]

  central pontine m., localized loss of myelin within the midbase of the pons; related to malnutrition and often to alcoholism.

my·e·lin·o·pa·thy (mī′ĕ-lin-op′ă-thē). A disorder affecting the myelin of peripheral nerve fibers, in contrast to one affecting axons (axonopathy).

my·e·lit·ic (mī-ĕ-lit′ik). Relating to or affected by myelitis.

my·e·li·tis (mī-ĕ-lī′tis). **1.** Inflammation of the spinal cord. **2.** Inflammation of the bone marrow. [myel- + G. *-itis*, inflammation]

my

acute necrotizing m., a spinal cord disorder, probably a demyelinating disease, which affects persons of all ages and either sex. Presents with abrupt or more gradual onset with sensory abnormalities and upper motor neuron weakness; soon a reflexic flaccid motor paralysis and sphincter paralysis supervenes, which is permanent. In some, but not all cases, bilateral or unilateral optic neuritis is associated. In the cerebrospinal fluid, the protein is increased, and mononuclear cells are present. After autopsy, the lesion has been identified as a necrotizing hemorrhagic leukomyelitis.

acute transverse m., acute inflammation and softening of the spinal cord; involves the entire thickness of the spinal cord but of limited longitudinal extent; multiple etiologies.

ascending m., progressive inflammation involving successively higher areas of the spinal cord.

bulbar m., inflammation of the medulla oblongata.

concussion m., traumatic myelopathy.

demyelinated m., acute multiple sclerosis presenting as a myelitis.

Foix-Alajouanine m., SYN subacute necrotizing m.

funicular m., (1) inflammation involving any of the columns of the spinal cord; (2) SYN subacute combined *degeneration* of the spinal cord.

postinfectious m., spinal cord inflammation that follows a viral infection, usually one of the exanthemas.

postvaccinal m., spinal cord inflammation that follows vaccination.

radiation m., SYN radiation *myelopathy*.

subacute necrotizing m., a disorder of the lower spinal cord in adult males resulting in progressive paraplegia. SYN angiodysgenetic myelomalacia, Foix-Alajouanine m.

systemic m., inflammation confined to special tracts of the spinal cord.

transverse m., an inflammatory process involving both gray and white matter of spinal cord.

myelo-. SEE myel-.

my·e·lo·ar·chi·tec·ton·ics (mī′ĕ-lō-ar′ki-tek-ton′iks). The pattern of myelinated nerve fibers in the brain, as distinguished from cytoarchitectonics.

my·e·lo·blast (mī′ĕ-lō-blast). An immature cell (10 to 18 μm in diameter) in the granulocytic series, occurring normally in bone marrow, but not in the circulating blood (except in certain diseases). When stained with the usual dyes, the cytoplasm is light blue, nongranular, and variable in amount, sometimes being only a thin rim around the nucleus; the latter is deep purple-blue with finely divided, punctate, threadlike chromatin that is somewhat condensed at the periphery. A few light blue nucleoli are usually present in the nucleus, and these generally disappear as the m. matures into a promyelocyte and then a myelocyte. M.'s ordinarily yield a negative reaction with peroxidase. [myelo- + G. *blastos,* germ]

my·e·lo·blas·te·mia (mī′ĕ-lō-blas-tē′mē-ă). The presence of myeloblasts in the circulating blood. [myeloblast + G. *haima,* blood]

my·e·lo·blas·to·ma (mī′ĕ-lō-blas-tō′mă). A nodular focus or fairly well-circumscribed accumulation of myeloblasts, as sometimes observed in acute myeloblastic leukemia and chlorosis. [myeloblast + G. *-oma,* tumor]

my·e·lo·blas·to·sis (mī′ĕ-lō-blas-tō′sis). The presence of unusually large numbers of myeloblasts in the circulating blood, or tissues, or both (as in acute leukemia).

my·e·lo·cele (mī′ĕ-lō-sēl). 1. Protrusion of the spinal cord in spina bifida. [myelo- + G. *kēlē,* hernia] 2. The central canal of the spinal cord. [G. *myelos,* marrow, + *koilia,* a hollow]

my·e·lo·cyst (mī′ĕ-lō-sist). Any cyst (usually lined with columnar or cuboidal cells) that develops from a rudimentary central canal in the central nervous system. [myelo- + G. *kystis,* bladder]

my·e·lo·cyst·ic (mī′ĕ-lō-sist′ik). Pertaining to or characterized by the presence of a myelocyst.

my·e·lo·cys·to·cele (mī′ĕ-lō-sis′tō-sēl). Spina bifida containing spinal cord substance. [myelo- + G. *kystis,* bladder, + *kēlē,* tumor]

my·e·lo·cys·to·me·ning·o·cele (mī′ĕ-lō-sis′tō-mĕ-ning′gō-sēl).

SYN meningomyelocele. [myelo- + G. *kystis,* bladder, + *mēninx* (*mēning-*), membrane, + *kēlē,* hernia]

my·e·lo·cyte (mī′ĕ-lō-sīt). 1. A young cell of the granulocytic series, occurring normally in bone marrow, but not in circulating blood (except in certain diseases). When stained with the usual dyes, the cytoplasm is distinctly basophilic and relatively more abundant than in myeloblasts or promyelocytes, even though m.'s are smaller cells; numerous cytoplasmic granules (i.e., neutrophilic, eosinophilic, or basophilic) are present in the more mature forms of m.'s, and the first two types are peroxidase-positive. The nuclear chromatin is coarser than that observed in myeloblasts, but it is relatively faintly stained and lacks a well defined membrane; the nucleus is fairly regular in contour (i.e., not indented), and seems to be "buried" beneath the numerous cytoplasmic granules. 2. A nerve cell of the gray matter of the brain or spinal cord. SYN medullocell. [myelo- + G. *kytos,* cell]

m. A, the youngest form of m., characterized by only a few (not more than ten) cytoplasmic granules, which are most reliably demonstrated by means of staining with neutral red; the mitochondria are numerous, and resemble those of the myeloblast.

m. B, the intermediate form of m., characterized by approximately 30–100 (or more) cytoplasmic granules scattered among the mitochondria; the latter are less numerous than in m.'s of the A stage, and they are frequently displaced toward the periphery of the cell.

m. C, the most mature of the m.'s characterized by numerous cytoplasmic granules that are recognizable as neutrophilic, eosinophilic, and basophilic; with neutral red these are stained, respectively, red, bright yellow, and deep maroon; C m.'s are frequently larger than earlier forms; if the nucleus is indented, the m. is maturing into a metamyelocyte.

my·e·lo·cy·the·mia (mī′ĕ-lō-sī-thē′mē-ă). The presence of myelocytes in the circulating blood, especially in persistently large numbers (as in myelocytic leukemia). [myelocyte + G. *haima,* blood]

my·e·lo·cyt·ic (mī′ĕ-lō-sit′ik). Pertaining to or characterized by myelocytes.

my·e·lo·cy·to·ma (mī′ĕ-lō-sī-tō′mă). A nodular focus or fairly well-circumscribed, relatively dense accumulation of myelocytes, as in certain tissues of persons with myelocytic leukemia. [myelocyte + G. *-oma,* tumor]

my·e·lo·cy·to·ma·to·sis (mī′ĕ-lō-sī′tō-mă-tō′sis). A form of tumor involving chiefly the myelocytes.

my·e·lo·cy·to·sis (mī′ĕ-lō-sī-tō′sis). The occurrence of abnormally large numbers of myelocytes in the circulating blood, or tissues, or both. [myelocyte + G. *-osis,* condition]

my·e·lo·di·as·ta·sis (mī′ĕ-lō-dī-as′tă-sis). Softening and destruction of the spinal cord. [myelo- + G. *diastasis,* separation]

my·e·lo·dys·pla·sia (mī′ĕ-lō-dis-plā′zē-ă). 1. An abnormality in development of the spinal cord, especially the lower part of the cord. 2. Inappropriate term for spina bifida occulta. [myelo- + G. *dys-,* difficult, + *plasis,* a molding]

my·e·lo·fi·bro·sis (mī′ĕ-lō-fī-brō′sis). Fibrosis of the bone marrow, especially generalized, associated with myeloid metaplasia of the spleen and other organs, leukoerythroblastic anemia, and thrombocytopenia, although the bone marrow often contains many megakaryocytes. SYN myelosclerosis, osteomyelofibrotic syndrome.

my·e·lo·gen·e·sis (mī′ĕ-lō-jen′ĕ-sis). 1. Development of bone marrow. 2. Development of the central nervous system. 3. Formation of myelin around an axon.

my·e·lo·ge·net·ic, my·e·lo·gen·ic (mī′ĕ-lō-jĕ-net′ik, -jen′ik). 1. Relating to myelogenesis. 2. Produced by or originating in the bone marrow. SYN myelogenous.

my·e·log·e·nous (mī-ĕ-loj′ĕ-nŭs). SYN myelogenetic (2).

my·e·lo·gone, my·e·lo·go·ni·um (mī′ĕ-lō-gōn, mī′ĕ-lō-gō′nē-ŭm). An immature white blood cell of the myeloid series that is characterized by a relatively large, fairly deeply stained, finely reticulated nucleus that contains palely stained nucleoli, and a scant amount of rimlike, nongranular, moderately basophilic cytoplasm. M.'s are difficult to distinguish from lymphoblasts and monoblasts, unless one evaluates them in relation to the more mature forms usually associated with the younger cells. [myelo- + G. *gonē*, seed]

my·e·lo·gram (mī′ĕ-lō-gram). Radiographic contrast study of the spinal subarachnoid space and its contents.

cervical m., contrast medium introduced directly into the cervical subarachnoid space, or moved with the help of gravity from the lumbar region, to outline the cervical cord and nerve roots.

lumbar m., most common study for herniated nucleus pulposus or intervertebral disc protrusion.

my·e·log·ra·phy (mī′ĕ-log′ră-fē). Radiography of the spinal cord and nerve roots after the injection of a contrast medium into the spinal subarachnoid space. [myelo- + G. *graphē*, a drawing]

my·e·lo·ic (mī-ĕ-lō′ik). Pertaining to the tissue and precursor cells from which neutrophils, eosinophils, and basophils are derived.

my·e·loid (mī′ĕ-loyd). 1. Pertaining to, derived from, or manifesting certain features of the bone marrow. 2. Sometimes used with reference to the spinal cord. 3. Pertaining to certain characteristics of myelocytic forms, but not necessarily implying origin in the bone marrow. [myel- + -oid]

my·e·loi·do·sis (mī′ĕ-loy-dō′sis). General hyperplasia of myeloid tissue.

myelokathexis. SYN kathexis.

my·e·lo·leu·ke·mia (mī′ĕ-lō-loo-kē′mē-ă). A form of leukemia in which the abnormal cells are derived from myelopoietic tissue.

my·e·lo·li·po·ma (mī′ĕ-lō-li-pō′mă). Nodular accumulations of cells derived from localized proliferation of reticuloendothelial tissue in the blood sinuses of the adrenal glands; grossly, the nodules may seem to be adipose tissue, but actually are foci of bone marrow containing erythropoietic or myeloid cells.

my·e·lo·lym·pho·cyte (mī′ĕ-lō-mon′ō-sīt). Obsolete term for an abnormal form of the lymphocytic series in the bone marrow, and presumed to be formed in that tissue.

my·e·lol·y·sis (mī-ĕ-lol′i-sis). Decomposition of myelin.

my·e·lo·ma (mī-ĕ-lō′mă). 1. A tumor composed of cells derived from hemopoietic tissues of the bone marrow. 2. A plasma cell tumor. [myelo- + G. *-oma*, tumor]

Bence Jones m., multiple m. in which the malignant plasma cells excrete only light chains of one type (either κ or λ); lytic bone lesions occur in about 60% of the cases, and light chains (Bence Jones protein) occur in the urine; amyloidosis and severe renal failure are more common than in multiple m. SYN L-chain disease, L-chain m.

endothelial m., SYN Ewing *tumor*.

giant cell m., SYN giant cell *tumor* of bone.

L-chain m., SYN Bence Jones m.

multiple m., m. mul′tiplex, an uncommon disease that occurs more frequently in men than in women and is associated with anemia, hemorrhage, recurrent infections, and weakness. Ordinarily, it is regarded as a malignant neoplasm that originates in bone marrow and involves chiefly the skeleton, with clinical features attributable to the sites of involvement and to abnormalities in formation of plasma protein; characterized by numerous diffuse foci or nodular accumulations of abnormal or malignant plasma cells in the marrow of various bones (especially the skull), causing palpable swellings of the bones, and occasionally in extraskeletal sites; radiologically, the bone lesions have a characteristic punched-out appearance. The myeloma cells produce abnormal proteins in the serum and urine; those formed in any one example of multiple m. are different from other m. proteins, as well as from normal serum proteins, the most frequent abnormalities in the metabolism of protein being: 1) the occurrence of Bence Jones proteinuria, 2) a great increase in monoclonal γ-globulin in the plasma, 3) the occasional formation of cryoglobulin, and 4) a form of primary amyloidosis. The Bence Jones protein is not a derivative of abnormal serum protein, but seems to be formed *de novo* from amino acid precursors. SEE ALSO plasma cell m. SYN multiple myelomatosis, myelomatosis multiplex, plasma cell m. (1).

nonsecretory m., multiple m. in which there is no detectable paraproteinemia or paraproteinuria.

plasma cell m., (1) SYN multiple m; **(2)** plasmacytoma of bone, which is usually a solitary lesion and not associated with the occurrence of Bence Jones protein or other disturbances in the metabolism of protein (as observed in multiple m.). Some observers emphasize that the solitary lesion probably represents an early phase of classic multiple m., or an example of the latter in which only one focus is recognized.

my·e·lo·ma·la·cia (mī′ĕ-lō-ma-lā′shē-ă). Softening of the spinal cord. [myelo- + G. *malakia*, a softness]

angiodysgenetic m., SYN subacute necrotizing *myelitis*.

my·e·lo·ma·to·sis (mī′ĕ-lō-mă-tō′sis). A disease characterized by the occurrence of myeloma in various sites.

multiple m., m. mul′tiplex, SYN multiple *myeloma*.

my·e·lo·me·ning·o·cele (mī′ĕ-lō-mĕ-ning′gō-sēl). SYN meningo-myelocele. [myelo- + G. *mēninx*, membrane, + *kēlē*, hernia]

my·e·lo·mere (mī′ĕ-lō-mēr). Neuromere of the brain or spinal cord. [myelo- + G. *meros*, part]

my·e·lo·mono·cyte (mī′ĕ-lō-mon′ō-sīt). A leukocyte that appears to resemble both myelocytes and monocytes in that nuclear chromatin is less condensed than in the myelocyte and the cytoplasm has few neutrophilic granules; such cells represent aberrant maturation, as occurs in myelomonocytic leukemia.

my·e·lo·neu·ri·tis (mī′ĕ-lō-noo-rī′tis). SYN neuromyelitis.

my·e·lon·ic (mī-ĕ-lon′ik). Relating to the spinal cord. [G. *myelon*, fr. *myelos*, marrow]

my·e·lo·pa·ral·y·sis (mī′ĕ-lō-pă-ral′i-sis). SYN spinal *paralysis*.

my·e·lo·path·ic (mī′ĕ-lō-path′ik). Relating to myelopathy.

my·e·lop·a·thy (mī-ĕ-lop′ă-thē). 1. Disorder of the spinal cord. 2. A disease of the myelopoietic tissues. [myelo- + G. *pathos*, suffering]

carcinomatous m., degeneration or necrosis of the spinal cord associated with a carcinoma. SYN paracarcinomatous m.

compressive m., destruction of spinal cord tissue caused by pressure from neoplasms, hematomas, or other masses.

diabetic m., degenerative changes in spinal cord tissue occurring as a complication of diabetes mellitus.

paracarcinomatous m., SYN carcinomatous m.

radiation m., damage to the spinal cord from exposure to x-rays or other high energy radiation; usually radiation myelitis. SYN radiation myelitis.

my·e·lo·per·ox·i·dase (mī′el-ō-per-oks′i-dās). A peroxidase occurring in phagocytic cells that can oxidize halogen ions (e.g., I⁻) to the free halogen; an autosomal recessive deficiency of m. leads to impaired bacterial killing.

my·e·lop·e·tal (mī-ĕ-lop′ĕ-tăl). Proceeding in a direction toward the spinal cord; said of different nerve impulses. [myelo- + L. *peto*, to seek]

my·e·lo·phthis·ic (mī′ĕ-lō-tiz′ik, -thiz′ik). Relating to or suffering from myelophthisis.

my·e·loph·thi·sis (mī′ĕ-lof′thi-sis, mī′ĕ-lō-tī′sis, -tē′sis). 1. Wasting or atrophy of the spinal cord as in tabes dorsalis. 2. Replacement of hemopoietic tissue in the bone marrow by abnormal tissue, usually fibrous tissue or malignant tumors that are most commonly metastatic carcinomas. SYN panmyelophthisis. [myelo- + G. *phthisis*, a wasting away]

my·e·lo·plast (mī′ĕ-lō-plast). Any of the leukocytic series of cells in the bone marrow, especially young forms. [myelo- + G. *plastos*, formed]

my·e·lo·ple·gia (mī′ĕ-lō-plē′jē-ă). SYN spinal *paralysis*. [myelo- + G. *plēgē*, a stroke]

my·e·lo·poi·e·sis (mī′ĕ-lō-poy-ē′sis). Formation of the tissue elements of bone marrow, or any of the types of blood cells derived from bone marrow; or both processes. [myelo- + G. *poiēsis*, a making]

my·e·lo·poi·et·ic (mī′ĕ-lō-poy-et′ik). Relating to myelopoiesis.

my·e·lo·pro·lif·er·a·tive (mī′ĕ-lō-prō-lif′er-ă-tiv). Pertaining to or characterized by unusual proliferation of myelopoietic tissue.

my·e·lo·ra·dic·u·li·tis (mī′ĕ-lō-ra-dik-ū-lī′tis). Inflammation of the spinal cord and nerve roots. [myelo- + L. *radicula*, root, + G. *-itis*, inflammation]

my·e·lo·ra·dic·u·lo·dys·pla·sia (mī′ĕ-lō-ra-dik′ū-lō-dis-plā-zē-

my

ă). Congenital maldevelopment of the spinal cord and spinal nerve roots. [myelo- + L. *radicula,* root, + dysplasia]

my·e·lo·ra·dic·u·lop·a·thy (mī′ĕ-lō-ră-dik′ū-lop′ă-thē). Disease involving the spinal cord and nerve roots. SYN radiculomyelopathy. [myelo- + L. *radicula,* root, + G. *pathos,* disease]

my·e·lo·ra·dic·u·lo·pol·y·neu·ron·i·tis (mī′ĕ-lō-ra-dik′ū-lō-pol′ē-noo-ron-ī′tis). SYN Guillain-Barré *syndrome.*

my·e·lor·rha·gia (mī′ĕ-lō-rā′jē-ă). SYN hematomyelia. [myelo- + G. *rhēgnymi,* to burst forth]

my·e·lor·rha·phy (mī-ĕ-lōr′ă-fē). Suture of a wound of the spinal cord. [myelo- + G. *rhaphē,* a seam]

my·e·los·chi·sis (mī-ĕ-los′ki-sis). Cleft spinal cord resulting from failure of the neural folds to close normally in the formation of the neural tube; inevitably spina bifida is a sequel. [myelo- + G. *schisis,* a cleaving]

my·e·lo·scle·ro·sis (mī′ĕ-lō-skle-rō′sis). SYN myelofibrosis. [myelo- + G. *sklērōsis,* induration]

my·e·lo·sis (mī-ĕ-lō′sis). **1.** A condition characterized by abnormal proliferation of tissue or cellular elements of bone marrow, e.g., multiple myeloma, myelocytic leukemia, myelofibrosis. **2.** A condition in which there is abnormal proliferation of medullary tissue in the spinal cord, as in a glioma.

aleukemic m., m. with absence of abnormal cellular elements in peripheral blood.

chronic nonleukemic m., a condition in which there is abnormal proliferation of leukopoietic tissue that results in immature white blood cells in the circulating blood, but the total count is within the normal range.

erythremic m., a neoplastic process involving the erythropoietic tissue, characterized by anemia, irregular fever, splenomegaly, hepatomegaly, hemorrhagic disorders, and numerous erythroblasts in all stages of maturation (with disproportionately large numbers of less mature forms) in the circulating blood; postmortem studies reveal primitive erythroblasts and reticuloendothelial cells, not only in hemopoietic organs, but also in the kidneys, adrenal glands, and other sites. Acute and chronic forms are recognized, but in the latter there is less prominence of the immature cells; the former is also called Di Guglielmo disease and acute erythremia.

funicular m., degeneration of spinal cord white matter.

leukemic m., (1) SYN granulocytic *leukemia;* **(2)** SYN myeloblastic *leukemia.*

leukopenic m., subleukemic m., SYN subleukemic *leukemia.*

my·e·lo·spon·gi·um (mī′ĕ-lō-spŭn′jē-ŭm). The fibrocellular meshwork in the spinal cord of the embryo, from which the neuroglia is developed. [myelo- + G. *spongos,* sponge]

my·e·lo·syph·i·lis (mī′ĕ-lō-sif′i-lis). SYN tabetic *neurosyphilis.*

my·e·lo·tome (mī′ĕ-lō-tōm). An instrument used in making serial sections of the spinal cord or for incising the spinal cord. [myelo- + G. *tomos,* cutting]

my·e·lo·to·mog·ra·phy (mī′ĕ-lō-tō-mog′ră-fē). Tomography of the spinal subarachnoid space opacified with contrast medium; an obsolete procedure.

my·e·lot·o·my (mī-ĕ-lot′ō-mē). Incision of the spinal cord. [myelo- + G. *tomē,* incision]

Bischof m., longitudinal incision of the spinal cord through the lateral column for treatment of spasticity of the lower extremities.

commissural m., SYN midline m.

midline m., section of the midline transverse fibers of the spinal cord for the treatment of intractable pain. SYN commissural m., commissurotomy (2).

T m., midline m. with lateral cuts into the anterior horns.

my·e·lo·tox·ic (mī′ĕ-lō-tok′sik). **1.** Inhibitory, depressant, or destructive to one or more of the components of bone marrow. **2.** Pertaining to, derived from, or manifesting the features of diseased bone marrow.

my·en·ter·ic (mī-en-ter′ik). Relating to the myenteron.

my·en·ter·on (mī-en′ter-on). The muscular coat, or muscularis, of the intestine. [G. *mys,* muscle, + *enteron,* intestine]

my·es·the·sia (mī-es-thē′zē-ă). SYN kinesthetic *sense.* [G. *mys,* muscle, + *aisthēsis,* sensation]

my·i·a·sis (mī-ī′ă-sis). Any infection due to invasion of tissues or cavities of the body by larvae of dipterous insects. [G. *myia,* a fly]

accidental m., gastrointestinal m. from ingestion of contaminated food.

African furuncular m., SYN cordylobiasis.

aural m., invasion of the external, middle, or inner ear by larvae of dipterous insects.

human botfly m., SYN dermatobiasis.

intestinal m., presence of larvae of certain dipterous insects in the gastrointestinal tract, as of *Musca domestica* (domestic housefly), the cheese mite, and *Fannia canicularis* (lesser housefly).

nasal m., fly larva invasion of the nasal passages, due most commonly in the U.S. to primary screw-worms, the larvae of *Cochliomyia hominivorax,* which develop in the nasal or aural cavity.

ocular m., invasion of the conjunctival sac or eyeball by larvae of flies, e.g., *Hypoderma bovis, H. lineata, Sarcophaga,* or *Gasterophilus intestinalis.* SYN ophthalmomyiasis.

tumbu dermal m., SYN cordylobiasis.

wound m., the infestation of a surface wound or other open lesion by fly larvae.

my·kol (mī′kol). SYN mycolic acids.

myl·a·bris (mil′ă-bris). The dried beetle, *Mylabris phalerata;* a vesicant similar to cantharis. [G. a cockroach found in mills and bakehouses, fr. *mylē,* mill]

my·lo·hy·oid (mī′lō-hī′oyd). Relating to the molar teeth, or posterior portion of the lower jaw, and to the hyoid bone; denoting various structures. SEE *nerve* to mylohyoid, muscle, region, sulcus. [G. *mylē,* a mill, in pl. *mylai,* molar teeth]

my·lo·hy·oi·de·us (mī-lō-hī-oy′dē-ŭs). SYN mylohyoid (*muscle*).

△**myo-.** Muscle. [G. *mys,* muscle]

my·o·aden·y·late de·am·i·nase (mī′ō-a-den-il-āt). Muscle AMP deaminase. SEE AMP deaminase.

my·o·al·bu·min (mī′ō-al-bū′min). Albumin in muscle tissue, possibly the same as serum albumin.

my·o·ar·chi·tec·ton·ic (mī′ō-ar′ki-tek-ton′ik). Relating to the structural arrangement of muscle or of fibers in general. [myo- + G. *architektonikos,* relating to construction]

my·o·at·ro·phy (mī-ō-at′rō-fē). SYN muscular *atrophy.*

my·o·blast (mī′ō-blast). A primitive muscle cell with the potentiality of developing into a muscle fiber. SYN sarcoblast, sarcogenic cell. [myo- + G. *blastos,* germ]

my·o·blas·tic (mī-ō-blas′tik). Relating to a myoblast or to the mode of formation of muscle cells.

my·o·blas·to·ma (mī′ō-blas-tō′mă). A tumor of immature muscle cells. [myo- + G. *blastos,* germ, + *-oma,* tumor]

granular cell m., obsolete term for granular cell *tumor.*

my·o·bra·dia (mī-ō-brā′dē-ă). Sluggish reaction of muscle to stimulation. [myo- + G. *bradys,* slow]

my·o·car·dia (mī-ō-kar′dē-ă). Plural of myocardium.

my·o·car·di·al (mī-ō-kar′dē-ăl). Relating to the myocardium.

my·o·car·di·o·graph (mī′ō-kar′dē-ō-graf). An instrument composed of a tambour with recording lever attachment, by means of which a tracing is made of the movements of the heart muscle. [myo- + G. *kardia,* heart, + *graphō,* to record]

my·o·car·di·op·a·thy (mī′ō-kar-dē-op′ă-thē). SYN cardiomyopathy. [myocardium + G. *pathos,* suffering]

alcoholic m., SYN alcoholic *cardiomyopathy.*

chagasic m. (chă′gă-sik), heart muscle disease due to Chagas disease (caused by *Trypanosoma cruzi*) in which right bundle branch block is common.

my·o·car·di·or·rha·phy (mī′ō-kar-dē-ōr′ă-fē). Suture of the myocardium. [myocardium + G. *rhaphē,* suture]

my·o·car·di·tic (mī-ō-kar′dī-ik). Related to myocarditis (adjective).

my·o·car·di·tis (mī′ō-kar-dī′tis). Inflammation of the muscular walls of the heart.

acute isolated m., an acute interstitial m. of unknown cause, the endocardium and pericardium being unaffected. SYN Fiedler m.

Fiedler m., SYN acute isolated m.

giant cell m., acute isolated m. characterized by infiltration by granulomas containing giant cells.

idiopathic m., inflammation of the heart muscle of unknown origin.

indurative m., chronic m. leading to hardening of the muscular wall of the heart.

toxic m., inflammation of heart muscle caused by any noxious chemical, e.g., alcohol, heavy metals.

my·o·car·di·um, pl. **my·o·car·dia** (mī-ō-kar′dē-ŭm, -kar′dē-ă) [TA]. The middle layer of the heart, consisting of cardiac muscle. [myo- + G. *kardia,* heart]

hibernating m., ventricular dysfunction following months or years of ischemia that is reversible when blood flow is restored. Must be carefully distinguished from dysfunction due to necrotic or scarred m.

stunned m., impaired myocardial contractile performance following a period of ischemia and ultimately reversible.

my·o·cele (mī′ō-sēl). **1.** Protrusion of muscle substance through a rent in its sheath. [myo- + G. *kēlē,* hernia] **2.** The small cavity that appears in somites. SYN somite cavity. [myo- + G. *koilia,* a cavity]

my·o·ce·li·al·gia (mī′ō-sē-lē-al′jē-ă). Obsolete term for celiomyalgia. [myo- + G. *koilia,* the belly, + *algos,* pain]

my·o·ce·li·tis (mī′ō-sē-lī′tis). Inflammation of the abdominal muscles. [myo- + G. *koilia,* belly, + -*itis,* inflammation]

my·o·cel·lu·li·tis (mī′ō-sel-ū-lī′tis). Inflammation of muscle and cellular tissue. [myo- + Mod. L. *cellularis,* cellular (tissue), + G. -*itis,* inflammation]

my·o·ce·ro·sis (mī′ō-sē-rō′sis). Waxy degeneration of the muscles. SYN myokerosis. [myo- + G. *kēros,* wax]

my·o·chrome (mī′ō-krōm). Rarely used term for cytochrome found in muscle tissue.

my·o·chron·o·scope (mī-ō-kron′ō-skōp). An instrument for timing a muscular impulse, i.e., the interval between the application of the stimulus and the muscular movement in response. [myo- + G. *chronos,* time, + *skopeō,* to examine]

my·o·cin·e·sim·e·ter (mī′ō-sin-ĕ-sim′ĕ-ter). SYN myokinesimeter.

my·o·clo·nia (mī′ō-klō′nē-ă). Any disorder characterized by myoclonus. [myo- + G. *klonos,* a tumult]

fibrillary m., the twitching of a limited part or group of fibers of a muscle.

my·o·clon·ic (mī-ō-klon′ik). Showing myoclonus.

my·oc·lo·nus (mī-ok′lō-nŭs, mī-ō-klo′nŭs). One or a series of shock-like contractions of a group of muscles, of variable regularity, synchrony, and symmetry, generally due to a central nervous system lesion. [myo- + G. *klonos,* tumult]

benign m. of infancy, SYN benign infantile m.

benign infantile m., a seizure disorder of infancy in which myoclonic movements occur in the neck, trunk, and extremities; the EEG is normal, and seizures do not persist beyond 2 years of age. SYN benign m. of infancy.

m. mul′tiplex, an ill-defined disorder marked by rapid and widespread muscle contractions. SYN paramyoclonus multiplex, polyclonia, polymyoclonus.

nocturnal m., frequently repeated muscular jerks occurring at the moment of dropping off to sleep.

palatal m., rhythmic contractions of the soft palate, the facial muscles, and the diaphragm, related to lesions of the olivocerebellar pathways. SEE ALSO palatal *nystagmus.*

stimulus sensitive m., m. induced by a variety of stimuli, e.g., talking, calculation, loud noises, tapping, etc.

my·o·col·pi·tis (mī-ō-kol-pī′tis). Inflammation of the muscular tissue of the vagina. [myo- + G. *kolpos,* bosom (vagina), + -*itis,* inflammation]

my·o·com·ma, pl. **my·o·com·ma·ta** (mī-ō-kom′ă, -kom′ă-tă). The connective tissue septum separating adjacent myotomes. SYN myoseptum. [myo- + G. *komma,* a coin or the stamp of a coin]

my·o·cris·mus (mī-ō-kris′mŭs). A creaking sound sometimes heard on auscultation of a contracting muscle. [myo- + G. *krizō,* to squeak]

my·o·cu·ta·ne·ous (mī-ō-kū-tā′nē-ŭs). SYN musculocutaneous. [myo- + L. *cutis,* skin]

my·o·cyte (mī′ō-sīt). A muscle cell. [myo- + G. *kytos,* cell]

Anitschkow m., SYN cardiac *histiocyte.*

my·o·cy·tol·y·sis (mī-ō-sī-tol′i-sis). Dissolution of muscle fiber. [myo- + G. *kytos,* cell, + *lysis,* a loosening]

m. of heart, local loss of myocardial syncytium as a result of a metabolic imbalance, insufficient in intensity or duration (or both) to cause stromal injury or to elicit any reactive exudation.

my·o·cy·to·ma (mī-ō-sī-tō′mă). A benign neoplasm derived from muscle.

my·o·de·gen·er·a·tion (mī′ō-dē-jen-ĕ-rā′shŭn). Muscular degeneration.

my·o·de·mia (mī-ō-dē′mē-ă). Fatty degeneration of muscle. [myo- + G. *dēmos,* tallow]

my·o·der·mal (mī-ō-der′mal). SYN musculocutaneous. [myo- + G. *derma,* skin]

my·o·di·as·ta·sis (mī′ō-dī-as′tă-sis). Separation of muscle. [myo- + G. *diastasis,* separation]

my·o·dy·na·mia (mī′ō-dī-nā′mē-ă). Muscular strength. [myo- + G. *dynamis,* power]

my·o·dy·nam·ics (mī′ō-dī-nam′iks). The dynamics of muscular action.

my·o·dy·na·mom·e·ter (mī′ō-dī-nă-mom′ĕ-ter). An instrument for determining muscular strength. [myo- + G. *dynamis,* force, + *metron,* measure]

my·o·dyn·ia (mī′ō-din′ē-ă). SYN myalgia. [myo- + G. *odynē,* pain]

my·o·dys·to·ny (mī′ō-dis′tō-nē). A condition of slow relaxation, interrupted by a succession of slight contractions, following electrical stimulation of a muscle. [myo- + G. *dys-,* difficult, + *tonos,* tone, tension]

my·o·dys·tro·phy, my·o·dys·tro·phia (mī-ō-dis′trō-fē, mī′-ō-dis-trō′fē-ă). SYN muscular *dystrophy.* [myo- + G. *dys-,* difficult, poor, + *trophē,* nourishment]

my·o·e·de·ma (mī′ō-e-dē′mă). A localized contraction of a degenerating muscle, occurring at the point of a sharp blow, independent of the nerve supply. SYN idiomuscular contraction, mounding, myoidema. [myo- + G. *oidēma,* swelling]

my·o·e·las·tic (mī′ō-ē-las′tik). Pertaining to closely associated smooth muscle fibers and elastic connective tissue.

my·o·e·lec·tric (mī′ō-ē-lek′trik). Relating to the electrical properties of muscle.

my·o·en·do·car·di·tis (mī-ō-en′dō-kar-dī′tis). Inflammation of the muscular wall and lining membrane of the heart. [myo- + G. *endon,* within, + *kardia,* heart, + -*itis,* inflammation]

my·o·ep·i·the·li·al (mī′ō-ep-i-thē′lē-ăl). Relating to myoepithelium.

my·o·ep·i·the·li·o·ma (mī′ō-ep-i-thē-lē-ō′mă). A benign tumor of myoepithelial cells. [myo- + epithelium, + G. -*ōma,* tumor]

my·o·ep·i·the·li·um (mī′ō-ep-i-thē′lē-ŭm). Spindle-shaped, contractile, smooth musclelike cells of epithelial origin that are arranged longitudinally or obliquely around sweat glands and the secretory alveoli of the mammary gland; stellate myoepithelial cells occur around lacrimal and some salivary gland secretory units. SYN muscle epithelium. [myo- + epithelium]

my·o·es·the·sis, my·o·es·the·sia (mī′ō-es-thē′sis, -thē′zē-ă). SYN kinesthetic *sense.*

my·o·fas·ci·al (mī-ō-fash′ē-ăl). Of or relating to the fascia surrounding and separating muscle tissue.

my·o·fas·ci·tis (mī′ō-fă-sī′tis). SYN *myositis* fibrosa.

my·o·fi·bril (mī-ō-fī′bril). One of the fine longitudinal fibrils occurring in a skeletal or cardiac muscle fiber comprising many regularly overlapped ultramicroscopic thick and thin myofilaments. SYN muscular fibril, myofibrilla. [myo- + Mod. L. *fibrilla,* fibril]

my·o·fi·bril·la, pl. **my·o·fi·bril·lae** (mī′ō-fī-bril′ă, -bril′ē). SYN myofibril.

my

my·o·fib·ril·lar (mī-ō-fī-bril-ar). Pertaining or relating to myofibril.

my·o·fi·bro·blast (mī-ō-fī′brō-blast). A cell thought to be responsible for contracture of wounds; such cells have some characteristics of smooth muscle, such as contractile properties and fibrils, and are also believed to produce, temporarily, type III collagen.

my·o·fi·bro·ma (mī′ō-fī-brō′mă). A benign neoplasm that consists chiefly of fibrous connective tissue, with variable numbers of muscle cells forming portions of the neoplasm.

my·o·fi·bro·ma·to·sis (mī-′yō-fī-brō-ma- tō′sis). Solitary or multiple tumors of muscle and fibrous tissue, or tumors composed by myofibroblasts. [myo- + L. *fibra*, fiber, + G. suffix, -*ōma*, tumor, + suffix -*osis*, condition]

infantile myofibromatosis, myofibromatosis seen at birth or in infants, with multiple lytic bone lesions and involving soft tissue, or with visceral involvement.

my·o·fi·bro·sis (mī′ō-fī-brō′sis). Chronic myositis with diffuse hyperplasia of the interstitial connective tissue pressing upon and causing atrophy of the muscular tissue.

m. cor′dis, m. of the heart walls.

my·o·fi·bro·si·tis (mī′ō-fī-brō-sī′tis). Inflammation of the perimysium.

my·o·fil·a·ments (mī-ō-fil′ă-ments). The ultramicroscopic threads of filamentous proteins making up myofibrils in striated muscle. Thick ones contain myosin and thin ones actin; thick and thin m.'s also occur in smooth muscle fibers but are not regularly arranged in discrete myofibrils and thus do not impart a striated appearance to these cells.

my·o·func·tion·al (mī′ō-fŭnk′shŭn-ăl). **1.** Relating to function of muscles. **2.** In dentistry, relating to the role of muscle function in the etiology or correction of orthodontic problems.

my·o·gen (mī′ō-jen). Proteins extracted from skeletal muscle with cold water, largely the enzymes promoting glycolysis; from the residue, alkaline 0.6 mol L^{-1} KCl extracts actin and myosin as actomyosin, with myosin further separable into two meromyosins by proteinase treatment. SYN myosinogen. [myo- + G. -*gen*, producing]

my·o·gen·e·sis (mī-ō-jen′ĕ-sis). Embryonic formation of muscle cells or fibers. [myo- + G. *genesis*, origin]

my·o·ge·net·ic, my·o·gen·ic (mī-ō-jĕ-net′ik, -jen′ik). **1.** Originating in or starting from muscle. **2.** Relating to the origin of muscle cells or fibers. SYN myogenous.

my·og·e·nous (mī-oj′ĕ-nŭs). SYN myogenetic.

my·o·glo·bin (Mb, MbCO, MbO₂) (mī-ō-glō′bin). The oxygen-carrying and storage protein of muscle, resembling blood hemoglobin in function but containing only one subunit and one heme as part of the molecule (rather than the four of hemoglobin), and with a molecular weight approximately one-quarter that of hemoglobin. SYN muscle hemoglobin, myohemoglobin. [myo- + hemoglobin]

carbonmonoxy m., SYN carboxyhemoglobin.

my·o·glo·bi·nu·ria (mī′ō-glō-bi-noo′rē-ă). Excretion of myoglobin in the urine; results from muscle degeneration, which releases myoglobin into the blood; occurs in certain types of trauma (crush syndrome), advanced or protracted ischemia of muscle, or as a paroxysmal process of unknown etiology. SYN idiopathic paroxysmal rhabdomyolysis, Meyer-Betz disease, Meyer-Betz syndrome.

my·o·glob·u·lin (mī-ō-glob′ū-lin). Globulin present in muscle tissue.

my·o·glob·u·li·nu·ria (mī′ō-glob′ū-li-noo′rē-ă). The excretion of myoglobulin in the urine.

my·og·na·thus (mī-og′nă-thŭs, mī-ō-nāth′ŭs). An unequal conjoined twin in which the rudimentary head of the parasite is attached to the lower jaw of the autosite by muscle and skin only. SEE conjoined *twins*, under *twin*. [myo- + G. *gnathos*, jaw]

my·o·gram (mī′ō-gram). The tracing made by a myograph. SYN muscle curve. [myo- + G. *gramma*, a drawing]

my·o·graph (mī′ō-graf). A recording instrument by which tracings are made of muscular contractions. [myo- + G. *graphō*, to write]

palate m., SYN palatograph.

my·o·graph·ic (mī-ō-graf′ik). Relating to a myogram, or the record of a myograph.

my·og·ra·phy (mī-og′ră-fē). **1.** The recording of muscular movements by the myograph. **2.** A description of or treatise on the muscles. SYN descriptive myology.

my·o·he·mo·glo·bin (mī′ō-hēm-ō-glō′bin). SYN myoglobin.

my·oid (mī′oyd). **1.** Resembling muscle. **2.** One of the fine, contractile, threadlike protoplasmic elements found in certain epithelial cells in lower animals. **3.** A contractile part of retinal cones in certain fish and amphibia. In mammals, the m. is the inner part of the inner segment of rods and cones; it contains microtubules, the Golgi apparatus, endoplasmic reticulum, and ribosomes, but no myofibrils. [myo- + G. *eidos,* appearance]

my·oi·de·ma (mī-oy-dē′mă). SYN myoedema. [myo- + G. *oidēma,* swelling]

my·o·i·no·si·tol (mī-ō-in-o′-si-tōl). SEE myo-inositol.

my·o·is·che·mia (mī′ō-is-kē′mē-ă). A condition of localized deficiency or absence of blood supply in muscular tissue.

my·o·ke·ro·sis (mī′ō-kē-rō′sis). SYN myocerosis.

my·o·ki·nase (mī-ō-kī′nās). SYN *adenylate* kinase.

my·o·kin·e·sim·e·ter (mī′ō-kin-ĕ-sim′ĕ-ter). A device for registering the exact time and extent of contraction of the larger muscles of the lower extremity in response to electric stimulation. SYN myocinesimeter. [myo- + G. *kinesis,* movement, + *metron,* measure]

my·o·ky·mia (mī-ō-kī′mē-ă). Continuous involuntary quivering or rippling of muscles at rest, caused by spontaneous, repetitive firing of groups of motor unit potentials. SYN fibrillary chorea, Morvan chorea. [myo- + G. *kyma,* wave]

facial m., m. that appears in the facial muscles, causing narrowing of the palpebral fissure and continuous undulation of the facial skin surface; the latter is referred to as "bag of worms" appearance and is best seen with reflected light; due to intrinsic brainstem lesion, such as a pontine glioma or multiple sclerosis.

generalized m., widespread m., present in multiple limbs and often the face; of various causes, including Isaac syndrome, uremia, thyrotoxicosis and gold toxicity (gold-m. syndrome).

hereditary m. [MIM*160100], a syndrome consisting of muscle contractions and night cramps; autosomal dominant inheritance.

limb m., m. present in one or more limbs; various causes, one of the more common being prior plexus radiation.

my·o·lem·ma (mī-ō-lem′ă). SYN sarcolemma.

my·o·li·po·ma (mī′ō-li-pō′mă). A benign neoplasm that consists chiefly of fat cells (adipose tissue), with variable numbers of muscle cells forming portions of the neoplasm.

my·o·lo·gia (mī′ō-lō′jē-ă). SYN myology.

my·ol·o·gist (mī-ol′ō-jist). One learned in the knowledge of muscles.

my·ol·o·gy (mī-ol′ō-jē). The branch of science concerned with the muscles and their accessory parts, tendons, aponeuroses, bursae, and fasciae. SYN myologia, sarcology (1). [myo- + G. *logos,* study]

descriptive m., SYN myography (2).

my·ol·y·sis (mī-ol′i-sis). Dissolution or liquefaction of muscular tissue, frequently preceded by degenerative changes such as infiltration of fat, atrophy, and fatty degeneration. [myo- + G. *lysis,* dissolution]

cardiotoxic m., cardiomalacia occurring in fever and various systemic infections.

my·o·ma (mī-ō′mă). A benign neoplasm of muscular tissue. SEE ALSO leiomyoma, rhabdomyoma. [myo- + G. -*oma,* tumor]

my·o·ma·la·cia (mī′ō-mă-lā′shē-ă). Pathologic softening of muscular tissue. [myo- + G. *malakia,* softness]

my·o·ma·tous (mī-ō′mă-tŭs). Pertaining to or characterized by the features of a myoma.

my·o·mec·to·my (mī-ō-mek′tō-mē). Operative removal of a myoma, specifically of a uterine myoma. SYN fibroidectomy, fibromectomy, hysteromyomectomy. [myoma + G. *ektomē,* excision]

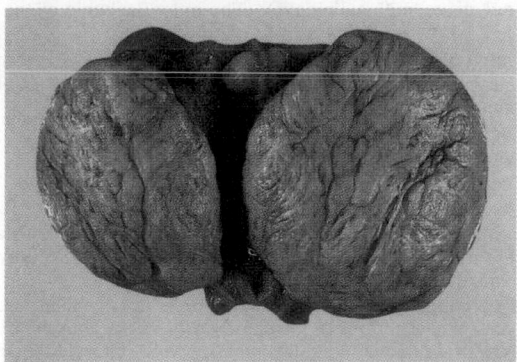

myoma of uterus: cross-section showing narrowing of uterine cavity

abdominal m., removal of a myoma of the uterus through an abdominal incision.

left ventricular m., resection of myocardial tissue used in cases of idiopathic hypertrophic subaortic stenosis.

vaginal m., removal of a myoma of the uterus through the vagina. SYN colpomyomectomy.

my·o·mel·a·no·sis (mī′ō-melă-nō′sis). Abnormal dark pigmentation of muscular tissue. SEE ALSO melanosis. [myo- + G. *melanōsis,* becoming black]

my·o·mere (mī′ō-mēr). SYN myotome (4). [myo- + G. *meros,* a part]

my·om·e·ter (mī-om′ĕ-ter). An instrument for measuring the extent of a muscular contraction. [myo- + G. *metron,* measure]

my·o·me·tri·al (mī-ō-mē′trē-ăl). Relating to the myometrium.

my·o·me·tri·tis (mī′ō-mē-trī′tis). Inflammation of the muscular wall of the uterus. [myo- + G. *mētra,* uterus, + *-itis,* inflammation]

my·o·me·tri·um (mī′ō-mē′trē-ŭm) [TA]. The muscular wall of the uterus. SYN tunica muscularis uteri [TA], muscular coat of uterus. [myo- + G. *mētra,* uterus]

my·o·mi·to·chon·dri·on, pl. **my·o·mi·to·chon·dri·a** (mī′ō-mī′tō-kon′drē-on, -drē-ă). A mitochondrion of a muscle fiber.

my·o·mot·o·my (mī-ō-mot′ō-mē). Incision of a myoma. [myoma + G. *tomē,* incision]

my·on (mī′on). An individual muscle unit. [G. *mys,* muscle]

my·o·ne·cro·sis (mī′ō-nĕ-krō′sis). Necrosis of muscle.

clostridial m., SYN gas *gangrene.*

my·o·neme (mī′ō-nēm). 1. A muscle fibril. 2. One of the contractile fibrils of certain protozoans; thought to function in an analogous fashion to metazoan muscle fibers. [myo- + G. *nēma,* thread]

my·o·neu·ral (mī-ō-noo′răl). Relating to both muscle and nerve; denoting specifically the synapse of the motor neuron with striated muscle fibers: myoneural junction or motor endplate. SEE ALSO neuromuscular. [myo- + G. *neuron,* nerve]

my·o·neu·ro·ma (mī′ō-noo-rō′mă). A tumefaction consisting chiefly of abnormally proliferating Schwann cells, with variable numbers of muscle cells forming portions of the mass; m.'s are probably malformations, rather than true neoplasms. [myo- + G. *neuron,* nerve, + *-oma,* tumor]

my·on·y·my (mī-on′i-mē). Nomenclature of the muscles. [myo- + G. *onyma* or *onoma,* name]

my·o·pa·chyn·sis (mī′ō-pă-kin′sis). Muscular hypertrophy. [myo- + G. *pachynsis,* a thickening]

my·o·pal·mus (mī-ō-pal′mŭs). Muscle twitching. [myo- + G. *palmos,* a quivering]

my·o·path·ic (mī-ō-path′ik). Denoting a disorder involving muscular tissue.

my·op·a·thy (mī-op′ă-thē). Any abnormal condition or disease of the muscular tissues; commonly designates a disorder involving skeletal muscle. [myo- + G. *pathos,* suffering]

carcinomatous m., SYN Lambert-Eaton *syndrome.*

centronuclear m., slowly progressive generalized muscle weak-

ness and atrophy beginning in childhood; on biopsy of skeletal muscle, the nuclei of most muscle fibers are seen to be located near the center of a small fiber (the normal position for a 10-week embryo) rather than at the periphery of the fiber; familial incidence. Autosomal dominant [MIM*160150] recessive [MIM*255200] and X-linked [310400] forms occur. The X-linked form is caused by mutation in the myotubular myopathy gene (MTM1) on Xq28. SYN myotubular m.

distal m., m. affecting predominantly the distal portions of the limbs; onset is usually after age 40, with weakness and wasting of small muscles of the hands; The infantile form [MIM*160300] and the Swedish later-onset [MIM*160500] are autosomal dominant. There is a Japanese late-onset type [MIM*254130] that is recessive and is caused by mutation in the gene encoding dysferlin on 2p13.

dysthyroid m., SYN thyrotoxic m.

minicore-multicore m., an uncommon nonprogressive m. with early onset, proximal weakness, and hypotonia. Muscle fibers show focal defects of oxidative and myofibrillar adenosine triphosphatase enzymes with disorganization of myofibril ultrastructure.

mitochondrial m., weakness and hypotonia of muscles, primarily those of the neck, shoulder, and pelvic girdles, with onset in infancy or childhood; on biopsy, giant, bizarre mitochondria are seen located between muscle fibrils just beneath the sarcolemma. There are autosomal dominant [MIM*251900] and recessive forms due to deletions or duplications of mitochondrial DNA, with one recessive form [MIM*252010] associated with a deficiency of complex 1 of the mitochondrial respiratory chain.

myotubular m., SYN centronuclear m.

nemaline m., congenital, nonprogressive muscle weakness most evident in the proximal muscles; named after the characteristic nemaline (threadlike) rods seen in the muscle cells composed of Z-band material. There are two forms, dominant [MIM*161800] caused by mutation in the tropomyosin-3 gene (TPM3) on 1q22–q23, and recessive [MIM*256030], that are clinically indistinguishable. SYN rod m.

ocular m., SYN chronic progressive external *ophthalmoplegia.*

proximal myotonic m. (PROMM), an autosomal dominant, multisystem disorder, with onset in young adult life, characterized by proximal myotonia and weakness, muscle pain, baldness, cataracts, cardiac conduction disturbances, and testicular atrophy. In contrast to myotonic dystrophy, features of this disorder do not include facial weakness and ptosis, distal limb weakness and wasting, and trinucleotide repeat expansion at the gene loci for myotonic dystrophy.

rod m., SYN nemaline m.

thyrotoxic m., extreme muscular weakness in severe thyrotoxicosis affecting muscles of limbs and trunk as well as those used in speech and swallowing. SYN dysthyroid m.

my·o·per·i·car·di·tis (mī′ō-per-i-kar-dī′tis). Inflammation of the muscular wall of the heart and of the enveloping pericardium; also, perimyocarditis--choice of term determined by whether the principal involvement is pericardial or myocardial. [myo- + pericarditis]

my·o·per·i·to·ni·tis (mī′ō-per-i-tō-nī′tis). Inflammation of the parietal peritoneum with myositis of the abdominal wall.

my·o·phone (mī′ō-fōn). An instrument to enable one to hear the murmur of muscular contractions. [myo- + G. *phōnē,* sound]

my·o·phos·phor·y·lase (mī-ō-fus-fōr′i-lās). Muscle phosphorylase

my·o·pia (M) (mī-ō′pē-ă). That optical condition in which only rays from a finite distance from the eye focus on the retina. SYN near sight, nearsightedness, short sight, shortsightedness. [G. fr. *myo,* to shut, + *ōps,* eye]

axial m., m. due to elongation of the globe of the eye.

curvature m., m. due to refractive errors resulting from excessive corneal curvature.

degenerative m., SYN pathologic m.

index m., m. arising from increased refractivity of the lens, as in nuclear sclerosis.

malignant m., SYN pathologic m.

my

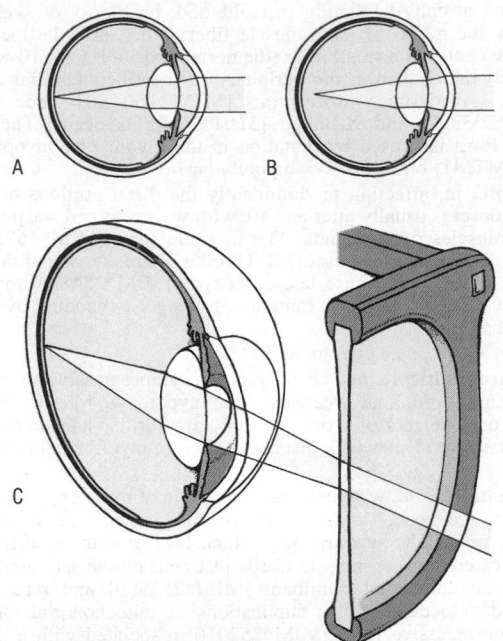

myopia: (A) normal (20/20) vision, light rays focus sharply on retina; (B) myopic (nearsighted) vision, light rays from a distance come to sharp focus in front of retina; (C) myopia corrected by eyeglasses with concave lenses

night m., in dark adaptation the eye becomes more sensitive to shorter wavelengths (Purkinje shift), and visual acuity depends on parafoveal blue cones. Shorter wavelengths come into focus in front of the retina, and this chromatic aberration accounts for some of the relative m. that a normal eye experiences at night; much of the remainder is due to an increase in accommodative tone in the dark.

pathologic m., progressive m. marked by fundus changes, posterior staphyloma, and subnormal corrected acuity. SYN degenerative m., malignant m.

prematurity m., m. observed in infants of low birthweight or in association with retrolental fibroplasia.

senile lenticular m., SYN second *sight*.

simple m., m. arising from failure of correlation of the refractive power of the anterior segment and the length of the eyeball.

space m., a type of m. arising when no contour is imaged on the retina.

transient m., m. observed in accommodative spasm secondary to iridocyclitis or ocular contusion.

my·o·pic (M) (mī-op′ik, -ō′pik). Relating to or suffering from myopia.

my·o·plasm (mī′ō-plazm). The contractile portion of the muscle cell, as distinguished from the sarcoplasm. [myo- + G. *plasma,* a thing formed]

my·o·plas·tic (mī-ō-plas′tik). Relating to the plastic surgery of the muscles, or to the use of muscular tissue to correct a defect.

my·o·plas·ty (mī′ō-plas-tē). Plastic surgery of muscular tissue. [myo- + G. *plastos,* formed]

my·o·po·lar (mī-ō-pō′lăr). Relating to muscular polarity, or to the portion of muscle between two electrodes.

my·o·pro·tein (mī-ō-prō′tēn). Protein occurring in muscle.

my·or·rha·phy (mī-ōr′ă-fē). Suture of a muscle. [myo- + G. *rhaphē,* seam]

my·or·rhex·is (mī-ō-rek′sis). Tearing of a muscle. [myo- + G. *rhēxis,* a rupture]

my·o·sal·pin·gi·tis (mī′ō-sal-pin-jī′tis). Inflammation of the muscular tissue of the uterine tube. [myosalpinx + G. *-itis* inflammation]

my·o·sal·pinx (mī′ō-sal′pingks). The muscular tunic of the uterine tube. [myo- + salpinx]

my·o·sar·co·ma (mī′ō-sar-kō′mă). A general term for a malignant neoplasm derived from muscular tissue. SEE ALSO leiomyosarcoma, rhabdomyosarcoma.

my·o·scle·ro·sis (mī′ō-skle-rō′sis). Chronic myositis with hyperplasia of the interstitial connective tissue.

my·o·sep·tum (mī-ō-sep′tŭm). SYN myocomma. [myo- + L. *saeptum,* a barrier]

my·o·sin (mī′ō-sin). A globulin present in muscle that has an ATPase activity; in combination with actin, it forms actomyosin; m. forms the thick filaments in muscle.

m. light chain kinase, a calcium/calmodulin-dependent enzyme that phosphorylates the light chains of smooth muscle m. and initiates contraction. In skeletal muscle, phosphorylation modulates tension during contraction.

my·o·sin·o·gen (mī-ō-sin′ō-jen). SYN myogen.

my·o·si·nose (mī′ō-si-nōs). A proteose formed by the partial hydrolysis of myosin.

my·o·sit·ic (mī-ō-sit′ik). Relating to myositis.

my·o·si·tis (mī-ō-sī′tis). Inflammation of a muscle. SYN initis (2). [myo- + G. *-itis,* inflammation]

cervical m., SEE posttraumatic neck *syndrome*.

epidemic m., m. epidem′ica acu′ta, SYN epidemic *pleurodynia.*

m. fibro′sa, induration of a muscle through an interstitial growth of fibrous tissue. SYN interstitial m., myofascitis.

infectious m., inflammation of the voluntary muscles, marked by swelling and pain, affecting usually the shoulders and arms, though almost the entire body may be involved.

interstitial m., SYN m. fibrosa.

m. ossif′icans, ossification or deposit of bone in muscle with fibrosis, causing pain and swelling in muscles.

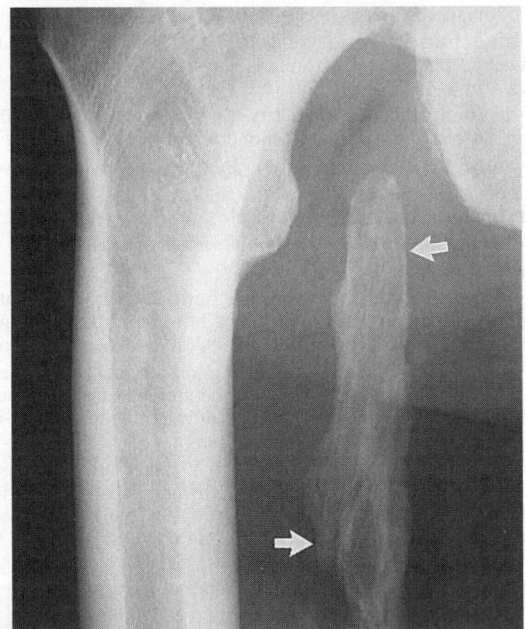

myositis ossificans: well-organized ossifying hematoma present in the adductor magnus muscle (arrows)

m. ossif′icans circumscrip′ta, local deposit of bone in a muscle, usually following prolonged trauma; e.g., riders' bone.

m. ossif′icans progressi′va, a rare and frequently fatal mutation, beginning in early life, characterized by progressive ossification of the muscles; it is not strictly a m., but a noninflammatory ossification.

proliferative m., a rapidly growing benign infiltrating fibrous nodule in skeletal muscle, containing characteristic giant cells resembling ganglion cells.

m. purulen′ta trop′ica, SYN tropical *pyomyositis.*

tropical m., SYN tropical *pyomyositis.*

my·o·spasm, my·o·spas·mus (mī′ō-spazm, mī-ō-spaz′mŭs). Spasmodic muscular contraction.

cervical m., SEE posttraumatic neck *syndrome.*

my·o·spher·u·lo·sis (mī′ō-sfēr-oo-lō′sis). A chronic granulomatous reaction to undetermined spherical structures frequently contained within a microscopic cyst; first reported in cystic lesions in skeletal muscle from eastern Africa and subsequently in nasal infections in the U.S. [myo- + L. *sphaerula,* small sphere, + G. *-osis,* condition]

my·o·sthe·nom·e·ter (mī′ō-sthĕ-nom′ĕ-ter). An instrument for measuring the power of muscle groups. [myo- + G. *sthenos,* strength, + *metron,* measure]

my·o·stro·ma (mī-ō-strō′mă). The supporting connective tissue or framework of muscular tissue. [myo- + G. *strōma,* mattress]

my·o·stro·min (mī-ō-strō′min). A protein found in muscle stroma.

my·o·tac·tic (mī-ō-tak′tik). Relating to the muscular sense. [myo- + L. *tactus,* a touching]

my·ot·a·sis (mī-ot′ă-sis). Stretching of a muscle. [myo- + G. *tasis,* a stretching]

my·o·tat·ic (mī-ō-tat′ik). Relating to myotasis.

my·o·ten·o·si·tis (mī′ō-te-nō-sī′tis). Inflammation of a muscle with its tendon. [myo- + G. *tenōn,* tendon, + *-itis,* inflammation]

my·o·te·not·o·my (mī′ō-te-not′ō-mē). Cutting through the principal tendon of a muscle, with division of the muscle itself in whole or in part. SYN tenomyotomy, tenontomyotomy. [myo- + G. *tenōn,* tendon, + *tomē,* incision]

my·o·ther·mic (mī-ō-ther′mik). Relating to the increased temperature in muscular tissue resulting from its contraction. [myo- + G. *thermē,* heat]

my·o·tome (mī′ō-tōm). **1.** A knife for dividing muscle. **2.** In embryos, that part of the somite that develops into skeletal muscle. SYN muscle plate. **3.** All muscles derived from one somite and innervated by one segmental spinal nerve. **4.** In primitive vertebrates, the muscular part of a metamere. SYN myomere. [myo- + G. *tomos,* a cut]

my·ot·o·my (mī-ot′ō-mē). **1.** Anatomy or dissection of the muscles. **2.** Surgical division of a muscle. [myo- + G. *tomē,* excision]

cricopharyngeal m., division of the cephalad portion of the cricopharyngeus muscle, usually for treatment of Zenker esophageal diverticulum.

Heller m., distal esophagomyotomy, usually for the treatment of achalasia.

my·o·tone (mī′ō-tōn). SYN myotony.

my·o·to·nia (mī-ō-tō′nē-ă). Delayed relaxation of a muscle after a strong contraction, or prolonged contraction after mechanical stimulation (as by percussion) or brief electrical stimulation; due to abnormality of the muscle membrane, specifically the ion channels. [myo- + G. *tonos,* tension, stretching]

m. acquisi′ta, acquired m. following exposure to certain toxins.

m. atroph′ica, SYN myotonic *dystrophy.*

m. congen′ita [MIM*160800], an uncommon muscle disorder, with onset in infancy or early childhood, characterized by muscle hypertrophy, myotonia, and a nonprogressive course; autosomal dominant inheritance; caused by mutations in the skeletal muscle chloride channel gene (CLCN1) on chromosome 7q. SYN Thomsen disease.

m. dystroph′ica, SYN myotonic *dystrophy.*

m. neonato′rum, SYN neonatal *tetany.*

my·o·ton·ic (mī-ō-ton′ik). Pertaining to or exhibiting myotonia.

my·ot·o·noid (mī-ot′ŏ-noyd). Denoting a muscular reaction, naturally or electrically excited, characterized by slow contraction and, especially, slow relaxation. [myo- + G. *tonos,* tone, tension, + *eidos,* resemblance]

my·ot·o·nus (mī-ot′ŏ-nŭs). A tonic spasm or temporary rigidity

of a muscle or group of muscles. [myo- + G. *tonos,* tension, stretching]

my·ot·o·ny (mī-ot′ŏ-nē). Muscular tonus or tension. SYN myotone. [myo- + G. *tonos,* tension]

my·ot·ro·phy (mī-ot′rō-fē). Nutrition of muscular tissue. [myo- + G. *trophē,* nourishment]

my·o·tube (mī′ō-toob). A skeletal muscle fiber formed by the fusion of myoblasts during a developmental stage; a few myofibrils occur at the periphery, and the central core is occupied by nuclei and sarcoplasm so that the fiber has a tubular appearance.

my·o·tu·bule (mī-ō-t;oo′bool). Former term for myotube.

My·o·vir·i·dae (mī-ō-vir′i-dē). A family of relatively large bacterial viruses with complex contractile tails, heads that are usually elongated but are isometric in some species, and a double-stranded DNA genome (MW 21–190 × 10⁶). It includes the T-even phage group and probably other genera.

myr·i·ca (mir′i-kă). The bark of *Myrica cerifera* (family Myricaceae); used in diarrhea and icterus, and externally in sore throat. SYN bayberry bark.

myr·i·cin (mir′i-sin). Myricyl palmitate, a white, almost odorless solid that is the chief constituent of beeswax.

△**myring-.** SEE myringo-.

my·rin·ga (mi-ring′gă). SYN tympanic *membrane.* [Mod. L. drum membrane]

myr·in·gec·to·my (mir-in-jek′tō-mē). Excision of the tympanic membrane. [myring- + G. *ektomē,* excision]

myr·in·gi·tis (mir-in-jī′tis). Inflammation of the tympanic membrane. SYN tympanitis. [myring- + G. *-itis,* inflammation]

m. bulbo′sa, SYN myringodermatitis.

bullous m., painful inflammation of the tympanic membrane accompanied by bullae.

△**myringo-, myring-.** The membrana tympani. [Mod. L. *myringa*]

my·rin·go·der·ma·ti·tis (mi-ring′gō-der-mă-tī′tis). Inflammation of the meatal or outer surface of the drum membrane and the adjoining skin of the external auditory canal. SYN myringitis bulbosa.

my·rin·go·plas·ty (mi-ring′gō-plas′tē). Operative repair of a damaged tympanic membrane. [myringo- + G. *plassō,* to form]

my·rin·go·scler·o·sis (mī-ring′gō-skler-ō′sis). Formation of dense connective tissue in the tympanic membrane, usually not associated with hearing loss. [myringo- + sclerosis]

my·rin·go·sta·pe·di·o·pexy (mi-ring′gō-stā-pē′dē-ō-pek′sē). A technique of tympanoplasty in which the tympanic membrane or grafted tympanic membrane is brought into functional connection with the stapes. [myringo- + L. *stapes,* stirrup (stapes), + G. *pēxis,* fixation]

my·rin·go·tome (mi-ring′gō-tōm). A knife used for paracentesis of the tympanic cavity. [myringo- + G. *tomē,* excision]

myr·in·got·o·my (mir-ing-got′ŏ-mē). Incision of the tympanic membrane. SYN tympanotomy. [myringo- + G. *tomē,* excision]

my·rinx (mī′ringks, mir′ringks). SYN tympanic *membrane.* [Mod. L. *myringa,* drum membrane]

my·ris·ti·ca (mi-ris′ti-kă). SYN nutmeg. [G. *myrizō,* to anoint, fr. *myron,* an unguent]

m. oil, SYN nutmeg oil.

my·ris·tic ac·id (mi-ris′tik). A saturated fatty acid present as an acylglycerol in milk, vegetable fats, cod liver oil, and waxes. SYN tetradecanoic acid.

my·ris·ti·cin (mī-ris′ti-sin). A constituent of nutmeg thought to be responsible, at least in part, for the bizarre central nervous system symptoms produced by the ingestion of large amounts of nutmeg.

my·ris·to·le·ic ac·id (mi-ris-tō-lē′ik). A 14-carbon unsaturated fatty acid with a double bond between carbons 9 and 10; the 14-carbon analog of oleic acid.

myr·me·cia (mĭr-mē′shē-ă). A form of viral wart in which the lesion has a domed surface (i.e., an ant hill configuration) and is associated with pale staining intranuclear and amphophilic intracytoplasmic inclusion bodies in the epidermal cells. [G. *murmex,* ant]

my

my·ro·si·nase (mī-rō'si-nās). SYN thioglucosidase.

myrrh (mer). A gum resin from *Commiphora molmol* and *C. abyssinica* (family Burseraceae) and other species of *C.*, a shrub of Arabia and eastern Africa; used as an astringent, tonic, and stimulant, and locally for diseases of the oral cavity and in mouthwashes; thought to have been used in ancient Egyptian medicine and embalming. [G. *myrrha*]

my·so·phil·ia (mī-sō-fil'ē-ă). SYN coprophilia (2). [G. *mysos*, defilement, + *philos*, fond]

my·so·pho·bia (mī-sō-fō'bē-ă). Morbid fear of dirt or defilement from touching familiar objects. SYN rhypophobia. [G. *mysos*, defilement, + *phobos*, fear]

my·ta·cism (mī'tă-sizm). A form of stammering in which the letter *m* is frequently substituted for other consonants. SYN mutacism. [G. *my*, the letter μ]

my·ur·ous (mī-ū'rŭs). Gradually decreasing in thickness, as a mouse's tail; rarely used term denoting certain symptoms in process of cessation, or the heartbeat in certain cases in which it grows feebler and feebler for a while and then strengthens. [G. *mys*, mouse, + *ouros*, tail]

myx·ad·e·ni·tis la·bi·a·lis. SYN *cheilitis* glandularis.

myx·as·the·nia (mik-sas-thē'nē-ă). Faulty secretion of mucus. [myx- + G. *astheneia*, weakness]

🔲 myx·e·de·ma (mik-se-dē'mă). Hypothyroidism characterized by a relatively hard edema of subcutaneous tissue, with increased content of mucins (proteoglycans) in the fluid; characterized by somnolence, slow mentation, dryness and loss of hair, increased fluid in body cavities such as the pericardial sac, subnormal temperature, hoarseness, muscle weakness, and slow return of a muscle to the neutral position after a tendon jerk; usually caused by removal or loss of functioning thyroid tissue. [myx- + G. *oidēma*, swelling]

congenital m., SYN infantile *hypothyroidism*.

infantile m., SYN infantile *hypothyroidism*.

operative m., m. developing after thyroidectomy.

pituitary m., m. resulting from inadequate secretion of the thyrotropic hormone; commonly occurs in association with inadequate secretion of other anterior pituitary hormones.

myx·e·de·ma·toid (mik-sĕ-dem'ă-toyd). Resembling myxedema.

myx·e·dem·a·tous (mik-sĕ-dem'ă-tŭs). Relating to myxedema.

myx·e·mia (mik-sē'mē-ă). SYN mucinemia. [myx- + G. *haima*, blood]

♺ myxo-, myx-. Mucus. SEE ALSO muci-, muco-. [G. *myxa*, mucus]

myx·o·chon·dro·fi·bro·sar·co·ma (mik'sō-kon'drō-fī'brō-sar-kō'mă). A malignant neoplasm derived from fibrous connective tissue, i.e., a fibrosarcoma, in which there are intimately associated foci of cartilaginous and myxomatous tissue. [myxo- + G. *chondros*, cartilage, + L. *fibra*, fiber, + G. *sarx*, flesh, + -*ōma*, tumor]

myx·o·chon·dro·ma (mik'sō-kon-drō'mă). A benign neoplasm of cartilaginous tissue, i.e., a chondroma, in which the stroma resembles relatively primitive mesenchymal tissue. SYN myxoma enchondromatosum. [myxo- + G. *chondros*, cartilage, + -*ōma*, tumor]

Myx·o·coc·cid·i·um steg·o·my·i·ae (mik'sō-kok-sid'ē-ŭm steg-ō-mī'ē-ē). A protozoon once found in the body of the mosquito, *Stegomyia calopus*, that had fed on the blood of a patient with yellow fever; the organism was then postulated, incorrectly, to be the causal agent of yellow fever.

myx·o·cyte (mik'sō-sīt). One of the stellate or polyhedral cells present in mucous tissue. [myxo- + G. *kytos*, cell]

myx·o·fi·bro·ma (mik'sō-fī-brō'mă). A benign neoplasm of fibrous connective tissue that resembles primitive mesenchymal tissue. SYN fibroma myxomatodes, myxoma fibrosum. [myxo- + L. *fibra*, fiber, + G. -*ōma*, tumor]

myx·o·fi·bro·sar·co·ma (mik'sō-fī'brō-sar-kō'mă). A malignant fibrous histiocytoma with a predominance of myxoid areas that resemble primitive mesenchymal tissue. [myxo- + L. *fibra*, fiber, + G. *sarx*, flesh, + -*ōma*, tumor]

myx·oid (mik'soyd). Resembling mucus. [myxo- + G. *eidos*, resemblance]

myx·o·li·po·ma (mik'sō-li-pō'mă). A benign neoplasm of adipose tissue in which portions of the tumor resemble mucoid mesenchymal tissue. SYN lipoma myxomatodes, myxoma lipomatosum. [myxo- + G. *lipos*, fat, + -*ōma*, tumor]

myx·o·ma (mik-sō'mă). A benign neoplasm derived from connective tissue, consisting chiefly of polyhedral and stellate cells that are loosely embedded in a soft mucoid matrix, thereby resembling primitive mesenchymal tissue; occurs frequently intramuscularly (where it may be mistaken for a sarcoma), also in the jaw bones, and encysted in the skin (focal mucinosis and dorsal wrist ganglion). [myxo- + G. -*ōma*, tumor]

atrial m., a primary cardiac neoplasm arising most commonly in the left atrium as a soft polypoid mass attached by a stalk to the atrial septum; it may resemble an organized mural thrombus, and the symptoms may include cardiac murmurs, which change with alteration of body position and signs of mitral stenosis or insufficiency, with continuous danger of embolism by fragments of the tumor or its entire mass.

m. enchondromato'sum, SYN myxochondroma.

m. fibro'sum, SYN myxofibroma.

m. lipomato'sum, SYN myxolipoma.

odontogenic m., a benign, expansile, multilocular radiolucent neoplasm of the jaws consisting of myxomatous fibrous connective tissue; presumably derived from the mesenchymal components of the odontogenic apparatus.

m. sarcomato'sum, SYN myxosarcoma.

myx·o·ma·to·sis (mik'sō-mă-tō'sis). 1. SYN mucoid *degeneration*. 2. Multiple myxomas.

myx·o·ma·tous (mik'sō-mă-tŭs). 1. Pertaining to or characterized by the features of a myxoma. 2. Said of tissue that resembles primitive mesenchymal tissue.

myx·o·my·cete (mik'sō-mī-sēt). A member of the class Myxomycetes.

Myx·o·my·ce·tes (mik'sō-mī-sē'tēz). A class of fungi containing the slime molds, which occur on rotting vegetation but are not pathogenic for humans. [myxo- + G. *mykēs*, fungus]

myx·o·neu·ro·ma (mik'sō-noo-rō'mă). 1. Obsolete term for a tumefaction resulting from abnormal proliferation of Schwann cells, in which focal or diffuse degenerative changes result in portions that resemble primitive mesenchymal tissue. 2. Obsolete term for a neurilemoma, meningioma, or glioma in which the stroma is myxomatous in nature. [myxo- + G. *neuron*, nerve, + -*ōma*, tumor]

myx·o·pap·il·lo·ma (mik'sō-pap-i-lō'mă). A benign neoplasm of epithelial tissue in which the stroma resembles primitive mesenchymal tissue. [myxo- + L. *papilla*, a nipple, + G. -*ōma*, tumor]

myx·o·poi·e·sis (mik'sō-poy-ē'sis). Mucus production. [myxo- + G. *poiēsis*, a making]

m. g. gas·'tri·ca. SYN gastromyxorrhea.

myx·o·sar·co·ma (mik'sō-sar-kō'mă). A sarcoma, usually a liposarcoma or malignant fibrous histiocytoma, with an abundant component of myxoid tissue resembling primitive mesenchyme containing connective tissue mucin. SYN myxoma sarcomatosum. [myxo- + G. *sarx*, flesh, + -*ōma*, tumor]

Myx·o·spo·ra (mik-sō-spō'ră). A subphylum of the phylum Protozoa, characterized by the presence of spores of multicellular origin, usually with two or three valves, two or more polar filaments, and an ameboid sporoplasm; parasitic in lower vertebrates, especially common in fishes. Important genera include *Ceratomyxa, Hanneguya, Leptotheca, Myxidium*, and *Myxobolus*. [myxo- + G. *sporos*, seed]

Myx·o·spo·rea (mik'sō-spō-rē'ă). A class of Myxozoa with spores containing one to six (usually two) polar capsules, each containing a coiled polar filament; parasitic in the celom or tissues of cold-blooded vertebrates, especially fishes. Important genera include *Ceratomyxa, Hanneguya, Leptotheca, Myxidium*, and *Myxobolus*.

myx·o·vi·rus (mik′sō-vī′rŭs). Term formerly used for viruses with an affinity for mucins, now included in the families Orthomyxoviridae and Paramyxoviridae. The m.'s included influenza virus, parainfluenza virus, respiratory syncytial virus, measles virus, and mumps virus.

Myx·o·zoa (mik-sō-zō′ă). A phylum of the subkingdom Protozoa, characterized by spores of multicellular origin (usually with two or three valves), one to six polar capsules or nematocysts (each with a coiled hollow filament), and a one- to many-nucleated ameboid sporoplasm; parasitic in annelids and other invertebrates (class Actinosporea; subclass Actinomyxa) and in lower vertebrates (class Myxosporea). [myxo- + G. *zōon,* animal]

ν 1. The 13th letter of the Greek alphabet, nu. **2.** Symbol for kinematic *viscosity*; frequency; stoichiometric *number*. **3.** In chemistry, denotes the position of a substituent located on the thirteenth atom from the carboxyl or other functional group.

N 1. Symbol for newton; nitrogen; asparagine; nucleoside; normal solution; haploid chromsome number. **2.** Designation for an inherited blood factor. See MNSs blood group, Blood Groups appendix.

N/2 Symbol for seminormal.

^{15}N Symbol for nitrogen-15.

^{13}N Symbol for nitrogen-13.

^{14}N Symbol for nitrogen-14.

N_A Symbol for Avogadro *number*.

n Symbol for nano- (2); reaction order.

N Symbol for normal *concentration*. SEE normal (3).

n 1. The number in a scientific study. Sample size. **2.** Symbol for refractive *index*.

n_0 Abbreviation for Loschmidt *number*.

NA Abbreviation for Nomina Anatomica.

N.A. Abbreviation for numerical *aperture*.

Na Symbol for sodium (natrium).

^{24}Na. Symbol for sodium-24.

nab·i·lone (nab'i-lōn). A synthetic cannabinoid used in the treatment of nausea and vomiting associated with cancer chemotherapy.

Naboth, Martin, German anatomist and physician, 1675–1721. SEE nabothian *cyst; follicle.

na·cre·ous (nā'krē-ŭs). Lustrous, like mother-of-pearl; descriptive term for bacterial colonies. [Fr. *nacre*, mother-of-pearl]

NAD Abbreviation for nicotinamide adenine dinucleotide.

N.A.D. Abbreviation for no appreciable disease; nothing abnormal detected (British).

NAD$^+$ Abbreviation for nicotinamide adenine dinucleotide (oxidized form).

NAD$^+$ nucleosidase, an enzyme hydrolyzing NAD$^+$ to nicotinamide and adenosine diphosphoribose. SYN NADase.

NAD$^+$ pyrophosphorylase, an enzyme that participates in the synthesis of NAD$^+$; it reacts nicotinamide mononucleotide with ATP to produce NAD$^+$ and pyrophosphate; it will also act on nicotinate mononucleotide.

NAD$^+$ synthetase, an enzyme that catalyzes the reaction of ATP, L-glutamine, and nicotinate adenine dinucleotide to form NAD$^+$, ADP, and L-glutamate.

NADase SYN *NAD$^+$ nucleosidase.*

NADH Abbreviation for nicotinamide adenine dinucleotide (reduced form).

NADH dehydrogenase, an iron-sulfur–containing flavoprotein reversibly oxidizing NADH to NAD$^+$; an inherited deficiency of this complex results in overwhelming acidosis. SYN cytochrome *c* reductase.

NADH dehydrogenase (quinone), an enzyme oxidizing NADH with quinones (e.g., menaquinone) as acceptors.

NADH-hydroxylamine reductase, an enzyme catalyzing the reaction of hydroxylamine and NADH to form ammonia, NAD$^+$, and water; used in a number of clinical assays.

na·dide (nā'dīd). A nicotinamide adenine dinucleotide compound used as an antagonist to alcohol and narcotics.

nadir (nā'dēr). The lowest value of blood counts after chemotherapy. [M.E., Med. L., lowest point, fr. Arabic *nazīr*, opposite (the zenith)]

Nadi re·ac·tion. See under reaction.

na·do·lol (nā'dō-lol). A β-adrenergic blocking agent with actions similar to those of propranolol.

NADP Abbreviation for nicotinamide adenine dinucleotide phosphate.

NADP$^+$ Abbreviation for nicotinamide adenine dinucleotide phosphate (oxidized form).

NAD(P)$^+$ nu·cle·o·si·dase. An enzyme hydrolyzing NAD(P)$^+$ to release free nicotinamide and adenosinediphosphoribose-(phosphate).

NADPH Abbreviation for nicotinamide adenine dinucleotide phosphate (reduced form).

NADPH-cytochrome c_2 reductase, an enzyme catalyzing the reduction of 2ferricytochrome c_2 to 2ferrocytochrome c_2 at the expense of NADPH. SYN cytochrome c_2 reductase.

NADPH dehydrogenase, a flavoprotein oxidizing NADPH to NADP$^+$. SYN NADPH diaphorase, old yellow enzyme, Warburg old yellow enzyme.

NADPH dehydrogenase (quinone), a flavoprotein oxidizing NADH or NADPH to NAD$^+$ or NADP$^+$ with quinones (e.g., menadione) as hydrogen acceptors. SYN DT-diaphorase, menadione reductase, phylloquinone reductase, quinone reductase.

NADPH diaphorase, SYN NADPH dehydrogenase.

NADPH-ferrihemoprotein reductase (fer'ī-hē-mō-prō'tēn, fer'ē-), an enzyme catalyzing the reduction of 2 ferricytochrome by NADPH to 2 ferrocytochrome; the physiologic acceptor is probably cytochrome P-450; hence, it has a role in steroid hydroxylations. SYN cytochrome reductase.

Naegeli, Otto, Swiss physician, 1871–1938. SEE N. type of monocytic *leukemia.*

Naegeli, Oskar, Swiss physician, 1885–1959. SEE N. *syndrome.*

Nae·gle·ria (nā-glē'rē-ă). A genus of free-living soil, water, and sewage ameba (order Schizopyrenida, family Vahlkampfiidae) one species of which, *N. fowleri*, has been implicated as the causative agent of the rapidly fatal primary amebic meningoencephalitis. Infection has been traced to swimming pools (including indoor chlorinated pools); entry is by the nasal mucosa, from which the amebae reach the meninges and brain through the cribriform plate and olfactory nerves. Other soil amebae that have been implicated, although of far less epidemiologic significance, include the genera *Acanthamoeba* and *Hartmanella*, the latter being a suspected but unproved causative agent.

naf·cil·lin (naf'sil'in). A semisynthetic penicillin derived from 6-aminopenicillanic acid; resistant to penicillinase, and effective against *Staphylococcus aureus.*

n. sodium, a penicillinase-resistant penicillin.

Naffziger, Howard C., U.S. surgeon, 1884–1961. SEE N. *operation, syndrome.*

naf·ti·fine hy·dro·chlo·ride (naf'ti-fēn). A broad-spectrum antifungal agent used in the topical treatment of tinea infections.

NAG Abbreviation for *N*-acetylglutamate.

na·ga·na (nah-gah'nah). An acute or chronic disease of cattle, dogs, pigs, horses, sheep, and goats in sub-Saharan Africa; marked by fever, anemia, and cachexia, varying in severity with the parasite and the host. A collective term for diseases caused by the protozoan parasites *Trypanosoma brucei brucei*, *T. congolense*, and *T. vivax.*

Nagel, Willibald A., German ophthalmologist and physiologist, 1870–1911. SEE N. *test.*

Nägele, Franz K., German obstetrician, 1777–1851. SEE N. *obliquity, pelvis, rule.*

Nägeli, Karl W. von, Swiss botanist, 1817–1891. SEE micelle.

Nageotte, Jean, French histologist, 1866–1948. SEE N. *cells,* under *cell.*

🔲 nail (nāl). **1.** One of the thin, horny, translucent plates covering

△ Combining Forms	☆ Official alternate Terminologia Anatomica term
🔲 Indicates term is illustrated, see Illustration Index	
	[MIM] Mendelian Inheritance in Man
SYN Synonym	
Cf. Compare	C.I. Colour Index
[NA] Nomina Anatomica	
[TA] Terminologia Anatomica	High Profile Term

CONTENTS

INDEX

Anatomy

Anatomical images provided by:

adam.com™

A.D.A.M.
Software, Inc.
1600 River Edge Parkway
Suite 800
Atlanta, GA 30328
(770) 980-0888
www.adam.com

Anatomy

Anatomy

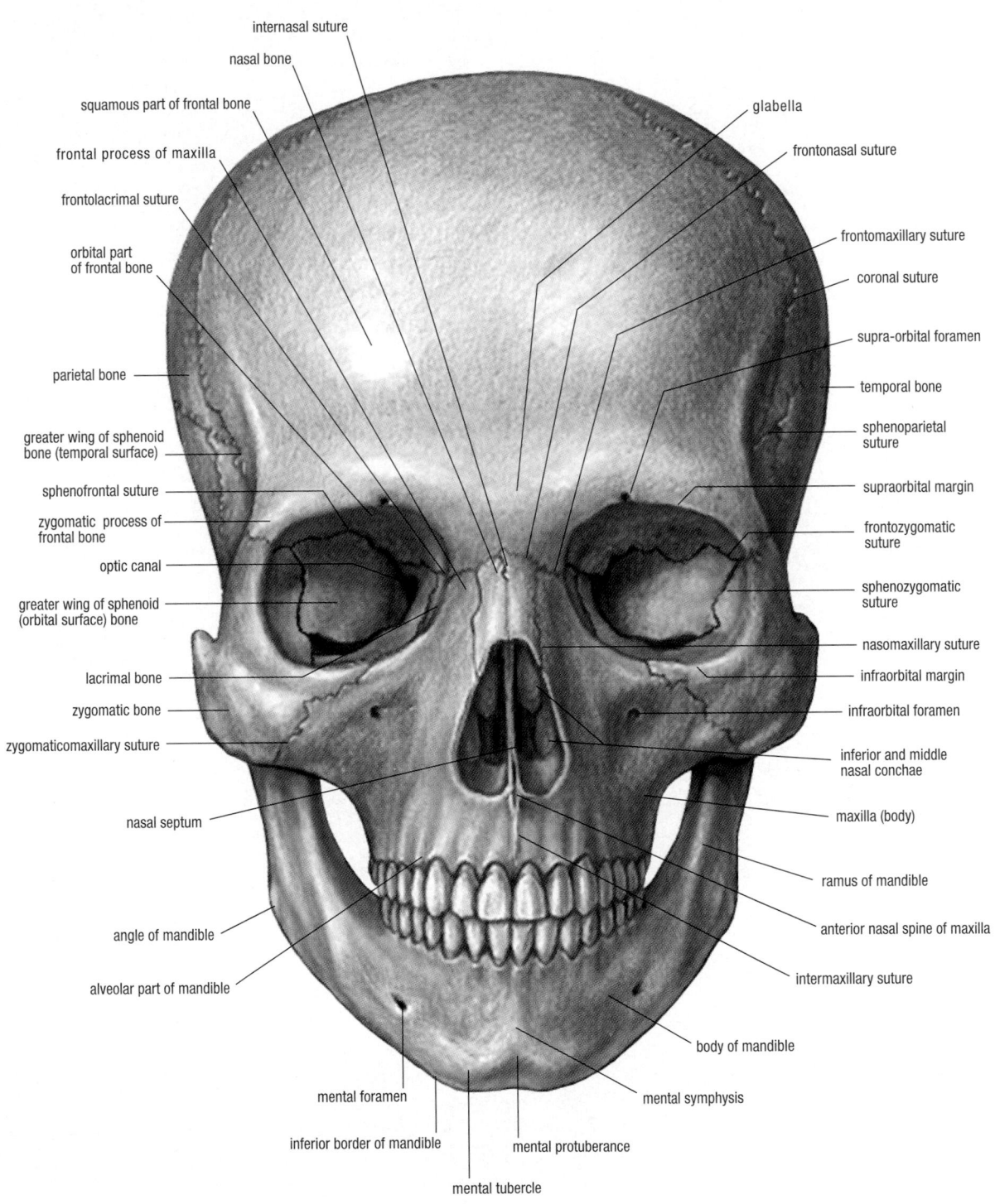

internasal suture

nasal bone

squamous part of frontal bone

frontal process of maxilla

frontolacrimal suture

orbital part
of frontal bone

parietal bone

greater wing of sphenoid
bone (temporal surface)

sphenofrontal suture

zygomatic process of
frontal bone

optic canal

greater wing of sphenoid
(orbital surface) bone

lacrimal bone

zygomatic bone

zygomaticomaxillary suture

nasal septum

angle of mandible

alveolar part of mandible

mental foramen

inferior border of mandible

mental tubercle

mental protuberance

mental symphysis

body of mandible

intermaxillary suture

anterior nasal spine of maxilla

ramus of mandible

maxilla (body)

inferior and middle
nasal conchae

infraorbital foramen

infraorbital margin

nasomaxillary suture

sphenozygomatic
suture

frontozygomatic
suture

supraorbital margin

sphenoparietal
suture

temporal bone

supra-orbital foramen

coronal suture

frontomaxillary suture

frontonasal suture

glabella

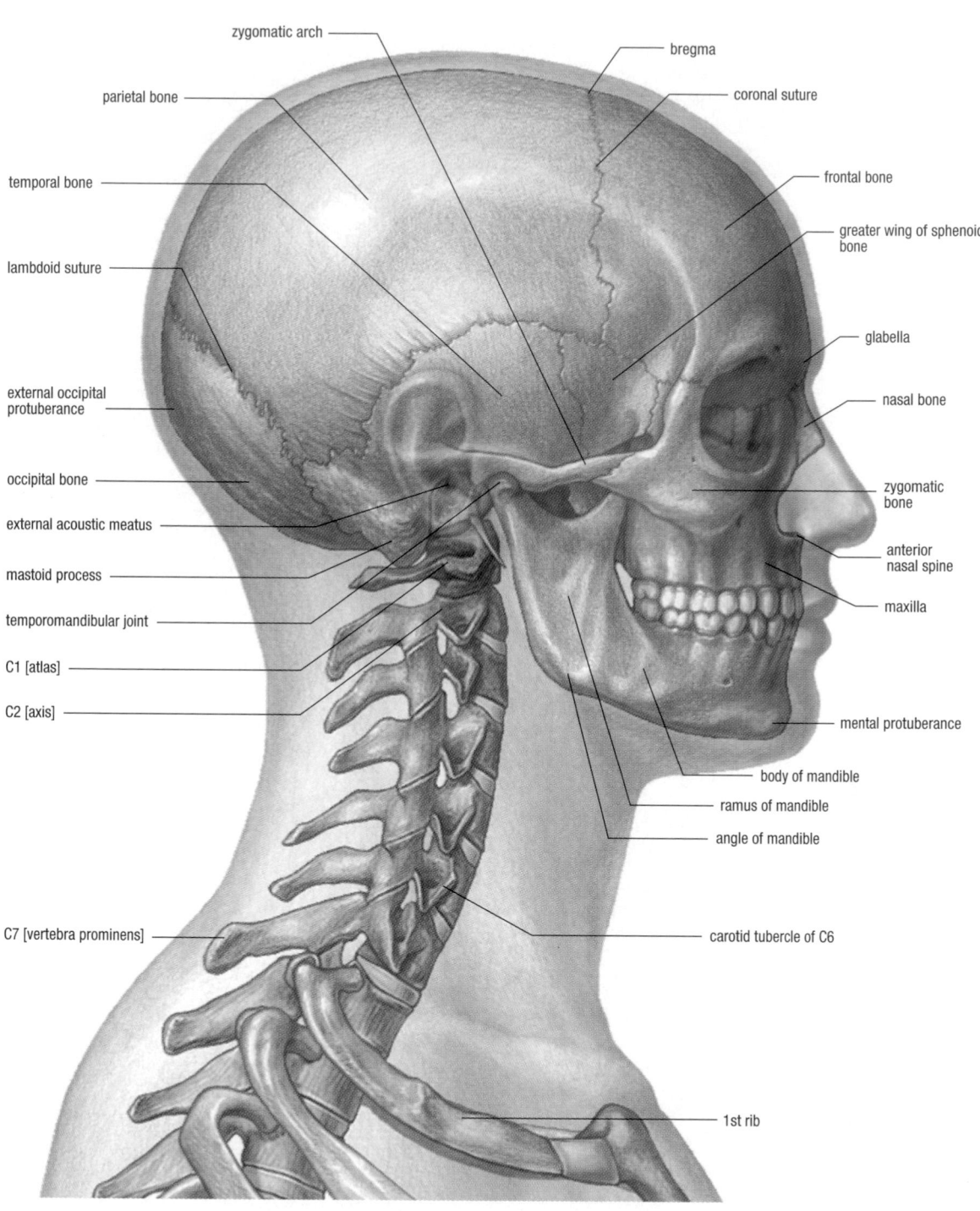

zygomatic arch

bregma

parietal bone

coronal suture

temporal bone

frontal bone

greater wing of sphenoid bone

lambdoid suture

glabella

external occipital protuberance

nasal bone

occipital bone

zygomatic bone

external acoustic meatus

anterior nasal spine

mastoid process

maxilla

temporomandibular joint

C1 [atlas]

mental protuberance

C2 [axis]

body of mandible

ramus of mandible

angle of mandible

C7 [vertebra prominens]

carotid tubercle of C6

1st rib

Anatomy

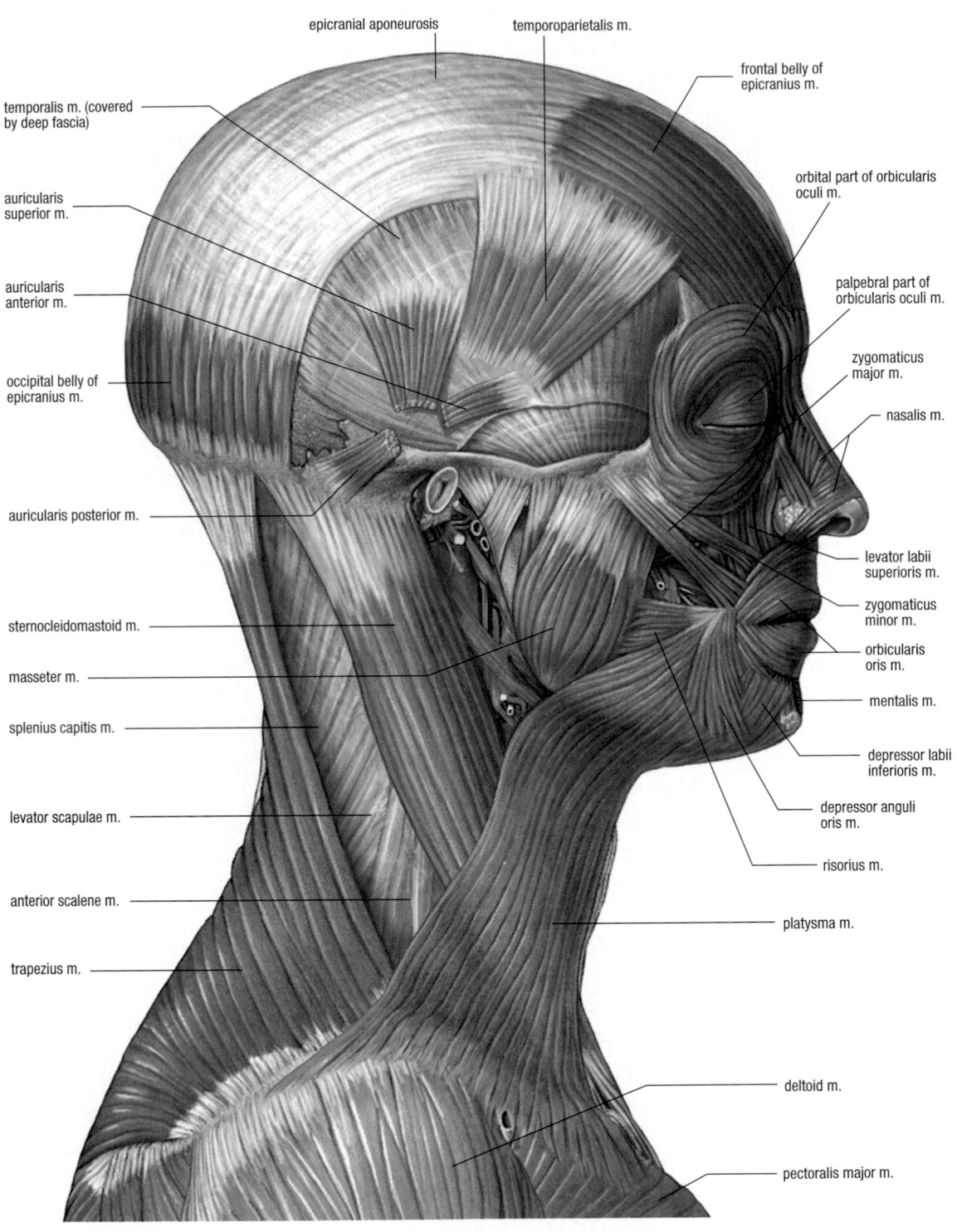

epicranial aponeurosis

temporoparietalis m.

frontal belly of epicranius m.

temporalis m. (covered by deep fascia)

orbital part of orbicularis oculi m.

auricularis superior m.

palpebral part of orbicularis oculi m.

auricularis anterior m.

zygomaticus major m.

nasalis m.

occipital belly of epicranius m.

auricularis posterior m.

levator labii superioris m.

zygomaticus minor m.

sternocleidomastoid m.

orbicularis oris m.

masseter m.

mentalis m.

splenius capitis m.

depressor labii inferioris m.

levator scapulae m.

depressor anguli oris m.

anterior scalene m.

risorius m.

trapezius m.

platysma m.

deltoid m.

pectoralis major m.

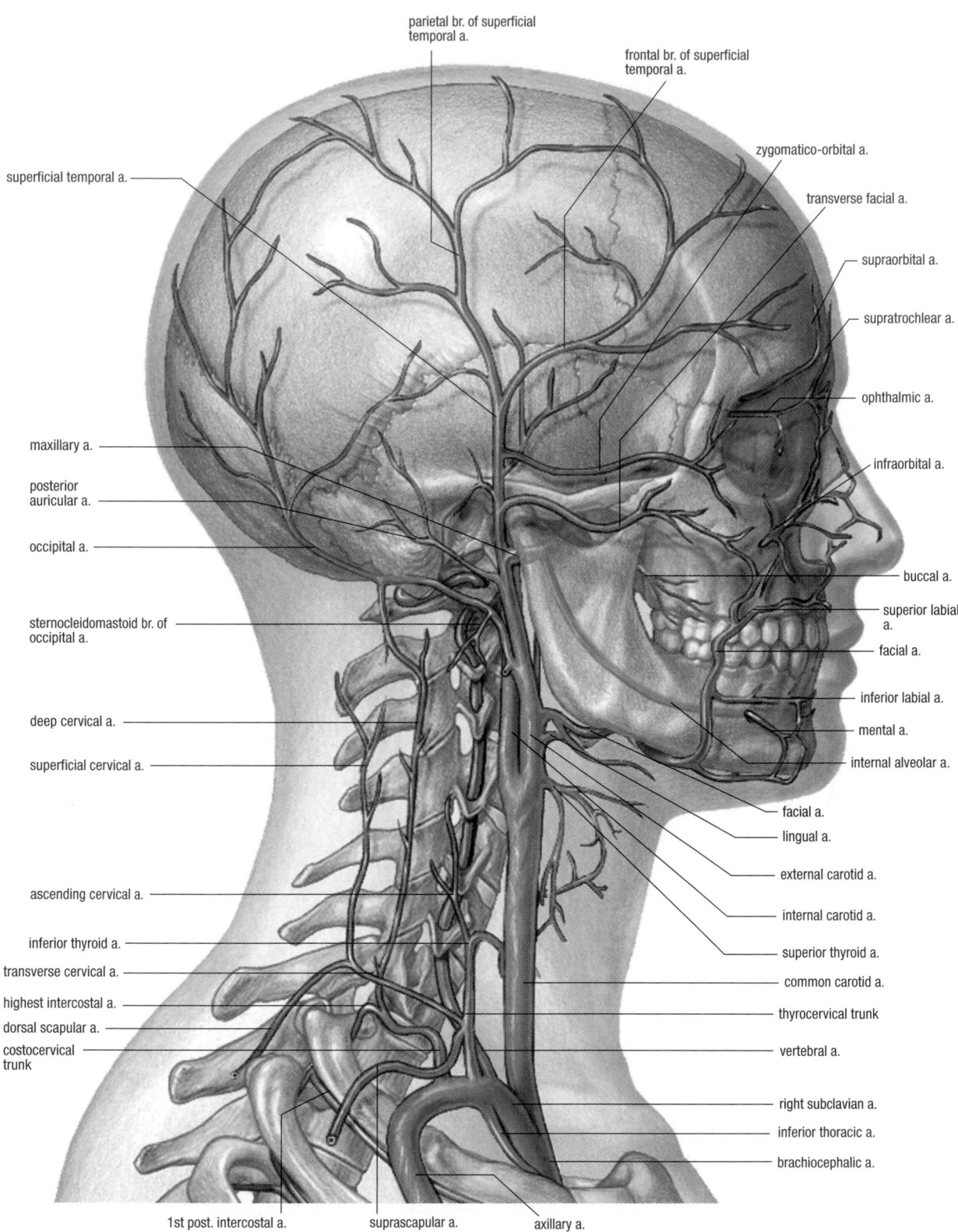

parietal br. of superficial
temporal a.

frontal br. of superficial
temporal a.

zygomatico-orbital a.

transverse facial a.

supraorbital a.

superficial temporal a.

supratrochlear a.

ophthalmic a.

maxillary a.

infraorbital a.

posterior
auricular a.

occipital a.

buccal a.

superior labial
a.

sternocleidomastoid br. of
occipital a.

facial a.

inferior labial a.

mental a.

deep cervical a.

internal alveolar a.

superficial cervical a.

facial a.

lingual a.

external carotid a.

ascending cervical a.

internal carotid a.

inferior thyroid a.

superior thyroid a.

transverse cervical a.

common carotid a.

highest intercostal a.

thyrocervical trunk

dorsal scapular a.

vertebral a.

costocervical
trunk

right subclavian a.

inferior thoracic a.

brachiocephalic a.

1st post. intercostal a.

suprascapular a.

axillary a.

Anatomy

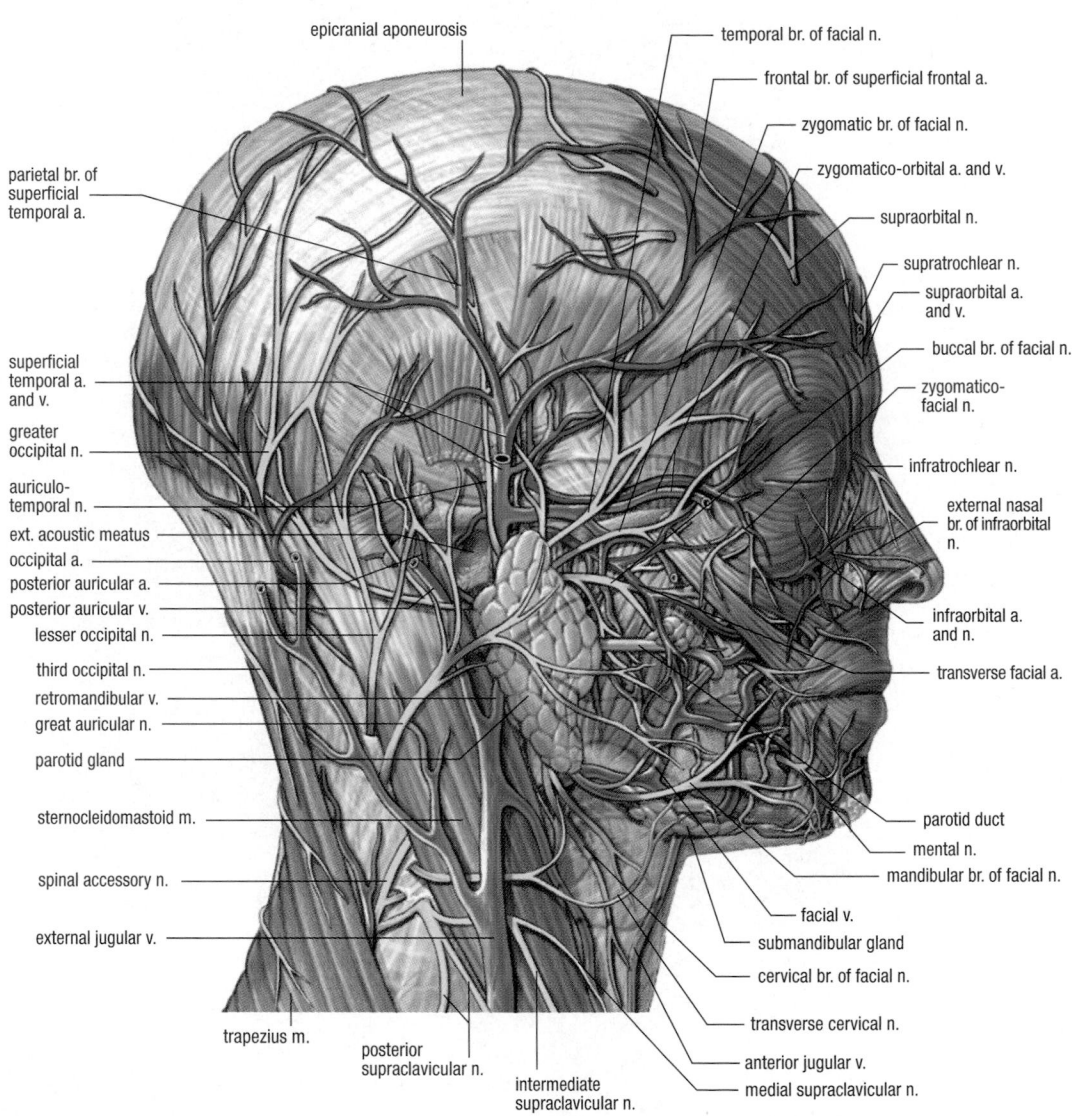

epicranial aponeurosis

temporal br. of facial n.

frontal br. of superficial frontal a.

zygomatic br. of facial n.

zygomatico-orbital a. and v.

parietal br. of superficial temporal a.

supraorbital n.

supratrochlear n.

supraorbital a. and v.

buccal br. of facial n.

superficial temporal a. and v.

zygomatico-facial n.

greater occipital n.

infratrochlear n.

auriculo-temporal n.

external nasal br. of infraorbital n.

ext. acoustic meatus

occipital a.

posterior auricular a.

posterior auricular v.

lesser occipital n.

infraorbital a. and n.

third occipital n.

retromandibular v.

transverse facial a.

great auricular n.

parotid gland

sternocleidomastoid m.

parotid duct

mental n.

mandibular br. of facial n.

spinal accessory n.

facial v.

external jugular v.

submandibular gland

cervical br. of facial n.

trapezius m.

transverse cervical n.

posterior supraclavicular n.

anterior jugular v.

medial supraclavicular n.

intermediate supraclavicular n.

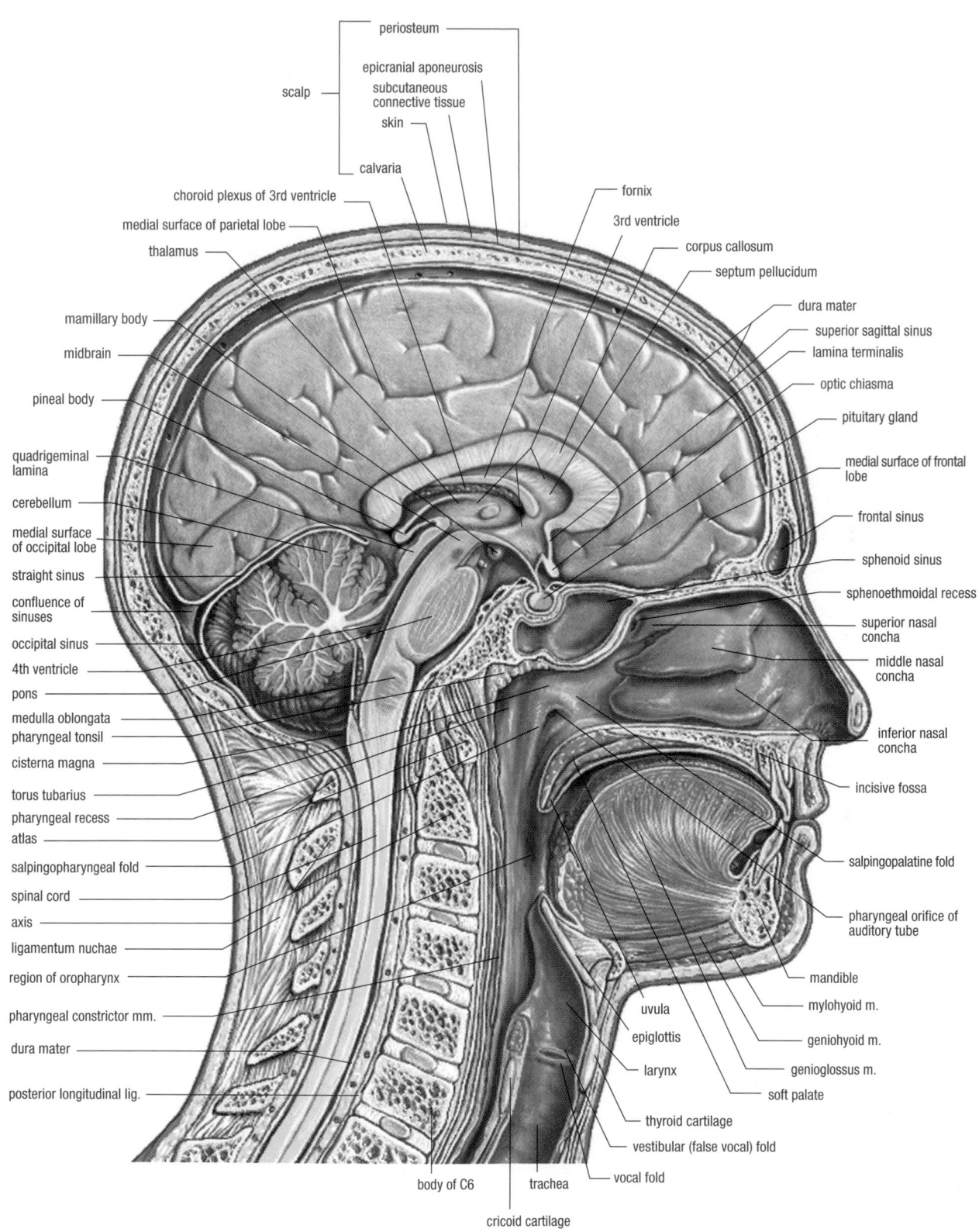

periosteum

epicranial aponeurosis

subcutaneous
connective tissue

scalp

skin

calvaria

choroid plexus of 3rd ventricle

medial surface of parietal lobe

thalamus

fornix

3rd ventricle

corpus callosum

septum pellucidum

dura mater

superior sagittal sinus

lamina terminalis

optic chiasma

pituitary gland

medial surface of frontal lobe

frontal sinus

sphenoid sinus

sphenoethmoidal recess

superior nasal concha

middle nasal concha

inferior nasal concha

incisive fossa

salpingopalatine fold

pharyngeal orifice of auditory tube

mandible

mylohyoid m.

geniohyoid m.

genioglossus m.

soft palate

thyroid cartilage

vestibular (false vocal) fold

vocal fold

uvula

epiglottis

larynx

body of C6

trachea

cricoid cartilage

mamillary body

midbrain

pineal body

quadrigeminal lamina

cerebellum

medial surface of occipital lobe

straight sinus

confluence of sinuses

occipital sinus

4th ventricle

pons

medulla oblongata

pharyngeal tonsil

cisterna magna

torus tubarius

pharyngeal recess

atlas

salpingopharyngeal fold

spinal cord

axis

ligamentum nuchae

region of oropharynx

pharyngeal constrictor mm.

dura mater

posterior longitudinal lig.

Anatomy

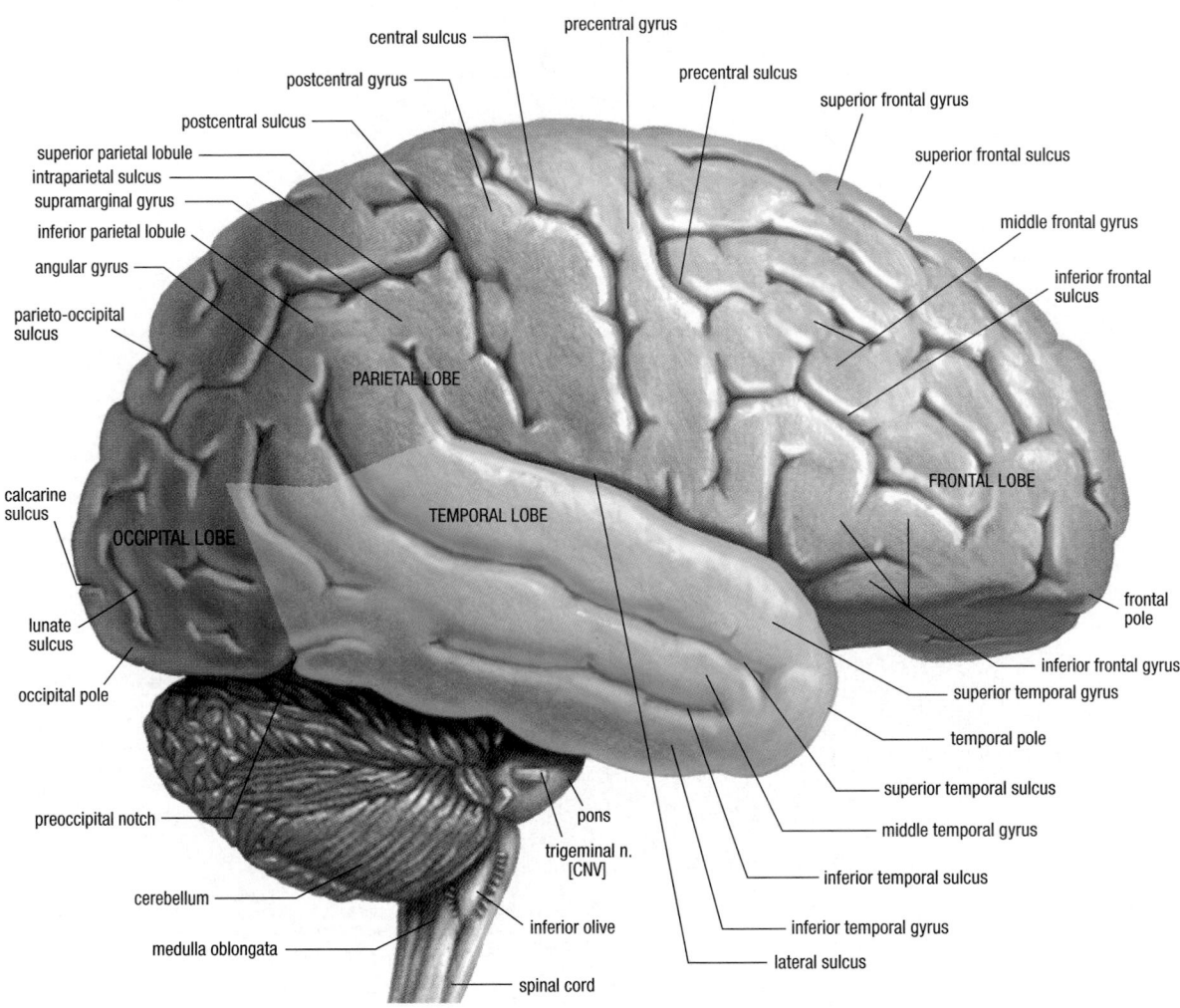

central sulcus

precentral gyrus

postcentral gyrus

precentral sulcus

postcentral sulcus

superior frontal gyrus

superior parietal lobule

superior frontal sulcus

intraparietal sulcus

supramarginal gyrus

middle frontal gyrus

inferior parietal lobule

inferior frontal sulcus

angular gyrus

parieto-occipital sulcus

PARIETAL LOBE

calcarine sulcus

TEMPORAL LOBE

FRONTAL LOBE

OCCIPITAL LOBE

frontal pole

lunate sulcus

inferior frontal gyrus

occipital pole

superior temporal gyrus

temporal pole

preoccipital notch

pons

superior temporal sulcus

trigeminal n. [CNV]

middle temporal gyrus

cerebellum

inferior temporal sulcus

medulla oblongata

inferior olive

inferior temporal gyrus

spinal cord

lateral sulcus

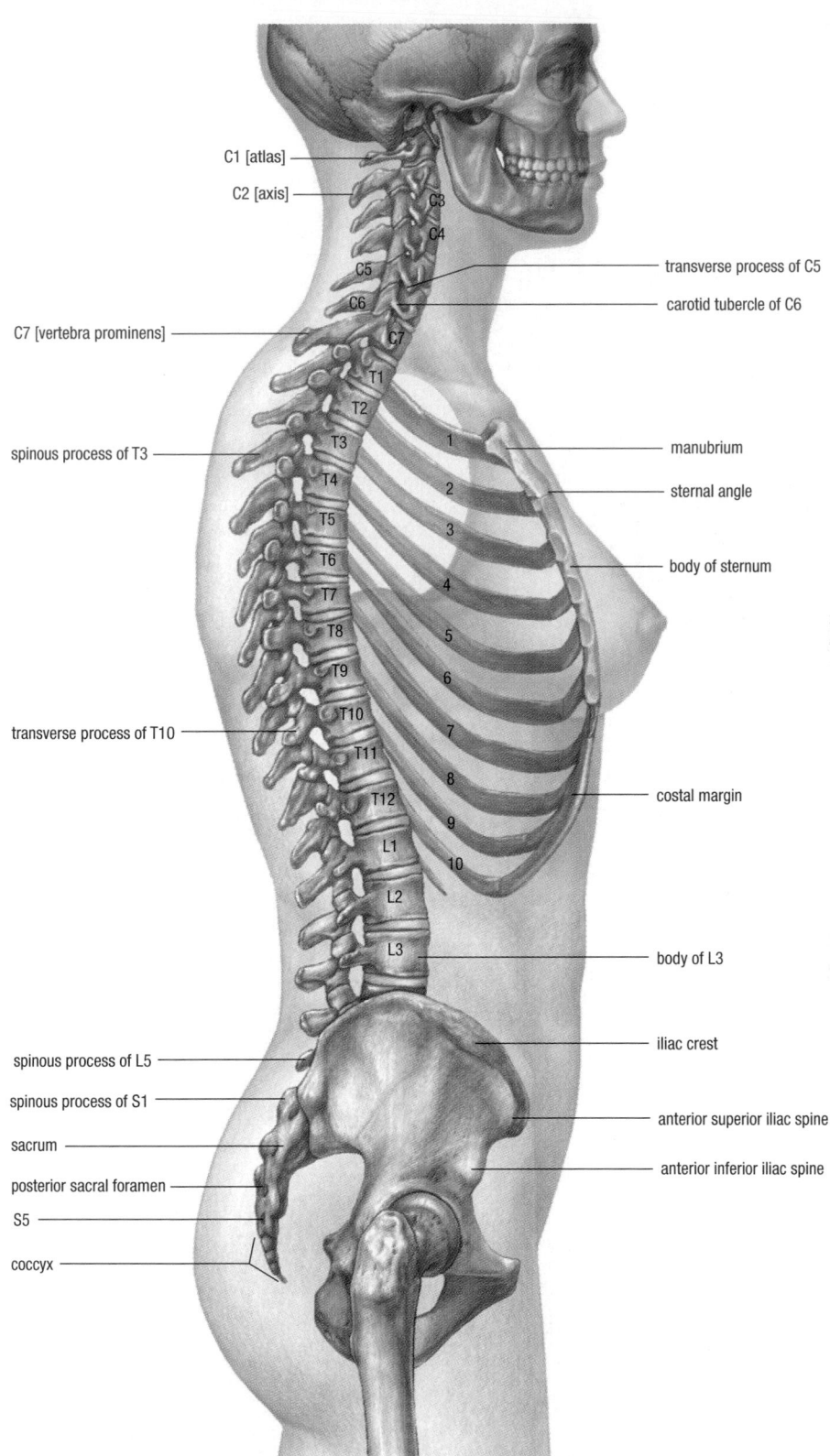

C1 [atlas]

C2 [axis]

C3

C4

transverse process of C5

C5

carotid tubercle of C6

C6

C7 [vertebra prominens]

C7

T1

T2

spinous process of T3

T3

1 — manubrium

T4

2 — sternal angle

T5

3

T6

4 — body of sternum

T7

5

T8

6

T9

7

transverse process of T10

T10

8

T11

9 — costal margin

T12

10

L1

L2

L3 — body of L3

iliac crest

spinous process of L5

spinous process of S1 — anterior superior iliac spine

sacrum — anterior inferior iliac spine

posterior sacral foramen

S5

coccyx

Anatomy

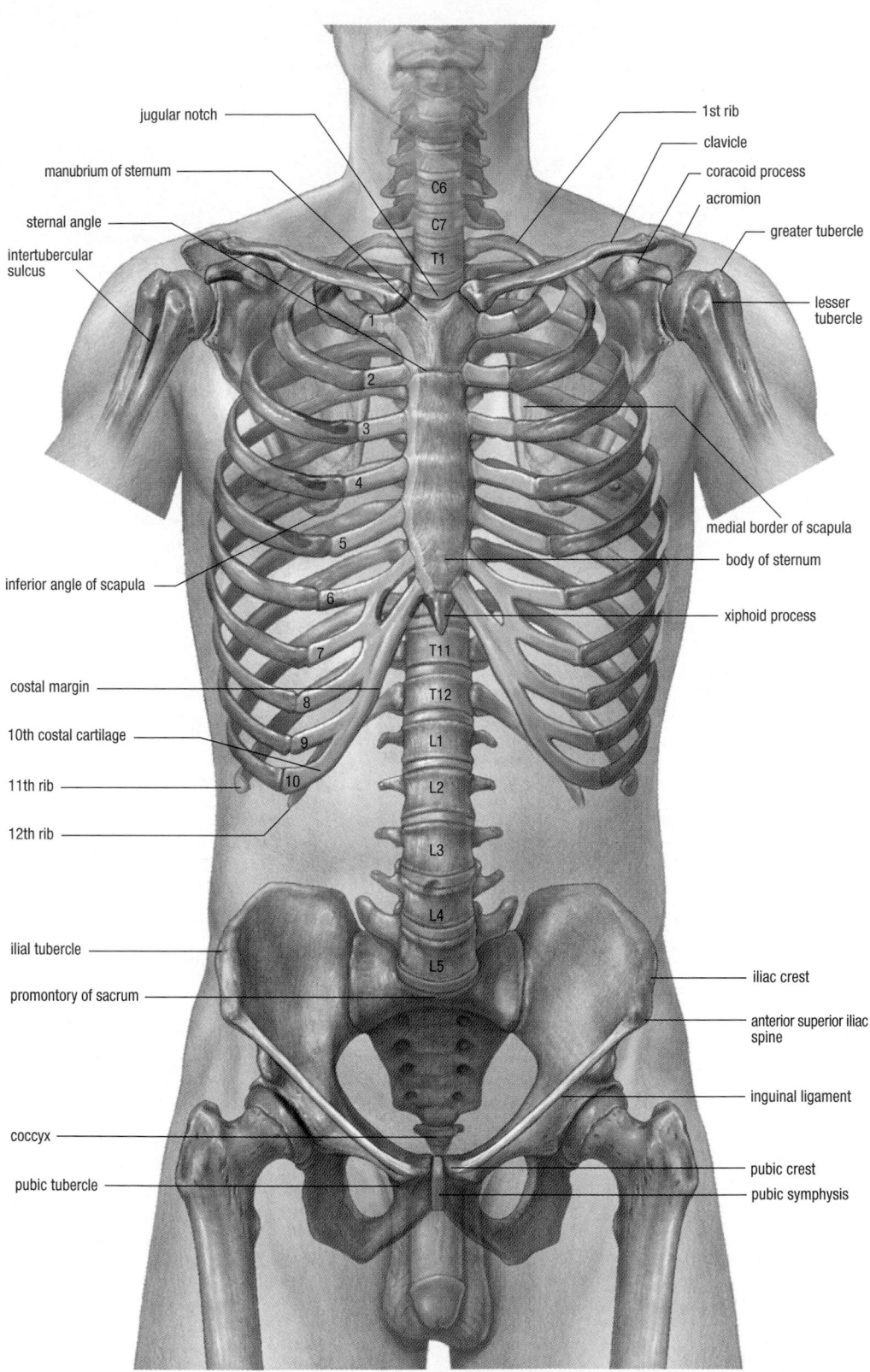

jugular notch

manubrium of sternum

sternal angle

intertubercular sulcus

inferior angle of scapula

costal margin

10th costal cartilage

11th rib

12th rib

ilial tubercle

promontory of sacrum

coccyx

pubic tubercle

1st rib

clavicle

coracoid process

acromion

greater tubercle

lesser tubercle

medial border of scapula

body of sternum

xiphoid process

iliac crest

anterior superior iliac spine

inguinal ligament

pubic crest

pubic symphysis

C6
C7
T1
1
2
3
4
5
6
7
8
9
10
T11
T12
L1
L2
L3
L4
L5

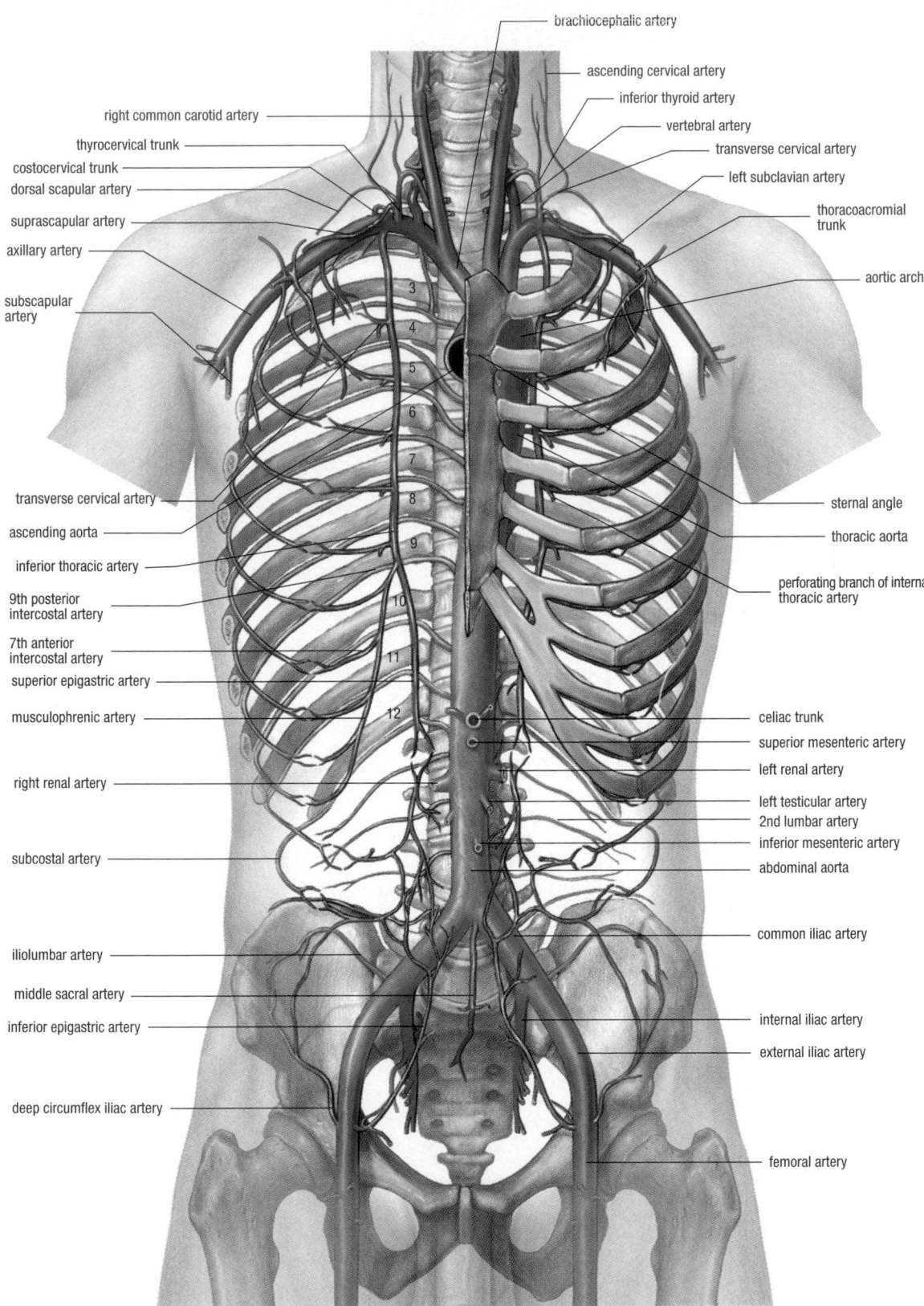

brachiocephalic artery

ascending cervical artery

inferior thyroid artery

vertebral artery

transverse cervical artery

left subclavian artery

thoracoacromial trunk

aortic arch

right common carotid artery

thyrocervical trunk

costocervical trunk

dorsal scapular artery

suprascapular artery

axillary artery

subscapular artery

transverse cervical artery

ascending aorta

inferior thoracic artery

9th posterior intercostal artery

7th anterior intercostal artery

superior epigastric artery

musculophrenic artery

right renal artery

subcostal artery

iliolumbar artery

middle sacral artery

inferior epigastric artery

deep circumflex iliac artery

sternal angle

thoracic aorta

perforating branch of internal thoracic artery

celiac trunk

superior mesenteric artery

left renal artery

left testicular artery

2nd lumbar artery

inferior mesenteric artery

abdominal aorta

common iliac artery

internal iliac artery

external iliac artery

femoral artery

Anatomy

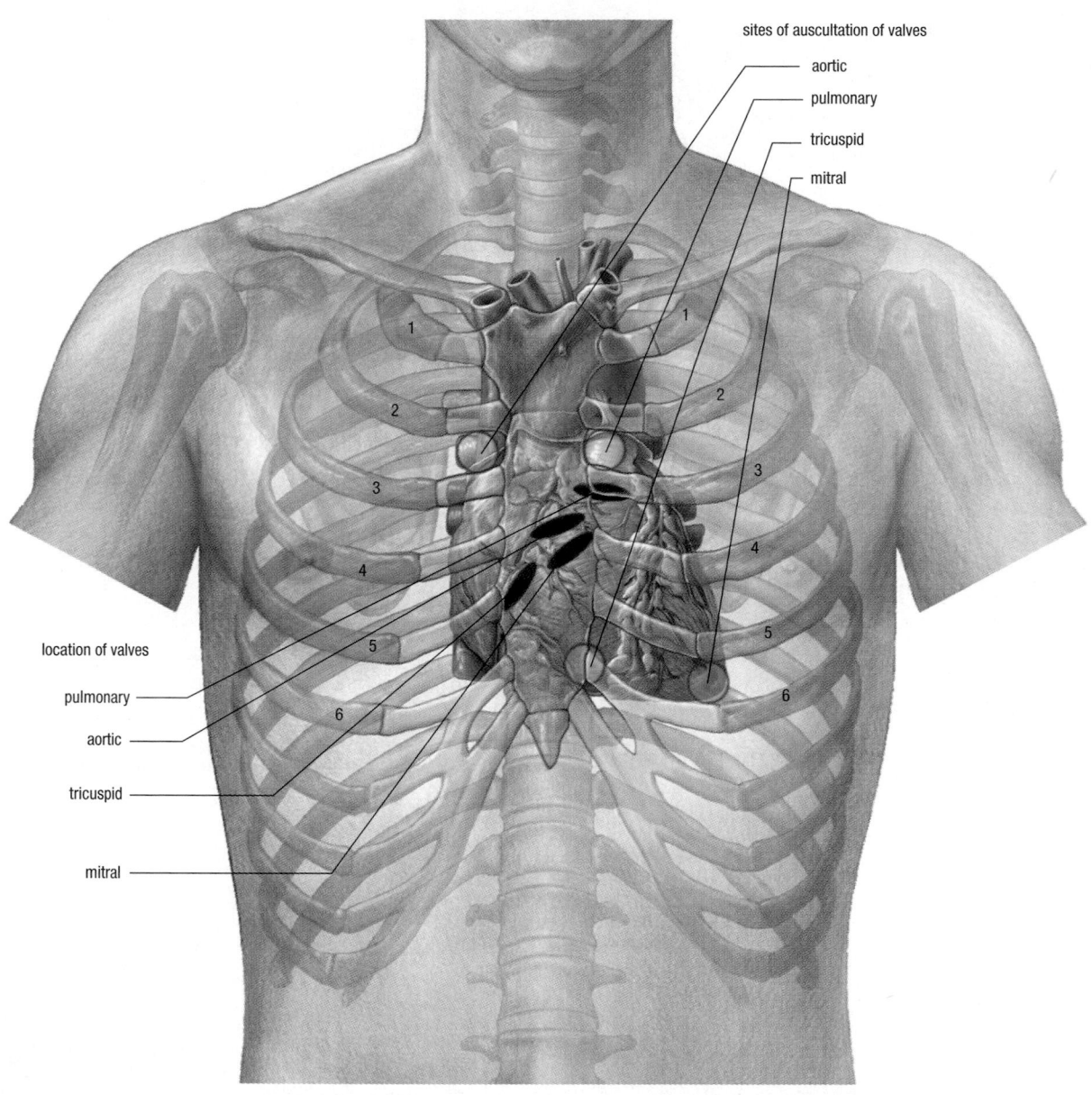

sites of auscultation of valves

aortic

pulmonary

tricuspid

mitral

location of valves

pulmonary

aortic

tricuspid

mitral

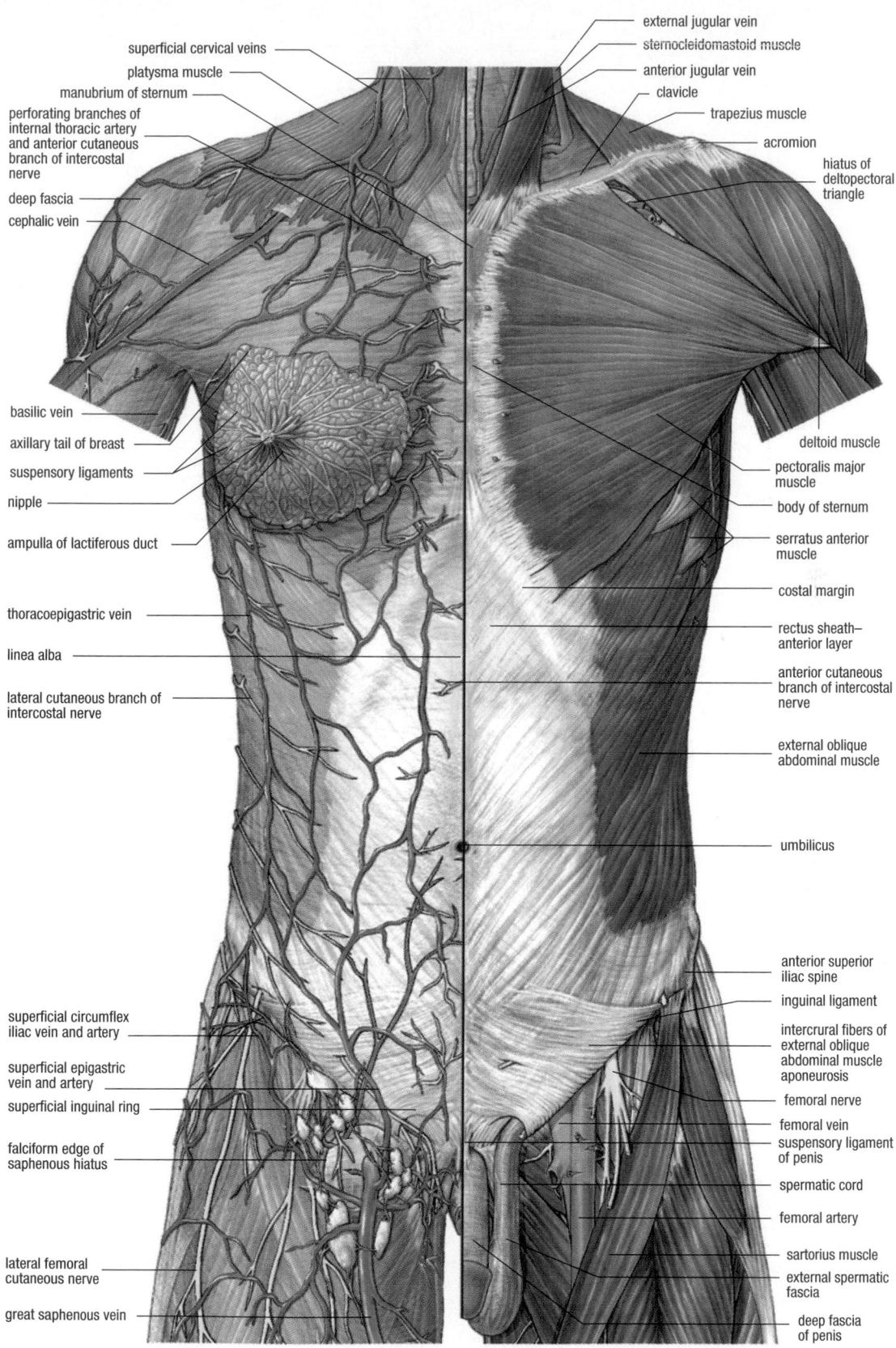

superficial cervical veins

platysma muscle

manubrium of sternum

perforating branches of
internal thoracic artery
and anterior cutaneous
branch of intercostal
nerve

deep fascia

cephalic vein

basilic vein

axillary tail of breast

suspensory ligaments

nipple

ampulla of lactiferous duct

thoracoepigastric vein

linea alba

lateral cutaneous branch of
intercostal nerve

superficial circumflex
iliac vein and artery

superficial epigastric
vein and artery

superficial inguinal ring

falciform edge of
saphenous hiatus

lateral femoral
cutaneous nerve

great saphenous vein

external jugular vein

sternocleidomastoid muscle

anterior jugular vein

clavicle

trapezius muscle

acromion

hiatus of
deltopectoral
triangle

deltoid muscle

pectoralis major
muscle

body of sternum

serratus anterior
muscle

costal margin

rectus sheath–
anterior layer

anterior cutaneous
branch of intercostal
nerve

external oblique
abdominal muscle

umbilicus

anterior superior
iliac spine

inguinal ligament

intercrural fibers of
external oblique
abdominal muscle
aponeurosis

femoral nerve

femoral vein

suspensory ligament
of penis

spermatic cord

femoral artery

sartorius muscle

external spermatic
fascia

deep fascia
of penis

Anatomy

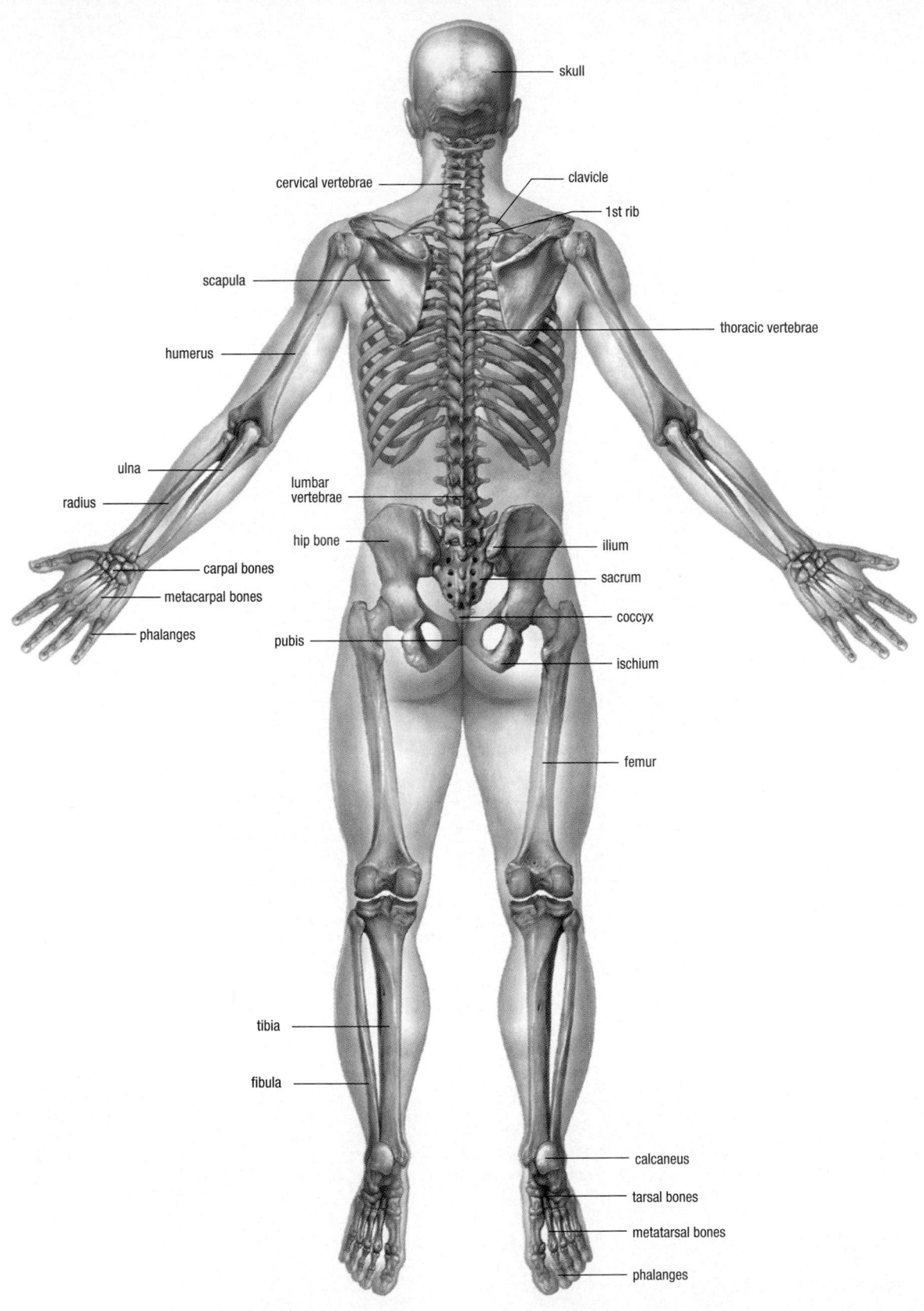

skull

cervical vertebrae

clavicle

1st rib

scapula

thoracic vertebrae

humerus

ulna

radius

lumbar
vertebrae

hip bone

ilium

carpal bones

sacrum

metacarpal bones

coccyx

phalanges

pubis

ischium

femur

tibia

fibula

calcaneus

tarsal bones

metatarsal bones

phalanges

A13

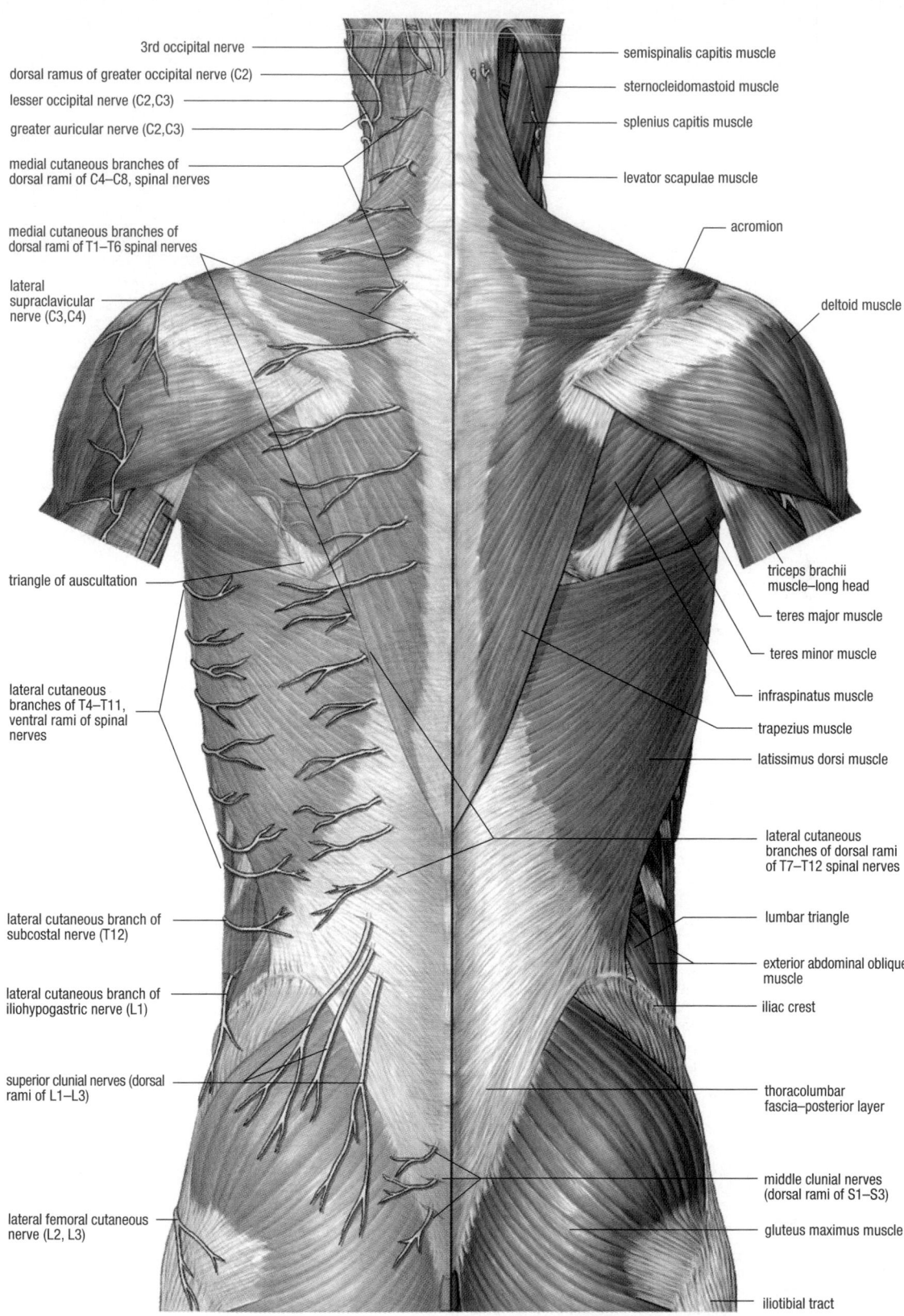

3rd occipital nerve

dorsal ramus of greater occipital nerve (C2)

lesser occipital nerve (C2,C3)

greater auricular nerve (C2,C3)

medial cutaneous branches of dorsal rami of C4–C8, spinal nerves

medial cutaneous branches of dorsal rami of T1–T6 spinal nerves

lateral supraclavicular nerve (C3,C4)

triangle of auscultation

lateral cutaneous branches of T4–T11, ventral rami of spinal nerves

lateral cutaneous branch of subcostal nerve (T12)

lateral cutaneous branch of iliohypogastric nerve (L1)

superior clunial nerves (dorsal rami of L1–L3)

lateral femoral cutaneous nerve (L2, L3)

semispinalis capitis muscle

sternocleidomastoid muscle

splenius capitis muscle

levator scapulae muscle

acromion

deltoid muscle

triceps brachii muscle–long head

teres major muscle

teres minor muscle

infraspinatus muscle

trapezius muscle

latissimus dorsi muscle

lateral cutaneous branches of dorsal rami of T7–T12 spinal nerves

lumbar triangle

exterior abdominal oblique muscle

iliac crest

thoracolumbar fascia–posterior layer

middle clunial nerves (dorsal rami of S1–S3)

gluteus maximus muscle

iliotibial tract

Anatomy

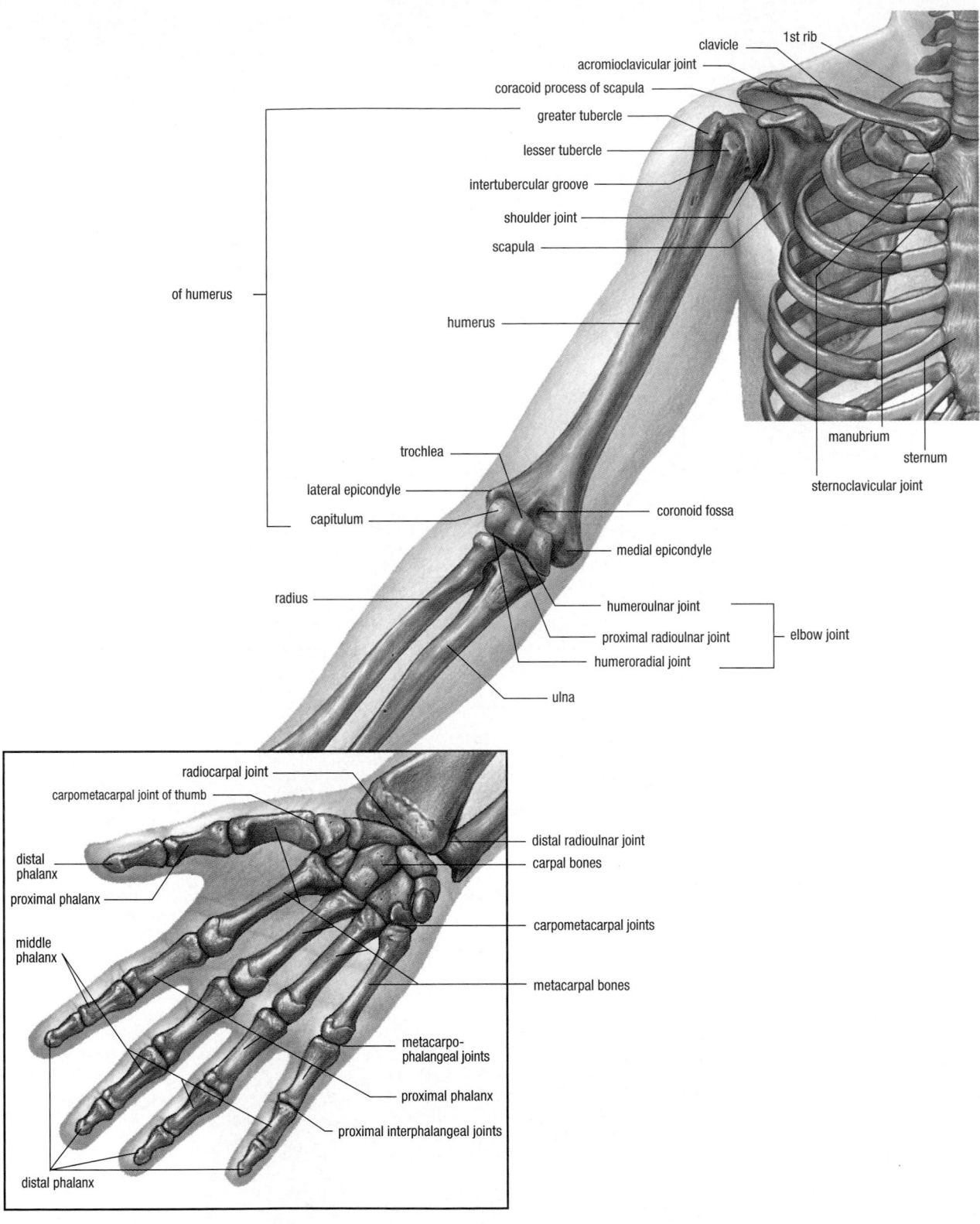

clavicle
1st rib
acromioclavicular joint
coracoid process of scapula
greater tubercle
lesser tubercle
intertubercular groove
shoulder joint
scapula

of humerus

humerus

manubrium

sternum

sternoclavicular joint

trochlea
lateral epicondyle
capitulum
coronoid fossa
medial epicondyle

radius

humeroulnar joint
proximal radioulnar joint
humeroradial joint

elbow joint

ulna

radiocarpal joint
carpometacarpal joint of thumb

distal radioulnar joint
carpal bones

distal
phalanx
proximal phalanx

carpometacarpal joints

middle
phalanx

metacarpal bones

metacarpo-
phalangeal joints

proximal phalanx

proximal interphalangeal joints

distal phalanx

A15

Imagery © adam.com

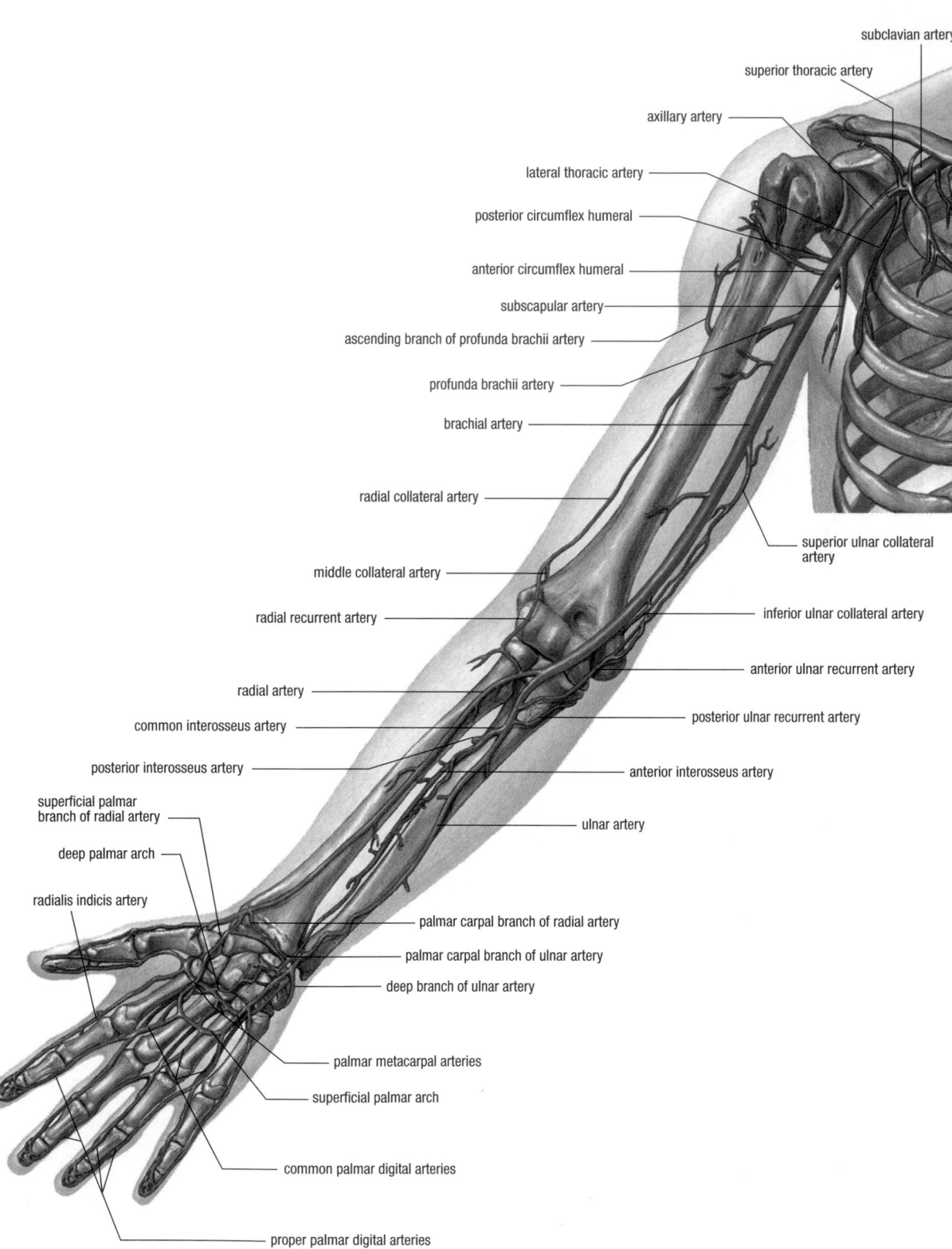

subclavian artery

superior thoracic artery

axillary artery

lateral thoracic artery

posterior circumflex humeral

anterior circumflex humeral

subscapular artery

ascending branch of profunda brachii artery

profunda brachii artery

brachial artery

radial collateral artery

superior ulnar collateral artery

middle collateral artery

radial recurrent artery

inferior ulnar collateral artery

anterior ulnar recurrent artery

radial artery

common interosseus artery

posterior ulnar recurrent artery

posterior interosseus artery

anterior interosseus artery

superficial palmar branch of radial artery

ulnar artery

deep palmar arch

radialis indicis artery

palmar carpal branch of radial artery

palmar carpal branch of ulnar artery

deep branch of ulnar artery

palmar metacarpal arteries

superficial palmar arch

common palmar digital arteries

proper palmar digital arteries

Anatomy

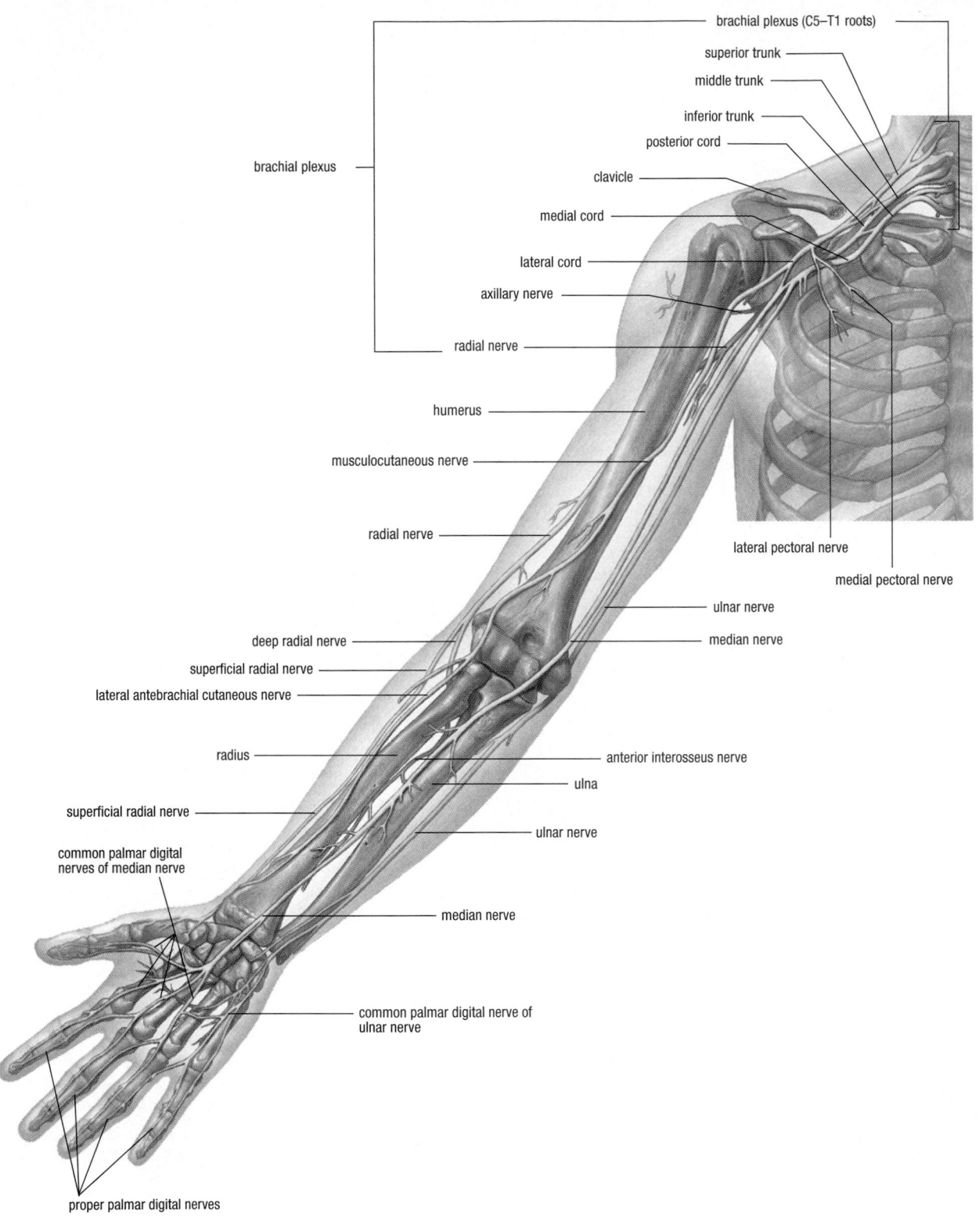

brachial plexus (C5–T1 roots)

superior trunk

middle trunk

inferior trunk

posterior cord

clavicle

medial cord

lateral cord

axillary nerve

radial nerve

brachial plexus

humerus

musculocutaneous nerve

radial nerve

lateral pectoral nerve

medial pectoral nerve

ulnar nerve

deep radial nerve

median nerve

superficial radial nerve

lateral antebrachial cutaneous nerve

radius

anterior interosseus nerve

ulna

superficial radial nerve

ulnar nerve

common palmar digital
nerves of median nerve

median nerve

common palmar digital nerve of
ulnar nerve

proper palmar digital nerves

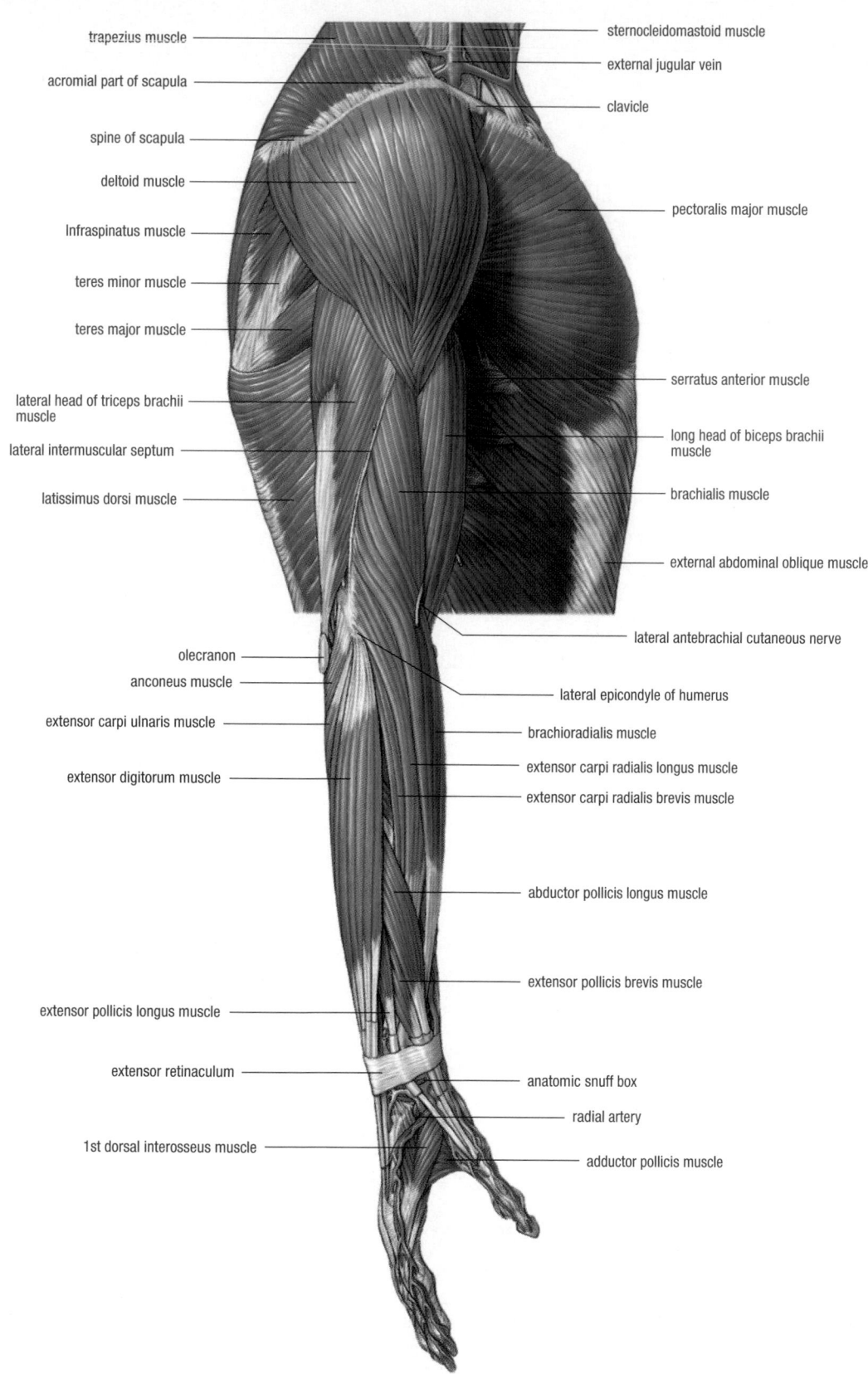

trapezius muscle

acromial part of scapula

spine of scapula

deltoid muscle

Infraspinatus muscle

teres minor muscle

teres major muscle

lateral head of triceps brachii muscle

lateral intermuscular septum

latissimus dorsi muscle

olecranon

anconeus muscle

extensor carpi ulnaris muscle

extensor digitorum muscle

extensor pollicis longus muscle

extensor retinaculum

1st dorsal interosseus muscle

sternocleidomastoid muscle

external jugular vein

clavicle

pectoralis major muscle

serratus anterior muscle

long head of biceps brachii muscle

brachialis muscle

external abdominal oblique muscle

lateral antebrachial cutaneous nerve

lateral epicondyle of humerus

brachioradialis muscle

extensor carpi radialis longus muscle

extensor carpi radialis brevis muscle

abductor pollicis longus muscle

extensor pollicis brevis muscle

anatomic snuff box

radial artery

adductor pollicis muscle

Anatomy

A18

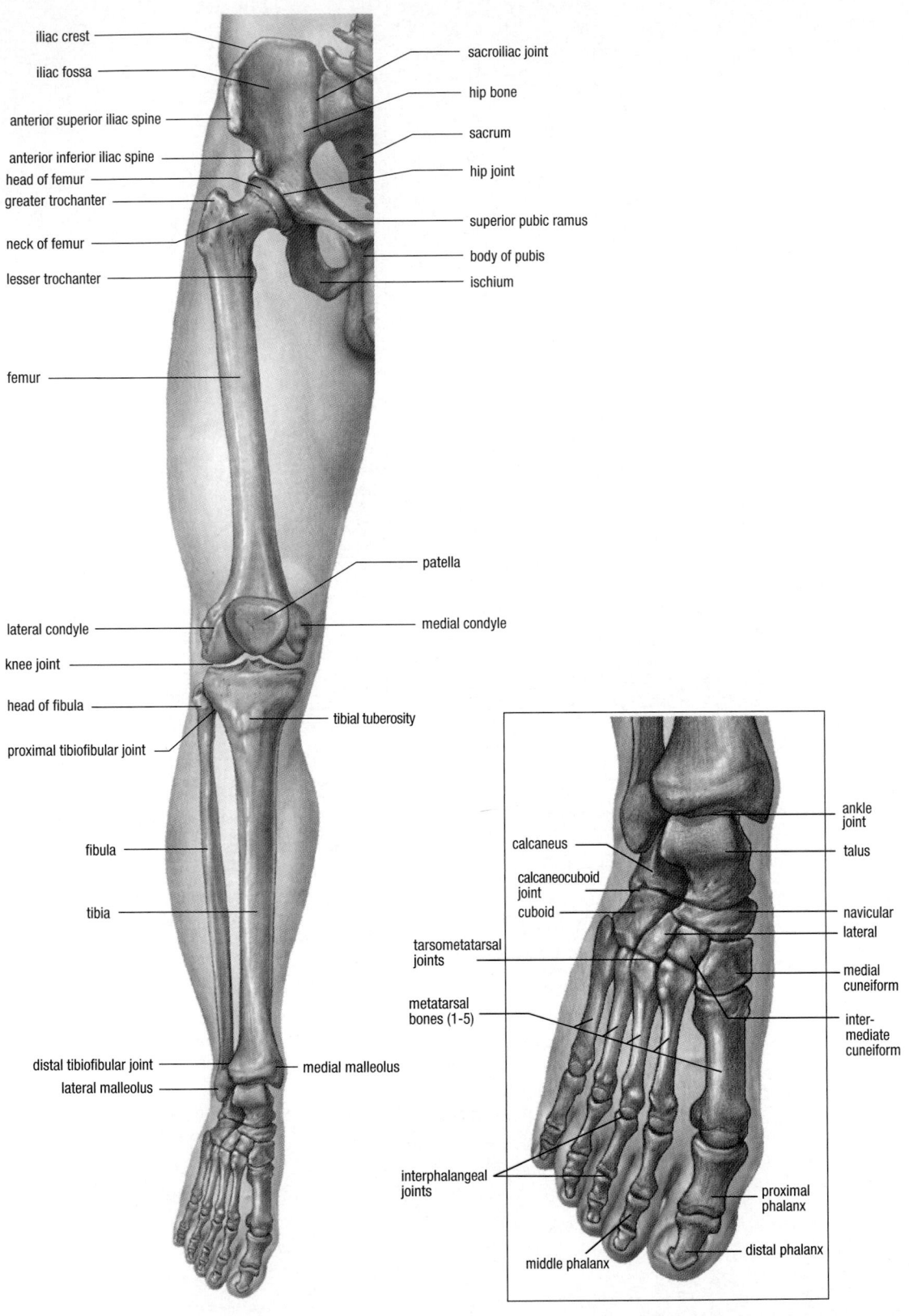

iliac crest

iliac fossa

anterior superior iliac spine

anterior inferior iliac spine

head of femur

greater trochanter

neck of femur

lesser trochanter

femur

lateral condyle

knee joint

head of fibula

proximal tibiofibular joint

fibula

tibia

distal tibiofibular joint

lateral malleolus

sacroiliac joint

hip bone

sacrum

hip joint

superior pubic ramus

body of pubis

ischium

patella

medial condyle

tibial tuberosity

medial malleolus

calcaneus

calcaneocuboid joint

cuboid

tarsometatarsal joints

metatarsal bones (1-5)

interphalangeal joints

middle phalanx

ankle joint

talus

navicular

lateral

medial cuneiform

inter- mediate cuneiform

proximal phalanx

distal phalanx

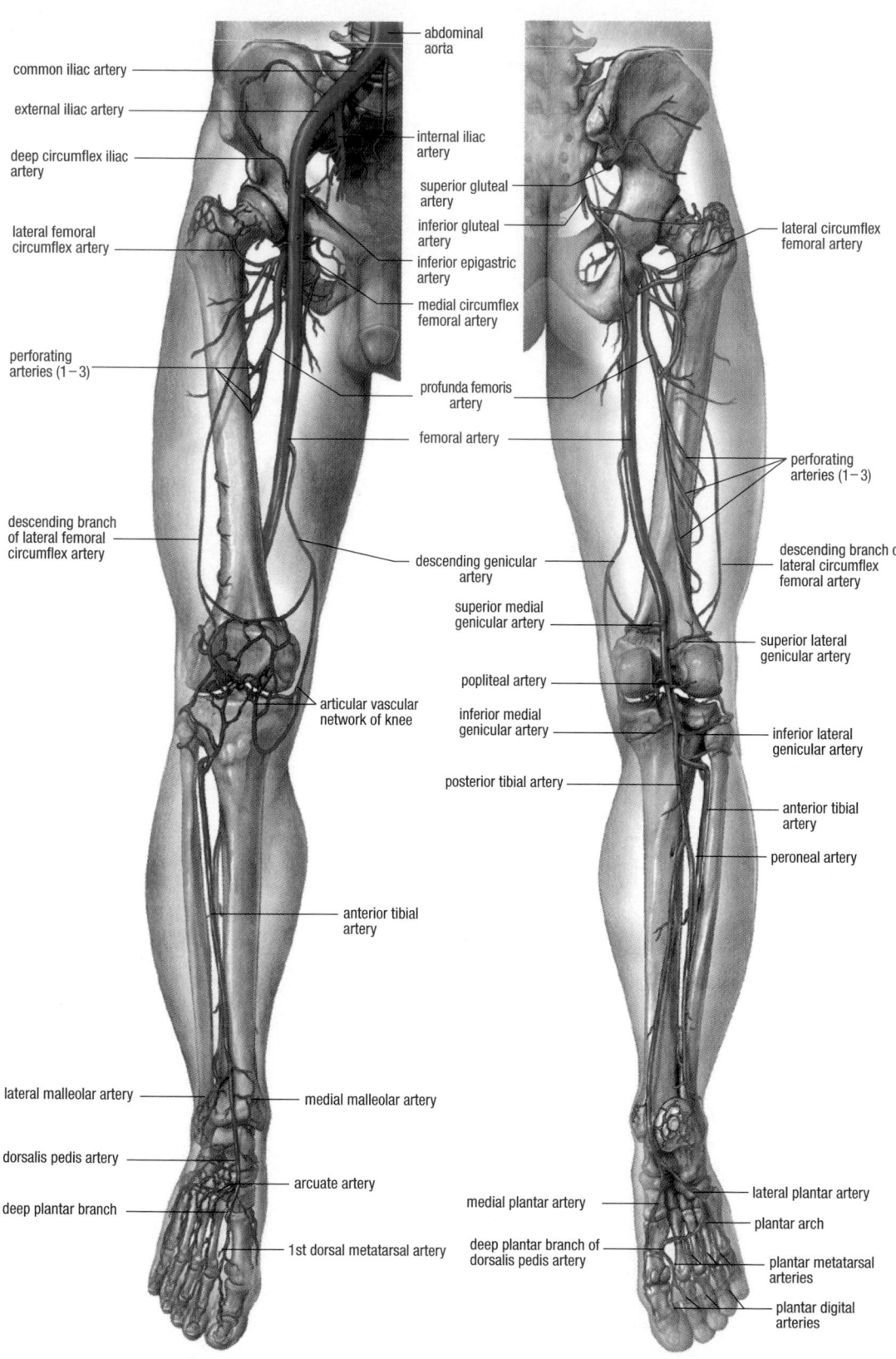

abdominal aorta

common iliac artery

external iliac artery

deep circumflex iliac artery

internal iliac artery

superior gluteal artery

inferior gluteal artery

lateral femoral circumflex artery

lateral circumflex femoral artery

inferior epigastric artery

medial circumflex femoral artery

perforating arteries (1−3)

profunda femoris artery

femoral artery

perforating arteries (1−3)

descending branch of lateral femoral circumflex artery

descending genicular artery

descending branch of lateral circumflex femoral artery

superior medial genicular artery

superior lateral genicular artery

popliteal artery

articular vascular network of knee

inferior medial genicular artery

inferior lateral genicular artery

posterior tibial artery

anterior tibial artery

peroneal artery

anterior tibial artery

lateral malleolar artery

medial malleolar artery

dorsalis pedis artery

arcuate artery

medial plantar artery

lateral plantar artery

plantar arch

deep plantar branch

1st dorsal metatarsal artery

deep plantar branch of dorsalis pedis artery

plantar metatarsal arteries

plantar digital arteries

Anatomy

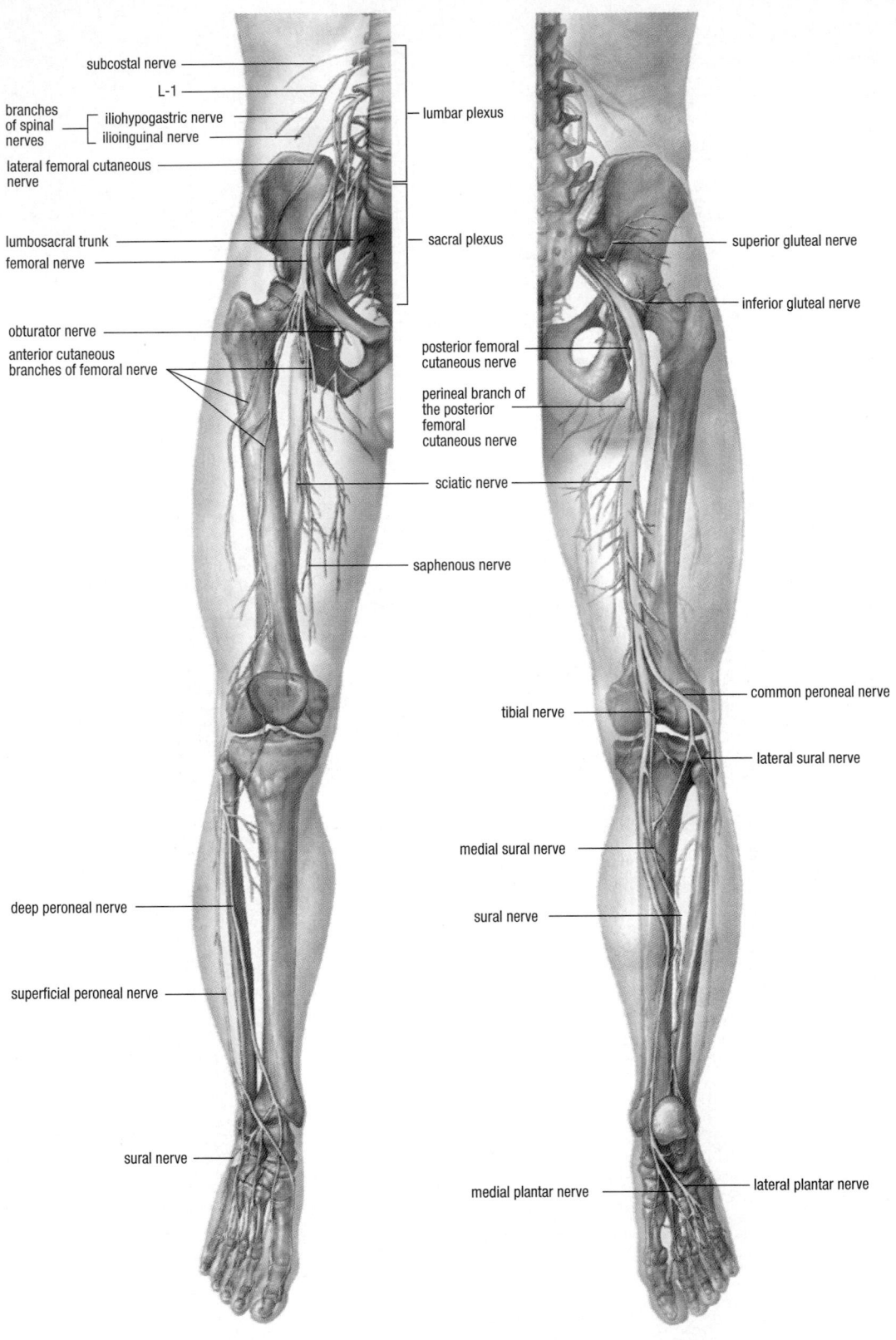

subcostal nerve

L-1

branches of spinal nerves

iliohypogastric nerve

ilioinguinal nerve

lateral femoral cutaneous nerve

lumbar plexus

sacral plexus

lumbosacral trunk

femoral nerve

obturator nerve

anterior cutaneous branches of femoral nerve

superior gluteal nerve

inferior gluteal nerve

posterior femoral cutaneous nerve

perineal branch of the posterior femoral cutaneous nerve

sciatic nerve

saphenous nerve

common peroneal nerve

tibial nerve

lateral sural nerve

medial sural nerve

sural nerve

deep peroneal nerve

superficial peroneal nerve

sural nerve

medial plantar nerve

lateral plantar nerve

A21

Imagery © adam.com

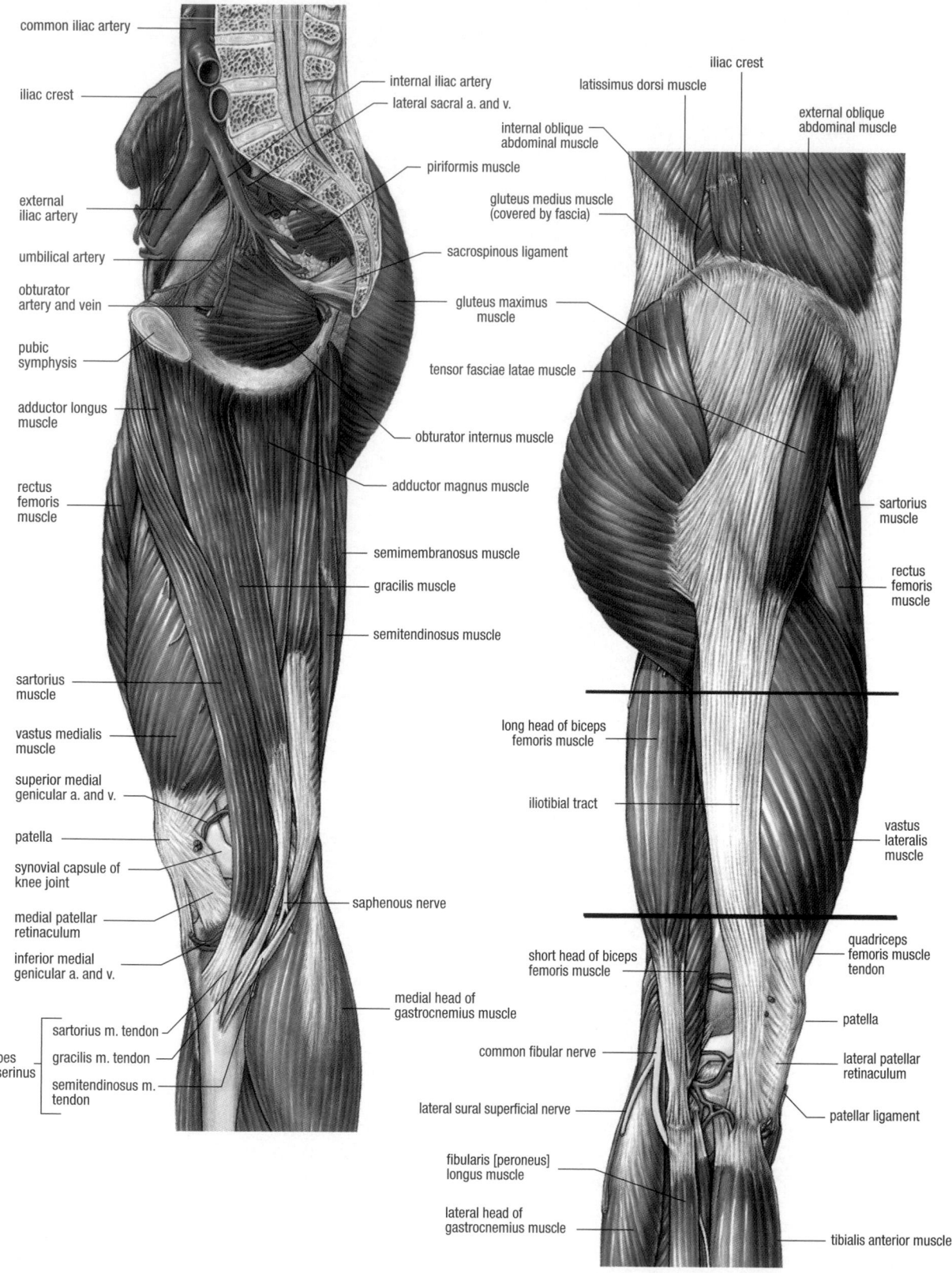

common iliac artery

iliac crest

external
iliac artery

umbilical artery

obturator
artery and vein

pubic
symphysis

adductor longus
muscle

rectus
femoris
muscle

sartorius
muscle

vastus medialis
muscle

superior medial
genicular a. and v.

patella

synovial capsule of
knee joint

medial patellar
retinaculum

inferior medial
genicular a. and v.

pes
anserinus

sartorius m. tendon

gracilis m. tendon

semitendinosus m.
tendon

internal iliac artery

lateral sacral a. and v.

piriformis muscle

sacrospinous ligament

gluteus maximus
muscle

obturator internus muscle

adductor magnus muscle

semimembranosus muscle

gracilis muscle

semitendinosus muscle

saphenous nerve

medial head of
gastrocnemius muscle

iliac crest

latissimus dorsi muscle

internal oblique
abdominal muscle

gluteus medius muscle
(covered by fascia)

tensor fasciae latae muscle

long head of biceps
femoris muscle

iliotibial tract

short head of biceps
femoris muscle

common fibular nerve

lateral sural superficial nerve

fibularis [peroneus]
longus muscle

lateral head of
gastrocnemius muscle

external oblique
abdominal muscle

sartorius
muscle

rectus
femoris
muscle

vastus
lateralis
muscle

quadriceps
femoris muscle
tendon

patella

lateral patellar
retinaculum

patellar ligament

tibialis anterior muscle

Anatomy

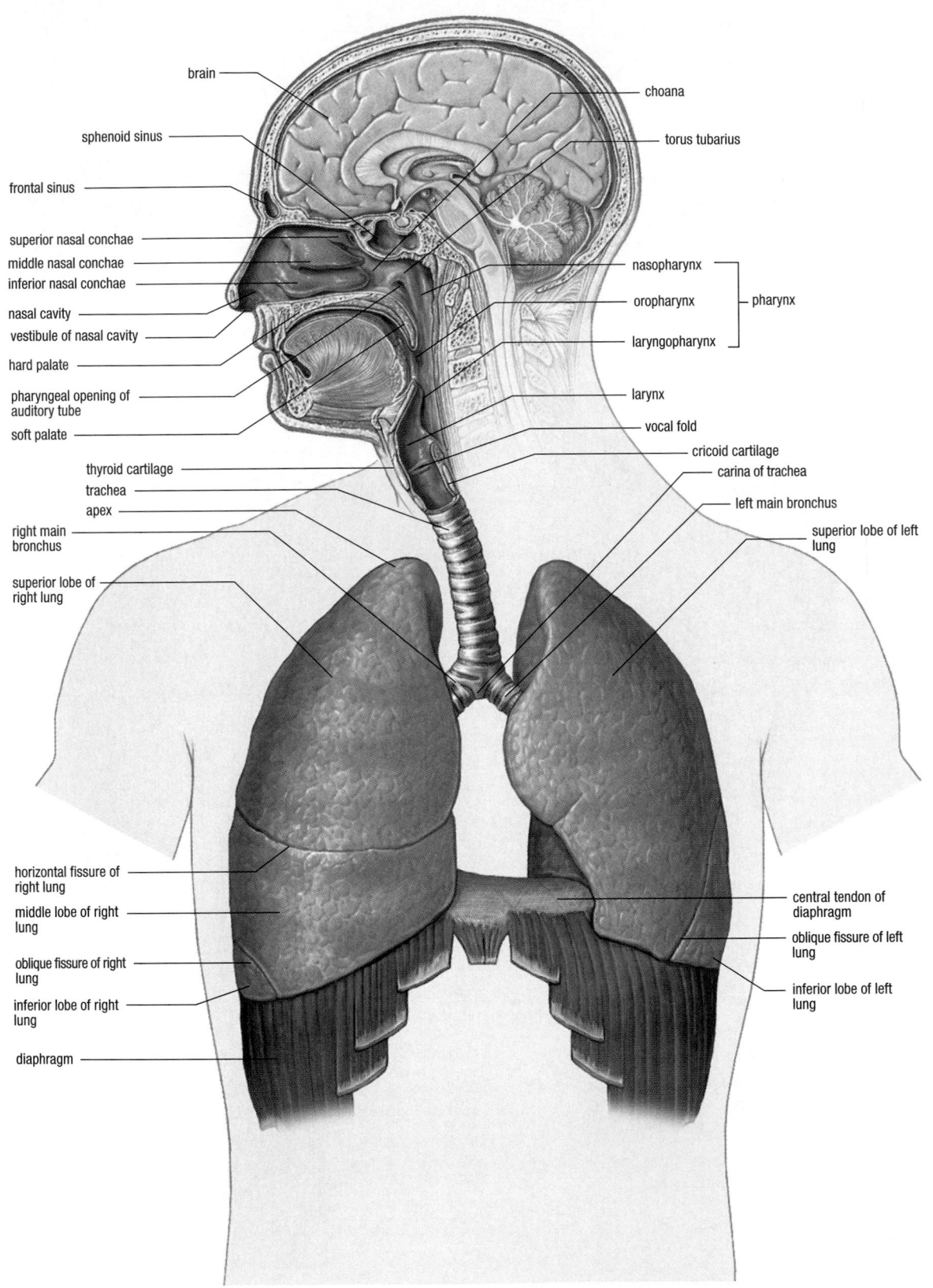

brain

choana

sphenoid sinus

torus tubarius

frontal sinus

superior nasal conchae

middle nasal conchae

inferior nasal conchae

nasopharynx

oropharynx

pharynx

nasal cavity

laryngopharynx

vestibule of nasal cavity

hard palate

larynx

pharyngeal opening of auditory tube

vocal fold

soft palate

cricoid cartilage

thyroid cartilage

carina of trachea

trachea

apex

left main bronchus

right main bronchus

superior lobe of left lung

superior lobe of right lung

horizontal fissure of right lung

central tendon of diaphragm

middle lobe of right lung

oblique fissure of left lung

oblique fissure of right lung

inferior lobe of left lung

inferior lobe of right lung

diaphragm

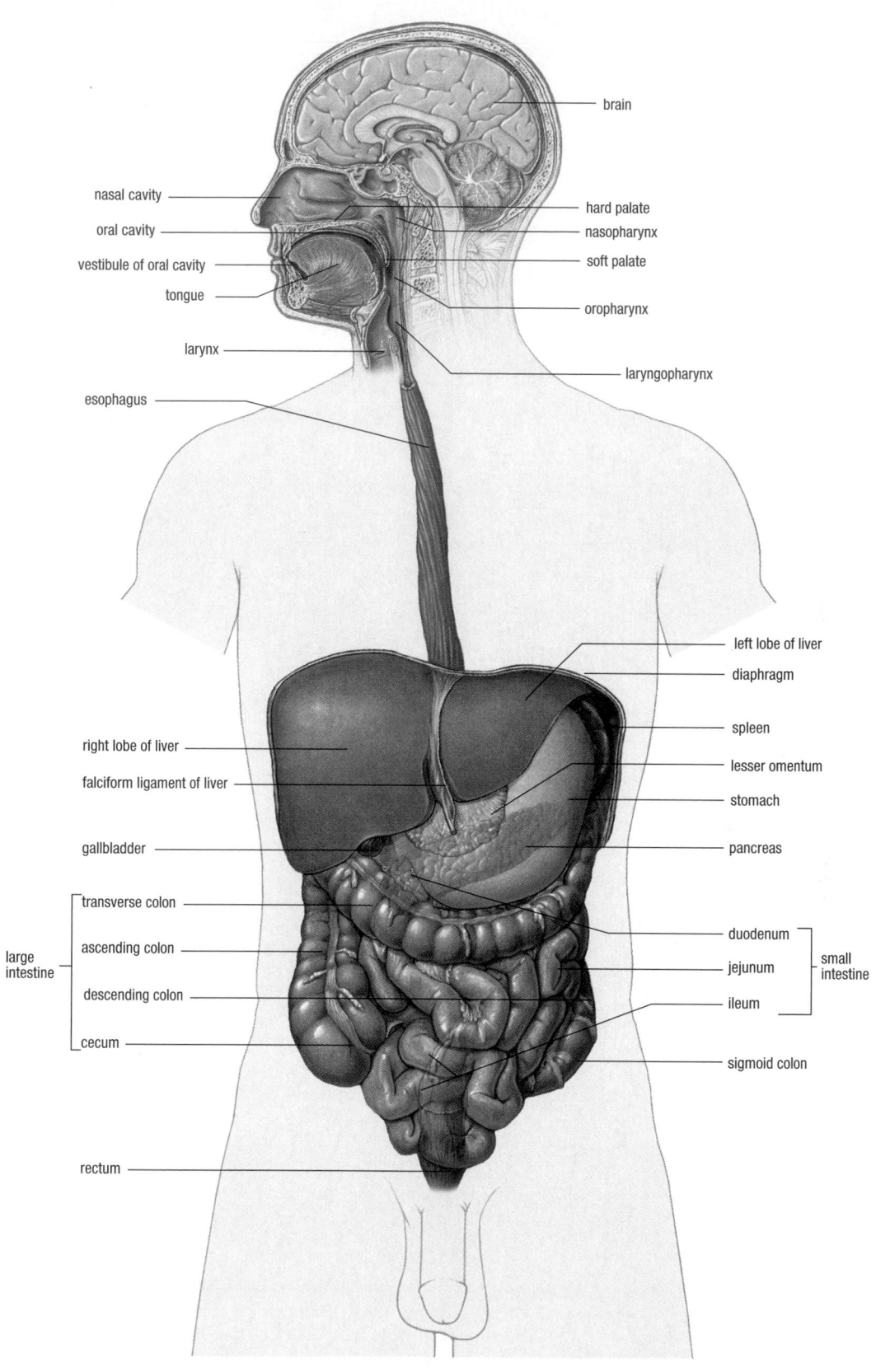

brain

nasal cavity

oral cavity

vestibule of oral cavity

tongue

larynx

esophagus

hard palate

nasopharynx

soft palate

oropharynx

laryngopharynx

left lobe of liver

diaphragm

spleen

lesser omentum

stomach

pancreas

right lobe of liver

falciform ligament of liver

gallbladder

transverse colon

ascending colon

descending colon

cecum

large
intestine

rectum

duodenum

jejunum

ileum

sigmoid colon

small
intestine

Anatomy

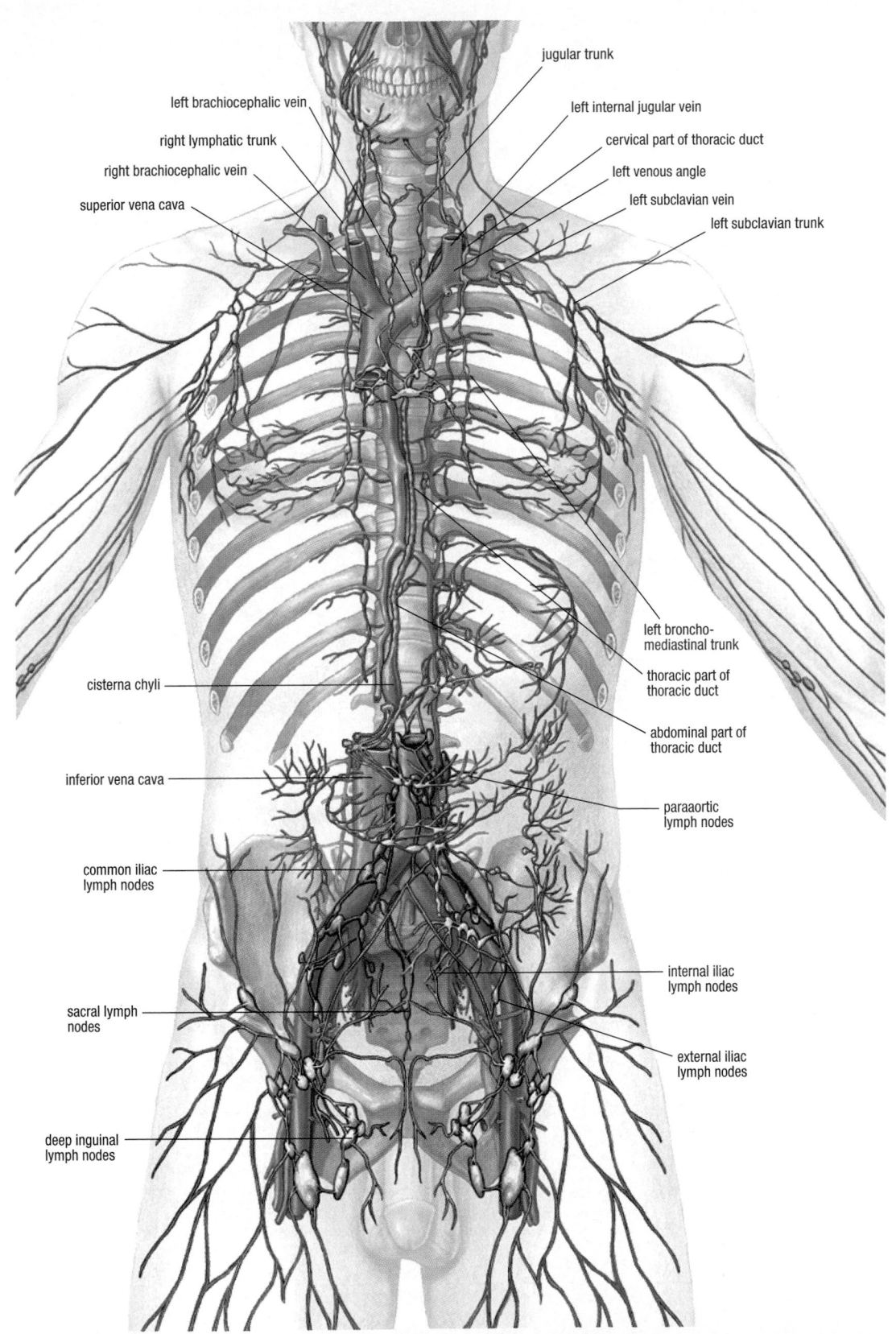

jugular trunk

left brachiocephalic vein

left internal jugular vein

right lymphatic trunk

cervical part of thoracic duct

right brachiocephalic vein

left venous angle

superior vena cava

left subclavian vein

left subclavian trunk

left broncho-mediastinal trunk

thoracic part of thoracic duct

cisterna chyli

abdominal part of thoracic duct

inferior vena cava

paraaortic lymph nodes

common iliac lymph nodes

internal iliac lymph nodes

sacral lymph nodes

external iliac lymph nodes

deep inguinal lymph nodes

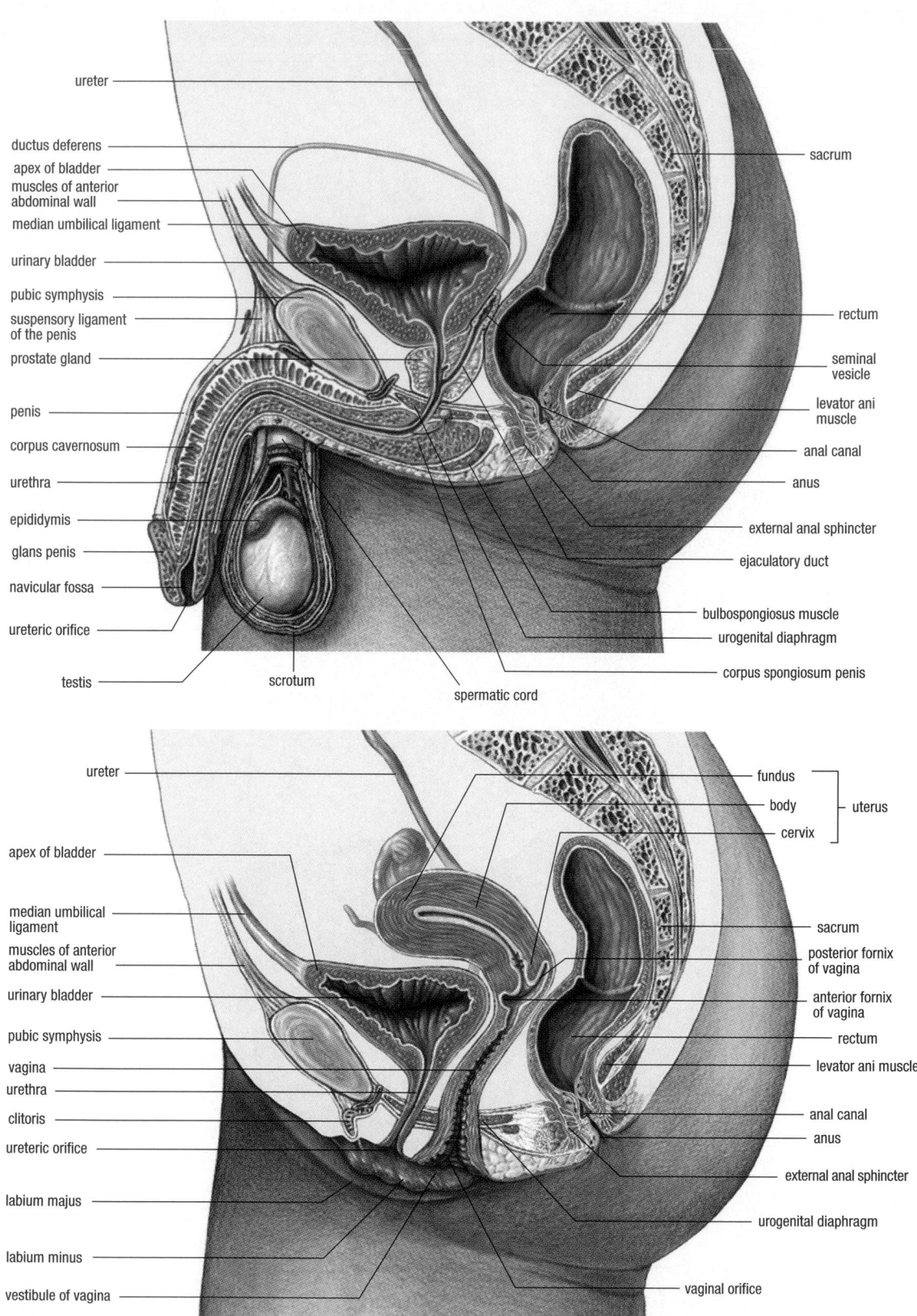

ureter

ductus deferens
apex of bladder
muscles of anterior abdominal wall
median umbilical ligament
urinary bladder
pubic symphysis
suspensory ligament of the penis
prostate gland
penis
corpus cavernosum
urethra
epididymis
glans penis
navicular fossa
ureteric orifice
testis
scrotum
spermatic cord

sacrum
rectum
seminal vesicle
levator ani muscle
anal canal
anus
external anal sphincter
ejaculatory duct
bulbospongiosus muscle
urogenital diaphragm
corpus spongiosum penis

ureter
apex of bladder
median umbilical ligament
muscles of anterior abdominal wall
urinary bladder
pubic symphysis
vagina
urethra
clitoris
ureteric orifice
labium majus
labium minus
vestibule of vagina

fundus
body
cervix
uterus
sacrum
posterior fornix of vagina
anterior fornix of vagina
rectum
levator ani muscle
anal canal
anus
external anal sphincter
urogenital diaphragm
vaginal orifice

Anatomy

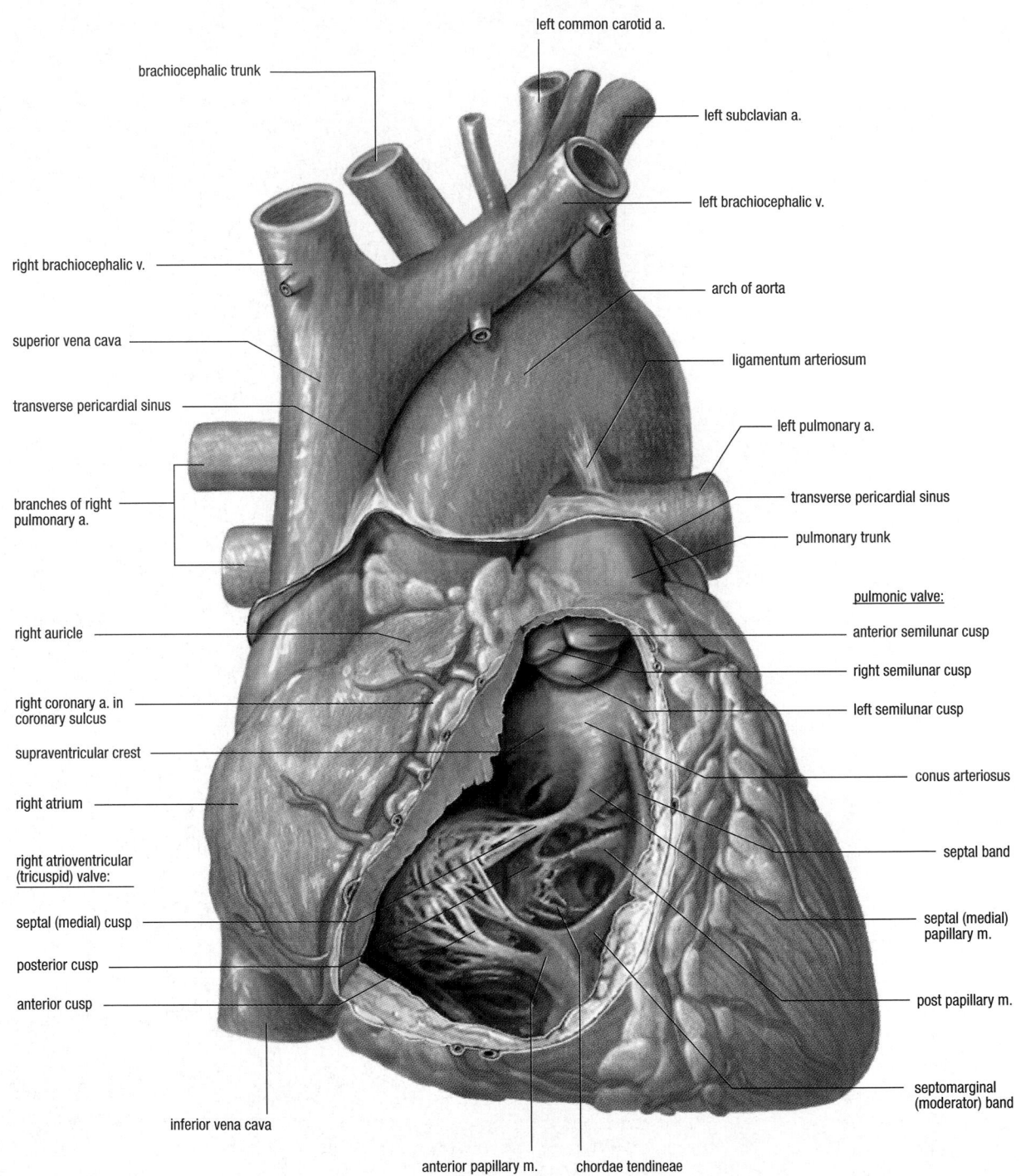

left common carotid a.

brachiocephalic trunk

left subclavian a.

left brachiocephalic v.

right brachiocephalic v.

arch of aorta

superior vena cava

ligamentum arteriosum

transverse pericardial sinus

left pulmonary a.

transverse pericardial sinus

branches of right pulmonary a.

pulmonary trunk

right auricle

pulmonic valve:

anterior semilunar cusp

right semilunar cusp

right coronary a. in coronary sulcus

left semilunar cusp

supraventricular crest

conus arteriosus

right atrium

septal band

right atrioventricular (tricuspid) valve:

septal (medial) cusp

septal (medial) papillary m.

posterior cusp

anterior cusp

post papillary m.

septomarginal (moderator) band

inferior vena cava

anterior papillary m.   chordae tendineae

the dorsal surface of the distal end of each terminal phalanx of fingers and toes. A nail consists of corpus or body, the visible part, and radix or root at the proximal end concealed under a fold of skin. The underpart of the nail is formed from the stratum germinativum of the epidermis, the free surface from the stratum lucidum, the thin cuticular fold overlapping the lunula representing the stratum corneum. SYN unguis [TA], nail plate, onyx. **2.** A slender rod of metal, bone, or other solid substance, used in operations to fasten together the fragments of a broken bone. [A.S. *naegel*]

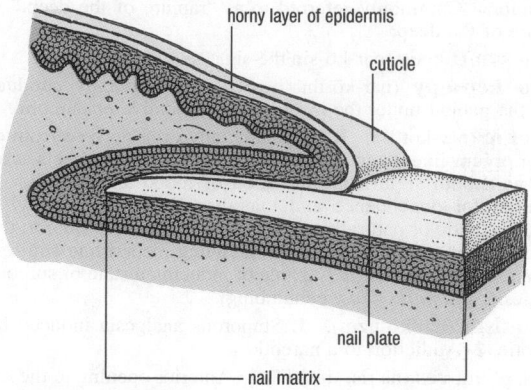

horny layer of epidermis

cuticle

nail plate

nail matrix

structure of the nail (unguis)

egg shell n., SYN hapalonychia.

half and half n., division of the n. by a transverse line into a proximal dull white part and a distal pink or brown part; seen in uremia.

Hippocratic n.'s, the coarse, curved n.'s capping clubbed digits.

ingrown n., a toenail, one edge of which is overgrown by the nailfold, producing a pyogenic granuloma; due to faulty trimming of the toenails or pressure from a tight shoe. SYN ingrowing toenail, onychocryptosis, unguis aduncus, unguis incarnatus.

Küntscher n., an intramedullary n. used for internal fixation of a fracture.

parrot-beak n., a markedly curved fingernail.

pincer n., transverse overcurvature of the n. that increases distally, causing the lateral borders of the n. to pinch the soft tissue with resulting tenderness; may result from a developmental anomaly or subungual exostosis.

racket n., a broad flat thumbnail resulting from a congenital shorter and wider distal phalanx of the thumb.

reedy n., a n. marked by longitudinal ridges and furrows.

shell n., nail dystrophy accompanying clubbing of digits in bronchiectasis, with excessive longitudinal curvature of the nail plate and atrophy of the nail bed and underlying bone.

Smith-Petersen n., a triflanged n. for internal fixation of a fracture of the neck of the femur.

spoon n., SYN koilonychia.

yellow n., the complete or almost complete cessation of all n. growth, with thickening of the n.'s, increase in the convexity, loss of cuticles, and yellowing; the resulting onycholysis can cause loss of some of the n.'s; the condition is often associated with pulmonary disease but differs from clubbing in that the soft tissues are not hypertrophic. Lymphatic drainage may be reduced, even in the absence of lymphedema. SYN yellow nail syndrome.

nail·ing (nāl'ing). Act of inserting or driving a nail into the ends of a fractured bone.

Najjar, Victor A., U.S. physician and biochemist, *1914. SEE Crigler-N. *syndrome*.

Nakanishi, Kazuhiro, Japanese physician, *1945. SEE N. *stain*.

nal·bu·phine hy·dro·chlo·ride (nal-bū'fēn). A synthetic opioid analgesic chemically related to oxymorphone, a narcotic, and to naloxone, a narcotic antagonist, with both agonist and antagonist narcotic properties.

na·li·dix·ic ac·id (nal-i-dik'sik). An orally effective antibacterial agent used in the treatment of genitourinary tract infections.

nal·or·phine (nal-ōr'fēn). An early antagonist of most of the depressant and stimulatory effects of morphine and related narcotic analgesics; precipitates severe withdrawal symptoms in morphine addicts; is used in the diagnosis of suspected morphine addiction, and counteracts the respiratory depression produced by morphine and related compounds; when administered in the absence of narcotics, n. has mild analgesic and respiratory depressant effects in nonaddicts; superseded by naloxone. SYN *N*-allyl-normorphine.

nal·ox·one hy·dro·chlo·ride (nal-ok'sōn). A potent antagonist of endorphins and narcotics, including pentazocine; devoid of pharmacologic action when administered without narcotics.

nal·trex·one (nal-treks'ōn). An orally active narcotic antagonist; devoid of pharmacologic action when administered in the absence of narcotics.

NAME Acronym for *n*evi, *a*trial myxoma, *m*yxoid neurofibromas, and *e*philides. SEE NAME *syndrome*.

NANDA. Acronym for North American Nursing Diagnosis Association.

nan·dro·lone (nan'drō-lōn). A semisynthetic, parenterally administered, anabolic, androgenic steroid.

  n. decanoate, an anabolic androgen.

  n. phenpropionate, a moderately long-acting synthetic anabolic androgen. SYN n. phenylpropionate.

  n. phenylpropionate, SYN n. phenpropionate.

nan·ism (nan'izm). Obsolete term for dwarfism. [G. *nanos;* L. *nanus,* dwarf]

  mulibrey n. (mŭ'li-brā), autosomal recessive disorder with defects of liver, brain, muscle, and eyes. [from *mu*scle, *li*ver, *br*ain, and *eyes*]

  renal n., infantile renal osteodystrophy.

  symptomatic n., dwarfism with defects in bone, dentition, and sexual development.

Nan·niz·zia (nă-niz'ē-ă). A genus of ascomycetous fungi composed of *Microsporum* species in their perfect state.

nano-. **1.** Combining form relating to dwarfism (nanism). **2 (n).** Prefix used in the SI and metric systems to signify submultiples of one-billionth (10^{-9}). [G. *nanos,* dwarf]

nan·o·ce·pha·lia (nan'ō-se-fā'lē-ă). SYN microcephaly.

nan·o·ceph·a·lous, nan·o·ce·phal·ic (nan-ō-sef'ă-lŭs, -se-fal'ik). SYN microcephalic.

nan·o·ceph·a·ly (nan-ō-sef'ă-lē). SYN microcephaly. [nano- + G. *kephalē,* head]

nan·o·cor·mia (nan-ō-kōr'mē-ă). SYN microsomia. [nano- + G. *kormos,* trunk]

nan·o·gram (ng) (nan'ō-gram). One-billionth of a gram (10^{-9} g).

nan·o·ka·tal (nkat) (nan-ō-ka-tăl'). One-billionth of a katal (10^{-9} kat).

nan·o·me·lia (nan-ō-mē'lē-ă). SYN micromelia. [nano- + G. *melos,* limb]

nan·o·me·ter (nm) (năn-om'ĕ-ter). One-billionth of a meter (10^{-9} m).

nan·oph·thal·mia, nan·oph·thal·mos (nan-of-thal'mē-ă, -mos). SYN microphthalmos. [nano- + G. *ophthalmos,* eye]

Na·no·phy·e·tus sal·min·co·la (na-nō'fī-ĕ-tŭs sal-min'kō-lă). A digenetic fish-borne fluke (family Nanophyetidae) of dogs and other fish-eating mammals; the vector of *Neorickettsia helmintheca,* the agent of salmon poisoning. SYN *Troglotrema salmincola.*

Nanta. SEE Gandy-Nanta *disease.*

na·nu·ka·ya·mi (nă-noo-kă-yah'mē). SYN nanukayami *fever.*

nape (nāp). SYN nucha.

na·pex (nā'peks). The area of the scalp just below the occipital protuberance.

naph·az·o·line hy·dro·chlo·ride (nă-faz'ō-lēn, naf-az'-). A sympathomimetic amine, used as a topical vasoconstrictor; available as n. h. nitrate, with the same uses. SYN naphthazoline hydrochloride.

naph·tha (naf′thă). SYN *petroleum* benzin. [G.]

  coal tar n., SYN benzene.

  wood n., SYN methyl *alcohol*.

naph·tha·lene (naf′thă-lēn). A carcinogenic and toxic hydrocarbon obtained from coal tar; used for many syntheses in industry and in some moth repellents; n. can cause an attack of hemolytic anemia in individuals with a deficiency of glucose-6-phosphate dehydrogenase. SYN naphthalin, tar camphor.

naph·thal·e·nol (naf-thal′ĕ-nol). SYN naphthol.

naph·tha·lin (naf′thă-lin). SYN naphthalene.

naph·thaz·o·line hy·dro·chlo·ride (naf-thaz′ŏ-lēn). SYN naphazoline hydrochloride.

naph·thol (naf′thol). A phenol of naphthalene, occurring in two forms: α-naphthol, a dye intermediate used in cytochemistry for L-arginine localization; β-naphthol, also known as isonaphthol, used as an anthelmintic and antiseptic. Both forms are also used in the manufacture of dyes, organic chemicals, and rubber products. SYN naphthalenol.

naph·tho·late (naf′thō-lāt). A compound of naphthol in which the hydrogen in the hydroxyl radical is substituted by a base.

naph·thol yel·low S [C.I. 10316]. An acid dye used as a stain for basic proteins in microspectrophotometry.

naph·tho·qui·none (naf-thō-kwin′ōn). **1.** A quinone derivative of naphthalene, reducible to naphthohydroquinone; 1,4-naphthoquinone derivatives have vitamin K activity (e.g., menaquinone). **2.** A class of compounds containing the n. (1) structure.

naph·thyl (naf′thil). The radical of naphthalene, $C_{10}H_7-$.

α-naph·thyl·thi·o·u·rea (ANTU) (naf′thil-thī′ō-ū-rē′ă). A derivative of thiourea; a highly toxic antithyroid agent, especially to small mammals, causing pulmonary edema, fatty degeneration of the liver, and low body temperature; used as a rat poison.

na·pi·er (nā′pē-er). SYN neper. [John *Napier,* Scottish mathematician, 1550–1617]

na·prox·en (nă-prok′sen). A nonsteroidal anti-inflammatory analgesic agent used in the treatment of rheumatoid conditions.

nap·syl·ate (nap′si-lāt). USAN-approved contraction for 2-naphthalenesulfonate.

nar·ce·ine (nar′sē-ēn). An alkaloid of opium; $C_{23}H_{27}NO_8$. Ethylnarceine is a narcotic, analgesic, and antitussive.

nar·cis·sism (nar-sis′izm, nar′si-sizm). **1.** A state in which one interprets and regards everything in relation to oneself and not to other persons or things. **2.** Self-love, which may include sexual attraction toward onself. SEE ALSO autoeroticism. SYN self-love. [*Narkissos,* G. myth. char.]

  primary n., in psychoanalysis, the original psychic energy embodied or invested in the ego.

  secondary n., in psychoanalysis, the psychic energy once attached to external objects, but now withdrawn from those objects and reinvested in the ego.

⌂narco-. Stupor, narcosis. [G. *narkoō,* to benumb, deaden]

nar·co·a·nal·y·sis (nar′kō-ă-nal′i-sis). Psychotherapeutic treatment under light anesthesia, originally used in acute combat cases during World War II; also has been used in the treatment of childhood trauma. SEE ALSO narcotherapy. SYN narcosynthesis.

nar·co·hyp·nia (nar-kō-hip′nē-ă). A general numbness sometimes experienced at the moment of waking. [narco- + G. *hypnos,* sleep]

nar·co·hyp·no·sis (nar′kō-hip-nō′sis). Stupor or deep sleep induced by hypnosis. [narco- + G. *hypnos,* sleep]

nar·co·lep·sy (nar′kō-lep-sē). A sleep disorder that usually appears in young adulthood, consisting of recurring episodes of sleep during the day and often disrupted nocturnal sleep; frequently accompanied by cataplexy, sleep paralysis, and hypnagogic hallucinations; a genetically determined disease. SYN Gélineau syndrome, paroxysmal sleep. [narco- + G. *lēpsis,* seizure]

nar·co·lep·tic (nar′kō-lep′-tik). **1.** A sleep-inducing drug. **2.** A person with narcolepsy.

nar·co·sis (nar-kō′sis). General and nonspecific reversible depression of neuronal excitability, produced by a number of physical and chemical agents, usually resulting in stupor rather than in

anesthesia (with which n. was once synonymous). [G. a benumbing]

CO_2 n., SYN hypoventilation *coma*.

intravenous n., administration of opiate medication intravenously.

nitrogen n., (1) n. produced by nitrogenous materials such as occurs in certain forms of uremia and hepatic coma; **(2)** the stuporous condition characterized by disorientation and by loss of judgment and skill, attributed to an increased partial pressure of nitrogen in the inspired air of deep-sea divers during underwater operations. Commonly referred to as "rapture of the deep." SYN rapture of the deep.

nar·co·syn·the·sis (nar-kō-sin′thĕ-sis). SYN narcoanalysis.

nar·co·ther·a·py (nar-kō-thār′ă-pē). Psychotherapy conducted with the patient under the influence of a sedative or narcotic.

nar·cot·ic (nar-kot′ik). **1.** Originally, any drug derived from opium or opium-like compounds with potent analgesic effects associated with both significant alteration of mood and behavior and potential for dependence and tolerance. **2.** More recently, any drug, synthetic or naturally occurring, with effects similar to those of opium and opium derivatives, including meperidine and fentanyl and its derivatives. **3.** Capable of inducing a state of stuporous analgesia. [G. *narkōtikos,* benumbing]

nar·co·tism (nar′kō-tizm). **1.** Stuporous analgesia induced by a narcotic. **2.** Addiction to a narcotic.

na·ris, pl. **na·res** (nā′ris, -res) [TA]. Anterior opening to the nasal cavity. SYN anterior n., external n., nostril, prenaris. [L.]

  anterior n., SYN naris.

  external n., SYN naris.

  internal n., obsolete term for choanae.

  posterior nares, SYN choanae.

NARP. Acronym for *n*europathy, *a*taxia, *r*etinitis *p*igmentosa syndrome, one of the inherited mitochondrial disorders, caused by a point mutation resulting in the substitution of a single amino acid in the mitochondrial DNA at position 8993. A more severe expression of the same point mutation manifests clinically as Leigh disease (q.v.).

nar·row·band. A limited band of sound frequencies, as opposed to the wideband of frequencies also known as white noise; used to mask hearing in the nontest ear in hearing measurement.

na·sal (nā′zăl). Relating to the nose. SYN rhinal. [L. *nasus,* nose]

nas·cent (nas′ent, nā′sent). **1.** Beginning; being born or produced. **2.** Denoting the state of a chemical element at the moment it is set free from one of its compounds. [L. *nascor,* pres. p. *nascens,* to be born]

na·si·o·in·i·ac (nā′zē-ō-in′ē-ak). Relating to the nasion and inion; denoting the distance in a straight line between the frontonasal suture and the external occipital protuberance.

na·si·on (nā′zē-on) [TA]. A point on the skull corresponding to the middle of the nasofrontal suture. SYN nasal point. [L. *nasus,* nose]

Nasmyth, Alexander, London dentist, 1789–1849. SEE N. *cuticle, membrane.*

⌂naso-. The nose. [L. *nasus*]

na·so·an·tral (nā′zō-an′trăl). Relating to the nose and the maxillary sinus.

na·so·cil·i·ary. Relating to nose and eyelids. SEE nasociliary *nerve.*

na·so·fron·tal (nā-zō-frŭn′tăl). Relating to the nose and forehead, or to the nasal cavity and frontal sinuses.

na·so·gas·tric (nā-zō-gas′trik). Pertaining to or involving both the nasal passages and the stomach, as in n. intubation.

na·so·la·bi·al (nā-zō-lā′bē-ăl). Relating to the nose and upper lip. [naso- + L. *labium,* lip]

na·so·lac·ri·mal (nā-zō-lak′ri-măl). Relating to the nasal and the lacrimal bones, or to the nasal cavity and the lacrimal ducts.

na·so-oral (nā-zō-ō′răl). Relating to the nose and mouth.

na·so·pal·a·tine (nā′zō-pal′ă-tēn, -tin). Relating to the nose and the palate.

na·so·pha·ryn·ge·al (nā′zō-fă-rin′jē-ăl). Relating to the nose or nasal cavity and the pharynx. SYN rhinopharyngeal (1).

na·so·pha·ryn·go·la·ryn·go·scope (nā′zō-fa-ring′gō-lā-ring′gō-skōp). An instrument, often of fiberoptic type, used to visualize the upper airways and pharynx.

na·so·pha·ryn·go·scope (nā′zō-fa-ring′gō-skōp). Telescopic instrument, electrically lighted, for examination of the nasal passages and the nasopharynx.

na·so·pha·ryn·gos·co·py (nā′zō-fa-ring-gos′kŏ-pē). Examination of the nasopharynx by flexible or rigid optical instruments, or with a mirror. [nasopharynx + G. skopeō, to view]

na·so·pha·rynx (nā′zō-far′ingks) [TA]. The part of the pharynx that lies above the soft palate; anteriorly it opens into the nasal cavities via the choanae; inferiorly, it communicates with the oropharynx via the pharyngeal isthmus; laterally it communicates with tympanic cavities via pharyngotympanic (auditory) tubes. SYN pars nasalis pharyngis [TA], epipharynx, nasal part of pharynx, nasal pharynx, pharyngonasal cavity, rhinopharynx.

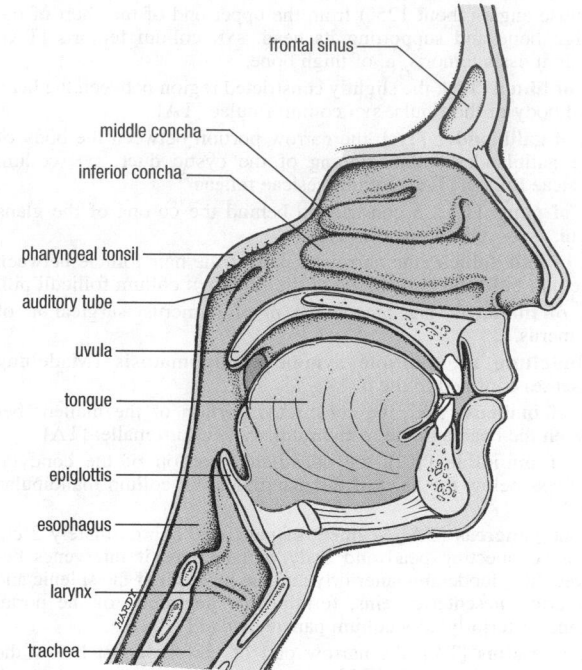

frontal sinus
middle concha
inferior concha
pharyngeal tonsil
auditory tube
uvula
tongue
epiglottis
esophagus
larynx
trachea

nasopharynx and surrounding structures

na·so·ros·tral (nā′zō-ros′trăl). Relating to the nasal cavity and the rostrum of the sphenoid bone.

na·so·si·nu·si·tis (nā′zō-sī-nŭ-sī′tis). Inflammation of the nasal cavities and of the accessory sinuses.

Nasse, Christian Friedrich, German physician, 1788–1851.

Nasse law. See under law.

na·sus (nā′sŭs). **1.** SYN external nose. **2.** SYN nose. [L.]

  n. exter′nus, SYN external nose.

na·tal (nā′tăl). **1.** Relating to birth. [L. natalis, fr. nascor, pp. natus, to be born] **2.** Relating to the buttocks or nates. [L. nates, buttocks]

na·tal·i·ty (nā-tal′i-tē). The birth rate; the ratio of births to the general population. [see natal (1)]

na·ta·my·cin (nā-tă-mī′sin). SYN pimaricin.

na·tes (nā′tēz) [TA]. SYN buttocks. [L. pl. of natis]

Na·tion·al For·mu·lary (NF). An official compendium formerly issued by the American Pharmaceutical Association but now published by the United States Pharmacopeial Convention for the purpose of providing standards and specifications which can be used to evaluate the quality of pharmaceuticals and therapeutic agents.

na·tre·mia, na·tri·e·mia (nā-trē′mē-ă, nā′trē-ē′mē-ă). The presence of sodium in the blood. [natrium, sodium, + G. haima, blood]

na·trex·one hy·dro·chlo·ride (nă-treks′on). An orally active narcotic antagonist used in maintenance therapy of detoxified, formerly opioid-dependent, patients.

na·trif·er·ic (nă-trif′er-ik). Tending to increase sodium transport. [natrium + L. fero, to carry]

na·tri·um (Na) (nā′trē-ŭm). SYN sodium. [Ar. natrūm, fr. G. nitron, carbonate of soda]

na·tri·u·re·sis (nā′trē-ū-rē′sis). Urinary excretion of sodium; commonly designates enhanced sodium excretion, which may occur in certain diseases or as a result of the administration of diuretic drugs. [natrium + G. ouron, urine]

na·tri·u·ret·ic (nā′trē-ū-ret′ik). **1.** Pertaining to or characterized by natriuresis. **2.** A substance that increases urinary excretion of sodium, usually as a result of decreased tubular reabsorption of sodium ions from glomerular filtrate.

Nattrassia mangiferae. A dematiaceous mold, previously known as *Hendersonula toruloidea*, that causes onychomycosis and phaeohyphomycosis. *Scytalidium dimidiatum* is a synanamorph. SYN *Hendersonula toruloidea*.

na·tur·o·path (nā′choor-ō-path). One who practices naturopathy.

na·tur·o·path·ic (nā′choor-ō-path′ik). Relating to or by means of naturopathy.

na·tur·op·a·thy (nā-choor-op′ă-thē). A system of therapeutics in which neither surgical nor medicinal agents are used, dependence being placed only on natural (nonmedicinal) forces.

nau·path·ia (naw-path′ē-ă). SYN seasickness. [G. naus, ship, + pathos, suffering]

nau·sea (naw′zē-ă, -zhă). An inclination to vomit. SYN sicchasia (1). [L. fr. G. nausia, seasickness, fr. naus, ship]

  epidemic n., SYN epidemic vomiting.

  n. gravida′rum, SYN morning sickness.

nau·se·ant (naw′zē-ănt). **1.** Nauseating; causing nausea. **2.** An agent that causes nausea.

nau·se·ate (naw′zē-āt). To cause an inclination to vomit.

nau·se·at·ed (naw′zē-ā-ted). Affected with nausea. SYN sick (2).

nau·seous (naw′zē-ŭs, naw′shŭs). **1.** Nauseated. **2.** Causing nausea.

Nauta, Walle J.H., U.S. neuroscientist, *1916. SEE N. stain.

na·vel (nā′vel). SYN umbilicus. [A.S. nafela]

na·vic·u·la (nă-vik′ū-lă). A small boat-shaped structure. [L. dim of navis, ship]

na·vic·u·lar (nă-vik′ū-lăr) [TA]. Flattened, medially placed tarsal bone, concave on its posterior surface to accommodate the head of the talus, and convex on its anterior surface to articulate with the three cuneiform bones. SYN os naviculare [TA], central bone of ankle, navicular (bone), os centrale tarsi. [L. navicularis, relating to shipping]

Nb Symbol for niobium.

NBT Abbreviation for nitroblue tetrazolium.

Nd Symbol for neodymium.

NDP Abbreviation for nucleoside diphosphate.

Ne Symbol for neon.

near·sight·ed·ness (nēr′sīt-ed-nes). SYN myopia.

ne·ar·thro·sis (nē-ar-thrō′sis). A new joint; e.g., a pseudarthrosis arising in an ununited fracture, or an artificial joint resulting from a total joint replacement operation. SYN neoarthrosis. [G. neos, new, + arthrōsis, a jointing]

neb·ra·my·cin (neb-ră-mī′sin). A complex of substances produced by *Streptomyces tenebrarius;* an antibacterial agent.

nebul. Abbreviation for nebula.

neb·u·la (nebul.), pl. **neb·′u·lae** (neb′ū-lă, -lē). **1.** A translucent foglike opacity of the cornea. **2.** A class of oily preparations, intended for application by atomization. SEE spray. **3.** A spray. [L. fog, cloud, mist]

ne

neb·u·la·rine (neb-ū-lār′in). A toxic nucleoside isolated from the mushroom *Agaricus nebularis* and from *Streptomyces* sp. SYN 9-β-ribofuranosylpurine, purine ribonucleoside, ribosylpurine.

neb·ul·in (neb′ū-lin). A very large protein, constituting about 3% of skeletal muscle protein; may aid in the organization of actin filaments as well as in actin polymerization. [L. *nebula*, mist, fog, fr. G. *nephelē*, + -in]

neb·u·li·za·tion (neb′ū-li-zā′shŭn). Spraying or vaporization. [L. *nebula*, mist]

neb·u·lize (neb′ū-līz). To break up a liquid into a fine spray or vapor; to vaporize. [L. *nebula*, mist]

neb·u·liz·er (neb′ū-līz-er). A device used to reduce liquid medication to extremely fine cloudlike particles; useful in delivering medication to deeper parts of the respiratory tract. SEE ALSO atomizer, vaporizer.

jet n., an atomizer that uses an air or gas stream to change a liquid into small particles.

spinning disk n., a n. in which water is changed into small particles as it is thrown by centrifugal force from a spinning disk.

ultrasonic n., a humidifier using high-frequency electricity to power a transducer that vibrates 1,350,000 times per second and changes water up into particles 0.5–3 μm in size in its nebulizing chamber; used in inhalation therapy.

⦿*Ne·ca·tor* (nē-kā′tŏr). A genus of nematode hookworms (family Ancylostomatidae, subfamily Necatorinae) distinguished by two chitinous cutting plates in the buccal cavity and fused male copulatory spicules. Species include *N. americanus*, the so-called New World hookworm (although it is also prevalent in the tropics of Africa, southern Asia, and Polynesia); the adults of this species attach to villi in the small intestine and suck blood, causing abdominal discomfort, diarrhea (usually with melena) and cramps, anorexia, loss of weight, and hypochromic microcytic anemia, which may occur in advanced disease. SEE ALSO *Ancylostoma*. [L. a murderer]

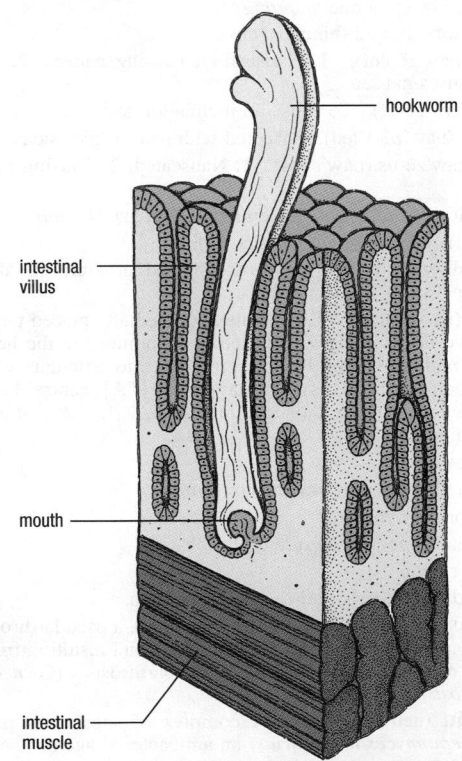

nematode: *(Necator americanus)* New World hookworm

ne·ca·to·ri·a·sis (nē-kā-tō-rī′ă-sis). Hookworm disease caused by

Necator, the resulting anemia being usually less severe than that from ancylostomiasis.

⦿neck (nek) [TA]. **1.** Part of body by which the head is connected to the trunk: it extends from the base of the cranium to the top of the shoulders. **2.** In anatomy, any constricted portion having a fancied resemblance to the n. of an animal. **3.** The germinative portion of an adult tapeworm which develops the segments or proglottids; the region of cestode segmentation behind the scolex. SYN cervix (1) [TA], collum☆. [A.S. *hnecca*]

anatomical n. of humerus [TA], a groove separating the head of the humerus from the tuberosities, giving attachment to the articular capsule. SYN collum anatomicum humeri [TA].

buffalo n., combination of moderate kyphosis with thick heavy fat pad on the n., seen especially in persons with Cushing disease or syndrome.

bull n., a heavy thick n. caused by hypertrophied muscles or enlarged cervical lymph nodes.

dental n., SYN n. of tooth.

n. of femur [TA], a short, constricted, strong bar projecting at an obtuse angle (about 125°) from the upper end of the shaft of the thigh bone and supporting its head. SYN collum femoris [TA], collum ossis femoris, n. of thigh bone.

n. of fibula [TA], the slightly constricted region between the head and body of the fibula. SYN collum fibulae [TA].

n. of gallbladder [TA], the narrow portion between the body of the gallbladder and beginning of the cystic duct. SYN collum vesicae biliaris [TA], collum vesicae felleae☆.

n. of glans [TA], a constriction behind the corona of the glans penis. SYN collum glandis [TA].

n. of hair follicle, the narrowed part of the hair follicle between the hair bulb and the surface of the skin. SYN collum folliculi pili.

n. of humerus, SEE anatomical n. of humerus, surgical n. of humerus.

Madelung n., multiple symmetric lipomatosis (Madelung disease) confined to the n.

n. of malleus [TA], the constricted portion of the malleus between the head and the manubrium. SYN collum mallei [TA].

n. of mandible [TA], the constricted portion of the condylar process below the head of the mandible. SYN collum mandibulae [TA].

n. of pancreas [TA], segment of pancreas, approximately 2 cm long, connecting head and body of pancreas; it intervenes between the duodenum anteriorly and the junction of the splenic and superior mesenteric veins, forming the beginning of the portal vein, posteriorly. SYN collum pancreaticus [TA].

n. of radius [TA], the narrow part of the shaft just below the head. SYN collum radii [TA].

n. of rib [TA], the flattened portion of a rib between the head and the tuberosity. SYN collum costae [TA].

n. of scapula [TA], a slight constriction marking the separation of that portion bearing the glenoid cavity and coracoid process from the remainder of the scapula. SYN collum scapulae [TA].

stiff n., nonspecific term for limited neck mobility, often due to muscle cramps and accompanied by pain.

surgical n. of humerus [TA], the narrow portion below the head and tuberosities. SYN collum chirurgicum humeri [TA].

n. of talus [TA], a constriction separating the head, or anterior portion, from the body of the talus. SYN collum tali [TA].

n. of thigh bone, SYN n. of femur.

n. of tooth [TA], the slightly constricted part of a tooth, between the crown and the root. SYN cervix dentis [TA], cervix of tooth☆, cervical margin of tooth, cervical zone of tooth, collum dentis, dental n.

turkey gobbler n., large skin folds hanging under the chin.

n. of (urinary) bladder [TA], the lowest part of the bladder formed by the junction of the fundus and the inferolateral surfaces. SYN cervix vesicae urinariae [TA], collum vesicae☆.

n. of uterus, SYN *cervix* of uterus.

webbed n., the broad n. due to lateral folds of skin extending from the clavicle to the head but containing no muscles, bones, or other structures; occurs in Turner syndrome and in Noonan syndrome.

n. of womb, SYN *cervix* of uterus.

wry n., SYN torticollis.

neck·lace (nek'lăs). Term used to describe a skin rash that encircles the neck.

Casal n., a dermatitis partly or completely encircling the lower part of the neck in pellagra.

△**necr-.** SEE necro-.

nec·rec·to·my (ne-krek'tō-mē). Operative removal of any necrosed tissue. [necr- + G. *ektomē,* excision]

△**necro-, necr-.** Death, necrosis. [G. *nekros,* corpse]

nec·ro·ba·cil·lo·sis (nek'rō-bas-il-ō'sis). Any disease with which the bacterium *Fusobacterium necrophorum* is associated.

nec·ro·bi·o·sis (nek'rō-bī-ō'sis). **1.** Physiologic or normal death of cells or tissues as a result of changes associated with development, aging, or use. **2.** Necrosis of a small area of tissue. [necro- + G. *biōs,* life]

n. lipoid'ica, n. lipoid'ica diabetico'rum, a condition, in many cases associated with diabetes, in which one or more yellow, atrophic, shiny lesions develop on the legs (typically pretibial); characterized histologically by indistinct areas of necrosis in the cutis.

nec·ro·bi·ot·ic (nek'rō-bī-ot'ik). Pertaining to or characterized by necrobiosis.

nec·ro·cy·to·sis (nek'rō-sī-tō'sis). A process that results in, or a condition that is characterized by, the abnormal or pathologic death of cells. [necro- + G. *kytos,* cell, + *-osis,* condition]

nec·ro·gen·ic (nek-rō-jen'ik). Relating to, living in, or having origin in dead matter. SYN necrogenous. [necro- + G. *genesis,* origin]

nec·rog·e·nous (ně-kroj'ě-nŭs). SYN necrogenic.

nec·ro·gran·u·lo·ma·tous (nek'rō-gran-ū-lō'mă-tŭs). Obsolete term for the characteristics of a granuloma with central necrosis.

ne·crol·o·gist (ně-krol'ō-jist). A student of, or a specialist in, necrology.

ne·crol·o·gy (ně-krol'ō-jē). The science of the collection, classification, and interpretation of mortality statistics. [necro- + G. *logos,* study]

ne·crol·y·sis (ně-krol'i-sis). Necrosis and loosening of tissue. [necro- + G. *lysis,* loosening]

🖾**toxic epidermal n. (TEN),** a syndrome in which a large portion of the skin becomes intensely erythematous with epidermal necrosis, and peels off in the manner of a second-degree burn, often simultaneous with the formation of flaccid bullae, resulting from drug sensitivity or of unknown cause; the level of separation is subepidermal, unlike staphylococcal scalded skin syndrome in which there is subcorneal change. SYN Lyell syndrome.

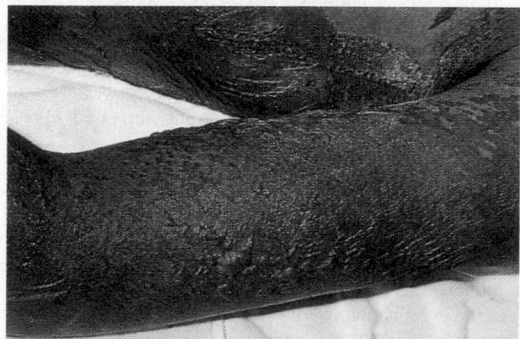

toxic epidermal necrolysis

nec·ro·ma·nia (nek-rō-mā'nē-ă). **1.** A morbid tendency to dwell with longing on death. **2.** A morbid attraction to dead bodies. [necro- + G. *mania,* frenzy]

ne·crom·e·ter (ně-krom'ě-ter). An instrument for measuring a

dead body or any of its parts or organs. [necro- + G. *metron,* measure]

nec·ro·par·a·site (nek-rō-par'ă-sīt). SYN saprophyte.

ne·crop·a·thy (ně-krop'ă-thē). A tendency to tissue death or gangrene. [necro- + G. *pathos,* disease]

ne·croph·a·gous (ně-krof'ă-gŭs). **1.** Living on carrion. **2.** SYN necrophilous. [necro- + G. *phagō,* to eat]

nec·ro·phil·ia, ne·croph·i·lism (nek-rō-fil'ē-ă, ně-krof'i-lizm). **1.** A morbid fondness for being in the presence of dead bodies. **2.** The impulse to have sexual contact, or the act of such contact, with a dead body, usually of males with female corpses. [necro- + G. *phileō,* to love]

ne·croph·i·lous (ně-krof'i-lŭs). Having a preference for dead tissue; denoting certain bacteria. SYN necrophagous (2). [necro- + G. *philos,* fond]

nec·ro·pho·bia (nek-rō-fō'bē-ă). Morbid fear of corpses. [necro- + G. *phobos,* fear]

ne·crop·sy (nek'rop-sē). SYN autopsy (1). [necro- + G. *opsis,* view]

nec·ro·sa·dism (nek-rō-sād'izm). Sexual gratification derived by mutilating corpses. [necro- + sadism]

ne·cros·co·py (ně-kros'kŏ-pē). Rarely used term for autopsy. [necro- + G. *skopeō,* to examine]

ne·crose (ně-krōz'). **1.** To cause necrosis. **2.** To become the site of necrosis.

nec·ro·sec·to·my (ně-krō'sek-tō-mē). Resection of necrotic tissue.

🖾**ne·cro·sis** (ně-krō'sis). Pathologic death of one or more cells, or of a portion of tissue or organ, resulting from irreversible damage; earliest irreversible changes are mitochondrial, consisting of swelling and granular calcium deposits seen by electron microscopy; most frequent visible alterations are nuclear: pyknosis, shrunken and abnormally dark basophilic staining; karyolysis, swollen and abnormally pale basophilic staining; or karyorrhexis, rupture and fragmentation of the nucleus. After such changes, the outlines of individual cells are indistinct, and affected cells may become merged, sometimes forming a focus of coarsely granular, amorphous, or hyaline material. [G. *nekrōsis,* death, fr. *nekroō,* to make dead]

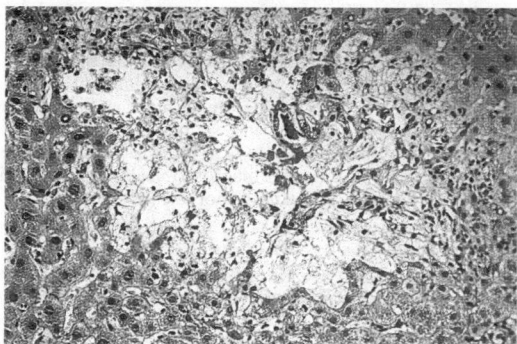

hepatic necrosis (centrilobular): microscopic section showing reticular transformation of cytoplasm, with cellular degeneration and fragmentation

acute massive liver n., a lesion in which there is extensive and rapid death of parenchymal cells of the liver, sometimes with fatty degeneration of the size of the organ; the necrosis may result from fulminant viral infection or chemical poisoning; associated with jaundice. SYN acute parenchymatous hepatitis, acute yellow atrophy of the liver, Rokitansky disease (1).

acute retinal n. (ARN), a viral syndrome occurring in immunocompetent patients, characterized by peripheral retinal destruction that becomes circumferential and leads to retinal *detachment.*

aseptic n., n. occurring in the absence of infection.

avascular n., n. due to deficient blood supply.

bridging hepatic n., area of liver n. that bridges adjacent portal areas and central veins; subsequent postnecrotic collapse and fibrosis is likely to result in cirrhosis.

caseous n., caseation n., n. characteristic of certain inflammations (e.g., tuberculosis, histoplasmosis), which represents n. with loss of separate structures of the various cellular and histologic elements; affected tissue manifests the friable, crumbly consistency and dull, opaque quality observed in cheese. SYN caseous degeneration.

central n., n. involving the deeper or inner portions of a tissue, or an organ or its units.

coagulation n., a type of n. in which the affected cells or tissue are converted into a dry, dull, fairly homogeneous eosinophilic mass without nuclear staining, as a result of the coagulation of protein as occurs in an infarct; microscopically, the necrotic process involves chiefly the cells, and remnants of histologic elements (e.g., elastin, collagen, muscle fibers) may be recognizable, as well as "ghosts" of cells and portions of cell membranes; may be caused by heat, ischemia, and other agents that destroy tissue, including enzymes that would continue to alter the devitalized cellular substance.

colliquative n., obsolete term for liquefactive n.

contraction band n., SYN contraction *band.*

cystic medial n., loss of elastic and muscle fibers in the aortic media, with accumulation of mucopolysaccharide, sometimes in cystlike spaces between the fibers; a disease of unknown cause, which may be inherited and which predisposes to dissecting aneurysms. SYN Erdheim disease, medionecrosis aortae idiopathica cystica, medionecrosis of the aorta, mucoid medial degeneration.

epiphysial aseptic n., aseptic n. of bony epiphyses in children or adults probably due to ischemia; it may affect the upper end of the femur (Legg-Calvé-Perthes disease), the tibial tubercle (Osgood-Schlatter disease), the tarsal navicular bone or the patella (Köhler disease), the second metatarsal head (Freiberg disease), vertebral bodies (Scheuermann disease), or the capitellum of the humerus (Panner disease).

fat n., the death of adipose tissue, characterized by the formation of small (1–4 mm), dull, chalky, gray or white foci; these represent small quantities of calcium soaps formed in the affected tissue when fat is hydrolyzed into glycerol and fatty acids. SYN steatonecrosis.

fibrinoid n., n. in which the necrotic tissue has some staining reactions resembling fibrin and becomes deeply eosinophilic, homogenous, and refractile.

focal n., occurrence of numerous, relatively small or tiny, fairly well-circumscribed, usually spheroidal portions of tissue that manifest coagulative, caseous, or gummatous n. and are characteristically associated with agents that are hematogenously disseminated; frequently observed only in histologic sections, but the foci may be as large as 1–3 mm and macroscopically visible; arbitrarily, foci larger than that are usually not termed focal n.

ischemic n., n. caused by hypoxia resulting from local deprivation of blood supply, as by infarction.

laminar cortical n., the breaking down of a definite cell layer in the cerebral cortex, encountered typically after temporary cardiac arrest or perinatal hypoxia.

liquefactive n., a type of n. characterized by a fairly well-circumscribed, microscopically or macroscopically visible lesion that consists of the dull, opaque or turbid, gray-white to yellow-gray, soft or boggy, partly or completely fluid remains of tissue that became necrotic and was digested by enzymes, especially proteolytic enzymes liberated from disintegrating leukocytes; it is classically observed in abscesses, and frequently in infarcts of the brain.

progressive emphysematous n., SYN gas *gangrene.*

progressive outer retinal n. (PORN), a viral syndrome occurring in AIDS patients, caused by herpesvirus and characterized by destruction of peripheral retina.

renal papillary n., n. of renal papillae, occurring in acute pyelonephritis, especially in diabetics, or in analgesic nephropathy; renal failure may result. SYN necrotizing papillitis.

simple n., a stage of coagulation n.; the occurrence of a coarsely granular or hyaline change in the cytoplasm, and the lack of a

recognizable nucleus, with the general configuration of the dead cells being relatively unchanged.

subcutaneous fat n. of newborn, indurated plaques and nodules appearing usually a few days or a few weeks after birth and usually resolving within a few months, characterized microscopically by birefringent needle-shaped crystals within necrotic fat cells; the condition remains localized, unlike sclerema neonatorum, although hypercalcemia may develop.

suppurative n., liquefactive n. with pus formation.

total n., (1) complete n. of the cytologic and histologic elements in a portion of tissue, as in caseous n.; (2) death of an entire organ or part.

zonal n., n. predominantly affecting or limited to an anatomical zone, especially parts of the hepatic lobules defined according to proximity to either the portal tracts or central (hepatic) veins.

nec·ro·sper·mia (nek-rō-sper′mē-ă). A condition in which there are dead or immobile spermatozoa in the semen. [necro- + G. *sperma,* seed]

ne·cros·te·on, ne·cros·te·o·sis (ně-kros′tē-on, ně-kros-tē-ō′sis). Gangrene of bone. [necro- + G. *osteon,* bone]

ne·crot·ic (ně-krot′ik). Pertaining to or affected by necrosis.

ne·crot·o·my (ne-krot′ō-mē). **1.** SYN dissection. **2.** Operation for the removal of a necrosed portion of bone (sequestrum). [necro- + G. *tomē,* cutting]

osteoplastic n., removal of a bone sequestrum through a hinged window of bone which is then replaced.

nee·dle (nē′dl). **1.** A slender, solid, usually sharp-pointed instrument used for puncturing tissues, suturing, or passing a ligature around or through a vessel. **2.** A hollow n. used for injection, aspiration, biopsy, or to guide introduction of a catheter into a vessel or other space. **3.** To separate the tissues by means of one or two n.'s, in the dissection of small parts. **4.** To perform discission of a cataract by means of a knife n. [M.E. *nedle,* fr. A.S. *nāedl*]

aneurysm n., artery n., a blunt-pointed, curved n., set in a handle, with the eye at the point, used for passing a ligature around an artery.

aspirating n., a hollow n. used for withdrawing fluid from a cavity, when combined with an aspirator tube attached to one end.

atraumatic n., an eyeless surgical n. with the suture permanently fastened into a hollow end.

biopsy n., a hollow n. used to obtain a core of tissue for histologic study.

cataract n., SYN knife n.

cutting n., a surgical n. with angulated surface designed to puncture tough tissue.

Deschamps n., a n. with a long shaft for passing sutures in the deep tissues.

Emmet n., a strong n. with the eye in the point, having a wide curve, and set in a handle, used to pass a ligature around an undissected structure.

exploring n., a strong n. with a longitudinal groove, which is thrust into a tumor or cavity to determine the presence of fluid, the latter escaping along the groove.

Francke n., a small lancet-shaped, spring-activated n., used to evacuate a small effusion of blood.

Frazier n., a n. for draining lateral ventricles of brain.

Gillmore n., a device for obtaining the setting time of dental cement.

Hagedorn n., a curved surgical n. flattened on the sides.

hypodermic n., a hollow n., similar to but smaller than an aspirating n., attached to a syringe; used primarily for injection.

knife n., a very narrow, needle-pointed knife used in discission of a cataract. SYN cataract n.

lumbar puncture n., a n., provided with a stylet, for entering the spinal canal or cisterna magna, with a bore of at least 1 mm and 40 mm or more in length.

Millner n., a fine, non-cutting n. with eye for thread frequently used for suture of skin.

Salah sternal puncture n., a wide-bore n. for obtaining samples of red marrow from the sternum.

spatula n., a minute n. with a flat (noncutting) concave surface, used by eye surgeons.

stop-n., a surgical n., with the eye at the tip, the shank of which has a projecting shelf to arrest the n. when it has passed the desired distance through the tissues.

Tuohy n., a n. with a lateral opening at the distal end, designed to cause a catheter passing through the needle's lumen to exit laterally at a 45° angle; used to place catheters into the subarachnoid or epidural space.

Veress n., a n. equipped with a spring loaded obturator that is used for insufflation of the abdomen in laparoscopic surgery.

nee·dle-hold·er, nee·dle-car·ri·er, nee·dle-driv·er. A hand-held instrument for grasping a needle in suturing. SYN needle forceps.

Needles, J.W., U.S. dentist. SEE N. split cast *method.*

Needles, Carl F., U.S. pediatrician, *1935. SEE Melnick-Needles *osteodysplasty;* Melnick-N. *syndrome.*

nee·dling (nēd′ling). Discission of a soft or secondary cataract.

Neelsen, Friedrich K.A., German pathologist, 1854–1894. SEE Ziehl-N. *stain.*

ne·en·ceph·a·lon (ne-en-sef′ă-lon). Edinger term for the higher levels of the central nervous system superimposed upon the metameric or propriospinal system (paleencephalon). SYN neoencephalon. [G. *neos,* new, + *enkephalos,* brain]

NEEP Abbreviation for negative end-expiratory *pressure.*

nef·o·pam hy·dro·chlo·ride (nef′ō-pam). An analgesic agent.

Neftel, William B., U.S. neurologist, 1830–1906.

ne·ga·tion (nĕ-gā′shŭn). SYN denial.

neg·a·tive (neg′ă-tiv). **1.** Not affirmative; refutative; not positive; not abnormal. **2.** Denoting failure of response, absence of a reaction, or absence of an entity or condition in question. [L. *negativus,* fr. *nego,* to deny]

neg·a·tive G. Gravity in a foot-to-head direction in flying, or in standing on one's head; opposite of positive G.

neg·a·tive S. SYN flotation *constant.*

neg·a·tiv·ism (neg′ă-tiv-izm). A tendency to do the opposite of what one is requested to do, or to stubbornly resist for no apparent reason; seen in catatonic states and in toddlers.

neg·a·tron (neg′ă-tron). Term used for an electron to emphasize its negative charge in contradistinction to the positive charge carried by the otherwise similar positron.

Negri, Adelchi, Italian physician, 1876–1912. SEE N. *bodies,* under *body, corpuscles,* under *corpuscle.*

Negro, Camillo, Italian neurologist, 1861–1927. SEE N. *phenomenon.*

Neisser, Albert L.S., German physician, 1855–1916. SEE *Neisseria;* N. *coccus, syringe.*

Neisser, Max, German bacteriologist, 1869–1938. SEE N. *stain.*

Neis·se·ria (nī-sē′rē-ă). A genus of aerobic bacteria (family Neisseriaceae) containing Gram-negative cocci which occur in pairs with the adjacent sides flattened. These organisms are parasites of animals. The type species is *N. gonorrhoeae.* [A. *Neisser*]

N. catarrhalis, former name for *Moraxella catarrhalis.*

N. ca′viae, a bacterial species found in the pharyngeal region of guinea pigs; may also be found in other animals.

N. fla′va, a bacterial species found in the mucous membranes of the human respiratory tract; easily confused with *N. meningitidis.* SYN *N. subflava.*

N. flaves′cens, a bacterial species found in cerebrospinal fluid in cases of meningitis; probably occurs in the mucous membranes of the human respiratory tract.

N. gonorrhoe′ae, a bacterial species that causes gonorrhea and other infections in humans; the type species of the genus *N.* SYN gonococcus, Neisser coccus.

N. haemol′ysans, former name for *Gemella haemolysans.* SEE *Gemella.*

N. meningi′tidis, a bacterial species found in the nasopharynx of humans but not in other animals; the causative agent of meningococcal meningitis and meningicoccemia; virulent organisms are strongly Gram negative and occur singly or in pairs; in the latter

case the cocci are elongated and are arranged with long axes parallel and facing sides kidney shaped; groups characterized by serologically specific capsular polysaccharides are designated by capital letters (the main serogroups being A, B, C, and D). SYN meningococcus, Weichselbaum coccus.

N. sic′ca, a bacterial species found in the mucous membranes of the human respiratory tract.

N. subfla′va, SYN *N. flava.*

neis·se·ria, pl. **neis·se·ri·ae** (nī-sē′rē-ă, nī-sē′rē-ē). A vernacular term used to refer to any member of the genus *Neisseria.*

Nélaton, Auguste, French surgeon, 1807–1873. SEE N. *catheter, fibers,* under *fiber, line, sphincter;* Roser-N. *line.*

Nelson, Don H., U.S. internist, *1925. SEE N. *syndrome, tumor.*

nem. A nutritional unit defined as 1 gram breast milk of specific nutritional components having a caloric value equivalent to $\frac{2}{3}$ calorie. [Ger. *Nahrungseinheit Milch,* milk nutrition unit]

nema-, nemat-, nemato-. Thread, threadlike. [G. *nēma*]

nem·a·thel·minth (nem-ă-thel′minth). A member of the former phylum Nemathelminthes.

Nem·a·thel·min·thes (nem′ă-thel-min′thēz). Formerly considered a phylum to incorporate the pseudocelomate organisms, which now are divided into the distinct phyla Acanthocephala, Entoprocta, Rotifera, Gastrotricha, Kinorhyncha, Nematoda, and Nematomorpha. [nemat- + G. *helmins, helminthos,* worm]

nem·a·ti·ci·dal, nem·a·to·ci·dal (nem′ă-tī-sī′dăl -tō-sī′ dăl). Destructive to nematode worms.

nem·a·ti·cide, nem·a·to·cide (nĕ-mat′ī-sīd -ō-sīd). An agent that kills nematodes. [nematode + L. *caedo,* to kill]

nem·a·ti·za·tion (nem′ă-tī-zā-shŭn). Infestation by nematodes.

nem·a·to·blast (nem′ah-to-blast). SYN spermatid. [G., *nēma,* thread + *blastos,* germ]

nem·a·to·cyst (nem′ă-tō-sist). A stinging cell of coelenterates consisting of a poison sac and a coiled barbed sting capable of being ejected and penetrating the skin of an animal on contact; of considerable consequence in large jellyfish and in the Portuguese man-of-war whose large numbers of these stinging cells can cause great pain and even death. SYN cnida, cnidocyst. [nemato- + G. *kystis,* bladder]

Nem·a·to·da (nem-ă-tō′dă). The roundworms, a large phylum that includes many of the helminths parasitic in humans and a far greater number of plant-parasitic and free-living soil and aquatic nonparasitic species. For practical purposes, the parasitic nematodes may be placed in two groups, based on their adult habitat in the human body: 1) the intestinal roundworms (e.g., the genera *Ascaris, Trichuris, Ancylostoma, Necator, Strongyloides, Enterobius,* and *Trichinella*); and 2) the filarial roundworms of the blood, lymphatic tissues, and viscera (e.g., the genera *Wuchereria, Mansonella, Loa, Onchocerca,* and *Dracunculus*). [nemat- + G. *eidos,* form]

nem·a·tode (nem′ă-tōd). A common name for any roundworm of the phylum Nematoda.

nem·a·to·di·a·sis (nem′ă-tō-dī′ă-sis). Infection with nematode parasites.

cerebrospinal n., invasion of the central nervous system by wandering nematode larvae; e.g., *Angiostrongylus cantonensis* in rats and humans.

Nem·a·to·di·rel·la lon·gi·spi·cu·la·ta (nē′mă-tō-di-rel′ă lon′gi-spik-ū-lā′tă). One of the thread-necked trichostrongyle nematodes in the small intestine of sheep, goats, reindeer, moose, musk ox, and pronghorn.

nem·a·toid (nem′ă-toyd). Relating to nematodes.

nem·a·tol·o·gist (nem-ă-tol′ŏ-jist). A specialist in nematology.

nem·a·tol·o·gy (nem-ă-tol′ŏ-jē). The science concerned with all aspects of nematodes, their biology, and their importance to humans. [nematode + G. *logos,* study]

nem·a·to·sper·mia (nem′ă-tō-sper′mē-ă). Spermatozoa with an elongated tail, as in humans, in contrast to spherospermia. [nemat- + G. *sperma,* seed]

Némethy, George, Hungarian-U.S. biochemist, *1934. SEE Adair-Koshland-Némethy-Filmer *model;* Koshland-N.-Filmer *model.*

△**neo-.** New, recent. [G. *neos*]

neoadjuvant (nē-ō-ad′joo-vant). Chemotherapy or radiation given before cancer surgery. [neo- + adjuvant]

ne·o·an·ti·gens (nē-ō-an′ti-jenz). SYN tumor *antigens*, under *antigen.*

ne·o·ars·phen·a·mine (nē′ō-ar-sfen′ă-mēn). Formerly used as an antisyphilitic agent.

ne·o·ar·thro·sis (nē-ō-ar-thrō′sis). SYN nearthrosis.

Ne·o·as·ca·ris vi·tu·lo·rum (nē-ō-as′kă-ris vit-ū-lō′rŭm). The large roundworm occurring in the small intestine of cattle, water buffalo, and (rarely) sheep; although uncommon in the U.S., it is a serious cattle parasite in many other areas. Experimental infection has been produced in rodents and humans.

ne·o·bi·o·gen·e·sis (nē′ō-bī-ō-jen′ĕ-sis). The theory that life can originate from nonliving matter. [neo- + G. *bios*, life, + *genesis*, origin]

neo·bladder (nē′ō-blad′er). Surgically constricted (usually using stomach or intestine) replacement for urinary bladder.

ne·o·blas·tic (nē-ō-blas′tik). Developing in or characteristic of new tissue. [neo- + G. *blastos*, germ, offspring]

ne·o·cer·e·bel·lum (nē′ō-ser-ĕ-bel′ŭm) [TA]. Phylogenetic term referring to the larger lateral portion of the cerebellar hemisphere receiving its dominant input from the pontine nuclei which, in turn, are dominated by afferent nerves originating from all parts of the cerebral cortex; phylogenetically, of more recent origin than the archicerebellum and paleocerebellum, q.v., the n. reaches its largest development in humans and other primates. SYN corticocerebellum.

ne·o·chy·mo·tryp·sin·o·gen (nē-ō-kī′mō-trip-sin′ō-jen). An intermediate in the conversion of chymotrypsin to α-chymotrypsin by chymotrypsin cleavage.

ne·o·cin·cho·phen (nē-ō-sin′kō-fen). The ethyl ester of 6-methyl-2-phenylquinolin-4-carboxylic acid; its action and uses are similar to those of cinchophen.

ne·o·cor·tex (nē-ō-kōr′teks) [TA]. SYN isocortex.

ne·o·cys·tos·to·my (nē′ō-sis-tos′tō-mē). SYN ureteroneocystostomy. [neo- + G. *kystis*, bladder, + *stoma*, mouth]

ne·o·dym·i·um (Nd) (nē-ō-dim′ē-ŭm). One of the rare earth elements; atomic no. 60, atomic wt. 144.24. [*neo-*, new, + G. *didymos*, twin (of lanthanum)]

ne·o·en·ceph·a·lon (nē-ō-en-sef′ă-lon). SYN neencephalon.

ne·o·fe·tal (nē-ō-fē′tăl). Relating to the neofetus or to the transition between the embryonic and fetal periods of development.

ne·o·fe·tus (nē-ō-fē′tŭs). The intrauterine organism at about 8 weeks of development.

ne·o·for·ma·tion (nē′ō-fōr-mā′shŭn). **1.** Formation of neoplasia, or a neoplasm. **2.** Sometimes used to indicate the process of regeneration, or a regenerated tissue or part.

ne·o·gen·e·sis (nē-ō-jen′ĕ-sis). SYN regeneration (1). [neo- + G. *genesis*, origin]

ne·o·ge·net·ic (nē′ō-je-net′ik). Pertaining to or characterized by neogenesis.

ne·o·ki·net·ic (nē′ō-ki-net′ik). Denoting one of the divisions of the motor system, the function of which is the transmission of isolated synergic movements of voluntary origin; it represents a more highly specialized form of movement than the paleokinetic function. [neo- + G. *kinetikos*, relating to movement]

ne·o·lal·lism (nē-ō-lal′izm). Abnormal use of neologisms in speech. [neo- + G. *laleō*, to chatter]

ne·ol·o·gism (nē-ol′ō-jizm). A new word or phrase of the patient's own making often seen in schizophrenia (e.g., headshoe to mean hat), or an existing word used in a new sense; in psychiatry, such usages may have meaning only to the patient or be indicative of the patient's condition. [neo- + G. *logos*, word]

ne·o·morph, ne·o·mor·phism (nē′ō-mōrf, nē′ō-mōr′fizm). A new formation; a structure found in higher organisms, only slight or no traces of which exist in lower orders. [neo- + G. *morphē*, form]

ne·o·my·cin sul·fate (nē-ō-mī′sin). The sulfate of an antibacterial antibiotic substance produced by the growth of *Streptomyces*

fradiae, active against a variety of Gram-positive and Gram-negative bacteria.

ne·on (Ne) (nē′on). An inert gaseous element in the atmosphere, separated from argon by W. Ramsay and M. Travers in 1898; atomic no. 10, atomic wt. 20.1797. [G. *neos*, new]

ne·o·na·tal (nē-ō-nā′tăl). Relating to the period immediately succeeding birth and continuing through the first 28 days of extrauterine life. SYN newborn. [neo- + L. *natalis*, relating to birth]

ne·o·nate (nē′ō-nāt). An infant aged 1 month or less. SYN newborn. [neo- + L. *natus*, born, fr. *nascor*, to be born]

ne·o·na·tol·o·gist (nē′ō-nā-tol′ō-jist). One who specializes in neonatology.

ne·o·na·tol·o·gy (nē′ō-nā-tol′ō-jē). The pediatric subspecialty concerned with disorders of the neonate. SYN neonatal medicine. [neo- + L. *natus*, pp. born, + G. *logos*, theory]

ne·o·neu·rot·i·za·tion (nē-ō-noo-rot′ĭ-zā′shun). Rarely observed phenomenon of return of facial motor function following deliberate transection of the facial nerve; believed to represent trigeminal reinnervation of the facial muscles.

ne·o·pal·li·um (nē-ō-pal′ē-ŭm). SYN isocortex.

ne·o·pho·bia (nē-ō-fō′bē-ă). Morbid aversion to, or dread of, novelty or the unknown. [neo- + G. *phobos*, fear]

🔟**ne·o·pla·sia** (nē-ō-plā′zē-ă). The pathologic process that results in the formation and growth of a neoplasm. [neo- + G. *plasis*, a molding]

cervical intraepithelial n., dysplastic changes beginning at the squamocolumnar junction in the uterine cervix that may be precursors of squamous cell carcinoma: grade 1, mild dysplasia involving the lower one-third or less of the epithelial thickness; grade 2, moderate dysplasia with one-third to two-thirds involvement; grade 3, severe dysplasia or carcinoma in situ, with two-thirds to full-thickness involvement.

lobular n., SYN noninfiltrating lobular *carcinoma.*

multiple endocrine n. (MEN), a group of disorders characterized by functioning tumors in more than one endocrine gland. SYN familial multiple endocrine adenomatosis, multiple endocrine adenomatosis.

multiple endocrine n. 1 [MIM*131100], syndrome characterized by tumors of the pituitary gland, pancreatic islet cells, and parathyroid glands and may be associated with Zollinger-Ellison syndrome; autosomal dominant inheritance, caused by mutation in the MEN1 gene on chromosome 11q.

multiple endocrine n. 2 [MIM*171400], syndrome associated with pheochromocytoma, parathyroid adenoma and medullary thyroid carcinoma; autosomal dominant inheritance, caused by mutation in the RET oncogene on chromosome 10q.

multiple endocrine n. 3 [MIM*162300], syndrome characterized by tumors found in MEN2, tall, thin habitus, prominent lips, and neuromas of the tongue and eyelids; autosomal dominant inheritance, caused by mutation in the RET oncogene on 10q. SYN multiple endocrine n. 2B.

multiple endocrine n. 2B, SYN multiple endocrine n. 3.

multiple endocrine n., type 1, SYN multiple endocrine neoplasia *syndrome*, type 1.

multiple endocrine n., type 2A (MEN2A), SYN multiple endocrine neoplasia *syndrome*, type 2A.

prostatic intraepithelial n. (PIN), dysplastic changes involving glands and ducts of the prostate that may be a precursor of adenocarcinoma; low grade (PIN 1), mild dysplasia with cell crowding, variation in nuclear size and shape, and irregular cell spacing; high grade (PIN 2 and 3), moderate to severe dysplasia with cell crowding, nucleomegaly and nucleolomegaly, and irregular cell spacing.

vaginal intraepithelial n., preinvasive squamous cell carcinoma (carcinoma in situ) limited to vaginal epithelium; like vulvar or cervical intraepithelial neoplasia, graded histologically on a scale from 1 to 3 or subdivided into low-grade and high-grade intraepithelial malignancy; usually related to human papilloma virus infection; may progress to invasive carcinoma.

vulvar intraepithelial n., preinvasive squamous cell carcinoma (carcinoma in situ) limited to vulvar epithelium; like vaginal or cervical intraepithelial neoplasia, graded histologically on a scale

---

International Lymphoma Study Group

B-cell neoplasms

I. precursor B-cell neoplasm; precursor B-lymphoblastic leukemia/lymphoma

II. peripheral B-cell neoplasms

  1. B-cell chronic lymphocytic leukemia/prolymphocytic leukemia/small lymphocytic lymphoma

  2. lymphoplasmacytoid lymphoma/immunocytoma

  3. mantle cell lymphoma

  4. follicle center lymphoma, follicular
    provisional cytologic grades: I (small cell), II (mixed small and large cell), III (large cell)
    provisional subtype: diffuse, predominantly small cell type

  5. marginal zone B-cell lymphoma
    extranodal (MALT-type +/– monocytoid B cells)
    provisional subtype: nodal (+/– monocytoid B cells)

  6. provisional entity: splenic marginal zone lymphoma (+/– villous lymphocytes)

  7. hairy cell leukemia

  8. plasmacytoma/plasma cell myeloma

  9. diffuse large B-cell lymphoma*
    subtype: primary mediastinal (thymic) B-cell lymphoma

  10. Burkitt lymphoma

  11. provisional entity: high-grade B-cell lymphoma, Burkittlike*

T-cell and putative natural killer (NK)-cell neoplasms

I. precursor T-cell neoplasm: precursor T-lymphoblastic lymphoma/leukemia

II. peripheral T-cell and NK-cell neoplasms

  1. T-cell chronic lymphocytic leukemia/prolymphocytic leukemia

  2. large granular lymphocyte leukemia (LGL)
    T-cell type
    NK-cell type

  3. mycosis fungoides/Sézary syndrome

  4. peripheral T-cell lymphomas, unspecified*
    provisional cytologic categories: medium-sized cell, mixed medium and large cell, large cell, lymphoepithelioid cell
    provisional subtype: hepatosplenic gd T-cell lymphoma
    provisional subtype: subcutaneous panniculitic T-cell lymphoma

  5. angioimmunoblastic T-cell lymphoma (AILD)

  6. angiocentric lymphoma

  7. intestinal T-cell lymphoma (+/– enteropathy-associated)

  8. adult T-cell lymphoma/leukemia (ATL/L)

  9. anaplastic large cell lymphoma (ALCL), CD30*, T-and null-cell types

  10. provisional entity: anaplastic large-cell lymphoma, Hodgkinlike

Hodgkin disease (HD)

I. lymphocyte predominance

II. nodular sclerosis

III. mixed cellularity

IV. lymphocyte depletion

V. provisional entity: lymphocyte-rich classical HD

* these categories are thought likely to include more than one disease entity

---

from 1 to 3 or subdivided into low-grade and high-grade intraepithelial malignancy; usually related to human papilloma virus infection; may progress to invasive carcinoma.

ne·o·plasm (nē′ō-plazm). An abnormal tissue that grows by cellular proliferation more rapidly than normal and continues to grow after the stimuli that initiated the new growth cease. N.'s show partial or complete lack of structural organization and func-

tional coordination with the normal tissue, and usually form a distinct mass of tissue that may be either benign (benign *tumor*) or malignant (cancer). SYN new growth, tumor (2). [neo- + G. *plasma,* thing formed]

  histoid n., old term for a n. characterized by a cytohistologic pattern that closely resembles the tissue from which the neoplastic cells are derived.

ne·o·plas·tic (nē-ō-plas′tik). Pertaining to or characterized by neoplasia, or containing a neoplasm.

ne·op·ter·in (nē-op′trin). A pteridine present in body fluids; elevated levels result from immune system activation, malignant disease, allograft rejection, and viral infections (especially as in AIDS). [neo- + G. *pteron,* wing, + -in]

ne·o·pyr·i·thi·a·min (nē′ō-pir-i-thī′ă-min). SYN pyrithiamin.

ne·o·ret·i·nal b (nē-ō-ret′in-al). SYN 11-*cis*-retinal.

ne·o·ret·i·nene B (nē-ō-ret′i-nēn). SYN 11-*cis*-retinol.

Ne·o·spo·ra ca·ni·um (nē-ō-spōr-ă kān′-ē-um). A protozoan parasite of dogs in the phylum Apicomplexa, an intracellular cyst-forming pathogen of neural and other tissues. Its epidemiology and life history are unknown.

ne·o·stig·mine (nē-ō-stig′min). A synthetic compound, similar in action to physostigmine (eserine); a reversible cholinesterase inhibitor, used as the bromide or methylsulfate salts in the treatment of myasthenia gravis, postoperative distention, urinary retention, and antagonist of stabilizing neuromuscular blocking drugs.

ne·os·to·my (nē-os′tō-mē). Surgical construction of a new or artificial opening. [neo- + G. *stoma,* mouth]

ne·o·stri·a·tum (nē-ō-strī-ā′tŭm). ☆official alternate term for striatum.

ne·ot·e·ny (nē-ot′e-nē). Prolongation of the larval state, as in the Mexican tiger salamander or axolotl, or in certain termite castes held in the larval stage as future replacements of the queen. Cf. pedogenesis. [neo- + G. *teinō,* to stretch]

Ne·o·tes·tu·di·na ro·sa·ti (nē′ō-tes-too-dī′nă rō-sā′tī). A species of fungus that causes white grain mycetoma in Somalia and elsewhere in Africa.

ne·o·thal·a·mus (nē-ō-thal′ă-mŭs). The portion of the thalamus projecting to the neocortex.

ne·o·ty·ro·sine (nē-ō-tī′rō-sēn). Dimethyltyrosine; a tyrosine antimetabolite.

ne·o·vas·cu·lar·i·za·tion (nē′ō-vas′kū-lar-i-zā′shŭn). Proliferation of blood vessels in tissue not normally containing them, or proliferation of blood vessels of a different kind than usual in tissue.

  choroidal n., ingrowth of new vessels from the choriocapillaris into the subretinal pigment epithelium and the retina; space associated with damage to the outer retina.

  classic choroidal n., well-demarcated areas of hyperfluorescence observed in the early phases of a retinal angiogram.

  occult choroidal n., area of leakage of undetermined source seen in the late phases of a retinal angiogram.

  Type 1 choroidal n., ingrowth of new vessels from the choriocapillaris into the subretinal pigment epithelial space; associated with damage to the outer retina.

  Type 2 choroidal n., ingrowth of new vessels from the choriocapillaris into the subretinal space; associated with damage to the outer retina.

ne·per (Np). A unit for comparing the magnitude of two powers, usually in electricity or acoustics; it is one half of the natural logarithm of the ratio of the two powers. SYN napier. [fr. *neperus,* latinized form of (John) *Napier*]

neph·e·lom·e·ter (nef-ĕ-lom′ĕ-ter). An instrument used in nephelometry. [G. *nephelē,* cloud, + *metron,* measure]

neph·e·lom·e·try (nef-ĕ-lom′ĕ-trē). A technique for estimation of the number and size of particles in a suspension by measurement of light scattered from a beam of light passed through the solution.

△**nephr-.** SEE nephro-.

ne·phral·gia (ne-fral′jē-ă). Rarely used term for pain in the kidney. [nephr- + G. *algos,* pain]

ne·phral·gic (ne-fral′jik). Relating to nephralgia.

ne·phrec·to·my (ne-frek′tō-mē). Removal of a kidney. [nephr- + G. *ektomē,* excision]

abdominal n., transperitoneal removal of the kidney by an incision through the anterior abdominal wall.

laparoscopic n., removal of a kidney by percutaneous endoscopic technique.

lumbar n., extraperitoneal n. through a flank, loin, or posterior lumbar incision.

morcellated n., removal of a kidney in pieces.

posterior n., retroperitoneal removal of a kidney through an incision in the posterior lumbar muscles, usually with the patient in a prone position. SYN lumbotomy incision.

neph·re·de·ma (nef-re-dē′mă). Edema caused by renal disease; rarely, edema of the kidney. [nephr- + G. *oidēma,* swelling]

neph·rel·co·sis (nef-rel-kō′sis). Ulceration of the mucous membrane of the pelvis or calices of the kidney. [nephr- + G. *helkōsis,* ulceration]

neph·ric (nef′rik). Relating to the kidney. SYN renal.

ne·phrid·i·um, pl. **ne·phrid·ia** (ne-frid′ē-ŭm, -ă). One of the paired, segmentally arranged excretory tubules of invertebrates such as the annelids. [G. *nephros,* kidney, + Mod. L. *-idium,* dim. suffix, fr. G. *-idion*]

ne·phrit·ic (ne-frit′ik). Relating to or suffering from nephritis.

ne·phri·tis, pl. **ne·phrit·i·des** (ne-frī′tis, -frit′i-dēz). Inflammation of the kidneys. [nephr- + G. *-itis,* inflammation]

acute n., SYN acute *glomerulonephritis.*

acute interstitial n., interstitial n. with variable tubular damage and infiltration by numerous neutrophils, due to bacterial infection, urinary tract obstruction, or other causes (including drugs), which may be hypersensitivity reactions; accompanied by renal failure, fever, blood or tissue eosinophilia, and rash.

analgesic n., chronic interstitial n. with renal papillary necrosis, occurring in patients with a long history of excessive consumption of analgesics, especially those containing phenacetin. SYN analgesic nephropathy.

anti–basement membrane n., glomerulonephritis produced by autologous or heterologous antibodies to the glomerular capillary basement membranes, the latter known as anti–kidney serum n.

anti–kidney serum n., experimental glomerulonephritis produced by injection of antiserum to kidney.

chronic n., SYN chronic *glomerulonephritis.*

focal n., SYN focal *glomerulonephritis.*

glomerular n., SYN glomerulonephritis.

n. gravida′rum, n. developing in pregnancy.

hemorrhagic n., acute glomerulonephritis accompanied by hematuria.

hereditary n. [MIM*161900], familial renal disease occurring in adulthood characterized by proteinuria, hematuria, and hypertension progressing to chronic renal failure. There is no ocular defect or deafness; autosomal dominant inheritance. SEE ALSO Alport *syndrome.*

immune complex n., an immune complex disease resulting from glomerular deposits, as in systemic lupus erythematosus.

interstitial n., a form of n. in which the interstitial connective tissue is chiefly affected.

lupus n., glomerulonephritis occurring in some patients with systemic lupus erythematosus, characterized by hematuria and a progressive course culminating in renal failure, often without hypertension; sometimes also applied to the nephrotic syndrome in patients with systemic lupus. Renal biopsies in patients with a progressive course show diffuse proliferative glomerulonephritis; in milder cases, there are focal proliferative glomerular lesions or mesangial nephritis.

mesangial n., glomerulonephritis with an increase in glomerular mesangial cells or matrix, or mesangial deposits.

salt-losing n., a rare disorder resulting from renal tubular damage of a variety of etiologies; mimics adrenocortical insufficiency in that abnormal renal loss of sodium chloride occurs, accompanied by hyponatremia, azotemia, acidosis, dehydration, and vascular collapse. SYN salt-losing syndrome, Thorn syndrome.

scarlatinal n., acute glomerulonephritis occurring as a complication of scarlet fever.

serum n., glomerulonephritis occurring in serum sickness or in animals injected with foreign serum protein.

subacute n., SYN subacute *glomerulonephritis.*

suppurative n., focal *glomerulonephritis* with abscess formation in the kidney.

syphilitic n., a rare complication of congenital and secondary syphilis, with the nephrotic syndrome, resulting from glomerular immune-complex deposits.

transfusion n., renal failure and tubular damage resulting from the transfusion of incompatible blood; the hemoglobin of the hemolyzed red cells is deposited as casts in the renal tubules.

tuberculous n., n., mainly interstitial, due to the tubercle bacillus.

tubulointerstitial n., n. affecting renal tubules and interstitial tissue, with infiltration by plasma cells and mononuclear cells; seen in lupus n., allograft rejection, and methicillin sensitization.

uranium n., an experimental n. produced by the administration of uranium nitrate.

ne·phrit·o·gen·ic (nef′ri-tō-jen′ik). Causing nephritis; said of conditions or agents. [nephritis + G. *genesis,* production]

♻**nephro-, nephr-.** The kidney. SEE ALSO reno-. [G. *nephros,* kidney]

neph·ro·blas·te·ma (nef′rō-blas-tē′mă). SYN nephric *blastema.* [nephro- + G. *blastēma,* a sprout]

neph·ro·blas·to·ma (nef′rō-blas-tō′mă). SYN Wilms *tumor.*

neph·ro·cal·ci·no·sis (nef′rō-kal-si-nō′sis). A form of renal lithiasis characterized by diffusely scattered foci of calcification in the renal parenchyma; deposits of calcium phosphate, calcium oxalate monohydrate, and similar compounds are usually demonstrable radiologically. [nephro- + calcinosis]

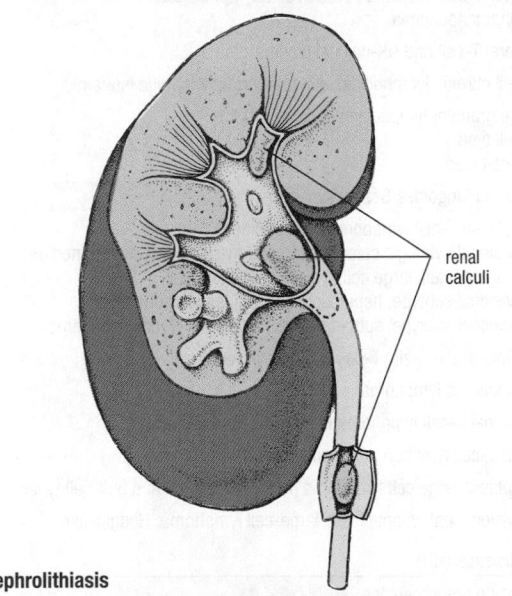

renal calculi

nephrolithiasis

neph·ro·cap·sec·to·my (nef′rō-kap-sek′tō-mē). Obsolete operation for decortication, or decapsulation, of the kidney. [nephro- + L. *capsula,* a small box, + G. *ektomē,* excision]

neph·ro·car·di·ac (nef′rō-kar′dē-ak). SYN cardiorenal. [nephro- + G. *kardia,* heart]

neph·ro·cele (nef′rō-sēl). **1.** Hernial displacement of a kidney. [nephro- + G. *kēlē,* hernia] **2.** Cavity of the nephrotome. SYN nephrotomic cavity. [nephro- + G. *koilōma,* a hollow (celom)]

neph·ro·cys·to·sis (nef′rō-sis-tō′sis). Formation of renal cysts. [nephro- + G. *kystis,* cyst, + *-osis,* condition]

neph·ro·ge·net·ic, neph·ro·gen·ic (nef′rō-jě-net′ik, -jen′ik). Developing into kidney tissue. [nephro- + G. *genesis,* origin]

ne·phrog·e·nous (ne-froj′ě-nŭs). Developing from kidney tissue.

neph·ro·gram (nef'rō-gram). **1.** Radiographic examination of the kidney after the intravenous injection of a water-soluble iodinated contrast material. **2.** The diffuse opacification of the renal parenchyma following such injection, an indication of renal blood flow and glomerular filtration. A persistent nephrogram indicates obstruction of kidney drainage.

ne·phrog·ra·phy (ne-frog'ră-fē). Radiography of the kidney. [nephro- + G. *graphō*, to write]

neph·roid (nef'royd). Kidney-shaped; resembling a kidney. SYN reniform. [nephro- + G. *eidos*, resemblance]

neph·ro·lith (nef'rō-lith). SYN renal *calculus*. [nephro- + G. *lithos*, stone]

neph·ro·li·thi·a·sis (nef'rō-li-thī'ă-sis). Presence of renal calculi.

neph·ro·li·thot·o·my (nef'rō-li-thot'ō-mē). Incision into the kidney for the removal of a renal calculus. [nephro- + G. *lithos*, stone, + *tomē*, incision]

ne·phrol·o·gy (ne-frol'ō-jē). The branch of medical science concerned with medical diseases of the kidneys. [nephro- + G. *logos*, study]

ne·phrol·y·sin (ne-frol'i-sin). An antibody that causes destruction of the cells of the kidneys, formed in response to the injection of an emulsion of renal substance; it is specific for the species from which the antigen was prepared.

ne·phrol·y·sis (ne-frol'i-sis). **1.** Freeing of the kidney from inflammatory adhesions, with preservation of the capsule. **2.** Destruction of renal cells. [nephro- + G. *lysis*, dissolution]

neph·ro·lyt·ic (nef-rō-lit'ik). Pertaining to, characterized by, or causing nephrolysis. SYN nephrotoxic (2).

ne·phro·ma (ne-frō'mă). A tumor arising from renal tissue. [nephro- + G. *-oma*, tumor]

mesoblastic n., a spindle cell neoplasm of the infant and, rarely, adult kidney with entrapped renal tubules.

neph·ro·ma·la·cia (nef'rō-mă-lā'shē-ă). Softening of the kidneys. [nephro- + G. *malakia*, softness]

neph·ro·meg·a·ly (nef-rō-meg'ă-lē). Extreme hypertrophy of one or both kidneys. [nephro- + G. *megas*, great]

neph·ro·mere (nef'rō-mēr). That portion of the intermediate mesoderm from which segmented kidney tubules develop. SEE nephrotome. [nephro- + G. *meros*, a part]

neph·ron (nef'ron). A long convoluted tubular structure in the kidney, consisting of the renal corpuscle, the proximal convoluted tubule, the nephronic loop, and the distal convoluted tubule. SEE ALSO uriniferous *tubule*. [G. *nephros*, kidney]

neph·ro·path·ia (nef'rō-path'ē-ă). SYN nephropathy.

n. epidemica, a generally benign form of epidemic hemorrhagic fever reported in Scandinavia.

neph·ro·path·ic (nef'rō-path'ik). Causing organic renal disease or impairment of renal function.

ne·phrop·a·thy (ne-frop'ă-thē). Any disease of the kidney. SYN nephropathia, nephrosis (1). [nephro- + G. *pathos*, suffering]

analgesic n., SYN analgesic *nephritis*.

Balkan n., interstitial chronic nephritis of unknown etiology, originally described as a disease endemic in the Balkans, characterized by insidious onset, scanty urinary findings, anemia, and acidosis. SYN Danubian endemic familial n.

Danubian endemic familial n., SYN Balkan n.

diabetic n., a syndrome occurring in people with diabetes mellitus and characterized by albuminuria, hypertension, and progressive renal insufficiency.

Diabetic nephropathy is a major cause of morbidity and mortality in people with diabetes mellitus (DM). People with diabetes make up the largest number (>25%) of those who start renal dialysis for end-stage renal disease (ESRD) each year in the U.S. The incidence of ESRD approaches 40% in people who have had type 1 DM for 20 years. The risk of diabetic nephropathy is higher in males, blacks, Hispanics, and Native Americans. Within 3 years after the diagnosis of DM is made, histologic study shows thickening of glomerular basement membrane and mesangial expansion, changes characteristic of diabetic glomeru-

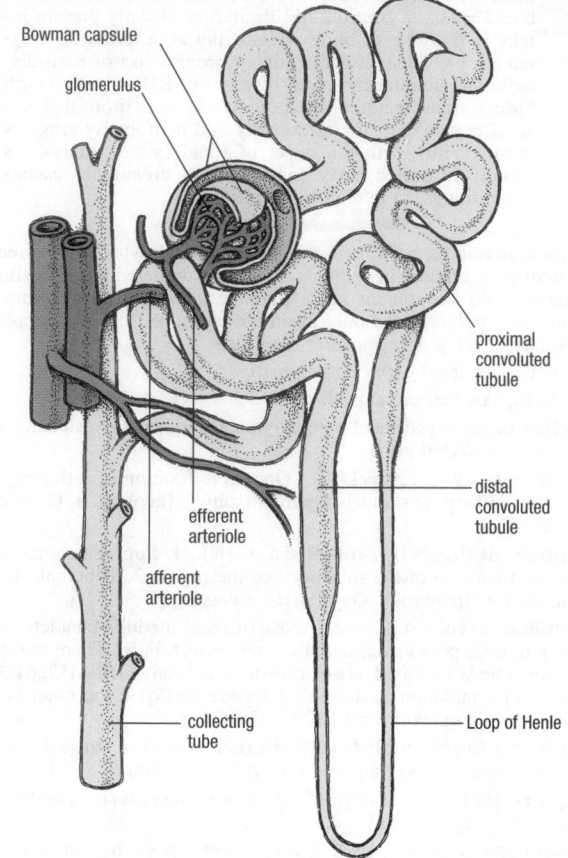

nephron

losclerosis (Kimmelstiel-Wilson disease). The kidneys increase in size and weight because of both hypertrophy and hyperplasia of parenchymal cells, and renal blood flow and glomerular filtration rate (GFR) are increased; as a result, serum creatinine and urea nitrogen are slightly reduced. After 10–15 years, the first evidence of renal damage may appear as microalbuminuria, a persistent excretion of albumin in concentrations not detected by routine tests for urinary protein. An albumin excretion rate of 20–200 µg/min (30–300 mg/day) heralds the onset of diabetic nephropathy and strongly predicts eventual ESRD. Further progression of renal damage leads to frank albuminuria and a decline in glomerular filtration rate and nitrogen clearance. The prevalence of hypertension is markedly greater in persons with microalbuminuria, and hypertension accelerates the progression of renal disease. Diabetic nephropathy can lead to hyperkalemia, metabolic acidosis, nephrotic syndrome, papillary necrosis, and increased susceptibility to acute renal failure after exposure to radiographic contrast media. Current practice guidelines for the treatment of DM call for annual assessment of 24-hour albumin excretion, prompt treatment of urinary tract infections, and avoidance of nephrotoxic drugs and radiographic dyes. No interventions have been shown to reverse clinical diabetic nephropathy. However, prospective randomized studies have established that improved metabolic control, maintaining plasma glucose as near normal as possible at all times, can markedly decrease the development and progression of diabetic nephropathy, as well as of other long-term microvascular complications of diabetes (retinopathy and neuropathy). In addition, aggressive management of hypertension with ACE inhibitors or angiotensin II receptor blockers has been shown to delay progression of nephropathy by mechanisms independent of blood pressure control, and limitation of daily protein intake to 0.8 g/kg of body weight (not appropriate in pregnancy) has been shown to delay progression of both diabetic and nondiabetic renal disease. ESRD is treated with kidney transplantation, hemodialysis, or peritoneal dialysis. Because diabetic retinopathy and neuropathy progress more rapidly with the onset of renal failure, dialysis is usually instituted early (when serum creatinine reaches about 6 mg/dL) in diabetic nephropathy.

---

hypokalemic n., vacuolation of the epithelial cytoplasm of renal convoluted tubules in patients seriously depleted of potassium; vacuoles do not contain fat or glycogen, concentrating ability is impaired, polyuria and polydipsia are common, and pyelonephritis may develop. SYN vacuolar nephrosis.

IgA n., SYN focal *glomerulonephritis.*

IgM n., SYN mesangial proliferative *glomerulonephritis.*

reflux n., damaged renal parenchyma secondary to vesicoureteral reflux of infected urine.

neph·ro·pexy (nef′rō-pek-sē). Operative fixation of a floating or mobile kidney. SEE ALSO nephrorrhaphy. [nephro- + G. *pēxis,* fixation]

neph·roph·thi·sis (nef-rof′thĭ-sis, -tĭ-sis). 1. Suppurative nephritis with wasting of the substance of the organ. 2. Tuberculosis of the kidney. [nephro- + G. *phthisis,* a wasting]

familial juvenile n., cystic disease of renal medulla characterized by polyuria, polydipsia, anemia, and renal failure. There are two forms: one is inherited as an autosomal recessive [MIM*256100], caused by mutation in the NPHP1 gene on 2q13; the other is an autosomal dominant form [MIM*174000].

neph·rop·to·sis, neph·rop·to·sia (nef-rop-tō′sis, -tō′sē-ă). Prolapse of the kidney. [nephro- + G. *ptōsis,* a falling]

neph·ro·py·o·sis (nef′rō-pī-ō′sis). SYN pyonephrosis. [nephro- + G. *pyōsis,* suppuration]

neph·ror·rha·phy (nef-rōr′ă-fē). Nephropexy by suturing the kidney. [nephro- + G. *rhaphē,* a suture]

neph·ros (nef′ros). SYN kidney.

neph·ro·scle·ro·sis (nef′rō-skle-rō′sis). Fibrosis of the kidney from overgrowth and contraction of the interstitial connective tissue. [nephro- + G. *sklērōsis,* hardening]

arterial n., patchy atrophic scarring of the kidney due to arteriosclerotic narrowing of the lumens of large branches of the renal artery, occurring in old or hypertensive persons and occasionally causing hypertension. SYN arterionephrosclerosis, senile n.

arteriolar n., renal scarring due to arteriolar sclerosis resulting from longstanding hypertension; the kidneys are finely granular and mildly or moderately contracted, with hyaline thickening of the walls of afferent glomerular arterioles and hyaline scarring of scattered glomeruli; chronic renal failure develops infrequently. SYN arteriolonephrosclerosis, benign n.

benign n., SYN arteriolar n.

malignant n., the renal changes in malignant hypertension; subcapsular petechiae, necrosis in the walls of scattered afferent glomerular arterioles, and red blood cells and casts in the urine, with uremia as a common termination.

senile n., SYN arterial n.

neph·ro·scle·rot·ic (nef′rō-skle-rot′ik). Pertaining to or causing nephrosclerosis.

neph·ro·scope (ne-frō′skōp). An endoscope passed into the renal pelvis to view it. Route of access may be percutaneous, through a surgically exposed kidney, or retrograde via the ureter.

ne·phro·sis (ne-frō′sis). 1. SYN nephropathy. 2. Degeneration of renal tubular epithelium. 3. SYN nephrotic *syndrome.* [nephro- + G. *-osis,* condition]

acute n., acute oliguric renal failure, especially that caused by certain poisons.

acute lobar n., a severe but localized bacterial infection of the renal parenchyma that may produce a mass effect simulating a renal abscess.

amyloid n., (1) SYN renal *amyloidosis;* (2) the nephrotic syndrome due to deposition of amyloid in the kidney.

familial n. [MIM*256300], the nephrotic syndrome appearing in siblings in infancy, without nerve deafness; inherited as an autosomal recessive, the Finnish type of which is due to mutation in the nephrin gene on chromosome 19q.

hemoglobinuric n., acute oliguric renal failure associated with hemoglobinuria, due to massive intravascular hemolysis, e.g., following an incompatible blood transfusion; the kidneys show the morphologic changes of hypoxic n.

hypoxic n., acute oliguric renal failure following hemorrhage, burns, shock, or other causes of hypovolemia and reduced renal blood flow; frequently associated with patchy tubular necrosis, tubulorrhexis, and distal tubular casts of hemoglobin.

lipoid n., idiopathic nephrotic syndrome occurring most commonly in children, in which glomeruli show minimal changes with no thickening of the basement membranes, fat vacuoles in the tubular epithelium, and fusion of glomerular foot processes. SYN minimal-change disease, nil disease.

osmotic n., swelling of renal tubular epithelium associated with glomerular filtration of sugars and dextrose; the swelling is due to formation of cytoplasmic vesicles by pinocytosis, and is reversible, probably with no dysfunction, when produced by glucose or mannitol.

toxic n., acute oliguric renal failure due to chemical poisons, septicemia, or bacterial toxemia; frequently associated with extensive necrosis of proximal convoluted tubules.

vacuolar n., SYN hypokalemic *nephropathy.*

ne·phros·to·gram (ne-fros′tō-gram). A radiograph of the kidney after opacification of the renal pelvis by injecting a contrast agent through a nephrostomy tube. [nephrostomy + G. *gramma,* writing]

ne·phros·to·ma, neph·ro·stome (ne-fros′tō-mă, nef′rō-stōm). One of the ciliated funnel-shaped openings by which pronephric and some primitive mesonephric tubules communicate with the celom. [nephro- + G. *stoma,* mouth]

ne·phros·to·my (ne-fros′tō-mē). Establishment of an opening between the collecting system of the kidney through its parenchyma to the exterior of the body; may be performed by surgical incision or be placed percutaneously. [nephro- + G. *stoma,* mouth]

percutaneous n., drainage of the collecting system through a catheter inserted through the skin of the flank under fluoroscopic control, usually using the Seldinger technique.

neph·rot·ic (nef-rot′ik). Relating to, caused by, or similar to nephrosis.

neph·ro·tome (nef′rō-tōm). The segmented intermediate mesoderm develops into nephric primordia. [nephro- + G. *tomē,* a cutting]

neph·ro·tom·ic (nef-rō-tom′ik). Relating to the nephrotome.

neph·ro·to·mo·gram (nef-rō-tō′mō-gram). A tomographic examination of the kidneys following the intravenous administration of contrast material for the purpose of improving demonstration of renal parenchymal abnormalities. [nephro- + G. *tomos,* a cutting + *gramma,* a writing]

neph·ro·to·mog·ra·phy (nef′rō-tō-mog′ră-fē). Tomographic examination of the kidney.

ne·phrot·o·my (ne-frot′ō-mē). Incision into the kidney. [nephro- + G. *tomē,* incision]

anatrophic n., an incision into the posterolateral renal parenchyma, gaining access to the calyceal system through an avascular plane between anterior and posterior branches of the renal artery; used for removal of calyceal and branched renal calculi, with maximum exposure yet minimal bleeding or parenchymal damage. SYN Smith-Boyce operation.

neph·ro·tox·ic (nef-rō-tok′sik). 1. Pertaining to nephrotoxin; toxic to renal cells. 2. SYN nephrolytic.

neph·ro·tox·ic·i·ty (nef′rō-tok-sis′i-tē). The quality or state of being toxic to kidney cells.

neph·ro·tox·in (nef-rō-tok′sin). A cytotoxin that is specific for cells of the kidney.

neph·ro·tro·phic (nef-rō-trof'ik). SYN renotrophic.

neph·ro·tro·pic (nef-rō-trop'ik). SYN renotrophic.

neph·ro·tu·ber·cu·lo·sis (nef'rō-too-ber-kū-lō'sis). Tuberculosis of the kidney.

neph·ro·u·re·ter·ec·ta·sis (nef'rō-ū-rē'ter-dk-ta'sis). SYN ureter-ohydronephrosis.

neph·ro·u·re·ter·ec·to·my (nef'rō-ū-rē'ter-ek'tō-mē). Surgical removal of a kidney and its ureter. SYN ureteronephrectomy. [nephro- + ureter + G. *ektomē*, excision]

neph·ro·u·re·ter·o·cys·tec·to·my (nef'rō-ū-rē'ter-ō-sis-tek'tō-mē). Removal of kidney, ureter, and part or all of the bladder. [nephro- + ureter + G. *kystis*, bladder, + *ektomē*, excision]

nep·tu·ni·um (Np) (nep-too'nē-ŭm). A radioactive element; atomic no. 93; first element of the transuranian series (not found in nature); ^{237}Np has a half-life of 2.14×10^6 years. [planet, *Neptune*]

ne·ral (nē'ral). *cis*-Citral. SEE citral.

Néri, Vincenzo, Italian neurologist, *1882. SEE Néri *sign*.

ne·ri·ine (nē'ri-ēn). SYN conessine.

Nernst, Walther, German physicist and Nobel laureate, 1864–1941. SEE N. *equation*.

NERVE

🅝 **nerve** (nerv) [TA]. A whitish cordlike structure composed of one or more bundles (fascicles) of myelinated or unmyelinated n. fibers, or more often mixtures of both, coursing outside the central nervous system, together with connective tissue within the fascicle and around the neurolemma of individual n. fibers (endoneurium), around each fascicle (perineurium), and around the entire n. and its nourishing blood vessels (epineurium), by which stimuli are transmitted from the central nervous system to a part of the body or the reverse. Nerve branches are given in the definition of the major nerve; many are also listed and defined under branch. SYN nervus [TA]. [L. *nervus*]

abdominopelvic splanchnic n.'s, visceral branches of the sympathetic trunks conveying presynaptic sympathetic fibers to and visceral afferent fibers from the prevertebral ganglia and para-aortic/hypogastric plexuses for the innervation of viscera located below the diaphragm. The greater, lesser, lowest, lumbar, and sacral splanchnic n.'s belong to this group.

abducens n., ⍟official alternate term for abducent n. [CN VI].

abducent n. [CN VI] [TA], a small motor n. supplying the lateral rectus muscle of the eye; its origin is in the dorsal part of the tegmentum of the pons just below the surface of the rhomboid fossa, and it emerges from the brain in the fissure between the medulla oblongata and the posterior border of the pons (medullopontine sulcus); it enters the dura of the clivus and passes through the cavernous sinus, entering the orbit through the superior orbital fissure. SYN nervus abducens [CN VI] [TA], abducens n.⍟, abducent (2), sixth cranial n. [CN VI].

accelerator n.'s, certain of the cardiopulmonary splanchnic n.'s establishing the sympathetic innervation of the heart; originating from ganglion cells of the superior, middle, and inferior cervical ganglion of the sympathetic trunk, the unmyelinated efferent fibers of the accelerator n.'s stimulate an increase in the heart rate.

accessory n. [CN XI] [TA], arises by two sets of roots: the presumed cranial, emerging from the side of the medulla, and spinal, emerging from the ventrolateral part of the first five cervical segments of the spinal cord; these roots unite to form the accessory n. trunk, which divides into two branches, internal and external; the internal branch, carrying fibers of the cranial root, unites with the vagus in the jugular foramen and supplies the muscles of the pharynx, larynx, and soft palate; the external branch continues independently through the jugular foramen to supply the sternocleidomastoid and trapezius muscles. While the accessory n. was originally believed to have cranial and spinal roots, it is now the general view that the so-called cranial root is actually a portion of the vagus nerve. SYN nervus accessorius [CN XI] [TA], accessorius willisii, eleventh cranial n. [CN XI], spinal accessory n.

accessory phrenic n.'s [TA], accessory n. strands that arise from the fifth cervical n., often as branches of the n. to the subclavius, passing downward to join the phrenic n. SYN nervi phrenici accessorii [TA].

acoustic n., an archaic term sometimes used to designate the vestibulocochlear n. [CN VIII].

afferent n., a n. conveying impulses from the periphery to the central nervous system. SYN centripetal n., esodic n.

Andersch n., SYN tympanic n.

anococcygeal n., small nerve arising from the coccygeal plexus, supplying the skin over the coccyx. SYN nervus anococcygeus.

anterior ampullary n. [TA], a branch of the utriculoampullar n. that supplies the crista ampullaris of the anterior semicircular duct. SYN nervus ampullaris anterior [TA].

anterior antebrachial n., SYN anterior interosseous n.

anterior auricular n.'s [TA], branches of the auriculotemporal n. that supply the tragus and upper part of the auricle. SYN nervi auriculares anteriores [TA].

anterior crural n., SYN femoral n.

anterior cutaneous n.'s of abdomen, SYN thoracoabdominal n.'s.

anterior ethmoidal n. [TA], a branch of the nasociliary n.; passes through anterior ethmoidal foramen on superomedial wall of orbit into cranial cavity, giving rise to anterior meningeal n.'s, then passes through cribriform plates into nasal cavity, supplying anterosuperior nasal mucosa. SYN nervus ethmoidalis anterior [TA].

anterior femoral cutaneous n.'s, SYN anterior cutaneous branches of femoral nerve, under branch.

anterior interosseous n. [TA], a branch of the median arising in the elbow region, running on interosseous membrane, supplying the flexor pollicis longus, part of flexor digitorum profundus and the pronator quadratus muscles, as well as radiocarpal and intercarpal joints. SYN nervus interosseus antebrachii anterior [TA], anterior antebrachial n., nervus antebrachii anterior, volar interosseous n.

anterior labial n.'s [TA], branches of the ilioinguinal n. distributed to the labia majora, mons pubis, and adjacent thigh. SYN nervi labiales anteriores [TA].

anterior scrotal n.'s [TA], the branches of the ilioinguinal n., distributed to the skin of the root of the penis, mons pubis, adjacent thigh, and anterior surface of the scrotum. SYN nervi scrotales anteriores [TA].

anterior superior alveolar n.'s [TA], the branches of the superior alveolar n. that supply the incisors, canines, premolars, and first molar by their contributions to the superior dental plexus. SYN anterior superior alveolar branches of infraorbital nerve, rami alveolares superiores anteriores nervi infraorbitalis.

anterior supraclavicular n., SYN medial supraclavicular n.

anterior tibial n., SYN deep fibular n.

aortic n., a branch of the vagus that ends in the aortic arch and base of the heart; composed entirely of afferent fibers; its stimulation elicits a brainstem reflex that causes slowing of the heart, dilation of the peripheral vessels, and a fall in blood pressure. SYN Cyon n., depressor n. of Ludwig, Ludwig n.

Arnold n., SYN auricular branch of vagus nerve.

articular n., a branch of a nerve supplying a joint. SYN nervus articularis.

auditory n., SYN cochlear n.

augmentor n.'s, SYN cervical splanchnic n.'s.

auriculotemporal n. [TA], a branch of the mandibular, usually arising by two roots embracing the middle meningeal artery; it passes through the parotid gland conveying postsynaptic parasympathetic secretomotor fibers from the otic ganglion, and continuing to terminate in the skin of the temple and scalp; also sends branches to the external acoustic meatus, tympanic membrane, and auricle as well as a communicating branch to the facial nerve. SYN nervus auriculotemporalis [TA].

autonomic n., a bundle of autonomic n. fibers outside of the central nervous system belonging or relating to the autonomic (visceral motor) nervous system. SYN nervus autonomicus [TA].

axillary n. [TA], arises from the posterior cord of the brachial plexus in the axilla, passes laterally and posteriorly through quadrangular space with the posterior circumflex humeral artery, winding round the surgical neck of the humerus to supply the deltoid and teres minor muscles, terminating as the superior lateral brachial cutaneous n. SYN nervus axillaris [TA], circumflex n.

baroreceptor n., SYN pressoreceptor n.

Bell respiratory n., SYN long thoracic n.

Bock n., SYN pharyngeal n.

buccal n. [TA], a sensory branch of the mandibular division of the trigeminal n.; it passes downward, emerging from beneath the ramus of the mandible to run forward on the buccinator muscle, piercing (but not supplying) it to supply the buccal mucous membrane and skin of the cheek near the angle of the mouth. SYN nervus buccalis [TA], buccinator n., long buccal n.

buccinator n., SYN buccal n.

cardiopulmonary splanchnic n.'s, visceral branches of the sympathetic trunks conveying postsynaptic sympathetic fibers to and visceral afferent fibers from viscera located above the diaphragm, mainly via the cardiac, pulmonary, and esophageal plexuses. The cervical and upper thoracic splanchnic n.'s are part of this group.

caroticotympanic n.'s, two sympathetic branches from the internal carotid plexus to the tympanic plexus. SYN nervi caroticotympanicus, small deep petrosal n.

carotid sinus n., SYN carotid *branch* of glossopharyngeal nerve (CN IX).

n. to carotid sinus, SYN carotid *branch* of glossopharyngeal nerve (CN IX).

cavernous n.'s of clitoris [TA], n.'s corresponding to the cavernous n.'s of penis in the male, arising from the vesicular portion of the pelvic plexus. SYN nervi cavernosi clitoridis [TA], cavernous plexus of clitoris.

cavernous n.'s of penis [TA], two n.'s, major and minor, derived from the prostatic portion of the pelvic plexus supplying sympathetic and parasympathetic fibers to the helicine arteries and arteriorvenous anastomoses of the corpus cavernosum stimulating erection. SYN nervi cavernosi penis [TA], cavernous plexus of penis.

centrifugal n., SYN efferent n.

centripetal n., SYN afferent n.

cervical n.'s [C1–C8], spinal n.'s arising from the cervical segments of the spinal cord. SYN nervi cervicales [C1–C8].

cervical splanchnic n.'s, visceral branches arising from the superior, middle, and inferior (stellate) cervical ganglia; they include the superior, middle, and inferior cervical cardiac nerves and are part of the cardiopulmonary splanchnic n.'s. SYN augmentor n.'s.

circumflex n., SYN axillary n.

coccygeal n. [Co] [TA], a small n., the lowest of the spinal n.'s, entering into the formation of the coccygeal plexus. SYN nervus coccygeus [Co] [TA].

cochlear n. [TA], the part of the vestibulocochlear n. [CN VIII] peripheral to the cochlear root; composed of the central n. processes of the bipolar neurons of the spiral ganglion, which have their peripheral processes on the four rows of neuroepithelial cells (hair cells) of the spiral organ. SEE ALSO cochlear *root* of VIII nerve. SYN nervus cochlearis [TA], auditory n., cochlear part of vestibulocochlear nerve, inferior part of vestibulocochlear nerve, pars cochlearis nervi vestibulocochlearis.

common fibular n. [TA], one of the terminal divisions of the sciatic n., diverging from the tibial n. at the upper end of the popliteal fossa, then coursing with the biceps tendon along the lateral portion of the popliteal space to wind around the neck of the fibula where it divides into the superficial and deep peroneal n.'s. The common peroneal n., or its deep branch, is the most commonly injured n., being located in a lateral subcutaneous position at the fibular neck; a lesion causes a loss of ability to dorsiflex the foot ("foot drop"). SYN nervus fibularis communis [TA], common peroneal n.⋆, nervus peroneus communis⋆.

common palmar digital n.'s [TA], four n.'s in the palm that send branches (proper palmar digital n.'s) to adjacent sides of two digits; three are branches of the median n., one is from the ulnar n. SYN nervi digitales palmares communes [TA].

common peroneal n., ⋆official alternate term for common fibular n.

common plantar digital n.'s [TA], three n.'s derived from the medial plantar n. and one from the lateral plantar n. that supply the skin overlying the metatarsals and terminate as proper plantar digital n.'s to the side of each toe. SYN nervi digitales plantares communes [TA].

cranial n.'s [TA], those n.'s that emerge from, or enter, the cranium or skull, in contrast to the spinal n.'s, which emerge from the spine or vertebral column. The twelve paired cranial n.'s are the olfactory [CN I], optic [CN II], oculomotor [CN III], trochlear [CN IV], trigeminal [CN V], abducent [CN VI], facial [CN VII], vestibulocochlear [CN VIII], glossopharyngeal [CN IX], vagal [CN X], accessory [CN XI], and hypoglossal [CN XII] n.'s. SYN nervi craniales [TA].

front

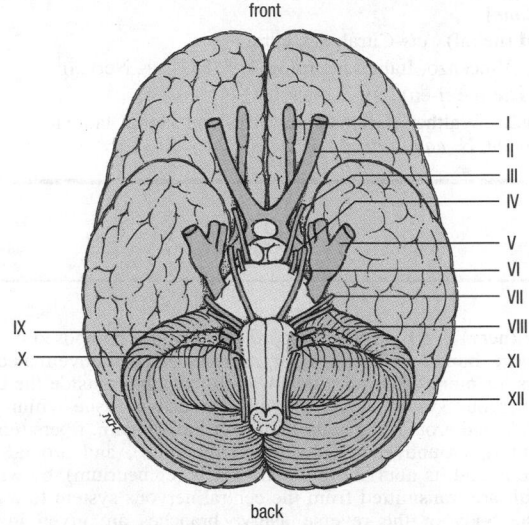

back

cranial nerves: (inferior view): (I) olfactory, (II) optic, (III) oculomotor, (IV) trochlear, (V) trigeminal, (VI) abducens, (VII) facial, (VIII) vestibulocochlear, (IX) glossopharyngeal, (X) vagus, (XI) accessory, (XII) hypoglossal

crural interosseous n. [TA], a n. given off from one of the muscular branches of the tibial n. which passes down over the posterior surface of the interosseous membrane supplying it and the two bones of the leg. SYN nervus interosseus cruris [TA], interosseous n. of leg.

cubital n., SYN ulnar n.

cutaneous n. [TA], a mixed n. supplying a region of the skin, including its sensory endings, blood vessels, smooth muscle and glands. SYN nervus cutaneus [TA].

cutaneous cervical n., SYN transverse cervical n.

Cyon n., SYN aortic n.

dead n., misnomer for nonvital dental pulp.

deep fibular n. [TA], one of the terminal branches of the common peroneal n., arising at the fibular neck and passing into the anterior compartment of the leg; it supplies the tibialis anterior, extensor hallucis longus, extensor digitorum longus, and peroneus tertius muscles in the leg, then crosses the ankle joint to supply the muscles on the dorsum of the foot (extensors hallucis and digitorum brevis), becoming cutaneous to innervate adjacent sides of the great and second toes. SYN nervus fibularis profundus [TA], deep peroneal n.⋆, nervus peroneus profundus⋆, anterior tibial n.

deep peroneal n., ⋆official alternate term for deep fibular n.

deep petrosal n. [TA], the deep petrosal branch of the internal carotid plexus, which joins the greater petrosal n. at the entrance of the pterygoid canal forming the nerve of the pterygoid canal and thus provides postsynaptic fibers to the pterygopalatine ganglion. SYN nervus petrosus profundus [TA], radix sympathica ganglii pterygopalatini⋆, sympathetic root of pterygopalatine ganglion⋆.

deep temporal n.'s [TA], two branches, anterior and posterior, from the mandibular n., supplying the temporalis muscle and periosteum of the temporal fossa. SYN nervi temporales profundi [TA].

dental n., (1) layperson's term for a dental pulp; (2) branches of the inferior and superior alveolar n.'s to the teeth. SEE inferior alveolar n., superior alveolar n.'s.

depressor n. of Ludwig, SYN aortic n.

dorsal n. of clitoris [TA], the deep terminal branch of the pudendal, supplying especially the glans clitoridis after passing through the deep perineal musculature, to run along the dorsum of the clitoral shaft. SYN nervus dorsalis clitoridis [TA].

dorsal digital n.'s, SYN dorsal digital n.'s of hand.

dorsal digital n.'s of deep fibular nerve [TA], terminal sensory portion of the deep fibular (peroneal) n. on the dorsum of the foot, remaining after the motor branches to the extensor digitorum brevis and extensor hallucis brevis muscles have been supplied; provides cutaneous innervation to a small, wedge-shaped area that includes the adjacent sides of the great and second toes. SYN nervi digitales dorsales nervi fibularis profundi [TA].

dorsal digital n.'s of foot [TA], n.'s supplying the skin of the dorsal aspect of the proximal and middle phalanges of the toes. SEE dorsal digital n.'s of superficial fibular nerve, dorsal digital n.'s of deep fibular nerve. SYN nervi digitales dorsales pedis [TA], dorsal n.'s of toes.

dorsal digital n.'s of hand [TA], terminal branches of the radial and ulnar n.'s in the hand supplying the skin of the dorsal surface of the proximal and middle phalanges of the fingers. SEE dorsal digital n.'s of ulnar nerve. SYN dorsal digital n.'s, nervi digitales dorsales.

dorsal digital n.'s of superficial fibular nerve [TA], n.'s arising in the lateral fibular/peroneal) compartment of the leg that pass to the dorsum of the foot, supplying the skin of most of the dorsum of the foot and dorsal aspect of the toes, with the exception of a small wedge-shaped area including the adjacent sides of the great and second toes. SYN nervi digitales dorsales nervi fibularis superficialis [TA].

dorsal digital n.'s of ulnar nerve [TA], n.'s arising from the dorsal branch of the ulnar n. supplying the skin of the dorsal aspect of the little and ulnar half of the ring fingers and adjacent area of the dorsum of the hand. SYN nervi digitales dorsales nervi ulnaris [TA].

dorsal interosseous n., SYN posterior interosseous n.

dorsal lateral cutaneous n., SYN lateral dorsal cutaneous n.

dorsal medial cutaneous n., SYN medial dorsal cutaneous n.

dorsal n. of penis [TA], the deep terminal branch of the pudendal nerves that runs through the deep perineal muscles giving branches, then runs along the dorsum of the penis, supplying the skin of the penis, the prepuce, the corpora cavernosa, and the glans. SYN nervus dorsalis penis [TA].

dorsal n. of scapula, SYN dorsal scapular n.

dorsal scapular n. [TA], arises from ventral primary rami of the fifth to seventh cervical n.'s and passes downward to supply the levator scapulae and the rhomboideus major and minor muscles. SYN nervus dorsalis scapulae [TA], dorsal n. of scapula, n. to rhomboid, posterior scapular n.

dorsal n.'s of toes, SYN dorsal digital n.'s of foot.

efferent n., a n. conveying impulses from the central nervous system to the periphery. SYN centrifugal n., exodic n.

eighth n., SYN vestibulocochlear n. [CN VIII].

eighth cranial n. [CN VIII], SYN vestibulocochlear n. [CN VIII].

eleventh cranial n. [CN XI], SYN accessory n. [CN XI].

esodic n., SYN afferent n.

excitor n., a n. conducting impulses that stimulate to increase function.

excitoreflex n., a visceral n. the special function of which is to cause reflex action.

exodic n., SYN efferent n.

n. to external acoustic meatus [TA], a branch of the auriculotemporal nerve supplying the lining of the external acoustic meatus. SYN nervus meatus acustici externi [TA].

external carotid n.'s [TA], cephalic arterial ramus of the sympathetic trunk, conveying a number of sympathetic nerve fibers extending from the superior cervical ganglion to the external carotid artery to form the external carotid plexus. SYN nervi carotici externi [TA].

external respiratory n. of Bell, SYN long thoracic n.

external saphenous n., SYN sural n.

external spermatic n., SYN genital *branch* of genitofemoral nerve.

facial n. [CN VII] [TA], n. with origin in the tegmentum of the lower portion of the pons; it emerges from the brain at the posterior border of the pons; it leaves the cranial cavity through the internal acoustic meatus where it is joined by the intermediate n., traverses the facial canal in the petrous portion of the temporal bone, and makes its exit through the stylomastoid foramen; after supplying the stapedius, occipitalis, auricular, stylohyoid, and posterior belly of the digastric muscles; its main trunk ramifies within the parotid gland forming the intraparotid plexus, the various branches of which pass to the muscles of facial expression. SYN nervus facialis [CN VII] [TA], motor n. of face, seventh cranial n. [CN VII].

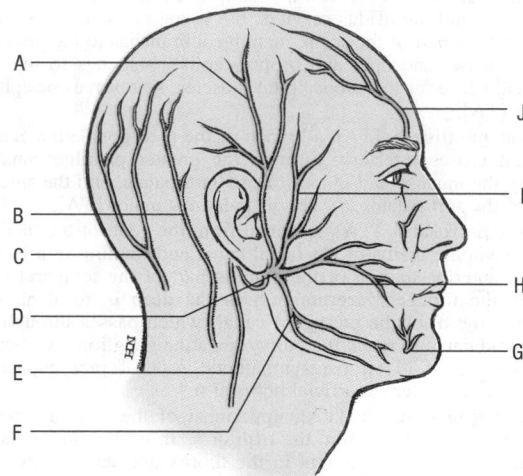

facial and other nerves supplying the head and neck: (A) auriculotemporal branch of facial nerve; (B) small occipital nerve; (C) greater occipital nerve; (D) facial nerve; (E) great auricular nerve; (F) mandibular branch of facial nerve; (G) mental nerve; (H) buccal branch of facial nerve; (I) temporal branch of facial nerve; (J) supraorbital nerve

femoral n. [TA], arises as a branch of the lumbar plexus, conveying fibers from the second, third, and fourth lumbar n.'s through the substance of the psoas muscle and enters the thigh via the retroinguinal muscular space posterior to the inguinal ligament, lateral to the femoral vessels; it arborizes within the femoral triangle into muscle branches to the sartorius, pectineus, and quadriceps muscles and anterior femoral cutaneous branches to the skin of the anterior and medial region of the thigh; its terminal branch is the saphenous n. by which it supplies the skin of the medial leg and foot. SYN nervus femoralis [TA], anterior crural n.

fifth cranial n. [CN V], SYN trigeminal n. [CN V].

first cranial n. [CN I], SYN olfactory n.'s [CN I].

fourth cranial n. [CN IV], SYN trochlear n. [CN IV].

fourth lumbar n. [L4] [TA], the ventral branch of the n. is forked to enter into the formation of both lumbar and sacral plexuses. SYN furcal n., nervus furcalis.

frontal n. [TA], a branch of the ophthalmic n. that divides within the orbit into the supratrochlear and the supraorbital n.'s. SYN nervus frontalis [TA].

furcal n., SYN fourth lumbar n. [L4].

Galen n., SYN communicating *branch* of internal laryngeal nerve with recurrent laryngeal nerve.

gangliated n., a sympathetic n.

genitocrural n., SYN genitofemoral n.

genitofemoral n. [TA], arises from the first and second lumbar n.'s, passes distally along the anterior surface of psoas major muscle and divides into genital and femoral branches. SYN nervus genitofemoralis [TA], genitocrural n.

glossopharyngeal n. [CN IX] [TA], ninth cranial nerve that emerges from the rostral end of the medulla and passes through the jugular foramen to supply sensation including taste to the pharynx and posterior third of the tongue; it also carries somatic motor fibers to the stylopharyngeus muscle and secretomotor presynaptic parasympathetic fibers to the otic ganglion for innervation of the parotid gland. SYN nervus glossopharyngeus [CN IX] [TA], ninth cranial n. [CN IX].

great auricular n. [TA], arises as a branch of the cervical plexus, conveying fibers from the ventral primary rami of the second and third cervical spinal n.'s; supplies the skin of part of the auricle, adjacent portion of the scalp, and that overlying the angle of the jaw; it also innervates the parotid sheath, conveying from it the pain fibers stimulated by stretching of the sheath during parotitis (mumps). SYN nervus auricularis magnus [TA].

greater occipital n. [TA], medial branch of the dorsal primary ramus of the second cervical n.; sends branches to the semispinalis capitis and multifidus cervicis, but is mainly sensory, supplying the back part of the scalp, meningeal branches to the posterior cranial fossa, and pain and proprioceptive branches to the first cervical nerve for the suboccipital muscles. SYN nervus occipitalis major [TA].

greater palatine n. [TA], a branch of the pterygopalatine ganglion that passes inferiorly through the greater palatine canal to supply the mucosa and glands of the hard palate, and the anterior part of the soft palate. SYN nervus palatinus major [TA].

greater petrosal n. [TA], a branch from the genu of the facial n. exiting via the hiatus of the facial canal and running in a groove on the anterior surface of the petrous part of the temporal bone beside the foramen lacerum to join the deep petrosal n., thus forming the n. of the pterygoid canal, which passes through the pterygoid canal to reach the pterygopalatine ganglion. SYN nervus petrosus major [TA], parasympathetic root of pterygopalatine ganglion★, greater superficial petrosal n.

greater splanchnic n. [TA], uppermost of the abdominopelvic splanchnic that arises from the fifth or sixth to the ninth or tenth thoracic sympathetic ganglia in the thorax and passes inferiorly along the bodies of the thoracic vertebrae, penetrating the diaphragm to join the celiac plexus; conveys presynaptic sympathetic fibers to the celiac ganglia and visceral afferent fibers from the celiac plexus. SYN nervus splanchnicus major [TA].

greater superficial petrosal n., SYN greater petrosal n.

great sciatic n., SYN sciatic n.

hemorrhoidal n.'s, SEE superior rectal (nervous) *plexus*, middle rectal (nervous) *plexus*, inferior anal n.'s.

Hering sinus n., SYN carotid *branch* of glossopharyngeal nerve (CN IX).

hypogastric n. [TA], one of the two n. trunks (right and left) that lead from the superior hypogastric plexus (presacral nerve) into the pelvis to join the inferior hypogastric plexuses. SYN nervus hypogastricus [TA].

hypoglossal n. [CN XII] [TA], arises from an oblong nucleus in the medulla and emerges by several root filaments between the pyramid and the olive via the preolivary groove; it passes through the hypoglossal canal, then courses downward and forward to supply the intrinsic and four of five extrinsic muscles of the tongue. SYN nervus hypoglossus [CN XII] [TA], twelfth cranial n. [CN XII].

iliohypogastric n. [TA], terminal branch, with ilioinguinal nerve, of the first lumbar n.; it supplies the abdominal muscles and the skin of the lower part of the anterior abdominal wall. SYN nervus iliohypogastricus [TA].

ilioinguinal n. [TA], terminal branch, with the iliohypogastric nerve, the first lumbar n., passes through the inguinal canal and superficial inguinal ring to supply the skin of the upper medial thigh, mons pubis, and scrotum or labia majora. SYN nervus ilioinguinalis [TA].

inferior alveolar n. [TA], one of the terminal branches of the

mandibular, it enters the mandibular canal to be distributed to the lower teeth, periosteum, and gingiva of the mandible; a branch, the mental n., passes through the mental foramen to supply the skin and mucosa of the lower lip and chin. SYN nervus alveolaris inferior [TA], inferior dental n.

inferior anal n.'s [TA], several branches of the pudendal n. that pass to the external anal sphincter anoderm and skin of the anal region. SYN nervi anales inferiores [TA], inferior rectal n.'s★, nervi rectales inferiores★, inferior hemorrhoidal n.'s.

inferior cervical cardiac n. [TA], a n. passing from the stellate ganglion to the cardiac plexus. SYN nervus cardiacus cervicalis inferior [TA].

inferior clunial n.'s [TA], branches of the posterior femoral cutaneous n. emerging from beneath the inferior border of the gluteus maximus to supply the skin of the lower half of the gluteal region. SYN nervi clunium inferiores [TA].

inferior dental n., SYN inferior alveolar n.

inferior gluteal n. [TA], arises as a branch of the sacral plexus, conveying fibers from the fifth lumbar and first and second sacral n.'s, and supplies the gluteus maximus muscle. It is subject to injury by compression and ischemia in sedentary individuals, resulting in difficulty in rising from a sitting position and difficulty climbing stairs. SYN nervus gluteus inferior [TA].

inferior hemorrhoidal n.'s, SYN inferior anal n.'s.

inferior laryngeal n. [TA], the terminal branch of the recurrent laryngeal n. as the latter passes deep to the inferior pharyngeal constrictor; it supplies the laryngeal mucosa inferior to the vocal folds and all laryngeal muscles except the cricothyroid. SYN nervus laryngeus inferior [TA].

inferior lateral brachial cutaneous n., ★official alternate term for inferior lateral cutaneous n. of arm.

inferior lateral cutaneous n. of arm [TA], cutaneous branch of the radial n. supplying the skin of the lower lateral aspect of the arm; it frequently arises as a branch of the posterior antebrachial n. SYN nervus cutaneus brachii lateralis inferior [TA], inferior lateral brachial cutaneous n.★.

inferior maxillary n., SYN mandibular n. [CN V3].

inferior rectal n.'s, ★official alternate term for inferior anal n.'s.

infraorbital n. [TA], the continuation of the maxillary n. [CN V2] after it has traversed the pterygopalatine fossa and enters the orbit, via the infraorbital fissure, it is then transmitted by the infraorbital canal to reach the face; it supplies the mucosa of the maxillary sinus, the upper incisors, canine and premolars, the upper gums, the inferior eyelid and conjunctiva, part of the nose, and the superior lip. SYN nervus infraorbitalis [TA].

infratrochlear n. [TA], a terminal branch of the nasociliary n. running beneath the pulley of the superior oblique muscle to the front of the orbit, and supplying the skin of the eyelids and root of the nose. SYN nervus infratrochlearis [TA].

inhibitory n., a n. conveying impulses that diminish functional activity in a part.

intercarotid n., SYN carotid *branch* of glossopharyngeal nerve (CN IX).

intercostal n.'s [TA], ventral primary rami of thoracic n.'s [T1–T11]. SYN nervi intercostales [TA].

intercostobrachial n.'s [TA], lateral cutaneous branches of the second and third intercostal n.'s that pass to the skin of the medial side of the arm. SYN nervi intercostobrachiales [TA], intercostohumeral n.'s.

intercostohumeral n.'s, SYN intercostobrachial n.'s.

intermediary n., SYN intermediate n.

intermediate n. [TA], a root of the facial nerve containing sensory fibers for taste from the anterior 2/3 of tongue whose cell bodies are located in the geniculate ganglion and presynaptic parasympathetic autonomic fibers whose cell bodies are located in the superior salivatory nucleus, i.e., the fibers are eventually conveyed via the chorda tympani branch of the facial n. to the lingual nerve. SYN nervus intermedius [TA], intermediary n., portio intermedia, Wrisberg n. (2).

intermediate dorsal cutaneous n. [TA], the lateral terminal branch of the superficial fibular (peroneal) n., supplying the dorsum of the foot and dorsal digital n.'s to the toes (except for adjacent parts of great and second toes). SYN nervus cutaneus dorsalis intermedius [TA].

intermediate supraclavicular n. [TA], one of several n.'s arising from the C-3–C-4 part of the cervical plexus that run across the top of the shoulder and pass down across the shaft of the clavicle to supply the skin of the top of the shoulder and in the infraclavicular region. SYN nervus supraclavicularis intermedius [TA], middle supraclavicular n.

internal carotid n. [TA], the cephalic arterial ramus conveying postsynaptic sympathetic fibers from the superior cervical ganglion to the internal carotid artery to form the internal carotid plexus. SYN nervus caroticus internus [TA].

internal saphenous n., SYN saphenous n.

interosseous n. of leg, SYN crural interosseous n.

Jacobson n., SYN tympanic n.

jugular n. [TA], a communicating branch between the superior cervical ganglion of the sympathetic n., the superior ganglion of the vagus n., and the inferior ganglion of the glossopharyngeal n. SYN nervus jugularis [TA].

lacrimal n. [TA], a branch of the ophthalmic n. [CN V1] supplying sensory fibers to the lateral part of the upper eyelid, conjunctiva, and lacrimal gland. The secretomotor fibers of the latter were conveyed to the lacrimal n. by the communicating branch of the zygomatic n. (a branch of the maxillary n. [CN V2]. SYN nervus lacrimalis [TA].

Latarget n., (1) SYN superior hypogastric (nervous) *plexus*; (2) terminal branch of anterior vagal trunk that runs along lesser curvature of the stomach to within a few centimeters of the gastroduodenal junction, but apparently never reaching the pyloric sphincter.

lateral ampullar n. [TA], a branch of the utriculoampullar n. that supplies the crista ampullaris of the lateral semicircular duct. SYN nervus ampullaris lateralis [TA].

lateral antebrachial cutaneous n., ⋆official alternate term for lateral cutaneous n. of forearm.

lateral anterior thoracic n., SYN lateral pectoral n.

lateral cutaneous n. of calf, SYN lateral sural cutaneous n.

lateral cutaneous n. of forearm [TA], the terminal cutaneous branch of the musculocutaneous n. that emerges between biceps brachii and brachialis muscles to supply the skin of the radial side of the forearm. SYN nervus cutaneus antebrachii lateralis [TA], lateral antebrachial cutaneous n.⋆.

lateral cutaneous n. of thigh [TA], arises from the lumbar plexus, conveying fibers from the second and third lumbar n.'s, supplies the skin of the anterolateral and lateral surfaces of the thigh. SYN nervus cutaneus femoris lateralis [TA], lateral femoral cutaneous n.⋆.

lateral dorsal cutaneous n. [TA], the continuation of the sural n. in the foot, supplying the lateral margin and dorsum. SYN nervus cutaneus dorsalis lateralis [TA], dorsal lateral cutaneous n.

lateral femoral cutaneous n., ⋆official alternate term for lateral cutaneous n. of thigh.

lateral pectoral n. [TA], a n. that arises from the lateral cord of the brachial plexus usually passing medial to pectoralis minor to supply the sternoclavicular head of pectoralis major. SYN nervus pectoralis lateralis [TA], lateral anterior thoracic n.

lateral plantar n. [TA], one of two terminal branches of the tibial n.; it courses along the lateral side of the sole, dividing into superficial and deep branches; it supplies the skin of the lateral aspect of the sole and the lateral one and one-half toes; it innervates the intrinsic muscles of the plantar part of the foot with the exception of the abductor hallucis and the flexor digitorum brevis; its distribution in the foot is very similar to that of the ulnar n. in the hand. SYN nervus plantaris lateralis [TA].

lateral supraclavicular n. [TA], one of several branches of the C-3–C-4 portion of the cervical plexus that descend to the skin over the acromion and deltoid region. SYN nervus supraclavicularis lateralis [TA], posterior supraclavicular n.

lateral sural cutaneous n. [TA], it arises from the common fibular (peroneal) in the popliteal space and is distributed to the skin of the inferolateral surface of the calf. SYN nervus cutaneus surae lateralis [TA], lateral cutaneous n. of calf.

least splanchnic n. [TA], one of the abdominopelvic splanchnic n.'s arising in the thorax and penetrating the diaphragm to supply presynaptic sympathetic fibers for the renal plexus; often combined with the lesser splanchnic n., but occasionally existing as an independent n. SYN nervus splanchnicus imus [TA], lowest splanchnic n.⋆, smallest splanchnic n.

lesser internal cutaneous n., SYN medial cutaneous n. of arm.

lesser occipital n. [TA], arises from cervical plexus, conveying fibers from the ventral primary rami of the second and third cervical n.'s; supplies the skin of the posterior surface of the auricle and the adjacent portion of the scalp posterior to the auricle. SYN nervus occipitalis minor [TA].

lesser palatine n.'s [TA], usually two, these n.'s emerge through the lesser palatine foramina and supply the mucosa and glands of the soft palate and uvula; they are branches of the pterygopalatine ganglion and contain postsynaptic parasympathetic and sensory fibers of the maxillary n. SYN nervi palatini minores [TA].

lesser petrosal n. [TA], the parasympathetic root of the otic ganglion, derived from the tympanic plexus; it leaves the tympanic cavity through the canal for the lesser petrosal n. and passes within the cranium to the sphenopetrosal fissure, or to the foramen ovale, or to the petrosal foramen through which it descends to reach the otic ganglion; conveys presynaptic parasympathetic fibers from the glossopharyngeal n. concerned with secretomotor innervation of the parotid gland. SYN nervus petrosus minor [TA], parasympathetic root of otic ganglion⋆, radix parasympathica ganglii otici⋆, lesser superficial petrosal n.

lesser splanchnic n. [TA], one of the abdominopelvic splanchnic n.'s arising in the thorax from the last two thoracic sympathetic ganglia and passing through the diaphragm to the aorticorenal ganglion; conveys presynaptic sympathetic fibers and visceral afferent fibers. SYN nervus splanchnicus minor [TA].

lesser superficial petrosal n., SYN lesser petrosal n.

lingual n. [TA], one of the branches of the mandibular n. [CN V3], passing medial to the lateral pterygoid muscle, between the medial pterygoid and the mandible, and beneath the mucous membrane of the floor of the mouth to the side of the tongue over the anterior two-thirds of which it is distributed: it supplies also the mucous membrane of the floor of the mouth. It passes close to the lingual side of the roots of the second and third lower molar teeth and is endangered during tooth extractions. SYN nervus lingualis [TA].

long buccal n., SYN buccal n.

long ciliary n. [TA], one of two or three branches of the nasociliary n., which bypass the ciliary ganglion, supplying postsynaptic sympathetic fibers for the dilator pupillae muscle and sensory fibers for the ciliary muscles, iris, and cornea. SYN nervus ciliaris longus [TA].

long saphenous n., SYN saphenous n.

long subscapular n., SYN thoracodorsal n.

long thoracic n. [TA], arises from the fifth, sixth, and seventh cervical n.'s (roots of brachial plexus), descends the neck behind the brachial plexus, and is distributed to the serratus anterior muscle; it is somewhat unusual in that it courses on the superficial aspect of the muscle it supplies; its paralysis results in "winged scapula." SYN nervus thoracicus longus [TA], Bell respiratory n., external respiratory n. of Bell, posterior thoracic n.

lowest splanchnic n., ⋆official alternate term for least splanchnic n.

Ludwig n., SYN aortic n.

lumbar n.'s [L1–L5], five bilaterally paired spinal n.'s emerging from the lumbar portion of the spinal cord; the first four n.'s enter into the formation of the lumbar plexus, the fourth and fifth into that of the sacral plexus. SYN nervi lumbales.

lumbar splanchnic n.'s [TA], branches arising from the medial aspect of the lumbar sympathetic trunks that pass anteriorly and medially to convey presynaptic sympathetic fibers to, and visceral afferents from, the celiac, intermesenteric, aortic, and superior hypogastric plexuses. SYN nervi splanchnici lumbales [TA].

lumboinguinal n., femoral branch of genitofemoral n. SEE genitofemoral n.

mandibular n. [CN V3] [TA], the third division of the trigeminal

n. formed by the union of sensory fibers from the trigeminal ganglion and the motor root of the trigeminal nerve in the foramen ovale, through which the n. emerges; its branches are: meningeal, masseteric, deep temporal, lateral and medial pterygoid, buccal, auriculotemporal, lingual, and inferior alveolar; its sensory fibers are distributed to the auricle, external acoustic meatus, tympanic membrane, temporal region, cheek, skin overlying the mandible (except its angle), anterior 2/3 of tongue, floor of mouth, lower teeth, and gingiva; its motor fibers innervate all the muscles of mastication plus the mylohyoid, anterior belly of the digestic, and the tensores veli palati and tympani. SYN nervus mandibularis [CN V3] [TA], inferior maxillary n.

masseteric n. [TA], a muscular branch of the mandibular n. [CN V3] passing through the mandibular notch to the medial surface of the masseter muscle that it supplies and the temporomandibular joint. SYN nervus massetericus [TA].

masticator n., SYN motor *root* of trigeminal nerve.

maxillary n. [CN V2], the second division of the trigeminal n., passing from the trigeminal ganglion in the middle cranial fossa through the foramen rotundum into the pterygopalatine fossa, where it gives off ganglionic branches to the pterygopalatine ganglion and continues forward to give off the zygomatic n. and enter the orbit, where it continues as the infraorbital nerve. Its sensory fibers are distributed to the skin and conjunctiva of the lower eyelid, the skin and mucosa of the upper lip and cheek, the palate, upper teeth and gingiva, the maxillary sinus, wings of the nose, and posterior/interior nasal cavity. SYN nervus maxillaris [CN V2] [TA], superior maxillary n.

medial antebrachial cutaneous n., ⋆official alternate term for medial cutaneous n. of forearm.

medial anterior thoracic n., SYN medial pectoral n.

medial brachial cutaneous n., ⋆official alternate term for medial cutaneous n. of arm.

medial clunial n.'s [TA], terminal branches of the dorsal primary rami of the sacral n.'s, supplying the skin of the midgluteal region. SYN nervi clunium medii [TA], middle cluneal n.'s.

medial crural cutaneous n., ⋆official alternate term for medial cutaneous n. of leg.

medial cutaneous n. of arm [TA], arises from the medial cord of the brachial plexus, unites in the axilla with the lateral cutaneous branch of the second intercostal n., and supplies the skin of the medial side of the arm. SYN nervus cutaneus brachii medialis [TA], medial brachial cutaneous n.⋆, lesser internal cutaneous n., Wrisberg n. (1).

medial cutaneous n. of forearm [TA], arises from the medial cord of the brachial plexus, passes downward in company with the brachial artery and then the basilic vein, and supplies the skin of the anterior and ulnar surfaces of the forearm. SYN nervus cutaneus antebrachii medialis [TA], medial antebrachial cutaneous n.⋆.

medial cutaneous n. of leg [TA], branches of saphenous nerve distributed to the skin of the medial side of the leg. SYN rami cutanei cruris mediales nervi sapheni [TA], medial crural cutaneous n.⋆, medial crural cutaneous branches of saphenous nerve.

medial dorsal cutaneous n. [TA], the medial terminal branch of the superficial fibular (peroneal) n., supplying the dorsum of the foot and dorsal n.'s to the toes (except adjacent sides of great and second toes). SYN nervus cutaneus dorsalis medialis [TA], dorsal medial cutaneous n.

medial pectoral n. [TA], a n. that arises from the medial cord of the brachial plexus to supply the pectoral muscles; usually pierces pectoralis minor, then continues to supply mainly the sternocostal portion of pectoralis major. SYN nervus pectoralis medialis [TA], medial anterior thoracic n.

medial plantar n. [TA], one of the two terminal branches of the tibial n.; it courses along the medial aspect of the sole to supply the abductor hallucis and flexor digitorum brevis and, by way of common and proper digital branches, to innervate the skin of the medial part of the foot and medial three and one-half toes. SYN nervus plantaris medialis [TA].

medial popliteal n., SYN tibial n.

medial supraclavicular n. [TA], one of several n.'s arising from the C3–C4 loop of the cervical plexus that supply the skin over the medial end of the clavicle and upper medial part of the thorax. SYN nervus supraclavicularis medialis [TA], anterior supraclavicular n.

medial sural cutaneous n. [TA], arises from the tibial n. in the popliteal space, passes down the calf between the two heads of the gastrocnemius and unites in the middle of the leg with the communicating branch of the common peroneal to form the sural n., distributed to the skin of the distal and lateral surfaces of the leg and ankle. SYN nervus cutaneus surae medialis [TA], popliteal communicating n., tibial communicating n.

median n. [TA], formed by the union of medial and lateral roots from the medial and lateral cords of the brachial plexus, respectively; it supplies all the muscles in the anterior compartment of the forearm with the exception of the flexor carpi ulnaris and ulnar half of the flexor digitorum profundus; it passes through the carpal tunnel to supply the thenar muscles (except adductor pollicis and the deep head of flexor pollicis brevis) via its recurrent thenar branch; its sensory fibers are distributed to the skin of the palmar and distal dorsal aspects of the radial three and one-half digits and adjacent palm. The median n. is most commonly injured through compression in carpal tunnel syndrome, resulting in a loss of ability to oppose the thumb ("ape hand") and loss of sensation over the radial portion of the hand. SYN nervus medianus [TA].

mental n. [TA], a branch of the inferior alveolar n., arising in the mandibular canal and passing through the mental foramen to the chin and lower lip. SYN nervus mentalis [TA].

middle cervical cardiac n. [TA], one of the cardiopulmonary splanchnic n.'s conveying postsynaptic sympathetic fibers running downward, from the middle cervical ganglion along the subclavian artery (on the left) or the brachiocephalic (on the right side) to join the cardiac plexus. SYN nervus cardiacus cervicalis medius [TA].

middle cluneal n.'s, SYN medial clunial n.'s.

middle meningeal n., SYN meningeal *branch* of maxillary nerve.

middle supraclavicular n., SYN intermediate supraclavicular n.

mixed n. [TA], a n. containing both afferent and efferent fibers. SYN nervus mixtus [TA].

motor n. [TA], a n. composed mostly or entirely of efferent (motor) n. fibers conveying impulses that excites muscular contraction; motor n.'s in the autonomic nervous system also elicit secretions from glandular epithelia.

motor n. of face, SYN facial n. [CN VII].

musculocutaneous n. [TA], arises from lateral cord of the brachial plexus, passes through the coracobrachialis muscle, and then downward between the brachialis and biceps, supplying these three muscles and being continued distally as the lateral cutaneous n. of the forearm. SYN nervus musculocutaneus [TA].

musculocutaneous n. of leg, SYN superficial fibular n.

musculospiral n., SYN radial n.

myelinated n., a peripheral n. whose axons are surrounded by layers of Schwann cell membranes that form the myelin sheath; also called medullated n.'s.

mylohyoid n., SYN n. to mylohyoid.

n. to mylohyoid [TA], a small branch of the inferior alveolar n. given off posteriorly just before the n. enters the mandibular foramen, distributed to the anterior belly of the digastric muscle and to the mylohyoid muscle. SYN nervus mylohyoideus [TA], mylohyoid n.

nasal n., SYN nasociliary n.

nasociliary n. [TA], a branch of the ophthalmic n. [CN V1]in the superior orbital fissure, passing through the orbit, giving rise to the communicating branch to the ciliary ganglion, the long ciliary n.'s, the posterior and anterior ethmoidal n.'s, and terminating as the infratrochlear and nasal branches, which supply the mucous membrane of the nose, the skin of the tip of the nose, and the conjunctiva. SYN nervus nasociliaris [TA], nasal n.

nasopalatine n. [TA], a branch from the pterygopalatine ganglion, passing through the sphenopalatine foramen, crossing to and then down the nasal septum, and through the incisive foramen to supply the mucous membrane of the hard palate. SYN nervus nasopalatinus [TA].

ninth cranial n. [CN IX], SYN glossopharyngeal n. [CN IX].

obturator n. [TA], arises from the lumbar plexus, conveying fibers from the second, third, and fourth lumbar n.'s in the psoas muscle, crosses the brim of the pelvis, and enters the thigh through the obturator canal; it supplies muscles of the medial compartment of the thigh (adductors of thigh at the hip joint) and terminates as the cutaneous branch of the obturator n., supplying a small area of medial thigh above knee. SYN nervus obturatorius [TA].

oculomotor n. [CN III] [TA], the third cranial nerve, it supplies all the extrinsic muscles of the eye, except the lateral rectus and superior oblique; it also supplies the levator palpebrae superioris and conveys presynaptic parasympathetic fibers to the ciliary ganglion for innervation of the ciliary muscle and sphincter pupillae; its origin is in the midbrain below the cerebral aqueduct; it emerges from the brain in the interpeduncular fossa, pierces the dura mater to the side of the posterior clinoid process, passes in the lateral wall of the cavernous sinus, and enters the orbit through the superior orbital fissure. SYN nervus oculomotorius [CN III] [TA], motor oculi, oculomotorius, third cranial n. [CN III].

olfactory n.'s [CN I] [TA], collective term denoting the numerous olfactory filaments: slender fascicles each composed of the thin, unmyelinated axons of 8 to 12 of the bipolar olfactory receptor cells in the olfactory portion of the nasal mucosa; the olfactory filaments pass through the cribriform plate of the ethmoid bone and enter the olfactory bulb, where they terminate in synaptic contact with mitral cells, tufted cells, and granule cells. SEE ALSO olfactory *tract.* SYN fila olfactoria [TA], nervus olfactorii [CN I] [TA], first cranial n. [CN I], n. of smell, olfactory fila.

ophthalmic n. [CN V1] [TA], a branch of the trigeminal n. that passes forward from the trigeminal ganglion in the lateral wall of the cavernous sinus, entering the orbit through the superior orbital fissure; through its branches, frontal, lacrimal, and nasociliary, it supplies sensation to the orbit and its contents, the anterior part of the nasal cavity, and the skin of the nose and forehead. SYN nervus ophthalmicus [CN V1] [TA].

optic n. [CN II] [TA], although classified as a cranial nerve, it is actually an extension of the forebrain; it conveys afferent fibers from the ganglion cells of the retina, it passes out of the orbit through the optic canal to the chiasm, where part of the fibers cross to the opposite side and pass through the optic tract to the geniculate bodies, superior colliculus, and the pretectum. SYN nervus opticus [CN II] [TA], second cranial n. [CN II].

orbital n., SYN zygomatic n.

parasympathetic n., one of the n.'s of the parasympathetic nervous system.

pathetic n., SYN trochlear n. [CN IV].

pelvic splanchnic n.'s [TA], visceral branches from the ventral primary rami of the second, third, and fourth sacral spinal n.'s that join the inferior hypogastric plexus to form the pelvic plexuses, to and from which they convey presynaptic parasympathetic and sensory fibers, respectively. SYN nervi pelvici splanchnici [TA], parasympathetic root of pelvic ganglia★, radices parasympathicae gangliorum pelvicorum★, nervi erigentes.

perineal n.'s [TA], the superficial terminal branches of the pudendal n., supplying most of the muscles of the perineum (deep branch) as well as the skin of that region (superficial branch). SYN nervi perineales [TA].

peroneal communicating n., SYN sural communicating *branch* of common fibular nerve.

pharyngeal n. [TA], branch of pterygopalatine ganglion passing posteriorly through pharyngeal canal to supply postsynaptic parasympathetic fibers to mucus glands of nasopharynx. SYN nervus pharyngeus [TA], Bock n., pharyngeal branch of pterygopalatine ganglion, ramus pharyngeus ganglii pterygopalatini.

phrenic n. [TA], arises from the cervical plexus, chiefly conveying fibers from the fourth cervical n., passes downward in front of the anterior scalene muscle and enters the thorax between the subclavian artery and vein behind the sternoclavicular articulation; it then passes in front of the root of the lung to the diaphragm; it is mainly the motor n. of the diaphragm but sends sensory fibers to the mediastinal parietal pleura, the pericardium,

the diaphragmatic pleura and peritoneum, and branches (phrenicoabdominales branches) that communicate with branches from the celiac plexus. SYN nervus phrenicus [TA].

pneumogastric n., SYN vagus n. [CN X].

popliteal communicating n., SYN medial sural cutaneous n.

posterior ampullar n. [TA], a branch of the vestibular part of the eighth n. that supplies the crista ampullaris of the posterior semicircular duct. SYN nervus ampullaris posterior [TA].

posterior antebrachial n., SYN posterior interosseous n.

posterior antebrachial cutaneous n., ★official alternate term for posterior cutaneous n. of forearm.

posterior auricular n. [TA], the first extracranial branch of the facial n., it passes behind the ear, supplying the auricularis posterior, intrinsic muscles of the auricle and, through its occipital branch, the occipital belly of the occipitofrontalis muscle. SYN nervus auricularis posterior [TA].

posterior brachial cutaneous n., ★official alternate term for posterior cutaneous n. of arm.

posterior cutaneous n. of arm [TA], a branch of the radial n. supplying the skin of the posterior surface of the arm. SYN nervus cutaneus brachii posterior [TA], posterior brachial cutaneous n.★.

posterior cutaneous n. of forearm [TA], a branch of the radial n. supplying the skin of the dorsal surface of the forearm. SYN nervus cutaneus antebrachii posterior [TA], posterior antebrachial cutaneous n.★.

posterior cutaneous n. of thigh [TA], arises as a branch of the sacral plexus, conveying fibers from the ventral rami of first three sacral n.'s; supplies the skin of the posterior surface of the thigh and of the popliteal region (S1 and S2 component); it gives off a perineal branch (S3 component) that passes to the lateral aspect of the scrotum or labia majora. SYN nervus cutaneus femoris posterior [TA], posterior femoral cutaneous n.★, small sciatic n.

posterior ethmoidal n. [TA], a branch of the nasociliary n. providing sensory innervation to the sphenoidal sinus and the posterior ethmoidal air cells. SYN nervus ethmoidalis posterior [TA].

posterior femoral cutaneous n., ★official alternate term for posterior cutaneous n. of thigh.

posterior inferior nasal n.'s [TA], branches of greater palatine nerve to posterior inferior lateral wall of nasal cavity, including posterior aspect of mucosa over posterior portion of inferior nasal concha and meatus; may arise independently from pterygopalatine ganglion. SYN rami nasales posteriores inferiores nervi palatini majoris [TA], posterior inferior nasal branches of greater palatine nerve.

posterior interosseous n. [TA], the terminal portion of the deep branch of the radial n.; arises in the cubital region, penetrating and supplying the supinator and continuing with the posterior interosseous artery to supply all the extensor muscles in the forearm. SYN nervus interosseous antebrachii posterior [TA], dorsal interosseous n., nervus antebrachii posterior, nervus interosseous dorsalis, nervus interosseus posterior, posterior antebrachial n.

posterior labial n.'s [TA], terminal branches of the superficial perineal n., supplying the skin of the posterior portion of the labia and the vestibule of the vagina, corresponding to the posterior scrotal n.'s in the male. SYN nervi labiales posteriores [TA].

posterior scapular n., SYN dorsal scapular n.

posterior scrotal n.'s [TA], several terminal branches of the superficial perineal n. supplying the skin of the posterior portion of the scrotum, corresponding to the posterior labial n.'s in the female. SYN nervi scrotales posteriores [TA].

posterior supraclavicular n., SYN lateral supraclavicular n.

posterior thoracic n., SYN long thoracic n.

presacral n., ★official alternate term for superior hypogastric (nervous) *plexus.*

pressor n., an afferent n., stimulation of which excites a reflex vasoconstriction, thereby raising the blood pressure.

pressoreceptor n., a n. composed of afferent fibers the endings of which are sensitive to increases in mechanical pressure; the term specifically refers to sensory n.'s innervating the walls of hollow organs. SYN baroreceptor n.

proper palmar digital n.'s [TA], the palmar n.'s of the digits of the hand derived from common palmar digital n.'s; each n. supplies a palmar quadrant of a digit and a part of the dorsal surface of the distal phalanx. SYN nervi digitales palmares proprii [TA].

proper plantar digital n.'s [TA], the ten n.'s derived from the common plantar digital n.'s; each n. supplies a plantar quadrant of a toe and part of the dorsal surface of the distal phalanx. SYN nervi digitales plantares proprii [TA].

pterygoid n. [TA], one of two motor branches, the nerves to the lateral and medial pterygoid muscles, from the mandibular n., supplying muscles with fibers of the motor root of the trigeminal n. SYN nervus pterygoideus [TA].

n. of pterygoid canal [TA], the n. constituting the parasympathetic and sympathetic root of the pterygopalatine ganglion; it is formed in the region of the foramen lacerum by the union of the greater and deep petrosal n.'s and runs through the pterygoid canal to the pterygopalatine fossa. SYN nervus canalis pterygoidei [TA], facial root, radix facialis, vidian n.

pterygopalatine n.'s, SYN sensory root of pterygopalatine ganglion.

pudendal n. [TA], branch of the sacral plexus formed by fibers from the ventral primary rami of the second, third, and fourth sacral spinal n.'s; it exits the pelvis via the greater sciatic foramen, passes posterior to the sacrospinous ligament, and accompanies the internal pudendal artery, into the perineum via the lesser sciatic foramen; it gives off inferior rectal n.'s, then courses through the pudendal canal in the lateral wall of the ischiorectal fossa, terminating as the dorsal n. of the penis or of the clitoris. SYN nervus pudendus [TA], plexus pudendus nervosus, pudic n.

pudic n., SYN pudendal n.

radial n. [TA], arises from the posterior cord of the brachial plexus conveying fibers from all roots of the plexus; it curves around the posterior surface of the humerus and passes down to the cubital fossa where it divides into its two terminal branches, the cutaneous superficial branch and the motor deep branch; it supplies the muscles of the posterior compartments of the arm and forearm and overlying skin. The radial n. is most commonly injured by fractures of the middle 1/3 of the humerus, resulting in a loss of extension at the wrist ("wrist drop"). SYN nervus radialis [TA], musculospiral n.

recurrent n., SYN recurrent laryngeal n.

recurrent laryngeal n. [TA], a branch of the vagus n. curving upward, on the right side around the root of the subclavian artery, on the left side around the arch of the aorta, then passing superiorly, posterior to the common carotid artery between the trachea and the esophagus to the larynx; it supplies cardiac, tracheal, and esophageal branches and terminates as the inferior laryngeal n. SYN nervus laryngeus recurrens [TA], recurrent n.

recurrent meningeal n., meningeal branches of 1) mandibular, 2) maxillary, 3) ophthalmic, and 4) spinal n.'s.

n. to rhomboid, SYN dorsal scapular n.

saccular n. [TA], a branch of the inferior part of the vestibular n. going to the macula of the sacculus. SYN nervus saccularis [TA].

sacral splanchnic n.'s [TA], branches from the sacral sympathetic trunk that pass to the inferior hypogastric plexus; part of the abdominopelvic (sympathetic) splanchnic n.'s, but their specific function is unclear. They tend to be confused with the pelvic splanchnic n.'s, which are much more significant structures. SYN nervi splanchnici sacrales [TA].

sacral n.'s [S1–S5], five n.'s issuing from the sacral foramina on either side; the ventral branches of the first three enter into the formation of the sacral plexus, and the last two into the coccygeal plexus. SYN nervi sacrales [S1–S5].

saphenous n. [TA], a branch of the femoral, extending from the femoral triangle to the foot, becoming subcutaneous on the medial side of the knee; it supplies cutaneous branches to the skin of the leg and foot, by way of infrapatellar and medial crural branches. SYN nervus saphenus [TA], internal saphenous n., long saphenous n.

sciatic n. [TA], arises as the major product of the sacral plexus, exits the pelvis via the greater sciatic foramen, and descends in the posterior compartment of the thigh, deep to the long head of biceps femoris n.; at the apex of the popliteal fossa it divides into the common peroneal and tibial n.'s, although the two may sepa-

rate at higher levels. SYN nervus ischiadicus [TA], great sciatic n., nervus sciaticus.

second cranial n. [CN II], SYN optic n. [CN II].

secretomotor n., SYN secretory n.

secretory n., a n. conveying impulses that excite functional activity in a gland. SYN secretomotor n.

sensory n., an afferent n. conveying impulses that are processed by the central nervous system so as to become part of the organism's perception of self and its environment.

seventh cranial n. [CN VII], SYN facial n. [CN VII].

short ciliary n. [TA], one of a number of branches passing from the ciliary ganglion to the eyeball, supplying the ciliary muscles, iris, and tunics of the eyeball. SYN nervus ciliaris brevis [TA].

short saphenous n., SYN sural n.

sinus n. of Hering, SYN carotid branch of glossopharyngeal nerve (CN IX).

sinuvertebral n.'s, SYN meningeal branch of spinal nerves.

sixth cranial n. [CN VI], SYN abducent n. [CN VI].

small deep petrosal n., SYN caroticotympanic n.'s.

smallest splanchnic n., SYN least splanchnic n.

small sciatic n., SYN posterior cutaneous n. of thigh.

n. of smell, SYN olfactory n.'s [CN I].

somatic n., one of the n.'s of parietal sensation or voluntary motion, as distinguished from the visceral sensory, involuntary motor, and secretory n.'s.

spinal n.'s [TA], the n.'s emerging from the spinal cord; there are 31 pairs, each arising from the cord by rootlets that converge to form two roots, anterior (ventral or motor) and posterior (dorsal or sensory); the latter type is provided with a circumscribed enlargement, the spinal (dorsal root) ganglion; the two roots unite in the intervertebral foramen, and the mixed spinal n. almost immediately divides again into anterior and posterior (primary) rami, the former supplying the anterolateral trunk and the limbs, the latter the true muscles and overlying skin of the back. SYN nervi spinales [TA].

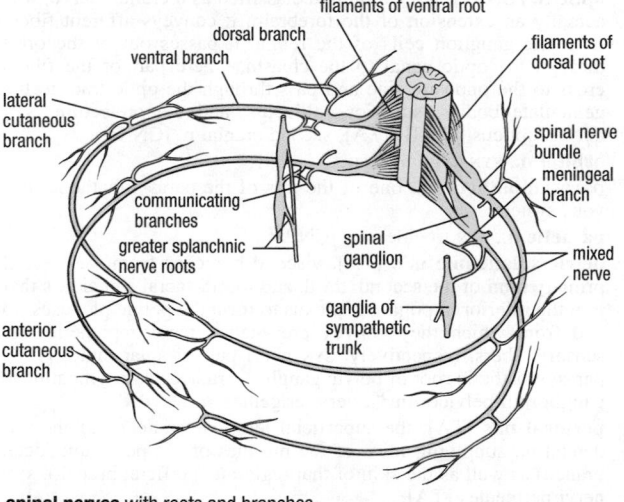

spinal nerves with roots and branches

spinal accessory n., SYN accessory n. [CN XI].

splanchnic n., one of the n.'s supplying the viscera. There are three groups of splanchnic n.'s: cardiopulmonary splanchnic n.'s that convey postsynaptic sympathetic fibers to thoracic viscera; abdominopelvic n.'s that convey presynpatic sympathetic fibers to the sympathetic ganglia of the abdominopelvic cavity; and pelvic splanchnic n.'s that convey presynaptic parasympathetic fibers to the pelvic ganglia. See also entries under the individual listings for the splanchnic n.'s mentioned.

n. to stapedius muscle [TA], a branch of the facial arising in the facial canal and innervating the stapedius muscle. SYN nervus stapedius [TA].

ne

statoacoustic n., SYN vestibulocochlear n. [CN VIII].

subclavian n. [TA], a branch from the superior trunk of the brachial plexus supplying the subclavius muscle. SYN nervus subclavius [TA].

subcostal n. [TA], the ventral ramus of the twelfth thoracic n.; it courses below the last rib paralleling the course of the intercostal nerves superior to it; it supplies parts of the abdominal muscles and gives off cutaneous branches to the skin of the lowermost ventrolateral abdominal wall and to the superolateral gluteal region. SYN nervus subcostalis [TA].

sublingual n. [TA], a branch of the lingual to the sublingual gland and mucosa of the floor of the mouth. SYN nervus sublingualis [TA].

suboccipital n. [TA], dorsal ramus of the first cervical n., passing through the suboccipital triangle and sending branches to the rectus capitis posterior major and minor, obliquus capitis superior and inferior, rectus capitis lateralis, and semispinalis capitis; the first cervical spinal n. is generally considered to have only motor fibers, but the suboccipital n. receives sensory fibers for proprioception via a communicating branch from the second cervical spinal n. SYN nervus suboccipitalis [TA].

subscapular n.'s [TA], two branches of the posterior cord of the brachial plexus, an upper and lower, supplying the subscapularis muscle; the lower subscapular n. also supplies the teres major muscle. SYN nervi subscapulares [TA].

sudomotor n.'s, n.'s containing autonomic (general visceral efferent–postganglionic) fibers that innervate sweat glands.

superficial cervical n., SYN transverse cervical n.

superficial fibular n. [TA], a branch of the common fibular (peroneal) n. that passes downward in the lateral compartment of the leg to supply the fibularis (peroneus) longus and brevis muscles and terminate as the intermediate and medial dorsal cutaneous n.'s supplying the skin of the dorsum of the foot and toes (except for adjacent sides of great and second toes). SYN nervus fibularis superficialis [TA], nervus peroneus superficialis★, superficial peroneal n.★, musculocutaneous n. of leg.

superficial peroneal n., ★official alternate term for superficial fibular n.

superior alveolar n.'s [TA], three branches (posterior, middle, and anterior) of the maxillary n. (or its continuation as the infraorbital n.) that enter the maxilla to supply the mucosa of the maxillary sinus, upper teeth, and gingiva. SYN nervi alveolares superiores [TA], superior dental n.'s.

superior cervical cardiac n. [TA], the uppermost of the cardiopulmonary splanchnic n.'s that arises from the lower part of the superior cervical ganglion and passes down to form, with branches of the vagus, the cardiac plexus. SYN nervus cardiacus cervicalis superior [TA].

superior clunial n.'s [TA], terminal branches of the dorsal primary rami of the lumbar n.'s, supplying the skin of the upper half of the gluteal region. SYN nervi clunium superiores [TA].

superior dental n.'s, SYN superior alveolar n.'s.

superior gluteal n. [TA], arises from sacral plexus, conveying fibers from the fourth and fifth lumbar and first sacral n.'s, and supplies the gluteus medius and minimus and tensor fasciae latae muscles (abductors and medial rotators of the hip joint). A lesion of this n. causes the pelvis to drop on the unsupported side when the foot is lifted off the ground (Trendelenburg sign). SYN nervus gluteus superior [TA].

superior laryngeal n. [TA], a branch of the vagus n. at the inferior ganglion; at the thyroid cartilage it divides into two branches: the internal laryngeal n., a sensory branch that supplies the mucous membrane of the larynx superior to the vocal folds, and the external laryngeal n., a motor branch that supplies the inferior pharyngeal constrictor and the cricothyroid muscle. SYN nervus laryngeus superior [TA].

superior lateral brachial cutaneous n., ★official alternate term for upper lateral cutaneous n. of arm.

superior maxillary n., SYN maxillary n. [CN V2].

supraorbital n. [TA], a branch of the frontal n. leaving the orbit through the supraorbital foramen or notch and dividing into branches distributed to the forehead and scalp, upper eyelid, and frontal sinus. SYN nervus supraorbitalis [TA].

suprascapular n. [TA], arises from the upper trunk of the brachial plexus (fifth and sixth cervical spinal n.'s), passes downward parallel to the cords of the brachial plexus, then through the scapular notch, supplying the supraspinatus and infraspinatus muscles, and also sending branches to the shoulder joint. It is vulnerable to injury in fractures of the middle 1/3 of the clavicle; a lesion of the suprascapular n. results in a loss of lateral rotation at the shoulder so that when relaxed the limb rotates medially (waiter's tip position); ability to initiate abduction is also affected. SYN nervus suprascapularis [TA].

supratrochlear n. [TA], a branch of the frontal n. supplying the medial part of the upper eyelid, the central part of the skin of the forehead, and the root of the nose. SYN nervus supratrochlearis [TA].

sural n. [TA], formed by the union of the medial sural cutaneous from the tibial and the peroneal communicating branch of the common peroneal n., usually about the middle of the calf, although this is highly variable; thence it accompanies the small saphenous vein around the lateral malleolus to the dorsum of the foot as the lateral dorsal cutaneous n. SYN nervus suralis [TA], external saphenous n., short saphenous n.

sympathetic n., one of the n.'s of the sympathetic nervous system.

temporomandibular n., SYN zygomatic n.

n. to tensor tympani (muscle) [TA], a branch of the mandibular n. conveying fibers from the motor root of the trigeminal n. that pass through the otic ganglion without synapse to supply the tensor tympani muscle. SYN nervus musculi tensoris tympani [TA].

n. to tensor veli palatini (muscle) [TA], a branch of the mandibular n. conveying fibers from the motor root of the trigeminal n. that pass through the otic ganglion without synapse to supply the tensor veli palatini muscle. SYN nervus musculi tensoris veli palatini [TA].

tenth cranial n. [CN X], SYN vagus n. [CN X].

tentorial n. [TA], the meningeal branch arising in a recurrent fashion from the intracranial portion of the ophthalmic n. supplying the tentorium cerebelli and supratentorial falx cerebri. SYN ramus meningeus recurrens nervi ophthalmici [TA], ramus tentorii★, nervus tentorii.

terminal n. [TA], delicate plexiform nerve strands passing parallel and medial to the olfactory tracts, distributing peripherally with the olfactory nerves and passing centrally into the anterior perforated substance; they are considered to have an autonomic function, but the exact nature of this is unknown. SYN nervus terminalis [TA].

third cranial n. [CN III], SYN oculomotor n. [CN III].

third occipital n. [TA], medial branch of the dorsal primary ramus of the third cervical n.; this is usually joined with the greater occipital, but may exist as an independent n. supplying cutaneous branches to the scalp and nucha. SYN nervus occipitalis tertius [TA].

thoracic cardiac n.'s, SYN thoracic cardiac *branches* of thoracic ganglia, under *branch*.

thoracic splanchnic n.'s, splanchnic n.'s arising from the thoracic portion of the sympathetic trunks; the upper thoracic splanchnic n.'s (from T1 to T4 or 5) pass to viscera above the diaphragm (mainly heart, lungs, and esophagus) and so are cardiopulmonary splanchnic n.'s; the lower thoracic splanchnic n.'s form the greater, lesser, and lowest splanchnic n.'s and supply viscera below the level of the diaphragm, and so are abdominopelvic splanchnic n.'s.

thoracic n.'s [T1–T12] [TA], twelve n.'s on each side, mixed motor and sensory, supplying the muscles and skin of the thoracic and abdominal walls. SYN nervi thoracici [T1–12].

thoracoabdominal n.'s, the ventral primary rami of spinal n.'s T7–T11 (seventh to eleventh intercostal n.'s), which supply the abdominal as well as the thoracic wall; innervate intercostal, subcostal, serratus posterior inferior, transversus abdominis, external and internal oblique, and rectus abdominis muscles, and provide sensory branches to the periphery of the diaphragm, and parietal pleura and peritoneum. SYN anterior cutaneous n.'s of abdomen, pectoral and abdominal anterior cutaneous branch of intercostal nerves, rami cutanei anteriores pectoralis et abdominalis nervorum intercostalium, ramus cutaneus anterior (pectoralis et abdominalis) nervorum thoracicorum.

thoracodorsal n. [TA], arises from the posterior cord of the brachial plexus; it contains fibers from the sixth, seventh, and eighth cervical n.'s and supplies the latissimus dorsi muscle. SYN nervus thoracodorsalis [TA], long subscapular n.

n. to thyrohyoid muscle, SYN thyrohyoid *branch* of ansa cervicalis.

tibial n. [TA], one of the two major divisions of the sciatic n., it courses down the back of the leg to terminate as the medial and lateral plantar n.'s in the foot; it supplies the hamstring muscles, the muscles of the back of the leg (the dorsiflexors and invertors of the foot), and the plantar aspect of the foot, as well as the skin on the back of the leg and sole of the foot. SYN nervus tibialis [TA], medial popliteal n.

tibial communicating n., SYN medial sural cutaneous n.

Tiedemann n., a sympathetic n. accompanying the central artery of the retina in the optic n.

transverse cervical n. [TA], a branch of the cervical plexus that supplies the skin over the anterior triangle of the neck. SYN nervus transversus colli [TA], nervus transversus cervicalis✗, cutaneous cervical n., nervus cervicalis superficialis, superficial cervical n., transverse n. of neck.

transverse n. of neck, SYN transverse cervical n.

trifacial n., SYN trigeminal n. [CN V].

ℹ trigeminal n. [CN V] [TA], the chief sensory n. of the face and the motor n. of the muscles of mastication; its nuclei are in the mesencephalon and in the pons and medulla oblongata extending down into the cervical portion of the spinal cord; it emerges by two roots, sensory and motor, from the lateral portion of the surface of the pons, and enters a cavity of the dura mater, the trigeminal cave, at the apex of the petrous portion of the temporal bone, where the sensory root expands to form the trigeminal ganglion; from there the three divisions (ophthalmic [CN V1], maxillary [CN V2], and mandibular [CN V3] n.'s) arise. SYN nervus trigeminus [CN V] [TA], fifth cranial n. [CN V], trifacial n.

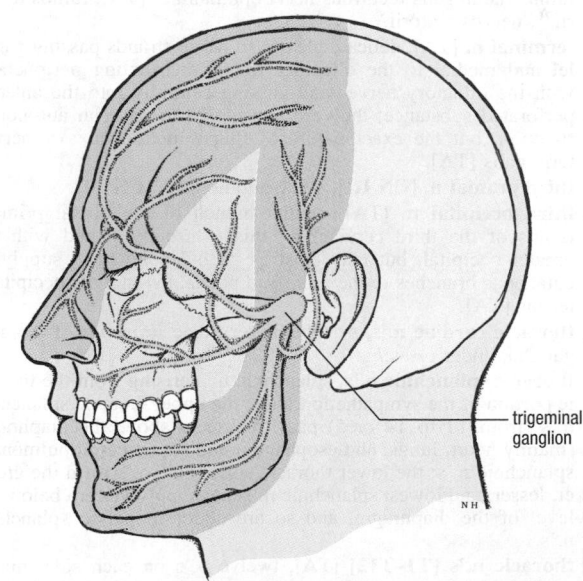

trigeminal ganglion

trigeminal nerve: the three sensory branches arise from the trigeminal ganglion and innervate the areas shown in color; (purple) ophthalmic nerve, CN V^1; (blue) maxillary nerve, CN V^2; (red) mandibular nerve, CN V^3

trochlear n. [CN IV] [TA], supplies the superior oblique muscle of the eye; its origin is in the midbrain below the cerebral aque-

duct, and its fibers decussate in the superior medullary velum, and emerge from the brain at the side of the frenulum, the only cranial n. to arise from the dorsal aspect of the brainstem; it therefore has the longest intracranial course, entering the dura in the free edge of the tentorium, close to the posterior clinoid process, and passing in the lateral wall of the cavernous sinus to enter the orbit through the superior orbital fissure. SYN nervus trochlearis [CN IV] [TA], fourth cranial n. [CN IV], pathetic n.

twelfth cranial n. [CN XII], SYN hypoglossal n. [CN XII].

tympanic n. [TA], a n. from the inferior ganglion of the glossopharyngeal n., passing through the tympanic canaliculus to the tympanic cavity, forming there the tympanic plexus that supplies the mucous membrane of the tympanic cavity, mastoid cells, and auditory tube; presynaptic parasympathetic fibers also pass through the tympanic n. via the lesser superficial petrosal n. to the otic ganglion, where they synapse with postsynaptic fibers that continue to supply the parotid gland. SYN nervus tympanicus [TA], Andersch n., Jacobson n.

n. of tympanic membrane, SYN *branches* of auriculotemporal nerve to tympanic membrane, under *branch*.

ulnar n. [TA], arises from the medial cord of the brachial plexus conveying fibers mainly from the C8 and T1 nerves; it passes down the arm, behind the medial epicondyle of the humerus, and down the ulnar side of the anterior compartment of the forearm to the hand; it gives off muscular branches in the forearm to the flexor carpi ulnaris muscle and the ulnar portion of flexor digitorum profundus and supplies the hypothenar, interosseous, medial lumbricals, adductor pollicis, and deep head of flexor hallucis brevis, and the intrinsic muscles of the hand and the skin of the small finger and medial side of the ring finger and adjacent portions of the palm of the hand. The ulnar n. is most vulnerable to injury where it passes subcutaneously behind the medial epicondyle of the humerus. Mild injury here produces "crazy bone" sensation. An ulnar n. lesion here results in loss of flexion of metacarpophalangeal joints and of extension at the interphalangeal joints ("claw hand"). SYN nervus ulnaris [TA], cubital n.

unmyelinated n., a n. made up largely, or exclusively, of unmyelinated fibers; a n. composed of axons having no myelin covering, but lying in troughs in Schwann cells; a slow conducting n.

upper lateral cutaneous n. of arm [TA], the terminal branch of the axillary n. supplying the skin over the lower portion of the deltoid and for a distance below its insertion. SYN nervus cutaneus brachii lateralis superior [TA], superior lateral brachial cutaneous n.✗

upper subscapular n., SEE subscapular n.'s.

upper thoracic splanchnic n.'s, SYN thoracic cardiac *branches* of thoracic ganglia, under *branch*.

utricular n. [TA], a branch of the utriculoampullar n., supplying the macula of the utricle. SYN nervus utricularis [TA].

utriculoampullar n. [TA], a division of the vestibular part of the eighth cranial n.; it gives off branches to the macula of the utricle (utricular n.) and to the cristae of the ampullae of the anterior and lateral semicircular ducts (anterior and lateral ampullary n.'s). SYN nervus utriculoampullaris [TA].

vaginal n.'s [TA], several n.'s passing from the uterovaginal plexus to the vagina. SYN nervi vaginales [TA].

vagus n. [CN X] [TA], a mixed n. that arises by numerous small roots from the side of the medulla oblongata, between the glossopharyngeal above and the accessory below; it leaves the cranial cavity by the jugular foramen and passes down to supply the pharynx, larynx, trachea, lungs, heart, and the gastrointestinal tract as far as the left colic (splenic) flexure; the only cranial nerve that does not arise from the brain, but is classified as such because it exits from the cranium. SYN nervus vagus [CN X] [TA], pneumogastric n., tenth cranial n. [CN X], vagus.

Valentin n., a n. that connects the pterygopalatine ganglion with the abducens n.

vascular n.'s [TA], a small n. filament that supplies the wall of a blood vessel. SYN nervi vasculorum [TA].

vasomotor n., a motor n. effecting or inhibiting contraction of the blood vessels.

vertebral n., a branch from the stellate ganglion that ascends along the vertebral artery to the level of the axis or atlas, giving branches to the cervical n.'s and meninges. SYN nervus vertebralis.

vestibular n. [TA], the part of the vestibulocochlear n. [CN VIII] peripheral to the vestibular root; it is composed of the central processes of bipolar neurons that have their terminals of their peripheral processes on the hair cells in the ampullae of the semicircular ducts and the maculae of the saccule and utricle, and cell bodies of the vestibular ganglion. SEE ALSO vestibular *root*. SYN nervus vestibularis [TA], pars vestibularis nervi vestibulo-cochlearis, superior part of vestibulocochlear nerve, vestibular part of vestibulocochlear nerve.

vestibulocochlear n. [CN VIII] [TA], a composite sensory n. innervating the receptor cells of the membranous labyrinth; it consists of two major, anatomically and functionally distinct components, each of which have different central connections: the vestibular n. and the cochlear n. SYN nervus vestibulocochlearis [CN VIII] [TA], eighth cranial n. [CN VIII], eighth n., nervus acusticus, nervus octavus, nervus statoacusticus, octavus, statoacoustic n.

vidian n., SYN n. of pterygoid canal.

visceral n., a term describing n.'s conveying autonomic (general visceral efferent) fibers.

volar interosseous n., SYN anterior interosseous n.

Wrisberg n., (1) SYN medial cutaneous n. of arm; **(2)** SYN intermediate n.

zygomatic n. [TA], a branch of the maxillary n. [CN V2] in the inferior orbital fissure through which it passes; it gives rise to two sensory branches, the zygomaticotemporal and zygomaticofacial, which supply the skin of the temporal and zygomatic regions and is continued as the communicating branch of the lacrimal n. with the zygomatic n. SYN nervus zygomaticus [TA], orbital n., temporomandibular n.

---

nerve root sleeve. In myelography, the funnel-shaped extension of the opacified subarachnoid space that surrounds each nerve root as it enters its neural foramen.

ner·vi (ner′vī). Plural of nervus. [L.]

ner·vi·mo·til·i·ty (ner-vi-mō-til′i-tē). Capability of movement in response to a nervous stimulus. SYN neurimotility.

ner·vi·mo·tion (ner-vi-mō′shŭn). Movement in response to a nervous stimulus.

ner·vi·mo·tor (ner-vi-mō′ter). Relating to a motor nerve. SYN neurimotor.

ner·vine (ner′vīn). Acting therapeutically, especially as a sedative, upon the nervous system.

ner·vone (ner′vōn). A cerebroside containing a nervonyl moiety.

ner·von·ic ac·id (ner-von′-ik). A 24-carbon straight-chain fatty acid unsaturated between C-15 and C-16; occurs in cerebrosides such as nervone.

ner·vous (ner′vŭs). **1.** Relating to a nerve or the nerves. **2.** Easily excited or agitated; suffering from mental or emotional instability; tense or anxious. **3.** Formerly, denoting a temperament characterized by excessive mental and physical alertness, rapid pulse, excitability, often volubility, but not always fixity of purpose. [L. *nervosus*]

ner·vous break·down. Nonmedical term for an emotional or mental illness; often a euphemism for a psychiatric disorder.

ner·vous·ness (ner′vŭs-nes). A condition of being nervous (2).

NERVUS

---

ner·vus, gen. and pl. **ner·vi** (ner′vŭs, -vī) [TA]. SYN nerve. [L.]
  n. abdu′cens [CN VI] [TA], SYN abducent *nerve* [CN VI].
  n. accesso′rius [CN XI] [TA], SYN accessory *nerve* [CN XI].
  n. acu′sticus, SYN vestibulocochlear *nerve* [CN VIII].

ner′vi alveola′res superio′res [TA], SYN superior alveolar *nerves*, under *nerve*.

nervi alveolares superiores anteriores [TA],

  n. alveola′ris infe′rior [TA], SYN inferior alveolar *nerve*.

  n. ampulla′ris ante′rior [TA], SYN anterior ampullary *nerve*.

  n. ampulla′ris latera′lis [TA], SYN lateral ampullar *nerve*.

  n. ampulla′ris poste′rior [TA], SYN posterior ampullar *nerve*.

nervi anales inferiores [TA], SYN inferior anal *nerves*, under *nerve*.

  n. anococcyg′eus, SYN anococcygeal *nerve*.

  n. antebra′chii anter′ior, SYN anterior interosseous *nerve*.

  n. antebra′chii poste′rior, SYN posterior interosseous *nerve*.

  n. articula′ris, SYN articular *nerve*.

ner′vi auricula′res anterio′res [TA], SYN anterior auricular *nerves*, under *nerve*.

  n. auricula′ris mag′nus [TA], SYN great auricular *nerve*.

  n. auricula′ris poste′rior [TA], SYN posterior auricular *nerve*.

  n. auriculotempora′lis [TA], SYN auriculotemporal *nerve*.

  n. autonomicus [TA], SYN autonomic *nerve*.

  n. axilla′ris [TA], SYN axillary *nerve*.

  n. bucca′lis [TA], SYN buccal *nerve*.

  n. cana′lis pterygoi′dei [TA], SYN *nerve* of pterygoid canal.

ner′vi cardi′aci thora′cici, SYN thoracic cardiac *branches* of thoracic ganglia, under *branch*.

  n. cardi′acus cervica′lis infe′rior [TA], SYN inferior cervical cardiac *nerve*.

  n. cardi′acus cervica′lis me′dius [TA], SYN middle cervical cardiac *nerve*.

  n. cardi′acus cervica′lis supe′rior [TA], SYN superior cervical cardiac *nerve*.

ner′vi carot′ici exter′ni [TA], SYN external carotid *nerves*, under *nerve*.

nervi caroticotympan′icus, SYN caroticotympanic *nerves*, under *nerve*.

  n. carot′icus inter′nus [TA], SYN internal carotid *nerve*.

ner′vi caverno′si clitor′idis [TA], SYN cavernous *nerves* of clitoris, under *nerve*.

ner′vi caverno′si pe′nis [TA], SYN cavernous *nerves* of penis, under *nerve*.

ner′vi cervica′les [C1–C8], SYN cervical *nerves* [C1–C8], under *nerve*.

  n. cervica′lis superficia′lis, SYN transverse cervical *nerve*.

  n. cilia′ris bre′vis, pl. **ner′vi cilia′res bre′ves** [TA], SYN short ciliary *nerve*.

  n. cilia′ris lon′gus, pl. **ner′vi cilia′res lon′gi** [TA], SYN long ciliary *nerve*.

ner′vi clu′nium inferio′res [TA], SYN inferior clunial *nerves*, under *nerve*.

ner′vi clu′nium me′dii [TA], SYN medial clunial *nerves*, under *nerve*.

ner′vi clu′nium superio′res [TA], SYN superior clunial *nerves*, under *nerve*.

  n. coccyg′eus [Co] [TA], SYN coccygeal *nerve* [Co].

  n. cochlea′ris [TA], SYN cochlear *nerve*; SEE ALSO cochlear *root* of VIII nerve.

  n. commu′nicans fibula′ris, SYN sural communicating *branch* of common fibular nerve.

  n. commu′nicans perone′us, SYN sural communicating *branch* of common fibular nerve.

ner′vi crania′les [TA], SYN cranial *nerves*, under *nerve*.

  n. cuta′neus [TA], SYN cutaneous *nerve*.

  n. cuta′neus antebra′chii latera′lis [TA], SYN lateral cutaneous *nerve* of forearm.

  n. cuta′neus antebra′chii media′lis [TA], SYN medial cutaneous *nerve* of forearm.

  n. cuta′neus antebra′chii poste′rior [TA], SYN posterior cutaneous *nerve* of forearm.

  n. cuta′neus bra′chii latera′lis infe′rior [TA], SYN inferior lateral cutaneous *nerve* of arm.

n. cuta′neus bra′chii latera′lis supe′rior [TA], SYN upper lateral cutaneous *nerve* of arm.

n. cuta′neus bra′chii media′lis [TA], SYN medial cutaneous *nerve* of arm.

n. cuta′neus bra′chii poste′rior [TA], SYN posterior cutaneous *nerve* of arm.

n. cuta′neus dorsa′lis interme′dius [TA], SYN intermediate dorsal cutaneous *nerve*.

n. cuta′neus dorsa′lis latera′lis [TA], SYN lateral dorsal cutaneous *nerve*.

n. cuta′neus dorsa′lis media′lis [TA], SYN medial dorsal cutaneous *nerve*.

n. cuta′neus fem′oris latera′lis [TA], SYN lateral cutaneous *nerve* of thigh.

n. cuta′neus fem′oris poste′rior [TA], SYN posterior cutaneous *nerve* of thigh.

n. cuta′neus su′rae latera′lis [TA], SYN lateral sural cutaneous *nerve*.

n. cuta′neus su′rae media′lis [TA], SYN medial sural cutaneous *nerve*.

ner′vi digita′les dorsa′les, SYN dorsal digital *nerves* of hand, under *nerve*.

nervi digitales dorsales nervi fibularis profundi [TA], SYN dorsal digital *nerves* of deep fibular nerve, under *nerve*.

nervi digitales dorsales nervi fibularis superficialis [TA], SYN dorsal digital *nerves* of superficial fibular nerve, under *nerve*.

nervi digitales dorsales nervi ulnaris [TA], SYN dorsal digital *nerves* of ulnar nerve, under *nerve*.

ner′vi digita′les dorsa′les pe′dis [TA], SYN dorsal digital *nerves* of foot, under *nerve*.

ner′vi digita′les palma′res commu′nes [TA], SYN common palmar digital *nerves*, under *nerve*.

ner′vi digita′les palma′res pro′prii [TA], SYN proper palmar digital *nerves*, under *nerve*.

ner′vi digita′les planta′res commu′nes [TA], SYN common plantar digital *nerves*, under *nerve*.

ner′vi digita′les planta′res pro′prii [TA], SYN proper plantar digital *nerves*, under *nerve*.

n. dorsa′lis clitor′idis [TA], SYN dorsal *nerve* of clitoris.

n. dorsa′lis pe′nis [TA], SYN dorsal *nerve* of penis.

n. dorsa′lis scap′ulae [TA], SYN dorsal scapular *nerve*.

ner′vi erigen′tes, SYN pelvic splanchnic *nerves*, under *nerve*.

n. ethmoida′lis ante′rior [TA], SYN anterior ethmoidal *nerve*.

n. ethmoida′lis poste′rior [TA], SYN posterior ethmoidal *nerve*.

n. facia′lis [CN VII] [TA], SYN facial *nerve* [CN VII].

n. femora′lis [TA], SYN femoral *nerve*.

n. fibula′ris commu′nis [TA], SYN common fibular *nerve*.

n. fibula′ris profun′dus [TA], SYN deep fibular *nerve*.

n. fibula′ris superficia′lis [TA], SYN superficial fibular *nerve*.

n. fronta′lis [TA], SYN frontal *nerve*.

n. furca′lis, SYN fourth lumbar *nerve* [L4].

n. genitofemora′lis [TA], SYN genitofemoral *nerve*.

n. glossopharyn′geus [CN IX] [TA], SYN glossopharyngeal *nerve* [CN IX].

n. glu′teus infe′rior [TA], SYN inferior gluteal *nerve*.

n. glu′teus supe′rior [TA], SYN superior gluteal *nerve*.

n. hemorrhoida′lis, SEE superior rectal (nervous) *plexus*, inferior anal *nerves*, under *nerve*.

n. hypogas′tricus [TA], SYN hypogastric *nerve*.

n. hypoglos′sus [CN XII] [TA], SYN hypoglossal *nerve* [CN XII].

n. iliohypogas′tricus [TA], SYN iliohypogastric *nerve*.

n. ilioinguina′lis [TA], SYN ilioinguinal *nerve*.

n. im′par, SYN terminal *filum*.

n. infraorbita′lis [TA], SYN infraorbital *nerve*.

n. infratrochlea′ris [TA], SYN infratrochlear *nerve*.

ner′vi intercosta′les [TA], SYN intercostal *nerves*, under *nerve*.

ner′vi intercostobrachia′les [TA], SYN intercostobrachial *nerves*, under *nerve*.

n. interme′dius [TA], SYN intermediate *nerve*.

n. interos′seus antebrachii ante′rior [TA], SYN anterior interosseous *nerve*.

n. interosseus antebrachii posterior [TA], SYN posterior interosseous *nerve*.

n. interos′seus cru′ris [TA], SYN crural interosseous *nerve*.

n. interos′seus dorsa′lis, SYN posterior interosseous *nerve*.

n. interos′seus poste′rior, SYN posterior interosseous *nerve*.

n. ischia′dicus [TA], SYN sciatic *nerve*.

n. jugula′ris [TA], SYN jugular *nerve*.

ner′vi labia′les anterio′res [TA], SYN anterior labial *nerves*, under *nerve*.

ner′vi labia′les posterio′res [TA], SYN posterior labial *nerves*, under *nerve*.

n. lacrima′lis [TA], SYN lacrimal *nerve*.

n. laryn′geus infe′rior [TA], SYN inferior laryngeal *nerve*.

n. laryn′geus recur′rens [TA], SYN recurrent laryngeal *nerve*.

n. laryn′geus supe′rior [TA], SYN superior laryngeal *nerve*.

n. lingua′lis [TA], SYN lingual *nerve*.

ner′vi lumba′les, SYN lumbar *nerves* [L1–L5], under *nerve*.

n. mandibula′ris [CN V3] [TA], SYN mandibular *nerve* [CN V3].

n. masseter′icus [TA], SYN masseteric *nerve*.

n. maxilla′ris [CN V2] [TA], SYN maxillary *nerve* [CN V2].

n. mea′tus acus′tici exter′ni [TA], SYN *nerve* to external acoustic meatus.

n. media′nus [TA], SYN median *nerve*.

n. menta′lis [TA], SYN mental *nerve*.

n. mixtus [TA], SYN mixed *nerve*.

n. musculi tenso′ris tym′pani [TA], SYN *nerve* to tensor tympani (muscle).

n. musculi tenso′ris ve′li palati′ni [TA], SYN *nerve* to tensor veli palatini (muscle).

n. musculocuta′neus [TA], SYN musculocutaneous *nerve*.

n. mylohyoi′deus [TA], SYN *nerve* to mylohyoid.

n. nasocilia′ris [TA], SYN nasociliary *nerve*.

n. nasopalati′nus [TA], SYN nasopalatine *nerve*.

ner′vi nervo′rum, nerves distributed to the sheaths of nerve trunks.

n. obturato′rius [TA], SYN obturator *nerve*.

n. occipita′lis ma′jor [TA], SYN greater occipital *nerve*.

n. occipita′lis mi′nor [TA], SYN lesser occipital *nerve*.

n. occipita′lis ter′tius [TA], SYN third occipital *nerve*.

n. octa′vus, SYN vestibulocochlear *nerve* [CN VIII].

n. oculomoto′rius [CN III] [TA], SYN oculomotor *nerve* [CN III].

n. olfacto′rii [CN I] [TA], SYN olfactory *nerves* [CN I], under *nerve*; SEE ALSO olfactory *tract*.

n. ophthal′micus [CN V1] [TA], SYN ophthalmic *nerve* [CN V1].

n. op′ticus [CN II] [TA], SYN optic *nerve* [CN II].

ner′vi palati′ni mino′res [TA], SYN lesser palatine *nerves*, under *nerve*.

n. palati′nus ma′jor [TA], SYN greater palatine *nerve*.

n. pectora′lis lateral′is [TA], SYN lateral pectoral *nerve*.

n. pectoral′is medial′is [TA], SYN medial pectoral *nerve*.

ner′vi pel′vici splanch′nici [TA], SYN pelvic splanchnic *nerves*, under *nerve*.

ner′vi perinea′les [TA], SYN perineal *nerves*, under *nerve*.

n. perone′us commu′nis, ✶official alternate term for common fibular *nerve*.

n. perone′us profun′dus, ✶official alternate term for deep fibular *nerve*.

n. perone′us superficia′lis, ✶official alternate term for superficial fibular *nerve*.

n. petro′sus ma′jor [TA], SYN greater petrosal *nerve*.

n. petro′sus mi′nor [TA], SYN lesser petrosal *nerve*.

n. petro′sus profun′dus [TA], SYN deep petrosal *nerve*.

n. pharyngeus [TA], SYN pharyngeal *nerve*.

ner′vi phren′ici accesso′rii [TA], SYN accessory phrenic *nerves*, under *nerve*.

n. phren′icus [TA], SYN phrenic *nerve*.

n. planta´ris latera´lis [TA], SYN lateral plantar *nerve.*

n. planta´ris media´lis [TA], SYN medial plantar *nerve.*

n. presacra´lis, ☆official alternate term for superior hypogastric (nervous) *plexus.*

n. pterygoi´deus [TA], SYN pterygoid *nerve.*

ner´vi pterygopalati´ni, SYN sensory *root* of pterygopalatine ganglion.

n. puden´dus [TA], SYN pudendal *nerve.*

n. radia´lis [TA], SYN radial *nerve.*

ner´vi recta´les inferio´res, ☆official alternate term for inferior anal *nerves,* under *nerve.*

n. saccula´ris [TA], SYN saccular *nerve.*

ner´vi sacra´les [S1–S5], SYN sacral *nerves* [S1–S5], under *nerve.*

n. saphe´nus [TA], SYN saphenous *nerve.*

n. sciaticus, SYN sciatic *nerve.*

ner´vi scrota´les anterio´res [TA], SYN anterior scrotal *nerves,* under *nerve.*

ner´vi scrota´les posterio´res [TA], SYN posterior scrotal *nerves,* under *nerve.*

n. spermat´icus exter´nus, SYN genital *branch* of genitofemoral nerve.

ner´vi sphenopalati´ni, SYN sensory *root* of pterygopalatine ganglion.

ner´vi spina´les [TA], SYN spinal *nerves,* under *nerve.*

n. spinosus, ☆official alternate term for meningeal *branch* of mandibular nerve.

ner´vi splanch´nici lumba´les [TA], SYN lumbar splanchnic *nerves,* under *nerve.*

ner´vi splanch´nici sacra´les [TA], SYN sacral splanchnic *nerves,* under *nerve.*

n. splanch´nicus i´mus [TA], SYN least splanchnic *nerve.*

n. splanch´nicus ma´jor [TA], SYN greater splanchnic *nerve.*

n. splanch´nicus mi´nor [TA], SYN lesser splanchnic *nerve.*

n. stape´dius [TA], SYN *nerve* to stapedius muscle.

n. statoacus´ticus, SYN vestibulocochlear *nerve* [CN VIII].

n. subcla´vius [TA], SYN subclavian *nerve.*

n. subcosta´lis [TA], SYN subcostal *nerve.*

n. sublingua´lis [TA], SYN sublingual *nerve.*

n. suboccipita´lis [TA], SYN suboccipital *nerve.*

nervi subscapula´res [TA], SYN subscapular *nerves,* under *nerve.*

n. supraclavicula´ris interme´dius [TA], SYN intermediate supraclavicular *nerve.*

n. supraclavicula´ris latera´lis [TA], SYN lateral supraclavicular *nerve.*

n. supraclavicula´ris media´lis [TA], SYN medial supraclavicular *nerve.*

n. supraorbita´lis [TA], SYN supraorbital *nerve.*

n. suprascapula´ris [TA], SYN suprascapular *nerve.*

n. supratrochlea´ris [TA], SYN supratrochlear *nerve.*

n. sura´lis [TA], SYN sural *nerve.*

ner´vi tempora´les profun´di [TA], SYN deep temporal *nerves,* under *nerve.*

n. tento´rii, SYN tentorial *nerve.*

n. termina´lis [TA], SYN terminal *nerve.*

ner´vi thora´cici [T1–12], SYN thoracic *nerves* [T1–T12], under *nerve.*

n. thora´cicus lon´gus [TA], SYN long thoracic *nerve.*

n. thoracodorsa´lis [TA], SYN thoracodorsal *nerve.*

n. tibia´lis [TA], SYN tibial *nerve.*

n. transversus cervicalis, ☆official alternate term for transverse cervical *nerve.*

n. transver´sus col´li [TA], SYN transverse cervical *nerve.*

n. trigem´inus [CN V] [TA], SYN trigeminal *nerve* [CN V].

n. trochlea´ris [CN IV] [TA], SYN trochlear *nerve* [CN IV].

n. tympan´icus [TA], SYN tympanic *nerve.*

n. ulna´ris [TA], SYN ulnar *nerve.*

n. utricula´ris [TA], SYN utricular *nerve.*

n. utriculoampulla´ris [TA], SYN utriculoampullar *nerve.*

ner´vi vagina´les [TA], SYN vaginal *nerves,* under *nerve.*

n. va´gus [CN X] [TA], SYN vagus *nerve* [CN X].

nervi vascula´rorum [TA], SYN vascular *nerves,* under *nerve.*

n. vertebra´lis, SYN vertebral *nerve.*

n. vestibula´ris [TA], SYN vestibular *nerve;* SEE ALSO vestibular *root* of vestibulocochlear nerve.

n. vestibulocochlea´ris [CN VIII] [TA], SYN vestibulocochlear *nerve* [CN VIII]; See entries under radix.

n. zygomat´icus [TA], SYN zygomatic *nerve.*

ne·sid·i·ec·to·my (nē-sid´ē-ek´tō-mē). Excision of islet tissue of the pancreas. [G. *nēsidion,* islet, dim. of *nēsos,* island, + *ektomē,* excision]

ne·sid·i·o·blast (nē-sid´ē-ō-blast). A pancreatic islet-forming cell. [G. *nēsidion,* dim. of *nēsos,* island, + *blastos,* germ]

ne·sid·i·o·blas·to·sis (ne-sid´ē-ō-blas-tō´sis). Hyperplasia of the cells of the islets of Langerhans. [nesidioblast + G. *-osis,* tumor]

Nessler, A., German chemist, 1827–1905. SEE N. *reagent.*

ness·ler·ize (nes´ler-īz). To treat with Nessler reagent; used in the determination of urea nitrogen in the blood and in the urine.

nest. A group or collection of similar objects. SEE ALSO nidus. [A.S.]

Brunn n., glandlike invagination of surface transitional epithelium in the epithelium of the lower urinary tract.

cell n., a small focus or accumulation of one type of cell that is different from the other cells in the tissue.

epithelial n., SYN keratin *pearl.*

isogenous n., a clone of cartilage cells all from one progenitor cell and occurring as a cluster.

net. SYN network (1).

Chiari n., abnormal fibrous or lacelike strands in the right atrium, extending from the margins of the coronary or caval valves and attaching to the atrial wall along the line of the crista terminalis; results when resorption of the septum spurium is markedly less than normal.

chromidial n., a reticulum of basophilic-staining material in the cytoplasm of certain cells.

Netherton, Earl W., 20th century U.S. dermatologist. SEE N. *syndrome.*

net·il·mi·cin sul·fate (net-il-mī´sin). A parenteral aminoglycoside antibiotic used for short-term treatment of serious or life-threatening bacterial infections.

net·tle (net´l). SYN urtica. [A.S. *netele*]

net·work (net´werk). **1.** A structure bearing a resemblance to a woven fabric. A network of nerve fibers or small vessels. SYN net, rete (1). SEE ALSO reticulum. **2.** The persons in a patient's environment, especially as significant for the course of the illness.

acromial arterial n., SYN acromial *anastomosis* of the thoracoacromial artery.

arteriolar n., SYN arterial *plexus.*

articular n., SYN articular vascular *plexus;* SEE plane *joint.*

articular vascular n., SYN articular vascular *plexus.*

articular vascular n. of elbow, SYN cubital *anastomosis.*

articular vascular n. of knee, SYN genicular *anastomosis.*

calcaneal arterial n., SYN calcaneal *anastomosis.*

chromatin n., the appearance of basophilic material in the nuclei of many cells after fixation. SEE ALSO chromatin.

dorsal carpal n., SYN dorsal carpal arterial *arch.*

dorsal venous n. of foot [TA], a superficial network of fine veins on the dorsum of the foot. SYN rete venosum dorsale pedis [TA].

dorsal venous n. of hand [TA], a superficial network of veins on the dorsum of the hand emptying into the cephalic and the basilic veins. SYN rete venosum dorsale manus [TA].

lateral malleolar n. [TA], a network over the lateral malleolus formed by branches of the posterior lateral malleolar, anterior lateral malleolar, peroneal, and lateral tarsal arteries. SYN rete malleolare laterale [TA].

linin n., SEE linin (3).

medial malleolar n. [TA], a network over the medial malleolus formed by branches from the anterior and posterior medial malleolar and medial tarsal arteries. SYN rete malleolare mediale [TA].

neurofibrillar n., the intertwined patterns formed by neurofibrils in the neuron.

patellar n., SYN patellar *anastomosis.*

peritarsal n., the lymphatic vessels along the margin of the eyelid.

plantar venous n. [TA], a fine superficial venous network in the sole of the foot. SYN rete venosum plantare [TA].

Purkinje n., the n. formed by Purkinje fibers beneath the endocardium.

subpapillary n., the capillary blood vessels in the deeper layers of the skin.

trabecular n., SYN trabecular *tissue* of sclera.

NeuAc Abbreviation for *N*-acetylneuraminic acid.

Neubauer, Johann E., German anatomist, 1742–1777. SEE N. *artery.*

Neufeld, Fred, German bacteriologist, 1869–1945. SEE N. *reaction,* capsular *swelling.*

Neumann, Ernst F.C., German histologist, anatomist, and pathologist, 1834–1918. SEE N. *sheath;* Rouget-N. *sheath.*

Neumann, Franz E., German physicist, 1798–1895. SEE N. *law.*

Neumann, Isidor Edler von Heilwart, Austrian dermatologist, 1832–1906. SEE N. *disease.*

△**neur-, neuri-, neuro-.** Nerve, nerve tissue, the nervous system. [G. *neuron*]

neu·ral (noor′ăl). **1.** Relating to any structure composed of nerve cells or their processes, or that on further development will evolve into nerve cells. **2.** Referring to the dorsal side of the vertebral bodies or their precursors, where the spinal cord is located, as opposed to hemal (2). [G. *neuron,* nerve]

neu·ral·gia (noo-ral′jē-ă). Pain of a severe, throbbing, or stabbing character in the course or distribution of a nerve. SYN neurodynia. [neur- + G. *algos,* pain]

atypical facial n., SYN atypical trigeminal n.

atypical trigeminal n., periodic pain in any region of the face, teeth, tongue, and occasionally in the occipital or shoulder area, which lasts several minutes to several days but has no trigger point and lacks the paroxysmal character of tic douloureux. SYN atypical facial n.

epileptiform n., SYN trigeminal n.

facial n., SYN trigeminal n.

n. facia′lis ve′ra, SYN geniculate n.

Fothergill n., SYN trigeminal n.

geniculate n., a severe paroxysmal lancinating pain deep in the ear, on the anterior wall of the external meatus, and on a small area just in front of the pinna. SYN geniculate otalgia, Hunt n., n. facialis vera.

glossopharyngeal n., paroxysmal lancinating pain in the throat or palate. SYN glossopharyngeal tic.

hallucinatory n., an impression of local pain persisting after an attack of n. has ceased.

Hunt n., SYN geniculate n.

idiopathic n., nerve pain not due to any apparent cause.

intercostal n., pain in the chest wall due to n. of one or more of the intercostal nerves.

mammary n., n. of the intercostal nerve or nerves supplying the breast.

Morton n., n. of an interdigital nerve, usually the anastomotic branch between the medial and lateral plantar nerves, resulting from compression of the nerve by the metatarsophalangeal joint. SYN Morton metatarsalgia, Morton neuroma.

occipital n., SEE posttraumatic neck *syndrome.*

periodic migrainous n., recurrent facial pain and headache, more common in men than in women. SYN Harris migraine.

sciatic n., SYN sciatica.

Sluder n., SYN sphenopalatine n.

sphenopalatine n., n. of the lower half of the face, with pain referred to the root of the nose, upper teeth, eyes, ears, mastoid, and occiput, in association with nasal congestion and rhinorrhea

occurring in infection of the nasal sinuses, and produced by lesions of the sphenopalatine ganglion; ocular hyperemia and excessive lacrimation may occur. SYN Sluder n.

stump n., pain experienced as coming from an absent part, caused by irritation of neuromas in the scarred tissue of an amputation stump.

suboccipital n., SEE posttraumatic neck *syndrome.*

supraorbital n., n. of the supraorbital nerve.

symptomatic n., n. occurring as a symptom of some local or systemic disease not involving primarily nerve structures.

trifacial n., SYN trigeminal n.

trigeminal n., severe, paroxysmal bursts of pain in one or more branches of the trigeminal nerve; often induced by touching trigger points in or about the mouth. SYN epileptiform n., facial n., Fothergill disease (1), Fothergill n., tic douloureux, trifacial n.

neu·ral·gic (noo-ral′jik). Relating to, resembling, or of the character of, neuralgia.

neu·ral·gi·form (noo-ral′ji-fōrm). Resembling or of the character of neuralgia.

neur·am·e·bim·e·ter (noor′am-ĕ-bim′ĕ-ter). An instrument for measuring the rapidity of response of a nerve to any stimulus. [neur- + G. *amoibē,* exchange, return, answer, + *metron,* measure]

neur·a·min·ic ac·id (noor′ă-min′ik). An aldol product of D-mannosamine and pyruvic acid, linking the C-1 of the former to the C-3 of the latter. The *N*- and *O*-acyl derivatives of n. a. are known as sialic acids and are constituents of gangliosides and of the polysaccharide components of muco- and glycoproteins from many tissues, secretions, and species. SYN prehemataminic acid.

neur·a·min·i·dase (noor-ă-min′i-dās). SYN sialidase.

α₂-**neur·a·mi·no·gly·co·pro·tein** (noor-ă-min′ō-glī-kō-prō′tēn). A glycoprotein that contains neuraminic acid and that during electrophoresis migrates with the α₂ portion of serum proteins. SEE ALSO C1 esterase *inhibitor.*

neur·an·a·gen·e·sis (noor′an-ă-jen′ĕ-sis). Regeneration of a nerve. [neur- + G. *ana,* up, again, + *genesis,* origin]

neur·a·poph·y·sis (noor-ă-pof′i-sis). SYN *lamina* of vertebral arch. [neur- + G. *apophysis,* offshoot]

neur·a·prax·ia (noor-ă-prak′sē-ă). The mildest type of focal nerve lesion that produces clinical deficits; localized loss of conduction along a nerve without axon degeneration; caused by a focal lesion, usually demyelinating, and followed by a complete recovery. Term is often misspelled (neuropraxia), and often used, incorrectly, as a synonym for nerve lesion. SEE ALSO axonotmesis. [neur- + G. a- priv. + *praxis,* action]

neur·ar·chy (noor′ar-kē). The dominant action of the nervous system over the physical processes of the body. [neur- + G. *archē,* dominion]

neur·as·the·nia (noor-as-thē′nē-ă). An ill-defined condition, commonly accompanying or following depression, characterized by vague fatigue believed to be brought on by psychological factors. [neur- + G. *astheneia,* weakness]

angiopathic n., angioparalytic n., an obsolete term for a form of mild n. in which the chief complaint is of a universal throbbing or sense of pulsation throughout the body.

gastric n., a condition marked by vague epigastric atony and distention, and mild neurasthenic symptoms.

n. gra′vis, obsolete term for a condition of extreme and lasting n.

n. prae′cox, obsolete term for a form of nervous exhaustion appearing in the adolescent period.

primary n., obsolete term for neurasthenia praecox.

pulsating n., obsolete term for angiopathic neurasthenia.

sexual n., obsolete term for a form in which sexual erethism, weakness, or perversion is a marked symptom.

traumatic n., obsolete term for posttraumatic syndrome.

neur·as·then·ic (noor-as-then′ik). Relating to, or suffering from, neurasthenia.

neur·ax·is (noo-rak′sis). The axial, unpaired part of the central nervous system: spinal cord, rhombencephalon, mesencephalon, and diencephalon, in contrast to the paired cerebral hemisphere, or telencephalon.

neur·ax·on, neur·ax·one (noo-rak′son, -sōn). Obsolete term for axon. [neur- + G. *axōn,* axis]

neur·ec·ta·sis, neur·ec·ta·sia, neur·ec·ta·sy (noo-rek′tă-sis, noor-ek-tā′zē-ă, -ek′tă-sē). The operation of stretching a nerve or nerve trunk. SYN neurotension. [neur- + G. *ektasis,* extension]

neu·rec·to·my (noo-rek′tō-mē). Excision of a segment of a nerve. SYN neuroectomy. [neur- + G. *ektomē,* excision]

occipital n., excision of greater occipital nerve for the treatment of occipital neuralgia.

presacral n., cutting of the presacral nerve to relieve severe dysmenorrhea. SYN Cotte operation, presacral sympathectomy.

retrogasserian n., SYN trigeminal *rhizotomy.*

vestibular n., transection of the vestibular division of the eighth cranial nerve.

neur·ec·to·pia, neur·ec·to·py (noor-ek-tō′pē-ă, -ek′tō-pē). A condition in which a nerve follows an anomalous course. [neur- + G. *ektopos,* fr. *ek,* out of, + *topos,* place]

neur·ep·i·the·li·um (noor′ep-i-thē′lē-ŭm). SYN neuroepithelium.

△**neuri-.** SEE neur-.

neu·ri·dine (noor′i-dēn). SYN spermine.

neu·ri·lem·ma (noor-i-lem′ă). A cell that enfolds one or more axons of the peripheral nervous system; in myelinated fibers its plasma membrane forms the lamellae of myelin. SYN neurolemma, sheath of Schwann. [neuri + G. *lemma,* husk]

neu·ri·le·mo·ma (noor′i-lē-mō′mă). SYN schwannoma. [neurilemma + G. *-oma,* tumor]

acoustic n., schwannoma arising from cranial nerve VIII.

Antoni type A n., relatively solid or compact arrangement of neoplastic tissue that consists of Schwann cells arranged in twisting bundles and associated with delicate reticulin fibers; the nuclei of the Schwann cells are frequently grouped in parallel rows (so-called palisades), and the nuclei and fibers sometimes form exaggerated tactile corpuscles, called Verocay bodies.

Antoni type B n., relatively soft or loose arrangement of neoplastic tissue that consists of Schwann cells in a haphazard or nondescript type of arrangement among reticulin fibers and tiny cystlike foci; fat-laden macrophages may be observed in some of the larger neoplasms.

neu·ril·i·ty (noo-ril′i-tē). The property, inherent in nerves, of conducting stimuli.

neu·ri·mo·til·i·ty (noor′i-mō-til′i-tē). SYN nervimotility.

neu·ri·mo·tor (noor-i-mō′ter). SYN nervimotor.

neu·rine (noor′ēn). A toxic amine that is a product of decomposing animal matter (dehydration of choline) and a poisonous constituent of mushrooms.

neu·ri·no·ma (noor-i-nō′mă). Obsolete term for schwannoma.

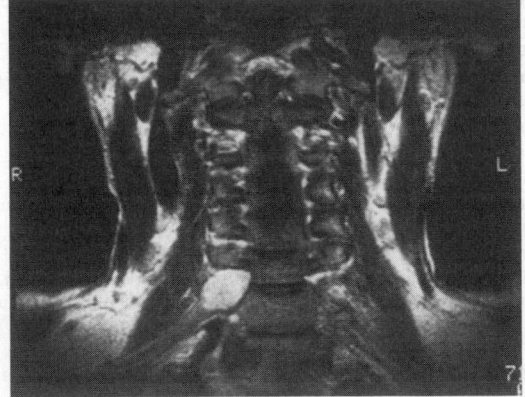

neurinoma of the nerve root of C₇: MRI, after injection of contrast medium

acoustic n., SYN vestibular *schwannoma.*

neu·rit·ic (noo-rit′ik). Relating to neuritis.

neu·ri·tis, pl. **neu·ri·ti·des** (noo-rī′tis, noo-rit′i-dēz). **1.** Inflam-

mation of a nerve. **2.** SYN neuropathy. [neuri- + G. *-itis,* inflammation]

adventitial n., inflammation of the sheath of a nerve. SEE ALSO perineuritis.

ascending n., inflammation progressing upward along a nerve trunk in a direction away from the periphery.

axial n., SYN parenchymatous n.

brachial n., SYN neuralgic *amyotrophy.*

central n., SYN parenchymatous n.

descending n., inflammation progressing along a nerve trunk toward the periphery.

Eichhorst n., SYN interstitial n.

endemic n., SYN beriberi.

fallopian n., SYN facial *paralysis.*

interstitial n., inflammation of the connective tissue framework of a nerve. SYN Eichhorst n.

intraocular n., inflammation of the retinal portion of the optic nerve.

Leyden n., fatty degeneration of the fibers of the affected nerve.

multiple n., SYN polyneuropathy.

occipital n., SEE posttraumatic neck *syndrome.*

optic n., inflammation of the optic nerve. SEE ALSO *neuromyelitis* optica, retrobulbar n., papillitis.

parenchymatous n., inflammation of the nervous substance proper, the axons, and myelin. SYN axial n., central n.

retrobulbar n., optic n. without swelling of the optic disk.

sciatic n., SYN sciatica.

segmental n., **(1)** inflammation occurring at several points along the course of a nerve; **(2)** segmental demyelinating neuropathy

suboccipital n., SEE posttraumatic neck *syndrome.*

toxic n., n. caused by an endogenous or exogenous toxin.

traumatic n., nerve lesion following an injury.

△**neuro-.** SEE neur-.

neu·ro·al·ler·gy (noor-ō-al′er-jē). An allergic reaction in nervous tissue.

neu·ro·an·as·to·mo·sis (noor′ō-an-as-tō-mō′sis). Surgical formation of a junction between nerves.

neu·ro·a·nat·o·my (noor′ō-ă-nat′ō-mē). The anatomy of the nervous system, usually specific to the central nervous system.

neu·ro·ar·throp·a·thy (noor′ō-ar-throp′ă-thē). A joint disorder caused by loss of joint sensation. SEE Charcot *joint.* [neuro- + G. *arthron,* joint, + *pathos,* suffering, disease]

neu·ro·aug·men·ta·tion (noor′ō-awg-men-tā′shoon). Use of electrical stimulation to supplement activity of the nervous system.

neu·ro·aug·men·tive (noor′ō-awg-men′tiv). Related to neuroaugmentation.

neur·o·bi·ol·o·gy. The biology of the nervous system.

neu·ro·bi·o·tax·is. The theory that nerve cell bodies may move toward, or their axons may grow toward, the area from which they receive the most stimuli. [G. *neuron,* nerve + *bios,* life + *taxis,* arrangement]

neu·ro·blast (noor′ō-blast). An embryonic nerve cell. [neuro- + G. *blastos,* germ]

neu·ro·blas·to·ma (noor′ō-blas-tō′mă). A malignant neoplasm characterized by immature, only slightly differentiated nerve cells of embryonic type, i.e., neuroblasts; typical cells are relatively small (10–15 μm in diameter) with disproportionately large, darkly staining, vesicular nuclei and scant, palely acidophilic cytoplasm; they may be arranged in sheets, irregular clumps, or cordlike groups, as well as occurring individually and in pseudorosettes (with nuclei arranged peripherally about the centrally directed cytoplasmic processes); ordinarily, the stroma is sparse, and foci of necrosis and hemorrhage are not unusual. N.'s occur frequently in infants and children in the mediastinal and retroperitoneal regions (approximately 30% associated with the adrenal glands); widespread metastases to the liver, lungs, lymph nodes, cranial cavity, and skeleton are very common.

olfactory n., a rare, often slowly growing malignant tumor of primitive nerve cells, usually arising in the olfactory area of the nasal cavity. SYN olfactory esthesioneuroblastoma.

neu·ro·bor·re·li·o·sis (noor'ō-bōr-rel'ē-ō'sis). Inflammation or disease caused by infection of the central nervous system by a member of the genus *Borrelia*. It is frequently a late stage in the disease process, particularly in immunosuppressed individuals, such as those suffering from AIDS.

neu·ro·car·di·ac (noor-ō-kar'dē-ak). **1.** Relating to the nerve supply of the heart. **2.** Relating to a cardiac neurosis. [neuro- + G. *kardia*, heart]

neu·ro·cele (noor'ō-sēl). Rarely used collective term for the central cavity of the cerebrospinal axis; the combined ventricles of the brain and central canal of the spinal cord. [neuro- + G. *koilos*, hollow]

neu·ro·chem·is·try (noor-ō-kem'is-trē). The science concerned with the chemical aspects of nervous system structure and function.

neu·ro·chi·tin (noor-ō-kī'tin). SYN neurokeratin. [neuro- + G. *chitōn*, tunic]

neu·ro·cho·ri·o·ret·i·ni·tis (noor-ō-kōr'ē-ō-ret-in-ī'tis). Inflammation of the choroid, the retina, and the optic nerve.

neu·ro·cho·roi·di·tis (noor'ō-kō-roy-dī'tis). Inflammation of the choroid and the optic nerve.

neu·roc·la·dism (noo-rok'lă-dizm). The outgrowth of axons from the central stump to bridge the gap in a cut nerve. SYN odogenesis. [neuro- + G. *klados*, a young branch]

neu·ro·cra·ni·um (noor-ō-krā'nē-ŭm) [TA]. Those bones of the skull enclosing the brain, as distinguished from the bones of the face. SYN brain box*, braincase, cranial vault, cranium cerebrale, cerebral cranium. [neuro- + G. *kranion*, skull]

cartilaginous n., in the embryo, that part of the base of the skull first laid down in cartilage and then ossified.

membranous n., the vault of the embryonic skull that is ossified in membrane.

neu·ro·cris·top·a·thy (noor'ō-kris-top'ă-thē). Developmental anomaly arising from maldevelopment of neural crest cells. [neuro- + L. *crista*, crest, + G. *pathos*, suffering]

neu·ro·cyte (noor'o-sīt). SYN neuron. [neuro- + G. *kytos*, cell]

neu·ro·cy·tol·y·sis (noor'ō-sī-tol'i-sis). Destruction of neurons. [neuro- + G. *kytos*, cell, + *lysis*, dissolution]

neu·ro·cy·to·ma (noor'ō-sī-tō'mă). A tumor of neuronal differentiation usually intraventricular in location, consisting of sheets of cells with uniform nuclei and occasional perivascular pseudorosette formation. [neuro- + G. *kytos*, cell, + *-oma*, tumor]

neu·ro·den·drite (noor-ō-den'drīt). SYN dendrite (1).

neu·ro·den·dron (noor-ō-den'dron). SYN dendrite (1).

neu·ro·der·ma·ti·tis (noor'ō-der-mă-tī'tis). A chronic lichenified skin lesion, localized or disseminated. [neuro- + G. *derma*, skin, + *-itis*, inflammation]

neu·ro·dy·nam·ic (noor'ō-dī-nam'ik). Pertaining to nervous energy. [neuro- + G. *dynamis*, force]

neu·ro·dyn·ia (noor-ō-din'ē-ă). SYN neuralgia. [neuro- + G. *odynē*, pain]

neu·ro·ec·to·derm (noor-ō-ek'tō-derm). That central region of the early embryonic ectoderm that on further development forms the brain and spinal cord, and the neural crest cells that become the nerve cells and neurilemma or Schwann cells of the peripheral nervous system.

neu·ro·ec·to·der·mal (noor'ō-ek-tō-der'măl). Relating to the neuroectoderm.

neu·ro·ec·to·my (noor-ō-ek'tō-mē). SYN neurectomy.

neu·ro·en·ceph·a·lo·my·e·lop·a·thy (noor'ō-en-sef'ă-lō-mī-ĕ-lop'ă-thē). Disease of the brain, spinal cord, and nerves.

neu·ro·en·do·crine (noor-ō-en'dō-krin). **1.** Pertaining to the anatomic and functional relationships between the nervous system and the endocrine apparatus. **2.** Descriptive of cells that release a hormone into the circulating blood in response to a neural stimulus. Such cells may compose a peripheral endocrine gland (e.g., the insulin-secreting beta cells of the islets of Langerhans in the pancreas and the adrenaline-secreting chromaffin cells of the

adrenal medulla); others are neurons in the brain (e.g., the neurons of the supraoptic nucleus that release antidiuretic hormone from their axon terminals in the posterior lobe of the hypophysis).

neu·ro·en·do·crin·ol·o·gy (noor-ō-en'dō-krin-ol'ō-jē). The specialty concerned with the anatomic and functional relationships between the nervous system and the endocrine apparatus.

neu·ro·ep·i·the·li·al (noor'ō-ep-i-thē'lē-ăl). Relating to the neuroepithelium.

neu·ro·ep·i·the·li·um (noor'ō-ep-i-thē'lē-oom). Epithelial cells specialized for the reception of external stimuli. Most neuroepithelial cells, notably the hair cells of the inner ear and the receptor cells of the taste buds, are not true neurons but transducer cells that stand in synaptic contact with the peripheral endings of sensory ganglion cells. The neuroepithelial receptor cells of the olfactory epithelium, by contrast, are true peripheral neurons whose extremely thin, unmyelinated axons compose the olfactory filaments that enter the olfactory bulb of the cerebral hemisphere. The NA also applies the term to the rods and cones of the retina. SYN neurepithelium, neuroepithelial cells.

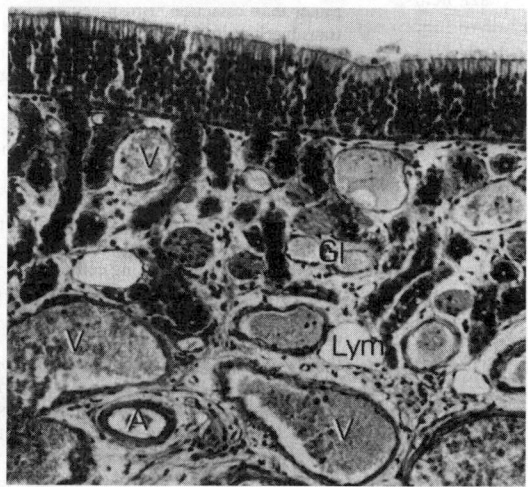

neuroepithelium: photomicrograph of olfactory mucosa including the olfactory epithelium and the underlying connective tissue that extends as far as the bone (not shown); A, artery; V, veins; Lym, lymphatic vessels; N, nerves; Gl, Bowman glands; × 160

n. of ampullary crest, the specialized sensory hair cells in the ampullary crest of the ampulla of each semicircular duct.

n. of macula, the specialized sensory hair cells of the epithelium of the macula sacculi and macula utriculi. SEE ALSO macula.

neu·ro·fi·bra.

neurofibrae autonomicae [TA], SYN autonomic nerve *fibers*, under *fiber*.

neurofibrae postganglionicae, SYN postganglionic.

neurofibrae preganglionicae, SYN preganglionic nerve *fibers*, under *fiber*.

neurofibrae somaticae [TA], SYN somatic nerve *fibers*, under *fiber*.

neu·ro·fi·bril (noor-ō-fī'bril). A filamentous structure seen with the light microscope in the nerve cell's body, dendrites, axon, and sometimes synaptic endings, as aggregations of much finer ultramicroscopic elements, the neurofilaments and microtubules; their functional significance remains to be established.

neu·ro·fi·bril·lar (noor-ō-fī'bri-lĕr). Relating to neurofibrils.

neu·ro·fi·bro·ma (noor'ō-fī-brō'mă). A moderately firm, benign, encapsulated tumor resulting from proliferation of Schwann cells in a disorderly pattern that includes portions of nerve fibers; in neurofibromatosis, n.'s are multiple. SYN fibroneuroma.

plexiform n., a type of n., representing an anomaly rather than a true neoplasm, in which the proliferation of Schwann cells occurs from the inner aspect of the nerve sheath, thereby resulting in an irregularly thickened, distorted, tortuous structure; in some instances, the process extends along the course of the nerve and may eventually involve the spinal roots and the spinal cord; seen most frequently in neurofibromatosis. SYN fibrillary neuroma, plexiform neuroma.

storiform n., SYN pigmented *dermatofibrosarcoma protuberans.*

neu·ro·fi·bro·ma·to·sis (noor'ō-fī-brō-mă-tō'sis). Under this heading are grouped two distinct hereditary disorders, formerly labeled peripheral and central n., but now entitled n. type 1 and type 2. Type 1 (peripheral) n., [MIM*162200] by far the most common of the two types, is characterized clinically by the combination of patches of hyperpigmentation and cutaneous and subcutaneous tumors. The hyperpigmented skin areas, present from birth and found anywhere on the body surface, can vary markedly in size and color—the dark brown ones are called café-au-lait spots. The multiple cutaneous and subcutaneous tumors, nerve sheath neoplasms, called neurofibromas, can develop anywhere along the peripheral nerve fibers, from the roots distally. Neurofibromas can become quite large, causing a major disfigurement, eroding bone, and compressing various peripheral nerve structures; a small hamartoma (Lisch nodule) can be found in the iris of almost all patients. Type 1 n., also called von Recklinghausen disease, has autosomal dominant inheritance, with the gene locus on chromosome 17q11, and is caused by mutation in the NF1 gene that encodes neurofibromin. Type 2 (central) n. [MIM*101000] has few cutaneous manifestations, and consists primarily of bilateral (less often, unilateral) acoustic neuromas, causing deafness, often accompanied by other intracranial and paraspinal neoplasms, such as meningiomas and gliomas. Type 2 n. also has autosomal dominant inheritance, but the gene locus is on 22q11, caused by mutation in the NF2 gene encoding the product merlin. SYN elephant man's disease (2).

abortive n., SYN incomplete n.

central type n., type 2 neurofibromatosis. SEE neurofibromatosis.

incomplete n., multiple neurofibromas with minimal manifestations, perhaps limited to café-au-lait spots; individuals with minimal lesions may have offspring with severe involvement. SYN abortive n.

neu·ro·fil·a·ment (noor-ō-fil'ă-ment). A class of intermediate filaments found in neurons.

neu·ro·gang·li·on (noor-ō-gang'lē-on). SYN ganglion (1).

neu·ro·gas·tric (noor-ō-gas'trik). Relating to the innervation of the stomach.

neu·ro·gen·e·sis (noor-ō-jen'ĕ-sis). Formation of the nervous system. [neuro- + G. *genesis,* production]

neu·ro·gen·ic, neu·ro·ge·net·ic (noor-ō-jen'ik, -jĕ-net'ik). **1.** Originating in, starting from, or caused by, the nervous system or nerve impulses. SYN neurogenous. **2.** Relating to neurogenesis.

neu·rog·e·nous (noo-roj'ĕ-nŭs). SYN neurogenic (1).

neu·rog·lia (noo-rog'lē-ă). Non-neuronal cellular elements of the central and peripheral nervous system; formerly believed to be merely supporting cells but now thought to have important metabolic functions, since they are invariably interposed between neurons and the blood vessels supplying the nervous system. In central nervous tissue they include oligodendroglia cells, astrocytes, ependymal cells, and microglia cells. The satellite cells of ganglia and the neurolemmal or Schwann cells around peripheral nerve fibers can be interpreted as the oligodendroglia cells of the peripheral nervous system. SYN reticulum (2) [TA], glia, Kölliker reticulum. [neuro- + G. *glia,* glue]

neu·rog·li·a·cyte (noo-rog'lē-ă-sīt). A neuroglia cell. SEE neuroglia. [neuro- + G. *glia,* glue, + *kytos,* cell]

neu·rog·li·al, neu·rog·li·ar (noo-rog'lē-ăl, -lē-ăr). Relating to neuroglia.

neu·rog·li·o·ma·to·sis (noo-rog'lē-ō-mă-tō'sis). SYN gliomatosis.

neu·ro·gram (noor'ō-gram). The imprint on the brain substance theoretically remaining after every mental experience, i.e., the engram or physical register of the mental experience, stimulation of which retrieves and reproduces the original experience, thereby producing memory. [neuro- + G. *gramma,* something written]

neu·rog·ra·phy (noo-rog'ră-fē). A method of depicting the state

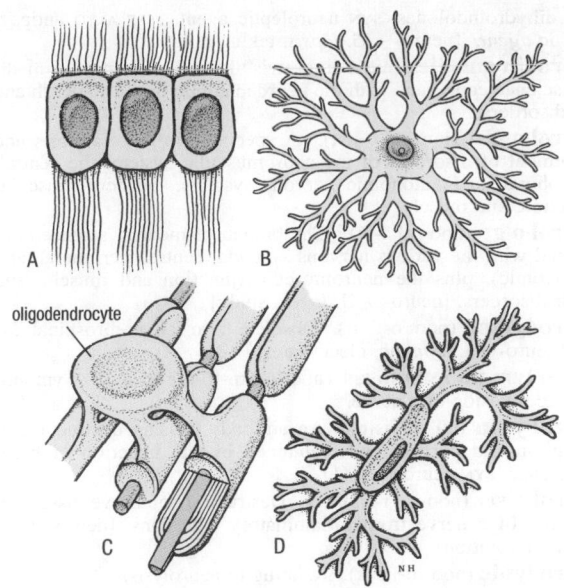

neuroglia: (A) ependymal cells, (B) astrocyte, (C) oligodendrocyte, (D) microglia

of a peripheral nerve, such as electrical recording or radiographic visualization by contrast media. [neuro- + G. *graphō,* to write]

neu·ro·he·mal (noor-ō-hē'măl). Descriptive of structures containing neurosecretory neurons, whose axons form no synapses with other neurons and whose axonal endings are modified to permit storage and release into the circulation of neurosecretory material. [neuro- + G. *haima,* blood + suffix -in, material]

neu·ro·his·tol·o·gy (noor-ō-his-tol'ō-jē). The microscopic anatomy of the nervous system. SYN histoneurology.

neu·ro·hor·mone (noor-ō-hōr'mōn). A hormone formed by neurosecretory cells and liberated by nerve impulses (e.g., norepinephrine).

neu·ro·hy·po·phys·i·al (noor'ō-hī-pō-fiz'ē-ăl). Relating to the neurohypophysis.

neu·ro·hy·poph·y·sis (noor'ō-hī-pof'i-sis) [TA]. It is composed of the infundibulum and the nervous lobe of the hypophysis. SEE ALSO pituitary *gland.* SYN lobus nervosus [TA], lobus posterior hypophyseos✶, pars nervosa hypophyseos✶, nervous lobe, neural part of hypophysis, posterior lobe of hypophysis. [neuro- + hypophysis]

neu·roid (noor'oyd). Resembling a nerve; nervelike. [neuro- + G. *eidos,* resemblance]

neu·ro·ker·a·tin (noor-ō-kār'ă-tin). **1.** The proteinaceous network that remains of the myelin sheath of axons following fixation and the removal of the fatty material; the reticular appearance is probably a fixation artifact. **2.** The insoluble protein matter of brain remaining after extraction with solvents following proteolytic digestion; it is unrelated to the keratins. SYN neurochitin. [neuro- + G. *keras,* horn]

neu·ro·lem·ma (noor-ō-lem'ă). SYN neurilemma. [neuro- + G. *lemma,* husk]

neu·ro·lept·an·al·ge·sia (noor'ō-lept-an-ăl-jē'zē-ă). An intense analgesic and amnesic state produced by administration of narcotic analgesics and neuroleptic drugs; unconsciousness may or may not occur, and cardiorespiratory function may be altered.

neu·ro·lept·an·es·the·sia (noor'ō-lept-an-es-thē'zē-ah). A technique of general anesthesia based upon intravenous administration of neuroleptic drugs, together with inhalation of a weak anesthetic with or without neuromuscular relaxants.

neu·ro·lep·tic (noor-ō-lep'tik). Any of a class of psychotropic drugs used to treat psychosis, particularly schizophrenia; includes the phenothiazine, thioxanthene, and butyrophenone derivates and the dihydroindolones. SYN neuroleptic agent. SEE ALSO antipsychotic *agent*. [neuro- + G. *lēpsis,* taking hold]

neu·ro·lin·guis·tics (nur′ō-ling-gwis′tiks). The branch of medical science concerned with the neuroanatomic basis of speech and its disorders.

neu·rol·o·gist (noo-rol′ō-jist). A specialist in the diagnosis and treatment of disorders of the neuromuscular system: the central, peripheral, and autonomic nervous systems, the neuromuscular junction, and muscle.

neu·rol·o·gy (noo-rol′ō-jē). The branch of medical science concerned with the various nervous systems (central, peripheral, and autonomic), plus the neuromuscular junction and muscle, and their disorders. [neuro- + G. *logos,* study]

neu·ro·lymph (noor′ō-limf). Obsolete term for cerebrospinal *fluid*. [neuro- + L. *lympha,* clear water]

neu·ro·lym·pho·ma·to·sis (noor′ō-lim-fō-mă-tō′sis). Lymphoblastic invasion of a nerve.

neu·rol·y·sin (nŭ-rol′i-sin). An antibody causing destruction of ganglion and cortical cells, obtained by the injection of brain substance. SYN neurotoxin (1).

neu·rol·y·sis (noo-rol′i-sis). **1.** Destruction of nerve tissue. **2.** Freeing of a nerve from inflammatory adhesions. [neuro- + G. *lysis,* dissolution]

neu·ro·lyt·ic (noor-ō-lit′ik). Relating to neurolysis.

neu·ro·ma (noo-rō′mă). General term for any neoplasm derived from cells of the nervous system; on the basis of newer knowledge pertaining to cytologic and histologic characteristics, a variety of neoplasms, formerly placed in the general category of n., may now be classified in more specific categories, e.g., ganglioneuroma, neurilemoma, pseudoneuroma, and others. [neuro- + G. *-oma,* tumor]

acoustic n., SYN vestibular *schwannoma.*

amputation n., SYN traumatic n.

n. cu′tis, neurofibroma of the skin.

false n., SYN traumatic n.

fibrillary n., SYN plexiform *neurofibroma.*

Morton n., SYN Morton *neuralgia.*

plexiform n., SYN plexiform *neurofibroma.*

n. telangiecto′des, a neurofibroma with a conspicuous number of blood vessels, some of which have unusually large lumens (in proportion to the thickness of the walls).

traumatic n., the nonneoplastic proliferative mass of Schwann cells and neurites that may develop at the proximal end of a severed or injured nerve. SYN amputation n., false n., pseudoneuroma.

neu·ro·ma·la·cia (noor′ō-mă-lā′shē-ă). Pathologic softening of nervous tissue. [neuro- + G. *malakia,* softness]

neu·ro·ma·to·sis (noor′ō-mă-tō′sis). The presence of multiple neuromas, as in neurofibromatosis.

neu·ro·mel·a·nin (noor-ō-mel′ă-nin). A modified form of melanin pigment normally found in certain neurons of the nervous system, especially in the substantia nigra and locus ceruleus.

neu·ro·men·in·ge·al (noor-ō-mĕ-nin′jē- ăl). Related to involvement of nervous tissue and the meninges.

neu·ro·mere (noor′ō-mēr). Elevations in the wall of the developing neural tube that divide the developing spinal cord (neuromere) into portions to which dorsal and ventral roots are attached, or that divide the developing rhombencephalon into portions associated primarily with motor portions of the cranial nerves of the medulla and pons. SYN encephalomere, neural segment, neurotome (2). [neuro- + G. *meros,* part]

neu·ro·mi·met·ic (noor′ō-mi-met′ik). Relating to the action of a drug that mimics the response of an effector organ to nerve impulses.

neu·ro·mus·cu·lar (noor-ō-mŭs′kū-lăr). Referring to the relationship between nerve and muscle, in particular to the motor innervation of skeletal muscles and its pathology (e.g., neuromuscular disorders). SEE ALSO myoneural.

neu·ro·my·as·the·ni·a (noor′ō-mī-as-thē′nē-ă). Obsolete term for muscular weakness, usually of emotional origin. [neuro- + G. *mys,* muscle, + *a-* priv. + *sthenos,* strength]

epidemic n., an epidemic disease characterized by stiffness of the neck and back, headache, diarrhea, fever, and localized muscular weakness; restricted almost exclusively to adults, affecting women more than men; probably viral in origin. SYN benign myalgic encephalomyelitis, epidemic myalgic encephalomyelitis, Iceland disease.

neu·ro·my·e·li·tis (noor′ō-mī-el-ī′tis). Neuritis combined with spinal cord inflammation. SYN myeloneuritis. [neuro- + G. *myelos,* marrow, + *-itis,* inflammation]

n. op′tica, a demyelinating disorder consisting of a transverse myelopathy and optic neuritis. SYN Devic disease.

neu·ro·my·op·a·thy (noor′ō-mī-op′ă-the). **1.** A disorder of muscle due to disorder of its nerve supply. **2.** Simultaneous disorders of nerve and muscles. [neuro- + G. *mys,* muscle, + *pathos,* disease]

carcinomatous n., n. associated with carcinoma, especially of the lung.

neu·ro·my·o·si·tis (noor′ō-mī-ō-sī′tis). Obsolete term for polymyositis. [neuro- + G. *mys,* muscle, + *-itis,* inflammation]

neu·ron (noor′on). The morphologic and functional unit of the nervous system, consisting of the nerve cell body, the dendrites, and the axon. SYN nerve cell, neurocyte, neurone. [G. *neuron,* a nerve]

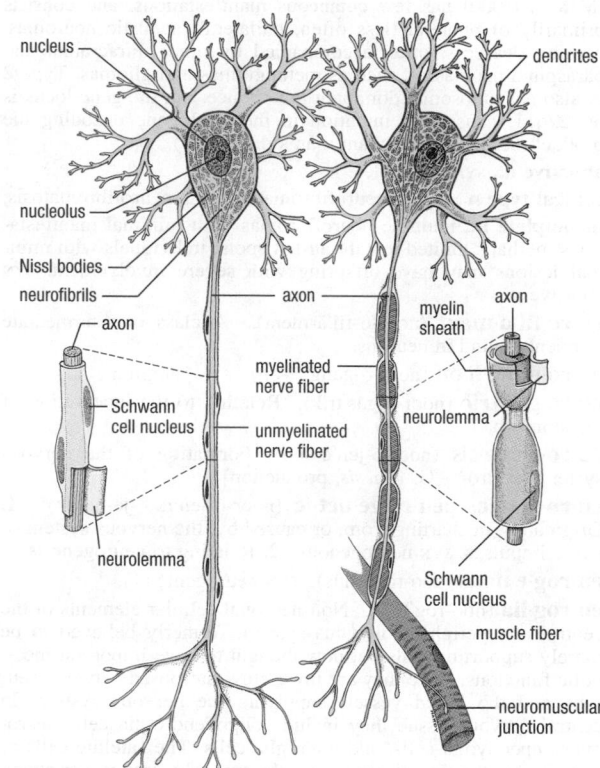

nucleus
dendrites
nucleolus
Nissl bodies
neurofibrils
axon
axon
myelin sheath
myelinated nerve fiber
Schwann cell nucleus
unmyelinated nerve fiber
neurolemma
neurolemma
Schwann cell nucleus
muscle fiber
neuromuscular junction

typical efferent neurons: (left) unmyelinated fiber, (right) myelinated fiber

autonomic motor n., SEE motor n.

bipolar n., a n. that has two processes arising from opposite poles of the cell body.

gamma motor n.'s, SYN gamma *loop.*

ganglionic motor n., SEE motor n.

Golgi type I n., nerve cells whose long axons leave the gray matter of which they form a part.

Golgi type II n., nerve cells with short axons that ramify in the gray matter.

intercalary n., SYN internuncial n.

internuncial n., a n. interposed between and connecting two other n.'s. SYN intercalary n.

lower motor n., clinical term used to indicate the final motor n.'s that innervate the skeletal muscles; distinguished from upper motor n.'s of the motor cortex that contribute to the corticospinal tract. SEE ALSO motor n.

motor n., a nerve cell in the spinal cord, rhombencephalon, or mesencephalon characterized by having an axon that leaves the central nervous system to establish a functional connection with an effector (muscle or glandular) tissue; **somatic motor n.'s** directly synapse with striated muscle fibers by motor endplates; **visceral motor n.'s** or **autonomic motor n.'s** (preganglionic m. n.'s), by contrast, innervate smooth muscle fibers or glands only by the intermediary of a second, peripheral, n. (postganglionic m. n.) located in an autonomic, or visceral motor, ganglion. SEE ALSO motor *endplate*, autonomic *division* of nervous system. SYN anterior horn cell, motoneuron.

multipolar n., a n. with several processes, usually an axon and three or more dendrites.

NANC n., abbreviation for nonadrenergic, noncholinergic n.

nonadrenergic, noncholinergic n. (NANC n.), autonomic efferent neuron whose transmission is not blocked by blocking adrenergic and cholinergic transmission. Nitric oxide may be the transmitter in some cases.

polymorphic n., occurring in many shapes. SEE ALSO multipolar *cell*.

postganglionic motor n., SEE motor n.

preganglionic motor n., SEE motor n.

pseudounipolar n., SYN unipolar n.

sensory n., a n. conveying information originating from sensory receptors or nerve endings; afferent neuron, may be general or special sensory.

somatic motor n., SEE motor n.

unipolar n., a n. whose cell body emits a single axonal process resulting from the fusion of two polar processes during development; at a variable distance from the cell body, the process divides into a peripheral axon branch extending outward as a peripheral afferent (sensory) nerve fiber and a central axon branch that enters into synaptic contact with n.'s in the spinal cord or brainstem. With the single known exception of the n.'s composing the mesencephalic nucleus of the trigeminus, unipolar n.'s are the exclusive neural elements of the sensory ganglia. The lack of dendritic processes of these primary sensory n.'s is only apparent: the dendritic pole of the unipolar n. is represented by the unmyelinated terminal ramifications of the peripheral axon branch. SYN pseudounipolar cell, pseudounipolar n., unipolar cell.

upper motor n., clinical term indicating those n.'s of the motor cortex that contribute to the formation of the corticospinal and corticonuclear (corticobulbar) tracts, as distinguished from the lower motor n.'s innervating the skeletal muscles. Although not motor n.'s in the strict sense, these cortical n.'s became colloquially classified as motor n.'s because their stimulation produces movement and their destruction causes moderate to severe disorders of movement. SEE ALSO motor n., motor *cortex*.

visceral motor n., SEE motor n.

neu·ro·nal (noor'ō-năl, noo-rō'năl). Pertaining to a neuron.

neu·rone (noor'ōn). SYN neuron.

neu·ro·neph·ric (noor-ō-nef'rik). Relating to the nerve supply of the kidney. [neuro- + G. *nephros,* kidney]

neu·ro·ne·vus (noor-ō-nē'vŭs). A variety of intradermal nevus in adults in which nests of atrophic nevus cells in the lower dermis are hyalinized and resemble nerve bundles.

neu·ron·i·tis (noor-ŏ-nī'tis). Inflammatory disorder of the neuron.

vestibular n., a paroxysmal attack of severe vertigo, not accompanied by deafness or tinnitus, which affects young to middle-aged adults, often following a nonspecific upper respiratory infection; due to unilateral vestibular dysfunction. SYN endemic paralytic vertigo, epidemic vertigo, Gerlier disease, kubisagari, kubisagaru, paralyzing vertigo.

neu·ro·nop·a·thy (noor-ō-nop'ă-thē). Disorder, often toxic, of the neuron (1).

sensory n., n. confined to dorsal root and gasserian ganglia.

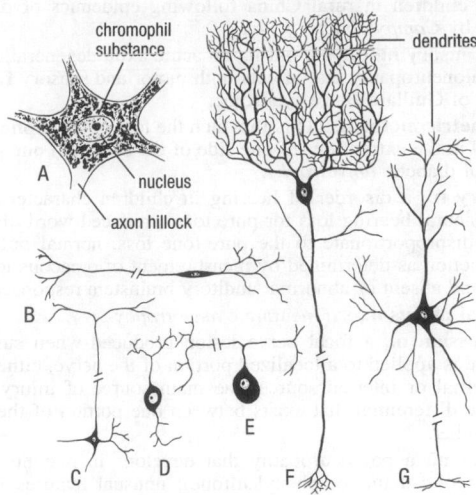

neuron types: (A) typical nerve cell body showing internal structure; (B) horizontal cell (of Cajal) from cerebral cortex; (C) Martinotti cell, (D) bipolar cell, (E) unipolar cell (posterior root ganglion), (F) Purkinje cell, (G) pyramidal cell of motor area of cerebral cortex. Sheaths are not shown

X-linked recessive bulbospinal n., SYN Kennedy *disease*.

neu·ron·o·phage (noo-ron'ō-fāj). A phagocyte that ingests neuronal elements. SEE microglia. [neuron + G. *phagō,* to eat]

neu·ron·o·pha·gia, neu·ro·noph·a·gy (noor'on'ō-fā'jē-ă, noor-ō-nof'ă-jē). Phagocytosis of nerve cells. [neuron + G. *phagō,* to eat]

neu·ro·nyx·is (noor-ō-nik'sis). Acupuncture of a nerve. [neuro- + G. *nyxis,* pricking]

neu·ro·on·col·o·gy (noor'ō-on-kol'ō-jē). The branch of medicine concerned with the direct and indirect effects of neoplasms on the nervous system, neuromuscular junction, and muscle. [neuro- + onco- + G. *logos,* study]

neu·ro·oph·thal·mol·o·gy (noor'ō-of-thal-mol'ō-jē). The branch of medicine concerned with the neurological aspects of the visual apparatus.

neu·ro·otol·o·gy (noor'ō-ō-tol'ō-jē). The branch of medicine concerned with the nervous system related to the auditory and vestibular systems.

neu·ro·pa·ral·y·sis (noor'ō-pă-ral'i-sis). Paralysis resulting from disease of the nerve supplying the affected part.

neu·ro·par·a·lyt·ic (noor'ō-pa-ră-lit'ik). Denoting or characterized by neuroparalysis.

neu·ro·path (noor'ō-path). One who suffers from or is predisposed to some disease of the nervous system.

neuropathia (noo-rō-path'ē-ă). SYN neuropathy.

n. epidemica, hemorrhagic fever with renal complications; due to Puumala virus.

neu·ro·path·ic (noor-ō-path'ik). Relating in any way to neuropathy.

neu·ro·path·o·gen·e·sis (noor'ō-path-ō-jen'ě-sis). The origin or causation of a disease of the nervous system. [neuro- + G. *pathos,* suffering, + *genesis,* origin]

neu·ro·pa·thol·o·gy (noor'ō-pa-thol'ō-jē). **1.** Pathology of the nervous system. **2.** That branch of pathology concerned with the nervous system.

neu·rop·a·thy (noo-rop'ă-thē). **1.** A classical term for any disorder affecting any segment of the nervous system. **2.** In contemporary usage, a disease involving the cranial nerves or the peripheral or autonomic nervous system. SYN neuritis (2), neuropathia. [neuro- + G. *pathos,* suffering]

acute motor axonal n., an acute, pure motor axon-degenerating type of polyradiculoneuropathy, a variant of Guillain-Barré syndrome; seen principally in a seasonal pattern (spring or summer) among children in rural China following epidemics of diarrhea caused by *Campylobacter jejuni.*

acute sensory motor axonal n., an acute axon-degenerating polyradiculoneuropathy that affects both motor and sensory fibers; a variant of Guillain-Barré syndrome.

asymmetric motor n., (1) n. in which the loss of function is more marked in the extremities of one side of the body; **(2)** one presentation of diabetic *amyotrophy.*

auditory n., a disorder of hearing in children characterized by sensorineural hearing loss for pure tones, reduced word discrimination disproportionate to the pure-tone loss, normal outer hair cell function as determined by measurement of otoacoustic emissions, and absent or abnormal auditory brainstem response.

brachial plexus n., SYN neuralgic *amyotrophy.*

compression n., a focal nerve lesion produced when sustained pressure is applied to a localized portion of the nerve, either from an external or internal source; the main source of injury is the pressure differential that exists between one portion of the nerve and another.

dapsone n., a polyneuropathy that develops in patients taking dapsone (4,4-diaminodiphenylsulfone); unusual features include being a pure motor n. and beginning in the hands, sometimes asymmetrically. SYN motor dapsone n.

diabetic n., a generic term for any diabetes mellitus–related disorder of the peripheral nervous system, autonomic nervous system, and some cranial nerves.

This most common of the chronic complications of diabetes can affect either the peripheral or the autonomic nervous system, or both. Peripheral neuropathies can cause bilaterally symmetric hypesthesia, hyperesthesia, paresthesia, loss of temperature and vibratory sense, or causalgia. Involvement of the autonomic nervous system may be manifested by postural hypotension, gastroparesis, alternating diarrhea and constipation, and impotence. The pathogenesis of chronic diabetic neuropathy is poorly understood. Symptoms tend to progress, and the response to treatment is unpredictable. In contrast, cranial nerve palsies due to microangiopathy in diabetes mellitus often resolve spontaneously.

diphtheritic n., a rapidly developing polyneuropathy caused by a toxin elaborated by *Corynebacterium diphtheriae.*

entrapment n., a focal nerve lesion produced by constriction or mechanical distortion of the nerve, within a fibrous or fibroosseous tunnel, or by a fibrous band; with these lesions, stretching and angulation of the nerve may be as important a source of injury as compression; entrapment n.'s tend to occur at particular sites in the body.

familial amyloid n. [MIM*105120, various kinds], a disorder in which various peripheral nerves are infiltrated with amyloid and their functions disturbed, an abnormal prealbumin is also formed and is present in the blood; characteristically, it begins during midlife and is found largely in persons of Portuguese descent; autosomal dominant inheritance. Other rare clinical types occur. SYN familial amyloidosis, hereditary amyloidosis.

giant axonal n., a rare disorder beginning at or after the third year of life, and presenting clinically with kinky hair, progressive painless clumsiness, muscle weakness and atrophy, sensory loss, and areflexia. Pathologically, both myelinated and unmyelinated nerve fibers contain axonal spheroids packed with neurofilaments; sporadic in nature.

Graves optic n., visual dysfunction due to optic nerve compression in Graves orbitopathy.

heavy metal n., peripheral nervous system disorders attributed to intoxication of one of the heavy metals: arsenic, gold, lead, mercury, platinum, and thallium.

hereditary hypertrophic n. [MIM*145900], SYN Dejerine-Sottas *disease.*

hereditary sensory radicular n. [MIM*162400], polyneuropathy characterized by the occurrence of severe, relapsing foot ulcerations of neuropathic origin, destruction of terminal digits of feet

and hands, and a loss of sensation; autosomal dominant inheritance is associated with onset in the second decade or later.

hypertrophic interstitial n., sensorimotor polyneuropathy characterized pathologically by collections of Schwann cell processes arranged concentrically around one or more nerve fibers. No genetic factors are known in its etiology. For hereditary types, see hereditary hypertrophic neuropathy.

ischemic n., n. resulting from acute or chronic ischemia of the involved nerves.

ischemic optic n., optic nerve n. secondary to hypoperfusion of the low pressure posterior ciliary arteries supplying the optic nerve head (nonarteritic) or to temporal arteritis (arteritic).

isoniazid n., axon loss; type of polyneuropathy seen in some patients treated with isoniazid.

lead n., a polyneuropathy reportedly seen in chronic lead intoxication; reputedly characterized by wrist-drop, but no convincing modern reports of this are available.

leprous n., a slowly developing granulomatous n., commonly seen in leprosy, caused by *Mycobacterium leprae.*

motor dapsone n., SYN dapsone n.

onion bulb n., designation for any of several demyelinating polyneuropathies in which the nerves are enlarged because of onion bulb formation—whorls of overlapping Schwann cell processes encircling bare medullated axons; e.g., progressive hypertrophic polyneuropathy. SEE hypertrophic interstitial n.

symmetric distal n., SYN polyneuropathy.

vitamin B$_{12}$ n., SYN subacute combined *degeneration* of the spinal cord.

neu·ro·pep·tide (noor-ō-pep'tīd). Any of a variety of peptides found in neural tissue; e.g., endorphins, enkephalins.

n. Y, a 36–amino acid peptide neurotransmitter found in the brain and autonomic nervous system. It augments the vasoconstrictor effects of noradrenergic neurons.

neu·ro·phar·ma·col·o·gy (noor'ō-far'mă-kol'ō-jē). The study of drugs that affect neuronal tissue.

neu·ro·phil·ic (noor-ō-fil'ik). SYN neurotropic. [neuro- + G. *philos,* fond]

neu·ro·pho·nia (noor-ō-fō'nē-ă). A spasm or tic of the muscles of phonation causing involuntary sounds or cries. [neuro- + G. *phōnē,* voice]

neu·ro·phy·sins (noor-ō-fiz'inz). A family of proteins synthesized in the hypothalamus as part of the large precursor protein that includes vasopressin and oxytocin in the neurosecretory granules; n. function as carriers in the transport and storage of neurohypophysial hormones.

neu·ro·phys·i·ol·o·gy (noor'ō-fiz-ē-ol'ō-jē). Physiology of the nervous system.

neu·ro·pil, neu·ro·pile (noor'ō-pil, -pīl). The complex, feltlike net of axonal, dendritic, and glial arborizations that forms the bulk of the central nervous system's gray matter, and in which the nerve cell bodies lie embedded. [neuro- + G. *pilos,* felt]

neu·ro·plasm (noor'ō-plazm). The protoplasm of a nerve cell.

neu·ro·plas·ty (noor'ō-plas-tē). Surgery of the nerves. [neuro- + G. *plastos,* formed]

neu·ro·ple·gic (noor-ō-plē'jik). Pertaining to paralysis due to nervous system disease. [neuro- + G. *plēgē,* a stroke]

neu·ro·plex·us (noo'rō-plek'sus). A plexus or network of nerve cells or fibers.

neu·ro·po·dia (noor-ō-pō'dē-ă). SYN axon *terminals,* under *terminal.* [pl. of *neuropodium* or *neuropodion,* fr. neuro- + G. *podion,* little foot]

neu·ro·pore (noor'ō-pōr). An opening in the embryo leading from the central canal of the neural tube to the exterior of the tube. [neuro- + G. *poros,* pore]

anterior n., SYN rostral n.

caudal n., the temporary opening at the extreme caudal end of the neural tube in early embryos; closes at approximately the 25th somite stage in humans. SYN posterior n.

cranial n., SYN rostral n.

posterior n., SYN caudal n.

rostral n., the temporary opening at the extreme rostral (cephalic) end of the early embryonic forebrain; closes at approximately the 20th somite stage in humans. SYN anterior n., cranial n.

neu·ro·prax·ia. Commonly used misspelling of neurapraxia.

neu·ro·psy·chi·a·try (noor′ō-sī-kī′ă-trē). The specialty dealing with both organic and psychic disorders of the nervous system; earlier term for psychiatry.

neu·ro·psy·cho·log·ic, neu·ro·psy·cho·log·i·cal (noor′ō-sī-kō-loj′ik, -loj′i-kăl). Pertaining to neuropsychology.

neu·ro·psy·chol·o·gy (noor′ō-sī-kol′ō-jē). A specialty of psychology concerned with the study of the relationships between the brain and behavior, including the use of psychological tests and assessment techniques to diagnose specific cognitive and behavioral deficits and to prescribe rehabilitation strategies for their remediation.

neu·ro·psy·cho·path·ic (noor′ō-sī-kō-path′ik). Relating to neuropsychopathy.

neu·ro·psy·chop·a·thy (noor′ō-sī-kop′ă-thē). An emotional illness of neurologic origin.

neu·ro·psy·cho·phar·ma·col·o·gy (noor′ō-sī′kō-far-mă-kol′ō-jē). SYN psychopharmacology.

neu·ro·ra·di·ol·o·gy (noor′rō-rā-dē-ol′ō-jē). The clinical subspecialty concerned with the diagnostic radiology of diseases of the central nervous system, head, and neck.

neu·ro·reg·u·la·tor (noor′ō-reg′ū-lā-tor). A chemical factor that extends a modulatory effect on a neuron.

neu·ro·re·lapse (noor′ō-rē-laps′). Obsolete term for the recurrence of neurological symptoms upon initiation of therapy, especially with antisyphilitic drugs.

neu·ro·ret·i·ni·tis (noor′ō-ret-i-nī′tis). An inflammation affecting the optic nerve head and the posterior pole of the retina, with cells in the nearby vitreous, usually producing a macular star. SYN papilloretinitis.

diffuse unilateral subacute n. (DUSN), inflammation of the neurosensory retina caused by infiltration by a roundworm such as *Baylisascaris* or *Ancylostoma* species.

Leber idiopathic stellate n., SYN stellate n.

stellate n., a unilateral n. with perifoveal exudates in Henle nerve fiber layer producing a macular star and spontaneous regression in a few months. SYN Leber idiopathic stellate n.

neu·ror·rha·phy (noor-ōr′ă-fē). Joining together, usually by suture, of the two parts of a divided nerve. SYN nerve suture, neurosuture. [neuro- + G. *rhaphē*, suture]

neu·ro·sar·co·clei·sis (noor′ō-sar-kō-klī′sis). An operation for the relief of neuralgia, consisting of resection of one of the walls of an osseous canal traversed by the nerve and transposition of the nerve into the soft tissues. [neuro- + G. *sarx*, flesh, + *kleisis*, closure]

neu·ro·sar·coid·o·sis (noor′ō-sar-koy-dō′sis). A granulomatous disease of unknown etiology involving the central nervous system, usually with concomitant systemic involvement.

neu·ro·sar·co·ma (noo′rō-sar-kō′mă). A sarcoma with neuromatous elements; includes neurofibrosarcoma, neurogenic sarcoma, and malignant schwannoma.

neu·ro·schwan·no·ma (noor′ō-shwah-nō′mă). SYN schwannoma.

neu·ro·sci·enc·es (noor-ō-sī′en-sez). The scientific disciplines concerned with the development, structure, function, chemistry, pharmacology, clinical assessments, and pathology of the nervous system.

neu·ro·se·cre·tion (noor′ō-sē-krē′shŭn). The release of a secretory substance from the axon terminals of certain nerve cells in the brain into the circulating blood. The secretory product may be a true hormone, e.g., the antidiuretic hormone released from the axon terminals of the neurons composing the supraoptic nucleus of the hypothalamus; in the case of the so-called releasing-factor neurons of the hypothalamus the cell product is not a systemic hormone in its own right but elicits the release of trophic hormones by the anterior lobe of the hypophysis, substances that in turn stimulate peripheral endocrine glands to release their systemically active hormones.

neu·ro·se·cre·to·ry (noor′ō-sē′krĕ-tōr-ē, -sē-krē′tōr-ē). Relating to neurosecretion.

neu·ro·sis, pl. **neu·ro·ses** (noo-rō′sis, -sēz). **1.** A psychological or behavioral disorder in which anxiety is the primary characteristic; defense mechanisms or any of the phobias are the adjustive techniques that an individual learns in order to cope with this underlying anxiety. In contrast to the psychoses, persons with a n. do not exhibit gross distortion of reality or disorganization of personality. **2.** A functional nervous disease, or one for which there is no evident lesion. **3.** A peculiar state of tension or irritability of the nervous system; any form of nervousness. SYN neurotic disorder. [neuro- + G. *-osis,* condition]

accident n., SYN traumatic n.

anxiety n., chronic abnormal distress and worry to the point of panic followed by a tendency to avoid or run from the feared situation, associated with overaction of the sympathetic nervous system.

cardiac n., anxiety concerning the state of the heart, as a result of palpitation, chest pain, or other symptoms not due to heart disease; a form of hypochondriasis. SYN cardioneurosis.

character n., a subclass of personality disorders.

combat n., SEE battle *fatigue,* posttraumatic stress *disorder.*

compensation n., the development of symptoms of n. believed to be motivated by the desire for, and hope of, monetary or interpersonal gain.

compulsive n., SYN obsessive-compulsive n.

conversion n., SYN conversion *hysteria.*

conversion hysteria n., SYN conversion *hysteria.*

depressive n., SEE depression, dysthymia.

experimental n., a behavior disorder produced experimentally, as when an organism is required to make a discrimination of extreme difficulty and "breaks down" in the process.

hypochondriacal n., SYN hypochondriasis.

hysterical n., a bona fide disorder characterized by an alteration or loss of physical functioning, such as blurred vision, numbness or paralysis of limbs, coordination difficulties, etc., that suggests a physical disorder, but that instead is apparently an expression of a psychological conflict or need. Also called conversion disorder. SEE ALSO hysteria.

noogenic n., in existential psychiatry, the neurotic symptomatology resulting from existential frustration.

obsessional n., SYN obsessive-compulsive n.

obsessive-compulsive n., a disorder characterized by the persistent and repetitive intrusion of unwanted thoughts, urges, or actions that the individual is unable to prevent; the compulsive thoughts may consist of single words, ideas, or ruminations often perceived by the sufferer as nonsensical; the repetitive urges or actions vary from simple movements to complex rituals; anxiety or distress is the underlying emotion or drive state, and the ritualistic behavior is a learned method of reducing the anxiety. SEE ALSO obsessive-compulsive *disorder.* SYN compulsive n., obsessional n.

oedipal n., continuation of the Oedipus complex into adulthood.

pension n., a type of compensation n., motivated by the desire for premature retirement on pension.

posttraumatic n., SYN traumatic n.

torsion n., SYN *dysbasia* lordotica progressiva.

transference n., in psychoanalysis, the phenomenon of the patient's developing a strong emotional relationship with the analyst, symbolizing an emotional relationship with a family figure; analysis of this n. constitutes an important part of psychoanalytic treatment.

traumatic n., any functional nervous disorder following an accident or injury. SEE posttraumatic stress *disorder.* SYN accident n., posttraumatic n.

neu·ro·splanch·nic (noor-ō-splangk′nik). SYN neurovisceral. [neuro- + G. *splanchnon,* a viscus]

neu·ro·spon·gi·um (noor-ō-spon′jē-ŭm, noor-ō-spŭn′jē-ŭm). **1.** Obsolete term for the plexus of neurofibrils within nerve cells. **2.** Obsolete designation for the reticular layer of the retina. [neuro- + G. *spongion,* small sponge]

Neu·ros·po·ra (noo-ros′pōr-ă). A genus of fungi (class Ascomycetes) grown in cultures and used in research in genetics and cellular biochemistry. SYN pink bread mold. [neuro- + G. *spora*, seed]

neurosteroid (nūr-ō-stēr′oyd). Steroid produced within the brain.

neu·ro·stim·u·la·tor (noor-ō-stim′ū-lā-ter). A device for electrical excitation of the central or peripheral nervous system.

neu·ro·sur·geon (noor-ō-ser′jŭn). A surgeon specializing in operations on the brain, spinal cord, spinal column, and peripheral nerves.

neu·ro·sur·gery (noor-ō-ser′jer-ē). Surgery of the nervous system.

functional n., destruction or chronic excitation of a part of the brain to treat disordered behavior or function.

neu·ro·su·ture (noor-ō-soo′choor). SYN neurorrhaphy.

neu·ro·syph·i·lis (noor-ō-sif′i-lis). Infection of the central nervous system by *Treponema pallidum*, or syphilis; there are several subdivisions, including asymptomatic n., meningeal n., meningovascular n., paretic n., and tabetic n.

asymptomatic n., clinically inapparent (except for possible abnormal pupils) syphilitic meningeal infection, diagnosed by examination of the cerebrospinal fluid; if untreated, often develops into some form of symptomatic n.

meningeal n., syphilitic meningeal infection producing an afebrile clinical meningitis, with headache, stiff neck, obtusion, etc., and abnormal CSF findings. Most often develops within 2 years of initial infection.

meningovascular n., syphilitic meningeal infection accompanied by changes (inflammation, fibrous thickening) in the walls of the subarachnoid arteries, manifested as a stroke, with sudden onset of symptoms such as hemiplegia, aphasia, visual disturbances, etc., and abnormal CSF findings.

paretic n., syphilitic infection manifested as dementia (often with delusional features), dysarthria, seizures, myoclonic jerks, action tremor, impaired walking and standing, pupillary abnormalities, and abnormal CSF findings. SYN chronic progressive syphilitic meningoencephalitis, general paresis.

tabetic n., type of n. in which the posterior roots of the spinal cord, especially in the lumbosacral area, are the principal sites of infection, resulting in ataxia, hypotonia, impotence, constipation, hypotonic bladder, areflexia, and Romberg sign; other findings include lancinating pains (most often in the legs), visceral crises, Argyll Robertson pupils, optic atrophy, and Charcot joints; in most patients, the CSF is abnormal. SYN myelosyphilis, posterior sclerosis, posterior spinal sclerosis.

neu·ro·tax·is (noor′ō-tak′sis). Neuronal elongation in the direction of a target. [neuro- + *taxis*, arrangement]

neu·ro·ten·di·nous (noor-ō-ten′di-nŭs). Relating to both nerves and tendons.

neu·ro·ten·sin (noo-rō-ten′sin). A 13–amino acid peptide neurotransmitter found in synapsomes in the hypothalamus, amygdala, basal ganglia, and dorsal gray matter of the spinal cord; it plays a role in pain perception, but its analgesic effects are not blocked by opioid antagonists; it also affects pituitary hormone release and gastrointestinal function.

neu·ro·ten·sion (noor-ō-ten′shŭn). SYN neurectasis.

neu·ro·the·ke·o·ma (noor-ō-thē-kē-ō′mă). A benign myxoma of cutaneous nerve sheath origin. [neuro- + G. *thēkē*, box, sheath, + *-oma*, tumor]

neu·ro·the·le (noor′ō-thēl). SYN nerve *papilla*. [neuro- + G. *thēlē*, nipple]

neu·ro·ther·a·peu·tics, neu·ro·ther·a·py (noor′ō-thār′ă-pū′ tiks, -thār′ă-pē). An older term for the treatment of psychological, psychiatric, and nervous disorders.

neu·rot·ic (noo-rot′ik). Relating to or suffering from a neurosis. SEE neurosis.

neu·rot·i·cism (noo-rot′i-sizm). The condition or psychological trait of being neurotic.

neu·rot·i·za·tion (noor′ō-ti-zā′shŭn). The acquisition of nervous substance; the regeneration of a nerve.

neu·ro·tize (noor′ō-tīz). To provide with nerve substance.

neu·rot·me·sis. A type of axon loss lesion resulting from focal peripheral nerve injury in which, at the lesion site, the nerve stroma is damaged to varying degrees, as well as the axon and myelin, which degenerate from that point distally; with the most severe n. lesions, the gross continuity of the nerve is disrupted. SEE axonotmesis, neurapraxia.

neu·ro·tome (noor′ō-tōm). **1.** A very slender knife or needle, used for teasing apart nerve fibers in microdissection. **2.** SYN neuromere. [neuro- + G. *tomē*, a cutting]

neu·rot·o·my (noo-rot′ō-mē). Operative division of a nerve. [neuro- + G. *tomē*, a cutting]

retrogasserian n., SYN trigeminal *rhizotomy*.

neu·ro·ton·ic (noor-ō-ton′ik). **1.** Relating to neurotony. **2.** Strengthening or stimulating impaired nervous action. **3.** An agent that improves the tone or force of the nervous system.

neu·ro·tox·ic (noor-ō-tok′sik). Poisonous to nervous substance.

neu·ro·tox·in (noor-ō-tok′sin). **1.** SYN neurolysin. **2.** Any toxin that acts specifically on nervous tissue.

neu·ro·trans·mis·sion (noor′ō-trans-mish′ŭn). SYN neurohumoral *transmission*.

neu·ro·trans·mit·ter (noor′ō-trans-mit′er). Any specific chemical agent (including acetylcholine, five amines, four amino acids, two purines, and more than 28 peptides) released by a presynaptic cell, upon excitation, that crosses the synapse to stimulate or inhibit the postsynaptic cell. More than one may be released at any given synapse. The n.'s released by presynaptic cells may modulate transmitter release from presynaptic cells. Nitric oxide may be a retrograde n., released from postsynaptic cells, to act on presynaptic cells. [neuro- + L. *transmitto*, to send across]

adrenergic n., a n. formed in sympathetic postganglionic synapses (e.g., norepinephrine).

cholinergic n., a n. formed in pre- and postganglionic synapses of the parasympathetic nervous system (e.g., acetylcholine).

neu·ro·trau·ma (noor-ō-traw′mă). **1.** Trauma of the nervous system. **2.** Trauma or wounding of a nerve. SYN neurotrosis. [neuro- + G. *trauma*, injury]

neu·ro·trip·sy (noor-ō-trip′sē). Operative crushing of a nerve. [neuro- + G. *tripsis*, a rubbing]

neu·ro·tro·phic (noor-ō-trof′ik). Relating to neurotrophy.

neu·rot·ro·phy (noo-rot′rō-fē). Nutrition and metabolism of tissues under nervous influence. [neuro- + G. *trophē*, nourishment]

neu·ro·tro·pic (noor-ō-trop′ik). Having an affinity for the nervous system. SYN neurophilic.

neu·rot·ro·py, neu·rot·ro·pism (noo-rot′rō-pē, -pizm). **1.** Affinity of basic dyes for nervous tissue. **2.** The attraction of certain pathogenic microorganisms, poisons, and nutritive substances toward the nerve centers. [neuro- + G. *tropē*, a turning]

neu·ro·tro·sis (noor-ō-trō′sis). SYN neurotrauma (2). [neuro- + G. *trōsis*, a wounding]

neu·ro·tu·bule (noor′ō-too-būl). One of the microtubules, about 24 nm in diameter, occurring in the cell body, dendrites, axon, and some synaptic endings of neurons.

neu·ro·vac·cine (noor-ō-vak′sēn). A fixed or standardized vaccine virus of definite strength, obtained by continued passage through the brain of rabbits; old way to prepare rabies vaccine.

neu·ro·var·i·co·sis, neu·ro·var·i·cos·i·ty (noor′ō-var-i-kō′sis, -var-i-kos′i-tē). A condition marked by multiple swellings along the course of a nerve. [neuro- + L. *varix*, varicosis]

neu·ro·vas·cu·lar (noor-ō-vas′kū-lăr). Relating to both nervous and vascular systems; relating to the nerves supplying the walls of the blood vessels, the vasomotor nerves.

neu·ro·veg·e·ta·tive (noor-ō-vej′ĕ-tā-tiv). SYN neurovisceral.

neu·ro·vi·rus (noor-ō-vī′rŭs). Vaccine virus modified by means of passage into and growth in nervous tissue.

neu·ro·vis·cer·al (noor-ō-vis′er-ăl). Referring to the innervation of the internal organs by the autonomic (visceral motor) nervous system. SYN neurosplanchnic, neurovegetative. [neuro- + L. *viscera*, the internal organs]

neu·ru·la, pl. **neu·ru·lae** (noor′oo-lă, -lē). Stage in embryonic development in which the prominent processes are the formation of the neural plate and the plate's closure to form the neural tube. [neur- + L. *-ulus,* small one]

neu·ru·la·tion (noor-oo-lā'shŭn). Formation of the neural plate and its closure to form the neural tube. [see neurula]

Neusser, Edmund von, Austrian physician, 1852–1912. SEE N. *granules,* under *granule.*

neu·tral (noo'trăl). 1. Exhibiting no positive properties; indifferent. 2. In chemistry, neither acid nor alkaline, i.e., [OH⁻] = [H⁺]. 3. Having the same number of positive and negative charges. [L. *neutralis,* fr. *neuter,* neither]

neu·tral·i·za·tion (noo'trăl-i-zā'shŭn). 1. The change in reaction of a solution from acid or alkaline to neutral by the addition of just a sufficient amount of an alkaline or of an acid substance, respectively. 2. The rendering ineffective of any action, process, or potential.

viral n., the elimination of viral infectivity as with specific antibodies.

neu·tra·lize (noo'tră-līz). To effect neutralization.

neu·tral red [C.I. 50040]. Used as an indicator (red at pH 6.8, yellow at 8.0), as a vital dye to stain granules and vacuoles in living cells, in testing the secretion of acid by the stomach (given with a test meal), and in general histologic staining. SYN toluylene red.

△**neutro-, neutr-.** Neutral. [L. *neutralis,* fr. *neuter,* neither]

neu·tro·clu·sion (noo-trō-kloo'zhŭn). A malocclusion in which there is a normal anteroposterior relationship between the maxilla and mandible; in Angle classification, a Class I malocclusion. SYN neutral occlusion (2). [neutro- + occlusion]

neu·tron (noo'tron). An electrically neutral particle in the nuclei of all atoms (except hydrogen-1) with a mass slightly larger than that of a proton; in isolation, it has a half-life of about 10.3 minutes. [L. *neuter,* neither]

epithermal n., a n. having an energy in the range immediately above the thermal range, i.e., having an energy between a few hundredths and approximately 100 ev.

neu·tro·pe·nia (noo-trō-pē'nē-ă). The presence of abnormally small numbers of neutrophils in the circulating blood. SYN neutrophilic leukopenia, neutrophilopenia. [neutrophil + G. *penia,* poverty]

cyclic n., SYN periodic n.

periodic n., n. recurring at regular intervals (14–45 days), in association with various types of infectious diseases, e.g., stomatitis, cutaneous ulcers, furuncles, arthritis, and others. SYN cyclic n.

▯**neu·tro·phil, neu·tro·phile** (noo'trō-fil, -fīl). 1. A mature white blood cell in the granulocytic series, formed by myelopoietic tissue of the bone marrow (sometimes also in extramedullary sites), and released into the circulating blood, where they normally represent 54–65% of the total number of leukocytes. When stained with the usual Romanovsky type of dyes, n.'s are characterized by 1) a nucleus that is dark purple-blue, lobated (three to five distinct lobes joined by thin strands of chromatin), and with a rather coarse network of fairly dense chromatin; and 2) a cytoplasm that is faintly pink (sharply contrasted with the nucleus) and contains numerous fine pink or violet-pink granules, i.e., not acidophilic or basophilic (as in eosinophils or basophils). The precursors of n.'s, in order of increasing maturity, are: myeloblasts, promyelocytes, myelocytes, metamyelocytes, and band forms. Although the terms neutrophilic leukocytes and neutrophilic granulocytes include younger cells in which neutrophilic granules are recognized, the two expressions are frequently used as synonyms for n.'s, which are mature forms unless otherwise indicated by a modifying term, such as immature n. SEE ALSO leukocyte, leukocytosis. 2. Any cell or tissue that manifests no special affinity for acid or basic dyes, i.e., the cytoplasm stains approximately equally with either type of dye. [neutro- + G. *philos,* fond]

band n., SYN band *cell.*

hypersegmented n., an aged and degenerated n. in which there may be 6 to 10 lobes in the nucleus.

immature n., a young n.; the term is usually used with reference to stab n.'s (or other "juvenile" n.'s), neutrophilic granulocytes in which the nucleus is indented but not distinctly segmented.

juvenile n., any cell of the granulocytic series in which the

neutrophilic granules are recognizable and the nucleus is indented (the first phase of segmentation).

mature n., SYN segmented n.

segmented n., a fully matured n. that has at least 2 (and as many as 5) distinct lobes in the nucleus and manifests active ameboid motion. SYN mature n.

stab n., SYN band *cell.*

neu·tro·phil·ia (noo-trō-fil'ē-ă). An increase of neutrophilic leukocytes in blood or tissues; also frequently used synonymously with leukocytosis, inasmuch as the latter is generally the result of an increased number of neutrophilic granulocytes in the circulating blood (or in the tissues, or both). N. is usually absolute, i.e., there is an increase in the total number of leukocytes as well as an increased percentage of neutrophils; in some instances, n. may be relative (i.e., there is an increased percentage of neutrophils), but the total number of all types of leukocytes may be within the normal range. SYN neutrophilic leukocytosis.

neu·tro·phil·ic (noo-trō-fil'ik). 1. Pertaining to or characterized by neutrophils, such as an exudate in which the predominant cells are n. granulocytes. 2. Characterized by a lack of affinity for acid or basic dyes, i.e., staining approximately equally with either type. SYN neutrophilous.

neu·tro·phil·o·pe·nia (noo'trō-fil-ō-pē'nē-ă). SYN neutropenia. [neutrophil + G. *penia,* poverty]

neu·troph·i·lous (noo-trof'i-lŭs). SYN neutrophilic (2).

neu·tro·tax·is (noo-trō-tak'sis). A phenomenon in which neutrophilic leukocytes are stimulated by a substance in such a manner that they are either attracted, and move toward it (**positive neutrotaxis**), or they are repelled, and move away from it (**negative neutrotaxis**); in some instances, there is no effect (sometimes called **indifferent neutrotaxis**). [neutrophil + G. *taxis,* arrangement]

ne·vi (nē'vī). Plural of nevus. [L.]

ne·vo·cyte (nē'vō-sīt). SYN nevus *cell.*

ne·void (nē'voyd). Resembling a nevus. [L. *naevus,* mole (nevus), + G. *eidos,* resemblance]

ne·vo·xan·tho·en·do·the·li·o·ma (nē'vō-zan'thō-en'dō-thē-lē-ō'mă). SYN juvenile *xanthogranuloma.* [nevus + G. *xanthos,* yellow, + endothelioma]

ne·vus, pl. **ne·vi** (nē'vŭs, -vī). 1. A circumscribed malformation of the skin, especially if colored by hyperpigmentation or increased vascularity; a n. may be predominantly epidermal, adnexal, melanocytic, vascular, or mesodermal, or a compound overgrowth of these tissues. 2. A benign localized overgrowth of melanin-forming cells of the skin present at birth or appearing early in life. SYN mole (1). [L. *naevus,* mole, birthmark]

acquired n., a melanocytic n. that is not visible at birth, but appears in childhood or adult life.

n. ane'micus, a functional developmental defect in vascular filling characterized by pale, round or oval, flat lesions, indistinguishable from surrounding normal skin on diascopy.

n. ara'neus, SYN spider *angioma.*

balloon cell n., a n. in which many of the cells are large, with clear cytoplasm.

basal cell n. [MIM*109400], a hereditary disease noted in infancy or adolescence, characterized by lesions of the eyelids, nose, cheeks, neck, and axillae, appearing as uneroded flesh-colored papules, some becoming pedunculated, and histologically indistinguishable from basal cell epithelioma; also noted are punctate keratotic lesions of the palms and soles; the lesions usually remain benign, but in some cases ulceration and invasion occur and are evidence of malignant change; autosomal dominant inheritance; caused by mutation in the human PTCH, the homolog of the "patched gene" of *Drosophila.* PTCH is found on chromosome 9q22.

bathing trunk n., a large hairy congenital pigmented n. with a predilection for the entire lower trunk; malignant melanoma may develop in childhood. SYN giant pigmented n.

Becker n., a n. first seen as an irregular pigmentation of the shoulders, upper chest, or scapular area, gradually enlarging irregularly and becoming thickened and hairy. SYN pigmented hair epidermal n.

blue n., a dark blue or blue-black n. covered by smooth skin and formed by heavily pigmented spindle-shaped or dendritic melanocytes in the reticular dermis.

blue rubber-bleb nevi, a syndrome characterized by erectile, easily compressible, thin-walled hemangiomatous nodules, present at birth, widely distributed in the skin and the alimentary canal and sometimes in other tissues; lesions in the gut may perforate or cause hemorrhage, and the patient may be anemic from continual bleeding.

capillary n., capillary hemangioma of the skin.

n. caverno'sus, SYN cavernous *angioma.*

cellular blue n., a large, acquired blue n. in which melanocytes are often clear and large, alternating with pigmented spindle cells and which may expand deeply into the subcutis; malignant change is very rare.

n. comedon'icus, congenital or childhood linear keratinous cystic invaginations of the epidermis, with failure of development of normal pilosebaceous follicles.

compound n., a n. in which there are nests of melanocytes in the epidermal-dermal junction and in the dermis.

congenital n., a melanocytic n. that is visible at birth, is often larger than an acquired n., and more frequently involves deeper structures. Congenital n. larger than 20.0 cm in diameter, termed giant congenital nevi, have a 6–12% lifetime risk of developing melanoma. SEE ALSO bathing trunk n.

dysplastic n., a n. exceeding 5 mm in diameter, with irregular, indistinct, or notched borders and mixed tan-to-black and pink-to-red color. Microscopically these are basally nested and scattered intraepidermal melanocytes with hyperchromatic nuclei larger than those of basal keratinocytes. If multiple and associated with a family history of melanoma, these nevi have a high risk of malignant change, but isolated dysplastic nevi in the absence of a family history of melanoma are less frequently premalignant. SEE ALSO malignant mole *syndrome.* SEE dysplastic nevus *syndrome.*

epithelioid cell n., SYN Spitz n.

faun tail n., a circumscribed growth of hair of the lumbosacral area, associated with diastematomyelia.

n. flam'meus, flame n., a large congenital vascular malformation n. having a purplish color; it is usually found on the head and neck and persists throughout life. SEE ALSO Sturge-Weber *syndrome.* SYN port-wine stain.

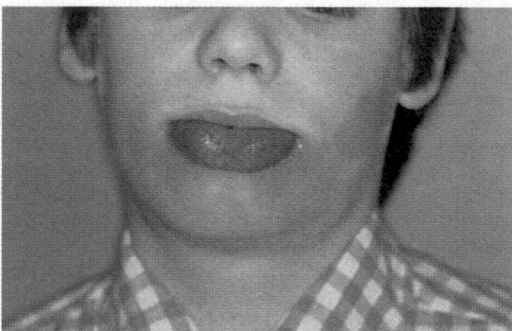

nevus flammeus

giant pigmented n., SYN bathing trunk n.

halo n., a benign, sometimes multiple, melanocytic n. in which involution occurs with a central brown mole surrounded by a uniformly depigmented zone or halo. SYN leukoderma acquisitum centrifugum, Sutton n.

inflammatory linear verrucous epidermal n., rare pruritic confluent scaly erythematous papules in linear array, usually appearing in early childhood on a limb and resolving before adulthood.

intradermal n., a n. in which nests of melanocytes are found in the dermis, but not at the epidermal-dermal junction; benign pigmented nevi in adults are most commonly intradermal.

Ito n., pigmentation of skin innervated by lateral branches of the supraclavicular nerve and the lateral cutaneous nerve of the arm,

due to scattered, heavily pigmented, dendritic melanocytes in the dermis.

Jadassohn n., SYN n. sebaceus.

junction n., a n. consisting of nests of melanocytes in the basal cell zone, at the junction of the epidermis and dermis, appearing as a slightly raised, small, flat, nonhairy pigmented (brown or black) tumor.

linear epidermal n., SYN n. unius lateris.

n. lymphat'icus, a cutaneous lymphangioma.

nape n., a pale vascular birthmark found on the nape of the neck in 25–50% of normal persons.

oral epithelial n., SYN white sponge n.

Ota n., SYN oculodermal *melanosis.*

n. papillomato'sus, a prominent wartlike mole.

pigmented hair epidermal n., SYN Becker n.

n. pigmento'sus, a benign pigmented melanocytic proliferation; raised or level with the skin, present at birth or arising early in life. SYN mole (2).

n. pilo'sus, a mole covered with an abundant growth of hair. SYN hairy mole.

n. seba'ceus, congenital papillary acanthosis of the epidermis, with hyperplasia of sebaceous glands developing at puberty and presence of apocrine glands in nonapocrine areas of the skin (commonly the scalp). A variety of epithelial tumors may arise from a n. sebaceus in adult life, most commonly basal cell carcinoma. SYN Jadassohn n.

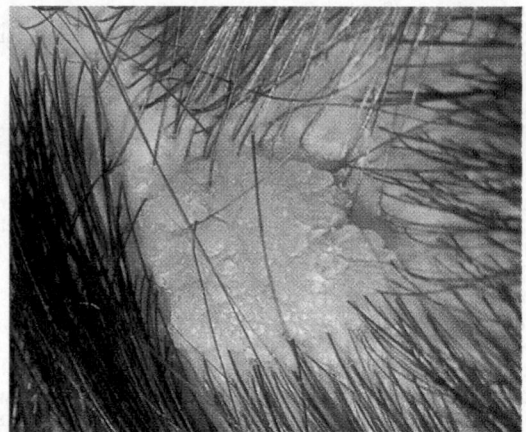

nevus sebaceus

spider n., SYN spider *angioma.*

n. spi'lus, a form of (flat) nevus pigmentosus. SYN spilus.

spindle cell n., SYN Spitz n.

Spitz n., a benign, slightly pigmented or red superficial small skin tumor composed of spindle-shaped, epithelioid, and multinucleated cells that may appear atypical; most common in children, but also appearing in adults. SYN benign juvenile melanoma, epithelioid cell n., spindle cell n.

strawberry n., a small n. vascularis (capillary hemangioma) resembling a strawberry in size, shape, and color; it usually disappears spontaneously in early childhood. SEE capillary *hemangioma.* SYN strawberry birthmark.

Sutton n., SYN halo n.

n. u'nius lat'eris, a congenital systematized linear n. limited to one side of the body or to portions of the extremities on one side; lesions are often extensive, forming wave-like bands on the trunk and spiraling streaks on the extremities. SYN linear epidermal n.

Unna n., capillary stain on nape of neck; persistent form of nevus flammeus nuchae. SYN erythema nuchae.

n. vascula'ris, n. vasculo'sus, SYN capillary *hemangioma.*

n. veno'sus, a n. formed of a patch of dilated venules.

verrucous n., a skin-colored or darker wartlike, often linear lesion appearing at birth or early in childhood and occurring in various sizes and locations, single or multiple.

white sponge n. [MIM*193900], an autosomal dominant condition of the oral cavity characterized by soft, white or opalescent, thickened, and corrugated folds of mucous membrane; other mucosal sites are occasionally involved simultaneously; caused by mutation in either the mucosal keratin gene K4 on chromosome 12 or keratin-13 gene on 17. SYN familial white folded dysplasia, oral epithelial n.

woolly hair n. [MIM*194300], a circumscribed patch of fine, curly hair in an otherwise normal scalp appearing during childhood and enlarging for a period of 2–3 years; autosomal dominant inheritance. There is another, mostly sporadic form that may be autosomal recessive [MIM*278150].

new·bery·ite (noo′ber-ē-īt). The trihydrate of magnesium hydrogen phosphate; found in some renal calculi. Cf. bobierrite, struvite. [J. Cosmo *Newberry*, Australian mineralogist, + -ite]

new·born (noo′bōrn). SYN neonatal, neonate.

Newcomer fix·a·tive. See under fixative.

Newton, Sir Isaac, English physicist, 1642–1727. SEE newton; newtonian *aberration;* Newtonian *constant* of gravitation; newtonian *flow;* newtonian *viscosity;* N. *disk, law.*

new·ton (N) (noo′tŏn). Derived unit of force in the SI system, expressed as meters-kilograms per second squared (m·kg s^{-2}); equivalent to 10^5 dynes in the CGS system. [I. *Newton*]

new·ton-me·ter. A unit of the MKS system, expressed as energy expended, or work done, by a force of 1 N acting through a distance of 1 m; equal to 1 J = 10^7 ergs.

nex·ins (neks′inz). Proteins that bridge adjacent microtubule doublets of the axoneme of cilia and flagella. [L. *nexus*, a binding, fr. *necto*, to bind + -in]

nex·us, pl. **nex·us** (nek′sŭs). SYN gap *junction.* [L. interconnection]

Nezelof, C., French pathologist, *1922. SEE N. *syndrome*, type of thymic *alymphoplasia.*

NF Abbreviation for National Formulary.

ng Abbreviation for nanogram.

NGF Abbreviation for nerve growth *factor.*

NHL Abbreviation for non-Hodgkin *lymphoma.*

N.H.S. Abbreviation for National Health Service (England).

NH$_2$-ter·mi·nal. SYN amino-terminal.

Ni Symbol for nickel.

ni·a·cin (nī′ă-sin). SYN nicotinic acid.

ni·a·cin·a·mide (nī′ă-sin-am′īd). SYN nicotinamide.

ni·al·a·mide (nī-al′ă-mīd). A monoamine oxidase inhibitor used in the treatment of depressive disorders.

nib. In dentistry, the portion of a condensing instrument that comes into contact with the restorative material being condensed; its end, the face, is smooth or serrated.

ni·car·di·pine (nī-kar′dē-pēn). A calcium channel blocker of the dihydropyridine series; used as an antihypertensive and antianginal agent.

niche (nitch, nēsh). **1.** In contrast radiography, an eroded or ulcerated area, especially gastrointestinal or vascular, which can be detected when it fills with contrast medium. **2.** An ecologic term for the position occupied by a species in a biotic community, particularly its relationships to various other competitor, predator, prey, and parasite species. [Fr.]

enamel n., SYN enamel *crypt.*

Haudek n., an archaic term for the radiographic appearance in profile of contrast material filling a gastric ulcer in the wall of the stomach.

nick (nik). In molecular biology, a hydrolytic cleavage of a phosphodiester bond in one strand of a double-stranded polynucleic acid. Cf. cut.

nick·el (Ni) (nik′l). A metallic bioelement, atomic no. 28, atomic wt. 58.6934, closely resembling cobalt and often associated with it. Protects ribosome structure against heat denaturation. A deficiency of n. causes changes in the ultrastructure of the liver. It is a cofactor in a number of enzymes (e.g., urease). [abbrev. fr. Ger.

kupfer-nickel, name of copper-colored ore from which nickel was first obtained; *nickel,* the Ger. word for a dwarfish imp]

Raney n., SEE Raney Nickel.

nick·el·o·plas·min (nik′l-ō-plas-mēn). A nickel-containing protein found in human sera.

Nickerson-Kveim test. See under test.

nick·ing (nik′ing). Localized constrictions in retinal blood vessels.

arteriovenous n., constriction of a retinal vein at an artery-vein crossing.

ni·clo·sa·mide (ni-klō′să-mīd). A teniacide effective against intestinal cestodes.

ni·co·fu·ra·nose (ni-kō-fū′ră-nōs). A peripheral vasodilator.

Nicol, William, Scottish physicist, 1768–1851. SEE N. *prism.*

Nicolas, Joseph, French physician, *1878. SEE N.-Favre *disease.*

Nicolle, Charles J.H., French microbiologist and Nobel laureate, 1866–1936. SEE N. *stain* for capsules.

nic·o·tin·a·mide (nik-ō-tin′ă-mīd). The biologically active amide of nicotinic acid, used in the prevention and treatment of pellagra. SYN niacinamide, nicotinic acid amide.

nic·o·tin·a·mide ad·e·nine di·nu·cle·o·tide (NAD, NAD$^+$, NADH). Ribosylnicotinamide 5′-phosphate (NMN) and adenosine 5′-phosphate (AMP) linked by phosphoanhydride linkage between the two phosphoric groups; binds as a coenzyme to proteins, serves in respiratory metabolism (hydrogen acceptor and donor) through alternate oxidation and reduction (NAD$^+$ ⇌ NADH). See also entries under NAD$^+$ and NADP$^+$.

nic·o·tin·a·mide ad·e·nine di·nu·cle·o·tide phos·phate (NADP, NADP$^+$, NADPH). A coenzyme of many oxidases (dehydrogenases), in which the reaction NADP$^+$ + 2H ⇌ NADPH + H$^+$ takes place; the third phosphoric group esterifies the 2′-hydroxyl of the adenosine moiety of NAD$^+$.

nic·o·tin·a·mide mon·o·nu·cle·o·tide (NMN). A condensation product of nicotinamide and ribose 5-phosphate, linking the N of nicotinamide to the (β) C-1 of the ribose; in NAD$^+$, the ring is linked by the 5′-phosphoryl residue of the ribose moiety to the 5′-phosphoryl residue of AMP; a precursor in the synthesis of NAD$^+$.

nic·o·tin·ate (nik′ō-ti-nāt). Salt or ester of nicotinic acid; some n.'s are used in ointments as rubefacients.

---

nic·o·tine (nik′ō-tēn). 1-Methyl-2-(3-pyridyl)pyrrolidine; a poisonous volatile alkaloid derived from tobacco (*Nicotiana* spp.) and responsible for many of the effects of tobacco; it first stimulates (small doses), then depresses (large doses) at autonomic ganglia and myoneural junctions; its principal urinary metabolite is cotinine. N. is an important tool in physiologic and pharmacologic investigation, is used as an insecticide and fumigant, and forms salts with most acids. SEE ALSO tobacco. [*Nicotiana*, genus name of botanical source, + - ine]

> Nicotine in inhaled tobacco smoke or in smokeless tobacco applied to buccal or nasal mucosa enters the circulation within seconds, causing an increase in heart rate, ventricular stroke volume, and myocardial oxygen consumption, as well as euphoria, heightened alertness, and a sense of relaxation. Nicotine use is powerfully addictive, readily leading to habituation, tolerance, and dependency. Withdrawal from nicotine causes restlessness, irritability, anxiety, difficulty concentrating, and craving for nicotine. Addiction to nicotine is the reason for most tobacco use and is thus directly responsible for the resulting morbidity and mortality.

---

nic·o·tine·hy·drox·am·ic ac·id me·thi·o·dide (nik′ō-tēn-hī′drok-sam′ik as′id mĕ-thī′ō-dīd). An effective cholinesterase reactivator, with actions that are most marked at the skeletal neuromuscular junction; antidotal effects are less striking at autonomic effector sites and insignificant in the central nervous system.

nic·o·tin·ic (nik-ō-tin′ik). Relating to the stimulating action of acetylcholine and other nicotine-like agents on autonomic ganglia, adrenal medulla, and the motor end-plate of striated muscle.

nic·o·tin·ic ac·id. Pyridine-3-carboxylic acid; a part of the vitamin B complex; used in the prevention and treatment of pellagra, as a vasodilator, and in hyperlipidemia, where it lowers cholesterol and acts as an HDL-raising agent. SYN anti–black-tongue factor, antipellagra factor, niacin, pellagra-preventing factor, vitamin PP.

nic·o·tin·ic ac·id am·ide. SYN nicotinamide.

nic·o·tin·ic al·co·hol. SYN nicotinyl alcohol.

nic·o·tin·o·mi·met·ic (nik-ō-tin′ō-mi-met′ik). Mimicking the action of nicotine.

nic·o·ti·nyl al·co·hol (nik-ō-tin′il). Same action and use as nicotinyl tartrate. SYN nicotinic alcohol.

nic·o·ti·nyl tar·trate. A relatively weak peripheral vasodilator related to nicotinic acid; used in peripheral vascular disorders such as Raynaud disease, acrocyanosis, and chilblains.

ni·cou·ma·lone (ni-koo′mă-lōn). SYN acenocoumarol.

nic·ta·tion (nik-tā′shŭn). SYN nictitation.

nic·ti·tate (nik′ti-tāt). To wink. [see nictitation]

nic·ti·ta·tion (nik-ti-tā′shŭn). Winking. SYN nictation. [L. *nicto*, pp. *-atus*, to wink, fr. *nico*, to beckon]

ni·dal (nī′dăl). Relating to a nidus, or nest.

ni·da·tion (nī-dā′shŭn). Embedding of the early embryo in the uterine endometrium. [L. *nidus*, nest]

NIDDM Abbreviation for non-insulin-dependent *diabetes* mellitus.

ni·do·gen (nī′dō-jen). SYN entactin. [L. *nidus*, nest, + -gen 1.]

ni·dus, pl. **ni·di** (nī′dŭs, nī′dī). **1.** A nest. **2.** The nucleus or central point of origin of a nerve. **3.** A focus of infection. **4.** The nucleus of a crystal; the coalescence of molecules or small particles that is the beginning of a crystal or similar solid deposit. **5.** The focus of reduced density at the center of an osteoid osteoma, on bone radiographs. [L. nest]

n. a′vis, a deep depression on each side of the inferior surface of the cerebellum, between the uvula and the biventral lobe, in which the tonsil rests. SYN n. hirundinis. [L. bird's nest]

n. hirun′dinis, SYN n. avis. [L. swallow's nest]

Niemann, Albert, German physician, 1880–1921. SEE N.-Pick *cell, disease;* N. *disease, splenomegaly.*

Niewenglowski, Gaston H., 19th century French scientist. SEE N. *rays,* under *ray.*

ni·fed·i·pine (ni-fed′i-pēn). A calcium channel-blocking agent of the dihydropyridine type; coronary vasodilator.

ni·fen·a·zone (ni-fen′ă-zōn). An analgesic and antipyretic.

ni·fur·al·de·zone (nī-fūr-al′dĕ-zōn). An antibacterial agent.

ni·fu·ra·tel (nī-fū′ră-tel). trichomonacide.

ni·fu·rox·ime (nī-fū-rok′sēm, -sim). A furan derivative, principally effective against *Candida albicans*.

ni·ge·rose (nī′jĕ-rōs). A disaccharide obtained by the hydrolysis of amylopectins, consisting of two D-glucose residues bound in an α1–3 linkage. [fr. *nigeran*, a polysaccharide synthesized by *Aspergillus niger*]

night·guard (nīt′gard). A device used to stabilize the teeth and reduce the traumatic effects of bruxism.

Nightingale, Florence, 1820-1910. English nurse; founder of modern nursing.

night·mare (nīt′mār). A terrifying dream, as in which one is unable to cry for help or to escape from a seemingly impending evil. SEE ALSO incubus, succubus. [A.S. *nyht*, night, + *mara*, a demon]

night·shade (nīt′shād). Any of a number of plants of the genus *Solanum* (family Solanaceae) and of some other genera of the family Solanaceae.

deadly n., SYN belladonna.

night ter·rors (nīt′tār-erz). A disorder occurring in children, in which the child awakes screaming with fright, the distress persisting for a time during a state of semiconsciousness. SYN pavor nocturnus, sleep terror.

nig·ra (nī′gră). In neuroanatomy, the *substantia* nigra. [L. fr. *niger,* black]

ni·gri·ti·es (nī-grish′i-ēz). A black pigmentation. [L. blackness, fr. *niger,* black]

n. lin′guae, SYN black *tongue.*

ni·gro·sin, ni·gro·sine (nī′grō-sin, -sēn) [C.I. 50420]. A variable mixture of blue-black aniline dyes; used as a histologic stain for nervous tissue and as a negative stain for studying bacteria and spirochetes; also used to discriminate between live and dead cells in dye-exclusion staining.

Ni·gros·po·ra (nī-gros′pōr-ă). A genus of rapidly growing fungi that produces shiny, black conidia in cultures; it is a common contaminant in laboratory cultures and is nonpathogenic for humans.

ni·gro·stri·a·tal (nī′grō-strī-ā′tăl). Referring to the efferent connection of the substantia nigra with the striatum. SEE *substantia nigra.*

NIH Abbreviation for National Institutes of Health (U.S. Public Health Service).

ni·hil·ism (nī′i-lizm, nī′hi-lizm). **1.** In psychiatry, the delusion of the nonexistence of everything, especially of the self or part of the self. **2.** Engagement in acts that are totally destructive to one's own purposes and those of one's group. [L. *nihil,* nothing]

therapeutic n., a disbelief in the efficacy or value of therapy, as of drugs, psychotherapy, etc.

ni·keth·a·mide (nī-keth′ă-mīd). Drug that acts mainly on the central nervous system, as a respiratory and cardiovascular stimulant.

Nikiforoff, Mikhail, Russian dermatologist, 1858–1915. SEE N. *method.*

Nikolsky, Pyotr V., Russian dermatologist, 1858–1940. SEE N. *sign.*

Nile blue A [C.I. 51180]. A basic oxazin dye, used as a fat and vital stain, and in Kittrich stain; as an indicator, it changes from blue to purplish red at pH 10–11.

ni·mo·di·pine (nī-mō′di-pēn). A calcium channel blocking drug of the dihydropyridine series used as a vasodilator.

ni·mus·tine (nī′mŭs-tīn). A nitrosourea antineoplastic similar to carmustine (BCNU)

nin·hy·drin (nin-hī′drin). Reacts with free amino acids to yield CO_2, NH_3, and an aldehyde, the NH_3 produced yielding a colored product (diketohydrindylidene-diketohydrinamine, a bi-indanedione derivative). SEE ALSO ninhydrin *reaction.*

ni·o·bi·um (Nb) (nī-ō′bē-ŭm). A rare metallic element, atomic no. 41, atomic wt. 92.90638, usually found with tantalum. [*Niobe,* daughter of Tantalus]

nip·ple (nip′l) [TA]. A wartlike projection at the apex of the breast on the surface of which the lactiferous ducts open; it is surrounded by a circular pigmented area, the areola. SYN papilla mammae [TA], mammilla (2), papilla of breast, teat (1), thele, thelium (3). [dim. of A.S. *neb,* beak, nose (?)]

accessory n., a supernumerary n. occurring on the mammary line.

aortic n., colloquial term for the radiographic appearance of the left superior intercostal or accessory hemiazygos vein as a bump on the aortic knob.

ni·ri·da·zole (nī-rid′ă-zōl). Used for the treatment of schistosomiasis, amebiasis, and dracontiasis.

nisin (nī′sin). A polypeptide antibiotic produced by *Streptococcus lactis;* active against certain streptococci, *Mycobacterium tuberculosis, Clostridium difficile,* and other bacteria.

nisol·di·pine (nī-sol′dī-pēn). A calcium channel blocker of the dihydropyridine series; used as an antihypertensive and antianginal agent.

Nissen, Rudolf, Swiss surgeon, 1896–1981. SEE Collis-Nissen *fundoplication;* Nissen *fundoplication;* N. *operation.*

Nissl, Franz, German neurologist, 1860–1919. SEE N. *bodies,* under *body, degeneration, granules,* under *granule, substance, stain.*

nit (nĭt). **1.** The ovum or hatched egg of a body, head, or crab louse; the egg is attached to human hair or clothing by a layer of chitin. **2.** A unit of luminance; a luminous intensity of 1 candela per square meter of orthogonally projected surface. [A.S. *knitu*]

Nitabuch, Raissa, 19th century German physician. SEE N. *layer, membrane, stria.*

ni·ter (nī′ter). SYN *potassium* nitrate. [G. *nitron,* soda, formerly not distinguished from potash]

cubic n., SYN *sodium* nitrate.

ni·ton (nī′ton). Archaic term for radon.

ni·trate (nī′trāt). A salt of nitric acid.

ni·tra·ze·pam (nī-trā′zĕ-pam). A hypnotic and sedative of the benzodiazepine class.

ni·tren·di·pine (nī-tren′-di-pēn). A calcium channel blocker of the dihydropyridine series; used as an antihypertensive.

ni·tric ac·id (nī′trik). A strong acid oxidant and corrosive.

fuming n. a., contains about 91% n. a.; used as a caustic.

ni·tric ox·ide (NO·). A colorless, radical-free gas that reacts rapidly with O_2 to form other nitrogen oxides (e.g., NO_2, N_2O_3, and N_2O_4) and ultimately is converted to nitrite (NO_2^-) and nitrate (NO_3^-); a gaseous mediator of cell-to-cell communication and potent vasodilator, formed from L-arginine in bone, brain, endothelium, granulocytes, pancreatic beta cells, and peripheral nerves by a constitutive nitric oxide synthase, and in hepatocytes, Kupffer cells, macrophages, and smooth muscle by an inducible nitric oxide synthase (e.g., induced by endotoxin). NO· activates soluble guanylate cyclase, mediates penile erection, and may be the first known retrograde neurotransmitter.

> The short-lived NO· molecule is a product of various tissues and plays a role in various processes. NO· elaborated by endothelium, which is identical to endothelium-derived relaxing factor, dilates vessels by relaxing vascular smooth muscle; nitrites used in coronary and peripheral vascular disease induce or mimic this action. The 1998 Nobel Prize in Medicine or Physiology was awarded to 3 U.S. pharmacologists, Robert F. Furchgott, Ferid Murad, and Louis J. Ignarro, for their independent discoveries of the role of nitric oxide in cardiovascular physiology. In the immune system, macrophages use NO· as a cytotoxic agent. Deficiency or inactivation of NO· may contribute to the pathogenesis of both hypertension and atherosclerosis. An excess of NO·, which is a free radical, is toxic to brain cells, and NO· is also responsible for the precipitate, often fatal, drop in blood pressure accompanying septic shock. Free NO· in the bloodstream is rapidly reduced by the iron of hemoglobin.

nitric oxide reductase, an enzyme oxidizing N_2 with some acceptor to 2NO·, a first step in the fixing of atmospheric nitrogen by bacteria.

nitric oxide synthase (NO synthase), an enzyme that catalyzes the reaction of L-arginine with $2O_2$ and 1.5NADPH to form NO, L-citrulline, $1.5NADP^+$, and $2H_2O$; there are an inducible and two constitutive forms of this enzyme: the constitutive forms play significant roles in regulating vascular tone, tissue blood flow, renal function, etc.; in bone, brain, endothelium, granulocytes, pancreatic Z-cells, and peripheral nerves, the constitutive forms are calcium-calmodulin dependent; in brain, the enzyme is cytosolic; in endothelium, it is membrane bound; the inducible form of the enzyme (e.g., by endotoxin) in hepatocytes, Kupffer cells, macrophages, and smooth muscle is not calmodulin dependent.

ni·trid·a·tion (nī-tri-dā′shŭn). Formation of nitrides; formation of nitrogen compounds through the action of ammonia (analogous to oxidation).

ni·tride (nī′trīd). A compound of nitrogen and one other element, e.g., magnesium nitride, Mg_3N_2.

ni·tri·fi·ca·tion (nī′tri-fi-kā′shŭn). **1.** Bacterial conversion of nitrogenous matter into nitrates. **2.** Treatment of a material with nitric acid.

ni·trile (nī′tril). An alkyl cyanide. Individual n.'s are named for the acid formed on hydrolysis; e.g., CH_3CN is acetonitrile rather than methyl cyanide.

nitrilo-. Prefix indicating a tervalent nitrogen atom attached to three identical groups; e.g., nitrilotriacetic acid, $N(CH_2COOH)_3$.

ni·tri·mu·ri·at·ic ac·id (nī′tri-mū-rē-at′ik). SYN nitrohydrochloric acid.

ni·trite (nī′trīt). A salt of nitrous acid.

ni·tri·tu·ria (nī-tri-too′rē-ă). The presence of nitrites in the urine, as a result of the action of *Escherichia coli, Proteus vulgaris,* and other microorganisms that may reduce nitrates.

nitro-. Prefix denoting the group $-NO_2$. [G. *nitron,* sodium carbonate.]

ni·tro·cel·lu·lose (nī-trō-sel′ū-lōs). SYN pyroxylin.

ni·tro·chlo·ro·form (nī-trō-klōr′ō-fōrm). SYN chloropicrin.

ni·tro·fu·rans (nī-trō-fū′ranz). Antimicrobials (e.g., nitrofurazone) effective against Gram-positive and Gram-negative organisms.

ni·tro·fu·ran·to·in (nī′trō-fū-ran′tō-in). A urinary antibacterial agent with a wide range of activity against both Gram-positive and Gram-negative organisms; also available as n. sodium for injection.

ni·tro·fu·ra·zone (nī-trō-fū′ră-zōn). A topical bacteriostatic and bactericidal agent often used in burns.

ni·tro·gen (N) (nī′trō-jen). **1.** A gaseous element, atomic no. 7, atomic wt. 14.00674; N_2 forms about 78.084% by volume of the dry atmosphere. **2.** The molecular form of n., N_2. **3.** Pharmaceutical grade N_2, containing not less than 99.0% by volume of N_2; used as a diluent for medicinal gases, and for air replacement in pharmaceutical preparations. [L. *nitrum,* niter, + *-gen,* to produce]

main components of nonprotein nitrogen		
(normal values given in mEq/100 mL)		
	whole blood	**plasma/serum**
total nonprotein nitrogen	20–40	18–29 (40)
nonprotein, nonurea nitrogen	16–26	6–18
unidentified nitrogen compounds	5–18	—
free amino acids (nonprotein amino acids)	4.6–6.8	3.4–5.9
ammonia	0.07–0.1	0.1–0.2
creatine	1.0–1.6	—
creatinine	—	0.5–1.3
ergothioneine	0.03	—
glutathione	4.6	—
uric acid	0.3–1.3	0.7–1.3
urea (BUN, blood urea nitrogen)	8.5–15	9.6–17.6
nucleotides	4.4–7.4	—

blood urea n. (BUN), n., in the form of urea, in the blood; the most prevalent of nonprotein nitrogenous compounds in blood; blood normally contains 10–15 mg of urea/100 mL. Measurements in the laboratory are commonly used as a measure of renal function. SEE ALSO urea n.

filtrate n., nonprotein n. in various compounds that normally pass through the glomerular filtration or through a filter in the laboratory (after proteins are precipitated).

heavy n., SYN nitrogen-15.

n. monoxide, SYN nitrous oxide.

nonprotein n. (NPN), the n. content of other than protein bodies; e.g., about one-half the nonprotein n. in the blood is contained in urea. SYN rest n.

rest n., SYN nonprotein n.

undetermined n., the n. of blood, urine, etc., other than urea, uric acid, amino acids, etc., that can be directly estimated; in blood it amounts to about 25 mg/100 mL.

urea n., the portion of n. in a biologic sample, such as blood or urine, that derives from its content of urea. SEE ALSO blood urea n.

urinary n., n. excreted as urea, amino acids, uric acid, etc., in the urine; 1 g of urinary n. indicates the breakdown in the body of 6.25 g of protein. SEE ALSO nitrogen *equivalent.*

ni·tro·gen-13 (^{13}N). A cyclotron-produced, positron-emitting radioisotope of nitrogen with a half-life of 9.97 minutes; used in protein metabolism studies and in positron-emission tomography.

ni·tro·gen-14 (^{14}N). The common nitrogen isotope, making up 99.63% of natural nitrogen.

ni·tro·gen-15 (^{15}N). The less common stable nitrogen isotope, making up 0.37% of natural nitrogen. SYN heavy nitrogen.

ni·tro·ge·nase (nī′trō-jĕ-nās). Formerly a general term used to describe enzyme systems that catalyze the reduction of molecular nitrogen to ammonia in nitrogen-fixing bacteria; now specifically applied to enzymes that carry out this reaction with reduced ferredoxin and ATP; typically n. consists of two components, the first of which reduces N_2 while the second transfers electrons.

ni·tro·gen dis·tri·bu·tion. SYN nitrogen partition.

ni·tro·gen group. Five trivalent or quinquivalent elements whose hydrogen compounds are basic and whose oxyacids vary from monobasic to tetrabasic: nitrogen, phosphorus, arsenic, antimony, and bismuth.

ni·tro·gen lag. The length of time after the ingestion of a given protein before the amount of nitrogen equal to that in the protein has been excreted in the urine.

ni·trog·e·nous (nī-troj′ĕ-nŭs). Relating to or containing nitrogen.

ni·tro·gen par·ti·tion. Determination of the distribution of nitrogen in the urine among the various constituents. SYN nitrogen distribution.

ni·tro·glyc·er·in (nī-trō-glis′er-in). An explosive yellowish oily fluid formed by the action of sulfuric and nitric acids on glycerin; used as a vasodilator, especially in angina pectoris; generates nitric oxide. SYN glyceryl trinitrate, trinitroglycerin.

ni·tro·hy·dro·chlo·ric ac·id (nī′trō-hī-drō-klōr′ik). An extremely caustic mixture that contains 18 parts nitric acid and 82 parts hydrochloric acid. SYN aqua regia, aqua regalis, nitrimuriatic acid.

ni·tro·man·ni·tol (nī-trō-man′i-tol). SYN *mannitol* hexanitrate.

ni·tro·mer·sol (nī-trō-mer′sol). The anhydride of 4-nitro-3-hydroxymercuriorthocresol; a synthetic organic mercurial compound, used as an antiseptic for skin and mucous membranes.

ni·trom·e·ter (nī-trom′ĕ-ter). A device for collecting and measuring the nitrogen set free in a chemical reaction. [nitrogen + G. *metron,* measure]

ni·tron (nī′tron). A reagent for the determination of nitric acid, perchlorate, and rhenium, as it is one of the few substances to form an insoluble nitrate.

ni·tro·phen·yl·sul·fen·yl (Nps) (nī′trō-fen′il-sŭl-fen′il). O_2N–C_6H_4–S–; nitrophenylthio; a radical easily attached to amino groups; used in peptide synthesis and protein chemistry.

ni·tro·prus·side (nī-trō-prŭs′īd). The anion $[Fe(CN)_5NO]^=$; as in sodium n.; used as a vasodilator by the intravenous route.

ni·tros·a·mines (nī-trōs′am-ēnz). Amines substituted by a nitroso (NO) group, usually on a nitrogen atom, to yield *N*-nitrosamines (R–NH–NO or R_2N–NO); can be formed by direct combination of an amine and nitrous acid (can be formed from nitrites in the acidic gastric juice); some are mutagenic and/or carcinogenic.

◇nitroso-. Prefix denoting a compound containing nitrosyl. [L. *nitrosus*]

***S*-nitrosohemoglobin** (nī-trō′sō-hē′mōglō′bin). A compound formed by the binding of nitric oxide with hemoglobin; release and uptake of the nitric oxide group produce changes in vascular resistance and blood flow, which assist in oxygen homeostasis.

ni·tro·sou·rea (nī-trō′sō-oor′ē-ă). Alkylating agent used in the treatment of many neoplasms; an example is BCNU [*N,N*′-bis(2-chloroethyl)-*N*-nitrosourea; carmustine].

ni·tro·syl (nī′trō-sil). A univalent radical or atom group, –N=O, forming the nitroso compounds.

ni·trous (nī′trŭs). Denoting a nitrogen compound containing one less atom of oxygen than the nitric compounds; one in which the nitrogen is present in its trivalent state.

ni·trous ac·id. HNO_2; a standard biologic and clinical laboratory reagent.

ni·trous ox·ide. N_2O; a nonflammable, nonexplosive gas that will support combustion; widely used as a rapidly acting, rapidly reversible, nondepressant, and nontoxic inhalation analgesic to supplement other anesthetics and analgesics; its anesthetic potency alone is inadequate to provide surgical anesthesia. SYN dinitrogen monoxide, nitrogen monoxide.

ni·tro·xan·thic ac·id (nī-trō-zan′thik). SYN picric acid.

ni·trox·o·line (nī-trok′sō-lēn). An antibacterial agent.

ni·troxy (nī-trok′sē). The –O–NO_2 radical. [contraction of nitryloxy]

ni·trox·yl (nī-trok′sil). The nitrosyl hydride, HNO.

ni·tryl (nī′tril). The radical –NO_2 of the nitro compounds.

ni·zat·i·dine (ni-zat′i-den). A histamine H_2 antagonist used to treat active duodenal ulcers.

njo·ve·ra (nyŏ-ver′ă). A nonvenereal disease of children in Zimbabwe, indistinguishable from syphilis, due to an organism apparently identical with *Treponema pallidum;* probably the same as bejel. [Zimbabwean]

N.K. Abbreviation for Nomenklatur Kommission.

nkat Abbreviation for nanokatal.

Nle Abbreviation for norleucine.

NLN. Abbreviation for National League for Nursing.

nM Abbreviation for nanomolar.

nm Abbreviation for nanometer.

NMDA Abbreviation for *N*-methyl D-aspartate; excitotoxic amino acid used to identify a specific subset of glutamate (an excitatory amino acid) receptors. SYN *N*-methyl D-aspartic acid.

NMN Abbreviation for nicotinamide mononucleotide.

NMP Abbreviation for nucleoside 5′-monophosphate.

NMR Abbreviation for nuclear magnetic *resonance.*

NO· Symbol for nitric oxide.

No Symbol for nobelium.

Noack, M., 20th century German physician. SEE N. *syndrome.*

no·bel·i·um (No) (nō-bel′ē-ŭm). An unstable transuranium element, atomic no. 102, prepared by bombardment of curium with carbon-12 nuclei and similar heavy ions on other elements of the transuranium series. [*Nobel* Institute for Physics and A.B. Nobel, Swedish inventor, 1833–1896]

Noble, Robert L., Canadian physiologist, *1910. SEE N.-Collip *procedure.*

Noble, Charles P., U.S. gynecologist, 1863–1935. SEE N. *position.*

Noble stain. See under stain.

Nocard, Edmund I.E., French veterinarian, 1850–1903. SEE *Nocardia; Nocardiaceae.*

No·car·dia (nō-kar′dē-ă). A genus of aerobic actinomycetes (family Nocardiaceae, order Actinomycetales), higher bacteria, containing weakly acid-fast, slender rods or filaments, frequently swollen and occasionally branched, forming a mycelium. Coccus or bacillary forms are produced by these organisms, which are mainly saprophytic but may be a cause of mycetoma or nocardiosis. [E. *Nocard*]

N. asteroi′des, a species of aerobic, Gram-positive, partially acid-fast, branching organisms causing nocardiosis and possibly mycetoma in humans.

N. brasilien′sis, a bacterial species that closely resembles *N. asteroides* and is a cause of mycetoma and nocardiosis in humans.

N. ca′viae, former name for *N. otitidiscaviarum.*

N. farci′nica, a species causing bovine farcy; it is the type species of the genus *Nocardia.*

N. gibso′nii, SYN *Streptomyces gibsonii.*

N. lu′rida, former name for *Amycolatopsis orientalis* subsp. *lurida.*

N. ma′durae, former name for *Actinomadura madurae.*

N. mediterra′nei, a bacterial species that produces rifamycin.

N. nova, a bacterial species commonly recovered from human infections.

N. orienta′lis, a bacterial species that produces vancomycin.

N. otitidiscaviarum, a higher bacteria (formerly *Nocardia caviae*) living in soil and one of the causes of nocardiosis and actinomycetoma.

N. transvalensis, an aerobic actinomycete; a cause of nocardiosis.

no·car·dia, pl. **no·car·di·ae** (nō-kar′dē-ă, nō-kar′dē-ē). A vernacular term used to refer to any member of the genus *Nocardia.*

No·car·di·a·ce·ae (nō-kar-dē-ā′sē-ē). A family of acid-fast, Gram-positive, aerobic bacteria (order Actinomycetales) that includes the genus *Nocardia.* [E. *Nocard*]

no·car·di·a·sis (nō-kar-dī′ă-sis). SYN nocardiosis.

no·car·di·o·form (nō-kar′dē-ō-fōrm). Denoting an organism that morphologically and culturally resembles members of the genus *Nocardia.*

Nocardiopsis (nō-kar-dē-op′sis). A genus of higher bacteria living in soil that cause subacute or chronic pneumonia, subcutaneous infection, or disseminated disease, usually in immunosuppressed patients.

N. dassonvillei, an aerobic actinomycete, formerly *Nocardia dassonvillei;* a cause of actinomycetoma.

no·car·di·o·sis (nō-kar-dē-ō′sis). A generalized disease in humans and other animals caused by *Nocardia asteroides, N. otitidiscaviarum, N. transvalensis,* and *N. brasiliensis* and characterized by primary pulmonary lesions that may be subclinical or chronic with hematogenous spread, to deep viscera, including the central nervous system; most commonly occurs in immunosuppressed patients. SYN nocardiasis.

> **granulomatous n.,** a form of n. characterized by emaciation, abdominal distention, and replacement of lymphoid tissue in lymph nodes and spleen by granulomatous tissue.

nocebo (nō-sē′bō). An unpleasant effect attributable to administration of a placebo; jargon. [L. I shall harm, fr. *noceo,* to harm, by analogy with *placebo,* I shall please]

△**noci-.** Hurt, pain, injury. [L. *noceo*]

no·ci·cep·tive (nō-si-sep′tiv). Capable of appreciation or transmission of pain. [see nociceptor]

no·ci·cep·tor (nō-si-sep′ter, -tōr). A peripheral nerve organ or mechanism for the reception and transmission of painful or injurious stimuli. [noci- + L. *capio,* to take]

no·ci·fen·sor (nō-si-fen′ser). Denoting processes or mechanisms that act to protect the body from injury; specifically, a system of nerves in the skin and mucous membranes that react to adjacent injury by causing vasodilation. [noci- + L. *fendo* (only in compounds), to strike, ward off]

△**noct-.** Nocturnal. SEE ALSO nycto-. [L. *nox,* night]

noc·tal·bu·min·ur·ia (nok′tal-boo′mi-nū′rē-ă). A pathologic increase of albumin in urine excreted during the evening, a rarely observed event. [L. *nox,* night, + albuminuria]

noc·ti·pho·bia (nok′tē-fō′bē-ă). Morbid dread of night and its darkness and silence. [noct- + phobia]

noct. maneq. Abbreviation for L. *nocte maneque,* at night and in the morning.

noc·to·graph (nok′tō-graf). SYN scotograph. [noct- + G. *graphō,* to write]

noc·tu·ria (nok-too′rē-ă). Purposeful urination at night, after waking from sleep; typically caused by increased nocturnal secretion of urine resulting from failure of suppression of urine production during recumbency or incomplete emptying of the bladder because of obstructive lesions in the lower urinary tract or detrusor instability. SYN nycturia. [noct- + G. *ouron,* urine]

noc·tur·nal (nok-ter′năl). Pertaining to the hours of darkness; opposite of diurnal (1). [L. *nocturnus,* of the night]

no·dal (nō′dăl). Relating to any node.

NODE

node (nōd) [TA]. **1.** A knob or nodosity; a circumscribed swelling; in anatomy, a circumscribed mass of tissue. **2.** A circumscribed mass of differentiated tissue. **3.** A knuckle, or finger joint. SYN nodus [TA]. [L. *nodus,* a knot]

anterior tibial n., SYN anterior tibial *lymph node.*

n. of Aschoff and Tawara, SYN atrioventricular n.

atrioventricular n. (AV n.) [TA], **(1)** a small node of modified cardiac muscle fibers located near the ostium of the coronary sinus; it gives rise to the atrioventricular bundle of the conduction system of the heart; **(2)** loosely circumscribed conduction tissue with sparse pacemakerlike (P) cells in the atrioventricular junction. SYN nodus atrioventricularis [TA], n. of Aschoff and Tawara, Tawara n.

Babès n.'s, collections of lymphocytes in the central nervous system found in rabies.

buccinator n., buccal n., SYN buccal *lymph node.*

n. of Cloquet, SYN proximal deep inguinal *lymph node.*

coronary n., the uppermost part of the atrioventricular n.

cystic n., SYN cystic *lymph node.*

delphian n., a midline prelaryngeal lymph node, adjacent to the thyroid gland, enlargement of which is indicative of thyroid disease or early metastasis from the subglottic larynx.

Dürck n.'s, perivascular chronic inflammatory infiltrates in the brain, occurring in human trypanosomiasis.

fibular n., SYN fibular *lymph node.*

Flack n., SYN sinuatrial n.

foraminal n., SYN *lymph node* of anterior border of omental foramen.

Haygarth n.'s, exostoses from the margins of the articular surfaces and from the periosteum and bone in the neighborhood of the joints of the fingers, leading to ankylosis and associated with lateral deflection of the fingers toward the ulnar side, which occur in rheumatoid arthritis.

🄸 **Heberden n.'s,** exostoses about the size of a pea or smaller, found on the terminal phalanges of the fingers in osteoarthritis, which are enlargements of the tubercles at the articular extremities of the distal phalanges. SYN tuberculum arthriticum (1).

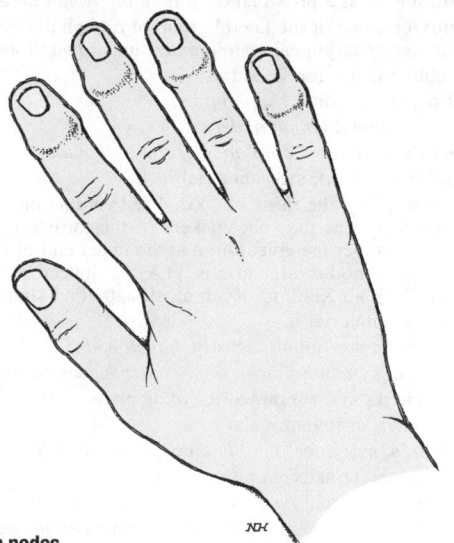

Heberden nodes

hemal n., a lymphoid structure in which the blood sinuses are present in place of lymph sinuses; hemal n.'s occur in ruminants and some other mammals, but their presence in humans is questioned. SYN hemal gland, hemolymph gland, hemolymph n., vascular gland.

hemolymph n., SYN hemal n.

Hensen n., SYN primitive n.

intermediate lacunar n., SYN intermediate lacunar *lymph node.*

jugulodigastric n., SYN jugulodigastric *lymph node.*

juguloomohyoid n., SYN juguloomohyoid *lymph node.*

Keith n., SYN sinuatrial n.

Keith and Flack n., SYN sinuatrial n.

Koch n., syn sinuatrial n.

lateral lacunar n., syn lateral lacunar *lymph node.*

n. of ligamentum arteriosum, syn *lymph node* of ligamentum arteriosum.

lymph n., see lymph node.

malar n., syn malar *lymph node.*

mandibular n.'s, syn mandibular *lymph node.*

medial lacunar n., syn medial lacunar *lymph node.*

middle rectal n., syn middle rectal *lymph node.*

milkers' n.'s, syn milkers' *nodules,* under *nodule.*

nasolabial n., syn nasolabial *lymph node.*

Osler n., in subacute bacterial endocarditis, circumscribed, painful erythematous swellings, ranging in size from that of a pinhead to that of a pea, in the skin and subcutaneous tissues of the hands and feet. syn Osler sign.

parietal n.'s, syn parietal *lymph nodes,* under *lymph node.*

posterior tibial n., syn posterior tibial *lymph node.*

primitive n., a local thickening of the blastoderm at the cephalic end of the primitive streak of the embryo. syn Hensen knot, Hensen n., Hubrecht protochordal knot, primitive knot, protochordal knot.

promontorial common iliac n.'s [TA], nodes of the common iliac group located at the promontory of the sacrum. syn nodi lymphoidei iliaci communes promontorii [TA], nodi lymphoidei promontorii.

n. of Ranvier, a short interval in the myelin sheath of a nerve fiber, occurring between each two successive segments of the myelin sheath; at the n., the axon is invested only by short, finger-like cytoplasmic processes of the two neighboring Schwann cells or, in the central nervous system, oligodendroglia cells. see also myelin *sheath.*

retropyloric n.'s, syn retropyloric *lymph nodes,* under *lymph node.*

Rosenmüller n., syn proximal deep inguinal *lymph node.*

n. of Rouviere, one of the lateral group of retropharyngeal lymph nodes. see retropharyngeal *lymph nodes,* under *lymph node.*

S-A n., abbreviation for sinoatrial n.

sentinel n., syn sentinel *lymph node.*

signal n., see signal *lymph node.*

singer's n.'s, syn vocal cord *nodules,* under *nodule.*

sinoatrial n. (S-A n.), syn sinuatrial n.

sinuatrial n. [TA], the mass of specialized cardiac muscle fibers that normally acts as the "pacemaker" of the cardiac conduction system; it lies under the epicardium at the upper end of the sulcus terminalis. syn nodus sinuatrialis [TA], atrionector, Flack n., Keith and Flack n., Keith n., Koch n., sinoatrial n., sinus n.

sinus n., syn sinuatrial n.

subdigastric n., syn jugulodigastric *lymph node.*

subpyloric n., syn subpyloric *lymph nodes,* under *lymph node.*

suprapyloric n., syn suprapyloric *lymph node.*

Tawara n., syn atrioventricular n.

teacher's n.'s, syn vocal cord *nodules,* under *nodule.*

Troisier n., syn Troisier *ganglion.*

Virchow n., syn signal *lymph node.*

visceral n.'s, syn visceral *lymph nodes,* under *lymph node.*

vital n., syn noeud vital.

---

no·di (nō′dī). Plural of nodus. [L.]

no·dose (nō′dōs). Having nodes or knotlike swellings. [L. *nodosus*]

nod·u·la·tion (nod-ū-lā′shŭn). The formation or the presence of nodules.

▋nod·ule (nod′ūl) [TA]. A small node; in skin, a node up to 1.0 cm in diameter, solid, with palpable depth. syn nodulus (1) [TA]. [L. *nodulus,* dim. of *nodus,* knot]

aggregated lymphatic n.'s, syn aggregated lymphoid n.'s of small intestine.

aggregated lymphoid n.'s [TA], masses of lymphoid tissue in the submucous coat of the vermiform appendix. syn noduli lymphoidei aggregati appendicis vermiformis [TA], aggregated lymphatic follicles of vermiform appendix, folliculi lymphatici aggregati appendicis vermiformis.

aggregated lymphoid n.'s of small intestine [TA], collections of many lymphoid follicles closely packed together, forming oblong elevations on the mucous membrane of the ileum opposite the attachment of mesentery. syn aggregate glands, aggregated lymphatic follicles of small intestine, aggregated lymphatic n.'s, agmen peyerianum, agminate glands, agminated glands, folliculi lymphatici aggregati, Peyer glands, Peyer patches.

Albini n.'s, minute fibrous n.'s on the margins of the mitral and tricuspid valves of the heart, sometimes present in the neonate and representing fetal tissue rests; described previously by Cruveilhier. Cf. n.'s of semilunar cusps.

apple jelly n.'s, descriptive term for the papular lesions of lupus vulgaris, as they appear on diascopy.

Arantius n., syn n.'s of semilunar cusps.

Aschoff n.'s, syn Aschoff *bodies,* under *body.*

benign rheumatoid n.'s, syn pseudorheumatoid n.'s.

Bianchi n., syn n.'s of semilunar cusps.

Bohn n.'s, tiny multiple cysts in newborns. They are found at the junction of the hard and soft palates and along buccal and lingual parts of the dental ridges and are derived from epithelial remnants of mucous gland tissue.

Busacca n.'s, inflammatory, granulomatous n.'s located away from the pupillary margin of the iris.

Caplan n.'s, syn Caplan *syndrome.*

cold n., a thyroid n. with a much lower uptake of radioactive iodine than the surrounding parenchyma; about one in four prove to be malignant.

Dalen-Fuchs n.'s, collections of epithelial cells lying between Bruch membrane and the retinal pigment epithelium in sympathetic ophthalmia and rarely in other granulomatous intraocular inflammations.

enamel n., syn enameloma.

Gamna-Gandy n.'s, syn Gamna-Gandy *bodies,* under *body.*

gastric lymphoid n.'s, lymphoid tissue within the lamina propria which, especially in early life, collect in small masses similar to intestinal solitary lymphatic follicles. syn folliculi lymphatici gastrici.

Hoboken n.'s, gross dilations on the outer surface of the umbilical arteries. see also Hoboken *valves,* under *valve.* syn Hoboken gemmules.

hot n., a thyroid n. with a much higher uptake of radioactive iodine than the surrounding parenchyma; usually benign but sometimes causing hyperthyroidism.

Jeanselme n.'s, a form of tertiary yaws that is characterized by the occurrence of n.'s on the arms and legs, situated usually near the joints. syn juxta-articular n.'s.

juxta-articular n.'s, syn Jeanselme n.'s.

laryngeal lymphoid n.'s, small follicles located on the posterior aspect of the epiglottis and in the ventricle of the larynx. syn folliculi lymphatici laryngei, laryngeal tonsils, lymphatic follicles of larynx.

Lisch n., iris hamartomas typically seen in type 1 neurofibromatosis. syn Sakurai-Lisch n.

lymph n., syn lymphoid n.

lymphatic n., syn lymphoid n.

lymphoid n., one of the spherical masses of lymphoid cells, frequently having a more lightly staining center. see solitary lymphatic n.'s, aggregated lymphoid n.'s of small intestine. syn folliculus lymphaticus, lymph n., lymphatic n., nodulus lymphaticus.

malpighian n.'s, syn splenic lymph *follicles,* under *follicle.*

milkers' n.'s, an infection of cows' udders by pseudocowpox virus, a member of the Poxviridae, that is transmitted to the fingers and hands of milkers, producing nodules and lymphangitis, and occasionally widespread papular or papulovesicular eruptions; human infection is transferable to uninfected cows. syn milkers' nodes, paravaccinia, pseudocowpox.

Morgagni n., syn n.'s of semilunar cusps.

picker's n.'s, lichenified skin n.'s seen in prurigo nodularis.

primary n., a lymphatic n. having small lymphocytes and lacking a germinal center.

pseudorheumatoid n.'s, benign subcutaneous n.'s of unknown etiology resembling rheumatoid n.'s but not associated with rheumatic disease; may occur in multiple sites, such as the dorsa of the feet or hands, elbows, scalp, and pretibial area. Serologic tests for collagen vascular disease are negative. SYN benign rheumatoid n.'s.

pulp n., SYN endolith.

rheumatoid n.'s, subcutaneous n.'s, occurring most commonly over bony prominences, in some patients with rheumatoid arthritis; microscopically, the n.'s are foci of fibrinoid necrosis, surrounded by a palisade of fibroblasts.

Sakurai-Lisch n., SYN Lisch n.

Schmorl n., prolapse of the nucleus pulposus through the vertebral body endplate into the spongiosa of an adjacent vertebra.

secondary n., a lymphatic n. having a germinal center.

n.'s of semilunar cusps [TA], a nodule at the center of the free border of each semilunar valve at the beginning of the pulmonary artery and aorta. SYN noduli valvularum semilunarium [TA], Arantius n., Bianchi n., corpus arantii, Morgagni n., n. of semilunar valve.

n. of semilunar valve, SYN n.'s of semilunar cusps.

siderotic n.'s, SYN Gamna-Gandy *bodies*, under *body*.

singer's n.'s, SYN vocal cord n.'s.

solitary n.'s of intestine, SYN solitary lymphatic n.'s.

solitary lymphatic n.'s [TA], minute collections of lymphoid tissue in the mucosa of the small and large intestines, being especially numerous in the cecum and appendix. SYN noduli lymphoidei solitarii [TA], folliculi lymphatici solitarii, solitary follicles, solitary glands, solitary lymphatic follicles, solitary n.'s of intestine.

splenic lymph n.'s, SYN splenic lymph *follicles*, under *follicle*.

vocal cord n.'s, small, circumscribed, bilateral, beadlike enlargements on the free edge of the vocal cords at the junction of the anterior one-third and the posterior two-thirds caused by overuse or abuse of the voice; often reversible by voice therapy. SYN singer's nodes, singer's n.'s, teacher's nodes.

no·du·lus, pl. **no·du·li** (nod′ū-lŭs, nod′ū-lī) [TA]. **1.** SYN nodule. **2.** The posterior extremity of the inferior vermis of the cerebellum, forming with the posterior medullary velum the central portion of the flocculonodular lobe. [L. dim. of *nodus*]

n. carot′icus, SYN carotid *body*.

n. lymphat′icus, SYN lymphoid *nodule*.

noduli lymphoidei aggregati appendicis vermiformis [TA], SYN aggregated lymphoid *nodules*, under *nodule*.

noduli lymphoidei solitarii [TA], SYN solitary lymphatic *nodules*, under *nodule*.

noduli val′vularum semiluna′rium [TA], SYN *nodules* of semilunar cusps, under *nodule*.

no·dus, pl. **no·di** (nō′dŭs, -dī) [TA]. SYN node. [L. a knot]

n. atrioventricula′ris [TA], SYN atrioventricular *node*.

n. buccinato′rius, SYN buccal *lymph node*.

n. sinuatria′lis [TA], SYN sinuatrial *node*.

n. tibia′lis ante′rior [TA], SYN anterior tibial *lymph node*.

NODUS LYMPHATICUS

---

no·dus lym·pha·ti·cus, pl. **no·di lym·pha·ti·ci** (nō′dŭs lim′fat′ē-kus, -nō′dī). ☆official alternate term for lymph node. [lympho- + L. *nodus,* node]

nodi lymphatici col′ici, SYN colic *lymph nodes*, under *lymph node*.

nodi lymphatici comitan′tes ner′vi accesso′rii, SYN accessory *lymph nodes*, under *lymph node*.

nodi lymphatici iliaci communes media′les, medial common iliac lymph nodes. SEE common iliac *lymph nodes*, under *lymph node*.

nodi lymphatici iliaci externi latera′les, SEE external iliac *lymph nodes*, under *lymph node*.

nodi lymphatici iliaci externi media′les, SEE external iliac *lymph nodes*, under *lymph node*.

nodi lymphatici pancrea′tici superio′res, superior pancreatic lymph nodes. SEE pancreatic *lymph nodes*, under *lymph node*.

nodi lymphatici paravesiculares, SEE paravesical *lymph nodes*, under *lymph node*.

nodi lymphatici postcavales, SEE right lumbar *lymph node*, under *lymph node*.

nodi lymphatici postvesiculares, SEE paravesical *lymph nodes*, under *lymph node*.

nodi lymphatici prevesiculares, SEE paravesical *lymph nodes*, under *lymph node*.

nodi lymphatici vesicales laterales, SEE paravesical *lymph nodes*, under *lymph node*.

---

nodus lymphoideus, pl. **nodi lymphoidei** [TA]. SYN lymph node.

nodi lymphoidei abdominis [TA], SYN abdominal *lymph nodes*, under *lymph node*.

nodi lymphoidei accessorii [TA], SYN accessory *lymph nodes*, under *lymph node*.

nodi lymphoidei anorecta′les, SYN pararectal *lymph nodes*, under *lymph node*.

nodi lymphoidei appendicula′res [TA], SYN appendicular *lymph nodes*, under *lymph node*.

n. l. ar′cus ve′nae az′ygos, SYN *lymph node* of arch of azygos vein.

nodi lymphoidei axilla′res [TA], SYN axillary *lymph nodes*, under *lymph node*.

nodi lymphoidei axillares anteriores, SYN pectoral axillary *lymph nodes*, under *lymph node*.

nodi lymphoidei axillares apicales [TA], SYN apical axillary *lymph nodes*, under *lymph node*.

nodi lymphoidei axillares centrales [TA], SYN central axillary *lymph nodes*, under *lymph node*.

nodi lymphoidei axillares humerales [TA], SYN humeral axillary *lymph nodes*, under *lymph node*.

nodi lymphoidei axillares laterales, ☆official alternate term for humeral axillary *lymph nodes*, under *lymph node*.

nodi lymphoidei axillares posteriores, ☆official alternate term for subscapular axillary *lymph nodes*, under *lymph node*.

nodi lymphoidei axillares subscapulares [TA], SYN subscapular axillary *lymph nodes*, under *lymph node*.

nodi lymphoidei axillares pectorales [TA], SYN pectoral axillary *lymph nodes*, under *lymph node*.

nodi lymphoidei brachia′les, SYN humeral axillary *lymph nodes*, under *lymph node*.

nodi lymphoidei brachiocephalici [TA], SYN brachiocephalic *lymph nodes*.

nodi lymphoidei bronchopulmona′les [TA], SYN bronchopulmonary *lymph nodes*, under *lymph node*.

n. l. buccinatorius [TA], SYN buccal *lymph node*.

nodi lymphoidei capitis et colli [TA], SYN *lymph nodes* of head and neck, under *lymph node*.

nodi lymphoidei centra′les, SYN superior mesenteric *lymph nodes*, under *lymph node*.

nodi lymphoidei cervicales anterio′res [TA], SYN anterior cervical *lymph nodes*, under *lymph node*.

nodi lymphoidei cervicales anterio′res profun′di, SYN deep anterior cervical *lymph nodes*, under *lymph node*.

nodi lymphoidei cervicales anterio′res superficia′les [TA], SYN anterior superficial cervical *lymph nodes*, under *lymph node*.

nodi lymphoidei cervicales laterales profundi [TA], SYN deep lateral cervical *lymph nodes*, under *lymph node*.

nodi lymphoidei cervicales laterales superficiales [TA], SYN superficial lateral cervical *lymph nodes*, under *lymph node*.

nodi lymphoidei coeliaci [TA], SYN celiac *lymph nodes*, under *lymph node*.

nodi lymphoidei col′ici dex′tri [TA], SYN right colic *lymph nodes*, under *lymph node*.

nodi lymphoidei col′ici me′dii [TA], SYN middle colic *lymph nodes*, under *lymph node*.

nodi lymphoidei col′ici sinis′tri [TA], SYN left colic *lymph nodes*, under *lymph node*.

nodi lymphoidei cubitales [TA], SYN cubital *lymph nodes*, under *lymph node*.

n. l. cys′ticus [TA], SYN cystic *lymph node*.

nodi lymphoidei epigastrici inferiores [TA], SYN inferior epigastric *lymph nodes*, under *lymph node*.

nodi lymphoidei faciales [TA], SYN facial *lymph nodes*, under *lymph node*.

n. l. fibula′ris [TA], SYN fibular *lymph node*.

n. l. foraminalis [TA], SYN *lymph node* of anterior border of omental foramen.

nodi lymphoidei gastrici dextri [TA], SYN right gastric *lymph nodes*, under *lymph node*.

nodi lymphoidei gastrici sinistri [TA], SYN left gastric *lymph nodes*, under *lymph node*.

nodi lymphoidei gastroomentales dextri [TA], SYN right gastro-omental *lymph nodes*, under *lymph node*.

nodi lymphoidei gastroomentales sinistri [TA], SYN left gastro-omental *lymph nodes*, under *lymph node*.

nodi lymphoidei gluteales [TA], SYN gluteal *lymph nodes*, under *lymph node*.

nodi lymphoidei hepatici [TA], SYN hepatic *lymph nodes*, under *lymph node*.

nodi lymphoidei ileocolici [TA], SYN ileocolic *lymph nodes*, under *lymph node*.

nodi lymphoidei iliaci communes [TA], SYN common iliac *lymph nodes*, under *lymph node*.

nodi lymphoidei iliaci communes promonto′rii [TA], SYN promontorial common iliac *nodes*, under *node*.

nodi lymphoidei iliaci externi [TA], SYN external iliac *lymph nodes*, under *lymph node*.

nodi lymphoidei iliaci interni [TA], SYN internal iliac *lymph nodes*, under *lymph node*.

nodi lymphoidei inguinales profundi, SYN deep inguinal *lymph nodes*, under *lymph node*.

nodi lymphoidei inguinales superficiales [TA], SYN superficial inguinal *lymph nodes*, under *lymph node*.

nodi lymphoidei intercostales [TA], SYN intercostal *lymph nodes*, under *lymph node*.

nodi lymphoidei interiliaci [TA], SYN interiliac *lymph nodes*, under *lymph node*.

nodi lymphoidei interpectorales [TA], SYN interpectoral *lymph nodes*, under *lymph node*.

nodi lymphoidei intrapulmonales [TA], SYN intrapulmonary *lymph nodes*, under *lymph node*.

nodi lymphoidei jugulares anteriores, SYN anterior superficial cervical *lymph nodes*, under *lymph node*.

nodi lymphoidei jugulares laterales, SYN lateral jugular *lymph nodes*, under *lymph node*.

n. l. jugulodigas′tricus [TA], SYN jugulodigastric *lymph node*.

n. l. juguloomohyoi′deus [TA], SYN juguloomohyoid *lymph node*.

nodi lymphoidei juxtaesophageales [TA], SYN juxtaesophageal *lymph nodes*, under *lymph node*.

nodi lymphoidei juxtaesophageales pulmonales, SYN juxtaesophageal *lymph nodes*, under *lymph node*.

nodi lymphoidei juxtaintestinales [TA], SYN juxta-intestinal mesenteric *lymph nodes*, under *lymph node*.

n. l. lacuna′ris interme′dius [TA], SYN intermediate lacunar *lymph node*.

n. l. lacuna′ris latera′lis [TA], SYN lateral lacunar *lymph node*.

n. l. lacuna′ris media′lis [TA], SYN medial lacunar *lymph node*.

nodi lymphoidei lienales, ✩official alternate term for splenic *lymph nodes*, under *lymph node*.

n. l. ligamen′ti arterio′si [TA], SYN *lymph node* of ligamentum arteriosum.

nodi lymphoidei linguales [TA], SYN lingual *lymph nodes*, under *lymph node*.

nodi lymphoidei lumbales dextri [TA], SYN right lumbar *lymph nodes*, under *lymph node*.

nodi lymphoidei lumbales intermedii [TA], SYN intermediate lumbar *lymph nodes*, under *lymph node*.

nodi lymphoidei lumbales sinistri [TA], SYN left lumbar *lymph nodes*, under *lymph node*.

nodi lymphoidei abdom′inis viscera′les [TA], SYN visceral *lymph nodes* of abdomen, under *lymph node*.

n. l. mala′ris [TA], SYN malar *lymph node*.

n. l. mandibula′ris [TA], SYN mandibular *lymph node*.

nodi lymphoidei mastoidei [TA], SYN mastoid *lymph nodes*, under *lymph node*.

nodi lymphoidei mediastinales anteriores, SYN brachiocephalic *lymph nodes*.

nodi lymphoidei mediastinales posteriores, SYN prevertebral *lymph nodes*, under *lymph node*.

nodi lymphoidei membri inferioris [TA], SYN *lymph nodes* of lower limb, under *lymph node*.

nodi lymphoidei membri superioris [TA], SYN *lymph nodes* of upper limb, under *lymph node*.

nodi lymphoidei mesenterici [TA], SYN mesenteric *lymph nodes*, under *lymph node*.

no′di lymphoidei mesenter′ici inferio′res [TA], SYN inferior mesenteric *lymph nodes*, under *lymph node*.

no′di lymphoidei mesenter′ici superio′res [TA], SYN superior mesenteric *lymph nodes*, under *lymph node*.

nodi lymphoidei mesocolici [TA], SYN mesocolic *lymph nodes*, under *lymph node*.

n. l. nasolabia′lis [TA], SYN nasolabial *lymph node*.

nodi lymphoidei obturatorii [TA], SYN obturator *lymph nodes*, under *lymph node*.

nodi lymphoidei occipitales [TA], SYN occipital *lymph nodes*, under *lymph node*.

nodi lymphoidei pancrea′tici [TA], SYN pancreatic *lymph nodes*, under *lymph node*.

nodi lymphoidei pancreaticoduodenales [TA], SYN pancreatico-duodenal *lymph nodes*, under *lymph node*.

nodi lymphoidei pancreaticolienales, SYN pancreaticosplenic *lymph nodes*, under *lymph node*.

nodi lymphoidei pancreaticosplenales [TA], SYN pancreatico-splenic *lymph nodes*, under *lymph node*.

nodi lymphoidei paracolici, SYN mesocolic *lymph nodes*, under *lymph node*.

nodi lymphoidei paramammarii [TA], SYN paramammary *lymph nodes*, under *lymph node*.

nodi lymphoidei pararectales [TA], SYN pararectal *lymph nodes*, under *lymph node*.

nodi lymphoidei parasternales [TA], SYN parasternal *lymph nodes*, under *lymph node*.

nodi lymphoidei paratracheales [TA], SYN paratracheal *lymph node*.

nodi lymphoidei parauterini [TA], SYN parauterine *lymph nodes*, under *lymph node*.

nodi lymphoidei paravaginales [TA], SYN paravaginal *lymph nodes*, under *lymph node*.

no′di lymphoidei parieta′les [TA], SYN parietal *lymph nodes*, under *lymph node*.

nodi lymphoidei parotid′ei intraglandulares [TA], SYN intraglandular deep parotid *lymph nodes*, under *lymph node*.

nodi lymphoidei parotid′ei profundi [TA], SYN deep parotid *lymph nodes*, under *lymph node*.

nodi lymphoidei parotid′ei profundi infra-auricula′res, SYN infraauricular deep parotid *lymph nodes*, under *lymph node*.

nodi lymphoidei parotidei profundi preauriculares [TA], SYN preauricular deep parotid *lymph nodes,* under *lymph node.*

nodi lymphoidei parotid'ei superficiales [TA], SYN superficial parotid *lymph nodes,* under *lymph node.*

nodi lymphoidei pelvis [TA], SYN pelvic *lymph nodes,* under *lymph node.*

nodi lymphoidei pericardiales laterales [TA], SYN lateral pericardial *lymph nodes,* under *lymph node.*

nodi lymphoidei phrenici inferiores [TA], SYN inferior phrenic *lymph nodes,* under *lymph node.*

nodi lymphoidei phrenici superiores [TA], SYN superior phrenic *lymph nodes,* under *lymph node.*

nodi lymphoidei popliteales [TA], SYN popliteal *lymph nodes,* under *lymph node.*

nodi lymphoidei precaecales [TA], SYN prececal *lymph nodes,* under *lymph node.*

nodi lymphoidei prelaryngeales [TA], SYN prelaryngeal *lymph nodes,* under *lymph node.*

nodi lymphoidei prepericardiaci [TA], SYN prepericardial *lymph nodes,* under *lymph node.*

nodi lymphoidei pretracheales [TA], SYN pretracheal *lymph nodes,* under *lymph node.*

nodi lymphoidei prevertebrales, ☆official alternate term for prevertebral *lymph nodes,* under *lymph node.*

nodi lymphoidei promontorii, SYN promontorial common iliac *nodes,* under *node.*

n. l. proximalis profundus [TA], SYN proximal deep inguinal *lymph node.*

nodi lymphoidei pulmonales, SYN intrapulmonary *lymph nodes,* under *lymph node.*

nodi lymphoidei pylorici, SYN pyloric *lymph nodes,* under *lymph node.*

nodi lymphoidei rectales superiores [TA], SYN superior rectal *lymph nodes,* under *lymph node.*

n. l. recta'lis me'dius, SYN middle rectal *lymph node.*

nodi lymphoidei retrocecales [TA], SYN retrocecal *lymph nodes,* under *lymph node.*

nodi lymphoidei retropharyngeales [TA], SYN retropharyngeal *lymph nodes,* under *lymph node.*

no'di lymphoidei retropylo'rici [TA], SYN retropyloric *lymph nodes,* under *lymph node.*

nodi lymphoidei sacrales [TA], SYN sacral *lymph nodes,* under *lymph node.*

nodi lymphoidei sigmoidei [TA], SYN sigmoid *lymph nodes,* under *lymph node.*

nodi lymphoidei splenici [TA], SYN splenic *lymph nodes,* under *lymph node.*

nodi lymphoidei subaortici [TA], SYN subaortic *lymph nodes,* under *lymph node.*

nodi lymphoidei submandibulares [TA], SYN submandibular *lymph nodes,* under *lymph node.*

nodi lymphoidei submentales [TA], SYN submental *lymph nodes,* under *lymph node.*

no'di lymphoidei subpylo'rici [TA], SYN subpyloric *lymph nodes,* under *lymph node.*

nodi lymphoidei superiores centrales [TA], SYN central superior mesenteric *lymph nodes,* under *lymph node.*

nodi lymphoidei supraclaviculares [TA], SYN supraclavicular *lymph nodes,* under *lymph node.*

n. l. suprapylo'ricus [TA], SYN suprapyloric *lymph node.*

nodi lymphoidei thoracis [TA], SYN thoracic *lymph nodes,* under *lymph node.*

nodi lymphoidei thyroidei [TA], SYN thyroid *lymph nodes,* under *lymph node.*

n. l. tibia'lis poste'rior [TA], SYN posterior tibial *lymph node.*

nodi lymphoidei tracheobronchiales inferiores, SYN inferior tracheobronchial *lymph nodes,* under *lymph node.*

nodi lymphoidei tracheobronchiales superiores [TA], SYN superior tracheobronchial *lymph nodes,* under *lymph node.*

nodi lymphoidei viscerales [TA], SYN visceral *lymph nodes,* under *lymph node.*

NOE Abbreviation for nuclear Overhauser *effect.*

no·e·mat·ic (nō-ē-mat′ik). Rarely used term relating to the mental processes. [G. *noēma,* perception, a thought]

no·e·sis (nō-ē′sis). Cognition, especially through direct and self-evident knowledge. [G. *noēsis,* thought, intelligence]

no·et·ic (nō-et′ik). Relating to noesis.

no·eud vi·tal (noo vē-tal′). A circumscript region in the lower part of the medulla oblongata, near the apex of the calamus scriptorius, interpreted by M. Flourens (1858) as a nerve center controlling respiration. SYN vital knot, vital node. [Fr.]

No·gu·chia (nō-goo′chē-ă). A genus of aerobic to facultatively anaerobic, motile, peritrichous bacteria (family Brucellaceae) containing small, slender, Gram-negative, encapsulated rods. These organisms are present in the conjunctiva of humans and other animals affected by a follicular type of disease. The type species is *N. granulosis.* [Hideyo *Noguchi,* Japanese bacteriologist, 1876–1928]

N. granulo'sis, a bacterial species regarded by some as a cause of trachoma in humans; it produces a granular conjunctivitis in monkeys and apes; it is the type species of the genus *N.*

noise (noyz). **1.** Unwanted sound, particularly complex sound that lacks a musical quality because the various frequencies of which it is composed are not whole or partial number multiples (harmonics) of each other. **2.** Unwanted additions to a signal not arising at its source; e.g., the 60-cycle frequency wave in an electrocardiogram; largely eliminated from modern (post-1980) machines (includes visual n. on imaging studies). SEE signal-to-noise *ratio.* **3.** Extraneous uncontrolled variables influencing the distibution of measurements in a set of data. [M.E., fr. O.Fr., fr. L.L. *nausea,* seasickness]

structured n., in radiology, the signals from anatomic structures that interfere with the detection of significant pathology.

white n., a complex sound consisting of many frequencies over a wide band of frequencies; often used for masking of hearing in the nontest ear in the measurement of hearing.

no·ma (nō′mă). A gangrenous stomatitis, usually beginning in the mucous membrane of the corner of the mouth or cheek, and then progressing fairly rapidly to involve the entire thickness of the lips or cheek (or both), with conspicuous necrosis and complete sloughing of tissue; usually observed in poorly nourished children and debilitated adults, especially in lower socioeconomic groups, and frequently preceded by another disease, e.g., kala azar, dysentery, or scarlet fever. A similar process (n. pudendi, n. vulvae) also may involve the labia majora. Several organisms are usually found in the necrotic material, but fusiform bacilli, *Borrelia* organisms, staphylococci, and anaerobic streptococci are most frequently observed. SYN cancrum oris, stomatonecrosis, water canker. [G. *nomē,* a spreading (sore)]

Nomarski, Georges, 20th century French optical inventor. SEE N. *optics.*

no·men·cla·ture (nō′men-klā-choor, nō-men′klă-choor). A system of names as of anatomic structures, organisms, used in any science. [L. *nomenclatura,* a listing of names, fr. *nomen,* name, + *calo,* to proclaim]

binary n., binomial n., SYN linnaean *system* of nomenclature.

Cleland n., a n. for representing the binding mechanisms of enzyme-catalyzed reactions; in this n., substrates are represented by the letters A, B, C, etc., while products are represented by P, Q, R, etc., enzyme by E, and modified forms of the enzyme by F, G, etc.; in addition, the number of substrates or products is represented by uni, bi, ter, etc.; thus, an aminotransferase reaction (e.g., alanine transaminase) has a ping-pong bi bi mechanism, and glutamine synthetase has been reported to have a random ter ter mechanism. See also entries under subentries under mechanism.

No·men·kla·tur Kom·mis·sion (N.K.). Committee on Nomenclature of the German Anatomical Society, appointed to revise or supplement the BNA (1895).

no·mi·fen·sine ma·le·ate (nō-mi-fen′sēn). An antidepressant.

Nom·i·na An·a·tom·i·ca (NA) (nom′i-nă an-ă-tom′i-kă, nō′mi-nă an′ă-tō′mi-kă). The modification of the Basle Nomina Anatomica or BNA system of anatomic terminology adopted in 1955 by the International Congress of Anatomists in Paris, France. The International Anatomical Nomenclature Committee was responsible for continued revisions of the NA that had been reviewed and adopted by the International Congress of Anatomists meeting at five-year intervals from 1955 to 1985. NA was replaced by Terminologia Anatomica [TA] in 1998, produced by the Federative Committee on Anatomical Terminology.

nom·o·gram (nōm′ō-gram). A form of line chart showing scales for the variables involved in a particular formula in such a way that corresponding values for each variable lie in a straight line intersecting all the scales. SYN nomograph (2). [G. *nomos,* law, + *gramma,* something written]

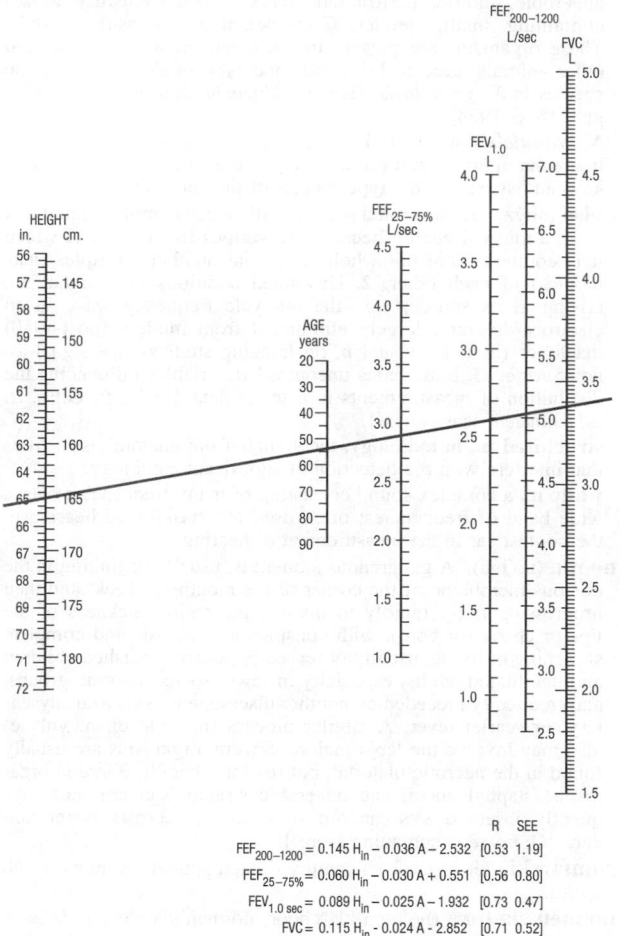

FEF$_{200-1200}$ = 0.145 H$_{in}$ − 0.036 A − 2.532 [0.53 1.19]

FEF$_{25-75\%}$ = 0.060 H$_{in}$ − 0.030 A + 0.551 [0.56 0.80]

FEV$_{1.0\ sec}$ = 0.089 H$_{in}$ − 0.025 A − 1.932 [0.73 0.47]

FVC = 0.115 H$_{in}$ − 0.024 A − 2.852 [0.71 0.52]

nomogram: predicting expiratory airflow (women)

blood volume n., a n. used to predict blood volume on the basis of the individual's weight and height.

cartesian n., a n. based on rectangular coordinates, representing two variables, on which a family of isopleths is superimposed for each of the additional variables involved. [from R. Descartes, French philosopher and mathematician, 1596–1650]

d'Ocagne n., an alignment chart consisting of an arrangement of three or more graduated lines (straight or curved), each constituting a scale of values of a variable, constructed so that any straight line crossing these scales connects the simultaneously compatible values; from values for any two variables, the values of all other variables can be determined.

Radford n., a n. used to predict necessary tidal volume for artificial respiration on the basis of respiratory rate, body weight, and

sex; correction factors are supplied for activity, fever, altitude, metabolic acidosis, and alterations in dead space.

Siggaard-Andersen n., a n. used to predict acid-base composition of blood by the slope and position of a buffer line constructed when P$_{CO_2}$ on a logarithmic scale is plotted against pH.

nom·o·graph (nom′ō-graf). **1.** A graph consisting of three coplanar curves, usually parallel, each graduated for a different variable so that a straight line cutting all three curves intersects the related values of each variable. **2.** SYN nomogram. [G. *nomos,* law, + *graphō,* to write]

nom·o·thet·ic (nom-ō-thet′ik). Denoting the generalizations pertaining to the behavior of groups of individuals as groups, as opposed to idiographic. [G. *nomos,* law, + *thesis,* a placing]

no·mo·top·ic (nō-mō-top′ik). Relating to, or occurring at, the usual or normal place. [G. *nomos,* law, custom, + *topos,* place]

non·al·lele (non-ă-lēl′). Used of genes that are not competitors at the same locus; how independently they will behave depends on whether their loci are linked. At least when first formed (for instance, as a result of unequal crossing-over), two nonalleles may be identical.

no·nan (nō′nan). Occurring on the ninth day. [L. *nonus,* ninth]

n-**non·a·no·ic ac·id** (non-ă-nō′ik). SYN pelargonic acid.

non·a·pep·tide (non-a-pep′tīd). An oligopeptide containing nine amino acid residues (e.g., oxytocin).

non·bur·sate (non-ber′sāt). Denoting a nontaxonomic division of Nematoda embracing those in which the male copulatory bursa is only a skin fold containing no fleshy ribs, as seen in hookworms and other bursate nematodes. [L. *non,* not, + Mediev. L. *bursa,* purse]

non·car·i·o·gen·ic (non-kā′rē-ō-jen′ik). Not caries-producing.

non·cel·lu·lar (non-sel′ū-lăr). **1.** Lacking cellular organization, as applied to viruses, which can only replicate within a cell, whether prokaryotic or eukaryotic. SYN subcellular. **2.** SYN acellular (1).

non·chro·mo·gens (non-krō′mō-jenz). SYN Runyon group III *mycobacteria.*

non·com·e·do·gen·ic (non-kom′ē-dō-jen′ik). Tending not to promote the formation of comedones.

non com·pos men·tis (non kom′pos men′tis). Not of sound mind; mentally incapable of managing one's affairs. [L. *non,* not, + *compos,* participating, competent, + *mens,* gen. *mentis,* mind]

non·dis·ease (non′dis-ēz). Absence of disease when a specific disease is suspected but not found.

non·dis·junc·tion (non-dis-jŭnk′shŭn). Failure of one or more pairs of chromosomes to separate at the meiotic stage of karyokinesis, with the result that both chromosomes are carried to the one daughter cell and none to the other.

primary n., n. occurring in a previously normal cell.

secondary n., n. occurring in an aneuploid cell that was the result of a primary n.

non·e·lec·tro·lyte (non-ē-lek′trō-līt). A substance with molecules that do not, in solution, dissociate to ions and, therefore, do not carry an electric current.

non·es·tro·gen·ic (non-es-trō-jen′ik). **1.** Not causing estrus in animals. **2.** Not having an action similar to that of an estrogen. Cf. nonuterotropic. SYN nonoestrogenic.

non·im·mune (non-i-mūn′). Pertaining to an individual that is not immune or to a serum from such an individual.

non·im·mun·i·ty (non-i-mūn′i-tē). SYN aphylaxis.

non·in·fec·tious (non′in-fek′shŭs). Not infectious; not able to spread disease.

non·in·va·sive (non-in-vā′siv). Denoting a procedure that does not require insertion of an instrument or device through the skin or a body orifice for diagnosis or treatment.

non·ion·ic (non-ī-on′ik). A class of radiographic contrast media that do not ionize in solution, thereby decreasing effective osmolarity and toxicity. SEE ALSO low osmolar contrast *agent.*

non·ma·lef·i·cence (non-mal′ef-ĭ-sens). The ethical principle of doing no harm, based on the Hippocratic maxim, *primum non nocere,* first do no harm. [non- + L. *maleficencia,* evildoing, fr. *male,* badly, wrongly, + *facio,* to do, act]

non·med·ul·lat·ed (non-med′ū-lāt-ed). SYN unmyelinated.

non·my·e·li·nat·ed (non-mī′ĕ-li-nāt′ed). SYN unmyelinated.

non·ne·o·plas·tic (non′nē-ō-plas′tik). Not neoplastic.

non·nu·cle·at·ed (non-noo′klē-ā-ted). Having no nucleus.

non·oc·clu·sion (non-ŏ-kloo′shŭn). Failure of a tooth to contact an opposing tooth.

non·oes·tro·gen·ic. SYN nonestrogenic.

non·ose (non′ōs). A sugar with nine carbon atoms. [L. *nonus*, ninth]

non·ox·y·nol 9 (non′noks-ĭ-nol). A group of compounds that are surface-acting agents, used in spermicidal preparations such as contraceptive foam and diaphragm jelly.

nonparametric (non-par′ă-met′rik). A group of statistical maneuvers that can be applied effectively to data nonnormal or non-Gaussian in distribution.

non·par·ous (non-par′ŭs). SYN nulliparous.

non·pen·e·trance (non-pen′ĕ-trans). The state in which a genetic trait, although present in the appropriate genotype (i.e., homozygous, hemizygous, or heterozygous according to the state of dominance and mode of inheritance), fails to manifest itself in the phenotype because of modifying factors. Cf. hypostasis.

non·pro·pri·e·tary name (non-prō-prī′ĕ-tār-ē). A short name (often called a generic name) of a chemical, drug, or other substance that is not subject to trademark (proprietary) rights but is, in contrast to a trivial name, recognized or recommended by government agencies (e.g., Federal Food and Drug Administration) and by quasi-official organizations (e.g., U.S. Adopted Names Council) for general public use. Like a proprietary name, it is almost always a coined designation derived without using set criteria. Cf. trivial name, proprietary name, semisystematic name, systematic name.

non·pro·te·o·gen·ic (non-prō′tē-ō-jen′ik). Not leading to the production of proteins.

non·re·set no·dus si·nu·a·tri·a·lis (non-rē′set nō′dŭs sī′noo-ā-trē-ā′lis). Nonreset of the sinoatrial node produced by a premature atrial depolarizaton when the sum of the duration of the premature cycle and the return cycle is fully compensatory, i.e., twice the duration of the spontaneous cycle length. Cf. reset nodus sinuatrialis.

non·ro·ta·tion (non-rō-tā′shŭn). Failure of normal rotation.

n. of intestine, a developmental anomaly resulting in the small intestine being on the right of the abdomen and the colon on the left.

n. of kidney, a developmental anomaly in which the hilum of the kidney retains its original position, with the renal pelvis lying ventrally.

non·sa·pon·i·fi·a·ble (non-să-pon-i-fī′a-bl). Not subject to saponification; e.g., triacylglycerols are saponifiable but cholesterol is n.

non·se·cre·tor (non-sē-krē′tŏr, -tōr). An individual whose saliva does not contain antigens of the ABO blood group. SEE ALSO secretor.

non·sense. As used in genetics, relating to a mutation that causes a sequence such that the growing peptide chain terminates, often after several incorrect amino acid residues are incorporated.

nonsense suppression, mutant tRNAs that read a chain termination codon as the signal for incorporation of a specific amino acid residue.

non·un·ion (non′ūn-yŭn). Failure of normal healing of a fractured bone.

non·uter·o·tro·pic (non-ū-ter-ō-trō′pik). Not causing an effect on the uterus. Cf. nonestrogenic.

non·va·lent (non-vā′lent). Having no valency; not capable of entering into chemical composition.

non·vas·cu·lar (non-vas′kū-lăr). SYN avascular.

non·ver·bal (non-ver′bl). Denoting communication without words, e.g., by signs, symbols, facial expressions, gestures, posture.

non·vi·a·ble (non-vī′ă-bl). **1.** Incapable of independent existence; often denoting a prematurely born fetus. **2.** Denoting a microorganism or parasite incapable of metabolic or reproductive activity.

Noonan, Jacqueline A., U.S. pediatric cardiologist, *1921. SEE N. *syndrome.*

♻**nor-.** **1.** Chemical prefix denoting 1) elimination of one methylene group from a chain, the highest permissible locant being used; 2) contraction of a (steroid) ring by one CH_2 unit, the locant being the capital letter identifying the ring. Elimination of two methylene groups is denoted by the prefix dinor-; three groups, by trinor-, etc. **2.** Chemical prefix denoting "normal," i.e., unbranched chain of carbon atoms in aliphatic compounds, as opposed to branched with the same number of carbon atoms; e.g., norleucine vs. leucine.

nor·a·dren·a·line (nor-ă-dren′ă-lin). SYN norepinephrine.

n. acid tartrate, SYN *norepinephrine* bitartrate.

n. bitartrate, SYN *norepinephrine* bitartrate.

nor·da·ze·pam (nor′daz-pam). An active sedative/hypnotic of the benzodiazepine class; an active metabolite of diazepam, chlorazepate, and several other benzodiazepines; has a long biologic half-life (40–80 hours).

nor·def·rin hy·dro·chlo·ride (nor-def′rin). A sympathomimetic and vasoconstrictor.

nor·ep·i·neph·rine (nor′ep-i-nef′rin). L-(−)-α-(aminomethyl)-3,4-dihydroxybenzyl alcohol; a catecholamine hormone of which the natural form is D, although the L form has some activity; the base is considered to be the postganglionic adrenergic mediator, acting on α and β receptors; it is stored in chromaffin granules in the adrenal medulla, in much smaller amounts than epinephrine, and secreted in response to hypotension and physical stress; in contrast to epinephrine it has little effect on bronchial smooth muscle, metabolic processes, and cardiac output, but has strong vasoconstrictive effects and is used pharmacologically as a vasopressor, primarily as the bitartrate salt. SYN levarterenol, noradrenaline.

n. bitartrate, (-)-α-(aminomethyl)-3,4-dihydroxybenzyl alcohol tartrate. For actions and uses, see n. SYN levarterenol bitartrate, noradrenaline acid tartrate, noradrenaline bitartrate.

nor·eth·an·dro·lone (nor-eth-an′drō-lōn). An androgenic steroid similar chemically and pharmacologically to testosterone.

nor·eth·in·drone (nor-eth′in-drōn). A potent orally effective progestational agent with some estrogenic and androgenic activity; used as a substitute for progesterone and, in combination with an estrogen, as an oral contraceptive. SYN norethisterone.

n. acetate, an orally active progestin with some estrogenic and androgenic activity, used to treat endometriosis and, with an estrogen, as an oral contraceptive.

nor·eth·is·ter·one (nor-eth-is′ter-ōn). SYN norethindrone.

nor·e·thyn·o·drel (nor-ĕ-thī′nō-drel). An orally active progestin with some estrogenic activity; used as a progestational agent and, in combination with mestranol, as an oral contraceptive.

nor·flox·a·cin (nor-floks′ă-sin). An oral broad-spectrum quinoline antibacterial agent used in the treatment of urinary tract infections.

nor·ges·trel (nor-jes′trel). A progestin used in oral contraceptive products.

nor·leu·cine (Nle) (nor-loo′sin). α-Amino-*n*-caproic acid; 2-aminohexanoic acid; an α-amino acid, isomer of leucine and isoleucine, but not found in proteins; a deamination product of L-lysine, to which it is linked in collagens. SYN glycoleucine.

norm. **1.** The usual value. **2.** The desirable value or behavior.

nor·ma, pl. **nor·mae** (nor′mă, nor′mē). **1.** SYN aspect. **2.** SYN profile (1). **3.** SYN projection. [L. a carpenter's square]

n. ante′rior, SYN facial *aspect.*

n. basilaris, SYN external *surface* of cranial base.

n. facia′lis [TA], SYN facial *aspect.*

n. fronta′lis, ✠official alternate term for facial *aspect.*

n. infe′rior, SYN external *surface* of cranial base.

n. latera′lis [TA], SYN lateral *aspect.*

n. occipita′lis [TA], SYN occipital *aspect.*

n. poste′rior, SYN occipital *aspect.*

n. sagitta′lis, the outline of a sagittal section through the skull.

n. supe′rior [TA], SYN superior *aspect*.

n. tempora′lis, SYN lateral *aspect*.

n. ventra′lis, SYN external *surface* of cranial base.

n. vertica′lis, ⋆official alternate term for superior *aspect*.

nor·mal (N) (nōr′măl). **1.** Typical; usual; according to the rule or standard. **2.** In bacteriology, nonimmune; untreated; denoting an animal, or the serum or substance contained therein, that has not been experimentally or naturally immunized against a microorganism or its products. **3.** Denoting a solution containing 1 eq of replaceable hydrogen or hydroxyl per liter; e.g., 1 mol/L HCl is 1 N, but 1 mol/L H_2SO_4 is 2 N. **4.** In psychiatry and psychology, denoting a level of effective functioning that is satisfactory both to persons and to their social milieus. **5.** Referring to a straight line (or plane) at a right angle to another line (or plane). **6.** Not diseased or having been subjected to an experimental procedure. [L. *normalis,* according to pattern]

nor·mal·i·za·tion (nōr′mal-i-zā′shŭn). **1.** Making normal or according to the standard. **2.** Reducing or strengthening of a solution to make it normal. **3.** Adjusting one curve to another by multiplication of the points of the one by some arbitrary factor.

nor·mal·ize (nōr′măl-īz). To effect normalization.

nor·ma·tive. Pertaining to the normal or usual.

nor·me·per·i·dine (nōr-mep′er-ĭ-dīn). A metabolite of meperidine in which the *N*-methyl group has been removed. The compound possesses convulsant properties.

nor·met·a·neph·rine (nōr-met′ă-nef′rin). A catabolite of norepinephrine found, together with metanephrine, in the urine and some tissues, resulting from the action of catechol-*O*-methyltransferase on norepinephrine; has no sympathomimetic actions.

nor·meth·a·done (nōr-meth′ă-dōn). An antitussive with narcotic properties.

△**normo-.** Normal, usual. [L. *normalis,* according to pattern]

nor·mo·bar·ic (nōr-mō-bar′ik). Denoting a barometric pressure equivalent to sea level pressure. [normo- + G. *baros,* weight]

nor·mo·blast (nōr′mō-blast). A nucleated red blood cell, the immediate precursor of a normal erythrocyte in humans. Its four stages of development are: 1) pronormoblast, 2) basophilic n., 3) polychromatic n., and 4) orthochromatic n. SEE erythroblast. [normo- + G. *blastos,* sprout, germ]

nor·mo·blas·to·sis. Excessive production of normoblasts by the bone marrow.

nor·mo·cap·nia (nōr-mō-kap′nē-ă). A state in which the arterial carbon dioxide pressure is normal, about 40 mm Hg. SEE ALSO eucapnia. [normo- + G. *kapnos,* vapor]

nor·mo·ce·phal·ic (nōr′mō-se-fal′ik). SYN mesocephalic. [normo- + G. *kephalē,* head]

nor·mo·chro·mia (nōr-mō-krō′mē-ă). Normal color; referring to blood in which the amount of hemoglobin in the red blood cells is normal. [normo- + G. *chrōma,* color]

nor·mo·chro·mic (nōr-mō-krō′mik). Being normal in color; referring especially to red blood cells that possess the normal quantity of hemoglobin.

nor·mo·cyte (nōr′mō-sīt). A nonnucleated erythrocyte of normal size (average 7.5 μm); a normal, healthy red blood cell. SYN normoerythrocyte. [normo- + G. *kytos,* cell]

nor·mo·cy·to·sis (nōr′mō-sī-tō′sis). A normal state of the blood with regard to its component formed elements.

nor·mo·e·ryth·ro·cyte (nōr′mō-ĕ-rith′rō-sīt). SYN normocyte.

nor·mo·gly·ce·mia (nōr′mō-glī-sē′mē-ă). SYN euglycemia.

nor·mo·gly·ce·mic (nōr′mō-glī-sē′mik). SYN euglycemic.

nor·mo·ka·le·mia, nor·mo·ka·li·e·mia (nōr′mō-kă-lē′mē-ă, -ka-lē-ē′mē-ă). A normal level of potassium in the blood.

nor·mo·sthe·nu·ria (nōr′mō-sthē-noo′rē-ă). Condition in which specific gravity of urine is normal. [normo- + G. *sthenos,* strength, + *ouron,* urine]

nor·mo·ten·sive (nōr-mō-ten′siv). Indicating a normal arterial blood pressure. SYN normotonic (2).

nor·mo·ther·mia (nōr-mō-ther′mē-ă). Environmental tempera-

ture that does not cause increased or depressed activity of body cells. [normo- + G. *thermē,* heat]

nor·mo·ton·ic (nōr-mō-ton′ik). **1.** Relating to or characterized by normal muscular tone. SYN eutonic. **2.** SYN normotensive.

nor·mo·to·pia (nōr-mō-tō′pē-ă). The state of being in the normal place; used in reference to normal placement of an organ. [normo- + G. *topos,* place]

nor·mo·top·ic (nōr-mō-top′ik). Relating to normotopia; in the right place.

nor·mo·vol·e·mia (nōr′mō-vol-ē′mē-ă). A normal blood volume. [normo- + volume, + G. *haima,* blood]

nor·mox·ia (nōr-mok′sē-ă). A state in which the partial pressure of oxygen in the inspired gas is equal to that of air at sea level, about 150 mm Hg. [normo- + oxygen]

nor·oph·thal·mic ac·id (nōr′of-thal-mik). A tripeptide analog of glutathione (L-cysteine replaced by L-alanine), found in the lens of the eye.

nor·pi·pa·none (nōr-pip′ă-nōn). An analgesic agent.

Norrie, Gordon, Danish ophthalmologist, 1855–1941. SEE N. *disease.*

Norris, Richard, English physiologist, 1830–1916. SEE N. *corpuscles,* under *corpuscle.*

nor·ster·oids (nōr-stēr′oydz). Steroids in which an angular methyl group is missing; most commonly, the group between the A and B rings (C-19).

nor·sym·pa·tol (nōr-sim′pă-tōl). SYN octopamine.

nor·sy·neph·rine (nōr-si-nef′rin). SYN octopamine.

Norton, U.F., U.S. obstetrician. SEE N. *operation.*

Norton, Larry, 20th century U.S. oncologist. SEE N.-Simon *hypothesis.*

nor·trip·ty·line hy·dro·chlo·ride (nōr-trip′ti-lēn). An antidepressant.

nor·val·ine (Nva) (nōr-val′ēn, -vā′lēn). α-Aminovaleric acid; the straight chain analog of valine; not found in proteins.

nos·ca·pine (nos′kă-pēn). An isoquinoline alkaloid, occurring in opium, with papaverine-like action on smooth muscle; suppresses the cough reflex and is used as an antitussive; it appears to be without addiction liability. SYN L-α-narcotine, opianine.

nose (nōz). That portion of the respiratory pathway above the hard palate; includes both the external nose and the nasal cavity. SYN nasus (2). [A.S. *nosu*]

    brandy n., SYN rhinophyma.

    cleft n., a n. with a furrow caused by failure of complete convergence of the embryonic primordia.

    copper n., SYN rhinophyma.

    dog n., SYN goundou.

    external n., the visible portion of the nose that forms a prominent feature of the face; it consists of a root, dorsum, and apex from above downward and is perforated inferiorly by two nostrils separated by a septum. SYN nasus externus, nasus (1).

    hammer n., SYN rhinophyma.

    potato n., SYN rhinophyma.

    rum n., SYN rhinophyma.

    saddle n., a n. with markedly depressed bridge, seen in congenital syphilis, after injury from trauma or operation, or infection of the nasal septum.

    toper's n., SYN rhinophyma.

nose·bleed (nōs′blēd). SYN epistaxis.

No·se·ma (nō-sē′mă). A protozoan genus (family Nosematidae, order Microsporida, phylum Microspora) with species (*N. apis, N. bombycis,* and others) pathogenic for invertebrates of economic importance (bees, silkworms); others are being studied as possible agents of biologic control of pest insects or other target invertebrates. *N. connori* infects human fat tissue, diaphragm, myocardium, liver, and other tissues of immunosuppressed individuals. [G. *nosēma,* plague, fr. *noseō,* to be sick, fr. *nosos,* disease]

N. corneum, a cause of keratoconjunctivitis and diffuse punctate keratopathy in AIDS patients.

No·se·mat·i·dae (nō-sē-mat′i-dē). A family of the class Microsporida that includes the genera *Encephalitozoon* and *Nosema,* containing several pathogenic and economically important species.

nose·ma·to·sis (nō-sē′ma-tō′sis). An infection of rabbits with the protozoan parasite *Encephalitozoon cuniculi* that can cause a focal interstitial nephritis; one case of n. has been reported in humans.

nose·piece (nōs′pēs). A microscope attachment, consisting of several objectives surrounding a central pivot.

nos·e·ti·ol·o·gy (nōs′ē-tē-ol′ŏ-jē). Rarely used term for the study of the causes of disease. [G. *nosos*, disease, + *aitia*, cause, + *logos*, study]

⊘**noso-.** Disease. SEE ALSO path-. [G. *nosos*]

no·so·ac·u·sis (nō-sō-ak-ū′sis). Hearing loss due to disease, as opposed to aging. [noso- + G. *akousis*, hearing]

nos·och·tho·nog·ra·phy (nos′ok-thō-nog′ră-fē). SYN geomedicine. [noso- + G. *chthōn*, the earth, + *graphē*, a description]

nos·o·co·mi·al (nos-ō-kō′mē-ăl). **1.** Relating to a hospital. **2.** Denoting a new disorder (not the patient's original condition) associated with being treated in a hospital, such as a hospital-acquired infection. [G. *nosokomeion*, hospital, fr. *nosos*, disease, + *komeō*, to take care of]

nos·o·gen·e·sis, no·sog·e·ny (nos-ō-jen′ĕ-sis, no-soj′ĕ-nē). Rarely used terms for pathogenesis. [noso- + G. *genesis*, production]

nos·o·gen·ic (nos-ō-jen′ik). SYN pathogenic.

nos·o·ge·og·ra·phy (nos′ō-jē-og′ră-fē). SYN geomedicine.

nos·o·graph·ic (nos-ō-graf′ik). Relating to nosography, or the description of diseases.

no·sog·ra·phy (nō-sog′ră-fē). **1.** Assignment of names to each disease entity in a group that has been classified according to a systematic nosology. **2.** A treatise on pathology or the practice of medicine. [noso- + G. *graphē*, description]

nos·o·log·ic (nos-ō-loj′ik). Relating to nosology.

no·sol·o·gy (nō-sol′ō-jē). The science of classification of diseases. SYN nosonomy, nosotaxy. [noso- + G. *logos*, study]

psychiatric n., SYN psychonosology.

nos·o·ma·nia (nos-ō-mā′nē-ă). A rarely used term for an unfounded morbid belief that one is suffering from some special disease. [noso- + G. *mania*, insanity]

nos·o·me·try (nō-som′ĕ-trē). Measurement of morbidity or of the sickness rate in occupations and social conditions. [noso- + G. *metron*, measure]

nos·o·my·co·sis (nos′ō-mī-kō′sis). Any disease caused by a fungus. [noso- + G. *mykēs*, fungus]

no·son·o·my (nō-son′ō-mē). SYN nosology. [noso- + G. *nomos*, law]

nos·o·phil·ia (nos-ō-fil′ē-ă). A morbid desire to be sick. [noso- + G. *phileō*, to love]

nos·o·pho·bia (nos-ō-fō′bē-ă). An inordinate dread and fear of disease. SYN pathophobia. [noso- + G. *phobos*, fear]

nos·o·phyte (nos′ō-fīt). A pathogenic microorganism of the plant kingdom. [noso- + G. *phyton*, plant]

nos·o·poi·et·ic (nos′ō-poy-et′ik). SYN pathogenic. [noso- + G. *poiēsis*, a making]

Nos·o·psyl·lus (nos-ō-sil′ŭs). A flea genus commonly found on rodents. *N. fasciatus*, the northern rat flea, is a species that infrequently transmits the plague bacillus to humans. [noso- + G. *psylla*, flea]

nos·o·taxy (nos′ō-tak-sē). SYN nosology. [noso- + G. *taxis*, arrangement]

nos·o·tox·ic (nos-ō-tok′sik). Relating to a nosotoxin or to nosotoxicosis.

nos·o·tox·i·co·sis (nos′ō-tok-si-kō′sis). A morbid state caused by a toxin. SEE ALSO toxicosis. [noso- + G. *toxikon*, poison]

nos·o·tox·in (nos-ō-tok′sin). Rarely used term for any toxin associated with a disease.

no·sot·ro·phy (nō-sot′rō-fē). Rarely used term for care of the sick. [noso- + G. *trophē*, nourishment]

nos·o·tro·pic (nos-ō-trop′ik). Directed against the pathologic changes or symptoms of a disease. [noso- + G. *tropē*, a turning]

nos·tal·gia (nos-tal′jē-ă). The longing to return home, to a former time in one's life, or to familiar people and surroundings. [G. *nostos*, a return (home), + *algos*, pain]

nos·to·ma·nia (nos-tō-mā′nē-ă). A rarely used term for an obsessive or abnormal interest in nostalgia, especially as an extreme manifestation of homesickness. [G. *nostos*, return, homecoming, + *mania*, frenzy]

nos·to·pho·bia (nos-tō-fō′bē-ă). Morbid fear of returning home. [G. *nostos*, return, homecoming, + *phobos*, fear]

nos·tril. SYN naris.

internal n., SYN secondary *choana*.

nos·trum (nos′trŭm). General term for a therapeutic agent, sometimes patented but usually of secret composition, offered to the general public as a specific remedy for any disease or class of diseases. Term presently carries pejorative connotation. [L. neuter of *noster*, our, "our own remedy"]

NO syn·thase Abbreviation for *nitric oxide* synthase.

no·tal (nō′tăl). Relating to the back. [G. *nōtos*, the back]

no·tan·ce·pha·lia (nō′tan-se-fā′lē-ă). Fetal malformation characterized by absence of the occipital bone of the cranium. [G. *nōtos*, back, + *an-* priv. + *kephalē*, head]

no·tan·en·ce·pha·lia (nō′tan-en-se-fā′lē-ă). Absence of the cerebellum. [G. *nōtos*, back, + *an-* priv. + *enkephalos*, brain]

no·ta·tin (nō-tā′tin). A protein (glucose oxidase) that has specifically been isolated from *Penicillium notatum*. [from *Penicillium notatum*]

NOTCH

notch [TA]. **1.** An indentation at the edge of any structure. **2.** Any short, narrow, V-shaped deviation, whether positive or negative, in a linear tracing. SYN incisura [TA], emargination, incisure.

acetabular n. [TA], a gap in the inferior the margin of the acetabulum. SYN incisura acetabuli [TA], cotyloid n.

angular n., SYN angular *incisure*.

antegonial n., the highest point of the n. or concavity of the lower border of the ramus where it joins the body of the mandible.

anterior n. of auricle [TA], a notch between the supratragic tubercle and the crus of the helix. SYN anterior auricular groove, anterior n. of ear, auricular n. (1), incisura anterior auris, sulcus auriculae anterior.

anterior cerebellar n., a wide, shallow notch on the anterior surface of the cerebellum occupied laterally by the superior cerebellar peduncles and the inferior quadrigeminal bodies medially. SYN anterior n. of cerebellum, incisura cerebelli anterior, semilunar n. (1).

anterior n. of cerebellum, SYN anterior cerebellar n.

anterior n. of ear, SYN anterior n. of auricle.

aortic n., the n. in a sphygmographic tracing caused by rebound following closure of the aortic valves.

n. of apex of heart, SYN n. of cardiac apex.

auricular n., (1) SYN anterior n. of auricle; **(2)** SYN terminal n. of auricle.

cardiac n., SYN cardial n.

n. of cardiac apex [TA], a slight notch near the apex of the heart where the anterior interventricular sulcus reaches the diaphragmatic surface of the heart. SYN incisura apicis cordis [TA], n. of apex of heart.

cardiac n. of left lung [TA], the notch in the anterior border of the superior lobe of the left lung that accommodates the pericardium. SYN incisura cardiaca pulmonis sinistri [TA].

cardial n. [TA], a deep notch between the esophagus and fundus of the stomach. SYN cardiac n., incisura cardiaca.

n. in cartilage of acoustic meatus [TA], (usually) two vertical fissures in the anterior portion of the cartilage of the external auditory meatus, filled by fibrous tissue. SYN incisura cartilaginis meatus acustici [TA], Duverney fissures, incisura santorini, Santorini fissures, Santorini incisures.

clavicular n. of sternum [TA], a hollow on either side of the upper surface of the manubrium sterni that articulates with the clavicle. SYN incisura clavicularis [TA], clavicular facet.

costal n.'s [TA], notches or facets on the lateral edge of the sternum for articulation with a costal cartilage. SYN incisurae costales [TA].

cotyloid n., SYN acetabular n.

dicrotic n. (dī-krot-ik), the acute drop followed by a rise in arterial pressure pulse curves following the systolic peak, corresponding to the incisura of the displacement pulse curve.

digastric n., SYN mastoid n.

ethmoidal n. [TA], an oblong gap between the orbital parts of the frontal bone in which the ethmoid bone is lodged. SYN incisura ethmoidalis [TA].

fibular n. [TA], a hollow on the lateral surface of the lower end of the tibia in which the fibula is lodged. SYN incisura fibularis [TA].

frontal n. [TA], a small notch, sometimes a foramen, on the orbital margin of the frontal bone medial to the supraorbital notch. SYN incisura frontalis [TA].

greater sciatic n. [TA], the deep indentation in the posterior border of the hip bone at the point of union of the ilium and ischium. SYN incisura ischiadica major [TA], iliosciatic n., sacrosciatic n.

hamular n., SYN groove of pterygoid hamulus.

Hutchinson crescentic n., the semilunar n. on the incisal edge of Hutchinson teeth, encountered in congenital syphilis.

iliosciatic n., SYN greater sciatic n.

inferior thyroid n. [TA], a shallow notch in the middle of the lower border of the thyroid cartilage. SYN incisura thyroidea inferior [TA].

interarytenoid n. [TA], the indentation of posterior portion of the aditus laryngeal inlet between the two arytenoid cartilages. SYN incisura interarytenoidea [TA].

interclavicular n., SYN jugular n. of sternum.

intercondyloid n., SYN intercondylar fossa.

intertragic n. [TA], the deep notch in the lower part of the auricle between the tragus and antitragus. SYN incisura intertragica [TA], incisura tragica.

intervertebral n., SYN vertebral n.

ischiatic n., SEE greater sciatic n., lesser sciatic n.

jugular n. of occipital bone [TA], the notch in the occipital bone that forms one boundary of the jugular foramen. SYN incisura jugularis ossis occipitalis [TA].

jugular n. of petrous part of temporal bone [TA], the notch in the petrous part of the temporal bone that forms one boundary of the jugular foramen. SYN incisura jugularis ossis temporalis [TA].

jugular n. of sternum [TA], the large notch in the superior margin of the sternum. SYN incisura jugularis sternalis [TA], suprasternal n.✩, interclavicular n., presternal n., sternal n.

Kernohan n., a n. in the cerebral peduncle caused by displacement of the brainstem against the incisura of the tentorium by a transtentorial herniation.

lacrimal n. [TA], the notch on the frontal process of the maxilla into which the lacrimal bone fits. SYN incisura lacrimalis [TA].

lesser sciatic n. [TA], the notch in the posterior border of the ischium below the ischial spine. SYN incisura ischiadica minor [TA].

n. for ligamentum teres [TA], the notch in the inferior border of the liver that accommodates the round ligament. SYN incisura ligamenti teretis hepatis [TA], incisura umbilicalis, n. for round ligament of liver, umbilical n.

mandibular n. [TA], the deep notch between the condylar and coronoid processes of the mandible. SYN incisura mandibulae [TA], sigmoid n.

marsupial n., SYN posterior cerebellar n.

mastoid n. [TA], the groove medial to the mastoid process of the temporal bone from which the digastric muscle originates. SYN incisura mastoidea [TA], digastric groove, digastric n., mastoid groove.

nasal n. [TA], the notch in the medial border of the maxilla anteriorly that, with its fellow, forms most of the piriform opening of the nasal cavity. SYN incisura nasalis [TA].

pancreatic n. [TA], a notch separating the uncinate process of the head of the pancreas from the neck. SYN incisura pancreatis [TA].

parietal n. [TA], the angle posteriorly between the squamous and petrous parts of the temporal bone. SYN incisura parietalis [TA].

parotid n., the space between the ramus of the mandible and the mastoid process of the temporal bone.

popliteal n., SYN intercondylar fossa.

posterior cerebellar n., a narrow notch between the cerebellar hemispheres posteriorly, occupied by the falx cerebelli. SYN incisura cerebelli posterior, marsupial n., posterior n. of cerebellum.

posterior n. of cerebellum, SYN posterior cerebellar n.

preoccipital n. [TA], an indentation in the ventrolateral border of the temporal lobe of the cerebral hemisphere. SYN incisura preoccipitalis [TA].

presternal n., SYN jugular n. of sternum.

pterygoid n. [TA], the cleft between the medial and lateral plates of the pterygoid process of the sphenoid into which the pyramidal process of the palatine bone is fitted. SYN fissura pterygoidea, incisura pterygoidea, pterygoid fissure.

pterygomaxillary n., SYN groove of pterygoid hamulus.

radial n. [TA], the concavity on the lateral aspect of the coronoid process of the ulna that articulates with the head of the radius. SYN incisura radialis [TA].

Rivinus n., SYN tympanic n.

n. for round ligament of liver, SYN n. for ligamentum teres.

sacrosciatic n., SYN greater sciatic n.

scapular n., SYN suprascapular n.

semilunar n., (1) SYN anterior cerebellar n; **(2)** SYN trochlear n.

sigmoid n., SYN mandibular n.

sphenopalatine n. [TA], the deep notch between the orbital and sphenoidal processes of the palatine bone that is converted into the foramen of the same name by the undersurface of the sphenoid bone. SYN incisura sphenopalatina [TA].

sternal n., SYN jugular n. of sternum.

superior thyroid n. [TA], a deep notch in the middle of the upper border of the thyroid cartilage. SYN incisura thyroidea superior [TA].

supraorbital n. [TA], a groove in the orbital margin of the frontal bone, about the junction of the medial and intermediate thirds, through which pass the supraorbital nerve and artery. SEE ALSO supraorbital foramen. SYN incisura supraorbitalis [TA].

suprascapular n., a n. on the superior border of the scapula through which the suprascapular nerve passes. SYN incisura scapulae, scapular n.

suprasternal n., ✩official alternate term for jugular n. of sternum.

tentorial n. [TA], the triangular opening in the tentorium cerebelli through which the brainstem extends from the posterior into the middle cranial fossa. SYN incisura tentorii [TA], incisura of tentorium✩, n. of tentorium.

n. of tentorium, SYN tentorial n.

terminal n. of auricle [TA], a deep notch separating the lamina tragi and cartilage of the external auditory meatus from the main auricular cartilage, the two being connected below by the isthmus. SYN incisura terminalis auricularis [TA], auricular n. (2), incisura terminalis auris.

trochlear n. [TA], the large semicircular notch at the proximal extremity of the ulna between the olecranon and coronoid processes that articulates with the trochlea of the humerus. SYN incisura trochlearis [TA], incisura semilunaris ulnae, semilunar n. (2).

tympanic n. [TA], the notch in the superior part of the tympanic ring bridged by the flaccid part of the tympanic membrane. SYN incisura tympanica [TA], incisura rivini, Rivinus incisure, Rivinus n., tympanic incisure.

ulnar n. [TA], the concave surface on the medial side of the distal end of the radius that articulates with the head of the ulna. SYN incisura ulnaris [TA].

umbilical n., SYN n. for ligamentum teres.

vertebral n. [TA], one of the two concavities above (superior) and below (inferior) the pedicle of a vertebra; the notches of two adjacent vertebrae (plus the intervertebral disc) form an intervertebral foramen. SYN incisura vertebralis [TA], intervertebral n.

---

notched. SYN emarginate.

no·ten·ceph·a·lo·cele (nō-ten-sef′ă-lō-sēl). Malformation in the occipital portion of the cranium with protrusion of brain substance. [G. *nōtos,* back, + *enkephalos,* brain, + *kēlē,* hernia]

Nothnagel, C.W. Hermann, Austrian physician, 1841–1905. SEE N. *syndrome.*

no·to·chord (nō′tō-kōrd). **1.** In primitive vertebrates, the primary axial supporting structure of the body, derived from the notochordal or head process of the early embryo; an important organizer for determining the final form of the nervous system and related structures. **2.** In embryos, the axial fibrocellular cord about which the vertebral primordia develop; vestiges of it persist in the adult as the nuclei pulposi of the intervertebral discs. SYN chorda dorsalis. [G. *nōtos,* back, + *chordē,* cord, string]

no·to·chor·dal (nō-tō-kōr′dăl). Relating to the notochord.

No·to·ed·res ca·ti (nō-tō-ed′rēz kā′tī). Sarcoptic mange mite of cats.

nou·men·al (noo′men-ăl). Intellectually, not sensuously or emotionally, intuitional; relating to the object of pure thought divorced from all concepts of time or space. [G. *nooumenos,* perceived, fr. *noeō,* to perceive, think]

nour·ish·ment (ner′ish-ment). A substance used to feed or to sustain life and growth of an organism. SYN aliment (1).

nous (noos, nows). A word originally used by Anaxagoras to mean an all-knowing, all-pervading spirit or force; in later Greek philosophy it came to mean simply mind, reason, or intellect. [G. mind, reason]

no·vo·bi·o·cin (nō-vō-bī′ō-sin). An antibiotic antibacterial substance produced by fermentation from cultures of *Streptomyces niveus* or *S. spheroides,* effective against penicillin-resistant *Staphylococcus* and *Proteus;* also available as n. calcium and n. sodium. SYN streptonivicin.

Novy, Frederick George, U.S. bacteriologist, 1864–1957. SEE N. and MacNeal blood *agar.*

noxa (nok′să). Anything that exerts a harmful influence, such as trauma, poison, etc. [L. injury, fr. *noceo,* to injure]

nox·ious (nok′shŭs). Injurious; harmful. [L. *noxius,* injurious, fr. *noceo,* to injure]

nox·y·thi·o·lin (nok-sē-thī′ō-lin). An antibacterial and antifungal agent.

Np 1. Symbol for neptunium. **2.** Abbreviation for neper.

NPC Abbreviation for Niemann-Pick C1 *disease.*

NPN Abbreviation for nonprotein *nitrogen.*

NPO, n.p.o.. Abbreviation for L. *non per os* or *nil per os,* nothing by mouth.

Nps Abbreviation for nitrophenylsulfenyl.

NREM Abbreviation for nonrapid eye movement.

nRNA Abbreviation for nuclear RNA.

NSAID Abbreviation for nonsteroidal anti-inflammatory *drugs,* under *drug;* e.g., aspirin, ibuprofen.

NSF Abbreviation for National Science Foundation.

NSILA Abbreviation for nonsuppressible insulinlike *activity.*

NTMI Abbreviation for nontransmural myocardial *infarction.*

NTNG Abbreviation for nontoxic nodular goiter.

NTP Abbreviation for nucleoside 5′-triphosphate.

nu (noo). Thirteenth letter of the Greek alphabet, ν (q.v.).

nu·bec·u·la (noo-bek′ū-lă). A faint cloud or cloudiness. [L. dim. of *nubes,* cloud]

Nuc Abbreviation for nucleoside.

nu·cha (noo′kă). The back of the neck. SYN nape. [Fr. *nuque*]

nu·chal (noo′kăl). Relating to the nucha.

Nuck, Anton, Dutch anatomist, 1650–1692. SEE N. *diverticulum, hydrocele; canal* of N.

△**nucl-.** SEE nucleo-.

nu·cle·ar (noo′klē-er). Relating to a nucleus, either cellular or atomic; in the latter sense, usually referring to radiation emanating from atomic nuclei (α, β, or γ) or to atomic fission.

Nuclear Regulatory Commission. The U.S. federal commission supervising the use of radioactive by-product material for commercial and medical purposes; successor to the Atomic Energy Commission along with the U.S. Department of Energy.

nu·cle·ase (noo′klē-ās). General term for enzymes that catalyze the hydrolysis of nucleic acid into nucleotides or oligonucleotides by cleaving phosphodiester linkages. For n.'s not listed below, see the specific term. Cf. exonuclease, endonuclease.

azotobacter n., endonuclease (*Serratia marcescens*).

micrococcal n., SYN micrococcal *endonuclease.*

mung bean n., endonuclease S_1 (*Aspergillus*).

nu·cle·ate (noo′klē-āt). A salt of a nucleic acid.

nu·cle·at·ed (noo′klē-ā-ted). Provided with a nucleus, a characteristic of all true cells.

nu·cle·a·tion (noo-klē-ā′shŭn). Process of forming a nidus (4).

heterogeneous n., n. about a nidus composed of material other than that precipitating.

homogeneous n., n. about a nidus composed of material identical with that precipitating.

nu·clei (noo′klē-ī). Plural of nucleus.

nu·cle·ic ac·id (noo-klē′ik, -klā′ik). A family of macromolecules, of molecular masses ranging upward from 25,000, found in the chromosomes, nucleoli, mitochondria, and cytoplasm of all cells, and in viruses; in complexes with proteins, they are called nucleoproteins. On hydrolysis they yield purines, pyrimidines, phosphoric acid, and a pentose, either D-ribose or D-deoxyribose; from the last, the n. a.'s derive their more specific names, ribonucleic acid and deoxyribonucleic acid. N. a.'s are linear (i.e., unbranched) chains of nucleotides in which the 5′-phosphoric group of each one is esterified with the 3′-hydroxyl of the adjoining nucleotide.

infectious n. a., viral n. a. that can infect cells and bring about the production of viruses.

nu·cle·i·form (noo′klē-i-fōrm). Shaped like or having the appearance of a nucleus. SYN nucleoid (1).

△**nucleo-, nucl-.** Nucleus, nuclear. SEE ALSO karyo-, caryo-. [L. *nucleus*]

nu·cle·o·cap·sid (noo′klē-ō-kap′sid). SEE virion.

nu·cle·o·chy·le·ma (noo-klē-ō-kī-lē′mă). SYN karyolymph. [nucleo- + G. *chylos,* juice]

nu·cle·o·chyme (noo′klē-ō-kīm). SYN karyolymph.

nu·cle·o·fil·a·ments (noo′klē-ō-fil′-a-ments). A filamentous form of chromosome formed in low ionic strength solutions; fibers are about 100 Å wide and have a string-of-beads appearance.

nu·cle·o·his·tone (noo′klē-ō-his′tōn). A complex of histone and deoxyribonucleic acid, the form in which the latter is usually found in the nuclei of cells; n. may be viewed as a salt between the basic protein and the acidic nucleic acid.

nu·cle·oid (noo′klē-oyd). **1.** SYN nucleiform. **2.** A nuclear inclusion body. **3.** SYN nucleus (2). [nucleo- + G. *eidos,* resemblance]

Lavdovsky n., SYN astrosphere.

nu·cle·o·lar (noo-klē′ō-lăr). Relating to a nucleolus.

nu·cle·o·li (noo-klē′ō-lī). Plural of nucleolus.

nu·cle·o·li·form (noo-klē′ō-le-fōrm). Resembling a nucleolus. SYN nucleoloid.

nu·cle·o·loid (noo-klē′ō-loyd). SYN nucleoliform. [nucleolus + G. *eidos,* resemblance]

nu·cle·o·lo·ne·ma (noo-klē′ō-lō-nē′mă). The irregular network or rows of fine ribonucleoprotein granules or microfilaments forming most of the nucleolus. [nucleolus + G. *nēma,* thread]

nu·cle·o·lus, pl. **nu·cle·o·li** (noo-klē′ō-lŭs, -lī). **1.** A small rounded mass within the cell nucleus where ribonucleoprotein is produced; it is usually single, but there may be several accessory nucleoli besides the principal one. The n. is composed of a meshwork (nucleolonema) of microfilaments and granules and the pars amorpha, now shown to have microfilaments also. **2.** A more or less central body in the vesicular nucleus of certain protozoa in which an endosome is lacking but one or more Feulgen-positive (DNA+) nucleoli are present; characteristic of certain sporozoans, flagellates, opalinids, dinoflagellates, and radiolarians among the Protozoa. The chromatin material is distributed throughout the nucleus rather than peripherally, as in the endosome type of nucleus of *Entamoeba*. [L. dim of *nucleus,* a nut, kernel]

chromatin n., SYN karyosome.

false n., SYN karyosome.

nu·cle·o·mi·cro·some (noo'klē-ō-mī'krō-sōm). SYN karyomicrosome.

nu·cle·on (noo'klē-on). **1.** One of the subatomic particles of the atomic nucleus; i.e., either a proton or a neutron. **2.** Slang term for specialist in nuclear medicine. [nucleus + -on]

Nu·cle·oph·a·ga (noo-klē-of'ă-gă). A microsporan parasite of amebae that destroys the nucleus of its host. [nucleo- + G. *phagō,* to eat]

nu·cle·o·phil, nu·cle·o·phile (noo'klē-ō-fil, -fīl). **1.** The electron pair donor atom in a chemical reaction in which a pair of electrons is picked up by an electrophil; any reagent or substance that is attracted to a region of low electron density. **2.** Relating to a nucleophil. SYN nucleophilic (1). [nucleo- + G. *philos,* fond]

nu·cle·o·phil·ic (noo'klē-ō-fil'ik). **1.** SYN nucleophil (2). **2.** A reaction involving a nucleophile.

nu·cle·o·phos·pha·tas·es (noo'klē-ō-fos'fă-tās-ez). SYN nucleotidases.

nu·cle·o·plasm (noo'klē-ō-plazm). The protoplasm of the nucleus of a cell.

nu·cle·o·plas·min (noo'klē-plas'min). Contents of resting (interphase) nucleus. [nucleo- + plasma + -in]

nu·cle·o·pro·tein (noo'klē-ō-prō'tēn). A complex of protein and nucleic acid, the form in which essentially all nucleic acids exist in nature; chromosomes and viruses are largely n.

nu·cle·o·re·tic·u·lum (noo'klē-ō-re-tik'ū-lŭm). The intranuclear network of chromatin or linin. [nucleo- + L. *reticulum,* dim. of *rete,* net]

nu·cle·or·rhex·is (noo'klē-ō-rek'sis). Fragmentation of a cell nucleus. [nucleo- + G. *rhēxis,* rupture]

nu·cle·o·si·das·es (noo'klē-ō-sī'dās-ez). Enzymes (particularly EC subgroup 3.2.2) that catalyze the hydrolysis or phosphorolysis of nucleosides, releasing the purine or pyrimidine base.

nu·cle·o·side (Nuc, N) (noo'klē-ō-sīd). A compound of a sugar (usually ribose or deoxyribose) with a purine or pyrimidine base by way of an *N*-glycosyl link.

n. bisphosphate, a n. that carries two independent (i.e., not linked to each other) phosphoric residues. Cf. n. diphosphate.

n. diphosphate (NDP), the pyrophosphoric ester of a n., i.e., a n. in which the H of one of the ribose hydroxyls (usually the 5′) is replaced by a pyrophosphoric (diphosphoric) radical; e.g., adenosine 5′-diphosphate. Cf. n. bisphosphate.

n. monophosphate, a nucleotide containing only one phosphoryl group, e.g., AMP.

n. triphosphate, a n. in which the H of one of the ribose hydroxyls (usually the 5′) is replaced by a triphosphoric group, $-PO(OH)-O-PO(OH)-O-PO(OH)_2$ or the corresponding conjugate base; e.g., adenosine triphosphate.

nu·cle·o·side di·phos·phate ki·nase. A phosphotransferase reversibly catalyzing the transfer of one phosphoryl group from ATP to a nucleoside diphosphate to yield a nucleoside triphosphate and ADP.

nu·cle·o·side di·phos·phate sug·ars. Nucleoside diphosphates linked through the 5′-diphosphoric group with simple or complex carbohydrates; e.g., GDPmannose, UDPglucose (UDPG), dTDPglucosamine.

nu·cle·o·skel·e·ton (nook'lē-ō-skel'ĕ-ton). Proteins forming a fibrillar substructure of the nuclear matrix to which DNA is bound.

nu·cle·o·some (noo'klē-ō-sōm). A localized aggregation of his-

tone and DNA that is evident when chromatin is in the uncondensed stage. SYN nu body. [nucleo- + G. *sōma,* body]

nu·cle·o·spin·dle (noo'klē-ō-spin'dl). The fusiform body in mitosis.

nu·cle·o·ti·da·ses (noo'klē-ō-tī-dās-ez). Enzymes (EC 3.1.3.x) that catalyze the hydrolysis of nucleotides into phosphoric acid and nucleosides; specificities are indicated by prefixes 3′- and 5′-. SYN nucleophosphatases.

nu·cle·o·tide (noo'klē-ō-tīd). Originally a combination of a (nucleic acid) purine or pyrimidine, one sugar (usually ribose or deoxyribose), and a phosphoric group; by extension, any compound containing a heterocyclic compound bound to a phosphorylated sugar by an *N*-glycosyl link (e.g., adenosine monophosphate, NAD^+). For individual n.'s see specific names. SYN mononucleotide.

cyclic n., a nucleoside monophosphate in which the phosphoryl group is linked twice to the sugar moiety; e.g., adenosine 3′,5′-cyclic monophosphate (cAMP).

flavin n., SEE flavin.

nu·cle·o·tid·yl·trans·fer·as·es (noo'klē-ō-tī'dil-trans'fer-ās-ez). Enzymes (EC 2.7.7.x) transferring nucleotide residues (nucleotidyls) from nucleoside di- or triphosphates into dimer or polymer forms. Some n.'s bear specific names (e.g., adenylyltransferases), trivial names indicating the linkage hydrolyzed in the synthesis (pyrophosphorylases, phosphorylases), or names of the material synthesized (RNA or DNA polymerase).

nu·cle·o·tox·in (noo'klē-ō-tok'sin). A toxin acting upon the cell nuclei.

NUCLEUS

nu·cle·us, pl. **nu·clei** (noo'klē-ŭs, noo'klē-ī). **1.** In cytology, typically a rounded or oval mass of protoplasm within the cytoplasm of a plant or animal cell; it is surrounded by a nuclear envelope, which encloses euchromatin, heterochromatin, and one or more nucleoli and undergoes mitosis during cell division. SYN karyon. **2.** By extension, because of similar function, the genome of microorganisms (microbes), which is relatively simple in structure, lacks a nuclear membrane and does not undergo mitosis during replication. SYN nucleoid (3). SEE ALSO virion. **3** [TA]. In neuroanatomy, a group of nerve cell bodies in the brain or spinal cord that can be demarcated from neighboring groups on the basis of either differences in cell type or the presence of a surrounding zone of nerve fibers or cell-poor neuropil. **4.** Any substance (e.g., foreign body, mucus, crystal) around which a urinary or other calculus is formed. **5.** The central portion of an atom (composed of protons and neutrons) where most of the mass and all of the positive charge are concentrated. **6.** A particle on which a crystal, droplet, or bubble forms. **7.** A characteristic arrangement of atoms in a series of molecules; e.g., the benzene n. is a series of aromatic compounds. [L. A little nut, the kernel, stone of fruits, the inside of a thing, dim. of *nux,* nut]

abducens n., n. abducen'tis, n. of abducens nerve, a group of motor neurons in the lower part of the pons, innervating the ipsilateral lateral rectus muscle of the eye; unique among motor cranial nerve nuclei in that it consists of two distinct populations of neurons: neurons that give rise to fibers forming the abducens nerve root and those internuclear neurons whose processes cross the midline, ascend in the opposite medial longitudinal fasciculus, and terminate upon specific oculomotor neurons; considered a primary center for mechanisms controlling conjugate horizontal gaze. SYN n. nervi abducentis [TA].

nuclei accessorii tractus optici [TA], SYN accessory nuclei of optic tract.

accessory cuneate n. [TA], a cell group lateral to the cuneate n. that receives posterior-root fibers corresponding to the proprioceptive innervation of the arm and hand; it projects to the cerebellum by way of the cuneocerebellar tract, and can be considered the upper-extremity equivalent of the thoracic n. SYN n. cuneatus accessorius [TA], external cuneate n., lateral cuneate n., Monakow n.

n. of accessory nerve, a slender column of motor neurons extending longitudinally through central and lateral parts of the ventral horn of the upper six segments of the spinal cord, giving origin to the accessory nerve. SYN n. nervi accessorii [TA].

accessory olivary nuclei, SEE dorsal accessory olivary n., medial accessory olivary n.

accessory nuclei of optic tract [TA], small groups of neuron cell bodies located along the trajectory of optic fibers in the mesencephalon. These consist of the posterior nucleus [TA] (nucleus posterior [TA]), medial nucleus [TA] (nucleus medialis [TA]), and lateral nucleus [TA] (nucleus lateralis [TA]), which are also called the posterior, medial and lateral terminal nuclei. The connections of these nuclei, along with the nucleus of the optic tract, comprise the accessory optic system that appears to be concerned with retinal slip in specific directions. SYN nuclei accessorii tractus optici [TA].

n. accum′bens [TA], the region of fusion between the head of the caudate n. and the putamen, covered on the ventral side by the olfactory tubercle. The former name nucleus accumbens septi ("a nucleus leaning against the septum") refers to a medial, hook-shaped expansion of this anteroventral region of the striatum, which curves under the floor of the frontal horn of the lateral ventricle and ascends for some distance into the ventral half of the septal region. Composed of a pars lateralis [TA] (lateral part [TA] or core region [TAalt]) and a pars medialis [TA] (medial part [TA] or shell region [TAalt]).

n. acu′sticus, obsolete term for the combined vestibular and cochlear nuclei.

n. a′lae cine′reae, SYN posterior n. of vagus nerve.

ambiguus n., SYN n. ambiguus.

n. ambig′uus [TA], a very slender, longitudinal column of motor neurons in the ventrolateral medulla oblongata; its efferent fibers leave with the vagus and glossopharyngeal nerve and innervate the striated muscle fibers of the pharynx (including the musculus levator veli palatini) and the vocal cord muscles of the larynx. SYN ambiguus n.

n. amyg′dalae, SYN amygdaloid *body.*

n. amygdalae basalis lateralis [TA], SYN basolateral amygdaloid n.

n. amygdalae basalis medialis [TA], SYN basomedial amygdaloid n.

n. amygdalae centralis [TA], SYN central amygdaloid n.

n. amygdalae corticalis [TA], SYN cortical amygdaloid n.

n. amygdalae interstitialis [TA], SYN interstitial amygdaloid n.

n. amygdalae lateralis [TA], SYN lateral amygdaloid n.

n. amygdalae medialis [TA], SYN medial amygdaloid n.

amygdaloid n., SYN amygdaloid *body.*

n. ansae lenticularis [TA], SYN n. of the ansa lenticularis; SEE dorsal hypothalamic *area.*

n. of the ansa lenticularis [TA], SEE dorsal hypothalamic *area.* SYN n. ansae lenticularis [TA].

n. anterior [TA], SEE anterior *horn.*

anterior n. [TA], SEE anterior *horn.*

n. anterior corporis trapezoidei [TA], SYN anterior n. of trapezoid body; SEE nuclei of trapezoid body.

nu′clei anterio′res thal′ami [TA], SYN anterior nu′clei of thalamus.

n. anterior hypothalami [TA], SYN anterior hypothalamic n; SEE anterior hypothalamic *area.*

anterior hypothalamic n. [TA], SEE anterior hypothalamic *area.* SYN n. anterior hypothalami [TA].

anterior interpositus n. [TA], one of two cerebellar nuclei interposed between the dentate and the fastigial nuclei. SYN n. interpositus anterior [TA].

anterior olfactory n. [TA], a n. located in the olfactory tract and prominent in microsmatic animals; receives input from the olfactory bulb and projects to the bulb, to other targets of olfactory fibers, and to its contralateral counterpart. SYN n. olfactorius anterior [TA].

anterior periventricular n. [TA], SEE anterior hypothalamic *area.* SYN n. periventricularis ventralis [TA].

anterior nuclei of thalamus [TA], collective term for three groups of nerve cells that together form the anterior thalamic tubercle: the anteroventral n. [TA], a relatively large n.; the anteromedial n. [TA]; and the anterodorsal n. [TA], a small (but large-celled) n. These nuclei receive the mamillothalamic tract from the mamillary body, and additional afferents by way of the fornix; they project collectively to the cortex of the cingulate and parahippocampal gyrus. SYN nuclei anteriores thalami [TA].

anterior n. of trapezoid body [TA], SEE nuclei of trapezoid body. SYN n. anterior corporis trapezoidei [TA].

n. anterodorsa′lis [TA], SYN anterodorsal n. of thalamus; SEE anterior nuclei of thalamus.

anterodorsal n. of thalamus, SYN n. anterodorsalis [TA]. SEE anterior nuclei of thalamus.

n. anterolateralis [TA], SEE anterior *horn.*

anteromedial n. [TA], SEE anterior *horn.*

n. anteromedia′lis [TA], SYN anteromedial n. of thalamus; SEE anterior nuclei of thalamus.

anteromedial n. of thalamus, SYN n. anteromedialis [TA]. SEE anterior nuclei of thalamus.

n. anteroventra′lis [TA], SYN anteroventral n. of thalamus; SEE anterior nuclei of thalamus.

anteroventral n. of thalamus, SYN n. anteroventralis [TA]. SEE anterior nuclei of thalamus.

arcuate n. [TA], **(1)** SYN n. arcuatus of intermediate hypothalamic area [TA], posterior periventricular n. [TA]. SYN arcuate n. of thalamus; **(2)** a cell group in the hypothalamus, located in the lowest part of the infundibulum adjacent to the median eminence. SYN n. arcuatus of medulla oblongata [TA]. **(3)** a variable assembly of small cell groups, probably outlying components of the ponting nuclei, on the ventral and medial aspects of the pyramid in the medulla oblongata. SYN n. arcuatus [TA].

arcuate n. of thalamus, the small ventral region of the ventral posteromedial n. of thalamus in which the fibers of the gustatory lemniscus and secondary trigeminal tracts terminate; it projects to the lower part of the postcentral gyrus of the cerebral cortex. SYN arcuate n. (1) [TA], n. arcuatus thalami, semilunar n. of Flechsig, thalamic gustatory n.

n. arcuatus [TA], SYN arcuate n; SEE intermediate hypothalamic *area.*

n. arcua′tus of intermediate hypothalamic area [TA], SYN arcuate n. (1).

n. arcuatus of medulla oblongata [TA], SYN arcuate n. (2).

n. arcua′tus thal′ami, SYN arcuate n. of thalamus.

auditory n., SEE nuclei nervi vestibulocochlearis.

autonomic (visceral motor) nuclei, nuclei located in the spinal cord (T1–L2, S2–S4) and in the brainstem (Edinger-Westphal n., superior and inferior salivatory nuclei, dorsal vagal n., and parts of the ambiguus n.) from which general visceral efferent preganglionic fibers arise; may be sympathetic (T1–L2) or parasympathetic (craniosacral); hypothalamic nuclei/areas function in concert with autonomic nuclei.

basal nuclei [TA], n. of the cerebral hemisphere that originally included the caudate and lenticular nuclei, the claustrum, and the amygdaloid body (complex); functionally the term basal nuclei now specifies the caudate and lenticular nuclei and adjacent cell groups having important connections therewith (subthalamic n.; substantia nigra and partes compacta and reticulata); amygdaloid complex now known to be part of the limbic system; SEE ALSO basal *ganglia,* under *ganglion.* SYN nuclei basales [TA].

nuclei basales [TA], SYN basal nuclei.

basal n. of Ganser, a large group of large cells in the innominate substance, ventral to the lentiform n. SYN n. basalis of Ganser.

n. basa′lis of Ganser, SYN basal n. of Ganser.

basket n., nuclear structure that may be seen in *Iodamoeba bütschlii* cysts and occasionally in trophozoites; in stained preparations, fibrils may be seen running between the karyosome and the chromatin granules.

basolateral amygdaloid n. [TA], SEE amygdaloid *body.* SYN n. amygdalae basalis lateralis [TA].

basomedial amygdaloid n. [TA], SEE amygdaloid *body*. SYN n. amygdalae basalis medialis [TA].

Bechterew n., (1) SEE vestibular nuclei; **(2)** SYN n. centralis tegmenti superior.

benzene n., the six conjugated carbon atoms of the benzene ring.

Blumenau n., the accessory cuneate n. [TA] of the medulla oblongata.

branchiomotor nuclei, collective term for those motoneuronal nuclei of the brainstem (n. ambiguus, facial motor n., motor n. of the trigeminus) that develop from the branchiomotor column of the embryo and innervate striated muscle fibers (muscles of mastication, facial musculature, pharynx, and vocal cord muscles) associated with the branchial arches. SYN special visceral efferent nuclei, special visceral motor nuclei.

Burdach n., SYN cuneate n.

caeruleun n. [TA], a widely used term designating the locus ceruleus; SEE *locus* caeruleus.

n. caeruleus [TA], a shallow depression, blue in the fresh brain, lying laterally in the most rostral portion of the rhomboidal fossa near the cerebral aqueduct; it lies near the lateral wall of the fourth ventricle and consists of about 20,000 melanin-pigmented neuronal cell bodies whose norepinephrine-containing axons have a remarkably wide distribution in the cerebral cortex, dorsal thalamus, amygdaloid complex and hippocampus, mesencephalic tegmentum, cerebellar nuclei and cortex, various nuclei in the pons and medulla, and the gray matter of the spinal cord.

n. campi dorsalis [TA], SYN n. of dorsal field; SEE nuclei of perizonal fields.

n. campi medialis [TA], SYN n. of medial field; SEE nuclei of perizonal fields.

nuclei camporum perizonalium [TA], SYN nuclei of perizonal fields.

n. campi ventralis [TA], SYN n. of ventral field; SEE nuclei of perizonal fields.

caudal pontine reticular n. [TA], SEE reticular nuclei of pons. SYN n. reticularis pontis caudalis [TA].

caudate n. [TA], an elongated curved mass of gray matter, consisting of an anterior thick portion, the caput [TA] or head [TA], which protrudes into the anterior horn of the lateral ventricle, a portion extending along the floor of the body of the lateral ventricle, known as the corpus [TA] or body [TA], and an elongated curved thin portion, the cauda [TA] or tail [TA], which curves downward, backward, and forward in the temporal lobe in the dorsolateral wall of the lateral ventricle. SYN n. caudatus [TA], caudate (2), caudatum.

n. cauda′tus [TA], SYN caudate n.

central n. [TA], SEE anterior *horn*.

central amygdaloid n. [TA], SEE amygdaloid *body*. SYN n. amygdalae centralis [TA].

n. centralis [TA], SEE anterior *horn*.

n. centra′lis latera′lis [TA], SYN central lateral n. of thalamus.

n. centra′lis tegmen′ti supe′rior, one of the nuclei raphes. SYN Bechterew n. (2).

central lateral n. of thalamus [TA], the most lateral of the intralaminar nuclei of the thalamus. SYN n. centralis lateralis [TA].

centromedian n. [TA], a large, lentil-shaped cell group, the largest and most caudal of the intralaminar nuclei, located within the lamina medullaris interna of the thalamus between the mediodorsal n. and ventrobasal n.; so called by Luys because of its prominent appearance on frontal sections midway between the anterior and posterior pole of the human thalamus. The n. receives numerous fibers from the internal segment of the globus pallidus by way of the thalamic fasciculus, ansa lenticularis, and lenticular fasciculus as well as projections from area 4 of the motor cortex; its major efferent connection is with the putamen although collaterals reach broad areas of the cerebral cortex. SYN n. centromedianus [TA], centre médian de Luys, centrum medianum.

n. centromedia′nus [TA], SYN centromedian n.

cerebellar nuclei [TA], collective term for the dentate, globosus, and emboliform nuclei, and the tectal and fastigial nuclei of the cerebellum. SYN nuclei cerebelli [TA].

nuclei cerebelli [TA], SYN cerebellar nuclei.

Clarke n., SYN posterior thoracic n.

cochlear nuclei [TA], SYN nuclei cochleares.

nu′clei cochlea′res [TA], the nucleus cochlearis posterior [TA] (posterior cochlear nucleus [TA] or dorsal cochlear nucleus [TAalt]) and nucleus cochlearis anterior [TA] (anterior cochlear nucleus [TA] or ventral cochlear nucleus [TAalt]) are located on the dorsal and lateral surface of the inferior cerebellar peduncle, in the floor of the lateral recess of the rhomboid fossa. The anterior cochlear nuclei may be divided into an anterior part [TA] (pars anterior [TA]) and a posterior part [TA] (pars posterior [TA]); they receive the incoming fibers of the cochlear part of the vestibulocochlear nerve and are the major source of origin of the lateral lemniscus or central auditory pathway. SYN cochlear nuclei [TA], nuclei nervi cochlearis.

n. cochlearis anterior [TA], SEE nuclei cochleares.

n. cochlearis posterior [TA], SEE nuclei cochleares.

nuclei colli′culi inferio′ris [TA], SYN nuclei of inferior colliculus.

n. commissurae posterioris [TA], SYN n. of posterior commissure.

convergence n. of Perlia, SYN Perlia n.

nuclei cor′poris genicula′ti media′lis [TA], SYN medial geniculate nuclei.

nu′clei cor′poris mamilla′ris, SYN nuclei of mammillary body.

n. corporis mammillaris lateralis [TA], SYN nuclei of mammillary body.

n. corporis mammillaris medialis [TA], SYN nuclei of mammillary body.

nuclei corporis trapezoidei [TA], SYN nuclei of trapezoid body.

cortical amygdaloid n. [TA], SEE amygdaloid *body*. SYN n. amygdalae corticalis [TA].

nuclei of cranial nerves, groups of nerve cells associated with the cranial nerves either as motor nuclei (nuclei originis) or sensory nuclei (nuclei terminationis). SYN n. nervi cranialis [TA].

cuneate n. [TA], the larger Burdach n.; one of the three nuclei of the posterior column of the spinal cord; located near the dorsal surface of the medulla oblongata at and below the level of the obex, the n. receives posterior root fibers corresponding to the sensory innervation of the arm and hand of the same side; it consists of a pars centralis [TA] (central part [TA], cell nest region [TAalt]) and a pars rostralis [TA] (rostral part [TA], shell region [TAalt]; together with its medial companion, the gracile n., it is the major source of origin of the medial lemniscus. SYN n. cuneatus pars, rostralis [TA], n. cuneatus, pars centralis [TA], n. cuneatus [TA], Burdach n., n. funiculi cuneati, n. of cuneate fasciculus.

n. of cuneate fasciculus, SYN cuneate n.

n. cunea′tus [TA], SYN cuneate n.

n. cunea′tus accesso′rius [TA], SYN accessory cuneate n.

n. cuneatus, pars centralis [TA], SYN cuneate n.

n. cuneatus pars, rostralis [TA], SYN cuneate n.

cuneiform n. [TA], SEE reticular nuclei of mesencephalon. SYN n. cuneiformis [TA].

n. cuneiformis [TA], SYN cuneiform n; SEE reticular nuclei of mesencephalon.

n. of Darkschewitsch, an ovoid cell group in the ventral central gray substance rostral to the oculomotor nucleus, receiving fibers from the vestibular nuclei by way of the medial longitudinal fasciculus; projections are not known, although some cross in the posterior commissure.

Deiters n., SEE vestibular nuclei.

dentate n. of cerebellum, the most lateral and largest of the cerebellar nuclei; it receives the axons of Purkinje cells from the lateral area of the cerebellar cortex (so-called neocerebellum) and input via collaterals of cerebellar afferent fibers en route to the overlying cerebellar cortex; together with the more medially located globosus and emboliform nuclei, it is the major source of fibers composing the massive superior cerebellar peduncle or brachium conjunctivum. SYN n. dentatus [TA], n. lateralis cerebelli ⋆, corpus dentatum, dentatum.

n. denta′tus [TA], SYN dentate n. of cerebellum.

descending n. of the trigeminus, SYN spinal n. of trigeminal nerve.

diploid n., a n. containing the diploid or normal double complement of chromosomes for one somatic cell.

dorsal n. [TA], SEE medial geniculate nuclei. SYN n. dorsalis hypothalami [TA], n. dorsalis [TA].

dorsal accessory olivary n., a detached part of the olivary n. dorsal to the latter's main body. SYN n. olivaris accessorius posterior [TA], posterior accessory olivary n. [TA].

n. dorsales thalami [TA], SYN dorsal n. of thalamus.

n. of dorsal field [TA], SEE nuclei of perizonal fields. SYN n. campi dorsalis [TA].

n. dorsalis [TA], SYN dorsal n; SEE medial geniculate nuclei.

n. dorsalis corporis geniculati lateralis [TA], SYN dorsal lateral geniculate n.

n. dorsa′lis cor′poris trapezoi′dei, SYN dorsal n. of trapezoid body.

n. dorsalis hypothalami [TA], SYN dorsal n; SEE intermediate hypothalamic *area*.

n. dorsalis lateralis [TA], SYN lateral dorsal n; SEE dorsal n. of thalamus.

n. dorsa′lis ner′vi va′gi, ✭official alternate term for posterior n. of vagus nerve.

dorsal lateral geniculate n. [TA], main division of the lateral geniculate *body*; consists of two magnocellular layers [TA] (strata magnocellularia [TA]) and four parvocellular layers [TA] (strata parvocellularia [TA]) and serves as a processing station in the major pathway from the retina to the cerebral cortex, receiving fibers from the optic tract and giving rise to the geniculocalcarine radiation to the visual cortex in the occipital lobe. SYN n. dorsalis corporis geniculati lateralis [TA].

dorsal motor n. of vagus, SYN posterior n. of vagus nerve.

dorsal premammillary n. [TA], SEE posterior hypothalamic *area*. SYN n. premammillaris dorsalis [TA].

dorsal septal n. [TA], SEE septal *area*.

dorsal n. of thalamus, one of the major subdivisions of the thalamus; the composite dorsal n. includes the n. lateralis anterior or dorsalis, n. lateralis intermedius, n. lateralis posterior, and pulvinar; together, these cell groups form most of the free dorsal surface of the posterior half of the thalamus and project to a very large region of parietal, occipitoparietal, and temporal cortex; its afferent connections are largely obscure, but the n. lateralis posterior and the pulvinar receive a projection from the superior colliculus. SYN n. dorsales thalami [TA].

dorsal thoracic n., ✭official alternate term for posterior thoracic n.

dorsal n. of trapezoid body, a term sometimes used to designate t6 superior olivary nucleus located ventrolaterally in the lower pontine tegmentum, immediately dorsal to the trapezoid body; the n. receives fibers from both the ipsilateral and contralateral cochlear nuclei and contributes fibers to the lateral (auditory) lemniscus of both sides. It is believed to be prominently involved in the function of spatial localization of sound. SYN n. dorsalis corporis trapezoidei, oliva superior, superior olive.

dorsal vagal n., SYN posterior n. of vagus nerve.

dorsal n. of vagus, SYN posterior n. of vagus nerve.

dorsolateral n., SEE anterior *horn*.

dorsomedial n. [TA], SEE dorsal hypothalamic *area*. SYN n. dorsomedialis [TA].

dorsomedial hypothalamic n., SYN dorsomedial n. of hypothalamus.

dorsomedial n. of hypothalamus [TA], an oval cluster of cells located dorsal to the ventromedial hypothalamic n. SYN n. dorsomedialis hypothalami [TA], dorsomedial hypothalamic n.

n. dorsomedialis [TA], SYN dorsomedial n; SEE intermediate hypothalamic *area*.

n. dorsomedia′lis hypothal′ami [TA], SYN dorsomedial n. of hypothalamus.

droplet nuclei, particles 1–10 μm in diameter, implicated in spread of airborne infection; the dried residue formed by evapora-tion of droplets coughed or sneezed into the atmosphere or by aerosolization of infective material.

Edinger-Westphal n., a small group of preganglionic parasympathetic motor neurons in the midline near the rostral pole of the oculomotor n. of the midbrain; the axons of these motor neurons leave the brain with the oculomotor nerve and synapse on the cells of the ciliary ganglion which in turn innervate the sphincter muscle of the pupil and ciliary muscle. Destruction of this n. or its efferent fibers causes maximal paralytic dilation of the pupil; also demonstrated to project fibers to lower levels of the brainstem and all spinal levels. SYN visceral nuclei of oculomotor nerve [TA].

emboliform n., one of two cerebellar nuclei interposed between the dentate and the fastigial nuclei; a small wedge-shaped n. in the central white substance of the cerebellum just internal to the hilus of the dentate n.; receives axons of Purkinje cells of the intermediate area of the cerebellar cortex; axons of these cells exit the cerebellum via the superior cerebellar peduncle. SYN n. emboliformis✭, embolus (2).

n. embolifor′mis, ✭official alternate term for emboliform n.

endolemniscal n. [TA], small clusters of neuron cell bodies located on the lateral aspect of the medial lemniscus in the medulla oblongata, or insinuated within the fascicles of this fiber bundle. SYN n. endolemniscalis [TA].

n. endolemniscalis [TA], SYN endolemniscal n.

endopeduncular n. [TA], SEE dorsal hypothalamic *area*. SYN n. endopeduncularis [TA].

n. endopeduncularis [TA], SYN endopeduncular n; SEE dorsal hypothalamic *area*.

external cuneate n., SYN accessory cuneate n.

facial n., a group of motor neurons located in the ventrolateral region of the lower pontine tegmentum and innervating the facial muscles, the stapedius muscle in the middle ear, the posterior limb of the musculus digastricus, and the stylohyoid muscle. SYN motor n. of facial nerve [TA], n. nervi facialis [TA], facial motor n., n. facialis.

n. facia′lis, SYN facial n.

facial motor n., SYN facial n.

n. fascic′uli gra′cilis, SYN gracile n.

fastigial n. [TA], the most medial of the cerebellar nuclei, lying medial to the interpositus n., near the midline, in the white matter underneath the vermis of the cerebellar cortex. It receives the axons of Purkinje cells from all parts of the vermis. Its major projection is to the vestibular nuclei and medullary reticular formation. SYN n. fastigii [TA], n. medialis cerebelli✭, fastigatum, n. tecti, roof n., tectal nucleus.

n. fasti′gii [TA], SYN fastigial n.

filiform n., SYN paraventricular n. [TA] of hypothalamus.

n. filifor′mis, SYN paraventricular n. [TA] of hypothalamus.

n. funic′uli cunea′ti, SYN cuneate n.

n. funic′uli gra′cilis, SYN gracile n.

gametic n., SYN micronucleus (2).

n. gelatino′sus, SYN n. pulposus.

gelatinous n., SYN n. pulposus.

geniculatus lateralis n., SEE lateral geniculate *body*.

germ n., SYN micronucleus (2).

n. gigantocellula′ris medul′lae oblonga′tae [TA], SYN gigantocellular n. of medulla oblongata.

gigantocellular n. of medulla oblongata [TA], one of the three major nuclei of the reticular formation of the brainstem; its small ventromedial portion is designated as pars alpha [TA]. SYN n. gigantocellularis medullae oblongatae [TA].

n. globo′sus, ✭official alternate term for globosus n.

globosus n., one of two cerebellar nuclei interposed between the fastigial and the dentate nuclei; a group of two or three small masses of gray substance in the white central core of the cerebellum, medial to the emboliform n.; receives axons of Purkinje cells of the intermediate area of the cerebellar cortex; axons of these cells exit the cerebellum via the superior cerebellar peduncle. SYN n. globosus✭, spherical n.

n. of Goll, SYN gracile n.

gonad n., SYN micronucleus (2).

gracile n. [TA], the medial one of the three nuclei of the dorsal column, the remaining two being the cuneate n. and the accessory cuneate n., which corresponds to the clava; it can be divided into a pars centralis [TA] (central part [TA]), cell nest region [TAalt]), a pars rostralis [TA] (rostral part [TA], shell region [TAalt]), and subnucleus rostrodorsalis [TA] (rostrodorsal subnucleus [TA], cell group z [TAalt]; it receives dorsal-root fibers conveying sensory innervation of the leg, and lower trunk, and projects, by way of the medial lemniscus, to the ventral posterolateral posterior n. of the thalamus. SYN n. gracilis [TA], n. fasciculi gracilis, n. funiculi gracilis, n. of Goll.

n. gra'cilis [TA], SYN gracile n.

Gudden tegmental nuclei, SYN tegmental nuclei.

gustatory n., SEE rhombencephalic gustatory n., thalamic gustatory n.

habenular nuclei, the gray matter of the habenula, composed of a small-celled medial habenular nucleus [TA] (nucleus habenularis medialis [TA]) and a large-celled lateral habenular nucleus [TA] (nucleus habenularis lateralis [TA]); both nuclei receive fibers from basal forebrain regions (septum, basal n., lateral preoptic n.); the lateral habenular n. receives an additional projection from the medial segment of the globus pallidus. Both nuclei project by way of the retroflex fasciculus to the interpeduncular n. and a medial zone of the midbrain tegmentum. SYN ganglion habenulae.

n. habenularis lateralis [TA], SYN lateral habenular n; SEE habenular nuclei.

n. habenularis medialis [TA], SYN medial habenular n; SEE habenular nuclei.

hypoglossal n., the motor n. innervating the intrinsic and four of the five extrinsic muscles of the tongue; it is located in the medulla oblongata near the midline, immediately beneath the floor of the inferior recess of the rhomboid fossa. SYN n. nervi hypoglossi [TA], n. of hypoglossal nerve [TA].

n. of hypoglossal nerve [TA], SYN hypoglossal n.

nuclei of inferior colliculus [TA], the nerve cell groups composing the colliculus inferior consisting of a central nucleus [TA] (nucleus centralis [TA]), an external nucleus [TA] (nucleus externus [TA] or nucleus lateralis [TAalt]), and a pericentral nucleus [TA] (nucleus pericentralis [TA]). SYN nuclei colliculi inferioris [TA].

inferior olivary n., a large aggregate of small densely packed nerve cells consisting of medial and dorsal accessory olivary nuclei and a principal olivary nucleus that is arranged in folded laminae shaped like a purse with the opening (hilum) directed medially. It corresponds in position to the oliva, projects to all parts of the contralateral half of the cerebellar cortex by way of the olivocerebellar tract, and is the only source of cerebellar climbing fibers. Its afferent connections include fibers from the spinal cord, dentate nucleus, and motor cortex, but its major input appears to be the central tegmental tract originating from multiple nuclei at midbrain levels. SYN n. olivaris inferior.

inferior salivary n., SYN inferior salivatory n.

inferior salivatory n. [TA], a group of preganglionic parasympathetic motor neurons located in the reticular formation of the medulla oblongata dorsal to the n. ambiguus; its axons leave the brain with the glossopharyngeal nerve and govern secretion from the parotid gland by the intermediary of the ganglion oticum; cells of the inferior and superior n. are scattered and overlapping in lateral regions of the reticular formation. SYN n. salivatorius inferior [TA], inferior salivary n.

inferior vestibular n. [TA], n. vestibularis inferior. SEE ALSO vestibular nuclei. SYN n. vestibularis inferior [TA].

intercalated n. [TA], a small collection of nerve cells in the medulla oblongata lying lateral to the hypoglossal n. SYN n. intercalatus, Staderini n.

n. intercala'tus [TA], SYN intercalated n.

intermediolateral n. [TA], the cell column that forms the lateral horn of the spinal cord's gray matter. Extending from the first thoracic through the second lumbar segment, the column contains the autonomic motor neurons that give rise to the preganglionic fibers of the sympathetic system. SYN n. intermediolateralis [TA], intermediolateral cell column of spinal cord.

n. intermediolatera'lis [TA], SYN intermediolateral n.

intermediomedial n. [TA], a small group of scattered visceral motor neurons immediately ventral to the thoracic n. in the thoracic and upper two lumbar segments of the spinal cord; considered to receive visceral afferent fibers at all spinal levels. SYN n. intermediomedialis [TA].

n. intermediomedia'lis [TA], SYN intermediomedial n.

interpeduncular n. [TA], a median, unpaired, ovoid cell group at the base of the midbrain tegmentum between the cerebral peduncles; it receives the retroflex fasciculus from the habenula and projects to the raphe region (raphe nuclei) and periaqueductal gray substance of the midbrain. SYN n. interpeduncularis [TA], ganglion isthmi, Gudden ganglion, intercrural ganglion, interpeduncular ganglion.

n. interpeduncula'ris [TA], SYN interpeduncular n.

n. interpos'itus, SYN interpositus n.

interpositus n., collective term denoting the globosus n. and emboliform n. of the cerebellum. SYN n. interpositus.

n. interpositus anterior [TA], SYN anterior interpositus n.

n. interpositus posterior [TA], SYN posterior interpositus n.

interstitial n. [TA], a group of widely spaced, medium-sized neurons in the dorsomedial region of the upper mesencephalic tegmentum, immediately lateral to the n. of Darkschewitsch; together with the latter, the interstitial n. is closely associated with the medial longitudinal fasciculus, via which it receives fibers from the vestibular nuclei and projects crossed fibers via the posterior commissure to the oculomotor n.; also projects fibers to all spinal levels. It is believed to be involved in the integration of head and eye movements, particularly eye movements of a vertical or oblique nature. SYN n. interstitialis [TA], interstitial n. of Cajal.

interstitial amygdaloid n. [TA], SEE amygdaloid *body*. SYN n. amygdalae interstitialis [TA].

interstitial nuclei of anterior hypothalamus [TA], SEE anterior hypothalamic *area*. SYN nuclei interstitiales hypothalami anterioris [TA].

interstitial n. of Cajal, SYN interstitial n.

n. interstitiales fasciculi longitudinalis medialis [TA], SYN interstitial n. of medial longitudinal fasciculus.

nuclei interstitiales hypothalami anterioris [TA], SYN interstitial nuclei of anterior hypothalamus; SEE anterior hypothalamic *area*.

n. interstitia'lis [TA], SYN interstitial n.

interstitial n. of medial longitudinal fasciculus [TA], small groups of cells located laterally adjacent to the medial longitudinal fasciculus in the area of the oculomotor nucleus; involved in eye movement through connections with the oculomotor and trochlear nuclei. These connections are primarily ipsilateral but have a bilateral component. SYN n. interstitiales fasciculi longitudinalis medialis [TA].

nu'clei intralamina'res thal'ami [TA], SYN intralaminar nuclei of thalamus.

intralaminar nuclei of thalamus [TA], collective term denoting several cell groups embedded in the internal medullary lamina of the thalamus: the central lateral n. [TA], paracentral n. [TA] (nucleus paracentralis [TA]), the central medial n. [TA] (nucleus centralis medialis [TA]), the centromedian n., and the parafascicular n. [TA] (nucleus parafascicularis [TA]). The central lateral and paracentral receive afferents from the cerebral cortex, brainstem, reticular formation, cerebellum, and spinal cord, and project more or less diffusely to large regions of the frontal and parietal cortex. The centromedian n. receives input from the internal segment of the globus pallidus and motor cortex and projects to the striatum and motor cortex. SEE ALSO centromedian n. SYN nuclei intralaminares thalami [TA].

Klein-Gumprecht shadow nuclei, shadow nuclei in degenerating lymphoidocytes and macrolymphocytes in leukemia.

lateral n. [TA], SEE accessory nuclei of optic tract. SYN n. lateralis [TA].

lateral amygdaloid n. [TA], SEE amygdaloid *body*. SYN n. amygdalae lateralis [TA].

lateral cervical n. [TA], diffusely arranged n. located in the dorsal portions of the lateral funiculus in about cervical levels C1–C3; synaptic station for the spinocervicothalamic tract.

lateral cuneate n., SYN accessory cuneate n.

lateral dorsal n. [TA], SEE dorsal n. of thalamus. SYN n. dorsalis lateralis [TA].

lateral geniculate n., SEE dorsal lateral geniculate n.

n. of lateral geniculate body, SEE dorsal lateral geniculate n.

lateral habenular n. [TA], SEE habenular nuclei. SYN n. habenularis lateralis [TA].

n. lateralis [TA], SYN lateral n; SEE accessory nuclei of optic tract.

n. lateralis cerebelli, ⁎official alternate term for dentate n. of cerebellum.

n. lateralis corporis trapezoidei [TA], SYN lateral n. of trapezoid body; SEE nuclei of trapezoid body.

n. lateralis medullae oblongatae, SYN lateral n. of medulla oblongata.

n. lateralis posterior [TA], SYN lateral posterior n; SEE dorsal n. of thalamus.

nuclei of lateral lemniscus [TA], a substantial cell mass embedded in the lateral lemniscus, immediately below the latter's entry into the inferior colliculus; may be divided into a posterior nucleus of lateral lemniscus [TA] (dorsal nucleus of lateral lemniscus [TAalt], nucleus posterior lemnisci lateralis [TA]), an intermediate nucleus of lateral lemniscus [TA] (nucleus intermedius lemnisci lateralis [TA]), and an anterior nucleus of lateral lemniscus [TA] (nucleus anterior lemnisci lateralis [TA], ventral nucleus of lateral lemniscus [TAalt]); the n. represents a synaptic way-station for part of the fibers of the lateral lemniscus. SYN nuclei lemnisci lateralis [TA].

lateral n. of mammillary body [TA], SEE posterior hypothalamic *area.*

lateral n. of medulla oblongata, SYN lateral reticular n. SYN n. lateralis medullae oblongatae.

n. of the lateral olfactory tract [TA], SEE amygdaloid *body.* SYN n. tractus olfactorii lateralis [TA].

lateral parabrachial n., a cell group located lateral to the brachium conjunctivum in rostral regions of the pons; may be divided into a pars lateralis [TA] (lateral part [TA]), a pars medialis [TA] (medial part [TA]), pars posterior [TA] (posterior part [TA]), and a pars anterior [TA] (anterior part [TA]). SEE ALSO parabrachial nuclei. SYN n. parabrachialis lateralis [TA].

lateral pericuneate n. [TA], a small flattened group of neuron cell bodies located ventrolateral to the cuneate nucleus and insinuated between the cuneate fasciculus and accessory cuneate n. and the spinal tract of the trigeminal nerve. SYN n. pericuneatus lateralis [TA].

lateral posterior n. [TA], SEE dorsal n. of thalamus. SYN n. lateralis posterior [TA].

lateral preoptic n. [TA], a vaguely defined group of nerve cells in the lateral zone of the preoptic region. SEE ALSO anterior hypothalamic *area.* SYN n. preopticus lateralis [TA].

lateral reticular n., group of cells in the medulla oblongata located between the inferior olive and the descending trigeminal n. and tract; composed of a magnocellular part [TA] (pars magnocellularis [TA]), a parvocellular part [TA] (pars parvocellularis [TA]), and a subtrigeminal part [TA] (pars subtrigeminalis [TA]); receives fibers from the spinal and motor cortex and projects to the cerebellum. SYN lateral n. of medulla oblongata.

lateral septal n. [TA], SEE septal *area.*

lateral superior olivary n. [TA], SEE superior olivary n. SYN n. olivaris superior lateralis [TA].

lateral n. of thalamus, SEE dorsal n. of thalamus.

lateral n. of trapezoid body [TA], SEE nuclei of trapezoid body. SYN n. lateralis corporis trapezoidei [TA].

lateral tuberal nuclei [TA], SEE intermediate hypothalamic *area.*

lateral vestibular n. [TA], n. vestibularis lateralis. SEE vestibular nuclei. SYN n. vestibularis lateralis [TA].

nuclei lemnisci lateralis [TA], SYN nuclei of lateral lemniscus.

n. of lens [TA], SYN n. lentis.

lenticular n.,

n. lentiformis [TA], SYN lentiform *nucleus.*

n. lentis [TA], the core or inner dense portion of the lens of the eye. SYN n. of lens [TA].

n. of Luys, SYN subthalamic n.

nucleus of mammillary body, located in the posterior hypothalamic area, this group of nuclei consists of a large-celled lateral nucleus of the mammillary body and larger medial nuclei of the mammillary body, dorsal and ventral premammillary nuclei, and supramammillary nucleus; the first two form the elevation seen on the ventral aspect of the diencephalon, the mammillary body. SYN n. corporis mammillaris lateralis [TA], n. corporis mammillaris medialis [TA], nuclei corporis mamillaris.

n. masticatorius, SYN motor n. of trigeminal nerve.

masticatory n., SYN motor n. of trigeminal nerve.

medial n. [TA], SEE accessory nuclei of optic tract. SYN n. medialis [TA].

medial accessory olivary n. [TA], a detached part of the olivary n. medial to the latter's main body, against the lateral side of the medial lemniscus and pyramidal tract. SYN n. olivaris accessorius medialis [TA].

medial amygdaloid n. [TA], SEE amygdaloid *body.* SYN n. amygdalae medialis [TA].

medial central n. of thalamus, a small cell group in the interthalamic adhesion of the thalamus, occupying the midline region of the internal medullary lamina, between the left and the right paracentral n. SYN n. medialis centralis thalami.

medial dorsal n. [TA] **of thalamus,** a large, composite cell group in the dorsomedial region of the thalamus having reciprocal connections with the entire extent of the frontal cortex anterior to the motor cortex (area 4) and premotor cortex (area 6). The afferent connections of the medial dorsal n. also include projections from the olfactory cortex and amygdala. Composed of a pars parvocellularis lateralis [TA] (lateral nucleus [TA] or parvocellular nucleus [TAalt]), a pars magnocellularis medialis [TA] (medial nucleus [TA] or magnocellular nucleus [TAalt]), and a pars paralaminaris [TA] (paralaminar part [TA] or pars laminaris [TAalt]). SYN mediodorsal n., n. medialis thalami, n. mediodorsalis.

nuclei mediales thalami [TA], SYN medial nuclei of thalamus.

n. of medial field [TA], SEE nuclei of perizonal fields. SYN n. campi medialis [TA].

medial geniculate nuclei, groups of cell bodies that function as the last of a series of processing stations along the auditory conduction pathway to the cerebral cortex, receiving the brachium of the inferior colliculus and giving rise to the auditory radiation to the auditory cortex in the superior temporal gyrus. SYN nuclei corporis geniculati medialis [TA], n. of medial geniculate body.

medial geniculate nuclei [TA], nerve cells that collectively form a surface elevation, the medial geniculate body; they comprise a ventral principal nucleus [TA], a dorsal nucleus [TA], and a small medial magnocellular nucleus; relay of auditory input to auditory cortex

n. of medial geniculate body, SYN medial geniculate nuclei.

medial habenular n. [TA], SEE habenular nuclei. SYN n. habenularis medialis [TA].

n. medialis [TA], SYN medial n; SEE accessory nuclei of optic tract.

n. medialis centralis thalami, SYN medial central n. of thalamus.

n. medialis cerebelli, ⁎official alternate term for fastigial n.

n. medialis corporis trapezoidei [TA], SYN medial n. of trapezoid body; SEE nuclei of trapezoid body.

n. medialis magnocellularis, SYN medial magnocellular n; SEE medial geniculate nuclei.

n. medialis thalami, SYN medial dorsal n. [TA] of thalamus.

medial magnocellular n., SEE medial geniculate nuclei. SYN n. medialis magnocellularis.

medial parabrachial n. [TA], a cell group located medial to the brachium conjunctivum in rostral areas of the pons; may be divided into a pars medialis [TA] (medial part [TA]) and a pars lateralis [TA] (lateral part [TA]). SEE ALSO parabrachial nuclei. SYN n. parabrachialis medialis [TA].

medial pericuneate n. [TA], a small group of neuron cell bodies located immediately ventromedial to the cuneate n., insinuated in a diffuse layer of cells, the pericuneate matrix. SYN n. pericuneatus medialis [TA].

medial preoptic n. [TA], a group of nerve cells forming the medial zone of the preoptic region. SYN n. preopticus medialis [TA].

medial septal n. [TA], SEE septal *area*.

medial superior olivary n. [TA], SEE superior olivary n. SYN n. olivaris superior medialis [TA].

medial nuclei of thalamus [TA], collective group of cells comprising the large medial dorsal nucleus (or dorsomedial nucleus) and its subdivisions (lateral nucleus or parvocellular nucleus, medial nucleus or magnocellular nucleus, paralaminar part or pars paralaminaris) and the medial ventral nucleus [TA] (nucleus medioventralis [TA]). SYN nuclei mediales thalami [TA].

medial n. of trapezoid body [TA], SEE nuclei of trapezoid body. SYN n. medialis corporis trapezoidei [TA].

medial ventral n. [TA], SEE medial nuclei of thalamus. SYN n. medioventralis [TA].

medial vestibular n. [TA], SEE vestibular nuclei. SYN n. vestibularis medialis [TA].

median preoptic n. [TA], SEE anterior hypothalamic *area*. SYN n. preopticus medianus [TA].

mediodorsal n., SYN medial dorsal n. [TA] of thalamus.

n. mediodorsalis, SYN medial dorsal n. [TA] of thalamus.

n. medioventralis [TA], SYN medial ventral n; SEE medial nuclei of thalamus.

mesencephalic n. of trigeminal nerve [TA], a long, narrow plate of unipolar neurons extending throughout the length of the midbrain, in and along the lateral angle of the central gray substance. The n. is the single known instance of primary sensory neurons enclosed in the central nervous system instead of in a peripheral sensory ganglion. Its peripheral axonal processes pass with the trigeminal nerve, give collaterals to the trigeminal motor n., and terminate in the muscles of mastication. SYN n. mesencephalicus nervi trigemini [TA].

n. mesenceph'alicus ner'vi trigem'ini [TA], SYN mesencephalic n. of trigeminal nerve.

Monakow n., SYN accessory cuneate n.

motor nuclei, SYN nuclei of origin.

motor n. of facial nerve [TA], SYN facial n.

n. moto'rius ner'vi trigem'ini [TA], SYN motor n. of trigeminal nerve.

motor n. of trigeminal nerve [TA], a group of motor neurons innervating the muscles of mastication (masseter, temporalis, and internal and external pterygoid muscles) and the musculi tensor tympani and tensor veli palatini. The n. lies in the upper pontine tegmentum medial to the principal sensory n. of the trigeminal nerve. SYN n. motorius nervi trigemini [TA], masticatory n., motor n. of trigeminus, n. masticatorius.

motor n. of trigeminus, SYN motor n. of trigeminal nerve.

n. ner'vi abducen'tis [TA], SYN abducens n.

n. ner'vi accesso'rii [TA], SYN n. of accessory nerve.

nu'clei ner'vi cochlea'ris, SYN nuclei cochleares.

n. nervi crania'lis [TA], SYN nuclei of cranial nerves.

n. ner'vi facia'lis [TA], SYN facial n.

n. ner'vi hypoglos'si [TA], SYN hypoglossal n.

n. ner'vi oculomoto'rii [TA], SYN oculomotor n.

n. nervi phrenici [TA], SYN n. of phrenic nerve.

n. ner'vi trochlea'ris [TA], SYN n. of trochlear nerve.

nu'clei ner'vi vestibulocochlea'ris, SYN vestibulocochlear nuclei.

n. ni'ger, SYN *substantia* nigra.

oculomotor n., the composite group of motor neurons innervating all of the external eye muscles except the musculus rectus lateralis and musculus obliquus superior, and including the musculus levator palpebrae superioris; the most rostral component of the n. is the Edinger-Westphal n., which innervates the musculi sphincter pupillae and ciliaris via the ciliary ganglion. The oculomotor n. lies in the rostral half of the midbrain, near the midline in the most ventral part of the central gray substance; fibers of the

medial longitudinal fasciculus form its lateral borders. SYN n. nervi oculomotorii [TA], n. of oculomotor nerve [TA].

n. of oculomotor nerve [TA], SYN oculomotor n.

n. olfactorius anterior [TA], SYN anterior olfactory n.

n. oliva'ris accesso'rius media'lis [TA], SYN medial accessory olivary n.

n. oliva'ris accesso'rius posterior [TA], SYN dorsal accessory olivary n.

n. oliva'ris inferior, SYN inferior olivary n.

n. olivaris principalis [TA], SYN principal olivary n.

n. olivaris superior [TA], SYN superior olivary n.

n. olivaris superior lateralis [TA], SYN lateral superior olivary n; SEE superior olivary n.

n. olivaris superior medialis [TA], SYN medial superior olivary n; SEE superior olivary n.

Onuf n., a group of small somatic motor neurons in the ventral horn of the spinal cord at sacral 2 level that innervate the vesicorectal sphincters, that is, the external anal and the urethral sphincter; Onuf n. has been identified in the cat, dog, and human. SYN n. of pudendal nerve [TA]. [Onufrowicz, Wladislaus, Swiss anatomist.]

oral pontine reticular n. [TA], SEE reticular nuclei of pons. SYN n. reticularis pontis oralis [TA].

nuclei of origin, collections of motor neurons (forming a continuous column in the spinal cord, discontinuous in the medulla and pons) giving origin to the spinal and cranial motor nerves. SYN n. originis [TA], motor nuclei.

n. ori'ginis [TA], SYN nuclei of origin.

parabigeminal n. [TA], a group of neuron cell bodies located in the lateral position of the midbrain in the area of spinothalamic fibers; ventrolaterally adjacent to the inferior colliculus with which it has interconnections. SYN n. parabigeminalis [TA].

n. parabigeminalis [TA], SYN parabigeminal n.

parabrachial nuclei [TA], the cell groups flanking the brachium conjunctivum at levels immediately caudal to the inferior colliculus; they serve as way-stations in the pathways ascending from the n. of solitary tract to the thalamus and hypothalamus and receive afferent fibers from the hypothalamus and amygdaloid body. SYN nuclei parabrachiales [TA].

nuclei parabrachia'les [TA], SYN parabrachial nuclei.

n. parabrachialis lateralis [TA], SYN lateral parabrachial n.

n. parabrachialis medialis [TA], SYN medial parabrachial n.

n. paracentra'lis thal'ami [TA], SYN paracentral n. of thalamus.

paracentral n. of thalamus [TA], one of the intralaminar nuclei of the thalamus, medial to the central lateral n. SYN n. paracentralis thalami [TA].

paralemniscal n. [TA], SEE reticular nuclei of pons. SYN n. paralemniscalis [TA].

n. paralemniscalis [TA], SYN paralemniscal n; SEE reticular nuclei of pons.

paramedial reticular n. [TA], SEE reticular nuclei of pons.

paranigral n. [TA], a small cell cluster located in the ventromedial regions of the midbrain and insinuated between the medial aspect of the substantia nigra and the interpeduncular nucleus. SYN n. paranigralis [TA].

n. paranigralis [TA], SYN paranigral n.

parapeduncular n. [TA], SEE reticular nuclei of mesencephalon. SYN n. parapeduncularis [TA].

n. parapeduncularis [TA], SYN parapeduncular n; SEE reticular nuclei of mesencephalon.

paraventricular n. [TA], SEE anterior hypothalamic *area*.

n. paraventricula'ris hypothalami, SYN paraventricular n. [TA] of hypothalamus.

paraventricular n. [TA] **of hypothalamus,** a triangular group of large magnocellular neurons in the periventricular zone of the anterior half of the hypothalamus. The cells of the n. are similar to those of the supraoptic n.; the axons of about 20% of their number join in the formation of the supraopticohypophysial tract and are functionally associated with the posterior lobe of the hypophysis; they project fibers to the brainstem nuclei (dorsal motor n. and solitary n.) and to the intermediolateral cell column of the spinal cord at thoracic, lumbar, and spinal levels; similar descending autonomic fibers arise from the lateral and posterior hypothalamic nuclei. SYN filiform n., n. filiformis, n. paraventricularis hypothalami.

pedunculopontine tegmental n. [TA], SEE reticular nuclei of mesencephalon. SYN n. tegmentalis pedunculopontinus [TA].

n. pericuneatus lateralis [TA], SYN lateral pericuneate n.

n. pericuneatus medialis [TA], SYN medial pericuneate n.

perifornical n. [TA], SEE lateral hypothalamic *area*. SYN n. perifornicalis [TA].

n. perifornicalis [TA], SYN perifornical n.

perihypoglossal nuclei [TA], nuclei found in the floor of the 4th ventricle in relation to the hypoglossal nucleus; term includes the prepositus and intercalated nuclei and the n. of Roller.

nuclei periolivares [TA], SYN periolivary nuclei; SEE superior olivary n.

periolivary nuclei [TA], SEE superior olivary n. SYN nuclei periolivares [TA].

peripeduncular n. [TA], a group of neuron cell bodies that form a thin, caplike configuration over the dorsolateral aspect of the crus cerebri; many of its cells are acetylcholinesterase-positive. SYN n. peripeduncularis [TA].

n. peripeduncularis [TA], SYN peripeduncular n.

peritrigeminal n. [TA], small diffuse clusters of cells located mainly on the lateral aspect of the spinal tract of the trigeminal nerve, or insinuated within this fiber bundle at the level of and caudal to the obex. SYN n. peritrigeminalis [TA].

n. peritrigeminalis [TA], SYN peritrigeminal n.

n. periventricularis posterior [TA], SYN posterior periventricular n; SEE intermediate hypothalamic *area*.

n. periventricularis ventralis [TA], SYN anterior periventricular n; SEE anterior hypothalamic *area*.

periventricular preoptic n. [TA], SEE anterior hypothalamic *area*. SYN n. preopticus periventricularis [TA].

nuclei of perizonal fields [TA], small groups of cells distributed along the course of, and insinuated within, pallidofugal fibers that form the lenticular fasciculus (nucleus of ventral field [TA], nucleus campi ventralis [TA], nucleus of field H2), that arch through the prerubral field (nucleus of medial field [TA], nucleus campi medialis [TA], nucleus of field H) and the thalamic fasciculus (nucleus of dorsal field [TA], nucleus campi dorsalis [TA], nucleus of field H1). SEE ALSO *fields* of Forel, under *field*. SYN nuclei camporum perizonalium [TA].

Perlia n., a small cell group located between the somatic cell columns of the oculomotor nuclei. Because it is placed between the groups of motor neurons innervating, respectively, the left and right medial rectus muscles, the n. is considered to represent possibly an integrating mechanism for ocular convergence. SYN convergence n. of Perlia, Spitzka n.

phenanthrene n., misnomer for tetracyclic steroid n.

phrenic n., ⋆official alternate term for n. of phrenic nerve.

n. of phrenic nerve [TA], neuron cell bodies located in the more medial portions of the anterior horn at cervical levels C3 to C7 that innervate the diaphragm via the phrenic nerve. SEE ALSO phrenic n. SYN n. nervi phrenici [TA], phrenic n.⋆.

pontine nuclei [TA], the massive gray matter, composed of individual nuclei, that fills the basilar pons. These nuclei are of fairly homogenous architecture and project primarily to the contralateral side of the cerebellum by way of the middle cerebellar peduncle; there is a modest ipsilateral pontocerebellar projection. Their main afferents come from the entire extent of the cerebral neocortex by way of the corticopontine fibers (longitudinal pontine bundles); thus, the pontine nuclei form a major way-station in the impulse conduction from the cerebral cortex off one hemisphere to the posterior lobe off the opposite cerebellum. The pontine nuclei consist of: nucleus anterior [TA] (anterior nucleus [TA], ventral nucleus [TAalt]), nucleus lateralis [TA] (lateral nucleus [TA]), nucleus medianus [TA] (median nucleus [TA]), nucleus paramedianus [TA] (paramedian nucleus [TA]), nucleus peduncularis [TA] (peduncular nucleus [TA], peripeduncular nucleus [TAalt]), nucleus posterior lateralis [TA] (posterolateral nucleus [TA], dorsolateral nucleus [TAalt]), and nucleus posterior media-

lis [TA] (posteromedial nucleus [TA], dorsomedial nucleus [TAalt]). The nucleus reticularis tegmenti pontis [TA] (reticulotegmental nucleus [TA]) is located at the interface of tegmental and basilar portions of the pons and is sometimes grouped with the pontine nuclei. SYN nuclei pontis [TA], pontine gray matter.

nu′clei pon′tis [TA], SYN pontine nuclei.

pontobulbar n. [TA], an irregularly shaped layer of cells located dorsal and lateral to the restiform body at mid to rostral levels of the medulla oblongata; becomes larger immediately ventrolateral to the restiform body at the medulla-pons junction; these cells are similar to those of the basilar pontine nuclei. SYN n. pontobulbaris [TA].

n. pontobulbaris [TA], SYN pontobulbar n.

n. posterior [TA], SYN posterior n; SEE accessory nuclei of optic tract.

posterior n. [TA], SEE accessory nuclei of optic tract. SYN n. posterior [TA].

posterior accessory olivary n. [TA], SYN dorsal accessory olivary n.

n. of posterior commissure [TA], a group of cells located immediately adjacent to the posterior commissure at the mesencephalon-diencephalon junction; may be divided into pars ventralis [TA] (ventral subdivision [TA]), pars dorsalis [TA] (dorsal subdivision [TA]), and pars interstitialis [TA] (interstitial subdivision [TA]). SYN n. commissurae posterioris [TA].

n. poste′rior hypothal′ami [TA], SYN posterior hypothalamic n.

posterior hypothalamic n. [TA], a large, periventricular hypothalamic n. located dorsal to the mamillary body, continuous with the central gray substance of the mesencephalon. SYN n. posterior hypothalami [TA].

n. posterior hypothalamic [TA], SYN posterior n. of hypothalamus.

posterior n. of hypothalamus [TA], SEE posterior hypothalamic *area*. SYN n. posterior hypothalamic [TA].

posterior interpositus n. [TA], one of two cerebellar nuclei interposed between the fastigial and the dentate nuclei. SEE ALSO globosus n. SYN n. interpositus posterior [TA].

n. posterior nervi vagi [TA], SYN posterior n. of vagus nerve.

posterior periventricular n. [TA], SYN arcuate n. (1). SYN n. periventricularis posterior [TA].

posterior thoracic n. [TA], a column of large neurons located in the base of the posterior gray column of the spinal cord, extending from the first thoracic through the second lumbar segment; it gives rise to the dorsal spinocerebellar tract of the same side. SYN n. thoracicus posterior [TA], dorsal thoracic n.⋆, Clarke column, Clarke n., Stilling column, Stilling n.

posterior n. of vagus nerve, the visceral motor n. located in the vagal trigone (ala cinerea) of the floor of the fourth ventricle. It gives rise to the parasympathetic fibers of the vagus nerve innervating the heart muscle and the smooth musculature and glands of the respiratory and intestinal tracts. SYN n. posterior nervi vagi [TA], n. dorsalis nervi vagi⋆, dorsal motor n. of vagus, dorsal n. of vagus, dorsal vagal n., n. alae cinereae.

posterolateral n. [TA], SEE anterior *horn*.

n. posterolateralis [TA], SEE anterior *horn*.

posteromedial n. [TA], SEE anterior *horn*.

n. posteromedialis [TA], SEE anterior *horn*.

precommissural septal n. [TA], the vertically oriented layer of neuron cell bodies located rostral to the anterior commissure in the base of the septum pellucidum. SYN n. septalis precommissuralis [TA].

pregeniculate n., ⋆official alternate term for ventral lateral geniculate n.

n. premammillaris dorsalis [TA], SYN dorsal premammillary n.

n. premammillaris ventralis [TA], SYN ventral premammillary n.

n. preop′ticus latera′lis [TA], SYN lateral preoptic n.

n. preop′ticus media′lis [TA], SYN medial preoptic n.

n. preopticus medianus [TA], SYN median preoptic n; SEE anterior hypothalamic *area*.

n. preopticus periventricularis [TA], SYN periventricular preoptic n; SEE anterior hypothalamic *area*.

prerubral n., the gray matter of field H$_2$; SEE *fields* of Forel, under *field*.

pretectal nuclei [TA], group of cells, constituting several subnuclei, located rostral to the superior colliculus in the "pretectal" area; receive input from retinal ganglion cells (via the optic tract) and project bilaterally to the Edinger-Westphal n.; relay center for pupillary light reflex pathway; they consist of the nucleus pretectalis anterior [TA] (anterior pretectal nucleus [TA]), nucleus pretectalis olivaris [TA] (olivary pretectal nucleus [TA]), and nucleus pretectalis posterior [TA] (posterior pretectal nucleus [TA]). The nucleus tractus optici [TA] (nucleus of optic tract) is also usually grouped as one of the pretectal nuclei. SYN nuclei pretectales [TA].

nuclei pretectales [TA], SYN pretectal nuclei.

n. principa'lis ner'vi trigem'ini [TA], SYN principal sensory n. of trigeminal nerve.

principal olivary n. [TA], the largest part of the inferior olivary complex, consisting of an undulating layer of cells formed by a dorsal lamella [TA] (lamella posterior [TA]) and a ventral lamella [TA] (lamella anterior [TA]) connected with each other laterally by a lateral lamella [TA] (lamella lateralis [TA]). The medially directed opening of this continuous cell layer is the hilum. SYN n. olivaris principalis [TA].

principal sensory n. of trigeminal nerve [TA], the term commonly used to designate the nucleus pontis nervi trigeminalis; located in pons lateral to the motor trigeminal n.; receives primary sensory (touch and pressure) input via the trigeminal nerve and projects to ventral posteromedial n. of thalamus. SYN n. principalis nervi trigemini [TA], n. sensorius superior nervi trigemini, principal sensory n. of the trigeminus.

principal sensory n. of the trigeminus, SYN principal sensory n. of trigeminal nerve.

n. of pudendal nerve [TA], SYN Onuf n.

n. pulpo'sus [TA], the soft fibrocartilage central portion of the intervertebral disk; regarded as a derivative of the notochord. SYN gelatinous n., n. gelatinosus, vertebral pulp.

pulvinar nuclei [TA], the large caudal portion of the lateral thalamic nuclear group; may be divided into four nuclei on the basis of cytoarchitecture and connections: nucleus pulvinaris anterior [TA] (anterior pulvinar nucleus [TA]), nucleus pulvinaris inferior [TA] (inferior pulvinar nucleus [TA]), nucleus pulvinaris lateralis [TA] (lateral pulvinar nucleus [TA]), and nucleus pulvinaris medialis [TA] (medial pulvinar nucleus [TA]); functionally related to the visual system. SYN nuclei pulvinares [TA].

nuclei pulvinares [TA], SYN pulvinar nuclei.

n. pyramida'lis, obsolete term for n. olivaris accessorius medialis.

pyrrole n., of porphyrins, a cyclic tetrapyrrole; four pyrrole groups joined into a ring structure by way of –CH= (methylidyne) bridges between the α (2) position of one pyrrole and the α' (5) position of another pyrrole, the fourth pyrrole being joined to the first. SEE ALSO porphin, porphyrin.

raphe nuclei [TA], collective term denoting a variety of nerve cell groups in and along the median plane of the medulla oblongata [n. raphes obscurus [TA] (obscure raphe n. [TA]), n. raphes pallidus [TA] (pallidal raphe n. [TA]), and caudal portions of the n. raphes magnus [TA] (magnus raphe n. [TA])]; of the pons [rostral portions of the n. raphes magnus [TA] (magnus raphe n. [TA]), n. raphes pontis [TA] (pontine raphe n. [TA]), n. raphes medianus [TA] (median raphe n. [TA] or superior central n. [TAalt]), and caudal portions of the n. raphes posterior [TA] (posterior raphe n. [TA]) or dorsal raphe n. [TAalt])]; and of the mesencephalon [rostral portions of the n. raphe posterior [TA] (posterior raphe n. [TA]), n. linearis inferioris [TA] (inferior linear n. [TA]), n. linearis intermedius [TA] (intermediate linear n. [TA]), and n. linearis superior [TA] (superior linear n. [TA])]. These nuclei include neurons characterized by their containing the indolamine transmitter agent serotonin; their serotonin-carrying axons extend rostrally to the hypothalamus, septum, hippocampus, and cingulate gyrus and include projections to brainstem, cerebellum, and spinal cord. SYN nuclei raphes [TA].

nu'clei raph'es [TA], SYN raphe nuclei.

red n., a large, well-defined, somewhat elongated cell mass, reddish-gray in the fresh brain, located in the rostral mesencephalic tegmentum. This n. is composed of a caudal pars magnocellularis [TA] (magnocellular part [TA]), a rostral pars parvocellularis [TA] (parvocellular part [TA]) and a small pars posteromedialis [TA] (posteromedial part [TA], dorsomedial part [TAalt]). The n. receives a massive projection from the contralateral half of the cerebellum by way of the superior cerebellar peduncle and an additional projection from the ipsilateral motor cortex. Projections from the anterior interposed n. and motor cortex to the red nucleus are somatopically organized. Its efferent connections are with the contralateral rhombencephalic reticular formation and spinal cord by way of the rubrobulbar and rubrospinal tracts. Rubrospinal fibers have somatotopic origin. SYN n. ruber [TA].

reduction n., a n. that degenerates in the cell during the changes incident to fertilization.

reproductive n., SYN micronucleus (2).

reticular nuclei of the brainstem, the vaguely delineated cell groups composing the gray matter of the reticular formation of the medulla oblongata, pons, and mesencephalon. In general, large-celled territories occupy the medial two-thirds of the reticular formation: some examples are gigantocellular n. of medulla oblongata, nuclei tegmenti pontis caudalis and oralis. Smaller groups of reticular nuclei are found laterally and in paramedian locations; lateral nuclei receive sensory collaterals and project medially; paramedian reticular nuclei largely project to the cerebellum. SEE ALSO reticular *formation*.

n. reticulares medullae oblongatae [TA], SYN reticular nuclei of medulla oblongata.

nuclei reticulares mesencephali [TA], SYN reticular nuclei of mesencephalon.

nuclei reticulares pontis [TA], SYN reticular nuclei of pons.

n. reticularis pontis caudalis [TA], SYN caudal pontine reticular n; SEE reticular nuclei of pons.

n. reticularis pontis oralis [TA], SYN oral pontine reticular n; SEE reticular nuclei of pons.

n. reticularis tegmenti pontis [TA], SEE reticular nuclei of pons.

n. reticula'ris thal'ami [TA], SYN reticular n. of thalamus.

reticular nuclei of medulla oblongata [TA], groups of neuron cell bodies located generally in the more central portions of each half of the medulla oblongata that are not all distinctly separated from each other yet may have specific connections. These nuclei are: gigantocellular reticular n. [TA] and its ventromedially located pars alpha [TA] (n. gigantocellularis [TA]), anterior gigantocellular reticular n. [TA] or ventral gigantocellular reticular n. [TAalt] (n. gigantocellularis anterior [TA]), lateral paragigantocellular reticular n. [TA] (n. paragigantocellularis lateralis [TA]), interfascicular n. of hypoglossal nerve (n. interfascicularis nervi hypoglossi [TA]), intermediate reticular n. [TA] (n. reticularis intermedius [TA]), parvocellular reticular n. [TA] (n. reticularis parvocellularis [TA]), posterior paragigantocellular reticular n. [TA] or dorsal paragigantocellular reticular n. [TAalt] (n. paragigantocellularis posterior [TA]) and medial reticular n. [TA] (n. reticularis medialis [TA]). The central reticular n. [TA] (n. reticularis centralis [TA]) can be divided into a dorsal part [TA] and a ventral part [TA] (pars dorsalis [TA], pars ventralis [TA]). The lateral reticular n. [TA] is located in the ventrolateral area of the medulla and can be divided into a magnocellular part [TA] (pars magnocellularis [TA]), a parvocellular part [TA] (pars parvocellularis [TA]), and a subtrigeminal part [TA] (pars subtrigeminalis [TA]). SEE ALSO reticular nuclei of the brainstem. SYN n. reticulares medullae oblongatae [TA].

reticular nuclei of mesencephalon [TA], diffusely arranged cell groups located in the dorsal and more medial area of the tegmentum of the mesencephalon. These nuclei are: cuneiform n. [TA] (n. cuneiformis [TA]), subcuneiform n. [TA] (n. subcuneiformis [TA]), parapeduncular n. [TA] (n. parapeduncularis [TA]), and the pedunculopontine tegmental n. [TA] (n. tegmentalis pedunculopontinus [TA]). This latter nucleus can be divided into a compact part [TA] or compact subnucleus [TAalt] (pars compacta [TA]) and a dissipated part [TA] or dissipated subnucleus

[TAalt] (pars dissipata [TA]). SYN nuclei reticulares mesencephali [TA].

reticular nuclei of pons [TA], groups of cells located in the pontine tegmentum that are not clearly separate one from the other, but that have in some instances distinct connections. These nuclei are: caudal pontine reticular n. [TA] (n. reticularis pontis caudalis [TA]), oral pontine reticular n. [TA] (n. reticularis pontis oralis [TA]), paralemniscal n. [TA] (n. paralemniscalis [TA]), and the paramedian reticular n. [TA] (n. reticularis paramedianus [TA]). The reticulotegmental n. [TA] (n. reticularis tegmenti pontis [TA]) is located in the ventromedial portion of the pontine tegmentum and is correctly a part of the reticular complex of the pons; it is sometimes also associated with the dorsal extent of the basilar pontine nuclei. SYN nuclei reticulares pontis [TA].

reticular n. of thalamus [TA], a sheet of fairly large neurons covering the lateral, ventral, and rostral surfaces of the thalamus; its reticular appearance is caused by the numerous fascicles of the thalamic peduncles that traverse the n. The n. receives numerous fibers from the cerebral cortex, but it has no cortical projection. SYN n. reticularis thalami [TA].

retroposterior lateral n., SEE anterior *horn.*

n. reuniens [TA], a small cell group belonging to the midline group of thalamic nuclei and extending into the interthalamic adhesion (massa intermedia) when the latter is present.

rhombencephalic gustatory n., the rostral one-third of the n. of solitary tract, receiving afferents from the facial, glossopharyngeal, and vagus nerves conveying impulses originating from the receptor cells of the taste buds.

Roller n., (1) lateral n. of the accessory nerve; **(2)** a small bulbar n. lying immediately anterior to the hypoglossal n., considered one of the perihypoglossal nuclei. SEE subhypoglossal nucleus.

roof n., SYN fastigial n.

n. ru'ber [TA], SYN red n.

n. saguli [TA], SYN sagulum n.

sagulum n. [TA], a group of neuron cell bodies located between the lateral lemniscus and lateral surface of the brainstem immediately caudal to the inferior colliculus; functionally associated with the auditory system. SYN n. saguli [TA].

n. salivato'rius infe'rior [TA], SYN inferior salivatory n.

n. salivato'rius supe'rior [TA], SYN superior salivatory n.

Schwalbe n., SEE vestibular nuclei.

secondary sensory nuclei, SYN terminal n.

segmentation n., (1) the compound n. in the impregnated ovum, formed by conjugation of the nuclei of the ovum and spermatozoon (female and male pronuclei); **(2)** the zygote nucleus after it commences the first cleavage division.

semilunar n. of Flechsig, SYN arcuate n. of thalamus.

n. senso'rius supe'rior ner'vi trigem'ini, SYN principal sensory n. of trigeminal nerve.

sensory nuclei, a group of cell bodies that receive afferent (sensory) input from the periphery.

n. septalis precommissuralis [TA], SYN precommissural septal n.

septofimbrial n. [TA], SEE septal *area.*

shadow n., a n. that has lost its pigment and staining properties.

sole nuclei, an accumulation of skeletal muscle fiber nuclei at the myoneural junction.

nuclei of solitary tract, a slender cell column extending sagittally through the dorsal part of the medulla oblongata, beneath the floor of the rhomboid fossa, immediately lateral to the limiting sulcus. This cell column is composed of smaller individual nuclei, and collectively they are the visceral sensory (visceral afferent) nuclei of the brainstem, receiving the afferent fibers of the vagus, glossopharyngeal, and facial nerves by way of the solitary tract. The caudal two-thirds of the n. processes impulses originating in the pharynx, larynx, intestinal and respiratory tracts, and heart and large blood vessels; its rostral one-third receives impulses from the taste buds and is known as the rhombencephalic gustatory n. The individual nuclei that collectively make up what is commonly called the solitary nucleus are: parasolitary n. [TA] (nucleus parasolitarius [TA]), commissural nucleus [TA] (nucleus commissuralis [TA]), gelatinous solitary nucleus [TA] (nucleus gelatinosus solitarius [TA]), intermediate solitary nucleus [TA] (nucleus intermedius solitarius [TA]), interstitial solitary nucleus [TA] (nucleus interstitialis solitarius [TA]), medial solitary nucleus [TA] (nucleus medialis solitarius [TA]), paracommissural solitary nucleus [TA] (nucleus paracommissuralis solitarius [TA]), posterior solitary nucleus [TA] or dorsal solitary nucleus [TAalt] (nucleus solitarius posterior [TA]), posterolateral solitary nucleus [TA] or dorsolateral solitary nucleus [TAalt] (nucleus solitarius posterolateralis [TA]), anterior solitary nucleus [TA] or ventral solitary nucleus [TAalt] (nucleus solitarius anterior [TA]), and naterolateral solitary nucleus [TA] or ventrolateral solitary nucleus [TA] (nucleus solitarius anterolateralis [TA]). SYN nuclei tractus solitarii [TA].

somatic n., SYN macronucleus (2).

somatic motor nuclei, collective term indicating the motor nuclei innervating the tongue musculature (hypoglossal n.) and the extraocular eye muscles (abducens n., trochlear n., and oculomotor n.), the sternocleidomastoid and trapezius muscles (accessory nerve) and the skeletal muscles of the body (ventral roots of spinal nerves).

special visceral efferent nuclei, SYN branchiomotor nuclei.

special visceral motor nuclei, SYN branchiomotor nuclei.

sperm n., the n. in the head of the spermatozoon, which becomes the male pronucleus after entering the ovum. SEE ALSO pronucleus.

spherical n., SYN globosus n.

n. spina'lis ner'vi trigem'ini [TA], SYN spinal n. of trigeminal nerve.

spinal trigeminal n., SEE spinal n. of trigeminal nerve.

spinal n. of trigeminal nerve [TA], the long sensory n. extending from the caudal border of the pontine sensory n. of the trigeminus down through the lateral region of the rhombencephalon into the upper three segments of the spinal cord's dorsal horn; it receives the fibers of the sensory root of the trigeminal nerve that descend along its lateral border as the spinal tract of trigeminal nerve [TA]. This n. is divided into a pars caudalis [TA] (caudal part [TA]), a pars interpolaris [TA] (interpolar part [TA]), and a subnucleus oralis [TA] (oral subnucleus [TA]). The pars caudalis is further organized into a subnucleus zonalis [TA] (zonal subnucleus [TA]), a subnucleus gelatinosus [TA] (gelatinosus subnucleus [TA]), and a subnucleus magnocellularis [TA] (magnocellular subnucleus [TA]). SYN n. spinalis nervi trigemini [TA], descending n. of the trigeminus, spinal n. of the trigeminus.

spinal n. of the trigeminus, SYN spinal n. of trigeminal nerve.

Spitzka n., SYN Perlia n.

Staderini n., SYN intercalated n.

steroid n., SYN tetracyclic steroid n.

Stilling n., SYN posterior thoracic n.

subcaeruleus n. [TA], diffusely organized n. of noradrenergic cells located ventral to the n. caerulea.

subcuneiform n. [TA], SEE reticular nuclei of mesencephalon. SYN n. subcuneiformis [TA].

n. subcuneiformis [TA], SYN subcuneiform n; SEE reticular nuclei of mesencephalon.

subhypoglossal n. [TA], a small bulbar n. lying immediately ventral (anterior) to the hypoglossal n.; considered one of the perihypoglossal nuclei. SYN n. subhypoglossalis [TA].

n. subhypoglossalis [TA], SYN subhypoglossal n.

n. subparabrachialis [TA], SYN subparabrachial n.

subparabrachial n. [TA], a cell group located ventral to the brachium conjunctivum in the general area where the medial and lateral parabrachial nuclei abut, shifting to the slightly more lateral position rostrally. SEE ALSO parabrachial nuclei. SYN n. subparabrachialis [TA].

subthalamic n. [TA], a circumscript n., shaped like a biconvex lens, located in the ventral part of the subthalamus on the dorsal surface of the peduncular part of the internal capsule immediately rostral to the substantia nigra. The n. receives a massive topographic projection from the lateral segment of the globus pallidus and a somatopically organized projection from the ipsilateral motor cortex; a smaller bundle of afferents from the centromedian n. of the thalamus terminates in the rostral part of the n. The subthalamic n. projects to both pallidal segments, to the pars reticulata of the substantia nigra, and in a small way to the ipsilateral pedunculopontine nucleus. SYN n. subthalamicus [TA], corpus luysi, Luys body, n. of Luys.

n. subthalam´icus [TA], SYN subthalamic n.

superior central tegmental n., SYN: median raphe nucleus. SEE raphe nuclei.

superior olivary n. [TA], a circumscript cell group located ventrolaterally in the lower pontine tegmentum, immediately dorsal to the trapezoid body; the n. receives fibers from the ipsilateral and contralateral cochlear nuclei, and contributes fibers to the lateral lemniscus of each side. It is prominently involved in the function of spatial localization of sound. The n. (also called the superior olivary complex) consists of a lateral superior olivary n. [TA] (n. olivaris superior lateralis [TA]), medial superior olivary n. [TA] (n. olivaris superior medialis [TA]), and the periolivary nuclei [TA] (nuclei periolivares [TA]), which are usually divided into medial nuclei [TA] and lateral nuclei [TA] (nuclei mediales [TA] and nuclei laterales [TA]). SYN n. olivaris superior [TA], superior olivary complex⋆.

superior salivary n., SYN superior salivatory n.

superior salivatory n. [TA], a group of preganglionic parasympathetic motor neurons situated rostral and lateral to the inferior salivatory n.; it governs secretion of the lacrimal, sublingual, and submaxillary glands by way of the facial nerve and the sphenopalatine and submandibular ganglia. SYN n. salivatorius superior [TA], superior salivary n.

superior vestibular n. [TA], n. vestibularis superior. SEE vestibular nuclei. SYN n. vestibularis superior [TA].

suprachiasmatic n. [TA], SEE anterior hypothalamic *area*.

n. suprachiasmaticus [TA], small n. located dorsal to the optic chiasm; receives input from retina and influences hypothalamic neuroendocrine function; closely associated with regulation of circadian rhythmicity. SEE ALSO anterior hypothalamic *area*.

supralemniscal n. [TA], a small group of neurons located dorsal to the medial lemniscus and insinuated among the fibers of the ventral trigeminothalamic tract at mid to rostral levels of the pons. SYN n. supralemniscalis [TA].

n. supralemniscalis [TA], SYN supralemniscal n.

n. supramammillaris [TA], SYN supramammillary n.

supramammillary n. [TA], SEE posterior hypothalamic *area*. SYN n. supramammillaris [TA].

supraoptic n. [TA], SYN supraoptic n. [TA] of hypothalamus.

supraoptic n. [TA] **of hypothalamus,** a large-celled neurosecretory n. in the hypothalamus, located over the lateral border of the optic tract, from which the supraopticohypophysial tract arises; its neurons produce and transport vasopressin released into the general circulation from the axon terminals in the supraopticohypophysial tract. This n. can be divided into a pars dorsolateralis [TA], pars dorsomedialis [TA], and pars ventromedialis [TA]. SYN n. supraopticus [TA], supraoptic n. [TA].

n. supraop´ticus [TA], SYN supraoptic n. [TA] of hypothalamus.

n. tec´ti, SYN fastigial n.

tegmental nuclei, collective term for cell groups in the caudal midbrain and mid-to-rostral pons, one of which (ventral tegmental nucleus) is associated with the mammillary nuclei by way of the mammillary peduncle and mammillotegmental tract. Neurons in these nuclei are acetylcholinesterase-rich. The anterior tegmental n. [TA], also called the ventral tegmental n. [TAalt] (n. tegmentalis anterior [TA]), is located in the pontine tegmentum adjacent to the medial longitudinal fasciculus at the level of the trigeminal motor nucleus. The posterior tegmental n. [TA], also called the dorsal tegmental n. [TAalt], is located in the rostral pons in the area of the central gray substance. The lateroposterior tegmental n. [TA], also known as the laterodorsal tegmental n. [TAalt] (n. tegmentalis posterolateralis [TA]), is a larger cell group located partially in the central gray and partially ventrolateral to it at rostral pontine levels. The pedunculopontine tegmental nucleus [TA] (nucleus tegmentalis pedunculopontinus [TA]) is located in the rostral pons and caudal midbrain and consists of a compact part [TA] (pars compacta [TA] or compact subnucleus [TAalt]) and a dissipated part [TA] (pars dissipata [TA] or dissipated subnucleus [TAalt]. SYN Gudden tegmental nuclei, nuclei tegmenti.

n. tegmentalis pedunculopontinus [TA], SYN pedunculopontine tegmental n; SEE reticular nuclei of mesencephalon.

nu´clei tegmen´ti, SYN tegmental nuclei.

terminal n., n. termina´lis, collective term indicating those nerve cell groups in the rhombencephalon and spinal cord in which the afferent fibers of the spinal and cranial nerves terminate. SYN n. terminationis [TA], secondary sensory nuclei.

n. terminatio´nis [TA], SYN terminal n.

tetracyclic steroid n., the group of four fused rings forming the framework or parent substance of the steroids. SYN perhydrocyclopenta[a]phenanthrene, steroid n.

thalamic gustatory n., SYN arcuate n. of thalamus.

n. thorac´icus posterior [TA], SYN posterior thoracic n.

n. tractus olfactorii lateralis [TA], SYN n. of the lateral olfactory tract.

nuclei trac´tus solita´rii [TA], SYN nuclei of solitary tract.

nuclei of trapezoid body [TA], small groups of neurons associated with the trapezoid body, forming the lateral n. of trapezoid body [TA] (n. lateralis corporis trapezoidei [TA]), medial n. of trapezoid body [TA] (n. medialis corporis trapezoidei [TA]), and the anterior n. of trapezoid body [TA] or ventral n. of trapezoid body [TA] (n. anterior corporis trapezoidei [TA]). These indistinct cell groups are involved in the relay of auditory input. SYN nuclei corporis trapezoidei [TA].

triangular n., alternative term for the medial vestibular nucleus.

triangular n. of septum [TA], SEE septal *area*.

trochlear n., SYN n. of trochlear nerve.

n. of trochlear nerve, a group of motor neurons innervating the superior oblique muscle of the contralateral eye. The n. lies in the caudal half of the midbrain, behind the oculomotor n., in the most ventral part of the central gray substance, near the midline. SYN n. nervi trochlearis [TA], trochlear n.

trophic n., SYN macronucleus (2).

tuberal nuclei, two or three small, encapsulated, round or ovoid clusters of cells in the lateral hypothalamic area along the surface of the tuber cinereum; their connections and functional significance are unknown. SYN nuclei tuberales laterales [TA].

nu´clei tubera´les laterales [TA], SYN tuberal nuclei.

n. tuberomammillaris [TA], SYN tuberomammillary n.

tuberomammillary n. [TA], SEE lateral hypothalamic *area*. SYN n. tuberomammillaris [TA].

ventral anterior n. [TA] **of thalamus,** the most rostral of the subdivisions of the ventral n., receiving projections from the globus pallidus and projecting to the premotor and frontal cortex. This nucleus is divisible into a magnocellular division [TA] (pars magnocellularis [TA]) and a principal division [TA] (pars principalis [TA]). SYN n. ventralis anterior [TA].

nuclei ventra´les thal´ami [TA], SYN ventral nuclei of thalamus.

n. of ventral field [TA], SEE nuclei of perizonal fields. SYN n. campi ventralis [TA].

ventral intermediate n. [TA] **of thalamus,** the composite middle third of the ventral n. receiving in its various parts distinctive projections from the contralateral half of the cerebellum (by way of the superior cerebellar peduncle) and the ipsilateral globus pallidus; nearly all parts of the n. project to the motor cortex. SYN n. ventralis intermedius [TA], n. ventralis lateralis, ventral lateral n. of thalamus.

n. ventralis [TA], SYN ventral principal n; SEE medial geniculate nuclei.

n. ventra´lis ante´rior [TA], SYN ventral anterior n. [TA] of thalamus.

n. ventralis corporis geniculi lateralis [TA], SYN ventral lateral geniculate n.

n. ventra´lis interme´dius [TA], SYN ventral intermediate n. [TA] of thalamus.

n. ventra´lis latera´lis, SYN ventral intermediate n. [TA] of thalamus.

n. ventra´lis poste´rior interme´dius thal´ami, intermediate part of the ventrobasal nuclear complex. SEE ventral posterior n. of thalamus. SYN ventral posterior intermediate n. of thalamus.

n. ventra´lis poste´rior thal´ami, SYN ventrobasal *complex*.

n. ventra′lis posterolatera′lis [TA], SYN ventral posterolateral n. [TA] of thalamus.

n. ventra′lis posteromedia′lis [TA], SYN ventral posteromedial n. [TA] of thalamus.

ventral lateral geniculate n. [TA], small cell group located rostral to the dorsal lateral geniculate n. SYN n. ventralis corporis geniculi lateralis [TA], pregeniculate n.✩.

ventral lateral n. of thalamus, SYN ventral intermediate n. [TA] of thalamus.

ventral posterior intermediate n. of thalamus, SYN n. ventralis posterior intermedius thalami; SEE ventral posterior n. of thalamus.

ventral posterior n. of thalamus, SEE ventrobasal *complex.*

ventral posterolateral n. [TA] of thalamus, **ventral posterior lateral n. of thalamus,** lateral part of the ventrobasal nuclear complex. SEE ventrobasal *complex.* SYN n. ventralis posterolateralis [TA].

ventral posteromedial n. [TA] of thalamus, **posterior medial n. of thalamus,** medial part of the ventrobasal nuclear complex. SEE ventrobasal *complex.* SYN n. ventralis posteromedialis [TA].

ventral premammillary n. [TA], SEE posterior hypothalamic *area.* SYN n. premammillaris ventralis [TA].

ventral principal n. [TA], SEE medial geniculate nuclei. SYN n. ventralis [TA].

ventral nuclei of thalamus [TA], a large, complex cell mass the external border of which forms the ventral and much of the lateral boundary, as well as the rostral border, of the thalamus; the nuclei making up this large area of the diencephalon are the ventral anterior nucleus [TA] (nucleus ventralis anterior [TA]), ventral lateral complex [TA] (nuclei ventrales laterales [TA]), ventral medial complex [TA] (nuclei ventrales medialis [TA]), ventral intermediate nucleus [TA] (nucleus ventralis intermedius [TA]), ventrobasal complex [TA] (nuclei ventrobasales [TA]), ventral posterior inferior nucleus [TA] (nucleus ventralis posterior internus [TA]), and ventral posterior parvocellular nucleus [TA] (nucleus ventroposterior parvocellularis [TA]). In general this area can be subdivided into an anterior, intermediate, and posterior part. SYN nuclei ventrales thalami [TA].

ventral tier thalamic nuclei, collective term for nuclei in the ventral part of the lateral nuclear group, e.g., ventral anterior, lateral, posterolateral, and posteromedial nuclei and the medial geniculate nuclei and the dorsal lateral geniculate n. The basoventral nuclear complex constitutes the caudal part of the ventral tier thalamic nuclei.

ventral n. of trapezoid body, a cell group embedded among the fibers of the trapezoid body, the major decussation of the central auditory pathway, in the lower pons. The n. receives fibers from the contralateral cochlear nuclei and contributes fibers to the ascending auditory system or lateral lemniscus.

ventrobasal nuclei (complex) [TA], SYN ventrobasal *complex.*

nuclei ventrobasales [TA], SYN ventrobasal *complex.*

ventrolateral n. [TA], SEE anterior *horn.*

ventromedial n. [TA], SEE intermediate hypothalamic *area.*

ventromedial n. of hypothalamus [TA], a circumscript ovoid group of small neurons in the medial zone of the tuberal region of the hypothalamus. Bilateral destruction of this n. in the rat leads to severe obesity. It receives numerous fibers from the amygdala via the terminal stria; its efferent connections are obscure. SYN n. ventromedialis hypothalami [TA].

n. ventromedia′lis hypothal′ami [TA], SYN ventromedial n. of hypothalamus; SEE intermediate hypothalamic *area.*

vestibular nuclei [TA], a group of four main nuclei that are located in the lateral region of the hindbrain beneath the floor of the rhomboid fossa. These nuclei are the inferior vestibular nucleus, medial vestibular nucleus (Schwalbe nucleus), lateral vestibular nucleus (Deiter nucleus), and superior vestibular nucleus (Bechterew nucleus). The inferior n. contains a group of large cells, the magnocellular part of inferior vestibular nucleus [TA] or cell group F [TAalt] (pars magnocellularis nuclei vestibularis inferioris [TA]), located caudally in the n. A group of medium-sized neurons is located in lateral portions of the lateral n., the parvocellular part [TA] or cell group I [TAalt] (pars parvocellu-

laris [TA]). These nuclei receive primary fibers of the vestibular nerve, are reciprocally connected with the flocculonodular lobe of the cerebellum, and project by way of the medial longitudinal fasciculus to the abducens, trochlear, and oculomotor nuclei and to the ventral horn of the spinal cord. The lateral vestibular n. projects to the ipsilateral ventral horn of the spinal cord by the vestibulospinal tract. SYN nuclei vestibulares [TA].

nu′clei vestibula′res [TA], SYN vestibular nuclei.

n. vestibularis inferior [TA], SYN inferior vestibular n; SEE vestibular nuclei.

n. vestibularis lateralis [TA], SYN lateral vestibular n; SEE vestibular nuclei.

n. vestibularis medialis [TA], SYN medial vestibular n; SEE vestibular nuclei.

n. vestibularis superior [TA], SYN superior vestibular n; SEE vestibular nuclei.

vestibulocochlear nuclei, the combined cochlear and vestibular nuclei in the brainstem that receive the incoming fibers of the eighth cranial nerve. SEE vestibular nuclei. SYN nuclei nervi vestibulocochlearis.

nuclei viscerales nervi oculomotorii, the visceral motor n. of the oculomotor nerve, also commonly called the Edinger-Westphal n., can be divided into an anterior medial n. [TA] (n. anteromedialis [TA]), and a posterior n. [TA] (n. dorsalis [TA]) SEE ALSO Edinger-Westphal n.

visceral nuclei of oculomotor nerve [TA], SYN Edinger-Westphal n.

nu·clide (noo′klīd). A particular (atomic) nuclear species with defined atomic mass and number. SEE ALSO isotope.

Nuel, Jean Pierre, Belgian ophthalmologist and otologist, 1847–1920. SEE N. *space.*

NUG Abbreviation for necrotizing ulcerative *gingivitis.*

Nuhn, Anton, German anatomist, 1814–1889. SEE N. *gland.*

nul·li·grav·i·da (nŭl-i-grav′i-dă). A woman who has never conceived a child. [L. *nullus,* none, + *gravida,* pregnant]

nul·lip·a·ra (nŭ-lip′ă-ră). A woman who has never borne a child. [L. *nullus,* none, + *pario,* to bear]

nul·li·par·i·ty (nŭl-i-par′i-tē). Condition of having borne no children.

nul·lip·a·rous (nŭl-ip′ă-rŭs). Never having borne a child. SYN nonparous.

num·ber (nŭm′ber). **1.** A symbol expressive of a certain value or of a specific quantity determined by count. **2.** The place of any unit in a series.

atomic n. (Z), the number of protons in the nucleus of an atom; it indicates the position of the element in the periodic system.

Avogadro n. (Λ, N_A), the n. of molecules in 1 gram-molecular weight (1 mol) of any compound; defined as the number of atoms in 0.0120 kg of pure carbon-12; equivalent to 6.0221367×10^{23}. SYN Avogadro constant.

Brinell hardness n. (BHN), a n. related to the size of the permanent impression made by a ball indenter of specified size (usually 10 mm in diameter) pressed into the surface of the material under a specified load:

$$BHN = \frac{P}{\frac{\pi D}{2}(D - \sqrt{D^2 - d^2})}$$

where P = applied load in kg, D = diameter of the ball in mm, and d = diameter of the impression in mm.

CT n., a normalized value of the calculated x-ray absorption coefficient of a pixel (picture element) in a computed tomogram, expressed in Hounsfield units, where the CT n. of air is −1000 and that of water is 0. SYN Hounsfield n.

electronic n., the n. of electrons in the outermost orbit (valence shell) of an element.

gold n., SYN gold *equivalent.*

Hehner n., the weight or percentage of the nonvolatile fatty acids yielded by 5 g of a saponified fat or oil. SYN Hehner value.

Hogben n., unique personal identifying number constructed by using a sequence of digits for birth date, sex, birthplace, and other identifiers; invented by and named for Lancelot Hogben, British mathematician; Hogben n.'s are the basis for identification n.'s in many primary care facilities and are used in many record linkage systems.

Hounsfield n., SYN CT n.

hydrogen n., the quantity of hydrogen that 1 g of fat will absorb; it is a measurement of the amount of unsaturated fatty acids in the fat. SEE ALSO iodine n.

iodine n., an indication of the quantity of unsaturated fatty acids present in a fat; it represents the number of grams of iodine absorbed by each 100 g of fat. SEE ALSO hydrogen n. SYN iodine value.

Kestenbaum n., the difference between the two pupil diameters when each eye is measured in bright light with the other eye tightly covered; an indicator of the relative afferent pupillary defect in patients with two normally innervated irises.

Knoop hardness n. (KHN), a n. obtained by dividing the load in kg applied to a pyramid-shaped diamond of specific size divided by the projected area of the impression: $KHN = L/A$, where $A=$ the projected area of the impression in mm^2 and L = the load in kg; used for measurements of hardness of any materials, especially very hard and brittle substances such as tooth dentin and enamel.

Koettstorfer n., SYN saponification n.

linking n. (L), a property of a long biopolymer (such as duplex DNA) equal to the number of twists (related to the frequency of turns around the central axis of the helix) plus the writhing n.

Loschmidt n. (n_0), the n. of molecules in 1 cm^3 of ideal gas at 0°C and 1 atm of pressure; Avogadro n. divided by 22,414 (i.e., 2.6868×10^{19} cm^{-3}).

Mach n., a n. representing the ratio between the speed of an object moving through a fluid medium, such as air, and the speed of sound in the same medium.

mass n., the mass of the atom of a particular isotope relative to hydrogen-1 (or to $\frac{1}{12}$ the mass of carbon-12), generally very close to the whole number represented by the sum of the protons and neutrons in the atomic nucleus of the isotope (indicated in the name or symbol of the isotope; e.g., oxygen-16, ^{16}O); not to be confused with the atomic weight of an element, which may include a number of isotopes in natural proportion.

MIM n., the catalog assignment for a mendelian trait in the MIM system. If the initial digit is 1, the trait is deemed autosomal dominant; if 2, autosomal recessive; if 3, X-linked. Wherever a trait defined in this dictionary has a MIM n., the n. from the 12th edition of MIM, is given in square brackets with or without an asterisk (asterisks indicate that the mode of inheritance is known; a number symbol (#) before an entry number means that the phenotype can be caused by mutation in any of 2 or more genes) as appropriate e.g., Pelizaeus-Merzbacher disease [MIM*169500] is a well-established, autosomal, dominant, mendelian disorder.

Polenské n., the n. of milliliters of 0.1 N KOH required to neutralize the nonvolatile fatty acids obtained from 5 g of a saponified fat or oil.

Reichert-Meissl n., an index of the volatile acid content of a fat; the n. of milliliters of 0.1 N KOH required to neutralize the soluble volatile fatty acids in 5 g of fat that has been saponified, acidified to liberate the fatty acids, and then steam-distilled. SYN volatile fatty acid n.

Reynolds n., a dimensionless n. that describes the tendency for a flowing fluid, such as blood, to change from laminar flow to turbulent flow or vice versa.

saponification n., the n. of milligrams of KOH required to saponify 1 g of fat; an approximate measure of the average molecular weight of a fat, with which it varies inversely. SYN Koettstorfer n.

stoichiometric n. (v), the n. associated with a reactant or product participating in a defined chemical reaction; usually an integer.

thiocyanogen n., the n. of grams of thiocyanogen taken up by 100 g of fat; analogous to the iodine n., except that thiocyanogen will not add to all the double bonds in polyunsaturated fatty acids, as will iodine. SYN thiocyanogen value.

transport n., the fraction of the total current carried through a solution by a particular type of ion present in that solution.

turnover n. (k_{cat}), the number of substrate molecules converted into product in an enzyme-catalyzed reaction under saturating conditions per unit time per unit quantity of enzyme; e.g., $k_{cat} = V_{max}/[E_{total}]$.

volatile fatty acid n., SYN Reichert-Meissl n.

wave n., the n. of waves (of any waveform such as light or sound) per unit length.

writhing n., the n. of times a DNA duplex axis crosses over itself in space.

numb·ness (nŭm'nes). Indefinite term for abnormal sensation, including absent or reduced sensory perception as well as paresthesias.

num·mi·form (nŭm'i-fōrm). SYN nummular.

num·mu·lar (nŭm'ū-ler). **1.** Discoid or coin-shaped; denoting the thick mucous or mucopurulent sputum in certain respiratory diseases, so called because of the disc shape assumed when it is flattened on the bottom of a sputum mug containing water or transparent disinfectant. **2.** Arranged like stacks of coins, denoting the lining up of the red blood cells into rouleaux formation. SYN nummiform. [L. *nummulus,* small coin, dim. of *nummus,* coin]

num·mu·la·tion (nŭm-ū-lā'shŭn). Formation of nummular masses.

nun·na·tion (nŭ-nā'shŭn). A speech disorder in which the *n* sound is given to other consonants. [Ar. *nūn,* the letter n.]

nurse (ners). **1.** To breast feed. **2.** To provide care of the sick. **3.** One who is educated in the scientific basis of nursing under defined standards of education and is concerned with the diagnosis and treatment of human responses to actual or potential health problems. [O. Fr. *nourice,* fr. L. *nutrix,* wet-nurse, nurse, fr. *nutrio,* to sucke, to tend]

certified registered n. anesthetist (C.R.N.A.), a registered professional nurse with additional education in the administration of anesthetics. Certification achieved through a program of study recognized by the American Association of Nurse Anesthetists.

charge n., a n. administratively responsible for a designated hospital unit, usually on an 8-hour basis. SYN head n. (2).

clinical n. specialist, a registered n. with at least a master's degree who has advanced education in a particular area of clinical practice such as oncology or psychiatry. Usually employed in a hands-on clinical setting such as a hospital.

community n., SYN public health n.

community health n., SYN public health n.

dry n., a woman who cares for newborn infants without breast feeding them, as opposed to a wet n.

n. epidemiologist, a registered n. with additional education in the monitoring and prevention of nosocomial infections in the client population in an agency. SYN infection control n.

flight n., a n. who cares for clients during transport in any type of aircraft.

general duty n., n. who accepts assignment to any unit of a hospital other than an intensive care unit.

graduate n., a n. who has received a degree, most often a bachelor's degree, from a school or college of nursing.

head n., **(1)** a n. administratively responsible for a designated hospital unit on a 24 hour basis; **(2)** SYN charge n.

home health n., a n. who is responsible for a group of clients in the home setting. Visits clients on a routine basis to assist client and family with care as needed and to teach family the care needed so that the client may remain in his/her home. SYN visiting n.

hospital n., a registered n. working in a hospital.

infection control n., SYN n. epidemiologist.

licensed practical n. (L.P.N.), a n. who has graduated from an accredited school of practical (vocational) nursing, passed the state examination for licensure, and been licensed to practice by a state authority. Program is generally 1 year in length. SYN licensed vocational n.

licensed vocational n. (L.V.N.), SYN licensed practical n.

practical n., a graduate of a specific educational program that prepares the individual for a career in nursing with less responsibility than a graduate or registered n.

private n., SYN private duty n.

private duty n., (1) a n. who is not a member of a hospital staff, but is hired by the client or his/her family on a fee-for-service basis to care for the client; **(2)** a n. who specializes in the care of patients with diseases of a particular class, e.g., surgical cases, tuberculosis, children's diseases. SYN private n.

public health n., a n. who provides care to individuals or groups in a community outside of institutions. Usually works through the auspices of a state or city health department. SYN community health n., community n.

registered n. (R.N.), a n. who has graduated from an accredited nursing program, has passed the state examination for licensure, and has been registered and licensed to practice by a state authority.

school n., a n., usually an RN, working in a school or similar institution.

scrub n., a n. who has scrubbed arms and hands, donned sterile gloves and, usually, a sterile gown, and assists an operating surgeon, primarily by passing instruments.

special n., a n., who might be a registered nurse or a practical nurse, assigned to limited, specialized functions; usually synonymous with private duty nurse.

student n., a student in a program leading to certification in a form of nursing; usually applied to students in an RN or practical n. program.

visiting n., SYN home health n.

wet n., a woman who breast feeds a child not her own.

---

nurse prac·ti·tion·er (ners prak-tish′ŭ-ner). A registered nurse with at least a master's degree in nursing and advanced education in the primary care of particular groups of clients; capable of independent practice in a variety of settings.

> Nurse practitioners have been recognized in the U.S. since 1955. State laws regulate their scope of practice and degree of autonomy. By assuming responsibility for preventive care, health education, routine surveillance, and the management of chronic disorders, nurse practitioners free physicians to render more sophisticated or elaborate diagnostic and therapeutic services. In thinly populated areas they enable patients to receive treatment for most medical problems without having to travel long distances. Some observers have noted that the pursuit by nurse practitioners of increasing autonomy and their popularity with managed care organizations threaten to diminish the quality of primary medical care.

---

nurs·ing (ner′sing). **1.** Feeding an infant at the breast; tending and caring for a child. **2.** The scientific application of principles of care related to prevention of illness and care during illness.

n. assignment, the method(s) by which the patient care load is distributed among the n. personnel available to provide care.

n. audit, a defined procedure used to evaluate the quality of n. care provided within an agency to its clients.

n. model, a set of abstract and general statements about the concepts that serve to provide a framework for organizing ideas about clients, their environment, health, and nursing.

n. plan of care, the written framework that provides direction for the delivery of n. care.

n. process, a five-part systematic decision-making method focusing on identifying and treating responses of individuals or groups to actual or potential alterations in health. Includes assessment, n. diagnosis, planning, implementation, and evaluation. The first phase of the n. process is assessment, which consists of data collection by such means as interviewing, physical examination, and observation. It requires collection of both objective and subjective data. The second phase is n. diagnosis, a clinical judgment about individual, family or community n. responses to actual or potential health problems/life processes. Provides the basis for selection of n. intervention to achieve outcomes for which the nurse is accountable (NANDA, 1990). The third phase is planning, which requires establishment of outcome criteria for the client's care. The fourth phase is implementation (intervention).

This phase involves demonstrating those activities that will be provided to and with the client to allow achievement of the expected outcomes of care. Evaluation is the fifth and final phase of the n. process. It requires comparison of client's current state with the stated expected outcomes and results in revision of the plan of care to enhance progress toward the stated outcomes.

nurs·ing home. A convalescent home or private facility for the care of individuals who do not require hospitalization and who cannot be cared for at home.

Nussbaum, Johann H.R. von, German surgeon, 1829–1890.

nu·ta·tion (noo-tā′shŭn). The act of nodding, especially involuntary nodding. [L. *annuo*, to nod]

nut·gall (nŭt′gahl). An excrescence on the oak, *Quercus infectoria* (family Fagaceae) and other species of *Quercus*, caused by the deposit of the ova of a fly, *Cynips gallae tinctorae;* an astringent and styptic, by virtue of the tannin it contains. SYN gall (3), galla, oak apple.

nut·meg (nŭt′meg). The dried ripe seed of *Myristica fragrans* (family Myristicaceae), deprived of its seed coat and arillode; an aromatic stimulant, carminative, condiment, and source of volatile and expressed nutmeg oils; it is consumed for its bizarre central nervous system effects. SEE ALSO myristicin. SYN myristica.

nut·meg oil. The volatile oil distilled from the dried kernels of the ripe seeds of *Myristica fragrans;* used as a flavoring agent and a carminative; in large quantities, it may produce narcosis and delirium; the fixed oil expressed from *M. fragrans* is used as a rubefacient. SYN myristica oil.

nu·tri·ent (noo′trē-ent). A constituent of food necessary for normal physiologic function. [L. *nutriens*, fr. *nutrio*, to nourish]

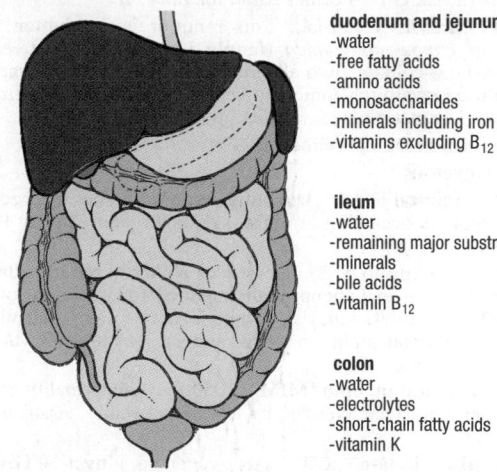

duodenum and jejunum
-water
-free fatty acids
-amino acids
-monosaccharides
-minerals including iron
-vitamins excluding B$_{12}$

ileum
-water
-remaining major substrates
-minerals
-bile acids
-vitamin B$_{12}$

colon
-water
-electrolytes
-short-chain fatty acids
-vitamin K

nutrient absorption: gastrointestinal tract sites

---

essential n.'s, nutritional substances required for optimal health. These must be in the diet, because they are not formed metabolically within the body.

trace n., SYN micronutrients.

nu·tri·lites (noo′tri-līts). Essential nutritional factors. [L. *nutrio,* to suckle, nourish]

nu·tri·tion (noo-trish′ŭn). **1.** A function of living plants and animals, consisting in the taking in and metabolism of food material whereby tissue is built up and energy liberated. SYN trophism (2). **2.** The study of the food and liquid requirements of human beings or animals for normal physiologic function, including energy, need, maintenance, growth, activity, reproduction, and lactation. [L. *nutritio,* fr. *nutrio,* to nourish]

total parenteral n. (TPN), n. maintained entirely by central intravenous injection or other nongastrointestinal route.

nu·tri·tive (noo′tri-tiv). **1.** Pertaining to nutrition. **2.** Capable of nourishing. SYN alible.

nu·tri·ture (noo′tri-choor). State or condition of the nutrition of

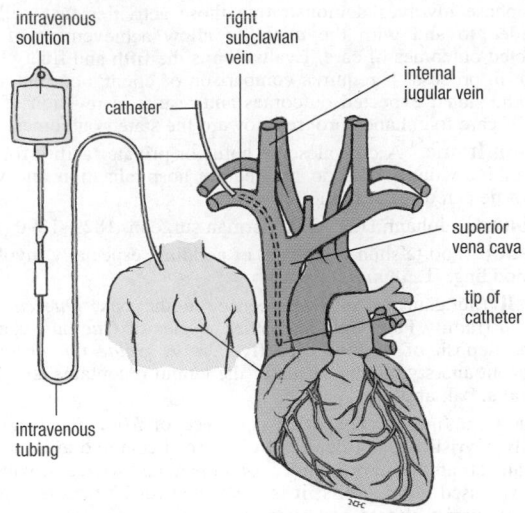

intravenous
solution

right
subclavian
vein

catheter

internal
jugular vein

superior
vena cava

tip of
catheter

intravenous
tubing

total parenteral nutrition: catheter enters the circulation at the right subclavian vein

---

the body; state of the body with regard to nourishment. [L. *nutritura*, a nursing, fr. *nutrio*, to nourish]

Nuttall, G. H. F., U.S. biologist, 1862–1937. SEE *Nuttallia*.

Nut·tal·lia (nŭ-tal'ē-ă). Former name for *Babesia*.

nux vom·i·ca (nŭks vom'i-kă). Poison nut or Quaker button, the seed of *Strychnos nux-vomica* (family Logeniaceae), a tree of tropical Asia; it contains two alkaloids, strychnine and brucine; it has been used as a bitter tonic and central nervous system stimulant. [Mod. L. emetic nut, fr. L. *nux*, nut, + *vomo*, to vomit]

Nva Abbreviation for norvaline.

⌂**nyct-.** SEE nycto-.

nyc·tal·gia (nik-tal'jē-ă). Denoting especially the osteocopic pains of syphilis occurring at night. SYN night pain. [nyct- + G. *algos*, pain]

nyc·ta·lo·pia (nik-tă-lō'pē-ă). Decreased ability to see in reduced illumination. Seen in patients with impaired rod function; often associated with a deficiency of vitamin A. SYN day sight, night blindness, nocturnal amblyopia, nyctanopia. [nyct- + G. *alaos*, obscure, + *ōps*, eye]

n. with congenital myopia [MIM*310500], an abnormality of X-linked inheritance characterized by low visual acuity, strabismus, or nystagmus.

nyc·ta·no·pia (nik-tă-nō'pē-ă). SYN nyctalopia. [nyct- + G. *an*-priv. + *opsis*, sight]

nyc·ter·ine (nik'ter-īn, -in). 1. By night. 2. Dark or obscure. [G. *nykterinos*]

nyc·ter·o·hem·er·al (nik'ter-ō-hē'mer-ăl). SYN nyctohemeral. [G. *nykteros*, by night, nightly, + *hēmera*, day]

⌂**nycto-, nyct-.** Night, nocturnal. SEE ALSO noct-. [G. *nyx*]

nyc·to·hem·e·ral (nik-tō-hē'mer-ăl). Both daily and nightly. SYN nycterohemeral. [nycto- + G. *hēmera*, day]

nyc·to·phil·ia (nik-tō-fil'ē-ă). Preference for the night or darkness. SYN scotophilia. [nycto- + G. *philos*, fond]

nyc·to·pho·bia (nik-tō-fō'bē-ă). Morbid fear of night or of the dark. SYN scotophobia. [nycto- + G. *phobos*, fear]

Nyc·to·the·rus (nik-tō-thē'rŭs). A genus of Ciliophora, one species of which, *N. faba*, has been reported, though rarely, from the human intestine; it is generally found in amphibia. [G. *nyktothēras*, one who hunts by night, fr. *thēraō*, to hunt, fr. *thēr*, wild beast]

nyc·tu·ria (nik-too'rē-ă). SYN nocturia.

Nyhan, William L. U.S. pediatrician, *1926. SEE Lesch-N. *syndrome*.

ny·li·drin hy·dro·chlo·ride (nī'li-drin, nil'). A sympathomimetic agent, similar to isoproterenol, that produces vasodilation of

---

arterioles of skeletal muscles and increases muscle blood flow; used in the treatment of peripheral vascular diseases.

nymph (nimf). 1. The earliest series of stages in metamorphosis following hatching in the development of hemimetabolous insects (e.g., locusts); the n. resembles the adult in many respects, but lacks full wing or genitalia development; it grows through successive instars without any intermediate or pupal stage into the imago or adult form. SEE ALSO incomplete *metamorphosis*, complete *metamorphosis*. 2. The third stage in the life cycle of a tick, between the larva and the adult. [G. *nymphē*, maiden]

nym·pha, pl. **nym·phae** (nim'fă, nim'fē). One of the labia minora. [Mod. L., fr. G. *nymphē*, a bride]

nym·phal (nim'făl). 1. Pertaining to a nymph. 2. Pertaining to the labia minora (nymphae).

nym·phec·to·my (nim-fek'tō-mē). Surgical removal of hypertrophied labia minora. [nympha + G. *ektomē*, excision]

nym·phi·tis (nim-fī'tis). Inflammation of the labia minora. [nympha + G. *-itis*, inflammation]

⌂**nympho-, nymph-.** The nymphae (labia minora). [L. *nympha*]

nym·pho·la·bi·al (nim'fō-lā'bē-ăl). Relating to the labia minora (nymphae) and the labia majora; denoting a furrow between the two labia on each side.

nym·pho·lep·sy (nim-fō-lep'sē). Demoniac frenzy, especially of an erotic nature. [nympho- + G. *lēpsis*, a seizure]

nym·pho·ma·nia (nim-fō-mā'nē-ă). An insatiable impulse to engage in sexual behavior in a female; the counterpart of satyriasis in a male. [nympho- + G. *mania*, frenzy]

nym·pho·ma·ni·ac (nim-fō-mā'nē-ak). A female exhibiting nymphomania.

nym·pho·ma·ni·a·cal (nim'fō-mă-nī'ă-kăl). Pertaining to, or exhibiting, nymphomania.

nym·phon·cus (nim-fong'kŭs). Swelling or hypertrophy of one or both labia minora. [nympho- + G. *onkos*, tumor]

nym·phot·o·my (nim-fot'ō-mē). Incision into the labia minora or the clitoris. [nympho- + G. *tomē*, incision]

nys·tag·mic (nis-tag'mik). Relating to or suffering from nystagmus.

nys·tag·mi·form (nis-tag'mi-fōrm). SYN nystagmoid.

nys·tag·mo·gram (nis-tag'mō-gram). The tracing produced by a nystagmograph.

nys·tag·mo·graph (nis-tag'mō-graf). An apparatus for measuring the amplitude, periodicity, and velocity of ocular movements in nystagmus, by measuring the change in the resting potential of the eye as the eye moves. [nystagmus + G. *graphō*, to write]

nys·tag·mog·ra·phy (nis-tag-mog'ră-fē). The technique of recording nystagmus.

nys·tag·moid (nis-tag'moyd). Resembling nystagmus. SYN nystagmiform. [nystagmus + G. *eidos*, resemblance]

▯**nys·tag·mus** (nis-tag'mŭs). Involuntary rhythmic oscillation of the eyeballs, either pendular or with a slow and fast component. [G. *nystagmos*, a nodding, fr. *nystazō*, to be sleepy, nod]

after-n., n. occurring after the abrupt cessation of rotation in the opposite direction of the rotatory n.

amaurotic n., SYN ocular n.

Bruns n., a fine, jerking (vestibular) n. on horizontal gaze in one direction, together with a slower, larger amplitude (gaze, paretic) n. on looking in the opposite direction; due to lateral brainstem compression, usually by a cerebellar-pontine angle mass such as an acoustic neuroma.

caloric n., n. with slow and fast components induced by labyrinthine stimulation with warm or cool water in the ear. SEE ALSO Bárány *sign*.

cervical n., n. arising from a lesion of the proprioceptive mechanism of the neck.

compressive n., a jerky n. resulting from unilateral changes of pressure in semicircular canals.

congenital n., (1) n. present at birth or caused by lesions sustained *in utero* or at the time of birth; (2) inherited n., usually X-linked, without associated neurologic lesions and nonprogressive; all three patterns of mendelian inheritance may occur: autosomal

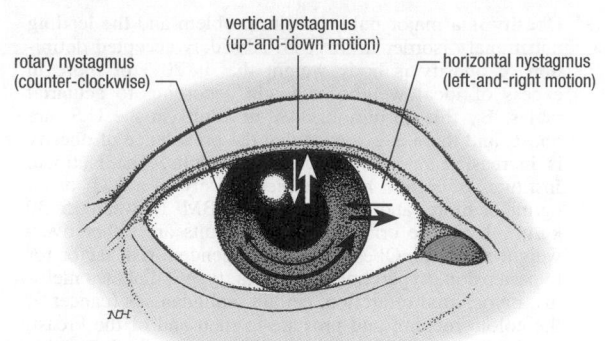

rotary nystagmus (counter-clockwise)

vertical nystagmus (up-and-down motion)

horizontal nystagmus (left-and-right motion)

nystagmus: thicker arrows indicate the slower, first phase

dominant [MIM*164100, *164150], autosomal recessive [MIM*257400], or X-linked recessive [MIM*310800, *310700]; (3) the n. associated with albinism, achromatopsia, and hypoplasia of the macula.

conjugate n., a n. in which the two eyes move simultaneously in the same direction.

convergence-retraction n., irregular, jerky n. combining convergence and retraction of the eye into the orbit, especially on attempting an upward gaze. SYN Koerber-Salus-Elschnig syndrome.

deviational n., SYN end-point n.

dissociated n., a n. in which the movements of the two eyes are dissimilar in direction, amplitude, and periodicity. SYN dysjunctive n., incongruent n., irregular n.

downbeat n., a vertical n. with a rapid component downward, occurring in lesions of the lower part of the brainstem or cerebellum.

dysjunctive n., SYN dissociated n.

end-point n., a jerky, physiologic n. occurring in a normal individual when attempts are made to fixate a point at the limits of the field of fixation. SYN deviational n.

fast component of n., compensatory movement of the eyes in the vestibuloocular reflex.

fixation n., n. aggravated or induced by ocular fixation, arising as optokinetic n., or resulting from midbrain lesions.

galvanic n., n. involving galvanic stimulation of the labyrinth.

gaze paretic n., a n. occurring in partial gaze paralysis when an attempt is made to look in the direction of the gaze paresis.

incongruent n., SYN dissociated n.

irregular n., SYN dissociated n.

jerky n., n. in which there is a slow drift of the eyes in one direction, followed by a rapid recovery movement, always described in the direction of the recovery movement; it usually arises from labyrinthine or neurologic lesions or stimuli.

labyrinthine n., SYN vestibular n.

latent n., jerky n. that is brought out by covering one eye. The fast phase is always away from the covered eye.

miner's n., n. occurring in 19th century coal miners and thought at the time to be related to lack of illumination as well as other factors. SYN miner's disease (1).

minimal amplitude n., SYN micronystagmus.

ocular n., the pendular or, rarely, jerky n. seen in severely reduced vision. SYN amaurotic n.

opticokinetic n., SYN optokinetic n.

optokinetic n., n. induced by looking at moving visual stimuli. SYN opticokinetic n., railroad n.

palatal n., a clonic spasm of the levator palati muscle, causing an audible click. SEE ALSO palatal *myoclonus*.

pendular n., a n. that, in most positions of gaze, has oscillations equal in speed and amplitude, usually arising from a visual disturbance.

positional n., n. occurring only when the head is in a particular position.

railroad n., SYN optokinetic n.

rotational n., jerky n. arising from stimulation of the labyrinth by rotation of the head around any axis and induced by change of motion.

rotatory n., a movement of the eyes around the visual axis.

seesaw n., a n. in which one eye moves upward as the other moves downward, often combined with a torsional rotation (down and out, up and in—as in a see-saw).

slow component of n., the fundamental movement of the eyes in the vestibuloocular reflex.

upbeat n., a vertical jerky n. with a rapid component upward, occurring with brainstem lesions.

vertical n., an up-and-down oscillation of the eyes.

vestibular n., n. resulting from physiological stimuli to the labyrinth that may be rotatory, linear, caloric, compressive, or galvanic, or due to labyrinthal lesions. SEE ALSO Bárány *sign*. SYN labyrinthine n.

voluntary n., pendular n. in which the individual causes an extremely fine and rapid horizontal oscillation of the eyes. The n. consists of back-to-back saccades and is seldom done for more than a few seconds at a time.

nys·tat·in (nī-stat′in, nis′tă-tin). An antibiotic substance isolated from cultures of *Streptomyces noursei*, effective in the treatment of all forms of candidiasis, particularly candidal infections of the intestine, skin, and mucous membranes. SYN fungicidin. [*New York State* + -in]

Nysten, Pierre H., French physician, 1771–1818. SEE N. *law*.

nyx·is (nik′sis). A pricking; paracentesis. [G.]

Ω **1.** The 24th and last letter of the Greek alphabet, omega. **2.** Symbol for ohm.

O 1. Symbol for oxygen; orotidine. **2.** Abbreviation for opening (in formulas for electrical reactions). **3.** Symbol for a blood group in the ABO system. See ABO blood group, Blood Groups appendix. **4.** An abbreviation derived from *ohne Hauch* (without a film), used as a designation for: 1) antigens that occur in the bacterial cell, in contrast to those in the flagella; 2) specific antibodies for such somatic antigens; 3) the agglutinative reaction between somatic antigen and its antibody.

^{15}**O** Symbol for oxygen-15.

^{16}**O** Symbol for oxygen-16.

^{17}**O** Symbol for oxygen-17.

^{18}**O** Symbol for oxygen-18.

o- In chemistry, the abbreviation for *ortho-* (2).

OA Abbreviation for occipitoanterior *position*.

oak ap·ple. SYN nutgall.

oari-, oario-. Obsolete term for an ovary. SEE oo-, oophor-, ovario-. [G. *ōarion*, a small egg, dim. of *ōon*, egg]

oath (ōth). A solemn affirmation or attestation.

OB Abbreviation for obstetrics.

O'Beirne, James, Irish surgeon, 1786–1862. SEE O'B. *sphincter.*

obe·li·ac (ō-bē′lē-ak). Relating to the obelion.

obe·li·ad (ō-bē′lē-ad). Toward the obelion.

obe·li·on (ō-bē′lē-on). A craniometric point on the sagittal suture between the parietal foramina near the lambdoid suture. [G. *obelos*, a spit]

Obermayer, Friedrich, Austrian physician, 1861–1925. SEE O. *test.*

Obermeier, Otto H.F., German physician, 1843–1873. SEE O. *spirillum.*

Obersteiner, Heinrich, Austrian neurologist, 1847–1922. SEE O.-Redlich *line, zone.*

obese (ō-bēs′). Excessively fat. SYN corpulent. [L. *obesus*, fat, partic. adj., fr. *ob-edo*, pp. *-esus*, to eat away, devour]

obe·si·ty (ō-bē′si-tē). An excess of subcutaneous fat in proportion to lean body mass. Excess fat accumulation is associated with increase in the size (hypertrophy) as well as the number (hyperplasia) of adipose tissue cells. O. is variously defined in terms of absolute weight, weight-height ratio, distribution of subcutaneous fat, and societal and esthetic norms. Measures of weight in proportion to height include relative weight (RW, body weight divided by median desirable weight for a person of the same height and medium frame according to actuarial tables), body mass index (BMI, kg/m^2) and ponderal index (kg/m^3). These do not differentiate between excess adiposity and increased lean body mass. In contrast, subscapular and triceps skinfold measurements and determination of the waist-to-hip ratio help define the regional deposition of fat and differentiate the more medically significant central o.from peripheral o. in adults. No single cause can explain all cases of o. Ultimately it results from an imbalance between energy intake and energy expenditure. While faulty eating habits related to failure of normal satiety feedback mechanisms may be responsible for some cases, many obese persons neither consume more calories nor eat different proportions of foodstuffs than nonobese persons. Contrary to popular belief, o. is not caused by disorders of pituitary, thyroid, or adrenal gland metabolism. However, it is often associated with hyperinsulinism and relative insulin resistance. Studies of obese twins strongly suggest the presence of genetic influences on resting metabolic rate, feeding behavior, changes in energy expenditures in response to overfeeding, lipoprotein lipase activity, and basal rate of lipolysis. Environmental factors associated with o. include socioeconomic status, race, region of residence, season, urban living, and being part of a smaller family. The prevalence of o. is greater when weight is measured during winter rather than summer. O. is much commoner in the northeastern and midwestern U.S. than in the south and west, a phenomenon independent of race, population density, and season. SYN adiposity (1), corpulence, corpulency. [L. *obesus*, pp. of *obedo*, to eat up, + -ity]

Obesity is a major public health problem and the leading nutritional disorder in the U.S. A widely accepted definition of obesity is body weight that is 20% or more in excess of ideal weight-for-height according to actuarial tables. By this definition, 34% of adults in the U.S. are obese, and there is evidence that the prevalence of obesity is increasing in both children and adults. The National Institutes of Health have defined obesity as a BMI of 30 kg/m^2 or more, and overweight as a BMI between 25–30 kg/m^2. By these criteria, 55% of adults are either overweight or obese. Obesity is an independent risk factor for hypertension, hypercholesterolemia, type 2 diabetes mellitus, myocardial infarction, certain malignancies (cancer of the colon, rectum, and prostate in men and of the breast, cervix, endometrium, and ovary in women), obstructive sleep apnea, hypoventilation syndrome, osteoarthritis and other orthopedic disorders, infertility, lower extremity venous stasis disease, gastroesophageal reflux disease, and urinary stress incontinence. Lesser degrees of obesity can constitute a significant health hazard in the presence of diabetes mellitus, hypertension, heart disease, or their associated risk factors. Body fat distribution in central (abdominal or male pattern, with an increased waist-to-hip ratio) versus peripheral (gluteal or female pattern) adipose tissue deposit is associated with higher risks of many of these disorders. Obese persons are more liable to injury, more difficult to examine by palpation and imaging techniques, and more likely to have unsuccessful outcomes and complications from surgical operations. Not least among the adverse effects of obesity are social stigmatization, poor self-image, and psychological stress. Weight reduction is associated with improvement in most of the health risks of obesity. All treatments for obesity (other than cosmetic surgical procedures in which subcutaneous fat is mechanically removed) require creation of an energy deficit by reducing caloric intake, increasing physical exercise, or both. Basic weight-reduction programs involve consumption of a restricted-calorie, low-fat diet and performance of at least 30 minutes of endurance-type physical activity of at least moderate intensity on most and preferably all days of the week. Behavior modification therapy, hypnosis, anorexiant drugs, and surgical procedures to reduce gastric capacity or intestinal absorption of nutrients are useful in selected cases, but the emphasis should be on establishing permanent changes in lifestyle. Weight reduction is not recommended during pregnancy or in patients with osteoporosis, cholelithiasis, severe mental illness including anorexia nervosa, or terminal illness.

android o., central o. (apple shape) with fat excess primarily in abdominal wall and visceral mesentery; associated with glucose intolerance, diabetes, decreased sex hormone–binding globulin, increased levels of free testosterone, and increased cardiovascular risk.

gynecoid o., o. with fat excess mainly in the femoral-gluteal region (pear shape).

hypothalamic o., o. caused by disease of the hypothalamus.

△ **Combining Forms**	☆ **Official alternate Terminologia Anatomica term**
Indicates term is illustrated, see Illustration Index	
	[MIM] Mendelian Inheritance in Man
SYN Synonym	
	C.I. Colour Index
Cf. Compare	
[NA] Nomina Anatomica	
[TA] Terminologia Anatomica	**High Profile Term**

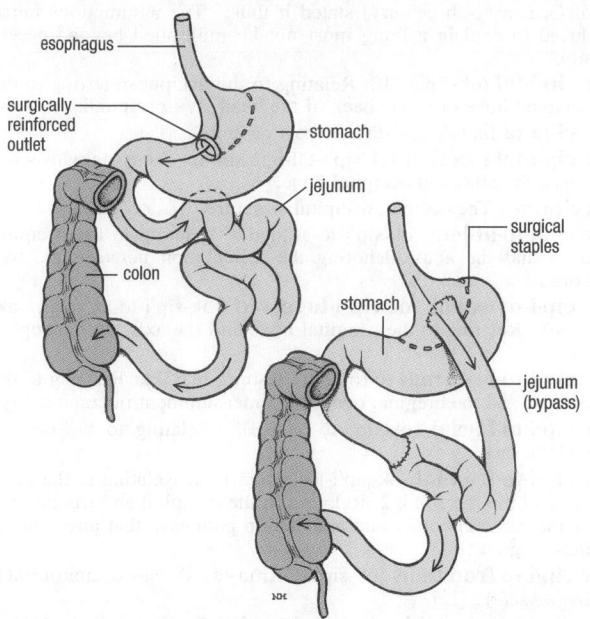

esophagus

surgically
reinforced
outlet

stomach

jejunum

surgical
staples

colon

stomach

jejunum
(bypass)

surgical procedures to control obesity: (A) vertical banded gastroplasty, (B) gastric bypass (gastrojejunostomy)

hypothalamic o. with hypogonadism, SYN adiposogenital *dystrophy.*

morbid o., o. sufficient to prevent normal activity or physiologic function, or to cause the onset of a pathologic condition.

simple o., o. resulting when caloric intake exceeds energy expenditure.

obex (ō′beks) [TA]. The point on the midline of the dorsal surface of the medulla oblongata that marks the caudal angle of the rhomboid fossa or fourth ventricle. It corresponds to a small, transverse medullary fold overhanging the calamus scriptorius. [L. barrier]

ob·fus·ca·tion (ob-fus-kā′shŭn). **1.** A rendering dark or obscure. **2.** A deliberate attempt to confuse or to prevent understanding. [L. *ob-fusco,* pp. *-atus,* to darken, fr. *fuscus,* dark, tawny]

OB/GYN Abbreviation for obstetrics and gynecology.

ob·i·dox·ime chlo·ride (ob′ē-dok-sēm). A cholinesterase reactivator much like 2-PAM.

ob·ject (ob′jekt). **1.** Anything to which thought or action is directed. **2.** In psychoanalysis, that through which an instinct can achieve its aim. **3.** In psychoanalysis, often used synonymously with person.

good o., in psychoanalysis, the good or supporting aspects of an important person in the patient's life, especially of a parent or parent-surrogate.

sex o., a person toward whom another is sexually attracted; a term most used by a female to indicate that a male narrowly views her as a vehicle for sex while completely disregarding the rest of her persona.

test o., (1) an o. having very fine surface markings, mounted on a slide, used to determine the defining power of the objective lens of a microscope; (2) the target in measurement of the visual field.

transitional o., an o. used by many children as a substitute for a parent who is absent (usually temporarily) to help them deal with separation; typically, a blanket or stuffed toy.

ob·ject choice. In psychoanalysis, the object (usually a person) upon which psychic energy is centered.

ob·jec·tive (ob-jek′tiv). **1.** The lens or lenses in the object end of the body tube of a microscope, by means of which the rays coming from the object examined are brought to a focus. SYN object glass. **2.** Viewing events or phenomena as they exist in the external world, impersonally, or in an unprejudiced way; open to

observation by oneself and by others. Cf. subjective. [L. *ob- jicio,* pp. *-jectus,* to throw before]

achromatic o., an o. that is corrected for two colors chromatically, and one color spherically.

apochromatic o., an o. in which chromatic aberration is corrected for three colors and spherical aberration is corrected for two.

immersion o., a high power o. used with a drop of oil between the lens and the specimen on the slide, allowing a greater numerical aperture; similar lenses are available for use with water as the immersing liquid.

ob·jec·tive as·sess·ment da·ta. Those facts that are observable and measurable by the nurse.

ob·li·gate (ob′li-gāt). Without an alternative system or pathway. [L. *ob-ligo,* pp. *-atus,* to bind to]

ob·lique (ob-lēk′). Slanting; deviating from the perpendicular, horizontal, sagittal, or coronal plane of the body. In radiography, a projection that is neither frontal nor lateral. [L. *obliquus*]

ob·liq·ui·ty (ob-lik′wi-tē). SYN asynclitism.

Litzmann o., inclination of the fetal head so that the biparietal diameter is oblique in relation to the plane of the pelvic brim, the posterior parietal bone presenting to the parturient canal. SYN posterior asynclitism.

Nägele o., inclination of the fetal head in cases of flat pelvis, so that the biparietal diameter is oblique in relation to the plane of the pelvic brim, the anterior parietal bone presenting to the parturient canal. SYN anterior asynclitism.

ob·li·qu·us (ob-lī′kwŭs). Denoting a structure having an oblique course or direction; a name given, with further qualification, to several muscles. SEE muscle. [L. slanting, oblique]

ob·lit·er·a·tion (ob-lit-er-ā′shŭn). Blotting out, especially by filling of a natural space or lumen by fibrosis or inflammation. In radiology, disappearance of the contour of an organ when the adjacent tissue has the same x-ray absorption. SEE silhouette *sign* of Felson. [L. *oblittero,* to blot out]

osteoplastic o. of the frontal sinus, operation to remove the diseased contents, including the mucous membrane, of the frontal sinus and to obliterate the sinus with a free fat graft without altering the external contour of the sinus.

ob·lon·ga·ta (ob-long-gah′tă). SYN *medulla* oblongata. [L. fem. of *oblongatus,* from *oblongus,* rather long]

ob·nu·bi·la·tion (ab-noo′bil-ā′shun). A clouded mental state. [L. *ob-nubilo,* to becloud, obscure, fr. *nubes,* cloud]

OBS Abbreviation for organic brain *syndrome.*

ob·ser·ver (ob-zer′ver). One who perceives, notices, or watches; in behavioral research with humans, the investigator or his/her surrogate. [L. *observo,* to watch]

nonparticipant o., an investigator who studies a group of subjects engaged in certain activities but does not directly participate in these activities, presumably being able to study them more objectively.

participant o., an investigator who while studying the activities of a group of subjects also participates in their activities, presumably being able to gain more detailed, relevant information but with less objectivity.

ob·ses·sion (ob-sesh′ŭn). A recurrent and persistent idea, thought, or impulse to carry out an act that is ego-dystonic, that is experienced as senseless or repugnant, and that the individual cannot voluntarily suppress. [L. *obsideo,* pp. *-sessus,* to besiege, fr. *sedeo,* to sit]

impulsive o., an o. accompanied by action, sometimes becoming a mania.

inhibitory o., an o. involving an impediment to action, usually representing a phobia.

ob·ses·sive-com·pul·sive. Having a tendency to perform certain repetitive acts or ritualistic behavior to relieve anxiety, as in obsessive-compulsive neurosis (e.g., a compulsive, ritualistic need to wash one's hands many dozens of times per day).

ob·so·les·cence (ob-sō-les′ens). Falling into disuse; denoting the abolition of a function. [L. *obsolesco,* to grow out of use]

ob·stet·ric, ob·stet·ri·cal (ob-stet′rik, -ri-kăl). Relating to obstetrics.

ob·ste·tri·cian (ob-stĕ-tri-sh′ŭn). A physician specializing in the medical care of women during pregnancy and childbirth. [see obstetrics]

ob·stet·rics (OB) (ob-stet′riks). The specialty of medicine concerned with the care of women during pregnancy, parturition, and the puerperium. SYN tocology. [L. *obstetrix,* a midwife, fr. *ob-sto,* to stand before, denoting the position formerly taken by the midwife]

ob·sti·nate (ob′sti-năt). **1.** Firmly adhering to one's own purpose or opinion, even when wrong; not yielding to argument, persuasion, or entreaty. SYN intractable (2), refractory (2). **2.** SYN refractory (1). [L. *obstinatus,* determined]

ob·sti·pa·tion (ob-sti-pā′shŭn). Intestinal obstruction; severe constipation. [L. *ob,* against, + *stipo,* pp. *-atus,* to crowd]

ob·struc·tion (ob-strŭk′shŭn). Blockage, clogging, or impeded flow, e.g., by occlusion or stenosis. [L. *obstructio*]

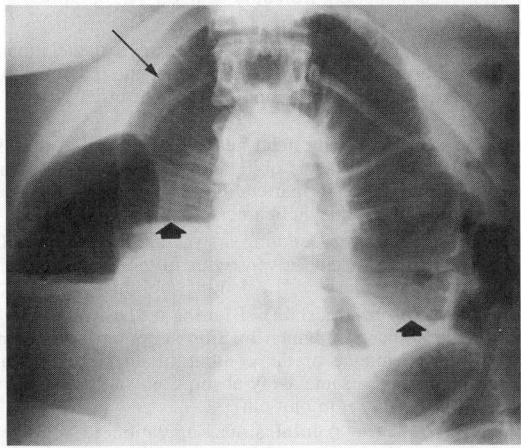

small bowel obstruction: plain, erect radiograph of the abdomen reveals dilated, air-filled loops of small bowel (arrows); the obstruction is due to adhesions

closed loop o., o. of a segment of intestine either rotated on a fixed point (volvulus) or herniated through a fibrous opening (as under an adhesion or into a hernia); frequently associated with impaired perfusion ultimately resulting in gangrene.

ureteropelvic junction o., an impediment to drainage of urine from kidney usually due to partial or intermittent blockage of renal collecting system at the junction of renal pelvis and ureter.

ureterovesical o., o. of the lower ureter at its entrance into the bladder.

ob·stru·ent (ob′stroo-ent). **1.** Rarely used term for obstructing or clogging. **2.** Rarely used term for an agent that obstructs or prevents a normal discharge, especially a discharge from the bowels. [L. *obstruo,* to build against, obstruct]

ob·tund (ob-tŭnd′). To dull or blunt, especially to blunt sensation or deaden pain. [L. *ob-tundo,* pp. *-tusus,* to beat against, blunt]

ob·tu·ra·tion (ob-too-rā′shŭn). Obstruction or occlusion. [see obturator]

intermittent self-o., passage of a blunt object in a lumen or meatus to occlude it or to dilate it.

ob·tu·ra·tor (ob′too-rā-tŏr). **1.** Any structure that occludes an opening. **2.** Denoting the obturator foramen, the obturator membrane, or any of several parts in relation to this foramen. **3.** A prosthesis used to close an opening of the hard palate, usually a cleft palate. **4.** The stylus or removable plug used during the insertion of many tubular instruments. [L. *obturo,* pp. *-atus,* to occlude or stop up]

ob·tuse (ob-toos′). **1.** Dull in intellect; of slow understanding. **2.** Blunt; not acute. [see obtund]

ob·tu·sion (ob-too′zhŭn). **1.** Dullness of sensibility. **2.** A dulling or deadening of sensibility.

Occam's ra·zor. The principle of scientific parsimony. William

of Occam (14th century) stated it thus: "The assumptions introduced to explain a thing must not be multiplied beyond necessity."

oc·cip·i·tal (ok-sip′i-tăl). Relating to the occiput; referring to the occipital bone or to the back of the head. SYN occipitalis.

oc·ci·pi·ta·lis (ok′sip-i-tā′lis). SYN occipital. [L.]

oc·cip·i·tal·i·za·tion (ok′sip′i-tăl-i-zā′shŭn). Bony ankylosis between the atlas and occipital bone.

occipito-. The occiput, occipital structures. [L. *occiput*]

oc·cip·i·to·at·loid (ok-sip′i-tō-at′loyd). Relating to the occipital bone and the atlas; denoting the articulation between the two bones.

oc·cip·i·to·ax·i·al, oc·cip·i·to·ax·oid (ok-sip′i-tō-ak′sē-ăl, -ak′soyd). Relating to the occipital bone and the axis, or epistropheus.

oc·cip·i·to·breg·mat·ic (ok-sip′i-tō-breg-mat′ik). Relating to the occiput and the bregma; denoting a measurement in craniometry.

oc·cip·i·to·fa·cial (ok-sip′i-tō-fā′shăl). Relating to the occiput and the face.

oc·cip·i·to·fron·tal (ok-sip′i-tō-frŭn′tăl). **1.** Relating to the occiput and the forehead. **2.** Relating to the occipital and frontal lobe of the cerebral cortex and association pathways that interconnect these regions.

oc·cip·i·to·fron·ta·lis (ok-sip′i-tō-frŭn-tā′lis). SEE occipitofrontalis (*muscle*). [L.]

oc·cip·i·to·mas·toid (ok-sip′i-tō-mas′toyd). Relating to the occipital bone and the mastoid process.

oc·cip·i·to·men·tal (ok-sip′i-tō-men′tăl). Relating to the occiput and the chin.

oc·cip·i·to·pa·ri·e·tal (ok-sip′i-tō-pă-rī′ĕ-tăl). Relating to the occipital and the parietal bones.

oc·cip·i·to·tem·po·ral (ok-sip′i-tō-tem′pŏ-răl). Relating to the occiput and the temple, or the occipital and the temporal bones.

oc·cip·i·to·tha·lam·ic (ok-sip′i-tō-tha-lam′ik). Relating to the nerve fibers leading from the occipital lobe of the cerebral cortex to the thalamus.

oc·ci·put, gen. **oc·cip·i·tis** (ok′si-put, ok-sip′i-tis) [TA]. The back of the head. [L.]

oc·clude (ŏ-klood). **1.** To close or bring together. **2.** To enclose, as in an occluded *virus*. [see occlusion]

oc·clud·er (ŏ-klood′er). In dentistry, a name given to some articulators.

oc·clu·sal (ŏ-kloo′zăl). **1.** Pertaining to occlusion or closure. **2.** In dentistry, pertaining to the contacting surfaces of opposing occlusal units (teeth or occlusion rims) or the masticating surfaces of the posterior teeth.

oc·clu·sion (ŏ-kloo′zhŭn). **1.** The act of closing or the state of being closed. **2.** In chemistry, the absorption of a gas by a metal or the inclusion of one substance within another (as in a gelatinous precipitate). **3.** Any contact between the incising or masticating surfaces of the upper and lower teeth. **4.** The relationship between the occlusal surfaces of the maxillary and mandibular teeth when they are in contact. [L. *oc- cludo,* pp. *-clusus,* to shut up, fr. *ob.,* against, + *claudo,* to close]

abnormal o., an arrangement of the teeth that is not considered to be within the normal range of variation.

afunctional o., a malocclusion that does not permit normal function of the dentition.

anterior o., (1) the o. of anterior teeth; (2) SYN mesial o. (1).

balanced o., the simultaneous contacting of the upper and lower teeth on the right and left and in the anterior and posterior occlusal areas in centric and eccentric positions within the functional range; used primarily in reference to the mouth, but also arranged and observed on articulators, developed to prevent a tipping or rotating of the denture bases in relation to the supporting structures. SYN balanced articulation, balanced bite.

bimaxillary protrusive o., an o. in which both the maxilla and mandible protrude, causing the long axes of the maxillary anterior teeth to be at an extremely acute angle to the mandibular teeth; may be secondary to a skeletal or dental deformity, or both; seen commonly in blacks.

buccal o., (1) malposition of a tooth toward the cheek; (2) the o. as seen from the buccal side of the teeth.

centric o., (1) the relation of opposing occlusal surfaces that provides the maximum planned contact and/or intercuspation; (2) the o. of the teeth when the mandible is in centric relation to the maxillae. SYN centric contact.

coronary o., blockage of a coronary vessel, usually by thrombosis or atheroma, often leading to myocardial infarction.

distal o., (1) a tooth occluding in a position distal to normal; SYN disto-occlusion, postnormal o., retrusive o. (2). (2) SYN distocclusion.

eccentric o., any o. other than centric.

edge-to-edge o., an o. in which the anterior teeth of both jaws meet along their incisal edges when the teeth are in centric o. SYN edge-to-edge bite, end-to-end bite, end-to-end o.

end-to-end o., SYN edge-to-edge o.

functional o., (1) any tooth contacts made within the functional range of the opposing teeth surfaces; (2) o. that occurs during function.

gliding o., SYN dental *articulation*.

hyperfunctional o., occlusal stress of tooth or teeth exceeding normal physiologic demands.

labial o., (1) malposition of a tooth in a labial direction; (2) the o. as seen from the labial side of the arches.

lateral o., malposition of a tooth or an entire dental arch in a direction away from the midline.

lingual o., (1) SYN linguoclusion; (2) interdigitation of the teeth as seen from the internal or lingual aspect.

mechanically balanced o., a balanced o. without reference to physiologic considerations, as on an articulator.

mesenteric artery o., obstruction of arterial flow in the mesenteric circulation by an embolus or thrombus; usually refers to o. of the superior mesenteric artery, although atherosclerotic narrowing may involve all three major splanchnic branches (celiac, superior, and inferior mesenteric).

mesial o., (1) o. in which the mandibular teeth articulate with the maxillary teeth in a position anterior to normal; SYN anterior o. (2), mesio-occlusion. (2) SYN mesioclusion.

neutral o., (1) an arrangement of teeth such that the maxillary and mandibular first permanent molars are in normal anteroposterior relation; SYN normal o. (2). (2) SYN neutroclusion.

normal o., (1) that arrangement of teeth and their supporting structure that is usually found in health and that approaches an ideal or standard arrangement; SYN normal bite. (2) SYN neutral o. (1).

pathogenic o., an occlusal relationship capable of producing pathologic changes in the supporting tissues.

physiologic o., o. in harmony with functions of the masticatory system.

physiologically balanced o., a balanced o. that is in harmony with the temporomandibular joints and the neuromuscular system.

posterior o., the most effective contact of the molar and bicuspid teeth of both jaws that allows for all the natural movements of the jaws essential to normal mastication and closure. SYN posteroclusion.

postnormal o., SYN distal o. (1).

protrusive o., o. that results when the mandible is protruded forward from centric position.

o. of pupil, the presence of an opaque membrane closing the pupillary area.

retrusive o., (1) a biting relationship in which the mandible is forcefully or habitually placed more distally than the patient's centric o.; (2) SYN distal o. (1).

spherical form of o., an arrangement of teeth that places their occlusal surfaces on the surface of an imaginary sphere (usually 8 inches in diameter) with its center above the level of the teeth. SEE ALSO Monson *curve*.

torsive o., SYN torsiversion.

traumatic o., SYN traumatogenic o.

traumatogenic o., a malocclusion capable of producing injury to the teeth and/or associated structures. SYN traumatic o.

working o., SYN working *contacts*, under *contact*.

oc·clu·sive (ŏ-kloo′siv). Serving to close; denoting a bandage or dressing that closes a wound and excludes it from the air.

oc·clu·som·e·ter (ok-loo-som′ĕ-ter). SYN gnathodynamometer.

oc·cult (ŏ-kŭlt′, ok′ŭlt). **1.** Hidden; concealed; not manifest. **2.** Denoting a concealed hemorrhage, the blood being inapparent or localized to a site where it is not visible. SEE occult *blood*. **3.** In oncology, a clinically unidentified primary tumor with recognized metastases. [L. *oc-culo*, pp. *-cultus*, to cover, hide]

Oce·an·o·spi·ril·lum (ō′shen-ō-spī-ril′ŭm). A genus of motile, nonsporeforming, aerobic bacteria (family Spirillaceae) containing Gram-negative, rigid, helical cells that are 0.3–1.2 μm in diameter. Motile cells contain bipolar fascicles of flagella. There is no growth anaerobically with nitrate. These organisms are chemoorganotrophic and possess a strictly respiratory metabolism; they neither oxidize nor ferment carbohydrates; found in marine environments. There are at present five species in this genus, of which the type species is *O. linum*. [L. *oceanus*, ocean, + *spirillum*, coil]

ocel·lus, pl. **ocel·li** (ō-sel′ŭs, -lī). **1.** The simple eye found in many invertebrates. SYN eyespot (2). **2.** Facet of the compound eye of an insect. [L. dim. of *oculus*, eye]

och·lo·pho·bia (ok-lō-fō′bē-ă). Morbid fear of crowds. [G. *ochlos*, a crowd, + *phobos*, fear]

Ochoa, Severo, Spanish-U.S. biochemist and Nobel laureate, 1905–1993. SEE O. *law*.

ochra·tox·in (ō-kra-toks′ins). A mycotoxin produced by *Aspergillus ochraceus* growing on stored cereal grains. Affects poultry and other animals fed the grain.

ochratoxin A, ochratoxin produced by some species of *Aspergillus* and *Penicillium* that can contaminate cereal grains and feeds, primarily following improper storage; a potent carcinogen in rodents.

Ochrobactrum (ō-krō-bak′trum). A Gram-negative genus of bacteria similar to *Alcaligenes* and *Pseudomonas* spp. in their distribution in environmental and water sources and their culture characteristics. These have been isolated from a number of clinical sources and appear to be a cause of nosocomial bacteremia.

ochro·der·mia (ō-krō-der′mē-ă). Yellow discoloration of the skin. [G. *ōchros*, pale yellow, + *derma*, skin]

ochrom·e·ter (ō-krom′ĕ-ter). An instrument for determining the capillary blood pressure; one of two adjacent fingers is compressed by a rubber balloon until blanching of the skin occurs, after which the force necessary to accomplish this color change is read in millimeters of mercury. [G. *ōchros*, pale yellow, + *metron*, measure]

ochro·no·sis (o-kron-ō′sis). A rare, autosomal recessive disease characterized by alkapton uria with pigmentation of the cartilages and sometimes tissues such as muscle, epithelial cells, and dense connective tissue; may affect also the sclera, mucous membrane of the lips, and skin of the ears, face, and hands, and cause standing urine to be dark-colored and contain pigmented casts; pigmentation is thought to result from oxidized homogentisic acid, and cartilage degeneration results in osteoarthritis, particularly of the spine. [G. *ōchros*, pale yellow, + *nosos*, disease]

exogenous o., pigmentation of the skin of the face and elsewhere from prolonged topical exposure to hydroquinone-containing bleaching creams.

ochro·not·ic (ō-kron-ot′ik). Relating to or characterized by ochronosis.

Ochsner, Albert John, U.S. surgeon, 1858–1925. SEE O. *clamp*, *method*.

oc·ry·late (ok′ri-lāt). A tissue adhesive for surgery.

△**oct-, octi-, octo-, octa-.** Eight. [G. *oktō*, L. *octo*]

OCTA (ok′ta). An eight–base-pair sequence in DNA that has a regulatory role; for example, if it is artificially appended to a gene, it will cause that gene to be preferentially expressed in cells of the β-lymphocyte lineage.

oc·tac·o·san·o·ic ac·id (ok-tă-kō′sān-ō-ik). A long-chain fatty acid; found in waxes. SYN montanic acid.

oc·tad (ok′tad). **1.** SYN octavalent. **2.** An octavalent element or radical. [L. *octo*, eight]

octafluoropropane (ok′ta-flōr′ō-prō-pān). A drug used for contrast enhancement during ultrasound imaging.

oc·ta·meth·yl py·ro·phos·phor·a·mide (OMPA) (ok-tă-meth′il pī′rō-fos-fōr′ă-mīd). SYN schradan.

oc·ta·myl·a·mine (ok-tă-mil′ă-mēn). An anticholinergic agent.

oc·tan (ok′tan). Applied to fever, the paroxysms of which recur every eighth day, the day of a paroxysm being counted as the first in the computation. [L. *octo*, eight]

oc·tan·di·o·ic ac·id. SYN suberic acid.

oc·ta·no·ate (ok′tă-nō′āt). SYN caprylate.

oc·ta·no·ic ac·id (ok′tă-nō′ik). SYN caprylic acid.

oc·ta·no·yl-CoA syn·the·tase (ok′tăn-ō-il sin′thē-tās). SYN butyrate-CoA ligase.

oc·ta·pep·tide (ok′tă-pep′tīd). A peptide made up of eight amino acid residues.

oc·ta·ploi·dy (ok′tă-ploy′dē). SEE polyploidy.

oc·ta·pres·sin (ok′tă-pres′in). SYN felypressin.

oc·ta·va·lent (ok′tă-vā′lent, ok-tav′ă-lent). Denoting a chemical element or radical having a combining power (valency) of eight. SYN octad (1).

oc·ta·vus (ok-tā′vŭs). SYN vestibulocochlear *nerve* [CN VIII]. [L.]

△**octi-.** SEE oct-.

△**octo-.** SEE oct-.

Oc·to·mit·i·dae (ok-tō-mit′i-dē). A family in the protozoan class Zoomastigophorea; flagellates with six to eight flagella arranged in pairs and a body that is bilaterally symmetric; it includes the common human intestinal parasite *G. lamblia*. [octo- + G. *mitos*, thread]

Oc·tom·i·tus hom·i·nis (ok-tom′i-tŭs hom′i-nis). *Pentatrichomonas hominis*.

oc·to·pa·mine (ok-tō′pă-mēn). A sympathomimetic amine; a false neurotransmitter produced by noradrenergic neurons in the presence of monoamine oxidase inhibitors. SYN norsympatol, norsynephrine.

oc·tose (ok′tōs). A sugar containing eight carbon atoms.

oc·tox·y·nol (ok-tok′si-nol). A surfactant.

oc·tu·lose (ok′too-lōs). An eight-carbon monoketose.

oc·tu·lo·son·ic ac·id (ok′too-lō-son′ik). The -onic acid formally formed by oxidation of carbon atom 1 of octulose to a carboxylic acid group; a condensation product of D-arabinose and phosphoenolpyruvate analogous to neuraminic acid. It forms part of the repeating unit of the polysaccharides of the complex lipopolysaccharides of the Enterobacteriaceae constituting the characteristic somatic octose antigens.

oc·tyl gal·late (ok′til gal′āt). An antioxidant.

oc·tyl·phe·noxy pol·y·eth·ox·y·eth·a·nol (ok′til-fe-nok′sē pol′ē-eth-ok′sē-eth′ă-nol). Mono-*p*-isooctyl phenyl ether of polyethylene glycol; a surface-active (wetting) agent.

oc·u·lar (ok′ū-lăr). **1.** SYN ophthalmic. **2.** The eyepiece of a microscope, the lens or lenses at the observer end of a microscope, by means of which the image focused by the objective is viewed. [L. *oculus*, eye]

compensating o., an o. that compensates and corrects for the effects of chromatic aberration in the objective.

Huygens o., the compound o. of a microscope, composed of two planoconvex lenses so arranged that the plane side of each is directed toward the observer.

o. motor, relating to or causing movements of the eyeball.

Ramsden o., an eyepiece of a microscope, consisting of two planoconvex lenses with convexities turned to each other.

wide field o., an o. that gives a larger than usual field of view and a high eyepoint.

oc·u·lar·ist (ok′ū-lăr-ist). One skilled in the design, fabrication, and fitting of artificial eyes and the making of prostheses associated with the appearance or function of the eyes. [L. *oculus*, eye]

o·cu·len·tum, pl. **o·cu·len·ta** (ok-ū-len′tŭm, -tă). SYN ophthalmic *ointment*. [Mod. L., fr. L. *oculus*, eye]

oc·u·li (ok′ū-lī). Plural of oculus. [L.]

oc·u·list (ok′ū-list). SYN ophthalmologist. [L. *oculus*, eye]

△**oculo-.** The eye, ocular. SEE ALSO ophthalmo-. [L. *oculus*]

oc·u·lo·au·ric·u·lo·ver·te·bral (ok′ū-lō-aw-rik′ū-lō-ver′tĕ-brăl). Relating to the eyes, ears, and vertebrae.

oc·u·lo·car·di·ac (ok′ū-lō-kar′dē-ak). Relating to the eyes and heart.

oc·u·lo·cer·e·bro·re·nal (ok′ū-lō-ser′ē-brō-rē′năl). Relating to the eyes, brain, and kidneys.

oc·u·lo·cu·ta·ne·ous (ok′ū-lō-kū-tā′nē-ŭs). Relating to the eyes and the skin.

oc·u·lo·den·to·dig·i·tal (ok′ū-lō-den′tō-dij′i-tăl). Relating to the eyes, teeth, and fingers.

oc·u·lo·der·mal (ok′ū-lō-der′măl). Relating to the eyes and skin.

oc·u·lo·dyn·ia. Pain in the eyeball. SYN ophthalmalgia. [ophthalmo- + G. *algos*, pain]

oc·u·lo·fa·cial (ok-ū-lō-fā′shăl). Relating to the eyes and the face.

oc·u·log·ra·phy (ok-ū-log′ră-fē). A method of recording eye position and movements. [oculo- + G. *graphē*, a writing]

photosensor o., o. in which photocells are directed to the surface of the eye to record rotations.

oc·u·lo·gy·ria (ok′ū-lō-jī′rē-ă). The limits of rotation of the eyeballs. [oculo- + G. *gyros*, circle]

oc·u·lo·gy·ric (ok′ū-lō-jī′rik). Referring to rotation of the eyeballs; characterized by oculogyria.

oc·u·lo·man·dib·u·lo·dys·ceph·a·ly (ok′ū-lō-man-dib′ū-lō-dis-sef′ă-lē). SYN *dyscephalia* mandibulo-oculofacialis.

oc·u·lo·mo·tor (ok′ū-lō-mō′tŏr). Pertaining to the o. cranial nerve. [L. *oculomotorius*, fr. oculo- + L. *motorius*, moving]

o·cu·lo·mo·to·ri·us (ok′ū-lō-mō-tō′rē-ŭs). SYN oculomotor *nerve* [CN III]. [L.]

oc·u·lo·na·sal (ok′ū-lō-nā′săl). Relating to the eyes and the nose. [oculo- + L. *nasus*, nose]

oc·u·lop·a·thy (ok-ū-lop′ă-thē). SYN ophthalmopathy.

oc·u·lo·pleth·ys·mog·ra·phy (ok′ū-lō-pleth-iz-mog′ră-fē). Indirect measurement of the hemodynamic significance of internal carotid artery stenosis or occlusion by demonstration of an ipsilateral delay in the arrival of ocular pressure transmitted from branches of the ophthalmic artery. [oculo- + G. *plēthymos*, increase, + *graphē*, to write]

oc·u·lo·pneu·mo·pleth·ys·mog·ra·phy (ok′ū-lō-noo′mō-pleth-iz-mog′ră-fē). A method of bilateral measurement of ophthalmic artery pressure that reflects pressure and flow in the internal carotid artery. SEE oculoplethysmography.

oc·u·lo·pu·pil·lary (ok′ū-lō-poo′pi-lār-ē). Pertaining to the pupil of the eye.

oc·u·lo·sym·pa·thet·ic (ok′oo-lō-sim-pa-the′tik). Pertaining to the sympathetic pathway to the eye, damage to which produces Horner *syndrome*.

oc·u·lo·ver·te·bral (ok′ū-lō-ver′tĕ-brăl). Relating to the eyes and vertebrae.

oc·u·lo·zy·go·mat·ic (ok′ū-lō-zī-gō-mat′ik). Relating to the orbit or its margin and the zygomatic bone.

oc·u·lus, gen. and pl. **oc·u·li** (ok′ū-lŭs, -lī) [TA]. SYN eye (1). [L.]

△**ocy-.** SEE oxy-.

ocy·toc·in (ō-si-tō′sin). SYN oxytocin. [G. *okytokos*, fast birth, prompt delivery]

OD Abbreviation for overdose; optic *density* (see absorbance).

O.D. 1. Abbreviation for L. *oculus dexter*, right eye. **2.** Abbreviation for Doctor of Optometry. SEE optometrist.

o.d. Abbreviation for L. *omni die*, every day.

odax·es·mus (ō′dak-sez′mŭs). A biting sensation; a form of paresthesia. [G. *odaxēsmos*, an irritation, fr. *odax* (adv.), by biting.]

odax·et·ic (ō′dak-set′ik). **1.** Causing formication or itching. **2.** A substance or agent that causes formication or itching. [G. *odaxēsmos*, an irritation]

Oddi, Ruggero, Italian physician; 1864–1913. SEE O. *sphincter.*

odds. The ratio of probability of occurrence to non-occurrence of an event. [pl. of *odd*, fr. M.E. *odde*, fr. O.Norse *oddi*, odd number]

△**-odes.** Having the form of, resembling. [G. *eidos*, form, resemblance]

Odland body. See under body.

odo·gen·e·sis (ō-dō-jen′ĕ-sis). SYN neurocladism. [G. *hodos*, path, + *genesis*, source]

△**odont-, odonto-.** A tooth, teeth. [G. *odous* (*odont-*)]

odon·tag·ra (ō-don-tag′ră). Obsolescent term for toothache thought to be of gouty origin. [odonto- + G. *agra*, seizure]

odon·tal·gia (ō-don-tal′jē-ă). SYN toothache. [odont- + G. *algos*, pain]

o. denta′lis, reflex pain in the ear due to dental disease, usually propagated along the auriculotemporal nerve.

odon·tal·gic (ō-don-tal′jik). Relating to or marked by toothache.

odon·tec·to·my (ō-don-tek′tō-mē). Removal of teeth by the reflection of a mucoperiosteal flap and excision of bone from around the root or roots before the application of force to effect the tooth removal. [odont- + G. *ektomē*, excision]

odon·ter·ism (ō-don′ter-izm). Chattering of the teeth. [odont- + G. *erismos*, quarrel]

odon·ti·a·sis (ō-don-tī′ă-sis). SYN teething.

odon·ti·noid (ō-don′ti-noyd). **1.** Resembling dentin. **2.** A small excrescence from a tooth, most common on the root or neck. **3.** Toothlike.

odon·ti·tis (ō-don-tī′tis). SYN pulpitis.

△**odonto-.** SEE odont-.

odon·to·am·e·lo·blas·to·ma (ō-don′tō-am′ĕ-lō-blas-tō′mă). SYN ameloblastic *odontoma.*

odon·to·blast (ō-don′tō-blast). One of the dentin-forming cells, derived from mesenchyme of neural crest origin, lining the pulp cavity of a tooth; o.'s are arranged in a peripheral layer in the dental pulp, each with an odontoblastic process extending through the thickness of the dentine; the cells generally are columnar in the coronal pulp but are more cuboidal in the radicular area and adjacent to tertiary dentin. [odonto- + G. *blastos*, sprout, germ]

odon·to·blas·to·ma (ō-don′tō-blas-tō′mă). **1.** A tumor composed of neoplastic epithelial and mesenchymal cells that may differentiate into cells able to produce calcified tooth substances. **2.** An odontoma in its early formative stage. [odontoblast + G. *-oma*, tumor]

odon·to·clast (ō-don′tō-klast). One of the cells believed to produce resorption of the roots of the deciduous teeth. [odonto- + G. *klastos*, broken]

odon·to·dyn·ia (ō-don-tō-din′ē-ă). SYN toothache. [odonto- + G. *odynē*, pain]

odon·to·dys·pla·sia (ō-don′tō-dis-plā′zē-ă). A developmental disturbance of one or of several adjacent teeth, of unknown etiology, characterized by deficient formation of enamel and dentin, which results in an abnormally large pulp chamber and imparts a ghostlike radiographic image to the teeth; such teeth exhibit delayed eruption into the oral cavity. SYN odontogenesis imperfecta, odontogenic dysplasia.

odon·to·gen·e·sis (ō-don-tō-jen′ĕ-sis). The process of development of the teeth. SYN odontogeny, odontosis. [odonto- + G. *genesis*, production]

o. imperfec′ta, SYN odontodysplasia.

odon·tog·e·ny (ō-don-toj′ĕ-nē). SYN odontogenesis.

odon·toid (ō-don′toyd). **1.** Shaped like a tooth. SYN dentoid. **2.** Relating to the toothlike o. process of the second cervical vertebra. [odont- + G. *eidos*, resemblance]

odon·tol·o·gy (ō-don-tol′ŏ-jē). SYN dentistry. [odonto- + G. *logos*, study]

forensic o., SYN forensic *dentistry.*

odon·to·lox·ia, odon·to·loxy (ō-don-tō-lok′sē-ă, ō-don-tol′ok-sē). SYN odontoparallaxis. [odonto- + G. *loxos*, slanting]

odon·tol·y·sis (ō-don-tol′i-sis). SYN erosion (3). [odonto- + G. *lysis*, dissolution]

odon·to·ma (ō-don-tō′mă). **1.** A tumor of odontogenic origin. **2.** A hamartomatous odontogenic tumor composed of enamel, dentin, cementum, and pulp tissue that may or may not be arranged in the form of a tooth. [odonto- + G. *-oma*, tumor]

ameloblastic o., a benign mixed odontogenic tumor composed of an undifferentiated component histologically identical to an ameloblastoma and a well-differentiated component identical to an odontoma; appears as a mixed radiolucent-radiopaque lesion and presents clinically as an ameloblastoma. SYN odontoameloblastoma.

complex o., an o. in which the various odontogenic tissues are organized in a haphazard arrangement with no resemblance to teeth.

compound o., an o. in which the odontogenic tissues are organized and resemble anomalous teeth.

odon·to·neu·ral·gia (ō-don′tō-noo-ral′jē-ă). Facial neuralgia caused by a carious tooth.

odon·ton·o·my (ō-don-ton′ō-mē). Dental nomenclature. [odonto- + G. *onoma*, name]

odon·to·no·sol·o·gy (ō-don′tō-nō-sol′ŏ-jē). SYN dentistry. [odonto- + G. *nosos*, disease, + *logos*, study]

odon·to·par·al·lax·is (ō-don′tō-par-ă-lak′sis). Irregularity of the teeth. SYN odontoloxia, odontoloxy. [odonto- + G. *parallax*, alternately]

odon·top·a·thy (ō-don-top′ă-thē). Any disease of the teeth or of their sockets. [odonto- + G. *pathos*, suffering]

odon·to·pho·bia (ō-don-tō-fō′bē-ă). Morbid fear of teeth. [odonto- + G. *phobos*, fear]

odon·to·plas·ty (ō-don′tō-plas-tē). Surgical contouring of tooth surface to enhance plaque control and gingival morphology. [odonto- + G. *plassō*, to mold]

odon·top·ri·sis (ō-don-top′ri-sis). Grinding together of the teeth. SEE ALSO bruxism. [odonto- + G. *prisis*, a sawing, a grinding]

odon·top·to·sis (ō-don-top-tō′sis, -tō-tō′sis). Downward movement of an upper tooth due to the loss of its lower antagonist(s). SEE ALSO supereruption. [odonto- + G. *ptōsis*, a falling]

odon·tor·rha·gia (ō-don-tō-rā′jē-ă). Profuse bleeding from the socket after the extraction of a tooth. [odonto- + G. *rhēgnymi*, to burst forth]

odon·to·schism (ō-don′tō-skizm, -sizm). Fissure of a tooth. [odonto- + G. *schisma*, a cleft]

odon·to·scope (ō-don′tō-skōp). An optical device, similar to a closed circuit television system, that projects a view of the oral cavity onto a screen for multiple viewing.

odon·tos·co·py (ō-don-tos′kŏ-pē). **1.** Examination of the oral cavity by means of the odontoscope. **2.** Examination of the markings in prints of the cutting edges of the teeth; used, like fingerprints, as a method of personal identification. [odonto- + G. *skopeō*, to view]

odon·to·sis (ō-don-tō′sis). SYN odontogenesis.

odon·to·ther·a·py (ō-don-tō-thar′ă-pē). Treatment of diseases of the teeth.

odon·tot·o·my (ō-don-tot′ō-mē). Cutting into the crown of a tooth. [odonto- + G. *tomē*, incision]

prophylactic o., a preventive operation in which imperfectly formed developmental grooves, pits, and fissures are opened up by means of a bur and filled to obviate future decay.

odor (ō′dŏr). Emanation from any substance that stimulates the olfactory sensory cells. SYN scent, smell (3). [L.]

odor·ant (ō′dŏr-ant). A substance with an odor.

odor·a·tism (ō′dŏr′ă-tizm). SEE lathyrism. [fr. *Lathyrus odoratus*, sweet pea]

odor·if·er·ous (ō-dŏ-rif′er-ŭs). Having a scent, perfume, or odor. SYN odorous. [odor + L. *fero*, to bear]

odor·im·e·ter (ō′dŏ-rim′ĕ-ter). Instrument for performing odorimetry.

odo·rim·e·try (ō′dŏ-rim′ĕ-trē). The determination of the comparative power of different substances in stimulating olfactory sensations. [odor + G. *metron*, measure]

od

odor·i·vec·tion (ō′dŏr-i-vek′shŭn). Conveying or bearing an odor, as in the air. [odor + L. *vector,* a carrier]

odor·og·ra·phy (ō′dŏ-rog′ră-fē). Description of odors. [odor + G. *graphē,* a description]

odor·ous (ō′dŏr-ŭs). SYN odoriferous.

O'Dwyer, Joseph P., U.S. physician, 1841–1898. SEE O'D. *tube.*

△**odyn-, odyno-.** Pain. [G. *odynē*]

odyn·a·cu·sis (ō-din′ă-koo′sis). Hypersensitiveness of the organ of hearing, so that sounds cause actual pain. [odyn- + G. *akouō,* to hear]

odyn·o·pha·gia (ō-din-ō-fā′jē-ă). Pain on swallowing. [odyno- + G. *phagō* to eat]

odyn·o·pho·nia (ō-din-ō-fō′nē-ă). Pain on using the voice. [odyno- + G. *phonē,* sound, voice]

Oe Symbol for oersted.

△**oe-.** For words so beginning and not found here, see e-.

oe·di·pism (ed′i-pizm). **1.** Manifestation of the Oedipus complex. **2.** Rarely used term for self-infliction of injury to the eyes, usually an attempt at evulsion. [*Oedipus,* G. myth. char.]

Oehl, Eusebio, Italian anatomist, 1827–1903. SEE O. *muscles,* under *muscle.*

oe·nan·thal (ē-nan′thăl). SYN heptanal.

oer·sted (Oe) (er′sted). A unit of magnetic field intensity; the magnetic field intensity that exerts a force of 1 dyne on a unit magnetic pole; equal to (1000/4π) A m⁻¹. [Hans-Christian *Oersted,* Danish physicist, 1777–1851]

oe·soph·a·go·sto·mi·a·sis (ē-sof′ă-gō-stō-mī′ă-sis). Infection with nematode parasites of the genus *Oesophagostomum.* SYN esophagostomiasis. [G. *oi-sophagos,* gullet (esophagus), + *stoma,* mouth, + *-iasis,* condition]

Oe·soph·a·gos·to·mum (ē-sof-ă-gos′tō-mŭm). A genus of strongyle nematodes (subfamily Oesophagostominae) that encyst in the intestinal wall of herbivores and primates, causing nodular disease. Larvae appear to stimulate a host reaction in the intestinal wall, forming nodules in which the worms complete their development (unless the host is immune); they then leave the nodule and feed as adults in the lumen of the large intestine. [G. *oisophagos,* gullet (esophagus), + *stoma,* mouth]

O. apios′tomum, a nematode species that has been reported in northern Nigeria and central Africa to encyst under the submucosa of the human intestine and occasionally cause dysentery; a common parasite of monkeys and apes, both in captivity and in the wild.

O. brevicau′dum, a nematode species that occurs in the cecum and colon of pigs in North America and India.

O. brump′ti, a nematode species described from African monkeys and reported occasionally in humans.

O. columbia′num, a nematode species that occurs in sheep, goats, and wild African antelopes; except when present in large numbers, it does not appear to seriously affect the health of the host.

O. denta′tum, a nematode species that affects the colon of swine; the lesions are similar to those in sheep.

O. georgia′num, a nematode species that occurs in the cecum and colon of pigs in the U.S.

O. quadrispinula′tum, a species that occurs in the cecum and colon of pigs in the Americas, Europe, and Southeast Asia.

O. radia′tum, a species that occurs worldwide in cattle and water buffalo; the lesions are similar to those of sheep.

O. stephanos′tomum, a species of nematode occurring in chimpanzees, monkeys, and gorillas in Africa, but also reported from humans and monkeys in Brazil.

O. venulo′sum, a species that occurs worldwide in the cecum and colon of cattle, sheep, goats, deer, and many other ruminants.

oest·ra·di·ol (es-tră-dī′ol). SYN estradiol.

oest·rids (est′ridz). Common name for botflies of the family Oestridae, such as *Oestrus.* [G. *oistros,* gadfly]

oes·tri·ol (es′trē-ol). SYN estriol.

oest·ro·gen (es′trō-jen). SYN estrogen.

oest·rone (es′tron). SYN estrone.

oes·tro·sis (es-trō′sis). Infection of small ruminants and, rarely, humans with larvae of the fly *Oestrus ovis.*

Oes·trus (es′tŭs). A genus of tissue-invading flies that cause myiasis in sheep; the head botflies in the family Oestridae. *O. ovis* (a nose fly) is a grayish brown, robust, hairy, beelike botfly, imported from Europe, and now a serious pest in parts of the U.S.; larvae are deposited by the adult fly in the nostrils of sheep, and inch-long larvae develop in the paranasal sinuses, causing considerable mucous discharge and distress in old or weak sheep. [G. *oistros,* gadfly]

of·fi·cial (ŏ-fish′ăl). Authoritative; denoting a drug or a chemical or pharmaceutical preparation recognized as standard in the pharmacopeia. Cf. officinal. [L. *officialis,* fr. *officium,* a favor, service, fr. *opus,* work, + *facio,* to do]

of·fic·i·nal (ŏ-fis′i-năl). Denoting a chemical or pharmaceutical preparation kept in stock, in contrast to magistral (prepared extemporaneously according to a physician's prescription); an o. preparation is often, though not necessarily, official. [L. *officina,* shop]

Ogino, Kyusaka, 20th century Japanese physician. SEE O.-Knaus *rule.*

Ogston, Sir Alexander, Scottish surgeon, 1844–1929. SEE O. *line;* O.-Luc *operation.*

Oguchi, Chita, Japanese ophthalmologist, 1875–1945. SEE O. *disease.*

Ogura, Joseph H., U.S. otolaryngologist, 1915–1983. SEE O. *operation.*

O'Hara, Michael, Jr., U.S. surgeon, 1869–1926. SEE O'H. *forceps.*

OHI Abbreviation for Oral Hygiene Index.

OHI-S Abbreviation for Simplified Oral Hygiene Index.

Ohm, Georg S., German physicist, 1787–1854. SEE ohm; O. *law.*

ohm (Ω) (ōm). The practical unit of electrical resistance; the resistance of any conductor allowing 1 A of current to pass under the electromotive force of 1 V. [G.S. *Ohm*]

ohm·am·me·ter (ōm-am′ĕ-ter). A combined ohmmeter and ammeter.

ohm·me·ter (ōm′ĕ-ter). An instrument for determining the resistance, in ohms, of a conductor.

oh·ne Hauch (ō′nă howch). Term used to designate the nonspreading growth of nonflagellated bacteria on agar media; also applied to somatic agglutination. SEE ALSO O *antigen.* [Ger. without breath]

Ohngren line. See under line.

OI Abbreviation for *osteogenesis* imperfecta.

△**oi-.** For words so beginning and not found here, see e-.

△**-oid.** Resemblance to, equivalent to Eng. -form. [G. *eidos,* form, resemblance]

oid·ia (ō-id′ēă). Plural of oidium.

oid·i·um, pl. **oid·ia** (ō-id′ē-ŭm, ō-id′ē-ă). Formerly used term for arthroconidium. [Mod. L. dim. of G. *ōon,* egg]

oil (oyl). An inflammable liquid, of fatty consistency and unctuous feel, which is insoluble in water, soluble or insoluble in alcohol, and freely soluble in ether. O.'s are variously classified as animal, vegetable, and mineral o.'s according to their source (the mineral o.'s probably being of remote animal and vegetable origin); into fatty (fixed) and volatile o.'s; and into drying and nondrying (fatty) o.'s, the former becoming gradually thicker when exposed to the air and finally drying to a varnish, the latter not drying but liable to become rancid on exposure. Many of the o.'s, both fixed and volatile, are used in medicine. For individual o.'s, see the specific names. [L. *oleum;* G. *elaion,* originally olive oil]

absolute o.'s, essential o.'s that are obtained by the removal of insoluble compounds from concrete oils.

o. of American wormseed, SYN o. of chenopodium.

o. of anise, volatile o. derived from the dried ripe fruit of *Pimpinella anisum* (family Umbelliferae) or of *Illicium verum,* (family Magnoliaceae) (Chinese star anise); has a characteristic anise aroma, resembling fennel. Used in manufacture of liqueurs, and as flavoring for candies, cookies, dentifrices. Pharmaceutical aid (flavor). Carminative.

o. of bay, volatile o. derived by steam distillation of the dried leaves of *Pimenta (Myrcia) acris* (family Myrtaceae); o. of myrcia; used as an aromatic in the manufacture of bay rum and as a pharmaceutical aid.

o. of bergamot, volatile o. derived by steam distillation from the rind of the fresh fruit of *Citrus aurantium* or *C. bergamia;* contains L-linalyl acetate, L-linalool; D-limonene, dipentene, bergaptene; used as a deodorant in preparations containing malodorous ingredients and as an aromatic in perfumes, hairdressings, and pomades.

betula o., o. of sweet birch, a volatile o. obtained by distillation from the bark of *Betula lenta* (sweet birch); used as a flavoring agent and as a counterirritant liniment. SEE ALSO methyl salicylate.

o. of bitter almond, volatile o. from the dried ripe kernels of bitter almonds or from other kernels containing amygdalin, such as apricots, peaches, plums, and cherries; obtained by steam distillation subsequent to maceration of the source with water. Formerly used as an antipruritic; poisonous—releases hydrocyanic acid (hydrogen cyanide). Only the oil free of hydrogen cyanide may be used to flavor liquors and foods.

o. of bitter orange, volatile o. obtained by steam distillation from the fresh peel of *Citrus aurantium* (family Rutaceae). Aromatic material used as a flavoring agent in pharmaceuticals and foods and liquors; also used in perfumes.

o. of cardamom, volatile o. obtained by steam distillation from the seeds of *Elettaria cardamomum* (family Zingiberacea.) A flavoring agent in pharmaceuticals (syrups), liquors, sauces, confections, and baked goods; formerly used as a carminative.

o. of chenopodium, volatile o. from the fresh above-ground part of the flower American wormseed, *Chenopodium ambrosioides,* or *C. anthelminticum.* Used as an anthelmintic. SYN o. of American wormseed.

o. of cherry laurel, volatile o. derived by steam distillation from *Prunus laurocerasus* (family Rosaceae); similar to o. of bitter almond; highly toxic because of hydrogen cyanide content.

o. of cinnamon, volatile o. obtained by steam distillation from the leaves and twigs of *Cinnamomum cassia* (family Lauracea). A flavor in foods and medicines.

o. of citronella, volatile o. obtained by steam distillation of fresh lemon grass. Contains citranellol; used as an insect repellent either on the skin or in the form of incense; also used as a perfume.

o. of clove, volatile o. obtained by steam distillation of the dried flower buds of *Eugenia caryophyllata* (family Myrtacea). Contains about 85% eugenol along with other constituents. Used in dentistry as a local anesthetic and component of temporary fillings of the teeth. Also used to flavor foods; strong, pungent odor. SYN clove oil.

concrete o.'s, essential o.'s obtained by extraction with organic solvents; contain waxes and paraffins.

o. of coriander, volatile o. from the dried ripe fruit of *Coriandrum sativum* (family Umbelliferae). Flavoring in foods and alcoholic beverages.

oil of crispmint, SYN o. of spearmint.

o. of cubeb, volatile o. of the unripe fruit of *Piper cubeba* (family Piperaceae). Formerly used as a urinary antiseptic.

oil of curled mint, SYN o. of spearmint.

o. of dwarf pine needles, volatile o. from the fresh leaves of *Pinus montana* (family Pinaceae). Pleasant pine odor; used as a pharmaceutical aid (flavor and perfume). Has been used as an expectorant.

essential o.'s, plant products, usually somewhat volatile, giving the odors and tastes characteristic of the particular plant, thus possessing the essence, e.g., citral, pinene, camphor, menthane, terpenes; usually, the steam distillates of plants or oils of plants obtained by pressing out the rinds of a particular plant. SEE ALSO volatile o.

ethereal o., SYN volatile o.

o. of eucalyptus, volatile o. from the fresh leaves of *Eucalyptus globulus* (family Myrtaceae) and some other species of *Eucalyp-*

tus; native to Australia; pungent o. with a spicy, cooling taste. Has been used as an aromatic in inhalants, as an expectorant, anthelmintic, and local antiseptic.

fatty o., an o. derived from both animals and plants; chemically, a glyceride of a fatty acid that, by substitution of the glycerine by an alkaline base, is converted into a soap; a fatty o., in contrast to a volatile o., is permanent, leaving a stain on an absorbent surface, and thus is not capable of distillation; it is obtained by expression or extraction; the consistency varies with the temperature, some being liquid (o.'s proper), others semisolid (fats), and others solid (tallows) at ordinary temperatures; both liquid and semisolid o.'s are congealed by cold and the solids are liquified by heat. SYN fixed o.

o. of fennel, volatile o. from the dried fruit of *Foeniculum vulgare* (family Umbelliferae). An aromatic o. with the odor and taste of fennel, similar to anise; used as a flavoring agent in pharmaceuticals. Has been used as a carminative.

fixed o., SYN fatty o.

fusel o., a mixture of side products of alcoholic fermentation; consists primarily of alcohols (e.g., amyl, propyl, isoamyl, and isobutyl alcohols).

joint o., SYN synovial *fluid.*

jojoba o., a liquid wax ester mixture extracted from ground or crushed seeds from *Simmondsia chinensis* and *S. californica* (family Buxaceae), desert shrubs native to Arizona, California, and northern Mexico. Used extensively in cosmetics for alleged skin softening and lubricating properties; other uses include as lubricant, fuel, chemical feedstock, substitute for sperm whale oil. SYN oil of jojoba.

oil of jojoba, SYN jojoba o.

o. of juniper, volatile o. from the dried ripe fruit (berries) of *Juniperus communis* (family Cupressaceae). Formerly used as a diuretic. Used in perfumery. SYN juniper berry oil.

o. of lavender, volatile o. from fresh flowering tops of *Lavandula officinalis* (family Labiatae). Aromatic o. used in perfume and as a flavoring agent. Has been used as a carminative.

o. of lemon, volatile o. expressed from fresh peel of *Citrus limonum* (family Rutaceae). Aromatic o. used for flavoring pharmaceuticals, liqueurs, pastry, foods, and beverages and in perfumes.

o. of lemon grass, volatile o. from *Cymbopogon citratus* and of *C. flexuosus* (family Gramineae). Used in perfumery and as a source of citral for the synthesis of vitamin A.

Lorenzo o., a mixture of four parts glyceryl trioleate and one part glyceryl trierucate; used in treatment of adrenoleukodystrophy. [for Lorenzo Odone, a child with adrenoleukodystrophy, whose family's discovery and support of this agent were dramatized in the U.S. film *Lorenzo's Oil* (1992)]

olive o., The expressed oil of the fruit of *Olea europaea;* used as a cholagogue, laxative, and emollient, in the preparation of liniments, and in the preparation of foods.

palm o., an o. obtained from the seeds of *Elaeis guineensis* (family Palmae); used in the manufacture of soap, liniments, and ointments and also in foods.

o. of pennyroyal, either American or European. The former is a volatile o. derived from the flowering tops and leaves of *Hedeoma pulegioides* (family Labiatae). Contains pulegone and ketones. European is o. of pulegium; a volatile o. from *Mentha pulegium* (family Labiatae); about 85% pulegone. Has been used as an aromatic carminative, abortifacient, and insect repellent.

o. of peppermint, a volatile o. containing menthol (not less than 50% of total) obtained by steam distillation from the fresh flowering plant *Mentha piperita* (family Labiatae). Used as a pharmaceutical aid (flavor) and in flavoring liqueurs; a carminative.

red o. [C.I. 26125], a weakly acid diazo oil-soluble dye, used in histologic demonstration of neutral fats.

rock o. (rok oyl), SYN petroleum.

o. of rose, a volatile o. from the fresh flowers of *Rosa gallica* and *R. damascena* and other members of the Rosaceae family. Used largely in perfumery, ointments, and toilet preparations. SYN attar of rose, essence of rose, otto of rose.

o. of spearmint, volatile o. from the flowering tops of *Mentha* *spicata* (family Labiatae, pharmaceutical aid (flavor) and a carminative. SYN oil of crispmint, oil of curled mint.

sweet birch o., SYN methyl salicylate.

o. of turpentine, volatile o. distilled from the oleoresin and obtained from *Pinus palastrus* (family Pinaceae) and other species of *Pinus* yielding terpene oils. Solvent for o.'s, resins, varnishes; also used as vehicle, thinner, and remover of o.-based paints; rubefacient; has been used as a counterirritant in liniments.

volatile o., a substance of oily consistency and feel, derived from a plant and containing the principles to which the odor and taste of the plant are due (essential o.); in contrast to a fatty o., a volatile o. evaporates when exposed to the air and thus is capable of distillation; it may also be obtained by expression or extraction; many volatile o.'s, identical to or closely resembling the natural o.'s, can be made synthetically. Volatile o.'s are used in medicine as stimulants, stomachics, correctives, and carminatives, and for purposes of flavoring (e.g., peppermint oil). SYN ethereal o.

o. of wormwood, volatile o. from leaves and tops of *Artemisia absinthium* (family Compositae). Thujol alcohol and acetate; thujone (a powerful convulsant), phellandrene, cadinene; also a blue o. Used in flavoring of vermouth and, formerly, in absinthe.

oil of vit·ri·ol. SYN sulfuric acid.

oint·ment (oynt′ment). A semisolid preparation usually containing medicinal substances and intended for external application. O. bases used as vehicles fall into four general classes: 1) Hydrocarbon bases (oleaginous o. bases) keep medicaments in prolonged contact with the skin, act as occlusive dressings, and are used chiefly for emollient effects. 2) Absorption bases either permit the incorporation of aqueous solutions with the formation of a water-in-oil emulsion or are water-in-oil emulsions that permit the incorporation of additional quantities of aqueous solutions; such bases permit better absorption of some medicaments and are useful as emollients. 3) Water-removable bases (creams) are oil-in-water emulsions containing petrolatum, anhydrous lanolin, or waxes; they may be washed from the skin with water and are thus more acceptable for cosmetic reasons; they favor absorption of serous discharges in dermatologic conditions. 4) Water-soluble bases (greaseless ointment bases) contain only water-soluble substances. SEE ALSO cerate. SYN salve, uncture, unguent. [O. Fr. *oignement;* L. *unguo,* pp. *unctus,* to smear]

blue o., a grease-based o. containing 20% finely divided metallic mercury, formerly widely used for local application to the skin for the destruction of body lice. Risk is associated with transdermal absorption of mercury and a local dermatitis. SYN mild mercurial ointment.

eye o., SYN ophthalmic o.

hydrophilic o., an o. base consisting of 25% each of white petrolatum and stearyl alcohol, 12% propyl glycol emulsified in 37% water by 1% of lauryl sulfate; preserved with paraben. Suitable for the incorporation of numerous drugs intended for local application; a washable o. base.

mild mercurial ointment, SYN blue o.

ophthalmic o., a special o. for application to the eye that must be free from particles and must be nonirritating to the eye. SYN eye o., oculentum.

Okazaki, Reiji (1930–1975) and Tuneko, 20th century Japanese molecular biologists. SEE O. *fragment.*

-ol. Suffix denoting that a substance is an alcohol or a phenol.

ol·a·mine (ōl′ă-mēn). USAN-approved contraction for ethanolamine.

Oldfield, Michael C., 20th century English physician. SEE O. *syndrome.*

o·le·ag·i·nous (ō-lē-aj′i-nŭs). Oily or greasy. [L. *oleagineus,* pertaining to *olea,* the olive tree]

ole·an·der (ō-lē-an′der). The bark and leaves of *Nerium oleander* (family Apocynaceae), a shrub of the eastern Mediterranean; formerly used as a diuretic and heart tonic.

ole·an·do·my·cin phos·phate (ō-lē-an-dō-mī′sin). An antibiotic substance produced by species of *Streptomyces antibioticus;* effective against staphylococci, streptococci, pneumococci, and some Gram-negative bacteria.

ole·ate (ō′lē-āt). **1.** A salt of oleic acid. **2.** A pharmacopeial preparation consisting of a combination or solution of an alkaloid or metallic base in oleic acid, used as an inunction.

olec·ra·non (ō-lek′ră-non, ō′lē-krā′non) [TA]. The prominent curved proximal extremity of the ulna, the upper and posterior surface of which gives attachment to the tendon of the triceps muscle, the anterior surface entering into the formation of the trochlear notch. SYN elbow bone, olecranon process, point of elbow, tip of elbow. [G. the head or point of the elbow, fr. *ōlenē,* ulna, + *kranion,* skull, head]

ole·fin (ō′lē-fin). SYN alkene.

ole·ic ac·id (ō-lē′ik). An unsaturated fatty acid that is the most widely distributed and abundant fatty acid in nature; used commercially in the preparation of oleates and lotions, and as a pharmaceutical solvent. Cf. elaidic acid. [L. *oleum,* oil]

ole·in (ō′lē-in). Trioleoyl glycerol; glyceryl trioleate; a triacylglycerol, solely containing oleoyl moieties, found in fats and oils. SYN triolein.

oleo-. Oil. SEE ALSO eleo-. [L. *oleum*]

ole·o·go·men·ol (ō′lē-ō-gō′men-ol). SYN gomenol.

ole·o·gran·u·lo·ma (ō′lē-ō-gran-ū-lō′mă). SYN lipogranuloma.

ole·o·ma (ō-lē-ō′mă). SYN lipogranuloma.

ole·om·e·ter (ō-lē-om′ĕ-ter). An instrument, similar to a hydrometer, for determining the specific gravity of oils. SYN eleometer. [oleo- + G. *metron,* measure]

ole·o·pal·mi·tate (ō′lē-ō-pal′mi-tāt). A double salt of oleic and palmitic acids.

ole·o·res·in (ō′lē-ō-rez′in). **1.** A compound of an essential oil and resin, present in certain plants. **2.** A pharmaceutical preparation. SEE aspidium, capsicum, ginger. **3.** SYN balsam.

ole·o·sac·cha·rum, pl. **ole·o·sac·cha·ra** (ō′lē-ō-sak′ă-rŭm). A class of preparations made by the trituration of a volatile oil (such as anise, fennel, or lemon) with sugar; used as a diluent or corrigent of powerful or bad-tasting drugs in powder form. SYN oil sugar. [oleo- + G. *saccharon,* sugar]

ole·o·ste·a·rate (ō′lē-ō-stē′ă-rāt). A double salt of oleic and stearic acids.

ole·o·sus (ō-lē-ō′sŭs). Greasy; relating to abnormality of the sebaceous apparatus. [L., fr. *oleum,* oil]

ole·o·ther·a·py (ō′lē-ō-thār′ă-pē). Treatment of disease by an oil given internally or applied externally. SYN eleotherapy. [oleo- + G. *therapeia,* therapy]

ole·o·vi·ta·min (ō′lē-ō-vī′tă-min). A solution of a vitamin in an edible oil.

o. A and D, a solution of vitamins A and D in fish liver oil or in an edible vegetable oil.

ole·um ter·e·bin·thin·ae (ō′lē-um ter-ē-ben′thin-ī). SYN turpentine oil.

ole·yl al·co·hol (ō-lē′il). A mixture of aliphatic alcohols consisting chiefly of $CH_3(CH_2)_7CH=CH(CH_2)_7CH_2OH$; used as an emulsifying aid and in the preparation of cold cream; found in fish oils.

ole·yl-CoA (ō-lē′il). A product of the Δ^9-desaturase enzyme system in the biosynthesis of monounsaturated fatty acids. SYN oleyl coenzyme A.

ole·yl-co·en·zyme A. SYN oleyl-CoA.

ol·fac·tie, ol·fac·ty (ol-fak′tē). The unit of smell; the threshold of olfactory stimulation, or the point at which the smell is just received in the olfactometer. [see olfaction]

ol·fac·tion (ol-fak′shŭn). **1.** The sense of smell. SYN smell (2). **2.** The act of smelling. SYN osmesis, osphresis. [L. *ol- facio,* pp. *-factus,* to smell]

ol·fac·tol·o·gy (ol′fak-tol′-ō-jē). Study of the sense of smell. [olfaction + G. *logos,* study]

ol·fac·tom·e·ter (ol′fak-tom′ĕ-ter). A device for estimating the sensitivity to odorants. [L. *olfactus,* smell, + G. *metron,* measure]

ol·fac·tom·e·try (ol′fak-tom′ĕ-trē). Determination of the degree of sensitivity to odorants.

ol·fac·to·pho·bia (ol-fak-tō-fō′bē-ă). Morbid fear of odors. SYN osmophobia, osphresiophobia. [L. *olfactus,* smell, + G. *phobos,* fear]

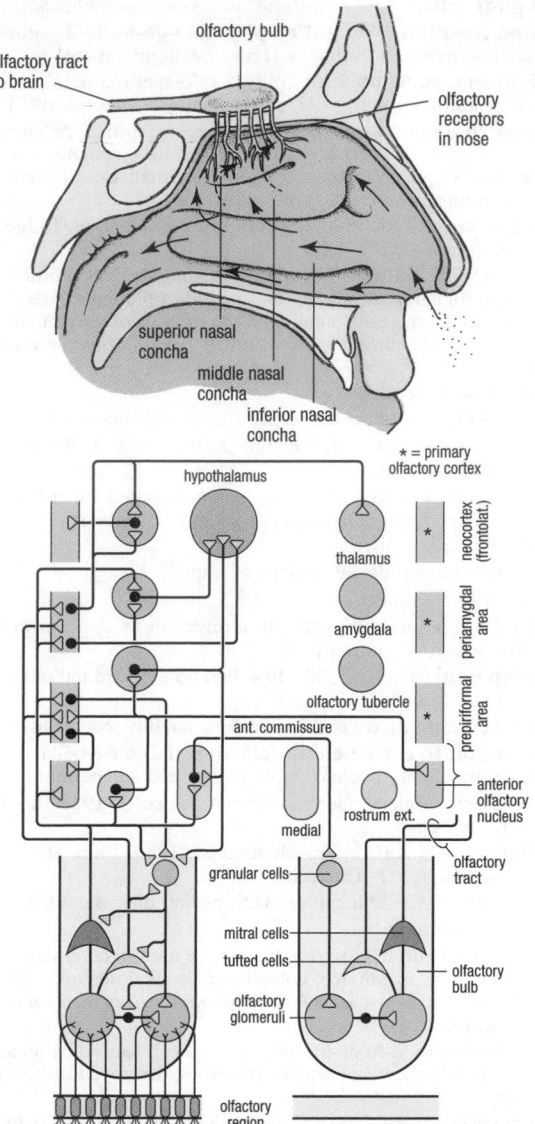

olfactory bulb

olfactory tract to brain

olfactory receptors in nose

superior nasal concha

middle nasal concha

inferior nasal concha

* = primary olfactory cortex

hypothalamus

thalamus

neocortex (frontolat.)

amygdala

periamygdal area

olfactory tubercle

prepiriform area

ant. commissure

medial

rostrum ext.

anterior olfactory nucleus

granular cells

olfactory tract

mitral cells

tufted cells

olfactory bulb

olfactory glomeruli

olfactory region

olfaction

ol·fac·to·ry (ol-fak′tŏ-rē). Relating to the sense of smell. SYN osmatic, osphretic. [see olfaction]

olib·a·num (ō-lib′ă-nŭm). A gum resin from several trees of the genus *Boswellia* (family Burseraceae); has been used as a stimulant expectorant in bronchitis, for fumigations, and as incense. SYN frankincense, thus. [Ar. *al,* the, + *lubān,* frankincense]

olig-. SEE oligo-.

ol·i·gam·ni·os (ol-i-gam′nē-os). SYN oligohydramnios.

ol·i·ge·mia (ol-i-gē′mē-ă). A deficiency in the amount of blood in the body or any organ or tissue. [oligo- + G. *haima,* blood]

ol·i·ge·mic (ol-i-gē′mik). Pertaining to or characterized by oligemia.

ol·ig·hid·ria, ol·ig·id·ria (ol-ig-hid′rē-ă, -id′rē-ă). Scanty perspiration. [oligo- + G. *hidrōs,* sweat]

oligo (ol′i-gō). In molecular genetics, oligonucleotide.

oligo-, olig-. **1.** A few, a little; too little, too few. **2.** In chemistry, used in contrast to "poly-" in describing polymers; e.g., oligosaccharide. [G. *oligos,* few]

ol·i·go·am·ni·os (ol′i-gō-am′nē-os). SYN oligohydramnios. [oligo- + amnion]

ol·i·go·cho·lia (ol′i-gō-kō′lē-ă). A deficient secretion of bile. [oligo- + G. *cholē,* bile]

ol·i·go·chy·li·a (ol′i-gō-kī′lē-ă). A deficiency of gastric juice. [oligo- + G. *chylos,* juice]

ol·i·go·chy·mia (ol′i-gō-kī′mē-ă). A deficiency of chyme. [oligo- + G. *chymos,* juice]

ol·i·go·cys·tic (ol′i-gō-sis′tik). Consisting of only a few cysts, as occasionally observed in certain examples of hydatidiform mole and other lesions that ordinarily have numerous cysts. [oligo- + G. *kystis,* bladder, cyst]

ol·i·go·dac·ty·ly, ol·i·go·dac·tyl·ia (ol′i-gō-dak′ti-lē, -dak-til′ē-ă). Presence of fewer than five digits on one or more limbs. [oligo- + G. *daktylos,* finger or toe]

ol·i·go·den·dria (ol′i-gō-den′drē-ă). SYN oligodendroglia.

ol·i·go·den·dro·blast (ol′i-gō-den′drō-blast). A primitive glial cell that is the normal precursor cell of the oligodendrocyte.

ol·i·go·den·dro·blas·to·ma (ol′i-gō-den′drō-blas-tō′mă). Obsolete term for oligodendroglioma. [oligo- + G. *dendron,* tree, + *blastos,* germ, + -oma]

ol·i·go·den·dro·cyte (ol′i-gō-den′drō-sīt). A cell of the oligodendroglia.

ol·i·go·den·drog·lia (ol′ī-gō-den-drog′lē-ă). One of the three types of glia cells (the other two being macroglia or astrocytes, and microglia) that, together with nerve cells, compose the tissue of the central nervous system. O. cells are characterized by variable numbers of veillike or sheetlike processes that are wrapped each around individual axons to form the myelin sheath of nerve fibers in the central nervous system (compared with Schwann cells in the peripheral nervous system); forms myelin in the central nervous system; accordingly, they are more numerous in white matter than in gray matter. SYN oligodendria. [oligo- + G. *dendron,* tree, + *glia,* glue]

ol·i·go·den·dro·gli·o·ma (ol′i-gō-den′drō-glī-ō′mă). A relatively rare, relatively slowly growing glioma derived from oligodendrocytes that occurs most frequently in the cerebrum of adult persons; the neoplasm is grossly homogeneous, fairly well circumscribed, moderately firm, and somewhat gritty in consistency with interstitial calcification sufficiently dense so as to be detected by x-ray imaging of the skull. Microscopically, an o. is characterized by numerous small, round or ovoid, oligodendroglial cells with small, deeply stained nuclei (rarely observed in mitosis), and palely stained, indistinct cytoplasm; the neoplastic cells are rather uniformly distributed in a sparse, fibrillary stroma with scattered calcific bodies and an often prominent arcuate vasculature. [oligo- + G. *dendron,* tree, + glia, + -oma]

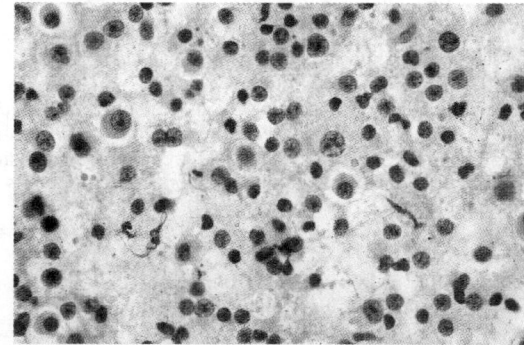

oligodendroglioma: section showing tumor cells with round uniform nuclei with no nucleoli or cell processes

anaplastic o., an aggressive o. characterized by prominent nuclear pleomorphism, mitoses, and increased cellularity. SYN pleomorphic o.

pleomorphic o., SYN anaplastic o.

ol·i·go·dip·sia (ol'i-gō-dip'sē-ă). Abnormal lack of thirst. SEE ALSO hypodipsia. [oligo- + G. *dipsa,* thirst]

ol·i·go·don·tia (ol'i-gō-don'shē-ă). SYN hypodontia. [oligo- + G. *odous,* tooth]

ol·i·go·dy·nam·ic (ol'i-gō-dī-nam'ik). Active in very small quantity; e.g., the germicidal effect of an exceedingly dilute solution (such as one to one hundred million) of copper in distilled water. [oligo- + G. *dynamis,* power]

ol·i·go·ga·lac·tia (ol'i-gō-gă-lak'tē-ă, -shē-ă). Slight or scant secretion of milk. [oligo- + G. *gala,* milk]

ol·i·go·glu·can·branch·ing gly·co·syl·trans·fer·ase (ol'i-gō-gloo'kan). SYN 1,4-α-D-glucan 6-α-D-glucosyltransferase.

ol·i·go-α-1,6-glu·co·si·dase. A glucanohydrolase cleaving α-1,6 links in isomaltose and dextrins produced from starch and glycogen by α-amylase; secreted into the duodenum; a deficiency of this enzyme leads to defects in intestinal digestion of limit dextrins. SEE ALSO sucrose α-D-glucohydrolase. SYN isomaltase, limit dextrinase (2).

ol·i·go·hy·dram·ni·os (ol'i-gō-hī-dram'nē-os). The presence of an insufficient amount of amniotic fluid (less than 300 mL at term). SYN hypamnion, hypamnios, oligamnios, oligoamnios. [oligo- + G. *hydōr,* water, + amnion]

ol·i·go·hy·dru·ria (ol'i-gō-hī-droo'rē-ă). Obsolete term for excretion of small quantities of urine, as seen in dehydration. [oligo- + G. *hydōr,* water, + *ouron,* urine]

ol·i·go·lec·i·thal (ol'i-gō-les'i-thal). Having little yolk; denoting an egg in which there is only a little scattered deutoplasm. [oligo- + G. *lekithos,* yolk]

ol·i·go·men·or·rhea (ol'i-gō-men-ō-rē'ă). Scanty menstruation. [oligo- + menorrhea]

ol·i·go·mer (ol'i-gō-mer). A polymer containing only a few repeating units, a "few" generally considered as fewer than 20.

ol·i·go·mor·phic (ol'i-gō-mōr'fik). Presenting few changes of form; not polymorphic. [oligo- + G. *morphē,* form]

ol·i·go·neph·ron·ic (ol'i-gō-nef-ron'ik). Characterized by a reduced number of nephrons.

ol·i·go·nu·cle·o·tide (ol'i-gō-noo'klē-ō-tīd). A compound made up of the condensation of a small number (typically fewer than 20) of nucleotides. Cf. polynucleotide.

ol·i·go·pep·sia (ol'i-gō-pep'sē-ă). SYN hypopepsia.

ol·i·go·pep·tide (ol'igō-pep-tīd). A peptide whose molecule contains a few amino acid residues up to about 20.

ol·i·go·phre·nia (ol'i-gō-frē'nē-ă). SYN mental *retardation.*
    phenylpyruvate oligophrenia, SYN phenylketonuria.

ol·i·go·plas·tic (ol'i-gō-plas'tik). Deficient in reparative power. [oligo- + G. *plassō,* to form]

ol·i·gop·nea (ol'i-gop-nē'ă, -gop'nē-ă). SYN hypopnea. [oligo- + G. *pnoē,* breath]

ol·i·go·pty·a·lism (ol'i-gō-tī'ă-lizm, ol'i-gop-tī'). A scanty secretion of saliva. SYN oligosialia. [oligo- + G. *ptyalon,* saliva]

ol·i·gor·ia (ol-i-gōr'ē-ă). A rarely used term for an abnormal indifference toward or dislike of persons or things. [G. *oligōria,* negligence, slight esteem, fr. *oligos,* little, + *ōra,* care, regard]

ol·i·go·sac·cha·ride (ol'i-gō-sak'ă-rīd). A compound made up of the condensation of a small number of monosaccharide units. Cf. polysaccharide.

ol·i·go·si·a·lia (ol'i-gō-sī-ā'lē-ă). SYN oligoptyalism. [oligo- + G. *sialon,* saliva]

ol·i·go·sper·mia, ol·i·go·sper·ma·tism (ol-i-gō-sper'mē-ă, -mă-tizm). SYN oligozoospermia. [oligo- + G. *sperma,* seed]

ol·i·go·symp·to·mat·ic (ol'i-gō-simp-tō-mat'ik). Having few or minor symptoms.

ol·i·go·sy·nap·tic (ol'i-gō-si-nap'tik). Referring to neural conduction pathways that are interrupted by only a few synaptic junctions, i.e., made up of a sequence of only few nerve cells, in contrast to polysynaptic pathways. SYN paucisynaptic.

ol·i·go·thy·mia (ol'i-gō-thī'mē-ă). Rarely used term for a poverty or loss of affect. [oligo- + -thymia]

ol·i·go·trich·ia (ol'i-gō-trik'ē-ă). SYN hypotrichosis.

ol·i·go·tri·cho·sis (ol'i-gō-tri-kō'sis). SYN hypotrichosis.

ol·i·go·tro·phia, ol·i·got·ro·phy (ol'i-gō-trō'fē-ă, -got'rō-fē). Deficient nutrition. [oligo- + G. *trophē,* nourishment]

ol·i·go·zo·o·sper·ma·tism (ol'i-gō-zō'ō-sper'mă-tizm). SYN oligozoospermia. [oligo- + G. *zōon,* animal, + *sperma,* seed]

ol·i·go·zo·o·sper·mia (ol'i-gō-zō'ō-sperm'ē-ă). A subnormal concentration of spermatozoa in the penile ejaculate. SYN oligospermia, oligospermatism, oligozoospermatism. [oligo- + G. *zōos,* living, + *sperma,* seed, semen, + -ia]

ol·i·gu·ria (ol-i-goo'rē-ă). Scanty urine production. [oligo- + G. *ouron,* urine]

oli·va, pl. **oli·'vae** (ō-lī'vă) [TA]. A smooth oval prominence of the ventrolateral surface of the medulla oblongata lateral to the pyramidal tract, corresponding to the inferior olivary nucleus. SYN corpus olivare, inferior olive, olivary body, olivary eminence, olive (1). [L.]
    o. infe'rior, the oliva.
    o. supe'rior, SYN dorsal *nucleus* of trapezoid body.

ol·i·vary (ol'i-vār-ē). **1.** Relating to the oliva. **2.** Relating to or shaped like an olive.

ol·ive (ol'iv). **1.** SYN oliva. **2.** Common name for a tree of the genus *Olea* (family Oleaceae) or its fruit. [L. *oliva*]
    inferior o., SYN oliva.
    superior o., SYN dorsal *nucleus* of trapezoid body.

ol·ive oil. See under oil.

ol·i·vif·u·gal (ol'i-vif'ū-găl). In a direction away from the olive. [oliva + L. *fugio,* to flee]

ol·i·vip·e·tal (ol'i-vip'ĕ-tăl). In a direction toward the olive. [oliva + L. *peto,* to seek]

ol·i·vo·co·chle·ar (ol'i-vō-kok'lē-ăr). SEE olivocochlear *tract.*

ol·i·vo·pon·to·cer·e·bel·lar (ol'i-vō-pon'tō-sār-ĕ-bel'ar). Relating to the olivary nucleus, basis pontis, and cerebellum.

Ollendorf, Helene, German dermatologist, fl. 1928. SEE Buschke-O. *syndrome.*

Ollier, Louis X.E.L., French surgeon, 1830–1900. SEE O. *graft, disease, theory;* O.-Thiersch *graft.*

Olmsted, H.C., 20th century U.S. pediatrician. SEE O. *syndrome.*

♻**-ology.** SEE -logia.

olo·liu·qui (ō-lō-lū'kē). A hallucinogen used in ceremonies by the Aztec Indians in Mexico; contains ergot alkaloids and derivatives of lysergic acid. SEE ALSO *Rivea corymbosa, Ipomoea rubrocoerulea* var. *praecox.*

olo·pho·nia (ol'ō-fō'nē-ă). Impaired speech caused by an anatomical defect in the vocal organs. [G. *oloos,* destroyed, lost, + *phōnē,* voice]

Olszewski, Jerzy, Polish-Canadian neuropathologist, 1913–1964. SEE Steele-Richardson-O. *disease, syndrome.*

♻**-oma.** A tumor or neoplasm. [G. *-ōma,* suffix forming nouns from some verb stems]

♻**-omata.** Plural of -oma.

Ombrédanne, Louis, French surgeon, 1871–1956. SEE O. *operation.*

om·bro·pho·bia (om-brō-fō'bē-ă). Morbid fear of rain. [G. *ombros,* rainstorm, + *phobos,* fear]

Omenn, Gilbert S., U.S. internist, *1941. SEE O. *syndrome.*

omen·tal (ō-men'tăl). Relating to the omentum. SYN epiploic.

omen·tec·to·my (ō-men-tek'tō-mē). Resection or excision of the omentum. SYN omentumectomy. [omentum + G. *ektomē,* excision]

omen·ti·tis (ō-men-tī'tis). Peritonitis involving the omentum. [L. *omentum* + G. *-itis,* inflammation]

♻**omento-, oment-.** The omentum. SEE ALSO epiplo-. [L. *omentum*]

omen·to·fix·a·tion (ō-men'tō-fik-sā'shŭn). SYN omentopexy.

omen·to·pexy (ō-men'tō-pek-sē). **1.** Suture of the greater omentum to the abdominal wall to induce collateral portal circulation. **2.** Suture of the omentum to another organ to increase arterial circulation. SEE ALSO omentoplasty. SYN omentofixation. [omento- + G. *pēxis,* fixation]

omen·to·plas·ty (ō-men′tō-plas-tē). Use of greater omentum to cover or fill a defect, augment arterial or portal venous circulation, absorb effusions, or increase lymphatic drainage. SEE ALSO omentopexy. [omento- + G. *plastos,* formed]

omen·tor·rha·phy (ō-men-tōr′ă-fē). Suture of an opening in the omentum. [omento- + G. *rhaphē,* suture]

omen·to·vol·vu·lus (ō-men-tō-vol′vū-lŭs). Twisting of the omentum on a pedicle.

omen·tu·lum (ō-men′tū-lŭm). SYN lesser *omentum.* [Mod. L. dim. of *omentum*]

omen·tum, pl. **omen·ta** (ō-men′tŭm, -tă) [TA]. A fold of peritoneum passing from the stomach to another abdominal organ. [L. the membrane that encloses the bowels]

gastrocolic o., SYN greater o.

gastrohepatic o., SYN lesser o.

gastrosplenic o., SYN gastrosplenic *ligament.*

greater o. [TA], an areolar, four-layer peritoneal fold, formed by the double-layer dorsal mesentery of the stomach (dorsal mesogastrium) descending from the greater curvature of the stomach to fold under on itself and ascend to the transverse colon; the descending and ascending portions fuse, obliterating the inferior recess of the omental bursa, resulting in the four-layer structure that usually hangs over the anterior aspect of the intestines like an apron; components include the following peritoneal ligaments: gastrophrenic, gastrosplenic, splenorenal, and gastrocolic. SYN o. majus [TA], caul (2), cowl, epiploon, gastrocolic o., pileus, velum (3).

lesser o. [TA], a thin, double-layer peritoneal fold formed by the ventral mesentery of the stomach (ventral mesogastrium) passing from the lesser curvature of the stomach and upper border to the proximal duodenum (2 cm distal to the pylorus) to the liver (margins of the porta hepatis and into the depth of the fissure of the ductus venosus); major subcomponents include the hepatogastric ligament (main sheetlike portion) and the hepatoduodenal ligament (thickened free right border, which encloses the hepatic artery, portal vein, and common bile duct. SYN o. minus [TA], gastrohepatic o., omentulum.

o. ma′jus [TA], SYN greater o.

o. mi′nus [TA], SYN lesser o.

omen·tum·ec·to·my (ō-men-tŭ-mek′tō-mē). SYN omentectomy.

ome·pra·zole (ō-mē′prā-zol). A drug that blocks the transport of hydrogen ions into the stomach and is used as an antiulcerative and in treatment of Zollinger-Ellison syndrome.

Ommaya, Ayub K., U.S. neurosurgeon, *1930. SEE O. *reservoir.*

omn. hor. Abbreviation for L. *omni hora,* every hour.

om·nip·o·tence of thought (om-nip′ō-tens). A childish or magical thought process whereby instantaneous gratification of fantasies and wishes is believed to be imminent.

om·niv·o·rous (om-niv′ŏ-rŭs). Living on food of all kinds, upon both animal and vegetable food. [L. *omnis,* all, + *voro,* to eat]

△**omo-.** The shoulder (sometimes including the upper arm). [G. *ōmos,* shoulder]

omo·cla·vic·u·lar (ō′mō-kla-vik′ū-lăr). Relating to the shoulder and the clavicle; denoting an anomalous muscle attached to the coracoid process or upper edge of the scapula and to the clavicle.

omo·hy·oid (ō-mō-hī′oyd). SYN omohyoid *(muscle).*

omo·pha·gia (ō-mō-fā′jē-ă). The eating of raw food, especially of raw flesh. [G. *ōmos,* raw, + *phagō,* to eat]

omo·thy·roid (ō-mō-thī′royd). Denoting a band of muscular fibers passing between the superior cornu of the thyroid cartilage and the omohyoid muscle.

OMP Abbreviation for oligo-N-methylmorpholinium propylene oxide; orotidylic acid; orotidylate; *orotidine* 5′-monophosphate.

OMPA Abbreviation for octamethyl pyrophosphoramide.

OMP de·car·box·yl·ase. SYN *orotidylic acid* decarboxylase.

△**omphal-, omphalo-.** The umbilicus, the navel. [G. *omphalos,* navel (umbilicus)]

om·pha·lec·to·my (om-fă-lek′tō-mē). Excision of the umbilicus or of a neoplasm connected with it. [omphal- + G. *ektomē,* excision]

om·phal·el·co·sis (om′fal-el-kō′sis). Ulceration at the umbilicus. [omphal- + G. *helkōsis,* ulceration]

om·phal·ic (om-fal′ik). SYN umbilical. [G. *omphalos,* umbilicus]

om·pha·li·tis (om-fă-lī′tis). Inflammation of the umbilicus and surrounding parts.

△**omphalo-.** SEE omphal-.

om·pha·lo·an·gi·op·a·gus (om′fă-lō-an-jē-op′ă-gŭs). Unequal conjoined twins in which the parasite derives its blood supply from the placenta of the autosite. SEE conjoined *twins,* under *twin.* SYN allantoidoangiopagus. [omphalo- + G. *angeion,* vessel, + *pagos,* something fixed]

om·pha·lo·cele (om′fal-ō-sēl, om′fă-lō-). Congenital herniation of viscera into the base of the umbilical cord, with a covering membranous sac of peritoneum-amnion. The umbilical cord is inserted into the sac here, in contradistinction to its attachment in gastroschisis. SEE ALSO umbilical *hernia.* SYN amniocele, exomphalos (3), exumbilication (3). [omphalo- + G. *kēlē,* hernia]

om·pha·lo·en·ter·ic (om′fă-lō-en-tār-ik). Relating to the umbilicus and the intestine.

om·pha·lo·mes·en·ter·ic (om′fă-lō-mez-en-tār′ik). **1.** Term denoting relationship of the midgut to the yolk sac. As the head and tail folds of the embryo continue to form, this relationship is diminished and is represented by a narrow yolk stalk or vitelline duct. **2.** Relating to the vitelline duct.

om·pha·lop·a·gus (om′fă-lop′ă-gŭs). Conjoined twins united at their umbilical regions. SEE conjoined *twins,* under *twin.* SYN monomphalus. [omphalo- + G. *pagos,* something fixed]

om·pha·lo·phle·bi·tis (om′fă-lō-fle-bī′tis). Inflammation of the umbilical veins. [omphalo- + G. *phleps,* vein, + *-itis,* inflammation]

om·pha·lor·rha·gia (om′fă-lō-rā′jē-ă). Bleeding from the umbilicus. [omphalo- + G. *rhēgnymi,* to burst forth]

om·pha·lor·rhea (om′fă-lō-rē′ă). A serous discharge from the umbilicus. [omphalo- + G. *rhoia,* flow]

om·pha·lor·rhex·is (om′fă-lō-rek′sis). Rupture of the umbilical cord during childbirth. [omphalo- + G. *rhēxis,* rupture]

om·pha·los (om′fă-los). Rarely used term for umbilicus. [G. navel]

om·pha·lo·site (om′fă-lō-sīt). Underdeveloped twin of allantoidangiopagous twin; joined by umbilical vessels. SYN placental parasitic twin. [omphalo- + G. *sitos,* food]

om·pha·lo·spi·nous (om′fă-lō-spī′nŭs). Denoting a line connecting the umbilicus and the anterior superior spine of the ilium, on which lies the McBurney point.

om·pha·lot·o·my (om-fă-lot′ō-mē). Cutting of the umbilical cord at birth. [omphalo- + G. *tomē,* incision]

om·pha·lo·trip·sy (om′fă-lō-trip′sē). Crushing, instead of cutting, the umbilical cord after childbirth. [omphalo- + G. *tripsis,* a rubbing]

om·pha·lo·ves·i·cal (om′fă-lō-ves′i-kăl). SYN vesicoumbilical.

om·pha·lus (om′fă-lŭs). Rarely used term for umbilicus. [G. *omphalos,* navel]

OMP py·ro·phos·pho·ryl·ase. SYN *orotate* phosphoribosyltransferase.

△**oncho-.** SEE onco-.

On·cho·cer·ca (ong-kō-ser′kă). A genus of elongated filariform nematodes (family Onchocercidae) that inhabit the connective tissue of their hosts, usually within firm nodules in which these parasites are coiled and entangled. SYN *Oncocerca.* [G. *onkos,* a barb, + *kerkos,* tail]

O. vol′vulus, the blinding nodular worm, a species that causes onchocerciasis.

on·cho·cer·ci·a·sis (ong′kō-ser-kī′ă-sis). Infection with *Onchocerca* (especially *O. volvulus,* a filarial nematode transmitted from person to person by black flies of the genus *Simulium*), marked by nodular swellings forming a fibrous cyst enveloping the coiled parasites (onchocercoma); microfilariae move freely out of the nodule and escape into the intercellular lymph in the dermis. Dermatologic changes often develop, especially in Africa, resulting in intense pruritus, scaly or lichenoid skin, depigmentation,

on

and destruction of elastic fibers. Most important are the ocular complications that may develop after a long chronic course, with blindness frequently occurring in advanced cases, caused by the presence of living or dead microfilariae seen by slitlamp biomicroscopy. SYN blinding disease, onchocercosis, volvulosis.

ocular o., ocular complications, such as keratitis, iridocyclitis, or retrobulbar neuritis, caused by the microfilariae of *Onchocerca volvulus.* SYN river blindness.

on·cho·cer·cid (ong-kō-ser'kid). Common name for members of the family Onchocercidae.

On·cho·cer·ci·dae (ong-kō-ser'ki-dē). A family of nematode parasites (superfamily Filarioidea) characterized by production of microfilariae; it includes the genera *Onchocerca, Wuchereria, Brugia, Loa,* and *Mansonella.*

onchocercoma (on'kō-ser-kō'ma). Nodule containing adult worms of *Onchocera volvulus.* [*Onchocerca,* taxonomic term, + -oma]

on·cho·cer·co·sis (ong'kō-ser-kō'sis). SYN onchocerciasis.

△ **onco-, oncho-.** A tumor. [G. *onkos,* bulk, mass]

On·co·cer·ca (ong-kō-ser'kă). SYN *Onchocerca.*

on·co·cyte (ong'kō-sīt). A large, granular, acidophilic tumor cell containing numerous mitochondria; a neoplastic oxyphil cell. [onco- + G. *kytos,* cell]

on·co·cy·to·ma (ong'kō-sī-tō'mă). A glandular tumor composed of large cells with cytoplasm that is granular and eosinophilic because of the presence of abundant mitochondria; occurs uncommonly in the kidney, salivary glands, and endocrine glands. SYN oxyphil adenoma. [onco- + G. *kytos,* cell, + -*oma,* tumor]

on·co·fe·tal (ong-kō-fē'tăl). Relating to tumor-associated substances present in fetal tissue, as o. antigens.

▬▬▬▬▬▬▬

🔲 **on·co·gene** (ong'kō-jēn). **1.** Any of a family of genes that normally encode proteins involved in cell growth or regulation (e.g., protein kinases, GTPases, nuclear proteins, growth factors) but that may foster malignant processes if mutated or activated by contact with retroviruses. Identified o.'s include *ras,* originally noted in bladder tumors, and p53, a mutated version of a gene on chromosome 17 that has been shown to be involved in more than half of all human cancers. O.'s can work in concert to produce cancer, and their action may be exacerbated by retroviruses, jumping genes, or inherited genetic mutations. SEE ALSO tumor suppressor *gene.* **2.** A gene found in certain DNA tumor viruses. It is required for viral replication. SYN transforming gene. [onco- + gene]

> Genes whose mutations can permit or induce uncontrolled cellular proliferation and malignant change are of 2 types: protooncogenes and tumor suppressor genes (antioncogenes). Protooncogenes encode proteins that stimulate DNA synthesis and cell division, including peptide growth factors and their cellular membrane receptors; second-messenger cascade proteins, which transmit information from cell membrane to nucleus; and nuclear transcription factors, which control gene expression by binding to DNA. Conversion of a protooncogene to an oncogene by amplification, translocation, or point mutation can lead to unrestrained cellular proliferation and malignant change. Only 1 copy (allele) of a protooncogene need undergo mutation to induce tumor formation. Protooncogenes are not involved in inherited cancer syndromes, with the exception of the RET protooncogene in multiple endocrine neoplasia. Tumor suppressor genes (antioncogenes), which encode proteins that normally serve to restrain cell proliferation, can be inactivated by point mutation, deletion, or loss of expression. An inherited mutation in 1 copy of a tumor suppressor gene is the basis of most familial predispositions to cancer. Malignant cellular proliferation does not occur until the remaining, functional copy of the gene is inactivated by mutation or by deletion of part or all of its chromosome. In a person born with 2 normal copies of a tumor suppressor gene, both must be inactivated by mutation before tumor formation occurs. BRCA1 and BRCA2, which are associated

with familial early-onset breast cancer and ovarian cancer, are tumor suppressor genes.

▬▬▬▬▬▬▬

ras o., point mutations first described in rat sarcoma cells that can be shown to have transforming activity in culture as well as in tumorigenesis models in mice; the ras gene family is composed of three closely related genes on three different chromosomes; abnormalities have been identified in a variety of human tumors.

on·co·gen·e·sis (ong-kō-jen'ĕ-sis). Origin and growth of a neoplasm. [onco- + G. *genesis,* production]

on·co·gen·ic (ong-kō-jen'ik). SYN oncogenous.

on·cog·en·ous (ong-koj'ĕ-nŭs). Causing, inducing, or being suitable for the formation and development of a neoplasm. SYN oncogenic.

on·co·graph (ong'kō-graf). A recording oncometer, or the recording portion of an oncometer. [onco- + G. *graphē,* a record]

on·cog·ra·phy (ong-kog'ră-fē). Graphic representation, by means of a special apparatus, of the size and configuration of an organ.

on·coi·des (ong-koy'dēz). Intumescence or turgescence. [onco- + G. *eidos,* resemblance]

on·col·o·gist (ong-kol'ō-jist). A specialist in oncology.

radiation o., SYN radiotherapist.

on·col·o·gy (ong-kol'ō-jē). The study or science dealing with the physical, chemical, and biologic properties and features of neoplasms, including causation, pathogenesis, and treatment. [onco- + G. *logos,* study]

radiation o., (1) the medical specialty concerned with the use of ionizing radiation in the treatment of disease; (2) the medical specialty of radiation *therapy;* (3) the use of radiation in the treatment of neoplasms. SYN radiotherapy, therapeutic radiology.

on·col·y·sis (ong-kol'i-sis). Destruction of a neoplasm; sometimes used with reference to the reduction of any swelling or mass. [onco- + G. *lysis,* dissolution]

on·co·lyt·ic (ong-kō-lit'ik). Pertaining to, characterized by, or causing oncolysis.

On·co·me·la·nia (ong'kō-mĕ-lā'nī-ă). A medically important genus of amphibious freshwater operculate snails of the family Hydrobiidae (subfamily Hydrobiinae; subclass Prosobranchiata). In Asia, several subspecies of *O. hupensis* serve as intermediate hosts of the oriental blood fluke, *Schistosoma japonicum.* [onco- + G. *melas (melan-),* black]

on·com·e·ter (ong-kom'ĕ-ter). **1.** An instrument for measuring the size and configuration of the kidneys and other organs. **2.** The measuring, as distinguished from the recording part of the oncograph. [onco- + G. *metron,* measure]

on·co·met·ric (ong-kō-met'rik). Relating to oncometry.

on·com·e·try (ong-kom'ĕ-trē). Measurement of the size of an organ.

on·co·sis (ong-kō'sis). A condition characterized by the formation of one or more neoplasms or tumors. [G. *onkōsis,* swelling, fr. *onkos,* bulk, mass]

on·co·sphere (ong'-kō-sfēr). SYN hexacanth. [onco- + G. *sphaira,* sphere]

oncostatin M (onk'ō-stat'in em). An interleukin 6. [onco- + -stat + -in]

on·co·ther·a·py (ong-kō-thār'ă-pē). Treatment of tumors.

on·cot·ic (ong-kot'ik). Relating to or caused by edema or any swelling (oncosis).

on·cot·o·my (ong-kot'ō-mē). Rarely used term for incision of an abscess, cyst, or other tumor. [onco- + G. *tomē,* incision]

on·co·tro·pic (ong'kō-trop'ik). Manifesting a special affinity for neoplasms or neoplastic cells. [onco- + G. *tropē,* a turning]

On·co·vir·i·nae (ong-kō-vir'i-nē). Term formerly used to designate a now obsolete subfamily of viruses (family Retroviridae) composed of the RNA tumor viruses that contain two identical plus-stranded RNA molecules. Subgroups are based on antigenicity, host range, and kind of malignancy induced (avian, feline, hamster, or murine leukemia-sarcoma complex; murine mammary tumor virus; primate oncoviruses). Like other retroviruses, they contain RNA-dependent DNA polymerases (reverse transcriptases). An important aspect of these viruses seems to be use of viral reverse transcriptase to make DNA that can be integrated into the DNA of the host cell and will replicate along with cellular DNA. SEE ALSO retrovirus.

on·co·vi·rus (ong'kō-vī'rŭs). Term formerly used to describe any virus of the subfamily Oncovirinae. SEE ALSO oncogenic *virus*.

on·dan·se·tron (ŏn-dan'sĕ-tron). A serotonin 5-HT$_3$ receptor antagonist used as an antiemetic, particularly in patients undergoing chemotherapy or radiation treatment for cancer.

Ondine, German mythological character. SEE Ondine *curse*.

△**-one.** Suffix indicating a ketone (–CO–) group.

onei·ric (ō-nī'rik). **1.** Pertaining to dreams. **2.** Pertaining to the clinical state of oneirophrenia. SYN oniric. [G. *oneiros,* dream]

onei·rism (ō-nī'rizm). A waking dream state. [G. *oneiros,* dream]

onei·ro·crit·i·cal (ō-nī-rō-krit'i-kăl). Rarely used term pertaining to the logic of dreams. [G. *oneiros,* dream, + *kritikos,* skilled in judgment]

onei·ro·dyn·ia (ō-nī-rō-din'ē-ă). Rarely used term for an unpleasant or painful dream. [G. *oneiros,* dream, + *odynē,* pain]
  o. acti′va, SYN somnambulism (1).

onei·rol·o·gy (ō-nī-rol'ō-jē). The study of dreams and their content. [G. *oneiros,* dream, + *logos,* study]

onei·ro·phre·nia (ō-nī-rō-frē'nē-ă). A rarely used term for a state

in which hallucinations occur, caused by such conditions as prolonged deprivation of sleep, sensory isolation, and a variety of drugs. [G. *oneiros,* dream, + *phrēn,* mind]

oni·o·ma·nia (ō'nē-ō-mā'nē-ă). Rarely used term for the morbidly exaggerated need or urge to buy beyond the realistic needs of the individual. [G. *ōnios,* for sale, + *mania,* insanity]

oni·ric (ō-nī'rik). SYN oneiric.

△**-onium.** Suffix indicating a positively charged radical; e.g., ammonium, NH$_4$+.

△**onko-.** SEE onco-.

on·lay (on'lā). **1.** A metal (usually gold) cast restoration of the occlusal surface of a posterior tooth or the lingual surface of an anterior tooth, the entire surface of which is in dentin without side walls; retention in the anterior tooth is by pins and in the posterior by pins and/or boxes in retentive grooves in the buccal and lingual walls. **2.** A graft applied on the exterior of a bone. **3.** A graft applied to skin in native urethra in hypospadias or stricture repair.

Onodi, Adolf, Hungarian laryngologist, 1857–1920. SEE Onodi *cell.*

on·o·mat·o·ma·nia (on'ō-mat-ō-mā'nē-ă). An abnormal impulse to dwell upon certain words and their supposed significance, or to frantically try to recall a particular word. [G. *onoma,* name, + *mania,* frenzy]

representative cellular oncogenes					
		origin		protein product	
general class	name of oncogene	prototype retrovirus	host species[1]	property	subcellular location
nonreceptor protein tyrosine kinases	*src*	Rous sarcoma virus	chicken	tyrosine kinase	plasma membrane
	abl	Abelson murine leukemia virus	mouse		plasma membrane, cytoplasm
	fes	ST feline sarcoma virus	cat		plasma membrane, cytoplasm
receptor protein tyrosine kinases	*fms*	McDonough feline sarcoma virus	cat	related to colony-stimulating factor receptor	plasma membrane, endoplasmic reticulum
	erb-B	avian erythroblastosis virus	chicken	epidermal growth factor receptor (truncated)	plasma membrane
	neu	none	rat (neuroglioblastomas)	related to epidermal growth factor receptor	plasma membrane, endoplasmic reticulum
serine/threonine protein kinase	*mos*	Moloney murine sarcoma virus	mouse		cytoplasm
growth factors	*sis*	simian sarcoma virus	woolly monkey	platelet-derived growth factor-like	cytoplasm, secreted
	int-2	none	mouse	related to fibroblast growth factor	
membrane associated G proteins	Ha-*ras*	Harvey murine sarcoma virus	rat	guanosine diphosphate/triphosphate binding; guanosine triphosphatase	plasma membrane
	Ki-*ras*	Kirsten murine sarcoma virus			
	N-*ras*	none	human (neuroblastomas)		
nuclear transcription factors	*myb*	avian myeloblastosis virus	chicken	DNA binding	nucleus
	myc	MC29 myelocytomatosis virus			
	fos	FBJ osteosarcoma virus	mouse	part of AP-1 transcription factor	
	jun	avian sarcoma virus-17	chicken	DNA binding; part of AP-1 transcription factor	
	erb-A	avian erythroblastosis virus	chicken	mutant thyroid hormone receptor	cytoplasm, nucleus

[1] Proto-oncogene sequences are conserved among many species; column indicates initial recovery of oncogene

on·o·mat·o·pho·bia (on′ō-mat-ō-fō′bē-ă). Abnormal dread of certain words or names because of their supposed significance. [G. *onoma*, name, + *phobos*, fear]

on·o·mat·o·poi·e·sis (on′ō-mat′ō-poy-ē′sis). The making of a name or word, especially to express or imitate a natural sound (e.g., hiss, crash, boom); in psychiatry, the tendency to make new words of this type is said to characterize some persons with schizophrenia. SEE ALSO neologism. [G. *onoma*, name, + *poiēsis*, making]

on·to·gen·e·sis (on-tō-jen′ĕ-sis). SYN ontogeny.

on·to·ge·net·ic, on·to·gen·ic (on′tō-jĕ-net′ik, -jen′ik). Relating to ontogeny.

on·tog·e·ny (on-toj′ĕ-nē). Development of the individual, as distinguished from phylogeny, which is evolutionary development of the species. SYN ontogenesis. [G. *ōn*, being, + *genesis*, origin]

on·tol·o·gy (on-tol′ō-jē). A traditional branch of metaphysics that deals with problems of being, existence, inner nature, meaning, etc. It is fundamental to problems involving normality and disease, individuality, responsibility, and the analysis of values. In recent years, it has been slowly assuming a place as a branch of medicine proper.

Onufrowicz, Wladislaus, Swiss anatomist, 1836–1900. SEE Onuf *nucleus.*

on·y·al·ai (on-i-al′ā). An acute disease affecting natives of Central Africa, characterized by bloody vesicles of the mouth and other mucous surfaces, hematuria, and melena; defective nutrition may be the cause. SYN akembe, kafindo.

△**onych-.** SEE onycho-.

on·y·chal·gia (on-i-kal′jē-ă). Pain in the nails. [onycho- + G. *algos*, pain]

on·y·cha·tro·phia, on·ych·at·ro·phy (on′i-kă-trō′fē-ă, on-ik-at′rō-fē). Atrophy of the nails. [onycho- + G. *atrophia*, atrophy]

on·y·chaux·is (on-i-kawk′sis). Marked overgrowth of the fingernails or toenails. [onycho- + G. *auxē*, increase]

on·y·chec·to·my (on-i-kek′tō-mē). Ablation of a toenail or fingernail. [onycho- + G. *ektomē*, excision]

onych·ia (ō-nik′ē-ă). Inflammation of the matrix of the nail. [onycho- + G. *-ia*, condition]

  o. malig′na, acute o. occurring spontaneously in debilitated patients, or in response to slight trauma.

  o. sic′ca, a condition characterized by brittle nails.

△**onycho-, onych-.** A finger nail, a toenail. [G. *onyx*, nail]

on·y·choc·la·sis (on-i-kok′lă-sis). Breaking of the nails. [onycho- + G. *klasis*, breaking]

on·y·cho·cryp·to·sis (on′i-kō-krip-tō′sis). SYN ingrown *nail.* [onycho- + G. *kryptō*, to conceal]

on·y·cho·dys·tro·phy (on′i-kō-dis′trō-fē). Dystrophic changes in the nails occurring as a congenital defect or due to any illness or injury that may cause a malformed nail. [onycho- + G. *dys-*, bad, + *trophē*, nourishment]

on·y·cho·graph (on′i-kō-graf). An instrument for recording the capillary blood pressure as shown by the circulation under the nail. [onycho- + G. *graphō*, to write]

on·y·cho·gry·po·sis (on′i-kō-gri-pō′sis). Enlargement with increased thickening and curvature of the fingernails or toenails. [onycho- + G. *grypōsis*, a curvature]

on·y·cho·het·er·o·to·pia (on′i-kō-het-er-ō-tō′pē-ă). Abnormal placement of nails.

on·y·choid (on′i-koyd). Resembling a fingernail in structure or form. [onycho- + G. *eidos*, resemblance]

on·y·chol·o·gy (on-i-kol′ō-jē). Study of the nails. [onycho- + G. *logos*, treatise]

on·y·chol·y·sis (on-i-kol′i-sis). Loosening of the nails, beginning at the free border, and usually incomplete. [onycho- + G. *lysis*, loosening]

on·y·cho·ma·de·sis (on′i-kō-mă-dē′sis). Complete shedding of the nails, usually associated with systemic disease. [onycho- + G. *madēsis*, a growing bald, fr. *madaō*, to be moist, (of hair) fall off]

on·y·cho·ma·la·cia (on′i-kō-mă-lā′shē-ă). Abnormal softness of the nails. [onycho- + G. *malakia*, softness]

on·y·cho·my·co·sis (on′i-kō-mī-kō′sis). Very common fungus infections of the nails, causing thickening, roughness, and splitting, often caused by *Trichophyton rubrum* or *T. mentagrophytes, Candida,* and occasionally molds. SYN ringworm of nails. [onycho- + G. *mykēs*, fungus, + *-ōsis*, condition]

on·y·cho·pa·thol·o·gy (on′i-kō-pă-thol′ō-jē). Study of diseases of the nails.

▣**on·y·chop·a·thy** (on-i-kop′ă-thē). Any disease of the nails. SYN onychosis. [onycho- + G. *pathos*, suffering]

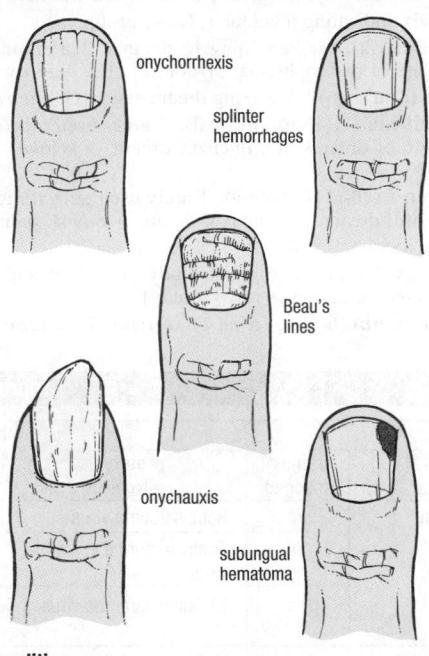

nail abnormalities

(labels: onychorrhexis; splinter hemorrhages; Beau's lines; onychauxis; subungual hematoma)

on·y·choph·a·gy, on·y·cho·pha·gia (on-i-kof′ă-jē, on′i-kō-fā′jē-ă). Habitual nailbiting. [onycho- + G. *phagō*, to eat]

on·y·cho·pho·sis (on′i-kō-fō′sis). A growth of horny epithelium in the nail bed. [onycho- + G. *phōs*, light, + *-osis*, condition]

on·y·chop·to·sis (on′i-kop-tō′sis). Falling off of the nails. [onycho- + G. *ptōsis*, a falling]

on·y·chor·rhex·is (on′i-kō-rek′sis). Abnormal brittleness of the nails with splitting of the free edge. [onycho- + G. *rhēxis*, a breaking]

on·y·cho·schiz·ia (on′i-kō-skiz′ē-ă). Splitting of the nails in layers. [onycho- + G. *schizō*, to divide, + *-ia*, condition]

on·y·cho·sis (on-i-kō′sis). SYN onychopathy.

on·y·cho·stro·ma (on′i-kō-strō′mă). SYN nail *matrix.* [onycho- + G. *strōma*, bedding]

on·y·chot·il·lo·ma·nia (on′i-kot′i-lō-mā′nē-ă). A tendency to pick at the nails. [onycho- + G. *tillō*, to pluck, + *mania*, insanity]

on·y·chot·o·my (on′i-kot′ō-mē). Incision into a toenail or fingernail. [onycho- + G. *tomē*, cutting]

on·y·chot·ro·phy (on-i-kot′rō-fē). Nutrition of the nails. [onycho- + G. *trophē*, nourishment]

on·yx (on′iks). SYN nail (1). [G. nail]

△**oo-.** Egg, ovary. SEE ALSO oophor-, ovario-, ovi-, ovo-. [G. *ōon*, egg]

oo·cy·e·sis (ō-ō-sī-ē′sis). SYN ovarian *pregnancy.* [G. *ōon*, egg, + *kyēsis*, pregnancy]

oo·cyst (ō′ō-sist). The encysted form of the fertilized macrogamete, or zygote, in coccidian Sporozoea in which sporogonic multiplication occurs; results in the formation of sporozoites, infectious agents for the next stage of the sporozoan life cycle. [G. *ōon*, egg, + *kystis*, bladder]

oo·cyte (ō′ō-sīt). The immature ovum. SYN ovocyte. [G. *ōon*, egg, + *kytos*, a hollow (cell)]

primary o., an o. during its growth phase and before it completes the first maturation division.

secondary o., an o. in which the first meiotic division is completed; the second meiotic division usually stops short of completion unless fertilization occurs.

oo·gen·e·sis (ō-ō-jen′ĕ-sis). Process of formation and development of the ovum. SYN ovigenesis, ovogenesis. [G. *ōon*, egg, + *genesis*, origin]

oo·ge·net·ic (ō-ō-jĕ-net′ik). Producing ova. SYN oogenic, oogenous, ovigenetic, ovigenic, ovigenous.

oo·gen·ic, oog·e·nous (ō-ō-jen′ik, ō-oj′ĕ-nŭs). SYN oogenetic.

oo·go·ni·um, pl. **oo·go·nia** (ō-ō-gō′nē-ŭm, -ă). **1.** Primitive germ cells; proliferate by mitotic division. All oogonia develop into primary oocytes prior to birth; no oogonia are present after birth. **2.** In fungi, the female gametangium bearing one or more oospores. [G. *ōon*, egg, + *gonē*, generation]

oo·ki·ne·sis, oo·ki·ne·sia (ō′ō-ki-nē′sis, -zē-ă). Chromosomal movements of the egg during maturation and fertilization. [G. *ōon*, egg, + *kinēsis*, movement]

oo·ki·nete (ō′ō-ki-ne′t, -kī′ne′t). The motile zygote of the malarial organism that penetrates the mosquito stomach to form an oocyst under the outer gut lining; the contents of the oocyst subsequently divide to produce numerous sporozoites. SYN vermicule (2). [G. *ōon*, egg, + *kinētos*, motile]

oo·lem·ma (ō-ō-lem′ă). Plasma membrane of the oocyte. [G. *ōon*, egg, + *lemma*, sheath]

oo·my·co·sis (ō′ō-mī-kō′sis). A mycosis caused by fungi belonging to the class Oomycetes; e.g., rhinosporidiosis.

oo·pha·gia, ooph·a·gy (ō-ō-fā′jē-ă, ō-of′ă-jē). The habitual eating of eggs; subsisting largely on eggs. [G. *ōon*, egg, + *phagō*, to eat]

△**oophor-, oophoro-.** The ovary. SEE ALSO oo-, ovario-. [Mod. L. *oophoron*, ovary, fr. G. *ōophoros*, egg-bearing]

ooph·or·al·gia (ō-of-ōr-al′jē-ă). SYN ovarialgia. [oophor- + G. *algos*, pain]

ooph·o·rec·to·my (ō-of-ōr-ek′tō-mē). SYN ovariectomy. [G. *ōon*, egg, + *phoros*, bearing, + *ektomē*, excision]

ooph·or·i·tis (ō-of-ōr-ī′tis). Inflammation of an ovary. SYN ovaritis. [G. *ōon*, egg, + *phoros*, a bearing, + *-itis*, inflammation]

△**oophoro-.** SEE oophor-.

ooph·or·o·cys·tec·to·my (ō-of′ōr-ō-sis-tek′tō-mē). Excision of an ovarian cyst.

ooph·or·o·cys·to·sis (ō-of′ōr-ō-sis-tō′sis). Ovarian cyst formation.

ooph·or·on (ō-of′ōr-on). Rarely used term for ovary. [G. *ōon*, egg, + *phoros*, bearing]

ooph·or·op·a·thy (ō-of-ōr-op′ă-thē). SYN ovariopathy.

ooph·or·o·pexy (ō-of′ōr-ō-pek-sē). Surgical fixation or suspension of an ovary. [oophoro- + G. *pēxis*, fixation]

ooph·or·o·plas·ty (ō-of′ōr-ō-plas-tē). Plastic operation upon an ovary. [oophoro- + G. *plastos*, formed, shaped]

ooph·o·ror·rha·phy (ō-of-ō-rōr′ă-fē). Suspension of the ovary by attachment to the pelvic wall. [oophoro- + G. *rhaphē*, suture]

ooph·or·o·sal·pin·gec·to·my (ō-of′ōr-ō-sal-pin-jek′tō-mē). SYN ovariosalpingectomy.

ooph·or·o·sal·pin·gi·tis (ō-of′ōr-ō-sal-pin-jī′tis). SYN ovariosalpingitis. [oophoro- + salpingitis]

ooph·or·ot·o·my (ō-of-ōr-ot′ō-mē). SYN ovariotomy. [oophoro- + G. *tomē*, incision]

ooph·or·rha·gia (ō-of-ōr-rā′jē-ă). Ovarian hemorrhage. [oophoro- + G. *rhēgnymi*, to burst forth]

oo·plasm (ō′ō-plazm). Protoplasmic portion of the ovum. [G. *ōon*, egg, + *plasma*, a thing formed]

oo·some (ō′ō-sōm). A cytoplasmic body in the ovum that passes into the germ cell. [G. *ōon*, egg + *sōma*, body]

oo·spo·ran·gi·um (ō′ō-spō-ran′jē-ŭm). Obsolete term for oogonium (2). [oospore + G. *angeion*, vessel]

oo·spore (ō′ō-spōr). A thick-walled fungus spore that develops from a female gamete either through fertilization or parthenogenesis in an oogonium. [see *Oospora*]

oo·the·ca (ō-oth-ē′kă). **1.** An egg case found in some lower animals. **2.** Rarely used term for ovary. [G. *ōon*, egg, + *thēkē*, box, case]

oo·tid (ō′ō-tid). The nearly mature ovum after the first meiotic division has been completed and the second initiated; in most higher mammals, the second meiotic division is not completed unless fertilization occurs. [G. *ōotidion*, a diminutive egg. See -id (2)]

oo·type (ō′ō-tūp). The central portion of the ovarian complex of trematodes and cestodes in which fertilization takes place and the vitellarian or eggshell materials are coated over the egg; this occurs in a rapid, stamping-mill sequence, after which eggs pass into the uterus for tanning of the shell, storage, and passage toward the genital pore. [G. *ōon*, egg, + *typos*, stamp, print]

OP Abbreviation for occipitoposterior *position.*

opac·i·fi·ca·tion (ō-pas′i-fi-kā′shŭn). **1.** The process of making opaque. **2.** The formation of opacities. [L. *opacus*, shady]

opac·i·ty (ō-pas′i-tē). **1.** A lack of transparency; an opaque or nontransparent area. **2.** On a radiograph, a more transparent area is interpreted as an o. to x-rays in the body. **3.** Mental dullness. [L. *opacitas*, shadiness]

nodular o., a solitary, round, circumscribed shadow found in the lung on chest radiograph; causes include granuloma, primary or metastatic carcinoma, benign tumor, vascular malformation. SYN coin lesion of lungs.

snowball o., a spherical, white body seen in the vitreous in asteroid hyalosis.

opal·es·cent (ō-pă-les′ent). Resembling an opal in the display of various colors; denoting certain bacterial cultures. [Fr. fr. L. *opalus*, opal]

Opalski, Adam, Polish physician, 1897–1963. SEE O. *cell.*

opaque (ō-pāk′). Impervious to light; not translucent or only slightly so. Cf. radiopaque. [Fr. fr. L. *opacus*, shady]

open (ō′pen). **1.** Not closed; exposed, said of a wound. **2.** To enter or expose, as a wound or cavity. [A.S.]

open·ing (ō′pen-ing) [TA]. A gap in or entrance to an organ, tube, or cavity. SEE ALSO aperture, fossa, ostium, orifice, pore.

access o., SYN access.

aortic o., SYN aortic *hiatus.*

o. of aqueduct of midbrain [TA], entrance to the cerebral aqueduct; point at which the caudal part of the third ventricle is continuous with the cerebral aqueduct of the midbrain; located on the midline immediately ventral to the posterior commissure. SYN apertura aqueductus mesencephali [TA], apertura aqueductus cerebri☆, o. of cerebral aqueduct☆, aditus ad aqueductum cerebri, Bartholin anus.

cardiac o., SYN cardial *orifice.*

o.'s of carotid canal [TA], the opening at each extremity of the carotid canal in the pyramidal petrous part of the temporal bone; the external opening of the carotid canal is on the inferior surface of the pyramid; the internal opening of the canal is at the apex of the petrous part. SYN carotid foramen.

caval o. of diaphragm [TA], an opening in the right lobe of the central tendon of the diaphragm that transmits the inferior vena cava and branches of the right phrenic nerve. SYN foramen of vena cava, foramen quadratum, foramen venae cavae, vena caval foramen.

o. of cerebral aqueduct, ☆official alternate term for o. of aqueduct of midbrain.

o. of coronary sinus [TA], orifice by which the coronary sinus enters and drains into the right atrium of the heart. SYN ostium sinus coronarii [TA].

esophageal o., SYN esophageal *hiatus.*

external o., SYN meatus.

o. of external acoustic meatus, SYN external acoustic *pore.*

external o. of cochlear canaliculus [TA], the external opening of the cochlear aqueduct on the temporal bone medial to the jugular fossa. SYN apertura canaliculi cochleae, external aperture of co-chlear canaliculus.

external o. of urethra, SYN external urethral *orifice*.

femoral o., SYN adductor *hiatus*.

o. of frontal sinus [TA], one of a pair of openings in the floor of the frontal sinuses in the nasal part of the frontal bone, through which the frontal sinuses communicate with the ethmoidal infundibulum via the frontonasal duct. SYN apertura sinus frontalis [TA], frontal sinus aperture.

ileocecal o., SYN ileal *orifice*.

o. of inferior vena cava [TA], the orifice through which the inferior vena cava opens into the right atrium. SYN ostium venae cavae inferioris [TA], orifice of inferior vena cava.

internal acoustic o. [TA], SYN internal acoustic *pore*.

o. of internal acoustic meatus, SYN internal acoustic *pore*.

internal urethral o., ✭official alternate term for internal urethral *orifice*.

lacrimal o., SYN lacrimal *punctum*.

oral o., ✭official alternate term for oral *fissure*.

orbital o. [TA], the somewhat quadrangular anterior entrance to the orbit that forms the base of the pyramid-shaped orbital cavity. It is bounded by the sharp supra-, infra-, and lateral orbital margins and a less obvious medial margin on each side of the upper nose. SYN aditus orbitae [TA], aperture of orbit.

o.'s of papillary ducts [TA], numerous minute openings, the apertures of the papillary ducts converging on the apical pole of each renal papilla. SYN foramina papillaria renis [TA], papillary foramina of kidney.

pharyngeal o. of eustachian tube, SYN pharyngeal o. of pharyngotympanic (auditory) tube.

pharyngeal o. of pharyngotympanic (auditory) tube [TA], an opening in the upper part of the nasopharynx about 1.2 cm behind the posterior extremity of the inferior concha on each side. SYN ostium pharyngeum tubae auditivae [TA], ostium pharyngeum tubae auditoriae✭, pharyngeal o. of eustachian tube.

piriform o., SYN piriform *aperture*.

o. of pulmonary trunk [TA], the o. of the pulmonary trunk from the right ventricle, guarded by the pulmonary valve. SYN ostium trunci pulmonalis [TA], pulmonary orifice.

o.'s of pulmonary veins [TA], the orifices of the pulmonary veins, usually two on each side, in the wall of the left atrium. SYN ostia venarum pulmonalium [TA].

saphenous o. [TA], the opening in the fascia lata inferior to the medial part of the inguinal ligament through which the saphenous vein passes to enter the femoral vein. SYN hiatus saphenus [TA], fossa ovalis (2), saphenous hiatus.

o.'s of smallest cardiac veins [TA], a number of fossae in the wall of the right atrium, containing the openings of minute intramural veins. SYN foramina of the smallest veins of heart, foramina of the venae minimae, foramina venarum minimarum cordis, Lannelongue foramina, thebesian foramina, Vieussens foramina.

o. of the sphenoidal sinus [TA], one of the pair of openings in the body of the sphenoid bone through which the sphenoid sinuses communicate with the sphenoethmoidal recess of the nasal cavity. SYN apertura sinus sphenoidalis [TA], sphenoidal sinus aperture.

o. of superior vena cava [TA], the point of entry of the superior vena cava into the right atrium. SYN ostium venae cavae superioris [TA], orifice of superior vena cava.

tendinous o., SYN adductor *hiatus*.

tympanic o. of canaliculus for chorda tympani, SYN tympanic *aperture* of canaliculus for chorda tympani.

tympanic o. of eustachian tube, SYN tympanic o. of pharyngotympanic (auditory) tube.

tympanic o. of pharyngotympanic (auditory) tube [TA], an opening in the anterior part of the tympanic cavity below the canal for the tensor tympani (muscle). SYN ostium tympanicum tubae auditivae [TA], tympanic o. of eustachian tube.

ureteral o., SYN ureteric *orifice*.

urethral o.'s, SEE external urethral *orifice*, internal urethral *orifice*.

uterine o. of uterine tubes, SYN uterine *ostium* of uterine tubes.

o. of uterus, SYN external *os* of uterus.

vaginal o., SYN vaginal *orifice*.

vertical o., SYN vertical *dimension*.

o. of vestibular canaliculus [TA], the external opening of the vestibular aqueduct on the posterior surface of the petrous part of the temporal bone near the groove for the sigmoid sinus. SYN apertura canaliculi vestibuli, external aperture of vestibular aqueduct.

op·er·a·ble (op′er-ă-bl). Denoting a patient or condition on which a surgical procedure can be performed with a reasonable expectation of cure or relief.

op·er·ant (op′er-ănt). In conditioning, any behavior or specific response chosen by the experimenter; its frequency is intended to increase or decrease by the judicious pairing with it of a reinforcer when it occurs. SYN target behavior (1), target response.

op·er·ate (op′er-āt). 1. To work upon the body by the hands or by means of cutting or other instrument. 2. To perform a surgical procedure. 3. To cause a movement of the bowels; said of a laxative or cathartic remedy. [L. *operor,* pp. *-atus,* to work, fr. *opus,* work]

OPERATION

op·er·a·tion (op-er-ā′shŭn). 1. Any surgical procedure. 2. The act, manner, or process of functioning. SEE ALSO method, procedure, technique.

Altemeier o., an o. for rectal prolapse that involves a sleeve resection of the prolapsed rectum and colon with a primary anastomosis performed transanally.

Arlt o., transplantation of the eyelashes back from the edge of the lid in trichiasis.

arterial switch o., o. for complete transposition of the great arteries; the most common way to repair this defect consists of switching the aorta and pulmonary arteries and implanting the coronary arteries into the neoaorta (the original pulmonary artery).

Ball o., division of the sensory nerve trunks supplying the anus, for relief of pruritus ani.

Barkan o., goniotomy for congenital glaucoma under direct observation of the anterior chamber angle.

Bassini o., SYN Bassini *herniorrhaphy*.

Battista o., SYN left ventricular volume reduction *surgery*.

Belsey Mark o., SYN Belsey *fundoplication*.

Billroth o. I, excision of the pylorus and antrum and partial closure of the gastric end with end-to-end anastomosis of stomach and duodenum.

Billroth o. II, excision of the pylorus and antrum with closure of the cut ends of the duodenum and stomach, followed by a gastrojejunostomy.

Blalock-Hanlon o., the creation of a large atrial septal defect as a palliative procedure for complete transposition of the great arteries.

Blalock-Taussig o., an o. for congenital malformations of the heart, in which an abnormally small volume of blood passes through the pulmonary circuit; blood from the systemic circulation is directed to the lungs by anastomosing the right or left subclavian artery to the right or left pulmonary artery.

bloodless o., an o. performed with negligible loss of blood.

Bozeman o., an o. for uterovaginal fistula, the cervix uteri being attached to the bladder and opening into its cavity.

Bricker o., an o. utilizing an isolated segment of ileum to collect urine from the ureters and conduct it to the skin surface.

Brock o., transventricular valvotomy for relief of pulmonic valvar stenosis. Obsolete procedure.

Brunschwig o., SYN total pelvic *exenteration*.

Caldwell-Luc o., an intraoral procedure for opening into the maxillary antrum through the supradental (canine) fossa above the maxillary premolar teeth. SYN intraoral antrostomy, Luc o.

Carmody-Batson o., reduction of fractures of the zygoma and zygomatic arch through an intraoral incision above the maxillary molar teeth.

cesarean o., SEE cesarean *section*, cesarean *hysterectomy*.

commando o., SYN commando *procedure*.

concrete o.'s, in the psychology of Piaget, a stage of development in thinking, occurring approximately between 7 and 11 years of age, during which a child becomes capable of reasoning about concrete situations.

Cotte o., SYN presacral *neurectomy*.

cricoid split o., an operation to repair subglottic stenosis by transecting the anterior and posterior aspects of the ring of the cricoid cartilage, with or without the insertion of grafts to reconstruct the subglottic lumen.

Dana o., SYN posterior *rhizotomy*.

Dandy o., SEE third *ventriculostomy*, trigeminal *rhizotomy*.

Daviel o., extracapsular cataract extraction.

debulking o., excision of a major part of a malignant tumor that cannot be completely removed.

decompression o.'s, SEE decompression.

Doyle o., paracervical uterine denervation.

Elliot o., trephining of the eyeball at the corneoscleral margin to relieve tension in glaucoma.

Emmet o., SYN trachelorrhaphy.

endolymphatic shunt o., an operation to establish a communication between the endolymphatic sac and the cerebrospinal fluid space for the treatment of Ménière disease.

Estes o., an o. for sterility in which a portion of an ovary is implanted on one uterine cornu.

fenestration o., a rarely used surgical procedure producing an opening from the external auditory canal to the membranous labyrinth to improve hearing in hearing impairment of the conduction type due to otosclerosis.

filtering o., a surgical procedure for creation of a fistula between the anterior chamber of the eye and the subconjunctival space in treatment of glaucoma.

Finney o., gastroduodenostomy that creates, by the technique of closure, a large opening to ensure free emptying from the stomach.

flap o., (**1**) SYN flap *amputation*; (**2**) in dental surgery, an o. in which a portion of the mucoperiosteal tissues is surgically detached from the underlying bone or impacted tooth for better access and visibility in exploring the area covered by the tissue. SEE ALSO flap.

Fontan o., SYN Fontan *procedure*.

formal o.'s, in the psychology of Piaget, a stage of development in thinking, occurring approximately between 11 and 15 years of age, during which a child becomes capable of reasoning about abstract situations; reasoning at this stage is comparable to that of normal adults but less sophisticated.

Fothergill o., SYN Manchester o.

Frazier-Spiller o., SEE trigeminal *rhizotomy*.

Fredet-Ramstedt o., SYN pyloromyotomy.

Freund o., (**1**) total abdominal hysterectomy for uterine cancer; (**2**) chondrotomy to relieve Freund anomaly.

Gilliam o., an o. for retroversion of the uterus by suturing round ligaments to abdominal wall fascia.

Gillies o., a technique for reducing fractures of the zygoma and the zygomatic arch through an incision in the temporal region above the hairline.

Gil-Vernet o., SYN extended *pyelotomy*.

Glenn o., anastomosis between the superior vena cava and the right main pulmonary artery to increase pulmonary blood flow as a palliative correction for tricuspid atresia.

Graefe o., (**1**) removal of cataract by a limbal incision with capsulotomy and iridectomy. Both operations were landmarks in the field of ophthalmic surgery; (**2**) iridectomy for glaucoma.

Gritti o., SYN Gritti-Stokes *amputation*.

Halsted o., (**1**) an o. for the radical correction of inguinal hernia; (**2**) SYN radical *mastectomy*.

Hartmann o., resection of the sigmoid colon beginning at or just above the peritoneal reflexion and extending proximally, with closure of the rectal stump and end-colostomy.

Heaney o., technique for vaginal hysterectomy.

Heller o., esophagomyotomy just above the gastroesophageal junction.

Hill o., repair of hiatus hernia; anchoring the esophagogastric junction within the abdomen by attaching it to the medial arcuate ligament.

Hoffa o., in congenital dislocation of the hip, a rarely used operation consisting of hollowing out the acetabulum and reduction of the head of the femur after severing the muscles inserted into the upper portion of the bone.

Hofmeister o., partial gastrectomy with closure of a portion of the lesser curvature and retrocolic anastomosis of the remainder to jejunum.

Hummelsheim o., transplantation of a normal ocular rectus muscle, to substitute for a paralyzed muscle.

Hunter o., ligation of an artery proximal and distal to an aneurysm.

interval o., an o. performed during a period of quiescence or of intermission in the condition necessitating surgery.

Jacobaeus o., obsolete term for pleurolysis.

Jansen o., an o. for frontal sinus disease; the lower wall and lower portion of the anterior wall are removed and the mucous membrane is curetted away.

Kasai o., SYN portoenterostomy.

Kazanjian o., surgical extension of the vestibular sulcus of edentulous ridges to increase their height and to improve denture retention. SEE ALSO ridge *extension*.

Keen o., removal of sections of the posterior branches of the spinal nerves to the affected muscles, and of the spinal accessory nerve, as a cure for torticollis.

Keller-Madlener o., an o. for treatment of gastric ulcer located in the proximal cardia that involves 75% gastrectomy and gastrojejunostomy.

Kelly o., (**1**) correction of retroversion of the uterus by plication of uterosacral ligaments; (**2**) correction of urinary stress incontinence by vaginally placing sutures beneath the bladder neck.

Killian o., an o. for frontal sinus disease in which the entire anterior wall is removed and the mucous membrane is curetted away; the ethmoid cells are removed through an opening in the nasal process of the maxillary bone, and the upper portion of the medial wall of the orbit is removed as well.

Koerte-Ballance o., operative anastomosis of the facial and hypoglossal nerves for the treatment of facial paralysis.

Kondoleon o., excision of strips of subcutaneous connective tissue for the relief of elephantiasis.

Kraske o., removal of the coccyx and excision of the left wing of the sacrum to afford approach for resection of the rectum for cancer or stenosis.

Krönlein o., orbital decompression through the anterior lateral wall of the orbit.

Ladd o., division of Ladd band to relieve duodenal obstruction in malrotation of the intestine.

Lambrinudi o., a form of triple arthrodesis done in such a manner as to prevent foot-drop such as occurs in poliomyelitis.

Laroyenne o., puncture of Douglas pouch to evacuate the pus and to secure drainage in cases of pelvic suppuration.

Lash o., removal of a wedge of the internal cervical os with suturing of the internal os into a tighter canal structure.

LeCompte o., SYN LeCompte *maneuver*.

Leriche o., SYN periarterial *sympathectomy*.

Lisfranc o., SYN Lisfranc *amputation*.

Longmire o., intrahepatic cholangiojejunostomy with partial hepatectomy for biliary obstruction.

Luc o., SYN Caldwell-Luc o.

Madlener o., tubal sterilization by clamp and tie.

major o., an extensive, relatively difficult surgical procedure involving vital organs and/or in itself hazardous to life.

Manchester o., a vaginal o. for prolapse of the uterus, consisting of cervical amputation and parametrial fixation (cardinal ligaments) anterior to the uterus. SYN Fothergill o. [*Manchester, England*]

Mann-Williamson o., an o. performed on experimental animals (dogs) in research on peptic ulcer, the duodenum with its alkaline secretions being transplanted into the ileum and the cut end of the jejunum anastomosed to the pylorus; the animals develop ulcers in the jejunum, which directly receives the gastric juice.

Marshall-Marchetti-Krantz o., an o. for urinary stress incontinence, performed retropubically.

Mayo o., an o. for the radical cure of umbilical hernia; the neck of the sac is exposed by two elliptical incisions, the gut is returned to the abdomen, the sac and adherent omentum are cut away, and the fascial edges of the opening are overlapped with mattress sutures.

McIndoe o., o. for the development of a neovagina using a split thickness skin graft over a vaginal mold.

McVay o., repair of inguinal and femoral hernias by suture of the transversus abdominis muscle and its associated fasciae (transversus layer) to the pectineal ligament.

mika o., the establishment of a permanent fistula in the bulbous portions of the urethra to render the man incapable of procreating; said to be a practice among certain Australian aborigines. [Australian native term]

Mikulicz o., excision of bowel in two stages: 1) exteriorizing the diseased area, suturing efferent and afferent limbs together, and closing the abdomen around them, after which the diseased part is excised; 2) at a later time, cutting the spur with an enterotome and closing the stoma extraperitoneally.

Miles o., combined abdominoperineal resection for carcinoma of the rectum.

minor o., a surgical procedure of relatively slight extent and not in itself hazardous to life.

morcellation o., vaginal hysterectomy in which the uterus is removed in multiple pieces after being split or partitioned.

Motais o., transplantation of the middle third of the tendon of the superior rectus muscle of the eyeball into the upper lid, between the tarsus and skin, to supplement the action of the levator muscle in ptosis.

Mules o., evisceration of the eyeball followed by the insertion within the sclera of a spherical prosthesis to support an artificial eye.

Mustard o., correction, at the atrial level, of hemodynamic abnormality caused by transposition of the great arteries by an intraatrial baffle to direct pulmonary venous blood through the tricuspid orifice into the right ventricle and the systemic venous blood through the mitral valve into the left ventricle. SYN Mustard procedure.

Naffziger o., orbital decompression for severe malignant exophthalmos by removal of the lateral and superior orbital walls.

Nissen o., SYN Nissen *fundoplication.*

Norton o., extraperitoneal cesarean section by a paravesical approach.

Norwood o., o. performed in infants with subaortic stenosis and tricuspid atresia; the pulmonary artery is divided and both ends are attached to the aorta, the distal end via a prosthetic graft.

Ogston-Luc o., an o. for frontal sinus disease; a skin incision is made from the inner third of the edge of the orbit toward the root of the nose or outward; the periosteum is pushed upward and outward, and the sinus is opened on the outer side of the median line; then a wide opening is made by curetting the nasofrontal duct, interior of the sinus, and anterior ethmoid cells.

Ogura o., orbital decompression by removal of the floor of the orbit through an opening made in the supradental (canine) fossa.

Ombrédanne o., a technique whereby the mobilized testis is brought down into the scrotum and through the scrotal septum, to be affixed to the tissues in the contralateral scrotal pouch. SYN transseptal orchiopexy.

Payne o., a jejunoileal bypass for morbid obesity utilizing end-to-side anastomosis of the upper jejunum to the terminal ileum, with closure of the proximal end of the bypassed intestine.

Pólya o., SYN Pólya *gastrectomy.*

Pomeroy o., excision of a ligated portion of the fallopian tubes.

Potts o., direct side-to-side anastomosis between aorta and pulmonary artery as a palliative procedure in congenital malformation of the heart. SYN Potts anastomosis.

pubovaginal o., operative procedure for urinary incontinence. A strip of tissue, usually autologous rectus abdominis fascia, is used to suspend or elevate bladder neck and posterior urethra toward pubic symphysis.

Putti-Platt o., a procedure for recurrent anterior dislocation of shoulder joint. SYN Putti-Platt procedure.

radical o. for hernia, an o. by which the hernia is not only reduced, but the hernial defect is also repaired.

Ramstedt o., SYN pyloromyotomy.

Rastelli o., for "anatomic" repair of transposition of the great arteries (ventriculoarterial discordance) with ventricular septal defect and left ventricular outflow tract obstruction; conduits are used to create left ventricular to aortic continuity and right ventricular to pulmonary artery continuity. All septal defects are obliterated, as are any previously constructed palliative shunts.

Récamier o., curettage of the uterus.

Ridell o., removal of the entire anterior and inferior walls of the frontal sinus, for chronic inflammation of that cavity.

Ripstein o., an o. for rectal prolapse that involves a transabdominal approach with dissection around the rectum and placement of a mesh sling to prevent the bowel from prolapsing through the anus.

Roux-en-Y o., anastomosis of the distal end of the divided upper jejunum to the stomach, esophagus, biliary tract, or other structure and anastomosis of the proximal end to the side of the jejunum a little further distal.

Saenger o., cesarean section followed by careful closure of the uterine wound by three tiers of sutures.

Schauta vaginal o., an extensive extirpation of the uterus and the adnexa, using the vaginal approach facilitated by Schuchardt o.

Schroeder o., excision of diseased endocervical mucosa.

Schuchardt o., a paravaginal rectal displacement incision, a surgical technique of making the upper vagina accessible for fistula closure or radical surgery via the vagina.

scleral buckling o., an o. performed in retinal detachment to indent the sclerochoroidal wall.

Scott o., a jejunoileal bypass for morbid obesity utilizing end-to-end anastomosis of the upper jejunum to the terminal ileum, with the bypassed intestine closed proximally and anastomosed distally to the colon.

second-look o., exploratory celiotomy within a year after apparently curative resection of intraabdominal cancer, in patients with no sign or symptom of recurrence, to resect an occult tumor if present.

Senning o., an atrial switch o. for patients with transposition of the great arteries that employs a septal flap instead of excising the atrial septum as in the Mustard o., thus minimizing foreign material and allowing for growth.

seton o., an o. for advanced glaucoma; passage of a tube or seton into the anterior chamber to act as a wick.

Shirodkar o., a cerclage procedure done by purse-string suturing of an incompetent cervical os with a nonabsorbent suture material.

Sistrunk o., excision of the thyroglossal cyst and duct including the midportion of the hyoid bone through, or near, which the duct traverses.

Smith o., SYN Smith-Indian o.

Smith-Boyce o., SYN anatrophic *nephrotomy.*

Smith-Indian o., a surgical technique for removal of cataract within the capsule. SYN Smith o.

Soave o., endorectal pull-through for treatment of congenital megacolon.

Spinelli o., an o. splitting the anterior wall of the prolapsed uterus and reversing the organ preliminary to reduction.

op

stapes mobilization o., now infrequently used o. involving fracture of otosclerotic tissue immobilizing the stapes to restore hearing.

Stoffel o., division of certain motor nerves for the relief of spastic paralysis.

Stookey-Scarff o., SEE third *ventriculostomy*.

Sturmdorf o., conical removal of the endocervix.

subcutaneous o., an o., as for the division of a tendon, performed without incising the skin other than by a minute opening made by the entering knife.

Syme o., SYN Syme *amputation*.

talc o., an obsolete o. in which magnesium silicate (talc) powder is applied to the epicardium to create a sterile granulomatous pericarditis and thus promote pericardial anastomoses with the coronary circulation. SYN poudrage (2).

TeLinde o., SYN modified radical *hysterectomy*.

Torek o., a two-stage o. for bringing down an undescended testicle.

Trendelenburg o., a pulmonary embolectomy.

Urban o., extended radical mastectomy, including *en bloc* resection of internal mammary lymph nodes, part of the sternum, and costal cartilages.

Waters o., an extraperitoneal cesarean section with a supravesical approach.

Waterston o., a surgically created anastomosis between the pulmonary artery and the ascending aorta to palliate adult tetralogy of Fallot.

Wertheim o., a radical o. for carcinoma of the uterus in which as much as possible of the vagina is excised and there is wide lymph node excision.

Whipple o., SYN pancreatoduodenectomy.

Whitehead o., excision of hemorrhoids by two circular incisions above and below involved veins, allowing normal mucosa to be pulled down and sutured to anal skin.

---

op·er·a·tive (op′er-ă-tiv). **1.** Relating to, or effected by means of an operation. **2.** Active or effective.

op·er·a·tor (op′er-ā-tor). **1.** One who performs an operation or operates equipment. **2.** In genetics, a sequence of DNA that interacts with a repressor of operon to control the expression of adjacent structural genes. SEE operator *gene*. **3.** A symbol representing a mathematical operation. [L. worker, fr *operor*, to work]

oper·cu·lar (ō-per′kū-lăr). Relating to an operculum.

oper·cu·lat·ed (ō-per′kū-lā-ted). Provided with a lid (operculum); denoting members of the mollusk class Gastropoda (the snails), subclass Prosobranchiata (operculate snails), and the eggs of certain parasitic worms such as the digenetic trematodes (except the schistosomes) and the broad fish tapeworm, *Diphyllobothrium latum*.

oper·cu·li·tis (ō-perk-ū-lī′tis). Originating under an operculum. [operculum + G. -*itis,* inflammation]

oper·cu·lum, gen. **oper·cu·li,** pl. **oper·cu·la** (ō-per′kū-lŭm, -lī, -lă). **1.** Anything resembling a lid or cover. **2** [TA]. In anatomy, the portions of the frontal (operculum frontale [TA], frontal operculum [TA]), parietal (operculum parietale [TA], parietal operculum [TA]), and temporal (operculum temporale [TA], temporal operculum [TA]) lobes bordering the lateral sulcus and covering the insula. **3.** In parasitology, the lid or caplike cover of the shell opening of operculated freshwater snails in the subclass Prosobranchiata, and of the eggs of certain trematode and cestode parasites. **4.** The attached flap in the tear of retinal detachment. **5.** The mucosal flap partially or completely covering an unerupted tooth. [L. cover or lid, fr. *operio,* pp. *opertus,* to cover]

o. il′ei, SYN ileal *sphincter*.

occipital o., a portion of the occipital lobe of the brain demarcated by the simian fissure (*sulcus* lunatus) when present in humans.

trophoblastic o., the mushroom-shaped plug of fibrin that fills the aperture in the endometrium made by the implanting ovum.

op·er·on (op′er-on). A genetic functional unit that controls production of a messenger RNA; it consists of an operator gene and two or more structural genes located in sequence in the *cis* position on one chromosome. [L. *operor,* to work, act, + -on]

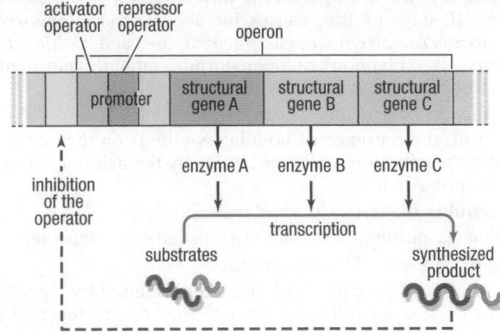

operon: the synthesized product exerts negative feedback to inhibit function of operon, in this way automatically controlling the concentration of the product itself

---

Lac o., a collection of adjacent bacterial genes responsible for the entry and metabolism of lactose; contains the genes coding for three enzymes and is flanked by a repressor and a promoter region to control expression.

ophi·a·sis (ō-fī′ă-sis). A form of alopecia areata in which the loss of hair occurs in bands along the scalp margin partially or completely encircling the head. [G., fr. *ophis,* snake]

Ophid·ia (ō-fid′ē-ă). The snakes, a suborder of the class Reptilia, including the families Colubridae, Crotalidae, Elapidae, Hydrophyidae, and Viperidae. [G. *ophidion,* dim. of *ophis,* a serpent]

ophi·di·a·sis (ō′fi-dī′ă-sis). Poisoning by a snake. SYN ophidism. [G. *ophidion,* dim. of *ophis,* a serpent]

ophid·i·o·pho·bia (ō-fid′ē-ō-fō′bē-ă). Morbid fear of snakes. [G. *ophidion,* a small snake, + *phobos,* fear]

ophid·ism (ō′fid-izm). SYN ophidiasis.

oph·ri·tis (of-rī′tis). Dermatitis in the region of the eyebrows. SYN ophryitis. [G. *ophrys,* eyebrow, + -*itis,* inflammation]

oph·ry·i·tis (of-rē-ī′tis). SYN ophritis.

oph·ry·og·e·nes (of′rē-yō-jen′enz). Related to the eyebrows. [Mod. L., fr. G. *ophrys,* eyebrow, + suffix -*genēs,* arising from]

oph·ry·on (of′rē-on). The point on the midline of the forehead just above the glabella (1). SYN supranasal point, supraorbital point. [G. *ophrys,* eyebrow]

Oph·ry·o·sco·lec·i·dae (of′rē-ō-skō-les′i-dē). A family of ciliate protozoa occurring in the rumen and reticulum of ruminant animals, characterized by having cilia arranged in spiral membranelles around the mouth (adoral) and in some genera also in a dorsal (metoral) position. The most important genera are *Entodinium, Diplodinium, Epidinium,* and *Ophryoscolex,* which are thought to contribute to ruminant nutrition by converting cellulose in plant material ingested by the ruminant into readily digestible animal protein of their own bodies. [G. *ophrys,* eyebrow, + *skōlēx,* a worm]

oph·ry·o·sis (of-rē-ō′sis). Spasmodic twitching of the upper portion of the orbicularis palpebrarum muscle causing a wrinkling of the eyebrow. [G. *ophrys,* eyebrow, + -*osis,* condition]

△**ophthalm-.** SEE ophthalmo-.

ophthalmalgia (of′thal-mal′jē-ă). SYN oculodynia. [ophthalmo- + G. *algos,* pain]

oph·thal·mia (of-thal′mē-ă). **1.** Severe, often purulent, conjunctivitis. **2.** Inflammation of the deeper structures of the eye. [G.]

catarrhal o., a mild form of conjunctivitis with mucopurulent secretion.

caterpillar-hair o., SYN o. nodosa.

Egyptian o., SYN trachoma.

gonorrheal o., acute purulent conjunctivitis excited by *Neisseria gonorrhoeae.* SYN blennophthalmia (2), blennorrhea conjunctivalis, gonorrheal conjunctivitis.

granular o., SYN trachoma.

metastatic o., (1) sympathetic o; **(2)** choroiditis in septicemia.

o. neonato′rum, a conjunctival inflammation occurring within the first 10 days of life; causes include *Neisseria gonorrhoeae, Staphylococcus, Streptococcus pneumoniae,* and *Chlamydia trachomatis.* SYN blennorrhea neonatorum, infantile purulent conjunctivitis, neonatal conjunctivitis.

o. niva′lis, SYN ultraviolet *keratoconjunctivitis.*

o. nodo′sa, the presence of nodular swellings on the conjunctiva, caused by penetration of ocular tissues by the hairs of caterpillars. SYN caterpillar-hair o.

phlyctenular o., SYN phlyctenular *conjunctivitis.*

purulent o., purulent conjunctivitis, usually of gonorrheal origin.

spring o., SYN vernal *conjunctivitis.*

sympathetic o., a serous or plastic uveitis caused by a perforating wound of the uvea followed by a similar severe reaction in the other eye that may lead to bilateral blindness. SYN transferred o.

transferred o., SYN sympathetic o.

oph·thal·mic (of-thal′mik). Relating to the eye. SYN ocular (1). [G. *ophthalmikos*]

oph·thal·mic ac·id. A tripeptide occurring in lens, similar to glutathione but differing in the replacement of cysteine by α-amino-*n*-butyric acid (i.e., in the replacement of –SH by –CH₃); a potent inhibitor of glyoxalase. Cf. norophthalmic acid.

△**ophthalmo-, ophthalm-.** Relationship to the eye. SEE ALSO oculo-. [G. *ophthalmos*]

oph·thal·mo·dy·na·mom·e·ter (of-thal′mō-dī-nă-mom′ĕ-ter). An instrument to measure the blood pressure in the retinal vessels. [ophthalmo- + G. *dynamis,* power, + *metron,* measure]

Bailliart o., an instrument used to measure the blood pressure of the central retinal artery; of value in diagnosing occlusion of the proximal carotid artery.

suction o., an o. with a suction disk that increases ocular pressure during ophthalmoscopic observation of the retinal artery.

oph·thal·mo·dy·na·mom·e·try (of-thal′mō-dī-nă-mom′ĕ-trē). The measurement of blood pressure in the retinal vessels by means of an ophthalmodynamometer. [ophthalmo- + G. *dynamis,* power, + *metron,* measure]

oph·thal·mo·lith (of-thal′mō-lith). SYN dacryolith. [ophthalmo- + G. *lithos,* stone]

oph·thal·mol·o·gist (of-thal-mol′ō-jist). A specialist in ophthalmology. SYN oculist.

oph·thal·mol·o·gy (of-thal-mol′ō-jē). The medical specialty concerned with the eye, its diseases, and refractive errors. [ophthalmo- + G. *logos,* study]

oph·thal·mo·ma·la·cia (of-thal′mō-mă-lā′shē-ă). Abnormal softening of the eyeball. [ophthalmo- + G. *malakia,* softness]

oph·thal·mo·mel·a·no·sis (of-thal′mō-mel-ă-nō′sis). Melanotic discoloration of the conjunctiva and adjoining tissues.

oph·thal·mom·e·ter (of-thal-mom′ĕ-ter). SYN keratometer. [ophthalmo- + G. *metron,* measure]

oph·thal·mo·my·co·sis (of-thal′mō-mī-kō′sis). Any disease of the eye or its appendages caused by a fungus. [ophthalmo- + G. *mykēs,* fungus, + *-osis,* condition]

oph·thal·mo·my·i·a·sis (of-thal′mō-mī-ī′ă-sis). SYN ocular *myiasis.*

oph·thal·mop·a·thy (of-thal-mop′ă-thē). Any disease of the eyes. SYN oculopathy. [ophthalmo- + G. *pathos,* suffering]

endocrine o., SYN Graves o.

external o., any disease of the conjunctiva, cornea, or adnexa of the eye.

Graves o., exophthalmos caused by increased water content of retroocular orbital tissues; associated with thyroid disease, usually hyperthyroidism. SYN endocrine o., Graves orbitopathy.

internal o., any disease of the internal structures of the eyeball.

oph·thal·mo·ple·gia (of-thal-mō-plē′jē-ă). Paralysis of one or more of the ocular muscles. [ophthalmo- + G. *plēgē,* stroke]

chronic progressive external o. (CPEO), a specific type of slowly worsening weakness of the ocular muscles, usually associated with a pigmentary retinopathy. SEE Kearns-Sayre *syndrome,* oculopharyngeal *dystrophy.* SYN ocular myopathy.

exophthalmic o., o. with protrusion of the eyeballs due to increased water content of orbital tissues incidental to thyroid disorders, usually hyperthyroidism.

o. exter′na, paralysis affecting one or more of the extrinsic eye muscles. SYN external o.

external o., SYN o. externa.

fascicular o., o. due to a lesion within the brainstem.

fibrotic o. [MIM*135700], o. that may be congenital in association with blepharoptosis; an autosomal dominant disorder.

o. inter′na, paralysis affecting only the sphincter muscle of the pupil and the ciliary muscle. SYN internal o.

internal o., SYN o. interna.

internuclear o. (INO), o. in lesions of the medial longitudinal fasciculus, with failure of adduction in horizontal gaze but with retention of convergence.

nuclear o., o. due to a lesion of the nuclei of origin of the motor nerves of the eye.

orbital o., o. due to a lesion within the orbit.

Parinaud o., SYN Parinaud *syndrome.*

o. partia′lis, incomplete o. involving only one or two of the extrinsic or intrinsic ocular muscles.

o. progressi′va, progressive upper bulbar palsy, due to degeneration of the nuclei of the motor nerves of the eye.

o. tota′lis, paralysis of both the extrinsic and intrinsic ocular muscles.

wall-eyed bilateral internuclear o. (WEBINO), a form of internuclear o. associated with an exotropia.

oph·thal·mo·ple·gic (of-thal-mō-plē′jik). Relating to or marked by ophthalmoplegia.

▪**oph·thal·mo·scope** (of-thal′mō-skōp). A device for studying the interior of the eyeball through the pupil. SYN funduscope. [ophthalmo- + G. *skopeō,* to examine]

binocular o., an o. that provides a stereoscopic view of the fundus.

demonstration o., an o. by which the fundus may be seen simultaneously by more than one observer.

direct o., an instrument designed to visualize the interior of the eye, with the instrument relatively close to the subject's eye and the observer viewing an upright magnified image.

indirect o., an instrument designed to visualize the interior of the eye, with the instrument at arm's length from the subject's eye and the observer viewing an inverted image through a convex lens located between the instrument and the subject's eye.

oph·thal·mo·scop·ic (of′thal-mō-skop′ik). Relating to examination of the interior of the eye.

▪**oph·thal·mos·co·py** (of-thal-mos′kŏ-pē). Examination of the fundus of the eye by means of the ophthalmoscope. SYN funduscopy.

direct o., o. performed with a direct ophthalmoscope.

indirect o., o. performed with an indirect ophthalmoscope.

o. with reflected light, examination of that part of the fundus adjacent to an area illuminated by a sharply focused light.

oph·thal·mo·trope (of-thal′mō-trōp). A model of the two eyes, to each of which are attached weighted cords pulling in the direction of the six extrinsic eye muscles; used to demonstrate the action of the ocular muscles singly or in various combinations. [ophthalmo- + G. *tropos,* a turning]

oph·thal·mo·vas·cu·lar (of-thal′mō-vas′kū-lăr). Relating to the blood vessels of the eye.

△**-opia.** Vision. [G. *ōps,* eye]

opi·a·nine (ō-pī′ă-nēn). SYN noscapine.

opi·a·nyl (ō′pī-ă-nil). SYN meconin.

opi·ate (ō′pē-āt). Any preparation or derivative of opium.

opine (ō′pēn). A derivative of basic amino acids, produced by crown-gall tumors in plants.

opi·o·cor·tin (ō′pē-ō-kōr′tin). SYN opiomelanocortin.

opi·oid (ō′pē-oyd). Originally, a term denoting synthetic narcotics

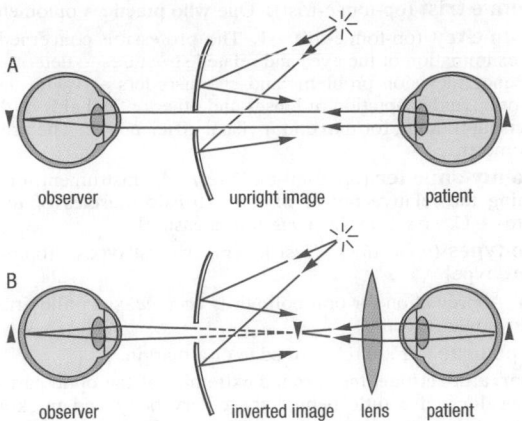

ophthalmoscopy: path of light rays in (A) direct and (B) indirect ophthalmoscopy, with upright or inverted image, respectively

resembling opiates but increasingly used to refer to both opiates and synthetic narcotics.

opi·o·mel·a·no·cor·tin (ō′pē-ō-mel′ă-nō-kōr′tin). A linear polypeptide of the pituitary gland that contains in its sequence the sequences of endorphins, MSH, ACTH, and the like, which are split off enzymically; the nucleotide sequence coding has been determined for several species. SYN opiocortin.

opip·ra·mol hy·dro·chlo·ride (ō-pip′ră-mōl). 4-[3-(5*H*-Dibenz[*b,f*]azepin-5-yl)propyl]-1-piperazineethanol dihydrochloride; an antidepressant agent.

opis·the·nar (ō-pis′thē-nar). Dorsum of the hand. [G. back of the hand, from *opisthen,* behind, + *thenar,* palm of the hand]

opis·thi·o·ba·si·al (ō-pis′thē-ō-bā′sē-ăl). Relating to both opisthion and basion; denoting a line connecting the two or the distance between them.

opis·thi·on (ō-pis′thē-on). The middle point on the posterior margin of the foramen magnum, opposite the basion. [G. *opisthios,* posterior]

opis·thi·o·na·si·al (ō-pis′thē-ō-nā′zē-ăl). Relating to the opisthion and the nasion; denoting the distance between the two points.

⌂**opistho-.** Backward, behind, dorsal. [G. *opisthen,* at the rear, behind]

op·is·tho·chei·lia, op·is·tho·chi·lia (op′is-thō-kī′lē-ă). Recession of the lips. [opistho- + G. *cheilos,* lip]

opis·tho·mas·ti·gote (ō-pis-thō-mas′ti-gōt). Term now used instead of herpetomonad for the stage of development of certain insect- and plant-parasitizing flagellates to avoid confusion between the stage and the genus *Herpetomonas.* In this stage the flagellum arises from the kinetoplast located behind the nucleus and emerges from the anterior end of the organism; an undulating membrane is absent. [opistho- + G. *mastix,* whip]

op·is·thor·chi·a·sis (op′is-thōr-kī′ă-sis). Infection with the Asiatic liver fluke, *Opisthorchis viverrini,* or other opisthorchids.

op·is·thor·chid (op-is-thōr′kid). Common name for members of the family Opisthorchiidae.

Opis·thor·chi·i·dae (op′is-thōr-kē′i-dē). A family of trematodes that includes the genera *Opisthorchis* and *Clonorchis.*

Opis·thor·chis (op-is-thōr′kis). Genus of digenetic trematodes (family Opisthorchiidae) found in the bile ducts or gallbladder of fish-eating mammals, birds, and fish. [opistho- + G. *orchis,* testis]

O. felin′eus, the cat liver fluke, a species frequently found as a human parasite in Eastern Europe, Siberia, India, Japan, and Southeast Asia; adults are lancet-shaped, thin, relatively transparent, and hermaphroditic, with sizes ranging from 7–12 by 2–3 mm; ingested eggs hatch in *Bithynia* snails, and cercariae encyst on various species of freshwater fish; humans acquire the infection by ingesting raw or inadequately cooked fish; the parasites sometimes cause no evidence of disease, but cholangitis, biliary cirrhosis, and chronic pancreatitis may occur.

O. sinen′sis, SYN *Clonorchis sinensis.*

O. viverri′ni, a species of fluke closely related to *O. felineus,* very common in humans in Thailand; causes opisthorchiasis.

op·is·thotic (op-is-thō′tik). Behind the ear. [opistho- + G. *ous* (*ōt-*), ear]

op·is·thot·on·ic (op-is-thot′ō-nik, ō-pis′thō-ton′ik). Relating to or characterized by opisthotonos.

op·is·thot·o·noid (op-is-thot′ō-noyd). Resembling opisthotonos.

op·is·thot·o·nos, op·is·thot·o·nus (op-is-thot′ō-nŭs). A tetanic spasm in which the spine and extremities are bent with convexity forward, the body resting on the head and the heels. [opistho- + G. *tonos,* tension, stretching]

Opitz, John M., U.S. pediatrician, *1935. SEE Smith-Lemli-O. *syndrome;* Opitz BBB *syndrome;* Opitz G *syndrome.*

opi·um (ō′pē-ŭm). The air-dried milky exudation obtained by incising the unripe capsules of *Papaver somniferum* (family Papveraceae) or its variety, *P. album.* Contains some 20 alkaloids, including morphine, 9–14%; noscapine, 4–8%; codeine, 0.8–2.5%; papaverine, 0.5–2.5%; and thebaine, 0.5–2%. Used as an analgesic, hypnotic, and diaphoretic, and in diarrhea and spasmodic conditions. SYN gum opium, meconium (2). [L. fr. G. *opion,* poppy-juice]

Boston o., o. so diluted after importation as barely to meet the official requirements. SYN pudding o.

deodorized o., denarcotized o., powdered o. treated with purified petroleum benzine that removes certain nauseating and odorous constituents.

granulated o., o. dried and reduced to a coarse powder; it contains 10–10.5% anhydrous morphine.

powdered o., dried and finely powdered o. containing 10% morphine.

pudding o., SYN Boston o.

⌂**opo-.** **1.** The face; an eye. SEE ALSO facio-. **2.** Juice, balm. [G. *ōps*]

op·o·bal·sa·mum (op-ō-bal′sa-mŭm). SYN *balm* of Gilead. [G. *opobalsamon,* the juice of the balsam tree, fr. *opos,* juice, + *balsamon*]

op·o·did·y·mus (op-ō-did′i-mŭs). Conjoined twins with a single body having two heads fused at the back with partially separated facial regions. SEE conjoined *twins,* under *twin.* [G. *ōps,* eye, face, + *didymos,* twin]

Oppenheim, Hermann, Berlin neurologist, 1858–1919. SEE O. *disease, reflex, syndrome;* Ziehen-O. *disease.*

op·pi·la·tive (op-i-lā′tiv). Obstructive to any secretion.

op·po·nens (ŏ-pō′nens). A name given to several muscles of the fingers or toes, by the action of which these digits are opposed to the others. The opponens muscles of the hands act at the carpometacarpal joints, cupping the palm; this enables flexion at the metacarpophalangeal joints to oppose the thumb to the small finger or vice versa. Although comparable muscles in the foot are called "opponens," no opposition occurs in the foot. [L. *op-pono* (*obp-*), pres. p. *-ens,* to place against, oppose]

op·por·tun·is·tic (op′ŏr-too-nis′tik). **1.** Denoting an organism capable of causing disease only in a host whose resistance is lowered, e.g., by other diseases or by drugs. **2.** Denoting a disease caused by such an organism.

op·po·sure (op′pō-shŭr). Bringing together of tissue during suturing.

op·sin. The protein portion of the rhodopsin molecule; at least three separate o.'s are located in cone cells.

op·sin·o·gen (op-sin′ō-jen). A substance that stimulates the formation of opsonin, such as the antigen contained in a suspension of bacteria used for immunization. SYN opsogen. [opsonin + -gen]

op·si·u·ria (op-sē-oo′rē-ă). A more rapid excretion of urine during fasting than after a full meal. [G. *opsi,* late, + *ouron,* urine]

op·so·clo·nus (op′sō-klō′nŭs). Rapid, irregular, nonrhythmic movements of the eye in horizontal and vertical directions. [G. *ōps, ōpos,* eye, + *klonos,* confused motion]

op·so·gen (op′sō-jen). SYN opsinogen.

op·so·ma·nia (op′sō-mā′nē-ă). A rarely used term for a longing for a particular article of diet, or for highly seasoned food. [G. *opson*, seasoning, + *mania*, frenzy]

op·son·ic (op-son′ik). Relating to opsonins or to their utilization.

op·so·nin (op′sŏ-nin). Any blood serum protein that binds to antigens, enhancing phagocytosis (e.g., C3b of the complement system, specific antibodies). [G. *opson*, boiled meat, provisions, fr. *hepsō*, to boil, + -in]

common o., SYN normal o.

immune o., SYN specific o.

normal o., o. normally present in the blood, i.e., without stimulation by a known, specific antigen such as certain complement components; it is relatively thermolabile and reacts with various organisms. SYN common o., thermolabile o.

specific o., antibodies formed in response to stimulation by a specific antigen, either as a result of an attack of a disease or as a result of injections with a suitably prepared suspension of the specific microorganism. SYN immune o., thermostable o.

thermolabile o., SYN normal o.

thermostable o., SYN specific o.

op·son·i·za·tion (op′sŏ-nī-zā′shŭn). The process by which bacteria and other cells are altered in such a manner that they are more readily and more efficiently engulfed by phagocytes.

op·so·no·cy·to·pha·gic (op′sŏ-nō-sī′tō-fā′jik). Pertaining to the increased efficiency of phagocytic activity of the leukocytes in blood that contains specific opsonin. [opsonin + G. *kytos*, a hollow (cell), + *phagō*, to eat]

op·so·nom·e·try (op-sŏ-nom′ĕ-trē). Determination of the opsonic index or the opsonocytophagic activity.

op·so·no·phil·ia (op-sŏ-nō-fil′ē-ă). The condition in which bacteria readily unite with opsonins, thereby sensitizing them for more effective phagocytosis. [opsonin + G. *phileō*, to love]

op·so·no·phil·ic (op-sŏ-nō-fil′ik). Pertaining to, characterized by, or resulting in opsonophilia.

op·tic, op·ti·cal (op′tik, op′ti-kăl). Relating to the eye, vision, or optics. [G. *optikos*]

op·ti·cian (op-tish′an). One who practices opticianry.

op·ti·cian·ry (op-tish′an-rē). The professional practice of filling prescriptions for ophthalmic lenses, dispensing spectacles, and making and fitting contact lenses.

△**optico-.** SEE opto-.

op·ti·co·cil·i·a·ry (op′ti-kō-sil′ē-ār-ē). Relating to the optic and ciliary nerves.

op·ti·co·pu·pil·lary (op′ti-kō-pū′pi-lār-ē). Relating to the optic nerve and the pupil.

op·tics (op′tiks). The science concerned with the properties of light, its refraction and absorption, and the refracting media of the eye in that relation. [G. *optikos*, fr. *ōps*, eye]

Nomarski o., an optical system for differential interference contrast microscopy.

schlieren o., an optical system, often used in diffusion and centrifugation studies, that observes the refractive index gradient in solutions containing macromolecules.

op·ti·mism (op′ti-mizm). The tendency to look on the bright side of everything, to believe that there is good in everything. [L. *optimus*, best]

therapeutic o., a belief in the efficacy of drugs and other therapeutic agents in the treatment of diseases.

op·ti·mum (op′ti-mŭm). The best or most suitable; e.g., denoting the dose of a remedy likely to give most benefit with fewest side effects, the temperature or pH at which an enzyme has maximal activity. [L. ntr. sing. of *optimus*, best]

△**opto-, optico-.** Optical; optic; ocular. [G. *optikos*, optical, from *ōps*, eye]

op·to·ki·net·ic (op′tō-ki-net′ik). SEE optokinetic *nystagmus*. [opto- + G. *kinēsis*, movement]

op·to·me·ninx (op′tō-mē′ninks). SYN retina. [opto- + G. *mēninx*, membrane]

op·tom·e·ter (op-tom′ĕ-ter). An instrument for determining the refraction of the eye. [opto- + G. *metron*, measure]

objective o., SYN refractometer.

op·tom·e·trist (op-tom′ĕ-trist). One who practices optometry.

op·tom·e·try (op-tom′ĕ-trē). **1.** The profession concerned with the examination of the eyes and related structures to determine the presence of vision problems and eye disorders and with the prescription and adaptation of lenses and other optical aids or the use of visual training for maximum visual efficiency. **2.** The use of an optometer.

op·to·my·om·e·ter (op′tō-mī-om′ĕ-ter). An instrument for determining the relative power of the extrinsic muscles of the eye. [opto- + G. *mys*, muscle, + *metron*, measure]

op·to·types (op′tō-tīps). Test letters. SEE test types. [opto- + G. *typos*, type]

OPV Abbreviation for oral poliovirus *vaccine*. SEE poliovirus *vaccines*, under *vaccine*.

ora, pl. **orae** (ō′ră, ō′rē). An edge or a margin. [L.]

o. serra′ta retinae, the serrated extremity of the optic part of the retina, located a little behind the ciliary body and marking the limits of the percipient portion of the membrane.

ora (ō′ră). Plural of L. *os*, the mouth. [L.]

or·ad (ōr′ad). **1.** In a direction toward the mouth. **2.** Situated nearer the mouth in relation to a specific reference point; opposite of aborad. [L. *os*, mouth, + *ad*, to]

oral (ōr′ăl). Relating to the mouth. [L. *os* (*or*-), mouth]

ora·le (ō-rā′lē). A point at the lingual side of the alveolar termination of the premaxillary suture. [Mod. L. punctum *orale*, oral point, fr. L. *os* (*or*-), mouth]

Oral Hy·giene In·dex (OHI). An index used in epidemiologic studies of dental disease to evaluate dental plaque and dental calculus separately.

oral·i·ty (ōr-al′i-tē). In freudian psychology, a term used to denote the psychic organization derived from, and characteristic of, the oral period of psychosexual development.

Oram, Samuel, 20th century English cardiologist. SEE Holt-O. *syndrome*.

or·ange (ōr′enj). **1.** The fruit of the orange tree, *Citrus aurantium* (family Rutaceae). **2.** A color between yellow and red in the spectrum. For individual orange dyes, see specific name. [O.F. *orenge*, fr. Ar. *nāranj*, the initial *n* being absorbed in Fr. article *une*]

bitter o. peel, the dried rind of the unripe but fully grown fruit; a flavoring agent.

bitter o. peel, dried, the dried outer part of the pericarp of the ripe, or nearly ripe, fruit; it contains not less than 2.5% v/w of volatile oil.

bitter o. peel, fresh, the outer part of the pericarp of the ripe, or nearly ripe, fruit; used to prepare the tincture and the syrup.

bitter o. peel oil, a volatile oil obtained by expression from the fresh peel of the bitter o.

or·ange G [C.I. 16230]. An azo dye, used as a cytoplasmic stain in histologic techniques.

or·ange wood. A soft wood used in dentistry for placement of bridges, crowns, etc. by biting pressure, also used as a burnishing point in the polishing of root surfaces.

Orbeli, Leon A., Russian physiologist, 1882–1958. SEE O. *effect*.

or·bic·u·lar (or-bik′ū-lăr). Similar in form to an orb; circular in form. [L. *orbiculus*, a small disk, dim. of *orbis*, circle]

or·bic·u·la·re (ōr-bik-ū-lā′rē). SYN lenticular *process* of incus. [L., fr. *orbiculus*, a small disk]

or·bi·cu·la·ris (ōr-bik′ū-lā′ris). **1.** Circular; denoting a circular or disk-shaped structure. **2.** SYN orbicular *muscle*. [L. fr. *orbiculus*, a small disk]

or·bi·cu·lus cil·i·ar·is (ōr-bik′ū-lŭs sil-ē-ār′is) [TA]. The darkly pigmented posterior zone of the ciliary body continuous with the retina at the ora serrata. SYN ciliary disk, ciliary ring, pars plana. [Mod. L.]

⬛**or·bit** (ōr′bit) [TA]. The bony cavity containing the eyeball and its adnexa; it is formed of parts of seven bones: the frontal, maxillary, sphenoid, lacrimal, zygomatic, ethmoid, and palatine bones. SYN orbita [TA], eye socket, orbital cavity.

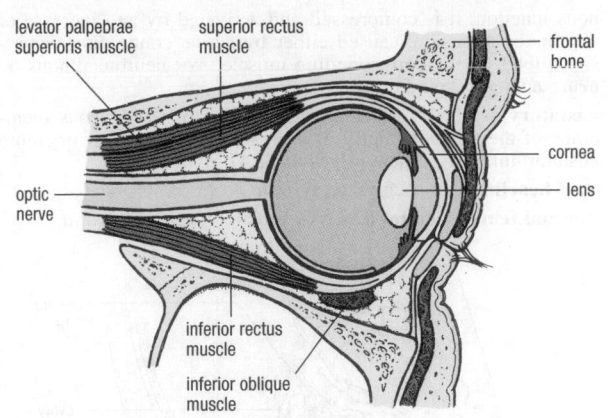

levator palpebrae
superioris muscle

superior rectus
muscle

frontal
bone

optic
nerve

cornea

lens

inferior rectus
muscle

inferior oblique
muscle

orbit: containing the eyeball and the ocular muscles

or·bi·ta, gen. **or·bi·tae** (ōr′bi-tă, -tē) [TA]. SYN orbit. [L. a wheel-track, fr. *orbis*, circle]

or·bi·tal (ōr′bi-tăl). Relating to the orbits.

or·bi·ta·le (ōr-bi-tā′lē). In cephalometrics, the lowermost point in the lower margin of the bony orbit that may be felt under the skin. [L. of an orbit]

or·bi·tog·ra·phy (ōr′bi-tog′ră-fē). Radiographic evaluation of the orbit. [L. *orbita*, orbit, + G. *graphō*, to write]

positive contrast o., o. with injection of a water soluble iodinated compound into the muscle cone or along the orbital floor.

or·bi·to·na·sal (ōr′bi-tō-nā′săl). Relating to the orbit and the nose or nasal cavity.

or·bi·to·nom·e·ter (ōr′bi-tō-nom′ĕ-ter). An instrument that measures the resistance offered to pressing the eyeball backwards into its socket. [L. *orbita*, orbit, + G. *metron*, measure]

or·bi·to·nom·e·try (ōr′bi-tō-nom′ĕ-trē). Measurement by means of the orbitonometer.

or·bi·top·a·gus (ōr-bi-top′ă-gŭs). Unequal conjoined twins in which the parasite, usually very imperfectly developed, is attached at an orbit of the autosite. SEE conjoined *twins*, under *twin*. SYN teratoma orbitae. [L. *orbita*, orbit, + G. *pagos*, something fixed]

or·bi·top·a·thy. Disease of the orbit and its contents.

dysthyroid orbitopathy, inflammation of the orbit in Graves *disease.*

Graves orbitopathy, SYN Graves *ophthalmopathy.*

or·bi·to·sphe·noid (ōr′bi-tō-sfe′noyd). Relating to the orbit and the sphenoid bone.

or·bi·tot·o·my (ōr-bi-tot′ō-mē). Surgical incision into the orbit. [L. *orbita*, orbit, + *tomē*, a cutting]

Or·bi·vi·rus (ōr′bi-vī-rŭs). A genus of viruses of vertebrates (family Reoviridae) that multiply in arthropods, including certain viruses formerly included with the arboviruses. They are antigenically distinct from other groups of viruses and are characterized by an indistinct but rather large outer layer of capsomeres that give the appearance of rings (hence the name). The genus includes, among others, bluetongue virus of sheep and African horse sickness virus. [L. *orbis*, ring, + virus]

or·ce·in (ōr′sē-in) [old C.I. 1242]. A natural dye derived from orcinol by treatment with air and ammonia, which as a purple dye complex is used in various histologic staining methods.

orch·al·gia (ork-al′-jē-ă). SYN orchialgia.

or·chec·to·my (ōr-kek′tō-mē). SYN orchiectomy.

or·chel·la (ōr-kel′ă) [old C.I. 1242]. SYN archil.

△**orcheo-.** SEE orchio-.

△**orchi-, orchido-, orchio-.** The testes. [G. *orchis*, testis]

or·chi·al·gia (ōr-kē-al′jē-ă). Pain in the testis. SYN orchalgia, orchiodynia, orchioneuralgia, testalgia. [orchi- + G. *algos*, pain]

or·chi·cho·rea (ōr′kē-kō-rē′ă). Involuntary rising and falling movements of the testis. [orchi- + G. *choreia*, a dance]

or·chi·dec·to·my (ōr-ki-dek′tō-mē). SYN orchiectomy.

or·chid·ic (ōr-kid′ik). Relating to the testis.

or·chi·di·tis (ōr-ki-dī′tis). SYN orchitis.

△**orchido-.** SEE orchi-.

or·chi·dom·e·ter (ōr-ki-dom′ĕ-ter). **1.** A caliper device used to measure the size of testes. **2.** A set of sized models of testes for comparison of testicular development. [orchido- + G. *metron*, measure]

or·chi·do·pexy (ōr-kid′ō-peks-e). SYN orchiopexy.

or·chi·dop·to·sis (ōr′ki-dop-tō′sis). Ptosis of the male gonads. [orchido- + G. *ptōsis*, a falling]

or·chi·dor·ra·phy (ōr-ki-dōr′ă-fē). SYN orchiopexy.

or·chi·ec·to·my (ōr-kē-ek′tō-mē). Removal of one or both testes. SYN orchectomy, orchidectomy, testectomy. [orchi- + G. *ektomē*, excision]

or·chi·ep·i·did·y·mi·tis (ōr′kē-ep′i-did′i-mī′tis). Inflammation of the testis and epididymis. [orchi- + epididymis, + G. *-itis*, inflammation]

or·chil (ōr′kil) [old C.I. 1242]. SYN archil.

△**orchio-.** SEE orchi-.

or·chi·o·cele (ōr′kē-ō-sēl). A testis retained in the inguinal canal. [orchio- + G. *kēlē*, hernia, tumor]

or·chi·o·dyn·ia (ōr′kē-ō-din′ē-ă). SYN orchialgia. [orchi- + G. *odynē*, pain]

or·chi·on·cus (ōr-kē-ong′kŭs). A neoplasm of the testis. [orchio- + G. *onkos*, bulk, mass]

or·chi·o·neu·ral·gia (ōr′kē-ō-noo-ral′jē-ă). SYN orchialgia. [orchio- + G. *neuron*, nerve, + *algos*, pain]

or·chi·op·a·thy (ōr-kē-op′ă-thē). Disease of a testis. [orchio- + G. *pathos*, suffering]

or·chi·o·pexy (ōr′kē-ō-pek′sē). **1.** Surgical treatment of an undescended testicle by freeing it and implanting it into the scrotum. **2.** Anchoring a testis susceptible to torsion in the scrotum. SYN orchidopexy, orchidorraphy, orchiorrhaphy. [orchio- + G. *pēxis*, fixation]

transseptal o., SYN Ombrédanne *operation.*

or·chi·o·plas·ty (ōr′kē-ō-plas-tē). Surgical reconstruction of the testis. [orchio- + G. *plastos*, formed]

or·chi·or·rha·phy (ōr-kē-ōr′ă-fē). SYN orchiopexy. [orchio- + G. *rhaphē*, a suture]

or·chi·o·ther·a·py (ōr′kē-ō-thār′ă-pē). Treatment with testicular extracts.

or·chi·ot·o·my (ōr-kē-ot′ō-mē). Incision into a testis. SYN orchotomy. [orchio- + G. *tomē*, incision]

or·chis, pl. **or·chis·es** (ōr′kis, ōr′ki-sēz). SYN testis. [G. testis, an orchid]

or·chit·ic (ōr-kit′ik). Denoting orchitis.

or·chi·tis (ōr-kī′tis). Inflammation of the testis. SYN orchiditis, testitis. [orchi- + G. *-itis*, inflammation]

o. parotid′ea, o. associated with mumps.

traumatic o., simple inflammation of the testis caused by mechanical injury.

o. variolo′sa, o. complicating smallpox.

or·chot·o·my (ōr-kot′ō-mē). SYN orchiotomy.

or·cin (ōr′sin). SYN orcinol.

or·cin·ol (ōr′sin-ol). 3,5-Dihydroxytoluene; the parent substance of the natural dye orcein, obtained from certain colorless lichens (*Lecanora tinctoria, Rocella tinctoria*) by treatment with boiling water; used as an external antiseptic in various skin diseases and in chemistry as a reagent for pentoses. SYN 5-methylresorcinol, orcin.

or·ci·pren·a·line sul·fate (ōr-si-pren′ă-lēn). SYN metaproterenol sulfate.

ORD Abbreviation for optic rotatory *dispersion.*

Ord Symbol for orotidine.

or·deal bean (ōr′dē-ăl). SYN physostigma.

or·der (ōr′der). **1.** In biologic classification, the division just below the class (or subclass) and above the family. **2.** In a reaction, o. is the sum of the exponents of all the concentration terms in that reaction's rate expression. For example, for the natural decomposition of nitrogen pentoxide, the rate expression is $v = -d[N_2O_5]/dt = k_1[N_2O_5]$. Thus, this is a first-order reaction. A reaction involving two different compounds is often a second-order reaction (but not necessarily so). Pseudo–first-order reactions are multiorder reactions in which one of the reactants is in substoichiometric amounts. Cf. molecularity. **3.** The sequence of residues in a heteropolymer. [L. *ordo*, regular arrangement]

pecking o., in some species of birds and primates, the establishment of a graded dominance in members of a group by the use of aggression.

or·dered (ord′erd). SYN ordered *mechanism*.

or·der·ly (ōr′der-lē). An attendant in a hospital unit who assists in the care of patients.

or·di·nate (ōr′di-nāt). In a plane cartesian coordinate system, the vertical axis (*y*). Cf. abscissa.

orec·tic (ō-rek′tik). Pertaining to or characterized by orexia.

orex·ia (ō-rek′sē-ă). **1.** The affective and conative aspects of an act, in contrast to the cognitive aspect. **2.** SYN appetite. [G. *orexis*, appetite]

orex·i·gen·ic (ŏ-rek-si-jen′ik). Appetite stimulating.

orf. A specific disease of sheep and goats, caused by the orf virus, family Poxviridae. This virus is transmissible to humans and characterized by vesiculation and ulceration of the infected site. SYN contagious ecthyma, scabby mouth, soremouth. [O.E. *orfcwealm*, murrain, fr. *orf*, cattle, + *cwealm*, destruction]

or·gan (ōr′găn) [TA]. Any part of the body exercising a specific function, as of respiration, secretion, or digestion. SYN organum [TA], organon. [L. *organum*, fr. G. *organon*, a tool, instrument]

accessory o.'s, (1) SYN accessory *structures*, under *structure*; **(2)** SYN supernumerary o.'s.

accessory o.'s of the eye, SYN accessory visual *structures*, under *structure*.

annulospiral o., SYN annulospiral *ending*.

auditory o., archaic term for Corti o.

Chievitz o., a normal epithelial structure, possibly a neurotransmitter, found at the angle of the mandible with branches of the buccal nerve.

circumventricular o.'s, four small areas in or near the base of the brain that have fenestrated capillaries and are outside the blood-brain barrier. They are neurohypophysis, area postrema [TA], organum vasculosum of lamina terminalis [TA], and subfornical organ [TA] (SFO). The neurohypophysis is a neurohemal organ. The other three are chemoreceptors: area postrema triggers vomiting in response to chemical changes in plasma, organum vasculosum of the lamina terminalis senses osmolality and alters vasopressin secretion, and SFO initiates drinking in response to angiotensin II.

Corti o., SYN spiral o.

critical o., the o. or physiologic system that for a given source of radiation would first reach its legally defined maximum permissible radiation exposure as the dose of radiation is increased; e.g., the kidney is the critical organ, receiving the most radiation, when Tc-99m dimethylsuccinic acid is given.

enamel o., a circumscribed mass of ectodermal cells budded off from the dental lamina; it becomes cup shaped and develops on its internal face the ameloblast layer of cells that produce the enamel cap of a developing tooth.

end o., the special structure containing the terminal of a nerve fiber in peripheral tissue such as muscle, tissue, skin, mucous membrane, or glands. SEE ALSO ending.

external female genital o.'s, SYN female external *genitalia*.

external male genital o.'s, SYN male external *genitalia*.

floating o., SYN wandering o.

flower-spray o. of Ruffini, SYN flower-spray *ending*.

genital o.'s, SYN genitalia.

Golgi tendon o., a proprioceptive sensory nerve ending embedded among the fibers of a tendon, often near the musculotendi-

nous junction; it is compressed and activated by any increase of the tendon's tension, caused either by active contraction or passive stretch of the corresponding muscle. SYN neurotendinous o., neurotendinous spindle.

gustatory o. [TA], located in the papillae of the mucous membrane of the tongue, chiefly in the vallate papillae. SYN organum gustatorium [TA], organum gustus [TA], o. of taste.

o. of hearing, SYN cochlear *labyrinth*.

internal female genital o.'s, SYN female internal *genitalia*.

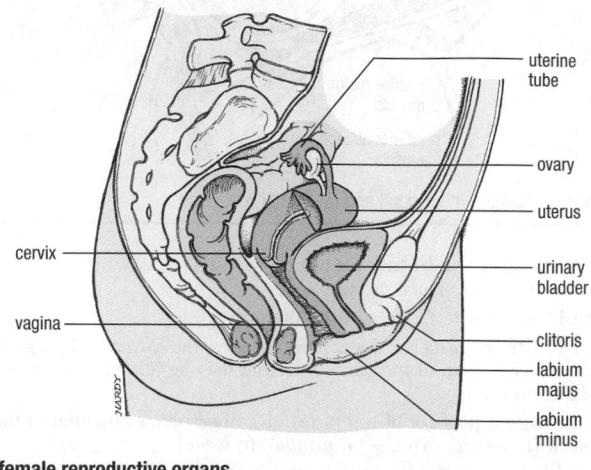

female reproductive organs

internal male genital o.'s, SYN male internal *genitalia*.

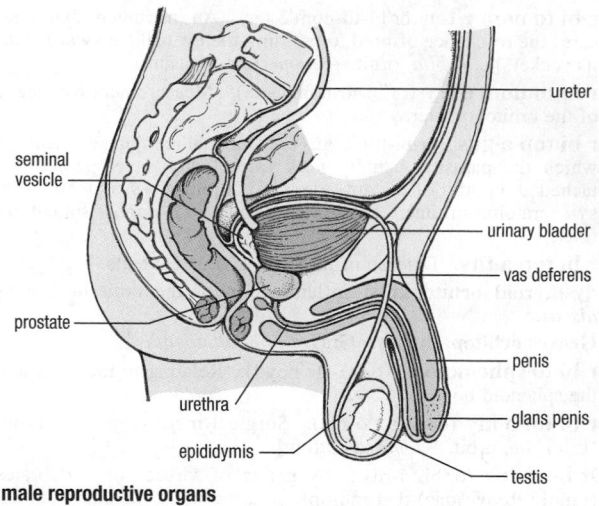

male reproductive organs

intromittent o., SYN penis.

Jacobson o., SYN vomeronasal o.

neurohemal o.'s, brain areas from which substances enter blood e.g., the neurohypophysis from which oxytocin and vasopressin enter blood.

neurotendinous o., SYN Golgi tendon o.

olfactory o. [TA], the olfactory region in the superior portion of the nasal cavity. SYN organum olfactus [TA], o. of smell.

otolithic o.'s, the utricle and saccule of the inner ear that possess otoliths and respond to linear acceleration and deceleration, including gravity.

ptotic o., SYN wandering o.

o. of Rosenmüller, SYN epoophoron.

sense o.'s [TA], the organs of special sense, including the eye, ear, olfactory organ, taste organs, and the accessory structures associated with these organs. SYN organa sensuum.

o. of smell, SYN olfactory o.

spiral o. [TA], a prominent ridge of highly specialized epithelium in the floor of the cochlear duct overlying the basilar membrane of cochlea, containing one inner row and three outer rows of hair cells, or cells of Corti (the auditory receptor cells innervated by the cochlear nerve) supported by various columnar cells: the pillars of Corti, cells of Hensen, and cells of Claudius; the spiral o. is partly overhung by an awninglike shelf, the tectorial membrane, the free marginal zone of which is covered by a gelatinous substance in which the stereocilia of the outer hair cells are embedded. SYN organum spirale [TA], acoustic papilla, Corti o.

subcommissural o. [TA], a microscopic organ, made up of columnar ciliated ependymal cells, located in the cerebral aqueduct beneath the posterior commissure of the brain; it is believed to have a neurosecretory function. SYN organum subcommissurale.

subfornical o. (SFO), the intercolumnar tubercle. One of the circumventricular o.'s. SFO has fenestrated capillaries and is outside the blood-brain barrier. It is thought to be a chemoreceptor zone involved in cardiovascular regulation. SYN organum subformicale [TA].

supernumerary o.'s, o.'s exceeding the normal number, which may develop from multiple foci of organization in an organformative field larger (originally) than that of the definitive main o.; such o.'s are aberrant but frequently not a cause of disease; illness may persist if they are left in the body after therapeutic removal of the main o., e.g., accessory spleen. SYN accessory o.'s (2).

tactile o., SYN o. of touch.

target o., a tissue or o. upon which a hormone exerts its action; generally, a tissue or organ with appropriate receptors for a hormone. SYN target (3).

o. of taste, SYN gustatory o.

o. of touch, any one of the sensory end o.'s. SYN organum tactus, tactile o.

urinary o.'s, organs involved with the formation, storage, and excretion of urine. SEE ALSO urinary *system*. SYN organa urinaria.

vascular o. of lamina terminalis [TA], SEE circumventricular o.'s. SYN organum vasculosum laminae terminalis [TA].

vestibular o., SYN vestibular *labyrinth*.

vestibulocochlear o. [TA], the external, middle, and internal ear. SYN organum vestibulocochleare [TA].

vestigial o., a rudimentary structure in humans corresponding to a functional structure or o. in the lower animals.

o. of vision, SYN visual o.

visual o., the eye and its adnexa. SYN o. of vision, organum visus.

vomeronasal o. [TA], a fine vestigal horizontal canal, ending in a blind pouch, in the mucous membrane of the nasal septum, beginning just behind and above the incisive duct; a structure that usually regresses after the 6th month of gestation. In many lower animals, it functions as an accessory olfactory organ. SYN organum vomeronasale [TA], Jacobson o.

wandering o., an o. with loose attachments, permitting its displacement. SYN floating o., ptotic o.

Weber o., SYN prostatic *utricle*.

o.'s of Zuckerkandl, SYN paraaortic *bodies*, under *body*.

or·ga·na (ōr′gă-nă). Plural of organum.

or·gan·elle (or′gă-nel). One of the specialized parts of a protozoan or tissue cell; these subcellular units include mitochondria, the Golgi apparatus, nucleus and centrioles, granular and agranular endoplasmic reticulum, vacuoles, microsomes, lysosomes, plasma membrane, and certain fibrils, as well as plastids of plant cells. SYN cell o., organoid (3). [G. *organon*, organ, + Fr. -*elle*, dim. suffix, fr. L. -*ella*]

cell o., SYN organelle.

paired o.'s, SYN rhoptry.

or·gan·ic (ōr-gan′ik). 1. Relating to an organ. 2. Relating to or formed by an organism. 3. Organized; structural. 4. SEE organic *compound*. [G. *organikos*]

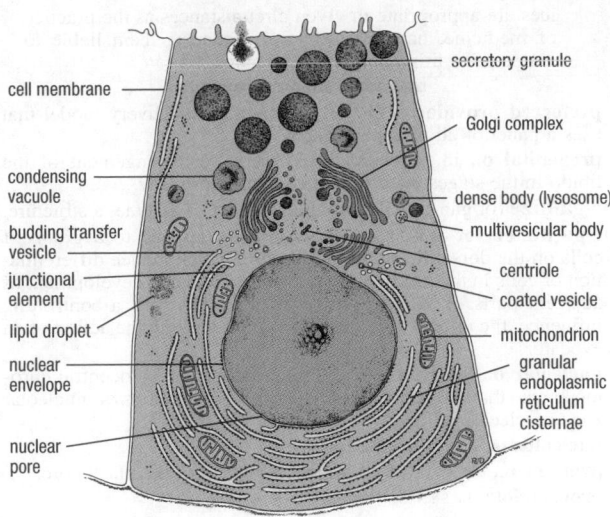

organelles: a secretory cell as it would appear in a thin section viewed in an electron microscope

Labels: cell membrane; condensing vacuole; budding transfer vesicle; junctional element; lipid droplet; nuclear envelope; nuclear pore; secretory granule; Golgi complex; dense body (lysosome); multivesicular body; centriole; coated vesicle; mitochondrion; granular endoplasmic reticulum cisternae

or·gan·i·cism (ōr-gan′i-sizm). A theory that attributes all diseases, in particular, all mental disorders, as organic in origin.

or·gan·i·cist (ōr-gan′i-sist). One who believes in, or subscribes to the views of, organicism.

or·gan·i·din. SYN iodinated *glycerol*.

or·ga·nism (ōr′gă-nizm). Any living individual, whether plant or animal, considered as a whole.

calculated mean o. (CMO), a hypothetical o. whose characters are the means of both the positive and negative characters of the o.'s which belong to the same taxon as the CMO, as opposed to the hypothetical mean. o.

defective o., SYN auxotrophic *mutant*.

fastidious o., a bacterial organism having complex nutritional requirements.

hypothetical mean o. (HMO), a hypothetical o. whose characters are the means of the positive characters of the organisms which belong to the same taxon as the HMO, as opposed to the calculated mean o.

pleuropneumonia-like o.'s (PPLO), the original name given to a group of bacteria that did not possess cell walls; these o.'s, isolated from humans and other animals, soil, and sewage, are now assigned to the order Mycoplasmatales.

or·ga·ni·za·tion (ōr′gan-i-zā′shŭn). 1. An arrangement of distinct but mutually dependent parts. 2. The conversion of coagulated blood, exudate, or dead tissue into fibrous tissue.

health maintenance o. (HMO), a comprehensive prepaid system of health care intended to have emphasis on the prevention and early detection of disease, and continuity of care; often used synonymously with "managed care plan."

The term HMO refers to a health care delivery system characterized by multiplicity of services (primary care physicians and specialists, laboratory, radiology, pharmacy, and hospitalization); restriction of services to subscribers, and of benefits to participating health care providers, both typically confined to a certain geographic area; and an accounting system based on prepayment rather than fee for service. An HMO may be a nonprofit institution or a commercial venture. During the last quarter of the 20th century, HMOs emerged as an important alternative to traditional medical indemnity insurance plans, and largely supplanted them. HMOs have had a profound effect on every aspect of the practice of medicine: professional, scientific, social, economic, and legal. Some state legislatures, seeing the HMO's determining which medical serv-

or

ices are appropriate in given circumstances as the practice of medicine, have passed laws rendering them liable to malpractice litigation. SEE ALSO managed care.

preferred provider o. (PPO), a health care delivery model that uses a panel of eligible physicians.

pregenital o., in psychoanalysis, the o. or arrangement of the libido in the stages prior to that of genital primacy.

or·ga·nize (ōr'gan-īz). To provide with, or to assume, a structure.

or·ga·niz·er (ōr'gan-ī-zer). **1.** Originally applied to a group of cells on the dorsal lip of the blastopore, which induce differentiation of cells in the embryo and control growth and development of adjacent parts. **2.** Any group of cells having such a controlling influence, the effects being brought about through the action of an evocator.

nucleolar o., the region of the satellites on the acrocentric chromosomes that is active in nucleolus formation. SYN nucleolar zone, nucleolus o.

nucleolus o., SYN nucleolar o.

primary o., the o. situated on the dorsal lip of the blastopore.

procentriole o., SYN deuterosome.

△**organo-.** Organ; organic. [G. *organon*]

or·ga·no·ax·i·al (ōr-gă'nō-aks'ē-ăl). Rotation around the long axis of the organ; a type of gastric volvulus.

or·gan·o·fer·ric (ōr'gă-nō-fār'ik). Relating to an organic compound containing iron.

or·gan·o·gel (ōr-gan'ō-jel). A hydrogel with an organic liquid instead of water as the dispersion means.

or·ga·no·gen·e·sis (ōr'gă-nō-jen'ĕ-sis). Formation of organs during development. SYN organogeny. [organo- + G. *genesis*, origin]

or·ga·no·ge·net·ic, *or* **or·ga·no·gen·ic** (ōr'gă-nō-jĕ-net'ik, -jen'ik). Relating to organogenesis.

or·ga·nog·e·ny (ōr-gan-oj'ĕ-nē). SYN organogenesis.

or·ga·nog·ra·phy (ōr'gă-nog'ră-fē). A treatise on, or description of, the organs of the body. [organo- + G. *graphē*, a writing]

or·gan·oid (ōr'gă-noyd). **1.** Resembling in superficial appearance or in structure any of the organs or glands of the body. **2.** Composed of glandular or organic elements and not of a single tissue; pertaining to certain neoplasms (e.g., an adenoma) that contain cytologic and histologic elements arranged in a pattern that closely resembles or is virtually identical to a normal organ. SEE ALSO histoid. **3.** SYN organelle. [organo- + G. *eidos*, resemblance]

or·ga·no·lep·tic (ōr'gă-nō-lep'tik). **1.** Stimulating any of the organs of sensation. **2.** Susceptible to a sensory stimulus. [organo- + G. *lēptikos*, disposed to accept]

or·ga·nol·o·gy (ōr-gă-nol'ō-jē). Branch of science concerned with the anatomy, physiology, development, and functions of the various organs. SEE ALSO splanchnology. [organo- + G. *logos*, study]

or·ga·no·meg·a·ly (ōr'gă-nō-meg'ă-lē). SYN visceromegaly.

or·gan·o·mer·cur·i·al (ōr-gan'ō-mer-kū'rē-ăl). Any organic mercurial compound; e.g., merbromin, thimerosal.

or·ga·no·me·tal·lic (ōr'gă-nō-me-tal'ik). Denoting an organic compound containing one or more metallic atoms in its structure.

or·ga·non, pl. **or·ga·na** (ōr'gă-non, ōr'gă-nă). SYN organ. [G. organ]

or·ga·non·o·my (ōr-gă-non'ō-mē). The body of laws regulating the life processes of organized beings. [organo- + G. *nomos*, law]

or·ga·non·y·my (ōr'gă-non'i-mē). The nomenclature of the organs of the body, as distinguished from toponymy. [organo- + G. *onyma*, name]

or·ga·nop·a·thy (ōr-gă-nop'ă-thē). Any disease especially affecting one of the organs of the body. [organo- + G. *pathos*, suffering]

or·ga·no·pexy, *or* **or·ga·no·pex·ia** (ōr'gă-nō-pek-sē, -pek'sē-ă). Fixation by suture or otherwise of a floating or ptotic organ. [organo- + G. *pēxis*, fixation]

or·ga·no·phil·ic (ōr'gă-nō-fil'ik). Pertaining to organophilicity.

or·ga·no·phi·lic·i·ty (ōr'gă-nō-fi-li'si-tē). Attraction of nonpolar substances (organic molecules) to each other.

or·ga·no·phos·phates (ōr-gă-nō-fos'fāts). A series of phospho-

rus-containing organic compounds usually also containing a halide ion that reacts with cholinesterase. Organophosphates phosphorylate cholinesterase and thus irreversibly inhibit it. Used as insecticides; have also been used as war gases.

or·gan·o·sol (ōr-gan'ō-sol). A hydrosol with an organic liquid instead of water as the dispersion means.

or·ga·no·tax·is (ōr'gă-nō-tak'sis). The tendency to migrate to a certain organ selectively. [organo- + G. *taxis*, orderly arrangement]

or·ga·no·ther·a·py (ōr'gă-nō-thār'ă-pē). Treatment of disease by preparations made from animal organs; now frequently by synthetic preparations instead of extracts of a gland.

or·ga·no·tro·phic (ōr'gă-nō-trof'ik). **1.** Pertaining to the nourishment of an organ. **2.** Pertaining to a microorganism that uses organic sources as a reducing power. [organo- + G. *trophē*, nourishment]

or·ga·no·tro·pic (ōr'gă-nō-trop'ik). Pertaining to or characterized by organotropism.

or·ga·not·ro·pism (ōr-gă-not'rō-pizm). The special affinity of particular drugs, pathogens, or metastatic tumors for particular organs or their component parts. Cf. parasitotropism. SYN organotropy. [organo- + G. *tropē*, a turning]

or·ga·not·ro·py (ōr-gă-not'rō-pē). SYN organotropism.

or·gan-spe·cif·ic. **1.** Denoting or pertaining to a serum produced by the injection of the cells of a certain organ or tissue that, when injected into another animal, destroys the cells of the corresponding organ. **2.** Denoting an antigen specific for a particular organ.

or·ga·num, pl. **or·ga·na** (ōr'gă-nŭm, ōr'gă-nă) [TA]. SYN organ, organ. [L. tool, instrument]

o. audi'tus, archaic term for vestibulocochlear *organ.*

or'gana genita'lia [TA], SYN genitalia.

organa genita'lia femini'na exter'na, SYN female external *genitalia.*

organa genita'lia femini'na inter'na, SYN female internal *genitalia.*

organa genita'lia masculi'na exter'na, SYN male external *genitalia.*

organa genita'lia masculi'na inter'na, SYN male internal *genitalia.*

o. gustatorium [TA], SYN gustatory *organ.*

o. gus'tus [TA], SYN gustatory *organ.*

or'gana oc'uli accesso'ria, SYN accessory visual *structures,* under *structure.*

o. olfac'tus [TA], SYN olfactory *organ.*

or'gana sen'suum, SYN sense *organs,* under *organ.*

o. spira'le [TA], SYN spiral *organ.*

o. subcommissurale, SYN subcommissural *organ.*

o. subformicale [TA], SYN subfornical *organ;* SEE circumventricular *organs,* under *organ.*

o. tac'tus, SYN *organ* of touch.

or'gana urina'ria, SYN urinary *organs,* under *organ.*

o. vasculosum laminae terminalis [TA], SYN vascular *organ* of lamina terminalis; SEE circumventricular *organs,* under *organ.*

o. vestibulocochlea're [TA], SYN vestibulocochlear *organ.*

o. vi'sus, SYN visual *organ.*

o. vomeronasa'le [TA], SYN vomeronasal *organ.*

or·gasm (ōr'gazm). The acme of the sexual act. SYN climax (2). [G. *orgaō*, to swell, be excited]

or·gas·mic, *or* **or·gas·tic** (ōr-gaz'mik, -gas'tik). Relating to, characteristic of, or tending to produce an orgasm.

or·i·en·ta·tion (ōr-ē-en-tā'shŭn). **1.** The recognition of one's temporal, spatial, and personal relationships and environment. **2.** The relative position of an atom with respect to one to which it is connected, i.e., the direction of the bond connecting them. [Fr. *orienter,* to set toward the East, therefore in a definite position]

sexual o., concept that includes the permutations among body morphology, gender identity, gender role, and sexual preference.

Orientia (ōr-ē-en'-ă). A member of the bacterial family Rickettsiae.

O. tsutsugamushi, the only member of its genus, this species is the causative agent of scrub typhus, transmitted by mites; formerly called *Rickettsia tsutsugamushi*.

or·i·en·to·my·cin (or′ē-en-tō-mī′sin). SYN cycloserine.

or·i·fice (or′i-fis) [TA]. Any aperture or opening. SEE ALSO aperture, opening, os, ostium, meatus. SYN orificium [TA]. [L. *orificium*]

anal o., SYN anus.

aortic o. [TA], the opening from the left ventricle into the ascending aorta; it is guarded by the aortic valve. SYN ostium aortae [TA], aortic ostium.

cardiac o., SYN cardial o.

cardial o. [TA], the trumpet-shaped opening of the esophagus into the stomach. SYN ostium cardiacum [TA], cardiac opening, cardiac o., esophagogastric o.

esophagogastric o., SYN cardial o.

o. of external acoustic meatus, SYN external acoustic *pore*.

external urethral o. [TA], **(1)** the slitlike opening of the urethra in the glans penis; **(2)** the external orifice of the urethra (in the female) in the vestibule, usually upon a slight elevation, the papilla urethrae. SYN ostium urethrae externum [TA], external urinary meatus⁎, external opening of urethra, meatus urinarius, orificium urethrae externum.

filling internal urethral o. [TA], the internal urethral orifice once the bladder begins to be distended with urine, when the trigonal muscles are contracted and the detrusor muscle is relaxed; during this stage the orifice occurs at a higher level, and is bounded by a different portion of the mucosa, than during voiding. SEE ALSO voiding internal urethral o. SYN ostium urethrae internum accipiens [TA].

gastroduodenal o., SYN pyloric o.

golf-hole ureteral o., a circular and often escessively lateral ureteral o. that may be associated with vesicoureteral reflux, previous bladder surgery, or tuberculosis.

ileal o. [TA], the opening of the terminal ileum into the large intestine at the transition between the cecum and the ascending colon. SYN ostium ileale [TA], o. of ileal papilla⁎, ileocecal opening, ileocecal o., ostium ileocecale.

o. of ileal papilla, ⁎official alternate term for ileal o.

ileocecal o., SYN ileal o.

o. of inferior vena cava, SYN *opening* of inferior vena cava.

o. of internal acoustic meatus, SYN internal acoustic *pore*.

internal urethral o. [TA], the internal opening or orifice of the urethra, at the anterior and inferior angle of the trigone. SYN ostium urethrae internum [TA], internal urethral opening⁎.

left atrioventricular o. [TA], an atrioventricular opening that leads from the left atrium into the left ventricle of the heart. SYN ostium atrioventriculare sinistrum [TA], mitral o., ostium arteriosum.

mitral o., SYN left atrioventricular o.

pulmonary o., SYN *opening* of pulmonary trunk.

pyloric o. [TA], the opening between the stomach and the superior part of the duodenum. SYN ostium pyloricum [TA], gastroduodenal o.

right atrioventricular o. [TA], an atrioventricular opening that leads from the right atrium into the right ventricle of the heart. SYN ostium atrioventriculare dextrum [TA], ostium venosum cordis, tricuspid o.

root canal o., an opening in the pulp chamber leading to the root canal.

o. of superior vena cava, SYN *opening* of superior vena cava.

tricuspid o., SYN right atrioventricular o.

ureteric o. [TA], the opening of the ureter in the bladder, situated one at each lateral angle of the trigone; wide gaping of the o. usually indicates vesicoureteral reflux. SYN ostium ureteris [TA], orificium ureteris, ureteral meatus, ureteral opening.

o. of uterus, SYN external *os* of uterus.

vaginal o. [TA], the narrowest portion of the canal, in the floor of the vestibule posterior to the urethral orifice. SYN ostium vaginae [TA], orificium vaginae, vaginal opening.

o. of vermiform appendix [TA], the opening of the vermiform appendix into the lumen of the cecum. SYN ostium appendicis vermiformis [TA], ostium of vermiform appendix.

voiding internal urethral o. [TA], the internal urethral orifice when the bladder is being emptied of urine, when the trigonal muscles are relaxed and the detrusor muscle is contracting; during this stage the orifice occurs at a lower level, and is bounded by a different portion of the mucosa, than during filling and reserving. SEE ALSO filling internal urethral o. SYN ostium urethrae internum evacuans [TA].

or·i·fi·cial (ōr-i-fish′ăl). Relating to an orifice of any kind.

or·i·fi·ci·um, pl. **or·i·fi·ci·a** (ōr-i-fish′ē-ŭm, -ă) [TA]. SYN orifice, orifice. [L.]

o. exter′num u′teri, SYN external *os* of uterus.

o. inter′num u′teri, SYN *isthmus* of uterus.

o. ure′teris, SYN ureteric *orifice*.

o. ure′thrae exter′num, SYN external urethral *orifice*.

o. vagi′nae, SYN vaginal *orifice*.

orig·a·num oil (ŏ-rig′ă-nŭm). The volatile oil (which contains carvacrol) obtained from various species of *Origanum* (family Labiatae); used as a rubefacient, as a constituent in veterinary liniments, and in microscopic techniques.

or·i·gin (ōr′i-jin). **1.** The less movable of the two points of attachment of a muscle, that which is attached to the more fixed part of the skeleton. **2.** The starting point of a cranial or spinal nerve. The former have two o.'s: the **ental o., deep o.,** or **real o.,** the cell group in the brain or medulla, whence the fibers of the nerve begin, and the **ectal o., superficial o.,** or **apparent o.,** the point where the nerve emerges from the brain. [L. *origo,* source, beginning, fr. *orior,* to rise]

o. of replication, a sequence of the bacterial genome required for the initiating of a replicating fork by leading strand synthesis.

ori·za·ba jal·ap root (ŏ-riz′ă-bă ja′lap). SYN ipomea.

Ormond, John K., U.S. urologist, *1886. SEE O. *disease*.

Orn Symbol for ornithine or its radical.

or·nate (ōr′nāt). A term that refers to the patterning of the scutum (gray or white markings on a dark background) in ixodid ticks. [L. *ornatus,* decorated]

Ornish, Dean, U.S. physician, *1953. SEE O. reversal *diet*.

or·ni·thine (Orn) (ōr′ni-thēn, -thin). 2,5-Diaminovaleric acid; the L-isomer is the amino acid formed when L-arginine is hydrolyzed by arginase; not a constituent of proteins, but an important intermediate in the urea cycle; elevated levels seen in certain defects of the urea cycle.

o. acetyltransferase, SYN *glutamate* acetyltransferase.

o. δ-aminotransferase, an enzyme that will reversibly catalyze the reaction of α-ketoglutarate and L-o. to form L-glutamate and L-glutamate γ-semialdehyde; a deficiency of this enzyme will result in gyrate atrophy of the choroid and retina. SYN o. transaminase.

o. carbamoyltransferase, an enzyme catalyzing formation of L-citrulline and orthophosphate from L-o. and carbamoyl phosphate; a part of the urea cycle; a deficiency of this enzyme will result in ammonia intoxication and impaired urea formation. SYN o. transcarbamoylase.

o. decarboxylase, an enzyme catalyzing the decarboxylation of L-o. to putrescine and CO_2; first step in polyamine biosynthesis.

o. transaminase, SYN o. δ-aminotransferase.

o. transcarbamoylase, SYN o. carbamoyltransferase.

or·ni·thi·ne·mia (ōr′ni-thi-nē′mē-ă). A toxic condition occasionally producing localized cerebral swelling, caused by abnormal amounts of ornithine in the blood. [ornithine + G. *haima,* blood]

or·ni·thi·nu·ria (ōr′ni-thi-noo′rē-ă). Excretion of excessive amounts of ornithine in the urine.

Or·ni·thod·o·ros (ōr-ni-thod′ŏ-rŭs). A genus of soft ticks (family Argasidae), several species of which are vectors of pathogens of various relapsing fevers. They are characterized by a capitulum hidden below the hood and by disks and mamillae of the integument that are continuous from dorsal to ventral surfaces in a variety of patterns. [G. *ornis* (ornith-), bird, + *doros,* a leather bag]

O. coria′ceus, a tick species common in the mountainous coastal areas of California; adults readily attack deer, cattle, and humans, and have an irritating, painful, sometimes toxic bite. Transmits epizootic bovine abortion to cattle. SYN pajaroello.

O. errat'icus, a species of tick the small variety of which is the vector of *Borrelia crocidurae* in Africa, the Near East, and Central Asia; the large variety is the vector of *B. hispanica* in the Spanish peninsula and adjacent north Africa.

O. herm'si, a tick species that is a rodent parasite and vector of relapsing fever spirochetes, such as *Borrelia hermsii,* in the western U.S. and Canada.

O. lahoren'sis, a species of tick that may transmit *Borrelia persica,* the agent of Persian relapsing fever.

O. mouba'ta complex, a group of four tick species in Africa; the taxonomy and ecology of this complex is of great significance because its members are vectors of relapsing fever spirochetes; members of the complex include *O. moubata* (various hosts), *O. compactus* (tortoises), *O. apertus* (porcupines), and *O. porcinus* (warthogs); a domestic subspecies of *O. porcinus,* in turn, forms three strains that feed chiefly on humans, fowl, and swine.

O. pappil'ipes, the "Persian bug," a tick species found in Central Asia and the Near East that transmits *Borrelia persica,* the pathogen in Iran of Persian relapsing fever.

O. par'keri, a tick species found in the western U.S. and a vector of *Borrelia parkeri.*

O. ru'dis, a tick species that is an important vector of relapsing fever spirochetes in Central and South America; possibly another complex similar to the *O. moubata* complex.

O. savi'gni, a tick species transmitting *Borrelia,* an agent of relapsing fever of eastern Africa, southern Egypt, Ethiopia, and southwestern Asia.

O. talajé, a tick species found in Mexico and in Central and South America, where it feeds on wild rodents, domestic animals, and humans; it delivers a painful, irritating bite and is a vector of *Borrelia mazzottii,* a cause of relapsing fever.

O. tholoza'ni, a species of tick that transmits *Borrelia persica,* an agent of relapsing fever in the Middle East and central Asia.

O. turica'ta, a species of tick that readily attacks humans and other animals in the southern portion of the U.S. and Mexico; it is a vector of *Borrelia turicatae,* an agent of relapsing fever; the bite is painful and irritating.

O. venezuelen'sis, a tick species that is the vector of *Borrelia venezuelensis,* agent of relapsing fever in Colombia, Venezuela, and mountainous parts of South America.

O. verruco'sus, a tick species, the vector of *Borrelia caucasica.*

Or·ni·tho·nys·sus (ōr-ni-thon′i-sŭs). A genus of bird and rodent mites; species include *O. bacoti,* the tropical rat mite, a possible vector of murine typhus and a cause of human dermatitis; *O. bursa,* the tropical fowl mite; and *O. sylviarum,* the northern fowl mite. [G. *ornis* (*ornith-*), bird, + *nyssus,* to prick]

or·ni·tho·sis (ōr-ni-thō′sis). Originally, a disease in nonpsittacine birds (domestic fowl, ducks, pigeons, turkeys, and many wild birds) caused by *Chlamydia psittaci;* now, generally referred to as psittacosis. [G. *ornis* (*ornith-*), bird, + *-osis,* condition]

Oro Symbol for orotic acid or orotate.

△**oro-.** **1.** The mouth. [L. *os, oris,* mouth] **2.** Obsolete alternative spelling is orrho-. SEE sero-. [G. *orrhos,* whey, serum]

or·o·dig·i·to·fa·cial (ōr′ō-dij′i-tō-fā′shăl). Relating to the mouth, fingers, and face.

or·o·fa·cial (ōr-ō-fā′shăl). Relating to the mouth and face.

or·o·lin·gual (ōr-ō-ling′gwăl). Relating to the mouth and tongue.

or·o·na·sal (ōr-ō-nā′săl). Relating to the mouth and nose.

or·o·pha·ryn·ge·al (ōr-ō-fă-rin′jē-ăl). Relating to the oropharynx.

or·o·phar·ynx (ōr′ō-far′ingks) [TA]. The portion of the pharynx that lies posterior to the mouth; it is continuous above with the nasopharynx via the pharyngeal isthmus and below with the laryngopharynx. SYN pars oralis pharyngis [TA], oral part of pharynx, oral pharynx. [L. *os* (*or-*), mouth]

or·o·so·mu·coid (ōr′ō-sō-mū′koyd). α₁-Acid glycoprotein; a subgroup of the α₁-globulin fraction of blood; increased plasma lev-

els are associated with inflammation. SYN α₁-acid glycoprotein, acid seromucoid.

or·o·tate (Oro) (ōr′ō-tāt). A salt or ester of orotic acid.

o. phosphoribosyltransferase, a phosphoribosyltransferase synthesizing orotidylate and pyrophosphate from orotate and 5-phospho-α-D-ribosyl-1-pyrophosphate; this enzyme is a part of pyrimidine biosynthesis; a deficiency of this enzyme is associated with orotic aciduria type I. Cf. *uridylic acid* synthase. SYN OMP pyrophosphorylase, orotidylic acid phosphorylase, orotidylic acid pyrophosphorylase.

orot·ic ac·id (Oro) (ōr-ot′ik). 6-Carboxyuracil; uracil-6-carboxylic acid; an important intermediate in the formation of the pyrimidine nucleotides; elevated in certain inherited defects of pyrimidine biosynthesis. SYN uracil-6-carboxylic acid.

orot·ic ac·i·du·ria [MIM*258900]. A rare disorder of pyrimidine metabolism characterized by hypochromic anemia with megaloblastic changes in bone marrow, leukopenia, retarded growth, and urinary excretion of orotic acid; autosomal recessive inheritance, caused by mutation in the uridine monophosphatate synthase gene (MMPS) on 3q13. [orotic acid + G. *ouron,* urine]

orot·i·dine (O, Ord) (ō-rot′i-dēn). Orotic acid-3-β-D-ribonucleoside; uridine-6-carboxylic acid; elevated in cases of orotidinuria. SYN 1-ribosylorotate.

o. 5′-monophosphate (OMP), SYN orotidylic acid.

orot·i·di·nu·ria (ō-rot′i-dēn-ū′rē-ă). Elevated levels of orotidine in the urine; has been observed in defects in and inhibition of orotidylic acid decarboxylase.

orot·i·dyl·ate (OMP) (ō-rot-i-dil′āt). A salt or ester of orotidylic acid.

orot·i·dyl·ic ac·id (OMP) (ō-rot-i-dil′ik). Orotidine 5′-monophosphate; an intermediate in the biosynthesis of the pyrimidine nucleosides (cytidine and uridine) that are found in nucleic acids. SYN orotidine 5′-monophosphate.

o. a. decarboxylase, an enzyme that catalyzes the conversion of OMP to UMP and CO₂; a defect or inhibition of this enzyme will result in orotic aciduria and orotidinuria; this enzyme is a part of pyrimidine biosynthesis. Cf. *uridylic acid* synthase. SYN OMP decarboxylase.

o. a. phosphorylase, SYN *orotate* phosphoribosyltransferase.

o. a. pyrophosphorylase, SYN *orotate* phosphoribosyltransferase.

or·phan (ōr′făn). SEE orphan *products,* under *product.* [G. *orphanos*]

or·phen·a·drine cit·rate (ōr-fen′ă-drēn). An antihistaminic that also has the same action and use as orphenadrine hydrochloride.

or·phen·a·drine hy·dro·chlo·ride. It reduces spasm of voluntary muscles, probably by action on the cerebral motor areas; used in the symptomatic treatment of paralysis agitans and drug-induced parkinsonism.

△**orrho-.** Serum. SEE sero-. [G. *orrhos, oros,* whey, serum]

or·ris (ōr′is). SYN iris.

Orsi, Francesco, Italian physician, 1828–1890. SEE O.-Grocco *method.*

Orth, Johannes J., German pathologist, 1847–1923. SEE O. *fixative, stain.*

△**orth-.** SEE ortho-.

or·the·sis (ōr-thē′sis). Rarely used term for an orthopedic brace, splint, or appliance. [ortho- + *-esis,* process]

or·thet·ics (ōr-thet′iks). SYN orthotics.

△**ortho-, orth-.** **1.** Prefix denoting straight, normal, in proper order. **2** (*o-*). In chemistry, italicized prefix denoting that a compound has two substitutions on adjacent carbon atoms in a benzene ring. For terms beginning *ortho-* or *o-,* see the specific name. **3.** The most hydrated of a series of oxoacids, e.g., orthophosphoric acid, H₃PO₄. [G. *orthos* correct]

or·tho·ac·id (ōr′thō-as′id). An acid in which the number of hydroxyl groups equals the valence of the acid-forming element; e.g., C(OH)₄, orthocarbonic acid. When there is no such acid, the one that most nearly approaches this condition is sometimes called an o.; e.g., OP(OH)₃, orthophosphoric acid.

or·tho·caine (ōr′thō-kān). The methyl ester of 3-amino-4-hydroxybenzoic acid; a surface anesthetic agent usually used in dusting powder form.

or·tho·ce·phal·ic (ōr-thō-sĕ-fal′ik). Having a head well proportioned to height; denoting a skull with a vertical index between 70 and 75. SEE ALSO metriocephalic. SYN orthocephalous. [ortho- + G. *kephalē*, head]

or·tho·ceph·a·lous (ōr-thō-sef′ă-lŭs). SYN orthocephalic.

or·tho·chro·mat·ic (ōr′thō-krō-mat′ik). Denoting any tissue or cell that stains the color of the dye used, i.e., the same color as the dye solution with which it is stained. SYN euchromatic (1), orthochromophil, orthochromophile. [ortho- + G. *chrōma*, color]

or·tho·chro·mo·phil, or·tho·chro·mo·phile (ōr-thō-krō′mō-fil, -fīl). SYN orthochromatic. [ortho- + G. *chrōma*, color, + *philos*, fond]

or·tho·cra·sia (ōr-thō-krā′sē-ă). Obsolete term for condition in which there is a normal reaction to drugs, articles of diet, etc. [ortho- + G. *krasis*, a mixing, temperament]

or·tho·cy·to·sis (ōr′thō-sī-tō′sis). A condition in which all of the cellular elements in the circulating blood are mature forms, irrespective of the proportions of various types and total numbers. [ortho- + G. *kytos*, cell, + *-osis*, condition]

or·tho·den·tin (ōr-thō-den′tin). Straight tubed dentin as seen in the teeth of mammals.

or·tho·de·ox·ia. Fall in arterial blood oxygen upon assuming the upright posture. Usually caused by right-to-left cardiac or vascular shunting with a posturally induced fall in left-sided pressure permitting a corresponding gradient across the shunt.

or·tho·di·gi·ta (or-tho-dij′ĭ-tah). Correction of malformations of fingers or toes. [ortho- + L. *digitus*, finger or toe]

or·tho·don·tia (ōr-thō-don′shē-ă). SYN orthodontics.

or·tho·don·tics (ōr-thō-don′tiks). That branch of dentistry concerned with the correction and prevention of irregularities and malocclusion of the teeth. SYN dental orthopedics, orthodontia. [ortho- + G. *odous*, tooth]

surgical o., the correction of occlusal abnormalities by the surgical repositioning of segments of the mandible or maxillae containing one to several teeth; or the bodily repositioning of entire jaws to improve function and esthetics. SYN orthognathic surgery.

or·tho·dont·ist. A dental specialist who practices orthodontics.

or·tho·dro·mic (ōr-thō-drō′mik). Denoting the propagation of an impulse along a conduction system (e.g., nerve fiber) in the direction it normally travels. Cf. antidromic. [ortho- + G. *dromos*, course]

or·tho·gen·e·sis (ōr-thō-jen′ĕ-sis). The doctrine that evolution is governed by intrinsic factors and occurs in predictable directions. [ortho- + G. *genesis*, origin]

or·tho·gen·ic (ōr-thō-jen′ik). Relating to orthogenesis.

or·tho·gen·ics (ōr-thō-jen′iks). SYN eugenics.

or·tho·gnath·ia (ōr-thō-nath′ē-ă, ōr-thog-nath′ē-ă). The study of the causes and treatment of conditions related to malposition of the bones of the jaws. [ortho- + G. *gnathos*, jaw]

or·tho·gnath·ic, or·thog·na·thous (ōr-thō-nath′ik, ōr-thog′năthŭs). **1.** Relating to orthognathia. **2.** Having a face without projecting jaw, one with a gnathic index below 98. [ortho- + G. *gnathos*, jaw]

or·tho·grade (ōr′thō-grād). Walking or standing erect; denoting the posture of humans; opposed to pronograde. [ortho- + L. *gradior*, pp. *gressus*, to walk]

or·tho·ker·a·tol·o·gy (ōr′thō-ker-ă-tol′ŏ-jē). A method of molding the cornea with contact lenses to improve unaided vision. [ortho- + G. *keras*, horn (cornea), + *logos*, science]

or·tho·ker·a·to·sis (ōr′thō-ker-ă-tō′sis). Formation of an anuclear keratin layer, as in the normal epidermis. [ortho- + G. *keras*, horn, + *-osis*, condition]

or·tho·ki·net·ics (ōr-thō-ki-net′iks). A method advocated for the treatment of hypertrophic osteoarthritis in which an attempt is made to change muscular action from one group of muscles to another set of muscles to protect the diseased joint. [ortho- + G. *kinētikos*, movable, fr. *kineō*, to move]

or·tho·me·chan·i·cal (ōr-thō-mĕ-kan′i-kăl). Pertaining to braces, prostheses, orthotic devices, and appliances. [ortho- + mechanical]

or·tho·me·chan·o·ther·a·py (ōr′thō-mĕ-kan-ō-thār′ă-pē). Treatment with braces, prostheses, orthotic devices, or appliances. [ortho- + G. *mēchanē*, machine, + *therapeia*, medical treatment]

or·tho·me·lic (ōr-thō-mē′lik). Correcting malformations of arms or legs. [ortho- + G. *melos*, limb]

or·thom·e·ter (ōr-thom′ĕ-ter). SYN exophthalmometer. [ortho- + G. *metron*, measure]

or·tho·mo·lec·u·lar (ōr′thō-mō-lek′ū-lăr). L.C. Pauling term denoting a therapeutic approach designed to provide an optimum molecular environment for body functions, with particular reference to the optimum concentrations of substances normally present in the human body, whether formed endogenously or ingested.

Or·tho·myx·o·vir·i·dae (ōr′thō-mik-sō-vir′i-dē). The family of viruses that contains the 3 genera of influenza viruses, types A and B, C, and "Thogoto-like viruses." Virions are roughly spherical or filamentous, and the former (the more common form) are 80–120 mm in diameter and ether-sensitive; envelopes are studded with surface projections; nucleocapsids are of helical symmetry, 6–9 nm in diameter, and contain single-stranded, segmented RNA. The nucleoprotein antigen of each type of virus is common to all strains of the type but is distinct from those of the other types; the mosaic of surface antigens varies from strain to strain. Nucleocapsids seem to be formed in the nuclei of infected cells, hemagglutinin, and neuraminidase in the cytoplasm; virus maturation occurs during budding of the cell membrane. Influenza virus types A and B are subject to mutation resulting in epidemics. Influenza virus C differs from types A and B (e.g., lacks neuraminidase) and belongs to a separate genus. SEE ALSO Influenza virus.

or·tho·pae·dic, or·tho·pe·dic (ōr-thō-pē′dik). Relating to orthopedics.

or·tho·pae·dics (ōr-thō-pē′diks). SYN orthopedics. [ortho- + G. *pais* (*paid-*), child]

or·tho·pae·dist, or·tho·pe·dist (ōr-thō-pē′dist). One who practices orthopaedics.

or·tho·pe·dics. The medical specialty concerned with the preservation, restoration, and development of form and function of the musculoskeletal system, extremities, spine, and associated structures by medical, surgical, and physical methods. SYN orthopaedics.

dental o., SYN orthodontics.

functional jaw o., utilization of muscle forces to effect changes in jaw position and tooth alignment by removable appliances. SYN functional orthodontic therapy.

or·tho·per·cus·sion (ōr′thō-per-kŭsh′ŭn). Very light percussion of the chest, made in a sagittal direction (i.e., anteroposteriorly, and not perpendicularly to the wall of the chest); used to determine the size of the heart, with the faint percussion sound disappearing when the heart is reached, even though that may be overlapped by a layer of the lung.

or·tho·pho·ria (ōr-thō-fōr′ē-ă). Absence of heterophoria; the condition of binocular fixation in which the lines of sight meet at a distant or near point of reference in the absence of a fusion stimulus. [ortho- + G. *phora*, motion]

or·tho·phor·ic (ōr-thō-fōr′ik). Pertaining to orthophoria.

or·tho·phos·phate (ōr-thō-fos′fāt). A salt or ester of orthophosphoric acid.

inorganic o. (P_i), any ion or salt form of phosphoric acid. SYN inorganic phosphate.

or·tho·phos·phor·ic ac·id (ōr′thō-fos-fōr′ik). Phosphoric acid, $O=P(OH)_3$, distinguished by ortho- from meta- and pyrophosphoric acids, $(HPO_3)_n$ and $OP(OH_2)OP(OH)_2O$, respectively, which are anhydrides of H_3PO_4; the ultimate anhydride is phosphorus pentoxide, P_2O_5.

or·tho·phre·nia (ōr-thō-frē′nē-ă). **1.** Rarely used term for soundness of mind. **2.** Rarely used term for a condition of normal interpersonal relationships. [ortho- + G. *phrēn*, mind]

or·thop·nea (ōr-thop-nē′ă, ōr-thop′nē-ă). Discomfort in breathing that is brought on or aggravated by lying flat. Cf. platypnea. [ortho- + G. *pnoē*, a breathing]

or·thop·ne·ic (or'thop-ne'ik). Relating to or characterized by orthopnea.

Or·tho·pox·vi·rus (ōr-thō-poks'vī-rŭs). The genus of the family Poxviridae, which comprises the viruses of alastrim, vaccinia, variola, cowpox, ectromelia, monkeypox, and rabbitpox.

or·tho·pros·the·sis (ōr'thō-pros'thĕ-sis, -pros-thē'sis). An appliance used in the management of prosthetic problems related to alignment of teeth.

or·tho·psy·chi·a·try (ōr'thō-sī-kī'ă-trē). A cross-disciplinary science combining child psychiatry, developmental psychology, pediatrics, and family care devoted to the discovery, prevention, and treatment of mental and psychological disorders in children and adolescents.

Or·thop·tera (ōr-thop'ter-ă). A large order of hemimetabolous insects that includes the locusts, grasshoppers, mantids, walking sticks, and related forms. [ortho- + G. *pteron*, a wing]

or·thop·tic (ōr-thop'tik). Relating to orthoptics.

or·thop·tics (ōr-thop'tiks). The study and treatment of defective binocular vision, of defects in the action of the ocular muscles, or of faulty visual habits. [*ortho*- straightened + G. *optikos*, sight]

or·thop·tist (ōr-thop'tist). One skilled in orthoptics.

Or·tho·re·o·vi·rus (ōr-thō-rē'ō-vī-rus). A genus in the family Reoviridae associated with a variety of respiratory and enteric diseases, but its causal relationship is not proven.

or·tho·scope (ōr'thō-skōp). **1.** An instrument by means of which one is able to draw the outlines of the various normas of the skull. [ortho- + G. *skopeō*, to view]

or·tho·sis (ōr-thō'sis, -sēz). An external orthopaedic appliance, as a brace or splint, that prevents or assists movement of the spine or the limbs. [G. *orthōsis*, a making straight]

ankle-foot o., an o. beginning at the toes, crossing the ankle, and terminating on the calf.

cervical o., an o. designed to limit cervical spine motion to varying degrees, e.g., a soft cervical collar.

cervicothoracic o., a device designed to limit cervical spine motion by extending to cover more of the upper torso than a standard cervical o.

knee-ankle-foot o., an o. extending from the upper portion of the thigh, crossing the knee and ankle, and terminating at the toes; designed to control knee and ankle motion.

thoracolumbosacral o., an external device applied to the trunk and extending from the upper portion of the thoracic spine to the pelvis; designed to provide immobilization of the thoracic spine.

wrist-hand o., an o. that begins at the fingers, crosses the wrist, and terminates on the distal portion of the forearm; used to provided grasp and release despite some degree of hand paralysis.

or·tho·stat·ic (ōr-thō-stat'ik). Relating to an erect posture or position.

or·tho·ster·e·o·scope (ōr'thō-ster'ē-ō-skōp). A rarely used instrument for viewing stereoscopic radiographs.

or·tho·tha·na·sia (ōr'thō-thă-nā'zē-ă). **1.** A normal or natural manner of death and dying. **2.** Sometimes used to denote the deliberate stopping of artificial or heroic means of maintaining life. [ortho- + G. *thanatos*, death]

or·thot·ics (ōr-thot'iks). The science concerned with the making and fitting of orthopaedic appliances. SYN orthetics.

or·tho·tist (ōr'thō'tist). A maker and fitter of orthopaedic appliances.

or·tho·tol·i·dine (ōr-thō-tō'li-dēn). In the presence of peroxidase, o. (like benzidine) is oxidized to a blue color; because hemoglobin behaves like a peroxidase, o. has been used as an in vitro aid for the detection of occult blood in feces.

or·thot·o·nos, or·thot·o·nus (ōr-thot'ŏ-nos, -ŏ-nŭs). A form of tetanic spasm in which the neck, limbs, and body are held fixed in a straight line. [ortho- + G. *tonos*, tension]

or·tho·top·ic (ōr-thō-top'ik). In the normal or usual position. [ortho- + G. *topos*, place]

or·tho·tro·pic (ōr-thō-trop'ik). Extending or growing in a straight, especially a vertical, direction. [ortho- + G. *trope*, a turn]

or·tho·vol·tage (ōr-thō-vōl'tij). In radiation therapy, a term for voltage between 400 and 600 kV.

Ortolani, Marius, 20th century Italian orthopaedic surgeon. SEE Ortolani *maneuver*, Ortolani *test*.

Orton, Samuel T., U.S. neurologist, 1879–1975. SEE Wolf-O. *bodies*, under *body*.

or·y·ce·nin (ōr-ē-sen'in). A glutelin in rice. [G. *oryza*, rice, + -in]

O.S. Abbreviation for L. *oculus sinister*, left eye.

Os Symbol for osmium.

OS

os, gen. **os·sis**, pl. **os·sa** (os, os'is, os'ă) [TA]. SYN bone. For histologic description, see bone. [L. bone]

o. acromia'le, an acromion that is joined to the scapular spine by fibrous rather than by bony union.

o. basila're, SYN basilar *bone*.

o. bre've [TA], SYN short *bone*.

o. cal'cis, SYN calcaneus (1).

o. capita'tum [TA], SYN capitate (1).

os'sa car'pi [TA], SYN carpal *bones*, under *bone*.

o. centra'le [TA], a small bone occasionally found at the dorsal aspect of the wrist between the scaphoid, capitate, and trapezoid; it is developed as an independent cartilage in early fetal life but usually becomes fused with the scaphoid; it occurs normally in most monkeys. SYN central bone.

o. centra'le tar'si, SYN navicular.

o. clitor'idis, a small bone located in the clitoris of many carnivorous mammals. It is homologous with the o. penis of many male mammals.

o. coc'cygis [TA], SYN coccyx.

o. costa'le, SYN Rib.

o. cox'ae [TA], SYN hip *bone*.

ossa cra'nii [TA], SYN *bones* of cranium, under *bone*.

o. cuboi'deum, SYN cuboid (*bone*).

o. cuneifor'me interme'dium, SYN intermediate cuneiform (*bone*).

o. cuneifor'me latera'le [TA], SYN lateral cuneiform (*bone*).

o. cuneifor'me media'le [TA], SYN medial cuneiform (*bone*).

os'sa digito'rum, ☆official alternate term for *bones* of digits, under *bone*; SEE ALSO phalanx (1).

o. ethmoida'le [TA], SYN ethmoid.

os'sa facie'i, SYN facial *bones*, under *bone*.

o. fem'oris, ☆official alternate term for thigh.

o. fronta'le [TA], SYN frontal *bone*.

o. hama'tum, SYN hamate (*bone*).

o. hyoi'deum, SYN hyoid *bone*; SEE ALSO hyoid *apparatus*.

o. iliacum, SYN ilium.

o. il'ium [TA], SYN ilium.

o. in'cae, SYN interparietal *bone*.

o. incisi'vum [TA], SYN incisive *bone*.

o. innomina'tum, SYN hip *bone*.

o. intermaxilla're, SYN incisive *bone*.

o. interme'dium, SYN lunate (*bone*).

o. intermetatar'seum, a supernumerary bone at the base of the first metatarsal, or between the first and second metatarsal bones, usually fused with one or the other or with the medial cuneiform bone. SYN intermetatarseum.

o. interparieta'le [TA], SYN interparietal *bone*.

o. irregula're [TA], SYN irregular *bone*.

o. is'chii [TA], SYN ischium.

o. japon'icum, a bipartite or tripartite zygomatic bone, found with greater frequency in the Japanese than in other races.

o. lacrima′le [TA], SYN lacrimal *bone.*

o. lon′gum [TA], SYN long *bone.*

o. luna′tum [TA], SYN lunate (*bone*).

o. mag′num, SYN capitate (1).

o. mala′re, SYN zygomatic *bone.*

os′sa mem′bri inferio′ris [TA], SYN *bones* of lower limb, under *bone.*

os′sa mem′bri superio′ris [TA], SYN *bones* of upper limb, under *bone.*

ossa metacarpalia I–V, SYN metacarpal (*bones*) [I–V], under *bone.*

ossa metacarpi, pl. **os′sa metacarpa′lia** [TA], SYN metacarpal (*bones*) [I–V], under *bone.*

ossa metatarsalia I–V, SYN metatarsal (*bones*) [I–V], under *bone.*

ossa metatarsi, pl. **os′sa metatarsa′lia** [TA], SYN metatarsal (*bones*) [I–V], under *bone.*

o. multan′gulum ma′jus, SYN trapezium *bone.*

o. multan′gulum mi′nus, SYN trapezoid (*bone*).

o. nasa′le [TA], SYN nasal *bone.*

o. navicula′re [TA], SYN navicular.

o. navicula′re ma′nus, SYN scaphoid (*bone*).

o. occipita′le [TA], SYN occipital *bone.*

o. odontoi′deum, the dens of the axis when anomalously not fused with the body of the axis.

o. orbicula′re, SYN lenticular *process* of incus.

o. palati′num [TA], SYN palatine *bone.*

o. parieta′le [TA], SYN parietal *bone.*

o. pisifor′me [TA], SYN pisiform (*bone*).

o. pla′num [TA], SYN flat *bone.*

o. pneumat′icum [TA], SYN pneumatized *bone.*

o. premaxilla′re, SYN incisive *bone.*

o. pterygoi′deum, SYN pterygoid *process* of sphenoid bone.

o. pu′bis, SYN pubis.

o. pyramida′le, SYN triquetrum.

o. sa′crum [TA], SYN sacrum.

o. scaphoi′deum [TA], SYN scaphoid (*bone*).

o. sesamoi′deum, pl. **os′sa sesamoi′dea** [TA], SYN sesamoid *bone.*

o. sphenoida′le [TA], SYN sphenoid (*bone*).

o. subtibia′le, an inconstant bone found very rarely in the distal articular end of the tibia.

ossa suprasterna′lia [TA], SYN suprasternal *bones,* under *bone.*

o. sutura′rum [TA], SYN sutural *bones,* under *bone.*

o. syl′vii, SYN lenticular *process* of incus.

ossa tarsalia, ✩official alternate term for tarsal *bones,* under *bone.*

os′sa tar′si [TA], SYN tarsal *bones,* under *bone.*

o. tempora′le [TA], SYN temporal *bone.*

o. tibia′le poste′rius, o. tibia′le posti′cum, a sesamoid bone in the tendon of the tibialis posterior muscle, occasionally fused with the tuberosity of the navicular. SYN tibiale posticum.

o. trape′zium, SYN trapezium *bone.*

o. trapezoi′deum [TA], SYN trapezoid (*bone*).

o. triangula′re, SYN triquetrum.

o. tribasila′re, the single bone resulting from the fusion in infancy of the occipital and temporal bones at the base of the cranial cavity.

o. trigo′num [TA], an independent ossicle sometimes present in the tarsus; usually it forms part of the talus, constituting the lateral tubercle of the posterior process. SYN triangular bone.

o. trique′trum [TA], SYN triquetrum.

o. un′guis, SYN lacrimal *bone.*

o. vesalia′num, the tuberosity of the fifth metatarsal bone sometimes existing as a separate bone. SYN vesalianum, Vesalius bone.

o. zygomat′icum [TA], SYN zygomatic *bone.*

---

os, gen. **o′ris,** pl. **ora. 1** [NA]. The mouth. **2.** Term applied sometimes to an opening into a hollow organ or canal, especially one with thick or fleshy edges. SEE ALSO mouth (2), ostium, orifice, opening. [L. mouth]

anatomical internal o. of uterus [TA], aperture at the narrowing of the uterine cavity demarcating and providing communication between the lumina of the body (uterine cavity) and of the cervix (cervical canal) of the uterus. SYN ostium anatomicum [TA].

external o. of uterus [TA], the vaginal opening of the uterus. SYN ostium uteri [TA], mouth of the womb, opening of uterus, orifice of uterus, orificium externum uteri, o. uteri externum, ostium uteri externum.

histological internal o. of uterus [TA], site of transition of mucosa of uterus (endometrium) to that of the cervix; it may or may not correspond to the anatomic internal os. SYN ostium histologicum [TA].

incompetent cervical o., a defect in the strength of the internal o. allowing premature dilation of the cervix.

ossa pedis [TA], SYN *bones* of foot, under *bone.*

o. u′teri exter′num, SYN external o. of uterus.

o. u′teri inter′num, SYN *isthmus* of uterus.

osa·zone (ō′să-zōn). The compound formed by certain sugars (e.g., glucose, galactose, fructose) with excess hydrazines, possessing two hydrazones on carbons 1 and 2 instead of only one at C-1, as in the ordinary hydrazone, thus, RNH–N=CR′–CR″=N–NHR‴; o.'s formed with phenylhydrazine (phenylosazones) are used to characterize and identify certain sugars. SYN dihydrazone.

osche-, oscheo-. The scrotum. [G. *oschē*]

os·che·al (os′kē-ăl). SYN scrotal.

os·che·o·plas·ty (os′kē-ō-plas-tē). SYN scrotoplasty. [oscheo- + *plastos,* formed]

os·cil·la·tion (os-i-lā′shŭn). **1.** A to-and-fro movement. **2.** A stage in the vascular changes in inflammation in which the accumulation of leukocytes in the small vessels arrests the passage of blood and there is simply a to-and-fro movement at each cardiac contraction. [L. *oscillatio,* fr. *oscillo,* to swing]

os·cil·la·tor (os′si-lā-ter). **1.** An apparatus somewhat like a vibrator, used to give a form of mechanical massage. **2.** An electric circuit designed to generate alternating current at a particular frequency. **3.** Any device that produces oscillation.

os·cil·lo·graph (ŏ-sil′ō-graf). An instrument that records oscillations, usually electrical.

os·cil·log·ra·phy (os-i-log′ră-fē). The study of the records made by an oscillograph.

os·cil·lom·e·ter (os-i-lom′ě-ter). An apparatus for measuring oscillations of any kind, especially those of the bloodstream in sphygmometry. SEE ALSO sphygmo-oscillometer. [L. *oscillo,* to swing, + G. *metron,* measure]

os·cil·lo·met·ric (os′i-lō-met′rik). Relating to the oscillometer or the records made by its use.

os·cil·lom·e·try (os-i-lom′ě-trē). The measurement of oscillations of any kind with an oscillometer.

os·cil·lop·sia (os-i-lop′sē-ă). The subjective sensation of oscillation of objects viewed. SYN oscillating vision. [L. *oscillo,* to swing, + G. *opsis,* vision]

os·cil·lo·scope (ŏ-sil′ō-skōp). An oscillograph in which the record of oscillations is continuously visible.

cathode ray o. (CRO), the common form of o., in which a varying electrical signal (*y*) vertically deflects an electron beam impinging on a fluorescent screen, while some other function (*x* or time) deflects the beam horizontally; the result is a visual graph of *y* plotted against *x* or time with negligible distortion by inertia.

storage o., a cathode ray o. in which the visual record of oscillations persists on the fluorescent screen until erased electrically.

os·ci·tate (os′i-tāt). To yawn; to gape. [L. *oscito,* fr. *os,* mouth, + *cieo,* to put in motion]

os·ci·ta·tion (os′i-tā′shŭn). SYN yawning. [L. *oscitatio*]

os·cu·lum, pl. **os·cu·la** (os′kū-lŭm, -lă). A pore or minute opening. [L. dim. of *os,* mouth]

-ose. 1. In chemistry, a terminator usually indicating a carbohydrate. **2.** Suffix appended to some Latin roots, with significance of the more common -ous (2). [L. *-osus,* full of, abounding]

-oses. Plural of -osis.

Osgood, Robert B., U.S. orthopedic surgeon, 1873–1956. SEE O.-Schlatter *disease*.

OSHA Abbreviation for Occupational Safety and Health Administration of the U.S. Department of Labor, responsible for establishing and enforcing safety and health standards in the workplace.

-osis, pl. **-oses.** Suffix meaning a process, condition, or state, usually abnormal or diseased; production or increase, physiologic or pathologic; an invasion or infestation; in the latter sense, it is similar to and often interchangeable with Greek *-iasis*, as seen in trichinosis, trichiniasis. [G.]

Osler, Sir William, Canadian physician in U.S. and England, 1849–1919. SEE O. *disease, node, sign;* Rendu-O.-Weber *syndrome.*

os·mate (os′māt). A salt of osmic acid.

os·mat·ic (oz-mat′ik). SYN olfactory. [G. *osmē,* smell]

OSMED SYN *chondrodystrophy* with sensorineural deafness.

os·me·sis (os-mē′sis). SYN olfaction. [G. *osmēsis,* smelling]

os·mic ac·id (oz′mik). OsO₄; a volatile caustic and strong oxidizing agent; colorless crystals, poorly soluble in water, but soluble in organic solvents; the aqueous solution is a fat and myelin stain and a general fixative for electron microscopy. SYN osmium tetroxide.

os·mi·cate (oz′mi-kāt). To stain or fix with osmic acid.

os·mi·ca·tion, os·mi·fi·ca·tion (os′mi-kā′shŭn, os′mi-fi-kā′shŭn). The fixation of tissue with an osmic acid solution; also serves as a stain for both light and electron microscopy.

os·mics (oz′miks). The science of olfaction. [G. *osmē,* smell]

os·mi·o·phil·ic (oz′mi-ō-fil′ik). Readily stained with osmic acid. [osmium + G. *phileō,* to love]

os·mi·o·pho·bic (oz′mi-ō-fō′bik). Not readily stained with osmic acid. [osmium + G. *phobos,* fear]

os·mi·um (Os) (oz′mē-ŭm). A metallic element of the platinum group, atomic no. 76, atomic wt. 190.2. [G. *osmē,* smell, because of the strong odor of the tetroxide]

o. tetroxide, SYN osmic acid.

osmo-. 1. Osmosis. [G. *ōsmos,* impulsion] 2. Smell, odor. [G. *osmē*]

os·mo·cep·tor (os-mō-sep′ter, tōr). SYN osmoreceptor.

os·mo·dys·pho·ria (oz′mō-dis-fōr′ē-ă). An abnormal dislike of certain odors. [G. *osmē,* smell, + *dys-,* bad, + *phora,* a carrying]

os·mo·gram (oz′mō-gram). SYN electroolfactogram. [G. *osmē,* smell, + *gramma,* a drawing]

os·mo·lal·i·ty (os-mō-lal′i-tē). The concentration of a solution expressed in osmoles of solute particles per kilogram of soluent.

calculated serum osmolality, the calculation of serum osmolality from serum sodium, glucose, and urea nitrogen values by a variety of formulae, the most common of which is: 1.86 × [Na] (mmol/L + glucose (mg/dL)/18 + BUN (mg/dL)/2.8.

os·mo·lar (os-mō′lăr). SYN osmotic.

os·mo·lar·i·ty (os-mō-lār′i-tē). The osmotic concentration of an osmotically active substance in solution, expressed as osmoles of solute particles per liter of solution.

os·mole (os′mōl). The molecular weight of a solute, in grams, divided by the number of ions or particles into which it dissociates in solution.

os·mol·o·gy (os-mol′ō-jē). 1. The study of odors, their production, and their effects. SYN osphresiology. 2. The study of osmosis.

os·mom·e·ter (os-mom′ĕ-ter). 1. An instrument for measuring osmolality by freezing point depression or vapor pressure elevation techniques. 2. An apparatus for measuring the acuteness of the sense of smell.

os·mom·e·try (os-mom′ĕ-trē). Measurement of osmolality by use of an osmometer.

os·mo·phil, os·mo·phil·ic (os′mō-fil, -fil′ik). Flourishing in a medium of high osmotic pressure. [osmo(sis) + G. *phileō,* to love]

os·mo·pho·bia (oz-mō-fō′bē-ă). SYN olfactophobia. [G. *osmē,* smell, + phobia]

os·mo·phore (oz′mō-fōr). The group of atoms in the molecule of a compound that is responsible for the compound's characteristic odor. [G. *osmē,* smell, + *phonos,* bearing]

os·mo·re·cep·tor (os′mō-rē-sep′ter, -tōr). 1. A receptor in the central nervous system (probably the hypothalamus) that responds to changes in the osmotic pressure of the blood. [G. *osmos,* impulsion] 2. A receptor that receives olfactory stimuli. [G. *osmē,* smell] SYN osmoceptor.

os·mo·reg·u·la·to·ry (os-mō-reg′ū-lă-tōr-ē). Influencing the degree and rapidity of osmosis.

os·mose (os′mōs). To move through a membrane by osmosis.

os·mo·sis (os-mō′sis). The process by which solvent tends to move through a semipermeable membrane from a solution of lower to a solution of higher osmolal concentration of the solutes to which the membrane is relatively impermeable. [G. *ōsmos,* a thrusting, an impulsion]

reverse o., movement of solvent in the opposite direction from o., i.e., pressure filtration of solvent through a semipermeable membrane that will hold back the solutes; commonly replaced by filtration or ultrafiltration when speaking of capillary membranes, as in the renal glomerulus.

os·mos·i·ty (os-mos′i-tē). An indirect measure of the osmotic characteristics of a solution, in terms of a comparable sodium chloride solution, now rendered obsolete by the more precisely defined term osmolality.

os·mo·ther·a·py (os′mō-thār′ă-pē). Dehydration by means of intravenous injections of hypertonic solutions of sodium chloride, dextrose, urea, mannitol, or other osmotically active substances, or by oral administration of glycerine, isosorbide, glycine, etc.; used in the treatment of cerebral edema and increased intracranial pressure. [osmosis + therapy]

os·mot·ic (os-mot′ik). Relating to osmosis. SYN osmolar.

osphresio-. Odor; sense of smell. [G. *osphrēsis,* smell]

os·phre·si·o·log·ic (os-frē-zē-ō-loj′ik). Relating to osphresiology.

os·phre·si·ol·o·gy (os-frē′zē-ol′ŏ-jē). SYN osmology (1). [osphresio- + G. *logos,* study]

os·phre·si·o·phil·ia (os-frē′zē-ō-fil′ē-ă). An unusual interest in odors. [osphresio- + G. *phileō,* to love]

os·phre·si·o·pho·bia (os-frē′zē-ō-fō′bē-ă). SYN olfactophobia. [osphresio- + G. *phobos,* fear]

os·phre·sis (os-frē′sis). SYN olfaction. [G. *osphrēsis,* smell]

os·phret·ic (os-fret′ik). SYN olfactory.

os·sa (os′ă). Plural of L. *os,* bone. [L.]

os·se·in, os·se·ine (os′ē-in). SYN collagen. [L. *os,* bone]

osseo-. Bony. SEE ALSO ossi-, osteo-. [L. *osseus*]

os·se·o·car·ti·lag·i·nous (os′ē-ō-kar-ti-laj′i-nŭs). Relating to, or composed of, both bone and cartilage. SYN osteocartilaginous, osteochondrous.

os·se·o·mu·cin (os′ē-ō-mū′sin). The ground substance of bony tissue.

os·se·o·mu·coid (os′ē-ō-mū′koyd). A mucoid derived from ossein.

os·se·ous (os′ē-ŭs). Bony, of bone-like consistency or structure. SYN osteal. [L. *osseus*]

ossi-. Bone. SEE ALSO osseo-, osteo-. [L. *os*]

os·si·cle (os′i-kl) [TA]. A small bone; specifically, one of the bones of the tympanic cavity or middle ear. SYN ossiculum [TA], bonelet. [L. *ossiculum,* dim. of *os,* bone]

Andernach o.'s, SYN sutural *bones,* under *bone.*

auditory o.'s [TA], the small bones of the middle ear; they are articulated to form a chain for the transmission of sound from the tympanic membrane to the oval window. SYN ossicula auditus [TA], ear bones, ossicular chain.

Bertin o.'s, SYN sphenoidal *conchae,* under *concha.*

epactal o.'s, SYN sutural *bones,* under *bone.*

Kerckring o., SYN Kerckring *center.*

os·sic·u·la (ŏ-sik′ū-lă). Plural of ossiculum. [L.]

os·sic·u·lar (ŏ-sik′ū-lăr). Pertaining to an ossicle.

os·sic·u·lec·to·my (os′i-kū-lek′tō-mē). Removal of one or more

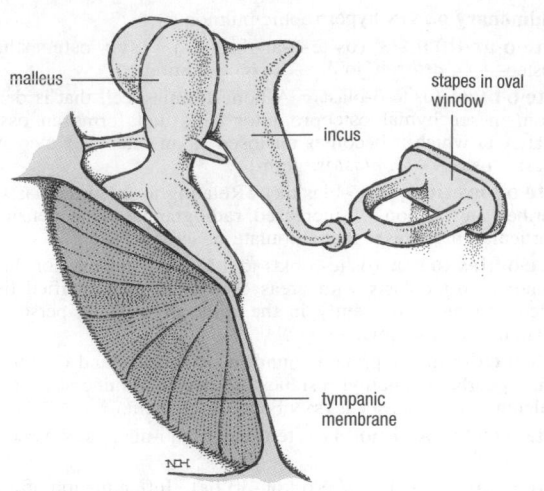

malleus

stapes in oval window

incus

tympanic membrane

auditory ossicles

of the ossicles of the middle ear. [L. *ossiculum,* ossicle, + G. *ektomē,* excision]

os·si·cu·lot·o·my (os'i-kū-lot'ō-mē). Division of one of the ossicles of the middle ear. [L. *ossiculum,* ossicle, + G. *tomē,* incision]

os·sic·u·lum, pl. **os·sic·u·la** (ŏ-sik'ū-lŭm, -lă) [TA]. SYN ossicle. [L. dim. of *os,* bone]

ossicula audi′tus [TA], SYN auditory *ossicles,* under *ossicle.*

ossic′ula menta′lia, small nodules of bone that appear at the symphysis menti shortly before birth and fuse with the mandible after birth.

os·sif·er·ous (ŏ-sif'er-ŭs). Containing or producing bone. [ossi- + L. *fero,* to bear]

os·sif·ic (o-sif'ik). Relating to a change into, or formation of, bone.

os·si·fi·ca·tion (os'i-fi-kā'shŭn). **1.** The formation of bone. **2.** A change into bone. [L. *ossificatio,* fr. *os,* bone, + *facio,* to make]

[i] endochondral o., formation of osseous tissue by the replacement of calcified cartilage; long bones grow in length by endochondral o. at the epiphysial cartilage plate where osteoblasts form bone trabeculae on a framework of calcified cartilage.

intramembranous o., SYN membranous o.

membranous o., development of osseous tissue within mesenchymal tissue without prior cartilage formation, such as occurs in the frontal and parietal bones. SYN intramembranous o.

metaplastic o., the formation of irregular foci of bone (sometimes including bone marrow) in various soft structures, such as the muscles, lungs, brain, and other sites where osseous tissue is abnormal.

os·si·form (os'i-fōrm). SYN osteoid (1). [ossi- + L. *forma,* form]

os·si·fy (os'i-fī). To form bone or convert into bone. [ossi- + L. *facio,* to make]

△ost-. SEE osteo-.

os·te·al (os'tē-ăl). SYN osseous. [G. *osteon,* bone]

os·te·al·gia (os-tē-al'jē-ă). Pain in a bone. SYN osteodynia. [osteo- + G. *algos,* pain]

os·te·an·a·gen·e·sis (os'tē-an-ă-jen'ĕ-sis). SYN osteoanagenesis.

os·te·a·naph·y·sis (os'tē-ă-naf'i-sis). SYN osteoanagenesis. [osteo- + G. *anaphysis,* a growing again]

os·tec·to·my (os-tek'tō-mē). **1.** Surgical removal of bone. **2.** In dentistry, resection of supporting osseous structure to eliminate periodontal pockets. SYN osteoectomy. [osteo- + G. *ektomē,* excision]

os·te·in, os·te·ine (os'tē-in). SYN collagen. [G. *osteon,* bone]

os·te·it·ic (os-tē-it'ik). Relating to or affected by osteitis. SYN ostitic.

os·te·i·tis (os-tē-ī'tis). Inflammation of bone. SYN ostitis. [osteo- + G. *-itis,* inflammation]

alveolar o., SYN alveoalgia.

caseous o., tuberculous caries in bone.

central o., (1) SYN osteomyelitis; **(2)** SYN endosteitis.

o. condensans ilii (con-den′sanz il′ē-ī), symmetric benign osteosclerosis of the portion of the iliac bones adjacent to the sacroiliac joints.

condensing o., SYN sclerosing o.

cortical o., periostitis with involvement of the superficial layer of bone.

o. defor′mans, SYN Paget *disease* (1).

o. fibro′sa cir′cumscrip′ta, SYN monostotic fibrous *dysplasia.*

o. fibro′sa cys′tica, increased osteoclastic resorption of calcified bone with replacement by fibrous tissue, caused by primary hyperparathyroidism or other causes of the rapid mobilization of mineral salts. SYN parathyroid osteosis, Recklinghausen disease of bone.

o. fibro′sa disseminat′a, SYN polyostotic fibrous *dysplasia.*

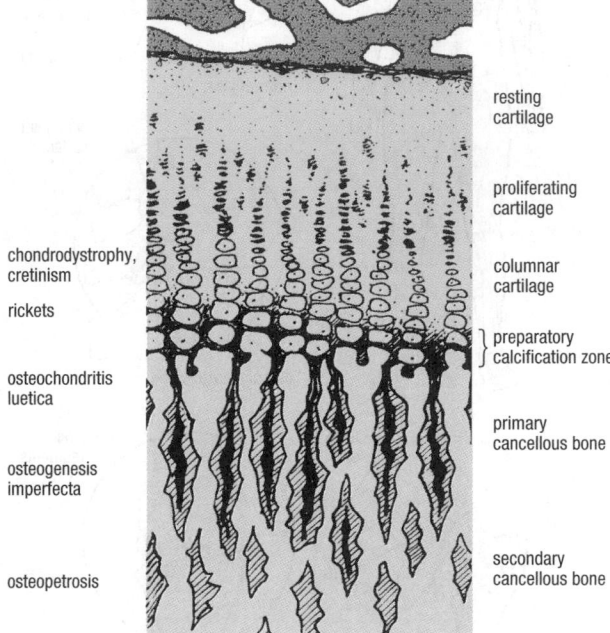

resting cartilage

proliferating cartilage

chondrodystrophy, cretinism

rickets

columnar cartilage

preparatory calcification zone

osteochondritis luetica

primary cancellous bone

osteogenesis imperfecta

osteopetrosis

secondary cancellous bone

ossification: endochondral ossification and sites of abnormalities in various disorders

focal condensing o., SYN chronic focal sclerosing *osteomyelitis.*

hematogenous o., any o. caused by infection carried in the bloodstream.

localized o. fibro′sa, SYN monostotic fibrous *dysplasia.*

multifocal o. fibro′sa, SYN polyostotic fibrous *dysplasia.*

o. pubis, osteosclerosis of the pubic bone next to the symphysis, caused by trauma to that region, from pregnancy or instrumentation.

renal o. fibro′sa, SYN renal *rickets.*

sclerosing o., fusiform thickening or increased density of bones, of unknown cause; it has been considered a form of chronic nonsuppurative osteomyelitis. SYN condensing o., Garré disease.

o. tuberculo′sa mul′tiplex cys′tica, an o. of tuberculous origin, marked by numerous small cavities in the osseous substance. SYN Jüngling disease.

os·te·mia (os-tē'mē-ă). Congestion or hyperemia of a bone. [osteo- + G. *haima,* blood]

os·tem·py·e·sis (os'tem-pī-ē'sis). Suppuration in bone. [osteo- + G. *empyēsis,* suppuration]

⌂**osteo-, ost-, oste-.** Bone. SEE ALSO osseo-, ossi-. [G. *osteon*]

os·te·o·an·a·gen·e·sis (os′tē-ō-an-ă-jen′ĕ-sis). Regeneration of bone. SYN osteanagenesis, osteanaphysis. [osteo- + G. *ana,* again, + *genesis,* generation]

ℹ️**os·te·o·ar·thri·tis** (os′tē-o-ar-thrī′tis). Arthritis characterized by erosion of articular cartilage, either primary or secondary to trauma or other conditions, which becomes soft, frayed, and thinned with eburnation of subchondral bone and outgrowths of marginal osteophytes; pain and loss of function result; mainly affects weight-bearing joints, is more common in older persons. SYN arthrosis (2), degenerative arthritis, degenerative joint disease, osteoarthrosis.

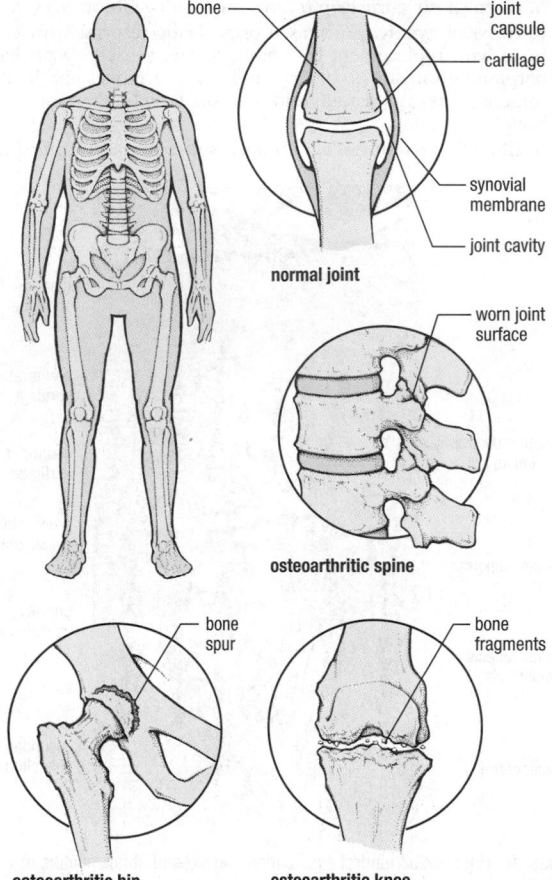

normal joint

osteoarthritic spine

osteoarthritic hip   **osteoarthritic knee**

osteoarthritis: problems associated with osteoarthritis and some sites where they commonly occur; a normal joint is shown in top right corner

---

    hyperplastic o., SYN hypertrophic pulmonary *osteoarthropathy.*

os·te·o·ar·throp·a·thy (os′tē-ō-ar-throp′ă-thē). A disorder affecting bones and joints. [osteo- + G. *arthron,* joint, + *pathos,* suffering]

    hypertrophic pulmonary o., expansion of the distal ends, or the entire shafts, of the long bones, sometimes with erosions of the articular cartilages and thickening and villous proliferation of the synovial membranes, and frequently clubbing of fingers; the disorder occurs in some chronic pulmonary diseases, in heart disease (most often congenital), and occasionally in other acute and chronic disorders. SYN Bamberger-Marie disease, Bamberger-Marie syndrome, hyperplastic osteoarthritis, pneumogenic o., pulmonary o.

    idiopathic hypertrophic o., o. not secondary to pulmonary or other progressive lesions, which may occur alone (acropathy) or as part of the syndrome of pachydermoperiostosis.

    pneumogenic o., SYN hypertrophic pulmonary o.

    pulmonary o., SYN hypertrophic pulmonary o.

os·te·o·ar·thro·sis (os′tē-ō-ar-thrō′sis). SYN osteoarthritis. [osteo- + G. *arthron,* joint, + *-osis,* condition]

os·te·o·blast (os′tē-ō-blast). A bone-forming cell that is derived from mesenchymal osteoprognitor cells and forms an osseous matrix in which it becomes enclosed as an osteocyte. SYN osteoplast. [osteo- + G. *blastos,* germ]

os·te·o·blas·tic (os′tē-ō-blas′tik). Relating to the osteoblasts; describes any region of increased radiographic bone density, in particular, metastases that stimulate o. activity.

os·te·o·blas·to·ma (os′tē-ō-blas-tō′mă). An uncommon benign tumor of osteoblasts with areas of osteoid and calcified tissue, occurring most frequently in the spine of a young person. SYN giant osteoid osteoma.

os·te·o·cal·cin. A protein found in osteoblasts and dentin; contains γ-carboxyglutamyl residues; has a role in mineralization and calcium ion homeostasis. SYN bone Gla protein.

os·te·o·car·ti·lag·i·nous (os′tē-ō-kar-ti-laj′i-nŭs). SYN osseocartilaginous.

os·te·o·chon·dri·tis (os′tē-ō-kon-drī′tis). Inflammation of a bone and its overlying articular cartilage. [osteo- + G. *chondros,* cartilage, + *-itis,* inflammation]

    o. defor′mans juveni′lis, SYN Legg-Calvé-Perthes *disease.*

    o. defor′mans juveni′lis dor′si, SYN Scheuermann *disease.*

    o. dis′secans, complete or incomplete separation of a portion of joint cartilage and underlying bone, usually involving the knee, associated with epiphyseal aseptic necrosis.

    syphilitic o., inflammation of the epiphysial line associated with congenital syphilis. SYN Wegner disease.

os·te·o·chondro·dys·pla·sia. SYN camptomelic *syndrome.*

os·te·o·chon·dro·dys·tro·phia de·for·mans (os′tē-ō-kon′drō-dis-trō′fē-ă dē-fōr′manz). SYN chondro-osteodystrophy.

os·te·o·chon·dro·dys·tro·phy (os′tē-ō-kon′drō-dis′trō-fē). SYN chondro-osteodystrophy.

os·te·o·chon·dro·ma (os′tē-ō-kon-drō′mă). A benign cartilaginous neoplasm that consists of a pedicle of normal bone (protruding from the cortex) covered with a rim of proliferating cartilage cells; may originate from any bone that is preformed in cartilage, but is most frequent near the ends of long bones, usually in patients 10–25 years of age; the lesion is frequently not noticed, unless it is traumatized or of large size; multiple o.'s are inherited and referred to as hereditary multiple exostoses. SYN solitary osteocartilaginous exostosis. [osteo- + G. *chondros,* cartilage, + *-oma,* tumor]

os·te·o·chon·dro·ma·to·sis (os′tē-ō-kon-drō-mă-tō′-sis). SYN hereditary multiple *exostoses,* under *exostosis.*

    synovial o., SYN synovial *chondromatosis.*

os·te·o·chon·dro·sar·co·ma (os′tē-ō-kon′drō-sar-kō′-mă). Chondrosarcoma arising in bone. Sarcomas in bone containing foci of neoplastic cartilage as well as bone are classified as osteogenic sarcomas. [osteo- + G. *chondros,* cartilage, + *sarx,* flesh, + *-oma,* tumor]

os·te·o·chon·dro·sis (os′tē-ō-kon-drō′sis). Any of a group of disorders of one or more ossification centers in children, characterized by degeneration or aseptic necrosis followed by reossification; includes the various forms of epiphysial aseptic necrosis. [osteo- + G. *chondros,* cartilage, + *-osis,* condition]

os·te·o·chon·drous (os′tē-ō-kon′drŭs). SYN osseocartilaginous. [osteo- + G. *chondros,* cartilage]

os·te·o·cla·sis, os·te·o·cla·sia (os′tē-ok′lă-sis, os′tē-ō-klā′zē-ă). Intentional fracture of a bone to correct deformity. SYN diaclasis, diaclasia. [osteo- + G. *klasis,* fracture]

os·te·o·clast (os′tē-ō-klast). **1.** A large multinucleated cell, possibly of monocytic origin, with abundant acidophilic cytoplasm, functioning in the absorption and removal of osseous tissue. SYN osteophage. **2.** An instrument used to fracture a bone to correct a deformity. [osteo- + G. *klastos,* broken]

os·te·o·clas·tic (os′tē-ō-klas′tik). Pertaining to osteoclasts, especially with reference to their activity in the absorption and removal of osseous tissue.

os·te·o·clas·to·ma (os'tē-ō-klas-tō'mă). SYN giant cell *tumor* of bone.

os·te·o·cra·ni·um (os'tē-ō-krā'nē-ŭm). The cranium of the fetus after ossification of the membranous cranium has made it firm. [osteo- + G. *kranion*, skull]

os·te·o·cys·to·ma (os'tē-ō-sis-tō'mă). SYN solitary bone *cyst*.

os·te·o·cyte (os'tē-ō-sīt). A cell of osseous tissue that occupies a lacuna and has cytoplasmic processes that extend into canaliculi and make contact by means of gap junctions with the processes of other osteocytes. SYN bone cell, bone corpuscle, osseous cell. [osteo- + G. *kytos,* cell]

os·te·o·den·tin (os'tē-ō-den'tin). Rapidly formed tertiary dentin that contains entrapped odontoblasts and few dentinal tubules, thereby superficially resembling bone. [osteo- + L. *dens,* tooth]

os·te·o·der·ma·to·poi·ki·lo·sis (os'tē-ō-der'mă-tō-poy-ki-lō'sis) [MIM*166700]. Osteopoikilosis with skin lesions, most commonly small elastic fibrous nodules on the posterior aspects of the thighs and buttocks; irregular autosomal dominant inheritance. SYN Buschke-Ollendorf syndrome. [osteo- + G. *derma,* skin, + *poikilos,* dappled, + *-osis,* condition]

os·te·o·des·mo·sis (os'tē-ō-dez-mō'sis). Transformation of tendon into bony tissue. [osteo- + G. *desmos,* a band (tendon), + *-osis,* condition]

os·te·o·di·as·ta·sis (os'tē-ō-dī-as'tă-sis). Separation of two adjacent bones, as of the cranium. [osteo- + G. *diastasis,* a separation]

os·te·o·dyn·ia (os-tē-ō-din'ē-ă). SYN ostealgia. [osteo- + G. *odynē,* pain]

os·te·o·dys·plas·ty (os'tē-ō-dis'plas-tē). SYN Melnick-Needles o. SYN Melnick-Needles syndrome. [osteo- + G. *dys-,* bad, + *plastos,* formed]

Melnick-Needles o., a generalized skeletal dysplasia with prominent forehead and small mandible; radiographically, there are irregular ribbonlike constrictions of the ribs and tubular bones; probably X-linked [MIM*309350]. Autosomal dominant and recessive inheritance [MIM*249420] have also been suggested. SYN osteodysplasty.

os·te·o·dys·tro·phia (os'tē-ō-dis-trō'fē-ă). SYN osteodystrophy.

os·te·o·dys·tro·phy (os'tē-ō-dis'trō-fē). Defective formation of bone. SYN osteodystrophia. [osteo- + G. *dys,* difficult, imperfect, + *trophē,* nourishment]

Albright hereditary o., an inherited form of hyperparathyroidism associated with ectopic calcification and ossification and skeletal defects, notably the small fourth metacarpals; intelligence may be normal or subnormal. Inheritance is heterogeneous; the autosomal form [MIM*103580] is caused by mutation in the guanine nucleotide-binding protein gene (GNAS1) on 20q. There are also the recessive [MIM*203330] and X-linked [MIM*300800] forms. SEE ALSO pseudohypoparathyroidism. SYN Albright syndrome (2).

renal o., generalized bone changes resembling osteomalacia and rickets or osteitis fibrosa, occurring in children or adults with chronic renal failure.

os·te·o·ec·to·my (os-tē-ō-ek'tō-mē). SYN ostectomy.

os·te·o·e·piph·y·sis (os'tē-ō-e-pif'i-sis). An epiphysis of a bone.

os·te·o·fi·bro·ma (os'tē-ō-fī-brō'mă). A benign lesion of bone, probably not a true neoplasm, consisting chiefly of fairly dense, moderately cellular, fibrous connective tissue in which there are small foci of osteogenesis. Most examples of this condition, especially in the maxilla and mandible, probably represent foci of fibrous dysplasia; a few examples of fibrous lesions with foci of osteogenesis, especially in vertebral bodies, may be neoplasms.

os·te·o·fi·bro·sis (os'tē-ō-fī-brō'sis). Fibrosis of bone, mainly involving red bone marrow.

periapical o., SYN periapical cemental *dysplasia*.

os·te·o·gen (os'tē-ō-jen). A bone matrix–producing tissue or layer. [osteo- + G. *-gen,* producing]

os·te·o·gen·e·sis (os'tē-ō-jen'ě-sis). The formation of bone. SYN osteogeny, osteosis (2), ostosis (2). [osteo- + G. *genesis,* production]

distraction o., a technique of inducing new bone formation by dividing a bone and applying tension through an external fixation device to lengthen the bone.

o. imperfec'ta (OI), a group of connective tissue disorders of type I collagen, characterized by bone fragility, fractures on trivial trauma, skeletal deformity, blue sclerae, ligament laxity, and hearing loss. The Sillence system, which is a clinical, radiographic, and genetic classification, shows four types; inherited as autosomal dominant, caused by mutation in either the collagen type I alpha-1 gene (COL1A1) on chromosome 17q or the alpha-2 gene (COL1A2) on 7q. SYN brittle bones.

o. imperfecta congenita, a severe form [MIM 166230], with fractures occurring before or at birth.

o. imperfecta tarda, a less severe form, with fractures occurring later in childhood.

Type I o. imperfecta [MIM*166200], a mild form characterized by blue sclerae, hearing loss, easy bruising, prepubertal bone fragility, and short stature.

Type II o. imperfecta [MIM*166210], a perinatal lethal form associated with stillbirth or lifespan less than 1 year; very fragile connective tissue, and radiographic findings of in utero fractures, large soft cranium, micromelia, tubular long bones, and beaded ribs.

Type III o. imperfecta [MIM*259420], a progressive deforming form with severe bone fragility, easy fractures, triangular facies with relative macrocephaly, skeletal deformities with scoliosis, pectus and bowing of limbs, dwarfism, and radiographic findings of metaphyseal flaring of long bones with sutural bone formation. Most cases are autosomal dominant disorders, but autosomal recessive inheritance has also been described.

Type IV o. imperfecta [MIM*166220], a moderately severe form, characterized by short stature, bone fragility, preambulatory fractures, and bowing of long bones.

os·te·o·gen·ic, os·te·o·ge·net·ic (os'tē-ō-jen'ik, -jě-net'ik). Relating to osteogenesis. SYN osteogenous, osteoplastic (1).

os·te·og·e·nous (os-tē-oj'ě-nŭs). SYN osteogenic.

os·te·og·e·ny (os-tē-oj'ě-nē). SYN osteogenesis.

os·te·og·ra·phy (os'tē-og'ră-fē). A treatise on or description of the bones. [osteo- + G. *graphē,* a writing]

os·te·o·ha·li·ste·re·sis (os'tē-ō-hal'is-ter-ē'sis). Softening of the bones through absorption or insufficient supply of the mineral portion. [osteo- + G. *hals,* salt, + *sterēsis,* privation]

os·te·o·hy·per·tro·phy (os'tē-ō-hī-per'trō-fē). Condition characterized by overgrowth of bones. [osteo- + G. *hyper-* over, + *trophē,* nourishment]

os·te·oid (os'tē-oyd). **1.** Relating to or resembling bone. SYN ossiform. **2.** Newly formed organic bone matrix prior to calcification. [osteo- + G. *eidos,* resemblance]

os·te·o·lip·o·chon·dro·ma (os'tē-ō-lip'ō-kon-drō'mă). A benign neoplasm of cartilaginous tissue, in which metaplasia occurs and foci of adipose cells and osseous tissue are formed. [osteo- + G. *lipos,* fat, + *chondros,* cartilage, + *-oma,* tumor]

os·te·o·lo·gia (os-tē-ō-lō'jē-ă). SYN osteology, osteology. [L.]

os·te·ol·o·gist (os-tē-ol'ŏ-jist). A specialist in osteology.

os·te·ol·o·gy (os'tē-ol'ŏ-jē). The anatomy of the bones; the science concerned with the bones and their structure. SYN osteologia. [osteo- + G. *logos,* study]

os·te·ol·y·sis (os-tē-ol'i-sis). Softening, absorption, and destruction of bony tissue, a function of the osteoclasts. [osteo- + G. *lysis,* dissolution]

os·te·o·lyt·ic (os-tē-ō-lit'ik). Pertaining to, characterized by, or causing osteolysis.

os·te·o·ma (os-tē-ō'mă). A benign, slow-growing mass of mature, predominantly lamellar bone, usually arising from the skull or mandible. [osteo- + G. *-oma,* tumor]

o. cu'tis, cutaneous ossification usually secondary to calcification in foci of degeneration in tumors or inflammatory lesions or, rarely, primary new bone formation in normal skin, often associated with Albright hereditary *ostrodystrophy*.

dental o., an exostosis arising from the root of a tooth.

giant osteoid o., SYN osteoblastoma.

o. medulla're, an o. containing spaces that are filled (or partly filled) with various elements of bone marrow.

osteoid o., a painful benign neoplasm that usually originates in one of the bones of the lower extremities, especially the femur or tibia of adolescent and young adult persons; characterized by a nidus (usually no larger than 1 cm in diameter) that consists of osteoid material, vascularized osteogenic stroma, and poorly formed bone; around the nidus there is a relatively large zone of reactive thickening of the cortex.

o. spongio′sum, an o. that consists chiefly of cancellous bone tissue.

os·te·o·ma·la·cia (os′tē-ō-mă-lā′shē-ă). A disease characterized by a gradual softening and bending of the bones with varying severity of pain; softening occurs because the bones contain osteoid tissue that has failed to calcify because of lack of vitamin D or renal tubular dysfunction; more common in women than in men, o. often begins during pregnancy. SYN adult rickets, late rickets, rachitis tarda. [osteo- + G. *malakia,* softness]

etiology of osteomalacia

vitamin D deficiency

malnutrition (in developing nations, slums, vegetarians, older persons)

reduced absorption due to impaired digestion (gastrectomy, reduced bile secretion, pancreatic insufficiency), malabsorption (sprue, intestinal resections)

reduced formation of vitamin D_3 due to lack of UV light (rickets in children)

impaired metabolism of vitamin D

inherited defects in the receptor for 1.25(OH)$_2$D in target tissues

impairment of calcidiol formation in liver (antiepileptic therapy, hepatic cirrhosis)

impairment of 1-hydroxylation in the kidneys (kidney failure, pseudovitamin D deficiency, rickets)

impaired phosphate metabolism

phosphaturia (phosphate diabetes, congenital and acquired)

cystinosis (congenital and acquired)

renal tubular acidosis

tumor-induced forms (with bone tumors and mesenchymal tumors)

phosphate deficiency

hypophosphatasia (congenital: autosomal recessive)

infantile o., juvenile o., SYN rickets.
senile o., osteoporosis in the aged.
os·te·o·ma·lac·ic (os′tē-ō-mă-lā′sik). Relating to, or suffering from, osteomalacia.
os·te·o·ma·toid (os-tē-ō′mă-toyd). An abnormal nodule or small mass of overgrowth of bone, usually occurring bilaterally and symmetrically, in juxtaepiphysial regions, especially in long bones of the lower extremities; lesions are not actually neoplasms, but represent anomalous developments in which there are outpouchings of the cortex (in contrast to a growth superimposed on the cortex), and are more properly termed exostoses. [osteoma + G. *eidos,* appearance, form]
os·te·o·mere (os′tē-ō-mēr). One of the series of bone segments, such as the vertebrae. [osteo- + G. *meros,* a part]
os·te·om·e·try (os-tē-om′ě-trē). The branch of anthropometry concerned with the relative size of the different parts of the skeleton. [osteo- + G. *metron,* measurement]
os·te·o·my·e·li·tis (os′tē-ō-mī-ě-lī′tis). Inflammation of the bone marrow and adjacent bone. SYN central osteitis (1). [osteo- + G. *myelos,* marrow, + -*itis,* inflammation]
chronic diffuse sclerosing o., a proliferative reaction of bone to a low-grade infection of the jaws; most often seen in middle-aged or older black women as extensive, often bilateral radio-opacities of the mandible and maxilla.
chronic focal sclerosing o., a reaction to a mild bacterial infection, often the result of a carious tooth, in persons with a high degree of tissue resistance; results in a localized radio-opacity. SYN focal condensing osteitis.

Garré o., chronic o. with proliferative periostitis. A focal gross thickening of the periosteum with peripheral reactive bone formation resulting from mild infection.
Pseudomonas **o.,** SYN malignant external *otitis.*
os·te·o·my·e·lo·dys·pla·sia (os′tē-ō-mī′ě-lō-dis-plā′-zē-ă). A disease characterized by enlargement of the marrow cavities of the bones, thinning of the osseous tissue, large, thin-walled vascular spaces, leukopenia, and irregular fever. [osteo- + G. *myelos,* marrow, + dysplasia]
os·te·on, os·te·one (os′tē-on, -ōn). A central canal containing blood capillaries and the concentric osseous lamellae around it occurring in compact bone. SYN haversian system. [G. *osteon,* bone]
os·te·on·cus (os-tē-ong′kŭs). An osteoma, sometimes used with reference to any neoplasm of a bone. [osteo- + G. *onkos,* bulk (swelling)]
os·te·o·ne·cro·sis (os′tē-ō-ne-krō′sis). The death of bone in mass, as distinguished from caries ("molecular death") or relatively small foci of necrosis in bone. [osteo- + G. *nekrōsis,* death]
os·te·o·nec·tin. A protein (MW 39,000–40,000) found in bone and nonmineralized tissues and believed to play a role in mineralization.
os·te·o·path (os′tē-ō-path). SYN osteopathic *physician.*
os·te·o·path·ia (os′tē-ō-path′e-ă). SYN osteopathy (1).
o. conden′sans, SYN osteopoikilosis.
o. hemorrha′gica infan′tum, SYN infantile *scurvy.*
o. stria′ta, linear striations seen radiographically in the metaphyses of long bones and also flat bones; it may be a variant of osteopoikilosis. SYN Voorhoeve disease.
os·te·o·path·ic (os-tē-ō-path′ik). Relating to osteopathy.
os·te·o·pa·thol·o·gy (os′tē-ō-pa-thol′ŏ-jē). Study of diseases of bone.
os·te·op·a·thy (os-tē-op′ă-thē). **1.** Any disease of bone. SYN osteopathia. **2.** A school of medicine based upon a concept of the normal body as a vital machine capable, when in correct adjustment, of making its own remedies against infections and other toxic conditions; practitioners use the diagnostic and therapeutic measures of conventional medicine in addition to manipulative measures. SYN osteopathic medicine. [osteo- + G. *pathos,* suffering]
alimentary o., bone disease due to dietary deficiency.
os·te·o·pe·di·on (os′tē-ō-pē′dē-on). Obsolete term for lithopedion. [osteo- + G. *paidion,* dim. of *pais,* a child]
os·te·o·pe·nia (os′tē-ō-pē′nē-ă). **1.** Decreased calcification or density of bone; a descriptive term applicable to all skeletal systems in which such a condition is noted; carries no implication about causality. **2.** Reduced bone mass due to inadequate osteoid synthesis. [osteo- + G. *penia,* poverty]
os·te·o·per·i·os·ti·tis (os′tē-ō-per′ē-os-tī′tis). Inflammation of the periosteum and of the underlying bone.
os·te·o·pe·tro·sis (os′tē-ō-pe-trō′sis) [MIM*166600]. Excessive formation of dense trabecular bone and calcified cartilage, especially in long bones, leading to obliteration of marrow spaces and to anemia with myeloid metaplasia and hepatosplenomegaly beginning in infancy, to bone fragility, and to progressive deafness and blindness; autosomal dominant inheritance. There are also autosomal recessive forms, which may be mild [MIM*259710], severe [MIM*259700], or lethal [MIM*259720], and sometimes involve a renal tubular defect [MIM*259730]. A milder, autosomal dominant form has onset in childhood and no neurologic sequelae. SYN Albers-Schönberg disease, marble bone disease, marble bones. [osteo- + G. *petra,* stone, + -*osis,* condition]
o. ac′ro-osteoly′tica, SYN pyknodysostosis.
o. with renal tubular acidosis, SYN carbonic anhydrase II deficiency *syndrome.*
os·te·o·pe·trot·ic (os′tē-ō-pe-trot′ik). Relating to osteopetrosis.
os·te·o·phage (os′tē-ō-fāj). SYN osteoclast (1). [osteo- + G. *phagō,* to eat]
os·te·o·phle·bi·tis (os′tē-ō-fle-bī′tis). Inflammation of the veins of a bone. [osteo- + G. *phleps,* vein, + -*itis,* inflammation]
os·te·oph·o·ny (os′tē-of′ō-nē). SYN bone *conduction.*

os·te·o·phyte (os'tē-ō-fīt).   A bony outgrowth or protuberance. [osteo- + G. *phyton,* plant]

os·te·o·plaque (os'tē-ō-plak).   Any osseous layer. [osteo- + Fr. *plaque,* plate]

os·te·o·plast (os'tē-ō-plast).   SYN osteoblast. [osteo- + G. *plastos,* formed]

os·te·o·plas·tic (os-tē-ō-plas'tik).   **1.** SYN osteogenic. **2.** Relating to osteoplasty.

os·te·o·plas·ty (os'tē-ō-plas-tē).   **1.** Bone grafting; reparative or plastic surgery of bones. **2.** In dentistry, resection of osseous structure to achieve acceptable gingival contour. [osteo- + G. *plastos,* formed]

os·te·o·poi·ki·lo·sis (os'tē-ō-poy-ki-lō'sis).   Mottled or spotted bones caused by widespread small foci of compact bone in the substantia spongiosa; autosomal dominant inheritance [MIM*166700]. SEE ALSO *osteopathia* striata, dermatofibrosis lenticularis disseminata. SYN osteopathia condensans. [osteo- + G. *poikilos,* dappled, + *-osis,* condition]

os·te·o·po·nin.   A protein produced by osteoblasts of unknown function.

os·te·o·pon·tin.   A secreted phosphoprotein, produced by many epithelial cell types, that is highly negatively charged and frequently associated with mineralization processes. It is found in plasma, urine, milk, and bile. Transformed cells express o. in elevated levels. SYN bone sialoprotein 1.

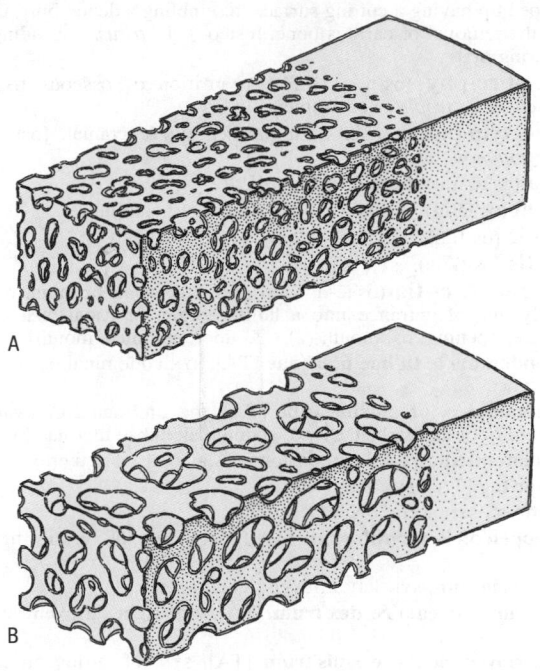

A

B

osteoporosis: (A) normal bone, (B) osteoporotic bone

os·te·o·po·ro·sis (os'tē-ō-pō-rō'sis).   Reduction in the quantity of bone or atrophy of skeletal tissue; an age-related disorder characterized by decreased bone mass and increased susceptibility to fractures. [osteo- + G. *poros,* pore, + *-osis,* condition]

> Osteoporosis affects 20 million Americans, about 80% of them women, and costs U.S. society as much as $3.8 billion annually. About 1.3 million fractures attributable to osteoporosis occur each year in people age 45 and older, and this condition is responsible for 50% of fractures occurring in women over age 50. Although all bones are affected, compression fractures of the vertebrae and traumatic fractures of the wrist and femoral neck are most common. Gradual asymptomatic vertebral compression may be detectable only on radiographic examination. Loss

of body height and development of kyphosis may be the only signs of vertebral collapse. After hip fracture, most elderly patients fail to recover normal activity, and mortality within 1 year approaches 20%. Fractures in the elderly often lead to loss of mobility and independence, social alienation, fear of further falls and fractures, and depression. Osteoporosis occurs when bone resorption outpaces bone formation. Mechanisms underlying osteoporosis are complex and probably diverse. Bone constantly undergoes cycles of resorption and formation (remodeling) to maintain the concentration of calcium and phosphate in the extracellular fluid. When serum calcium concentration drops, parathyroid hormone secretion increases, and this hormone stimulates bone resorption by osteoclasts to restore serum calcium levels to normal. Bone mass declines with age and is influenced by sex, race, menopause, and body weight-for-height. Dietary intake of calcium and vitamin D as well as intestinal and renal function affect calcium and phosphate homeostasis. The risk of osteoporosis is highest in postmenopausal women. Asian or white race, underweight, dietary calcium deficiency, sedentary lifestyle, alcohol use, and cigarette smoking appear to be independent risk factors. The decline of vitamin D_3 level with aging results in calcium malabsorption, which, in turn, stimulates bone resorption. Estrogen deficiency exacerbates this problem by increasing the sensitivity of bone to resorbing agents. Women who become amenorrheic because of rigorous athletic exercise and dietary restriction or eating disorders are at risk of osteoporosis. The formation and resorption of bone are also influenced by external physical factors such as body weight and exercise. Immobilization and prolonged bed rest produce rapid bone loss, while exercise involving weight-bearing has been shown both to reduce bone loss and to increase bone mass. Osteoporosis is common in young adults with cystic fibrosis, particularly those treated with long-term corticosteroid therapy. The diagnosis of primary osteoporosis is established by documentation of reduced bone density after exclusion of known causes of excessive bone loss. Radiographs are insensitive indicators of bone loss, since bone density must be decreased by at least 20–30% before the reduction can be appreciated. Standard diagnostic procedures are determination of bone mineral density at the ultradistal radius and midshaft radius by single-photon absorptiometry, and at the hip and lumbar spine by dual-energy x-ray absorptiometry (DEXA). A quantitative ultrasound procedure recently approved by the FDA is comparable to bone density measurements by DEXA in predicting fractures due to osteoporosis. The goal of therapy in osteoporosis is prevention of fractures in susceptible patients. The appropriate timing and proper use of agents such as calcium, vitamin D, estrogen, bisphosphonates, calcitonin, and raloxifene and the role of exercise have generated major research efforts and considerable controversy. Intake of adequate amounts of calcium and vitamin D, and continuing moderate weight-bearing exercise, are basic preventive measures for persons of all ages. Administration of estrogen at and after menopause does not simply halt the loss of bone, but actually increases bone mass. Hormone replacement with estrogen remains the most effective prevention and treatment for postmenopausal osteoporosis. It is believed to be most appropriate to start estrogen at the earliest sign of the menopause, since bone loss probably begins before the cessation of menses. Estrogen therapy must be continued through later life to maintain optimal bone density. There is no convincing evidence that initiating estrogen therapy in elderly women will prevent osteoporosis. The benefits of estrogen therapy must be weighed against the increased risk of endometrial hyperplasia and endometrial carcinoma (which can be offset by concomitant administration of progestogen) and possibly of carcinoma of the breast. The selective estrogen receptor modulator raloxifene has been approved for prevention of osteoporosis. It does not cause endometrial hyperplasia but is less effective than estrogen in conserv-

OS

ing bone mass. The hormone calcitonin, administered by injection or nasal spray, inhibits bone resorption and has other effects on mineral metabolism. Bisphosphonates such as alendronate and etidronate, which bind to bone crystals, rendering them resistant to enzymatic hydrolysis and inhibiting the action of osteoclasts, have been shown to increase bone mineral density. Strategies to prevent falls are important in elderly patients. SEE ALSO estrogen replacement therapy, raloxifene.

o. circumscrip′ta cra′nii, localized cranial o. often seen in Paget disease.

juvenile o., idiopathic o. with onset before puberty, leading to pain or fractures, with spontaneous remission within a few years.

posttraumatic o., SYN Sudeck *atrophy.*

os·te·o·po·rot·ic (os′tē-ō-pŏ-rot′ik). Pertaining to, characterized by, or causing a porous condition of the bones.

osteoprotegerin (os′tē-ō-prō-teg′er-in). A secreted protein that inhibits osteoclast differentiation.

os·te·o·ra·di·ol·o·gist (os′tē-ō-rā-dē-ol′ō-jist). A physician who specializes in radiology of the bones and joints. [osteo- + radiologist]

os·te·o·ra·di·ol·o·gy. The clinical subspecialty of diagnostic bone radiology.

os·te·o·ra·di·o·ne·cro·sis (os′tē-ō-rā′dē-ō-ne-krō′sis). Necrosis of bone produced by ionizing radiation; may be planned or unplanned. [osteo- + radionecrosis]

os·te·or·rha·phy (os-tē-ōr′ă-fē). Wiring together the fragments of a broken bone. SYN osteosuture. [osteo- + G. *rhaphē,* suture]

os·te·o·sar·co·ma (os′tē-ō-sar-kō′mă). SYN osteogenic *sarcoma.*

parosteal o., low-grade o. arising on the surface of bone without involvement of the underlying marrow, usually occurring as a heavily ossified mass of the distal femur in women in the third and fourth decades of life.

periosteal o., chondroblastic o. occurring on the surface of bones without involvement of the marrow; usually presents in adolescents and young adults as a lucent defect with bone spicules extending into soft tissues. Histologically, the tumor is intermediate to high grade, and the cartilage is lobulated.

os·te·o·scle·ro·sis (os′tē-ō-skle-rō′sis). Abnormal hardening or eburnation of bone. [osteo- + G. *sklērōsis,* hardness]

os·te·o·scle·rot·ic (os′tē-ō-skle-rot′ik). Relating to, due to, or marked by hardening of bone substance.

os·te·o·sis (os-tē-ō′sis). **1.** A morbid process in bone. SYN ostosis (1). **2.** SYN osteogenesis. [osteo- + G. *-osis,* condition]

parathyroid o., SYN *osteitis* fibrosa cystica.

renal fibrocystic o., SYN renal *rickets.*

os·te·o·spon·gi·o·ma (os′tē-ō-spon′jē-ō′mă). General nonspecific term for a neoplasm in bone that results in thinning and fragmentation (thus, in softening) of the cortex. [osteo- + G. *spongos,* sponge, + *-oma,* tumor]

os·te·o·ste·a·to·ma (os′tē-ō-stē′ă-tō′mă). A benign mass, usually a lipoma or sebaceous cyst, in which small foci of bony elements are present. [osteo- + G. *stear,* suet, fat, + *-oma,* tumor]

os·te·o·su·ture (os-tē-ō-soo′cher). SYN osteorrhaphy.

os·te·o·syn·the·sis (os-tē-ō-sin′thē-sis). Internal fixation of a fracture by means of a mechanical device, such as a pin, screw, or plate.

os·te·o·throm·bo·sis (os′tē-ō-throm-bō′sis). Thrombosis in one or more of the veins of a bone.

os·te·o·tome (os′tē-ō-tōm). An instrument for use in cutting bone. [osteo- + G. *tomē,* incision]

os·te·ot·o·my (os-tē-ot′ō-mē). Cutting a bone, usually by means of a saw or osteotome. [osteo- + G. *tomē,* incision]

"C" sliding o., an extraoral o. in the shape of a "C" performed bilaterally in the mandibular rami for the correction of retrognathia and/or apertognathia.

Dwyer o., a procedure for clubfoot.

horizontal o., an o. performed intraorally for genioplasty; the inferior aspect of the anterior mandible is advanced or retruded by movement of the free segment.

Le Fort o., an o. performed along the classic lines of fracture as described by Le Fort to correct a maxillary skeletal deformity; classified as Le Fort o. I, lower maxillary; II, pyramidal nasoorbitomaxillary; or III, high maxillary, depending upon the location.

sagittal split mandibular o., an intraoral surgical procedure for correction of retrognathism, apertognathia, and prognathism; the mandibular rami and posterior body are sectioned in the sagittal plane.

segmental alveolar o., an intraoral surgical procedure in which segments of alveolar bone containing teeth are sectioned between, and apically to, the teeth for the repositioning of the alveolus and teeth; it may be maxillary or mandibular, and may be combined with ostectomy.

sliding oblique o., an oral surgical procedure in which the mandibular ramus is cut vertically from the sigmoid notch to the angle to facilitate posterior repositioning of the mandible in correction of mandibular prognathism; it may be performed extraorally or intraorally, and is similar to vertical o.

vertical o., an oral surgical procedure similar to sliding oblique o.

os·te·o·tribe (os′tē-ō-trīb). An instrument for crushing off bits of necrosed or carious bone. [osteo- + G. *tribō,* to bruise, to grind down]

os·te·o·trite (os′tē-ō-trīt). An instrument with conical or olive-shaped tip having a cutting surface, resembling a dental burr, used for the removal of carious bone. [osteo- + L. *tritus,* a grinding, a wearing off]

os·te·ot·ro·phy (os-tē-ot′rō-fē). Nutrition of osseous tissue. [osteo- + G. *trophē,* nourishment]

os·te·o·tym·pan·ic (os′tē-ō-tim-pan′ik). SYN otocranial. [osteo- + G. *tympanon,* drum]

os·tia (os′tē-ă). Plural of ostium. [L.]

os·ti·al (os′tē-ăl). Relating to any orifice, or ostium.

os·ti·tic (os-tī′tik). SYN osteitic.

os·ti·tis (os-tī′tis). SYN osteitis.

os·ti·um, pl. **os·tia** (os′tē-ŭm, -ă) [TA]. A small opening, especially one of entrance into a hollow organ or canal. SEE ALSO orifice, opening, os, mouth (2). [L. door, entrance, mouth]

o. abdomina′le tu′bae uteri′nae [TA], SYN abdominal o. of uterine tube.

abdominal o. of uterine tube [TA], the fimbriated or ovarian extremity of an oviduct. SYN o. abdominale tubae uterinae [TA].

o. anatomicum [TA], SYN anatomical internal *os* of uterus.

o. aor′tae [TA], SYN aortic *orifice.*

aortic o., SYN aortic *orifice.*

o. appen′dicis vermifor′mis [TA], SYN *orifice* of vermiform appendix.

o. arterio′sum, SYN left atrioventricular *orifice.*

o. atrioventricula′re dex′trum [TA], SYN right atrioventricular *orifice.*

o. atrioventricula′re sinis′trum [TA], SYN left atrioventricular *orifice.*

o. cardi′acum [TA], SYN cardial *orifice.*

o. histologicum [TA], SYN histological internal *os* of uterus.

o. ileale [TA], SYN ileal *orifice.*

o. ileoceca′le, SYN ileal *orifice.*

o. inter′num, SYN uterine o. of uterine tubes.

o. pharyn′geum tu′bae auditi′vae [TA], SYN pharyngeal *opening* of pharyngotympanic (auditory) tube. ☆

o. pharyngeum tubae auditoriae, ☆official alternate term for pharyngeal *opening* of pharyngotympanic (auditory) tube.

o. pri′mum, SYN interatrial *foramen* primum.

o. pylor′icum [TA], SYN pyloric *orifice.*

o. secun′dum, SYN interatrial *foramen* secundum.

o. sinus coronarii [TA], SYN *opening* of coronary sinus.

o. trun′ci pulmona′lis [TA], SYN *opening* of pulmonary trunk.

o. tympan′icum tu′bae auditi′vae [TA], SYN tympanic *opening* of pharyngotympanic (auditory) tube.

ot

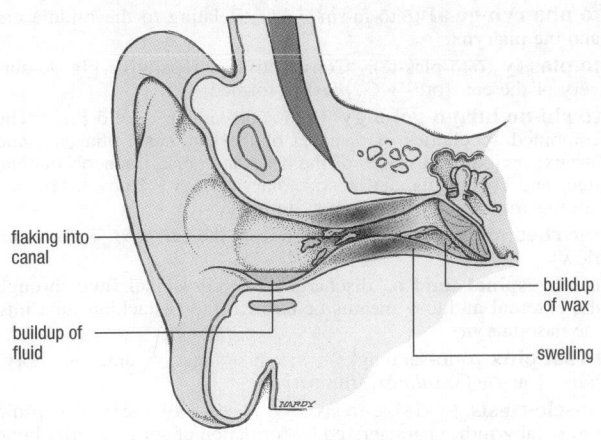

flaking into canal
buildup of wax
buildup of fluid
swelling

otitis externa

o. ure′teris [TA], SYN ureteric *orifice.*

o. ure′thrae exter′num [TA], SYN external urethral *orifice.*

o. ure′thrae inter′num [TA], SYN internal urethral *orifice.*

o. urethrae internum accipiens [TA], SYN filling internal urethral *orifice.*

o. urethrae internum evacuans [TA], SYN voiding internal urethral *orifice.*

o. u′teri [TA], SYN external *os* of uterus.

o. u′teri exter′num, SYN external *os* of uterus.

o. u′teri inter′num, SYN *isthmus* of uterus.

uterine o. of uterine tubes [TA], the uterine opening of the oviduct. SYN o. uterinum tubae uterinae [TA], o. internum, uterine opening of uterine tubes.

o. uteri′num tu′bae uteri′nae [TA], SYN uterine o. of uterine tubes.

o. vagi′nae [TA], SYN vaginal *orifice.*

o. ve′nae ca′vae inferio′ris [TA], SYN *opening* of inferior vena cava.

o. ve′nae ca′vae superio′ris [TA], SYN *opening* of superior vena cava.

os′tia vena′rum pulmona′lium [TA], SYN *openings* of pulmonary veins, under *opening.*

o. veno′sum cordis, SYN right atrioventricular *orifice.*

o. of vermiform appendix, SYN *orifice* of vermiform appendix.

os·to·mate (os′tō-māt). Term for one who has an ostomy. [L. *ostium,* mouth]

os·to·my (os′tō-mē). **1.** An artificial stoma or opening into the urinary or gastrointestinal canal, or the trachea. **2.** Any operation by which a permanent opening is created between two hollow organs or between a hollow viscus and the skin externally, as in tracheostomy. [L. *ostium,* mouth]

△**-ostomy.** SEE -stomy.

os·to·sis (os-tō′sis). **1.** SYN osteosis (1). **2.** SYN osteogenesis.

os·tra·ceous (os-trā′shŭs). Denoting the heaping up of scales seen in psoriasis, which resembles the stratification of oyster shells. [*Ostraeacea,* group including the oysters]

os·tre·o·tox·ism (os′trē-ō-tok′sizm). Poisoning from eating infected or contaminated oysters. [G. *ostreon,* oyster, + *toxikon,* poison]

Ostwald, Friedrich Wilhelm, German physical chemist and Nobel laureate, 1853–1932. SEE O. solubility *coefficient.*

OT Abbreviation for occupational therapist or therapy; Koch old *tuberculin.*

△**ot-.** The ear. SEE ALSO auri-. [G. *ous*]

Ota, Masao T., Japanese dermatopathologist, 1885–1945. SEE Ota *nevus.*

otal·gia (ō-tal′jē-ă). SYN earache. [ot- + G. *algos,* pain]
geniculate o., SYN geniculate *neuralgia.*

reflex o., pain referred to the ear from disease in another part, most commonly teeth, maxillary sinus, nasopharynx, tonsil, pharynx, or larynx.

otal·gic (ō-tal′jik). **1.** Relating to otalgia, or earache. **2.** A remedy for earache.

OTC Abbreviation for *over the counter,* pertaining to a drug available without a prescription.

oth·er·di·rect·ed (odh′er-di-rek′ted). Pertaining to a person readily influenced by the attitudes of others.

otic (ō′tik). Relating to the ear. [G. *otikos,* fr. *ous,* ear]

Otis, Arthur Brooks, U.S. respiratory physiologist, *1913. SEE Rahn-O. *sample.*

otit·ic (ō-tit′ik). Relating to otitis.

oti·tis (ō-tī′tis). Inflammation of the ear. [ot- + G. *-itis,* inflammation]

adhesive o., inflammation of the middle ear caused by prolonged eustachian tube dysfunction resulting in permanent retraction of the eardrum and obliteration of the middle ear space.

o. desquamati′va, o. externa with a copious desquamation.

▣**o. exter′na,** inflammation of the external auditory canal. SYN swimmer's ear.

o. inter′na, SYN labyrinthitis.

malignant external o., a life-threatening *Pseudomonas* osteomyelitis of the temporal bone in elderly diabetics that begins with ear pain and swelling of and discharge from the external auditory canal. SYN *Pseudomonas* osteomyelitis.

▣**o. me′dia,** inflammation of the middle ear, or tympanum.

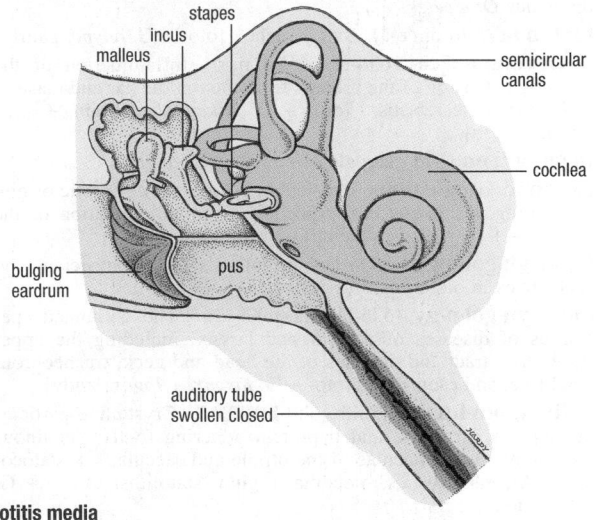

stapes
incus
malleus
semicircular canals
cochlea
bulging eardrum
pus
auditory tube swollen closed

otitis media

reflux o. me′dia, o. media caused by passage of an ingested liquid (usually milk) or nasopharyngeal secretions through the eustachian tube.

secretory o. media, SYN middle-ear *effusion.*

serous o. media, SYN middle-ear *effusion.*

△**oto-.** The ear. SEE ALSO auri-. [G. *ous*]

oto·acous·tic (ō′tō-a-koo-stik). Referring to the very faint sounds produced by the ear; thought to represent mechanical vibrations in the cochlea.

oto·bi·o·sis (ō′tō-bī-ō′sis). Presence of larvae and the characteristic spiny nymphs of the tick *Otobius megnini* in the external auditory canal of cattle, horses, cats, dogs, deer, coyotes, and other domestic and wild animals; they may remain in the ear for several months before dropping out to pupate and mature. Several records of human infestation are known.

Oto·bi·us (ō-tō′bē-ŭs). A genus of argasid ticks similar to *Ornithodoros* but characterized by a granulated integument, a hypostome that is vestigial in the adult but well developed in the spiny nymphs, and the absence of eyes and hood. Two species are recognized: *O. lagophilus* (the face tick of rabbits) and *O. megnini,* the spinose ear tick that causes otobiosis in horses, cattle, sheep, dogs, and some wild animals; it occurs in southwestern parts of the U.S., where it is an important pest, and is also distributed worldwide.

oto·ceph·a·ly (ō-tō-sef′ă-lē). Malformation characterized by markedly defective development of the lower jaw (micrognathia or agnathia) and the union or close approach of the ears (synotia) on the front of the neck. [oto- + G. *kephalē,* head]

oto·cer·e·bri·tis (ō-tō-ser-ĕ-brī′tis). SYN otoencephalitis.

oto·co·nia, sing. **oto·co·ni·um** (ō-to-kō′nē-ă, -ŭm). SYN otoliths.

oto·cra·ni·al (ō-tō-krā′nē-ăl). Relating to the otocranium. SYN osteotympanic.

oto·cra·ni·um (ō′tō-krā′nē-um). The bony case of the internal and middle ear, consisting of the petrous portion of the temporal bone. [oto- + G. *kranion,* cranium]

oto·cyst (ō′tō-sist). **1.** Embryonic auditory vesicle. **2.** A balancing organ, analogous to the utricle of mammals, possessed by certain invertebrates and containing grains of calcareous material or of sand. [oto- + G. *kystis,* a bladder]

Oto·dec·tes (ō-tō-dek′tēz). A genus of ear mites (family Psoroptidae) consisting of a single species, *O. cynotis,* the cause of otodectic mange in dogs, cats, and other carnivores; the entire lifespan of this mite is spent in the ears (rarely on the body) of the host, where it feeds on epidermal debris; it can be found in the encrusted material scraped from infected ears. [oto- + *dektēs,* beggar, receiver]

oto·dec·tic (ō-tō-dek′tik). Of, relating to, or caused by mites of the genus *Otodectes.*

oto·dyn·ia (ō-tō-din′ē-ă). SYN earache. [oto- + G. *odynē,* pain]

oto·en·ceph·a·li·tis (ō′tō-en-sef-ă-lī′tis). Inflammation of the brain by extension of the process from the middle ear and mastoid cells. SYN otocerebritis. [oto- + G. *enkephalos,* brain, + *-itis,* inflammation]

oto·gang·li·on (ō′tō-gang′glē-on). SYN otic *ganglion.*

oto·gen·ic, otog·e·nous (ō′tō-jen′ik, ō-toj′ĕ-nŭs). Of otic origin; originating within the ear, especially from inflammation of the ear. [oto- + G. *-gen,* producing]

oto·lar·yn·gol·o·gist (ō′tō-lar-ing-gol′ŏ-jist). A physician who specializes in otolaryngology.

oto·lar·yn·gol·o·gy (ō′tō-lar-ing-gol′ŏ-jē). The combined specialties of diseases of the ear and larynx, including the upper respiratory tract and diseases of the head and neck, tracheobronchial tree, and esophagus. [oto- + G. *larynx,* + *logos,* study]

oto·liths, oto·lites (ō′tō-lith, ō′tō-līt) [TA]. Crystalline particles of calcium carbonate and a protein adhering to the gelatinous membrane of the maculae of the utricle and saccule. SYN statoconia [TA], ear crystals, otoconia, sagitta, statoliths. [oto- + G. *lithos,* stone]

oto·log·ic (ō′tō-loj′ik). Relating to otology.

otol·o·gist (ō-tol′ŏ-jist). A specialist in otology.

otol·o·gy (ō-tol′ŏ-jē). The branch of medical science concerned with the study, diagnosis, and treatment of diseases of the ear and related structures. [oto- + G. *logos,* study]

oto·mu·cor·my·co·sis (ō-tō-mū′kōr-mī-kō′sis). Mucormycosis of the ear.

△**-otomy.** SEE -tomy.

▯**oto·my·co·sis** (ō′tō-mī-kō′sis). An infection in which fungal mycelia are seen in cerumen and desquamated cells in the external auditory canal, usually unilateral, with scaling, itching, and pain as the primary symptoms. The fungus does not invade tissue and plays little role in pathogenicity.

oto·neu·ral·gia (ō′tō-noo-ral′jē-ă). Earache of neuralgic origin, not caused by inflammation. [oto- + G. *neuron,* nerve, + *algos,* pain]

oto·pal·a·to·dig·i·tal (ō′tō-pal′ă-tō-dij′i-tăl). Relating to the ears, palate, and fingers.

otop·a·thy (ō-top′ă-thē). Any disease of the ear. [oto- + G. *pathos,* suffering]

oto·pha·ryn·ge·al (ō′tō-fa-rin′jē-ăl). Relating to the middle ear and the pharynx.

oto·plas·ty (ō′tō-plas-tē). Constructive or reparative plastic surgery of the ear. [oto- + G. *plastos,* formed]

oto·rhi·no·lar·yn·gol·o·gy (ō′tō-rī′nō-lar-ing -gol′ŏ-jē). The combined specialties of diseases of the ear, nose, pharynx, and larynx; including diseases of the head and neck, tracheobronchial tree, and esophagus. SEE ALSO otolaryngology. [oto- + G. *rhis,* nose, + *larynx,* larynx, + *logos,* study]

otor·rhea (ō-tō-rē′ă). A discharge from the ear. [oto- + G. *rhoia,* flow]

cerebrospinal fluid o., discharge of cerebrospinal fluid through the external auditory meatus or through the eustachian tube into the nasopharynx.

oto·sal·pinx (ō-tō-sal′pingks). SYN pharyngotympanic (auditory) *tube.* [oto- + G. *salpinx,* trumpet]

oto·scle·ro·sis (ō′tō-sklē-rō′sis). A disease of the otic capsule (bony labyrinth) characterized by formation of soft, vascular bone and resulting in progressive conductive hearing loss because of fixation of the stapes and sensory hearing loss because of involvement of the cochlear duct. [oto- + G. *sklērōsis,* hardening]

▯**oto·scope** (ō′tō-skōp). An instrument for examining the eardrum. [oto- + G. *skopeō,* to view]

Siegle o., an o. with a bulb attachment by which the air pressure can be varied, thus imparting movement to the tympanic membrane, if intact, while under inspection.

▯**otos·co·py** (ō-tos′kŏ-pē). Inspection of the ear, especially of the eardrum. [oto- + G. *skopeō,* to view]

pneumatic o., inspection of the ear with a device capable of varying air pressure against the eardrum. Imparting movement to the tympanic membrane suggests normal middle ear compliance; the lack of movement indicates either increased impedance, as with fluid in the middle ear, or perforation of the tympanic membrane.

oto·spon·gi·o·sis (ot-ō-spun-jē-ō′sis). A more accurately descriptive term for the pathologic changes in otosclerosis.

otos·te·al (ō-tos′tē-ăl). Relating to the ossicles of the ear. [oto- + G. *osteon,* bone]

oto·tox·ic (ō′tō-tok′sik). Relating to ototoxicity.

oto·tox·ic·i·ty (ō-tō-tok-sis′i-te). The property of being injurious to the ear. [oto- + G. *toxikon,* poison]

familial aminoglycoside o., inherited susceptibility to sensory hearing loss upon administration of aminoglycoside antibiotics due to a mutation in the mitochondrial genome.

Otto, Adolph W., German surgeon, 1786–1845. SEE O. *pelvis, disease.*

ot·to of rose. SYN *oil* of rose.

Ottoson, David, Swedish physiologist, *1918. SEE O. *potential.*

O.U. Abbreviation for Latin *oculus uterque,* each eye or both eyes.

oua·ba·gen·in (wă′bă-jen-in). The aglycon obtained from the hydrolysis of the cardiac glycoside, ouabain; exerts cardiotonic activity.

oua·ba·in (wah′bān, wah′bah-in). A glycoside and African arrow poison from ouabaio, obtained from the wood of *Acocanthera ouabaio* or from the seeds of *Strophanthus gratus;* its action is qualitatively identical to that of strophanthus and the digitalis glycosides; used for rapid digitalization; often used in pharmacological studies because of water solubility.

Ouchterlony, Orjan, Swedish bacteriologist, *1914. SEE O. method, *technique, test, technique.*

△**oul-.** For words beginning thus, see ulo-.

ounce (oz.) (owns). A weight containing 480 g, or ¹/₁₂ pound troy and apothecaries' weight, or 437.5 g, ¹/₁₆ pound avoirdupois. The apothecary oz (used in the USP) contains 8 dram and is equivalent to 31.10349 g; the avoirdupois oz is equivalent to 28.35 g. [L. *uncia,* the twelfth part (of a pound or foot) hence also inch]

△**-ous.** **1.** Chemical suffix attached to the name of an element in one of its lower valencies. Cf. -ic (1). **2.** Having much of. [L. *-osus,* full of, abounding]

out·let (owt′let) [TA]. An exit or opening of a passageway. SEE ALSO aperture.

  pelvic o. [TA], the lower opening of the true pelvis, bounded anteriorly by the pubic arch, laterally by the rami of the ischium and the sacrotuberous ligament on either side, and posteriorly by these ligaments and the tip of the coccyx. SYN apertura pelvis inferior [TA], apertura pelvis minoris, fourth parallel pelvic plane, inferior pelvic aperture, pelvic plane of outlet, plane of outlet.

  thoracic o., (1) SYN inferior thoracic *aperture*; **(2)** SYN superior thoracic *aperture*.

out·li·er (owt′lē-er). An observation that differs so widely from all others in a set as to justify the conclusion that a gross error has occurred or that it comes from a different population.

out·pa·tient (owt′pā′shent). A patient treated in a hospital dispensary or clinic instead of in an overnight room or ward.

out of phase. Not in phase, moving in opposite directions at the same time; 180° out of phase; a possible characteristic of two simultaneous oscillations of similar frequency.

out·put (owt′poot). The quantity produced, ejected, or excreted of a specific entity in a specified period of time or per unit time, e.g., urinary sodium o.; the opposite of intake or input.

  cardiac o., the amount of blood ejected by the heart in a unit of time (i.e., the minute volume), usually expressed in liters per minute. SYN minute o.

  maximum power o., the greatest sound resulting from amplification that the instrument can produce; an indication of hearing aid performance.

  minute o., SYN cardiac o.

  pacemaker o., electrical energy delivered into a standard load (500 Ω resistance).

  stroke o., SYN stroke *volume*.

ova (ō′vă). Plural of ovum. [L.]

oval (ō′văl). **1.** Relating to an ovum. **2.** Egg-shaped, resembling in outline the longitudinal section of an egg.

ov·al·bu·min (ō-văl-bū′min). The chief protein occurring in the white of egg and resembling serum albumin; also found in phosphorylated form. SYN albumen, egg albumin.

oval·o·cy·to·sis (ō′vă-lō-sī-tō′sis). SYN elliptocytosis.

ovar·i·al·gia (ō-var-ē-al′jē-ă). Pain in an ovary. SYN oophoralgia. [ovario- + G. *algos*, pain]

ovar·i·an (ō-var′ē-an). Relating to the ovary.

ovar·i·ec·to·my (ō-var-ē-ek′tō-mē). Excision of one or both ovaries. SYN oophorectomy. [ovario- + G. *ektomē*, excision]

ovario-, ovari-. Ovary. SEE ALSO oo-, oophor-. [L. *ovarium*]

ovar·i·o·cele (ō-var′ē-ō-sēl). Hernia of an ovary. [ovario- + G. *kēlē*, hernia]

ovar·i·o·cen·te·sis (ō-var′ē-ō-sen-tē′sis). Puncture of an ovary or an ovarian cyst. [ovario- + G. *kentēsis*, puncture]

ovar·i·o·cy·e·sis (ō-var′ē-ō-sī-ē′sis). SYN ovarian *pregnancy*. [ovario- + G. *kyēsis*, pregnancy]

ovar·i·o·dys·neu·ria (ō-var′ē-ō-dis-noo′rē-ă). Ovarian pain or neuralgia. [ovario- + G. *dys-*, bad, + *neuron*, nerve]

ovar·i·o·gen·ic (ō-var′ē-ō-jen′ik). Originating in the ovary. [ovario- + G. *-gen*, producing]

ovar·i·o·lyt·ic (ō-var′ē-ō-lit′ik). Destructive to the ovary. [ovario- + G. *lysis*, dissolution]

ovar·i·op·a·thy (ō-var-ē-op′ă-thē). Any disease of the ovary. SYN oophoropathy. [ovario- + G. *pathos*, suffering]

ovar·i·or·rhex·is (ō-var′ē-ō-rek′sis). Rupture of an ovary. [ovario- + G. *rhēxis*, rupture]

ovar·i·o·sal·pin·gec·to·my (ō-var′ē-ō-sal-pin-jek′tō-mē). Operative removal of an ovary and the corresponding oviduct. SYN oophorosalpingectomy. [ovario- + salpingectomy]

ovar·i·o·sal·pin·gi·tis (ō-var′ē-ō-sal-pin-jī′tis). Inflammation of ovary and oviduct. SYN oophorosalpingitis. [ovario- + salpingitis]

ovar·i·os·to·my (ō-var-ē-os′tō-mē). Establishment of a temporary fistula for drainage of a cyst of the ovary. [ovario- + G. *stoma*, mouth]

ovar·i·ot·o·my (ō-var-ē-ot′ō-mē). An incision into an ovary, e.g.,

a biopsy or a wedge excision. SYN oophorotomy. [ovario- + G. *tomē*, incision]

ova·ri·tis (ō-vă-rī′tis). SYN oophoritis.

ovar·i·um, pl. **ova·ria** (ō-vār′ē-ŭm, -ă) [TA]. SYN ovary. [Mod. L. fr. *ovum*, egg]

  o. biparti′tum, an ovary separated into two distinct parts.

  o. disjunc′tum, an ovary partially or completely divided into two sections.

  o. gyra′tum, an ovary showing curved or irregular grooves or furrows.

  o. loba′tum, an ovary demarcated by deep furrows into two or more lobes.

  o. masculi′num, SYN *appendix* of testis.

ova·ry (ō′vă-rē) [TA]. One of the paired female reproductive glands containing the ova or germ cells; the o.'s stroma is a vascular connective tissue containing numbers of ovarian follicles enclosing the ova; surrounding this stroma is a more condensed layer of stroma called the tunica albuginea. SYN ovarium [TA], female gonad, genital gland (2). [Mod. L. *ovarium*, fr. *ovum*, egg]

  mulberry o., the type of o. produced by the administration of anterior pituitary extracts to immature rats; such an o. contains many more follicles than normal, with the follicles in various stages of development and with prominent corpora lutea on their surfaces, thus the perceived resemblance to a mulberry.

  polycystic o., enlarged cystic o.'s, pearl white in color, with thickened tunica albuginea, characteristic of the Stein-Leventhal syndrome; clinical features are abnormal menses, obesity, and evidence of masculinization, such as hirsutism.

  third o., an accessory o.

over·bite (ō′ver-bīt). SYN vertical *overlap*.

over·clo·sure (ō′ver-klō-zher). A decrease in occlusal vertical dimension.

over·com·pen·sa·tion (ō′ver-kom-pen-sā′shŭn). **1.** An exaggeration of personal capacity by which one overcomes a real or imagined inferiority. **2.** The process in which a psychologic deficiency inspires exaggerated correction. SEE compensation.

over·cor·rec·tion (ō′ver-kŏ-rek′shŭn). In behavior modification treatment programs, especially those involving mentally retarded individuals, overlearning the desired target behavior beyond the set criterion to assure that the behavior will continue to meet the established criterion when the post-learning decrements and forgetting occur.

over·den·ture (ō-ver-den′choor). SYN overlay *denture*.

over·de·ter·mi·na·tion (o′ver-dē-ter′min-ā′shŭn). In psychoanalysis, ascribing the cause of a single behavioral or emotional reaction, mental symptom, or dream to the operation of two or more forces, that is, it is overdetermined (e.g., ascribing the nature of an emotional outburst not only to the immediate precipitant but also to a lingering inferiority complex).

over·dom·i·nance (ō-ver-dom′i-năns). That state in which the heterozygote has greater phenotype value and perhaps is more fit than the homozygous state for either of the alleles that it comprises. Cf. balanced *polymorphism*.

over·dom·i·nant (ō-ver-dom′i-nănt). Denoting heterozygous states that exhibit overdominance.

over·drive (ō-ver-drīv). **1.** An electrophysiologic pacing technique to exceed the rate of an abnormal pacemaker and so capture the territory controlled by that pacemaker (usually atrial). **2.** A state of eukaryotic RNA polymerase wherein it is resistant to pause, arrest, or termination signals. SEE ALSO hesitant, antitermination.

over·e·rup·tion (ō′ver-ē-rŭp′shŭn). Occlusal projection of a tooth beyond the line of occlusion.

over·ex·ten·sion (ō-ver-eks-ten′shŭn). SYN hyperextension.

over·graft·ing (ō′ver-graft′ing). Placing a second or additional grafts over a previously healed graft from which the epithelium has been removed, as with dermabrasion, to strengthen and thicken a split-thickness *graft*.

over·hang (ō′ver-hang). An excess of dental filling material beyond the cavity margin or normal tooth contour.

over·head pro·jec·tor. SYN epidiascope.

OV

over·hy·dra·tion (ō′ver-hī-drā′shŭn). SYN hyperhydration.

over·jet, over·jut (ō′ver-jet, ō′ver-jŭt). SYN horizontal *overlap*.

over·lap (ō′ver-lap). **1.** Suturing of one layer of tissue above or under another to gain strength. **2.** An extension or projection of one tissue over another.

horizontal o., the projection of the upper anterior and/or posterior teeth beyond their antagonists in a horizontal direction. SYN overjet, overjut.

vertical o., (1) the extension of the upper teeth over the lower teeth in a vertical direction when the opposing posterior teeth are in contact in centric occlusion; (2) the distance that teeth lap over their antagonists vertically, especially for the distance that the upper incisal edges drop below the lower ones, but may also describe the vertical relations of opposing cusps; (3) the relationship of the maxillary incisors to the mandibular incisors when the incisal edges pass each other in centric occlusion. SYN overbite.

over·lay (ō′ver-lā). An addition to an already existing condition.

emotional o., the emotional or psychologic concomitant of an organic disability.

over·learn·ing (ō′ver-lern′ing). In the psychology of memory, continuation of practice beyond the point at which one is able to perform according to the specified criterion; typically, retention is longer after o. as compared with retention after practice only to the point of performance meeting the specified criterion.

over·re·sponse (ō′ver-rē-spons′). An abnormally strong reaction to a stimulus.

over·rid·ing (ō′ver-rī′ding). **1.** Slippage of the lower fragment of a broken long bone upward and alongside the proximal portion. **2.** Obsolete term denoting a fetal head that is palpable above the symphysis because of cephalopelvic disproportion. **3.** The slippage of fetal bones of the skull that occurs after an interutero fetal death.

over·sens·ing (ō′ver-sen′sing). Sensing of electrical or magnetic signals, which normally should not be sensed by a pacemaker, but result in inappropriate inhibition of the pacemaker's output.

over·shoot (ō′ver-shoot). **1.** Generally, any initial change, in response to a sudden step change in some factor, that is greater than the steady-state response to the new level of that factor; common in systems in which inertia or a time lag in negative feedback outweighs any damping that may be present. Changes in a negative direction are sometimes distinguished by the term undershoot, and the two may alternate in an oscillatory fashion, as in the transient oscillations of a pendulum when released from an initial displacement. **2.** Momentary reversal of the membrane potential of a cell (inside becoming positive rather than negative relative to the outside) during an action potential; considered a form of overshoot (1) because, before discovery of overshoot (2), excitation was thought merely to depolarize the membrane to zero transmembrane potential.

Overton, Charles E., German biologist in Sweden, 1865–1933. SEE Meyer-O. *rule, theory* of narcosis.

over·tone (ō′ver-tōn). Any of the tones, other than the lowest or fundamental tone, of which a complex sound is composed.

psychic o., the mental associations related to any stimulus.

over·ven·ti·la·tion (ō′ver-ven-ti-lā′shŭn). SYN hyperventilation.

over·win·ter·ing (ō′ver-win′ter-ing). Persistence of an infectious agent in its vector for extended periods, such as the cooler winter months, during which the vector has no opportunity to be reinfected or to infect another host.

△**ovi-.** Egg. SEE ALSO oo-, ovo-. [L. *ovum*]

ovi·ci·dal (ō-vi-sī′dăl). Causing death of the ovum. [ovi- + L. *caedo,* to kill]

ovi·du·cal (ō-vi-doo′kăl). SYN oviductal.

ovi·duct (ō′vi-dŭkt). SYN uterine *tube.* [ovi- + L. *ductus,* a leading, fr. *duco,* pp. *ductus,* to lead]

ovi·duc·tal (ō-vi-dŭk′tăl). Relating to a uterine tube. SYN oviducal.

ovif·er·ous (ō-vif′er-ŭs). Carrying, containing, or producing ova. SYN ovigerous. [ovi- + L. *fero,* to carry]

ovi·form (ō′vi-fōrm). SYN ovoid (2).

ovi·gen·e·sis (ō-vi-jen′ĕ-sis). SYN oogenesis.

ovi·ge·net·ic, ovi·gen·ic (ō-vi-jĕ-net′ik, -jen′ik). SYN oogenetic.

ovig·e·nous (ō-vij′ĕ-nŭs). SYN oogenetic.

ovig·er·ous (ō-vij′er-ŭs). SYN oviferous.

ovi·ge·rus. SYN *cumulus* oöphorus.

ovine (ō′vīn). Relating to sheep; sheeplike. [L. *ovinus,* relating to a sheep]

ovi·par·i·ty (ō-vi-par′i-tē). The quality of being oviparous. [ovi- + L. *pario,* to bear]

ovip·a·rous (ō-vip′ă-rŭs). Egg-laying; denoting those birds, fish, amphibians, reptiles, monotreme mammals, and invertebrates whose young develop in eggs outside of the maternal body. [L. *oviparus,* fr. *ovum,* egg, + *pario,* to bear]

ovi·pos·it (ō′vi-poz′it). To lay eggs; applied especially to insects. [ovi- + L. *pono,* pp. *positus,* to place]

ovi·po·si·tion (ō′vi-pō-zish′ŭn). Act of laying or depositing eggs by insects.

ovi·pos·i·tor (ō-vi-poz′i-tŏr, -tōr). A specialized female organ especially well developed in insects for laying or depositing eggs.

ovist (ō′vist). A preformationist who believed that the female sex cell contained a miniature body susceptible to growth when stimulated by semen. Cf. spermist.

△**ovo-.** Egg. SEE ALSO oo-, ovi-. [L. *ovum*]

ovo·cyte (ō′vō-sīt). SYN oocyte. [ovo- + G. *kytos,* a hollow (cell)]

ovo·fla·vin (ō-vō-flā′vin). Riboflavin found in eggs.

ovo·gen·e·sis (ō-vō-jen′ĕ-sis). SYN oogenesis.

ovo·glob·u·lin (ō-vō-glob′ū-lin). Globulin in the white of egg.

ovoid (ō′voyd). **1.** An oval or egg-shaped form. **2.** Resembling an egg. SYN oviform. [ovo- + G. *eidos,* resemblance]

fetal o., the form of the fetus *in utero;* its length is about one-half of the length of the extended fetus.

Manchester o., an egg-shaped radium applicator for placement in the lateral vaginal fornices. [University of *Manchester,* England]

ovo·lar·vip·a·rous (ō′vō-lar-vip′ă-rŭs). Denoting certain nematodes and other invertebrates in which the eggs are hatched within the female, and the larvae developed or protected within the uterus until the correct time for their emergence. [ovo- + L. *larva,* a mask, + *pario,* to bear]

ovo·mu·cin (ō-vō-mū′sin). A glycoprotein in the white of egg.

ovo·mu·coid (ō-vō-mū′koyd). A mucoprotein obtained from the white of egg.

ovo·plasm (ō′vō-plazm). Protoplasm of an unfertilized egg.

ovo·pro·to·gen (ō-vō-prō′tō-jen). SYN lipoic acid.

ovo·sis·ton (ō-vō-sis′ton). An oral contraceptive that consists of a mixture of a progestin and an estrogen.

ovo·tes·tis (ō′vō-tes′tis). Gonad in which both testicular and ovarian components are present; a form of hermaphroditism.

ovo·trans·fer·rin (ō′vō-trans-fār′in). SYN conalbumin.

ovo·vi·tel·lin (ō′vō-vī-tel′in). SYN vitellin. [ovo- + L. *vitellus,* yolk]

ovo·vi·vip·ar·ous (ō′vō-vī-vip′ă-rŭs). Denoting those fish, amphibians, and reptiles that produce eggs that hatch within the body of the parent. [ovo- + L. *viviparus,* bringing forth alive, fr. *vivus,* alive, + *pario,* to bear]

o·vu·lar (ov′ū-lăr, ō′vū-). Relating to an ovule.

■**o·vu·la·tion** (ov′ū-lā′shŭn, ō′vū-). Release of an ovum from the ovarian follicle.

anestrous o., discharge of ova occurring in animals without estrus.

paracyclic o., obsolete term for o. occurring in the menstrual cycle at any time other than the normally anticipated time.

o·vu·la·to·ry (ov′ū-lă-tō-rē, ō′vū-). Relating to ovulation.

o·vule (ov′ūl, ō′vū-). **1.** The ovum of a mammal, especially while still in the ovarian follicle. **2.** A small beadlike structure bearing a fancied resemblance to an o. SYN ovulum. [Mod. L. *ovulum,* dim. of L. *ovum,* egg]

o·vu·lo·cy·clic (ov′ū-lō-sī′klik, ō′vū-). Denoting any recurrent phenomenon associated with and occurring at a certain time

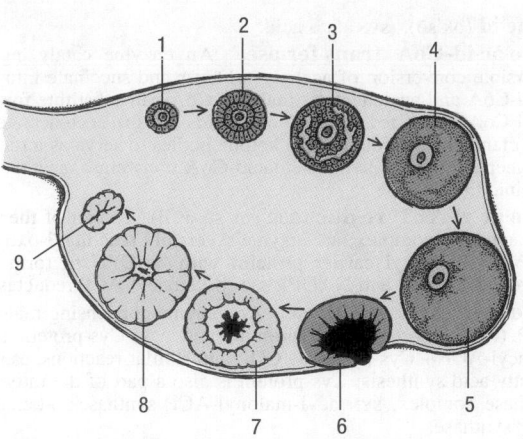

ovulation: (1) primary follicle; (2) double-layered follicle; (3) follicle at beginning of antrum formation; (4) follicle approaching maturity; (5) mature follicle; (6) corpus hemorrhagicum; (7) young corpus luteum; (8) corpus luteum; (9) corpus albicans

within the ovulatory cycle, as, for example, ovulocyclic porphyria.

o·vu·lum, pl. **ovu·la** (ov′ū-lŭm, ō′vū-; -lă). SYN ovule.

ovum, gen. **ovi**, pl. **ova** (ō′vŭm, -vī, -vă). The female sex cell. When fertilized by a spermatozoon, an o. is capable of developing into a new individual of the same species; during maturation, the o., like the spermatozoon, undergoes a halving of its chromosomal complement so that, at its union with the male gamete, the species number of chromosomes (46 in humans) is maintained; yolk contained in the ova of different species varies greatly in amount and distribution, which influences the pattern of the cleavage divisions. [L. egg]

alecithal o., an o. in which the yolk is nearly absent, consisting of only a few particles.

blighted o., a fertilized o. whose development has ceased at an early stage.

centrolecithal o., one in which the yolk is mostly located near the center of the egg, as in arthropods.

fertilized o., an o. impregnated by a spermatozoon.

isolecithal o., an o. in which the yolk is evenly distributed throughout the cytoplasm.

Peters o., an o. with a presumptive fertilization age of about 13 days; for many years, it was one of very few young human embryos recovered in good condition and its study furnished many facts regarding early embryonic changes.

telolecithal o., an o. in which there is a large amount of yolk massed at the vegetative pole, as in the eggs of birds and reptiles.

Owen, Sir Richard, English anatomist, 1804–1892. SEE O. *lines*, under *line;* contour *lines* of O., under *line;* interglobular *space* of O.

Owren, Paul A., Norwegian hematologist, *1905. SEE O. *disease.*

oxa-. Combining form inserted in names of organic compounds to signify the presence or addition of oxygen atom(s) in a chain or ring (as in ethers), not appended to either (as in ketones and aldehydes). SEE ALSO hydroxy-, oxo-, oxy-. [English. *oxygen*]

ox·a·cil·lin so·di·um (ok-să-sil′in). A semisynthetic penicillin used in the oral therapy of penicillin-resistant staphylococcal infections.

ox·al·al·de·hyde (ok-să-lal′dĕ-hīd). SYN glyoxal.

ox·a·late (ok′să-lāt). A salt of oxalic acid.

ox·a·le·mia (ok-să-lē′mē-ă). The presence of an abnormally large amount of oxalates in the blood. [oxalate + G. *haima,* blood]

ox·al·ic ac·id (ok-sal′ik). An acid, HOOC—COOH, found in many plants and vegetables, particularly in buckwheat (family Polygoniaceae) and *Oxalis* (family Oxalidaceae); used as a hemostatic in veterinary medicine, but toxic in elevated levels when ingested by humans; also used in the removal of ink and other stains, and as a general reducing agent; salts of o. a. are found in renal calculi; accumulates in cases of primary hyperoxaluria.

ox·a·lo (ok′să-lō). The monoacyl radical, HOOC—C(O)–.

ox·a·lo·ac·e·tate trans·ac·e·tase (ok′să-lō-as′ĕ-tāt trans-as′ĕ-tās). SYN *citrate* synthase.

ox·a·lo·a·ce·tic ac·id (ok′să-lō-ă-sē′tik). A ketodicarboxylic acid and important intermediate in the tricarboxylic acid cycle; the product formed when L-aspartic acid acts as an amine donor in transamination reactions. SYN ketosuccinic acid, oxosuccinic acid.

ox·a·lo·sis (ok-să-lō′sis). Widespread deposition of calcium oxalate crystals in the kidneys, bones, arterial media, and myocardium, with increased urinary excretion of oxalate; may be an acquired disorder, as in oxalate poisoning, or represent one aspect of primary hyperoxaluria and o. [oxalate + -osis, condition]

ox·a·lo·suc·cin·ic ac·id (ok-să-lō-sŭk-sin′ik). The product of the dehydrogenation of isocitric acid under the catalytic influence of isocitrate dehydrogenase; an enzyme-bound intermediate of the tricarboxylic acid cycle.

ox·a·lo·suc·cin·ic car·box·yl·ase. SYN *isocitrate* dehydrogenase.

ox·a·lo·u·rea (ok′să-lō-ū-rē′ă). SYN oxalylurea.

ox·a·lu·ria (ok-să-loo′rē-ă). SYN hyperoxaluria. [oxalate + G. *ouron,* urine]

ox·a·lur·ic ac·id (ok-să-loor′ik). The ureide of oxalic acid, derived from uric acid or oxalylurea.

ox·a·lyl (ok′să-lil). The diacyl radical, –CO—CO– .

ox·a·lyl·u·rea (ok′să-lil-ū-rē′ă). The cyclic (end-to-end) amide anhydride of oxaluric acid; an oxidation product of uric acid. SYN oxalourea, parabanic acid.

ox·am·ni·quine (oks-am′ni-quin). A tetrahydroquinoline derivative, similar to hycanthone and lucanthone, effective against *Schistosoma mansoni;* now largely superseded by the broad-spectrum anthelmintic drug praziquantel.

ox·an·a·mide (ok-san′ă-mīd). A sedative.

ox·an·dro·lone (ok-san′drō-lōn). 17β-Hydroxy-17α-methyl-2-oxa-5α-androstan-3-one (C-2 replaced by O in the androstane nucleus); an androgenic anabolic steroid.

ox·a·phen·a·mide (ok-să-fen′ă-mīd). A choleretic.

ox·a·ze·pam (ok-sā′zĕ-pam). A benzodiazepine chemically and pharmacologically related to chlordiazepoxide and diazepam; an antianxiety agent.

ox·a·zin (ok′să-zin). Parent substance of a series of biologic dyes, e.g., gallocyanin, brilliant cresyl blue, cresyl violet acetate.

ox·a·zole (ok′să-zōl). The fundamental ring system of pyranoses.

ox·a·zo·li·dine·di·ones (ok-să-zō-lid′īn-dē-onz). An obsolescent chemical class of antiepileptic drugs useful in the treatment of absence (petit mal) seizures; examples include trimethadione and paramethadione.

oxazolidinones (oks′ă-zō-lid′i-nōnz). A new class of antibacterial antibiotics.

ox·el·a·din (ok-sel′ă-din). An antitussive agent.

ox·i·con·a·zole (ok′sē-kō′nă-zōl). Broad-spectrum antifungal agent resembling ketoconazole.

ox·i·dant (ok′si-dant). The substance that is reduced and that, therefore, oxidizes the other component of an oxidation-reduction system.

ox·i·dase (ok′si-dās). Classically, one of a group of enzymes, now termed oxidoreductases (EC class 1), that bring about oxidation by the addition of oxygen to a metabolite or by the removal of hydrogen or of one or more electrons. O. is now used for those cases in which O_2 acts as an acceptor (of H or of electrons); those removing hydrogen are now termed dehydrogenases. For individual o.'s, see the specific names.

direct o., originally, an o. catalyzing the transfer of O_2 directly to other bodies; now termed oxygenase.

indirect o., originally, an o. that acts by reducing a peroxide; now termed peroxidase.

terminal o., the last protein in the electron transport, respiratory chain. In mammals this is cytochrome *c* oxidase.

OX

ox·i·da·sis (ok-si-dā′sis). Oxidation by an oxidase.

ox·i·da·tion (ok-si-dā′shŭn). **1.** Combination with oxygen. **2.** Increasing the valence of an atom or ion by the loss from it of hydrogen or of one or more electrons thus rendering it more electropositive, as when iron is changed from the ferrous (2+) to the ferric (3+) state. **3.** In bacteriology, the aerobic dissimilation of substrates with the production of energy and water; in contrast to fermentation, the transfer of electrons in the o. process is accomplished via the respiratory chain, which utilizes oxygen as the final electron acceptor.

alpha-o., α-oxidation, a form of o. of fatty acids in which carbons are removed one at a time in the form of CO_2; the α-carbon is first hydroxylated and then converted into a carbonyl; a deficiency of this pathway is associated with Refsum disease.

beta-o., β-oxidation, (1) o. of the β-carbon (carbon 3) of a fatty acid, forming the β-keto (β-oxo) acid analog; of importance in fatty acid catabolism; **(2)** the entire pathway for the catabolism of saturated fatty acids containing an even number of carbon atoms; beta-o. (1) is a part of this pathway; acetyl-CoA is a major product of this pathway.

end o., the last o. step in a catabolic pathway. SYN terminal o.

omega-o., ω-oxidation, o. at the carbon atom farthest removed (ω-carbon) from the carboxyl group (carbon 1); thus, in this pathway, a dicarboxylic acid is formed; an important pathway in the degradation of prostaglandins.

terminal o., SYN end o.

ox·i·da·tion-re·duc·tion. Any chemical oxidation or reduction reaction, which must, in toto, comprise both oxidation and reduction; the basis for calling all oxidative enzymes (formerly oxidases) oxidoreductases. Often shortened to "redox."

ox·i·da·tive (ok-si-dā′tiv). Having the power to oxidize; denoting a process involving oxidation.

ox·ide (ok′sīd). A compound of oxygen with another element or a radical; e.g., mercuric o., HgO.

acid o., an acid anhydride; an o. of an electronegative element or radical; it can combine with water to form an acid.

basic o., a base anhydride; an o. of an electropositive element or radical; it can combine with water to form a base.

indifferent o., SYN neutral o.

neutral o., an o. that is neither an acid nor a base; e.g., water (hydrogen oxide, H_2O). SYN indifferent o.

ox·i·dize (ok′si-dīz). To combine or cause an element or radical to combine with oxygen or to lose electrons.

ox·i·do·re·duc·tase (ok′si-dō-rē-dŭk′tās). An enzyme (EC class 1) catalyzing an oxidation-reduction reaction. Trivial names for o.'s include dehydrogenase, reductase, oxidase (where O_2 is the H acceptor), oxygenase (where O_2 is incorporated into the substrate), peroxidase (H_2O_2 is the acceptor; catalase is an exception), and hydroxylase (coupled oxidation of two donors). SEE ALSO oxidase.

ox·ime (ok′sēm). A compound resulting from the action of hydroxylamine, NH_2OH, on a ketone or an aldehyde to yield the group =N–OH attached to the former carbonyl carbon atom.

amide o.'s, SYN amidoximes.

ox·im·e·ter (ok-sim′ĕ-ter). An instrument for determining photoelectrically the oxygen saturation of a sample of blood.

cuvette o., an o. that reads the percentage of oxygen saturation of the blood as it passes through a cuvette outside the body.

ox·im·e·try (oks-ĭm-a-tree). Procedure using a device to measure oxygen saturation by fluctations of light absorption in well-vascularized tissue during systole and diastole. The underlying principle is Beer law, or the relationship between the amount of light absorbed by a solute in solution and the concentration of the unknown solute.

pulse o., o. performed noninvasively, usually on the finger or ear lobe, in which the small increase in absorption of light during the systolic pulse is used to calculate oxygen saturation.

oxi·rane (oks′ē-rān). SYN *ethylene* oxide.

△**oxo-.** Prefix denoting addition of oxygen; used in place of keto- in systematic nomenclature. SEE ALSO hydroxy-, oxa-, oxy-.

oxo·ace·tic ac·id (ok′sō-a-sē′tik). SYN glyoxylic acid.

oxo ac·id (ok′sō). SYN keto acid.

3-ox·o·ac·id-CoA trans·fer·ase. An enzyme catalyzing the reversible conversion of acetoacetyl-CoA and succinate into succinyl-CoA and acetoacetate; malonyl-CoA can substitute for succinyl-CoA and a few other 3-oxo acids for the acetoacetate; an important step in order for the ketone bodies to serve as a fuel for extrahepatic tissues. SYN 3-ketoacid-CoA transferase, acetoacetyl-succinic thiophorase.

3-ox·o·ac·yl-ACP re·duc·tase (ok′sō-as′il). A part of the fatty acid synthase complex; an enzyme reversibly reacting 3-oxoacyl-ACP (ACP = acyl carrier protein) with NADPH to form D-3-hydroxyacyl-ACP and $NADP^+$. SYN β-ketoacyl-ACP reductase.

3-ox·o·ac·yl-ACP syn·thase. An enzyme condensing malonyl-ACP (ACP = acyl carrier protein) and acyl-Cys-protein to 3-oxoacyl-ACP + Cys-protein + CO_2, and similar reactions, as steps in fatty acid synthesis; Cys-protein is also a part of the fatty acid synthase complex. SYN acyl-malonyl-ACP synthase, β-ketoacyl-ACP synthase.

2-ox·o·glu·tar·ate de·hy·dro·gen·ase (ok′sō-gloo-tar′āt). SYN α-*ketoglutarate* dehydrogenase.

2-ox·o·glu·tar·ic ac·id (oks′-ō-gloo-tar-ik). SYN α-ketoglutaramic acid.

2-oxo-5-guanidovaleric ac·id (gwan-ē′dō-va-ler′ik). The deaminated derivative of arginine.

ox·ol·a·mine (ok-sol′ă-mēn). Used for treatment of bronchopulmonary infections.

ox·o·lin·ic ac·id (ok-sō-lin′ik). A quinolone antibacterial agent used in the treatment of urinary tract infections.

ox·o·phen·ar·sine hy·dro·chlo·ride (ok′sō-fen-ar′sēn). An antisyphilitic and antitrypanosomal agent.

5-ox·o·pro·lin·ase. An enzyme that catalyzes the ATP-dependent hydrolysis of L-5-oxoproline (ATP + L-5-oxoproline → ADP + orthophosphate + L-glutamate); a deficiency of this enzyme will result in 5-oxoprolinuria.

5-ox·o·pro·line (Glp) (oks′ō-prō′lēn). A keto derivative of proline that is formed nonenzymatically from glutamate, glutamine, and γ-glutamylated peptides; it is also produced by the action of γ-glutamylcyclotransferase; elevated levels of 5-o. are often associated with problems of glutamine or glutathione metabolism. SYN 5-pyrrolidone-2-carboxylic acid, pyroglutamic acid, pyrrolidone-5-carboxylate.

4-ox·o·pro·line re·duc·tase. SYN 4-*hydroxyproline* oxidase.

5-ox·o·pro·lin·ur·ia (oks′ō-prō′lēn-ūr-ē-ă). Elevated levels of 5-oxoproline in the urine.

17-ox·o·ste·roids (ok-sō-stēr′oydz). SYN 17-ketosteroids.

ox·o·suc·cin·ic ac·id (ok′sō-sŭk-sin′ik). SYN oxaloacetic acid.

ox·o·tre·mo·rine (ok′sō-trem′er-ēn). An active metabolite of tremorine. Used as a pharmacologic tool for producing a parkinsonian tremor.

ox·pren·o·lol hy·dro·chlo·ride (oks-pren′ō-lol). A β-receptor blocking agent with coronary vasodilator activity.

OXT Abbreviation for oxytocin.

ox·tri·phyl·line (oks-trī′fi-lin, oks′trī-fil′in). A true salt of theophylline; it has mild diuretic, myocardial stimulating vasodilator, and bronchodilator actions, with the same uses as theophylline, but is better absorbed and less irritating. SYN choline theophyllinate.

△**oxy-. 1.** Combining form denoting shrill; sharp, pointed; quick (incorrectly used for ocy-, from G. *ōkys,* swift). **2.** In chemistry, combining form denoting the presence of oxygen, either added or substituted, in a substance. SEE ALSO hydroxy-, oxa-, oxo-. [G. *oxys,* keen]

ox·y·a·coia, ox·y·a·koia (ok′sē-ă-koy′ă). Increased sensitiveness to sounds, occurring in facial paralysis, especially when the stapedius muscle is paralyzed. [G. *oxys,* acute, + *akoē,* hearing]

ox·y·a·phia (ok-sē-ā′fē-ă). SYN hyperaphia. [G. *oxys,* acute, + *haphē,* touch]

ox·y·bar·bi·tu·rates (ok′sē-bar-bit′ūr-āts). Hypnotics of the barbiturate group in which the atom attached at the carbon-2 position is oxygen; virtually all hypnotic barbituates are o.'s.

ox·y·ben·zone (ok-sē-ben′zōn). An ultraviolet screen for use in skin ointments and lotions.

ox·y·bi·o·tin (ok-sē-bī′ō-tin). An analog and antimetabolite of biotin, in which the sulfur atom is replaced by oxygen.

ox·y·bu·ty·nin chlo·ride (ok-sē-bū′ti-nin). An intestinal antispasmodic.

ox·y·cal·o·rim·e·ter (ok′sē-kal-ō-rim′ĕ-ter). A calorimeter measuring energy content of substances in terms of oxygen consumed.

ox·y·cel·lu·lose (ok-sē-sel′ū-lōs). Cellulose that has been oxidized by NO_2 or other oxidizing agents to the point at which all or most of the glucose residues have been converted to glucuronic acid residues; used as an adsorbent in chromatography or other adsorption processes. SEE ALSO oxidized *cellulose.*

ox·y·ce·pha·lia (ok′sē-se-fā′lē-ă). SYN oxycephaly.

ox·y·ce·phal·ic, ox·y·ceph·a·lous (ok-sē-se-fal′ik, -sef′ă-lŭs). Relating to or characterized by oxycephaly. SYN acrocephalic, acrocephalous.

ox·y·ceph·a·ly (ok-sē-sef′ă-lē). A type of craniosynostosis in which there is premature closure of the lambdoid and coronal sutures, resulting in an abnormally high, peaked, or conical skull. SYN acrocephalia, acrocephaly, hypsicephaly, hypsocephaly, oxycephalia, steeple skull, tower skull, turricephaly. [G. *oxys,* pointed, + *kephalē,* head]

ox·y·chlo·ride (ok-sē-klōr′īd). A compound of oxygen with a metallic chloride; e.g., a chlorate or perchlorate.

ox·y·chro·mat·ic (ok′sē-krō-mat′ik). SYN acidophilic. [G. *oxys,* sour, acid, + *chrōma,* color]

ox·y·chro·ma·tin (ok-sē-krō′mă-tin). Chromatin that stains with acid dyes, as in interphase nuclei. SYN oxyphil chromatin.

ox·y·co·done (ok-sē-kō′dōn). A narcotic analgesic often combined with aspirin or acetaminophen.

11-ox·y·cor·ti·coids (ok-sē-kōr′ti-koydz). Corticosteroids bearing an alcohol or ketonic group on carbon-11; e.g., cortisone, cortisol.

ox·y·gen (O) (ok′sē-jen). **1.** A gaseous element, atomic no. 8, atomic wt. 15.9994 on the basis of $^{12}C = 12.0000$; an abundant and widely distributed chemical element, which combines with most of the other elements to form oxides and is essential to animal and plant life. **2.** The molecular form of o., O_2. **3.** A medicinal gas that contains not less than 99.0%, by volume, of O_2. [G. *oxys,* sharp, acid and *genes,* forming]

heavy o., SYN oxygen-18.

hyperbaric o., high pressure o., o. at a pressure greater than 1 atm. SEE ALSO hyperbaric *oxygenation.*

singlet o., an excited or higher-energy form of o. characterized by the spin of a pair of electrons in opposite directions, whereas electron spin is unidirectional in normal molecular o. Because of its great reactivity, singlet o. is a probable intermediate in most photo-oxidation reactions. Although it exists for no more than 0.1 second, it may react with atmospheric pollutants to foster smog formation and may have harmful biologic effects.

triplet o., the normal unexcited state of O_2 in the atmosphere, in which the unpaired pair of electrons are so displaced that their magnetic fields are oriented in the same direction, resulting in paramagnetism; each of the heat-generated spectral lines of such o. can be split by a magnetic field into a triplet. Cf. singlet o.

ox·y·gen-15 (^{15}O). A cyclotron-produced, positron-emitting radioisotope of oxygen with a half-life of 122.2 seconds; used in studies of respiratory function and in positron emission tomography.

ox·y·gen-16 (^{16}O). The common oxygen isotope, making up 99.76% of natural oxygen.

ox·y·gen-17 (^{17}O). The rarest of the stable oxygen isotopes, making up 0.04% of natural oxygen.

ox·y·gen-18 (^{18}O). A stable oxygen isotope making up 0.20% of natural oxygen; used in mass spectrometry and in NMR studies of tissue. SYN heavy oxygen.

ox·y·gen·ase (ok′sē-jĕ-nās). One of a group of enzymes (EC subclass 1.13) catalyzing direct incorporation of O_2 into substrates; e.g., tryptophan 2,3-dioxygenase (tryptophan pyrrolase)

catalyzing reaction between O_2 and L-tryptophan to form *N*-L-formylkynurenine. Cf. dioxygenase, monooxygenases.

mixed function o., any monooxygenase that catalyzes AH + O_2 + DH_2 → AOH + H_2O + D.

ox·y·gen·ate (ok′sē-jĕ-nāt). To accomplish oxygenation.

ox·y·gen·a·tion (ok′sē-jĕ-nā′shŭn). Addition of oxygen to any chemical or physical system.

apneic o., SYN diffusion *respiration.*

hyperbaric o., an increased amount of oxygen in organs and tissues resulting from the administration of oxygen in a compression chamber at an ambient pressure greater than 1 atm.

ox·y·gen·ic (ok-sē-jen′ik). Pertaining to or containing oxygen.

ox·y·gen·ize (ok′sē-jen-īz). To oxidize with oxygen.

ox·y·heme (ok′sē-hēm). SYN hematin.

ox·y·he·mo·chro·mo·gen (ok′sē-hēm′ō-krō′mō-jen). SYN hematin.

ox·y·he·mo·glo·bin (HbO₂) (ok′sē-hē-mō-glō′bin). Hemoglobin in combination with oxygen, the form of hemoglobin present in arterial blood, scarlet or bright red when dissolved in water. SYN oxygenated hemoglobin.

ox·y·i·o·dide (ok-sē-ī′ō-dīd). A compound of oxygen with a metallic iodide, e.g., an iodate or periodate.

ox·y·krin·in (ok-sē-krin′in). SYN secretin.

ox·y·lu·ci·fer·in (oks′ē-loo-si′fer-in). The activated derivative of luciferin formed in bioluminescence.

ox·y·mes·ter·one (ok-sē-mes′te-rōn). An anabolic steroid.

ox·y·met·az·o·line hy·dro·chlo·ride (ok′sē-mĕ-taz′ō-lēn). A vasoconstrictor used topically to reduce swelling and congestion of the nasal mucosa.

ox·y·meth·o·lone (ok-sē-meth′ŏ-lōn). An androgenic anabolic steroid.

ox·y·mor·phone hy·dro·chlo·ride (ok-sē-mōr′fōn). A semisynthetic narcotic analgesic closely related chemically to hydromorphone hydrochloride; its actions are similar to those of morphine, but more potent.

ox·y·my·o·glo·bin (MbO₂) (ok′sē-mī-ō-glō′bin). Myoglobin in its oxygenated form, analogous in structure to oxyhemoglobin.

ox·y·ner·vone (ok′sē-ner′vōn). SYN hydroxynervone.

ox·yn·tic (ok-sin′tik). Acid forming, e.g., the parietal cells of the gastric glands. [G. *oxynō,* to sharpen, make sour, acid]

ox·y·per·tine (ok-sē-per′tēn). An antianxiety agent; also available as the hydrochloride.

ox·y·phen·bu·ta·zone (ok′sē-fen-boo′tă-zōn). An orally effective analgesic and anti-inflammatory agent used (usually in short courses) for rheumatoid arthritis and gout.

ox·y·phen·cy·cli·mine hy·dro·chlo·ride (ok′sē-fen-sī′klī-mēn). The hydrochloride of 1,4,5,6-tetrahydro-1-methylpyrimidin-2-ylmethyl-α-cyclohexyl-α-hydroxy-α-phenylacetate; an anticholinergic agent.

ox·y·phe·ni·sa·tin ac·e·tate (ok′sē-fe-nī′să-tin). A cathartic with pharmacologic properties resembling those of phenolphthalein, except that it is not absorbed from the gastrointestinal tract.

ox·y·phe·no·ni·um bro·mide (ok′sē-fe-nō′nē-ŭm). A quaternary ammonium compound with anticholinergic action.

ox·y·phil, ox·y·phile (ok′sē-fil, -fīl). **1.** Oxyphil *cell.* **2.** SYN eosinophilic *leukocyte.* **3.** SYN oxyphilic. [G. *oxys,* sour, acid, + *philos,* fond]

ox·y·phil·ic (ok-sē-fil′ik). Having an affinity for acid dyes; denoting certain cell or tissue elements. SYN oxyphil (3), oxyphile.

ox·y·pho·nia (ok-sē-fō′nē-ă). Shrillness or high pitch of the voice. [G. *oxys,* sharp, + *phōnē,* voice]

ox·y·pol·y·gel·a·tin (ok′sē-pol-ē-jel′ă-tin). A modified gelatin used as a plasma extender in transfusions.

ox·y·pu·rine (ok-sē-pūr′ēn). A purine containing oxygen; e.g., hypoxanthine, xanthine, uric acid.

ox·y·pu·ri·nol (ok′sē-poor′ĭ-nol). Alloxanthine and inhibitor of xanthine oxidase; an active metabolite of allopurinol. The drug inhibits the formation of uric acid and is used in the treatment of gout.

ox·y·rhine (ok′sē-rīn). Having a sharp-pointed nose. [G. *oxys,* sharp, + *rhis* (*rhin-*), nose]

ox·y·ryg·mia (ok-sē-rig′mē-ă). Obsolete term for eructation of acid fluid. [G. *oxys,* acid, + *erygmos,* eructation]

Ox·y·spi·ru·ra man·so·ni (ok′-sē-spī-roo′ră man-sō′nī). A widely distributed spiruroid nematode parasite found under the nictitating membrane in the eye of turkeys, chickens, peafowl, quail, and grouse; larvae develop to the infective stage in cockroaches. SYN Manson eye worm.

ox·y·ta·lan (ok-sit′ă-lan). A type of connective tissue fiber histochemically distinct from collagen or elastic fibers described in the periodontal ligament and gingivae. [G. *oxys,* acid, + *talas,* suffering, resisting; coined term probably intended to mean "resistant to acid hydrolysis"]

ox·y·tet·ra·cy·cline (ok′sē-tet-ră-sī′klēn). An antibiotic produced by the actinomycete, *Streptomyces rimosus,* present in the soil; its actions and uses are similar to those of tetracycline; available as the dihydrate, hydrochloride, and calcium.

ox·y·thi·a·min (ok-sē-thī′ă-min). A molecule similar to that of thiamin but with a hydroxyl group replacing the amino group on the pyrimidine ring; a thiamin antagonist capable of inducing symptoms of thiamin deficiency on administration; increases thiamin excretion.

ox·y·to·cia (ok-sē-tō′sē-ă). Rapid parturition. [G. *okytokos,* swift birth]

ox·y·to·cic (ok-sē-tō′sik). **1.** Hastening childbirth. **2.** SYN parturifacient (2).

ox·y·to·cin (OXT) (ok-sē-tō′sin). A nonapeptide neurohypophysial hormone, differing from human vasopressin in having leucine at position 8 and isoleucine at position 3, that causes myometrial contractions at term and promotes milk release during lactation; used for the induction or stimulation of labor, in the management of postpartum hemorrhage and atony, and to relieve painful breast engorgement. SYN ocytocin. [G. *okytokos,* swift birth]

arginine o., o. with arginine at position 8 (identical to arginine vasotocin). SEE ALSO arginine *vasopressin.*

ox·y·u·ri·cide (ok′sē-ū′ri-sīd). An agent that destroys pinworms. [oxyurid + L. *caedo,* to kill]

ox·y·u·rid (ok-sē-ū′rid). Common name for members of the family Oxyuridae. [see *Oxyuris*]

Ox·y·u·ri·dae (ok-sē-ū′ri-dē). A family of parasitic nematodes (superfamily Oxyuroidea) found in the large intestine or cecum of vertebrates and the intestine of invertebrates, especially insects and millipedes; it includes the genera *Aspiculurus, Enterobius, Oxyuris, Passalurus, Syphacia,* and *Thelandros.*

Ox·y·u·ris (ok′sē-ū′ris). A genus of nematodes commonly called seatworms or pinworms (although the pinworm of humans is the closely related form, *Enterobius vermicularis*). *O. equi,* the horse pinworm, is a common parasite of horses in all parts of the world, inhabiting the large intestine. [G. *oxys,* sharp, + *oura,* tail]

♻**-oyl.** Suffix denoting an acyl radical; -yl replaces -ic in acid names.

oz. Abbreviation for ounce.

oze·na (ō-zē′nă). SYN atrophic *rhinitis.* [G. *ozaina,* a fetid polypus, fr. *ozō,* to smell]

oze·nous (ō′zē-nŭs). Relating to ozena.

ozo·ce·rite (ō-zō-sē′rīt). SYN ozokerite.

ozo·ker·ite (ō-zō-kēr′īt). A mixture of paraffinic and cycloparaffinic hydrocarbons occurring in nature; it has a higher melting point than synthetic paraffin, and is used as a substitute for beeswax. SYN ozocerite.

purified o., SYN ceresin.

ozon·a·tor (ō′zō-nā-ter, -tōr). An apparatus for generating ozone and diffusing it in the atmosphere of a room.

ozone (ō′zōn). O_3; a powerful oxidizing agent; air containing a perceptible amount of O_3 formed by an electric discharge or by the slow combustion of phosphorus, and has an odor suggestive of Cl_2 or SO_2; also formed by the action of solar UV radiation on atmospheric O_2. [G. *ozō,* to smell]

ozo·nide (ō′zō-nīd). The unstable intermediate formed by the reaction of ozone with an unsaturated organic compound, especially with unsaturated fatty acids.

ozon·ol·y·sis (ō-zō-nol′ĭ-sis). The splitting of a double bond in a hydrocarbon chain upon treatment with ozone, with the formation of two aldehydes (an ozonide is the unstable intermediate); has been used to determine the structure of unsaturated fatty acids. [ozone + G. *lysis,* dissolution]

ozon·om·e·ter (ō-zō-nom′ĕ-ter). A modified form of ozonoscope, in which by a series of test papers the amount of ozone in the atmosphere may be estimated.

ozo·no·scope (ō-zō′nō-skōp). Filter paper saturated with starch and potassium iodide or with litmus and potassium iodide; turns blue in the presence of ozone.

ozo·sto·mia (ō-zō-stō′mē-ă). SYN halitosis. [G. *ozō,* to smell, + *stoma,* mouth]

π. **1.** The 16th letter of the Greek alphabet, pi. **2.** Symbol for the ratio of the circumference of a circle to its diameter, approximately 3.14159; symbol for osmotic *pressure* (Π).

Π. SEE π.

Φ The 21st letter of the Greek alphabet, phi. Symbol for phenyl; symbol for quantum *yield* (π).

φ SEE Φ.

Ψ, Ψrd. 1. Capital psi, the 23rd letter of the Greek alphabet. **2.** Symbol for pseudouridine; psychology.

P-170. SYN P-glycoprotein.

P 1. Symbol for peta-; phosphorus; proline; product; poise; power; frequently with subscripts indicating location and/or chemical species. **2.** Followed by a subscript, 1) refers to the plasma concentration of the substance indicated by the subscript; 2) permeability *constant*. **3.** A blood group designation. See P blood group, Blood Groups appendix. **4.** Symbol for probability; when followed by the sign for "less than" (<), this indicates that a test statistic, e.g., a chi-square test, gives a result unlikely to occur by chance.

P_{O_2}, pO_2 Symbol for the partial pressure (tension) of oxygen. SEE partial *pressure*.

P **1.** In nucleic acid terminology, symbol for phosphoric residue. **2.** Symbol for pressure; partial *pressure*.

p 1. Abbreviation for pupil; optic *papilla*. **2.** In polynucleotide symbolism, phosphoric ester or phosphate. **3.** Symbol for pico- (2); the negative decadic logarathm; proton; protein; momentum (in italics). **4.** In cytogenetics, symbol for the short arm of a chromosome. [fr. Fr. *petit*, small]

P_{CO_2}, pCO_2 Symbol for partial pressure (tension) of carbon dioxide. SEE partial *pressure*.

P_i Symbol for inorganic *orthophosphate* (should not be used when covalently linked to another moiety).

P_1 Abbreviation for parental *generation*.

^{32}P Symbol for phosphorus-32.

^{33}P Symbol for phosphorus-33.

P_{700} The pigment in chloroplasts bleached by light of wavelengths about 700 nm.

P_B Symbol for barometric *pressure*.

p53. A tumor suppressor gene located on the short arm of chromosome 17 that encodes a nucleophosphoprotein that binds DNA and negatively regulates cell division; frequently measured as a marker of malignant diseases.

p_{870} The pigment in bacterial chromatophores bleached by light of wavelengths about 870 nm.

△*p-* Abbreviation for *para-* (4).

P.A. Abbreviation for physician assistant.

Pa Symbol for pascal; protactinium.

Paas, H.R., German physician, *1900. SEE P. *disease*.

PABA Abbreviation for *p*-aminobenzoic acid.

pab·lum (pab'lŭm). A precooked infant food, a mixture of wheat, oat, and corn meals, wheat embryo, alfalfa leaves, brewers' yeast, iron, and sodium chloride. [L. *pabulum*, nourishment, fr. *pasco*, to nourish]

pab·u·lar (pab'ū-lăr). Relating to, or of the nature of, pabulum.

pab·u·lum (pab'ū-lŭm). Food or nutriment. [L.]

Pacchioni, Antonio, Italian anatomist, 1665–1726. SEE pacchionian *bodies*, under *body*, pacchionian *corpuscles*, under *corpuscle*, pacchionian *depressions*, under *depression*, pacchionian *glands*, under *gland*, pacchionian *granulations*, under *granulation*.

pac·chi·o·ni·an (pak-ē-ō'nē-an). Attributed to or described by Antonio Pacchioni (1665–1726).

pace·fol·low·er (pās'fawl-ō-er). Any cell in excitable tissue that responds to stimuli from a pacemaker.

pace·mak·er (pās'mā-ker). **1.** Biologically, any rhythmic center that establishes a pace of activity. **2.** An artificial regulator of rate activity. **3.** In chemistry, the substance of which the rate of reaction sets the pace for a series of chain reactions; the rate-limiting reaction itself; e.g., in a metabolic pathway, the enzyme catalyz-

ing the slowest or rate-limiting reaction in that pathway. [L. *passus*, step, pace]

artificial p., any device that substitutes for the normal p. and controls the rhythm of the organ; especially an electronic cardiac p., which may be implanted in the chest, with electrodes attached to the external cardiac surface, or passed through the venous circulation into the right side of the heart (pervenous p.).

demand p., a form of artificial p. usually implanted into cardiac tissue because its output of electrical stimuli can be inhibited by endogenous cardiac electrical activity.

diaphragmatic p., a device that paces the diaphragm, used in patients with chronic ventilatory insufficiency resulting from quadriplegia or certain types of phrenic nerve malfunction.

ectopic p., any p. other than the sinus node.

electric cardiac p., an electric device that can substitute for the normal cardiac p., controlling the heart's rhythm by artificial electric discharges. SYN electronic p.

electronic p., SYN electric cardiac p.

external p., an artificial cardiac p. of which the electrodes for delivering rhythmic electric stimuli to the heart are placed on the chest wall. SYN transthoracic p.

fixed-rate p., an artificial p. that emits electrical stimuli at a constant frequency.

nuclear p., a nuclear-powered unit used to generate the electrical current for artificially pacing the heart; replaced by units using long-life nickel-cadmium and other power sources.

pervenous p., an artificial p. passed through the venous circulation into the right side of the heart.

runaway p., rapid heart rates over 140/min caused by electronic circuit instability in an implanted pulse generator.

shifting p., SYN wandering p.

subsidiary atrial p., secondary source for rhythmic control of the heart, available for controlling cardiac activity if the sinoatrial pacemaker fails; usually located within the crista terminalis and atrial free wall near the inferior vena cava.

transthoracic p., SYN external p.

wandering p., a disturbance of the normal cardiac rhythm in which the site of the controlling p. shifts from beat to beat, usually between the sinus and AV nodes, often with gradual sequential changes in P waves between upright and inverted in a given ECG lead. SYN shifting p.

pa·chom·e·ter (pa-kom'ĕ-ter). SYN pachymeter.

Pachon, Michel V., French physiologist, 1867–1938. SEE P. *method*, *test*.

△**pachy-.** Thick. [G. *pachys*, thick]

pach·y·bleph·a·ron (pak'ē-blef'ă-ron). Thickening of the tarsal border of the eyelid. SYN tylosis ciliaris. [pachy- + G. *blepharon*, eyelid]

pach·y·ce·pha·lia (pak'ē-se-fā'lē-ă). SYN pachycephaly.

pach·y·ce·phal·ic, pach·y·ceph·a·lous (pak'ē-se-fal'ik, -sef'ă-lŭs). Relating to or marked by pachycephaly.

pach·y·ceph·a·ly (pak-i-sef'ă-lē). Abnormal thickness of the skull. SYN pachycephalia. [pachy- + G. *kephalē*, head]

pach·y·chei·lia, pach·y·chi·lia (pak-i-kī'lē-ă). Swelling or abnormal thickness of the lips. [pachy- + G. *cheilos*, lip]

pach·y·cho·lia (pak-i-kō'lē-ă). Inspissation of the bile. [pachy- + G. *cholē*, bile]

pa

△ **Combining Forms**	☆ **Official alternate**
	Terminologia Anatomica
🖻 **Indicates term is illustrated,**	**term**
see Illustration Index	
	[MIM] Mendelian Inheritance
	in Man
SYN **Synonym**	
Cf. **Compare**	C.I. **Colour Index**
[NA] **Nomina Anatomica**	
	High Profile Term
[TA] **Terminologia Anatomica**	

pach·y·chro·mat·ic (pak'ē-krō-mat'ik). Having a coarse chromatin reticulum.

pach·y·chy·mia (pak-i-kī'mē-ă). Inspissation of the chyme. [pachy- + G. *chymos*, juice]

pach·y·dac·tyl·ia (pak'ē-dak-til'ē-ă). SYN pachydactyly.

pach·y·dac·ty·lous (pak-i-dak'ti-lŭs). Relating to or characterized by pachydactyly.

pach·y·dac·ty·ly (pak-i-dak'ti-lē). Enlargement of the fingers or toes, especially extremities; often seen in neurofibromatosis. SYN pachydactylia. [pachy- + G. *daktylos*, finger or toe]

pach·y·der·ma (pak-i-der'mă). Abnormally thick skin. SEE ALSO elephantiasis. SYN pachydermatosis. [pachy- + G. *derma*, skin]

p. laryn'gis, a circumscribed epithelial hyperplasia at the posterior commissure of the larynx.

p. lymphangiectat'ica, elephantiasis due to lymph stasis.

p. verruco'sa, chronic wartlike elephantiasis.

p. vesi'cae, elephantiasis with nodules composed of lymph vesicles on the skin surface.

pach·y·der·ma·to·sis (pak'i-der'mă-tō'sis). SYN pachyderma.

pachydermodactyly. Digital swelling due to diffuse fibromatosis occurring on the proximal interphalangeal joints of the index, middle, and ring fingers (sometimes involving the fifth finger, rarely the thumb); a familial form exists [MIM 600356].

pach·y·der·mo·per·i·os·to·sis (pak-i-der'mō-per'ē-os-tō'sis) [MIM*167100]. A syndrome of clubbing of the digits, periosteal new bone formation, especially over the distal ends of the long bones (idiopathic hypertrophic osteoarthropathy), and coarsening of the facial features with thickening, furrowing, and oiliness of the skin of the face and forehead (cutis verticis gyrata); there is seborrheic hyperplasia with open sebaceous pores filled with plugs of sebum; often of autosomal dominant inheritance, usually more severe in males. SYN acropachyderma. [pachy- + G. *derma*, skin, + periostosis]

pach·y·glos·sia (pak-i-glos'ē-ă). An enlarged, thick tongue. [pachy- + G. *glōssa*, tongue]

pa·chyg·na·thous (pă-kig'nath-ŭs). Characterized by a large or thick jaw. [pachy- + G. *gnathos*, jaw]

pach·y·gy·ria (pak-i-jī'rē-ă). Condition in which the convolutions of the cerebral cortex are abnormally large; there are fewer sulci than normal and in some cases the amount of brain substance is somewhat increased. SYN macrogyria. [pachy- + G. *gyros*, circle]

pach·y·lep·to·men·in·gi·tis (pak'i-lep'tō-men-in-jī'tis). Inflammation of all the membranes of the brain or spinal cord. [G. *pachys*, thick, + *leptos*, thin, + *mēninx* (*mēning-*), membrane, + *-itis*, inflammation]

pach·y·men·in·gi·tis (pak'i-men'in-jī'tis). Inflammation of the dura mater. SYN perimeningitis. [pachy- + G. *mēninx*, membrane, + *-itis*, inflammation]

p. exter'na, inflammation of the outer surface of the dura mater. SYN epidural meningitis, external meningitis.

hemorrhagic p., subdural *hemorrhage* associated with pachymeningitis. SEE ALSO subdural *hemorrhage*.

hypertrophic cervical p., a fibrotic and inflammatory thickening of spinal pachymeninges, particularly in the cervical region, resulting in spinal nerve radiculopathy; believed to be of syphilitic etiology.

p. inter'na, inflammation of the inner surface of the dura mater. SYN internal meningitis.

pyogenic p., suppurative inflammation of the dura, often spreading from a neighboring osteomyelitis.

pach·y·me·nin·gop·a·thy (pak'ē-mĕ-ning-gop'ă-thē). Disease of the dura mater. [pachy- + G. *mēninx* (*mēning-*), membrane, + *pathos,* disease]

pach·y·me·ninx (pak'i-mē'ningks) [TA]. SYN dura mater. [pachy- + G. *mēninx,* membrane]

pa·chym·e·ter (pă-kim'ĕ-ter). An instrument for measuring the thickness of any object, especially of thin objects such as a plate of bone or a membrane. SYN pachometer. [pachy- + G. *metron,* measure]

optical p., a lens and/or mirror used to measure corneal thickness.

pach·y·ne·ma (pak-ē-nē'mă). SYN pachytene. [pachy- + G. *nēma,* thread]

pa·chyn·sis (pă-kin'sis). Obsolete term for any pathologic thickening. [G. a thickening]

pa·chyn·tic (pă-kin'tic). Relating to pachynsis.

pach·y·o·nych·ia (pak'ē-ō-nik'ē-ă). Abnormal thickness of the fingernails or toenails. [pachy- + G. *onyx,* nail]

p. congen'ita [MIM*167200], a syndrome of ectodermal dysplasia of abnormal thickness and elevation of nail plates with palmar and plantar hyperkeratosis; the tongue is whitish and glazed owing to papillary atrophy; autosomal dominant inheritance caused by mutation in the keratin 16 gene (KRT16) on chromosome 17q or the keratin 6A gene (KRT6A) on 12q. SYN Jadassohn-Lewandowski syndrome.

pach·y·o·tia (pak-i-ō'shē-ă). Thickness and coarseness of the auricles of the ears. [pachy- + G. *ous,* ear]

pach·y·per·i·os·ti·tis (pak'i-per'ē-ōs-tī'tis). Proliferative thickening of the periosteum caused by inflammation. [pachy- + periostitis]

pach·y·per·i·to·ni·tis (pak'i-per'i-tō-nī'tis). Obsolete term for inflammation of the peritoneum with thickening of the membrane. SYN productive peritonitis. [pachy- + peritonitis]

pach·y·pleu·ri·tis (pak'ē-ploo-rī'tis). Obsolete term for inflammation of the pleura with thickening of the membrane. SYN productive pleurisy. [pachy- + pleura + G. *-itis,* inflammation]

pa·chyp·o·dous (pă-kip'ō-dŭs). Having large thick feet. [pachy- + G. *pous,* foot]

pach·y·so·mia (pak-i-sō'mē-ă). Pathologic thickening of the soft parts of the body, notably in acromegaly. [pachy- + G. *sōma,* body]

pach·y·tene (pak'i-tēn). The stage of prophase in meiosis in which pairing of homologous chromosomes is complete and the paired homologues may twine about each other as they continue to shorten; longitudinal cleavage occurs in each chromosome to form two sister chromatids so that each homologous chromosome pair becomes a set of four intertwined chromatids. SYN pachynema. [pachy- + G. *tainia,* band, tape]

pach·y·vag·i·nal·i·tis (pak'i-vaj'i-năl-ī'tis). Obsolete term for chronic inflammation with thickening of the tunica vaginalis testis. [pachy- + Mod. L. (tunica) *vaginalis,* + G. *-itis,* inflammation]

pach·y·vag·i·ni·tis (pak'i-vaj'i-nī'tis). Obsolete term for chronic vaginitis with thickening and induration of the vaginal walls. [pachy- + vagina + G. *-itis,* inflammation]

p. cys'tica, SYN *vaginitis* emphysematosa.

Pacini, Filippo, Italian anatomist, 1812–1883. SEE pacinian *corpuscles,* under *corpuscle;* Vater-P. *corpuscles,* under *corpuscle.*

pa·ci·ni·an (pa-sin'ē-an, pa-chin'). Attributed to or described by Pacini.

pa·cin·i·tis (pa-sin-ī'tis, pa-chin-). Inflammation of the pacinian corpuscles.

pack (pak). **1.** To fill, stuff, or tampon. **2.** To enwrap or envelop the body in a sheet, blanket, or other covering. **3.** To apply a dressing or covering to a surgical site. **4.** The items used for wound dressing. [M.E. *pak,* fr. Germanic]

cold p., a p. of cloth or other material soaked in cold water or encasing ice.

dry p., a p. enveloping one in dry, warmed blankets to induce profuse perspiration.

hot p., a p. of cloth or other material soaked in hot water or producing moist heat by another means.

wet p., the usual form of p. using hot or cold moisture.

pack·er (pak'er). **1.** An instrument for tamponing. **2.** SYN plugger.

pack·ing (pak'ing). **1.** Filling a natural cavity, a wound, or a mold with some material. **2.** The material so used. **3.** The application of a pack.

denture p., filling and compressing a denture base material into a mold in a flask.

pac·li·tax·el (pac-lē-taks'ĕl). Antitumor agent that promotes microtubule assembly by preventing depolymerization; currently used in salvage therapy for metastatic carcinoma of ovary.

PACS Acronym for *picture archive and communication system,* a computer network for digitized radiologic images and reports.

pad. **1.** Soft material forming a cushion, used in applying or relieving pressure on a part, or in filling a depression so that dressings can fit snugly. **2.** A more or less encapsulated body of fat or some other tissue serving to fill a space or act as a cushion in the body. (i.e., heel pad).

abdominal p., SYN laparotomy p.

dinner p., a p. of moderate thickness placed over the pit of the stomach before the application of a plaster jacket; after the plaster has set the p. is removed, leaving space for varying degrees of abdominal distention.

fat p., SEE fat-pad.

fat p. of ischioanal fossa,

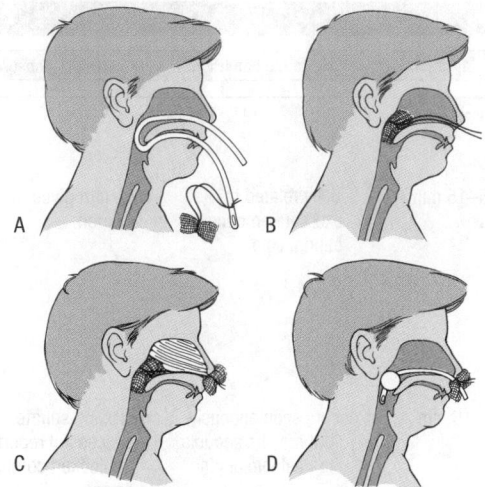

nasal packing: packing to control bleeding from the posterior nose, (A) catheter inserted and packing attached; (B) packing drawn into position as catheter is removed; (C) strip tied over bolster to hold packing in place with anterior pack installed "accordion pleat" style; (D) alternative method, using balloon catheter instead of gauze packing

heel p., an encapsulated body of fat beneath the plantar surface of the calcaneus, which cushions during weight bearing and walking.

knuckle p.'s, (1) an autosomal dominant trait, in which thick p.'s of skin appear over the proximal phalangeal joints; occasionally associated with leukonychia and deafness or Dupuytren contracture; **(2)** a callus reaction resulting from occupational or self-inflicted trauma.

laparotomy p., a p. made from several layers of gauze folded into a rectangular shape; used as a sponge, for packing off the viscera in abdominal operations, and in other ways. SYN abdominal p.

Passavant p., SYN Passavant *ridge.*

periarterial p., SYN juxtaglomerular *body.*

pharyngoesophageal p.'s, SYN pharyngoesophageal *cushions,* under *cushion.*

retromolar p., a cushioned mass of tissue, frequently pear-shaped, located on the alveolar process of the mandible behind the area of the last natural molar tooth; of particular concern in fitting full dentures. SYN pear-shaped area.

sucking p., suctorial p., SYN buccal *fat-pad.*

threshold p.'s of anal canal, SYN anal *cushions,* under *cushion.*

Padykula-Herman stain for my·o·sin ATPase. See under stain.

Pae·ci·lo·my·ces (pē-sil-ō-mī′sēz). A genus of saprophytic imperfect fungi whose conidia-bearing hyphae superficially resemble the penicillus of *Penicillium;* isolated as contaminants, occasional pathogen.

P. lilacinus, a mold; a rare cause of paecilomycosis; has been implicated in human eye infections due to contaminated implanted intraocular lenses. SYN Penicillium lilacinum.

pae·ci·loy·co·sis (pē-sil′ō-ē-cō′sis). A systemic (mainly pulmonary) mycosis of humans and various lower animals caused by fungi of the genus *Paecilomyces.*

△**paed-.** SEE ped-.

PAF Abbreviation for platelet-activating *factor.*

PAGE Abbreviation for polyacrylamide gel *electrophoresis.*

Pagenstecher, Alexander, German ophthalmologist, 1828–1879. SEE P. *circle.*

Paget, Sir James, English surgeon, 1814–1899. SEE P. *cells,* under *cell, disease;* extramammary P. *disease;* Paget-von Schrötter *syndrome.*

Paget-Eccleston stain. See under stain.

pa·get·ic (pa-jet′ik). Relating to or suffering from Paget disease.

pag·et·oid (paj′ĕ-toyd). Resembling or characteristic of Paget disease.

pa·go·pha·gia (pā-gō-fā′jē-ă). Compulsive and repeated ingestion of ice; sometimes associated with iron-deficiency anemia. [G. *pagos,* frost, + *phagō,* to eat]

△**-pagus.** Conjoined twins, the first element of the word denoting the parts fused. SEE ALSO -didymus, -dymus. [G. *pagos,* something fixed, fr. *pēgnymi,* to fasten together]

PAH Abbreviation for *p*-aminohippuric acid.

pain (pān). **1.** An unpleasant sensation associated with actual or potential tissue damage and mediated by specific nerve fibers to the brain where its conscious appreciation may be modified by various factors. **2.** Term used to denote a painful uterine contraction occurring in childbirth. [L. *poena,* a fine, a penalty]

after-p.'s, SEE afterpains.

bearing-down p., a uterine contraction accompanied by straining and tenesmus; usually appearing in the second stage of labor.

expulsive p.'s, effective labor p.'s, associated with contraction of the uterine muscle.

false p.'s, ineffective uterine contractions, preceding and sometimes resembling true labor, but distinguishable from it by the lack of progressive effacement and dilation of the cervix.

girdle p., a painful sensation encircling the body like a belt, occurring in tabes dorsalis or other spinal cord disease.

growing p.'s, aching p.'s, frequently felt at night, in the limbs of children; cause is unclear, but the condition is benign.

hunger p., cramp in the epigastrium associated with hunger.

intermenstrual p., (1) pelvic discomfort occurring approximately at the time of ovulation, usually at the midpoint of the menstrual cycle; SYN midpain. **(2)** SYN mittelschmerz.

intractable p., p. resistant or refractory to ordinary analgesic agents.

labor p.'s, rhythmic uterine contractions that under normal conditions increase in intensity, frequency, and duration, culminating in vaginal delivery of the infant. SYN parodynia.

middle p., SYN mittelschmerz.

night p., SYN nyctalgia.

organic p., pain caused by an organic lesion.

periodic bone p., SYN periodic *arthralgia.*

phantom limb p., the sensation that an amputated p. is still present, often associated with painful paresthesia. SYN phantom limb, pseudesthesia (3), pseudoesthesia (3), stump hallucination.

postprandial p., p. occurring after eating, typical of malignancy in esophagus or stomach.

psychogenic p., somatoform p.; p. that is associated or correlated with a psychologic, emotional, or behavioral stimulus. SYN psychalgia (2), somatoform p.

referred p., p. from deep structures perceived as arising from a surface area remote from its actual origin; the area where the pain is appreciated is innervated by the same spinal segment(s) as the deep structure. SYN telalgia.

respirophasic p., p., often mistakenly termed pleuritic, that occurs or worsens synchronously with the respiratory cycle. [L. *re-*

pa

spiro, to breathe, + G. *phasis,* recurring appearance, as of a star, fr. *phaino,* to appear, + -ic]

rest p., p. occurring, usually in the extremities, during rest in the sitting or lying position.

somatoform p., SYN psychogenic p.

paint (pānt). A solution or suspension of one or more medicaments applied to the skin with a brush or large applicator; usually used in the treatment of widespread eruptions.

carbol-fuchsin p., a p. containing boric acid, phenol, resorcinol, fuchsin, acetone, and alcohol in water; used in the treatment of superficial mycotic infections. SYN Castellani p.

Castellani p., SYN carbol-fuchsin p.

pair (pār). Two objects considered together because of similarity, for a common purpose, or because of some attracting force between them.

base p. (b.p.), the complex of two heterocyclic nucleic acid bases,

one a pyrimidine and the other a purine, brought about by hydrogen bonding between the purine and the pyrimidine; base pairing is the essential element in the structure of DNA proposed by J. Watson and F. Crick in 1953; usually guanine is paired with cytosine (G·C), and adenine with thymine (A·T) or uracil (A·U). SYN nucleoside p., nucleotide p.

buffer p., an acid and its conjugate base (anion).

chromosome p., two chromosomes of the full diploid karyotype that are similar in form and function but that usually differ in content, one normally being inherited from each parent and one being transmitted to each progeny; in the heteromorphic sex (in humans, the male), one pair, the sex chromosomes, differ markedly in appearance, content, and function.

conjugate acid-base p., in prototonic solvents (e.g., H_2O, NH_3, acetic acid), two molecular species differing only in the presence

assessment of chest pain				
ailment	character, location, and radiation	duration	precipitating conditions	relieving measures
angina pectoris	substernal or retrosternal pain spreading across chest may radiate to inside of arm, neck, or jaws	5–15 min	usually related to exertion, emotion, eating, cold	rest, nitroglycerin, oxygen
myocardial infarction	substernal pain or pain over precordium may spread widely throughout chest painful disability of shoulders and hands may be present	>15 min	occurs spontaneously but may be sequela to unstable angina	morphine sulfate, successful reperfusion of blocked coronary artery
pericarditis	sharp, severe substernal pain or pain to the left of stenum may be felt in epigastrium and may be referred to neck, arms, and back	intermittent	sudden onset pain increases with inspiration, swallowing, coughing, and rotation of trunk	sitting upright, analgesia, anti-inflammatory medications
pulmonary pain	pain arises from inferior portion of pleura may be referred to costal margins or upper abdomen patient may be able to localize the pain	30+ min	often occurs spontaneously pain occurs or increases with inspiration	rest, time treatment of underlying cause, bronchodilation
esophageal pain (hiatus hernia, reflux esophagitis, or spasm)	substernal pain may be projected around chest to shoulders	5–60 min	recumbency, cold liquids, exercise may occur spontaneously	food, antacid nitroglycerin relieves spasm
anxiety	pain over left chest may be variable does not radiate patient may complain of numbness and tingling of hands and mouth	2–3 min	stress, emotional tachypnea	removal of stimulus, relaxation

or absence of a hydrogen ion (e.g., carbonic acid/bicarbonate ion or ammonium ion/ammonia); the basis of buffer action.

line p.'s, a unit of resolution of radiographic screens and films or photographic films; greatest number of line p.'s per cm that can be resolved.

nucleoside p., nucleotide p., SYN base p.

p. production, creation of a positron and electron, each of mass 0.511 MeV, when an incident photon of energy greater than 1.02 MeV is absorbed by matter; occurs in high-energy radiotherapy.

pa·ja·roe·llo (pah-har-wā′ō). SYN *Ornithodoros coriaceus.* [Am. Sp. *pajahuello,* fr. Sp. *paja,* straw, + *huello,* undersurface of hoof]

Palade, George E., Romanian-U.S. cell biologist and Nobel laureate, *1912. SEE P. *granule;* Weibel-P. *bodies,* under *body.*

pal·a·tal (pal′ă-tăl). Relating to the palate or the palate bone. SYN palatine.

pal·ate (pal′ăt) [TA]. The bony and muscular partition between the oral and nasal cavities. SYN palatum [TA], roof of mouth, uraniscus. [L. *palatum,* palate]

bony p. [TA], a concave elliptical bony plate, constituting the roof of the oral cavity, formed of the palatine process of the maxilla and the horizontal plate of the palatine bone on either side. SYN palatum osseum [TA].

Byzantine arch p., incomplete fusion of the palatal process with the nasal spine.

cleft p., a congenital fissure in the median line of the p., often associated with cleft lip. Often occurs as a feature of a syndrome or generalized condition, e.g., diastrophic dwarfism or spondyloepiphyseal dysplasia congenita; its general genetic behavior resembles that of cleft *lip.* SYN palatoschisis, palatum fissum.

falling p., SYN uvuloptosis.

Gothic p., an abnormally highly arched p.

hard p. [TA], **(1)** the anterior part of the palate, consisting of the bony p. covered above by the mucous membrane of the floor of the nasal cavity and below by the mucoperiosteum of the roof of the mouth, which contains the palatine vessels, nerves, and mucous glands; SYN palatum durum [TA]. **(2)** in cephalometrics, a line connecting the anterior and posterior nasal spines to represent the position of the bony p.

pendulous p., SYN *uvula* of soft palate.

primary p., in the early embryo, the shelf, formed from the medial nasal processes, that anteriorly separates the oral cavity below from the primitive nasal cavities above. SYN primitive p.

primitive p., SYN primary p.

secondary p., the portion of the embryonic p., posterior to the primary palate that forms from the palatal processes of the embryonic maxilla and develops into the hard and soft p.'s.

soft p. [TA], the posterior muscular portion of the palate, forming an incomplete septum between the mouth and the oropharynx, and between the oropharynx and the nasopharynx. SYN palatum molle [TA], velum palatinum★, velum pendulum palati.

pa·lat·i·form (pă-lat′i-fōrm). Palate-shaped; resembling the palate.

pa·lat·i·nase (pă-lat′i-nās). A maltase in the intestinal mucosa that hydrolyzes palatinose; probably oligo-1,6-glucosidase.

pal·a·tine (pal′ă-tīn). SYN palatal.

pa·lat·i·nose (pă-lat′i-nōs). A disaccharide consisting of D-glucose and D-fructose in α-1,6 linkage (sucrose is α-1,2).

pal·a·ti·tis (pal-ă-tī′tis). Inflammation of the palate. SYN uranisconitis.

△**palato-.** Palate. [L. *palatum,* palate]

pal·a·to·glos·sal (pal′ă-tō-glos′ăl). Relating to the palate and the tongue or to the palatoglossus muscle.

pal·a·to·glos·sus (pal-ă-tō-glos′ŭs). SYN palatoglossus (*muscle*).

pal·a·tog·na·thous (pal′ă-tog′nă-thŭs). Having a cleft palate. [palato- + G. *gnathos,* jaw]

pal·a·to·gram (pal′ă-tō-gram). A registration of tongue action against the palate made by placing soft wax or powder on a baseplate.

pal·a·to·graph (pal′ă-tō-graf). An instrument used in recording

the movements of the soft palate in speaking and during respiration. SYN palate myograph, palatomyograph. [palato- + G. *graphō,* to record]

pal·a·to·max·il·lary (pal′ă-tō-mak′si-lār-ē). Relating to the palate and the maxilla.

pal·a·to·my·o·graph (pal′ă-tō-mī′ō-graf). SYN palatograph. [G. palato- + *mys,* muscle, + *graphō,* to record]

pal·a·to·na·sal (pal-ă-tō-nā′sal). Relating to the palate and the nasal cavity.

pal·a·to·pha·ryn·ge·al (pal′ă-tō-fa-rin′jē-ăl). Relating to palate and pharynx.

pal·a·to·pha·ryn·ge·us (pal′ă-tō-far-in-jē′ŭs). SYN palatopharyngeus (*muscle*). [L.]

pal·a·to·pha·ryn·go·plas·ty (pal′ă-tō-fa-rin′gō-plas-tē). Surgical resection of unnecessary palatal and oropharyngeal tissue in selected cases of snoring, with or without sleep apnea. SYN uvulopalatopharyngoplasty. [palato- + pharynx, + *plastos,* formed]

pal·a·to·pha·ryn·gor·rha·phy (pal′ă-tō-far′in-gōr′ă-fē). SYN staphylopharyngorrhaphy. [palato- + pharynx + G. *rhaphē,* suture]

pal·a·to·plas·ty (pal′ă-tō-plas-tē). Surgery of the palate to restore form and function. SYN staphyloplasty, uraniscoplasty, uranoplasty, uvulopalatoplasty. [palato- + G. *plassō,* to form]

pal·a·to·ple·gia (pal′ă-tō-plē′jē-ă). Paralysis of the muscles of the soft palate. [palato- + G. *plēgē,* stroke]

pal·a·tor·rha·phy (pal-ă-tōr′ă-fē). Suture of a cleft palate. SYN staphylorrhaphy, uraniscorrhaphy, uranorrhaphy, velosynthesis. [palato- + G. *rhaphē,* suture]

pal·a·tos·chi·sis (pal-ă-tos′ki-sis). SYN cleft *palate.* [palato- + G. *schisis,* fissure]

pa·la·tum, pl. **pa·la·′ti** (pă-lā′tŭm) [TA]. SYN palate. [L.]

p. du′rum [TA], SYN hard *palate* (1).

p. fis′sum, SYN cleft *palate.*

p. mol′le [TA], SYN soft *palate.*

p. os′seum [TA], SYN bony *palate.*

pa·le·en·ceph·a·lon (pā′lē-en-sef′ă-lon). L. Edinger term for the metameric nervous *system.* Excludes cerebral cortex. [paleo- + G. *enkephalos,* brain]

△**paleo-, pale-.** Old, primitive, primary, early. [G. *palaios,* old, ancient]

pa·le·o·cer·e·bel·lum (pā′lē-ō-ser′ĕ-bel′ŭm) [TA]. Phylogenetic term referring to the portion of the cerebellum including most of the vermis and the adjacent zones of the cerebellar hemispheres rostral to the primary fissure; p. is equated with the anterior lobe and corresponds to the zone of distribution of the spinocerebellar tracts and is sometimes called spinocerebellum; in phylogenetic age, it is thought to be intermediate between the archicerebellum [TA] and the neocerebellum [TA]. SYN spinocerebellum [TA]. [paleo- + L. *cerebellum*]

pa·le·o·cor·tex (pā′lē-ō-kōr′teks) [TA]. The phylogenetically oldest part of the cortical mantle of the cerebral hemisphere, represented by the olfactory cortex.

pa·le·o·ki·net·ic (pā′lē-ō-ki-net′ik). Denoting the primitive motor mechanisms underlying muscular reflexes and automatic, stereotyped movements. [paleo- + G. *kinētikos,* relating to movement]

pa·le·o·pa·thol·o·gy (pā′lē-ō-pa-thol′ō-jē). The science of disease in prehistoric times as revealed in bones, mummies, and archaeologic artifacts. [paleo- + pathology]

pa·le·o·stri·a·tal (pā′lē-ō-strī-ā′tăl). Relating to the paleostriatum.

pa·le·o·stri·a·tum (pā′lē-ō-strī-ā′tŭm). Term denoting the globus pallidus and expressing the hypothesis that this component of the striate body developed earlier in evolution than the "neostriatum" or striatum (caudate nucleus and putamen) and that it is a diencephalic derivative. SEE ALSO *globus* pallidus. [paleo- + L. *striatum*]

pa·le·o·thal·a·mus (pā′lē-ō-thal′ă-mŭs). The intralaminar nuclei, believed to have been the earliest components of the thalamus to evolve; they lack reciprocal connections with the isocortex.

Palfyn (Palfin), Jean, Belgian surgeon and anatomist, 1650–1730. SEE P. *sinus.*

pal·i·ki·ne·sia, pal·i·ci·ne·sia (pal-i-ki-nē′zē-ă, -si-nē′zē-ă). Involuntary repetition of movements. [G. *palin,* again, + *kinēsis,* movement]

pal·i·nal (pal′i-năl). Moving backward. [G. *palin,* backward]

pal·in·drome (pal′in-drōm). In molecular biology, a self-complementary nucleic acid sequence; a sequence identical to its complementary strand, if both are "read" in the same 5′ to 3′ direction, or inverted repeating sequences running in opposite directions (e.g., 5′-AGT–TGA-3′) on either side of an axis of symmetry; p.'s occur at sites of important reactions (e.g., binding sites, sites cleaved by restriction enzymes); imperfect p.'s exist, as do interrupted p.'s that allow the formation of loops. [G. *palindromos,* a running back]

pal·in·dro·mia (pal-in-drō′mē-ă). A relapse or recurrence of a disease. [G. *palindromos,* a running back, + *-ia,* condition]

pal·in·drom·ic (pal-in-drom′ik). Recurring.

pal·i·sade (pal′i-sād). In pathology, a row of elongated nuclei parallel to each other. [Fr. *palissade,* fr. L. *palus,* a pale, stake]

pal·la·di·um (Pd) (pă-lā′dē-ŭm). A metallic element resembling platinum, atomic no. 46, atomic wt. 106.42. [fr. the asteroid, Pallas; G. *Pallas,* goddess of wisdom]

pall·an·es·the·sia (pal′an-es-thē′zē-ă). Absence of pallesthesia. SYN apallesthesia. [G. *pallō,* to quiver, + *anaisthēsia,* insensibility]

pall·es·the·sia (pal′es-thē′zē-ă). The appreciation of vibration, a form of pressure sense; most acute when a vibrating tuning fork is applied over a bony prominence. SYN bone sensibility, pallesthetic sensibility, vibratory sensibility. [G. *pallō,* to quiver, + *aisthēsis,* sensation]

pall·es·thet·ic (pal-es-thet′ik). Pertaining to pallesthesia.

pal·li·al (pal′ē-ăl). Relating to the pallium.

pal·li·ate (pal′ē-āt). To reduce the severity of; to relieve slightly. SYN mitigate. [L. *palliatus* (adj.), dressed in a *pallium,* cloaked]

pal·li·a·tive (pal′ē-ă-tiv). Reducing the severity of; denoting the alleviation of symptoms without curing the underlying disease.

pal·li·dal (pal′i-dăl). Relating to the pallidum.

pal·li·dec·to·my (pal′i-dek′tō-mē). Excision or destruction of the globus pallidus, usually by stereotaxy; a prefix may indicate the method used, e.g., chemopallidectomy (destruction by a chemical agent), cryopallidectomy (destruction by cold). [pallidum + G. *ektomē,* excision]

pal·li·do·a·myg·da·lot·o·my (pal′i-dō-ă-mig′dă-lot′ō-mē). Production of lesions in the globus pallidus and amygdaloid nuclei. [pallidum + amygdala (1) + G. *tomē,* a cutting]

pal·li·do·an·sot·o·my (pal′i-dō-an-sot′ō-mē). Production of lesions in the globus pallidus and ansa lenticularis.

pal·li·dot·o·my (pal-i-dot′ō-mē). A destructive operation on the globus pallidus, done to relieve involuntary movements or muscular rigidity. [pallidum + G. *tomē,* incision]

pal·li·dum (pal′i-dŭm) [TA]. SYN *globus* pallidus. [L. *pallidus,* pale]

dorsal p. [TA], those parts of the globus pallidus located generally dorsal to the plane of the anterior commissure; along with the dorsal striatum, functions in motor activities with cognitive origins; also form part of the dorsal basal ganglia. SYN p. dorsale [TA].

p. dorsale [TA], SYN dorsal p.

ventral p. [TA], those parts of the globus pallidus located ventral to the anterior commissure; includes portions of the substantia innominata; along with the ventral striatum believed to function in motor activities with strong motivational or emotional contructs. SYN p. ventrale [TA].

p. ventrale [TA], SYN ventral p.

pal·li·um (pal′ē-ŭm) [TA]. SYN cerebral *cortex.* [L. cloak]

pal·lor (pal′ŏr). Paleness, as of the skin. [L.]

cachectic p., SYN achromasia (1).

palm (pahm, pawlm) [TA]. The flat of the hand; the flexor or anterior surface of the hand, exclusive of the thumb and fingers; the opposite of the dorsum of the hand. SYN palma [TA]. [L. *palma*]

liver p., exaggerated erythema of the thenar and hypothenar eminences.

pal·ma, pl. **pal·mae** (pawl′mă, pawl′mē) [TA]. SYN palm, palm. [L.]

p. ma′nus, palm of the hand. SEE palm.

pal·mar (pawl′mār) [TA]. Referring to the palm of the hand; volar. SYN palmaris [TA]. [L. *palmaris,* fr. *palma*]

pal·mar·is (pawl-mār′is) [TA]. SYN palmar, palmar. [L.]

pal·mel·lin (pal′mel-in). A red coloring matter formed by an alga, *Palmella cruenta.*

Palmer, Walter L., U.S. physician, *1896. SEE P. acid *test* for peptic ulcer.

palm·ic (pal′mik). Beating; throbbing; relating to a palmus.

pal·mi·tal·de·hyde (pal-mi-tal′dĕ-hīd). Hexadecanal; the 16-carbon aldehyde analog of palmitic acid; a constituent of plasmalogens.

pal·mi·tate (pal′mi-tāt). A salt of palmitic acid.

pal·mit·ic ac·id (pal-mit′ik). A common saturated fatty acid occurring in palm oil and olive oil as well as many other fats and waxes; the end product of mammalian fatty acid synthase. SYN hexadecanoic acid.

pal·mi·tin (pal′mi-tin). The triglyceride of palmitic acid occurring in palm oil. SYN tripalmitin.

pal·mit·o·le·ic ac·id (pal′mi-tō-lē′ik). 9-Hexadecenoic acid; a monounsaturated 16-carbon acid; one of the common constituents of the triacylglycerols of human adipose tissue. SYN zoomaric acid.

pal·mi·tyl al·co·hol (pal′mi-til). SYN *cetyl* alcohol.

pal·mod·ic (pal-mod′ik). Relating to palmus (1).

pal·mos·co·py (pal-mos′kŏ-pē). Examination of the cardiac pulsation. [G. *palmos,* pulsation, + *skopeō,* to examine]

pal·mus, pl. **pal·mi** (pal′mŭs, -mī). 1. SYN facial *tic.* 2. Rhythmic fibrillary contractions in a muscle. SEE ALSO jumping *disease.* 3. The heart beat. [G. *palmos,* pulsation, quivering]

pal·pa·ble (pal′pă-bl). 1. Perceptible to touch; capable of being palpated. 2. Evident; plain. [see palpation]

pal·pate (pal′pāt). To examine by feeling and pressing with the palms of the hands and the fingers.

pal·pa·tion (pal-pā′shŭn). 1. Examination with the hands, feeling for organs, masses, or infiltration of a part of the body, feeling the heart or pulse beat, vibrations in the chest, etc. 2. Touching, feeling, or perceiving by the sense of touch. [L. *palpatio,* fr. *palpo,* pp. *-atus,* to touch, stroke]

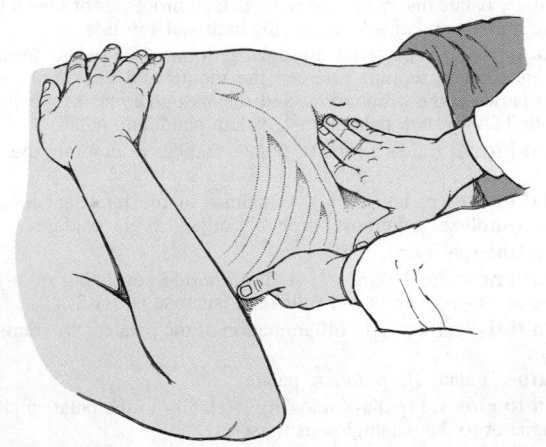

palpation of liver

bimanual p., use of both hands to feel organs or masses, especially in the abdomen or pelvis.

light-touch p., a method of determining the outlines of organs or masses by lightly palpating the surface with the tip of a finger.

pal·pa·to·per·cus·sion (pal′pă-tō-per-kŭsh′ŭn). Examination by means of combined palpation and percussion.

pal·pe·bra, pl. **pal·pe·brae** (pal-pē′bră, pē′brē) [TA]. SYN eyelid. [L.]

p. III, SYN *plica semilunaris* of conjunctiva (2).

p. infe′rior [TA], SYN inferior *eyelid.*

p. supe′rior [TA], SYN superior *eyelid.*

p. ter′tia, SYN *plica semilunaris* of conjunctiva (2).

pal·pe·bral (pal′pē-brăl). Relating to an eyelid or the eyelids.

pal·pe·bra·lis (pal′pē-brā′lis). SYN levator palpebrae superioris (*muscle*). [L.]

pal·pe·brate (pal′pē-brāt). **1.** Having eyelids. **2.** To wink. [L. *palpebra,* eyelid]

pal·pe·bra·tion (pal-pē-brā′shŭn). Winking. [L. *palpebratio*]

pal·pi·ta·tio cor·dis (pal-pi-tā′shē-ō kōr′dis). Palpitation of the heart.

pal·pi·ta·tion (pal-pi-tā′shŭn). Forcible or irregular pulsation of the heart, perceptible to the patient, usually with an increase in frequency or force, with or without irregularity in rhythm. SYN trepidatio cordis. [L. *palpito,* to throb]

PALS Abbreviation for periarterial lymphatic *sheath.*

pal·sy (pawl′zē). Paralysis or paresis. [a corruption of O. Fr. fr. L. and G. *paralysis*]

Bell p., paresis or paralysis, usually unilateral, of the facial muscles, caused by dysfunction of the 7th cranial nerve; probably due to a viral infection; usually demyelinating in type. SYN peripheral facial paralysis.

birth p., motor and sensory deficits that result from nerve fiber injury associated with delivery; the brachial plexus is the region most commonly affected. Examples include Erb p. and Klumpke p.

brachial birth p., SYN obstetric p.

bulbar p., SYN progressive bulbar *paralysis.*

cerebral p., a generic term for various types of nonprogressive motor dysfunction present at birth or beginning in early childhood. Causes are both hereditary and acquired; depending upon cause, classified as intrauterine, natal, and early postnatal; motor disturbances include diplegia, hemiplegia, quadriplegia, choreoathetosis, and ataxia.

crutch p., SYN crutch *paralysis.*

Dejerine-Klumpke p., SYN Klumpke p.

diver′s p., SYN decompression *sickness.*

double elevator p., limited elevation of an eye in abduction and adduction, implying paresis of the superior rectus and inferior oblique muscles, although many cases are due to restriction of the inferior rectus muscle.

Erb p., a type of obstetric p. in which there is paralysis of the muscles of the upper arm and shoulder girdle (deltoid, biceps, brachialis, and brachioradialis muscles) caused by a lesion of the upper trunk of the brachial plexus or of the roots of the fifth and sixth cervical roots. SYN Duchenne-Erb paralysis, Erb paralysis.

extrapyramidal cerebral p., SYN athetosis.

facial p., SYN facial *paralysis.*

Klumpke p., a type of obstetric p. in which there is paralysis of the muscles of the distal forearm and hand (all ulnar innervated muscles, plus more distal radial and median-innervated muscles), caused by a lesion of the lower trunk of the brachial plexus, or of the C8 and T1 cervical roots. SYN Dejerine-Klumpke p., Dejerine-Klumpke syndrome, Klumpke paralysis.

lead p., a peculiar type of reputedly toxic neuropathy, resulting from lead intoxication, consisting of bilateral weakness of wrist and finger extensor muscles that is presumably due to bilateral radial neuropathies. Although often mentioned, apparently no verified cases have been described in the modern medical literature. SYN lead paralysis.

obstetric p., a brachial plexus lesion sustained by the infant during the birthing process; three types are recognized: 1) upper plexus type, affecting the shoulder and upper arm (Erb p., q.v., by far the most common form); 2) total plexus type, involving the whole arm; 3) lower plexus type, involving the forearm and hand (Klumpke p., q.v.). SYN brachial birth p., obstetric paralysis.

posticus p., paralysis of the cricoarytenoideus posticus muscle, resulting in the vocal cord being held in or near the midline.

pressure p., SYN pressure *paralysis.*

progressive bulbar p., one of the subgroups of motor neuron disease; a progressive degenerative disorder of the motor neurons of primarily the brainstem, manifested as weakness (and wasting) of the various bulbar muscles, resulting in dysarthria and dysphagia—fluid regurgitation is an outstanding symptom and can cause aspiration; tongue weakness and wasting are usually evident, and often the fasciculation potentials are present in the tongue and facial muscles. SYN glossopalatolabial paralysis, glossopharyngeolabial paralysis.

progressive supranuclear p., a progressive neurologic disorder in the sixth decade characterized by a supranuclear paralysis of vertical gaze, retraction of eyelids, exophoria under cover, dysarthria, and dementia. SYN Steele-Richardson-Olszewski disease, Steele-Richardson-Olszewski syndrome.

scrivener′s p., SYN writer′s *cramp.*

shaking p., trembling p., SYN parkinsonism (1).

pal·u·dal (pal′oo-dăl). Obsolete term for malarial. [L. *palus,* marsh]

PAM Acronym for potential acuity *meter.*

2-PAM Abbreviation for 2-pralidoxime.

pam·a·quine (pam′ă-kwēn). An antimalarial agent, active against avian malaria and against the gametocytes of all malarial forms in humans; it is more toxic than chloroquine or primaquine and has been replaced by primaquine.

pam·o·ate (pam′ō-āt). USAN-approved contraction for 4,4′-methylenebis(3-hydroxy-2-naphthoate).

pam·pin·i·form (pam-pin′i-fōrm). Having the shape of a tendril; denoting a vinelike structure. [L. *pampinus,* a tendril, + *forma,* form]

pam·pin·o·cele (pam-pin′ō-sēl). SYN varicocele. [L. *pampinus,* tendril, + G. *kēlē,* tumor]

Pan. Genus of anthropoid apes including the gorilla and chimpanzee. *P. panisus* and *P. troglodytes* are chimpanzee species used in biologic experiments. [G. myth. god of forest]

pan-. All, entire. SEE ALSO pant-. [G. *pas,* all]

pan·a·cea (pan-ă-sē′ă). A cure-all; a remedy claimed to be curative of all diseases. [G. *panakeia,* universal remedy, fr. Panacea, Aesculapius′ daughter]

pan·ag·glu·ti·na·ble (pan-ă-gloo′ti-nă-bl). Agglutinable with all types of human serum; denoting erythrocytes having this property.

pan·ag·glu·ti·nins (pan-ă-gloo′ti-ninz). Agglutinins that react with all human erythrocytes. [pan + L. *agglutino,* to glue]

pan·an·gi·i·tis (pan′an-jē-ī′tis). Inflammation involving all the coats of a blood vessel. [pan- + angiitis]

pan·ar·ter·i·tis (pan′ar-ter-ī′tis). An inflammatory disorder of the arteries characterized by involvement of all structural layers of the vessels. SYN endoperiarteritis. [pan- + L. *arteria,* artery, + G. *-itis,* inflammation]

pan·ar·thri·tis (pan-ar-thrī′tis). **1.** Inflammation involving all the tissues of a joint. **2.** Inflammation of all the joints of the body.

pan·at·ro·phy (pan-at′rō-fē). **1.** Atrophy of all the parts of a structure. **2.** General atrophy of the body. SYN pantatrophia, pantatrophy.

pan·blas·tic (pan-blas′tik). Relating to all the primary germ layers. [pan- + G. *blastos,* germ]

pan·bron·chi·ol·i·tis (pan′bron-kē-ō-lī′tis). Idiopathic inflammation and obstruction of bronchioles, eventually accompanied by bronchiectasis; cases reported are almost all from Japan. SYN diffuse panbronchiolitis.

diffuse panbronchiolitis, SYN panbronchiolitis.

pan·car·di·tis (pan-kar-dī′tis). SYN endoperimyocarditis.

Pancoast, Henry K., U.S. roentgenologist, 1875–1939. SEE P. *syndrome, tumor.*

pan·co·lec·to·my (pan′kō-lek′tō-mē). Extirpation of the entire colon.

pan·cre·as, pl. **pan·cre·a·ta** (pan′krē-as, pan-krē-ā′tă) [TA]. An elongated lobulated retroperitoneal gland, devoid of capsule, extending from the concavity of the duodenum to the spleen; it consists of a flattened head (caput) within the duodenal concavity, an elongated three-sided body extending transversely across the abdomen, and a tail in contact with the spleen. The gland secretes from its exocrine part pancreatic juice that is discharged into the intestine, and from its endocrine part the internal secretions insulin and glucagon. [G. *pankreas*, the sweetbread, fr. *pas* (*pan*), all, + *kreas*, flesh]

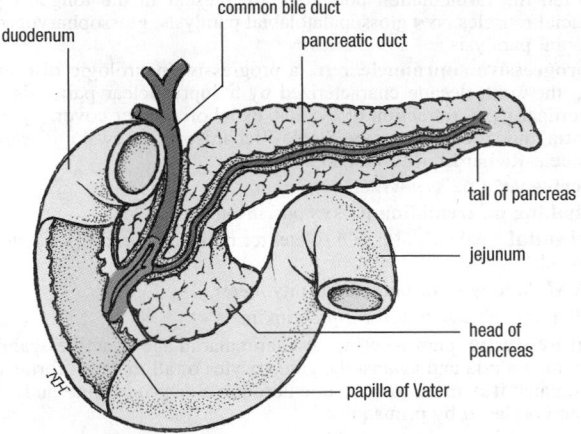

pancreas (and part of duodenum)

p. accesso′rium [TA], SYN accessory p.

accessory p. [TA], a detached portion of pancreatic tissue, usually the uncinate process, and hence most often found in the vicinity of the head of the pancreas, but may occur within the gut wall (stomach or duodenum). SYN p. accessorium [TA].

anular p., a ring of p. encircling the duodenum, caused by a failure of the embryologic ventral pancreas to migrate to the right of the duodenum.

Aselli p., SYN Aselli *gland.*

p. divi′sum, a bifid, or divided, p. resulting from a congenital failure of the embryonic primordia to unite completely; each of the portions has its own duct.

dorsal p., that portion of the pancreatic primordium of the embryo that arises as a dorsal bud from the foregut endoderm above the hepatic diverticulum.

lesser p., SYN uncinate *process* of pancreas.

p. mi′nus, SYN uncinate *process* of pancreas.

small p., SYN uncinate *process* of pancreas.

uncinate p., unciform p., SYN uncinate *process* of pancreas.

ventral p., that portion of the primordium of the pancreas that develops, together with the hepatic diverticulum, as a ventral bud from the foregut endoderm.

Willis p., SYN uncinate *process* of pancreas.

Winslow p., SYN uncinate *process* of pancreas.

⌂**pancreat-, pancreatico-, pancreato-, pancreo-.** The pancreas. [G. *pankreas*, pancreas]

pan·cre·a·tal·gia (pan′krē-ă-tal′jē-ă). Rarely used term for pain arising from the pancreas or felt in or near the region of the pancreas. [pancreat- + G. *algos,* pain]

pan·cre·a·tec·to·my (pan′krē-ă-tek′tō-mē). Excision of the pancreas. SYN pancreectomy. [pancreat- + G. *ektomē,* excision]

pan·cre·at·em·phrax·is (pan′krē-at-em-frak′sis). Obstruction in the pancreatic duct, causing swelling of the gland. [pancreat- + G. *emphraxis,* a stoppage]

pan·cre·at·ic (pan-krē-at′ik). Relating to the pancreas.

⌂**pancreatico-.** SEE pancreat-.

pan·cre·at·i·co·du·o·de·nal (pan-krē-at′i-kō-doo′ō-dē′năl, -doo-od′ĕ-năl). Relating to the pancreas and the duodenum.

pancreaticoduodenectomy (pan-krē-at′ĭ-kō-doo-od′en- ek′tō-mē). SYN pancreatoduodenectomy.

pylorus-preserving p., excision of all or part of the pancreas and the duodenum with preservation of the distal stomach and the innervated pylorus; usually limited to the head and neck of the pancreas and most often performed for pancreatic carcinoma.

pan·cre·a·tin (pan′krē-ă-tin). A mixture of the enzymes from the pancreas of the ox or hog, used internally as a digestive, and also as a peptonizing agent in preparing predigested foods; it contains the proteolytic trypsin, the amylolytic amylopsin, and the lipolytic steapsin.

ℹ**pan·cre·a·ti·tis** (pan′krē-ă-tī′tis). Inflammation of the pancreas.

acute pancreatitis: frequency of etiologic factors	
I.	**principal causes**
1.	cholecystolithiasis, choledocholithiasis
2.	alcoholism
3.	abdominal surgery — postoperative pancreatitis
4.	endoscopy of biliary and pancreatic ducts
5.	blunt abdominal injury
II.	**less frequent causes**
1.	endocrine diseases (polyadenomatosis, hyperparathyroidism, Cushing syndrome)
2.	pregnancy, hyperlipoproteinemia, pancreatitis due to ingestion of birth-control pills
3.	drug effects (corticosteroids, diuretics)
4.	immunologic-allergic causes
5.	neurogenic pancreatitis
6.	hereditary pancreatitis
7.	viral pancreatitis
8.	parasitic pancreatitis
III.	**pancreatitis due to shock and acidosis**

acute hemorrhagic p., an acute inflammation of the pancreas accompanied by the formation of necrotic areas and hemorrhage into the substance of the gland; clinically marked by sudden severe abdominal pain, nausea, fever, and leukocytosis; areas of fat necrosis are present on the surface of the pancreas and in the omentum because of the action of the escaped pancreatic enzyme (trypsin and lipase).

calcareous p., chronic p. with appearance of areas of calcification, seen by x-ray. SYN calcific p.

calcific p. (kal′sif-ik), SYN calcareous p.

chronic p., recurrent bouts of inflammatory disease of the pancreas characterized by fibrosis and varying degrees of irreversible loss of exocrine and ultimately endocrine function.

chronic fibrosing p., inflammation of the pancreas consisting of fibrosis, acinar atrophy, and calcification. Clinically, it follows a protracted course with relapses and remissions, and is usually due to alcohol abuse or malnutrition.

chronic relapsing p., repeated exacerbations of p. in patient with chronic inflammation of that organ. Relapses are usually due to persistence of etiologic factor or repeated exposure to it, such as occurs with partial ductal obstruction or chronic alcoholism.

⌂**pancreato-.** SEE pancreat-.

pan·cre·at·o·cho·le·cys·tos·to·my (pan-krē-at′ō-kō-lē-sis-tos′tō-mē, pan′krē-ă-tō-). A rarely performed surgical anastomosis between a pancreatic cyst or fistula and the gallbladder.

ℹ**pan·cre·at·o·du·o·de·nec·to·my** (pan-krē-at′ō-doo-ō-dē-nek′tō-mē, pan′krē-ă-tō-). Excision of all or part of the pancreas together with the duodenum and usually the distal stomach. SYN pancreaticoduodenectomy, Whipple operation.

pan·cre·at·o·du·o·de·nos·to·my (pan-krē-at′ō-doo-ō-dē-nos′tō-mē, pan′krē-ă-tō-). Surgical anastomosis of a pancreatic duct, cyst, or fistula to the duodenum.

pan·cre·at·o·gas·tros·to·my (pan-krē-at′ō-gas-tros′tō-mē, pan′krē-ă-tō-). Surgical anastomosis of a pancreatic cyst or fistula to the stomach.

pan·cre·a·to·gen·ic, pan·cre·a·tog·en·ous (pan′krē-ă-tō-jen′ik, -toj′ĕ-nŭs). Of pancreatic origin; formed in the pancreas. [pancreato- + G. *genesis,* origin]

pan·cre·a·tog·ra·phy (pan′krē-ă-tog′ră-fē). Radiographic demonstration of the pancreatic ducts, after retrograde injection of radiopaque material into the distal duct. [pancreato- + G. *graphō,* to write]

pan·cre·a·to·je·ju·nos·to·my (pan-krē-at′ō-je-joo-nos′tō-mē, pa-n′krē-ă-tō-). Surgical anastomosis of a pancreatic duct, cyst, or fistula to the jejunum.

pan·cre·at·o·lith (pan-krē-at′ō-lith). SYN pancreatic *calculus.* [pancreato- + G. *lithos,* stone]

pan·cre·at·o·li·thec·to·my (pan-krē-at′ō-li-thek′tō-mē, pan′krē-ă-tō-). SYN pancreatolithotomy. [pancreato- + G. *lithos,* stone, + *ektomē,* excision]

pan·cre·at·o·li·thi·a·sis (pan-krē-at′ō-li-thī′ă-sis, pan′krē-ă-tō-). Stones in the pancreas, usually found in the pancreatic duct system.

pan·cre·at·o·li·thot·o·my (pan-krē-at′ō-li-thot′ō-mē, pan′krē-ă-tō-). Removal of a pancreatic concretion. SYN pancreatolithectomy. [pancreato- + G. *lithos,* stone, + *tomē,* incision]

pan·cre·a·tol·y·sis (pan′krē-ă-tol′i-sis). Destruction of the pancreas. [pancreato- + G. *lysis,* dissolution]

pan·cre·a·to·lyt·ic (pan′krē-ă-tō-lit′ik). Denoting pancreatolysis.

pan·cre·a·to·meg·a·ly (pan′krē-ă-tō-meg′ă-lē). Abnormal enlargement of the pancreas. [pancreato- + G. *megas,* great]

pan·cre·at·o·my (pan′krē-at′ō-mē). SYN pancreatotomy.

pan·cre·a·top·a·thy (pan′krē-ă-top′ă-thē). Any disease of the pancreas. SYN pancreopathy. [pancreato- + G. *pathos,* suffering]

pan·cre·a·to·pep·ti·dase E (pan′krē-ă-tō-pep′ti-dās). SEE elastase.

pan·cre·a·tot·o·my (pan′krē-ă-tot′ō-mē). Incision of the pancreas. SYN pancreatomy. [pancreato- + G. *tomē,* incision]

pan·cre·a·tro·pic (pan′krē-ă-trop′ik). Exerting an action on the pancreas. [pancreat- + G. *tropikos,* relating to a turning]

pan·cre·ec·to·my (pan-krē-ek′tō-mē). SYN pancreatectomy.

pan·cre·li·pase (pan-krē-lip′ās, -lī′pās). A concentrate of pancreatic enzymes standardized for lipase content; a lipolytic used for substitution therapy. SYN lipancreatin.

pancreo-. SEE pancreat-.

pan·cre·o·lith (pan′krē-ō-lith). SYN pancreatic *calculus.* [pancreo- + G. *lithos,* stone]

pan·cre·op·a·thy (pan-krē-op′ă-thē). SYN pancreatopathy.

pan·cre·o·zy·min (pan′krē-ō-zī′min). SYN cholecystokinin.

pan·cu·ro·ni·um bro·mide (pan-kūr-ō′nē-ŭm). A nondepolarizing steroidal neuromuscular blocking agent resembling curare but without its potential for ganglionic blockade, histamine release, or hypotension.

pan·cy·to·pe·nia (pan′sī-tō-pē′nē-ă). Pronounced reduction in the number of erythrocytes, all types of white blood cells, and the blood platelets in the circulating blood. [pan- + G. *kytos,* cell, + *penia,* poverty]

congenital p., SYN Fanconi *anemia.*

Fanconi p., SYN Fanconi *anemia.*

pan·dem·ic (pan-dem′ik). Denoting a disease affecting or attacking the population of an extensive region, country, continent, global; extensively epidemic. [pan- + G. *dēmos,* the people]

pan·de·mic·i·ty (pan-dĕ-mis′i-tē). The state or condition of being pandemic.

pan·dic·u·la·tion (pan-dik-ū-lā′shŭn). The act of stretching, as when awaking. [L. *pandiculor,* to stretch oneself, fr. *pando,* to spread out]

Pandy, Kalman, Hungarian neurologist, 1868–1945. SEE P. *test, reaction.*

pan·en·ceph·a·li·tis (pan′en-sef-ă-lī′tis). A diffuse inflammation of the brain.

nodular p., probably a form of subacute sclerosing p. SYN Pette-Döring disease.

subacute sclerosing p. (SSPE), a rare chronic, progressive encephalitis that affects primarily children and young adults, caused by the measles virus. Characterized by a history of primary measles infection before the age of 2 years, followed by several asymptomatic years, and then gradual, progressive psychoneurological deterioration, consisting of personality change, seizures, myoclonus, ataxia, photosensitivity, ocular abnormalities, spasticity, and coma. Characteristic periodic activity is seen on EEG; pathologically, the white matter of both the hemispheres and brainstem are affected, as well as the cerebral cortex, and eosinophilic inclusion bodies are present in the cytoplasm nuclei of neurons and glial cells. Death usually occurs within 3 years. SYN Bosin disease, Dawson encephalitis, inclusion body encephalitis, sclerosing leukoencephalitis, subacute inclusion body encephalitis, subacute sclerosing leukoencephalitis, van Bogaert encephalitis.

pan·en·do·scope (pan-en′dō-skōp). An illuminated instrument for inspection of the interior of the urethra as well as the bladder

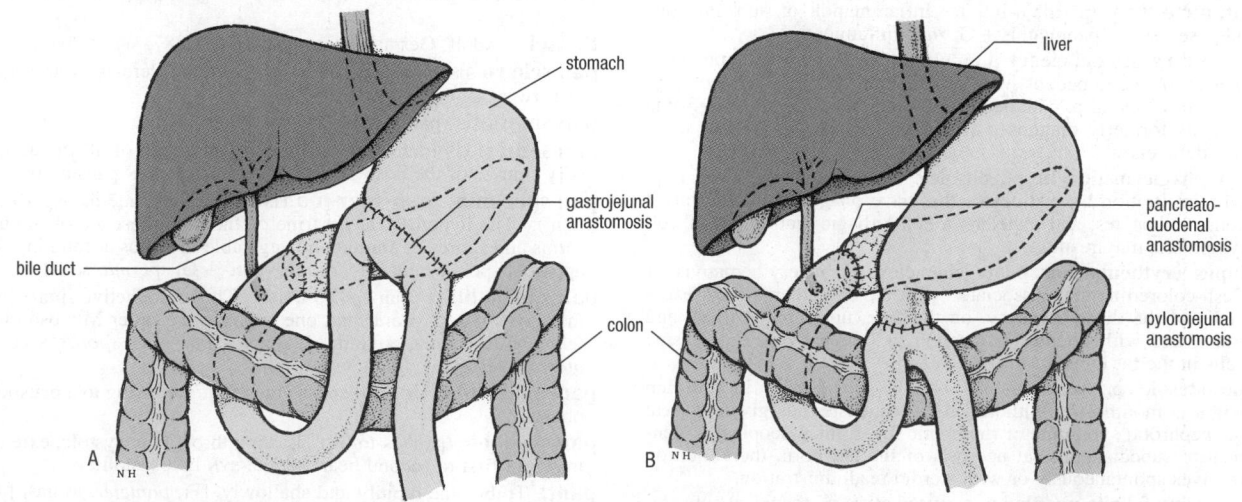

pancreatoduodenectomy: (A) Whipple operation, (B) pylorus-saving Whipple procedure

by means of a telescopic lens system. [pan- + G. *endon*, within, + *skopeō*, to view]

pan·es·the·sia (pan-es-thē'zē-ă). The sum of all the sensations experienced by a person at one time. SEE ALSO cenesthesia. [pan- + G. *aisthēsis*, sensation]

Paneth, Josef, Austrian physician, 1857–1890. SEE P. granular *cells*, under *cell*.

pang (pang). A sudden sharp, brief pain.

breast p., SYN *angina* pectoris.

pan·hi·dro·sis (pan-hi-drō'sis). SYN panidrosis.

pan·hy·drom·e·ter (pan-hī-drom'ĕ-ter). A hydrometer for determining the specific gravity of any liquid. [pan- + G. *hydōr*, water, + *metron*, measure]

pan·hy·per·e·mia (pan'hī-per-ē'mē-ă). Universal congestion or hyperemia. [pan- + G. *hyper*, over, + *haima*, blood]

pan·hy·po·pi·tu·i·tar·ism (PHP) (pan-hī'pō-pi-too'i-tă-rizm). A state in which the secretion of all anterior pituitary hormones is inadequate or absent; caused by a variety of disorders that result in destruction or loss of function of all or most of the anterior pituitary gland. Rare forms of PHP are inherited as autosomal recessive [MIM*262600] or as X-linked recessive [MIM*312000]. SYN ateliotic dwarfism, hypophyseal cachexia, hypophysial cachexia.

pan·ic (pan'ik). Extreme and unreasoning anxiety and fear, often accompanied by disturbed breathing, increased heart activity, vasomotor changes, sweating, and a feeling of dread. SEE anxiety. [fr. G. myth. char., *Pan*]

homosexual p., an acute, severe attack of anxiety based on unconscious conflicts regarding homosexuality.

pan·i·dro·sis (pan-i-drō'sis). Sweating of the entire surface of the body. SYN panhidrosis. [pan- + G. *hidros*, sweat]

pan·im·mu·ni·ty (pan-i-mū'ni-tē). A general immunity to many infectious diseases.

pan·mix·is (pan-mik'sis). SYN random *mating*. [pan- + G. *mixis*, intercourse]

pan·my·e·loph·thi·sis (pan'mī-ĕ-lof'thi-sis). SYN myelophthisis (2).

pan·my·e·lo·sis (pan'mī-ĕ-lō'sis). Myeloid metaplasia with abnormal immature blood cells in the spleen and liver, associated with myelofibrosis. [pan- + G. *myelos*, marrow, + *-osis*, condition]

Panner, H.J., Danish radiologist, 1871–1930. SEE P. *disease*.

pan·ni (pan'ī). Plural of pannus.

pan·nic·u·lec·to·my (pa-nik-ū-lek'tō-mē). Surgical excision of redundant paniculus adiposus, usually of the abdomen. [panniculus + G. *ektomē*, a cutting out]

pan·nic·u·li·tis (pă-nik'ū-lī'tis). Inflammation of subcutaneous adipose tissue. [panniculus + G. *-itis*, inflammation]

α₁-antitrypsin deficiency p., multiple painful subcutaneous nodules occurring in patients with severe antitrypsin deficiency; biopsies show lobular p. with neutrophils and foamy histiocytes. Some patients formerly diagnosed with Weber-Christian disease show this deficiency.

cytophagic histiocytic p., obsolete term for chronic lobular p. with infiltration by histiocytes that have phagocytized red blood cells, leukocytes, and platelets; a hemorrhagic diathesis or T cell lymphoma may result.

lupus erythematosus p., p. characterized by erythematous or flesh-colored nodules associated with lupus erythematosus, especially of the discoid variety, on the face, upper extremities, and trunk, and with nodular infiltration of lymphocytes and plasma cells in the fat lobules.

poststeroid p., subcutaneous nodules developing in children within a month after withdrawal of corticosteroids given to treat the nephrotic syndrome or rheumatic fever; microscopically identical to subcutaneous fat necrosis of the newborn, the condition resolves spontaneously or with steroid readministration.

relapsing febrile nodular nonsuppurative p., recurrent subcutaneous nodules accompanied by fever and followed by depression of the skin on involution. The nodules show a neutrophilic lobular p. with necrosis, lipid phagocytosis, and subsequent fibrosis. A

majority of cases can be classified as factitious, or secondary to α₁-antitrypsin deficiency, lupus profundus, pancreatic (enzymatic) fat necrosis, or cytophagic histiocytic p. Cases of undetermined cause have been called Weber-Christian *disease* or syndrome. SYN Christian disease (2), Weber-Christian disease.

subacute migratory p., nonscarring plaques of changing configuration on the lateral aspect of one or both legs, of many months duration. Biopsy shows septal p. with fibrosis and giant cells. SYN erythema nodosum migrans.

pan·nic·u·lus, pl. **pan·nic·u·li** (pă-nik'ū-lŭs, -lī). SYN layer. [L. dim. of *pannus*, cloth]

p. adiposus [TA], SYN fatty *layer* of subcutaneous tissue.

p. adiposus telae subcutaneae abdominis [TA], SYN fatty *layer* of subcutaneous tissue of abdomen.

p. carno'sus, the skeletal muscle layer in the superficial fascia represented in humans by the platysma muscle; it is much more extensive in lower mammals.

pan·ning (pan'ing). Use of plastic plates or surfaces coated with either antigen or antibody to separate or concentrate specific cells with appropriate receptors.

pan·nus, pl. **pan·ni** (pan'ŭs, pan'ī). A membrane of granulation tissue covering a normal surface: **1.** The inflammatory synovial tissue found in rheumatoid joints that covers the articular cartilages that progressively destroys the underlying articular cartilages; also found in other chronic granulomatous disease, including tuberculosis. **2.** The cornea in trachoma. SEE ALSO corneal p. [L. cloth]

corneal p., fibrovascular connective tissue that proliferates in the anterior layers of the peripheral cornea in inflammatory corneal disease, particularly trachoma in which the p. involves the superior cornea. Three forms occur: **p. crassus** (thick), in which there are many blood vessels and the opacity is very dense; **p. siccus** (dry), p. with dry, glossy surface; and **p. tenuis** (thin), in which there are few blood vessels and the opacity is slight.

phlyctenular p., p. occurring in phlyctenular conjunctivitis.

trachomatous p., p. of the superior cornea associated with trachoma.

pan·oph·thal·mitis (pan'of-thal-mī'-tĭs). Purulent inflammation of all layers of the eye. [pan- + G. *ophthalmos*, eye]

pan·op·tic (pan-op'tik). All-revealing, denoting the effect of multiple or differential staining. [pan- + G. *optikos*, relating to vision]

pan·o·ste·i·tis. Inflammation of an entire bone.

pan·o·ti·tis (pan'ō-tī'tis). General inflammation of all parts of the ear; specifically, a disease that begins as an otitis interna, the inflammation subsequently extending to the middle ear and neighboring structures. [pan- + G. *ous*, ear, + *-itis*, inflammation]

pan·pho·bia (pan-fō'bē-ă). Fear of everything. [pan- + G. *phobos*, fear]

Pansch, Adolf, German anatomist, 1841–1887. SEE P. *fissure*.

pan·scle·ro·sis (pan-skle-rō'sis). Universal sclerosis of an organ or part.

pan·sin·u·i·tis (pan-sin-ū-ī'tis). SYN pansinusitis.

pan·si·nu·si·tis (pan-sī-nŭ-sī'tis). Inflammation of all the accessory sinuses of the nose on one or both sides. SYN pansinuitis.

pan·sper·mia, pan·sper·ma·tism (pan-sper'mē-ă, -sper'mă-tizm). The hypothetical doctrine of the omnipresence of minute forms and spores of animal and vegetable life, thus accounting for apparent spontaneous generation. [pan- + G. *sperma*, seed]

pan·spor·o·blast (pan-spō'rō-blast). The reproductive sporoblast that gives rise to more than one spore in the order Myxosporida (class Myxosporea, phylum Myxozoa). [pan- + G. *sporos*, seed, + *blastos*, germ]

pan·spo·ro·blas·tic (pan'spō-rō-blas'tik). Referring to a pansporoblast.

pan·sys·tol·ic (pan'sis-tol'ik). Lasting throughout systole, extending from first to second heart sound. SYN holosystolic.

pant. To breathe rapidly and shallowly. [Fr. *panteler*, to gasp]

△**pant-, panto-.** Entire. SEE ALSO pan-. [G. *pas*, all]

pan·tal·gia (pan-tal'jē-ă). Pain involving the entire body. [pant- + G. *algos*, pain]

pan·ta·mor·phia (pan-tă-mōr′fē-ă). Shapelessness; general or overall malformation. [pant- + G. *a-* priv. + *morphē,* shape]

pan·ta·mor·phic (pan-tă-mōr′fik). Relating to or characterized by pantamorphia.

pan·tan·en·ceph·a·ly, pan·tan·en·ce·pha·lia (pan′tan-en-sef′ă-lē, -se-fā′lē-ă). Congenital absence of the brain. [pant- + G. *an-* priv. + *enkephalos,* brain]

pan·ta·pho·bia (pan-tă-fō′bē-ă). Absolute fearlessness. [pant- + G. *a-* priv. + *phobos,* fear]

pan·ta·tro·phia, pan·tat·ro·phy (pan-tă-trō′fē-ă, pan-tat′rō-fē). SYN panatrophy. [pant- + atrophy]

pan·te·the·ine (pan-tĕ-thē′in). The condensation product of pantothenic acid and aminoethanethiol; *N*-pantothenyl-2-aminoethanethiol; an intermediate in biosynthesis of coenzyme A via 4′-phosphopantetheine (a phosphoryl on the terminal –CH₂O group) and ATP. SYN *Lactobacillus bulgaricus* factor.

p. kinase, an enzyme that catalyzes the phosphorylation of pantetheine by ATP to pantetheine 4′-phosphate; a step in coenzyme A biosynthesis.

p. 4′-phosphate, SYN 4′-phosphopantetheine.

pan·te·thine (pan′tĕ-thin). The disulfide formed from two pantetheines.

pan·the·nol (pan′thĕ-nol). SYN dexpanthenol.

△**panto-.** SEE pant-.

pan·to·ate (pan′tō-āt). A salt or ester of pantoic acid.

pan·to·graph (pan′tō-graf). **1.** An instrument for reproducing drawings by a system of levers whereby a recording pencil is made to follow the movements of a stylet passing along the lines of the original. **2.** In dentistry, an instrument used to record mandibular border movements that may be transferred to make equivalent settings on an articulator. [panto- + G. *graphō,* to record]

pan·to·ic ac·id (pan-tō′ik). A coenzyme A precursor, the β-alanine amide of which is pantothenic acid.

pan·to·mo·gram (pan′tō-mō-gram). A panoramic radiographic record of the maxillary and mandibular dental arches and their associated structures, obtained by a pantomograph. [pan- + tomogram]

pan·to·mo·graph (pan′tō-mō-graf). A panoramic radiographic instrument that permits visualization of the entire dentition, alveolar bone, and contiguous structures on a single extraoral film.

pan·to·mog·ra·phy (pan-tō-mog′ră-fē). A method of radiography by which a radiograph (pantomogram) of the maxillary and mandibular dental arches and their contiguous structures may be obtained on a single film.

pan·to·mor·phia (pan-to-mōr′fē-ă). **1.** The condition of an organism, such as an ameba, that is capable of assuming all shapes. **2.** Perfect shapeliness or symmetry. [panto- + G. *morphē,* shape]

pan·to·mor·phic (pan-tō-mōr′fik). Capable of assuming all shapes.

pan·to·nine (pan′tō-nēn). An amino acid identified in *Escherichia coli* that may be an intermediate in the biosynthesis of pantothenic acid by that organism, containing NH₂ in place of the α-OH group of pantothenic acid.

pan·to·scop·ic (pan-tō-skop′ik). Designed for observing objects at all distances; denoting bifocal lenses. [panto- + G. *skopeō,* to view]

pan·to·the·nate (pan-tō-then′āt). A salt or ester of pantothenic acid.

p. synthetase, an enzyme that converts pantoate and β-alanine to p. with cleavage of ATP to AMP and pyrophosphate; a key step in coenzyme A biosynthesis. SYN pantoate-activating enzyme.

pan·to·then·ic ac·id (pan-tō-then′ik). The β-alanine amide of pantoic acid. A growth substance widely distributed in plant and animal tissues, and essential for growth of a number of organisms; deficiency in diet causes a dermatitis in chicks and rats and achromotrichia in the latter; a precursor to coenzyme A. SYN antidermatitis factor.

pan·to·then·yl (pan-tō-then′il). The acyl radical of pantothenic acid.

p. alcohol, SYN dexpanthenol.

pan·to·yl (pan′tō-il). The acyl radical of pantoic acid.

pan·to·yl·tau·rine (pan′tō-il-taw′rin, -rēn). Pantothenic acid in which the carboxyl group is replaced by a sulfonic acid group; analogous to pantothenic acid in structure, except that taurine replaces β-alanine in the molecule. SYN thiopanic acid.

Panum, Peter L., Danish physiologist, 1820–1885. SEE P. *area.*

pan·zer·herz (pahn′zer-hārtz). SYN armored *heart.* [Ger. *Panzerherz*]

PAP Acronym for *p*eroxidase *a*nti*p*eroxidase complex. Abbreviation for 3′-phosphoadenosine 5′-phosphate. SEE PAP *technique.*

pap. A food of soft consistency, like that of breadcrumbs soaked in milk or water.

pa·pa·in, pa·pa·in·ase (pa-pā′in, -ās). A cysteine endopeptidase, or a crude extract containing it, obtained from papaya latex. It has esterase, thiolase, transamidase, and transesterase activities, and is used as a protein digestant, meat tenderizer, and to prevent adhesions. It had been used to liquify contents of herniated intervertebral discs so that these contents could be removed by aspiration. SYN papayotin.

Papanicolaou, George N., Greek-U.S. physician, anatomist, and cytologist, 1883–1962. SEE Pap *smear;* Pap *test;* P. *examination, smear,* smear *test,* stain.

Pa·pav·er (pă-pā′ver, pă-pav′er). A genus of plants, one species of which, *P. somniferum* (family Papaveraceae), furnishes opium. SYN poppy. [L. poppy]

pa·pav·er·e·tum (pă-pav-er-ē′tŭm). A preparation of water soluble opium alkaloids, including 50% anhydrous morphine. [L. *papaver,* poppy]

pa·pav·er·ine (pa-pav′er-ēn). A benzylisoquinoline alkaloid of opium that is not a narcotic but has mild analgesic action and is a powerful spasmolytic; does not evoke tolerance and has no addiction liability; used to treat male impotence by local injection. Also available as p. hydrochloride. [L. *papaver,* poppy]

pa·paw (pă-paw′). SEE papaya.

pa·pa·ya (pă-pī′yah, pă-pā′yah). The fruit of the papaw (pawpaw), *Carica papaya* (family Caricaceae), a tree of tropical America; it possesses a proteolytic action and is the source of papain. SYN carica. [Sp.]

pap·a·yo·tin (pap-ā′yō-tin). SYN papain.

pa·per (pā′per). **1.** A substance manufactured in thin sheets from wood, rags, or other materials. **2.** A square of p. folded over so as to form an envelope containing a dose of any medicinal powder. **3.** A piece of blotting p. or filter p. impregnated with a medicinal solution, dried, and burned; formerly, the fumes were inhaled in the treatment of asthma and other respiratory affections. [L. *papyrus;* G. *papyros,* a kind of rush, from which writing paper was made]

articulating p., SYN occluding p.

chromatography p., used in p. chromatography. SYN high-quality filter p.

Congo red p., p. impregnated with Congo red; used as a pH indicator, changing from blue-violet at 3.0 to red at 5.0.

filter p., an unsized p. used in pharmacy and chemistry for filtering solutions; many varieties are used for p. chromatography.

high-quality filter p., SYN chromatography p.

niter p., p. impregnated with potassium nitrate that is ignited to produce fumes inhaled as treatment for asthma. SYN potassium nitrate p., saltpeter p.

occluding p., an inked p. or ribbon interposed between natural or artificial teeth to determine tooth contacts. SYN articulating p.

potassium nitrate p., SYN niter p.

saltpeter p., SYN niter p.

Papez, James W., U.S. anatomist, 1883–1958. SEE P. *circuit.*

PAPILLA

pa·pil·la, pl. **pa·pil·lae** (pă-pil′ă, -pil′ē) [TA]. Any small, nipple-like process. SYN teat (3). [L. a nipple, dim. of *papula,* a pimple]

acoustic p., SYN spiral *organ.*

basilar p., the auditory sense organ of birds, amphibians, and reptiles; homologous to the organ of Corti in mammals.

Bergmeister p., a small mass of glial tissue that forms during fetal life a temporary conical investment of the hyaloid artery at its emergence into the vitreous chamber; vestiges of it may persist as a prepapillary membrane.

bile p., SYN major duodenal p.

p. of breast, SYN nipple.

circumvallate papillae, SYN vallate papillae.

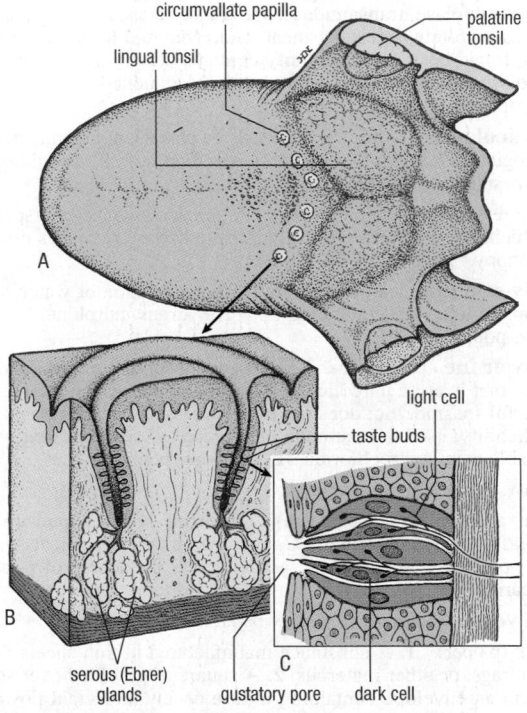

circumvallate papilla
lingual tonsil
palatine tonsil
A
light cell
taste buds
B
serous (Ebner) glands
gustatory pore
dark cell
C

circumvallate papilla of tongue: (A) superior view of tongue, (B) circumvallate papilla in detail, (C) taste bud in detail

clavate papillae, SYN fungiform papillae.

conic papillae, SYN conical papillae.

papil′lae con′icae, SYN conical papillae.

conical papillae, numerous projections on the dorsum of the tongue, scattered among the filiform papillae and similar to them, but shorter. SYN conic papillae, papillae conicae.

papil′lae co′rii, ✫official alternate term for p. of dermis.

papillae of corium, ✫official alternate term for p. of dermis.

dental p. [TA], a projection of the mesenchymal tissue of the developing jaw into the cup of the enamel organ; its outer layer becomes a layer of specialized columnar cells, the odontoblasts, that form the dentin of the tooth. SYN p. dentis [TA], dentinal p.

dentinal p., SYN dental p.

p. den′tis [TA], SYN dental p.

dermal papillae, SYN p. of dermis.

papil′lae der′mis [TA], SYN p. of dermis.

p. of dermis [TA], the superficial projections of the dermis (corium) that interdigitate with recesses in the overlying epidermis;

they contain vascular loops and specialized nerve endings, and are arranged in ridgelike lines best developed in the hand and foot. SYN papillae dermis [TA], papillae corii✫, papillae of corium✫, dermal papillae.

p. ductus parotidei [TA], SYN p. of parotid gland.

p. duode′ni ma′jor [TA], SYN major duodenal p.

p. duode′ni mi′nor [TA], SYN minor duodenal p.

filiform papillae [TA], numerous elongated conical keratinized projections on the dorsum of the tongue. SYN papillae filiformes [TA].

papil′lae filifor′mes [TA], SYN filiform papillae.

papil′lae folia′tae [TA], SYN foliate papillae.

foliate papillae [TA], numerous projections arranged in several transverse folds upon the lateral margins of the tongue just in front of the palatoglossus muscle. SYN papillae foliatae [TA], folia linguae.

fungiform papillae [TA], numerous minute elevations on the dorsum of the tongue, of a fancied mushroom shape, the tip being broader than the base; the epithelium of many of these papillae has taste buds. SYN papillae fungiformes [TA], clavate papillae.

papil′lae fungifor′mes [TA], SYN fungiform papillae.

gingival p. [TA], thickening (seen as an elevation) of the gingiva that fills the interproximal space between two adjacent teeth. SYN p. gingivalis [TA], interdental p.✫, p. interdentalis✫, gingival septum, interproximal p.

p. gingivalis [TA], SYN gingival p.

hair p., a knoblike indentation of the bottom of the hair follicle, upon which the hair bulb fits like a cap; it is derived from the corium and contains vascular loops for the nourishment of the hair root. SYN p. pili.

ileal p. [TA], seen in the cadaver as a bilabial prominence of the terminal ileum protruding into the large intestine at the cecocolic junction; in the living individual, it appears as a truncated cone with a star-shaped orifice. SYN p. ilealis [TA], valva ileocecalis [TA], Bauhin valve, ileocecal eminence, ileocecal valve, ileocolic valve, Tulp valve, Tulpius valve, valve of Varolius.

p. ilealis [TA], SYN ileal p.

p. incisi′va [TA], SYN incisive p.

incisive p. [TA], a slight elevation of the mucosa at the anterior extremity of the raphe of the palate. SYN p. incisiva [TA], palatine p.

interdental p., ✫official alternate term for gingival p.

p. interdentalis, ✫official alternate term for gingival p.

interproximal p., SYN gingival p.

lacrimal p. [TA], a slight projection from the margin of each eyelid near the medial commissure, in the center of which is the lacrimal punctum (opening of the lacrimal duct). SYN p. lacrimalis [TA].

p. lacrima′lis [TA], SYN lacrimal p.

lenticular papillae, SYN *folliculi* linguales, under *folliculus.*

lingual papillae, (1) SYN papillae of tongue; **(2)** SYN lingual gingival p.

lingual gingival p., the lingual portions of the gingiva filling the interproximal space between adjacent teeth; in molar and premolar areas, there may be separate lingual and buccal interdental papillae. SYN lingual interdental p., lingual papillae (2).

lingual interdental p., SYN lingual gingival p.

p. lingua′lis, pl. **papil′lae lingua′les,** SYN papillae of tongue.

major duodenal p. [TA], point of opening of the common bile duct and pancreatic duct into the duodenum; it is located posteriorly in the descending part of the duodenum. SYN p. duodeni major [TA], bile p., p. of Vater, Santorini major caruncle.

p. mam′mae [TA], SYN nipple.

minor duodenal p. [TA], the site of the opening of the accessory pancreatic duct into the duodenum, located anterior to and slightly superior to the major p. SYN p. duodeni minor [TA], Santorini minor caruncle.

nerve p., one of the papillae in the dermis containing a tactile corpuscle or other form of end organ. SYN neurothele.

p. ner′vi op′tici, SYN optic *disk.*

optic p. (p), SYN optic *disk.*

palatine p., SYN incisive p.

parotid p., SYN p. of parotid gland.

p. parotid′ea, SYN p. of parotid gland.

p. of parotid gland [TA], the projection at the opening of the parotid duct into the vestibule of the mouth opposite the neck of the upper second molar tooth. SYN p. ductus parotidei [TA], p. parotidea, parotid p.

p. pi′li, SYN hair p.

renal p. [TA], the apex of a renal pyramid that projects into a minor calyx; some 10–25 openings of papillary ducts occur on its tip, forming the area cribrosa. SYN p. renalis [TA].

p. rena′lis, pl. **papil′lae rena′les** [TA], SYN renal p.

retrocuspid p., a small tissue tag located on the mandibular gingiva lingual to the cuspid teeth; usually occurs bilaterally, is more commonly identified in children, and is considered a normal anatomic structure.

tactile p., one of the papillae of the dermis containing a tactile cell or corpuscle.

papillae of tongue [TA], numerous variously shaped projections of the mucous membrane of the dorsum of the tongue; includes filiform, foliate, fungiform, and vallate papillae. SYN lingual papillae (1), p. lingualis.

urethral p., p. urethra′lis, the slight projection often present in the vestibule of the vagina marking the urethral orifice.

papillae valla′tae, pl. **papil′lae valla′tae** [TA], SYN vallate papillae.

vallate papillae [TA], one of eight or ten projections from the dorsum of the tongue forming a row anterior to and parallel with the sulcus terminalis; each p. is surrounded by a circular trench (fossa) having a slightly raised outer wall (vallum); on the sides of the vallate p. and the opposed margin of the vallum are numerous taste buds. SYN papillae vallatae [TA], circumvallate papillae.

vascular papillae, dermal papillae containing vascular loops.

p. of Vater, SYN major duodenal p.

---

pap·il·lary, pap·il·late (pap′i-lār-ē, -i-lāt). Relating to, resembling, or provided with papillae.

pap·il·lec·to·my (pap-i-lek′tō-mē). Surgical removal of any papilla. [papilla + G. *ektomē,* excision]

pa·pil·le·de·ma (pă-pil-e-dē′mă). Edema of the optic disk, often due to increased intracranial pressure. SYN choked disk. [papilla + edema]

pap·il·lif·er·ous (pap-i-lif′er-ŭs). Provided with papillae. [papilla + L. *fero,* to bear]

pa·pil·li·form (pă-pil′i-fōrm). Resembling or shaped like a papilla.

pap·il·li·tis (pap-i-lī′tis). **1.** Optic neuritis with swelling of the optic disk. **2.** Inflammation of the renal papilla. [papilla + G. *-itis,* inflammation]

foliate p., inflamed vestigial foliate papillae on the posterior lateral tongue.

necrotizing p., SYN renal papillary *necrosis.*

△**papillo-.** A papilla, papillary. [L. *papilla*]

pap·il·lo·ad·e·no·cys·to·ma (pap′i-lō-ad′ĕ-nō-sis-tō′mă). A benign epithelial neoplasm characterized by glands or glandlike structures, formation of cysts, and fingerlike projections of neoplastic cells covering a core of fibrous connective tissue.

pap·il·lo·car·ci·no·ma (pap′i-lō-kar-si-nō′mă). A carcinoma that is characterized by papillary, fingerlike projections of neoplastic cells in association with cores of fibrous stroma as a supporting structure. [papilla + G. *karkinōma,* cancer]

pap·il·lo·ma (pap-i-lō′mă). A circumscribed, benign epithelial tumor projecting from the surrounding surface; more precisely, a benign epithelial neoplasm consisting of villous or arborescent outgrowths of fibrovascular stroma covered by neoplastic cells. SYN papillary tumor. [papilla + G. *-oma,* tumor]

basal cell p., SYN seborrheic *keratosis.*

p. canalic′ulum, a papillomatous benign tumor arising within the duct of a gland.

p. diffu′sum, widespread occurrence of p.'s.

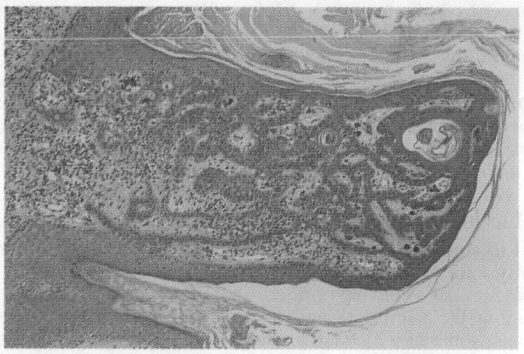

basal cell papilloma of skin: tumor is composed of cells resembling those in basal layer of epidermis; exophytic tumor forms papillae projecting above surface of skin

---

duct p., SYN intraductal p.

p. du′rum, a wart, corn, or cutaneous horn. SYN hard p.

hard p., SYN p. durum.

Hopmann p., a papillomatous overgrowth of the nasal mucous membrane. SYN Hopmann polyp.

p. inguina′le trop′icum, a cutaneous eruption, occurring in Colombia, characterized by numerous slender pink vegetations in the inguinal region.

intracystic p., a p. growing within a cystic adenoma, filling the cavity with a mass of branching epithelial processes.

intraductal p., a small, often nonpalpable, benign p. arising in a lactiferous duct and frequently causing bleeding from the nipple. SYN duct p.

inverted p., an epithelial tumor of the urinary bladder or nasal cavity in which proliferating epithelium is invaginated beneath the surface and is more smoothly rounded than in other p.'s.

p. mol′le, SYN skin *tag.*

Shope p., a papillomatous growth found in wild cottontail rabbits originally described by Shope that is caused by a virus in the family Papovaviridae and can be transferred to domestic rabbits where it will cause similar growths. A high percentage of these growths may become malignant.

soft p., SYN skin *tag.*

transitional cell p., SYN urothelial p.

urothelial p., a benign papillary tumor of urothelium. SYN transitional cell p.

villous p., a p. composed of slender, fingerlike excrescences occurring in the bladder or large intestine, or from the choroid plexus of the cerebral ventricles; villous p. of the colon is usually sessile and frequently becomes malignant. SYN villous tumor.

zymotic p., SYN yaws.

pap·il·lo·ma·to·sis (pap′i-lō-mă-tō′sis). **1.** The development of numerous papillomas. **2.** Papillary projections of the epidermis forming an undulating surface.

confluent and reticulate p., discrete and confluent gray-brown papules of the anterior and posterior mid-chest, spreading gradually; *Malassezia furfur* has been found in the keratin layer. SYN Gougerot-Carteaud syndrome.

florid oral p., diffuse involvement of the lips and oral mucosa with benign squamous papillomas; microscopically, it resembles verrucous carcinoma, but it is not invasive or localized to a specific area of the oral mucosa.

juvenile p., a form of fibrocystic disease of the breast in young women, with florid and sclerosing adenosis that microscopically may suggest carcinoma.

laryngeal p., multiple squamous-cell papillomas of the larynx, seen most commonly in young children, usually due to infection by the human papilloma virus, which may be transmitted at birth from the maternal condylomata; recurrences are common, with remission after several years. SEE ALSO recurrent respiratory p.

palatal p., SYN inflammatory papillary *hyperplasia.*

pa

recurrent respiratory p., a disease of the respiratory tract caused by the human papilloma virus; characterized by rapid recurrence of papillomas after surgical removal, airway obstruction, and hoarseness to aphonia when the larynx is involved. SEE ALSO laryngeal p.

subareolar duct p., a benign tumor that may clinically resemble Paget disease, but that is a papillary or solid growth of columnar and myoepithelial cells producing a florid pseudoinfiltrative pattern. SYN adenoma of nipple, erosive adenomatosis of nipple.

pap·il·lo·ma·tous (pap-i-lō′mă-tŭs). Relating to a papilloma.

Pa·pil·lo·ma·vi·rus (pap-i-lō′mă-vī-rŭs). A genus of viruses (family Papovaviridae) containing double-stranded circular DNA (MW 5×10^6), having virions about 55 nm in diameter, and including the papilloma and wart viruses of humans and other animals, some of which are associated with inductions of carcinoma. More than 70 types are known to infect humans and are differentiated by DNA homology. SYN papilloma virus.

Papillon, M.M., 20th century French dermatologist. SEE P.-Lefèvre *syndrome.*

Papillon-Léage, E., 20th century French dentist. SEE Papillon-Léage and Psaume *syndrome.*

pap·il·lo·ret·i·ni·tis (pap′i-lō-ret-i-nī′tis). SYN neuroretinitis.

pap·il·lot·o·my (pă-pi-lot′ō-mē). An incision into a papilla; usually in reference to the major duodenal papilla. [papilla + G. *tomē,* incision]

pa·pil·lu·la pl. **pa·pil·lu·lae** (pă-pil′ū-lă, -lē). A small papilla. [Mod. L. dim. of L. *papilla*]

Pa·po·va·vir·i·dae (pă-po′vă-vir′i-dē). A family of small, antigenically distinct viruses that replicate in nuclei of infected cells; most have oncogenic properties. Virions are 45–55 nm in diameter, nonenveloped, and ether-resistant; capsids are icosahedral with 72 capsomeres, and they contain double-stranded circular DNA (MW $3–5 \times 10^6$). The family includes 2 genera Papillomavirus and Polyomavirus. [*pap*illoma + *pol*yoma + *va*cuolating]

pa·po·va·vi·rus (pă-pō′vă-vī′rŭs). An old name for any virus of the family Papovaviridae.

PAPP Abbreviation for *p*-aminopropiophenone.

Pappenheim, Artur, German physician, 1870–1916. SEE P. *stain;* Unna-P. *stain.*

Pap·pen·hei·mer, A.M., U.S. pathologist, 1878–1955. His work in experimental pathology was extensive and included studies of the thymus, identification of the role of lice transmission in trench *fever,* development of an experimental model for rickets, and evaluation of viral infections in animals. SEE Pappenheimer *bodies,* under *body.*

pap·pus (pap′ŭs). The first downy growth of beard. [G. *pappos,* down]

PAPS Abbreviation for adenosine 3′-phosphate 5′-phosphosulfate; 3′-phosphoadenosine 5′-phosphosulfate.

pap·u·lar (pap′ū-lăr). Relating to papules.

pap·ule (pap′ūl). A circumscribed, solid elevation up to 100 cm in diameter on the skin. A p. may be pedunculated, sessile, or filiform. [L. *papula,* pimple]

follicular p., a papular lesion arising about a hair follicle; not specific for any condition.

moist p., mucous p., SYN *condyloma* latum.

piezogenic pedal p., pressure-induced papules of the heel, occurring probably as a result of herniation of fat tissue.

pruritic urticarial p.'s and plaques of pregnancy (PUPPP), intensely pruritic papulovesicles that begin on the abdomen in the third trimester and spread peripherally, resolves rapidly after delivery, and does not affect the fetus.

split p.'s, p.'s at commissures of the mouth seen in some cases of secondary syphilis.

papulo-. Papule. [L. *papula,* papule]

pap·u·lo·er·y·them·a·tous (pap′ū-lō-er-i-them′ă-tŭs, -thē′mă-tŭs). Denoting an eruption of papules on an erythematous surface.

pap·u·lo·pus·tu·lar (pap′ū-lō-pŭs′too-lăr). Denoting an eruption composed of papules and pustules.

pap·u·lo·pus·tule (pap′ū-lō-pŭs′tūl). A small semisolid skin elevation that rapidly evolves into a pustule.

pa·pu·lo·sis (pap-ū-lō′sis). The occurrence of numerous widespread papules.

bowenoid p., a clinically benign form of intraepithelial neoplasia that microscopically resembles Bowen disease or carcinoma in situ, occurring in young individuals of both sexes on the genital or perianal skin usually as multiple well-demarcated pigmented warty papules.

lymphomatoid p., a chronic papular and ulcerative variant of pityriasis lichenoides et varioliformis acuta characterized by dermal perivascular infiltration by atypical T lymphocytes suggestive of a lymphoma; it is usually benign, but transformation to lymphoma has been reported.

malignant atrophic p., a cutaneovisceral syndrome characterized by pathognomonic umbilicated porcelain-white papules with elevated telangiectatic annular borders, followed by the development of intestinal ulcers that perforate, causing peritonitis; arterioles in the lesions are occluded by thrombosis without inflammatory cells, leading to infarction, progressive neurological disability, and death. SYN Degos disease, Degos syndrome.

pap·u·lo·squa·mous (pap′ū-lō-skwā′mŭs). Denoting an eruption composed of both papules and scales. [papulo- + L. *squamosus,* scaly (squamous)]

pap·u·lo·ves·i·cle (pap′ū-lō-ves′i-kl). A small skin elevation that evolves into a blister.

pap·u·lo·ve·sic·u·lar (pap′ū-lō-ve-sik′ū-lăr). Denoting an eruption composed of papules and vesicles.

PAPVR Abbreviation for partial anomalous pulmonary venous return. SEE anomalous pulmonary venous *connections,* total or partial, under *connection.*

pap·y·ra·ceous (pap-i-rā′shŭs). Like parchment or paper. [L. *papyraceus,* made of *papyrus*]

par. A pair; specifically a pair of cranial nerves, e.g., p. nonum, ninth pair, glossopharyngeal; p. vagum, the vagus or tenth pair. [L. equal]

para (par′ă). A woman who has given birth to one or more infants. Para followed by a roman numeral or preceded by a Latin prefix (primi-, secundi-, terti-, quadri-, etc.) designates the number of times a pregnancy has culminated in a single or multiple birth; e.g., **para I**, primipara, a woman who has given birth for the first time; **para II**, secundipara, a woman who has given birth for the second time to one or more infants. Cf. gravida. [L. *pario,* to bring forth]

para-. 1. Prefix denoting a departure from the normal. 2. Prefix denoting involvement of two like parts or a pair. 3. Prefix denoting adjacent, alongside, near, etc. 4 (*p*-). In chemistry, an italicized prefix denoting two substitutions in the benzene ring arranged symmetrically, i.e., linked to opposite carbon atoms in the ring. For words beginning with *para*- or *p*-, see the specific name. [G. alongside of, near]

para-ac·ti·no·my·co·sis (par-ă-ak′ti-nō-mī- kō′sis). Chronic infection, usually pulmonary, resembling actinomycosis; ordinarily caused by nocardiosis. SYN pseudoactinomycosis.

par·a·ami·no·ben·zo·ic ac·id (par′ă-mē′nō). SYN *p*-aminobenzoic acid.

para-ap·pen·di·ci·tis (par′ă-ă-pen-di-sī′tis). SYN periappendicitis.

par·a·ban·ic ac·id (par′ă-ban-ik). SYN oxalylurea.

par·a·bi·o·sis (par-ă-bī-ō′sis). 1. Fusion of whole eggs or embryos, as occurs in some forms of conjoined twins. 2. Surgical joining of the vascular systems of two organisms. [para- + G. *biōsis,* life]

par·a·bi·ot·ic (par-ă-bī-ot′ik). Relating to, or characterized by, parabiosis.

par·a·bu·lia (par-ă-boo′lē-ă). Perversion of volition or will in which one impulse is checked and replaced by another. [para- + G. *boulē,* will]

par·ac·an·tho·ma (par′ak-an-thō′mă). A neoplasm arising from abnormal hyperplasia of the prickle cell layer of the skin. [para- + G. *akantha,* a thorn, + -*oma,* tumor]

par·ac·an·tho·sis (par′ak-an-thō′sis). **1.** The development of paracanthomas. **2.** A division of tumors that includes the cutaneous epitheliomas.

par·a·car·mine. SEE paracarmine *stain.*

par·a·ca·se·in (par-ă-kā′sē-in). The compound produced by the action of rennin upon κ-casein (which liberates a glycoprotein), and that precipitates with calcium ion as the insoluble curd.

Paracelsus, Aureolus Theophrastus Bombastus von Hohenheim, Swiss physician, 1493–1541. SEE paracelsian *method.*

par·a·ce·nes·the·sia (par′ă-sē-nes-thē′zē-ă). Deterioration in one's sense of bodily well-being, i.e., of the normal functioning of one's organs. [para- + G. *koinos,* common, + *aisthēsis,* feeling]

par·a·cen·te·sis (par′ă-sen-tē′sis). The passage into a cavity of a trocar and cannula, needle, or other hollow instrument for the purpose of removing fluid; variously designated according to the cavity punctured. SYN tapping (2). [G. *parakentēsis,* a tapping for dropsy, fr. *para,* beside, + *kentēsis,* puncture]

par·a·cen·tet·ic (par-ă-sen-tet′ik). Relating to paracentesis.

par·a·cen·tral (par-ă-sen′trăl). Close to or beside the center or some structure designated "central."

par·a·cer·vi·cal (par-ă-ser′vi-kăl). Connective tissue adjacent to the uterine cervix.

par·a·cer·vix (par-ă-ser′viks) [TA]. The connective tissue of the pelvic floor extending from the fibrous subserous coat of the cervix of the uterus laterally between the layers of the broad ligament.

par·ac·e·tal·de·hyde (par-as-ĕ-tal′dĕ-hīd). SYN paraldehyde.

par·a·cet·a·mol (par-ă-set′ă-mol). SYN acetaminophen.

par·a·chlo·ro·phe·nol (par′ă-klōr-ō-fē′nol). A disinfectant effective against most Gram-negative organisms; also available as camphorated p. SYN *p*-chlorophenol.

par·a·chol·er·a (par-ă-kol′er-ă). A disease clinically resembling Asiatic cholera but due to a vibrio specifically different from *Vibrio cholerae.*

par·a·chor·dal (par-ă-kōr′dăl). Alongside the anterior portion of the notochord in the embryo; designating the bilateral cartilaginous bars that enter into the formation of the base of the skull. [para- + G. *chordē,* cord]

par·a·chro·ma (par-ă-krō′mă). Abnormal coloration of the skin. [para- + G. *chrōma,* color]

par·a·chy·mo·sin (par-ă-kī′mō-sin). An enzyme resembling chymosin.

par·a·ci·ne·sia, par·a·ci·ne·sis (par′ă-si-nē′zē-ă, -nē′sis). SYN parakinesia.

par·ac·ma·sis (par-ak′mă-sis). SYN paracme.

par·ac·mas·tic (par-ak-mas′tik). Relating to the paracme.

par·ac·me (par-ak′mē). **1.** The stage of subsidence of a fever. **2.** The period of life beyond the prime; the decline or stage of involution of an organism. SYN paracmasis. [G. the point at which the prime is past; fr. *para,* beyond, + *akmē,* highest point, prime]

Par·a·coc·cid·i·oi·des bra·sil·i·en·sis (par′ă-kok-sid-ē-oy′dēz bră-sil-ē-en′sis). A dimorphic fungus that causes paracoccidioidomycosis. In tissues and on enriched culture medium at 37°C, it grows as large spherical or oval cells that bear single or several buds and usually is identified by this characteristic; at lower temperatures, it grows slowly as a white mold with minimal sporulation.

par·a·coc·cid·i·oi·din (par′ă-kok-sid-ē-oy′din). A filtrate antigen prepared from the filamentous form of the pathogenic fungus, *Paracoccidioides brasiliensis;* used for demonstrating delayed type dermal hypersensitivity in populations and useful in demonstrating endemic areas in different geographic regions.

par·a·coc·cid·i·oi·do·my·co·sis (par′ă-kok-sid-ē-oy′dō-mī-kō′sis). A chronic mycosis characterized by primary pulmonary lesions with dissemination to many visceral organs, conspicuous ulcerative granulomas of the buccal and nasal mucosa with extensions to the skin, and generalized lymphangitis; caused by *Paracoccidioides brasiliensis.* SYN Almeida disease, Lutz-Splendore-Almeida disease, paracoccidioidal granuloma, South American blastomycosis.

par·a·co·li·tis (par′ă-kō-lī′tis). Inflammation of the peritoneal coat of the colon.

par·a·col·pi·tis (par′ă-kol-pī′tis). SYN paravaginitis. [para- + G. *kolpos,* vagina, + *-itis,* inflammation]

par·a·col·pi·um (par-ă-kol′pē-ŭm). The tissues alongside the vagina. [para- + G. *kolpos,* vagina]

par·a·cone (par′ă-kōn). The mesiobuccal cusp of an upper molar tooth. [para- + G. *kōnos,* cone]

par·a·co·nid (par-ă-kon′id). The mesiobuccal cusp of a lower molar tooth.

par·a·cor·tex (par-ă-kōr′teks). The area of a lymph node between the subcapsular cortex and the medullary cords; it contains mostly the long-lived lymphocytes derived from the thymus. SYN deep cortex, tertiary cortex, thymus-dependent zone.

par·a·cou·sis (par-ă-koo′sis). SYN paracusis.

par·a·crine (par′ă-krin). Relating to a kind of hormone function in which the effects of the hormone are restricted to the local environment. Cf. endocrine. [para- + G. *krinō,* to separate]

par·a·cu·sis, par·a·cu·sia (par′ă-koo′sis, -koo′sē-ă). **1.** Impaired hearing. **2.** Auditory illusions or hallucinations. SYN paracousis. [para- + G. *akousis,* hearing]

false p., the apparent increase in hearing of a person with a conductive hearing loss in conversation in noisy surroundings because of others speaking more loudly. SYN Willis p.

p. loci, loss or diminution of the power of determining the direction of sound.

Willis p., SYN false p.

par·a·cy·e·sis (par-ă-sī-ē′sis). SYN ectopic *pregnancy.* [para- + G. *kyēsis,* pregnancy]

par·a·cys·tic (par-ă-sis′tik). Alongside or near a bladder, specifically the urinary bladder. SYN paravesical. [para- + G. *kystis,* bladder]

par·a·cys·ti·tis (par′ă-sis-tī′tis). Inflammation of the connective tissue and other structures about the urinary bladder. [para- + G. *kystis,* bladder, + *-itis,* inflammation]

par·a·cys·ti·um (par-ă-sis′tē-ŭm). The tissues adjacent to the urinary bladder. [para- + G. *kystis,* bladder]

par·a·cy·tic (par-ă-sī′tik). **1.** Relating to cells other than those normal to the part where they are found. **2.** Between or among, but independent of, cells. [para- + G. *kytos,* cell]

par·ad·e·ni·tis (par′ad′ĕ-nī′tis). Inflammation of the tissues adjacent to a gland. [para- + G. *adēn,* gland, + *-itis,* inflammation]

par·a·den·tal (par-ă-den′tăl). SYN periodontal.

par·a·den·ti·um (par-ă-den′tē-oom). SYN periodontium.

par·a·did·y·mal (par-ă-did′i-măl). **1.** Relating to the paradidymis. **2.** Alongside the testis.

par·a·did·y·mis, pl. **par·a·did·y·mi·des** (par′ă-did′i-mis, -didim′i-dēz) [TA]. A small body sometimes attached to the front of the lower part of the spermatic cord above the head of the epididymis; the remnants of tubules of the mesonephros. Its equivalent in the female is the paroöphoron. SYN parepididymis. [para- + G. *didymos,* twin, in pl. *didymoi,* testes]

par·a·dip·sia (par-ă-dip′sē-ă). A perverted appetite for fluids, ingested without relation to bodily need. [para- + G. *dipsa,* thirst]

par·a·dox (par′ă-doks). That which is apparently, though not actually, inconsistent with or opposed to the known facts in any case. [G. *paradoxos,* incredible, beyond belief, fr. *doxa,* belief]

Weber p., if a muscle is loaded beyond its power to contract it may elongate.

par·a·es·the·sia (par-es-thē′zē-ă). SYN paresthesia.

par·af·fin (par′ă-fin). **1.** One of the methane series of acyclic hydrocarbons. **2.** SYN hard p. [L. *parum,* little, + *affinis,* neighboring, akin, so called because of its slight tendency to chemical reaction]

chlorinated p., a solvent for dichloramine-T.

hard p., a purified mixture of solid hydrocarbons derived from petroleum. SYN paraffin (2).

liquid p., SYN mineral oil.

white soft p., SYN white *petrolatum.*

yellow soft p., SYN petrolatum.

par·af·fi·no·ma (par'ă-fi-nō'mă). A tumefaction, usually a granuloma, caused by the prosthetic or therapeutic injection of paraffin into the tissues; sometimes used with reference to similar lesions resulting from the injection of any oil, wax, or the like. SEE ALSO lipogranuloma. SYN paraffin tumor.

Par·a·fi·lar·ia mul·ti·pa·pil·lo·sa (par'ă-fi-lā'rē-ă mul'ti-pap-i-lō' să). A common filarial parasite that causes dermatorrhagia parasitica.

par·a·fla·gel·la (par'ă-fla-jel'ă). Plural of paraflagellum.

par·a·flag·el·late (par-ă-flaj'ě-lāt). 1. Having one or more paraflagella. 2. SYN paramastigote.

par·a·fla·gel·lum, pl. **par·a·fla·gel·la** (par'ă-fla-jel'ŭm, -ă). A minute accessory flagellum sometimes present in addition to the ordinary flagellum of certain protozoans.

paraflocculus ventralis. SYN ventral paraflocculus.

par·a·fol·lic·u·lar (par-ă-fo-lik'ū-lăr). Associated spatially with a follicle.

par·a·for·mal·de·hyde (par-ă-fōr-mal'dě-hīd). A polymer of formaldehyde, used as a disinfectant. SYN trioxymethylene.

par·a·fuch·sin (par-ă-fuk'sin). SYN pararosanilin.

par·a·gam·ma·cism (par'ă-gam'ă-sizm). Substitution of another letter sound for the g sound. SEE ALSO gammacism. [para- + G. *gamma,* the letter g]

par·a·gan·glia (par-ă-gang'glē-ă). Plural of paraganglion.

par·a·gan·gli·o·ma (par'ă-gang-glē-ō'mă). A neoplasm usually derived from the chromoreceptor tissue of a paraganglion, such as the carotid body, or the medulla of the adrenal gland; the latter is usually termed a chromaffinoma or pheochromocytoma.

   nonchromaffin p., SYN chemodectoma.

par·a·gan·gli·on, pl. **par·a·gan·glia** (par-ă-gang'glē-on, -ă). A small, roundish body containing chromaffin cells; a number of such bodies may be found retroperitoneally near the aorta and in organs such as the kidney, liver, heart, and gonads. SYN chromaffin body.

par·a·gene (par'ă-jēn). SYN plasmid.

par·a·gen·i·tal (par-ă-jen'i-tal). Alongside the gonads.

par·a·geu·sia (par-ă-gū'sē-ă, -joo'sē-ă). SYN dysgeusia. [para- + G. *geusis,* taste]

par·a·geu·sic (par-ă-gū'sik). Relating to parageusia.

pa·rag·na·thus (pa-rag'na-thŭs). 1. A developmental defect resulting in an individual with an accessory lower jaw. 2. A parasitic fetus attached to the jaw of the autosite. [para- + G. *gnathos,* jaw]

par·ag·no·men (par-ag-nō'men). An unexpected reaction. [para- + G. *gnōmēn, gnōmē,* judgment]

par·a·gon·i·mi·a·sis (par'ă-gon-i-mī'ă-sis). Infection with a worm of the genus *Paragonimus,* especially *P. westermani.* SYN pulmonary distomiasis.

Par·a·gon·i·mus (par-ă-gon'i-mŭs). A genus of lung flukes, parasitic in humans and a wide variety of mammals, that feed upon crustacea carrying the metacercariae. [para- + G. *gonimos,* with generative power]

   P. kellicot'ti, a species of fluke prevalent in certain wild animals, such as raccoons, and occurring in dogs, in the Great Lakes region of the U.S.; it is morphologically similar to *P. westermani.*

   P. rin'geri, SYN *P. westermani.*

   P. westermani, the bronchial or lung fluke; a species that causes paragonimiasis, found chiefly in Japan, Korea, Taiwan, China, the Philippines, and Thailand; eggs are coughed up in sputum or swallowed and passed in the feces; miracidia invade *Melania* snails, and produce large numbers of stumpy-tailed cercariae that leave the snail and crawl into muscles and viscera of crayfish or crabs and encyst; in humans the excysted worms invade the wall of the gut and migrate through the diaphragm into the lungs; the developing parasites cause an intense inflammatory reaction and eventually induce fibrous-walled nodules that usually contain a pair of adult worms, along with exudate, eggs, and remains of red blood cells; the fibroparasitic nodules may become contiguous and form multiloculated cystlike structures; in some instances, the

flukes involve the brain, liver, peritoneum, intestine, or skin. SYN *P. ringeri.*

par·a·gon·or·rhe·al (par'ă-gon-ō-rē'ăl). Indirectly related to or consequent to gonorrhea.

par·a·gram·ma·tism (par-ă-gram'ă-tizm). SYN paraphasia.

par·a·graph·ia (par-ă-graf'ē-ă). 1. Loss of the power of writing from dictation, although the words are heard and comprehended. 2. Writing one word when another is intended. [para- + G. *graphō,* to write]

par·a·he·pat·ic (par-ă-he-pat'ik). Adjacent to the liver.

par·a·hi·dro·sis (par'ă-hi-drō'sis). SYN paridrosis.

par·a·hor·mone (par-ă-hōr'mōn). A substance, product of ordinary metabolism, not produced for a specific purpose, that acts like a hormone in modifying the activity of some distant organ; e.g., the action of carbon dioxide on the control of breathing.

par·a·hy·poph·y·sis (par'ă-hī-pof'i-sis). A small mass of pituitary tissue, or tissue resembling in structure the anterior lobe of the hypophysis, occasionally found in the dura mater lining of the sella turcica.

par·a·kap·pa·cism (par'ă-kap'ă-sizm). Substitution of another letter sound for that of k. SEE ALSO kappacism. [para- + G. *kappa,* the letter k]

par·a·ker·a·to·sis (par'ă-ker-ă-tō'sis). Retention of nuclei in the cells of the stratum corneum of the epidermis, observed in many scaling dermatoses such as psoriasis and subacute or chronic dermatitis.

   p. pustulo'sa, idiopathic subungual keratosis with nail deformity or pitting and with pustular or well-demarcated scaling eczematous changes of the fingertips; usually seen in young girls.

   p. scutula'ris, a disease of the scalp marked by the formation of crusts that envelop the hairs.

par·a·ki·ne·sia, par·a·ki·ne·sis (par'ă-ki-nē'zē-ă, -ki-nē'sis). Any motor abnormality. SYN paracinesia, paracinesis. [para- + G. *kinēsis,* movement]

par·a·la·lia (par-ă-lā'lē-ă). Any speech defect; especially one in which one letter is habitually substituted for another. [para- + G. *lalia,* talking]

   p. litera'lis, SYN stammering.

par·a·lamb·da·cism (par-ă-lam'dă-sizm). Mispronunciation of the letter l, or the substitution of some other letter for it. SEE ALSO lambdacism. [para- + G. *lambda,* letter l]

par·al·de·hyde (par-al'dě-hīd). $(CH_3CHO)_3$; a cyclic polymer of acetaldehyde; a potent hypnotic sedative, and anticonvulsant suitable for oral, rectal, intravenous, and intramuscular administration; its offensive odor limits its use; effective in suppressing abstinence from alcohol dependence. SYN paracetaldehyde.

par·a·lep·ro·sis (par-ă-lě-prō'sis). Presence of certain trophic or nerve changes suggesting an attenuated form of leprosy in regions where the disease has long prevailed.

par·a·lep·sy (par'ă-lep-sē). 1. A rarely used term for a temporary attack of mental inertia and hopelessness. 2. A sudden alteration in mood or emotional tension. [G. para- + *lēpsis,* seizure]

par·a·lex·ia (par-ă-lek'sē-ă). Misapprehension of written or printed words, other meaningless words being substituted for them in reading. [para- + G. *lexis,* speech]

par·al·ge·sia (par-al-jē'zē-ă). Painful paresthesia; any disorder or abnormality of the sense of pain. [para- + G. *algēsis,* the sense of pain]

par·al·gia (par-al'jē-ă). Abnormal or unusual pain. [para- + G. *algos,* pain]

par·a·lip·o·pho·bia (par'ă-lip-ō-fō'bē-ă). Morbid fear of neglect of duty. [G. *paraleipō,* to omit, pass over, + *phobos,* fear]

par·al·lac·tic (par-ă-lak'tik). Relating to a parallax.

par·al·lax (par'ă-laks). 1. The apparent displacement of an object that follows a change in the position from which it is viewed. 2. SEE phi *phenomenon.* [G. alternately, fr. *par-allassō,* to make alternate, fr. *allos,* other]

   binocular p., the difference in the angles formed by the lines of sight to two objects situated at different distances from the eyes; a factor in the visual perception of depth. SYN stereoscopic p.

heteronymous p., the apparent movement of an object toward the closed eye; noted in exophoria.

homonymous p., the apparent movement of an object toward the open eye when one is closed; noted in esophoria.

stereoscopic p., SYN binocular p.

vertical p., the relative vertical displacement of the image when each eye is closed in turn; seen in vertical diplopia, or heterophoria.

par·al·lel·ism (par′ă-lel-izm). **1.** The state of being structurally parallel. **2.** In psychology, the mind-body doctrine that for every conscious process there is a corresponding or parallel organic process, without asserting a causal interrelation between the two. [para- + G. *allēlōn,* of one another, fr. *allos,* other]

par·al·lel·om·e·ter (par′ă-lel-om′ĕ-ter). An apparatus used for paralleling the attachments and abutments for fixed or removable partial dentures.

par·al·ler·gic (par-ă-ler′jik). Denoting an allergic state in which the body becomes predisposed to nonspecific stimuli following original sensitization with a specific allergen.

par·a·lo·gia, pa·ral·o·gism, pa·ral·o·gy (par-ă-lō′jē-ă, pă-ral′ō-jizm, -ral′ō-jē). False reasoning, involving self-deception. [G. *paralogia,* a fallacy, fr. *para,* beside, + *logos,* reason]

thematic p., false reasoning in relation chiefly to one theme or subject, upon which the mind dwells insistently.

pa·ral·y·sis, pl. **pa·ral·y·ses** (pă-ral′i-sis, -sēz). **1.** Loss of power of voluntary movement in a muscle through injury or disease of it or its nerve supply. **2.** Loss of any function, as sensation, secretion, or mental ability. [G. fr. para- + *lysis,* a loosening]

acute ascending p., a p. of rapid course beginning in the legs and involving progressively the trunk, arms, and neck, ending sometimes in death in 1–3 weeks; generally due to either a fulminant Guillain-Barré syndrome or an ascending necrotizing myelopathy. SYN ascending p.

p. ag′itans, obsolete term for parkinsonism (1).

ascending p., SYN acute ascending p.

Brown-Séquard p., SYN Brown-Séquard *syndrome.*

bulbar p., SYN progressive bulbar p.

central p., p. due to a lesion in the brain or spinal cord.

compression p., p. due to external presure on a nerve.

crossed p., SYN alternating *hemiplegia.*

crutch p., a form of pressure p. affecting the arm and caused by compression of the infraclavicular brachial plexus or radial nerve by the crosspiece of a crutch. SYN crutch palsy.

diphtheritic p., SYN postdiphtheritic p.

diver's p., lay term for decompression *sickness.*

Duchenne-Erb p., SYN Erb *palsy.*

Erb p., SYN Erb *palsy.*

facial p., paresis or p. of the facial muscles, usually unilateral, due to either 1) a lesion involving either the nucleus or the facial nerve peripheral to the nucleus (peripheral facial paralysis) or 2) a supranuclear lesion in the cerebrum or upper brainstem (central facial paralysis); with the latter, facial weakness is usually partial and the upper portion of the face is relatively spared, because of bilateral cortical connections. SYN facial palsy, facioplegia, fallopian neuritis.

familial periodic p., one of the inherited muscle disorders manifested as recurrent episodes of marked generalized weakness. SEE hyperkalemic periodic p., hypokalemic periodic p., normokalemic periodic p.

faucial p., SYN isthmoparalysis.

flaccid p., p. with a loss of muscle tone. Cf. spastic *diplegia.*

generalized p., SYN global p.

ginger p., SYN jake p.

global p., p. of both whole sides of the body. SYN generalized p.

glossolabiolaryngeal p., glossolabiopharyngeal p., SYN progressive bulbar p.

glossopalatolabial p., SYN progressive bulbar *palsy.*

glossopharyngeolabial p., SYN progressive bulbar *palsy.*

Gubler p., SYN Gubler *syndrome.*

hyperkalemic periodic p. [type II MIM*170500], a form of periodic p. in which the serum potassium level is elevated during attacks; onset occurs in infancy, attacks are frequent but relatively mild, and myotonia is often present; autosomal dominant inheritance caused by mutation in the sodium channel gene (SCN4A) on chromosome 17q.

hypokalemic periodic p. [type I MIM*170400], a form of periodic p. in which the serum potassium level is low during attacks; onset usually occurs between the ages of 7–21 years; attacks may be precipitated by exposure to cold, high carbohydrate meal, or alcohol, may last hours to days, and may cause respiratory p.; autosomal dominant caused by mutation in the muscle dihydropyridine (DHP)-sensitive calcium channel α-1-subunit (CACNL1A3) on chromosome 1q, or X-linked inheritance.

hysterical p., a psychosomatic numbness of a limb sometimes to the point of p. SEE hysteria.

immune p., the induction of tolerance due to injection of large amounts of antigen. The antigen is poorly metabolized and the p. remains only during the persistence of the above. SEE immunologic *tolerance.* SYN immunologic p.

immunologic p., SYN immune p.

jake p., polyneuropathy produced by drinking synthetic Jamaican ginger (or "jake" in the vernacular) containing tri-orthocresylphosphate. SYN ginger p.

Klumpke p., SYN Klumpke *palsy.*

Landry p., SYN Guillain-Barré *syndrome.*

lead p., SYN lead *palsy.*

mimetic p., p. of the facial muscles.

mixed p., combined motor and sensory p.

motor p., loss of the power of muscular contraction.

musculospiral p., p. of the muscles of the forearm due to injury of the radial (musculospiral) nerve.

normokalemic periodic p. [type III MIM 170600], a form of periodic p. in which the serum potassium level is within normal limits during attacks; onset usually occurs between the ages of 2–5 years; there is often severe quadriplegia, usually improved by the administration of sodium salts; autosomal dominant inheritance. SYN sodium-responsive periodic p.

obstetric p., SYN obstetric *palsy.*

ocular p., p. of extraocular and intraocular muscles.

periodic p., term for a group of diseases characterized by recurring episodes of muscular weakness or flaccid p. without loss of consciousness, speech, or sensation; attacks begin when the patient is at rest, and there is apparent good health between attacks. SEE hyperkalemic periodic p., hypokalemic periodic p., normokalemic periodic p.

peripheral facial p., SYN Bell *palsy.*

postdiphtheritic p., p. affecting the uvula most frequently, but also any other muscle, due to toxic neuritis; usually appears in the second or third week following the beginning of the attack of diphtheria. SYN diphtheritic p.

posti′cus p., p. of the posterior cricoarytenoid muscles.

Pott p., SYN Pott *paraplegia.*

pressure p., p. due to compression of a nerve, nerve trunk, plexus, or spinal cord. SYN pressure palsy.

progressive bulbar p., progressive weakness and atrophy of the muscles of the tongue, lips, palate, pharynx, and larynx, usually occurring in later life; most often caused by motor neuron disease. SYN bulbar palsy, bulbar p., Erb disease, glossolabiolaryngeal p., glossolabiopharyngeal p.

pseudobulbar p., p. of the lips and tongue, simulating progressive bulbar p., but due to supranuclear lesions with bilateral involvement of the upper motor neurons; characterized by speech and swallowing difficulties, emotional instability, and spasmodic, mirthless laughter.

sensory p., loss of sensation; anesthesia.

sleep p., brief episodic loss of voluntary movement that occurs when falling asleep (hypnagogic sleep p.) or when awakening (hypnopompic sleep p.). One of the narcoleptic tetrad. SYN sleep dissociation.

sodium-responsive periodic p., SYN normokalemic periodic p.

spastic spinal p., SYN spastic *diplegia.*

pa

spinal p., loss of motor power due to a lesion of the spinal cord. SYN myeloparalysis, myeloplegia, rachioplegia.

supranuclear p., p. due to lesions above the primary motor neurons.

tick p., an ascending flaccid p. caused by the continuing presence of gravid *Dermacentor* and *Ixodes* ticks; reported from North America and Australia; affects humans (mainly children) and other animals.

Todd p., p. of temporary duration (normally not more than a few days) that occurs in the limb or limbs involved in jacksonian epilepsy after the seizure. SYN Todd postepileptic p.

Todd postepileptic p., SYN Todd p.

vasomotor p., SYN vasoparesis.

Zenker p., paresthesia and p. in the area of the external popliteal nerve.

pa·ra·lys·sa (par'ă-lis'ă). A paralytic form of rabies caused by the bite of the vampire bat (*Desmodus*). [paralysis + G. *lyssa*, madness (rabies)]

par·a·lyt·ic (par-ă-lit'ik). Relating to paralysis or suffering from paralysis.

par·a·lyze (par'ă-līz). To render incapable of movement.

par·a·mag·net·ic (par'ă-mag-net'ik). Having the property of paramagnetism; in magnetic resonance imaging, contrast media are chosen for their p. property, which shortens relaxation time.

par·a·mag·ne·tism (par-ă-mag'nĕ-tizm). The property of having a strong magnetic moment from one or more unpaired electrons, causing orientation in a magnetic field; most significant in imaging are ions of certain transition metals such as gadolinium, iron, and manganese, or organic compounds that are stable free radicals; molecular oxygen also exhibits p.

par·a·mas·ti·gote (par-ă-mas'ti-gōt). A mastigote having two flagella, one long and one short. SYN paraflagellate (2). [para- + G. *mastix*, whip]

par·a·mas·toid (par-ă-mas'toyd). Near the mastoid process.

Par·a·me·ci·um (par-ă-mē'shē-ŭm, -sē-ŭm). An abundant genus of freshwater holotrichous ciliates, characteristically slipper-shaped and often large enough to be visible to the naked eye; commonly used for genetic and other studies. [G. *paramēkes*, rather long, fr. *mēkos*, length]

par·a·me·di·an (par-ă-mē'dē-an). Near the middle line. SYN paramesial.

par·a·med·ic (par-ă-med'ik). A person trained and certified to provide emergency medical care.

par·a·med·i·cal (par-ă-med'i-kăl). **1.** Related to the medical profession in an adjunctive capacity, e.g., denoting allied health fields such as physical therapy, speech pathology, etc. **2.** Relating to a paramedic.

par·a·me·nia (par-ă-mē'nē-ă). Any disorder or irregularity of menstruation. [para- + G. *mēn*, month]

par·a·me·si·al (par-ă-mē'sē-ăl). SYN paramedian.

par·a·mes·o·neph·ric (par-ă-mes-ō-nef'rik). Close to or alongside the embryonic mesonephros. SEE paramesonephric *duct*.

pa·ram·e·ter (pă-ram'ĕ-ter). One of many dimensions or ways of measuring or describing an object or evaluating a subject: **1.** In a mathematical expression, an arbitrary constant that can possess different values, each value defining other expressions, and can determine the specific form but not the general nature of the expression; e.g., in the equation $y = a + bx$, a and b are p.'s. **2.** In statistics, a term used to define a characteristic of a population, in contrast to a sample from that population; e.g., the mean and standard deviation of a total population. **3.** In psychoanalysis, any tactic, other than interpretation, used by the analyst to further the patient's progress. [para- + G. *metron*, measure]

enzyme p.'s, those factors and constants that govern the rate of an enzyme-catalyzed reaction, e.g., V_{max} and K_m.

infection transmission p., the proportion of total possible contacts between infectious cases and susceptibles that lead to new infections. SEE ALSO serial *interval*, mass action *principle*.

practice p.'s, SYN practice guidelines, under guideline.

par·a·meth·a·di·one (par'ă-meth-ă-dī'ōn). An anticonvulsant used in petit mal epilepsy.

par·a·meth·a·sone (par-ă-meth'ă-sōn). A glucocorticoid with anti-inflammatory effects and toxicity similar to those of prednisone.

p. acetate, acetic ester of p. at C-21; a glucocorticoid useful in the treatment of rheumatoid arthritis and other collagen diseases, allergic conditions, and certain hematologic disorders.

par·a·me·tri·al (par-ă-mē'trē-ăl). Pertaining to the parametrium.

par·a·met·ric (par-ă-met'rik). Relating to the parametrium, or structures immediately adjacent to the uterus.

par·a·me·trit·ic (par'ă-me-trit'ik). Relating to parametritis.

par·a·me·tri·tis (par'ă-me-trī'tis). Inflammation of the tissue adjacent to the uterus, particularly in the broad ligament. SYN pelvic cellulitis. [parametrium + G. *-itis*, inflammation]

par·a·me·tri·um, pl. **par·a·me·tria** (par-ă-mē'trē-ŭm, -ă) [TA]. The connective tissue of the pelvic floor extending from the fibrous subserous coat of the supracervical portion of the uterus laterally between the layers of the broad ligament. [para- + G. *mētra*, uterus]

par·a·mim·ia (par-ă-mim'ē-ă). The use of gestures unsuited to the words that they accompany. [para- + G. *mimia*, imitation]

par·am·ne·sia (par-am-nē'zē-ă). False recollection, as of events that have never occurred or partial forgetting of events that have occurred. [para- + G. *amnēsia*, forgetfulness]

Par·a·moe·ba (par-ă-mē'bă). Former name for *Entamoeba*.

par·a·mo·lar (par-ă-mō'lăr). A supernumerary tooth lying among, lingual, or buccal to the maxillary or mandibular molars.

par·a·mor·phine (par-ă-mōr'fēn). SYN thebaine.

Par·am·phis·to·mat·i·dae (par'am-fis-tō-mat'i-dē). A family of parasitic trematodes characterized by large fleshy bodies with a large posterior sucker; included are the genera *Paramphistomum*, *Gastrodiscoides*, and *Watsonius*.

par·am·phis·to·mi·a·sis (par'am-fis-tō-mī'ă-sis). Infection of animals and humans with trematodes of the family Paramphistomatidae; human disease is caused by *Gastrodiscoides hominis* in Asia and *Watsonius watsoni* in Africa.

Par·am·phis·to·mum (par-am-fis'tō-mŭm). The rumen fluke, a genus of digenetic trematodes (family Paramphistomatidae) parasitic in the rumen or paunch of cattle; species include *P. microbothrioides*, *P. cervi*, and *P. liorchis*. [para- + G. *amphistomos*, having a double mouth, fr. *amphi*, two-sided, + *stoma*, mouth]

par·a·mu·sia (par-ă-moo'zē-ă). Loss of the ability to read or to render music correctly. [para- + G. *mousa*, music, + -ia]

par·am·y·loi·do·sis (par-am'ĭ-loy-dō'sis). **1.** Deposition in tissues of an amyloid-like protein resembling light chains of immunoglobulins in primary amyloidosis or (particularly) in atypical amyloidosis of multiple myeloma. **2.** Various hereditary amyloidoses (Portuguese amyloidosis, Indiana amyloidosis) characterized by progressive hypertrophic polyneuritis with sensory changes, ataxia, paresis, and muscle atrophy due to amyloid deposits in peripheral and visceral nerves.

par·a·my·oc·lo·nus mul·ti·plex (par'ă-mī-ok'lō-nŭs). SYN myoclonus multiplex. [para- + G. *mys*, muscle, + *klonos*, a tumult]

par·a·my·o·to·nia (par'ă-mī-ō-tō'nē-ă). An atypical form of myotonia. SYN paramyotonus.

ataxic p., a disorder characterized by a tonic muscular spasm on attempted movement, associated with slight paresis and ataxia.

congenital p., p. congen'ita [MIM*168300], a nonprogressive myotonia induced by exposure of muscles to cold; there are episodes of intermittent flaccid paralysis, but no atrophy or hypertrophy of muscles; autosomal dominant inheritance caused by mutation in the sodium channel gene (SCN4A) on chromosome 17q. This is a disorder allelic to hyperkalemic periodic *paralysis*. There is a variant autosomal dominant form [MIM*168350] in which cold is not a provoking factor. SYN Eulenburg disease.

par·a·my·ot·o·nus (par-ă-mī-ot'ō-nŭs). SYN paramyotonia.

Par·a·myx·o·vir·i·dae (par-ă-mik'sō-vir'i-dē). A family of RNA-containing viruses about twice the size of the influenza viruses (Orthomyxoviridae) but similar to them in morphology. Virions are 150–300 nm in diameter, enveloped and ether-sensitive and contain RNA-dependent RNA polymerase. Nucleocapsids are helical, considerably larger than those of the influenza viruses, and contain single-stranded unsegmented RNA. Four genera are recognized: Paramyxovirus, Morbillivirus, Rubulavirus, and Pneumovirus, all of which cause cell fusion and produce cytoplasmic eosinophilic inclusions. Diseases associated with these viruses include croup and other upper respiratory infections, measles, mumps, and pneumonia.

Par·a·myx·o·vi·rus (par-ă-mik′sō-vī-rŭs). A genus of viruses (family Paramyxoviridae) that includes parainfluenza viruses (types 1 and 3).

par·an·al·ge·sia (par-an-ăl-jē′zē-ă). Analgesia of the lower half of the body. [para- + analgesia]

par·a·na·sal (par-ă-nā′săl). Alongside the nose.

par·a·ne·o·pla·sia (par′ă-nē-ō-plā′zē-ă). Hormonal, neurologic, hematologic, and other clinical and biochemical disturbances associated with malignant neoplasms but not directly related to invasion by the primary tumor or its metastases.

par·a·ne·o·plas·tic (par′ă-nē-ō-plas′tik). Relating to or characteristic of paraneoplasia.

par·a·neph·ric (par-ă-nef′rik). 1. Relating to the paranephros. 2. SYN pararenal.

par·a·neph·ros, pl. **par·a·neph·roi** (par-ă-nef′ros, -nef′roy). SYN suprarenal *gland*. [para- + G. *nephros*, kidney]

par·an·es·the·sia (par-an-es-thē′zē-ă). Anesthesia of the lower half of the body. [para- + anesthesia]

par·a·neu·rone (par-ă-noor′ōn). A gland or aggregate of cells containing neurosecretory granules. SYN neuroendocrine cell (2).

pa·ran·gi (pă-rang′gē, -ran′jē). A disease similar to yaws, occurring in Sri Lanka.

par·a·noia (par-ă-noy′ă). A severe but relatively rare mental disorder characterized by the presence of systematized delusions, often of a persecutory character involving being followed, poisoned, or harmed by other means, in an otherwise intact personality. SEE ALSO paranoid *personality*. [G. derangement, madness, fr. para- + *noeō*, to think]

acute hallucinatory p., a form in which periods of hallucination occur in addition to the delusions.

litigious p., a form of p. in which one is inclined to initiate lawsuits.

par·a·noi·ac (par-ă-noy′ak). 1. Relating to or affected with paranoia. 2. One who is suffering from paranoia.

par·a·noid (par′ă-noyd). 1. Relating to or characterized by paranoia. 2. Having delusions of persecution.

par·a·no·mia (par-ă-nō′mē-ă). A form of aphasia in which objects are called by the wrong names. [para- + G. *onoma*, name]

par·a·nu·cle·ar (par-ă-noo′klē-ăr). 1. SYN paranucleate. 2. Outside, but near the nucleus.

par·a·nu·cle·ate (par′ă-noo′klē-āt). Relating to or having a paranucleus. SYN paranuclear (1).

par·a·nu·cle·o·lus (par′ă-noo-klē′ō-lŭs). SEE sex *chromatin*.

par·a·nu·cle·us (par-ă-noo′klē-ŭs). An accessory nucleus or small mass of chromatin lying outside, though near, the nucleus.

par·a·om·phal·ic (par′ă-om-fal′ik). SYN paraumbilical. [para- + G. *omphalos*, umbilicus]

par·a·op·er·a·tive (par′ă-op′er-ă-tiv). SYN perioperative.

par·a·o·ral (par-ă-ō′răl). Near or adjacent to the mouth. [para- + L. *os* (*or*-), mouth]

par·a·o·var·i·an (par′ă-ō-var′ē-an). SYN parovarian (2).

par·a·ox·on (par-ă-ok′son). An organophosphorous cholinesterase inhibitor used in insecticides; parathion is converted in the liver to p.

par·a·pan·cre·at·ic (par′ă-pan-krē-at′ik). Near or alongside of the pancreas.

par·a·pa·re·sis (par-ă-pă-rē′sis). Weakness affecting the lower extremities. [para- + paresis]

par·a·pa·ret·ic (par′ă-pă-ret′ik). 1. Relating to paraparesis. 2. A person with paraparesis.

par·a·pe·de·sis (par′ă-pĕ-dē′sis). Excretion or secretion through an abnormal channel. [para- + G. *pēdēsis*, a bending, deflection]

par·a·per·i·to·ne·al (par′ă-per′i-tō-nē′ăl). Outside of or alongside the peritoneum.

par·a·pes·tis (par-ă-pes′tis). SYN ambulant *plague*. [para- + L. *pestis*, plague]

par·a·pha·sia (par-ă-fā′zē-ă). A form of aphasia in which a person has lost the ability to speak correctly, substituting one word for another and jumbling words and sentences unintelligibly. SEE ALSO jargon. SYN paragrammatism, paraphrasia, pseudoagrammatism. [para- + G. *phasis*, speech]

thematic p., incoherent speech that wanders from the theme or subject under discussion.

par·a·pha·sic (par-ă-fā′sik). Relating to paraphasia.

pa·ra·phia (pa-rā′fē-ă). Any disorder of the sense of touch. SYN pseudesthesia (1), pseudoesthesia (1). [para- + G. *haphē*, touch]

par·a·phil·ia (par-ă-fil′ē-ă). 1. A condition, in either men or women, of compulsive responsivity and obligatory dependence on an unusual or personally or socially unacceptable external stimulus or internal fantasy for sexual arousal or orgasm. 2. In legal parlance, a perversion or deviancy. [para- + G. *philos*, fond]

par·a·phi·mo·sis (par′ă-fī-mō′sis). 1. Painful constriction of the glans penis by a phimotic foreskin, which has been retracted behind the corona. 2. SEE p. palpebrae. [para- + G. phimosis]

p. palpe′brae, total spastic eversion of the upper and lower eyelids.

par·a·pho·nia (par-ă-fō′nē-ă). Any disorder of the voice, especially a change in its tone. [para- + G. *phōnē*, voice]

par·a·phra·sia (par-ă-frā′zē-ă). SYN paraphasia. [para- + G. *phrasis*, speech]

par·a·phys·i·al, par·a·phys·e·al (par-ă-fiz′ē-ăl). Pertaining to the paraphysis.

pa·raph·y·sis, pl. **pa·raph·y·ses** (pă-raf′i-sis, -sēz). A median organ developing from the roofplate of the diencephalon in certain lower vertebrates. Present in the human embryo and fetus for a short time. SYN paraphysial body. [G. an offshoot]

par·a·pin·e·al (par-ă-pin′ē-ăl). Beside the pineal; denoting the visual or photoreceptive portion of the pineal body present, if not functioning, in certain lizards.

par·a·plasm (par′ă-plazm). 1. Obsolete term for hyaloplasm. 2. Malformed or abnormal tissue. [para- + G. *plasma*, a thing formed]

par·a·plas·tic (par-ă-plas′tik). Relating to paraplasm.

par·a·ple·gia (par-ă-plē′jē-ă). Paralysis of both lower extremities and, generally, the lower trunk. [para- + *plēgē*, a stroke]

ataxic p., progressive ataxia and paresis of the leg muscles due to sclerosis of the lateral and posterior funiculi of the spinal cord.

congenital spastic p., a spastic paralysis of the lower extremities occurring in the infant. SYN infantile spastic p.

p. doloro′sa, paralysis of the lower extremities in which the affected parts, in spite of loss of motion and sensation, are the seat of excruciating pain; occurs in certain cases of cancer of the spinal cord. SYN painful p.

p. in extension, paralysis of the legs, maintained in an extended position by hypertonic extensor muscles.

p. in flexion, the fixation of the paralyzed legs in a flexed posture; usually in transection of the spinal cord.

infantile spastic p., SYN congenital spastic p.

painful p., SYN p. dolorosa.

Pott p., paralysis of the lower part of the body and the extremities, due to pressure on the spinal cord as the result of tuberculous spondylitis. SYN Pott paralysis.

spastic p., paresis of the lower extremities with increased muscle tone and spasmodic contraction of the muscles. SYN Erb-Charcot disease (2).

superior p., paralysis of both arms.

par·a·ple·gic (par-ă-plē′jik). Relating to or suffering from paraplegia.

Par·a·pox·vi·rus (par-ă-poks′vī-rŭs). The genus of viruses (family Poxviridae) that includes the contagious ecthyma of sheep, bovine papular stomatitis, and paravaccinia viruses. They possess the nucleoprotein antigen common to all viruses included in the family but differ from other poxviruses in morphology (e.g., virions are smaller and have thicker external coats) and by not multiplying in embryonated eggs.

par·a·prax·ia (par-ă-prak′sē-ă). A condition analogous to paraphasia and paragraphia in which there is a defective performance of purposive acts; e.g., slips of the tongue, or mislaying of objects. [para- + G. *praxis,* a doing]

par·a·proc·ti·tis (par′ă-prok-tī′tis). Inflammation of the cellular tissue surrounding the rectum. [para- + G. *prōktos,* anus, + *-itis,* inflammation]

par·a·proc·ti·um, pl. **par·a·proc·tia** (par′ă-prok′shē-um, -tē-ŭm; -ă). The cellular tissue surrounding the rectum. [para- + G. *prōktos,* anus]

par·a·pros·ta·ti·tis (par′ă-pros-tă-tī′tis). Obsolete term for inflammation of the tissue around the prostate gland. [para- + L. *prostata,* prostate, + *-itis,* inflammation]

par·a·pro·tein ((par-a-prō′tēn). **1.** A monoclonal immunoglobulin of blood plasma, observed electrophoretically as an intense band in γ, β, or α regions, due to an isolated increase in a single immunoglobulin type as a result of a clone of plasma cells arising from the abnormal rapid multiplication of a single cell. The finding of a paraprotein in a patient's serum indicates the presence of a proliferating clone of immunoglobulin-producing cells and may be seen in a variety of malignant, benign, or nonneoplastic diseases. **2.** SYN monoclonal *immunoglobulin.* [para + protein, fr. G. *protos,* first]

par·a·pro·tein·e·mia (par′ă-prō-tēn-ē′mē-ă). The presence of a monoclonal gammopathy in the blood.

par·a·pso·ri·a·sis (par′ă-sō-rī′ă-sis). A heterogenous group of skin disorders unrelated to psoriasis, including pityriasis lichenoides and small and large plaque p.

p. en plaque, a form of large plaque parapsoriasis in middle age that frequently develops into mycosis fungoides. Affecting the trunk and proximal extremities, the lesions exceed 5 cm in diameter and are often symmetric. Small plaques p. en plaque is a benign variant, also called digitate dermatosis.

p. gutta′ta, SYN *pityriasis* lichenoides.

p. lichenoi′des, SYN *poikiloderma* atrophicans vasculare.

p. lichenoi′des et variolifor′mis acu′ta, SYN *pityriasis* lichenoides et varioliformis acuta.

small plaque p., SYN digitate *dermatosis.*

p. variolifor′mis, SYN *pityriasis* lichenoides et varioliformis acuta.

par·a·psy·chol·o·gy (par′ă-sī-kol′ō-jē). The study of extrasensory perception, such as thought transference (telepathy) and clairvoyance.

par·a·quat (par′ă-kwaht). A weedkiller that produces delayed toxic effects on the liver, kidneys, and lungs when ingested; progressive interstitial pneumonia with proliferation of alveolar lining cells may develop.

par·a·ra·ma (par-ă-rā′mă). Painful or crippling disease of the fingers, first described in Brazilian rubber workers, produced by accidental contact with setae of the larva of the moth, *Premolis semirufa;* immediate pruritus, hyperemia, and local edema may be followed by chronic swelling and immobility that may lead to loss of one or more fingers, presenting a clinical picture corresponding to ankylosis.

par·a·rec·tal (par-ă-rek′tăl). Near the rectum or rectus muscle.

par·a·re·nal (par-ă-rē′năl). Near or adjacent to the kidneys. SYN paranephric (2).

par·a·rho·ta·cism (par′ă-rō′tă-sizm). Substitution of another sound for that of r. SEE ALSO rhotacism. [para- + G. *rho,* letter r]

par·a·ro·san·i·lin (par′ă-rō-san′i-lin) [C.I. 42500]. A tri-(aminophenyl)methane hydrochloride; an important red biologic stain used in Schiff reagent to detect cellular DNA (Feulgen stain), mucopolysaccharides (PAS stain), and proteins (ninhydrin-Schiff stain). SYN parafuchsin.

par·ar·rhyth·mia (par-ă-ridh′mē-ă). A cardiac dysrhythmia in which two independent rhythms coexist, but not as a result of A-V block; p. thus includes parasystole and A-V dissociation (2), but not complete A-V block. [para- + G. *rhythmos,* rhythm]

par·a·sac·ral (par-ă-sā′krăl). Alongside the sacrum.

par·a·sal·pin·gi·tis (par′ă-sal-pin-jī′tis). Inflammation of the tissues surrounding the fallopian or the eustachian tube. [para- + salpinx + G. *-itis,* inflammation]

Par·as·ca·ris equo·rum (pa-ras′ka-ris ē-kwō′rŭm). A large, heavy-bodied ascarid nematode extremely common in the small intestine of horses and other equids. Larvae may develop in humans or mice, but do not reach the adult stage. SYN *Ascaris equorum.*

par·a·scar·la·ti·na (par′ă-skar-lă-tē′nă). SYN Filatov-Dukes *disease.*

par·a·sex·u·al·i·ty (par′ă-sek-shŭ-al′i-tē). Abnormal or perverted sexuality.

par·a·sig·ma·tism (par-ă-sig′mă-tizm). SYN lisping. [para- + G. *sigma,* the letter s]

par·a·si·noi·dal (par′ă-sī-noy′dăl). Near a sinus, particularly a cerebral sinus.

par·a·site (par′ă-sīt). **1.** An organism that lives on or in another and draws its nourishment therefrom. **2.** In the case of a fetal inclusion or conjoined twins, the usually incomplete twin that derives its support from the more nearly normal autosite. [G. *parasitos,* a guest, fr. *para,* beside, + *sitos,* food]

accidental p., SYN incidental p.

autistic p., a p. descended from the tissues of the host. SYN autochthonous p.

autochthonous p., SYN autistic p.

commensal p., SEE commensal (2).

euroxenous p., a p. with a broad or nonspecific host range.

facultative p., an organism that may either lead an independent existence or live as a p., in contrast to obligate p.

heterogenetic p., a p. whose life cycle involves an alternation of generations.

heteroxenous p., a p. that has more than one obligatory host in its life cycle.

incidental p., a p. that normally lives on a host other than its normal host. SYN accidental p.

inquiline p., SEE inquiline.

malignant tertian malarial p., SYN *Plasmodium falciparum.*

obligate p., a p. that cannot lead an independent nonparasitic existence, in contrast to facultative p.

quartan p., SYN *Plasmodium malariae.*

specific p., a p. that habitually lives in its present host and is particularly adapted for the host species.

spurious p., organisms that parasitize other hosts that pass through the human intestine and are detected in the stool after ingestion (e.g., *Capillaria* sp. eggs in animal liver).

stenoxous p., a p. with a narrow or specific host range.

temporary p., an organism accidentally ingested that survives briefly in the intestine.

tertian p., SYN *Plasmodium vivax.*

par·a·si·te·mia (păr′ă-sī-tē′mē-ă). The presence of parasites in the circulating blood; used especially with reference to malarial and other protozoan forms, and microfilariae.

par·a·sit·ic (par-ă-sit′ik). **1.** Relating to or of the nature of a parasite. **2.** Denoting organisms that normally grow only in or on the living body of a host.

par·a·sit·i·ci·dal (par′ă-sit-i-sī′dăl). Destructive to parasites.

par·a·sit·i·cide (par-ă-sit′i-sīd). An agent that destroys parasites. [parasite + L. *caedo,* to kill]

par·a·sit·ism (par′ă-si-tizm). A symbiotic relationship in which one species (the parasite) benefits at the expense of the other (the host). Cf. mutualism, commensalism, symbiosis, metabiosis.

multiple p., a condition in which parasites of different species parasitize a single host, in contrast to superparasitism (2) or hyperparasitism.

par·a·si·tize (par′ă-si-tīz). To invade as a parasite.

par·a·si·to·ce·nose (par-ă-sī′tō-sē-nōz). Complex of all parasite species and individuals associated with a specific host. SYN parasite-host ecosystem. [parasite + G. *koinos,* common, together]

par·a·si·to·gen·e·sis (par′ă-sī-tō-jen′ĕ-sis). The evolution of relationships between parasite and host.

par·a·si·to·gen·ic (par′-ă-sī-tō-jen′ik). **1.** Caused by certain parasites. **2.** Favoring parasitism. [parasite + G. -gen, producing]

par·a·si·toid (par-ă-sī′toyd). Denoting a feeding relationship intermediate between predation and parasitism, in which the p. eventually destroys its host; refers especially to parasitic wasps (order Hymenoptera) whose larvae feed on and finally destroy a grub or other arthropod host stung by the mother wasp prior to laying its egg(s) on the host. [parasite + G. eidos, appearance]

par·a·si·tol·o·gist (par′ă-sī-tol′ŏ-jist). One who specializes in the science of parasitology.

par·a·si·tol·o·gy (par′ă-sī-tol′ō-jē). The branch of biology and of medicine concerned with all aspects of parasitism. [parasite + G. logos, study]

par·a·si·tome (par′ă-sī-tōm). The total mass or number of individuals of all developmental stages of a single parasite species in one host. [parasite + -ome (fr. G. -ōma), group, mass]

par·a·si·to·pho·bia (par′ă-sī-tō-fō′bē-ă). Morbid fear of parasites. [parasite + G. phobos, fear]

par·a·sit·o·sis (par′ă-sī-tō′sis). Infestation or infection with parasites.

par·a·si·to·tro·pic (par′ă-sī-tō-trop′ik). Pertaining to or characterized by parasitotropism.

par·a·si·tot·ro·pism (par′ă-sī-tot′rō-pizm). The special affinity of particular drugs or other agents for parasites rather than for their hosts, including microparasites that infect a larger parasite. Cf. organotropism. SYN parasitotropy. [parasite + G. tropē, a turning]

par·a·si·tot·ro·py (par′ă-sī-tot′rō-pē). SYN parasitotropism.

par·a·som·nia (par-ă-som′nē-ă). Any dysfunction associated with sleep, e.g., somnabulism, pavor nocturnus, enureseis, or nocturnal seizures.

par·a·sta·sis (par-ă-stā′sis). A reciprocal relationship among causal mechanisms that can compensate for, or mask defects in, each other; in genetics, a relationship between nonalleles (classified by some as a form of epistasis). [G. standing shoulder to shoulder]

par·a·ster·nal (par-ă-ster′năl). Alongside the sternum.

Par·a·stron·gy·lus (par′a-stron′ji-lus). SYN *Angiostrongylus.*

parasubiculum. A narrow region of cortex located between the entorhinal area (or cortex) and the subiculum.

par·a·sym·pa·thet·ic (par-ă-sim-pa-thet′ik). Pertaining to a division of the autonomic nervous system. SEE autonomic *division* of nervous system.

par·a·sym·pa·tho·lyt·ic (par-ă-sim′pă-thō-lit′ik). Relating to an agent that annuls or antagonizes the effects of the parasympathetic nervous system; e.g., atropine.

par·a·sym·pa·tho·mi·met·ic (par-ă-sim′pă-thō-mi-met′ik). Relating to drugs or chemicals having an action resembling that caused by stimulation of the parasympathetic nervous system. SEE ALSO cholinomimetic. [para- + G. sympatheia, sympathy, + mimētikos, imitative]

par·a·sym·pa·tho·to·nia (par-ă-sim′pă-thō-tō′nē-ă). SYN vagotonia.

par·a·sy·nap·sis (par′ă-si-nap′sis). Union of chromosomes side to side in the process of reduction. [para- + G. synapsis, a connection, junction]

par·a·sy·no·vi·tis (par′ă-si-nō-vī′tis). Inflammation of the tissues immediately adjacent to a joint. [para- + synovitis]

par·a·syph·i·lis (par-ă-sif′i-lis). Any condition indirectly due to syphilis. SYN metasyphilis (2), parasyphilosis, quaternary syphilis.

par·a·syph·i·lit·ic (par′ă-sif-i-lit′ik). Denoting certain diseases supposed to be indirectly due to syphilis but presenting none of the recognized lesions of that infection. SYN metaluetic (3). SYN metasyphilitic (3).

par·a·syph·i·lo·sis (par′ă-sif-i-lō′sis). SYN parasyphilis.

par·a·sys·to·le (par-ă-sis′tō-lē). A second automatic rhythm existing simultaneously with normal sinus or other dominant rhythm, the parasystolic center being protected from the dominant rhythm's impulses so that its basic rhythm is undisturbed, although it may be manifest in the ECG only at various multiples of its basic periodicity. SYN parasystolic beat. [para- + G. systolē, a contracting]

par·a·tax·ia (par-ă-tak′sē-ă). SYN parataxis.

par·a·tax·ic (par-ă-tak′sik). Pertaining to parataxis.

par·a·tax·is (par-ă-tak′sis). An older term for the psychologic state or repository of attitudes, ideas, and experiences accumulated during personality development that are not effectively assimilated or integrated into the growing mass and residue of the other attitudes, ideas, and experiences of an individual's personality. SYN parataxia. [para- + G. taxis, orderly arrangement]

par·a·te·ne·sis (par-ă-te-nē′sis). Passage of an infective agent by one or a series of paratenic hosts in which the agent is transported between hosts but does not undergo further development. [parasite + L. teneo, to hold, maintain]

par·a·ten·on (par-ă-ten′on). The tissue, fatty or synovial, between a tendon and its sheath. [para- + G. tenōn, tendon]

par·a·ter·mi·nal (par-ă-ter′mi-năl). Near or alongside any terminus.

par·a·thi·on (par-ă-thī′on). An organic phosphate insecticide, highly toxic to animals and humans, that is an irreversible inhibitor of cholinesterases.

par·a·thor·mone (par-ă-thōr′mōn). SYN parathyroid *hormone.*

par·a·thy·mia (par-ă-thī′mē-ă). Misdirection of the emotional faculties; disordered mood. [para- + G. thymos, soul, mind]

par·a·thy·rin (par-ă-thī′rin). SYN parathyroid *hormone.*

par·a·thy·roid (par-ă-thī′royd). **1.** Adjacent to the thyroid gland. **2.** SYN parathyroid *gland.*

par·a·thy·roid·ec·to·my (pa′ră-thī-roy-dek′to-mē). Excision of the parathyroid glands. [parathyroid + G. ektomē, excision]

par·a·thy·ro·tro·pic, par·a·thy·ro·tro·phic (par′ă-thī-rō-trop′ik, -trof′ik). Influencing the growth or activity of the parathyroid glands. [parathyroid + G. tropē, a turning; trophē, nourishment]

par·a·tope (par′a-tōp). That part of an antibody molecule composed of the variable regions of both the light and heavy chains that combine with the antigen. SYN antibody-combining site, antigen-binding site. [para- + -tope]

par·a·tri·cho·sis (par′ă-tri-kō′sis). Any disorder in the growth of the hair, with particular reference to quantity. [para- + G. trichōsis, making or being hairy, fr. thrix (trich-), hair]

par·a·trip·sis (par-ă-trip′sis). Chafing. [G. friction, fr. para, beside, + tripsis, rubbing]

par·a·tro·phic (par-ă-trof′ik). Deriving sustenance from living organic material. SEE ALSO metatrophic, prototrophic. [para- + G. trophē, nourishment]

par·a·typh·li·tis (par′ă-tif-lī′tis). Inflammation of the connective tissue adjacent to the cecum. [para- + G. typhlon, cecum, + -itis, inflammation]

par·a·ty·phoid (par-ă-tī′foyd). SYN paratyphoid *fever.*

par·a·um·bil·i·cal (par′ă-ŭm-bil′i-kal). Near the umbilicus. SYN paraomphalic, parumbilical.

par·a·u·re·thral (par′ă-ū-rē′thrăl). Alongside the urethra.

par·a·vac·cin·ia (par′ă-vak-sin′ē-ă). Former name for Pseudo-cowpox virus. SYN milkers' *nodules,* under *nodule.*

par·a·vag·i·nal (par-ă-vaj′i-năl). Alongside the vagina.

par·a·vag·i·ni·tis (par′ă-vaj-i-nī′tis). Inflammation of the connective tissue alongside the vagina. SYN paracolpitis.

par·a·val·vu·lar (par-ă-val′vū-lăr). Alongside or in the vicinity of a valve.

par·a·ve·nous (par′ă-vē′nŭs). Beside a vein.

par·a·ver·te·bral (par-ă-ver′tĕ-brăl). Alongside a vertebra or the vertebral column.

par·a·ves·i·cal (par-ă-ves′i-kăl). SYN paracystic.

par·ax·i·al (par-ak′sē-ăl). By the side of the axis of any body or part.

par·ax·on (par-ak′son). A collateral branch of an axon. [para- + G. axōn, axis]

Par·a·zoa (par-ă-zō′ă). A subkingdom that includes the sponges (phylum Porifera), considered by many zoologists to be intermediate between the subkingdoms Protozoa and Metazoa.

par·a·zo·on (par-ă-zō'on). **1.** An animal parasite. **2.** A member of the subkingdom Parazoa. [para- + G. *zōon,* animal]

parch·ment crack·ling (parch'ment krak'ling). The sensation as of the crackling of stiff paper or parchment, noted on palpation of the skull in cases of craniotabes.

Paré, Ambroïse, French surgeon, 1510–1590. SEE P. *suture.*

par·e·gor·ic (par-ĕ-gōr'ik). Camphorated opium tincture, an antiperistaltic agent containing powdered opium, anise oil, benzoic acid, camphor, glycerin, and diluted alcohol. [G. *parēgorikos,* soothing]

pa·rei·ra (pă-rā'-ră). Pareira brava, the root of *Chondodendron tomentosum* and other species of *Chondodendron* (family Menispermaceae), a vine of tropical America; one of the chief sources of D-tubocurarine; it has diuretic and urinary antiseptic properties. [Pg. *parreira,* vine trained against a wall]

par·e·lec·tro·nom·ic (par'ĕ-lek-trō-nom'ik). Not subject to the laws of electricity, i.e., not excited by an electric stimulus. [para- + G. *ēlektron,* amber (electricity), + *nomos,* law]

par·en·ce·pha·lia (par'en-se-fā'lē-ă). Congenital defect of brain. [para- + G. *enkephalos,* brain]

par·en·ceph·a·li·tis (par'en-sef-ă-lī'tis). Inflammation of the cerebellum. [parencephalon + G. *-itis,* inflammation]

par·en·ceph·a·lo·cele (par-en-sef'ă-lō-sēl). Protrusion of the cerebellum through a defect in the cranium. [parencephalon + G. *kēlē,* hernia]

par·en·ceph·a·lous (par-en-sef'ă-lŭs). Relating to parencephalia.

pa·ren·chy·ma (pă-reng'ki-mă) [TA]. **1.** The distinguishing or specific cells of a gland or organ, contained in and supported by the connective tissue framework, or stroma. **2.** The endoplasm of a protozoan cell. [G. anything poured in beside, fr. *parencheō,* to pour in beside]

p. glandulae thyroideae [TA], SYN p. of thyroid gland.

p. prostatae [TA], SYN p. of prostate.

p. of prostate [TA], the basis cellular tissue (substance) composing the prostate. SYN p. prostatae [TA].

p. tes'tis [TA], SYN p. of testis.

p. of testis [TA], the basic cellular tissue substance composing the testis, consisting of the seminiferous tubules and interstitial cells (Leydig and Sertoli cells) located within the lobules. SYN p. testis [TA].

p. of thyroid gland [TA], the basic cellular tissue (substance) composing the thyroid gland, organized as follicles. SYN p. glandulae thyroideae [TA].

pa·ren·chy·mal (pă-reng'ki-măl). SYN parenchymatous.

pa·ren·chy·ma·ti·tis (pă-reng'ki-mă-tī'tis). Inflammation of the parenchyma or differentiated substance of a gland or organ.

par·en·chym·a·tous (par'eng-kim'ă-tŭs). Relating to the parenchyma. SYN parenchymal.

par·ent (par'ent). **1.** An individual who has produced at least one offspring through sexual reproduction. **2.** Any source or basis, as for the elaboration of a substance. [L. *parens,* fr. *pario,* to bring forth]

par·en·ter·al (pă-ren'ter-ăl). By some other means than through the gastrointestinal tract; referring particularly to the introduction of substances into an organism by intravenous, subcutaneous, intramuscular, or intramedullary injection. [para- + G. *enteron,* intestine]

Parenti, Gian Carlo, Italian physician. SEE Parenti-Fraccaro *syndrome.*

par·ep·i·cele (par-ep'i-sēl). The lateral recess of the fourth ventricle of the brain. [para- + G. *epi,* upon, + *koilia,* a hollow]

par·ep·i·did·y·mis (par'ep'i-did'i-mis). SYN paradidymis.

par·ep·i·thy·mia (par'ep-i-thī'mē-ă). An older term for a morbid longing; an abnormal desire or craving. [para- + G. *epithymia,* desire]

par·e·re·thi·sis (par-ĕ-rēth'i-sis). An older term for abnormal or morbid excitement. [para- + G. *erethizō,* to excite]

pa·re·sis (pă-rē'sis, par'ĕ-sis). Partial or incomplete paralysis. [G. a letting go, slackening, paralysis, fr. *paritēmi,* to let go]

divergence p., an esodeviation of the eyes that is greater in the distance than near, which may be a sign of central nervous system disease or a mild bilateral 6th nerve palsy.

general p., SYN paretic *neurosyphilis.*

par·es·the·sia (par-es-thē'zē-ă). An abnormal sensation, such as of burning, pricking, tickling, or tingling. SYN paraesthesia. [para- + G. *aisthēsis,* sensation]

par·es·thet·ic (par-es-thet'ik). Relating to or marked by paresthesia; denoting numbness and tingling in an extremity that usually occurs on the resumption of the blood flow to a nerve following temporary pressure or mild injury.

pa·ret·ic (pa-ret'ik). Relating to or suffering from paresis.

pa·reu·nia (par-ū'nē-ă). SYN coitus. [G. *pareunos,* lying beside, fr. *para,* beside, + *eunē,* a bed]

par·gy·line hy·dro·chlo·ride (par'ji-lēn). A nonhydrazine monoamine oxidase inhibitor, used as an antihypertensive agent.

par·i·dro·sis (par-i-drō'sis). Any derangement of perspiration. SYN parahidrosis. [para- + G. *hidrōsis,* sweating]

par·i·es, gen. **pa·ri·e·tis,** pl. **pa·ri·e·tes** (par'i-ēz, pā'rī-ēz; pă-rī'ĕ-tēz) [TA]. SYN wall. [L. wall]

p. ante'rior gas'tris [TA], SYN anterior *wall* of stomach.

p. ante'rior vagi'nae [TA], SYN anterior *wall* of vagina.

p. carot'icus ca'vi tym'pani [TA], SYN carotid *wall* of tympanic cavity.

p. exter'nus duc'tus cochlea'ris [TA], SYN external *surface* of cochlear duct.

p. infe'rior or'bitae [TA], SYN *floor* of orbit.

p. jugula'ris ca'vi tym'pani [TA], SYN jugular *wall* of middle ear.

p. labyrin'thicus ca'vi tym'pani [TA], SYN labyrinthine *wall* of tympanic cavity.

p. latera'lis or'bitae [TA], SYN lateral *wall* of orbit.

p. mastoi'deus ca'vi tym'pani [TA], SYN mastoid *wall* of tympanic cavity.

p. media'lis or'bitae [TA], SYN medial *wall* of orbit.

p. membrana'ceus ca'vi tym'pani [TA], SYN membranous *wall* of tympanic cavity.

p. membrana'ceus tra'cheae [TA], SYN membranous *wall* of trachea.

p. poste'rior gas'tris [TA], SYN posterior *wall* of stomach.

p. poste'rior vagi'nae [TA], SYN posterior *wall* of vagina.

p. supe'rior or'bitae [TA], SYN *roof* of orbit.

p. tegmenta'lis ca'vi tym'pani [TA], SYN tegmental *wall* of tympanic cavity.

p. tympan'icus duc'tus cochlea'ris [TA], SYN tympanic *surface* of cochlear duct.

p. vestibula'ris duc'tus cochlea'ris [TA], SYN vestibular *surface* of cochlear duct.

pa·ri·e·tal (pă-rī'ĕ-tăl). **1.** Relating to the wall of any cavity. **2.** SYN somatic (1). **3.** SYN somatic (2). **4.** Relating to the parietal bone.

pa·ri·e·tes (pă-rī'ĕ-tēz). Plural of paries. [L.]

△**parieto-.** A wall (of the body, e.g., the abdominal wall); a parietal bone. [L. *paries,* wall]

pa·ri·e·to·fron·tal (pa-rī'ĕ-tō-fron'tăl). Relating to the parietal and the frontal bones or the parts of the cerebral cortex corresponding thereto.

pa·ri·e·tog·ra·phy (pa-rī'ĕ-tog'ră-fē). Rarely used term for a radiographic examination of the wall of the stomach using a combination of pneumoperitoneum and intraluminal air and barium. [parieto- + G. *graphē,* a writing]

pa·ri·e·to·mas·toid (pă-rī'ĕ-to-mas'toyd). Relating to the parietal bone and the mastoid portion of the temporal bone.

pa·ri·e·to·oc·cip·i·tal (pă-rī'ĕ-tō-ok-sip'i-tăl). Relating to the parietal and occipital bones or to the parts of the cerebral cortex corresponding thereto.

pa·ri·e·to·sphe·noid (pă-rī'ĕ-tō-sfē'noyd). Relating to the parietal and the sphenoid bones.

pa·ri·e·to·splanch·nic (pă-rī'ĕ-tō-splangk'nik).   SYN parietovisceral.

pa·ri·e·to·squa·mo·sal (pă-rī'ĕ-tō-skwā-mō'săl).   Relating to the parietal bone and the squamous portion of the temporal bone.

pa·ri·e·to·tem·po·ral (pă-rī'ĕ-tō-tem'pŏ-răl).   Relating to the parietal and the temporal bones.

pa·ri·e·to·vis·cer·al (pă-rī'ĕ-tō-vis'er-ăl).   Relating to the wall of a cavity and to the contained viscera.   SYN parietosplanchnic.

Parinaud, Henri, French ophthalmologist, 1844–1905.   SEE P. *conjunctivitis*, *ophthalmoplegia*, *syndrome*, oculoglandular *syndrome*.

Par·is green. Cupric acetoarsenite, used as an insecticide and as a pigment.

Par·is yel·low [C.I. 77600].   SYN chrome yellow.

par·i·ty (par'ĭ-tē).   The condition of having given birth to an infant or infants, alive or dead; a multiple birth is considered as a single parous experience. [L. *pario*, to bear]

Park, William H., U.S. bacteriologist, 1863–1939.   SEE P.-Williams *fixative*.

Park, Henry, British surgeon, 1745–1831.   SEE P. *aneurysm*.

Parker, Edward Mason, U.S. surgeon, 1860–1941.   SEE P.-Kerr *suture*.

Parkinson, Sir John, British cardiologist, 1885–1976.   SEE Wolff-P.-White *syndrome*.

Parkinson, James, British physician, 1755–1824.   SEE parkinsonism (1); P. *disease*, *facies*.

par·kin·so·ni·an (par-kin-sō'nē-an).   Relating to or the suffering from parkinsonism (1).

par·kin·son·ism (par'kin-son-izm).   **1.** A neurologic syndrome usually resulting from deficiency of the neurotransmitter dopamine as the consequence of degenerative, vascular, or inflammatory changes in the basal ganglia; characterized by rhythmic muscular tremors, rigidity of movement, festination, droopy posture, and masklike facies.   SYN Parkinson disease, shaking palsy, trembling palsy.   **2.** A syndrome similar to p. appearing as a side effect of certain antipsychotic drugs. [J. *Parkinson*]

Parnas, Jakob Karol, Polish physiologic chemist, 1884–1955.   SEE Embden-Meyerhof-P. *pathway*.

par·oc·cip·i·tal (par'ok-sip'i-tăl).   Near or beside the occipital bone or the occiput. [para- + occipital]

par·o·don·ti·tis (par'ō-don-tī'tis).   Obsolete term for periodontitis.

pa·ro·don·ti·um (par-ō-don'shē-ŭm).   SYN periodontium. [para- + G. *odous*, tooth]

par·o·dyn·ia (par-ō-din'ē-ă).   SYN labor *pains*, under *pain*. [L. *pario*, to bear, + G. *odynē*, pain]

pa·role (pă-rōl').   In psychiatry, term for conditional release of a formally committed patient from a mental hospital prior to formal discharge, so that the patient may be returned to the hospital if necessary without fresh legal action. [Fr., fr. L. *parabola*, discourse, fr G. *parabolē*]

par·ol·fac·to·ry (par-ol-fak'tōr-ē).   Associated with or related to the olfactory system.

par·ol·i·vary (par-ol'i-văr-ē).   By the side of or near the oliva. [para- + L. *oliva*, olive]

par·o·mo·my·cin sul·fate (par'ō-mō-mī'sin).   A broad-spectrum antibiotic produced by *Streptomyces rimosus* forma *paromomycinus;* used in the treatment of bacterial enteritis and amebiasis, and for preoperative suppression of intestinal bacteria.

par·om·pha·lo·cele (par-om'fă-lō-sēl).   **1.** A tumor near the umbilicus.   **2.** A hernia through a defect in the abdominal wall near the umbilicus. [para- + G. *omphalos*, umbilicus, + *kēlē*, tumor, hernia]

Parona, Francesco, 19th century Italian surgeon.   SEE P. *space*.

▣ **par·o·nych·ia** (par-ō-nik'ē-ă).   Suppurative inflammation of the nail fold surrounding the nail plate; may be due to bacteria or fungi, most commonly staphylococci and streptococci. [para- + G. *onyx*, nail]

par·o·oph·o·ri·tis (par'ō-of'ō-rī'tis).   Inflammation of tissues adjacent to the ovaries. [paroophoron + G. *-itis*, inflammation]

par·o·öph·o·ron (par-ō-of'ōr-on) [TA].   Remnants of the tubules

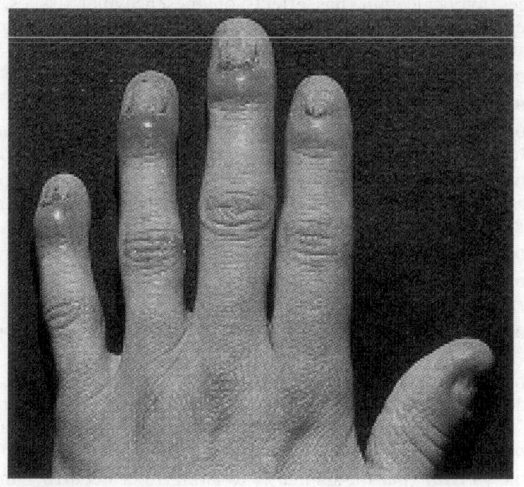

paronychia: chronic form

and glomeruli of the lower part of the mesonephros appearing as a few scattered tubules in the broad ligament between the epoöphoron and the uterus. Its equivalent in the male is the paradidymis.   SYN parovarium. [para- + oophoron, ovary]

par·or·chid·i·um (par-ōr-kid'ē-ŭm).   SYN testis *ectopia*. [para- + G. *orchis*, testis]

par·or·chis (par-ōr'kis).   SYN epididymis. [para- + G. *orchis*, testis]

par·o·rex·ia (par-ō-rek'sē-ă).   An abnormal or disordered appetite. [para- + G. *orexis*, appetite]

par·os·mia (par-oz'mē-ă).   SYN dysosmia. [para + G. *osmē*, sense of smell]

par·os·phre·sia (par-os-frē'zē-ă).   SYN dysosmia. [para- + G. *osphrēsis*, smell]

par·os·te·al (par-os'tē-ăl).   Relating to the tissues immediately adjacent to the periosteum of a bone.

par·os·te·i·tis (păr-os-tē-ī'tis).   Inflammation of the tissues immediately adjacent to a bone.   SYN parostitis. [para- + G. *osteon*, bone, + *-itis*, inflammation]

par·os·te·o·sis, par·os·to·sis (par'os-tē-ō'sis, -os-tō'sis).   **1.** Development of bone in an unusual location, as in the skin.   **2.** Abnormal or defective ossification. [para- + G. *osteon*, bone, + *-osis*, condition]

par·os·ti·tis (par-os-tī'tis).   SYN parosteitis.

pa·rot·ic (pă-rot'ik).   Near or beside the ear. [para- + G. *ous*, ear]

pa·rot·id (pă-rot'id).   Situated near the ear; denoting several structures in this neighborhood. Usually refers to the p. salivary gland. [G. *parōtis* (*parōtid-*), the gland beside the ear, fr. *para*, beside, + *ous* (*ōt-*), ear]

pa·rot·i·dec·to·my (pă-rot'i-dek'tō-mē).   Surgical removal of the parotid gland. [parotid + G. *ektomē*, excision]

pa·rot·i·di·tis (pă-rot-i-dī'tis).   Inflammation of the parotid gland.   SYN parotitis.

epidemic p., SYN mumps.

postoperative p., an acute inflammation of the parotid gland occurring in the postoperative period, especially in debilitated or dehydrated patients; frequently results in abscess formation and rapidly spreading cellulitis that may become fatal.

punctate p., recurrent or chronic p. with terminal sialectasis, giving a punctate pattern on sialography; associated with epithelial hyperplasia of intralobular ducts, atrophy of acini, and lymphocytic infiltration, characteristic in Sjögren *disease*.

pa·ro·ti·do·au·ri·cu·la·ris (pă-rot'i-dō-aw-rik-ū-lā'ris).   **1.** An occasional band of muscle fibers passing from the surface of the parotid gland to the auricle.   **2.** Relating to the parotid gland and the external ear.

par·o·tin (par'ō-tin).   A globulin obtained from parotid glands that causes hypocalcemia, has effects on mesenchymal tissues, produces first leukopenia and then leukocytosis, and promotes calcification of dentin. SYN salivary gland hormone.

par·o·ti·tis (par-o-tī'tis). SYN parotiditis.

par·ous (par'ŭs). Pertaining to parity. [L. *pario,* to bear]

par·o·var·i·an (par-ō-var'ē-an). **1.** Relating to the paroöphoron. **2.** Beside or in the neighborhood of the ovary. SYN paraovarian.

par·o·var·i·ot·o·my (par'ō-var-ē-ot'ō-mē). Incision into or removal of a tumor of the parovarium. [parovarium + G. *tomē,* incision]

par·o·va·ri·tis (par'ō-var-ī'tis). Inflammation of the parovarium.

par·o·var·i·um (par-ō-var'ē-ŭm). SYN paroöphoron. [para- + L. *ovarium,* ovary]

par·ox·y·pro·pi·one (par-ok-si-prō'pē-ōn). An inhibitor of pituitary gonadotropic hormone.

par·ox·ysm (par'ok-sizm). **1.** A sharp spasm or convulsion. **2.** A sudden onset of a symptom or disease, especially one with recurrent manifestations such as the chills and rigor of malaria. [G. *paroxysmos,* fr. *paroxynō,* to sharpen, irritate, fr. *oxys,* sharp]

par·ox·ys·mal (par-ok-siz'măl). Relating to or occurring in paroxysms.

par·ri·cide (par'i-sīd). **1.** The killing of one's parent (patricide or matricide). **2.** One who commits such an act. [L. *parricidium,* killing of close kin]

Parrot, Jules, French physician, 1829–1883. SEE P. *disease.*

Parry, Caleb H., English physician, 1755–1822. SEE P. *disease.*

PARS

pars, pl. **par·tes** (pars, par'tēz) [TA]. SYN part. [L. *pars* (*part-*) a part]

p. abdomina'lis aor'tae [TA], SYN abdominal *aorta.*

p. abdomina'lis duc'tus thora'cici [TA], SYN abdominal *part* of thoracic duct.

p. abdomina'lis esoph'agi [TA], SYN abdominal *part* of esophagus.

p. abdominalis musculi pectorales majoris [TA], SYN abdominal *part* of pectoralis major (muscle).

p. abdominalis plexus visceralis et ganglii visceralis [TA], SYN abdominal *part* of peripheral autonomic plexuses and ganglia.

p. abdomina'lis ure'teris [TA], SYN abdominal *part* of ureter.

p. acromialis musculi deltoidei [TA], SYN acromial *part* of deltoid (muscle).

p. ala'ris mus'culi nasa'lis [TA], SYN alar *part* of nasalis muscle; SEE nasalis (*muscle*).

p. alveola'ris mandib'ulae [TA], SYN alveolar *part* of mandible.

p. amor'pha, the part of the nucleolus that occupies irregular spaces in the nucleolonema and contains finely filamentous substance. SEE ALSO p. granulosa.

p. ante'rior [TA], SYN anterior *part.*

p. ante'rior commissu'rae anterio'ris [TA], SYN anterior *part* of anterior commissure of brain.

p. ante'rior commissu'rae rostra'lis, SYN anterior *part* of anterior commissure of brain.

p. ante'rior facie'i diaphrag'matis hepa'tis [TA], SYN anterior *part* of diaphragmatic surface of liver.

p. ante'rior for'nicis vagi'nae [TA], SYN anterior *part* of fornix of vagina.

p. anterior linguae [TA], SYN anterior *part* of tongue.

p. anula'ris vagi'nae fibro'sae digitorum manus et pedis [TA], SYN anular *part* of fibrous digital sheath of digits of hand and foot.

p. aryepiglottica musculi arytenoidei obliqui [TA], SYN aryepiglottic *part* of oblique arytenoid muscle.

p. ascen'dens aor'tae [TA], SYN ascending *aorta.*

p. ascen'dens duode'ni [TA], SYN ascending *part* of duodenum.

p. ascendens musculi trapezii [TA], SYN ascending *part* of trapezius (muscle).

p. atlantica arteriae vertebralis [TA], SYN atlantic *part* of vertebral artery.

p. autonom'ica systematis nervosi peripherici [TA], SYN autonomic *division* of nervous system.

p. basalis [TA], SYN basal *part.*

p. basalis arteriarum lobarium inferiorum pulmonis sinistri et dextri [TA], SYN basal *part* of left and right inferior pulmonary arteries.

p. basa'lis arte'riae pulmona'lis, SEE right pulmonary *artery,* left pulmonary *artery.*

p. basilaris [TA], SYN basal *part.*

p. basilaris pontis [TA], SYN basilar *part* of pons.

p. basila'ris os'sis occipita'lis [TA], SYN basilar *part* of occipital bone.

p. buccopharyn'gea mu'sculi constricto'ris phary'ngei superio'ris, SYN buccopharyngeal *part* of superior pharyngeal constrictor; SEE superior pharyngeal constrictor (*muscle*).

p. canalis ner'vi op'tici [TA], SYN *part* of optic nerve in canal.

p. cardi'aca gas'tricae [TA], SYN cardia.

p. cardi'aca ventric'uli, SYN cardia.

p. cartilagin'ea sep'ti na'si, SYN septal nasal *cartilage.*

p. cartilaginea systema'tis skeleta'lis [TA], SYN cartilaginous *part* of skeletal system.

p. cartilagin'ea tu'bae auditi'vae [TA], SYN cartilaginous *part* of pharyngotympanic (auditory) tube.

p. cartilaginea tubae auditoriae, SYN cartilaginous *part* of pharyngotympanic (auditory) tube.

p. caverno'sa, SYN spongy *urethra.*

p. caverno'sa arte'riae caro'tidis inter'nae [TA], SYN cavernous *part* of internal carotid artery.

p. ce'ca ret'inae, the embryologic anterior part of the retina that evolves into the p. ciliaris retinae and p. iridica retinae.

p. centra'lis systematis nervosi [TA], SYN central nervous *system.*

p. centra'lis ventric'uli latera'lis [TA], the body of the lateral ventricle of the brain, extending from the interventricular foramen (of Monro) to the collateral trigone (i.e., junction of posterior and inferior horns). SYN body of lateral ventricle, cella media, central part of lateral ventricle.

p. ceratopharyn'gea mu'sculi constricto'ris phary'ngis me'dii [TA], SYN ceratopharyngeal *part* of middle constrictor muscle of pharynx; SEE middle constrictor (*muscle*) of pharynx.

p. cerebra'lis arte'riae caro'tidis inter'nae [TA], SYN cerebral *part* of internal carotid artery.

p. cervica'lis arte'riae caro'tidis inter'nae [TA], SYN cervical *part* of internal carotid artery.

p. cervicalis arteriae vertebralis [TA], SYN cervical *part* of vertebral artery.

p. cervica'lis duc'tus thora'cici [TA], SYN cervical *part* of thoracic duct.

p. cervica'lis esoph'agi [TA], SYN cervical *part* of esophagus.

p. cervica'lis medul'lae spina'lis [TA], SYN cervical *part* of spinal cord.

p. chondropharyn'gea muscu'li constricto'ris pharyn'gei medi'i [TA], SYN chondropharyngeal *part* of middle constrictor muscle of pharynx; SEE middle constrictor (*muscle*) of pharynx.

p. cilia'ris ret'inae [TA], SYN ciliary *part* of retina; SEE retina.

p. clavicularis musculi deltoidei [TA], SYN clavicular *part* of deltoid (muscle).

p. clavicula'ris mus'culi pectoral'is major'is [TA], SYN clavicular *head* of pectoralis major muscle; SEE pectoralis major (*muscle*).

p. coccyg'ea medul'lae spina'lis [TA], SYN coccygeal *part* of spinal cord.

p. cochlea'ris ner'vi vestibulocochlea'ris, SYN cochlear *nerve.*

p. coeliacoduodenalis musculi (ligamenti) suspensorii duodeni [TA], SYN celiacoduodenal *part* of suspensory muscle (ligament) of duodenum.

p. convolu′ta lo′buli cortica′lis re′nis, SYN convoluted *part* of kidney lobule.

p. corneoscle′ra′lis reti′culi trabecula′ris sclerae [TA], SYN corneoscleral *part* of trabecular tissue of sclera.

par′tes cor′poris huma′ni [TA], SYN *parts* of human body, under *part*.

p. cortica′lis, SYN cortical *part*; SEE middle cerebral *artery*, posterior cerebral *artery*.

p. cortica′lis arteri′ae cerebra′lis medi′ae, SEE terminal *branches* of middle cerebral artery, under *branch*.

p. costa′lis diaphrag′matis [TA], SYN costal *part* of diaphragm.

p. costalis pleurae parietalis [TA], SYN costal *part* of parietal pleura.

p. cranialis partis parasympathetici divisionis autonomici systematis nervosi [TA], SYN cranial *part* of parasympathetic part of autonomic division of nervous system.

p. craniocervicalis plexuum et gangliorum visceralium [TA], SYN craniocervical *part* of peripheral autonomic plexuses and ganglia.

p. cricopharyn′gea mus′culi constricto′ris pharyn′gis inferio′ris [TA], SYN cricopharyngeal *part* of inferior constrictor (muscle) of pharynx; SEE inferior constrictor (*muscle*) of pharynx.

p. crucifor′mis vagi′nae fibro′sae [TA], SYN cruciform *part* of fibrous digital sheath.

p. cuneiformis vomeris [TA], SYN cuneiform *part* of vomer.

p. cupula′ris reces′sus epitympan′ici [TA], SYN cupular *part* of epitympanic recess.

p. cys′tica, the smaller caudal division of the primitive embryonic hepatic bud, developing into the gallbladder and cystic duct.

p. descen′dens aor′tae [TA], SYN descending *aorta*.

p. descen′dens duode′ni [TA], SYN descending *part* of duodenum; SEE duodenum.

p. descendens ligamenti iliofemoralis [TA], SYN descending *part* of iliofemoral ligament.

p. descendens musculi trapezii [TA], SYN descending *part* of trapezius (muscle).

p. dex′tra facie′i diaphragma′ticae hepa′tis [TA], SYN right *part* of diaphragmatic surface of liver.

p. diaphragmatica pleurae parietalis [TA], SYN diaphragmatic *part* of parietal pleura.

p. dista′lis adenohypophyseos [TA], SYN distal *part* [TA] of anterior lobe of hypophysis.

p. distalis prostatae [TA], SYN distal *part* of prostate.

p. distalis urethrae prostaticae [TA], SYN distal *part* of prostatic urethra.

partes dorsales musculorum intertransversariorum lateralium lumborum [TA], SYN dorsal *part* of intertransversarii laterales lumborum (muscles).

p. dorsa′lis pon′tis, SYN dorsal *part* of pons.

p. duralis fili terminalis [TA], SEE terminal *filum*.

p. endocri′na pancrea′tis [TA], SYN endocrine *part* of pancreas. SEE pancreas.

p. exocri′na pancrea′tis [TA], SYN exocrine *part* of pancreas; SEE pancreas.

p. extraocularis arteriae et venae centralis retinae [TA], SYN extraocular *part* of central retinal artery and vein.

p. feta′lis placen′tae, SYN fetal *placenta*.

p. flac′cida membra′nae tym′panae [TA], SYN flaccid *part* of tympanic membrane.

p. fronta′lis cor′poris callo′si, SYN minor *forceps*.

p. funicularis ductus deferentis [TA], SYN funicular *part* of ductus deferens.

par′tes genita′les femini′nae exter′nae, outmoded term for external female genital *organs*, under *organ*.

par′tes genita′les masculi′nae exter′nae, outmoded term for external male genital *organs*, under *organ*.

p. glossopharyn′gea mus′culi constricto′ris pharyn′gis superio′ris, SYN glossopharyngeal *part* of superior pharyngeal constrictor; SEE superior pharyngeal constrictor (*muscle*).

p. granulo′sa, the granular and filamentous part of the nucleolonema of the nucleolus.

p. hepat′ica, the larger cranial division of the primitive embryonic hepatic bud, developing into the liver proper.

p. hepatis dextra [TA], SYN right *liver*.

p. hepatis sinistra [TA], SYN left *liver*.

p. horizonta′lis duode′ni [TA], SYN inferior *part* of duodenum; SEE duodenum.

p. iliaca fasciae iliopsoaticae [TA], SYN iliac *fascia*.

p. infe′rior [TA], SYN inferior *part*.

p. inferior alae lobuli centralis [TA], SYN ala central *lobule*.

p. infe′rior duode′ni, ✩ official alternate term for inferior *part* of duodenum.

p. infe′rior gang′lii vestibula′ris [TA], SYN inferior *part* of vestibular ganglion.

p. infe′rior venae lingularis venae pulmonalis superioris sinistrae [TA], SYN inferior *part* of lingular vein (of left superior pulmonary vein).

p. infraclavicula′ris plex′us brachia′lis [TA], SYN infraclavicular *part* of brachial plexus.

p. infraloba′ris venae posterio′ris ve′nae pulmona′lis superioris dex′trae [TA], SYN infralobar *part* of posterior vein (of right superior pulmonary vein).

p. infundibula′ris, SYN p. tuberalis.

p. inguinalis ductus deferentis [TA], SYN inguinal *part* of ductus deferens.

p. insula′ris, SYN *lobus* insula.

p. insularis arte′riae cerebri mediae [TA], SYN insular *part* of middle cerebral artery; SEE middle cerebral *artery*.

p. interarticula′ris (in-ter-ar-tik′u-lar-is), the segment of bone between the superior and inferior articular facets, especially in the lumbar spine.

p. intercartilagin′ea ri′mae glot′tidis [TA], SYN intercartilaginous *part* of rima glottidis.

p. interme′dia [TA], SYN intermediate *part*.

p. interme′dia adenohypophys′eos [TA], SYN intermediate *part* of adenohypophysis.

p. interme′dia commissurae bulbo′rum, SYN *commissure* of bulbs.

p. intermedia urethrae masculinae [TA], SYN intermediate *part* of male urethra.

p. intermembrana′cea ri′mae glot′tidis [TA], SYN intermembranous *part* of rima glottidis.

partes intersegmenta′les venarum pulmonum [TA], SYN intersegmental *vein*.

p. intracrania′lis arte′riae vertebra′lis [TA], SYN intracranial *part* of vertebral artery. SEE vertebral *artery*.

p. intracrania′lis ner′vi op′tici [TA], SYN intracranial *part* of optic nerve.

p. intralamina′ris ner′vi op′tici intralocularis [TA], SYN intralaminar *part* of intralocular part of optic nerve.

p. intraloba′ris (intersegmentalis) venae posterioris lobi superioris pulmonis dextri [TA], SYN intralobar *part* of the posterior vein (of the right superior pulmonary vein).

p. intramuralis urethrae masculinae [TA], SYN intramural *part* of male urethra.

p. intraocula′ris ner′vi op′tici [TA], SYN intraocular *part* of optic nerve.

p. intrasegmenta′lis venae pulmonum [TA], SYN intrasegmental *part* of pulmonary veins.

p. irid′ica ret′inae [TA], SYN iridial *part* of retina; SEE retina.

p. labia′lis mus′culi orbicula′ris o′ris [TA], SYN labial *part* of orbicularis oris (muscle).

p. lacrima′lis mus′culi orbicula′ris oc′uli [TA], SYN lacrimal *part* of orbicularis oculi muscle; SEE orbicularis oculi (*muscle*).

p. laryn′gea pharyn′gis [TA], SYN laryngopharynx.

p. latera′lis ar′cus pe′dis longitudina′lis [TA], SYN lateral *part* of longitudinal arch of foot; SEE longitudinal *arch* of foot.

p. lateralis compartimenti antebrachii posterioris (extenso-

pa

rum) [TA], SYN lateral *part* of posterior (extensor) compartment of forearm.

p. latera′lis for′nicis vagi′nae [TA], SYN lateral *part* of vaginal fornix; SEE vaginal *fornix*.

p. latera′lis mus′culorum intertransversa′riorum posterio′rum cer′vicis [TA], SEE posterior cervical intertransversarii (*muscles*), under *muscle*.

p. lateralis nuclei accumbentis [TA], SEE *nucleus* accumbens.

p. latera′lis os′sis occipita′lis [TA], SYN lateral *part* of occipital bone.

p. latera′lis os′sis sa′cri [TA], SYN lateral *part* of sacrum.

p. latera′lis venae lo′bi medi′i ve′nae pulmona′lis dex′tri superi′oris, SYN lateral *part* of middle lobe vein (of right superior pulmonary vein).

p. libera membri inferioris [TA], SYN free *part* of lower limb.

p. libera membri superioris [TA], SYN free *part* of upper limb.

p. lumba′lis diaphrag′matis [TA], SYN lumbar *part* of diaphragm.

p. lumba′lis medul′lae spina′lis [TA], SYN lumbar *part* of spinal cord.

p. margina′lis mus′culi orbicula′ris o′ris [TA], SYN marginal *part* of orbicularis oris (muscle).

p. mastoi′dea os′sis tempora′lis, SYN mastoid *process* of petrous part of temporal bone.

p. media′lis ar′cus pe′dis longitudina′lis [TA], SYN medial *part* of longitudinal arch of foot; SEE longitudinal *arch* of foot.

p. media′lis mus′culorum intertransversa′riorum posterior′um cer′vicis, SEE posterior cervical intertransversarii (*muscles*), under *muscle*.

p. medialis nuclei accumbentis [TA], SEE *nucleus* accumbens.

p. media′lis venae lo′bi me′dii ve′nae pulmo′nis dex′tri superio′ris [TA], SYN medial *part* of middle lobe vein (of right superior pulmonary vein).

p. mediastinalis pleurae parietalis [TA], SYN mediastinal *part* of parietal pleura.

p. mediastina′lis pulmo′nis, SYN mediastinal *surface* of lung.

p. membrana′cea sep′ti interventricula′ris [TA], SYN membranous *part* of interventricular septum.

p. membrana′cea sep′ti na′si [TA], SYN membranous *part* of nasal septum.

p. membrana′cea ure′thrae masculi′nae, ⋆official alternate term for intermediate *part* of male urethra.

p. mo′bilis sep′ti na′si [TA], SYN mobile *part* of nasal septum.

p. muscula′ris sep′ti interventricula′ris (cor′dis) [TA], SYN muscular *part* of interventricular septum (of heart).

p. mylopharyn′geus mus′culi constricto′ris pharyn′gis superio′ris [TA], SYN mylopharyngeal *part* of superior constrictor muscle of pharynx; SEE superior pharyngeal constrictor (*muscle*).

p. nasa′lis os′sis fronta′lis [TA], SYN nasal *part* of frontal bone.

p. nasa′lis pharyn′gis [TA], SYN nasopharynx.

p. nervo′sa hypophys′eos, ⋆official alternate term for neurohypophysis.

p. nervo′sa ret′inae, SYN nervous *part* of retina; SEE retina.

p. obli′qua mus′culi cricothyroi′dei [TA], SYN oblique *part* of cricothyroid (muscle); SEE cricothyroid *muscle*.

p. occipita′lis cor′poris callo′si, SYN major *forceps*.

p. olfactoria tunicae mucosae [TA], SYN olfactory *region* of nasal mucosa.

p. opercula′ris [TA], SYN opercular *part*.

p. op′tica ret′inae [TA], SYN cerebral *layer* of retina; SEE retina.

p. ora′lis pharyn′gis [TA], SYN oropharynx.

p. orbitalis [TA], SYN orbital *part* [TA] of inferior frontal gyrus.

p. orbita′lis glan′dulae lacrima′lis [TA], SYN orbital *part* of lacrimal gland. SEE lacrimal *gland*.

p. orbita′lis mus′culi orbicula′ris oc′uli [TA], SYN orbital part of orbicularis oculi (muscle) [TA]. SEE orbicularis oculi (*muscle*).

p. orbita′lis ner′vi op′tici [TA], SYN orbital *part* of optic nerve.

p. orbita′lis os′sis fronta′lis [TA], SYN orbital *part* of frontal bone.

p. os′sea sep′ti na′si [TA], SYN bony *part* of nasal septum.

p. os′sea syste′matis skeleta′lis [TA], SYN bony *part* of skeletal system.

p. os′sea tu′bae auditi′vae [TA], SYN bony *part* of pharyngotympanic (auditory) tube.

p. ossea tubae auditoriae, SYN bony *part* of pharyngotympanic (auditory) tube.

p. palpebra′lis glan′dulae lacrima′lis [TA], SYN palpebral *part* of lacrimal gland; SEE lacrimal *gland*. SEE lacrimal *gland*.

p. palpebra′lis mus′culi orbicula′ris oc′uli [TA], SYN palpebral *part* of orbicularis oculi (muscle); SEE orbicularis oculi (*muscle*).

p. parasympath′ica divisionis automaticae systematis nervosi peripherici [TA], SYN parasympathetic *part* of autonomic division of peripheral nervous system.

p. patens arteriae umbilicalis [TA], SYN patent *part* of umbilical artery.

p. pel′vica [TA], SYN pelvic *part*.

p. pelvica ductus deferentes [TA], SYN pelvic *part* of ductus deferens.

p. pel′vica ure′teris [TA], SYN pelvic *part* of ureter.

p. peripher′ica systematis nervosi [TA], SYN peripheral nervous *system*.

p. perpendicula′ris, SYN perpendicular *plate*.

p. petro′sa arte′riae caro′tidis inter′nae [TA], SYN petrous *part* of internal carotid artery; SEE internal carotid *artery*.

p. petro′sa os′sis tempora′lis [TA], SYN petrous *part* of temporal bone; SEE temporal *bone*.

p. phal′lica, the lower portion of the urogenital sinus, related to the base of the genital tubercle.

p. pharyn′gea hypophys′eos, SYN pharyngeal *hypophysis*.

p. phrenicocoeliaca musculi (ligamenti) suspensorii duodeni [TA], SYN phrenicoceliac *part* of suspensory muscle (ligament) of duodenum.

p. pialis fili terminalis [TA], SYN pial *part* of filum terminale.

p. pigmento′sa, SYN pigmented *part* of retina; SEE retina.

p. pla′na, SYN orbiculus ciliaris.

p. postcommunicalis arteriae cerebri anterioris [TA], SYN postcommunicating *part* of anterior cerebral artery.

p. posterior commissurae anterioris [TA], SYN posterior *part* of anterior commissure of brain.

p. poste′rior facie′i diaphrag′matis hep′atis [TA], SYN posterior *part* of the diaphragmatic surface of the liver.

p. posterior fornicis vaginae [TA], SYN posterior *part* of vaginal fornix.

p. posterior linguae [TA], SYN posterior *part* of tongue.

p. postlamina′ris ner′vi op′tici intraocularis [TA], SYN postlaminar *part* of intraocular part of optic nerve.

p. postsulcalis linguae, ⋆official alternate term for posterior *part* of tongue.

p. precommunica′lis arteri′ae cere′bri anteri′oris [TA], SYN precommunicating *part* of anterior cerebral artery; SEE anterior cerebral *artery*.

p. precommunica′lis arteri′ae cere′bri posteri′oris [TA], SYN precommunicating *part* of posterior cerebral artery.

p. prelamina′ris ner′vi op′tici intraocularis [TA], SYN prelaminar *part* of intraocular part of optic nerve.

p. preprostatica urethrae masculinae, ⋆official alternate term for intramural *part* of male urethra.

p. presulca′lis, ⋆official alternate term for anterior *part* of tongue.

p. presulcalis linguae, ⋆official alternate term for anterior *part* of tongue.

p. prevertebralis arteriae prevertebralis [TA], SYN prevertebral *part* of vertebral artery; SEE vertebral *artery*.

p. proximalis prostatae [TA], SYN proximal *part* of prostate.

p. prima duodeni, SYN superior *part* of duodenum.

p. profunda compartimenti antebrachii anterioris [TA], SYN deep *part* of anterior compartment of forearm.

p. profunda compartimenti cruris posterioris [TA], SYN deep *part* of posterior (flexor) compartment of leg.

p. profun′da glan′dulae parotid′eae, SEE parotid *gland*.

p. profunda glandulae parotidis [TA], SYN deep *part* of parotid gland.

p. profun'da mus'culi masse'teri [TA], SYN deep *part* of masseter (muscle).

p. profun'da mus'culi sphinc'teri a'ni exter'ni, SYN deep *part* of external anal sphincter. SEE external anal *sphincter*.

p. profunda partis palpebralis musculi orbicularis oculi [TA], SYN deep *part* of palpebral part of orbicularis oculi (muscle).

p. prostat'ica ure'thrae [TA], SYN prostatic *urethra*.

p. proximalis urethrae prostaticae [TA], SYN proximal *part* of prostatic urethra.

p. psoatica fasciae iliopsoaticae [TA], SYN psoatic *part* of iliopsoas fascia.

p. pterygopharyn'gea mus'culi constricto'ris pharyn'gis superio'ris, SYN pterygopharyngeal *part* of superior constrictor muscle of pharynx; SEE superior pharyngeal constrictor (*muscle*).

p. pylo'rica gas'tris [TA], SYN pyloric *part* of stomach.

p. pylo'rica ventric'uli, SYN pyloric *part* of stomach.

p. quadra'ta hep'atis, SYN anterior *portion* of left medial segment IV of liver.

p. radia'ta lo'buli cortica'lis re'nis, SYN medullary *ray*.

p. rec'ta mus'culi cricothyroi'dei, SEE cricothyroid *muscle*.

p. respiratoria tunicae mucosae [TA], SYN respiratory *region* of mucosa of nasal cavity.

p. retrolentifor'mis cap'sulae inter'nae [TA], SYN retrolenticular *part* of internal capsule.

p. retrolentiformis cruris posterior [TA], SYN retrolentiform *limb* of internal capsule.

p. sacra'lis medul'lae spina'lis [TA], SYN sacral *part* of spinal cord.

p. scrotalis ductus deferentis [TA], SYN scrotal *part* of ductus deferens.

p. secundum duodeni, SYN descending *part* of duodenum.

p. sella'ris, SYN *sella* turcica.

p. solealis compartimenti cruris posterioris [TA], SYN soleal *part* of posterior (plantar flexor) compartment of leg.

p. sphenoida'lis arte'riae cerebra'lis me'diae [TA], SYN sphenoid *part* of middle cerebral artery; SEE middle cerebral *artery*.

p. spinalis fili terminalis [TA], SYN spinal *part* of filum terminale.

p. spinalis musculi deltoidei [TA], SYN spinal *part* of deltoid (muscle).

p. spina'lis ner'vi accesso'rii, ☆official alternate term for spinal *root* of accessory nerve.

p. spongio'sa ure'thrae masculi'nae [TA], SYN spongy *urethra*.

p. squamo'sa os'sis tempora'lis [TA], SYN squamous *part* of temporal bone.

p. sterna'lis diaphrag'matis [TA], SYN sternal *part* of diaphragm.

p. sternocosta'lis mus'culi pectora'lis majo'ris [TA], SYN sternocostal *head* of pectoralis major (muscle).

p. subcuta'nea mus'culi sphinc'teri a'ni exter'ni [TA], SYN subcutaneous *part* of external anal sphincter; SEE external anal *sphincter*.

p. sublentifor'mis cap'sulae inter'nae [TA], SYN sublenticular *part* of internal capsule.

p. sublentiformis cruris posterioris [TA], SYN sublentiform *limb* of internal capsule.

p. superficialis compartimenti antebrachii anterioris [TA], SYN superficial *part* of anterior (flexor) compartment of forearm.

p. superficialis compartimenti cruris posterioris [TA], SYN superficial *part* of posterior (plantar flexor) compartment of leg.

p. superficia'lis glan'dulae parotid'eae [TA], SYN superficial *part* of parotid gland; SEE parotid *gland*.

p. superficia'lis mus'culi masse'teri [TA], SYN superficial *part* of masseter muscle; SEE masseter (*muscle*).

p. superficia'lis mus'culi sphinc'teri a'ni exter'ni [TA], SYN superficial *part* of external anal sphincter; SEE external anal *sphincter*.

p. superior ali lobuli centralis [TA], SYN ala central *lobule*.

p. supe'rior duode'ni [TA], SYN superior *part* of duodenum.

p. supe'rior facie'i diaphrag'maticae hep'atis [TA], SYN superior *part* of diaphragmatic surface of liver.

p. supe'rior gan'glii vestibula'ris [TA], SYN superior *part* of vestibular ganglion.

p. supe'rior venae lingula'ris ve'nae pulmo'nis superioris sin'istri [TA], SYN superior *part* of lingular vein (of left superior pulmonary vein).

p. supraclavicula'ris plex'us brachia'lis [TA], SYN supraclavicular *part* of brachial plexus.

p. sympath'ica (divisionis autonomicae systematis nervosi peripherici) [TA], SYN sympathetic *part* of autonomic division of peripheral nervous system.

p. tec'ta, obsolete term; **p. tecta pancreatis**, hidden portion of the pancreas; part of the pancreas covered by the root of the transverse mesocolon, the coalescence of the ascending mesocolon, and the root of the mesentery; **p. tecta renalis**, hidden portion of the kidney; part of the kidney covered by the root of the transverse mesocolon; **p. tecta ureteralis**, hidden portion of the ureter; part of the right ureter covered (crossed) by the root of the mesentery, and of the left ureter covered (crossed) by the root of the sigmoid mesocolon. SYN hidden part.

p. tec'ta duode'ni, SYN hidden *part* of duodenum.

p. ten'sa membra'nae tym'pani [TA], SYN tense *part* of the tympanic membrane.

p. termina'lis, SEE middle cerebral *artery*, posterior cerebral *artery*. SYN terminal part.

p. terminalis ilei [TA], SYN terminal *ileus*.

p. thorac'ica aor'tae [TA], SYN thoracic *aorta*.

p. thorac'ica duc'tus thorac'ici [TA], SYN thoracic *part* of thoracic duct; SEE thoracic *duct*.

p. thorac'ica esoph'agi [TA], SYN thoracic *part* of esophagus.

p. thorac'ica medul'lae spina'lis [TA], SYN thoracic *part* of spinal cord.

p. thoracica muscularis iliocostalis lumborum [TA], SYN thoracic *part* of iliocostalis lumborum (muscle).

p. thoracica plexum et ganglionorum visceralium [TA], SYN thoracic *part* of peripheral autonomic plexuses and ganglia.

p. thoracica tracheae [TA], SYN thoracic *part* of trachea.

p. thyroepiglottica musculi thyroarytenoidei [TA], SYN thyroepiglottic *part* of thyroarytenoid (muscle).

p. thyropharyn'gea mus'culi constricto'ris pharyn'gis inferio'ris [TA], SYN thyropharyngeal *part* of inferior constrictor muscle of pharynx; SEE inferior constrictor (*muscle*) of pharynx.

p. tibiocalcanea ligamenti deltoidei, ☆official alternate term for tibiocalcaneal *part* of medial ligament of ankle joint.

p. tibiocalca'nea ligamen'ti collateralis media'lis articulationis talocruralis [TA], SYN tibiocalcaneal *part* of medial ligament of ankle joint.

p. tibionavicula'ris ligamen'ti collateralis media'lis articulationis talocrucalis [TA], SYN tibionavicular *part* of medial ligament of ankle joint.

p. tibiotala'ris ante'rior ligamen'ti collateralis media'lis articulationis talocruralis [TA], SYN anterior tibiotalar *part* of medial ligament of ankle joint.

p. tibiotala'ris poste'rior ligamen'ti collateralis media'lis articulationis talocruralis [TA], SYN tibiotalar *part* of medial ligament of ankle joint.

p. transversa ligamenti iliofemoralis [TA], SYN transverse *part* of iliofemoral ligament.

p. transver'sa mus'culi nasa'lis [TA], SYN transverse *part* of nasalis muscle; SEE nasalis (*muscle*).

p. transversa musculi trapezii [TA], SYN transverse *part* of trapezius (muscle).

p. transver'sa ra'mi si'nistri ve'nae por'tae hepa'tis [TA], SYN transverse *part* of left branch of portal vein.

p. transversa'ria arte'riae vertebra'lis, SEE vertebral *artery*.

p. triangula'ris [TA], SYN triangular *part*.

p. tricipitalis compartimenti cruris posterioris, ☆official alternate term for superficial *part* of posterior (plantar flexor) compartment of leg.

p. tubera'lis [TA], the upward extension of the anterior lobe that wraps around the infundibular stalk; its cells, mostly gonadotropic, are arranged in cords and clusters; it is supplied by the superior hypophyseal arteries and contains the first capillary bed and the venules of a portal system that carries neurosecretory factors from the hypothalamus to a second capillary bed in the adenohypophysis where they regulate the release of hormones. SEE ALSO pituitary *gland*. SYN infundibular part, p. infundibularis.

p. tympan′ica os′sis tempora′lis [TA], SYN tympanic *plate* of temporal bone.

p. umbilica′lis ra′mi si′nistri ve′nae por′tae hepa′tis [TA], SYN umbilical *part* of left branch of portal vein.

p. uteri′na placen′tae, the part of the placenta derived from the uterine tissue. SEE ALSO placenta. SYN maternal placenta, placenta uterina.

p. uteri′na tu′bae uteri′nae [TA], SYN uterine *part* of uterine tube.

p. uvea′lis reti′culi trabecula′ris sclerae [TA], SYN uveal *part* of trabecular tissue of sclera.

p. vaga′lis ner′vi accesso′rii, ☆official alternate term for cranial *root* of accessory nerve.

p. ventralis musculi intertransversarii lateralium lumborum [TA], SYN ventral *part* of intertransversarii laterales lumborum (muscles).

p. ventralis pontis, SYN basilar *part* of pons.

p. vertebra′lis facie′i costa′lis pulmo′nis [TA], SYN vertebral *part* of the costal surface of the lungs.

p. vestibula′ris ner′vi vestibulocochlea′ris, SYN vestibular *nerve*.

---

pars·pla·ni·tis (parz′plā-nī′tis). A clinical syndrome consisting of inflammation of the peripheral retina and/or pars plana, exudation into the overlying vitreous base, and edema of the optic disk and adjacent retina.

part. A portion. SYN pars [TA].

abdominal p. of aorta, SYN abdominal *aorta*.

abdominal p. of esophagus [TA], the portion of the esophagus from where it passes through the diaphragm to the stomach. SEE esophagus. SYN pars abdominalis esophagi [TA], epicardia.

abdominal p. of pectoralis major (muscle) [TA], portion of pectoralis major originating from the rectus sheath. SYN pars abdominalis musculi pectorales majoris [TA].

abdominal p. of peripheral autonomic plexuses and ganglia [TA], portion of the autonomic nervous system (networks composed largely of autonomic nerve fibers—but also including visceral afferent fibers—and ganglia associated with blood vessels and organs) that occur both retro- and intraperitoneally in the abdominal cavity. SYN pars abdominalis plexus visceralis et ganglii visceralis [TA].

abdominal p. of thoracic duct [TA], the part of the thoracic duct between the cisterna chyli and the aortic hiatus of the diaphragm. SYN pars abdominalis ductus thoracici [TA].

abdominal p. of ureter [TA], the part of the ureter between the renal pelvis and the brim of the pelvis. SYN pars abdominalis ureteris [TA].

acromial p. of deltoid (muscle) [TA], portion of deltoid (muscle) originating from the acromion. SYN pars acromialis musculi deltoidei [TA].

alar p. of nasalis muscle [TA], SEE nasalis (*muscle*). SYN pars alaris musculi nasalis [TA].

alveolar p. of mandible [TA], the portion of the body of the mandible that surrounds and supports the lower teeth. SYN pars alveolaris mandibulae [TA].

anterior p. [TA], the portion of a structure that lies most forward, or closest to the front surface relative to other parts; in human anatomy, the ventral portion of a structure. SEE anterior part of: anterior commissure of brain; guadrangular lobule of cerebellum; central lobule of cerebellum; culmen; lateral parabranchial nucleus; diaphragmatic surface of liver; tongue; formix of vagina. SYN pars anterior [TA].

anterior p. of anterior commissure of brain [TA], the anterior part of the anterior or rostral commissure of the brain; SYN pars anterior commissurae anterioris [TA], pars anterior commissurae rostralis.

anterior p. of diaphragmatic surface of liver [TA], the part of the diaphragmatic surface of the liver deep to the costal arches and the xiphoid process. SYN pars anterior faciei diaphragmatis hepatis [TA].

anterior p. of fornix of vagina [TA], the portion of the fornix of the vagina anterior to the uterine cervix. SYN pars anterior fornicis vaginae [TA].

anterior p. of pons, SYN basilar p. of pons.

anterior tibiotalar p. of deltoid ligament, SYN anterior tibiotalar p. of medial ligament of ankle joint.

anterior tibiotalar p. of medial ligament of ankle joint [TA], the part of the medial or deltoid ligament that extends from the medial malleolus to the neck of the talus. SYN pars tibiotalaris anterior ligamenti collateralis medialis articulationis talocruralis [TA], anterior talotibial ligament, anterior tibiotalar ligament, anterior tibiotalar p. of deltoid ligament, ligamentum mediale, ligamentum talotibiale anterius.

anterior p. of tongue [TA], portion of the tongue (≈2/3) anterior to the sulcus terminalis, distinct from the posterior part in embryologic origin and innervation. SYN pars anterior linguae [TA], pars presulcalis linguae☆, pars presulcalis☆, presulcal p. of tongue☆.

anular p. of fibrous digital sheath of digits of hand and foot [TA], one of the five circular fibrous bands or pulleys (A1–A5) of the fibrous sheaths of the fingers and the corresponding structures of the toes attached to the shaft of the proximal and middle phalanges and associated joint capsules. SYN pars anularis vaginae fibrosae digitorum manus et pedis [TA], anular pulley, anulus of fibrous sheath, ligamentum anulare digitorum.

aryepiglottic p. of oblique arytenoid muscle [TA], fibers of the oblique arytenoid muscle that continue past the summit of the arytenoid cartilage to the side of the epiglottis; *action*, constricts the laryngeal aperture in a "purse-string" manner. SYN pars aryepiglottica musculi arytenoidei obliqui [TA], aryepiglottic muscle, musculus aryepiglotticus.

ascending p. of aorta, SYN ascending *aorta*.

ascending p. of duodenum [TA], the terminal or fourth p. of the duodenum, ascending from the horizontal p. to the jejunum. SYN pars ascendens duodeni [TA].

ascending p. of trapezius (muscle) [TA], lower third of trapezius that ascends to insert on the spine of the scapula; acts independently of other parts to depress scapula (lower shoulders); acts with other parts to retract and rotate scapula. SYN pars ascendens musculi trapezii [TA], inferior p. of trapezius (muscle)☆.

atlantic p. of vertebral artery [TA], suboccipital part of vertebral artery. SEE vertebral *artery*. SYN pars atlantica arteriae vertebralis [TA], suboccipital p. of vertebral artery.

autonomic p. of peripheral nervous system, ☆official alternate term for autonomic *division* of nervous system.

basal p. [TA], portion of a structure which forms its base—the bottom part or part opposite the apex of the structure—or a branch serving that portion of the structure; e.g., the basal part of the lungs (formed by the four basal bronchopulmonary segments of each side) served by basal parts of the right and left pulmonary arteries. SYN basilar p.'s [TA], pars basalis [TA], pars basilaris [TA].

basal p. of left and right inferior pulmonary arteries [TA], SEE right pulmonary *artery*, left pulmonary *artery*. SYN pars basalis arteriarum lobarium inferiorum pulmonis sinistri et dextri [TA]. SEE right pulmonary *artery*, left pulmonary *artery*.

basal p. of occipital bone, SYN basilar p. of occipital bone.

basilar p.'s [TA], SYN basal p.

basilar p. of occipital bone [TA], the wedgelike part of the occipital bone that lies anterior to the foramen magnum and joins with the body of the sphenoid bone. SYN pars basilaris ossis occipitalis [TA], basal p. of occipital bone, basilar apophysis, basilar process of occipital bone, basilar process, basiocciput.

basilar p. of pons [TA], the large bulbous portion of the pons seen on the ventral portion of the brainstem and ventral to the medial lemniscus in a cross section: contains longitudinally oriented fibers (corticospinal, corticopontine, corticoreticular, and others) and the transversely oriented pontocerebellar fibers. SYN pars basilaris pontis [TA], pons basilaris pontis [TA], anterior p. of pons, pars ventralis pontis, ventral p. of pons.

bony p. of external acoustic meatus, the medial two-thirds of the external acoustic meatus, that is formed as the tympanic plate of the temporal bone develops; it extends approximately 16 mm from its junction with the cartilaginous part to the tympanic membrane.

bony p. of nasal septum [TA], the major portion of the nasal septum including (supported by) the vomer and the perpendicular plate of the ethmoid. SYN pars ossea septi nasi [TA].

bony p. of pharyngotympanic (auditory) tube [TA], the portion of the pharyngotympanic (auditory) tube formed by the petrous part of the temporal bone passing from the tympanic cavity anteromedially through the semicanal for auditory tube. SYN pars ossea tubae auditivae [TA], pars ossea tubae auditoriae.

bony p. of skeletal system [TA], portion of the skeleton composed of cortical, compact, or spongy bone. SYN pars ossea systematis skeletalis [TA], osseous p. of skeletal system.

buccopharyngeal p. of superior pharyngeal constrictor, SEE superior pharyngeal constrictor (*muscle*). SYN pars buccopharyngea musculi constrictoris pharyngei superioris.

cardiac p. of stomach, SYN cardia.

cardial p. of stomach, SYN cardia.

cartilaginous p. of external acoustic meatus, the lateral third of the external acoustic meatus, which is continuous with the auricular cartilage and attached to the circumference of the bony part.

cartilaginous p. of nasal septum [TA], portion of the nasal septum supported by cartilage (instead of bone).

cartilaginous p. of pharyngotympanic (auditory) tube, that portion of the auditory tube that is supported by cartilage; it continues anteromedially from the osseous part to open into the nasopharynx. SYN pars cartilaginea tubae auditivae [TA], pars cartilaginea tubae auditoriae.

cartilaginous p. of skeletal system [TA], the part of the skeleton composed of cartilage. SYN pars cartilaginea systematis skeletalis [TA].

cavernous p. of internal carotid artery [TA], the more tortuous portion of the internal carotid artery that traverses the cavernous sinus; it has numerous small branches. SYN pars cavernosa arteriae carotidis internae [TA].

celiacoduodenal p. of suspensory muscle (ligament) of duodenum [TA], fibromuscular band of smooth muscle passing from the terminal duodenum and duodenojejunal flexure to end in connective tissue in the vicinity of the celiac trunk. SYN pars coeliacoduodenalis musculi (ligamenti) suspensorii duodeni [TA].

central p. of lateral ventricle, SYN *pars* centralis ventriculi lateralis.

ceratopharyngeal p. of middle constrictor muscle of pharynx [TA], SEE middle constrictor (*muscle*) of pharynx. SYN pars ceratopharyngea musculi constrictoris pharyngis medii [TA], ceratopharyngeal p. of middle pharyngeal constrictor (muscle) of pharynx.

ceratopharyngeal p. of middle pharyngeal constrictor (muscle) of pharynx, SYN ceratopharyngeal p. of middle constrictor muscle of pharynx.

cerebral p. of arachnoid, SYN cranial *arachnoid* mater.

cerebral p. of dura mater, SYN cranial *dura mater*.

cerebral p. of internal carotid artery [TA], the portion of the internal carotid artery that lines in contact with and directly supplies the brain; its branches are: superior hypophyseal, clival, ophthalmic, anterior choroidal, anterior cerebral, and middle cerebral. SYN pars cerebralis arteriae carotidis internae [TA].

cervical p. of esophagus [TA], the p. of the esophagus located in the neck. SEE esophagus. SYN pars cervicalis esophagi [TA].

cervical p. of internal carotid artery [TA], the unbranched portion located in the neck. SYN pars cervicalis arteriae carotidis internae [TA].

cervical p. of spinal cord [TA], the p. of the spinal cord located in the neck consisting of eight cervical segments [C1–C8] and giving rise to the first eight pairs of spinal nerves [C1–C8]. SYN

pars cervicalis medullae spinalis [TA], segmenta cervicalia medullae spinalis [TA], segmenta medullae spinalis cervicalia C1–C8 [TA], cervical segments of spinal cord [C1–C8]*, segmenta cervicalia C1–C5.

cervical p. of thoracic duct [TA], the portion of the thoracic duct above the first rib. SYN pars cervicalis ductus thoracici [TA].

cervical p. of vertebral artery [TA], portion of vertebral artery that traverses the transverse foramina of cervical vertebrae C1–C6 and gives rise to spinal and muscular branches. SYN pars cervicalis arteriae vertebralis [TA], transversarial p. of vertebral artery [TA].

chondropharyngeal p. of middle constrictor muscle of pharynx [TA], SEE middle constrictor (*muscle*) of pharynx. SYN pars chondropharyngea musculi constrictoris pharyngei medii [TA], chondropharyngeal p. of middle pharyngeal constrictor (muscle) of pharynx.

chondropharyngeal p. of middle pharyngeal constrictor (muscle) of pharynx, SYN chondropharyngeal p. of middle constrictor muscle of pharynx.

ciliary p. of retina [TA], SEE retina. SYN pars ciliaris retinae [TA].

clavicular p. of deltoid (muscle) [TA], anterior portion of the deltoid originating from the clavicle; acts independently of other parts to contribute to flexion at the shoulder joint. SYN pars clavicularis musculi deltoidei [TA].

clavicular p. of pectoralis major (muscle), SYN clavicular *head* of pectoralis major muscle. SEE pectoralis major (*muscle*).

coccygeal p. of spinal cord [TA], the terminal part of the spinal cord consisting of the three coccygeal segments of the spinal cord from which the three pairs of coccygeal nerves originate. SYN pars coccygea medullae spinalis [TA], segmenta coccygea medullae spinalis [TA].

cochlear p. of vestibulocochlear nerve, SYN cochlear *nerve*.

convoluted p. of kidney lobule, proximal and distal convoluted tubules and the associated renal corpuscles supplied by branches of the interlobular arteries. SYN labyrinthus, Ludwig labyrinth, pars convoluta lobuli corticalis renis, renal labyrinth.

corneoscleral p. of trabecular tissue of sclera [TA], the anterior part of the trabecular reticulum, located between the sinus venosus sclerae, the scleral spur, and the posterior limiting membrane of the cornea. SYN pars corneoscleralis reticuli trabecularis sclerae [TA].

cortical p., SYN pars corticalis. SEE middle cerebral *artery*, posterior cerebral *artery*.

cortical p. of middle cerebral artery, SEE middle cerebral *artery*.

costal p. of diaphragm [TA], the part of the diaphragm that arises from the inner aspect of the lower six costal cartilages and the lower four ribs and inserts on the anterolateral part of the central tendon. SYN pars costalis diaphragmatis [TA].

costal p. of parietal pleura [TA], portion of the parietal pleura that lines the internal aspect of the ribs and intercostal muscles. SYN pars costalis pleurae parietalis [TA], costal pleura, pleura costalis.

cranial p. of parasympathetic part of autonomic division of nervous system [TA], the roots and branches of the parasympathetic ganglia (ciliary, pterygopalatine, otic, and submandibular/sublingual) of the head. SYN pars cranialis partis parasympathetici divisionis autonomici systematis nervosi [TA].

craniocervical p. of peripheral autonomic plexuses and ganglia [TA], networks of postsynaptic sympathetic nerve fibers accompanying the carotid arteries and branches thereof within the head and neck. SYN pars craniocervicalis plexuum et gangliorum visceralium [TA].

cricopharyngeal p. of inferior constrictor (muscle) of pharynx [TA], SEE inferior constrictor (*muscle*) of pharynx. SYN pars cricopharyngea musculi constrictoris pharyngis inferioris [TA], cricopharyngeus muscle*.

cruciform p. of fibrous digital sheath [TA], the fibers of the fibrous sheath of the fingers and toes that constitute three X-shaped pulleys (C1–C3) over the proximal and middle phalanx. SYN pars cruciformis vaginae fibrosae [TA], crucial ligament (4), cruciform p. of fibrous sheath, cruciform pulley, ligamenta cruciata digitorum.

cruciform p. of fibrous sheath, SYN cruciform p. of fibrous digital sheath.

cuneiform p. of vomer [TA], the wedge-shaped thin anterior portion of the vomer. SYN pars cuneiformis vomeris [TA].

cupular p. of epitympanic recess [TA], the dome-shaped, highest portion of the epitympanic recess. SYN pars cupularis recessus epitympanici [TA].

deep p. of anterior compartment of forearm [TA], portion of anterior (flexor) compartment of forearm that includes the flexor pollicis longus, flexor digitorum profundus, and pronator quadratus muscle. SYN pars profunda compartimenti antebrachii anterioris [TA].

deep p. of external anal sphincter [TA], SEE external anal *sphincter.* SYN pars profunda musculi sphincteri ani externi.

deep p. of flexor retinaculum, SYN flexor *retinaculum.*

deep p. of masseter (muscle) [TA], SEE masseter *(muscle).* SYN pars profunda musculi masseteri [TA].

deep p. of palpebral part of orbicularis oculi (muscle) [TA], portion of the palpebral part of orbicularis oculi arising from the posterior aspect of the medial palpebral ligament and adjacent bone. SYN pars profunda partis palpebralis musculi orbicularis oculi [TA].

deep p. of parotid gland [TA], that portion of the parotid salivary gland that is located behind the mandible and occupies the space between the ramus of the mandible and the mastoid process extending as far medially as the pharyngeal wall. SYN pars profunda glandulae parotidis [TA], processus retromandibularis glandulae parotidis, processus retromandibularis, retromandibular process of parotid gland. SEE parotid *gland.*

deep p. of posterior (flexor) compartment of leg [TA], portion of posterior (flexor) compartment of leg including flexor digitorum longus, flexor hallucis longus, and tibialis posterior (muscles). SYN pars profunda compartimenti cruris posterioris [TA].

descending p. of aorta, SYN descending *aorta.*

descending p. of duodenum [TA], SEE duodenum. SYN pars descendens duodeni [TA], pars secundum duodeni, second p. of duodenum.

descending p. of facial canal, second portion of the facial canal, after the horizontal parts, beginning at the posterior end of the lateral crus where the canal begins to descend. It runs vertically downward, ending at the stylomastoid foramen. Anteriorly, the descending part of the facial canal communicates with the tympanic cavity via the canaliculus for the nerve to the stapedius muscle and the posterior canaliculus of the chorda tympani. SEE ALSO facial *canal.*

descending p. of iliofemoral ligament [TA], the more vertical of the limbs of the inverted Y-shaped iliofemoral ligament (vs. the more horizontal transverse part). SYN pars descendens ligamenti iliofemoralis [TA].

descending p. of trapezius (muscle) [TA], the upper third of the trapezius (muscle) that descends to insert on the clavicle and acromion; acting independently of the other parts, it acts to elevate the scapula (shrug shoulders). SYN pars descendens musculi trapezii [TA].

diaphragmatic p. of parietal pleura [TA], portion of the outer (parietal) layer of pleura that lines the superior aspect of the diaphragm on each side of the pericardium. SYN pars diaphragmatica pleurae parietalis [TA], diaphragmatic pleura, phrenic pleura, pleura diaphragmatica, pleura phrenica.

distal p. of prostate [TA], portion of the prostate derived from the more caudal anlage; includes the right, left, and posterior lobes of prostate. SYN pars distalis prostatae [TA].

distal p. of prostatic urethra [TA], portion of prostatic urethra inferior to the merging of the urinary and genital tracts at the openings of the ejaculatory ducts. SYN pars distalis urethrae prostaticae [TA].

distal p. [TA] of anterior lobe of hypophysis, the larger part of the adenohypophysis composed of cords of epithelial cells individually specialized to secrete various tropic hormones that exert their effect on several target organs in the body. The secretory activity of these cells is under the control of either releasing or inhibiting factors elaborated by hypothalamic neurons and transported to the adenohypophysis by the hypothalamo-hypophysial portal system. SYN pars distalis adenohypophyseos [TA].

dorsal p. of intertransversarii laterales lumborum (muscles) [TA], portion of the lateral intertransversarii of the lumbar region connecting the accessory processes of one vertebra to the transverse processes of the vertebra above. SYN partes dorsales musculorum intertransversariorum lateralium lumborum [TA].

dorsal p. of pons, the part of the pons bounded laterally by the middle cerebellar peduncles and anteriorly by the ventral part of pons; it is continuous with the tegmentum of the mesencephalon and contains long tracts such as the medial and lateral lemnisci, cranial nerve nuclei, and reticular formation. SYN tegmentum of pons [TA], tegmentum pontis [TA], pars dorsalis pontis.

dural p. of filum terminale [TA], the threadlike termination of the spinal dura mater, surrounding and fused to the filum terminale of the cord, and attached to the deep dorsal sacrococcygeal ligament; extends from S2–3 to Co2 vertebral levels. SEE ALSO terminal *filum.* SYN coccygeal ligament✭, filum terminale externum✭, filum durae matris spinalis, filum of spinal dura mater.

endocrine p. of pancreas [TA], SEE pancreas. SYN pars endocrina pancreatis [TA].

exocrine p. of pancreas [TA], SEE pancreas. SYN pars exocrina pancreatis [TA].

extraocular p. of central retinal artery and vein [TA], orbital portion of central retinal artery and vein external (posterior) to the eyeball. SYN pars extraocularis arteriae et venae centralis retinae [TA].

first p. of duodenum, SYN superior p. of duodenum.

flaccid p. of tympanic membrane [TA], triangular loose p. of tympanic membrane between the malleolar folds. SYN pars flaccida membranae tympanae [TA], flaccid membrane, membrana flaccida, Rivinus membrane, Shrapnell membrane.

free p. of lower limb [TA], portion of the appendicular skeleton of the lower limb distal to the hip joint; the pelvic girdle is excluded. SYN pars libera membri inferioris [TA].

free p. of upper limb [TA], portion of the appendicular skeleton of the upper limb distal to the shoulder joint; the pectoral girdle is not included. SYN pars libera membri superioris [TA].

frontal p. of corpus callosum, SYN minor *forceps.*

funicular p. of ductus deferens [TA], portion of the ductus deferens contained within the spermatic cord. SYN pars funicularis ductus deferentis [TA].

glossopharyngeal p. of superior pharyngeal constrictor, SEE superior pharyngeal constrictor *(muscle).* SYN pars glossopharyngea musculi constrictoris pharyngis superioris.

hidden p., SYN *pars* tecta.

hidden p. of duodenum, the part of duodenum covered by the root of the transverse mesocolon, the coalescence of the ascending mesocolon, and the root of the mesentery. SYN pars tecta duodeni.

horizontal p. of duodenum, ✭official alternate term for inferior p. of duodenum. SEE duodenum.

horizontal p. of facial canal, first portion of facial canal, between beginning of canal (at the introitus of the facial canal at the end of the internal auditory meatus) and the point at which it turns to descend, beginning the *descending part.* There are two components (crura) of the horizontal part: the medially located, anteriorly directed medial crus and the laterally placed, posteriorly directed lateral crus, the two being continuous at a sharp bend, the genu of the facial canal. This lateral part is where the genicular ganglion is located and communicates with the middle cranial fossa via the hiatus of the facial canal, through which the greater superficial petrosal nerve passes.

p.'s of human body [TA], the head, neck, trunk, limbs, and cavities. SYN partes corporis humani [TA].

inferior p. [TA], the lowermost portion of a structure relative to the other parts; portion closest to the soles of the feet. SEE inferior part of: duodenum, lingular branch of left pulmonary vein, and vestibular ganglion. SYN pars inferior [TA].

inferior p. of duodenum [TA], third section of duodenum inferior to head of pancreas that lies between the superior mesenteric vessels anteriorly and the aorta and inferior vena cava posteriorly.

syn pars horizontalis duodeni [TA], horizontal p. of duodenum✫, pars inferior duodeni✫, third p. of duodenum.

inferior p. of lingular vein (of left superior pulmonary vein) [TA], the vein draining the inferior lingular bronchopulmonary segment of the left lung. syn pars inferior venae lingularis venae pulmonalis superioris sinistrae [TA].

inferior p. of trapezius (muscle), ✫official alternate term for ascending p. of trapezius (muscle).

inferior p. of vestibular ganglion [TA], the lower part of the vestibular ganglion that receives fibers from the macula of the saccule and the ampulla of the posterior semicircular duct. syn pars inferior ganglii vestibularis [TA].

inferior p. of vestibulocochlear nerve, syn cochlear nerve.

infraclavicular p. of brachial plexus [TA], the part of the brachial plexus that extends from the level of the clavicle downward into the axilla; it includes the cords of the plexus and their branches. syn pars infraclavicularis plexus brachialis [TA].

infralobar p. of posterior vein (of right superior pulmonary vein) [TA], the vein draining the posterior segment of the right lung that emerges inferior to the superior lobe; tributary to the posterior branch of the right superior pulmonary vein. syn pars infralobaris venae posterioris venae pulmonalis superioris dextrae [TA].

infrasegmental p., syn intersegmental vein.

infundibular p., syn pars tuberalis.

inguinal p. of ductus deferens [TA], portion of ductus deferens located within the inguinal canal, i.e., between superficial and deep inguinal rings. syn pars inguinalis ductus deferentis [TA].

insular p., syn lobus insula.

insular p. of middle cerebral artery [TA], see middle cerebral artery. syn pars insularis arteriae cerebri mediae [TA].

intercartilaginous p. of glottic opening, syn intercartilaginous p. of rima glottidis.

intercartilaginous p. of rima glottidis [TA], the opening between the vocal processes of the arytenoid cartilages; this part is open during whispering and is closed during phonation and the Valsalva maneuver. syn pars intercartilaginea rimae glottidis [TA], glottis respiratoria, intercartilaginous p. of glottic opening.

intermediate p. [TA], central portion; the portion located between extreme portions of a structure; an interposed or intervening part. see intermediate p. of adenohypophysis, intermediate p. of male urethra. syn pars intermedia [TA].

intermediate p. of adenohypophysis [TA], the part of the adenohypophysis located between the pars distalis and the nervous lobe; poorly developed in humans. syn pars intermedia adenohypophyseos [TA].

intermediate p. of male urethra [TA], the shortest and narrowest portion of the male urethra, about 1 cm in length, extending from the prostate to the beginning of the urethra in the corpus spongiosum just beyond the bulb. syn pars intermedia urethrae masculinae [TA], membranous urethra✫, pars membranacea urethrae masculinae✫, membranous p. of male urethra.

intermediate p. of vestibular bulb, syn commissure of bulbs.

intermembranous p. of glottic opening, syn intermembranous p. of rima glottidis.

intermembranous p. of rima glottidis [TA], the portion of the opening anterior to the vocal processes of the arytenoid cartilages bounded by the vocal ligaments; this portion is closed by contraction of the lateral cricoarytenoid (muscle) only during whispering. syn pars intermembranacea rimae glottidis [TA], glottis vocalis, intermembranous p. of glottic opening.

intersegmental p. of pulmonary vein [TA], syn intersegmental vein.

intracranial p. of optic nerve [TA], the portion of the optic nerve between the optic canal and the optic chiasm. syn pars intracranialis nervi optici [TA].

intracranial p. of vertebral artery [TA], see vertebral artery. syn pars intracranialis arteriae vertebralis [TA].

intralaminar p. of intralocular part of optic nerve [TA], the portion of the intraocular part of the optic nerve as it passes through the lamina cribrosa of the sclera. syn pars intralaminaris nervi optici intralocularis [TA].

intralobar p. of the posterior vein (of the right superior pulmonary vein) [TA], the vein draining the apical and posterior segments of the right lung; tributary to the posterior branch of the right superior pulmonary vein. syn pars intralobaris (intersegmentalis) venae posterioris lobi superioris pulmonis dextri [TA].

intramural p. of male urethra [TA], initial portion of male urethra traversing the wall (floor) of the bladder. syn pars intramuralis urethrae masculinae [TA], pars preprostatica urethrae masculinae✫, preprostatic p. of male urethra✫.

intraocular p. of optic nerve [TA], the part of the optic nerve within the eyeball; it is divided into intralaminar, postlaminar, and prelaminar parts. syn pars intraocularis nervi optici [TA].

intrasegmental p. of pulmonary veins [TA], a p. emerging from the bronchopulmonary segment it drains; a tributary to a branch of a pulmonary p. syn pars intrasegmentalis venae pulmonum [TA], intrasegmental veins.

iridial p. of retina [TA], see retina. syn pars iridica retinae [TA].

labial p. of orbicularis oris (muscle) [TA], the major p. of the orbicularis oris muscle within the body of the lips. syn pars labialis musculi orbicularis oris [TA].

lacrimal p. of orbicularis oculi muscle [TA], part of orbicularis oculi (muscle) arising from lacrimal bone. see orbicularis oculi (muscle). syn pars lacrimalis musculi orbicularis oculi [TA], Duverney muscle, Horner muscle, musculus tensor tarsi.

laryngeal p. of pharynx, syn laryngopharynx.

lateral p. of longitudinal arch of foot [TA], portion of longitudinal arch of foot formed by the calcaneus, cuboid, and lateral two metatarsals (N–V); it is lower and less mobile than the medial part; it functions in the transmission of weight while the medial part of the arch functions to absorb the shock of the foot in locomotion. syn pars lateralis arcus pedis longitudinalis [TA].

lateral p. of middle lobe vein (of right superior pulmonary vein) [TA], the vein draining the lateral bronchopulmonary segment of the middle lobe of the right lung. syn pars lateralis venae lobi medii venae pulmonalis dextri superioris.

lateral p. of occipital bone [TA], the part of the occipital bone that lies on either side of the foramen magnum. syn pars lateralis ossis occipitalis [TA], exoccipital bone.

lateral p. of posterior cervical intertransversarii (muscles), see posterior cervical intertransversarii (muscles), under muscle.

lateral p. of posterior (extensor) compartment of forearm [TA], portion of the posterior fascial compartment of the forearm that includes the "lateral wad" muscles; brachioradialis and extensors radialis. syn pars lateralis compartimenti antebrachii posterioris (extensorum) [TA], radial p. of posterior compartment of forearm✫.

lateral p. of sacrum [TA], the mass of the sacrum lateral to the sacral foramina formed by the fused costal elements. syn pars lateralis ossis sacri [TA].

lateral p. of vaginal fornix [TA], see vaginal fornix. syn pars lateralis fornicis vaginae [TA].

left p. of liver, ✫official alternate term for left liver.

lumbar p. of diaphragm [TA], the portion of the diaphragm that arises from the upper lumbar vertebrae and from the medial and lateral arcuate ligaments. see right crus of diaphragm, left crus of diaphragm, lateral arcuate ligament, medial arcuate ligament. syn pars lumbalis diaphragmatis [TA], vertebral p. of diaphragm.

lumbar p. of spinal cord [TA], portion of spinal cord that consists of the five lumbar segments (L1–L5) and from which five pairs of lumbar spinal nerves originate; in the adult it is located in the T10–L1 portion of the vertebral canal, and is enlarged relative to other parts of the cord because of its involvement in innervation of the lower limb. syn pars lumbalis medullae spinalis [TA], lumbar segments L1–L5 of spinal cord, segmenta lumbalia L1–L5, segmenta lumbalia medullae spinalis.

marginal p. of orbicularis oris (muscle) [TA], the p. of the orbicularis oris muscle located in the margin of the lips, i.e., the red area. syn pars marginalis musculi orbicularis oris [TA].

mastoid p. of the temporal bone, syn mastoid process of petrous part of temporal bone.

medial p. of longitudinal arch of foot [TA], portion of longitudinal arch of foot formed by the calcaneus, talus, mavicular, cuneiforms, and medial metatarsals [I–III]. SEE longitudinal *arch* of foot. SYN pars medialis arcus pedis longitudinalis [TA]. SEE longitudinal *arch* of foot.

medial p. of middle lobe vein (of right superior pulmonary vein) [TA], the vein draining the medial bronchopulmonary segment of the middle lobe of the right lung. SYN pars medialis venae lobi medii venae pulmonis dextri superioris [TA].

mediastinal p. of lung, SYN mediastinal *surface* of lung.

mediastinal p. of parietal pleura [TA], the continuation of the costal and diaphragmatic pleura of each side that passes from the vertebral column and sternum covering the sides of the mediastinum. SYN pars mediastinalis pleurae parietalis [TA], mediastinal pleura, pleura mediastinalis.

membranous p. of interventricular septum [TA], p. of the fibrous skeleton of the heart that is seen as a small, thin, round or oval nonmuscular area at the superior end of the interventricular septum; it lies just below and is continuous with the portion of the fibrous ring of the aortic valve supporting the anterior and posterior cusps, and with the right fibrous trigone; the atrioventricular bundle of conducting tissue courses along its dorsal margin and bifurcates at its inferior margin into the right and left crura. SYN pars membranacea septi interventricularis [TA], membranous septum (2), septum membranaceum ventriculorum.

membranous p. of male urethra, SYN intermediate p. of male urethra.

membranous p. of nasal septum [TA], the small portion of the nasal septum anterior and inferior to the portion supported by the cartilage of the nasal septum. SYN pars membranacea septi nasi [TA], membranous septum (1).

mobile p. of nasal septum [TA], the anteroinferior movable part of the nasal septum formed by the membranous part and the medial crus of the greater alar cartilage on each side. SYN pars mobilis septi nasi [TA], septum mobile nasi.

muscular p. of interventricular septum (of heart) [TA], the thick muscular portion that composes most of the interventricular septum of the heart. SYN pars muscularis septi interventricularis (cordis) [TA], septum musculare ventriculorum.

mylopharyngeal p. of superior constrictor muscle of pharynx [TA], SEE superior pharyngeal constrictor (*muscle*). SYN pars mylopharyngeus musculi constrictoris pharyngis superioris [TA], mylopharyngeal p. of superior pharyngeal constrictor (muscle) of pharynx.

mylopharyngeal p. of superior pharyngeal constrictor (muscle) of pharynx, SYN mylopharyngeal p. of superior constrictor muscle of pharynx.

nasal p. of frontal bone [TA], nasal portion of the frontal bone which lies between the two orbital parts anteriorly and forms part of the roof of the nasal cavity. SYN pars nasalis ossis frontalis [TA].

nasal p. of pharynx, SYN nasopharynx.

nervous p. of retina, SYN optic p. of retina. SYN pars nervosa retinae.

neural p. of hypophysis, SYN neurohypophysis.

oblique p. of cricothyroid (muscle) [TA], SEE cricothyroid *muscle*. SYN pars obliqua musculi cricothyroidei [TA].

occipital p. of corpus callosum, SYN major *forceps*.

opercular p. [TA], one of the three small cortical convolutions together forming a cover for the insular region. Opercular convolutions are frontal, temporal, and parietal. SYN pars opercularis [TA].

p. of optic nerve in canal [TA], the part of the optic nerve lying within the optic canal. SYN pars canalis nervi optici [TA].

optic p. of retina [TA], SEE retina. SYN nervous p. of retina.

oral p. of pharynx, SYN oropharynx.

orbital p. of frontal bone [TA], the portion of the frontal bone that contributes to the formation of the orbits. SYN pars orbitalis ossis frontalis [TA].

orbital p. of lacrimal gland [TA], SEE lacrimal *gland*. SYN pars orbitalis glandulae lacrimalis [TA].

orbital p. of optic nerve [TA], the part of the optic nerve between the eyeball and the optic canal, i.e., within the orbit. SYN pars orbitalis nervi optici [TA].

orbital p. of orbicularis oculi (muscle) [TA], SYN *pars* orbitalis musculi orbicularis oculi; SEE orbicularis oculi (*muscle*).

orbital p. [TA] of inferior frontal gyrus, the rostral and slightly ventral portion of the inferior frontal gyrus. SYN pars orbitalis [TA].

osseous p. of skeletal system, SYN bony p. of skeletal system.

palpebral p. of lacrimal gland [TA], SEE lacrimal *gland*. SYN pars palpebralis glandulae lacrimalis [TA].

palpebral p. of orbicularis oculi (muscle) [TA], SEE orbicularis oculi (*muscle*). SYN pars palpebralis musculi orbicularis oculi [TA].

parasympathetic p. of autonomic division of peripheral nervous system [TA], the presynaptic (preganglionic) autonomic neurons having cell bodies located in the brain, associated with the motor nuclei of certain cranial nerves [CN III, VII, IX, and X], or in the gray matter of spinal cord segments S2–S4, and the postsynaptic neurons with which the presynaptic fibers connect (synapse); in the head, there are four discrete parasympathetic ganglia: ciliary, pterygopalatine, otic, and submandibular/sublingual; in the trunk, the postsynaptic cells occur as isolated intrinsic ganglia. SEE autonomic *division* of nervous system. SYN pars parasympathica divisionis automaticae systematis nervosi peripherici [TA], bulbosacral system, craniosacral division of autonomic nervous system, craniosacral nervous system.

patent p. of umbilical artery [TA], portion of umbilical artery between its origin as a branch of the internal iliac artery and its postnatal occlusion distal to the origin of the superior vesicle arteries. SYN pars patens arteriae umbilicalis [TA].

pelvic p. [TA], the portion of a structure that is located within or is related to the pelvis. SEE pelvic part of ductus deferens, of parasympathetic part of autonomic division of nervous system, and of ureter. SYN pars pelvica [TA].

pelvic p. of ductus deferens [TA], portion of ductus deferens extending between the deep inguinal ring and the ampulla. SYN pars pelvica ductus deferentes [TA].

pelvic p. of peripheral autonomic plexuses and ganglia [TA], portion of the autonomic nerve plexuses which extend into and lie within the lesser pelvis, i.e., inferior to the plane of the pelvic inlet; included are the superior and inferior hypogastric plexuses, and the plexuses of the pelvic viscera: middle and inferior rectal, vesical, uterovaginal, prostatic and deferential; although technically they exit the pelvis and course within the erectile bodies of the perineum, the cavernous nerves of the penis and clitoris are also included. SYN pars pelvica plexus visceralis et ganglii visceralis [TA].

pelvic p. of ureter [TA], the p. of the ureter between the brim of the pelvis and the urinary bladder. SYN pars pelvica ureteris [TA].

pelvic p. of the urogenital sinus, the upper pelvic portion of the embryologic urogenital sinus.

peripheral p. of nervous system, SYN peripheral nervous *system*.

petrous p. of internal carotid artery [TA], the part of the internal carotid artery in the carotid canal; its branches are carotidotympanic arteries and the artery of the pterygoid canal. SYN pars petrosa arteriae carotidis internae [TA], petrous bone.

petrous p. of temporal bone [TA], the part of the temporal bone that contains the structures of the inner ear and the second part of the internal carotid artery; in antenatal life it appears as a separate ossification center. SYN pars petrosa ossis temporalis [TA], periotic bone, petrosal bone, petrous pyramid.

phrenicoceliac p. of suspensory muscle (ligament) of duodenum [TA], slip of skeletal muscle arising from the right crus of the diaphragm near the esophageal hiatus and joining the celiacoduodenal part to attach to the terminal duodenum and duodenojejunal flexure. SYN pars phrenicocoeliaca musculi (ligamenti) suspensorii duodeni [TA].

pial p. of filum terminale [TA], portion of the filum terminale within the dural sac; it is composed of a prolongation of the pia caudal to the termination of the spinal cord at the tip of the conus medullaris. SEE ALSO terminal *filum*. SYN pars pialis fili terminalis [TA], filum terminale internum✶, pial filament✶.

pigmented p. of retina, SYN pars pigmentosa. SEE retina.

postcommunicating p. of anterior cerebral artery [TA], portion of anterior cerebral artery distal to the anterior communicating artery. SYN pars postcommunicalis arteriae cerebri anterioris [TA], A2 segment of anterior cerebral artery★, segmentum A2 arteriae cerebri anterioris★.

postcommunicating p. of posterior cerebral artery [TA], portion of posterior cerebral artery distal to the posterior communicating artery. SYN pars postcommunicalis arteriae cerebri posterioris [TA], P2 segment of posterior cerebral artery★.

posterior p. [TA], the posterior portion of the anterior commissure of the brain.

posterior p. of anterior commissure of brain [TA], major, posterior portion of the connection between the paired olfactory bulbs and adjacent portions of the cortex of the frontal and temporal lobes. SYN pars posterior commissurae anterioris [TA].

posterior p. of the diaphragmatic surface of the liver [TA], that portion of the diaphragmatic surface of the liver that includes the bare area and the caudate lobe. SYN pars posterior faciei diaphragmatis hepatis [TA].

posterior p. of liver, ★official alternate term for posterior hepatic *segment* I.

posterior tibiotalar p. of deltoid ligament, SYN tibiotalar p. of medial ligament of ankle joint.

posterior tibiotalar p. of medial ligament of ankle joint [TA], SEE medial *ligament* of ankle joint.

posterior p. of tongue [TA], portion (posterior third) of tongue that lies posterior to the terminal sulcus, it is distinct from the anterior part (anterior two-thirds) of tongue in both its embryologic origin and its innervation. SEE ALSO *dorsum* of tongue. SYN pars posterior linguae [TA], pars postsulcalis linguae★, postsulcal p. of tongue★.

posterior p. of vaginal fornix [TA], SYN pars posterior fornicis vaginae [TA].

postlaminar p. of intraocular part of optic nerve [TA], the portion of the intraocular part of the optic nerve immediately posterior to the lamina cribrosa of the sclera. SYN pars postlaminaris nervi optici intraocularis [TA].

postsulcal p. of tongue, ★official alternate term for posterior p. of tongue.

precommunicating p. of anterior cerebral artery [TA], portion of anterior cerebral artery proximal to the anterior communicating artery. SYN pars precommunicalis arteriae cerebri anterioris [TA], A1 segment of anterior cerebral artery★, segmentum A1 arteriae cerebri anterioris★, precommunical segment of anterior cerebral artery.

precommunicating p. of posterior cerebral artery [TA], portion of posterior cerebral artery proximal to the posterior communicating artery. SYN pars precommunicalis arteriae cerebri posterioris [TA], P1 segment of posterior cerebral artery, precommunical segment of posterior cerebral artery.

prelaminar p. of intraocular part of optic nerve [TA], the portion of the intraocular part of the optic nerve immediately anterior to the lamina cribrosa of the sclera. SYN pars prelaminaris nervi optici intraocularis [TA].

preprostatic p. of male urethra, ★official alternate term for intramural p. of male urethra.

presulcal p. of tongue, ★official alternate term for anterior p. of tongue.

prevertebral p. of vertebral artery [TA], SEE vertebral *artery*. SYN pars prevertebralis arteriae prevertebralis [TA].

proximal p. of prostate [TA], portion of prostate derived from the more rostral anlage; includes anterior and middle lobes of mature prostate. SYN pars proximalis prostatae [TA].

proximal p. of prostatic urethra [TA], portion of prostatic urethra superior to the merging of the urinary and genital tracts at the openings of the ejaculatory ducts. SYN pars proximalis urethrae prostaticae [TA].

psoatic p. of iliopsoas fascia [TA], portion of the fascia overlying the iliopsoas (muscle), the specific portion directly related to the psoatic portion. SYN pars psoatica fasciae iliopsoaticae [TA].

pterygopharyngeal p. of superior constrictor muscle of pharynx [TA], SEE superior pharyngeal constrictor (*muscle*). SYN pars pterygopharyngea musculi constrictoris pharyngis superioris.

pyloric p. of stomach [TA], that portion of the stomach between the angular notch and the pylorus; its mucosa contains pyloric glands. SYN pars pylorica gastris [TA], pars pylorica ventriculi.

quadrate p. of liver [TA], SYN anterior *portion* of left medial segment IV of liver.

radial p. of posterior compartment of forearm, ★official alternate term for lateral p. of posterior (extensor) compartment of forearm.

retrolenticular p. of internal capsule, that portion of the capsule caudal to the lentiform nucleus that contains occipitopontine fibers [TA], occipitiotectal fibers [TA], optic radiations [TA] (geniculocalcarine fibers [TA], posterior thalamic radiation [TA], and other fiber systems. SEE ALSO retrolenticular *limb* of internal capsule. SYN pars retrolentiformis capsulae internae [TA].

right p. of diaphragmatic surface of liver [TA], the part of the diaphragmatic surface of the liver deep to the bodies of the lower ribs on the right side. SYN pars dextra faciei diaphragmaticae hepatis [TA].

right p. of liver, ★official alternate term for right *liver*.

sacral p. of spinal cord [TA], the part of the cord from which consists of the five sacral segments of the spinal cord (S1–S5) and from which five pairs of sacral nerves originate. SYN pars sacralis medullae spinalis [TA], segmenta sacralia medullae spinalis [TA].

scrotal p. of ductus deferens [TA], initial portion of ductus deferens, between the epididymis and the spermatic cord, as the ductus runs parallel to the epididymis and the testis. SYN pars scrotalis ductus deferentis [TA].

second p. of duodenum, SYN descending p. of duodenum.

soft p.'s, the nonbony and noncartilaginous tissues of the body.

soleal p. of posterior (plantar flexor) compartment of leg [TA], portion of posterior osteofascial compartment of leg that includes the soleus muscle. SYN pars solealis compartimenti cruris posterioris [TA].

sphenoid p. of middle cerebral artery [TA], SEE middle cerebral *artery*. SYN pars sphenoidalis arteriae cerebralis mediae [TA].

spinal p. of accessory nerve, ★official alternate term for spinal *root* of accessory nerve.

spinal p. of arachnoid, SYN spinal *arachnoid* mater.

spinal p. of deltoid (muscle) [TA], portion of deltoid (muscle) originating from the spine of the scapula. SYN pars spinalis musculi deltoidei [TA].

spinal p. of filum terminale [TA], initial (superiormost) portion of filum terminale at the tip of the conus medullaris that still includes a central canal. SYN pars spinalis fili terminalis [TA].

spongy p. of the male urethra, SYN spongy *urethra*.

squamous p. of frontal bone [TA], the broad, curved portion of the frontal bone forming the forehead. SYN squama frontalis [TA].

squamous p. of occipital bone [TA], the tabular or squamous portion of occipital bone. SYN squama occipitalis, occipital squama [TA], frontal squama.

squamous p. of temporal bone [TA], the broad, flat, thin (scale-like) anterior and superior portion of the temporal bone forming part of the lateral wall of the cranial vault. SYN pars squamosa ossis temporalis [TA], squama temporalis, temporal squama.

sternal p. of diaphragm [TA], the small slip on each side that arises from the inner surface of the xiphoid process and inserts on the central tendon. SYN pars sternalis diaphragmatis [TA].

sternocostal p. of pectoralis major muscle, SYN sternocostal *head* of pectoralis major (muscle). SEE pectoralis major (*muscle*).

straight p. of cricothyroid muscle [TA], SEE cricothyroid *muscle*.

subcutaneous p. of external anal sphincter [TA], SEE external anal *sphincter*. SYN pars subcutanea musculi sphincteri ani externi [TA], subcutaneous portion of external anal sphincter.

sublenticular p. of internal capsule, the part of the internal capsule below the caudal third of the lentiform nucleus that contains the acoustic radiation [TA] (geniculotemporal fibers [TA]), corticotectal fibers [TA], temporopontine fibers [TA], and corticothalamic fibers as well as that part of the optic radiation representing the upper part of the contralateral half of the binocular visual field. SEE ALSO sublentiform *limb* of internal capsule. SYN pars sublentiformis capsulae internae [TA].

pa

suboccipital p. of vertebral artery, SYN atlantic p. of vertebral artery.

superficial p. of anterior (flexor) compartment of forearm [TA], portion of anterior (flexor) compartment of forearm including the superficial (and intermediate) layers of pronator and flexor muscles: pronator teres, flexor carpi radialis, palmaris longus, flexor carpi ulnaris, and flexor digitorum superficialis. SYN pars superficialis compartimenti antebrachii anterioris [TA].

superficial p. of external anal sphincter [TA], SEE external anal *sphincter.* SYN pars superficialis musculi sphincteri ani externi [TA].

superficial p. of masseter muscle [TA], SEE masseter (*muscle*). SYN pars superficialis musculi masseteri [TA].

superficial p. of parotid gland [TA], SEE parotid *gland.* SYN pars superficialis glandulae parotideae [TA].

superficial p. of posterior (plantar flexor) compartment of leg [TA], portion of posterior (plantar flexor) compartment of leg including the gastrocnemius and soleus (muscles); it is separated from the deep part by the transverse intermuscular septum of leg. SYN pars superficialis compartimenti cruris posterioris [TA], pars tricipitalis compartimenti cruris posterioris✖.

superior p. of diaphragmatic surface of liver [TA], the convex superior portion of the diaphragmatic surface of the liver. SYN pars superior faciei diaphragmaticae hepatis [TA].

superior p. of duodenum, initial (first) part of duodenum immediately distal to the pylorus and proximal to the descending (second) part. SEE duodenum. SYN pars superior duodeni [TA], first p. of duodenum, pars prima duodeni. SEE duodenum.

superior p. of lingular vein (of left superior pulmonary vein) [TA], the vein that drains the superior lingular bronchopulmonary segment of the left lung. SYN pars superior venae lingularis venae pulmonis superioris sinistri [TA].

superior p. of vestibular ganglion [TA], rostral part, the superior part of the vestibular ganglion that receives fibers from the maculae of the utricle and the saccule and the ampullae of the anterior and lateral semicircular ducts. SYN pars superior ganglii vestibularis [TA].

superior p. of vestibulocochlear nerve, SYN vestibular *nerve.*

supraclavicular p. of brachial plexus [TA], the part of the brachial plexus that lies superior to the clavicle; it includes the roots, trunks, and divisions that give rise to the dorsal scapular, long thoracic, suprascapular and subclavian nerves. SYN pars supraclavicularis plexus brachialis [TA].

supravaginal p. of cervix [TA], the part of the cervix of the uterus lying above the attachment of the vagina. SYN portio supravaginalis cervicis [TA].

sympathetic p. of autonomic division of peripheral nervous system [TA], the sympathetic part of the autonomic division of the nervous system. SEE ALSO autonomic *division* of nervous system. SYN pars sympathica (divisionis autonomicae systematis nervosei peripherici) [TA], sympathetic nervous system, thoracolumbar nervous system.

tense p. of the tympanic membrane [TA], the greater portion of the tympanic membrane that is tense and firm, contrasting with the small triangular flaccid part of tympanic membrane. SYN pars tensa membranae tympani [TA], membrana tensa, membrana vibrans.

terminal p., SYN *pars* terminalis; SEE terminal *branches* of middle cerebral artery, under *branch*, posterior cerebral *artery.*

third p. of duodenum, SYN inferior p. of duodenum.

thoracic p. of aorta, SYN thoracic *aorta.*

thoracic p. of esophagus [TA], the p. of the esophagus between the superior thoracic aperture and the diaphragm. SYN pars thoracica esophagi [TA].

thoracic p. of iliocostalis lumborum (muscle) [TA], portion of the iliocostalis muscle which extends superiorly from the costal angles of the lower six ribs to the costal angles of the upper six ribs and the transverse process of vertebra C7, between iliocostalis lumborum inferiorly and laterally and iliocostalis cervicis superiorly and medially. SYN pars thoracica muscularis iliocostalis lumborum [TA].

thoracic p. of peripheral autonomic plexuses and ganglia [TA], autonomic plexuses of the thoracic viscera: heart/aorta, lungs/bronchi, and esophagus, and associated parasympathetic ganglia. SYN pars thoracica plexuum et ganglionorum visceralium [TA].

thoracic p. of spinal cord [TA], the p. of the spinal cord that consists of the twelve thoracic segments [T1–T12] of the spinal cord from which the twelve pairs of thoracic nerves [T1–T12] originate. SYN pars thoracica medullae spinalis [TA], segmenta thoracica medullae spinalis [TA].

thoracic p. of thoracic duct [TA], portion of the thoracic duct within the thorax, from aortic hiatus to the level of the first thoracic vertebra. SYN pars thoracica ductus thoracici [TA].

thoracic p. of trachea [TA], portion of trachea that lies within the thorax, that is, the portion between the plane of the superior thoracic aperture above and the bifurcation of the trachea at the level of the sternal angle below. SYN pars thoracica tracheae [TA].

thyroepiglottic p. of thyroarytenoid (muscle) [TA], intrinsic muscle of larynx; *origin,* inner surface of thyroid cartilage in common with the thyroarytenoideus p.; *insertion,* aryepiglottic fold and margin of epiglottis; *action,* depresses base of epiglottis; *nerve supply,* recurrent laryngeal. SYN pars thyroepiglottica musculi thyroarytenoidei [TA], depressor muscle of epiglottis, musculus thyroepiglotticus, thyroepiglottic muscle, thyroepiglottidean muscle, ventricularis (2).

thyropharyngeal p. of inferior constrictor muscle of pharynx [TA], SEE inferior constrictor (*muscle*) of pharynx. SYN pars thyropharyngea musculi constrictoris pharyngis inferioris [TA], thyropharyngeal p. of inferior pharyngeal constrictor (muscle) of pharynx.

thyropharyngeal p. of inferior pharyngeal constrictor (muscle) of pharynx, SYN thyropharyngeal p. of inferior constrictor muscle of pharynx.

tibiocalcaneal p. of deltoid ligament, ✖official alternate term for tibiocalcaneal p. of medial ligament of ankle joint.

tibiocalcaneal p. of medial ligament of ankle joint [TA], the part of the medial or deltoid ligament that extends from the medial malleolus to the sustentaculum tali of the calcaneus. SYN pars tibiocalcanea ligamenti collateralis medialis articulationis talocruralis [TA], pars tibiocalcanea ligamenti deltoidei✖, tibiocalcaneal p. of deltoid ligament✖, calcaneotibial ligament, ligamentum calcaneotibiale, tibiocalcaneal ligament.

tibionavicular p. of deltoid ligament, SYN tibionavicular p. of medial ligament of ankle joint.

tibionavicular p. of medial ligament of ankle joint [TA], the part of the medial or deltoid ligament that extends from the medial malleolus to the navicular bone. SEE ALSO medial *ligament* of ankle joint. SYN pars tibionavicularis ligamenti collateralis medialis articulationis talocrucalis [TA], ligamentum tibionaviculare, tibionavicular ligament, tibionavicular p. of deltoid ligament.

tibiotalar p. of medial ligament of ankle joint [TA], the part of the medial or deltoid ligament that extends from the medial malleolus to the posterior process of the talus. SYN pars tibiotalaris posterior ligamenti collateralis medialis articulationis talocruralis [TA], ligamentum talotibiale posterius, posterior talotibial ligament, posterior tibiotalar ligament, posterior tibiotalar p. of deltoid ligament.

transversarial p. of vertebral artery [TA], SYN cervical p. of vertebral artery.

transverse p. of iliofemoral ligament [TA], the more horizontal limb of the inverted Y-shaped iliofemoral ligament. SYN pars transversa ligamenti iliofemoralis [TA].

transverse p. of left branch of portal vein [TA], the long unbranched portion of the left branch of the portal vein. SYN pars transversa rami sinistri venae portae hepatis [TA].

transverse p. of nasalis muscle [TA], SEE nasalis (*muscle*). SYN pars transversa musculi nasalis [TA].

transverse p. of trapezius (muscle) [TA], middle third of trapezius with muscle fibers running transversely to the spine of the scapula; acts to retract the scapulae (shoulders) at the conceptual scapulothoracic joint. SYN pars transversa musculi trapezii [TA].

triangular p. [TA], the middle one of three small convolutions that together compose the inferior frontal gyrus of the cerebral cortex, the other two being the orbital part and opercular part. SYN pars triangularis [TA].

tympanic p. of temporal bone, SYN tympanic *plate* of temporal bone.

umbilical p. of left branch of portal vein [TA], the highly branched part of the left branch of the portal vein; the round and venous ligaments attach to this part. SYN pars umbilicalis rami sinistri venae portae hepatis [TA].

uterine p. of uterine tube [TA], the part of the uterine tube located within the wall of the uterus. SYN pars uterina tubae uterinae [TA].

uveal p. of trabecular reticulum, SYN uveal p. of trabecular tissue of sclera.

uveal p. of trabecular tissue of sclera [TA], the posterior part of the trabecular reticulum, located between the scleral spur, the ciliary body, and the anterior surface of the iris. SYN pars uvealis reticuli trabecularis sclerae [TA], uveal p. of trabecular reticulum.

vagal p. of accessory nerve, ☆official alternate term for cranial *root* of accessory nerve; SEE accessory *nerve* [CN XI].

vaginal p. of cervix [TA], the part of the cervix uteri contained within the vagina. SYN portio vaginalis cervicis [TA].

ventral p. of intertransversarii laterales lumborum (muscles) [TA], portions of the lateral intertransversarii of the lumbar region connecting the costal elements of the transverse processes of the lumbar vertebrae. SYN pars ventralis musculi intertransversarii lateralium lumborum [TA].

ventral p. of pons, SYN basilar p. of pons.

vertebral p. of the costal surface of the lungs [TA], the p. of the medial surface of the lung in contact with the vertebral bodies. SYN pars vertebralis faciei costalis pulmonis [TA].

vertebral p. of diaphragm, SYN lumbar p. of diaphragm.

vestibular p. of vestibulocochlear nerve, SYN vestibular *nerve*.

part. aeq. Abbreviation for L. *partes aequales,* in equal parts (amounts).

par·tes (par′tēz). Plural of pars.

par·the·no·gen·e·sis (par′the-nō-jen′ĕ-sis). A form of nonsexual reproduction, or agamogenesis, in which the female reproduces its kind without fecundation by the male. SYN apogamia, apogamy, apomixia, virgin generation. [G. *parthenos,* virgin, + *genesis,* product]

par·the·no·pho·bia (par′the-nō-fō′bē-ă). Morbid fear of girls. [G. *parthenos,* virgin, + *phobos,* fear]

par·ti·cle (par′ti-kl). 1. A very small piece or portion of anything. 2. An elementary p. such as a proton or electron. [L. *particula,* dim. of *pars,* part]

alpha p. (α), a p. consisting of two neutrons and two protons, with a positive charge $(2e^+)$; emitted energetically from the nuclei of unstable isotopes of high atomic number (elements of mass number from 82 up); identical to the helium nucleus. SYN alpha ray.

beta p., an electron, either positively (positron, β^+) or negatively (negatron, β^-) charged, emitted during beta decay of a radionuclide. SEE ALSO cathode *rays,* under *ray.* SYN beta ray.

chromatin p.'s, fine bluish dots thought to represent remnants of the nucleus, occasionally seen in stained erythrocytes.

core p., released by partial enzymatic digestion of chromatin.

Dane p.'s, the larger spherical forms of hepatitis-associated antigens; they compose the virion of hepatitis B virus, containing a 27-nm "core" in which DNA-dependent DNA polymerase and circular, double-stranded DNA have been found.

defective interfering p., an incomplete virus that is unable to replicate and interferes with replication of an infectious virus.

D.I. p., abbreviation for defective interfering p.

electron transport p.'s (ETP), fragments of mitochondria still capable of transporting electrons. SYN submitochondrial p.'s.

elementary p., (1) SYN platelet; (2) one of the units occurring on the matrical surface of mitochondrial cristae; the head of the p., which measures about 9 nm, attaches to the membrane of the crista by a stalk 5 nm long; the p.'s may be concerned with the electron transport system.

kappa p.'s, inheritable cytoplasmic symbionts, once thought to be

p.'s mainly or exclusively of DNA, occurring in some strains of *Paramecium;* capable of producing a product lethal to other strains.

signal recognition p. (SRP), a small RNA-protein complex that interacts with the signal sequence of nascent secretory proteins. Binding of the signal recognition p. results in arrest of translation until interaction with docking protein, an integral part of the endoplasmic reticulum membrane.

submitochondrial p.'s, SYN electron transport p.'s.

Zimmermann elementary p., obsolete term for platelet.

par·tic·u·late (par-tik′ū-lāt). Relating to or occurring in the form of fine particles.

par·tic·u·lates (par-tik′ū-lats). Formed elements, discrete bodies, as contrasted with the surrounding liquid or semiliquid material; e.g., granules or mitochondria in cells.

partogram (par′tō-gram). Graph of labor parameters of time and dilation with alert and action lines to prompt intervention if the curve deviates from expected. SYN Friedman curve, labor curve. [L. *partus,* childbirth, + -gram]

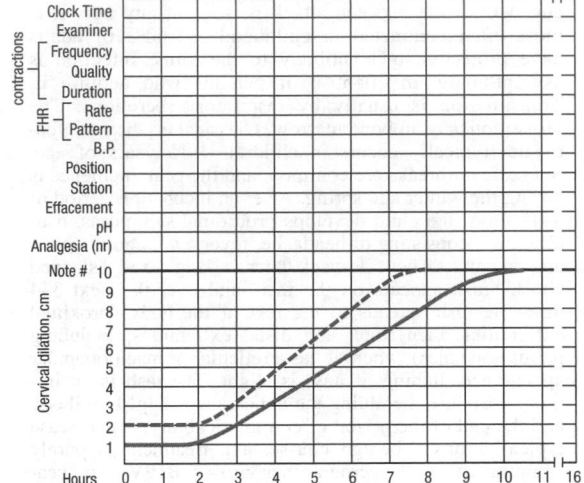

partogram: flowsheet for charting labor progress, FHR = fetal heart rate

par·tu·ri·ent (par-too′rē-ent). Relating to or in the process of childbirth. [L. *parturio,* to be in labor]

par·tu·ri·fa·cient (par-toor-ē-fā′shent). 1. Inducing or accelerating labor. 2. An agent that induces or accelerates labor. SYN oxytocic (2). [L. *parturio,* to be in labor, + *facio,* to make]

par·tu·ri·tion (par-toor-ish′ŭn). SYN childbirth. [L. *parturitio,* fr. *parturio,* to be in labor]

part. vic. Abbreviation for L. *partes vicibus,* in divided doses.

pa·ru·lis, pl. **pa·ru·li·des** (pă-roo′lis, -li-dēz). SYN gingival *abscess.* [G. *paroulis,* gumboil, fr. *para,* beside, + *oulon,* gum]

par·um·bil·i·cal (par′ŭm-bil′i-kăl). SYN paraumbilical.

par·u·re·sis (par-ū-rē′sis). Inhibited urination, especially in the presence of strangers. [para- + G. *ourēsis,* urination]

par·val·bu·min (par-val-bū′min). Any of a group of small water-soluble calcium-binding proteins distinct from calmodulin and other calcium-binding proteins; found in the brain, skeletal muscle, and retina, but not in the heart, liver, or spleen, of various species. [L. *parvus,* small, + albumin]

Par·vo·bac·te·ri·a·ce·ae (par′vō-bak-tēr-ē-ā′sē-ē). A family name regarded as a former name for the bacterial family Brucellaceae. No type genus has ever been proposed for the family P.

par·vo·cel·lu·lar (par-vō-sel′ū-lăr). Relating to or composed of cells of small size. [L. *parvus,* small, + Mod. L. *cellularis,* cellular]

par·vo·line (par′vō-lēn). A ptomaine, $C_9H_{13}N$, from decaying fish.

Par·vo·vir·i·dae (par-vō-vir′i-dē). A family of small viruses containing single-stranded DNA. Virions are 18–26 nm in diameter, are not enveloped, and are ether-resistant. Capsids are of cubic symmetry, with 32 capsomeres. Replication and assembly occur in the nucleus of infected cells. Three genera in the subfamily Parvovirinae are recognized: Parvovirus, Erythrovirus, and Dependovirus, which includes the adeno-associated virus. A second subfamily, Densovirinae, has 3 additional genera, all of which infect arthropods.

Par·vo·vi·rus (par′vō-vī-rŭs). A genus of viruses (family Parvoviridae) that replicate autonomously in suitable cells. Strain B19 infects humans, causing erythema infectiosum and aplastic crisis in hemolytic anemia. [L. *parvus,* small, + virus]

Par·vo·vi·rus B19. A single-stranded DNA virus belonging to the family Parvoviridae; the cause of erythema infectiosum (fifth disease) and aplastic crises.

Parvovirus B19 (B19V) was first isolated in 1975 from a specimen of healthy donor blood. In 1983 it was linked to erythema infectiosum, also called fifth disease, a generally benign febrile exanthem of children. B19V infection occurs worldwide and can attack persons of any age. It is most often contracted in childhood; 30–60% of adults have protective IgG antibody to the virus. Infection is asymptomatic in 20–50% of persons who acquire it. Transmission is usually by respiratory secretions. The virus replicates in bone marrow. Classical erythema infectiosum typically occurs in children 4–15 years of age. Sporadic outbreaks are common, and the peak incidence is during the winter and spring. After an incubation period of 4–14 days, the child develops prodromal symptoms, usually mild, consisting of headache, fever, chills, joint pains, and malaise. About 1 week later, a bright red "slapped cheek" rash appears on the face, and over the next 3–4 days the rash spreads to the rest of the body (proximal extremities, then trunk and distal extremities, including palms and soles), where it has a reticular or maculopapular appearance. Itching, if any, is slight. The rash is an immune response, heralding the appearance of IgM antibody and the end of the period of communicability. The disease typically runs a benign course, and treatment is purely symptomatic. (Like certain other viruses, B19V also occasionally causes a benign exanthem known as papular-purpuric gloves-and-socks syndrome.) Infection in adults follows a different pattern: the "slapped cheek" appearance does not occur, and the rash on the trunk and limbs tends to be milder and more subtle, but 15–20% of adult patients, virtually all of them women, develop significant joint involvement. Deposition of immune complexes in joint membranes leads to sudden onset of symmetric polyarthritis, affecting particularly the metacarpophalangeal and proximal interphalangeal joints, the wrists, and the knees. Swelling may or may not occur. Pain and disability can be severe, and symptoms can persist for weeks or months, although eventual spontaneous resolution is the rule. Because B19V infects the bone marrow, most patients experience a transient decline in red blood cells, white blood cells, and platelets. Generally this is of no consequence, but occasionally it progresses to a transient aplastic crisis (TAC), in which red blood cell production virtually stops and the red blood cell count falls rapidly. The risk of this complication is much greater in sickle cell anemia, autoimmune hemolytic anemias, immunodeficiency, and pregnancy. With the formation of IgG antibody by the immune system, red blood cell formation resumes and the anemia resolves. In patients with congenital or acquired immune deficiency, however, failure to form antibody can lead to prolonged anemia. Infection in a pregnant woman has about 1 chance in 3 of being passed to the fetus and inducing a fetal aplastic crisis. This in turn can result in congestive heart failure and fetal hydrops. Spontaneous recovery is typical, but fetal death occurs in as many as 10% of cases. Fetal infection with B19V apparently does not cause congenital anomalies. Acute B19V infection can be confirmed by a rapid rise and fall of IgM

antibody. Diagnosis can also be established by culturing the virus from bone marrow or by ELISA detection of the antigen in serum. The treatment of all forms of B19V infection is purely symptomatic and supportive, since specific antiviral therapy is not available. Hospitalized patients with B19V are isolated, and pregnant workers are advised to avoid contact with them. Severe anemia may require blood transfusions. When prolonged anemia results from inability to form IgM antibody, intravenous immune globulin may help.

par·vule (par′vool). A very small pill. [L. *parvulus,* very small, fr. *parvus,* small]

par·vus (par′vŭs). Small. [L.]

PAS Abbreviation for *p*-aminosalicylic acid; periodic acid-Schiff *stain.*

PASA Abbreviation for *p*-aminosalicylic acid.

Pascal, Blaise, French scientist, 1623–1662. SEE pascal; P. *law.*

pas·cal (Pa) (pas′kăl). A derived unit of pressure or stress in the SI system, expressed in newtons per square meter; equal to 10^{-5} bar or 7.50062×10^{-3} torr. [B. *Pascal*]

Pascheff (Pashev), Konstantin M., Bulgarian ophthalmologist, 1873–1961. SEE P. *conjunctivitis.*

Paschen, Enrique, German pathologist, 1860–1936. SEE P. *bodies,* under *body.*

Pashev. SEE Pascheff.

Pasini, Augustine, 20th century Argentinian dermatologist. SEE *atrophoderma* of P. and Pierini.

pas·pal·ism (pas′păl-izm). Poisoning by seeds of a species of grass, *Paspalum scrobiculatum.* [G. *paspalos,* a kind of millet, fr. *pas,* all, + *palē,* meal]

pas·sage (pas′ij). **1.** The act of passing. **2.** A discharge, as from the bowels or of urine. **3.** Inoculation of a series of animals with the same strain of a pathogenic microorganism whereby the virulence usually is increased, but is sometimes diminished. **4.** A channel, duct, pore, or opening. [Mediev. L. *passo,* to pass]

blind p., successive transfer of an agent through cultures or animals without apparent replication or disease.

nasopharyngeal p., SYN nasopharyngeal *meatus.*

oropharyngeal p., SYN fauces.

serial p., successive transfer of an infectious agent through a series of cultures or experimental animals, usually to attenuate pathogenicity.

Pas·sal·u·rus am·big·u·us (pa-sal′ū-rŭs am-big′ū-ŭs). The rabbit pinworm, an oxyurid nematode found abundantly in the cecum and large intestine of rabbits.

Passavant, Philippas G., German physician, 1815–1893. SEE P. *bar, cushion, pad, ridge.*

Passey, R.D., 20th century British pathologist. SEE Harding-P. *melanoma.*

pas·si·flo·ra (pas-i-flō′ră). The passion-flower, *Passiflora incarnata* (family Passifloraceae), a climbing herb of the southern U.S.; the dried flowering and fruiting top has been used in neuralgia, dysmenorrhea, and insomnia, and as an application to hemorrhoids and for burns. [L. *passio,* passion, + *flos (flor-),* flower]

pas·sion (pash′ŭn). **1.** Intense emotion. **2.** Obsolete term for suffering or pain. [L. *passio,* fr. *patior,* pp. *passus,* to suffer]

pas·sive (pas′iv). Not active; submissive. [L. *passivus,* fr. *patior,* to endure]

pas·siv·ism (pas′iv-izm). **1.** An attitude of submission. **2.** A sexual practice in which the subject is submissive to the will of the partner in behavior that usually requires the consent of both participants (e.g., anal intercourse). SEE ALSO pathic. [see passive]

pas·siv·i·ty (pas-iv′i-tē). **1.** The condition of a metal having formed a protective oxide coating; e.g., rustless metals and aluminum become passive in air. **2.** In dentistry, the quality or condition of inactivity or rest assumed by the teeth, tissues, and denture when a removable partial denture is in place but not under masticatory pressure.

pas·ta, gen. and pl. **pas·tae** (pas′tă, -tē). SYN paste. [L.]

paste (pāst). A soft semisolid of firmer consistency than pap, but soft enough to flow slowly and not to retain its shape. SYN pasta. [L. *pasta*]

dermatologic p., a class of preparations consisting of starch, dextrin, sulfur, calcium carbonate, or zinc oxide made into a p. with glycerin, soft soap, petrolatum, or some fat, with which is incorporated some medicinal substance.

desensitizing p., an ointment, usually caustic, coagulating or cytotoxic, formulated to be applied to the cervix of a tooth for the purpose of obtunding pain from sensitive, exposed cementum or dentin.

past·er (pā′ster). The segment forming the part for near vision in two-piece bifocal lenses.

Pasteur, Louis, French chemist and bacteriologist, 1822–1895. SEE P. *vaccine, effect, pipette.*

Pas·teu·rel·la (pas-ter-el′ă). A genus of aerobic to facultatively anaerobic, nonmotile bacteria (family Brucellaceae) containing very small, Gram-negative, cocci or ellipsoidal to elongated rods which, with special methods, may show bipolar staining. These organisms are parasites of humans and other animals, including birds. The type species is *P. multocida.* [L. *Pasteur*]

P. aerogenes, a species found in swine that may cause human wound infections following pig bites.

P. multoci′da, a bacterial species that causes fowl cholera and hemorrhagic septicemia in warm-blooded animals and may infect dog or cat bites or scratches and cause cellulitis and septicemia in humans with chronic disease. Most common pathogen associated with cat and dog bites. Cause of pasteurellosis. It is the type species of the genus *P.*

P. pes′tis, SYN *Yersinia pestis.*

P. pseudotuberculo′sis, SYN *Yersinia pseudotuberculosis.*

P. "SP", a rarely encountered organism of problematic taxonomy that can cause infections after a guinea pig bite; human infections are quite rare, probably because the bacterium is not widespread and is of low virulence.

P. tularen′sis, SYN *Francisella tularensis.*

pas·teu·rel·la, pl. **pas·teu·rel·lae** (pas-ter-el′ă, pas-ter-el′ē). A vernacular term used to refer to any member of the genus *Pasteurella.*

pas·teur·el·lo·sis (pas′ter-ĕ-lō′sis). Infection with bacteria of the genus *Pasteurella.*

pas·teur·i·za·tion (pas′ter-i-zā′shŭn). The heating of milk, wines, fruit juices, etc., for about 30 minutes at 68°C (154.4°F) whereby living bacteria are destroyed, but the flavor or bouquet is preserved; the spores are unaffected, but are kept from developing by immediately cooling the liquid to 10°C (50°F) or lower. SEE ALSO sterilization. [L. *Pasteur*]

pas·teur·ize (pas′ter-īz). To treat by pasteurization.

pas·teur·iz·er (pas′ter-ī-zer). An apparatus used in pasteurization.

Pastia, Constantin C., Roumanian physician, 1883–1926. SEE P. *sign.*

pas·til, pas·tille (pas′til, pas-tēl′). **1.** A small mass of benzoin and other aromatic substances to be burned for fumigation. **2.** SYN troche. [Fr. *pastille;* L. *pastillus,* a roll (of bread), dim. of *panis,* bread]

Sabouraud p.'s, disks containing barium platinocyanide that undergo a color change when exposed to x-rays; previously used to indicate the administered dose.

past-point·ing (past′poynt′ing). A test of the integrity of the vestibular system: the subject, seated in a revolving chair, is rotated to the right 10 times with eyes closed; then with the arm held horizontal, the right index finger is brought in touch with the tip of the examiner's finger; the arm is then raised vertically and the subject is instructed to touch the examiner's finger on bringing the arm once more to the horizontal; if the vestibular apparatus is normal, the finger will be brought down several inches to the right of the examiner's finger; the reverse is true on rotation to the left. In cerebellar disease, a patient attempting to reach a point with the finger will overshoot it. The test is also used in connec-

tion with caloric stimulation. In some vestibular disorders, p.-p. occurs without rotation or caloric stimulation.

pa·ta·gi·um, pl. **pa·ta·gia** (pă-tā′jē-ŭm, -ă). A winglike membrane. [L. a gold edging on a woman's gown]

Patau, Klaus, 20th century U.S. cytogeneticist. SEE P. *syndrome.*

patch. 1. A small circumscribed area differing in color or structure from the surrounding surface. **2.** In dermatology, a flat area greater than 1.0 cm in diameter. **3.** An intermediate stage in the formation of a cap on the surface of a cell.

butterfly p., SYN butterfly (2).

p. clamping, a technique used in the study of ion channels in which the movement of ions across a small p. of isolated membrane is measured when the membrane is electrically polarized or hyperpolarized and maintained at that potential. SYN patch clamp.

cotton-wool p.'s, white, fuzzy areas on the surface of the retina (accumulations of cellular organelles) caused by damage (usually infarction) of the retinal fiber layer. SYN cotton-wool spots.

herald p., the initial rapidly enlarging oval-shaped red papulosquamous lesion, usually on the trunk, heralding the widespread eruption of pityriasis rosea, and preceding the latter by 7–14 days.

Hutchinson p., SYN salmon p.

mucous p., an oval to round, yellow-gray to white, membrane-covered lesion or lesions occurring on the mucous membranes; usually seen in secondary syphilis.

Peyer p.'s, SYN aggregated lymphoid *nodules* of small intestine, under *nodule.*

salmon p., (1) an intraretinal hemorrhage seen in sickle cell *retinopathy;* **(2)** the appearance of an orbital lymphoid tumor as seen in the subconjunctival space; **(3)** a common macular orange-pink to red vascular malformation present at or near birth on the head and neck that involutes during childhood. SYN Hutchinson p.

shagreen p., SYN shagreen *skin.*

smoker's p.'s, SYN leukoplakia.

soldier's p.'s, SYN milk *spots* (1), under *spot.*

Patein, G., French physician, 1857–1928. SEE P. *albumin.*

pa·tel·la, gen. and pl. **pa·tel·lae** (pa-tel′ă, -ē) [TA]. The large sesamoid bone in the combined tendon of the extensors of the leg, covering the anterior surface of the knee. SYN kneecap. [L. a small plate, the kneecap, dim. of *patina,* a shallow disk, fr. *pateo,* to lie open]

p. alta, term used to describe a somewhat more proximal position of the p. than anticipated when it is visualized on a lateral radiograph of the knee. [patella + L. *alta,* high]

p. baja, term used to describe a somewhat more distal position of the p. than anticipated when it is visualized on a lateral radiograph of the knee. [patella + Sp. *baja,* low]

floating p., a p. elevated by the presence of a knee effusion.

slipping p., spontaneous or easily provoked dislocation of the p.

pa·tel·lar (pa-tel′ăr). Relating to the patella.

pat·el·lec·to·my (pat′ĕ-lek′tō-mē). Excision of the patella. [patella + G. *ektomē,* excision]

pa·tel·li·form (pa-tel′i-fōrm). Of the shape of the patella.

pa·ten·cy (pā′ten-sē). The state of being freely open or exposed.

probe p., (of foramen ovale), a term introduced by B.M. Patten to cover incomplete fibrous adhesion of an adequate valvula foraminis ovalis in the postnatal closure of the foramen ovale.

pa·tent (pā′tent, pā′tent). Open or exposed. SYN patulous. [L. *patens,* pres. p. of *pateo,* to lie open]

pa·tent blue V. SYN leuco patent blue.

Paterson, Donald R., English otolaryngologist, 1863–1939. SEE P.-Kelly *syndrome;* Paterson-Brown-Kelly *syndrome.*

path. A road or way; the course taken by an electric current or by nervous impulses. SEE ALSO pathway. [A.S. *paeth*]

clinical p., a map that outlines the entire track or p. a patient is expected to follow throughout the course of treatment and beyond.

condyle p., the p. traveled by the mandibular condyle in the temporomandibular joint during the various mandibular movements.

generated occlusal p., a registration of the p.'s of movement of

pa

the occlusal surfaces of mandibular teeth on a plastic or abrasive surface attached to the maxillary arch. SEE ALSO functional chew-in *record*.

incisal p., SYN incisal *guidance.*

p. of insertion, the direction in which a dental prosthesis is placed upon or removed from the supporting tissues or abutment teeth.

milled-in p.'s, (1) contours carved by various mandibular movements into the occluding surface of an occlusion rim, by teeth or studs placed in the opposing occlusion rim; the curves or contours may be carved into wax, modeling plastic, or plaster of Paris; **(2)** occlusal curves developed by masticatory or gliding movements of occlusion rims that are composed of materials including abrasives. SEE ALSO functional chew-in *record.* SYN milled-in curves.

occlusal p., (1) a gliding occlusal contact; **(2)** the p. of movement of an occlusal surface.

△**path-, -pathy, patho-, path·ic.** Disease. [G. *pathos,* feeling, suffering, disease]

pa·the·ma (pă-thē′mă). Obsolete term for a disease or morbid condition. [G. *pathēma,* suffering]

path·er·gy (path′er-jē). Those reactions resulting from a state of altered activity, both allergic (immune) and nonallergic. [G. *pathos,* disease, + *ergon,* work]

pa·thet·ic (pă-thet′ik). **1.** Denoting the fourth cranial nerve (pathetic nerve), the trochlear nerve. **2.** Denoting that which arouses sorrow or pity. [G. *pathētikos,* relating to the feelings]

path·find·er (path′fīn-der). A filiform bougie for introduction through a narrow stricture end to serve as a guide for the passage of a larger sound or catheter.

path·ic (path′ik). A person who assumes the passive role in less frequently engaged sexual acts. SEE ALSO passivism (2). [G. *pathikos,* remaining passive]

△**patho-.** SEE path-.

path·o·am·ine (path-ō-am′ēn). A ptomaine; a toxic amine causing disease or resulting from a disease process.

path·o·bi·ol·o·gy (path′ō-bī-ol′ō-jē). Pathology with emphasis more on the biologic than on the medical aspects.

path·o·ci·din (path-ō-sī′din). 8-Azaguanine.

path·o·clis·is (path-ō-klis′is). A specific tendency to sensitivity to special toxins; a tendency for toxins to attack certain organs. [patho- + G. *klisis,* bending, proneness]

path·o·crin·ia (path-ō-krin′ē-ă). Obsolete term for any disorder of the endocrine glands. [patho- + G. *krinō,* to separate]

path·o·don·tia (path-ō-don′shē-ă). The science concerned with diseases of the teeth. [patho- + G. *odous,* tooth]

path·o·for·mic (path-ō-fōr′mik). Relating to the beginning of disease; denoting especially certain symptoms occurring in the transition period between a normal and a diseased state. [patho- + L. *formo,* to form]

path·o·gen (path′ō-jen). Any virus, microorganism, or other substance causing disease. [patho- + G. *-gen,* to produce]

behavioral p., the personal habits and lifestyle behaviors of an individual which are associated with an increased risk of physical illness and dysfunction. SEE ALSO risk *factor.*

opportunistic p., an organism that is capable of causing disease only when the host's resistance is lowered, e.g., by other diseases or drugs.

path·o·gen·e·sis (path-ō-jen′ĕ-sis). The pathologic, physiologic, or biochemical mechanism resulting in the development of a disease or morbid process. Cf. etiology. [patho- + G. *genesis,* production]

drug p., the production of morbid symptoms by drugs.

path·o·gen·ic, path·o·ge·net·ic (path-ō-jen′ik, -jĕ-net′ik). Causing disease or abnormality. SYN morbific, morbigenous, nosogenic, nosopoietic.

path·o·ge·nic·i·ty (path′ō-jĕ-nis′i-tē). The condition or quality of being pathogenic, or the ability to cause disease.

pa·thog·e·ny (pă-thoj′ĕ-nē). Rarely used synonym for pathogenesis.

path·og·no·mon·ic (path′og-nō-mon′ik). Characteristic or indicative of a disease; denoting especially one or more typical symptoms, findings, or pattern of abnormalities specific for a given disease and not found in any other condition. [see pathognomy]

path·og·no·my (pă-thog′nō-mē). Rarely used term for diagnosis by means of a study of the typical symptoms of a disease, or of the subjective sensations of the patient. [patho- + G. *gnōmē,* a mark, a sign]

path·og·nos·tic (path-og-nos′tik). Rarely used synonym for pathognomonic. [patho- + G. *gnōstikos,* pertaining to knowledge]

path·o·log·ic, path·o·log·i·cal (path-ō-loj′ik, -i-kăl). **1.** Pertaining to pathology. **2.** Morbid or diseased; resulting from disease.

pa·thol·o·gist (pa-thol′ō-jist). A specialist in pathology; a physician who practices, evaluates, or supervises diagnostic tests, using materials removed from living or dead patients, and functions as a laboratory consultant to clinicians, or who conducts experiments or other investigations to determine the causes or nature of disease changes.

speech-language p., a practitioner concerned with the diagnosis and rehabilitation of persons with voice, speech, and language disorders.

pa·thol·o·gy (pa-thol′ō-jē). The medical science, and specialty practice, concerned with all aspects of disease, but with special reference to the essential nature, causes, and development of abnormal conditions, as well as the structural and functional changes that result from the disease processes. [patho- + G. *logos,* study, treatise]

anatomic p., the subspecialty of p. that pertains to the gross and microscopic study of organs and tissues removed for biopsy or during postmortem examination, and also the interpretation of the results of such study. SYN pathological anatomy.

cellular p., (1) the interpretation of diseases in terms of cellular alterations, i.e., the ways in which cells fail to maintain homeostasis; **(2)** sometimes used as a synonym for cytopathology (1).

clinical p., (1) any part of the medical practice of p. as it pertains to the care of patients; **(2)** the subspecialty in p. concerned with the theoretical and technical aspects (i.e., the methods or procedures) of chemistry, immunohematology, microbiology, parasitology, immunology, hematology, and other fields as they pertain to the diagnosis of disease and the care of patients, as well as to the prevention of disease.

comparative p., the p. of diseases of animals, especially in relation to human p.

dental p., SYN oral p.

functional p., p. pertaining to abnormalities in function of a tissue, organ, or part, with or without associated changes in structure.

humoral p., the thesis that disorders in the fluids of the body, especially the blood, are the basic factors in disease.

medical p., p. pertaining to various diseases not suitable for treatment by surgery.

molecular p., the study of biochemical and biophysical cellular mechanisms as the basic factors in disease.

oral p., the branch of dentistry concerned with the etiology, pathogenesis, and clinical, gross, and microscopic aspects of oral and paraoral disease, including oral soft tissues, the teeth, jaws, and salivary glands. SYN dental p.

speech p., the science concerned with functional and organic speech defects and disorders. SYN speech-language p.

speech-language p., SYN speech p.

surgical p., a field in anatomical p. concerned with examination of tissues removed from living patients for the purpose of diagnosis of disease and guidance in the care of patients.

path·o·met·ric (path-ō-met′rik). Relating to pathometry.

pa·thom·e·try (pă-thom′ĕ-trē). Rarely used term for the determination of the proportionate number of individuals affected with a certain disease at a given time, and of the conditions leading to an increase or decrease in this number. [patho- + G. *metron,* measure]

path·o·mi·me·sis (path′ō-mi-mē′sis). Mimicry of a disease or dysfunction, whether intentional or unconscious. SYN pathomimicry. [patho- + G. *mimēsis,* imitation]

path·o·mim·ic·ry (path-ō-mim′i-krē). SYN pathomimesis.

path·o·mi·o·sis (path-ō-mī-ō′sis). The attitude that leads a patient to minimize his or her disease. [patho- + G. *meiōsis,* a lessening]

path·o·mor·phism (path-ō-mōr′fizm). Abnormal morphology.

path·o·no·mia, pa·thon·o·my (path-ō-nō′mē-ă, pă-thon′ō-mē). The science of the laws of morbid changes. [patho- + G. *nomos,* law]

path·o·pho·bia (path-ō-fō′bē-ă). SYN nosophobia. [patho- + G. *phobos,* fear]

path·o·phys·i·ol·o·gy (path′ō-fiz-ē-ol′ō-jē). Derangement of function seen in disease; alteration in function as distinguished from structural defects.

path·o·poi·e·sis (path′ō-poy-ē′sis). Rarely used term for the mode of production of disease. [patho- + G. *poiēsis,* making]

pa·tho·sis (pă-thō′sis). Rarely used term for a state of disease, diseased condition, or disease entity. [patho- + G. *-osis,* condition]

pa·thot·ro·pism (pa-thot′rō-pizm). Attraction of drugs toward diseased structures. [patho- + G. *tropos,* a turning]

path·way (path′wā). **1.** A collection of axons establishing a conduction route for nerve impulses from one group of nerve cells to another group or to an effector organ composed of muscle or gland cells. **2.** Any sequence of chemical reactions leading from one compound to another; if taking place in living tissue, usually referred to as a **biochemical p.**

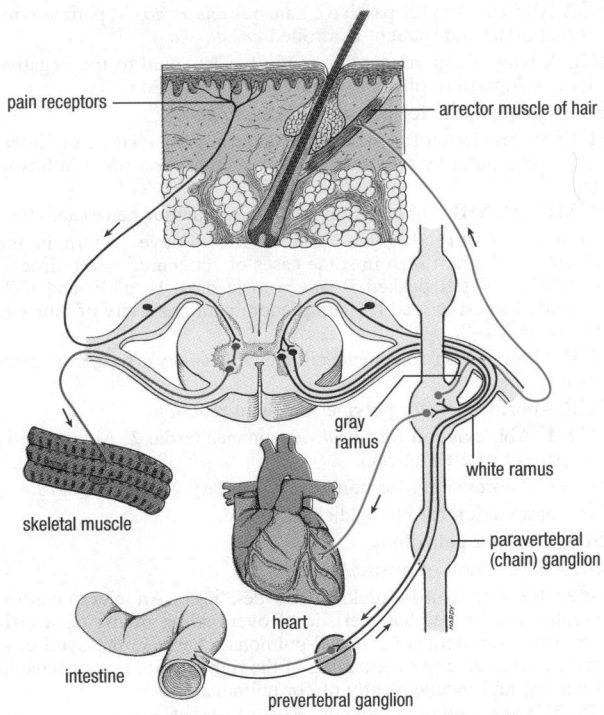

somatic and visceral reflex pathways: diagrammatic representation; arrows indicate the direction of impulse transmission; visceral afferent neurons, shown on the right, are preganglionic (red lines) and postganglionic (green lines); synapses occur either in paravertebral ganglia or in prevertebral ganglia

4-aminobutyrate p., the p. that ultimately converts 4-aminobutyrate to succinate; succinate is then converted to α-ketoglutarate, via the tricarboxylic acid cycle, which is then acted upon by glutamate dehydrogenase; glutamate is then decarboxylated to reform 4-aminobutyrate; an important p. for those cells that make this neuroactive molecule. SYN GABA p.

auditory p., neural paths and connections within the central nervous system, beginning at the organ of Corti hair cells, continuing along the eighth nerve, and terminating at the auditory cortex.

critical p., outline or diagram that documents the process of

diagnosis or treatment deemed appropriate for a condition based on practice guidelines.

Embden-Meyerhof p., the anaerobic glycolytic p. by which D-glucose (most notably in muscle) is converted to lactic acid. Cf. glycolysis. SYN Embden-Meyerhof-Parnas p.

Embden-Meyerhof-Parnas p., SYN Embden-Meyerhof p.

Entner-Douderoff p., a degradative p. for carbohydrates in certain microorganisms (e.g., *Pseudomonas* sp.) that lack hexokinase, phosphofructokinase, and glyceraldehyde-3-phosphate dehydrogenase.

GABA p., SYN 4-aminobutyrate p.

hexose monophosphate p., SYN pentose phosphate p.

lacrimal p. [TA], a space between the closed lids and the eyeball through which the tears flow to the punctum lacrimale. SYN rivus lacrimalis [TA], Ferrein canal.

mercapturic acid p., a glutathione-dependent p. for the detoxification of a number of compounds, including arene oxides; an *S*-substituted glutathione is formed and ultimately converted to a mercapturic acid (an *S*-substituted *N*-acetylated L-cysteine), which is excreted; the leukotrienes are believed to be degraded through this p.

pentose phosphate p., a secondary p. for the oxidation of D-glucose (not occurring in skeletal muscle), generating reducing power (NADPH) in the cytoplasm outside the mitochondria and synthesizing pentoses and a few other sugars. It also provides a means of converting pentoses and certain other sugars into intermediates of the glycolytic p. It proceeds from D-glucose 6-phosphate to D-ribulose and D-ribose phosphates, thence (with D-xylulose 5-phosphate) to D-sedoheptulose 7-phosphate and D-glyceraldehyde 3-phosphate; carbon dioxide is released in the gluconate-ribulose step. In plants, it participates in the formation of D-glucose from carbon dioxide in the dark reactions of photosynthesis. This p. is defective in certain inherited diseases, e.g., glucose-6-phosphate dehydrogenase deficiency. SYN Dickens shunt, hexose monophosphate p., hexose monophosphate shunt, pentose monophosphate shunt, pentose phosphate cycle, phosphogluconate p., Warburg-Dickens-Horecker shunt, Warburg-Lipmann-Dickens-Horecker shunt.

phosphogluconate p., SYN pentose phosphate p.

polyol p., SYN sorbitol p.

salvage p., the utilization of preformed purine and pyrimidine bases to synthesize nucleotides.

sorbitol p., a p. responsible for D-fructose formation from sorbitol; increases in activity as the glucose concentration rises in diabetes. SYN polyol p.

ubiquitin-protease p., p. in which a small protein cofactor, ubiquitin, couples with protein substrate to catalyze proteolytic destruction by proteases; this p. is highly selective and tightly regulated and is responsible for protein degradation seen in muscle-wasting diseases.

visual p., neural paths and connections within the central nervous system, beginning with the retina and terminating in the occipital cortex.

-pathy. SEE path-.

pa·tient (pā′shent). One who is suffering from any disease or behavioral disorder and is under treatment for it. Cf. case (1). [L. *patiens,* pres. p. of *patior,* to suffer]

target p., in group therapy, the p. being analyzed in turn by another member p.

pat·ri·cide (pat′ri-sīd). **1.** The killing of one's father. **2.** One who commits such an act. SEE parricide. Cf. matricide. [L. *pater,* father, + *caedo,* to kill]

Patrick, Hugh T., U.S. neurologist, 1860–1938. SEE P. *test.*

pat·ri·lin·e·al (pat-ri-lin′ē-ăl). Related to descent through the male line; inheritance of the Y chromosome is exclusively patrilineal. [L. *pater,* father, + *linea,* line]

pat·tern (pat′ern). **1.** A design; often refers to chest radiographic findings. **2.** In dentistry, a form used in making a mold, as for an inlay or partial denture framework.

airspace-filling p., SYN alveolar p.

airway p., chest radiographic appearance of thickened bronchial walls, bronchiectasis, bronchiolitis, or acinar consolidation.

alveolar p., cloudy to dense opacities, obscuring vascular markings, on chest radiographs. SYN airspace-filling p.

ballerina-foot p., a vigorous posteromedial contraction of the left ventricle coupled with convexity anteriorly sometimes resulting from poor contraction of the opposing anterior wall; it is the most frequent dyssynergy observed in the prolapsed mitral valve leaflet syndrome (even with a normal anterior wall) and produces a configuration of angiographic dye in the right anterior oblique projection resembling a ballerina's foot; sometimes called dancer's foot malformation.

butterfly p., bilateral, symmetric, pulmonary alveolar opacities sparing the periphery, on chest radiographs; usually caused by pulmonary edema.

ground-glass p., radiographic or CT appearance of hazy opacity that fails to obscure pulmonary vascular markings.

honeycomb p., dense, slightly irregular circular shadows, most common next to the pleura at the lung base, on chest radiographs or CT; caused by chronic interstitial fibrosis of diverse causes.

hourglass p., a vigorous ringlike contraction observed angiographically in the left ventricular angiogram in the right anterior oblique projection, resembling an hourglass; it is seen in the prolapsed mitral valve leaflet syndrome.

interstitial p., one of several chest radiographic patterns associated with interstitial infiltration or thickening, including honeycomb p., miliary p., reticulonodular p., or septal lines.

juvenile p., a precordial T-wave inversion, sometimes with J-ST elevations in an electrocardiogram, resembling that seen in normal children, which occurs as a normal variant in some adults, especially black persons, and especially in leads V_1, V_2, and V_3.

miliary p., a chest radiographic pattern of fine, rounded opacities, typical of hematogenous dissemination of tuberculosis; size has some relationship to that of a millet seed.

mosaic p., on high-resolution CT scans of the lungs, a p. of brighter and darker regions corresponding to differences in perfusion or aeration; found in some cases of chronic thromboembolism or of bronchiolitis obliterans. Cf. oligemia.

occlusal p., SYN occlusal *form.*

reticulonodular p. (re-tik′ū-lō-nod′ū-lăr), a somewhat netlike chest radiographic p., with nodular thickening at the intersections of the lines; a nonspecific interstitial p.

wax p., a p. of wax that, when invested and burned out or otherwise eliminated, will produce a mold in which a casting may be made. SYN wax form.

pat·u·lin (pat′ū-lin). An antibiotic derived from metabolites of fungi, such as species of *Aspergillus, Penicillium,* and *Gymnoascus;* has carcinogenic activity.

pat·u·lous (pat′ū-lŭs). SYN patent. [L. *patulus,* fr. *pateo,* to lie open]

pau·ci·ar·ti·cu·lar (paw-sē-ar-tik′ū-lar). A joint condition in which only a few (>1, <5) joints are involved [L. *pauci,* few, + articular]

pau·ci·bac·il·lary (paw-sē-bas′i-lār-ē). Made up of, or denoting the presence of, few bacilli.

pau·ci·sy·nap·tic (paw′sē-si-nap′tik). SYN oligosynaptic. [L. *paucus,* few, + synapse]

Paul, Gustav, Austrian physician, 1859–1935. SEE P. *reaction, test;* P.-Bunnell *test.*

Pauli, Wolfgang, Austrian-U.S. physicist and Nobel laureate, 1900–1958. SEE P. exclusion *principle.*

Pauling, Linus C., U.S. chemist and Nobel laureate, 1901–1994. SEE P. *theory;* P.-Corey *helix.*

pause (pawz). Temporary stop. [G. *pausis,* cessation]

apneic p., cessation of air flow for more than 10 seconds. SEE sleep *apnea.*

compensatory p., the p. following an extrasystole, when the p. is long enough to compensate for the prematurity of the extrasystole; the short cycle ending with the extrasystole plus the p. following the extrasystole together equal two of the regular cycles.

postextrasystolic p., the somewhat prolonged cycle immediately following an extrasystole.

preautomatic p., a temporary p. in cardiac activity before an automatic pacemaker escapes. SEE ALSO escape.

respiratory p., cessation of air flow for less than 10 seconds. SEE sleep *apnea.*

sinus p., a spontaneous interruption in the regular sinus rhythm, the p. lasting for a period that is not an exact multiple of the sinus cycle. SEE ALSO sinus *arrest,* sinus *standstill.*

Pautrier, Lucien M.A., French dermatologist, 1876–1959. SEE P. *abscess, microabscess.*

Pauzat, Jean E., 19th century French physician.

Pavlov, Ivan P., Russian physiologist and Nobel laureate, 1849–1936. SEE pavlovian *conditioning;* P. *method, pouch, stomach, reflex.*

pav·or noc·tur·nus (pā′vōr nok-ter′nŭs). SYN night terrors. [L.]

Pavy, Frederick W., English physician, 1829–1911. SEE P. *disease.*

paw·paw. SEE papaya.

Payne, J. Howard, U.S. surgeon, *1916. SEE P. *operation.*

Payr, Erwin, German surgeon, 1871–1946. SEE P. *clamp, membrane, sign.*

Pb Symbol for lead (plumbum).

PBG Abbreviation for porphobilinogen.

PBI Abbreviation for protein-bound *iodine.*

p. c. Abbreviation for L. *post cibum,* after a meal.

PCA Abbreviation for passive cutaneous *anaphylaxis;* patient-controlled *analgesia;* patient-controlled *anesthesia.*

pCa A way of reporting calcium ion levels; equal to the negative decadic logarithm of the calcium ion concentration.

PCB Abbreviation for polychlorinated *biphenyl.*

PCIS Abbreviation for patient *care* information *system,* the interactive computer system used to store medical records in a hospital.

PCMB, *p*CMB Abbreviation for *p*-chloromercuribenzoate.

P con·gen·i·ta·le (kon-jen-i-tā′lē). The P-wave pattern in the electrocardiogram seen in some cases of congenital heart disease, consisting of tall peaked P waves in leads I, II, aVF, and aVL (usually largest in lead II) with predominant positivity of diphasic waves in V1–2.

PCP Abbreviation for phencyclidine; *Pneumocystis carinii* pneumonia.

PCR Abbreviation for polymerase chain *reaction.*

PCT 1. Abbreviation for *porphyria* cutanea tarda. **2.** Abbreviation for patient care technician.

PCWP Abbreviation for pulmonary capillary wedge *pressure.*

PD Abbreviation for phenyldichloroarsine.

Pd Symbol for palladium.

p.d. Abbreviation of prism *diopter.*

P-dex·tro·car·di·a·le (deks′trō-kar-dē-ā′lē). An electrocardiographic syndrome characteristic of overloading of the right atrium, often erroneously called P-pulmonale because the syndrome can result from any overloading of the right atrium (e.g., tricuspid stenosis) and independently of cor pulmonale.

PDGF Abbreviation for platelet-derived growth *factor.*

PDI Abbreviation for Periodontal Disease Index.

PDL. Abbreviation for pulsed dye *laser.*

PEA Abbreviation for pulseless electrical *activity.*

peach ker·nel oil (pēch ker′něl). SEE persic oil.

peak (pēk). The top or upper limit of a graphic tracing or of any variable. [M.E. *peke, pike,* fr. Sp. *pico,* beak, fr. L. *picus,* magpie]

biclonal p., two narrow electrophoretic bands thought to represent immunoglobulins of two cell lines.

juxtaphrenic p. (jŭks-tă-fren′ik pēk), on chest radiograph, a triangular density on top of the right diaphragmatic shadow, probably caused by tension of the phrenic nerve on the pleura over the diaphragm.

monoclonal p., a narrow band visible on electrophoresis or an abnormal arc seen on immunoelectrophoresis, thought to represent immunoglobulin of one cell clone.

pea·nut oil (pē'nŭt). Oil extracted from the kernels of one or more cultivated varieties of *Arachis hypogaea* (family Leguminosae); used as a solvent for intramuscular injections and in the preparation of foods. SYN arachis oil.

Pearl, Raymond, U.S. biologist, 1879–1940. SEE P. *index.*

pearl (perl). **1.** A concretion formed around a grain of sand or other foreign body within the shell of certain mollusks. **2.** One of a number of small tough masses, such as mucus occurring in the sputum in asthma. **3.** SYN keratin p.

Elschnig p.'s, focal retention of lens fibers that have undergone proliferative and degenerative changes surrounded by lens capsular fragments seen after extracapsular cataract extraction.

enamel p., SYN enameloma.

epithelial p., SYN keratin p.

Epstein p.'s, multiple small, white, epithelial inclusion cysts found in the midline of the palate in newborn infants.

gouty p., SYN tophus.

keratin p., a focus of central keratinization within concentric layers of abnormal squamous cells; seen in squamous cell carcinoma. SYN epithelial nest, epithelial p., pearl (3), squamous p.

Laënnec p.'s, obsolete term for small, round, translucent, tenacious bodies in the sputum of some persons with asthma; when floated in water, they become unfurled and are then recognizable as Curschmann spirals.

squamous p., SYN keratin p.

pearl-ash. SYN potash.

Pearson, Karl, English mathematician, 1857–1936. SEE Poisson-P. *formula;* McArdle-Schmid-P. *disease.*

peau d'orange (pō-dŏ-rahnj'). A swollen pitted skin surface overlying carcinoma of the breast in which there is both stromal infiltration and lymphatic obstruction with edema. [Fr. orange peel]

pec·cant (pek'ant). Unhealthy; producing disease. [L. *peccans* (-*ant*-), pres. p. of *pecco,* to sin]

pec·ca·ti·pho·bia (pek'kă-ti-fō'bē-ă). Morbid fear of sinning. [L. *peccatum,,* sin, + G. *phobos,* fear]

⚠**pecilo-.** SEE poikilo-.

pe·cil·o·cin (pĕ-sil'ō-sin). An antifungal agent.

Pecquet, Jean, French anatomist, 1622–1674. SEE P. *cistern, duct; receptaculum* pecqueti; P. *reservoir.*

pec·tase (pek'tās). An enzyme that converts pectin to D-galacturonic acid (pectic acid); used in the treatment of certain foodstuffs. SYN pectinesterase.

pec·ten (pek'ten). **1** [NA]. A structure with comblike processes or projections. **2.** SYN anal p. [L. comb]

anal p. [TA], the middle third of the surgical anal canal; upper half of anatomic anal canal extends between pectinate line and the intersphincteric groove, and is lined with anoderm. SYN p. analis [TA], pecten (2).

p. ana'lis [TA], SYN anal p.

p. os'sis pu'bis [TA], SYN p. pubis.

p. pu'bis [TA], the continuation on the superior ramus pubis of the linea terminalis, forming a sharp ridge. SYN p. ossis pubis [TA], pectineal line of pubis.

pec·ten·i·tis (pek-ten-ī'tis). Inflammation of the sphincter ani. [L. *pecten,* a comb, + G. *-itis,* inflammation]

pec·ten·o·sis (pek-ten-ō'sis). Exaggerated enlargement of the pecten band.

pec·tic (pek'tik). Relating to any of the substances or materials now referred to as pectin. [G. *pēktos,* stiff, curdled]

pec·tic ac·id. SYN D-galacturonic acid.

pec·tin (pek'tin). **1.** Broad generic term for what are now called pectic substances or materials; specifically, a gelatinous substance, consisting largely of long chains of mostly D-galacturonic acid units (typically α-1,4 linkages and sometimes present as methyl esters), that is extracted from fruits where it is presumed to exist as protopectin (pectose). **2.** Commercial p.'s, sometimes called pectinic acid, are whitish, soluble powders prepared from the rinds of citrus fruits. They are used in the preparation of jams, jellies, and similar food products where they enhance viscosity;

therapeutically, they are used to control diarrhea (usually in conjunction with other agents), as a plasma expander, and as a protectant; p.'s bind calcium ions and are highly hydrated.

p. lyase, an enzyme that catalyzes the elimination of 6-methyl-Δ-4,5-D-galacturonate residues from pectin; thus, it brings about depolymerization; it does not act on deesterified p.; used in the treatment of certain foodstuffs.

pec·tin·ase (pek'tin-ās). SYN polygalacturonase.

pec·ti·nate (pek'ti-nāt). **1.** Combed; comb-shaped. SYN pectiniform. **2.** In fungi, used to describe a particular type of branching hyphae in cultures of dermatophytes.

pec·tin·e·al (pek-tin'ē-ăl). Ridged; relating to the os pubis or to any comblike structure. SYN pectineus (1).

pec·tin·es·ter·ase (pek-tin-es'ter-ās). SYN pectase.

pec·ti·ne·us (pek'ti-nē'ŭs). **1.** SYN pectineal. **2.** SEE pectineus (*muscle*). [L.]

pec·tin·ic ac·ids (pek-tin'ik). Term sometimes used for commercial pectins.

pec·tin·i·form (pek-tin'i-fōrm). SYN pectinate (1).

pec·ti·za·tion (pek-ti-zā'shŭn). In colloidal chemistry, coagulation. [G. *pēktikos,* curdling]

pec·to·ral (pek'tō-răl). Relating to the chest. [L. *pectoralis;* fr. *pectus,* breast bone]

pec·to·ral·gia (pek-tō-ral'jē-ă). Pain in the chest. [L. *pectus* (*pector*-), chest, + G. *algos,* pain]

pec·to·ril·o·quy (pek-tō-ril'ō-kwē). Increased transmission of the voice sound through the pulmonary structures, so that it is clearly audible on auscultation of the chest; usually indicates consolidation of the underlying lung parenchyma. SYN pectorophony. [L. *pectus,* chest, + *loquor,* to speak]

aphonic p., SYN Baccelli *sign.*

whispered p., whispering p., p. of whispered sounds in the same fashion as that of voice sounds. SYN whispered bronchophony.

pec·to·roph·o·ny (pek-tō-rof'ō-nē). SYN pectoriloquy. [L. *pectus,* chest, + G. *phōnē,* voice]

pec·tose (pek'tōs). SEE pectin, protopectin.

pec·tous (pek'tŭs). **1.** Relating to or consisting of pectin or pectose. **2.** Denoting a firm coagulated condition sometimes assumed by a gel, which is permanent in that the substance cannot be made to reassume the gel form.

pec·tus, gen. **pec·to·ris,** pl. **pec·to·ra** (pek'tŭs, pek'tō-ris, pek'tō-ră). SYN chest. [L.]

p. carina'tum, flattening of the chest on either side with forward projection of the sternum resembling the keel of a boat. SYN chicken breast, keeled chest, pigeon breast, pigeon chest.

p. excava'tum, a hollow at the lower part of the chest caused by a backward displacement of the xiphoid cartilage. SYN foveated chest, funnel chest, funnel breast, koilosternia, p. recurvatum, trichterbrust.

p. recurva'tum, SYN p. excavatum.

⚠**ped-, pedi-, pedo-.** **1.** Child. [G. *pais,* child] **2.** Foot, feet. [L. *pes,* foot]

ped·al (ped'ăl). Relating to the feet, or to any structure called pes. [L. *pedalis,* fr. *pes* (*ped*-), a foot]

pe·da·tro·phia, pe·dat·ro·phy (ped-ă-trō'fē-ă, -at'rō-fē). SYN marasmus. [G. *pais* (*paid*-), child, + atrophy]

ped·er·ast (ped'er-ast). One who practices pederasty.

ped·er·as·ty (ped'er-as-tē). Homosexual anal intercourse, especially when practiced on boys. [G. *paiderastia;* fr. *pais* (*paid*-), boy, + *eraō,* to long for]

Pedersen spec·u·lum. See under speculum.

pe·de·sis (pē-dē'sis). SYN brownian *movement.* [G. *pēdēsis,* a leaping]

⚠**pedi-.** SEE ped-.

pe·di·at·ric (pē-dē-at'rik). Relating to pediatrics. [G. *pais* (*paid*-), child, + *iatrikos,* relating to medicine]

pe·di·a·tric·ian (pē'dē-ă-trish'ăn). A specialist in pediatrics. SYN pediatrist.

pe·di·at·rics (pē-dē-at'riks). The medical specialty concerned with the study and treatment of children in health and disease during development from birth through adolescence. [G. *pais* (*paid-*), child, + *iatreia*, medical treatment]

pe·di·at·rist (pē-dē-at′rist). SYN pediatrician.

ped·i·at·ry (pē′dē-at-rē, pē-dī′ă-trē). A rarely used term for pediatrics

ped·i·cel (ped′i-sel). The secondary process of a podocyte, which helps form the visceral capsule of a renal corpuscle. SYN footplate (2), foot-plate★, foot process. [Mod. L. *pedicellus*, dim. of L. *pes*, foot]

ped·i·cel·late (ped′i-sel-lāt). SYN pediculate.

ped·i·cel·la·tion (ped′i-sĕ-lā′shŭn). Formation of a pedicle or peduncle.

ped·i·cle (ped′ĭ-kl) [TA]. **1.** A constricted portion or stalk. SYN pediculus (1) [TA]. **2.** A stalk by which a nonsessile tumor is attached to normal tissue. SYN pedunculus [TA], peduncle (2). **3.** A stalk through which a flap of tissue is vascularized, permitting transfer to another site. [L. *pediculus*, dim. of *pes*, foot]

p. of arch of vertebra [TA], the constricted portion of the arch on either side extending from the body to the lamina; bound intervertebral foramina superiorly and inferiorly. SYN pediculus arcus vertebrae [TA], radix arcus vertebrae.

vascular p., the tissues containing arteries and veins of an organ; specifically in chest radiology, the (width of the) mediastinum at the level of the aortic arch and superior vena cava.

pe·dic·u·lar (pĕ-dik′ū-lăr). Relating to pediculi, or lice. [L. *pedicularis*]

pe·dic·u·late (pĕ-dik′ū-lāt). Not sessile, having a pedicle or peduncle. SYN pedicellate, pedunculate. [L. *pediculatus*]

pe·dic·u·li (pĕ-dik′ū-lī). Plural of pediculus. [L.]

pe·dic·u·li·cide (pĕ-dik′ū-li-sīd). An agent used to destroy lice. [L. *pediculus*, louse, + *caedo*, to kill]

Pe·dic·u·loi·des ven·tri·co·sus (pĕ-dik-ū-loy′dēz ven-tri-kō′sŭs). SYN *Pyemotes tritici*. [Mod. L., fr. L. *pediculus*, louse, + *venter*, belly]

pe·dic·u·lo·pho·bia (pē-dik′ū-lō-fō′bē-ă). Morbid fear of infestation with lice. SYN phthiriophobia. [L. *pediculus*, louse, + G. *phobos*, fear]

pe·dic·u·lo·sis (pĕ-dik′ū-lō′sis). The state of being infested with lice. [L. *pediculus*, louse, + G. *-osis*, condition]

p. cap′itis, the presence of lice on the scalp, seen especially in children, with nits attached to hairs.

p. cor′poris, the presence of body lice that live in the seams of clothing. Biting causes pruritus and excoriations.

p. palpebra′rum, the presence of lice in the eyelashes.

p. pu′bis, infestation with the pubic or crab louse, *Pthirus pubis*, especially in pubic hair, causing pruritus and maculae ceruleae.

pe·dic·u·lous (pĕ-dik′ū-lŭs). Infested with lice. SYN lousy.

Pe·dic·u·lus (pĕ-dik′ū-lŭs). A genus of parasitic lice (family Pediculidae) that live in the hair and feeds periodically on blood. Important species include *P. humanus*, the species of louse infecting humans; *P. humanus* var. *capitis*, the head louse of humans; *P. humanus* var. *corporis* (also called *P. vestimenti* or *P. corporis*), the body louse or clothes louse, which lives and lays eggs (nits) in clothing and feeds on the human body; and *P. pubis*. [L.]

pe·dic·u·lus, pl. **pe·dic·u·li** (pĕ-dik′ū-lŭs, -lī) [TA]. **1.** SYN pedicle (1). [L. pedicle] **2.** A louse. SEE *Pediculus*. [L.]

p. ar′cus ver′tebrae [TA], SYN *pedicle* of arch of vertebra.

ped·i·cure (ped′i-kūr). Care and treatment of the feet. [L. *pes* (*ped-*), foot, + *cura*, treatment]

ped·i·gree (ped′i-grē). Ancestral line of descent, especially as diagrammed on a chart to show ancestral history; used in genetics to analyze inheritance. [M.E. *pedegra* fr. O.Fr. *pie de grue*, foot of crane]

pe·di·o·pho·bia (pē′dē-ō-fō′bē-ă). Morbid fear aroused by the sight of a child or of a doll. [G. *paidion*, a little child, + *phobos*, fear]

ped·i·pha·lanx (ped′i-fā′langks). A phalanx of the foot, distinguished from maniphalanx. [L. *pes* (*ped-*), foot, + phalanx]

♻**pedo-.** SEE ped-.

pe·do·don·tia (pē-dō-don′shē-ă). SYN pedodontics.

pe·do·don·tics (pē-dō-don′tiks). The branch of dentistry concerned with the dental care and treatment of children. SYN pediatric dentistry, pedodontia. [G. *pais*, child, + *odous*, tooth]

pe·do·don·tist (pē-dō-don′tist). A dentist who practices pedodontics.

pe·do·dy·na·mom·e·ter (ped′ō-dī-nă-mom′ĕ-ter). An instrument for measuring the strength of the leg muscles. [L. *pes* (*ped-*), foot, + G. *dynamis*, force, + G. *metron*, measure]

pe·do·gen·e·sis (pē-dō-jen′ĕ-sis). Permanent larval stage with sexual development, as in certain gall midges (genus *Miastor*). Cf. neoteny. [G. *pais* (*paid-*), child, + *genesis*, origin]

ped·o·gram (ped′ō-gram). A record made by the pedograph.

ped·o·graph (ped′ō-graf). An instrument for recording and studying the gait. [L. *pes* (*ped-*), foot, + G. *graphō*, to write]

pe·dog·ra·phy (pĕ-dog′ră-fē). Production of a record as made by a pedograph.

pe·dom·e·ter (pĕ-dom′ĕ-ter). An instrument for measuring the distance covered in walking. SYN podometer. [L. *pes* (*ped-*), foot]

pe·do·mor·phism (pē-dō-mōr′fizm). Description of adult behavior in terms appropriate to child behavior. [G. *pais* (*paid*), child, + *morphē*, form]

pe·do·phil·ia (pē-dō-fil′ē-ă). In psychiatry, an abnormal attraction to children by an adult for sexual purposes. [G. *pais*, child, + *philos*, fond]

pe·do·phil·ic (pē-dō-fil′ik). Relating to or exhibiting pedophilia.

pe·dun·cle (pe-dŭng′kl, pē′dŭng-kl). **1.** In neuroanatomy, term loosely applied to a variety of stalklike connecting structures in the brain, composed either exclusively of white matter (e.g., cerebellar p.) or of white and gray matter (e.g., cerebral p. **2.** SYN pedicle (2). [Mod. L. *pedunculus*, dim. of *pes*, foot]

cerebral p. [TA], originally denoting either of the two halves of the midbrain (a relatively narrow "neck" connecting the forebrain to the hindbrain); this term has been variably used to designate only those large bundles of corticofugal fibers forming the crus cerebri or to designate the crus cerebri plus the midbrain tegmentum; this latter, more inclusive, usage (crus cerebri and midbrain tegmentum) is preferred; the substantia nigra, while a part of the base of the p. (basis pedunculi), is considered a structure separating the midbrain tegmentum from the crus cerebri. SEE ALSO *crus cerebri*. SYN pedunculus cerebri [TA].

p. of corpus callosum, SYN subcallosal *gyrus*.

p. of flocculus [TA], the bundle of afferent and efferent nerve fibers connecting the flocculus and the nodule of the cerebellum; part of its course is in the inferior medullary velum. SYN pedunculus flocculi [TA].

inferior cerebellar p., large paired bundles of nerve fibers that develop on the dorsolateral surfaces of the upper medulla, extend under the lateral recesses of the rhomboid fossa and curve dorsally into the cerebellum caudomedial to the middle cerebellar peduncle; composed of a larger (lateral) bundle, the restiform body [TA], and a small (medial) bundle, the juxtarestiform body [TA]. Fibers forming this composite bundle originate from spinal neurons and medullary relay nuclei. The largest constituent (restiform body) contains crossed fibers from the inferior olive; it also contains the dorsal spinocerebellar tract and cerebellar projections from the lateral reticular nucleus, the accessory cuneate nucleus, the paramedian reticular nuclei, the perihypoglossal nuclei, and other nuclei. Vestibulocerebellar fibers are placed medially in the inferior cerebellar p. and are separately identified as the juxtarestiform body. SYN pedunculus cerebellaris inferior [TA].

inferior thalamic p., a large fiber bundle emerging from the anterior part of the thalamus in the ventral direction, in part joining the medial fibers of the internal capsule, in other part curving laterally around the medial margin of the capsule into the innominate substance. Many of its fibers establish a reciprocal connection of the mediodorsal nucleus of the thalamus with the orbital gyri of the frontal lobe, but numerous other fibers constitute a conduction system from the amygdala and olfactory cortex to the mediodorsal nucleus. SEE ALSO *ansa* peduncularis. SYN inferior thalamic radiation [TA], radiatio inferior thalami [TA], pedunculus thalami inferior.

lateral thalamic p., the massive group of fibers that emerges from the laterodorsal side of the thalamus to join the corona radiata; it reciprocally connects the lateral nucleus and the geniculate bodies of the thalamus with the corresponding regions of the cerebral cortex. SEE ALSO central thalamic *radiation.* SYN pedunculus thalami lateralis.

p. of mammillary body, a fascicle of nerve fibers passing to the mamillary body along the ventral surface of the midbrain; it consists of fibers that originate from the dorsal and ventral tegmental nuclei. SYN fasciculus pedunculomammillaris, pedunculomammillary fasciculus, pedunculus corporis mammillaris.

middle cerebellar p. [TA], the largest of three paired cerebellar p.'s, composed mainly of fibers that originate in the pontine nuclei, cross the midline in the basilar pons, and emerge on the opposite side as a massive bundle arching dorsally along the lateral side of the pontine tegmentum into the cerebellum; there are some uncrossed pontocerebellar fibers in this p.; its fibers are distributed chiefly to the cortex of the cerebellar hemisphere with some collateral fibers passing to the cerebellar nuclei. SYN pedunculus cerebellaris medius [TA], brachium pontis.

olfactory p., SYN olfactory *tract.*

superior cerebellar p. [TA], a large bundle of nerve fibers that originates from the dentate and interpositus nuclei and emerges from the cerebellum in the rostral direction, along the lateral wall of the fourth ventricle. The bundle submerges from the dorsal surface of the brainstem into the mesencephalic tegmentum, where most of its fibers cross in the massive decussation of the superior cerebellar p.'s. Part of the bundle terminates in the contralateral red nucleus; the bulk of the fibers continue rostrally to parts of the ventral intermediate nucleus of thalamus, ventral posterolateral nucleus of thalamus, and central lateral nucleus of thalamus. SYN pedunculus cerebellaris superior [TA], brachium conjunctivum cerebelli.

ventral thalamic p., the massive system of fiber bundles emerging through the ventral, lateral, and anterior borders of the thalamus to join the internal capsule and parts of the corona radiata; it contains the fibers reciprocally connecting the ventral thalamic nuclei with the precentral and postcentral gyri of the cerebral cortex. SYN pedunculus thalami ventralis.

pe·dun·cu·lar (pĕ-dŭng′kū-lăr). Relating to a pedicle or peduncle.

pe·dun·cu·late (pĕ-dŭng′kū-lāt). SYN pediculate.

pe·dun·cu·lot·o·my (pe-dŭng′kū-lot′ō-mē). 1. A total or partial section of a cerebral peduncle. 2. A mesencephalic pyramidal tractotomy. [peduncle + G. *tomē,* incision]

pe·dun·cu·lus, pl. **pe·dun·cu·li** (pe-dŭng′kū-lŭs, -kū-lī) [TA]. SYN pedicle (2). [Mod. L. dim. of *pes,* foot]

p. cerebella′ris infe′rior [TA], SYN inferior cerebellar *peduncle.*

p. cerebella′ris me′dius [TA], SYN middle cerebellar *peduncle.*

p. cerebella′ris supe′rior [TA], SYN superior cerebellar *peduncle.*

p. cer′ebri [TA], SYN cerebral *peduncle.*

p. cor′poris callo′si, SYN subcallosal *gyrus.*

p. cor′poris mammilla′ris, SYN *peduncle* of mammillary body.

p. floc′culi [TA], SYN *peduncle* of flocculus.

p. of pineal body, SEE habenula (2).

p. thal′ami infe′rior, SYN inferior thalamic *peduncle.*

p. thal′ami latera′lis, SYN lateral thalamic *peduncle.*

p. thal′ami ventra′lis, SYN ventral thalamic *peduncle.*

p. vitelli′nus, obsolete term for yolk *stalk.*

peel. To remove the outer layer of.

face p., removal of skin blemishes such as wrinkles, freckles, or acne scars by chemical agents producing injury (trichloracetic, phenol, or other organic acids) or solid carbon dioxide.

peel·ing (pēl′ing). A stripping off or loss of epidermis, as in sunburn. [M.E. *pelen*]

chemical p., SYN chemexfoliation.

pee·nash (pē′nash). Rhinitis caused by insect larvae in the nasal passages. [East Indian]

PEEP Abbreviation for positive end-expiratory *pressure.*

peer re·view. Process of p. r. of research proposals, manuscripts submitted for publication, and abstracts submitted for presentation at a scientific meeting, whereby these are judged for technical and scientific merit by other scientists in the same field.

peg. A cylindrical projection.

rete p.'s, SYN rete *ridge.*

PEGs Abbreviation for polyethylene glycols.

Peiffer, J., German physician, *1922. SEE Hirsch-P. *stain.*

pe·jor·ism (pē′jŏr-izm). A pessimistic attitude. [L. *pejor,* worse]

PEL. Abbreviation for permissible exposure *limit.*

Pel, Pieter K., Dutch physician, 1852–1919. SEE P.-Ebstein *disease, fever.*

pe·lade (pĕ-lad′, -lahd′). SYN alopecia. [Fr. *peler,* to remove the hair from a hide]

pel·ar·gon·ic ac·id (pel-ar-gon′ik). Used in the manufacture of lacquers and plastics; produced in the oxidative cleavage of oleic acid. SYN *n*-nonanoic acid.

Pelger, Karel, Dutch physician, 1885–1931. SEE P.-Huët nuclear *anomaly.*

pe·li·o·sis (pē-lē-ō′sis, pel-). SYN purpura. [G. *peliōsis,* a livid spot, livor]

bacterial p., bacterial infection of hemorrhagic cysts of the liver, spleen, or lymph nodes, seen in immunocompromised persons, caused by *Rochalimaea henselae.*

p. hep′atis, the presence throughout the liver of blood-filled cavities that may become lined by endothelium or become organized.

Pelizaeus, Friedrich, German neurologist, 1850–1917. SEE Merzbacher-P. *disease;* P.-Merzbacher *disease.*

pel·lag·ra (pĕ-lag′ră, pĕ-lā′gră). An affection characterized by gastrointestinal disturbances, erythema (particularly of exposed areas) followed by desquamation, and nervous and mental disorders; may occur because of a poor diet, alcoholism, or some other disease causing impairment of nutrition; commonly seen when corn (maize) is a main nutrient in the diet, resulting in a deficiency of niacin. SYN Alpine scurvy, maidism, mal de la rosa, mal rosso, mayidism, psychoneurosis maidica, Saint Ignatius itch. [It. *pelle,* skin, + *agra,* rough]

infantile p., SYN kwashiorkor.

secondary p., p. resulting from any morbid condition that impairs nutrition by increasing the requirement or reducing the available supply of vitamins.

p. si′ne p., p. without the characteristic skin lesions.

pel·lag·roid (pĕ-lag′royd). Resembling pellagra.

pel·lag·rous (pĕ-lag′rŭs). Relating to or suffering from pellagra.

Pellegrini, Augusto, Italian surgeon, *1877. SEE P. *disease;* P.-Stieda *disease.*

pel·let (pel′et). 1. A pilule, or very small pill. 2. A small rod-shaped or ovoid dosage form that is sterile and is composed essentially of pure steroid hormones in compressed form, intended for subcutaneous implantation in body tissues; serves as a depot providing for the slow release of the hormone over an extended period of time. [Fr. *pelote;* L. *pila,* a ball]

pel·li·cle (pel′i-kl). 1. Literally and nonspecifically, a thin skin. 2. A film or scum on the surface of a liquid. 3. Cell boundary of sporozoites and merozoites among members of the protozoan subphylum Apicomplexa (Sporozoa), consisting of an outer unit membrane and an inner layer of two unit membranes. [L. *pellicula,* dim of *pellis,* skin]

acquired p., a thin film (about 1 μm), derived mainly from salivary glycoproteins, that forms over the surface of a cleansed tooth crown when it is exposed to the saliva. SYN acquired cuticle, acquired enamel cuticle, brown p., posteruption cuticle.

brown p., SYN acquired p.

pel·lic·u·lar, pel·lic·u·lous (pe-lik′ū-lăr, -lŭs). Relating to a pellicle.

Pellizzari, Pietro, Italian dermatologist, 1823–1892. SEE Jadassohn-P. *anetoderma.*

Pellizzi, G.B., 19th–20th century Italian physician. SEE P. *syndrome.*

pe·llo·te (pā-yō′tā). SYN peyote. [Aztec, *peyotl*]

pel·lu·cid (pe-loo′sid). Allowing the passage of light. [L. *pellucidus*]

pe

pel·ma (pel'mă). SYN sole. [G.]

pel·mat·ic (pel-mat'ik). Relating to the sole of the foot. [G. *pelma*, sole]

pel·mat·o·gram (pel-mat'ō-gram). An imprint of the sole of the foot, made by resting the inked foot on a sheet of paper, or by pressing the greased foot on a plaster of Paris paste. [G. *pelma* (*pelmat*-), sole of the foot, + *gramma*, a picture]

pe·lop·a·thy (pē-lop'ă-thē). SYN pelotherapy. [G. *pēlos*, mud, + *pathos*, suffering]

pel·o·ther·a·py (pē'lō-thār-ă-pē). Application of peloids, such as mud, peat, or clay, to all or part of the body. SYN pelopathy. [G. *pēlos*, mud, + *therapeia*, treatment]

pel·ta (pel'tă). A crescentic, silver-staining, membranous organelle located anteriorly near the base of the flagella in certain flagellate protozoa, as in *Trichomonas*. [L. a shield]

pel·ta·tion (pel-tā'shŭn). Protection provided by inoculation with an antiserum or with a vaccine. [L. *pelta*, a light shield, fr. G. *peltē*]

pelvi-, pelvio-, pelvo-. The pelvis. Cf. pyelo-, pelyco-. [L. *pelvis*, basin (pelvis)]

pel·vic (pel'vik). Relating to a pelvis.

pel·vic di·rec·tion (pel'vik dī-rek'shŭn). The direction of the axis of the pelvis.

pel·vi·ceph·a·log·ra·phy (pel'vi-sef-ă-log'ră-fē). SYN cephalopelvimetry. [pelvi- + G. *kephalē*, head, + *graphō*, to write]

pel·vi·ceph·a·lom·e·try (pel'vi-sef-ă-lom'ĕ-trē). Measurement of the female pelvic diameters in relation to those of the fetal head. [pelvi- + G. *kephalē*, head, + *metron*, measure]

pel·vi·fix·a·tion (pel-vi-fik-sā'shŭn). Surgical attachment of a floating pelvic organ to the wall of the pelvic cavity.

pel·vi·li·thot·o·my (pel'vi-li-thot'ō-mē). SYN pyelolithotomy. [pelvi- + G. *lithos*, stone, + *tomē*, incision]

pel·vim·e·try (pel-vim'ĕ-trē). Measurement of the diameters of the pelvis. SYN radiocephalpelvimetry. [pelvi- + G. *metron*, measure]

CT p., procedure for measurement of the bony pelvis and fetal head through use of CT images; currently the more accurate imaging technique.

manual p., measurement of the essential diameters of the bony pelvis using the hands.

radiographic p., procedure for measurement of the bony pelvis and fetal head using anteroposterior and lateral radiographs, with a device for the correction of magnification.

pelvio-. SEE pelvi-.

pel·vi·o·li·thot·o·my (pel-vē-ō-li-thot'ō-mē). SYN pyelolithotomy.

pel·vi·o·per·i·to·ni·tis (pel'vē-ō-per-i-tō-nī'tis). SYN pelvic *peritonitis*.

pel·vi·o·plas·ty (pel'vē-ō-plas-tē). SYN pyeloplasty. [pelvio- + G. *plastos*, formed]

pel·vi·os·co·py (pel-vē-os'kŏ-pē). Examination of the pelvis for any purpose, usually by endoscopy. SYN pelvoscopy. [pelvio- + G. *skopeō*, to view]

pel·vi·per·i·to·ni·tis (pel-vē-per-i-tō-nī'tis). SYN pelvic *peritonitis*.

PELVIS

pel·vis, pl. **pel·ves** (pel'vis, pel'vēz) [TA]. **1** [NA]. The massive cup-shaped ring of bone, with its ligaments, at the lower end of the trunk, formed of the hip bone (the pubic bone, ilium, and ischium) on either side and in front, and the of sacrum and coccyx posteriorly. **2.** Any basinlike or cup-shaped cavity, as the p. of the kidney. [L. basin]

android p., a masculine or funnel-shaped p.

anthropoid p., p. with a long anteroposterior diameter and a narrow transverse diameter.

assimilation p., a deformity in which the transverse processes of the last lumbar vertebra are fused with the sacrum, or the last sacral with the first coccygeal body.

beaked p., SYN osteomalacic p.

brachypellic p., a p. in which the transverse diameter is more than 1 cm longer but less than 3 cm longer than the anteroposterior diameter. SYN transverse oval p.

caoutchouc p., in osteomalacia, a p. in which the bones are still soft. SYN rubber p.

contracted p., a p. with less than normal measurements in any diameter.

cordate p., cordiform p., a p. with sacrum projecting forward between the ilia, giving to the brim a heart shape. SYN heart-shaped p.

Deventer p., a p. with shortened anteroposterior diameter.

dolichopellic p., a p. in which the anteroposterior diameter is longer than the transverse. SYN longitudinal oval p.

dwarf p., a very small p., in which the several bones are united by cartilage as in the infant. SYN p. nana.

false p., SYN greater p.

flat p., a p. in which the anteroposterior diameter is uniformly contracted, the sacrum being dislocated forward between the iliac bones. SYN p. plana.

frozen p., a condition in which the true p. is indurated throughout, especially by carcinoma. SYN hardened p.

funnel-shaped p., a p. in which the pelvic inlet dimensions are normal, but the outlet is contracted in the transverse or in both transverse and anteroposterior diameters.

p. of gallbladder, SYN Hartmann *pouch*.

greater p. [TA], the expanded portion of the p. above the brim. SYN p. major [TA], false p., large p., p. spuria.

gynecoid p., the normal female p.

hardened p., SYN frozen p.

heart-shaped p., SYN cordate p.

inverted p., split p. with separation at pubis.

p. jus'to ma'jor, a symmetrical p. with greater than normal measurements in all diameters.

p. jus'to mi'nor, a p. of the female type, but with all its diameters smaller than normal.

juvenile p., a p. justo minor in which the bones are slender.

kyphoscoliotic p., a p. with marked anteroposterior curvature of the spine combined with lateral spinal curvature, usually due to severe rickets.

kyphotic p., a deformed pelvis associated with a kyphotic deformity of the spine.

large p., SYN greater p.

lesser p. [TA], the cavity of the p. below the brim or superior aperture. SYN p. minor [TA], p. vera, small p., true p.

longitudinal oval p., SYN dolichopellic p.

lordotic p., a deformed p. associated with a lordotic curvature of the spine.

p. ma'jor [TA], SYN greater p.

masculine p., (**1**) a p. justo minor in which the bones are large and heavy; (**2**) a slight degree of funnel-shaped p. in the woman, in which the shape approximates that of the male p.

mesatipellic p., obsolete term for one in which the anteroposterior and transverse diameters are equal or the transverse diameter is not more than 1 cm longer than the anteroposterior diameter. SYN round p.

p. mi'nor [TA], SYN lesser p.

Nägele p., an obliquely contracted or unilateral synostotic p., marked by arrest of development of one lateral half of the sacrum, usually ankylosis of the sacroiliac joint on that side, rotation of the sacrum toward the same side, and deviation of the symphysis pubis to the opposite side.

p. na'na, SYN dwarf p.

p. obtec'ta, a form of kyphotic p. in which the angular curvature of the spine is low and extreme so that the spinal column projects horizontally across the inlet of the p.

~~osteomalacic p.,~~ a pelvic deformity in osteomalacia; the pressure of the trunk on the sacrum and lateral pressure of the femoral heads produce a pelvic aperture that is three-cornered or has the shape of a heart or a cloverleaf, while the pubic bone becomes beak shaped. SYN beaked p., rostrate p.

Otto p., SYN Otto *disease.*

p. pla′na, SYN flat p.

platypellic p., flat oval p., in which the transverse diameter is more than 3 cm longer than the anteroposterior diameter.

platypelloid p., simple flat p.

Prague p., SYN spondylolisthetic p.

pseudoosteomalacic p., an extreme degree of rachitic p., resembling the puerperal osteomalacic p., in which the pelvic canal is obstructed by a forward projection of the sacrum, and an approximation of the acetabula.

rachitic p., a contracted and deformed p.; most commonly, a flat p. occurring from rachitic softening of the bones in early life.

renal p. [TA], a flattened funnel-shaped expansion of the upper end of the ureter receiving the calices, the apex being continuous with the ureter. SYN p. renalis [TA], ureteric p.

p. rena′lis [TA], SYN renal p.

reniform p., a modified cordate p., with a long transverse diameter, giving the brim a kidney shape.

Robert p., obsolete term for a p. that is narrowed transversely in consequence of the almost entire absence of the alae of the sacrum.

Rokitansky p., SYN spondylolisthetic p.

rostrate p., SYN osteomalacic p.

round p., SYN mesatipellic p.

rubber p., SYN caoutchouc p.

scoliotic p., a deformed p. associated with lateral curvature of the spine.

small p., SYN lesser p.

spider p., narrow calices of renal p.

split p., a p. in which the symphysis pubis is absent, the pelvic bones being separated by quite an interval; usually associated with exstrophy of the bladder.

spondylolisthetic p., a p. whose brim is more or less occluded by a forward dislocation of the body of the lower lumbar vertebra. SYN Prague p., Rokitansky p.

p. spu′ria, SYN greater p.

transverse oval p., SYN brachypellic p.

true p., SYN lesser p.

ureteric p., SYN renal p.

p. ve′ra, SYN lesser p.

---

pel·vi·sa·cral (pel-vi-sā′krăl). Relating to both the pelvis, or hip bones, and the sacrum.

pel·vi·scope (pel′vi-skōp). Endoscopic instrument for examining the interior of the pelvis. [pelvi- + G. *skopeō,* to view]

pel·vi·therm (pel′vi-therm). Instrument for applying heat to the pelvic organs. [pelvi- + G. *thermē,* heat]

pel·vi·u·re·ter·og·ra·phy (pel-vi-ū-rē-ter-og′ră-fē). SYN pyelography.

△**pelvo-.** SEE pelvi-.

pel·vo·ca·li·ec·ta·sis (pel′vō-kal-ē-ek-tā′sis). SYN hydronephrosis.

pel·vo·ceph·a·log·ra·phy (pel′vō-sef-ă-log′ră-fē). SYN cephalopelvimetry.

pel·vos·co·py (pel-vos′cŏ-pē). SYN pelvioscopy.

pel·vo·spon·dy·li·tis os·sif·i·cans (pel′vō-spon-di-lī′tis os-if′i-kanz). Deposit of bony substance between the vertebrae of the sacrum. [L. *pelvis,* basin, + G. *spondylos,* vertebra, + *-itis;* L. *os,* bone, + *facio,* to make]

△**pelyco-.** The pelvis. SEE pelvi-. [G. *pelyx,* bowl (pelvis)]

pem·o·line (pem′ō-lēn). A psychostimulant used in the treatment of attention deficit disorder (hyperactivity) in children.

pem·phi·goid (pem′fi-goyd). **1.** Resembling pemphigus. **2.** A disease resembling pemphigus but significantly distinguishable histologically (nonacantholytic) and clinically (generally benign course). [G. *pemphix,* blister, + *eidos,* resemblance]

benign mucosal p., SYN ocular cicatricial p.

bullous p., a chronic, generally benign disease, most commonly of old age, characterized by tense nonacantholytic bullae in which serum antibodies are localized to hemidesmosomal components of the epidermal basement membrane, causing detachment of the entire thickness of the epidermis.

localized p. of Brunsting-Perry, a variant of p., primarily on the scalp and face, with some scar formation.

ocular p., SYN ocular cicatricial p.

ocular cicatricial p., a chronic disease that produces adhesions and progressive cicatrization and shrinkage of the conjunctival, oral, and vaginal mucous membranes. SYN benign mucosal p., ocular p.

pem·phi·gus (pem′fi-gŭs). **1.** Autoimmune bullous diseases with acantholysis: p. vulgaris, p. foliaceus, p. erythematosus, or p. vegetans. **2.** A nonspecific term for blistering skin diseases. [G. *pemphix,* a blister]

benign familial chronic p. [MIM*169600], recurrent eruption of vesicles and bullae that become scaling and crusted lesions with vesicular borders, predominantly of the neck, groin, and axillary regions; autosomal dominant inheritance, presenting in late adolescence or early adult life. SYN Hailey-Hailey disease.

Brazilian p., SYN fogo selvagem.

p. erythemato′sus, an eruption involving sun-exposed skin, especially the face; the lesions are scaling erythematous macules and blebs, combining the clinical features of both lupus erythematosus and p. vulgaris; bullae are subcorneal; probably a variant of p. foliaceus, occasionally penicillamine-induced. SYN Senear-Usher disease, Senear-Usher syndrome.

p. folia′ceus, a generally chronic form of p., rarely affecting mucosal surfaces, in which extensive exfoliative dermatitis, with no perceptible blistering, may be present in addition to the bullae; serum autoantibodies induce bullae and crusted acantholytic superficial epidermal lesions.

p. gangreno′sus, **(1)** SYN *dermatitis* gangrenosa infantum; **(2)** SYN bullous *impetigo* of newborn.

paraneoplastic p., painful mucosal erosions and polymorphous skin eruptions with biopsy findings resembling p. vulgaris, associated with neoplasm and serum antibodies reactive with intercellular substance of all epithelia; usually rapidly fatal.

p. veg′etans, **(1)** a rare, verrucous form of p. vulgaris in which vegetations develop on the eroded surfaces left by ruptured bullae; new bullae continue to form; SYN Neumann disease. **(2)** a chronic benign vegetating form of p., with lesions commonly in the axillae and perineum; spontaneous remissions and occasionally permanent healing to occur. SYN Hallopeau disease.

p. vulga′ris, a serious form of p., occurring in middle age, in which cutaneous flaccid acantholytic suprabasal bullae and oral mucosal erosions may be localized a few months before becoming generalized; blisters break easily and are slow to heal; results from the action of autoimmune antibodies that localize to intercellular sites of stratified squamous epithelium.

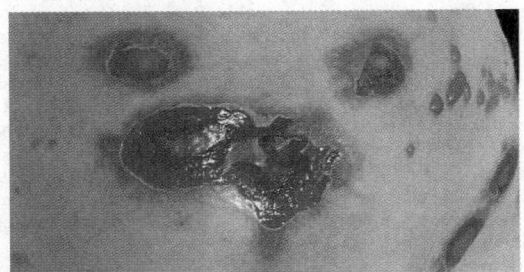

pemphigus vulgaris

---

pem·pi·dine (pem′pi-dēn). Secondary amine of the mecamylamine group, effective as a ganglionic blocking agent; also available as p. tartrate, with the same uses.

pen·del·luft (pen-del-lŭft'). Transient movement of gas out of some alveoli and into others when flow has just stopped at the end of inspiration, or such movement in the opposite direction just at the end of expiration; occurs when regions of the lung differ in compliance, airway resistance, or inertance so that the time constants of their filling (or emptying) in response to a change of transpulmonary pressure are not the same. [Ger. *Pendel,* pendulum, + *Luft,* air]

Pendred, Vaughan, English surgeon, 1869–1946. SEE P. *syndrome.*

pe·nec·to·my (pē-nek'tō-mē). SYN phallectomy. [L. *penis* + G. *ektomē,* excision]

pe·nes. Plural of penis, as in diphallus.

pen·e·trance (pen'ĕ-trans). The frequency, expressed as a fraction or percentage, of individuals who are phenotypically affected, among persons of an appropriate genotype (i.e., homozygous or hemizygous for recessives, heterozygous or hemozygous for dominants); for an autosomal dominant disorder, if only a proportion of individuals carrying the mutant allele display the abnormal phenotype, the trait is said to show incomplete penetrance. If all with the mutant allele show the abnormal phenotype, the trait is said to have complete or full penetrance. SEE penetration.

genetic p. (pen'ĕ-trans), the extent to which a genetically determined condition is expressed in an individual.

pen·e·trate (pen'ĕ-trāt). To pierce; to pass into the deeper tissues or into a cavity.

pen·e·tra·tion (pen-ĕ-trā'shŭn). **1.** A piercing or entering. **2.** Mental acumen. **3.** SYN focal *depth.* [L. *penetratio,* fr. *penetro,* pp. *-atus,* to enter]

pen·e·trom·e·ter (pen-ĕ-trom'ĕ-ter). An obsolete instrument for measuring the penetrating power of x-rays from any given source. [penetration + G. *metron,* measure]

△**-penia.** Deficiency. [G. *penia,* poverty]

pe·ni·al (pē'nē-ăl). SYN penile.

pe·ni·a·pho·bia (pē'nē-ă-fō'bē-ă). Morbid fear of poverty. [G. *penia,* poverty, + *phobos,* fear]

pen·i·cil·la·mine (pen-i-sil'ă-mēn). A degradation product of penicillin; a chelating agent used in the treatment of lead poisoning, hepatolenticular degeneration, and cystinuria, and in the removal of excess copper in Wilson disease; also available as p. hydrochloride. SYN β,β-dimethylcysteine.

pen·i·cil·la·nate (pen-i-sil'ă-nāt). A salt of penicillanic acid.

pen·i·cil·lan·ic ac·id (pen-i-si-lan'ik). A penicillin without the characterizing R group (with H– replacing ROONH–) of penicillin.

pen·i·cil·lar·y (pen-i-sil'ă-rē). Denoting a penicillus (1).

pen·i·cil·late (pen-i-sil'āt). **1.** Pertaining to a penicillus. **2.** Having a tuftlike structure.

pen·i·cil·lic ac·id (pen-i-sil'ik). An antibiotic produced by *Penicillium puberulum,* a mold found on maize, and from *P. cyclopium;* active against Gram-positive and Gram-negative bacteria but toxic to animal tissues.

pen·i·cil·lin (pen-i-sil'in). **1.** Originally, an antibiotic substance obtained from cultures of the molds *Penicillium notatum* or *P. chrysogenum;* interferes with cell wall synthesis in bacteria. **2.** One of a family of natural or synthetic variants of penicillic acid. They are mainly bactericidal in action, are especially active against Gram-positive organisms, and, with the exception of hypersensitivity reactions, show a particularly low toxic action on animal tissue. [see penicillus]

aluminum p., the trivalent aluminum salt of an antibiotic substance or substances produced by the growth of the molds *Penicillium notatum* or *P. chrysogenum;* used for oral or sublingual administration.

p. amidase, an enzyme that catalyzes the hydrolysis of the amide bond in the p.'s, producing a carboxylic acid anion and penicin; penicin is the precursor of many synthetic p.'s.

p. B, SYN phenethicillin potassium.

benzyl p., SYN p. G.

buffered crystalline p. G, crystalline potassium p. G or crystalline sodium p. G buffered with not less than 4% and not more than 5% of sodium citrate.

chloroprocaine p. O, a crystalline salt of 2-chloroprocaine and p. O, insoluble in water; the level of the antibiotic in the blood persists for 24 hours; its antibacterial activity is similar to that of p. O and G.

p. G, a commonly used p. compound; it comprises 85% of the p. salts: sodium, potassium, aluminum, and procaine, with the latter exerting prolonged action on intramuscular injection, because of limited solubility. An antibiotic obtained from the mold *Penicillium chrysogenum* used orally and parenterally; primarily active against Gram-positive staphylococci and streptococci; destroyed by bacterial β-lactamase. SYN benzyl p., benzylpenicillin.

p. G benzathine, a relatively insoluble preparation that may remain in the body for 1–2 weeks.

p. G hydrabamine, a dipenicillin compound, a mixture of p. G salts consisting chiefly of the salt of the diacidic base *N,N'*-bis-(dehydroabietyl) ethylenediamine.

p. G potassium, the potassium salt of p. G, containing 85–90% p. G.

p. G procaine, the procaine salt of p. G; it has a more prolonged action than p. G.

p. G sodium, the sodium salt of p. G, containing not less than 85% p. G.

p. N, SYN *cephalosporin N.*

p. O, produced by growing the mold in a medium containing allylmercaptomethylacetic acid; also available as the potassium and sodium salts. SYN allylmercaptomethylpenicillin.

p. phenoxymethyl, SYN p. V.

p. V, a p. derivative containing a phenoxyacetyl group; obtained from *Penicillium chrysogenum* Q 176; a crystalline nonhydroscopic acid, very stable even in high humidity; it resists destruction by gastric juice; the potassium salt is used orally; precursor for the synthesis of analogs of cephalosporin C. SYN p. phenoxymethyl, phenoxymethylpenicillin.

p. V benzathine, p. for oral use.

p. V hydrabamine, a compound with preparation and uses analogous to those of p. G hydrabamine.

pen·i·cil·li·nase (pen-i-sil'i-nās). **1.** SYN β-lactamase. **2.** A purified enzyme preparation obtained from cultures of a strain of *Bacillus cereus;* formerly used in the treatment of slowly developing or delayed penicillin reactions. Used by bacteria to develop penicillin resistance.

pen·i·cil·li·nate (pen-i-sil'i-nāt). A salt of a penicillic acid (i.e., of a penicillin).

penicilliosis. Invasive infection by a species of *Penicillium.*

Pen·i·cil·li·um (pen-i-sil'ē-ŭm). A genus of fungi (class Ascomycetes, order Aspergillales), species of which yield various antibiotic substances and biologicals; e.g., *citrinum* yields citrinin; *P. claviforme, P. expansum,* and *P. patulum* yield patulin; *P. chrysogenum* yields penicillin; *P. griseofulvum* yields griseofulvin; *P. notatum* yields penicillin and notatin; *P. cyclopium* and *P. puberulum* yield penicillic acid; *P. purpurogenum* and *P. rubrum* yield rubratoxin. *P. marneffei* is a true pathogen in Southeast Asia and in bamboo rats. [see penicillus]

P. lilacinum, SYN *Paecilomyces lilacinus.*

pen·i·cil·lo·ic ac·id (pen'i-si-lō'ik). Alkali and bacterial degradation product of a penicillin, resulting from hydrolysis of the 1,7 bond.

pen·i·cil·lo·yl pol·y·ly·sine (pen-i-sil'ō-il). A preparation of polylysine and a penicillic acid, used intradermally in the diagnosis of penicillin sensitivity; sensitive persons may react with systemic manifestations, including generalized cutaneous eruptions.

pen·i·cil·lus, pl. **pe·ni·cil·li** (pen-i-sil'ŭs, -sil'ī) [TA]. **1** [NA]. One of the tufts formed by the repeated subdivision of the minute arterial twigs in the spleen. **2.** In fungi, one of the branched conidiophores bearing chains of conidia in *Penicillium* species. [L. paint brush]

pen·i·cin (pen'i-sin). SYN 6-aminopenicillanic acid.

pe·nile (pē'nīl). Relating to the penis. SYN penial.

pe·nil·lic ac·ids (pe-nil′ik). Acid degradation products of penicillins, produced by cleavage of the 1,7 bond, forming penicilloic acid, and formation of a bond between the exocyclic carbonyl carbon and N-1 with elimination of H_2O from those two positions and the exocyclic NH.

pen·in (pen′in). 6-Aminopenicillanic acid; an intermediate in the synthesis of penicillins.

pe·nis, pl. **pe·nes** (pē′nis) [TA]. The organ of copulation and urination in the male; it is formed of three columns of erectile tissue, two arranged laterally on the dorsum (corpora cavernosa p.) and one median below (corpus spongiosum); the urethra traverses the latter; the extremity (glans p.) is formed by an expansion of the corpus spongiosum, and is more or less completely covered by a free fold of skin (preputium). SYN intromittent organ, membrum virile, phallus, priapus, virga. [L. tail]

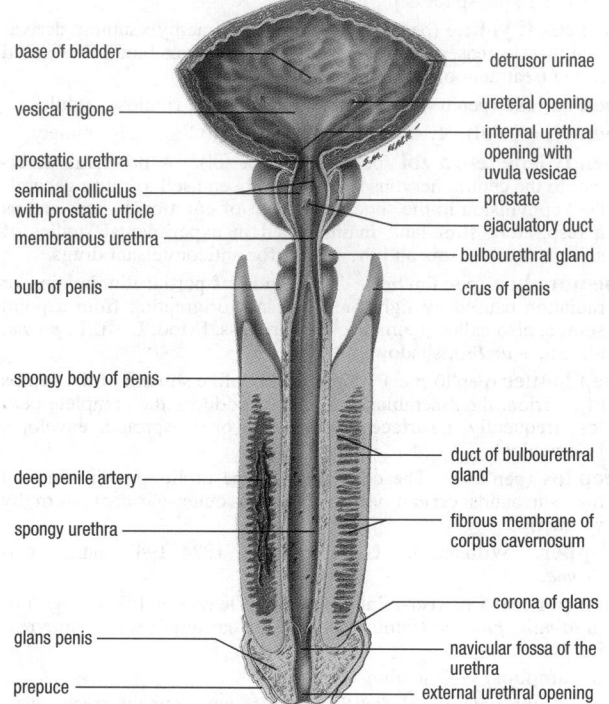

base of bladder
vesical trigone
prostatic urethra
seminal colliculus
with prostatic utricle
membranous urethra
bulb of penis

spongy body of penis

deep penile artery

spongy urethra

glans penis
prepuce

detrusor urinae
ureteral opening
internal urethral
opening with
uvula vesicae
prostate
ejaculatory duct
bulbourethral gland
crus of penis

duct of bulbourethral
gland
fibrous membrane of
corpus cavernosum

corona of glans

navicular fossa of the
urethra
external urethral opening

penis, base of bladder and urethra: longitudinal section (skin of penis removed as far as prepuce)

bifid p., SYN diphallus.

buried p., normal p. obscured by suprapubic fat.

clubbed p., a deformity of the erect p. marked by a curve to one side or toward the scrotum.

concealed p., usually a complication of circumcision wherein the anastomotic line between shaft skin and preputial collar closes like an iris or cicatrix over glans (some equate this to buried penis).

p. femin′eus, obsolete term for clitoris.

gryposis p., SYN chordee (1).

p. mulie′bris, obsolete term for clitoris.

webbed p., deficient ventral penile shaft skin that is buried in scrotum or tethered to scrotal midline by a fold or web of skin. The urethra and erectile bodies are usually normal.

pe·nis·chi·sis (pē-nis′ki-sis). A fissure of the penis resulting in an abnormal opening into the urethra, either above (epispadias), below (hypospadias), or to one side (paraspadias). [L. *penis* + G. *schisis*, fissure]

pen·nate (pen′āt). Feathered; resembling a feather. SYN penniform. [L. *pennatus,* fr. *penna,* feather]

pen·ni·form (pen′i-fōrm). SYN pennate. [L. *penna,* feather, + *forma,* form]

pen·ny·roy·al (pen′ē-roy-ăl). A name in folk medicine given to *Mentha pulegium* (an aromatic p.), or to *Hedeoma pulegeoides* (American p.) (family Labiatae); an aromatic stimulant formerly used as an emmenagogue.

pe·no·scro·tal (pē′nō-skrō′tăl). Relating to both penis and scrotum.

pe·not·o·my (pē-not′o-mē). SYN phallotomy. [L. *penis* + G. *tomē,* a cutting]

Penrose, Charles B., U.S. gynecologist, 1862–1925. SEE P. *drain.*

penta-. Combining form denoting five. [G. *pente,* five]

pen·ta·ba·sic (pen-tă-bā′sik). Denoting an acid having five replaceable hydrogen atoms. [penta- + G. *basis,* base]

pen·ta·chlo·ro·phe·nol (pen-tă-klōr-ō-fen′ol). Insecticide for termite control; preharvest defoliant; general herbicide. Has been used extensively for use in the preservation of wood, wood products, starches, dextrins, glues. No longer available for consumer use; a powerful irritant.

pen·tad. **1.** A collection of five things in some way related. **2.** In chemistry, a pentavalent element. [G. *pentas,* the number five]

Reynolds p., abdominal pain, fever, jaundice, shock, and depression of central nervous system function; usually indicative of acute suppurative cholangitis.

pen·ta·dac·tyl, pen·ta·dac·tyle (pen-tă-dak′til). Having five fingers or toes on each hand or foot. SYN quinquedigitate. [penta- + G. *daktylos,* finger]

pen·ta·e·ryth·ri·tol (pen-tă-ĕ-rith′ri-tol). The tetranitrate is a coronary vasodilator with action similar to that of other slow-acting organic nitrates.

pen·ta·e·ryth·ri·tol tet·ra·ni·trate. An organic nitrate used as a vasodilator in the treatment of angina pectoris; exerts a longer duration of action than nitroglycerin; acts via conversion to nitric oxide.

pen·ta·gas·trin (pen-tă-gas′trin). The substituted pentapeptide, BOC-β-Ala-Trp-Met-Asp-Phe(NH_2); a gastric acid stimulator.

pen·tal·o·gy (pen-tal′ō-jē). A rarely used term for a combination of five elements, such as five concurrent symptoms. [penta- + G. *logos,* treatise, word]

p. of Cantrell, a congenital defect involving a cleft lower sternum, an anterior diaphragmatic defect, absence of the parietal pericardium, a connected or separate omphalocele, and a major cardiac anomaly, most often *tetralogy* of Fallot and left ventricular diverticulum. SYN thoracoabdominal ectopia cordis.

p. of Fallot, tetralogy of Fallot with, in addition, a patent foramen ovale or atrial septal defect.

pen·ta·mer (pen′tă-mer). SEE virion. [penta- + G. *meros,* part]

pen·tam·i·dine is·e·thi·o·nate (pen-tam′i-dēn). A toxic but effective drug used in the prophylaxis and treatment of early stages of both types of African sleeping sickness (Gambian and Rhodesian trypanosomiasis). It does not cross the blood-brain barrier and is not effective in the treatment of the advanced (neurologic) stage of the disease. Also used to treat leishmaniasis that does not respond to therapy with pentavalent antimonials and in the treatment of pneumonia caused by *Pneumocystis carinii*.

pen·ta·no·ic ac·id (pen-tă-nō′ik). SYN valeric acid.

pen·ta·pep·tide (pen′tă-pep′tīd). A compound containing five amino acid residues linked via peptide bonds.

pen·ta·pip·er·ide fu·ma·rate (pen-tă-pip′er-īd). An intestinal antispasmodic.

pen·ta·pi·per·i·um meth·yl·sul·fate (pen′tă-pī-per′ē-ŭm). An anticholinergic agent.

pen·ta·quine (pen′tă-kwīn). An antimalarial agent closely related chemically to pamaquine but less toxic and more effective; it is administered with quinine, the two drugs acting synergically; active against *Plasmodium vivax* infections.

Pen·tas·to·ma (pen-tas′tō-mă). Older name for a genus of Pentastomida, now called *Linguatula*. The species described as *P. denticulatum* proved to be the larva of *Linguatula rhinaria*, sometimes parasitic in the nose of humans and other mammals; adults are found in the lungs of reptiles. [penta- + G. *stoma,* mouth]

pen·ta·sto·mi·a·sis (pen'tă-stō-mī'ă-sis). Infection of herbivorous animals, swine, and humans with larval tongue worms; lesions occur principally in the lymph nodes of the digestive tract, where they often resemble those of tuberculosis.

Pen·ta·stom·i·da (pen-tă-stom'i-dă). The tongue worms, a group of parasitic wormlike animals considered to form a distinct phylum thought to be descended from primitive arthropods, though modified by parasitism to form elongate, pseudosegmented, wormlike organisms with two to three pairs of budlike degenerate limbs in the larva and anterior, hollow, fanglike hooks in the adult. Adults are usually parasitic in the lungs or respiratory tract of vertebrates, usually in snakes and other reptiles, though one group parasitizes the air sacs of birds and one family (Linguatulidae) has become adapted to the lungs of mammal carnivores (families Felidae and Canidae). Larvae are found in the viscera of many hosts that serve as prey of the final hosts (insects, fish, amphibians, chiefly frogs, and mammals, chiefly rodents). Dogs may develop adult *Linguatula serrata* in their nasal passages from infective larvae (nymphs) in the viscera of sheep, cattle, or rabbits, which became infected from water or vegetation contaminated with eggs passed by infected dogs; humans also can develop a larval infection from this source. Human infection of liver, spleen, and lungs has been reported in Africa from *Armillifer armillatus* and in China by *A. moniliformis* from contaminated water or vegetation or from handling infected snakes. [see *Pentastoma*]

pent·a·tom·ic (pent'ă-tom-ik). Denoting five atoms per molecule. [penta- + atomic]

Pen·ta·trich·o·mon·as (pen'tă-trik-ŏ-mō'nas, pen'tă-trī-kom'ŏ-nas). A genus of parasitic protozoan flagellates, formerly part of the genus *Trichomonas* but now separated as a distinct genus by the presence of five anterior flagella and a granular parabasal body. The species *Pentatrichomonas hominis* lives as a commensal in the colon of humans and other primates, dogs, cats, oxen, and various rodents. [penta- + *Trichomonas*]

pen·ta·va·lent (pen-tă-vā'lent, pen-tav'ă-lent). Having a combining power (valence) of five. SYN quinquevalent.

pen·taz·o·cine (pen-taz'ō-sēn). An opioid agonist/antagonist analgesic with some addiction liability but only rare withdrawal syndrome and tolerance; very irritating to tissues on local injection; available as the hydrochloride and lactate salts.

pen·te·tate tri·so·di·um cal·ci·um (pen'tě-tāt). The calcium trisodium salt of pentetic acid. SYN calcium trisodium pentetate.

pen·tet·ic ac·id (pen-tet'ik). A pentaacetic acid triamine with affinity for heavy metals; used as the calcium sodium chelate in the treatment of iron-storage disease and poisoning from heavy metals and radioactive metals. SEE ALSO ethylenediaminetetraacetic acid.

pen·thi·e·nate bro·mide (pen-thī'ě-nāt). An anticholinergic agent.

pen·tif·yl·line (pen-tif'i-lēn). A vasodilator; has more lipid solubility than theobromine.

pen·ti·tol (pen'ti-tol). A reduced pentose; e.g., ribitol, lyxitol, xylitol.

pen·to·bar·bi·tal (pen-tō-bar'bi-tahl). An oral and intravenous sedative and short-acting hypnotic barbiturate; largely replaced by benzodiazepines.

pen·to·lin·i·um tar·trate (pen-tō-lin'ē-ŭm). A quaternary ammonium compound with potent ganglionic blocking action; used in the management of severe and malignant hypertension and peripheral vasospastic diseases.

pen·ton (pen'tŏn). The pentagonal capsomere (p. base) along with the protruding fiber at each of the 12 vertices of the adenovirus capsid; antigenically, the p. base differs from the fiber, and both differ from the other (hexagonal) capsomeres.

pen·to·san (pen'tō-san). A poly- or oligosaccharide of a pentose; e.g., arabans, xylans.

pen·tose (pen'tōs). A monosaccharide containing five carbon atoms in the molecule; e.g., arabinose, lyxose, ribose, xylose, xylulose.

p. nucleotide, a nucleotide having a p. as the sugar component.

pen·to·sta·tin (pen'tō-stat'in). An antineoplastic; a potent inhibitor of adenosine deaminase; interferes with the synthesis of nicotinamide adenine dinucleotide. SYN 2-deoxycoformycin.

pen·to·su·ria (pen-tō-soo'rē-ă). The excretion of one or more pentoses in elevated amounts in the urine.

alimentary p., the urinary excretion of L-arabinose and L-xylose, as the result of the excessive ingestion of fruits containing these pentoses.

essential p. [MIM*260800], a benign heritable disorder in which the urinary output of L-xylulose is 1–4 g/24 h; it occurs principally in Ashkenazi Jewish individuals; autosomal recessive inheritance. SYN L-xylulosuria, primary p.

primary p., SYN essential p.

pen·tox·ide (pen-tok'sīd). An oxide containing five oxygen atoms; e.g., phosphorus p., P_2O_5.

pen·tox·if·yl·line (pen-toks-if'i-lēn). A dimethylxanthine derivative that decreases blood viscosity and improves blood flow; used in the treatment of intermittent claudication.

pen·tu·lose (pen'tū-lōs). A ketopentose; e.g., ribulose, xylulose.

pen·tyl (pen'til). **1.** SYN amyl. **2.** The $CH_3(CH_2)_4CH_2$– moiety.

pen·ty·lene·tet·ra·zol (pen'ti-lēn-tet'ră-zol). A powerful stimulant to the central nervous system; has been used to cause generalized convulsion in the shock treatment of emotional states and as a respiratory stimulant; mainly used in experimental studies of seizure mechanisms and the search for anticonvulsant drugs.

pe·num·bra (pe-nŭm'bră). The region of partial illumination or radiation caused by light or x-rays not originating from a point source; also called geometric unsharpness. [Mod. L., fr. L. *paene,* almost, + *umbra,* shadow]

pep·lo·mer (pep'lō-mer). A part or knoblike subunit of the peplos of a virion, the assemblage of which produces the complete peplos; frequently a surface glycoprotein on lipoprotein envelope. [see peplos]

pep·los (pep'lōs). The coat or envelope of lipoprotein material that surrounds certain virions. [G. an outer garment worn by women]

Pepper, William, Jr., U.S. physician, 1874–1947. SEE P. *syndrome.*

pep·per·mint (pep'er-mint). The dried leaves and flowering tops of *Mentha piperita* (family Labiatae); a carminative and antiemetic.

p. camphor, SYN menthol.

p. oil, the volatile oil distilled with steam from the fresh, overground parts of the flowering plant of *Mentha piperita,* rectified by distillation and neither partially nor wholly dementholized; a flavor.

pep·sic (pep'sik). SYN peptic.

pep·sin (pep'sin). A group of closely related aspartic proteinases. P. A is the principal digestive enzyme of gastric juice, formed from pepsinogen; it hydrolyzes peptide bonds at low pH values (is alkali-labile), preferably adjacent to phenylalanyl and leucyl residues, thus reducing proteins to smaller molecules (referred to as proteoses and peptones); p. B (gelatinase) is similar to p. A, formed from porcine pepsinogen B and has a more restricted specificity; p. C (gastricsin is human p. C) is also similar to p. A, and structurally related to it, having a more restricted specificity. [G. *pepsis,* digestion]

pep·si·nate (pep'si-nāt). To mix pepsin with.

pep·si·nif·er·ous (pep-si-nif'er-ŭs). SYN pepsinogenous.

pep·sin·o·gen (pep-sin'ō-jen). A proenzyme or zymogen formed and secreted by the chief cells of the gastric mucosa; the acidity of the gastric juice and pepsin itself remove 44 amino acyl residues from p. to form active pepsin. SYN propepsin. [pepsin + G. -*gen,* producing]

pep·sin·og·e·nous (pep-sin-oj'ě-nŭs). Producing pepsin. SYN pepsiniferous.

pep·si·nu·ria (pep-si-noo'rē-ă). Excretion of pepsin in the urine. [pepsin + G. *ouron,* urine]

pep·sta·tin (pep-sta′tin). An inhibitor peptide from actinomycetes that inhibits pepsin and cathepsin D.

pep·tic (pep′tik). Relating to the stomach, to gastric digestion, or to pepsin A. SYN pepsic. [G. *peptikos*, fr. *peptō*, to digest]

pep·ti·dase (pep′ti-dās). Any enzyme capable of hydrolyzing a peptide bond of a peptide; e.g., carboxypeptidases, aminopeptidases. SYN peptide hydrolase.

p. D, SYN *proline* dipeptidase.

p. P, SYN peptidyl dipeptidase A.

pep·tide (pep′tīd). A compound of two or more amino acids in which a carboxyl group of one is united with an amino group of another, with the elimination of a molecule of water, thus forming a peptide bond, –CO–NH–; i.e., a substituted amide. Cf. eupeptide *bond*, isopeptide *bond*.

adrenocorticotropic p., a p. with ACTH activity, isolated from pituitary extracts.

anionic neutrophil-activating p. (ANAP), SYN interleukin-8.

antigen p.'s, the protein fragments that bind to MHC molecules.

atrial natriuretic p. (ANP) (na′trē-oo-ret′ik), a 28–amino acid p. (α-ANP), derived from cardiac atria, several smaller fragments of α-ANP, and a dimer of α-ANP with 56 amino acids (β-ANP) that are present in plasma in heart failure. ANP actions include increasing capillary filtration, and renal salt and water excretion, and decreasing arterial pressure and the secretion of renin, angiotensin, aldosterone, and antidiuretic hormone. SYN atriopeptin, cardionatrin.

bitter p.'s, p.'s that have a bitter taste and may spoil certain foods; often contain high proportions of leucyl, valyl, and aromatic amino acyl residues.

bradykinin-potentiating p., SYN teprotide.

calcitonin gene-related p. (CGRP), a second product transcribed from the calcitonin gene. CGRP is found in a number of tissues including nervous tissue. It is a vasodilator that may participate in the cutaneous triple response.

cyclic p., a p. that forms a ring structure; e.g., tyrocidin A, an antibiotic, is a cyclic decapeptide; valinomycin is a cyclic depsipeptide.

gastric inhibitory p. (GIP), SYN gastric inhibitory *polypeptide*.

glucagonlike p., a gut hormone that slows gastric emptying and stimulates insulin secretion. It may become useful in the future in the treatment of noninsulin-dependent diabetes mellitus, perhaps administered by patch, inhaler, or buccal pellet formulation.

glucagonlike insulinotropic p., an insulinotropic substance originating in the gastrointestinal tract and released into the circulation following ingestion of a meal containing glucose.

heterodetic p., a p. that contains p. bonds as well as covalent linkages between certain amino acyl residues that are not p. bonds; e.g., valinomycin, oxytocin. [hetero- + G. *detos*, bound, fr. *deō*, to bind, + -ic]

heteromeric p., a p. that, on hydrolysis, yields substances other than amino acids in addition to amino acids; e.g., pteroylglutamic acid.

homodetic p., a p. in which all of the covalent linkages between the constituent amino acids are p. bonds; e.g., bradykinin. [homo- + G. *detos*, bound, fr. *deō*, to bind, + -ic]

homomeric p., **(1)** a p. that, on hydrolysis, yields only amino acids; e.g., glutathione; **(2)** a p. that consists of only one particular amino acid; e.g., alanylalanylalanine.

p. hydrolase [EC subclass 3.4], SYN peptidase.

parathyroid hormone-related p., a hormone that can be produced by tumors, especially of the squamous cell type; massive overproduction can lead to hypercalcemia and other manifestations of hyperparathyroidism. PTHrP exerts a biologic action similar to that of parathyroid hormone (PTH), acting via the same receptor, which is expressed in many tissues but most abundantly in kidney, bone, and growth plate cartilage. It apparently has significant actions during development, but it is uncertain whether PTHrP circulates at all or has any function in normal human adults. The structure of the gene for human PTHrP is more complex than that of PTH, and varying molecular forms exist, including proteins of 141, 139, and 173 amino acids, which share a significant homology with parathyroid hormone.

phenylthiocarbamoyl p., PTC p., the p. formed by combination of phenylisothiocyanate and an α-amino group of a peptide. SEE ALSO phenylthiohydantoin.

S p., SEE S *protein*.

sigma p., a p. with one end bonded to a point within the chain, usually by means of the disulfide group of a cystine residue, so that only one end of the p. is free; so called since the p. chain has then the rough shape of the Greek letter sigma; e.g., oxytocin.

p. synthetase [EC 6.3.2.x], any enzyme that catalyzes the synthesis of peptide bonds, with the concomitant hydrolysis of a nucleoside triphosphate.

vasoactive intestinal p., SYN vasoactive intestinal *polypeptide*.

pep·ti·der·gic (pep-ti-der′jik). Referring to nerve cells or fibers that are believed to employ small peptide molecules as their neurotransmitter. [peptide + G. *ergon*, work]

pep·ti·do·gly·can (pep′ti-dō-glī′kan). A compound containing amino acids (or peptides) linked to sugars, with the latter preponderant. Cf. glycopeptide. SYN mucopeptide (2).

pep·ti·doid (pep′ti-doyd). A condensation product of two amino acids involving at least one condensing group other than the α-carboxyl or α-amino group; e.g., glutathione.

pep·ti·do·lyt·ic (pep′ti-dō-lit′ik). Causing the cleavage or digestion of peptides. [peptide + G. *lytikos*, solvent]

pep·ti·dyl di·pep·ti·dase A (pep′ti-dil). A zinc-containing hydrolase cleaving C-terminal dipeptides from a variety of substrates, including angiotensin I, which is converted to angiotensin II and histidylleucine (an important step in the metabolism of certain vasopressor agents). Drugs that inhibit it are used to treat hypertension and congestive heart failure. SYN angiotensin-converting enzyme, carboxycathepsin, dipeptidyl carboxypeptidase, kinase II, peptidase P.

pep·tid·yl·trans·fer·ase (pep-tī′dil-trans′fer-ās). The enzyme responsible for the formation of the peptide bond on the ribosome during protein biosynthesis, peptidyl-tRNA^1 + aminoacyl-tRNA^2 → tRNA^1 + peptidylaminoacyl-tRNA^2.

pep·ti·za·tion (pep-ti-zā′shŭn). In colloid chemistry, an increase in the degree of dispersion, tending toward a uniform distribution of the dispersed phase.

Pep·to·coc·ca·ce·ae (pep′tō-kok-ā′sē-ē). A family of nonmotile, nonsporeforming, anaerobic bacteria (order Eubacteriales) containing Gram-positive (staining may be equivocal) cocci, 0.5–1.6 μm in diameter, which occur singly, in pairs, chains, tetrads, and irregular masses but not in three-dimensional, cubic packets. These organisms are chemoorganotrophic and have complex nutritional requirements. Carbohydrates may or may not be fermented by these organisms, which produce gas, principally CO_2 and usually H_2, from amino acids, or carbohydrates, or both. They are found in the mouth and intestinal and respiratory tracts of humans and other animals; they are frequently found in normal and pathologic human female urogenital tracts.

Pep·to·coc·cus (pep′tō-kok′ŭs). A genus of nonmotile, anaerobic, chemoorganotrophic bacteria (family Peptococcaceae) containing Gram-positive, spherical cells that occur singly, in pairs, tetrads, or irregular masses, and rarely in short chains. They are frequently found in association with pathologic conditions. The type species is *P. niger*. [G. *peptō*, to digest, + *kokkos*, berry]

P. aero′genes, former name for *Peptostreptococcus asaccharolyticus*.

P. constellatus, a bacterial species found in tonsils, purulent pleurisy, appendix, the nose, throat, and gums, and infrequently on the skin and in the vagina.

P. ni′ger, a bacterial species found once, in the urine of an aged woman; type species of the genus *P*.

pep·to·crin·ine (pep-tō-krin′ēn). An extract of the intestinal mucosa resembling secretin.

pep·to·gen·ic, pep·tog·e·nous (pep-tō-jen′ik, pep-toj′ĕ-nŭs). **1.** Producing peptones. **2.** Promoting digestion.

pep·toid (pep′tōyd). A peptide with one or more non—amino acyl groups (e.g., sugar, lipid, etc.) covalently linked to the peptide.

pep·to·lide (pep′tō-līd). **1.** A cyclic depsipeptide; e.g., valinomycin. **2.** A heteromeric depsipeptide.

pep·tol·y·sis (pep-tol′i-sis). The hydrolysis of peptones.

pep·to·lyt·ic (pep-tō-lit′ik). **1.** Pertaining to peptolysis. **2.** Denoting an enzyme or other agent that hydrolyzes peptones.

pep·tone (pep′tōn). Descriptive term applied to intermediate polypeptide products, formed in partial hydrolysis of proteins, that are soluble in water, diffusible, and not coagulable by heat; used in bacterial culture media.

pep·ton·ic (pep-ton′ik). Relating to or containing peptone.

pep·to·ni·za·tion (pep′ton-i-zā′shŭn). Conversion by enzymic action of native protein into soluble peptone.

Pep·to·strep·to·coc·cus (pep′tō-strep-tō-kok′ŭs). A genus of nonmotile, anaerobic, chemoorganotrophic bacteria (family Peptococcaceae) containing spherical to ovoid, Gram-positive cells that occur in pairs and short or long chains. These organisms are found in normal and pathologic female genital tracts and blood in puerperal fever, in respiratory and intestinal tracts of normal humans and other animals, in the oral cavity, and in pyogenic infections, putrefactive war wounds, and appendicitis; they may be pathogenic. The type species is *P. anaerobius.* [G. *peptō,* to digest, + *streptos,* curved, + *kokkos,* berry]

P. anaero′bius, a bacterial species found in the mouth, intestinal and respiratory tracts, and cavities, especially the vagina, of humans and other animals; it may be pathogenic; it is the type species of the genus *P.*

P. asaccharoly′ticus, a bacterial species found in the human large intestine, buccal cavity, pleura, uterus, and vagina; also found in cases of puerperal fever; characterized by its inability to metabolize sugars.

P. evolu′tus, a bacterial species found in the human respiratory tract, mouth, and vagina.

P. foe′tidus, a bacterial species found in abscesses, blood, the intestinal tract, vagina, and mouth of humans and other animals; it is sometimes fatal.

P. interme′dius, SYN *Streptococcus intermedius.*

P. mag′nus, a bacterial species found in putrefying butcher's meat and in a case of appendicitis.

P. mi′cros, a bacterial species found in natural cavities of humans and other animals; it has been isolated from various pathologic conditions.

P. morbillo′rum, a bacterial species found in the nose, throat, eyes, ears, mucous secretions, and blood in cases of measles, being irrelevant, however, to the etiology of measles; probably present normally, developing as a secondary invader. SYN *Streptococcus morbillorum.*

P. paleopneumo′niae, a bacterial species found in the buccal pharyngeal cavity and the upper respiratory tract of humans.

P. par′vulus, former name for *Atopobium parvulus.*

P. plagarumbel′li, a bacterial species commonly found in septic war wounds.

P. produc′tus, former name for *Ruminococcus productus.*

P. pu′tridus, a bacterial species found in the human mouth and intestinal tract but especially in the vagina.

⌂**per-.** **1.** Through, conveying intensity. **2.** In chemistry, a prefix denoting either 1) more or most, with respect to the amount of a given element (usually oxygen, as in perchloric acid) or radical contained in a compound, or 2) the degree of substitution for hydrogen, as in peroxides, peroxy acids (e.g., hydrogen peroxide, peroxyformic acid). SEE ALSO peroxy-. [L. through, throughout, extremely]

per·a·ceph·a·lus (per-ă-sef′ă-lŭs). An omphalosite lacking head and arms, and with a defective thorax; typically, the body consists of little more than pelvis and legs. [per- + G. *a-* priv. + *kephalē,* head]

per·ac·id (per-as′id). An acid containing a peroxide group (–O–OH); e.g., peracetic acid. SYN peroxy acid.

per·a·cute (per-ă-kyut′). Very acute; said of a disease. [L. *peracutus,* very sharply]

per an·um (per ā′nŭm). By or through the anus. [L.]

per·ar·tic·u·la·tion (per′ar-tik′ū-lā′shŭn). SYN synovial *joint.* [per- + L. *articulatio,* joint]

per·a·to·dyn·ia (per′ă-tō-din′ē-ă). Obsolete term for pyrosis. [G. *peratos,* on the opposite side, + *odynē,* pain]

per·ax·il·lary (per-ak′si-lār-ē). Through the axilla.

per·a·zine (per′ă-zēn). An antipsychotic.

per·cen·tile (per-sen′tīl). The rank position of an individual in a serial array of data, stated in terms of what percentage of the group the individual equals or exceeds.

per·cept (per′sept). **1.** That which is perceived; the complete mental image, formed by the process of perception, of an object or idea. **2.** In clinical psychology, a single unit of perceptual report, such as one of the responses to an inkblot in the Rorschach test. [L. *perceptum,* a thing perceived]

per·cep·tion (per-sep′shun). The mental process of becoming aware of or recognizing an object or idea; primarily cognitive rather than affective or conative, although all three aspects are manifested. SYN esthesia (1).

depth p., the visual ability to judge depth or distance.

extrasensory p. (ESP), p. by means other than through the ordinary senses; e.g., telepathy, clairvoyance, precognition.

simultaneous p., a combination of two slightly dissimilar images into a single image.

per·cep·tive (per-sep′tiv). Relating to or having a higher than normal power of perception.

per·cep·tiv·i·ty (per-sep-tiv′i-tē). The power of perception.

per·cep·to·ri·um (per-sep-tōr′ē-ŭm). SYN sensorium (2).

per·co·la·tion (per-kō-lā′shŭn). **1.** SYN filtration. **2.** Extraction of the soluble portion of a solid mixture by passing a solvent liquid through it. **3.** Passage of saliva or other fluids into the interface between tooth structure and restoration; sometimes induced by thermal changes. [L. *percolatio,* fr. per- + *colare,* to strain]

per·co·la·tor (per′kō-lā-ter). A funnel-shaped vessel used for the process of percolation in pharmacy.

per·co·morph oil (per-kō-mōrf). A liver oil from fish of the order Percomorphi, with a standardized amount of vitamins A and D.

per con·tig·u·um (per kon-tig′ū-ŭm). In contiguity; denoting the mode by which an inflammation or other morbid process spreads into an adjacent contiguous structure. [per- + L. *contiguus,* touching, fr. *tango,* to touch]

per con·tin·u·um (per kon-tin′ū-ŭm). In continuity; continuous; denoting the mode by which an inflammation or other morbid process spreads from one part to another through continuous tissue. [per- + L. *continuus,* holding together, continuous, fr. *teneo,* to hold]

per·cuss (per-kŭs′). To perform percussion.

per·cus·sion (per-kŭsh′ŭn). **1.** A diagnostic procedure designed to determine the density of a body part by the sound produced by tapping the surface with the finger or a plessor; performed primarily over the chest to determine presence of normal air content in the lungs and over the abdomen to evaluate air in the loops of intestine and the size of solid organs such as the liver and spleen. **2.** A form of massage, consisting of repeated blows or taps of varying force. [L. *percussio,* fr. *per-cutio,* pp. *-cussus,* to beat, fr. *quatio,* to shake, beat]

auscultatory p., auscultation of the chest or other part at the same time that p. is made, to aid in hearing the sound made by p.

bimanual p., immediate p. in which the finger of one hand taps the other hand; a form of mediate p.

clavicular p., p., usually direct, along the entire clavicle to demonstrate dullness, particularly in apical pulmonary tuberculosis.

deep p., heavy p. to obtain information about deeply situated organs or structures.

direct p., SYN immediate p.

finger p., p. in which a finger of one hand is used as a plessimeter and one of the other hand as a plessor.

immediate p., the striking of the part under examination directly with the finger or a plessor, without the intervention of another finger or plessimeter. SYN direct p.

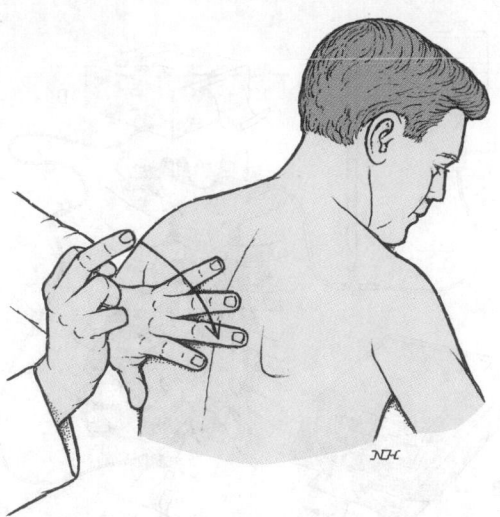

bimanual percussion: distal phalanx of left middle finger is pressed firmly against chest wall parallel with ribs; a short, quick blow is struck at the base of the distal phalanx of the middle finger with the tip of the middle finger of the right hand

mediate p., p. effected by the intervention of a finger or a plessimeter between the striking finger or plessor and the part percussed.

Murphy p., examination for dullness by striking the chest wall directly with the fingertips of one hand successively, beginning with the fifth finger. SYN piano p.

palpatory p., finger p. in which attention is focused upon the resistance and reverberation of the tissues under the finger as well as upon the sound elicited. SYN plessesthesia.

piano p., SYN Murphy p.

threshold p., p. effected by means of a glass rod as a plessimeter, the rod being inclined to the wall of the chest or abdomen and touching it only by one extremity.

per·cus·sor (per-kŭs′er). SYN plessor.

per·cu·ta·ne·ous (per-kū-tā′nē-ŭs). Denoting the passage of substances through unbroken skin, as in absorption by inunction; also passage through the skin by needle puncture, including introduction of wires and catheters by Seldinger *technique.* SYN transcutaneous, transdermic.

per·en·ceph·a·ly (per-en-sef′ă-lē). A condition marked by one or more cerebral cysts. [G. *pēra,* a purse, a wallet, + *enkephalos,* brain]

Perez, George V., Spanish physician, †1920. SEE P. *sign.*

Perez, Bernard, French physician, 1836–1903. SEE P. *reflex.*

per·fec·tion·ism (per-fek′shŭn-izm). A tendency to set rigid high standards of performance for oneself.

per·fla·tion (per-flā′shŭn). Blowing air into or through a cavity or canal to force apart its walls or to expel any contained material. [L. *per-flo,* pp, *-flatus,* to blow through]

per·flu·bron (per-floo′bron). Generic name for perfluorooctyl bromide.

per·flu·o·ro·octyl bro·mide (PFOB) (per-floo′rō-ok-til brō′mĭd). A bromine-substituted fluorocarbon, prepared as a particulate emulsion, used as a CT, MR, and ultrasound contrast medium.

per·fo·rans (per′fō-rans). A term applied to several muscles and nerves that, in their course, perforate other structures. [L. perforating]

per·fo·rat·ed (per′fō-rāt-ed). Pierced with one or more holes. [L. *perforatus,* fr. *per-foro,* pp. *-atus,* to bore through]

per·fo·ra·tion (per-fō-rā′shŭn). Abnormal opening in a hollow organ or viscus. SYN tresis. [see perforated]

per·fo·ra·tor (per′fōr-ā-ter). An instrument for making a bony opening through the cranium. SYN trephine (1).

per·fo·rin (per′fōr-in). A protein found in the cytoplasmic granules of both T cytotoxic lymphocytes and natural killer cells. This protein is implicated in target cell lysis by the above cells. [L. *per-foro,* to bore, pierce, + -in]

per·for·mic ac·id (per-fōr′mik). An organic peracid used in cleaving disulfide links in peptides by oxidizing cystinyl residues to cysteic acid. SYN peroxyformic acid.

per·frig·er·a·tion (per-frij-er-ā′shŭn). A minor degree of frostbite. [L. *per-frigero,* pp. -atus, to make cold, fr. *frigus,* cold]

per·fus·ate (per′fū-sāt). The fluid used for perfusion; sometimes more broadly applied to fluid that has been forced through any more or less porous membrane or material. [see perfuse]

per·fuse (per-fyŭs′). To force blood or other fluid to flow from the artery through the vascular bed of a tissue or to flow through the lumen of a hollow structure (e.g., an isolated renal tubule). Cf. perifuse, superfuse. [L. *perfusio,* fr. per- + *fusio,* a pouring]

per·fu·sion (per-fū′zhŭn). 1. The act of perfusing. 2. The flow of blood or other perfusate per unit volume of tissue, as in ventilation/perfusion ratio.

regional p., p. of part of the body, especially a limb, and particularly with chemotherapeutic agents, for treatment of a malignant tumor, primary, recurrent, or metastatic.

per·go·lide mes·y·late (per′go-līd). An ergot derivative with dopaminergic properties; used in parkinsonism.

per·hex·i·line ma·le·ate (per-hek′si-lēn). A coronary vasodilator and diuretic.

per·hy·dro·cy·clo·pen·ta[a]phen·an·threne. SYN tetracyclic steroid *nucleus.*

⌂**peri-.** Around, about, near. Cf. circum-. [G. around]

per·i·ac·cre·tio pe·ri·car·dii (per′i-ă-krē′shē-ō per-i-kar′dē-ī). Adhesion of the p. p. or part of it to the cardiac surface due to antecedent inflammation.

per·i·ac·i·nal, per·i·ac·i·nous (per-ē-as′i-năl, -i-nŭs). Surrounding an acinus.

per·i·ad·e·ni·tis (per′ē-ad-ě-nī′tis). Inflammation of the tissues surrounding a gland. [peri- + G. *adēn,* gland, + *-itis,* inflammation]

p. muco′sa necrot′ica recur′rens, SYN *aphthae* major, under *aph-tha.*

per·i·a·nal (per-ē-ā′năl). SYN circumanal.

per·i·an·gi·o·cho·li·tis (per′ē-an′jē-ō-kō-lī′tis). SYN pericholangitis. [peri- + G. *angeion,* vessel, + *cholē,* bile, + *-itis,* inflammation]

per·i·an·gi·tis (per′ē-an-jī′tis). Inflammation of the adventitia of a blood vessel or of the tissues surrounding it or a lymphatic vessel. SEE ALSO periarteritis, periphlebitis, perilymphangitis. SYN perivasculitis. [peri- + G. *angeion,* a vessel, + *-itis,* inflammation]

per·i·a·or·tic (per′ē-ā-ōr′tik). Surrounding or adjacent to the aorta.

per·i·a·or·ti·tis (per′ē-ā-ōr-tī′tis). Inflammation of the adventitia of the aorta and of the tissues surrounding it.

per·i·a·pex (per′ē-ā′peks). The periapical structures, particularly periodontal membrane and adjacent bone. [peri- L. *apex,* tip]

per·i·ap·i·cal (per-ē-ap′i-kăl). 1. At or around the apex of a root of a tooth. 2. Denoting the periapex.

per·i·ap·pen·di·ci·tis (per′ē-ă-pen-di-sī′tis). Inflammation of the tissue surrounding the vermiform appendix. SYN para-appendicitis.

p. decidua′lis, the presence of decidual cells in the peritoneum of the vermiform appendix in cases of right tubal pregnancy with adhesions between the fallopian tube and the appendix.

per·i·ap·pen·dic·u·lar (per′ē-ap-en-dik′ū-lăr). Surrounding an appendix, especially the vermiform appendix.

per·i·ar·te·ri·al (per′ē-ar-tē′rē-ăl). Surrounding an artery.

per·i·ar·te·ri·tis (per′ē-ar-ter-ī′tis). Inflammation of the adventitia of an artery. SYN exarteritis.

p. nodo′sa, SYN *polyarteritis* nodosa.

per·i·ar·thric (per′ē-ar′thrik). SYN circumarticular.

pe

per·i·ar·thri·tis (per'ē-ar-thrī'tis). Inflammation of the parts surrounding a joint. [peri- + arthritis]

per·i·ar·tic·u·lar (per'ē-ar-tik'ū-lăr). SYN circumarticular.

per·i·a·tri·al (per'ē-ā'trē-ăl). Surrounding the atrium of the heart. SYN periauricular (1).

per·i·au·ric·u·lar (per'ē-aw-rik'ū-lăr). **1.** SYN periatrial. **2.** SYN periconchal. **3.** Around the external ear.

per·i·ax·i·al (per'ē-ak'sē-ăl). Surrounding an axis.

per·i·ax·il·lary (per'ē-ak'sē-lār-ē). SYN circumaxillary.

per·i·ax·o·nal (per'ē-ak'sō-năl). Surrounding the axon of a nerve. [peri- + G. *axōn,* axis]

per·i·blast (per'i-blast). A specialized region of yolk surface immediately peripheral to the blastoderm in telolecithal eggs. [peri- + G. *blastos,* germ]

per·i·bron·chi·al (per-i-brong'kē-ăl). Surrounding a bronchus or the bronchi.

per·i·bron·chi·o·lar (per-i-brong'kē-ō'lăr). Surrounding the bronchioles.

per·i·bron·chi·o·li·tis (per'i-brong'kē-ō-lī'tis). Inflammation of the tissues surrounding the bronchioles.

per·i·bron·chi·tis (per'i-brong-kī'tis). Inflammation of the tissues surrounding the bronchi or bronchial tubes.

per·i·buc·cal (per'i-bŭk'ăl). Surrounding the cheek.

per·i·bul·bar (per-i-bŭl'băr). Surrounding any bulb, especially the eyeball or the bulb of the urethra. SYN circumbulbar.

per·i·bur·sal (per-i-ber'săl). Surrounding a bursa.

per·i·can·a·lic·u·lar (per'i-kan-ă-lik'oo-lăr). Surrounding a canaliculus.

per·i·car·dec·to·my (per'i-kar-dek'tō-mē). SYN pericardiectomy.

per·i·car·dia (per-i-kar'dē-ă). Plural of pericardium.

per·i·car·di·ac, per·i·car·di·al (per-i-kar'dē-ak, -dē-ăl). **1.** Surrounding the heart. **2.** Relating to the pericardium.

per·i·car·di·cen·te·sis (per-i-kar'dē-sen-tē'sis). SYN pericardiocentesis.

per·i·car·di·ec·to·my (per'i-kar-dē-ek'tō-mē). Excision of a portion of the pericardium. SYN pericardectomy. [pericardium + G. *ektomē,* excision]

 radical p., excision of almost the entire pericardium.

per·i·car·di·o·cen·te·sis (per-i-kar'dē-ō-sen-tē'sis). Needle or catheter drainage of the pericardium. SYN pericardial tap, pericardicentesis. [peri- + G. *kardia,* heart, + *kentēsis,* puncture]

per·i·car·di·ol·ogy (per-ē-kar-dē-ol'ō-jē). The science or study of the pericardium, its physiology, and diseases.

per·i·car·di·o·per·i·to·ne·al (per-i-kar'dē-ō-per-i-tō-nē'ăl). Relating to the pericardial and peritoneal cavities.

per·i·car·di·o·phren·ic (per-i-kar'dē-ō-fren'ik). Relating to the pericardium and the diaphragm. [pericardium + G. *phrēn,* diaphragm]

per·i·car·di·o·pleur·al (per-i-kar'dē-ō-ploor'ăl). Relating to the pericardial and pleural cavities.

per·i·car·di·or·rha·phy (per'i-kar-dē-ōr'ă-fē). Suture of the pericardium. [pericardium + G. *rhaphē,* suture]

per·i·car·di·os·to·my (per'i-kar-dē-os'tō-mē). Establishment of an opening into the pericardium. [pericardium + G. *stoma,* mouth]

per·i·car·di·ot·o·my (per'i-kar-dē-ot'ō-mē). Incision into the pericardium. SYN pericardotomy. [pericardium + G. *tomē,* incision]

per·i·car·dit·ic (per'i-kar-dit'ik). Relating to pericarditis.

per·i·car·di·tis (per'i-kar-dī'tis). Inflammation of the pericardium.

 acute fibrinous p., the usual lesion of acute p. in which inflammation produces large quantities of fibrin.

 adhesive p., p. with adhesions between the two pericardial layers, between the pericardium and heart, or between the pericardium and neighboring structures. SYN adherent pericardium.

 bacterial p., p. produced by bacterial infection.

 p. calculosa, pericardial calcification owing to antecedent p.

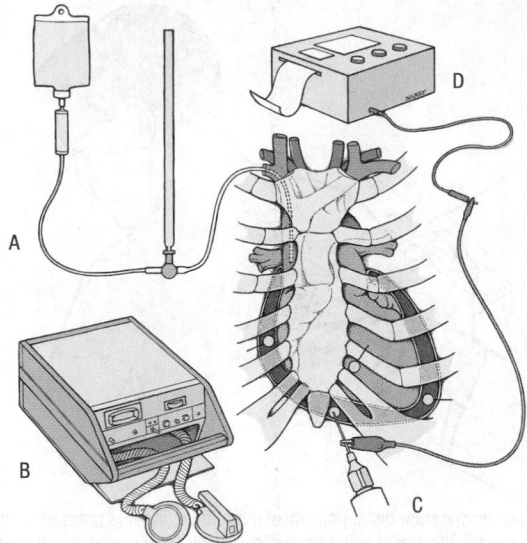

pericardiocentesis: support for patient, (A) central venous pressure monitoring IV line open for emergency drugs, (B) defibrillator and resuscitation equipment ready, (C) pericardiocentesis, with syringe and needle to which ECG has been attached, (D) ECG monitoring, (small circles indicate sites for pericardial aspiration)

 carcinomatous p., p. due to infiltration of carcinomatous cells, usually from surrounding structures.

 chronic constrictive p., scarring of the pericardium with thickening of the membrane and prolonged constriction of the cardiac chambers.

 constrictive p., postinflammatory thickening and scarring of the membrane producing constriction of the cardiac chambers; may be acute, subacute, or chronic. Formerly called chronic constrictive p.

 dry p., pericardial inflammation in the absence of demonstrable pericardial effusion.

 epistenocardiac p., p. accompanying transmural myocardial infarction and limited to the area over the infarct. SYN p. epistenocardica.

 p. epistenocardica, SYN epistenocardiac p.

 fibrinous p., acute p. with fibrinous exudate. SEE ALSO bread-and-butter *pericardium.* SYN hairy heart, p. villosa, shaggy pericardium.

 fibrous p., scarring, usually with adhesions, of all or most of the pericardium.

 hemorrhagic p., p. with bloodstained effusion.

 internal adhesive p., SYN concretio cordis.

 p. oblit'erans, inflammation of the pericardium leading to adhesion of the two layers, obliterating the sac. SEE ALSO adhesive p.

 obliterative p., complete obliteration by postinflammatory adhesions of the pericardial cavity.

 postmyocardial infarction p., an acute form of p. usually developing 1 week after a myocardial infarction.

 postpericardiotomy p., a syndrome characterized by fever, substernal chest pain, and pericardial rub following cardiac surgery.

 posttraumatic p., pericardial inflammation developing following injury to the chest.

 purulent p., p., usually bacterial, with pus in the sac. SYN empyema of the pericardium, pyopericardium.

 rheumatic p., fibrinous p. occurring in acute rheumatic fever.

 p. sic'ca, fibrinous p. without significant pericardial effusion.

 tuberculous p., p. caused by tuberculosis infection.

 uremic p., fibrinous p. seen in chronic renal failure.

 p. villo'sa, SYN fibrinous p.

viral p., p. due to a viral infection.

p. with effusion, pericardial inflammation producing excess pericardial fluid.

per·i·car·di·um, pl. **per·i·car·dia** (per-i-kar′dē-ŭm, -ă) [TA]. The fibroserous membrane, consisting of mesothelium and submesothelial connective tissue, covering the heart and beginning of the great vessels. It is a closed sac having two layers: the visceral layer (epicardium), immediately surrounding and applied to all the heart's surfaces, and the outer parietal layer, forming the sac, composed of strong fibrous tissue lined with a serous membrane. The phrenic nerves pass to the diaphragm through the anterior p. and divide the p. into antephrenic and retrophrenic portions; the pulmonary hilum divides both of these portions into suprahilar, hilar, and infrahilar portions. SYN capsula cordis, heart sac, membrana cordis, theca cordis. [L. fr. G. *pericardion,* the membrane around the heart]

adherent p., SYN adhesive *pericarditis.*

bread-and-butter p., fibrinous pericarditis in which the visceral and parietal surfaces of the p. resemble those of two pieces of buttered bread that have been pressed together and then pulled apart, when they are separated at surgery or necropsy.

p. fibro′sum [TA], SYN fibrous p.

fibrous p. [TA], SEE pericardium. SYN p. fibrosum [TA].

p. sero′sum, SYN serous p.

serous p. [TA], SEE pericardium. SYN p. serosum.

shaggy p., SYN fibrinous *pericarditis.*

visceral p., the layer of the pericardial sac on the epicardial surface of the heart. It is composed mainly of a single layer of mesothelium.

per·i·car·dot·o·my (per-i-kar-dot′ō-mē). SYN pericardiotomy.

per·i·ce·cal (per′i-sē′kăl). Surrounding the cecum. SYN perityphlic.

per·i·cel·lu·lar (per-i-sel′ū-lăr). Surrounding a cell. SYN pericytial.

per·i·ce·men·tal (per′i-sē-men′tăl). SYN periodontal.

per·i·cen·tral (per-i-sen′trăl). Surrounding the center.

per·i·cho·lan·gi·tis (per′i-kō-lan-jī′tis). Inflammation of the tissues around the bile ducts. SYN periangiocholitis. [peri- + G. *cholē,* bile, + *angeion,* vessel, + *-itis,* inflammation]

per·i·chon·dral, per·i·chon·dri·al (per-i-kon′drăl, -kon′drē-ăl). Relating to the perichondrium.

per·i·chon·dri·tis (per′i-kon-drī′tis). Inflammation of the perichondrium.

peristernal p., SYN Tietze *syndrome.*

relapsing p., SYN relapsing *polychondritis.*

per·i·chon·dri·um (per-i-kon′drē-ŭm) [TA]. The dense irregular connective tissue membrane around cartilage. [peri- + G. *chondros,* cartilage]

per·i·chord (per′i-kōrd). Sheath of the notochord.

per·i·chor·dal (per-i-kōr′dăl). Relating to the perichord.

per·i·cho·roi·dal (per-i-kŏ-roy′dăl). Surrounding the choroid coat of the eye.

per·i·chrome (per′i-krōm). Denoting a nerve cell in which the chromophil substance, or stainable material, is scattered throughout the cytoplasm. [peri- + G. *chrōma,* a color]

per·i·col·ic (per′i-kol′ik). Surrounding or encircling the colon.

per·i·co·li·tis (per′i-kō-lī′tis). Inflammation of the connective tissue or peritoneum surrounding the colon. SYN pericolonitis, serocolitis.

p. dex′tra, p. involving the ascending colon.

p. sinis′tra, SYN perisigmoiditis.

per·i·co·lon·i·tis (per′i-kō-lon-ī′tis). SYN pericolitis.

per·i·col·pi·tis (per′i-kol-pī′tis). SYN perivaginitis. [peri- + G. *kolpos,* bosom (vagina), + *-itis,* inflammation]

per·i·con·chal (per′i-kong′kăl). Surrounding the concha of the auricle. SYN periauricular (2).

per·i·cor·ne·al (per-i-kōr′nē-ăl). Surrounding the cornea. SYN circumcorneal, perikeratic.

per·i·cor·o·nal (per-i-kōr′ŏ-năl). Around the crown of a tooth.

per·i·cor·o·ni·tis (per-i-kōr-ŏ-nī′tis). Inflammation around the crown of a tooth, usually one that is incompletely erupted into the oral cavity. [peri- + L. *corona,* crown, + G. *-itis,* inflammation]

per·i·cra·ni·al (per-i-krā′nē-ăl). Relating to the pericranium; surrounding the skull.

per·i·cra·ni·tis (per′i-krā-nī′tis). Inflammation of the pericranium.

per·i·cra·ni·um (per′i-krā′nē-ŭm) [TA]. The periosteum of the skull. SYN periosteum cranii [TA]. [peri- + G. *kranion,* skull]

per·i·cy·a·zine (per-i-sī′ă-zēn). An antipsychotic.

per·i·cys·tic (per′i-sis′tik). 1. Surrounding the urinary bladder. 2. Surrounding the gallbladder. 3. Surrounding a cyst. SYN perivesical. [peri- + G. *kystis,* bladder]

per·i·cys·ti·tis (per′i-sis-tī′tis). Inflammation of the tissues surrounding a bladder, especially the urinary bladder.

per·i·cys·ti·um (per-i-sis′tē-ŭm). 1. The tissues surrounding the urinary bladder or gallbladder. 2. A vascular investment of a cystic tumor. [peri- + G. *kystis,* bladder, cyst]

per·i·cyte (per′i-sīt). One of the slender mesenchymal-like cells found in close association with the outside wall of postcapillary venules; it is relatively undifferentiated and may become a fibroblast, macrophage, or smooth muscle cell. SYN adventitial cell, pericapillary cell, perithelial cell. [peri- + G. *kytos,* cell]

per·i·cy·ti·al (per′i-sish′ē-ăl, -sit′ē-ăl). SYN pericellular.

per·i·dens (per′i-denz). A supernumerary tooth appearing elsewhere than the midline of the dental arch. [peri- + L. *dens,* tooth]

per·i·den·tal (per-i-den′tăl). SYN periodontal.

per·i·den·ti·tis (per′i-den-tī′tis). Obsolete term for periodontitis.

per·i·den·ti·um (per′i-den′tē-ŭm). SYN periodontium.

per·i·derm, per·i·der·ma (per′i-derm, -i-der′mă). The outermost layer of the epidermis of the embryo and fetus to the sixth month of intrauterine life; desquamated peridermal cells are a considerable component of the vernix caseosa. SYN epitrichium. [peri- + G. *derma,* skin]

per·i·der·mal, per·i·der·mic (per-i-der′măl, -mik). Relating to the periderm.

per·i·des·mic (per-i-dez′mik). 1. Surrounding a ligament. 2. Relating to the peridesmium. SYN periligamentous.

per·i·des·mi·tis (per′i-dez-mī′tis). Inflammation of the connective tissue surrounding a ligament. [peri- + G. *desmos,* band, + *-itis,* inflammation]

per·i·des·mi·um (per′i-dez′mē-ŭm). The connective tissue membrane surrounding a ligament. [peri- + G. *desmion (desmos),* band]

per·i·did·y·mis (per-i-did′i-mis). SYN *tunica* albuginea of testis. [G. *didymos,* twin, pl. *didymoi,* testes]

per·i·did·y·mi·tis (per′i-did-i-mī′tis). Inflammation of the perididymis.

pe·rid·i·um (pe-rid′ē-ŭm). In fungi, the hyphal structure that surrounds the asci. [G. *pēridion,* dim. of *pēra,* leather pouch]

per·i·di·ver·tic·u·li·tis (per′i-dī′ver-tik′ū-lī′tis). Inflammation of the tissues around an intestinal diverticulum.

per·i·du·o·de·ni·tis (per′i-doo′ō-dē-nī′tis). Inflammation around the duodenum.

per·i·du·ral (per-i-doo′răl). SYN epidural.

per·i·en·ceph·a·li·tis (per′ē-en-sef-ă-lī′tis). Inflammation of the cerebral membranes, particularly leptomeningitis or inflammation of the pia mater with involvement of the underlying cortex. [peri- + G. *enkephalos,* brain]

per·i·en·ter·ic (per-ē-en-ter′ik). Surrounding the intestine. SYN circumintestinal.

per·i·en·ter·i·tis (per′ē-en-ter-ī′tis). Inflammation of the peritoneal coat of the intestine. SYN seroenteritis.

per·i·e·pen·dy·mal (per′ē-e-pen′di-măl). Surrounding the ependyma.

per·i·e·soph·a·ge·al (per′ē-e-sof′ă-jē′ăl). Surrounding the esophagus.

per·i·e·soph·a·gi·tis (per′ē-e-sof′ă-jī′tis). Inflammation of the tissues surrounding the esophagus.

pe

per·i·fo·cal (per-i-fō'kăl). Surrounding a focus; denoting tissues, or the blood that they contain, in the vicinity of an infective focus.

per·i·fol·lic·u·lar (per'i-fŏ-lik'ū-lăr). Surrounding a hair follicle; usually used to describe the histopathologic appearance of the infiltrate surrounding a hair follicle.

per·i·fol·lic·u·li·tis (per'i-fŏ-lik'ū-lī'tis). The presence of an inflammatory infiltrate surrounding hair follicles; frequently occurs in conjunction with folliculitis.
p. absce'dens et suffo'diens, a chronic dissecting folliculitis of the scalp. SYN dissecting cellulitis.

per·i·fuse (per'i-fūs). To flush a fresh supply of bathing fluid around all of the outside surfaces of a small piece of tissue immersed in it. Cf. perfuse, superfuse. [peri- + L. *fusio,* a pouring]

per·i·fu·sion (per-i-fū'shŭn). The act of perifusing.

per·i·gan·gli·on·ic (per'i-gang-glē-on'ik). Surrounding a ganglion, especially a nerve ganglion.

per·i·gas·tric (per-i-gas'trik). Surrounding the stomach. [peri- + G. *gastēr,* belly, stomach]

per·i·gas·tri·tis (per'i-gas-trī'tis). Inflammation of the peritoneal coat of the stomach.

per·i·gem·mal (per'i-jem'ăl). SYN circumgemmal. [peri- + L. *gemma,* bud]

per·i·glan·du·li·tis (per'i-glan-doo-lī'tis). Inflammation of the tissues surrounding a gland.

per·i·glot·tic (per-i-glot'ik). Around the tongue, especially around the base of the tongue and the epiglottis, or around the glottis (laryngis), the rima glottidis. [peri- + G. *glōssa* or *glōtta,* tongue]

per·i·glot·tis (per-i-glot'is). The mucous membrane of the tongue. [G. *periglōttis,* covering of the tongue]

per·i·he·pat·ic (per-i-he-pat'ik). Surrounding the liver. [peri- + G. *hēpar,* liver]

per·i·hep·a·ti·tis (pĕr'i-hep-ă-tī'tis). Inflammation of the serous, or peritoneal, covering of the liver. SYN hepatic capsulitis, hepatitis externa, hepatoperitonitis. [peri- + G. *hēpar,* liver, + *-itis,* inflammation]

per·i·her·ni·al (per-i-her'nē-ăl). Surrounding a hernia.

peri-im·plan·to·cla·sia (per'ē-im-plan'tō-klā'zē-ă). In dentistry, a general term implying disease of the supporting bone involving an implant; the disease may be exfoliative, resorptive, traumatic, or ulcerative in nature. [peri- + L. *im,* in, + *planto,* to plant, + G. *klasis,* breaking up]

per·i·je·ju·ni·tis (per'i-jĕ-joo-nī'tis). Inflammation around the jejunum.

per·i·kar·y·on, pl. **per·i·kar·ya** (per-i-kar'ē-on, -ă). 1. The cytoplasm around the nucleus, such as that of the cell body of nerve cells. 2. The body of the odontoblast, excluding the dentinal fiber. 3. The cell body of the nerve cell, as distinguished from its axon and dendrites. [peri- + G. *karyon,* kernel]

per·i·ke·rat·ic (per-i-ke-rat'ik). SYN pericorneal. [peri- + G. *keras,* horn]

per·i·ky·ma·ta, sing. **per·i·ky·ma** (per-i-kī'mă-tă, -kī'mă). The transverse ridges and grooves on the surface of tooth enamel. [peri- + G. *kyma,* wave]

per·i·lab·y·rin·thi·tis (per'i-lab'ĭ-rin-thī'tis). Inflammation of the parts about the labyrinth.

per·i·la·ryn·ge·al (per'i-lă-rin'jē-ăl). Surrounding the larynx.

per·i·len·tic·u·lar (per-i-len-tik'ū-lăr). Surrounding the lens of the eye. SYN circumlental.

per·i·lig·a·men·tous (per'i-lig-ă-men'tŭs). SYN peridesmic.

per·i·lymph (per'i-limf) [TA]. The fluid contained within the osseous labyrinth, surrounding and protecting the membranous labyrinth; perilymph resembles extracellular fluid in composition (sodium salts are the predominate positive electrolyte) and, via the perilymphatic duct, is in continuity with cerebrospinal fluid. SYN perilympha [TA], Cotunnius liquid, liquor cotunnii.

per·i·lym·pha (per'i-lim'fă) [TA]. SYN perilymph. [peri- + L. *lympha,* a clear fluid (lymph)]

per·i·lym·phan·gi·al (per'i-lim-fan'jē-ăl). Surrounding a lymphatic vessel.

per·i·lym·phan·gi·tis (per'i-lim-fan-jī'tis). Inflammation of the tissues surrounding a lymphatic vessel.

per·i·lym·phat·ic (per'i-lim-fat'ik). 1. Surrounding a lymphatic structure (node or vessel). 2. The spaces and tissues surrounding the membranous labyrinth of the inner ear.

per·i·men·in·gi·tis (per'i-men-in-jī'tis). SYN pachymeningitis.

per·i·men·o·pause (per'i-men'ō-paws). The 3–5-year period prior to menopause during which estrogen levels begin to drop.

pe·rim·e·ter (pe-rim'ĕ-ter). 1. A circumference, edge, or border. 2. An instrument, usually half a circle or sphere, used to measure the field of vision. [G. *perimetros,* circumference, fr. *peri,* around, + *metron,* measure]
arc p., a p. consisting of a semicircular frame at the center of which the patient looks while a white object is moving along the arc, the exact point where it becomes visible or invisible being noted and recorded on a chart.
Goldmann p., a projection p. that adds further precision by controlling the surrounding illumination.
projection p., a p. that uses as target a spot of light that can be adjusted rapidly as to size, brightness, and color, and moves silently at any desired speed.
Tübinger p., a bowl p. in which a static stimulus was increased in intensity until detected. [*Tübingen,* German city]

per·i·met·ric (per-i-met'rik). 1. Surrounding the uterus; relating to the perimetrium. SYN periuterine. [G. *peri,* around, + *mētra,* uterus] 2. Relating to the circumference of any part or area. [G. *perimetros,* circumference] 3. Relating to perimetry.

per·i·me·trit·ic (per-i-me-trit'ik). Relating to or marked by perimetritis.

per·i·me·tri·tis (per'i-me-trī'tis). Inflammation of the uterus involving the perimetreal covering. SYN metroperitonitis. [perimetrium + G. *-itis,* inflammation]

per·i·me·tri·um, pl. **per·i·me·tria** (per-i-mē'trē-ŭm, -ă) [TA]. The serous (peritoneal) coat of the uterus. SYN tunica serosa uteri [TA]. [peri- + G. *mētra,* uterus]

pe·rim·e·try (pe-rim'ĕ-trē). 1. The determination of the limits of the visual field. 2. The mapping of the sensitivity contours of the visual field. [G. *perimetros,* circumference]
computed p., determination of the visual field by means of a programmed routine of static stimuli.
flicker p., a technique of p. using the criterion of critical fusion frequency. SYN flicker fusion frequency technique.
kinetic p., mapping of the visual field by using a moving rather than a static test object.
mesopic p., exploration of the visual field in dim illumination.
objective p., determination of the visual field by pupillary constriction, electroencephalography, or eye movements.
quantitative p., a plotting of the visual field in isopters of equal retinal sensitivity.
scotopic p., p. of a dark-adapted eye.
static p., determination of the visual field by using test objects at fixed positions and gradually increasing luminance to the threshold of visibility.

per·i·mol·y·sis (per-ē-mol'i-sis). Decalcification of the teeth from exposure to gastric acid in individuals with chronic vomiting. [=perimylolysis, fr. peri- + G. *mylos,* molar + *lysis,* loosening, dissolving, fr. *luō,* to loosen]

per·i·my·e·lis (per-i-mī'ĕ-lis). SYN endosteum. [peri- + G. *myelos,* marrow]

per·i·my·e·li·tis (per'i-mī-ĕ-lī'tis). SYN endosteitis.

per·i·my·o·car·di·tis (per-i-mī'ō-kar-dī'tis). Simultaneous pericarditis and myocarditis usually due to the same etiologic agent.

per·i·my·o·si·tis (per'i-mī-ō-sī'tis). Inflammation of the loose cellular tissue surrounding a muscle. SYN perimysiitis (2), perimysitis.

per·i·my·si·al (per-i-mis'ē-ăl, -miz'ē-ăl). Relating to the perimysium; surrounding a muscle.

per·i·my·si·i·tis, per·i·my·si·tis (per′i-mis-ē-ī′tis, -mī-sī′tis). **1.** Inflammation of the perimysium. **2.** SYN perimyositis.

per·i·my·si·um, pl. **per·i·my·sia** (per-i-mis′ē-ŭm, -miz′ē-ŭm; -ē-ă) [TA]. The fibrous sheath enveloping each of the fascicles of skeletal muscle fibers. [peri- + G. *mys,* muscle]

p. exter′num, SYN epimysium.

p. inter′num, in the older literature, a term referring to the connective tissue around secondary and tertiary fascicles and individual fibers and also to the supporting framework of the myocardium.

per·i·na·tal (per-i-nā′tăl). Occurring during, or pertaining to, the periods before, during, or after the time of birth; i.e., before delivery from the 22nd week of gestation through the first 28 days after delivery. [peri- + L. *natus,* pp. of *nascor,* to be born]

per·i·nate (per′i-nāt). An infant in the perinatal period.

per·i·na·tol·o·gist (per-i-nā-tol′ō-jist). An obstetrician who subspecializes in perinatology.

per·i·na·tol·o·gy (per-i-nā-tol′ō-jē). A subspeciality of obstetrics concerned with care of the mother and fetus during pregnancy, labor, and delivery, particularly when the mother and/or fetus are at a high risk for complications. SYN perinatal medicine.

per·i·ne·al (per′i-nē′ăl). Relating to the perineum.

⊘**perineo-.** The perineum. [L. fr. G. *perineos, perinaion*]

per·i·ne·o·cele (per-i-nē′ō-sēl). A hernia in the perineal region, either between the rectum and the vagina or the rectum and the bladder, or alongside the rectum. [perineo- + G. *kēlē,* hernia]

per·i·ne·om·e·ter (per′i-nē-om′ĕ-ter). Instrument used to measure the strength of voluntary muscle contractions of the perineum. [perineo- + G. *metron,* measure]

per·i·ne·o·plas·ty (per-i-nē′ō-plas-tē). Plastic surgery of the perineum. [perineum + G. *plastos,* formed]

per·i·ne·or·rha·phy (per-i-nē-ōr′ă-fē). Suture of the perineum, performed in perineoplasty. [perineum + G. *rhaphē,* a sewing]

per·i·ne·o·scro·tal (per-i-nē′ō-skrō′tăl). Relating to the perineum and the scrotum.

per·i·ne·os·to·my (per-i-nē-os′tō-mē). Urethrostomy through the perineum. [perineo- + G. *stoma,* mouth]

per·i·ne·o·syn·the·sis (per′i-nē-ō-sin′thĕ-sis). Rarely used term for perineoplasty in a case of extensive laceration of the perineum.

per·i·ne·ot·o·my (per-i-nē-ot′ō-mē). Incision into the perineum to facilitate childbirth. SEE ALSO episiotomy.

per·i·ne·o·vag·i·nal (per-i-nē′ō-vaj′i-năl). Relating to the perineum and the vagina.

per·i·neph·ri·al (per′i-nef′rē-ăl). Relating to the perinephrium.

per·i·neph·ric (per′i-nef′rik). Surrounding the kidney in whole or part. SYN circumrenal, perirenal.

per·i·neph·ri·tis (per′i-ne-frī′tis). Inflammation of perinephric tissue.

per·i·neph·ri·um, pl. **per·i·neph·ria** (per′i-nef′rē-ŭm, -nef′rē-ă). The connective tissue and fat surrounding the kidney. [peri- + G. *nephros,* kidney]

per·i·ne·um, pl. **per·i·nea** (per′i-nē′ŭm, -nē′ă) [TA]. **1** [NA]. The area between the thighs extending from the coccyx to the pubis and lying below the pelvic diaphragm. **2.** The external surface of the central tendon of the perineum, lying between the vulva and the anus in the female and the scrotum and the anus in the male. [L. fr. G. *perineon, perinaion*]

watering-can p., a p. riddled with fistulas resulting from urethral stricture.

per·i·neu·ral (per′i-noo′răl). Surrounding a nerve. [peri- + G. *neuron,* nerve]

per·i·neu·ri·al (per′i-noo′rē-ăl). Relating to the perineurium.

per·i·neu·ri·tis (per′i-noo-rī′tis). Inflammation of the perineurium. SEE ALSO adventitial *neuritis.*

per·i·neu·ri·um, pl. **per·i·neu·ria** (per-i-noo′rē-ŭm, -rē-ă). One of the supporting structures of peripheral nerve trunks, consisting of layers of flattened cells and collagenous connective tissue, which surround the nerve fasciculi and form the major diffusion barrier within the nerve; with the endoneurium and epineurium,

composes the peripheral nerve stroma. [L. fr. peri- + G. *neuron,* nerve]

per·i·nu·cle·ar (per-i-noo′klē-ăr). Surrounding a nucleus. SYN circumnuclear.

per·i·oc·u·lar (per-i-ok′ū-lăr). SYN circumocular.

pe·ri·od (pēr′ē-ŏd). **1.** A certain duration or division of time. **2.** One of the stages of a disease, e.g., p. of incubation, p. of convalescence. SEE ALSO stage, phase. **3.** Colloquialism for menses. **4.** Any of the horizontal rows of chemical elements in the periodic table. [G. *periodos,* a way round, a cycle, fr. *peri,* around, + *hodos,* way]

absolute refractory p., the p. following excitation when no response is possible regardless of the intensity of the stimulus.

amblyogenic p., p. during early visual development when the visual neurosensory system is vulnerable to developing amblyopia from blurred retinal image formation, bilateral cortical suppression (as in strabismic *amblyopia*), or both. SYN critical p. (3).

critical p., (1) in the first hours after birth, the p. of maximum imprintability; the period before and after which imprinting is difficult or impossible; (2) in animals, a p. following birth when the processes underlying the capacity for socialization are activated or stamped in; (3) SYN amblyogenic p.

eclipse p., the time between infection by (or induction of) a bacteriophage, or other virus, and the appearance of mature virus within the cell; an interval of time during which viral infectivity cannot be recovered. SYN eclipse phase.

effective refractory p., the p. during which impulses may appear but are too weak to be conducted; the longest interval between adequate stimuli, falling just short of the time necessary to allow a propagated response to be evoked in a tissue by the second stimulus; it differs from the functional refractory p. in that it is a measure of stimulus interval rather than response interval of time.

ejection p., SYN sphygmic *interval.*

extrinsic incubation p. (eks-trin′sik), time required for the development of a disease agent in a vector, from the time of uptake of the agent to the time when the vector is infective.

fertile p., the p. in a regularly menstruating woman's cycle, during which conception is most likely.

functional refractory p., the minimum interval possible between successive responses to stimulation of a tissue.

gap₁ p., the p. of the cell cycle after cell division when there is synthesis of RNA and protein; it may last for a few hours in rapidly growing tissue or a lifetime in non-renewing cells such as nerve cells. SYN gap₁ phase, postmitotic phase.

gap₂ p., the p. in the cell cycle when synthesis of DNA is completed but before mitosis begins. SYN gap₂ phase, premitotic phase.

gap₀ p., phase of a cell no longer in the cell cycle and thus at least temporarily incapable of division. SYN gap₀ phase.

incubation p., (1) time interval between invasion of the body by an infecting organism and the appearance of the first sign or symptom it causes; SYN incubative stage, latent p. (2), latent stage, stage of invasion. (2) in a disease vector, the p. between entry of the disease organism and the time at which the vector is capable of transmitting the disease to another human host.

induction p., the p. required for a specific agent to produce a disease; the interval from the causal action of a factor to initiation of disease, e.g., the interval between exposure to radiation and the onset of leukemia; the interval between an initial injection of antigen and the appearance of demonstrable antibodies in the blood.

intrapartum p., in obstetrics, the p. from the onset of labor to the end of the third stage of labor.

isoelectric p., an abnormal p. occurring in the electrocardiogram between the end of the S wave and the beginning of the T wave during which electrical forces are acting in directions so as to neutralize each other so that there is no difference in potential under the electrodes. SYN abnormal ST segment.

isometric p. of cardiac cycle, that p. in which the muscle fibers do not shorten although the cardiac muscle is excited and the pressure in the ventricles rises, extending from the closure of the atrioventricular valves to the opening of the semilunar valves (isovolumic constriction) or the reverse (isovolumic relaxation). SYN isovolumic p.

isometric contraction p., the time between closure of the atrioventricular valves and opening of the semilunar valves.

isometric relaxation p., early ventricular diastole beginning with closure of the aortic and pulmonic valves and preceding opening of the atrioventricular valves.

isovolumic p., SYN isometric p. of cardiac cycle.

latency p., SYN latency *phase*.

latent p., (1) the p. elapsing between the application of a stimulus and the response, e.g., contraction of a muscle; **(2)** SYN incubation p. (1).

masticatory silent p., a pause in electromyographic patterns associated with tooth contacts during chewing and biting; a part of the complex feedback mechanism of mandibular control involving receptors in the periodontal ligament and muscles.

menstrual p., SYN menses.

missed p., the failure of menstruation to occur in any month at the expected time.

mitotic p., the p. of the cell cycle in which all phases of mitosis occur. SYN M phase.

oedipal p., SYN oedipal *phase*.

preejection p., the interval between onset of QRS complex and cardiac ejection; electromechanical systole minus ejection time.

prepatent p., in parasitology, the p. equivalent to the incubation period of microbial infections; it is biologically different, however, because the parasite is undergoing developmental stages in the host.

prodromal p., the time during which a disease process has begun but is not yet clinically manifest.

puerperal p., the p. elapsing between the termination of labor and the return of the generative tract to its normal condition; the 6 weeks following the completion of labor.

pulse p., the reciprocal of the repetition rate; e.g., the interval between leading edges of successive pulses.

quarantine p., the time during which an infected individual or an area is kept isolated, avoiding contact with uninfected individuals; can be any specified p. of time, varying with the disease in question. The term is derived from the Italian word for 40, since the period of isolation of individuals suspected of plague in the Middle Ages was 40 days.

refractory p., (1) the p. following effective stimulation, during which excitable tissue such as heart muscle and nerve fails to respond to a stimulus of threshold intensity (i.e., excitability is depressed); **(2)** a period of temporary psychophysiologic resistance to further sexual stimulation that occurs immediately following orgasm.

refractory p. of electronic pacemaker, the time required to restore full sensitivity after detecting cardiac activity or delivering a pacing impulse.

relative refractory p., the p. between the effective refractory p. and the end of the refractory p.; fibers then respond only to high-intensity stimuli and the impulses conduct more slowly than normally.

silent p., (1) the time during which there is no electrical activity in a muscle following its rapid unloading; **(2)** any pause in an otherwise continuous series of electrophysiologic events.

synthesis p., the p. of the cell cycle when there is synthesis of DNA and histone; it occurs between Gap_1 and Gap_2. SYN S phase.

total refractory p., the absolute refractory p. plus the relative refractory p.

vulnerable p., vulnerable p. of heart, a brief time during the cardiac cycle when stimuli are particularly likely to induce repetitive activity like tachycardia, flutter, or fibrillation which persists after the stimulus has ceased; for the ventricle, it occurs during the latter part of systole, during the relative refractory period coincident with the inscription of the latter half of the T wave of the electrocardiogram.

Wenckebach p., a sequence of cardiac cycles in the electrocardiogram ending in a dropped beat due to AV block, the preceding cycles showing progressively lengthening PR intervals; the PR interval following the dropped beat is again shortened.

per·i·o·date (per-ī′ō-dāt). A salt of periodic acid.

pe·ri·od·ic (pēr-ē-od′ik). **1.** Recurring at regular intervals. **2.** Denoting a disease with regularly recurring exacerbations or paroxysms. **3.** Denoting any of several oxoacids of iodine.

pe·ri·od·ic ac·id (per-ī′ō-dik). **1.** HIO_4, but existing in solution usually in hydrated form; used in carbohydrate detection and analysis. SYN metaperiodic acid. **2.** Any of several iodic(VII) acids formed by the combination of iodine heptoxide, I_2O_7, with water.

per·i·o·dic·i·ty (pēr′ē-ō-dis′i-tē). Tendency to recurrence at regular intervals.

diurnal p., a circadian rhythm with primary expression of the p. during daylight hours, as in the release of microfilariae of *Loa loa* into the peripheral blood during the day, with far fewer released at night; associated with the day-biting habits of the vector, *Chrysops* species.

filarial p., the circadian rhythm observed in the appearance of filarial microfilariae in the peripheral blood. SEE ALSO diurnal p., nocturnal p.

lunar p., any rhythmic phenomenon that follows a lunar or monthly cycle.

malarial p., a clinical rhythmicity reflected in periodic fevers and chills recurring at approximately 48-hour intervals in tertian malaria (*Plasmodium vivax* or *P. ovale*) or at 72-hour intervals in quartan malaria (*P. malariae*); the rhythm of tertian or 48-hour cycles is frequently modified in malignant tertian or falciparum malaria (*P. falciparum*); associated with release of merozoites from red cells during erythrocytic schizogony, although the controlling mechanism for the synchronous release is unknown.

nocturnal p., a circadian rhythm with the p. expressed during nighttime hours, as in the night release of microfilariae of the human filaria *Wuchereria bancrofti* into the peripheral blood; this type of p. is found in regions where the vector mosquito is a night-biting species.

subperiodic p., a modified circadian rhythm in which the p. is not clearcut, as in certain zoonotic strains of Malayan filariasis caused by *Brugia malayi;* as in examples of strict filarial p., this response is correlated with the biting habits of the vector insect (mosquito), although the precise mechanism inducing this microfilarial response is not clearly established.

per·i·o·don·tal (per′ē-ō-don′tăl). Around a tooth. SYN paradental, pericemental, peridental. [peri- + G. *odous,* tooth]

Per·i·o·don·tal Dis·ease In·dex (PDI). An index used for estimating the degree of periodontal disease based on the measurement of six representative teeth for gingival inflammation, pocket depth, calculus and plaque, attrition, mobility, and lack of contact.

Per·i·o·don·tal In·dex (PI). An index for the epidemiologic classification of periodontal disease.

per·i·o·don·tia (per′ē-ō-don′shē-ă). **1.** Plural of periodontium. **2.** SYN periodontics.

per·i·o·don·tics (per′ē-ō-don′tiks). The branch of dentistry concerned with the study of the normal tissues and the treatment of abnormal conditions of the tissues immediately about the teeth. SYN periodontia (2). [peri- + G. *odous,* tooth]

per·i·o·don·tist (per′ē-ō-don′tist). A dentist who specializes in periodontics.

per·i·o·don·ti·tis (per′ē-ō-don-tī′tis). **1.** Inflammation of the periodontium. **2.** A chronic inflammatory disease of the periodontium occurring in response to bacterial plaque on the adjacent teeth; characterized by gingivitis, destruction of the alveolar bone and periodontal ligament, apical migration of the epithelial attachment resulting in the formation of periodontal pockets, and ultimately loosening and exfoliation of the teeth. [periodontium + G. *-itis,* inflammation]

apical p., inflammation of the periodontal ligament surrounding the root apex of a tooth; usually a consequence of pulpal inflammation or necrosis.

p. com′plex, vertical resorption of the alveolar process with pockets of uneven depth on adjacent teeth, and with traumatic occlusion as a factor.

juvenile p., a degenerative periodontal disease of adolescents in which the periodontal destruction is out of proportion to the local irritating factors present on the adjacent teeth; inflammatory changes become superimposed, and bone loss, migration, and extrusion are observed. Two forms are recognized: 1) localized, in which the destruction is limited to the incisors and first molars; 2) generalized, involving all of the teeth. SYN periodontosis.

p. sim'plex, horizontal resorption of the alveolar process with pockets of even depth on adjacent teeth; traumatic occlusion is not a factor.

suppurative p., p. accompanied by purulent exudate.

per·i·o·don·ti·um, pl. **per·i·o·don·tia** (per'ē-ō-don'shē-ŭm, -shē-ă) [TA]. The connective tissue that surrounds the tooth root and attaches it to its bony socket; it consists of fibers anchored in the cementum and extending into the alveolar bone; the tissues that surround and support the teeth, including the gingivae, cementum, desmodentium, periodontal fibrs, and alveolar and supporting bone. SYN periodontal ligament [TA], periodontal membrane ☆, alveolar periosteum, periosteum alveolare, alveolodental ligament, alveolodental membrane, gingivodental ligament, paradentium, parodontium, peridental ligament, peridental membrane, peridentium, tapetum alveoli. [L. fr. peri- + G. *odous,* tooth]

per·i·o·don·to·cla·sia (per'ē-ō-don-tō-klā'zē-ă). Destruction of periodontal tissues, gingiva, pericementum, alveolar bone, and cementum. SYN periodontolysis. [periodontium + *klasis,* breaking]

per·i·o·don·tol·y·sis (per'ē-ō-don-tol'i-sis). SYN periodontoclasia. [periodontium + G. *lysis,* dissolution]

per·i·o·don·to·sis (per'ē-ō-don-tō'sis). SYN juvenile *periodontitis.* [periodontium + G. *-osis,* condition]

per·i·om·phal·ic (per'ē-om-fal'ik). SYN periumbilical. [peri- + G. *omphalos,* umbilicus]

per·i·o·nych·ia (per-ē-ō-nik'ē-ă). **1.** Inflammation of the perionychium. **2.** Plural of perionychium.

per·i·o·nych·i·um, pl. **per·i·o·nych·ia** (per-ē-ō-nik'ē-ŭm, -nik'ē-ă). SYN eponychium (2). [peri- + G. *onyx,* nail]

per·i·on·yx (per-ē-on'iks) [TA]. Remnant of the eponychium remaining in the narrow fold overlapping the proximal part of the lunula found beginning in the eighth month of pregancy and remaining throughout life. [peri- + G. *onyx,* nail]

per·i·o·o·pho·ri·tis (per'ē-ō-of'ō-rī'tis). Inflammation of the peritoneal covering of the ovary. SYN periovaritis. [peri- + Mod. L. *oophoron,* ovary, + *-itis,* inflammation]

per·i·o·o·pho·ro·sal·pin·gi·tis (per'ē-ō-of'ō-rō-sal-pin-jī'tis). Inflammation of the peritoneum and other tissues around the ovary and oviduct. SYN perisalpingoovaritis. [peri- + Mod. L. *oophoron,* ovary, + *salpinx,* trumpet, + *-itis,* inflammation]

per·i·op·er·a·tive (per-ē-op'er-ă-tiv). Around the time of operation. SYN paraoperative.

per·i·oph·thal·mic (per'ē-of-thal'mik). SYN circumocular. [peri- + G. *ophthalmos,* eye]

per·i·oph·thal·mi·tis (per'ē-of-thal-mī'tis). Inflammation of the tissues surrounding the eye.

per·i·o·ral (per-ē-ō'răl). Around the mouth. SYN circumoral, peristomal, peristomatous.

per·i·or·bit (per-ē-ōr'bit). SYN periorbita.

pe·ri·or·bi·ta (per'ē-ōr'bi-tă) [TA]. The periosteum of the orbit. SYN periorbit, periorbital membrane. [peri- + L. *orbita,* orbit]

per·i·or·bi·tal (per-ē-ōr'bi-tăl). **1.** Relating to the periorbita. **2.** SYN circumorbital.

per·i·or·chi·tis (per'ē-ōr-kī'tis). Inflammation of the tunica vaginalis testis. [peri- + G. *orchis,* testis, + *-itis,* inflammation]

p. hemorrha'gica, chronic hematocele of the tunica vaginalis testis.

per·i·ost (per'ē-ost). SYN periosteum.

pe·ri·os·tea (per-ē-os'tē-ă). Plural of periosteum.

per·i·os·te·al (per-ē-os'tē-ăl). Relating to the periosteum. SYN periosteous.

per·i·os·te·i·tis (per'ē-os-tē-ī'tis). SYN periostitis.

△**periosteo-.** The periosteum. [Mod. L. *periosteum*]

per·i·os·te·o·ma (per'ē-os'tē-ō'mă). A neoplasm derived from the periosteum. SYN periosteophyte, periostoma.

per·i·os·te·o·med·ul·li·tis (per-ē-os'tē-ō-med-ū-lī'tis). SYN periosteomyelitis. [periosteo- + L. *medulla,* marrow, + G. *-itis,* inflammation]

per·i·os·te·o·my·e·li·tis (per-ē-os'tē-ō-mī-ĕ-lī'tis). Inflammation of the entire bone, with the periosteum and marrow. SYN periosteomedullitis. [periosteo- + G. *myelos,* marrow, + *-itis,* inflammation]

per·i·os·te·op·a·thy (par'ē-os-tē-op'ă-thē). Any disease of the periosteum.

per·i·os·te·o·phyte (per-ē-os'te-ō-fīt). SYN periosteoma. [periosteo- + G. *phyton,* growth]

per·i·os·te·o·sis (per'ē-os-tē-ō'sis). The formation of a periosteoma. SYN periostosis.

per·i·os·te·o·tome (per'ē-os'tē-ō-tōm). A strong scalpel-shaped knife, for cutting the periosteum. SYN periostotome.

per·i·os·te·ot·o·my (per'ē-os-tē-ot'ō-mē). The operation of cutting through the periosteum to the bone. SYN periostotomy. [periosteo- + G. *tomē,* incision]

per·i·os·te·ous (per-ē-os'tē-ŭs). SYN periosteal.

▣**per·i·os·te·um,** pl. **pe·ri·os·tea** (per-ē-os'tē-ŭm, -ă) [TA]. The thick fibrous membrane covering the entire surface of a bone except its articular cartilage. In young bones, it consists of two layers: an inner cellular layer that is osteogenic, forming new bone tissue, and an outer fibrous connective tissue layer conveying the blood vessels and nerves supplying the bone; in older bones, the osteogenic layer is reduced. SEE ALSO perichondral *bone.* SYN periost. [Mod. L. fr. G. *periosteon,* ntr. of adj. *periosteos,* around the bones, fr. *peri,* around, + *osteon,* bone]

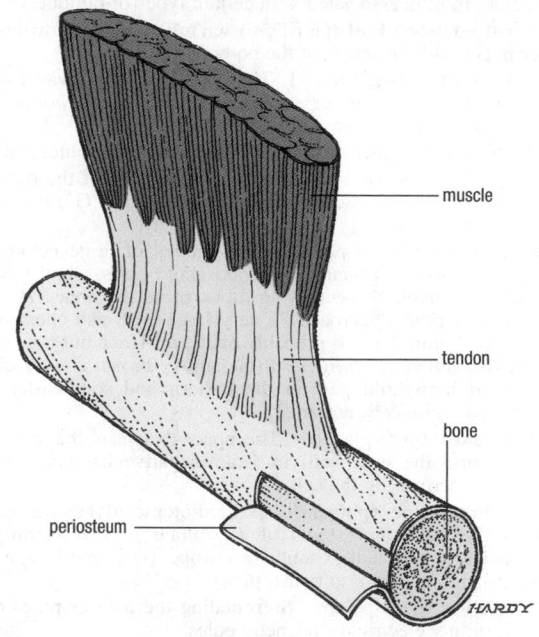

— muscle

— tendon

bone

periosteum —

HARDY

periosteum

---

alveolar p., p. alveola're, SYN periodontium.

p. cra'nii [TA], SYN pericranium.

per·i·os·ti·tis (per'ē-os-tī'tis). Inflammation of the periosteum. SYN periosteitis.

per·i·os·to·ma (per'ē-os-tō'mă). SYN periosteoma.

per·i·os·to·sis, pl. **per·i·os·to·ses** (per'ē-os-tō'sis, -sēz). SYN periosteosis.

per·i·os·tos·te·i·tis (per-ē-os'tos-tē-ī'tis). Inflammation of a bone with involvement of the periosteum. [periosteum + G. *osteon,* bone, + *-itis,* inflammation]

per·i·os·to·tome (per-ē-os'tō-tōm). SYN periosteotome.

per·i·os·tot·o·my (per-ē-os-tot'ō-mē). SYN periosteotomy.

per·i·o·tic (per'ē-ō'tik, -ot'ik). Surrounding the internal ear; referring to the petrous portion of the temporal bone, or the spaces and tissues in the bony labyrinth that surround the membranous labyrinth. [peri- + G. *ous,* ear]

per·i·o·va·ri·tis (per'ē-ō-vă-rī'tis). SYN perioophoritis.

per·i·o·vu·lar (per'ē-ō'vū-lăr). Surrounding the ovum.

per·i·pach·y·men·in·gi·tis (per'i-pak'ē-men-in-jī'tis). Inflammation of the area between the dura and bony covering of the central nervous system. [peri- + pachymeninx (dura mater) + G. *-itis,* inflammation]

per·i·pan·cre·a·ti·tis (per'i-pan'krē-ă-tī'tis). Inflammation of the peritoneal coat of the pancreas.

per·i·pap·il·lary (per-i-pap'i-lār-ē). Surrounding a papilla.

per·i·pa·tet·ic (per'i-pă-tet'ik). Walking around; formerly used to describe a patient with "walking" (i.e., mild) typhoid fever. [G. *peripatēsis,* a walking about]

per·i·pe·ni·al (per-i-pē'nē-ăl). Surrounding the penis.

per·i·pha·ryn·ge·al (per'i-fă-rin'jē-ăl). Surrounding the pharynx.

pe·riph·er·ad (pĕ-rif'ĕ-rad). In a direction toward the periphery. [G. *periphereia,* periphery, + L. *ad,* to]

pe·riph·e·ral (pĕ-rif'ĕ-răl) [TA]. **1.** Relating to or situated at the periphery. **2.** Situated nearer the periphery of an organ or part of the body in relation to a specific reference point; opposite of central (centralis). SYN peripheralis [TA], eccentric (3).

pe·ri·phe·ra·lis (pĕ-rif-ĕ-rā'lis) [TA]. SYN peripheral, peripheral.

per·i·phe·rin (pĕri-fer-in). A glycoprotein that apparently is needed to maintain the shape of the outer segment disk membranes of rods and cones; it is thought by many investigators that a defect in p. is associated with certain types of blindness.

pe·riph·e·ro·cen·tral (pĕ-rif'ĕ-rō-sen'trăl). Relating to both the periphery and the center of the body or any part.

pe·riph·e·ry (pĕ-rif'ĕ-rē). **1.** The part of a body away from the center; the outer part or surface. **2.** SYN denture *border.* [G. *periphereia,* fr. *peri,* around, + *pherō,* to carry]

per·i·phle·bit·ic (per'i-fle-bit'ik). Relating to periphlebitis.

per·i·phle·bi·tis (per'i-fle-bī'tis). Inflammation of the outer coat of a vein or of the tissues surrounding it. [peri- + G. *phleps,* vein, + *-itis,* inflammation]

Per·i·pla·ne·ta (per-i-pla-nē'tă). A genus of large cockroaches including several cosmopolitan household pests found wherever food is available, especially in moist protected areas. *P. americana* (American cockroach), a very large brownish-chestnut species, 30–40 mm long, is probably native to Africa but now universally distributed; *P. fuliginosa* (the smoky-brown cockroach) is a common household pest in the eastern and southeastern U.S. [peri- + G. *planētēs,* a roamer]

per·i·plasm (per'i-plazm). The space between the cell membranes and the cell wall, in Gram-negative bacteria; contains proteins secreted by the cell.

pe·rip·lo·cin (pe-rip'lō-sin). A cardiotonic glycoside obtained from the bark and stems of *Periploca graeca* (family Asclepiadaceae), a plant of southern Europe. [G. *peri-plokē,* a winding around, fr. *plekō,* to twine, plait]

per·i·po·lar (per-i-pō'lăr). Surrounding the pole or poles of any body, or any electric or magnetic poles.

per·i·po·le·sis (per'i-pō-lē'sis). Penetration of migrating cells between fixed tissue cells that are normally in close contact. [peri- + G. *poleomai,* to wander]

per·i·po·ri·tis (per'i-pŏ-rī'tis). Miliary papules and papulovesicles with staphylococcic infection; most frequently on the face and in infants. [peri- + G. *poros,* pore, + *-itis,* inflammation]

per·i·por·tal (per-i-pōr'tăl). Surrounding the portal vein. SYN peripylic.

per·i·proc·tic (per'ē-prok'tik). SYN circumanal. [peri- + G. *prōktos,* anus]

per·i·proc·ti·tis (per'i-prok-tī'tis). Inflammation of the areolar tissue about the rectum. SYN perirectitis.

per·i·pros·tat·ic (per'i-pros-tat'ik). Surrounding the prostate.

per·i·pros·ta·ti·tis (per'i-pros-tă-tī'tis). Obsolete term for inflammation of the tissues surrounding the prostate.

per·i·py·le·phle·bi·tis (per-i-pī'lĕ-fle-bī'tis). Inflammation of the tissues around the portal vein. [peri- + G. *pylē,* gate, + *phleps,* vein, + *-itis,* inflammation]

per·i·py·lic (per-i-pī'lik). SYN periportal. [peri- + G. *pylē,* portal, gate]

per·i·py·lor·ic (per'i-pī-lōr'ik, -pĕ-lōr'ik). Surrounding the pylorus.

per·i·rec·tal (per'i-rek'tăl). Surrounding the rectum.

per·i·rec·ti·tis (per'i-rek-tī'tis). SYN periproctitis.

per·i·re·nal (per'i-rē'năl). SYN perinephric. [peri- + L. *ren,* kidney]

per·i·rhi·nal (per'i-rī'năl). Around the nose or nasal cavity. [peri- + G. *rhis,* nose]

per·i·rhi·zo·cla·sia (per'ē-rī-zō-klā'zē-ă). Inflammatory destruction of tissues immediately around the root of a tooth, i.e., pericementum, cementum, and approximating layers of alveolar bone. [peri- + G. *rhiza,* root, + *klasis,* destruction]

per·i·sal·pin·gi·tis (per-i-sal-pin-jī'tis). Inflammation of the peritoneum covering the fallopian tube. [peri- + G. *salpinx,* trumpet, + *-itis,* inflammation]

per·i·sal·pin·go·ova·ri·tis (per'i-sal-ping'gō-ō-vă-rī'tis). SYN perioophorosalpingitis. [peri- + G. *salpinx,* trumpet, + ovary + G. *-itis,* inflammation]

per·i·sal·pinx (per'i-sal'pingks). The peritoneal covering of the uterine tube. [peri- + G. *salpinx* (*salping-*), trumpet]

per·i·scop·ic (per'i-skop'ik). Denoting that which gives the ability to see objects to one side as well as in the direct axis of vision. [peri- + G. *skopeō,* to view]

per·i·sig·moi·di·tis (per'i-sig-moy-dī'tis). Inflammation of the connective tissues surrounding the sigmoid flexure, giving rise to symptoms, referable to the left iliac fossa, similar to those of perityphlitis in the right iliac fossa. SYN pericolitis sinistra.

per·i·sin·u·ous (per'i-sin'ū-ŭs). Surrounding a sinus, especially a sinus of the dura mater.

per·i·sper·ma·ti·tis (per'i-sper-mă-tī'tis). Inflammation of the tissues around the spermatic cord.

p. sero'sa, hydrocele of the spermatic cord.

per·i·splanch·nic (per'i-splangk'nik). Surrounding any viscus or viscera. SYN perivisceral. [peri- + G. *splanchna,* viscera]

per·i·splanch·ni·tis (per'i-splangk-nī'tis). Inflammation surrounding any viscus or viscera. [peri- + G. *splanchna,* viscera, + *-itis,* inflammation]

per·i·splen·ic (per-i-splen'ik). Around the spleen.

per·i·sple·ni·tis (per'i-sple-nī'tis). Inflammation of the peritoneum covering the spleen.

per·i·spon·dyl·ic (per-i-spon-dil'ik). SYN perivertebral. [peri- + G. *spondylos,* vertebra]

per·i·spon·dy·li·tis (per-i-spon-di-lī'tis). Inflammation of the tissues about a vertebra. [peri- + G. *spondylos,* vertebra, + *-itis,* inflammation]

per·i·stal·sis (per-i-stal'sis). The movement of the intestine or other tubular structure, characterized by waves of alternate circular contraction and relaxation of the tube by which the contents are propelled onward. SYN vermicular movement. [peri- + G. *stalsis,* constriction]

mass p., forcible peristaltic movements of short duration, occurring only three or four times a day, which move the contents of the large intestine from one division to the next, as from the ascending to the transverse colon. SYN mass movement.

reversed p., a wave of intestinal contraction in a direction the reverse of normal, by which the contents of the intestine are forced backward. SYN antiperistalsis.

per·i·stal·tic (per-i-stal'tik). Relating to peristalsis.

pe·ris·ta·sis (pĕ-ris'tă-sis). Phases of inactivity of vasoconstriction in inflammation. SYN peristatic hyperemia. [peri- + G. *stasis,* a standing still]

pe·ris·to·le (pĕ-ris'tō-lē). The tonic activity of the walls of the stomach whereby the organ contracts about its contents; contrasting with the peristaltic waves passing from the cardia toward the pylorus (peristalsis). [peri- + G. *stellō*, to contract]

per·i·stol·ic (per-i-stol′ik). Relating to peristole.

pe·ris·to·ma (pe-ris′tō-mă, per-i-stō′mă). SYN peristome.

per·i·sto·mal, per·i·sto·ma·tous (per′i-stō′măl, -stō′mă-tŭs). SYN perioral.

per·i·stome (per′i-stōm). A groove leading from the cytostome in ciliates and certain other forms of protozoa. SYN peristoma. [peri- + G. *stoma*, mouth]

per·i·stru·mous (per′i-stroo′mŭs). Situated about or near a goiter. [peri- + L. *struma*, goiter]

per·i·syn·o·vi·al (per′i-si-nō′vē-ăl). Around a synovial membrane.

per·i·sys·tol·ic (per-i-sis-tol′ik). Descriptive of events occurring before and after ventricular systole.

per·i·tec·to·my (per′i-tek′tō-mē). **1.** The removal of a paracorneal strip of the conjunctiva for the relief of corneal disease. **2.** SYN circumcision (2). [peri- + G. *ektomē*, excision]

pe·ri·ten·di·ne·um, pl. **pe·ri·ten·di·nea** (per-i-ten-din′ē-ŭm, -ē-ŭ). One of the fibrous sheaths surrounding the primary bundles of fibers in a tendon. [L. fr. peri- + G. *tenōn*, tendon]

per·i·ten·di·ni·tis (per′i-ten-di-nī′tis). Inflammation of the sheath of a tendon. SYN peritenonitis, peritenontitis.

p. calca′rea, a calcium (chalky) deposit around a tendon.

p. sero′sa, SYN ganglion (2).

per·i·ten·on (per′i-ten-on). SYN tendinous *sheath* of extensor carpi ulnaris muscle. [peri- + G. *tenōn*, tendon]

per·i·ten·on·ti·tis (per′i-ten-on-tī′tis). SYN peritendinitis.

per·i·the·ci·um, pl. **per·i·the·cia** (per-i-thē′sē-ŭm, -sē-ă). In fungi, a flask-shaped ascocarp, one of the many shapes of structures that bear asci and ascospores; useful as an aid in identifying a fungus. [peri- + G. *thēkē*, flask]

per·i·the·li·um, pl. **per·i·the·lia** (per-i-thē′lē-ŭm, -ă). The connective tissue that surrounds smaller vessels and capillaries. [peri- + G. *thēlē*, nipple]

Eberth p., an incomplete layer of connective tissue cells encasing the blood capillaries.

per·i·tho·rac·ic (per-i-thō-ras′ik). Surrounding or encircling the thorax.

per·i·thy·roi·di·tis (per′i-thī-roy-dī′tis). Inflammation of the capsule or tissues surrounding the thyroid gland.

pe·rit·o·mist (pe-rit′ō-mist). One who performs circumcision.

pe·rit·o·my (pe-rit′ō-mē). A circumcorneal incision through the conjunctiva. [G. *peritomē*, fr. *peri*, around, + *tomē*, incision]

per·i·to·ne·al (per′i-tō-nē′ăl). Relating to the peritoneum.

per·i·to·ne·al·gia (per′i-tō-nē-al′jē-ă). A rarely used term for pain in the peritoneum. [peritoneum + G. *algos*, pain]

♻**peritoneo-.** The peritoneum. [L. *peritoneum*]

per·i·to·ne·o·cen·te·sis (per′i-tō-nē′ō-sen-tē′sis). Paracentesis of the abdomen. [peritoneum + G. *kentēsis*, puncture]

per·i·to·ne·oc·ly·sis (per′i-tō-nē-ok′li-sis). Irrigation of the abdominal cavity. [peritoneum, + G. *klysis*, a washing out]

per·i·to·ne·op·a·thy (per′i-tō-nē-op′ă-thē). A rarely used term for inflammation or other disease of the peritoneum. [peritoneum, + *pathos*, suffering]

per·i·to·ne·o·per·i·car·di·al (per′i-tō-nē′ō-per′i-kar′dē-ăl). Relating to the peritoneum and the pericardium.

per·i·to·ne·o·pexy (per′i-tō-nē′ō-pek-sē). A suspension or fixation of the peritoneum. [peritoneum + G. *pēxis*, fixation]

per·i·to·ne·o·plas·ty (per′i-tō-nē′ō-plas-tē). Loosening adhesions and covering the raw surfaces with peritoneum to prevent reformation. [peritoneum + G. *plastos*, formed]

per·i·to·ne·o·scope (per′i-tō-nē′ō-skōp). SYN laparoscope. [peritoneum + G. *skopeō*, to view]

per·i·to·ne·os·co·py (per′i-tō-nē-os′kŏ-pē). Examination of the contents of the peritoneum with a peritoneoscope passed through the abdominal wall. SEE laparoscopy. SYN celioscopy, ventroscopy.

per·i·to·ne·ot·o·my (per′i-tō-nē-ot′ō-mē). Incision of the peritoneum. [peritoneum + G. *tomē*, incision]

per·i·to·ne·um, pl. **pe·ri·to·nea** (per′i-tō-nē′ŭm, -ă) [TA]. The serous sac, consisting of mesothelium and a thin layer of irregular connective tissue, that lines the abdominal cavity and covers most of the viscera contained therein; it forms two sacs: the peritoneal (or greater) sac and the omental bursa (lesser sac) connected by the epiploic foramen. SYN membrana abdominis. [Mod. L. fr. G. *peritonaion*, fr. *periteinō*, to stretch over]

parietal p. [TA], the layer of p. lining the abdominal walls. SYN p. parietale [TA].

p. parieta′le [TA], SYN parietal p.

urogenital p. [TA], peritoneum of the pelvic cavity, including the folds and fossae formed by it. SYN p. urogenitale [TA].

p. urogenitale [TA], SYN urogenital p.

visceral p. [TA], the layer of p. investing the abdominal organs. SYN p. viscerale [TA].

p. viscera′le [TA], SYN visceral p.

per·i·to·ni·tis (per′i-tō-nī′tis). Inflammation of the peritoneum.

adhesive p., a form of p. in which a fibrinous exudate occurs, matting together the intestines and various other organs.

benign paroxysmal p., SYN familial paroxysmal *polyserositis*.

bile p., inflammation of the peritoneum caused by the escape of bile into the free peritoneal cavity. SYN choleperitonitis.

chemical p., p. due to the escape of bile, contents of the gastrointestinal tract, or pancreatic juice into the peritoneal cavity; the contents of the fluid causes chemical injury, shock, and peritoneal exudation prior to occurrence of any associated infection.

chyle p., p. due to free chyle in the peritoneal cavity.

circumscribed p., SYN localized p.

p. defor′mans, a chronic p. in which thickening of the membrane and contracting adhesions cause shortening of the mesentery and kinking and retraction of the intestines.

diaphragmatic p., p. affecting mainly the peritoneal surface of the diaphragm.

diffuse p., SYN general p.

p. encap′sulans, a localized fibrous or adhesive p. remaining after a generalized p. has nearly disappeared; it is marked by pain, constipation, and a palpable tumor.

fibrocaseous p., p. characterized by caseation and fibrosis, usually caused by the tubercle bacillus.

gas p., inflammation of the peritoneum accompanied by an intraperitoneal accumulation of gas.

general p., p. throughout the peritoneal cavity. SYN diffuse p.

localized p., p. confined to a demarcated region of the peritoneal cavity. SYN circumscribed p.

meconium p., p. caused by intestinal perforation in the fetus or newborn; associated with congenital obstruction or due to cystic fibrosis.

pelvic p., generalized inflammation of the peritoneum surrounding the uterus and fallopian tubes. SYN pelvioperitonitis, pelviperitonitis.

periodic p., SYN familial paroxysmal *polyserositis*.

productive p., SYN pachyperitonitis.

tuberculous p., p. caused by the tubercle bacillus.

per·i·ton·sil·lar (per′i-ton′si-lăr). Around a tonsil or the tonsils.

per·i·ton·sil·li·tis (per′i-ton′si-lī′tis). Inflammation of the connective tissue above and behind the tonsil.

per·i·tra·che·al (per-i-trā′kē-ăl). About the trachea.

pe·rit·ri·chal, pe·rit·ri·chate, per·i·trich·ic (pe-rit′ri-kăl, -rit′ri-kāt, per-i-trik′ik). SYN peritrichous (2).

Per·i·trich·i·da (per-i-trik′i-dă). An order of ciliates (subclass Peritrichia, phylum Ciliophora) characterized by a cylindrical shape with the cilia usually limited to the zone surrounding the mouth opening; includes the suborder Mobilina, whose members are all ecto- or endoparasites of aquatic invertebrates and vertebrates, of which the genus *Trichodina* includes economically important gill parasites of fish. [peri- + G. *thrix*, hair]

pe·rit·ri·chous (pe-rit′ri-kŭs). **1.** Relating to cilia or other appendicular organs projecting from the periphery of a cell. **2.** Having flagella uniformly distributed over a cell; used especially with reference to bacteria. SYN peritrichal, peritrichate, peritrichic. [peri- + G. *thrix,* hair]

per·i·tro·chan·ter·ic (per′i-trō′kan-ter′ik). Around a trochanter.

per·i·typh·lic (per′i-tif′lik). SYN pericecal. [peri- + G. *typhlon,* cecum]

per·i·typh·li·tis (per′ĭ-tif-lī′tis). Inflammation of the peritoneum surrounding the cecum.

perityphlitis p. (per′ĭ-tif-lī′tis ak′ti-nō-mī-kot-ĭ-kă), abdominal infection, predominantly around the cecum, with Actinomycetes, usually *Actinomyces israelii.*

per·i·um·bil·i·cal (per′i-ŭm-bil′i-kăl). Around or near the umbilicus. SYN periomphalic.

per·i·un·gual (per′i-ŭng′gwăl). Surrounding a nail; involving the nail folds. [peri- + L. *unguis,* nail]

per·i·u·re·ter·al, per·i·u·re·ter·ic (per′i-ū-rē′ter-ăl, -ū′rē-ter′ik). Surrounding one or both ureters.

per·i·u·re·ter·i·tis (per′i-ū-rē′ter-ī′tis). Inflammation of the tissues about a ureter. [peri- + ureter + G. *-itis,* inflammation]

p. plas′tica, SYN retroperitoneal *fibrosis.*

per·i·u·re·thral (per′i-ū-rē′thrăl). Surrounding the urethra.

per·i·u·re·thri·tis (per′i-ū-rē-thrī′tis). Inflammation of the tissues about the urethra. [peri- + urethra + G. *-itis,* inflammation]

per·i·u·ter·ine (per′i-ū′ter-in). SYN perimetric (1).

per·i·u·vu·lar (per′i-ū′vū-lăr). Around the uvula.

per·i·vag·i·ni·tis (per′i-vaj-i-nī′tis). Inflammation of the connective tissue around the vagina. SYN pericolpitis.

per·i·vas·cu·lar (per′i-vas′kū-lăr). Surrounding a blood or lymph vessel. SYN circumvascular. [peri- + L. *vasculum,* vessel]

per·i·vas·cu·li·tis (per′i-vas-koo-lī′tis). SYN periangitis.

per·i·ve·nous (per-i-vē′nŭs). Surrounding a vein.

per·i·ver·te·bral (per-i-ver′te-brăl). Around a vertebra or vertebrae. SYN perispondylic.

per·i·ves·i·cal (per-i-ves′i-kăl). SYN pericystic. [peri- + L. *vesica,* bladder]

per·i·vis·cer·al (per-i-ivis′er-ăl). SYN perisplanchnic.

per·i·vis·cer·i·tis (per′i-vis-er-ī′tis). Inflammation surrounding any viscus or viscera. [peri- + L. *viscera,* internal organs, + G. *-itis,* inflammation]

per·i·vi·tel·line (per′i-vi-tel′in, -īn). Surrounding the vitellus or yolk. [peri- + L. *vitellus,* yolk]

per·i·win·kle (per′i-wing-kl). SYN *Vinca rosea.*

per·kin·ism (per′kin-izm). A form of quackery purporting to treat disease by applying metals with magnetic and magic properties.

Perkins, Elisha, U.S. physician, 1741–1799. SEE perkinism.

per·lèche (per-lesh′). SYN angular *cheilitis.* [Fr. *per,* intensive, + *lécher,* to lick]

Perlia, Richard, 19th century German ophthalmologist. SEE P. *nucleus;* convergence *nucleus* of P.

per·lin·gual (per-ling′gwăl). Through or by way of the tongue, denoting a method of medication. [L. *per,* through, + *lingua,* tongue]

Perls, Max, German pathologist, 1843–1881. SEE P. Prussian blue *stain, test.*

per·man·ga·nate (per-mang′gă-nāt). A salt of permanganic acid. Formerly used in efforts (probably unsuccessful) to oxidize and thus detoxify alkaloidal poisons.

per·man·gan·ic ac·id (per-mang-gan′ik). An acid, $HMnO_4$, derived from manganese, forming permanganates with bases. SEE ALSO *potassium* permanganate.

per·me·a·bil·i·ty (per′mē-ă-bil′i-tē). The property of being permeable.

per·me·a·ble (per′mē-ă-bl). Permitting the passage of substances (e.g., liquids, gases, heat), as through a membrane or other structure. SYN pervious. [L. *permeabilis* (see permeate)]

per·me·ant (per′mē-ănt). Able to pass through a particular semipermeable membrane. [L. *permeabilis* (see permeate)]

per·me·ase (per′mē-ās). Any of a group of membrane-bound carriers (enzymes) that effect the transport of solute through a

semipermeable membrane; this term is not typically used with eukaryotes.

per·me·ate (per′mē-āt). **1.** To pass through a membrane or other structure, typically by diffusion. **2.** That which can so pass. [L. *permeo,* to pass through]

per·me·a·tion (per-mē-ā′shŭn). The process of spreading through or penetrating, as the extension of a malignant neoplasm by proliferation of the cells continuously along the blood vessels or lymphatics. [L. *per-meo,* pp. *-meatus,* to pass through]

per·nic·i·o·si·form (per-nish′ē-o′si-fōrm). Rarely used term meaning apparently pernicious, denoting a condition or disease that appears to be pernicious or malignant.

per·ni·cious (per-nish′ŭs). Destructive; harmful; denoting a disease of severe character and usually fatal without appropriate treatment. [L. *perniciosus,* destructive, fr. *pernicies,* destruction]

per·ni·o·sis (per-nē-ō′sis). SYN chilblain. [L. *pernio,* chilblain, + G. *-osis,* condition]

△**pero-.** Maimed, malformed. [G. *pēros*]

pe·ro·bra·chi·us (pē-rō-brā′kē-ŭs). An individual with a congenital malformation of one or both hands and forearms. [pero- + G. *brachiōn,* arm]

pe·ro·ceph·a·lus (pē-rō-sef′ă-lŭs). An individual with congenitally defective face and head. [pero- + G. *kephalē,* head]

pe·ro·chi·rus (pē-rō-kī′rŭs). An individual with a congenital malformation of one or both hands. [pero- + G. *cheir,* hand]

pe·ro·dac·ty·ly, pe·ro·dac·tyl·ia (pē-rō-dak′ti-lē, -dak-til′ē-ă). Congenitally malformed fingers or toes. [pero- + G. *daktylos,* finger or toe]

per·o·gen (per′ō-jen). A preparation of sodium perborate that, when mixed with the accompanying catalyzer, liberates 10% of the oxygen in the salt.

pe·ro·me·lia, pe·rom·e·ly (pē-rō-mē′lē-ă, pĕ-rom′ĕ-lē). Severe congenital malformations of extremities, including absence of hand or foot. [pero- + G. *melos,* limb]

per·o·ne (per-ō′nē). SYN fibula. [G. *peronē,* brooch, the small bone of the arm or leg, the fibula, fr. *peirō,* to pierce]

per·o·ne·al (per-ō-nē′ăl). SYN fibular. [L. *peroneus,* fr. G. *peronē,* fibula]

per·o·ne·o·tib·i·al (per′ō-nē′ō-tib′ē-ăl). SYN tibiofibular.

pe·ro·pus (pē′rō-pŭs). A person with a congenital malformation of one or both feet. [pero- + G. *pous,* foot]

per·o·ral (per-ō′răl). Through the mouth, denoting a method of medication or an approach. [L. *per,* through, + *os* (*or-*), mouth]

per os (PO). By or through the mouth, denoting a method of medication. [L.]

pe·ro·splanch·nia (pē-rō-splank′nē-ă). Congenital malformation of the viscera. [pero- + G. *splanchnon,* viscus]

per·os·se·ous (per-os′ē-ŭs). Through bone. [L. *per,* through, + *os,* bone]

△**peroxi-.** SEE peroxy-.

per·ox·i·das·es (per-ok′si-dās-ez) [EC subclass 1.11]. Hydrogen peroxide–reducing oxidoreductases; enzymes in animal and plant tissues that catalyze the dehydrogenation (oxidation) of various substances in the presence of hydrogen peroxide, which acts as hydrogen acceptor, being converted to water in the process.

horseradish p., a p. isolated from horseradish that is used in immunohistochemistry to label the antigen-antibody complex.

per·ox·ide (per-ok′sīd). **1.** That oxide of any series that contains the greatest number of oxygen atoms; applied most correctly to compounds containing an –O–O– link, as in hydrogen peroxide (H–O–O–H); a hydroperoxide is R–O–O–H. **2.** The O_2^{2-} ion. **3.** Any member of a class of metallic oxides that contain the peroxide ion.

per·ox·i·some (per-ok′si-sōm). A membrane-bound organelle occurring in many eukaryotic cells that often has an electron-dense crystalline inclusion containing catalase, urate oxidase, and other oxidative enzymes relating to the formation and degradation of H_2O_2; thought to be important in detoxifying various molecules and in catalyzing the breakdown of fatty acids to acetyl-CoA; an absence of p.'s is found in individuals with Zellweger syndrome. [peroxide + G. *sōma,* body]

peroxy-. Prefix denoting the presence of an extra O atom, as in peroxides, peroxy acids (e.g., hydrogen peroxide, peroxyformic acid). Often shortened to per-.

per·ox·y·a·ce·tyl ni·trate (per-ok-sē-ă-sē′til). The major pollutant responsible for eye and nose irritation in smog.

per·oxy ac·id (per-ok′sē). SYN peracid.

per·ox·y·for·mic ac·id (per-ok′sē-fōr′mik). SYN performic acid.

per·ox·yl (per-ok′sil). H–O–O; one of the free radicals presumed formed as a result of the bombardment of tissue by high-energy radiation.

per·phe·na·zine (per-fen′ă-zēn). An antipsychotic of the phenothiazine type.

per pri·mam (per prī′mam in-ten-shē-ō′nem). By first intention. SEE *healing* by first intention. [L.]

per rec·tum (per rek′tŭm). By or through the rectum, denoting a method of medication. [L.]

per·salt (per′sawlt). In chemistry, any salt that contains the greatest possible amount of the acid radical.

per sal·tum (per sal′tŭm). At a leap; at one bound; not gradually or through different stages. [L.]

per·sev·er·a·tion (per-sev-er-ā′shŭn). **1.** The constant repetition of a meaningless word or phrase. **2.** The duration of a mental impression, measured by the rapidity with which one impression follows another as determined by the revolving of a two-colored disk. **3.** In clinical psychology, the uncontrollable repetition of a previously appropriate or correct response, even though the repeated response has since become inappropriate or incorrect. [L. *persevero,* to persist]

per·sic oil (per′sik). The fixed oil expressed from the kernels of varieties of *Prunus armeniaca* (apricot kernel oil) or *Prunus persica* (peach kernel oil); used as a vehicle.

per·sis·tence (per-sis′tens). Obstinate continuation of characteristic behavior, or of existence in spite of treatment or adverse environmental conditions. [L. *persisto,* to abide, stand firm]

    lactase p., an inherited trait (autosomal dominant) in which the levels of lactase do not decline after weaning. Cf. lactase *restriction.*

    microbial p., the phenomenon of survival, in high concentration of an antimicrobial substance, of microbes that seem not to be resistant variants (mutants) since their progeny are fully susceptible.

per·sist·er (per-sis′ter). That which, or one who, is capable of persistence; especially a bacterium that exhibits microbial persistence.

per·so·na (per-sō′nă). A term that embodies the totality of the individual, the total constellation of the physical, psychological, and behavioral attributes of each unique individual; in jungian psychology, the outer aspect of character, as opposed to anima (2); the assumed personality used to mask the true one. [L. *per,* through, + *sonare,* to sound: from the small megaphone in ancient dramatic masks, to aid in projecting the actor's voice]

per·son·al·i·ty (per-sŏn-al′i-tē). **1.** The unique self; the organized system of attitudes and behavioral predispositions by which one feels, thinks, acts, and impresses and establishes relationships with others. **2.** An individual with a particular p. pattern.

    affective p., a chronic behavioral pattern in an enduring disturbance of feelings or mood expressed as a form of depression and related emotional features that color the whole of the psychic life.

    antisocial p., SEE psychopath, sociopath, antisocial personality *disorder.* SYN psychopathic p.

    asthenic p., an older term for a p. type characterized by low energy level, easy fatigability, incapacity for enjoyment, lack of enthusiasm, and oversensitivity to physical and emotional stress. SYN asthenic personality disorder.

    authoritarian p., a cluster of p. traits reflecting a desire for security and order, e.g., rigidity, highly conventional outlook, unquestioning obedience, scapegoating, desire for structured lines of authority.

    avoidant p., SYN avoidant personality *disorder.*

    basic p., SEE basic personality *type.*

    borderline p., SEE borderline personality *disorder.*

    compulsive p., SYN obsessive-compulsive personality *disorder.*

    cyclothymic p., a p. disorder in which a person experiences regularly alternating periods of elation and depression, less severe than seen in bipolar disorder, usually not related to external circumstances. SYN cyclothymic personality disorder.

    dependent p., SYN dependent personality *disorder.*

    dual p., an older term for a mental disturbance in which a person assumes alternately two different identities without either p. being consciously aware of the other. SEE ALSO multiple p.

    hysterical p., SYN histrionic personality *disorder.*

    inadequate p., a p. disorder, characterized by personal and social ineptness plus emotional and physical instability, that renders the individual unable to cope with the normal vicissitudes of life.

    masochistic p., a p. disorder in which the individual accepts exploitation and sacrifices self-interest while at the same time feeling morally superior or feigning moral superiority, attempting to elicit sympathy, and inducing guilt in others.

    multiple p., SYN dissociative identity *disorder.*

    neurasthenic p., an obsolete term for a condition characterized by some of the following features: poor appetite or overeating, insomnia or hypersomnia, low energy or fatigue, low self esteem, poor concentration or difficulty making decisions, and feelings of hopelessness. In its most severe form it may become a chronic disturbance of mood called dysthymia (depressive neurosis) in which a depressive mood accompanies the features listed above.

    obsessive p., SYN obsessive-compulsive personality *disorder*; SEE obsessive-compulsive p., obsessive-compulsive *disorder.*

    obsessive-compulsive p., SYN obsessive-compulsive personality *disorder.*

    paranoid p., SYN paranoid personality *disorder.*

    passive-aggressive p., a p. disorder characterized by a pervasive and enduring pattern of behavior in which aggressive feelings are manifested in passive ways, especially through mild obstructionism and stubbornness.

    perfectionistic p., a p. characterized by rigidity, extreme inhibition, and excessive concern with conformity and adherence to often unique standards.

    psychopathic p., SYN antisocial p.

    schizoid p., SYN schizoid personality *disorder.*

    schizotypal p., SYN schizotypal personality *disorder.*

    shut-in p., a rarely used term for a person who responds inadequately to contacts with other people.

    syntonic p., a rarely used term for a stable p., one characterized by even temperament.

    type A p., type B p., SEE type A *behavior,* type B *behavior.*

per·son-years. The product of the number of years times the number of members of a population who have been affected by a certain condition; e.g., years of treatment with a certain drug.

pers·pi·ra·tion (pers-pi-rā′shŭn). **1.** The excretion of fluid by the sweat glands of the skin. SYN diaphoresis, sudation, sweating. SEE ALSO sweat. **2.** All fluid loss through normal skin, whether by sweat gland secretion or by diffusion through other skin structures. **3.** The hypotonic fluid excreted by the sweat glands; it consists of water containing sodium chloride and phosphate, urea, ammonia, ethereal sulfates, creatinine, fats, and other waste products; the average daily quantity is estimated at about 1500 g. SYN sudor. SEE ALSO sweat (1). [L. *per-spiro,* pp. *-atus,* to breathe everywhere]

    insensible p., p. that evaporates before it is perceived as moisture on the skin; the term sometimes includes evaporation from the lungs.

    sensible p., the p. excreted in large quantity, or when there is much humidity in the atmosphere, so that it appears as moisture (sweat) on the skin.

per·stil·la·tion (per-sti-lā′shŭn). SEE pervaporation. [L. *per,* through, + *stillo,* to trickle, distil]

per·sua·sion (per-swā′zhŭn). The act of influencing the mind of another, by authority, argument, reason, or personal insight; an important element in most types of psychotherapy. [L. *persuasio*, fr. *persuadeo*, to persuade]

per·sul·fate (per-sŭl'fāt). A salt of persulfuric acid.

per·sul·fide (per-sŭl'fīd). 1. The compound of a series of sulfides that contains more atoms of sulfur than any other. 2. The sulfur analog of a peroxide.

per·sul·fu·ric ac·id (per-sŭl-fūr'ik). H_2SO_5; peroxymonosulfuric acid; an oxidizing agent.

pertactin (per-tak'tin). An antigenic material produced by *Bordetella pertussis* used to improve the effectiveness of pertussis vaccines. [*pert*ussis + *act* + -*in*]

per·tech·ne·tate (per-tek-ne-tāt). Anionic form of technetium used widely in nuclear scanning; $^{99m}TcO_4$.

Perthes, Georg C., German surgeon, 1869–1927. SEE P. *disease, test;* Calvé-P. *disease;* Legg-Calvé-P. *disease.*

♻**perthio-.** Prefix denoting substitution of sulfur for every oxygen in a compound; e.g., perthiocarbonic acid, H_2CS_3.

Pertik, Otto, Hungarian pathologist, 1852–1913. SEE P. *diverticulum.*

per tu·bam (per too'băm). Through a tube. [L.]

per·tus·sis (per-tŭs'is). An acute infectious inflammation of the larynx, trachea, and bronchi caused by *Bordetella pertussis;* characterized by recurrent bouts of spasmodic coughing that continues until the breath is exhausted, then ending in a noisy inspiratory stridor the "whoop") caused by laryngeal spasm. SYN pertussis syndrome, whooping cough. [L. *per,* very (intensive), + *tussis,* cough]

Pe·ru·vi·an bark. SYN cinchona.

per·vap·o·ra·tion (per'vap-ōr-ā'shŭn). The heating of a liquid within a dialyzing bag suspended over a hot plate, evaporation taking place rapidly through the membrane; any colloids in solution remain within the bag while crystalloids diffuse out and crystallize on the outer surface of the bag (perstillation). [L. *per,* through, + *vapor,* steam]

per·ver·sion (per-ver'zhŭn). A deviation from the norm, especially concerning sexual interests or behavior. [L. *perversio,* fr. *per-verto,* pp. -*versus,* to turn about]

   polymorphous p., (1) in psychoanalytic theory, a child's variegated sexual activity and interests; (2) in general, the manifold p.'s shown by an adult.

   sexual p., SYN sexual *deviation.*

per·vert (per'vert). One who practices perversions. SEE ALSO deviant (2).

per·vert·ed (per-ver'ted). Abnormal, deviant, or disordered.

per vi·as na·tu·ra·les (per vī'as nach'er-ā'lēz). Through the natural passages; e.g., denoting a normal delivery, as opposed to cesarean section, or the passage in stool of a foreign body instead of its surgical removal. [L.]

per·vi·ous (per'vē-ŭs). SYN permeable. [L. *pervius,* fr. *per,* through, + *via,* a way]

pes, gen. **pe·dis,** pl. **pe·des** (pes, pē'dis, -dēz). 1 [TA]. SYN foot (1). 2. Any footlike or basal structure or part. 3. Talipes. In this sense, p. is always qualified by a word expressing the specific type. [L.]

   p. abduc'tus, SYN talipes valgus.

   p. adduc'tus, SYN talipes varus.

   p. anseri'nus, (1) SYN parotid *plexus* of facial nerve; (2) the combined tendinous expansions of the sartorius, gracilis, and semitendinosus muscles at the medial border of the tuberosity of the tibia.

   p. ca'vus, SYN talipes cavus.

   p. equi'noval'gus, SYN talipes equinovalgus.

   p. equi'nova'rus, SYN talipes equinovarus.

   p. gi'gas, SYN macropodia.

   p. hippocam'pi [TA], SYN *foot* of hippocampus.

   p. pla'nus, a condition in which the longitudinal arch is broken down, the entire sole touching the ground. SYN flatfoot, talipes planus.

   p. prona'tus, SYN talipes valgus.

   p. val'gus, SYN talipes valgus.

p. va'rus, SYN talipes varus.

pes·co·veg·e·tar·i·an. A vegetarian who consumes dairy products, eggs, and fish, but does not consume other animal flesh.

pes·sa·ry (pes'ă-rē). 1. An appliance of varied form, introduced into the vagina to support the uterus or to correct any displacement. 2. A medicated vaginal suppository. [L. *pessarium,* fr. G. *pessos,* an oval stone used in certain games]

   cube p., plastic or rubber p. in a cube shape particularly suitable for elderly women with uterine prolapse.

   diaphragm p., a ring with a covered opening, used as a platform to support uterus, bladder, or rectum.

   doughnut p., SYN ring p.

   Dumontpallier p., an elastic ring p. SYN Mayer p.

   Gariel p., a hollow inflatable rubber p. made in the form of a ring or a pear.

   Hodge p., a double-curve oblong p. employed for the correction of retrodeviations of the uterus.

   Mayer p., SYN Dumontpallier p.

   Menge p., a ring p. with a central horizontal bar into which a detachable handle is inserted.

   ring p., a ring of rubber, plastic, or metal in which the cervix rests; designed to support the uterus and to correct prolapse of that organ. SYN doughnut p.

pes·si·mism (pes'i-mizm). A tendency to see or anticipate the worst. [L. *pessimus,* worst, irreg. superl. of *malus,* bad]

   therapeutic p., a disbelief in the curative virtues of remedies in general and especially of drugs.

pest. SYN plague (2). [L. *pestis*]

pes·ti·ce·mia (pes-ti-sē'mē-ă). Bacteremia due to *Yersinia pestis.* [L. *pestis,* plague, + G. *haima,* blood]

pes·ti·cide (pes'ti-sīd). General term for an agent that destroys fungi, insects, rodents, or any other pest.

pes·tif·er·ous (pes-tif'ĕ-rŭs). SYN pestilential.

pes·ti·lence (pes'ti-lens). 1. SYN plague (2). 2. A virulent outbreak of any disease. [L. *pestilentia*]

pes·ti·len·tial (pes-ti-len'shăl). Relating to or tending to produce a pestilence. SYN pestiferous.

pes·tis. SYN plague (2). [L.]

   p. am'bulans, SYN ambulant *plague.*

   p. bubonica (pes'tis boo'bōn'ik-ă), SYN bubonic *plague.*

   p. ful'minans, SYN bubonic *plague.*

   p. ma'jor, SYN bubonic *plague.*

   p. mi'nor, SYN ambulant *plague.*

   p. sid'erans, SYN septicemic *plague.*

Pes·ti·vi·rus (pes'ti-vī'rŭs). A genus of viruses (family Flaviviridae) composed of the hog cholera virus and related viruses. [L. *pestis,* plague, + virus]

pes·tle (pes'l). An instrument in the shape of a rod with one rounded and weighted extremity, used for bruising, breaking, grinding, and mixing substances in a mortar. [L. *pistillum,* fr. *pinso,* or *piso,* to pound]

PET Abbreviation for positron emission *tomography.*

♻**peta- (P).** Prefix used in the SI and metric system to signify multiples of one quadrillion (10^{15}).

♻**-petal.** Seeking; movement toward the part indicated by the main portion of the word. [L. *peto,* to seek, strive for]

▣**pe·te·chi·ae,** sing. **pe·te·chia** (pe-tē'kē-ē, pē-tek'-; pe-tē'kē-ă). Minute hemorrhagic spots, of pinpoint to pinhead size, in the skin, which are not blanched by pressure. [Mod. L. form of It. *petecchie*]

   calcaneal p., traumatic hemorrhage into the stratum corneum of the heel that may persist for several weeks as centrally confluent black dots. SYN black heel.

   Tardieu petechiae, SYN Tardieu *ecchymoses,* under *ecchymosis.*

pe·te·chi·al (pē-tē'kē-ăl, pē-tek'-). Relating to, accompanied by, or characterized by petechiae.

Peters, Albert, German physician, 1862–1938. SEE P. *anomaly.*

Peters, Hubert, Austrian obstetrician, 1859–1934. SEE P. *ovum.*

Petersen, C.F., German surgeon, 1845–1908.

peth·i·dine (peth′ĭ-dēn). SYN meperidine hydrochloride.

pet·i·o·late, pet·i·o·lat·ed (pet′ē-ō-lāt, -lāt-ed). Having a stem or pedicle. SYN petioled. [L. *petiolus*]

pet·i·ole (pet′ē-ōl). SYN petiolus.

pet·i·oled (pet′ē-ōld). SYN petiolate.

pe·ti·o·lus (pe-tī′ō-lŭs). A stem or pedicle. SYN petiole. [L. dim. of *pes* (foot), the stalk of a fruit]

p. epiglot′tidis, SYN *stalk* of epiglottis.

Petit, Francois du, French surgeon and anatomist, 1664–1741. SEE P. *canals,* under *canal, sinus.*

Petit, Paul, French anatomist, *1889. SEE P. *aponeurosis.*

Petit, Jean L., Paris surgeon, 1674–1750. SEE P. *hernia, herniotomy,* lumbar *triangle.*

Petit, Alexis T., French physicist, 1791–1820. SEE Dulong-P. *law.*

Petri, Julius, German bacteriologist, 1852–1921. SEE P. *dish;* Petri dish *culture.*

pet·ri·fac·tion (pet-ri-fak′shŭn). Fossilization, as in conversion into stone. [L. *petra,* rock + *facio,* to make]

pé·tris·sage (pā-trē-sazh′). A manipulation in massage, consisting in a kneading of the muscles. [Fr. kneading]

△**petro-.** Stone; stone-like hardness. [L. *petra,* rock; G. *petros,* stone]

pet·roc·cip·i·tal (pet′rok-sip′i-tăl). SYN petrooccipital.

pe·tro·la·tum (pet-rō-lā′tŭm). A yellowish mixture of the softer members of the paraffin or methane series of hydrocarbons, obtained from petroleum as an intermediate product in its distillation; used as a soothing application to burns and abrasions of the skin and as a base for ointments. SYN petroleum jelly, yellow soft paraffin.

heavy liquid p., SYN mineral oil.

hydrophilic p., p. composed of cholesterol 30 g, stearyl alcohol 30 g, white wax 80 g, and white p. 860 g, to make 1000 g.

light liquid p., light mineral oil.

white p., of the same composition as p. except that it is decolorized by treatment with activated charcoal; used for the same purposes as p. SYN white soft paraffin.

pe·tro·le·um (pĕ-trō′lē-ŭm). A mixture of liquid hydrocarbons found in the earth in various parts of the world and believed to be derived from fossilized animal and plant remains; the source of petrolatum, in addition to its use for lighting and heating purposes. SYN coal oil, rock oil. [L. *petra,* rock, + *oleum,* oil]

p. benzin, purified, low boiling fractions distilled from p. consisting of hydrocarbons, chiefly of the methane series; it is highly flammable, and its vapors, when mixed with air and ignited, may explode; used as a solvent. SYN benzin, benzine, naphtha, p. ether.

p. ether, SYN p. benzin.

liquid p., SYN mineral oil.

pe·tro·le·um jel·ly. SYN petrolatum.

pet·ro·mas·toid (pet′rō-mas′toyd). Relating to the petrous and the squamous portions of the temporal bone, which are usually united at birth by the petrosquamosal suture. SYN petrosomastoid.

pet·ro·oc·cip·i·tal (pet′rō-ok-sip′i-tăl). Denoting the cranial suture between the occipital bone and the petrous portion of the temporal. SYN petroccipital.

pet·ro·pha·ryn·ge·us. SEE *musculus* petropharyngeus.

pe·tro·sa, pl. **pe·tro·sae** (pe-trō′să, -sē). The petrous portion of the temporal bone. [L. fr. *petra,* rock]

pe·tro·sal (pe-trō′săl). Relating to the petrosa. SYN petrous (2).

pe·tro·sal·pin·go·sta·phy·li·nus (pet′rō-sal′pin-gō-staf-i-lī′nŭs). Obsolete term for the levator veli palatini muscle. [petrosa + G. *salpinx,* trumpet, + *staphylē,* uvula]

pet·ro·si·tis (pet-rō-sī′tis). An inflammation involving the petrous portion of the temporal bone and its air cells. SYN petrousitis.

pet·ro·so·mas·toid (pet-rō′sō-mas′toyd). SYN petromastoid.

pet·ro·sphe·noid (pet′rō-sfē′noyd). Relating to the petrous portion of the temporal bone and to the sphenoid bone.

pet·ro·squa·mo·sal, pet·ro·squa·mous (pet′rō-skwā-mō′săl, -skwā′mŭs). Relating to the petrous and the squamous portions of the temporal bone. SYN squamopetrosal.

pe·tro·sta·phy·li·nus (pet′rō-staf-i-lī′nŭs). Obsolete term for the levator veli palatini (*muscle*). [G. *petra,* stone, + *staphylē,* uvula]

pet·rous (pet′rŭs, pē′trŭs). **1.** Of stony hardness. **2.** SYN petrosal. [L. *petrosus,* fr. *petra,* a rock]

pet·rou·si·tis (pet-roo-sī′tis). SYN petrositis.

Pette, H.H. German neuropathologist, 1887–1964. SEE P.-Döring *disease.*

Pettit, Auguste, French physician, 1869–1939. SEE Bachman-P. *test.*

Peutz, J.L.A., Dutch physician. SEE P.-Jeghers *syndrome;* Jeghers-P. *syndrome.*

pex·in (pek′sin). SYN chymosin.

pex·in·o·gen (pek-sin′ō-jen). SYN prochymosin.

pex·is (pek′sis). Fixation of substances in the tissues. [G. *pēxis,* fixation]

△**-pexy.** Fixation, usually surgical. [G. *pēxis,* fixation]

Peyer, Johann K., Swiss anatomist, 1653–1712. SEE P. *glands,* under *gland;* aggregated lymphoid *nodules* of small intestine, under *nodule.*

pe·yo·te, pe·yo·tl (pā-yō′tē, pā-yō′tl). Aztec name for *Lophophora williamsii,* a small cactus indigenous to Mexico and the southwestern United States and used in Native American tribal ceremonies, where it produces a trance and hallucinations; principal active component of peyote is mescaline. SYN pellote. [Sp.]

Peyronie, Francois de la, French surgeon, 1678–1747. SEE P. *disease.*

Peyrot, Jean J., French surgeon, 1843–1918. SEE P. *thorax.*

Pezzer, O. de. SEE de Pezzer.

Pfannenstiel, Hermann Johann, German gynecologist, 1862–1909. SEE P. *incision.*

Pfaundler, Meinhard von, German physician, 1872–1947. SEE P.-Hurler *syndrome.*

Pfeiffer, Richard F.J., German physician, 1858–1945. SEE *Pfeifferella;* P. *phenomenon, syndrome.*

Pfeif·fer·el·la (fī-fer-el′lä). An obsolete genus of bacteria, the type species of which, *P. mallei,* formerly was placed in the genus *Actinobacillus* and now is in the genus *Pseudomonas.* [R. F. J. *Pfeiffer*]

PFFD Abbreviation for proximal femoral focal *deficiency.*

Pflüger, Eduard F.W., German anatomist and physiologist, 1829–1910. SEE P. *law.*

PFOB Abbreviation for perfluorooctyl bromide.

Pfuhl, Eduard, German physician, 1852–1905. SEE P. *sign.*

PG Abbreviation for prostaglandin.

pg Symbol for picogram.

PGA, PGB, PGC, PGD Abbreviations, with numeric subscripts according to structure, often used for prostaglandins. Letters A, B, etc., indicate the nature of the cyclopentane ring (substituents, double bonds, orientation); numerical subscripts indicate the number of double bonds in the alkyl chains.

P-glycoprotein (glī-kō-prō′tēn). Protein associated with tumor multidrug resistance; acts as energy-requiring efflux pump for many classes of natural products and chemotherapeutic drugs. SYN P-170.

PGR Abbreviation for psychogalvanic *response.*

P₂Gri Symbol for diphosphoglycerate.

1,3-P₂Gri Symbol for 1,3-bisphosphoglycerate.

2,3-P₂Gri Symbol for 2,3-bisphosphoglycerate.

Ph Symbol for phenyl.

Ph1. Abbreviation for Philadelphia *chromosome.*

pH Symbol for the negative decadic logarithm of the H^+ ion concentration (measured in moles per liter); a solution with pH 7.00 (1×10^{-7} g molecular weight of hydrogen per liter) is neutral at 22°C (i.e., $[H^+] = [OH^-]$), one with a pH value of more than 7.00 is alkaline, one with a pH lower than 7.00 is acid. At a temperature of 37°C, neutrality is at a pH value of 6.80. Cf. dissociation *constant* of water. [p (power or potency) of $[H^+]$]

blood pH, pH of arterial blood; normal is 7.4 (normal range 7.36–7.44).

critical pH, the pH range, about 5.5, at which saliva ceases to be saturated with respect to calcium and phosphate, and below which tooth mineral will dissolve.

optimum pH, the pH at which an enzymatic or any other reaction or process is most effective under a given set of conditions.

PHA Abbreviation for phytohemagglutinin.

△**phaco-.** **1.** Lens-shaped, relating to a lens; **2.** Birthmark; as in phacomatosis. [G. *phakos*, lentil (lens), anything shaped like a lentil]

phac·o·an·a·phy·lax·is (fak′ō-an-ă-fī-lak′sis). Hypersensitivity to protein of the lens of the eye.

phac·o·cele (fak′ō-sēl). Hernia of the lens of the eye through the sclera. [phaco- + G. *kēlē*, hernia]

phac·o·cyst (fak′ō-sist). SYN *capsule* of lens. [phaco- + G. *kystis*, bladder]

phac·o·cys·tec·to·my (fak′ō-sis-tek′tō-mē). Rarely used term for surgical removal of a portion of the capsule of the lens of the eye. [phaco- + G. *kystis*, bladder, + *ektomē*, excision]

phac·o·don·e·sis (fak′ō-don-ē′sis). Tremulousness of the lens of the eye. [phaco- + G. *doneō*, to shake to and fro]

phac·o·e·mul·si·fi·ca·tion (fak′ō-ē-mŭl-si-fi-kā′shŭn). A method of emulsifying and aspirating a cataract with a low-frequency ultrasonic needle.

phac·o·er·y·sis (fak-ō-er′i-sis). Extraction of the lens of the eye by means of a suction cup called the erysophake. [phaco- + G. *erysis*, pulling, drawing off]

phac·o·frag·men·ta·tion (fak′ō-frag′men-tā′shŭn). Rupture and aspiration of the lens.

pha·coid (fak′oyd). Of lentil shape. [phaco- + G. *eidos*, resemblance]

pha·col·y·sis (fă-kol′i-sis). Operative breaking down and removal of the lens. [phaco- + G. *lysis*, dissolution]

pha·co·lyt·ic (fak-ō-lit′ik). Characterized by or referring to phacolysis.

pha·co·ma (fa-kō′mă). A hamartoma found in phacomatosis; often refers to a retinal hamartoma in tuberous sclerosis. SYN phakoma. [phaco- + G. *-oma*, tumor]

pha·co·ma·la·cia (fak′ō-mă-lā′shē-ă). Softening of the lens, as may occur in hypermature cataract. [phaco- + G. *malakia*, softness]

phac·o·ma·to·sis (fak′ō-mă-tō′sis). A generic term for a group of hereditary diseases characterized by hamartomas involving multiple tissues; e.g., von Hippel-Lindau disease, neurofibromatosis, Sturge-Weber syndrome, tuberous sclerosis. SYN phakomatosis. [Van der Hoeve's coinage fr. G. *phakos*, mother-spot]

phac·o·scope (fak′ō-skōp). An instrument in the form of a dark chamber for observing the changes in the lens during accommodation. [phaco- + G. *skopeō*, to view]

Phae·ni·cia ser·i·ca·ta (fen-ī′sē-ă ser-i-kā′tă). A common species of yellowish or metallic green blowfly (family Calliphoridae, order Diptera); an abundant scavenger feeding on carrion or excrement, and implicated in sheep strike and other forms of myiasis. SYN *Lucilia sericata.*

△**phaeo-.** SEE pheo-.

phae·o·hy·pho·my·co·sis (fē′ō-hī′fō-mī-kō′sis). A group of superficial and deep infections caused by fungi that form pigmented hyphae and yeastlike cells in tissue, i.e., dematiaceous fungal infections other than chromoblastomycosis and mycetomas. In humans, cats, and horses, p. is caused by many species. [G. *phaios*, dusky, + *hyphē*, web, + mycosis]

phage (fāj). SYN bacteriophage.
    β p., SYN β *corynebacteriophage.*
    defective p., SYN defective *bacteriophage.*
    Lambda p., a bacteriophage used extensively in experimental systems.

△**-phage, -phagia, -phagy.** Eating, devouring. [G. *phagō*, to eat]

phag·e·de·na (faj-ě-dē′nă). Obsolete term for an ulcer that rapidly spreads peripherally, destroying the tissues as it increases in size. [G. *phagedaina*, a canker]
    p. gangreno′sa, severe gangrene with sloughing.

p. nosocomia′lis, gangrene arising in a hospital from cross infection.

p. trop′ica, the tropical ulcer of Old World cutaneous leishmaniasis.

phag·e·den·ic (faj-ě-den′ik). Obsolete term for relating to or having the characteristics of phagedena.

△**phago-.** Eating, devouring. [G. *phagō*, to eat]

phag·o·cyte (fag′ō-sīt). A cell possessing the property of ingesting bacteria, foreign particles, and other cells. P.'s are divided into two general classes: 1) microphages, polymorphonuclear leukocytes that ingest chiefly bacteria; 2) macrophages, mononucleated cells (histiocytes and monocytes) that are largely scavengers, ingesting dead tissue and degenerated cells. SYN carrier cell, scavenger cell. [phago- + G. *kytos*, cell]

phag·o·cyt·ic (fag-ō-sit′ik). Relating to phagocytes or phagocytosis.

phag·o·cy·tin (fag-ō-sī′tin). A very labile bactericidal substance that may be isolated from polymorphonuclear leukocytes.

phag·o·cy·tize (fag′ō-si-tīz). SYN phagocytose.

phag·o·cy·to·blast (fag-ō-sī′tō-blast). A primitive cell developing into a phagocyte. [phagocyte + G. *blastos*, germ]

phag·o·cy·tol·y·sis (fag′ō-sī-tol′i-sis). **1.** Destruction of phagocytes, or leukocytes, occurring in the process of blood coagulation or as the result of the introduction of certain antagonistic foreign substances into the body. SYN phagolysis. **2.** A spontaneous breaking down of the phagocytes, preliminary (according to Metchnikoff) to the liberation of cytase, or complement. [phagocyte + G. *lysis*, dissolution]

phag·o·cy·to·lyt·ic (fag′ō-sī-tō-lit′ik). Relating to phagocytolysis. SYN phagolytic.

phag·o·cy·tose (fag′ō-si-tōz). To perform phagocytosis, denoting the action of phagocytic cells. SYN phagocytize.

ℹ**phag·o·cy·to·sis** (fāg-ō-sī-tō′sis). The process of ingestion and digestion by cells of solid substances, e.g., other cells, bacteria, bits of necrosed tissue, foreign particles. SEE ALSO endocytosis. [phagocyte + G. *-osis*, condition]

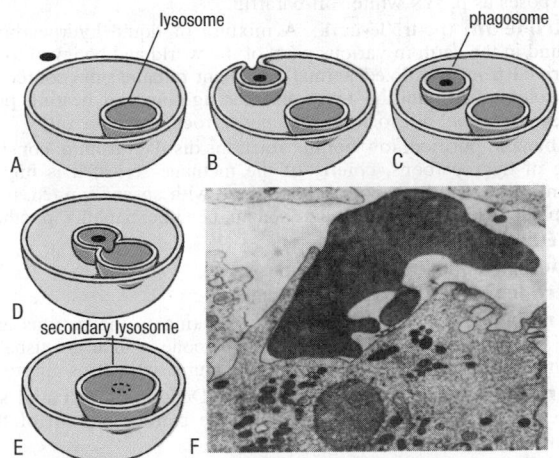

phagocytosis: (A) cell and foreign particle converging; (B) particle endocytized; (C) phagosome approaching lysosome; (D) phagosome and lysosome fused; (E) particle digested in secondary lysosome; (F) initial stage of phagocytosis of erythrocyte by neutrophilic granulocyte (guinea pig)

induced p., p. occurring when bacteria are subjected to the action of opsonins in blood and then brought in contact with leukocytes.

spontaneous p., p. occurring when a culture of bacteria is brought in contact with washed leukocytes in an indifferent medium, such as a physiologic salt solution.

phag·o·dy·na·mom·e·ter (fag′ō-dī-nă-mom′ě-ter). A device for measuring the force required to chew various foods. [phago- + G. *dynamis*, force, + *metron*, measure]

pha·gol·y·sis (fa-gol′i-sis). SYN phagocytolysis (1).

phag·o·ly·so·some (fag-ō-līʹsō-sōm). A body formed by union of a phagosome or ingested particle with a lysosome having hydrolytic enzymes.

phag·o·lyt·ic (fag-ō-litʹik). SYN phagocytolytic.

phag·o·pho·bia (fag-ō-fōʹbē-ă). Morbid fear of eating. [phago- + G. *phobos*, fear]

phag·o·some (fagʹō-sōm). A vesicle that forms around a particle (bacterial or other) within the phagocyte that engulfed it, separates from the cell membrane, and then fuses with and receives the contents of cytoplasmic granules (lysosomes), thus forming a phagolysosome in which digestion of the engulfed particle occurs. [phago- + G. *sōma*, body]

phag·o·type (fagʹō-tīp). In microbiology, a subdivision of a species distinguished from other strains therein by sensitivity to a certain bacteriophage or set of bacteriophages. [phago- + G. *typos*, type]

-phagy. SEE -phage.

phako-. For words so beginning and not listed here, see phaco-.

pha·ko·ma (fa-kōʹmă). SYN phacoma.

phak·o·ma·to·sis (fakʹō-mă-tōʹsis). SYN phacomatosis.

pha·lan·ge·al (fă-lanʹjē-ăl). Relating to a phalanx.

phal·an·gec·to·my (fal-an-jekʹtō-mē). Excision of one or more of the phalanges of hand or foot. [phalang- + G. *ektomē*, excision]

pha·lan·ges (fă-lanʹjēz). Plural of phalanx. [L.]

pha·lanx, gen. **pha·lan·gis**, pl. **pha·lan·ges** (fāʹlangks, fă-langksʹ; fă-lanʹjis; -jēz) [TA]. **1** [NA]. One of the long bones of the digits, 14 in number for each hand or foot, two for the thumb or great toe, and three each for the other four digits; designated as proximal, middle, and distal, beginning from the metacarpus. **2.** One of a number of cuticular plates, arranged in several rows, on the surface of the spiral organ (of Corti), which are the heads of the outer row of pillar cells and of phalangeal cells; between them are the free ends of the hair cells. [L. fr. G. *phalanx* (*-ang-*), line of soldiers, bone between two joints of the fingers and toes]

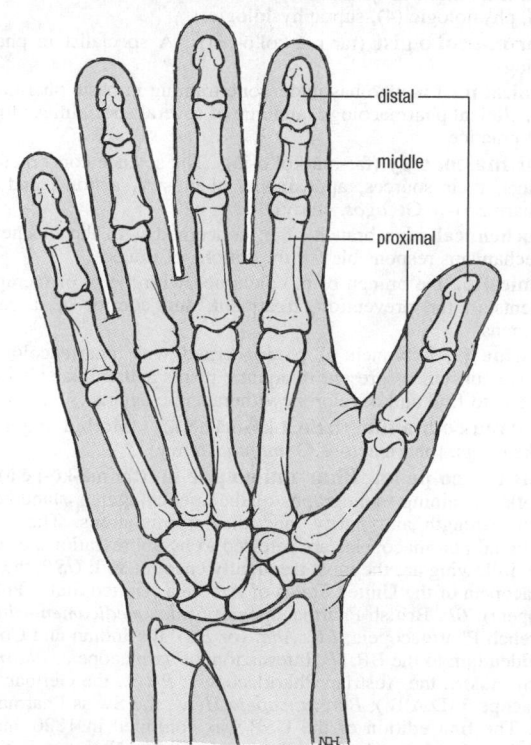

distal —
middle —
proximal —

phalanges of the fingers

distal p. of foot [TA], small, relatively flat bone of the toes underlying the nail bed, each of which bears a tuberosity on its distal plantar aspect from which connective tissue strands (skin ligaments) radiate through the pulp; the bases of the phalanges of the lateral four toes articulate proximally with the heads of middle phalanges; whereas that of the great toe articulates with a proximal phalanx. SYN p. distalis pedis [TA].

distal p. of hand [TA], small, spade-shaped bone in the ends of the fingers underlying the nail bed, each of which bears a tuberosity on its distal palmar aspect from which connective tissue strands (skin ligaments) radiate through the pulp; the bases of the phalanges of the medial four fingers articulate proximally with the heads of middle phalanges; that of the thumb articulates with a proximal phalanx. SYN p. distalis manus [TA].

p. distalis manus [TA], SYN distal p. of hand.

p. distalis pedis [TA], SYN distal p. of foot.

p. media pedis et manus [TA], SYN middle phalanges of foot and hand.

middle phalanges of foot and hand [TA], the small, long bone in the middle of the lateral four toes and medial four fingers, lying between and articulating with a distal and a proximal phalanx. SYN p. media pedis et manus [TA].

proximal p. of foot [TA], the relatively larger bone of the toes that articulates proximally with the head of a metatarsal; those of the lateral four toes articulate distally with a middle phalanx; that of the great toe articulates distally with a distal phalanx. SYN p. proximalis pedis [TA].

proximal p. of hand [TA], the relatively larger bone of the fingers that articulates proximally with the head of a metacarpal; those of the medial four fingers articulate distally with a middle phalanx; that of the thumb articulates distally with a distal phalanx. SYN p. proximalis manus [TA].

p. proximalis manus [TA], SYN proximal p. of hand.

p. proximalis pedis [TA], SYN proximal p. of foot.

tufted p., one of the terminal phalanges of the fingers in acromegaly; it has an expanded extremity resembling a sheaf of wheat.

ungual p., the distal p. of each of the digits; so called because of the flattened tuberosity at its termination that supports the nail.

phall-, phalli-, phallo-. The penis. [G. *phallos*]

phal·lal·gia (fal-alʹjē-ă). SYN phallodynia. [phall- + G. *algos*, pain]

phal·lec·to·my (fal-ekʹtō-mē). Surgical removal of the penis. SYN penectomy. [phall- + G. *ektomē*, excision]

phal·lic (falʹik). **1.** Relating to the penis. **2.** In psychoanalysis, relating to the penis, especially during the phases of infantile psychosexuality. SEE ALSO phallic *phase*. [G. *phallos*, penis]

phal·li·cism (falʹi-sizm). Worship of the male genitalia. SYN phallism.

phal·li·form (falʹi-fōrm). SYN phalloid.

phal·lism (falʹizm). SYN phallicism.

phallo-. SEE phall-.

phal·lo·camp·sis (fal-ō-kampʹsis). Curvature of the erect penis. SEE ALSO chordee. [phallo- + G. *kampsis*, a bending]

phal·lo·cryp·sis (fal-ō-kripʹsis). Dislocation and retraction of the penis. [phallo- + G. *krypsis*, concealment]

phal·lo·dyn·ia (fal-ō-dinʹē-ă). Pain in the penis. SYN phallalgia. [phallo- + G. *odynē*, pain]

phal·loid (falʹoyd). Resembling in shape a penis. SYN phalliform. [phallo- + G. *eidos*, resemblance]

phal·loi·din (fă-loyʹdin). Best known of the toxic cyclic peptides produced by the poisonous mushroom, *Amanita phalloides*; closely related to amanitin.

phal·lol·y·sin (fă-lolʹi-sin). A glycoprotein that is the heat-sensitive (destroyed in cooking) toxin of the mushroom *Amanita phalloides*.

phal·lon·cus (fal-ongʹkŭs). A tumor or swelling of the penis. [phallo- + G. *onkos*, mass]

phal·lo·plas·ty (falʹō-plas-tē). Surgical reconstruction of the penis. [phallo- + G. *plastos*, formed]

phal·lot·o·my (fal-otʹō-mē). Surgical incision into the penis. SYN penotomy. [phallo- + G. *tomē*, a cutting]

phal·lo·tox·ins (falʹō-toksʹins). A class of heterodetic cyclic heptapeptides present in *Amanita phalloides;* together with the amatoxins, the main toxin components of this fungus.

phal·lus, pl. **phalli** (fal′ŭs, fal′ī). SYN penis. [L.; G. *phallos*]

△**phanero-.** Visible, obvious. [G. *phaneros*]

phan·er·o·gen·ic (fan′er-ō-jen′ik). Denoting a disease, the etiology of which is manifest. Cf. cryptogenic. [phanero- + G. *genesis,* origin]

phan·er·o·ma·nia (fan′er-ō-mā′nē-ă). Obsolete term for constant preoccupation with some external part, as plucking the beard, pulling the lobe of the ear, picking at a pimple, etc. [phanero- + G. *mania,* frenzy]

phan·er·o·scope (fan′er-ō-skōp). A lens used to concentrate the light from a lamp upon the skin, to facilitate examination of lesions of the skin and subcutaneous tissues. [phanero- + G. *skopeō,* to view]

phan·er·o·sis (fan-er-ō′sis). The act or process of becoming visible. [phanero- + G. *osis,* condition]

fatty p., presumed unmasking of previously invisible fat in the cytoplasm of cells; marked fatty metamorphosis is associated with an absolute increase in the fat content of cells, so that the occurrence of p. is doubted.

phan·er·o·zo·ite (fan′er-ō-zō′īt). An exoerythrocytic tissue stage of malaria infection other than the primary exoerythrocytic stages (cryptozoite and metacryptozoite generations); consists chiefly of reinfection of the liver by merozoites produced by a blood infection (not found in falciparum malaria). [phanero- + G. *zōon,* animal]

phan·quone (fan′kwōn). An amebicide.

phan·ta·sia (fan-tā′zē-ă). SYN fantasy. [G. appearance]

phan·tasm (fan′tazm). The mental imagery produced by fantasy. SYN phantom (1). [G. *phantasma,* an appearance]

phan·tas·ma·go·ria (fan-taz-mă-gōr′ē-ă). A fantastic sequence of haphazardly associative imagery.

phan·tas·mol·o·gy (fan-tas-mol′ō-jē). The study of spiritualistic manifestations and of apparitions. [G. *phantasma,* an appearance, + *logos,* study]

phan·tas·mo·sco·pia, phan·tas·mos·co·py (fan-taz-mō-skō′ pē-ă, -mos′kō-pē). A rarely used term for the delusion of seeing phantoms. [G. *phantasma,* an appearance, + *skopeō,* to view]

phan·tom (fan′tŏm). **1.** SYN phantasm. **2.** A model, especially a transparent one, of the human body or any of its parts. SEE ALSO manikin. **3.** In radiology, a mechanical or computer-originated model for predicting irradiation dosage deep in the body. [G. *phantasma,* an appearance]

Schultze p., a model of a female pelvis used in demonstrating the mechanism of childbirth and the application of forceps.

sensory p., a perceived sensation unrelated to or distinct from any actual stimulus, which can occur in any of the senses.

phan·tom·ize (fan′tŏm-īz). In psychiatry, to create mental imagery by fantasy.

phar·ma·cal (far′mă-kăl). SYN pharmaceutic.

phar·ma·ceu·tic, phar·ma·ceu·ti·cal (far-mă-soo′tik, soo′ti-kăl). Relating to pharmacy or to pharmaceutics. SYN pharmacal. [G. *pharmakeutikos,* relating to drugs]

phar·ma·ceu·tics (far-mă-soo′tiks). **1.** SYN pharmacy (1). **2.** The science of pharmaceutical systems, i.e., preparations, dosage forms, etc.

phar·ma·ceu·tist (far-mă-soo′tist). SYN pharmacist.

phar·ma·cist (far′mă-sist). One who is licensed to prepare and dispense drugs and compounds and is knowledgeable concerning their properties. SYN pharmaceutist. [G. *pharmakon,* a drug]

△**pharmaco-.** Drugs. [G. *pharmakon,* medicine]

phar·ma·co·chem·is·try (far′mă-kō-kem′is-trē). SYN pharmaceutical chemistry.

phar·ma·co·di·ag·no·sis (far′mă-kō-dī-ag-nō′sis). Use of drugs in diagnosis.

phar·ma·co·dy·nam·ic (far′mă-kō-dī-nam′ik). Relating to drug action.

phar·ma·co·dy·nam·ics (far′mă-kō-dī-nam′iks). The study of uptake, movement, binding, and interactions of pharmacologically

active molecules at their tissue site(s) of action. [pharmaco- + G. *dynamis,* force]

phar·ma·co·en·do·cri·nol·o·gy (far′mă-kō-en′dō-krin-ol′ō-jē). The pharmacology of endocrine function.

phar·ma·co·ep·i·dem·i·ol·o·gy (far′mă-kō-ep-i-dē-mē- ol′ō-jē). The study of the distribution and determinants of drug-related events in populations, and the application of this study to efficacious drug treatment.

phar·ma·co·ge·net·ics (far′mă-kō-jĕ-net′iks). The study of genetically determined variations in responses to drugs in humans or in laboratory organisms. SYN pharmacogenomics.

pharmacogenomics (far′mă-kō-jēn-om′iks). SYN pharmacogenetics.

phar·ma·cog·no·sist (far-ma-kog′nō-sist). One skilled in pharmacognosy.

phar·ma·cog·no·sy (far-mă-kog′nō-sē). A branch of pharmacology concerned with the physical characteristics and botanical and animal sources of crude drugs. SYN pharmaceutical biology. [pharmaco- + G. *gnōsis,* knowledge]

phar·ma·cog·ra·phy (far-mă-kog′ră-fē). A treatise on or description of drugs. [pharmaco- + G. *graphē,* description]

phar·ma·co·ki·net·ic (far′mă-kō-ki-net′ik). Relating to the disposition of drugs in the body (i.e., their absorption, distribution, metabolism, and elimination).

phar·ma·co·ki·net·ics (far′mă-kō-ki-net′iks). Movements of drugs within biologic systems, as affected by uptake, distribution, binding, elimination, and biotransformation; particularly the rates of such movements. [pharmaco- + G. *kinēsis,* movement]

phar·ma·co·log·ic, phar·ma·co·log·i·cal (far′mă-kō-loj′ik, -loj′ i-kăl). **1.** Relating to pharmacology or to the composition, properties, and actions of drugs. **2.** Sometimes used in physiology to denote a dose (of a chemical agent that either is or mimics a hormone, neurotransmitter, or other naturally occurring agent) that is so much larger or more potent than would occur naturally that it might have qualitatively different effects. Cf. homeopathic (2), physiologic (4), supraphysiologic.

phar·ma·col·o·gist (far-mă-kol′ō-jist). A specialist in pharmacology.

clinical p., a p. who has undergone training in basic pharmacology, clinical pharmacology, and one of several specialities of medical practice.

phar·ma·col·o·gy (far-mă-kol′ō-jē). The science concerned with drugs, their sources, appearance, chemistry, actions, and uses. [pharmaco- + G. *logos,* study]

biochemical p., a branch of p. concerned with the biochemical mechanisms responsible for the actions of drugs.

clinical p., the branch of p. concerned with the p. of therapeutic agents in the prevention, treatment, and control of disease in humans.

marine p., a branch of p. concerned with pharmacologically active substances present in aquatic plants and animals; its objective is to find and develop new therapeutic agents.

phar·ma·co·ma·nia (far′mă-kō-mā′nē-ă). Morbid impulse to take drugs. [pharmaco- + G. *mania,* frenzy]

Phar·ma·co·pe·ia, Phar·ma·co·poe·ia (far′mă-kō-pē′ă). A work containing monographs of therapeutic agents, standards for their strength and purity, and their formulations. The various national pharmacopeias are referred to by abbreviations, of which the following are the most frequently encountered: *USP,* the Pharmacopeia of the United States of America (United States Pharmacopeia); *BP,* British Pharmacopoeia; *Codex medicamentarius,* the French Pharmacopeia; *I.C. Add.* (or *BA*), the Indian and Colonial Addendum to the BP; *IP,* International Pharmacopeia; *Pharmacopeia Austr.,* the Austrian Pharmacopeia; *Ph.G.,* the German Pharmacopeia (D.A.B.); *Pharmacopeia Helv.,* the Swiss Pharmacopeia. The first edition of the USP was compiled in 1820 and was made a legal standard by the terms of the National Food and Drugs Act in January, 1907. [G. *pharmakopoiia,* fr. *pharmakon,* a medicine, + *poieo,* to make]

phar·ma·co·pe·ial (far′mă-kō-pē′ăl). Relating to the Pharmacopeia; denoting a drug in the list of the Pharmacopeia. SEE ALSO official.

phar·ma·co·phi·lia (far′mă-kō-fil′ē-ă). Morbid fondness for taking drugs. [pharmaco- + G. *phileō*, to love]

phar·ma·co·pho·bia (far′mă-kō-fō′bē-ă). Morbid fear of taking drugs. [pharmaco- + G. *phobos*, fear]

phar·ma·co·psy·cho·sis (far′mă-kō-sī-kō′sis). Rarely used term for a psychosis causally related to taking a drug. [pharmaco- + psychosis]

phar·ma·co·ther·a·py (far′mă-kō-thār′ă-pē). Treatment of disease by means of drugs. SEE ALSO chemotherapy. [pharmaco- + G. *therapeia*, therapy]

phar·ma·cy (far′mă-sē). **1.** The practice of preparing and dispensing drugs. SYN pharmaceutics (1). **2.** A drugstore. [G. *pharmakon*, drug]

  clinical p., a branch of p. practice that emphasizes the therapeutic use of drugs rather than the preparation and dispensing of drugs.

Pharm. D. Abbreviation for Doctor of Pharmacy.

pharyng-. SEE pharyngo-.

pha·ryn·ge·al (fă-rin′jē-ăl). Relating to the pharynx. SYN pharyngeus. [Mod. L. *pharyngeus*]

phar·yn·gec·to·my (far′in-jek′tō-mē). Resection of the pharynx. [pharyng- + G. *ektomē*, excision]

phar·yn·gei (far-in′jē-ī). SYN pharyngeal *branches,* under *branch.*

pha·ryn·ges (fă-rin′jēz). Plural of pharynx.

pha·ryn·ge·us (far-in-jē′ŭs). SYN pharyngeal. [Mod. L.]

phar·yn·gis·mus (far-in-jiz′mŭs). Spasm of the muscles of the pharynx. SYN pharyngospasm.

phar·yn·git·ic (far-in-jit′ik). Relating to pharyngitis.

phar·yn·gi·tis (far-in-jī′tis). Inflammation of the mucous membrane and underlying parts of the pharynx. [pharyng- + G. *-itis,* inflammation]

  atrophic p., chronic p. accompanied by a varying degree of atrophy of the mucous glands and absence of their secretion. SYN p. sicca.

  gangrenous p., gangrenous inflammation of the pharyngeal mucous membrane.

  membranous p., inflammation accompanied by a fibrinous exudate, forming a nondiphtheritic false membrane.

  p. sic′ca, SYN atrophic p.

  ulcerative p., inflammation of the pharynx marked by ulceration of the mucosa; may have a viral etiology.

  ulceromembranous p., inflammation of the pharyngeal mucosa with membranous debris overlying the ulcerative lesions.

pharyngo-, pharyng-. The pharynx. [Mod. L. fr. G. *pharynx*]

pha·ryn·go·cele (fă-ring′gō-sēl). A diverticulum from the pharynx. [pharyngo- + G. *kēlē,* hernia]

pha·ryn·go·ep·i·glot·tic, pha·ryn·go·ep·i·glot·tid·e·an (fă-ring′gō-ep′i-glot′ik, -glo-tid′ē-an). Relating to the pharynx and the epiglottis.

pha·ryn·go·e·soph·a·ge·al (fă-ring′gō-ē-sof′ă-jē′ăl). Relating to the pharynx and the esophagus.

pha·ryn·go·e·soph·a·go·plas·ty (fă-ring′gō-ē-sof′ă-gō-plas-tē). Plastic surgery of the pharynx and esophagus. [pharyngo- + esophago- + G. *plastos,* formed]

pha·ryn·go·glos·sal (fă-ring′gō-glos′ăl). Relating to the pharynx and the tongue.

pha·ryn·go·glos·sus (fă-ring-gō-glos′ŭs). SEE superior pharyngeal constrictor (*muscle*).

pha·ryn·go·la·ryn·ge·al (fă-ring′gō-lă-rin′jē-ăl). Relating to both the pharynx and the larynx.

pha·ryn·go·lar·yn·gi·tis (fă-ring′gō-lar-in-jī′tis). Inflammation of both the pharynx and the larynx.

pha·ryn·go·lith (fă-ring′gō-lith). A concretion in the pharynx. SYN pharyngeal calculus. [pharyngo- + G. *lithos,* stone]

pha·ryn·go·max·il·lary (fă-ring′gō-mak′si-lār-ē). Relating to the pharynx and the maxilla.

pha·ryn·go·na·sal (fă-ring′gō-nā′săl). Relating to the pharynx and the nasal cavity.

pha·ryn·go-oral (fă-ring′gō-ō′răl). Relating to the pharynx and the mouth; oropharyngeal. [pharyngo- + L. *os* (or-), mouth]

pha·ryn·go·pal·a·tine (fă-ring′gō-pal′ă-tīn). Relating to the pharynx and the palate.

pha·ryn·go·pa·la·ti·nus (fă-ring′gō-pal-ă-tī′nŭs). SYN palatopharyngeus (*muscle*). [L.]

pha·ryn·go·plas·ty (fă-ring′gō-plas-tē). Plastic surgery of the pharynx, a procedure designed to correct velopharyngeal dysfunction. [pharyngo- + G. *plastos,* formed]

pha·ryn·go·ple·gia (fă-ring′gō-plē′jē-ă). Paralysis of the muscles of the pharynx. [pharyngo- + G. *plēgē,* stroke]

pha·ryn·go·rhi·nos·co·py (fă-ring′gō-rī-nos′kŏ-pē). Inspection of the nasopharynx and posterior nares by means of the rhinoscopic mirror. [pharyngo- + G. *rhis,* nose, + *skopeō,* to view]

pha·ryn·go·scope (fă-ring′gō-skōp). An instrument like a laryngoscope, used for inspection of the pharynx. [pharyngo- + G. *skopeō,* to view]

phar·yn·gos·co·py (far′ing-gos′kŏ-pē). Inspection and examination of the pharynx. [pharyngo- + G. *skopeō,* to view]

pha·ryn·go·spasm (fă-ring′gō-spazm). SYN pharyngismus.

pha·ryn·go·sta·phy·li·nus (fă-ring′gō-staf-i-lī′nŭs). SYN palatopharyngeus (*muscle*). [L. fr. pharyngo- + G. *staphylē,* uvula]

pha·ryn·go·ste·no·sis (fă-ring′gō-ste-nō′sis). Stricture of the pharynx. [pharyngo- + G. *stenōsis,* a narrowing]

phar·yn·got·o·my (far′ing-got′ō-mē). Any cutting operation upon the pharynx either from without or from within. [pharyngo- + G. *tomē,* incision]

pha·ryn·go·ton·sil·li·tis (fă-ring′gō-ton-si-lī′tis). Inflammation of the pharynx and tonsils. [pharyngo- + tonsillitis]

phar·ynx, gen. **pha·ryn·gis,** pl. **pha·ryn·ges** (far′ingks, fă-rin′jis, fă-rin′jēz) [TA]. The upper expanded portion of the digestive tube, between the esophagus below and the mouth and nasal cavities above and in front; it is distinct from the rest of the digestive tube in that it is composed exclusively of skeletal (voluntary) muscle arranged in outer circular and inner longitudinal layers. [Mod. L. fr. G. *pharynx* (*pharyng-*), the throat, the joint opening of the gullet and windpipe]

  laryngeal p., SYN laryngopharynx.

  nasal p., SYN nasopharynx.

  oral p., SYN oropharynx.

phase (fāz). **1.** A stage in the course of change or development. **2.** A homogeneous, physically distinct, and separable portion of a heterogeneous system; e.g., oil, gum, and water are three p.'s of an emulsion. **3.** The time relationship between two or more events. **4.** A particular part of a recurring time pattern or wave form. SEE ALSO stage, period. [G. *phasis,* an appearance]

  anal p., in psychoanalytic personality theory, the stage of psychosexual development, occurring when a child is between 1 and 3 years of age, during which activities, interests, and concerns are centered around the anal zone.

  aqueous p., the water portion of a system consisting of two liquid p.'s, one mainly water, the other a liquid immiscible with water (e.g., benzene, ether).

  cis p., SEE coupling p.

  continuous p., SYN external p.

  coupling p., the physical relationship of two syntenic genes. If they are on the same chromosome, they are said to be "in coupling" or "in the cis p."; if on opposite members of a chromosome pair, "in repulsion" or "in the trans p."

  discontinuous p., SYN internal p.

  dispersed p., SYN internal p.

  dispersion p., SYN external p.

  eclipse p., SYN eclipse *period.*

  p. encoding, in magnetic resonance imaging, the technique of inducing a gradient in the magnetic field in the *x* or *y* axis to induce phase differences with location. SYN gradient encoding.

  eruptive p., that period in the tooth formation that includes the development of the roots, periodontal ligament, and dentogingival junction of the tooth.

  external p., the medium or fluid in which a disperse is suspended. SYN continuous p., dispersion medium, dispersion p., external medium.

gap₁ p., SYN gap₁ period.

gap₂ p., SYN gap₂ period.

gap₀ p., SYN gap₀ period.

genital p., in psychoanalytic personality theory, the final stage of psychosexual development, occurring during puberty, in which the individual's psychosexual development is so organized that sexual gratification can be achieved from genital-to-genital contact and the capacity exists for a mature affectionate relationship with an individual of the opposite sex. SEE phallic p.

horizontal growth p., an early stage of development of cutaneous melanoma by intraepidermal spread of atypical melanocytes.

internal p., the particles contained in a colloid solution. SYN discontinuous p., dispersed p.

lag p., a brief period in the course of the growth of a bacterial culture, especially at the beginning, during which the growth is very slow or scarcely appreciable.

latency p., in psychoanalytic personality theory, the period of psychosexual development in children, extending from about age 5 to the beginning of adolescence at age 12, during which the apparent cessation of sexual preoccupation stems from a strong, aggressive blockade of libidinal and sexual impulses in an effort to avoid oedipal relationships; during this p., boys and girls are inclined to choose friends and join groups of their own sex. SYN latency period.

logarithmic p., exponential, a period in the course of growth of a bacterial culture in which maximal multiplication is occurring by geometrical progression; thus, if the logarithms of their numbers are plotted against time, they will form a straight upward line.

luteal p., that portion of the menstrual cycle extending from the time of formation of the corpus luteum to the onset of menses, usually 14 days long; **short luteal p.,** a period of 10 days or fewer between ovulation and the onset of menses, frequently associated with infertility.

M p., SYN mitotic period.

meiotic p., the stage of nuclear changes in the sexual cells during which reduction of the chromosomes takes place; it embraces the cell generations of the spermatocytes and oocytes. SYN reduction p.

negative p., the period during which the opsonic index is lowered following the injection of a vaccine.

oedipal p., in psychoanalysis, a stage in the psychosexual development of the child, characterized by erotic attachment to the parent of the opposite sex, repressed because of fear of the parent of the same sex; usually occurring between the ages of 3 and 6 years. SYN oedipal period.

oral p., in psychoanalytic personality theory, the earliest stage in psychosexual development, lasting through the first 18 months of life, during which the oral zone is the center of the infant's needs, expression, gratification, and pleasurable erotic experiences; has a strong influence on the organization and development of the child's psyche.

phallic p., in psychoanalytic personality theory, the stage in psychosexual development, occurring when a child is between 2 and 6 years of age, during which interest, curiosity, and pleasurable experiences are centered around the penis in boys and the clitoris in girls. SEE genital p.

positive p., the period following the negative p., during which the opsonic index rises.

postmeiotic p., the stage following that of reduction of the chromosomes in the sexual cells, representing the mature forms of these cells, ending with the conjugation of the nuclei in the impregnated ovum. SYN postreduction p.

postmitotic p., SYN gap₁ period.

postreduction p., SYN postmeiotic p.

poststationary p., the period in the growth of a bacterial culture in which growth is declining.

pregenital p., in psychoanalysis, the collective psychosexual development p.'s preceding the genital p.

premeiotic p., the stage of nuclear changes in the sexual cells before the reduction of the chromosomes, embracing the cell generations up to that of the spermatogonia and oogonia. SYN prereduction p.

premitotic p., SYN gap₂ period.

pre-oedipal p., in psychoanalysis, the collective p.'s of psychosexual development preceding the oedipal p.

prereduction p., SYN premeiotic p.

radial growth p., the early pattern of growth of cutaneous malignant melanoma, in which tumor cells spread laterally in the epidermis.

reduction p., SYN meiotic p.

S p., SYN synthesis period.

stationary p., (1) the period in the course of growth of a bacterial culture during which the multiplication of the organisms becomes gradually less and the bacteria undergoing division are in equilibrium with those dying; (2) referring to the usually solid, nonmobile component in partition chromatography.

supernormal recovery p., a brief period during the recovery of cardiac muscle following excitation when diseased muscle is more (i.e., less abnormally) excitable; corresponds to the end of the T wave in the ECG.

synaptic p., SYN synapsis.

trans p., SEE coupling p.

vertical growth p., spread of melanoma cells from the epidermis into the dermis and later the subcutis, from which site metastasis may take place.

vulnerable p., a period in the cardiac cycle during which an ectopic impulse may lead to repetitive activity such as flutter or fibrillation of the affected chamber.

phas·mid (faz′mid). **1.** One of a pair of caudal chemoreceptors seen in nematodes of the class Secernentasida (Phasmidia). **2.** Common name for a member of the class Phasmidia, now Secernentasida.

Phas·mid·ia (faz-mid′ē-ă). SYN Secernentasida. [G. *phasma*, appearance]

phas·mo·pho·bia (fas-mō-fō′bē-ă). Morbid fear of ghosts. [G. *phasma*, apparition, + *phobos*, fear]

phat·nor·rha·gia (fat-nō-rā′jē-ă). Hemorrhage from a dental alveolus. [G. *phatnōma*, manger (alveolus), + G. *rhēgnymi*, to burst forth]

Ph.D. Abbreviation for Doctor of Philosophy.

Phe Symbol for phenylalanine or phenylalanyl.

Phemister, Dallas B., American surgeon, 1882–1951.

△**phen-, pheno-.** **1.** Combining form denoting appearance. **2.** In chemistry, combining form denoting derivation from benzene (phenyl-). [fr. G. *phainō*, to appear, show forth]

phen·a·caine hy·dro·chlo·ride (fen′ă-kān). A potent local surface anesthetic used in ophthalmology.

phen·ac·e·mide (fe-nas′ĕ-mīd). An anticonvulsant used in the treatment of epilepsy. SYN phenylacetylurea.

phen·ac·e·tin (APC) (fĕ-nas′ĕ-tin). An analgesic and antipyretic; the "P" in APC, an analgesic combination also containing aspirin and caffeine; biotransformed to acetaminophen. SYN acetophenetidin.

phen·ac·e·to·lin (fen′ă-set′ō-lin). A red powder, $(C_{16}H_{12})_2$; used as an indicator. It has a pH range of 5 to 6, being yellow at 5 and red at 6.

phen·ac·e·tur·ic ac·id (fĕ-nas-ĕ-toor′ik). An end product of the metabolism of phenylated fatty acids with even numbers of carbon atoms. SYN phenylaceturic acid.

phen·ac·ri·dane chlo·ride (fe-nas′ri-dān). Topical antiseptic.

phen·a·cy·cla·mine (fen-ă-sī′klă-mēn). SYN phenetamine.

phen·a·gly·co·dol (fen-ă-glī′kō-dol). A central nervous system depressant used in the treatment of anxiety and simple neuroses.

phen·an·threne (fĕ-nan′thrēn). A compound isomeric with anthracene, derived from coal tar; a major component of steroids, as cyclopenta[α]phenanthrene. Used as a basis for the synthesis of various dyes and drugs.

phen·ar·sen·a·mine (fen-ar-sen-am′ēn). SYN arsphenamine.

phen·ar·sone sulf·ox·y·late (fen-ar′sōn sŭl-fok′si-lāt). A pentavalent arsenical used in trichomonal vaginitis.

phe·nate (fē′nāt). A salt or ester of phenol (carbolic acid). SYN carbolate (1).

phe·naz·o·cine (fen-ā′zō-sēn). A potent analgesic when given intramuscularly or intravenously, less effective orally.

phen·az·o·line hy·dro·chlo·ride (fen-az′ŏ-lēn). SYN antazoline hydrochloride.

phen·az·o·pyr·i·dine hy·dro·chlo·ride (fen-ā-zō-pēr′i-dēn). An orally administered urinary tract analgesic.

phen·cy·cli·dine (PCP) (fen-sī′kli-dēn). A substance of abuse, used for its hallucinogenic properties, which can produce profound psychologic and behavioral disturbances; the hydrochloride has analgesic and anesthetic properties.

phen·di·me·tra·zine tar·trate (fen-di-met′ră-zēn). An anorexic agent.

phen·el·zine sul·fate (fen′el-zēn). A monoamine oxidase inhibitor used as an antidepressant.

phe·net·a·mine (fĕ-net′ă-mēn). An intestinal antispasmodic. SYN phenacyclamine.

phe·neth·i·cil·lin po·tas·si·um (fĕ-neth-i-sil′in). A penicillin preparation that is stable in gastric acid and is rapidly but only partially absorbed from the gastrointestinal tract. SYN α-phenoxyethylpenicillin potassium, penicillin B.

phen·eth·yl al·co·hol (fĕ-neth′il). SYN phenylethyl alcohol.

phe·net·sal (fĕ-net′sal). SYN acetaminosalol.

phe·net·u·ride (fĕ-net′ū-rīd). An antiepileptic similar in action to phenacemide.

phen·for·min hy·dro·chlo·ride (fen-fōr′min). An oral hypoglycemic agent no longer used in the U.S. because of the high incidence of fatal lactic acidosis associated with its use. Metformin, a chemically related agent, is presently in use.

phen·glu·tar·i·mide hy·dro·chlo·ride (fen-gloo-tar′i-mīd). The hydrochloride of α-2-diethylaminoethyl-α-phenylglutarimide; an antihistaminic used to decrease or prevent motion sickness, and to control Ménière disease and vomiting.

phen·go·pho·bia (fen-gō-fō′bē-ă). Morbid fear of daylight. [G. *phengos,* daylight, + *phobos,* fear]

phen·i·car·ba·zide (fen-i-kar′bă-zīd). An antipyretic.

phe·nin·da·mine tar·trate (fĕ-nin′dă-mēn). An antihistaminic.

phen·in·di·one (fĕ-nin-dī′ōn). 2-Phenyl-1,3-indanedione: a synthetic anticoagulant with action and uses similar to those of bishydroxycoumarin. SYN phenylindanedione.

phen·ir·a·mine ma·le·ate (fĕ-nir′ă-mēn, -min). An H₁ antihistaminic. SYN prophenpyridamine maleate.

phen·meth·y·lol (fen-meth′il-ol). SYN *benzyl* alcohol.

phen·met·ra·zine hy·dro·chlo·ride (fen-met′ră-zēn). An anorexic agent with sympathomimetic properties.

◇**pheno-.** SEE phen-.

phe·no·bar·bi·tal (fē-nō-bar′bi-tahl). A long-acting oral or parenteral sedative, anticonvulsant, and hypnotic; also available as a soluble sodium salt; also used in therapeutic management of epilepsy and induction of hepatic microsomal enzymes. SYN phenylethylbarbituric acid, phenylethylmalonylurea.

phe·no·bu·ti·o·dil (fen′ō-bū-tī′ō-dil). A radiographic contrast medium formerly used for cholecystography.

phe·no·copy (fē′nō-kop′ē). An environmentally induced mimic of a disease that is characteristically produced by a specific gene. [G. *phainō,* to display, + copy]

phe·no·din (fē′nō-din). SYN hematin.

phe·nol (fē′nol). Hydroxybenzene; an antiseptic, anesthetic, and disinfectant; locally escharotic in concentrated form and neurolytic in 3–4% solutions; internally, a powerful escharotic poison. SYN carbolic acid, phenyl alcohol.

camphorated p., camphorated carbolic acid, consisting of p., camphor, and liquid petrolatum; used as a local anesthetic and for the relief of toothache.

liquefied p., liquefied carbolic acid, p. liquefied by the addition of 10% of water.

p. oxidase, SYN laccase.

phe·no·lase (fē′nō-lās). SYN laccase.

phe·no·lat·ed (fē′nō-lāt-ed). Impregnated or mixed with phenol. SYN carbolated.

phe·nol·e·mia (fē-nol-ē′mē-ă). The presence of phenols in the blood. [phenol + G. *haima,* blood]

phe·nol·o·gy (fe-nol′ō-jē). The study of the biologic rhythms of plants and animals, particularly those rhythms showing seasonal variation. [G. *phainō,* to appear, + *logos,* study]

phe·nol·phthal·e·in (fē-nol-thal′ē-in, -thal′ēn). Obtained by the action of phenol on phthalic anhydride; used as a hydrogen ion indicator and formerly used as a laxative.

phe·nol red. SYN phenolsulfonphthalein.

phe·nol·sul·fon·phthal·e·in (PSP) (fē′nol-sŭl-fōn-thal′ē-in, -thal′ēn). Occurs as a bright to dark red crystalline powder; used as an indicator in tissue culture media (yellow at pH 6.8, red at pH 8.4); in the past given by parenteral injection as a test for renal function. SYN phenol red.

phe·nol·u·ria (fē-nol-ū′rē-ă). The excretion of phenols in the urine.

phe·nom·e·nol·o·gy (fē-nom-ĕ-nol′ō-jē). **1.** The systematic description and classification of phenomena without attempt at explanation or interpretation. **2.** The study of human experiences, irrespective of objective-subjective distinctions. SEE ALSO existential *psychology.* [phenomenon, + G. *logos,* study]

PHENOMENON

phe·nom·e·non, pl. **phe·nom·e·na** (fĕ-nom′ĕ-non, -nă). **1.** A symptom; an occurrence of any sort, whether ordinary or extraordinary, in relation to a disease. **2.** Any unusual fact or occurrence. [G. *phainomenon,* fr. *phainō,* to cause to appear]

adhesion p., a p. manifested by the adherence of antigen-antibody-complement complex to "indicator cells" (microorganisms, platelets, leukocytes, or erythrocytes), the reaction being sensitive and specific for the antigen and antibody in the complex. SYN erythrocyte adherence p., immune adherence p., red cell adherence p.

AFORMED p., as induced pulsus alternans progresses, a state in which alternating heart depolarizations fail to eject any blood, thus allowing longer diastolic filling; the subsequent beat is then able to produce a significant ejection; at high rates the cardiac minute volume and blood pressure may appear normal. [Alternating, *f*ailure *o*f *r*esponse, *m*echanical, to *e*lectrical *d*epolarization]

Anrep p., homeometric autoregulation of the heart whereby cardiac performance improves as the afterload (systolic wall stress) is increased.

aqueous influx p., the filling of the aqueous vein, which normally carries blood and aqueous, with aqueous, when the junction of the aqueous vein and the recipient vein is partially occluded. SYN Ascher aqueous influx p.

Arias-Stella p., focal, unusual, decidual changes in endometrial epithelium, consisting of intraluminal budding, and nuclear enlargement and hyperchromatism with cytoplasmic swelling and vacuolation; may be associated with ectopic or uterine pregnancy. SYN Arias-Stella effect, Arias-Stella reaction.

arm p., SYN Pool p. (2).

Arthus p., a form of immediate hypersensitivity resulting in erythema, edema, hemorrhage, and necrosis observed in rabbits after injection of antigen to which the animal has already been sensitized and has specific IgG antibodies. The reaction is caused by the inflammation that results from the deposition of antigen-antibody complexes in tissue spaces and in blood vessel walls that activate complement, most of the damage seemingly being due to the polymorphonuclear leukocytes that phagocytize the deposits and release lysosomal enzymes. The p., described by Arthus, was in rabbits, but similar reactions (Arthus-type reactions) are observed in guinea pigs, rats, and dogs, as well as in humans. SEE ALSO Arthus *reaction* (2). SYN Arthus reaction (1).

Ascher aqueous influx p., SYN aqueous influx p.

Aschner p., SYN oculocardiac *reflex.*

Ashman p., aberrant ventricular conduction of a beat ending a

ph

short cycle that is preceded by a longer cycle most commonly during atrial fibrillation.

Aubert p., a p. in which a bright perpendicular line appears to incline to one side when the observer turns the head to the opposite side in a dark room.

Austin Flint p., the murmur of relative mitral stenosis during significant aortic regurgitation owing to narrowing of the mitral orifice by pressure of the aortic regurgitant flow on the anterior mitral leaflet. SYN Austin Flint murmur.

autoscopic p., the encountering of an image of oneself, the image being an illusion, a hallucination, or a vivid fantasy.

Babinski p., SYN Babinski sign (1).

Bell p., reflex upper deviation of the eye on attempted eye closure; seen with several disorders, including facial mononeuropathies, Guillain-Barré syndrome, and myasthenia gravis.

Bombay p., a rare recessive trait at a locus that ordinarily manufactures H substance, the precursor from which the A and B phenotypes are elaborated; the mutant causes failure to produce H substance and no matter what the genotype at the ABO locus, the phenotype is O. The Bombay p. is epistatic to the ABO locus. [*Bombay,* India, where first reported]

Bordet-Gengou p., the p. of complement fixation; when complement-containing serum is added to a mixture of bacteria and specific antibody, the complement is removed (fixed) and is not available to lyse subsequently added erythrocytes sensitized with specific antibody. SEE ALSO Gengou p.

breakoff p., breakaway p., the occurrence, during high-altitude flight, of a sensation of being totally detached from the earth and from other people.

Brücke-Bartley p., the sensation of glare in response to successive stimuli at frequencies just below the fusion point.

Capgras p., SYN Capgras syndrome.

centralization p., the relatively rapid change in the perceived location of pain, from more peripheral, or distal, to a more proximal, or central, location; commonly occurs during initial evaluation of patients with low back and radiating limb pain; helpful in determining the type and prognosis of physical therapy.

cervicolumbar p., a sense of weakness in the lower extremities on movement of the neck when a lesion is present in the upper portion of the spinal cord; or sensations referred to the neck when a lesion exists in the lower portion of the cord.

cogwheel p., a sudden brief halt in usually smooth respiration or other motor activity. SYN Negro p.

constancy p., in perception, the tendency for brightness, color, size, or shape to remain relatively perceptually constant despite real changes in color, size, shape or other conditions of observation.

crowding p., a characteristic of amblyopic vision in which vision is better for single optotype presentation than multiple, simultaneous optotype presentation.

Cushing p., a rise in systemic blood pressure when the intracranial pressure acutely increases, usually in excess of 50% of the systolic arterial pressure. SYN Cushing effect, Cushing response.

Danysz p., reduction of the neutralizing effect of an antitoxin when toxin is mixed with it in divided portions, rather than adding the same total quantity of toxin in one step.

dawn p., abrupt increases in fasting levels of plasma glucose concentrations between 5 and 9 a.m., in the absence of antecedent hypoglycemia; occurs in diabetic patients receiving insulin therapy.

Debré p., in measles, the failure of the rash to develop at the site of immune serum injection.

declamping p., shock or hypotension following abrupt release of clamps from a large portion of the vascular bed, as from the aorta; apparently caused by transient pooling of blood in a previously ischemic area. SYN declamping shock.

déjà vu p., the mental impression that a new experience (e.g., a scene, sight, sound, or action) has happened before; a common p. in normal persons that may occur more frequently or continuously in certain emotional or organic disorders. Also variously referred to as déjà entendu, déjà éprouvé, déjà fait, déjà pensé, déjà racon-

té, déjà vécu, or déjà voulu, depending on the experience or sense that is evoked.

Dejerine hand p., clonic contractions of the flexors of the hand (wrist) on tapping the dorsum of the hand or the volar side of the forearm near the wrist; occurs in normal persons but is exaggerated in pyramidal tract lesions. SYN Dejerine reflex.

Denys-Leclef p., enhanced phagocytosis by leukocytes of microorganisms in the presence of immune serum.

d'Herelle p., SYN Twort-d'Herelle p.

dip p., complete disappearance of ventricular excitability followed by progressive recovery within a few microseconds at the end of excitation; the muscle as a whole repolarizes somewhat inhomogeneously, so that this period is one of special sensitivity to exogenous or endogenous stimuli and reentry.

Donath-Landsteiner p., the hemolysis that results in a sample of blood of a subject with paroxysmal hemoglobinuria when the sample is cooled to around 5°C and then warmed again.

Doppler p., SYN Doppler effect.

Duckworth p., respiratory arrest before cardiac arrest as a result of intracranial disease.

Ehret p., a sudden throb felt by the finger on the brachial artery, as the pressure in the cuff falls during a blood pressure estimation; said to indicate fairly accurately the diastolic pressure.

Ehrlich p., the difference between the amount of diphtheria toxin that will exactly neutralize one unit of antitoxin and that which, added to one unit of antitoxin, will leave one lethal dose free is greater than one lethal dose of toxin; i.e., it is necessary to add more than one lethal dose of toxin to a neutral mixture of toxin and antitoxin to make the mixture lethal (the basis of the L_+ dose).

erythrocyte adherence p., SYN adhesion p.

escape p., failure of the pupil in an eye with optic neuritis to maintain constriction as both eyes are alternately stimulated with light.

facialis p., facial spasm produced by light rubbing of the skin or a tap on the zygoma; sometimes percussion above the zygoma causes contraction of the lip only; observed in tetany and sometimes in exophthalmic goiter.

finger p., a sign of organic hemiplegia; with the patient's elbow resting on a table, the patient's wrist is grasped by the examiner's hand, the thumb of which is used to exert pressure on the radial side of the patient's pisiform bone; if the hemiplegia is organic, some or all of the patient's fingers become extended and spread out in a fanlike form. SYN Gordon sign.

Flynn p., SYN paradoxical pupillary reflex.

Friedreich p., the tympanitic percussion sound over a pulmonary cavity is slightly raised in pitch on deep inspiration.

Galassi pupillary p., SYN eye-closure pupil reaction.

Gallavardin p., dissociation between the noisy and musical elements of the ejection murmur of aortic stenosis, the musical element being better heard at the left sternal border and at the cardiac apex while the noisy element is better heard at the aortic area; projection of the aortic stenotic murmur to the low left sternal edge.

gap p., a short period in the cycle of the atrioventricular or intraventricular conduction allowing passage of an impulse which at other times would be blocked in transit. SYN excitable gap.

Gärtner vein p., fullness of the veins of the arm and hand held below heart level and collapse at a certain variable distance above that level. An unreliable test for venous pressure.

generalized Shwartzman p., when both the primary injection of endotoxin-containing filtrate and the secondary injection are given intravenously 24 hours apart, the animal usually dies within 24 hours after the second inoculation; the characteristic lesions in the rabbit include widespread hemorrhages in the lung, liver, and other organs and bilateral cortical necrosis of the kidney. This reaction has no immunologic basis. SYN Sanarelli p., Sanarelli-Shwartzman p.

Gengou p., an extension of the Bordet-Gengou p.; noncellular antigens, when mixed with specific antibody, also fix complement.

gestalt p., SEE gestalt.

Glover p., nonrandom (i.e., haphazard) variation among communities in rates of performing common elective procedures, such as tonsillectomy, hysterectomy, attributable to local variations in medical and surgical practices.

Grasset p., in organic paralysis of the lower extremity, the supine patient can raise either limb separately, but not both together. SYN Grasset-Gaussel p.

Grasset-Gaussel p., SYN Grasset p.

Gunn p., SYN jaw-winking *syndrome.*

Hamburger p., SYN chloride *shift.*

Hill p., SYN Hill *sign.*

hip p., SYN Joffroy *reflex.*

hip-flexion p., when a hemiplegic attempts to rise from a lying posture, the hip on the paralyzed side is flexed first; the same movement takes place on lying down.

Hoffmann p., excessive irritability of the sensory nerves to electrical or mechanical stimuli in tetany.

Houssay p., SEE Houssay *animal.*

Hunt paradoxic p., in dystonia musculorum deformans, if an attempt is made at plantar flexion of the foot when the foot is in dorsal spasm the only response is an increase of the extensor, or dorsal, spasm; if, however, the patient is told to extend the foot that is already in a state of strong dorsal flexion, there will be a sudden movement of plantar flexion; the same p., *mutatis mutandis,* is observed when there is a condition of strong plantar flexion.

immune adherence p., SYN adhesion p.

jaw-winking p., SYN jaw-winking *syndrome.*

Jod-Basedow p., induction of thyrotoxicosis in a previously euthyroid individual as a result of exposure to large quantities of iodine; occurs most often in areas of endemic iodine-deficient goiter and in patients with multinodular goiter; also can develop following use of iodine-containing agents for diagnostic studies. SYN iodine-induced hyperthyroidism.

Köbner p., SYN isomorphic *response.*

Koch p., **(1)** the p. of infection immunity; living tubercle bacilli (*Mycobacterium tuberculosis*) do not cause reinfection when inoculated into tuberculous guinea pigs (i.e., the animals are "immune" to reinfection) even though the original infections continue to develop and eventually cause death of the animals; **(2)** rise of temperature and increase of the local lesion, in a tuberculous subject, following an injection of tuberculin.

Kohnstamm p., SYN aftermovement.

Kühne p., when a constant current is passed through a muscle, an undulation is seen to pass from the positive to the negative pole.

LE p., the formation of LE cells in bone marrow or blood on adding serum from patients with disseminated lupus erythematosus.

Leede-Rumpel p., Rumpel-Leede p. (q.v.).

leg p., SYN Pool p. (1).

Lucio leprosy p., SYN Lucio *leprosy.*

Marcus Gunn p., SYN jaw-winking *syndrome.*

misdirection p., SYN aberrant *regeneration.*

Mitsuo p., restoration of the normal color of the fundus with dark adaptation in Oguchi disease.

Negro p., SYN cogwheel p.

no reflow p., lack of blood flow, at the microcirculation level, in a damaged area of the brain after reperfusion.

on-off p., a state in the treatment of Parkinson disease by L-dopa, in which there is a rapid fluctuation of akinetic (off) and choreoathetotic (on) movements.

orbicularis p., SYN eye-closure pupil *reaction.*

paradoxical diaphragm p., in pyopneumothorax, hydropneumothorax, and some cases of injury, the diaphragm on the affected side rises during inspiration and falls during expiration.

paradoxical pupillary p., SYN paradoxical pupillary *reflex.*

peroneal p., tapping the peroneal nerve below the head of the fibula causes dorsiflexion and abduction of the foot.

Pfeiffer p., the alteration and complete disintegration of cholera vibrios when introduced into the peritoneal cavity of an immunized guinea pig, or into that of a normal one if immune serum is

injected at the same time; extended to include bacteriolysis in general.

phi p., an illusion of movement, which occurs by means of successive visual impressions at intervals of $\frac{1}{15}$ to $\frac{1}{20}$ sec; when an occluder is passed from one eye to the other while a small distant light is observed, the light seems to move with the occluder in exophoria, but in an opposite direction in esophoria.

Pool p., **(1)** in tetany, spasm of both the quadriceps and calf muscles when the extended leg is flexed at the hip; SYN leg p., Pool-Schlesinger sign, Schlesinger sign. **(2)** in tetany, contraction of the arm muscles following the stretching of the brachial plexus by elevation of the arm above the head with the forearm extended, resembles the contraction resulting from stimulation of the ulnar nerve. SYN arm p.

pseudo-Graefe p., retraction of the upper eyelid on downward movement of the eyes.

psi p., a p. that includes both psychokinesis and extrasensory perception; the extrasensory mental processes involved in the alleged ability to send or receive telepathic messages.

Pulfrich p., the binocular perception that an small target oscillating in the frontal plane is moving in an elliptical path seen when one eye is covered by a filter or in the presence of a unilateral optic neuropathy.

Purkinje p., in the light-adapted eye, the region of maximal brightness is in the yellow; in the dark-adapted eye, the region of maximal brightness is in the green. SYN Purkinje effect, Purkinje shift.

quellung p., SYN Neufeld capsular *swelling.*

radial p., dorsal flexion of the hand occurring involuntarily with palmar flexion of the fingers.

Raynaud p., spasm of the digital arteries, with blanching and numbness or pain of the fingers, often precipitated by cold. Fingers become variably red, white, and blue.

rebound p., **(1)** SYN Stewart-Holmes *sign;* **(2)** generally, any p. in which a variable that has been displaced from its normal state by a disturbing influence temporarily deviates from normal in the opposite direction when the disturbing influence is suddenly removed, before finally stabilizing at its normal state, i.e., a p. involving undershoot; e.g., the subsequent hypoglycemia that may follow injection of glucose, because the initial hyperglycemia caused excessive secretion of insulin.

reclotting p., SYN thixotropy.

red cell adherence p., SYN adhesion p.

reentry p., SEE reentry.

release p., the increased tonus and hyperirritability of muscle-stretch reflexes that occur following damage of the upper portions of the extrapyramidal system.

Riddoch p., ability to appreciate a small moving object in an area of the visual field blind to static objects; particularly associated with occipital lobe lesions.

Ritter-Rollet p., on equal electrical stimulation of motor nerve trunks, the flexor and abductor muscle groups react more readily than the extensors and adductors.

R-on-T p., a premature ventricular (QRS) complex in the electrocardiogram interrupting the T wave of the preceding beat; often predisposes to serious ventricular arrhythmias.

Rumpel-Leede p., appearance of petechiae in an area following application of vascular constriction, such as by a tourniquet, usually after 10 minutes but can appear after shorter period, such as following application of tourniquet to draw blood specimen or use of blood pressure cuff; due to capillary fragility or abnormal platelet numbers (e.g. thrombocytopenia) or function.

Rust p., in cancer or caries of the upper cervical vertebrae, the patient will always support the head by the hands when changing from the recumbent to the sitting posture or the reverse.

Sanarelli p., SYN generalized Shwartzman p.

Sanarelli-Shwartzman p., SYN generalized Shwartzman p.

Schellong-Strisower p., a reduction of the systolic blood pressure, accompanied sometimes by vertigo, on rising from the horizontal to the erect posture.

Schiff-Sherrington p., when the spinal cord is transected in the midthoracic region or a little lower, the stretch and other postural

ph

reflexes of the upper extremity become exaggerated; if the transection is made in the sacral cord, a similar effect is observed in the lower limbs. The effect is regarded as a release p., i.e., release from an inhibitory influence normally exerted by the spinal segments below the transection.

Schüller p., when patients with hemiplegia walk, if the disorder is functional they turn to the unaffected side; if it is organic, they turn to the affected side.

Schultz-Charlton p., SYN Schultz-Charlton *reaction.*

Sherrington p., after the muscles of the leg have been deprived of their motor innervation by sectioning the ventral roots containing fibers for the sciatic nerve, and allowing time for the degeneration of the fibers to occur, stimulation of the sciatic nerve causes slow contraction of the muscles.

shot-silk p., SYN shot-silk *retina.*

Shwartzman p., a rabbit is injected intradermally with a small quantity of lipopolysaccharide (endotoxin) followed by a second intravenous injection 24 hours later and will develop a hemorrhagic and necrotic lesion at the site of the first injection. SEE ALSO generalized Shwartzman p. SYN Shwartzman reaction.

Somogyi p., a rebound p. of reactive hyperglycemia following a period of relative hypoglycemia, which may be subclinical and difficult to detect; the hyperglycemia induces use of more insulin, thus aggravating the problem. SYN posthypoglycemic hyperglycemia.

Soret p., in a solution kept in a long, upright tube at room temperature, the upper part, being the warmer, is also the more concentrated.

sparing p., SYN sparing *action.*

Splendore-Hoeppli p., radiating or annular eosinophilic deposits of host-derived materials, and possibly of parasite antigens, which form around fungi, helminths, or bacterial colonies in tissue.

staircase p., SYN treppe.

Staub-Traugott p., the increased rate of removal of loads of glucose given shortly after administration of an initial glucose load.

steal p., SEE steal.

Strümpell p., dorsal flexion of the great toe, sometimes of the entire foot, in a paralyzed limb when the extremity is drawn up against the body, flexing both knee and hip. SYN tibial p.

symbiotic fermentation p., "two organisms, neither of which alone produces gas fermentation in certain carbohydrates, may do so when living in symbiosis or when artificially mixed" (Castellani).

Theobald Smith p., a p. observed in guinea pigs that had survived use for diphtheria antitoxin standardization, the animals having been rendered highly susceptible to subsequent inoculation of horse serum.

tibial p., SYN Strümpell p.

toe p., SYN Babinski *sign* (1).

tongue p., SYN Schultze *sign.*

Tournay p., dilation of the pupil in the abducting eye on extreme lateral gaze. This is present in only a small percentage of the normal popupation and has no known association with disease. SYN Tournay sign.

Tullio p., momentary vertigo caused by any loud sound, notably occurring in cases of active labyrinthine fistula.

two-dimension–three-dimension p., an experience in telescopic endoscopy in which a two-dimensional image appears to be three-dimensional because of the movement of the endoscope in and out of the view of the object.

Twort p., SYN Twort-d'Herelle p.

Twort-d'Herelle p., the lysis of bacteria by bacteriophage. SYN d'Herelle p., Twort p.

Tyndall p., the visibility of floating particles in gases or liquids when illuminated by a ray of sunlight and viewed at right angles to the illuminating ray. SYN Tyndall effect.

vacuum disk p., the appearance of a radiolucent stripe in an intervertebral disk, a manifestation of disk degeneration; a misnomer since there is gas present.

warmup p., progressive diminution of the myotonic response of a muscle, during repeated contraction of the muscle.

Wenckebach p., progressive lengthening of conduction time in any cardiac tissue (most often the AV node or junction) with ultimate dropping of a beat (AV Wenckebach) or reversion to the initial conduction time (as in QRS Wenckebach).

Westphal-Piltz p., SYN eye-closure pupil *reaction.*

Wever-Bray p., SYN cochlear microphonic.

phe·no·per·i·dine (fĕ-nō-per'i-dēn). An analgesic.

phe·no·thi·a·zine (fĕ-nō-thī'ă-zēn). A compound formerly used extensively for the treatment of intestinal nematodes in animals; without central nervous system depressant activity itself, it serves as the parent compound for synthesis of a large number of antipsychotic compounds, including chlorpromazine, thioridazine, perphenazine, and fluphenazine. SYN dibenzothiazine, thiodiphenylamine.

phe·no·type (fē'nō-tīp). The observable characteristics, at the physical, morphologic, or biochemical level, of an individual, as determined by the genotype and environment. [G. *phainō,* to display, + *typos,* model]

phe·no·typ·ic (fē'nō-tip'ik, fen-ō-). Relating to phenotype.

phen·ox·a·zine (fe-nok'să-zēn). Phenothiazine in which S is replaced by O; as the 3-oxo derivative (phenoxazone), p. is the chromophore of actinomycins.

phen·ox·a·zone (fe-nok'să-zōn). SEE phenoxazine.

phe·nox·y·ben·za·mine hy·dro·chlo·ride (fĕ-nok'si-ben'ză-mēn). A potent nonselective adrenergic (α-receptor) blocking agent of the β-haloalkylamines; blocks the excitatory response of smooth muscle and exocrine glands to epinephrine; used in the treatment of peripheral vascular diseases and in pheochromocytoma.

2-phe·nox·y·eth·a·nol (fĕ-nok-si-eth'ă-nol). An antibacterial agent used in the topical treatment of wound infections; it is active against Gram-negative bacteria that are resistant to most other antiseptics.

α-phe·nox·y·eth·yl·pen·i·cil·lin po·tas·si·um (fē-nok'sē-eth'il-pen-i-sil'in). SYN phenethicillin potassium.

phe·nox·y·meth·yl·pen·i·cil·lin (fĕ-nok'si-meth'il-pen-i-sil'in). SYN *penicillin* V.

α-phe·nox·y·pro·pyl·pen·i·cil·lin po·tas·si·um (fē'nok-sē-prō' pil-pen-i-sil'in). SYN propicillin.

phe·no·zy·gous (fē'nō-zī'gŭs, fe-noz'i-gŭs). Having a narrow cranium as compared with the width of the face, so that when the skull is viewed from above, the zygomatic arches are visible. [G. *phainō,* to show, + *zygon,* yoke]

phen·pen·ter·mine tar·trate (fen-pen'ter-mēn). An anorexigenic agent.

phen·pro·ba·mate (fen-prō'bă-māt). A skeletal muscle relaxant with antianxiety action similar to meprobamate. SYN proformiphen.

phen·pro·cou·mon (fen-prō-koo'mon). A long-acting orally effective anticoagulant.

phen·pro·pi·o·nate (fen-prō'pē-ō-nāt). USAN-approved contraction for 3-phenylpropionate.

phen·sux·i·mide (fen-sŭk'si-mīd). An anticonvulsant drug used in the treatment of absence (petit mal) epilepsy.

phen·ter·mine (fen'ter-mēn). An anorexic agent resembling amphetamine; also available as the hydrochloride.

phen·tol·a·mine hy·dro·chlo·ride (fen-tol'ă-mēn). A nonselective adrenergic (α-receptor) blocking agent.

phen·tol·a·mine mes·y·late. The same actions as phentolamine hydrochloride, for intravenous use only.

phen·yl (Ph, Φ) (fen'il). The univalent moiety, C_6H_5-, of benzene.

p. alcohol, SYN phenol.

p. aminosalicylate, a second-line antituberculosis drug with a high incidence of hypersensitivity reactions and gastrointestinal upset.

p. salicylate, the salicylic ester of phenol; the phenylic ester of salicylic acid; an intestinal analgesic and antipyretic; it has been used in the treatment of rheumatism, diarrhea, and pharyngitis, as an enteric coating for tablets, and in ointments for sunburn prevention. SYN salol.

phen·yl·a·ce·tic ac·id (fen'il-ă-se'tik). An abnormal product of phenylalanine catabolism, appearing in the urine in individuals with phenylketonuria.

phen·yl·a·ce·tur·ic ac·id (fen'il-as-ĕ-toor'ik). SYN phenaceturic acid.

phen·yl·a·ce·tyl·u·rea (fen-il-as'ĕ-til-ū-rē'ă). SYN phenacemide.

phen·yl·a·cryl·ic ac·id (fen'il-ă-kril'ik). SYN cinnamic acid.

phen·yl·al·a·nin·ase (fen-il-al'ă-nin-ās). Phenylalanine 4- monooxygenase.

phen·yl·al·a·nine (Phe, F) (fen-il-al'ă-nēn). 2-Amino-3-phenyl-propionic acid; the L-isomer is one of the common amino acids in proteins; a nutritionally essential amino acid.

p. ammonia-lyase, a nonmammalian enzyme that catalyzes the conversion of L-p. to *trans*-cinnamate and ammonia; it has been used in the treatment of phenylketonuria.

p. 4-hydroxylase, SYN p. 4-monooxygenase.

p. 4-monooxygenase, an enzyme that catalyzes the oxidation of L-phenylalanine to L-tyrosine with O_2 and tetrahydrobiopterin (the latter forming the dihydro derivative) which is, in turn, reduced by NADPH and a reductase to the active form; a deficiency of either of these enzymes will result in phenylketonuria. SYN p. 4-hydroxylase.

phen·yl·a·mine (fe-nil'ă-mēn). SYN aniline.

phen·yl·ben·zene (fen-il-ben'zēn). SYN diphenyl.

phen·yl·bu·ta·zone (fen-il-bū'tă-zōn). An analgesic, antipyretic, anti-inflammatory, and uricosuric agent.

phen·yl·car·bi·nol (fen-il-kar'bi-nol). SYN *benzyl* alcohol.

phen·yl·di·chlo·ro·ar·sine (PD) (fen'il-dī-klōr-ō-ar'sēn). A toxic liquid that has been used as a blister and vomiting agent by certain military and police organizations; it was first used in a limited manner in World War I.

phen·yl·eph·rine hy·dro·chlo·ride (fen-il-ef'rin). A powerful vasoconstrictor, used as a nasal decongestant and mydriatic.

phen·yl·eth·a·no·la·mine *N*-meth·yl·trans·fer·ase (PNMT) (fē'nil-eth-an-ol'a-mēn). A key enzyme in catecholamine biosynthesis that catalyzes the conversion of norepinephrine to epinephrine, using *S*-adenosyl-L-methionine; found in the adrenal medulla and some neurons; this enzyme's biosynthesis is induced by cortisol.

phen·yl·eth·yl al·co·hol (fen-il-eth'il). A natural constituent of some volatile oils (rose, geranium, neroli); used as an antibacterial agent in ophthalmic solutions. SYN benzyl carbinol, phenethyl alcohol.

phen·yl·eth·yl·bar·bi·tur·ic ac·id (fen'il-eth'il-bar-bi-tūr'ik). SYN phenobarbital.

phen·yl·eth·yl·ma·lo·na·mide (fen'il-eth'il-mal-on-ă-mīd). A metabolite of primidone, an antiepileptic agent. P. has anticonvulsant activity in animals but has not been evaluated as an antiepileptic agent in humans.

phen·yl·eth·yl·mal·o·nyl·u·rea (fen'il-eth'il-mal'ō-nil-ū-rē'ă). SYN phenobarbital.

phen·yl·gly·col·ic ac·id (fen'il-glī-kol'ik). SYN mandelic acid.

phen·yl·in·dane·di·one (fen'il-in-dān'dī-ōn). SYN phenindione.

phen·yl·i·so·thi·o·cy·a·nate (PITC, PhNCS) (fen'il-ī'sō-thī-ō-sī'ă-nāt). A reagent that condenses with the free N-terminal amino group of a peptide chain to form a phenylthiohydantoin in the Edman method of identifying N-terminal amino acids. SYN Edman reagent.

phen·yl·ke·to·nu·ria (PKU) (fen'il-kē'tō-noo'rē-ă). Autosomal recessively inherited inborn error of metabolism of phenylalanine characterized by deficiency of 1) phenylalanine hydroxylase [MIM*261600] caused by mutation in the phenylalanine hydroxylase gene (PAH) on 12q; 2) occasionally, dihydropteridine reductase [MIM*261630], caused by mutation in the dihydropteridine reductase gene (DHPR) on 4p; 3) rarely, dihydrobiopterin synthetase [MIM*261640], caused by mutation in the pyruvoyl tetrahydropterin synthase gene (PTS) on 11q; or 4) even more rarely, guanidine triphosphate cyclohydrolase 1 [MIM*233910]. The disorder is characterized by inadequate formation of L-tyro-

sine, elevation of serum L-phenylalanine, urinary excretion of phenylpyruvic acid and other derivatives, and accumulation of phenylalanine and its metabolites, which can produce brain damage resulting in severe mental retardation, often with seizures, other neurologic abnormalities such as retarded myelination and deficient melanin formation leading to hypopigmentation of the skin and eczema. Cf. hyperphenylalaninemia. SYN Folling disease, phenylpyruvate oligophrenia. [phenyl + ketone + G. *ouron*, urine]

nonclassical p., SYN malignant *hyperphenylalaninemia.*

phen·yl·lac·tic ac·id (fen-il-lak'tik). A product of phenylalanine catabolism, appearing prominently in the urine in individuals with phenylketonuria.

phen·yl·mer·cu·ric ac·e·tate (fen'il-mer-kū'rik). A bacteriostatic preservative, fungicide, and herbicide (especially for crabgrass).

phen·yl·mer·cu·ric ni·trate. A mixture of phenylmercuric nitrate and phenylmercuric hydroxide; an antiseptic used for the prophylactic disinfection of the intact skin or of minor wounds.

phen·yl·pro·pa·nol·a·mine (fen'il-prō-pă-nol'ă-mēn). A sympathomimetic amine, used as a nasal decongestant, bronchodilator, and appetite suppressant.

phe·nyl·py·ru·vic ac·id (fen'il-pī-roo'vik). The transaminated product of the action of phenylalanine aminotransferase; elevated in the urine in individuals with phenylketonuria.

phen·yl·thi·o·car·ba·mide (fen'il-thī-ō-kar'bă-mīd). SYN phenylthiourea.

phen·yl·thi·o·car·bam·o·yl (PTC). SEE phenylthiocarbamoyl *peptide.*

phen·yl·thi·o·hy·dan·to·in (PTH) (fen'il-thī'ō-hī-dan'tō-in). The compound formed from an amino acid in the Edman method of protein degradation, in which phenylisothiocyanate reacts with the amino moiety of the N-terminal amino acid to form a phenyl-thiocarbamoyl peptide or protein, on which weak acids act to release the p. containing the N-terminal amino acid.

phen·yl·thi·o·u·rea (fen'il-thī'ō-ū-rē'ă) [MIM*171200]. A substance that tastes bitter to some persons but is tasteless to others. The ability to taste it is thought to be an autosomal dominant trait. P. contains the N–C=S group upon which the taste peculiarity apparently depends; goitrogenic or antithyroid substances (e.g., thiourea and thiouracil), which also contain this group, possess the same property with respect to taste. SYN phenylthiocarbamide.

phen·yl·to·lox·a·mine (fen'il-tol-ok'să-mēn). An antihistaminic.

phen·yl·tri·meth·yl·am·mo·ni·um (PTMA) (fen'il-trī-meth'il-ă-mō'nē-ŭm). A highly selective stimulant of the motor endplates of skeletal muscle.

phen·y·ram·i·dol hy·dro·chlo·ride (fen-i-ram'i-dol). An analgesic and a muscle relaxant.

phen·yt·o·in (fen'i-tō-in). An anticonvulsant used in the treatment of generalized tonic clonic and complex partial epilepsy. Also available as p. sodium, with the same uses as p. SYN 5,5-diphenylhydantoin.

△**pheo-.** 1. Prefix denoting the same substituents on a phorbin or phorbide (porphyrin) residue as are present in chlorophyll, excluding any ester residues and Mg. 2. Combining form meaning gray, dark-colored. [G. *phaios*, dusky]

phe·o·chrome (fē'ō-krōm). 1. SYN chromaffin. 2. Staining darkly with chromic salts. [G. *phaios*, dusky, + *chrōma*, color]

phe·o·chro·mo·blast (fē-ō-krō'mō-blast). A primitive chromaffin cell that, with sympathetoblasts, enters into the formation of the adrenal gland. [G. *phaios*, dusky, + *chrōma*, color, + *blastos*, germ]

phe·o·chro·mo·cyte (fē-ō-krō'mō-sīt). A chromaffin cell of a sympathetic paraganglion, medulla of an adrenal gland, or a pheochromocytoma. [pheochrome + G. *kytos*, cell]

phe·o·chro·mo·cy·to·ma (fē'ō-krō'mō-sī-tō'mă). A functional chromaffinoma, usually benign, derived from adrenal medullary tissue cells and characterized by the secretion of catecholamines, resulting in hypertension, which may be paroxysmal and associated with attacks of palpitation, headache, nausea, dyspnea, anxiety, pallor, and profuse sweating. P. is often hereditary, not only in phacomas such as Hippel-Lindau disease, neurofibromatosis, and familial endocrine neoplasia, but also as an isolated defect [MIM*171300] as an autosomal dominant trait. SEE ALSO paraganglioma.

phe·o·mel·a·nin (fē-ō-mel′ă-nin). A type of melanin found in red hair; it contains sulfur and is alkali-soluble; elevated levels are found in the rufous type of oculocutaneous albinism. Cf. eumelanin. [G. *phaios,* dusky, + *melos* (*melan-*), black]

phe·o·mel·a·no·gen·e·sis (fē′ō-mel′ă-nō-jen′ĕ-sis). The formation of pheomelanin by living cells.

phe·o·mel·a·no·some (fē-ō-mel′ā-nō-sōm). A spherical melanosome of pheomelanin in red hair.

phe·re·sis (fe-rē′sis). A procedure in which blood is removed from a donor, separated, and a portion retained, with the remainder returned to the donor. SEE ALSO leukapheresis, plateletpheresis, plasmapheresis. [G. *aphairesis,* a taking away, a withdrawal]

pher·o·mones (fer′ō-mōnz). A type of ectohormone secreted by an individual and perceived by a second individual of the same or similar species, thereby producing a change in the sexual or social behavior of that individual. Cf. allelochemicals, allomones, kairomones. [G. *pherō,* to carry, + *hormaō,* to excite, stimulate]

Ph.G. **1.** Abbreviation for *Pharmacopoeia Germanica;* German Pharmacopoeia. **2.** Abbreviation for Graduate in Pharmacy, a degree no longer offered in the U.S.

phi (φ, Φ) (fī). **1.** The 21st letter of the Greek alphabet. **2.** (Φ) Symbol for phenyl; potential energy; magnetic flux. **3.** (φ) Symbol for plane angle; volume fraction; quantum yield; the dihedral angle of rotation about the N–C$_\alpha$ bond associated with a peptide bond.

phi·al (fī′ăl). SYN vial. [G. *phialē,* a broad flat vessel]

phi·a·lide (fī′ă-līd). In fungi, a conidiogenous cell in which the meristematic end remains unchanged as successive conidia are extruded out to form chains. [G. *phialē,* a broad, flat vessel]

phi·a·lo·co·nid·i·um, pl. **phi·a·lo·co·nid·ia** (fī′ă-lō-ko-nid′ē-ŭm, fī′ă-lō-kō-nid′ē-ă). A conidium produced by a phialide.

Phi·a·loph·o·ra (fī-ă-lof′ŏ-ră). A genus of fungi of which at least two species, *P. verrucosa* and *P. dermatitidis* (*Exophiala dermatitides*), cause chromoblastomycosis. [G. *phialē,* a broad, flat vessel, + *phoreō,* to carry]

-phil, -phile, -philic, -philia. Affinity for, craving for. SEE ALSO philo-. [G. *philos,* fond, loving; *phileō,* to love]

phil·i·a·ter (fil′ē-ā′ter, fi-lī′ă-ter). Rarely used term for one interested in the study of medicine. [G. *philos,* fond, + *iatreia,* practice of medicine]

Philip, Sir Robert W., Scottish physician, 1857–1939. SEE P. *glands,* under *gland.*

Philippe, Claudien, French pathologist, 1866–1903. SEE P. *triangle.*

Phillips, Charles, French urologist, 1809–1871. SEE P. *catheter.*

Phillipson re·flex. See under reflex.

philo-. SEE -phil. [G. *philos,* fond, loving; *phileō,* to love]

phi·lo·mi·me·sia (fil′ō-mĭ-mē′sē-ă). Rarely used term for a morbid impulse to imitate or mimic. [philo- + G. *mimēsis,* imitation]

Phil·o·pia ca·sei (fil-ō′pē-ă kā′sē-ī). A species that may cause temporary intestinal myiasis. SYN cheese maggot.

phil·o·pro·gen·i·tive (fil′ō-prō-jen′i-tiv). **1.** Procreative, producing offspring. **2.** In psychiatry, an obsolete term for pedophilia. [philo- + L. *progenies,* offspring, progeny]

phil·trum, pl. **phil·tra** (fil′trŭm, -tră) [TA]. **1.** A philter or love potion. **2** [NA]. The infranasal depression; the groove in the midline of the upper lip. [L., fr. G. *philtron,* a love-charm, depression on upper lip, fr. *phileō,* to love]

phi·mo·sis, pl. **phi·mo·ses** (fī-mō′sis, -sēz). Narrowness of the opening of the prepuce, preventing its being drawn back over the glans. [G. a muzzling, fr. *phimos,* a muzzle]

p. clitor′idis, agglutination of the clitoral folds.

p. vagina′lis, narrowness of the vagina.

phi·mot·ic (fī-mot′ik). Pertaining to phimosis.

phleb-. SEE phlebo-.

phle·bal·gia (flĕ-bal′jē-ă). Pain originating in a vein. [phlebo- + G. *algos,* pain]

phleb·ec·ta·sia (fleb-ek-tā′zē-ă). Vasodilation of the veins. SYN venectasia. [phlebo- + G. *ektasis,* a stretching]

phle·bec·to·my (fle-bek′tō-mē). Excision of a segment of a vein, performed sometimes for the cure of varicose veins. SEE ALSO strip (2). SYN venectomy. [phlebo- + G. *ektomē,* excision]

phleb·eu·rysm (fleb′ū-rizm). Pathologic dilation (varix) of a vein. [phlebo- + G. *eurys,* wide]

phle·bit·ic (fle-bit′ik). Relating to phlebitis.

phle·bi·tis (fle-bī′tis). Inflammation of a vein. [phlebo- + G. *-itis,* inflammation]

adhesive p., a form of p. in which the walls adhere, leading to obliteration of the vessel.

p. nodula′ris necroti′sans, obsolete term for p. in which tuberculous nodules are formed in the skin; the lesions spread peripherally and undergo central necrosis.

septic p., inflammation of a vein due to infection.

phlebo-, phleb-. Vein [G. *phleps*]

phleb·o·cly·sis (flĕ-bok′li-sis). Intravenous injection of an isotonic solution of dextrose or other substances in quantity. SYN venoclysis. [phlebo- + G. *klysis,* a washing out]

drip p., intravenous injection of a liquid drop by drop, by the drip method.

phleb·o·dy·nam·ics (fleb′ō-dī-nam′iks). Laws and principles governing blood pressures and flow within the venous circulation. [phlebo- + G. *dynamis,* force]

phleb·o·gram (fleb′ō-gram). A tracing of the jugular or other venous pulse. SYN venogram (2). [phlebo- + G. *gramma,* something written]

phleb·o·graph (fleb′ō-graf). A venous sphygmograph; an instrument for making a tracing of the venous pulse. [phlebo- + G. *graphō,* to write]

phle·bog·ra·phy (fle-bog′ră-fē). **1.** The recording of the venous pulse. **2.** SYN venography. [phlebo- + G. *graphē,* a writing]

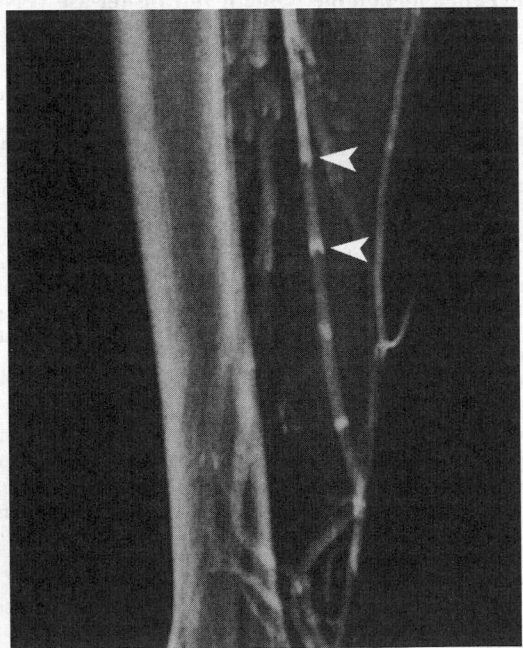

phlebography: lateral view of left leg; venous valves are clearly visible (arrows)

phleb·oid (fleb′oyd). **1.** Resembling a vein. **2.** SYN venous. **3.** Containing many veins. [phlebo- + G. *eidos,* resemblance]

phleb·o·lite (fleb′ō-līt). SYN phlebolith.

phleb·o·lith (fleb′ō-lith). A calcific deposit in a venous wall or thrombus; commonly seen on abdominal radiographs in the lower pelvic region. SYN phlebolite, vein stone. [phlebo- + G. *lithos*, stone]

phleb·o·li·thi·a·sis (fleb'ō-li-thī'ă-sis). The formation of phleboliths.

phle·bol·o·gy (flĕ-bol'ō-jē). The branch of medical science concerned with the anatomy and diseases of the veins. [phlebo- + G. *logos*, study]

phle·bo·ma·nom·e·ter (fleb'ō-mă-nom'ĕ-ter). A manometer for measuring venous blood pressure.

phleb·o·me·tri·tis (fleb'ō-mē-trī'tis). Inflammation of the uterine veins. [phlebo- + G. *mētra*, uterus, + -*itis*, inflammation]

phleb·o·my·o·ma·to·sis (fleb'ō-mī-ō-mă-tō'sis). Thickening of the walls of a vein by an overgrowth of muscular fibers arranged irregularly, intersecting each other without any definite relation to the axis of the vessel. [phlebo- + myoma + G. -*osis*, condition]

phleb·o·phle·bos·to·my (fleb'ō-fle-bos'tō-mē). SYN venovenostomy.

phleb·o·plas·ty (fleb'ō-plas-tē). Repair of a vein. [phlebo- + G. *plastos*, formed]

phle·bor·rha·phy (fle-bōr'ă-fē). Suture of a vein. [phlebo- + G. *rhaphē*, seam]

phleb·o·scle·ro·sis (fleb'ō-skle-rō'sis). Fibrous hardening of the walls of the veins. SYN venofibrosis, venosclerosis. [phlebo- + G. *sklērōsis*, hardening]

phle·bos·ta·sis (fle-bos'tă-sis). **1.** Abnormally slow motion of blood in veins, usually with venous distention. **2.** Treatment of congestive heart failure by compressing proximal veins of the extremities with tourniquets. SYN bloodless phlebotomy. SYN venostasis. [phlebo- + G. *stasis*, a standing still]

phleb·o·ste·no·sis (fleb'ō-stĕ-nō'sis). Narrowing of the lumen of a vein from any cause. [phlebo- + G. *stenōsis*, a narrowing]

phleb·o·throm·bo·sis (fleb'ō-throm-bō'sis). Thrombosis, or clotting, in a vein without primary inflammation. [phlebo- + thrombosis]

phle·bot·o·mine (flĕ-bot'ō-mēn). Relating to sand flies of the genus *Phlebotomus*.

phle·bot·o·mist (fle-bot'ō-mist). An individual trained and skilled in phlebotomy.

phle·bot·o·mize (fle-bot'ō-mīz). **1.** To draw blood from. **2.** To achieve iron overload reduction by repeated removal of blood, as in hemochromatosis.

Phle·bot·o·mus (fle-bot'ō-mŭs). A genus of very small bloodsucking sandflies of the subfamily Phlebotominae, family Psychodidae. [phlebo- + G. *tomos*, cutting]

P. argen'tipes, the vector of kala azar in India.

P. chinen'sis, the vector of kala azar in China.

P. flaviscutel'latus, SYN *Lutzomyia flaviscutellata*.

P. longipal'pis, a vector of kala azar in South America. SYN *Lutzomyia longipalpis*.

P. ma'jor, a vector of kala azar in the Mediterranean region.

P. nogu'chi, the transmitter of *Bartonella* organisms, the causal agent of Oroya fever.

P. orienta'lis, a vector of kala azar in the Sudan.

P. papata'sii, transmitter of the virus of phlebotomus fever; also a vector of *Leishmania tropica* in the Mediterranean area.

P. pernicio'sus, a vector of kala azar in the Mediterranean region.

P. sergen'ti, a vector of *Leishmania tropica*, the cause of anthroponotic cutaneous leishmaniasis.

P. verruca'rum, a form found in Peru that transmits *Bartonella* organisms, the causal agent of Oroya fever.

phle·bot·o·my (fle-bot'ō-mē). Incision into or needle puncture of a vein for the purpose of drawing blood. SYN venesection, venotomy. [phlebo- + G. *tomē*, incision]

bloodless p., SYN phlebostasis (2).

Phleb·o·vi·rus (fleb'ō-vī-rŭs). A genus of the family Bunyaviridae that contains more than 40 viruses that cross-react; transmitted by arthropods primarily of the genus *Phlebotomus;* causes sandfly fever and Rift Valley fever.

phlegm (flem). **1.** Abnormal amounts of mucus, especially as expectorated from the mouth. **2.** One of the four humors of the body, according to the ancient Greek humoral *doctrine*. [G. *phlegma*, inflammation]

phleg·ma·sia (fleg-mā'zē-ă). Obsolete term for inflammation, especially when acute and severe. [G. fr. *phlegma*, inflammation]
p. ceru'lea do'lens, thrombosis of the veins of a limb, with sudden severe pain with swelling, cyanosis, and edema of the part, followed by circulatory collapse and shock.

phleg·mat·ic (fleg-mat'ik). Relating to the heavy one of the four ancient Greek humors (see phlegm), and therefore calm, apathetic, unexcitable. [G. *phlegmatikos*, relating to phlegm]

phleg·mon·ous (fleg'mon-ŭs). Denoting phlegmon.

phlo·gis·ton (flō-jis'ton). A hypothetical substance of negative mass that, according to the theory of G.E. Stahl, was given off by a substance when it underwent combustion, thus accounting for the decrease in mass of the ash over the original substance; abandoned after the discoveries of Priestley and Lavoisier concerning oxygen. [G. *phlogistos*, inflammable]

phlo·go·sin (flō'gō-sin). A substance, isolated from cultures of pus-producing cocci, injections of sterilized solutions of which will excite suppuration. [G. *phlogōsis*, inflammation]

phlo·go·ther·a·py (flō'gō-thār'ă-pē). SYN nonspecific *therapy*. [G. *phlogōsis*, inflammation, + therapy]

phlo·rid·zin. A dihydrochalcone occurring in many parts of the apple tree; used experimentally to produce glycosuria in animals. SYN phlorizin.

phlo·ri·zin. SYN phloridzin.

phlor·o·glu·cin, phlor·o·glu·cin·ol, phlor·o·glu·col (flōr-ō-gloo'sin, -gloo'sin-ol, -gloo'kol). An isomer of pyrogallol, obtained from resorcinol by fusion with caustic soda; used as a reagent with vanillin, as a decalcifier of bone specimens, and as an antispasmodic. [phloridzin + G. *glykys*, sweet, + -in]

phlox·ine (flok-sēn, -sin) [C.I. 45405]. A red acid dye used as a cytoplasmic stain in histology.

phlyc·ten·u·la, pl. **phlyc·ten·u·lae** (flik-ten'ū-lă). A small red nodule of lymphoid cells, with ulcerated apex, occurring in the conjunctiva. SYN phlyctenule. [Mod. L. dim. of G. *phlyktaina*, blister]

phlyc·ten·u·lar (flik-ten'ū-lăr). Relating to a phlyctenula.

phlyc·ten·ule (flik'ten-ūl). SYN phlyctenula.

phlyc·ten·u·lo·sis (flik-ten'ū-lō'sis). A nodular hypersensitive affection of corneal and conjunctival epithelium due to endogenous toxin.

PhNCS Symbol for phenylisothiocyanate.

PHOBIA

pho·bia (fō'bē-ă). Any objectively unfounded morbid dread or fear that arouses a state of panic. The word is used as a combining form in many terms expressing the object that inspires the fear. [G. *phobos*, fear]

alcoholism, alcoholophobia.

animals, zoophobia.

bees, apiphobia, melissophobia.

being beaten, rhabdophobia.

being buried alive, taphophobia.

being dirty, automysophobia.

being locked in, clithrophobia.

being stared at, scopophobia.

birth of malformed fetus, teratophobia.

blood, hemophobia.

blushing, ereuthophobia.

cancer, cancerophobia, carcinophobia.

cats, ailurophobia.

childbirth, tocophobia.

children, pediophobia.

choking, pnigophobia.

ph

climbing, climacophobia.
cold, psychrophobia.
colors, chromatophobia, chromophobia.
confinement, claustrophobia.
corpses, necrophobia.
crossing a bridge, gephyrophobia.
crowds, ochlophobia.
dampness, hygrophobia.
darkness, nyctophobia, scotophobia.
dawn, eosophobia.
daylight, phengophobia.
death, thanatophobia.
deep places, bathophobia.
deserted places, eremophobia.
dirt, mysophobia, rhypophobia.
disease, nosophobia, pathophobia.
disorder, ataxiophobia.
dogs, cynophobia.
dolls, pediophobia.
drafts, aerophobia, anemophobia.
drugs, pharmacophobia.
eating, phagophobia.
electricity, electrophobia.
enclosed space, claustrophobia.
error, hamartophobia.
everything, panphobia.
excrement, coprophobia.
fatigue, ponophobia, kopophobia.
fever, pyrexiophobia.
filth, rhypophobia.
fire, pyrophobia.
fish, ichthyophobia.
food, cibophobia.
forests, hylephobia.
fur, doraphobia.
germs, microphobia.
ghosts, phasmophobia.
girls, parthenophobia.
glare of light, photaugiaphobia.
glass, crystallophobia, hyalophobia.
God, theophobia.
hair, trichophobia, trichopathophobia.
heart disease, cardiophobia.
heat, thermophobia.
heights, acrophobia.
home, returning to, nostophobia.
human companionship, anthropophobia, phobanthropy.
ideas, ideophobia.
infection, molysmophobia.
insects, entomophobia.
itching, acarophobia.
jealousy, zelophobia.
lice, pediculophobia, phthiriophobia.
light, photophobia.
lightning, astrapophobia, keraunophobia.
machinery, mechanophobia.
malignancy, cancerophobia, carcinophobia.
many things, polyphobia.
marriage, gamophobia.
men, (males), androphobia.
metal objects, metallophobia.
microorganisms, microphobia.
minute objects, microphobia.
mirrors, spectrophobia.
missiles, ballistophobia.
moisture, hygrophobia.
movements, kinesophobia.

nakedness, gymnophobia.
names, nomatophobia, onomatophobia.
neglect of duty, omission of duty, paralipophobia.
night, nyctophobia.
novelty, neophobia.
odors, olfactophobia, osmophobia, osphresiophobia, bromidosiphobia.
open spaces, agoraphobia.
pain, algophobia.
parasites, parasitophobia.
phobias, phobophobia.
places, topophobia.
pleasure, hedonophobia.
pointed objects, aichmophobia.
poisoning, toxicophobia, iophobia.
poverty, peniaphobia.
precipices, cremnophobia.
pregnancy, maieusiophobia.
radiation, radiophobia.
rain, ombrophobia.
rectal disease, proctophobia, rectophobia.
religious objects, sacred objects, hierophobia.
responsibility, hypengyophobia.
rivers, potamophobia.
robbers, harpaxophobia.
school p., a young child's sudden aversion to or fear of attending school, usually considered a manifestation of separation anxiety.
sea, thalassophobia.
self, autophobia.
semen, loss of, spermatophobia.
sexual intercourse, coitophobia, cypridophobia.
sexual love, erotophobia.
sharp objects, belonephobia.
simple p., SYN specific p.
sin, hamartophobia.
sinning, peccatiphobia.
skin of animals, doraphobia.
skin diseases, dermatophobia.
sleep, hypnophobia.
snakes, ophidiophobia.
social p., (1) a persistent pattern of significant fear of a social or performance situation, manifesting in anxiety or panic on exposure to the situation or in anticipation of it, which the person realizes is unreasonable or excessive and interferes significantly with the person's functioning; (2) a DSM diagnosis that is established when specific criteria are met.
solitude, eremophobia, autophobia, monophobia.
sounds, acousticophobia, phonophobia.
speaking, laliophobia.
specific p., (1) a persistent pattern of significant fear of specific objects or situations, manifesting in anxiety or panic on exposure to the object or situation or in anticipation of them, which the person realizes is unreasonable or excessive and which interferes significantly with the person's functioning; (2) a DSM diagnosis that is established when the specific criteria are met. SYN simple p.
spiders, arachnephobia.
stairs, climacophobia
stealing, kleptophobia.
strangers, xenophobia.
stuttering, laliophobia.
sun, heliophobia.
teeth, odontophobia.
thirteen, triskaidekaphobia.
thunder, keraunophobia, tonitrophobia, brontophobia.
time, chronophobia.
touching, being touched, aphephobia, haphephobia.
traveling, hodophobia.
trembling, tremophobia.

uncleanliness, automysophobia.
vaccination, vaccinophobia.
vehicles, amaxophobia, hamaxophobia.
venereal disease, cypridophobia, venereophobia.
voices, phonophobia.
walking, basiphobia.
water, aquaphobia.
wind, anemophobia.
women, (females), gynephobia.
work, ergasiophobia.
worms, helminthophobia.
writing, graphophobia.

---

pho·bic (fō′bik). Pertaining to or characterized by phobia.

pho·bo·pho·bia (fō-bō-fō′bē-ă). Morbid dread of developing some phobia. [G. *phobos,* fear]

pho·co·me·lia, pho·com·e·ly (fō-kō-mē′lē-ă, fō-kom′ĕ-lē). Defective development of arms or legs, or both, so that the hands and feet are attached close to the body, resembling the flippers of a seal. [G. *phōkē,* a seal, + *melos,* extremity]

phol·co·dine (fol′kō-dēn). A narcotic with little or no analgesic or euphorigenic activity, used mainly as an antitussive.

phol·e·drine (fōl′ĕ-drēn). A sympathomimetic agent for the treatment of shock; also an adrenergic and vasopressor.

Pho·ma (fō′mă). A genus of rapidly growing fungi that are common laboratory contaminants and common plant pathogens; rare cause of infection in immunosuppressed patients.

phon (fōn). A unit of loudness of sound.

phon-. SEE phono-.

pho·nac·o·scope (fō-nak′ō-skōp). An instrument for increasing the intensity of the percussion note or of the voice sounds, the examiner's ear or the stethoscope being placed on the opposite side of the chest. [phon- + G. *akouō,* to listen, + *skopeō,* to view]

pho·na·cos·co·py (fō-nă-kos′kŏ-pē). Examination of the chest by means of the phonacoscope.

pho·nal (fō′năl). Relating to the voice or to sound. [G. *phōnē,* voice]

pho·nar·te·ri·o·gram (fōn-ar-tēr′ē-ō-gram). An obsolete technique for recording sound created in arteries.

pho·nar·ter·i·og·ra·phy (fōn-ar-tēr′ē-og′ră-fē). The procedure of obtaining a phonarteriogram.

phon·as·the·nia (fō-nas-thē′nē-ă). Weak voice production, which may be due to fatigue. SYN functional vocal fatigue. [phon- + G. *astheneia,* weakness]

pho·na·tion (fō-nā′shŭn). The production of sounds by vibration of the vocal folds. [G. *phōnē,* voice]

pho·na·tory (fō′nă-tōr-ē). Relating to phonation.

pho·neme (fō′nēm). The smallest speech sound that provides meaning. [G. *phōnēma,* a voice]

pho·ne·mic (fō-nē′mik). Pertaining to or having the characteristics of a phoneme.

pho·nen·do·scope (fō-nen′dō-skōp). A stethoscope that intensifies the auscultatory sounds by means of two parallel resonating plates, one resting on the patient's chest or attached to a stethoscope tube, the other vibrating in unison with it. [phon- + G. *endon,* within, + *skopeō,* to view]

pho·net·ic (fō-net′ik). Relating to speech or to the voice. SEE ALSO phonic. [G. *phōnētikos*]

pho·net·ics (fō-net′iks). The science of speech and of pronunciation. SYN phonology.

pho·ni·at·rics (fō-nē-at′riks). The study of speech; the science of speech. [phon- + G. *iatrikos,* of the healing art]

phon·ic (fon′ik, fō′nik). Relating to the voice or to sound. SEE ALSO phonetic.

phono-, phon-. Sound, speech, or voice sounds. [G. *phōnē*]

pho·no·an·gi·og·ra·phy (fō′nō-an-jē-og′ră-fē). Recording and analysis of the frequency-intensity components of the bruit of turbulent arterial blood flow through a stenotic lesion. [phono- + G. *angeion,* vessel, + *graphō,* to write]

pho·no·car·di·o·gram (fō-nō-kar′dē-ō-gram). A record of the heart sounds made by means of a phonocardiograph.

pho·no·car·di·o·graph (fō-nō-kar′dē-ō-graf). An instrument, utilizing microphones, amplifiers, and filters, for graphically recording the heart sounds, which are displayed on an oscilloscope or analog tracing.

linear p., a p. that records all chest wall vibrations resulting from cardiac activity, with emphasis on low-frequency vibrations due to its filter characteristics.

logarithmic p., a p. that records only theoretically audible vibrations with emphasis on the higher frequencies due to filter characteristics designed to imitate the logarithmic frequency-intensity response of the human auditory apparatus.

spectral p., an instrument for recording the heart sounds in which the electrical changes created by the latter pass from a microphone through a series of filters, each of which is tuned to a particular frequency band; output from each filter activates a separate light source of brightness proportional to the intensity of the sound transmitted through that filter; the lights are arranged vertically in descending order of frequencies. A record is obtained by photographing the vertical row of lights.

stethoscopic p., a p. that records all sound vibrations, audible and inaudible, conveyed by the stethoscope; however, very low-frequency vibrations (in the range of body movements) are filtered out.

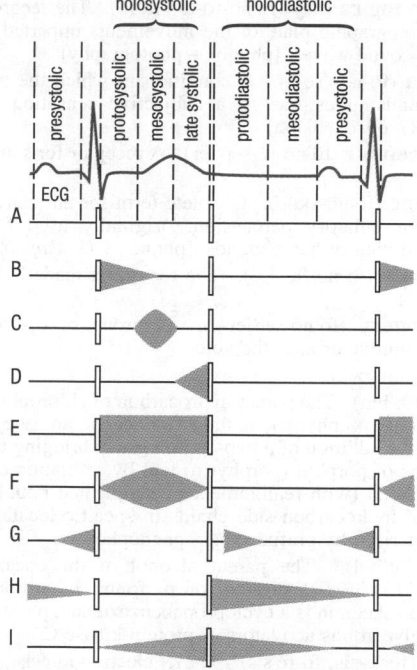

phonocardiography (showing timing and intensity of various cardiac murmurs): (A) temporal sequence of first and second heart sounds; (B) protosystolic decrescendo murmur (e.g., in mitral and tricuspid insufficiency); (C) mesosystolic spindle murmur (e.g., in aortic stenosis); (D) late systolic crescendo murmur (e.g., vestigial pericardial friction rub; in mitral valve insufficiency); (E) holosystolic band-shaped murmur (e.g., in ventricular septal defect, mitral valve insufficiency); (F) holosystolic diamond-shaped murmur (e.g., in pulmonary stenosis); (G) presystolic crescendo and early diastolic decrescendo murmurs – latter is separated from the second heart sound by a brief interval (Flint murmur, in mitral stenosis); (H) holodiastolic decrescendo murmur beginning immediately after second heart sound (as in aortic insufficiency); (I) continuous murmur (e.g., with patent ductus arteriosus or atrioventricular aneurysm)

---

pho·no·car·di·og·ra·phy (fō′nō-kar-dē-og′ră-fē). **1.** Recording of the heart sounds with a phonocardiograph. **2.** The science of interpreting phonocardiograms. [phono- + G. *kardia*, heart, + *graphō*, to record]

pho·no·cath·e·ter (fō-nō-kath′ĕ-ter). A cardiac catheter with diminutive microphone in its tip, for recording sounds and murmurs from within the heart and great vessels.

pho·no·gram (fō′nō-gram). A graphic curve depicting the duration and intensity of a sound. [phono- + G. *gramma*, diagram]

pho·nol·o·gy (fō-nol′ō-jē). SYN phonetics. [phono- + G. *logos*, study]

pho·no·ma·nia (fō-nō-mā′nē-ă). Rarely used term for a homicidal mania. [G. *phonos*, murder, + *mania*, frenzy]

pho·nom·e·ter (fō-nom′ĕ-ter). An instrument for measuring the frequency and intensity of sounds. [phono- + G. *metron*, measure]

pho·no·my·oc·lo·nus (fō′nō-mī-ok′lō-nŭs). Clonic spasms of muscles in response to aural stimuli. [phono- + G. *mys*, muscle, + *klonos*, tumult]

pho·no·my·og·ra·phy (fō′nō-mī-og′ră-fē). The recording of the varying sounds made by contracting muscular tissue. [phono- + G. *mys*, muscle, + *graphē*, drawing]

pho·nop·a·thy (fō-nop′ă-thē). Any disease of the vocal system affecting speech. [phono- + G. *pathos*, suffering]

pho·no·pho·bia (fō-nō-fō′bē-ă). Morbid fear of one's own voice, or of any sound. [phono- + G. *phobos*, fear]

pho·no·phore (fō′nō-fōr). A form of binaural stethoscope with a bell-shaped chest piece into which project the recurved extremities of the sound tubes. [phono- + G. *phoros*, carrying]

pho·no·pho·tog·ra·phy (fō′nō-fō-tog′ră-fē). The recording on a moving photographic plate of the movements imparted to a diaphragm by sound waves. [phono- + photography]

pho·nop·sia (fō-nop′sē-ă). A condition in which the hearing of certain sounds gives rise to a subjective sensation of color. [phono- + G. *opsis*, vision]

pho·no·re·cep·tor (fō′nō-rē-sep′ter). A receptor for sound stimuli.

pho·no·scope (fō′nō-skōp). Obsolete term for an instrument for recording ausculatory percussion; originally used for photographic recording of heart sounds. [phono- + G. *skopeō*, to view]

pho·nos·co·py (fō-nos′kŏ-pē). The recording made by a phonoscope.

pho·no·sur·gery (fō′nō-ser′jer-ē). A group of operations designed to improve or alter the voice.

△**phor-.** SEE phoro-.

phor·bin (fōr′bin). The parent hydrocarbon of chlorophyll; differs from porphin (porphyrin) in the presence of an isocyclic ring formed by the addition of a two-carbon group bridging the 13 and 15 positions of porphin (porphyrin) and by saturation of the 17–18 double bond (with realignment of conjugated double bonds). Addition of hydrocarbon side chains in specific locations yields p.'s characterized by prefixes; e.g., phenophorbin.

phor·bol (fōr′bol). The parent alcohol of the cocarcinogens, which are 12,13(9,9a) diesters of p. found in croton oil; the hydrocarbon skeleton is a cyclopropabenzazulene; p. esters mimic 1,2-diacylglycerol as activators of protein kinase C.

pho·re·sis (fōr′ē-sis, fō-rē′sis). **1.** SYN electrophoresis. **2.** A biologic association in which one organism is transported by another, as in the attachment of the eggs of *Dermatobia hominis*, a human and cattle botfly, to the legs of a mosquito, which transports them to the human, cattle, or other host in which the botfly larvae can develop. SYN epizoic commensalism, phoresy. [G. *phorēsis*, a being borne]

phor·e·sy (fōr′ĕ-sē). SYN phoresis (2).

phor·ia (fōr′ē-ă). The relative directions assumed by the eyes during binocular fixation of a given object in the absence of an adequate fusion stimulus. SEE cyclophoria, esophoria, exophoria, heterophoria, hyperphoria, hypophoria, orthophoria. [G. *phora*, a carrying, motion]

Phor·mia re·gi·na (fōr′mē-ă re·jī′nă). The black blowfly, the larvae of which were formerly used in the treatment of septic wounds because they secrete a proteolytic enzyme that aids in the removal of dead tissue; it is a frequent cause of maggot infestation of sheep, depositing eggs in the wool, and is a widely distributed cold weather species that lays its eggs on dead or decaying tissues.

△**phoro-, phor-.** Carrying, bearing; a carrier, a bearer; phobia. [G. *phoros*, carrying, bearing]

Pho·rop·tor (fŏ-rop′ter). A device containing different lenses that is used for refraction of the eye.

phor·o·zo·on (fōr-ō-zō′on). The nonsexual stage in the life history of an animal that passes through several phases in its life cycle. [phoro- + G. *zōon*, animal]

△**phos-.** Light. [G. *phōs*]

phos·gene (CG) (fos′jēn). Carbonyl chloride; a colorless liquid below 8.2°C, but an extremely poisonous gas at ordinary temperatures; it is an insidious gas, since it is not immediately irritating, even when fatal concentrations are inhaled; more than 80% of World War I chemical agent fatalities were caused by p.

p. oxime (CX), a blister agent stored by the military of some governments; a powerful irritant that produces immediate pain. SYN dichloroformoxime.

△**phosph-, phospho-, phosphor-, phosphoro-.** Prefixes indicating the presence of phosphorus in a compound. See phospho- for specific usage of that prefix. [G. *phōs*, light; *phoros*, carrying]

phos·pha·gen (fos′fă-jen). Energy-rich guanidinium or amidine phosphate, serving as an energy store in muscle and brain; e.g., phosphocreatine in mammals, phosphoarginine in invertebrates. Other p.'s include phosphoagmatine, phosphoglycocyamine, and phospholombricine.

phos·pha·gen·ic (fos-fă-jen′ik). Phosphate-producing.

phos·pham·ic ac·id (fos-fam′ik). $R–NH–PO_3H_2$, one of the three types of high-energy phosphates (the others being phosphophosphoric acids and phosphosulfuric acids).

phos·pham·i·dase (fos-fam′i-dās). SYN phosphoamidase.

phos·pha·stat (fos′fă-stat). A conceptual mechanism whereby the parathyroid hormone is increased when the levels of phosphorus rise to an above-normal level; there is as yet no satisfactory evidence for its existence. [phosphate + L. *status*, a standing]

phos·pha·tase (fos′fă-tās). Any of a group of enzymes (EC 3.1.3.x) that liberate orthophosphate from phosphoric esters. SEE ALSO phosphohydrolases.

acid p., a p. with an optimum pH of less than 7.0 (for several isozymes, it is 5.4), notably present in the prostate gland; demonstrable in lysosomes with Gomori nonspecific acid p. stain; it hydrolyzes many orthophosphoric monoesters.

alkaline p., a p. with an optimum pH of above 7.0 (e.g., 8.6), present ubiquitously; localized cytochemically in membranes by modifications of Gomori nonspecific alkaline p. stain; it hydrolyzes many orthophosphoric monoesters; low levels of this enzyme are seen in cases of hypophosphatasia.

phos·phate (fos′fāt). **1.** A salt or ester of phosphoric acid. For individual p.'s not listed here, see under the name of the base. **2.** The trivalent ion, PO_4^{3-}.

bone p., SYN tribasic *calcium* phosphate.

codeine p., a water-soluble salt of codeine often used in the pharmaceutical preparation of codeine-containing liquid medications.

cyclic p., SYN adenosine 3′,5′-cyclic monophosphate.

dihydrogen p., one-third-neutralized phosphoric acid; e.g., NaH_2PO_4, KH_2PO_4.

disodium p., na_2HPO_4.

energy-rich p.'s, SYN high-energy p.'s.

high-energy p.'s, those p. esters and phosphoanhydrides that, on hydrolysis, yield an unusually large amount of energy; e.g., nucleotide polyphosphates such as ATP, enol p.'s such as phospho*enol*pyruvate. SEE ALSO high-energy *compounds*, under *compound*. SYN energy-rich p.'s.

inorganic p. (Pi), SYN inorganic *orthophosphate*.

monopotassium p., KH_2PO_4; a dihydrogen p. used as a reagent; commonly used in buffers.

monosodium p., NaH_2PO_4; a dihydrogen p. used as a reagent; commonly used in buffers.

normal p., a salt of phosphoric acid or pyrophosphoric acid in which all the hydrogen atoms are displaced; e.g., Na_3PO_4, $Na_4P_2O_7$.

organic p., an ester of phosphoric acid; e.g., glycerol p., adenosine p., hexose p.

triple p., (1) magnesium ammonium p., $MgNH_4PO_4$; **(2)** a crude phosphate fertilizer product from phosphate rock and phosphoric acid.

trisodium p., Na_3PO_4; used to emulsify fats, oil, and grease; an irritant.

phos·phate ace·tyl·trans·fer·ase. An enzyme-catalyzing transfer of an acetyl moiety from acetyl-CoA to orthophosphate, forming acetyl phosphate and coenzyme A. SYN phosphoacylase, phosphotransacetylase.

phos·phat·ed (fos′fāt-ed). Containing phosphates.

phos·pha·te·mia (fos-fă-tē′mē-ă). An abnormally high concentration of inorganic phosphates in the blood. [phosphate + G. *haima,* blood]

phos·phat·ic (fos-fat′ik). Relating to or containing phosphates.

phos·pha·ti·dal (fos-fă-tī′dăl). Older trivial name for alk-1-enylglycerophospholipid; plasmenyl.

phos·pha·ti·dase (fos-fă-tī′dās). SYN *phospholipase* A_2.

phos·pha·ti·date (fos-fă-tī′dāt). A salt or ester of a phosphatidic acid.

    p. phosphatase, an enzyme that catalyzes the hydrolysis of p. producing orthophosphate and 1,2-diacylglycerol; this enzyme participates in phospholipid and triacylglycerol metabolism.

phos·pha·tide (fos′fă-tīd). Former name for 1) phosphatidic acid and 2) phosphatidate.

phos·pha·tid·ic ac·id (fos′fă-tid′ik). 1,2-Diacylglycerol phosphate; a derivative of glycerophosphoric acid in which the two remaining hydroxyl groups of the glycerol are esterified with fatty acids; e.g., phosphatidic acids attached to choline are phosphatidylcholines (lecithins).

phos·pha·ti·do·lip·ase (fos′fă-tī-dō-lip′ās). SYN *phospholipase* A_2.

phos·pha·ti·dyl (Ptd) (fos-fă-tī′dĭl). The radical of a phosphatidic acid; e.g., phosphatidylcholine.

phos·pha·ti·dyl·cho·line (PtdCho) (fos-fă-tī′dĭl-kō′lēn). SEE lecithin.

phos·pha·ti·dyl·eth·a·nol·a·mine (PtdEth) (fos-fă-tī′dĭl-eth-ă-nol′ă-mēn). The condensation product of a phosphatidic acid and ethanolamine; found in biomembranes. SEE ALSO cephalin.

    p. cytidylyltransferase, a key enzyme in the biosynthesis of cephalin; it catalyzes the reaction of phosphoethanolamine and CTP to form CDP-ethanolamine and pyrophosphate.

phos·phat·i·dyl·glyc·er·ol (fos-fă-tī′dĭl-glis′er-ol). A phosphatidic acid in which a second glycerol molecule replaces the usual choline, or ethanolamine or serine; a constituent in human amniotic fluid that denotes fetal lung maturity when present in the last trimester.

phos·pha·ti·dyl·in·o·si·tol (PtdIns) (fos-fă-tī′dĭl-in-ō′si-tol). A phosphatidic acid combined with inositol found in biomembranes and a precursor to certain cellular signals. Sometimes referred to as inositide. SYN phosphoinositide.

    p. 4,5-bisphosphate (PIP₂, PtdIns(4,5)P₂), p. with two additional sites of phosphorylation; an important constituent of cell membrane phospholipids as well as a precursor of the second messengers, diacylglycerol and inositol 1,4,5-trisphosphate.

    p. 4-phosphate, the intermediate in the biosynthesis of p. 4,5-bisphosphate from p.

    p. synthase, an enzyme that catalyzes the reaction of CDP-diacylglycerol with inositol to form CMP and p.; found in the endoplasmic reticulum.

phos·pha·ti·dyl·ser·ine (PtdSer) (fos-fă-tī′dĭl-ser′ēn). The condensation product of phosphatidic acid and serine; found in biomembranes. SEE ALSO cephalin.

phos·pha·tu·ria (fos-fă-too′rē-ă). Excessive excretion of phosphates in the urine. SYN phosphoruria, phosphuria. [phosphate + G. *ouron,* urine]

phos·phene (fos′fēn). Sensation of light produced by mechanical or electrical stimulation of the peripheral or central optic pathway of the nervous system. [G. *phōs,* light, + *phainō,* to show]

    accommodation p., a p. occurring during accommodation, caused by sudden relaxation of the ciliary muscle.

phos·phide (fos′fīd). A compound of phosphorus with valence −3; e.g., sodium phosphide, Na_3P.

phos·phine (fos′fēn, -fin). A colorless poisonous war gas with a characteristic garlic-like odor; also the active agent in some rodenticides; formed in small quantities in the putrefaction of organic matter containing phosphorus. SYN hydrogen phosphide, phosphureted hydrogen.

phosphinico-. In chemistry, symmetrically doubly substituted phosphinic acid, $R_2P(O)OH$.

phos·phite (fos′fīt). A salt of phosphorous acid.

phospho-. Prefix for *O*-phosphono-, which may replace the suffix phosphate; e.g., glucose phosphate is *O*-phosphonoglucose or phosphoglucose. SEE ALSO phosph-, phosphoryl-.

phos·pho·ac·y·lase (fos-fō-as′i-lās). SYN phosphate acetyltransferase.

3′-phos·pho·aden·o·sine 5′-phos·phate (PAP) (fos′fō-a-den′ō-sēn). A product in sulfuryl transfer reactions.

3′-phos·pho·aden·o·sine 5′-phos·pho·sul·fate (PAPS). SEE adenosine 3′-phosphate 5′-phosphosulfate.

phos·pho·am·i·dase (fos-fō-am′i-dās). An enzyme catalyzing the hydrolysis of phosphorus-nitrogen bonds, notably the hydrolysis of *N*-phosphocreatine to creatine and orthophosphate. SYN phosphamidase.

phos·pho·am·ides (fos-fō-am′īdz). Amides of phosphoric acid (phosphoramidic acids) and their salts or esters (phosphoramidates), of the general formula $(HO)_2P(O)–NH_2$; e.g., creatine phosphate.

phos·pho·ar·gi·nine (fos-fō-ar′gi-nēn). A compound (in particular, a phosphagen) of L-arginine with phosphoric acid containing the phosphoamide bond; a source of energy in the contraction of muscle in invertebrates, corresponding to phosphocreatine in the muscles of vertebrates. Cf. phosphocreatine. SYN arginine phosphate.

phos·pho·cho·line (fos-fō-kō′lēn). Choline *O*-phosphate; important in choline metabolism, e.g., in the biosynthesis of lecithins. SYN phosphorylcholine.

    p. cytidylyltransferase, an enzyme that catalyzes the reaction of p. with CTP to form pyrophosphate and CDP-choline; the rate-limiting step of lecithin biosynthesis; the cytosolic form of the enzyme is inactive (a phosphorylated form of the enzyme).

    p. diacylglycerol transferase, an enzyme in lecithin biosynthesis that catalyzes the reaction of 1,2-diacylglycerol with CDP-choline to form CMP and phosphatidylcholine.

phos·pho·cre·a·tine (fos-fō-krē′ă-tēn). A phosphagen; a compound of creatine (through its NH_2 group) with phosphoric acid; a source of energy in the contraction of vertebrate muscle, its breakdown furnishing phosphate for the resynthesis of ATP from ADP by creatine kinase. Cf. phosphoarginine. SYN creatine phosphate, N^ω-phosphonocreatine.

phos·pho·di·es·ter (fos′fō-dī-es′ter). A diesterified orthophosphoric acid, $RO–(PO_2H)–OR′$, as in the nucleic acids.

    p. hydrolases, SYN phosphodiesterases.

phos·pho·di·es·ter·as·es (fos′fō-dī-es′ter-ās-ez). Enzymes (EC 3.1.4.x) cleaving phosphodiester bonds, such as those in cAMP or between nucleotides in nucleic acids, liberating smaller poly- or oligonucleotide units or mononucleotides but not orthophosphate. SYN phosphodiester hydrolases.

    spleen p., SYN micrococcal *endonuclease.*

phos·pho·dis·mu·tase (fos-fō-dis′mū-tās). SYN phosphomutase.

phos·pho·enol·py·ru·vate car·box·y·kin·ase. SYN *phosphoenolpyruvic acid* carboxykinase.

phos·pho·*e·nol*·pyr·u·vic ac·id (fos′fō-ē′nol-pī-roo′vik). The phosphoric ester of pyruvic acid in the latter's enol form; an intermediate in the conversion of D-glucose to pyruvic acid and an example of a high-energy phosphate ester.

    p. a. carboxykinase, an enzyme that catalyzes the reaction of oxaloacetate and GTP to form p. a., CO_2, and GDP; a key enzyme

ph

in gluconeogenesis; the biosynthesis of this enzyme is decreased by insulin. SYN phospho*enol*pyruvate carboxykinase.

phos·pho·eth·a·no·la·mine (fos′fō-eth-an-ol′a-mēn). A key intermediate in the formation of cephalins; formed in liver and brain by phosphorylation of ethanolamine.
p. cytidylyltransferase, a key enzyme in the biosynthesis of cephalins; it catalyzes the reaction of p. and CTP to form CDP-ethanolamine and pyrophosphate.

1-phos·pho·fruc·tal·do·lase (fos′-fō-frŭk-tal′dō-lās). SYN fructose-bisphosphate aldolase.

1-phos·pho·fruc·to·ki·nase (fos′fō-frŭk-tō-kī′nās). Fructose-1-phosphate kinase; an enzyme catalyzing phosphorylation of D-fructose 1-phosphate by ATP (or other NTP) to D-fructose 1,6-bisphosphate and ADP (or other NDP); a key step in the metabolism of D-fructose; a deficiency of the muscle enzyme can result in glycogen storage disease type VII.

6-phos·pho·fruc·to·ki·nase. Phosphofructokinase I; an enzyme that catalyzes the phosphorylation of D-fructose 6-phosphate by ATP (or other NTP) to fructose 1,6-bisphosphate and ADP (or other NDP); this enzyme catalyzes a step in glycolysis; it is inhibited by elevated levels of either ATP or citrate; a deficiency of this enzyme can lead to hemolytic anemia. SYN phosphohexokinase.

phos·pho·ga·lac·to·i·som·er·ase (fos′fō-gă-lak′tō-ī-som′er-ās). SYN UDPglucose-hexose-1-phosphate uridylyltransferase.

phos·pho·glu·co·ki·nase (fos′fō-gloo-kō-kī′nās). An enzyme that, in the presence of ATP, catalyzes the phosphorylation of D-glucose 1-phosphate to form D-glucose 1,6-bisphosphate and ADP; found in yeast and muscle; D-glucose 1,6-bisphosphate is a required cofactor of one of the enzymes in glycogenolysis. SYN glucose-1-phosphate kinase.

phos·pho·glu·co·mu·tase (fos′fō-gloo-kō-mū′tās). An enzyme that catalyzes the reversible reaction, α-D-glucose 1-phosphate ⇌ α-D-glucose 6-phosphate, with glucose 1,6-bisphosphate a necessary cofactor; one of the steps in glycogenolysis. SYN glucose phosphomutase.

phos·pho·glu·co·nate de·hy·dro·gen·ase (fos-fō-gloo′kŏ-nāt). 6-phosphogluconic dehydrogenase; an enzyme catalyzing the reaction of 6-phospho-D-gluconate and NAD(P)+ to form 6-phospho-2-keto-D-gluconate and NAD(P)H; a deficiency of this enzyme has been reported, but no cell disruption has been observed.

phos·pho·glu·co·nate de·hy·dro·gen·ase (de·car·box·y·lat·ing). An enzyme, which is part of the pentose phosphate shunt, that catalyzes the reaction of 6-phospho-D-gluconate and NADP+ to produce CO_2, NADPH, and D-ribulose 5-phosphate.

6-phos·pho·glu·co·no·lac·to·nase (fos′fō-gloo′kŏ-nō-lak′tō-nās). A hydrolase that catalyzes the hydrolysis of 6-phospho-D-glucono δ-lactone to 6-phospho-D-gluconate; this enzyme is a part of the pentose phosphate shunt.

6-phos·pho·D-glu·co·no-δ-lac·tone. An intermediate in the pentose phosphate pathway that is synthesized from D-glucose 6-phosphate.

phos·pho·glyc·er·ac·e·tals (fos′fō-glis-er-as′ĕ-tălz). SYN plasmalogens.

phos·pho·glyc·er·ate ki·nase (fos′fō-glis′er-āt). An enzyme catalyzing the formation of 3-phospho-D-glyceroyl phosphate and ADP from 3-phospho-D-glycerate and ATP; this enzyme is a part of the glycolytic pathway; a deficiency of p. k. (an X-linked disorder) results in impaired glycolysis in most cells.

phos·pho·gly·cer·ic ac·id (fos′fō-gli-ser′ik, -glis′er-ik). **1.** Glyceroyl phosphoric acid; glyceroyl phosphate; an acid anhydride between glyceric acid and phosphoric acid. **2.** 2-Phosphoglyceric acid; the deprotonated form, 2-phosphoglycerate, is an intermediate in glycolysis. **3.** 3-Phosphoglyceric acid; the deprotonated form, 3-phosphoglycerate, is an intermediate in glycolysis.

phos·pho·glyc·er·ides (fos-fō-glis′er-īdz). Acylglycerol and diacylglycerol phosphates; constituents of nerve tissue, and involved in fat transport and storage.

phos·pho·glyc·er·o·mu·tase (fos′fō-glis′er-ō-mū′tās). An isomerizing enzyme catalyzing the reversible interconversion of

2-phosphoglycerate and 3-phosphoglycerate with 2,3-bisphosphoglycerate present as a cofactor; a deficiency of this enzyme, which plays a role in glycolysis, is an inherited disorder that results in an intolerance for strenuous exercise.

phos·pho·hex·o·ki·nase (fos′fō-hek-sō-kī′nās). SYN 6-phosphofructokinase.

phos·pho·hex·o·mu·tase (fos′fō-hek-sō-mū′tās). SYN glucosephosphate isomerase.

phos·pho·hex·ose isom·er·ase (fos-fō-hek′sōs). SYN glucosephosphate isomerase.

phos·pho·hy·dro·las·es (fos-fō-hī′drō-lās-ez). Phosphoric monoester hydrolases; enzymes (EC 3.1.3.x) cleaving phosphoric acid (as orthophosphate) from its esters; trivial names usually end in phosphatase.

phos·pho·in·o·si·tide (fos′fō-in-ō′si-tīd). SYN phosphatidylinositol.

phos·pho·ki·nase (fos-fō-kī′nās). A phosphotransferase or a kinase.

phos·pho·li·pase (fos-fō-lip′ās). An enzyme that catalyzes the hydrolysis of a phospholipid. SYN lecithinase.
p. A_1, an enzyme that hydrolyzes a lecithin (1,2-diacylglycerophosphocholine) to a 2-acylglycerophosphocholine and a fatty acid anion.
p. A_2, an enzyme that catalyzes the hydrolysis of a lecithin to a lysolecithin by removing the 2-acyl group; also acts on other phospholipids by removing a fatty acid from the 2-position; this enzyme has an important role in prostaglandin and leukotriene biosynthesis. SYN lecithinase A, phosphatidase, phosphatidolipase.
p. B, (1) SYN lysophospholipase; (2) a mixture of p. A_1 and p. A_2.
p. C, *Clostridium welchii* α-toxin; *Clostridium oedematiens* β- and γ-toxins; an enzyme that catalyzes the hydrolysis of phosphatidylcholine (and perhaps other phospholipids) to produce choline phosphate and 1,2-diacylglycerol; also acts on sphingomyelin; a key enzyme in the formation of inositol 1,4,5-trisphosphate. SYN lecithinase C, lipophosphodiesterase I.
p. D, an enzyme that hydrolyzes phosphatidylcholine to produce choline and a phosphatidate; also acts on other phosphatidyl esters. SYN choline phosphatase, lecithinase D, lipophosphodiesterase II.

phos·pho·lip·id (fos-fō-lip′id). A lipid containing phosphorus, thus including the lecithins and other phosphatidyl derivatives, sphingomyelin, and plasmalogens; the basic constituents of biomembranes.

phos·pho·mu·tase (fos-fō-mū′tās). One of a number of enzymes (mutases) (EC 5.4.2.x) that apparently catalyze intramolecular transfer because the donor is regenerated (e.g., phosphoglyceromutase, phosphoglucomutase). SYN phosphodismutase.

phos·pho·ne·cro·sis (fos-fō-ne-krō′sis). Necrosis of the bone of the jaw, a result of poisoning by inhalation of phosphorus fumes, occurring especially in persons who work with the element. [phosphorus + G. *nekrōsis*, death (necrosis)]

phos·pho·ni·um (fos-fō′nē-ŭm). The radical, $(PR_4)^+$.

⚛*O*-**phosphono-.** Prefix indicating a phosphonic acid radical $(-PO_3H_2)$ attached through an oxygen atom, hence a phosphoric ester. SEE ALSO phospho-.

N^ω-**phosphonocreatine.** SYN phosphocreatine.

4′-phos·pho·pan·te·the·ine (fos′fō-pan-tĕ-thē′in). The prosthetic group of the acyl carrier protein in the fatty acid synthase complex. SYN pantetheine 4′-phosphate.

phos·pho·pen·ia (fos′fō-pē′nē-ă). Low serum phosphate levels. SYN phosphorpenia. [phospho- + G. *penia*, poverty]

phos·pho·pen·tose ep·i·mer·ase (fos-fō-pen′tōs ē-pim-er-ās). An enzyme that catalyzes the reversible epimerization of a number of phosphorylated, five-carbon sugars; most notably ribulose 5-phosphate to xylulose 5-phosphate in the pentose phosphate pathway.

phos·pho·pen·tose isom·er·ase (fos-fō-pen′tōs). SYN ribose 5-phosphate isomerase.

phos·pho·pho·rin (fos-fō-fōr′in). A protein (MW 155,000) found in dentin that is believed to have a role in mineralization.

phos·pho·pro·tein (fos-fō-prō′tēn). A protein containing phosphoryl groups attached directly to the side chains of some of its constituent amino acids, usually to the hydroxyl group of an L-seryl residue or an L-threonyl residue; e.g., casein, vitellin, ovalbumin.

phos·pho·py·ru·vate hy·dra·tase (fos-fō-pī′roo-vāt). SYN enolase.

phos·phor (fos′fŏr). **1.** A chemical substance that transforms incident electromagnetic or radiation energy into light, as in scintillation radioactivity determinations or radiographic intensifying screens or image amplifiers. **2.** Any substance capable of exhibiting phosphorescence. [G. *phōs*, light, + *phoros*, bearing]

photostimulable p., the chemical coating the p. plate in a computed radiography system; the latent image is recovered by laser scanning.

⌂**phosphor-, phosphoro-.** SEE phosph-.

phos·phor·at·ed (fos′fŏr-āt-ed). Forming a compound with phosphorus.

phos·pho·res·cence (fos-fŏ-res′ens). The quality or property of emitting light without active combustion or the production of heat, generally as the result of prior exposure to radiation, which persists after the inciting cause is removed. [G. *phōs*, light, + *phoros*, bearing]

phos·pho·res·cent (fos′fŏ-res′ent). Having the property of phosphorescence.

phos·phor·hi·dro·sis (fos′fŏr-hī-drō′sis). The excretion of luminous sweat. SYN phosphoridrosis. [G. *phōs*, light, + *phoros*, bearing, + *hidrōsis*, sweating]

phos·pho·ri·bo·i·som·er·ase (fos′fŏ-rī′bō-ī-som′er-ās). SYN *ribose 5-phosphate* isomerase.

5-phos·pho·ri·bose 1-di·phos·phate. SYN 5-phospho-α-D-ribosyl-1-pyrophosphate.

5-phos·pho·ri·bo·syl·am·ine (fos′fŏ-rī-bō-sil-a-mēn). An intermediate in purine biosynthesis.

phos·pho·ri·bo·syl·gly·cine·a·mide syn·the·tase (fos′fŏ-rī′bō-sil-gli-sin′ă-mīd). Glycinamide ribonucleotide synthetase; an enzyme that reacts glycine with ribosylamine 5-phosphate and ATP to form ADP, orthophosphate, and phosphoribosylglycineamide in the course of purine biosynthesis.

5-phos·pho-α-D-ri·bo·syl-1-py·ro·phos·phate (PPRibp, PPRP, PRPP). 5-Phosphoribosyl 1-diphosphate; D-ribose carrying a phosphate group on ribose carbon-5 and a pyrophosphate group on ribose carbon-1; an intermediate in the formation of the pyrimidine and purine nucleotides as well as NAD$^+$. SYN 5-phosphoribose 1-diphosphate.

phos·pho·ri·bo·syl·trans·fer·ase (fos′fŏ-rī′bō-sil-trans′fer-ās). One of a group of enzymes (EC 2.4.2.x, pentosyltransferases) that transfers D-ribose 5-phosphate from 5-phospho-α-D-ribosyl pyrophosphate to a purine, pyrimidine, or pyridine acceptor, forming a 5′-nucleotide and pyrophosphate, or D-ribose from D-ribosyl phosphate to a base, forming a nucleoside, or similar pentose transfers; important in nucleotide biosynthesis. Specific p.'s are preceded by the name of the acceptor base, e.g., uracil phosphoribosyltransferase (i.e., uracil + PRPP ⇌ UMP + pyrophosphate).

phos·pho·ri·bu·lo·ki·nase (fos′fŏ-rī′bū-lō-kī′nās). An enzyme that, in the presence of ATP, catalyzes the phosphorylation of D-ribulose 5-phosphate to D-ribulose 1,5-bisphosphate and ADP, a reaction of importance in the carbon dioxide fixation cycle of photosynthesis.

phos·pho·ri·bu·lose ep·i·mer·ase (fos-fō-rī′bū-lōs). SYN ribulose-phosphate 3-epimerase.

phos·phor·ic ac·id (fos-fōr′ik). Orthophosphoric acid; a strong acid of industrial importance; m.p. 42.35°C; dilute solutions have been used as urinary acidifiers and as dressings to remove necrotic debris. In dentistry, it constitutes about 60% of the liquid used in zinc phosphate and silicate cements; solutions in varying concentrations are used for etching enamel and dentin surfaces prior to applications of various types of resins.

cyclic p. a., (1) in general, a linear polymer of phosphoric acid residues in pyrophosphate linkage in which the α and ω residues are similarly linked to make one endless loop or cyclic compound; (2) specifically, a generic term applied to compounds in which one phosphoric acid residue is esterified to two hydroxyl

groups of a single carbon chain, as in adenosine 3′,5′-phosphoric acid, adenosine 2′,3′-phosphoric acid, etc.

dilute p. a., a solvent containing 10% H$_3$PO$_4$.

glacial p. a., an anhydride of phosphoric acid used as a reagent and in the manufacture of zinc oxyphosphate cement for dentistry. SYN metaphosphoric acid.

phos·phor·i·dro·sis (fos′fŏr-i-drō′sis). SYN phosphorhidrosis.

phos·phor·ism (fos′fŏr-izm). Chronic poisoning with phosphorus.

phos·phor·ized (fos′fŏr-īzd). Containing phosphorus.

phos·pho·rol·y·sis (fos-fŏ-rol′i-sis). A reaction analogous to hydrolysis except that the elements of phosphoric acid, rather than of water, are added in the course of splitting a bond; e.g., the formation of glucose 1-phosphate from glycogen. SYN phosphoroclastic cleavage.

phos·pho·rous (fos′fŏr-ŭs, fos-fōr′ŭs). **1.** Relating to, containing, or resembling phosphorus. **2.** Referring to phosphorus in its lower (+3) valence state.

phos·pho·rous ac·id. H$_3$PO$_3$; its salts are phosphites.

phos·phor·pen·ia (fos′fŏr-pē′nē-ă). SYN phosphopenia.

phos·phor·u·ria (fos-fō-roo′rē-ă). SYN phosphaturia.

phos·pho·rus (P) (fos′fŏr-ŭs). A nonmetallic chemical element, atomic no. 15, atomic wt. 30.973762, occurring extensively in nature always in combination as phosphates, phosphites, etc., and as the phosphate in every living cell; the elemental form is extremely poisonous, causing intense inflammation and fatty degeneration; repeated inhalation of p. fumes may cause necrosis of the jaw (phosphonecrosis); the approximate fatal dose is 50–100 mg. [G. *phosphoros*, fr. *phōs*, light, + *phoros*, bearing]

amorphous p., red p., an allotropic form of p. formed by heating ordinary p., in the absence of oxygen, to 260°C; it occurs as an amorphous dark red mass or powder, nonpoisonous, and much less flammable than ordinary p.; it may be reconverted to the latter by heating to 454.4°C in nitrogen gas.

p. pentoxide, the ultimate anhydride of orthophosphoric acid; a drying and dehydrating agent; corrosive.

phos·pho·rus-32 (^{32}P). Radioactive phosphorus isotope; beta emitter with half-life of 14.28 days; used as tracer in metabolic studies and in the treatment of certain diseases of the osseous and hematopoietic systems.

phos·pho·rus-33 (^{33}P). A radioactive isotope of phosphorus with a half-life of 25.3 days; used as a tracer in metabolic studies.

phos·pho·ryl (fos′fŏ-ril). The radical, O=P–, as in phosphoryl chloride, POCl$_3$.

⌂**phosphoryl-.** Prefix incorrectly used to signify a phosphate (e.g., phosphorylcholine) in place of the correct *O*-phosphono- or phospho-.

phos·pho·ryl·ase (fos-fōr′i-lās). A phosphorylated enzyme cleaving poly(1,4-α-D-glucosyl)$_n$ with orthophosphate to form poly(1,4-α-D-glucosyl)$_{n-1}$ and α-D-glucose 1-phosphate. SYN α-glucan phosphorylase, glycogen phosphorylase, P enzyme, p. *a*, polyphosphorylase.

p. *a*, SYN phosphorylase.

p. *b*, dephosphorylated p. *a*. Under most conditions, the inactive form of p.; active in the presence of AMP. SEE p. phosphatase.

p. kinase, an enzyme that uses ATP to phosphorylate p. *b* and thus reform p. *a*, the active form of p.; the active form of p. kinase is itself a phosphorylated protein; upon dephosphorylation of p. kinase, the enzyme is inactivated; it can be rephosphorylated with a cAMP-dependent protein kinase; p. kinase is deficient in certain types of glycogen storage disease.

p. phosphatase, an enzyme catalyzing the conversion of one p. *a* into two p. *b*, with the release of four orthophosphates. SYN phosphorylase-rupturing enzyme.

phos·pho·ryl·as·es (fos-fōr′i-lās-ez). **1.** General term for enzymes transferring a phosphoryl group to some organic acceptor, hence belonging to the transferases. **2.** Specifically, enzymes that release a single glucosyl residue from a polyglucose as D-glucose 1-phosphate, the phosphate coming from orthophosphate; e.g., phosphophorylase, sucrose p., cellobiose p.

nucleoside p., enzymes that catalyze the phosphorolysis of a nucleoside, forming the free purine or pyrimidine plus ribose (or deoxyribose 1-phosphate); e.g., purine-nucleoside phosphorylases.

phos·pho·ryl·a·tion (fos'fōr-i-lā'shŭn). Addition of phosphate to an organic compound, such as glucose to produce glucose monophosphate, through the action of a phosphotransferase (phosphorylase) or kinase.

oxidative p., formation of high-energy phosphoric bonds (e.g., in pyrophosphates) from the energy released by the flow of electrons to O_2 and the dehydrogenation (*i.e.*, oxidation) of various substrates, most notably isocitric acid, α-ketoglutaric acid, succinic acid, and malic acid in the tricarboxylic acid cycle.

substrate-level p., the synthesis of ATP (or other NTP) not involving electron transport coupled with oxidative p. or with photophosphorylation.

phos·pho·ryl·cho·line (fos'fōr-il-kō'lēn). SYN phosphocholine.

phos·pho·ryl·eth·a·nol·a·mine glyc·er·ide·trans·fer·ase (fos'fōr-il-eth-ă-nol'ă-mēn). SYN ethanolaminephosphotransferase.

***O*-phos·pho·ser·ine** (fos-fō-ser'ēn). The phosphoric ester of serine; found as a constituent in many proteins (e.g., phosphorylase *a* and phosvitin).

phos·pho·sphin·go·sides (fos-fō-sfing'gō-sīdz). SYN sphingomyelins.

phos·pho·sug·ar (fos-fō-shug'er). A phosphorylated saccharide; any sugar containing an alcoholic group esterified with phosphoric acid.

phos·pho·trans·a·cet·y·lase (fos'fō-trans-ă-set'i-lās). SYN phosphate acetyltransferase.

phos·pho·trans·fer·as·es (fos-fō-trans'fer-ās-ez). A subclass of transferases (EC subclass 2.7) transferring phosphorus-containing groups. P. include the "kinases" (2.7.1) transferring phosphate to alcohols, to carboxyl groups (2.7.2), to nitrogenous groups (2.7.3), or to another phosphate group (2.7.4). Phosphomutases (5.4.2) catalyze apparent intramolecular transfers; pyrophosphokinases (2.7.6) catalyze transfer of the pyrophosphate group; nucleotidyltransferases (2.7.7) catalyze transfer of the nucleotide (nucleotidyl) groups (including polyribonucleotide nucleotidyltransferase) and other similar groups (2.7.8). SYN transphosphatases.

phos·pho·tri·ose isom·er·ase (fos-fō-trī'ōs). SYN triosephosphate isomerase.

phos·pho·tung·stic ac·id (PTA) (fos-fō-tŭng'stik). A mixture of phosphoric and tungstic acids; a protein precipitant and reagent for arginine, lysine, histidine, and cystine; used with hematoxylin for nuclear and muscle staining; also used in electron microscopy as a stain for collagen and as a negative stain.

phos·pho·vi·tin. SYN phosvitin.

phos·phu·re·sis (fos'foo-rē'sis). Excretion of excessive amounts of phosphate in the urine. [phospho- + G. *ourēsis,* urination]

phos·phu·ria (fos-foo'rē-ă). SYN phosphaturia.

phos·vi·tin (fos-vī'tin). A phosphated protein constituting about 7% of the protein of egg yolk; it is about 60% serine, largely as *O*-phosphoserine, and has anticoagulant properties; an anticoagulant. SYN phosphovitin.

phot (fōt). A unit of illumination; 1 p. equals 1 lumen/cm^2 of surface. [G. *phōs* (*phōt-*), light]

△phot-. SEE photo-.

pho·tal·gia (fō-tal'jē-ă). Light-induced pain, especially of the eyes; for example, in uveitis, the light-induced movement of the iris may be painful. SYN photodynia, photophobia. [phot- + G. *algos,* pain]

pho·tau·gi·a·pho·bia (fō-taw'jē-a-fō'bē-ă). Morbid fear of, or overreaction to, a glare of light. [G. *phōtaugeia,* glare of light, + *phobos,* fear]

pho·tes·the·sia (fō-tes-thē'zē-ă). Perception of light. [photo- + G. *aisthēsis,* sensation]

pho·tic (fō'tik). Relating to light.

pho·tism (fō'tizm). Production of a sensation of light or color by a stimulus to another sense organ, such as of hearing, taste, or touch. SYN pseudophotesthesia.

△**photo-, phot-.** Light. [G. *phōs* (*phōt-*)]

pho·to·ab·la·tion (fō'tō-ab-lā'shun). The process of photoablative decomposition of tissue by laser light, e.g., in photorefractive keratectomy.

pho·to·ac·tin·ic (fō'tō-ak-tin'ik). Denoting radiation that produces both luminous and chemical effects. [photo- + G. *aktis,* ray]

photoaging (fō'tō-āj'ing). Damage from years of sun exposure, particularly wrinkling of skin. [[photo- + aging]]

pho·to·al·ler·gy (fō'tō-al'er-jē). SEE photosensitization.

pho·to·au·to·troph (fō'tō-aw'tō-trōf). An organism that depends solely on light for its energy and principally on carbon dioxide for its carbon. Cf. photoheterotroph, photolithotroph, phototroph. [photo- + G. *autos,* self, + *trophē,* nourishment]

pho·to·au·to·tro·phic (fō-tō-aw'tō-trof'ik). Pertaining to a photoautotroph.

pho·to·bac·te·ria (fō'tō-bak-tēr'ē-ă). Plural of photobacterium.

Pho·to·bac·te·ri·um (fō'tō-bak-tēr'ē-ŭm). A genus of motile and nonmotile, aerobic to facultatively anaerobic bacteria (family Pseudomonadaceae) containing Gram-negative coccobacilli and occasional rods; under adverse conditions pleomorphic forms frequently occur. Motile cells have polar flagella. The metabolism of these organisms is fermentative. They are usually luminescent and occur symbiotically in tissues of luminous organs of cephalopods and deep-sea fishes and on the skin and in the intestines of some marine fish. The type species is *P. phosphoreum.*

P. phospho'reum, a luminescent species found on dead fish and in sea water; it is the type species of the genus *P.*

pho·to·bac·te·ri·um, pl. **pho·to·bac·te·ria** (fō'tō-bak-tēr'ē-ŭm, -bak-tēr'ē-ă). A vernacular term used to refer to any member of the genus *Photobacterium.*

pho·to·bi·ol·o·gy (fō'tō-bī-ol'ō-jē). The study of the effects of light upon plants and animals.

pho·to·bi·ot·ic (fō'tō-bī-ot'ik). Living or flourishing only in the light. [photo- + G. *bios,* life]

pho·to·bleach (fō'tō-blēch). To lose color or make white by the action of light; e.g., the use of a laser to bleach a fluorescent dye covalently linked to a macromolecule.

pho·to·cat·a·lyst (fō-tō-kat'ă-list). A substance that helps bring about a light-catalyzed reaction; e.g., chlorophyll. [photo- + G. *katalysis,* dissolution (catalysis)]

pho·to·cep·tor (fō'tō-sep'ter, -tōr). SYN photoreceptor.

pho·to·chem·i·cal (fō-tō-kem'i-kăl). Denoting chemical changes caused by or involving light.

pho·to·chem·is·try (fō-tō-kem'is-trē). The branch of chemistry concerned with the chemical changes caused by or involving light.

pho·to·che·mo·ther·a·py (fō'tō-kem-ō-thār'ă-pē, -kē-mō-). SYN photoradiation.

pho·to·chro·mo·gens (fō'tō-krō'mō-jenz). SYN Runyon group I mycobacteria. [photo- + G. *chrōma,* color, + *-gen,* producing]

pho·to·co·ag·u·la·tion (fō'tō-kō-ag'ū-lā'shŭn). A method by which a beam of electromagnetic energy is directed to a desired tissue under visual control; localized coagulation results from absorption of light energy and its conversion to heat or conversion of tissue to plasma (atoms stripped of electrons). [photo- + L. *coagulo,* pp. *-atus,* to curdle]

pho·to·co·ag·u·la·tor (fō'tō-kō-ag'ū-lā'ter, tōr). The apparatus used in photocoagulation.

laser p., a high-energy source of electromagnetic radiation. SEE laser.

xenon-arc p., a p. in which a xenon-arc bulb delivers radiation from the visible and near-infrared spectrum.

▪**pho·to·der·ma·ti·tis** (fō'tō-der-mă-tī'tis). Dermatitis caused or elicited by exposure to sunlight; may be phototoxic or photoallergic, and can result from topical application, ingestion, inhalation, or injection of mediating phototoxic or photoallergic material. SEE ALSO photosensitization. SYN actinic dermatitis. [photo- + G. *derma,* skin, + *-itis,* inflammation]

pho·to·dis·tri·bu·tion (fō'tō-dis-tri-bū'shŭn). Areas on the skin that receive the greatest amount of exposure to sunlight, and which are involved in eruptions due to photosensitivity.

pho·tod·ro·my (fō-tod′rō-mē). In the induced or spontaneous clarification of certain suspensions, the settlement of particles on the side nearest the light (**positive p.**) or on the dark side (**negative p.**). [photo- + G. *dromos*, a running]

pho·to·dy·nam·ic (fō′tō-dī-nam′ik). Relating to the energy or force exerted by light. [photo- + G. *dynamis*, force]

pho·to·dyn·ia (fō-tō-din′ē-ă). SYN photalgia. [photo- + G. *odynē*, pain]

pho·to·dys·pho·ria (fō′tō-dis-fōr′ē-ă). Extreme photophobia. [photo- + G. *dysphoria*, extreme discomfort]

pho·to·e·lec·tric (fō′tō-ē-lek′trik). Denoting electronic or electric effects produced by the action of light. SEE photoelectric *effect*, photoelectric *absorption*.

pho·to·e·lec·trom·e·ter (fō′tō-ē-lek-trom′ĕ-ter). A device employing a photoelectric cell for measuring the concentration of substances in solution.

pho·to·e·lec·tron (fō′tō-ē-lek′tron). An electron freed by the action of light.

pho·to·er·y·the·ma (fō′tō-er-i-thē′mă). Erythema caused by exposure to light. [photo- + G. *erythēma*, flush]

pho·to·es·thet·ic (fō′tō-es-thet′ik). Sensitive to light. [photo- + G. *aisthēsis*, sensation]

pho·to·flu·o·rog·ra·phy (fō′tō-flōr-og′ră-fē). Miniature radiographs made by contact photography of a fluoroscopic screen, formerly used in mass radiographic examination of the lungs. SYN fluorography, fluororoentgenography. [photo- + L. *fluor*, a flow, + G. *graphē*, a writing]

pho·to·gas·tro·scope (fō′tō-gas′trō-skōp). An instrument for taking photographs of the interior of the stomach. [photo- + G. *gastēr*, stomach, + *skopeō*, to view]

pho·to·gen (fō′tō-jen). A microorganism that produces luminescence. [photo- + G. *gen-*, producing]

pho·to·gen·e·sis (fō-tō-jen′ē-sis). Production of light, as by bacteria, insects, or phosphorescence. [photo- + G. *genesis*, production]

pho·to·gen·ic, pho·tog·e·nous (fō-tō-jen′ik, fō-toj′ĕ-nŭs). Denoting or capable of photogenesis.

pho·to·he·mo·ta·chom·e·ter (fō′tō-hē′mō-tă-kom′ĕ-ter). An appliance for recording photographically the rapidity of the blood current. [photo- + G. *haima*, blood, + *tachos*, speed, + *metron*, measure]

pho·to·het·er·o·troph (fō′tō-het′er-ō-trof, -trōf). An organism that depends on light for most of its energy and principally on organic compounds for its carbon. Cf. photoautotroph, photolithotroph, phototroph. [photo- + G. *heteros*, other, + *trophē*, nourishment]

pho·to·het·er·o·tro·phic (fō′tō-het′er-ō-trof′ik). Pertaining to a photoheterotroph.

pho·to·in·ac·ti·va·tion (fō′tō-in-ak-ti-vā′shŭn). Inactivation by light; e.g., as in the treatment of herpes simplex by local application of a photoactive dye followed by exposure to a fluorescent lamp.

pho·to·ker·a·to·scope (fō′tō-ker′ah-tō-skōp). A keratoscope fitted with a still film camera.

pho·to·ki·ne·sis (fō′tō-ki-nē′sis). Alteration of random movements of motile organisms in response to light. [photo- + G. *kinēsis*, movement]

pho·to·ki·net·ic (fō′tō-ki-net′ik). **1.** Pertaining to photokinesis. **2.** Pertaining to photokinetics.

pho·to·ki·net·ics (fō′tō-ki-net′iks). The changes in rate of a chemical reaction in response to light. [photo- + G. *kinētikos*, relating to movement]

pho·to·ky·mo·graph (fō′tō-kī′mō-graf). A device for moving film at a constant speed so that a continuous record of a physiologic event may be obtained, as by a beam of light shining on the film. [photo- + G. *kyma*, wave, + *graphō*, to record]

pho·to·lith·o·troph (fō′tō-lith′ō-trof). An organism that requires inorganic compounds and that uses light for most of its energy

needs. Cf. photoautotroph, photoheterotroph, phototroph. [photo- + G. *lithos*, stone, mineral, + *trophē*, nourishment]

pho·to·lu·mi·nes·cent (fō′tō-loo-mi-nes′ent). Having the ability to become luminescent upon exposure to visible light. [photo- + L. *lumen*, light]

pho·to·ly·ase (fō-tō-lī′ās). SEE deoxyribodipyrimidine photolyase. [photo- + G. *lyo*, to loosen, + -ase]

pho·tol·y·sis (fō-tol′i-sis). Decomposition of a chemical compound or cleavage of a chemical bond by the action of light. [photo- + G. *lysis*, dissolution]

pho·to·lyte (fō′tō-līt). Any product of decomposition by light.

pho·to·lyt·ic (fō-tō-lit′ik). Pertaining to photolysis.

pho·to·mac·rog·ra·phy (fō′tō-mă-krog′ră-fē). A technique for investigating and recording conditions and procedures involving small objects that ordinarily would be inspected through a loupe rather than a microscope. [photo- + G. *makros*, large, + *graphō*, to write]

pho·to·ma·nia (fō-tō-mā′nē-ă). Morbid or exaggerated desire for light. [photo- + G. *mania*, frenzy]

pho·tom·e·ter (fō-tom′ĕ-ter). An instrument designed to measure the intensity of light or to determine the light threshold. [photo- + G. *metron*, measure]

flame p., an instrument that uses flame emission spectrophotometry to measure the intensity and other properties of light.

flicker p., an instrument that compares two variable visual stimuli through control of the frequency of a flickering light.

pho·tom·e·try (fō-tom′ĕ-trē). The measurement of the intensity of light.

pho·to·mi·cro·graph (fō′tō-mī′krō-graf). An enlarged photograph of an object viewed with a microscope, as distinguished from microphotograph. SYN micrograph (2). [photo- + G. *mikros*, small, + *graphē*, a record]

pho·to·mi·crog·ra·phy (fō′tō-mī-krog′ră-fē). The production of a photomicrograph. SYN micrography (3).

pho·to·my·oc·lo·nus (fō′tō-mī-ok′lō-nŭs). Clonic spasms of muscles in response to visual stimuli. [photo- + G. *mys*, muscle, + *klonos*, confused motion]

hereditary p. [MIM*172500], p. associated with diabetes mellitus, deafness, nephropathy, and cerebral dysfunction; autosomal dominant inheritance.

pho·ton (hν, γ) (fō′ton). In physics, a corpuscle of energy or particle of light; a quantum of light or other electromagnetic radiation.

pho·top·a·thy (fō-top′ă-thē). Any disease caused by exposure to light. [photo- + G. *pathos*, suffering]

pho·to·peak (fō′tō-pēk). The characteristic energies of photons emitted by a radionuclide, used to set scanning parameters.

pho·to·per·cep·tive (fō′tō-per-sep′tiv). Capable of both receiving and perceiving light.

pho·to·pe·ri·od·ism (fō′tō-pēr′ē-ō-dizm). The periodic (seasonal or diurnal) activities, behavior, or changes in plants or animals brought about by the action of light.

pho·to·pho·bia (fō-tō-fō′bē-ă). SYN photalgia. [photo- + G. *phobos*, fear]

pho·to·pho·bic (fō-tō-fō′bik). Relating to or suffering from photophobia.

pho·to·phore (fō′tō-fōr). In bacteriology, the organ producing intracellular bioluminescence in certain organisms. [photo- + G. *phoros*, bearing]

pho·to·pho·re·sis. SEE extracorporeal p.

extracorporeal p., destruction of cells separated from blood in an extracorporeal flow system by ultraviolet activation of chemotherapeutic agents such as psoralens.

pho·to·phos·pho·ry·la·tion (fō-tō-fos′fōr-i-lā′shŭn). Formation of ATP as a result of absorption of light.

pho·toph·thal·mia (fō′tof-thal′mē-ă). Keratoconjunctivitis caused by ultraviolet energy, as in snow blindness, exposure to an ultraviolet lamp, arc welding, or the short circuit of a high-tension electric current. SEE ALSO photoretinopathy. [photo- + G. *ophthalmos*, eye]

pho·to·pia (fō-tō'pē-ă). SYN photopic *vision*. [photo- + G. *opsis,* vision]

pho·top·ic (fō-top'ik). Pertaining to photopic vision.

pho·top·sia (fō-top'sē-ă). A subjective sensation of lights, sparks, or colors due to electrical or mechanical stimulation of the ocular system. SEE ALSO Moore lightning *streaks,* under *streak.* SYN photopsy. [photo- + G. *opsis,* vision]

pho·top·sin (fō-top'sin). The protein moiety (opsin) of the pigment (iodopsin) in the cones of the retina.

pho·top·sy (fō-top'sē). SYN photopsia.

pho·to·ptar·mo·sis (fō'tō-tar-mō'sis). Sneezing on looking at a light, especially a bright light (e.g., sunlight), a reflex of which the neuroanatomic pathways are debated; autosomal dominant transmission. SYN photic-sneeze reflex. [photo- + G. *ptarmos,* a sneezing, + *-osis,* condition]

pho·to·ra·di·a·tion (fō'tō-rā-dē-ā'shŭn). Treatment of cancer by intravenous injection of a photosensitizing agent, such as hematoporphyrin, followed by exposure to visible light of superficial tumors or of deep tumors by a fiberoptic probe. SYN photochemotherapy, photodynamic therapy, photoradiation therapy.

pho·to·re·ac·tion (fō'tō-rē-ak'shŭn). A reaction caused or affected by light; e.g., a photochemical reaction, photolysis, photosynthesis, phototropism, thymine dimer formation.

pho·to·re·ac·ti·va·tion (fō'tō-rē-ak-ti-vā'shŭn). Activation by light of something or of some process previously inactive or inactivated; e.g., pyrimidine dimers, formed in polynucleic acids by the action of UV light, can be monomerized by UV light of a different wavelength via DNA photolyase.

pho·to·re·cep·tive (fō'tō-rē-sep'tiv). Functioning as a photoreceptor.

pho·to·re·cep·tor (fō'tō-rē-sep'ter, tōr). A receptor that is sensitive to light, e.g., a retinal rod or cone. SYN photoceptor. [photo- + L. *re-cipio,* pp. *-ceptus,* to receive, fr. *capio,* to take]

pho·to·res·pir·a·tion (fō'tō-res-pir-ā'shŭn). Light-enhanced respiration in photosynthetic organisms; i.e., light increases O_2 utilization.

pho·to·ret·i·ni·tis (fō'tō-ret'i-nī'tis). SEE photoretinopathy.

pho·to·ret·i·nop·a·thy (fō'tō-ret'i-nop'ă-thē). A macular burn from excessive exposure to sunlight or other intense light (e.g., the flash of a short circuit); characterized subjectively by reduced visual acuity. SEE ALSO solar *maculopathy.* SYN electric retinopathy, solar retinopathy. [photo- + retina, + G. *pathos,* suffering]

pho·to·scan (fō'tō-skan). SYN scintiscan.

pho·to·sen·si·tive (fō-tō-sen'si-tiv). **1.** An abnormally heightened reactivity of the skin to sunlight. **2.** Responding to light, e.g., as by a photocell. [photo + L. *sensus,* a feeling, fr. *sentio,* to feel]

pho·to·sen·si·tiv·i·ty (fō'tō-sen-si-tiv'i-tē). Abnormal sensitivity to light, especially of the eyes. For example, light may irritate the eyelids, conjunctiva, cornea or, in excess, the retina; when scattered by a cataractous lens light may produce glare; it can produce a migraine headache or a temporary exotropia. SEE photophobia, photalgia, photesthesia.

pho·to·sen·si·ti·za·tion (fō'tō-sen-si-ti-zā'shŭn). **1.** Sensitization of the skin to light, usually due to the action of certain drugs, plants, or other substances; may occur shortly after administration of the drug (phototoxic sensitivity), or may occur only after a latent period of from days to months (photoallergic sensitivity, or photoallergy). **2.** SYN photodynamic *sensitization.*

pho·to·sen·sor (fō'tō-sen'ser, sōr). A device designed to respond to light and to transmit resulting impulses for interpretation, movement, or operating control. SEE sensor.

pho·to·sta·ble (fō'tō-stā-bl). Not subject to change upon exposure to light.

pho·to·steth·o·scope (fō-tō-steth'ō-skōp). Device that converts sound into flashes of light; used for continuous observation of the fetal heart.

pho·to·stress (fō'tō-stres). Exposure to intense illumination. SEE ALSO photostress *test.*

pho·to·syn·the·sis (fō-tō-sin'thĕ-sis). **1.** The compounding or building up of chemical substances under the influence of light. **2.** The process by which green plants, using chlorophyll and the energy of sunlight, produce carbohydrates from water and carbon dioxide, liberating molecular oxygen in the process. [photo- + G. *synthesis,* a putting together]

  bacterial p., a primitive form of p. observed in some bacteria using only one photosystem and some reducing agent other than water.

pho·to·tax·is (fō-tō-tak'sis). Reaction of living protoplasm to the stimulus of light, involving bodily motion of the whole organism toward (**positive p.**) or away from (**negative p.**) the stimulus. Cf. phototropism. [photo- + G. *taxis,* orderly arrangement]

pho·to·ther·a·py (fō-tō-thăr'ă-pē). Treatment of disease by means of light rays. SYN light treatment.

pho·to·ther·mal (fō-tō-ther'măl). Relating to radiant heat. [photo- + G. *therme,* heat]

pho·to·tim·er (fō-tō-tīm'ĕr). An electronic device in radiography that measures the radiation that has passed through the patient and terminates the x-ray exposure when it is sufficient to form an image.

pho·to·tox·ic (fō-tō-tok'sik). Relating to, characterized by, or causing phototoxicity.

pho·to·tox·ic·i·ty (fō-tō-tok-sis'i-tē). The condition resulting from an overexposure to ultraviolet light, or from the combination of exposure to certain wavelengths of light and a phototoxic substance. SEE ALSO photosensitization. [photo- + G. *toxikon,* poison]

pho·to·troph (fō'tō-trōf). An organism that uses light for its energy needs. Cf. photoautotroph, photoheterotroph, photolithotroph.

pho·tot·ro·pism (fō-to'trō-pizm). Movement of a part of an organism toward (**positive p.**) or away from (**negative p.**) the stimulus of light. Cf. phototaxis. [photo- + G. *trope,* a turning]

pho·tu·ria (fō-too'rē-ă). The passage of phosphorescent urine. [photo- + G. *ouron,* urine]

PHP Abbreviation for panhypopituitarism.

phrag·mo·plast (frag'mō-plast). Barrel-shaped enlargement of the spindle associated with formation of the new cell membrane during telophase in plant cells. [G. *phragma,* hedge, enclosure, + *plasso,* to form]

phren (fren). **1.** SYN diaphragm (1). **2.** The mind. [G. *phren,* the diaphragm, mind, heart (as seat of emotions)]

phren-. SEE phreno-.

phre·nal·gia (fre-nal'jē-ă). **1.** SYN psychalgia (1). **2.** Pain in the diaphragm. [phren- + G. *algos,* pain]

phre·nec·to·my (fre-nek'tō-mē). SYN phrenicectomy.

phren·em·phrax·is (fren'em-frak'sis). SYN phreniclasia. [phren- + G. *emphraxis,* a stoppage]

phre·net·ic (frĕ-net'ik). **1.** Frenzied; maniacal. **2.** An individual exhibiting such behavior. [G. *phrenitikos,* frenzied]

phreni-. SEE phreno-.

-phrenia. **1.** The diaphragm. **2.** The mind. SEE phreno-. [G. *phren,* the diaphragm, mind, heart (as seat of emotions)]

phren·ic (fren'ik). **1.** SYN diaphragmatic. **2.** Relating to the mind.

phren·i·cec·to·my (fren-i-sek'tō-mē). Exsection of a portion of the phrenic nerve, to prevent reunion such as may follow phrenicotomy. SYN phrenectomy, phrenicoexeresis, phreniconeurectomy. [phreni- + G. *ektome,* excision]

phren·i·cla·sia (fren-i-klā'zē-ă). Crushing of a section of the phrenic nerve to produce a temporary paralysis of the diaphragm. SYN phrenemphraxis, phrenicotripsy. [phreni- + G. *klasis,* a breaking away]

phren·i·co·col·ic (fren'i-kō-kol'ik). Relating to the diaphragm and the colon. SYN phrenocolic.

phren·i·co·ex·er·e·sis (fren'i-kō-ek-ser'ĕ-sis). SYN phrenicectomy. [phrenico- + G. *exairesis,* a taking out, fr. *haireo,* to take, grasp]

phren·i·co·gas·tric (fren'i-kō-gas'trik). Relating to the diaphragm and the stomach. SYN phrenogastric.

phren·i·co·glot·tic (fren'i-kō-glo'tik). Relating to the diaphragm and the glottis; denoting a spasm involving the diaphragm and the vocal cords.

phren·i·co·he·pa·tic (fren′i-kō-he-pa′tik). Relating to the diaphragm and the liver. SYN phrenohepatic.

phren·i·co·neu·rec·to·my (fren′i-kō-noo-rek′tō-mē). SYN phrenicectomy.

phren·i·co·splen·ic (fren′i-kō-splen′ik). Relating to the diaphragm and the spleen.

phren·i·cot·o·my (fren-i-kot′ō-mē). Section of the phrenic nerve in order to induce unilateral paralysis of the diaphragm, which is then pushed up by the abdominal viscera and exerts compression upon a diseased lung. [phrenico- + G. *tomē,* incision]

phren·i·co·trip·sy (fren′i-kō-trip′sē). SYN phreniclasia. [phrenico- + G. *tripsis,* a rubbing]

△**phreno-, phren-, phreni-, phrenico-.** **1.** The diaphragm. **2.** The mind. **3.** The phrenic nerve. [G. *phrēn,* diaphragm, mind, heart (as seat of emotions)]

phren·o·car·dia (fren-ō-kar′dē-ă). Precordial pain and dyspnea of psychogenic origin, often a symptom of anxiety neurosis. SEE cardiac *neurosis.* SYN cardiophrenia. [phreno- + G. *kardia,* heart]

phren·o·col·ic (fren′ō-kol′ik). SYN phrenicocolic. [phreno- + G. *kolon,* colon]

phren·o·gas·tric (fren-ō-gas′trik). SYN phrenicogastric. [phreno- + G. *gastēr,* stomach]

phren·o·graph (fren′ō-graf). An instrument for recording graphically the movements of the diaphragm. [phreno- + G. *graphō,* to record]

phren·o·he·pat·ic (fren′ō-hĕ-pat′ik). SYN phrenicohepatic. [phreno- + G. *hepar,* liver]

phre·nol·o·gist (frĕ-nol′ō-jist). One who claims to be able to diagnose mental and behavioral characteristics by a study of the external configuration of the skull. [see phrenology]

phre·nol·o·gy (frĕ-nol′ō-jē). An obsolete doctrine that each of the mental faculties is located in a definite part of the cerebral cortex, the size of which part varies in a direct ratio with the development and strength of the corresponding faculty, this size being indicated by the external configuration of the skull. SYN craniognomy. [phreno- + G. *logos,* study]

phren·o·ple·gia (fren-ō-plē′jē-ă). Paralysis of the diaphragm. [phreno- + G. *plēgē,* stroke]

phren·op·to·sia (fren-op-tō′sē-ă). An abnormal sinking down of the diaphragm. [phreno- + G. *ptōsis,* a falling]

phren·o·sin (fren′ō-sin). A cerebroside abundant in white matter of the brain, composed of cerebronic acid, D-galactose, and sphingosine. SYN cerebron.

phren·o·sin·ic ac·id (fren-ō-sin′ik). SYN cerebronic acid.

phren·o·spasm (fren′ō-spazm). Diaphragmatic spasm, as in hiccup. [phreno- + G. *spasmos,* spasm]

phren·o·tro·pic (fren-ō-trop′ik). Affecting or working through the mind or brain. [phreno- + G. *tropē,* a turning]

phryn·o·der·ma (frin-ō-der′mă). A follicular hyperkeratotic eruption thought to be due to deficiency of vitamin A. SYN toad skin. [G. *phrynos,* toad, + *derma,* skin]

phry·nol·y·sin (frĭ-nol′ĭ-sin). The poison of the fire-toad (*Bombinator igneus*). [G. *phrynos,* toad, + *lysis,* solution]

PHS Abbreviation for Public Health Service.

pH-stat. A device for continuously sensing the pH of a solution and automatically adding acid or alkali as necessary to keep the pH constant; used to follow the time course of reactions that liberate an acid or alkali.

o-**phtha·lal·de·hyde** (thal-al′de-hīd). A reagent used in the identification and the detection of amino acid.

phthal·ein (thal′ē-in). One of a group of highly colored compounds based on a triphenylmethyl base; e.g., phenolphthalein.

phthal·ic ac·id (thal′ik). *o*-Benzenedicarboxylic acid.

phthal·o·yl (thal′ō-il). The diacyl radical of phthalic acid.

phthal·yl (thal′il). The monoacyl radical of phthalic acid.

phthal·yl·sul·fa·cet·a·mide (thal′il-sŭl-fă-set′ă-mīd). N^1-acetyl-N^4-phthalylsulfanilamide; a sulfonamide used in the treatment of enteric infections.

phthal·yl·sul·fa·thi·a·zole (thal′il-sŭl-fă-thī′ă-zōl). A sulfonamide used in the treatment of enteric infections.

phthi·ri·o·pho·bia (thī′rē-ō-fō′bē-ă). SYN pediculophobia. [G. *phtheir,* louse, + *phobos,* fear]

Phthi·rus (thī′rŭs). SEE *Pthirus.* [L. *phthir;* G. *phtheir,* a louse]

△**phthisio-.** Phthisis (tuberculosis). [G. *phthisis,* a wasting]

phthis·i·ol·o·gist (thī-zē-ol′ō-jist). Obsolete term for specialist in tuberculosis.

△**phyco-.** Seaweed. [G. *phykos*]

Phy·co·my·ce·tes (fī′kō-mī-sē′tēz). SYN Zygomycetes. [phyco- + G. *mykēs,* fungus]

phy·co·my·ce·to·sis (fī′kō-mī-sē-tō′sis). SYN zygomycosis.

phy·co·my·co·sis (fī′kō-mī′kō-sis). SYN zygomycosis. **subcutaneous p.,** SYN *entomophthoramycosis* basidiobolae.

phy·lac·a·gog·ic (fī-lak-ă-goj′ik). Stimulating the production of protective antibodies. [G. *phylaxis,* a guarding, protection, + *agogos,* leading]

phy·lax·is (fī-lak′sis). Protection against infection. [G. a guarding, protection]

phy·let·ic (fī-let′ik). Denoting the evolution of sequential changes in a line of descent by which one species is transformed into a new species. [G. *phyletikos,* tribal, fr. *phylē,* a tribe]

△**phyllo-.** A leaf; leaf-like; chlorophyll. [G. *phyllon,* foliage]

phyl·lode (fil′ōd). A flattened leaflike petiole; applied to any structure resembling a leaf, especially to a cross section of a neoplasm with a foliated structure, such as cystosarcoma phyllodes. [G. *phyllōdēs,* like leaves, fr. *phyllon,* leaf, + *eidos,* resemblance]

phyl·lo·qui·none (K), phyl·lo·qui·none K (fil-ō-kwin′ōn, -kwī′nōn). Isolated from alfalfa; also prepared synthetically; major form of vitamin K found in plants. SYN phytomenadione, phytonadione, vitamin K_1, vitamin K_1(20).

p. reductase, SYN *NADPH* dehydrogenase (quinone).

△**phylo-.** Tribe, race; a taxonomic phylum. [G. *phylon,* tribe]

phy·lo·a·nal·y·sis (fī′lō-ă-nal′i-sis). **1.** The study of bioracial origins. **2.** A rarely used term for a method of investigating individual and collective behavioral disorders putatively arising from impaired tensional processes. [phylo- + analysis]

phy·lo·gen·e·sis (fī-lō-jen′ĕ-sis). SYN phylogeny. [phylo- + G. *genesis,* origin]

phy·lo·ge·net·ic, phy·lo·gen·ic (fī′lō-jĕ-net′ik, -jen′ik). Relating to phylogenesis.

phy·log·e·ny (fī-loj′ĕ-nē). The evolutionary development of species, as distinguished from ontogeny, development of the individual. SYN phylogenesis.

phy·lum, pl. **phy·la** (fī′lŭm, fī′lă). A taxonomic division below the kingdom and above the class. [Mod. L. fr. G. *phylon,* tribe]

phy·ma·toid (fī′mă-toyd). Resembling a neoplasm. [G. *phyma,* a tumor, + *eidos,* resemblance]

phy·ma·tor·rhy·sin (fī′mă-tōr′i-sin). A variety of melanin obtained from certain melanotic neoplasms, and from hair and other heavily pigmented parts. [G. *phyma* (phymat-), tumor, + *rhysis,* a flowing]

Phy·sa (fī′să). Type genus of the freshwater pulmonate snails (family Physidae), which includes several common American species such as *P. parkeri, P. gyrina,* and *P. integra;* they are intermediate hosts of a number of bird and animal trematodes, including several that cause schistosome dermatitis in humans. [G. a pair of bellows; an air bubble; bladder]

Physalia. A genus of the invertebrate phylum Cnidaria that includes the Portuguese man-of-war.

P. physalis, the Portuguese man-of-war, a jellyfishlike animal consisting of a complex colony of individual members that can inflict extremely painful stings. SYN Portuguese man-of-war.

phys·a·lif·er·ous (fis-ă-lif′er-ŭs). SYN physaliphorous.

phy·sal·i·form (fi-sal′i-fōrm). Like a bubble or small bleb. [G. *physallis,* bladder, bubble, + L. *forma,* form]

phy·sal·i·phore (fi-sal′i-fōr). A mother cell, or giant cell containing

ing a large vacuole, in a malignant growth. [G. *physallis,* bladder, bubble, + *phoros,* bearing]

phys·a·liph·or·ous (fis-ă-lif′ŏr-ŭs). Having bubbles or vacuoles. SYN physaliferous. [G. *physallis,* bladder, bubble, + *phoros,* bearing]

phys·a·lis (fis′ă-lis). A vacuole in a giant cell found in certain malignant neoplasms, such as chordoma. [G. *physallis,* a bladder]

Phy·sa·lop·tera (fī′să-lop′ter-ă, fis-). A large genus of spiruroid roundworms parasitic in the stomach and duodenum of vertebrates, especially birds and mammals; they are transmitted via insect and annelid intermediate hosts and are frequently pathogenic, causing erosions and catarrhal gastritis. *P. caucasica* is a species reported in humans in the southern part of the USSR; *P. mordens* is a species from tropical Africa found only rarely in the esophagus, stomach, and intestine of humans (probably cases of temporary infection from ingestion of infected insects). [G. *physallis,* bladder, + *pteron,* wing]

phy·sa·lop·ter·i·a·sis (fī′să-lop-ter-ī′ă-sis). Infection of animals and humans with nematodes of the genus *Physaloptera.*

phys·e·al (fiz′ē-ăl). Pertaining to the physis, or growth cartilage area, separating the metaphysis and the epiphysis in skeletally immature bones.

⌂**physi-.** SEE physio-.

phys·i·at·ri·cian (fiz′ē-ă-trish′ŭn). A physician who specializes in physiatry (rehabilitation medicine).

phys·i·at·rics (fiz-ē-at′riks). **1.** Old term for physical *therapy.* **2.** Rehabilitation management. [G. *physis,* nature, + *iatrikos,* healing]

phys·i·a·trist (fiz-ī′ă-trist). A physician who specializes in physical medicine.

phys·i·a·try (fi-zī′ă-trē; fiz-ē-at′rē). SYN physical *medicine.*

phys·ic (fiz′ik). **1.** The art of medicine. **2.** A medicine; often a lay term for a cathartic. [G. *physikos,* natural, physical]

phys·i·cal (fiz′i-kăl). Relating to the body, as distinguished from the mind. [Mod. L. *physicalis,* fr. G. *physikos*]

phy·si·cian (fi-zish′ŭn). **1.** A doctor; a person who has been educated, trained, and licensed to practice the art and science of medicine. **2.** A practitioner of medicine, as contrasted with a surgeon. [Fr. *physicien,* a natural philosopher]

attending p., (1) p. responsible for the care of a patient; **(2)** p. supervising the care of patients by interns, residents, and/or medical students. **(3)** a doctor who has completed internship and residency.

family p., a p. who specializes in family practice.

hospital-based p., SYN hospitalist (1).

osteopathic p., a practitioner of osteopathy. SYN osteopath.

resident p., SYN resident.

phy·si·cian as·sis·tant (P.A.). A person who is trained, certified, and licensed to perform history taking, physical examination, diagnosis, and treatment of commonly encountered medical problems, and certain technical skills, under the supervision of a licensed physician, and who thereby extends the physician's capacity to provide medical care. Many subspecialties exist, such as orthopedist's assistant, sports injury assistant, pediatrician's assistant, etc.

Physick, Philip Syng, U.S. surgeon, 1768–1837. SEE P. *pouches,* under *pouch.*

phys·i·co·chem·i·cal (fiz′i-kō-kem′i-kăl). Relating to the field of physical chemistry.

phys·ics (fiz′iks). The branch of science concerned with the phenomena of matter and energy and their interactions. SEE physic.

radiation p., the scientific discipline of the application of p. to the use of ionizing radiation in therapy and in diagnostic radiology; including, by extension, nuclear medicine applications, ultrasound, and magnetic resonance imaging.

⌂**physio-, physi-. 1.** Physical, physiological. **2.** Natural, relating to physics. [G. *physis,* nature]

phys·i·o·gen·ic (fiz′ē-ō-jen′ik). Related to or caused by physiologic activity. [physio- + G. *genesis,* origin]

phys·i·og·no·my (fiz-ē-og′nō-mē). **1.** The physical appearance of one's face, countenance, or habitus, especially regarded as an indication of character. **2.** Estimation of one's character and mental qualities by a study of the face and other external bodily features. [physio- + G. *gnōmōn,* a judge]

phys·i·og·no·sis (fiz-ē-og-nō′sis). Diagnosis of disease based upon a study of the facial appearance or bodily habitus. [physio- + G. *gnōsis,* knowledge]

phys·i·o·log·ic, phys·i·o·log·i·cal (fiz-ē-ō-loj′ik, -loj′i-kăl). **1.** Relating to physiology. **2.** Normal, as opposed to pathologic; denoting the various vital processes. **3.** Denoting something that is apparent from its functional effects rather than from its anatomical structure; e.g., a p. sphincter. **4.** Denoting a dose or the effects of such a dose (of a chemical agent that either is or mimics a hormone, neurotransmitter, or other naturally occurring agent) that is within the range of concentrations or potencies that would occur naturally. Cf. homeopathic (2), pharmacologic (2), supraphysiologic.

phys·i·o·log·i·co·an·a·tom·i·cal (fiz′ē-ō-loj′i-kō-an-ă-tom′i-kăl). Relating to both physiology and anatomy.

phys·i·ol·o·gist (fiz-ē-ol′ō-jist). A specialist in physiology.

phys·i·ol·o·gy (fiz-ē-ol′ō-jē). The science concerned with the normal vital processes of animal and vegetable organisms, especially as to how things normally function in the living organism rather than to their anatomical structure, their biochemical composition, or how they are affected by drugs or disease. [L. or G. *physiologia,* fr. G. *physis,* nature, + *logos,* study]

comparative p., the science concerned with the differences in the vital processes in different species of organisms, particularly with a view to the adaptation of the processes to the specific needs of the species, to illuminating the evolutionary relationships among different species, or to establishing other interspecific generalizations and relationships.

general p., the science of the functions or vital processes common to almost all living things, whether animal or plant, as opposed to aspects of p. peculiar to particular types of animals or plants, or to the application of p. to applied sciences such as medicine and agriculture.

hominal p., p. as applied to the elucidation of the normal functions of the human being.

pathologic p., that part of the science of disease concerned with disordered function, as distinguished from anatomical lesions. SYN physiopathology.

phys·i·o·path·o·log·ic (fiz′ē-ō-path-ō-loj′ik). Relating to pathologic physiology.

phys·i·o·pa·thol·o·gy (fiz′ē-ō-pă-thol′ō-jē). SYN pathologic *physiology.*

phys·i·o·psy·chic (fiz′ē-ō-sī′kik). Pertaining to both mind and body.

phys·i·o·py·rex·ia (fiz′ē-ō-pī-rek′sē-ă). Fever produced by a physical agent. [physio- + G. *pyrexis,* feverishness]

phys·i·o·ther·a·peu·tic (fiz′ē-ō-thār-ă-pū′tik). Pertaining to physical *therapy.*

phys·i·o·ther·a·pist (fiz′ē-ō-thār′ă-pist). A physical therapist. SEE physical *therapy* (2).

phys·i·o·ther·a·py (fiz′ē-ō-thār′ă-pē). SYN physical *therapy* (1). [physio- + G. *therapeia,* treatment]

oral p., the use of a toothbrush, interdental stimulator, floss, irrigating device, or other adjunctive aid to maintain oral health.

phy·sique (fi-zēk′). constitutional type; the physical or bodily structure; the "build." [Fr.]

phy·sis (fī′sis). A term sometimes used in referring to the epiphysial cartilage. [G. growth]

⌂**physo-. 1.** Tendency to swell or inflate. **2.** Relation to air or gas. [G. *physaō,* to inflate, distend]

phy·so·cele (fī′sō-sēl). **1.** A circumscribed swelling due to the presence of gas. **2.** A hernial sac distended with gas. [physo- + G. *kēlē,* tumor, hernia]

Phy·so·ceph·a·lus sex·a·la·tus (fī′sō-sef′ă-lŭs sek′să-lā′tŭs). A small species of spiruroid nematodes (family Spiruridae) found in the stomach of pigs, horses, camels, rabbits, and hares; worldwide in distribution, and especially prevalent in hogs. [G. *physa*, bellows, + *kephalē*, head]

phy·so·ceph·a·ly (fī-sō-sef′ă-lē). Swelling of the head resulting from introduction of air into the subcutaneous tissues. [physo- + G. *kephalē*, head]

phy·so·me·tra (fī-sō-mē′tră). Distention of the uterine cavity with air or gas. SYN uterine tympanites. [physo- + G. *mētra*, uterus]

Phy·sop·sis (fī-sop′sis). A subgenus of the genus *Bulinus*, most species of which transmit the human blood fluke, *Schistosoma haematobium*, and some animal schistosomes in Africa south of the Sahara. [G. *physis*, growth, + *opsis*, aspect, appearance]

phy·so·py·o·sal·pinx (fī′sō-pī-ō-sal′pingks). Pyosalpinx accompanied by a formation of gas in a uterine tube. [physo- + G. *pyon*, pus, + *salpinx*, trumpet]

phy·so·stig·ma (fī-sō-stig′mă). The dried seed of *Physostigma venenosum* (family Leguminosae), a vine of western Africa; it contains the alkaloids physostigmine (eserine), eseramine, eseridine (geneserine) and physovenine; in toxic doses it causes vomiting, colic, salivation, diarrhea, convulsions, sweating, dyspnea, vertigo, slow pulse, and extreme prostration. SYN Calabar bean, ordeal bean. [G. *physa*, bellows, + *stigma*, a mark, spot; so called because of the shape of the stigma]

phy·so·stig·mine (fī-sō-stig′mēn, -min). An alkaloid of physostigma; it is a reversible inhibitor of the cholinesterases, and prevents destruction of acetylcholine; used as a cholinergic agent, and experimentally to enhance the action of acetylcholine at any of its sites of liberation. SYN eserine.

  p. salicylate, used by conjunctival instillation to reduce tension in glaucoma, in the treatment of postoperative intestinal atony and urinary retention, in the management of myasthenia gravis, and to counteract excessive doses of tubocurarine; also available as p. sulfate, with the same uses. SYN eserine salicylate.

phyt-. SEE phyto-.

phy·tan·ate (fī′tan-āt). The anion of phytanic acid.

  p. α-oxidase, an enzyme that oxidizes phytanic acid, removing the carboxyl group.

phy·tan·ic ac·id (fī-tan′ik). A branched-chain fatty acid that accumulates in the serum and tissues in Refsum disease and attributed to the hereditary absence of phytanate α-oxidase; arises from phytol and acts as an inhibitor of the α-oxidation of palmitic (hexadecanoic) acid; it also accumulates in a number of other disorders, notably peroxisomal disorders.

6-phy·tase (fī′tās). Phytate 6-phosphate; an enzyme-hydrolyzing phytic acid, removing the 6-phosphoric group, thus producing orthophosphate and 1L-*myo*-1,2,3,4,5-pentakisphosphate.

phy·tate (fī′tāt). A salt or ester of phytic acid.

phy·tic ac·id (fī′tik). The hexakisphosphoric ester of *myo*-inositol; the mixed salt with magnesium and calcium is phytin.

phy·tin (fī′tin). The calcium magnesium salt of phytic acid; a dietary supplement used to provide calcium, organic phosphorus, and *myo*-inositol.

phyto-, phyt-. Plants. [G. *phyton*, a plant]

phy·to·ag·glu·ti·nin (fī′tō-ă-gloo′ti-nin). A lectin that causes agglutination of erythrocytes or of leukocytes.

phy·to·be·zoar (fī-tō-bē′zōr). A gastric concretion formed of vegetable fibers, with the seeds and skins of fruits, and sometimes starch granules and fat globules. SYN food ball. [phyto- + bezoar]

phy·to·chem·is·try (fī-tō-kem′is-trē). The biochemical study of plants; concerned with the identification, biosynthesis, and metabolism of chemical constituents of plants; especially used in regard to natural products.

phy·to·der·ma·ti·tis (fī′tō-der-mă-tī′tis). Dermatitis caused by various mechanisms, including mechanical and chemical injury, allergy, or photosensitization (phytophotodermatitis) at skin sites previously exposed to plants.

Phy·to·fla·gel·la·ta (fī′tō-flaj-ĕ-lā′tă). A subclass of Phytomastigophorea, the members of which have yellow or green chromatophores. [phyto- + L. *flagellum*, a whip]

phy·to·hem·ag·glu·ti·nin (PHA) (fī′tō-hēm-ă-gloo′ti-nin). A phytomitogen from plants that agglutinates red blood cells. The

term is commonly used specifically to refer to the lectin obtained from the red kidney bean (*Phaseolus vulgaris*), which is also a mitogen that stimulates T lymphocytes more vigorously than B lymphocytes. SYN phytolectin.

phy·toid (fī′toyd). Resembling a plant; denoting an animal having many of the biologic characteristics of a vegetable. [G. *phytōdēs*, fr. *phyton*, plant, + *eidos*, resemblance]

phy·tol (fī′tol). An unsaturated primary alcohol derived from the hydrolysis of chlorophyll; a constituent of vitamins E and K₁. SYN phytyl alcohol.

phy·to·lec·tin (fī-tō-lek′tin). SYN phytohemagglutinin.

Phy·to·mas·ti·gi·na (fī′tō-mas-ti-jī′nă). Former term for plant-like flagellates, originally classified as a suborder or order, raised to the class Phytomastigophorea (Phytomastigophorasida) in recent classifications. [phyto- + G. *mastix*, whip]

Phy·to·mas·ti·go·pho·ras·i·da (fī′tō-mas′ti-gō-fō-ras′i-dă). SYN Phytomastigophorea.

Phy·to·mas·ti·goph·o·rea (fī′tō-mas′ti-gof-ō-rē′ă). A class of the subphylum Mastigophora (flagellates) within the phylum Sarcomastigophora (flagellate and ameboid protozoans), consisting mostly of free-living plantlike flagellates with or without chloroplasts, and usually with one or two flagella. Cf. Zoomastigophorea. SYN Phytomastigophorasida. [phyto- + G. *mastix*, whip, + *phoros*, bearing]

phy·to·men·a·di·one (fī′tō-men-ă-dī′ōn). SYN phylloquinone.

phy·to·mi·to·gen (fī-tō-mī′tō-jen). A mitogenic lectin causing lymphocyte transformation accompanied by mitotic proliferation of the resulting blast cells identical to that produced by antigenic stimulation; e.g., phytohemagglutinin, concanavalin A.

phy·to·na·di·one (fī′tō-nā-dī′ōn). SYN phylloquinone.

phy·toph·a·gous (fī-tof′ă-gŭs). Plant-eating; vegetarian. [phyto- + G. *phagō*, to eat]

phy·to·pho·to·der·ma·ti·tis (fī′tō-fō′tō-der-mă-tī′tis). Phytodermatitis resulting from photosensitization.

phy·to·pneu·mo·co·ni·o·sis (fī′tō-noo′mō-kō-nē-ō′sis). A chronic fibrous reaction in the lungs due to the inhalation of particles of vegetable origin. [phyto- + pneumoconiosis]

phy·to·por·phy·rin (fī-tō-pōr′fī-rin). **1.** A porphyrin similar to the pheophorbide of the chlorophylls but with the vinyl group replaced by an ethyl group, with no methoxycarbonyl group, and minus two hydrogen atoms, producing one more double bond in ring D. **2.** Any plant porphyrin.

phy·to·sis (fī-tō-sis). A disease process caused by infection with a vegetable organism, such as a fungus.

phy·to·sphin·go·sine (fī-tō-sfing′gō-sēn, -sin). A sphingosine derivative isolated from various plants.

phy·to·ste·rol (fi-tō-stēr′ol). Generic term for the sterols of plants.

phy·to·ste·ro·lem·ia (fī-tō-stēr′ol-ē-mē-ă). An inherited disorder in which there is a hyperabsorption of phytosterols and shellfish sterols resulting in tendon and tuberous xanthomata. SYN sitosterolemia.

phy·to·tox·ic (fī-tō-tok′sik). **1.** Poisonous to plant life. **2.** Pertaining to a phytotoxin.

phy·to·tox·in (fī-tō-tok′sin). A toxic substance of plant origin. SYN plant toxin. [phyto- + G. *toxikon*, poison]

phy·to·trich·o·be·zoar (fī′tō-trik′ō-bē′zōr). SYN trichophytobezoar.

phy·tyl (fī′til). The radical found in phylloquinone (vitamin K₁); a tetraprenyl radical, reduced in 3 of the 4 prenyl groups.

phy·tyl al·co·hol. SYN phytol.

PI Abbreviation for Periodontal Index.

Pi Abbreviation for inorganic *phosphate*.

p*I* The pH value for the isoelectric *point* of a given substance.

pi (π, Π) (pī). **1.** The 16th letter of the Greek alphabet. **2.** (Π). Symbol for osmotic pressure; in mathematics, symbol for the product of a series. **3.** (π). Symbol for the ratio of the circumference of a circle to its diameter (approximately 3.14159). **4.** Symbol for *pros*.

pia (pī′ă, pē′ă). SYN pia mater. [L. fem. of *pius*, tender]

pia·a·rach·ni·tis (pī′ă-ă-rak-nī′tis). SYN leptomeningitis.

pia·a·rach·noid (pī′ă-ă-rak′noyd, pē′ă-). SYN leptomeninx.

pi·al (pī′al, pē′al). Relating to the pia mater.

pia mat·er (pī′ă mā′ter, pē′ă mah′ter) [TA]. A delicate vasculated fibrous membrane firmly adherent to the glial capsule of the brain (**p. m. cranialis** [TA]) and spinal cord (pia mater spinalis [TA] or membrana limitans gliae); following exactly the outer markings of the cerebrum and also the ependymal lining circumference of the choroid membranes and plexus, it invests the cerebellum but not so intimately as it does the cerebrum, not dipping down into all the smaller sulci. The p. m. and the arachnoid are collectively called leptomenin [TA], as distinguished from dura mater or pachymeninx. SYN pia. [L. tender, affectionate mother]

pi·an (pē-an′, pī′an). SYN yaws.

p. bois, a form of New World cutaneous leishmaniasis caused by *Leishmania braziliensis guyanensis* in the Amazon delta; a small proportion of cases are said to metastasize to the nasal mucosa with espundia-like involvement. SYN bosch yaws, bush yaws.

pi·a·rach·noid (pī′ă-rak′noyd). SYN leptomeninx.

pi·blok·to, pi·blok·tog (pib-lok′tō). A hysterical dissociative state, usually occurring in Innit women, in which the individual screams, tears off clothes, and runs out into the snow; afterward, there is no memory of the episode. [Native]

pi·ca (pī′kă, pē′kă). A perverted appetite for substances not fit as food or of no nutritional value; e.g., clay, dried paint, starch, ice. [L. *pica,* magpie]

Picchini. Luigi, late 19th century Italian physician. SEE Picchini *syndrome.*

Pick, Arnold, Czechoslovakian psychiatrist, 1851–1924. SEE P. *atrophy, bundle, disease.*

Pick, Friedel, German physician, 1867–1926. SEE P. *bodies,* under *body, disease, syndrome.*

Pick, Ludwig, German physician, 1868–1935. SEE P. *cell;* Niemann-P. *cell, disease.*

Pickles, William, British general practitioner, researcher in transmission of infections in isolated communities, 1885–1969. SEE P. *chart.*

pick·ling (pik′ling). In dentistry, the process of cleansing metallic surfaces of the products of oxidation and other impurities by immersion in acid.

Pickworth, Frederick A., *1889. SEE Lepehne-P. *stain.*

♻**pico-.** **1.** Combining form meaning small. **2 (p).** Prefix used in the SI and metric system to signify submultiples of one-trillionth (10^{-12}). SYN bicro-. [It. *piccolo*]

pi·co·gram (pg) (pī′kō-gram, pē′kō-gram). One-trillionth of a gram.

pi·co·ka·tal (pkat) (pī′kō-kat′ăl; pē′ko-kat′ăl). One trillionth of a katal (10^{-12} katal).

pi·co·lin·ic ac·id (pik-ō-lin′ik). Pyridine-4-carboxylic acid; an isomer of nicotinic acid.

pi·co·li·nur·ic ac·id (pik-ō-li-noor′ik). *N*-Picolinoylglycine; the amide, with glycine, of picolinic acid; a hippuric acid analog in which picolinic acid, rather than benzoic acid, is conjugated with glycine and excreted.

pi·com·e·ter (pm) (pī′kō-me-ter). One-trillionth of a meter. SYN bicron.

pi·co·mole (pmol) (pē′kō-mōl; pī′kō-mōl). One-trillionth of a mole (10^{-12} mol).

Pi·cor·na·vir·i·dae (pi-kōr-nă-vir′i-dē). A family of very small (20–30 nm) ether-resistant, nonenveloped viruses having a core of positive sense single-stranded infectious RNA enclosed in a capsid of icosahedral symmetry with 60 capsomeres. Numerous species (including the polioviruses, coxsackieviruses, and echoviruses) are included in the family. There are five accepted genera: Enterovirus, Rhinovirus, Hepatovirus, Cardiovirus, and Aphthovirus. [It. *piccolo,* very small, + RNA + -viridae]

pi·cor·na·vi·rus (pi-kōr-nă-vī′rŭs). A virus of the family Picornaviridae.

pic·ram·ic ac·id (pī-kram′ik). Red crystals sometimes found in the blood of persons poisoned with picric acid; the crystals are formed as a result of partial reduction of picric acid.

Pic·ras·ma (pi-kraz′mă). SEE quassia. [L., fr. G. *pikrasmos,* bitterness]

pic·rate (pik′rāt). A salt of picric acid.

pic·ric ac·id (pik′rik). Has been used as an application in burns, eczema, erysipelas, and pruritus. SYN carbazotic acid, nitroxanthic acid. [G. *pikros,* bitter]

pic·ro·car·mine (pik-rō-kar′min, -mēn). SEE picrocarmine *stain.*

pic·ro·for·mol (pik′rō-fōr′mol). SEE picroformol *fixative.*

pic·ro·ni·gro·sin (pik′rō-nī′grō-sin). SEE picronigrosin *stain.*

pic·ro·tox·in (pik′rō-tok′sin). A very bitter neutral principle derived from the fruit of *Anamirta cocculus* (family Menispermaceae); a central nervous system stimulant, used as an antidote for poisoning by barbiturates and certain other CNS-depressant drugs; a convulsant and GABA antagonist used extensively in experimental procedures studying seizure mechanisms. SYN cocculin. [G. *pikros,* bitter, + *toxicon,* poison]

pic·ro·tox·in·in (pik-rō-tok′si-nin). A lactone breakdown product of picrotoxin; pharmacologic properties resemble those of picrotoxin.

pic·ryl (pik′ril). The organic radical derived from picric acid by removal of the hydroxyl group.

pic·to·graph (pik′tō-graf). A vision test chart for illiterates.

PID Abbreviation for pelvic inflammatory *disease.*

Pidgin Sign English (PSE) (pij′in). A system of communication that is a manual representation of English in which American Sign Language signs are used in English word order; there are no inflectional signs, and finger spelling is used for proper names.

pie·bald·ism (pī′bawld-izm) [MIM*172800]. Patchy absence of the pigment of scalp hair, giving a streaked appearance; patches of vitiligo may be present in other areas due to absence of melanocytes; often transmitted as an autosomal dominant trait caused by mutation in the KIT protooncogene on 4q and may be associated with neurologic defects [MIM*172850] or eye changes [MIM*172870]. Cf. Waardenburg *syndrome.* SYN cutaneous albinism, piebald skin, piebaldness.

pie·bald·ness (pī′bawld-ness). SYN piebaldism.

piece (pēs). A part or portion.

end p., a part of the spermatozoon consisting of an axoneme surrounded only by the flagellar membrane.

Fab p., SYN Fab *fragment.*

Fc p., SYN Fc *fragment.*

middle p., a part of the spermatozoon characterized by an axoneme and by a sheath of mitochondria arranged in a tight helix.

principal p., the principal part of the spermatozoon, which is about 45 μm long and has a characteristic fibrous sheath surrounding the axoneme.

pie·dra (pē-ā′dră). A fungus disease of the hair characterized by the formation of numerous waxy, small, firm, nodular masses on the hair shaft. SEE ALSO trichosporosis. [Sp. a stone]

black p., p. involving the hairs of the scalp, caused by *Piedraia hortae* and characterized by firmly adherent black, hard, gritty nodules composed of an organized, firmly cemented mass of fungus cells; the fungal growth is always located above the level of the hair follicles; the disease occurs in humid tropical areas of the Americas, Africa, and Asia, and attacks chimpanzees and other primates as well as humans.

p. nos′tras, a condition similar to p., but affecting the hair of the beard.

white p., p. of the beard, moustache, and genital areas, as well as the scalp, caused by *Trichosporon beigelii* and found in South America, Europe, and Japan; characterized by soft, mucilaginous, white to light brown nodules, within as well as on the hairs.

Pi·e·dra·ia (pī′ě-drī′ă). A genus of fungi, based on *P. hortae,* which is probably the only species and which causes black piedra. [see piedra]

pieds ter·mi·naux (pē-e′ter-mē-nō′). SYN axon *terminals,* under *terminal.* [Fr., end feet]

Pierini, Luigi, 20th century Argentinian dermatologist. SEE *atrophoderma* of Pasini and P.

Pierre Robin. SEE Robin.

pi·e·sim·e·ter, pi·e·som·e·ter (pī-ĕ-sim′ĕ-ter, pī-ĕ-som′ĕ-ter). An instrument for measuring the pressure of a gas or a fluid. SYN piezometer. [G. *piesis,* pressure]

Hales p., a glass tube inserted into an artery at right angles to its axis, the pressure being shown by the height to which the blood ascends in the tube.

pi·e·sis (pī′ĕ-sis). SYN blood *pressure.* [G. pressure]

pi·e·zo·chem·is·try (pī-ĕ-zō-kem′is-trē). The study of the effect of very high pressures on chemical reactions.

pi·e·zo·e·lec·tric (pī′ĕ-zō-ē-lek′trik). Pertaining to piezoelectricity.

pi·e·zo·e·lec·tric·i·ty (pī′ĕ-zō-ē-lek-tris′i-tē). Electric currents generated by pressure upon certain crystals, e.g., quartz, mica, calcite. [G. *piezō,* to press, squeeze, + electricity]

pi·e·zo·gen·ic (pī′ĕ-zō-jen′ik). Resulting from pressure. [G. *piezo,* to press, squeeze, + *genesis,* origin]

pi·e·zom·e·ter (pī-ĕ-zom′ĕ-ter). SYN piesimeter.

pig. A container, usually made of lead, used for shielding vials or syringes containing radioactive materials. [jargon]

pig·bel. A type of necrotizing enteritis endemic in the Papua New Guinea highlands caused by the B toxin of *Clostridium perfringens* type C; occurs predominantly in children because of poor immunity to B toxin and a low level of intestinal proteases resulting from a diet low in protein and high in sweet potatoes.

pig·ment. 1. Any coloring matter, as that of the red blood cells, hair, iris, etc., or the stains used in histologic or bacteriologic work, or that in paints. **2.** A medicinal preparation for external use, applied to the skin like paint, or coloring agents used in paints. [L. *pigmentum,* paint]

bile p.'s, coloring matter in the bile derived from porphyrins by rupture of a methane bridge; e.g., bilirubin, biliverdin.

chymotropic p., a p. dissolved in the vacuole of a plant cell. [G. *chymos,* juice, + *tropē,* turning, inclination, + -ic]

formalin p., a p. formed when acid aqueous solutions of formaldehyde act on blood-rich tissues; characterized by rotation of the plane of polarized light, withstanding extraction in aqueous and lipid solvents, being bleached in acids and hydrogen peroxide; not formed when tissue is fixed with formaldehyde buffered to pH levels above 6.

hematogenous p., a p. derived from the hemoglobin of the red blood cells.

hepatogenous p., bile p. derived from the destruction of hemoglobin in the liver.

malarial p., a dark brown, granular p. that rotates the plane of polarized light and has other properties similar to formalin p.; occurs in parasites, such as *Plasmodium malariae,* around brain capillaries, and in fixed macrophages of spleen, liver, bone marrow, and lymph nodes; composed of excess protein, an iron porphyrin, and hematin left over from the metabolism of hemoglobin by the malarial parasite within the red blood cell. SEE malarial pigment *stain.*

melanotic p., SYN melanin.

natural p., a naturally occurring colored compound; absorbs light in the visible range of the electromagnetic spectrum. Cf. structural *color.* SYN biochrome.

respiratory p.'s, the oxygen-carrying (colored) substances in blood and tissues (hemoglobin, myoglobin, hemocyanin, etc.).

visual p.'s, the photopigments in the retinal cones and rods that absorb light and initiate the visual process.

wear-and-tear p., lipofuscin that accumulates in aging or atrophic cells as a residue of lysosomal digestion.

pig·men·tary (pig′men-tār-ē). Relating to a pigment.

pig·men·ta·tion (pig-men-tā′shŭn). Coloration, either normal or pathologic, of the skin or tissues resulting from a deposit of pigment.

arsenic p., generalized but spotty increased melanin p. of the skin in chronic arsenic poisoning.

exogenous p., discoloration of the skin or tissues by a pigment introduced from without.

pig·ment·ed (pig′men-ted). Colored as the result of a deposit of pigment.

pig·men·to·ly·sin (pig-men-tol′i-sin). An antibody causing destruction of pigment. [L. *pigmentum,* pigment, + G. *lysis,* a loosening]

pig·men·tum ni·grum (pig-men′tŭm nī′grŭm). Melanin of the choroid coat of the eye.

pig·my (pig′mē). SYN pygmy.

Pignet, Maurice-C.J., French surgeon, *1871. SEE P. *formula.*

pi·lar, pi·la·ry (pī′lăr, pil′ă-rē). SYN hairy. [L. *pilus,* hair]

pile (pīl). **1.** A series of plates of two different metals imposed alternately one on the other, separated by a sheet of material moistened with a dilute acid solution, used to produce a current of electricity. [L. *pīla,* pillar] **2.** An individual hemorrhoidal tumor. SEE hemorrhoids. [L. *pīla,* ball]

sentinel p., a circumscribed thickening of the mucous membrane at the lower end of a fissure of the anus.

thermoelectric p., SYN thermopile.

piles (pīlz). SYN hemorrhoids. [L. *pila,* a ball]

pi·le·us (pī′lē-ŭs). SYN greater *omentum.* [L. *pileum* or *pileus,* a felt cap]

pi·li (pī′lī). Plural of pilus. [L.]

pi·li·mic·tion (pī-li-mik′shŭn). Passage of hairs in the urine, as in cases of dermoid tumors, or of threads of mucus in the urine. [L. *pilus,* hair, + *mictio,* urination]

pil·in (pī′lin). The protein component of bacterial adhesive appendages that help the bacterium to stick to tissue or container surfaces, often the glycoproteins on the surface of eukaryotic cells. [pilus 2. + -in]

pill. 1. A small globular mass of some coherent, but soluble, substance containing a medicinal substance to be swallowed. SEE ALSO tablet. **2.** The Pill; a colloquial term for oral contraceptives. [L. *pilula;* dim. of *pila,* ball]

bread p., a placebo made of bread crumbs or other inactive substances.

morning after p., an oral drug that, when taken by a woman within 2–3 days after intercourse, reduces the probability that she will become pregnant. SYN emergency hormonal contraception.

Usually the term refers to oral contraceptive tablets (birth control pills) taken briefly in higher-than-usual dosage. Use of oral contraceptives has been approved by the U.S. Food and Drug Administration as a means of "emergency contraception" after rape or unplanned and unprotected intercourse, but not as a regular means of preventing pregnancy. The Yupze regimen consists of a combination of progestogen (levonorgestrel 0.25 mg or norgestrel 0.5 mg) and estrogen (ethinyl estradiol 0.05 mg) taken at once and repeated in 12 hours. Depending on the product used, this regimen requires taking 2–4 tablets of a standard oral contraceptive. The first dose should preferably be taken within 24 hours after intercourse, and no later than 72 hours after. The method reduces the likelihood of pregnancy by about 75%. About 50% of women experience uterine bleeding within 1 week and most of the rest within 3 weeks unless conception has occurred. If taken early enough, the hormones may prevent fertilization from taking place by altering tubal function or exerting toxicity against the ovum. Probably, however, they usually act by preventing implantation of a fertilized ovum. At this hormone dosage the incidence of nausea is about 50% and of vomiting about 20%; headache, fluid retention, and breast tenderness may also occur. (Levonorgestrel administered alone has been reported to cause less nausea than combination therapy and to yield comparable or better protection against pregnancy.) This procedure is contraindicated in women for whom oral contraceptives are contraindicated, such as those with hypertension or a history of stroke or thromboembolic disease. The short course of high-dose hormones probably does not interrupt a pregnancy once implantation has occurred, and there is no evidence that fetal harm has occurred when such a pregnancy has continued to term. However, hormone use is contraindicated in known pregnancy or if the woman has had unprotected intercourse within the preceding 3–10 days.

pep p.'s, colloquialism for tablets containing a central nervous system stimulant, especially amphetamine.

pil·lar (pil'ăr). A structure or part having a resemblance to a column or pillar. [L. *pila*]

anterior p. of fauces, ⋆official alternate term for palatoglossal *arch.*

anterior p. of fornix, SYN *column* of fornix.

Corti p.'s, SYN pillar *cells,* under *cell.*

p.'s of fauces, SEE palatoglossal *arch,* palatopharyngeal *arch.*

p.'s of fornix, the columna fornicis [TA] and crus fornicis [TA].

p. of iris, SYN trabecular *tissue* of sclera.

posterior p. of fauces, ⋆official alternate term for palatopharyngeal *arch.*

posterior p. of fornix, SYN *crus* fornicis.

pil·let (pil'et). A small pill.

pill mass. SYN pilular *mass.*

pill-roll·ing (pil'rōl'ing). A circular movement of the opposed tips of the thumb and the index finger appearing as a form of tremor in paralysis agitans.

△**pilo-.** Hair. [L. *pilus*]

pi·lo·car·pine (pī-lō-kar'pēn). An alkaloid obtained from the leaves of *Pilocarpus; Microphyllus* or *P. jaborandi* (family Rutaceae), shrubs of the West Indies and tropical America; a parasympathomimetic agent used as a diaphoretic, sialogogue, and stimulant of intestinal motility, and externally as a miotic and in the treatment of glaucoma; used as the hydrochloride and the nitrate salts. [G. *pilos,* a felt hat, + *karpos,* fruit]

pi·lo·car·pus (pil'ō-kar-pŭs). A genus of trees and shrubs found in Central and South America and in the West Indies. Constitutes the botanical source for pilocarpine, an alkaloid that activates cholinergic muscarinic receptors. Pilocarpine is used in the treatment of glaucoma, in which it is instilled in the eye. Sudorific; miotic. SYN Jaborandi.

pi·lo·cys·tic (pi'lō-sis'tik). Denoting a dermoid cyst containing hair. [pilo- + G. *kystis,* bladder]

pi·lo·e·rec·tion (pī'lō-ē-rek'shŭn). Erection of hair due to action of arrectores pilorum muscles.

pi·loid (pī'loyd). Hairlike; resembling hair. [pilo- + G. *eidos,* resemblance]

pi·lo·ma·trix·o·ma (pī'lō-mā-trik-sō'mă). A benign solitary hair follicle tumor, often starting in childhood, containing cells resembling basal cell carcinoma and areas of epithelial necrosis forming eosinophilic ghost cells with variable calcification and foreign body giant cell reaction in the fibrous stroma. SYN Malherbe calcifying epithelioma. [pilo- + matrix + G. *-oma,* tumor]

pi·lo·mo·tor (pī'lō-mō'ter). Moving the hair; denoting the arrectores pilorum muscles of the skin and the postganglionic sympathetic nerve fibers innervating these small smooth muscles. [pilo- + L. *motor,* mover]

pi·lo·ni·dal (pī-lō-nī'dăl). Denoting the presence of hair in a dermoid cyst or in a sinus opening on the skin. [pilo- + L. *nidus,* nest]

pi·lose (pī'lōs). SYN hairy. [L. *pilosus*]

pi·lo·se·ba·ceous (pī'lō-sē-bā'shŭs). Relating to the hair follicles and sebaceous glands. [pilo- + L. *sebum,* suet]

pi·lo·sis (pī-lō'sis). SYN hirsutism. [pilo- + G. *-osis,* condition]

Piltz, Jan, Polish neurologist, 1870–1931. SEE P. *sign;* Westphal-P. *phenomenon.*

pil·u·la, gen. and pl. **pil·u·lae** (pil'ū-lă, -lē). A pill or pilule. [L. dim. of *pila,* a ball]

pil·u·lar (pil'ū-lăr). Relating to a pill.

pil·ule (pil'ūl). A small pill. [L. *pilula*]

pi·lus, pl. **pi·li** (pī'lŭs, pī'lī) [TA]. **1** [TA]. SYN hair (1). **2.** A fine filamentous appendage, somewhat analogous to the flagellium,

that occurs on some bacteria. Pili consist only of protein and are shorter, straighter, and much more numerous and may be chemically similar to flagella; specialized pili (F pili, I pili, and other conjugative pili) seem to mediate bacterial conjugation. SYN fimbria (2). SEE ALSO conjugative *plasmid.* [L.]

pi'li annula'ti, SYN ringed *hair.*

F pili, SEE pilus (2).

F p., a structure responsible for attachment of individual male (F⁺) to female (F⁻) bacteria, forming conjugal pairs.

I pili, SEE pilus (2).

pi'li multigem'ini, the presence of several hairs in a single follicle.

R pili, specialized pili found on bacterial cells, similar to F pili and associated with R plasmids.

pi'li tor'ti, a condition in which many hair shafts are twisted on the long axis, congenital or acquired as a result of distortion of the follicles from a scarring inflammatory process, mechanical stress, or cicatrizing alopecia; the hair shafts resemble spangles in reflected light, are brittle, and break at varying lengths with many areas appearing bald with a dark stubble; as a developmental defect it can be manifested in such syndromes as Bjornstad, Crandall, and Menkes. SYN twisted hairs.

pi·mar·i·cin (pi-mar'i-sin). An antifungal antibiotic for topical use, produced by *Streptomyces natalensis;* effective against *Aspergillus, Candida,* and *Mucor* species. SYN natamycin.

pi·mel·ic ac·id (pĭ-mel'ik). Heptanedioic acid; an intermediate in the oxidation of oleic acid in some microorganisms; a precursor of biotin.

△**pimelo-.** Fat, fatty. [G. *pimelē,* soft fat, lard, fr. *piar,* fat]

pim·e·lor·rhea (pim'ĕ-lō-rē'ă). SYN fatty *diarrhea.* [pimelo- + G. *rhoia,* a flux]

pim·e·lor·thop·nea (pim'ĕ-lōr-thop'nē-ă, -nē'ă). Orthopnea; difficulty breathing in any but the erect posture, due to obesity. SYN piorthopnea. [pimelo- + G. *orthos,* straight, + *pnoē,* breath]

pi·men·ta, pi·men·to (pi-men'tă, -tō). The dried fruit of *Pimenta officinalis* (family Myrtaceae), a tree native in Jamaica and other parts of tropical America, used as a carminative and aromatic spice; p. oil comprises 3 to 4% of the dried fruit. [Sp. fr. L. *pigmentum,* paint (Mediev. L. spice)]

p. oil, comprises 3–4.5% of the dried fruit. SYN allspice oil.

pim·o·zide (pim'ō-zīd). A tranquilizing antipsychotic drug.

pim·ple (pim'pl). A papule or small pustule; usually meant to denote an inflammatory lesion of acne.

PIN Abbreviation for prostatic intraepithelial *neoplasia.*

pin. A metallic implant used in surgical treatment of bone fractures. SEE ALSO nail. [O.E. *pinn,* fr. L. *pinna,* feather]

Steinmann p., a p. that is used to transfix bone for traction or fixation.

pin·a·cy·a·nol (pin-ă-sī'ă-nol) [old C.I. 808]. A basic dye, used as a color sensitizer (violet red in water, blue in alcohol) in photography and for vital staining of leukocytes.

Pinard, Adolphe, French obstetrician, 1844–1934. SEE P. *maneuver.*

pince·ment (pans-mon'). A pinching manipulation in massage. [Fr. pinching]

🖑**pinch.** OCCUPATIONAL THERAPY Grip between fingers at the most distal joints.

Pindborg, Jens J., Danish oral pathologist, 1921–1995. SEE P. *tumor.*

pin·do·lol (pin'dō-lol). A β-adrenergic blocking agent used in the treatment of hypertension; also possesses intrinsic sympathomimetic activity.

pine (pīn). An evergreen coniferous tree of the genus *Pinus* (family Pinaceae), various species of which yield tar, turpentine, resin, and volatile oils. [L. *pinus,* a pine tree]

p.-needle oil, a volatile oil distilled with steam from the fresh leaf of *Pinus mugo;* has been used by inhalation and spray in catarrhal affections of the air passages, and locally in rheumatism; also used as a flavoring and in perfumery.

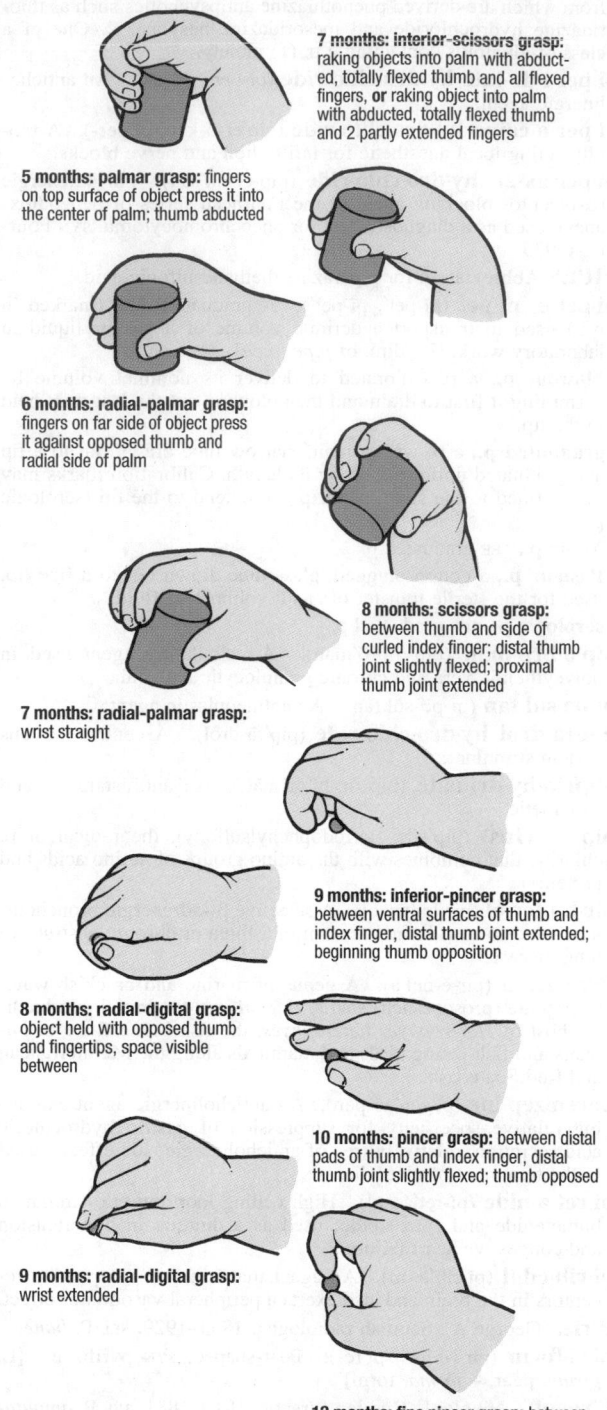

7 months: interior-scissors grasp: raking objects into palm with abducted, totally flexed thumb and all flexed fingers, **or** raking object into palm with abducted, totally flexed thumb and 2 partly extended fingers

5 months: palmar grasp: fingers on top surface of object press it into the center of palm; thumb abducted

6 months: radial-palmar grasp: fingers on far side of object press it against opposed thumb and radial side of palm

7 months: radial-palmar grasp: wrist straight

8 months: scissors grasp: between thumb and side of curled index finger; distal thumb joint slightly flexed; proximal thumb joint extended

9 months: inferior-pincer grasp: between ventral surfaces of thumb and index finger, distal thumb joint extended; beginning thumb opposition

8 months: radial-digital grasp: object held with opposed thumb and fingertips, space visible between

10 months: pincer grasp: between distal pads of thumb and index finger, distal thumb joint slightly flexed; thumb opposed

9 months: radial-digital grasp: wrist extended

12 months: fine pincer grasp: between fingertips or fingernails; distal thumb joint flexed

pinch and grasp patterns

p. oil, the volatile oil from the wood of *Pinus palustris* and other species of *Pinus;* used as a deodorant and disinfectant.

p. tar, obtained by the destructive distillation of the wood of *Pinus palustris* and other species of *Pinus;* used internally as an expectorant and externally in the treatment of skin diseases. SYN liquid pitch.

white p., the dried inner bark of *Pinus strobus,* used as an ingredient in cough syrups.

pin·e·al (pin′ē-ăl). **1.** Shaped like a pine cone. SYN piniform. **2.** Pertaining to the pineal body. [L. *pineus,* relating to the pine, *pinus*]

pin·e·al·ec·to·my (pin′ē-ă-lek′tō-mē). Removal of the pineal body. [pineal + G. *ektomē,* excision]

pin·e·a·lo·cyte (pin-ē′al-ō-sīt). A cell of the pineal body with long processes ending in bulbous expansions. P.'s receive a direct innervation from sympathetic neurons that form recognizable synapses. The club-shaped endings of pinealocyte processes terminate in perivascular spaces surrounding capillaries. SYN chief cell of corpus pineale, parenchymatous cell of corpus pineale. [pineal + G. *kytos,* cell]

pin·e·a·lo·ma (pin′ē-ă-lō′mă). A term that has been variably used to designate germ cell tumors, pineocytomas, and pineoblastomas of the pineal gland. [pineal + G. *-oma,* tumor]

ectopic p., an obsolete term for an undifferentiated neoplasm resembling a p., usually found near the pituitary gland; believed by some to be an undifferentiated teratoma.

extrapineal p., obsolete term for ectopic p.

pin·e·a·lop·a·thy (pin′ē-ă-lop′ă-thē). Disease of the pineal gland. [pineal + G. *pathos,* disease]

pine·ap·ple (pīn′ap-ĕl). The fruit of *Ananas sativa* or *Bromelia ananas* (family Bromeliaceae); it contains a proteolytic and milk-clotting enzyme, bromelain.

Pinel, Philippe, French psychiatrist, 1745–1826. SEE P. *system.*

pin·e·o·blas·to·ma (pin′ē-ō-blas-tō′mă). A poorly differentiated tumor of the pineal gland most frequently occurring in the first three decades of life consisting of small cells with a scant amount of cytoplasm and often forming pseudorosettes; histologically resembles a medulloblastoma; a type of primitive neuroectodermal tumor. [pineal + G. *blastos,* germ, + *-oma,* tumor]

pin·e·o·cy·to·ma (pin′ē-ō-cī′tō′mă). A tumor arising in the pineal gland that resembles normal pineal parenchyma.

ping-pong (ping′pong). SEE ping-pong *mechanism.* [Ping-Pong, trademark for table tennis]

pin·guec·u·la, pin·guic·u·la (ping-gwek′ū-lă). A yellowish accumulation of connective tissue that thickens the conjunctiva; occurs in the aged. [L. *pinguiculus,* fattish, fr. *pinguis,* fat]

pin·i·form (pin′i-fōrm, pī′ni-). SYN pineal (1). [L. *pinus,* pine, + *forma,* form]

pink·eye (pink′ī). SYN acute contagious *conjunctivitis.*

pin·ledge (pin′ledj). A cast metal dental restoration or technique that employs parallel pins as part of the casting to increase retention of the restoration.

pin·na, pl. **pin·nae** (pin′ă, pin′ē). **1.** SYN auricle (1). **2.** A feather, wing, or fin. [L. *pinna* or *penna,* a feather, in pl. a wing]

p. na′si, SYN *ala* of nose.

pin·nal (pin′ăl). Relating to the pinna.

pin·ni·ped (pin′i-ped). A member of the suborder Pinnipedia, aquatic carnivorous mammals with all four limbs modified into flippers (e.g., seal, walrus). [L. *pinna,* feather (wing), + *pes* (*ped-*), foot]

pin·o·cyte (pin′ō-sīt, pī′nō-). A cell that exhibits pinocytosis. [G. *pineō,* to drink, + *kytos,* cell]

pin·o·cy·to·sis (pin′ō-sī-tō′sis, pī′nō-). The cellular process of actively engulfing liquid, a phenomenon in which minute incuppings or invaginations are formed in the surface of the cell membrane and close to form fluid-filled vesicles; it resembles phagocytosis. [pinocyte + G. *-osis,* condition]

pin·o·some (pin′ō-sōm, pī′nō-). A fluid-filled vacuole formed by pinocytosis. [G. *pineō,* to drink, + *sōma,* body]

Pins, Emil, Austrian physician, 1845–1913. SEE P. *sign,* *syndrome.*

pint (pīnt). A measure of quantity (U.S. liquid), containing 16 fluid ounces, 28.875 cubic inches; 473.1765 cc. An imperial p. contains 20 British fluid ounces, 34.67743 cubic inches; 568.2615 cc.

pin·ta (pin′tă, pēn′tă). A disease caused by a spirochete, *Trepone-*

ma carateum, endemic in Mexico and Central America, and characterized by a small primary papule followed by an enlarging plaque and disseminated secondary macules of varying color called pintids that finally become white. SEE ALSO nonvenereal *syphilis.* SYN azul, carate, mal del pinto. [Sp. painted]

pin·tids. Eruptions of plaque-like lesions in the secondary phase of pinta; the lesions, which vary in color (hypochromic, hyperchromic, and erythematosquamous), result in depigmentation. [pinta + -id(1)]

pi·nus (pī'nŭs). SYN pineal *body.* [L. a pine tree]

🔲 **pin·worm** (pin'werm). A member of the genus *Enterobius* or related genera of nematodes in the family Oxyuridae, abundant in a large variety of vertebrates, including such species as *Oxyuris equi* (the horse p.), *Enterobius vermicularis* (the human p.), *Syphacia* and *Aspiculuris* species (the mouse p.), *Passalurus ambiguus* (the rabbit p.), and *Syphacia muris* (the rat p.). SYN seatworm.

Pi·oph·i·la ca·sei (pī-of'i-lă kā'sē-ī). The cheese fly, a species of muscoid flies whose eggs are deposited on exposed cheese, cured meats, and other foods and are thus ingested, sometimes giving rise to temporary intestinal myiasis, with diarrhea, colicky pains, and vomiting. [L., fr. G. *piōn,* fat, + *philos,* fond; L. *caseus,* cheese]

pi·or·thop·nea (pī-ōr-thop'nē-ă, -nē'ă). SYN pimelorthopnea. [G. *piōn,* fat, + *orthos,* straight, + *pnoē,* breath]

PIP₂ Abbreviation for *phosphatidylinositol* 4,5-bisphosphate.

pi·pam·a·zine (pi-pam'ă-zēn). A phenothiazine analogue with antiemetic and tranquilizing properties.

pi·pam·per·one (pi-pam'per-ōn). An antipsychotic tranquilizer.

pi·paz·e·thate (pi-paz'ě-thāt). An antitussive agent.

pip·e·co·lic ac·id (pip'ě-kō'lik, -kol'ik). Dihydrobaikiaine; 2-piperidinecarboxylic acid; saturated picolinic acid; the L-isomers of the Δ¹- and Δ⁶-dehydropipecolic acids are intermediates in the catabolism of L-lysine; p. a. accumulates in disorders of the peroxisomes. SYN homoproline, pipecolinic acid.

pip·e·co·lin·ic ac·id (pip-ě-kō-lin'ik, -kol'i-nik). SYN pipecolic acid.

pip·e·cur·o·ni·um (pip'ě-kūr-ō'nē-ŭm). A nondepolarizing steroid muscle relaxant structurally related to pancuronium and characterized by long duration of action.

pip·e·cu·ron·i·um bro·mide (pī-pě-kur-ō'nē-ŭm brō'mīd). A neuromuscular blocking agent with nondepolarizing properties, thus resembling D-tubocurarine but having a shorter duration of paralytic action.

pi·pen·zo·late meth·yl·bro·mide (pi-pen'zō-lāt). An anticholinergic drug.

Piper, E.B., U.S. obstetrician-gynecologist, 1881–1935. SEE P. *forceps.*

pip·er (pī'per). Black pepper, the dried unripe fruit of *Piper nigrum* (family Piperaceae), a climbing plant of the East Indies; used as a condiment, diaphoretic, stimulant, and carminative, and locally as a counterirritant. [L. pepper]

pi·per·a·cil·lin so·di·um (pi-per'ă-sil'in). A semisynthetic extended spectrum penicillin active against a wide variety of Gram-positive and Gram-negative bacteria.

pi·per·a·zine (pī-per'ă-zēn, -zin). Its former use in gout was based upon its property of dissolving uric acid in vitro, but it is ineffective in increasing uric acid excretion; its compounds are now used as anthelmintics in oxyuriasis and ascariasis. SYN diethylenediamine.
  p. adipate, a veterinary anthelmintic and filaricide.
  p. calcium edetate, an anthelmintic.
  p. citrate, a vermifuge for pinworms and roundworms.
  p. estrone sulfate, a purified preparation of natural estrone sulfate; the p. acts as a buffer to increase the stability of estrone sulfate.
  p. tartrate, an anthelmintic useful in the treatment of nematode infestation.

pi·per·a·zine di·eth·ane·sul·fon·ic ac·id (PIPES). One of several aminosulfonic acids (like HEPES) used in biologic buffers; active range, 6.0–8.5.

pi·per·i·dine (pī'per-i-dēn). **1.** Hexahydropyridine; a compound

from which are derived phenothiazine antipsychotics such as thioridazine hydrochloride and mesoridazine besylate. **2.** One of a class of alkaloids containing a p. (1) moiety.

pi·per·i·do·late hy·dro·chlo·ride (pi-per'i-dō-lāt). An anticholinergic agent.

pi·per·o·caine hy·dro·chlo·ride (pip'er-ō-kān, pī'per-). A rapidly acting local anesthetic for infiltration and nerve blocks.

pi·per·ox·an hy·dro·chlo·ride (pip-er-ok'san). An adrenergic (α-receptor blocking agent of the Fourneau series of benzodioxanes); used as a diagnostic test for pheochromocytoma. SYN Fourneau 933.

PIPES Abbreviation for piperazine diethanesulfonic acid.

pi·pette, pi·pet (pĭ-pet', pī-pet'). A graduated tube (marked in mL) used to transport a definite volume of a gas or liquid in laboratory work. [Fr. dim. of *pipe,* pipe]
  blowout p., a p. calibrated to deliver its nominal volume by permitting it first to drain and then blowing out the last drop held in the tip.
  graduated p., a p. with a plain, narrow tube drawn out to a tip and graduated uniformly along its length. Calibration marks may be confined to the stem (Mohr p.) or extend to the tip (serologic p.).
  Mohr p., SEE graduated p.
  Pasteur p., a cotton-plugged, glass tube drawn out to a fine tip, used for the sterile transfer of small volumes of fluid.
  serologic p., SEE graduated p.

pip·o·bro·man (pip-ō-brō'man). An alkylating agent used in polycythemia vera and chronic granulocytic leukemia.

pi·po·sul·fan (pi-pō-sŭl'fan). An antineoplastic agent.

pi·pra·drol hy·dro·chlo·ride (pip'ră-drol). A central nervous system stimulant.

pi·prin·hy·dri·nate (pip-rin-hī'dri-nāt). An antihistaminic and antiemetic.

pip·syl (Ips) (pip'sil). *p*-Iodophenylsulfonyl, the radical of p. chloride that combines with the amino groups of amino acids and proteins.

pir·bu·ter·ol (pir-bū'ter-ol). A selective β₂-adrenergic bronchodilator used to treat bronchospasm in asthma or chronic obstructive lung disease.

Pi·re·nel·la (pir-ě-nel'ă). A genus of marine and brackish water operculate (prosobranch) snails. *P. conica* is the initial intermediate host of *Heterophyes heterophyes,* the fish-borne fluke of humans and fish-eating birds and mammals along the Mediterranean and Red Sea coasts.

pi·ren·zep·ine (pĭ-ren'zě-pēn). An anticholinergic agent exhibiting relative specificity for suppression of gastric hydrochloric acid secretion; relatively free of anticholinergic side effects; used in the treatment of ulcer disease.

pi·ret·a·nide (pĭ-ret'ă-nīd). High ceiling loop diuretic similar to bumetanide and furosemide; used as a diuretic in hypertension and congestive heart failure.

pi·rib·ed·il (pĭ-rib'ě-dil). An agent that stimulates dopamine receptors in the brain and also exerts a peripheral vasodilator effect.

Pirie, George A., Scottish radiologist, 1864–1929. SEE P. *bone.*

pir·i·form (pir'i-fōrm, pī'rē-). Pear-shaped. SYN pyriform. [L. *pirum,* pear, + *forma,* form]

Pirogoff, Nikolai I., Russian surgeon, 1810–1881. SEE P. *amputation, angle, triangle.*

pir·o·men (pir'ō-men, pī'rō-). A sterile, nonprotein, nonanaphylactogenic extract of *Pseudomonas aeruginosa* and *Proteus vulgaris.* The active components are bacterial polysaccharides of low toxicity; used in the treatment of certain allergic, dermatologic, and ophthalmic disorders. SYN pyromen.

Pi·ro·plas·ma (pir'ō-plaz'mă, pī'rō-). Former name for *Babesia.* [L. *pirum,* pear, + G. *plasma,* a thing formed]

Pi·ro·plas·mi·da (pi'rō-plaz-mī'dă). An order of sporozoan protozoa (subclass Piroplasmia, class Sporozoea) consisting of the families Habesiidae, Theileriidae, and Dactylosomatidae; includes heteroxenous tick-borne blood parasites of vertebrates with reduced apical complex, lacking spores, and with asexual reproduction by binary fission or schizogony.

pir·o·plas·mo·sis (pir′ō-plas-mō′sis). SYN babesiosis.

pir·ox·i·cam ol·a·mine (pir-oks′i-kam). A long-acting nonsteroidal anti-inflammatory agent with analgesic and antipyretic actions.

pir·pro·fen (pir-prō′fen). An anti-inflammatory used in the treatment of rheumatoid arthritis.

Pirquet von Cesenatico, Clemens P., Austrian physician, 1874–1929. SEE Pirquet *reaction;* Pirquet *test.*

Pis·ces (pis′ēz, pī′sēz). A superclass of vertebrates, generally known as fish; the term is sometimes confined to the bony fishes. [L. pl. of *piscis,* a fish]

pis·i·form (pis′i-fōrm) [TA]. Pea-shaped or pea-sized. [L. *pisum,* pea, + *forma,* appearance]

pit. 1. SYN fovea. 2. One of the pinhead-sized depressed scars following the pustule of acne, chickenpox, or smallpox (pockmark). 3. A sharp-pointed depression in the enamel surface of a tooth, due to faulty or incomplete calcification or formed at the confluent point of two or more lobes of enamel. 4. To indent, as by pressure of the finger on the edematous skin; to become indented, said of the edematous tissues when pressure is applied with the fingertip. [L. *puteus*]

anal p., SYN proctodeum (1).

articular p. of head of radius, SYN articular *facet* of radial head.

p. of atlas for dens, SYN *facet* (of atlas) for dens.

auditory p.'s, SYN otic p.'s.

buccal p., a structural depression found on the buccal enamel of molars.

central p., SYN central retinal *fovea.*

coated p., specialized depressions on the cell surface involved in receptor-mediated endocytosis; the visible proteinaceous layer on the cytosolic side of the depression provides the coated appearance.

⊞commisural p.'s, similar to lip p.'s but found at the labial commisures.

costal p. of transverse process, SYN transverse costal *facet.*

gastric p. [TA], one of the numerous small pits in the mucous membrane of the stomach that are the mouths of the gastric glands. SYN foveola gastrica [TA].

granular p.'s, SYN granular *foveolae,* under *foveola.*

p. of head of femur, SYN *fovea* for ligament of head of femur.

inferior articular p. of atlas, SYN inferior articular *surface* of atlas.

inferior costal p., SYN inferior costal *facet.*

iris p.'s, colobomas affecting the stroma of the iris with pigment epithelium intact.

lens p.'s, the paired depressions formed in the superficial ectoderm of the embryonic head as the lens placodes sink in toward the optic cup; the external openings of the p.'s are closed as the lens vesicles are formed.

lip p.'s, malformations of the lip seen in unilateral or bilateral depressions or fistulae. May be hereditary or associated with cleft lip and/or palate.

Mantoux p., shallow 2–3-mm depressions of the palms and soles in basal cell nevus syndrome.

nail p.'s, small punctate depressions on the surface of the nail plate due to defective nail formation; seen in psoriasis and other disorders. SEE ALSO geographic *stippling* of nails.

nasal p.'s, the paired depressions formed when the nasal placodes come to lie below the general external contour of the developing face as a result of the rapid growth of the adjacent nasal elevations; the p.'s are the primordia of the rostral portions of the nasal chambers. SYN olfactory p.'s.

oblong p. of arytenoid cartilage, SYN oblong *fovea* of arytenoid cartilage.

olfactory p.'s, SYN nasal p.'s.

optic p., a congenital anomaly characterized by a focal depression of the temporal optic nerve head.

otic p.'s, paired depression, one on either side of the head of the embryo, marking the location of the future auditory vesicles. SYN auditory p.'s.

preauricular p., SYN preauricular *sinus.*

primitive p., the depression in the primitive node that serves to connect the notochordal canal with the surface ectoderm.

pterygoid p., SYN pterygoid *fovea.*

p. of stomach, SYN epigastric *fossa.*

sublingual p., SYN sublingual *fossa.*

superior articular p. of atlas, SYN superior articular *surface* of atlas.

superior costal p., SYN superior costal *facet.*

suprameatal p., SYN suprameatal *triangle.*

triangular p. of arytenoid cartilage, SYN triangular *fovea* of arytenoid cartilage.

trochlear p., SYN trochlear *fovea.*

pit-1. A nuclear binding transcriptional factor found in many cells in normal human pituitary glands and expressed in a large percentage of pituitary adenomas, in particular those positive for growth hormone, or thyrotropin.

PITC Abbreviation for phenylisothiocyanate.

pitch (pich). A resinous substance obtained from tar after the volatile substances have been expelled by boiling. SYN pix. [L. *pix*]

Burgundy p., a resinous exudation from the spruce fir or Norway spruce, *Picea excelsa;* has been used as a counterirritant in the form of a plaster. SYN white p.

liquid p., SYN *pine* tar.

white p., SYN Burgundy p.

pitch·blende (pich′blend). A mineral of pitchlike appearance, chiefly uranium dioxide, the main source of uranium and elements, such as radium, produced as a result of the radioactive breakdown of that element. SYN uraninite.

pith. 1. The center of a hair. 2. The spinal cord and medulla oblongata. 3. To pierce the medulla of an animal with a sharp instrument introduced at the base of the skull. [A.S. *pitha*]

pith·e·coid (pith′ĕ-koyd). Resembling an ape. [G. *pithēkos,* ape, + *eidos,* resemblance]

pith·ode (pith′ōd). The nuclear spindle in karyokinesis. [G. *pithōdēs,* like a jar, fr. *pithos,* earthenware wine-jar, + *eidos,* resemblance]

Pitot, Henri, French engineer, 1695–1771. SEE P. *tube.*

Pitres, Jean A., French physician, 1848–1927. SEE P. *area, sign.*

Pi·tressin (pi-tres′in). SYN vasopressin.

pit·ting. In dentistry, the formation of well defined, relatively deep depressions in a surface, usually used in describing defects in surfaces (often golds, solder joints, or amalgam). It may arise from a variety of causes, although the clinical occurrence is often associated with corrosion. SEE ALSO pitting *edema,* nail *pits,* under *pit.*

pi·tu·i·cyte (pi-too′i-sīt). The primary cell of the posterior lobe of the pituitary gland, a fusiform cell closely related to neuroglia. [pituitary + G. *kytos,* cell]

pi·tu·i·cy·to·ma (pi-too′i-sī-tō′mă). A rare gliogenous neoplasm derived from pituicytes, occurring in the posterior lobe of the pituitary gland and characterized by cells with relatively small, round or oval nuclei and long branching processes that form a complex network of cytoplasmic material, in which numerous small droplets of fat may be demonstrated. [pituicyte + G. *-oma,* tumor]

pi·tu·i·ta (pi-too′i-tă). A thick nasal secretion. SYN glairy mucus. [L. phlegm or thick mucous secretion]

pi·tu·i·tar·ism (pi-too′i-tār-izm). Pituitary dysfunction. SEE hyperpituitarism, hypopituitarism.

pi·tu·i·ta·ri·um (pi-too-i-tā′rē-ŭm). SYN pituitary. [Mod. L.]

pi·tu·i·tary (pi-too′i-tār-ē). Relating to the pituitary gland (hypophysis). SYN pituitarium. [L. *pituita,* a phlegm]

anterior p., the dried, partially defatted, and powdered anterior lobe of the p. gland of cattle, sheep, or swine; now rarely used therapeutically.

desiccated p., SYN posterior p.

pharyngeal p., the embryonic remnant of the oral end of Rathke pouch that is cut off from the adenohypophysis by the developing sphenoid bone; composed chiefly of chromophobes and, under normal conditions, considered physiologically inactive. SEE pituitary *gland*.

posterior p., the cleaned, dried, and powdered posterior lobe obtained from the p. body of domestic animals used for food by humans; an oxytocic, vasoconstrictor, antidiuretic, and stimulant of intestinal motility. SYN desiccated p., hypophysis sicca.

pi·tu·i·tous (pi-too′i-tŭs). Relating to pituita.

pit·y·ri·a·sis (pit-i-rī′ă-sis). A dermatosis marked by branny desquamation. [G. fr. *pityron*, bran, dandruff]

p. al′ba, patchy hypopigmentation of the skin resulting from mild dermatitis.

p. al′ba atroph′icans, a scaling condition of the skin followed by atrophy.

p. cap′itis, SYN dandruff.

p. circina′ta, SYN p. rosea.

p. lichenoi′des, a self-limited skin disorder of children and adults, usually divided into p. lichenoides et varioliformis acuta and p. lichenoides chronica. SYN parapsoriasis guttata.

p. lichenoi′des et variolifor′mis acu′ta (PLEVA), an acute dermatitis affecting children and young adults that runs a relatively mild course and is self-limited, although persistence of lesions and recurrence of attacks are not uncommon; vesicles, papules, and crusted lesions eventually produce smallpox-like scars. SYN Mucha-Habermann disease, parapsoriasis lichenoides et varioliformis acuta, parapsoriasis varioliformis.

p. linguae, SYN geographic *tongue*.

p. macula′ta, SYN p. rosea.

p. ni′gra, SYN *tinea* nigra.

p. ro′sea, a self-limited eruption of macules or papules involving the trunk and, less frequently, extremities, scalp, and face; the lesions are usually oval and follow the crease lines of the skin; occurs most commonly in children and young adults and is frequently preceded by a single larger scaling lesion known as the herald patch. SYN p. circinata, p. maculata.

p. ru′bra pila′ris, an uncommon chronic pruritic eruption of the hair follicles, which become firm, red, surmounted with a horny plug, and often confluent to form scaly plaques; it is most conspicuously noted on the dorsa of the fingers and on the elbows and knees and is associated with erythema, thickening of the palms and soles, and opaque thickening of the nails.

p. versic′olor, SYN *tinea* versicolor.

pit·y·ri·a·sis li·che·noi·des chron·i·ca (līk′en-noyd′dēz kron′ik-ă). An eruption, lasting up to a few years, of reddish-brown papules with central scaling; it clears without scarring. [lichenoides Mod. L., fr. G. *leichēn*, lichen, a lichen-like eruption, + *eidos*, resemblance chronica Mod. L. chronic, fr. G. *chronikos*, pertaining to time; fr. *chronos*, time]

pit·y·roid (pit′i-royd). SYN furfuraceous. [G. *pityrōdēs*, branlike, fr. *pityron*, bran, + *eidos*, resemblance]

Pit·y·ro·spo·rum (pit-i-ros′pō-rŭm, pit′i-rō-spō′rŭm). A genus of fungi of disputed pathogenicity found in dandruff and seborrheic dermatitis. [G. *pityron*, bran, + *sporos*, seed]

P. orbicula′re, SYN *Malassezia furfur*.

P. ova′le, SYN *Malassezia furfur*.

piv·a·late (piv′ă-lāt). USAN-approved contraction for trimethylacetate, $(CH_3)_3C–CO_2^-$.

piv·ot (piv′ŏt). A post upon which something hinges or turns.

adjustable occlusal p., an occlusal p. that may be adjusted vertically by means of a screw or by other means.

occlusal p., an elevation contrived on the occlusal surface, usually in the molar region, designed to act as a fulcrum and to induce sagittal mandibular rotation.

pix, gen. **pi·cis** (piks, pī′sis). SYN pitch. [L]

pix·el (pik′sel). A contraction for picture element, a two-dimensional representation of a volume element (voxel) in the display of the CT or MR image, usually 512×512 or 256×256 pixels, respectively.

PK Abbreviation for *pyruvate* kinase.

pKₐ. The negative decadic logarithm of the ionization constant (K_a) of an acid; equal to the pH value at which equal concentrations of the acid and conjugate base forms of a substance (often a buffer) are present.

pkat Abbreviation for picokatal.

PKU Abbreviation for phenylketonuria.

pkV Abbreviation for peak kilovoltage, the nominal voltage setting of an x-ray machine.

PL Abbreviation for placental lactogen.

pla·ce·bo (plă-sē′bō). **1.** An inert substance given as a medicine for its suggestive effect. **2.** An inert compound identical in appearance to material being tested in experimental research, which may or may not be known to the physician and/or patient, administered to distinguish between drug action and suggestive effect of the material under study. SYN active p. [L. I will please, future of *placeo*]

active p., SYN placebo.

PLACENTA

pla·cen·ta (plă-sen′tă). Organ of metabolic interchange between fetus and mother. It has a portion of embryonic origin, derived from a highly developed area of the outermost embryonic membrane (chorion frondosum), and a maternal portion formed by a modification of the part of the uterine mucosa (decidua basalis) in which the chorionic vesicle is implanted. Within the p., the chorionic villi, with their contained capillaries carrying blood of the embryonic circulation, are exposed to maternal blood in the intervillous spaces in which the villi lie; no direct mixing of fetal and maternal blood occurs, but the intervening tissue (the placental membrane) is sufficiently thin to permit the absorption of nutritive materials, oxygen, and some harmful substances, like viruses, into the fetal blood and the release of carbon dioxide and nitrogenous waste from it. At term, the human p. is disk shaped, about 4 cm in thickness and 18 cm in diameter, and averages about ⅙ to ⅐ the weight of the fetus; its fetal surface is smooth, being formed by the adherent amnion, with the umbilical cord normally attached near its center; the maternal surface of a detached p. is rough because of the torn decidual tissue adhering to the chorion and shows lobular elevations called cotyledons or lobes. [L. cake]

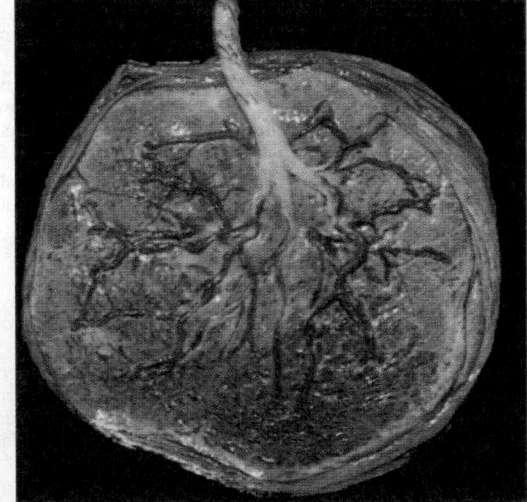

placenta: amniotic surface, with umbilical cord

accessory p., a mass of placental tissue distinct from the main p. SYN succenturiate p., supernumerary p.

p. accre′ta, the abnormal adherence of the chorionic villi to the myometrium, associated with partial or complete absence of the decidua basalis and, in particular, the stratum spongiosum. SEE ALSO p. percreta.

p. accre′ta ve′ra, the term applied when villi are juxtaposed to the myometrium.

adherent p., a p. that fails to separate cleanly from the uterus after delivery.

anular p., a p. in the form of a band encircling the interior of the uterus. SYN ring-shaped p., zonary p.

battledore p., a p. in which the umbilical cord is attached at the border; so called because of the fancied resemblance to the racquet (racket) used in battledore, a precursor to badminton.

bidiscoidal p., a p. with two separate disc-shaped portions attached to opposite walls of the uterus, normal for certain monkeys and shrews, and occasionally found in humans.

p. bilo′ba, a p. duplex in which the two parts are separated by a constriction. SYN p. bipartita.

p. biparti′ta, SYN p. biloba.

central p. pre′via, SYN p. previa centralis.

chorioallantoic p., a p. (such as that of primates) in which the chorion is formed by the fusion of the allantoic mesoderm and vessels to the inner face of the serosa.

chorioamnionic p., a form of placentation in which the amnion is fused to the inside of the chorion, thus permitting interchange of water and electrolytes between mother and fetus.

p. circumvalla′ta, a cup-shaped p. with raised edges, having a thick, round, white, opaque ring around its periphery; a portion of the decidua separates the margin of the p. from its chorionic plate; the remainder of the chorionic surface is normal in appearance, but the fetal vessels are limited in their course across the p. by the ring. SEE ALSO p. marginata, p. reflexa.

cotyledonary p., a p. in which the substance is divided into lobes or cotyledons.

deciduate p., a p. in which the maternal decidua is cast off with the fetal p.

dichorionic diamnionic p., SEE twin p.

p. diffu′sa, SYN p. membranacea.

p. dimidia′ta, SYN p. duplex.

disperse p., a p. in which the umbilical arteries divide dichotomously before entering the placental substance.

Duncan p., a separated p. that appears at the vulva with the chorionic surface outward.

p. du′plex, a p. consisting of two parts, almost entirely detached, being united only at the point of attachment of the cord. SEE p. biloba. SYN p. dimidiata.

endotheliochorial p., a p. in which the chorionic tissue penetrates to the endothelium of the maternal blood vessels.

endothelio-endothelial p., a p. in which the endothelium of the maternal vessels comes in direct contact with the endothelium of the fetal vessels to form the placental barrier.

epitheliochorial p., a p. in which the chorion is merely in contact with, and does not erode, the endometrium.

p. extrachora′les, a p. in which the chorionic plate is limited by a thin membranous fold at the edge.

p. fenestra′ta, a p. in which there are areas of thinning, sometimes extending to entire absence of placental tissue.

fetal p., p. feta′lis, the chorionic portion of the placenta, containing the fetal blood vessels, from which the umbilical cord develops; specifically, in humans, it develops from the chorion frondosum. SYN pars fetalis placentae.

hemochorial p., the type of p., as in humans and some rodents, in which maternal blood is in direct contact with the chorion.

hemoendothelial p., the type of p., as in rabbits, in which the trophoblast becomes so attenuated that, by light microscopy, maternal blood appears to be separated from fetal blood only by the endothelium of the chorionic capillaries.

horseshoe p., an exaggerated p. reniformis curved in the form of a horseshoe; present in some twin pregnancies.

incarcerated p., SYN retained p.

p. incre′ta, a form of p. accreta in which the chorionic villi invade the myometrium.

labyrinthine p., a p. in which maternal blood circulates through channels within the fetal syncytiotrophoblast.

p. margina′ta, a p. with raised edges, less pronounced than the p. circumvallata. SEE ALSO p. reflexa.

maternal p., SYN pars uterina placentae.

p. membrana′cea, an abnormally thin p. covering an unusually large area of the uterine lining. SYN p. diffusa.

monochorionic diamnionic p., SEE twin p.

monochorionic monoamnionic p., SEE twin p.

p. multilo′ba, a p. having more than three lobes separated from each other by simple constrictions, the fetus being single. SYN p. multipartita.

p. multiparti′ta, SYN p. multiloba.

nondeciduous p., a p. in which the fetal p. is cast off, leaving the uterine mucosa intact (e.g., an epitheliochorial p.).

p. panduraor′mis, a form of p. dimidiata with the two halves placed side by side in a shape suggestive of a lutelike musical instrument (pandura).

p. percre′ta, the term applied when the villi have invaded the full thickness of myometrium to or through the serosa of the uterus, causing incomplete or complete uterine rupture, respectively. SEE ALSO p. accreta.

p. pre′via, the condition in which the p. is implanted in the lower segment of the uterus, extending to the margin of the internal os of the cervix or partially or completely obstructing the os. SYN placental presentation.

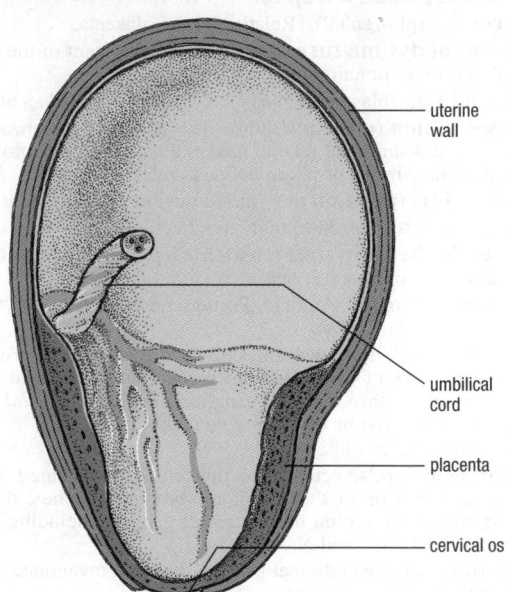

uterine wall

umbilical cord

placenta

cervical os

central placenta previa: the placenta entirely covers the internal cervical os; fetus is not shown

p. pre′via centra′lis, p. previa in which the p. entirely covers the internal os of the cervix. SYN central p. previa, total p. previa.

p. pre′via margina′lis, p. previa in which the p. comes to the margin of, but does not occlude, the internal os of the cervix.

p. pre′via partia′lis, p. previa in which the internal os of the cervix is partially covered by placental tissue.

p. reflex′a, an anomaly of the p. in which the margin is thickened so as to appear turned back upon itself. SEE ALSO p. circumvallata, p. marginata.

p. renifor′mis, a kidney-shaped p.

retained p., incomplete separation of the p. and its failure to be expelled at the usual time after delivery of the child. SYN incarcerated p.

ring-shaped p., SYN anular p.

Schultze p., a p. that appears at the vulva with the glistening fetal surface (amnion) presenting.

p. spu′ria, a mass of placental tissue that has no vascular connection with the main p.

succenturiate p., SYN accessory p.

supernumerary p., SYN accessory p.

total p. pre′via, SYN p. previa centralis.

p. tri′loba, SYN p. tripartita.

p. triparti′ta, a p. consisting of three parts almost entirely separate, being joined together only by the blood vessels of the umbilical cord; the fetus is single. SYN p. triloba, p. triplex.

p. tri′plex, SYN p. tripartita.

twin p., the placenta(s) of a twin pregnancy; if dizygotic, the p.'s may be separate or fused, the latter retaining two amnionic and two chorionic sacs (dichorionic diamnionic p.); if monozygotic, the p. may be a **monochorionic monoamnionic p.** or monochorionic diamnionic p., depending on the stage at which twinning took place; if twinning occurs early, there may be a fused p. with two chorionic and two amnionic membranes.

p. uteri′na, SYN *pars* uterina placentae.

p. velamento′sa, a p. in which the umbilical cord is attached to the adjoining membranes, with the umbilical vessels spread out and entering the p. independently.

villous p., a p. in which the chorion forms villi.

zonary p., SYN anular p.

---

pla·cen·ta·go·nad·o·trop·in. SYN chorionic *gonadotropin.*

pla·cen·tal (pla-sen′tăl). Relating to the placenta.

pla·cen·tal dys·ma·ture. Immature development of the placenta so that normal function does not occur.

Pla·cen·ta·lia (plas-en-tā′lē-ă). SEE Eutheria. [L. *placenta*]

plac·en·ta·tion (plas-en-tā′shŭn). The structural organization and mode of attachment of fetal to maternal tissues in the formation of the placenta. Types of p. are defined under placenta.

plac·en·ti·tis (plas-en-tī′tis). Inflammation of the placenta.

plac·en·to·ma (plas-en-tō′mă). SYN deciduoma.

pla·cen·to·ther·a·py (plă-sen′tō-thār′ă-pē). Therapeutic use of an extract of placental tissue.

Placido da Costa, Antonio, Portuguese ophthalmologist, 1848–1916. SEE P. da C. *disk.*

plac·ode (plak′ōd). Local thickening in the embryonic ectoderm layer; the cells of the p. ordinarily constitute a primordial group from which a sense organ or ganglion develops. [G. *plakōdēs,* fr. *plax,* anything flat or broad, + *eidos,* like]

auditory p.'s, SYN otic p.'s.

epibranchial p.'s, ectodermal thickenings associated with the more dorsal parts of the embryonic branchial arches; their cells contribute to formation of the cranial ganglia, including those of nerves V, VII, IX, and X.

lens p.'s, paired ectodermal p.'s that become invaginated to form the embryonic lens vesicles. SYN optic p.'s.

nasal p.'s, SYN olfactory p.'s.

olfactory p.'s, paired ectodermal p.'s that come to lie in the bottom of the olfactory pits as the pits are deepened by the growth of the surrounding medial and lateral nasal processes. SYN nasal p.'s.

optic p.'s, SYN lens p.'s.

otic p.'s, paired ectodermal p.'s that sink below the general level of the superficial ectoderm to form the auditory vesicles. SYN auditory p.'s.

pla·fond (plă-fon′d). A ceiling, especially the ceiling of the ankle joint, i.e., the articular surface of the distal end of the tibia. [Fr. ceiling]

△**plagio-.** Oblique, slanting. [G. *plagios*]

pla·gi·o·ce·phal·ic (plă′jē-ō-se-fal′ik). Relating to or marked by plagiocephaly. SYN plagiocephalous.

pla·gi·o·ceph·a·lism (plă′jē-ō-sef′ă-lizm). SYN plagiocephaly.

pla·gi·o·ceph·a·lous (plă′jē-ō-sef′ă-lŭs). SYN plagiocephalic.

pla·gi·o·ceph·a·ly (plă′jē-ō-sef′ă-lē). An asymmetric craniostenosis due to premature closure of the lambdoid and coronal sutures on one side; characterized by an oblique deformity of the skull, plagiocephalism. [G. *plagios,* oblique, + *kephalē,* head]

plague (plāg). **1.** Any disease of wide prevalence or of excessive mortality. **2.** An acute infectious disease caused by the bacterium *Yersinia pestis* and marked clinically by high fever, toxemia, prostration, a petechial eruption, lymph node enlargement, and pneumonia, or hemorrhage from the mucous membranes; primarily a disease of rodents, transmitted to humans by fleas that have bitten infected animals. In humans the disease takes one of four clinical forms: bubonic p., septicemic p., pneumonic p., or ambulant p. SYN pest, pestilence (1), pestis. [L. *plaga,* a stroke, injury]

ambulant p., ambulatory p., a mild form of bubonic p. characterized by symptoms such as mild fever and lymphadenitis. SYN larval p., parapestis, pestis ambulans, pestis minor.

black p., SEE black *death.*

bubonic p., the usual form of p. of which manifestations include inflammatory enlargement of the lymphatic glands in the groin, axillae, or other parts. SYN glandular p., pestis bubonica, pestis fulminans, pestis major, polyadenitis maligna.

glandular p., SYN bubonic p.

hemorrhagic p., the hemorrhagic form of bubonic p.

larval p., SYN ambulant p.

Pahvant Valley p., SYN tularemia.

pneumonic p., a rapidly progressive and frequently fatal form of p. in which there are areas of pulmonary consolidation, with chill, pain in the side, bloody expectoration, high fever, and possible human-to-human transmission. SYN plague pneumonia, pulmonic p.

pulmonic p., SYN pneumonic p.

septicemic p., a generally fatal form of p. in which there is an intense bacteremia with symptoms of profound toxemia. SYN pestis siderans.

sylvatic p., bubonic p. in rats and other wild animals.

plak·al·bu·min (plak-al-bū′min). The product of the action of subtilisin upon egg albumin, removing a hexapeptide.

pla·kins (plă′kinz). Bactericidal substances similar to leucins extracted from blood platelets. [G. *plax, plakos,* anything flat, + -in]

△**plan-.** SEE plano-.

pla·na (plă′nă). Plural of planum. [L.]

plan·chet (plan′shet). A small, flat plate or dish used to support a sample for radioactivity determination; the sample is usually evaporated on (in) the p. [Fr. *planchette,* dim. of *planche,* plank]

Planck, Max, German physicist and Nobel laureate, 1858–1947. SEE P. *constant, theory.*

PLANE

---

plane (plān) [TA]. **1.** A two-dimensional flat surface. SEE planum. **2.** An imaginary surface formed by extension of a point through any axis or two definite points, in reference especially to craniometry and to pelvimetry. SYN planum. [L. *planus,* flat]

Addison clinical p.'s, a series of p.'s used as landmarks in thoracoabdominal topography; the trunk is divided vertically by a *median p.* from the upper border of the manubrium of the sternum to the pubic symphysis, by a *lateral p.* drawn vertically on either side through a point halfway between the anterior superior iliac spine and the median p. at the interspinal p., and by an *interspinal p.* passing vertically through the anterior superior iliac spine on either side; transversely the trunk is divided by a *transthoracic p.* passing across the thorax 3.2 cm above the lower border of the body of the sternum, by a *transpyloric p.* midway between the jugular notch of the sternum and the pubic symphysis, corresponding to the disk between the first and second lumbar verte-

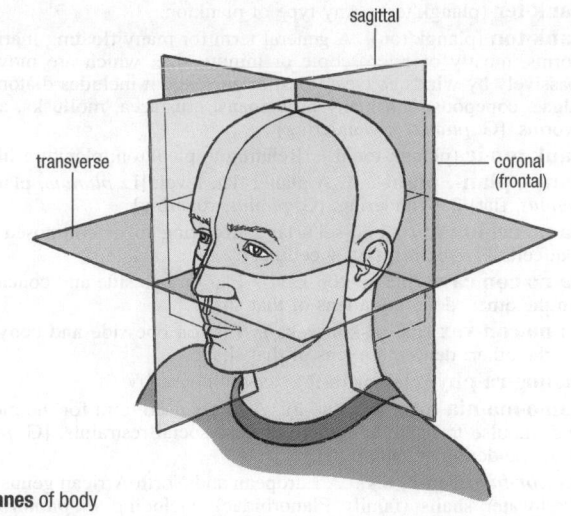

planes of body

brae, and by an *intertubercular p.* passing through the iliac tubercles and cutting usually the fifth lumbar vertebra; the p.'s formed on these lines, and also on transverse p.'s cutting the upper edge of the manubrium and the upper edge of the pubic symphysis, constitute the clinical p.'s of Addison.

Aeby p., in craniometry, a p. perpendicular to the median p. of the cranium, cutting the nasion and the basion.

auriculoinfraorbital p., SYN orbitomeatal p.

axial p., transverse plane at right angles to long axis of body, as in CT scanning. SYN transaxial p.

axiolabiolingual p., a p. parallel to the long axis of a tooth and extending in a labiolingual direction.

axiomesiodistal p., a p. parallel to the long axes of the teeth and extending in a mesiodistal direction.

bite p., SYN occlusal p.

Broca visual p., a p. drawn through the visual axes of each eye.

Camper p., a p. running from the tip of the anterior nasal spine (acanthion) to the center of the bony external auditory meatus on the right and left sides.

canthomeatal p., p. passing through the two lateral angles of the eye and the center of the external acoustic meatus; this p. lies approximately midway between the Frankfort and the supraorbitomeatal p.'s.

coronal p., SYN frontal p.

cove p., a classic description of terminal inversion of the electrocardiographic T wave with the initial portion arched above the baseline and the terminal portion below it, the former being rounded and the latter pointed.

datum p., an arbitrary p. used as a base from which to make craniometric measurements.

Daubenton p., the p. of the foramen magnum. SEE ALSO Daubenton *angle,* Daubenton *line.*

equatorial p., in metaphase of mitosis, the p. that touches all of the centromeres and their spindle attachments.

eye-ear p., SYN orbitomeatal p.

facial p., a measurement of the bony profile of the face. SYN nasion-pogonion measurement.

first parallel pelvic p., SYN pelvic *inlet.*

fourth parallel pelvic p., SYN pelvic *outlet.*

Frankfort p., SYN orbitomeatal p.

Frankfort horizontal p., SYN orbitomeatal p.

frontal p. [TA], a vertical p. at right angles to a sagittal p., dividing the body into anterior and posterior portions, or any plane parallel to the central coronal plane. SYN plana frontalia [TA], coronal p., plana coronalia.

guide p., a fixed or removable device used to displace a single tooth, an arch segment, or an entire arch toward an improved relationship.

horizontal p.'s [TA], plane parallel and relative to the horizon; in the anatomic position, horizontal planes are transverse planes; in the supine or prone positions, horizontal planes are frontal (coronal planes). SYN plana horizontalia [TA].

p. of incidence, the p. perpendicular to a lens surface that contains the incident light ray.

infraorbitomeatal p., SYN orbitomeatal p.

p. of inlet, SYN pelvic *inlet.*

interspinal p., SYN interspinous p.

interspinous p. [TA], a transverse plane passing through the anterior superior iliac spines; it marks the boundary between the lateral and umbilical regions superiorly and the inguinal and pubic regions inferiorly. SYN planum interspinale [TA], interspinal p., Lanz line.

intertubercular p. [TA], a transverse plane passing through the iliac tubercles. SYN planum intertuberculare [TA].

labiolingual p., a p. parallel to the labial and lingual surfaces of the teeth.

p. of least pelvic dimensions, SYN pelvic p. of least dimensions.

mean foundation p., the mean of the various irregularities in form and inclination of the basal seat; the ideal condition for denture stability exists when the mean foundation p. is most nearly at right angles to the direction of force.

Meckel p., a craniometric p. cutting the alveolar and the auricular points.

median p. [TA], a p. vertical in the anatomic position, through the midline of the body that divides the body into right and left halves. SEE ALSO Addison clinical p.'s. SYN planum medianum [TA].

p. of midpelvis, SYN pelvic p. of least dimensions.

midsagittal p., obsolete term for median p.

Morton p., a p. passing through the summits of the parietal and occipital protuberances.

nasion-postcondylar p., a p. passing through the nasion anteriorly and to a point immediately behind each condylar process of the mandible, posteriorly.

nodal p., the p. corresponding to the optical center of a simple lens. SEE nodal *point.*

nuchal p., the external surface of the squamous part of the occipital bone below the superior nuchal line, giving attachment to the muscles of the back of the neck.

occipital p. [TA], the external surface of the occipital bone above the superior nuchal line. SYN planum occipitale [TA].

occlusal p., p. of occlusion, an imaginary surface that is related anatomically to the cranium and that theoretically touches the incisal edges of the incisors and the tips of the occluding surfaces of the posterior teeth; it is not a p. in the true sense of the word but represents the mean of the curvature of the surface. SEE ALSO *curve* of occlusion. SYN bite p.

orbital p., the orbital surface of the maxilla, lying perpendicular to the orbitomeatal p. at the orbitale. SYN planum orbitale.

orbitomeatal p., (1) a line approximating the base of the skull, passing from the infraorbital ridge to the midline of the occiput, intersecting the superior margin of the external auditory meatus; the skull is in the anatomical position when the base line lies in the horizontal plane and right and left sides are level. (2) a standard craniometric reference p. passing through the right and left porion and the left orbitale; drawn on the profile radiograph or photograph from the superior margin of the acoustic meatus to the orbitale. SYN auriculoinfraorbital p., eye-ear p., Frankfort horizontal p., Frankfort p., infraorbitomeatal p.

p. of outlet, SYN pelvic *outlet.*

parasagittal p., obsolete term for sagittal p.

p. of pelvic canal, SYN *axis* of pelvis.

pelvic p. of greatest dimensions, the p. extending from the middle of the posterior surface of the pubic symphysis to the junction of the second and third sacral vertebrae, and laterally passing through the ischial bones over the middle of the acetabulum. SYN second parallel pelvic p., wide p.

pelvic p. of inlet, SYN pelvic *inlet.*

pelvic p. of least dimensions, the p. that extends from the end of the sacrum to the inferior border of the pubic symphysis; it is bounded posteriorly by the end of the sacrum, laterally by the ischial spines, and anteriorly by the inferior border of the pubic symphysis. SYN midplane, p. of least pelvic dimensions, p. of midpelvis, third parallel pelvic p.

pelvic p. of outlet, SYN pelvic *outlet.*

popliteal p. of femur, SYN popliteal *surface* of femur.

principal p., the theoretic p. of a compound lens system. SEE principal *point.*

p.'s of reference, p.'s that act as a guide to the location of other p.'s.

p. of regard, an imaginary p. through which the point of regard moves as the eyes are turned from side to side.

sagittal p. [TA], plane parallel to the median plane; sagittal planes are vertical planes in the anatomic position. SYN plana sagittalia [TA].

second parallel pelvic p., SYN pelvic p. of greatest dimensions.

spectacle p., the p. at which spectacles are worn.

sternal p., a p. indicated by the front surface of the sternum. SYN planum sternale.

subcostal p. [TA], a transverse plane passing through the inferior limits of the costal margin, i.e., the tenth costal cartilages; it marks the boundary between the hypochondriac and epigastric regions superiorly and the lateral and umbilical regions inferiorly. SYN planum subcostale [TA], infracostal line.

supracrestal p., SYN supracristal p.

supracristal p. [TA], a transverse plane passing through the summits of the iliac crests; it usually passes through the fourth lumbar spinous process. SYN planum supracristale [TA], supracrestal p.

supraorbitomeatal p., a p. passing the superior orbital margins and the superior margin of the external acoustic meatuses; it makes an angle of approximately 25°–30° with the Frankfort p.; routine CT scans of the brain are made parallel to this plane to limit exposure of eyeball to ionizing radiation.

suprasternal p., a transverse p. passing through the body at the level of the superior margin of the manubrium of the sternum.

temporal p. [TA], a slightly depressed area on the side of the cranium, below the inferior temporal line, formed by the temporal and parietal bones, the greater wing of the sphenoid, and a part of the frontal bone. SYN planum temporale [TA].

third parallel pelvic p., SYN pelvic p. of least dimensions.

tooth p., any one of the imaginary p.'s of section of a tooth, such as the axial, horizontal, or vertical.

transaxial p., SYN axial p.

transpyloric p. [TA], a transverse plane midway between the superior margins of the manubrium sterni and the symphysis pubis; the pylorus may be located on this plane in the supine or prone positions, but in the erect (anatomic) position it descends to a lower level. SYN planum transpyloricum [TA].

transverse p. [TA], a p. across the body at right angles to the coronal and sagittal p.'s; transverse planes are perpendicular to the long axis of the body or limbs, regardless of the position of the body or limb; in the anatomic position, transverse planes are horizontal planes; otherwise the two terms are not synonymous. SYN plana transversalia [TA].

wide p., SYN pelvic p. of greatest dimensions.

⌂**plani-.** SEE plano-.

pla·nig·ra·phy (pla-nig′ră-fē). SYN tomography. [L. *planum,* plane, + G. *graphē,* a writing]

pla·nim·e·ter (plă-nim′ĕ-ter). An instrument formed of jointed levers with a recording index, used for measuring the area of any surface, by tracing its boundaries. [L. *planum,* plane, + G. *metron,* measure]

pla·nim·et·ry (plă-nim′e-trē). The measurement of surface areas and perimeters by tracing the boundaries. Planimetry on photomicrographs or projected images may be used to evaluate the size of cells.

plan·i·tho·rax (plan′i-thō′raks). A diagram of the chest showing the front and back in plane projection, after the manner of Mercator projection of the earth's surface.

plank·ter (plangk′ter). Any type of plankton.

plank·ton (plangk′ton). A general term for many floating marine forms, mostly of microscopic or minute size, which are moved passively by winds, waves, tides, or currents; it includes diatoms, algae, copepods, and many protozoans, crustacea, mollusks, and worms. [G. *planktos,* wandering]

plank·ton·ic (plangk-ton′ik). Relating to plankton; plankton-like.

⌂**plano-, plan-, plani-.** **1.** A plane; flat, level. [L. *planum,* plane; *planus,* flat] **2.** Wandering. [G. *planos,* roaming]

pla·no·cel·lu·lar (plă-nō-sel′ū-lăr). Relating to or composed of flat cells. [L. *planus,* flat, + cellular]

pla·no·con·cave (plă′nō-kon-kāv′). Flat on one side and concave on the other; denoting a lens of that shape.

pla·no·con·vex (plă′nō-kon-veks′). Flat on one side and convex on the other; denoting a lens of that shape.

pla·nog·ra·phy (pla-nog′ră-fē). SYN tomography.

plan·o·ma·nia (plan-ō-mā′nē-ă). A rarely used term for the morbid impulse to leave home and discard social restraints. [G. *planos,* wandering, + *mania,* frenzy]

Pla·nor·bis (plan-ōr′bis). A European and North African genus of freshwater snails (family Planorbidae), including *P. planorbis,* intermediate host of the sheep and cattle fluke, *Paramphistoma cervi.* [G. *planos,* wandering, + L. *orbis,* circle, ring]

pla·no·val·gus (plă-nō-val′gŭs). A condition in which the longitudinal arch of the foot is flattened and the hindfoot is everted. [plano- + L. *valgus,* turned outward]

plan·ta, gen. and pl. **plan·tae** (plan′tă, plan′tē) [TA]. SYN sole. [L.]

p. pe′dis [TA], SYN *sole* of foot.

plan·ta·go (plan-tā′gō). The root and leaves of the common or large-leaved plantain, *Plantago major* (family Plantaginaceae). [L. plantain]

p. ovata coating, the separated outer mucilaginous layers of *Plantago ovata* seeds; used in simple constipation associated with lack of sufficient bulk.

p. seed, SYN psyllium seed.

plan·tain seed. SYN psyllium seed.

plan·tal·gia (plan-tal′jē-ă). Pain on the plantar surface of the foot over the plantar fascia. [L. *planta,* sole of foot, + G. *algos,* pain]

plan·tar (plan′tăr) [TA]. Relating to the sole of the foot. SYN plantaris [TA]. [L. *plantaris*]

plan·tar·is (plan-tār′is) [TA]. SYN plantar, plantar. [L.]

plan·ti·grade (plan′ti-grād). Walking with the entire sole and heel of the foot on the ground, as do humans and bears. [L. *planta,* sole, + *gradior,* to walk]

plan·u·la, pl. **plan·u·lae** (plan′ū-lă, -lē). Name given by Lankester to a coelenterate embryo when it consists of the two primary germ layers only, the ectoderm and endoderm. [L. dim. of *planum,* flat surface]

invaginate p., SYN gastrula.

pla·num, pl. **pla·na** (plă′nŭm, plă′nă). SYN plane. [L. plane]

plana coronalia, SYN frontal *plane.*

plana frontalia [TA], SYN frontal *plane.*

horizontal planes [TA], plane parallel and relative to the horizon; in the anatomic position, horizontal planes are transverse planes; in the supine or prone positions, horizontal planes are frontal (coronal planes). SYN plana horizontalia [TA].

plana horizontalia [TA], SYN horizontal planes.

p. interspina′le [TA], SYN interspinous *plane*; SEE ALSO Addison clinical *planes,* under *plane.*

p. intertubercula′re [TA], SYN intertubercular *plane*; SEE ALSO Addison clinical *planes,* under *plane.*

p. medianum [TA], SYN median *plane.*

p. occipita′le [TA], SYN occipital *plane.*

p. orbita′le, SYN orbital *plane.*

p. poplit′eum, SYN popliteal *surface* of femur.

plana sagittalia [TA], SYN sagittal *plane.*

p. semiluna′tum, the area of epithelium bounding the sensory area of the crista ampullaris.

p. sphenoida'le [TA], SYN *jugum* sphenoidale.

p. sterna'le, SYN sternal *plane.*

p. subcosta'le [TA], SYN subcostal *plane.*

p. supracrista'le [TA], SYN supracristal *plane.*

p. tempora'le [TA], SYN temporal *plane.*

p. transpylo'ricum [TA], SYN transpyloric *plane;* SEE Addison clinical *planes,* under *plane.*

plana transversalia [TA], SYN transverse *plane.*

pla·nu·ria (plă-noo'rē-ă). **1.** Extravasation of urine. **2.** The voiding of urine from an abnormal opening. [G. *planos,* wandering, + *ouron,* urine]

plaque (plak). **1.** A patch or small differentiated area on a body surface (e.g., skin, mucosa, or arterial endothelium) or on the cut surface of an organ such as the brain; in skin, a circumscribed, elevated, superficial, and solid area greater than 1.0 cm in diameter. **2.** An area of clearing in a flat confluent growth of bacteria or tissue cells, such as is caused by the lytic action of bacteriophage in an agar plate culture of bacteria, by the cytopathic effect of certain animal viruses in a sheet of cultured tissue cells, or by antibody (hemolysin) produced by lymphocytes cultured in the presence of erythrocytes and to which complement has been added. **3.** A sharply defined zone of demyelination characteristic of multiple sclerosis. **4.** SEE dental p. [Fr. a plate]

atheromatous p., a well-demarcated yellow area or swelling on the intimal surface of an artery; produced by intimal lipid deposit.

bacterial p., in dentistry, a mass of filamentous microorganisms and a large variety of smaller forms attached to the surface of a tooth that, depending on bacterial activity and environmental factors, may give rise to caries, calculus, or inflammatory changes in adjacent tissue. SYN dental p. (2), mucous p., mucinous p.

bacteriophage p., a clear circular zone in an otherwise confluent growth of bacteria on an agar surface resulting from bacterial lysis by bacterial viruses.

dental p., (1) the noncalcified accumulation mainly of oral microorganisms and their products that adheres tenaciously to the teeth and is not readily dislodged; **(2)** SYN bacterial p.

Hollenhorst p.'s, glittering, orange-yellow, atheromatous emboli in the retinal arterioles that contain cholesterol crystals and originate in the carotid artery or great vessels.

mucous p., mucinous p., SYN bacterial p.

neuritic p., SYN senile p.

pleural p., fibrous thickening of the parietal pleura, characteristically caused by inhalation exposure to asbestos; both microscopic and macroscopic calcification in this lesion is common.

Randall p.'s, mineral concentrations on renal papillae.

senile p., a spherical mass composed primarily of amyloid fibrils and interwoven neuronal processes, frequently, although not exclusively, observed in Alzheimer disease. SYN neuritic p.

Plaque In·dex. An index for estimating the status of oral hygiene by measuring dental plaque that occurs in the areas adjacent to the gingival margin.

-plasia. Formation (especially of cells). SEE plasma-. [G. *plassō,* to form]

plasm (plazm). SYN plasma.

plas·ma (plaz'mă). **1.** The proteinaceous fluid (noncellular) portion of the circulating blood, as distinguished from the serum obtained after coagulation. SYN blood p. **2.** The fluid portion of the lymph. **3.** The fluid in which the fat droplets of milk are suspended. **4.** A "fourth state of matter" in which, owing to elevated temperature, atoms have broken down to form free electrons and more or less stripped nuclei; produced in the laboratory in connection with hydrogen fusion (thermonuclear) research. SYN plasm. [G. something formed]

antihemophilic p., human p. in which the labile antihemophilic globulin component, present in fresh p., has been preserved; it is used to temporarily relieve dysfunction of the hemostatic mechanism in hemophilia.

blood p., SYN plasma (1).

p. expander (plaz'mă eks-pan'der), SYN plasma *substitute.*

fresh frozen p. (FFP), separated p., frozen within 6 hours of

blood plasma		
selected components of plasma or serum: normal ranges		
ammonia nitrogen (whole blood)	53–143	μmol/l
bicarbonate	21–25	mmol/l
bilirubin (total)	5.1–18.8	μmol/l
bilirubin (direct)	up to 6.8	μmol/l
calcium	2.2–2.7	mmol/l
chloride	94–111	mmol/l
cholesterol	3.36–5.20*	mmol/l
copper	♂ 11.0–22.0 ♀ 13.4–24.4	μmol/l
creatine	♂ 23–61 ♀ 23–92	μmol/l
creatinine	♂ 62–106 ♀ 44–88	μmol/l
fat, total	3.6–8.2*	g/l
fatty acids, free	200–900	μmol/l
fructose	up to 0.55	mmol/l
galactose	up to 0.24	mmol/l
glucose	3.33–5.55*	mmol/l
iron	♂ 16.1–25.1 ♀ 14.3–21.5	μmol/l
iron binding capacity —total	♂ 53.7–71.6 ♀ 44.8–62.7	μmol/l
—free	♂ 35.8–53.7 ♀ 26.9–44.8	μmol/l
lactate	1.00–1.78	mmol/l
LDL cholesterol		
lead (whole blood)	up to 2.0	μmol/l
lithium	0.4–6.3	μmol/l
magnesium	0.66–0.90	mmol/l
phosphorus, inorganic	0.81–1.55	mmol/l
potassium	4.1–5.6	mmol/l
protein, total	67–87	g/l
sodium	137–148	mmol/l
thyroxine	66–187	nmol/l
triglyceride	0.4–15	g/l
uric acid (enzymatic)	♂ 155–404 ♀ 119–375	μmol/l
urea	3.33–6.66	mmol/l

*age-dependent

collection, used in hypovolemia and coagulation factor deficiency.

p. hydrolysate, an artificial digest of protein derived from bovine blood p. prepared by a method of hydrolysis sufficient to provide more than half of the total nitrogen present in the form of α-amino nitrogen; used when high protein intake is indicated and cannot be accomplished through ordinary foods. SEE ALSO protein hydrolysate.

p. mari'num, sea water diluted to make it isotonic with p.

muscle p., an alkaline fluid in muscle that is spontaneously coagulable, separating into myosin and muscle serum.

normal human p., sterile p. obtained by pooling approximately equal amounts of the liquid portion of citrated whole blood from eight or more adult humans who have been certified as free from any disease that is tranmissible by transfusion, and treating it with ultraviolet irradiation to destroy possible bacterial and viral contaminants.

salted p., the fluid portion of blood drawn from the vessels, which is prevented from coagulating by being drawn into a solution of sodium or magnesium sulfate. SYN salted serum.

plasma-, plasmat-, plasmato-, plasmo-. Formative, organized; plasma. [G. *plasma,* something formed]

plas·ma·blast (plaz'mă-blast). Precursor of the plasma cell. SYN plasmacytoblast. [plasma + G. *blastos,* germ]

plas·ma cell dys·cra·sia. A diverse group of diseases characterized by the proliferation of a single clone of cells producing a monoclonal immunoglobulin or immunoglobulin fragment (a serum M component). The cells usually have plasma cell morphology, but may have lymphocytic or lymphoplasmacytic morphology. This group includes multiple myeloma, Waldenström macroglobulinemia, the heavy chain disease, benign monoclonal gammopathy, and immunocytic amyloidosis.

plas·ma·crit (plaz′mă-krit). A measure of the percentage of the volume of blood occupied by plasma, in contrast to a hematocrit. [plasma + G. *krino̅*, to separate]

plas·ma·cyte (plaz′mă-sīt). SYN plasma *cell*.

plas·ma·cy·to·blast (plas-mă-sī′tō-blast). SYN plasmablast.

plas·ma·cy·to·ma (plaz′mă-sī-tō′mă). A discrete, presumably solitary mass of neoplastic plasma cells in bone or in one of various extramedullary sites; in humans, such lesions are probably the initial phase of developing plasma cell myeloma. [plasmacyte + G. *-oma*, tumor]

plas·ma·cy·to·sis (plaz′mă-sī-tō′sis). **1.** Presence of plasma cells in the circulating blood. **2.** Presence of unusually large proportions of plasma cells in the tissues or exudates. [plasmacyte + G. *-osis*, condition]

plas·ma·gene (plaz′mă-jēn). A determinant of an inherited character located in the cytoplasm. SYN cytogene. [plasma + gene]

plas·ma·ki·nins (plaz′mă-kīn′inz). A group of highly active oligopeptides found in sera that act upon smooth muscle of blood vessels, uterus, bronchi, etc.; e.g., bradykinin, kallidin.

plas·ma·lem·ma (plaz-mă-lem′ă). SYN cell *membrane*. [plasma + G. *lemma*, husk]

plas·mal·o·gens (plaz-mal′ō-jenz). Generic term for glycerophospholipids in which the glycerol moiety bears a 1-alkenyl ether group (on rarer occasions, a 1-alkyl ether group); e.g., alk-1-enylglycerophospholipid; p. synthesis is reduced in disorders of the peroxisome. SYN phosphoglyceracetals.

plas·mals (plaz′mălz). Long-chain aldehydes occurring in plasmalogens; e.g., stearaldehyde, palmitaldehyde.

plas·ma·phe·re·sis (plaz′mă-fĕ-rē′sis). Removal of whole blood from the body, separation of its cellular elements by centrifugation, and reinfusion of them suspended in saline or some other plasma substitute, thus depleting the body's own plasma without depleting its cells. [plasma + G. *aphairesis*, a withdrawal]

plas·ma·phe·ret·ic (plaz′mă-fĕ-ret′ik). Relating to plasmapheresis.

⌂**plasmat-**. SEE plasma-.

plas·mat·ic (plaz-mat′ik). Relating to plasma. SYN plasmic.

plas·ma·tog·a·my (plaz-mă-tog′ă-mē). SYN plasmogamy.

plas·men·ic ac·id (plaz′men-ik). Proposed name for phosphatidates such as 2-acyl-1-alk-1-enylglycerol 3-phosphate.

plas·mic (plaz′mik). SYN plasmatic.

ⓘ**plas·mid** (plaz′mid). A genetic particle physically separate from the chromosome of the host cell (chiefly bacterial) that can stably function and replicate and usually confer some advantage to the host cell; not essential to the cell's basic functioning. SYN extrachromosomal element, extrachromosomal genetic element, paragene. [cyto*plasm* + -id]

bacteriocinogenic p.'s, bacterial p.'s responsible for the elaboration of bacteriocins. SYN bacteriocin factors, bacteriocinogens.

conjugative p., a p. that can effect its own intercellular transfer by means of conjugation; this transfer is accomplished by a bacterium being rendered a donor, usually with specialized pili. SYN infectious p., transmissible p.

F p., the prototype conjugative p. associated with conjugation in the K-12 strain of *Escherichia coli.* SYN fertility factor, sex factor.

infectious p., SYN conjugative p.

nonconjugative p., a p. that cannot effect conjugation and self-transfer to another bacterium (bacterial strain); transfer depends upon mediation of another (and conjugative) p.

R p.'s, SYN resistance p.'s.

resistance p.'s, p.'s carrying genes responsible for antibiotic (or antibacterial drug) resistance among bacteria (notably Enterobacteriaceae); they may be conjugative or nonconjugative p.'s, the former possessing transfer genes (resistance transfer factor) lack-

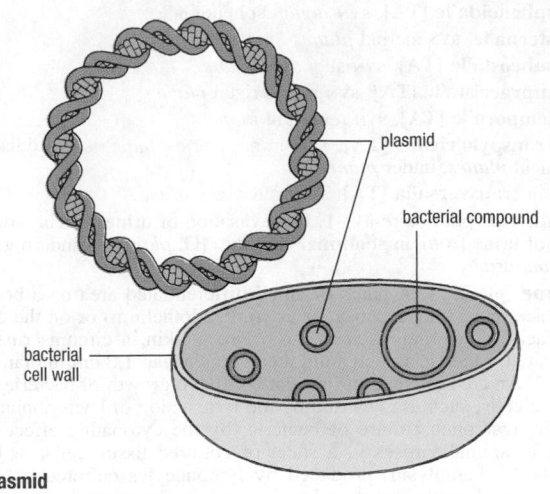

plasmid
bacterial compound
bacterial cell wall

plasmid

ing in the latter. SYN R factors, R p.'s, resistance factors, resistance-transferring episomes.

transmissible p., SYN conjugative p.

plas·min (plaz′min). A serine proteinase hydrolyzing peptides and esters of L-arginine and L-lysine and converting fibrin to soluble products; occurs in plasma as the precursor plasminogen (profibrinolysin) and is activated to plasmin by organic solvents, which remove an inhibitor, and by streptokinase, trypsin, and plasminogen activator, all cleaving a single arginyl-valyl bond; p. is responsible for the dissolution of blood clots. SYN fibrinase (2), fibrinolysin.

plas·min·o·gen (plaz-min′ō-jen). A precursor of plasmin. There is an autosomal dominant deficiency of p. [MIM*173350] that may promote thrombosis. SEE plasmin.

plas·min·o·ki·nase (plaz′min-ō-kī′nās). SYN streptokinase.

plas·min·o·plas·tin (plaz′min-ō-plas′tin). Term proposed for activator agents that produce plasmin by direct action on plasminogen; e.g., staphylokinase, plasminogen activator.

⌂**plasmo-**. SEE plasma-.

plas·mo·dia (plaz-mō′dē-ă). Plural of plasmodium. [L.]

plas·mo·di·al (plaz-mō′dē-ăl). **1.** Relating to a plasmodium. **2.** Relating to any species of the genus *Plasmodium.*

plas·mo·di·o·tro·pho·blast (plaz-mō′dē-ō-trō′fō-blast). SYN syncytiotrophoblast. [plasmodium + G. *trophē*, nourishment, + *blastos*, germ]

ⓘ***Plas·mo·di·um*** (plaz-mō′dē-ŭm). A genus of the protozoan family Plasmodiidae (suborder Haemosporina, subclass Coccidia), blood parasites of vertebrates, characterized by separate microgametes and macrogametes, a motile ookinete, sporogony in the invertebrate host, and merogony (schizogony) in the vertebrate host; includes the causal agents of malaria in humans and other animals, with an asexual cycle occurring in liver and red blood cells of vertebrates and a sexual cycle in mosquitoes, the latter cycle resulting in the production of large numbers of infective sporozoites in the salivary glands of the vector, which are transmitted when the mosquito bites and draws blood. Primate malaria is transmitted by various species of *Anopheles* mosquitoes, bird malaria by species of *Aedes, Culex, Anopheles,* and *Culiseta.* [Mod. L. from G. *plasma*, something formed, + *eidos*, appearance]

P. aethio′picum, SYN *P. falciparum.*

P. ber′ghei, a species of protozoan that is the etiologic agent of rodent malaria from central Africa; an important source of experimental nonprimate mammal malaria.

P. brazilian′um, a protozoan species found in New World monkeys of the family Cebidae in northern South America and Panama, which can cause mild malaria in humans.

P. cynomol′gi, a protozoan species similar to *P. vivax* occurring

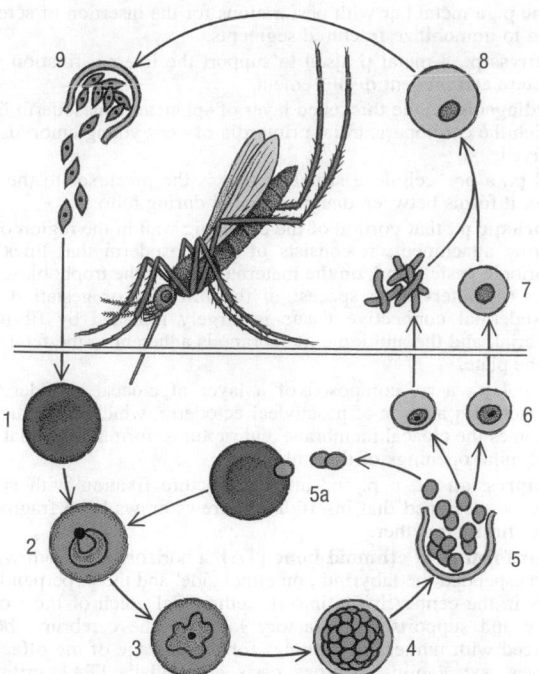

plasmodium: life cycle; (1) sporozoite invading red blood cell; (2) "ring" stage of development; (3) ameboid stage of development; (4) asexual division; (5) cell rupture with release of spore; (5a) reinfection of red blood cell by some spores; (6) development of other spores into sexual forms; (7) development into egg and sperm cells after mosquito sucks them in; (8) fertilized cell developing into cyst; (9) ruptured cyst releasing sporozoites

naturally in the macaque, but infecting humans both accidentally and experimentally; it produces a *P.-vivax* type of malaria.

P. falcip′arum, *Laverania falciparum,* a species that is the causal agent of falciparum (malignant tertian) malaria; a young trophozoite is about one-fifth the size of an erythrocyte, but developing erythrocytic stages are rarely seen in circulating blood, as they render infected cells sticky and cause them to concentrate in capillaries in the vital organs, particularly the brain and the heart; a schizont occupies about one-half to two-thirds of the red blood cell and has fine, sparse granules (observed in peripheral blood only from moribund patients); infected erythrocytes are normal or contracted in size and are likely to contain basophilic granules and red dots (Maurer clefts or dots); multiple infection is extremely frequent and causes bouts of fever somewhat irregularly, since the parasite's cycles of multiplication are usually asynchronous. SYN malignant tertian malarial parasite, *P. aethiopicum.*

P. knowles′i, a species of protozoan from Southeast Asia that causes monkey malaria with a quotidian fever cycle; highly fatal in rhesus monkeys; naturally acquired by a human in Malaysia, and also transmitted to humans experimentally.

P. ko′chi, a *P.* species now recognized as *Hepatocystis kochi.*

P. mala′riae, a protozoan species that is the causal agent of quartan malaria; a ring-stage trophozoite is triangular, ovoid, or slightly bean shaped, with fine or coarse black granules, approximately one-third the size of an eythrocyte; the schizont is oval or rounded and nearly fills the red blood cell; infected erythrocytes are normal or slightly contracted in size, usually with no stippling (the two most important characteristics that distinguish it from *P. vivax*), although extremely fine Ziemann dots may be observed; multiple infection is extremely rare; thus, bouts of fever occur fairly regularly at 72-hour intervals; prolonged asymptomatic parasitemia is characteristic of the species, and recrudescence of fever may occur 10 years or more after the initial episode. SYN quartan parasite.

P. ova′le, a protozoan species that is the agent of the least com-

mon form of human malaria; resembles *P. vivax* in its earlier stages but often modifies the cell membrane, causing it to form a fimbriated outline and, often assume an oval shape; Schüffner dots are abundant and appear early, host cells are normal or only slightly enlarged, and only about 8–10 grapelike merozoites are produced; fever is tertian (every 48 hours), and relapses are infrequent.

P. vi′vax, a protozoan species that is the most common malarial parasite of humans (except in West Africa, where the form of the Duffy antigen (FyFy) protects most of the resident populations, which has permitted *P. ovale* to replace *P. vivax*); the early trophozoite is irregular and ameboid in shape, one-fourth to one-third the size of a red blood cell, and contains several fine granules; the schizont is irregular in shape, fills the enlarged erythrocyte, and contains numerous yellow-brown pigment granules; affected red blood cells are pale, enlarged, and contain Schüffner dots in the later stages of growth; characteristically causes bouts of fever fairly regularly at 48-hour intervals, but multiple infection, causing irregular fever patterns, is common. SYN tertian parasite.

plas·mo·di·um, pl. **plas·mo·dia** (plaz-mō′dē-ŭm, -dē-ă). A protoplasmic mass containing several nuclei, resulting from multiplication of the nucleus with cell division. [Mod. L. fr. G. *plasma,* something formed, + *eidos,* appearance]

placental p., SYN syncytiotrophoblast.

Plas·mo·dro·ma·ta (plaz-mō-drō′mă-tă). A former taxonomic category that included ameboid and flagellate Protozoa in which the nucleus is not separated into reproductive (micro-) and vegetative (macro-) portions; equivalent to the present phylum Sarcomastigophora. [plasmo- + G. *dromos,* a running, a course]

plas·mog·a·my (plaz-mog′ă-mē). Union of two or more cells with preservation of the individual nuclei; formation of a plasmodium. SYN plasmatogamy, plastogamy. [plasmo- + G. *gamos,* marriage]

plas·mo·gen (plaz′mō-jen). SYN protoplasm. [plasmo- + G. -*gen,* producing]

plas·mo·ki·nin (plaz-mō-kī′nin). Obsolete term for *factor* VIII.

plas·mo·lem·ma (plaz-mō-lem′ă). SYN cell *membrane.*

plas·mol·y·sis (plaz-mol′i-sis). Shrinking of plant cells by osmotic loss of cytoplasmic water. SYN protoplasmolysis. [plasmo- + G. *lysis,* dissolution]

plas·mo·lyt·ic (plaz-mō-lit′ik). Relating to plasmolysis.

plas·mo·lyze (plaz′mō-līz). To subject to plasmolysis.

plas·mon (plaz′mon). The total of the extrachromosomal genetic determinants of the eukaryotic cell cytoplasm. SYN plasmotype. [cyto*plasm* + -*on*]

plas·mor·rhex·is (plaz-mō-rek′sis). The splitting open of a cell from the pressure of the protoplasm.

plas·mos·chi·sis (plaz-mos′ki-sis). The splitting of protoplasm into fragments. [plasmo- + G. *schisis,* a cleaving]

plas·mo·sin (plaz′mō-sin). A highly viscous substance in cytoplasm containing discrete fibers of considerable length; a nucleoprotein regarded as the structural foundation of the cell.

plas·mot·o·my (plaz-mot′ō-mē). A form of mitosis in multinuclear protozoan cells in which the cytoplasm divides into two or more masses, later reproducing, in some cases by sporulation. [plasmo- + G. *tomē,* incision]

plas·mo·tro·pic (plaz-mō-trop′ik). Pertaining to or manifesting plasmotropism.

plas·mot·ro·pism (plaz-mot′rō-pizm). A condition in which the bone marrow, spleen, and liver are sites for the destruction of the erythrocytes, as opposed to destruction in the circulating blood. [plasmo- + G. *tropē,* a turning]

plas·mo·type (plaz′mō-tīp). SYN plasmon.

plas·mo·zyme (plaz′mō-zīm). Obsolete term for prothrombin. [plasmo- + G. *zymē,* leaven]

plas·tein (plas′tē-in). **1.** Insoluble polypeptide formed through the random condensation of amino acids or peptides under the catalytic influence of a proteinase-like chymotrypsin; molecular weights as high as 500,000 are reported. **2.** A gel that is formed on treating a partial hydrolysate of a protein with an endopeptidase.

plas·ter. **1.** A solid preparation that can be spread when heated and that becomes adhesive at the temperature of the body; used to keep the edges of a wound in apposition, to protect raw surfaces, and, when medicated, to redden or blister the skin, as in mustard p., or to apply drugs to the surface to obtain their systemic effects. **2.** In dentistry, colloquialism for p. of Paris. [L. *emplastrum;* G. *emplastron,* plaster or mold]

p. of Paris, exsiccated calcium sulfate from which the water of crystallization has been expelled by heat, but which, when mixed with water, will form a paste which subsequently sets.

plas·tic (plas′tik). **1.** Capable of being formed or molded. **2.** A material that can be shaped by pressure or heat to the form of a cavity or mold. [G. *plastikos,* relating to molding]

Bingham p., a material that, in the idealized case, does not flow until a critical stress (yield stress) is exceeded, and then flows at a rate proportional to the excess of stress over the yield stress; real materials probably only approach this ideal model.

modeling p., a thermoplastic material usually composed of gum damar and prepared chalk, used especially for making dental impressions. SYN impression compound, modeling composition, modeling compound.

plas·tic·i·ty (plas-tis′i-tē). The capability of being formed or molded; the quality of being plastic.

plas·tid (plas′tid). **1.** One of the differentiated structures in cytoplasm of plant cells where photosynthesis or other cellular processes are carried on; p.'s contain DNA and are self-replicating. SYN trophoplast. **2.** One of the granules of foreign or differentiated matter, food particles, fat, waste material, chromatophores, trichocysts, etc., in cells. **3.** A self-duplicating viruslike particle that multiplies within a host cell, such as κ particles in certain paramecia. [G. *plastos,* formed, + -id]

blood p., any basic, morphologic unit in the biologic composition of blood, e.g., an erythrocyte.

plas·to·chro·man·ol-3, plas·to·chro·ma·nol E₃ (plas-tō-krō′man-ol). A γ-tocotrienol. SEE tocotrienol.

plas·to·chro·men·ol-8 (plas-tō-krō′men-ol). The chromenol (isomeric) form of plastoquinone-9. SYN solanochromene.

plas·tog·a·my (plas-tog′ă-mē). SYN plasmogamy.

plas·to·quin·one (PQ) (plas-tō-kwin′ōn, -kwī′nōn). 2,3-Dimethyl-1,4-benzoquinone with a multiprenyl side chain; a trivial name sometimes used for plastoquinone-9.

plas·to·quin·one-9 (PQ-9), plas·to·quin·one E₉. 2,3-Dimethyl-6-nonaprenyl-1,4-benzoquinone; one of a group of vitamins E and K and coenzymes Q; the isomeric form is plastochromenol-8; a participant in photosynthetic electron transport.

plas·tron. The sternum with costal cartilages attached. [Fr. a breastplate]

△**-plasty.** Molding, shaping or the result thereof, as of a surgical procedure. [G. *plastos,* formed, shaped]

-plas·ty (plas′tē). Surgical procedure for repair of a defect or restoration of form and/or function of a part. [G. *plastos,* formed]

plate (plāt). **1** [TA]. In anatomy, a thin, relative flat, structure. SYN lamina [TA]. **2.** A metal bar perforated for screws applied to a fractured bone to maintain the ends in apposition. **3.** The agar layer within a Petri dish or similar vessel. **4.** To form a very thin layer of a bacterial culture by streaking it on the surface of an agar p. (usually within a Petri dish) to isolate individual organisms from which a colonial clone will develop. **5.** Any one of the horizontal perforated p.'s that comprise the fractionating component of a column in fractional distillation (or, the theoretic equivalent of such a p.). [O.Fr. *plat,* a flat object, fr. G. *platys,* flat, broad]

alar p. of neural tube, SYN alar *lamina* of neural tube.

amorphous selenium p., SYN selenium p.

anal p., the anal portion of the cloacal p.

axial p., the primitive streak of an embryo.

basal p. of neural tube, SYN basal *lamina* of neural tube.

base p., SEE baseplate.

blood p., obsolete term for platelet.

bone p., a metal bar with perforations for the insertion of screws; used to immobilize fractured segments.

buttress p., a metal p. used to support the internal fixation of a fracture and prevent displacement.

cardiogenic p., the thickened layer of splanchnic mesoderm from which the cardiopericardial primordia of very young embryos are derived.

cell p., a non-cellulose structure that is the precursor to the cell wall; it forms between daughter nuclei during mitosis.

chorionic p., that portion of the chorionic wall in the region of its uterine attachment; it consists of the mesoderm that lines the chorionic vesicle and, on the maternal side, of the trophoblast that lines the intervillous spaces; in the last half of gestation, the mesodermal connective tissue is largely replaced by fibrinoid material, and the amnionic membrane is adherent to the fetal side of the plate.

cloacal p., a p., composed of a layer of cloacal endoderm in contact with a layer of proctodeal ectoderm, which subsequently becomes the cloacal membrane and ruptures, forming the anal and urogenital openings of the embryo.

compression p., a p. for internal fracture fixation with screw holes so designed that insertion of screws draws bone fragments more firmly together.

cribriform p. of ethmoid bone [TA], a horizontal p. from which are suspended the labyrinth, on either side, and the p. perpendicularis in the center; it fits into the ethmoidal notch of the frontal bone and supports the olfactory lobes of the cerebrum, being pierced with numerous openings for the passage of the olfactory nerves. SYN lamina cribrosa ossis ethmoidalis [TA], cribrum, sieve bone, sieve p.

cutis p., SYN dermatome (2).

dorsal p. of neural tube, SYN roof p.

dorsolateral p. of neural tube, SYN alar *lamina* of neural tube.

end p., SEE endplate.

epiphysial p. [TA], the disc of cartilage between the metaphysis and the epiphysis of an immature long bone permitting growth in length. SYN lamina epiphysialis [TA], growth p.

equatorial p., the assembly of chromosomes in mitosis.

ethmovomerine p., the central portion of the ethmoid bone, forming a distinct element at birth.

flat p., jargon for plain *film.*

floor p., ventral midline thinning of the developing neural tube, a continuity between the basal laminae of either side; opposite of roof plate. SYN ventral p.

foot p., SEE footplate.

frontal p., in the fetus, a cartilage p. between the lateral parts of ethmoid cartilage and the developing sphenoid bone.

growth p., SYN epiphysial p.

horizontal p. of palatine bone [TA], the part of the palatine bone that forms the posterior part (approximately one-third) of the bony palate. SYN lamina horizontalis ossis palatini [TA].

Kühne p., the endplate of a motor nerve fiber in a muscle spindle.

lateral p., a nonsegmented mass of mesoderm on the lateral periphery of the embryonic disk; it forms the somatopleuric (parietal) and splanchnopleuric (visceral) mesoderm.

lateral cartilaginous p., SYN lateral *lamina* of cartilage of pharyngotympanic (auditory) tube.

lateral p. of cartilaginous auditory tube, SYN lateral *lamina* of cartilage of pharyngotympanic (auditory) tube.

lateral pterygoid p. [TA], the larger and more lateral of the two bony plates extending downward from the point of union of the body and greater wing of the sphenoid bone on either side; forms medial wall of infratemporal fossa and gives origin to pterygoi muscles. SYN lamina lateralis processus pterygoidei [TA], lateral p. of pterygoid process.

lateral p. of pterygoid process, SYN lateral pterygoid p.

lingual p., SYN linguoplate.

medial cartilaginous p., SYN medial *lamina* of cartilage of pharyngotympanic (auditory) tube.

medial p. of cartilaginous auditory tube, SYN medial *lamina* of cartilage of pharyngotympanic (auditory) tube.

medial pterygoid p. [TA], the smaller and more medial of the two bony plates extending downward from the point of union of the body and greater wing of the sphenoid bone on either side, ending inferiorly in the pterygoid hamulus. SYN lamina medialis processus pterygoidei [TA], medial p. of pterygoid process.

medial p. of pterygoid process, SYN medial pterygoid p.

medullary p., SYN neural p.

p. of modiolus, SYN lamina of modiolus of cochlea.

motor p., a motor endplate.

muscle p., SYN myotome (2).

nail p., SYN nail (1).

neural p., the neuroectodermal region of the early embryo's dorsal surface that in later development is transformed into the neural tube and neural crest. SYN medullary p.

neutralization p., a metal p. used for the internal fixation of a bone fracture to neutralize the forces producing displacement.

notochordal p., the sheet of notochordal cells that are intercalated in the endodermal roof of the primitive yolk sac. SEE ALSO head process.

oral p., a circumscribed area of fusion of foregut endoderm and stomodeal ectoderm in the embryo that breaks through early in development to establish the oral opening. SEE ALSO buccopharyngeal membrane.

orbital p., SYN orbital p. of ethmoid bone.

orbital p. of ethmoid bone [TA], a thin plate of ethmoid bone forming part of the medial wall of the orbit and the lateral wall for the ethmoidal labyrinth. SYN lamina orbitalis ossis ethmoidalis [TA], lamina papyracea, orbital lamina of ethmoid bone, orbital layer of ethmoid bone, orbital p., paper p., papyraceous p.

palatal p., a partial denture major connector that has an anteroposterior width in excess of two maxillary premolars.

palmar p.'s, SYN palmar ligaments of metacarpophalangeal joints, under ligament.

paper p., papyraceous p., SYN orbital p. of ethmoid bone.

parachordal p., the cartilage primordia of the base of the skull situated on either side of the cephalic part of the notochord.

parietal p., (1) the outer of the two layers of the lateral plate mesoderm, which becomes associated with the ectoderm; the ectoderm and parietal plate mesoderm together constitute the somatopleure; **(2)** the lamina of the ethmoid bone that forms part of the nasal septum.

perpendicular p. [TA], flat portion of a bone that lies within or closely approximates a vertical plane. SEE perpendicular p. of ethmoid bone, perpendicular p. of palatine bone. SYN lamina perpendicularis [TA], pars perpendicularis, vertical p.

perpendicular p. of ethmoid bone [TA], a thin plate of bone projecting downward from the crista galli of the ethmoid; it forms part of the nasal septum. SYN lamina perpendicularis ossis ethmoidalis [TA].

perpendicular p. of palatine bone [TA], the part of the palatine bone that extends vertically upward from the horizontal lamina; it forms part of the lateral wall of the nasal cavity. SYN lamina perpendicularis ossis palatini [TA].

phosphor p., the coated p. used in place of a radiographic film cassette in a computed radiography system. SEE ALSO selenium p., amorphous silicon.

polar p.'s, condensed platelike bodies at the ends of the spindle during mitosis of certain types of cells.

prechordal p., SYN prochordal p.

prochordal p., a small area immediately rostral to the cephalic tip of the notochord where ectoderm and endoderm are in contact; when turned under the growing head, it forms the buceopharyngeal membrane. SEE ALSO oral p. SYN prechordal p.

pterygoid p.'s, SEE lateral pterygoid p., medial pterygoid p.

quadrigeminal p., SYN lamina of mesencephalic tectum.

roof p., the thin layer of the embryonic neural tube connecting the alar p.'s dorsally. SYN dorsal p. of neural tube.

secondary spiral p., SYN secondary spiral lamina.

segmental p., SYN segmental zone.

selenium p., a radiation-sensitive material used in directed digital

radiography. SEE ALSO digital radiography. SYN amorphous selenium p.

sieve p., SYN cribriform p. of ethmoid bone.

spiral p., SYN osseous spiral lamina.

stigmal p.'s, area in arthropod larvae where the tracheal system opens to the outside; morphology of this area is used to identify various arthropod larvae. SEE ALSO spiracle.

suction p., in dentistry, a p. held in place by atmospheric pressure.

tarsal p.'s, SEE superior tarsus, inferior tarsus.

tectal p. [TA], SYN lamina of mesencephalic tectum.

terminal p., SYN lamina terminalis of cerebrum.

tympanic p. of temporal bone [TA], the bony p. forming the greater part of the anterior wall of the bony part of the external acoustic meatus and the tympanic cavity, and the posterior wall of the mandibular fossa. SYN pars tympanica ossis temporalis [TA], tympanic part of temporal bone.

urethral p., the endodermal lining of the urethral groove that forms the lining of the penile urethra.

ventral p., SYN floor p.

ventral p. of neural tube, SYN basal lamina of neural tube.

vertical p., SYN perpendicular p.

visceral p., the inner of the two layers of the lateral mesoderm; the splanchnic mesoderm that becomes associated with the endoderm and together with it constitutes the splanchnopleure.

wing p., SYN alar lamina of neural tube.

Plateau, Joseph Antoine Ferdinand, Belgian physicist, 1801–1883. SEE P.-Talbot law.

pla·teau (plă-tō). A flat elevated segment of a graphic record. [Fr.]

    ventricular p., a level diastolic portion of the intraventricular blood pressure curve, representing graphically an equilibrium or final state of filling.

plate·let (plāt′let). An irregularly shaped disklike cytoplasmic fragment of a megakaryocyte that is shed in the marrow sinus and subsequently found in the peripheral blood, where it functions in clotting. A p. contains granules in the central part (granulomere) and, peripherally, clear protoplasm (hyalomere), but no definite nucleus; is about one-third to one-half the size of an erythrocyte; and contains no hemoglobin. SYN Bizzozero corpuscle, blood disk, elementary bodies (2), elementary particle (1), third corpuscle, thrombocyte, thromboplastid (1), Zimmermann corpuscle. [see plate]

plate·let·phe·re·sis (plāt′let-fĕ-rē′sis). Removal of blood from a donor with replacement of all blood components except platelets. [platelet + G. aphairesis, a withdrawal]

plat·ing (plāt′ing). **1.** Sowing of bacteria on a solid medium in a Petri dish or similar container; the making of a plate culture. **2.** Application of a metal bar to keep the ends of a fractured bone in apposition. **3.** Electrolytic deposition of a metal.

    compression p., a technique for internal fixation using a compression plate.

    replica p., a procedure for producing an accurate copy of bacterial colonies from one agar plate to another.

pla·tin·ic (pla-tin′ik). Relating to platinum; denoting a compound containing platinum in its higher valency.

plat·i·nous (plat′i-nŭs). Relating to platinum; denoting a compound containing platinum in its lower valency.

plat·i·num (Pt) (plat′i-nŭm). A metallic element, atomic no. 78, atomic wt. 195.08, used for making small parts for chemical apparatus because of its resistance to acids; in powdered form (**p. black**), it is an important catalyst in hydrogenation. Some of its salts have been used in the treatment of syphilis. A derivative, cisplatin, is used as an antineoplastic agent. [Mod. L., originally platina, fr. Sp. plata, silver]

plat·i·num foil. Pure platinum rolled into extremely thin sheets; its high fusing point makes it suitable as a matrix for various soldering procedures in dentistry and also suitable for providing internal form to porcelain restorations during their fabrication.

plat·i·num group. A group of six amphoteric elements: iridium, osmium, palladium, platinum, rhodium, and ruthenium.

pl

Platt, Sir Harry, British surgeon, *1886. SEE Putti-P. *operation*, *procedure*.

△**platy-.** Width; flatness. [G. *platys*, flat, broad]

plat·y·ba·sia (plat-i-bā′sē-ă). A developmental anomaly of the skull or an acquired softening of the skull bones so that the floor of the posterior cranial fossa bulges upward in the region about the foramen magnum. SYN basilar invagination. [*platy-* + G. *basis*, ground]

plat·y·ceph·a·ly (plat′i-sef′ă-lē). Flatness of the skull, a condition in which the vertical cranial index is below 70. SYN platycrania. [*platy-* + G. *kephalē*, head]

plat·yc·ne·mia (plat′ik-nē′mē-ă). A condition in which the tibia is abnormally broad and flat. SYN platycnemism. [*platy-* + G. *knēmē*, leg]

plat·yc·ne·mic (plat′ik-nē′mik). Relating to or marked by platycnemia.

plat·yc·ne·mism (plat′ik-nē′mizm). SYN platycnemia.

plat·y·cra·nia (plat′i-krā′nē-ă). SYN platycephaly. [*platy-* + G. *kranion*, skull]

plat·y·cyte (plat′i-sīt). Obsolete term for a relatively small giant cell sometimes formed in tubercles. [*platy-* + G. *kytos*, cell]

plat·y·glos·sal (plat′i-glos′ăl). Having a broad, flattened tongue. [*platy-* + G. *glōssa*, tongue]

plat·y·hel·minth (plat-i-hel′minth). Common name for any flatworm of the phylum Platyhelminthes; any cestode (tapeworm) or trematode (fluke). [*platy-* + G. *helmins*, worm]

Plat·y·hel·min·thes (plat′i-hel-min′thēz). A phylum of flatworms that are bilaterally symmetric, flattened, and acelomate. There is no digestive tract in some platyhelminths (Cestoda), or the gut may be incomplete (without an anus), as in the Trematoda; most of the forms are hermaphroditic. There are three major classes, but the parasitic species of medical and veterinary importance are in the subclass Cestoda (the true tapeworms) of the class Cestoidea, and in the subclass Digenea (the digenetic flukes) of the class Trematoda.

plat·y·hi·er·ic (plat-i-hī-er′ik). Having a broad sacrum. [*platy-* + G. *heiron*, sacrum]

plat·y·me·ric (plat-i-mē′rik, -mer′ik). Having a broad femur. [*platy-* + G. *mēros*, thigh]

plat·y·mor·phia (plat′i-mōr′fē-ă). Having a flat shape; term denoting an eye with a short anteroposterior axis. [*platy-* + G. *morphē*, shape]

plat·y·o·pia (plat′i-ō′pē-ă). Broadness of the face; denoting a condition in which the orbitonasal index is less than 107.5. [*platy-* + G. *ōps*, eye, face]

plat·y·op·ic (plat′i-op′ik, -ō′pik). Relating to or characterized by platyopia.

plat·y·pel·lic (plat-i-pel′ik). Having a broad pelvis, with an index below 90°. SEE platypellic *pelvis*. SYN platypelloid. [*platy-* + G. *pellis*, bowl (pelvis)]

plat·y·pel·loid (plat-ē-pel′oyd). SYN platypellic.

pla·typ·nea (plă-tip′nē-ă). Difficulty in breathing when erect, relieved by recumbency. Cf. orthopnea. [*platy-* + G. *pnoē*, a breathing]

plat·yr·rhine (plat′i-rīn). **1.** Characterized by a nose of large width in proportion to its length. **2.** Denoting a skull with a nasal index between 53 and 58. [*platy-* + G. *rhis*, nose]

plat·yr·rhi·ny (plat′i-rī-nē). A condition in which the nose is wide in proportion to its length.

pla·tys·ma, pl. **pla·tys·mas, pla·tys·ma·ta** (plă-tiz′mă, -tiz′mă-tă) [TA]. SYN platysma (*muscle*). [G. *platysma*, a flatplate]

plat·y·spon·dyl·ia, plat·y·spon·dyl·i·sis (plat-i-spon-dil′ē-ă, plat′i-spon-dil′i-sis). Flatness of the bodies of the vertebrae. [*platy-* + G. *spondylos*, vertebra]

pla·tys·ten·ceph·a·ly (plă-tis′ten-sef′ă-lē). Extreme width of the skull in the occipital region, with narrowing anteriorly and prognathism. [G. *platystos*, widest, superl. of *platys*, wide, + *enkephalē*, brain]

Pleasure, Max A., U.S. dentist, 1903–1965. SEE P. *curve*.

plec·trid·i·um (plek-trid′ē-ŭm). A bacterial rod-shaped cell that contains a spore at one end, imparting a drumstick shape to the cell, such as the spore-containing cells in the organism causing tetanus, *Clostridium tetani*. [Mod. L. dim. of G. *plēktron*, an instrument to strike with]

pled·get (plej′et). A tuft of wool, cotton, or lint.

△**-plegia.** Paralysis. [G. *plēgē*, stroke]

△**pleio-.** Rarely used alternative spelling for pleo-.

plei·o·tro·pic (plī-ō-trop′ik). Denoting, or characterized by, pleiotropy. SYN polyphenic.

plei·ot·ro·py, plei·o·tro·pia (plī-ot′rō-pē, plī′ō-trō′pē-ă). Production by a single mutant gene of apparently unrelated multiple effects at the clinical or phenotypic level. [*pleio-* + G. *tropos*, turning]

functional p., the p. due to the participation of the same allelic change in multiple otherwise distinct processes; e.g., heparin is active in many body reactions including coagulation and the metabolism of fat.

structural p., a p. that occurs when two or more regions of a polypeptide may have quite distinct and unrelated biologic functions that share nothing in common except that they are transcribed and translated at the same time.

Pleis·to·pho·ra (plīs-tof′er-ah). A genus of microsporidians in the protozoan phylum Microspora, commonly found in fish and insects, with mononucleate, thick-walled spores in clusters of more than eight. An undescribed but distinct species of P. was implicated as the cause of a disseminated microsporidial myositis in an immunocompromised male patient.

△**pleo-.** more. [G. *pleiōn*]

ple·o·chro·ic (plē-ō-krō′ik). SYN pleochromatic. [*pleo-* + G. *chroa*, color]

ple·och·ro·ism (plē-ok′rō-izm). SYN pleochromatism.

ple·o·chro·mat·ic (plē-ō-krō-mat′ik). Relating to pleochromatism. SYN pleochroic.

ple·o·chro·ma·tism (plē-ō-krō′mă-tizm). Property of showing changes of color when illuminated along different axes, as certain crystals or liquids. SYN pleochroism. [*pleo-* + G. *chrōma*, color]

ple·o·cy·to·sis (plē′ō-sī-tō′sis). Presence of more cells than normal, often denoting leukocytosis and especially lymphocytosis or round cell infiltration; orginally applied to the lymphocytosis of the cerebrospinal fluid present in syphilis of the central nervous system. [*pleo-* + G. *kytos*, cell, + *-ōsis*, condition]

ple·o·mas·tia, ple·o·ma·zia (plē-ō-mas′tē-ă, -mā′zē-ă). SYN polymastia. [*pleo-* + G. *mastos*, breast]

ple·o·mor·phic (plē-ō-mōr′fik). **1.** SYN polymorphic. **2.** Among fungi, having two or more spore forms; also used to describe a sterile mutant dermatophyte resulting from degenerative changes in culture.

ple·o·mor·phism (plē-ō-mōr′fizm). SYN polymorphism. [*pleo-* + G. *morphē*, form]

ple·o·mor·phous (plē-ō-mōr′fŭs). SYN polymorphic.

ple·o·nasm (plē′ō-nazm). Excess in number or size of parts. [G. *pleonasmos*, exaggeration, excessive, fr. *pleiōn*, more]

ple·on·os·te·o·sis (plē′on-os-tē-ō′sis). Superabundance of bone formation. [*pleo-* + G. *osteon*, bone, + *-osis*, condition]

Leri′ p., SYN dyschondrosteosis.

ple·op·tics (plē-op′tiks). A term introduced by Bangerter to include all forms of treatment for amblyopia, particularly that associated with eccentric fixation. [*pleo-* + optics]

ple·op·to·phor (plē-op′tō-fōr). An instrument for the treatment of amblyopia. [*pleo-* + G. *optos*, visible, + *phoros*, bearing]

ple·ro·cer·coid (plē-rō-ser′koyd). A stage in the development of a tapeworm following the procercoid stage, which develops in an animal serving as the second or subsequent intermediate host; a wormlike nonsegmented larva with an invaginated scolex at one end, usually unencysted in the flesh of various fishes, reptiles, or amphibians, the ingestion of which transmits the parasite to the final host. SEE ALSO *Diphyllobothrium latum*. [G. *plērēs*, full, complete, + *kerkos*, tail]

△**plesio-.** Nearness, similarity. [G. *plēsios*, close, near]

Ples·i·o·mo·nas. A genus of Gram-negative, facultatively anaerobic, chemoorganotropic, rod-shaped, motile bacteria. It possesses the enterobacterial common antigen. This genus is found in fish and other aquatic animals and in some other animals. Associated with diarrhea and occasional opportunistic infection in humans.

P. shigelloides, species that is an enteric pathogen and an etiologic agent of various extraintestinal infections transmitted to humans in contaminated food or water or as a colonizer of various animals. This is the only species in the genus and has also been referred to as *Pseudomonas s.,* *Aeromonas s.,* C57, and *Vibrio s.*

ple·si·o·mor·phic (plē′sē-ō-mōr′fik). Similar in form. SYN plesiomorphous.

ple·si·o·mor·phism (plē′sē-ō-mōr′fizm). Similarity in form. [plesio- + G. *morphē,* form]

ple·si·o·mor·phous (plē′sē-ō-mōr′fŭs). SYN plesiomorphic.

△**pless-, plessi-.** A striking, especially percussion. [G. *plēssō,* to strike]

ples·ses·the·sia (ples-es-thē′zē-ă). SYN palpatory *percussion.* [G. *plēssō,* to strike, + *aisthēsis,* sensation]

ples·sim·e·ter (ple-sim′ĕ-ter). An oblong flexible plate used in mediate percussion by being placed against the surface and struck with the plessor. SYN pleximeter, plexometer. [G. *plēssō,* to strike, + *metron,* measure]

ples·si·met·ric (ples-i-met′rik). Relating to a plessimeter.

ples·sor (ples′er). A small hammer, usually with soft rubber head, used to tap the part directly, or with a plessimeter, in percussion of the chest or other part. SYN percussor, plexor. [G. *plēssō,* to strike]

pleth·o·ra (pleth′ŏ-ră). **1.** SYN hypervolemia. **2.** An excess of any of the body fluids. [G. *plēthōrē,* fullness, fr. *plēthō,* to become full]

pleth·o·ric (ple-thōr′ik, pleth′ŏ-rik). Relating to plethora. SYN sanguine (1), sanguineous (2).

ple·thys·mo·graph (plĕ-thiz′mō-graf). A device for measuring and recording changes in volume of a part, organ, or whole body. [G. *plēthysmos,* increase, + *graphō,* to write]

  body p., a chamber apparatus surrounding the entire body, commonly used in studies of respiratory function.

  digital p., p. applied to a digit of a hand or foot to measure skin blood flow.

  pressure p., (1) a p. applied to part of the body, e.g., a limb segment, and arranged so that volume is measured during temporary application of sufficient pressure to the part to empty its blood vessels; **(2)** a body p. in which changes of body volume are measured in terms of the consequent changes in air pressure in the body p.

  volume-displacement p., a p., usually a body p., in which changes in volume displace a corresponding volume into or out of a very compliant measuring device, such as a Krogh spirometer or integrating flowmeter.

pleth·ys·mog·ra·phy (pleth-iz-mog′ră-fē). Measuring and recording changes in volume of an organ or other part of the body by a plethysmograph. [G. *plēthysmos,* increase, + *graphē,* a writing]

  impedance p., recording changes in electrical impedance between electrodes placed on opposite sides of a part of the body, as a measure of volume changes in the path of the current. SYN dielectrography.

  venous occlusion p., measurement of the rate of arterial inflow into an organ or limb segment by measuring its initial rate of increase in volume when its venous outflow is suddenly occluded.

pleth·ys·mom·e·try (pleth-iz-mom′ĕ-trē). Measuring the fullness of a hollow organ or vessel, as of the pulse. [G. *plēthysmos,* increase, + *metron,* measure]

△**pleur-, pleura-, pleuro-.** Rib, side, pleura. [G. *pleura;* a rib, the side]

pleu·ra, gen. and pl. **pleu·rae** (ploor′ă, ploor′ē) [TA]. The serous membrane enveloping the lungs and lining the walls of the pleural cavity. SYN membrana succingens. [G. *pleura,* a rib, pl. the side]

  cervical p. [TA], the dome-shaped roof of the pleural cavity extending up through the superior aperture of the thorax. SYN cupula pleurae [TA], dome of pleura⭐, pleural cupula⭐.

  costal p., SYN costal *part* of parietal pleura.

  p. costa′lis, SYN costal *part* of parietal pleura.

  diaphragmatic p., SYN diaphragmatic *part* of parietal pleura.

  p. diaphragmat′ica, SYN diaphragmatic *part* of parietal pleura.

  mediastinal p., SYN mediastinal *part* of parietal pleura.

  p. mediastina′lis, SYN mediastinal *part* of parietal pleura.

  parietal p. [TA], that which lines the different parts of the wall of the pleural cavity; called costal, diaphragmatic, and mediastinal, according to the parts invested. SYN p. parietalis [TA].

  p. parieta′lis [TA], SYN parietal p.

  p. pericardi′aca, pericardial p., that portion of the mediastinal p. that is fused with the pericardium.

  phrenic p., SYN diaphragmatic *part* of parietal pleura.

  p. phren′ica, SYN diaphragmatic *part* of parietal pleura.

  p. pulmona′lis, ⭐official alternate term for visceral p.

  pulmonary p., ⭐official alternate term for visceral p.

  visceral p. [TA], the layer investing the lungs and dipping into the fissures between the several lobes. SYN p. visceralis [TA], p. pulmonalis⭐, pulmonary p.⭐.

  p. viscera′lis [TA], SYN visceral p.

pleu·ra·cen·te·sis (ploor′ă-sen-tē′sis). SYN thoracentesis.

pleu·ral (ploor′ăl). Relating to the pleura.

pleu·ral crac·kles (krăk′lz). Sounds heard on auscultation of the chest as a result of inflammation of the pleura with fibrinous exudate.

pleu·ral·gia (ploo-ral′jē-ă). Rarely used synonym for pleurodynia (2). [pleur- + G. *algos,* pain]

pleur·a·poph·y·sis (ploor′ă-pof′i-sis). A rib, or the process on a cervical or lumbar vertebra corresponding thereto. Cf. superior articular *process.* [pleur- + G. *apophysis,* process, offshoot]

pleur·ec·to·my (ploo-rek′tō-mē). Excision of pleura, usually parietal. [pleur- + G. *ektomē,* excision]

pleu·ri·sy (ploor′i-sē). Inflammation of the pleura. SYN pleuritis. [L. *pleurisis,* fr. G. *pleuritis*]

  adhesive p., SYN dry p.

  benign dry p., SYN epidemic *pleurodynia.*

  bilateral p., inflammation of the pleura on both sides of the thorax. SYN double p.

  chronic p., vague or indefinite term for long-standing inflammation of the pleura of any etiology (e.g., tuberculosis).

  costal p., inflammation of the pleura lining the thoracic walls.

  diaphragmatic p., SYN epidemic *pleurodynia.*

  double p., SYN bilateral p.

  dry p., p. with a fibrinous exudation, without an effusion of serum, resulting in adhesion between the opposing surfaces of the pleura. SYN adhesive p., fibrinous p., plastic p.

  encysted p., a form of serofibrinous p., in which adhesions occur at various points, circumscribing the serous effusion.

  epidemic benign dry p., SYN epidemic *pleurodynia.*

  epidemic diaphragmatic p., SYN epidemic *pleurodynia.*

  fibrinous p., SYN dry p.

  hemorrhagic p., p. with an effusion of blood-stained serum.

  interlobular p., inflammation limited to the pleura in the sulci between the pulmonary lobes.

  mediastinal p., inflammation of the portion of the pleura lining the mediastinal surface of the lung.

  plastic p., SYN dry p.

  productive p., SYN pachypleuritis.

  proliferating p., p. with a tendency for the proliferation of inflammatory exudate.

  pulmonary p., inflammation of the pleura covering the lungs. SYN visceral p.

  purulent p., p. with empyema. SYN suppurative p.

  sacculated p., p. with the inflammatory exudate divided into separate regions by adhesions or inflammatory changes.

  serofibrinous p., the more common form of p., characterized by a fibrinous exudate on the surface of the pleura and an extensive effusion of serous fluid into the pleural cavity.

  serous p., SYN p. with effusion.

pl

suppurative p., SYN purulent p.

typhoid p., obsolete term for acute or subacute p. with typhoid symptoms (confusion or dementia).

visceral p., SYN pulmonary p.

wet p., SYN p. with effusion.

p. with effusion, p. accompanied by serous exudation. SYN serous p., wet p.

pleu·rit·ic (ploo-rit′ik). Pertaining to pleurisy.

pleu·ri·tis (ploo-rī′tis). SYN pleurisy. [G. fr. *pleura,* side, + *-itis,* inflammation]

pleur·i·tog·e·nous (ploor-i-toj′ĕ-nŭs). Tending to produce pleurisy. [G. *pleuritis,* pleurisy, + *genesis,* origin]

⟁**pleuro-.** SEE pleur-.

pleu·ro·cele (ploor′ō-sēl). SYN pneumonocele. [pleuro- + G. *kēlē,* hernia]

pleu·ro·cen·te·sis (ploor′ō-sen-tē′sis). SYN thoracentesis. [pleuro- + G. *kentēsis,* puncture]

pleu·ro·cen·trum (ploor′ō-sen′trŭm). One of the lateral halves of the body of a vertebra. [pleuro- + G. *kentron,* center]

pleu·roc·ly·sis (ploor-ok′li-sis). Washing out of the pleural cavity. [pleuro- + G. *klysis,* a washing out]

pleu·rod·e·sis (ploor-od′e-sis). The creation of a fibrous adhesion between the visceral and parietal layers of the pleura, thus obliterating the pleural cavity; it is performed surgically by abrading the pleura or by inserting a sterile irritant into the pleural space, and applied as treatment in cases of malignant pleural effusion, recurrent spontaneous pneumothorax, and chylothorax. [pleuro- + G. *desis,* a binding together]

pleu·ro·dyn·ia (ploor-ō-din′ē-ă). **1.** Pleuritic pain in the chest. **2.** A painful affection of the tendinous attachments of the thoracic muscles, usually of one side only. SYN costalgia. [pleuro- + G. *odynē,* pain]

epidemic p., an acute infectious disease usually occurring in epidemic form, characterized by paroxysms of pain, usually in the chest, and associated with strains of Enterovirus coxsackievirus type B. SYN benign dry pleurisy, Bornholm disease, Daae disease, devil grip, diaphragmatic pleurisy, epidemic benign dry pleurisy, epidemic diaphragmatic pleurisy, epidemic myalgia, epidemic myositis, myositis epidemica acuta, epidemic transient diaphragmatic spasm, Sylvest disease.

pleu·ro·gen·ic (ploor-ō-jen′ik). Of pleural origin; beginning in the pleura. SYN pleurogenous (1). [pleuro- + G. *-gen,* producing]

pleu·rog·e·nous (ploor-oj′ĕ-nŭs). **1.** SYN pleurogenic. **2.** In fungi, denoting spores or conidia developed on the sides of a conidiophore or hypha.

pleu·rog·ra·phy (ploor-og′ră-fē). Radiography of the pleural cavity after injecting contrast medium. [pleuro- + G. *graphō,* to write]

pleu·ro·hep·a·ti·tis (ploor′ō-hep-ă-tī′tis). Hepatitis with extension of the inflammation to the neighboring portion of the pleura. [pleuro- + G. *hēpar,* liver, + *-itis,* inflammation]

pleu·ro·lith (ploor′ō-lith). A concretion in the pleural cavity. SYN pleural calculus. [pleuro- + G. *lithos,* stone]

pleu·rol·y·sis (ploor-ol′i-sis). Locating pleural adhesions by the aid of an endoscope and then dividing them with the electric cautery. [pleuro- + G. *lysis,* dissolution]

pleu·ro·per·i·car·di·al (ploor′ō-per-i-kar′dē-ăl). Relating to both pleura and pericardium.

pleu·ro·per·i·car·di·tis (ploor′ō-per-i-kar-dī′tis). Combined inflammation of the pericardium and of the pleura. [pleuro- + pericardium + G. *-itis,* inflammation]

pleu·ro·per·i·to·ne·al (ploor′ō-per-i-tō-nē′ăl). Relating to both pleura and peritoneum.

pleuropneumonectomy. Surgical resection of an entire lung along with the parietal pleura; formerly used mainly for destroyed lung due to tuberculosis; currently, a method of treating malignant mesothelioma.

pleu·ro·pul·mo·nary (ploor-ō-pul′mō-ner-ē). Relating to both pleura and the lungs.

pleu·ros·co·py (ploor-ōs′kō-pē). SYN thoracoscopy. [pleuro- + G. *skopeō,* to inspect]

pleu·rot·o·my (ploo-rot′ō-mē). SYN thoracotomy. [pleuro- + G. *tomē,* incision]

pleu·ro·ty·phoid (plur-ō-tī′foyd). Typhoid fever in which the early stage is masked by the physical signs of pleurisy.

pleu·ro·vis·cer·al (ploor′ō-vis′er-ăl). SYN visceropleural.

PLEVA. Acronym for *pityriasis* lichenoides et varioliformis acuta.

plex·al (plek′săl). Relating to a plexus.

plex·ect·o·my (plek-sek′tō-mē). Surgical excision of a plexus. [plexus + G. *ektomē,* excision]

plex·i·form (plek′si-fōrm). Weblike, or resembling or forming a plexus. [plexus + L. *forma,* form]

plex·im·e·ter (plek-sim′i-ter). SYN plessimeter. [G. *plēxis,* stroke]

plex·i·tis (plek-sī′tis). Inflammation of a plexus.

brachial p., SYN neuralgic *amyotrophy.*

plex·o·gen·ic (plek′sō-jen-ik). Giving rise to weblike or plexiform structures. [plexus + G. *-gen,* producing]

plex·om·e·ter (plek-som′ĕ-ter). SYN plessimeter.

plex·o·path·y (pleks-op′a-thē). Disorder involving one of the major peripheral neural plexuses: cervical, brachial, or lumbosacral. [plexus + G. *pathos,* disease]

plex·or (plek′ser). SYN plessor. [G. *plēxis,* a stroke]

PLEXUS

plex·us, pl. **plex·us, plex·us·es** (plek′sŭs, -sŭs-ez) [TA]. A network or interjoining of nerves and blood vessels or of lymphatic vessels. [L. a braid]

abdominal aortic (nervous) p. [TA], an autonomic p. surrounding the abdominal aorta, directly continuous with the thoracic aortic p. superiorly and continuing inferiorly to the bifurcation of the aorta as the superior hypogastric plexus. SYN p. nervosus aorticus abdominalis [TA].

acromial p., SYN acromial *anastomosis* of the thoracoacromial artery.

p. annula′ris, SYN anular p.

anterior coronary periarterial p., the part of the cardiac p. that accompanies the coronary arteries on the anterior aspect of the heart.

anular p., a nerve p. near the corneoscleral junction from which myelinated and unmyelinated nerves pass to the cornea. SYN p. annularis.

aortic lymphatic p., a p. of lymph nodes and connecting vessels lying along the lower portion of the abdominal aorta. SYN p. aorticus.

p. aor′ticus, SYN aortic lymphatic p.

areolar venous p. [TA], a venous p. in the areola surrounding the nipple, formed by the mammary veins, and sending its blood to the lateral thoracic vein; erectile tissue of the areola of the nipple. SYN p. venosus areolaris [TA], circulus venosus halleri, Haller circle (2), vascular circle (2), venous circle of mammary gland.

p. arte′riae choroi′deae, SYN periarterial p. of choroid artery.

arterial p. [TA], a vascular network formed by anastomoses between minute arteries just before they become capillaries. SYN rete arteriosum [TA], arteriolar network.

articular vascular p. [TA], a vascular rete in the neighborhood of a joint, where such arrangements are common, enabling a collateral circulation by which blood will be supplied distal to the joint regardless of compromises resulting from joint position. SYN rete vasculosum articulare [TA], articular network, articular vascular circle, articular vascular network, circulus articularis vasculosus.

ascending pharyngeal p., SYN periarterial p. of ascending pharyngeal artery.

Auerbach p., SYN myenteric (nervous) p.

autonomic plexuses [TA], plexuses of nerves in relation to blood vessels and viscera, the component fibers of which are sympathetic, parasympathetic, and sensory. SYN plexus viscerales.

p. autonomicus brachialis [TA], SYN brachial autonomic p.

axillary p., SYN axillary lymphatic p.

axillary lymphatic p., a lymphatic p. formed of the lymph nodes, with their afferent and efferent vessels, in the axilla. SYN axillary p., p. lymphaticus axillaris.

basilar venous p. [TA], a venous p. on the clivus, connected with the cavernous and petrosal sinuses and the internal vertebral (epidural) venous p. SYN p. venosus basilaris [TA], basilar sinus.

Batson p., SYN vertebral venous *system*.

brachial p. [TA], major nerve p. formed of the ventral primary rami of the fifth cervical to first thoracic spinal nerves for innervation of the upper limb. The ventral primary rami entering into formation of the p. constitute the roots of the p.; the roots are located in the posterior triangle of the neck, converging to emerge from the scalenus anterior and medius muscles. As they emerge from the scalene hiatus, the C5 and C6 roots combine to form the superior trunk, C7 remains alone as the middle trunk, and the C8 and T1 roots combine to form the inferior trunk of the p. The trunks pass beneath the clavicle, passing from the neck into the axilla through the cervicoaxillary canal. As they cross the first rib, all three trunks divide into anterior and posterior divisions of the p. Nerve fibers contained within anterior divisions are destined for the anterior aspect of the limb; those contained within the posterior divisions are destined for the posterior aspect of the limb. Within the axilla, the anterior divisions of the superior and middle trunks merge to form the lateral cord of the p.; the anterior division of the inferior trunk becomes the medial cord of the p., and the posterior divisions of all three trunks become the posterior cord, the cords being named for their position in relation to the axillary artery, to which they run parallel and which they surround. The cords of the brachial p. give rise to most of the named peripheral nerves that are the products of the p. formation. The major nerves of the lateral cord are the musculocutaneous nerve and the lateral root of the median nerve. The medial cord gives rise to the ulnar and medial root of the median nerve. The lateral and medial roots of the median nerve merge to form the medial nerve. The posterior cord of the p. gives rise to the radial and axillary nerves. SYN p. brachialis [TA].

brachial autonomic p. [TA], periarterial automic plexus of the brachial artery. SYN p. autonomicus brachialis [TA].

p. brachia'lis [TA], SYN brachial p.

cardiac (nervous) p. [TA], a wide-meshed network formed by anastomosing cardiopulmonary and splanchnic nerves conveying afferent and autonomic nerve fibers (sympathetic and parasympathetic), surrounding the arch of the aorta, the pulmonary artery, and continuing to the atria, ventricles, and coronary vessels. SYN p. nervosus cardiacus [TA].

p. cardi'acus profun'dus, SYN deep cardiac p.

p. carot'icus inter'nus, SYN internal carotid venous p.

cavernous p. of clitoris, SYN cavernous *nerves* of clitoris, under *nerve*.

cavernous nervous p. [TA], the portion of the internal carotid p. in the cavernous sinus. SYN p. nervosus cavernosus [TA], intracavernous p., Walther p.

cavernous p. of penis, SYN cavernous *nerves* of penis, under *nerve*.

cavernous (vascular) p. of conchae [TA], erectile tissue in the mucous membrane covering the conchae of the nasal cavity. SYN p. vascularis cavernosus conchae [TA], corpus cavernosum conchae.

celiac p., a network related to the celiac trunk. SEE celiac (nervous) p., celiac (lymphatic) p.

celiac (lymphatic) p., a network formed of the efferent and afferent lymphatic vessels of the celiac lymph nodes and related to the celiac trunk; the afferent lymphatic vessels bring lymph primarily from structures served by the celiac artery (stomach, duodenum, pancreas, and visceral aspect of the liver); the efferent vessels drain into the cisterna chyli/thoracic duct via the intestinal lymph trunks.

celiac (nervous) p. [TA], the most substantial, superior portion of the abdominal aortic plexus lying anterior to the aorta at the level of origin of the celiac trunk (vertebral level T-12); the celiac ganglia lie within the plexus; it is formed by contributions from the greater splanchnic and vagus (especially the posterior or right vagus) nerves and communicating branches to and from the superior mesenteric and renal plexuses and ganglia; most sympathetic, parasympathetic and visceral afferent fibers serving the abdominal viscera pass through this plexus. SYN plexus coeliacus [TA], p. nervosus celiacus [TA], solar p.

cervical p., formed by loops joining the adjacent ventral primary rami of the first four cervical nerves and receiving gray communicating rami from the superior cervical ganglion; it lies deep to the sternocleidomastoid muscle and sends out numerous cutaneous, muscular, and communicating rami. SYN p. cervicalis.

p. cervica'lis, SYN cervical p.

choroid p. [TA], a vascular proliferation or fringe of the tela choroidea in the third, fourth, and lateral cerebral ventricles; it secretes cerebrospinal fluid, thereby regulating to some degree the intraventricular pressure. SYN p. choroideus [TA], tela vasculosa.

p. choroi'deus [TA], SYN choroid p.

p. choroi'deus ventric'uli latera'lis [TA], SYN choroid p. of lateral ventricle.

p. choroi'deus ventric'uli quar'ti [TA], SYN choroid p. of fourth ventricle.

p. choroi'deus ventric'uli ter'tii [TA], SYN choroid p. of third ventricle.

choroid p. of fourth ventricle [TA], one of two vascular fringes of pia mater projecting on either side from the lower part of the roof of the fourth cerebral ventricle. SYN p. choroideus ventriculi quarti [TA].

choroid p. of lateral ventricle [TA], the vascular fringe that projects from the choroidal fissure into each lateral ventricle. SYN p. choroideus ventriculi lateralis [TA].

choroid p. of third ventricle [TA], the double row of vascular projections from the undersurface of the tela choroidea, where it roofs over the third ventricle. SYN p. choroideus ventriculi tertii [TA].

ciliary ganglionic p., an autonomic p. lying on the ciliary muscle, derived from the oculomotor, trigeminal, and sympathetic. SYN p. gangliosus ciliaris.

coccygeal p. [TA], a small p. formed by the fifth sacral and the coccygeal nerves; it gives origin to the anococcygeal nerves. SYN p. coccygeus [TA].

p. coccyg'eus [TA], SYN coccygeal p.

common carotid p., SYN common carotid nervous p.

common carotid nervous p. [TA], an autonomic p. accompanying the artery of the same name formed by fibers from the middle cervical ganglion. SYN p. nervosus caroticus communis [TA], common carotid p.

p. corona'rii cor'dis, SYN periarterial plexuses of coronary arteries.

coronary p., SYN periarterial plexuses of coronary arteries.

Cruveilhier p., a nerve p. formed by communication between the dorsal primary rami of the first three cervical nerves; it lies deep to the semispinalis capitis muscle.

deep cardiac p., the deeper part of the cardiac p. inferior to the arch of the aorta. SYN p. cardiacus profundus.

deferential (nervous) p. [TA], an autonomic p. on the seminal vesicle and ampulla of the ductus deferens on each side, derived from the inferior hypogastric p. SYN p. nervosus deferentialis [TA], p. of ductus deferens.

p. of ductus deferens, SYN deferential (nervous) p.

enteric (nervous) p. [TA], the autonomic p. in the wall of the intestine; it consists of three parts, submucosal, myenteric, and subserosal; ganglionic cells are scattered through the myenteric and submucosal plexus. SYN p. nervosus entericus [TA].

esophageal (nervous) p. [TA], one of two nervous plexuses, posterior and anterior on the walls of the esophagus; the first is formed by branches from the right vagus and left recurrent, the second by the anastomosing trunks of the vagus after leaving the pulmonary plexuses; branches supply the mucous and muscular coats of the esophagus. SYN p. nervosus esophageus [TA], p. gulae.

Exner p., a p. formed by tangential nerve fibers in the superficial plexiform or molecular layer of the cerebral cortex.

external carotid (nervous) p. [TA], an autonomic p. formed by the external carotid nerves surrounding the artery of the same name and giving origin to a number of secondary plexuses along the branches of this artery and to branches to the carotid body. SYN p. nervosus caroticus externus [TA].

external iliac lymphatic p., a lymphatic p. formed by the lymph nodes along the external iliac artery on either side, and their afferent and efferent vessels. SYN p. lymphaticus iliacus externus.

external maxillary p., SYN periarterial p. of facial artery.

facial p., SYN periarterial p. of facial artery.

femoral (nervous) p. [TA], an autonomic p. surrounding the femoral artery, derived from the iliac p. SYN p. nervosus femoralis [TA].

p. ganglio′sus cilia′ris, SYN ciliary ganglionic p.

gastric plexuses of autonomic system, SYN gastric nervous plexuses.

p. gas′trici syste′matis autono′mici, SYN gastric nervous plexuses.

gastric nervous plexuses [TA], the plexuses along the greater and lesser curvatures of the stomach derived from the celiac p.; also known as inferior and superior p. SYN p. nervorum gastricorum [TA], gastric plexuses of autonomic system, p. gastrici systematis autonomici.

p. gu′lae, SYN esophageal (nervous) p.

Haller p., a nervous p. of sympathetic filaments and branches of the external laryngeal nerve on the surface of the inferior constrictor muscle of the pharynx.

Heller p., p. of small arteries in the wall of the intestine.

hemorrhoidal p., SYN rectal venous p; SEE ALSO inferior rectal (nervous) p., middle rectal (nervous) p., superior rectal (nervous) p.

hepatic (nervous) p. [TA], an unpaired autonomic p. lying on the hepatc artery and its branches in the liver. SYN p. nervosus hepaticus [TA].

iliac (nervous) p. [TA], the autonomic p. lying on the iliac arteries, derived from the aortic p. SYN p. nervosus iliacus [TA].

inferior dental (nervous) p. [TA], formed by branches of the inferior alveolar nerve interlacing before they supply the teeth; it gives off interior dental branches to the teeth and inferior gingival branches to the gums. SYN p. nervosus dentalis inferior [TA].

inferior hemorrhoidal plexuses, SYN inferior rectal (nervous) p.

inferior hypogastric (nervous) p. [TA], one of the bilateral autonomic p. in the pelvis distributed to the pelvic viscera; it receives the hypogastric nerves and the pelvic splanchnic nerves. SYN p. nervosus hypogastricus inferior [TA], pelvic (nervous) p.✫, p. nervosus pelvicus✫.

inferior mesenteric (nervous) p. [TA], an autonomic p., derived from the abdominal aortic p., surrounding the inferior mesenteric artery and sending branches to the descending colon, sigmoid, and rectum. SYN p. nervosus mesentericus inferior [TA].

inferior rectal (nervous) p. [TA], the autonomic plexuses along the anus derived from the inferior hypogastric p. SYN p. nervosus rectalis inferiores [TA], inferior hemorrhoidal plexuses.

inferior thyroid p., SYN periarterial p. of inferior thyroid artery.

inferior vesical venous p., a venous p. in the female corresponding to the prostatic venous p. in the male. SYN p. venosus vesicalis inferior.

inguinal lymphatic p., a lymphatic p. formed of 10–15 lymph nodes with their connecting vessels lying superficially near the termination of the great saphenous vein and more deeply along the femoral artery and vein. SEE superficial inguinal *lymph nodes*, under *lymph node*. SYN p. lymphaticus inguinalis.

intermesenteric (nervous) p. [TA], the part of the abdominal aortic p. lying between the superior and inferior mesenteric plexuses. SYN p. nervosus intermesentericus [TA].

internal carotid (nervous) p. [TA], an autonomic nervous p. surrounding the internal carotid artery in the carotid canal and cavernous sinus, and sending branches to the tympanic p., sphenopalatine ganglion, abducens and oculomotor nerves, the cerebral vessels, and the ciliary ganglion. SYN p. nervosus arteriae carotidis internae.

internal carotid venous p., a venous network around the internal carotid artery in the carotid canal of the temporal bone, connecting with the cavernous sinus and internal jugular vein. SYN p. caroticus internus, p. venosus caroticus internus.

internal mammary p., SYN periarterial p. of internal thoracic artery.

internal maxillary p., SYN periarterial p. of maxillary artery.

internal thoracic p., SYN periarterial p. of internal thoracic artery.

internal thoracic lymphatic p., a lymphatic p., including the parasternal; (internal thoracic) lymph nodes, with their vessels, situated along the course of the internal thoracic veins. SYN mammary p., p. mammarius.

intracavernous p., SYN cavernous nervous p.

p. intraparoti′deus nervi facialis, SYN parotid p. of facial nerve.

intraparotid p. of facial nerve, SYN parotid p. of facial nerve.

ischiadic p., SYN sacral p.

Jacobson p., SYN tympanic (nervous) p.

Jacques p., a nerve p. within the muscular coat of the uterine (fallopian) tube.

jugular lymphatic p., a lymphatic p. that includes the deep cervical group of lymph nodes, with their afferent and efferent vessels, extending along the internal jugular vein (carotid sheath). SYN p. lymphaticus jugularis.

Leber p., a small venous p. in the eye between the venous sinuses of the sclera (of Schlemm) and the spaces of the iridocorneal angle (of Fontana).

lingual p., SYN periarterial p. of lingual artery.

lumbar lymphatic p., a lymphatic p. formed of about 20 lymph nodes and connecting vessels situated along the lower portion of the aorta and the common iliac vessels. SYN p. lymphaticus lumbalis.

lumbar (nervous) p., a nervous p., formed by the ventral rami of the first four lumbar nerves; it lies in the substance of the psoas muscle. SYN p. nervorum lumbalium.

lumbosacral (nervous) p. [TA], formed by the union of the anterior rami of the lumbar and sacral nerves; it is divided into lumbar and sacral plexuses. SYN p. nervosus lumbosacralis [TA].

lymphatic p., a p. of lymphatic capillaries, usually without valves, that opens into one or more larger lymphatic vessels. SYN p. lymphaticus.

p. lymphat′icus, SYN lymphatic p.

p. lymphaticus axilla′ris, SYN axillary lymphatic p.

p. lymphaticus ili′acus exter′nus, SYN external iliac lymphatic p.

p. lymphaticus inguina′lis, SYN inguinal lymphatic p.

p. lymphaticus jugula′ris, SYN jugular lymphatic p.

p. lymphaticus lumbalis, SYN lumbar lymphatic p.

p. lymphaticus sacra′lis me′dius, SYN middle sacral lymphatic p.

p. mamma′rius, SYN internal thoracic lymphatic p.

p. mamma′rius inter′nus, SYN periarterial p. of internal thoracic artery.

mammary p., SYN internal thoracic lymphatic p.

p. maxilla′ris exter′nus, SYN periarterial p. of facial artery.

p. maxilla′ris inter′nus, SYN periarterial p. of maxillary artery.

maxillary p., SYN periarterial p. of maxillary artery.

Meissner p., SYN submucosal (nervous) p.

meningeal p., a nerve p. on the cerebral meninges, derived from the external carotid p. SYN p. meningeus.

p. menin′geus, SYN meningeal p.

middle hemorrhoidal plexuses, SYN middle rectal (nervous) p.

middle rectal (nervous) p. [TA], the autonomic plexuses along the rectum derived from the inferior hypogastric p. SYN middle hemorrhoidal plexuses, p. nervosus rectalis medius.

middle sacral lymphatic p., a lymphatic p. formed of lymph nodes and connecting vessels situated chiefly in the mesorectum,

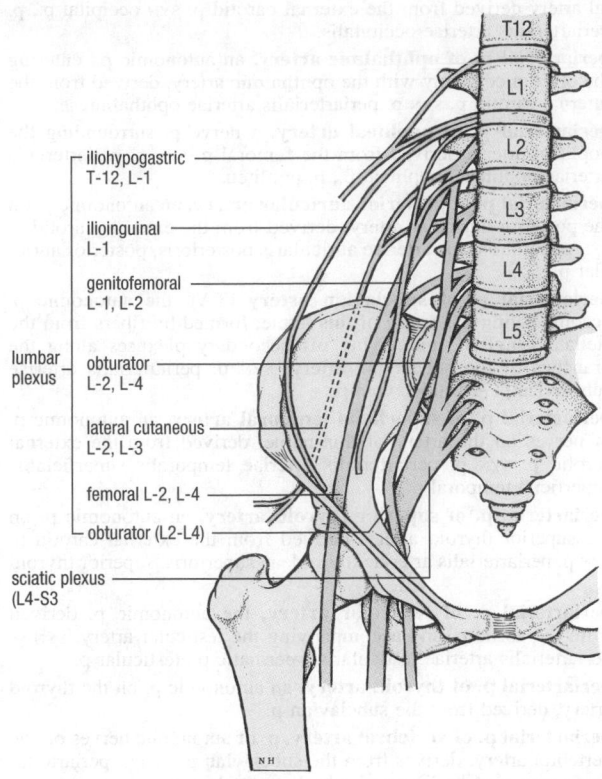

iliohypogastric
T-12, L-1

ilioinguinal
L-1

genitofemoral
L-1, L-2

lumbar plexus

obturator
L-2, L-4

lateral cutaneous
L-2, L-3

femoral L-2, L-4

obturator (L2-L4)

sciatic plexus
(L4-S3)

T12
L1
L2
L3
L4
L5

lumbosacral plexus and **sciatic plexus**

anterior and inferior to the sacral promontory. SYN p. lymphaticus sacralis medius.

myenteric (nervous) p. [TA], a p. of unmyelinated fibers and postganglionic autonomic cell bodies lying in the muscular coat of the esophagus, stomach, and intestines; it communicates with the subserous and submucous plexuses, all subdivisions of the enteric p. SYN p. (nervosus) myentericus [TA], Auerbach p.

nerve p. [TA], a p. formed by the interlacing of nerves or nerve fibers by means of numerous communicating branches or fibers. SYN p. nervosus [TA].

p. nervorum gastricorum [TA], SYN gastric nervous plexuses.

p. nervorum lumba′lium, SYN lumbar (nervous) p.

p. nervo′rum spina′lium [TA], SYN spinal nerve p.

p. nervo′sus [TA], SYN nerve p.

p. nervosus aor′ticus abdomina′lis [TA], SYN abdominal aortic (nervous) p.

p. (nervosus) aor′ticus thora′cicus [TA], SYN thoracic aortic (nervous) p.

p. nervosus arteriae carotidis internae, SYN internal carotid (nervous) p.

p. nervosus cardi′acus [TA], SYN cardiac (nervous) p.

p. (nervosus) cardi′acus superficia′lis [TA], SYN superficial cardiac (nervous) p.

p. nervosus carot′icus commu′nis [TA], SYN common carotid nervous p.

p. nervosus carot′icus exter′nus [TA], SYN external carotid (nervous) p.

p. nervosus caverno′sus [TA], SYN cavernous nervous p.

p. nervosus celi′acus [TA], SYN celiac (nervous) p.

p. nervosus cervicalis posterior [TA], SYN posterior cervical (nervous) p.

p. nervosus deferentia′lis [TA], SYN deferential (nervous) p.

p. nervosus denta′lis infe′rior [TA], SYN inferior dental (nervous) p.

p. (nervosus) denta′lis supe′rior [TA], SYN superior dental (nervous) p.

p. nervosus enter′icus [TA], SYN enteric (nervous) p.

p. nervosus esopha′geus [TA], SYN esophageal (nervous) p.

p. nervosus femora′lis [TA], SYN femoral (nervous) p.

p. nervosus hepat′icus [TA], SYN hepatic (nervous) p.

p. nervosus hypogas′tricus infe′rior [TA], SYN inferior hypogastric (nervous) p.

p. (nervosus) hypogas′tricus supe′rior [TA], SYN superior hypogastric (nervous) p.

p. nervosus ili′acus [TA], SYN iliac (nervous) p.

p. nervosus intermesenter′icus [TA], SYN intermesenteric (nervous) p.

p. (nervosus) liena′lis, ☆official alternate term for splenic (nervous) p.

p. nervosus lumbosacra′lis [TA], SYN lumbosacral (nervous) p.

p. nervosus mesenter′icus infe′rior [TA], SYN inferior mesenteric (nervous) p.

p. (nervosus) mesenter′icus supe′rior [TA], SYN superior mesenteric (nervous) p.

p. (nervosus) myenter′icus [TA], SYN myenteric (nervous) p.

p. (nervosus) ova′ricus [TA], SYN ovarian (nervous) p.

p. (nervosus) pancreat′icus [TA], SYN pancreatic (nervous) p.

p. nervosus pel′vicus, ☆official alternate term for inferior hypogastric (nervous) p.

p. nervosus pharyn′geus [TA], SYN pharyngeal (nervous) p.

p. nervosus prostat′icus [TA], SYN prostatic (nervous) p.

p. (nervosus) pulmona′lis [TA], SYN pulmonary (nervous) p.

p. nervosus recta′lis inferio′res [TA], SYN inferior rectal (nervous) p.

p. nervosus recta′lis me′dius, SYN middle rectal (nervous) p.

p. (nervosus) recta′lis supe′rior [TA], SYN superior rectal (nervous) p.

p. (nervosus) rena′lis [TA], SYN renal (nervous) p.

p. (nervosus) sple′nicus [TA], SYN splenic (nervous) p.

p. (nervosus) submuco′sus [TA], SYN submucosal (nervous) p.

p. (nervosus) subsero′sus [TA], SYN subserous (nervous) p.

p. (nervosus) suprarena′lis [TA], SYN suprarenal (nervous) p.

p. (nervosus) tympan′icus [TA], SYN tympanic (nervous) p.

p. (nervosus) ureter′icus [TA], SYN ureteric (nervous) p.

p. (nervosus) uterovagina′lis [TA], SYN uterovaginal (nervous) p.

p. vesica′lis [TA], SYN vesical (nervous) p.

plexus viscerales, SYN autonomic plexuses.

occipital p., SYN periarterial p. of occipital artery.

ovarian (nervous) p. [TA], an autonomic p. derived from the aortic p. and accompanying the ovarian artery to the ovary, broad ligament, and uterine tube. SYN p. (nervosus) ovaricus [TA].

pampiniform venous p., a p. formed, in the male, by veins from the testicle and epididymis, consisting of 8 or 10 veins lying in front of the ductus deferens and forming part of the spermatic cord; in the female the ovarian veins form this p. between the layers of the broad ligament; in the male it is part of the thermoregulatory system of the testis, helping to keep the testis at a constant temperature slightly lower than the other body temperature. SYN p. venosus pampiniformis [TA].

pancreatic (nervous) p. [TA], the autonomic p. that accompanies the pancreatic arteries. SYN p. (nervosus) pancreaticus [TA].

parotid p. of facial nerve [TA], the diverging branches of the facial nerve passing through the substance of the parotid gland, connected by numerous looped anastomoses. SYN intraparotid p. of facial nerve, pes anserinus (1), p. intraparotideus nervi facialis.

pelvic (nervous) p., ☆official alternate term for inferior hypogastric (nervous) p.

periarterial p. [TA], an autonomic p. that accompanies an artery, surrounding it in a network of autonomic nerve fibers. SYN p. periarterialis [TA].

periarterial p. of anterior cerebral artery, an autonomic p. accompanying the anterior cerebral artery, derived from the internal carotid p. SYN p. periarterialis arteriae cerebri anterioris.

periarterial p. of ascending pharyngeal artery, an autonomic p.

pl

on the ascending pharyngeal artery, formed of fibers from the superior cervical ganglion. SYN ascending pharyngeal p., p. periarterialis arteriae pharyngeae ascendentis.

periarterial p. of choroid artery, an autonomic p. accompanying the artery of the same name, derived from the internal carotid p. SYN p. arteriae choroideae, p. periarterialis arteriae choroideae.

periarterial plexuses of coronary arteries, the continuation of the cardiac p. onto the coronary arteries. SYN coronary p., p. coronarii cordis.

periarterial p. of facial artery, an autonomic p. on the facial artery derived from the external carotid p.; it sends a branch to the submandibular ganglion. SYN external maxillary p., facial p., p. maxillaris externus, p. periarterialis arteriae facialis.

periarterial p. of inferior phrenic artery, an autonomic p. surrounding the inferior phrenic artery. SYN phrenic p., p. phrenicus, p. periarterialis arteriae phrenicae inferioris.

periarterial p. of inferior thyroid artery, an autonomic plexus on the inferior thyroid artery derived from the subclavian plexus. SYN inferior thyroid p., p. thyroideus inferior.

periarterial p. of internal thoracic artery, an autonomic p. on the internal thoracic artery derived from the subclavian p. SYN internal mammary p., internal thoracic p., p. mammarius internus, p. periarterialis arteriae thoracicae internae.

p. periarteria'lis [TA], SYN periarterial p.

p. periarterialis arteriae auricula'ris poste'rioris, SYN periarterial p. of posterior auricular artery.

p. periarterialis arte'riae cer'ebri anterio'ris, SYN periarterial p. of anterior cerebral artery.

p. periarterialis arte'riae cer'ebri me'diae, SYN periarterial p. of middle cerebral artery.

p. periarterialis arteriae choroideae, SYN periarterial p. of choroid artery.

p. periarterialis arteriae facialis, SYN periarterial p. of facial artery.

p. periarterialis arteriae lingualis, SYN periarterial p. of lingual artery.

p. periarterialis arteriae maxillaris, SYN periarterial p. of maxillary artery.

p. periarterialis arteriae occipita'lis, SYN periarterial p. of occipital artery.

p. periarterialis arteriae ophthal'micae, SYN periarterial p. of ophthalmic artery.

p. periarterialis arteriae pharyn'geae ascen'dentis, SYN periarterial p. of ascending pharyngeal artery.

p. periarterialis arteriae phrenicae inferioris, SYN periarterial p. of inferior phrenic artery.

p. periarterialis arteriae popliteae, SYN periarterial p. of popliteal artery.

p. periarterialis arteriae subcla'viae [TA], SYN periarterial p. of subclavian artery.

p. periarterialis arteriae tempora'lis superficia'lis, SYN periarterial p. of superficial temporal artery.

p. periarterialis arteriae testicula'ris, SYN periarterial p. of testicular artery.

p. periarterialis arteriae thoracicae internae, SYN periarterial p. of internal thoracic artery.

p. periarterialis arteriae thyroi'deae superio'ris, SYN periarterial p. of superior thyroid artery.

p. periarterialis arteriae vertebralis, SYN periarterial p. of vertebral artery.

periarterial p. of lingual artery, an autonomic p. on the lingual artery, derived from the external carotid p. SYN lingual p., p. periarterialis arteriae lingualis.

periarterial p. of maxillary artery, an autonomic p. on the maxillary artery derived from the external carotid p. SYN internal maxillary p., maxillary p., p. maxillaris internus, p. periarterialis arteriae maxillaris.

periarterial p. of middle cerebral artery, an autonomic p. accompanying the middle cerebral artery, derived from the internal carotid p. SYN p. periarterialis arteriae cerebri mediae.

periarterial p. of occipital artery, an autonomic p. on the occipi-

tal artery derived from the external carotid p. SYN occipital p., p. periarterialis arteriae occipitalis.

periarterial p. of ophthalmic artery, an autonomic p., entering the orbit in company with the ophthalmic artery, derived from the internal carotid p. SYN p. periarterialis arteriae ophthalmicae.

periarterial p. of popliteal artery, a nerve p. surrounding the popliteal artery, derived from the femoral p. SYN p. periarterialis arteriae popliteae, popliteal p., p. popliteus.

periarterial p. of posterior auricular artery, an autonomic p. on the posterior auricular artery, derived from the external carotid p. SYN p. periarterialis arteriae auricularis posterioris, posterior auricular p.

periarterial p. of subclavian artery [TA], the autonomic p. accompanying the artery of this name, formed by fibers from the stellate ganglion, and giving off secondary plexuses along the branches of the subclavian artery. SYN p. periarterialis arteriae subclaviae [TA], subclavian p.

periarterial p. of superficial temporal artery, an autonomic p. of nerves on the artery of this name, derived from the external carotid p. SYN p. periarterialis arteriae temporalis superficialis, superficial temporal p.

periarterial p. of superior thyroid artery, an autonomic p. on the superior thyroid artery, derived from the external carotid p. SYN p. periarterialis arteriae thyroideae superioris, superior thyroid p.

periarterial p. of testicular artery, the autonomic p. derived from the aortic p. and accompanying the testicular artery. SYN p. periarterialis arteriae testicularis, spermatic p., testicular p.

periarterial p. of thyroid artery, an autonomic p. on the thyroid artery, derived from the subclavian p.

periarterial p. of vertebral artery, p. of autonomic nerves on the vertebral artery, derives from the subclavian p. SYN p. periarterialis arteriae vertebralis, p. vertebralis, vertebral p.

pharyngeal (nervous) p., (1) the p. of nerves, including branches of the glossopharyngeal, vagus, and accessory nerves (cranial root), that lies along the posterior wall of the pharynx; (2) [TA], a venous p. on the posteriolateral walls of the pharynx, emptying through the pharyngeal veins into the internal jugular. SYN p. nervosus pharyngeus [TA].

phrenic p., p. phren'icus, SYN periarterial p. of inferior phrenic artery.

popliteal p., p. poplit'eus, SYN periarterial p. of popliteal artery.

posterior auricular p., SYN periarterial p. of posterior auricular artery.

posterior cervical (nervous) p. [TA], not traditionally described with the major nerve plexuses, all of which are formed by ventral rami, this refers to the dorsal rami of the upper cervical spinal nerves and the relatively small communicating branches that extend between them. SYN p. nervosus cervicalis posterior [TA].

posterior coronary p., the portion of the cardiac p. that accompanies branches of the coronary arteries on the posteroinferior surface of the heart.

prostatic (nervous) p. [TA], an autonomic p. of nerves intimately associated with the capsule of the prostate, derived from the inferior hypogastric p., and giving rise to the cavernous nerves to the erectile tissue of the penis; surgical injury of this plexus often results in impotence. SYN p. nervosus prostaticus [TA].

prostaticovesical venous p., a venous p. that includes the prostatic venous plexus around the prostate gland and that of the neck of the bladder; it communicates with the vesical and pudendal plexuses, receives the deep dorsal vein of the penis, and empties, by one or more efferent vessels, into the internal iliac (hypogastric) vein; it corresponds to the inferior vesical p. in the female. SYN p. venosus prostaticovesicalis.

prostatic venous p. [TA], a venous p., arising chiefly from the dorsal vein of the penis, situated below the base of the bladder at the sides of the prostate. SEE ALSO prostaticovesical venous p. SYN p. venosus prostaticus [TA], p. pudendalis, Santorini labyrinth.

pterygoid venous p. [TA], a venous p. occupying the infratemporal fossa receiving veins accompanying the branches of the maxillary artery, and terminating posteriorly in the maxillary vein;

anteriorly the pterygoid plexus drains via the deep facial vein into the facial vein. SYN p. venosus pterygoideus.

p. pudenda′lis, SYN prostatic venous p.

p. puden′dus nervo′sus, SYN pudendal *nerve.*

pulmonary (nervous) p. [TA], one of two autonomic plexuses, anterior and posterior, at the hilus of each lung, formed by cardiopulmonary splanchnic nerves of the sympathetic trunk and bronchial branches of the vagus nerve; from them various branches accompany the bronchi and arteries into the lung. SYN p. (nervosus) pulmonalis [TA].

Quénu hemorrhoidal p., lymphatic plexuses in the skin about the anus.

Ranvier p., a subbasal stroma p. of the cornea. SEE stroma p.

rectal plexuses, SEE inferior rectal (nervous) p., middle rectal (nervous) p., superior rectal (nervous) p.

rectal venous p. [TA], a venous p. resting upon the posterior and lateral walls of the rectum; it drains into the superior rectal vein to the portal, the middle rectal to the internal iliac, and the inferior rectal to the internal pudendal. SYN p. venosus rectalis [TA], hemorrhoidal p.

Remak p., SYN submucosal (nervous) p.

renal (nervous) p. [TA], the autonomic p. surrounding the renal artery and extending with it into the substance of the kidney. SYN p. (nervosus) renalis [TA].

sacral p. [TA], p. formed by the fourth and fifth lumbar (lumbosacral trunk) and first, second, and third sacral nerves; it lies on the inner surface of the posterior wall of the pelvis usually embedded in the piriformis muscle; its nerves supply the lower limbs, its major product being the sciatic nerve. SYN p. sacralis [TA], ischiadic p., sciatic p.

p. sacra′lis [TA], SYN sacral p.

sacral venous p., a venous p. on the pelvic surface of the sacrum, formed by tributaries to the lateral sacral veins. SYN p. venosus sacralis.

Santorini p., venous p. on ventral and lateral prostatic surfaces.

Sappey p., a network of lymphatics in the areola of the nipple.

sciatic p., SYN sacral p.

solar p., SYN celiac (nervous) p.

spermatic p., SYN periarterial p. of testicular artery.

spinal nerve p. [TA], an intermingling of fiber fascicles from adjacent spinal nerves to form a network; the major plexuses are the cervical, brachial, and lumbosacral. SYN p. nervorum spinalium [TA], p. of spinal nerves [TA].

p. of spinal nerves [TA], SYN spinal nerve p.

splenic (nervous) p. [TA], the p. of autonomic nerves along the splenic artery. SYN p. (nervosus) splenicus [TA], p. (nervosus) lienalis☆.

Stensen p., the venous network surrounding the parotid (Stensen) duct.

stroma p., a p. of nerves in the parenchyma of the cornea consisting of the primary or deep p., in the substance of the cornea, and the subbasal or superficial p. just beneath the anterior limiting membrane.

subclavian p., SYN periarterial p. of subclavian artery.

submucosal (nervous) p. [TA], a gangliated p. of unmyelinated nerve fibers, derived chiefly from the superior mesenteric p., ramifying in the intestinal submucosa. SYN p. (nervosus) submucosus [TA], Meissner p., Remak p.

suboccipital venous p. [TA], the extensive p. of veins in the suboccipital region. SYN p. venosus suboccipitalis [TA].

subserous (nervous) p. [TA], the subserous part of the enteric plexus of autonomic nerves. SYN p. (nervosus) subserosus [TA].

superficial cardiac (nervous) p. [TA], the superficial and smaller subdivision of the cardiac p., formed by the left superior cardiac nerves from the left vagus and cervical sympathetic trunk; it is found beneath the aortic arch, between the arch and the bifurcation of the pulmonary trunk. SYN p. (nervosus) cardiacus superficialis [TA].

superficial temporal p., SYN periarterial p. of superficial temporal artery.

superior dental (nervous) p. [TA], formed by branches of the infraorbital nerve, it gives off superior dental branches to the upper and superior gingival branches to the gums. SYN p. (nervosus) dentalis superior [TA].

superior hemorrhoidal p., SYN superior rectal (nervous) p.

superior hypogastric (nervous) p. [TA], the continuation of the aortic p. inferior to the aortic bifurcation across the fifth lumbar vertebra into the pelvis where it divides into two hypogastric nerves at the sides of the rectum; these join the pelvic splanchnic nerves to form the inferior hypogastric plexuses supplying pelvic viscera. SYN p. (nervosus) hypogastricus superior [TA], nervus presacralis☆, presacral nerve☆, Latarget nerve (1).

superior mesenteric (nervous) p. [TA], an autonomic p., a continuation of the abdominal aortic p., sending nerves to the intestines and forming with the vagus the subserous, myenteric, and submucous plexuses; this periarterial plexus is so dense that it results in the appearance of a characteristic perivascular "collar" distinguishing the superior mesenteric artery from the superior mesenteric vein in several imaging modalities such as with ultrasound. SYN p. (nervosus) mesentericus superior [TA].

superior rectal (nervous) p. [TA], the autonomic p. derived as a continuation of the inferior mesenteric p. that accompanies the superior rectal artery. SYN p. (nervosus) rectalis superior [TA], superior hemorrhoidal p.

superior thyroid p., SYN periarterial p. of superior thyroid artery.

suprarenal (nervous) p. [TA], an autonomic p. formed mainly by branches from the celiac ganglion, lying at the hilus of the suprarenal gland. SYN p. (nervosus) suprarenalis [TA].

sympathetic plexuses [TA], autonomic plexuses, in which postsynaptic sympathetic nerve fibers are predominant.

testicular p., SYN periarterial p. of testicular artery.

thoracic aortic (nervous) p. [TA], an autonomic p. surrounding the thoracic aorta and passing with it through the aortic opening in the diaphragm to become continuous with the abdominal aortic p. SYN p. (nervosus) aorticus thoracicus [TA].

p. thyroi′deus infe′rior, SYN periarterial p. of inferior thyroid artery.

tympanic (nervous) p. [TA], a p. on the promontory of the labyrinthine wall of the tympanic cavity, formed by the tympanic nerve, an anastomotic branch of the facial, and sympathetic branches from the internal carotid p.; it supplies the mucosa of the middle ear, mastoid cells, and auditory (eustachian) tube and gives off the lesser superficial petrosal nerve to the otic ganglion. SYN p. (nervosus) tympanicus [TA], Jacobson p.

unpaired thyroid venous p. [TA], a venous p. in front of the lower portion of the trachea formed by anastomoses between the inferior laryngeal veins and veins emerging from the caudal border of the thyroid; it terminates in the unpaired inferior thyroid vein. SYN p. venosus thyroideus impar.

ureteric (nervous) p. [TA], the autonomic p. derived from the celiac p. that accompanies the ureter. SYN p. (nervosus) uretericus [TA].

uterine venous p. [TA], the plexiform veins that lie along the sides of the uterus in the broad ligament. SYN p. venosus uterinus [TA].

uterovaginal (nervous) p. [TA], a gangliated autonomic p. on each side of the cervix of the uterus, derived from the inferior hypogastric p. SYN p. (nervosus) uterovaginalis [TA], Frankenhäuser ganglion, Lee ganglion.

vaginal venous p. [TA], the p. of veins that surrounds the vagina. SYN p. venosus vaginalis [TA].

vascular p. [TA], a vascular network formed by frequent anastomoses between the blood vessels (arteries or veins) of a part. SYN p. vasculosus [TA].

p. vascularis cavernosus conchae [TA], SYN cavernous (vascular) p. of conchae.

p. vasculo′sus [TA], SYN vascular p.

p. veno′sus [TA], SYN venous p.

p. veno′sus areola′ris [TA], SYN areolar venous p.

p. venosus basila′ris [TA], SYN basilar venous p.

p. veno′sus cana′lis hypoglos′si [TA], SYN venous p. of canal of hypoglossal nerve.

p. veno′sus carot′icus inter′nus, SYN internal carotid venous p.

p. veno′sus foram′inis ova′lis [TA], SYN venous p. of foramen ovale.

p. venosus pampinifor′mis [TA], SYN pampiniform venous p.

p. venosus prostaticovesica′lis, SYN prostaticovesical venous p.

p. veno′sus prostat′icus [TA], SYN prostatic venous p.

p. venosus pterygoi′deus, SYN pterygoid venous p.

p. veno′sus recta′lis [TA], SYN rectal venous p.

p. veno′sus sacra′lis, SYN sacral venous p.

p. veno′sus suboccipita′lis [TA], SYN suboccipital venous p.

p. venosus thyroi′deus im′par, SYN unpaired thyroid venous p.

p. veno′sus uteri′nus [TA], SYN uterine venous p.

p. veno′sus vagina′lis [TA], SYN vaginal venous p.

p. veno′sus vertebra′lis, SYN vertebral venous *system*.

p. veno′sus vesica′lis [TA], SYN vesicular venous p.

p. venosus vesica′lis infe′rior, SYN inferior vesical venous p.

venous p. [TA], a vascular network formed by numerous anastomoses between veins. SYN p. venosus [TA].

venous p. of bladder, SYN vesicular venous p.

venous p. of canal of hypoglossal nerve [TA], a small venous network around the hypoglossal nerve, connecting with the occipital sinus, inferior petrosal sinus, and internal jugular vein. SYN p. venosus canalis hypoglossi [TA], circellus venosus hypoglossi, rete canalis hypoglossi.

venous p. of foramen ovale [TA], a venous network around the mandibular nerve connecting the cavernous sinus and the pterygoid p. SYN p. venosus foraminis ovalis [TA], rete foraminis ovalis.

vertebral p., SYN periarterial p. of vertebral artery.

p. vertebra′lis, SYN periarterial p. of vertebral artery.

vertebral venous p., SYN vertebral venous *system*.

vesical (nervous) p. [TA], an autonomic p. on the bladder, derived from the inferior hypogastric p. SYN p. vesicalis [TA].

vesicular venous p. [TA], a p. of veins around the fundus and sides of the bladder. SYN p. venosus vesicalis [TA], venous p. of bladder.

Walther p., SYN cavernous nervous p.

PLICA

---

pli·ca, gen. and pl. **pli·cae** (plī′kă, plī′sē). [TA] SYN fold (1). [Mod. L. a plait or fold]

pli′cae adipo′sae pleurae, SYN fatty *folds* of pleura, under *fold*.

pli′cae ala′res plicae synovialis infrapatellaris, SYN alar *folds* of intrapatellar synovial fold, under *fold*.

pli′cae ampulla′res tu′bae uteri′nae, SYN ampullary *folds* of uterine tube, under *fold*.

p. anterior faucium, ☆official alternate term for palatoglossal *arch*.

p. aryepiglot′tica [TA], SYN aryepiglottic *fold*.

p. axilla′ris, SYN axillary *fold*.

pli′cae ceca′les [TA], SYN cecal *folds*, under *fold*.

p. ceca′lis vascula′ris [TA], SYN vascular *fold* of the cecum.

p. chor′dae tym′pani, SYN *fold* of chorda tympani.

p. choroi′dea, in the embryo, an infolding of the pia mater from which the choroid plexus develops.

pli′cae cilia′res [TA], SYN ciliary *folds*, under *fold*.

pli′cae circula′res intestini tenuis [TA], SYN circular *folds* of small intestine, under *fold*.

p. duodena′lis infe′rior [TA], SYN inferior duodenal *fold*.

p. duodena′lis supe′rior [TA], SYN superior duodenal *fold*.

p. duodenojejuna′lis, ☆official alternate term for superior duodenal *fold*.

p. duodenomesocol′ica, ☆official alternate term for inferior duodenal *fold*.

p. epigas′trica, SYN lateral umbilical *fold*.

pli′cae epiglot′ticae, SYN epiglottic *folds*, under *fold*.

p. fimbria′ta faciei inferioris linguae [TA], SYN fimbriated *fold* of inferior surface of tongue.

pli′cae gas′tricae [TA], SYN gastric *folds*, under *fold*.

pli′cae gastropancreat′icae [TA], SYN gastropancreatic *folds*, under *fold*.

p. glossoepiglot′tica latera′lis [TA], SYN lateral glossoepiglottic *fold*.

p. glossoepiglot′tica media′na [TA], SYN median glossoepiglottic *fold*.

p. guberna′trix, SYN genitoinguinal *ligament*.

p. hypogas′trica, SYN medial umbilical *fold*.

p. ileoceca′lis [TA], SYN ileocecal *fold*.

p. incu′dis, SYN incudal *fold*.

p. inguina′lis, an embryonic mesodermal thickening that joins the caudal end of the urogenital ridge to the anterior abdominal wall; the gubernaculum of the testis develops in it. SYN inguinal fold.

p. interdigita′lis, SYN *web* of fingers/toes.

p. interureter′ica [TA], SYN interureteric *crest*.

pli′cae ir′idis [TA], SYN *folds* of iris, under *fold*.

p. lacrima′lis [TA], SYN lacrimal *fold*.

p. longitudina′lis duode′ni [TA], SYN longitudinal *fold* of duodenum.

p. luna′ta, SYN p. semilunaris of conjunctiva.

plicae mallea′res (anterior et posterior) [TA], SYN mallear *folds*, under *fold*.

p. membra′nae tym′pani, SYN mallear *folds*, under *fold*.

pli′cae muco′sae vesi′cae biliaris [TA], SYN mucosal *folds* of gallbladder, under *fold*.

p. ner′vi laryn′gei superioris [TA], SYN *fold* of superior laryngeal nerve.

p. palati′na transver′sa [TA], SYN transverse palatine *fold*.

pli′cae palma′tae canalis cervicis uteri [TA], SYN palmate *folds* of cervical canal, under *fold*.

p. palpebronasa′lis [TA], SYN palpebronasal *fold*.

p. paraduodena′lis [TA], SYN paraduodenal *fold*.

p. posterior faucium, ☆official alternate term for palatopharyngeal *arch*.

pli′cae rec′ti, SYN transverse *folds* of rectum, under *fold*.

p. rectouteri′na [TA], SYN rectouterine *fold*.

p. rectovagina′lis, SYN sacrovaginal *fold*.

p. salpingopalatin′a [TA], SYN salpingopalatine *fold*.

p. salpingopharyn′gea [TA], SYN salpingopharyngeal *fold*.

plicae semilunares coli [TA], SYN semilunar *folds* of colon, under *fold*.

plicae semiluna′res of colon, SYN semilunar *folds* of colon, under *fold*.

p. semiluna′ris [TA], SYN semilunar *fold*.

p. semiluna′ris of conjuncti′va [TA], **(1)** [NA], the semilunar fold formed by the palpebral conjunctiva at the medial angle of the eye; **(2)** a fold of the conjunctival mucous membrane found in many animals; normally partially hidden in the medial canthus of the eye when at rest, it may be extended to cover part or all of the cornea in a winking-like action to clean the cornea, as in birds. SYN membrana nictitans, nictitating membrane, palpebra III, palpebra tertia, third eyelid. SYN p. semilunaris conjunctivae [TA], p. lunata, p. semilunaris of eye, semilunar conjunctival fold.

p. semilunaris conjunctivae [TA], SYN p. semilunaris of conjunctiva.

p. semilunaris of eye, SYN p. semilunaris of conjunctiva.

p. spira′lis duc′tus cys′tici [TA], SYN spiral *fold* of cystic duct.

p. stapedialis, SYN *fold* of stapes.

p. sublingua′lis [TA], SYN sublingual *fold*.

p. synovia′lis, SYN synovial *fold*.

p. synovia′lis infrapatella′ris [TA], SYN infrapatellar synovial *fold*.

p. synovia′lis patella′ris, SYN infrapatellar synovial *fold.*

pli′cae transversa′les rec′ti [TA], SYN transverse *folds* of rectum, under *fold.*

p. triangula′ris [TA], SYN triangular *fold.*

pli′cae tuba′riae tu′bae uteri′nae [TA], SYN *folds* of uterine tubes, under *fold.*

p. tubopalati′na, SYN salpingopalatine *fold.*

p. umbilica′lis latera′lis [TA], SYN lateral umbilical *fold.*

p. umbilica′lis media′lis [TA], SYN medial umbilical *fold.*

p. ura′chi, SYN median umbilical *fold.*

p. ureter′ica, SYN interureteric *crest.*

p. uterovesica′lis, SYN uterovesical *ligament.*

p. ve′nae ca′vae sinis′trae [TA], SYN *fold* of left vena cava.

p. ventricula′ris, SYN vestibular *fold.*

p. vesica′lis transver′sa, SYN transverse vesical *fold.*

p. vesicouteri′na, SYN uterovesical *ligament.*

p. vestibula′ris [TA], SYN vestibular *fold.*

p. vestib′uli, a fold of mucous membrane forming a ridge on the septum of the nose.

p. villo′sa, one of the ridges of the mucous membrane of the stomach in the region of the pylorus.

p. voca′lis [TA], SYN vocal *fold.*

---

pli·cate (plī′kāt). Folded; pleated; tucked.

pli·ca·tion (plī-kā′shŭn, pli-). A folding or putting together in pleats; specifically, an operation for reducing the size of a hollow viscus by taking folds or tucks in its walls. [L. *plico,* pp. *-atus,* to fold]

pli·cot·o·my (plī-kot′ō-mē). Division of the posterior malleolar fold. [plica + G. *tomē,* incision]

⟡**-ploid.** Multiple in form; its combinations are used both adjectivally and substantively of a (specified) multiple of chromosomes. [G. *-plo-, -ides,* in form; L. *-ploïdeus*]

ploi·dy (ploy′dē). The number of haploid sets in a cell. Gametes normally contain one; somatic cells two. SEE ALSO polyploidy. [-ploid + *-y,* condition]

plom·bage (plom-bahzh′). Formerly, the use of an inert material in collapse of the lung in the surgical treatment of pulmonary tuberculosis. [Fr. lit. lead-work]

plo·sive (plō′siv). Speech sound made by impounding the air stream for a moment and then suddenly releasing it.

plot (plot). A graphical representation.

double-reciprocal p., a graphic representation of enzyme kinetic data in which $1/v$ (on the vertical axis), where v is the initial velocity, is plotted as a function of the reciprocal of the substrate concentration (1/[S]). SYN Lineweaver-Burk p., Woolf-Lineweaver-Burk p.

Eadie-Hofstee p., a graphic representation of enzyme kinetic data in which velocities, v, are plotted on the vertical axis as a function of the $v/[S]$ ratio on the horizontal axis. On occasion, these axes are reversed. Sometimes referred to as the Eadie-Augustinsson p. or Woolf-Eadie-Augustinsson-Hofstee p.

funnel p., a graphic method of detecting publication bias. The estimate of risk derived from a set of epidemiologic studies used in a metaanalysis is plotted against sample size. If there is no publication bias, the p. is funnel-shaped; if studies giving significant results are more likely to be published than negative studies, the p. is asymmetric. SEE ALSO metaanalysis.

Hanes p., a graphic representation of enzyme kinetic data in which the substrate concentration divided by the velocity (i.e., the [S]/v ratio) is plotted on the vertical axis as a function of [S]. Sometimes referred to as the Hanes-Wilkinson p.

Hill p., a graphic representation of enzyme kinetic data or of binding phenomena to assess the degree of cooperativity of a system; the vertical axis in a Hill plot is log $[Y/(1 - Y)]$, in which Y is the degree of saturation (for enzymes, the vertical axis is log $[v/(V_{max} - v)]$, where v is the initial velocity and V_{max} is the maximum velocity, and the horizontal axis is the logarithm of the ligand concentration.

Lineweaver-Burk p., SYN double-reciprocal p.

Ramachandran p., a graphic representation in which the dihedral angle of rotation about the α-carbon-to-carbonyl-carbon bond in polypeptides is plotted against the dihedral angle of rotation about the α-carbon-to-nitrogen bond. SYN conformational map.

Scatchard p., (1) a graphic representation used in the analysis of binding phenomena in which the concentration of bound ligand divided by the concentration of free ligand is plotted against the concentration of bound ligand; (2) similar to (1), except the concentration of the bound ligand is on the vertical axis.

Woolf-Lineweaver-Burk p., SYN double-reciprocal p.

PLP Abbreviation for *pyridoxal* 5-phosphate; parathyroid hormonelike *protein.*

plug (plŭg). Any mass filling a hole or closing an orifice.

Dittrich p.'s, minute, dirty-grayish, ill-smelling masses of bacteria and fatty acid crystals in the sputum in pulmonary gangrene and fetid bronchitis. SYN Traube p.'s.

epithelial p., a mass of epithelial cells temporarily occluding an embryonic opening; the term is most commonly used with reference to the external nares.

laminated epithelial p., SYN *keratosis* obturans.

meconium p., a p. of thick, inspissated meconium that may cause intestinal obstruction.

mucous p., a mass of mucus and cells filling the cervical canal between periods or during pregnancy; a mass of mucous occluding a main or lobar bronchus.

Traube p.'s, SYN Dittrich p.'s.

plug·ger. A dental instrument used for condensing gold (foil), amalgam, or any plastic material in a cavity; operated by hand or by mechanical means. SYN packer (2), plugging instrument.

automatic p., a mechanically or electrically activated device used to provide condensing pressure in the placement of amalgam or gold foil in a cavity preparation. SYN automatic condenser.

back-action p., an instrument for condensing gold foil or amalgam in areas that cannot be reached directly.

foot p., a p. the shape of which resembles a foot, used for condensing gold foil; the working surface may be flat or curved in the heel-toe direction.

root canal p., fine-tapered root canal instrument, blunt at the tip, used for pressing or forcing a gutta percha cone into a root canal.

plum·ba·go (plŭm-bā′gō). SYN graphite. [L. *plumbago,* black lead]

plum·bic (plŭm′bik). **1.** Relating to or containing lead. **2.** Denoting the higher valence of the lead ion, Pb^{4+}. [L. *plumbum,* lead]

plum·bism (plŭm′bizm). SYN lead *poisoning.* [L. *plumbum,* lead]

plum·bum (plŭm′bŭm). SYN lead. [L.]

Plummer, Henry S., U.S. physician, 1874–1937. SEE P. *disease;* P.-Vinson *syndrome.*

plu·mose (ploo′mōs). Feathery. [L. *pluma,* feather]

⟡**pluri-.** Several, more. SEE ALSO multi-, poly-. [L. *plus, pluris*]

plu·ri·cau·sal (ploor-i-kaw′zăl). Having two or more causes; used in reference to the etiology of a disease; often indicates that a given disease develops only when two or more causative factors are operative simultaneously.

plu·ri·glan·du·lar (ploo-ri-glan′doo-lăr). Denoting several glands or their secretions. SYN multiglandular, polyglandular.

plu·ri·loc·u·lar (ploo-ri-lok′ū-lăr). SYN multilocular.

plu·ri·nu·cle·ar (ploo-ri-noo′klē-ăr). SYN multinuclear.

plu·rip·o·tent, plu·ri·po·ten·tial (ploo-rip′ō-tent, ploo′rē-pō-ten′shăl). **1.** Having the capacity to affect more than one organ or tissue. **2.** Not fixed as to potential development. SEE ALSO pluripotent *cells,* under *cell.*

plu·ri·re·sis·tant (ploo′ri-rē-sis′tănt). Having multiple aspects of resistance.

plu·to·ma·nia (ploo-tō-mā′nē-ă). A delusion that one has great wealth. [G. *ploutos,* wealth, + *mania,* frenzy]

plu·to·nism (ploo′ton-izm). Effects produced, as demonstrated in experimental animals, by means of exposure to the radioactive element plutonium present in atomic piles; they consist of hepatic damage, bone changes, and graying of the hair.

plu·to·ni·um (**Pu**) (ploo-tō′nē-ŭm). A transuranium artificial radioactive element, atomic no. 94, atomic wt. 244.064. The best-known α-emitting isotope is ^{239}Pu (half-life 24,110 years) which, like ^{235}U, is fissionable and can be used in atomic bombs and nuclear power plants; ^{238}Pu (half-life 87.74 years) is used as an energy source in pacemakers. Pu ions are bone-seekers; ingestion is a radiation hazard, as with radium and radiostrontium. [planet, *Pluto*]

Pm Symbol for promethium.

pM Abbreviation for picomolar (10^{-12} M).

pm Symbol for picometer.

P mit·ra·le (mī-trā′lē). Broad, notched P waves in several or many leads of the electrocardiogram with a prominent late negative component to the P wave in lead V$_1$, presumed to be characteristic of mitral valvular disease. (Although this term is extensively used in electrocardiographic literature, it is actually a misnomer and would be more appropriately called P-sinistrocardiale, as it results from overload of the left atrium regardless of the cause and may occur independently of disease of the mitral valve.)

PML Abbreviation for progressive multifocal *leukoencephalopathy*.

pmol Abbreviation for picomole.

PMR Abbreviation for proportional mortality ratio.

PMS Abbreviation for premenstrual *syndrome*.

△**-pnea.** Breath, respiration. [G. *pneō*, to breathe]

△**pneo-.** Combining form denoting breath or respiration. SEE ALSO pneum-, pneumo-. [G. *pneō*, to breathe]

△**pneum-, pneuma-, pneumat-, pneumato-.** Presence of air or gas, the lungs, or breathing. SEE ALSO pneo-, pneumo-. [G. *pneuma, pneumatos*, air, breath]

pneu·ma (noo′mă). In ancient Greek philosophy and medicine: **1.** Air or an all-pervading fiery essence in the air (which today would be identified with oxygen), which was the creative and animating spirit of the universe; drawn into the body through the lungs, it generated and sustained the innate heat in the left ventricle of the heart and was distributed by the arteries to the brain and all parts of the body. **2.** Soul or psyche. [G. *pneuma*, air, breath]

pneu·marth·ro·gram (noo-marth′rō-gram). Film records of pneumarthrography.

pneu·marth·rog·ra·phy (noo-marth-rog′ră-fē). Radiographic examination of a joint following the introduction of air, with or without another contrast medium.

pneu·mar·thro·sis (noo-mar-thrō′sis). Presence of air in a joint. [G. *pneuma*, air, + *arthron*, joint, + *-osis*, condition]

pneu·mat·ic (noo-mat′ik). **1.** Relating to air or gas, or to a structure filled with air. **2.** Relating to respiration. [G. *pneumatikos*]

pneu·mat·ic an·ti·shock gar·ment. An inflatable suit used to apply pressure to the peripheral circulation, thus reducing blood flow and fluid exudation into tissues, to maintain central blood flow in the presence of shock. SYN military antishock trousers.

pneu·mat·ics (noo-mat′iks). The science concerned with the physical properties of air or gases. [G. *pneuma*, air or gas]

pneu·ma·tism (noo′mă-tizm). The doctrine of the pneumatists.

pneu·ma·tists (noo′mă-tists). Followers of the school whose physiology centered on the pneuma and who conceived the causes of disease as disturbances of this vital principle.

pneu·ma·ti·za·tion (noo′mă-ti-zā′shŭn). The development of air cells such as those of the mastoid and ethmoidal bones. [G. *pneuma*, air]

pneu·ma·tized (noo′mă-tīzd). Containing air.

△**pneumato-.** SEE pneum-.

pneu·ma·to·car·dia (noo′mă-tō-kar′dē-ă). Presence of air bubbles or gas in the blood of the heart; produced by air embolism.

pneu·ma·to·cele (noo′măt′ō-sēl). **1.** An emphysematous or gaseous swelling. **2.** SYN pneumonocele. **3.** A thin-walled cavity within the lung, one of the characteristic sequelae of staphylococcus pneumonia and *Pneumocystis carinii* pneumonia. [G. *pneuma*, air, + *kēlē*, tumor, hernia]

extracranial p., collection of gas beneath the galea aponeurotica, usually due to fracture into the paranasal sinuses. SYN extracranial pneumocele.

intracranial p., a collection of gas within the skull, in the brain, or in the meninges. SYN intracranial pneumocele.

pneu·ma·to·en·ter·ic. SYN celomic *bay*.

pneu·ma·to·he·mia (noo′mă-tō-hē′mē-ă). SYN pneumohemia.

pneu·ma·tom·e·ter (noo-mă-tom′ĕ-ter). Obsolete term for spirometer.

pneu·ma·tor·rha·chis (noo-mă-tōr′ă-kis). SYN pneumorrhachis. [G. *pneuma*, air, + *rhachis*, spine]

pneu·ma·to·scope (noo′mă-tō-skōp, noo-mat′ō-skōp). **1.** Obsolete term for an instrument for measuring the extent of the respiratory excursions of the chest. **2.** Obsolete term for an instrument for use in auscultatory percussion, the percussion sounds of the chest being heard at the mouth. SYN pneumoscope. [G. *pneuma*, air, + *skopeō*, to examine]

pneu·ma·to·sis (noo-mă-tō′sis). Abnormal accumulation of gas in any tissue or part of the body. [G. a blowing out]

p. coli, a usually benign condition in which gas is seen radiographically in the wall of the colon; sometimes associated with obstructive lung disease.

ⓘ **p. cystoi′des intestina′lis,** a condition of unknown cause characterized by the occurrence of gas cysts in the intestinal mucous membrane; may produce intestinal obstruction. SYN intestinal emphysema.

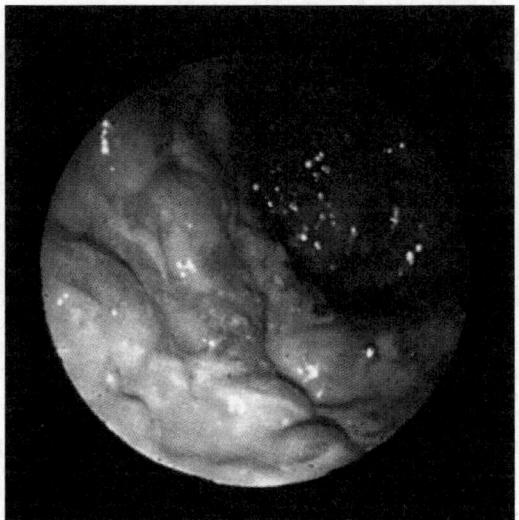

pneumatosis cystoides intestinalis: endoscopic view of gas cysts

pneu·ma·tu·ria (noo-mă-too′rē-ă). The passage of gas or air from the urethra during or after urination, resulting from infected urine or, more commonly, from an intestinal fistula. [G. *pneuma*, air, + *ouron*, urine]

pneu·ma·type (noo′mă-tīp). A device for determining the patency of the nasal fossae by exhaling through the nose against a plate of cooled glass. [G. *pneuma*, breath, + *typos*, type]

△**pneumo-, pneumon-, pneumono-.** The lungs, air or gas, respiration, or pneumonia. SEE ALSO aer-, pneo-, pneum-. [G. *pneumōn, pneumonos*, lung]

pneu·mo·ar·throg·ra·phy (noo′mō-ar-throg′ră-fē). Radiography of a joint after injection of air and usually a water-soluble contrast medium. [G. *pneuma*, air, + *arthron*, joint, + *graphō*, to write]

pneu·mo·ba·cil·lus (noo′mō-bă-sil′ŭs). SYN *Klebsiella pneumoniae*.

pneu·mo·bul·bar (noo′mō-bŭl′bar). Relating to the lungs and their connection with the medulla oblongata by way of the vagus nerve. [G. *pneumōn*, lung, + L. *bulbus*, bulb]

pneu·mo·car·di·al (noo′mō-kar′dē-ăl). SYN cardiopulmonary.

pneu·mo·cele (noo′mō-sēl). SYN pneumonocele.

extracranial p., SYN extracranial *pneumatocele.*

intracranial p., SYN intracranial *pneumatocele.*

pneu·mo·cen·te·sis (noo′mō-sen-tē′sis). SYN pneumonocentesis.

pneu·mo·ceph·a·lus (noo-mō-sef′ă-lŭs). Presence of air or gas within the cranial cavity. [G. *pneuma,* air, + *kephalē,* head]

pneu·mo·cho·le·cys·ti·tis (noo′mō-kō′lē-sis-tī′tis). Cholecystitis with gas-forming organisms giving rise to gas in the gallbladder.

pneu·mo·coc·cal (noo-mō-kok′ăl). Pertaining to or containing the pneumococcus.

pneu·mo·coc·ce·mia (noo′mō-kok-sē′mē-ă). The presence of pneumococci in the blood. [pneumococcus + G. *haima,* blood]

pneu·mo·coc·ci·dal (noo′mō-kok-sī′dăl). Destructive to pneumococci. [pneumococcus + L. *caedo,* to kill]

pneu·mo·coc·col·y·sis (noo′mō-kok-ol′i-sis). Lysis or destruction of pneumococci. [pneumococcus + G. *lysis,* dissolution]

pneu·mo·coc·co·sis (noo′mō-kok-ō′sis). Rarely used term for infection with pneumococci.

pneu·mo·coc·co·su·ria (noo′mō-kok-o-soo′rē-ă). The presence of pneumococci or their specific capsular substance in the urine. [pneumococcus + G. *ouron,* urine]

pneu·mo·coc·cus, pl. **pneu·mo·coc·ci** (noo-mō-kok′ŭs, -kok′sī). SYN *Streptococcus pneumoniae.* [G. *pneumōn,* lung, + *kokkos,* berry (coccus)]

Fraenkel p., SYN *Streptococcus pneumoniae.*

pneu·mo·co·lon (noo-mō-kō′lŏn). Gas in the colon or interstitial gas in the wall of the colon. [G. *pneuma,* air, + *kolon,* colon]

pneu·mo·co·ni·o·sis, pneu·mo·ko·ni·o·sis, pl. **pneu·mo·co·ni·o·ses** (noo′mō-kō-nē-ō′sis, -sēz). Inflammation commonly leading to fibrosis of the lungs caused by the inhalation of dust incident to various occupations; characterized by pain in the chest, cough with little or no expectoration, dyspnea, reduced thoracic excursion, sometimes cyanosis, and fatigue after slight exertion; degree of disability depends on the types of particles inhaled, as well as the level of exposure to them. SYN anthracotic tuberculosis, pneumonoconiosis, pneumonokoniosis. [G. *pneumōn,* lung, + *konis,* dust, + *-osis,* condition]

bauxite p., a condition due to the occupational inhalation of bauxite fumes emitted during the manufacture of alumina abrasives; characterized by cough, shortness of breath, a combined obstructive and restrictive breathing pattern, and impairment of diffusing capacity. SYN Shaver disease.

coal worker's p., SYN anthracosilicosis.

collagenous p., a disease of the lungs, characterized by interstitial fibrosis, caused by inhalation of dusts or toxins in the workplace.

p. siderotica (sid-er-ot′ĭ-kă), p. caused by inhalation of iron dust. SYN pulmonary siderosis.

pneu·mo·cra·ni·um (noo-mō-krā′nē-ŭm). Air present between the cranium and the dura mater; the term is commonly used to indicate extradural or subdural air. [G. *pneuma,* air, + *kranion,* skull]

⊞ *Pneu·mo·cys·tis ca·ri·nii* (noo-mō-sis′tis kă-rī′nē-ī). The eukaryotic microorganism responsible for interstitial pneumonia in immunocompromised patients. The exact taxonomic position remains unclear, as the organism has morphologic similarities to protozoa but shares substantial 16S ribosomal RNA and mitochondrial DNA with some species of the Ascomycetes. *P. carinii* fails to grow on fungal culture media but takes up fungal stains, and infections from it respond to antiprotozoal as well as to some antifungal drugs. [G. *pneuma,* air, breathing, + *kystis,* bladder, pouch]

pneu·mo·cys·tog·ra·phy (noo′mō-sis-tog′ră-fē). Radiography of the bladder following injection of air. [G. *pneuma,* air, + *kystis,* bladder, + *graphō,* to write]

pneu·mo·cys·to·sis (noo′mō-sis-tō′sis). SYN *Pneumocystis carinii* pneumonia.

pneu·mo·cyte (noo′mō-sīt). SYN alveolar *cell.* [pneumo- + G. *kytos,* cell]

pneu·mo·der·ma (noo-mō-der′mă). SYN subcutaneous *emphysema.* [G. *pneuma,* air, + *derma,* skin]

pneu·mo·dy·nam·ics (noo′mō-dī-nam′iks). The mechanics of respiration. [G. *pneuma,* breath, + *dynamis,* force]

pneu·mo·em·py·e·ma (noo′mō-em′pī-ē′mă). A rarely used term for pyopneumothorax.

pneu·mo·en·ceph·a·lo·gram (noo′mō-en-sef′ă-lō-gram). Radiographs obtained by pneumoencephalography.

pneu·mo·en·ceph·a·log·ra·phy (noo′mō-en-sef′ă-log′ră-fē). Radiographic visualization of cerebral ventricles and subarachnoid spaces by use of gas such as air; no longer used because of CT and MRI. [G. *pneuma,* air, + *enkephalos,* brain, + *graphō,* to write]

pneu·mo·gas·tric (noo-mō-gas′trik). **1.** Relating to the lungs and the stomach. **2.** Obsolete term denoting the nervus vagus. SYN gastropneumonic, gastropulmonary. [G. *pneumōn,* lung, + *gastēr,* stomach]

pneu·mo·gas·trog·ra·phy (noo′mō-gas-trog′ră-fē). Rarely used radiographic study of stomach after injection of air. [G. *pneuma,* air, + *gastēr,* stomach, + *graphō,* to write]

pneu·mo·gram (noo′mō-gram). **1.** The record or tracing made by a pneumograph. **2.** Radiographic record of pneumography. [G. *pneumōn,* lung, + *gramma,* a drawing]

pneu·mo·graph (noo′mō-graf). Generic term for any device that records respiratory excursions from movements on the body surface; e.g., an impedance p., which applies the principles of impedance plethysmography to the chest. [G. *pneumōn,* lung, + *graphō,* to write]

pneu·mog·ra·phy (noo-mog′ră-fē). **1.** Examination with a pneumograph. **2.** A general term indicating radiography after injection of air. SYN pneumoradiography, pneumoroentgenography. [G. *pneumōn,* lung, + *graphō,* to write]

pneu·mo·he·mia (noo-mō-hē′mē-ă). Presence of air in blood vessels. SEE ALSO air *embolism.* SYN pneumatohemia. [G. *pneuma,* air, + *haima,* blood]

pneu·mo·he·mo·per·i·car·di·um (noo′mō-hē-mō-per-i-kar′dē-ŭm). SYN hemopneumopericardium.

pneu·mo·he·mo·thor·ax (noo′mō-hē-mō-thōr′aks). SYN hemopneumothorax.

pneu·mo·hy·dro·me·tra (noo′mō-hī-drō-mē′tră). The presence of gas and serum in the uterine cavity. [G. *pneuma,* air, + *hydōr* (hydr-), water, + *mētra,* uterus]

pneu·mo·hy·dro·per·i·car·di·um (noo′mō-hī′drō-pār-i-kar′dē-ŭm). SYN hydropneumopericardium.

pneu·mo·hy·dro·per·i·to·ne·um (noo′mō-hī-drō-per-i-tō-nē′ŭm). SYN hydropneumoperitoneum.

pneu·mo·hy·dro·thor·ax (noo-mō-hī-drō-thōr′aks). SYN hydropneumothorax.

pneu·mo·hy·po·der·ma (noo′mō-hī-pō-der′mă). SYN subcutaneous *emphysema.* [G. *pneuma,* air, + *hypo,* beneath, + *derma,* skin]

pneu·mo·ko·ni·o·sis. SEE pneumoconiosis.

pneu·mo·lith (noo′mō-lith). A calculus in the lung. SYN pulmolith. [G. *pneumōn,* lung, + *lithos,* stone]

pneu·mo·li·thi·a·sis (noo-mō-li-thī′ă-sis). Formation of calculi in the lungs.

pneu·mol·o·gy (noo-mol′ō-jē). A rarely used term for the study of diseases of the lung and air passages. [G. *pneuma,* lung, + *logos,* study]

pneu·mol·y·sis (noo-mol′i-sis). Surgical separation of the lung and costal pleura from the endothoracic fascia; formerly used in collapse therapy for tuberculosis. [G. *pneumōn,* lung, + *lysis,* a loosening]

pneu·mo·ma·la·cia (noo-mō-mă-lā′shē-ă). Softening of the lung tissue. [G. *pneumōn,* lung, + *malakia,* softness]

pneu·mo·mas·sage (noo′mō-mă-sahzh′). Compression and rarefaction of the air in the external auditory meatus, causing movement of an intact tympanic membrane. [G. *pneuma,* air, + *massage*]

pneu·mo·me·di·as·ti·num (noo′mō-mē′dē-ă-stī′nŭm). Abnormal presence of air in mediastinal tissues; multiple causes include pulmonary interstitial emphysema, ruptured bleb, perforation of the cervical or thoracic esophagus or airways, cervicomediastinal infection, and perforated abdominal viscus. SYN mediastinal emphysema. [G. *pneuma*, air, + mediastinum]

pneu·mo·mel·a·no·sis (noo′mō-mel-ă-nō′sis). Blackening of the lung tissue from the inhalation of coal dust or other black particles. SEE ALSO anthracosis. SYN pneumonomelanosis. [G. *pneumōn*, lung, + *melanosis*, a becoming black]

pneu·mo·my·co·sis (noo′mō-mī-kō′sis). Obsolete term denoting any disease of the lungs caused by the presence of fungi. [G. *pneumōn*, lung, + *mykēs*, fungus]

pneu·mo·my·e·log·ra·phy (noo′mō-mī′ĕ-log′ră-fē). Rarely used radiographic examination of spinal canal after injection of air or gas into the subarachnoid space. [G. *pneuma*, air, + *myelos*, marrow, + *graphō*, to write]

△**pneumon-.** SEE pneumo-.

pneu·mo·nec·to·my (noo′mō-nek′tō-mē). Removal of an entire lung. SYN pulmonectomy. [G. *pneumōn*, lung, + *ektomē*, excision]

pneu·mo·nia (noo-mō′nē-ă). Inflammation of the lung parenchyma characterized by consolidation of the affected part, the alveolar air spaces being filled with exudate, inflammatory cells, and fibrin. Most cases are due to infection by bacteria or viruses, a few to inhalation of chemicals or trauma to the chest wall, and a small minority to rickettsiae, fungi, and yeasts. Distribution may be lobar, segmental, or lobular; when lobular and in associated with bronchitis, it is termed bronchopneumonia. SEE ALSO pneumonitis. [G. fr. *pneumōn*, lung, + *-ia*, condition]

acute interstitial p., a severe and usually fatal form of p. occurring primarily in infants; usually considered a form of hypersensitivity *pneumonitis*.

alcoholic p., p. occurring in patient with alcoholism, usually after a period of intoxication with stupor, resulting in aspiration.

anaerobic p., p. caused by bacteria usually originating in the mouth, especially in the presence of periodontal disease; cavitation common.

apex p., apical p., p. of the apex or apices.

aspiration p., bronchopneumonia resulting from the inhalation of foreign material, usually food particles or vomit, into the bronchi; p. developing secondary to the presence in the airways of fluid, blood, saliva, or gastric contents. SYN deglutition p.

atypical p., p. caused by a nonbacterial pathogen, classically caused by *Mycoplasma pneumoniae*, but generally used to refer to any nonbacterial p. with mild systemic symptoms, including viral. SEE primary atypical p.

bacterial p., infection of the lung with any of a large variety of bacteria, especially *Streptococcus pneumoniae* (pneumococcus).

bilious p., p. following aspiration of gastric contents containing bile.

bronchial p., SYN bronchopneumonia.

caseous p., a form of severe pulmonary tuberculosis in which tubercles are not prominent, but with a diffuse extensive cellular infiltration that undergoes caseation affecting large areas of lung.

central p., a form of p. in which exudation is confined for a time to the central portion of a lobe or the hilar region. SYN core p.

chemical p., p. caused by inhalation of toxic gas, such as the war gases phosgene or chlorine; exudation into alveoli causes the lungs to be edematous and hemorrhagic; large amounts of fluid that fill the air passages block gaseous exchange; recovery occurs, permanent damage of the lungs remains, and recurrent pulmonary infections are common.

chronic p., vague or indefinite term for long-standing inflammation of pulmonary tissue of any etiology.

chronic eosinophilic p., a disease characterized by night sweats, exertional dyspnea, occasional wheezing, and peripheral eosinophilia. X-rays show peripheral, nonsegmental pulmonary infiltrates that can be nodular with cavitation. Responds to treatment with corticosteroids. SYN Carrington disease.

community-acquired p., p. caused by any organism found regularly outside the hospital; common organisms include *Streptoccum pneumoniae, Haemophilus influenza, Mycoplasma*, as opposed to hospital-acquired or nosocomial p.

congenital p., p. in the newborn, infection being contracted prenatally.

core p., SYN central p.

deglutition p., SYN aspiration p.

desquamative p., relatively rare form of p. with homogeneous filling of alveolar air spaces with macrophages and a few type II epithelial lining cells, some alveolar septal infiltration with inflammatory and connective tissue cells; usually idiopathic, but some cases have been reported in association with drugs or underlying systemic connective tissue disease; rarely progresses to end-stage lung disease.

desquamative interstitial p. (D.I.P.), diffuse proliferation of alveolar epithelial cells, which desquamate into the air sacs and become filled with macrophages, accompanied by interstitial cellular infiltration and fibrosis; gradual onset of dyspnea and nonproductive cough occurs.

p. dis′secans, SYN p. interlobularis purulenta.

double p., lobar p. involving both lungs.

embolic p., infarction following embolization of a pulmonary artery or arteries.

eosinophilic p., SYN Loeffler *syndrome* I. SYN eosinophilic pneumonopathy.

fibrous p., a process affecting pulmonary tissue and leading to deposition of collagen, either interstitially or in alveolar sacs.

Friedländer p., a form of p. caused by infection with *Klebsiella pneumoniae* (Friedländer bacillus), characteristically severe and lobar in distribution.

Friedländer bacillus p., p. caused by *Klebsiella pneumoniae*, the Friedländer bacillus.

gangrenous p., gangrene of the lungs.

giant cell p., a rare complication of measles, with the postmortem finding of multinucleated giant cells lining alveoli. SYN Hecht p., interstitial p.

Hecht p., SYN giant cell p.

hospital-acquired p., p. in a patient in a hospital, or hospital-like setting, such as a rehabilitation facility. Often caused by Gram-negative or staphylococcal organisms. SYN nosocomial p.

hypostatic p., p. resulting from infection developing in the dependent portions of the lungs due to decreased ventilation of those areas, with resulting failure to drain bronchial secretions; occurs primarily in the aged or those debilitated by disease who lie in the same position for long periods.

influenza p., p. complicating influenza.

influenzal virus p., serious, often fatal form of p. caused by a virus of the influenzal type; occurs in epidemics and pandemics.

p. interlobula′ris purulen′ta, p. in which the lobules of the lung are separated by collections of purulent exudate. SYN p. dissecans.

interstitial p., SYN giant cell p.

interstitial plasma cell p., SYN *Pneumocystis carinii* p.

intrauterine p., fetal p. contracted *in utero* and manifesting itself in the early neonatal period.

lipid p., lipoid p., pulmonary condition marked by inflammatory and fibrotic changes in the lungs due to the inhalation of various oily or fatty substances, particularly liquid petrolatum, or resulting from accumulation in the lungs of endogenous lipid material, either cholesterol from obstructive pneumonitis or following fracture of a bone; phagocytes containing lipid are usually present. SYN oil p.

lobar p., p. affecting one or more lobes, or part of a lobe, of the lung in which the consolidation is virtually homogeneous; often due to infection by *Streptococcus pneumoniae;* sputum is scanty and usually of a rusty tint from altered blood.

lymphocytic interstitial p. (LIP), SYN lymphocytic interstitial *pneumonitis.*

lymphoid interstitial p. (LIP), SYN lymphocytic interstitial *pneumonitis.*

p. malleosa (ma-lē′ō-să), p. associated with glanders.

metastatic p., a purulent inflammation in the lungs due to infected emboli.

migratory p., a form of p. in which successive areas of the lung are affected; may occur in bronchopulmonary aspergillosis. SYN wandering p.

nosocomial p., SYN hospital-acquired p.

obstructive p., infection of lung resulting from obstruction of

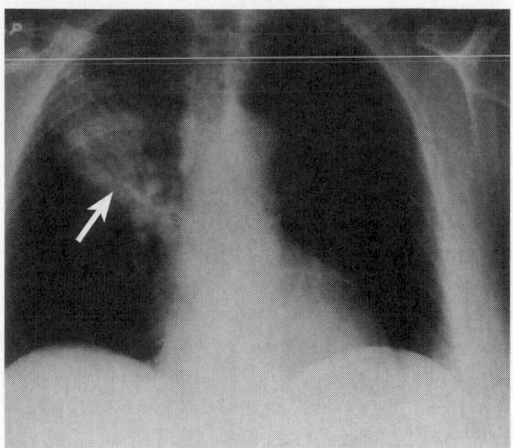

lobar pneumonia: chest radiograph showing pulmonary infiltrates (arrow) in upper lobe of right lung

airway, by narrowing resulting from previous disease process, persistent bronchospasm, or thick secretions or by aspiration of a foreign body.

oil p., SYN lipid p.

Pittsburgh p., a variant of Legionnaires disease caused by *Legionella micdadei.*

plague p., SYN pneumonic *plague.*

pleuritic p., p. associated with inflammation of the overlying pleura. SYN pneumonopleuritis.

***Pneumocystis carinii* p. (PCP),** pneumonia resulting from infection with *Pneumocystis carinii,* frequently seen in the immunologically compromised, such as persons with AIDS, or steroid-treated individuals, the elderly, or premature or debilitated babies during their first 3 months. In AIDS patients the tissue damage is usually restricted to the pulmonary parenchyma, whereas in the infantile form of the disease the alveoli are filled with a honeycomb-like or foamy network of acidophilic material, apparently not fibrin and not stainable with silver, within which the organisms, individually or in aggregates, are enmeshed; throughout the alveolar walls and pulmonary septa there is a diffuse infiltration of mononuclear inflammatory cells, chiefly plasma cells and macrophages, as well as a few lymphocytes. Patients may be only slightly febrile (or even afebrile), but are likely to be extremely weak, dyspneic, and cyanotic. This is a major cause of morbidity among patients with AIDS. SYN interstitial plasma cell p., pneumocystosis.

postobstructive p., p. occurring distally to a bronchial obstruction.

primary atypical p., an older term referring to an acute systemic disease with involvement of the lungs, usually caused by *Mycoplasma pneumoniae* and marked by fever, cough, relatively few physical signs, and scattered densities on x-rays; usually associated with development of cold agglutinins and antibodies to the infectious agent.

purulent p., p. caused by an organism that produces pus, implying that there can be destruction of lung tissue with permanent changes; usually sputum contains pus. *Staphylococci,* hemolytic *streptococci,* under *streptococcus,* and Friedländer *bacillus* are typical causes, as opposed to *Streptococcus pneumoniae,* which is rarely a cause of purulent p.

rheumatic p., p. rarely occurring in severe acute rheumatic fever, even when the disease was common; consolidation occurs, the lungs being of a rubbery consistency, with fibrin exudate and small hemorrhages, as well as edema from left ventrical failure.

septic p., SYN suppurative p.

staphylococcal p., p., usually caused by *Staphylococcus aureus,* usually commencing as a bronchopneumonia, and frequently leading to suppuration and destruction of lung tissue.

streptococcal p., p. due to *Streptococcus pyogenes.*

suppurative p., any p. associated with the formation of pus and destruction of pulmonary tissue; abscess formation may occur. SYN septic p.

terminal p., p. occurring in the course of some other disease near its fatal termination.

tularemic p., tularemia with pulmonary lesions.

typhoid p., p. complicating typhoid fever.

unresolved p., p. in which the alveolar exudate persists and eventually undergoes fibrosis.

uremic p., (1) SYN uremic *lung;* **(2)** terminal infective p. occurring in a patient with uremia.

usual interstitial p. of Liebow (UIP), a progressive inflammatory condition starting with diffuse alveolar damage and resulting in fibrosis and honeycombing over a variable time period; also a common feature of collagen-vascular diseases.

wandering p., SYN migratory p.

woolsorter's p., SYN pulmonary *anthrax.*

pneu·mon·ic (noo-mon'ik). **1.** SYN pulmonary. **2.** Relating to pneumonia.

pneu·mo·ni·tis (noo-mō-nī'tis). Inflammation of the lungs. SEE ALSO pneumonia. SYN pulmonitis. [G. *pneumōn,* lung, + *-itis,* inflammation]

acute interstitial p., usually considered a form of hypersensitivity p.

hypersensitivity p., chronic progressive form of pneumonia with wheezing, dyspnea, diffuse infiltrates seen on radiographs; occurs following exposure to any of a variety of antigens, sometimes occupational, and many names are given to cases with known types of exposure (such as farmer's lung, maple bark stripper's lung, chicken plucker's lung, bagassosis, byssinosis, and humidifier lung); biopsy findings usually show patchy infiltration of alveolar walls with lymphocytes, plasma cells, and other inflammatory cells; can progress to irreversible interstitial fibrotic disease with restrictive pattern on pulmonary function, but in early disease most manifestations are reversible if offending antigen is identified and removed from environment.

lymphocytic interstitial p., a rare disease characterized by interstitial accumulation of lymphocytes in the lungs and late fibrosis; usually a result of a lymphoma, occasionally seen in AIDS, especially in children; sometimes seen as an autoimmune disorder. SYN lymphocytic interstitial pneumonia, lymphoid interstitial pneumonia.

radiation p., the interstitial pneumonia and fibrosis that follow pulmonary irradiation at radiotherapeutic doses.

uremic p., SYN uremic *lung.*

⌂**pneumono-.** SEE pneumo-.

pneu·mo·no·cele (noo-mōn'ō-sēl). Protrusion of a portion of the lung through a defect in the chest wall. SYN pleurocele, pneumatocele (2), pneumocele.

pneu·mo·no·cen·te·sis (noo'mō-nō-sen-tē'sis). Rarely used term for paracentesis of the lung. SYN pneumocentesis. [G. *pneumōn,* lung, + *kentēsis,* puncture]

pneu·mo·no·coc·cal (noo'mō-nō-kok'ăl). Relating to or associated with *Streptococcus pneumoniae.*

pneu·mo·no·coc·cus (noo'mō-nō-kok'ŭs). SYN *Streptococcus pneumoniae.*

pneu·mo·no·co·ni·o·sis, pneu·mo·no·ko·ni·o·sis (noo'mō-nō-kō-nē-ō'sis). SYN pneumoconiosis.

pneu·mo·no·cyte (noo'mō-nō-sīt). Nonspecific term referring to cells lining alveoli in the respiratory part of the lung. [G. *pneumōn,* lung, + *kytos,* cell]

granular p.'s, SYN great alveolar *cells,* under *cell.*

phagocytic p., an alveolar phagocyte containing hemosiderin, carbon, or other foreign particles.

pneu·mo·no·ko·ni·o·sis. SEE pneumonoconiosis.

pneu·mo·no·mel·a·no·sis (noo'mō-nō-mel-ă-nō'sis). SYN pneumomelanosis.

pneu·mo·nop·a·thy (noo'mō-nop'ă-thē). Disease of the lung.

eosinophilic p., SYN eosinophilic *pneumonia.*

pneu·mo·no·pexy (noo'mō-nō-pek-sē). Fixation of the lung by suturing the parietal and visceral pleurae or otherwise causing adhesion of the two layers. SYN pneumopexy. [G. *pneumōn*, lung, + *pēxis*, fixation]

pneu·mo·no·pleur·i·tis (noo′mō′nō-ploo-rī′tis). SYN pleuritic *pneumonia*.

pneu·mo·nor·rha·phy (noo-mō-nōr′ă-fē). Suture of the lung. [G. *pneumōn*, lung, + *rhaphē*, suture]

pneu·mo·not·o·my (noo-mō-not′ō-mē). Incision of the lung. SYN pneumotomy. [G. *pneumōn*, lung, + *tomē*, incision]

pneu·mo·or·bi·tog·ra·phy (noo′mō-ōr′bi-tog′ră-fē). Radiographic visualization of the orbital contents following injection of a gas, usually air.

pneu·mo·per·i·car·di·um (noo′mō-per-i-kar′dē-ŭm). Presence of gas (usually air) in the pericardial sac. [G. *pneuma*, air, + pericardium]

tension p., the presence of air under pressure in the pericardial space, with the potential for cardiac tamponade.

pneu·mo·per·i·to·ne·um (noo′mō-per-i-tō-nē′ŭm). Presence of air or gas in the peritoneal cavity as a result of disease, or produced artificially in the abdomen to achieve exposure during laporoscopic surgery. [G. *pneuma*, air, + peritoneum]

pneu·mo·per·i·to·ni·tis (noo′mō-per-i-tō-nī′tis). Inflammation of the peritoneum with an accumulation of gas in the peritoneal cavity. [G. *pneuma*, air, + peritonitis]

pneu·mo·pexy (noo′mō-pek-sē). SYN pneumonopexy.

pneu·mo·pha·gia (noo-mō-fā′jē-ă). SYN aerophagia.

pneu·mo·pleu·ri·tis (noo′mō-ploo-rī′tis). Pleurisy with air or gas in the pleural cavity. [G. *pneuma*, air, + pleur- + -*itis*, inflammation]

pneu·mo·py·e·log·ra·phy (noo′mō-pī-ĕ-log′ră-fē). Radiography of the kidney after air or gas has been injected into the renal pelvis. [G. *pneuma*, air, + *pyelos*, pelvis, + *graphō*, to write]

pneu·mo·ra·di·og·ra·phy (nu′mo-ra-dĭ-og′ră-fī). SYN pneumography (2).

pneu·mo·re·sec·tion (noo′mō-rē-sek′shŭn). Excision of part of a lung. [G. *pneumōn*, lung, + resection]

pneu·mo·ret·ro·per·i·to·ne·um (noo′mō-ret′rō-per-i-tō-nē′ŭm). Pathologic presence of air in the retroperitoneal tissues.

pneu·mo·roent·gen·og·ra·phy (noo′mō-rent′gĕ-nog′ră-fē). SYN pneumography (2).

pneu·mor·rha·chis (noo-mō-rā′kis, noo-mōr′ă-kis). The presence of gas in the spinal canal. SYN pneumatorrhachis. [G. *pneuma*, air, + *rhachis*, spinal column]

pneu·mo·scope (noo′mō-skōp). SYN pneumatoscope.

pneu·mo·ser·o·thor·ax (noo′mō-sēr-ō-thōr′aks). SYN hydro-pneumothorax.

pneu·mo·sil·i·co·sis (noo′mō-sil′i-kō′sis). SYN silicosis.

pneu·mo·tach·o·gram (noo-mō-tak′ō-gram). A recording of respired gas flow as a function of time, produced by a pneumotachograph. [G. *pneuma*, air, + *tachys*, swift, + *gramma*, something written]

pneu·mo·tach·o·graph (noo-mō-tak′ō-graf). An instrument for measuring the instantaneous flow of respiratory gases. SYN pneumotachometer.

Fleisch p., a p. that measures flow in terms of the proportional pressure drop across a resistance consisting of numerous capillary tubes in parallel.

Silverman-Lilly p., a p. that measures flow in terms of the proportional pressure drop across a resistance consisting of a very fine mesh screen.

pneu·mo·ta·chom·e·ter (noo′mō-tă-kom′ĕ-ter). SYN pneumotachograph. [G. *pneuma*, air, + *tachys*, swift, + *metron*, measure]

pneu·mo·ther·mo·mas·sage (noo-mō-ther′mō-mă-sahzh′). Application to the body of hot air under varying degrees of pressure. [G. *pneuma*, air, + *thermē*, heat, + Fr. *massage*]

▯ pneu·mo·thor·ax (noo-mō-thōr′aks). The presence of free air or gas in the pleural cavity. [G. *pneuma*, air, + *thorax*]

artificial p., p. produced by the injection of air, or a more slowly absorbed gas such as nitrogen, into the pleural space; formerly used for collapse therapy of tuberculosis. SYN therapeutic p.

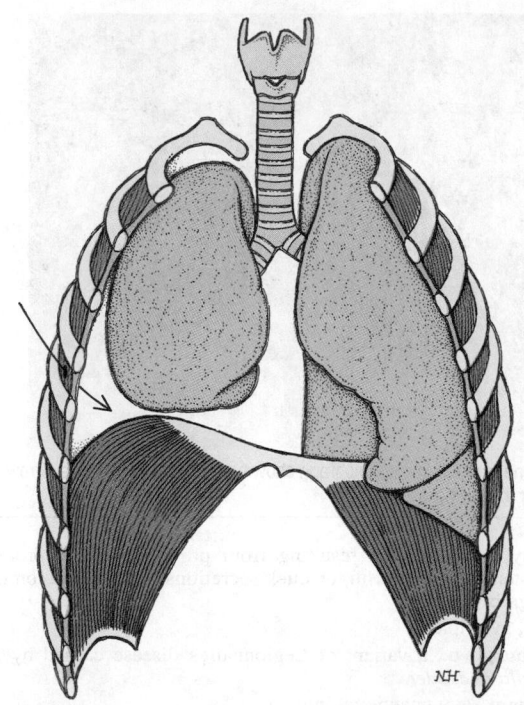

pneumothorax: caused by penetrating wound of chest wall

catamenial p., p. occurring in young women during menstruation, usually on the right side.

extrapleural p., the presence of a gas between the endothoracic fascia-pleural layer and the adjacent chest wall.

iatrogenic p., p. caused by a medical procedure, most often central venous *catheter* insertion, thoracentesis, or transbronchial and transthoracic lung biopsy.

open p., a free communication between the atmosphere and the pleural space either via the lung or through the chest wall. SYN sucking chest wound.

pressure p., SYN tension p.

p. sim′plex, p., without known cause, in an otherwise healthy person.

spontaneous p., p. occurring without iatrogenic or other trauma; primary spontaneous p. generally occurs in young people with apical blebs but otherwise normal lungs; secondary spontaneous p. occurs in people with underlying lung disease, most commonly chronic obstructive pulmonary disease and, less often, interstitial lung disease, pneumonia, lung abscess, and lung tumors.

tension p., a p. in which air enters the pleural cavity and is trapped during expiration; intrathoracic pressure builds to levels higher than atmospheric pressure, compresses the lung, and may displace the mediastinum and its structures toward the opposite side, with consequent cardiopulmonary impairment. SYN pressure p.

therapeutic p., SYN artificial p.

traumatic p., p. caused by blunt or penetrating chest injury.

pneu·mot·o·my (noo-mot′ō-mē). SYN pneumonotomy.

pneu·mo·ven·tri·cle (noo-mō-ven′tri-kl). Air in the ventricular system of the brain; occurs as a complication of a fracture of the skull that passes through the accessory nasal sinuses.

Pneu·mo·vi·rus (noo′mō-vī′rŭs). A genus of viruses (family Paramyxoviridae) including respiratory syncytial virus, which causes severe lower respiratory tract disease in infants. Nucleocapsids are 13–15 nm in diameter and thus intermediate in size between other Paramyxoviridae and the Orthomyxoviridae; cytoplasmic inclusions are considerably more dense than those of other viruses in the family.

pneu·sis (noo'sis). SYN breathing. [G. *pneō*, to breathe]

pni·go·pho·bia (nī-gō-fō'bē-ă). Morbid fear of choking. [G. *pnigos*, choking, + *phobos*, fear]

PNMT Abbreviation for phenylethanolamine *N*-methyltransferase.

PNP Abbreviation for psychogenic nocturnal *polydipsia*.

PNPB Abbreviation for positive-negative pressure *breathing*.

PO Abbreviation for per os.

Po Symbol for polonium.

pock (pok). The specific pustular cutaneous lesion of smallpox. [A.S. *poc*, a pustule]

pock·et (pok'et). **1.** A cul-de-sac or pouchlike cavity. **2.** A diseased gingival attachment; a space between the inflamed gum and the surface of a tooth, limited apically by an epithelial attachment. **3.** To enclose within a confined space, as the stump of the pedicle of an ovarian or other abdominal tumor between the lips of the external wound. **4.** A collection of pus in a nearly closed sac. **5.** To approach the surface at a localized spot, as with the thinned-out wall of an abscess that is about to rupture. [Fr. *pochette*]

gingival p., a diseased gingival attachment in which the increased depth of the sulcus is due to an increase in the bulk of its gingival wall.

infrabony p., intrabony p., SYN subcrestal p.

periodontal p., a pathologic deepening of the gingival sulcus resulting from detachment of the gingiva from the tooth.

Rathke p., SYN pituitary *diverticulum*.

retraction p.'s, small areas of retraction of the tympanic membrane due to chronic negative pressure in the middle ear that can lead to formation of cholesteatoma.

rheumatoid p., SYN susceptibility *cassette*.

Seessel p., the part of the embryonic foregut extending cephalad to the level of the oral plate and caudal to the pituitary diverticulum (Rathke pouch). SYN preoral gut.

subcrestal p., a p. extending apically below the level of the adjacent alveolar crest. SYN infrabony p., intrabony p.

Tröltsch p.'s, SYN anterior *recess* of tympanic membrane, posterior *recess* of tympanic membrane.

pock·mark (pok'mark). The small depressed scar left after the healing of the smallpox pustule.

po·cu·lum (pok'ū-lŭm). SYN cup (1). [L.]

p. diog'enis, SYN *cup* of palm.

△**pod-, podo-.** Foot, foot-shaped. Cf. ped-. [G. *pous, podos*]

po·dag·ra (pō-dag'ră). Severe pain in the foot, especially that of typical gout in the great toe. [G. fr. *pous*, foot, + *agra*, a seizure]

po·dag·ral, po·dag·ric, po·dag·rous (pod'ă-grăl, pō-dag'rik, pod'ă-grŭs). Relating to or characterized by podagra.

po·dal·gia (pō-dal'jē-ă). Pain in the foot. SYN pododynia, tarsalgia. [pod- + G. *algos*, pain]

po·dal·ic (pō-dal'ik). Relating to the foot. [G. *pous* (*pod-*), foot]

pod·ar·thri·tis (pod-ar-thrī'tis). Inflammation of any of the tarsal or metatarsal joints. [pod- + arthritis]

pod·e·de·ma (pod-e-dē'mă). Edema of the feet and ankles.

po·di·a·tric (pō-dī'ă-trik). Relating to podiatry.

po·di·a·trist (pō-dī'ă-trist). A practitioner of podiatry. SYN chiropodist, podologist. [pod- + G. *iatros*, physician]

po·di·a·try (pō-dī'ă-trē). The specialty concerned with the diagnosis and/or medical, surgical, mechanical, physical, and adjunctive treatment of the diseases, injuries, and defects of the human foot. SYN chiropody, podiatric medicine, podology. [pod- + G. *iatreia*, medical treatment]

po·dis·mus (pō-diz'mŭs). SYN podospasm.

po·di·tis (pō-dī'tis). An inflammatory disorder of the foot. [pod- + G. *-itis*, inflammation]

tourniquet p., postischemic acute inflammatory edema in the foot (or paw), as the result of complete obstruction of the circulation to that member by use of a tourniquet; produced experimentally in animals as a means of evaluating the anti-inflammatory efficacy of drugs.

△**podo-.** SEE pod-.

pod·o·bro·mi·dro·sis (pod'ō-brō-mi-drō'sis). Foul-smelling perspiration of the feet. [podo- + G. *brōmos*, a foul smell, + *hidrōs*, sweat]

pod·o·cyte (pod'ō-sīt). An epithelial cell of the visceral layer of Bowman capsule in the renal corpuscle, attached to the outer surface of the glomerular capillary basement membrane by cytoplasmic foot processes (pedicels); believed to play a role in the ultrafiltration of blood. [podo- + G. *kytos*, a hollow (cell)]

pod·o·dy·na·mom·e·ter (pod'ō-dī'nă-mom'ĕ-ter). An instrument for measuring the strength of the muscles of the foot or leg. [podo- + G. *dynamis*, force, + *metron*, measure]

pod·o·dyn·ia (pod-ō-din'ē-ă). SYN podalgia. [podo- + G. *odynē*, pain]

podofilox (pō-dof'il-oks). An antimitotic agent derived from species of *Juniperus* and *Podophyllum;* used to treat external genital and perianal warts.

pod·o·gram (pod'ō-gram). An imprint of the sole of the foot, showing the contour and the condition of the arch, or an outline tracing. [podo- + G. *gramma*, written]

pod·o·graph (pod'ō-graf). A device for taking an outline at the foot and an imprint of the sole. [podo- + G. *graphō*, to write]

pod·o·lite (pod'ō-līt). SYN dahllite.

po·dol·o·gist (pō-dol'ō-jist). SYN podiatrist.

po·dol·o·gy (pō-dol'ō-jē). SYN podiatry. [podo- + G. *logos*, study]

pod·o·mech·a·no·ther·a·py (pod-ō-mek'ă-nō-thār'ă-pē). Treatment of foot conditions with mechanical devices; e.g., arch supports, orthoses.

po·dom·e·ter (pō-dom'ĕ-ter). SYN pedometer. [podo- + G. *metron*, measure]

pod·o·phyl·lin (pod-ō-fil'in). SYN podophyllum *resin*.

pod·o·phyl·lo·tox·in (pod'ō-fil-ō-tok'sin). A toxic polycyclic substance, $C_{22}H_{22}O_8$, with cathartic properties present in podophyllum; has antineoplastic action.

pod·o·phyl·lum (pod-ō-fil'ŭm). The rhizome of *Podophyllum peltatum* (family Berberidaceae), used as a powerful laxative. SYN May apple, vegetable calomel.

Indian p., the dried rhizome and roots of *P. emodi*, a Himalayan plant; a cholagogue and cathartic.

pod·o·spasm, pod·o·spas·mus (pod'ō-spazm, -spaz-mŭs). Spasm of the foot. SYN podismus. [podo- + G. *spasmos*, spasm]

Po·do·vir·i·dae (po-dō-vir'i-dē). Name for a family of bacterial viruses with short tails and genomes of double-stranded DNA (MW $12–73 \times 10^6$); heads may be isometric or elongated. The family includes the T-7 phage group and probably other genera.

POEMS Acronym for *p*olyneuropathy, *o*rganomegaly, *e*ndocrinopathy, *m*onoclonal gammopathy, and *s*kin changes. SEE POEMS *syndrome*. SYN Crow-Fukase syndrome.

po·go·ni·a·sis (pō-gō-nī'ă-sis). A rarely used term for the growth of a beard on a woman, or excessive hairiness of the face in men. SEE ALSO hirsutism. [G. *pōgōn*, beard, + *-iasis*, condition]

po·go·ni·on (pō-gō'ni-on). In craniometry, the most anterior point on the mandible in the midline; the most anterior, prominent point on the chin. SYN mental point. [G. dim. of *pōgōn*, beard]

Po·go·no·myr·mex (pō-gō'nō-mir'meks, -mer'meks). A genus of ants that attack humans and small animals. SYN harvester ant. [G. *pōgōn*, beard, + *myrmex*, ant]

pOH. The negative decadic logarithm of the OH⁻ concentration (in moles per liter).

△**-poiesis.** Production; producing. [G. *poiēsis*, a making]

poi·e·tin. Suffix used with words to indicate an agent with a stimulatory effect on growth or multiplication of cells, such as erythropoietin, and others. [G. *poietēs*, maker, + *-in*]

△**poikilo-.** Irregular, varied. [G. *poikilos*, many colored, varied]

poi·ki·lo·blast (poy'ki-lō-blast). A nucleated red blood cell of irregular shape. [poikilo- + G. *blastos*, germ]

poi·ki·lo·cyte (poy'ki-lō-sīt). A red blood cell of irregular shape. [poikilo- + G. *kytos*, cell]

poi·ki·lo·cy·the·mia (poy'ki-lō-sī-thē'mē-ă). SYN poikilocytosis. [poikilocyte + G. *haima*, blood]

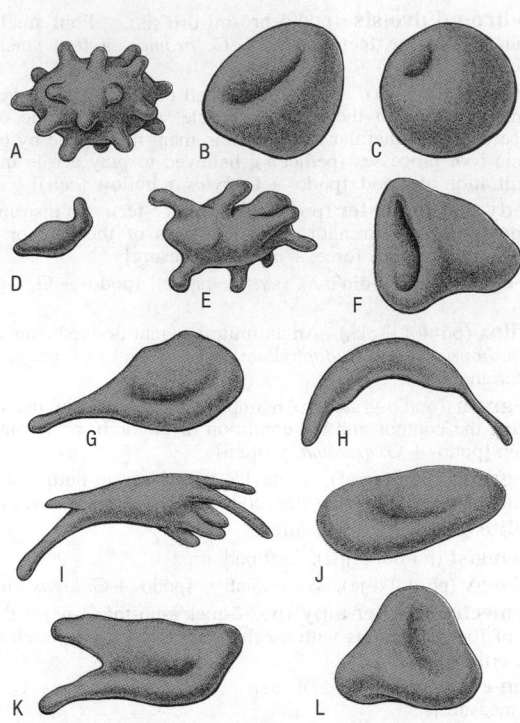

poikilocytes: (A) echinocyte, (B) stomatocyte, (C) spherocyte, (D) schistocyte, (E) acanthocyte, (F) codocyte (target cell), G) dacryocyte (teardrop), (H) drepanocyte (sickle cell), (I) drepanocyte (holly leaf), (J) elliptocyte, (K) keratocyte (helmet cell), (L) knizocyte

poi·ki·lo·cy·to·sis (poy′ki-lō-sī-tō′sis). The presence of poikilocytes in the peripheral blood. SYN poikilocythemia. [poikilocyte + G. -osis, condition]

poi·ki·lo·den·to·sis (poy′ki-lō-den-tō′sis). Hypoplastic defects or mottling of enamel due to excessive fluoride in the water supply. [poikilo- + L. dens, tooth, + G. -osis, condition]

poi·ki·lo·der·ma (poy′ki-lō-der′mǎ). A variegated hyperpigmentation and telangiectasia of the skin, followed by atrophy. [poikilo- + G. derma, skin]

p. atroph′icans and cataract, SYN Rothmund syndrome.

p. atroph′icans vascula′re, a rare condition that simulates chronic radiodermatitis in appearance; may eventuate as mycosis fungoides. SYN parapsoriasis lichenoides.

p. of Civatte, reticulated pigmentation and telangiectasia of the sides of the cheeks and neck; common in middle-aged women.

p. congenita′le, SYN Rothmund syndrome.

poi·ki·lo·therm (poy′ki-lō-therm). A poikilothermic animal. SYN allotherm, cold-blooded animal.

poi·ki·lo·ther·mic, poi·ki·lo·ther·mal, poi·ki·lo·ther·mous (poy′ki-lō-ther′mic, -măl, -mŭs). **1.** Varying in temperature according to the temperature of the surrounding medium; denoting the so-called cold-blooded animals, such as the reptiles and amphibians, and the plants. **2.** Capable of existence and growth in media of varying temperatures. Cf. heterothermic, homeothermic. **3.** Causing a disruption of normal hypothalamic thermoregulatory function, as seen with drugs such as phenothiazines. SYN cold-blooded, hematocryal. [poikilo- + G. thermē, heat]

poi·ki·lo·ther·my, poi·ki·lo·ther·mism (poy′ki-lō-ther′mē, -therm′izm). The condition of plants and cold-blooded animals, the temperature of which varies with the changes in the temperature of the surrounding medium. [poikilo- + G. thermē, heat]

poi·ki·lo·throm·bo·cyte (poy′ki-lō-throm′bō-sīt). A blood platelet of abnormal shape. [poikilo- + G. thrombos, clot, + kytos, cell]

poi·ki·lo·thy·mia (poy′ki-lō-thī′mē-ǎ). A rarely used term for a mental state marked by abnormal variations in mood. [poikilo- + G. thymos, mind]

POINT

point (poynt). **1.** SYN punctum. **2.** A sharp end or apex. **3.** A slight projection. **4.** A stage or condition reached, as the boiling p. **5.** To become ready to open, said of an abscess or boil the wall of which is becoming thin and about to rupture. **6.** In mathematics, a dimensionless geometric element. **7.** A location or position on a graph, plot, or diagram. **8.** Decimal point. [Fr.; L. punctum, fr. pungo, pp. punctus, to pierce]

p. A, SYN subspinale.

absorbent p.'s, cones of paper or paper products used for drying or maintaining medicaments during root canal therapy.

alveolar p., SYN prosthion.

anterior focal p., the p. where parallel rays from the retina are focused.

apophysary p., apophysial p., (1) SYN subnasal p; **(2)** SYN Trousseau p.

auricular p., SYN auriculare.

axial p., SYN nodal p.

p. B, SYN supramentale.

boiling p. (b.p.), the temperature at which the vapor pressure of a liquid equals the ambient atmospheric pressure.

Cannon p., the location in the mid–transverse colon at which innervation by superior and inferior mesenteric plexuses overlaps at the junction of the primitive midgut and hindgut, frequently resulting in narrowing evident on barium enema. SEE Cannon ring. SYN Cannon ring.

Capuron p.'s, the iliopubic eminences and the sacroiliac joints, constituting four fixed p.'s in the pelvic inlet.

cardinal p.'s, (1) the four p.'s in the pelvic inlet toward one of which the occiput of the baby is usually directed in case of head presentation: two sacroiliac articulations and the two iliopectineal eminences corresponding to the acetabula; **(2)** six p.'s of a compound optical system: the anterior focal p., the posterior focal p., the two principal p.'s, and the two nodal p.'s.

central-bearing p., the contact p. of a central-bearing device.

Clado p., a p. at the junction of the interspinous and right semilunar lines, at the lateral border of the rectus abdominis muscle, where marked tenderness on pressure is felt in some cases of appendicitis.

clinical end p., traditional medical measures of a diagnostic or therapeutic impact that may or may not be perceived by the patient.

cold-rigor p., the degree of lowered temperature at which the activity of a cell ceases and the cell passes into the narcotic or hibernating state.

congruent p.'s, the p. in each retina referred to the same external stimulus.

conjugate p., a p. so related to another that an object at one is imaged at the other.

contact p., SYN contact area.

p.'s of convergence, SEE convergence.

craniometric p.'s, fixed p.'s on the skull used as landmarks in craniometry.

critical p., a p. at which two phases become identical; thus, at a given critical temperature and critical pressure, the liquid and gaseous state of a particular substance can no longer be differentiated.

dew p., the temperature at and below which moisture will condense for a specific humidity.

p. of elbow, SYN olecranon.

end p., the completion of a reaction; usually evident by the first perceptible alteration of the color of an added indicator.

equivalence p., SYN equivalence zone.

far p., that p. in conjugate focus with the retina when the eye is not accommodating. SYN punctum remotum.

p. of fixation, the p. on the retina at which the rays coming from an object regarded directly are focused. SYN p. of regard.

flash p., the lowest temperature at which vapors of a liquid may be ignited by a flame.

focal p., SEE anterior focal p., posterior focal p.

freezing p., the temperature at which a liquid solidifies.

fusing p., SEE fusion *temperature* (wire method).

Guéneau de Mussy p., a p., painful on pressure, at the junction of a line prolonging the left border of the sternum and a horizontal line at the level of end of the bony portion of the tenth rib; it is present in cases of diaphragmatic pleurisy.

gutta-percha p.'s, cones of a gutta percha compound used for filling root canals in conjunction with a cement, paste, or plastic.

Hallé p., a p. at the intersection of a horizontal line touching the anterior superior spine of the ilium and a perpendicular line drawn from the spine of the pubis; here the ureter can be most readily palpated.

heat-rigor p., the degree of elevated temperature at which coagulation of protoplasm occurs with death of the cell.

incident p., the p. at which a light ray enters an optical system.

incisal p., the p. located between the incisal edges of the lower central incisors; the graphic projection of the excursions of the incisal p. in certain planes is generally used to illustrate the envelope of motion of mandibular movement.

isoelectric p. (p*I***, IEP, I.P., i.p.),** the pH at which an amphoteric substance, such as protein or an amino acid, is electrically neutral.

isoionic p., the pH at which a zwitterion has an equal number of positive and negative charges; in water and in the absence of other solutes, this is the isoelectric p.

isosbestic p., in applied spectroscopy, a wavelength at which absorbance of two substances, one of which can be converted into the other, is the same.

J p., the p. marking the end of the QRS complex and the beginning of the S or T wave in the electrocardiogram. SYN ST junction.

jugal p., SYN jugale.

lower alveolar p., SYN infradentale.

malar p., apex of the tuberosity of the zygomatic (malar) bone.

p. of maximal impulse, the p. on the chest wall at which the maximal cardiac impulse is seen and/or felt.

maximum occipital p., the p. on the squama of the occipital bone farthest from the glabella.

Mayo-Robson p., a p. just above and to the right of the umbilicus, where tenderness on pressure exists in disease of the pancreas.

McBurney p., a p. between 1½ and 2 inches superomedial to the anterior superior spine of the ilium, on a line joining that process and the umbilicus, where pressure elicits tenderness in acute appendicitis.

median mandibular p., a p. on the anteroposterior center of the mandibular ridge in the median sagittal plane.

melting p. (m.p., T_m), (1) the temperature at which a solid becomes a liquid; **(2)** the temperature at which 50% of a macromolecule becomes denatured.

mental p., SYN pogonion.

metopic p., SYN metopion.

motor p., a p. on the skin overlying the endplates of an underlying muscle; the application of an electrical stimulus, via an electrode, will cause contraction of the muscle.

Munro p., a p. at the right edge of the rectus abdominis muscle, between the umbilicus and the anterior superior spine of the ilium, where pressure elicits tenderness in appendicitis.

nasal p., SYN nasion.

near p., that p. in conjugate focus with the retina when the eye exerts maximal accommodation. SYN punctum proximum.

neutral p., the p. at which a solution is neither acid nor alkaline (pH 7 at 22°C for aqueous solutions).

nodal p., one of two p.'s in a compound optical system so related

that a ray directed toward the first p. will appear to have passed through the second p. parallel to its original direction. SYN axial p.

occipital p., the most prominent posterior p. on the occipital bone above the inion.

p. of ossification, SYN ossification *center*.

painful p., SEE Valleix p.'s.

posterior focal p., the p. of a compound optical system where parallel rays entering the system are focused.

power p., in dentistry, the vertical dimension at which the greatest masticatory force may be registered.

preauricular p., a p. of the posterior root of the zygomatic arch lying immediately in front of the upper end of the tragus.

pressure p., a cutaneous locus having pressure-sensitive elements that, when compressed, yield a sensation of pressure.

primary p. of ossification, SYN primary ossification *center*.

principal p., one of two p.'s on an optic axis so related that an object at one is exactly imaged at the other without magnification, minification, or inversion.

p. of proximal contact, SYN contact *area*.

p. of regard, SYN p. of fixation.

retention p., a provision made within a cavity preparation of a tooth to hold in place the first pieces of gold when placing a direct gold restoration.

secondary p. of ossification, SYN secondary ossification *center*.

silver p., a solid core cone of silver used in filling root canals in conjunction with a cement or paste.

spinal p., SYN subnasal p.

subnasal p., the center of the root of the anterior nasal spine. SYN apophysary p. (1), apophysial p., spinal p.

Sudeck critical p., region in the colon between the supply of the sigmoid arteries and that of the superior rectal artery.

supra-auricular p., a craniometric p. on the posterior root of the zygomatic process of the temporal bone directly above the auricular p.

supranasal p., SYN ophryon.

supraorbital p., SYN ophryon.

sylvian p., the nearest p. on the skull to the lateral (sylvian) fissure, about 30 mm behind the zygomatic process of the frontal bone.

tender p.'s, SYN Valleix p.'s.

trigger p., a specific p. or area where stimulation by touch, pain, or pressure induces a painful response. SYN dolorogenic zone, trigger area, trigger zone.

triple p., the temperature at which all three phases (i.e., solid, liquid, and gas) are in equilibrium; the triple p. of water (273.16 K) is a fundamental fixed point in temperature scales.

Trousseau p., a painful p., in neuralgia, at the spinous process of the vertebra below which arises the offending nerve. SYN apophysary p. (2), apophysial p.

Valleix p.'s, various p.'s in the course of a nerve, pressure upon which is painful in cases of neuralgia; these p.'s are: 1) where the nerve emerges from the bony canal; 2) where it pierces a muscle or aponeurosis to reach the skin; 3) where a superficial nerve rests upon a resisting surface where compression is easily made; 4) where the nerve gives off one or more branches; and 5) where the nerve terminates in the skin. SYN tender p.'s.

Weber p., a p. situated 1 cm below the promontory of the sacrum; believed by Weber to represent the center of gravity of the body.

zygomaxillary p., SYN zygomaxillare.

---

poin·til·lage (pwan-tē-yazh′). A massage manipulation with the tips of the fingers. [Fr. dotting, stippling]

point·ing (poynt′ing). Preparing to open spontaneously, said of an abscess or a boil.

point source. In photometry, a very small source of light that is regarded as a geometric point from which light emanates in straight lines in all directions.

Poirier, Paul J., French surgeon, 1853–1907. SEE P. *gland, line.*

poise (P) (poyz, pwahz). In the CGS system, the unit of viscosity equal to 1 dyne-second per square centimeter and to 0.1 pascal-second. [J.-L. M. *Poiseuille*]

Poiseuille, Jean Léonard Marie, French physiologist and physicist, 1799–1869. SEE poise; P. viscosity *coefficient, law, space.*

poi·son (poy′zŭn). Any substance, either taken internally or applied externally, that is injurious to health or dangerous to life. [Fr., fr. L. *potio,* potion, draught]

acrid p., a p. that causes a destructive local irritation as well as systemic effects.

arrow p., (1) SYN curare; **(2)** any natural toxin used for coating arrows, spears, and darts (e.g., extracts containing aconitin, ouabain, cardiac glycosides, batrachotoxin, curare).

fish p., (1) SYN ichthyotoxicon; **(2)** SYN fugu p.

fugu p. (foo′goo), a p. in the roe and other parts of various species of *Diodon, Triodon,* and *Tetradon,* fishes of eastern Asiatic waters. SYN fish p. (2). [Jap. *fugu,* a poisonous fish]

respiratory p., SYN respiratory *inhibitor.*

poi·son·ing (poy′zŏn-ing). **1.** The administering of poison. **2.** The state of being poisoned. SYN intoxication (1).

ackee p., an acute and frequently fatal vomiting disease associated with central nervous system symptoms and marked hypoglycemia, caused by eating unripe ackee fruit of *Blighia spaida,* a tree common in Jamaica. SYN Jamaican vomiting sickness.

bacterial food p., a term commonly used to refer to conditions limited to enteritis or gastroenteritis (excluding the enteric fevers and the dysenteries) caused by bacterial multiplication per se or by a soluble bacterial exotoxin.

blood p., SEE septicemia, pyemia.

carbon disulfide p., acute or chronic intoxication by CS_2, an industrial disease encountered among rubber workers and makers of artificial silk (rayon) by the viscose process; characterized by insomnia, listlessness, and irritability, followed by paralyses, impaired vision, peptic ulcer, and psychoses.

carbon monoxide p., a potentially fatal acute or chronic intoxication caused by inhalation of carbon monoxide gas, which has an affinity 210 times that of oxygen for binding with hemoglobin (carboxyhemoglobinemia) and thus interferes with the transportation of oxygen and carbon dioxide by the blood.

crotalaria p., p. of humans and animals with alkaloids of the plants *Senecio* (ragwort), *Crotalaria* (rattlebox), and *Heliotropum;* produces a veno-occlusive disease of the liver similar to Chiari disease. SYN crotalism.

cyanide p., a fairly common disease of herbivorous animals, caused by eating cyanogenic plants containing glucosides that are hydrolyzed, yielding hydrocyanic acid; some farm chemicals, such as fungicides or insecticides, may be causes of cyanide p.; hydrogen cyanide and its salts are extremely poisonous to humans, either by inhalation or by ingestion.

Datura p., p. resulting from ingestion of plants of the genus *Datura;* symptoms are parasympatholytic in nature and in severe p. include central nervous system depression, circulatory failure, and respiratory depression.

djenkol p., p. believed to result from eating excessive amounts of a bean, *Pitecolobium lobatum;* symptoms are pain in the renal region, dysuria, and later anuria; the djenkol bean has a high vitamin B content and is used for food despite its toxic qualities.

ergot p., a syndrome brought on by the consumption of bread (notably rye) contaminated by the ergot fungus, *Claviceps purpurea* (rye smut), the source of numerous ergot alkaloids. The effects observed include peripheral vascular constriction leading to gangrene, partial paralysis with numbing, tingling, and burning in the limbs, feeble pulse, restlessness, stupor, or delirium; can prove fatal.

food p., poisoning in which the active agent is contained in ingested food.

lead p., acute or chronic intoxication by lead or any of its salts; symptoms of **acute lead p.** usually are those of acute gastroenteritis in adults or encephalopathy in children; **chronic lead p.** is manifested chiefly by anemia, constipation, colicky abdominal pain, neuropathy with paralysis with wrist-drop involving the extensor muscles of the forearm, bluish lead line of the gums, and

interstitial nephritis; saturnine gout, convulsions, and coma may occur. SYN plumbism, saturnism.

mercury p., a disease usually caused by the ingestion or inhalation of mercury or mercury compounds, which are toxic in relation to their ability to produce mercuric ions; usually **acute mercury p.** is associated with ulcerations of the mouth (including loosening of teeth), stomach, and intestine and toxic changes in the renal tubules; anuria and anemia may occur; respiratory distress and pneumonia can follow inhalation; usually **chronic mercury p.** is a result of industrial p. and causes gastrointestinal or central nervous system manifestations including stomatitis, diarrhea, headaches, ataxia, tremor, hyperreflexia, sensorineural impairment, and emotional instability and sometimes delirium (Mad Hatter syndrome). SYN hydrargyria, hydrargyrism, mercurialism.

mushroom p., SEE mycetism.

oxygen p., SYN oxygen *toxicity.*

radiation p., SYN radiation *sickness.*

Salmonella food p., gastroenteritis caused by various strains of *Salmonella* that multiply freely in the gastrointestinal tract but do not produce septicemia; symptoms usually begin within 8–24 hours and include fever, headache, nausea, vomiting, diarrhea, and abdominal pain.

scombroid p., p. from ingestion of heat-stable toxins produced by bacterial action on inadequately preserved dark-meat fish of the order Scombroidea (tuna, bonito, mackerel, albacore, skipjack); characterized by epigastric pain, nausea and vomiting, headache, thirst, difficulty in swallowing, and urticaria.

silver p., SYN argyria.

***Staphylococ′cus* food p.,** outbreaks commonly caused by staphylococcal enterotoxin and characterized by an abrupt onset of gastroenteritis within several hours after ingestion of the food contaminated with the preformed exotoxin; vomiting is usually more severe and diarrhea less severe than in infectious forms of bacterial food p.

systemic p., SYN toxicosis.

tetraethyl p., SEE tetraethyllead.

thallium p., a condition characterized by vomiting, diarrhea, leg pains, and severe sensorimotor polyneuropathy; about 3 weeks after p., temporary extensive loss of hair typically occurs; usually occurs after accidental ingestion of a rodenticide.

turpentine p., p. from oil of turpentine; symptoms include hematuria, albuminuria, and coma; the urine may have an odor of violets. SYN terebinthinism.

poi·son ivy, poi·son oak, poi·son su·mac. 1. SEE *Toxicodendron.* **2.** Common name for the cutaneous eruption (rhus dermatitis) caused by contact with these species of *Toxicodendron.*

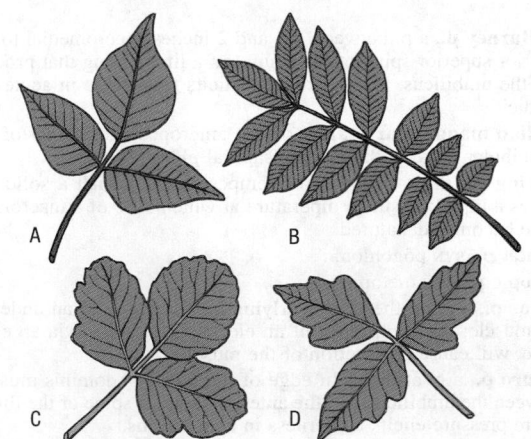

Toxicodendron: (A) poison ivy, (B) poison sumac, (C) poison oak (Western), (D) poison oak, (Eastern)

poi·son·ous (poy′zŭn-ŭs). Characterized by, having the characteristics of, or containing a poison. SYN toxic (1), toxicant (1), toxiferous, venenous.

Poisson, Siméon Denis, French mathematician, 1781–1840. SEE P. *distribution;* P.-Pearson *formula.*

po·lar (pō′lăr). **1.** Relating to a pole. **2.** Having poles, said of certain nerve cells having one or more processes. [Mod. L. *polaris,* fr. *polus,* pole]

po·lar·im·e·ter (pō′lăr-im′ĕ-ter). An instrument for measuring the angle of rotation in polarization or the amount of polarized light. [Mod. L. *polaris,* polar, + G. *metron,* measure]

po·lar·im·e·try (pō′lăr-im′ĕ-trē). Measurement by polarimeter.

po·lar·i·scope (pō-lar′i-skōp). An instrument for studying the phenomena of the polarization of light. [Mod. L. *polaris,* polar, + G. *skopeō,* to examine]

po·lar·i·scop·ic (pō-lar-i-skop′ik). Relating to the polariscope or to polariscopy.

po·lar·is·co·py (pō′lă-ris′kŏ-pē). Use of the polariscope in studying properties of polarized light.

po·lar·i·ty (pō-lar′i-tē). **1.** The property of having two opposite poles, as that possessed by a magnet. **2.** The possession of opposite properties or characteristics. **3.** The direction or orientation of positivity relative to negativity. **4.** The direction along a polynucleotide chain, or any biopolymer or macrostructure (e.g., microtubules). **5.** With respect to solvents, ionizing power. **6.** The tendency of an organism to develop differentially along an axis. [Mod. L. *polaris,* polar]

po·lar·i·za·tion (pō′lăr-i-zā′shŭn). **1.** In electricity, coating of an electrode with a thick layer of hydrogen bubbles, with the result that the flow of current is weakened or arrested. **2.** A change effected in a ray of light passing through certain media, whereby the transverse vibrations occur in one plane only, instead of in all planes as in an ordinary light ray. **3.** Development of differences in potential between two points in living tissues, as between the inside and outside of a cell wall.

po·lar·ize (pō′lăr-īz). To put into a state of polarization.

po·la·riz·er (pō′lă-rīz′er). The first element of a polariscope that polarizes the light, as distinguished from the analyzer, the second polarizing element.

po·lar·og·ra·phy (pō′lă-rog′ră-fē). That branch of electrochemistry concerned with the variation in current flowing through a solution as the voltage is varied; this will vary with the ionic concentration of reducible substances so that p. can be used in chemical analysis. P. is commonly employed in the form of a reduction at a dropping mercury electrode. [Mod. L. *polaris,* polar, + G. *graphō,* to write]

pol·dine meth·yl·sul·fate (pōl′dēn). An anticholinergic agent.

pole (pōl) [TA]. **1.** One of the two points at the extremities of the axis of any organ or body. **2.** Either of the two points on a sphere at the greatest distance from the equator. **3.** One of the two points in a magnet or an electric battery or cell having extremes of opposite properties; the negative p. is a cathode, the positive p. an anode. **4.** Either end of a spindle. **5.** Either of the differentiated zones at opposite ends of an axis in a cell, organ, or organism. SYN polus [TA]. [L. *polus,* the end of an axis, pole, fr. G. *polos*]

abapical p., in an ovum, the p. opposite the animal p. (i.e., vegetal p.).

animal p., the point in a telolecithal egg opposite the yolk, where most of the protoplasm is concentrated and where the nucleus is located; from this region, the polar bodies are extruded during maturation. SYN germinal p.

anterior p. of eyeball [TA], the center of the corneal curvature of the eye. SYN polus anterior bulbi oculi [TA].

anterior p. of lens [TA], the central point on the anterior surface of the lens of the eye. SYN polus anterior lentis [TA].

cephalic p., the head end of the fetus.

frontal p. [TA], SYN frontal p. [TA] of cerebrum.

frontal p. [TA] **of cerebrum,** the most anterior promontory of each cerebral hemisphere. SYN frontal p. [TA], polus frontalis [TA].

germinal p., SYN animal p.

inferior p. [TA], for a structure having a vertically oriented long

axis, the point at the lower end of the axis, nearest the soles of the feet; the lowest point of a structure's surface. SEE inferior p. of kidney, lower p. of testis. SYN extremitas inferior [TA], lower p. [TA], inferior extremity (1)⋆, polus inferior⋆.

inferior p. of kidney [TA], the inferior end of the kidney. SYN extremitas inferior renis [TA], inferior extremity of kidney⋆, polus inferior renis⋆.

inferior p. of testis, ⋆official alternate term for lower p. of testis.

lateral p., SYN tubal *extremity* of ovary.

lower p. [TA], SYN inferior p.

lower p. of testis [TA], the inferior end of the testis. SYN extremitas inferior testis [TA], inferior p. of testis⋆, polus inferior testis⋆.

medial p. of ovary, SYN uterine *extremity* of ovary.

occipital p. [TA], SYN occipital p. [TA] of cerebrum.

occipital p. [TA] **of cerebrum,** the most posterior promontory of each cerebral hemisphere; the apex of the occipital lobe. SYN occipital p. [TA], polus occipitalis [TA].

pelvic p., the breech end of the fetus.

posterior p. of eyeball [TA], the center of the posterior curvature of the eye. SYN polus posterior bulbi oculi [TA].

posterior p. of lens [TA], the central point on the posterior surface of the lens. SYN polus posterior lentis [TA].

superior p. [TA], for a structure having a vertically oriented long axis, the point at the upper end of the axis, furthest from the soles of the feet; the highest point of a structure's surface. SEE superior p. of kidney, upper p. of testis. SYN extremitas superior [TA], upper p. [TA], polus superior⋆, superior extremity (1)⋆.

superior p. of kidney [TA], the superior end of the kidney. SYN extremitas superior renis [TA], polus superior renis⋆, superior extremity of kidney⋆.

superior p. of testis, ⋆official alternate term for upper p. of testis.

temporal p. [TA], SYN temporal p. [TA] of cerebrum.

temporal p. [TA] **of cerebrum,** the most prominent part of the anterior extremity of the temporal lobe of each cerebral hemisphere, a short distance below the fissure of Sylvius. SYN polus temporalis [TA], temporal p. [TA].

upper p. [TA], SYN superior p.

upper p. of testis [TA], the superior end of the testis. SYN extremitas superior testis [TA], polus superior testis⋆, superior p. of testis⋆.

vegetal p., vegetative p., the part of a telolecithal egg where the bulk of the yolk is situated.

vitelline p., the vegetative p. of an ovum.

Polenské num·ber. See under number.

po·lice·man (pō-lēs′man). An instrument, usually a rubber-tipped rod, for removing solid particles from a container, particularly the walls of that container.

po·lio (pō′lē-ō). Abbreviated term for poliomyelitis.

△**polio-.** Gray; gray matter (substantia grisea). [G. *polios*]

po·li·o·clas·tic (pō′lē-ō-klas′tik). Destructive to gray matter of the nervous system. [polio- + G. *klastos,* broken]

po·li·o·dys·tro·phia (pō′lē-ō-dis-trō′fē-ă). SYN poliodystrophy.

p. cer′ebri progressi′va infan′tilis [MIM*203700], autosomal recessively inherited progressive spastic paresis of extremities with progressive mental deterioration, with development of seizures, blindness, and deafness, beginning during the first year of life, and with destruction and disorganization of nerve cells of the cerebral cortex. SYN Alpers disease, Christensen-Krabbe disease, progressive cerebral poliodystrophy.

po·li·o·dys·tro·phy (pō′lē-ō-dis′trō-fē). Wasting of the gray matter of the nervous system. SYN poliodystrophia. [polio- + G. *dys-,* bad, + *trophē,* nourishment]

progressive cerebral p., SYN *poliodystrophia* cerebri progressiva infantilis.

po·li·o·en·ceph·a·li·tis (pō′lē-ō-en-sef′ă-lī′tis). Inflammation of the gray matter of the brain, either of the cortex or of the central nuclei; as contrasted to inflammation of the white matter. [polio- + G. *enkephalos,* brain, + -*tis,* inflammation]

p. infecti′va, SYN von Economo *disease.*

inferior p., p. with predominantly bulbar paralysis.

superior p., p. with ophthalmoplegia.

superior hemorrhagic p., SYN Wernicke *syndrome*.

po·li·o·en·ceph·a·lo·me·nin·go·my·e·li·tis (pō'lē-ō-en-sef'ă-lō-mě-ning'gō-mī-ĕ-lī'tis). Inflammation of the gray matter of the brain and spinal cord and of the meningeal covering of the parts. [polio- + G. *enkephalos*, brain, + *mēninx*, membrane, + *myelon*, marrow, + *-itis*, inflammation]

po·li·o·en·ceph·a·lo·my·e·li·tis (pō'lē-ō-en-sef'ă-lō-mī'ĕ-lī'tis). Inflammation of the gray matter of the brain and spinal cord.

po·li·o·en·ceph·a·lop·a·thy (pō'lē-ō-en-sef'ă-lop'ă-thē). Any disease of the gray matter of the brain. [polio- + G. *enkephalos*, brain, + *pathos*, suffering]

po·li·o·my·e·li·tis (pō'lē-ō-mī'ĕ-lī'tis). An inflammatory process involving the gray matter of the cord. [polio- + G. *myelos*, marrow, + *-itis*, inflammation]

acute anterior p., a disease that results in death or irreversible damage of motor cells in the cerebrum, brainstem, and spinal cord, caused by infection with small RNA enteroviruses of the Picornaviridae group; formerly due almost solely to one of three types of polio virus, but now more often caused by coxsackieviruses A and B, or echoviruses.

acute bulbar p., poliomyelitis virus infection affecting nerve cells in the medulla oblongata and producing paralysis of the lower motor cranial nerves.

chronic anterior p., muscular atrophy of the upper extremities and neck, in which there are long intermissions of quiescence or improvement; not to be confused with poliomyelitis virus infections.

po·li·o·my·e·lo·en·ceph·a·li·tis (pō'lē-ō-mī'ĕ-lō-en-sef'ă-lī'tis). Acute anterior poliomyelitis with pronounced cerebral signs. [polio- + G. *myelon*, marrow, + *enkephalos*, brain, + *-itis*, inflammation]

po·li·o·my·e·lop·a·thy (pō'lē-ō-mī'ĕ-lop'ă-thē). Any disease of the gray matter of the spinal cord. [polio- + G. *myelon*, marrow, + *pathos*, suffering]

po·li·o·sis (po-lē-ō'sis). A patchy absence or lessening of melanin in hair of the scalp, brows, or lashes, due to lack of pigment in the epidermis; it occurs in several hereditary syndromes but may be caused by inflammation, irradiation, or infection such as herpes zoster. SYN trichopoliosis. [G., fr. *polios*, gray]

ciliary p., SYN piebald *eyelash*.

po·li·o·vi·rus. An enterovirus in the family Picornaviridae. There are 3 distinct serotypes, with Type 1 responsible for 85% of the cases of paralytic polio and most epidemics.

po·li·o·vi·rus hom·i·nis (pō'lē-ō-vī'rŭs hom'i-nis). SYN poliomyelitis *virus*.

pol·ish·ing. In dentistry, the act or process of making a restoration smooth and glossy.

Politzer, Adam, Austrian otologist, 1835–1920. SEE P. *bag*, *method*, luminous *cone*.

pol·itz·er·i·za·tion (pol'it-zer-i-zā'shŭn). Inflation of the eustachian tube and middle ear by the Politzer method.

negative p., withdrawal of secretions from a cavity by suction, effected by attaching a compressed Politzer bag or rubber bulb to a tube inserted in the cavity.

pol·kis·sen of Zimmermann (pōl'kis-en). SYN extraglomerular *mesangium*. [Ger. *Polkissen*, pole + cushion]

pol·la·ki·dip·sia (pol'ă-ki-dip'sē-ă). Rarely used term for unduly frequent thirst. [G. *pollakis*, often, + *dipsa*, thirst]

pol·la·ki·u·ria (pol'ă-kē-ū'rē-ă). Rarely used term for extraordinary urinary frequency. [G. *pollakis*, often, + *ouron*, urine]

pol·len (pol'en). Microspores of seed plants carried by wind or insects prior to fertilization; important in the etiology of hay fever and other allergies. [L. fine dust, fine flour]

pol·le·no·sis (pol-ĕ-nō'sis). SYN pollinosis.

pol·lex, gen. **pol·li·cis,** pl. **pol·li·ces** (pol'eks, pol'i-sis, -sēz) [TA]. SYN thumb. [L.]

p. pe'dis, SYN great *toe* I.

pol·li·ci·za·tion (pol'i-si-zā'shŭn). Construction of a substitute thumb. [L. *pollex*, thumb, + *-ize*, to make like, + *-ation*, state]

pol·li·no·sis (pol-i-nō'sis). Hay fever excited by the pollen of various plants. SYN pollenosis. [L. *pollen*, pollen, + G. *-osis*, condition]

pol·lu·tant (pŏ-loo'tănt). An undesired contaminant that results in pollution.

pol·lu·tion (pŏ-loo'shŭn). Rendering unclean or unsuitable by contact or mixture with an undesired contaminant. [L. *pollutio*, fr. *pol-luo*, pp. *-lutus*, to defile]

air p., contamination of air by smoke and harmful gases, mainly oxides of carbon, sulfur, and nitrogen, as from automobile exhausts, industrial emissions, or burning rubbish. SEE ALSO smog.

noise p., annoying or damaging environmental noise levels, as from automobile engines, industrial machinery, or amplified music.

po·lo·cyte (pō'lō-sīt). SYN polar *body*. [G. *polos*, pole, + *kytos*, cell]

po·lo·ni·um (Po) (pō-lō'nē-ŭm). A radioactive element, atomic no. 84, isolated from pitchblende; the longest-lived isotope is ^{209}Po (half-life 102 years); ^{210}Po is radium F (half-life 138.38 days), the only readily accessible isotope. [L. fr. *Polonia*, Poland, native country of Mme. M.S. Curie who with her husband, P. Curie, discovered the substance]

pol·ox·a·lene (pōl-ok'să-lēn). An oxyalkylene polymer, nonionic surface-active agent similar in actions and uses to dioctyl sodium sulfosuccinate; used in constipation due to hard dry stools. SYN poloxalkol.

pol·ox·al·kol (pōl-ok'sal-kol). SYN poloxalene.

pol·ster (pōl'ster). A bulge of smooth muscle cells, as in the penile arteries and veins, formerly thought to regulate blood flow. [G. cushion, bolster]

po·lus, pl. **po·li** (pō'lŭs, -lī) [TA]. SYN pole. [L. pole]

p. ante'rior bul'bi oc'uli [TA], SYN anterior *pole* of eyeball.

p. ante'rior len'tis [TA], SYN anterior *pole* of lens.

p. fronta'lis [TA], SYN frontal *pole* [TA] of cerebrum.

p. inferior, ✫official alternate term for inferior *pole*.

p. inferior renis, ✫official alternate term for inferior *pole* of kidney.

p. inferior testis, ✫official alternate term for lower *pole* of testis.

po'li liena'lis infe'rior et supe'rior, SEE anterior *extremity* of spleen, posterior *extremity* of spleen.

p. occipita'lis [TA], SYN occipital *pole* [TA] of cerebrum.

p. poste'rior bul'bi oc'uli [TA], SYN posterior *pole* of eyeball.

p. poste'rior len'tis [TA], SYN posterior *pole* of lens.

poli rena'les infe'rior et supe'rior, SEE superior *pole* of kidney, inferior *pole* of kidney.

p. superior, ✫official alternate term for superior *pole*.

p. superior renis, ✫official alternate term for superior *pole* of kidney.

p. superior testis, ✫official alternate term for upper *pole* of testis.

p. tempora'lis [TA], SYN temporal *pole* [TA] of cerebrum.

poly (pol'ē). Abbreviated form and colloquialism for polymorphonuclear *leukocyte*.

♻**poly-.** 1. Prefix denoting many; multiplicity. Cf. multi-, pluri-. 2. In chemistry, prefix meaning "polymer of," as in polypeptide, polysaccharide, polynucleotide; often used with symbols, as in poly(A) for poly(adenylic acid), poly(Lys) for poly(L-lysine). [G. *polys*, much, many]

Pólya, Jenö (Eugene), Hungarian surgeon, 1876–1944. SEE Pólya *gastrectomy*; P. *operation*; Reichel-P. stomach *procedure*.

pol·y·(A) 1. Abbreviation for poly(adenylic acid). 2. Iridoid indole alkaloid isolated from *Vinca* sp.; may have pharmacologic applications; falling in this class are vinblastine and vincristine. 3. Excretion of D-glyceric acid in the urine; found in renal calculi. 4. An inborn error in metabolism resulting in D-glyceric aciduria (1). 5. A class of basic antibiotic peptides, found in neutrophils, that apparently kill bacteria by causing membrane damage.

poly(A) polymerase, an enzyme that catalyzes the formation of a poly(adenylic acid) sequence.

pol·y·ac·id (pol-ē-as'id). An acid capable of liberating more than one hydrogen ion per molecule; e.g., H_2SO_4, citric acid. [G. *polys*, much, many + acid]

pol·y·ac·ry·la·mide (pol-ē-a-kril-a-mīd). A branched polymer of acrylamide ($H_2C=CHCONH_2$) that is used in gel electrophoresis; e.g., $R–CH_2–CH(CONH_2)–CH(CONHR)CH(CONHR')–R''$.

pol·y·ad·e·ni·tis (pol'ē-ad-ĕ-nī'tis). Inflammation of many lymph nodes, especially with reference to the cervical group.

    p. malig'na, SYN bubonic *plague*.

pol·y·ad·e·nop·a·thy (pol'ē-ad-ĕ-nop'ă-thē). Adenopathy affecting many lymph nodes. SYN polyadenosis.

pol·y·ad·e·no·sis (pol'ē-ad-ĕ-nō'sis). SYN polyadenopathy.

pol·y·ad·e·nous (pol-ē-ad'ĕ-nŭs). Pertaining to or involving many glands.

pol·y·ad·e·nyl·a·tion. **1.** The process of formation of poly-(adenylic acid). **2.** The covalent modification of a macromolecule (e.g., mRNA) by the formation of a polyadenylyl moiety covalent linked to the macromolecule.

pol·y·(ad·en·yl·ic ac·id) (pol·y·(A)) (pol-ē-ă-dē-nil'ik). A homopolymer of adenylic acid; often seen at the 3' end of many eukaryotic mRNAs.

pol·y·al·co·hol (pol-ē-al'kō-hol). An aliphatic or alicyclic molecule characterized by the presence of two or more hydroxyl groups; e.g., glycerol, inositol. [G. *polys*, much, many + alcohol]

pol·y·al·lel·ism (pol'ē-ă-lēl'izm). The existence of multiple alleles at a genetic locus.

pol·y·a·mine (pol-ē-am'ēn). Class name for substances of the general formula $H_2N(CH_2)_nNH_2$, $H_2N(CH_2)_nNH(CH_2)_nNH_2$, $H_2N(CH_2)_nNH(CH_2)_nNH(CH_2)_nNH_2$, where $n = 3, 4,$ or 5. Many p.'s arise by bacterial action on protein; many are normally occurring body constituents of wide distribution or are essential growth factors for microorganisms. [G. *polys*, much, many + amine]

    p. oxidase, an enzyme of liver peroxisomes that uses molecular oxygen to oxidize spermine to spermidine and spermidine to putrescine, in both cases also producing H_2O_2 and β-aminopropionaldehyde; a part of the catabolic pathway of p.'s.

pol·y(ami·no ac·ids). Polypeptides that are polymers of aminoacyl groups, i.e., of –NH–CHR–CO–; typically, a term used with homopolymers. SEE poly- (2).

pol·y·an·gi·i·tis (pol'ē-an-jē-ī'tis). Inflammation of multiple blood vessels involving more than one type of vessel, e.g., arteries and veins, or arterioles and capillaries.

    microscopic p., systemic, nongranulomatous small-vessel vasculitis, associated with glomerulonephritis, pulmonary capillaritis, palpable purpura, and antineutrophil cytoplasmic autoantibodies.

pol·y·an·i·on (pol-ē-an'ī-on). Anionic sites on proteoglycans in the renal glomeruli that restrict filtration of anionic molecules and facilitate filtration of cationic proteins; loss of p. may cause albuminuria in lipoid nephrosis.

pol·y·ar·ter·i·tis (pol'ē-ar-ter-ī'tis). Simultaneous inflammation of a number of arteries.

    p. nodo'sa, segmental inflammation, with infiltration by eosinophils, and necrosis of medium-sized or small arteries, more common in males, with varied symptoms related to involvement of arteries in the kidneys, muscles, gastrointestinal tract, and heart. SYN arteritis nodosa, Kussmaul disease, periarteritis nodosa.

pol·y·ar·thric (pol-ē-ar'thrik). SYN multiarticular.

pol·y·ar·thri·tis (pol'ē-ar-thrī'tis). Simultaneous inflammation of several joints. [poly- + G. *arthron*, joint, + *-itis*, inflammation]

    p. chron'ica, obsolete term for rheumatoid *arthritis*.

    p. chron'ica villo'sa, a chronic inflammation confined to the synovial membrane, involving a number of joints; it occurs in women at the menopause and in children.

    epidemic p., a mild febrile illness of humans in Australia characterized by polyarthralgia and rash, caused by the Ross River virus, a member of the family Togaviridae, and transmitted by mosquitoes. SYN epidemic exanthema, Murray Valley rash, Ross River fever.

p. rheumat'ica acu'ta, obsolete term for p. associated with rheumatic fever.

vertebral p., inflammation of a number of the intervertebral disks without involvement of the vertebral bodies.

pol·y·ar·tic·u·lar (pol-ē-ar-tik'ū-lăr). SYN multiarticular. [poly- + L. *articulus,* joint]

pol·y·a·sple·nia. SYN polysplenia. [blend of *polysplenia* and *asplenia*]

pol·y·aux·o·troph (pol-ē-awks'ō-trōf). A mutant organism that requires several nutrients that are not required by the wild-type organism. Cf. auxotroph, monoauxotroph.

pol·y·a·vi·ta·min·o·sis (pol'ē-ā'vī-tă-mi-nō'sis). Avitaminosis with multiple deficiencies.

pol·y·ba·sic (pol-ē-bās'ik). Having more than one replaceable hydrogen atom, denoting an acid with a basicity greater than 1.

pol·y·blen·nia (pol-ē-blen'ē-ă). Excessive production of mucus. [poly- + G. *blennos,* mucus]

pol·y·car·bo·phil (pol-ē-kar'bō-fil). A polyacrylic acid crosslinked with divinyl glycol; used as a gastrointestinal absorbent.

pol·y·car·dia (pol-ē-kar'dē-ă). SYN tachycardia.

pol·y·cen·tric (pol-ē-sen'trik). Having several centers.

pol·y·chei·ria, pol·y·chi·ria (pol-ē-kī'rē-ă). Presence of supernumerary hands. [poly- + G. *cheir,* hand]

pol·y·chon·dri·tis (pol'ē-kon-drī'tis). Inflammation of cartilage. [poly- + G. *chondros,* cartilage, + *-itis,* inflammation]

    chronic atrophic p., SYN relapsing p.

    relapsing p., a degenerative disease of cartilage producing a bizarre form of arthritis, with collapse of the ears, the cartilaginous portion of the nose, and the tracheobronchial tree; death may occur from chronic infection or suffocation because of loss of stability in the tracheobronchial tree; of autosomal origin. SYN chronic atrophic p., generalized chondromalacia, Meyenburg disease, Meyenburg-Altherr-Uehlinger syndrome, relapsing perichondritis, systemic chondromalacia.

pol·y·chro·ma·sia (pol'ē-krō-mā'zē-ă). SYN polychromatophilia.

pol·y·chro·mat·ic (pol-ē-krō-mat'ik). Multicolored.

pol·y·chro·mat·o·cyte (pol'ē-krō-mat'ō-sīt). SYN polychromatophil (2).

pol·y·chro·ma·to·phil, pol·y·chro·ma·to·phile (pol-ē-krō'mă-tō-fil, -fīl). **1.** Staining readily with acid, neutral, and basic dyes; denoting certain cells, especially certain red blood cells. SYN polychromatophilic. **2.** A young or degenerating erythrocyte that manifests acidic and basic staining affinities. SYN polychromatocyte. SYN polychromophil. [poly- + G. *chrōma,* color, + *phileō,* to love]

pol·y·chro·ma·to·phil·ia (pol-ē-krō'mă-tō-fil'ē-ă). **1.** A tendency of certain cells, such as the red blood cells in pernicious anemia, to stain with basic and also acid dyes. **2.** Condition characterized by the presence of many red blood cells that have an affinity for acid, basic, or neutral stains. SYN polychromasia, polychromatosis, polychromophilia.

pol·y·chro·ma·to·phil·ic (pol-ē-krō'mă-tō-fil'ik). SYN polychromatophil (1).

pol·y·chro·ma·to·sis (pol'ē-krō-mă-tō'sis). SYN polychromatophilia.

pol·y·chro·me·mia (pol-ē-krō-mē'mē-ă). An increase in the total amount of hemoglobin in the blood.

pol·y·chro·mia (pol-ē-krō'mē-ă). Increased pigmentation in any part.

pol·y·chro·mo·phil (pol-ē-krō'mō-fil). SYN polychromatophil.

pol·y·chro·mo·phil·ia (pol-ē-krō-mō-fil'ē-ă). SYN polychromatophilia.

pol·y·chy·lia (pol-ē-kī'lē-ă). An increased production of chyle. [poly- + G. *chylos,* chyle, + *-ia,* condition]

pol·y·cis·tron·ic (pol-ē-sis-tron'ik). Pertaining to mRNA carrying information for the synthesis of more than one protein.

pol·y·clin·ic (pol-ē-klin'ik). A dispensary for the treatment and study of diseases of all kinds. [poly- + G. *klinē,* bed]

pol·y·clo·nal (pol-ē-klō'năl). In immunochemistry, pertaining to

po

proteins (i.e., antibodies) from more than a single clone of cells, in contradistinction to monoclonal.

pol·y·clo·nia (pol'ē-klō'nē-ă). SYN *myoclonus* multiplex. [poly- + G. *klonos,* tumult]

pol·y·co·ria (pol-ē-kō'rē-ă). The presence of two or more pupils in one iris. [poly- + G. *korē,* pupil]

pol·y·crot·ic (pol-ē-krot'ik). Relating to or marked by polycrotism.

po·lyc·ro·tism (pol-ik'rō-tizm). A condition in which the sphygmographic tracing shows several upward breaks in the descending wave. [poly- + G. *krotos,* a beat]

pol·y·cy·e·sis (pol'ē-sī-ē'sis). SYN multiple *pregnancy.* [poly- + G. *kyēsis,* pregnancy]

pol·y·cys·tic (pol-ē-sis'tik). Composed of many cysts.

pol·y·cy·the·mia (pol'ē-sī-thē'mē-ă). An increase above the normal in the number of red cells in the blood. SYN erythrocythemia. [poly- + G. *kytos,* cell, + *haima,* blood]

compensatory p., a secondary p. resulting from anoxia, e.g., in congenital heart disease, pulmonary emphysema, or prolonged residence at a high altitude.

p. hyperton'ica, p. associated with hypertension, but without splenomegaly. SYN Gaisböck syndrome.

relative p., a relative increase in the number of red blood cells as a result of loss of the fluid portion of the blood.

p. ru'bra, SYN p. vera.

p. ru'bra ve'ra, SYN p. vera.

p. ve'ra, a chronic form of polycythemia of unknown cause; characterized by bone marrow hyperplasia, an increase in blood volume as well as in the number of red cells, redness or cyanosis of the skin, and splenomegaly. SYN erythremia, Osler disease, Osler-Vaquez disease, p. rubra vera, p. rubra, Vaquez disease.

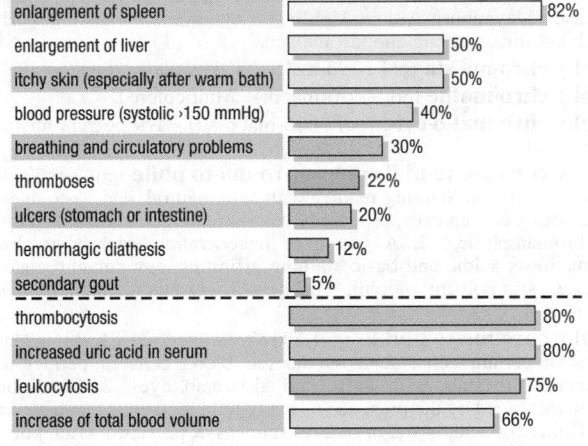

enlargement of spleen	82%
enlargement of liver	50%
itchy skin (especially after warm bath)	50%
blood pressure (systolic ›150 mmHg)	40%
breathing and circulatory problems	30%
thromboses	22%
ulcers (stomach or intestine)	20%
hemorrhagic diathesis	12%
secondary gout	5%
thrombocytosis	80%
increased uric acid in serum	80%
leukocytosis	75%
increase of total blood volume	66%

polycythemia vera: relative frequency of major symptoms

pol·y·dac·tyl·ism (pol-ē-dak'ti-lizm). SYN polydactyly.

pol·y·dac·tyl·ous (pol-ē-dak'til-ŭs). Relating to polydactyly.

pol·y·dac·ty·ly (pol-ē-dak'ti-lē). Presence of more than five digits on hand or foot. SYN polydactylism. [poly- + G. *daktylos,* finger]

pol·y·den·tia (pol-ē-den'shē-ă). SYN polyodontia. [poly- + L. *dens,* tooth]

pol·y·dip·sia (pol-ē-dip'sē-ă). Excessive thirst that is relatively prolonged. [poly- + G. *dipsa,* thirst]

hysterical p., SYN psychogenic p.

psychogenic p., excessive fluid consumption resulting from a disorder of the personality, without demonstrable organic lesion. SYN hysterical p.

psychogenic nocturnal p. (PNP), SEE psychogenic nocturnal polydipsia *syndrome.*

pol·y·dis·per·soid (pol'ē-dis-per'soyd). A colloid system in which the dispersed phase is composed of particles having different degrees of dispersion.

pol·y·dys·pla·sia (pol'ē-dis-plā'zē-ă). Tissue development abnormal in several respects. [poly- + G. *dys-,* bad, + *plasis,* a molding]

pol·y·dys·tro·phic (pol'ē-dis-trof'ik). Relating to polydystrophy.

pol·y·dys·tro·phy (pol-ē-dis'trō-fē). A condition characterized by the presence of many congenital anomalies. [poly- + dystrophy]

pseudo-Hurler p., SYN *mucolipidosis* III.

pol·y·em·bry·o·ny (pol-ē-em-brē'ō-nē). Condition of a zygote's giving rise to two or more embryos. [poly- + G. *embryon,* embryo]

pol·y·en·do·crin·op·athy (pol'ē-en'dō-krī- nop'ă-thē). A disease usually caused by insufficiency of multiple endocrine glands. SEE multiple endocrine deficiency *syndrome.*

pol·y·ene (pol-ē-ēn'). A chemical compound having a series of conjugated (alternating) double bonds; e.g., the carotenoids.

pol·y·e·nic ac·ids (pol-ē-ē'nik). SYN polyenoic acids.

pol·y·e·no·ic ac·ids (pol-ē-en'ik). Fatty acids with more than one double bond in the carbon chain; e.g., linoleic, linolenic, and arachidonic acids. SYN polyenoic acids.

pol·y·er·gic (pol-ē-er'jik). Capable of acting in several different ways. [poly- + G. *ergon,* work]

pol·y·es·the·sia (pol-ē-es-thē'zē-ă). A disorder of sensation in which a single touch or other stimulus is felt as several. [poly- + G. *aisthēsis,* sensation]

pol·y·es·tra·di·ol phos·phate (pol'ē-es-tră-dī'ol). An estradiol phosphate polymer, used as a long-acting estrogen for treatment of prostatic carcinoma.

pol·y·es·trous (pol-ē-es'trŭs). Having two or more estrous cycles in a mating season.

pol·y·eth·y·lene gly·cols (PEGs) (pol-ē-eth'i-lēn). Condensation polymers of ethylene oxide and water, of the general formula $HO(CH_2CH_2O)_nH$, where *n* equals the average number of oxyethylene groups (300–6,000); they vary in consistency based on molecular size; PEG 300 is a viscous liquid; PEG 6000 is a waxlike solid; PEGs are soluble in water and are used as pharmaceutic aids.

pol·y·fruc·tose (pol-ē-fruk'tōs). SYN fructosan (1).

pol·y·ga·lac·tia (pol'ē-gă-lak'tē-ă, -shē-ă). Excessive secretion of breast milk, especially at the weaning period. [poly- + G. *gala,* milk]

pol·y·ga·lac·tu·ro·nase (pol'ē-gă-lak'too-ron-ās). Pectin depolymerase; an enzyme catalyzing the random hydrolysis of 1,4-α-D-galactosiduronic linkages in pectate and other galacturonans. SYN pectinase.

pol·y·gan·gli·on·ic (pol'ē-gang-glē-on'ik). Containing or involving many ganglia.

pol·y·gene (pol'ē-jēn). One of many genes that contribute to the phenotypic value of a measurable phenotype.

pol·y·gen·ic (pol-ē-jen'ik). Relating to a hereditary disease or normal characteristic controlled by the added effects of genes at multiple loci.

polyglactin 910 (pol'ē-glak'tin). A synthetic absorbable suture for wound support of superficial approximation of the skin and mucosa.

pol·y·glan·du·lar (pol-ē-glan'doo-lăr). SYN pluriglandular.

poly-β-glu·co·sa·min·i·dase. SYN chitinase.

pol·y·glu·ta·mate (pol-ē-gloo'tă-māt). SYN poly(glutamic acid).

pol·y·(glu·tam·ic ac·id) (pol'ē-gloo-tam'ik). A polymer of glutamic acid residues in the usual peptide linkage (α-carboxyl to α-amino). SEE poly- (2). SEE ALSO poly(γ-glutamic acid). SYN polyglutamate.

pol·y·(γ-glu·tam·ic ac·id). A polypeptide formed of glutamic acid residues, the γ-carboxyl group of one glutamic acid being condensed to the amino group of its neighbor; occurs naturally in the anthrax bacillus capsule.

poly(gly·col·ic ac·id) (pol'ē-glī-kol'ik). A polymer of glycolic acid, used in absorbable surgical sutures. [see poly- (2)]

pol·y·gna·thus (pol-ē-nath'ŭs, pŏ-lig'na-thŭs). Unequal conjoined twins in which the parasite is attached to the jaw of the autosite. SEE conjoined *twins*, under *twin*. [poly- + G. *gnathos*, jaw]

pol·y·graph (pol'ē-graf). **1.** An instrument to obtain simultaneous tracings from several different sources; e.g., radial and jugular pulse, apex beat of the heart, phonocardiogram, electrocardiogram. The ECG is nearly always included for timing. **2.** An instrument for recording changes in respiration, blood pressure, galvanic skin response, and other physiologic changes while the person is questioned about some matter or asked to give associations to relevant and irrelevant words; the physiologic changes are presumed to be indicators of emotional reactions, and thus whether the person is telling the truth. SYN lie detector. [poly- + G. *graphō*, to write]

Mackenzie p., an instrument consisting of a system of tambours and a time-marker for recording simultaneously the jugular and arterial pulses and the apex beat; formerly used in the clinical investigation of cardiac arrhythmias.

pol·y·gy·ria (pol-ē-jī're-ă). Condition in which the brain has an excessive number of convolutions. [poly- + G. *gyros*, circle, gyre]

pol·y·he·dral (pol-ē-hē'drăl). Having many sides or facets. [G. *polyedros*, many-sided, fr. poly- + G. *hedra*, seat, facet]

pol·y·hex·os·es (pol-ē-heks'ōs-ez). SYN hexosans.

pol·y·hi·dro·sis (pol'ē-hī-drō'sis). SYN hyperhidrosis.

pol·y·hy·brid (pol-ē-hī'brid). The offspring of parents differing from each other in more than three characters.

pol·y·hy·dram·ni·os (pol'ē-hī-dram'nē-os). SYN hydramnios.

pol·y·hy·dric (pol-ē-hī'drik). Containing more than one hydroxyl group, as in polyhydric alcohols (glycerol, $C_3H_5(OH)_3$) or polyhydric acids (*o*-phosphoric acid, $OP(OH)_3$).

pol·y·hy·per·men·or·rhea (pol-ē-hī'per-men-ō-rē'ă). Frequent and excessive menstruation. [poly- + G. *hyper*, above, + *mēn*, month, + *rhoia*, flow]

pol·y·hy·po·men·or·rhea (pol-ē-hī'pō-men-ō-rē'ă). Frequent but scanty menstruation. [poly- + G. *hypo*, below, + *mēn*, month, + *rhoia*, a flow]

pol·y·iso·pre·nes (pol-ē-ī'sō-prēnz). SYN polyterpenes.

pol·y·iso·pre·noids (pol-ē-i-sō-prē-nōydz). SYN polyterpenes.

pol·y·kar·y·o·cyte (pol-ē-kar'ē-ō-sīt). A cell containing many nuclei, such as the osteoclast. [poly- + G. *karyon*, kernel, + *kytos*, cell]

pol·y·lac·to·sa·mines (pol-ē-lak-tōs'a-mēnz). A class of glycoproteins containing repeating lactosamine units in their oligosaccharide components; the I/i blood group substances belong to this class.

pol·y·lep·tic (pol-ē-lep'tik). Denoting a disease occurring in many paroxysms, e.g., malaria, epilepsy. [poly- + G. *lēpsis*, a seizing]

pol·y·link·er (pol-ē-link'er). An inserted sequence of DNA in recombinant DNA vectors consisting of a cluster of numerous restriction endonuclease sites unique in the plasmid; also called restriction site bank and polycloning site.

pol·y·lo·gia (pol-ē-lō'jē-ă). Continuous and often incoherent speech. [poly- + G. *logos*, word]

pol·y·mas·tia (pol-ē-mas'tē-ă). In humans, a condition in which more than two breasts are present. SYN hypermastia (1), multimammae, pleomastia, pleomazia. [poly- + G. *mastos*, breast]

pol·y·mas·ti·gote (pol-ē-mas'ti-gōt). A mastigote having several grouped flagella. [poly- + G. *mastix*, a whip]

pol·y·meg·eth·ism (pol'ē-meg'-ĕ-thism). A greater than normal variation in the size of the cells of the human corneal endothelium.

pol·y·me·lia (pol-ē-mē'lē-ă). A developmental defect in which there are supernumerary limbs or parts of limbs. [poly- + G. *melos*, limb]

pol·y·men·or·rhea (pol-ē-men-ō-rē'ă). Occurrence of menstrual cycles of greater than usual frequency. [poly- + G. *mēn*, month, + *rhoia*, flow]

pol·y·mer (pol'i-mer). A substance of high molecular weight,

made up of a chain of repeated units sometimes called "mers." SEE ALSO biopolymer. [see -mer (1)]

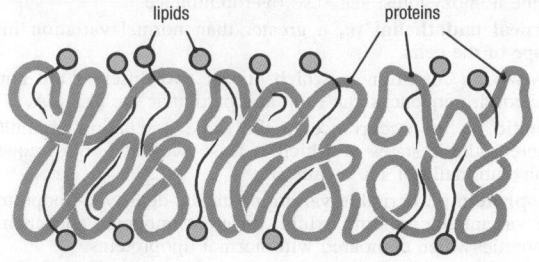

polymer membrane (structure)

cross-linked p., a p. in which long-chain molecules are attached to each other, forming a two- or three-dimensional network. SYN cross-linked resin.

pol·y·mer·ase (po-lim'er-ās). General term for any enzyme catalyzing a polymerization, as of nucleotides to polynucleotides, thus belonging to EC class 2, the transferases.

p. alpha, a class of mammalian DNA p.'s in the nucleus that function in chromosome replication. SYN polymerase α.

p. beta, a class of mammalian DNA p.'s in the nucleus that do not have a role in replication but may function in DNA repair. SYN polymerase β.

p. gamma, a class of mammalian DNA p.'s in the mitochondria responsible for replication of the mitochondrial genome. SYN polymerase γ.

Taq p., a temperature-resistant DNA polymerase isolated from *Thermus aquaticus* that can extend primers at high temperatures; used in the p. chain reaction.

pol·y·mer·ase γ. SYN *polymerase* gamma.

pol·y·mer·ase α. SYN *polymerase* alpha.

pol·y·mer·ase β. SYN *polymerase* beta.

pol·y·me·ria (pol-ē-mēr'ē-ă). Condition characterized by an excessive number of parts, limbs, or organs of the body. [poly- + G. *meros*, part]

pol·y·mer·ic (pol-i-mer'ik). **1.** Having the properties of a polymer. **2.** Relating to or characterized by polymeria. **3.** Rarely used synonym for polygenic.

po·lym·er·i·za·tion (po-lim'er-i-za'shŭn). A reaction in which a high molecular weight product is produced by successive additions to or condensations of a simpler compound; e.g., polystyrene may be produced from styrene, or rubber from isoprene, or a polynucleotide from mononucleotides, or microtubules from tubulin.

po·lym·er·ize (pol'i-mer-īz, po-lim'er-īz). To bring about polymerization.

pol·y·met·a·car·pa·lia, pol·y·met·a·car·pa·lism (pol'ē-met-ă-kar-pā'lē-ă, -kar'pă-lizm). Congenital anomaly characterized by the presence of supernumerary metacarpal bones.

pol·y·met·a·tar·sa·lia, pol·y·met·a·tar·sa·lism (pol'ē-met-ă-tar-sā'lē-ă, -tar'să-lizm). Congenital anomaly characterized by the presence of supernumerary metatarsal bones.

pol·y·mi·cro·lip·o·ma·to·sis (pol-ē-mī'krō-lip'ō-mă-tō'sis). The occurrence of multiple small, nodular, fairly discrete masses of lipid in the subcutaneous connective tissue. [poly- + G. *mikros*, small, + lipoma + G. *-osis*, condition]

po·lym·i·tus (pŏ-lim'i-tŭs). SYN exflagellation. [poly- + G. *mitos*, thread]

pol·y·morph (pol'ē-mōrf). Colloquial term for polymorphonuclear *leukocyte*.

pol·y·mor·phic (pol-ē-mōr'fik). Occurring in more than one morphologic form. SYN multiform, pleomorphic (1), pleomorphous, polymorphous. [G. *polymorphos*, multiform]

pol·y·mor·phism (pol-ē-mōr'fizm). Occurrence in more than one form; existence in the same species or other natural group of more than one morphologic type. SYN pleomorphism.

balanced p., a unilocal trait in which two alleles are maintained at stable frequencies because the heterozygote is more fit than either of the homozygotes. SEE ALSO overdominance.

corneal endothelial p., a greater than normal variation in the shape of the cells.

DNA p., a condition in which one of two different but normal nucleotide sequences can exist at a particular site in DNA.

genetic p., the occurrence in the same population of multiple discrete allelic states of which at least two have high frequency (conventionally of 1% or more).

lipoprotein p., heritable variations in low-density β-lipoproteins; the variant lipoproteins exhibit different antigenic and chemical properties when compared with normal lipoproteins.

restriction fragment length p. (RFLP), used in genetic analysis of populations or individual relationships. In regions of the human genome not coding for proteins there is often wide sequence variety between individuals that can be measured; in effect, the distance (in nucleotides on the chromosome) can be different, usually because of repeated base patterns.

restriction length p., fragment length p., the existence of allelic forms recognizable by the length of fragments that result when the nucleotide chain is treated by a specific restriction enzyme that cleaves wherever a particular sequence of nucleotides occurs. A mutation in this sequence changes cleaving and hence the number of fragments.

restriction-site p., DNA p. in which the sequence of one form of the p. contains a recognition site for a particular endonuclease, but the sequence of the other form lacks such a site.

pol·y·mor·pho·cel·lu·lar (pol-ē-mōr′fō-sel′ū-lăr). Relating to or formed of cells of several different kinds. [G. *polymorphos,* multiform, + L. *cellula,* cell]

pol·y·mor·pho·nu·cle·ar (pol′ē-mōr-fō-noo′klē-ăr). Having nuclei of varied forms; denoting a variety of leukocyte. [G. *polymorphos,* multiform, + L. *nucleus,* kernel]

pol·y·mor·phous (pol-ē-mōr′fŭs). SYN polymorphic.

pol·y·my·al·gia (pol′ē-mī-al′jē-ă). Pain in several muscle groups. [poly- + G. *mys,* muscle, + *algos,* pain]

p. arterit′ica, p. rheumatica resulting from arteritis, especially disseminated giant cell arteritis.

p. rheumat′ica, a syndrome within the group of collagen diseases different from spondylarthritis or from humeral scapular periarthritis by the presence of an elevated sedimentation rate; much commoner in women than in men.

pol·y·my·oc·lo·nus (pol′ē-mī-ok′lō-nŭs). SYN *myoclonus* multiplex.

pol·y·my·o·si·tis (pol′ē-mī-ō-sī′tis). Inflammation of a number of voluntary muscles simultaneously. [poly- + G. *mys,* muscle, + -*itis,* inflammation]

pol·y·myx·in (pol-ē-mik′sin). A mixture of antibiotic substances obtained from cultures of *Bacillus polymyxa* (*B. serosporus*), an organism found in water and soils and obtainable as a crystalline hydrochloride; all are polypeptides containing various amino acids and a branched-chain fatty acid, usually (+)-6-methyloctanoic acid. There are several p.'s, (e.g., designated A, B₁, C, D, E, M, T), which are about equally effective against Gram-negative bacteria, but which differ in toxicity, p. E (colistin) and p. B being the least toxic. SEE ALSO *colistin* sulfate, colistimethate sodium.

p. B sulfate, an antibacterial effective in tularemia, brucellosis, *Pseudomonas* infections, and urinary tract infections, but used systemically only for severe infections not responsive to less toxic agents; it is also used locally. P. B is a mixture of p. B₁ and p. B₂.

pol·y·ne·sic (pol-i-nē′sik). Occurring in many separate foci; denoting certain forms of inflammation or infection. [poly- + G. *nēsos,* island]

pol·y·neu·ral (pol-ē-noo′răl). Relating to, supplied by, or affecting several nerves. [poly- + G. *neuron,* nerve]

pol·y·neu·ral·gia (pol′ē-noo-ral′jē-ă). Neuralgia of several nerves simultaneously.

pol·y·neu·ri·tis (pol′ē-noo-rī′tis). SYN polyneuropathy (2).

acute idiopathic p., SYN Guillain-Barré *syndrome.*

chronic familial p., inflammation of nerves related to infiltration by amyloid.

infectious p., SYN Guillain-Barré *syndrome.*

postinfectious p., SYN Guillain-Barré *syndrome.*

pol·y·neu·ro·ni·tis (pol′ē-noo-rō-nī′tis). Inflammation of several groups of nerve cells.

pol·y·neu·rop·a·thy (pol′ē-noo-rop′ă-thē). **1.** A disease process involving a number of peripheral nerves (literal sense). **2.** A nontraumatic generalized disorder of peripheral nerves, affecting the distal fibers most severely, with proximal shading (e.g., the feet are affected sooner or more severely than the hands), and typically symmetrically; most often affects motor and sensory fibers almost equally, but can involve either one solely or very disproportionately; classified as axon degenerating (axonal), or demyelinating; many causes, particularly metabolic and toxic; familial or sporadic in nature. SYN polyneuritis. SYN multiple neuritis, symmetric distal neuropathy. [poly- + G. *neuron,* nerve, + *pathos,* disease]

acute inflammatory p., SYN Guillain-Barré *syndrome.*

alcoholic p., a nutritional axon loss p. associated with chronic alcoholism.

arsenical p., an axon loss p. that results from subacute or chronic arsenic poisoning; almost always preceded by gastrointestinal symptoms; one of the heavy metal neuropathies.

axonal p., SYN axon loss p.

axon loss p., a type of p. in which axon degeneration is the sole/predominant feature; many etiologies, particularly toxic and metabolic; on nerve conduction studies, affects amplitudes of the responses, but does not cause conduction slowing or block. SYN axonal p.

buckthorn p., ascending p. resulting from ingestion of the fruit of *Karwinskia humboldtiana.*

chronic inflammatory demyelinating p. (CIDP), an uncommon, acquired, demyelinating sensorimotor p. clinically characterized by insidious onset, slow evolution, (either steady progression or stepwise), and chronic course; symmetric weakness is a predominant symptom, often involving proximal leg muscles, accompanied by paresthesias, but not pain; CSF examination shows elevated protein, while electrodiagnostic studies reveal evidence of a demyelinating process, primarily conduction slowing rather than block; sometimes responds to prednisone.

critical illness p., a diffuse axon loss sensorimotor p. seen in severely ill patients, usually in the intensive care unit; most patients have been on multiple drugs and cannot be weaned from ventilatory support; electrodiagnostic studies show evidence of an axon loss p., predominantly motor; of unknown etiology.

demyelinating p., a type of p. in which almost solely the peripheral nerve myelin is affected; can be familial (e.g., Charcot-Marie-Tooth disease, type 1) or acquired (e.g., Guillain-Barré syndrome); on motor nerve conduction studies, manifested as conduction slowing or block. SYN segmental demyelinating p.

diabetic p., a distal, symmetric, generally sensorimotor p. that is a frequent complication of diabetes mellitus.

isoniazid p., an axonal loss p. seen in some patients treated with isoniazid.

nitrofurantoin p., an axon loss p., often severe, seen in some patients treated with nitrofurantoin, particularly patients with chronic renal failure.

nutritional p., an axon loss p. noted in beriberi, chronic alcoholism, and other clinical states, resulting from thiamin deficiency.

progressive hypertrophic p., SYN Dejerine-Sottas *disease.*

segmental demyelinating p., SYN demyelinating p.

uremic p., a distal sensory and motor p. without conspicuous inflammation and ascribed to the metabolic effects of chronic renal failure.

pol·y·nox·y·lin (pol-ē-nok′si-lin). Poly{methylenebis[*N,N*′-di(hydroxymethyl)urea]}; a polymer of urea with formaldehyde, used as a topical antiseptic.

pol·y·nu·cle·ar, pol·y·nu·cle·ate (pol-ē-noo′klē-ăr, -klē-āt). SYN multinuclear.

pol·y·nu·cle·o·sis (pol′ē-noo-klē-ō′sis). The presence of numbers of polynuclear, or multinuclear, cells in the peripheral blood. SYN multinucleosis.

pol·y·nu·cle·o·ti·das·es (pol′ē-noo′klē-ō-ti′dās-ez). **1.** Enzymes catalyzing the hydrolysis of polynucleotides to oligonucleotides or to mononucleotides; e.g., phosphodiesterases, nucleases. **2.** Terms once applied to the two polynucleotide phosphatases, 2′(3′)- and 5′-, which do not cleave internucleotide links.

pol·y·nu·cle·o·tide (pol-ē-noo′klē-ō-tīd). A linear polymer containing an indefinite (usually large) number of nucleotides, linked from one ribose (or deoxyribose) to another via phosphoric residues. Cf. oligonucleotide.

p. methyltransferases, enzymes that catalyze the methylation of purine and/or pyrimidine bases of p.'s or of the sugars of p.'s. SYN polynucleotide methylases.

p. phosphorylase, SYN polyribonucleotide nucleotidyltransferase.

p. thioltransferases, enzymes that catalyze specific thiolation reaction of purine and/or pyrimidine bases in p.'s.

pol·y·nu·cle·o·tide meth·yl·ases. SYN *polynucleotide* methyl-transferases.

pol·y·o·don·tia (pol-ē-ō-don′shē-ă). Presence of supernumerary teeth. SYN polydentia. [poly- + G. *odous*, tooth]

pol·y·ol (pol′ē-ol). Polyhydroxy alcohol; a sugar that contains many –OH (-ol) groups, such as the sugar alcohols and inositols.

p. dehydrogenases, oxidizing enzymes that catalyze the dehydrogenation of sugar alcohols to monosaccharides (in EC class 1.1), e.g., L-iditol dehydrogenase and aldose reductase.

Pol·y·o·ma·vi·rus (pol-ē-ō′mă-vī′rŭs). A genus of viruses (family Papovaviridae) containing DNA (MW 3×10^6), having virions about 45 nm in diameter, and including viruses oncogenic for animals; includes the polyoma virus of rodents, vacuolating viruses (SV40) of primates, and the BK and JC viruses of humans. [poly- + G. *-ōma*, tumor]

pol·y·on·co·sis, pol·y·on·cho·sis (pol′ē-ong-kō′sis). Formation of multiple tumors. [poly- + G. *onkos*, tumor, + *-osis*, condition]

pol·y·o·nych·ia (pol-ē-ō-nik′ē-ă). Presence of supernumerary nails on fingers or toes. SYN polyunguia. [poly- + G. *onyx*, nail]

pol·y·o·pia, pol·y·op·sia (pol′ē-ō′pē-ă, -op′sē-ă). The perception of several images of the same object. SYN multiple vision. [poly- + G. *ōps*, eye]

pol·y·or·chism, pol·y·or·chid·ism (pol-ē-ōr′kizm, -ōr′kid-izm). Presence of one or more supernumerary testes. [poly- + G. *orchis*, testis]

pol·y·os·tot·ic (pol′ē-os-tot′ik). Involving more than one bone. [poly- + G. *osteon*, bone]

pol·y·o·tia (pol-ē-ō′shē-ă). Presence of a supernumerary auricle on one or both sides of the head. [poly- + G. *ous*, ear]

pol·y·ov·u·lar (pol-ē-ō′vū-lăr). Containing more than one ovum.

pol·y·ov·u·la·tory (pol-ē-ō′vū-lă-tōr-ē). Discharging several ova in one ovulatory cycle. SYN polyzygotic.

pol·y·ox·yl 40 ste·a·rate (pol-ē-ok′sil). A mixture of the monostearate and distearate esters of a condensation polymer, $H(OCH_2CH_2)_n \cdot OCOC_{16}H_{32}CH_3$ (*n* is approximately 40); it is a nonionic surface-active agent used as an emulsifying agent in hydrophilic ointment and other emulsions.

pol·yp (pol′ip). A general descriptive term used with reference to any mass of tissue that bulges or projects outward or upward from the normal surface level, thereby being macroscopically visible as a hemispheroidal, spheroidal, or irregular moundlike structure growing from a relatively broad base or a slender stalk; p.'s may be neoplasms, foci of inflammation, degenerative lesions, or malformations. SYN polypus. [L. *polypus*; G. *polypous*, contr. fr. G. *polys*, many, + *pous*, foot]

adenomatous p., a p. that consists of benign neoplastic tissue derived from glandular epithelium. SYN cellular p., polypoid adenoma.

bleeding p., SYN vascular p.

bronchial p., a p. growing from the bronchial mucosa.

cardiac p., usually a rounded thrombus attached to the endocardium.

cellular p., SYN adenomatous p.

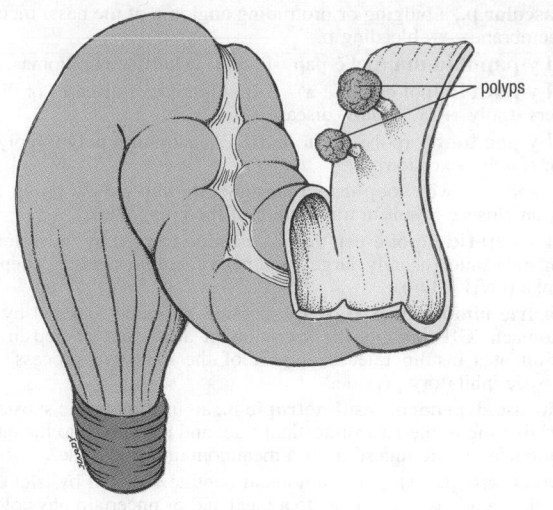

polyps: in sigmoid region of large intestine

choanal p., an antral-choanal p. that extends into the nasopharynx; originates in the maxillary sinus.

cystic p., a pedunculated cyst. SYN hydatid p.

dental p., SYN hyperplastic *pulpitis*.

fibroepithelial p. (fī′brō-ep-the′lē- ăl), SYN skin *tag*.

fibrous p., a p. consisting chiefly of cellular fibrous tissue, frequently with foci of fairly dense collagen or hyaline material (or both).

fleshy p., SYN myomatous p.

gelatinous p., (1) a p. that consists of delicate, loose, edematous connective tissue; (2) a polypoid myxoma.

Hopmann p., SYN Hopmann *papilloma*.

hydatid p., SYN cystic p.

hyperplastic p., a benign small sessile p. of the large bowel showing lengthening and cystic dilation of mucosal glands; also applied to nonneoplastic gastric mucosal p.'s. SYN metaplastic p.

inflammatory p., SYN pseudopolyp.

juvenile p., a smoothly rounded mucosal hamartoma of the large bowel, which may be multiple and cause rectal bleeding, especially in the first decade of life; it is not precancerous. SYN retention p.

laryngeal p., a p. projecting from the surface of one of the vocal cords.

lipomatous p., (1) a p. consisting chiefly of adipose tissue; (2) lipoma that bulges from the surface or is attached by means of a stalk.

lymphoid p., benign p. consisting of aggregates of lymphocytes in the rectum.

metaplastic p., SYN hyperplastic p.

mucous p., (1) an adenomatous p. in which conspicuous amounts of mucin are formed; (2) a polypoid cyst that contains mucus.

myomatous p., a p. that consists of benign neoplastic tissue derived from nonstriated (smooth) muscle. SYN fleshy p.

nasal p., an inflammatory or allergic p., arising from the ostium or cavity of one of the paranasal sinuses, which projects into the nasal cavity.

osseous p., a p. consisting in part of bony tissue.

pedunculated p., any form of p. that is attached to the base tissue by means of a slender stalk.

placental p., a p. developed from a piece of retained placenta.

pulp p., SYN hyperplastic *pulpitis*.

regenerative p., a hyperplastic p. of the gastric mucosa.

retention p., SYN juvenile p.

sessile p., any form of p. that has a relatively broad base.

tooth p., SYN hyperplastic *pulpitis*.

po

vascular p., a bulging or protruding angioma of the nasal mucous membrane. SYN bleeding p.

pol·y·pap·il·lo·ma (pol′ē-pap-i-lō′mă). Multiple papillomas.

pol·y·path·ia (pol-ē-path′ē-ă). A multiplicity of diseases or disorders. [poly- + G. *pathos*, disease]

pol·y·pec·to·my (pol-i-pek′tō-mē). Excision of a polyp. [polyp + G. *ektomē*, excision]

p. snare, a wire loop device designed to slip over a polyp and, upon closure, result in transection of the polyp stalk.

pol·y·pep·tide (pol-ē-pep′tīd). A peptide formed by the union of an indefinite (usually large) number of amino acids by peptide links (–NH–CO–).

gastric inhibitory p. (GIP), a peptide hormone secreted by the stomach; GIP inhibits the secretion of acids and of pepsin and stimulates insulin release as part of the digestive process. SYN gastric inhibitory peptide.

glucose-dependent insulinotropic p., an insulinotropic substance originating in the gastrointestinal tract and released into the circulation following ingestion of a meal containing glucose.

pancreatic p., (1) a 36-amino acid peptide secreted by islet cells of the pancreas in response to a meal and of uncertain physiologic function; **(2)** a family of gastrointestinal peptides, which includes pancreatic polypeptide, neuropeptide Y, and peptide YY.

trefoil p., a group of p.'s that share the trefoil moiety of a highly stable three-loop structure held together by disulfide bonds based on cysteine residues; they are widely expressed in gastrointestinal tissues and secreted by mucous cells; their functions are as yet unknown.

vasoactive intestinal p. (VIP), a p. hormone secreted most commonly by non-β islet cell tumors of the pancreas; VIP increases the rate of glycogenolysis and stimulates pancreatic bicarbonate secretion; excess production causes copious watery diarrhea and fecal electrolyte loss, with hypokalemia and hypochlorhydria. SYN vasoactive intestinal peptide.

pol·y·pha·gia (pol-ē-fā′jē-ă). Excessive eating; gluttony. [poly- + G. *phagō*, to eat]

pol·y·pha·lan·gism (pol′ē-fă-lan′jizm). SYN hyperphalangism.

pol·y·phal·lic (pol-ē-fal′ik). Pertaining to the fantasy of possessing multiple penises.

pol·y·phar·ma·cy (pol-ē-far′mă-sē). The administration of many drugs at the same time. SEE ALSO shotgun *prescription*.

pol·y·phen·ic (pol-ē-phēn′ik). SYN pleiotropic. [poly- + G. *phainō*, to display]

pol·y·phe·nol ox·i·dase (pol-ē-fē′nol). SYN laccase.

pol·y·pho·bia (pol-ē-fō′bē-ă). Morbid fear of many things; a condition marked by the presence of many phobias. [poly- + G. *phobos*, fear]

pol·y·phos·phor·y·lase (pol′ē-fos-fōr′i-lās). SYN phosphorylase.

pol·y·phra·sia (pol-ē-frā′zē-ă). Extreme talkativeness. SEE logorrhea. [poly- + G. *phrasis*, speech]

pol·y·phy·let·ic (pol′ē-fī-let′ik). **1.** Derived from more than one source, or having several lines of descent, in contrast to monophyletic. **2.** In hematology, relating to polyphyletism.

pol·y·phy·le·tism (pol-ē-fī′lĕ-tizm). In hematology, the theory that blood cells are derived from several different stem cells, depending on the particular cell type. SYN polyphyletic theory. [poly- + G. *phylē*, tribe]

pol·y·phy·o·dont (pol-ē-fī′ō-dont). Having several sets of teeth formed in succession throughout life. [poly- + G. *phyō*, to produce, + *odous* (*odont-*), tooth]

po·ly·pi (pol′i-pī). Plural of polypus.

pol·yp·i·form (po-lip′i-fōrm). SYN polypoid.

pol·y·plas·mia (pol-ē-plaz′mē-ă). SYN hydremia.

pol·y·plas·tic (pol-ē-plas′tik). **1.** Formed of several different structures. **2.** Capable of assuming several forms. [poly- + G. *plastikos*, plastic]

Pol·y·plax (pol′ē-plaks). A sucking louse (order Anoplura) of rats and mice. The species *P. serratus* (the mouse louse) has been shown experimentally to be capable of transmitting tularemia and may also be a vector for murine typhus and *Trypanosoma lewisi*. [poly- + G. *plax*, plate, plaque]

pol·yp·loid (pol′ē-ployd). Characterized by or pertaining to polyploidy.

pol·y·ploi·dy (pol′ē-ploy′dē). The state of a cell nucleus containing three or more haploid sets. Cells containing three, four, five, or six multiples are referred to, respectively, as triploid, tetraploid, pentaploid, or hexaploid. [poly- + G. *ploidēs*, in form]

pol·yp·nea (pol-ip-nē′ă). SYN tachypnea. [poly- + G. *pnoia*, breath]

pol·y·po·dia (pol-i-pō′dē-ă). Presence of supernumerary feet.

pol·yp·oid (pol′i-poyd). Resembling a polyp in gross features. SYN polypiform. [polyp + G. *eidos*, resemblance]

po·lyp·or·ous (pol-ip′ōr-ŭs). SYN cribriform. [poly- + G. *poros*, pore]

Pol·y·po·rus (po-lip′ŏ-rŭs). A genus of mushrooms. SEE agaric. [poly- + G. *poros*, pore]

pol·y·po·sia (pol-ē-pō′zē-ă). Rarely used term for sustained, excessive consumption of liquids. [poly- + G. *posis*, drinking]

pol·yp·o·sis (pol′i-pō′sis). Presence of several polyps. [polyp + G. *-osis*, condition]

adenomatous p. coli, SYN familial adenomatous p.

familial adenomatous p. (FAP) [MIM*175100], p. that usually begins in childhood; polyps increase in number, causing symptoms of chronic colitis; pigmented retinal lesions are frequently found; carcinoma of the colon almost invariably develops in untreated cases; autosomal dominant inheritance, caused by mutation in the adenomatous polyposis coli gene (APC) on 5q. In Gardner syndrome, which is allelic to FAP, there are extracolonic changes (desmoid tumors, osteomas, jaw cysts). SYN adenomatous p. coli, familial p. coli, multiple intestinal p. (1).

familial p. coli, SYN familial adenomatous p.

lymphomatoid p., multifocal mantle cell lymphoma, producing numerous lymphoid polyps in the intestines.

multiple intestinal p. [MIM*175100], **(1)** SYN familial adenomatous p; **(2)** hamartomatous p. of the small or large intestine, Peutz-Jeghers syndrome [MIM*175200] with melanin spots on the lips, less common.

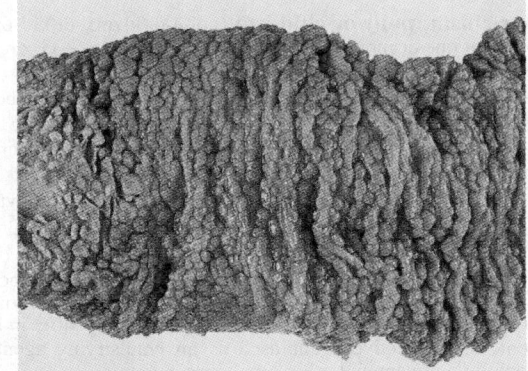

polyposis (multiple intestinal)

po·lyp·o·tome (po-lip′ō-tōm). An instrument used for cutting away a polyp. [polyp + G. *tomos*, cutting]

pol·yp·o·trite (pol-ip′ō-trīt). An instrument for crushing polyps. [polyp + L. *tero*, pp. *tritus*, to rub]

pol·y·pous (pol′i-pŭs). Pertaining to, manifesting the gross features of, or characterized by the presence of a polyp or polyps.

pol·y·prag·ma·sy (pol-ē-prag′mă-sē). Administration of many different remedies at the same time. [poly- + G. *pragma*, a thing]

pol·y·pre·nols (pol-ē-prēn-olz). Acyclic polyisoprene alcohols.

pol·yp·tych·i·al (pol-ē-tik′ē-ăl). Folded or arranged so as to form more than one layer. [G. *polyptychos*, having many folds or layers, fr. poly- + *ptychē*, fold or layer]

pol·y·pus, pl. **po·ly·pi** (pol′i-pŭs, -pī). SYN polyp. [L.]

pol·y·ra·dic·u·li·tis (pol'ē-ra-dik'ū-lī'tis). SYN polyradiculopathy.

pol·y·ra·dic·u·lo·my·op·a·thy (pol'ē-ra-dik'ū-lō-mī-op'ă-thē). Coexisting polyradiculopathy and myopathy.

pol·y·ra·dic·u·lo·neu·rop·a·thy (pol-ē-ra-dik'ū-lō-noo-rop'ă-thē). 1. Literally, a disease process that affects roots and peripheral nerves. 2. A nontraumatic, usually sporadic, generalized disorder of nerve roots and peripheral nerves, which may affect motor fibers or sensory fibers, but usually both, although often not to the same degree; classified as axon degenerating (axonal) or demyelinating. This disorder has many causes, primarily immune mediated, and includes Guillain-Barré syndrome and chronic inflammatory polyneuropathy.

acute inflammatory demyelinating p., the classic type of Guillain-Barré syndrome, in which the predominant type of underlying nerve fiber pathology is demyelination. SEE ALSO acute motor axonal *neuropathy*.

pol·y·ra·dic·u·lop·a·thy (pol-ē-ra-dik'ū-lop'ă-thē). Diffuse root involvement; seen with, among other disorders, diabetic neuropathy (diabetic polyradiculopathy). SYN polyradiculitis.

diabetic p., an inclusive term for several types of diabetic neuropathy other than a polyneuropathy; includes diabetic amyotrophy and diabetic thoracic radiculopathy; attributed to diabetes-induced injury of one or more roots, often sequential, in the lumbar, thoracic, or occasionally, cervical region; affects primarily older males.

pol·y·ri·bo·nu·cle·o·tide nu·cle·o·tid·yl·trans·fer·ase (pol'ē-rī-bō-noo'klē-ō-tīd). An enzyme-catalyzing phosphorolysis of polyribonucleotides or of RNA, yielding nucleoside diphosphates (or the reverse, the first artificial polynucleotide formation discovered). SYN polynucleotide phosphorylase.

pol·y·ri·bo·somes (pol-ē-rī'bō-sōmz). Conceptually, two or more ribosomes connected by a molecule of messenger RNA; structures satisfying this concept can be seen in electron micrographs and can be sedimented at rates consistent with aggregates of ribosomes (whence it is often, sometimes incorrectly, assumed that aggregates containing ribosomes are true p.); p. are active in protein synthesis. SYN polysomes.

pol·yr·rhea (pol-i-rē'ă). Profuse discharge of serous or other fluid. [poly- + G. *rhoia,* a flow]

pol·y·sac·char·ide (pol-ē-sak'ă-rīd). A carbohydrate containing a large number of saccharide groups; e.g., starch. Cf. oligosaccharide. SYN glycan.

pneumococcal p., SYN specific capsular *substance.*

specific soluble p., SYN specific capsular *substance.*

pol·y·sce·lia (pol-ē-sē'lē-ă). A form of polymelia involving the presence of more than two legs. [poly- + G. *skelos,* leg]

pol·y·scope (pol'ē-skōp). SYN diaphanoscope.

pol·y·ser·o·si·tis (pol'ē-sēr-ō-sī'tis). Chronic inflammation with effusions in several serous cavities; can result in fibrous thickening of the serosa, including constrictive pericarditis. SYN Bamberger disease (2), Concato disease, multiple serositis. [poly- + L. *serum,* serum, + G. *-itis,* inflammation]

familial paroxysmal p. [MIM*249100], transient recurring attacks of abdominal pain, fever, pleurisy, arthritis, and rash; the condition is asymptomatic between attacks; autosomal recessive inheritance, caused by mutation in the marenostrin gene on 16p. There is an autosomal dominant form [MIM*134610] in which amyloidosis in common. SYN benign paroxysmal peritonitis, familial Mediterranean fever, familial recurrent p., Mediterranean fever (2), periodic peritonitis, periodic p.

familial recurrent p., SYN familial paroxysmal p.

periodic p., SYN familial paroxysmal p.

recurrent p., familial Mediterranean *fever.*

pol·y·si·nu·si·tis (pol'ē-sī-nŭ-sī'tis). Simultaneous inflammation of two or more sinuses.

pol·y·somes (pol'ē-sōmz). SYN polyribosomes.

pol·y·so·mia (pol-ē-sō'mē-ă). Fetal malformation involving two or more imperfect and partially fused bodies. [poly- + G. *sōma,* body]

pol·y·so·mic (pol-ē-sō'mik). Pertaining to or characterized by polysomy.

pol·y·som·no·gram (pol-ē-som'nō-gram). The recorded physiologic function(s) obtained in polysomnography. [poly- + L. *somnus,* sleep, + G. *gramma,* diagram]

pol·y·som·nog·ra·phy (pol'ē-som-nog'ră-fē). Simultaneous and continuous monitoring of relevant normal and abnormal physiologic activity during sleep. [poly- + L. *somnus,* sleep, + G. *graphō,* to write]

pol·y·so·my (pol-ē-sō'mē). State of a cell nucleus in which a specific chromosome is represented more than twice. Cells containing three, four, or five homologous chromosomes are referred to, respectively, as trisomic, tetrasomic, or pentasomic. Cf. polyploidy. [poly- + G. *sōma,* body (chromosome)]

pol·y·sor·bate 80 (pol-ē-sōr'bāt). A mixture of polyoxethylene ethers of mixed partial oleic esters of sorbitol anhydrides; used as an emulsifier, as in the preparation of pharmacologic products.

pol·y·sper·mia, pol·y·sper·mism (pol-ē-sper'mē-ă, -sper'mizm). 1. SYN polyspermy. 2. An abnormally profuse spermatic secretion.

pol·y·sper·my (pol'ē-sper-mē). The entrance of more than one spermatozoon into the ovum. SYN polyspermia (1), polyspermism.

pol·y·sple·nia (pol-ē-sple'nē-ă) [MIM*208530]. A condition in which splenic tissue is divided into nearly equal masses or totally absent; congenital heart disease and malposition and maldevelopment of abdominal organs are common; may be related to situs inversus. Most cases are sporadic, although some suggest autosomal recessive inheritance. SEE ALSO bilateral *left-sidedness.* SYN asplenia with cardiovascular anomalies, Ivemark syndrome, polyasplenia. [poly- + G. *splēn,* spleen]

pol·y·ster·ax·ic (pol'ē-ster-ak'sik). A rarely used term for behavior characterized by its socially provocative quality.

pol·y·stich·ia (pol-ē-stik'ē-ă). Arrangement of the eyelashes in two or more rows. [poly- + G. *stichos,* row]

pol·y·sul·fide rub·ber (pol-ē-sŭl'fīd). Synthetic rubber used as a dental impression material.

pol·y·sus·pen·soid (pol-ē-sŭs-pen'soyd). A colloid system of solid phases having different degrees of dispersion.

pol·y·sym·brach·y·dac·ty·ly (pol'ē-sim-brak-ē-dak'ti-lē). Malformation of the hand or foot in which the shortened digits are syndactylous and polydactylous. [poly- + symbrachydactyly]

pol·y·syn·ap·tic (pol'ē-si-nap'tik). Referring to neural pathways formed by a chain of a large number of synaptically connected nerve cells, as distinguished from oligosynaptic conduction systems. SYN multisynaptic.

pol·y·syn·dac·ty·ly (pol'ē-sin-dak'ti-lē). Syndactyly of several fingers or toes. There are several forms: a simple one [MIM*174300] and one with abnormal skull shape, Grieg cephalopolysyndactyly syndrome [MIM*175700], both inherited as an autosomal dominant trait; a recessive form is associated with cardiac defects [MIM*263630].

pol·y·ten·di·ni·tis (pol'ē-ten-di-nī'tis). Inflammation of several tendons.

pol·y·tene (pol'i-tēn). Consisting of many filaments of chromatin as the result of repeated division of chromonema without separation of filaments.

pol·y·ten·i·za·tion (pol'ē-ten-i-zā'shŭn). The process of polytene formation without separation.

pol·y·ter·penes (pol-ē-ter'pēnz). Acyclic polymers containing a large number of isoprene subunits, usually unsaturated. SYN polyisoprenes, polyisoprenoids.

pol·y·the·lia (pol-ē-thē'lē-ă). Presence of supernumerary nipples, either on the breast or elsewhere on the body. SYN hyperthelia. [poly- + G. *thēlē,* nipple]

pol·y·thi·a·zide (pol-ē-thī'ă-zīd). A diuretic and antihypertensive of the benzothiadiazine group.

po·lyt·o·cous (pŏ-lit'ŏ-kŭs). Producing multiple young at a birth. [poly- + G. *tokos,* birth]

pol·y·to·mog·ra·phy (pol-i-tō-mog'ră-fē). Body section radiography using a machine designed to effect complex hypocycloidal motion; images a thinner tissue plane than does simple linear or circular tomography.

po

pol·y·trich·ia (pol-ē-trik′ē-ă). Excessive hairiness. SYN polytri-chosis. [poly- + G. *thrix* (*trich-*), hair]

pol·y·tri·cho·sis (pol′ē-tri-kō′sis). SYN polytrichia.

pol·y·tro·phic (pol′ē-trō-fik). Exhibiting an attraction, trophism, for multiple organs; usually used for a virus that affects multiple organ systems.

pol·y·(U) Abbreviation for poly(uridylic acid).

pol·y·un·guia (pol-ē-ŭng′gwē-ă). SYN polyonychia. [poly- + L. *unguis,* nail]

pol·y·u·ria (pol-ē-ū′rē-ă). Excessive excretion of urine resulting in profuse and frequent micturition. [poly- + G. *ouron,* urine]

pol·y·(uri·dyl·ic ac·id) (pol·y·(U)). A homopolymer of uridyl-ic acids.

pol·y·uro·nides (pol-ē-ūr′ō-nīdz). Polymers of uronic acids (e.g., glucuronic acid, galacturonic acid); the pectins are p.

pol·y·va·lent (pol-ē-vā′lent). **1.** SYN multivalent. **2.** Pertaining to a polyvalent antiserum.

pol·y·vi·done (pol-ē-vī′dŏn). SYN povidone.

pol·y·vi·nyl (pol-ē-vī′năl). Referring to a compound containing a number of vinyl groups in polymerized form.

pol·y·vi·nyl al·co·hol. A compound, $CH_2(CHOH)_n$, that is solu-ble in water; an adhesive and emulsifier.

pol·y·vi·nyl chlo·ride (PVC). A substance used as a rubber substitute in many industrial applications and suspected of being carcinogenic in humans. SYN chlorethene homopolymer.

pol·y·vi·nyl·pyr·rol·i·done (PVP) (pol-ē-vī′nil-pi-rol′i-dŏn). SYN povidone.

pol·y·vi·nyl·pyr·rol·i·done-io·dine com·plex. SYN povidone *iodine.*

pol·y·zo·ic (pol-ē-zō′ik). Segmented body form, as in the higher tapeworms, subclass Cestoda. SEE ALSO strobila, monozoic.

pol·y·zy·got·ic (pol-ē-zī-got′ik). SYN polyovulatory. [poly- + G. *zygōtos,* yoked]

po·made (pō-mād′, pō-mahd′). An ointment or cream containing medicaments; usually used on the hair. SYN pomatum. [Fr. *po-made,* fr. L. *pomum,* apple]

po·ma·tum (pō-mā′tŭm). SYN pomade. [Mod. L.]

POMC Abbreviation for proopiomelanocortin.

pome·gran·ate (pom′gran-at). Fruit of *Punica granatum* (family Punicaceae), a reddish yellow fruit the size of an orange, contain-ing many seeds enclosed in a reddish acidic pulp; used in diarrhea for its astringent properties; the bark of the tree and of the root contains pelletierine and other alkaloids and has been used as a teniacide. SYN granatum. [L. *pomum,* apple, + *granatus,* many seeded, fr. *granum,* grain or seed]

Pomeroy, Ralph H., U.S. obstetrician-gynecologist, 1867–1925. SEE P. *operation.*

POMP Abbreviation for Purinethol (6-mercaptopurine), Oncovin (vincristine sulfate), methotrexate, and prednisone, a cancer che-motherapy regimen.

Pompe, J.C., 20th century Dutch physician. SEE P. *disease.*

pom·pho·lyx (pom′fō-liks). SYN dyshidrosis. [G. a bubble, fr. *pomphos,* a blister]

pon·ceau de xy·li·dine (pon-sō′ dĕ zī′li-dēn) [C.I.-16151]. A monoazo acid dye originally employed as a red histologic coun-terstain in Masson trichrome stain.

Ponfick, Emil, German pathologist, 1844–1913. SEE P. *shadow.*

⚠**pono-.** Bodily exertion, fatigue, overwork, pain. [G. *ponos,* toil, fatigue, pain]

po·no·graph (pō′nō-graf). An instrument for recording graphi-cally the progressive fatigue of a contracting muscle. [pono- + G. *graphō,* to write]

po·no·pal·mo·sis (pō′nō-pal-mō′sis). Rarely used term for a con-dition of irritable heart in which palpitation is excited by slight exertion. [pono- + G. *palmos,* palpitation]

po·no·pho·bia (pō-nō-fō′bē-ă). Morbid fear of overwork or of becoming fatigued. [pono- + G. *phobos,* fear]

po·nos (pō′nos). A disease occurring in young children in certain of the islands of Greece, characterized by enlargement of the spleen, hemorrhages, fever, and cachexia; possibly the infantile form of visceral leishmaniasis. [G. toil, fatigue, pain]

pons, pl. **pon·tes** (ponz, pon′tēz). **1** [TA]. In neuroanatomy, the pons varolii or pons cerebelli; that part of the brainstem between the medulla oblongata caudally and the mesencephalon rostrally, composed of the basilar part of pons and the tegmentum of pons. On the ventral surface of the brain the basilar part of pons, the white pontine protuberance, is demarcated from both the medulla oblongata and the mesencephalon by distinct transverse grooves. SYN p. cerebelli, p. varolii. **2.** Any bridgelike formation connect-ing two more or less disjoined parts of the same structure or organ. [L. bridge]

p. basilaris pontis [TA], SYN basilar *part* of pons.

p. cerebel′li, SYN pons (1).

pontes grisei caudolenticulares [TA], SYN caudolenticular gray *bridges,* under *bridge.*

p. hep′atis, a bridge of liver tissue that sometimes overlaps the fossa of the inferior vena cava, converting it into a canal. SYN ponticulus hepatis.

p. varo′lii, SYN pons (1).

pon·tes (pon′tēz). Plural of pons. [L.]

pon·tic (pon′tik). An artificial tooth on a fixed partial denture; it replaces the lost natural tooth, restores its functions, and usually occupies the space previously occupied by the natural crown. SYN dummy.

pon·ti·cu·lus (pon-tik′ū-lŭs). A vertical ridge on the eminentia conchae giving insertion to the auricularis posterior muscle. [L. dim. of *pons,* bridge]

p. hep′atis, SYN *pons* hepatis.

p. na′si, bridge of the nose.

p. promonto′rii, SYN *subiculum* promontorii.

pon·tile, pon·tine (pon′tīl, -tīn; -tēn). Relating to a pons.

pontocerebellum. Those areas of the cerebellar cortex that receive input from cells of the basilar pontine nuclei; includes all cortical regions; projections to the hemisphere greater than to the vermis; pontocerebellar fibers send collaterals to the cerebellar nuclei enroute to the overlying cortex.

Pool, Eugene H., U.S. surgeon, 1874–1949. SEE P. *phenomenon;* P.-Schlesinger *sign.*

pool (pool). **1.** A collection of blood or other fluid in any region of the body; p. of blood results from dilation and retardation of the circulation in the capillaries and veins of the region. **2.** A combi-nation of resources. [A.S. *pōl*]

abdominal p., the volume of blood within the abdomen.

gene p., the set of the genes that are available for inheritance in a particular mating population.

metabolic p., the quantity of a given chemical compound or group of related compounds participating in metabolic reactions; may constitute only a portion of the total bodily content of such compounds.

vaginal p., the secretions and material that accumulate in the posterior fornix of the vagina; used for sampling, principally for evaluation after premature rupture of the membranes.

pop·les (pop′lēz). SYN popliteal *fossa.* SEE ALSO popliteal *fossa.* [L. the ham of the knee]

pop·lit·e·al (pop-lit′ē-ăl, pop-li-tē′ăl). Relating to the popliteal fossa. SYN popliteus (1).

pop·li·te·us (pop-li-tē′ŭs). **1.** SYN popliteal. **2.** SYN popliteal *fossa.* **3.** SYN popliteus (*muscle*). [L.]

POPOP Abbreviation for 1,4-bis(5-phenyloxazol-2-yl)benzene, a liquid scintillator.

pop·py (pop′ē). SYN Papaver.

p. oil, a fixed (drying) oil expressed from the seed of *Papaver somniferum;* sometimes used in the preparation of liniments and as a solvent of iodine in iodized oil.

pop·u·la·tion (pop-ū-lā′shŭn). Statistical term denoting all the objects, events, or subjects in a particular class. Cf. sample. [L. *populus,* a people, nation]

POR Abbreviation for problem-oriented *record.*

⚠**por-.** SEE poro-.

por·ce·lain (pōr'sĕ-lin). A powder composed of a clay, silica, and a flux that, when mixed with water, forms a paste that is molded to form artificial teeth, inlays, jacket crowns, and dentures. When heated, the materials fuse to form a ceramic.

por·cine (pōr'sīn, -sin). Relating to pigs. [L. *porcinus*, fr. *porcus*, a hog]

pore (pōr) [TA]. **1.** An opening, hole, perforation, or foramen. A pore, meatus, or foramen. SEE ALSO opening. **2.** SYN sweat p. SEE ALSO opening, meatus, foramen. [G. *poros*, passageway]

alveolar p.'s, openings in the interalveolar septa of the lung that permit air flow between adjacent alveoli.

dilated p., an enlarged follicular opening of the skin, with a keratinous plug and occasional lanugo or mature hair.

external acoustic p., external auditory p. [TA], the orifice of the external acoustic meatus in the tympanic portion of the temporal bone. SYN porus acusticus externus [TA], external acoustic aperture, external acoustic foramen, external auditory foramen, opening of external acoustic meatus, orifice of external acoustic meatus.

gustatory p., SYN taste p.

interalveolar p.'s, openings in the interalveolar septa of the lung. SYN Kohn p.'s.

internal acoustic p., auditory p., the inner opening of the internal acoustic meatus on the posterior surface of the petrous part of the temporal bone. SYN internal acoustic opening [TA], internal acoustic foramen, internal auditory foramen, opening of internal acoustic meatus, orifice of internal acoustic meatus, porus acusticus internus.

Kohn p.'s, SYN interalveolar p.'s.

nuclear p., an octagonal opening, about 70 nm across, where the inner and outer membranes of the nuclear envelope are continuous.

skin p., SYN sweat p.

slit p.'s, the intercellular clefts between the interdigitating pedicels of podocytes; they are part of the filtration barrier of renal corpuscles. SYN filtration slits.

sweat p. [TA], the surface opening of the duct of a sweat gland. SYN pore (2) [TA], porus sudoriferus, porus, skin p.

taste p. [TA], the minute opening of a taste bud on the surface of the oral mucosa through which the gustatory hairs of the specialized neuroepithelial gustatory cells project. SYN porus gustatorius [TA], gustatory p.

por·en·ce·pha·lia (pōr'en-se-fā'lē-ă). SYN porencephaly.

por·en·ce·phal·ic (pōr'en-se-fal'ik). Relating to or characterized by porencephaly. SYN porencephalous.

por·en·ceph·a·li·tis (pōr'en-sef-ă-lī'tis). Chronic inflammation of the brain with the formation of cavities in the organ's substance. [G. *poros*, pore, + *enkephalos*, brain, + *-itis*, inflammation]

por·en·ceph·a·lous (pōr-en-sef'ă-lŭs). SYN porencephalic.

por·en·ceph·a·ly (pōr-en-sef'ă-lē). The occurrence of cavities in the brain substance, communicating usually with the lateral ventricles. SYN porencephalia, spelencephaly. [G. *poros*, pore, + *enkephalos*, brain]

Porges, Otto, Austrian bacteriologist, 1879–1968. SEE P. *method*; P.-Meier *test*.

po·ri (pō'rī). Plural of porus.

po·ria (pō'rē-ă). Plural of porion.

Po·rif·era (pō-rif'er-ă). The sponges; a phylum of the Metazoa, comprising a group of sessile, aquatic animals possessing an endoskeleton and many branching canals, lined by flagellated collar cells; communication of the canals with the surface is made through many pores or through larger openings and oscula. SEE ALSO Parazoa. [L. *porus*, pore, + *fero*, to bear]

po·rins (pōr'inz). Proteins found in the outer membrane of a double membrane that allow permeability in most small molecules. [G. *poros*, passageway, + *-in*]

por·i·o·ma·nia (pōr'ē-ō-mā'nē-ă). A morbid impulse to wander or journey away from home. [G. *poreia*, a journey, + *mania*, frenzy]

por·i·on, pl. **po·ria** (pōr'ē-on, -ē-ă). The central point on the upper margin of the external auditory meatus; as a cephalometric landmark, it is located in the middle of the metal rods of the cephalometer. [G. *poros*, a passage]

PORN Acronym for progressive outer retinal *necrosis*.

por·no·lag·nia (pōr-nō-lag'nē-ă). A rarely used term for sexual attraction toward prostitutes. [G. *pornē*, prostitute, + *lagneia*, lust]

⊘**poro-, por-.** **1.** A pore, a duct, an opening. [G. *poros* (L. *porus*), passageway] **2.** A going through, a passing through. [G. *poreia*, a journey, passage] **3.** A callus; an induration. [G. *poros*, a kind of marble, a stone]

po·ro·ceph·a·li·a·sis (pō'rō-sef-ă-lī'ă-sis). Infection with a species of the tongue worms *Porocephalus*. SYN porocephalosis.

Po·ro·ce·phal·i·dae (pō'rō-se-fal'i-dē). A family of parasitic tongue worms (order Porocephalida, phylum Pentastomida) characterized by four hooks arranged in a curved line on either side of the mouth. Adults are found in the lungs of reptiles, and larvae or nymphs are found in the tissues of a great variety of vertebrates, including humans. SEE ALSO Linguatulidae, *Armillifer*, *Linguatula*. [G. *poros*, pore, + *kephalē*, head]

po·ro·ceph·a·lo·sis (pō'rō-sef-ă-lō'sis). SYN porocephaliasis.

Po·ro·ceph·a·lus (pō-rō-sef'ă-lŭs). A genus of tongue worms of the family Porocephalidae, of which the adult worms or larvae cause porocephaliasis in a number of animal species, including humans. [G. *poros*, pore, + *kephalē*, head]

P. armilla'tus, SYN *Armillifer armillatus*.

po·ro·co·nid·i·um (pōr'ō-kŏ-nid'ē-ŭm). In fungi, a conidium produced through the microscopic pore of the conidiophore. SYN porospore.

po·ro·ker·a·to·sis (pō'rō-ker-ă-tō'sis). A rare dermatosis in which there is a thickening of the stratum corneum with an annular keratotic rim or cornoid lamella surrounding progressive centrifugal atrophy; cutaneous carcinoma has been reported to arise in the lesions. SYN Mibelli disease. [G. *poros*, pore, + keratosis]

actinic p., a lesion that occurs on exposed areas of extremities primarily; bears a resemblance to actinic keratosis, but the histologic features are those of p.

po·ro·ma (pō-rō'mă). **1.** SYN callosity. **2.** SYN exostosis. **3.** Induration following a phlegmon. **4.** A tumor of cells lining the skin openings of sweat glands. [G. *pōrōma*, callus, fr. *pōros*, stone]

eccrine p., a p. or acrospiroma of the eccrine sweat glands, usually occurring on the sole of the foot. as a soft reddish nodule composed of basaloid cells and fibrovascular tissue.

po·ro·sis, pl. **po·ro·ses** (pō-rō'sis, -sēz). A porous condition. SYN porosity (1). [L. *porosus*, porous]

cerebral p., a porous condition of the brain caused by postmortem growth of *Clostridium perfringens* or other gas-forming organisms in the tissue.

po·ros·i·ty (pō-ros'i-tē). **1.** SYN porosis. **2.** A perforation. [G. *poros*, pore]

por·o·spore (pōr'ō-spōr). SYN poroconidium.

po·rot·ic (pō-rot'ik). Porous, as in osteoporotic.

po·rous (pō'rŭs). Having openings that pass directly or indirectly through the substance.

por·phin, por·phine (pōr'fin). The unsubstituted cyclic tetrapyrrole nucleus that is the basis of the porphyrins. SEE ALSO porphyrins. Cf. chlorin, phorbin, corrin. SYN porphyrin.

por·pho·bi·lin (pōr'fō-bī'lin). General term denoting intermediates between the monopyrrole, porphobilinogen, and the cyclic tetrapyrrole of heme (a porphin derivative). SEE ALSO bilin.

por·pho·bi·lin·o·gen (PBG) (pōr'fō-bī-lin'ō-jen). A porphyrin precursor of porphyrinogens, porphyrins, and heme; found in the urine in large quantities in cases of acute or congenital porphyria.

p. synthase, a liver enzyme catalyzing the formation of porphobilinogen and water from two molecules of δ-aminolevulinate, an important reaction in porphyrin biosynthesis; inhibited by lead in cases of lead poisoning; a deficiency of this enzyme results in elevated levels of δ-aminolevulinate and results in neurologic disturbances. SYN δ-aminolevulinate dehydratase.

por·phyr·ia (pōr-fir'ē-ă). A group of disorders involving heme biosynthesis, characterized by excessive excretion of porphyrins or their precursors; may be inherited or may be acquired, as from the effects of certain chemical agents (e.g., hexachlorobenzene).

acute intermittent p., acute p., SYN intermittent acute p.

δ-aminolevulinate dehydratase p., an inherited disorder in which there is a deficiency of porphobilinogen synthase; δ-aminolevulinate levels are elevated, leading to neurologic disturbances. SYN porphobilinogen synthase p.

congenital erythropoietic p. [MIM*263700], enhanced porphyrin formation by erythroid cells in bone marrow, leading to severe porphyrinuria, often with hemolytic anemia and persistent cutaneous photosensitivity; caused by a deficiency of uroporphyrinogen III cosynthetase; autosomal recessive inheritance, caused by mutation in the uroporphyrinogen III synthase gene (UROS) on chromosome 10q; there is an overproduction of type I porphyrin isomers.

p. cuta′nea tar′da (PCT) [MIM*176090, MIM*176100], familial or sporadic p. characterized by liver dysfunction and photosensitive cutaneous lesions, with bullae, hyperpigmentation, and scleroderma-like changes in the skin and increased excretion of uroporphyrin; caused by a deficiency of uroporphyrinogen decarboxylase induced in sporadic cases by chronic alcoholism; autosomal dominant inheritance in familial cases. SYN symptomatic p.

p. cuta′nea tar′da heredita′ria, SEE p. cutanea tarda.

p. cuta′nea tar′da symptoma′tica, SEE p. cutanea tarda.

erythropoietic p., a classification of p. that includes congenital erythropoietic p. and erythropoietic protoporphyria.

hepatic p. [MIM*176100.0002], a category of p. that includes p. cutanea tarda, variegate p., and coproporphyria. SYN p. hepatica.

p. hepatica (he-pat′ĭ-kă), SYN hepatic p.

hepatoerythropoietic p., an autosomal recessive disorder in which there is a deficiency or absence of uroporphyrinogen decarboxylase; results in photosensitivity and excessive hepatic production of 8- and 7-carboxylate porphyrins.

intermittent acute p. (IAP) [MIM*176000], p. caused by hepatic overproduction of δ-aminolevulinic acid, with greatly increased urinary excretion of it and of porphobilinogen, and some increase of uroporphyrin, due to a deficiency of porphobilinogen deaminase; characterized by intermittent acute attacks of hypertension, abdominal colic, psychosis, and polyneuropathy, but with no photosensitivity; autosomal dominant inheritance, caused by mutation in the human porphobilinogen deaminase gene on 11q24; exacerbation caused by ingestion of certain drugs (e.g., barbiturates). SYN acute intermittent p., acute p.

ovulocyclic p., acute episodic exacerbations of p. occurring in the premenstrual period.

porphobilinogen synthase p., SYN δ-aminolevulinate dehydratase p.

South African type p., SYN variegate p.

symptomatic p., SYN p. cutanea tarda.

variegate p. (VP) [MIM*176200], porphyria characterized by abdominal pain and neuropsychiatric abnormalities, by dermal sensitivity to light and mechanical trauma, by increased fecal excretion of proto- and coproporphyrin, and by increased urinary excretion of δ-aminolevulinic acid, porphobilinogen, and porphyrins; due to a deficiency of protoporphyrinogen oxidase; autosomal dominant inheritance, caused by mutation in the gene for protoporphyrinogen oxidase (PPOX) on chromosome 1q. SYN protocoproporphyria hereditaria, South African type p.

por·phy·rin (pōr′fi-rin). SYN porphin.

por·phy·rin·o·gens (pōr-fi-rin′ō-jenz). Intermediates in the biosynthesis of heme, as follows: four porphobilinogens condense to form uroporphyrinogens I and III (giving rise to side products uroporphyrins I and III) which are decarboxylated to form coproporphyrinogens I and III (giving rise to side products coproporphyrins I and III); coproporphyrinogen III is oxidized to protoporphyrinogen III (IX), which is then oxidized to form protoporphyrin III (IX) (this last intermediate adds ferrous iron to yield heme); certain p. are elevated in certain porphyrias.

por·phy·ri·nop·a·thy (pōr′fir-in-op′ă-thē). A syndrome that results from abnormal porphyrin metabolism such as acute porphyria. SYN porphyrism. [porphyrin + G. *pathos*, disease]

por·phy·rins (pōr′fi-rinz). Pigments widely distributed through-

out nature (e.g., heme, bile pigments, cytochromes) consisting of four pyrroles joined in a ring (porphin) structure. They are substitution products of porphin (porphyrin) and comprise several varieties, differing for the most part in the side chains (methyl, ethyl, vinyl, formyl, carboxyethyl, carboxymethyl, etc.) present at the eight available positions on the pyrrole rings. Depending on the nature of the side chains, the prefixes dentero-, etio-, meso-, proto-, etc., are attached to p.; distribution within each class is given by type I, II, III, and IV. P. combine with various metals (iron, copper, magnesium, etc.) to form metalloporphyrins, and with nitrogenous substances.

por·phy·ri·nu·ria (pōr′fir-i-noo′rē-ă). Excretion of porphyrins and related compounds in the urine. SYN porphyruria, purpurinuria.

por·phy·rism. SYN porphyrinopathy.

por·phy·ri·za·tion (pōr′fi-ri-zā′shŭn). Grinding in a mortar (formerly on a slab of porphyry).

Por·phy·ro·mo·nas (pōr′fir-ō-mōn′as). A genus of small anaerobic Gram-negative nonmotile cocci and usually short rods that produce smooth, gray to black pigmented colonies the size of which varies with the species. In humans, they are found as part of the normal flora in the oropharynx, including gingival crevices, and in the vaginal and intestinal tracts. The type species is *P. asaccharolytica*.

P. asaccharolytica, a species that rarely causes infections independently but is an important component of mixed infections associated with oral, genitourinary, and intra-abdominal abscesses, as well as in infectious associated with impaired circulation and diabetic gangrene.

por·phy·ru·ria (pōr-fi-roo′rē-ă). SYN porphyrinuria.

Porro, Edoardo, Italian obstetrician, 1842–1902. SEE *P. hysterectomy.*

port (port). SYN portal.

ancillary p.'s, during endoscopic surgery, the placement of more than one entry site to allow insertion of instruments other than the endoscope.

por·ta, pl. **por·tae** (pōr′tă, -tē). **1.** SYN hilum (1). **2.** SYN interventricular *foramen.* [L. gate]

p. hep′atis [TA], a transverse fissure on the visceral surface of the liver between the caudate and quadrate lobes, lodging the portal vein, hepatic artery, hepatic nerve plexus, hepatic ducts, and lymphatic vessels. SYN caudal transverse fissure, portal fissure.

p. lie′nis, SYN splenic *hilum.*

p. pulmo′nis, SYN *hilum* of lung.

p. re′nis, SYN *hilum* of kidney.

Port-a-Cath (port′ă-kath). A long-term central venous catheter with subcutaneous port(s). [brand name]

por·ta·ca·val (pōr′tă-kā′văl). Concerning the portal vein and the inferior vena cava.

por·tal (pōr′tăl). **1.** Relating to any porta or hilus, specifically to the porta hepatis and the p. vein. **2.** The point of entry into the body of a pathogenic microorganism. SYN port. [L. *portalis,* pertaining to a porta (gate)]

anterior intestinal p., SYN *fovea* cardiaca.

posterior intestinal p., in young embryos, the communications from the midgut to the hindgut.

Porter, Curt C., U.S. biochemist, *1914. SEE P.-Silber *chromogens,* under *chromogen, reaction,* chromogens *test.*

Porter, Thomas C., British scientist, 1860–1933. SEE Ferry-P. *law.*

Porter, William H., Irish surgeon, 1790–1861. SEE *P. fascia.*

por·tio, pl. **por·ti·o·nes** (pōr′shē-ō, -ō′nēz). A part. [L. portion]

p. interme′dia, SYN intermediate *nerve.*

p. ma′jor ner′vi trigem′ini, SYN sensory *root* of trigeminal nerve.

p. mi′nor ner′vi trigem′ini, SYN motor *root* of trigeminal nerve.

p. supravagina′lis cervicis [TA], SYN supravaginal *part* of cervix.

p. vagina′lis cervicis [TA], SYN vaginal *part* of cervix.

por·tion (pōr′shun). Part or division.

accessory p. of spinal accessory nerve, SYN cranial *root* of accessory nerve.

anterior p. of left medial segment IV of liver [TA], the part of the medial segment of the liver that includes the quadrate lobe. SYN quadrate part of liver [TA], pars quadrata hepatis.

mesenteric p. of small intestine, the freely movable portion of the small intestine supplied with a mesentery, comprising the jejunum and ileum. SYN intestinum tenue mesenteriale.

subcutaneous p. of external anal sphincter, SYN subcutaneous *part* of external anal sphincter; SEE external anal *sphincter*.

por·ti·plex·us (pōr-ti-plek′sŭs). The union of the choroid plexus of the lateral ventricle with that of the third ventricle at the interventricular foramen (of Monro).

○**porto-.** Portal. [L. *porta,* gate]

por·to·bil·i·o·ar·te·ri·al (pōr′tō-bil′ē-ō-ar-tēr′ē-ăl). Relating to the portal vein, biliary ducts, and hepatic artery, which have similar distributions. SEE ALSO portal *triad*.

por·to·en·ter·os·to·my (pōr′tō-en-ter-os′tō-mē). An operation for biliary atresia in which a Roux-en-Y loop of jejunum is anastomosed to the hepatic end of the divided extravascular portal structures, including rudimentary bile ducts. SYN Kasai operation.

por·to·gram (pōr′tō-gram). Radiographic record of portography. [porto- + G. *gramma,* a writing]

por·tog·ra·phy (pōr-tog′ră-fē). Delineation of the portal circulation by radiography, using radiopaque material, usually introduced into the spleen or into the portal vein at operation. SYN portovenography. [porto- + G. *graphō,* to write]

por·to·sys·tem·ic (pōr′tō-sis-tem′ik). Relating to connections between the portal and systemic venous systems.

por·to·ve·nog·ra·phy (pōr′tō-vē-nog′ră-fē). SYN portography.

po·rus, pl. **po·ri** (pō′rŭs, -rī). SYN sweat *pore.* SEE ALSO opening. [L. fr. G. *poros,* passageway]

p. acus′ticus exter′nus [TA], SYN external acoustic *pore.*

p. acus′ticus inter′nus, SYN internal acoustic *pore.*

p. crotaphy′tico-buccinato′rius, an occasional foramen in the sphenoid bone through which passes the motor portion of the trigeminal nerve; it is formed by ossification of a ligament below and lateral to the foramen ovale. SYN Hyrtl foramen.

p. gustato′rius [TA], SYN taste *pore.*

p. op′ticus, SYN optic *disk.*

p. sudorif′erus, SYN sweat *pore.*

Posadas, Alejandro, Argentinian parasitologist, 1870–1902. SEE P. *disease.*

POSITION

🅸**po·si·tion** (pŏ-zish′ŭn). **1.** An attitude, posture, or place occupied. **2.** Posture or attitude assumed by a patient for comfort and to facilitate the performance of diagnostic, surgical, or therapeutic procedures. **3.** In obstetrics, the relation of an arbitrarily chosen portion of the fetus to the right or left side of the mother; with each presentation there may be a right or left p.; the fetal occiput, chin, and sacrum are the determining points of p. in vertex, face, and breech presentations, respectively. Cf. presentation. [L. *positio,* a placing, position, fr. *pono,* to place]

🅸**anatomic p.,** the erect. of the body with the face directed forward (skull aligned in orbitomeatal or Frankfort plane), the arms at the side, and the palms of the hands directed forward; the terms posterior, anterior, lateral, medial, etc., are applied to the parts as they stand related to each other and to the axis of the body when in this p.

Bozeman p., knee-elbow p., the patient being strapped to supports.

Casselberry p., a prone p. that allows an intubated patient to drink without risking entry of the liquid into the tube.

centric p., the p. of the mandible in its most retruded unstrained relation to the maxillae. SEE ALSO centric jaw *relation*.

condylar hinge p., (1) the p. of the condyles in the temporomandibular joints from which a hinge movement is possible; **(2)** the maxillomandibular relation from which a consciously stimulated true hinge movement can be executed.

dorsal p., SYN supine p.

dorsosacral p., SYN lithotomy p.

eccentric p., SYN eccentric *relation.*

electrical heart p., a description of the heart's assumed electrical habitus based upon the form of the QRS complexes in leads aVL, aVF, V_1, and V_6. Sometimes loosely (and inaccurately) used to describe the frontal plane electric axis. SYN heart p.

Elliot p., a supine p. upon a double inclined plane or on a single inclined plane, with a cushion under the back at the level of the liver; used to facilitate abdominal section.

English p., SYN Sims p.

flank p., a lateral recumbent p., but with the lower leg flexed, the upper leg extended, and convex extension of the upper side of the body; used for nephrectomy.

Fowler p., an inclined p. obtained by raising the head of the bed about 20–30 inches to promote collection of intraabdominal fluid in the lower part of the abdomen.

frog leg p., supine with soles of feet together and knees apart to expose the perineum.

frontoanterior p., a cephalic presentation of the fetus with its forehead directed toward the right (**right frontoanterior,** RFA) or to the left (**left frontoanterior,** LFA) of the acetabulum of the mother.

frontoposterior p., a cephalic presentation of the fetus with its forehead directed toward the right (**right frontoposterior,** RFP) or to the left (**left frontoposterior,** LFP) sacroiliac articulation of the mother.

frontotransverse p., a cephalic presentation of the fetus with its forehead directed toward the right (**right frontotransverse,** RFT) or to the left (**left frontotransverse,** LFT) iliac fossa of the mother.

genucubital p., SYN knee-elbow p.

genupectoral p., SYN knee-chest p.

heart p., SYN electrical heart p.

hinge p., in dentistry, the orientation of parts in a manner permitting hinge movement between them.

intercuspal p., the p. of the mandible when the cusps and sulci of the maxillary and mandibular teeth are in their greatest contact and the mandible is in its most closed position.

knee-chest p., a prone posture resting on the knees and upper part of the chest, assumed for gynecologic or rectal examination. SYN genupectoral p.

knee-elbow p., a prone p. resting on the knees and elbows, assumed for gynecologic or rectal examination or operation. SYN genucubital p.

lateral recumbent p., SYN Sims p.

leapfrog p., a stooping p., such as that taken by children in playing leapfrog, assumed for rectal examination.

lithotomy p., a supine p. with buttocks at the end of the operating table, the hips and knees being fully flexed with feet strapped in p. SYN dorsosacral p.

mandibular hinge p., any p. of the mandible that exists when the condyles are so situated in the temporomandibular joints that opening or closing movements can be made on the hinge axis.

Mayo-Robson p., a supine p. with a thick pad under the loins, causing a marked lordosis in this region; used in operations on the gallbladder.

mentoanterior p. (MA), a cephalic presentation of the fetus with its chin pointing to symphysis or rotated to the right (**right mentoanterior,** RMA) or to the left (**left mentoanterior,** LMA) acetabulum of the mother.

mentoposterior p. (MP), a cephalic presentation of the fetus with its chin pointing to the sacrum or rotated to the right (**right mentoposterior,** RMP) or to the left (**left mentoposterior,** LMP) sacroiliac articulation of the mother.

mentotransverse p., a cephalic presentation of the fetus with its chin pointing to the right (**right mentotransverse,** RMT) or to the left (**left mentotransverse,** LMT) iliac fossa of the mother.

Noble p., patient standing and bent slightly forward; useful for inspection of a swelling of the loin that may occur with pyelonephritis.

obstetric p., the p. assumed by the parturient woman, either dorsal recumbent or lateral recumbent.

occipitoanterior p. (OA), a cephalic presentation of the fetus with its occiput under the symphysis or rotated toward the right (**right occipitoanterior**, ROA) or to the left (**left occipitoanterior**, LOA) acetabulum of the mother.

occipitoposterior p. (OP), a cephalic presentation of the fetus with its occiput turned toward the sacrum or rotated to the right (**right occipitoposterior**, ROP) or to the left (**left occipitoposterior**, LOP) sacroiliac joint of the mother.

occipitotransverse p., a cephalic presentation of the fetus with its occiput turned toward the right (**right occipitotransverse**, ROT) or to the left (**left occipitotransverse**, LOT) iliac fossa of the mother.

occlusal p., the relationship of the mandible and maxillae when the jaws are closed and the teeth are in contact; it may or may not coincide with centric occlusion.

orthopnea p., SYN orthopneic p.

orthopneic p., the p. assumed by patients with orthopnea, namely sitting propped up in bed by several pillows. SYN orthopnea p.

physiologic rest p., the usual p. of the mandible when the patient is resting comfortably in the upright p. and the condyles are in a neutral unstrained p. in the glenoid fossae. SEE ALSO rest *relation*. SYN postural p., postural resting p., rest p.

postural p., postural resting p., SYN physiologic rest p.

prone p., lying face down.

protrusive p., a forward p. of the mandible produced by muscular effort.

rest p., SYN physiologic rest p.

reverse Trendelenburg p., supine position without flexing or extending, in which the head is higher than the feet.

Rose p., supine p. with the head off the end of the table, the neck in extension; used in operations within the mouth or pharynx.

sacroanterior p. (SA), a breech presentation of the fetus with the sacrum under the symphysis or rotated to the right (**right sacroanterior**, RSA) or to the left (**left sacroanterior**, LSA) acetabulum of the mother.

sacroposterior p. (SP), a breech presentation of the fetus with the sacrum next to maternal sacrum or rotated pointing to the right (**right sacroposterior**, RSP) or to the left (**left sacroposterior**, LSP) sacroiliac articulation of the mother.

sacrotransverse p., a breech presentation of the fetus with its sacrum pointing to the right (**right sacrotransverse**, RST) or to the left (**left sacrotransverse**, LST) sacroiliac articulation of the mother.

Scultetus p., a supine p. on an inclined plane with head low, recommended by Scultetus for herniotomy and castration.

semi-Fowler p., an inclined p. obtained by raising the head of the bed 10–15 inches, flexing the hips, and placing a support under the knees so that they are bent at approximately 90°, thereby allowing fluid in the abdominal cavity to collect in the pelvis.

semiprone p., SYN Sims p.

Simon p., a p. for vaginal examination; a supine p. with hips elevated, thighs and legs flexed, and thighs widely separated.

Sims p., a p. to facilitate a vaginal examination, with the patient lying on her side with the lower arm behind the back, the thighs flexed, the upper one more than the lower. SYN English p., lateral recumbent p., semiprone p.

supine p., lying upon the back. SYN dorsal p.

terminal hinge p., the mandibular hinge p. from which further opening of the mandible would produce translatory rather than hinge movement.

Trendelenburg p., a supine p. on the operating table, which is inclined at varying angles so that the pelvis is higher than the head; used during and after operations in the pelvis or for shock.

Valentine p., a supine p. on a table with double inclined plane so as to cause flexion at the hips; used to facilitate urethral irrigation.

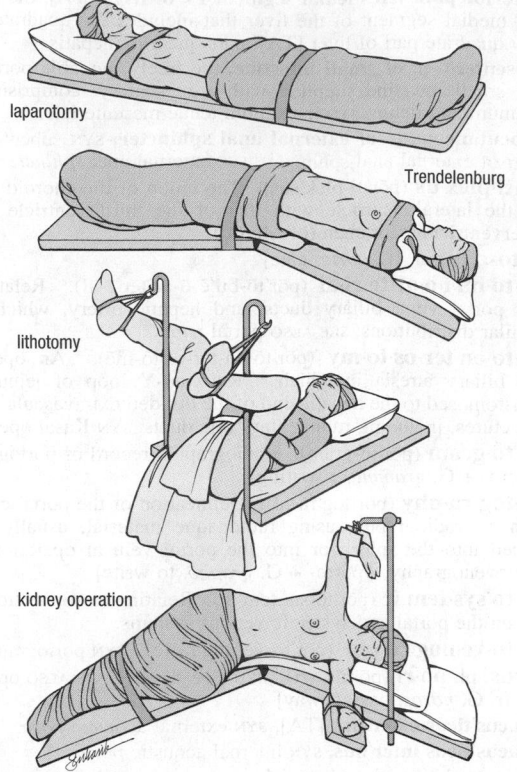

laparotomy

Trendelenburg

lithotomy

kidney operation

positions on the operating table

Walcher p., obsolete term for a supine p. of the parturient woman with the lower extremities falling over the edge of the table.

po·si·tion·er (pŏ-zish′ŭn-er). A resilient elastoplastic or rubber removable appliance fitting over the occlusal surface of the teeth, to obtain limited tooth movement and/or stabilization, usually used at the end of orthodontic treatment.

pos·i·tive (poz′i-tiv). **1.** Affirmative; definite; not negative. **2.** Denoting a response, the occurrence of a reaction, or the existence of the entity or condition in question. **3.** Having a value greater than zero. [L. *positivus*, settled by arbitrary agreement, fr. *pono*, pp. *positus*, to set, place]

pos·i·tive G. Gravity or acceleration in the usual head-to-foot direction in flying or in standing upright; the reverse of negative G.

pos·i·tron (β^+) (poz′i-tron). A subatomic particle of mass and charge equal to the electron but of opposite (i.e., positive) charge. SYN positive electron.

po·so·log·ic (pō-sō-loj′ik). Relating to posology.

po·sol·o·gy (pō-sol′ō-jē). The branch of pharmacology and therapeutics concerned with a determination of the doses of remedies; the science of dosage. [G. *posos*, how much, + *logos*, study]

post (pōst). In dentistry, a dowel or pin inserted into the root canal of a natural tooth as an attachment for an artificial crown.

△**post-.** After, behind, posterior; opposite of anti-. Cf. meta-. [L. *post*]

post·ac·e·tab·u·lar (pōst′as-ĕ-tab′ū-lăr). Posterior to the acetabular cavity.

post·ad·o·les·cence (pōst-ad-ō-les′ens). The period after adolescence or puberty.

post·a·nal (pōst-ā′năl). Posterior to the anus.

post·an·es·thet·ic (pōst′an-es-thet′ik). Occurring after anesthesia.

post·ap·o·plec·tic (pōst′ap-ŏ-plek′tik). Occurring after an attack of apoplexy.

post·ax·i·al (pōst-ak′sē-ăl). **1.** Posterior to the axis of the body or any limb, the latter being in the anatomic position. **2.** Denoting the portion of a limb bud that lies caudal to the axis of the limb: the ulnar aspect of the upper limb and the fibular aspect of the lower limb.

post·bra·chi·al (pōst′brā′kē-ăl). On or in the posterior part of the upper arm.

post·car·di·nal (pōst′kar′di-năl). Relating to the posterior cardinal veins.

post·ca·va (pōst′kā′vă). SYN inferior *vena* cava.

post·ca·val (pōst′kā′văl). Relating to the inferior vena cava.

post·cen·tral (pōst-sen′trăl). Referring to the cerebral convolution forming the posterior bank of the central sulcus: the postcentral gyrus.

post·chrom·ing (pōst′krōm′ing). SYN afterchroming.

post·ci·bal (pōst-sī′băl). After a meal or the taking of food. [L. *cibum*, food]

post·cla·vic·u·lar (pōst′kla-vik′ū-lăr). Posterior to the clavicle.

post·co·i·tal (pōst-kō′i-tăl). After coitus.

post·co·i·tus (pōst-kō′i-tŭs). The time immediately after coitus.

post·cor·di·al (pōst′kōr′jăl). Posterior to the heart. [L. *cor* (*cord-*), heart]

post·cos·tal (pōst-kos′tăl). Behind the ribs.

post·crown. A crown, replacing the natural crown, which is retained on the stump of the root of a tooth from which the pulp has been removed, by a post or pin integral with the crown and sealed in the treated root canal with a cement.

post·cu·bi·tal (pōst′kū′bi-tăl). On or in the posterior or dorsal part of the forearm.

post·dam. SYN posterior palatal *seal*.

post·di·a·stol·ic (pōst′dī-ă-stol′ik). Following diastole.

post·di·crot·ic (pōst-dī-krot′ik). Following the dicrotic wave in a sphygmogram; denoting an additional variation in the descending line of the pulse tracing.

post·diph·the·rit·ic (pōst′dif-the-rit′ik). Following or occurring as a sequel of diphtheria.

post·dor·mi·tal (pōst′dōr′mi-tăl). Relating to the postdormitum.

post·dor·mi·tum (pōst′dōr′mi-tŭm). The period of increasing consciousness between sound sleep and waking. [L. *dormio*, to sleep]

post·duc·tal (pōst-dŭk′tăl). Relating to that part of the aorta distal to the aortic opening of the ductus arteriosus.

post·en·ceph·a·lit·ic (pōst-en-sef′ă-lit′ik). Following encephalitis.

post·ep·i·lep·tic (pōst′ep-i-lep′tik). Following an epileptic seizure.

pos·te·ri·or (pos-tēr′ē-ŏr) [TA]. **1.** After, in relation to time or space. **2** [NA]. In human anatomy, denoting the back surface of the body. Often used to indicate the position of one structure relative to another, i.e., nearer the back of the body. SYN dorsal (2) [TA], dorsalis [TA], posticus. **3.** Near the tail or caudal end of certain embryos. **4.** An undesirable and confusing substitute for caudal in quadrupeds; in veterinary anatomy, p. is used only to denote some structures of the head. [L. comparative of *posterus*, following]

pos·te·ri·us (pos-tēr′ē-ŭs). Neuter of posterior. [L.]

postero-. Posterior; at the back of. [L. *posterior*]

pos·ter·o·an·te·ri·or (pos′ter-ō-an-tēr′ē-ŏr). A term denoting the direction of view or progression, from posterior to anterior, through a part.

pos·ter·o·clu·sion (pos′ter-ō-kloo′shŭn). SYN posterior *occlusion*.

pos·ter·o·ex·ter·nal (pos′ter-ō-ek-ster′năl). SYN posterolateral.

pos·ter·o·in·ter·nal (pos′ter-ō-in-ter′năl). SYN posteromedial.

pos·ter·o·lat·er·al (pos′ter-ō-lat′e-răl). Behind and to one side, specifically to the outer side. SYN posteroexternal.

pos·ter·o·me·di·al (pos′ter-ō-mē′dē-ăl). Behind and to the inner side. SYN posterointernal.

pos·ter·o·me·di·an (pos′ter-ō-mē′dē-an). Occupying a central position posteriorly.

pos·ter·o·pa·ri·e·tal (pos′ter-ō-pa-rī′e-tăl). Relating to the posterior portion of the parietal lobe of the cerebrum.

pos·ter·o·su·pe·ri·or (pos′ter-ō-soo-pē′rē-ŏr). Situated behind and at the upper part.

pos·ter·o·tem·po·ral (pos′ter-ō-tem′po-răl). Relating to or lying in the posterior portion of the temporal lobe of the cerebrum.

post·e·soph·a·ge·al (pōst′ē-sof′ă-jē′ăl, ē-sŏ-faj′ē-ăl). Behind the esophagus.

post·es·trus, post·es·trum (pōst-es′trŭs, -trŭm). The period in the estrus cycle following estrus; characterized by the growth of the corpus luteum and physiologic changes related to the production of progesterone.

post·feb·rile (pōst-fē′brĭl). Occurring after a fever. SYN metapyretic.

post·gan·gli·on·ic (pōst′gang-glē-on′ik). Distal to or beyond a ganglion; referring to the unmyelinated nerve fibers originating from cells in an autonomic ganglion. SYN neurofibrae postganglionicae.

post·hem·i·ple·gic (pōst′hem-i-plē′jik). Following hemiplegia.

post·hem·or·rha·gic (pōst-hem-ŏ-raj′ik). Following a hemorrhage.

post·he·pat·ic (pōst-he-pat′ik). Behind the liver.

pos·thet·o·my (pos-thet′ō-mē). Dorsal slit of foreskin. [G. *posthē*, prepuce, + *tomē*, incision]

pos·thi·o·plas·ty (pos′thē-ō-plas-tē). Surgical reconstruction of the prepuce. [G. *posthion*, dim. form of *posthē*, prepuce, + *plastos*, formed]

pos·thi·tis (pos-thī′tis). Inflammation of the prepuce. [G. *posthē*, prepuce, + *-itis*, inflammation]

pos·tho·lith (pos′thō-lith). SYN preputial *calculus*. [G. *posthē*, prepuce, + *lithos*, stone]

post·hy·oid (pōst-hī′oyd). Behind the hyoid bone.

post·hyp·not·ic (pōst-hip-not′ik). Following hypnotism; denoting an act suggested during hypnosis that is to be carried out at some time after the hypnotized subject is awakened.

post·ic·tal (pōst-ik′tăl). Following a seizure, e.g., epileptic.

pos·ti·cus (pos-tī′kŭs). SYN posterior (2). [L. fr. *post*, after]

post·in·flu·en·zal (pōst′in-floo-en′zăl). Occurring as a sequel to influenza.

post·is·chi·al (pōst-is′kē-ăl). Posterior to the ischium.

post·ma·lar·i·al (pōst-mă-lār′ē-ăl). Occurring as a sequel to malaria.

post·mas·toid (pōst′mas′toyd). Posterior to the mastoid process.

post·ma·ture (pōst-mă-toor′, mă-tūr′). Referring to a fetus that remains in the uterus longer than the normal gestational period; i.e., longer than 42 weeks (288 days) in humans.

post·me·di·an (pōst′mē′dē-an). Posterior to the median plane.

post·me·di·as·ti·nal (pōst′mē′dē-as′ti-năl, -mē′dē-ă-stī′năl). **1.** Posterior to the mediastinum. **2.** Relating to the posterior mediastinum.

post·me·di·as·ti·num (pōst′mē′dē-ă-stī′nŭm). SYN posterior *mediastinum*.

post·men·o·pau·sal (pōst-men-ō-paw′săl). Relating to the period following the menopause.

post·min·i·mus (pōst-min′i-mŭs). A small accessory appendage attached to the side of the fifth finger or toe; it may resemble a normal digit or be merely a fleshy mass. [post- + L. *minimus*, smallest (finger)]

post·mor·tem (pōst-mōr′tem). **1.** Pertaining to or occurring during the period after death. **2.** Colloquialism for autopsy (1). [post- + L. acc. case of *mors* (*mort-*), death]

post·na·ri·al (pōst′nā′rē-ăl). Relating to the posterior nares or choanae.

post·na·ris (pōst′nā′ris). SYN choanae.

post·na·sal (pōst′nā′săl). **1.** Posterior to the nasal cavity. **2.** Relating to the posterior portion of the nasal cavity.

post·na·tal (pōst-nā′tăl). Occurring after birth. [L. *natus*, birth]

post·ne·crot·ic (post-ne-krot'ik). Subsequent to the death of a tissue or part of the body.

post·neu·rit·ic (pōst-noo-rit'ik). Following neuritis.

post·oc·u·lar (pōst'ok'ū-lăr). Posterior to the eyeball. [L. *oculus*, eye]

post·op·er·a·tive (pōst-op'er-ă-tiv). Following an operation.

post·o·ral (pos-tō'răl). In the posterior part of, or posterior to, the mouth. [L. *os* (*or-*), mouth]

post·or·bi·tal (pōst'ōr'bi-tăl). Posterior to the orbit.

post·pal·a·tine (pōst'pal'ă-tīn). Posterior to the palatine bones. Usually used to refer to the soft palate.

post·par·a·lyt·ic (pōst'par-ă-lit'ik). Following or consequent upon paralysis.

post·par·tum (pōst-par'tŭm). After childbirth. Cf. antepartum, intrapartum. [L. *partus*, birth (noun), fr. *pario*, pp. *partus*, to bring forth]

post·pha·ryn·ge·al (pōst'fă-rin'jē-ăl). Posterior to the pharynx.

post·pneu·mon·ic (pōst-noo-mon'ik). Following or occurring as a sequel to pneumonia.

post·pran·di·al (pōst-pran'dē-ăl). Following a meal. [L. *prandium*, breakfast]

post·pu·ber·al, post·pu·ber·tal (pōst-poo'ber-ăl, -ber-tăl). SYN postpubescent.

post·pu·ber·ty (pōst-poo'ber-tē). The period after puberty.

post·pu·bes·cent (pōst-poo-bes'ent). Subsequent to the period of puberty. SYN postpuberal, postpubertal.

post·pyk·not·ic (pōst-pik-not'ik). Following the stage of pyknosis in a red cell, denoting the disappearance of the nucleus (chromatolysis).

post·ro·lan·dic (pos'trō-lan'dik). Behind the fissure of Rolando, or central sulcus. SEE postcentral.

post·sa·cral (pōst'sā'krăl). Referring to the coccyx.

post·scap·u·lar (pōst-skap'ū-lăr). Posterior to the scapula.

post·scar·la·ti·nal (pōst'skar-lă-tē'năl). Occurring as a sequel to scarlatina.

post·sphyg·mic (pōst-sfig'mik). Occurring after the pulse wave. [G. *sphygmos*, pulse]

post·splen·ic (pōst'splen'ik). Posterior to the spleen.

post·syn·ap·tic (pōst-si-nap'tik). Pertaining to the area on the distal side of a synaptic cleft.

post·tar·sal (pōst'tar'săl). Relating to the posterior portion of the tarsus.

post·tec·ta (pōst'tek'tă). Aboral to the hidden part of the duodenum.

post·tib·i·al (pōst'tib'ē-ăl). Posterior to the tibia; situated in the posterior portion of the leg.

post·trans·crip·tion·al (pōst-tran-skrip'shŭn-al). Referring to events that occur after transcription.

post·trans·la·tion·al (pōst-trans-lā'shŭn-al). Referring to events that occur after translation.

post·trans·verse (pōst-tranz'vers). Behind a transverse process.

post·trau·mat·ic (pōst-traw-mat'ik). Occurring after trauma and, by implication, caused by it.

post·tre·mat·ic (pōst-trē-mat'ik). Relating to the caudal surface of a branchial cleft. [post- + G. *trēma*, perforation]

post·tus·sis (pōst-tŭs'is). After coughing; referring usually to certain auscultatory sounds. [L. *tussis*, cough]

post·ty·phoid (pōst-tī'foyd). Occurring as a sequel of typhoid fever.

pos·tu·late (pos'tū-lăt). A proposition that is taken as self-evident or assumed without proof as a basis for further analysis. SEE ALSO hypothesis, theory. [L. *postulo*, pp. *-atus*, to demand]

Ampère p., SYN Avogadro *law*.

Avogadro p., SYN Avogadro *law*.

Ehrlich p., SYN side-chain *theory*.

Koch p.'s, to establish the specificity of a pathogenic microorganism, it must be present in all cases of the disease, inoculations of its pure cultures must produce disease in animals, and from these it must be again obtained and be propagated in pure cultures. SYN Koch law.

pos·tur·al (pos'tū-răl, pos'cher-ăl). Relating to or affected by posture.

pos·ture (pos'choor, pos'cher). The position of the limbs or the carriage of the body as a whole. [L. *positura*, fr. *pono*, pp. *positus*, to place]

Stern p., a supine position with the head extended and lowered over the end of the table, by which the murmur is developed or made more distinct in cases of tricuspid insufficiency.

pos·tur·og·ra·phy (pos-tyur-og'ra-fē). SYN dynamic p. [posture + G. *graphō*, to write]

dynamic p., a measurement of postural stability under varying visual and proprioceptive inputs. SYN posturography.

post·u·ter·ine (pōst-ū'ter-in). Posterior to the uterus.

post·vac·ci·nal (pōst-vak'si-năl). After vaccination.

post·val·var, post·val·vu·lar (pōst-val'văr, -val'vū-lăr). Relating to a position distal to the pulmonary or aortic valves.

po·ta·ble (pō'tă-bl). Drinkable; fit to drink. [L. *potabilis*, fr. *poto*, to drink]

Potain, Pierre C.E., French physician, 1825–1901. SEE P. *sign*.

pot·a·mo·pho·bia (pot'ă-mō-fō'bē-ă). Morbid fears aroused by the sight, and sometimes thought, of a river or any flow of water. [G. *potamos*, river, + *phobos*, fear]

pot·ash. Impure potassium carbonate. SYN pearl-ash. [E. pot-ashes]

caustic p., SYN *potassium* hydroxide.

sulfurated p., a mixture composed chiefly of potassium polysulfides and potassium thiosulfate; used externally in scabies, acne, and psoriasis; used in the manufacture of "white lotion." SYN liver of sulfur.

po·tas·sic (pŏ-tas'ik). Relating to or containing potassium.

po·tas·si·um (K) (pō-tas'ē-ŭm). An alkaline metallic element, atomic no. 19, atomic wt. 39.0983, occurring abundantly in nature but always in combination; its salts are used medicinally. For organic p. salts not listed below, see the name of the anion. SYN kalium. [Mod. L., fr. Eng. potash (fr. pot + ashes) + *-ium*]

p. acetate, a diuretic, diaphoretic, and systemic and urinary alkalizer. SYN sal diureticum.

p. acid tartrate, SYN p. bitartrate.

p. alum, SYN *aluminum* potassium sulfate.

p. aminosalicylate, SEE *p*-aminosalicylic acid.

p. antimonyltartrate, SYN *antimony* potassium tartrate.

p. atractylate, the p. salt of atractylic acid, the natural source of the latter.

p. bicarbonate, used as a diuretic to decrease the acidity of the urine and as an electrolyte replenisher.

p. bitartrate, a diuretic and laxative. SYN cream of tartar, p. acid tartrate.

p. bromide, KBr; an obsolescent sedative and hypnotic (sodium bromide is usually preferred).

p. chlorate, chlorate of potash, $KClO_3$, used as a mouthwash and gargle in stomatitis and follicular pharyngitis; it is incompatible in the dry state with all easily oxidizable substances.

p. chloride, used to correct p. deficiency.

p. citrate, a deliquescent powder, soluble in water; used as a diuretic, diaphoretic, expectorant, and systemic and urinary alkalizer. SYN Rivière salt.

p. cyanide, a commercial fumigant.

dibasic p. phosphate, SYN p. phosphate.

p. dichromate, p. bichromate, used externally as an astringent, antiseptic, and caustic; a strong oxidizing agent to be handled with care.

effervescent p. citrate, a mixture of p. citrate, citric acid, sodium bicarbonate, and tartaric acid; used as a gastric antacid and urinary alkalizer.

p. ferrocyanide, yellow prussiate of potash, used in the preparation of various cyanides and in medicine as an antidote to copper sulfate.

p. gluconate, gluconic acid p. salt, used in hypokalemia as a replenisher.

p. guaiacolsulfonate, used as an expectorant.

p. hydroxide, KOH; a strong, penetrating caustic. SYN caustic potash.

p. hypophosphite, formerly believed to have a tonic effect upon the nervous system; may be explosive if triturated or heated with oxidizing agents.

p. iodate, an oxidizing agent and disinfectant.

p. iodide, KI; used as an alterative and expectorant, and in certain mycoses.

p. metaphosphate, a pharmaceutic aid (buffer).

monobasic p. phosphate, used as a urinary acidifier and buffer.

p. nitrate, sometimes used as a diuretic and diaphoretic; formerly it was included in asthmatic powders containing stramonium leaves. SYN niter, saltpeter.

penicillin G p., SEE *penicillin* G potassium.

p. perchlorate, occasionally used, as an alternative to a thiouracil derivative, in the control of hyperthyroidism.

p. permanganate, a strong oxidizing agent, used in solution as an antiseptic and deodorizing application for foul lesions, and formerly as a gastric lavage in poisoning from morphine, strychnine, aconite, and picrotoxin; in electron microscopy, it stains cytomembranes well and gives results similar to lead hydroxide staining; also used as a fixative (Luft).

p. phosphate, a mild saline cathartic and diuretic. SYN dibasic p. phosphate, dipotassium phosphate.

p. rhodanate, SYN p. thiocyanate.

p. sodium tartrate, a mild saline cathartic, used as an ingredient in compound effervescent powders. SYN Rochelle salt, Seignette salt, sodium potassium tartrate.

p. sorbate, 2,4-hexadienoic acid potassium salt; a mold and yeast inhibitor, used as a preservative.

p. succinate, a deliquescent powder used as a hemostatic.

p. sulfate, an obsolete laxative.

p. sulfocyanate, SYN p. thiocyanate.

p. tartrate, a mild purgative and diuretic. SYN soluble tartar.

p. thiocyanate, formerly used in the treatment of essential hypertension and as a reagent in the detection of copper, iron, and silver. SYN p. rhodanate, p. sulfocyanate.

potassium-39 (^{39}**K**). Most abundant, nonradioactive isotope of potassium; accounts for 93.1% of natural potassium.

po·tas·si·um-40 (^{40}**K**). A naturally occurring (0.0117%) radioactive potassium isotope; beta emitter with half-life of 1.26 billion years; chief source of natural radioactivity of living tissue.

po·tas·si·um-42 (^{42}**K**). An artificial potassium isotope; beta emitter with half-life of 12.36 hr, used as a tracer in studies of potassium distribution in body fluid compartments and in localization of brain tumors.

po·tas·si·um-43 (^{43}**K**). An artificial potassium isotope; a beta emitter with a half-life of 22.3 hr, used as a tracer in myocardial perfusion studies.

po·ten·cy (pō'ten-sē). **1.** Power, force, or strength; the condition or quality of being potent. **2.** Specifically, sexual p. **3.** In therapeutics, the relative pharmacologic activity of a dose of a compound compared with the dose of a different agent producing the same effects; e.g., aspirin and acetaminophen are of equal potency in alleviating headache (same dose required), but ketorolac exhibits greater potency than ibuprofen, as 20 mg of the former is as effective as 400 mg of the latter. [L. *potentia,* power]

sexual p., the ability to carry out and consummate sexual intercourse, usually referring to the male.

po·tent (pō'tent). **1.** Possessing force, power, strength. **2.** Indicating the ability of a primitive cell to differentiate. SEE ALSO totipotent, pluripotent, unipotent. **3.** In psychiatry, possessing sexual potency.

po·ten·tial (pō-ten'shăl). **1.** Capable of doing or being, although not yet doing or being; possible, but not actual. **2.** A state of tension in an electric source enabling it to do work under suitable conditions; in relation to electricity, p. is analogous to the temperature in relation to heat. [L. *potentia,* power, potency]

action p., the change in membrane p. occurring in nerve, muscle, or other excitable tissue when excitation occurs.

after-p., SEE afterpotential.

bioelectric p., electrical p.'s occurring in living organisms.

biotic p., a theoretical measurement of the capacity of a species to survive or to compete successfully.

brain p., the electrical charge of the brain as compared to a point on the body; the p. may be steady (DC p.) or may fluctuate at specific frequencies when recorded against time, giving rise to the electroencephalogram.

brainstem auditory evoked p., responses triggered by click stimuli, which are generated in the acoustic nerve and brainstem auditory pathways; recorded over the scalp.

chemical p. (μ), a measure of how the Gibbs free energy of a phase depends on any change in the composition of that phase.

cochlear p., SYN cochlear microphonic.

compound action p., the combined p.'s resulting from activation of the auditory division of the eighth cranial nerve.

demarcation p., the difference in p. recorded when one electrode is placed on intact nerve fibers or muscle fibers and the other electrode is placed on the injured ends of the same fibers; the intact portion is positive with reference to the injured portion. SYN injury p.

early receptor p. (ERP), a voltage arising across the eye from a charge displacement within photoreceptor pigment, in response to an intense flash of light.

endocochlear p., the standing direct current p. in the endolymph relative to the perilymph, measuring positive 80 mV.

evoked p., an event-related potential, elicited by, and time-locked to, a stimulus. SEE ALSO evoked *response.*

excitatory junction p. (EJP), discrete partial depolarization of smooth muscle produced by stimulation of excitatory nerves; similar to small end-plate p.'s. summate with repeated stimuli.

excitatory postsynaptic p. (EPSP), the change in p. that is produced in the membrane of the next neuron when an impulse that has an excitatory influence arrives at the synapse; it is a local change in the direction of depolarization; summation of these p.'s can lead to discharge of an impulse by the neuron.

generator p., local depolarization of the membrane p. at the end of a sensory neurone in graded response to the strength of a stimulus applied to the associated receptor organ, e.g., a pacinian corpuscle; if the generator p. becomes large enough (because the stimulus is at least of threshold strength), it causes excitation at the nearest node of Ranvier and a propagated action p.

inhibitory junction p. (IJP), hyperpolarization of smooth muscle produced by stimulation of inhibitory nerves.

inhibitory postsynaptic p. (IPSP), the change in p. produced in the membrane of the next neuron when an impulse that has an inhibitory influence arrives at the synapse; it is a local change in the direction of hyperpolarization; the frequency of discharge of a given neuron is determined by the extent to which impulses that lead to excitatory postsynaptic p.'s predominate over those that cause inhibitory postsynaptic p.'s.

injury p., SYN demarcation p.

membrane p., the p. inside a cell membrane, measured relative to the fluid just outside; it is negative under resting conditions and becomes positive during an action p. SYN transmembrane p.

myogenic p., action p. of muscle.

oscillatory p., the variable voltage in the positive deflection of the electroretinogram (β-wave) of the dark-adapted eye arising from amacrine cells.

Ottoson p., SYN electroolfactogram.

oxidation-reduction p. (E_0^+), the p. in volts of an inert metallic electrode measured in a system of an arbitrarily chosen ratio of [oxidant] to [reductant] and referred to the normal hydrogen electrode at absolute temperature; it is calculated from the following equation; where R is the gas constant expressed in electrical units, T the absolute temperature (Kelvin), n the number of electrons transferred, F the faraday, and E_0 the normal symbol for the p. of the system at pH 0; for biologic systems, E_0' is often used (in which pH = 7). Cf. Nernst *equation.* SYN redox p.

po

pacemaker p., the voltage inscribed by impulses from an artificial electronic pacemaker.

redox p., SYN oxidation-reduction p.

S p., prolonged, slow, depolarizing or hyperpolarizing responses to illumination; initiated between the photoreceptor and ganglion cell layers of the retina.

somatosensory evoked p., the computer-averaged cortical and subcortical responses to repetitive stimulation of peripheral nerve sensory fibers.

spike p., the main wave in the action p. of a nerve; it is followed by negative and positive afterpotentials.

summating p.'s, alternating current responses of the organ of Corti to acoustic stimulation.

thermodynamic p., SEE free *energy.*

transmembrane p., SYN membrane p.

ventricular late p., high-frequency microvolt electrocardiogram signals at the end of the QRS complex.

visual evoked p., voltage fluctuations that may be recorded from the occipital area of the scalp as the result of retinal stimulation by a light flashing at $1/4$-s intervals; commonly summated and averaged by computer.

zeta p., the degree of negative charge on the surface of a red blood cell; i.e., the p. difference between the negative charges on the red cell and the cation in the fluid portion of the blood.

zoonotic p., the p. for infections of subhuman animals to be transmissible to humans.

po·ten·ti·a·tion (pō-ten′shē-ā′shŭn). Interaction between two or more drugs or agents resulting in a pharmacologic response greater than the sum of individual responses to each drug or agent.

po·ten·ti·a·tor (pō-ten′shē-ā-ter, -tōr). In chemotherapy, a drug used in combination with other drugs to produce deliberate potentiation.

po·ten·ti·om·e·ter (pō-ten-shē-om′ĕ-ter). **1.** An instrument used for measuring small differences in electrical potential. **2.** An electrical resistor of fixed total resistance between two terminals, but with a third terminal attached to a slider that can make contact at any desired point along the resistance. [L. *potentia,* power, + G. *metron,* measure]

po·tion (pō′shŭn). A draft or large dose of liquid medicine. [L. *potio, potus,* fr. *poto,* to drink]

Pott, Sir Percivall, English surgeon, 1714–1788. SEE P. *abscess, aneurysm, curvature, disease, fracture, paralysis, paraplegia.*

Potter, Edith L., U.S. perinatal pathologist, *1901. SEE P. *disease, facies, syndrome.*

Potter, Irving White, U.S. obstetrician, 1868–1956. SEE P. *version.*

Potts, Willis J., U.S. pediatric surgeon, 1895–1968. SEE P. *anastomosis, clamp, operation.*

pouch (powch). A pocket or cul-de-sac. SEE ALSO fossa, recess, sac.

antral p., a p. made in the antrum of the stomach of experimental animals.

branchial p.'s, SYN pharyngeal p.'s.

Broca p., SYN pudendal *sac.*

deep perineal p., SYN deep perineal *space.*

Denis Browne p., a pocket formed between Scarpa and external oblique fascia adjacent to external inguinal ring; a common lodging site for undescended testes (as in cryptorchism). SYN superficial inguinal p.

p. of Douglas, SYN rectouterine p.

Douglas p., SYN rectouterine p.

endodermal p.'s, SYN pharyngeal p.'s.

Hartmann p., a spheroid or conical p. at the junction of the neck of the gallbladder and the cystic duct. SYN ampulla of gallbladder, fossa provesicalis, pelvis of gallbladder.

Heidenhain p., a small sac or p. of the stomach, vagally denervated and closed off from the main cavity but with an opening through the abdominal wall, fashioned for the purpose of obtaining gastric juice and for studying gastric secretion in physiologic experiments.

hepatorenal p., SYN hepatorenal *recess* of subhepatic space.

hypophyseal p., SYN pituitary *diverticulum.*

ileoanal p. (il′ē-ō-ā′nal), a p. constructed from the ileum and anastomosed to the proximal anus for restoration of continence after proctocolectomy.

Kock p., a continent ileostomy with a reservoir and valved opening fashioned from doubled loops of ileum. SYN Kock ileostomy.

laryngeal p., SYN laryngeal *saccule.*

Morison p., SYN hepatorenal *recess* of subhepatic space.

paracystic p., SYN paravesical *fossa.*

pararectal p., SYN pararectal *fossa.*

paravesical p., SYN paravesical *fossa.*

Pavlov p., a section of the stomach of a dog, retaining its vagal innervation but shut off from all communication with the main part of the organ and connected with the outside by a fistula; used in studies of gastric secretions. SYN miniature stomach, Pavlov stomach.

pharyngeal p.'s, paired evaginations of embryonic pharyngeal endoderm, between the branchial arches, extending toward the corresponding ectodermally lined branchial grooves; during development they evolve into epithelial tissues and organs, such as thymus and thyroid glands. SYN branchial p.'s, endodermal p.'s.

Physick p.'s, proctitis with mucous discharge and burning pain, involving especially the sacculations between the rectal valves.

Prussak p., SYN superior *recess* of tympanic membrane.

Rathke p., SYN pituitary *diverticulum.*

rectouterine p. [TA], a pocket formed by the deflection of the peritoneum from the rectum to the uterus. SYN excavatio rectouterina [TA], cavum douglasi, cul-de-sac (2), Douglas cul-de-sac, Douglas p., p. of Douglas, rectovaginouterine p.

rectovaginouterine p., SYN rectouterine p.

rectovesical p. [TA], a pocket formed by the deflection of the peritoneum from the rectum to the bladder in the male. SYN excavatio rectovesicalis [TA], Proust space.

Seessel p., SEE Seessel *pocket.*

superficial inguinal p., SYN Denis Browne p.

superficial perineal p., SYN superficial perineal *space.*

ultimobranchial p., a transient fifth pharyngeal p.; it is now considered to be incorporated into the caudal pharyngeal complex, the cells of which become the parafollicular cells (C cells) of the thyroid.

uterovesical p., SYN vesicouterine p.

vesicouterine p. [TA], a pocket formed by the deflection of the peritoneum from the bladder to the body of the uterus in the female. SYN excavatio vesicouterina [TA], cavum vesicouterinum, uterovesical p.

Willis p., obsolete term for lesser *omentum*

pouch·i·tis (pow-chī′tis). Acute inflammation of the mucosa of an ileal reservoir or pouch that has been surgically created, usually following total colectomy for inflammatory bowel disease or multiple polyposis. [pouch + -*itis,* inflammation]

pou·drage (poo-drahzh′). **1.** Powdering. **2.** SYN talc *operation.* [F.]

pleural p., covering the opposing pleural surfaces with a slightly irritating powder in order to secure adhesion.

poul·tice (pōl′tis). A soft magma or mush prepared by wetting various powders or other absorbent substances with oily or watery fluids, sometimes medicated, and usually applied hot to the surface; it exerts an emollient, relaxing, or stimulant, counterirritant effect upon the skin and underlying tissues. SYN cataplasm. [L. *puls* (*pult-*), a thick pap; G. *poltos*]

pound (pownd). A unit of weight, containing 12 ounces, apothecaries' weight, or 16 ounces, avoirdupois. [A.S. *pund;* L. *pondus,* weight]

pound·al (pownd′ăl). The force required to give a mass of 1 lb an acceleration of 1 ft/s^2; equal to 0.138255 N.

Poupart, François, French anatomist, 1616–1708. SEE P. *ligament, line.*

po·vi·done (pō′vi-dōn). A synthetic polymer consisting mainly of linear 1-vinyl-2-pyrrolidone groups, with mean molecular weights ranging from 10,000 to 70,000; used as a dispersing and suspending agent; p. with molecular weight between 20,000 and 40,000 has been used as a plasma extender. It is not metabolized, but is excreted unchanged by the kidney. SYN polyvidone, polyvinylpyrrolidone.

po·vi·done-io·dine. SYN povidone *iodine.*

pow·der. 1. A dry mass of minute separate particles of any substance. **2.** In pharmaceutics, a homogenous dispersion of finely divided, relatively dry, particulate matter consisting of one or more substances; the degree of fineness of a p. is related to passage of the material through standard sieves. **3.** A single dose of a powdered drug, enclosed in an envelope of folded paper. **4.** To reduce a solid substance to a state of very fine division. [Fr. *poudre;* L. *pulvis*]

bleaching p., SYN chlorinated *lime.*

pow·er (pŏw'er). **1.** In optics, the refractive vergence of a lens. **2.** In physics and engineering, the rate at which work is done. **3.** The exponent of a number or expression that provides the number of times that number has to be multiplied by itself.

back vertex p., the effective p. of a lens as measured from a surface toward the eye; a standard for measurement of ophthalmic lenses.

carbon dioxide combining p., a measurement of the total CO_2 that can be bound as HCO_3^- at a PCO_2 of 40 mmHg at 25°C by serum, plasma, or whole blood.

equivalent p., the p. equal to an infinitely thin lens as measured on an optical bench.

resolving p., (1) definition of a lens; in a microscope objective lens it is calculated by dividing the wavelength of the light used by twice the numerical aperture of the objective. SEE ALSO definition; **(2)** analogies to other modalities, e.g., two-point discrimination in neurologic examination. Commonly misinterpreted as random error, although it has none of its properties. **(3)** SYN resolution (2).

statistical p., in Neyman-Pearson hypothesis testing, the probability of rejecting the null hypothesis when it is false; the complement of an *error* of the second kind.

pox (poks). **1.** An eruptive disease, usually qualified by a descriptive prefix; e.g., smallpox, cowpox, chickenpox. See the specific term. **2.** Archaic or colloquial term for syphilis. [var. of pl. *pocks*]

Kaffir p., SYN alastrim.

Pox·vir·i·dae (poks-vir'i-dē). A family of large complex viruses, with a marked affinity for skin tissue, that are pathogenic for humans and other animals. Virions are large, up to 250×400 nm, and enveloped (double membranes). Replication occurs entirely in the cytoplasm of infected cells. Capsids are of complex symmetry and contain double-stranded DNA (MW 160×10^6), the nucleoprotein antigen being common to all members of the family. A number of genera are recognized, including: Orthopoxvirus, Avipoxvirus, Capripoxvirus, Leporipoxvirus, and Parapoxvirus.

pox·vi·rus (poks'vī-rŭs). Any virus of the family Poxviridae.

p. officina'lis, SYN vaccinia *virus.*

Pozzi, Samuel J., French gynecologist and anatomist, 1846–1918. SEE P. *muscle.*

PP Abbreviation for pyrophosphate.

PP$_i$ Abbreviation for inorganic pyrophosphate (diphosphate).

P.p. Abbreviation for *punctum* proximum.

ppb Abbreviation for parts per billion.

PPCA Abbreviation for proserum prothrombin conversion *accelerator.*

PPCF Abbreviation for plasmin prothrombins conversion *factor.*

PPD Abbreviation for purified protein derivative of *tuberculin.*

PPLO Abbreviation for pleuropneumonia-like *organisms,* under *organism.*

ppm Abbreviation for parts per million.

PPO Abbreviation for 2,5-diphenyloxazole, a liquid scintillator; preferred provider *organization.*

PPPPPP A mnemonic of 6 Ps designating the symptom complex of acute arterial occlusion. [*p*ain, *p*allor, *p*aresthesia, *p*ulselessness, *p*aralysis, *p*rostration]

PPRibp, PPRP Abbreviation for 5-phospho-α-D-ribosyl-1-pyrophosphate.

P pul·mo·na·le (pul-mō-nā'lā). Tall, narrow, peaked P waves in electrocardiographic leads II, III, and aVF, and often a prominent initial positive P wave component in V_1, presumed to be characteristic of cor pulmonale. (Although this term is extensively used in the electrocardiographic literature, it is actually a misnomer and would be more appropriately called P-dextrocardiale, since it results from overload of the right atrium regardless of the cause, as in tricuspid stenosis, and may occur independently of cor pulmonale.) In lung disease, P-pulmonale is usually transient, occurring during exacerbations, usually asthmatic.

PQ Abbreviation for plastoquinone.

PQ-9 Abbreviation for plastoquinone-9.

P.r. Abbreviation for *punctum* remotum.

Pr 1. Abbreviation for presbyopia. **2.** Symbol for praseodymium; propyl.

PRA Abbreviation for plasma renin *activity;* phosphoribosylamine.

prac·tice (prak'tis). The exercise of the profession of medicine or one of the allied health professions. [Mediev. L. *practica,* business, G. *praktikos,* pertaining to action]

extramural p., delivery of health care services by university faculties or full-time hospital staff to persons beyond the physical confines of their respective medical centers.

family p., a specialty of medicine in which the physician takes responsibility for the health and medical care of all members of a family group, regardless of age or gender, but usually does limited amounts of obstetrics and surgery.

general p., a relatively obsolete term for physicians who care for all types of medical problems, including internal medical, pediatric, obstetrical, and surgical diseases. Postgraduate training for general practitioners was limited and there was no specialty certification; the field has been replaced by more extensively trained family practitioners.

group p., the cooperative p. of medicine by a group of physicians, each of whom as a rule specializes in some particular field; such a group often shares a common suite of consulting rooms, laboratories, staff, equipment, etc.

intramural p., delivery of health care services by university faculties or full-time hospital staff conducted within the physical confines of their respective medical centers.

prac·ti·tion·er (prak-tish'ŭn-er). A person who practices medicine or one of the allied health care professions.

Prader, Andrea, Swiss pediatrician, *1919. SEE P.-Willi *syndrome.*

△**prae-.** SEE pre-.

prag·mat·ics (prag-mat'iks). A branch of semiotics; the theory that deals with the relation between signs and their users, both senders and receivers. [G. *pragmatikos,* fr. *pragma,* thing done]

prag·ma·tism (prag'mă-tizm). A philosophy emphasizing practical applications and consequences of beliefs and theories, that the meaning of ideas or things is determined by the testability of the idea in real life. [G. *pragma* (*pragmat-*), thing done]

2-pra·li·dox·ime (2-PAM). One of several oximes that are effective in reversing cholinesterase inhibition by organophosphates. The 2-PAM facilitates the hydrolysis of the phosphorylated enzyme so as to regenerate active cholinesterase.

pral·i·dox·ime chlo·ride (pral-i-dok'sēm, prā-li-). Used to restore the inactivated cholinesterase activity resulting from organophosphate poisoning; has some limited value as an antagonist of the carbamate type of cholinesterase inhibitors that are used in the treatment of myasthenia gravis. Dizziness, blurred vision, drowsiness, nausea, tachycardia, and muscular weakness may occur.

pra·mox·ine hy·dro·chlo·ride (pră-mok'sēn, -sin). A nonester, nonamide local anesthetic for dermal and rectal use.

pran·di·al (pran'dē-ăl). Relating to a meal. [L. *prandium,* breakfast]

pra·se·o·dym·i·um (Pr) (prā-sē-ō-dim'ē-ŭm). An element of the lanthanide or "rare earth" group; atomic no. 59, atomic wt.

140.90765. [G. *prasios,* leekgreen, fr. *prason,* a leek, + *didymos,* twin]

Pratt, Joseph H., U.S. physician, 1872–1956. SEE P. *symptom.*

Prausnitz, Otto Carl, German hygienist, 1876–1963. SEE P.-Küstner *antibody, reaction;* reversed P. *reaction.*

prav·a·sta·tin. An inhibitor of the enzyme 3-hydroxy-3-methyglutaryl coenzyme A (HMG-CoA), the rate-limiting enzyme in the biosynthesis of cholesterol; used in the treatment of hypercholesteremia; similar to lovastatin and simvastatin.

prax·i·ol·o·gy (prak-sē-ol′ō-jē). The science or study of behavior; it excludes the study of consciousness and similiar nonobjective metaphysical concepts. [G. *praxis,* action, + *logos,* study]

prax·is (prak′sis). The performance of an action. [G. *praxis,* action]

pra·ze·pam (prā′zē-pam). An antianxiety agent of the benzodiazepine class; a prodrug for nordiazepam.

pra·zi·quan·tel (prā-zi-kwahn′tel). A pyrazinoisoquinoline derivative; a synthetic heterocyclic broad-spectrum anthelmintic agent effective against all schistosome species parasitic of humans as well as most other trematodes and adult cestodes.

pra·zo·sin hy·dro·chlo·ride (prā′zō-sin). An antihypertensive agent, which is an α_1-specific adrenergic blocking drug.

△**pre-.** Anterior; before (in time or space). SEE ALSO ante-, pro- (1). [L. *prae*]

pre·ag·o·nal (prē-ag′ō-năl). Immediately preceding death. [pre- + G. *agōn,* struggle (agony)]

pre·al·bu·min (prē-al-bū′min). **1.** A protein component of plasma having a molecular weight of about 55,000 and containing 1.3% carbohydrate; estimated plasma concentration is 0.3 g per 100 mL; abnormal levels of p. are found in cases of familial amyloidosis. SYN transthyretin. **2.** The protein-containing zone observed in zone electrophoresis of serum that migrates more rapidly than serum albumin.

thyroxine-binding p. (TBPA), a protein located in the "prealbumin" zone upon electrophoretic analysis of plasma proteins; its affinity for binding thyroxine is less than that of thyroxine-binding globulin but greater than that of albumin. SYN thyroxine-binding protein (2).

pre·a·nal (prē-ā′năl). Anterior to the anus.

pre·an·es·thet·ic (prē-an-es-thet′ik). Before anesthesia.

pre·an·ti·sep·tic (prē′an-ti-sep′tik). Denoting the period, especially in relation to surgery, before the adoption of the principles of antisepsis.

pre·a·or·tic (prē′ā-ōr′tik). Anterior to the aorta; denoting certain lymph nodes so situated.

pre·a·sep·tic (prē-ă-sep′tik). Denoting the period, especially the early antiseptic period in relation to surgery, before the principles of asepsis were known or adopted.

pre·au·ric·u·lar (prē-aw-rik′ū-lăr). Anterior to the auricle of the ear; denoting lymphatic nodes so situated.

pre·ax·i·al (prē-ak′sē-ăl). **1.** Anterior to the axis of the body or a limb, the latter being in the anatomical position. **2.** Denoting the portion of a limb bud that lies cranial to the axis of the limb: the radial aspect of the upper limb and the tibial aspect of the lower limb.

pre·cal·cif·er·ol (prē-kal-si′fer-ol). The immediate precursor of ergocalciferol and lumisterol.

ℹ**pre·can·cer** (prē-kan′ser). A lesion from which a malignant neoplasm is believed to develop in a significant number of instances, and which may or may not be recognizable clinically or by microscopic changes in the affected tissue.

pre·can·cer·ous (prē-kan′ser-ŭs). Pertaining to any lesion that is interpreted as precancer. SYN premalignant.

pre·cap·il·lary (prē-kap′i-lār-ē). Preceding a capillary; an arteriole or venule.

pre·car·di·ac (prē-kar′dē-ak). Anterior to the heart.

pre·car·di·nal (prē-kar′di-năl). Relating to the anterior cardinal veins.

pre·car·ti·lage (prē-kar′ti-lij). A closely packed aggregation of

precancers		
organ or tissue system	**preneoplasm**	**later malignancy**
A) chronic irritation		
skin	photodermatitis	"light cancer"
	x-ray dermatitis	x-ray cancer
	tar dermatitis	pitch-worker's cancer
	arsenic dermatitis	arsenic cancer
	lupus dermatitis	lupus cancer
	senile keratosis	
	Paget disease	skin cancer
	condylomata	
scars	burn scar	
	syphilitic scar	scar cancer
	fistula scar	
	ulcus cruris scar	
ulcers	chronic ulcer	ulcer cancer
	varicose ulcer	
	bone fistula	fistula cancer
	rectal fistula	
esophagus	Barrett esophagus	squamous metaplasia
stomach	gastric ulcer	carcinoma ex ulcere
	gastritis	
liver, gallbladder	cholelithiasis	adenocarcinoma, scirrhous carcinoma, gallbladder carcinoma
vagina	kraurosis vulvae	vulvar carcinoma
B) systemic diseases, tissue deformities, benign neoplasms		
skin	nevus pigmentosus	malignant melanoma
	Bowen dermatosis	
	xeroderma pigmentosum	skin carcinomas and sarcomas
	erythroplasia	
mucous membrane	leukoplakia	tongue cancer
		cheek cancer
		palate cancer
		penis cancer
bones	Paget disease of bone	osteosarcoma
	exostoses	chondrosarcoma
	ecchondroma	
	osteitis fibrosa	osteosarcoma
	leontiasis ossea	osteosarcoma
nervous system	neurofibromatosis	fibrosarcoma
stomach/intestine	polyposis	adenocarcinoma
uterus	hydatidiform mole	chorionic epithelioma
	adenomatous hyperplasia	cancers of uterus and cervix
	carcinoma *in situ*	
thyroid gland	struma nodosa	thyroid cancer

mesenchymal cells just prior to their differentiation into embryonic cartilage.

precautions.

pre·ca·va (prē-kā′vă). SYN superior *vena cava.*

pre·cen·tral (prē-sen′trăl). Referring to the cerebral convolution immediately anterior to the central sulcus: precentral gyrus.

pre·chor·dal (prē-kōr′dăl). SYN prochordal.

pre·chrom·ing (prē-krōm′ing). Treatment of a tissue or fabric first with a metal mordant, followed by a dye.

pre·cip·i·ta·ble (prē-sip′i-tă-bl). Capable of being precipitated.

pre·cip·i·tant (prē-sip′i-tant). Anything causing a precipitation from a solution.

pre·cip·i·tate (prē-sip′i-tāt). **1.** To cause a substance in solution to separate as a solid. **2.** A solid separated out from a solution or suspension; a floc or clump, such as that resulting from the mixture of a specific antigen and its antibody. **3.** Accumulation of inflammatory cells on the corneal endothelium in uveitis (keratic precipitates). [L. *praecipito,* pp. *-atus,* to cast headlong]

keratic p.'s, inflammatory cells on the corneal endothelium. SYN punctate keratitis, keratitis punctata.

mutton-fat keratic p.'s, coalescent p.'s forming small plaques that gradually become more translucent.

pigmented keratic p.'s, p.'s that occur in eyes with brown irides or after prolonged inflammation.

red p., SYN mercuric oxide, red.

sweet p., SYN calomel.

white mercuric p., SYN ammoniated *mercury.*

yellow p., SYN mercuric oxide, yellow.

pre·cip·i·ta·tion (prē-sip-i-tā′shŭn). **1.** The process of formation of a solid previously held in solution or suspension in a liquid. **2.** The phenomenon of clumping of proteins in serum produced by the addition of a specific precipitin. [see precipitate]

double antibody p., a method of separating antibody-bound antigen (e.g., insulin) from free antigen by precipitating the former with antibody specific for immunoglobulin. SYN double antibody immunoassay, double antibody method.

immune p., SYN immunoprecipitation.

pre·cip·i·tin (prē-sip′i-tin). An antibody that under suitable conditions combines with and causes its specific and soluble antigen to precipitate from solution. SYN precipitating antibody.

pre·cip·i·tin·o·gen (prē-sip-i-tin′ō-jen). **1.** An antigen that stimulates the formation of specific precipitin when injected into an animal body. **2.** A precipitable soluble antigen. SYN precipitogen. [precipitin + G. -*gen,* producing]

pre·cip·i·tin·o·ge·noid (prē-sip-i-tin′ō-jĕ-noyd). A precipitinogen that is altered by means of heating, thereby resulting in a substance that combines with the specific precipitin, but does not lead to the formation of a precipitate.

pre·cip·i·to·gen (prē-sip′i-tō-jen). SYN precipitinogen.

pre·cip·i·toid (prē-sip′i-toyd). A heat-treated precipitin that when mixed with specific precipitinogen does not cause a precipitate and also interferes with the precipitating effect of additional nonheated precipitin. [precipitin + G. *eidos,* resemblance]

pre·cip·i·to·phore (prē-sip′i-tō-fōr). In Ehrlich side chain theory, the portion of a precipitin molecule that is required in the formation of a precipitate, as distinguished from the haptophore group. [precipitin + G. *phoros,* bearing]

pre·ci·sion (prē-sĭ′zhun). **1.** The quality of being sharply defined or stated; one measure of precision is the number of distinguishable alternatives to a measurement. **2.** In statistics, the inverse of the variance of a measurement or estimate. **3.** Reproducibility of a quantifiable result; an indication of the random error.

pre·clin·i·cal (prē-klin′i-kăl). **1.** Before the onset of disease. **2.** A period in medical education before the student becomes involved with patients and clinical work.

pre·co·cious (prē-kō′shŭs). Developing unusually early or rapidly. [L. *praecox,* premature]

pre·coc·i·ty (prē-kos′i-tē). Unusually early or rapid development of mental or physical traits. [see precocious]

pre·cog·ni·tion (prē-kog-nish′ŭn). Advance knowledge, by means other than the normal senses, of a future event; a form of extrasensory perception. [L. *praecogito,* to ponder before]

pre·con·scious (prē-kon′shŭs). In psychoanalysis, one of the three divisions of the psyche according to Freud's topographic psychology, the other two being the conscious and unconscious; includes all ideas, thoughts, past experiences, and other memory impressions that with effort can be consciously recalled. Cf. foreconscious.

pre·con·vul·sive (prē-kon-vŭl′siv). Denoting the stage in an epileptic paroxysm preceding convulsions (e.g., aura).

pre·cor·dia (prē-kōr′dē-ă). The epigastrium and anterior surface of the lower part of the thorax. SYN antecardium. [L. *praecordia* (ntr. pl. only), the diaphragm, the entrails, fr. *prae,* before, + *cor* (*cord-*), heart]

pre·cor·di·al (prē-kōr′dē-ăl). Relating to the precordia.

pre·cor·di·al·gia (prē′kōr-dē-al′jē-ă). Pain in the precordial region. [precordia + G. *algos,* pain]

pre·cor·di·um (prē-kōr′dē-ŭm). Singular of precordia.

pre·cos·tal (prē-kos′tăl). Anterior to the ribs. [pre- + L. *costa,* rib]

pre·crit·i·cal (prē-krit′i-kăl). Relating to the phase before a crisis.

pre·cu·ne·al (prē-koo′nē-ăl). Anterior to the cuneus.

pre·cu·ne·ate (prē-koo′nē-āt). Relating to the precuneus.

pre·cu·ne·us (prē-koo′nē-ŭs) [TA]. A division of the medial surface of each cerebral hemisphere between the cuneus and the paracentral lobule; it lies above the subparietal sulcus and is bounded anteriorly by the marginal branch of the cingulate sulcus and posteriorly by the parietooccipital sulcus. SYN lobulus quadratus (2), quadrate lobe (3), quadrate lobule (2). [pre- + L. *cuneus,* a wedge]

pre·cur·sor (prē-ker′ser). That which precedes another or from which another is derived, applied especially to a physiologically inactive substance that is converted to an active enzyme, vitamin, hormone, etc., or to a chemical substance that is built into a larger structure in the course of synthesizing the latter. [L. *praecursor,* fr. *prae-,* pre- + *curro,* to run]

pre·den·tin (prē-den′tin). The organic fibrillar matrix of the dentin before its calcification.

pre·di·a·be·tes (pre′dī-ă-bē′tēz). A state of potential diabetes mellitus, with normal glucose tolerance but with an increased risk of developing diabetes, (e.g., family history). Term declared obsolete by American Diabetes Association.

pre·di·as·to·le (prē-dī-as′tō-lē). The interval in the cardiac rhythm immediately preceding diastole. SYN late systole.

pre·di·a·stol·ic (prē-dī-ă-stol′ik). Late systolic, relating to the interval preceding cardiac diastole.

pre·di·crot·ic (prē-dī-krot′ik). Preceding the dicrotic notch.

pre·di·ges·tion (prē-dī-jes′chŭn). The artificial initiation of digestion of proteins (proteolysis) and starches (amylolysis) before they are eaten.

pre·dis·pose (prē′dis-pōz). To render susceptible.

pre·dis·po·si·tion (prē′dis-pō-zish′ŭn). A condition of special susceptibility to a disease.

pred·nis·o·lone (pred-nis′ō-lōn). A dehydrogenated analog of cortisol with the same actions and uses as cortisol; a potent glucocorticoid.

p. acetate, same uses as p.; suitable for intramuscular administration.

p. butylacetate, SYN p. tebutate.

p. sodium phosphate, more soluble than p. and the other p. esters and useful when a rapid onset or a short duration of action is desired; suitable for intrasynovial, parenteral, and topical administration.

p. succinate, p. compound suitable for intramuscular, intravenous, or rectal administration.

p. tebutate, same actions and uses as p. but with longer duration of action and suitable for intrasynovial and soft tissue injection. SYN p. butylacetate.

pred·ni·sone (pred′ni-sōn). A dehydrogenated analogue of cortisone with the same actions and uses; must be converted to prednisolone before active; inhibits proliferation of lymphocytes.

pred·nyl·i·dene (prĕd-nil′i-dēn). A glucocorticoid.

pre·dor·mi·tal (prē-dōr′mi-tăl). Pertaining to the predormitum.

pre·dor·mi·tum (prē-dōr′mi-tŭm). The stage of semi-unconsciousness preceding actual sleep. [pre- + L. *dormio,* to sleep]

pre·duc·tal (prē-dŭk′tăl). Relating to that part of the aorta proximal to the aortic opening of the ductus arteriosus.

pre·e·clamp·sia (prē-ē-klamp′sē-ă). Development of hypertension with proteinuria or edema, or both, due to pregnancy or the influence of a recent pregnancy; it usually occurs after the 20th week of gestation, but may develop before this time in the presence of trophoblastic disease. [pre- + G. *eklampsis,* a shining forth (eclampsia)]

superimposed p., the development of p. in a patient with chronic hypertensive vascular or renal disease; when the hypertension antedates the pregnancy as established by previous blood pressure recordings, a rise in the systolic pressure of 30 mmHg or a rise in the diastolic pressure of 15 mmHg and the development of proteinuria or edema, or both, are required during pregnancy to establish the diagnosis.

pre·ep·i·glot·tic (prē′ep-i-glot′ik). Anterior to the epiglottis.

pre·e·rup·tive (prē-e-rŭp′tiv). Denoting the stage of an exanthematous disease preceding the eruption.

pre·ex·ci·ta·tion (prē′ek-sī-tā′shŭn). Premature activation of part of the ventricular myocardium by an impulse that travels by an anomalous path and so avoids physiologic delay in the atrioventricular junction; an intrinsic part of the Wolff-Parkinson-White syndrome.

ventricular p., SEE Wolff-Parkinson-White *syndrome*.

pre·for·ma·tion. SEE preformation *theory*.

pre·fron·tal (prē-fron′tăl). **1.** Denoting the anterior portion of the frontal lobe of the cerebrum. **2.** Denoting the granular frontal cortex rostral to the premotor area.

pre·gan·gli·on·ic (prē′gang-glē-on′ik). Situated proximal to or preceding a ganglion; referring specifically to the preganglionic motor neurons of the autonomic nervous system (located in the spinal cord and brainstem) and the preganglionic, myelinated nerve fibers by which they are connected to the autonomic ganglia.

preg·nan·cy (preg′nan-sē). The state of a female after conception and until the termination of the gestation. SYN fetation, gestation, gravidism, graviditas. [L. *praegnans* (*praegnant-*), pregnant, fr. *prae,* before, + *gnascor,* pp. *natus,* to be born]

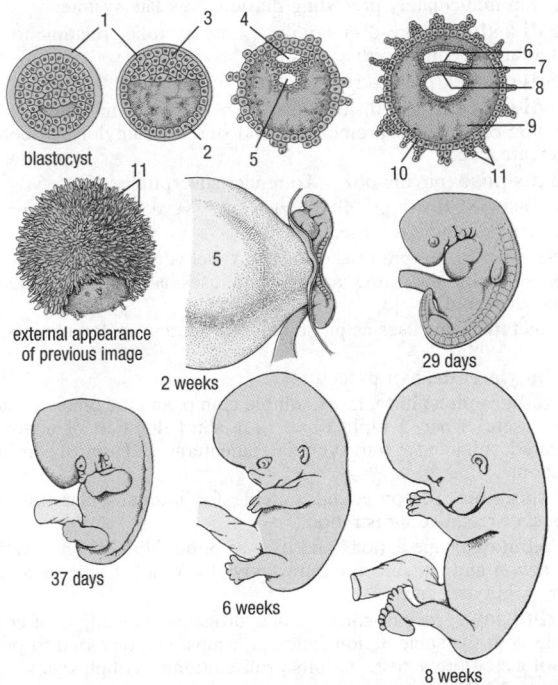

blastocyst

external appearance of previous image

2 weeks

29 days

37 days

6 weeks

8 weeks

development: from blastocyst to fetus; (1) zona pellucida, (2) trophectoderm, (3) inner cell mass, (4) amniotic cavity, (5) yolk sac, (6) ectoderm, (7) mesoderm, (8) entoderm, (9) mesoderm, (10) trophectoderm, (11) chorionic villi

abdominal p., the implantation and development of the ovum in the peritoneal cavity, usually secondary to an early rupture of a tubal p.; very rarely, primary implantation may occur in the peritoneal cavity. SYN abdominocyesis (1), intraperitoneal p.

aborted ectopic p., SYN tubal *abortion*.

ampullar p., tubal p. situated near the midportion of the oviduct.

cervical p., the implantation and development of the impregnated ovum in the cervical canal.

chemical p., slight, unsustained rise in HCG levels.

combined p., coexisting uterine and ectopic p.

compound p., development of a uterine p. in addition to a previously existing ectopic pregnancy (usually a lithopedion).

cornual p., the implantation and development of the impregnated ovum in one of the cornua of the uterus.

ectopic p., the development of an impregnated ovum outside the cavity of the uterus. SYN eccyesis, extrauterine p., heterotopic p., paracyesis.

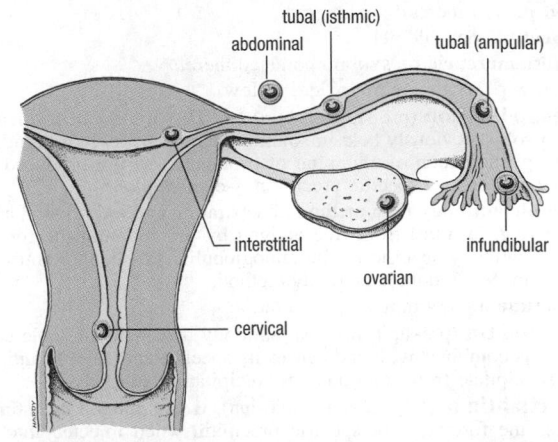

tubal (isthmic)
abdominal
tubal (ampullar)
interstitial
infundibular
ovarian
cervical

sites of ectopic pregnancy

extraamniotic p., a p. in which the chorion is intact, but the amnion has ruptured and shrunk. SYN graviditas examnialis.

extrachorial p., p. in which the membranes rupture and shrink, causing the fetus to develop outside the chorionic sac but within the uterus. SYN graviditas exochorialis.

extramembranous p., a p. in which during the course of gestation the fetus has broken through its envelopes, coming directly in contact with the uterine walls.

extrauterine p., SYN ectopic p.

fallopian p., SYN tubal p.

false p., a condition in which some signs and symptoms suggest pregnancy, although the woman is not pregnant. SYN hysterical p., pseudocyesis, pseudopregnancy (1), spurious p.

heterotopic p., SYN ectopic p.

heterotropic p.'s, p.'s occurring simultaneously in different sites, e.g., intrauterine and ampullary.

higher order p., a p. that has three fetuses (triplets) or more.

hydatid p., the presence of a hydiform mole in the pregnant uterus.

hysterical p., SYN false p.

interstitial p., SYN intramural p.

intraligamentary p., p. within the broad ligament.

intramural p., development of the fertilized ovum in the uterine portion of the fallopian tube. SYN interstitial p., tubouterine p.

intraperitoneal p., SYN abdominal p.

molar p., p. marked by a neoplasm within the uterus, whereby part or all of the chorionic villi are converted into a mass of clear vesicles.

multiple p., condition of bearing two or more fetuses simultaneously. SYN polycyesis.

mural p., p. in uterine muscular wall.

ovarian p., development of an impregnated ovum in an ovarian follicle. SEE ALSO Spiegelberg *criteria,* under *criterion.* SYN oocyesis, ovariocyesis.

ovarioabdominal p., ovarian p. that, as the result of the embryo's growth, becomes abdominal.

persistent ectopic p., an ectopic p. that has persistent viable tissue, secreting hCG after conservative surgery.

postdate p., a p. of more than 294 days or 42 completed weeks. SYN prolonged p.

prolonged p., SYN postdate p.

secondary abdominal p., a condition in which the embryo or fetus continues to grow in the abdominal cavity after its expulsion from the fallopian tube or other seat of its primary development. SYN abdominocyesis (2).

spurious p., SYN false p.

tubal p., development of an impregnated ovum in the fallopian tube. SYN fallopian p., salpingocyesis.

tuboabdominal p., development of an ectopic p. partly in the fallopian tube and partly in the abdominal cavity.

tuboovarian p., development of the ovum at the fimbriated extremity of the fallopian and involving the ovary.

tubouterine p., SYN intramural p.

twin p., a p. that may result from the fertilization of two separate ova or of a single ovum. SEE ALSO twin.

uterine p., development of fetus within the uterus.

uteroabdominal p., development of the ovum primarily in the uterus and later, in consequence of the rupture of the uterus, in the abdominal cavity.

preg·nane (preg′nān). Parent hydrocarbon of two series of steroids stemming from 5α-pregnane (originally allopregnane) and 5β-pregnane (17β-ethyletiocholane). 5β-Pregnane is the parent of the progesterones, pregnane alcohols, ketones, and several adrenocortical hormones and is found largely in urine as a metabolic product of 5β-pregnane compounds. For structure, see steroids.

preg·nane·di·ol (preg-nān-dī′ol). 5β-Pregnane-3α,20α-diol; the chief steroid metabolite of progesterone that is biologically inactive and occurs as p. glucuronate in the urine.

preg·nane·di·one (preg-nān-dī′ōn). 5β-Pregnane-3,20-dione; a metabolite of progesterone, formed in relatively small quantities, that occurs in 5α and 5β isomeric forms.

preg·nane·tri·ol (preg-nān-trī′ol). 5β-Pregnane-3α,17α,20α-triol; a urinary metabolite of 17-hydroxyprogesterone and a precursor in the biosynthesis of cortisol; its excretion is enhanced in certain diseases of the adrenal cortex and following administration of corticotropin.

preg·nant. Denoting a gestating female. SYN gravid. [see pregnancy]

preg·nene (preg′nēn). An unsaturated steroid of primarily terminologic importance; utilized in systematic nomenclature of appropriate 21-carbon steroids.

preg·nen·in·o·lone (preg-nēn-in′ō-lōn, preg-nēn′in-). SYN ethisterone.

preg·nen·o·lone (preg-nēn′ō-lōn). 3β-Hydroxy-5-pregnen-20-one; a steroid that serves as an intermediate in the biosynthesis of numerous hormones, including progesterone.

p. succinate, a corticosteroid used for the treatment of rheumatoid arthritis.

pre·hal·lux (prē-hal′ŭks). A supernumerary digit, usually only partial, attached to the medial border of the great toe. [pre- + Mod. L. *hallux,* great toe]

pre·hel·i·cine (prē-hel′i-sēn). In front of the helix of the pinna.

pre·he·ma·ta·min·ic ac·id (prē′hēm-tă-min′ik). SYN neuraminic acid.

pre·hen·sile (prē-hen′sil). Adapted for taking hold of or grasping. [L. *prehendo,* pp. -*hensus,* to lay hold of, seize]

pre·hen·sion (prē-hen′shŭn). The act of grasping, or taking hold of.

pre·hor·mone (prē-hōr′mōn). A glandular secretory product, having little or no inherent biologic potency, that is converted peripherally to an active hormone. Cf. prohormone (1).

pre·hy·oid (prē-hī′oyd). Anterior or superior to the hyoid bone; denoting certain accessory thyroid glands lying superior to the mylohyoid muscle.

pre·ic·tal (prē-ik′tăl). Occurring before a seizure or stroke. [pre- + L. *ictus,* a stroke]

pre·in·duc·tion (prē-in-dŭk′shŭn). An effect from the action of environment on the germ cells of progenitors upon their grand-

children. [L. *prae,* before, + *inductio,* a bringing in, fr. *induco,* to lead in]

Preisz, Hugo von, Hungarian bacteriologist, 1860–1940.

pre·kal·li·kre·in (prē-kal-ĭ-krē′in). A plasma glycoprotein that in complex with kininogen serves as a cofactor in the activation of factor XII. P. also serves as the proenzyme for plasma kallikrein. SYN Fletcher factor.

pre·lac·ri·mal (prē-lak′ri-măl). Anterior to the lacrimal sac.

pre·la·ryn·ge·al (prē-lă-rin′jē-ăl). Anterior to the larynx; denoting especially one or two small lymphatic nodes.

pre·lep·to·tene (prē-lep′tō-tēn). The earliest stage of prophase in meiosis, characterized by physiochemical changes in cytoplasm and karyoplasm and beginning contraction of chromosomes. [pre- + leptotene, fr. G. *leptos,* slender, + *tainia,* band]

pre·leu·ke·mia (prē-loo-kē′mē-ă). A syndrome that in time may develop into overt leukemia. It is characterized by bone marrow dysfunction manifested by anemia, neutropenia, and thrombocytopenia. SYN myelodysplastic syndrome.

pre·lim·bic (prē-lim′bik). Anterior to the limbus of the fossa ovalis.

pre·load (prē′lōd). **1.** The load to which a muscle is subjected before shortening. **2.** SYN ventricular p.

ventricular p., formerly, the end-diastolic pressure stretching the ventricular walls, which determines the end-diastolic fiber length at the onset of ventricular contraction, or some other measure of this load on the muscle fibers before contraction; now, more rigorously expressed in terms of the wall stress at this moment, related to the tension per unit cross-sectional area in the ventricular muscle fibers (calculated by Laplace law from internal radius and pressure modified by wall thickness) that balances this transmural pressure at the moment before contraction begins. SYN preload (2).

pre·ma·lig·nant (prē-mă-lig′nănt). SYN precancerous.

pre·ma·ni·a·cal (prē-mă-nī′ă-kăl). Preceding a manic attack.

pre·ma·ture (prē-mă-toor′, -choor). **1.** Occurring before the usual or expected time. **2.** Denoting an infant born at a gestational age of less than 37 weeks; birth weight is no longer considered a critical criterion for use of this designation. [L. *praematurus,* too early, fr. *prae-,* pre- + *maturus,* ripe (mature)]

pre·ma·tu·ri·ty (prē-mă-toor′i-tē, -choor′i-tē). **1.** The state of being premature. **2.** In dentistry, deflective occlusal *contact.*

pre·max·il·la (prē-mak-sil′ă). **1.** ☆official alternate term for incisive *bone.* **2.** The central isolated bony part in a complete bilateral cleft of the lip. [pre- + L. *maxilla,* jawbone]

pre·max·il·lary (prē-mak′si-lār-ē). **1.** Anterior to the maxilla. **2.** Denoting the premaxilla.

pre·med·i·ca·tion (prē′med-i-kā′shŭn). **1.** Administration of drugs prior to anesthesia to allay apprehension, produce sedation, and facilitate the administration of anesthesia. **2.** Drugs used for such purposes.

pre·mel·a·no·some (prē-mel′ă-nō-sōm). A nonpigmented membrane-bound vesicle in a melanocyte that contains tyrosine and matures into the melanin-filled melanosome; prominent in melanocytes of albinos.

pre·men·stru·al (prē-men′stroo-ăl). Relating to the period of time preceding menstruation.

pre·men·stru·um (prē-men′stroo-ŭm). The few days preceding menstruation. [pre- + L. *menstruum,* ntr. of *menstruus,* monthly, pertaining to menstruation]

pre·mi·to·chond·ria (prē-mī-tō-kon′drē-ă). SYN promitochondria.

pre·mo·lar (prē-mō′lăr). **1.** Anterior to a molar tooth. **2.** A bicuspid tooth.

pre·mon·o·cyte (prē-mon′ō-sīt). An immature monocyte not normally seen in the circulating blood. SYN promonocyte.

pre·mor·bid (prē-mōr′bid). Preceding the occurrence of disease. [pre- + L. *morbidus,* ill, fr. *morbus,* disease]

pre·mu·ni·tion (prē-moo-nish′ŭn). A state of existing resistance of a host to infection or reinfection with a parasite; used espe-

pr

cially in malaria epidemiology. [L. *praemunitio,* fortification in advance, fr. *prae-,* + *munio,* to fortify]

pre·mu·ni·tive (prē-moo′ni-tiv). Relating to premunition.

pre·my·e·lo·blast (prē-mī′ĕ-lō-blast). The earliest recognizable precursor of the myeloblast.

pre·my·e·lo·cyte (prē-mī′ĕ-lō-sīt). SYN promyelocyte.

pre·na·ris, pl. **pre·na·res** (prē-nā′ris, nā′rēz). SYN naris.

pre·na·tal (prē-nā′tăl). Preceding birth. SYN antenatal. [pre- + L. *natus,* born]

pre·ne·o·plas·tic (prē′nē-ō-plas′tik). Preceding the formation of any neoplasm, benign or malignant; a p. condition is not always precancerous, although the term is frequently used erroneously in that sense. [pre- + G. *neos,* new, + *plastikos,* formative]

Prentice, Charles F., U.S. optician, 1854–1946. SEE P. *rule.*

pren·yl (pren′il). Poly- or multiprenyl residues or derivatives thereof, apparently formed by end-to-end polymerization of isoprene molecules; found in the isoprenoids in nature.

pre·nyl·a·mine (pre-nil′ă-mēn). An antianginal agent.

pre·nyl·a·tion (pren′il-ā′shŭn). The covalent addition of prenyl and multiprenyl residues to a macromolecule.

pre·op·er·a·tive (prē-op′er-ă-tiv). Preceding an operation.

pre·op·tic (prē-op′tik). Referring to the preoptic *region.*

pre·o·ral (prē-ō′răl). In front of the mouth. [pre- + L. *os (or-),* mouth]

pre·os·te·o·blast (prē-os′tē-ō-blast). SYN osteoprogenitor *cell.*

pre·ox·y·gen·a·tion (prē′ok-sĕ-jĕ-nā′shŭn). Denitrogenation with 100% oxygen prior to induction of general anesthesia.

prep (prep). To prepare the skin or other body surface for an operative procedure, usually by cleaning and application of antiseptic solutions. [slang for preparation or prepare]

pre·pal·a·tal (prē-pal′ă-tăl). Relating to the anterior part of the palate, or anterior to the palate bone.

prep·a·ra·tion (prep-ă-rā′shŭn). 1. A getting ready. 2. Something made ready, as a medicinal or other mixture, or a histologic specimen. [L. *praeparatio,* fr. *prae,* before, + *paro,* pp. *-atus,* to get ready]

cavity p., (1) removal of dental caries and surgical p. of the remaining tooth structure to receive a dental restoration; **(2)** the final form of an excavation in a tooth resulting from such p.

corrosion p., a p. in which the hollow parts such as ducts, vessels, or alveoli of the lung are filled with a substance that hardens and persists after dissolving the tissues by digestion.

cytologic filter p., a cytologic specimen made by depositing a watery sample (obtained by a variety of methods from many body sites) upon a filter having pores of uniform size smaller than the cellular material to be concentrated; this is followed by fixation and staining, usually with 95% ethyl alcohol and Papanicolaou stain.

heart-lung p., an animal p. in which blood (rendered incoagulable) circulates through the heart and lungs and through an artificial system of vessels representing the systemic circulation; the latter is connected with the divided aorta on the one hand and with the superior vena cava on the other; used in physiologic studies of the heart and circulation.

pre·par·tu·ri·ent (prē-par-too′rē-ent). Relating to the period before birth.

pre·pa·tel·lar (prē-pă-tel′ăr). Anterior to the patella.

pre·per·i·to·ne·al (prē′per-i-tō-nē′ăl). Denoting a fatty layer between the peritoneum and the transversalis fascia in the lower anterior abdominal wall.

pre·phe·nic ac·id (prē-fē′nik, -fen′ik). An intermediate in the microbial conversion of shikimic acid to L-phenylalanine and L-tyrosine.

pre·pla·cen·tal (prē-pla-sen′tăl). Before formation of a placenta.

preponderance (prē-pon′der-ans). Quality of outweighing, or exceeding in extent or importance.

directional p., a right or left predominance of nystagmus calculated from the responses to the binaural, bithermal caloric test.

pre·po·ten·tial (prē-pō-ten′shăl). A gradual rise in potential between action potentials as a phasic swing in electric activity of the cell membrane, which establishes its rate of automatic activity, as in the ureter or cardiac pacemaker.

pre·pro·col·la·gen (prē-prō-kol-ō-jen). The precursor of collagen that is synthesized on ribosomes; procollagen with a leader or signal sequence that directs the polypeptide chain into the vesicular space of the endoplasmic reticulum.

pre·pro·in·su·lin (prē-prō-in′soo-lin). The precursor protein to proinsulin. SEE preprotein.

pre·pro·pro·tein (prē-prō-prō′tēn). A precursor to an inactive secretory proprotein.

pre·pro·tein (prē-prō′tēn). A secretory protein with a signal peptide region attached.

pre·psy·chot·ic (prē-sī-kot′ik). **1.** Relating to the period antedating the onset of psychosis. **2.** Denoting a potential for a psychotic episode, one that appears imminent under continued stress.

pre·pu·ber·al, pre·pu·ber·tal (prē-pū′ber-ăl, -ber-tăl). Before puberty.

pre·pu·bes·cent (prē-pū-bes′ent). Immediately prior to the commencement of puberty.

pre·puce (prē′poos) [TA]. A free fold of skin that covers. SYN preputium [TA], foreskin✵. [L. *praeputium,* foreskin]

p. of clitoris [TA], the external fold of the labia minora, forming a cap over the clitoris. SYN preputium clitoridis.

hooded p., incomplete circumferential formation of foreskin with a dorsal component (the dorsal hood) but an absent or incomplete ventral portion. Typically seen in boys with hypospadias or isolated chordee. In the rare condition of epispadias, the incomplete portion may be ventral.

p. of penis [TA], the free fold of skin that covers, more or less completely, the glans penis. SYN foreskin of penis [TA], preputium penis [TA].

ventral apron p., the incomplete foreskin seen in epispadias patients typically such that a ventral apron remains.

pre·pu·ti·al (pre-pū′shē-ăl). Relating to the prepuce.

pre·pu·ti·ot·o·my (prē-pū′shē-ot′ō-mē). Incision of prepuce. [preputium + G. *tomē,* incision]

pre·pu·ti·um, pl. **pre·pu·tia** (prē-pū′shē-ŭm, shē-ă) [TA]. SYN prepuce. [L. *praeputium*]

p. clitor′idis, SYN *prepuce* of clitoris.

p. penis [TA], SYN *prepuce* of penis.

pre·py·lor·ic (prē-pī-lōr′ik). Anterior to or preceding the pylorus; denoting a temporary constriction of the wall of the stomach separating the fundus from the antrum during digestion.

pre·rec·tal (prē-rek′tăl). Anterior to or preceding the rectum.

pre·re·duced (prē-rē-doosd′). Pertaining to bacteriologic media that are boiled, tubed under oxygen-free gas with chemical reducing agents and colorimetric redox indicator in stoppered tubes or bottles, and then sterilized.

pre·re·nal (prē-rē′năl). Anterior to a kidney. [L. *ren,* kidney]

pre·ret·i·nal (prē-ret′i-nal). Anterior to the retina.

pre·sa·cral (prē-sā′krăl). Anterior to or preceding the sacrum.

△**presby-, presbyo-.** Old age. SEE ALSO gero-. [G. *presbys,* old man]

pres·by·a·cou·sia (prez-bē-ă-koo′sē-ă). SYN presbyacusis.

pres·by·a·cu·sis, pres·by·a·cu·sia (prez′bē-ă-koo′sis). Loss of ability to perceive or discriminate sounds associated with aging; the pattern and age of onset vary. SYN presbyacousia, presbycusis. [presby- + G. *akousis,* hearing]

pres·by·a·sta·sis (prez′bĭ-ă-stā′sis). Impairment of vestibular function associated with aging. [presby- + G. *a-* priv. + *stasis,* standing]

pres·by·at·rics (prez-bē-at′riks). Rarely used terms for geriatrics. [presby- + G. *iatreia,* medical treatment]

pres·by·cu·sis (prez-bē-koo′sis). SYN presbyacusis.

pres·by·o·pia (Pr) (prez-bē-ō′pē-ă). The physiologic loss of accommodation in the eyes in advancing age, said to begin when the near point has receded beyond 22 cm (9 inches). [presby- + G. *ōps,* eye]

pres·by·op·ic (prez′bē-op′ik, -ō′pik). Relating to or suffering from presbyopia.

pre·scribe (prē-skrīb′). To give directions, either orally or in writing, for the preparation and administration of a remedy to be used in the treatment of any disease. [L. *prae-scribo,* pp. *-scriptus,* to write before]

pre·scrip·tion (prē-skrip′shŭn). **1.** A written formula for the preparation and administration of any remedy. **2.** A medicinal preparation compounded according to formulated directions, said to consist of four parts: 1) *superscription,* consisting of the word *recipe,* take, or its sign, ℞; 2) *inscription,* the main part of the p., containing the names and amounts of the drugs ordered; 3) *subscription,* directions for mixing the ingredients and designation of the form (pill, powder, solution, etc.) in which the drug is to be made, usually beginning with the word, *misce,* mix, or its abbreviation, M.; 4) *signature,* directions to the patient regarding the dose and times of taking the remedy, preceded by the word *signa,* designate, or its abbreviation, S. or Sig. [L. *praescriptio;* see prescribe]

shotgun p., a p. containing many ingredients, some of which may be useless, in an attempt to cover all possible types of therapy that may be needed; a pejorative term.

pre·se·nile (prē-sē′nīl). Prior to the usual onset of senility, as in the milder, presenile *dementia.*

pre·se·nil·i·ty (prē-sĕ-nil′i-tē). Premature old age; the condition of an individual, not old in years, who displays the physical and mental characteristics of old age but not to the extent of senility. [pre- + L. *senilis,* old]

pre·se·ni·um (prē-sē′nē-ŭm). The period preceding old age.

pre·sent (prē-zent′). **1.** To precede or appear first at the os uteri, said of the part of the fetus first felt during examination. **2.** To appear for examination, treatment, etc., said of a patient. [L. *praesens* (*-sent-*), pres. p. of *prae-sum,* to be before, be at hand]

pre·sen·ta·tion (prē′zen-tā′shŭn, prez′). That part of the fetus presenting at the superior strait of the maternal pelvis; occiput, chin, and sacrum are, respectively, the determining points in vertex, face, and breech p. SEE ALSO position (3). See also entries under position. [see present]

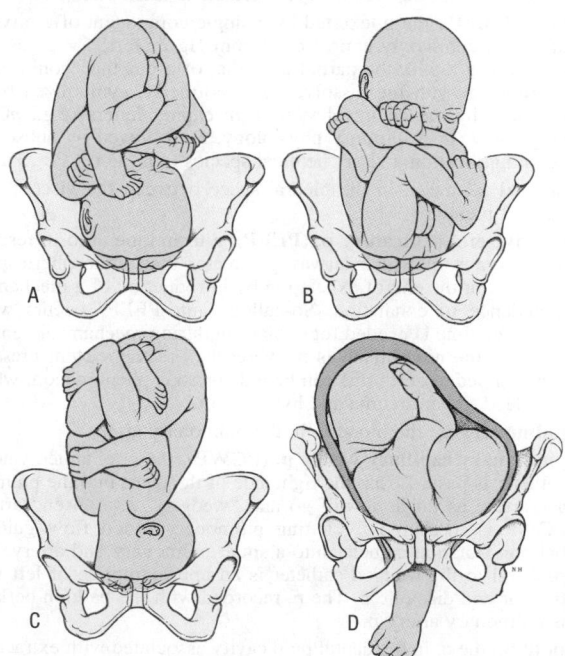

fetal presentations: (A) cephalic, (B) breech, (C) face, (D) transverse

acromion p., SYN shoulder p.
breech p., p. of any part of the pelvic extremity of the fetus, the nates, knees, or feet; more properly only of the nates; frank breech p. occurs when the fetus presents by the pelvic extremity; the thighs may be flexed and the legs extended over the anterior surfaces of the body; in **full breech p.,** the thighs may be flexed on the abdomen and the legs upon the thighs; and in **footling p.,** **foot p.,** the feet may be the lowest part; in **incomplete foot p.,** **incomplete knee p.,** one leg may retain the position that is typical of one of the above-mentioned presentations, while the other foot or knee may present. SYN pelvic p.

brow p., SEE cephalic p.
cephalic p., p. of any part of the fetal head, usually the upper and back part, as a result of flexion such that the chin is in contact with the thorax in vertex p.; there may be degrees of flexion so that the presenting part is the large fontanel in sincipital p., the brow in brow p., or the face in face p. SYN head p.

compound p., prolapse of an extremity, usually a hand, along the presenting part, with both in the pelvis simultaneously.

face p., SEE cephalic p.
footling p., SEE breech p.
frank breech p., SEE breech p.
head p., SYN cephalic p.
incomplete foot p., SEE breech p.
knee p., SEE breech p.
pelvic p., SYN breech p.
placental p., SYN *placenta* previa.
polar p., the p. of either pole of the fetal oval; may be either a cephalic or breech p., or a longitudinal lie.
shoulder p., transverse p. with the shoulder as the presenting part. SYN acromion p.
sincipital p., SEE cephalic p.
transverse p., an abnormal p., neither head nor breech, in which the fetus lies transversely in the uterus across the axis of the parturient canal.
vertex p., SEE cephalic p.

pre·ser·va·tive (prē-zer′vă-tiv). A substance added to food products or to an organic solution to prevent chemical change or bacterial action.

pre·so·mite (prē-sō′mīt). Relating to the embryonic stage before the appearance of somites (before day 19 in the human).

pre·sphe·noid (prē-sfē′noyd). In front of the sphenoid bone or cartilage.

pre·sphyg·mic (prē-sfig′mik). Preceding the pulse beat; denoting a brief interval following the filling of the ventricles with blood before their contraction forces open the semilunar valves, corresponding to the isovolumic contraction period. [pre- + G. *sphygmos,* pulse]

pre·spi·nal (prē-spī′năl). Anterior to the spine.

pre·spon·dy·lo·lis·the·sis (prē-spon-di-lō-lis′thē-sis). A condition predisposing to spondylolisthesis, consisting of a defect in the laminae of a lumbar vertebra but before development of any displacement of the vertebral body. SEE spondylolysis.

pres·sor (pres′er, -ōr). Exciting to vasomotor activity; producing increased blood pressure; denoting afferent nerve fibers that, when stimulated, excite vasoconstrictors, which increase peripheral resistance. SYN hypertensor. [L. *premo,* pp. *pressus,* to press]

pres·so·re·cep·tive (pres′ō-rē-sep′tiv). Capable of receiving as stimuli changes in pressure, especially changes of blood pressure. SYN pressosensitive.

pres·so·re·cep·tor (pres′ō-rē-sep′ter, -tōr). SYN baroreceptor.

pres·so·sen·si·tive (pres-ō-sen′si-tiv). SYN pressoreceptive.

pres·so·sen·si·tiv·i·ty (pres′ō-sen-si-tiv′i-tē). The state of being able to perceive changes in pressure. SEE ALSO pressoreceptive.

reflexogenic p., p. also capable of initiating the regulation of heart rate, vascular tone, and blood pressure.

pres·sure (P, *P*) (presh′ŭr). **1.** A stress or force acting in any direction against resistance. **2** (*P,* frequently followed by a subscript indicating location). In physics and physiology, the force per unit area exerted by a gas or liquid against the walls of its container or that would be exerted on a wall immersed at that spot in the middle of a body of fluid.

$$p = \frac{\text{force}}{\text{unit area}}$$
pressure

The p. can be considered either relative to some reference p., such as that of the ambient atmosphere (imagined to be on the other side of the wall), or in absolute terms (relative to a perfect vacuum). [L. *pressura,* fr. *premo,* pp. *pressus,* to press]

pressure: various units expressed in pascals (Pa)				
pounds per square inch	1 psi	=	6894.76	Pa
atmosphere (standard)	1 atm	=	101325.0	Pa
atmosphere (technical)	1 kg/cm²	=	98066.5	Pa
water column	1 in H₂0 (60° F)	=	248.84	Pa
mercury column	1 mmHg (0° C)	=	133.32	Pa
torr	1 torr	=	133.32	Pa
bar	1 bar	=	100 000	Pa
dynes per square centimeter	1 dyn/cm²	=	0.10	Pa

abdominal p., p. surrounding the bladder; estimated from rectal, gastric, or intraperitoneal p.

absolute p., p. measured with respect to zero p. Cf. gauge p.

acoustic p., in ultrasound, the instantaneous value of the total pressure minus the ambient pressure; unit is pascal (Pa).

atmospheric p., SYN barometric p.

back p., p. exerted upstream in the circulation as a result of obstruction to forward flow, as when congestion in the pulmonary circulation results from stenosis of the mitral valve or failure of the left ventricle.

barometric p. (P_B), the absolute p. of the ambient atmosphere, varying with weather, altitude, etc.; expressed in millibars (meteorology) or mm Hg or torr (respiratory physiology); at sea level, one atmosphere (atm, 760 mm Hg or torr) is equivalent to: 14.69595 lb/sq in, 1013.25 millibars, 1013.25×10^6 dynes/cm², and, in SI units, 101,325 pascals (Pa). SYN atmospheric p.

biting p., SYN occlusal p.

blood p. (BP), the p. or tension of the blood within the systemic arteries, maintained by the contraction of the left ventricle, the resistance of the arterioles and capillaries, the elasticity of the arterial walls, as well as the viscosity and volume of the blood; expressed as relative to the ambient atmospheric p. SYN piesis.

central venous p. (CVP), the p. of the blood within the venous system in the superior and inferior vena cava cephalad to the diaphragm, normally between 4 and 10 cm of water; it is depressed in circulatory shock and deficiencies of circulating blood volume and increased with cardiac failure and congestion of the venous circulation.

cerebrospinal p., the p. of the cerebrospinal fluid, normally 100–150 mm of water, relative to the ambient atmospheric p.

continuous positive airway p. (CPAP), a technique of respiratory therapy, in either spontaneously breathing or mechanically ventilated patients, in which airway p. is maintained above atmospheric p. throughout the respiratory cycle by pressurization of the ventilatory circuit.

coronary perfusion p., the p. at which blood proceeds through the coronary circulation, mainly in diastole.

critical p., the minimum p. required to liquefy a gas at the critical temperature.

detrusor p., that component of intravesical pressure created by the tension (active and passive) exerted by the bladder wall; the transmural p. across the bladder wall estimated by subtracting abdominal p. from intravesical p.

diastolic p., the intracardiac p. during or resulting from diastolic relaxation of a cardiac chamber; the lowest arterial blood p. reached during any given ventricular cycle.

differential blood p., the arterial blood p. at corresponding points on the two sides of the body.

Donders p., an increase of about 6 mm Hg shown by a manometer connected with the trachea when the thorax of a dead body is opened; it is caused by the collapse of the lungs when air is admitted to the thorax.

effective osmotic p., that part of the total osmotic p. of a solution that governs the tendency of its solvent to pass across a boundary, usually a semipermeable membrane; it is commonly represented by the product of the total osmotic p. of the solution and the ratio (corrected for activities) of the number of dissolved particles that do not permeate the bounding membrane to the total number of particles in the solution; equivalent in meaning to tonicity; commonly expressed in equivalent units of osmolality rather than p. per se.

gauge p., p. measured relative to ambient atmospheric p.; at sea level, it is 1 atm less than the p. in the atmosphere. Cf. absolute p.

hydrostatic p., the p. exerted by a liquid as a result of its potential energy, ignoring its kinetic energy; frequently used to distinguish a true p. from an osmotic p. or to emphasize the variation in p. in a column of fluid due to the effect of gravity.

intracranial p. (ICP), p. within the cranial cavity.

intraocular p., the p. (usually measured in millimeters of mercury) of the intraocular fluid within the eye, measured by means of a manometer.

leak point p., storage p. in bladder at which leakage occurs passively, usually in patients with neuropathic bladder.

negative p., p. less than that of the ambient atmosphere.

negative end-expiratory p. (NEEP), a subatmospheric p. at the airway at the end of expiration.

occlusal p., any force exerted upon the occlusal surfaces of teeth. SYN biting p.

oncotic p., osmotic p. exerted by colloids in solution.

osmotic p. (Π), the p. that must be applied to a solution to prevent the passage into it of solvent when solution and pure solvent are separated by a membrane permeable only to the solvent (sometimes less correctly viewed as the force with which the solution attracts solvent through the semipermeable membrane).

partial p. (P), the p. exerted by a single component of a mixture of gases, commonly expressed in mm Hg or torr; for a gas dissolved in a liquid, the partial p. is that of a gas that would be in equilibrium with the dissolved gas. Formerly, symbolized by p, followed by the chemical symbol in capital letters (e.g., pCO_2, pO_2); now, in respiratory physiology, P, followed by subscripts denoting location and/or chemical species (e.g., P_{CO_2}, P_{O_2}, P_{aCO_2}).

pleural p., the p. in the pleural space between the visceral and parietal pleurae.

positive end-expiratory p. (PEEP), a technique used in respiratory therapy in which airway p. greater than atmospheric p. is achieved at the end of exhalation by introduction of a mechanical impedance to exhalation. So-called "auto-PEEP" occurs when increased time is needed for expiration during mechanical ventilation and the next breath is delivered before the system pressure has dropped to zero; this can be a dangerous phenomenon, which may lead to barotrauma and hypotension.

pulmonary p., the blood p. in the pulmonary artery.

pulmonary capillary wedge p. (PCWP), the p. obtained when a catheter is passed from the right side of the heart into the pulmonary artery as far as it will go and "wedged" into an end artery. PCWP is measured by letting pulmonary blood flow guide a balloon-flotation catheter into a small pulmonary end artery. The p. distal to the wedged catheter is an approximation of left ventricular end diastolic p. The p. recorded with the balloon deflated is pulmonary artery p.

pulp p., the p. in the dental pulp cavity associated with extracellular fluid p., but showing pulsatile variations during the cardiac cycle because of the encasement of the pulp within the tooth.

pulse p., the variation in blood p. occurring in an artery during the cardiac cycle; it is the difference between the systolic or maximum and diastolic or minimum p.'s.

selection p., impact of effective reproduction due to environmental impact on the phenotype.

solution p., the force driving atoms or molecules to leave a solid particle and enter into solution (i.e., to dissolve).

standard p., the absolute p. to which gases are referred under standard conditions (STPD), i.e., 760 mmHg, 760 torr, or 101,325 N/m² (i.e., 101,325 Pa).

⊞ **systolic p.,** the intracardiac p. during or resulting from systolic contraction of a cardiac chamber; the highest arterial blood pressure reached during any given ventricular cycle.

intracardial pressure (mmHg)					
	A wave	X trough	V wave	Y trough	average
right atrium	up to 5	0	up to 5	0	up to 4
left atrium	ca. 8	0	ca. 10	0	ca. 6–8
	systolic		early diastolic		late diastolic
right ventricle	20–30		0		up to 5
left ventricle	ca. 120		0		ca. 7–10

transmural p., p. across the wall of a cardiac chamber or of a blood vessel. In the heart, transmural p. is the resultant of the intracavitary p. minus the extracavitary (i.e., pericardial) p. and is the distending, i.e., true filling, p. of the cardiac chamber of measurement when this is done during diastole. Since the pericardial p. normally approximates zero, the filling p. usually equals ventricular diastolic mean p., obviating the complexities of measuring pericardial p.

transpulmonary p., the difference between the p. of the respired gas at the mouth and the pleural p. around the lungs, measured when the airway is open; thus, it includes not only the transmural p. of the lung but also any drop in p. along the tracheobronchial tree during flow.

transthoracic p., the p. in the pleural space measured relative to the p. of the ambient atmosphere outside the chest; the transmural p. across the chest wall.

vapor p., the partial p. exerted by the vapor phase of a liquid.

ventricular filling p., the p. in the ventricle as it fills with blood, ordinarily equivalent to the mean atrial p. when there is no AV valvular gradient. Atrial p. can be used in place of transmural p. because pericardial pressure usually varies between −2 and +2 mm Hg and hence is negligible. During cardiac tamponade, pericardial and atrial p.'s equilibrate so that transmural p. is zero and the high atrial p.'s cannot be "filling" p.'s.

wedge p., the intravascular pressure reading obtained when a fine catheter is advanced until it completely occludes a small blood vessel or is sealed in place by inflation of a small cuff; commonly measured in the lung (pulmonary artery) to estimate left atrial pressure.

zero end-expiratory p. (ZEEP), airway p. that, at the end of expiration, equals atmospheric p.

pre·ster·num (prē′ster′nŭm). SYN *manubrium* of sternum.

pre·sup·pu·ra·tive (prē-sŭp′ū-rā-tiv). Denoting an early stage in an inflammation prior to the formation of pus.

pre·syn·ap·tic (prē′si-nap′tik). Pertaining to the area on the proximal side of a synaptic cleft.

pre·sys·to·le (prē-sis′tō-lē). That part of diastole immediately preceding systole. SYN late diastole.

pre·sys·tol·ic (prē-sis-tol′ik). Late diastolic, relating to the interval immediately preceding systole.

pre·tar·sal (prē-tar′săl). Denoting the anterior, or inferior, portion of the tarsus.

pre·tec·ta (prē-tek′tă). Orad to the hidden part of the duodenum.

pre·tec·tum (prē-tek′tŭm). SYN pretectal *area*.

pre·thy·roid, pre·thy·roi·de·al, pre·thy·roi·de·an (prē-thī′royd, -thī-roy′dē-ăl, -thī-roy′dē-an). Anterior to or preceding the thyroid gland or cartilage.

pre·tib·i·al (prē-tib′ē-ăl). Relating to the anterior portion of the leg; denoting especially certain muscles.

pre·tra·che·al (prē-trā′kē-al). Anterior to the trachea; denoting especially the middle layer of deep cervical fascia.

pre·tre·mat·ic (prē-trē-mat′ik). Relating to the cranial surface of a branchial cleft. [pre- + G. *trēma*, perforation]

pre·tym·pan·ic (prē-tim-pan′ik). Anterior to the drum of the ear.

prev·a·lence (prev′ă-lens). The number of cases of a disease existing in a given population at a specific period of time (*period p.*) or at a particular moment in time (*point p.*).

pre·ven·tive (prē-ven′tiv). SYN prophylactic (1). [L. *prae-venio*, pp. -*ventus*, to come before, prevent]

pre·ver·te·bral (prē-ver′tĕ-brăl). Anterior to the body of a vertebra or of the vertebral column; denoting especially the deepest layer of deep cervical fascia and the muscles on the anterior aspect of the vertebral column.

pre·ves·i·cal (prē-ves′i-kăl). Anterior to the bladder; denoting especially the retropubic space. [pre- + L. *vesica*, bladder]

Pre·vo·tel·la (prev′ō-tel′ah). Genus of Gram-negative, nonmotile, nonsporeforming, obligately anaerobic, chemoorganotrophic, and pleomorphic rods; contains many species previously classified in the genus Bacteroides.

P. bivia, the species of *Prevotella* in highest concentration in the human vaginal tract.

P. denticola, a bacterial species found in the human mouth; a cause of infections of the oral cavity and adjacent structures.

P. di'siens, a bacterial species associated with human infections, primarily of the female genital tract. SYN *Bacteroides disiens.*

P. heparinolytica, a bacterial species associated with human periodontal disease.

P. intermedia, a species found in gingival crevices, especially associated with gingivitis, and other oral infections.

P. melani'noge'nica, a species found in the mouth, feces, infections of the mouth, soft tissue, respiratory tract, urogenital tract, and intestinal tract; implicated in periodontal disease; seen in aspiration. The type species of *Pretovella.* SYN *Bacteroides melaninogenicus.*

P. ora'lis, a bacterial species found in the gingival crevice of humans and in infections of the oral cavity and upper respiratory and genital tracts.

P. o'ris, a bacterial species isolated from the gingival crevice, systemic infections, face, neck, and chest abscesses, wound drainages, and blood and various bodily fluids.

pre·zone (prē′zōn). SYN prozone.

pri·a·pism (prī′ă-pizm). Persistent erection of the penis, accompanied by pain and tenderness, resulting from a pathologic condition rather than sexual desire; a term loosely used as a synonym for satyriasis. [see priapus]

pri·a·pus (prī′ă-pŭs). SYN penis. [L. fr. *Priapus* (G. *Priapos*), god of procreation]

Prib·now (prib′now). David, 20th-century U.S. molecular biologist. SEE Pribnow *box.*

Price, Ernest Arthur, English biochemist, *1882. SEE Carr-P. *reaction.*

Price-Jones, Cecil, English hematologist, 1863–1943. SEE Price-Jones *curve.*

Priestley, John Gillies, British physiologist, 1880–1941. SEE Haldane-P. *sample.*

pril·o·caine hy·dro·chlo·ride (pril′ō-kān). A local anesthetic of the amide type, related chemically and pharmacologically to lidocaine hydrochloride; used for peridural, caudal, and nerve blocks, and for regional and infiltration anesthesia. SYN propitocaine hydrochloride.

pri·ma·cy (prī′mă-sē). The state of being primary, or foremost in rank or importance. [see primary]

genital p., in psychoanalysis, the primary characteristic of the genital phase of psychosexual development, i.e., the libido becomes preponderantly concentrated in the penis.

oral p., in psychoanalysis, the primary characteristic of the oral phase of psychosexual development, i.e., the libido is concentrated mainly in the oral zone.

pri·mal (prī′măl). 1. First or primary. 2. SYN primordial (2).

pri·ma·quine phos·phate (prī′mă-kwin). An antimalarial agent

pr

especially effective against *Plasmodium vivax*, terminating relapsing vivax malaria; usually administered with chloroquine.

p. p. sensitivity, a sensitivity to p. p. observed in individuals with glucose-6-phosphate dehydrogenase deficiency.

pri·mary (prī′mār-ē). **1.** The first or foremost, as a disease or symptoms to which others may be secondary or occur as complications. **2.** Relating to the first stage of growth or development. SEE primordial. [L. *primarius,* fr. *primus,* first]

pri·mary re·nin·ism (ren′in-izm). Overproduction of renin by juxtaglomerular cells in the absence of a stimulus (such as decreased renal perfusion); leads to hyperaldosteronism, hypertension, hypokalemia, and edema.

pri·mase (prī′māz). A polymerase that acts on a template DNA strand to produce RNA, resulting in the formation of an RNA primer needed in RNA replication. SYN dnaG. [*prim*er + -ase]

pri·mate (prī′māt). An individual of the order Primates. [L. *primus,* first]

Pri·ma·tes (prī-ma′tēz). The highest order of mammals, including humans, monkeys, and lemurs. [L. *primus,* first]

prim·er (prī′mer). **1.** A molecule (which may be a small polymer) that initiates the synthesis of a larger structure. SYN starter. **2.** A pheromone that causes a long-term physiologic change.

pri·mer·ite (prī′mĕ-rīt). SYN protomerite. [L. *primus,* first, + G. *meros,* part]

pri·mi·done (prī′mi-dōn). An anticonvulsant drug used in the management of generalized tonic clonic and complex partial epilepsy.

pri·mi·grav·i·da (prī-mi-grav′i-dă). SEE gravida. [L. fr. *primus,* first, + *gravida,* a pregnant woman]

elderly p., dated term referring to a woman older than 35 years who is pregnant for the first time.

pri·mip·a·ra (prī-mip′ă-ră). SEE para. [L. fr. *primus,* first, + *pario,* to bring forth]

pri·mi·par·i·ty (prī-mi-par′i-tē). Condition of being a primipara.

pri·mip·a·rous (prī-mip′ă-rŭs). Denoting a primipara.

pri·mite (prī′mīt). The anterior member of a pair of gregarine gamonts in syzygy.

prim·i·tive (prim′i-tiv). SYN primordial (2). [L. *primitivus,* fr. *primus,* first]

pri·mor·dia (prī-mōr′dē-ă). Plural of primordium.

pri·mor·di·al (prī-mōr′dē-ăl). **1.** Relating to a primordium. **2.** Relating to a structure in its first or earliest stage of development. SYN primal (2), primitive.

pri·mor·di·um (prī-mōr′-dē-ŭm). An aggregation of cells in the embryo indicating the first trace of an organ or structure. SYN anlage (1). [L. origin, fr. *primus,* first, + *ordior,* to begin]

genital p., ovoid clump of cells seen in the rhabditiform larvae of *Strongyloides stercoralis* and hookworm that becomes the reproductive system.

prim·o·some (prī-mō-sōm). A complex of proteins that bind with primase at specific sequences of DNA that serve as the sites for the formation of RNA primers; a part of the replisome. [*prim*er + -some]

prim·u·la (prim′ū-lă). The rhizome and roots of a number of species of *Primula* (family Primulaceae), primrose or cowslip; has been used as expectorant, diuretic, and anthelmintic. In some sensitive persons contact with the plant causes a rash. [Mediev. L. primrose, fem. of L. *primulus,* first]

pri·mu·lin (prī′mū-lin) [C.I. 49000]. An acid yellow thiazole dye used as a fluorescent vital stain.

pri·mus (prī′mŭs). First; denoting the first of a series of similar structures. [L.]

prin·ceps, pl. **prin·ci·pes** (prin′seps, -si-pēz). Principal; in anatomy, term used to distinguish the largest and most important of several arteries. [L. chief, fr. *primus,* first, + *capio,* to take, choose]

p. cervi′cis, SYN descending *branch* of occipital artery.

p. pol′licis, SYN princeps pollicis *artery.*

Princeteau, L.R., French physician, *1884. SEE P. *tubercle.*

prin·ci·ple (prin′si-pl). **1.** A general or fundamental doctrine or

tenet. SEE ALSO law, rule, theorem. **2.** The essential ingredient in a substance, especially one that gives it its distinctive quality or effect. [L. *principium,* a beginning, fr. *princeps,* chief]

active p., a constituent of a drug, usually an alkaloid or glycoside, upon the presence of which the characteristic therapeutic action of the substance largely depends.

antianemic p., the material in liver (and certain other tissues) that stimulates hemopoiesis in pernicious anemia; for practical purposes, the antianemic effect of extracts from such tissues is approximately equivalent to the content of vitamin B_{12}.

Bernoulli p., SYN Bernoulli *law.*

bitter p.'s, a class of plant substances with a bitter taste that produce a reflexive increase in saliva secretion as well as secretion of digestive juices.

closure p., in psychology, the p. that when one views fragmentary stimuli forming a nearly complete figure (e.g., an incomplete rectangle) one tends to ignore the missing parts and perceive the figure as whole. SEE gestalt.

consistency p., in psychology, the desire of the human being to be consistent, especially in attitudes and beliefs; theories of attitude formation and change based on the consistency p. include balance theory, which suggests that one seeks to avoid incongruity in one's various attitudes. SEE ALSO cognitive dissonance *theory.*

Fick p., SYN Fick *method.*

follicle-stimulating p., SYN follitropin.

founder p., the conditional probabilities of the frequencies of a set of genes at any future date depend on the initial composition of the founders of the population and have in general no tendency to revert to the composition of the population from which the founders were themselves derived.

hematinic p., the p. previously thought to be produced by the action of Castle intrinsic factor upon an extrinsic factor in food, now recognized as vitamin B_{12}.

Huygens p., used in ultrasound technology; the p. that any wave phenomenon can be analyzed as the sum of many simple sources properly chosen with regard to phase and amplitude.

p. of inertia, SYN repetition-compulsion p.

Le Chatelier p., SYN Le Chatelier *law.*

luteinizing p., SYN lutropin.

mass action p., the fundamental p. in epidemic theory: the incidence of an infectious disease is determined by the product of the current prevalence and the number of susceptibles in the population. SEE ALSO serial *interval,* infection transmission *parameter.*

melanophore-expanding p., SYN melanotropin.

Mitrofanoff p., use of a catheterizable channel (appendix, bowel, ureter) to drain the bladder as an alternative to the urethra. SEE ALSO appendicovesicostomy.

nirvana p., in psychoanalysis, the p. that expresses the tendency to attain a conflict-free state of freedom from pain or worry.

organic p., SYN proximate p.

pain-pleasure p., a psychoanalytic concept that, in human psychic functioning, the person tends to seek pleasure and avoid pain; a term borrowed by experimental psychology to denote the same tendency of an animal in a learning situation. SYN pleasure p.

Pauli exclusion p., the theory limiting the number of electrons in the orbit or shell of an atom; that it is not possible for any two electrons to have all four quantum numbers identical.

pleasure p., SYN pain-pleasure p.

proximate p., in chemistry, an organic compound that may exist already formed as a part of some other more complex substance (e.g., various sugars, starches, and albumins). SYN organic p.

reality p., the concept that the pleasure p. in personality development is modified by the demands of external reality; the p. or force that compels the growing child to adapt to the demands of external reality.

repetition-compulsion p., in psychoanalysis, the impulse to redramatize or reenact earlier emotional experiences or situations. SYN p. of inertia.

ultimate p., one of the chemical elements.

Pringle, John J., English dermatologist, 1855–1922. SEE P. *disease;* Bourneville-Pringle *disease.*

Prinzmetal, Myron, U.S. cardiologist, 1908–1994. SEE P. *angina.*

pri·on (prī′on). Small, infectious proteinaceous particle, of non-nucleic acid composition because of its resistance to nucleases; the causative agent, either on a sporadic, genetic, or infectious basis, of six neurodegenerative diseases in animals, and four in humans; the latter include the spongiform encephalopathies of kuru, Creutzfeldt-Jakob disease, Gerstmann-Straussler-Scheinker syndrome and fatal familial insomnia. The gene encoding for the PrP is found on chromosome 20. SYN prion protein. [proteinaceous infectious particle]

> Stanley B. Prusiner received the Nobel Prize in Physiology or Medicine in 1997 for his discovery of prions. Prusiner began his research in 1972 to identify the infectious agent of Creutzfeldt-Jakob disease. In 1982 he and his colleagues isolated a protein that was capable of transmitting infection but, unlike all other known pathogens, contained neither DNA nor RNA. Prusiner's term for this protein, *prion,* was derived from the phrase *proteinaceous infectious particle.* A gene encoding this protein has been found in all animals tested, including humans. The prion protein can occur in either of 2 structural conformations, one that is normal (but of unknown function), designated PrPc, and one that results in disease, called PrPSc. The normal prion protein is a component of lymphocytes and other cells and is particularly abundant on the cell membranes of CNS neurons. The PrPSc prion protein is extremely stable and is resistant to proteolysis, organic solvents, and high temperatures. Once produced or acquired by a suitable host, it can initiate a chain reaction whereby normal PrPc protein is converted into the more stable PrPSc form. After a long, asymptomatic incubation period, the disease-causing PrPSc accumulates to reach neurotoxic levels. Symptoms of prion diseases vary with the parts of the brain affected. All known prion diseases lead to the death of those affected. Prion diseases are called spongiform encephalopathies because of the histologic appearance of affected cerebral cortex and cerebellum, which display large vacuoles. Probably most mammalian species develop these diseases. Prions are not living, are smaller than viruses, and do not elicit an immune response in either their normal or disease-causing form. Prion diseases besides Creutzfeldt-Jakob disease include kuru (once prevalent among the Fore people of New Guinea, who practiced ritual cannibalism), bovine spongiform encephalopathy (BSE, mad cow disease), and scrapie, a disease of sheep. A new variant of CJD may have arisen through transmission of prions to human beings from cattle infected with BSE. Prion diseases are unique in being both infectious and hereditary. Hereditary forms are due to transmitted mutations in the prion gene, located on chromosome 20 in human beings. Gertsmann-Sträussler-Scheinker (GSS) disease is a hereditary dementia resulting from a mutation in this gene. Approximately 50 families with GSS mutations have been identified. About 10–15% of cases of CJD are caused by inherited mutations in the prion protein gene. Strains of mice from which this gene has been abolished are immune to prion-caused disease. See Creutzfeldt-Jakob disease, bovine spongiform encephalopathy.

prism (prizm). A transparent solid, with sides that converge at an angle, that deflects a ray of light toward the thickest portion (the base) and splits white light into its component colors; in spectacles, a p. corrects ocular muscle imbalance. [G. *prisma*]

enamel p.'s, SYN *prismata* adamantina, under *prisma.*

Fresnel p., a p. composed of concentric annular rings.

Nicol p., a p. that transmits only polarized light.

Risley rotary p., a p. with a circular base that is rotated in a metal frame marked with a scale; used in examination of ocular muscle imbalance.

pris·ma, pl. **pris·ma·ta** (priz′mă, priz′mah-tă). A structure resembling a prism. [G. something sawed, a prism]

pris′mata adamanti′na, the calcified, microscopic rods radiating from the surface of the dentin, forming the substance of the enamel of a tooth. SYN enamel fibers, enamel prisms, enamel rods.

pris·mat·ic (priz-mat′ik). Relating to or resembling a prism.

pri·va·cy (prī′vă-sē). **1.** Being apart from others; seclusion; secrecy. **2.** Especially in psychiatry and clinical psychology, respect for the confidential nature of the therapist-patient relationship.

PRK Acronym for photorefractive *keratectomy.*

PRL Abbreviation for prolactin.

p.r.n. Abbreviation for L. pro re nata, as the occasion arises; when necessary.

Pro Symbol for proline or prolyl.

△**pro-.** **1.** Prefix denoting before, forward. SEE ALSO ante-, pre-. **2.** In chemistry, prefix indicating precursor of. SEE ALSO -gen. [L. and G. *pro*]

pro·ac·cel·er·in (prō-ak-sel′er-in). SYN *factor* V.

pro·ac·ro·sin (prō-ak′rō-sin). A precursor protein of acrosin.

pro·ac·ro·so·mal (prō-ak-rō-sō′mǎl). Relating to an early stage in the development of the acrosome.

pro·ac·tin·i·um (prō-ak-tin′ē-ŭm). SYN protactinium.

pro·ac·ti·va·tor (prō-ak′ti-vā-ter). A substance that, when chemically split, yields a fragment (activator) capable of rendering another substance enzymatically active.

pro·al (prō′ăl). Relating to a forward movement.

pro·am·ni·on (prō-am′nē-on). An area of the extraembryonic membranes beneath, and in front of, the developing head of a young embryo that remains without mesoderm for some time.

prob·a·bil·i·ty (P) (pro-bă-bil′i-tē). **1.** A measure, ranging from 0 to 1, of the likelihood of truth of a hypothesis or statement. **2.** The limit of the relative frequency of an event in a sequence of N random trials as N approaches infinity.

conditional p., a p. quoted when the range of choices admitted is restricted, i.e., conditional; thus, the p. of the child of a color-blind man inheriting the gene is 1/2 if the child is female and almost 0 if the child is male.

joint p., the p. that two or more outcomes are realized jointly.

objective p., a p. of an outcome based either on unassailable theory or extensive empiric experience of exactly the same combination of circumstances; the notion also implies that the realization concerned has not been effected and therefore even in principle not known with certainty.

personal p., an idiosyncratic judgment about the outcome of an event; it may include evidence too subtle to be disposed of in a subjective p.

posterior p., the best rational assessment of the p. of an outcome on the basis of established knowledge modified and brought up to date. SEE ALSO prior p., Bayes *theorem.* Cf. Bayes *theorem.*

prior p., the best rational assessment of the p. of an outcome on the basis of established knowledge before the present experiment is performed. For instance, the prior p. of the daughter of a carrier of hemophilia being herself a carrier of hemophilia is 1/2. But if the daughter already has an affected son, the posterior p. that she is a carrier is unity, whereas if she has a normal child, the posterior p. that she is a carrier is 1/3. SEE Bayes *theorem.*

subjective p., a fair statement of the odds that a rational, well-informed person would give or take for the outcome of an experiment. The experiment may be unique and not rationally understood (precluding both theoretically sound predication and empirical experience). The formulation is applicable to experiments that have been carried out but the outcome unknown. (For instance, a certain statement about the sex of the fetus early in pregnancy is established but perhaps not accessible until amniocentesis can be done.) Unlike personal p., the subjective p. should be the same from all competent counselors in possession of the same evidence.

pro·bac·te·ri·o·phage (prō-bak-tēr′ē-ō-fāj). The stage of a temperate bacteriophage in which the genome is incorporated in the genetic apparatus of the bacterial host. SYN prophage.

defective p., SEE defective *bacteriophage*.

pro·band (prō'band). In human genetics, the patient or member of the family that brings a family under study. SYN index case. [L. *probo,* to test, prove]

pro·bang (prō-bang'). A flexible rod with some soft material at the distal end used injudiciously to try to advance or retrieve foreign bodies from the esophagus; a practice to be condemned as dangerous. [alteration of *provang,* (a term of unknown etymology coined by the inventor, Walter Rumsey) under the influence of *probe*]

probe (prōb). **1.** A slender rod of rigid or flexible material, with a blunt bulbous tip, used for exploring sinuses, fistulas, other cavities, or wounds. **2.** A device or agent used to detect or explore a substance; e.g., a molecule used to detect the presence of a specific fragment of DNA or RNA or of a specific bacterial colony. **3.** To enter and explore, as with a p. [L. *probo,* to test]

> Probes are essential tools for DNA analysis. Every DNA molecule possesses some unique nucleotide sequences that differentiate it from all others. A probe is a relatively short fabricated fragment of DNA that matches, in lock-and-key fashion, a nucleotide sequence unique to the material that is being sought. Probes are used to test for the presence of cloned genes in bacterial or yeast colonies, for specific nucleotide sequences in samples of DNA, or for specific genes on chromosomes.

Bowman p., a double-ended p. for the lacrimal duct.

nucleic acid p., a nucleic acid fragment, labeled by a radioisotope, biotin, etc., that is complementary to a sequence in another nucleic acid (fragment) and that will, by hydrogen binding to the latter, locate or identify it and be detected; a diagnostic technique based on the fact that every species of microbe possesses some unique nucleic acid sequences that differentiate it from all others, and thus can be used as identifying markers or "fingerprints."

periodontal p., a calibrated instrument used to measure the depth and topography of periodontal pockets.

radioactive p., SEE nucleic acid p.

vertebrated p., a p. made up of a series of short sections hinged together for flexibility in penetrating convoluted tracts.

viral p., SEE nucleic acid p.

pro·ben·e·cid (prō-ben'ĕ-sid). A competitive inhibitor of the secretion of penicillin or *p*-aminohippurate by kidney tubules; a uricosuric agent used in chronic gouty arthritis.

pro·bil·i·fus·cins (prō-bil'i-fŭs'in). SEE bilirubinoids.

pro·bi·o·sis (prō-bī-ō'sis). An association of two organisms that enhances the life processes of both. Cf. antibiosis (1), symbiosis, mutualism. [pro- + G. *biōsis,* life]

pro·bi·ot·ic (prō-bī-ot'ik). Relating to probiosis.

prob·lem. In the mental health professions, a term often used to denote life problems (the difficulties or challenges of life); sometimes used in preference to the terms mental illness or mental disorder. [G. *problēma,* proposition, topic, fr. *proballo,* to put forward]

pro·bos·cis, pl. **pro·bos·ci·des, pro·bos·ci·ses** (prō-bos'is, prō-bos'i-dēz, -sēz). **1.** A long flexible snout, such as that of a tapir or an elephant. **2.** In teratology, a cylindric protuberance of the face that, in cyclopia or ethmocephaly, represents the nose. [G. *proboskis,* a means of providing food, fr. pro- + *boskein,* to feed]

Prob·sty·may·ria vi·vip·a·ra (prob-sti-mā'rē-ă vi-vip'ă-ră). A nematode (family Atractidae) closely related to the true pinworms (family Oxyuridae) and still commonly considered the horse pinworm; it is distributed worldwide and is found often in tremendous numbers, because of internal autoreinfection, in the colon of horses and other equids.

pro·bu·col (prō'bū-kōl). An antihyperlipoproteinemic agent.

pro·cain·a·mide hy·dro·chlo·ride (pro-kān'ă-mīd, pro'kān-am'īd, -id). Differs chemically from procaine by containing the amide group (CONH) instead of the ester group (COO). It de-presses the irritability of the cardiac muscle, having a quinidine-like action upon the heart, and is used in ventricular arrhythmias.

pro·caine hy·dro·chlo·ride (prō'kān). A local anesthetic for infiltration and spinal anesthesia; previously widely used but now infrequently employed.

pro·cap·sid (prō-kap'sid). A protein shell lacking a virus genome.

pro·car·ba·zine hy·dro·chlo·ride (prō-kar'bă-zēn). An antineoplastic agent.

pro·car·box·y·pep·ti·dase (prō'kar-bok-sē-pep'ti-dās). Inactive precursor of a carboxypeptidase.

pro·car·cin·o·gens (prō-kar-sin'-ō-jens). Inactive xenobiotics that are converted to carcinogens in the organism.

Pro·car·y·o·tae (pro-kar-ē-ō'tē). SYN Prokaryotae. [pro- + G. *karyon,* kernel, nut]

pro·car·y·ote (pro-kar'ē-ōt). SYN prokaryote. [pro- + G. *karyon,* kernel, nut]

pro·car·y·ot·ic (prō'kar-ē-ot'ik). SYN prokaryotic.

pro·cat·arc·tic (prō-kă-tark'tik). Rarely used term for denoting the exciting cause of a disease. [G. *prokatarktikos,* beginning beforehand]

pro·cat·arx·is (prō-kă-tark'sis). **1.** SYN exciting *cause.* **2.** The beginning of a disease under the influence of the exciting cause, a predisposing cause already existing. [G. a beginning beforehand, fr. *prokatararchomi,* to begin first, fr. *pro,* before, + *kata,* upon, + *archō,* to begin]

pro·ce·dure (prō-sē'jŭr). Act or conduct of diagnosis, treatment, or operation. SEE ALSO method, operation, technique.

back table p., p. performed on an organ that has been removed from a patient before it is replaced.

Batista p., surgical reduction of one or both ventricles when they are excessively dilated; incompletely investigated as of 1999. SYN ventricular reduction surgery.

Belsey p., SYN Belsey *fundoplication.*

Chamberlain p., a limited left anterior thoracostomy for biopsy of the mediastinal nodes out of reach by cervical mediastinoscopy. SEE ALSO anterior *mediastinoscopy.* SYN anterior mediastinotomy.

Clagett p. for empyema, a two-stage surgical p. for treatment of postpneumonectomy empyema without bronchopleural fistula.

Collis-Belsey p., SYN Collis-Nissen *fundoplication.*

commando p., an operation for malignant tumors of the floor of the oral cavity, involving resection of portions of the mandible in continuity with the oral lesion and radical neck dissection. SYN commando operation.

Damus-Kaye-Stancel p., a p. for subaortic stenosis, entails the creation of an end-to-side pulmonary trunk/aortic anastomosis, performed along with a Fontan p., particularly for patients with a double inlet left ventricle. SYN Damus-Stancel-Kaye anastomosis.

dideoxy p. (di'dē-ōks-ē), an enzymatic procedure for sequencing of DNA employing dideoxy nucleotides as chain terminators. SEE Sanger *method.*

Dor p., SYN Jatene p.

Eloesser p., transposition of a tonguelike pedicled skin flap from the chest wall into the depths of an incision that communicates with an empyema or peripheral lung abscess; used to prevent scar closure of the tract to ensure long-term mandatory dependent drainage. SEE ALSO Eloesser *flap.*

endorectal pull-through p., removal of diseased rectal mucosa along with resection of the lower bowel, followed by anastomosis of the proximal stump to the anus, to spare the function of the anus.

Ewart p., elevation of the larynx between the thumb and forefinger to elicit tracheal tugging.

Fontan p., placement of a conduit (usually valved) from the right atrium to the main pulmonary artery as a bypass to a hypoplastic right ventricle, as in tricuspid atresia. SYN Fontan operation.

Girdlestone p., complete resection or excision of the head and neck of the femur.

Harada-Ito p., a p. designed to correct ocular extorsion due to

4th nerve palsy by selectively tightening the anterior fibers of the superior oblique tendon.

Hummelsheim p., surgical p. to correct an ocular deviation due to a 6th nerve palsy by which the superior and inferior rectus tendons are split and transferred laterally.

Jatene p., a method of repairing congenital tunnel-type subaortic stenosis and narrowing of the left ventricular-aortic junction by aortoventriculoplasty and prosthetic valve replacement. SYN Dor p.

Kestenbaum p., surgical p. on the extraocular *muscles*, under *muscle* indicated for patients with torticollis associated with nystagmus.

Konno p., a method of repairing congenital tunnel-type subaortic stenosis and narrowing of the left ventricular-aortic junction by aortoventriculoplasty and prosthetic valve replacement.

Konno-Rastan p., an aortoventriculoplasty used to enlarge the aortic annular size, especially when subaortic fibromuscular stenosis is present.

lateral tarsal strip p., a p. designed to correct lower eyelid malposition due to horizontal lid laxity by shortening it at the lateral canthal end.

loop electrocautery excision p. (LEEP), electrocautery excisional biopsy of abnormal cervical tissue.

loop electrosurgical excision p. (LEEP), SYN loop *excision.*

McCall culdoplasty p., method of supporting the vaginal cuff during a vaginal hysterectomy by attaching the uterosacral and cardinal ligaments to the peritoneal surface with suture material that, when tied, draws toward the midline, helping to close off the cul-de-sac.

Mitchell p., surgical p. to correct a hallux valgus by combining a bunionectomy and soft tissue correction of the first metatarsophalangeal joint with an osteotomy of the proximal portion of the first metatarsal.

Mustard p., SYN Mustard *operation.*

Nick p., enlarges the aortic annulus by incising the noncoronary sinus and the roof of the left atrium.

Noble-Collip p., obsolete p. in which shock in rats is induced by rotating them in a drum.

Norwood p., a complex p. designed to treat aortic atresia with hypoplastic left heart syndrome; sometimes performed in two stages.

Puestow p., longitudinal pancreaticojejunostomy for treatment of chronic pancreatitis.

push-back p., a surgical maneuver designed to reposition the soft palate posteriorly to reestablish velopharyngeal competence.

Putti-Platt p., SYN Putti-Platt *operation.*

Reichel-Pólya stomach p., retrocolic anastomosis of the full circumference of the open stomach to the jejunum.

Rittenhouse-Manogian p., enlarges the aortic annulus by incising the left coronary-noncoronary commissure down unto the anterior leaflet of the mitral valve.

Ross p., p. for aortic valve stenosis or regurgitation in which the aortic valve is replaced with the patient's own pulmonic valve (autograft) and the pulmonic valve is in turn replaced with a homograft valve.

sacrocolpopexy p., support of the vaginal vault by affixing it to the periosteum of the sacrum following a hysterectomy. [sacro- + colpo- + -pexy]

sacrospinous vaginal vault suspension p., surgical repair of prolapsed vaginal vault by suturing to the sacrospinous ligament; done either vaginally or abdominally.

shelf p., insertion of a graft from the ilium into the roof of the acetabulum for congenital dislocation of the hip.

Sugiura p., esophageal transection with paraesophageal devascularization, for esophageal varices.

Thal p., correction of a benign stricture of the lower esophagus in which the narrowed area is opened longitudinally and the adjacent external gastric wall is patch sutured over this defect.

Vineberg p., obsolete operation for myocardial ischemia in which the internal mammary artery is implanted into the myocardium to improve blood flow to the heart.

Walsh p., anatomic (nerve-sparing) radical retropubic prostatectomy.

pro·ce·lia (prō-sē′lē-ă). A lateral ventricle of the brain; the hollow of the prosencephalon. [pro- + G. *koilia,* a hollow]

pro·ce·lous (prō-sē′lŭs). Concave anteriorly. [pro- + G. *koilos,* hollow]

pro·cen·tri·ole (prō-sen′trē-ōl). The early phase in development *de novo* of centrioles or basal bodies from the centrosphere; p.'s form in relation to deuterosomes (p. organizers).

pro·ce·phal·ic (prō-se-fal′ik). Relating to the anterior part of the head. [pro- + G. *kephalē,* head]

pro·cer·coid (prō-ser′koyd). The first stage in the aquatic life cycle of certain tapeworms, such as the pseudophyllideans (family Diphyllobothriidae), following ingestion of the newly hatched larva (coracidium) by a copepod (water flea). The p. develops into a tailed larva in the body cavity of the crustacean first intermediate host; when the p. and its host are ingested by a fish, the p. enters the new host's tissues and becomes a plerocercoid. SEE ALSO *Diphyllobothrium latum,* Pseudophyllidea. [pro- + G. *kerkos,* tail, + *eidos,* resemblance]

pro·ce·rus (prō-sē′rŭs). SYN procerus (*muscle*). [L. long, stretched out]

PROCESS

pro·cess (pros′es, prō′ses) [TA]. **1.** In anatomy, a projection or outgrowth. SYN processus [TA]. **2.** A method or mode of action used in the attainment of a certain result. **3.** An advance, progress, or method, as of a disease. SEE processus. **4.** A pathologic condition or disease. **5.** In dentistry, a series of operations that convert a wax pattern, such as that of a denture base, into a solid denture base of another material. SEE dental *curing.* [L. *processus,* an advance, progress, process, fr. *pro-cedo,* pp. *-cessus,* to go forward]

A.B.C. p., purification of water or deodorization of sewage by a mixture of *alum, blood,* and *charcoal.*

accessory p. of lumbar vertebra [TA], a small apophysis at the posterior part of the base of the transverse process of each of the lumbar vertebrae. SYN processus accessorius vertebrae lumbalis [TA], accessory tubercle.

acromial p., SYN acromion.

agene p., bleaching of flour with nitrogen trichloride (prohibited in the United States).

alar p., SYN *ala* of crista galli.

alveolar p. of maxilla [TA], the projecting ridge on the inferior surface of the body of the maxilla containing the tooth sockets; the term is also applied to the superior aspect of the body of the mandible, containing the tooth sockets of the lower jaw. SYN alveolar body, alveolar bone (1), alveolar border (2), alveolar ridge, basal ridge (1), dental p., processus alveolaris maxillae.

anterior clinoid p. [TA], the posteriorly directed projection that is the medial end of the sphenoidal ridge (lesser wing of sphenoid); it provides attachment for the free edge of the tentorium cerebelli. SYN processus clinoideus anterior [TA].

anterior p. of malleus [TA], a slender spur running anteriorly from the neck of the malleus toward the petrotympanic fissure. SYN processus anterior mallei [TA], Folli p., follian p., long p. of malleus, processus gracilis, processus ravii, Rau p., Ravius p., slender p. of malleus.

apical p., the dendritic p. extending from the apex of a pyramidal cell of the cerebral cortex toward the surface. SYN apical dendrite.

articular p. [TA], one of the bilateral small flat projections on the surfaces of the arches of the vertebrae, at the point where the pedicles and laminae join, forming the zygapophysial joint surfaces. SYN processus articularis [TA], zygapophysis.

ascending p., SYN *processus* ascendens.

auditory p., the roughened edge of the tympanic plate giving attachment to the cartilaginous portion of the external acoustic meatus.

basilar p., SYN basilar *part* of occipital bone.

basilar p. of occipital bone, SYN basilar *part* of occipital bone.

binary p., a random event with two exhaustive and mutually exclusive outcomes; a Bernoulli p.

Budde p., a method of milk sterilization; to the fresh milk, hydrogen peroxide is added in the proportion of 15 mL of a 3% solution to 1 liter of milk, and the mixture is heated to 51° or 52°C (124°F) for 3 hours, by which time the peroxide is decomposed and the nascent oxygen acts as an efficient germicide; the milk is then rapidly cooled and put into sealed bottles.

Burns falciform p., SYN superior *horn* of falciform margin of saphenous opening.

calcaneal p. of cuboid [TA], the process projecting posteriorly from the plantar surface of the cuboid; it supports the anterior end of the calcaneus. SYN processus calcaneus ossis cuboidei [TA].

caudate p. [TA], a narrow band of hepatic tissue connecting the caudate and right lobes of the liver posterior to the porta hepatis. SYN processus caudatus [TA].

ciliary p. [TA], one of the radiating pigmented ridges, usually 70 in number, on the inner surface of the ciliary body, increasing in thickness as they advance from the orbiculus ciliaris to the external border of the iris; these, together with the folds (plicae) in the furrows between them, constitute the corona ciliaris. SYN processus ciliaris [TA].

Civinini p., SYN pterygospinous p.

clinoid p. [TA], one of three pairs of bony projections from the sphenoid bone; the anterior and posterior pairs of which surround the hypophysial fossa like bedposts. SYN processus clinoideus [TA], clinoid (2).

cochleariform p., SYN *processus* cochleariformis.

complex learning p.'s, those p.'s that require the use of symbolic manipulations, as in reasoning.

condylar p. of mandible [TA], the articular process of the ramus of the mandible; it includes the head of the mandible, the neck of the mandible and pterygoid fovea. SYN processus condylaris mandibulae [TA], condyloid p., mandibular condyle.

condyloid p., SYN condylar p. of mandible.

conoid p., SYN conoid *tubercle* (of clavicle).

coracoid p. [TA], a long, curved projection resembling a flexed finger arising from the neck of the scapula overhanging the glenoid cavity; it gives attachment to the short head of the biceps, the coracobrachialis, and the pectoralis minor muscles, and the conoid and coracoacromial ligaments. SYN processus coracoideus [TA].

coronoid p., a sharp triangular projection from a bone. SYN processus coronoideus.

coronoid p. of the mandible [TA], the triangular anterior process of the mandibular ramus, giving attachment to the temporal muscle. SYN processus coronoideus mandibulae [TA].

coronoid p. of the ulna [TA], a bracketlike projection from the anterior portion of the proximal extremity of the ulna; its anterior surface gives attachment to the brachialis, and its proximal surface enters into the formation of the trochlear notch. SYN processus coronoideus ulnae [TA].

costal p. [TA], an apophysis extending laterally from the transverse process of a lumbar vertebra; it is the homolog of the rib. SYN processus costalis [TA].

dendritic p., SYN dendrite (1).

dental p., SYN alveolar p. of maxilla.

ensiform p., SYN xiphoid p.

ethmoidal p. of inferior nasal concha [TA], a projection of the inferior concha, situated behind the lacrimal process and articulating with the uncinate process of the ethmoid. SYN processus ethmoidalis conchae nasalis inferioris [TA].

falciform p. of sacrotuberous ligament [TA], a continuation of the inner border of the sacrotuberous ligament upward and forward on the inner aspect of the ramus of the ischium. SYN processus falciformis ligamenti sacrotuberalis [TA], falciform ligament, ligamentum falciforme.

Folli p., SYN anterior p. of malleus.

follian p., SYN anterior p. of malleus.

foot p., SYN pedicel.

frontal p. of maxilla [TA], the upward extension from the body of the maxilla, which articulates with the frontal bone. SYN processus frontalis maxillae [TA], nasal p.

frontal p. of zygomatic bone [TA], the p. of the zygomatic bone that extends upward to form the lateral margin of the orbit and articulates with the frontal bone and greater wing of the sphenoid bone. SYN processus frontalis ossis zygomatici [TA], frontosphenoidal p.

frontonasal p., SYN frontonasal *prominence*.

frontosphenoidal p., SYN frontal p. of zygomatic bone.

funicular p., the tunica vaginalis surrounding the spermatic cord.

globular p., obsolete term for intermaxillary *segment*.

hamular p. of lacrimal bone, SYN lacrimal *hamulus*.

hamular p. of sphenoid bone, SYN pterygoid *hamulus*.

head p., the primordium for the notochord. SEE ALSO notochordal p.

inferior articular p. [TA], one of the articular processes on the inferior surface of the vertebral arch. SYN zygapophysis inferior [TA].

Ingrassia p., SYN lesser *wing* of sphenoid (bone).

intrajugular p. [TA], a small, pointed process of bone extending from the middle of the jugular notch in both the occipital and the temporal bones, the two being joined by a ligament and dividing the jugular foramen into two portions. SYN processus intrajugularis [TA].

jugular p. of occipital bone [TA], a short process jutting out from the posterior part of the condyle of the occipital bone, its anterior border forming the posterior boundary of the jugular foramen. SYN processus jugularis ossis occipitalis [TA].

lacrimal p. of inferior nasal concha [TA], a projection from the anterior edge of the inferior concha that articulates with the lower border of the lacrimal bone. SYN processus lacrimalis conchae nasalis inferioris [TA].

lateral p. of calcaneal tuberosity [TA], the lateral projection from the posterior part of the calcaneus. SYN processus lateralis tuberis calcanei [TA].

lateral p. of malleus [TA], a short projection from the base of the manubrium of the malleus, attached firmly to the drum membrane. SYN processus lateralis mallei [TA], processus brevis, short p. of malleus, tuberculum mallei.

lateral nasal p., SYN lateral nasal *prominence*.

lateral p. of septal nasal cartilage [TA], the flat process of the septal nasal cartilage located in the lateral wall of the nose above the alar cartilage. SYN cartilago nasi lateralis, lateral cartilage of nose.

lateral p. of talus [TA], a projection on the lateral side of the talus below the malleolar articular surface. SYN processus lateralis tali [TA].

Lenhossék p.'s, short p.'s ("aborted axons") possessed by some ganglion cells.

lenticular p. of incus [TA], a knob at the tip of the long limb of the incus that articulates with the stapes. SYN processus lenticularis incudis [TA], lenticular apophysis, lenticular bone, orbicular bone, orbicular p., orbiculare, os orbiculare, os sylvii.

long p. of malleus, SYN anterior p. of malleus.

malar p., SYN zygomatic p. of maxilla.

mammillary p. of lumbar vertebra [TA], a small apophysis or tubercle on the dorsal margin of the superior articular process of each of the lumbar vertebrae and usually of the twelfth thoracic vertebra. SYN processus mammillaris vertebrae lumbalis [TA], mammillary tubercle, metapophysis.

mandibular p., SYN mandibular *arch*.

Markov p., a stochastic p. such that the conditional probability distribution for the state at any future instant, given the present state, is unaffected by any additional knowledge of the past history of the system.

mastoid p. [TA], the nipplelike projection of the petrous part of the temporal bone. SYN processus mastoideus [TA], mastoid bone, temporal apophysis.

mastoid p. of petrous part of temporal bone [TA], the portion of the petrous part of the temporal bone bearing the mastoid process. SYN processus mastoideus partis petrosae ossis temporalis [TA], mastoid part of the temporal bone, pars mastoidea ossis temporalis.

maxillary p. of embryo, the proximal part of the first pharyngeal arch that develops in most of the upper jaw.

maxillary p. of inferior nasal concha [TA], a thin plate of irregular form projecting from the middle of the upper border of the inferior concha, articulating with the maxilla bone and partly closing the orifice of the maxillary sinus. SYN processus maxillaris conchae nasalis inferioris [TA].

medial p. of calcaneal tuberosity [TA], the medial projection from the posterior part of the calcaneus. SYN processus medialis tuberis calcanei [TA].

medial nasal p., SYN medial nasal *prominence*.

mental p., SYN mental *protuberance*.

middle clinoid p. [TA], an inconstant, small spur of bone on the body of the sphenoid, posterolateral to (and occasionally continuous with) the tuberculum sellae; it is around this point that the internal carotid artery makes a 180° turn, changing direction from anterior to posterior to join the cerebral arterial circle. SYN processus clinoideus medius [TA].

muscular p. of arytenoid cartilage [TA], the blunt lateral projection of the arytenoid cartilage giving attachment to the lateral and posterior cricoarytenoid muscles of the larynx. SYN processus muscularis cartilaginis arytenoideae [TA].

nasal p., SYN frontal p. of maxilla.

notochordal p., in the embryo, a midline column of cells that are rostral to the primitive node and form the notochord. SEE ALSO head p.

odontoblastic p., the extension of the odontoblast that lies within the dentinal tubule; application of stimuli to dentin may cause aspiration of odontoblast contents into the p.

odontoid p., SYN dens (2).

odontoid p. of epistropheus, SYN dens (2).

olecranon p., SYN olecranon.

orbicular p., SYN lenticular p. of incus.

orbital p. of palatine bone [TA], the anterior and larger of the two processes at the upper extremity of the vertical plate of the palatine bone, articulating with the maxilla, ethmoid, and sphenoid bones. SYN processus orbitalis ossis palatini [TA].

packing p., the method of placing denture base material in a flask for processing.

palatine p. of maxilla [TA], medially directed shelves from the maxillae that, with the horizontal plate of the palatine bone, form the bony palate. SYN processus palatinus ossis maxillae [TA].

papillary p. of caudate lobe of liver [TA], the left lower angle of the caudate lobe of the liver, opposite the caudate process. SYN processus papillaris lobi caudati hepatis [TA].

paramastoid p. [TA], an occasional process of bone extending downward from the jugular process of the occipital bone in humans. SYN processus paramastoideus [TA], paroccipital p.

paroccipital p., SYN paramastoid p.

posterior clinoid p. [TA], the sharp superolateral corners of the dorsum sella that provide attachment for connective tissue fibers that radiate within the tentorium cerebelli. SYN processus clinoideus posterior [TA].

posterior p. of septal cartilage [TA], the tapering extension of the septal cartilage that lies between the perpendicular plate of the ethmoid and the vomer. SYN processus posterior cartilaginis septi nasi [TA], sphenoid p. of septal nasal cartilage [TA], processus sphenoidalis cartilaginis septi nasi*.

posterior p. of talus [TA], a projection of the talus bearing medial and lateral tubercles; it is posterior and inferior to the trochlea. SYN processus posterior tali [TA], Stieda p.

primary p., in psychoanalysis, the mental p. directly related to the functions of the primitive life forces associated with the id and characteristic of unconscious mental activity; marked by unorganized, illogical thinking and by the tendency to seek immediate discharge and gratification of instinctual demands. Cf. secondary p.

progressive p.'s, p.'s that continue after they no longer serve the needs of the organism, and after cessation of the stimulus that evoked the p.

pterygoid p. of sphenoid bone [TA], a long p. extending downward from the junction of the body and greater wing of the sphenoid bone on either side; it is formed of two plates (lateral and medial), united anteriorly but separated below to form the pterygoid notch; the pterygoid fossa is formed by the divergence of these two plates posteriorly. SYN processus pterygoideus ossis sphenoidalis [TA], os pterygoideum.

pterygospinous p. [TA], a sharp projection from the posterior edge of the lateral pterygoid plate of the sphenoid bone. SYN processus pterygospinosus [TA], Civinini p.

pyramidal p. of palatine bone [TA], the portion of the palatine bone passing lateral and posterior from the angle formed by the vertical and horizontal plates. SYN processus pyramidalis ossis palatini [TA].

Rau p., SYN anterior p. of malleus.

Ravius p., SYN anterior p. of malleus.

retromandibular p. of parotid gland, SYN deep *part* of parotid gland.

secondary p., in psychoanalysis, the mental p. directly related to the learned and acquired functions of the ego and characteristic of conscious and preconscious mental activities; marked by logical thinking and by the tendency to delay gratification by regulation of the discharge of instinctual demands. Cf. primary p.

sheath p. of sphenoid bone, SYN vaginal p. of sphenoid bone.

short p. of malleus, SYN lateral p. of malleus.

slender p. of malleus, SYN anterior p. of malleus.

sphenoid p., SYN sphenoidal p. of palatine bone.

sphenoidal p. of palatine bone [TA], the posterior and smaller of the two processes at the extremity of the vertical plate of the palatine bone. SYN processus sphenoidalis ossis palatini [TA], sphenoid p.

sphenoid p. of septal nasal cartilage [TA], SYN posterior p. of septal cartilage.

spinous p. of sphenoid, SYN spine of sphenoid bone.

spinous p. of tibia, SYN intercondylar *eminence*.

spinous p. of vertebra [TA], the dorsal projection from the center of a vertebral arch. SYN processus spinosus vertebrae [TA].

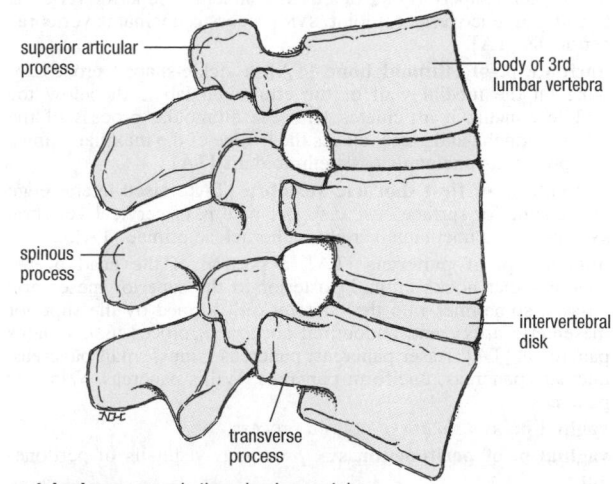

superior articular process

body of 3rd lumbar vertebra

spinous process

intervertebral disk

transverse process

vertebral processes in three lumbar vertebrae

Stieda p., SYN posterior p. of talus.

stochastic p., a p. that incorporates some element of randomness. [G. *stochastikos*, pertaining to guessing, fr. *stochazomai*, to guess]

styloid p. of fibula, SYN *apex* of head of fibula.

styloid p. of radius [TA], a thick, pointed, palpable projection on the lateral side of the distal extremity of the radius. SYN processus styloideus radii [TA].

styloid p. of temporal bone [TA], a slender needlelike pointed

pr

projection running downward and slightly forward from the base of the inferior surface of the petrous portion of the temporal bone where it joins the tympanic portion; it gives attachment to the styloglossus, stylohyoid, and stylopharyngeus muscles and the stylohyoid and stylomandibular ligaments. SYN processus styloideus ossis temporalis [TA].

styloid p. of third metacarpal bone [TA], a pointed projection from the dorsolateral angle of the base of the third metacarpal bone; it sometimes exists as a separate ossicle. SYN processus styloideus ossis metacarpalis III [TA].

styloid p. of ulna [TA], a cylindrical, pointed palpable projection from the medial and posterior aspect of the head of the ulna, to the tip of which is attached the ulnar collateral ligament of the wrist. SYN processus styloideus ulnae [TA].

superior articular p. [TA], one of the articular processes on the superior surface of the vertebral arch. SYN zygapophysis superior [TA], diapophysis.

superior articular p. of sacrum [TA], the large process on each side of the sacrum posteriorly that articulates with the corresponding inferior articular process of the fifth lumbar vertebra. SYN processus articularis superior ossis sacri [TA].

supracondylar p. of humerus [TA], an occasional spine projecting from the anteromedial surface of the humerus about 5 cm above the medial epicondyle to which it is joined by a fibrous band. The supracondylar foramen thus formed transmits the brachial artery and median nerve. SYN processus supraepicondylaris humeri [TA], supraepicondylar p.

supraepicondylar p., SYN supracondylar p. of humerus.

temporal p. of zygomatic bone [TA], the posterior projection of the zygomatic bone articulating with the zygomatic process of the temporal bone to form the zygomatic arch. SYN processus temporalis ossis zygomatici [TA].

Tomes p.'s, apical p.'s of ameloblasts.

transverse p. of vertebra [TA], a bony protrusion on either side of the arch of a vertebra, from the junction of the lamina and pedicle, which functions as a lever for attached muscles. SYN processus transversus vertebrae [TA].

trochlear p., SYN fibular *trochlea* of calcaneus.

uncinate p. of cervical vertebra [TA], raised lateral margins of the superior surface of the cervical vertebrae; with aging they often extend superiorly sufficient to contact the superior vertebra, forming an uncovertebral joint. SYN processus uncinatus vertebrae cervicalis [TA].

uncinate p. of ethmoid bone [TA], a sickle-shaped process of bone on the medial wall of the ethmoidal labyrinth below the middle concha; it articulates with the ethmoidal process of the inferior concha and partly closes the orifice of the maxillary sinus. SYN processus uncinatus ossis ethmoidalis [TA].

uncinate p. of first thoracic vertebra [TA], raised lateral edge of the superior surface. SEE ALSO uncinate p. of cervical vertebra. SYN processus uncinatus vertebrae thoracicae primae [TA].

uncinate p. of pancreas [TA], a portion of the head of the pancreas that hooks around posterior to the superior mesenteric vessels, sometimes into the "nutcracker" formed by the superior mesenteric artery and abdominal aorta. SYN processus uncinatus pancreatis [TA], lesser pancreas, pancreas minus, small pancreas, uncinate pancreas, unciform pancreas, Willis pancreas, Winslow pancreas.

vaginal p., SYN *sheath* of styloid process.

vaginal p. of peritoneum, SYN *processus* vaginalis of peritoneum.

vaginal p. of sphenoid bone [TA], a thin lamina of bone that extends medially under the body of the sphenoid bone from the medial lamina of the pterygoid process; it articulates with the vomer and the palatine bone. SYN processus vaginalis ossis sphenoidalis [TA], sheath p. of sphenoid bone.

vaginal p. of testis, SYN *processus* vaginalis of peritoneum.

vermiform p., SYN appendix (2).

vocal p., SYN vocal p. of arytenoid cartilage.

vocal p. of arytenoid cartilage [TA], the lower end of the anterior margin of the arytenoid cartilage to which the vocal cord is attached. SYN processus vocalis cartilaginis arytenoideae [TA], vocal p.

xiphoid p. [TA], the cartilage at the lower end of the sternum. SYN processus xiphoideus [TA], ensiform p., ensisternum, metasternum, mucro sterni, xiphisternum, xiphoid cartilage.

zygomatic p. of frontal bone [TA], the massive projection of the frontal bone that joins the zygomatic bone to form the lateral margin of the orbit. SYN processus zygomaticus ossis frontalis [TA].

zygomatic p. of maxilla [TA], the rough projection from the maxilla that articulates with the zygomatic bone. SYN processus zygomaticus maxillae [TA], malar p.

zygomatic p. of temporal bone [TA], the anterior process of the temporal bone that articulates with the temporal process of the zygomatic bone to form the zygomatic arch. SYN processus zygomaticus ossis temporalis [TA].

---

pro·cess·ing (pros′es-ing). **1.** Posttranslational modification of proteins, particularly secretory proteins and proteins targeted for membranes or specific cellular locations. SYN trafficking. **2.** Posttranscriptional modification of polynucleic acids.

pro·ces·sor (pră′ses-sōr). A device that converts one form of energy into another form of energy or one form of material into another form of material.

speech p., the part of a cochlear implant that converts speech into electrical impulses that are used to stimulate the neurons of the auditory division of the eighth cranial nerve.

PROCESSUS

---

pro·ces·sus, pl. **pro·ces·sus** (prō-ses′ŭs) [TA]. SYN process (1). [L. see process]

p. accesso′rius vertebrae lumbalis [TA], SYN accessory *process* of lumbar vertebra.

p. alveola′ris maxillae, SYN alveolar *process* of maxilla; SEE ALSO alveolar *bone* (2).

p. ante′rior mal′lei [TA], SYN anterior *process* of malleus.

p. articula′ris [TA], SYN articular *process.*

p. articula′ris supe′rior os′sis sa′cri [TA], SYN superior articular *process* of sacrum.

p. ascen′dens, an upward extension of the embryonic pterygoquadrate cartilage; it develops into the greater wing of the sphenoid bone. SYN ascending process.

p. bre′vis, SYN lateral *process* of malleus.

p. calca′neus os′sis cuboi′dei [TA], SYN calcaneal *process* of cuboid.

p. cauda′tus [TA], SYN caudate *process.*

p. cilia′ris [TA], SYN ciliary *process.*

p. clinoi′deus [TA], SYN clinoid *process.*

p. clinoideus anterior [TA], SYN anterior clinoid *process.*

p. clinoideus medius [TA], SYN middle clinoid *process.*

p. clinoideus posterior [TA], SYN posterior clinoid *process.*

p. cochlearifor′mis [TA], a bony angular process (the termination of the septum of the pharyngotympanic (auditory) tube) above the anterior end of the vestibular window, forming a pulley over which the tendon of the tensor tympani muscle plays. SYN cochleariform process, p. trochleariformis.

p. condyla′ris mandibulae [TA], SYN condylar *process* of mandible.

p. coracoi′deus [TA], SYN coracoid *process.*

p. coronoi′deus, SYN coronoid *process.*

p. coronoideus mandibulae [TA], SYN coronoid *process* of the mandible.

p. coronoideus ulnae [TA], SYN coronoid *process* of the ulna.

p. costa′lis [TA], SYN costal *process.*

p. ethmoida′lis conchae nasalis inferioris [TA], SYN ethmoidal *process* of inferior nasal concha.

p. falcifor′mis ligamenti sacrotuberalis [TA], SYN falciform *process* of sacrotuberous ligament.

p. ferrei′ni, SYN medullary *ray.*

p. fronta′lis maxil′lae [TA], SYN frontal *process* of maxilla.

p. fronta′lis os′sis zygomat′ici [TA], SYN frontal *process* of zygomatic bone.

p. grac′ilis, SYN anterior *process* of malleus.

p. intrajugula′ris [TA], SYN intrajugular *process.*

p. jugula′ris ossis occipitalis [TA], SYN jugular *process* of occipital bone.

p. lacrima′lis conchae nasalis inferioris [TA], SYN lacrimal *process* of inferior nasal concha.

p. latera′lis mal′lei [TA], SYN lateral *process* of malleus.

p. latera′lis ta′li [TA], SYN lateral *process* of talus.

p. latera′lis tu′beris calca′nei [TA], SYN lateral *process* of calcaneal tuberosity.

p. lenticula′ris incu′dis [TA], SYN lenticular *process* of incus.

p. mammilla′ris vertebrae lumbalis [TA], SYN mammillary *process* of lumbar vertebra.

p. mastoi′deus [TA], SYN mastoid *process.*

p. mastoideus partis petrosae ossis temporalis [TA], SYN mastoid *process* of petrous part of temporal bone.

p. maxilla′ris conchae nasalis inferioris [TA], SYN maxillary *process* of inferior nasal concha.

p. media′lis tu′beris calca′nei [TA], SYN medial *process* of calcaneal tuberosity.

p. muscula′ris cartila′ginis arytenoi′deae [TA], SYN muscular *process* of arytenoid cartilage.

p. orbita′lis ossis palatini [TA], SYN orbital *process* of palatine bone.

p. palati′nus ossis maxillae [TA], SYN palatine *process* of maxilla.

p. papilla′ris lobi caudati hepatis [TA], SYN papillary *process* of caudate lobe of liver.

p. paramastoi′deus [TA], SYN paramastoid *process.*

p. poste′rior cartila′ginis sep′ti na′si [TA], SYN posterior *process* of septal cartilage.

p. poste′rior ta′li [TA], SYN posterior *process* of talus.

p. pterygoi′deus ossis sphenoidalis [TA], SYN pterygoid *process* of sphenoid bone.

p. pterygospino′sus [TA], SYN pterygospinous *process.*

p. pyramida′lis ossis palatini [TA], SYN pyramidal *process* of palatine bone.

p. ra′vii, SYN anterior *process* of malleus.

p. retromandibula′ris, SYN deep *part* of parotid gland.

p. retromandibula′ris glan′dulae paro′tidis, SYN deep *part* of parotid gland.

p. sphenoida′lis cartila′ginis sep′ti na′si, ✩official alternate term for posterior *process* of septal cartilage.

p. sphenoida′lis ossis palatini [TA], SYN sphenoidal *process* of palatine bone.

p. spino′sus [TA], SYN *spine* of sphenoid bone.

p. spinosus vertebrae [TA], SYN spinous *process* of vertebra.

p. styloi′deus os′sis metacarpa′lis III [TA], SYN styloid *process* of third metacarpal bone.

p. styloi′deus os′sis tempora′lis [TA], SYN styloid *process* of temporal bone.

p. styloi′deus ra′dii [TA], SYN styloid *process* of radius.

p. styloi′deus ul′nae [TA], SYN styloid *process* of ulna.

p. supraepicondyla′ris hu′meri [TA], SYN supracondylar *process* of humerus.

p. tempora′lis ossis zygomatici [TA], SYN temporal *process* of zygomatic bone.

p. transver′sus vertebrae [TA], SYN transverse *process* of vertebra.

p. trochleariform′is, SYN p. cochleariformis.

p. trochlea′ris, SYN fibular *trochlea* of calcaneus.

p. uncina′tus os′sis ethmoida′lis [TA], SYN uncinate *process* of ethmoid bone.

p. uncina′tus pancrea′tis [TA], SYN uncinate *process* of pancreas.

p. uncinatus vertebrae cervicalis [TA], SYN uncinate *process* of cervical vertebra.

p. uncinatus vertebrae thoracicae primae [TA], SYN uncinate *process* of first thoracic vertebra.

p. vagina′lis os′sis sphenoida′lis [TA], SYN vaginal *process* of sphenoid bone.

p. vagina′lis peritone′i, SYN p. vaginalis of peritoneum.

p. vaginalis of peritoneum, a peritoneal diverticulum in the embryonic lower anterior abdominal wall that traverses the inguinal canal; in the male it forms the tunica vaginalis testis and normally loses its connection with the peritoneal cavity; a persistent p. vaginalis in the female is known as the canal of Nuck. SYN Nuck diverticulum, p. vaginalis peritonei, vaginal process of peritoneum, vaginal process of testis.

p. vermifor′mis, SYN appendix (2).

p. voca′lis cartila′ginis arytenoi′deae [TA], SYN vocal *process* of arytenoid cartilage.

p. xiphoi′deus [TA], SYN xiphoid *process.*

p. zygomat′icus maxil′lae [TA], SYN zygomatic *process* of maxilla.

p. zygomat′icus os′sis fronta′lis [TA], SYN zygomatic *process* of frontal bone.

p. zygomat′icus os′sis tempora′lis [TA], SYN zygomatic *process* of temporal bone.

---

pro·chei·lia, pro·chi·lia (prō-kī′lē-ă). Protruding lips. [pro- + G. *cheilos,* lip]

pro·chei·lon, pro·chi·lon (prō-kī′lon). SYN *tubercle* of upper lip.

pro·chi·ral (prō-kī′ral). Refers to an atom in a molecule (usually a carbon atom) that would become chiral if one of two identical substituents is replaced by a new ligand; i.e., an atom that has two enantiotopic groups linked to it. For example, carbon-1 of ethanol is a prochiral carbon.

pro·chi·ral·i·ty (prō-ki-ral′i-tē). The property of being prochiral.

pro·chlor·per·a·zine (prō-klōr-per′ă-zēn). A phenothiazine compound similar in structure, actions, and uses to chlorpromazine; used as a tranquilizer and antiemetic; available as the edisylate for oral and intramuscular administration and as the maleate for oral administration.

pro·chon·dral (prō-kon′drăl). Denoting a developmental stage prior to the formation of cartilage. [pro- + G. *chondros,* cartilage]

pro·chor·dal (prō-kōr′dăl). Located cephalic to the notochord. SYN prechordal.

pro·chy·mo·sin (prō-kī′mō-sin). The precursor of chymosin. SYN chymosinogen, pexinogen, prorennin, renninogen, rennogen.

pro·ci·den·tia (pros-i-den′shē-ă, prō′si-). A sinking down or prolapse of any organ or part; usually related to prolapse of the uterus. [L. a falling forward, fr. *procido,* to fall forward]

p. u′teri, SEE *prolapse* of the uterus.

pro·col·la·gen (prō-kol′ă-jen). Soluble precursor of collagen formed by fibroblasts and other cells in the process of collagen synthesis; unstable type III p. is associated with Ehlers-Danlos syndrome type IV.

p. aminoproteinase, an extracellular enzyme that participates in the processing of collagen, removing the extension peptide at the amino-terminal end of p.

p. carboxyproteinase, an extracellular enzyme that participates in the processing of collagen, removing the extension peptide at the carboxy-terminal end of p.

pro·con·ver·tin (prō-kon-ver′tin). SYN *factor* VII.

pro·cre·ate (prō′krē-āt). To beget; to produce by the sexual act; said usually of the male parent. [L. *pro-creo,* pp. *-creatus,* to beget]

pro·cre·a·tion (prō-krē-ā′shŭn). SYN reproduction (1).

pro·cre·a·tive (prō′krē-ā-tiv). Having the power to beget or procreate.

pr

△**proct-.**   SEE procto-.

proc·tal·gia (prok-tal′jē-ă). Pain at the anus, or in the rectum. SYN proctodynia, rectalgia. [proct- + G. *algos*, pain]

p. fu′gax, painful spasm of the muscle about the anus without known cause; probably a neurosis. SYN anorectal spasm.

proc·ta·tre·sia (prok-tă-trē′zē-ă). SYN anal *atresia.* [proct- + G. *a-* priv. + *trēsis*, a boring]

proc·tec·ta·sia (prok′tek-tā′zē-ă). Obsolete term for dilation of the anus or rectum. [proct- + G. *ektasis*, extension]

proc·tec·to·my (prok-tek′tō-mē). Surgical resection of the rectum. SYN rectectomy. [proct- + G. *ektomē*, excision]

proc·ti·tis (prok-tī′tis). Inflammation of the mucous membrane of the rectum. SYN rectitis. [proct- + G. *-itis*, inflammation]

chronic ulcerative p., SYN idiopathic p.

epidemic gangrenous p., a generally fatal disease affecting chiefly children in the tropics, characterized by gangrenous ulceration of the rectum and anus, accompanied by frequent watery stools and tenesmus. SYN bicho, caribi, Indian sickness.

idiopathic p., probably a variant of ulcerative colitis involving the rectum; some cases progress to involve the remainder of the colon as well. SYN chronic ulcerative p.

△**procto-, proct-.** Anus; (more frequently) rectum; Cf. recto-. [G. *prōktos*]

proc·to·cele (prok′tō-sēl). Prolapse or herniation of the rectum. SYN rectocele. [procto- + G. *kēlē*, tumor]

proc·to·cly·sis (prok-tok′li-sis). Slow continuous administration of saline solution by instillation into the rectum and sigmoid colon. SYN Murphy drip, rectoclysis. [procto- + G. *klysis*, a washing out]

proc·to·coc·cy·pexy (prok-tō-kok′si-pek-sē). Suture of a prolapsing rectum to the tissues anterior to the coccyx. SYN rectococcypexy. [procto- + G. *kokkyx*, coccyx, + *pēxis*, fixation]

proc·to·co·lec·to·my (prok′tō-kō-lek′tō-mē). Surgical removal of the rectum together with part or all of the colon. [procto- + G. *kolon*, colon, + *ektomē*, excision]

proc·to·co·li·tis (prok′tō-kō-lī′tis). SYN coloproctitis.

proc·to·co·lo·nos·co·py (prok′tō-kō′lō-nos′kŏ-pē). Inspection of interior of rectum and colon. [procto- + G. *kolon*, colon, + *skopeō*, to view]

proc·to·col·po·plas·ty (prok′tō-kol′pō-plas-tē). Surgical closure of a rectovaginal fistula. [procto- + G. *kolpos*, bosom (vagina), + *plastos*, formed]

proc·to·cys·to·cele (prok′tō-sis′tō-sēl). Herniation of the bladder into the rectum. [procto- + G. *kystis*, bladder, + *kēlē*, hernia]

proc·to·cys·to·plas·ty (prok′tō-sis′tō-plas-tē). Surgical closure of a rectovesical fistula. [procto- + G. *kystis*, bladder, + *plastos*, formed]

proc·to·cys·tot·o·my (prok′tō-sis-tot′ō-mē). Incision into the bladder from the rectum. [procto- + G. *kystis*, bladder, + *tomē*, incision]

proc·to·de·al (prok′tō-dē-ăl). Relating to the proctodeum.

proc·to·de·um, pl. **proc·to·dea** (prok-tō-dē′ŭm, -dē′ă). **1.** An ectodermally lined depression under the root of the tail, adjacent to the terminal part of the embryonic hindgut; at its bottom, proctodeal ectoderm and cloacal endoderm form the cloacal plate. When this epithelial plate ruptures, the anal and urogenital external orifices are established. SYN anal pit. **2.** Terminal portion of the insect alimentary canal, extending from the pylorus (area of malpighian tubule attachment) to the anal opening; in certain diptera (flies) and other insects, the p. is divided into a tubular anterior intestine and an enlarged posterior intestine, or rectum, ending at the anus. [L. fr. G. *prōktos*, anus + *hodaios*, on the way, fr. *hodos*, a way]

proc·to·dyn·ia (prok′tō-din′ē-ă). SYN proctalgia. [procto- + G. *odynē*, pain]

proc·to·log·ic (prok′tō-loj′ik). Relating to proctology.

proc·tol·o·gist (prok-tol′ō-jist). A specialist in proctology.

proc·tol·o·gy (prok-tol′ō-jē). Surgical specialty concerned with the anus and rectum and their diseases. [procto- + G. *logos*, study]

proc·to·pa·ral·y·sis (prok′tō-pa-ral′i-sis). Paralysis of the anus, leading to incontinence of feces.

proc·to·per·i·ne·o·plas·ty (prok′tō-per-i-nē′ō-plas-tē). Plastic surgery of the anus and perineum. SYN rectoperineorrhaphy. [procto- + perineum, + G. *plastos*, formed]

proc·to·pexy (prok′tō-pek-sē). Surgical fixation of a prolapsing rectum. SYN rectopexy. [procto- + G. *pēxis*, fixation]

proc·to·pho·bia (prok-tō-fō′bē-ă). A morbid fear of rectal disease. SYN rectophobia. [procto- + G. *phobos*, fear]

proc·to·plas·ty (prok′tō-plas-tē). Plastic surgery of the anus or rectum. SYN rectoplasty. [procto- + G. *plastos*, formed]

proc·to·ple·gia (prok′tō-plē′jē-ă). Paralysis of the anus and rectum occurring with paraplegia. [procto- + G. *plēgē*, stroke]

proc·to·pol·y·pus (prok-tō-pol′i-pŭs). Polypus of the rectum.

proc·top·to·sia, proc·top·to·sis (prok-top-tō′sē-ă, -tō′sis). Prolapse of the rectum and anus. [procto- + G. *ptōsis*, a falling]

proc·tor·rha·gia (proc-tō-rā′jē-ă). State characterized by having a bloody discharge from the anus. [procto- + G. *rhēgnymi*, to burst forth]

proc·tor·rha·phy (prok-tōr′ă-fē). Repair by suture of a lacerated rectum or anus. SYN rectorrhaphy. [procto- + G. *rhaphē*, suture]

proc·tor·rhea (prok-tō-rē′ă). A mucoserous discharge from the rectum. [procto- + G. *rhoia*, a flow]

proc·to·scope (prok′tō-skōp). A rectal speculum. SYN rectoscope. [procto- + G. *skopeō*, to view]

Tuttle p., a tubular rectal speculum illuminated at its distal extremity; after introduction, the obturator is withdrawn and a glass window is inserted in the proximal end; then, by means of a rubber bulb and tube connected with the p., the rectal ampulla may be inflated.

proc·tos·co·py (prok-tos′kŏ-pē). Visual examination of the rectum and anus, as with a proctoscope. SYN rectoscopy.

proc·to·sig·moid (prok′tō-sig′moyd). The area of the anal canal and sigmoid colon, usually used to describe the region visualized by sigmoidoscopy.

proc·to·sig·moi·dec·to·my (prok′tō-sig-moy-dek′tō-mē). Excision of the rectum and sigmoid colon. [procto- + sigmoid, + G. *ektomē*, excision]

proc·to·sig·moi·di·tis (prok′tō-sig-moy-dī′tis). Inflammation of the sigmoid colon and rectum. [procto- + sigmoid + G. *-itis*, inflammation]

proc·to·sig·moi·do·scope (prok′-tō-sig-moid′ō-skōp). Instrument used for examination of the sigmoid colon and rectum.

proc·to·sig·moi·dos·co·py (prok′tō-sig-moy-dos′kŏ-pē). Direct inspection through a sigmoidoscope of the rectum and sigmoid colon. [procto- + sigmoid + G. *skopeō*, to view]

proc·to·spasm (prok′tō-spazm). **1.** Spasmodic contraction of the anus. **2.** Spasmodic contraction of the rectum. [procto- + G. *spasmos*, spasm]

proc·tos·ta·sis (prok-tos′tă-sis). Constipation with stasis in the rectum. [procto- + G. *stasis*, a standing]

proc·to·stat (prok′tō-stat). A tube containing radium for insertion through the anus in the treatment of rectal cancer; obsolete. [procto- + G. *statos*, standing]

proc·to·ste·no·sis (prok′tō-stĕ-nō′sis). Stricture of the rectum or anus. SYN rectostenosis. [procto- + G. *stenōsis*, a narrowing]

proc·tos·to·my (prok-tos′tō-mē). The formation of an artificial opening into the rectum. SYN rectostomy. [procto- + G. *stoma*, mouth]

proc·to·tome (prok′tō-tōm). An instrument for use in proctotomy. SYN rectotome.

proc·tot·o·my (prok-tot′ō-mē). An incision into the rectum. SYN rectotomy. [procto- + G. *tomē*, incision]

proc·to·tre·sia (prok-tō-trē′zē-ă). Operation for correction of an imperforate anus. [procto- + G. *trēsis*, a boring]

proc·to·val·vot·o·my (prok′tō-val-vot′ō-mē). Incision of rectal valves.

pro·cum·bent (prō-kŭm′bent). Rarely used term denoting in a prone position; lying face down. [L. *procumbens*, falling or leaning forward]

pro·cur·va·tion (prō-ker-vā′shŭn). Rarely used term for a bending forward. [L. *pro-curvo,* to bend forward]

pro·cy·cli·dine hy·dro·chlo·ride (prō-sī′kli-dēn). An anticholinergic agent used in the treatment of paralysis agitans and drug-induced parkinsonism.

pro·cy·cli·dine meth·o·chlo·ride. An anticholinergic drug used in the treatment of functional gastrointestinal spasm. SYN tricyclamol chloride.

pro·dig·i·os·in (prō-dij′ē-ō-sin). A red pigment synthesized by the bacterium *Serratia marcescens;* an antifungal agent.

α-pro·dine hy·dro·chlo·ride. SEE alphaprodine.

pro·dro·mal (prō-drō′măl, prod′rō′măl). Relating to a prodrome. SYN prodromic, prodromous, proemial.

pro·drome (prō′drōm). An early or premonitory symptom of a disease. SYN prodromus. [G. *prodromos,* a running before, fr. pro- + *dromos,* a running, a course]

pro·dro·mic, pro·dro·mous (prō-drō′-mik, prod′rō-; -mŭs). SYN prodromal.

prod·ro·mus, pl. **prod·ro·mi** (prod′rō-mŭs, -mī). SYN prodrome.

pro·drug (prō′drŭg). A class of drugs, the pharmacologic action of which results from conversion by metabolic processes within the body (biotransformation).

pro·duct (prod′ŭkt). **1.** Anything produced or made, either naturally or artificially. **2.** In mathematics, the result of multiplication. [L. *productus,* fr. *pro-duco,* pp. *-ductus,* to lead forth]

cleavage p., a substance resulting from the splitting of a molecule into two or more simpler molecules.

double p., the p. of systolic blood pressure multiplied by the heart frequency; a measure of heart work load. SEE Robinson *index.*

end p., the final p. in a metabolic pathway.

fibrin/fibrinogen degradation p.'s (FDP), several poorly characterized small peptides, designated X, Y, D, and E, that result following the action of plasmin on fibrinogen and fibrin in the fibrinolytic process.

fission p., an atomic species produced in the course of the fission of a larger atom such as ^{235}U.

natural p.'s, naturally occurring compounds that are end p.'s of secondary metabolism; often, they are unique compounds for particular organisms or classes of organisms.

orphan p.'s, drugs, biologicals, and medical devices (including diagnostic in vitro tests) that may be useful in either common or rare diseases but that are not considered commercially viable. SYN orphan drugs.

spallation p., an atomic species produced in the course of the spallation of any atom.

substitution p., a p. obtained by replacing one atom or group in a molecule with another atom or group.

pro·duc·tive (prō-dŭk′tiv). Producing or capable of producing; denoting especially an inflammation leading to the production of new tissue with or without an exudate. [see product]

pro·elas·tase (prō-ĕ-las′tās). The precursor protein of elastase; formed in the pancreas (in vertebrates) and converted to elastase by the action of trypsin.

pro·e·mi·al (prō-ē′mē-ăl). SYN prodromal. [L. *prooemium,* fr. G. *prooimion,* prelude]

pro·en·ceph·a·lon (prō-en-sef′ă-lon). SYN prosencephalon.

pro·en·keph·a·lin (prō-en-kef′ă-lin). A precursor protein that contains several enkephalin sequences. Cf. propiocortin.

pro·en·zyme (prō-en′zīm). The precursor of an enzyme, requiring some change (usually the hydrolysis of an inhibiting fragment that masks an active grouping) to render it active; e.g., pepsinogen, trypsinogen, profibrolysin. SYN zymogen.

pro·e·ryth·ro·blast (prō-ĕ-rith′rō-blast). SYN pronormoblast.

pro·e·ryth·ro·cyte (prō-ĕ-rith′rō-sīt). The precursor of an erythrocyte; an immature red blood cell with a nucleus.

pro·es·tro·gen (prō-es′trō-jen). A substance that acts as an estrogen only after it has been metabolized in the body to an active compound.

pro·es·trum (prō-es′trŭm). SYN proestrus.

pro·es·trus (prō-es′trŭs). The period in the estrus cycle preceding estrus, characterized by the growth of the graafian follicles and physiologic changes related to estrogen production. SYN proestrum.

pro·fen·a·mine hy·dro·chlo·ride (pro-fen′ă-mēn). SYN ethopropazine hydrochloride.

Profeta, Giuseppe, Italian dermatologist, 1840–1910. SEE P. *law.*

pro·fi·bri·nol·y·sin (prō′fī-bri-nol′i-sin). SEE plasmin.

pro·fi·lac·tin (prō-fil-ak′tin). A complex of actin and profilin. Cf. profilin.

pro·file (prō′fīl). **1.** An outline or contour, especially one representing a side view of the human head. SYN norma (2). **2.** A summary, brief account, or record. [It. *profilo,* fr. L. *pro,* forward, + *filum,* thread, line (contour)]

biochemical p., SYN test p.

biophysical p., technique for evaluating fetal status using fetal heart rate monitoring and ultrasound assessment of amniotic fluid volume, fetal movement, and fetal breathing motion.

facial p., (1) the outline form of the face from a lateral view; (2) the sagittal outline form of the face.

personality p., (1) a method by which the results of psychologic testing are presented in graphic form; (2) a vignette or brief personality description.

test p., a combination of laboratory tests usually performed by automated methods and designed to evaluate organ systems of patients upon admission to a hospital or clinic. SYN biochemical p.

urethral pressure p., the continual recording of pressure through a hole in the side of a small catheter as it is pulled (at a constant rate while either water or a gas is infused through the hole) from a point within the bladder, through the vesical neck, and down the entire urethra; a form of resistance measurement which gives a tracing indicative of the functional length of the urethra and the points of maximal urethral resistance.

pro·fi·lin (prō-fil′in). A small protein that binds to monomeric actin (thus becoming profilactin), preventing premature polymerization of actin. It also participates in the inhibition of one isoform of phospholipase C.

pro·fi·lom·e·ter (prō′fi-lom′ĕ-ter). An instrument for measuring the roughness of a surface, e.g., of teeth.

pro·fla·vine (hem·i)sul·fate (prō-flā′vin, -vēn). The neutral sulfate of 3,6-diaminoacridine; a compound closely allied to acriflavine, having similar antiseptic properties.

pro·for·mi·phen (prō-fōr′mi-fen). SYN phenprobamate.

pro·fun·da (prō-fŭn′dă). The deep one; a term applied to structures (muscles, nerves, veins, and arteries, etc.) that lie deep in the tissues, especially when contrasted with a similar, more superficial (sublimis) structure. [L. fem. of *profundus,* deep]

pro·fun·dus (prō-fŭn′dŭs) [TA]. SYN deep. [L.]

pro·fu·sion (prō-fū′zhŭn). A score reflecting the number of visible lesions in a region on chest radiographs of individuals with pneumoconiosis. SEE International Labour Organization *Classification.* [L. *profusio,* a pouring forth, fr. *profundo,* to pour forth]

pro·ga·bide (prō′gă-bīd). An anticonvulsant that is a lipid-soluble derivative of the amidated form of γ-aminobutyric acid (GABAmide) that, unlike γ-aminobutyric acid (GABA) itself, is able to cross the blood-brain barrier. Once inside the brain the drug is converted to several metabolites, some of which are active forms of GABA or related compounds that act on GABA receptors to increase inhibition in the brain.

pro·gas·trin (prō-gas′trin). Precursor of gastric secretion in the mucous membrane of the stomach.

pro·ge·nia (prō-jē′nē-ă). SYN prognathism. [pro- + L. *gena,* cheek]

pro·gen·i·ta·lis (prō-jen-i-tā′lis). On any of the exposed surfaces of the genitalia. [L. prefix *pro-,* before, in front of, + *genitalis,* pertaining to the reproductive organs, fr. *gigno,* to bear]

pro·gen·i·tor (prō-jen′i-ter, -tōr). A precursor, ancestor; one who begets. [L.]

prog·e·ny (proj′ĕ-nē). Offspring; descendants. [L. *progenies,* fr. *progigno,* to beget]

pro·ge·ria (prō-jēr′ē-ă) [MIM*176670]. A condition of precocious aging with onset at birth or early childhood; characterized by growth retardation, a senile appearance with dry wrinkled skin, total alopecia, and birdlike facies; early occurrence of atherosclerosis in blood vessels and premature death due to coronary artery disease; genetics unclear. SYN Hutchinson-Gilford disease, Hutchinson-Gilford syndrome, premature senility syndrome. [pro- + G. *gēras*, old age]

p. with cataract, p. with microphthalmia, SYN *dyscephalia* mandibulo-oculofacialis.

pro·ges·ta·tion·al (prō′jes-tā′shŭn-ăl). **1.** Favoring pregnancy; conducive to gestation; capable of stimulating the uterine changes essential for implantation and growth of a fertilized ovum. **2.** Referring to progesterone, or to a drug with progesterone-like properties.

pro·ges·ter·one (prō-jes′ter-ōn). An antiestrogenic steroid, believed to be the active principle of the corpus luteum, isolated from the corpus luteum and placenta or synthetically prepared; used to correct abnormalities of the menstrual cycle and as a contraceptive and to control habitual abortion. SYN luteohormone, pregnancy hormone, progestational hormone.

pro·ges·tin (prō-jes′tin). **1.** A hormone of the corpus luteum. **2.** Generic term for any substance, natural or synthetic, that effects some or all of the biologic changes produced by progesterone. **3.** SYN gestagen. [pro- + gestation + -in]

pro·ges·to·gen (prō-jes′tō-jen). **1.** Any agent capable of producing biologic effects similar to those of progesterone; most p.'s are steroids like the natural hormones. **2.** A synthetic derivative from testosterone or progesterone that has some of the physiologic activity and pharmacologic effects of progesterone; progesterone is antiestrogenic, whereas some p.'s have estrogenic or androgenic properties in addition to progestational activity. [pro- + gestation + G. *-gen*, producing]

pro·glos·sis (prō-glos′is). The anterior portion, or tip, of the tongue. [pro- + G. *glōssa*, tongue]

pro·glot·tid (prō-glot′id). One of the segments of a tapeworm, containing the reproductive organs. SYN proglottis. [pro- + G. *glōssa*, tongue]

pro·glot·tis, pl. **pro·glot·ti·des** (prō-glot′is, -i-dēz). SYN proglottid.

prog·nath·ic (prog-nath′ik, -nā′thik). **1.** Having a projecting jaw; having a gnathic index above 103. **2.** Denoting a forward projection of either or both of the jaws relative to the craniofacial skeleton. SYN prognathous. [pro- + G. *gnathos,* jaw]

prog·na·thism (prog′nă-thizm). The condition of being prognathic; abnormal forward projection of one or of both jaws beyond the established normal relationship with the cranial base; the mandibular condyles are in their normal rest relationship to the temporomandibular joints. SYN progenia.

basilar p., the concave facial profile, or forward position of the chin, resembling mandibular p., created by the prominence of the bone of the mandible at the chin or menton.

prog·na·thous (prog′nă-thŭs). SYN prognathic.

prog·nose (prog-nōs′, -nōz′). SYN prognosticate.

prog·no·sis (prog-nō′sis). A forecast of the probable course and/or outcome of a disease. [G. *prognōsis,* fr. *pro,* before, + *gignōskō,* to know]

denture p., an opinion or judgment, given in advance of treatment, of the prospects for success in the construction and usefulness of a denture or restoration.

prog·nos·tic (prog-nos′tik). **1.** Relating to prognosis. **2.** A symptom upon which a prognosis is based, or one indicative of the likely outcome. [G. *prognōstikos*]

prog·nos·ti·cate (prog-nos′ti-kāt). To give a prognosis. SYN prognose.

prog·nos·ti·cian (prog-nos-tish′ŭn). One skilled in prognosis.

pro·gon·o·ma (prō-gon-ō′mă). A nodule or mass resulting from displacement of tissue when atavism occurs in embryonic development; represents a reversion to structures not normally occurring in the individuals of a species, but observed in ancestral forms of that species. [pro- + G. *gonos,* offspring, + *-oma,* tumor]

p. of jaw, SYN melanotic neuroectodermal *tumor* of infancy.

melanotic p., a pigmented hairy nevus.

pro·grade. In the normal direction of flow.

pro·gram. **1.** A formal set of procedures for conducting an activity. **2.** An ordered list of instructions directing a computer to carry out a desired sequence of operations required to solve a problem.

pro·gram·ming (prō′gram-ing). Sequential instruction; a method of training in discrete segments.

neurolinguistic p., a branch of cognitive-behavioral psychology employing specific techniques, that use language to access the unconscious in order to change a client's internal states or external behaviors.

pro·gran·u·lo·cyte (prō-gran′ū-lō-sīt). SYN promyelocyte.

pro·gress. **1** (prog′res). An advance; the course of a disease. **2** (prō-gres′). To advance; to go forward; said of a disease, especially when unqualified, of one taking an unfavorable course. [L. *pro-gredior,* pp. *-gressus,* to go forth, fr. *gradior,* to step, go, fr. *gradus,* a step]

pro·gress·ive (prō-gres′iv). Going forward; advancing; denoting the course of a disease, especially, when unqualified, an unfavorable course.

pro·gua·nil hy·dro·chlo·ride (prō-gwah′nil). SYN chloroguanide hydrochloride.

pro·hor·mone (prō-hōr′mōn). **1.** An intraglandular precursor of a hormone; e.g., proinsulin. Cf. prehormone. **2.** Obsolete term formerly used to designate a substance developed in serum that antagonizes a specific antihormone, and thus enhances the action of the corresponding hormone.

pro·in·su·lin (prō-in′sŭ-lin). A single-chain precursor of insulin.

pro·jec·tion (prō-jek′shŭn). **1.** A pushing out; an outgrowth or protuberance. **2.** The referring of a sensation to the object producing it. **3.** A defense mechanism by which a repressed complex in the individual is denied and conceived as belonging to another person, as when faults that the person tends to commit are perceived in or attributed to others. **4.** The conception by the consciousness of a mental occurrence belonging to the self as of external origin. **5.** Localization of visual impressions in space. **6.** In neuroanatomy, the system or systems of nerve fibers by which a group of nerve cells discharges its nerve impulses ("projects") to one or more other cell groups. **7.** The image of a three-dimensional object on a plane, as in a radiograph. **8.** In radiography, standardized views of parts of the body, described by body part position, the direction of the x-ray beam through the body part, or by eponym. SYN norma (3), salient (1), view. [L. *projectio;* fr. *pro- jicio,* pp. *-jectus,* to throw before]

anteroposterior p., SYN AP p.

AP p., the alternative frontal radiographic p., used mainly in bedside or portable radiography. SYN anteroposterior p.

apical lordotic p., SYN backprojection.

axial p., radiographic p. devised to obtain direct visualization of the base of the skull. SYN axial view, base p., submental vertex p., submentovertical p., verticosubmental view.

base p., SYN axial p.

Caldwell p., inclined PA radiographic p. devised to permit visualization of orbital structures unobstructed by the petrous ridges. SYN Caldwell view.

cross-table lateral p., lateral p. radiography of a supine subject using a horizontal x-ray beam.

enamel p., extension of enamel into furcation.

erroneous p., SYN false p.

false p., the faulty visual sensation arising secondarily to underaction of an ocular muscle. SYN erroneous p.

Fischer p., SEE sugars.

frog-leg lateral p., a lateral p. of the femoral neck made with the thigh maximally abducted.

Granger p., view, reversed half-axial view; uncommonly used PA view of the skull.

half-axial p., SYN Towne p.

Haworth p., SEE sugars.

lateral p., radiographic p. with the x-ray beam in a coronal plane.

maximum intensity p. (MIP), a computerized image display method, used in MR angiography and helical computed tomography; a series of slices are combined with display of the brightest pixel on any slice at each location, and suppression of the background; simulates a projection *angiogram.*

oblique p., any radiographic p. between frontal and lateral.

occipitomental p., SYN Waters p.

PA p., the standard frontal chest film p.; radiographic skull p. with the petrous ridge superimposed on the orbits. SYN posteroanterior p.

posteroanterior p., SYN PA p.

Rhese p., oblique radiographic view of the skull to show the optic foramen.

Stenvers p., oblique radiographic p. of the skull devised to provide an unobstructed view of the petrous bone, bony labyrinth, internal auditory canal, and meatus. SYN Stenvers view.

submental vertex p., SYN axial p.

submentovertical p., SYN axial p.

Towne p., reverse tilted AP radiographic p. devised to permit demonstration of the entire occipital bone, foramen magnum, and dorsum sellae, as well as the petrous ridges. SYN half axial view, half-axial p., Towne view.

visual p., a perceptual synthesis involving visual mechanisms.

Waters p., a PA radiographic view of the skull made with the orbitomeatal line at an angle of 37° from the plane of the film, to show the orbits and maxillary sinuses. SYN occipitomental p., Waters view.

Pro·kar·y·o·tae (pro-kar-ē-ō'tē). A superkingdom of cellular organisms that includes the kingdom Monera (bacteria and blue-green algae) and is characterized by the prokaryotic condition, minute size (0.2–10 μm for bacteria), and absence of the nuclear organization, mitotic capacities, and complex organelles that typify the superkingdom Eukaryotae. SYN Procaryotae.

pro·kar·y·ote (prō-kar'ē-ōt). A member of the superkingdom Prokaryotae; an organismic unit consisting of a single and presumably primitive moneran cell, or a precellular organism, which lacks a nuclear membrane, paired organized chromosomes, a mitotic mechanism for cell division, microtubules, and mitochondria. SEE ALSO Prokaryotae, Monera, eukaryote. SYN procaryote.

pro·kar·y·ot·ic (prō'kar-ē-ot'ik). Pertaining to or characteristic of a prokaryote. SYN procaryotic.

pro·la·bi·al (prō-lā'bē-ăl). Denoting the isolated central soft-tissue segment of the upper lip in the embryonic state and in an unrepaired bilateral cleft palate.

pro·la·bi·um (prō-lā'bē-ŭm). **1.** The exposed carmine margin of the lip. **2.** The isolated central soft-tissue segment of the upper lip in the embryonic state and in an unrepaired bilateral cleft palate. [pro- + L. *labium,* lip]

pro·lac·tin (PRL) (prō-lak'tin). A protein hormone of the anterior lobe of the hypophysis that stimulates the secretion of milk and possibly, during pregnancy, breast growth. SYN galactopoietic hormone, lactation hormone, lactogenic hormone, lactotropin, mammotropic factor, mammotropic hormone. [pro- + L. *lac, lact-,* milk, + -in]

pro·lac·ti·no·ma (prō-lak-ti-nō'mă). SYN prolactin-producing *adenoma.*

pro·lam·ines (prō-lam'ēnz, prō'lă-mēnz, -minz). Proteins insoluble in water or neutral salt solutions, soluble in dilute acids or alkalies, and in 50–90% alcohol; e.g., gliadin, zein, hordein; all have relatively high proline contents.

pro·lapse (prō-laps'). **1.** To sink down, said of an organ or other part. **2.** A sinking of an organ or other part, especially its appearance at a natural or artificial orifice. SEE ALSO procidentia, ptosis. [L. *prolapsus,* a falling]

p. of the corpus luteum, ectropion of the corpus luteum, due to eversion of the granulosa membrane through the opening in the ruptured follicle; this occurs normally in certain animals.

mitral valve p., excessive retrograde movement of one or both mitral valve leaflets into the left atrium during left ventricular systole, often allowing mitral regurgitation; responsible for the click-murmur of Barlow syndrome, and rarely may be due to rheumatic carditis, a connective tissue disorder such as Marfan syndrome, or ruptured chorda tendinea ("flail mitral leaflet").

Morgagni p., chronic inflammation of Morgagni ventricle.

p. of umbilical cord, presentation of part of the umbilical cord ahead of the fetus; it may cause fetal death due to compression of

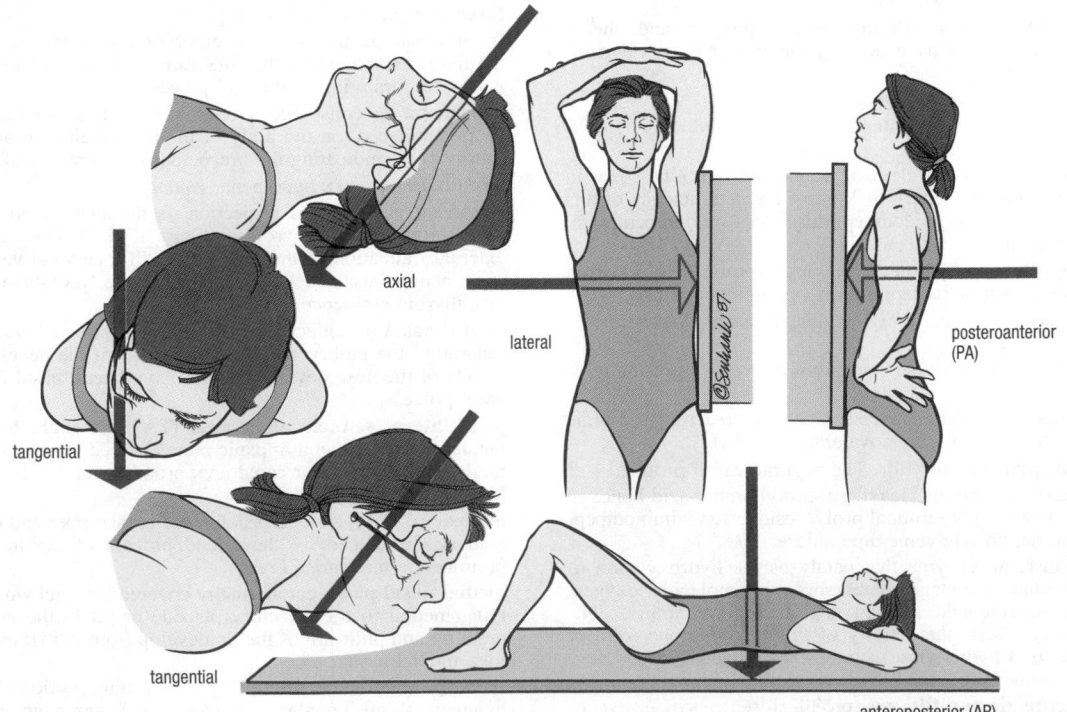

axial

lateral

posteroanterior (PA)

tangential

tangential

anteroposterior (AP)

radiographic projections

the cord between the presenting part of the fetus and the maternal pelvis.

p. of the uterus, downward movement of the uterus due to laxity and atony of the muscular and fascial structures of the pelvic floor, usually resulting from injuries of childbirth or advanced age; p. occurs in three forms; **first degree p.,** the cervix of the prolapsed uterus is well within the vaginal orifice; **second degree p.,** the cervix is at or near the introitus; **third degree p.** (procidentia uteri), the cervix protrudes well beyond the vaginal orifice. SYN descensus uteri, falling of the womb.

valvular p., p. that may involve any valve or combination of valves, but usually the mitral valve. Pulmonic valve p. is extremely rare.

pro·lec·tive (prō′lek-tiv). Pertaining to data collected by planning in advance proportional mortality ratio. Number of deaths from a given cause in a specified period, per 100 or per 1000 total deaths. [pro- + L. *lego,* pp. *lectum,* to gather]

pro·lep·sis (prō-lep′sis). Recurrence of the paroxysm of a periodical disease at regularly shortening intervals. [G. *prolēpsis,* anticipation]

pro·lep·tic (prō-lep′tik). Relating to prolepsis. SYN subintrant.

pro·leu·ko·cyte (prō-loo′kō-sīt). SYN leukoblast.

pro·li·dase (prō′li-dās). SYN *proline* dipeptidase.

pro·lif·er·ate (prō-lif′ĕ-rāt). To grow and increase in number by means of reproduction of similar forms. [L. *proles,* offspring, + *fero,* to bear]

pro·lif·er·a·tion (prō-lif-ĕ-rā′shŭn). Growth and reproduction of similar cells.

diffuse mesangial p., SYN mesangial proliferative *glomerulonephritis.*

gingival p., SYN gingival *hyperplasia.*

pro·lif·er·a·tive, pro·lif·er·ous (prō-lif′er-ă-tiv, -er-ŭs). Increasing the numbers of similar forms.

pro·lif·ic (prō-lif′ik). Fruitful; bearing many children. [L. *proles,* offspring, + *facio,* to make]

pro·lig·er·ous (prō-lij′er-ŭs). Germinating; producing offspring. [L. *proles,* offspring, + *gero,* to bear]

pro·li·nase (prō′li-nās). SYN *prolyl* dipeptidase.

pro·line (Pro) (prō′lēn). Pyrrolidine-2-carboxylic acid; the L-isomer is found in proteins, especially the collagens. SYN pyrrolidine-2-carboxylate.

p. aminopeptidase, SYN p. iminopeptidase.

p. dehydrogenase, SYN pyrroline-2-carboxylate reductase, pyrroline-5-carboxylate reductase.

p. dipeptidase, an enzyme cleaving aminoacyl-L-proline bonds in dipeptides containing a C-terminal p. residue; a deficiency of this enzyme results in hyperimidodipeptiduria. SYN imidodipeptidase, peptidase D, prolidase.

p. iminopeptidase, a hydrolase cleaving L-prolyl residues from the N-terminal position in peptides. SYN p. aminopeptidase.

p. oxidase, SYN pyrroline-2-carboxylate reductase, pyrroline-5-carboxylate reductase.

p. racemase, an enzyme that reversibly converts D-proline to L-proline.

D-p. reductase, an oxidoreductase reversibly reacting D-proline with NADH to produce 5-aminovalerate and NAD^+.

pro·lyl (Pro, pro·lyl) (prō′lil). The acyl radical of proline.

p. dipeptidase, an enzyme cleaving L-prolyl-amino acid bonds in dipeptides containing N-terminal prolyl residues. SYN iminodipeptidase, prolinase, prolylglycine dipeptidase.

p. hydroxylase, an enzyme that catalyzes the hydroxylation of certain p. residues in collagen precursors using molecular oxygen, ferrous ion, ascorbic acid, and α-ketoglutarate; a vitamin C deficiency directly affects the activity of this enzyme; one form of this enzyme (p. 4-hydroxylase) synthesizes 4-hydroxyprolyl residues while another produces 3-hydroxyprolyl residues.

pro·lyl·gly·cine di·pep·ti·dase (prō′lil-glī′sēn). SYN *prolyl* dipeptidase.

pro·mas·ti·gote (prō-mas′ti-gōt). Term now generally used instead of "leptomonad" or "leptomonad stage," to avoid confusion

with the flagellate genus *Leptomonas.* It denotes the flagellate stage of a trypanosomatid protozoan in which the flagellum arises from a kinetoplast in front of the nucleus and emerges from the anterior end of the organism; usually an extracellular phase, as in the insect intermediate host (or in culture) of *Leishmania* parasites. [pro- + G. *mastix,* whip]

pro·meg·a·lo·blast (prō-meg′ă-lō-blast). The earliest of four maturation stages of the megaloblast. SEE erythroblast. SYN pernicious anemia type rubriblast.

pro·met·a·phase (prō-met′ă-fāz). The stage of mitosis or meiosis in which the nuclear membrane disintegrates and the centrioles reach the poles of the cell, while the chromosomes continue to contract.

pro·meth·a·zine hy·dro·chlo·ride (prō-meth′ă-zēn). An antihistaminic with antiemetic properties, often used to enhance the efficacy of narcotics.

pro·meth·a·zine the·o·clate (prō-meth′ă-zēn). Promethiazine salt of 8-chlorotheophylline; an antihistaminic drug used for motion sickness.

pro·meth·es·trol di·pro·pi·o·nate (prō-meth′es-trol dī-prō′pē-ō-nāt). A synthetic estrogen derived from stilbene.

pro·me·thi·um (Pm) (prō-mē′thē-ŭm). A radioactive element of the rare earth series, atomic no. 61; first chemically identified in 1945; ^{145}Pm has the longest known half-life (17.7 years). [*Prometheus,* a Titan of G. myth who stole fire to give to mortals]

prom·i·nence (prom′i-nens) [TA]. In anatomy, tissues or parts that project beyond a surface. SYN prominentia [TA]. [L. *prominentia*]

Ammon p., an external p. in the posterior pole of the eyeball during early embryogenesis.

canine p., SYN canine *eminence.*

cardiac p., the conspicuous external bulge appearing on the ventral aspect of the human embryo as early as at the fourth week, indicative of the precocious development of the heart.

p. of facial canal [TA], the prominence on the medial wall of the tympanic cavity above the vestibular (oval) window produced by the presence of the facial canal. SYN prominentia canalis facialis [TA].

forebrain p., SYN frontonasal p.

frontonasal p., the unpaired embryonic prominence formed by the tissues surrounding the forebrain vesicle. SYN forebrain eminence, forebrain p., frontonasal process.

hepatic p., the conspicuous external bulge appearing dorsocaudal to the cardiac p. on the body of the human embryo at about the fourth week, indicating the precocious development of the liver.

hypothenar p., SYN hypothenar *eminence.*

laryngeal p. [TA], the projection on the anterior portion of the neck formed by the thyroid cartilage of the larynx; serves as an external indication of the level of the fifth cervical vertebra. SYN prominentia laryngea [TA], Adam's apple, protuberantia laryngea, thyroid eminence.

lateral nasal p., an ectodermally covered mesenchymal swelling separating the embryonic olfactory pit from the developing eye; the ala of the nose develops from it. SYN lateral nasal fold, lateral nasal process.

p. of lateral semicircular canal [TA], the slight bulge in the medial wall of the epitympanic recess caused by the proximity of the lateral semicircular canal. SYN prominentia canalis semicircularis lateralis [TA].

mallear p. [TA], a small prominence at the upper end of the stria mallearis produced by the lateral process of the malleus. SYN prominentia mallearis [TA].

medial nasal p., an ectodermally covered mesenchymal swelling lying medial to the olfactory placode or pit in the embryo; the nasal tip and philtrum of the lip develop from it. SYN medial nasal fold, medial nasal process.

spiral p. of cochlear duct [TA], a projecting portion of the spiral ligament of the cochlea, bounding the lower edge of the stria vascularis and containing within it a blood vessel, the vas prominens. SYN prominentia spiralis ductus cochlearis [TA].

styloid p. [TA], a rounded eminence on the posterior (mastoid) wall of the tympanic cavity corresponding to the base of the styloid process. SYN prominentia styloidea [TA].

thenar p., SYN thenar *eminence.*

tubal p., SYN *torus* tubarius.

p. of venous valvular sinus, a slight eminence on the external wall of a vein correlating with the valvular sinus immediately proximal to the leaflets of the venous valve. SYN agger valvae venae.

pro·mi·nens (prom'i-nens). Prominent; in anatomy, denoting a prominence. [L.]

prom·i·nen·tia, pl. **prom·i·nen·ti·ae** (prom-i-nen'shē-ă, -shē-ē) [TA]. SYN prominence. [L. fr. *promineo,* to jut out, be prominent]

p. cana'lis facia'lis [TA], SYN *prominence* of facial canal.

p. cana'lis semicircula'ris latera'lis [TA], SYN *prominence* of lateral semicircular canal.

p. laryn'gea [TA], SYN laryngeal *prominence.*

p. mallea'ris [TA], SYN mallear *prominence.*

p. spira'lis ductus cochlearis [TA], SYN spiral *prominence* of cochlear duct.

p. styloi'dea [TA], SYN styloid *prominence.*

pro·mi·to·chon·dria (prō-mī-tō-kon'drē-ă). Mitochondrial precursors with little internal structure (e.g., no cristae) and no proteins of electron transport. SYN premitochondria.

PROMM Acronym for proximal myotonic *myopathy.*

pro·mon·o·cyte (prō-mon'ō-sīt). SYN premonocyte.

prom·on·to·ri·um, pl. **prom·on·to·ria** (prom'on-tō'rē-ŭm, -rē-ă) [TA]. SYN promontory. [L. a mountain ridge, a headland, fr. *promineo,* to jut out]

p. ca'vi tym'pani [TA], SYN *promontory* of tympanic cavity.

p. os'sis sa'cri [TA], SYN sacral *promontory.*

prom·on·to·ry (prom'on-tō-rē) [TA]. An eminence or projection; a projection of a part. SYN promontorium [TA]. [L. *promontorium*]

pelvic p., SYN sacral p.

sacral p. [TA], the most prominent anterior projection of the base of the sacrum. SYN promontorium ossis sacri [TA], pelvic p., p. of the sacrum.

p. of the sacrum, SYN sacral p.

tympanic p., SYN p. of tympanic cavity.

p. of tympanic cavity [TA], a rounded eminence on the labyrinthine wall of the middle ear, caused by the first coil of the cochlea. SYN promontorium cavi tympani [TA], tuber cochleae, tympanic p.

pro·mot·er (prō-mō'ter). **1.** In chemistry, a substance that increases the activity of a catalyst. **2.** In molecular biology, a DNA sequence at which RNA polymerase binds and initiates transcription.

pro·mo·tion (prō-mō'shŭn). Stimulation of tumor induction, following initiation, by a promoting agent that may of itself be noncarcinogenic.

health p., according to the World Health Organization, the process of enabling people to increase control over and improve their health; it involves the population as a whole in the context of their everyday lives, rather than focusing on people at risk for specific diseases and is directed toward action on the determinants or causes of health.

pro·my·e·lo·cyte (prō-mī'ě-lō-sīt). **1.** The developmental stage of a granular leukocyte between the myeloblast and myelocyte, when a few specific granules appear in addition to azurophilic ones. **2.** A large uninuclear cell occurring in the circulating blood of persons with myelocytic leukemia. SYN premyelocyte, progranulocyte. [pro- + G. *myelos,* marrow, + *kytos,* cell]

pro·na·si·on (prō-nā'zē-on). The point of the angle between the septum of the nose and the surface of the upper lip, found at the point where a tangent applied to the nasal septum meets the upper lip. [pro- + L. *nasus,* nose]

pro·nate (prō'nāt). **1.** To perform pronation of the forearm or foot. **2.** To assume, or to be placed in, a prone position. [L. *pronatus,* fr. *prono,* pp. *-atus,* to bend forward, fr. *pronus,* bent forward]

pro·na·tion (prō-nā'shŭn) [TA]. The condition of being prone; the act of assuming or of being placed in a prone position; a specific rotational motion of the forearm that moves the palm into a downfacing position, a specific rotational motion of the foot in which the plantar surface is rotated outward.

p. of foot, eversion and abduction of the foot, raising the lateral edge.

p. of forearm, rotation of the forearm in such a way that the palm of the hand faces backward when the arm is in the anatomic position, or downward when the arm is extended at a right angle to the body.

pro·na·tor (prō-nā'ter, tōr) [TA]. A muscle that turns a part into the prone position. SEE muscle. [L.]

prone (prōn). Denoting: **1.** The body when lying face downward. **2.** Pronation of the forearm or of the foot. [L. *pronus,* bending down or forward]

pro·neph·ros, pl. **pro·neph·roi** (prō-nef'ros, -roy). **1.** The definitive excretory organ of primitive fishes. SYN head kidney. **2.** In the embryos of higher vertebrates, a vestigial structure consisting of a series of tortuous tubules emptying into the cloaca by way of the primary nephric duct; in the human embryo, the p. is a very rudimentary and temporary structure, followed by the mesonephros and still later by the metanephros. SYN forekidney, primordial kidney. [pro- + G. *nephros,* kidney]

pro·no·grade (prō'nō-grād). Walking or resting with the body horizontal, denoting the posture of quadrupeds; opposed to orthograde. [L. *pronus,* inclined forward, + *gradior,* to walk]

pro·nom·e·ter (prō-nom'ě-ter). SYN goniometer (3).

pro·nor·mo·blast (prō-nōr'mō-blast). The earliest of four stages in development of the normoblast. SEE ALSO erythroblast. SYN proerythroblast, rubriblast.

pro·nu·cle·us, pl. **pro·nu·clei** (prō-noo'klē-ŭs, -klē-ī). **1.** One of a pair of nuclei undergoing fusion in karyogamy. **2.** In embryology, the nuclear material of the head of the spermatozoon (**male p.**) or of the ovum (**female p.**), after the ovum has been penetrated by the spermatozoon; each p. normally carries a haploid set of chromosomes, so that the merging of the pronuclei in fertilization reestablishes diploidy.

proof·read·ing (pruf'rēd-ing). The property of certain polymerases, e.g., DNA polymerase, to use their exonuclease activity to remove erroneously introduced bases and to replace them with the correct bases.

pro·opi·o·mel·a·no·cor·tin (POMC) (prō-ō'pē-ō-mel'ă-nō-kōr'tin). A large molecule found in the anterior and intermediate lobes of the pituitary gland, the hypothalamus, and other parts of the brain as well as in the lungs, gastrointestinal tract, and placenta; the precursor of ACTH, CLIP, β-LPH, γ-MSH, β-endorphin, and met-enkephalin.

pro·o·tic (prō-ō'tik). In front of the ear. [pro- + G. *ous,* ear]

pro-ox·i·dants (prō-oks'i-dănts). Compounds or agents capable of generating toxic oxygen species. Cf. antioxidant.

pro·pa·fen·one (prō-paf'ě-nōn). Antiarrhythmic agent classified as a class I_C type, thus resembling flecainide and encainide. Blocks fast sodium channels and has been used in the treatment of ventricular cardiac arrhythmias.

prop·a·gate (prop'ă-gāt). **1.** To reproduce; to generate. **2.** To move along a fiber, e.g., propagation of the nerve impulse. [L. *propago,* pp. *-atus,* to generate, reproduce]

prop·a·ga·tion (prop-ă-gā'shŭn). The act of propagating.

prop·a·ga·tive (prop-ă-gā'tiv). Relating to or concerned in propagation; denoting the sexual part of an animal or plant as distinguished from the soma.

pro·pal·i·nal (prō-pal'i-năl). Back and forth; denoting a forward and backward movement. [pro- + G. *palin,* backward]

pro·pam·i·dine (prō-pam'i-dēn). Active against *Trypanosoma gambiense* infections; also markedly bacteriostatic; used as a local antiinfective agent in 0.1% aqueous solution and against systemic fungal infections such as blastomycosis; also used to treat *Acanthamoeba* keratitis.

pro·pane (prō'pān). One of the alkane series of hydrocarbons.

pro·pane·di·o·ic ac·id (prō-pān-dī'ō-ik). SYN malonic acid.

1,2,3-pro·pane·tri·ol (prō-pān-trī′ol). SYN glycerol.

pro·pan·i·did (prō-pan′i-did). A short-acting eugenol used intravenously for induction of general anesthesia.

pro·pa·no·ic ac·id (prō-pă-nō′ik). SYN propionic acid.

pro·pa·nol (prō′pă-nol). SYN *propyl* alcohol.

pro·pa·no·yl (prō′pă-nō-ĭl). SYN propionyl.

pro·pan·the·line bro·mide (prō-pan′thĕ-lēn). The isopropyl analogue of methantheline bromide; an anticholinergic agent.

pro·par·a·caine hy·dro·chlo·ride (prō-par′ă-kān). A surface anesthetic agent used in ophthalmology. SYN proxymetacaine hydrochloride.

pro·pa·tyl ni·trate (prō′pă-til). A coronary vasodilator.

pro·pene (prō′pēn). SYN propylene.

pro·pent·dy·o·pents (prō-pent-dī′ō-pentz). SEE bilirubinoids.

pro·pe·nyl (prō′pē-nil). The radical, –CH=CH–CH₃.

pro·pep·sin (prō-pep′sin). SYN pepsinogen.

pro·pep·tone (prō-pep′tōn). A nondescript mixture of intermediate products in the conversion of native protein into peptone.

pro·per·din (prō-per′din). A globulin in normal serum involved in resistance to infection that participates, in conjunction with other factors, in an alternative pathway to the activation of the terminal components of complement; a deficiency of p. results in the lack of stabilization of the alternative C3-convertase enzyme (an X-linked recessive disorder). SEE ALSO properdin *system, component* of complement, *factor* P. [pro- + L. *perdo,* to destroy]

pro·per·i·to·ne·al (prō′per-i-tō-nē′ăl). In front of the peritoneum.

pro·phage (prō′fāj). SYN probacteriophage.

   defective p., SEE defective *bacteriophage.*

pro·phase (prō′fāz). The first stage of mitosis or meiosis, consisting of linear contraction and increase in thickness of the chromosomes (each composed of two chromatids) accompanied by migration of the two daughter centrioles and their asters toward the poles of the cell. In meiosis, p. is complex and can be subdivided into stages: preleptotene, leptotene, zygotene, pachytene, diplotene, and diakinesis. [G. *prophasis,* from *prophainō,* to foreshadow]

pro·phen·py·rid·a·mine ma·le·ate (prō′fen-pi-rid′ă-mēn). SYN pheniramine maleate.

pro·phy·lac·tic (prō-fi-lak′tik). **1.** Preventing disease; relating to prophylaxis. SYN preventive. **2.** An agent that acts to prevent a disease. [G. *prophylaktikos;* see prophylaxis]

pro·phy·lax·is, pl. **pro·phy·lax·es** (prō-fi-lak′sis, -sēz). Prevention of disease or of a process that can lead to disease. [Mod. L. fr. G. *pro-phylassō,* to guard before, take precaution]

   active p., use of an antigenic (immunogenic) agent to actively stimulate the immunologic mechanism.

   chemical p., the administration of chemicals or drugs to members of a community to reduce the number of carriers of a disease and to prevent others contracting the disease.

   dental p., a series of procedures whereby calculus, stain, and other accretions are removed from the clinical crowns of the teeth, and the enamel surfaces are polished.

   passive p., use of an antiserum from another person or animal to provide temporary protection against a specific infectious or toxic agent.

pro·pi·cil·lin (prō-pi-sil′in). A semisynthetic acid-stable penicillin that may be more effective than penicillin G. SYN α-phenoxypropylpenicillin potassium.

pro·pi·o·cor·tin (prō-pē-ō-kōr′ten). An endogenous polypeptide that might be a precursor to the enkephalins. Cf. proenkephalin.

pro·pi·o·lac·tone (prō′pē-ō-lak′tōn). Used to sterilize plasma, vaccines, and tissue grafts.

pro·pi·o·nate (prō′pē-ō-nāt). A salt or ester of propionic acid.

Pro·pi·on·i·bac·te·ri·um (prō-pē-on-i-bak-tēr′ē-ŭm). A genus of nonmotile, non–spore-forming, anaerobic to aerotolerant bacteria (family Propionibacteriaceae) containing Gram-positive rods that are usually pleomorphic, diphtheroid, or club shaped, with one end rounded, the other tapered or pointed. Some cells may be coccoid, elongate, bifid, or even branched. The cells usually occur singly, in pairs, in V and Y configurations, short chains, or clumps in "Chinese character" arrangement. The metabolism of these organisms is fermentative, and the products of fermentation include combinations of propionic and acetic acids. These organisms occur in dairy products, on human skin, and in the intestinal tracts of humans and other animals. They may be pathogenic. The type species is *P. freudenreichii.*

   P. ac′nes, a species of bacteria commonly found in acne pustules, although it occurs in other types of lesions in humans and even as a saprophyte in the intestine, skin, hair follicles, and in sewage.

   P. freudenrei′chii, a bacterial species found in raw milk, Swiss cheese, and other dairy products; it is the type species of the genus *P.*

   P. jensen′ii, a bacterial species found in dairy products, silage, and occasionally in infections.

   P. propion′icus, SYN *Arachnia propionica.*

pro·pi·on·ic ac·id (prō-pē-on′ik). Methylacetic acid; ethylformic acid; found in sweat; elevated in cases of ketotic hyperglycinemia and in cases of biotin deficiency. SYN propanoic acid.

pro·pi·on·ic ac·i·de·mia (prō-pē-on′ik-as-i-dē′mē-ă). SYN ketotic *hyperglycinemia.*

pro·pi·o·nyl (prō′pē-ō-nil). CH₃CH₂CO–; the acyl radical of propionic acid. SYN propanoyl.

pro·pi·o·nyl-CoA (prō′pē-ō-nil-kō-ā). The coenzyme A thioester derivative of propionic acid; an intermediate in the degradation of L-valine, L-isoleucine, L-threonine, L-methionine, and odd-chain fatty acids; a precursor for the synthesis of odd-chain fatty acids; it accumulates in individuals with a deficiency of p.-CoA carboxylase.

   p.-CoA carboxylase, an enzyme that catalyzes the reaction of p.-CoA with CO₂ and ATP to produce ADP, orthophosphate, and D-methylmalonyl-CoA; a biotin-dependent enzyme; an inherited deficiency of this enzyme will lead to propionic acidemia and developmental retardation.

pro·pi·o·nyl·gly·cine (prō′pē-ō-nil-glī′sēn). A minor metabolite that accumulates in individuals with propionic acidemia.

pro·pit·o·caine hy·dro·chlo·ride (prō-pit′ō-kān). SYN prilocaine hydrochloride.

pro·pla·sia (prō-plā′zē-ă). That state of cell or tissue in which activity is increased above that of euplasia, i.e., characterized by stimulation, repair, or regeneration. [pro- + G. *plassō,* to form]

pro·plas·ma·cyte (prō-plaz′mă-sīt). A cell in the process of differentiating from a plasmablast to a mature plasma cell.

pro·plex·us (prō-plek′sŭs). The choroid plexus in the lateral ventricle of the brain.

pro·po·fol (prō′pō-fōl). An oil-in-water emulsion of 1,6-diisopropylphenol, a hypnotic with rapid onset and short duration of action; used intravenously for induction and maintenance of general anesthesia. SYN 2,6-diisopropyl phenol.

pro·pos·i·tus, pl. **pro·po·si·ti** (prō′poz′i-tŭs, -tī). **1.** Proband, usually referring to the first index case to be ascertained. Cf. consultand. **2.** A premise; an argument. [L. fr. *propono,* pp. *-positus,* to lay out, propound]

pro·pox·y·phene hy·dro·chlo·ride (prō-pok′si-fēn). A nonantipyretic, orally effective weak narcotic analgesic structurally related to methadone and used for the relief of mild to moderate pain; it is less effective than codeine. SYN dextropropoxyphene hydrochloride.

pro·pox·y·phene nap·syl·ate (prō-pok′si-fēn). A weak narcotic analgesic. SYN dextropropoxyphene napsylate.

pro·pran·o·lol hy·dro·chlo·ride (prō-pran′ō-lōl). An adrenergic β-receptor blocking agent; used in the treatment of angina pectoris, hypertension, cardiac arrhythmias, and other conditions.

pro·pri·e·tary name (prō-prī′ĕ-tār-ē). The protected brand name or trademark, registered with the U.S. Patent Office, under which a manufacturer markets its product. It is written with a capital initial letter and is often further distinguished by a superscript R in a circle (®). Cf. generic name, nonproprietary name. [L. *proprietas,* ownership]

pro·pri·o·cep·tion (prō-prē-ō-sep′shun). A sense or perception, usually at a subconscious level, of the movements and position of the body and especially its limbs, independent of vision; this sense is gained primarily from input from sensory nerve terminals in muscles and tendons (muscle spindles) and the fibrous capsule of joints combined with input from the vestibular apparatus.

pro·pri·o·cep·tive (prō′prē-ō-sep′tiv). Capable of receiving stimuli originating in muscles, tendons, and other internal tissues. [L. *proprius,* one's own, + *capio,* to take]

pro·pri·o·cep·tor (prō′prē-ō-sep′ter). One of a variety of sensory end organs (such as the muscle spindle and Golgi tendon organ) in muscles, tendons, and joint capsules that sense position or state of contraction.

pro·pri·o·spi·nal (prō′prē-ō-spī′năl). Relating especially or wholly to the spinal cord; specifically, denoting those nerve cells and their fibers that connect the different segments of the spinal cord with each other (e.g., spino-spinalis).

pro·pro·teins (prō′prō-tenz). Inactive protein precursors; e.g., proinsulin.

prop·tom·e·ter (prop-tom′ĕ-ter). SYN exophthalmometer. [pro- + G. *ptōsis,* a falling, + *metron,* measure]

prop·to·sis (prop-tō′sis). SYN exophthalmos. [G. *proptōsis,* a falling forward]

prop·tot·ic (prop-tot′ik). Referring to proptosis.

pro·pul·sion (prō-pŭl′shŭn). The tendency to fall forward; responsible for the festination in paralysis agitans. [G. *pro-pello,* pp. -*pulsus,* to drive forth]

pro·pyl (Pr) (prō′pil). The alkyl radical of propane, $CH_3CH_2CH_2-$.
p. alcohol, a solvent for resins and cellulose esters. SYN propanol.
p. gallate, an antioxidant for emulsions.
p. hydroxybenzoate, SYN propylparaben.

pro·pyl·car·bi·nol (prō-pil-kar′bi-nol). Primary butyl alcohol. SEE *butyl* alcohol.

pro·py·lene (prō′pi-lēn). Methylethylene; a gaseous olefinic hydrocarbon. SYN propene.
p. glycol, a solvent for several water-insoluble drugs intended for parenteral administration; an ingredient of hydrophilic ointment; a viscous organic solvent frequently used in pharmaceutical preparations to dissolve drug substances with limited aqueous solubility; used in part for preparing injectable solutions of diazepam, phenytoin, pentobarbital, and other drugs.

pro·pyl·hex·e·drine (prō-pil-hek′se-drēn). A sympathomimetic and local vasoconstrictor; often used by inhalation.

pro·pyl·i·o·done (prō-pil-ī′ō-dōn). A radiopaque medium formerly used for bronchography.

pro·pyl·par·a·ben (prō-pil-par′ă-ben). An antifungal agent and pharmaceutical preservative. SYN propyl hydroxybenzoate.

pro·pyl·thi·o·ur·a·cil (PTU) (prō′pil-thī-ō-ū′ră-sil). An antithyroid agent that inhibits the synthesis of thyroid hormones; used in the treatment of hyperthyroidism; a goitrogen.

pro·py·ro·ma·zine (prō-pi-rō′mă-zēn). An intestinal antispasmodic with anticholinergic properties.

pro rat. aet. Abbreviation for L. *pro ratione aetatis,* according to (patient's) age.

pro re na·ta (p.r.n.) (prō rē nā′tă). As the occasion arises; as necessary. [L.]

pro·ren·nin (prō-ren′in). SYN prochymosin.

pror·sad (prōr′sad). In a forward direction. [L. *prorsum,* forward, + *ad,* to]

pro·ru·bri·cyte (prō-roo′bri-sīt). Basophilic normoblast. SEE erythroblast. [pro- + rubricyte]
pernicious anemia type p., basophilic megaloblast. SEE erythroblast, megaloblast.

pros (pros). **1.** (π) Referring to the nitrogen atom in the imidazole ring in histidine that is closest to the β-carbon. Cf. *tele.* **2.** pros-; Prefix for near or in front. [G. near]

pro·scil·lar·i·din (prō-si-lar′i-din). Prepared from squill, the sea onion *Urginea maritima;* a cardiotonic agent, used for the treatment of congestive heart failure.

pro·sco·lex (prō-skō′leks). Seldom used term for the embryonic form of a tapeworm. [pro- + G. *skōlēx,* a worm]

pro·se·cre·tin (prō-sē-krē′tin). Unactivated secretin.

pro·sect (prō-sekt′). To dissect a cadaver or any part, that it may serve for a demonstration of anatomy before a class. [L. *pro-seco,* pp. -*sectus,* to cut]

pro·sec·tor (prō-sek′ter). One who prosects, or prepares the material for a demonstration of anatomy before a class.

pro·sec·to·ri·um (prō′sek-tō′rē-ŭm). A dissecting room; a place in which anatomical preparations are made for demonstration or for preservation in a museum. [L.]

pros·en·ceph·a·lon (pros-en-sef′ă-lon) [TA]. The anterior primitive cerebral vesicle and the most rostral of the three primary brain vesicles of the embryonic neural tube; it subdivides to form the diencephalon and telencephalon. SYN forebrain vesicle⋆, forebrain⋆, proencephalon. [G. *prosō,* forward, + *enkephalos,* brain]

Proskauer, Bernhard, German bacteriologist, 1851–1915. SEE Voges-P. *reaction.*

pros·o·dem·ic (pros-ō-dem′ik). Denoting a disease that is transmitted directly from person to person. [G. *prosō,* forward, + *dēmos,* people]

pros·o·dy (proz′ŏ-dē). The varying rhythm, stress, and frequency of speech that aids meaning transmission.

⌓**prosop-.** SEE prosopo-.

pros·o·pag·no·sia (pros′ō-pag-nō′sē-ă). Difficulty in recognizing familiar faces. [prosop- + G. *a-* priv. + *gnōsis,* recognition]

pro·sop·a·gus (pro-sop′ă-gŭs). SYN prosopopagus.

pros·o·pec·ta·sia (pros′ō-pek-tā′zē-ă). Enlargement of the face, as in acromegaly. [prosop- + G. *ektasis,* extension]

pros·o·pla·sia (pros-ō-plā′zē-ă). Progressive transformation, such as the change of cells of the salivary ducts into secreting cells. SEE cytomorphosis. [G. *prosō,* forward, + *plasis,* a molding]

⌓**prosopo-, prosop-.** The face. SEE ALSO facio-. [G. *prosopon*]

pros·o·po·a·nos·chi·sis (pros′ō-pō-ă-nos′ki-sis). SYN facial *cleft.* [prosopo- + G. *anō,* upward, + *schisis,* fissure]

pros·o·pop·a·gus (pros-ō-pop′ă-gŭs). Unequal conjoined twins in which the parasite, in the form of a tumorlike mass, is attached to the orbit or cheek of the autosite. SEE conjoined *twins,* under *twin.* SYN prosopagus. [prosopo- + G. *pagos,* something fastened]

pros·o·pos·chi·sis (pros-ō-pos′ki-sis). Congenital facial cleft from mouth to the inner canthus of the eye. SYN oblique facial cleft. [prosopo- + G. *schisis,* fissure]

pros·o·po·thor·a·cop·a·gus (pros′ō-pō-thōr-ă-kop′ă-gŭs). Conjoined twins attached by the face and chest; a variety of cephalothoracopagus. SEE conjoined *twins,* under *twin.* [prosopo- + G. *thōrax,* chest, + *pagos,* something fastened]

pros·ta·cy·clin (pros-tă-sī′klin). A potent natural inhibitor of platelet aggregation and a powerful vasodilator. SYN epoprostenol, epoprostenol sodium.

pros·ta·glan·din (PG) (pros-tă-glan′din). Any of a class of physiologically active substances present in many tissues, with effects such as vasodilation, vasoconstriction, stimulation of intestinal or bronchial smooth muscle, uterine stimulation, and antagonism to hormones influencing lipid metabolism. P.'s are prostanoic acids with side chains of varying degrees of unsaturation and varying degrees of oxidation. Often abbreviated PGA, PGB, PGC, PGD, etc. with numeric subscripts, according to structure. [fr. genital fluids and accessory glands where discovered]
p. E_1, SYN alprostadil.
p. E_2, SYN dinoprostone.
p. endoperoxide synthase, a protein complex that catalyzes two steps in p. biosynthesis; the cyclooxygenase activity (which is inhibited by aspirin and indomethacin) converts arachidonate and $2O_2$ to p. G_2; the hydroperoxidase activity uses glutathione to convert p. G_2 to p. H_2. SYN cyclooxygenase.
p. $F_{2\alpha}$, SYN dinoprost.
p. $F_{2\alpha}$ tromethamine, SYN *dinoprost* tromethamine.

pros·ta·no·ic ac·id (pros′tă-nō-ik). The 20-carbon acid that is the skeleton of the prostaglandins, with various hydroxyl and keto substitutions at positions 9, 11, and 15, and double bonds in the long aliphatic chains.

pros·ta·noids (pros′tă-nōids). Derivatives of prostanoic acid; e.g., prostaglandins, thromboxanes, etc.

⚠**prostat-.** SEE prostato-.

pros·ta·ta (pros′tah-tă) [TA]. SYN prostate. [Mod. L. from G. *prostatēs,* one standing before]

pros·ta·tal·gia (pros-tă-tal′jē-ă). A rarely used term for pain in the area of the prostate gland. [prostat- + G. *algos,* pain]

❶prostate (pros′tāt) [TA]. A chestnut-shaped body, surrounding the beginning of the urethra in the male, that consists of two lateral lobes connected anteriorly by an isthmus and posteriorly by a middle lobe lying above and between the ejaculatory ducts. In structure, the prostate consists of 30–50 compound tubuloalveolar glands between which is abundant stroma consisting of collagen and elastic fibers and many smooth muscle bundles. The secretion of the glands is a milky fluid that is discharged by excretory ducts into the prostatic urethra at the time of the emission of semen. SYN prostata [TA], glandula prostatica, prostate gland.

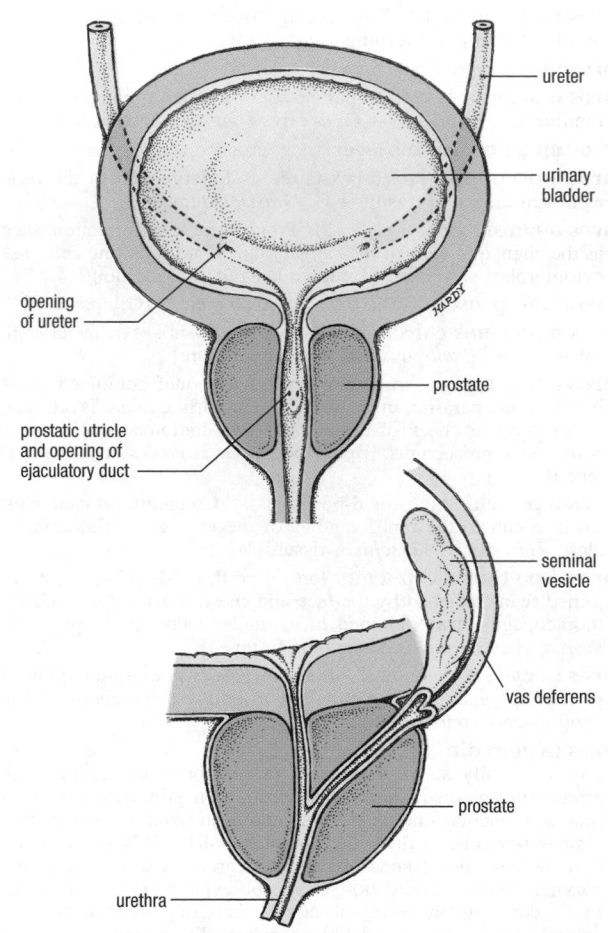

prostate and surrounding structures

female p., term sometimes applied to the periurethral glands in the upper part of the urethra in the female.

pros·ta·tec·to·my (pros-tă-tek′tō-mē). Removal of a part or all of the prostate. [prostat- + G. *ektomē,* excision]

pros·tat·ic (pros-tat′ik). Relating to the prostate.

pros·tat·i·co·ves·i·cal (pros-tat′i-kō-ves′i-kăl). Relating to the prostate and the bladder.

pros·ta·tism (pros′tă-tizm). A clinical syndrome, occurring mostly in older men, usually caused by enlargement of the prostate gland and manifested by irritative (nocturia, frequency, de-

creased voided volume, sensory urgency, and urgency incontinence) and obstructive (hesitancy, decreased stream, terminal dribbling, double voiding, and urinary retention) symptoms.

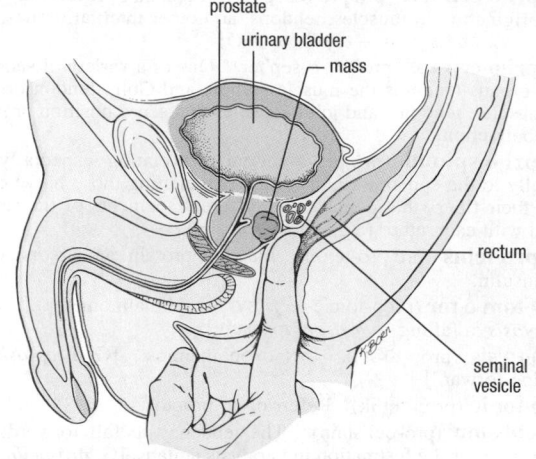

palpation of the prostate gland

pros·ta·ti·tis (pros-tă-tī′tis). Inflammation of the prostate. The NIH consensus designates 4 categories of p.: I, acute bacterial p.; II, chronic bacterial p.; III, chronic p./chronic pelvic pain syndrome: A, inflammatory and B, noninflammatory; and IV, asymptomatic inflammatory p. [prostat- + G. *-itis,* inflammation]

⚠**prostato-, prostat-.** The prostate gland. [Med. L. *prostata* fr. G. *prostatēs,* one who stands before, protects]

pros·ta·to·cys·ti·tis (pros′tă-tō-sis-tī′tis). Inflammation of the prostate and the bladder; cystitis by extension of inflammation from the prostatic urethra. [prostato- + G. *kystis,* bladder, + *-itis,* inflammation]

pros·ta·to·dyn·ia (pros′tă-tō-din′ē-ă). A rarely used term for prostatalgia. [prostato- + G. *odynē,* pain]

pros·tat·o·lith (pros-tat′ō-lith). SYN prostatic *calculus.* [prostato- + G. *lithos,* stone]

pros·ta·to·li·thot·o·my (pros′tă-tō-li-thot′ō-mē, pros-tat′ō-). Incision of the prostate for removal of a calculus. [prostato- + G. *lithos,* stone, + *tomē,* incision]

pros·ta·to·meg·a·ly (pros′tă-tō-meg′ă-lē). Enlargement of the prostate gland. [prostato- + G. *megas,* large]

pros·tat·o·my (pros-tat′ō-mē). SYN prostatotomy.

pros·ta·tor·rhea (pros′tă-tō-rē′ă). An abnormal discharge of prostatic fluid. [prostato- + G. *rhoia,* a flow]

pros·ta·to·sem·i·nal·ve·sic·u·lec·to·my (pros′tă-tō-sem′i-năl-ve-sik-ū-lek′tō-mē). SYN prostatovesiculectomy.

pros·ta·tot·o·my (pros′tă-tot′ō-mē). An incision into the prostate. SYN prostatomy. [prostato- + G. *tomē,* incision]

pros·ta·to·ve·sic·u·lec·to·my (pros′tă-tō-ve-sik′ū-lek′tō-mē). Surgical removal of the prostate gland and seminal vesicles. SYN prostatoseminalvesiculectomy.

pros·ta·to·ve·sic·u·li·tis (pros′tă-tō-ve-sik′ū-lī′tis). Inflammation of the prostate gland and seminal vesicles.

pros·ter·na·tion (pros-ter-nā′shŭn). SYN camptocormia.

pros·the·on (pros′thē-on). SYN prosthion.

pros·the·sis, pl. **pros·the·ses** (pros′thē-sis, -sēz; pros-thē′sis). Fabricated substitute for a damaged or missing part of the body. [G. an addition]

auditory p., generic term for implantable devices to restore sound perception to the deaf, the most common of which is the cochlear implant; a brainstem implant to stimulate the neurons of the cochlear nucleus is under development.

cardiac valve p., SEE valve (2).

cochlear p., SYN cochlear *implant.*

definitive p., a dental p. to be used over a prescribed period of time.

dental p., an artificial replacement of one or more teeth and/or associated structures. SEE ALSO denture.

heart valve p., replacement of a cardiac valve removed for disease by either a mechanical or a biologically derived artificial valve.

hybrid p., SYN overlay *denture.*

mandibular guide p., a p. with an extension designed to direct a resected mandible into a functional relation with the maxilla.

ocular p., an artificial eye or implant.

penile p., device placed inside penis to correct erectile failure.

provisional p., an interim dental p. worn for varying periods of time.

surgical p., an appliance prepared as an aid or as a part of a surgical procedure, such as a heart valve, cranial plate, or artificial joint replacement.

testicular p., SYN testicular *implant.*

tilting disk valve p., a low-profile artificial heart valve employing a caged disk that tilts to open during systole.

pros·thet·ic (pros-thet'ik). **1.** Relating to a prosthesis or to an artificial part. **2.** SEE prosthetic *group.*

pros·thet·ics (pros-thet'iks). The art and science of making and adjusting artificial parts of the human body, SEE anaplastology.

dental p., SYN prosthodontics.

maxillofacial p., that branch of dentistry that provides prostheses or devices to treat or restore tissues of the stomatognathic system and associated facial structures that have been affected by disease, injury, surgery, or congenital defect, to provide all possible function and esthetics.

pros·the·tist (pros'the-tist). One skilled in constructing and fitting prostheses.

pros·the·to·phac·os (pros'the-tō-fak'ōs). SYN lenticulus. [G. *prosthesis,* an addition, + *phakos,* lens]

pros·thi·on (pros'the-on). The most anterior point on the maxillary alveolar process in the midline. SYN alveolar point, prostheon. [G. ntr. of *prosthios,* foremost]

pros·tho·don·tia (pros-thō-don'shē-ă). SYN prosthodontics. [L.]

pros·tho·don·tics (pros-thō-don'tiks). The science of and art of providing suitable substitutes for the coronal portions of teeth, or for one or more lost or missing teeth and their associated parts, in order that impaired function, appearance, comfort, and health of the patient may be restored. SYN dental prosthetics, prosthetic dentistry, prosthodontia. [L. *prosthodontia,* fr. G. *prosthesis* + *odous (odont-),* tooth]

pros·tho·don·tist (pros-thō-don'tist). A dentist engaged in the practice of prosthodontics.

Pros·tho·gon·i·mus ma·cror·chis (pros'thō-gon'i-mŭs mak-rōr'kis). A digenetic trematode (family Prosthogonimidae) located in the oviduct and bursa fabricii of poultry in North America, particularly common in states bordering the Great Lakes. [G. *prosthe,* in front of, + *gonos,* seed, offspring; macro- + *orchis,* testicle]

pros·tho·ker·a·to·plas·ty (pros'thō-ker'ă-tō-plas-tē). The surgical technique involved in utilizing a keratoprosthesis.

pros·tra·tion (pros-trā'shŭn). A marked loss of strength, as in exhaustion. [L. *pro-sterno,* pp. *-stratus,* to strew before, overthrow]

heat p., SEE heat *exhaustion.*

⌒**prot-.** SEE proteo-, proto-.

prot·ac·tin·i·um (Pa) (prō-tak-tin'ē-ŭm). A radioactive element, atomic no. 91, atomic wt. 231.03588, formed in the decay of uranium and thorium; its most long-lived isotope, ^{231}Pa, has a half-life of 32,500 years. SYN proactinium, protoactinium. [G. *prōtos,* first]

pro·tal·bu·mose (prō-tal'bū-mōs). Intermediate products of protein digestion, derived from hemialbumose; soluble in water and not coagulable by heat, but precipitated by ammonium sulfate, cupric sulfate, and sodium chloride. SYN protoalbumose.

pro·tam·i·nase (prō-tam'i-nās). SYN carboxypeptidase B.

prot·a·mine (prō'tă-mēn, -min). Any of a class of proteins, highly basic because rich in L-arginine and simpler in constitution than the albumins and globulins, etc., found in fish spermatozoa in combination with nucleic acid; the p.'s have a histonelike function and are present in the sperm of all mammals; neutralizes anticoagulant action of heparin; used in the preparation of several long-acting insulin preparations.

p. sulfate, a purified mixture of simple protein principles from the sperm or testes of suitable species of fish; it is a heparin antagonist used in certain hemorrhagic states associated with increased amounts of heparin-like substances in the circulation and for the treatment of heparin overdosage.

pro·ta·nom·a·ly (prō'tă-nom'ă-lē). A deficiency of color perception in which the red-sensitive pigment in cones is decreased. [G. *prōtos,* first, + *anōmalia,* anomaly]

pro·ta·no·pia (prō'tă-nō'pē-ă). A form of dichromatism characterized by absence of the red-sensitive pigment in cones, decreased luminosity for long wavelengths of light, and confusion in recognition of red and green. [G. *prōtos,* first, + *a-* priv. + *ōps (ōp-)* eye]

pro·te·an (prō'tē-an). Changeable in form; having the power to change body form, like the ameba. [G. *Prōteus,* a god having the power to change his form]

pro·te·ase (prō'tē-ās). Descriptive term for proteolytic enzymes, both endopeptidases and exopeptidases; enzymes that hydrolize (break) polypeptide chains.

Lon p. (prō'tē-ās), an enzyme that degrades a bacterial protein and stops cell division until chromosomal repair is completed.

tricorn p., a p. found in organisms lacking membrane-bound compartments that forms the core of a modular proteolytic system used to generate multicatalytic activities in a controlled manner.

pro·tec·tion (prō-tek'shŭn). SYN protective *block.* [see protective]

protector. A cover or shield. [L.L. *protectus* from pp. *protegere,* to protect, to cover over]

hearing p.'s, occlusive devices for the external auditory canal made of pliable material or fluid (usually glycerin)-filled ear muffs for protection against noise-induced hearing loss.

Pro·tee·ae (prō'tē-ē). A tribe within the bacterial family Enterobacteriaceae that includes the three genera: *Proteus, Morganella,* and *Providencia.*

pro·tein (p) (prō'tēn, prō'tē-in). Macromolecules consisting of long sequences of α-amino acids [H₂N–CHR–COOH] in peptide (amide) linkage (elimination of H_2O between the α-NH₂ and α-COOH of successive residues). P. is three-fourths of the dry weight of most cell matter and is involved in structures, hormones, enzymes, muscle contraction, immunologic response, and essential life functions. The amino acids involved are generally the 20 α-amino acids (glycine, L-alanine, etc.) recognized by the genetic code. Cross-links yielding globular forms of p. are often effected through the –SH groups of two L-cysteinyl residues, as well as by noncovalent forces (hydrogen bonds, lipophilic attractions, etc.). [G. *prōtos,* first, + -in]

p. 4.1, a peripheral p. that binds tightly to spectrin in the red cell membrane; it also binds to certain glycophorins and helps determine the shape and flexibility of the red blood cell.

p. A, a component of some strains of *Staphyloccocus aureus.*

acute phase p., plasma p.'s associated with inflammation including C-reactive p. (CRP), mannose-binding p., serum amyloid P component, α₁-antitrypsin, fibrinogen, ceruloplasmin, and complement components C9 and factor B, the concentrations of which increase in response to interleukins 1, 6, and 11.

acyl carrier p. (ACP), one of the p.'s of the complex in cytoplasm that contains all of the enzymes required to convert acetyl-CoA (and, in certain cases, butyryl-CoA or propionyl-CoA) and malonyl-CoA to palmitic acid. This complex is tightly bound together in mammalian tissues and in yeast, but that from *Escherichia coli* is readily dissociated. The ACP thus isolated is a heatstable p. with a molecular weight of about 10,000. It contains a free –SH that binds the acyl intermediates in the synthesis of fatty acids as thioesters. This –SH group is part of a 4'-phosphopantetheine, added to the apoprotein by ACP phosphodiesterase, which

pr

thus plays the same role that it does in coenzyme A. ACP is involved in every step of the fatty acid synthetic process.

amyloid p., SEE amyloid.

androgen binding p. (ABP), a p. secreted by testicular Sertoli cells along with inhibin and müllerian inhibiting substance. Androgen binding p. probably maintains a high concentration of androgen in the seminiferous tubules.

antitermination p., a p. that permits RNA polymerase to transcribe through certain termination sites.

antitumor p., a p. that inhibits tumor growth.

antiviral p. (AVP), a human or animal factor, induced by interferon in virus-infected cells, which mediates interferon inhibition of virus replication.

autologous p., any p. found normally in the fluids or tissues of the body.

basic p.'s, p.'s that are rich in basic amino acids; e.g., histones.

Bence Jones p.'s, p.'s with unusual thermosolubility found in the urine of patients with multiple myeloma, consisting of monoclonal immunoglobulin light chains. SEE Bence Jones *reaction*; SEE ALSO immunoglobulin. [H. Bence Jones, English physician, 1813–1873]

bone Gla p. (BGP), SYN osteocalcin.

p. C, a vitamin K–dependent glycoprotein that inhibits coagulation by enzymatic cleavage of the activated forms of factors V and VIII, and thus interferes with the regulation of intravascular clot formation; a deficiency of p. C leads to impaired regulation of blood coagulation. There is an autosomal dominant deficiency [MIM*176860] that, like antithrombin III deficiency and plasminogen deficiency, is associated with an increased risk of severe or premature thrombosis.

cAMP receptor p. (CRP), SYN catabolite (gene) activator p.

capping p.'s, p.'s that bind to one end of actin filaments, preventing both addition and loss of actin monomers.

catabolite (gene) activator p. (CAP), a p. that can be activated by cAMP, whereupon it affects the action of RNA polymerase by binding it with it or near it on the DNA to be transcribed. SYN cAMP receptor p., catabolite gene activator.

cholesterol ester transport p.'s, a p. that transports cholesterol esters from HDL to VLDL and LDL; a deficiency of this protein is associated with elevated HDL cholesterol.

circumsporozoite p., one of two p.'s (the other is thrombospondin-related adhesive p.) involved in sporozoite recognition of host cells in malaria.

cis-**acting p.,** a p. that acts on the molecule of DNA from which it was expressed.

compound p., SYN conjugated p.

conjugated p., p. attached to some other molecule or molecules (not amino acid in nature) otherwise than as a salt; e.g., flavoproteins; chromoproteins, hemoglobins. SEE ALSO prosthetic *group*; Cf. simple p. SYN compound p.

copper p., a p. containing one or more copper ions; e.g., cytochrome *c* oxidase, phenol oxidase.

corticosteroid-binding p., SYN transcortin.

C-reactive p. (CRP), a β-globulin found in the serum of various persons with certain inflammatory, degenerative, and neoplastic diseases; although the p. is not a specific antibody, it precipitates in vitro the C polysaccharide present in all types of pneumococci.

denatured p., a p. whose characteristics or properties have been altered in some way, as by heat, enzyme action, or chemicals, and in so doing has lost its biologic activity.

derived p., a derivative of p. effected by chemical change, e.g., hydrolysis.

docking p., in the process of translating p.'s that are to be secreted from the cell, translation is arrested until the growing polypeptide chain that is complexed by a specific particle (signal recognition particle) comes in contact with this integral p. of the endoplasmic reticulum.

encephalithogenic p., an important protein in the central nervous system. SYN myelin p. A1.

eosinophil cationic p. (ECP), p. the level of which in serum of clotted blood reflects the rate of activation of circulating eosinophils.

extrinsic p.'s, SYN peripheral p.'s.

fatty acid–binding p., SYN Z-p.

fibrous p., any insoluble p., including the collagens, elastins, and keratins, involved in structural or fibrous tissues.

foreign p., a p. that differs from any p. normally found in the organism in question. SYN heterologous p.

G p.'s, intracellular membrane-associated p.'s activated by several (e.g., β-adrenergic) receptors; they serve as second messengers or transducers of the receptor-initiated response to intracellular elements such as enzymes to initiate an effect. These p.'s have a high affinity for guanine nucleotides and hence are named G p.'s. SYN G-p., GTP binding p.'s.

G-p., SYN G p.'s.

glial fibrillary acidic p., a cytoskeletal p. of 51 kd found in fibrous astrocytes; stains for this p. are frequently used to assist in the differential diagnosis of neurologic lesions.

globular p., any p. soluble in water, usually with added acid, alkali, salt, or ethanol, and roughly so classified (albumins, globulins, histones, and protamines), in contrast to fibrous p.

GTP binding p.'s, SYN G p.'s.

heat shock p.'s (hsp), specific p.'s whose synthesis is increased immediately after sudden elevation of temperature; their function is to help diminish the harmful effects of high temperature.

heterologous p., SYN foreign p.

homologous p.'s, p.'s having a very similar primary, secondary, and tertiary structure.

immune p., SYN antibody.

integral p.'s, p.'s that cannot be easily separated from a biomembrane. SYN intrinsic p.'s.

intrinsic p.'s, SYN integral p.'s.

iron-sulfur p.'s, p.'s containing one or more iron atoms that are linked to sulfur bridges and/or sulfur of cysteinyl residues; e.g., certain p.'s in the electron transport pathway.

p. kinase C, any of a number of cytoplasmic calcium-activated kinases involved in numerous processes, including hormonal binding, platelet activation, and tumor promotion.

p. kinases, a class of enzymes that phosphorylates other p.'s; many of these kinases are responsive to other effectors (e.g., cAMP, cGMP, insulin, epidermal growth factor, calcium and calmodulin, calcium and phospholipids).

latent membrane p. (LMP), gene product of Epstein-Barr virus.

low molecular weight p.'s (LMP), gene products that are components of proteosomes.

M p., (1) SYN Streptococcus M *antigen*; SEE ALSO β-hemolytic *streptococci*, under *streptococcus, Streptococcus pneumoniae*; (2) SYN monoclonal *immunoglobulin*.

macrophage inflammatory p. (MIP) (mak′rō-fāj in′flam-mă-tor-ē), a member of the chemokine family that is chemotactic for certain lymphocyte subsets such as T cytotoxic cells.

mannose-binding p., a p. involved in innate immunity that can bind mannosylated microorganisms and activate the complement pathway.

matrix Gla p. (MGP), a calcium binding p.

microtubule-associated p.'s (MAPs), p.'s that have a specific association with α- and/or β-tubulin; e.g., tau, MAP1, MAP2; several have been found in the plaques observed in Alzheimer disease.

monoclonal p., SYN monoclonal *immunoglobulin*.

monocyte chemoattractant p., a cytokine involved in monocyte migration.

monocyte chemoattractant p.-1 (MCP-1), secreted by endothelial cells of a blood vessel wall; it induces extravasation of monocytes.

muscle p.'s, p.'s present in muscle.

myelin p. A1, SYN encephalithogenic p.

native p., the concept of a p. in its natural state, in the cell, unaltered by heat, chemicals, enzyme action, or the exigencies of extraction.

neutrophil-activating p., old term for interleukin-8.

non-heme iron p., any p. containing iron but not any heme iron; e.g., NADH dehydrogenase.

pr

nonspecific p., a p. substance that elicits a response not mediated by specific antigen-antibody reaction.

odorant binding p., p.'s in nasal mucus that bind lipophilic odor-producing molecules and transfer them to the olfactory receptors. Similar p.'s may mediate taste.

p. p53, a multifunctional p. that modulates gene transcription and controls DNA repair, apoptosis, and the cell cycle.

parathyroid hormonelike p. (PLP), SYN parathyroid hormone-related p.

parathyroid hormone-related p., a 140–amino acid p. secreted by some cancer cells; it causes hypercalcemia. SYN parathyroid hormonelike p.

pathologic p.'s, SEE paraprotein.

peripheral p.'s, p.'s that can be easily removed from a biomembrane (e.g., by altering the pH or the ionic strength). SYN extrinsic p.'s.

phenylthiocarbamoyl p., formed by the reaction of phenylisothiocyanate with a terminal α-amino group of a peptide or p. SEE ALSO phenylisothiocyanate, phenylthiohydantoin. SYN PhNCS p., PTC p.

PhNCS p., SYN phenylthiocarbamoyl p.

p. phosphatases, a class of enzymes that catalyze the dephosphorylation of specific phosphorylated p.'s.

placenta p., SYN human placental *lactogen*.

▪ **plasma p.'s,** dissolved p.'s (>100) of blood plasma, mainly albumins and globulins (normally 6–8 g/100 mL); they hold fluid in blood vessels by osmosis and include antibodies and blood-clotting p.'s. SYN serum p.'s.

prion p. (PrP), SYN prion.

protective p., SYN antibody.

PTC p., SYN phenylthiocarbamoyl p.

purified placental p., SYN human placental *lactogen*.

receptor p., an intracellular p. (or p. fraction) that has a high specific affinity for binding a known stimulus to cellular activity, such as a steroid hormone or adenosine 3′,5′-cyclic phosphate.

retinol-binding p., a plasma p. that binds and transports retinol.

S p., the major fragment produced from pancreatic ribonuclease by the limited action of subtilisin, which cleaves the ribonuclease between residues 20 and 21; the smaller fragment (residues 1–20) is S peptide.

p. S, a vitamin K–dependent antithrombotic p. that functions as a cofactor with activated p. C.

serum p.'s, SYN plasma p.'s.

simple p., p. that yields only α-amino acids or their derivatives by hydrolysis; e.g., albumins, globulins, glutelins, prolamines, albuminoids, histones, protamines. Cf. conjugated p.

stimulatory p. 1 (SP1), an RNA polymerase II transcription factor in vertebrates; binds to DNA in regions rich in G and C residues; a general promoter-binding factor necessary for the activation of many genes.

structure p.'s, p.'s whose role is for structure and support in tissue and within the cell; e.g., the collagens.

surfactant-specific p.'s, the p. components of pulmonary surfactant, including surfactant p. A, B, C.

Tamm-Horsfall p., SEE Tamm-Horsfall *mucoprotein*.

thrombospondin-related adhesive p., one of two p.'s (the other is circumsporozoite p.) involved in sporozoite recognition of host cells in malaria.

thyroxine-binding p. (TBP), (1) SYN thyroxine-binding *globulin*; **(2)** SYN thyroxine-binding *prealbumin*.

unwinding p.'s, enzymes that uncoil the DNA allowing recombination events to occur.

vitamin D–binding p. (DBP), a plasma p. that binds vitamin D.

whey p., the soluble p. contained in the whey of milk clotted by rennin; e.g., lactoglobulin, α-lactalbumin, lactoferrin.

Z-p., a fatty acid–binding protein that participates in the intracellular movement of fatty acids. SYN fatty acid–binding p.

pro·tein·a·ceous (prō′tē-nā′shŭs, prō′tē-i-nā′shŭs). Resembling a protein; possessing, to some degree, the physicochemical properties characteristic of proteins.

pro·tein·ase. SYN endopeptidase.

pro·tein hy·drol·y·sate. A sterile solution of amino acids and soft-chain peptides prepared from a suitable protein by acid or enzymatic hydrolysis; used intravenously for the maintenance of positive nitrogen balance in severe illness, and after surgery involving the alimentary tract; or used orally in the diets of infants allergic to milk or as a supplement when high protein intake from ordinary foods cannot be accomplished.

pro·tein·o·gen·ic (prō′ten-ō-jen′ik). SYN proteogenic.

pro·tein·oids (prō′tēn-oydz; prō′tē-in-oyds). Artificially synthesized heteropoly(amino acids).

pro·tein·o·sis (pro-tē-nō′sis, prō′tē-i-nō′sis). A state characterized by disordered protein formation and distribution, particularly as manifested by the deposition of abnormal proteins in tissues. [protein + G. *-osis,* condition]

lipoid p. [MIM*247100], a disturbance of lipid metabolism in which there are deposits of a protein-lipid complex on the tongue and sublingual and faucial areas leading to hoarseness, and translucent keratotic papillomatous eyelid lesions; autosomal recessive inheritance, frequently with specific intracranial calcifications. SYN hyalinosis cutis et mucosae, lipoidosis cutis et mucosae, Urbach-Wiethe disease.

pulmonary alveolar p., a chronic progressive lung disease of adults, characterized by alveolar accumulation of granular proteinaceous material that is PAS-positive and lipid- rich, with little inflammatory cellular exudate; the cause is unknown.

pro·tein·u·ria (prō-tē-noo′rē-ă, prō′tē-i-noo′rē-ă). **1.** Presence of urinary protein in amounts greater than 0.3 g in a 24-hour urine collection or in concentrations greater than 1 g/L (1+ to 2+ by standard turbidometric methods) in a random urine collection on two or more occasions at least 6 hours apart; specimens must be clean, voided midstream, or obtained by catheterization. **2.** SYN albuminuria. [protein + G. *ouron,* urine]

Bence Jones p., presence of Bence Jones proteins in the urine, usually indicative of a neoplastic process such as multiple myeloma, amyloidosis, or Waldenström macroglobulinemia.

gestational p., the presence of p. during or under the influence of pregnancy in the absence of hypertension, edema, renal infection, or known intrinsic renovascular disease.

isolated p., p. in a patient who is asymptomatic, has normal renal function and urinary sediment, and has no manifestation of systemic disease upon initial examination.

nonisolated p., p. associated with other abnormalities.

orthostatic p., postural p., SYN orthostatic *albuminuria*.

pro·ten·si·ty (prō-ten′si-tē). The time attribute of a mental process; the attribute of a mental process characterized by its temporality or movement forward in time. [L. *protendo (-tensum),* to extend]

⌂ **proteo-, prot-.** Protein.

pro·te·o·clas·tic (prō′tē-ō-klas′tik). SYN proteolytic. [proteo- + G. *klastos,* broken]

pro·te·o·gen·ic (prō′tē-ō-jen-ik). Capable of producing proteins. SYN proteinogenic.

pro·te·o·gly·can I. SYN biglycan.

pro·te·o·gly·cans (prō′tē-ō-glī′kanz). Glycoaminoglycans (mucopolysaccharides) bound to protein chains in covalent complexes; occur in the extracellular matrix of connective tissue.

pro·te·o·hor·mone (prō′tē-ō-hōr′mōn). Obsolete term for a hormone possessing a protein structure.

pro·te·o·lip·ids (prō′tē-ō-lip′idz). A class of lipid-soluble proteins found in brain tissue, insoluble in water but soluble in chloroform-methanol-water mixtures.

pro·te·ol·y·sis (prō-tē-ol′i-sis). The decomposition of protein; primarily via the hydrolysis of peptide bonds, both enzymatically and nonenzymatically. [proteo- + G. *lysis,* dissolution]

pro·te·o·lyt·ic (prō′tē-ō-lit′ik). Relating to or effecting proteolysis. SYN proteoclastic.

pro·te·o·met·a·bol·ic (prō′tē-ō-met′ă-bol′ik). Relating to the metabolism of proteins.

pro·te·o·me·tab·o·lism (prō′tē-ō-mě-tab′ō-lizm). SYN protein *metabolism*.

plasma proteins				
	physiologic function	concentration in plasma or serum (mg/L)	electrophoretic activity	molecular weight (daltons)
transport proteins				
albumin	oncotic pressure, transport of many substances	35,000–55,000	5.92	66,300
prealbumin	thyroxine binding	100–400	7.6	55,000
transcortin	cortisone binding	70	α_1	55,700
haptoglobin (types 1-1, 2-1, 2-2)	hemoglobin binding, acute phase protein	410–2,460	α_2 4.5	100,000–400,000
hemopexin	binds heme	500–1,150	β_1 3.1	57,000
retinol-binding protein	binds vitamin A	30–60	α_2	21,000
transcobalamins I–III	vitamin B_{12} transport		α_1–β_1	
α_2-macroglobulin	hormone transport, enzyme inhibition, acute phase protein	1,500–4,200	α_2 4.2	725,000
transferrin	iron transport	2,000–4,000	β_1 3.1	76,500
acidic α_1-glycoprotein	acute phase protein	550–1,400	α_1 5.7	41,000
C-reactive protein	acute phase protein, stimulation of phagocytosis	<1		135,000–140,000
immunoglobulins (Ig)				
IgM	early antibodies	600–2,800	β/γ 2.1	950,000
IgG	late antibodies	8,000–18,000	γ 1.2	150,000
IgA	secretory antibodies	900–4,500	β/γ 2.1	160,000 and multiples
IgD	regulatory antibodies	<150	β/γ < 2.1	175,000
IgE	reagins, allergic antibodies	0.3	β/γ 2.3	190,000
complement system				
C1q		190	γ_2	400,000
C1r		100	β	190,000
C1s		120	α_2	85,000
C2		30	β_2	117,000
C3		1,300	β_1	180,000
C4	(see under "complement")	430	β_1	206,000
C5		75	β_1	180,000
C6		60	β_2	128,000
C7		10	β_2	121,000
C8		10	γ_1	153,000
C9		10	α_2	79,000
activators of alternate pathways				
properdin	complement activation	10–20	β–$\gamma2$	224,000
C3-proactivator (C3-PA)	through surface-bonded polysaccharides	225	$\beta2$	93,000
C3-PA convertase		trace		22,000
enzyme				
cholinesterase	hydrolysis of choline esters	5–15	α_2 3.1	348,000
ceruloplasmin	oxidase, Cu-binding	150–600	α_2 4.6	132,000
plasminogen	fibrinolysis (proenzyme)	100–300	β_1 3.7	91,000
lysozyme	protease	5–15	α_1	~15,000
lipoprotein lipase	fat transport	varies	?	?
adenosine desaminase	nucleotide metabolism	trace	α/β	?

continued

plasma proteins (continued)				
	physiologic function	concentration in plasma or serum (mg/L)	electrophoretic activity	molecular weight (daltons)
enzyme inhibitors				
C1-esterase inhibitor	inactivation	150–350	α_2	104,000
α_1-antitrypsin	trypsin inhibition	2,000–4,000	α_1 5.42	45,000–54,000
inter-α-trypsin inhibitor	trypsin inhibition	200–700	α_1/α_2	~160,000
antichymotrypsin	chymotrypsin inhibition	300–600	α_1	68,000
antithrombin III	thrombin inhibition	170–300	α_2	65,000
coagulation factors				
factor I, fibrinogen	formation of coagulants, endphase	2,000–4,500	$\beta/\gamma = \phi\ 2.1$	340,000
factor II, prothrombin	proenzyme	50–100	α	69,000
factors III–XIII	see under coagulation (diagram); see also factor...			
lipoproteins				
α_1-lipoprotein, HDL$_2$	lipid transport	400–1,200	α_1	
α_1-lipoprotein, HDL$_3$	lipid transport	220–2,700	α_1	
α_2-lipoprotein, pre-β, very low density lipoprotein, VLDL	lipid transport	150–2,300	α_2	
β-lipoprotein, low density lipoprotein, LDL	lipid transport	250–8,000	β	

Pro·te·o·myx·id·ia (prō′tē-ō-mik-sid′ē-ă). Former name for Eumycetozoea. [*Proteus* + G. *myxa,* mucus]

pro·te·o·pec·tic, pro·te·o·pex·ic (prō′tē-ō-pek′tik, -pek′sik). Relating to proteopexis.

pro·te·o·pep·sis (prō′tē-ō-pep′sis). The digestion of protein. [proteo- + G. *pepsis,* digestion]

pro·te·o·pex·is (prō′tē-ō-pek′sis). The fixation of protein in the tissues. [proteo- + G. *pēxis,* fixation]

pro·te·ose (prō′tē-ōs). A nondescript mixture of intermediate products of proteolysis between protein and peptone.

primary p., the first result of hydrolysis of metaprotein; two stages, protoproteose and heteroproteose, have been distinguished.

secondary p., p. derived from primary p. by further hydrolysis.

proteosome (prō′tē-ō-sōm). A cluster of genes that encode components of the cell cytosolic proteolytic complex, a set of proteins thought to be involved in cellular processing and transport of peptides in the formation of the major histocompatibility complex class I molecules. [proteo- + G. *sōma,* body]

Pro·teus (prō′tē-ŭs). **1.** A former genus of the Sarcodina, now termed *Amoeba.* **2.** A genus of motile, peritrichous, nonsporeforming, aerobic to facultatively anaerobic bacteria (family Enterobacteriaceae) containing Gram-negative rods; coccoid forms, large irregular involution forms, filaments, and spheroplasts occur under certain conditions. The metabolism is fermentative, producing acid or acid and visible gas from glucose; lactose is not fermented, and they rapidly decompose urea and deaminate phenylalanine. *P.* occurs primarily in fecal matter and in putrefying materials. The type species is *P. vulgaris.* [G. *Proteus,* a sea god, who had the power to change his form]

P. incon′stans, a bacterial species found in urinary tract infections and in sporadic cases of diarrhea in humans; some strains cause gastroenteritis.

P. mirab′ilis, a bacterial species found in putrid meat, infusions, and abscesses; a cause of urinary tract infections associated with formation of renal and bladder calculi.

P. morgan′ii, former name for *Morganella morganii,* a bacterial species found in the intestinal canal, and in nosocomial infections.

P. rettge′ri, SYN *Providencia rettgeri.*

P. vulgar′is, the type species of the bacterial genus *P.,* found in putrefying materials and in abscesses; it is pathogenic for fish, dogs, guinea pigs, and mice; certain strains, the X strains of Weil and Felix, are agglutinated by typhus serum and are therefore of great importance in the diagnosis of typhus; strain X-19 is strongly agglutinated. SEE ALSO Weil-Felix *reaction.*

pro·thi·pen·dyl (prō-thī′pen-dil). An antipsychotic.

pro·throm·base (prō-throm′bās). SEE *factor* X.

pro·throm·bin (prō-throm′bin). A glycoprotein, molecular weight approximately 72,500, formed and stored in the parenchymal cells of the liver and present in blood in a concentration of approximately 20 mg/100 mL. In the presence of thromboplastin and calcium ion, p. is converted to thrombin, which in turn converts fibrinogen to fibrin, this process resulting in coagulation of blood; a deficiency of p. leads to impaired blood coagulation. SYN serozyme, thrombinogen, thrombogen.

pro·throm·bin·ase (prō-throm′bi-nās). SYN *factor* X.

pro·throm·bi·no·gen (prō-throm′bi-nō-jen). SYN *factor* VII.

pro·throm·bi·no·pe·nia (prō-throm′bi-nō-pē′nē-ă). SYN hypoprothrombinemia.

pro·throm·bo·ki·nase (prō′throm-bō-kī′nās). SYN *factor* V, *factor* VIII.

pro·ti·re·lin (prō-tī′rĕ-lin). A synthetic form of thyroliberin.

pro·tist (prō′tist). A member of the kingdom Protista.

Pro·tis·ta (prō-tis′ta). A kingdom of both plantlike and animallike eucaryotic unicellular organisms, either in the form of solitary organisms, e.g., protozoa, or colonies of cells lacking true tissues. [G. ntr. pl. of *prōtistos,* the first of all]

pro·ti·um (prō′tē-ŭm). SYN hydrogen-1.

△**proto-, prot-.** The first in a series; the highest in rank. [G. *prōtos,* first]

pro·to·ac·tin·i·um (prō′tō-ak-tin′ē-um). SYN protactinium.

pro·to·al·bu·mose (prō-tō-al′bū-mōs). SYN protalbumose.

pro·to·al·ka·loid (prō-tō-al′kă-loyd). A biogenic amine serving as a precursor of an alkaloid.

pro·to·bi·ol·o·gy (prō′tō-bī-ol′ō-jē). SYN bacteriophagology.

pro·to·cat·e·chu·ic ac·id (prō'tō-kat'ĕ-choo'ik, -koo'ik). Oxidation product of epinephrine.

pro·to·col (prō'tō-kol). A precise and detailed plan for the study of a biomedical problem or for a regimen of therapy.

Bruce p., a method of graduated, increasingly strenuous exercise testing to determine the severity of coronary artery disease.

Bruce p., a standardized p. for electrocardiogram-monitored exercise using increasing speeds and elevations of the treadmill; a test for ischemia usually due to coronary artery disease. SEE ALSO stress *test*.

pro·to·cone (prō'tō-kōn). The mesiolingual cusp of an upper molar tooth in a mammal. [proto- + G. *kōnos*, cone]

pro·to·co·nid (prō-tō-kon'id). The mesiolingual cusp of a lower molar tooth in a mammal.

pro·to·cop·ro·por·phyr·ia (prō'tō-kop'rō-pōr-fir'ē-ă). Enhanced fecal excretion of proto- and coproporphyrins.

p. heredita·ria, SYN variegate *porphyria*.

Pro·toc·tis·ta (prō-tok-tis'tă). A kingdom of eukaryotes incorporating the algae and the protozoans that comprise the presumed ancestral stocks of the fungi, plant, and animal kingdoms; they lack the developmental pattern stemming from a blastula, typical of animals, the pattern of embryo development typical of plants, and development from spores as in the fungi. Included in P. are the nucleated algae and seaweeds, the flagellated water molds, slime molds, and slime nets, and the protozoa; unicellular, colonial, and multicellular organisms are included, but the complex development of tissues and organs of plants and animals is absent. The term P. replaces the term Protista, which connotes single-celled or acellular organisms, whereas the basal pre-plant (Protophyta) and pre-animal (Protozoa) assemblages incorporated in P. include many multicellular forms, since multicellularity appears to have evolved independently a number of times within these primitive groups. [G. *prōtos*, the first, + *ktizō*, to establish]

pro·to·derm (prō'tō-derm). The undifferentiated cells of very young embryos, from which the primary germ layers will evolve. [proto- + G. *derma*, skin]

pro·to·di·a·stol·ic (prō'tō-dī-ă-stol'ik). Early diastolic, relating to the beginning of cardiac diastole.

pro·to·du·o·de·num (prō'tō-doo-ō-dē'nŭm, -doo-od'ĕ-nŭm). The first part of the duodenum, which extends from the gastroduodenal pylorus as far as the major duodenal papilla and develops from the caudal foregut of the embryo; it has no plicae circulares and is the seat of the duodenal glands.

pro·to·e·ryth·ro·cyte (prō'tō-ĕ-rith'rō-sīt). A primitive erythroblast.

pro·to·fil·a·ment (prō-tō-fil'ă-ment). Basic element of a contractile flagellar microtubule, approximately 5 nm thick. [proto- + L. *filum*, a thread]

pro·to·gen, pro·to·gen A (prō'tō-jen). SYN lipoic acid.

pro·to·gon·o·plasm (prō-tō-gon'ō-plazm). A differentiated mass of cytoplasm in a protozoan, which forms the substance of later developing reproductive bodies. [proto- + G. *gonos*, seed, + *plasma*, a thing formed]

pro·to·ky·lol hy·dro·chlo·ride (prō-tō-kī'lōl). A derivative of isoproterenol with the selective β-receptor–stimulating activity of the parent compound; it is effective orally and is more stable in the body than isoproterenol; used as a bronchodilator in the treatment of bronchial asthma and status asthmaticus.

pro·to·leu·ko·cyte (prō-tō-loo'kō-sīt). A primitive leukocyte; a leukocyte of the bone marrow.

pro·tol·y·sate (prō-tol'i-sāt). Rarely used term for a protein hydrolysate.

pro·tom·er (prō'tō-mer). A structural subunit of a larger structure. P.'s may themselves consist of subunits. For example, tubulin, an αβ dimer, is the protomer for microtubules. [G. *protos*, first, + -mer 1]

pro·tom·e·rite (prō-tom'ĕ-rīt, prō'tō-mēr'īt). The second segment (lacking a nucleus) of a septate gregarine, between the epimerite and the deutomerite; it becomes the anterior end of the gamont after it has broken free of its host cell, leaving the epimerite

embedded (usually in the gut wall of an infected invertebrate). SYN primerite. [proto- + G. *meros*, part]

pro·to·me·tro·cyte (prō-tō-mē'trō-sīt). The ancestor cell of the protoleukocyte and protoerythrocyte, or of the cells of the leukocytic and erythrocytic series. [proto- + G. *mētēr*, mother, + *kytos*, cell]

pro·ton (p) (prō'ton). The positively charged unit of the nuclear mass; p.'s form part (or in hydrogen-1 the whole) of the nucleus of the atom around which the negative electrons revolve. [G. ntr. of *prōtos*, first]

pro·to·neu·ron (prō-tō-noor'on). Hypothetical primitive neuron lacking polarization. [proto- + G. *neuron*, nerve]

pro·to·nymph (prō'tō-nimf). In mites, the second instar.

pro·to·on·co·gene (prō-tō-on'kō-jēn). A gene conserved long on the evolutionary scale present in the normal human genome, that appears to have a role in normal cellular physiology and is often involved in regulation of normal cell growth or proliferation; as a result of somatic mutations, these genes may become oncogenic; products of p.-o.'s may have important roles in normal cellular differentiation.

pro·to·path·ic (prō-tō-path'ik). Denoting a supposedly primitive set or system of peripheral sensory nerve fibers conducting a low order of pain and temperature sensibility that is poorly localized. Cf. epicritic. [proto- + G. *pathos*, suffering]

pro·to·pec·tin (prō-tō-pek'tin). SEE pectin.

pro·to·pi·an·o·ma (prō'tō-pē-an-ō'mă). SYN mother *yaw*.

pro·to·plasm (prō'tō-plazm). **1.** Living matter, the substance of which animal and vegetable cells are formed. SEE ALSO cytoplasm, nucleoplasm. **2.** The total cell material, including cell organelles. Cf. cytoplasm, cytosol, hyaloplasm. SYN plasmogen. [proto- + G. *plasma*, thing formed]

totipotential p., living matter with the least recognizable differentiation of structure but with the greatest potential, all cell organs being formable by it.

pro·to·plas·mat·ic, pro·to·plas·mic (prō'tō-plaz-mat'ik, -plaz'mik). Relating to protoplasm.

pro·to·plas·mol·y·sis (prō'tō-plaz-mol'i-sis). SYN plasmolysis.

pro·to·plast (prō'tō-plast). **1.** Archaic term meaning the first individual of a type or race. **2.** A bacterial cell from which the rigid cell wall has been completely removed; the bacterium loses its characteristic form. [proto- + G. *plastos*, formed]

pro·to·por·phyr·ia (prō'tō-pōr-fir'ē-ă). Enhanced fecal excretion of protoporphyrin.

erythropoietic p. [MIM*177000], a benign disorder of porphyrin metabolism due to a deficiency of ferrochelatase associated with enhanced fecal excretion of protoporphyrin, red-purple urine, and increased protoporphyrin IX in red blood cells, plasma, and feces; characterized by acute solar urticaria or more chronic solar eczema develops quickly on exposure to sunlight; autosomal dominant inheritance.

pro·to·por·phy·rin·o·gen type III (prō-tō-pōr'fi-rin'ō-jen). The immediate precursor of protoporphyrin III in heme biosynthesis; elevated in cases of variegate porphyria.

p. t. III oxidase, a mitochondrial enzyme that uses O_2 to convert p. t. III to protoporphyrin type III in heme biosynthesis; a deficiency of this enzyme is associated with variegate porphyria.

pro·to·por·phy·rin type III (prō-tō-pōr'fi-rin). The principal protoporphyrin found in nature (one of 15 possible isomers), characterized by the presence of four methyl groups, two vinyl groups, and two propionic acid side chains; a porphyrin derivative that, with iron, forms the heme of hemoglobin and the prosthetic groups of myoglobin, catalase, cytochromes, etc.

pro·to·pro·te·ose (prō-tō-prō'tē-ōs). SEE primary *proteose*.

pro·to·salt (prō'tō-sawlt). SYN acid *salt*.

pro·to·spore (prō'tō-spōr). The initial product of progressive cleavage, in which a multinucleate spore is produced. [proto- + G. *sporos*, seed]

pro·to·sto·ma (prō'tō-stō'ma). SYN blastopore.

pro·tos·tome (prō'tō-stōm). SYN blastopore. [proto- + G. *stoma*, mouth]

pr

pro·to·sul·fate (prō-tō-sŭl′fāt). A compound of sulfuric acid with a protoxide of the metal.

pro·to·tax·ic (prō-tō-tak′sik). In interpersonal psychiatry, a term referring to the earliest form of experience characteristic of the infant that is undifferentiated, global, and unorganized. [proto- + G. *taxis*, order, arrangement]

Pro·to·the·ca (prō-tō-thē′kă). A genus of an achlorophyllous alga; two species, *P. zopfii* and *P. wickerhamii*, cause protothecosis.

pro·to·the·co·sis (prō′tō-thē-kō′sis). A rare verrucous cutaneous infection, olecranon bursitis, or disseminated disease caused by *Prototheca zopfii* and *Prototheca wickerhamii*.

pro·to·troph (prō′tō-trof, -trōf). A bacterial strain that has the same nutritional requirements as the wild-type strain from which it was derived. SEE ALSO wild-type *strain*. [proto- + G. *trophē*, nourishment]

pro·to·tro·phic (prō-tō-trof′ik). 1. Pertaining to a prototroph. 2. Denoting the ability to undertake anabolism or to obtain nourishment from a single source, as with iron, sulfur, or nitrifying bacteria or photosynthesizing plants.

pro·to·tro·phism (prō-tō-trōf-izm). The property of being prototrophic.

pro·to·type (prō′tō-tīp). The primitive form; the first form to which subsequent individuals of the class or species conform. [proto- + G. *typos*, type]

pro·to·ver·a·trine A and B (prō-tō-ver′ă-trēn). A mixture of two alkaloids isolated from *Veratrum album;* they exert their main effect upon the cardiovascular system through the carotid sinus receptors and vagal sensory endings in the heart; they cause vasodilation and are thought to bring about a redistribution to all vascular beds and thus to induce a fall in blood pressure; used in certain forms of hypertension; the maleates have the same actions.

pro·to·ver·te·bra (prō′tō-ver′tĕ-bră). 1. In the older literature, a somite. 2. More recently applied to the sclerotomal concentration that becomes the centrum of a vertebra. SYN provertebra.

pro·to·ver·te·bral (prō-tō-ver′tĕ-brăl). Relating to a protovertebra.

prot·ox·ide (prō-tok′sīd). SYN suboxide.

Pro·to·zoa (prō-tō-zō′ă). Formerly considered a phylum, now regarded as a subkingdom of the animal kingdom, including all of the so-called acellular or unicellular forms. They consist of a single functional cell unit or aggregation of nondifferentiated cells, loosely held together and not forming tissues, as distinguishes the Animalia or Metazoa, which include all other animals. P. were formerly divided into four classes: Sarcodina, Mastigophora, Sporozoa, and Ciliata; new classifications employ higher taxa (phyla, subphyla, and superclasses) and a number of major subdivisions. [proto- + G. *zōon*, animal]

pro·to·zo·al (prō-tō-zō′ăl). SYN protozoan (2).

pro·to·zo·an (prō-tō-zō′an). 1. A member of the phylum Protozoa. SYN protozoon. 2. Relating to protozoa. SYN protozoal.

pro·to·zo·i·a·sis (prō′tō-zō-ī′ă-sis). Infection with protozoans.

pro·to·zo·i·cide (prō-tō-zō′i-sīd). An agent used to kill protozoa. [protozoa + L. *caedo*, to kill]

pro·to·zo·ol·o·gist (prō′tō-zō-ol′ō-jist). A biologist who specializes in protozoology.

pro·to·zo·ol·o·gy (prō′tō-zō-ol′ō-jē). The science concerned with all aspects of the biology and human interest in protozoa. [protozoa + G. *logos*, study]

pro·to·zo·on, pl. **pro·to·zoa** (prō-tō-zō′on, -zō′ă). SYN protozoan (1).

pro·to·zo·o·phage (prō-tō-zō′ō-fāj). A phagocyte that ingests protozoa. [protozoa + G. *phagō*, to eat]

pro·trac·tion (prō-trak′shŭn). In dentistry, the extension of teeth or other maxillary or mandibular structures into a position anterior to normal. [see protractor]

    mandibular p., a type of facial anomaly in which the gnathion lies anterior to the orbital plane.

    maxillary p., a type of facial anomaly in which the subnasion lies anterior to the orbital plane.

pro·trac·tor (prō-trak′ter, -tōr). A muscle drawing a part forward, as antagonistic to a retractor; e.g., the serratus anterior muscle is a protractor of the scapula; the lateral pterygoid muscle is a protractor of the mandible. [L. *pro-traho*, pp. -*tractus,* to draw forth]

pro·trip·ty·line hy·dro·chlo·ride (prō-trip′ti-lēn). An antidepressant.

pro·trude (prō-trood′). To thrust forward or project.

pro·tru·sio ac·e·tab·u·li (prō-troo′sē-ō as-ĕ-tab′ū-lī). SYN Otto *disease.*

pro·tru·sion (prō-troo′zhŭn). 1. The state of being thrust forward or projected. 2. In dentistry, a position of the mandible forward from centric relation. [L. *protrusio*]

    bimaxillary p., the excessive forward projection of both the maxilla and the mandible in relation to the cranial base. SYN double p.

    bimaxillary dentoalveolar p., the positioning of the entire dentition forward with respect to the facial profile.

    double p., SYN bimaxillary p.

pro·tryp·sin (prō-trip′sin). SYN trypsinogen.

pro·tu·ber·ance (prō-too′ber-ans) [TA]. A swelling or knoblike outgrowth. A bulging, swelling, or protruding part. SEE ALSO protuberance. SYN protuberantia [TA]. [Mod. L. *protuberantia*]

    Bichat p., SYN buccal *fat-pad.*

    external occipital p. [TA], a prominence about the center of the outer surface of the squamous portion of the occipital bone, giving attachment to the ligamentum nuchae. SYN protuberantia occipitalis externa [TA].

    internal occipital p. [TA], a projection from about the center of the cruciform eminence on the inner surface of the occipital bone. SYN protuberantia occipitalis interna [TA].

    mental p. [TA], the prominence of the chin at the anterior part of the mandible. SYN protuberantia mentalis [TA], mental process.

pro·tu·be·ran·tia (prō-too-ber-an′shē-ă) [TA]. SYN protuberance. SEE ALSO protuberance, prominence, eminence. [Mod. L. fr. *protubero,* to swell out, fr. *tuber,* a swelling]

    p. laryn′gea, SYN laryngeal *prominence.*

    p. menta′lis [TA], SYN mental *protuberance.*

    p. occipita′lis exter′na [TA], SYN external occipital *protuberance.*

    p. occipita′lis inter′na [TA], SYN internal occipital *protuberance.*

pro·ur·o·kin·ase (prō-ūr-ō-kī′nās). The precursor of an activator of plasminogen, urokinase.

Proust, Louis J., French chemist, 1755–1826. SEE P. *law.*

Proust, T., 19th century French physician. SEE P. *space.*

pro·ver·te·bra (prō-ver′tĕ-bră). SYN protovertebra.

Pro·vi·den·cia (prov′i-den′sē-ă). A genus of motile, peritrichous, nonsporeforming, aerobic or facultatively anaerobic bacteria (family Enterobacteriaceae) containing Gram-negative rods. These organisms do not hydrolyze urea or produce hydrogen sulfide; they produce indole and grow on Simmons citrate medium. They do not decarboxylate lysine, arginine, or ornithine. These organisms occur in specimens from extraintestinal sources, particularly urinary tract infections; they have also been isolated from small outbreaks and sporadic cases of diarrheal disease. The type species is P. alcalifaciens.

    P. alcalifa′ciens, a bacterial species found in extraintestinal sources, particularly in urinary tract infections; it has also been isolated from small outbreaks and sporadic cases of diarrheal disease; it is the type species of the genus P.

    P. rettger′i, bacterial species that is found in chicken cholera and human gastroenteritis. SYN *Proteus rettgeri.*

    P. stuar′tii, a bacterial species isolated from urinary tract infections and from small outbreaks and sporadic cases of diarrheal disease.

pro·vi·rus (prō-vī′rŭs). The precursor of an animal virus, usually a retrovirus; theoretically analogous to the prophage in bacteria, the p. is integrated in the nucleus of infected cells, and can be activated in response to certain stimuli.

pro·vi·ta·min (prō-vī′tă-min). A substance that can be converted into a vitamin; e.g., β-carotene.

    p. A, trivial name for carotenoids exhibiting qualitatively the biologic activity of β-carotene, i.e., vitamin A precursors (α-, β-, and γ-carotene and cryptoxanthin); contained in fish liver oils, spinach, carrots, egg yolk, milk products, and other green leaf or yellow vegetables and fruits.

p. D₂, any substance that can give rise to ergocalciferol (vitamin D_2); e.g., ergosterol.

p. D₃, SYN 7-dehydrocholesterol.

Prowazek, Stanislas J.M. von, German protozoologist, 1876–1915. SEE *Prowazekia;* P. *bodies,* under *body;* P.-Greeff *bodies,* under *body;* Halberstaedter-P. *bodies,* under *body.*

Pro·wa·ze·kia (prō-vă-zē′kē-ă). A genus of coprozoic flagellate protozoans, formerly part of the genus *Bodo;* the organisms may be parasitic but are not, so far as is known, pathogenic. [S. *Prowazek*]

Prower. Surname of a patient in whom the Stuart-Prower *factor* was first discovered.

⌂**prox-.** SEE proximo-.

prox·em·ics (prok-sem′iks). The scientific discipline concerned with the various aspects of urban overcrowding. [L. *proximus,* nearest, next]

⌂**proxi-.** SEE proximo-.

prox·i·mad (prok′si-mad). In a direction toward a proximal part, or toward the center; not distad. [L. *proximus,* nearest, next, + *ad,* to]

prox·i·mal (prok′si-măl). **1.** Nearest the trunk or the point of origin, said of part of a limb, of an artery or a nerve, etc., so situated. Toward the median plane following the curvature of the dental arch, in contrast to distal (2). SYN proximalis. **2.** In dental anatomy, denoting the surface of a tooth in relation with its neighbor, whether mesial or distal, i.e., nearer to or farther from the anteroposterior median plane. SYN mesial [TA]. [Mod. L. *proximalis,* fr. L. *proximus,* nearest, next]

prox·i·ma·lis (prok-si-mā′lis). SYN proximal (1). [Mod. L.]

prox·i·mate (prok′si-māt). Immediate; next; proximal.

⌂**proximo-, prox-, proxi-.** Proximal. [L. *proximus,* nearest, next (to)]

prox·i·mo·a·tax·ia (prok′si-mō-ă-tak′sē-ă). Ataxia or lack of muscular coordination in the proximal portions of the extremities, i.e., arms and forearms, thighs and legs. Cf. acroataxia. [proximo- + ataxia]

prox·i·mo·buc·cal (prok′si-mō-bŭk′ăl). Relating to the proximal and buccal surfaces of a tooth; denoting the angle formed by their junction.

prox·i·mo·la·bi·al (prok′si-mō-lā′bē-ăl). Relating to the proximal and labial surfaces of a tooth; denoting the angle formed by their junction.

prox·i·mo·lin·gual (prok′si-mō-ling′gwăl). Relating to the proximal and lingual surfaces of a tooth; denoting the angle formed by their junction.

prox·y·met·a·caine hy·dro·chlo·ride (prok-si-met′ă-kān). SYN proparacaine hydrochloride.

pro·zone (prō′zōn). In the case of agglutination and of precipitation, the phenomenon in which visible reaction does not occur in mixtures of specific antigen and antibody because of antibody excess. SYN prezone.

pro·zy·go·sis (prō-zī-gō′sis). SYN syncephaly. [G. *pro,* before, + *zygōsis,* a yoking]

PrP Abbreviation for prion *protein.*

PRPP Abbreviation for 5-phospho-α-D-ribosyl-1-pyrophosphate.

PRPP syn·the·tase. An enzyme that catalyzes the reaction of α-D-ribose 5-phosphate and ATP to produce PRPP and AMP; a regulatory enzyme in purine and pyrimidine biosynthesis; enhanced activity of this enzyme results in an increase in purine biosynthesis leading to gout.

prune (proon). The dried ripe fruit of *Prunus domestica* (family Rosaceae), a tree cultivated in warm, temperate regions; a food with laxative properties.

Pru·nus (proo′nŭs). A genus of trees (family Rosaceae) including the cherry, plum, peach, and apricot trees. [L. a plum-tree]

P. seroti′na, the wild black cherry; a botanical source of wild cherry. SEE *P. virginiana.*

P. virginia′na, **(1)** wild black cherry bark, the bark of *P. serotina,* used as a tonic and in cough mixtures as a bronchial sedative; **(2)** the choke cherry; the chief substitute and adulterant of *P. serotina.*

pru·ri·go (proo-rī′gō). A chronic disease of the skin marked by a persistent eruption of papules that itch intensely. [L. itch, fr. *prurio,* to itch]

actinic p., SYN p. aestivalis.

p. aestiva′lis, p. recurring each summer, becoming very severe as long as the hot weather continues. SYN actinic p., summer p.

Besnier p., European term for p., possibly atopic.

p. gestatio′nis, a pruritic papular skin disease occurring in pregnant women, without adversely affecting pregnancy or the fetus.

Hebra p., a severe form of chronic dermatitis with secondary infection in which there are constantly recurring, intensely itchy papules and nodules, often associated with atopy.

p. mi′tis, a mild form of a chronic dermatitis characterized by recurring, intensely itching papules and nodules, probably atopic.

p. nodula′ris, an eruption of hard, dome-shaped nodules (Picker nodules) in the skin caused by rubbing and accompanied by intense itching; occasionally due to mycobacterial infection, the cause is usually unknown.

p. sim′plex, a mild form of p. having a pronounced tendency to relapse.

summer p., SYN p. aestivalis.

pru·rit·ic (proo-rit′ik). Relating to pruritus.

pru·ri·tus (proo-rī′tŭs). **1.** SYN itching. **2.** SYN itch (1). [L. an itching, fr. *prurio,* to itch]

p. aestiva′lis, p. occurring during hot weather; may be associated with prickly heat. SYN summer itch.

p. a′ni, itching of varying intensity at the anus; may be paroxysmal or constant, associated with seborrheic dermatitis or moniliasis, with irritated and enlarged hemorrhoidal veins, or may occur independently of any cutaneous lesions in association with systemic disease.

aquagenic p., intense itching produced by brief contact with water at any temperature without visible changes in the skin.

bath p., itching produced by inadequate rinsing off of soap or by overdrying of skin from excessive bathing. SYN bath itch.

essential p., itching that occurs independently of skin lesions.

p. gravidarum, severe p. without associated rash occurring during pregnancy secondary to intrahepatic cholestasis and bile salt retention.

p. hiema′lis, SYN winter *itch.*

p. seni′lis, senile p., itching associated with dryness of the skin in the aged.

symptomatic p., itching occurring as a symptom of some systemic disease.

p. vul′vae, itching of the external female genitalia, caused by a variety of factors, e.g., seborrheic dermatitis, allergy to local contactants, senile atrophy of the vulva, and occasionally systemic disease.

Prussak, Alexander, Russian otologist, 1839–1897. SEE P. *fibers,* under *fiber, pouch, space.*

Prus·sian blue [C.I. 77510]. SYN Berlin blue.

prus·si·ate (prŭsh′ē-āt, prŭs′ē-āt). **1.** A cyanide; a salt of hydrocyanic acid. **2.** A ferricyanide or ferrocyanide.

prus·sic ac·id (prŭs′ik). SYN hydrocyanic acid.

PSA Abbreviation for prostate-specific *antigen.*

psal·ter·i·al (sawl-ter′ē-ăl). Relating to the psalterium.

psal·ter·i·um, pl. **psal·ter·ia** (sawl-ter′ē-ŭm, sawl-ter′ē-ă). SYN *commissura* fornicis. [G. *psaltērion,* harp]

⌂**psammo-.** Sand. [G. *psammos*]

psam·mo·car·ci·no·ma (sam′ō-kar-si-nō′mă). Obsolete term for a carcinoma that contains calcified foci resembling psammoma bodies.

psam·mo·ma (sa-mō′mă). Obsolete term for psammomatous *meningioma* or meningioma. [psammo- + G. *-oma,* tumor]

Virchow p., SYN psammomatous *meningioma.*

psam·mo·ma·tous (sa-mō′mă-tŭs). Possessing or characterized by the presence of psammoma bodies; refers usually to certain types of meningioma or to meningeal hyperplasia with psammoma bodies.

psam·mous (sam′ŭs). Sandy. [G. *psammos,* sand]

Psaume, J., 20th century French physician. SEE Papillon-Léage and P. *syndrome.*

PSE Abbreviation for Pidgin Sign English.

psel·lism (sel′izm). SYN stammering. [G. *psellismos,* a stammering]

⊘**pseud-.** SEE pseudo-.

pseud·ac·ro·meg·a·ly (soo-dak-rō-meg′ă-lē). Enlargement of the extremities and face, not caused by acromegaly.

pseud·a·graph·ia (soo-dă-graf′ē-ă). Partial agraphia in which one can do no original writing, but can copy correctly. SYN pseudoagraphia. [pseud- + G. *a-* priv. + *graphō,* to write]

pseud·al·bu·min·u·ria (soo′dal-bū-mi-noo′rē-ă). Albuminuria that is not associated with renal disease. SYN pseudoalbuminuria.

Pseud·al·les·che·ria boy·dii (sood′al-es-kē′rē-ă boy′dē-ī). A species of fungus that causes eumycotic mycetoma and pseudallescheriasis; its conidial (asexual) state is *Scedosporium apiospermum;* formerly called *Allescheria boydii.*

pseud·al·les·che·ri·a·sis (sood′al-es-kē′ri-ă-sis). A variety of clinical diseases resulting from infection with *Pseudallescheria boydii;* e.g., bronchial colonization, and invasive pneumonitis, as well as mycotic keratitis, endophthalmitis, endocarditis, meningitis, sinusitis, brain abscesses, cutaneous and subcutaneous infections, and disseminated systemic infections.

Pseu·dam·phis·to·mum (soo-dam-fis′tō-mŭm). A genus of digenetic flukes of the family Opisthorchiidae; *P. truncatum* is a species that infects the bile ducts of the dog and cat (rarely of humans) in Europe and India. [pseud- + G. *amphi,* two-sided, + *stoma,* mouth]

pseud·an·gi·na (soo′dan-jī′nă, soo-dan′ji-nă). SYN *angina* pectoris vasomotoria.

pseud·an·ky·lo·sis (soo-dang′ki-lō′sis). SYN fibrous *ankylosis.*

pseud·ar·thro·sis (soo-dar-thrō′sis). A new, false joint arising at the site of an ununited fracture. SYN false joint, pseudoarthrosis. [pseud- + G. *arthrōsis,* a joint]

pseu·del·minth (soo-del′minth). Anything having the appearance of an intestinal worm. [pseud- + G. *helmins,* worm]

pseud·es·the·sia (soo-des-thē′zē-ă). 1. SYN paraphia. 2. A subjective sensation not arising from an external stimulus. SYN pseudoesthesia (2). 3. SYN phantom limb *pain.* [pseud- + G. *aisthēsis,* sensation]

⊘**pseudo- (psi), pseud-.** False (often used about a deceptive resemblance). [G. *pseudēs*]

pseu·do·ac·an·tho·sis ni·gri·cans (soo′dō-ak-an-thō′sis nī′gri-kanz). Acanthosis nigricans secondary to maceration of the skin from excessive sweating, or occurring in obese and dark-complexioned adults, or in association with endocrine disorders; not associated with visceral cancer.

pseu·do·a·ceph·a·lus (soo′dō-ă-sef′ă-lŭs). An apparently headless placental parasitic twin that, however, has rudimentary cephalic structures that can be demonstrated by dissection. [pseudo- + G. *a-* priv. + *kephalē,* head]

pseu·do·a·chon·dro·pla·sia (soo′dō-ă-kon-drō-plā′sē-ă). A skeletal dysplasia characterized by short-limb dwarfism with leg deformities associated with genu varum or genu valgum and ligamentous laxity, allowing the joints to telescope; normal appearing head and face. Autosomal dominant inheritance [MIM*177150 and MIM*177170] caused by mutation in the cartilage oligomeric matrix protein gene (COMP) on 19p. SYN pseudoachondroplastic spondyloepiphysial dysplasia.

pseu·do·ac·tin·o·my·co·sis (soo′dō-ak′ti-nō-mī- kō′sis). SYN para-actinomycosis.

pseu·do·ag·glu·ti·na·tion (soo′dō-ă-gloo-ti-nā′shŭn). 1. Agglomeration of particles in solution that does not involve antigen-antibody combination. SYN false agglutination. 2. SYN rouleaux *formation.*

pseu·do·a·gram·ma·tism (soo′dō-ă-gram′ă-tizm). SYN parapha-

sia. [pseudo- + G. *a-* priv. + *gramma,* writing, + *-ismos,* condition]

pseu·do·a·graph·ia (soo′dō-ă-graf′ē-ă). SYN pseudagraphia.

pseu·do·ai·nhum (soo′dō-in′ŭm). Nonspontaneous amputation of a digit, caused by a variety of disorders such as neural leprosy, syringomyelia, and palmoplantar keratoderma.

pseu·do·al·bu·mi·nu·ria (soo′dō-al-bū′mi-noo′rē-ă). SYN pseudalbuminuria.

pseu·do·al·ka·loids (soo′dō-al-kă-loydz). A group of compounds that are structurally similar to alkaloids.

pseu·do·al·lel·ic (soo′dō-ă-le′lik). Relating to pseudoallelism.

pseu·do·al·lel·ism (soo-dō-ă-lē′lizm). Relationship of two or more loci that are difficult to distinguish from a single locus by classical genetic analysis. For instance, the states of the D, D, and E components of the Rh blood locus [MIM*111700] are so far unresolved.

pseu·do·al·o·pe·cia ar·e·a·ta (soo′dō-al-ō-pē′shē-ă ar-ē-ā′tă). Alopecia in which mild inflammatory changes develop at the orifices of the affected hair follicles.

pseu·do·an·a·phy·lac·tic (soo′dō-an-ă-fī-lak′tik). SYN anaphylactoid.

pseu·do·an·a·phy·lax·is (soo′dō-an-ă-fī-lak′sis). A condition resembling anaphylaxis, but not due to specific antigen-antibody reaction. SYN anaphylactoid crisis (2).

pseu·do·a·ne·mia (soo′dō-ă-nē′mē-ă). Pallor of the skin and mucous membranes without the blood changes of anemia. SYN false anemia.

pseu·do·an·eu·rysm (soo-dō-an′ū-rizm). 1. Pulsating, encapsulated hematoma in communication with the lumen of a ruptured vessel. 2. Ventricular pseudoaneurysm, a cardiac rupture contained and loculated by pericardium, which forms its external wall. 3. An p. whose walls consist of adventitia and periarterial fibrous tissue and hematoma. SYN communicating hematoma, false aneurysm, pulsatile hematoma.

pseu·do·an·gi·na (soo′dō-an′ji-nă, -an-jī′nă). SYN *angina* pectoris vasomotoria.

pseu·do·an·o·don·tia (soo′dō-an-ō-don′shē-ă). Clinical absence of teeth due to a failure in eruption. [pseudo- + G. *an-* priv. + *odous,* tooth]

pseu·do·ap·pen·di·ci·tis (soo′dō-ă-pen-di-sī′tis). A symptom complex simulating appendicitis without inflammation of the appendix.

pseu·do·a·prax·ia (soo′dō-ă-prak′sē-ă). A condition of exaggerated awkwardness in which the person makes wrong use of objects.

pseu·do·ar·thro·sis (soo′dō-ar-thrō′sis). SYN pseudarthrosis.

pseu·do·au·then·tic·i·ty (soo′dō-aw-then-ti′si-tē). False or copied expression of thoughts and feelings. [pseudo- + G. *authentikos,* original]

pseu·do·ba·cil·lus (soo′dō-bă-sil′ŭs). Any microscopic object, such as a poikilocyte, resembling a bacillus.

pseu·do·bac·te·ri·um (soo′dō-bak-tēr′ē-ŭm). Any microscopic object resembling a small bacillary organism or other bacterial form.

pseu·do·bul·bar (soo-dō-bŭl′bar). Denoting a supranuclear paralysis of the bulbar nerves.

pseu·do·car·ti·lage (soo-dō-kar′ti-lij). SYN chondroid *tissue* (1).

pseu·do·car·ti·lag·i·nous (soo′dō-kar-ti-laj′i-nŭs). Composed of a substance resembling cartilage in texture.

pseu·do·cast (soo′dō-kast). SYN false *cast.*

pseu·do·cele (soo′dō-sēl). SYN *cavity* of septum pellucidum. [pseudo- + G. *koilia,* cavity]

pseu·do·ce·lom (soo-dō-sē′lom). A partial or false celom, typical of Nematoda (roundworms) and related phyla, in which the body cavity is lined by mesoderm along only one surface (hypodermis, under the cuticular body wall). Cf. celom, acelom. [pseudo- + G. *koilōma,* hollow]

pseu·do·ceph·a·lo·cele (soo-dō-sef′ă-lō-sēl). Acquired herniation of intracranial tissues caused by injury or disease. [pseudo- + G. *kephalē,* head, + *kēlē,* tumor]

ps

pseu·do·chan·cre (soo-dō-shang′ker). A nonspecific indurated sore, usually located on the penis, resembling a chancre.

pseu·do·cho·lin·es·ter·ase (soo′dō-kol-in-es′ter-ās). SYN butyro-cholinesterase.

atypical p. [MIM*177400, MIM*177500, MIM*177600], a genetic variant of cholinesterase that fails to catalyze the hydrolysis of succinylcholine. SEE ALSO dibucaine number, fluoride number.

typical p., a cholinesterase formed in the liver and present in plasma; it catalyzes the hydrolysis of succinylcholine, first into succinylmonocholine and choline and then into choline and succinic acid.

pseu·do·cho·rea (soo-dō-kōr-ē′ă). A spasmodic affection or extensive tic resembling chorea.

pseu·do·chro·mes·the·sia (soo′dō-krō-mes-thē′zē-ă). An anomaly in which each vowel in the printed word is seen as colored. SEE ALSO photism, color *hearing*. [pseudo- + G. *chrōma,* color, + *aisthēsis,* sensation]

pseu·do·chro·mi·dro·sis, pseu·do·chrom·hi·dro·sis (soo′dō-krō-mi-drō′sis, -hi-drō′sis). The presence of pigment on the skin in association with sweating, but due to the local action of pigment-forming bacteria and not to the excretion of colored sweat. [pseudo- + G. *chrōma,* color, + *hidrōs,* sweat]

pseu·do·chy·lous (soo-dō-kī′lŭs). Resembling chyle.

pseu·do·cir·rho·sis (soo′dō-si-rō′sis). SYN cardiac *cirrhosis.*

pseu·do·clo·nus (soo-dō-klō′nŭs). Unsustained clonic response despite continued force to elicit it.

pseu·do·co·arc·ta·tion (soo′dō-kō-ark-tā′shŭn). Distortion, often with slight narrowing, of the aortic arch at the level of insertion of the ligamentum arteriosum. SYN buckled aorta, kinked aorta.

pseu·do·col·loid (soo-dō-kol′oyd). A colloid-like or mucoid substance found in ovarian cysts and elsewhere.

pseu·do·col·lu·sion (soo′dō-co-loo′zhŭn). In psychoanalysis, a merely apparent sense of closeness emanating from a transference. [pseudo- + Fr. *collusion,* fr. L. *colludo,* to play together]

pseu·do·co·ma (soo-dō-kō′mă). SYN locked-in *syndrome.*

pseu·do·cow·pox (soo-dō-kow′poks). SYN milkers′ *nodules,* under *nodule.*

pseu·do·cox·al·gia (soo′dō-kok-sal′jē-ă). SYN Legg-Calvé-Perthes *disease.* [pseudo- + L. *coxa,* hip, + G. *algos,* pain]

pseu·do·cri·sis (soo-dō-krī′sis). A temporary fall of the temperature in a disease usually ending by crisis; not a true crisis.

pseu·do·croup (soo-dō-kroop′). SYN *laryngismus* stridulus.

pseu·do·cryp·tor·chism (soo-dō-krip′tōr-kizm). SYN retractile *testis.* [pseudo- + G. *kryptos,* hidden, + *orchis,* testis]

pseu·do·cu·mene (soo-dō-koo′mēn). A colorless liquid obtained from coal tar; used in the sterilization of catgut. SYN pseudocumol.

pseu·do·cu·mol (soo-dō-koo′mol). SYN pseudocumene.

pseu·do·cy·e·sis (soo′dō-sī-ē′sis). SYN false *pregnancy.* [pseudo- + G. *kyēsis,* pregnancy]

pseu·do·cyl·in·droid (soo-dō-sil′in-droyd). A shred of mucus or other substance in the urine resembling a renal cast.

▪ **pseu·do·cyst** (soo′dō-sist). **1.** An accumulation of fluid in a cystlike loculus, but without an epithelial or other membranous lining. SYN adventitious cyst, false cyst. **2.** A cyst whose wall is formed by a host cell and not by a parasite. **3.** A mass of 50 or more *Toxoplasma* bradyzoites, found within a host cell, frequently in the brain; formerly called a p., but now considered a true cyst enclosed in its own membrane within the host cell that may rupture to release particles that form new cysts, and apparently is infective to another vertebrate host. SEE ALSO bradyzoite. [pseudo- + G. *kystis,* bladder]

pseu·do·de·cid·u·o·sis (soo′dō-de-sid-ū-ō′sis). A decidual response of endometrium in the absence of pregnancy. [pseudo- + L. *deciduus,* falling off]

pseu·do·de·men·tia (soo′dō-dē-men′shē-ă). A condition resembling dementia but usually due to a depressive disorder rather than brain dysfunction.

pseu·do·dex·tro·car·dia (soo′dō-deks′trō-kar′dē-ă). Displace-

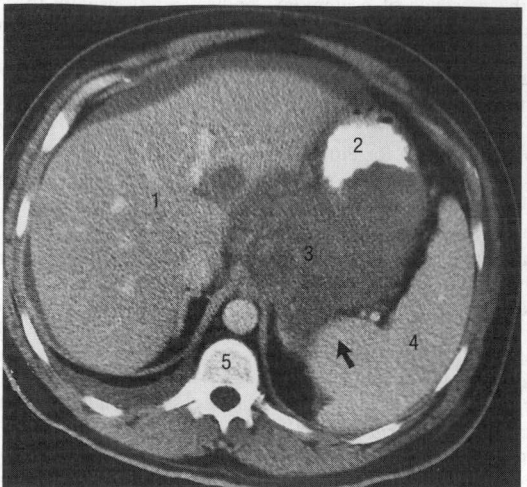

pancreatic pseudocyst: CT image shows pseudocyst compressing the posterior gastric wall (arrow); (1) liver, (2) air in stomach, (3) stomach, (4) pancreas, (5) vertebra

ment of the heart to the right, either congenital or due to trauma, with all the chambers and vessels in their correct positions.

pseu·do·di·a·be·tes (soo′dō-dī-ă-bē′tēz). A condition in which a false positive test for sugar in the urine occurs.

pseu·do·di·a·stol·ic (soo′dō-dī-as-tol′ik). Seemingly associated with cardiac diastole.

pseu·do·dig·i·tox·in (soo′dō-dij-i-tok′sin). SYN gitoxin.

pseu·do·diph·the·ria (soo′dō-dif-thēr′ē-ă). SYN diphtheroid (1).

pseu·do·dip·sia (soo-dō-dip′sē-ă). SYN false *thirst.* [pseudo- + G. *dipsa,* thirst]

pseu·do·di·ver·tic·u·lum (soo′dō-dī-ver-tik′ū-loom). An outpouching from the lumen into an area of central necrosis within a large smooth muscle tumor, along any part of the intestinal wall.

pseu·do·dom·i·nance (soo-dō-dom′ĭ-nans). SYN quasidominance.

pseu·do·dys·en·tery (soo-dō-dis′en-tār-ē). Occurrence of symptoms indistinguishable from those of bacillary dysentery, due to causes other than the presence of the specific microorganisms of bacillary dysentery.

pseu·do·e·phed·rine hy·dro·chlo·ride (soo′dō-e-fed′rin). The naturally occurring isomer of ephedrine; a sympathomimetic amine with actions and uses similar to those of ephedrine.

pseu·do·er·y·sip·e·las (soo′dō-er-i-sip′ĕ-lăs). SYN erysipeloid.

pseu·do·es·the·sia (soo-dō-es-thē′zē-ă). **1.** SYN paraphia. **2.** SYN pseudesthesia (2). **3.** SYN phantom limb *pain.*

pseu·do·ex·fo·li·a·tion (soo′dō-eks-fō-lē-ā′shŭn). A condition simulating exfoliation in some respects, but in which the surface layer is not actually detached.

p. of lens capsule, deposition in all parts of the eye, including the lens capsule, of a material derived from basement membranes. If this material clogs the trabecular meshwork, impeding the outflow of aqueous humor from the eye, glaucoma may result. SEE exfoliation *syndrome,* pseudoexfoliative *glaucoma.*

pseu·do·fluc·tu·a·tion (soo′dō-flŭk-choo-ā′shŭn). A wavelike sensation, resembling fluctuation, obtained by tapping muscular tissue.

pseu·do·fol·lic·u·li·tis (soo′dō-fo-lik-ū-lī′tis). Erythematous follicular papules or, less commonly, pustules resulting from close shaving of very curly hair; growing tips of hairs consequently reenter the skin adjacent to the follicle producing ingrown hairs; p. of the beard area is very common in blacks.

pseu·do·frac·ture (soo-dō-frak′choor). A condition in which a radiograph shows formation of new bone with thickening of periosteum at site of an injury to bone.

pseu·do·fruc·tose (soo-dō-fruk′tōs). SYN psicose.

pseu·do·gan·gli·on (soo-dō-gang′glē-on). A localized thickening of a nerve trunk having the appearance of a ganglion.

pseu·do·gene (soo′dō-jēn). **1.** A sequence of nucleotides that is not transcribed and therefore has no phenotypic effect. **2.** An inactive DNA segment that arose by a mutation of a parental active gene.

pseu·do·geu·ses·the·sia (soo′dō-gū-ses-thē′zē-ă). SYN color taste. [pseudo- + G. *geusis,* taste, + *aisthēsis,* sensation]

pseu·do·geu·sia (soo-dō-gū′sē-ă). A subjective taste sensation not produced by an external stimulus. [pseudo- + G. *geusis,* taste]

pseu·do·glan·ders (soo-dō-glan′derz). SYN melioidosis.

pseu·do·gli·o·ma (soo′dō-glī-ō′mă). Any intraocular opacity liable to be mistaken for retinoblastoma.

pseu·do·glob·u·lin (soo-dō-glob′oo-lin). The fraction of the serum globulin that is more soluble in an ammonium sulfate solution than is the euglobulin fraction.

pseu·do·glo·mer·u·lus (soo′dō-glō-mer′ū-lŭs). A structure within a neoplasm microscopically resembling a renal glomerulus but not representing renal glomerular differentiation.

pseu·do·glu·co·sa·zone (soo′dō-gloo-kō′să-zōn). A substance sometimes present in normal urine that gives a reaction in the phenylhydrazine test.

pseu·do·gout (soo′dō-gowt) [MIM*118600]. Acute episodic synovitis caused by deposits of calcium pyrophosphate crystals rather than urate crystals as in true gout; associated with articular chondrocalcinosis; the genetics is unclear. SYN calcium gout.

pseu·do·gy·ne·co·mas·tia (soo′dō-gī-ně-kō-mas′tē-ă, -jin-ě-kō-). Enlargement of the male breast by an excess of adipose tissue without any increase in breast tissue. [pseudo- + G. *gynē,* woman, + *mastos,* breast]

pseu·do·he·ma·tu·ria (soo′dō-hem-ă-too′rē-ă). A red pigmentation of urine caused by certain foods or drugs, and thus not actually hematuria. SYN false hematuria.

pseu·do·he·mop·ty·sis (soo′dō-hē-mop′ti-sis). Spitting of blood that does not come from the lungs or bronchial tubes. [pseudo- + G. haima, blood, + *ptysis,* a spitting]

pseu·do·her·maph·ro·dite (soo′dō-her-maf′rō-dīt). An individual exhibiting pseudohermaphroditism.

pseu·do·her·maph·ro·dit·ism (soo′dō-her-maf′rō-dī-tizm). A state in which the individual is of an unambiguous gonadal sex (i.e., possesses either testes or ovaries) but has ambiguous external genitalia. Cf. *steroid* 5α-reductase. SYN false hermaphroditism.
　　female p. [MIM*264270], p. with skeletal and genital anomalies but with female gonads and an XX karyotype. SYN androgynism, androgyny (1).
　　male p. [MIM*261550, MIM*264300, MIM*312100], p. in which the gonads are male and the karyotype is XY but with genital anomalies.

pseu·do·her·nia (soo-dō-her′nē-ă). Inflammation of the scrotal tissues or of an inguinal gland, simulating a strangulated hernia.

pseu·do·het·er·o·to·pia (su′dō-het-er-o-tō′pē-ă). A seeming displacement of certain tissues observed postmortem; actually an artifact, rather than a true heterotopia.

pseu·do·hy·dro·ceph·a·ly (soo′dō-hī-drō-sef′ă-lē). Condition characterized by an enlargement of the head without concomitant enlargement of the ventricular system.

pseu·do·hy·dro·ne·phro·sis (soo′dō-hī-drō-ne-frō′sis). Presence of a cyst near the kidney, simulating hydronephrosis.

pseu·do·hy·per·kal·e·mia (soo′dō-hī′per-kal-ē′ē-ă). A spurious elevation of the serum concentration of potassium occurring when potassium is released in vitro from cells in a blood sample collected for a potassium measurement. This may be a consequence of disease (i.e., myeloproliferative disorders with marked leukocytosis or thrombocytosis) or as a result of improper collection technique with in vitro hemolysis. [pseudo + G. *hyper,* above + L. *kalium,* potassium, G. *haima,* blood]

pseu·do·hy·per·par·a·thy·roid·ism (soo′dō-hī′per-par-ă-thī′roy-dizm). Hypercalcemia in a patient with a malignant neoplasm in the absence of skeletal metastases or primary hyperparathyroid-

ism; believed to be due to formation of parathyroid-like hormone by nonparathyroid tumor tissue.

pseu·do·hy·per·tel·or·ism (soo′dō-hī-per-tel′ōr-izm). An appearance of excessive distance between the eyes (ocular telorism) due to lateral displacement of the inner canthi. SEE Waardenburg *syndrome.*

pseu·do·hy·per·tro·phic (soo′dō-hī-per-trof′ik). Relating to or marked by pseudohypertrophy.

pseu·do·hy·per·tro·phy (soo′dō-hī-per′trō-fē). Increase in size of an organ or a part, due not to increase in size or number of the specific functional elements but to that of some other tissue, fatty or fibrous. SYN false hypertrophy.

pseu·do·hy·pha (soo-dō-hī′fă). A chain of easily disrupted fungal cells that is intermediate between a chain of budding cells and a true hypha, marked by constrictions rather than septa at the junctions. [pseudo- + G. *hyphē,* a web (hypha)]

pseu·do·hy·po·na·tre·mia (soo′dō-hī-pō-nă-trē′mē-ă). A low serum sodium concentration due to volume displacement by massive hyperlipidemia or hyperproteinemia; also used to describe the low serum sodium concentration that may occur with high blood glucose.

pseu·do·hy·po·par·a·thy·roid·ism (soo′dō-hī′pō-par-ă-thī′roydizm) [MIM*103580]. A disorder resembling hypoparathyroidism, with high serum phosphate and low calcium levels but with normal or elevated serum parathyroid hormone levels; the defect is due to lack of end-organ responsiveness to parathyroid hormone. There are two types: type I shows lack of renal tubular response to exogenous parathyroid hormone with increase in urinary cAMP, type Is has type I skeletal defects (SYN Albright hereditary osteodystrophy), and type II is associated with a defect at a locus after cAMP production. X-linked dominant inheritance caused by mutation in the gene encoding guanine nucleotide-binding protein α-stimulating activity polypeptide 1 (GNAS1), which regulates adenyl cyclase on chromosome 20q. Cf. thyrotropin *resistance.*
　　p. type Ia, p. believed to be due to a defect in the G protein associated with adenylate cyclase (probably autosomal dominant).
　　p. type Ib, p. due to a defect in the adenylate cyclase complex.

pseu·do·ic·ter·us (soo-dō-ik′ter-ŭs). Yellowish discoloration of the skin not due to bile pigments, as in Addison disease. SYN pseudojaundice.

pseu·do·il·e·us (soo-dō-il′ē-ŭs). Absolute obstipation, stimulating ileus, due to paralysis of the intestinal wall.

pseu·do·in·farc·tion (soo-dō-in-fark′shŭn). Any condition mimicking myocardial infarction, for example, acute pericarditis, dissecting aneurysm of the aorta, etc.

pseu·do·in·flu·en·za (soo′dō-in-floo-en′ză). An epidemic catarrh simulating influenza, but less severe.

pseu·do·in·tra·lig·a·men·tous (soo′dō-in′tră-lig-ă-men′tŭs). Falsely giving the impression of lying within the broad ligament; e.g., a p. tumor.

❚**pseu·do·i·so·chro·mat·ic** (soo′dō-ī-sō-krō-mat′ik). Apparently of the same color; denoting certain charts containing colored spots mixed with figures printed in confusion colors; used in testing for color vision deficiency.

pseu·do·iso·en·zymes (soo′dō-ī-sō-en′zīmz). Multiple forms of enzymes that catalyze the same reaction and have the same amino acid sequence; differences are due to effects of some posttranslational modification.

pseu·do·jaun·dice (soo-dō-jawn′dis). SYN pseudoicterus.

pseu·do·ker·a·tin (soo-dō-kār′ă-tin). A protein extracted from epidermis and nervous tissue (glial fibrils), probably involved in keratinization.

pseu·do·li·po·ma (soo′dō-li-pō′mă). Any circumscribed, soft, smooth, usually movable swelling or tumefaction that grossly resembles a lipoma.

pseu·do·li·thi·a·sis (soo′dō-li-thī′ă-sis). A disorder resembling one of the syndromes associated with a stone in a hollow viscus or elsewhere. [pseudo- + G. *lithos,* stone]

pseu·do·lo·gia (soo-dō-lō′jē-ă). Pathologic lying in speech or writing. [pseudo- + G. *logos,* word]

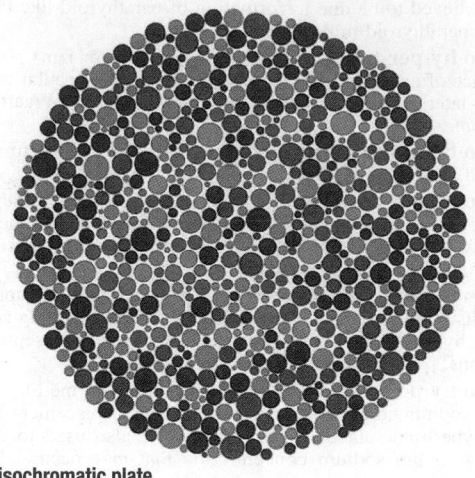

pseudoisochromatic plate

p. phantas′tica, an elaborate and often fantastic account of a patient's exploits, which are completely false but which the patient appears to believe.

pseu·do·lym·pho·cyte (soo-dō-lim′fō-sīt). A small neutrophilic leukocyte with a single round nucleus, characteristic of the rare homozygous Pelger-Huët anomaly.

pseu·do·lym·pho·ma (soo′dō-lim-fō′mă). A benign infiltration of lymphoid cells or histiocytes that microscopically resembles a malignant lymphoma.

cutaneous p., SYN benign *lymphocytoma* cutis.

pseu·do·ly·so·gen·ic (soo′dō-lī-sō-jen′ik). Pertaining to pseudolysogeny.

pseu·do·ly·sog·e·ny (soo′dō-lī-soj′ĕ-nē). The condition in which a bacteriophage is maintained (carried) in a culture of a bacterial strain by infecting susceptible variants of the strain, in contradistinction to true lysogeny in which the bacteriophage genome multiplies as an integral part of the bacterial genome.

pseu·do·ma·lig·nan·cy (soo′dō-mă-lig′nan-sē). A benign tumor that appears, clinically or histologically, to be a malignant neoplasm. SEE ALSO pseudotumor.

pseu·do·mam·ma (soo-dō-mam′ă). Obsolete term for a glandular structure resembling the mammary gland, occurring in dermoid cysts.

pseu·do·ma·nia (soo-dō-mā′nē-ă). **1.** A factitious mental disorder. **2.** A mental disorder in which the patient falsely claims to have committed a crime. **3.** Generally, the morbid impulse to falsify or lie, as in pseudologia.

pseu·do·mas·tur·ba·tion (soo′dō-mas-ter-bā′shŭn). A behavior that simulates genital stimulation.

pseu·do·meg·a·col·on. Enlargement of the distal colon with sluggish muscular function without the neurologic abnormalities of congenital megacolon (Hirschsprung *disease*).

pseu·do·mel·a·no·sis (soo′dō-mel-ă-nō′sis). A dark greenish or blackish postmortem discoloration of the surface of the abdominal viscera, resulting from the action of sulfureted hydrogen upon the iron of disintegrated hemoglobin. [pseudo- + G. *melas,* black]

pseu·do·mem·brane (soo-dō-mem′brān). SYN false *membrane.*

pseu·do·men·in·gi·tis (soo′dō-men-in-jī′tis). SYN meningism.

pseu·do·men·stru·a·tion (soo′dō-men-stroo-ā′shŭn). Uterine bleeding without the typical premenstrual endometrial changes.

pseu·do·met·a·pla·sia (soo′dō-met-ă-plā′zē-ă). SYN histologic *accommodation.*

pseu·dom·ne·sia (soo-dom-nē′zē-ă). A subjective impression of memory of events that have not occurred. [pseudo- + G. *mnēsis,* memory]

pseu·do·mo·nad (soo-dō-mō′nad). A vernacular term used to refer to any member of the genus *Pseudomonas.*

■*Pseu·do·mo·nas* (soo·dō-mō′nas). A genus of motile, polar-flag-

ellate, non–spore-forming, strictly aerobic bacteria (family Pseudomonadaceae) containing straight or curved, but not helical, Gram-negative rods that occur singly. The metabolism is respiratory, never fermentative. They occur commonly in soil and in freshwater and marine environments. Some species are plant pathogens. Others are involved in human infections. The type species is *P. aeruginosa.* [pseudo- + G. *monas,* unit, monad]

P. acido′vorans, a bacterial species found in water, soil, and occasionally in clinical specimens.

P. aerugino′sa, a bacterial species found in soil, water, and commonly in clinical specimens (wound infections, infected burn lesions, urinary tract infections); the causative agent of blue pus; occasionally pathogenic for plants; usually causes infections in humans in whom there is a defect in host defense mechanisms. It is the type species of the genus *P.* SYN blue pus bacillus.

P. cepa′cia, SYN *Burkholderia cepacia.*

P. diminu′ta, a bacterial species found primarily in clinical specimens, rarely in water.

P. fluores′cens, a bacterial species found in soil and water; it is frequently found in clinical specimens and is commonly associated with food spoilage (eggs, cured meats, fish, and milk).

P. mallei, SYN *Burkholderia mallei.*

P. maltophil′ia, species now called *Xanthomonas maltophilia.* SEE *Stenotrophomonas maltophilia.*

P. piscici′da, a bacterial species pathogenic for fish.

P. pseudoalcalig′enes, a bacterial species found in a sinus discharge.

P. pseudomal′lei, SYN *Burkholderia pseudomallei.* SYN Whitmore bacillus.

P. putrefa′ciens, former term for *Alteromonas putrefaciens.*

P. stut′zeri, a bacterial species found in soil and water, frequently in clinical specimens.

P. vesicula′ris, a bacterial species found in the medicinal leech (*Hirudo medicinalis*) and in water from a stream.

pseudomonilethrix (soo′dō-mō-nil′ĕ-thriks). A nodal trichodystrophy similar to monilethrix but with fractures within the nodal swellings; autosomal dominant inheritance with late onset.

pseu·do·mon·o·mo·lec·u·lar (soo-dō-mon-ō-mol-ek′koo-lar). SYN pseudounimolecular.

pseu·do·morph (soo′dō-mōrf). A mineral found crystallized in a form that is not proper to it but to some other mineral. [pseudo- + G. *morphē,* form]

pseu·do·my·ce·li·um (soo′dō-mī-se′lē-ŭm). A mycelium-like mass of pseudohyphae.

pseu·do·my·o·pia (soo′dō-mī-ō′pē-ă). A condition simulating myopia and due to spasm of the ciliary muscle.

pseu·do·myx·o·ma (soo′dō-mik-sō′mă). A gelatinous mass resembling a myxoma but composed of mucus.

p. peritone′i, the accumulation of large quantities of mucinous material in the peritoneal cavity, as a result of malignant cystic neoplasms of the ovary or appendix; it frequently persist because of the growth of mucus-secreting cells scattered on serosal surfaces. SYN gelatinous ascites.

pseu·do·nar·cot·ic (soo′dō-nar-kot′ik). Inducing sleep by reason of a sedative effect, but not directly narcotic.

pseu·do·ne·o·plasm (soo-dō-nē′ō-plazm). SYN pseudotumor.

pseu·do·neu·ro·ma (soo′dō-noo-rō′mă). SYN traumatic *neuroma.*

pseu·do·nit (soo′dō-nit). SYN hair *cast.*

pseu·do·os·te·o·ma·la·cia (soo′dō-os′tē-ō-mă-lā′shē-ă). Rachitic softening of bone.

pseu·do·os·te·o·ma·la·cic (soo′dō-os′tē-ō-mă-lā′sik). Marked by pseudo-osteomalacia.

pseu·do·pap·il·le·de·ma (soo′dō-pap-il-e-dē′mă). Anomalous elevation of the optic disk; seen in severe hyperopia and optic nerve drusen.

pseu·do·pa·ral·y·sis (soo′dō-pă-ral′i-sis). Apparent paralysis due to voluntary inhibition of motion because of pain, incoordination, or other cause, but without actual paralysis. SYN pseudoparesis (1).

arthritic general p., a disease, occurring in arthritic subjects, having symptoms resembling those of general paresis, the lesions of which consist of diffuse changes of a degenerative and noninflammatory character due to intracranial atheroma.

congenital atonic p., SYN *amyotonia* congenita.

pseu·do·par·a·ple·gia (soo′dō-par-ă-plē′jē-ă). Apparent paralysis in the lower extremities, in which the tendon and skin reflexes and the electrical reactions are normal; the condition is sometimes observed in rickets.

Basedow p., weakness of the thigh muscles in thyrotoxicosis; may occur suddenly and cause the patient to fall.

pseu·do·par·a·site (soo-dō-par′ă-sīt). A false parasite; may be either a commensal or a temporary parasite (the latter being an organism accidentally ingested and surviving briefly in the intestine).

pseu·do·pa·ren·chy·ma (soo′dō-pă-reng′ki-mă). In fungi, a tissue-like mass of modified hyphae.

pseu·do·pa·re·sis (soo′dō-pa-rē′sis, -par′ē-sis). **1.** SYN pseudoparalysis. **2.** A condition marked by the pupillary changes, tremors, and speech disturbances suggestive of early paretic neurosyphilis, in which, however, the serologic test results are negative.

pseu·do·pe·lade (soo′dō-pĕ-lahd′). A scarring type of alopecia; usually occurs in scattered irregular patches; of uncertain cause. SYN p. of Brocq. [pseudo- + Fr. *pelade,* disease that causes sporadic falling of hair]

p. of Brocq, SYN pseudopelade.

pseu·do·per·i·car·di·tis (soo′dō-per-i-kar-dī′tis). An artifact of auscultation resembling a friction rub, but due to movement of the tissue in the intercostal space when the diaphragm of the stethoscope is placed over the apex beat.

pseu·do·per·ox·i·dase (soo′dō-per-oks-i-dās). Referring to the nonenzymatic, heat-stable peroxidase activity associated with hemeproteins.

pseu·do·phac·os (soo′dō-fak′ōs). SYN lenticulus. [pseudo- + G. *phakos,* lens]

pseu·do·pha·kia (soo-dō-fak′ē-ă). An eye in which the natural lens is replaced with an intraocular lens. [pseudo- + *phakos,* lentil (lens)]

pseu·do·pha·ko·do·ne·sis (soo-dō-fā′kō-dō-nē′sis). Excessive mobility of an intraocular lens implant.

pseu·do·pho·tes·the·sia (soo′dō-fō-tes-thē′zē-ă). SYN photism. [pseudo- + G. *phōs,* light, + *aisthēsis,* sensation]

pseu·do·phyl·lid (soo-dō-fī′lid). Common name for members of the order Pseudophyllidea.

Pseu·do·phyl·lid·ea (soo′dō-fi-lid′ē-ă). An order of tapeworms with an aquatic life cycle, passing through coracidium, procercoid, and plerocercoid stages before developing into adults in fish, marine mammals, or fish-eating mammals; includes the broad fish tapeworm of humans, *Diphyllobothrium latum.* [pseudo- + G. *phyllon,* leaf]

pseu·do·plate·let (soo-dō-plāt′let). Any of the fragments of neutrophils that may be mistaken for platelets, especially in peripheral blood smears of leukemic patients.

pseu·do·pock·et (soo′dō-pok′et). A pocket, adjacent to a tooth, resulting from gingival hyperplasia and edema but without apical migration of the epithelial attachment.

pseu·do·pod (soo′dō-pod). SYN pseudopodium.

pseu·do·po·di·um, pl. **pseu·do·po·dia** (soo-dō-pō′dē-ŭm, -pō′dē-ă). A temporary protoplasmic process, put forth by an ameboid stage or amebic protozoan for locomotion or for prehension of food. SYN pseudopod. [pseudo- + G. *pous,* foot]

pseu·do·pol·y·dys·tro·phy (soo′dō-pol-ē-dis′trō-fē). SYN *mucolipidosis* III.

pseu·do·pol·yp (soo-dō-pol′ip). A projecting mass of granulation tissue, large numbers of which may develop in ulcerative colitis; may become covered by regenerating epithelium. SYN inflammatory polyp.

pseu·do·por·phyr·ia (soo′dō-pōr-fir′ē-ă). A condition clinically identical to porphyria but with no abnormality in porphyrin excretion, consequent to drug ingestion or hemodialysis.

pseu·do·preg·nan·cy (soo-dō-preg′nan-sē). **1.** SYN false *pregnancy.* **2.** A condition in which symptoms resembling those of

pregnancy are present, but which is not pregnancy; occurs after sterile copulation in mammalian species in which copulation induces ovulation, and also in dogs, in which the estrous cycle includes a marked luteal phase.

pseu·do·prog·na·thism (soo-dō-prog′nă-thizm). An acquired projection of the mandible due to occlusal disharmonies that force the mandible forward; the mandibular condyles are forward of their expected functional position.

pseu·do·pte·ryg·i·um (soo′dō-tĕ-rij′ē-ŭm). Adhesion of the conjunctiva to the cornea, occurring after injury.

pseu·dop·to·sis (soo-dō-tō′sis, soo-dop′tō-sis). A condition resembling an inability to elevate the eyelid, due to blepharophimosis, blepharochalasis, or some other affection. SYN false blepharoptosis. [pseudo- + G. *ptōsis,* a falling]

pseu·do·pu·ber·ty (soo′dō-pū′ber-tē). Condition characterized by the precocious development of a varying number of the somatic and functional changes typical of puberty; commonly caused by the hormonal secretions of an ovarian tumor (especially ovarian or testicular) and typically arises before the chronologic age of puberty. It does not represent the normal pubertal sequence intiated with hypothalamic-pituitary gonadotropins.

precocious p., the development of p. in very young children; commonly characterized by secretion of gonadal hormones, without stimulation of gametogenesis.

pseu·do·re·ac·tion (soo′dō-rē-ak′shŭn). A false reaction; one not due to specific causes in a given test.

pseu·do·rep·li·ca (soo-dō-rep′li-kă). A specimen for electron microscopic examination obtained by depositing particles from a virus-containing suspension on an agarose surface, covering the surface with a plastic-containing solution, and, after evaporation of the solvent, removing the film along with enmeshed particles by floating it onto the surface of a uranyl acetate solution.

pseu·do·ret·i·ni·tis pig·men·to·sa (soo′dō-ret-i-nī′tis pig-men-tō′să). A widespread pigmentary mottling of the retina that may follow severe eye trauma, especially from a penetrating injury.

pseu·do·rheu·ma·tism (soo-dō-roo′mă-tizm). **1.** Joint or muscle symptoms without objective findings and with no apparent underlying causes. **2.** Feigned joint symptoms (obsolete).

pseu·do·rick·ets (soo-dō-rik′ets). SYN renal *rickets.*

pseu·do·ro·sette (soo′dō-rō-zet′). Perivascular radial arrangement of neoplastic cells around a small blood vessel. SEE rosette (2).

pseu·do·ru·bel·la (soo′dō-roo-bel′ă). SYN *exanthema* subitum.

pseu·do·sar·co·ma (soo-dō-sar-kō′mă). A bulky polyploid malignant tumor of the esophagus, composed of spindle cells with a focus of squamous cell carcinoma; spindle cells may be epithelial or metaplastic malignant fibroblasts.

pseu·do·scar·la·ti·na (soo′dō-skar-lă-tē′nă). Erythema with fever, due to causes other than *Streptococcus pyogenes.*

pseu·do·scle·ro·sis (soo′dō-sklēr-ō′sis). Inflammatory induration or fatty or other infiltration simulating fibrous thickening. [pseudo- + G. *sklērōsis,* hardening]

pseu·do·sei·zure (soo′dō-sē′zher). A psychogenic seizure.

pseu·do·small·pox (soo-dō-smawl′poks). SYN alastrim.

pseu·dos·mia (soo-doz′mē-ă). Subjective sensation of an odor that is not present. [pseudo- + G. *osmē,* smell]

Pseu·do·ster·ta·gia bul·lo·sa (soo′dō-ster-tā′jē-ă bŭl-ō′să). One of the medium stomach worms located in the abomasum of sheep, goats, and pronghorn; it is found chiefly in the western U.S.

pseu·do·sto·ma (soo-dos′tō-mă). An apparent opening in a cell, membrane, or other tissue, due to a defect in staining or other cause. [pseudo- + G. *stoma,* mouth]

pseu·do·stra·bis·mus (soo′dō-stra-biz′mŭs). The appearance of strabismus caused by epicanthus, abnormality in interorbital distance, or corneal light reflex not corresponding to the center of the pupil. [pseudo- + G. *strabismos,* a squinting]

pseu·do·ta·bes (soo-dō-tā′bēz). A syndrome having the characteristics of tabetic neurosyphilis but not due to syphilis. SYN Leyden ataxia.

pupillotonic p., SYN Adie *syndrome.*

pseu·do·trun·cus ar·te·ri·o·sus (soo-dō-trŭng′kŭs ar-tēr-ē-ō′

sŭs). Congenital cardiovascular malformation with atresia of the pulmonic valve and absence of the main pulmonary artery; the lungs are supplied with blood either through a patent ductus or via bronchial arteries arising from the aorta; a characteristic of the most severe form of tetralogy of Fallot.

pseu·do·tu·ber·cle (soo-dō-too′ber-kl). A nodule histologically similar to a tuberculous granuloma, but due to infection by some microorganism other than *Mycobacterium tuberculosis*.

pseu·do·tu·ber·cu·lo·sis (soo′dō-too-ber′kū-lō′sis). A disease of a wide variety of animal species caused by the bacterium *Yersinia pseudotuberculosis*. Epizootics of p. are commonly seen in birds and rodents, often with high case fatality rates. In humans, seven clinical entities are recognized: primary focalized infections (pseudoappendicitis, acute mesenteric lymphadenitis, or acute terminal ileitis), primary generalized infections (septicemia or scarlatiniform fever), and secondary immunologic phenomena (erythema nodosum or arthralgia). SYN pseudotubercular yersiniosis.

pseu·do·tu·mor (soo′dō-too-mer). An enlargement of nonneoplastic character that clinically resembles a true neoplasm so closely as to often be mistaken for such. SYN pseudoneoplasm.

p. cer′ebri, a disorder, commonly associated with obesity in young females, consisting of cerebral edema with narrowed small ventricles but with increased intracranial pressure and, frequently, papilledema.

inflammatory p., a tumor-like mass in the lungs or other sites, composed of fibrous or granulation tissue infiltrated by inflammatory cells.

pseu·do·uni·mo·lec·u·lar (soo′dō-oo-nē-mō-lek-oo-lar). Referring to a reaction whose rate appears to be dependent on the concentration of only one substrate; usually due to a constant, saturating level of the other compounds. SYN pseudomonomolecular.

pseu·do·u·ri·dine (Ψ, Q) (soo-dō-ū′ri-dēn, -din). 5-β-D-Ribosyluracil; a naturally occurring isomer of uridine found in transfer ribonucleic acids; unique in that the ribosyl is attached to carbon (C-5) rather than to nitrogen; excreted in urine.

pseu·do·vac·u·ole (soo-dō-vak′ū-ōl). An apparent vacuole in a cell, either an artifact or an intracellular parasite.

pseu·do·va·ri·o·la (soo′dō-vă-rī′ō-lă). SYN alastrim. [pseudo- + L. *variola,* smallpox]

pseu·do·ven·tri·cle (soo-dō-ven′tri-kl). SYN *cavity* of septum pellucidum.

pseu·do·vi·ta·min (soo-dō-vī′tă-min). A substance having a chemical structure very similar to that of a given vitamin, but lacking the usual physiologic action.

p. B₁₂, cobamide cyanide phosphate, 3′-ester with 7-α-D-ribofuranosyladenine, inner salt; vitamin B_{12} with adenine replacing dimethylbenzimidazole; one of several substances produced during anaerobic fermentation by certain organisms in bovine rumen contents; it is chemically closely similar to vitamin B_{12} (cyanocobalamin) but without, in humans, the physiologic action of the vitamin.

pseu·do·vom·it·ing (soo-dō-vom′i-ting). Regurgitation of matter from the esophagus or stomach without expulsive effort.

pseu·do·xan·tho·ma elas·ti·cum (soo′dō-zan-thō′mă e-las′ti-kŭm) [MIM*177850, MIM*177860, MIM*264800,]. An inherited disorder of connective tissue characterized by slightly elevated yellowish plaques on the neck, axillae, abdomen, and thighs, developing in the second or third decade, associated with angioid streaks of the retina and similar elastic tissue degeneration and calcification in arteries; autosomal dominant and autosomal recessive types have been described, with much milder systemic complications in the latter.

psi (sī) 1. The 23rd letter of the Greek alphabet (ψ). 2. (ψ) Symbol for pseudouridine; pseudo-; wave function; the dihedral angle of rotation about the C_1–C_α bond associated with a peptide bond. 3. Pounds per square inch.

psi·cose (sī′kōs). A ketohexose; D-p. is epimeric with D-fructose. SYN pseudofructose, ribo-2-hexulose.

psi·lo·cin (sī′lō-sin). A hallucinogenic agent related to psilocybin.

Psil·o·cy·be (sī-lō-sī′bē). A genus of mushrooms (family Agaricaceae) containing many species with psychotropic or hallucino-

genic properties, including *P. mexicana,* of which the fruiting bodies are a source of the hallucinogen, psilocybin.

psi·lo·cy·bin (sī-lō-sī′bin, -sib′in). The *N′,N′* -dimethyl derivative of 4-hydroxytryptamine; obtained from the fruiting bodies of the fungus *Psilocybe mexicana* and other species of *Psilocybe* and *Stropharia.* P. is a congener of 5-hydroxytryptamine, with striking central nervous system effects, and is readily hydrolyzed to 4-hydroxybufotenine; used as a hallucinogenic agent (and by Mexican aborigines to induce trances). SYN indocybin.

psi·lo·sis (sī-lō′sis). Falling out of the hair. [G. *psilōsis,* a stripping, fr. *psilos,* bare]

psil·o·thin (sil′ō-thin). A depilatory plaster applied when warm to a hairy surface, and ripped off when cool, causing removal of the hairs. [see psilosis]

psi·lot·ic (sī-lot′ik). 1. Relating to psilosis. 2. SYN epilatory (1).

P-sin·is·tro·car·di·a·le (sin-is-trō-kar-dē-ā′lē). An electrocardiographic P-wave characteristic of overloading of the left atrium; often erroneously called P-mitrale, as the syndrome can result from any overloading of the left atrium from any cause.

psit·ta·cine (sit′ă-sēn). Referring to birds of the parrot family (parrots, parakeets, and budgerigars).

psit·ta·co·sis (sit-ă-kō′sis). An infectious disease in psittacine birds and humans caused by the bacterium *Chlamydia psittaci.* Avian infections are mainly inapparent or latent, although acute disease does occur; human infections may result in mild disease with a flulike syndrome or in severe disease, especially in older persons, with symptoms of bronchopneumonia. SYN Parrot disease (3), parrot fever. [G. *psittakos,* a parrot, + -*osis,* condition]

pso·as (sō′as). SEE psoas major (*muscle*), psoas minor (*muscle*). [G. *psoa,* the muscles of the loins]

pso·mo·pha·gia, pso·moph·a·gy (sō-mō-fā′jē-ă, sō-mof′ă-jē). The practice of swallowing food without thorough mastication. [G. *psōmos,* morsel, bit, + *phagō,* to eat]

psor·a·len (sōr′ă-len). A phototoxic drug used by topical or oral administration for the treatment of vitiligo and psoriasis. Also present in oil of bergamot perfume and in fruits and vegetables such as limes, which may cause photosensitization. SEE ALSO PUVA.

psor·en·ter·i·tis (sōr′en-ter-ī′tis). Inflammatory swelling of the solitary lymphatic follicles of the intestine. [G. *psōra,* itch (scabies), + *enteron,* intestine, + -*itis,* inflammation]

Psor·er·ga·tes (psō-rer′gă-tēz). A genus of itch mites (family Cheyletidae) parasitic on cattle, sheep, and goats. *P. bos* is the itch mite of cattle, described in New Mexico; *P. ovis* is the small itch mite of sheep in the U.S., Australia, New Zealand, and South Africa. [G. *psōra,* itch]

pso·ri·a·si·form (sō-rī′ă-si-fōrm). Resembling psoriasis.

pso·ri·a·sis (sō-rī′ă-sis). A common multifactorial inherited condition characterized by the eruption of circumscribed, discrete and confluent, reddish, silvery-scaled maculopapules; the lesions occur predominantly on the elbows, knees, scalp, and trunk, and microscopically show characteristic parakeratosis and elongation of rete ridges with shortening of epidermal keratinocyte transit time due to decreased cyclic guanosine monophosphate. [G. *psōriasis,* fr. *psōra,* the itch]

p. annula′ris, p. annula′ta, SYN p. circinata.

p. arthrop′ica, p. associated with severe arthritis resembling rheumatoid arthritis, although serum rheumatoid factor is absent.

p. circina′ta, p. in which healing is taking place at the center of the lesion while the process continues at the periphery, producing a ring-shaped or annular lesion. SYN p. annularis, p. annulata.

p. diffu′sa, diffused p., a form of p. with extensive coalescence of the lesions.

exfoliative p., exfoliative dermatitis developing from chronic p., sometimes resulting from overtreatment of p.

flexural p., p. involving intertriginous folds, e.g., axillary and inguinal skin, which may resemble seborrheic dermatitis.

generalized pustular p. of Zambusch, SYN pustular p. (1).

p. geograph′ica, p. gyrata in which the lesions suggest the coast outline on a map.

p. gutta′ta, p. occurring abruptly in round patches of small size; seen in young persons following streptococcal infections.

p. gyra′ta, p. circinata in which there is a coalescence of the rings giving rise to figures of various outlines.

p. nummula′ris, p. in which the lesions are discrete and discoid.

palmar p., patchy, hyperkeratotic p. affecting contact points of the volar surface of fingers and palms, alone or with mild p. elsewhere; believed to be an isomorphic response, it may affect one palm involved in a sport or occupation.

p. puncta′ta, p. in which the individual lesions are papules, each red in color and tipped with a single white scale.

pustular p., (1) an extensive exacerbation of p., with pustule formation in the normal and psoriatic skin, fever, and granulocytosis; sometimes precipitated by oral steroids; SYN generalized pustular p. of Zambusch. (2) a local pustular eruption of the palms and soles, occurring most commonly in a patient with p.; difficult to distinguish from acrodermatitis continua.

pso·ri·at·ic (sō-rē-at′ik). Relating to psoriasis.

Pso·rop·tes (sō-rop′tēz). A genus of itch or mange mites (family Cheyletidae), including the species *P. cuniculi* (the scab mite of rabbits), *P. equi* (the mange or body mite of horses), and *P. ovis* (the common scab mite of sheep and cattle). [G. *psōra,* itch]

PSP Abbreviation for phenolsulfonphthalein.

psych-. SEE psycho-.

psy·chal·ga·lia (sī-kal-gā′lē-ă). SYN psychalgia (1).

psy·chal·gia (sī-kal′jē-ă). **1.** Distress attending a mental effort, noted especially in melancholia. SYN phrenalgia (1), psychalgalia. **2.** SYN psychogenic *pain.* [psych- + G. *algos,* pain]

psy·cha·lia (sī-kā′lē-ă). A rarely used term for an emotional condition characterized by auditory and visual hallucinations.

psy·cha·nop·sia (sī′kă-nop′sē-ă). SYN mind *blindness.* [psych- + G. *an-* priv, + *opsis,* vision]

psy·cha·tax·ia (sī-kă-tak′sē-ă). Mental confusion; inability to fix one's attention or to make any continued mental effort. [psych- + G. *ataxia,* confusion]

psy·che (sī′kē). Term for the subjective aspects of the mind, self, soul; the psychologic or spiritual as distinct from the bodily nature of persons. [G. mind, soul]

psyche-. SEE psycho-.

psy·che·del·ic (sī-kĕ-del′ik). **1.** Pertaining to a rather imprecise category of drugs with mainly central nervous system action, and with effects said to be the expansion or heightening of consciousness, e.g., LSD, hashish, mescaline. **2.** A hallucinogenic substance, visual display, music, or other sensory stimulus having such action. SYN hallucinogenic. [psyche- + G. *dēloō,* to manifest]

psy·chi·at·ric (sī-kē-at′rik). Relating to psychiatry.

psy·chi·at·rics (sī-kē-at′riks). SYN psychiatry.

psy·chi·a·trist (sī-kī′ă-trist). A physician who specializes in psychiatry.

psy·chi·a·try (sī-kī′ă-trē). **1.** The medical specialty concerned with the diagnosis and treatment of mental disorders. **2.** The diagnosis and treatment of mental disorders. For some types of p. not listed below, see also subentries under therapy, psychotherapy, psychoanalysis. SYN psychiatrics. [psych- + G. *iatreia,* medical treatment]

analytic p., SYN psychoanalytic p.

biologic p., a branch of p. that emphasizes molecular, genetic, and pharmacologic approaches in the diagnosis and treatment of mental disorders.

child p., the branch of p. that deals with the emotional and mental disorders of children.

community p., p. focusing on the detection, prevention, early treatment, and rehabilitation of individuals with emotional disorders and social deviance as they develop in the community rather than as encountered one-on-one, in private practice, or at larger centralized psychiatric facilities; particular emphasis is placed on the social-interpersonal-environmental factors that contribute to mental illness.

contractual p., an older term for psychiatric intervention voluntarily assumed by the patient, who is prompted by personal difficulties or suffering and who retains control over participation with the psychiatrist.

cross-cultural p., a field of p. with interest in the study of psychologic and psychiatric phenomena as differentially expressed in the cultures of different countries.

descriptive p., that aspect of the practice of psychiatry that deals with the diagnosis of mental disorders.

dynamic p., SYN psychoanalytic p.

existential p., SYN existential *psychotherapy.*

forensic p., legal p., the application of p. in courts of law, e.g., in determinations for commitment, competency, fitness to stand trial, responsibility for crime.

industrial p., the application of the principles of p. to problems in business and industry.

orthomolecular p., an approach to p. that focuses on the use of megavitamins and nutrition in the treatment of such mental illnesses as the schizophrenic disorders.

psychoanalytic p., psychiatric theory and practice emphasizing the principles of psychoanalysis. SYN analytic p., dynamic p.

social p., an approach to psychiatric theory and practice emphasizing the cultural and sociologic aspects of mental disorder and treatment; the application of p. to social problems. SEE ALSO community p.

psy·chic (sī′kik). **1.** Relating to the phenomena of consciousness, mind, or soul. SYN psychical. **2.** A person supposedly endowed with the power of communicating with spirits; a spiritualistic medium. [G. *psychikos*]

psy·chi·cal (sī′ki-kăl). SYN psychic (1).

psy·chism (sī′kizm). The theory that a principle of life pervades all nature. [G. *psychē,* soul]

psycho-, psych-, psyche-. The mind; mental; psychologic. [G. *psychē,* soul, mind]

psy·cho·a·cous·tics (sī′kō-ă-koos′tiks). **1.** A discipline combining experimental psychology and physics that deals with the physical features of sound as related to audition, as well as with the physiology and psychology of sound recepter processes. **2.** The science pertaining to the psychologic factors that influence one's awareness of sound. [psycho- + G. *akoustikos,* relating to hearing]

psy·cho·ac·tive (sī-kō-ak′tiv). Possessing the ability to alter mood, anxiety, behavior, cognitive processes, or mental tension; usually applied to pharmacologic agents.

psy·cho·al·ler·gy (sī-kō-al′er-jē). A rarely used term for a sensitization to emotionally charged symbols.

psy·cho·a·nal·y·sis (sī′kō-ă-nal′i-sis). **1.** A method of psychotherapy, originated by Freud, designed to bring preconscious and unconscious material to consciousness primarily through the analysis of transference and resistance. SYN psychoanalytic therapy. SEE ALSO freudian p. **2.** A method of investigating the human mind and psychologic functioning, interpretations of resistances, and the patient's emotional reactions to the analyst plus use of free association and dream analysis in the psychoanalytic situation. **3.** An integrated body of observations and theories on personality development, motivation, and behavior. **4.** An institutionalized school of psychotherapy, as in jungian or freudian p. [psycho- + analysis]

active p., an older term for p. in which the analyst intervenes directly and actively in the patient's life, e.g., by making prohibitions, assigning tasks.

adlerian p., SYN individual *psychology.*

freudian p., the theory and practice of p. and psychotherapy as developed by Freud, based on: 1) his theory of personality, which postulates that psychic life is made up of instinctual and socially acquired forces, or the id, the ego, and the superego, each of which must constantly accommodate to the other; 2) his discovery that the free-association technique of verbalizing for the analyst all thoughts without censoring any of them is the therapeutic tactic that reveals the areas of conflict within a patient's personality; and 3) that the vehicle for gaining this insight and next, on this basis, readjusting one's personality is the learning a patient does in first developing a stormy emotional bond with the analyst (transference relationship) and next successfully breaking this bond.

jungian p., the theory of psychopathology and the practice of psychotherapy, according to the principles of Jung, which utilizes a system of psychology and psychotherapy emphasizing the human being's symbolic nature, and differs from freudian p. especially in placing less significance upon instinctual (sexual) urges. SYN analytical psychology.

psy·cho·an·a·lyst (sī-kō-an'ă-list). A psychotherapist, usually a psychiatrist or clinical psychologist, trained in psychoanalysis and employing its methods in the treatment of emotional disorders.

psy·cho·an·a·lyt·ic (sī'kō-an-ă-lit'ik). Pertaining to psychoanalysis.

psy·cho·au·di·to·ry (sī-kō-aw'di-tōr-ē). Relating to the mental perception and interpretation of sounds. SEE psychoacoustics. [psycho- + L. *auditorius,* relating to hearing]

psy·cho·bi·ol·o·gy (sī'kō-bī-ol'ō-jē). 1. The study of the interrelationships of the biology and psychology in cognitive functioning, including intellectual, memory, and related neurocognitive processes. 2. Adolf Meyer term for psychiatry.

psy·cho·ca·thar·sis (sī'kō-kă-thar'sis). SYN catharsis (2).

psy·cho·chrome (sī'kō-krōm). A certain color mentally conceived in response to a sense impression. SEE ALSO psychochromesthesia. [psycho- + G. *chrōma,* color]

psy·cho·chro·mes·the·sia (sī'kō-krō-mes-thē'zē-ă). A form of synesthesia in which a certain stimulus to one of the special organs of sense produces the mental image of a color. SEE ALSO photism, color *taste,* pseudogeusesthesia. [psycho- + G. *chrōma,* color, + *aisthēsis,* sensation]

psy·cho·di·ag·no·sis (sī'kō-dī-ag-nō'sis). 1. Any method used to discover the factors that underlie behavior, especially maladjusted or abnormal behavior. 2. A subspecialty within clinical psychology that emphasizes the use of psychologic tests and techniques for assessing psychopathology.

Psy·chod·i·dae (sī-kod'i-dē). A family of small flies or gnats characterized by hairy mothlike body and the presence of 7–11 long parallel wing veins lacking cross-veins; includes the sandflies, *Phlebotomus* and *Lutzomyia,* vectors of all known forms of leishmaniasis. [G. *Psychē,* a Greek nymph, sometimes represented as a butterfly]

psy·cho·dom·e·try (sī-kō-dom'ě-trē). The measurement of the rapidity of mental action. [psycho- + G. *hodos,* way, + *metron,* measure]

psy·cho·dra·ma (sī'kō-drah-mā). A method of psychotherapy in which patients act out their personal problems by spontaneously enacting without rehearsal diagnostically specific roles in dramatic performances put on before their patient peers.

psy·cho·dy·nam·ics (sī'kō-dī-nam'iks). The systematized study and theory of the psychologic forces that underlie human behavior, emphasizing the interplay between unconscious and conscious motivation and the functional significance of emotion. SEE role-playing. [psycho- + G. *dynamis,* force]

psy·cho·en·do·cri·nol·o·gy (sī'kō-en'dō-krĭ-nol'ō-jē). Study of the interrelationships between endocrine function and mental states.

psy·cho·ex·plor·a·tion (sī'kō-eks-plōr-ā'shŭn). Study of the attitudes and emotional life of a person.

psy·cho·gal·van·ic (sī'kō-gal-van'ik). Relating to changes in electric properties of the skin; e.g., a change in skin resistance induced by psychologic stimulus.

psy·cho·gal·va·nom·e·ter (sī'kō-gal-vă-nom'ě-ter). A galvanometer that records changes in skin resistance related to emotional stress.

psy·cho·gen·der (sī-kō-jen'der). The attitudes adopted by a person related to his or her identification as either a male or a female. SEE ALSO gender *role.*

psy·cho·gen·e·sis (sī-kō-jen'ě-sis). The origin and development of the psychic processes including mental, behavioral, emotional, personality, and related psychologic processes. SYN psychogeny. [psycho- + G. *genesis,* origin]

psy·cho·gen·ic, psy·cho·ge·net·ic (sī-kō-jen'ik, -jě-net'ik). 1. Of mental origin or causation. 2. Relating to emotional and related psychologic development or to psychogenesis.

psy·chog·e·ny (sī-koj'ě-nē). SYN psychogenesis.

psy·cho·geu·sic (sī-kō-goo'sik). Pertaining to the mental perception and interpretation of taste. [psycho- + G. *geusis,* taste]

psy·cho·gog·ic (sī-kō-goj'ik). Acting as a stimulant to the emotions. [psycho- + G. *agōgos,* a leading away]

psy·cho·graph·ic (sī-kō-graf'ik). Relating to psychography.

psy·chog·ra·phy (sī-kog'ră-fē). The literary characterization of an individual, real or fictional, that uses psychoanalytic and psychologic categories and theories; a psychologic biography or character description. [psycho- + G. *graphē,* a writing]

psy·cho·his·to·ry (sī-kō-his'tōr-ē). The combined use of psychology (especially psychoanalysis) and history in the writing, especially of biography, as in the work of Erik Erikson. SEE ALSO psychography.

psy·cho·ki·ne·sis, psy·cho·ki·ne·sia (sī'kō-ki-nē'sis, -nē'zē-ă). 1. The influence of mind upon matter, as the use of mental "power" to move or distort an object. 2. Impulsive behavior. [psycho- + G. *kinēsis,* movement]

psy·cho·lin·guis·tics (sī'kō-ling-gwi'stiks). Study of a host of psychological factors associated with speech, including voice, attitudes, emotions, and grammatical rules, that affect communication and understanding of language. [psycho- + L. *lingua,* tongue]

psy·cho·log·ic, psy·cho·log·i·cal (sī-kō-loj'ik, -loj'i-kăl). 1. Relating to psychology. 2. Relating to the mind and its processes. SEE psychology.

psy·chol·o·gist (sī-kol'ō-jist). A specialist in psychology licensed to practice professional psychology (e.g., clinical p.), or qualified to teach psychology as a scholarly discipline (academic p.), or whose scientific specialty is a subfield of psychology (research p.).

psy·chol·o·gy (sī-kol'ō-jē). The profession (e.g., clinical p.), scholarly discipline (academic p.), and science (research p.) concerned with the behavior of humans and animals, and related mental and physiologic processes. [psycho- + G. *logos,* study]

adlerian p., SYN individual p.

analytical p., SYN jungian *psychoanalysis.*

animal p., a branch of p. concerned with the study of the behavior and physiologic responses of animal organisms as a means of understanding human behavior; some synonyms include comparative psychology, experimental psychology, and physiologic psychology.

atomistic p., any psychologic system based on the doctrine that mental processes are built up through the combination of simple elements; e.g., psychoanalysis, behaviorism.

behavioral p., SYN behaviorism.

behavioristic p., a branch of psychology that uses behavioral approaches such as desensitization and flooding in contrast to counseling and other psychodynamic approaches to the treatment of psychologic disorders. SEE ALSO behavior *therapy.*

child p., a branch of p. the theories and applications of which focus on the cognitive and intellectual development of the child in contrast to the adult; subspecialties include developmental psychology, child clinical psychology, pediatric psychology, and pediatric neuropsychology.

clinical p., a branch of p. that specializes in both discovering new knowledge and in applying the art and science of p. to persons with emotional or behavioral disorders; subspecialties include clinical child p. and pediatric p.

cognitive p., a branch of p. that attempts to integrate into a whole the disparate knowledge from the subfields of perception, learning, memory, intelligence, and thinking.

community p., the application of p. to community programs, e.g., in the schools, correctional and welfare systems, and community mental health centers.

comparative p., a branch of p. concerned with the study and comparison of the behavior of organisms at different levels of phylogenic development to discover developmental trends.

constitutional p., the p. of the individual as related to body habitus.

counseling p., p. with emphasis on facilitating the normal development and growth of the individual in coping with important problems of everyday living, as initally contrasted with clinical p.

criminal p., the study of the mind and its workings in relation to crime. SEE forensic p.

depth p., the p. of the unconscious, especially in contrast with older (19th century) academic p. dealing only with conscious mentation; sometimes used synonymously with psychoanalysis.

developmental p., the study of the psychologic, physiologic, and behavioral changes in an organism that occur from birth to old age.

dynamic p., a psychologic approach that concerns itself with the causes of behavior.

educational p., the application of p. to education, especially to problems of teaching and learning.

environmental p., the study and application by behavioral scientists and architects of how changes in physical space and related physical stimuli impact upon the behavior of individuals. SEE ALSO personal *space.*

existential p., a theory of p., based on the philosophies of phenomenology and existentialism, which holds that the proper study of p. is a person's experience of the sequence, spatiality, and organization of his or her existence in the world.

experimental p., (1) a subdiscipline within the science of p. that is concerned with the study of conditioning, learning, perception, motivation, emotion, language, and thinking; (2) also used in relation to subject-matter areas in which experimental, in contrast to correlational or socioexperiential, methods are emphasized.

forensic p., the application of p. to legal matters in a court of law.

genetic p., a science dealing with the evolution of behavior and the relation to each other of the different types of mental activity.

gestalt p., SEE gestaltism.

health p., the aggregate of the specific educational, scientific, and professional contributions of the discipline of p. to the promotion and maintenance of health, the prevention and treatment of illness, the identification of etiologic and diagnostic correlates of health, illness, and related dysfunction, and the analysis and improvement of the health care system.

holistic p., any psychologic system that postulates that the human mind or any mental process must be studied as a unit; e.g., gestaltism, existential p.

humanistic p., an existential approach to psychology that emphasizes human uniqueness, subjectivity, and capacity for psychologic growth.

individual p., a theory of human behavior emphasizing humans' social nature, strivings for mastery, and drive to overcome, by compensation, feelings of inferiority. SYN adlerian psychoanalysis, adlerian p.

industrial p., the application of the principles of p. to problems in business and industry.

medical p., the branch of p. concerned with the application of psychologic principles to the practice of medicine; the application of clinical p. or clinical health p., usually in a hospital setting.

objective p., p. as studied by observation of the behavior and mental functions in others.

subjective p., the study of one's own mind and its various modes of action as a basis for psychologic deductions.

psy·cho·met·rics (sī-kō-met′riks). SYN psychometry.

psy·chom·e·try (sī-kom′ĕ-trē). The discipline pertaining to psychological and mental testing, and to any quantitative analysis of an individual's psychological traits or attitudes or mental processes. SYN psychometrics. [psycho- + G. *metron,* measure]

psy·cho·mo·tor (sī-kō-mō′ter). **1.** Relating to the psychologic processes associated with muscular movement and to the production of voluntary movements. **2.** Relating to the combination of psychic and motor events, including disturbances. [psycho- + L. *motor,* mover]

psy·cho·neu·ro·im·mun·o·logy (sī′kō-noo-rō-im′ū-nol′ō-jē). An area of study that focuses on emotional and other psychologic states that affect the immune system, rendering the individual less or more susceptible to disease or the course of a disease. [psycho- + neuro- + immunology]

psy·cho·neu·ro·sis (sī′kō-noo-rō′sis). **1.** A mental or behavioral disorder of mild or moderate severity. **2.** Formerly a classification of neurosis that included hysteria, psychasthenia, neurasthenia, and the anxiety and phobic disorders. [psycho- + G. *neuron,* nerve, + *-osis,* condition]

p. mai′dica, SYN pellagra.

psy·cho·neu·rot·ic (sī′kō-noo-rot′ik). Pertaining to or suffering from psychoneurosis.

psy·cho·nom·ic (sī-kō-nom′ik). Relating to psychonomy.

psy·chon·o·my (sī-kon′ō-mē). A rarely used term referring to the branch of psychology concerned with the laws of behavior. [psycho- + G. *nomos,* law]

psy·cho·no·sol·o·gy (sī′kō-nō-sol′ō-jē). The classification of mental illnesses and behavioral disorders. SYN psychiatric nosology. [psycho- + G. *nosos,* disease, + *logos,* study]

psy·cho·nox·ious (sī-kō-nok′shŭs). Rarely used term for: **1.** Having an unfavorable effect on the emotional life and reactions mediated by higher levels of the central nervous system; may be endogenous or exogenous. **2.** Denoting persons or situations that elicit fear, pain, anxiety, or anger in an individual. [psycho- + L. *noxius,* harmful]

psy·cho·on·col·o·gy (sī-kō-ong-kol′ō-jē). The psychologic aspects of the treatment and management of the patient with cancer; it combines elements of psychiatry, psychology, and medicine with special concern for the psychosocial needs of the patient and his/her family.

psy·cho·path (sī′kō-path). Former designation for an individual with an antisocial type of personality disorder. SEE ALSO antisocial *personality,* sociopath. [psycho- + G. *pathos,* disease]

psy·cho·path·ic (sī-kō-path′ik). Relating to or characteristic of psychopathy.

psy·cho·pa·thol·o·gist (sī′kō-pă-thol′ō-jist). One who specializes in psychopathology.

psy·cho·pa·thol·o·gy (sī′kō-pă-thol′ō-jē). **1.** The science concerned with the pathology of the mind and behavior. **2.** The science of mental and behavioral disorders, including psychiatry and abnormal psychology. [psycho- + G. *pathos,* disease, + *logos,* study]

psy·chop·a·thy (sī-kop′ă-thē). An older and inexact term referring to a pattern of antisocial or manipulative behavior engaged in by a psychopath. SEE ALSO personality *disorder.* [psycho- + G. *pathos,* disease]

psy·cho·phar·ma·ceu·ti·cals (sī′kō-far-mă-soo′ti-kălz). Drugs used in the treatment of emotional disorders.

---

psy·cho·phar·ma·col·o·gy (sī′kō-far′mă-kol′ō-jē). **1.** The use of drugs to treat mental and psychologic disorders. **2.** The science of drug-behavior relationships. SYN neuropsychopharmacology. [psycho- + G. *pharmakon,* drug, + *logos,* study]

> With the explosive advance of brain science since 1970 has come fuller understanding of the role that neurotransmitters play in emotion, mood, and psychologic states and of how errors in the synthesis or metabolism of these agents can cause or contribute to neurologic disease and mental illness. Using nucleotide-tagged molecules as probes, neurochemists have identified the major neural pathways and functions of many neurotransmitters, more than 60 of which are currently known. Building on this knowledge, neuropsychopharmacologists have succeeded in designing potent new psychoactive drugs. Most successful to date have been those for treating psychoses, obsessive-compulsive disorders, anxiety states, and clinical depression.

---

psy·cho·phys·i·cal (sī-kō-fiz′i-kăl). **1.** Relating to the mental perception of physical stimuli. SEE psychophysics. **2.** SYN psychosomatic.

psy·cho·phys·ics (sī-kō-fiz′iks). The science of the relation between the physical attributes of a stimulus and the measured, quantitative attributes of the mental perception of that stimulus (e.g., the relationship between changes in decibel level and the corresponding changes in the human's perception of the sound).

psy·cho·phys·i·o·log·ic (sī′kō-fiz-ē-ō-loj′ik). **1.** Pertaining to psychophysiology. **2.** Denoting a so-called psychosomatic illness. **3.** Denoting a somatic disorder with significant emotional or psychologic etiology.

psy·cho·phys·i·ol·o·gy (sī′kō-fiz-ē-ol′ō-jē). The science of the relation between psychologic and physiologic processes; e.g., elements of autonomic nervous system activity activated by emotion.

psy·cho·pro·phy·lax·is (sī′kō-prō-fi-lak′sis). Psychotherapy directed toward the prevention of emotional disorders and the maintenance of mental health. [psycho- + prophylaxis]

psy·cho·re·lax·a·tion (sī′kō-rē-lak-sā′shŭn). A method of treating anxiety and tension by practicing general bodily relaxation, as in systematic desensitization.

psy·chor·mic (sī-kōr′mik). SYN psychostimulant. [psycho- + G. *hormaō*, to set in motion]

psy·cho·sen·so·ry, psy·cho·sen·so·ri·al (sī′kō-sen′sōr-ē, -sen-sōr′ē-ăl). **1.** Denoting the mental perception and interpretation of sensory stimuli. **2.** Denoting a hallucination which by effort the mind is able to distinguish from reality.

psy·cho·sex·u·al (sī-kō-sek′shoo-ăl). Pertaining to the relationships among the emotional, mental physiologic, and behavioral components of sex or sexual development.

psy·cho·sine (sī′kō-sēn). Galactosylsphingosine, a constituent of cerebrosides, formed from UDPgalactose and sphingosine by UDPgalactose-sphingosine β-D-galactosyltransferase.

psy·cho·sis, pl. **psy·cho·ses** (sī-kō′sis, -sēz). **1.** A mental and behavioral disorder causing gross distortion or disorganization of a person's mental capacity, affective response, and capacity to recognize reality, communicate, and relate to others to the degree of interfering with the person's capacity to cope with the ordinary demands of everyday life. The psychoses are divided into two major classifications according to their origins: 1) those associated with organic brain syndromes (e.g., Korsakoff syndrome); 2) those less clearly organic and having some functional component(s) (e.g., the schizophrenias, bipolar disorder). **2.** Generic term for any of the so-called insanities, the most common forms being the schizophrenias. **3.** A severe emotional and behavioral disorder. SYN psychotic disorder. [G. an animating]

affective p., p. with predominant affective features. SYN manic p.

alcoholic psychoses, mental disorders that result from alcoholism and that involve organic brain damage, as in delirium tremens and Korsakoff syndrome.

bipolar p., a mental disorder characterized by one or more episodes of mania (manic depression) which is usually accompanied by one or more episodes of depression (major depressive episode). SEE endogenous *depression*, manic-depressive.

Cheyne-Stokes p., a mental state characterized by anxiety and restlessness, accompanying Cheyne-Stokes respiration.

psychopharmacology

antipsychotic agents

traditional (typical) low-potency agents chlorpromazine, mesoridazine, thioridazine	exert their therapeutic effect, putatively, by blocking D_2 (dopamine) receptors, but also produce an impact on a number of other receptors, causing anticholinergic side effects, sedation, and orthostatic hypotension
high-potency agents fluphenazine, haloperidol, loxapine,* molindone, perphenazine, pimozide, thiothixene, trifluoperazine	exert their therapeutic effect, putatively, by blocking D_2 (dopamine) receptors; are more likely than low-potency agents to cause neurologic side effects (e.g., extrapyramidal symptoms, acute dystonia, akisthesia, tardive dyskinesia)
atypical agents clozapine, risperidone, olanzapine, quetiapine	exert their therapeutic effect, putatively, by their generally greater blocking of $5\text{-}HT_2$ (serotonin) receptors relative to D_2 (dopamine) receptors; are less likely than typical agents to cause neurologic side effects

antidepressant agents

heterocyclic agents amitriptyline, amoxapine, clomipramine, desipramine, doxepin, imipramine, maprotiline, nortriptyline, protriptyline, trimipramine	exert their therapeutic effect, putatively, by blocking the reuptake of serotonin and/or norepinephrine, at presynaptic neurons, increasing the availability of these neurotransmitters; recent evidence suggests significant effects on postsynaptic neurons may also be responsible for the therapeutic effect
selective serotonin reuptake inhibitors citalopram, fluoxetine, fluvoxamine, paroxetine, sertraline	exert their therapeutic effect, putatively, by selectively (relative to other neurotransmitters) blocking the reuptake of serotonin
monoamine oxidase inhibitors isocarboxazid, phenelzine, tranylcypromine	exert their therapeutic effect, putatively, by irreversibly limiting the activity of monoamine oxidase, leading to an increase in the availability of norepinephrine and serotonin at the synapse
currently novel agents bupropion, mirtazepine, nefazodone, trazodone, venlafaxine	exert their therapeutic effect by a variety of actions, putatively increasing the availability of serotonin, norepinephrine, and/or dopamine at the synapse
antimanic agents lithium, carbamazepine, gabapentin,** lamotrigine,** valproic acid	exert their therapeutic effect of mood stabilization by actions that are not yet fully understood

antianxiety agents

benzodiazepines alprazolam, chlorazepate, chlordiazepoxide, clonazepam, diazepam, lorazepam, oxazepam	exert their therapeutic effect by their agonist activity at the γ-aminobutyric acid–receptor site, and in high enough dosage, this will result in excessive sedation or sleep; all have potential for habituation. Other benzodiazepines, because of their pharmacologic properties, are primarily useful as hypnotics

* also has ability to block $5\text{-}HT_2$ (serotonin receptors)
** relatively recently available anticonvulsants that have off-label efficacy in mood stabilization

depressive p., a major disorder of mood in which biologic factors are believed to play a prominent role. SEE depression.

drug p., p. following or precipitated by ingestion of a drug, e.g., LSD.

febrile p., SYN infection-exhaustion p.

functional p., an obsolete term once used to denote schizophrenia and other severe mental disorders before modern science discovered a biological component to some aspects of each of the disorders.

hysterical p., (1) a psychotic disturbance with predominantly hysterical symptoms; (2) a mental disorder resembling conversion hysteria but of psychotic severity; (3) a brief reactive p., often culture bound.

ICU p., psychotic episode(s), classically occurring in coronary care patients, occurring within 24 hours after entering the ICU in individuals with no previous history of p.; related to sleep deprivation, overstimulation in the ICU, and time spent on life support systems, and should be distinguished from exacerbation of a preexisting p. or an organic p. such as delirium.

infection-exhaustion p., an obsolete term for a p. following an acute infection, shock, or chronic intoxication; begins as delirium followed by pronounced mental confusion with hallucinations and unsystematized delusions, and sometimes stupor. SYN febrile p.

Korsakoff p., SYN Korsakoff *syndrome.*

manic p., SYN affective p; SEE bipolar *disorder*, manic-depressive *disorder*, endogenous *depression.*

manic-depressive p., SYN bipolar *disorder.*

posthypnotic p., p. following or precipitated by hypnosis.

postinfectious p., psychotic disturbance dementia following acute febrile disease such as pneumonia or typhoid fever.

postpartum p., an acute mental disorder with depression in the mother following childbirth. SYN puerperal p.

posttraumatic p., p. following trauma, especially to the head. Cf. traumatic p.

pseudo p., a condition resembling p.; may be a factitious or malingering disorder.

puerperal p., SYN postpartum p.

schizo-affective p., psychotic disturbance in which there is a mixture of schizophrenic and manic-depressive symptoms.

senile p., mental disturbance occurring in old age and related to degenerative cerebral processes.

situational p., a transitory but severe emotional disorder caused in a predisposed person by a seemingly unbearable situation.

toxic p., a p. caused by some toxic substance, whether endogenous or exogenous.

traumatic p., a p. resulting from physical injury or emotional shock. Cf. posttraumatic p.

Windigo p., Wittigo p., severe anxiety neurosis with special reference to food, manifested in melancholia, violence, and obsessive cannibalism, occurring among Canadian Indians.

psy·cho·so·cial (sī-kō-sō′shăl). Involving both psychologic and social aspects; e.g., age, education, marital and related aspects of a person's history.

psy·cho·so·mat·ic (sī′kō-sō-mat′ik). Pertaining to the influence of the mind or higher functions of the brain (e.g., emotions, fears, desires) upon the functions of the body, especially in relation to bodily disorders or disease. SEE psychophysiologic. SYN psychophysical (2). [psycho- + G. *sōma*, body]

psy·cho·so·mi·met·ic (sī-kō′sō-mi-met′ik). SYN psychotomimetic.

psy·cho·stim·u·lant (sī-kō-stim′ū-lant). An agent with antidepressant or mood-elevating properties. SYN psychormic.

psy·cho·sur·gery (sī-kō-ser′jer-ē). The treatment of mental disorders by operation upon the brain, e.g., lobotomy.

psy·cho·syn·the·sis (sī-kō-sin′thĕ-sis). Term for an older style of therapy, posited as the opposite of psychoanalysis, stressing the restoration of useful inhibitions and of the id to its rightful place in relation to the ego. [psycho- + synthesis]

psy·cho·tech·nics (sī-kō-tek′niks). An older term denoting the practical application of psychologic methods in the study of eco-

nomics, sociology, and other subjects. [psycho- + G. *technē*, art, skill]

psy·cho·ther·a·peu·tic (sī′kō-thār-ă-pū′tik). Relating to psychotherapy.

psy·cho·ther·a·peu·tics (sī′kō-thār-ă-pū′tiks). SYN psychotherapy.

psy·cho·ther·a·pist (sī-kō-thār′ă-pist). A person, usually a psychiatrist or clinical psychologist, professionally trained and engaged in psychotherapy. Currently, the term is also applied to social workers, nurses, and others whose state-licensed practice acts include psychotherapy.

psy·cho·ther·a·py (sī-kō-thār′ă-pē). Treatment of emotional, behavioral, personality, and psychiatric disorders based primarily upon verbal or nonverbal communication and interventions with the patient, in contrast to treatments utilizing chemical and physical measures. See entries under psychoanalysis; psychiatry; psychology; therapy. SYN psychotherapeutics. [psycho- + G. *therapeia*, treatment]

anaclitic p., a psychotherapeutic method characterized by encouragement and utilization of the patient's tendency to depend and lean upon the therapist as an authority figure.

autonomous p., a type of psychoanalytic p. placing special emphasis on the value of the patient's self-determination in both the therapeutic situation and in real life.

brief p., any form of psychotherapy or counseling designed to produce emotional or behavioral therapeutic change within a minimal amount of time (generally not more than 20 sessions). Brief therapy is usually active and directive; it is more clearly indicated when there are clearly defined symptoms or problems, and where the goals are limited and specific.

contractual p., p. based on a firm agreement, or "contract," between therapist and patient as to the role of each in the therapeutic situation.

directive p., p. utilizing the authority of the therapist to direct the course of the patient's therapy, as contrasted with nondirective p.

dyadic p., a psychotherapeutic session involving only two persons, the therapist and the patient. Cf. group p. SYN individual therapy.

dynamic p., SYN psychoanalytic p.

existential p., a type of therapy, based on existential philosophy, emphasizing confrontation, primarily spontaneous interaction, and feeling experiences rather than rational thinking, with less attention given to patient resistances; the therapist is involved on the same level and to the same degree as the patient. SYN existential psychiatry.

group p., a type of psychologic treatment involving several patients participating together in the presence of one or more psychotherapists who facilitate both emotional and rational cognitive interaction to effect targeted changes in the maladaptive behavior of the individual patient in his or her everyday interpersonal exchanges. See also entries under group.

heteronomous p., term embracing all forms of p. that foster the patient's dependence on others, especially dependence on the psychotherapist, in contrast to autonomous p.

hypnotic p., p. based on hypnosis.

intensive p., p. involving thorough exploration of the patient's life history, conflicts, and related psychodynamics; often contrasted with supportive p.

marathon group p., a type of group p. characterized by uninterrupted sessions for periods of hours or days, with minimal interruptions for food and rest.

nondirective p., p. in which the therapist follows the lead of the patient during the interview rather than introducing the therapist's own theories and directing the course of the interview. SEE ALSO client-centered *therapy.*

psychoanalytic p., p. utilizing freudian principles. SEE ALSO psychoanalysis. SYN dynamic p.

reconstructive p., a form of therapy, such as psychoanalysis, that seeks not only to alleviate symptoms but also to produce alterations in maladaptive character structure and to expedite new adaptive potentials; this aim is achieved by bringing into conscious-

ps

ness an awareness of and insight into conflicts, fears, inhibitions, and their manifestations.

suggestive p., an older term for p. using the influence and authority of the therapist. SEE ALSO directive p.

supportive p., p. aiming at bolstering the patient's psychologic defenses and providing reassurance, as in crisis intervention, rather than probing provocatively into the patient's conflicts.

transactional p., p. with central emphasis on the actual day-to-day interactions (transactions) between the patient and other people in the patient's life.

psy·chot·ic (sī-kot'ik). Relating to or affected by psychosis.

psy·chot·o·gen (sī-kot'ŏ-jen). A drug that produces psychotic manifestations. [psychotic + G. -gen, producing]

psy·chot·o·gen·ic (sī-kot-ō-jen'ik). Capable of inducing psychosis; particularly referring to drugs of the LSD series and similar substances.

psy·chot·o·mi·met·ic (sī-kot'ō-mi-met'ik). **1.** A drug or substance that produces psychologic and behavioral changes resembling those of psychosis; e.g., LSD. **2.** Denoting such a drug or substance. SYN psychosomimetic. [psychosis + G. *mimetikos*, imitative]

psy·cho·tro·pic (sī-kō-trop'ik). Capable of affecting the mind, emotions, and behavior; denoting drugs used in the treatment of mental illnesses. [psycho- + G. *tropē*, a turning]

△**psychro-.** Cold. SEE ALSO cryo-, crymo-. [G. *psychros*]

psy·chro·al·gia (sī-krō-al'jē-ă). A painful sensation of cold. [psychro- + G. *algos*, pain]

psy·chro·es·the·sia (sī'krō-es-thē'zē-ă). **1.** The form of sensation that perceives cold. **2.** A sensation of cold although the body is warm; a chill. [psychro- + G. *aisthēsis*, sensation]

psy·chrom·e·ter (sī-krom'ĕ-ter). A device for measuring the humidity of the atmosphere by the difference in temperature between two thermometers, the bulb of one kept moist, the other dry. Evaporation from the moist bulb lowers the reading of that thermometer; the greater the difference in readings, the drier the air; no difference indicates 100% relative humidity. SYN wet and dry bulb thermometer. [psychro- + G. *metron*, measure]

sling p., wet and dry bulb thermometers mounted on a hand sling, for use when a small portable psychrometer is required.

psy·chrom·e·try (sī-krom'ĕ-trē). The calculation of relative humidity and water vapor pressures from wet and dry bulb temperatures and barometric pressure; whereas relative humidity is the value ordinarily employed, the vapor pressure is the measurement of physiologic significance. SYN hygrometry. [psychro- + G. *metron*, measure]

psy·chro·phile, psy·chro·phil (sī'krō-fīl). An organism which grows best at a low temperature (0–32°C; 32–86°F), with optimum growth occurring at 15–20°C (59–68°F). [psychro- + G. *phileō*, to love]

psy·chro·phil·ic (sī-krō-fil'ik). Pertaining to a psychrophile. [psychro- + G. *phileō*, to love]

psy·chro·pho·bia (sī-krō-fō'bē-ă). **1.** Extreme sensitiveness to cold. **2.** A morbid dread of cold. [psychro- + G. *phobos*, fear]

psy·chro·phore (sī'krō-fōr). A double catheter through which cold water is circulated to apply cold to the urethra or another canal or cavity. [psychro- + G. *phoros*, bearing]

psyl·li·um hy·dro·phil·ic mu·cil·loid (sil'ē-ŭm). SEE *plantago* seed.

psyl·li·um seed (sil'ē-ŭm). The cleaned, dried ripe seed of *Plantago indica* or of *P. ovata*. A mild cathartic that acts by absorbing water and providing indigestible mucilaginous bulk for the intestines. Must not be used in intestinal obstruction. SYN plantago seed, plantain seed.

PT Abbreviation for physical *therapy*, physical therapist, and pro-thrombin *time*.

Pt Symbol for platinum.

PTA Abbreviation for plasma thromboplastin *antecedent*; phosphotungstic acid; percutaneous transluminal *angioplasty*.

PTAH Abbreviation for phosphotungstic acid *hematoxylin*.

ptar·mic (tar'mik). SYN sternutatory. [G. *ptarmikos*, causing to sneeze, fr. *ptarmos*, a sneezing]

ptar·mus (tar'mŭs). Sneezing. [G. *ptarmos*, a sneezing]

PTC Abbreviation for plasma thromboplastin *component*; phenyl-thiocarbamoyl.

PTCA Abbreviation for percutaneous transluminal coronary *angioplasty.*

Ptd Abbreviation for phosphatidyl.

PtdCho Abbreviation for phosphatidylcholine.

PtdEth Abbreviation for phosphatidylethanolamine.

PtdIns Abbreviation for phosphatidylinositol.

PtdIns(4,5)P$_2$. Symbol for *phosphatidylinositol* 4,5-bisphosphate.

PtdSer Abbreviation for phosphatidylserine.

PTE Abbreviation for pulmonary thromboembolism or pulmonary thromboendarterectomy.

PTEA Abbreviation for pulmonary thromboendarterectomy.

△**pter-, ptero-.** Combining form meaning wing; feather. [G. *pteron*, wing, feather]

pter·i·dine (ter'i-dēn, -din). Azinepurine; benzotetrazine; pyrazino[2,3-*d*]pyrimidine; a two-ring heterocyclic compound found as a component of pteroic acid and the pteroylglutamic acids (folic acids, pteropterin, etc.); simple p. derivatives (e.g., xanthopterin, leucopterin) occur as pigments in butterfly wings, whence the name.

pter·in (ter'in). Term loosely used for any of the compounds containing pteridine; specifically, 2-amino-4-hydroxypteridine. Some pteridines (e.g., xanthopterin, leucopterin) still retain the pterin root.

p. deaminase, an aminohydrolase catalyzing hydrolytic deamination of 2-amino-4-hydroxypteridine to form 2,4-dihydroxypteridine and ammonia.

pter·i·on (tē'rē-on) [TA]. A craniometric point in the region of the sphenoid fontanelle, at the junction of the greater wing of the sphenoid, the squamous temporal, the frontal, and the parietal bones; it intersects the course of the anterior division of the middle meningeal artery. [G. *pteron*, wing]

pte·ro·ic ac·id (tĕ-rō'ik). A constituent of folic acid, containing *p*-aminobenzoic acid and pteridine linked by a –CH$_2$– group between the amino group of the former and C-6 of the latter.

pter·op·ter·in (ter-op'ter-in). A folic acid conjugate, a principle chemically similar to folic acid except that it contains three molecules of glutamic acid instead of one, in γ linkage. SYN fermentation *Lactobacillus casei* factor, pteroyltriglutamic acid.

pter·o·yl·mon·o·glu·tam·ic ac·id (ter'ō-il-mon-ō'gloo-tam'ik). SYN folic acid (2).

pter·o·yl·tri·glu·tam·ic ac·id (ter'ō-il-trī'gloo-tam'ik). SYN pteropterin.

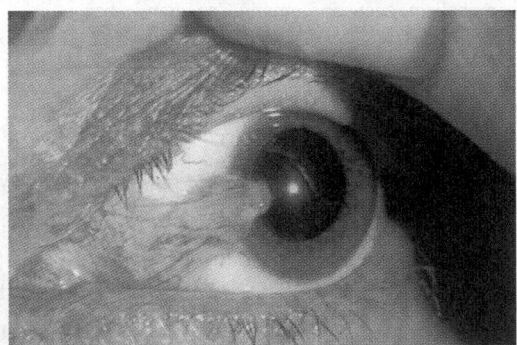

pterygium: vessels and tissue have grown from the conjunctiva over the edge of the cornea

pte·ryg·i·um (tĕ-rij'ē-ŭm). **1.** A triangular patch of hypertrophied bulbar subconjunctival tissue, extending from the medial canthus to the border of the cornea or beyond, with apex pointing toward the pupil. SYN web eye. **2.** Forward growth of the cuticle over the nail plate, seen most commonly in lichen planus. SYN p. unguis. **3.** An abnormal skin web. [G. *pterygion,* anything like a wing, a disease of the eye, dim. of *pteryx,* wing]

p. col′li, a congenital, usually bilateral, web or tight band of skin of the neck extending from the acromion to the mastoid seen in Turner's syndrome and Noonan syndrome.

p. un′guis, SYN pterygium (2).

△**pterygo-.** Wing-shaped, usually relating to the pterygoid process. [G. *pteryx, pterygos,* wing]

pter·y·goid (ter′i-goyd). Wing-shaped; resembling a wing; a term applied to various anatomical parts relating to the sphenoid bone. [G. *pteryx* (*pteryg-*), wing, + *eidos,* resemblance]

pter·y·go·man·dib·u·lar (ter′i-gō-man-dib′ū-lăr). Relating to the pterygoid process and the mandible.

pte·ry·go·max·il·la·re (ter′i-gō-mak-si-lār′ē). The point where the pterygoid process of the sphenoid bone and the pterygoid process of the maxilla begin to form the pterygomaxillary fissure; the lowest point of the opening is used in cephalometrics.

pter·y·go·max·il·lary (ter′i-gō-mak′si-lār-ē). Relating to the pterygoid process and the maxilla.

pter·y·go·pal·a·tine (ter′i-gō-pal′ă-tīn). Relating to the pterygoid process and the palatine bone.

PTF Abbreviation for plasma thromboplastin *factor.*

PTH Abbreviation for parathyroid *hormone*; phenylthiohydantoin.

PTHC Abbreviation for percutaneous transhepatic *cholangiography.*

pthi·ri·a·sis (thī-rī′a-sis). SYN *pediculosis* pubis. [G. *phtheiriasis,* fr. *phtheir,* a louse]

p. pu′bis, presence of crab lice in the pubis and other hairy areas of the trunk, and in the eyelashes of infants and young children.

🗎*Pthir·us* (thī′rŭs). A genus of lice (family Pediculidae) formerly grouped in the genus *Pediculus.* The main species is *P. pubis* (formerly *Pediculus pubis*), the crab or pubic louse, a parasite that infests the pubis and neighboring hairy parts of the body. Often incorrectly spelled *Phthirus* or *Phthirius.* [irreg. fr. G. *phtheir,* louse]

PTHrP Abbreviation for parathyroid hormone-related *peptide.*

PTK Acronym for phototherapeutic *keratectomy.*

PTMA Abbreviation for phenyltrimethylammonium.

pto·maine (tō′mān). An indefinite term applied to poisonous substances, e.g., toxic amines, formed in the decomposition of protein by the decarboxylation of amino acids by bacterial action. SYN ptomatine. [G. *ptōma,* a corpse]

pto·mai·ne·mia (tō-mā-nē′mē-ă). A condition resulting from the presence of a ptomaine in the circulating blood. [ptomaine + G. *haima,* blood]

pto·ma·tine (tō′mă-tēn). SYN ptomaine.

pto·mat·ro·pine (tō-mat′rō-pēn). A ptomaine characterized by poisonous properties similar to those of atropine; formed by the action of bacteria in the decarboxylation of amino acids.

ptosed (tōzd). SYN ptotic.

🗎**pto·sis,** pl. **pto·ses** (tō′sis, tō′sēz). **1.** A sinking down or prolapse of an organ. **2.** SYN blepharoptosis. [G. *ptōsis,* a falling]

p. adipo′sa, SYN blepharochalasis.

aponeurogenic p., drooping of the eyelid caused by dehiscence of the tendon of the levator muscle.

p. sympathet′ica, SYN Horner *syndrome.*

△**-ptosis.** A sinking down or prolapse of an organ. [G. *ptōsis,* a falling]

pto·tic (tot′ik). Relating to or marked by ptosis. SYN ptosed.

6-PTS Abbreviation for 6-pyruvoyltetrahydropterin synthase.

PTT Abbreviation for partial thromboplastin *time.*

PTU Abbreviation for propylthiouracil.

△**ptyal-, ptyalo-.** The salivary glands, saliva. SEE ALSO sialo-. [G. *ptyalon*]

pty·al·a·gogue (tī-al′ă-gog). SYN sialagogue.

pty·a·lec·ta·sis (tī′ă-lek′tă-sis). SYN sialectasis. [ptyal- + G. *ektasis,* a stretching out]

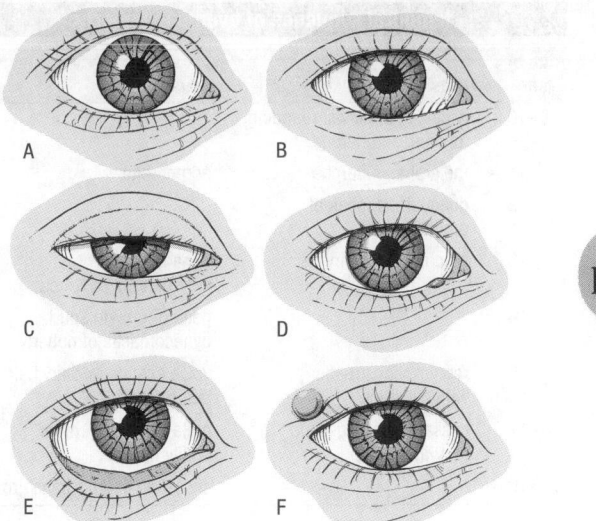

structural alterations and disorders of the eye: (A) exopthalmos, (B) entropion (C) ptosis, (D) sty, (E) ectropion, (F) chalazion

pty·a·lin (tī′ă-lin). SYN α-amylase.

pty·a·lism (tī′al-izm). SYN sialorrhea. [G. *ptyalismos,* spitting]

pty·a·lo·cele (tī′ă-lō-sēl). SYN ranula (2).

pty·a·log·ra·phy (tī-ă-log′ră-fē). SYN sialography.

pty·a·lo·lith (tī′ă-lō-lith). SYN sialolith.

pty·a·lo·li·thi·a·sis (tī′ă-lō-li-thī′ă-sis). SYN sialolithiasis.

pty·a·lo·li·thot·o·my (tī′ă-lō-li-thot′ō-mē). SYN sialolithotomy.

pty·cho·tis oil (tī-kō′tis). SYN ajowan oil.

pty·oc·ri·nous (tī-ok′ri-nŭs). Secreting by discharge of the contents of the cell, as in mucous cells. [G. *ptyō,* to spit out, + *krinō,* to separate]

Pu Symbol for plutonium.

pu·bar·che (pū-bar′kē). Onset of puberty, particularly as manifested by the appearance of pubic hair. [puberty + G. *archē,* beginning]

pu·ber·al, pu·ber·tal (pū′ber-ăl, -ber-tăl). Relating to puberty.

🗎**pu·ber·ty** (pū′ber-tē). Sequence of events by which a child becomes a young adult, characterized by the beginning of gametogenesis, secretion of gonadal hormones, development of secondary sexual characteristics and reproductive functions; sexual dimorphism is accentuated. In girls, the first signs of p. may be evident at age 8 with the process largely completed by age 16; in boys, p. commonly begins at ages 10–12 and is largely completed by age 18. Ethnic and geographic factors may influence the time at which various events typical of p. occur. [L. *pubertas,* fr. *puber,* grown up]

delayed p., lack of any signs of p. by age 14 years in either sex.

precocious p., condition in which pubertal changes begin at an unexpectedly early age. This can involve the initiation of the normal hypothalamic-pituitary axis changes before the age of 8. Idiopathic is the most common reason.

true precocious p., SYN hyperovarianism.

pu·bes (pū′bis) [TA]. **1** [NA]. SYN pubic *hair.* **2.** SYN *mons* pubis. [L. *pubes,* the hair on the genitals; the genitals]

pu·bes·cence (pū-bes′ens). **1.** The approach of the age of puberty or sexual maturity. [L. *pubesco,* to attain puberty] **2.** Presence of downy or fine, short hair. [L. *pubes,* pubic hair]

pu·bes·cent (pū-bes′ent). Pertaining to pubescence.

pu·bic (pū′bik). Relating to the os pubis.

pu·bi·ot·o·my (pū-bē-ot′ō-mē). Severance of the pubic bone a few centimeters lateral to the symphysis, in order to increase the capacity of a contracted pelvis sufficiently to permit the passage of a living child. [L. *pubis,* pubic bone, + G. *tomē,* incision]

temporal sequence of events in puberty		
age in years	girls	boys
9–10	widening of pelvis, rounding of hips, adrenarche	
11	thelarche, pubarche	adrenarche
12	gonadarche, peak of growth spurt	
13	menarche, axillary hair	gonadarche, enlargement of testes
14		peak of growth spurt, gynecomastia of puberty
15	regular menstruation, with ovulation	voice change, axillary hair, beard growth
16–17	cessation of long-bone growth	male pubic hair, more bodily hair
18–19		cessation of long-bone growth

pubis. The anteroinferior portion of the hip bone, distinct at birth but later becoming fused with the ilium and ischium; it is composed of a body that articulates with its fellow at the symphysis pubis, and two rami; the superior ramus enters into the formation of the acetabulum, and the inferior ramus fuses with the ramus of the ischium to form the ischiopubic ramus. SYN os pubis.

Pub·lic Health Ser·vice (PHS). SEE United States Public Health Service.

⌂**pubo-.** Pubic, pubes. [L. *pubes*]

pu·bo·cap·su·lar (pū′bō-kap′soo-lăr). Relating to the pubis and the capsule of the hip joint.

pu·bo·coc·cy·ge·al (pū-bō-kok-sij′ē-ăl). Relating to the pubis and the coccyx.

pu·bo·fem·o·ral (pū′bō-fem′ŏ-răl). Relating to the os pubis and the femur.

pu·bo·pros·tat·ic (pū′bō-pros-tat′ik). Relating to the pubic bone and the prostate.

pu·bo·rec·tal (pū′bō-rek′tăl). Relating to the pubic bone and the rectum.

pu·bo·ves·i·cal (pū′bō-ves′i-kăl). Relating to the pubic bone and the bladder.

Puchtler-Sweat stains. SEE Puchtler-Sweat *stain* for basement membranes, Puchtler-Sweat *stain* for hemoglobin and hemosiderin.

pu·den·da (pū-den′dă). Plural of pudendum. [L.]

pu·den·dal (pū-den′dăl). Relating to the external genitals. SYN pudic.

pu·den·dum, pl. **pu·den·da** (pū-den′dŭm, -dă) [TA]. The external genitals, especially the female genitals (vulva). Used also in the plural. [L. ntr. of *pudendus,* particip. adj. of *pudeo,* to feel ashamed]

p. femini′num, SYN vulva.

p. mulieb′re, obsolete term for vulva.

Pudenz, Robert H., U.S. neurosurgeon, *1911. SEE Heyer-P. *valve.*

pu·dic (pū′dik). SYN pudendal. [L. *pudicus,* modest]

Pud·lak, P., 20th century Czech physician. SEE Hermansky-Pudlak *syndrome.*

pu·er·pera, pl. **pu·er·per·ae** (pū-er′per-ă, -per-ē). A woman who has just given birth. [L., fr. *puer,* child, + *pario,* to bring forth]

pu·er·per·al (pū-er′per-ăl). Relating to the puerperium, or period after childbirth. SYN puerperant (1).

pu·er·per·ant (pū-er′per-ant). 1. SYN puerperal. 2. A puerpera.

pu·er·pe·ri·um, pl. **pu·er·pe·ria** (pū-er-pēr′ē-ŭm, -ē-ă). Period from the termination of labor to complete involution of the uterus,

usually defined as 42 days. [L. childbirth, fr. *puer,* child, + *pario,* to bring forth]

Puestow, Charles B., U.S. surgeon, 1902–1973. SEE P. *procedure.*

puff (pŭf). A short blowing sound heard on auscultation, usually a systolic murmur heard over the heart. SEE ALSO *chromosome* puffs.

veiled p., a faint pulmonary murmur, simulating the muffled flapping of a cloth in the wind.

puff·ball (pŭf′bal). SYN *Lycoperdon.*

Pu·lex (pū′leks). A genus of fleas (family Pulicidae, order Siphonaptera). [L. flea]

P. che′opis, former name for *Xenopsylla cheopis.*

P. fascia′tus, former name for *Nosopsyllus fasciatus.*

P. ir′ritans, the human flea, a common flea that infests humans, many domestic animals (especially swine), and wild mammals and birds; a poor vector of plague.

P. pen′etrans, incorrect name for *Tunga penetrans.*

P. serra′ticeps, former name for *Ctenocephalides canis.*

pu·lic·i·cide, pu·li·cide (pū-lis′i-sīd, pū′li-sīd). A chemical agent destructive to fleas. [L. *pulex* (*pulic-*), flea, + *caedo,* to kill]

pul·ley (pŭl′ē). SEE trochlea.

anular p., SYN anular *part* of fibrous digital sheath of digits of hand and foot.

cruciform p., SYN cruciform *part* of fibrous digital sheath.

p. of humerus, SYN *trochlea* of humerus.

muscular p., SYN muscular *trochlea.*

peroneal p., SYN fibular *trochlea* of calcaneus.

p. of talus, SYN *trochlea* of the talus.

pul·lu·la·nase (pul′yŭ-lă-nās). SYN α-dextrin endo-1,6-α-glucosidase.

pul·lu·late (pŭl′ū-lāt). To undergo pullulation.

pul·lu·la·tion (pŭl-ū-lā′shŭn). The act of sprouting, or of budding as seen in yeast. [L. *pullulo,* pp. *-atus,* to sprout forth]

pul·mo, gen. **pul·mo·nis,** pl. **pul·mo·nes** (pŭl′mō, pŭl-mō′nis, -mō′nēz) [TA]. SYN lung. [L.]

p. dex′ter, right lung.

p. sinis′ter, left lung.

⌂**pulmo-, pulmon-, pulmono-.** The lungs. SEE ALSO pneum-, pneumo-. [L. *pulmo,* lung]

pul·mo·a·or·tic (pŭl′mō-ā-ōr′tik). Relating to the pulmonary artery and the aorta.

pul·mo·lith (pŭl′mō-lith). SYN pneumolith. [L. *pulmo,* long, + G. *lithos,* stone]

pul·mo·nary (pŭl′mō-nār-ē). Relating to the lungs, to the pulmonary artery, or to the aperture leading from the right ventricle into the pulmonary artery. SYN pneumonic (1), pulmonic (1). [L. *pulmonarius,* fr. *pulmo,* lung]

pul·mo·nec·to·my (pŭl-mō-nek′tō-mē). SYN pneumonectomy. [L. *pulmo* (*pulmon-*), lung, + G. *ektomē,* excision]

pul·mon·ic (pŭl-mon′ik). 1. SYN pulmonary. 2. Obsolete term for a remedy for diseases of the lungs.

pul·mo·ni·tis (pŭl-mō-nī′tis). SYN pneumonitis.

pulp (pŭlp) [TA]. 1. A soft, moist, coherent solid. SYN pulpa [TA]. 2. SYN dental p. 3. SYN chyme. [L. *pulpa,* flesh]

coronal p., SYN crown p.

crown p. [TA], that portion of the dental p. contained within the pulp chamber or crown cavity of the tooth. SYN pulpa coronalis [TA], coronal p.

dead p., SYN necrotic p.

dental p. [TA], the soft tissue within the pulp cavity, consisting of connective tissue containing blood vessels, nerves and lymphatics, and at the periphery a layer of odontoblasts capable of internal repair of the dentin. SYN pulp (2) [TA], pulpa dentis [TA], dentinal p., tooth p.

dentinal p., SYN dental p.

digital p., SYN p. of finger.

digital p. of hand, SYN p. of finger.

enamel p., a layer of stellate cells in the enamel organ.

exposed p., p. that has been exposed or laid bare by a pathologic process, trauma, or a dental instrument.

p. of finger, the fleshy mass on the palmar aspect of the extremity of the finger. SYN digital p. of hand, digital p., pulpa digiti manus.

mummified p., a misnomer for a p. treated with a formaldehyde derivative.

necrotic p., necrosis of the dental p. that clinically does not respond to thermal stimulation; the tooth may be asymptomatic or sensitive to percussion and palpation. SYN dead p., nonvital p.

nonvital p., SYN necrotic p.

putrescent p., a decomposed p., often infected.

radicular p., SYN root p.

red p., splenic p. seen grossly as a reddish-brown substance, because of its abundance of red blood cells, consisting of splenic sinuses and the tissue intervening between them (splenic cords).

red p. of spleen [TA], bluish-red tissue that constitutes about 75% of the parenchyma of the spleen; contains a large number of venous sinuses separated by a fibrocellular reticulum rich in fibroblasts and macrophages; on section, has a corded appearance. SYN pulpa rubra splenica [TA].

root p. [TA], that part of the dental p. contained within the apical or root portion of the tooth. SYN pulpa radicularis [TA], radicular p.

splenic p. [TA], the soft cellular substance of the spleen. SYN pulpa splenica [TA], pulpa lienis.

p. of toe [TA], the fleshy mass of the plantar aspect of the distal part of the toe.

tooth p., SYN dental p.

vertebral p., SYN *nucleus* pulposus.

vital p., a p. composed of viable tissue, either normal or diseased, that responds to electric stimuli and to heat and cold.

white p., that part of the spleen that consists of nodules and other lymphatic concentrations.

white p. of spleen [TA], aggregations of β lymphocytes visible macroscopically when the fresh spleen is sectioned; they appear as white translucent dots of 1 mm or less that contrast with the surrounding matrix of red pulp. SYN pulpa alba splenica [TA].

pul·pa (pŭl′pă) [TA]. SYN pulp (1). [L. pulp]

p. alba splenica [TA], SYN white *pulp* of spleen.

p. corona′lis [TA], SYN crown *pulp*.

p. den′tis [TA], SYN dental *pulp*.

p. digiti manus, SYN *pulp* of finger.

p. lie′nis, SYN splenic *pulp*.

p. radicula′ris [TA], SYN root *pulp*.

p. rubra splenica [TA], SYN red *pulp* of spleen.

p. splen′ica [TA], SYN splenic *pulp*; SEE ALSO red *pulp*, white *pulp*.

pul·pal (pŭl′păl). Relating to the pulp.

pul·pal·gia (pŭl-pal′jē-ă). Pain arising from the dental pulp. [L. pulpa, pulp, + G. algos, pain]

pulp·ec·to·my (pŭl-pek′tō-mē). Removal of the entire pulp structure of a tooth, including the pulp tissue in the roots. [L. pulpa, pulp, + G. ektomē, excision]

pul·pi·fac·tion (pŭl-pi-fak′shŭn). Reduction to a pulpy condition. [L. pulpa, pulp, + facio, pp. factus, to make]

pulp·i·form (pŭl′pi-fōrm). Resembling pulp; pulpy.

pulp·i·fy (pŭl′pi-fī). To reduce to a pulpy state.

pulp·i·tis (pŭl-pī′tis). Inflammation of the pulp of a tooth. SYN odontitis. [L. pulpa, pulp, + G. -itis, inflammation]

hyperplastic p., hyperplastic granulation tissue growing out of the exposed pulp chamber of a grossly decayed tooth. SYN dental polyp, pulp polyp, tooth polyp.

hypertrophic p., a misnomer for hyperplastic p.

irreversible p., inflammation of the dental pulp from which the pulp is unable to recover; clinically, may be asymptomatic or characterized by pain that persists after thermal stimulation; microscopically, characterized by marked acute or chronic inflammation, sometimes with partial pulpal necrosis.

reversible p., minor inflammation from which the pulp is able to recover; characterized clinically by pain that disappears rapidly

upon removal of thermal stimulation; characterized microscopically by vasodilation, hyperemia, and edema with minimal diapedesis of leukocytes.

suppurative p., obsolete term for a purulent irreversible p.

pulp·less. 1. Without a pulp. **2.** Denoting a tooth in which the pulp has died or from which the pulp has been removed. **3.** Denoting a tooth that gives no response to an electric pulp test or thermal test.

pulp·o·don·tia (pŭl-pō-don′shē-ă). The science of root canal therapy. SEE ALSO endodontics. [L. pulpa, pulp, + G. odous, tooth]

pul·po·sus (pŭl-pō′sŭs). SYN pulpy. [L.]

pulp·ot·o·my (pŭl-pot′ō-mē). Removal of a portion of the pulp structure of a tooth, usually the coronal portion. SYN pulp amputation. [L. pulpa, pulp, + G. tomē, incision]

pulpy (pŭl′pē). In the condition of a soft, moist solid. SYN pulposus.

pul·sate (pŭl′sāt). To throb or beat rhythmically; said of the heart or an artery. [L. pulso, pp. -atus, to beat]

pul·sa·tile (pŭl′să-til). Throbbing or beating.

pul·sa·tion (pŭl-sā′shŭn). A throbbing or rhythmic beating, as of a pulse or the heart. [L. pulsatio, a beating]

balloon counter p., a form of circulatory assistance in which a balloon inflates in the aorta during diastole to improve diastolic pressure and deflates during systole to reduce left ventricular afterload. Cf. intraaortic balloon *pump*.

suprasternal p., any p. in the suprasternal notch at the anterior route of the neck.

pul·sa·tor (pŭl-sā′ter, -tōr). A machine or device that operates in a throbbing, vibrating, or rhythmic manner.

🔲 **pulse** (pŭls). Rhythmic dilation of an artery, produced by the increased volume of blood thrown into the vessel by the contraction of the heart. A p. may also at times occur in a vein or a vascular organ, such as the liver. SYN pulsus. [L. pulsus]

abdominal p., the soft, compressible aortic p. occurring in certain abdominal disorders. SYN pulsus abdominalis.

alternating p., mechanical alternation; a pulse regular in time but with alternate beats stronger and weaker, often detectable only with the sphygmomanometer or other pressure measurement and usually indicating serious myocardial disease. SYN pulsus alternans.

anacrotic p., anadicrotic p., a p. wave showing one or more notches or indentations on its rising limb that are sometimes detectable by palpation. SYN pulsus anadicrotus.

bigeminal p., a p. in which the beats occur in pairs. SYN bigemina, coupled p., pulsus bigeminus.

bisferious p. (bis-fer′ē-ŭs), an arterial p. with peaks that may be palpable. SYN pulsus bisferiens.

bulbar p., a jugular p. supposed to indicate tricuspid insufficiency.

cannonball p., SYN water-hammer p.

capillary p., the alternate rhythmic blanching and reddening of a capillary area, as seen under the nails or in the lip, upon gentle compression; a sign of arteriolar dilation, well seen in aortic insufficiency. SEE ALSO Quincke p.

carotid p., the p. of the carotid arteries in the neck.

catacrotic p., a p. in which there is an upward notch interrupting the descending limb of the sphygmogram. SYN pulsus catacrotus.

catadicrotic p., a catacrotic p. in which there are two interrupting upward notches. SYN pulsus catadicrotus.

collapsing p., SYN water-hammer p.

cordy p., SYN tense p.

Corrigan p., SYN Corrigan *sign*.

coupled p., SYN bigeminal p.

dicrotic p., a p. that is marked by a double beat, the second, due to a palpable dicrotic wave, being weaker than the first. SYN pulsus duplex.

entoptic p., an intermittent phose synchronous with the p.

filiform p., a thready p.

gaseous p., a soft, full, but feeble p.

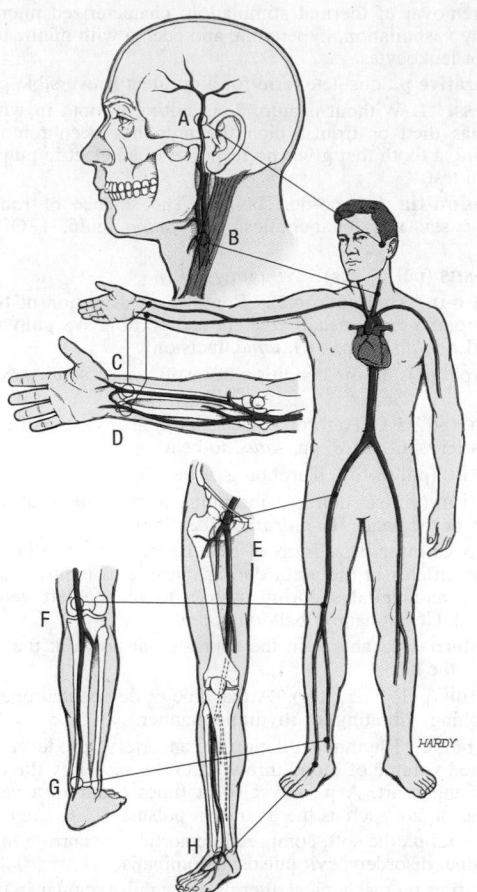

peripheral pulses: (A) temporal, (B) carotid, (C) radial, (D) ulnar, (E) femoral, (F) popliteal, (G) posterior tibial, (H) dorsalis pedis

guttural p., a pulsation felt in the throat.

hard p., a p. that strikes forcibly against the tip of the finger and is with difficulty compressed, suggesting hypertension. SYN pulsus durus.

intermittent p., irregularity of the heart due to extrasystoles that are too weak to open the semilunar valves; often owing to the long pause following the premature beat, extra long pauses equal to two regular cycles occur from time to time between p. beats. SYN pulsus intercidens.

irregular p., variation in rate of impulses in an artery due to cardiac arrhythmia.

jugular p., the venous p. as observed in the jugular veins of the neck, usually the deep jugular veins.

labile p., frequent changes in p. rate.

long p., a p. in which the impact is felt longer than usual. SYN sustained p.

monocrotic p., a p. without any perceptible dicrotism. SYN pulsus monocrotus.

mousetail p., SYN *pulsus* myurus.

movable p., the lateral movement of a strongly pulsating tortuous artery.

nail p., a capillary p. seen through the nail.

paradoxic p., an exaggeration of the normal variation in the systemic arterial p. volume with respiration, becoming weaker with inspiration and stronger with expiration; characteristic of cardiac tamponade, rare in constrictive pericarditis; so called because these changes are independent of changes in the cardiac rate as measured directly or by electrocardiogram. SYN pulsus paradoxus, pulsus respiratione intermittens.

piston p., SYN water-hammer p.

plateau p., a slow, sustained p.

quadrigeminal p., a p. in which the beats are grouped in fours, a pause following every fourth beat. SYN pulsus quadrigeminus.

Quincke p., the capillary p. as appreciated in the finger nails and toenails during aortic regurgitation; ebb and flow is seen. SYN Quincke sign.

radial p., the p. as appreciated at the radial artery usually in the wrist.

radiofrequency p., in nuclear magnetic resonance, a short electromagnetic signal used to change the direction of the magnetic field. SEE sequence p.

respiratory p., waxing and waning of any pulsation produced by respiration.

reversed paradoxical p., a p. in which the amplitude increases with inspiration and decreases with expiration, as observed in some cases of tricuspid insufficiency and of AV dissociation with sinus arrhythmia. SYN Riegel p.

Riegel p., SYN reversed paradoxical p.

sequence p., in magnetic resonance imaging, the series of radiofrequency signals used to shift the magnetic field to change proton orientation.

soft p., a p. that is readily extinguished by pressure with the finger.

sustained p., SYN long p.

tense p., a hard, full p. but without very wide excursions, resembling the vibration of a thick cord. SYN pulsus cordy p.

thready p., a small fine p., feeling like a small cord or thread under the finger. SYN pulsus filiformis.

trigeminal p., a p. in which the beats occur in trios, a pause following every third beat. SYN pulsus trigeminus.

triphammer p., SYN water-hammer p.

undulating p., a toneless p. in which there is a succession of waves without character or force. SYN pulsus fluens.

unequal p., differing strength of p. in the same artery between the right and left of the circulation.

vagus p., a slow p. due to the inhibitory action of the vagus nerve on the heart.

venous p., a pulsation occurring in the veins, especially the internal jugular vein. SYN pulsus venosus.

vermicular p., a small rapid p., giving a wormlike sensation to the finger.

water-hammer p., a p. with forcible impulse but immediate collapse, characteristic of aortic incompetency. SEE ALSO Corrigan *sign.* SYN cannonball p., collapsing p., piston p., pulsus celerrimus, triphammer p.

wiry p., a small, fine, incompressible p.

pul·sel·lum (pŭl-sel′ŭm). A posterior flagellum constituting the organ of locomotion in certain protozoa. [Mod. L. dim. of L. *pulsus,* a stroking]

pul·sim·e·ter, pul·som·e·ter (pŭl-sim′ĕ-ter, -som′ĕ-ter). An instrument for measuring the force and rapidity of the pulse. [L. *pulsus,* pulse, + *metron,* measure]

pul·sion (pŭl′shŭn). A pushing outward or swelling. [L. *pulsio*]

pul·sus (pŭl′sŭs). SYN pulse. [L. a stroke, pulse]

 p. abdomina′lis, SYN abdominal *pulse.*

 p. alter′nans, SYN alternating *pulse.*

 p. anadic′rotus, SYN anacrotic *pulse.*

 p. bigem′inus, SYN bigeminal *pulse.*

 p. bisfer′iens, SYN bisferious *pulse.*

 p. cap′risans, a bounding leaping pulse, irregular in both force and rhythm.

 p. catac′rotus, SYN catacrotic *pulse.*

 p. catadic′rotus, SYN catadicrotic *pulse.*

 p. cel′er, a pulse beat swift to rise and fall.

 p. celer′rimus, SYN water-hammer *pulse.*

 p. cor′dis, the apex beat of the heart.

 p. deb′ilis, a weak pulse.

 p. dif′ferens, a condition in which the pulses in the two radial or other corresponding arteries differ in strength. SYN p. incongruens.

 p. du′plex, SYN dicrotic *pulse.*

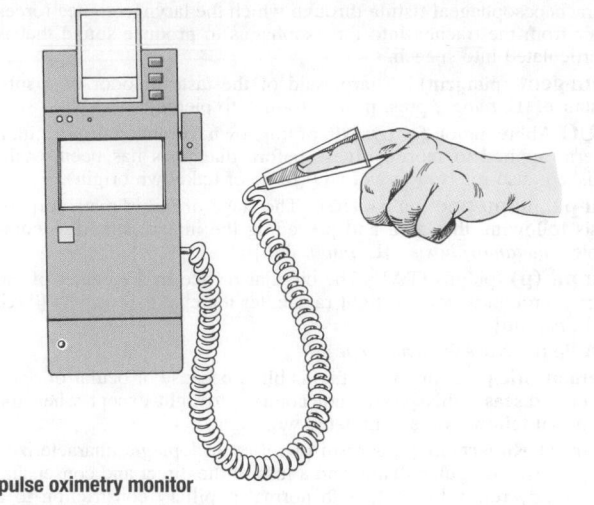

pulse oximetry monitor

p. du'rus, SYN hard *pulse.*

p. filifor'mis, SYN thready *pulse.*

p. flu'ens, SYN undulating *pulse.*

p. for'micans, a very small, nearly imperceptible pulse, the impression it gives to the finger being compared to formication.

p. for'tis, a full strong pulse.

p. fre'quens, a rapid pulse.

p. heterochron'icus, an arrhythmic pulse.

p. inaequa'lis, a pulse irregular in rhythm and force.

p. incon'gruens, SYN p. differens.

p. infre'quens, a slow pulse.

p. inter'cidens, SYN intermittent *pulse.*

p. intercur'rens, an occasional strong dicrotic pulse wave giving the impression of an intercurrent ventricular contraction.

p. irregula'ris perpet'uus, permanently irregular pulse often caused by, or characteristic of, atrial fibrillation; it may also be produced by a wide variety of other chaotic rhythms.

p. mag'nus, a large, full pulse.

p. mol'lis, a soft, easily compressible pulse.

p. monoc'rotus, SYN monocrotic *pulse.*

p. myu'rus, a pulse marked by a wave, the apex of which is reached suddenly and which then subsides very gradually. SYN mousetail pulse.

p. paradoxus (pŭl'sŭs par'ă-doks-ŭs), SYN paradoxic *pulse.*

p. par'vus, a pulse of small amplitude, as in aortic stenosis.

p. par'vus et tar'dus (pŭl'sŭs par'vŭs ā tar'dŭs), small, late pulse considered typical of severe aortic stenosis.

p. quadrigem'inus, SYN quadrigeminal *pulse.*

p. respiratio'ne intermit'tens, SYN paradoxic *pulse.*

p. tar'dus, a pulse with pathologically gradual upstroke typical of severe aortic stenosis. SEE ALSO plateau *pulse.*

p. trem'ulus, a feeble fluttering pulse.

p. trigem'inus, SYN trigeminal *pulse.*

p. vac'uus, a very weak pulse hardly distending the arterial wall.

p. veno'sus, SYN venous *pulse.*

pul·ta·ceous (pŭl-tā'shŭs). Macerated; pulpy. [G. *poltos,* porridge]

pul·ver·i·za·tion (pŭl'ver-i-zā'shŭn). Reduction to powder.

pul·ver·ize (pŭl'ver-īz). To reduce to a powder. [L. *pulverizo,* fr. *pulvis, pulveris,* dust]

pul·ver·u·lent (pŭl-ver'ū-lent). In a state of powder; powdery.

pul·vi·nar (pŭl-vī'năr). The expanded posterior extremity of the thalamus that forms a cushionlike prominence overlying the geniculate bodies. This structure, called nuclei pulvinares [TA] (pulvinar nuclei [TA]), is a composite cell group made up of anterior, inferior, lateral, and medial nuclei. [L. a couch made from cushions, fr. *pulvinus,* cushion]

pul·vi·nate (pŭl'vi-nāt). Raised or convex, denoting a form of surface elevation of a bacterial culture. [L. *pulvinus,* cushion]

pum·ice (pŭm'is). Volcanic cinders ground to particles of varying sizes; used in dentistry for polishing restorations or teeth; an abrasive. [L. *pumex (pumic-),* a pumice stone]

pump (pŭmp). **1.** An apparatus for forcing a gas or liquid from or to any part. **2.** Any mechanism for using metabolic energy to accomplish active transport of a substance.

breast p., a suction instrument for withdrawing milk from the breast.

calcium p., a membranal protein that can transport calcium ions across the membrane using energy from ATP.

calf p., muscular activity of calf that promotes venous flow towards the heart.

Carrel-Lindbergh p., a perfusion device designed for use in culture of whole organs.

constant infusion p., an electrically driven device for delivery from a reservoir of a constant, often very small, volume of solution over a prolonged period of time.

dental p., SYN saliva *ejector.*

hydrogen p., molecular mechanism for acid secretion from gastric parietal cells based on the activity of a H^+-K^+-ATPase.

intraaortic balloon p., an externally actuated and intermittently inflatable balloon placed into the descending aorta and that, on activation during diastole, augments blood pressure and organ perfusion by its pulsatile thrust; then, on deflation, decreases the cardiac work with each systole—the so-called counterpulsation principle—by reducing cardiac afterload.

ion p., a membranal complex of proteins that is capable of transporting ions against a concentration gradient using the energy from ATP.

jet ejector p., a suction p. in which fluid under high pressure is forced through a nozzle into an abruptly larger tube where a high-velocity jet, at a low pressure in accordance with the Bernoulli law, entrains gas or liquid from a side tube opening just beyond the end of the nozzle to create suction; e.g., the p. by which steam is used to evacuate an autoclave, a water aspirator.

proton p., molecular mechanism for the net transport of protons across a membrane; usually involves the activity of an ATPase.

saliva p., SYN saliva *ejector.*

sodium p., a biologic mechanism that uses metabolic energy from ATP to achieve active transport of sodium across a membrane; sodium p.'s expel sodium from most cells of the body, sometimes coupled with the transport of other substances, and also serve to move sodium across multicellular membranes such as renal tubule walls.

sodium-potassium p., a membrane-bound transporter found in nearly all mammalian cells that transports potassium ions into the cytoplasm from the extracellular fluid while simultaneously transporting sodium ions from the cytoplasm to the extracellular fluid. The p. transports both ions against large electrochemical potential gradients and maintains the potassium concentration of the cytoplasm far above, and the sodium concentration far below, their extracellular values. The p. is an enzyme that transports two potassium ions in exchange for three sodium ions in a reaction driven by hydrolysis of one molecule of ATP to form ADP plus one inorganic phosphate ion.

stomach p., an apparatus for removing the contents of the stomach by means of suction.

pump·ox·y·gen·a·tor (pŭmp-ok'si-je-nā'ter). A mechanical device that can substitute for both the heart (pump) and the lungs (oxygenator) during open heart surgery.

pu·na (poo'nä). SYN altitude *sickness.* [Sp., fr. Quechua *puna,* a high, dry Andean plateau]

punch (pŭnch). An instrument for making a hole or indentation in some solid material or for driving out a foreign body in such material. [L. *pungo,* pp. *punctus,* to stick, to punch]

punch card. A card on which data are stored by means of holes made in specified positions so that data can be sorted, processed, and analyzed.

punch·drunk (pŭnch'drŭnk). SEE punchdrunk *syndrome.*

pu

punc·ta (pŭngk′tă). Plural of punctum. [L.]

punc·tate (pŭngk′tāt). Marked with points or dots differentiated from the surrounding surface by color, elevation, or texture. [L. *punctum,* a point]

punc·ti·form (pŭngk′ti-fōrm). Very small but not microscopic, having a diameter of less than 1 mm. [L. *punctum,* a point, + *forma,* shape]

punc·tum, gen. **punc·ti,** pl. **punc·ta** (pŭngk′tŭm, -tī, -tă) [TA]. **1.** The tip or end of a sharp process. **2.** A minute round spot differing in color or otherwise in appearance from the surrounding tissues. **3.** A point on the optic axis of an optical system. SEE ALSO point. SYN point (1). SEE ALSO point, tip, end, center. [L. a prick, point, pp. ntr. of *pungo,* to prick, used as noun]

p. ce′cum, the blind spot in the visual field corresponding to the location of the optic disk.

p. coxa′le, the highest point of the crest of the ilium.

p. doloro′sum, SEE Valleix *points,* under *point.*

p. fixa [TA], SYN fixed *end.*

kissing puncta, a condition in which the upper p. is apposed to the lower p. when the eyes are open.

lacrimal p. [TA], the minute circular opening of the lacrimal canaliculus, on the margin of each eyelid near the medial commissure. SYN p. lacrimale [TA], lacrimal opening.

p. lacrima′le [TA], SYN lacrimal p.

p. lu′teum, SYN *macula* of retina.

p. mobile [TA], SYN mobile *end.*

p. ossificatio′nis, SYN ossification *center.*

p. ossificatio′nis prima′rium, SYN primary ossification *center.*

p. ossificatio′nis secunda′rium, SYN secondary ossification *center.*

p. prox′imum (P.p.), SYN near *point.*

p. remo′tum (P.r.), SYN far *point.*

p. vasculo′sum, one of the minute dots seen on section of the brain, due to small drops of blood at the cut extremities of the arteries.

punc·ture (pŭnk′choor). **1.** To make a hole with a small pointed object, such as a needle. **2.** A prick or small hole made with a pointed instrument. [L. *punctura,* fr. *pungo,* pp. *punctus,* to prick]

Bernard p., SYN diabetic p.

cisternal p., passage of a hollow needle through the posterior atlantooccipital membrane into the cerebellomedullary *cistern.*

diabetic p., a p. at a point in the floor of the fourth ventricle of the brain that causes glycosuria. SYN Bernard p.

▯lumbar p., a p. into the subarachnoid space of the lumbar region to obtain spinal fluid for diagnostic or therapeutic purposes. SYN Quincke p., rachicentesis, rachiocentesis, spinal p., spinal tap.

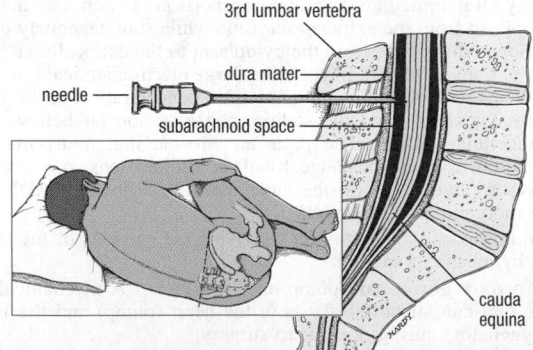

lumbar puncture: technique

Quincke p., SYN lumbar p.

spinal p., SYN lumbar p.

sternal p., removal of bone marrow from the manubrium by needle.

tracheoesophageal p., a surgical procedure to restore vocal function in patients who have had a laryngectomy by creating a tracheoesophageal fistula through which the laryngectomee forces air from the trachea into the esophagus to produce sound that is articulated into speech.

pun·gent (pŭn′jent). Sharp; said of the taste or odor of a substance. [L. *pungo,* pres. p. *-ens (-ent-),* to pierce]

PUO Abbreviation for pyrexia of unknown (or uncertain) origin, a term applied to febrile illness before diagnosis has been established; also referred to as FUO (fever of unknown origin).

pu·pa, pl. **pu·pae** (pū′pă, -pē). The stage of insect metamorphosis following the larva and preceding the imago. SEE ALSO complete *metamorphosis.* [L. *pupa,* doll]

pu·pil (p) (pū′pĭl) [TA]. The circular orifice in the center of the iris, through which the light rays enter the eye. SYN pupilla [TA]. [L. *pupilla*]

Adie p., SYN Adie *syndrome.*

amaurotic p., p. in an eye that is blind because of ocular or optic nerve disease; this p. will not contract to light except when the normal fellow eye is stimulated with light.

Argyll Robertson p., a form of reflex iridoplegia characterized by miosis, irregular shape, and a loss of the direct and consensual pupillary reflex to light, with normal pupillary constriction to a near vision effort (light-near dissociation); often present in tabetic neurosyphilis. SYN Robertson p.

artificial p., an opening made by excision of a portion of the iris in order to improve the vision in cases of central opacity of the cornea or lens.

Bumke p., dilation of the p. in response to anxiety or other psychic stimuli.

catatonic p., transient pupillary dilation with absence of pupillary reaction to light and convergence.

cat's-eye p., a distorted, elongated p.; usually due to anterior segment anomaly.

fixed p., a stationary pupil unresponsive to all stimuli.

Gunn p., SYN Marcus Gunn p.

Holmes-Adie p., SYN Adie *syndrome.*

Horner p., constricted p. due to impairment of sympathetic nerve innervation of the dilator muscle of the pupil. SEE ALSO Horner *syndrome.*

Hutchinson p., dilation of the p. on the side of the lesion as part of a third nerve palsy; often due to herniation of the uncus of the temporal lobe through the tentorial notch.

keyhole p., a p. with a coloboma.

Marcus Gunn p., relative afferent *pupillary* defect. SYN Gunn p.

paradoxical p., SEE paradoxical pupillary *reflex.*

pinhole p., an extremely constricted p.

Robertson p., SYN Argyll Robertson p.

seclusion of p. (se-kloo′zhŭn), the condition resulting from posterior annular synechia, in which the iris is bound down throughout the entire pupillary margin, but the pupil is not occluded. SYN exclusion of pupil.

tadpole-shaped p., an intermittent, brief distortion and dilation of a pupil that draws one part of the iris into a peak so that the p. resembles a tadpole; a temporary, benign condition associated with migraine that may leave the patient with Horner syndrome.

tonic p., a general term for a p. with delayed, slow, long-lasting contractions to light and to a near vision effort, often with light-near dissociation; due to denervation and aberrant reinnervation of the iris sphincter; seen in various autonomic neuropathies and in Adie *syndrome.*

pu·pil·la, pl. **pu·pil·lae** (pū-pil′ă, pū-pil′ē) [TA]. SYN pupil. [L. dim. of *pupa,* a girl or doll]

pu·pil·lary (pū′pi-lār-ē). Relating to the pupil.

p. light-near dissociation, a stronger near pupil response than light response; due to weak pupillomotor input, Argyll Robertson *pupil,* dorsal midbrain syndrome, or to misdirection of ciliary muscle fibers into the iris sphincter. SYN light-near dissociation.

relative afferent p. defect, an asymmetry of the pupillomotor input between the two eyes; tested by alternating the light from one eye to the other and comparing the direct light reactions.

△**pupillo-.** The pupils. [L. *pupilla,* pupil]

pu·pil·log·ra·phy (pū'pi-log'ră-fē). The recording of pupillary reactions. [pupillo- + G. *graphō*, to write]

pu·pil·lom·e·ter (pū'pi-lom'ĕ-ter). An instrument for measuring and recording the diameter of the pupil. [pupillo- + G. *metron*, measure]

pu·pil·lom·e·try (pū'pi-lom'ĕ-trē). Measurement of the pupil.

pu·pil·lo·mo·tor (pū'pĭ-lō-mō'ter). Relating to the autonomic nerve fibers that supply the smooth muscle of the iris. SYN iridomotor. [pupillo- + L. *motor*, mover]

pu·pil·lo·sta·tom·e·ter (pū'pi-lō-stă-tom'ĕ-ter). An instrument for measuring the distance between the centers of the pupils. [pupillo- + G. *statos*, placed, + *metron*, measure]

pu·pip·a·rous (pū-pip'ă-rŭs). Pupae-bearing; denoting those insects that give birth to late-stage larvae that have already passed their larval development within the body of the female, as in flies of the family Hippoboscidae and in the Glossinidae (tsetse flies). [pupa + L. *pario*, to give birth]

PUPPP Acronym for *p*ruritic *u*rticarial *p*apules and *p*laques of *p*regnancy, an intensely pruritic, occasionally vesicular, eruption appearing in the third trimester of pregnancy, without effect on the fetus; spontaneous involution occurs within 10 days of term, and recurrence is rare in subsequent pregnancies. Negative lesional immunofluorescence microscopy helps to exclude herpes gestationis.

Pur Abbreviation for purine.

pure (pūr). Unadulterated; free from admixture or contamination with any extraneous matter. [L. *purus*]

pur·ga·tion (per-gā'shŭn). Evacuation of the bowels with the aid of a purgative or cathartic. SYN catharsis (1). [L. *purgatio*]

pur·ga·tive (per'gă-tiv). An agent used for purging the bowels. SEE ALSO cathartic (2). [L. *purgativus*, purging]

    saline p., epsom salt, Rochelle salt, or any salt having p. properties.

purge (perj). **1.** To cause a copious evacuation of the bowels. **2.** A cathartic remedy. [L. *purgo*, to cleanse, fr. *purus*, pure, + *ago*, to do]

purg·ing cas·sia (perj'ing kash'yă). SYN cassia fistula.

pu·ri·form (pū'ri-fōrm). Resembling pus. [L. *pus (pur-)*, pus, + *forma*, form]

pu·rine (Pur) (pūr'ēn, -rin). The parent substance of adenine, guanine, and other naturally occurring p. "bases"; not known to exist as such in mammals.

    p.-nucleoside phosphorylase, a ribosyltransferase that reversibly catalyzes the phosphorolysis of a p. nucleoside with orthophosphate to produce a p. and α-D-ribose 1-phosphate; an inherited deficiency of this enzyme leads to cellular immunodeficiency.

    p. ribonucleoside, SYN nebularine.

pu·ri·ne·mia (pū-ri-nē'mē-ă). The presence of purine or xanthine bases in the circulating blood. [purine + G. *haima*, blood]

pu·ri·ty (pūr'i-tē). The state of being pure, free from contaminants or pollutants. [L. *puritas*, fr. *purus*, clean, undefiled]

    radiochemical p., the proportion of the total activity of a specific radionuclide in a specific chemical or biological form.

    radioisotopic p., a loose term commonly used to denote radionuclidic p.

    radionuclidic p., the proportion of the total radioactivity that is present as a specific radionuclide.

    radiopharmaceutical p., the sterility and apyrogenicity of a radioactive tracer for human use.

Purkinje, Johannes E. von (Jan E. Purkyne), Bohemian anatomist and physiologist, 1787–1869. SEE P. *conduction*, *images*, under *image*, *shift;* subendocardial conducting *system* of heart; P. *cells*, under *cell*, *corpuscles*, under *corpuscle*, *fibers*, under *fiber*, *figures*, under *figure*, cell *layer*, *network*, *phenomenon;* P.-Sanson *images*, under *image*.

Purmann, Matthaeus G., German surgeon, 1649–1721. SEE P. *method*.

pu·ro·mu·cous (pū-rō-mū'kŭs). SYN mucopurulent. [L. *pus (pur-)*, pus, + *mucus*, mucus]

pu·ro·my·cin (pū-rō-mī'sin). An antibiotic produced by the growth of *Streptomyces alboniger;* formerly used in the treatment of amebiasis and trypanosomiasis.

pur·ple (per'pl). A color formed by a mixture of blue and red. For individual purple dyes see specific name. [L. *purpura*]

    visual p., SYN rhodopsin.

pur·pu·ra (pŭr'poo-ră). A condition characterized by hemorrhage into the skin. Appearance of the lesions varies with the type of p., the duration of the lesions, and the acuteness of the onset. The color is first red, gradually darkens to purple, fades to a brownish yellow, and usually disappears in 2 or 3 weeks; color of residual permanent pigmentation depends largely on the type of unabsorbed pigment of the extravasated blood; extravasations may occur also into the mucous membranes and internal organs. SYN peliosis. [L. fr. G. *porphyra*, purple]

    allergic p., nonthrombocytopenic p. due to sensitization to foods, drugs, and insect bites. SYN anaphylactoid p. (1).

    anaphylactoid p., (1) SYN allergic p; (2) SYN Henoch-Schönlein p.

    p. angioneurot'ica, an eruption marked by angioneurotic edema, petechiae, and hyperesthesia of the skin and gastric mucous membrane.

    p. annula'ris telangiecto'des, asymptomatic annular lesions, principally of the lower extremities of adolescent males, in which the peripheral portion is composed of purpura or petechiae with brawny staining of hemosiderin deposits and minute telangiectasia.

    factitious p., self-induced, often painful, ecchymoses.

    fibrinolytic p., p. in which the bleeding is associated with rapid fibrinolysis of the clot.

    p. ful'minans, a severe and rapidly fatal form of p. hemorrhagica, occurring especially in children, with hypotension, fever, and disseminated intravascular coagulation, usually following an infectious illness.

    Henoch p., SYN Henoch-Schönlein p.

    Henoch-Schönlein p., an eruption of nonthrombocytopenic, palpable purpuric lesions due to dermal leukocytoclastic vasculitis with IgA in vessel walls associated with joint pain and swelling, colic, and passage of bloody stools, and occurring characteristically in young children; glomerulonephritis may occur during an initial episode or develop later. SYN anaphylactoid p. (2), Henoch p., Henoch-Schönlein syndrome, p. rheumatica, Schönlein p., Schönlein-Henoch syndrome.

    hyperglobulinemic p., SYN Waldenström *macroglobulinemia*.

    idiopathic thrombocytopenic p. (ITP), a systemic illness characterized by extensive ecchymoses and hemorrhages from mucous membranes and very low platelet counts; resulting from platelet destruction by macrophages due to an antiplatelet factor; childhood cases are usually brief and rarely present with intracranial hemorrhages, but adult cases are often recurrent and have a higher incidence of grave bleeding, especially intracranial. SYN immune thrombocytopenic p., thrombopenic p.

    immune thrombocytopenic p., SYN idiopathic thrombocytopenic p.

    nonthrombocytopenic p., SYN p. simplex.

    psychogenic p., a psychosomatic condition similar to autoerythrocyte sensitization syndrome.

    p. pu'licans, p. pulico'sa, petechiae caused by the bites of insects and animal parasites.

    p. rheumat'ica, SYN Henoch-Schönlein p.

    Schönlein p., SYN Henoch-Schönlein p.

    p. seni'lis, the occurrence of petechiae and ecchymoses on the atrophic skin of the legs in aged and debilitated subjects.

    p. sim'plex, the eruption of petechiae or larger ecchymoses, usually unaccompanied by constitutional symptoms and not associated with systemic illness. SYN nonthrombocytopenic p.

    p. symptomat'ica, a petechial eruption in scarlet fever and other exanthemas.

    thrombocytopenic p., SEE idiopathic thrombocytopenic p.

    thrombopenic p., SYN idiopathic thrombocytopenic p.

    thrombotic thrombocytopenic p., a rapidly fatal or occasionally protracted disease with varied symptoms in addition to p., includ-

pu

ing signs of central nervous system involvement, due to formation of fibrin or platelet thrombi in arterioles and capillaries in many organs.

p. urti′cans, p. simplex accompanied by an urticarial eruption.

Waldenström p., SYN Waldenström *macroglobulinemia.*

pur·pu·rea gly·co·sides A, pur·pu·rea gly·co·sides B (per′ pŭ-rē′ă glī′kō-sīdz). The cardioactive precursor glycosides of *Digitalis purpurea;* they are structurally identical with desacetyl-lanatosides A and B, respectively. SEE ALSO lanatosides A, B, and C.

pur·pu·ric (pŭr-poo′rik). Relating to or affected with purpura.

pur·pu·rin (per′pū-rin). **1.** SYN uroerythrin. **2.** A violet stain related to alizarin by addition of a 4-OH group to alizarin; found in madder root and other members of the *Rubiaceae;* used to detect calcium salts, boron, and as a histologic stain. SYN alizarin purpurin.

pur·pu·ri·nu·ria (per′pū-ri-noo′rē-ă). SYN porphyrinuria.

purr (per). A low vibratory murmur.

Purtscher, Otmar, German ophthalmologist, 1852–1927. SEE P. *disease.*

pu·ru·lence, pu·ru·len·cy (pūr′ŭ-lens, -len-sē; pūr′ū-lens). The condition of containing or forming pus. [L. *purulentia,* a festering, fr. *pus (pur-),* pus]

pu·ru·lent (pūr′ŭ-lent, pūr′ū-). Containing, consisting of, or forming pus.

pu·ru·loid (pū′rŭ-loyd). Resembling pus.

pus (pŭs). A fluid product of inflammation, consisting of a liquid containing leukocytes and the debris of dead cells and tissue elements liquefied by the proteolytic and histolytic enzymes (e.g., leukoprotease) that are elaborated by polymorphonuclear leukocytes. [L.]

blue p., p. tinged with pyocyanin, a product of *Pseudomonas aeruginosa.*

cheesy p., a very thick almost solid p. resulting from the absorption of the liquor puris.

curdy p., p. containing flakes of caseous matter.

green p., blue p. when, as sometimes happens, it has more of a green hue.

ichorous p., thin p. containing shreds of sloughing tissue, and sometimes of a fetid odor.

laudable p., an obsolete term used when suppuration was considered unlikely to lead to pyemia (blood poisoning) but more likely to remain localized.

sanious p., ichorous p. stained with blood.

pus·tu·lant (pŭs′choo-lant). **1.** Causing a pustular eruption. **2.** An agent producing pustules.

pus·tu·lar (pŭs′choo-lăr). Relating to or marked by pustules.

pus·tu·la·tion (pŭs′choo-lā′shŭn). The formation or the presence of pustules.

▣**pus·tule** (pŭs′chool). A circumscribed, superficial elevation of the skin, up to 1.0 cm in diameter, containing purulent material. [L. *pustula*]

malignant p., SYN cutaneous *anthrax.*

spongiform p. of Kogoj, an epidermal p. formed by infiltration of neutrophils into necrotic epidermis in which the cell walls persist as a spongelike network; seen in pustular psoriasis.

pus·tu·lo·crus·ta·ceous (pŭs′choo-lō-krŭs-tā′shŭs). Marked by pustules crusted with dry pus.

pus·tu·lo·sis (pŭs-choo-lō′sis). **1.** An eruption of pustules. **2.** Term occasionally used to designate acropustulosis. [L. *pustula,* pustule, + G. *-osis,* condition]

p. palmar′is et plantar′is, a sterile pustular eruption of the fingers and toes, variously attributed to dyshidrosis, pustular psoriasis, and unidentified bacterial infection. SYN acrodermatitis continua, acrodermatitis perstans, dermatitis repens.

p. vaccinifor′mis acu′ta, SYN *eczema* herpeticum.

pu·ta·men (pū-tā′men) [TA]. The outer, larger, and darker gray of the three portions into which the lenticular nucleus is divided by laminae of white fibers; it is connected with the caudate nucleus by bridging bands of gray substance that penetrate the internal capsule. Its histologic structure is similar to that of the caudate nucleus together with which it composes the striatum. SEE ALSO striate *body,* lenticular *nucleus.* [L. that which falls off in pruning, fr. *puto,* to prune]

Putnam, James J., U.S. neurologist, 1846–1918. SEE P.-Dana *syndrome.*

pu·tre·fac·tion (pū-tri-fak′shŭn). Decomposition or rotting, the breakdown of organic matter usually by bacterial action, resulting in the formation of other substances of less complex constitution with the evolution of ammonia or its derivatives and hydrogen sulfide; characterized usually by the presence of toxic or malodorous products. SYN decay (2), decomposition. [L. *putre-facio,* pp. *-factus,* to make rotten]

pu·tre·fac·tive (pū-tri-fak′tiv). Relating to or causing putrefaction.

pu·tre·fy (pū′tri-fī). To cause to become, or to become, putrid.

pu·tres·cence (pū-tres′ens). The state of putrefaction.

pu·tres·cent (pū-tres′ent). Denoting, or in the process of, putrefaction. [L. *putresco,* to grow rotten, fr. *puter,* rotten]

pu·tres·cine (pū-tres′ēn). 1,4-Diaminobutane; a poisonous polyamine formed from the amino acid arginine during putrefaction; found in urine and feces; in certain cells, p. is a precursor to γ-aminobutyrate.

pu·trid (pū′trid). **1.** In a state of putrefaction. **2.** Denoting putrefaction. [L. *putridus*]

Putti, Vittorio, Italian surgeon, 1880–1940. SEE P.-Platt *operation, procedure.*

PUVA Acronym for oral administration of *psoralen and subsequent exposure to long-wavelength ultraviolet light (*uv-a*); used to treat psoriasis.

PVC Abbreviation for polyvinyl chloride.

PVP Abbreviation for polyvinylpyrrolidone.

PVS Abbreviation for persistent vegetative *state.*

PWM Abbreviation for pokeweed *mitogen.*

py·ar·thro·sis (pī-ar-thrō′sis). SYN suppurative *arthritis.* [G. *pyon,* pus, + *arthrōsis,* a jointing]

△**pycno-.** SEE pykno-.

△**pyel-.** SEE pyelo-.

py·e·lec·ta·sis, py·e·lec·ta·sia (pī-ě-lek′tă-sis, pī-ě-lek-tā′zē-ă). Dilation of the pelvis of the kidney. [pyel- + G. *ektasis,* extension]

py·e·lit·ic (pī-ě-lit′ik). Relating to pyelitis.

py·e·li·tis (pī-ě-lī′tis). Inflammation of the renal pelvis. [pyel- + G. *-itis,* inflammation]

△**pyelo-, pyel-.** Pelvis, usually the renal pelvis. [G. *pyelos,* trough, tub, vat]

py·e·lo·cal·i·ce·al (pī′ě-lō-kal′i-sē′ăl). Relating to the renal pelvis and calices. SYN pyelocalyceal.

py·e·lo·cal·i·ec·ta·sis (pī′ě-lō-kal′ē-ek′tă-sis). SYN caliectasis.

py·e·lo·cal·y·ce·al (pī′ě-lō-kal′i-sē′ăl). SYN pyelocaliceal.

py·e·lo·cys·ti·tis (pī-ě-lō-sis-tī′tis). Inflammation of the renal pelvis and the bladder. [pyelo- + G. *kystis,* bladder, + *-itis,* inflammation]

py·e·lo·flu·o·ros·co·py (pī′ě-lō-flōr-os′kŏ-pē). Fluoroscopic examination of the renal pelves and ureters, following administration of contrast medium. [pyelo- + L. *fluo,* to flow, + G. *skopeō,* to view]

py·el·o·gram (pī′el-ō-gram). A radiograph or series of radiographs of the renal pelvis and ureter, following injection of contrast medium.

▣**py·e·log·ra·phy** (pī′ě-log′ră-fē). Radiologic study of the kidney, ureters, and usually the bladder, performed with the aid of a contrast agent injected either intravenously, or directly through a ureteral or nephrostomy catheter, or percutaneously. SYN pelviureterography, pyeloureterography, ureteropyelography. [pyelo- + G. *graphō,* to write]

antegrade p., antegrade urography in which the contrast medium is injected into the renal calices or pelvis.

intravenous p. (IVP), former name for intravenous *urography.*

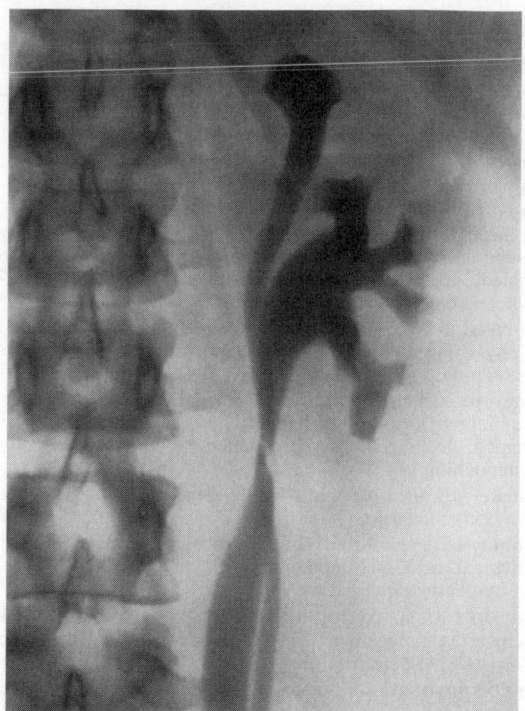

pyelography (antegrade urography): postpartum pyelogram of patient with pyelonephritis gravidarum showing reduplication of left renal pelvis and ureter

retrograde p., p. in which contrast material is injected into the ureters from an endoscope in the bladder.

py·e·lo·li·thot·o·my (pī′ĕ-lō-li-thot′ō-mē). Operative removal of a calculus from the kidney through an incision in the renal pelvis. SYN pelvilithotomy, pelviolithotomy. [pyelo- + G. *lithos*, stone, + *tomē*, incision]

py·e·lo·lym·phat·ic (pī′ĕ-lō-lim-fat′ik). Pertaining to the lymphatics of the renal pelvis.

py·e·lo·ne·phri·tis (pī′ĕ-lō-ne-frī′tis). Inflammation of the renal parenchyma, calices, and pelvis, particularly due to local bacterial infection. [pyelo- + G. *nephros*, kidney, + *-itis*, inflammation]

acute p., acute inflammation of the renal parenchyma and pelvis characterized by small cortical abscesses and yellowish streaks in the medulla due to pus in the collecting tubules and interstitial tissue.

ascending p., p. due to bacterial infection from the lower urinary tract, particularly by reflux of infected urine.

chronic p., chronic inflammation of the renal parenchyma and pelvis resulting from bacterial infection, characterized by calyceal deformities and overlying large flat renal scars with patchy distribution.

xanthogranulomatous p., a chronic inflammatory condition diffusely involving the entire kidney and usually resulting in a grossly enlarged and functionless kidney that can grossly resemble a neoplasm or tuberculosis; histologically, it is characterized by an inflammatory reaction with numerous lipid-laden, foamy histiocytes mixed with lymphocytes and plasma cells to form multiple granulomas.

py·e·lo·ne·phro·sis (pī′ĕ-lō-ne-frō′sis). Obsolete term for any disease of the pelvis of the kidney. [pyelo- + G. *nephros*, kidney, + *-osis*, condition]

py·e·lo·plas·ty (pī′e-lō-plas-tē). Surgical reconstruction of the renal pelvis and ureter to correct an obstruction at the ureteropelvic junction. SYN pelvioplasty. [pyelo- + G. *plastos*, formed]

capsular flap p., a reconstructive procedure for correction of uteropelvic obstruction, whereby a flap of renal capsule is swung down from the renal hilus to enlarge an obstructed intrarenal pelvis and upper ureter; used to correct situations involving loss of renal pelvic tissue that preclude the use of renal pelvis for the reconstruction.

Culp p., a reconstructive technique for correction of uteropelvic obstruction, whereby a spiral flap of renal pelvis is brought down and interposed into a vertical incision in the ureter. SEE ALSO Scardino vertical flap p.

disjoined p., dismembered p., a reconstructive procedure for correction of ureteropelvic obstruction, whereby the obstructed segment is resected and the upper ureter reanastomosed into the lower renal pelvis, usually utilizing a modified elliptical anastomotic technique.

Foley Y-plasty p., a reconstructive procedure for correction of ureteropelvic obstruction, whereby a V-shaped flap of renal pelvis is advanced downward into a vertical incision in the upper ureter, thereby widening the ureteropelvic junction.

Scardino vertical flap p., a reconstructive technique for correction of uteropelvic obstruction, whereby a vertical flap of renal pelvis is brought down and interposed into a vertical incision in the ureter. Cf. Culp p.

py·e·lo·pli·ca·tion (pī′ĕ-lō-pli-kā′shŭn). An obsolete procedure of taking tucks in the wall of the renal pelvis when unduly dilated by a hydronephrosis. [pyelo- + L. *plico*, to fold]

py·e·los·co·py (pī-ĕ-los′kŏ-pē). Endoscopic or fluoroscopic observation of the pelvis and calices of the kidney. [pyelo- + G. *skopeō*, to view]

py·e·los·to·my (pī-ĕ-los′tō-mē). Formation of an opening into the kidney pelvis to establish urinary drainage. [pyelo- + G. *stoma*, mouth]

py·e·lot·o·my (pī-ĕ-lot′ō-mē). Incision into the pelvis of the kidney. [pyelo- + G. *tomē*, incision]

extended p., extension of a standard p. into the lower pole infundibulum through the avascular plane between the posterior and basilar segmental renal arteries. SYN Gil-Vernet operation.

py·e·lo·u·re·ter·ec·ta·sis (pī′ĕ-lō-ū-rē′ter-ek′tă-sis). SYN hydronephrosis. [pyelo- + ureter + G. *ektasis*, a stretching]

py·e·lo·u·re·ter·og·ra·phy (pī′ĕ-lō-ū-rē′ter-og′ră-fē). SYN pyelography.

py·e·lo·ve·nous (pī′ĕ-lō-vē′nŭs). Denoting the phenomenon of drainage from the renal pelvis into the renal veins from increased intrapelvic pressure. [pyelo- + venous]

py·em·e·sis (pī-em′ĕ-sis). The vomiting of pus. [G. *pyon*, pus, + *emesis*, vomiting]

py·e·mia (pī-ē′mē-ă). Septicemia due to pyogenic organisms causing multiple abscesses. SYN pyogenic fever. [G. *pyon*, pus, + *haima*, blood]

cryptogenic p., p. whose source is not evident.

portal p., suppurative pylephlebitis.

py·e·mic (pī-ē′mik). Relating to or suffering from pyemia.

Py·e·mo·tes tri·ti·ci (pī-ĕ-mō′tēz tri-tī′kī, -sē). The straw or grain itch mite, a common parasite of insects in stored grain and a frequent cause of straw or grain itch from their bites; not to be confused with *P. t. ventricosus*, often called the straw itch mite, which is associated with the furniture beetle *Anobium punctatum* and is harmless to humans. SYN *Pediculoides ventricosus*.

py·en·ceph·a·lus (pī-en-sef′ă-lŭs). SYN pyocephalus. [G. *pyon*, pus, + *enkephalos*, brain]

py·e·sis (pī-ē′sis). SYN suppuration. [G. *pyon*, pus, + *-esis*, condition or process]

△**pyg-.** SEE pygo-.

py·gal (pī′găl). Relating to the buttocks. [G. *pygē*, buttocks]

py·gal·gia (pī-gal′jē-ă). Rarely used term meaning pain in the buttocks. [pyg- + G. *algos*, pain]

pyg·ma·li·on·ism (pig-māl′yon-izm). Rarely used term for the state of being in love with an object of one's own creation. [Pygmalion, G. myth. char.]

pyg·my (pig′mē) [MIM*265850]. A physiologic dwarf with normal serum levels of growth hormone and somatomedin and refractoriness to exogenous hormone; especially one of a race of similar people, such as the p.'s of central Africa. SYN pigmy. [G.

pygmaios, dwarfish, fr. *pygmē,* fist, also a measure of length from elbow to knuckles]

⌂**pygo-, pyg-.** The buttocks. [G. *pygē*]

py·go·a·mor·phus (pī′gō-ă-mōr′fŭs). Conjoined twins in which the parasite, attached to the buttocks of the autosite, is reduced to a formless mass or embryoma. SEE conjoined *twins,* under *twin.* [pygo- + G. *a-* priv. + *morphē,* form]

py·go·did·y·mus (pī-gō-did′i-mŭs). Conjoined twins with a single cephalothoracic region but with the buttocks and parts below doubled. SEE conjoined *twins,* under *twin.* SEE ALSO *duplicitas posterior.* [pygo- + G. *didymos,* twin]

py·gom·e·lus (pī-gom′ĕ-lŭs). Unequal conjoined twins in which the parasite is represented by a fleshy mass, or by a more fully developed limb, attached to the sacral or coccygeal region of the autosite. SEE conjoined *twins,* under *twin.* [pygo- + G. *melos,* part]

py·gop·a·gus (pī-gop′ă-gŭs). Conjoined twins in which the two individuals are joined at the buttocks, most often back to back. SEE conjoined *twins,* under *twin.* [pygo- + G. *pagos,* something fixed]

⌂**pyk-.** SEE pykno-.

pyk·nic (pik′nik). Denoting a constitutional body type characterized by well-rounded external contours and ample body cavities; virtually synonymous with endomorphic. [G. *pyknos,* thick]

⌂**pykno-, pyk-.** Thick, dense, compact. [G. *pyknos*]

pyk·no·dys·os·to·sis (pik′nō-dis-os-tō′sis). A condition characterized by short stature, delayed closure of the fontanels, and hypoplasia of the terminal phalanges. Autosomal recessive inheritance. SYN osteopetrosis acro-osteolytica. [pykno- + G. *dys-,* difficult, + *osteon,* bone, + *-osis,* condition]

pyk·no·ep·i·lep·sy, pyk·no·lep·sy (pik′nō-ep-i-lep-sē, pik′nō-lep-sē). Obsolete terms for absence. [pykno- + G. *lepsis,* seizure]

pyk·no·lep·sy. SYN childhood absence *epilepsy.*

pyk·no·mor·phous (pik′nō-mōr′fŭs). Denoting a cell or tissue that stains deeply because the stainable material is closely packed. [pykno- + G. *morphē,* form, shape]

pyk·no·phra·sia (pik′nō-frā′zē-ă). Thickness of speech. [pykno- + G. *phrasis,* speech]

pyk·no·sis (pik-nō′sis). A thickening or condensation; specifically, a condensation and reduction in size of the cell or its nucleus, usually associated with hyperchromatosis; nuclear p. is a stage of necrosis. [pykno- + G. *-osis,* condition]

pyk·not·ic (pik-not′ik). Relating to or characterized by pyknosis.

py·la (pī′lă). The orifice of communication between the third ventricle and cerebral aqueduct (of Sylvius). [G. *pylē,* gate]

py·lar (pī′lăr). Relating to the pyla.

py·le·phle·bi·tis (pī′lē-fle-bī′tis). Inflammation of the portal vein or any of its branches. [G. *pylē,* a gate, + *phleps,* vein, + *-itis,* inflammation]

py·le·throm·bo·phle·bi·tis (pī-lē-throm′bō-phle-bī′tis). Inflammation of the portal vein with the formation of a thrombus. [G. *pylē,* gate, + *thrombos,* a clot, + *phleps,* vein, + *-itis,* inflammation]

py·le·throm·bo·sis (pī′lē-throm-bō′sis). Thrombosis of the portal vein or its branches. [G. *pylē,* gate, + *thrombos,* a clot, + *-osis,* condition]

py·lic (pī′lik). Relating to the portal vein.

py·lon (pī′lon). A simple prosthesis, usually without joints, for a lower limb amputation. [G. gateway]

⌂**pylor-.** SEE pyloro-.

py·lo·ral·gia (pī-lō-ral′jē-ă). Rarely used term for pain in the pyloric region of the stomach. [pylor- + G. *algos,* pain]

py·lo·rec·to·my (pī′lōr-ek′tō-mē). Excision of the pylorus. [pylor- + G. *ektomē,* excision]

py·lo·ri (pī-lōr′ī). Plural of pylorus. [L.]

py·lor·ic (pī-lōr′ik). Relating to the pylorus.

py·lo·ri·ste·no·sis (pī-lōr′i-ste-nō′sis). Stricture or narrowing of the orifice of the pylorus. SYN pylorostenosis. [pylor- + G. *stenosis,* a narrowing]

py·lo·ri·tis (pī-lō-rī′tis). Inflammation of the pyloric end of the stomach. [pylor- + G. *-itis,* inflammation]

⌂**pyloro-, pylor-.** The pylorus. [G. *pyloros,* gatekeeper]

py·lo·ro·du·o·de·ni·tis (pī-lōr′ō-doo′od-ĕ-nī′tis). Inflammation involving the pyloric outlet of the stomach and the duodenum. [pyloro- + duodenitis]

py·lo·ro·gas·trec·to·my (pī-lōr′ō-gas-trek′tō-mē). Resection of the pylorus and a portion of the distal stomach.

py·lo·ro·my·ot·o·my (pī-lōr′ō-mī-ot′ō-mē). Longitudinal incision through the anterior wall of the pyloric canal to the level of the submucosa, to treat hypertrophic pyloric stenosis. SYN Fredet-Ramstedt operation, Ramstedt operation. [pyloro- + G. *mys,* muscle, + *tomē,* incision]

py·lo·ro·plas·ty (pī-lōr′ō-plas-tē). Widening of the pyloric canal and any adjacent duodenal stricture by means of a longitudinal incision closed transversely. [pyloro- + G. *plastos,* formed]

Finney p., a long, full-thickness incision from the duodenum, through the pylorus and proximally into the gastric antrum, with a C-shaped closure to provide a wider opening between stomach and duodenum.

Heineke-Mikulicz p., p. in which a short (2–3 inch), longitudinal incision is made through the pylorus and closed transversely.

Jaboulay p., a side-to-side gastroduodenostomy, useful when the pylorus and proximal duodenum are extensively scarred or indurated by peptic ulcer disease.

py·lor·op·to·sis, py·lor·op·to·sia (pī-lōr-ō-tō′sis, -tō′sē-ă). Downward displacement of the pyloric end of the stomach. [pyloro- + G. *ptōsis,* a falling]

py·lo·ro·spasm (pī-lōr′ō-spazm). Spasmodic contraction of the pylorus.

py·lo·ro·ste·no·sis (pī-lōr′ō-stĕ-nō′sis). SYN pyloristenosis.

py·lo·ros·to·my (pī-lō-ros′tō-mē). Establishment of a fistula from the abdominal surface into the stomach near the pylorus. [pyloro- + G. *stoma,* mouth]

py·lo·rot·o·my (pī-lō-rot′ō-mē). Incision of the pylorus. [pyloro- + G. *tomē,* incision]

py·lo·rus, pl. **py·lo·ri** (pī-lōr′ŭs, pī-lōr′ī) [TA]. **1.** A muscular or myovascular device to open (musculus dilator) and to close (musculus sphincter) an orifice or the lumen of an organ. **2.** The muscular tissue surrounding and controlling the aboral outlet of the stomach. [L. fr. G. *pylōros,* a gatekeeper, the pylorus, fr. *pylē,* gate, + *ouros,* a warder]

Pym, Sir William, English physician, 1772–1861. SEE P. *fever.*

⌂**pyo-.** Suppuration, accumulation of pus. [G. *pyon,* pus]

py·o·cele (pī′ō-sēl). An accumulation of pus in the scrotum. [pyo- + G. *kēlē,* tumor, hernia]

py·o·ce·lia (pī′ō-sē′lē-ă). SYN pyoperitoneum. [pyo- + G. *koilia,* a cavity]

py·o·ceph·a·lus (pī′ō-sef′ă-lŭs). A purulent effusion within the cranium. SYN pyencephalus. [pyo- + G. *kephalē,* head]

circumscribed p., abscess of the brain.

external p., meningeal suppuration.

internal p., intraventricular suppuration.

py·o·che·zia (pī-ō-kē′zē-ă). A discharge of pus from the bowel. [pyo- + G. *chezō,* to defecate]

py·o·cin (pī′ō-sin). Bacteriocin produced by strains of *Pseudomonas pyocyaneus.*

py·o·coc·cus (pī′ō-kok′ŭs). One of the cocci causing suppuration, especially *Streptococcus pyogenes.* [pyo- + G. *kokkos,* berry (coccus)]

py·o·col·po·cele (pī-ō-kol′pō-sēl). A vaginal tumor or cyst containing pus. [pyo- + G. *kolpos,* bosom (vagina), + *kēlē,* tumor, hernia]

py·o·col·pos (pī-ō-kol′pos). Accumulation of pus in the vagina. [pyo- + G. *kolpos,* bosom (vagina)]

py·o·cy·an·ic (pī′ō-sī-an′ik). Relating to blue pus or the organism that causes blue pus, *Pseudomonas aeruginosa.* [pyo- + G. *kyanos,* blue]

py·o·cy·a·no·gen·ic (pī′ō-sī′ă-nō-jen′ik). Causing blue pus. [pyo- + G. *kyanos,* blue, + *-gen,* producing]

py·o·cy·a·nol·y·sin (pī'ō-sī-ă-nol'i-sin). A hemolysin formed by *Pseudomonas aeruginosa*.

py·o·cyst (pī'ō-sist). A cyst with purulent contents. [pyo- + G. *kystis*, bladder]

py·o·cys·tis (pī-ō-sis'tis). Chronic development and retention of excessive amounts of purulent matter in a urinary bladder that may have been defunctionalized by prior supravesical diversion. [pyo- + G. *kystis*, bladder]

py·o·cyte (pī'ō-sīt). SYN pus *corpuscle*. [pyo- + G. *kytos*, cell]

py·o·der·ma (pī-ō-der'mă). Any pyogenic infection of the skin; may be primary, as impetigo, or secondary to a previously existing condition. [pyo- + G. *derma*, skin]

p. gangreno'sum, a chronic, noninfective eruption of spreading, undermined ulcers showing central healing, with diffuse dermal neutrophil infiltration; often associated with ulcerative colitis.

secondary p., a p. in which an existing skin lesion (e.g., eczema, herpes, seborrheic dermatitis) becomes secondarily infected.

p. veg'etans, SYN *dermatitis* vegetans.

py·o·gen (pī'ō-jen). An agent that causes pus formation. [pyo- + G. *-gen*, producing]

py·o·gen·e·sis (pī'ō-jen'ĕ-sis). SYN suppuration. [pyo- + G. *genesis*, production]

py·o·gen·ic, py·o·ge·net·ic (pī-ō-jen'ik, -jĕ-net'ik). Pus-forming; relating to pus formation. SYN pyogenous.

py·og·e·nous (pī-oj'ĕ-nŭs). SYN pyogenic.

py·o·he·mia (pī-ō-hē'mē-ă). A rarely used term for pyemia.

py·o·he·mo·tho·rax (pī'ō-hē-mō-thōr'aks). Presence of pus and blood in the pleural cavity. [pyo- + G. *haima*, blood, + thorax]

py·oid (pī'oyd). Resembling pus. [G. *pyōdēs*, fr. *pyon*, pus, + *eidos*, resemblance]

py·o·me·tra (pī-ō-mē'tră). Accumulation of pus in the uterine cavity. [pyo- + G. *mētra*, uterus]

py·o·me·tri·tis (pī'ō-mē-trī'tis). Inflammation of uterine musculature associated with pus in the uterine cavity. [pyo- + G. *mētra*, womb, + *-itis*, inflammation]

py·o·my·o·si·tis (pī'ō-mī-ō-sī'tis). Abscesses, carbuncles, or infected sinuses lying deep in muscles. [pyo- + G. *mys*, muscle, + *-itis*, inflammation]

tropical p., a disease observed in Samoa and in tropical Africa, marked by pains in the extremities, fever of a remittent or intermittent type, and abscesses in the muscles in various parts of the body (may result in death from sepsis); causative organisms are *Staphylococcus aureus* and *Streptococcus pyogenes*, but usually the disease is associated with parasitic infections. SYN bungpagga, lambo lambo, myositis purulenta tropica, tropical myositis.

py·o·ne·phri·tis (pī-ō-ne-frī'tis). Suppurative inflammation of the kidney. [pyo- + G. *nephros*, kidney, + *-itis*, inflammation]

py·o·neph·ro·li·thi·a·sis (pī'ō-nef'rō-li-thī'ă-sis). Presence in the kidney of pus and calculi. [pyo- + G. *nephros*, kidney, + *lithos*, stone, + *-iasis*, condition]

py·o·ne·phro·sis (pī'ō-ne-frō'sis). Distention of the pelvis and calices of the kidney with pus, usually associated with obstruction. SYN nephropyosis. [pyo- + G. *nephros*, kidney, + *-osis*, condition]

pyo-ova·ri·um (pī'ō-ō-var'ē-ŭm). Presence of pus in the ovary; an ovarian abscess.

py·o·per·i·car·di·tis (pī'ō-per-i-kar-dī'tis). Suppurative inflammation of the pericardium.

py·o·per·i·car·di·um (pī'ō-per-i-kar'dē-ŭm). SYN purulent *pericarditis*.

py·o·per·i·to·ne·um (pī'ō-per-i-tō-nē'ŭm). An accumulation of pus in the peritoneal cavity. SYN pyocelia. [G. *pyon*, pus]

py·o·per·i·to·ni·tis (pī'ō-per-i-tō-nī'tis). Suppurative inflammation of the peritoneum. [pyo- + peritonitis]

py·o·phy·so·me·tra (pī'ō-fī-sō-mē'tră). Presence of pus and gas in the uterine cavity. [pyo- + G. *physa*, air, + *mētra*, uterus]

py·o·pneu·mo·cho·le·cys·ti·tis (pī'ō-noo'mō-kō'lē-sis-tī'tis). Combination of pus and gas in an inflamed gallbladder caused by gas-producing organisms or by the entry of air from the duodenum through the biliary tree. [pyo- + G. *pneuma*, air, + cholecystitis]

py·o·pneu·mo·hep·a·ti·tis (pī'ō-noo'mō-hep-ă-tī'tis). Combination of pus and air in the liver, usually in association with an abscess. [pyo- + G. *pneuma*, air, + hepatitis]

py·o·pneu·mo·per·i·car·di·um (pī'ō-noo'mō-per-i-kar'dē-ŭm). Presence of pus and gas in the pericardial sac. [pyo- + G. *pneuma*, air, + pericardium]

py·o·pneu·mo·per·i·to·ne·um (pī'ō-noo'mō-per-i-tō-nē'ŭm). Presence of pus and gas in the peritoneal cavity. [pyo- + G. *pneuma*, air, + peritoneum]

py·o·pneu·mo·per·i·to·ni·tis (pī'ō-noo'mō-per-i-tō-nī'tis). Peritonitis with gas-forming organisms or with gas introduced from a ruptured bowel. [pyo- + G. *pneuma*, air, + peritonitis]

py·o·pneu·mo·tho·rax (pī'ō-noo-mō-thōr'aks). The presence of gas together with a purulent effusion in the pleural cavity. [pyo- + G. *pneuma*, air, + thorax]

subdiaphragmatic p., subphrenic p., subphrenic abscess associated with perforation of one of the hollow viscera, with gas in the chest and abdomen.

py·o·poi·e·sis (pī'ō-poy-ē'sis). SYN suppuration. [pyo- + G. *poiēsis*, a making]

py·o·poi·et·ic (pī'ō-poy-et'ik). Pus-producing.

py·o·py·e·lec·ta·sis (pī'ō-pī-ĕ-lek'tă-sis). Dilation of the renal pelvis with pus-producing inflammation. [pyo- + G. *pyelos*, pelvis, + *ektasis*, a stretching]

py·or·rhea (pī-ō-rē'ă). A purulent discharge. [pyo- + G. *rhoia*, a flow]

py·o·sal·pin·gi·tis (pi'ō-sal-pin-ji'tis). Suppurative inflammation of the uterine (fallopian) tube. [pyo- + salpingitis]

py·o·sal·pin·go-ooph·o·ri·tis (pī-ō-sal'pin-gō-ō-of'ō-rī'tis). Suppurative inflammation of the uterine (fallopian) tube and the ovary. SYN pyosalpingo-oothecitis. [pyo- + G. *salpinx*, trumpet (tube), + oophoritis]

py·o·sal·pin·go-oo·the·ci·tis (pī-ō-sal'ping-gō-ō'ō-thē-sī'tis). SYN pyosalpingo-oophoritis. [pyo- + G. *salpinx*, trumpet (tube), + Mod. L. *ootheca*, ovary, + G. *-itis*, inflammation]

py·o·sal·pinx (pī-ō-sal'pingks). Distention of a uterine (fallopian) tube with pus. SYN pus tube. [pyo- + G. *salpinx*, trumpet (tube)]

py·o·se·mia (pī-ō-sē'mē-ă). Presence of pus in seminal fluid, often associated with chronic prostatitis or other inflammatory conditions of the male genital tract. SYN pyospermia. [pyo- + L. *semen*, seed (of man)]

py·o·sep·ti·ce·mia (pī'ō-sep-ti-sē'mē-ă). Infection of the blood with several forms of bacteria, so-called pyogenic and also nonpyogenic organisms. [pyo- + G. *sēptikos*, putrefying, + *haima*, blood]

py·o·sis (pī-ō'sis). SYN suppuration. [G.]

py·o·sper·mia (pī-ō-sper'mē-ă). SYN pyosemia. [pyo- + G. *sperma*, seed, + *ia*, condition]

py·o·stat·ic (pī-ō-stat'ik). **1.** Arresting the formation of pus. **2.** An agent that arrests the formation of pus. [pyo- + G. *statikos*, causing to stand]

py·o·sto·ma·ti·tis (pī'ō-stō-mă-tī'tis). A suppurating inflammatory eruption of the mouth. [pyo- + G. *stoma*, mouth, + *-itis*, inflammation]

p. veg'etans, confluent pustular lesions of the mouth, with proliferative and verrucose eruptions of the buccal mucous membrane; associated with ulcerative colitis and other wasting diseases.

py·o·tho·rax (pī-ō-thōr'aks). Empyema in a pleural cavity.

py·o·u·ra·chus (pī-ō-ū'ră-kŭs). A purulent accumulation in the urachus.

py·o·u·re·ter (pī-ō-ū-rē'ter). Distention of a ureter with pus.

Pyr Abbreviation for pyrimidine; pyroglutamic acid.

△pyr-. Fire, heat. SEE ALSO pyreto-, pyro- (1). [G. *pyr*]

pyr·a·cin (pir'ă-sin). Pyridoxolactone, the lactone of 4-pyridoxic acid.

pyr·a·mid (pir'ă-mid) [TA]. **1.** A term applied to a number of anatomic structures having a more or less pyramidal shape. SYN pyramis [TA]. **2.** A term denoting the petrous portion of the temporal bone. [G. *pyramis* (*pyramid-*), a pyramid]

anterior p., SYN p. of medulla oblongata.

cerebellar p., SYN p. of vermis.

Ferrein p., SYN medullary *ray.*

Lallouette p., SYN pyramidal *lobe* of thyroid gland.

p. of light, SYN light *reflex* (3).

Malacarne p., a lobule on the undersurface of the cerebellum, the posterior portion of the vermis.

malpighian p., SYN renal p.'s.

p. of medulla oblongata, an elongated, white prominence on the ventral surface of the medulla oblongata on either side along the anterior median fissure, corresponding to the position of fibers forming the corticospinal tracts. SYN pyramis medullae oblongatae [TA], anterior column of medulla oblongata, anterior p.

medullary p., SYN renal p.'s.

olfactory p., a small area of gray matter situated between the roots of the olfactory tracts; it is continuous caudally with the anterior perforated substance.

petrous p., SYN petrous *part* of temporal bone.

population p., graphic representation of the age and sex composition of a population, constructed by computing the percentage distribution of the population in each age and sex class.

posterior p. of the medulla, SYN gracile *fasciculus.*

renal p.'s [TA], pyramidal masses seen on longitudinal section of the kidney; collectively, they constitute the renal medullae and contain part of the secreting tubules and the collecting tubules. SYN malpighian p., medullary p., pyramides renales, pyramis renalis.

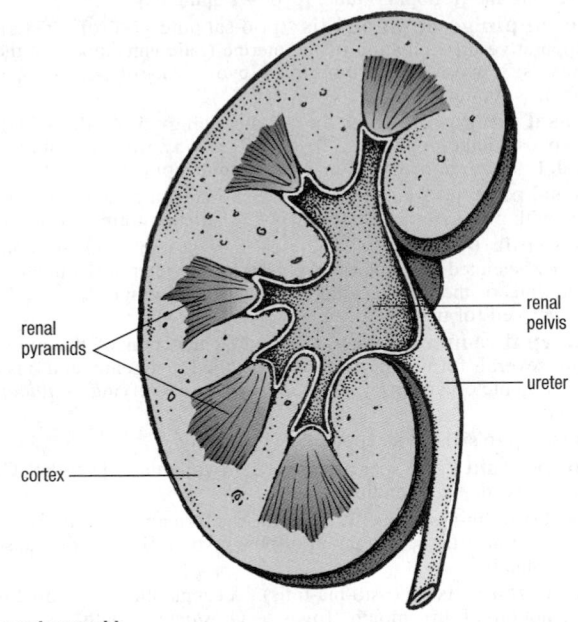

renal pelvis

ureter

renal pyramids

cortex

renal pyramid

p. of thyroid, SYN pyramidal *lobe* of thyroid gland.

p. of tympanum, SYN eminentia pyramidalis.

p. of vermis [TA], a subdivision of the inferior vermis of the cerebellum between the tuber and the uvula; vermis lobule VIII. SYN cerebellar p., pyramis [TA] of cerebellum.

p. of vestibule [TA], the upper triangular extremity of the crista vestibuli. SYN pyramis vestibuli [TA].

py·ram·i·dal (pi-ram′i-dal). **1.** Of the shape of a pyramid. **2.** Relating to any anatomical structure called pyramid.

py·ra·mi·da·le (pi-ram′i-dā′lē). SYN triquetrum. [Mod. L.]

py·ra·mi·da·lis. SEE pyramidalis (*muscle*).

py·ram·i·dot·o·my (pi-ram′i-dot′ŏ-mē). Section of pyramidal

tracts, in the spinal cord, for the relief of involuntary movements. [G. *pyramis,* pyramid, + *tomē,* incision]

medullary p., a medullary pyramidal tractotomy.

spinal p., a spinal pyramidal tractotomy.

pyr·a·min, pyr·a·mine (pir′ă-min). SYN toxopyrimidine.

pyr·a·mis, pl. **py·ra·mi·des** (pir′ă-mis, pi-ram′i-dēz) [TA]. SYN pyramid (1). [Mod. L. fr. G. pyramid]

p. medul′lae oblonga′tae [TA], SYN *pyramid* of medulla oblongata.

p. rena′lis, pl. **pyram′ides rena′les,** SYN renal *pyramids,* under *pyramid.*

p. [TA] of cerebellum, SYN *pyramid* of vermis.

p. tym′pani, SYN *eminentia* pyramidalis.

p. vestib′uli [TA], SYN *pyramid* of vestibule.

py·ran (pī′ran). A cyclic compound that may be considered the formal parent of sugars with an oxygen bridge from carbon atoms 1–5 (the pyranoses).

pyr·a·none (pir′ă-nōn, pī′-). SYN pyrone.

pyr·a·nose (pir′ă-nōs, pī′-). A cyclic form of a sugar in which the oxygen bridge forms a pyran.

py·ran·tel pam·o·ate (pi-ran′tel). An anthelmintic, especially useful drug for single or mixed intestinal nematode infections such as *Ascaris,* hookworm, pinworm, and *Trichostrongylus* species.

pyr·a·thi·a·zine hy·dro·chlo·ride (pir-ă-thī′ă-zēn). An antihistaminic.

pyr·a·zin·a·mide (pir-ă-zin′ă-mīd). First-line antituberculosis drug, particularly active against *Mycobacterium tuberculosis* in macrophages. Like all antituberculosis drugs, it must be given with other drugs to be effective in active disease. Its major toxicity is hepatic.

pyr·az·o·lone (pir-ă-zō′lōn). A class of nonsteroidal anti-inflammatory agents used in the treatment of arthritic conditions; e.g., phenylbutazone.

py·rec·tic (pī-rek′tik). SYN febrile.

py·re·ne·mia (pī-rĕ-nē′mē-ă). A condition characterized by the presence of nucleated red cells in the blood. [G. *pyrēn,* the pit of a fruit, + *haima,* blood]

Py·re·no·chae·ta ro·me·roi (pī′rĕ-nō-kē′tă rō′mĕ-roy). One of the numerous species of true fungi capable of causing mycetoma in humans.

py·re·noid (pī′rē-noyd). One of the minute luminous bodies sometimes visualized in the chromatophores of some protozoa, such as *Euglena viridis.* [G. *pyrēn,* pit of a fruit, + *eidos,* resemblance]

py·re·thrins (pī-reth′rinz). Insecticidal constituents of pyrethrum flowers.

py·re·throids. Synthetic pyrethrin derivatives that are used as insecticides; as a class these agents are less toxic to mammals than are other effective insecticides.

py·re·thro·lone (pī-reth′rō-lōn). 2-Methyl-4-oxo-3-(2,4-pentanedienyl)-2-cyclopentenol, a constituent of the pyrethrins.

py·re·thrum (pī-rē′thrŭm). The root of *Anacyclus pyrethrum* (family Compositae), a shrub native to Morocco; has been used as a sialogogue; its flowers are a source of pyrethrins. [G. *pyrethron,* feverfew, fr. *pyr,* fire, from the hot-tasting root]

py·ret·ic (pī-ret′ik). SYN febrile. [G. *pyretikos*]

pyreto-. Fever. SEE ALSO pyr-, pyro- (1). [G. *pyretos,* fever, fr. *pyr,* fire]

py·ret·o·gen (pī-ret′ō-jen). Rarely used term for pyrogen. [pyreto- + G. *-gen,* producing]

py·re·to·gen·e·sis (pī′rĕ-tō-jen′ĕ-sis, pir′ĕ-tō-). Rarely used term for the origin and mode of production of fever. [pyreto- + G. *genesis,* origin]

py·re·to·ge·net·ic, py·re·to·gen·ic (pī′rĕ-tō-jĕ-net′ik, -jen′ik). SYN pyrogenic.

py·re·tog·e·nous (pī-rĕ-toj′ĕ-nŭs). SYN pyrogenic.

py·re·to·ther·a·py (pī′rĕ-tō-thār′ă-pē). **1.** Obsolete synonym for pyrotherapy. **2.** Treatment of fever. SYN artificial fever, induced fever. [pyreto- + G. *therapeia,* treatment]

py·rex·ia (pī-rek′sē-ă). SYN fever. [G. *pyrexis*, feverishness]

py·rex·i·al (pī-rek′sē-ăl). Relating to fever.

py·rex·i·o·pho·bia (pī-rek′sē-ō-fō′bē-ă). Morbid fear of fever. [G. *pyrexis*, feverishness, + *phobos*, fear]

pyr·i·ben·zyl meth·yl sul·fate (pir-i-ben′zil). SYN bevonium methyl sulfate.

pyr·i·dine (pir′i-dēn, -din). C_5H_5N; a colorless volatile liquid of empyreumatic odor and burning taste, resulting from the dry distillation of organic matter containing nitrogen; used as an industrial solvent, in analytic chemistry, and for denaturing alcohol.

pyridinium. A breakdown product of bone collagen, excreted in urine, and assayed as a measure of osteoclast activity; increased in disease states such as Paget's disease, primary hyperparathyroidism, and osteoporosis.

pyridinoline. Hydroxypyridinium; a. breakdown product of bone collagen, assayed as is pyridinium (q.v.) to gauge osteoclastic activity.

pyr·i·dof·yl·line (pir-i-dof′i-lin). 7-(2-Hydroxyethyl)theophylline hydrogen sulfate compound with pyridoxol; a coronary vasodilator.

pyr·i·do·stig·mine bro·mide (pir′i-dō-stig′mēn). A cholinesterase inhibitor useful in the treatment of myasthenia gravis and to reverse the neuromuscular block produced by curare and similar agents at the termination of a surgical procedure.

pyr·i·dox·al (pir′i-dok′săl). The 4-aldehyde of pyridoxine, having a similar physiologic action. SEE ALSO pyridoxine.

p. kinase, an enzyme that catalyzes the phosphorylation by ATP of p. to p. 5-phosphate and ADP, thus converting the nutrient to the active coenzyme.

p. 5-phosphate (PLP), a coenzyme essential to many reactions in tissue, notably transaminations and amino acid decarboxylations.

pyr·i·dox·a·mine (pir-i-dok′să-mēn). The amine of pyridoxine ($–CH_2NH_2$ replacing $–CH_2OH$ at position 4), having a similar physiologic action. SEE pyridoxine.

p. 5-phosphate, the amine of pyridoxal 5-phosphate ($–CH_2NH_2$ replacing –CHO at position 4), it is the intermediate formed in many enzyme-catalyzed reactions that utilize pyridoxal 5-phosphate.

pyr·i·dox·a·mine-phos·phate ox·i·dase. An oxidoreductase catalyzing oxidative deamination of pyridoxamine 5-phosphate (with O_2 and H_2O) to form pyridoxal 5-phosphate, H_2O_2, and NH_3.

4-pyr·i·dox·ic ac·id (pir-i-dok′sik). The principal product of the metabolism of pyridoxal (–COOH replaces –CHO at position 4), appearing in the urine.

pyr·i·dox·ine (pir-i-dok′sēn, -sin). The original vitamin B_6, which term now includes pyridoxal and pyridoxamine, associated with the utilization of unsaturated fatty acids. In rats, deficiency produces a nutritional dermatitis and acrodynia; in humans, deficiency may result in increased irritability, convulsions, and peripheral neuritis. The hydrochloride is used in pharmaceutic preparations; found in vegetables.

pyr·i·dox·ine 4-de·hy·dro·gen·ase. An oxidoreductase catalyzing oxidation of pyridoxine with $NADP^+$ to pyridoxal and NADPH.

pyr·i·form (pir′i-fōrm). SYN piriform. [L. *pyrum* (prop. *pirum*), pear, + *forma*, form]

py·ril·a·mine ma·le·ate (pī-ril′ă-mēn, pir′i-lă-). An antihistaminic. SYN mepyramine maleate.

py·ri·meth·a·mine (pir-i-meth′ă-mēn). A potent folic acid antagonist used as an antimalarial agent effective against *Plasmodium falciparum;* a valuable suppressant, active against the asexual erythrocytic and tissue forms; also used in the treatment of toxoplasmosis.

py·rim·i·dine (Pyr) (pī-rim′i-dēn). 1,3-Diazine; a heterocyclic substance, the formal parent of several "bases" present in nucleic acids (uracil, thymine, cytosine) as well as of the barbiturates.

p. 5′-nucleotidase, an enzyme that catalyzes the hydrolysis of a pyrimidine-nucleoside 5′-monophosphate to produce orthophosphate and the pyrimidine nucleoside; a deficiency of this enzyme

results in accumulation of pyrimidine nucleotides leading to hemolytic anemia.

p. transferase, SYN *thiamin* pyridinylase.

pyrin. An abnormal neutrophil protein encoded by the MEFV gene in familial Mediterranean fever. SYN marenostrin.

pyr·i·thi·a·min (pir′i-thī′ă-min). A thiamin antimetabolite, differing from thiamin in that the thiazole ring of the thiamin molecule is replaced by a pyridine ring. SYN neopyrithiamin.

⌂ **pyro-.** **1.** Combining form denoting fire, heat, or fever. SEE ALSO pyr-, pyreto-. **2.** In chemistry, combining form denoting derivatives formed by removal of water (usually by heat) to form anhydrides. SEE ALSO anhydro-. [G. *pyr*, fire]

py·ro·bo·ric ac·id (pī-rō-bōr′ik). SYN tetraboric acid.

py·ro·cal·cif·er·ol (pī′ro-kal-sif′er-ol). A thermal decomposition product of calciferol.

py·ro·cat·e·chase (pī-rō-kat′ĕ-kās). SYN catechol 1,2-dioxygenase.

py·ro·cat·e·chin (pī-rō-kat′ĕ-kin). SYN pyrocatechol.

py·ro·cat·e·chol (pī-rō-kat′ĕ-kol). 1,2-Benzenediol; a constituent of the catecholamines, epinephrine and norepinephrine, and dopa; used externally as an antiseptic. SYN catechol (1), pyrocatechin.

py·ro·gal·lic ac·id (pī-rō-gal′ik). SYN pyrogallol.

py·ro·gal·lol (pī-rō-gal′ol). Used externally in the treatment of psoriasis, ringworm, and other skin affections. SYN pyrogallic acid.

py·ro·gal·lol·phthal·e·in (pī′rō-gal-ō-thal′ē-in, -thāl′ē-in). SYN gallein.

py·ro·gen (pī′rō-jen). A fever-inducing agent; p.'s are produced by bacteria, molds, viruses, and yeasts. [pyro- + G. *-gen*, producing]

endogenous p. (EP), proteins that induce fever. Several (about 11) have been identified, including cytokines formed by components of the immune system, especially macrophages (e.g., interleukins 1 and 6, interferons and tumor necrosis factors). SYN leukocytic p.'s.

exogenous p.'s, drugs or substances that are formed by microorganisms and induce fever. Among the latter are lipopolysaccharides and lipoteichoic acid.

leukocytic p.'s, SYN endogenous p.

py·ro·gen·ic (pī-rō-jen′ik). Causing fever. SEE ALSO febrifacient. SYN pyretogenetic, pyretogenic, pyretogenous.

py·ro·glob·u·lins (pī-rō-glob′ū-linz). Serum proteins (immunoglobulins), usually associated with multiple myeloma or macroglobulinemia, which precipitate irreversibly when heated to 56°C.

py·ro·glu·tam·ic ac·id (Pyr) (pī′rō-gloo-ta′mik). SYN 5-oxoproline.

py·ro·lig·ne·ous (pī-rō-lig′nē-ŭs). Relating to or produced by the dry distillation of wood. [pyro- + L. *lignum*, wood]

py·rol·y·sis (pī-rol′i-sis). Decomposition of a substance by heat. [pyro- + G. *lysis*, dissolution]

py·ro·ma·nia (pī-rō-mā′nē-ă). A morbid impulse to set fires. SYN incendiarism. [pyro- + G. *mania*, frenzy]

py·ro·ma·ni·ac (pī-rō-mā′nē-ak). One affected with pyromania; arsonist.

py·ro·men (pī′rō-men). SYN piromen.

py·rom·e·ter (pī-rom′ĕ-ter). An instrument for measuring very high degrees of heat, beyond the capacity of a mercury or gas thermometer. [pyro- + G. *metron*, measure]

resistance p., SYN resistance *thermometer*.

py·rone (pī′rōn). A keto derivative of pyran. SYN pyranone.

py·ro·nin (pī′rō-nin). A fluorescent red basic xanthene dye, the chloride of tetramethyldiaminoxanthene, **p. Y** or **p. G** (C.I. 45005), or of tetraethyldiaminoxanthene, **p. B** (C.I. 45010). These dyes, especially p. Y, are used in combination with methyl green for differential staining of RNA (red) and DNA (green); difference in staining result is probably due to the higher degree of polymerization of DNA; p. Y is also used as a tracking dye for RNA in electrophoresis.

py·ro·ni·no·phil·ia (pī′rō-nin-ō-fil′ē-ă). An affinity for the basic pyronin dyes; a useful indicator of intense protein synthesis accompanying RNA synthesis, as in the cytoplasm of an active plasma cell. [pyronin + G. *philos,* fond]

py·ro·pho·bia (pī-rō-fō′bē-ă). Morbid dread of fire. [pyro- + G. *phobos,* fear]

py·ro·phos·pha·tase (pī-rō-fos′fă-tās). Any enzyme cleaving a pyrophosphate bond between two phosphoric groups, leaving one on each of the two fragments; e.g., inorganic p., NAD$^+$ p. (cleaves NAD, etc., to mononucleotides), ATP p. (cleaves inorganic pyrophosphate from ATP, leaving AMP). SEE ALSO *flavin* adenine dinucleotide. SYN diphosphatase.

inorganic p., a phosphohydrolase catalyzing hydrolysis of inorganic pyrophosphate to two orthophosphates. SYN inorganic diphosphatase.

py·ro·phos·phate (PP, PP$_i$) (pī-rō-fos′fāt). A salt of pyrophosphoric acid; accumulates in cases of hypophosphatasia; sometimes referred to as inorganic p. (PP$_i$). SYN diphosphate.

^{99m}Tc p., a radionuclide tracer used for imaging ischemic myocardium in nuclear medicine. SEE technetium-99m.

py·ro·phos·pho·ki·nas·es (pī′rō-fōs-fō-kī′nās-ez). Enzymes (EC 2.7.6.x) transferring a pyrophosphoric group (e.g., phospho-α-D-ribosyl-pyrophosphate synthetase). SYN pyrophosphotransferases.

py·ro·phos·phor·ic ac·id (pī′rō-fos-fōr′ik). An anhydride of phosphoric acid obtained by heating phosphoric acid to 213°C; it forms pyrophosphates with bases, and its esters are important in energy metabolism and in biosynthesis.

py·ro·phos·pho·ryl·as·es (pī′rō-fos-fōr′il-ās-ez). Trivial name applied to the nucleotidyltransferases that catalyze the transfer of the AMP of ATP to another residue with the release of inorganic pyrophosphate, or the attachment of a nucleoside pyrophosphate to a polynucleotide with release of inorganic orthophosphate.

py·ro·phos·pho·trans·fer·as·es (pī′rō-fos-fō-trans′fer-ās-ez). SYN pyrophosphokinases.

py·ro·poi·ki·lo·cy·to·sis (pī′rō-pōy-kil-ō-si-tō-sis). A rare recessive disorder manifested by severe hemolysis, marked poikilocytosis, and a characteristic sensitivity of the red cells to heat-induced fragmentation in vitro; apparently due to a defect in spectrin self-association. SYN hereditary pyropoikilocytosis.

hereditary pyropoikilocytosis, SYN pyropoikilocytosis.

py·ro·scope (pī′rō-skōp). An instrument for measuring temperature by comparing the light of a heated object with a light standard. [pyro- + G. *skopeō,* to view]

py·ro·sis (pī-rō′sis). Substernal pain or burning sensation, usually associated with regurgitation of acid-peptic gastric juice into the esophagus. SYN heartburn. [G. a burning]

py·ro·ther·a·py (pī′rō-thār′ă-pē). Treatment of disease by inducing an artificial fever in the patient. SYN therapeutic fever.

py·rot·ic (pī-rot′ik). **1.** Relating to pyrosis. **2.** SYN caustic.

py·ro·tox·in (pī′rō-tok′sin). Obsolete term for a toxic substance produced in the tissues during the progress of a fever.

pyr·ox·y·lin (pī-rok′si-lin). Consists chiefly of cellulose tetranitrate, obtained by the action of nitric and sulfuric acids on cotton; used in the preparation of collodion. SYN colloxylin, dinitrocellulose, nitrocellulose, soluble gun cotton, xyloidin. [pyro- + G. *xylon,* wood]

pyr·ro·bu·ta·mine phos·phate (pir-ō-bū′tă-mēn). An antihistamine.

pyr·ro·lase (pir′ō-lās). SYN *tryptophan* 2,3-dioxygenase.

pyr·rol blue (pir′ol) [C.I. 42700]. An acid triarylmethane dye employed as a vital dye and as an elastin stain. SYN Isamine blue.

pyr·role (pir′ōl). Divinylenimine; a heterocyclic compound found in many biologically important substances. SYN azole, imidole.

pyr·rol·i·dine (pi-rol′i-dēn). **1.** Tetrahydropyrrole; pyrrole to which four H atoms have been added; the structural basis of proline and hydroxyproline. **2.** A class of alkaloids containing a p. (1) moiety or a p. derivative.

pyr·rol·i·dine-2-car·box·yl·ate. SYN proline.

pyr·rol·i·done-5-car·box·yl·ate (pi-rol′i-dōn). SYN 5-oxoproline.

5-pyr·ro·li·done-2-car·box·yl·ic ac·id. SYN 5-oxoproline.

pyr·ro·line (pir′ō-lēn). A group of isomers of pyrrole to which

two H atoms have been added; 1-p. has a double bond between the nitrogen and an adjacent carbon.

1-pyr·ro·line-5-car·box·y·late de·hy·dro·gen·ase. An enzyme that catalyzes the reversible reaction of 1-pyrroline 5-carboxylate and NAD$^+$ to form L-glutamate and NADH; this enzyme plays a role in proline and ornithine metabolism; 1-pyrroline 5-carboxylate is in equilibrium with glutamate γ-semialdehyde; a deficiency of this enzyme is associated with type II hyperprolinemia.

pyr·ro·line-2-car·box·yl·ate re·duc·tase. An oxidoreductase reducing 1-pyrroline-2-carboxylate to L-proline with NAD(P)H. SYN proline dehydrogenase, proline oxidase.

pyr·ro·line-5-car·box·y·late re·duc·tase. An oxidoreductase reversibly reducing 1-pyrroline-5-carboxylate to L-proline with NAD(P)H; a deficiency of this enzyme is associated with type I hyperprolinemia. SYN proline dehydrogenase, proline oxidase.

py·ru·val·dox·ine (pī′roo-văl-dok′sēn). SYN isonitrosoacetone.

py·ru·vate (pī′roo-vāt). A salt or ester of pyruvic acid.

active p., an intermediate formed in the oxidative decarboxylation of pyruvate. Cf. p. dehydrogenase (lipoamide). SYN α-lactylthiamin pyrophosphate.

p. carboxylase, ligase catalyzing reaction of ATP, p., and HCO$_3$$^{2-}$, to form ADP, orthophosphate, and oxaloacetate; biotin and acetyl-CoA are involved; an absence of this enzyme results in neuronal loss in the cerebral cortex, leading to mental retardation.

p. decarboxylase, α-carboxylase; α-ketoacid carboxylase; a thiamin-pyrophosphate–dependent carboxylase of yeast catalyzing decarboxylation of a 2-oxoacid (e.g., p.) to an aldehyde (e.g., acetaldehyde) without oxidoreduction and without lipoamide, in contrast to p. dehydrogenase (lipoamide).

p. dehydrogenase, a structurally distinct collection of enzymes containing p. dehydrogenase (lipoamide), dihydrolipoyl transacetylase, and dihydrolipoyl dehydrogenase.

p. dehydrogenase (cytochrome), an oxidoreductase catalyzing reaction between ferricytochrome b_1 and p. to yield acetate and CO$_2$, and ferrocytochrome b_1.

p. dehydrogenase (lipoamide), an oxidoreductase catalyzing conversion of p. and (oxidized) lipoamide to CO$_2$ and S^6-acetyldihydrolipoamide in two successive reactions: the first between p. and thiamin pyrophosphate to yield CO$_2$ and α-hydroxyethylthiamin pyrophosphate (active p.); the second between the last named and lipoamide to regain the thiamin pyrophosphate and yield S^6-acetylhydrolipoamide. Cf. α-ketodecarboxylase.

p. kinase (PK), phospho*enol*pyruvate kinase; a phosphotransferase catalyzing transfer of phosphate from phospho*enol*pyruvate to ADP, forming ATP and p.; other nucleoside phosphates can participate in the reaction; a key step in glycolysis; a deficiency in p. kinase will lead to hemolytic anemia.

p. oxidase, an oxidoreductase catalyzing the reaction of p., phosphate, and O$_2$ to yield acetyl phosphate, CO$_2$, and H$_2$O$_2$.

py·ru·vic ac·id (pī-roo′vik). 2-Oxopropanoic acid; α-ketopropionic acid; acetylformic acid; pyroacemic acid; the simplest α-keto acid; an intermediate compound in the metabolism of carbohydrate; in thiamin deficiency, its oxidation is retarded and it accumulates in the tissues, especially in nervous structures. The enol form, *enol* pyruvic acid, when phosphorylated, plays an important metabolic role. SEE phospho*enol*pyruvic acid.

py·ru·vic al·de·hyde. SYN methylglyoxal.

py·ru·vic-mal·ic car·box·yl·ase. SYN *malate* dehydrogenase.

6-py·ru·vo·yl·tet·ra·hy·drop·ter·in syn·thase (6-PTS). An enzyme that catalyzes a step in the synthesis of tetrahydrobiopterin; a deficiency of this enzyme will result in one form of hyperphenylalaninemia.

pyr·vin·i·um pam·o·ate (pir-vin′i-ŭm). A highly effective drug used in the eradication of human pinworms. SYN viprynium embonate.

Pyth·i·um in·si·di·o·sum (pith′ē-ŭm in-sid′ē-um). A species of fungi found in water or wet soil, and a cause of hyphomycosis or pythiosis.

py·tho·gen·e·sis (pī-thō-jen′ĕ-sis). **1.** Origination from decaying matter. **2.** The causation of decay. [G. *pythō,* to decay, + *genesis,* origin]

py·tho·gen·ic, py·thog·e·nous (pī-thō-jen′ik, pī-thoj′ĕ-nŭs). Originating from filth or putrescence.

py·u·ria (pī-ū′rē-ă). Presence of pus in the urine when voided. [G. *pyon,* pus, + *ouron,* urine]

Q Symbol for coulomb; quantity; quaternary; glutamine; glutaminyl; pseudouridine; coenzyme Q; electric charge; the second product formed in an enzyme-catalyzed reaction.

Q̇ Symbol for blood flow. SEE flow (3). [quantity + an overdot denoting the time derivative]

Q_O, Q_{O2}. Symbols for oxygen consumption (1).

Q_{10} Symbol for the increase in rate of a process produced by raising the temperature 10°C; rate of contraction of an excised heart approximately doubles for every 10°C (i.e., Q_{10} = 2).

Q_{CO} Symbol for the microliters STPD of CO_2 given off per milligram of tissue per hour.

△**-Q_6.** Symbol for ubiquinone-6.

△**-Q_{10}.** Symbol for ubiquinone-10.

q 1. In cytogenetics, symbol for long arm of a chromosome (in contrast to p for the short arm). **2.** Abbreviation for [L.] quodque, each; every. **3.** *q.* Symbol for heat.

QALY Acronym for quality-adjusted life years, an adjustment that allows for prevalence of activity limitation.

Q-band·ing. SEE Q-banding *stain*.

q.d. Abbreviation for L. *quaque die*, every day.

QF Abbreviation for quality *factor*, the same as relative biologic effectiveness in radiation protection.

QH_2 Symbol for ubiquinol.

q.h. Abbreviation for L. *quaque hora*, every hour.

q.i.d. Abbreviation for L. *quater in die*, four times a day.

q.l. Abbreviation for L. *quantum libet*, as much as desired.

QNB Abbreviation for quinuclidinyl benzilate.

Q.R. Abbreviation for [L] quantum rectum, however much is correct.

q.s. Abbreviation for L. *quantum sufficiat* or *satis*, as much as suffices.

Q-TWiST Time without symptoms or toxicity; a quality of life measurement. [acronym, *q*uality *t*ime *wi*thout *s*ymptoms or *t*oxicity]

quack (kwak). SYN charlatan. [Abbreviation of quacksalver, Dutch *quack*, to boast + *salf*, cream]

quack·ery (kwak'er-ē). SYN charlatanism.

qua·dran·gu·lar (kwah-drang'ū-lăr). Having four angles. [L. *quadrangularis*, fr. *quadrangulum*, quadrangle]

🔲**quad·rant** (kwah'drant). One quarter of a circle. In anatomy, roughly circular areas are divided for descriptive purposes into q.'s. The abdomen is divided into right upper and lower and left upper and lower q.'s by a horizontal and a vertical line intersecting at the umbilicus. Q.'s of the ocular fundus (superior and inferior nasal, superior and inferior temporal) are demarcated by a horizontal and a vertical line intersecting at the optic disk. The tympanic membrane is divided into anterosuperior, anteroinferior, posterosuperior, and posteroinferior q.'s by a line drawn across the diameter of the drum in the axis of the handle of the malleus and another intersecting the first at right angles at the umbo. [L. *quadrans*, a quarter]

quad·rant·an·o·pia (kwah'drant-an-op'ē-ă). Loss of vision in a quarter section of the visual field of one or both eyes; if bilateral, it may be homonymous or heteronymous, binasal or bitemporal, or crossed, e.g., involving the upper quadrant in one eye and the lower quadrant in the other. SYN quadrantic hemianopia.

quad·rate (kwah'drāt). Having four equal sides; square. [L. *quadratus*, square]

qua·dra·tus (kwah'drā-tŭs).
quadratus lumborum fascia, ✭official alternate term for anterior *layer* of thoracolumbar fascia.

△**quadri-.** Four. [L. *quattuor*]

quad·ri·ba·sic (kwah-dri-bā'sik). Denoting an acid having four hydrogen atoms that are replaceable by atoms or radicals of a basic character.

quad·ri·ceps (kwah'dri-seps). SYN four-headed *muscle*. [L. fr. quadri- + *caput*, head]

quad·ri·ceps·plas·ty (kwah-dri-seps'plas-tē). A corrective surgical procedure on the quadriceps femoris muscle and tendon to release adhesions and improve mobility. [quadriceps + G. *plastos*, formed]

quad·ri·cus·pid (kwah-dri-kŭs'pid). SYN tetracuspid.

quad·ri·dig·i·tate (kwah'dri-dij'i-tāt). SYN tetradactyl. [quadri- + L. *digitus*, digit]

quad·ri·gem·i·nal (kwah'dri-jem'i-năl). Four-fold. [quadri- + L. *geminus*, twin]

quad·ri·ge·mi·num (kwah'dri-jem'i-nŭm). One of the quadrigeminal bodies.

quad·ri·ge·mi·nus (kwah'dri-jem'i-nŭs). SYN quadruplet. [L.]

quad·ri·ge·mi·ny (kwah'dri-jem'i-nē). SYN quadrigeminal *rhythm*.

quad·ri·pa·re·sis (kwah'dri-pă-rē'sis). SYN tetraparesis.

quad·ri·ple·gia (kwah'dri-plē'jē-ă). Paralysis of all four limbs. SYN tetraplegia. [quadri- + G. *plēgē*, stroke]

quad·ri·ple·gic (kwah'dri-plē'jik). Pertaining to or afflicted with quadriplegia. SYN tetraplegic.

quad·ri·po·lar (kwah'dri-pō'lăr). Having four poles.

quad·ri·sect (kwah'dri-sekt). To divide into four parts. SYN quartisect. [quadri- + L. *seco*, pp. *sectus*, to cut]

quad·ri·sec·tion (kwah'dri-sek'shŭn). Division into four parts.

quad·ri·tu·ber·cu·lar (kwah'dri-too-ber'kū-lăr). Having four tubercles or cusps, as a molar tooth. [quadri- + L. *tuberculum*, tubercle]

quad·ri·va·lent (kwah-dri-vā'lent). Having the combining power (valency) of four. SYN tetravalent.

quad·ru·ped (kwah'droo-ped). A four-footed animal. [L. *quattuor*, four, + *pes* (*ped*-), foot]

quad·rup·let (kwah'drŭp-let, kwă-droo'plet). One of four children born at one birth. SYN quadrigeminus. [L. *quadruplus*, four-fold]

qual·i·ty as·sur·ance. Programs of regular assessment of medical and nursing activities to evaluate the quality of medical care.

Quant, C. A. J., early 20th century Dutch physician. SEE Quant *sign*.

quan·ta (kwahn'tă). Plural of quantum. [L.]

quan·ti·le (kwon'til). Division of a distribution into equal, ordered subgroups; deciles are tenths, quartiles are quarters, quintiles are fifths, terciles are thirds, centiles are hundredths. [L. *quantum*, how much, + -*ilis*, adj. suffix]

quan·tum, pl. **quan·ta** (kwahn'tŭm, -tă). **1.** A unit of radiant energy (ε) varying according to the frequency (ν) of the radiation. **2.** A certain definite amount. [L. how much]

q. mottle, SEE quantum *mottle*. See entries under under *mottle*.

q. rectum, SEE Q.R. [L. however much is correct]

q. satis, SEE q.s. [L. however much is enough]

q. sink, in radiologic imaging, the stage at which statistical information reaches its lowest level because of a low photon flux.

q. sufficiat, SEE q.s. [L. however much is enough]

q. vis (q.v.), SEE q.v. [L. however much you wish]

quar·an·tine (kwar'an-tēn). **1.** A period (originally 40 days) of detention of vessels and their passengers coming from an area where an infectious disease prevails. **2.** To detain such vessels and their passengers until the incubation period of an infectious disease has passed. **3.** A place where such vessels and their

---

△ Combining Forms	✭ Official alternate Terminologia Anatomica term
🔲 Indicates term is illustrated, see Illustration Index	
	[MIM] Mendelian Inheritance in Man
SYN Synonym	
Cf. Compare	C.I. Colour Index
[NA] Nomina Anatomica	
[TA] Terminologia Anatomica	**High Profile Term**

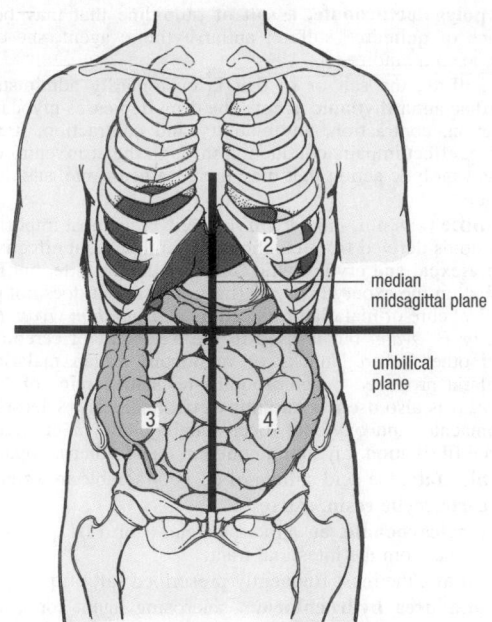

quadrants: (1) right upper, (2) left upper, (3) right lower, (4) left lower

passengers are detained. **4.** The isolation of a person with a known or possible contagious disease. [It. *quarantina* fr. L. *quadraginta,* forty]

quark (qwark). A fundamental particle believed to be the primary constituent of all mesons and baryons; q.'s have a charge that is a fraction of 1 electron charge and interact through electromagnetic and nuclear forces. Six varieties are thought to exist with the unusual names of up, down, strange, charmed, bottom, and top. [a word of indeterminate sense used by James Joyce in his novel *Finnegans Wake*]

quart (kwŏrt). **1.** A measure of fluid capacity; the fourth part of a gallon; the equivalent of 0.9468 liter. An imperial q. contains about 20% more than the ordinary q., or 1.1359 liters. **2.** A dry measure holding a little more than the fluid measure. [L. *quartus,* fourth]

quar·tan (kwŏr′tan). Recurring every fourth day, including the first day of an episode in the computation, i.e., after a free interval of two days. [L. *quartanus,* relating to a fourth (thing)]

double q., denoting malaria infection with two independent groups of q. parasites, so that paroxysms occur on two successive days followed by one day without fever.

triple q., denoting malaria infection with three independent groups of q. parasites, so that a paroxysm occurs every day, resembling a double tertian or a quotidian fever.

quar·ti·sect (kwŏr′ti-sekt). SYN quadrisect. [L. *quartus,* fourth, + *seco,* pp. *sectus,* to cut]

quartz (kwŏrts). A crystalline form of silicon dioxide used in chemical apparatus and in optical and electric instruments.

qua·si·dom·i·nance (kwā-si-dom′i-nans). Simulation of dominant inheritance of a recessive trait, e.g., a heterozygote mating with an affected homozygote resulting in the manifestation of the recessive trait generation after generation. SYN false dominance, pseudodominance.

qua·si·dom·i·nant (kwā-si-dom′i-nănt). Denoting a trait in an inbred pedigree that exhibits quasidominance.

quas·sa·tion (kwah-sā′shŭn). The breaking up of crude drug materials, such as bark and woody stems, into small pieces to facilitate extraction and other treatment. [L. *quassatio,* fr. *quasso,* pp. *-atus,* to shake violently, fr. *quatio,* to shake]

quas·sia (kwah′shē-ă). Bitterwood, the heartwood of *Picrasma excelsa* (*Picraena excelsa*), known as Jamaica q., or of *Quassia amara* (family Simarubaceae), known as Surinam q.; a bitter

tonic; the infusion has been administered by enema in the treatment of threadworms. [*Quassi,* a resident of Surinam who used it as a tonic]

quater in die (kua′ter-in-dē-ā). SEE q.i.d. [L. four times a day]

qua·ter·na·ry (Q) (kwah′ter-nār-ē, kwah-ter′nĕ-rē). **1.** Denoting a chemical compound containing four elements; e.g., $NaHSO_4$. Cf. quaternary *structure.* **2.** Fourth in a series. **3.** Relating to organic compounds in which some central atom is attached to four functional groups; applied to the usually trivalent nitrogen in its "onium" state, R_4N^+, "quaternary nitrogen." **4.** Referring to a level of structure of macromolecules in which more than one biopolymer is present. Cf. quaternary *structure.* [L. *quaternarius,* fr. *quaterni,* four each, fr. *quattuor,* four, + *-arius,* adj. suffix]

Quatrefages de Breau, Jean L.A. de, French naturalist, 1810–1892. SEE Quatrefages *angle.*

qua·ze·pam (kwā′zĕ-pam). A benzodiazepine derivative used as a sedative and hypnotic.

que·brach·ine (kē-brah′chēn). An alkaloid, $C_{21}H_{26}N_2O_3$, from quebracho and identical with yohimbine; formerly used in cardiac dyspnea.

que·bra·cho (kē-brah′chō). The dried bark of a genus of trees, *Aspidosperma quebrachoblanco* (family Apocynaceae); has been used as a respiratory stimulant in emphysema, dyspnea, and chronic bronchitis; the two chief alkaloids are aspidospermine and quebrachine. [Port. *quebrahacho,* fr. *quebrar,* to break, + *hacha,* axe, referring to the hardness of the wood]

Queckenstedt, Hans, German neurophysiologist, 1876–1918. SEE Q.-Stookey *test.*

quench·ing (kwench′ing). **1.** The process of extinguishing, removing, or diminishing a physical property such as heat or light; e.g., the cooling of a hot metal rapidly by plunging it into water or oil. **2.** In beta liquid scintillation counting, the shifting of the energy spectrum from a true to a lower energy; it is caused by a variety of interfering materials in the counting solution, including foreign chemicals and coloring agents. **3.** The process of stopping a chemical or enzymatic reaction. [M. E. *quenchen,* fr. O.E. *āc-wencan*]

fluorescence q., a technique used in investigations dealing with binding of antigens (haptens) by purified antibodies, applicable in cases in which the bound antigen (hapten) absorbs (quenches) light emitted during fluorescence of protein (antibody) excited by ultraviolet light.

Quénu, Eduard A.V.A., French surgeon and anatomist, 1852–1933. SEE Q. hemorrhoidal *plexus;* Q.-Muret *sign.*

quer·ce·tin (kwer′sē-tin). An aglycon of quercitrin, rutin, and other glycosides; occurs usually as the 3-rhamnoside; used in the treatment of abnormal capillary fragility. SYN meletin, sophoretin.

quer·cus (kwer′kŭs). The bark of *Quercus alba,* white oak or stone oak; formerly used as an astringent. [L. oak]

quer·u·lent (kwer′ŭ-lent). Denoting one who is ever suspicious, always opposing any suggestion, complaining of ill treatment and of being slighted or misunderstood, easily enraged, and dissatisfied; characteristic of paranoid personalities. [L. *querulus,* complaining, fr. *queror,* to complain]

Quervain, Fritz de. SEE de Quervain.

ques·tion·naire (kwes-chŭn-ār′). A list of questions submitted orally or in writing to obtain personal information or statistically useful data.

Holmes-Rahe q., a survey to measure in life change units the stressfulness of various life events such as an acute illness, bankruptcy, death of a loved one, etc.

Quetelet, Lambert Alphonse Jacques, 1796–1857. Belgian astronomer and mathematician.

Queyrat, Auguste, French dermatologist, *1872. SEE *erythroplasia* of Q.

Quick, Armand J., U.S. physician, 1894–1978. SEE Q. *method, test.*

quick (kwik). **1.** Pregnant with a child whose fetal movements are recognizable. **2.** A sensitive part, painful to touch. [A.S. *cwic,* living]

quick·en·ing (kwik′ĕn-ing). Signs of life felt by the mother as a result of fetal movements, usually noted from 16 to 20 weeks of pregnancy. [A.S. *cwic*, living]

quick·lime (kwik′līm). Unslaked lime. SEE lime (2).

quick·sil·ver (kwik′sil′ver). SYN mercury.

qui·es·cent (kwi-es′ent). At rest or inactive.

quin-2. (2-[(2-bis-[carboxymethyl]aono-5-methoxyphenyl)-methyl-6- methoxy-8-bis[carboxymethyl]aminoquinoline); a fluorescent compound that binds Ca^{++} tightly. The wavelengths of light that cause fluorescence when Ca^{++} is bound are longer than the wavelengths that cause fluorescence when Ca^{++} is not bound. When excited at two different wavelengths, the ratio of the fluorescence intensities at the two wavelengths gives the ratio of the concentrations of bound to free Ca^{++}. Free quin-2 concentration can be measured precisely, so free Ca^{++} concentration can be calculated precisely. Quin-2 may be injected into cells to measure moment-to-moment changes in intracellular Ca^{++} concentration. SEE ALSO aequorin, fura-2.

quin-, quino-. Root of quinoline and quinone, hence used in many names of substances containing these structures (e.g., quinine, quinol).

qui·na (kē′nă, kwē′nă). SYN cinchona. [Sp., fr. Peruv. *quina* or *kina*, cinchona]

quin·a·crine hy·dro·chlo·ride (kwin′ă-krēn, -krin). An acridine derivative, used as an antimalarial that destroys the trophozoites of *Plasmodium vivax* and *P. falciparum*, but does not affect the gametocytes, sporozoites, or exoerythrocytic stage of parasites; also used as an anthelmintic. As a dihydrochloride, it is used as a stain in cytogenetics to demonstrate Y chromatin by fluorescent microscopy. Q. h. intercalates with DNA and also uncouples oxidation and photophosphorylation. SYN atabrine hydrochloride, mepacrine hydrochloride.

quin·al·dic ac·id (kwin-al′dik). Quinoline-2-carboxylic acid; a product of L-tryptophan catabolism, via kynurenic acid, found in human urine. SYN quinaldinic acid.

quin·al·dine red (kwin′al-dēn). A styrene-quinolinium iodide; used as a pH indicator (turns red at pH 3.2) in a 1% ethanol solution.

quin·al·din·ic ac·id (kwin-al-din′ik). SYN quinaldic acid.

qui·na·qui·na (kē′nă-kē′nă, kwin′ă-kwin′ă). SYN cinchona. [a reduplication of Sp. *quina*, cinchona]

qui·nate (kwī′nāt, kwin′āt). A salt or ester of quinic acid.

q. dehydrogenase, an oxidoreductase catalyzing reaction of quinate and NAD$^+$ to form 3-dehydroquinate and NADH.

quin·a·zo·lines (kwin-a-zōl′ēns). A class of alkaloids that are derived biosynthetically from anthranilic acid.

quince (kwints). The edible fruit of *Cydonia oblongata* (family Rosaceae); the seeds have demulcent properties.

Quincke, Heinrich I., German physician, 1842–1922. SEE Q. *pulse, puncture, sign.*

quin·es·tra·di·ol, quin·es·tra·dol (kwin′es-tră-dī′ol, kwin-es′ tră-dol). An estrogen.

quin·es·trol (kwin-es′trōl). The 3-cyclopentyl ether of ethinyl estradiol; used as the estrogenic component in oral contraceptive preparations; the compound is stored in fat and can be taken weekly; an estrogen.

quin·eth·a·zone (kwin-eth′ă-zōn). A diuretic and antihypertensive agent.

quin·ges·ta·nol ac·e·tate (kwin-jes′tă-nol). A progestational agent.

quin·hy·drone (kwin-hī′drōn). A mixture of equimolecular quantities of quinone and hydroquinone; used in pH determinations (i.e., via a q. electrode).

quin·ic ac·id (kwin′ik). L-quinic acid; the (−) isomer is an acid found in cinchona bark and elsewhere in plants; 5-dehydroquinic acid is an intermediate in the biosynthesis of L-phenylalanine, L-tyrosine, and L-tryptophan from carbohydrate precursors; q. a. forms a γ-lactone upon heating. SYN kinic acid.

quin·i·dine (kwin′i-dēn, -din). β-Quinine; one of the alkaloids of cinchona, a stereoisomer of quinine (the C-9 epimer); used as an antimalarial; also used in the treatment of atrial fibrillation and flutter, and paroxysmal ventricular tachycardia. SYN conquinine.

q. polygalacturonate, a salt of quinidine that may be used in place of quinidine sulfate; antiarrhythmic agent. SEE q. sulfate; SEE ALSO quinidine.

q. sulfate, the salt of q. that is customarily administered as a cardiac antiarrhythmic agent. The drug depresses myocardial conduction, contraction, automaticity and contraction; it also by a direct effect impairs conduction through the atrioventricular node. Has vagolytic action that may increase heart rate. SEE ALSO quinidine.

qui·nine (kwī′nīn, -nēn, kwin′-īn, -ēn). The most important of the alkaloids derived from cinchona; an antimalarial effective against the asexual and erythrocytic forms of the parasite, but having no effect on the exoerythrocytic (tissue) forms. It does not produce a radical cure of malaria produced by *Plasmodium vivax*, *P. malariae*, or *P. ovale*, but is used in the treatment of cerebral malaria and other severe attacks of malignant tertian malaria, and in malaria produced by chloroquine-resistant strains of *P. falciparum;* it is also used as an antipyretic, analgesic, sclerosing agent, stomachic, and oxytocic (occasionally), and in the treatment of atrial fibrillation, myotonia congenita, and other myopathies.

q. bisulfate, the acid sulfate of q., very soluble in water.

q. carbacrylic resin, SEE resin.

q. ethylcarbonate, an almost tasteless form of q. that is poorly absorbed from the intestinal tract.

q. sulfate, the most frequently prescribed salt of q.

q. and urea hydrochloride, sclerosing agent for treatment of internal hemorrhoids, hydrocele, and varicose veins, containing not less than 58% and not more than 65% of anhydrous q.

q. urethan, a mixture of urethan and q. hydrochloride; a sclerosing agent for the treatment of varicose veins.

qui·nin·ism (kwī′ni-nizm, kwin′i-). SYN cinchonism.

Quinlan test. See under test.

quino-. SEE quin-.

quin·o·cide hy·dro·chlo·ride (kwin′ō-sīd). An antimalarial comparable to primaquine in effectiveness and scope.

quin·ol (kwin′ol). SYN hydroquinone.

quin·o·line (kwin′ō-lēn, -lin). **1.** Benzo[*b*]pyridine; 1-benzazine; a volatile nitrogenous base obtained by the distillation of coal tar, bones, alkaloids, etc.; a basic structure of many dyes and drugs; also used as an antimalarial. SYN chinoleine, leucoline. **2.** One of a class of alkaloids based on the q. (1) structure.

quin·o·lin·ic ac·id (kwin-ō-lin′ik). A catabolite of L-tryptophan and a precursor of NAD$^+$.

quin·o·lin·ol (kwin-ol′in-ol). SYN 8-hydroxyquinoline.

quin·o·li·zi·dines (kwin-ol-i-za-dēns). A class of alkaloids based on the quinolizidine (norlupinane) structure.

qui·nol·o·gy (kwin-ol′ō-jē). The botany, chemistry, pharmacology, and therapeutics of cinchona and its alkaloids. [Sp. *quina*, cinchona, + G. *logos*, study]

quin·o·lones (kwin′ō-lōnz). A class of synthetic broad-spectrum antibacterial agents that exhibit bactericidal action (e.g., ciprofloxacin). SYN fluoroquinolone.

qui·none (kwin′ōn, kwī′nōn). **1.** General name for aromatic compounds bearing two oxygens in place of two hydrogens, usually in the *para* position; the oxidation product of a hydroquinone. **2.** SYN 1,4-benzoquinone (1).

q. reductase, SYN *NADPH* dehydrogenase (quinone).

qui·no·vose (kwin′ō-vōs). SYN D-epirhamnose.

quin·que·dig·i·tate (kwin′kwē-dij′i-tāt). SYN pentadactyl. [L. *quinque*, five, + *digitus*, digit]

quin·que·tu·ber·cu·lar (kwin′kwĕ-too-ber′kū-lăr). Having five tubercles or cusps, as certain molar teeth. [L. *quinque*, five, + *tuberculum*, tubercle, dim. of *tuber*, a swelling]

quin·que·va·lent (kwin-kwĕ-vā′lent). SYN pentavalent. [L. *quinque*, five, + *valentia*, strength]

quin·qui·na (kwin-kwi′nă). SYN cinchona.

quin·sy (kwin′zē). Obsolete term for peritonsillar *abscess*. [M.E. *quinsie* (*quinesie*), a corruption of L. *cynanche*, sore throat]

lingual q., phlegmonous inflammation of the lingual tonsil and neighboring structures.

quin·tan (kwin′tan). Recurring every fifth day, including the first day of an episode in the computation, i.e., after a free interval of three days. [L. *quintus,* fifth]

quin·tu·plet (kwin-tŭp′let). One of five children born at one birth. [L. *quintuplex,* fivefold]

qui·nuc·li·din·yl ben·zi·late (QNB) (kwin-oo′-kli-di-nil ben′-zil-āt). A highly potent anticholinergic agent exhibiting 50- to 100-fold greater potency over atropine in binding with and blocking muscarinic cholinergic receptors. Originally developed as a potential military incapacitating agent, it is currently extensively used as a radioactive agent (usually tritiated –H3 –QNB) to identify and label muscarinic receptors in pharmacologic studies.

quis·qua·late (kwiz′kwa-lāt). An agonist at glutamate receptors of the amino-3-hydroxy-5-methyl-isoxazole-4-propionic acid (AMPA) type. The anion formed when quisqualic acid is dissolved in water. SEE quisqualic acid.

quis·qual·ic ac·id (kwiz′kwa-lik). Excitatory amino acid (EAA) obtained from the seeds of *Quisqualis chinensis.* Used to identify a specific subset of non–*N*-methyl *D*-aspartate (NMDA) EAA receptor; has anthelmintic properties.

quod·que (q). Each, every. [L.]

quo·tid·i·an (kwō-tid′ē-ăn). Daily; occurring every day. [L. *quotidianus,* daily, fr. *quot,* as many as, + *dies,* day]

quo·tient (kwo′shĕnt). The number of times one amount is contained in another; the ratio of two numbers. SEE ALSO index (2), ratio. [L. *quoties,* how often]

achievement q., a ratio, percentile rating, or related q. denoting the amount a child has learned in relation to peers of his or her age or level of education.

Ayala q., SYN Ayala *index.*

cognitive laterality q. (CLQ), test for difference in cognitive performance of left and right sides of the brain.

extremal q., the ratio of the rate in the jurisdiction with the highest rate of interventions such as surgical procedures to the rate in the jurisdiction with the lowest rate.

intelligence q. (IQ), the psychologist's index of measured intelligence as one part of a two-part determination of intelligence, the other part being an index of adaptive behavior and including such criteria as school grades or work performance. IQ is a score, or similar quantitative index, used to denote a person's standing relative to age peers on a test of general ability, ordinarily expressed as a ratio between the person's score on a given test and the score that the average individual of comparable age attained on the same test, the ratio being computed by the psychologist or determined from a table of age norms, such as the various Wechsler intelligence scales.

Meyerhof oxidation q., an index for the effect of oxygen on glycolysis and on fermentation (i.e., on the Pasteur effect); equal to the rate of anaerobic fermentation minus the rate of aerobic respiration divided by the rate of oxygen uptake.

P/O q., SYN P/O *ratio.*

protein q., the number obtained by dividing the quantity of globulin of the blood plasma by the quantity of albumin.

respiratory q. (R.Q.), the steady-state ratio of carbon dioxide produced by tissue metabolism to oxygen consumed in the same metabolism; for the whole body, normally about 0.82 under basal conditions; in the steady state, the respiratory q. is equal to the respiratory exchange ratio. SYN respiratory coefficient.

spinal q., SYN Ayala *index.*

quot. op. sit. Abbreviation for quoties opus sit, as often as necessary.

q.v. Abbreviation for [L] *quantum>* vis, as much as you wish.

qu

ρ **1.** The 17th letter of the Greek alphabet, rho. **2.** Symbol for population correlation coefficient; density.

R Abbreviation or symbol for electrical resistance; radical (usually an alkyl or aryl group, e.g., ROH is an alcohol, RNH_2 an amine); Réaumur; respiration; respiratory exchange *ratio*; roentgen; the remainder of a chemical formula; the calculated unit representing vascular resistance in the cardiovascular system; arginine; arginyl; purine nucleoside.

℞ Symbol for *recipe* in a prescription. SEE prescription (2).

R$_f$, R$_F$ Symbol denoting movement of a substance in paper chromatography *r*elative to the solvent *f*ront (i.e., retardation factor); equal to the migration distance of a substance divided by the migration distance of the solvent front.

R. Abbreviation or symbol for (in italics) molar gas *constant*; one of two stereochemical designations in the Cahn, Ingold, and Prelog system; the third product formed in an enzyme-catalyzed reaction.

r Abbreviation for roentgen; radius.

***r.* 1.** Symbol for correlation *coefficient*. **2.** Abbreviation for racemic, occasionally used in naming compounds in place of the more common DL or (±), as "*r*-alanine" (more often as the prefix *rac*-).

Ra Symbol for radium.

rab·bet·ing (rab′et-ing). Obsolete term for making congruous stepwise cuts on apposing bone surfaces for stability after impaction. [Fr. *raboter*, to plane]

rab·id. Relating to or suffering from rabies. [L. *rabidus*, raving, mad]

🔢**ra·bies** (rā′bēz). Highly fatal infectious disease that may affect all species of warm-blooded animals, including humans; transmitted by the bite of infected animals including dogs, cats, skunks, wolves, foxes, raccoons, and bats, and caused by a neurotropic species of Lyssavirus, a member of the family Rhabdoviridae, in the central nervous system and the salivary glands. The symptoms are characteristic of a profound disturbance of the nervous system, e.g., excitement, aggressiveness, and madness, followed by paralysis and death. Characteristic cytoplasmic inclusion bodies (Negri bodies) found in many of the neurons are an aid to rapid laboratory diagnosis. SYN hydrophobia. [L. rage, fury, fr. *rabio*, to rave, to be mad]

dumb r., SYN paralytic r.

furious r., the form or stage of r. in which the animal is markedly hyperactive, characterized by periods of agitation, thrashing, running, snapping, or biting.

paralytic r., a form or stage of r. marked by paralytic symptoms. SYN dumb r.

ra·bi·form (rā′bi-fōrm). Resembling rabies.

△***rac-.*** Prefix for racemic.

ra·ce·fem·ine (rā-sě-fem′ēn). Used as a uterine relaxant for relief of postpartum pain.

rac·e·mase (rā′sě-mās). An enzyme capable of catalyzing racemization, i.e., inversions of asymmetric groups; when more than one center of asymmetry is present, "epimerase" is used (e.g., hydroxyproline, ribulose phosphate).

rac·e·mate (rā′sě-māt). A racemic compound, or the salt or ester of such a compound. SEE ALSO racemic.

ra·ceme (rā-sēm′). An optically inactive chemical compound. SEE ALSO racemic.

ra·ce·mic (*r*) (rā-sē′mik, -sem′ik). Denoting a mixture of opti-

△ **Combining Forms**	☆ **Official alternate Terminologia Anatomica term**
🔢 **Indicates term is illustrated, see Illustration Index**	
	[MIM] Mendelian Inheritance in Man
SYN Synonym	
Cf. Compare	**C.I. Colour Index**
[NA] Nomina Anatomica	
[TA] Terminologia Anatomica	__**High Profile Term**__

rabies postexposure prophylaxis guide

animal type	evaluation of animal	treatment of exposed person[1]
domestic dogs and cats	healthy and available for 10 days of observation	none, unless animal develops symptoms of rabies[2]
	rabid or suspected rabid	HRIG[3] and HDCV or RVA[4] immediately
	unknown (escaped)	consult public health officials; if treatment is indicated, give HRIG[3] and HDCV or RVA
wild skunks, raccoons, bats, foxes, coyotes, and other carnivores	regard as rabid unless geographic area is known to be free of rabies or until animal is proved negative for rabies by laboratory tests[5]	HRIG[3] and HDCV or RVA[4] immediately
other livestock, rodents, and lagomorphs (rabbits and hares)	consider individually; local and state public health officials should be consulted about the need for rabies prophylaxis; bites of squirrels, hamsters, guinea pigs, gerbils, chipmunks, rats, mice, other rodents, rabbits, and hares almost never require antirabies prophylaxis	

the preceding recommendations are only a guide; in applying them, take into account the animal species involved, the circumstances of the bite or other exposure, the vaccination status of the animal, and the presence of rabies in the region; *note:* local or state public health officials should be consulted if questions arise about the need for rabies prophylaxis

[1] All bites and wounds should *immediately be thoroughly cleansed with soap and water*; if antirabies treatment is indicated, both human rabies immune globulin (HRIG) and human diploid cell rabies vaccine (HDCV) or rabies vaccine, absorbed (RVA) should be given as soon as possible, *regardless* of the interval from exposure

[2] During the usual holding period of 10 days, begin treatment with HRIG and vaccine at first sign of rabies in a dog or cat that has bitten someone; the symptomatic animal should be killed immediately and tested

[3] If HRIG is not available, use antirabies serum, equine; do not use more than the recommended dosage

[4] Local reactions to vaccines are common and do not contradict continuing treatment; discontinue vaccine if fluorescent antibody test results of the animal are negative

[5] The animal should be killed and tested as soon as possible; holding for observation is not recommended

cally active compounds that is itself optically inactive, being composed of an equal number of dextro- and levorotatory substances, which are separable. Those compounds internally compensated (i.e., having an internal plane of symmetry) and therefore not separable into D and L (or + and −) forms, are termed "*meso*."

rac·e·mi·za·tion (rā′sē-mi-zā′shŭn, ras-mi-). Partial conversion of one enantiomorph into another (as an L-amino acid to the corresponding D-amino acid) so that the specific optical rotation is decreased, or even reduced to zero, in the resulting mixture.

rac·e·mose (ras′ĕ-mōs). Branching, with nodular terminations; resembling a bunch of grapes. [L. *racemosus*, full of clusters]

rac·e·phed·rine hy·dro·chlo·ride (rās-ĕ-fed′rin). A sympathomimetic drug with peripheral effects similar to those of epinephrine and with the same actions and uses as ephedrine.

♲**rachi-, rachio-.** The spine. [G. *rhachis*, spine, backbone]

ra·chi·al (rā′kē-ăl). SYN spinal.

ra·chi·cen·te·sis (rā-kē-sen-tē′sis). SYN lumbar *puncture*. [rachi- + G. *kentēsis*, puncture]

ra·chid·i·al (rā-kid′ē-ăl). SYN spinal.

ra·chid·i·an (rā-kid′ē-an). SYN spinal.

ra·chil·y·sis (ră-kil′i-sis). Forcible correction of lateral curvature of the spine by lateral pressure against the convexity of the curve. [rachi- + G. *lysis*, a loosening]

♲**rachio-.** SEE rachi-.

ra·chi·o·cen·te·sis (rā-kē-ō-sen-tē′sis). SYN lumbar *puncture*. [rachio- + G. *kentēsis*, puncture]

ra·chi·och·y·sis (rā-kē-ok′i-sis). A subarachnoid effusion of fluid in the spinal canal. [rachio- + G. *chysis*, a pouring out]

ra·chi·op·a·gus (rā-kē-op′ă-gŭs). Conjoined twins united back to back with union of their spinal columns. SEE conjoined *twins*, under *twin*. SYN rachipagus. [rachio- + G. *pagos*, something fixed]

ra·chi·o·ple·gia (rā′kē-ō-plē′jē-ă). SYN spinal *paralysis*. [rachio- + G. *plēgē*, stroke]

ra·chi·o·tome (rā′kē-ō-tōm). A specially devised instrument for dividing the laminae of the vertebrae. SYN rachitome. [rachio- + G. *tomē*, incision]

ra·chi·ot·o·my (rā-kē-ot′ō-mē). SYN laminotomy. [rachio- + G. *tomē*, incision]

ra·chip·a·gus (ră-kip′ă-gŭs). SYN rachiopagus.

ra·chis, pl. **rach·i·des, ra·chis·es** (rā′kis, rā′ki-dēz, rak-). SYN vertebral *column*. [G. spine, backbone]

ra·chis·chi·sis (ră-kis′ki-sis). 1. Embryologic failure of fusion of vertebral arches and neural tube with consequent exposure of neural tissue at the surface; spina bifida cystica with myelocele or myeloschisis. 2. Spinal dysraphism. [G. *rhachis*, spine, + *schisis*, division]

r. partia′lis, SYN merorachischisis.

r. tota′lis, SYN holorachischisis.

ra·chit·ic (ră-kit′ic). Relating to or suffering from rickets (rachitis). SYN rickety.

ra·chi·tis (ră-kī′tis). SYN rickets. [G. *rhachitis*]

r. feta′lis, congenital rickets. SYN r. intrauterina, r. uterina.

r. feta′lis annula′ris, congenital enlargement of the epiphyses of the long bones.

r. feta′lis micromel′ica, a congenital condition in which development of the long bones is deficient.

r. intrauteri′na, r. uteri′na, SYN r. fetalis.

r. tar′da, SYN osteomalacia.

ra·chi·tism (rak′i-tizm). A rachitic state or tendency.

rach·i·to·gen·ic (ră-kit-ō-jen′ik). Producing or causing rickets. [rachitis + G. *genesis*, production]

ra·chi·tome (rak′i-tōm). SYN rachiotome.

rad 1. The unit for the dose absorbed from ionizing radiation, equivalent to 100 ergs per gram of tissue; 100 rad = 1 Gy. **2.** Symbol for radian.

ra·dar·ky·mog·ra·phy (rā′dar-kī-mog′ră-fē). An obsolete procedure involving the video tracking of heart motion by means of

image intensification and closed circuit television during fluoroscopy; enabled cardiac motion to be measured by reproducible linear graphic tracing.

ra·dec·to·my (rā-dek′tō-mē). SYN root *amputation*. [L. *radix*, root, + G. *ektomē*, excision]

Radford, Edward P., Jr., U.S. physiologist, *1922. SEE R. *nomogram.*

ra·di·a·bil·i·ty (rā′dē-ă-bil′i-tē). The property of being radiable.

ra·di·a·ble (rā′dē-ă-bl). Capable of being penetrated or examined by rays, especially by x-rays.

ra·di·ad (rā′dē-ad). In a direction toward the radial side.

ra·di·al (rā′dē-ăl). **1.** Relating to the radius (bone of the forearm), to any structures named from it, or to the radial or lateral aspect of the upper limb as compared to the ulnar or medial aspect. SYN radialis [TA]. **2.** Relating to any radius. **3.** Radiating; diverging in all directions from any given center. [L. *radialis*, fr. *radius*, ray, lateral bone of the forearm]

ra·di·a·lis (rā-dē-ā′lis) [TA]. SYN radial (1). [Mod. L.]

ra·di·an (rad) (rā′dē-ăn). A supplementary SI unit of plane angle. [L. *radius*, ray]

ra·di·ant (rā′dē-ant). **1.** Giving out rays. **2.** A point from which light radiates to the eye.

ra·di·ate (rā′dē-āt). **1.** To spread out in all directions from a center. **2.** To emit radiation. [L. *radio*, pp. -*atus*, to shine]

ra·di·a·tio, pl. **ra·di·a·ti·o·nes** (rā-dē-ā′shē-ō, -shē-ō′nēz). In neuroanatomy, a term applied to any one of the thalamocortical fiber systems that together compose the corona radiata of the cerebral hemisphere's white matter (e.g., optic radiation, acoustic radiation, etc.). SYN radiation (3). [L.]

r. acus′tica [TA], SYN acoustic *radiation*.

r. cor′poris callo′si [TA], SYN *radiation* of corpus callosum.

r. inferior thalami [TA], SYN inferior thalamic *peduncle*.

r. op′tica [TA], SYN optic *radiation*.

r. pyramida′lis, SYN pyramidal *radiation*.

r. thalami anterior [TA], SYN anterior thalamic *radiation*.

r. thalami centralis [TA], SYN central thalamic *radiation*.

r. thalamica posterior [TA], SYN posterior thalamic *radiation*.

ra·di·a·tion (rā′dē-ā′shŭn). **1.** The act or condition of diverging in all directions from a center. **2.** The sending forth of light, short radio waves, ultraviolet or x-rays, or any other rays for treatment or diagnosis or for other purpose. Cf. irradiation (2). **3.** SYN radiatio. **4.** A ray. **5.** Radiant energy or a radiant beam. [L. *radiatio*, fr. *radius*, ray, beam]

acoustic r. [TA], the fibers that pass from the medial geniculate body to the transverse temporal gyri of the cerebral cortex by way of the sublentiform part of the internal capsule. SYN radiatio acustica [TA].

afterloading r., method of administering r. that involves initial placement of local catheters with later installation of the r. source.

alpha r., an emission of a nucleus of high kinetic energy from the nucleus of an atom undergoing radioactive decay or fission.

annihilation r., the r. resulting when a positron from beta positive decay comes to rest. It encounters an electron, and they annihilate each other and convert their rest mass into two 0.51-MeV gamma rays emitted in exactly opposite directions. SEE *pair* production.

anterior thalamic r. [TA], r. formed by fibers interconnecting, via the anterior limb of the internal capsule, the anterior and medial thalamic nuclei and the cerebral cortex of the frontal lobe (excluding the precentral gyrus bordering on the central sulcus). SYN radiatio thalami anterior [TA].

background r., irradiation from environmental sources, including the earth's crust, the atmosphere, cosmic rays, and ingested radionuclides.

Natural sources account for the largest amount of radiation received by most persons each year (average annual dose, 3.00 mSv), with medical and occupational sources providing only a fraction (average less than 0.60 mSv). It is currently believed that radon, a gas produced by radium decay within crystal rock, constitutes the major source of background radiation throughout many parts of the U.S.

ra

Radon buildup in inadequately ventilated homes may pose a long-term health hazard. The deleterious effects of background radiation, estimated as causing 1–6% of spontaneous genetic mutations, rise with dose.

beta r., radiant energy from a source of beta rays.

central thalamic r. [TA], r. formed by fibers interconnecting, through the posterior limb of the internal capsule, the ventral lateral, ventral posterolateral and posteromedial, lateral dorsal, and lateral posterior nuclei and the precentral gyrus and parietal lobe of the cerebral cortex. SYN radiatio thalami centralis [TA].

Cerenkov r., light given off by a transparent medium when a high-energy particle speeds through it at a velocity greater than that of light in that medium.

characteristic r., monochromatic r. that is produced when an electron is ejected from an atom and another takes its place by jumping from another shell; the energy of the emitted photon is the difference between that of the two shell positions. SEE photoelectric *effect.* SYN characteristic emission.

r. of corpus callosum [TA], the spreading out of the fibers of the corpus callosum in the centrum semiovale of each cerebral hemisphere. SYN radiatio corporis callosi [TA].

corpuscular r., r. consisting of streams of subatomic particles such as protons, electrons, neutrons, etc.

electromagnetic r., r. originating in a varying electromagnetic field; e.g., long and short radio waves; light, visible and invisible; x-radiation and gamma rays.

gamma r., ionizing electromagnetic r. resulting from nuclear processes, such as radioactive decay or fission.

geniculocalcarine r., SYN optic r.

Gratiolet r., SYN optic r.

hemibody r., a palliative cancer therapy involving r. to one-half of the body. [hemi- + body]

heterogeneous r., r. consisting of different frequencies, various energies, or a variety of particles. SEE ALSO polychromatic r.

homogeneous r., r. consisting of a narrow band of frequencies, the same energy, or a single type of particle.

hyperfractionated r., smaller fractions of a dose of r. given more frequently than daily.

hypofractionated r., larger fractions of a dose of r. given less frequently than daily.

inferior thalamic r. [TA], SYN inferior thalamic *peduncle.*

ionizing r., corpuscular (e.g., neutrons, electrons) or electromagnetic (e.g., gamma) r. of sufficient energy to ionize the irradiated material.

K-r., usually a very penetrating form of x-r. excited by cathode rays (high-speed electrons) impinging upon a metal anode such as tungsten; the energy of the r. is a function of the binding energy of the K-shell electrons of the metal anode.

L-r., an x-r. of slight penetrating power excited by cathode rays (high-speed electrons) impinging on a metal anode; the energy of the r. is a function of the binding energy of the L-shell electrons of the metal anode.

monochromatic r., light rays or ionizing r. of a very narrow band of wavelengths (ideally, of a single wavelength). Cf. photopeak, characteristic r.

neutron r., an emission of neutrons from the nucleus of an atom by decay or fission.

occipitothalamic r., SYN optic r.

optic r. [TA], the massive, fanlike fiber system passing from the lateral geniculate body of the thalamus to the visual cortex (striate or calcarine cortex, area 17 of Brodmann); the fibers follow the retrolenticular and sublenticular limbs of the internal capsule into the corona radiata but they curve back along the lateral wall of the temporal and occipital horns of the lateral ventricle to the striate cortex on the medial surface and pole of the occipital lobe. SYN radiatio optica [TA], geniculocalcarine r., geniculocalcarine tract, Gratiolet fibers, Gratiolet r., occipitothalamic r., Wernicke r.

polychromatic r., r. containing gamma *rays,* under *ray* of many different energies; in diagnostic radiology, typically bremsstrahlung.

posterior thalamic r. [TA], r. formed by fibers interconnecting through the retrolenticular part of the posterior limb of the internal capsule, the pulvinar complex and lateral geniculate nucleus, and the posterior parietal and occipital lobes of the cerebral cortex. SYN radiatio thalamica posterior [TA].

primary r., an incident x-ray beam.

pyramidal r., corticospinal fibers passing from the cortex into the pyramid. SYN radiatio pyramidalis.

scattered r., secondary r. emitted from the interaction of x-rays with matter; generally lower in energy, with a directional distribution that depends on the energy of the incident r. SYN secondary r.

secondary r., SYN scattered r.

Wernicke r., SYN optic r.

rad·i·cal (rad′i-kăl). **1.** In chemistry, a group of elements or atoms usually passing intact from one compound to another, but usually incapable of prolonged existence in a free state (e.g., methyl, CH_3); in chemical formulas, a r. is often distinguished by being enclosed in parentheses or brackets. **2.** Thorough or extensive; relating or directed to the extirpation of the root or cause of a morbid process; e.g., a r. operation. **3.** Denoting treatment by extreme, drastic, or innovative, as opposed to conservative, measures. **4.** SYN free r. [L. *radix* (*radic-*), root]

acid r., a r. formed from an acid by loss of one or more hydrogen ions; e.g., SO_4^-, NO_3^-.

color r., SYN chromophore.

free r., a r. in its (usually transient) uncombined state; an atom or atom group carrying an unpaired electron and no charge; e.g., hydroxyl $(\cdot\underset{\cdot\cdot}{O}:H)$ and methyl

$$\left(H:\underset{\cdot\cdot}{\overset{H}{\underset{H}{C}}}\cdot \right)$$

Free r.'s may be involved as short-lived, highly active intermediates in various reactions in living tissue, notably in photosynthesis. The free r. nitric oxide, NO, plays an important role in vasodilation. SYN radical (4).

Free radicals occur naturally within the body as a result of metabolic processes and can also be introduced from without (through smoking, inhaling environmental pollutants, or exposure to UV radiation). They interact readily with nearby molecules and may cause cellular damage, including genetic alterations. It has been theorized that they are involved in plaque formation in atherosclerosis, in cancer, and in degenerative disorders such as Alzheimer dementia and parkinsonism. Natural enzymes such as superoxide dismutase and peroxidase are thought to counteract free radicals, and there is evidence that many nutrients, including vitamins C and E and β-carotene, also exert an antioxidant effect. SEE ALSO antioxidant.

oxygen-derived free r.'s, an atom or atom group having an unpaired electron on an oxygen atom, typically derived from molecular oxygen. For example, one-electron reduction of O_2 produces the superoxide radical, $\bar{O}_2\cdot$; other examples include the hydroperoxyl radical (HOO·), the hydroxyl radical (HO·), and nitric oxide (NO·). These apparently have a role in reprofusion injury.

ra·di·ces (ra-dī′sēz). Plural of radix.

rad·i·cle (rad′i-kl). A rootlet or structure resembling one, as the r. of a *vein,* a minute veinlet joining with others to form a vein, or the r. of a *nerve,* a nerve fiber that joins others to form a nerve. [L. *radicula,* dim. of *radix,* root]

rad·i·cot·o·my (rad-i-kot′ō-mē). SYN rhizotomy. [L. *radix* (*radic-*), root, + G. *tomē,* incision]

△**radicul-.** SEE radiculo-.

ra·dic·u·la (ră-dik′ū-lă). A spinal nerve root. [L. dim of *radix,* root]

ra·dic·u·lal·gia (ra-dik′ū-lal′jē-ă). Neuralgia due to irritation of the sensory root of a spinal nerve. [radicul- + G. *algos,* pain]

ra·dic·u·lar (ra-dik′ū-lăr). **1.** Relating to a radicle. **2.** Pertaining to the root of a tooth.

ra·dic·u·lec·to·my (ra-dik′ū-lek′tō-mē). SYN rhizotomy. [radicul- + G. *ektomē*, excision]

ra·dic·u·li·tis (ra-dik-ū-lī′tis). SYN radiculopathy. [radicul- + G. *-itis*, inflammation]

   acute brachial r., SYN neuralgic *amyotrophy.*

⌂**radiculo-, radicul-.** Radicle; radicular. [L. *radicula,* radicle, dim. of *radix,* root]

ra·dic·u·lo·gang·li·o·ni·tis (ra-dik′ū-lō-gang′glē-ō-nī′tis). Involvement of roots and ganglia.

ra·dic·u·lo·me·nin·go·my·e·li·tis (ra-dik′ū-lō-mĕ-ning′gō-mī-ĕ-lī′tis). SYN rhizomeningomyelitis.

ra·dic·u·lo·my·e·lop·a·thy (ra-dik′ū-lō-mī′ĕ-lop′ă-thē). SYN myeloradiculopathy.

ra·dic·u·lo·neu·rop·a·thy (ra-dik′ū-lō-noo-rop′ă-thē). Disease of the spinal nerve roots and nerves.

ra·dic·u·lop·a·thy (ra-dik′ū-lop′ă-thē). Disorder of the spinal nerve roots. SYN radiculitis. [radiculo- + G. *pathos,* suffering]

   diabetic thoracic r., a type of diabetic neuropathy that affects primarily elderly patients with diabetes mellitus; clinically characterized by thoracic or abdominal pain, mainly anterior, but sometimes with radiation around the trunk from the midline; usually unilateral; may extend over several segments; probably due to ischemic injury of two or more contiguous roots; one type of diabetic polyradiculopathy.

ra·di·ec·to·my (rā-dē-ek′tō-mē). SYN root *amputation.* [L. *radix,* root, + G. *ektomē,* excision]

ra·dif·er·ous (rā-dif′er-ŭs). Containing radium.

ra·dii (rā′dē-ī). Plural of radius. [L.]

⌂**radio-.** **1.** Radiation, chiefly (in medicine) gamma or x-ray. **2.** SYN radioactive. **3.** SYN radius. [L. *radius,* ray]

ra·di·o·ac·tive (rā′dē-ō-ak′tiv). Possessing radioactivity. SYN radio- (2).

ra·di·o·ac·tive cow. Colloquialism for radionuclide *generator.* SEE ALSO COW.

ra·di·o·ac·tiv·i·ty (rā′dē-ō-ak-tiv′i-tē). The property of some atomic nuclei of spontaneously emitting gamma rays or subatomic particles (α and β rays) by the process of nuclear disintegration and measured in disintegrations per second (dps). One dps is equal to 1 becquerel, and 3.7×10^{10} dps equals 1 curie.

   artificial r., the r. of isotopes created by the bombardment of naturally occurring isotopes by subatomic particles, or high levels of x- or gamma radiation. SYN induced r.

   induced r., SYN artificial r.

ra·di·o·au·to·gram (rā′dē-ō-aw′tō-gram). Older term for autoradiograph.

ra·di·o·au·tog·ra·phy (rā′dē-ō-aw-tog′ră-fē). SYN autoradiography.

ra·di·o·bi·cip·i·tal (rā′dē-ō-bī-sip′i-tăl). Relating to the radius and the biceps muscle.

ra·di·o·bi·ol·o·gy (rā′dē-ō-bī-ol′ō-jē). The study of the biologic effects of ionizing radiation upon living tissue. Cf. radiopathology.

ra·di·o·cal·ci·um (rā′dē-ō-kal′sē-ŭm). A radioisotope of calcium, particularly calcium-45.

ra·di·o·car·bon (rā′dē-ō-kar′bŏn). A radioactive isotope of carbon; e.g., ^{14}C.

ra·di·o·car·di·o·gram (rā′dē-ō-kar′dē-ō-gram). A graphic record of the concentration of injected radioisotope within the cardiac chambers.

ra·di·o·car·di·og·ra·phy (rā′dē-ō-kar-dē-og′ră-fē). The technique of recording or interpreting radiocardiograms.

ra·di·o·car·pal (rā′dē-ō-kar′păl). **1.** Relating to the radius and the bones of the carpus. **2.** On the radial or lateral side of the carpus.

ra·di·o·ceph·al·pel·vim·e·try (rā′dē-ō-sef-ăl-pel-vim′ĕ-trē). SYN pelvimetry. [radio- + cephal- + pelvimetry]

ra·di·o·chem·is·try (rā′dē-ō-kem′is-trē). **1.** The science of using radionuclides to synthesize labeled compounds for biochemical or biologic research, or radiopharmaceuticals for clinical diagnostic studies. **2.** The study of methods of labeling compounds with

radionuclides. **3.** The science concerned with the effects of ionizing or nuclear radiation on chemical reactions or materials.

ra·di·o·chlo·rine (rā′dē-ō-klōr′ēn). A radioactive isotope of chlorine, e.g., ^{36}Cl.

ra·di·o·chol·an·gi·og·ra·phy (rā′dē-ō-kō-lan-jē-og′ră-fē). Cholangiography obtained by the intravenous administration of an excreted radiopharmaceutical. [radio- + cholangiography]

ra·di·o·cho·le·cys·tog·ra·phy (rā′dē-ō-kō-lē-sis-tog′ră-fē). Visualization of the gallbladder by scintigraphic means using a radiopharmaceutical such as technetium-99m–labeled iminodiacetic acid derivative. [radio- + cholecysography]

ra·di·o·cin·e·an·gi·o·car·di·og·ra·phy (rā′dē-ō-sin′ē-an′jē-ō-kar-dē-og′ră-fē). Scintigraphic motion picture of the passage of a radiopharmaceutical through the heart and great vessels. [radio- + cineangiography]

ra·di·o·cin·e·an·gi·og·ra·phy (rā′dē-ō-sin′ē-an′jē-og′ră-fē). Scintigraphic motion pictures of the passage of a radiopharmaceutical through blood vessels.

ra·di·o·cin·e·ma·tog·ra·phy (rā′dē-ō-sĭ-nē-mă-tog′ră-fē). Taking a motion picture of the movements of organs or other structures as revealed by x-ray fluoroscopic examination. [radio- + G. *kinēma,* motion, + *graphō,* to write]

ra·di·o·co·balt (rā′dē-ō-kō′balt). A radioactive isotope of cobalt; e.g., ^{60}Co.

ra·di·o·cur·a·ble (rā′dē-ō-kūr′ă-bl). Curable by irradiation therapy.

ra·di·o·dense (rā′dē-ō-dens). SYN radiopaque.

ra·di·o·den·si·ty (rā′dē-ō-den′si-tē). SYN radiopacity.

ℹ**ra·di·o·der·ma·ti·tis** (rā′dē-ō-der-mă-tī′tis). Dermatitis due to exposure to x-rays or gamma rays causing ionization of tissue water with acute changes resembling thermal injury.

ra·di·o·di·ag·no·sis (rā′dē-ō-dī-ag-nō′sis). Diagnosis using x-rays; or, more broadly, diagnostic imaging, including radiology, ultrasound, and magnetic resonance.

ra·di·o·dig·i·tal (rā′dē-ō-dij′i-tăl). Relating to the fingers on the radial or lateral side of the hand.

ra·di·o·e·lec·tro·phys·i·ol·o·gram (ra′dē-ō-e-lek′trō-fiz-ē-ol′ō-gram). The record obtained by means of the radioelectrophysiolograph.

ra·di·o·e·lec·tro·phys·i·ol·o·graph (rā′dē-ō-ē-lek′trō-fiz-ē-ol′ō-graf). Formerly, an apparatus carried by a mobile individual by means of which changes in electrical potential from the brain or heart can be picked up and radio-transmitted to an electroencephalograph or an electrocardiograph. SEE telemeter.

ra·di·o·e·lec·tro·phys·i·o·log·ra·phy (rā′dē-ō-ē-lek′trō-fiz′ē-ō-log′ră-fē). Formerly, recording the changes in the electrical potential of the brain or heart by means of the radioelectrophysiolograph. SEE telemetry.

ra·di·o·e·le·ment (rā′dē-ō-el′ĕ-ment). Any element possessing radioactivity.

ra·di·o·ep·i·the·li·tis (rā′dē-ō-ep′i-thē-lī′tis). Destructive changes in epithelium produced by ionizing radiation.

ra·di·o·fre·quen·cy (rā′dē-o-frē′kwen-sē). **1.** Radiant energy of a certain frequency range; e.g., radio and television employ radiant energy having a frequency between 10^5–10^{11} Hz, while diagnostic x-rays have a frequency in the range of 3×10^{18} Hz. **2.** In magnetic resonance imaging, the energy applied to switch or create a gradient in the magnetic field.

ra·di·o·gal·li·um (rā′dē-ō-gal′ē-ŭm). Gallium that is radioactive. SEE gallium-67, gallium-68.

ra·di·o·gen·e·sis (rā′dē-ō-jen′ĕ-sis). The formation or production of radioactivity resulting from radioactive transformation or disintegration of radioactive substances. [radio- + G. *genesis,* production]

ra·di·o·gen·ic (rā′dē-ō-jen′ik). **1.** Producing rays of any sort, especially electromagnetic rays. **2.** Caused by x- or gamma rays.

ra·di·o·gen·ics (rā′dē-ō-jen′iks). The science of radiation.

ra·di·o·gold col·loid (rā′dē-ō-gōld kol′oyd). A radioactive isotope of gold emitting negative beta particles and gamma radiation, with a half-life of 2.7 days; formerly used for irradiation of closed serous cavities in the palliative treatment of ascites and pleural effusion due to metastatic malignancies, and for liver scans. SYN [198]Au colloid, colloidal radioactive gold.

ra·di·o·gram (rā′dē-ō-gram). Obsolete term for radiograph. [radio- + G. *gramma,* something written]

ra·di·o·graph (rā′dē-ō-graf). A negative image on photographic film made by exposure to x-rays or gamma rays that have passed through matter or tissue. SYN roentgenogram, roentgenograph, x-ray (3). [radio- + G. *graphō,* to write]

bitewing r., intraoral dental film adapted to show the coronal portion and cervical third of the root of the teeth in near occlusion; especially useful in detecting interproximal caries and determining alveolar septal height.

cephalometric r., a radiographic view of the jaws and skull permitting measurement. SYN cephalogram.

decubitus r., a r. of a recumbent subject on his side, made in the frontal projection with a horizontal x-ray beam. SYN lateral decubitus r.

lateral decubitus r., SYN decubitus r.

lateral oblique r., a radiographic view of the mandible, revealing one side of the mandible from symphysis to condyle by displacing the other side upwards.

lateral ramus r., a radiographic view of the mandibular ramus and condyle.

lateral skull r., a true lateral projection r. of facial bones and calvarium, showing bone structures and air-containing passages.

maxillary sinus r., a radiographic frontal view of the maxillary sinuses, orbits, nasal structures and zygomas; permits direct comparison of the sides. SYN Waters view r.

occlusal r., intraoral section film positioned on the occlusal plane and used in visualizing entire sections of the jaw; especially useful in exploring calcifications of the sublingual salivary glands.

panoramic r., a radiographic view of the maxillae and mandible extending from the left to the right glenoid fossae.

periapical r., a r. demonstrating tooth apices and surrounding structures in a particular intraoral area.

scout r., SYN scout *film.*

submental vertex r., SYN submentovertex r.

submentovertex r., a radiographic projection showing the base of the skull, positions of the mandibular condyles, and zygomatic arches. SYN base view, submental vertex r.

Towne projection r., SEE Towne *projection.*

transcranial r., a radiographic view of the temporomandibular articulation.

Trendelenburg r., r. of a subject tilted head downwards, usually in the decubitus position; used to detect small pleural effusions.

Waters view r., SYN maxillary sinus r.

ra·di·og·raph·er (rā-dē-og′ră-fĕr). A technician trained to position patients and take radiographs or perform other radiodiagnostic procedures.

ra·di·og·ra·phy (rā′dē-og′ră-fē). Examination of any part of the body for diagnostic purposes by means of x-rays with the record of the findings usually impressed upon a photographic film. SYN roentgenography.

advanced multiple-beam equalization r. (AMBER), a variant of scanning equalization r. using several x-ray beams.

air-gap r., chest r. with a space (at least 10 inches) between the subject and film. Instead of using a grid, this method uses the geometry and x-ray absorption by the air to remove scattered radiation.

bedside r., SYN portable r.

computed r. (CR), converting transmitted x-rays into light, using a solid-state imaging device such as a photostimulable phosphor plate, and recovering and processing the image using a digital computer; the image may then be printed on film or displayed on a computer screen.

digital r. (DR), direct conversion of transmitted x-rays into a digital image using an array of solid-state detectors such as amorphous selenium or silicon, with computer processing and display of the image. SEE DSA.

electron r., radiographic imaging in which x-radiation incident on the receptor is converted to a latent charge image and subsequently recovered by a special printing process; advantages include wider latitude of exposure and greater sensitivity than conventional film-screen combinations. SEE xeroradiography, phosphor *plate.*

filmless r., electronic acquisition and distribution of radiographic images, eliminating the handling and storage of film. SEE ALSO PACS.

magnification r., r. using a microfocal x-ray tube and increased subject-film distance to provide geometric magnification of the subject without unacceptable loss of sharpness and resolution.

mucosal relief r., radiographic technique showing fine detail of gastrointestinal mucosa after coating it with a barium suspension and distending the organ with air or gas released from an ingested powder.

portable r., making a radiographic film of a patient confined to bed by taking a movable x-ray machine to the room. SYN bedside r.

scanning equalization r., an electronically enhanced method of radiography in which a narrow x-ray beam is scanned over the patient while its attenuation is measured, providing feedback to modulate beam intensity in order to equalize regional x-ray film exposure.

sectional r., SYN tomography.

serial r., making several x-ray exposures of a single region over a period of time, as in angiography.

spot-film r., an x-ray of a localized region, usually under study by fluoroscopy.

ra·di·o·hu·mer·al (rā′dē-ō-hū′mer-ăl). Relating to the radius and the humerus; denoting the articulation between them.

ra·di·o·im·mu·ni·ty (rā′dē-ō-i-mū′ni-tē). Lessened sensitivity to radiation.

ra·di·o·im·mu·no·as·say (RIA) (rā′dē-ō-im′u-nō-as′sā). An immunologic (immunochemical) procedure that uses the competition between radioisotope-labeled antigen or other substance and unlabeled antigen for antiserums, resulting in quantitation of the unlabeled antigen; any method for detecting or quantitating antigens or antibodies using radiolabeled reactants. Minute quantities of enzymes, hormones, or other substances can be assayed.

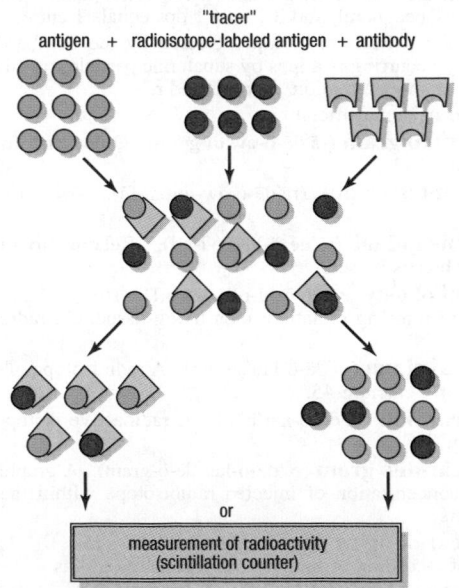

radioimmunoassay

ra·di·o·im·mu·no·dif·fu·sion (rā′dē-ō-im′u-nō-di-fū′zhŭn). A method for the study of antigen-antibody reactions by gel diffusion using radioisotope-labeled antigen or antibody.

ra·di·o·im·mu·no·elec·tro·pho·re·sis (rā′dē-ō-im′u-nō-ē-lek′

trō-fō-rē′sis). Immunoelectrophoresis in which the antigen or antibody is labeled with a radioisotope; e.g., in testing for insulin-binding antibodies by treating the test serum with radioactive iodine-labeled insulin, subjecting the mixture (antigen) to electrophoresis, precipitating the separated immunoglobulins with immunoglobulin-specific antiserum, and, then, with radiosensitive film (autoradiography), testing for bound insulin in the precipitates.

ra·di·o·im·mu·no·pre·cip·i·ta·tion (RIP) (rā′dē-ō-im′ū-nō-prē-sip-i-tā′shŭn). Immunoprecipitation utilizing a radioisotope-labeled antibody or antigen.

ra·di·o·i·o·din·at·ed (rā′dē-ō-ī′ō-din-ā-ted). Treated or combined with radioiodine.

ra·di·o·i·o·dine (rā′dē-ō-i′ō-dīn). A radioactive isotope of iodine; e.g., ^{123}I.

ra·di·o·i·ron (rā′dē-ō-i′ern). A radioactive isotope of iron; e.g., ^{59}Fe.

ra·di·o·i·so·tope (rā′dē-ō-i′sō-tōp). An isotope that changes to a more stable state by emitting radiation.

ra·di·o·la·beled (rā′dē-ō-lā′bld). SEE tag (1).

ra·di·o·lead (rā′dē-ō-led′). A radioactive isotope of lead, usually 210 Pb. SEE lead.

ra·di·o·le·sion (rā′dē-ō-lē′zhŭn). A lesion produced by ionizing radiation.

ra·di·o·li·gand (rā′dē-ō-lig′and). A molecule with a radionuclide tracer attached; usually used for radioimmunoassay procedures. [radio- + L. *ligandus,* that which is to be bound, fr. *ligo,* to bind]

ra·di·o·log·ic, ra·di·o·log·i·cal (rā-dē-ō-log′ik, -loj′i-kăl). Pertaining to radiology.

ra·di·ol·o·gist (rā-dē-ol′ō-jist). A physician trained in the diagnostic and/or therapeutic use of x-rays and radionuclides, radiation physics and biology; a diagnostic r. would also be trained in diagnostic ultrasound and magnetic resonance imaging and applicable physics.

ra·di·ol·o·gy (rā-dē-ol′ō-jē). **1.** The science of high-energy radiation and of the sources and the chemical, physical, and biologic effects of such radiation; the term usually refers to the diagnosis and treatment of disease. **2.** The scientific discipline of medical imaging using ionizing radiation, radionuclides, nuclear magnetic resonance, and ultrasound. SYN diagnostic r. [radio- + G. *logos,* study]

cardiovascular r., the clinical subspecialty of r. concerned with diagnosis and treatment of diseases of the vascular system.

chest r., the clinical subspecialty concerned with the diagnostic r. of diseases of the thorax, especially of the heart and lungs.

diagnostic r., SYN radiology (2).

interventional r., the clinical subspecialty that uses fluoroscopy, CT, and ultrasound to guide percutaneous procedures such as performing biopsies, draining fluids, inserting catheters, or dilating or stenting narrowed ducts or vessels.

pediatric r., the clinical subspecialty concerned with the radiologic manifestations of diseases of children.

therapeutic r., SYN radiation *oncology.*

ra·di·o·lu·cen·cy (rā-dē-ō-loo′sen-sē). A region of a radiograph showing increased exposure, either because of greater transradiancy of the corresponding portion of the subject or because of inhomogeneity in the source of radiation, such as off-center positioning.

ra·di·o·lu·cent (rā-dē-ō-loo′sent). Relatively penetrable by x-rays or other forms of radiation. Cf. radiopaque. [radio- + L. *lucens,* shining]

ra·di·o·lus (rā-dē′ō-lŭs). A probe or sound. [L. dim. of *radius,* spoke]

ra·di·om·e·ter (rā-dē-om′ĕ-ter). A device for determining the penetrative power of x-rays. SYN roentgenometer. [radio- + G. *metron,* measure]

ra·di·o·mi·crom·e·ter (rā′dē-ō-mī-krom′ĕ-ter). A sensitive thermopile designed for the measurement of minute changes in radiant energy.

ra·di·o·mi·met·ic (rā′dē-ō-mi-met′ik). Imitating the biologic ef-

fects of radiation, as in the case of chemicals such as nitrogen mustards. [radio- + G. *mimētikos,* imitative]

ra·di·o·mus·cu·lar (rā′dē-ō-mŭs′kū-lăr). Relating to the radius and the neighboring muscles; denoting certain nerves and muscular branches of the radial artery.

ra·di·o·ne·cro·sis (rā′dē-ō-ne-krō′sis). Necrosis due to radiation; e.g., after excessive exposure to x- or gamma rays. SEE radiation *burn.*

ra·di·o·neu·ri·tis (rā′dē-ō-noo-rī′tis). Neuritis caused by prolonged or repeated exposure to x-rays or radium.

ra·di·o·ni·tro·gen (rā′dē-ō-nī′trō-jen). A radioactive isotope of nitrogen; e.g., ^{13}N.

ra·di·o·nu·clide (rā′dē-ō-noo′klīd). An isotope of artificial or natural origin that exhibits radioactivity.

ra·di·o·pac·i·ty (rā′dē-ō-pas′i-tē). The x-ray shadow of a radiopaque object. SYN radiodensity.

ra·di·o·pal·mar (rā′dē-ō-pal′măr). Relating to the radial or lateral side of the palm.

ra·di·o·paque (rā-dē-ō-pāk′). Exhibiting relative opacity to, or impenetrability by, x-rays or any other form of radiation. Cf. radiolucent. SYN radiodense. [radio- + Fr. opaque fr. L. *opacus,* shady]

ra·di·o·pa·thol·o·gy (rā′dē-ō-path-ol′ō-jē). A branch of radiology or pathology concerned with the effects of radiation on cells and tissues. Cf. radiobiology.

ra·di·o·pel·vim·e·try (rā′dē-ō-pel-vim′ĕ-trē). Radiographic measurement of the pelvis. SEE pelvimetry.

ra·di·o·phar·ma·ceu·ti·cal (rā′dē-ō-far-mă-soo′ti-kal). A radioactive chemical or pharmaceutic preparation, labeled with a radionuclide in tracer or therapeutic concentration, used as a diagnostic or therapeutic agent.

ra·di·o·pho·bia (rā′dē-ō-fō′bē-ă). Morbid fear of radiation, as from x-rays or nuclear energy. [radio- + G. *phobos,* fear]

ra·di·o·phos·pho·rus (rā′dē-ō-fos′fōr-ŭs). A radioactive isotope of phosphorus; e.g., ^{32}P.

ra·di·o·pill (rā′dē-ō-pil). SYN radiotelemetering *capsule.*

ra·di·o·po·tas·si·um (rā′dē-ō-pō-tas′ē-ŭm). A radioactive isotope of potassium; e.g., ^{40}K.

radioprotectant (rā′dē-ō-prō-tek′tant). Substance that prevents or lessens the effects of radiation.

ra·di·o·re·cep·tor (rā′dē-ō-rē-sep′ter). **1.** A receptor that normally responds to radiant energy such as light or heat. **2.** A receptor used as a binding agent for unlabeled and radiolabeled analyte in a type of competitive binding assay called radioreceptor assay.

ra·di·o·re·sis·tant (rā′dē-ō-rē-zis′tant). Indicates cells or tissues that are less affected than average mammalian cells on exposure to radiation; when applied to neoplasms, indicates less susceptibility to damage from therapeutic radiation than the surrounding host tissues.

ra·di·os·co·py (rā′dē-os′kŏ-pē). Obsolete term for fluoroscopy. [radio- + G. *skopeō,* to view]

ra·di·o·sen·si·tive (rā′dē-ō-sen′si-tiv). Readily affected by radiation. Cf. radioresistant.

ra·di·o·sen·si·tiv·i·ty (rā′dē-ō-sen-si-tiv′i-tē). The condition of being readily affected by radiant energy.

ra·di·o·sen·si·ti·za·tion (rā′dē-ō-sen-sĭ-tĭ-zā′shun). The use of chemotherapy or other agents that increase the sensitivity of tissue to the effects or radiation therapy, usually by inhibiting cellular repair or increasing the percentage of cells in mitotic phases of the growth cycle.

ra·di·o·sen·si·tiz·er (rā′dē-ō-sen-si-tī′zĕr). A chemical substance that increases the radiosensitivity of tissues; restoring normal tissue oxygen tension to an anoxic region is also an effective r.

ra·di·o·so·di·um (rā′dē-ō-sō′dē-ŭm). A radioactive isotope of sodium; e.g., ^{24}Na.

ra·di·o·ster·e·os·co·py (rā′dē-ō-ster-ē-os′kŏ-pē). Simultaneous viewing of two radiographs made in slightly different projections, usually with a device that reflects the image of one on each eye, allowing three-dimensional visualization of an object in relation

ra

to others. SEE stereoradiography, stereoscope. [radio- + G. *stereos*, solid, + *skopeō*, to view]

ra·di·o·stron·ti·um (rā'dē-ō-stron'tē-ŭm). A radioactive isotope of strontium; e.g., ⁹⁰Sr.

ra·di·o·sul·fur (rā'dē-ō-sŭl'fŭr). A radioactive isotope of sulfur; e.g., ³⁵S.

ra·di·o·sur·gery (rā'dē-ō-sŭr-gĕ-rē). Radiotherapy with a sharply delimited field, optimistically considered to be equivalent to resecting the irradiated region.

ra·di·o·te·lem·e·try (rā'dē-ō-tĕ-lem'ĕ-trē). SEE telemetry, biotelemetry.

ra·di·o·ther·a·peu·tic (rā'dē-ō-thār-ă-pū'tik). Relating to radiotherapy or to radiotherapeutics.

ra·di·o·ther·a·peu·tics (rā'dē-ō-thār-ă-pū'tiks). The study and use of radiotherapeutic agents.

ra·di·o·ther·a·pist (rā'dē-ō-thār'ă-pist). One who practices radiotherapy or is versed in radiotherapeutics. SYN radiation oncologist.

ra·di·o·ther·a·py (rā'dē-ō-thār'ă-pē). SYN radiation *oncology*.
   mantle r., r. with shielding of uninvolved radiosensitive structures or organs.

ra·di·o·ther·my (rā'dē-ō-ther'mē). Diathermy effected by heat from radiant sources. [radio- + G. *thermē*, heat]

ra·di·o·thy·roid·ec·to·my (rā'dē-ō-thī'roy-dek'-tō-mē). The destruction of thyroid tissue by administration of radioactive iodine.

ra·di·o·thy·rox·in (rā'dē-ō-thī-rok'sin). SYN radioactive *thyroxine*.

ra·di·o·tox·e·mia (rā'dē-ō-tok-sē'mē-ă). Radiation sickness caused by the products of disintegration produced by the action of x-rays or other forms of radioactivity and by the depletion of certain cells and enzyme systems from the organism. [radio- + G. *toxikon*, poison, + *haima*, blood]

ra·di·o·trac·er (rā'dē-ō-trā'sĕr). A radionuclide or radiolabeled chemical; a radioactive tracer.

ra·di·o·trans·par·ent (rā'dē-ō-trans-par'ent). Allowing relatively free transmission of radiant energy. Cf. radiolucent.

ra·di·o·trop·ic (rā'dē-ō-trop'ik). Affected by radiation. [radio- + G. *tropē*, a turning]

ra·di·o·ul·nar (rā'dē-ō-ŭl'năr). Relating to both radius and ulna.

ra·di·sec·to·my (rā-dē-sek'tō-mē). SYN root *amputation*. [L. *radix*, root, + G. *ektomē*, excision]

ra·di·um (Ra) (rā'dē-ŭm). A metallic element, atomic no. 88, extracted in very minute quantities from pitchblende; ²²⁶Ra, its longest-lived isotope, is produced as an intermediate in the uranium series by the emission of an α particle from thorium-230 (ionium); ²²⁶Ra emits α particles and gamma rays with a half-life of 1,599 years breaking down to ²²²Rn; chemically, it is an alkaline earth metal with properties similar to those of barium. Its therapeutic action is similar to that of x-rays, since the α emission is filtered out. [L. *radius*, ray]

ra·di·us, gen. and pl. **ra·dii** (rā'dē-ŭs, rā'dē-ī) [TA]. **1** [NA]. The lateral and shorter of the two bones of the forearm. **2.** A straight line passing from the center to the periphery of a circle. SYN radio- (3). [L. spoke of a wheel, rod, ray]
   r. fix'us, a line passing from the hormion to the inion.
   radii of lens [TA], 9–12 faint lines on the anterior and posterior surfaces of the lens that radiate from the poles toward the equator; they mark the lines along which the ends of lens fibers abut. SYN radii lentis [TA], lens stars (1), lens sutures.
   ra'dii len'tis [TA], SYN radii of lens.

ra·dix, gen. **ra·di·cis**, pl. **ra·di·ces** (rā'diks, rā-di'sis, rā'di-sēz or rā-dī'sēz) [TA]. **1.** SYN root (1). **2.** SYN *root* of tooth. **3.** The hypothetical size of the birth cohort in a life table, commonly 1,000 or 100,000. [L.]
   r. accessoria [TA], SYN accessory *root* of tooth.
   r. ante'rior nervi spinalis [TA], SYN anterior *root* of spinal nerve.
   r. ar'cus ver'tebrae, SYN *pedicle* of arch of vertebra.
   r. bre'vis gan'glii cilia'ris, SYN parasympathetic *root* of ciliary ganglion.
   r. buccalis [TA], SYN buccal *root* of tooth.
   r. clin'ica dentis [TA], SYN clinical *root* of tooth.

r. crania'lis nervi accessorii [TA], SYN cranial *root* of accessory nerve.
   r. den'tis [TA], SYN *root* of tooth.
   r. dorsa'lis nervi spinalis, SYN posterior *root* of spinal nerve.
   r. facia'lis, SYN *nerve* of pterygoid canal.
   r. infe'rior an'sae cervica'lis [TA], SYN inferior *root* of ansa cervicalis.
   r. infe'rior ner'vi vestibulocochlea'ris, SYN cochlear *root* of VIII nerve.
   r. latera'lis ner'vi media'ni [TA], SYN lateral *root* of median nerve.
   r. latera'lis trac'tus op'tici [TA], SYN lateral *root* of optic tract.
   r. lin'guae [TA], SYN *root* of tongue.
   r. lon'ga gan'glii cilia'ris, SYN sensory *root* of ciliary ganglion.
   r. media'lis ner'vi media'ni [TA], SYN medial *root* of median nerve.
   r. media'lis trac'tus op'tici [TA], SYN medial *root* of optic tract.
   r. mesenter'ii [TA], SYN *root* of mesentery.
   r. moto'ria nervi spinalis, ⋆official alternate term for anterior *root* of spinal nerve.
   r. moto'ria ner'vi trigem'ini [TA], SYN motor *root* of trigeminal nerve.
   r. na'si [TA], SYN *root* of nose.
   r. nasocilia'ris ganglii ciliaris, ⋆official alternate term for sensory *root* of ciliary ganglion.
   r. ner'vi facia'lis, SYN *root* of facial nerve.
   r. nervi oculomotorii ad ganglion ciliare, ⋆official alternate term for parasympathetic *root* of ciliary ganglion.
   ra'dices ner'vi trigem'ini, SYN *roots* of trigeminal nerve, under *root*.
   r. oculomoto'ria gan'glii cilia'ris, ⋆official alternate term for parasympathetic *root* of ciliary ganglion.
   r. parasympathica ganglii submandibularis, SYN *chorda* tympani.
   radices parasympathicae gangliorum pelvicorum, ⋆official alternate term for pelvic splanchnic *nerves*, under *nerve*.
   r. parasympath'ica gan'glii cilia'ris [TA], SYN parasympathetic *root* of ciliary ganglion.
   r. parasympathica ganglii otici, ⋆official alternate term for lesser petrosal *nerve*.
   r. pe'nis [TA], SYN *root* of penis.
   r. pi'li, SYN hair *root*.
   r. poste'rior nervi spinalis [TA], SYN posterior *root* of spinal nerve.
   r. pulmo'nis [TA], SYN *root* of lung.
   r. senso'ria gan'glii cili'aris [TA], SYN sensory *root* of ciliary ganglion.
   r. senso'ria gan'glii pterygopalatini [TA], SYN sensory *root* of pterygopalatine ganglion.
   r. sensoria ganglii sublingualis [TA], SYN sensory *root* of sublingual ganglion.
   r. sensoria ganglii submandibularis [TA], SYN sensory *root* of submandibular ganglion.
   r. senso'ria nervi spinalis, ⋆official alternate term for posterior *root* of spinal nerve.
   r. senso'ria ner'vi trigem'ini [TA], SYN sensory *root* of trigeminal nerve.
   r. spina'lis nervi accessorii [TA], SYN spinal *root* of accessory nerve.
   r. supe'rior an'sae cervica'lis [TA], SYN superior *root* of ansa cervicalis.
   r. supe'rior ner'vi vestibulocochlea'ris, SYN vestibular *root*.
   r. sympath'ica gan'glii cilia'ris [TA], SYN sympathetic *root* of ciliary ganglion.
   r. sympathica ganglii otici [TA], SYN sympathetic *root* of otic ganglion.
   r. sympathica ganglii pterygopalatini, ⋆official alternate term for deep petrosal *nerve*.
   r. sympathica ganglii sublingualis [TA], SYN sympathetic *root* of sublingual ganglion.

r. sympathica ganglii submandibularis [TA], SYN sympathetic *root* of submandibular ganglion.

r. un′guis, SYN *root* of nail.

r. ventra′lis nervi spinalis, SYN anterior *root* of spinal nerve.

r. vestibula′ris, SYN vestibular *root.*

ra·don (Rn) (rā′don). A gaseous radioactive element, atomic no. 86, resulting from the breakdown of radium; of the isotopes with mass numbers between 198 and 228, only ^{222}Rn is medically significant as an alpha-emitter, with a half-life of 3.8235 days; it is used in the treatment of certain malignancies. Poorly ventilated homes in some parts of the country accumulate a dangerous amount of naturally occurring radon gas. [from radium]

Raeder, Georg Johann, Norwegian ophthalmologist, 1889–1956. SEE R. paratrigeminal *syndrome.*

raf·fi·nose (raf′i-nōs). A dextrorotatory trisaccharide, occurring in cotton seed and in the molasses of beet root, composed of D-galactose, D-glucose, and D-fructose and formed by transfer of D-galactose from UDP-D-galactose to sucrose; many seeds are rich in r. SYN gossypose, melitose, melitriose.

rage (rāj). Violent anger; a total discharge of the sympathetic portion of the autonomic nervous system. [Fr., fr. L. *rabies,* violent anger, fr. *rabo,* to rave]

sham r., a quasiemotional state, characterized by manifestations of fear and anger upon trifling provocation; produced in animals by the removal of the cerebral cortex (decortication).

Rahe, Richard H., U.S. psychiatrist, *1936. SEE Holmes-R. *questionnaire.*

Rahn, Hermann, U.S. respiratory physiologist, 1912–1990. SEE R.-Otis *sample.*

Rail·li·e·ti·na (rī-li-ě-tē′nă). A genus of tapeworms (family Davaineidae, order Cyclophyllidea), three species of which, *R. madagascariensis* or *R. demerariensis, R. asiatica,* and *R. formsana,* have been found in humans. However, the identification of many of these worms found in humans has been questioned.

rail·li·e·ti·ni·a·sis (rī′li-ě-ti-nī′ă-sis). Infection of rodents and monkeys, and occasionally humans, with tapeworms of the genus *Raillietina.*

Rainey, George, English anatomist, 1801–1884. SEE R. *corpuscles,* under *corpuscle.*

rale (rahl). Ambiguous term for an added sound heard on auscultation of breath sounds; used by some to denote rhonchus and by others for crepitation. SYN crackle. [Fr. rattle]

amphoric r., sound heard through the stethoscope associated with the movement of fluid in a lung cavity communicating with a bronchus.

atelectatic r., transitory light crackling sound that disappears after deep breathing or coughing.

bubbling r., moist sound heard through the stethoscope as a result of air entering portions of lung tissue containing exudate and thus creating bubbles; sometimes associated with resolving pneumonia or small lung cavities.

cavernous r., a resonating, bubbling sound caused by air entering a cavity partly filled with fluid. SYN cavernous rhonchus.

clicking r., short, sticking sound usually associated with opening of small bronchi on deep breathing, sometimes heard in early pulmonary tuberculosis.

consonating r., a resonant r. produced in a bronchial tube and heard through consolidated lung tissue.

crackling r. (krak′ling), very fine sounds produced by fluid in very small airways in pneumonia or congestive heart *failure.*

crepitant r., a fine bubbling or crackling sound produced by air mixing with very thin secretions in the smaller bronchial tubes. SYN vesicular r.

dry r., a harsh or musical breath sound produced by a constriction in a bronchial tube or the presence of a viscid secretion narrowing the lumen.

gurgling r., coarse sound heard over large cavities or over trachea nearly filled with secretions.

guttural r., sound heard over the lung but resulting from upper airway obstruction.

metallic r., a r. of metallic quality caused by resonance in a large cavity.

moist r., a bubbling r. caused by air mixing with a fluid exudate in the bronchial tubes or a cavity.

mucous r., a bubbling r. heard on auscultation over bronchial tubes containing mucus.

palpable r., a vibration that can be felt accompanying a low-pitched, hard, musical, or sonorous r.

pleural r., SYN pleural *rub.*

sibilant r., a whistling sound caused by air moving through a viscid secretion narrowing the lumen of a bronchus. SYN whistling r.

Skoda r., a r. in a bronchus heard through an area of consolidated tissue in pneumonia.

sonorous r., a cooing or snoring sound often produced by the vibration of a projecting mass of viscid secretion in a large bronchus.

subcrepitant r., a very fine crepitant r.

vesicular r., SYN crepitant r.

whistling r., SYN sibilant r.

ral·ox·i·fene (ral-ox′ĭ-fēn). A selective estrogen receptor modulator (SERM) that has estrogen-agonistic effects on bone and lipid metabolism but estrogen-antagonistic effects on breast and uterus; used in the prophylaxis of osteoporosis after menopause.

> Raloxifene is a benzothiophene derivative that binds to estrogen receptor sites. Besides conferring protection against osteoporosis after menopause, it has been shown to improve bone mineral density and reduce the risk of fractures in established osteoporosis. The reduction in fracture risk is greater than would be expected from the increase in bone density. Unlike tamoxifen, which also reduces osteoporosis risk, raloxifene does not heighten the risk of endometrial cancer. Although raloxifene increases bone mineral density to a lesser degree than estrogen, it reduces the risk of breast cancer rather than increasing it as estrogen may perhaps do. Hence it may be preferred for women who fear breast cancer or are at high risk for it. Like hormone replacement therapy with estrogen-progestogen, raloxifene decreases LDL cholesterol, fibrinogen, and lipoprotein(a), increasing HDL cholesterol without raising triglycerides. It does not relieve hot flashes; in fact, it causes them in 25% of patients. Like estrogen replacement therapy, it is contraindicated in pregnancy and in women with a history of thromboembolism. Whether it protects against cardiovascular disease and Alzheimer dementia as estrogen does has not yet been determined.

ra·mal (rā′măl). Relating to a ramus.

Raman, Sir Chandrasekhara V., Indian physicist and Nobel laureate, 1888–1970. SEE R. *effect, spectrum.*

Rambourg stains. SEE Rambourg chromic acid-phosphotungstic acid *stain,* Rambourg periodic acid-chromic methenamine-silver *stain.*

ra·mi (rā′mī). Plural of ramus. [L.]

ram·i·cot·o·my (ram-i-kot′ō-mē). SYN ramisection. [L. *ramus,* branch, + G. *tomē,* incision]

ram·i·fi·ca·tion (ram′i-fi-kā′shŭn). The process of dividing into a branchlike pattern.

ram·i·fy (ram′i-fī). To split into a branchlike pattern. [L. *ramus,* branch, + *facio,* to make]

ram·i·sec·tion (ram-i-sek′shŭn). Section of the rami communicantes of the sympathetic nervous system. SYN ramicotomy. [L. *ramus,* branch, + L. *sectio,* section]

ram·i·tis (ram-ī′tis). Inflammation of a ramus. [L. *ramus,* branch, + G. *-itis,* inflammation]

Ramón y Cajal, SEE Cajal.

ra·mose, ra·mous (rā′mōs, rā′mŭs). SYN branching. [L. *ramosus,* fr. *ramus,* a branch]

ramp. In electrical recording, a uniformly rising voltage or current. If reset to zero at regular intervals, it forms a sawtooth

ra

pattern used to provide the time sweep of a cathode ray oscilloscope beam; if reset to zero by a periodic event (e.g., heart beats), the recorded height of the r.'s represents time between events.

Ramsay Hunt. SEE Hunt.

Ramsden, Jesse, English optician, 1735–1800. SEE R. *ocular.*

Ramstedt, Conrad, German surgeon, 1867–1962. SEE R. *operation;* Fredet-R. *operation.*

ram·u·lus, pl. **ram·u·li** (ram′ū-lŭs, -lī). A small branch or twig; one of the terminal divisions of a ramus. [L. dim. of *ramus,* a branch]

RAMUS

ra·mus, pl. **ra·mi** (rā′mŭs, rā′mī) [TA]. **1.** SYN branch. **2.** One of the primary divisions of a nerve or blood vessel. Arterial and nerve branches are also given under the major nerve or artery. SEE artery, nerve. **3.** A part of an irregularly shaped bone (less slender than a "process") that forms an angle with the main body (e.g., ramus of mandible). **4.** One of the primary divisions of a cerebral sulcus. [L.]

r. accessorius arteriae meningeae mediae [TA], SYN accessory *branch* of middle meningeal artery.

r. acetabula′ris [TA], SYN acetabular *branch.*

r. acromia′lis arte′riae suprascapula′ris [TA], SYN acromial *branch* of suprascapular artery.

r. acromia′lis arte′riae thoracoacromia′lis [TA], SYN acromial *branch* of thoracoacromial artery.

ra′mi ad pon′tem, SYN pontine *arteries,* under *artery.*

ra′mi alveola′res superio′res anterio′res ner′vi infraorbita′lis, SYN anterior superior alveolar *nerves,* under *nerve.*

ra′mi alveola′res superio′res posterio′res ner′vi maxilla′ris [TA], SYN posterior superior alveolar *branches* of maxillary nerve, under *branch.*

r. alveola′ris supe′rior me′dius ner′vi infraorbita′lis [TA], SYN middle superior alveolar *branch* of infraorbital nerve.

r. anastomot′icus [TA], SYN anastomotic *branch;* SEE ALSO communicating *branch.*

r. anastomot′icus arte′riae menin′geae me′diae cum arteriae lacrima′li [TA], SYN anastomotic *branch* of middle meningeal artery with lacrimal artery.

r. ante′rior [TA], SYN anterior *branch.*

r. anterior arteriae renalis [TA], SEE segmental *arteries* of kidney, under *artery.*

anterior rami of cervical nerves [TA], SEE anterior r. of spinal nerve. SYN rami anteriores nervorum cervicalium [TA], ventral rami of cervical nerves[*], rami ventrales nervorum cervicalium, ventral primary rami of cervical spinal nerves.

r. ante′rior descen′dens, SYN descending *branch* of anterior segmental artery of left and right lungs.

rami anteriores nervorum cervicalium [TA], SYN anterior rami of cervical nerves.

rami anteriores nervorum lumbalium [TA], SYN anterior rami of lumbar nerves.

rami anteriores nervorum sacralium [TA], SYN anterior rami of sacral nerves.

rami anteriores nervorum thoracis [TA], SYN anterior rami of thoracic nerves.

r. ante′rior latera′lis, the lateral anterior branch, the former name for the ascending anterior branch of the left pulmonary artery.

anterior r. of lateral sulcus of cerebrum [TA], SYN r. anterior sulci lateralis cerebri [TA].

anterior rami of lumbar nerves [TA], SEE anterior r. of spinal nerve. SYN rami anteriores nervorum lumbalium [TA], ventral rami of lumbar nerves[*], rami ventrales nervorum lumbalium, ventral primary rami of lumbar spinal nerves.

r. anterior nervi spinalis [TA], SYN anterior r. of spinal nerve.

anterior rami of sacral nerves [TA], SEE anterior r. of spinal

nerve. SYN rami anteriores nervorum sacralium [TA], ventral rami of sacral nerves[*], rami ventrales nervorum sacralium, ventral primary rami of sacral spinal nerves.

anterior r. of spinal nerve [TA], the larger, anterolaterally directed major terminal branch (with the posterior ramus) of all 31 pairs of mixed spinal nerves, formed at the intervertebral foramen. Most anterior rami, especially those involved in the innervation of the limbs, participate in the formation of the major nerve plexuses (cervical, brachial, and lumbosacral) and lose their identities. Most in the thoracic region, however, remain separate from adjacent rami to become the intercostal and subcostal nerves. Anterior rami provide innervation to the anterolateral body wall and trunk. Terminologia Anatomica lists anterior rami for each group of spinal nerves: 1) cervical (nervorum cervicalium [TA]), 2) thoracic (nervorum thoracicorum [TA]), 3) lumbar (nervorum lumbalium [TA]), 4) sacral (nervorum sacralium [TA]), and 5) coccygeal (nervi coccygei [TA]). SYN r. anterior nervi spinalis [TA], r. ventralis nervi spinalis[*], ventral r. of spinal nerve[*], anterior primary division, ventral primary r. of spinal nerve.

r. anterior sulci lateralis cerebri [TA], SYN anterior r. of lateral sulcus of cerebrum.

anterior rami of thoracic nerves [TA], SEE anterior r. of spinal nerve. SYN rami anteriores nervorum thoracis [TA], rami ventrales nervorum thoracis[*], ventral rami of thoracic nerves[*], ventral primary rami of thoracic spinal nerves.

r. apica′lis lo′bi inferio′ris arte′riae pulmona′lis dex′trae, [*]official alternate term for apical segmental *artery* of superior lobar artery of right lung.

r. apicalis venae pulmonalis dextrae superioris, [*]official alternate term for apical *vein.*

r. apicoposte′rior ve′nae pulmona′lis sinis′trae supe′rioris, [*]official alternate term for apicoposterior *vein.*

ra′mi articula′res [TA], SYN articular *branches,* under *branch.*

rami articulares arte′riae descenden′tis genicular′is, SEE articular *branches,* under *branch.*

r. ascen′dens [TA], SYN ascending *branch.*

r. ascendens arteriae superficialis cervicalis [TA], SYN ascending *branch* of superficial cervical artery.

r. ascendens sulci lateralis cerebri [TA], SYN ascending r. of lateral sulcus of cerebrum.

ascending r. of lateral sulcus of cerebrum [TA], SYN r. ascendens sulci lateralis cerebri [TA].

ra′mi atria′les [TA], SYN atrial *branches,* under *branch.*

r. atrialis anastomoticus ramus circumflexus arteriae coronariae sinistrae [TA], SYN atrial anastomotic *branch* of circumflex branch of left coronary artery.

r. atrialis intermedius arteriae coronariae dextrae [TA], SYN intermediate atrial *branch* of right coronary artery.

ra′mi auricula′res anterio′res arte′riae tempora′lis superficia′lis [TA], SYN anterior auricular *branches* of superficial temporal artery, under *branch.*

r. auricularis arteriae auricularis posterioris [TA], SYN auricular *branch* of posterior auricular artery.

r. auricula′ris arte′riae occipita′lis [TA], SYN auricular *branch* of occipital artery.

r. auricula′ris nervi va′gi, SYN auricular *branch* of vagus nerve.

r. basa′lis ante′rior, SYN anterior basal segmental *artery.*

r. basalis anterior venae basalis superioris, [*]official alternate term for anterior basal *vein.*

r. basa′lis latera′lis, SYN lateral basal segmental *artery.*

r. basa′lis media′lis, SYN medial basal segmental *artery.*

r. basa′lis poste′rior, SYN posterior basal segmental *artery* of left / right lung.

r. basalis tento′rii arte′riae caro′tidis inter′nae [TA], SYN tentorial basal *branch* of internal carotid artery.

ra′mi bronchia′les, SYN bronchial *branches* of thoracic aorta, under *branch.*

ra′mi bronchia′les segmento′rum, SYN intrasegmental *bronchi,* under *bronchus.*

ra′mi bucca′les ner′vi facia′lis [TA], SYN buccal *branches* of facial nerve, under *branch.*

ra′mi calca′nei [TA], SYN calcaneal *branches*, under *branch*.

ra′mi calca′nei latera′les ner′vi sura′lis [TA], SYN lateral calcaneal *branches* of sural nerve, under *branch*.

ra′mi calca′nei media′les ner′vi tibia′lis [TA], SYN medial calcaneal *branches* of tibial nerve, under *branch*.

r. calcari′nus arte′riae occipita′lis media′lis [TA], SYN calcarine *branch* of medial occipital artery.

ra′mi cap′sulae inter′nae, the internal capsular branches, the branches of the anterior choroid artery to the internal capsule. SYN branches to internal capsule, genu [TA], branches to internal capsule, posterior limb [TA], rami cruris posterioris capsulae internae [TA], rami genus capsulae internae [TA], rami partis retrolentiformis capsulae internae [TA], branches to internal capsule, retrolentiform limb.

rami capsulares arteriorum intrarenalium [TA], SYN capsular *branches* of intrarenal arteries, under *branch*.

ra′mi capsula′res arte′riae rena′lis [TA], SYN capsular *branches* of renal artery, under *branch*.

ra′mi cardi′aci cervica′les inferio′res ner′vi va′gi [TA], SYN inferior cervical cardiac *branches* of vagus nerve, under *branch*.

ra′mi cardi′aci cervica′les superio′res ner′vi va′gi [TA], SYN superior cervical cardiac *branches* of vagus nerve, under *branch*.

rami cardiaci thoracici gangliorum thoracicorum [TA], SYN thoracic cardiac *branches* of thoracic ganglia, under *branch*.

ra′mi cardi′aci thora′cici ner′vi va′gi [TA], SYN thoracic cardiac *branches* of vagus nerve, under *branch*.

r. cardi′acus, obsolete term for medial basal *branch* of pulmonary artery.

ra′mi caroticotympan′ici, SYN caroticotympanic *arteries* (of internal carotid artery), under *artery*.

r. carpa′lis dorsa′lis arte′riae radia′lis [TA], SYN dorsal carpal *branch* of radial artery.

r. carpa′lis dorsa′lis arte′riae ulna′ris [TA], SYN dorsal carpal *branch* of ulnar artery.

r. carpa′lis palma′ris arte′riae radia′lis [TA], SYN palmar carpal *branch* of radial artery.

r. carpa′lis palma′ris arte′riae ulna′ris [TA], SYN palmar carpal *branch* of ulnar artery.

r. car′peus dorsa′lis arte′riae radia′lis, SYN dorsal carpal *branch* of radial artery.

r. car′peus dorsa′lis arte′riae ulna′ris, SYN dorsal carpal *branch* of ulnar artery.

r. car′peus palma′ris arte′riae radia′lis, SYN palmar carpal *branch* of radial artery.

r. car′peus palma′ris arte′riae ulna′ris, SYN palmar carpal *branch* of ulnar artery.

ra′mi cau′dae nu′clei cauda′ti [TA], branches to the tail of the caudate nucleus. **(1)** branches from either the anterior choroid or the posterior communicating artery, or both, to supply the tail of the caudate nucleus; **(2)** a branch from the middle cerebral artery to the tail of the caudate nucleus.

ra′mi celi′aci ner′vi va′gi, SYN celiac *branches* of posterior vagal trunk, under *branch*.

rami celiaci trunci vagi posterioris [TA], SYN celiac *branches* of posterior vagal trunk, under *branch*.

ra′mi centra′les anteromedia′les [TA], SYN anteromedial central *branches*, under *branch*.

cephalic arterial rami, parietal branches of the sympathetic trunks conveying postsynaptic sympathetic fibers from the superior cervical ganglion to the carotid arteries for distribution within the head.

r. cervicalis ner′vi facia′lis, ✩official alternate term for cervical *branch* of facial nerve.

r. chiasmat′icus [TA], the chiasmatic branch, a branch of the anterior cerebral artery to the optic chiasm.

ra′mi choroi′dei, SYN choroid *branches*, under *branch*.

rami choroidei posteriores arteriae cerebri posteriores laterales et mediales [TA], SYN lateral and medial posterior choroidal *branches* of posterior cerebral artery, under *branch*.

r. choroi′dei posterio′res latera′les [TA], posterior lateral cho-

roid branches [TA] of posterior cerebral artery. SEE choroid *branches*, under *branch*.

r. choroi′dei posterio′res media′les [TA], posterior medial choroid branches [TA] of posterior cerebral artery. SEE choroid *branches*, under *branch*.

r. choroi′dei ventric′uli latera′lis [TA], choroidal branches to lateral ventricle [TA] of anterior choroid artery. SEE choroid *branches*, under *branch*.

r. choroi′dei ventric′uli ter′tii, third ventricle choroid branch of anterior artery. SEE choroid *branches*, under *branch*.

r. choroi′deus ventric′uli quar′ti [TA], choroidal branch to fourth ventricle [TA] of posterior inferior cerebellar artery. SEE choroid *branches*, under *branch*.

r. cingula′ris [TA], cingular branch [TA], a branch of the callosomarginal artery supplying the gyrus cinguli.

r. cingularis arteriae callosomarginalis [TA], SYN cingular *branch* of callosomarginal artery.

r. circumflex′us arte′riae corona′riae sinis′trae [TA], SYN circumflex *branch* of left coronary artery.

r. circumflex′us fibula′ris arte′riae tibia′lis posterio′ris [TA], SYN circumflex fibular *branch* (of posterior tibial artery).

r. circumflexus peronealis arteriae tibialis posterioris, ✩official alternate term for circumflex fibular *branch* (of posterior tibial artery).

r. clavicula′ris arte′riae thoracoacromia′lis [TA], SYN clavicular *branch* of thoracoacromial artery.

rami cli′vales [TA], clivus branches [TA], the branch to the clivus, a branch of the cerebral part of the internal carotid artery supplying the clivus.

rami clivales partis cerebralis arteriae carotidis internae [TA], SYN clivus *branches* of cerebral part of internal carotid artery, under *branch*.

r. cochlea′ris arte′riae labyrin′thi, SYN cochlear *branch* of vestibulocochlear artery.

r. cochlearis arteriae vestibulocochlearis [TA], SYN cochlear *branch* of vestibulocochlear artery.

r. colicus arteriae ileocolicae [TA], SYN colic *branch* of ileocolic artery.

r. collatera′lis arte′riarum intercosta′lium posterio′rum III–XI [TA], SYN collateral *branches* of posterior intercostal arteries 3–11, under *branch*.

r. collateralis nervorum intercostalium [TA], SYN collateral *branch* of intercostal nerves.

r. col′li ner′vi facia′lis, SYN cervical *branch* of facial nerve.

r. commu′nicans, pl. **ra′mi communican′tes** [TA], SYN communicating *branch*.

r. commu′nicans arte′riae fibula′ris [TA], SYN communicating *branch* of fibular artery.

r. commu′nicans arte′riae perone′ae, ✩official alternate term for communicating *branch* of fibular artery.

r. commu′nicans cum chor′da tym′pani [TA], **(1)** SYN communicating *branch* of chorda tympani with lingual nerve; **(2)** SYN communicating *branch* of otic ganglion with chorda tympani.

r. commu′nicans cum ner′vo glossopharyn′geo, **(1)** SYN communicating *branch* of facial nerve with glossopharyngeal nerve; **(2)** SYN communicating *branch* of tympanic plexus with auricular branch of vagus nerve.

r. commu′nicans fibula′ris ner′vi fibula′ris commu′nis [TA], SYN sural communicating *branch* of common fibular nerve.

r. communicans ganglii otici cum chorda tympani, SYN communicating *branch* of otic ganglion with chorda tympani.

r. commu′nicans gang′lii o′tici cum ner′vo auriculotempora′li, SYN communicating *branch* of otic ganglion to auriculotemporal nerve.

r. commu′nicans gang′lii o′tici cum ner′vo pterygoi′deo media′li, SYN communicating *branch* of otic ganglion with medial pterygoid nerve.

r. commu′nicans gang′lii o′tici cum ra′mo menin′geo nervi mandibularis, SYN communicating *branch* of otic ganglion with meningeal branch of mandibular nerve.

ra′mi communican′tes ner′vi auriculotempora′lis cum ner′vo

facia′li [TA], SYN communicating *branches* of auriculotemporal nerve with facial nerve, under *branch*.

r. communicans nervi facialis cum nervo glossopharyngeo [TA], SYN communicating *branch* of facial nerve with glossopharyngeal nerve.

r. commu′nicans ner′vi facia′lis cum plex′u tympan′ico, SYN communicating *branch* of intermediate nerve with tympanic plexus.

r. communicans nervi fibularis communis cum nervo cutaneo surae mediali, ☆official alternate term for sural communicating *branch* of common fibular nerve.

r. commu′nicans ner′vi glossopharyn′gei cum ra′mo auricula′ri ner′vi vagi, SYN communicating *branch* of tympanic plexus with auricular branch of vagus nerve.

r. communicans nervi intermedii cum plexu tympanico [TA], SYN communicating *branch* of intermediate nerve with tympanic plexus.

r. communicans nervi interossei antebrachii anterioris cum nervi ulnari [TA], SYN communicating *branch* of anterior interosseous nerve with ulnar nerve.

r. commu′nicans ner′vi lacrima′lis cum ner′vo zygomat′ico [TA], SYN communicating *branch* of lacrimal nerve with zygomatic nerve.

r. communicans nervi laryngei interni cum nervo laryngeo recurrente [TA], SYN communicating *branch* of internal laryngeal nerve with recurrent laryngeal nerve.

r. commu′nicans ner′vi laryn′gei recurren′tis cum ra′mo laryn′geo inter′no, SYN communicating *branch* of internal laryngeal nerve with recurrent laryngeal nerve.

r. commu′nicans ner′vi laryn′gei superio′ris cum ner′vo laryn′geo recurrenti, SYN communicating *branch* of internal laryngeal nerve with recurrent laryngeal nerve.

r. communicans nervi lingualis cum chorda tympani, SYN communicating *branch* of chorda tympani with lingual nerve.

ra′mi communican′tes ner′vi lingua′lis cum ner′vo hypoglos′so [TA], SYN communicating *branches* of lingual nerve with hypoglossal nerve, under *branch*.

r. commu′nicans ner′vi media′ni cum ner′vo ulna′ri, SYN communicating *branch* of median nerve with ulnar nerve.

r. commu′nicans ner′vi nasocilia′ris cum gan′glio cilia′ri, ☆official alternate term for sensory *root* of ciliary ganglion.

r. communicans nervi peronei communis cum nervo cutaneo surae mediali, ☆official alternate term for sural communicating *branch* of common fibular nerve.

r. communicans nervi radialis cum nervi ulnari [TA], SYN communicating *branch* of radial nerve with ulnar nerve.

ra′mi communican′tes nervo′rum spina′lium, SYN white rami communicantes.

r. commu′nicans perone′us ner′vi pero′nei commu′nis, ☆official alternate term for sural communicating *branch* of common fibular nerve.

r. communicans plexus tympanici cum ramo auriculari nervi vagi [TA], SYN communicating *branch* of tympanic plexus with auricular branch of vagus nerve.

r. commu′nicans ulna′ris ner′vi radia′lis, SYN communicating *branch* of superficial radial nerve with ulnar nerve.

rami communicantes albi [TA], SYN white rami communicantes.

rami communicantes ganglii sublingualis cum nervo linguali, ☆official alternate term for sensory *root* of sublingual ganglion.

rami communicantes grisei [TA], SYN gray rami communicantes.

rami communicantes of sympathetic part of autonomic division of nervous system, the communicating branches of the spinal nerves and sympathetic trunk, small bundles of nerve fibers connecting spinal nerves with sympathetic ganglia; the fibers passing from the ganglion to the spinal nerve are nonmyelinated and are called gray rami communicantes, those passing in the reverse direction are myelinated and are called white rami communicantes.

communicating rami of sympathetic trunk, SYN gray rami communicantes.

ra′mi cor′poris amygdaloi′dei [TA], branches to amygdaloid body [TA], branches of the anterior choroid artery to the amygdaloid body.

r. cor′poris callo′si dorsa′lis [TA], dorsal branch to corpus callosum [TA], branches of the medial occipital artery to the dorsum of the corpus callosum.

ra′mi cor′poris genicula′ti latera′lis [TA], branches to lateral geniculate body [TA] branches, branches of the anterior choroid artery to the lateral geniculate body.

r. costa′lis latera′lis arte′riae thora′cicae inter′nae [TA], SYN lateral costal *branch* of internal thoracic artery.

r. cricothyroi′deus (arteriae thyroideae superioris), SYN cricothyroid *branch* of superior thyroid artery.

rami cruris posterioris capsulae internae [TA], SYN rami capsulae internae.

ra′mi cuta′nei anterio′res ner′vi femora′lis [TA], SYN anterior cutaneous *branches* of femoral nerve, under *branch*.

rami cuta′nei anteriores pectora′lis et abdominalis nervorum intercostalium, SYN thoracoabdominal *nerves*, under *nerve*.

ra′mi cuta′nei cru′ris media′les ner′vi saphe′ni [TA], SYN medial cutaneous *nerve* of leg.

r. cutaneus anterior abdominalis nervi intercostalis [TA], SYN anterior abdominal cutaneous *branch* of intercostal nerve.

r. cutaneus anterior pectoralis nervi intercostalis [TA], SYN anterior pectoral cutaneous *branch* of intercostal nerves.

r. cuta′neus ante′rior ner′vi iliohypogas′trici [TA], SYN anterior cutaneous *branch* of iliohypogastric nerve.

r. cuta′neus ante′rior (pectora′lis et abdomina′lis) nervo′rum thoracico′rum, SYN thoracoabdominal *nerves*, under *nerve*.

r. cuta′neus latera′lis [TA], SYN lateral cutaneous *branch*.

r. cutaneus lateralis abdominalis/pectoralis nervorum intercostalium, SYN lateral abdominal/pectoral cutaneous *branches* of intercostal nerves, under *branch*.

r. cuta′neus latera′lis ner′vi iliohypogas′trici, lateral cutaneous branch of iliohypogastric nerve. SEE lateral cutaneous *branch*.

r. cuta′neus latera′lis ramor′um posterior′um arte′riae intercostal′ium, lateral cutaneous branch of dorsal branch of posterior intercostal arteries. SEE lateral cutaneous *branch*.

r. cutaneus medialis rami dorsalis arteriarum intercostalium posteriorum III–XI, SYN medial cutaneous *branch* of dorsal branch of posterior intercostal arteries; SEE medial cutaneous *branch* of dorsal branch of posterior intercostal arteries.

r. cuta′neus media′lis ramor′um dorsa′lium nervo′rum thoracico′rum, medial cutaneous branch of dorsal branch of thoracic nerves. SEE medial cutaneous *branch* of dorsal branch of posterior intercostal arteries.

r. cutaneus nervi mixti [TA], SYN cutaneous *branch* of mixed nerve.

r. cuta′neus ra′mi anterio′ris ner′vi obturato′rii [TA], SYN cutaneous *branch* of anterior branch of obturator nerve.

r. deltoi′deus [TA], SYN deltoid *branch*.

r. deltoideus arteriae profundae brachii [TA], SYN profunda brachii *artery*.

r. deltoideus arteriae thoracoacromialis [TA], SYN thoracoacromial *artery*.

dental rami, SYN dental *branches*, under *branch*.

ra′mi denta′les [TA], SYN dental *branches*, under *branch*.

rami denta′les arte′riae alveola′ris inferio′ris, dental branches of inferior alveolar artery. SEE dental *branches*, under *branch*.

rami denta′les arte′riae alveola′ris superio′ris posterio′ris, dental branch of the posterior superior alveolar artery. SEE dental *branches*, under *branch*.

ra′mi denta′les inferio′res [TA], SYN inferior dental *branches* of inferior dental plexus, under *branch*; SEE dental *branches*, under *branch*.

rami denta′les inferio′res plex′us denta′lis inferio′ris [TA], SYN inferior dental *branches* of inferior dental plexus, under *branch*.

ra′mi denta′les superio′res [TA], SYN superior dental *branches* of superior dental plexus, under *branch*.

rami denta′les superio′res plex′us denta′lis superio′ris [TA], SYN superior dental *branches* of superior dental plexus, under *branch*.

r. descen′dens [TA], sʏɴ descending *branch.*

r. descen′dens arteri′ae circumflex′ae femo′ris latera′lis [TA], sʏɴ descending *branch* of lateral circumflex femoral artery.

r. descendens arteriae circumflexae femoris medialis [TA], sʏɴ descending *branch* of medial circumflex femoral artery.

r. descen′dens arte′riae occipita′lis [TA], sʏɴ descending *branch* of occipital artery.

r. descendens arteriae segmentalis anterioris pulmonis dextri et sinistri [TA], sʏɴ descending *branch* of anterior segmental artery of left and right lungs.

r. descendens arteriae segmentalis posterioris pulmonis dextri et sinistri [TA], sʏɴ descending *branch* of posterior segmental artery of left and right lungs.

r. descendens rami superficialis arteriae transversae cervicis [TA], sʏɴ descending *branch* of superficial cervical artery.

r. dex′ter [TA], sʏɴ right *branch.*

r. dex′ter arte′riae hepat′icae propri′ae [TA], sʏɴ right *branch* of hepatic artery proper.

r. dex′ter ve′nae por′tae hepa′tis [TA], sʏɴ right *branch* of portal vein.

r. digas′tricus ner′vi facia′lis [TA], sʏɴ digastric *branch* of facial nerve.

rami dorsales arteriarum intercostalium posteriorum primae et secundae [TA], sʏɴ dorsal *branches* of first and second posterior intercostal artery, under *branch.*

rami dorsa′les arte′riae intercosta′lis supre′mae, sʏɴ dorsal *branches* of first and second posterior intercostal artery, under *branch.*

rami dorsa′les arte′riae subcosta′lis, sʏɴ dorsal *branch* of the subcostal artery.

r. dorsales arteriae subcostalis [TA], sʏɴ dorsal *branch* of the subcostal artery.

ra′mi dorsa′les lin′guae arte′riae lingua′lis [TA], sʏɴ dorsal lingual *branches* of lingual artery, under *branch.*

rami dorsa′les ner′vi ulna′ris [TA], sʏɴ dorsal *branch* of the ulnar nerve.

r. dorsa′lis, sʏɴ posterior r. of spinal nerve.

r. dorsa′lis arte′riae lumba′lis [TA], sʏɴ dorsal *branch* of the lumbar artery.

r. dorsa′lis arteria′rum intercostal′ium posterior′um III–XI [TA], sʏɴ dorsal *branch* of the posterior intercostal arteries 3–11.

r. dorsa′lis ner′vi spina′lis, ⋆official alternate term for posterior r. of spinal nerve.

r. dorsa′lis vena′rum intercostal′ium posterior′um IV–XI [TA], sʏɴ dorsal *branch* of the posterior intercostal veins 4–11.

dorsal primary r. of spinal nerve, ⋆official alternate term for posterior r. of spinal nerve.

rami duodenales arteriae pancreaticoduodenalis superioris anterioris [TA], sʏɴ duodenal *branches* of anterior superior pancreaticoduodenal artery, under *branch.*

ra′mi epiplo′icae, sʏɴ omental *branches,* under *branch.*

ra′mi esophagea′les, ⋆official alternate term for esophageal *branches,* under *branch.*

ra′mi esophagea′les aor′tae thora′cicae, ⋆official alternate term for esophageal *branches* of the thoracic aorta, under *branch.*

ra′mi esophagea′les arte′riae gas′tricae sinis′trae [TA], sʏɴ esophageal *branches* of the left gastric artery, under *branch.*

ra′mi esophagea′les arte′riae thyroi′deae inferio′ris [TA], sʏɴ esophageal *branches* of the inferior thyroid artery, under *branch.*

rami esophageales gangliorum thoracicorum [TA], sʏɴ esophageal *branches* of thoracic ganglia, under *branch.*

rami esophageales partis thoracicae aortae [TA], sʏɴ esophageal *branches* of the thoracic aorta, under *branch.*

ra′mi esopha′gei [TA], sʏɴ esophageal *branches,* under *branch.*

ra′mi esopha′gei ner′vi laryn′gei recurren′tis [TA], sʏɴ esophageal *branches* of the recurrent laryngeal nerve, under *branch.*

ra′mi esopha′gei ner′vi va′gi, sʏɴ esophageal *branches* of the vagus nerve, under *branch.*

r. exter′nus ner′vi laryn′gei superio′ris [TA], sʏɴ external *branch* of superior laryngeal nerve.

r. externus trunci nervi accessorii [TA], sʏɴ external *branch* of trunk of accessory nerve.

ra′mi faucia′les ner′vi lingua′lis, sʏɴ *branches* of lingual nerve to isthmus of fauces, under *branch.*

r. femora′lis ner′vi genitofemora′lis [TA], sʏɴ femoral *branch* of genitofemoral nerve.

r. fronta′lis anteromedia′lis [TA], anteromedial frontal branch [TA] of the callosomarginal artery.

r. frontalis anteromedialis arteriae callosomarginalis [TA], sʏɴ anteromedial frontal *branch* of callosomarginal artery.

r. frontalis arteriae meningeae mediae [TA], sʏɴ frontal *branch* of middle meningeal artery.

r. fronta′lis arte′riae tempora′lis superficia′lis [TA], sʏɴ frontal *branch* of superficial temporal artery.

r. fronta′lis intermediomedia′lis [TA], intermediomedial frontal branch [TA] of the callosomarginal artery.

r. frontalis intermediomedialis arteriae callosomarginalis [TA], sʏɴ intermediomedial frontal *branch* of callosomarginal artery.

r. fronta′lis posteromedia′lis [TA], posteromedial frontal branch [TA] of the callosomarginal artery.

r. frontalis posteromedialis arteriae callosomarginalis [TA], sʏɴ posteromedial frontal *branch* of callosomarginal artery.

rami gang′lii submandibula′ris, sʏɴ glandular *branches* of submandibular ganglion, under *branch.*

ra′mi communican′tes gang′lii submandibula′ris cum ner′vo lingua′li, ⋆official alternate term for sensory *root* of submandibular ganglion.

r. gang′lii trigemina′lis, sʏɴ *branches* of internal carotid artery to trigeminal ganglion, under *branch.*

ra′mi gangliona′res, sʏɴ sensory *root* of pterygopalatine ganglion.

r. ganglionares trigeminales arteriae carotidis internae [TA], sʏɴ *branches* of internal carotid artery to trigeminal ganglion, under *branch.*

rami ganglio′nici ner′vi maxilla′ris, ⋆official alternate term for sensory *root* of pterygopalatine ganglion.

ra′mi gas′trici anterio′res ner′vi va′gi, sʏɴ anterior gastric *branches* of anterior vagal trunk, under *branch.*

rami gastrici anteriores trunci vagalis anterioris [TA], sʏɴ anterior gastric *branches* of anterior vagal trunk, under *branch.*

ra′mi gas′trici posterio′res ner′vi va′gi, sʏɴ gastric *branches* of posterior vagal *trunk,* under *branch.*

rami gastrici posteriores trunci vagalis posterioris [TA], sʏɴ posterior gastric *branches* of posterior vagal trunk, under *branch.*

r. genita′lis ner′vi genitofemora′lis [TA], sʏɴ genital *branch* of genitofemoral nerve.

rami genus capsulae internae [TA], sʏɴ rami capsulae internae.

ra′mi gingiva′les inferio′res plex′us denta′lis inferio′ris [TA], sʏɴ inferior gingival *branches* of inferior dental plexus, under *branch.*

ra′mi gingiva′les superio′res plex′us denta′lis superio′ris [TA], sʏɴ superior gingival *branches* of superior dental plexus, under *branch.*

ra′mi glandula′res [TA], sʏɴ glandular *branches,* under *branch.*

r. glandula′res ante′rior/latera′lis/poste′rior arte′riae thyroi′de-ae superio′ris, sʏɴ anterior/lateral/posterior glandular *branches* of superior thyroid artery, under *branch.*

rami glandula′res arte′riae facia′lis, sʏɴ glandular *branches* of facial artery, under *branch.*

rami glandula′res arte′riae thyroi′deae inferio′ris [TA], sʏɴ glandular *branches* of inferior thyroid artery, under *branch.*

rami glandular′es gang′lii submandibular′is, sʏɴ glandular *branches* of submandibular ganglion, under *branch.*

r. glandularis anterior arteriae thyroideae superioris [TA], sʏɴ anterior glandular *branch* of superior thyroid artery.

r. glandularis posterior arteriae thyroideae superioris [TA], sʏɴ posterior glandular *branch* of superior thyroid artery.

ra′mi glo′bi pal′lidi [TA], branches to globus pallidus [TA], branches of the anterior choroid artery to the globus pallidus.

gray rami communicantes [TA], short nerves arising from the lateral aspect of the sympathetic trunk conducting nonmyelinated postsynaptic sympathetic nerve fibers from the sympathetic trunk to the initial portions of all 31 pairs of ventral primary rami of spinal nerves for distribution by all parts (including the dorsal primary ramus) of the spinal nerve. The gray rami are the parietal branches of the sympathetic trunks since all postsynaptic fibers to be distributed to the body wall (including limbs) must pass through them. SYN rami communicantes grisei [TA], communicating branches of sympathetic trunk, communicating rami of sympathetic trunk.

ra'mi hepat'ici ner'vi va'gi, SYN hepatic *branches* of anterior vagal trunk, under *branch.*

rami hepatici trunci vagi anterior [TA], SYN hepatic *branches* of anterior vagal trunk, under *branch.*

r. hypothalam'icus [TA], the hypothalamic branch, a branch of the anterior cerebral artery to the hypothalamus.

r. ili'acus arte'riae iliolumba'lis [TA], SYN iliacus *branch* of iliolumbar artery.

r. infe'rior [TA], SYN inferior *branch.*

r. infe'rior arte'riae glu'teae superio'ris [TA], SYN inferior *branch* of superior gluteal artery.

inferior dental rami, SYN inferior dental *branches* of inferior dental plexus, under *branch.*

ra'mi inferio'res ner'vi transver'si cervicalis [col'li], SYN inferior *branches* of transverse cervical nerve, under *branch.*

rami inferiores nervi transversi colli, ⋆official alternate term for inferior *branches* of transverse cervical nerve, under *branch.*

r. infe'rior ner'vi oculomoto'rii [TA], SYN inferior *branch* of oculomotor nerve.

r. inferior ossis pubis [TA], SYN inferior pubic r.

inferior pubic r. [TA], inferior extension from body of pubic bone that meets with the ramus of the ischium to form the ischiopubic ramus. SYN r. inferior ossis pubis [TA].

r. infrahyoi'deus arte'riae thyroi'deae superio'ris [TA], SYN infrahyoid *branch* of superior thyroid artery.

r. infrapatella'ris ner'vi saphe'ni [TA], SYN infrapatellar *branch* of saphenous nerve.

ra'mi inguina'les arte'riarum puden'darum exter'narum profundarum [TA], SYN inguinal *branches* of deep external pudendal arteries, under *branch.*

ra'mi intercosta'les anterio'res, SYN anterior intercostal *branches* of internal thoracic artery, under *branch.*

rami intercostal'es anterior'es arter'iae thora'cicae inter'nae [TA], SYN anterior intercostal *branches* of internal thoracic artery, under *branch.*

ra'mi intergangliona'res trunci sympathici [TA], SYN interganglionic *branches* of sympathetic trunk, under *branch.*

r. intermedius arteriae hepaticae propriae [TA], SYN intermediate *branch* of hepatic artery proper.

internal r. of accessory nerve, SYN internal *branch* of trunk of accessory nerve; SEE ALSO accessory *nerve* [CN XI].

r. inter'nus trunci ner'vi accesso'rii [TA], SYN internal *branch* of trunk of accessory nerve; SEE ALSO accessory *nerve* [CN XI].

r. inter'nus ner'vi laryn'gei superio'ris [TA], SYN internal *branch* of superior laryngeal nerve.

ra'mi interventricula'res septa'les, SYN interventricular septal *branches* of left/right coronary artery, under *branch.*

rami interventriculares septales arteriae coronariae sinistrae/dextrae, SYN interventricular septal *branches* of left/right coronary artery, under *branch.*

r. interventricula'ris ante'rior arte'riae corona'riae sinis'trae [TA], SYN anterior interventricular *branch* of left coronary artery.

r. interventricula'ris poste'rior arte'riae corona'riae dex'trae [TA], SYN posterior interventricular branch of right coronary *artery.*

ischial r., SYN r. of ischium.

ischiopubic r., the inferior r. of the pubis and the r. of the ischium continuous with it, forming the inferomedial boundary of the obturator foramen.

r. of ischium [TA], the branch of the ischial bone, formerly called inferior branch of the ischium; the portion of the bone that passes

forward from the ischial tuberosity to join the inferior r. of the pubic bone, thus forming the ischiopubic r. SYN r. ossis ischii [TA], ischial r.

ra'mi isth'mi fau'cium ner'vi lingua'lis [TA], SYN *branches* of lingual nerve to isthmus of fauces, under *branch.*

ra'mi labia'les anterio'res arte'riae puden'dae exter'nae profundae [TA], SYN anterior labial *branches* of deep external pudendal artery, under *branch.*

ra'mi labia'les inferio'res ner'vi menta'lis, SYN labial *branches* of mental nerve, under *branch.*

rami labiales nervi mentalis [TA], SYN labial *branches* of mental nerve, under *branch.*

rami labiales posteriores arteriae perinealis [TA], SYN posterior labial branches of internal perineal *artery.*

ra'mi labia'les posterio'res arte'riae puden'dae inter'nae, SYN posterior labial branches of internal perineal *artery.*

ra'mi labia'les superio'res ner'vi infraorbita'lis [TA], SYN superior labial *branches* of infraorbital nerve, under *branch.*

r. labialis inferior arteriae facialis, SYN inferior labial *branch* of facial artery.

r. labialis superior arteriae facialis, SYN superior labial *branch* of facial artery.

ra'mi laryngopharyn'gei gang'lii cervica'lis superio'ris [TA], SYN laryngopharyngeal *branches* of superior cervical ganglion, under *branch.*

ra'mi latera'les [TA], SYN lateral *branches,* under *branch.*

rami laterales arteriae pontis [TA], SYN lateral *branches* of pontine arteries, under *branch.*

rami latera'les arteria'rum centra'lium anterolatera'lium, lateral branch of anterolateral central arteries.

rami laterales arteriarum tuberis cinerei [TA], SYN lateral *branches* of artery of tuber cinereum, under *branch.*

rami latera'les ra'mi sinis'tri ve'nae por'tae hep'atis, lateral branch of left branch of portal vein. SEE lateral *branches,* under *branch.*

rami laterales ramorum dorsalium nervorum spinalis, lateral branch of dorsal primary rami of spinal nerves. SEE lateral *branches,* under *branch.*

r. latera'lis duc'tus hepa'tici sinis'tri, lateral branch left hepatic duct. SEE lateral *branches,* under *branch.*

r. lateralis interventricularis anterioris arteriae coronariae sinistrae, lateral branch of anterior interventricular artery. SEE lateral *branches,* under *branch.*

r. lateralis nasi arteriae facialis [TA], SYN lateral nasal *branch* of facial artery.

r. latera'lis ner'vi supraorbita'lis, lateral branch of supraorbital nerve. SEE lateral *branches,* under *branch.*

r. latera'lis ramor'um dorsa'lium nervo'rum thoracico'rum, lateral cutaneous branch of dorsal branch of thoracic nerves.

r. latera'lis rami lobar'is me'dii arteriae pulmona'lis dextrae, lateral branch of middle lobe branch of right pulmonary artery. SEE lateral *branches,* under *branch.*

rami liena'les arte'riae liena'lis, ⋆official alternate term for splenic *branches* of splenic artery, under *branch.*

rami lingua'les ner'vi glossopharyn'gei, lingual branch of glossopharyngeal nerve. SEE lingual *branches,* under *branch.*

rami lingua'les ner'vi hypoglos'si, lingual branch of hypoglossal nerve. SEE lingual *branches,* under *branch.*

rami lingua'les ner'vi lingua'lis, lingual branch of lingual nerve. SEE lingual *branches,* under *branch.*

ra'mi lingua'les, SYN lingual *branches,* under *branch.*

r. lingual'is ner'vi facia'lis, SYN lingual *branch* of facial nerve.

r. lingula'ris infe'rior, SYN inferior lingular *artery.*

r. lingula'ris supe'rior, SYN superior lingular *artery.*

r. lingularis venae pulmonis sinistrae superioris, ⋆official alternate term for lingular *vein.*

ra'mi lobi cauda'ti rami sinistri venae portae hepatis [TA], SYN caudate *branches* of left branch of portal vein, under *branch.*

r. lobi medii arteriae pulmonalis dextrae, middle lobe branch of right pulmonary artery. SEE middle lobe *vein.*

r. lo′bi me′dii ve′nae pulmona′lis dex′trae superio′ris, SYN middle lobe *vein*; SEE middle lobe *vein*.

r. lumba′lis arte′riae iliolumba′lis [TA], SYN lumbar *branch* of iliolumbar artery.

ra′mi malleola′res latera′les arteriae fibularis (peronei) [TA], SYN lateral malleolar *branch* (of fibular peroneal artery).

ra′mi malleola′res media′les arteriae tibialis posterioris [TA], SYN medial malleolar *branches* (of posterior tibial artery), under *branch*.

ra′mi mamma′rii, SEE lateral mammary *branches*, under *branch*, medial mammary *branches*, under *branch*.

ra′mi mamma′rii latera′les, SYN lateral mammary *branches*, under *branch*.

rami mamma′rii latera′les arte′riae thora′cicae latera′lis [TA], SYN lateral mammary *branches* of lateral thoracic artery, under *branch*.

rami mamma′rii latera′les ramo′rum cutaneo′rum latera′lium nervo′rum intercosta′lium, SYN lateral mammary *branches* of lateral cutaneous branches of thoracic spinal nerves, under *branch*.

rami mamma′rii latera′les ramo′rum cuta′neorum latera′lis nervo′rum thoracico′rum, SYN lateral mammary *branches* of lateral cutaneous branches of thoracic spinal nerves, under *branch*.

ra′mi mamma′rii media′les, SYN medial mammary *branches*, under *branch*.

rami mammari′i media′les ramo′rum cutaneo′rum anterio′rum nervo′rum intercostal′ium, medial mammary branches of anterior cutaneous branches of ventral primary rami of thoracic spinal nerves. SEE medial mammary *branches*, under *branch*.

rami mamma′rii media′les ra′mi cuta′nei anterio′ris ramor′um ventral′ium nervo′rum thoraci′corum, medial mammary branches of anterior cutaneous branches of ventral primary rami of thoracic spinal nerves. SEE medial mammary *branches*, under *branch*.

rami mamma′rii media′les ramo′rum perforan′tium arte′riae thora′cicae inter′nae, medial mammary branches of perforating branches of internal thoracic artery. SEE medial mammary *branches*, under *branch*.

r. of mandible [TA], the upturned perpendicular extremity of the mandible on either side; it gives attachment on its lateral surface to the masseter muscle. SYN r. mandibulae [TA].

r. mandib′ulae [TA], SYN r. of mandible.

r. marginalis [TA], SYN marginal *sulcus*.

r. marginalis dexter (arteriae coronariae dextrae) [TA], SYN right marginal *branch* (of right coronary artery).

r. margina′lis mandib′ulae ner′vi facia′lis [TA], SYN marginal mandibular *branch* of facial nerve.

r. marginalis sinister arteriae coronariae sinistrae [TA], SYN left marginal *artery*.

r. marginalis sulci cinguli [TA], SYN marginal *branch* of cingulate sulcus.

r. marginalis sulci parietooccipitalis [TA], SYN marginal *branch* of parietooccipital sulcus.

r. margina′lis tento′rii arte′riae caro′tidis inter′nae, SYN tentorial marginal *branch* of cavernous part of internal carotid artery.

r. marginalis tentorii partis cavernosae arteriae carotidis internae [TA], SYN tentorial marginal *branch* of cavernous part of internal carotid artery.

ra′mi mastoi′dei arte′riae auricula′ris posterio′ris, SYN mastoid *branches* of posterior tympanic artery, under *branch*.

rami mastoidei arteriae tympanicae posterioris [TA], SYN mastoid *branches* of posterior tympanic artery, under *branch*.

r. mastoi′deus arte′riae occipita′lis [TA], SYN mastoid *branch* of occipital artery.

r. mea′tus acus′tici inter′ni, SYN labyrinthine *artery*.

ra′mi media′les [TA], SYN medial *branches*, under *branch*.

rami mediales arteriae pontis [TA], SYN medial *branches* of pontine arteries, under *branch*.

rami media′les arteria′rum centra′lium anterolatera′lium, me-

dial branch of anterolateral central arteries. SEE medial *branches*, under *branch*.

rami mediales arteriarum tuberis cinerei [TA], SYN medial *branches* of artery of tuber cinereum, under *branch*.

r. media′lis duc′tus hepa′tici sinis′tri, medial branch of left hepatic duct. SEE medial *branches*, under *branch*.

r. media′lis ner′vi supraorbita′lis, medial branch of supraorbital nerve. SEE medial *branches*, under *branch*.

r. media′lis ra′mi loba′ris me′dii arteriae pulmona′lis dextrae, medial branch of middle lobar branch of right pulmonary artery. SEE medial *branches*, under *branch*.

rami media′les ra′mi sinis′tri ve′nae por′tae hepa′tis, medial branch of left branch of portal vein. SEE medial *branches*, under *branch*.

r. media′lis ramor′um dorsa′lium nervo′rum spinalis, SYN medial *branch* of posterior rami of spinal nerves; SEE medial *branches*, under *branch*.

ra′mi mediastina′les [TA], SYN mediastinal *branches*, under *branch*.

rami mediastina′les aor′tae thora′cicae [TA], SYN mediastinal *branches* of thoracic aorta, under *branch*.

rami mediastina′les arte′riae thora′cicae inter′nae [TA], SYN mediastinal *branches* of internal thoracic artery, under *branch*.

ra′mi medulla′res latera′les, lateral medullary branches [TA], branches of the posterior inferior cerebellar artery to the lateral part of the medulla oblongata.

rami medullares laterales (partis intracranialis) arteriae vertebralis [TA], SYN lateral medullary *branches* of (intracranial part of) vertebral artery, under *branch*.

ra′mi medulla′res media′les, medial medullary branches [TA], branches of the posterior inferior cerebellar artery to the medial part of the medulla oblongata.

rami medullares mediales arteriae vertebralis [TA], SYN medial medullary *branches* of vertebral artery, under *branch*.

rami membra′nae tym′pani ner′vi auriculotempora′lis, SYN *branches* of auriculotemporal nerve to tympanic membrane, under *branch*.

rami menin′gei [TA], SYN meningeal *branches*, under *branch*.

r. meningeus accessorius, SYN pterygomeningeal *artery*.

r. menin′geus accesso′rius arte′riae menin′geae me′diae, SYN accessory *branch* of middle meningeal artery.

r. menin′geus anterior arteriae ethmoidalis anterioris [TA], SYN anterior meningeal *branch* (of anterior ethmoidal artery).

r. menin′geus ante′rior arte′riae vertebra′lis, meningeal branch of the vertebral artery.

r. menin′geus arte′riae carot′idis inter′nae, SYN meningeal *branch* of cavernous part of internal carotid artery.

r. menin′geus arte′riae occipita′lis [TA], SYN meningeal *branch* of occipital artery.

r. menin′geus me′dius ner′vi maxilla′ris, SYN meningeal *branch* of maxillary nerve.

r. menin′geus ner′vi mandibula′ris [TA], SYN meningeal *branch* of mandibular nerve.

r. meningeus nervi maxillaris [TA], SYN meningeal *branch* of maxillary nerve.

r. menin′geus ner′vi va′gi [TA], SYN meningeal *branch* of vagus nerve.

r. menin′geus nervo′rum spina′lium [TA], SYN meningeal *branch* of spinal nerves.

r. meningeus partis cavernosae arteriae carotidis internae [TA], SYN meningeal *branch* of cavernous part of internal carotid artery.

r. meningeus partis cerebralis arteriae carotidis internae [TA], SYN meningeal *branch* of cerebral part of internal carotid artery.

r. meningeus (partis intracranialis) arteriae vertebralis [TA], SYN meningeal *branch* of (intracranial part of) vertebral artery.

r. menin′geus poste′rior, the posterior meningeal branch of the vertebral artery.

r. meningeus recurrens nervi ophthalmici [TA], SYN tentorial *nerve*.

ra

ra'mi menta'les ner'vi menta'lis [TA], SYN mental *branches* of mental nerve, under *branch*.

r. mentalis arteriae alveolaris inferioris [TA], SYN mental *branch* (of inferior alveolar artery).

ra'mi muscula'res [TA], SYN muscular *branches*, under *branch*.

rami musculares arteriae vertebralis [TA], SEE muscular *branches*, under *branch*.

rami musculares nervi accessorii [TA], SEE muscular *branches*, under *branch*.

rami musculares nervi axillaris [TA], SEE muscular *branches*, under *branch*.

rami musculares nervi fibularis profundi [TA], SEE muscular *branches*, under *branch*.

rami musculares nervi fibularis superficialis [TA], SEE muscular *branches*, under *branch*.

rami musculares nervi interossei antebrachii anterior [TA], SEE muscular *branches*, under *branch*.

rami musculares nervi mediani [TA], SEE muscular *branches*, under *branch*.

rami musculares nervi musculocutanei [TA], SEE muscular *branches*, under *branch*.

rami musculares nervi radialis [TA], SEE muscular *branches*, under *branch*.

rami musculares nervi tibialis [TA], SEE muscular *branches*, under *branch*.

rami musculares nervi ulnaris [TA], SEE muscular *branches*, under *branch*.

rami musculares nervorum intercostalium [TA], SEE muscular *branches*, under *branch*.

rami musculares nervorum perinealium [TA], SEE muscular *branches*, under *branch*.

rami musculares nervorum spinalium [TA], SEE muscular *branches*, under *branch*.

rami musculares partis supraclavicularis plexus brachialis [TA], SEE muscular *branches*, under *branch*.

rami musculares rami anterioris nervi obturatorii [TA], SEE muscular *branches*, under *branch*.

rami musculares rami posterioris nervi obturatorii [TA], SEE muscular *branches*, under *branch*.

r. mus'culi stylopharyn'gei ner'vi glossopharyn'gei [TA], SYN stylopharyngeal *branch* of glossopharyngeal nerve.

r. mylohyoi'deus arte'riae alveola'ris inferio'ris [TA], SYN mylohyoid *branch* (of inferior alveolar artery).

rami nasales anteriores laterales arteriae ethmoidalis anterioris [TA], SYN anterior lateral nasal *branches* of anterior ethmoidal artery, under *branch*.

ra'mi nasa'les exter'ni ner'vi ethmoida'lis anterio'ris, external nasal branch of nasociliary nerve; SEE external nasal *branches* of infraorbital nerve, under *branch*.

ra'mi nasa'les exter'ni ner'vi infraorbita'lis, SYN external nasal *branches* of infraorbital nerve, under *branch*; SEE external nasal *branches* of infraorbital nerve, under *branch*.

ra'mi nasa'les inter'ni [TA], SYN internal nasal *branches*, under *branch*.

rami nasa'les inter'ni ner'vi ethmoida'lis anterio'ris, internal nasal branch of nasociliary nerve. SEE internal nasal *branches*, under *branch*.

rami nasa'les inter'ni ner'vi infraorbita'lis, internal nasal branch of infraorbital nerve. SEE internal nasal *branches*, under *branch*.

ra'mi nasa'les latera'les ner'vi ethmoida'lis anterio'ris [TA], SYN lateral nasal *branches* of anterior ethmoidal nerve, under *branch*.

ra'mi nasa'les media'les ner'vi ethmoida'lis anterio'ris [TA], SYN medial nasal *branches* of anterior ethmoidal nerve, under *branch*.

ra'mi nasa'les posterio'res inferio'res ner'vi palati'ni majo'ris [TA], SYN posterior inferior nasal *nerves*, under *nerve*.

ra'mi nasa'les posterio'res superio'res latera'les gang'lii pterygopalati'ni, SYN posterior superior lateral nasal *branches* of maxillary nerve, under *branch*.

rami nasales posteriores superiores laterales nervi maxillaris, SYN posterior superior lateral nasal *branches* of maxillary nerve, under *branch*.

ra'mi nasa'les posterio'res superio'res media'les gang'lii pterygopalati'ni, SYN posterior superior medial nasal *branches* of maxillary nerve, under *branch*.

rami nasales posteriores superiores mediales nervi maxillaris [TA], SYN posterior superior medial nasal *branches* of maxillary nerve, under *branch*.

r. ner'vi oculomoto'rii arte'riae communican'tis posterio'ris, the branch to the oculomotor nerve, a branch of the posterior communicating artery to the oculomotor nerve.

r. no'di atrioventricula'ris [TA], SYN atrioventricular nodal *branch*.

r. no'di sinuatria'lis arte'riae corona'riae dex'trae [TA], SYN sinuatrial (S-A) nodal *branch* of right coronary artery.

ra'mi nucleo'rum hypothalamico'rum [TA], branches to hypothalamic nuclei [TA], branches of the anterior choroid artery to the nuclei of the hypothalamus.

r. obturato'rius arte'riae epigas'tricae inferio'ris, SYN accessory obturator *artery*.

r. obturatorius rami pubici arteriae epigastricae inferioris [TA], SYN obturator *branch* of pubic branch of inferior epigastric vein.

rami occipita'les arte'riae auricula'ris posterio'ris, occipital branch of posterior auricular artery. SEE occipital *branch*.

rami occipita'les arte'riae occip'itis, occipital branch of occipital artery. SEE occipital *branch*.

rami occipita'les ner'vi auricula'ris posterio'ris, occipital branch posterior auricular nerve. SEE occipital *branch*.

r. occipita'lis [TA], SYN occipital *branch*.

r. occipitotempora'lis [TA], occipitotemporal branch [TA], a branch of the medial occipital artery to the occipital and temporal regions of the cerebral cortex.

ra'mi omenta'les [TA], SYN omental *branches*, under *branch*.

rami orbitales nervi maxillaris [TA], SYN orbital *branches* of maxillary nerve, under *branch*.

r. orbita'lis arte'riae menin'geae me'diae [TA], SYN orbital *branch* of middle meningeal artery.

r. orbita'lis gang'lii pterygopalati'ni, SYN orbital *branches* of maxillary nerve, under *branch*.

r. os'sis is'chii [TA], SYN r. of ischium.

rami ova'rici arte'riae uteri'nae [TA], SYN ovarian *branches* of uterine artery, under *branch*.

r. palmaris nervi interossei antebrachii anterioris [TA], SYN palmar *branch* of anterior interosseous nerve.

r. palma'ris ner'vi media'ni, SYN palmar *branch* of anterior interosseous nerve.

r. palma'ris ner'vi ulna'ris [TA], SYN palmar *branch* of ulnar nerve.

r. palma'ris profun'dus arte'riae ulna'ris [TA], SYN deep palmar *branch* of ulnar artery.

r. palma'ris superficia'lis arte'riae radia'lis [TA], SYN superficial palmar *branch* of radial artery.

ra'mi palpebra'les ner'vi infratrochlea'ris [TA], SYN palpebral *branches* of infratrochlear nerve, under *branch*.

ra'mi pancrea'tici [TA], SYN pancreatic *branches*, under *branch*.

rami pancrea'tici arte'riae pancreaticoduodena'lis superio'ris, pancreatic branch of superior pancreaticoduodenal arteries. SEE pancreatic *branches*, under *branch*.

rami pancrea'tici arte'riae sple'nicae, pancreatic branch splenic artery. SEE pancreatic *branches*, under *branch*.

r. paracentrales [TA], SYN paracentral *branches* (of pericallosal artery), under *branch*.

rami paracentrales arteriae callosomarginalis [TA], SYN paracentral *branches* of callosomarginal artery, under *branch*.

ra'mi parieta'les [TA], SYN parietal *branch*.

r. parietal'is arte'riae menin'geae me'diae [TA], SYN parietal *branch* of middle meningeal artery.

r. parietal'is arte'riae occipita'lis media'lis [TA], SYN parietal *branch* of medial occipital artery.

r. parietal'is arte'riae tempora'lis superficia'lis [TA], SYN parietal *branch* of superficial temporal artery.

r. pari'eto-occipita'lis [TA], parieto-occipital branch [TA] of medial occipital artery.

r. parieto-occipitalis arteriae occipitalis medialis [TA], SYN parieto-occipital *branch* (of posterior cerebral artery).

ra'mi parotid'ei [TA], SYN parotid *branches*, under *branch*.

r. parotid'ei arte'riae tempora'lis superficia'lis, parotid branch of superficial temporal artery. SEE parotid *branches*, under *branch*.

rami parotid'ei ner'vi auriculotempora'lis, parotid branch of auriculotemporal nerve. SEE parotid *branches*, under *branch*.

rami parotid'ei ve'nae facia'lis, parotid branch of facial vein. SEE parotid *branches*, under *branch*.

rami partis retrolentiformis capsulae internae [TA], SYN rami capsulae internae.

ra'mi pectora'les arteri'ae thoracoacromia'lis [TA], SYN pectoral *branch* of thoracoacromial artery, under *branch*.

ra'mi peduncula'res [TA], peduncular branches [TA], branches of the posterior cerebral artery to the cerebral peduncles.

r. per'forans [TA], SYN perforating *branches*, under *branch*.

r. per'forans arte'riae fibula'ris [TA], SYN perforating *branch* of fibular artery.

r. perforans arteriae interossei anterioris [TA], SYN perforating *branch* of anterior interosseous artery.

rami perforantes arcus palmaris profundi [TA], SYN perforating *branches* of deep palmar arch.

rami perforan'tes arte'riae thorac'icae inter'nae [TA], SYN perforating *branches* of internal thoracic artery, under *branch*.

rami perforan'tes arteria'rum metacarpa'lium palma'rium, SEE perforating *branches* of deep palmar arch.

rami perforan'tes arteria'rum metatarsea'rum planta'rium [TA], SYN perforating *branches* (of plantar metatarsal arteries), under *branch*.

ra'mi pericardi'aci aor'tae thora'cicae [TA], SYN pericardial *branch* of thoracic aorta, under *branch*.

r. pericardi'acus ner'vi phren'ici [TA], SYN pericardial *branch* of phrenic nerve.

ra'mi perinea'les ner'vi cuta'nei fem'oris posterio'ris [TA], SYN perineal *branches* of posterior cutaneous nerve of thigh, under *branch*.

peroneal anastomotic r., SYN sural communicating *branch* of common fibular nerve.

r. petro'sus arte'riae menin'geae med'iae [TA], SYN petrosal *branch* of middle meningeal artery.

ra'mi pharyngea'les, *official alternate term for pharyngeal *branches*, under *branch*.

rami pharyngea'les arte'riae pharyn'geae ascenden'tis [TA], SYN pharyngeal *branch* of the ascending pharyngeal artery.

rami pharyngea'les arte'riae thyroi'deae inferio'ris [TA], SYN pharyngeal *branch* of inferior thyroid artery.

rami pharyngei [TA], SYN pharyngeal *branches*, under *branch*.

rami pharyn'gei ner'vi glossopharyn'gei [TA], SYN pharyngeal *branch* of glossopharyngeal nerve.

rami pharyngei nervi laryngei recurrentis [TA], SYN pharyngeal *branches* of recurrent laryngeal nerve, under *branch*.

rami pharyn'gei ner'vi va'gi [TA], SYN pharyngeal *branch* of vagus nerve.

r. pharyn'geus arte'riae cana'lis pterygoi'dei [TA], SYN pharyngeal *branch* of the artery of pterygoid canal.

r. pharyn'geus arte'riae palati'nae descen'dentis [TA], SYN pharyngeal *branch* of descending palatine artery.

r. pharyn'geus gan'glii pterygopalati'ni, SYN pharyngeal *nerve*.

ra'mi phrenicoabdomina'les ner'vi phre'nici, SYN phrenicoabdominal *branches* of phrenic nerve, under *branch*.

r. planta'ris profun'dus arte'riae dorsa'lis pe'dis, SYN deep plantar *artery*.

r. poste'rior arte'riae obturato'riae [TA], SYN posterior *branch* of obturator artery.

r. poste'rior arte'riae pancreaticoduodena'lis inferio'ris [TA], SYN posterior *branch* of inferior pancreaticoduodenal artery.

r. poste'rior arte'riae recurren'tis ulna'ris [TA], SYN posterior *branch* of ulnar recurrent artery.

r. poste'rior arte'riae rena'lis [TA], SYN posterior *branch* of renal artery; SEE segmental *arteries* of kidney, under *artery*.

r. poste'rior arte'riae thyroi'deae superio'ris, SYN posterior glandular *branch* of superior thyroid artery.

r. poste'rior descen'dens, SYN descending *branch* of posterior segmental artery of left and right lungs.

r. poste'rior duc'tus hepa'tici dex'tri [TA], SYN posterior *branch* of right hepatic duct.

rami posterio'res [TA], SYN posterior *branches*, under *branch*.

r. poste'rior nervi spina'lis [TA], SYN posterior r. of spinal nerve.

posterior r. of lateral cerebral sulcus [TA], the long, posteriorly-directed continuation of the lateral cerebral sulcus which extends between the temporal lobe inferiorly and the parietal lobe superiorly, its termination surrounded by the supramarginal gyrus. SYN posterior branch of lateral cerebral sulcus, r. posterior sulci lateralis cerebri.

posterior r. of lateral sulcus of cerebrum [TA], SYN r. posterior sulci lateralis cerebri [TA].

r. poste'rior ner'vi auricula'ris mag'ni [TA], SYN posterior *branch* of great auricular nerve.

r. posterior nervi cutanei antebrachii medialis [TA], SYN posterior *branch* of medial cutaneous nerve of forearm.

r. poste'rior ner'vi obturato'rii [TA], SYN posterior *branch* of obturator nerve.

r. poste'rior ra'mi dex'tri ve'nae por'tae hepa'tis [TA], SYN posterior *branch* of right branch of portal vein.

posterior r. of spinal nerve [TA], the smaller, posteriorly directed major terminal branch (with the anterior r.) of all 31 pairs of mixed spinal nerves, formed at the intervertebral foramen and turning abruptly posteriorly to divide into lateral and medial branches, both of which will supply the deep (true) muscles of the back. The medial branch (rami medialis [TA]) of the dorsal primary r. also supplies articular branches to the zygapophyseal joints and the periosteum of the vertebral arch. In the neck and upper back, the medial branch continues through the deep and superficial back muscles to supply overlying skin; in the lower back, the lateral branch does this. Terminologia Anatomica lists posterior rami (rami dorsales) for each group of spinal nerves: 1) cervical (nervorum cervicalium [TA]), 2) thoracic (nervorum thoracicorum [TA]), 3) lumbar (nervorum lumbalium [TA]), 4) sacral (nervorum sacralium [TA]), and 5) coccygeal (nervi coccygei [TA]). SYN r_i posterior nervi spinalis [TA], dorsal primary r. of spinal nerve*, r. dorsalis nervi spinalis*, dorsal branch (1), posterior primary division, r. dorsalis.

r. poste'rior sul'ci latera'lis cere'bri, SYN posterior r. of lateral cerebral sulcus.

r. posterior sulcus lateralis cerebri [TA], SYN posterior r. of lateral sulcus of cerebrum.

r. poste'rior ve'nae pulmona'lis dex'trae superio'ris [TA], SYN posterior *branch* of right superior pulmonary vein.

rami precuneales arteriae cerebri anterioris [TA], SYN precuneal *branches* (of anterior cerebral artery), under *branch*.

r. prelaminaris rami spinalis rami dorsalis arteriae intercostalis posterioris [TA], SYN prelaminar *branch* of spinal branch of dorsal branch of posterior intercostal artery.

rami profun'di arte'riae transver'sae cervi'cis [TA], SYN dorsal scapular *artery*.

r. profun'dus [TA], SYN deep *branch*.

r. profun'dus arte'riae circumflex'ae fem'oris media'lis [TA], SYN deep *branch* of the medial circumflex femoral artery.

r. profundus arteriae gluteae superioris [TA], SYN deep *branch* of the superior gluteal artery.

r. profun'dus arte'riae plantaris media'lis [TA], SYN deep *branch* of the medial plantar artery.

r. profun'dus arte'riae scapula'ris descenden'tis, SYN dorsal scapular *artery*.

r. profun′dus arte′riae transver′sae col′li [TA], SYN dorsal scapular *artery*.

r. profun′dus ner′vi plantar′is latera′lis [TA], SYN deep *branch* of the lateral plantar nerve.

r. profundus nervi radialis [TA], SYN deep *branch* of radial nerve.

r. profun′dus ner′vi ulna′ris [TA], SYN deep *branch* of the ulnar nerve.

rami prostatici arteriae rectalis mediae [TA], SYN prostatic *branches* of middle rectal artery, under *branch*.

rami prostatici arteriae vesicalis inferioris [TA], SYN prostatic *branches* of inferior vesical artery, under *branch*.

ra′mi pterygoi′dei arte′riae maxilla′ris, SYN pterygoid *branch* of posterior deep temporal artery.

r. pterygoideus arteriae temporalis profundae posterioris [TA], SYN pterygoid *branch* of posterior deep temporal artery.

pubic rami, SEE pubic *hair*.

r. pu′bicus arte′riae epigas′tricae inferio′ris [TA], SYN pubic *branch* of inferior epigastric artery.

r. pu′bicus arte′riae obturato′riae [TA], SYN pubic *branch* of obturator artery.

r. pubicus venae epigastricae inferioris [TA], SYN pubic *branch* of inferior epigastric vein.

rami pulmonales plexi nervosi pulmonalis [TA], SYN pulmonary *branches* of pulmonary nerve plexus, under *branch*.

ra′mi pulmona′les syste′matis autono′mici, SYN pulmonary *branch* of autonomic nervous system, under *branch*.

rami pulmonales thoracici gangliorum thoracicorum [TA], SYN thoracic pulmonary *branches* of thoracic ganglia, under *branch*.

r. pyloricus trunci vagalis anterioris [TA], SYN pyloric *branch* of anterior vagal trunk.

ra′mi radicula′res, SYN spinal *arteries*, under *artery*.

r. atrialis intermedius arteriae coronariae sinistrae [TA], SYN intermediate atrial *branch* of left coronary artery.

ra′mi rena′les ner′vi va′gi [TA], SYN renal *branch* of vagus nerve, under *branch*.

r. rena′lis ner′vi splanch′nici mino′ris [TA], SYN renal *branch* of lesser splanchnic *nerve*.

rami sacrales laterales arteriae sacralis medianae [TA], SYN lateral sacral *branches* of median sacral artery, under *branch*.

r. saphe′nus arte′riae descenden′tis genicula′ris [TA], SYN saphenous *branch* of descending genicular artery.

ra′mi scrota′les anterio′res arte′riae puden′dae exter′nae profundae [TA], SYN anterior scrotal *branch* of deep external pudendal artery.

rami scrotales posteriores arteriae perinealis [TA], SYN posterior scrotal *branches* of perineal artery, under *branch*.

ra′mi scrota′les posterio′res arte′riae puden′dae inter′nae, SYN posterior scrotal *branches* of perineal artery, under *branch*.

ra′mi septa′les, rami interventricularis septales.

rami septales anteriores arteriae ethmoidalis anterioris [TA], SYN anterior septal *branches* of anterior ethmoidal artery, under *branch*.

r. septi nasi arteriae labialis superioris [TA], SYN nasal septal *branch* of superior labial branch of facial artery.

r. septi posterioris nasalis [TA], SYN posterior septal *branch* of nose.

r. sinis′ter [TA], SYN left *branch*.

r. sinis′ter arte′riae hepat′icae pro′priae [TA], SYN left *branch* of hepatic artery proper.

r. sinis′ter ve′nae por′tae hepa′tis, left branch of hepatic portal vein.

r. si′nus carot′ici [TA], SYN carotid *branch* of glossopharyngeal nerve (CN IX).

r. sinus carotici nervi glossopharyngei CN IX [TA], SYN carotid *branch* of glossopharyngeal nerve (CN IX).

r. si′nus caverno′si, the cavernous sinus branch, a branch of the cavernous part of the internal carotid artery supplying the walls of the cavernous sinus.

r. si′nus caverno′si arte′riae caro′tidis arte′riae, SYN cavernous *branch* of cavernous part of internal carotid artery.

r. sinus cavernosi arteriae carotidis internae, SYN cavernous *branch* of cavernous part of internal carotid artery.

r. sinus cavernosi partis cavernosae arteriae carotidis internae [TA], SYN cavernous *branch* of cavernous part of internal carotid artery.

ra′mi spina′les [TA], spinal branches (**1**) SYN spinal *branches*, under *branch*; (**2**) veins draining the meninges and spinal cord, tributaries of the intervertebral veins.

ra′mi sple′nici arte′riae sple′nicae [TA], SYN splenic *branches* of splenic artery, under *branch*.

r. stape′dius arte′riae stylomastoi′deae, SYN stapedial *branch* of posterior tympanic artery.

r. stapedius arteriae tympanicae posterioris [TA], SYN stapedial *branch* of posterior tympanic artery.

ra′mi sterna′les arte′riae thora′cicae inter′nae [TA], SYN sternal *branches* of internal thoracic artery, under *branch*.

ra′mi ster′noclei′domastoi′dei arte′riae occipita′lis, SYN sternocleidomastoid *branches* of occipital artery, under *branch*.

r. ster′noclei′domastoi′deus arte′riae thyroi′deae superio′ris [TA], SYN sternocleidomastoid *branch* of superior thyroid artery.

r. stylohyoi′deus ner′vi facia′lis [TA], SYN stylohyoid *branch* of facial nerve.

rami subendocardiales fasciculi atrioventricularis [TA], SYN subendocardial *branches* of atrioventricular bundles, under *branch*.

ra′mi subscapula′res arte′riae axilla′ris [TA], SYN subscapular *branches* of axillary artery, under *branch*.

ra′mi substan′tiae ni′grae [TA], branches to substantia nigra [TA], the branches of the anterior choroid artery to the substantia nigra.

r. superficia′lis [TA], SYN superficial *branch*.

r. superficialis arteriae circumflexae femoris medialis [TA], SYN superficial *branch* of medial circumflex femoral artery.

r. superficia′lis arte′riae glu′teae superio′ris [TA], SYN superficial *branch* of the superior gluteal artery.

r. superficia′lis arte′riae plantar′is media′lis [TA], SYN superficial *branch* of the medial plantar artery.

r. superficialis arteriae transversae cervicis [TA], SYN superficial cervical *artery*.

r. superficialis arteriae transversae colli [TA], SYN superficial *branch* of the transverse cervical artery.

r. superficia′lis ner′vi plantar′is latera′lis [TA], SYN superficial *branch* of the lateral plantar nerve.

r. superficia′lis ner′vi radia′lis [TA], SYN superficial *branch* of the radial nerve.

r. superficia′lis ner′vi ulna′ris [TA], SYN superficial *branch* of the ulnar nerve.

r. supe′rior [TA], SYN superior *branch*.

r. supe′rior arte′riae glute′ae superio′ris [TA], SYN superior *branch* of the superior gluteal artery.

superior dental rami, SYN superior dental *branches* of superior dental plexus, under *branch*.

r. supe′rior ner′vi oculomoto′rii [TA], SYN superior *branch* of the oculomotor nerve.

r. supe′rior ner′vi transversa′lis cervica′lis (col′li) [TA], SYN superior *branch* of the transverse cervical nerve.

r. supe′rior os′sis pu′bis [TA], SYN superior pubic r.

superior pubic r. [TA], a bar of bone, triangular in section, which extends posterosuperiorly from the body of the pubis to form the superior boundary of the obturator foramen; developmentally, it contributes about one-fifth of the articular surface of the acetabulum. SYN r. superior ossis pubis [TA], superior branch of the pubic bone.

r. supe′rior ve′nae pulmona′lis dex′trae/sinis′trae inferio′ris, SYN superior *branch* of the right and left inferior pulmonary veins.

r. suprahyoi′deus arte′riae lingua′lis [TA], SYN suprahyoid *branch* of lingual artery.

r. sympath′icus (sympathe′ticus) ad gang′lion submandibula′re, SYN sympathetic *root* of submandibular ganglion.

ra′mi tempora′les anterio′res [TA], anterior temporal branches [TA] of lateral occipital artery, giving arterial supply to the cortex of the anterior part of the temporal lobe of the brain.

ra′mi tempora′les interme′dii [TA], intermediate temporal branches [TA] of lateral occipital artery, giving arterial supply to the cortex of the intermediate and medial part of the temporal lobe of the brain.

rami temporales intermedii arteriae occipitalis lateralis [TA], SYN intermediate temporal *branches* of lateral occipital artery, under *branch*.

rami temporales medii arteriae occipitalis lateralis, ✫official alternate term for intermediate temporal *branches* of lateral occipital artery, under *branch*.

ra′mi tempora′les ner′vi facia′lis [TA], SYN temporal *branch* of facial nerve, under *branch*.

ra′mi tempora′les posterio′res [TA], posterior temporal branches [TA] of lateral occipital artery giving arterial supply to the cortex of the posterior part of the temporal lobe of the brain.

ra′mi tempora′les superficia′les ner′vi auriculotempora′lis [TA], SYN superficial temporal *branch* of auriculotemporal nerve, under *branch*.

r. temporalis anterior [TA], SYN anterior temporal *branch*.

r. temporalis medius partis insularis arteriae cerebrae mediae [TA], SYN middle temporal *branch* of insular part of middle cerebral artery.

r. temporalis posterior arteriae cerebri mediae [TA], SYN posterior temporal *branch* of middle cerebral artery.

r. tentor′ii, ✫official alternate term for tentorial *nerve*.

rami terminales arteriae cerebri medii [TA], SYN terminal *branches* of middle cerebral artery, under *branch*.

ra′mi thalam′ici, branches of the posterior cerebral artery to the thalamus, such as the thalamoperforating and thalamogeniculate arteries.

r. thalam′icus, a branch of the middle cerebral artery to the thalamus.

ra′mi thy′mici, SYN mediastinal *branches* of internal thoracic artery, under *branch*.

rami thymici arteriae thoracicae internae [TA], SYN thymic *branches* of internal thoracic artery, under *branch*.

r. thyrohyoi′deus an′sae cervica′lis [TA], SYN thyrohyoid *branch* of ansa cervicalis.

r. tonsil′lae cerebel′lae [TA], cerebellar tonsillar branch [TA], the branch to the cerebellar tonsil, a branch from the posterior inferior cerebellar artery supplying the tonsil of the cerebellum.

ra′mi tonsilla′res ner′vi glossopharyn′gei, SYN tonsillar *branches* of glossopharyngeal nerve, under *branch*.

rami tonsillares nervi palatini minores [TA], SYN tonsillar *branches* of lesser palatine nerves, under *branch*.

r. tonsilla′ris arte′riae facia′lis [TA], SYN tonsillar *branch* of the facial artery.

ra′mi trachea′les [TA], SYN tracheal *branches*, under *branch*.

rami trachea′les arte′riae thyroi′deae inferio′ris, tracheal branches of inferior thyroid artery. SEE tracheal *branches*, under *branch*.

rami trachea′les ner′vi laryn′gei recurren′tis, tracheal branches of recurrent laryngeal nerve. SEE tracheal *branches*, under *branch*.

ra′mi trac′tus op′tici [TA], branches to optic tract [TA] branches, branches of the anterior choroid artery to the optic tract.

r. transversus arteriae circumflexae femoris lateralis [TA], SYN transverse *branch* of lateral femoral circumflex artery.

r. transver′sus arte′riae circumflex′ae fem′oris media′lis, transverse branches of medial femoral circumflex artery.

r. tuba′rius [TA], SYN tubal *branch*.

r. tubarius arteriae ovaricae [TA], SYN tubal *branch* of ovarian artery.

r. tubari′us arte′riae uteri′nae [TA], SYN tubal *branch* of the uterine artery.

r. tuba′rius plex′us tympan′ici [TA], SYN tubal *branch* of the tympanic plexus.

ra′mi tu′beris cine′rei [TA], branches to tuber cinereum [TA], the branches of the anterior choroid artery to the tuber cinereum.

r. ulna′ris ner′vi cuta′nei antebra′chii media′lis, SYN posterior *branch* of medial cutaneous nerve of forearm.

ra′mi ureter′ici [TA], SYN ureteric *branches*, under *branch*.

rami urete′rici arte′riae ovar′icae [TA], SYN ureteric *branches* of the ovarian artery, under *branch*.

rami urete′rici arte′riae rena′lis, SYN ureteric *branches* of the renal artery, under *branch*.

rami ureterici arteriae suprarenalis inferioris [TA], SYN ureteric *branches* of the inferior suprarenal artery, under *branch*.

rami urete′rici arte′riae testicula′ris [TA], SYN ureteric *branches* of the testicular artery, under *branch*.

rami urete′rici par′tis paten′tis arte′riae umbilica′lis [TA], SYN ureteric *branches* of the patent part of umbilical artery, under *branch*.

ventral rami of cervical nerves, ✫official alternate term for anterior rami of cervical nerves.

rami ventrales nervorum thoracis, ✫official alternate term for anterior rami of thoracic nerves.

ra′mi ventra′les nervo′rum cervica′lium, SYN anterior rami of cervical nerves; SEE anterior r. of spinal nerve.

ra′mi ventra′les nervo′rum lumba′lium, SYN anterior rami of lumbar nerves; SEE anterior r. of spinal nerve.

ra′mi ventra′les nervo′rum sacra′lium, SYN anterior rami of sacral nerves; SEE anterior r. of spinal nerve.

r. ventralis, SYN ventral *branch*.

r. ventra′lis ner′vi spina′lis, ✫official alternate term for anterior r. of spinal nerve.

ventral rami of lumbar nerves, ✫official alternate term for anterior rami of lumbar nerves.

ventral primary rami of cervical spinal nerves, SYN anterior rami of cervical nerves.

ventral primary rami of lumbar spinal nerves, SYN anterior rami of lumbar nerves.

ventral primary rami of sacral spinal nerves, SYN anterior rami of sacral nerves; SEE anterior r. of spinal nerve.

ventral primary r. of spinal nerve, SYN anterior r. of spinal nerve.

ventral primary rami of thoracic spinal nerves, SYN anterior rami of thoracic nerves.

ventral rami of sacral nerves, ✫official alternate term for anterior rami of sacral nerves.

ventral r. of spinal nerve, ✫official alternate term for anterior r. of spinal nerve.

ventral rami of thoracic nerves, ✫official alternate term for anterior rami of thoracic nerves.

r. vermis superior [TA], SYN superior vermian *branch* (of superior cerebellar artery).

ra′mi vestibula′res arte′riae labyrin′thi, vestibular branches of labyrinthine artery.

r. vestibularis posterior arteriae vestibulocochlearis [TA], SYN posterior vestibular *branch* of vestibulocochlear artery.

white rami communicantes [TA], short nerves arising from the initial portion of the ventral primary rami of the thoracic and upper lumbar spinal nerves through which all presynaptic sympathetic nerve fibers must pass to reach the sympathetic trunks; also conveyed by the white rami communicans are visceral afferent (sensory) fibers that were conveyed to the sympathetic trunks in splanchnic nerves. Most fibers conveyed by the white rami communicantes are myelinated. SYN rami communicantes albi [TA], communicating branches of spinal nerves, rami communicantes nervorum spinalium.

ra′mi zygomat′ici ner′vi facia′lis, SYN zygomatic *branches* of facial nerve, under *branch*.

r. zygomaticofacia′lis ner′vi zygoma′tici [TA], SYN zygomaticofacial *branch* of zygomatic nerve.

r. zygomaticotempora′lis ner′vi zygoma′tici [TA], SYN zygomaticotemporal *branch* of zygomatic nerve.

ra·my·cin (ră-mī′sin). SYN fusidic acid.

ran·cid (ran′sid). Having a disagreeable odor and taste, usually

ra

characterizing fat undergoing oxidation or bacterial decomposition to more volatile odoriferous substances. [L. *rancidus,* stinking, rank]

ran·cid·i·fy (ran-sid′i-fī). To make or become rancid.

ran·cid·i·ty (ran-sid′i-tē). The state of being rancid.

Rand, M.J., 20th century pharmacologist. SEE Burn and R. *theory.*

Rand, Gertrude, U.S. visual psychologist, 1886–1970. SEE Hardy-R.-Ritter *test.*

Randall, Alexander, U.S. urologist, *1883. SEE R. stone *forceps.*

ran·dom (ran′dom). Governed by chance; used of a process in which the outcome is indeterminate but may assume any of a set of values (the domain) with probabilities specifiable in advance. While the random process is widely used in probability theory, empiric justification for the term is more complicated. The minimum requirement is that repeated realization of the process will settle down to a stable distribution or, if not metrical, a stable set of frequencies if the trait is classifiable only. SEE random *mechanism.* [M.E. *randon,* speed, errancy, fr. O. Fr. *randir,* to run, fr. Germanic]

ran·dom·i·za·tion. Allocation of individuals to groups, e.g., for experimental and control regimens, by chance.

Raney Nic·kel. Proprietary name for a finely powdered nickel catalyst made from Raney alloy by dissolving out the aluminum with alkali; used in the hydrogenation of organic substances. SYN Raney catalyst.

range (rānj). A statistical measure of the dispersion or variation of values determined by the endpoint values themselves or the difference between them; e.g., in a group of children aged 6, 8, 9, 10, 13, and 16, the r. would be from 6 to 16 or, alternately, 10 (16 minus 6). [O.Fr. *rang,* line fr. Germanic]

therapeutic r., refers to either the dosage r. or blood plasma or serum concentration usually expected to achieve desired therapeutic effects. Some patients will require doses (or concentrations) above or below this r. Some patients will experience drug toxicity within this r.

ra·nine (rā′nīn). 1. Relating to the frog. 2. Relating to the undersurface of the tongue. [L. *rana,* a frog]

ra·ni·ti·dine (ră-nī′ti-dēn). A histamine H₂ antagonist used in the treatment of duodenal and gastric ulcers and gastroesophageal reflux, where it reduces hydrochloric acid secretion.

rank. 1. The ordinal position of an observation in the set of observations of which it is a member. 2. To order a set of observations according to their r.

Ranke, Johannes, German anthropologist and physician, 1836–1916. SEE R. *angle.*

Ranke, Karl E. von, German chemist, 1870–1926. SEE R. *formula.*

Rankin, Fred Wharton, U.S. surgeon, 1886–1954. SEE R. *clamp.*

Rankine, William J. McQ., Scottish physicist, 1820–1870. SEE R. *scale.*

Ransohoff, Joseph, U.S. surgeon, 1853–1921. SEE R. *sign.*

RANTES. A member of the interleukin-8 superfamily of cytokines. This cytokine is an 8-kD protein that is a selective chemoattractant for memory T lymphocytes and monocytes. [*R*egulated on *a*ctivation, *n*ormal *T* *e*xpressed and *s*ecreted]

ran·u·la (ran′ū-lă). 1. Hypoglottis. 2. Obsolete term for any cystic tumor of the undersurface of the tongue or floor of the mouth, especially one of the floor of the mouth due to obstruction of the duct of the sublingual glands. SYN ptyalocele, ranine tumor, sialocele, sublingual cyst. [L. tadpole, dim. of *rana,* frog]

ran·u·lar (ran′ū-lăr). Relating to a ranula.

Ranvier, Louis A., French pathologist, 1835–1922. SEE R. *crosses,* under *cross, disks,* under *disk; node* of R.; R. *plexus, segment.*

RAO Abbreviation for right anterior oblique, a radiographic projection.

Raoult, François, M., French physicist, 1830–1899. SEE R. *law.*

RAPD Abbreviation for rapid analysis of polymorphic DNA.

rape (rāp). 1. Sexual intercourse by force, duress, intimidation, or without legal consent (as with a minor). 2. The performance of such an act. [L. *rapio,* to seize, to drag away]

rape·seed oil (rāp′sēd). The compressed oil from the seeds of *Brassica campestris* (family Cruciferae); used in the manufacture of soaps, margarine, and lubricants. [L. *rapa,* turnip]

ra·pha·nia (ră-fā′nē-ă). A spasmodic disease supposed to be due to poisoning by the seeds of *Rhaphanus rhaphanistrum,* the wild radish. SYN rhaphania.

ra·phe (rā′fē) [TA]. The line of union of two contiguous, bilaterally symmetrical structures. SYN rhaphe. [G. *rhaphē,* suture, seam]

amnionic r., the line of fusion of the amnionic folds over the embryo in reptiles, birds, and certain mammals.

r. anococcyg′ea, SYN anococcygeal *ligament.*

anogenital r., in the male embryo the line of closure of the genital folds and swellings extending from the anus to the glans of the penis; it is differentiated in the adult into three regions: perineal r., scrotal r., and penile r.

r. cor′poris callo′si, a slight anteroposterior furrow on the median line of the upper surface of the corpus callosum.

iliococcygeal r. [TA], portion of anococcygeal body formed by the attachment of the right and left halves of the iliococcygeus (muscle) to each other in the midline, posterior to the anal canal. SYN r. musculi iliococcygeus [TA].

lateral palpebral r., a narrow fibrous band in the lateral part of the orbicularis oculi muscle formed by the interlacing of fibers passing through the upper and lower eyelids. SYN palpebral r., r. palpebralis lateralis.

r. lin′guae, SYN median *sulcus* of tongue.

median longitudinal r. of tongue, SYN median *sulcus* of tongue.

r. of medulla oblongata, SYN r. medullae oblongatae.

r. medul′lae oblonga′tae [TA], the seamlike median zone of the medulla oblongata, marked by intercrossing fiber bundles among which lie scattered neuronal cell bodies. SYN r. of medulla oblongata.

r. musculi iliococcygeus [TA], SYN iliococcygeal r.

r. pala′ti [TA], SYN palatine r.

palatine r. [TA], a rather narrow, low elevation in the center of the hard palate that extends from the incisive papilla posteriorly over the entire length of the mucosa of the hard palate. SYN r. palati [TA], palatine ridge.

palpebral r., SYN lateral palpebral r.

r. palpebra′lis latera′lis, SYN lateral palpebral r.

penile r., SYN r. of penis.

r. pe′nis [TA], SYN r. of penis.

r. of penis [TA], the continuation of the r. of the scrotum onto the underside of the penis. SYN r. penis [TA], penile r.

perineal r. [TA], the central anteroposterior line of the perineum, most marked in the male, being continuous with the r. of the scrotum. SYN r. perinei [TA].

r. perine′i [TA], SYN perineal r.

pharyngeal r. [TA], the central line of the pharynx posteriorly where the muscular fibers meet and partly interlace. SYN r. pharyngis [TA].

r. pharyn′gis [TA], SYN pharyngeal r.

r. of pons, SYN r. pontis.

r. pon′tis [TA], the continuation of the r. medullae oblongatae into the pars dorsalis (or tegmentum) pontis. SYN r. of pons.

pterygomandibular r. [TA], a tendinous thickening of the buccopharyngeal fascia, separating and giving origin to the buccinator muscle anteriorly and the superior constrictor of the pharynx posteriorly. SYN r. pterygomandibularis [TA], pterygomandibular ligament.

r. pterygomandibula′ris [TA], SYN pterygomandibular r.

r. ret′inae, the horizontal line separating the superior and inferior portions of the temporal retina over which the retinal nerve fibers do not course.

scrotal r., SYN r. of scrotum.

r. scro′ti [TA], SYN r. of scrotum.

r. of scrotum [TA], a central line, like a cord, running over the scrotum from the anus to the root of the penis; it marks the position of the septum scroti. SYN r. scroti [TA], scrotal r., Vesling line.

Stilling r., the transverse interdigitations of fiber bundles across the anterior median fissure of the medulla oblongata at the decussation of the pyramidal tracts.

Rapoport, Abraham, Canadian urologist, *1926. SEE R. *test*.

Rapoport, Samuel Mitja, Russian biochemist, 1912–1977. SEE R.-Luebering *shunt*.

Rappaport, Henry, U.S. pathologist, *1913. SEE Rappaport *classification*.

rap·port (rap-ōr′). **1.** A feeling of relationship, especially when characterized by emotional affinity. **2.** A conscious feeling of harmonious accord, trust, empathy, and mutual responsiveness between two or more persons (e.g., physician and patient) that fosters the therapeutic process. [Fr.]

rap·ture of the deep (rap′choor). SYN nitrogen *narcosis* (2).

rar·e·fac·tion (rār-ĕ-fak′shŭn). **1.** The process of becoming light or less dense; the condition of being light; opposed to condensation. **2.** In vascular physiology, the process that results in a reduction in the density of capillaries in a tissue. [L. *rarus*, thin, scanty + *facio*, to make]

rar·e·fy (rār′ĕ-fī). To become light or less dense.

RAS Abbreviation for reticular activating *system*.

ra·sce·ta (ră-sē′tă). The transverse wrinkling on the anterior surface of the wrist. [Mod. L. *raseta*, fr. Ar. *rāhah*, the palm of the hand]

rash. Lay term for a cutaneous eruption. [O. Fr. *rasche*, skin eruption, fr. L. *rado*, pp. *rasus*, to scratch, scrape]

antitoxin r., a cutaneous manifestation of serum sickness.

black currant r., the cutaneous eruption of lentigines seen in xeroderma pigmentosum.

butterfly r., SYN butterfly (2).

caterpillar r., SYN caterpillar *dermatitis*.

crystal r., SYN *miliaria* crystallina.

diaper r., SYN diaper *dermatitis*.

heat r., SYN *miliaria* rubra.

hydatid r., a toxic eruption occasionally following the rupture of a hydatid cyst.

Murray Valley r., SYN epidemic *polyarthritis*.

serum r., a cutaneous manifestation of serum sickness.

summer r., SYN *miliaria* rubra.

wildfire r., SYN *miliaria* rubra.

ra·sion (rā′zhŭn). The subdivision of a crude drug by a rasp to prepare it for extraction. [L. *rasio*, a scraping, fr. *rado*, pp. *rasus*, to scrape, shave]

Rasmussen, Grant L., American neuroanatomist, *1904. SEE *bundle* of Rasmussen, rasmussen *encephalitis*, Rasmussen *syndrome*.

Rasmussen, Fritz W., Danish physician, 1834–1881. SEE R. *aneurysm*.

ras·pa·to·ry (ras′pă-tōr-ē). A surgical instrument used to smooth the edges of a divided bone. [L. *raspatorium*]

RAST Acronym for radioallergosorbent *test*.

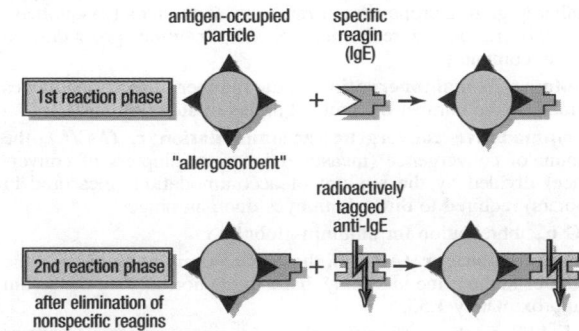

antigen-occupied particle — specific reagin (IgE)

1st reaction phase

"allergosorbent"

radioactively tagged anti-IgE

2nd reaction phase

after elimination of nonspecific reagins

radioallergosorbent test (RAST)

Rastelli, Gian C. SEE R. *operation*.

rat. A rodent of the genus *Rattus* (family Muridae), involved in the spread of some diseases, including bubonic plague.

albino r.'s, r.'s with white fur and pink eyes; used extensively in laboratory experiments.

Wistar r.'s, an inbred strain of rats, homozygous at most loci, produced by strict brother-sister inbreeding over many generations to develop animals for research with the same general genetic composition. [*Wistar* Institute]

rate (rāt). **1.** A record of the measurement of an event or process in terms of its relation to some fixed standard; measurement is expressed as the ratio of one quantity to another (e.g., velocity, distance per unit time). **2.** A measure of the frequency of an event in a defined population; the components of a r. are: the numerator (number of events); the denominator (population at risk of experiencing the event); and the specified time in which the events occur. [L. *ratum*, a reckoning (see ratio)]

abortion r., (1) the number of induced abortions per 1000 pregnancies that resulted in a livebirth, stillbirth, or induced termination. (2) the number of terminations ×1000 ÷ the female population ages 15–44 years.

age-specific r., a r. for a specified age group, in which the numerator and denominator refer to the same age group.

attack r., a cumulative incidence rate used for particular groups observed for limited periods under special circumstances, such as during an epidemic.

average flow r., the flow r. determined by dividing the total volume of urine passed by the time of voiding.

basal metabolic r. (BMR), SYN basal *metabolism*.

baseline fetal heart r., the average heart r. for a particular fetus during the diastolic phase of uterine contractions.

birth r., a summary r. based on the number of live births in a population over a given period, usually 1 year; the numerator is the number of live births, the denominator is the midyear population.

case fatality r., the proportion of individuals contracting a disease that die of that disease.

concordance r., the proportion of a random sample of pairs that are concordant for a trait of interest. A high r. of concordance may be generated in several ways, many of which may result from irrelevant bias; but broadly it is taken as evidence of causal connection (e.g., in the case of identical twins, a genetic component or in spouses of assortative mating).

critical r., a heart r. at which aberration or incomplete block will occur; a result of shortening of cycle length so that it barely includes the refractory period.

death r., an estimate of the proportion of the population that dies during a specified period, usually a year; the numerator is the number of people dying, the denominator is the number in the population, usually an estimate of the number at the midperiod. SYN crude death rate, lethality r., mortality r., mortality (2).

erythrocyte sedimentation r. (ESR), the rate of settling of red blood cells in anticoagulated blood; increased r.'s are often associated with anemia or inflammatory states.

fatality r., the death r. observed in a designated series of persons affected by a simultaneous event such as a disaster.

fetal death r., the number of fetal deaths divided by the sum of live births and fetal deaths occurring in the same population during the same time period. SYN stillbirth r.

fetal heart r., in the fetus, the number of heart beats per minute, normally 120–160.

five-year survival r., the proportion of patients still alive five years after a diagnosis or form of treatment is completed. Usually applied to statistics of survival of cancer patients, since, after five years, recurrences are much less likely to occur.

general fertility r., a refined measure of fertility in a population; the numerator is the number of live births in a year, the denominator is the number of females of child-bearing age, usually defined as ages 15–44 (but increasingly recognized as extending to age 49).

glomerular filtration r. (GFR), the volume of water filtered out of the plasma through glomerular capillary walls into Bowman capsules per unit time; it is considered to be equivalent to inulin clearance.

gross reproduction r., the average number of female children a woman would have if she survived to the end of her childbearing years and if, throughout that period, she were subject to a given set of age-specific fertility r.'s and a given sex ratio at birth; this r. provides a measure of the replacement fertility of a population in the absence of mortality.

growth r., absolute or relative growth increase, expressed per unit of time.

growth r. of population, a measure of population change in the absence of migration, comprising addition of newborns and subtraction of deaths; the result is known as the natural r. of increase of the population; it is the difference between the crude birth r. and the crude death r.

hazard r., theoretical measure of the risk of occurrence of an event, e.g., death, new disease, at a point in time.

heart r., r. of the heart's beat, recorded as the number of beats per minute.

inception r., the r. at which new spells of illness or cases of a condition occur in a population.

incidence r., the r. at which new events occur in a population. The numerator is the number of new events occurring in a defined period; the denominator is the population at risk of experiencing the event during this period.

infant mortality r., a measure of the r. of deaths of liveborn infants before their first birthday; the numerator is the number of infants under one year of age born alive in a defined region during a calendar year who die before they are one year old; the denominator is the total number of live births; often quoted as a useful indicator of the level of health in a community.

initial r., SYN initial *velocity.*

lethality r., SYN death r.

maternal death r., the number of maternal deaths that occur as the direct result of the reproductive process per 100,000 live births. SEE rate; SEE ALSO maternal *death.* SYN maternal mortality ratio.

mitotic r., the proportion of cells in a tissue that are undergoing mitosis, expressed as a mitotic index or, roughly, as the number of cells in mitosis in each microscopic high-power field in tissue sections.

morbidity r., the proportion of patients with a particular disease during a given year per given unit of population.

mortality r., SYN death r.

mucociliary clearance r., velocity of movement of the mucus blanket over respiratory epithelium, usually expressed in mm/hour.

mutation r., the probability (or proportion) of progeny genes with a particular component of the genome not present in either biologic parent; usually expressed as the number of mutants per generation occurring at one gene or locus.

neonatal mortality r., the number of deaths in the first 28 days of life divided by the number of live births occurring in the same population during the same period of time.

peak flow r., maximum urinary flow r. during voiding as measured by a uroflowmeter.

perinatal mortality r., the number of stillborn infants of 24 completed weeks or more plus the number of deaths occurring under 28 days of life divided by the number of stillborn infants of 24 weeks or more gestation plus all liveborn infants in the same population, regardless of the period of gestation.

pulse r., r. of the pulse as observed in an artery; recorded as beats per minute.

recurrence r., in genetic counseling, the risk that a future offspring will be affected given some specific set of relatives of whom at least one is already affected.

repetition r., the number of pulses per minute, describing an energy output, e.g., ultrasound pulses in echocardiography rather than vascular pulses.

respiratory r., frequency of breathing, recorded as the number of breaths per minute.

sedimentation r., the r. at which a sediment is deposited from a solution. SEE ALSO erythrocyte sedimentation r.

shear r., the change in velocity of parallel planes in a flowing fluid separated by unit distance; its units expressed in seconds^{-1}.

slew r., in electronic pacemaker function, the maximum rate of change of an amplifier output voltage; important variable affecting heart function as controlled by an electronic pacemaker. Sensing circuits in the pacemaker often respond to the slew r. rather than to the absolute amplitude of the voltage pulse.

steady-state r., SYN steady-state *velocity.*

steroid metabolic clearance r. (MCR), a measure of the r. of metabolism of a given steroid within the body, usually expressed as liters of body fluid that contain the amount of steroid metabolized per day.

steroid production r., the total quantity of a given steroid formed in the body, usually expressed as milligrams per day; represents the sum of the glandular secretion of the steroid and extraglandular formation of it from various steroid precursors.

steroid secretory r., the r. of glandular secretion of a given steroid, usually expressed as milligrams per day; does not include any amount of the steroid that might be formed extraglandularly.

stillbirth r., SYN fetal death r.

voiding flow r., urinary flow as a function of time during micturition, as graphically recorded by a flow meter.

Rathke, Martin H., German anatomist, physiologist, and pathologist, 1793–1860. SEE R. *bundles,* under *bundle,* cleft *cyst, diverticulum, pocket, pouch,* pouch *tumor.*

rating of perceived exertion. Subjective numerical rating (range 6–19) of exercise intensity based on how an individual feels in relation to level of physiologic stress. An RPE of 13 or 14 (exercise that feels "somewhat hard") coincides with an exercise heart rate of about 70% maximum.

rating of perceived exertion (RPE)	
6	
7	very, very light
8	
9	very light
10	
11	fairly light
12	
13	somewhat hard
14	
15	hard
16	
17	very hard
18	
19	very, very hard

ra·tio (rā′shē-ō). An expression of the relation of one quantity to another (e.g., of a proportion or rate). SEE ALSO index (2), quotient. [L. *ratio* (*ration-*) a reckoning, reason, fr. *reor,* pp. *ratus,* to reckon, compute]

absolute terminal innervation r., the number of motor endplates divided by the number of terminal axons related to them.

accommodative convergence-accommodation r. (AC/A), the amount of convergence (measured in prism diopters of convergence) divided by the amount of accommodation (measured in diopters) required to direct both eyes upon an object.

A/G r., abbreviation for albumin-globulin r.

albumin-globulin r. (A/G r.), the r. of albumin to globulin in the serum or in the urine in kidney disease; the normal r. in the serum is approximately 1.55.

ALT:AST r., the r. of serum alanine aminotransferase to serum aspartate aminotransferase; elevated serum levels of both enzymes characterize hepatic disease; when both levels are abnormally elevated and the ALT:AST r. is greater than 1.0, severe hepatic necrosis or alcoholic hepatic disease is likely; when the r.

is less than 1.0, an acute nonalcoholic hepatic condition is favored.

amylase-creatinine clearance r., a test for the diagnosis of acute pancreatitis; it is determined by measuring amylase and creatinine in serum and urine; in apparently healthy individuals the renal clearance of amylase is less than 5% that of creatinine; in acute pancreatitis the r. is said to be greater than 5%.

body-weight r., body weight (in grams) divided by stature (in centimeters).

cardiothoracic r., the r. of the horizontal diameter of the heart to the inner diameter of the rib cage at its widest point as determined on a chest roentgenogram.

case fatality r., the mortality rate of a disease, usually expressed per 100 cases.

r. of decayed and filled surfaces (RDFS), an index of decayed and filled permanent surfaces per person, per full complement of 122 tooth surfaces.

r. of decayed and filled teeth (RDFT), an index of decayed and filled permanent teeth per person, per full complement of 28 teeth.

extraction r. (E), the fraction of a substance removed from the blood flowing through the kidney; it is calculated from the formula $(A - V)/A$, where A and V, respectively, are the concentrations of the substance in arterial and renal venous plasma.

fertility r., a measure of the fertility of a population based on the female population in the child-bearing age group, defined as ages 15–49 years.

flux r., the r. of the two unidirectional fluxes through a particular boundary layer or membrane.

functional terminal innervation r., the number of muscle fibers divided by the number of axons that innervate them.

grid r., in a radiographic scatter-absorbing grid, the r. of the height to the width of the gaps between lead strips; a higher grid r. removes more scattered radiation but requires more careful x-ray tube positioning to avoid grid cutoff of the primary radiation beam.

gyromagnetic r., in nuclear magnetic resonance, the r. of the magnetic dipole moment of the nucleus to the nuclear spin angular momentum; the gyromagnetic r. is a unique value for each type of nucleus. SYN magnetogyric r.

hand r., the r. of the length of the hand (measured on the dorsum from the styloid process of the ulna to the tip of the third finger) to the width across the knuckles.

international normalized r. (INR), the prothrombin time r. that would have been obtained if a standard reagent had been used in a prothrombin time determination; the prothrombin time r. is expressed as the patient prothrombin time divided by the mean of the prothrombin time reference interval; the prothrombin time r. is obtained for a working reagent in the laboratory through use of a parameter designated the international sensitivity index. SEE ALSO international sensitivity *index*.

IRI/G r., the r. of immunoreactive insulin to serum or plasma glucose; in hypoglycemic states a r. of less than 0.3 is usual, with the exception of the hypoglycemia due to insulinoma, where the r. is often higher than 0.3.

K:A r., abbreviation for ketogenic-antiketogenic r.

ketogenic-antiketogenic r. (K:A r.), the proportion between substances that form ketones in the body and those that form D-glucose.

lecithin/sphingomyelin r. (L/S r.), a r. used to determine fetal pulmonary maturity, found by testing the amniotic fluid; when the lungs are mature, lecithin exceeds sphingomyelin by 2 to 1.

L/S r., abbreviation for lecithin/sphingomyelin r.

magnetogyric r. (mag′nĕ-tō-gy-rik), SYN gyromagnetic r.

mass-action r., the ratio of the product of all of the product concentrations divided by the product of all of the reactant concentrations of a particular reaction; when the reaction has been completed (i.e., $t = \infty$), then this r. is equal to the equilibrium constant.

maternal mortality r., SYN maternal death *rate*.

M:E r., the r. of myeloid to erythroid precursors in bone marrow; normally it varies from 2:1 to 4:1; an increased r. is found in

infections, chronic myelogenous leukemia, or erythroid hypoplasia; a decreased r. may mean a depression of leukopoiesis or normoblastic hyperplasia depending on the overall cellularity of the bone marrow.

mendelian r., the r. of progeny with particular phenotypes or genotypes expected in accordance with Mendel law among the offspring of matings specified as to genotype or phenotype.

molecular weight r. (M_r), SYN molecular *weight*.

nuclear-cytoplasmic r., r. of volume of nucleus to volume of cytoplasm, fairly constant for a particular cell type and usually increased in malignant neoplasms.

nucleolar-nuclear r., r. of volume of nucleolus to volume of nucleus, usually increased in malignant neoplasms.

P/O r., a measure of oxidative phosphorylation; the r. of phosphate radicals esterified (forming adenosine 5′-triphosphate from adenosine 5′-diphosphate) to atoms of oxygen consumed by mitochondria; normally, the r. is 3 (starting from NADH). SYN P/O quotient.

respiratory exchange r., the r. of the net output of carbon dioxide to the simultaneous net uptake of oxygen at a given site, both expressed as moles or STPD volumes per unit time; in the steady state, respiratory exchange r. is equal to the respiratory quotient of metabolic processes.

segregation r., in genetics, the proportion of progeny of a particular genotype or phenotype from actual matings of specified genotypes. The test of a mendelian hypothesis is the comparison of the segregation r. with the mendelian r.

sex r., (1) the r. of male to female progeny at some specified stage of the life cycle, notably at conception (primary), at birth (secondary), or at any stage between birth and death (tertiary); **(2)** the r. of the numbers of males to females affected by a particular disease or trait.

signal-to-noise r., the relative intensity of a signal to the random variation in signal intensity, or noise; used to evaluate many imaging techniques and electronic systems.

standardized mortality r., the r. of the number of events observed in a population to the number that would be expected if the population had the same distribution as a standard or reference population.

systolic/diastolic r., a calculation from pulsed Doppler ultrasound determinations of blood flow velocities that reflects intrinsic resistance in an arterial blood vessel.

therapeutic r., the r. of the maximally tolerated dose of a drug to the minimal curative or effective dose; LD_{50} divided by ED_{50}.

variance r. (F), the distribution of the r. of two independent estimates of the same variance from a gaussian distribution based on samples of sizes $(n + 1)$ and $(m + 1)$, respectively. Estimates are usually based on one such sample analyzed in such a way as to make them independent, e.g., analysis of variance, and F may be used to test a null hypothesis that the observed differences among sample means is no greater than could readily be accounted for by chance.

ventilation/perfusion r. ($\dot{V}a/\dot{Q}$), the r. of alveolar ventilation to simultaneous alveolar capillary blood flow in any part of the lung; because both ventilation and perfusion are expressed per unit volume of tissue and per unit time, which cancel, the units become liters of gas per liter of blood.

waist-hip r., r. of the abdominal circumference at the navel to maximum hip and buttocks circumference.

zeta sedimentation r. (ZSR), the r. of the zetacrit to the hematocrit, normally 0.41–0.54 (41–54%); it is a sensitive indicator of the erythrocyte sedimentation rate (ESR) and, unlike the latter, is unaffected by anemia, which tends to elevate the ESR.

ra·tion·al (rash′ŭn-ăl). **1.** Pertaining to reasoning or to the higher thought processes; based on objective or scientific knowledge, in contrast to empiric (1). **2.** Influenced by reasoning rather than by emotion. **3.** Having the reasoning faculties; not delirious or comatose. [L. *rationalis*, fr. *ratio,* reason]

ra·tion·al·i·za·tion (ra-shŭn-ăl-i-zā′shŭn). A postulated psychoanalytic defense mechanism through which irrational behavior, motives, or feelings are made to appear reasonable. [L. *ratio,* reason]

Ratner. SEE Kurzrok-Ratner *test*.

rats·bane (rats′bān). SYN arsenic.

rat·tle·snake (rat′l-snāk). A member of the crotalid genera *Crotalus* and *Sistrurus*, characterized by possession of cuticular warning rattles at the tip of the tail.

Rat·tus (rat′ŭs). The rats, a genus of rodents, family Muridae. *R. rattus*, the black r., is the species most commonly responsible for transmitting plague to humans by means of the flea, *Xenopsylla cheopis;* it is smaller and darker than the Norwegian, sewer, or brown rat (*Rattus norvegicus*) and has longer ears and tail. SEE rat.

Rau (Ravius, Raw), Johann J., Dutch anatomist, 1668–1719. SEE R. *process; processus ravii*.

Rauber, August A., German anatomist, 1841–1917. SEE R. *layer*.

Rauscher, Frank J., 20th century U.S. oncologist. SEE R. *virus*.

Rau·wol·fia (row-wool′fē-ă, raw-, rah-). A genus of tropical trees and shrubs (family Apocynaceae). The powdered whole root of *R. serpentina* contains alkaloids that produce a sedative-antihypertensive-bradycardiac action; approximately 50% of the total activity is due to reserpine. [L. *Rauwolf*, German botanist, 16th century]

RAV Abbreviation for Rous-associated *virus*.

Ravius, SEE Rau.

ray (rā). **1.** A beam of light, heat, or other form of radiation. The r.'s from radium and other radioactive substances are produced by a spontaneous disintegration of the atom; they are electrically charged particles or electromagnetic waves of extremely short wavelength. **2.** A part or branch that extends radially from a structure. [L. *radius*]

actinic r., a light r. toward and beyond the violet end of the spectrum that acts upon a photographic plate and produces other chemical effects. SYN chemical r.

alpha r., SYN alpha *particle*.

anode r.'s, those originating in a gas discharge tube and moving in a direction opposite to that of cathode r.'s; made up of positively charged ions. SYN positive r.'s.

Becquerel r.'s, obsolete term for radiation given off by uranium and other radioactive substances; these include α, β, and γ r.'s.

beta r., SYN beta *particle*.

cathode r.'s, a stream of electrons emitted from the negative electrode (cathode) in a Crookes tube; their bombardment of the anode or the glass wall of the tube gives rise to x-r.'s.

chemical r., SYN actinic r.

cosmic r.'s, high-velocity particles of enormous energies, bombarding earth from outer space; the "primary radiation" consists of protons and more complex atomic nuclei that, on striking the atmosphere, give rise to neutrons, mesons, and other less energetic "secondary radiation."

direct r.'s, SYN primary r.'s (2).

gamma r.'s, electromagnetic radiation emitted from radioactive substances; they are high-energy x-rays but originate from the nucleus rather than the orbital shell and are not deflected by a magnet.

glass r.'s, those formed by cathode r.'s striking the wall of an x-ray tube; a special case of indirect r.'s and soft x-rays. Obsolete.

grenz r. (grents), very soft x-r.'s, closely allied to the ultraviolet r.'s in their wavelength (i.e., relatively long) and in their biologic action upon tissues; they are produced by a specially built vacuum tube with a hot cathode operating from a transformer delivering not more than 8 kw. [Ger. *Grenze*, borderline, boundary]

H r.'s, a stream of hydrogen nuclei; i.e., protons.

hard r.'s, r.'s of short wavelength and great penetrability.

incident r., the r. that strikes the surface before reflection.

indirect r.'s, x-r.'s generated at a surface other than the anode target.

infrared r., SEE infrared.

intermediate r.'s, those between ultraviolet and x-r.'s. SYN W r.'s.

marginal r.'s, in geometric optics, those r.'s originating from the periphery.

medullary r., the center of the renal lobule, which has the shape of a small, steep pyramid, consisting of straight tubular parts; these may be either ascending or descending limbs of the nephronic loop or collecting tubules. SYN Ferrein pyramid, pars radiata lobuli corticalis renis, processus ferreini.

Niewenglowski r.'s, radiation emitted from a phosphorescent body after exposure to sunlight.

parallel r.'s, r.'s parallel to the axis of an optical system.

paraxial r.'s, in geometric optics, those r.'s focused at the principal point.

positive r.'s, SYN anode r.'s.

primary r.'s, (1) cosmic r.'s in the form in which they first strike the atmosphere; **(2)** x-r.'s generated at the focal spot of the tube. SYN direct r.'s.

reflected r., a r. of light or other form of radiant energy which is thrown back from a nonpermeable or nonabsorbing surface; the r. which strikes the surface before reflection is the incident r.

roentgen r., SYN x-ray (1).

secondary r.'s, x-r.'s generated when primary x-r.'s impinge upon matter; scattered radiation.

soft r.'s, x-r.'s of relatively long wavelength and slight penetrability.

supersonic r.'s, r.'s with a wavelength higher than that perceptible to the human ear, above 20,000 Hz.

ultrasonic r.'s, SEE ultrasonic.

ultraviolet r.'s, SEE ultraviolet.

W r.'s, SYN intermediate r.'s.

x-r., SEE x-ray.

Rayer, Pierre F., French physician, 1793–1867. SEE R. *disease*.

rayl (rāl). Unit of acoustic impedance. $1 \text{ rayl} = 1 \text{ kg} \times \text{m}^{-2} \times \text{sec}^{-1}$. [Baron *Rayleigh* (John W. Strutt), Eng. physicist]

Rayleigh, Lord John William Strutt, British physicist and Nobel laureate, 1842–1919. SEE R. *equation, test*.

Raynaud, Maurice, French physician, 1834–1881. SEE R. *syndrome, disease, phenomenon, sign*.

Rb Symbol for rubidium.

R-band·ing. SEE R-banding *stain*.

rbc, RBC Abbreviation for red blood *cell*; red blood count.

RBE Abbreviation used in radiation protection for relative biologic effectiveness; Cf. quality factor, QF.

RBF Abbreviation for renal blood flow. SEE effective renal blood *flow*.

R.C.P. Abbreviation for Royal College of Physicians (of England).

R.C.P.(E), R.C.P.(Edin) 1. Abbreviation for Royal College of Physicians (Edinburgh). **2.** Symbol for reactivity.

R.C.P.(I) Abbreviation for Royal College of Physicians (Ireland).

R.C.P.S.C. Abbreviation for Royal Colleges of Physicians and Surgeons of Canada.

R.C.S. Abbreviation for Royal College of Surgeons (England).

R.C.S.(E), R.C.S.(Edin) Abbreviation for Royal College of Surgeons (Edinburgh).

R.C.S.(I) Abbreviation for Royal College of Surgeons (Ireland).

RCT Abbreviation for randomized controlled *trial*.

R.D. Abbreviation for registered dietician.

RDA Abbreviation for recommended daily *allowance*.

RDFS Abbreviation for *ratio* of decayed and filled surfaces.

RDFT Abbreviation for *ratio* of decayed and filled teeth.

R.D.H. Abbreviation for Registered Dental Hygienist.

RDPA Abbreviation for right descending pulmonary *artery*.

R.E. Abbreviation for right eye.

Re Symbol for rhenium.

△**re-.** Prefix meaning again or backward. [L.]

re·act (rē-akt′). To take part in or to undergo a chemical reaction. [Mod. L. *reactus*]

re·ac·tance (X) (rē-ak′tans). The weakening of an alternating electric current by passage through a coil of wire or a condenser. SYN inductive resistance.

re·ac·tant (rē-ak′tant). A substance taking part in a chemical reaction.

acute phase r.'s, a group of proteins that are produced and/or released in increased concentrations during the acute phase reaction, including fibrinogen; C-reactive protein; complement proteins B, C3, C4; α_2-acid glycoprotein, serum amyloid A, proteinase inhibitors, etc.

REACTION

re·ac·tion (rē-ak′shŭn). **1.** The response of a muscle or other living tissue or organism to a stimulus. **2.** The color change effected in litmus and certain other organic pigments by contact with substances such as acids or alkalies; also the property that such substances possess of producing this change. **3.** In chemistry, the intermolecular action of two or more substances upon each other, whereby these substances are caused to disappear, new ones being formed in their place (chemical r.). **4.** In immunology, in vivo or in vitro action of an antibody on a specific antigen, with or without the involvement of a complement or other components of the immunologic system. [L. *re-*, again, backward, + *actio*, action]

accelerated r., a response occurring in a shorter time than expected; the cutaneous manifestations occurring during the period between the second and tenth day following smallpox vaccination; because it is intermediate between a primary r. and an immediate r., it is regarded as evidence of some degree of resistance. SYN vaccinoid r.

acid r., (1) any test by which an acid r. is recognized, such as the change of blue litmus paper to red; **(2)** an excess of hydrogen ions over hydroxide ions in aqueous solution indicated by a pH value less than 7 (at 22°C). Cf. dissociation *constant* of water.

acute phase r., refers to the changes in synthesis of certain proteins within the serum during an inflammatory response; this response provides rapid protection for the host against microorganisms via nonspecific defense mechanisms. SYN acute phase response.

acute situational r., SYN stress r.

acute stress r., SYN anxiety r.

adverse r., any undesirable or unwanted consequence of a preventive, diagnostic, or therapeutic procedure or regimen.

alarm r., the various phenomena, e.g., stimulated endocrine activity, which the body exhibits as an adaptive response to injury or stress; first phase of the general adaptation syndrome.

aldehyde r., the r. of the indole derivatives with aromatic aldehydes; e.g., tryptophan and *p*-dimethylaminobenzaldehyde in H_2SO_4 give a red-violet color useful in assaying proteins for tryptophan content. SYN Ehrlich r.

alkaline r., (1) any test by which an alkaline r. is recognized, such as the change of red litmus paper to blue; **(2)** an excess of hydroxide ions over hydrogen ions in aqueous solution as indicated by a pH value >7 (at 22°C). Cf. dissociation *constant* of water. SYN basic r.

allergic r., a local or general r. of an organism following contact with a specific allergen to which it has been previously exposed and sensitized; immunologic interaction of endogenous or exogenous antigen with antibody or sensitized lymphocytes gives rise to inflammation or tissue damage. Allergic r.'s are classified into four major types: type I, anaphylactic and IgE dependent; type II, cytotoxic; type III, immune-complex mediated; type IV, cell mediated (delayed). SYN hypersensitivity r.

amphoteric r., a double r. possessed by certain fluids that have a combination of acid and alkaline properties.

anamnestic r., augmented production of an antibody due to previous exposure of the subject to the same antigen.

anaphylactic r. (an′a-fĭ-lak′tik), SYN anaphylaxis.

anaplerotic r., SEE anaplerotic.

antigen-antibody r. (AAR), the reversible phenomenon, occur-

ring in vitro or in vivo, of an antibody combining with an antigen of the type that stimulated the formation of the antibody, thereby resulting in agglutination, precipitation, complement fixation, greater susceptibility to ingestion and destruction by phagocytes, or neutralization of exotoxin. SEE ALSO skin *test*.

anxiety r., a psychologic r. or experience involving the apprehension of danger accompanied by a feeling of dread and such physical symptoms as an increase in the rate of breathing, sweating, and tachycardia, in the absence of a clearly identifiable fear stimulus; when chronic, it is called generalized anxiety *disorder*. SEE ALSO panic *attack*. SYN acute stress r.

Arias-Stella r., SYN Arias-Stella *phenomenon*.

arousal r., change in pattern of the brain waves when the subject is suddenly awakened and becomes alert.

Arthus r., (1) SYN Arthus *phenomenon*; **(2)** Arthus-type r.; r. in humans and other species that results from the same basic immunologic (allergic) mechanism that evokes, in the rabbit, the typical Arthus phenomenon. SEE ALSO immune complex *disease*.

Ascoli r., a method for confirming the diagnosis of anthrax by means of a precipitin r., which indicates the presence of heat-stable *Bacillus anthracis* antigen in the extracted tissue.

associative r., a secondary or side r.

basic r., SYN alkaline r.

Bence Jones r., the classic means of identifying Bence Jones protein, which precipitates when urine (from patients with this type of proteinuria) is gradually warmed to 45–70°C and redissolves as the urine is heated to near boiling; as the specimen cools, the Bence Jones protein precipitates in the indicated range of temperature and redissolves as the temperature of the specimen becomes less than 30–35°C.

Berthelot r., the r. of ammonia with phenol-hypochlorite to give indophenol; the principle is used to analyze ammonia concentration in body fluids.

bi bi r., a r. catalyzed by a single enzyme in which two substrates and two products are involved; the ping-pong mechanism may be involved in such a r. Cf. mechanism.

Bittorf r., in cases of renal colic, pain radiating to the kidney upon squeezing the testicle or pressing the ovary.

biuret r., the formation of biuret that gives a violet color as a result of the r. of a polypeptide of more than three aminoacyl residues with $CuSO_4$ in strongly alkaline solution; dipeptides and amino acids (except histidine, serine, and threonine) do not so react; used for the detection and quantification of polypeptides, or proteins, in biologic fluids.

Bloch r., SYN dopa r.

Bordet and Gengou r., SEE complement *fixation*.

Brunn r., the increased absorption of water through the skin of the frog when the animal is injected with pituitrin and immersed in water; one of the physiologic reactions used to study and classify posterior pituitary polypeptides and their analogues.

Burchard-Liebermann r., a blue-green color produced by acetic anhydride with cholesterol (and other sterols) dissolved in chloroform, when a few drops of concentrated sulfuric acid are added. SEE Liebermann-Burchard *test*.

Cannizzaro r., formation of an acid and an alcohol by the simultaneous oxidation of one aldehyde molecule and reduction of another; a dismutation: $2RCHO \rightarrow RCOOH + RCH_2OH$; when the aldehydes are not identical, this is referred to as a crossed Cannizzaro reaction.

capsular precipitation r., SYN quellung r. (2).

Carr-Price r., the r. of antimony trichloride with vitamin A to yield a brilliant blue color; this r. forms the basis of several quantitative techniques for the determination of vitamin A.

catalatic r., decomposition of H_2O_2 to O_2 and H_2O, as in the action of catalase; analogous to peroxidase r.

catastrophic r., the disorganized behavior that is the response to a severe shock or threatening situation with which the person cannot cope.

cell-mediated r., immunologic r. of the delayed type, involving chiefly T lymphocytes, important in host defense against infection, in autoimmune diseases, and in transplant rejection. SEE ALSO skin *test*.

re

chain r., a self-perpetuating r. in which a product of one step in the r. itself serves to bring about the next step in the r. Cf. autocatalysis.

Chantemesse r., a conjunctival r., especially as applied to typhoid.

cholera-red r., a test for cholera vibrio whereby the addition of 3 or 4 drops of sulfuric acid (concentrated, chemically pure) to an 18-hour-old bouillon or peptone culture of the organism produces a color from rose-pink to claret.

chromaffin r., production of a yellow-brown to brown coloration in normal and abnormal cells containing epinephrine and norepinephrine, when fresh tissue slices are placed in a dichromate-chromate mixture overnight; useful for detection of pheochromocytoma (adrenal medulla) and other tumors which produce catecholamines.

circular r., in sensorimotor theory, the tendency of an organism to repeat novel experiences.

cocarde r., cockade r., SEE Römer *test.*

colloidal gold r., a test (now obsolete) based on precipitation of cerebrospinal fluid protein when mixed with colloidal gold. Abnormalities in this reaction were observed in patients with syphilis, multiple *sclerosis,* poliomyelitis, and encephalitis.

complement-fixation r., SEE complement *fixation.*

consensual r., contraction of the pupil of the fellow eye in consensus with the pupil of the illuminated eye. SYN consensual light reflex, indirect pupillary r.

constitutional r., a generalized r. in contrast to a focal or local r.; in allergy the immediate or delayed response, following the introduction of an allergen, occurring at sites remote from that of injection.

conversion r., SYN conversion *hysteria.*

cross-r., a specific r. between an antiserum and an antigen complex other than the antigen complex that evoked the various specific antibodies of the antiserum. It is due to at least one antigenic determinant that is included among the determinants of the other complex.

cutaneous graft versus host r., an acute erythematous maculopapular r. with bulla formation in the most severe cases; chronic changes may resemble lichen planus or scleroderma.

cytotoxic r., an immunologic (allergic) r. in which noncytotropic IgG or IgM antibody combines with specific antigen on cell surfaces; the resulting complex initiates the activation of complement which causes cell lysis or other damage, or which, in the absence of complement, may lead to phagocytosis or enhance T lymphocyte involvement leading to cellular cytotoxicity.

Dale r., SEE Schultz-Dale r.

dark r., in photosynthesis, the fixation of CO_2 into carbohydrate, which is independent in place and time of the absorption of light.

decidual r., the cellular and vascular changes occurring in the endometrium at the time of implantation.

delayed r., a local or generalized response that begins 24–48 hours after exposure to an antigen involving T cells. SEE cell-mediated r. SYN contact hypersensitivity (2), delayed hypersensitivity (2), late r., tuberculin-type hypersensitivity.

depot r., reddening of the skin at the point where the needle entered, in the subcutaneous tuberculin test.

depressive r., SYN depression (4).

dermotuberculin r., SYN Pirquet *test.*

diazo r., the r. of diazotized sulfanilic acid with bilirubin to form azobilirubin, which forms the basis of quantitating the amount of bilirubin in biologic fluids. SEE van den Bergh *test.* SYN Ehrlich diazo r.

digitonin r., the r. of naturally occurring steroids with 3β-hydroxyl groups with digitonin, a steroid glycoside, resulting in the formation of an insoluble precipitate; useful in determining the presence of cholesterol and ergosterol.

Dische r., the assay of DNA by means of the blue color formed with diphenylamine in acid (Dische reagent).

dissociative r., r. characterized by such dissociative behavior as amnesia, fugues, sleepwalking, and dream states.

dopa r., a dark staining observed in fresh tissue sections to which a solution of dopa has been applied, presumably due to the pres-

ence of dopa oxidase in the protoplasm of certain cells. SYN Bloch r.

dystonic r., a state of abnormal tension or muscle tone, similar to dystonia, produced as a side effect of certain antipsychotic medication; a severe form, in which the eyes appear to roll up into the head, is called oculogyric crisis.

early r., SYN immediate r.

echo r., SYN echolalia.

Ehrlich r., SYN aldehyde r.

Ehrlich benzaldehyde r., a test for urobilinogen in the urine, by dissolving 2 g of dimethyl-*p*-aminobenzaldehyde in 100 mL of 5% hydrochloric acid and adding this reagent to urine; a red color in the cold indicates the presence of an excessive amount of urobilinogen.

Ehrlich diazo r., SYN diazo r.

eosinopenic r., reduction in the numbers of circulating eosinophils by ACTH or by adrenal corticoids.

error-prone polymerase chain r., use of PCR under conditions in which misincorporation of bases is favored, e.g., where random mutants are sought for a portion of amplified DNA.

eye-closure pupil r., a constriction of both pupils when an effort is made to close eyelids forcibly held apart; a variant of the pupil response to near vision. SYN Galassi pupillary phenomenon, Gifford reflex, lid-closure r., orbicularis phenomenon, orbicularis pupillary reflex, Piltz sign, Westphal pupillary reflex, Westphal-Piltz phenomenon.

false-negative r., an erroneous or mistakenly negative response.

false-positive r., an erroneous or mistakenly positive response.

Fenton r., (1) the use of H_2O_2 and ferrous salts (Fenton reagent) to oxidize α-hydroxy acids to α-keto acids or to convert 1,2-glycols to α-hydroxy aldehydes; (2) the formation of OH·, OH⁻, and Fe^{3+} from the nonenzymatic r. of Fe^{2+} with H_2O_2; a r. of importance in the oxidative stress in blood cells and various tissues.

Fernandez r., a delayed hypersensitivity lepromin r., similar to a tuberculin r., at the site of intradermal injection of Dharmendra antigen in a lepromin test.

ferric chloride r. of epinephrine, an intense emerald green color in a neutral or slightly acid solution of epinephrine when ferric chloride is added to it; a r. typical of catechols.

Feulgen r., SEE Feulgen *stain.*

fight or flight r., the theory advanced by Walter Cannon, that in the autonomic nervous system and the effectors connected with it, the organism in situations of danger requiring either fight or flight is provided with a check-and-drive mechanism that puts it in readiness to meet emergencies with undivided energy output. Also known as the emergency *theory.*

first-order r., a r. the rate of which is proportional to the concentration of the single substance undergoing change; radioactive decay is a first-order process, defined by the equation $dN/dt = kN$, where N is the number of atoms subject to decay (reaction), t is time, and k is the first-order decay (reaction) constant, i.e., the fraction of all atoms decaying per unit of time. SEE ALSO decay *constant,* order.

fixation r., SEE complement *fixation.*

flocculation r., a form of precipitin r. in which precipitation occurs over a narrow range of antigen-antibody ratio, owing chiefly to peculiarities of the antibody (precipitin).

focal r., a r. that occurs at the point of entrance of an infecting organism or of an injection, as in the Arthus phenomenon. SYN local r.

Folin r., the r. of amino acids in alkaline solution with 1,2-naphthoquinone-4-sulfonate (Folin reagent) to yield a red color; useful for quantitative assay. SYN Folin reagent.

Forssman r., SYN Forssman antigen-antibody r.

Forssman antigen-antibody r., the combination of Forssman antibody with heterogenetic antigen of the Forssman type, as in the agglutination of sheep erythrocytes (which contain Forssman antigen) by serum from a person with infectious mononucleosis that contains Forssman antibody. SYN Forssman r.

fragment r., a r. used to assay the activity of peptidyl transferase.

Frei-Hoffmann r., SYN Frei *test.*

fright r., after section and degeneration of the facial nerve of an animal, the denervated facial muscles contract if the animal is frightened or becomes angry; caused by the release of acetylcholine into the circulation.

fuchsinophil r., the property possessed by certain elements, when stained with acid fuchsin, of retaining the stain when treated with picric acid alcohol.

furfurol r., production of a red color on addition of furfurol to a solution of aniline.

galvanic skin r., SYN galvanic skin *response*.

gel diffusion r.'s, SYN gel diffusion precipitin *tests,* under *test*.

Gell and Coombs r.'s, SEE allergic r.

gemistocytic r., a r. to injury resulting in the proliferation of reactive, protoplastic, or gemistocytic astrocytes.

general adaptation r., SEE general adaptation *syndrome*.

Gerhardt r., SYN Gerhardt *test* for acetoacetic acid.

graft versus host r. (GVHR), clinical and histologic changes of graft versus host disease occurring in a specific organ.

group r., a r. with an agglutinin or other antibody that is common (though usually in varying concentrations) to an entire group of related bacteria, e.g., the coli group.

Gruber r., SYN Widal r.

Gruber-Widal r., SYN Widal r.

Günning r., the formation of iodoform from acetone by iodine and ammonia in alcohol.

Haber-Weiss r., the reaction of superoxide ($O_2^{·-}$) with hydrogen peroxide to produce molecular oxygen (O_2), hydroxide radical ($OH·$), and OH^-; often, iron-catalyzed; a source of oxidative stress in blood cells and various tissues.

harlequin r., sudden blanching of the lower half of the body of an infant lying on its side, leaving the remaining half of the body the normal color.

heel-tap r., SEE heel *tap*.

hemoclastic r., hemolysis as observed in the laking of the blood.

Henle r., dark brown staining of the medullary cells of the adrenal bodies when treated with the salts of chromium, the cortical cells remaining unstained.

Herxheimer r., an inflammatory r. in syphilitic tissues (skin, mucous membrane, nervous system, or viscera) induced in certain cases by specific treatment with Salvarsan, mercury, or antibiotics; believed to be due to a rapid release of treponemal antigen with an associated allergic reaction in the patient. SYN Jarisch-Herxheimer r.

Hill r., that portion of the photosynthesis r. that involves the photolysis of water and the liberation of oxygen and does not include carbon dioxide fixation. It involves the addition of oxidants (quinones or ferricyanide) to chloroplasts; upon illumination, O_2 is evolved and the added oxidant is reduced.

homograft r., rejection of an allogenic graft by the host.

hunting r., an unusual r. of digital blood vessels exposed to cold; vasoconstriction is alternated with vasodilation in irregular repeated sequences, in an apparent hunting of equilibrium of skin temperature.

hypersensitivity r., SYN allergic r.

id r., an allergic manifestation of candidiasis, the dermatophytoses, and other mycoses characterized by itching, vesicular lesions that appear in response to superficial infections that are distant from the id r. itself. SEE ALSO dermatophytid, -id (1).

r. of identity, SEE gel diffusion precipitin *tests* in two dimensions, under *test*.

immediate r., local or generalized response that begins within a few minutes to about an hour after exposure to an antigen to which the individual has been sensitized. SEE ALSO skin *test,* wheal-and-erythema r. SYN early r.

immediate hypersensitivity r., an immune response mediated by antibody, usually IgE, which occurs within minutes after a second encounter with an antigen, resulting in the release of histamine and subsequent swelling and vasodilation.

immune r., antigen-antibody r. indicating a certain degree of resistance, usually in reference to the 36- to 48-hour reaction in vaccination against smallpox; because the degree of resistance indicated by the r. is not true immunity and may disappear relatively rapidly there is a tendency to refer to the immune r. as an allergic r.

incompatible blood transfusion r., a syndrome due to intravascular hemolysis of transfused blood by serum antibodies of the recipient, which react with an antigen of the donor red cells; characterized by chills, fever, backache or muscle cramps, hemoglobinemia, hemoglobinuria, and oliguria, which may result in acute renal failure, DIC, and death.

indirect pupillary r., SYN consensual r.

intracutaneous r., intradermal r., a r. following the injection of antigen into the skin of a sensitive subject, such as in the case of the tuberculin test.

iodate r. of epinephrine, a r. dependent upon the oxidation of epinephrine by iodine liberated from iodate, which is decomposed by the hormone; a faint pink color results.

iodine r. of epinephrine, a r. resulting from the oxidation of the hormone, a faint pink color appearing upon the addition of iodine.

irreversible r., a r. or response by the tissues to a pathogenic agent characterized by a permanent pathologic change.

Jaffe r., a bright orange-red complex resulting from the treatment of creatinine with alkaline picrate solution; the basis of most routine creatinine tests.

Jarisch-Herxheimer r., SYN Herxheimer r.

Jolly r., rapid loss of response to faradic stimulation of a muscle with the galvanic response and the power of voluntary contraction retained; an obsolete method for detecting myasthenia gravis. SYN myasthenic r.

Kiliani-Fischer r., SEE Kiliani-Fischer *synthesis*.

late r., SYN delayed r.

lengthening r., in the decerebrate animal, the rather sudden relaxation with lengthening of the extensor muscles when a limb is passively flexed; associated with clasp-knife spasticity.

lepromin r., a delayed hypersensitivity r. at the site of an intradermal injection of a lepromin, such as the Dharmendra antigen or Mitsuda antigen, in a lepromin test; the r.'s, such as the Fernandez or Mitsuda r., are variable, occurring in 48 hours or 3–5 weeks, but are uniformly negative in lepromatous leprosy, borderline leprosy, and mid-borderline leprosy.

leukemoid r., SEE leukemoid reaction.

lid-closure r., SYN eye-closure pupil r.

Liebermann-Burchard r., SEE Burchard-Liebermann r.

ligase chain r., a technique for target amplification of DNA in which DNA ligase is used to join two complementary oligonucleotide probes that have bound to a target sequence in vitro. The ligation product is used as a template for ligation of complementary oligonucleotides that, through repeated enzymatic processing, allow for logarithmic accumulation of products that can be used to determine the presence of the target of interest.

local r., SYN focal r.

local anesthetic r., a toxic r. due to absorption of local anesthetic drug during regional anesthesia, ranging from drowsiness to convulsions and cardiovascular collapse.

Loewenthal r., the agglutinative r. in relapsing fever.

Lohmann r., the r. catalyzed by creatine kinase.

magnet r., a r. seen in an animal deprived of its cerebellum; when the animal is placed upon its back and the head strongly flexed, the four limbs become flexed in all their joints. Because of stimulation of receptors in the deep layers of the skin, light pressure made upon a toe-pad with the finger causes reflex contraction of the limb extensors; the limb is thus pressed gently against the finger, and when the finger is withdrawn slightly, the experimenter has the sensation that the finger is raising the limb or drawing it out as by a magnet.

Marchi r., failure of the myelin sheath of a nerve to blacken when submitted to the action of osmic acid.

Mazzotti r., SYN Mazzotti *test*.

Millon r., the r. of phenolic compounds (e.g., tyrosine in protein) with $Hg(NO_3)_2$ in HNO_3 (and a trace of HNO_2) to give a red color.

miostagmin r., a physiochemical immunity test, designed by Ascoli, consisting in determination of the surface tension of an immune serum to which its specific antigen has been added, before and after incubation at 37°C for 2 hours; in a positive r. the surface tension, as measured by the stalagmometer, is lowered.

Mitsuda r., a delayed hypersensitivity lepromin r., in the form of erythematous papular nodules, at the site of intradermal injection of Mitsuda antigen in a lepromin test.

mixed agglutination r., immune agglutination in which the aggregates contain cells of two different kinds but with common antigenic determinants; when used to identify isoantigens, the test cells are exposed to appropriate isoantibody, washed, and then mixed with indicator erythrocytes that combine with free sites on the test cell-attached isoantibody.

mixed lymphocyte culture r., SEE mixed lymphocyte culture *test*.

monomolecular r., a r. involving a single molecule (e.g., decomposition, intramolecular rearrangement, intramolecular oxidation or reduction), even if a catalytic agent, such as acid or alkali, is present in large excess, on a molecular basis, or is not rate-determining; such r.'s are usually first-order r.'s. Cf. molecularity. SYN unimolecular r.

myasthenic r., SYN Jolly r.

Nadi r., SYN peroxidase r.

near r., the pupillary constriction associated with a near vision effort, i.e., with accommodation and convergence.

nested polymerase chain r., use of the PCR in series such that a specified piece of DNA is amplified, then a portion contained within the first piece is amplified further; used where extremely low amounts of DNA are present, or where there are problems with background or contaminating DNA.

Neufeld r., SYN Neufeld capsular *swelling*.

neurotonic r., muscular contraction continuing well after cessation of stimulation.

neutral r., pH of 7.00; H^+ and OH^- ion concentrations equal at 10^{-7} mol/L at 22°C. Cf. dissociation *constant* of water.

ninhydrin r., a test for proteins, peptones, peptides, and amino acids possessing free carboxyl and α-amino groups that is based upon the r. with triketohydrinene hydrate; a blue color r. is used to quantitate free amino acids (e.g., after hydrolysis and separation of the amino acids of a protein). SYN triketohydrindene r.

nitritoid r., a severe r. resembling that following the administration of nitrites, sometimes following intravenous administration of arsphenamine or other drugs; consists of flushing of the face, edema of the tongue and lips, vomiting, profuse sweating, a fall in blood pressure, and sometimes death.

r. of nonidentity, SEE gel diffusion precipitin *tests* in two dimensions, under *test*.

nuclear r., the interaction of two atomic nuclei or of one such with a subatomic particle, or of the subatomic particles within an atomic nucleus, resulting in a change in the nature of the nuclei concerned or in the energy content of the nuclei or both, usually manifested by transmutation (accompanied by emission of alpha-, beta-, and/or gamma-rays) or by fission or fusion of the nuclei.

oxidase r., (1) the formation of indol blue when a blood smear containing myeloid leukocytes is treated with a mixture of α-naphthol and *p*-dimethylaniline sulfate; the myeloid leukocytes contain an oxidase that catalyzes this r., and the lymphoid leukocytes do not; **(2)** in bacteriology, a r. that depends on the presence of certain oxidases in some bacteria that catalyze the transport of electrons between electron donors in the bacteria and an oxidation reduction dye, such as tetramethyl-*p*-phenylenediamine; the dye is reduced to a blue or black color.

oxidation-reduction r., SEE oxidation-reduction.

pain r., dilation of the pupil or any other involuntary act occurring in response to a stimulus causing sharp pain anywhere.

Pandy r., a test to determine the presence of proteins (chiefly globulins) in the spinal fluid, by adding one drop of spinal fluid to 1 mL of solution (e.g., carbolic acid crystals in distilled water, cresol, or pyrogallic acid); the r. varies from a faint turbidity to a dense "milky" precipitate according to the degree of protein content. SYN Pandy test.

r. of partial identity, SEE gel diffusion precipitin *tests* in two dimensions, under *test*.

passive cutaneous anaphylactic r., SEE passive cutaneous *anaphylaxis*.

Paul r., pus is rubbed into a scarification on a rabbit's eye; if the pus is from a variolous or vaccinal pustule a condition of epitheliosis develops in 36–48 hours; the sputum of a smallpox patient is said to cause the same r. SYN Paul test.

performic acid r., oxidative destruction of the ethylene double bond (–HC=CH–) which is converted to a Schiff-reactive double aldehyde; used to indicate the presence of unsaturated lipids, such as phospholipids and cerebrosides, as well as cystine-rich substances, such as keratin, in tissue sections.

periosteal r., radiographically detectable new subperiosteal bone formed as a r. to soft tissue or osseous disease.

peroxidase r., formation of indophenol blue by the action of an oxidizing enzyme present in certain cells and tissues when they are treated with a solution of α-naphthol and dimethylparaphenylenediamine; by this method, cells of the myelocyte series, which give a positive r., may be distinguished from those of the lymphocyte series, which give a negative r. SYN Nadi r.

phosphoroclastic r., cleavage of C–C bonds that involves phosphate transfer but not, as in phosphorolysis, directly to one of the products; e.g., the decomposition of pyruvate to acetate + CO_2, in which orthophosphate is added to ADP to form ATP.

Pirquet r., SYN Pirquet *test*.

plasmal r., a histochemical technique that uses mercuric chloride to unmask the aldehyde group of acetalphosphatides and permit Schiff staining.

pleural r., thickening of the pleural stripe on chest radiographs, representing pleuritis, pleural effusion, or pleural fibrosis.

polymerase chain r. (PCR) (po-lim′er-ās), an enzymatic method for the repeated copying of the two strands of DNA of a particular gene sequence. It is widely used to amplify minute quantities of biological material so as to provide adequate specimens for laboratory study.

> The replication of DNA in the living cell is facilitated by polymerases. The two DNA chains of the double helix first unzip from one another, and DNA polymerase then generates a copy of each strand by adding free nucleotides to form a sequence of base pairs complementary with the sequence in the strand. The laboratory technique known as polymerase chain reaction, for which the American biochemist Kary Mullis won a Nobel Prize in Chemistry in 1993, exploits the capacity of DNA polymerase to assemble new DNA. Taq polymerase, named for its source, *Thermus aquaticus*, a thermophilic bacterium, is added to a mixture of free nucleotides and primers. (Primers are specially prepared units containing both RNA and DNA with a free terminus where the polymerase will react.) The short sequence of DNA to be amplified is flanked by two primers. Once the reaction begins, the polymerase generates numerous copies of the target sequence. The sequential phases of the reaction are initiated simply by making a series of strategic changes in the temperature of the system. Millions of copies of the target sequence can be generated by cyclically repeating these temperature changes as many as 30 times, each DNA strand produced by one cycle giving rise to many more in the next. The technique is used to amplify specimens for diagnosis of both infectious and genetic diseases, to carry out DNA fingerprinting, and in genomic research.

Porter-Silber r., the basis of the 17-hydroxycorticosteroid test; C-21 adrenocorticosteroids, which contain a dihydroxyacetone group at carbons 19, 20, and 21, react with phenylhydrazine.

Prausnitz-Küstner r., a test for the presence of immediate hypersensitivity in humans; test serum from an atopic individual is injected intradermally into a normal subject; the normal subject is challenged 24–48 hours later with the antigen suspected of causing the immediate hypersensitivity r. in the atopic individual, usually in the form of a wheal flare. SYN P-K test.

precipitin r., SEE precipitin, precipitin *test*.

primary r., SYN vaccinia.

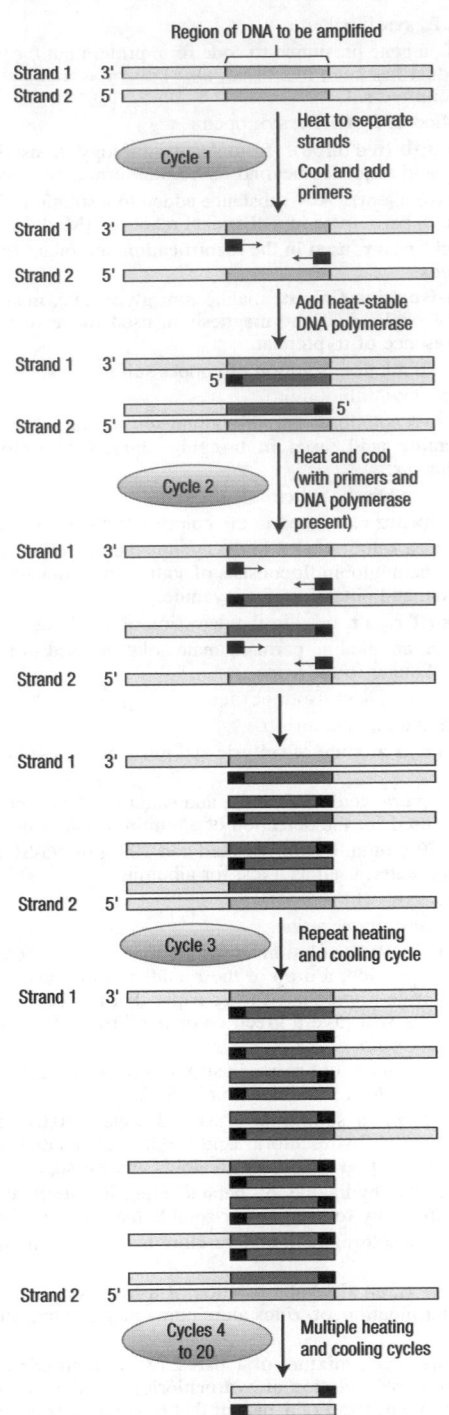

Region of DNA to be amplified

Strand 1   3'

Strand 2   5'

Cycle 1 — Heat to separate strands / Cool and add primers

Strand 1   3'

Strand 2   5'

Add heat-stable DNA polymerase

Strand 1   3'   5'

Strand 2   5'   5'

Cycle 2 — Heat and cool (with primers and DNA polymerase present)

Strand 1   3'

Strand 2   5'

Strand 1   3'

Strand 2   5'

Cycle 3 — Repeat heating and cooling cycle

Strand 1   3'

Strand 2   5'

Cycles 4 to 20 — Multiple heating and cooling cycles

Amplified DNA present in about 10^6 copies

polymerase chain reaction (PCR)

prozone r., SEE prozone.

psychogalvanic r., psychogalvanic skin r., SYN galvanic skin *response.*

quellung r., (1) SYN Neufeld capsular *swelling;* **(2)** if pneumococcal organisms, India ink, and specific antisera are mixed, the antibodies present in the sera will bind to the polysaccharide antigens of the pneumococcal capsule and the capsule will appear more opaque and swollen. This test will identify the organism as being pneumococci as well as the specific capsular types. SYN capsular precipitation r. [Ger. *Quellung,* swelling]

reversed Prausnitz-Küstner r., the appearance of an urticarial r. at the site of injection when serum containing reaginic antibody is injected into the skin of a person in whom the allergen is already present.

reverse transcriptase polymerase chain r. (RT-PCR), a process for specific mRNA amplification wherein reverse transcriptase added to the in vitro reaction uses mRNA as a template to produce one cDNA, which is then amplified by the usual PCR.

reversible r., a chemical r. that takes place in either direction, i.e., from the forward or reverse direction; ionization is such a r., as are r.'s involving racemases, isomerases, mutases, transferases, etc.

Sakaguchi r., guanidines in alkaline solution develop an intense red color when treated with α-naphthol and sodium hypochlorite; a qualitative test for arginine, free or in a protein.

Schardinger r., the reduction of methylene blue to methylene white by formaldehyde is rapidly catalyzed by fresh milk but not by boiled milk, the catalyzing agent being xanthine oxidase (Schardinger enzyme); an example of oxidation in the absence of O_2 with an organic hydrogen acceptor (the dye).

Schultz r., SEE Schultz *stain.*

Schultz-Charlton r., the specific blanching of a scarlatinal rash at the site of intracutaneous injection of scarlatina antiserum. SYN Schultz-Charlton phenomenon.

Schultz-Dale r., the contraction of an excised intestinal loop (Schultz) or of an excised strip of virginal uterus (Dale) from a sensitized animal (guinea pig) that occurs when the tissue is exposed to the specific antigen.

serum r., SYN serum *sickness.*

shortening r., the adaptive shortening of the extensor muscles of the limb of a decerebrate animal when the limb is extended after it has been flexed. Cf. lengthening r.

Shwartzman r., SYN Shwartzman *phenomenon.*

skin r., SYN skin *test.*

specific r., the phenomena produced by an agent that is identical with or immunologically related to the one that has already caused an alteration in capacity of the tissue to react.

startle r., SYN startle *reflex.*

Straus r., a diagnostic test for glanders. Male guinea pigs are inoculated intraperitoneally with suspected material; if the glanders organism is present, it will usually set up a necrotizing inflammation in the scrotal sac within a few days and the specific organism can be confirmed bacteriologically.

stress r., an acute emotional r. related to extreme environmental threat or challenge. SYN acute situational r.

supporting r.'s, described by Magnus, who distinguished two types: **positive supporting r.'s,** consisting of those reflex muscular contractions whereby the body is supported against gravity; seen in an exaggerated form in the decerebrate animal; **negative supporting r.,** consisting of inhibition of the extensor muscles and unfixing of the joints that thus enable the limb to be flexed and moved into a new position. SYN supporting reflexes.

symptomatic r., an allergic response similar to the original one, but occurring after the use of a test or therapeutic dose of an allergen or atopen.

thermoprecipitin r., the throwing down of a precipitate on the application of heat, as in the case of proteinaceous urine.

transcription-based chain r., a technique for target amplification of DNA or RNA in which reverse transcriptase is used to produce a single-stranded DNA molecule for each DNA or RNA target; this molecule is used as a template for further amplification.

***Treponema pallidum* immobilization r.,** SYN *Treponema pallidum* immobilization *test.*

triketohydrindene r., SYN ninhydrin r.

type III hypersensitivity r., SYN immune complex *disease.*

unimolecular r., SYN monomolecular r.

vaccinoid r., SYN accelerated r.

Voges-Proskauer r., a chemical r. used in testing for the production of acetyl methyl carbinol by various bacteria; potassium hydroxide is added to a 24-hour culture in a suitable medium and thoroughly mixed; the treated culture is exposed to air and is observed at intervals of 2, 12, and 24 hours; a positive r. consists of the development of an eosin-like pink color, due to the production of acetylmethylcarbinol, which in the presence of alkali and oxygen is oxidized to diacetyl.

Wassermann r. (W.r.), SYN Wassermann *test*.

Weidel r., a r. showing the presence of xanthine; a solution of the suspected substance in chlorine water with a little nitric acid is evaporated in a water bath, and then exposed to the vapor of ammonia; the presence of xanthine is indicated when a red or purple color develops.

Weil-Felix r., SYN Weil-Felix *test*.

Weinberg r., a complement fixation test of the presence of hydatid disease.

Wernicke r., in hemianopia, a r. due to damage of the optic tract, consisting in loss of pupillary constriction when the light is directed to the blind side of the retina; pupillary constriction is maintained when light stimulates the normal side. This sign cannot be seen with a bright light because of intraocular scatter onto the seeing half of the retina. SYN Wernicke sign.

wheal-and-erythema r., the characteristic immediate r. observed in the skin test; within 10–15 minutes after injection of antigen (allergen), an irregular, blanched, elevated wheal appears, surrounded by an area of erythema (flare). SYN wheal-and-flare r.

wheal-and-flare r., SYN wheal-and-erythema r.

white r., the response seen in many individuals after the skin is lightly stroked with a blunt instrument; it is attributed to capillary action.

whitegraft r., an immune r. to a incompatible tissue graft that results in failure of graft vascularization and ensuing rejection.

Widal r., agglutination r. as applied to the diagnosis of typhoid. SYN Gruber r., Gruber-Widal r.

xanthoprotein r., a qualitative test for proteins; a yellow product is formed by reacting proteins with hot, concentrated nitric acid.

Yorke autolytic r., a test for paroxysmal hemoglobinuria; serum is placed in an ice chest and kept at 0°C for 5–7 minutes, then in an incubator at 37°C with erythrocytes for 1 hour, at which time, if the r. is positive, hemolysis occurs; if the serum is kept at 1°C for an hour and then placed in the incubator with erythrocytes there is little hemolysis.

zero-order r., a r. that proceeds at a particular rate independently of the concentration of the reactant or reactants.

Zimmermann r., a chemical r. between an alkaline solution of *meta*-dinitrobenzene and an active methylene group (carbon-16) of 17-ketosteroids; it is the basis of the 17-ketogenic steroid assay test; more generally, a r. between methylene ketones and aromatic polynitro compounds in alkaline solutions. SYN Zimmermann test.

---

re·ac·ti·vate (rē-ak′ti-vāt). **1.** To render active again. **2.** In particular, of an inactivated immune serum to which normal serum (complement) is added.

re·ac·ti·va·tion (rē′ak-ti-vā′shŭn). **1.** Restoration of the lytic activity of an inactivated serum by means of the addition of complement. **2.** Restoration of activity in an inactivated enzyme.

re·ac·tiv·i·ty (rē-ak-tiv′i-tē). **1.** The property of reacting, chemically or in any other sense. **2.** The process of reacting.

read·ing (rēd′ing). **1.** The perception and understanding of the meaning of visual symbols (e.g., letters or words) by the scanning of writing or print with the eyes. **2.** Any of several alternative ways of interpreting symbols, such as Braille or the close observation of a speaker's facial movements.

lip r., SYN speech r.

speech r., used by people with hearing impairment of nonauditory clues as to what is being said through observing the speaker's facial expressions, lip and jaw movements, and other gestures. SYN lip r.

read·ing frame. The grouping of nucleotides by threes into codons. SEE frame-shift *mutation*.

blocked r. f., a sequence of DNA that cannot be translated into a viable protein; usually due to the interruption by one or more termination codons. SYN closed r. f.

closed r. f., SYN blocked r. f.

open r. f., a gene presumed to code for a protein but for which no gene product has been identified; also known as unidentified r. f. SYN unidentified r. f.

unidentified r. f. (URF), SYN open r. f.

read·through (rēd′throo). In molecular biology, transcription of a nucleic acid sequence beyond its normal termination sequence.

re·a·gent (rē-ā′jent). Any substance added to a solution of another substance to participate in a chemical reaction. [Mod. L. *reagens*]

amino acid r., a r. used in the identification and quantification of amino acids.

Benedict-Hopkins-Cole r., magnesium glyoxalate, made from a mixture of oxalic acid and magnesium, used for testing proteins for the presence of tryptophan.

biuret r., an alkaline solution of copper sulfate.

Cleland r., SYN dithiothreitol.

diazo r., two solutions, one of sodium nitrite, the other of acidified sulfanilic acid, used in bringing about diazotization. SYN Ehrlich diazo r.

Dische r., SEE Dische *reaction*.

Dische-Schwarz r., r. used in the colorimetric detection of RNA.

Drabkin r., a solution used in the cyanmethemoglobin method of measuring hemoglobin. It consists of sodium bicarbonate, potassium cyanide, and potassium ferricyanide.

Dragendorff r., a r. used in the detection of alkaloids.

Edlefsen r., an alkaline permanganate solution used in the determination of sugar in the urine.

Edman r., SYN phenylisothiocyanate.

Ehrlich diazo r., SYN diazo r.

Erdmann r., a mixture of sulfuric and nitric acids, used in testing alkaloids.

Esbach r., picric acid, citric acid, and water (in the proportions 1, 2, and 97) used for the detection of albumin in the urine.

Exton r., 50 g of sulfosalicylic acid and 200 g of $Na_2SO_4·10H_2O$ in a liter of water, used as a test for albumin.

Fehling r., SYN Fehling *solution*.

Folin r., SYN Folin *reaction*.

Fouchet r., a 25% solution of trichloroacetic acid, containing 0.9% ferric chloride; a drop of the r. added at the surface line of barium chloride-impregnated filter paper that has been dipped in urine for 10 s will give a green color if bilirubin is present. SEE ALSO Fouchet *stain*.

Froehde r., sodium molybdate in strong sulfuric acid; this reagent gives various color reactions with alkaloids.

Frohn r., bismuth subnitrate (1.5) and water (20.0) heated to boiling, to which hydrochloric acid (10.0) and potassium iodide (7.0) are added; used to test for alkaloids and for sugar.

Girard r., the hydrazine of betaine chloride, used to extract ketonic steroids by forming water-soluble hydrazones with them.

Günzberg r., phloroglucin and vanillin used as a r. in Günzberg test.

Hahn oxine r., an alcoholic solution of 8-hydroxyquinoline used in the determination of zinc, aluminum, magnesium, and other minerals.

Hammarsten r., a mixture of 1 part 25% solution of nitric acid and 19 parts 25% solution of hydrochloric acid; the addition of a few drops to a mixture of 1 part of this r. and 4 parts alcohol will give a green color if bile is present.

Ilosvay r., sulfanilic acid 0.5, dissolved in dilute acetic acid 150, mixed with naphthylamine 1, and dissolved in boiling water 20; the blue sediment that forms is dissolved in dilute acetic acid 150; a few drops of this r. added to water, saliva, or other fluid to be tested will produce a red color if nitrites are present.

Kasten fluorescent Schiff r.'s, fluorescent analogs of Schiff r. that are fluorescent basic dyes lacking acidic side groups and containing one or more primary amine groups; used in cytochemical detection of DNA in Kasten fluorescent Feulgen stain, polysaccharides in Kasten fluorescent PAS stain, and proteins in the ninhydrin-Schiff stain; such analogs include acriflavine, auramine O, and flavophosphine N.

Lloyd r., precipitated aluminum silicate, used in the determination of alkaloids.

Mandelin r., a solution of ammonium vanadate in sulfuric acid, used in color tests for alkaloids.

Marme r., a solution of potassium iodide and cadmium iodide used in testing for alkaloids.

Marquis r., a solution of formaldehyde in sulfuric acid used in color tests for formaldehyde.

Mecke r., a solution of selenous acid in sulfuric acid, used for color tests of alkaloids.

Meyer r., a solution of phenolphthalein with sodium hydroxide, in water (glass-distilled); in the presence of minute traces of blood, the solution becomes purple or blue-red.

Millon r., mercuric nitrate and nitric acid as used in the Millon reaction.

Nessler r., a solution of potassium hydroxide, mercuric iodide, and potassium iodide; it yields a yellow color with ammonia (a brown precipitate with larger amounts) that can be used for quantitative assay.

Rosenthaler-Turk r., a solution of potassium arsenate in sulfuric acid used in obtaining color tests for various opium alkaloids.

Sanger r., SYN fluoro-2,4-dinitrobenzene.

Schaer r., an alcoholic or aqueous solution of chloral hydrate used as an extraction medium in investigations of alkaloids.

Scheibler r., a solution of sodium tungstate in phosphoric acid used in tests for alkaloids.

Schiff r., an aqueous solution of basic fuchsin or pararosaniline that is decolorized by sulfur dioxide, commonly prepared by addition of hydrochloric acid to a dye solution containing a metabisulphite or bisulphite salt; used for aldehydes and in histochemistry to detect polysaccharides, DNA, and proteins. SEE Feulgen *stain*, periodic acid-Schiff *stain*, ninhydrin-Schiff *stain* for proteins.

Scott-Wilson r., an alkaline solution of mercuric cyanide and silver nitrate used in the detection of acetone.

sulfhydryl r., r. that reacts with thiol groups, particularly those in proteins.

Sulkowitch r., a r. for the detection of calcium in the urine, consisting of 2.5 g of oxalic acid, 2.5 g of ammonium oxalate, 5 mL of glacial acetic acid, and distilled water to make 150 mL; a milky precipitate of calcium oxalate is formed when the r. is added to urine that contains calcium.

Uffelmann r., a solution prepared by adding a 2% solution of phenol in water to aqueous ferric chloride until the solution becomes violet in color; this turns lemon yellow in the presence of lactic acid, assumes an opaline tint in butyric acid, and is decolorized by hydrochloric acid.

Wurster r., filter paper impregnated with tetramethyl-*p*-phenylenediamine, which turns blue in the presence of ozone or hydrogen peroxide.

re·a·gin (rē-ā′jin). 1. Wolff-Eisner term for antibody. 2. Old term for the "Wassermann" antibody; not to be confused with the Prausnitz-Küstner antibody. 3. Antibodies that mediate immediate hypersensitivity reactions (IgE in humans). 4. SYN homocytotropic *antibody.*

atopic r., SYN Prausnitz-Küstner *antibody.*

re·a·gin·ic (rē-ā-jin′ik). Pertaining to a reagin.

REAL Abbreviation for Revised European-American Classification of Lymphoid Neoplasms. SEE REAL *classification* .

re·al·i·ty (rē-al′i-tē). That which exists objectively and in fact, and can be consensually validated. [L. *res,* thing, fact]

real·i·ty aware·ness. The ability to distinguish external objects as being different from oneself.

ream·er (rē′mer). A rotating finishing or drilling tool used to shape or enlarge a hole in bone or a tooth. [A.S. *ryman,* to widen]

engine r., an engine-mounted spirally bladed instrument, used for enlarging the root canals of teeth.

intramedullary r., a rasp used for shaping the intramedullary canal of a large bone before inserting an appliance or prosthesis.

re·ar·range·ment (rē-a-rānj-ment). A restructuring; e.g., in a molecule.

Amadori rearrangement, a rearrangement that occurs in cross-linking reactions seen in collagen and in protein glycosylations; e.g., conversion of *N*-glycosides of aldoses to *N*-glycosides of the corresponding ketoses.

reassignment.

sex r., a process whereby the sex of an individual is changed by a combination of psychiatric, psychologic, pharmacologic, and surgical procedures, usually as a part of the treatment of hermaphroditism transexualism. SYN sex reversal.

re·at·tach·ment (rē-ă-tach′ment). New epithelial or connective tissue attachment to the surface of a tooth that was surgically detached and not exposed to oral environment.

Réaumur, René A.F. de, French physicist, 1683–1757. SEE R. *scale.*

re·base (rē′bās). In dentistry, to refit a denture by replacing the denture base material without changing the occlusal relationship of the teeth. SEE ALSO reline.

re·breath·ing (rē-brēdh′ing). Inhalation of part or all of gases previously exhaled.

Rebuck skin win·dow tech·nique. See under technique.

RecA. An *Escherichia coli* protein that specifically recognizes single-stranded DNA and anneals it to a complementary sequence in a duplex that is homologous. This results in the displacement of the original complementary strand of the duplex.

re·cal·ci·fi·ca·tion (rē-kal′si-fi-kā′shŭn). Restoration to the tissues of lost calcium salts.

re·call (rē′kawl). The process of remembering thoughts, words, and actions of a past event in an attempt to recapture actual happenings.

Récamier, Joseph C.A., French gynecologist, 1774–1852. SEE R. *operation.*

re·ca·nal·i·za·tion (rē-kan′ăl-i-zā′shŭn). 1. Restoration of a lumen in a blood vessel following thrombotic occlusion, by organization of the thrombus with formation of new channels. 2. Spontaneous restoration of the continuity of the lumen of any occluded duct or tube, as with postvasectomy r.

re·ca·pit·u·la·tion (rē′kă-pit′ū-lā′shŭn). SEE recapitulation *theory.*

re·ceiv·er (rē-sē′ver). In chemistry, a vessel attached to a condenser to receive the product of distillation. [L. *receptor,* fr. *recipio,* to receive]

re·cep·tac·u·lum, pl. **re·cep·tac·u·la** (rē′sep-tak′ū-lŭm, -lă). A receptacle. SYN reservoir. [L. fr. *re-cipio,* pp. *-ceptus,* to receive, fr. *capio,* to take]

r. chy′li, SYN *cisterna* chyli.

r. gan′glii petro′si, SYN petrosal *fossula.*

r. pecquet′i, SYN *cisterna* chyli.

re·cep·tive (rē-sep′-tĭv). Sensitive or responsive to stimulus.

r. field, that part of the retina of which the photoreceptors (rods and cones) pertain to a single optic nerve fiber. The response of a neuron to stimulation of its receptive field depends on the type of neuron and the part of the field that is illuminated; an "on-center" neuron is stimulated by light falling at the center of its r. field and inhibited by light falling at the periphery; an "off-center" neuron reacts in exactly the opposite fashion; that is, it is inhibited by light falling at the center of its receptive field. In either case, the net response depends on a complex switching action in the retina. When an entire receptive field is equally illuminated, the response of receptors at the center of the field predominates.

re·cep·tor (rē-sep′tŏr, tōr). 1. A structural protein molecule on the cell surface or within the cytoplasm that binds to a specific factor, such as a drug, hormone, antigen, or neurotransmitter. 2. C. Sherrington term for any one of the various sensory nerve endings in the skin, deep tissues, viscera, and special sense organs. [L. receiver, fr. *recipio,* to receive]

adrenergic r.'s, reactive components of effector tissues, most of which are innervated by adrenergic postganglionic fibers of the sympathetic nervous system. Such r.'s can be activated by norepinephrine and/or epinephrine and by various adrenergic drugs; r. activation results in a change in effector tissue function, such as contraction of arteriolar muscles or relaxation of bronchial muscles; adrenergic r.'s are divided into α-r.'s and β-r.'s, on the basis

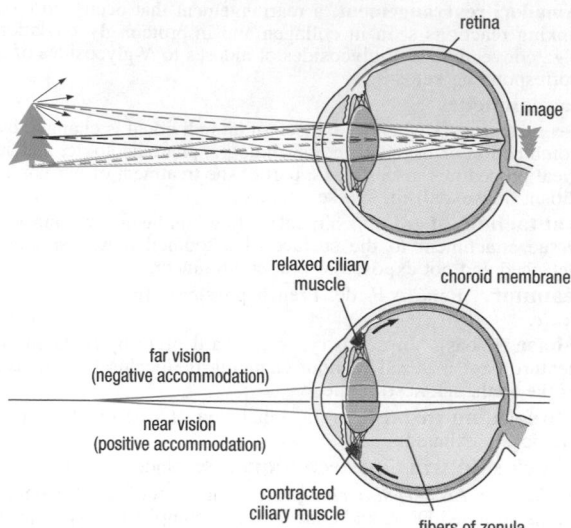

formation of image on retina: every part of object corresponds to part of image on retina; image is inverted miniature of object

of their response to various adrenergic activating and blocking agents. SYN adrenoceptor, adrenoreceptors.

α-adrenergic r.'s, adrenergic r.'s in effector tissues capable of selective activation and blockade by drugs; conceptually derived from the ability of certain agents, such as phenoxybenzamine, to block only some adrenergic r.'s and of other agents, such as methoxamine, to activate only the same adrenergic r.'s. Such r.'s are designated as α-receptors. Their activation results in physiologic responses such as increased peripheral vascular resistance, mydriasis, and contraction of pilomotor muscles.

β-adrenergic r.'s, adrenergic r.'s in effector tissues capable of selective activation and blockade by drugs; conceptually derived from the ability of certain agents, such as propranolol, to block only some adrenergic r.'s and of other agents, such as isoproterenol, to activate only the same adrenergic r.'s. Such r.'s are designated as β-receptors. Their activation results in physiologic responses such as increases in cardiac rate and force of contraction (β_1), and relaxation of bronchial and vascular smooth muscle (β_2) contained in skeletal muscle.

β-adrenergic receptors

	the principal effects on organs of various β-receptor subtypes	
	organ	function of receptor
β_1 type	heart	increase heart rate, contractility, speed of conduction
	kidney	increase release of renin
	fatty tissue	increase lipolysis
β_2 type	bronchial passages	dilate constricted bronchial passages
	blood vessels	produce vasodilation in blood vessels of skeletal muscles
	uterus	relaxe uterine smooth muscle
	pancreas (β cells)	increase release of insulin
	liver, skeletal muscles	increase glycogenolysis
	fatty tissue	increase lipolysis

AMPA r., a type of glutamate r. that participates in excitatory neurotransmission and also binds α-amino-3-hydroxy-5-methyl-4-isoxazole propionic acid and acts as a cation channel. SYN quisqualate r.

angiotensin r., cell-surface G-protein–coupled r.'s that mediate the effects of angiotensin II. Two types are recognized: AT_1 and AT_2; the former mediates the powerful vascular smooth-muscle contraction responsible for the hypertensive response produced by angiotensin II; the latter is not sufficiently understood to be assigned any physiologic function.

ANP r.'s, cell surface r.'s for atrial natriuretic peptide that have a single transmembrane spanning element; these have integral kinase and guanylate cyclase domains.

ANP clearance r.'s, cell surface proteins that bind atrial natriuretic peptide and ANP fragments without initiating biologic action.

asialoglycoprotein r., a surface r. found in hepatocytes that binds galactose-terminal glycoproteins; thus, this r. removes those proteins from circulation and they are in turn acted upon by hepatocyte lysosomes.

B cell r.'s, a complex comprising a membrane-bound immunoglobulin molecule and two associated signal-transducing α and β chains.

cholinergic r.'s, chemical sites in effector cells or at synapses through which acetylcholine exerts its action.

epidermal growth factor r. (EGFR), r. often upregulated in epithelial tumors.

estrogen r., r. for estrogens; its presence conveys a better prognosis for breast cancers.

Fas r., SEE Fas.

Fc r., r.'s present on a variety of cells for the Fc fragment of immunoglobulins. These r.'s recognize immunoglobulins of the IgG and IgE class.

kainate r., a type of glutamate r. that participates in excitatory neurotransmission and also binds kainate and acts as a cation channel; injection of kainate causes death of neurons but preserves glial cells and axons.

laminin r., a r. found in many cell types that binds laminin and has a role in cell attachment and neurite outgrowth.

L-AP$_4$ r., a type of glutamate receptor that also binds a particular synthetic agonist and acts as a cation channel.

low-density lipoprotein r.'s, r.'s on the surface of cells, especially liver cells, which bind to low-density lipoprotein and promote clearance of LDL from the plasma.

mannose-6-phosphate r.'s (MPR), r.'s in Golgi apparatus to which newly synthesized proteins that are destined to enter lysosomes bind.

metabotropic r., a type of r. that is linked to intracellular production of 1,2-diacylglycerol and inositol 1,4,5-trisphosphate. [metabolism + G. *tropē*, turning, inclination, + -ic]

muscarinic r.'s, membrane-bound proteins whose extracellular domain contains a recognition site for acetylcholine (ACh); combination of Ach with the r. initiates a physiologic change (slowing of heart rate, increased glandular secretory activity, and stimulation of smooth muscle contractions); changes are observed after treatment with the mushroom alkaloid muscarine. Muscarinic r.'s are to be distinguished from nicotinic r.'s.

nicotinic r.'s, a class of cholinergic r.'s on skeletal muscle cells that are linked to ion channels in the cell membrane.

nicotinic cholinergic r., a class of r.'s responsive to acetylcholine that also are activated by nicotine; ganglionic (including the adrenal medulla) and neuromuscular r.'s. Two classes exist: nicotinic-neuronal and nicotinic-muscular.

NMDA r., a type of glutamate r. that participates in excitatory neurotransmission and also binds *N*-methyl-D-aspartate; may be particularly involved in the cell damage observed in individuals with Huntington disease.

opiate r.'s, regions of the brain that have the capacity to bind morphine; some, along the aqueduct of Sylvius and in the center median, are in areas related to pain, but others, as in the striatum, are not related.

orphan r., a nuclear r. for which no ligand has yet been identified.

progesterone r., intracellular r. for progesterone; often over-expressed in breast cancer.

quisqualate r., SYN AMPA r.

retinoic acid r., nuclear r. for retinoic acid.

retinoid X r., r. for retinoic acids; has less affinity for retinoic acid than the retinoic acid r.'s; function is not yet well understood.

ryanodine r., r. associated with a calcium conductance channel in the sacroplasmic or endoplasmic reticulum of cells, which when bound to ryanodine, causes the channel to remain in a subconductive state, allowing slow continuing release of calcium ions from the sarcoplasmic reticulum into the cytoplasm. The channels are normally sensitive to calcium ions and not sensitive to inositol triphosphate.

scavenger r., a r. on macrophages that binds preferentially to oxidized LDL, causing macrophages to internalize the LDL.

sensory r.'s, peripheral endings of afferent neurons.

stretch r.'s, r.'s that are sensitive to elongation, especially those in Golgi tendon organs and muscle spindles, but also those found in visceral organs such as the stomach, small intestine, and urinary bladder; these r.'s have the function of detecting elongation, and this distinguishes them from baroreceptors, which actually are activated by stretching of the wall of the blood vessel but whose function is to elicit central reflex mechanism reducing the arterial blood pressure.

T cell antigen r.'s, r.'s present on T cells that interact with both processed antigen and major histocompatibility antigens simultaneously; these are heterodimers, each consisting of either an α and β chain or a γ and δ chain.

re·cep·to·somes (rē-sep′tō-sōms). Vesicles that avoid lysosomes and deliver their contents to other intracellular sites.

re·cess (rē′ses) [TA]. A small hollow or indentation. SYN recessus [TA]. [L. *recessus*]

anterior r., a circumscript deepening of the interpeduncular fossa in the direction of the mamillary bodies. SYN recessus anterior [TA].

anterior r. of tympanic membrane [TA], a slitlike space on the tympanic wall between the anterior malleolar fold and the tympanic membrane. SYN recessus anterior membranae tympanicae [TA], Tröltsch pockets, Tröltsch r.'s.

azygoesophageal r., the region below the azygos vein arch in which the right lung intrudes into the mediastinum between the heart and vertebral column, bordered on the left by the esophagus.

cecal r., SYN retrocecal r.

cerebellopontine r., SEE cerebellopontine *angle.*

cochlear r. [TA], a small depression on the inner wall of the vestibule of the labyrinth at the portion of the pyramid of vestibule, between the two limbs into which the vestibular crest divides posteriorly; it is perforated by foramina giving passage to fibers that the cochlear branch of the vestibulocochlear nerve sends to the posterior extremity of the cochlear duct. SYN recessus cochlearis [TA], Reichert cochlear r.

costodiaphragmatic r. [TA], the cleftlike extension of the pleural cavity between the diaphragm and the rib cage; pleural effusions collect here when in the upright position, and since the lung only partially enters, this is the site of thoracocentesis. SYN recessus costodiaphragmaticus [TA], phrenicocostal sinus.

costomediastinal r. [TA], the recess of the pleural cavity between the costal cartilages and the mediastinum. SYN recessus costomediastinalis [TA], costomediastinal sinus.

duodenojejunal r., SYN superior duodenal *fossa.*

elliptical r. of bony labyrinth [TA], an oval depression in the roof and inner wall of the vestibule of the labyrinth, lodging the utriculus. SYN recessus ellipticus labyrinthi ossei [TA], recessus utricularis labyrinthi ossei★, utricular r. of bony labyrinth★, fovea elliptica, fovea hemielliptica.

epitympanic r. [TA], the upper portion of the tympanic cavity above the tympanic membrane; it contains the head of the malleus and the body of the incus. SYN recessus epitympanicus [TA], attic, epitympanic space, epitympanum, Hyrtl epitympanic r., tympanic attic.

hepatoenteric r., a peritoneal r. at the caudal end of the embryonic pneumatoenteric r.; it separates the developing liver and stomach.

hepatorenal r. of subhepatic space [TA], the deep recess of the subhepatic space of the peritoneal cavity on the right side extending upward between the liver in front and the kidney and suprare-

nal behind; this is a gravity-dependent portion of the peritoneal cavity when in the supine position; fluids draining from the omental bursa drain here. SYN recessus hepatorenalis recessus subhepatici [TA], hepatorenal pouch, Morison pouch.

Hyrtl epitympanic r., SYN epitympanic r.

inferior duodenal r., SYN inferior duodenal *fossa.*

inferior ileocecal r. [TA], a deep fossa sometimes found between the ileocecal fold, the mesoappendix, and the cecum. SYN recessus ileocecalis inferior [TA].

inferior omental r., SYN inferior r. of omental bursa.

inferior r. of omental bursa [TA], a recess of the omental bursa extending between anterior and posterior layers of the great omentum. SYN recessus inferior omentalis [TA], inferior omental r.

infundibular r. [TA], a funnel-shaped diverticulum leading from the anterior portion of the third ventricle down into the infundibulum of the hypophysis. SYN aditus ad infundibulum [TA], recessus infundibuli [TA].

intersigmoid r. [TA], a triangular peritoneal recess posterior and inferior to the sigmoid colon created by the attachment of the sigmoid mesocolon ascending across the left psoas, then turning sharply to descend into the pelvis; the left ureter descends the posterior wall of this recess. SYN recessus intersigmoideus [TA].

Jacquemet r., a pouch of peritoneum between the gallbladder and the liver.

lateral r. of fourth ventricle [TA], the narrow r. of the ventricle that extends laterally over, and down along the side of, the inferior cerebellar peduncle and the overlying cochlear nuclei; at its tip it opens by way of Luschka foramen into the interopeduncular cistern of the subarachnoid space. By way of this r., part of the choroid plexus of the fourth ventricle protrudes into the subarachnoid space. SYN recessus lateralis ventriculi quarti [TA].

mesentericoparietal r., SYN parajejunal *fossa.*

optic r., SEE supraoptic r.

pancreaticoenteric r., a r. of the embryonic peritoneal cavity that develops into the adult omental bursa.

paracolic r.'s, SYN paracolic *gutters,* under *gutter.*

paraduodenal r. [TA], an occasional recess in the peritoneum to the left of the terminal portion of the duodenum located posterior to a fold containing the inferior mesenteric vein. SYN recessus paraduodenalis [TA], fossa venosa, paraduodenal fossa.

parotid r., SYN parotid *space.*

pharyngeal r. [TA], a slitlike depression in the lateral membranous (nonmuscular) pharyngeal wall extending posterior to the opening of the pharyngotympanic (auditory) tube. SYN recessus pharyngeus [TA], recessus infundibuliformis, Rosenmüller fossa, Rosenmüller r.

phrenicomediastinal r. [TA], the recess of the pleural cavity between the diaphragm and the mediastinum. SYN recessus phrenicomediastinalis [TA].

pineal r. [TA], a diverticulum from the posterior part of the third ventricle extending back between the posterior commissure and the habenular commissure; sometimes extending into the stalk of the pineal. SYN recessus pinealis [TA].

piriform r., ★official alternate term for piriform *fossa.*

pleural r.'s [TA], four recesses of the pleural cavity, one behind the sternum and costal cartilages (costomediastinal r.), one between the diaphragm and chest wall (costodiaphragmatic r.), one between the diaphragm and mediastinum (phrenicomediastinal r.), and one between the vertebral bodies and mediastinum (vertebromediastinal r.). SYN recessus pleurales [TA], pleural sinuses.

pneumatoenteric r., pneumoenteric r., a r. of the embryonic celom between the right lung bud and the gut; it is normally largely obliterated before birth, leaving only the superior r. of the vestibule of the lesser peritoneal sac as a vestige.

pontocerebellar r., SYN cerebellopontine *angle.*

posterior r. [TA], a deepening of the interpeduncular fossa toward the pons. SYN recessus posterior [TA].

posterior r. of tympanic membrane [TA], a narrow pocket in the tympanic wall between the posterior malleolar fold and the

re

tympanic membrane. SYN recessus posterior membranae tympanicae [TA], Tröltsch pockets, Tröltsch r.'s.

Reichert cochlear r., SYN cochlear r.

retrocecal r. [TA], one of several small pockets sometimes found extending alongside the right margin of the ascending colon near the cecum. SYN recessus retrocecalis [TA], cecal r.

retroduodenal r. [TA], a peritoneal recess occasionally found behind the third part of the duodenum, between it and the aorta. SYN recessus retroduodenalis [TA], infraduodenal fossa, retroduodenal fossa.

Rosenmüller r., SYN pharyngeal r.

sacciform r. of distal radioulnar joint [TA], an extension of the cavity of the distal radioulnar articulation proximad between the two bones; SYN recessus sacciformis articulationis radioulnaris distalis [TA].

sacciform r. of elbow joint [TA], an extension of the capsule of the elbow joint at the neck of the radius. SYN recessus sacciformis articulationis [TA].

saccular r. of bony labyrinth, ☆official alternate term for spherical r. of bony labyrinth.

sphenoethmoidal r. [TA], a small cleftlike pocket of the nasal cavity above the superior concha into which the sphenoid sinuses drain. SYN recessus sphenoethmoidalis [TA].

spherical r. of bony labyrinth [TA], a rounded depression on the inner wall of the vestibule of the labyrinth, lodging the sacculus. SYN recessus saccularis larbyrinthi ossei☆, saccular r. of bony labyrinth☆, fovea hemispherica, fovea spherica, recessus sphericus labyrinthi ossei.

splenic r. [TA], the extension of the omental bursa toward the hilum of the spleen. SYN recessus splenicus [TA], recessus lienalis☆.

subhepatic r., SYN subhepatic *space*.

subphrenic r.'s, SYN subphrenic *space*.

subpopliteal r. [TA], the extension of the cavity of the knee joint between the tendon of the popliteus and lateral condyle of the femur. SYN recessus subpopliteus [TA], bursa of popliteus.

superior azygoesophageal r., the region above the azygos vein arch in which the right lung is in contact with the esophagus.

superior duodenal r., ☆official alternate term for superior duodenal *fossa*.

superior ileocecal r. [TA], a shallow pouch occasionally existing between the terminal ileum, the cecum, and the ileocolic artery when the latter is present. SYN recessus ileocecalis superior [TA].

superior r. of lesser peritoneal sac, SEE pneumatoenteric r.

superior omental r., SYN superior r. of omental bursa.

superior r. of omental bursa [TA], a portion of the vestibule of the bursa omentalis that extends upward between the inferior vena cava and the esophagus. SYN recessus superior bursae omentalis [TA], superior omental r.

superior r. of tympanic membrane [TA], a space in the mucous membrane on the inner surface of the tympanic membrane between the flaccid part of the membrane and the neck of the malleus. SYN recessus superior membranae tympanicae [TA], Prussak pouch, Prussak space.

supraoptic r., a diverticulum extending forward from the anterior part of the third ventricle above the optic chiasm. SYN recessus supraopticus [TA], recessus supraaopticus [TA].

suprapineal r. [TA], a variable diverticulum from the posterior portion of the third ventricle of the brain, running backward some distance above and beyond the pineal r. SYN recessus suprapinealis [TA].

supratonsillar r., SYN supratonsillar *fossa*.

triangular r., an occasional evagination of the anterior wall of the third ventricle of the brain between the anterior commissure and the diverging pillars of the fornix. SYN recessus triangularis.

Tröltsch r.'s, SYN anterior r. of tympanic membrane, posterior r. of tympanic membrane.

tubotympanic r., the dorsal portion of the embryonic first endodermal pharyngeal pouch; it develops into the middle ear cavity.

r.'s of tympanic cavity [TA], spaces of the tympanic wall around

the tympanic membrane. SYN recessus membranae tympanicae [TA].

utricular r. of bony labyrinth, ☆official alternate term for elliptical r. of bony labyrinth.

utricular r. of membranous labyrinth [TA], part of the utricle that forms a blind-ended pouch that extends into the ellipsoid (utricular) recess of the bony labyrinth. SYN recessus utricularis labyrinthi membranacei [TA].

vertebromediastinal r. [TA], pleural recess formed by the reflection of the mediastinal part of the parietal pleura onto the vertebral bodies. SYN recessus vertebromediastinalis [TA].

re·ces·sion (rē-sesh′ŭn). A withdrawal or retreating. SEE ALSO retraction. [L. *recessio* (see recessus)]

angle r., tearing of the iris root between the longitudinal and circular ciliary muscles; often leading to glaucoma.

clitoral r., operative procedure to reduce the visual prominence of the clitoris that often occurs in females with congenital adrenal hyperplasia; distinct from clitoral amputation (clitorectomy) or clitoral reduction. SEE ALSO clitoroplasty.

gingival r., apical migration of the gingiva along the tooth surface, with exposure of the tooth surface. SYN gingival atrophy, gingival resorption.

tendon r., surgical displacement of the tendon of an eye muscle posterior to its anatomic insertion. SYN curb tenotomy.

re·ces·si·tiv·i·ty (rē′ses-i-tiv′i-tē). The state of being recessive (2).

re·ces·sive (rē-ses′iv). 1. Drawing away; receding. 2. In genetics, denoting a trait due to a particular allele or alleles at a single locus that does not manifest itself unless mutant alleles are present on both homologous chromosomes of a pair.

re·ces·sus, pl. **re·ces·sus** (rē-ses′sŭs) [TA]. SYN recess. [L. a withdrawing, a receding]

r. ante′rior [TA], SYN anterior *recess*.

r. anterior membra′nae tympa′nicae [TA], SYN anterior *recess* of tympanic membrane.

r. cochlea′ris [TA], SYN cochlear *recess*.

r. costodiaphragmat′icus [TA], SYN costodiaphragmatic *recess*.

r. costomediastina′lis [TA], SYN costomediastinal *recess*.

r. duodena′lis infe′rior [TA], SYN inferior duodenal *fossa*.

r. duodena′lis supe′rior [TA], SYN superior duodenal *fossa*.

r. ellip′ticus labyrinthi ossei [TA], SYN elliptical *recess* of bony labyrinth.

r. epitympan′icus [TA], SYN epitympanic *recess*.

r. hepatorena′lis recessus subhepatici [TA], SYN hepatorenal *recess* of subhepatic space.

r. ileoceca′lis infe′rior [TA], SYN inferior ileocecal *recess*.

r. ileoceca′lis supe′rior [TA], SYN superior ileocecal *recess*.

r. infe′rior omenta′lis [TA], SYN inferior *recess* of omental bursa.

r. infundib′uli [TA], SYN infundibular *recess*.

r. infundibulifor′mis, SYN pharyngeal *recess*.

r. intersigmoi′deus [TA], SYN intersigmoid *recess*.

r. latera′lis ventric′uli quar′ti [TA], SYN lateral *recess* of fourth ventricle.

r. liena′lis, ☆official alternate term for splenic *recess*.

r. membranae tympanicae [TA], SYN *recesses* of tympanic cavity, under *recess*.

r. paraduodena′lis [TA], SYN paraduodenal *recess*.

r. parotid′eus, SYN parotid *space*.

r. pharyn′geus [TA], SYN pharyngeal *recess*.

r. phrenicomediastina′lis [TA], SYN phrenicomediastinal *recess*.

r. pinea′lis [TA], SYN pineal *recess*.

r. pirifor′mis [TA], SYN piriform *fossa*.

r. pleura′les [TA], SYN pleural *recesses*, under *recess*.

r. poste′rior [TA], SYN posterior *recess*.

r. posterior membra′nae tym′panicae [TA], SYN posterior *recess* of tympanic membrane.

r. retroceca′lis [TA], SYN retrocecal *recess*.

r. retroduodena′lis [TA], SYN retroduodenal *recess*.

r. sacciformis articulationis [TA], SYN sacciform *recess* of elbow joint.

r. sacciformis articulationis radioulnaris distalis [TA], SYN sacciform *recess* of distal radioulnar joint.

r. saccularis larbyrinthi ossei, ☆official alternate term for spherical *recess* of bony labyrinth.

r. sphenoethmoida′lis [TA], SYN sphenoethmoidal *recess*.

r. spher′icus labyrinthi ossei, SYN spherical *recess* of bony labyrinth.

r. splenicus [TA], SYN splenic *recess*.

r. subhepat′icus [TA], SYN subhepatic *space*.

r. subphren′icus [TA], SYN subphrenic *space*.

r. subpoplit′eus [TA], SYN subpopliteal *recess*.

r. supe′rior bursae omenta′lis [TA], SYN superior *recess* of omental bursa.

r. superior membra′nae tympa′nicae [TA], SYN superior *recess* of tympanic membrane.

r. supraop′ticus [TA], SYN supraoptic *recess*.

r. supraopticus [TA], SYN supraoptic *recess*.

r. suprapinea′lis [TA], SYN suprapineal *recess*.

r. triangula′ris, SYN triangular *recess*.

r. utricularis labyrinthi membranacei [TA], SYN utricular *recess* of membranous labyrinth.

r. utricularis labyrinthi ossei, ☆official alternate term for elliptical *recess* of bony labyrinth.

r. vertebromediastinalis [TA], SYN vertebromediastinal *recess*.

re·cid·i·va·tion (rē-sid-i-vā′shŭn). Relapse of a disease, a symptom, or a behavioral pattern such as an illegal activity for which one was previously imprisoned. [L. *recidivus,* falling back, recurring, fr. *re- cido,* to fall back]

re·cid·i·vism (rē-sid′i-vizm). The tendency of an individual toward recidivation. [L. *recidivus,* recurring]

re·cid·i·vist (rē-sid′i-vist). A person who tends toward recidivation.

rec·i·pe (℞) (res′i-pē) 1. The superscription of a prescription, usually indicated by the sign ℞. 2. A prescription or formula. [L. imperative *recipio,* to receive]

re·cip·i·ent (rē-sip′ē-ent). One who receives, as in blood transfusion or tissue or organ transplant. [L. *recipiens,* fr. *recipio,* to receive]

re·cip·i·o·mo·tor (rē-sip′ē-ō-mō′ter). Relating to the reception of motor stimuli. [L. *recipio,* to receive, + *motor,* mover]

re·cip·ro·ca·tion (rē-sip-rō-kā′shŭn). In prosthodontics, the means by which one part of an appliance is made to counter the effect created by another part. [L. *reciprocare,* pp. *reciprocatus,* to move back and forth]

re·cir·cu·la·tion (rē-ser-kū-lā′shun). Circular movement of the mucus blanket in a paranasal sinus due to the presence of an accessory ostium or failure to include the natural ostium in sinusotomy.

Recklinghausen, Friedrich D. von, German histologist and pathologist, 1833–1910. SEE R. *disease* of bone; von R. *disease*.

rec·li·na·tion (rek-li-nā′shŭn). Turning the cataractous lens over into the vitreous to displace it from the line of vision; distinguished from couching, in which the lens is simply depressed into the vitreous. [L. *reclino,* pp. *-atus,* to bend back]

rec·ol·lec·tion (rē-kŏ-lek′shŭn). In renal physiology, a technique in which a known fluid is infused into a renal tubule lumen at one point and collected for analysis by a second micropipette further downstream. [re- + L. *collectus,* pp. of *colligo,* to collect]

re·com·bi·nant (rē-kom′bi-nant). 1. A cell or organism that has received genes from different parental strains. 2. Pertaining to or denoting such organisms. 3. In linkage analysis, the change of coupling phase at two loci during meiosis. If two syntenic, nonallelic genes are inherited from the same parent, they must be in coupling. An offspring that inherits only one of them is r. and indicates an odd number of cross-overs between the loci; an offspring that inherits neither or both is nonrecombinant and may indicate an even number of cross-overs or none.

re·com·bi·na·tion (rē-kom-bi-nā′shŭn). 1. The process of reuniting of parts that had become separated. 2. The reversal of coupling phase in meiosis as gauged by the resulting phenotype. SEE ALSO recombinant. 3. The formation of new combinations of genes.

genetic r., (1) the presence in progeny of combinations of genotypes and perhaps phenotypes, not present in either parent, resulting from crossing-over; (2) in microbial genetics, the inclusion of a chromosomal part or extrachromosomal element of one microbial strain in the chromosome of another; the interchange of chromosomal parts or genes between different microbial strains.

homologous r., the exchange of corresponding stretches of DNA between two sister chromosomes.

site-specific r., integration of foreign DNA into a particular site in the host genome.

re·con (rē′kon). Obsolete term for the smallest unit (corresponding to a single DNA nucleotide) of recombination or crossing-over between two homologous chromosomes.

re·con·sti·tu·tion (rē′kon-sti-too′shŭn). 1. The restitution or return to an original state of a substance, or combination of parts to make a whole. 2. In the case of a lower organism, the restoration of a part of the body by regeneration.

re·con·struc·tion (rē-cŏn-strŭk′shun). The computerized synthesis of one or more two-dimensional images from a series of x-ray projections in computed tomography, or from a large number of measurements in magnetic resonance imaging; several methods are used; the earliest was back-projection, and the most common is 2D Fourier transformation.

ossicular r., generic term denoting a number of surgical techniques to restore the continuity of the ossicular chain from the tympanic membrane to the oval window for sound pressure transmission and, thereby, improved hearing.

rec·ord (rek′erd). 1. In medicine, a chronologic written account that includes a patient's initial complaint(s) and medical history, physical findings, results of diagnostic tests and procedures, any therapeutic medicines and/or procedures, and subsequent developments during the course of the illness. 2. In dentistry, a registration of desired jaw relations in a plastic material or on a device to permit these relationships to be transferred to an articulator. [M.E. *recorden,* fr. O.Fr. *recorder,* fr. L. *recordor,* to remember, fr. *re-,* back, again, + *cor,* heart]

anesthesia r., a written or electronic account of drugs administered, procedures undertaken, and physiologic responses during the course of surgical or obstetric anesthesia.

face-bow r., a registration utilizing a face-bow of the position of the hinge axis and/or the condyles; the face-bow r. is used to orient the maxillary cast to the opening and closing axis of the articulator.

functional chew-in r., a r. of the natural chewing movements of the mandible made on an occlusion rim by teeth or scribing studs.

hospital r., the medical r. generated during a period of hospitalization, usually including written accounts of consultants' opinions, physicians' and nurses' observations, treatments, and the results of all tests and/or procedures performed.

interocclusal r., a r. of the positional relationship of the teeth or jaws to each other, recorded by placing a plastic material that hardens (such as plaster of Paris or wax) between the occlusal surfaces of the rims or teeth; the hardened material serves as the r.; it may be registered in centric or eccentric positions, as **centric interocclusal r.,** a r. of centric jaw relation; **eccentric interocclusal r.,** a r. of jaw position in other than centric relation; **lateral interocclusal r.,** a r. of a lateral eccentric jaw position; and **protrusive interocclusal r.,** a r. of a protruded eccentric jaw position. SYN checkbite.

maxillomandibular r., (1) a r. of the relation of the mandible to the maxillae; (2) the act of recording the relation of the mandible to the maxillae. SYN biscuit bite, maxillomandibular registration.

medical r., SEE record (1).

occluding centric relation r., a registration of centric relation made at the established occlusal vertical dimension.

preextraction r., SYN preoperative r.

preoperative r., in dentistry, any r. made for the purpose of study

re

or treatment planning. SEE ALSO diagnostic *cast.* SYN preextraction r.

problem-oriented r. (POR), a system of record keeping in which a list of the patient's problems is made and all history, physical findings, laboratory data, etc. pertinent to each problem are placed under that heading; especially useful for outpatient records of patients with multiple problems who are followed for long periods.

profile r., a registration or r. of the profile of a patient.

protrusive r., a registration of a forward position of the mandible with reference to the maxillae.

terminal jaw relation r., a r. of the relationship of the mandible to the maxillae made at the vertical relation of occlusion and at the centric position.

three-dimensional r., a maxillomandibular r. made at the occluding relation.

re·cord·ing (rē-kōrd′ing). Preserving the results of a study.

clinical r., SYN charting.

depth r., study of subcortical cerebral electrical activity after placing electrodes in these areas.

re·cov·ery (rē-kŏv′er-ē). **1.** A getting back or regaining; recuperation. **2.** Emergence from general anesthesia. **3.** In nuclear magnetic resonance, refers to relaxation. [M.E., fr. O.Fr. *recoverer,* fr. L. *recupero,* to recover, get back, fr. *re-,* again, + *capio,* to take]

creep r., the time-dependent portion of the decrease in strain in a material or object following removal of the stress that has deformed it.

inversion r., a magnetic resonance pulse sequence in which a series of 180° magnetic field inversions is followed by a spin echo sequence for signal detection; of note, during r., the longitudinal magnetization vector passes through zero.

short TI inversion r. (STIR), an inversion r. sequence that uses a short inversion time, about 100 ms, between 180° pulses; by proper selection of TI, the signal from water or fat can be suppressed.

spontaneous r., the return of the conditioned response, after apparent extinction, in the presence of the conditioned stimulus without the unconditioned stimulus also being present. SEE classical *conditioning.*

ultrasonic egg r., obtaining an egg for in vitro fertilization by means of an ultrasonically guided needle aspiration of ovarian follicles; may be performed transvesically or via the cul-de-sac.

re·cov·ery room. A hospital facility with special equipment and personnel for the immediate postoperative care of patients as they recover from anesthesia and/or surgery.

re·cru·des·cence (rē-kroo-des′ens). Resumption of a morbid process or its symptoms after a period of remission. [L. *re-crudesco,* to become raw again, break out afresh, fr. *crudus,* raw, harsh]

re·cru·des·cent (rē-kroo-des′ent). Becoming active again, relating to a recrudescence.

re·cruit·ment (rē-kroot′ment). **1.** In the testing of hearing, the abnormally greater increase in loudness in response to increments in intensity of the acoustic stimulus in an ear with a sensory hearing loss compared with a normal ear. **2.** In neurophysiology, the activation of additional neurons (spatial recruitment) or an increase in their firing rate (temporal recruitment). SYN recruiting response. SEE ALSO irradiation. **3.** The adding of parallel channels of flow in any system. [Fr. *recrutement,* fr. L. *re-cresco,* pp. *-cretus,* to grow again]

△**rect-.** SEE recto-.

rec·tal (rek′tăl). Relating to the rectum.

rec·tal·gia (rek-tal′jē-ă). SYN proctalgia.

rec·tec·to·my (rek-tek′tō-mē). SYN proctectomy.

rec·ti·fi·er (rek′ti-fī-ĕr). An electronic device for converting alternating to direct voltage, part of the circuit of an x-ray machine. [Mediev. L. *rectifico,* to make right, fr. *rectus,* right + *facio* to make]

rec·ti·fy (rek′ti-fī). **1.** To correct. **2.** To purify or refine by distillation; usually implies repeated distillations. [L. *rectus,* right, straight]

rec·ti·tis (rek-tī′tis). SYN proctitis.

△**recto-, rect-.** The rectum. SEE ALSO procto-. [L. *rectum,* fr. *rectus,* straight]

rec·to·ab·dom·i·nal (rek′tō-ab-dom′i-năl). Relating to the rectum and the abdomen; denoting a bimanual method of examination with one hand on the abdominal wall and a finger of the other hand in the rectum.

rec·to·cele (rek′tō-sēl). SYN proctocele. [recto- + G. *kēlē,* tumor, hernia]

rec·toc·ly·sis (rek-tok′li-sis). SYN proctoclysis.

rec·to·coc·cyg·e·al (rek-tō-kok-sij′ē-ăl). Relating to the rectum and the coccyx.

rec·to·coc·cy·pexy (rek-tō-kok′si-pek-sē). SYN proctococcypexy.

rec·to·co·li·tis (rek′tō-kō-lī′tis). SYN coloproctitis.

rec·to·per·i·ne·al (rek′tō-per-i-nē′ăl). Relating to the rectum and perineum.

rec·to·per·i·ne·or·rha·phy (rek′tō-per-i-nē-ōr′a-fē). SYN proctoperineoplasty. [recto- + perineo- + G. *rhaphē,* a sewing]

rec·to·pexy (rek′tō-pek-sē). SYN proctopexy.

rec·to·pho·bia (rek-tō-fō′bē-ă). SYN proctophobia. [recto- + G. *phobos,* fear]

rec·to·plas·ty (rek′tō-plas-tē). SYN proctoplasty.

rec·tor·rha·phy (rek-tōr′ă-fē). SYN proctorrhaphy.

rec·to·scope (rek′tō-skōp). SYN proctoscope.

rec·tos·co·py (rek-tos′kŏ-pē). SYN proctoscopy.

rec·to·sig·moid (rek′tō-sig′moyd). The rectum and sigmoid colon considered as a unit; the term is also applied to the junction of the sigmoid colon and rectum.

rec·to·ste·no·sis (rek′tō-stě-nō′sis). SYN proctostenosis.

rec·tos·to·my (rek-tos′tō-mē). SYN proctostomy.

rec·to·tome (rek′tō-tōm). SYN proctotome.

rec·tot·o·my (rek-tot′ō-mē). SYN proctotomy.

rec·to·u·re·thral (rek-tō-ū-rē′thrăl). Relating to the rectum and the urethra.

rec·to·u·ter·ine (rek-tō-ū′ter-in). Relating to the rectum and the uterus.

rec·to·vag·i·nal (rek-tō-vaj′i-năl). Relating to the rectum and the vagina.

rec·to·ves·i·cal (rek-tō-ves′i-kăl). Relating to the rectum and the bladder.

rec·to·ves·tib·u·lar (rek′tō-ves-tib′ū-lăr). Relating to the rectum and the vestibule of the vagina.

rec·tum, pl. **rec·tums, rec·ta** (rek′tŭm, rek′tă). The terminal portion of the digestive tube, extending from the rectosigmoid junction to the anal canal. (Perineal flexure). [L. *rectus,* straight, pp. of *rego,* to make straight]

re·cum·bent (rē-kŭm′bent). Leaning; reclining; lying down. [L. *recumbo,* to lie back, recline, fr. *re-,* back, + *cubo,* to lie]

re·cu·per·ate (rē-koo′per-āt). To undergo recuperation. [L. *recupero* (or *recip-*), pp. *-atus,* to take again, recover]

re·cu·per·a·tion (rē-koo-per-ā′shŭn). Recovery of or restoration to the normal state of health and function. [L. *recuperatio* (see recuperate)]

re·cur·rence (rē-kŭr′ens). **1.** A return of the symptoms, occurring as a phenomenon in the natural history of the disease, as seen in recurrent fever. **2.** SYN relapse. **3.** Appearance of a genetic trait in a genetic relative of a proband. [L. *re-curro,* to run back, recur]

re·cur·rent (rē-kŭr′ent). **1.** In anatomy, turning back on itself. **2.** Denoting symptoms or lesions reappearing after an intermission or remission.

re·cur·va·tion (rē-ker-vā′shŭn). A backward bending or flexure. [L. *re-curvus,* bent back]

red. One of the primary colors, occupying the lower extremity of the spectrum at the other end from violet. For individual red dyes, see specific name. [A.S. *reád*]

Red Cross. A red Geneva cross on a white background, an international sign to identify medical and other personnel caring for the sick and wounded and facilities devoted to their care in times of war, also the emblem of the American Red Cross.

re·dia, pl. **re·di·ae** (rē′dē-ă, -dē-ē). Intramolluscan development stage of a digenetic trematode, following the primary sporocyst stage, which forms after penetration of the snail tissues by the miracidium. Rediae are produced from cells within the sporocyst, are liberated from the latter, and develop in the tissues of the host snail as elongated, saclike, muscular organisms with a mouth and gut. The rediae may produce one or a number of additional generations in the snail, but they ultimately produce the final development stage, the cercaria. SEE ALSO sporocyst (1), miracidium. [F. *Redi*, Italian physician, 1626–1697]

re·dif·fer·en·ti·a·tion (rē-dif′er-en′shē-ā′shŭn). The return to a fully specialized condition for the performance of a particular function after a period of nonspecific activity.

re·din·te·gra·tion (rē′din-tĕ-grā′shŭn). 1. The restoration of lost or injured parts. 2. Restoration to health. 3. The recalling of a whole experience on the basis only of some item or portion of the original stimulus or circumstances of the experience. [L. *red-integro*, pp. *-atus*, to make whole again, renew, fr. *integer*, untouched, entire]

Redlich, Emil, Austrian neurologist, 1866–1930. SEE Obersteiner-R. *line, zone.*

re·dox (red′oks). Contraction of oxidation-reduction. SEE oxidation-reduction *potential.*

re·dresse·ment for·cé (rĕ-dres-mon′ fōr-sā′). Obsolete term for straightening by force of a deformed part, as of knock-knee. [Fr.]

re·dress·ment (rē-dres′ment). 1. Obsolete term for correction of a deformity; putting a part straight. 2. A renewed dressing of a wound.

re·duce (rē-doos′). 1. To place back into a preferred position; to perform reduction (1). 2. In chemistry, to initiate reduction (2). [L. *re-duco*, to lead back, restore, reduce]

re·duc·i·ble (rē-doos′i-bl). Capable of being reduced.

re·duc·tant (rē-dŭk′tant). The substance that is oxidized in the course of reduction.

re·duc·tase (rē-dŭk′tās). An enzyme that catalyzes a reduction; since all enzymes catalyze reactions in either direction, any r. can, under the proper conditions, behave as an oxidase and vice versa, hence the term oxidoreductase. For individual r.'s, see the specific names. SYN reducing enzyme.

re·duc·tic ac·id (rē-dŭk′tik). A strong reducing product (antioxidant) formed in hot alkaline sugar solutions.

re·duc·tion (rē-dŭk′shŭn). 1. The restoration, by surgical or manipulative procedures, of a part to its normal anatomic relation. SYN repositioning (2). 2. In chemistry, a reaction involving a gain of one or more electrons by a substance, such as when iron passes from the ferric (3+) to the ferrous (2+) state, or when hydrogen is added to the double bond of an organic compound, or when an aldehyde is converted to an alcohol. [L. *reductio*, fr. *re-duco*, pp. *ductus*, to lead back]

r. of chromosomes, the process during meiosis whereby one member of each homologous pair of chromosomes is distributed to a sperm or ovum; the diploid set of chromosomes (46 in humans) is thus reduced to the haploid set in each gamete; union of the sperm and ovum then restores the diploid or somatic number in the one-cell zygote.

closed r. of fractures, r. by manipulation of bone, without incision in the skin.

r. en masse, r. of hernial sac and contents, so that intestinal obstruction is still present.

open r. of fractures, r. by manipulation of bone, after surgical exposure of the site of the fracture.

selective r., a technique for intrauterine termination of one or more fetuses while leaving one or more fetuses undisturbed, usually in pregnancies with fetal anomalies or with multiple gestations. SYN selective termination.

tuberosity r., the surgical excision of excessive fibrous or bony tissue in the area of the maxillary tuberosity prior to the construction of prosthetic appliances.

re·dun·dan·cy (rē-dun′dăns-ē). Occurrence of linearly arranged, largely identical, repeated sequences of DNA.

terminal r., the condition in a viral chromosome in which identical genetic information occurs at each end of the chromosome.

re·du·pli·ca·tion (rē′doo′pli-kā′shŭn). 1. A redoubling. 2. A duplication or doubling, as of the sounds of the heart in certain morbid states or the presence of two instead of a normally single part. 3. A fold or duplicature. [L. *reduplicatio*, fr. *re-*, again, + *duplico*, to double, fr. *duplex*, two-fold]

re·du·vid, re·du·vi·id (rē-doo′vĭd -vid). A member of the family Reduviidae.

Red·u·vi·i·dae (rē-doo-vī′i-dē). A family (order Hemiptera) of predatory insects, the assassin bugs, which attack animals and humans. It includes the subfamily Triatominae, the kissing or cone-nosed bugs, whose type genus *Triatoma* includes species that are vectors of *Trypanosoma cruzi*.

Reed, Dorothy M., U.S. pathologist, 1874–1964. SEE R. *cell;* R.-Sternberg *cell;* Sternberg-R. *cell.*

Reed, Walter, 1851–1902. U.S. Army surgeon, elucidated epidemiology of yellow fever. SEE Reed-Frost *model.*

reef·ing (rēf′ing). Surgically reducing the extent of a tissue by folding it and securing with sutures, as in plication.

stomach r., SYN gastroplication.

re·en·act·ment (rē-en-akt′ment). In psychodrama, the acting out of a past experience.

re·en·try (rē-en′trē). Return of the same impulse into a zone of heart muscle that it has recently activated, sufficiently delayed that the zone is no longer refractory, as seen in most ectopic beats, reciprocal rhythms, and most tachycardias.

Rees, H. Maynard, 20th century U.S. physician. SEE R.-Ecker *fluid.*

Reese, Algernon B., U.S. ophthalmologist, 1896–1981. SEE Cogan-R. *syndrome.*

re·fect (rē-fekt′). To induce refection.

re·fec·tion (rē-fek′shŭn). A restoring to the normal state. [L. *refectio*, fr. *reficere*, to restore, fr. *re-* + *facio*, to do]

Refetoff, S., 20th century U.S. endocrinologist. SEE R. *syndrome.*

re·fine (rē-fīn′). To free from impurities.

re·flect (rē-flekt′). 1. To bend back. 2. To throw back, as of radiant energy from a surface. 3. To meditate; to think over a matter. 4. To send back a motor impulse in response to a sensory stimulus. [L. *re- flecto*, pp. *-flexus*, to bend back]

re·flec·tance. A measure of reflected acoustic energy as a function of immittance, as in middle ear impedance.

re·flec·tion (rē-flek′shŭn). 1. The act of reflecting. 2. That which is reflected. 3. In psychotherapy, a technique in which a patient's statements are repeated, restated, or rephrased in order that the patient will continue to explore and expound on emotionally significant content. [L. *reflexio*, a bending back]

re·flec·tor (rē-flek′ter). Any surface that reflects light, heat, or sound.

REFLEX

re·flex (rē′fleks). 1. An involuntary reaction in response to a stimulus applied to the periphery and transmitted to the nervous centers in the brain or spinal cord. Most of the deep r.'s listed as subentries are stretch or myotatic r.'s, elicited by striking a tendon or bone, causing stretching, even slight, of the muscle, which then contracts as a result of the stimulus applied to its proprioceptors. SEE ALSO phenomenon. 2. A reflection. [L. *reflexus*, pp. of *reflecto*, to bend back]

abdominal r.'s, contraction of the muscles of the abdominal wall upon stimulation of the skin (superficial a. r.'s) or tapping neighboring bony structures (deep a. r.'s). SYN supraumbilical r. (2).

abdominocardiac r., mechanical stimulation (usually distention) of abdominal viscera causing changes (usually a slowing) in the heart rate or the occurrence of extrasystoles.

re (in margin tab)

locations of neuronal cell bodies of the afferent and efferent limbs of representative reflexes			
reflex	cell of origin/afferent limb	cell of origin/efferent limb	functional response
abdominal	dorsal root ganglia at spinal cord levels T_8–T_{11}	ventral horn motor neurons at spinal cord levels T_6–T_{11}	contraction of abdominal muscles with deflection of umbilicus toward stimulus
Achilles (ankle jerk)	dorsal root ganglia at spinal cord levels L_5–S_1	ventral horn motor neurons at spinal cord levels L_5–S_1	contraction of the gastrocnemius and soleus muscles with plantar flexion of foot
Babinski (Babinski sign)	dorsal root ganglia at spinal cord levels L_5–S_1 (usually only the latter)	ventral horn motor neurons at spinal cord levels L_4–S_1	dorsiflexion of the large toe and fanning of the other toes subsequent to a firm stroke on the bottom of the foot; considered indicative of CNS disease after about 14–15 months of age, suggesting damage in the corticospinal system
carotid sinus	inferior ganglion of the glossopharyngeal nerve	preganglionic cells in the dorsal motor vagal nucleus, postganglionic cells in ganglia of heart that act on atrial muscle	regulation of (arterial) blood pressure
corneal (blink)	trigeminal ganglion	facial motor nucleus	contraction of muscles of the eyelids and closure of the palpebral fissure in response to touching the cornea
crossed extension	dorsal root ganglia at about C_7–T_1 (for hand) and L_5–S_1 (for foot)	contralateral ventral horn cells at about C_5–T_1 (for arm) and L_2–S_1 (for leg)	extension of the extremity on the side opposite a noxious stimulus to help stabilize the body, works in concert with the withdrawal reflex
flexor (withdrawal)	dorsal root ganglia at about C_7–T_1 (for hand) and L_5–S_1 (for foot)	ipsilateral ventral horn cells at about C_5–T_1 (for arm) and L_2–S_1 (for leg)	sudden withdrawal of the extremity from a noxious stimulus
gag	inferior ganglion of glossopharyngeal and/or vagus nerves	bilateral cells in ambiguous nuclei	constriction of pharyngeal muscles and elevation of the soft palate and uvula
Hoffmann (Hoffmann sign)	dorsal root ganglia at spinal cord levels C_7–C_8	ventral horn motor neurons at spinal cord levels C_7–T_1	brisk flicking of the distal phalanx on the third digit produces a flexion of the thumb and index finger or thumb and all other fingers
jaw (jaw jerk)	mesencephalic nucleus of trigeminal nerve	trigeminal motor nucleus	bilateral contraction of temporal and masseter muscles in response to a slightly downward tap on the chin
patellar (knee jerk)	dorsal root ganglia at spinal cord levels L_2–L_4	ventral horn motor neurons at spinal cord levels L_2–L_4	contraction of quadriceps muscle with extension of the leg at the knee
pupillary (light)	ganglion cells in retina	preganglionic cells in Edinger-Westphal nucleus, postganglionic cells in ciliary ganglion	contraction of the sphincter pupillae muscles and decrease in the size of the pupil in response to light shone in eye; *direct reaction* is contraction of pupil ipsilateral to stimulus, *consensual reaction* is contraction of opposite pupil
rooting	trigeminal ganglion	facial motor nucleus	pursing of the lips and rotation of the mouth toward the source of the stimulus, elicited by rubbing corner of mouth or cheek, seen in infants during early months
salivatory	geniculate ganglion (CN VII) and inferior ganglion of glossopharyngeal and (possibly) vagus nerves	preganglionic cells in superior salivatory nucleus (CN VII) and in inferior salivatory nucleus (CN IX), postganglionic cells in ganglia found in (or on) the sublingual and submandibular glands and the parotid gland	vasodilation and increased secretions of salivary glands in response to food in oral cavity and consequent stimulation of taste receptors
snout	trigeminal ganglion	facial motor nucleus	pursing or puckering of the muscles around the mouth in response to a tap to the upper lip, usually considered indicative of damage in the corticospinal system
swallowing	inferior ganglia of glossopharyngeal and vagus nerves	nucleus ambiguus for pharyngeal muscles, preganglionic cells in dorsal motor vagal nucleus and postganglionic cells in myenteric ganglia in the esophagus	contraction of pharyngeal muscles, wavelike contractions of esophageal muscles, together move food through pharynx and into (and down) esophagus
vomiting (pharyngeal)	inferior ganglia of glossopharyngeal and vagus nerves	nucleus ambiguus for constriction of pharyngeal muscles and closure of epiglottis; dorsal motor vagal nucleus supplies preganglionic fibers to postganglionic cells in esophagus and stomach; intermediolateral cell column at upper thoracic levels supplies preganglionic fibers to postganglionic cells in esophagus and stomach and pyloric sphincter, ventral horn motor neurons innervate skeletal muscles of abdominal wall	vomiting; retrograde movement of stomach contents up the esophagus and into the oral cavity; closure of epiglottis prevents movement of vomitus into lungs; contraction of abdominal muscles assists emptying of stomach; the vomiting reflex is essentially a gag reflex that has spread wider in the neuraxis and influenced a wider range of visceral and somatic centers

reflex related to brainstem and cranial nerves   reflex related to spinal cord   reflex with brainstem and spinal components

Abrams heart r., a contraction of the myocardium when the skin of the precordial region is irritated.

accommodation r., increased convexity of the lens, due to contraction of the ciliary muscle and relaxation of the suspensory ligament, to maintain a distinct retinal image.

Achilles r., Achilles tendon r., a contraction of the calf muscles when the tendo calcaneus is sharply struck. SYN ankle jerk, ankle r., tendo Achillis r., triceps surae r.

acoustic r., contraction of the stapedius muscle in response to intense sound, increasing impedance of the middle ear and thereby protecting the inner ear from the sound. SYN cochleostapedial r., stapedial r.

acousticopalpebral r., SYN cochleopalpebral r.

acquired r., SYN conditioned r.

acromial r., contraction of the biceps muscle caused by a tap on the acromion or the coracoid process.

adductor r., contraction of the adductors of the thigh caused by tapping the tendon of the adductor magnus muscle while the thigh is abducted.

allied r.'s, r.'s that, acting toward a common purpose, can traverse the final common path together.

anal r., contraction of the internal sphincter gripping the finger passed into the rectum.

ankle r., SYN Achilles r.

antagonistic r.'s, r.'s that do not act toward a common purpose, and cannot together traverse the final common path.

aortic r., SYN cardiac depressor r.

aponeurotic r., plantar flexion of the foot and toes elicited by tapping the sole near its outer edge; has the same significance as the Rossolimo toe flexion r. SYN Guillain-Barré r., sole tap r., Weingrow r.

Aschner r., SYN oculocardiac r.

Aschner-Dagnini r., SYN oculocardiac r.

attitudinal r.'s, SYN statotonic r.'s.

auditory r., any r. occurring in response to a sound, e.g., cochleopalpebral r.

auditory oculogyric r., rotation of the eyes toward the source of a sudden sound.

auricular r., a movement of the ears in animals in response to a sound; part of the investigatory r.

auriculopalpebral r., SYN Kisch r.

auriculopressor r., peripheral vasoconstriction and a rise in blood pressure in response to a fall in pressure in the great veins. SYN Pavlov r.

auropalpebral r., SYN cochleopalpebral r.

axon r., a response elicited by peripheral nerve stimulation; attributed to impulses traveling proximally from the stimulation site along motor axons, encountering a branch point, and then passing distally down the other branch to activate local arterioles (to cause vasodilation) or muscle (to cause contractions). Latency of the response decreases with more proximal stimulation; axon r. is eliminated by axon degeneration or strong stimuli but not by proximal anesthetic blocks of the nerve.

Babinski r., SYN Babinski sign (1).

back of foot r., dorsum of foot r., SYN Mendel instep r.

Bainbridge r., an increase in heart rate caused by a rise in pressure of the blood in the right atrium due to increased flow and/or pressure in the great veins at its entrance.

Barkman r., contraction of the ipsilateral rectus muscle in response to a stimulus applied to the skin below a nipple.

basal joint r., opposition and adduction of the thumb with flexion at its metacarpophalangeal joint and extension at its interphalangeal joint, when firm passive flexion of the third, fourth, or fifth finger is made; the r. is present normally but is absent in pyramidal lesions. SYN finger-thumb r., Mayer r.

Bechterew-Mendel r., plantar flexion of the toes caused by percussion of the dorsum of the foot; present in a pyramidal lesion. SYN dorsum pedis r., Mendel-Bechterew r.

behavior r., SYN conditioned r.

Benedek r., plantar flexion of the foot caused by tapping the anterior margin of the lower part of the fibula, while the foot is slightly dorsiflexed.

Bezold-Jarisch r., a r. with afferent and efferent pathways in the vagus, originating in unidentified chemoreceptors in the heart and resulting in sinus bradycardia, hypotension, and probable peripheral vasodilation.

biceps r., contraction of the biceps muscle when its tendon is struck.

biceps femoris r., contraction of the biceps femoris upon tapping its lower part, just above its attachment to the head of the fibula, while the limb is partly flexed at hip and knee.

Bing r., when the foot is passively dorsiflexed, plantar flexion occurs if any point on the ankle between the two malleoli is tapped.

bladder r., SYN micturition r.

blink r., SEE blink response.

body righting r.'s, r. effects upon the neck muscles that bring the head into the correct position in space caused by stimulation of pressoreceptors in the body wall by contact with the ground.

brachioradial r., with the arm supinated to 45°, a tap near the lower end of the radius causes contraction of the brachioradial (supinator longus) muscle. SYN radioperiosteal r., styloradial r., supination r., supinator jerk, supinator r., supinator longus r.

Brain r., SYN quadripedal extensor r.

bregmocardiac r., in infants, pressure upon the anterior fontanelle causing cardiac slowing.

Brissaud r., tickling the sole causes a contraction of the tensor fasciae latae muscle, even when there is no responsive movement of the toes.

bulbocavernosus r., a sharp contraction of the bulbocavernosus and ischiocavernosus muscles when the glans penis is suddenly compressed or tapped.

bulbomimic r., in a case of coma from severe apoplexy, pressure on the eyeballs causes contraction of the facial muscles of expression on the side opposite to the lesion; if coma due to diabetes, uremia, or other toxic cause the r. is present on both sides. SYN facial r., Mondonesi r.

Capps r., obsolete eponym for vasomotor collapse at the time of crisis in pneumonia.

cardiac depressor r., a fall in blood pressure due to peripheral vasodilation and cardiac inhibition by stimulations of terminations of a cardiac depressor nerve in the aortic arch and base of the heart. SYN aortic r., depressor r.

carotid sinus r., a normal r. relating to the carotid sinus syndrome, which results from hypersensitivity or hyperactivation of the carotid sinus.

celiac plexus r., arterial hypotension coincident with surgical manipulations in the upper abdomen during general anesthesia.

cephalopalpebral r., contraction of the orbicularis muscle elicited by tapping the vertex of the skull.

Chaddock r., SYN Chaddock sign.

chain r., a series of r.s, each serving as a stimulus for the next.

chin r., SYN jaw r.

Chodzko r., contractions of several muscles of the shoulder girdle and arm when the manubrium sterni is percussed.

ciliospinal r., SYN pupillary-skin r.

clasping r., the strong flexion of the forelimbs of amphibia and certain other animals during the mating season when the chest or abdomen is stimulated; it is dependent upon the male sex hormone.

cochleo-orbicular r., SYN cochleopalpebral r.

cochleopalpebral r., a form of the wink r. in which there is a contraction, sometimes very slight, of the orbicularis palpebrarum muscle to an intense sound. SEE ALSO startle r. SYN acousticopalpebral r., auropalpebral r., cochleo-orbicular r.

cochleopupillary r., mydriasis in response to a sudden and unexpected loud noise; a normal response.

cochleostapedial r., SYN acoustic r.

conditioned r. (CR), a r. that is gradually developed by training and association through the frequent repetition of a definite stimulus. SEE conditioning. SYN acquired r., behavior r., trained r.

conjunctival r., closure of the eyes in response to irritation of the conjunctiva.

consensual light r., SYN consensual *reaction*.

contralateral r., SYN Brudzinski *sign* (1).

corneal r., (1) a contraction of the eyelids when the cornea is lightly touched with a camel-hair pencil; SYN lid r. (2) reflection of light from the surface of the cornea.

costal arch r., contraction of the rectus abdominis muscle by tapping the costal margin inside the mammary line.

costopectoral r., SYN pectoral r.

cough r., the r. that mediates coughing in response to irritation of the larynx or tracheobronchial tree. SYN laryngeal r.

craniocardiac r., stimulation of nerve endings of certain cranial nerves (e.g., olfactory, ophthalmic branch of trigeminal), with resultant cardiac depressor r., manifested by bradycardia and hypotension, through the cardiac branch of the vagus.

cremasteric r., a drawing up of the scrotum and testicle of the same side when the skin over the Scarpa triangle or on the inner side of the thigh is scratched.

crossed r., a r. movement on one side of the body in response to a stimulus applied to the opposite side. SYN crossed jerk.

crossed adductor r., contraction of the adductors of the thigh and inward rotation of the limb elicited by tapping the sole. SYN crossed adductor jerk.

crossed extension r., extension of the contralateral hind limb when the paw of an animal is painfully stimulated or the central cut end of an afferent nerve, e.g., the peroneal, is stimulated; sometimes occurs in humans upon tapping the skin.

crossed knee r., contraction of the contralateral quadriceps when a patellar r. is elicited. SYN crossed knee jerk.

crossed r. of pelvis, contraction of the contralateral adductors of the thigh upon tapping the anterior superior iliac spine. SYN crossed spino-adductor r.

crossed spino-adductor r., SYN crossed r. of pelvis.

cuboidodigital r., flexion of the toes on tapping over the cuboid bone; almost identical with Guillain-Barré r., and fundamentally similar to Rossolimo r. SYN metatarsal r.

cutaneous r., wrinkling of the skin, caused by a cutaneous stimulus, due to contraction of arrectores pilorum muscles.

cutaneous pupil r., cutaneous-pupillary r., SYN pupillary-skin r.

darwinian r., the tendency of young infants to grasp a bar and hang suspended. Cf. grasping r.

deep r., an involuntary muscular contraction following percussion of a tendon or bone. SYN jerk (2).

deep abdominal r.'s, contraction of abdominal muscles elicited by stimulation, such as tapping a deep structure; e.g., the costal margin. SEE ALSO Galant r., upper abdominal periosteal r.

deep tendon r. (DTR), SYN myotatic r.

defense r., (1) SYN flexor r; (2) automatic reactions of an animal, e.g., raising of hair or feathers, dilation of the pupils, or baring of claws, when alarmed.

deglutition r., SYN swallowing r.

Dejerine r., SYN Dejerine hand *phenomenon*.

delayed r., a r. in which a little time elapses between stimulus and response. SEE ALSO trace conditioned r.

depressor r., SYN cardiac depressor r.

diffused r., one of several r.'s occurring in association with the main r.

digital r., SYN Hoffmann *sign* (2).

diving r., a r. by which immersing the face or body in water, especially cold water, tends to cause bradycardia and peripheral vasoconstriction; mean aortic pressure is little affected because the reduction in cardiac output tends to balance the increased peripheral resistance that reduces peripheral blood flow. Although relatively minor in most humans, the changes can be profound in some diving species of animal, e.g., ducks and seals.

dorsal r., contraction of the muscles of the back elicited by cutaneous stimulation over the erector spinal muscle.

dorsum pedis r., SYN Bechterew-Mendel r.

elbow r., SYN triceps r.

enterogastric r., peristaltic contraction of the small intestine in-

duced by the entrance of food into the stomach. SEE ALSO gastrocolic r.

epigastric r., a contraction of the upper portion of the rectus abdominis muscle when the skin of the epigastrium above is scratched. SYN supraumbilical r. (1).

erector-spinal r., a contraction of part of the erector spinae muscle following scratching of the skin on its outer border.

esophagosalivary r., salivation caused by irritation of the lower end of the esophagus, as by carcinoma. SYN Roger r.

external oblique r., contraction of the external oblique and rectus abdominis muscles upon tapping the anterior and outer part of the lower thoracic wall.

eye r., SYN light r. (2).

eyeball compression r., SYN eyeball-heart r.

eyeball-heart r., slowing of the heart rate due to the vagal effects of compressing an eyeball. SYN eyeball compression r.

eye-closure r., SYN wink r.

facial r., SYN bulbomimic r.

faucial r., SYN gag r.

femoral r., scratching the skin of the upper part of the front of the thigh causes extension of the knee and flexion of the foot.

femoroabdominal r., contraction of the abdominal muscles upon stroking the inner aspect of the thigh; in association with the cremasteric r. SYN hypogastric r.

Ferguson r., enhancement of uterine activity due to mechanical stretching of the lower uterine segment and cervix.

finger-thumb r., SYN basal joint r.

flexor r., flexion of ankle, knee, and hip when the foot is painfully stimulated; the crossed extension r. occurs in association with it. SYN defense r. (1), nociceptive r., withdrawal r.

forced grasping r., SYN grasping r.

front-tap r., contraction of the gastrocnemius muscle when the shin is struck. SYN periosteal r. (1).

fundus r., SYN light r. (2).

gag r., contact of a foreign body with the mucous membrane of the fauces causes retching or gagging. SYN faucial r.

Galant r., a deep abdominal r. in which there is a contraction of the abdominal muscles on tapping the anterior superior iliac spine. SYN lower abdominal r.

galvanic skin r., SYN galvanic skin *response*.

gastrocolic r., a mass movement of the contents of the colon, frequently preceded by a similar movement in the small intestine, that sometimes occurs immediately following the entrance of food into the stomach.

gastroileac r., opening of the ileocolic valve induced by entrance of food into the stomach.

Geigel r., in the female, a contraction of the muscular fibers at the upper edge of the Poupart ligament on gently stroking the inner side of the thigh; analogue of the cremasteric r. in males.

Gifford r., SYN eye-closure pupil *reaction*.

gluteal r., contraction of the gluteal muscles following irritation of the skin of the buttocks.

Gordon r., dorsal flexion of the great toe produced by firm lateral pressure on the calf muscles. SYN paradoxical flexor r.

grasp r., SYN grasping r.

grasping r., an involuntary flexion of the fingers to tactile or tendon stimulation on the palm of the hand, producing an uncontrollable grasp; usually associated with frontal lobe lesions. Cf. darwinian r. SYN forced grasping r., grasp r.

great-toe r., SYN Babinski *sign* (1).

Guillain-Barré r., SYN aponeurotic r.

gustatory-sudorific r., sweating, especially over the face, when chewing food. SEE ALSO auriculotemporal nerve *syndrome*.

H r., a monosynaptic r. consistently obtained in normal adults only by stimulating the tibial nerve, generally in the popliteal fossa, while recording from the gastrocnemius-soleus muscle group; similar to the Achilles r., except the neuromuscular spindles are bypassed; widely used in the EMG laboratory to diagnose S1 radiculopathies and polyneuropathies.

hepatojugular r., SEE hepatojugular *reflux*.

Hering-Breuer r., the effects of afferent impulses from the pulmonary vagi in the control of respiration; e.g., inflation of the lungs arrests inspiration with expiration then ensuing, whereas deflation of the lungs brings on inspiration.

Hoffmann r., SYN Hoffmann *sign* (2).

hypochondrial r., a quick inspiration induced by sharp pressure beneath the costal margin.

hypogastric r., SYN femoroabdominal r.

inborn r., SYN innate r.

innate r., an unlearned or instinctive r. such as sucking, which is present at birth. SYN inborn r.

interscapular r., SYN scapular r.

intrinsic r., a r. muscular contraction elicited by the application of a stimulus, usually stretching, to the muscle itself as opposed to a muscular contraction caused by an extrinsic stimulus, e.g., skin, as in the abdominal skin r.'s.

inverted r., SYN paradoxical r.

inverted radial r., flexion of the fingers without flexion of the forearm, on tapping the lower end of the radius; regarded as indicating a lesion of the fifth cervical segment of the spinal cord.

investigatory r., SYN orienting r.

ipsilateral r., a r. in which the response occurs on the side of the body that is stimulated.

Jacobson r., flexion of the fingers elicited by tapping the flexor tendons over the wrist joint or the lower end of the radius.

jaw r., a spasmodic contraction of the temporal muscles following a downward tap on the loosely hanging mandible. SYN chin jerk, chin r., jaw jerk, mandibular r., masseter r.

jaw-working r., SYN jaw-winking *syndrome*.

Joffroy r., twitching of the glutei muscles when firm pressure is made on the nates, in cases of spastic paralysis. SYN hip phenomenon.

Kisch r., closure of the eye in response to stimulation of the skin at the depth of the external auditory meatus. SYN auriculopalpebral r.

knee r., SYN patellar r.

knee-jerk r., SYN patellar r.

labyrinthine r.'s, r.'s initiated through stimulation of receptors in the utricle or semicircular canals. SEE ALSO statotonic r.'s, statokinetic r., righting r.'s.

labyrinthine righting r.'s, stimulation of the receptors of the labyrinth causes changes in tone of the neck muscles that bring the head into position.

lacrimal r., discharge of tears when the conjunctiva is irritated.

lacrimogustatory r., chewing of food causing secretion of tears. SEE ALSO crocodile tears *syndrome*.

laryngeal r., SYN cough r.

laryngospastic r., SYN laryngospasm.

latent r., a r. that must be considered normal but that usually appears only under some pathologic circumstance that lowers its threshold.

laughter r., uncontrollable laughter excited by tickling.

let-down r., SYN milk-ejection r.

lid r., SYN corneal r. (1).

Liddell-Sherrington r., SYN myotatic r.

light r., **(1)** SYN pupillary r; **(2)** a red glow reflected from the fundus of the eye when a light is cast upon the retina, as in retinoscopy; SYN eye r., fundus r. **(3)** a triangular area at the anterior inferior part of the tympanic membrane, extending from the umbo to the periphery, where there is seen a reflection of light. SYN cone of light, Politzer luminous cone, pyramid of light, red r., Wilde triangle.

lip r., a pouting movement of the lips provoked in young infants by tapping near the angle of the mouth.

Lovén r., a reaction in which a local dilation of vessels accompanies a general vasoconstriction; e.g., when the central end of an afferent nerve to an organ is suitably stimulated, its efferent vasomotor fibers remaining intact, a general rise in blood pressure occurs together with a dilation of the vessels of the organ.

lower abdominal periosteal r., SYN Galant r.

magnet r., SEE magnet *reaction*.

mandibular r., SYN jaw r.

mass r., in cases of gross injury to the spinal cord, as the stage of r. activity follows the primary flaccidity of the shock, a condition arises in which a strong stimulus to any part of one of the paralyzed limbs will be followed by contraction of the hip, knee, and ankle of the same side and often, when the stimulus is applied to the middle line of the body, of both sides, as well as of the abdominal wall, and even evacuation of the bladder and sweating over an area corresponding to the level of the lesion.

masseter r., SYN jaw r.

Mayer r., SYN basal joint r.

McCarthy r.'s, (1) SYN spinoadductor r; **(2)** SYN supraorbital r.

mediopubic r., contraction of the adductors of the thigh upon tapping the pubic bone near the symphysis.

Mendel-Bechterew r., SYN Bechterew-Mendel r.

Mendel instep r., the foot being firmly supported on its inner side, a sharp tap on the dorsal tendons causes extension of the second to the fifth toes. SYN back of foot r., dorsum of foot r.

metacarpohypothenar r., flexion of the little finger on tapping the dorsum of the hand; seen in pyramidal tract lesions; similar to Starling r.

metacarpothenar r., SYN thumb r.

metatarsal r., SYN cuboidodigital r.

micturition r., contraction of the walls of the bladder and relaxation of the trigone and urethral sphincter in response to a rise in pressure within the bladder; the r. can be voluntarily inhibited and the inhibition readily abolished to control micturition. SYN bladder r., urinary r., vesical r.

milk-ejection r., release of milk from the breast following tactile stimulation of the nipple; the afferent path is postulated to exist from the nipple to the hypothalamus; the efferent limb is represented by the neurohypophysial release of oxytocin into the systemic circulation; contraction of myoepithelial elements within the breast, caused by oxytocin, moves milk into the collecting ducts and toward the nipple. SYN let-down r., milk let-down r.

milk let-down r., SYN milk-ejection r.

Mondonesi r., SYN bulbomimic r.

Moro r., SYN startle r.

muscular r., SYN myotatic r.

myenteric r., contraction above and relaxation below a stimulated point in the intestine. SYN law of intestine.

myotatic r., tonic contraction of the muscles in response to a stretching force, due to stimulation of muscle proprioceptors. SYN deep tendon r., Liddell-Sherrington r., muscular r., stretch r.

nasal r., sneezing caused by irritation of the nasal mucous membrane.

nasomental r., contraction of the mentalis muscle following a tap on the side of the nose.

near r., pupillary constriction with a near vision effort, with ocular convergence, or with accommodation; an associated reaction, not a true r.

neck r.'s, changes in position of the head cause alterations in tone of the neck muscles through stimulation of proprioceptors in the labyrinth which bring the head into its correct position in space; stimulation of proprioceptors in the neck muscles causes in turn r. movements of the limbs which bring the animal into the normal position in relation to the head.

nociceptive r., SYN flexor r.

nocifensor r., vascular dilation in a part surrounding an injury or in its neighborhood.

nose-bridge-lid r., SYN orbicularis oculi r.

nose-eye r., SYN orbicularis oculi r.

oculocardiac r., a decrease in pulse rate associated with traction on extraocular muscles or compression of the eyeball; especially sensitive in children; may produce asystolic cardiac arrest. SYN Aschner phenomenon, Aschner r., Aschner-Dagnini r.

oculocephalic r., SYN oculocephalogyric r.

oculocephalogyric r., turning of the eyes and head toward the source of an auditory, visual, or other form of stimulation. SYN oculocephalic r.

oculovagal r., SEE oculocardiac r.

re

olecranon r., flexion of the forearm caused by tapping the olecranon. SYN paradoxical triceps r.

Oppenheim r., extension of the toes induced by scratching of the inner side of the leg or by following sudden flexion of the thigh on the abdomen and the leg on the thigh; a sign of cerebral irritation.

optical righting r.'s, visual stimuli that enable an animal to maintain the correct position of the head in space, by bringing about movements of the muscles of the neck and limbs.

orbicularis oculi r., contraction of the orbicularis oculi muscles upon tapping the margin of the orbit, or the bridge or tip of the nose. SYN nose-bridge-lid r., nose-eye r.

orbicularis pupillary r., SYN eye-closure pupil *reaction.*

orienting r., an aspect of attending in which an organism's initial response to a change or to a novel stimulus is such that the organism becomes more sensitive to the stimulation; e.g., dilation of the pupil of the eye in response to dim light. SYN investigatory r., orienting response.

palatal r., palatine r., swallowing r. induced by stimulation of the palate.

palmar r., flexion of the fingers following tickling of the palm.

palm-chin r., SYN palmomental r.

palmomental r., unilateral (sometimes bilateral) contraction of the mentalis and orbicularis oris muscles caused by a brisk scratch made on the palm of the ipsilateral hand. SYN palm-chin r.

parachute r., SYN startle r.

paradoxical r., any r. in which the usual response is reversed or does not conform to the pattern characteristic of the particular r. SYN inverted r.

paradoxical extensor r., SYN Babinski sign (1).

paradoxical flexor r., SYN Gordon r.

paradoxical patellar r., (1) a tap on the patellar tendon causes contraction of the adductor; (2) sudden passive extension of the leg causes a contraction of the extensor muscles of the leg.

paradoxical pupillary r., constriction of pupils in darkness, the reverse of that expected. SYN Flynn phenomenon, paradoxical pupillary phenomenon.

paradoxical triceps r., SYN olecranon r.

ⓘ **patellar r.,** a sudden contraction of the anterior muscles of the thigh, caused by a smart tap on the patellar tendon while the leg hangs loosely at a right angle with the thigh. SYN knee jerk, knee r., knee-jerk r., patellar tendon r., quadriceps r.

patellar tendon r., SYN patellar r.

patelloadductor r., crossed adduction of the leg on tapping the quadriceps tendon.

Pavlov r., SYN auriculopressor r.

pectoral r., contraction of the pectoralis major muscle elicited by tapping the seventh rib between the anterior and the medial axillary lines while the arm is abducted; contraction of the deltoid and biceps may also occur. SYN costopectoral r.

Perez r., running a finger down the spine of an infant held supported in a prone position will normally cause the whole body to become extended.

pericardial r., a vagal r. seen during operations involving pericardial manipulation; characterized by signs of vagal stimulation (bradycardia and arterial hypotension).

periosteal r., (1) SYN front-tap r; (2) a muscular contraction in the arm following a tap on the radius or ulna.

pharyngeal r., (1) SYN swallowing r; (2) SYN vomiting r.

phasic r., a coordinated complex response such as the scratch r. in the spinal animal.

Phillipson r., a contraction of the extensors of the knee when the extensors of the opposite knee are inhibited.

photic-sneeze r., SYN photoptarmosis.

pilomotor r., contraction of the smooth muscle of the skin resulting in "gooseflesh" caused by mild application of a tactile stimulus or by local cooling.

plantar r., the response to tactile stimulation of the ball of the foot, normally plantar flexion of the toes; the pathologic response is Babinski *sign* (1). SYN sole r.

plantar muscle r., SYN Rossolimo r.

pneocardiac r., a modification in the blood pressure or heart rhythm caused by the inhalation of an irritating vapor.

pneopneic r., a modification of the respiratory rhythm caused by the inhalation of an irritating vapor.

postural r., responses that control the position of the trunk and extremities. SEE ALSO righting r.'s. SYN static r. (1).

pressoreceptor r., a normal r. related to the carotid sinus *syndrome.*

pronator r., SYN ulnar r.

proprioceptive r.'s, any r. brought about by stimulation of proprioceptors. SEE ALSO proprioceptor.

proprioceptive-oculocephalic r., SYN vestibuloocular r.

protective laryngeal r., closure of the glottis to prevent entry of foreign substances into the respiratory tract.

psychocardiac r., a change in the circulatory rate and subjective heart consciousness (often "thumping") resulting from a memory of, or a subconscious dream state recollection of, an emotional impression or experience.

psychogalvanic r., psychogalvanic skin r., SYN galvanic skin *response.*

pulmonocoronary r., r. constriction of the coronary arteries as a result of vagal stimuli arising in the lungs, as in pulmonary embolism.

pupillary r., change in diameter of the pupil as a reflex response to any type of stimulus; e.g., constriction caused by light. SYN light r. (1).

pupillary-skin r., dilation of the pupil following scratching of the skin of the neck. SYN ciliospinal r., cutaneous pupil r., cutaneous-pupillary r., skin-pupillary r.

quadriceps r., SYN patellar r.

important deep tendon reflexes

type	biceps tendon r.	triceps r.	patellar r.	Achilles r.
stimulus	percussion of finger resting on biceps tendon	tap on triceps tendon directly above olecranon	tap on the patellar tendon	Achilles tendon
effect	flexion of elbow joint	extension of elbow joint	extension of knee joint	plantar flexion of foot
spinal segment	C5–C6	C6–C8	L2–L4	S1–S2

quadripedal extensor r., extension of the arm of a hemiplegic patient when turned prone as if on all fours. SYN Brain r.

radial r., on tapping the lower end of the radius, flexion of the forearm occurs, and sometimes, on strong percussion, flexion of the fingers. SEE ALSO inverted radial r.

radiobicipital r., contraction of the biceps muscle that sometimes occurs in the elicitation of the brachioradial r.

radioperiosteal r., SYN brachioradial r.

rectal r., the entrance of fecal matter into the rectum from the sigmoid colon causes an impulse to defecate.

rectocardiac r., a parasympathetic r. producing bradycardia and hypotension upon stimulation of the pelvic nerve, the afferent limb being the sacral outflow of the parasympathetic division of the autonomic nervous system, and the efferent limb, the cardiac vagus; said to accompany proctologic examinations.

rectolaryngeal r., laryngeal spasm precipitated by stretching the anal sphincter.

red r., SYN light r. (3).

Remak r., plantar flexion of the first three toes and, sometimes, the foot with extension of the knee induced by stroking of the upper anterior surface of the thigh; it occurs when the conducting paths in the cord are interrupted.

renal r., anuria caused by injury to a remote part of the body or by disease or injury to one kidney or ureter.

righting r.'s, r.'s that through various receptors, in labyrinth, eyes, muscles, or skin tend to bring an animal's body into its normal position in space and that resist any force acting to put it into a false position, e.g., on its back. SEE ALSO body righting r.'s, labyrinthine righting r.'s, neck r.'s, optical righting r.'s. SYN static r. (2).

Roger r., SYN esophagosalivary r.

rooting r., in infants, rubbing or scratching about the mouth causes a puckering of the lips.

Rossolimo r., flicking the tops of the toes from the plantar surface causes flexion of the toes; a stretch r. of the flexors of the toes seen in lesions of the pyramidal tracts. SEE ALSO Starling r. SYN plantar muscle r., Rossolimo sign.

scapular r., contraction of the upper muscles of the back by stimulation between the scapulae. SYN interscapular r.

scapulohumeral r., contraction of muscles of the shoulder girdle and arm caused by tapping the lower part of the unilateral border of the scapula; the muscles that respond vary according to their degree of stretching at the time. SYN scapuloperiosteal r.

scapuloperiosteal r., SYN scapulohumeral r.

Schäffer r., in cases of injury to the corticospinal tract, the great toe is dorsiflexed when the skin over the Achilles tendon is pinched.

semimembranosus r., semitendinosus r., contraction of these muscles by tapping in the region of the tuberosity of the tibia.

shot-silk r., SYN shot-silk *retina.*

sinus r., SEE carotid sinus *syndrome.*

skin r.'s, SYN skin-muscle r.'s.

skin-muscle r.'s, superficial or cutaneous r.'s, such as the superficial abdominal r.'s. SYN skin r.'s.

skin-pupillary r., SYN pupillary-skin r.

snapping r., SYN Hoffmann *sign* (2).

snout r., pouting or pursing of the lips induced by light tapping of the closed lips in the midline; considered a sign of frontal lobe dysfunction.

sole r., SYN plantar r.

sole tap r., SYN aponeurotic r.

spinal r., a r. arc involving the spinal cord. SEE reflex *arc.*

spinoadductor r., contraction of the adductors of the thigh upon tapping the spinal column. SYN McCarthy r.'s (1).

stapedial r., SYN acoustic r.

Starling r., tapping the volar surfaces of the fingers causes flexion of the fingers; analogous to Rossolimo r., for the toes.

startle r., the r. response of an infant (contraction of the limb and neck muscles) when allowed to drop a short distance through the air or startled by a sudden noise or jolt; SYN Moro r., parachute r., startle reaction. SEE ALSO cochleopalpebral r.

static r., (**1**) SYN postural r; (**2**) SYN righting r.'s.

statokinetic r., a r. that, through stimulation of the receptors in the neck muscles and semicircular canals, brings about movements of the limbs and eyes appropriate to a given movement of the head in space.

statotonic r.'s, r.'s in which utricular receptors in the vestibular apparatus sense changes in the head's position in space in terms of linear acceleration and the earth's gravitational field while receptors in the neck muscles sense changes in the position of the head relative to the trunk; input from these receptors reflexly controls the tone of the limb muscles to maintain or regain the desired posture. SYN attitudinal r.'s.

sternobrachial r., contraction of the adductors of the arm when the sternum is tapped.

stretch r., SYN myotatic r.

Strümpell r., stroking the abdomen or thigh causes flexion of the leg and adduction of the foot.

styloradial r., SYN brachioradial r.

suckling r., the r. liberation of prolactin from the anterior lobe of the hypophysis evoked by stimulation of nerves in the nipple during the act of suckling by the newborn animal.

superficial r., any r., e.g., the abdominal or cremasteric r., that is elicited by stimulation of the skin.

supination r., SYN brachioradial r.

supinator r., supinator longus r., SYN brachioradial r.

supporting r.'s, SYN supporting *reactions,* under *reaction.*

supraorbital r., contraction of the orbicularis oculi muscle induced by electrical or mechanical stimulation of the supraorbital nerve. SYN McCarthy r.'s (2), trigeminofacial r.

suprapatellar r., the patella rises when a tap is given on the quadriceps tendon above the patella.

supraumbilical r., (**1**) SYN epigastric r; (**2**) SYN abdominal r.'s.

swallowing r., the act of swallowing (second stage) induced by stimulation of the palate, fauces, or posterior pharyngeal wall. SYN deglutition r., pharyngeal r. (1).

synchronous r., subsidiary r. actions occurring in association with the main or leading r.

tarsophalangeal r., extension of all the toes except the first, when the outer part of the tarsus is tapped; in certain cerebral diseases the reverse takes place, the toes being flexed.

tendo Achillis r., SYN Achilles r.

tendon r., a myotatic or deep r. in which the muscle stretch receptors are stimulated by percussing the tendon of a muscle.

tensor tympani r., contraction of the tensor tympani muscle in response to intense sound, increasing impedance of the middle ear and thus protecting the inner ear from exposure.

thumb r., flexion of the thumb upon tapping the dorsum of the hand. SYN metacarpothenar r.

tonic r., the occurrence of an appreciable interval after the production of a r. before relaxation, e.g., the leg remains up for a time after a knee jerk. SYN Gordon symptom.

trace conditioned r., a conditioned r. established by applying the stimulus a short time before reinforcement; in the conditioned r. of the animal so prepared, the response occurs at the same interval of time after the application of the stimulus as during the period of training.

trained r., SYN conditioned r.

triceps r., a sudden contraction of the triceps muscle caused by a smart tap on its tendon when the forearm hangs loosely at a right angle with the arm. SYN elbow jerk, elbow r.

triceps surae r., SYN Achilles r.

trigeminofacial r., SYN supraorbital r.

trochanter r., contraction of the adductor muscles of the thigh elicited by a tap on the trochanter.

Trömner r., a modified Rossolimo r. in which, with the fingers of the patient partially flexed, the tapping of the volar aspect of the tip of the middle or index finger causes flexion of all four fingers and thumb; seen in pyramidal tract lesions with moderate spasticity.

ulnar r., pronation and adduction of the hand caused by tapping the styloid process of the ulna. SYN pronator r.

re

unconditioned r., an instinctive r. not dependent on previous learning or experience.

upper abdominal periosteal r., percussing the lower margin of the costal cartilages in the nipple line causes a contraction of the ipsilateral abdominal muscles (inconstant).

urinary r., SYN micturition r.

utricular r.'s, SEE statotonic r.'s.

vagovagal r., bradycardia with arterial hypotension, often with supraventricular arrhythmias; ascribed to stimulation, especially mechanical, of afferent vagal pathways in the abdomen, thorax, or airway, the efferent arc being vagal cardioinhibitory fibers.

vasopressor r., vasoconstriction caused by stimulation of certain afferent fibers, e.g., in vagus nerve.

venorespiratory r., stimulation of respiration and increased pulmonary ventilation in response to an increase in pressure in the right atrium.

vesical r., SYN micturition r.

vestibuloocular r., generic term for the r. control of the vestibular system over extraocular motility manifest as nystagmus in clinical testing. SYN proprioceptive-oculocephalic r.

vestibulospinal r., the influence of vestibular stimulation on body posture.

visceral traction r., laryngeal spasm precipitated during an operation by traction on the stomach, gallbladder, or appendiceal mesentery.

viscerogenic r., any of a number of r.'s, such as headache, cough, disturbed pulse, etc., caused by disordered conditions of any of the viscera.

visceromotor r., contraction of the muscles of the thorax or abdomen in response to a stimulus from one of the viscera therein.

viscerosensory r., an area of pain or sensitivity to pressure in the external body wall due to disease of one of the viscera. SEE ALSO Head *lines*, under *line*.

viscerotrophic r., a degenerative change in the skeletal soft tissues consequent upon a chronic inflammatory condition of any of the thoracic or abdominal viscera.

visual orbicularis r., contraction of the orbicularis oculi muscle caused by a sudden visual stimulus. SEE ALSO wink r.

vomiting r., vomiting (contraction of the abdominal muscles with relaxation of the cardiac sphincter of the stomach and of the muscles of the throat) elicited by a variety of stimuli, especially one applied to the region of the fauces. SYN pharyngeal r. (2).

Weingrow r., SYN aponeurotic r.

Westphal pupillary r., SYN eye-closure pupil *reaction*.

white pupillary r., SYN leukocoria.

wink r., general term for r. closure of eyelids caused by any stimulus. SYN eye-closure r.

withdrawal r., SYN flexor r.

wrist clonus r., sudden extension of the wrist induces a sustained clonic movement.

---

re·flex·o·gen·ic (rē-flek-sō-jen′ik). Causing a reflex. SYN reflexogenous.

re·flex·og·e·nous (rē-flek-soj′ĕ-nŭs). SYN reflexogenic.

re·flex·o·graph (rē-flek′sō-graf). An instrument for graphically recording a reflex. [reflex + G. *graphō*, to write]

re·flex·ol·o·gy (rē-flek-sol′ō-jē). The study of reflexes. [reflex + G. *logos*, study]

re·flex·om·e·ter (rē-flek-som′ĕ-ter). An instrument for measuring the force necessary to excite a reflex. [reflex + G. *metron*, measure]

re·flex·o·phil, re·flex·o·phile (rē-flek′sō-fil, -fīl). Having exaggerated reflexes. [reflex + G. *phileō*, to love]

re·flex·o·ther·a·py (rē-flek′sō-thār′ă-pē). SYN reflex *therapy*.

re·flux (rē′flŭks). 1. A backward flow. SEE ALSO regurgitation. 2. In chemistry, to boil without loss of vapor because of the presence of a condenser that returns vapor as liquid. [L. *re-*, back, + *fluxus*, a flow]

abdominojugular r., SYN hepatojugular r.

esophageal r., gastroesophageal r., regurgitation of the contents of the stomach into the esophagus, possibly into the pharynx where they can be aspirated between the vocal cords and down into the trachea; symptoms of burning pain and acid taste result; pulmonary complications of aspiration are dependent upon the amount, content, and acidity of the aspirate.

hepatojugular r., an elevation of venous pressure visible in the jugular veins and measurable in the veins of the arm, produced in active or impending congestive heart failure and constrictive pericarditis by firm pressure with the flat hand over the abdomen. Often called hepatojugular reflux when pressure is exclusively over the liver. SYN abdominojugular r.

intrarenal r., urinary r. from renal pelvis and calices into the collecting ducts. This is seen as a blush of the renal pyramid on voiding cystourethrography. SYN pyelotubular r.

pyelotubular r., SYN intrarenal r.

ureterorenal r., backward flow of urine from ureter into renal pelvis.

vesicoureteral r., backward flow of urine from bladder into ureter.

re·for·mat (rē-for′mat). In computed tomography, when data from a series of contiguous transverse scan images are recombined to produce images in a different plane, such as sagittal or coronal.

re·fract (rē-frakt′). 1. To change the direction of a ray of light. 2. To detect an error of refraction and to correct it by means of lenses. [L. *refringo*, pp. *-fractus*, to break up]

re·frac·ta·ble (ri-frak′ta-bil). Subject to refraction. SYN refrangible.

re·frac·tion (rē-frak′shŭn). 1. The deflection of a ray of light when it passes from one medium into another of different optical density; in passing from a denser into a rarer medium it is deflected away from a line perpendicular to the surface of the refracting medium; in passing from a rarer to a denser medium it is bent toward this perpendicular line. 2. The act of determining the nature and degree of the refractive errors in the eye and correction of the same by lenses. SYN refringence. [L. *refractio* (see refract)]

double r., the property of having more than one refractive index according to the direction of the transmitted light. SYN birefringence.

dynamic r., r. of the eye during accommodation.

static r., r. without accommodation.

re·frac·tion·ist (rē-frak′shŭn-ist). A person trained to measure the refraction of the eye and to determine the proper corrective lenses.

re·frac·tion·om·e·ter (rē-frak-shŭn-om′ĕ-ter). SYN refractometer.

re·frac·tive (rē-frak′tiv). 1. Pertaining to refraction. 2. Having the power to refract. SYN refringent.

re·frac·tiv·i·ty (rē-frak-tiv′i-tē). Refractive power. SYN refringency.

re·frac·tom·e·ter (rē-frak-tom′ĕ-ter). An instrument for measuring the degree of refraction in translucent substances, especially the ocular media. SEE refractive *index*. SYN objective optometer, refractionometer. [refraction + G. *metron*, measure]

re·frac·tom·e·try (rē-frak-tom′ĕ-trē). 1. Measurement of the refractive index. 2. Use of a refractometer to determine the refractive error of the eye.

re·frac·to·ry (rē-frak′tōr-ē). 1. Resistant to treatment, as of a disease. SYN intractable (1), obstinate (2). 2. SYN obstinate (1). [L. *refractarius*, fr. *refringo*, pp. *-fractus*, to break in pieces]

re·frac·ture (rē-frak′choor). Breaking a bone that has united after a previous fracture with the new fracture occurring at or near the previous fracture site. [re- + fracture]

re·fran·gi·ble (rē-fran′ji-bl). SYN refractable. [L. *refringo*, to break in pieces]

re·fresh (rē-fresh′). 1. To renew; to cause to recuperate. 2. To perform revivification (2). [O. Fr. *re-frescher*]

re·frig·er·ant (rē-frij′er-ănt). 1. Cooling; reducing slight fever. 2. An agent that gives a sensation of coolness or relieves feverishness. [L. *re-frigero*, pp. *-atus*, pr. p. *-ans*, to make cold, fr. *frigus* (*frigor-*), cold]

re·frig·er·a·tion (rē-frij-er-ā′shŭn). The act of cooling or reducing fever. [L. *refrigeratio* (see refrigerant)]

re·frin·gence (rē-frin′jens). SYN refraction.

re·frin·gen·cy (rē-frin′jen-sē). SYN refractivity.

re·frin·gent (rē-frin′jent). SYN refractive.

Refsum, Sigvald, Norwegian neurologist, *1907. SEE R. *disease,* *syndrome.*

re·fu·sion (rē-foo′zhŭn). Return of the circulation of blood which has been temporarily cut off by ligature of a limb. [L. *re-fundo,* pp. *-fusus,* to pour back]

re·gain·er (rē-gān′er). An appliance used in an attempt to regain space in the dental arches.

Regaud, Claude, French radiologist, 1870–1940. SEE R. *fixative;* residual *body* of R.

re·gen·er·ate (rē-jen′er-āt). To renew; to reproduce. [L. *re-genero,* pp. *-atus,* to reproduce, fr. *genus* (*gener-*), birth, race]

re·gen·er·a·tion (rē′jen-er-ā′shŭn). **1.** Reproduction or reconstitution of a lost or injured part. SYN neogenesis. **2.** A form of asexual reproduction; e.g., when a worm is divided into two or more parts, each segment is regenerated into a new individual. [L. *regeneratio* (see regenerate)]

    aberrant r., misdirected regrowth of nerve fibers seen, for example, after oculomotor nerve injury. SYN misdirection phenomenon.

    guided tissue r., r. of tissue directed by the physical presence and/or chemical activities of a biomaterial; often involves placement of barriers to exclude one or more cell types during healing or r. of tissue.

reg·i·men (rej′i-men). A program, including drugs, which regulates aspects of one's lifestyle for a hygienic or therapeutic purpose; a program of treatment; sometimes mistakenly called regime. [L. direction, rule]

REGIO

re·gio, gen. **re·gi·o·nis,** pl. **re·gi·o·nes** (rē′jē-ō, -ō′nis, -ō′nēz) [TA]. SYN region. [L.]

regio′nes abdo′minis [TA], SYN abdominal *regions,* under *region.*

r. abdominis latera′lis, ✶official alternate term for flank.

r. ana′lis [TA], SYN anal *triangle.*

r. antebrachia′lis ante′rior, ✶official alternate term for anterior *region* of forearm.

r. antebrachia′lis poste′rior, ✶official alternate term for posterior *region* of forearm.

r. antebrachii anterior [TA], SYN anterior *region* of forearm.

r. antebrachii posterior [TA], SYN posterior *region* of arm.

r. axilla′ris [TA], SYN axillary *region.*

r. brachia′lis ante′rior, ✶official alternate term for anterior *region* of arm.

r. brachia′lis poste′rior, ✶official alternate term for posterior *region* of arm.

r. brachii anterior [TA], SYN anterior *region* of arm.

r. bucca′lis [TA], SYN buccal *region.*

r. calca′nea [TA], SYN heel *region.*

regio′nes cap′itis [TA], SYN *regions* of head, under *region.*

r. carpa′lis ante′rior, SYN anterior *region* of wrist.

r. carpa′lis poste′rior, SYN posterior *region* of wrist.

regio′nes cervica′les [TA], SYN *regions* of neck, under *region.*

r. cervica′lis ante′rior, SYN anterior cervical *region.*

r. cervica′lis latera′lis [TA], SYN lateral cervical *region.*

r. cervica′lis poste′rior, SYN posterior cervical *region.*

r. colli posterior, ✶official alternate term for posterior cervical *region.*

regio′nes cor′poris, SYN *regions* of body, under *region.*

r. crura′lis poste′rior, SYN posterior *region* of leg.

r. cruris ante′rior, SYN anterior *region* of leg.

r. cubita′lis ante′rior [TA], SYN anterior *region* of elbow.

r. cubita′lis poste′rior, ✶official alternate term for posterior *region* of elbow.

r. deltoi′dea [TA], SYN deltoid *region.*

regio′nes dorsa′les [TA], SYN *regions* of back, under *region.*

regiones dorsi, ✶official alternate term for *regions* of back, under *region.*

r. epigas′trica, ✶official alternate term for epigastric *region.*

r. facialis [TA], SYN face *region.*

r. femora′lis poste′rior, SYN posterior *region* of thigh.

r. femoris [TA], SYN femoral *region.*

r. femoris ante′rior [TA], SYN anterior *region* of thigh.

r. femoris posterior [TA], SYN posterior *region* of thigh.

r. fronta′lis cap′itis [TA], SYN frontal *region* of head.

r. ge′nus ante′rior [TA], SYN anterior *region* of knee.

r. ge′nus poste′rior [TA], SYN posterior *region* of knee.

r. glutea′lis [TA], SYN gluteal *region.*

r. hypochondri′aca, ✶official alternate term for hypochondriac *region.*

r. infraclavicula′ris, SYN infraclavicular *fossa.*

r. inframamma′ria [TA], SYN inframammary *region.*

r. infraorbita′lis [TA], SYN infraorbital *region.*

r. infrascapula′ris [TA], SYN infrascapular *region.*

r. inguina′lis, ✶official alternate term for groin (1).

r. lateralis abdominis, ✶official alternate term for flank.

r. lumba′lis [TA], SYN lumbar *region.*

r. mamma′ria [TA], SYN mammary *region.*

regio′nes mem′bri inferio′ris [TA], SYN *regions* of lower limb, under *region.*

regio′nes mem′bri superio′ris [TA], SYN *regions* of upper limb, under *region.*

r. menta′lis [TA], SYN mental *region.*

r. nasa′lis [TA], SYN nasal *region.*

r. nucha′lis, SYN posterior cervical *region.*

r. occipita′lis cap′itis [TA], SYN occipital *region* of head.

r. olfacto′ria tu′nicae muco′sae na′si, SYN olfactory *region* of nasal mucosa.

r. ora′lis [TA], SYN oral *region.*

r. orbita′lis [TA], SYN orbital *region.*

r. parieta′lis cap′itis [TA], SYN parietal *region.*

r. pectora′lis [TA], SYN pectoral *region.*

r. perinea′lis [TA], SYN perineal *region.*

r. plantaris, ✶official alternate term for *sole* of foot.

r. presterna′lis [TA], SYN presternal *region.*

r. pu′bica, ✶official alternate term for pubic *region.*

r. respirato′ria tu′nicae muco′sae na′si, SYN respiratory *region* of mucosa of nasal cavity.

r. sacra′lis [TA], SYN sacral *region.*

r. scapula′ris [TA], SYN scapular *region.*

r. sternocleidomastoi′dea [TA], SYN sternocleidomastoid *region.*

r. sura′lis [TA], SYN sural *region,* sural *region.*

r. talocrura′lis, SYN ankle *region.*

r. tarsalis [TA], SYN ankle *region.*

r. tempora′lis cap′itis [TA], SYN temporal *region* of head.

regiones thoracicae anteriores et laterales [TA], SYN anterior and lateral thoracic *regions,* under *region.*

r. umbilica′lis [TA], SYN umbilical *region.*

r. urogenita′lis [TA], SYN urogenital *triangle.*

r. vertebra′lis [TA], SYN vertebral *region.*

r. zygomat′ica [TA], SYN zygomatic *region.*

re·gion (rē′jŭn) [TA]. **1.** An often arbitrarily limited portion of the surface of the body. SEE ALSO space, zone. **2.** A portion of the body having a special nervous or vascular supply, or a part of an organ having a special function. SEE ALSO area, space, spatium, zone. SYN regio [TA]. [L. *regio*]

abdominal r.'s [TA], the topographic subdivisions of the abdomen; based on subdividing the abdomen by the transpyloric, inter-

re

spinous, and midclavicular planes; including the right and left hypochondrium, right and left flank or lateral, right and left groin or inguinal, and the unpaired epigastric, umbilical, and pubic regions. SYN regiones abdominis [TA], abdominal zones.

anal r., SYN anal *triangle*.

ankle r. [TA], the region of the lower limb between the leg (crus) and the foot (pes). SYN regio tarsalis [TA], regio talocruralis.

anterior antebrachial r., SYN anterior r. of forearm.

anterior r. of arm [TA], area between deltoid region superiorly and anterior region of elbow inferiorly. SYN regio brachii anterior [TA], regio brachialis anterior✶, anterior surface of arm, facies anterior brachii, facies brachialis anterior.

anterior brachial r., the anterior region of the arm.

anterior carpal r., SYN anterior r. of wrist.

anterior cervical r. [TA], the area of the neck bounded by the mandible, the anterior border of the sternocleidomastoid muscle, and the anterior midline of the neck; it is subdivided into carotid, muscular, submandibular, and submental r.'s. SYN regio cervicalis anterior [TA], anterior triangle of neck✶, trigonum cervicale anterius✶, trigonum colli anterius✶, anterior r. of neck.

anterior crural r., SYN anterior r. of leg.

anterior cubital r., SYN anterior r. of elbow.

anterior r. of elbow [TA], the area in front of the elbow, including the cubital fossa. SYN regio cubitalis anterior [TA], anterior cubital r., anterior surface of elbow, facies cubitalis anterior.

anterior r. of forearm [TA], the area between the radial and ulnar borders of the forearm anteriorly. SYN regio antebrachii anterior [TA], regio antebrachialis anterior✶, anterior antebrachial r., anterior surface of forearm, facies antebrachialis anterior, facies anterior antebrachii.

anterior hypothalamic r., ✶official alternate term for anterior hypothalamic *area*.

anterior knee r., SYN anterior r. of knee.

anterior r. of knee [TA], the anterior region of the knee. SYN regio genus anterior [TA], anterior knee r.

anterior and lateral thoracic r.'s [TA], the topographic divisions of the chest: presternal, pectoral, and axillary. SYN regiones thoracicae anteriores et laterales [TA], r.'s of chest.

anterior r. of leg [TA], the anterior surface of the inferior limb between the knee and the ankle. SYN regio cruris anterior [TA], anterior crural r., anterior surface of leg, facies anterior cruris, facies cruralis anterior.

anterior r. of neck, SYN anterior cervical r.

anterior r. of thigh [TA], the front of the thigh, including the femoral triangle. SYN regio femoris anterior [TA], anterior surface of thigh, facies femoralis anterior.

anterior r. of wrist [TA], the anterior part of the wrist. SYN regio carpalis anterior [TA], anterior carpal r.

axillary r. [TA], the region of the axilla, including the axillary fossa. SYN regio axillaris [TA].

r.'s of back [TA], the topographic regions of the back of the trunk, including the vertebral r., sacral r., scapular r., infrascapular r., and lumbar r. SYN regiones dorsales [TA], regiones dorsi✶.

r.'s of body, the topographic divisions of the body. SYN regiones corporis.

buccal r. [TA], the region of the cheek, corresponding approximately to the outlines of the underlying buccinator muscle. SYN regio buccalis [TA].

calcaneal r., SYN heel r.

r.'s of chest, SYN anterior and lateral thoracic r.'s.

chromosomal r., that part of a chromosome defined either by anatomical details, notably banding, or by its linkages (linkage group).

complementarity determining r.'s, that part of an antibody or T cell receptor variable r. that binds with antigen or antigen/major histocompatibility molecule.

constant r., SEE immunoglobulin.

deltoid r. [TA], the lateral aspect of the shoulder demarcated by the outlines of the deltoid muscle. SYN regio deltoidea [TA].

dorsal hypothalamic r., ✶official alternate term for dorsal hypothalamic *area*.

epigastric r. [TA], the region of the abdomen located between the costal margins and the subcostal plane. (TA lists this term as synonymous with epigastric *fossa*. SYN epigastrium [TA], regio epigastrica✶.

r.'s of face, SYN face r.

face r. [TA], the topographic subdivisions of the face, including nasal, oral, mental, orbital, infraorbital, buccal, parotid, and zygomatic. SYN regio facialis [TA], r.'s of face.

femoral r. [TA], the region of the thigh between hip and knee. SYN regio femoris [TA].

framework r., in immunology, a conserved sequence of amino acids on either side of the hypervariable regions in the variable domains of an immunoglobulin chain.

frontal r. of head [TA], the surface region of the head corresponding to the outlines of the frontal bone. SYN regio frontalis capitis [TA].

gluteal r. [TA], the region of the buttocks. SYN regio glutealis [TA].

r.'s of head [TA], the topographic division of the cranium in relation to the bones of the cranial vault; the regions include frontal, parietal, occipital, temporal, auricular, mastoid, and facial. SYN regiones capitis [TA].

heel r. [TA], the region of the heel. SYN regio calcanea [TA], calcaneal r.

hinge r., (1) that part of a tRNA structure that is deformed, bending a "cloverleaf" (two-dimensional) model to form an "L" model (crystal form, as seen by electron microscopy); **(2)** in an immunoglobulin, a short sequence of amino acids that lies between two longer sequences and allows the latter to bend about the former.

hypervariable r.'s (hī-per′var-ĭ-a-ble), the r.'s of the immunoglobulin molecule that contain most of the residues involved in the antibody binding site.

hypochondriac r., the region on each side of the abdomen covered by the costal cartilages; it is lateral to the epigastric region. SYN hypochondrium [TA], regio hypochondriaca✶.

I r., that area of the H-2 complex of mice that contains Class II major histocompatibility complex genes.

iliac r., SYN groin (1).

r.'s of inferior limb, SYN r.'s of lower limb.

inframammary r. [TA], the region of the chest (portion of pectoral region) inferior to the mammary gland. SYN regio inframammaria [TA].

infraorbital r. [TA], the facial region below the orbit and lateral to the nose on each side. SYN regio infraorbitalis [TA].

infrascapular r. [TA], the region of the back lateral to the vertebral region and below the scapula. SYN regio infrascapularis [TA].

inguinal r., ✶official alternate term for groin (1).

r. of interest, in computed tomography or other computerized imaging, an interactively selected portion of the image, the individual or average pixel values of which can be displayed numerically.

intermediate r. [TA], SYN intermediate *column*.

intermediate hypothalamic r., ✶official alternate term for intermediate hypothalamic *area*.

K r., carbons 9 and 10 of the phenanthrene ring system; thought by some to be the reactive spot in the various hydrocarbon carcinogens.

lateral abdominal r., ✶official alternate term for flank.

lateral r. of abdominal r., ✶official alternate term for flank.

lateral cervical r. [TA], the region of the neck bounded by the sternocleidomastoid muscle, the trapezius muscle, and the upper border of the clavicle, including the omoclavicular triangle. SYN regio cervicalis lateralis [TA], posterior triangle of neck✶, trigonum cervicale posterius✶, trigonum colli laterale✶, lateral r. of neck.

lateral hypothalamic r., extends throughout most of the rostrocaudal extent of the hypothalamus lateral to the column of the fornix; includes lateral tuberal nuclei, tuberomamillary nuclei, and diffuse populations of cells.

lateral r. of neck, SYN lateral cervical r.

r.'s of lower limb [TA], the topographic divisions of the lower limb: gluteal, hip, femoral, knee, leg, ankle, and foot. SYN regiones membri inferioris [TA], r.'s of inferior limb.

lumbar r. [TA], the region of the back lateral to the vertebral region and between the rib cage and the pelvis. SYN regio lumbalis [TA].

mammary r. [TA], the region of the chest (pectoral region) that includes the breast. SYN regio mammaria [TA].

mental r. [TA], the region of the chin. SYN regio mentalis [TA].

nasal r. [TA], the region of the nose. SYN regio nasalis [TA].

r.'s of neck [TA], the topographic subdivisions of the neck. SYN regiones cervicales [TA].

nuchal region, SYN posterior cervical r.

nucleolus organizer r., an arrangement of the DNA coding for the production of ribosomal RNA (rRNA).

occipital r. of head [TA], the surface region of the head corresponding to the outlines of the occipital bone. SYN regio occipitalis capitis [TA].

r. of olfactory mucosa, SYN olfactory r. of nasal mucosa.

olfactory r. of mucosa of nose [TA], epithelium containing nerve cells whose axons form the filaments of the olfactory nerve; the lamina propria contains numerous olfactory glands (Bowman) that open to the surface. SYN olfactory mucosa.

olfactory r. of nasal mucosa [TA], the specialized olfactory receptive area that includes the upper one-third of the nasal septum and the lateral wall above the superior concha; it is lined with olfactory mucosa. SYN pars olfactoria tunicae mucosae [TA], olfactory r. of tunica mucosa of nose, regio olfactoria tunicae mucosae nasi, r. of olfactory mucosa, Schultze membrane.

olfactory r. of nose [TA], that part of the nasal mucosa having olfactory receptor cells and glands of Bowman. SYN olfactory membrane.

olfactory r. of tunica mucosa of nose, SYN olfactory r. of nasal mucosa.

oral r. [TA], the region of the face including the lips and mouth. SYN regio oralis [TA].

orbital r. [TA], the region about the orbit. SYN regio orbitalis [TA].

parietal r. [TA], the surface region of the head corresponding to the outlines of the underlying parietal bone. SYN regio parietalis capitis [TA].

pectoral r. [TA], the region of the chest demarcated by the outline of the pectoralis major muscle; includes lateral pectoral, mammillary, and inframammary regions. SEE ALSO anterior and lateral thoracic r.'s. SYN regio pectoralis [TA].

perineal r. [TA], the r. at the lower end of the trunk, anterior to the sacral region and posterior to the pubic region between the thighs; it is divided into the anal triangle posteriorly and the urogenital triangle anteriorly. SYN regio perinealis [TA].

plantar r., ☆official alternate term for *sole* of foot.

popliteal r., SYN popliteal *fossa*.

posterior antebrachial r., SYN posterior r. of forearm.

posterior r. of arm [TA], the back of arm. SYN regio antebrachii posterior [TA], regio brachialis posterior☆, facies brachialis posterior, posterior brachial r., posterior surface of arm.

posterior brachial r., SYN posterior r. of arm.

posterior carpal r., SYN posterior r. of wrist.

posterior cervical r. [TA], the back of neck, including the suboccipital region. SYN regio cervicalis posterior [TA], regio colli posterior☆, nuchal region, posterior neck r., posterior r. of neck, regio nuchalis.

posterior crural r., SYN posterior r. of leg.

posterior cubital r., SYN posterior r. of elbow.

posterior r. of elbow [TA], the back of the elbow. SYN regio cubitalis posterior☆, facies cubitalis posterior, posterior cubital r., posterior surface of elbow.

posterior r. of forearm [TA], the area between the radial and ulnar borders of the forearm posteriorly. SYN regio antebrachialis posterior☆, facies antebrachialis posterior, posterior antebrachial r., posterior surface of forearm.

posterior hypothalamic r., caudal portions of the hypothalamus located internally in the area of the mamillary body, includes medial, intermediate, and lateral mamillary nuclei and the posterior hypothalamic nuclei. SEE ALSO posterior hypothalamic *area.*

posterior knee r., SYN posterior r. of knee.

posterior r. of knee [TA], the posterior region of the knee, including the popliteal fossa. SYN regio genus posterior [TA], posterior knee r.

posterior r. of leg [TA], the back of the leg. SYN regio cruralis posterior [TA], facies cruralis posterior, facies posterior cruris, posterior crural r., posterior surface of leg.

posterior r. of neck, SYN posterior cervical r.

posterior neck r., SYN posterior cervical r.

posterior r. of thigh [TA], the back of the thigh. SYN regio femoris posterior [TA], facies femoralis posterior, posterior surface of thigh, regio femoralis posterior.

posterior r. of wrist [TA], the posterior part of the wrist. SYN regio carpalis posterior [TA], posterior carpal r.

preoptic r., the most anterior part of the hypothalamus surrounding the anterior or preoptic part of the third ventricle and including the lamina terminalis; containing the lateral and medial preoptic nucleus continuous caudally with, respectively, the lateral and anterior hypothalamic nucleus; rostrally the preoptic r. is continuous with the precommissural septum, laterally with the innominate substance. SYN area preoptica [TA], preoptic area [TA].

presternal r. [TA], the part of the chest over the sternum. SYN regio presternalis [TA].

presumptive r., in experimental embryology, an area of the blastula from which a specific tissue or organ may be expected to develop.

pretectal r., SYN pretectal *area.*

pubic r. [TA], the lower central region of the abdomen below the umbilical region and superior to the mons pubis. SYN hypogastrium [TA], regio pubica☆.

r. of respiratory mucosa, SYN respiratory r. of mucosa of nasal cavity.

respiratory r. of mucosa of nasal cavity [TA], the area commencing at the vestibule of the nose lined with respiratory mucosa; with the exception of the olfactory mucusa, it includes the entire nasal cavity. SYN pars respiratoria tunicae mucosae [TA], regio respiratoria tunicae mucosae nasi, r. of respiratory mucosa, respiratory r. of tunica mucosa of nose.

respiratory r. of tunica mucosa of nose, SYN respiratory r. of mucosa of nasal cavity.

sacral r. [TA], the area of the back overlying the sacrum. SYN regio sacralis [TA].

scaffold-associated r.'s (SAR), sites in DNA that bind topoisomerase II and other scaffold proteins; found in introns.

scapular r. [TA], the area of the back corresponding to the outlines of the scapula. SYN regio scapularis [TA].

sternocleidomastoid r. [TA], the region overlying the sternocleidomastoid muscle, including the lesser supraclavicular fossa. SYN regio sternocleidomastoidea [TA].

suboccipital r., upper back of neck, inferior to occipital region of head and above the level of the second cervical vertebra; overlies (or includes, deeply) the suboccipital triangle.

r.'s of superior limb, SYN r.'s of upper limb.

sural r. [TA], the muscular swelling of the back of the leg below the knee, formed chiefly by the bellies of the gastrocnemius and soleus muscles. SYN regio suralis [TA].

temporal r. of head [TA], the surface region of the head corresponding approximately to the outlines of the temporal bone. SYN regio temporalis capitis [TA].

umbilical r. [TA], the central region of the abdomen about the umbilicus. SYN regio umbilicalis [TA].

r.'s of upper limb [TA], the topographic divisions of the upper limb: deltoid, arm, brachial, cubital, antebrachial, carpal, and hand. SYN regiones membri superioris [TA], r.'s of superior limb.

urogenital r., SYN urogenital *triangle.*

variable r., SEE immunoglobulin.

re

vertebral r. [TA], the central region of the back, corresponding to the underlying vertebral column. SYN regio vertebralis [TA].

Wernicke r., SYN Wernicke *center.*

zygomatic r. [TA], the region of the face outlined by the zygomatic bone; the prominence above the cheek. SYN regio zygomatica [TA].

re·gion·al (rē′jŭn-ăl). Relating to a region.

re·gi·o·nes (rē′jē-ō′nēz). Plural of regio. [L.]

reg·is·ter (rej′is-ter). The file of data concerning all cases of a specified condition, such as cancer, occurring in a defined population; the register is the actual document, and the registry is the system of ongoing registration. [Mediev. L. *registrum,* fr. L.L. *regero,* pp. *regestum* to record]

reg·is·tra·tion (rej-is-trā′shŭn). In dentistry, a record.

maxillomandibular r., SYN maxillomandibular *record.*

tissue r., in dentistry, (1) the accurate r. of the shape of tissues under any condition by means of a suitable material; (2) an impression.

reg·is·try (rej′is-trē). 1. An organization that lists professionals in certain fields. 2. An agency for the collection of pathologic material and related information and the organization of these materials for the purpose of study. 3. An agency for the collection of data on individuals who have had a certain disease to allow follow-up and evaluation of response to therapy.

reg·nan·cy (reg′nan-sē). The briefest unit of experience; the unit composed of the total physiologic processes occurring at a single moment, which constitute dominant configurations in the brain. A single process constituting part of the r. is referred to as a regnant process. [L. *regnant-, regnans,* pres. p. of *regno,* to rule]

re·gres·sion (rē-gresh′ŭn). 1. A subsidence of symptoms. 2. A relapse; a return of symptoms. 3. Any retrograde movement or action. 4. A return to a more primitive mode of behavior due to an inability to function adequately at a more adult level. 5. The tendency for offspring of exceptional parents to possess characteristics closer to those of the general population. 6. An unconscious defense mechanism by which there occurs a return to earlier patterns of adaptation. 7. The distribution of one random variable given particular values of other variables relevant to it, e.g., a formula for the distribution of weight as a function of height and chest circumference. The method was formulated by Galton in his study of quantitative genetics. [L. *regredior,* pp. *-gressus,* to go back]

phonemic r., a decrease in intelligibility of speech associated with aging.

re·gres·sive (rē-gres′iv). Relating to or characterized by regression.

reg·u·la·tion (reg′ū-lā′shŭn). 1. Control of the rate or manner in which a process progresses or a product is formed. 2. In experimental embryology, the power of a pregastrula embryo to continue approximately normal development after a part or parts have been manipulated or destroyed. [L. *regula,* a rule]

enzyme r., control of the rate of a reaction catalyzed by an enzyme by some effector (e.g., inhibitors or activators) or by alteration of some condition (e.g., pH or ionic strength).

gene r., control of protein synthesis by means of activation or inhibition of that protein synthesis.

reg·u·la·tor (reg-ū-lā′tōr). A substance or process that controls another substance or process.

growth r.'s, substances that can alter the growth of a living organism.

humoral r., a substance whose action is a result of contact with targets for activity through blood or body fluids.

reg·u·lon (reg′ū-lon). A set of structural genes, all with the same gene regulation, whose gene products are involved in the same reaction pathway.

re·gur·gi·tant (rē-ger′ji-tant). Regurgitating; flowing backward.

re·gur·gi·tate (rē-ger′ji-tāt). 1. To flow backward. 2. To expel the contents of the stomach in small amounts, short of vomiting. [L. *re-,* back, + *gurgito,* pp. *-atus,* to flood, fr. *gurges* (*gurgit-*), a whirlpool]

re·gur·gi·ta·tion (rē-ger′ji-tā′shŭn). 1. A backward flow, as of blood through an incompetent valve of the heart. 2. The return of gas or small amounts of food from the stomach. [L. *regurgitatio* (see regurgitate)]

aortic r., reflux of blood through an incompetent aortic valve into the left ventricle during ventricular diastole. SYN Corrigan disease.

ischemic mitral r., a r. of the mitral valve caused by ischemic heart disease.

mitral r., reflux of blood through an incompetent mitral valve.

pulmonic r., incompetence of the pulmonic valve permitting retrograde flow.

valvular r., a leaky state of one or more of the cardiac valves, the valve not closing tightly and blood therefore regurgitating through it. SYN valvular incompetence, valvular insufficiency.

re·ha·bil·i·ta·tion (rē′hă-bil-i-tā′shŭn). Restoration, following disease, illness, or injury, of the ability to function in a normal or near-normal manner. [L. *rehabilitare,* pp. *-tatus,* to make fit, fr. *re-* + *habilitas,* ability]

mouth r., restoration of the form and function of the masticatory apparatus to as nearly a normal condition as possible.

re·hears·al (rē-her′săl). A process associated with enhancing short-term and long-term memory wherein newly presented information, such as a name or a list of words, is repeated to oneself one or more times in order not to forget it.

Rehfuss, Martin E., U.S. physician, 1887–1964. SEE R. *method,* stomach *tube.*

re·hy·dra·tion (rē-hī-drā′shŭn). The return of water to a system after its loss.

Reichel, Friedrich P., German gynecologist and surgeon, 1858–1934. SEE R.-Pólya stomach *procedure.*

Reichert, Karl B., German anatomist, 1811–1883. SEE R. *cartilage,* cochlear *recess;* R.-Meissl *number.*

Reid, Robert W., Scottish anatomist, 1851–1939. SEE R. base *line.*

Reifenstein, Edward C. Jr., U.S. endocrinologist, 1908–1975. SEE R. *syndrome.*

Reil, Johann C., German physician, neurologist, and histologist, 1759–1813. SEE R. *ansa, band, ribbon, triangle;* limiting *sulcus* of R.; circular *sulcus* of R.; *island* of R.

re·im·plan·ta·tion (rē′im-plan-tā′shŭn). SYN replantation.

extravesical r., SYN detrusorrhaphy.

ureteral r., SYN ureteroneocystostomy.

re·in·fec·tion (rē-in-fek′shŭn). A second infection by the same microorganism, after recovery from or during the course of a primary infection.

re·in·force·ment (rē-in-fōrs′ment). 1. An increase of force or strength; denoting specifically the increased sharpness of the patellar reflex when the patient at the same time closes the fist tightly or pulls against the flexed fingers or contracts some other set of muscles. SEE ALSO Jendrassik *maneuver.* 2. In dentistry, a structural addition or inclusion used to give additional strength in function; e.g., bars in plastic denture base. 3. In conditioning, the totality of the process in which the conditioned stimulus is followed by presentation of the unconditioned stimulus, which itself elicits the response to be conditioned. SEE ALSO reinforcer, *schedules* of reinforcement, under *schedule,* classical *conditioning,* operant *conditioning.*

primary r., satisfaction of physiologic needs or drives, such as that supplied by food or sleep.

secondary r., r. through something which, while it does not satisfy the need directly, has been associated with direct satisfaction of the need, such as the effect on behavior of a food or beer commercial on television.

re·in·forc·er (rē-in-fōrs′er). In conditioning, a pleasant or satisfaction-yielding (**positive r.**) or painful or unsatisfying (**negative r.**), stimulus, object, or stimulus event that is obtained upon the performance of a desired or predetermined operant. SEE ALSO reinforcement (3). SYN reward.

Reinke, Friedrich B., German anatomist, 1862–1919. SEE R. *crystalloids,* under *crystalloid.*

re·in·ner·va·tion (rē-in-ner-vā′shŭn). Restoration of nerve control of a paralyzed muscle or other effector organ by means of regrowth of nerve fibers, either spontaneously or after anastomosis.

re·in·oc·u·la·tion (rē'i-nok-ū-lā'shŭn). Reinfection by means of inoculation.

Reinsch, Adolf, German physician, 1862–1916. SEE R. *test*.

re·in·te·gra·tion (rē'in-tĕ-grā'shŭn). In the mental health professions, the return to well-adjusted functioning following disturbances due to mental illness.

re·in·ver·sion (re-in-ver'shŭn). The correction, spontaneous or operative, of an inversion, as of the uterus.

Reis, Heinrich Maria Wilhelm, German ophthalmologist, *1872. SEE Reis-Bücklers corneal *dystrophy*. SEE ALSO Reis-Bücklers corneal *dystrophy*.

Reisseisen, Franz D., German anatomist, 1773–1828. SEE R. *muscles*, under *muscle*.

Reissner, Ernst, German anatomist, 1824–1878. SEE R. *fiber, membrane*.

Reitan, Ralph M., U.S. psychologist, *1922. SEE Halstead-R. *battery*.

Reiter, Hans, German bacteriologist, 1881–1969. SEE R. *test, disease, syndrome;* Fiessinger-Leroy-R. *syndrome*.

re·jec·tion (rē-jek'shŭn). **1.** The immunologic response to incompatibility in a transplanted organ. **2.** A refusal to accept, recognize, or grant; a denial. **3.** Elimination of small ultrasonic echoes from display. [L. *rejectio,* a throwing back]

accelerated r., a transplant r. manifested in less than 3 days.

acute r., SYN acute cellular r.

acute cellular r., graft r. that usually begins within 10 days after a graft has been transplanted into a genetically dissimilar host. Lesions at the site of the graft characteristically are infiltrated with large numbers of lymphocytes and macrophages that cause tissue damage. SEE primary r. SYN acute r.

allograft r. (al'lō-graft), the r. of tissue transplanted between two genetically different individuals of the same species. R. is caused by T lymphocytes responding to the foreign major histocompatibility complex of the graft.

chronic r., a transplant r. occurring gradually, sometimes months later.

chronic allograft r., immunologically mediated damage to the allograft, typically occurring months or years after transplantation.

first-set r., allograft transplantation between two organisms not previously sensitized to the graft tissue. Necrosis of the graft usually begins within 10 days of transplantation.

hyperacute r., (1) a r. that usually develops immediately after the implantation of a vascular graft; may be caused by preformed, cytotoxic antibodies to the graft; **(2)** a form of antibody-mediated, usually irreversible damage to a transplanted organ, particularly the kidney, manifested predominantly by diffuse thrombotic lesions, usually confined to the organ itself and only rarely disseminated.

parental r., (1) withholding of affection from or denial of attention to one's child; **(2)** child's withholding of affection from its parent.

primary r., a r. occurring more than 7 days after transplantation, mainly from a cellular immune response.

second set r., an accelerated r. of a transplant that occurs when an individual has been previously sensitized to the graft.

re·ju·ve·nes·cence (rē-joo-vĕ-nes'ens). A renewal of youth; return of a cell or tissue to a state in which it was in an earlier stage of existence. [L. *re-,* again, + *juvenesco,* to grow young, fr. *juvenis,* a youth]

re·lapse (rē'laps). Return of the manifestations of a disease after an interval of improvement. SYN recurrence (2). [L. *re-labor,* pp. *-lapsus,* to slide back]

re·laps·ing (rē-lap'sing). Recurring; said of a disease or its manifestations that returns in a new attack after an interval of improvement.

re·la·tion (rē-lā'shŭn). **1.** An association or connection between or among people or objects. SEE ALSO relationship. **2.** In dentistry, the mode of contact of teeth or the positional relationship of oral structures. [L. *relatio,* a bringing back]

acquired centric r., SEE centric jaw r.

acquired eccentric r., an eccentric r. that is assumed by habit in order to bring the teeth into occlusion.

buccolingual r., the position of a space or tooth in r. to the tongue and the cheek.

centric jaw r., centric r., (1) the most retruded physiologic r. of the mandible to the maxillae to and from which the individual can make lateral movements; it is a condition that can exist at various degrees of jaw separation, and it occurs around the terminal hinge axis; **(2)** the most posterior r. of the mandible to the maxillae at the established vertical r. SEE ALSO eccentric r. SYN median retruded r., median r.

dynamic r.'s, relative movements between two objects, e.g., the relationship of the mandible to the maxillae.

eccentric r., any r. of the mandible to the maxillae other than centric r. SYN eccentric position.

intermaxillary r., SYN maxillomandibular r.

maxillomandibular r., any one of the many r.'s of the mandible to the maxillae, e.g., centric jaw r., eccentric r. SYN intermaxillary r.

median retruded r., median r., SYN centric jaw r.

occluding r., the jaw r. at which the opposing teeth occlude.

protrusive r., the r. of the mandible to the maxillae when the lower jaw is thrust forward.

protrusive jaw r., a jaw r. resulting from a protrusion of the mandible.

rest r., the postural r. of the mandible to the maxillae when the patient is resting comfortably in the upright position and the condyles are in a neutral unstrained position in the glenoid fossa. SYN rest jaw r., unstrained jaw r.

rest jaw r., SYN rest r.

ridge r., the positional r. of the mandibular ridge to the maxillary ridge.

static r., relationship between two parts that are not in motion.

unstrained jaw r., SYN rest r.

re·la·tion·ship (rē-lā'shŭn-ship). The state of being related, associated, or connected.

dose-response r., r. in which a change in the amount, intensity, or duration of exposure is associated with a change in risk of a specified outcome.

dual r.'s, r.'s in which a health service provider is concurrently participating in two or more role categories with a patient; such dual r.'s may be benign (as when both are members of the same social group) or exploitive (a sexual r.).

Haldane r., a mathematical r. between the equilibrium constant of an enzyme-catalyzed reaction and all of that enzyme's kinetic parameters (e.g., V_{max} and K_m's).

hypnotic r., r. between hypnotist and the hypnotized.

object r., in the behavioral sciences, the emotional bond between an individual and another person (or between two groups), as opposed to the individual's (or group's) interest in him or herself (itself).

sadomasochistic r., a r. characterized by the complementary enjoyment of inflicting and suffering cruelty.

re·lax (rē-laks'). **1.** To loosen; to slacken. **2.** To cause a movement of the bowels. [L. *re-laxo,* to loosen]

re·lax·ant (rē-lak'sănt). **1.** Relaxing; causing relaxation; reducing tension, especially muscular tension. **2.** An agent that reduces muscular tension or produces skeletal muscle paralysis, usually referred to as a muscle r.

depolarizing r., an agent, e.g., succinylcholine, that induces depolarization of the motor endplate and so paralyzes skeletal muscle by a phase I block.

muscle r., a drug with the capacity to reduce muscle tone; may be either a peripherally acting muscle r. such as curare and act to produce blockade at the neuromuscular junction (and thus useful in surgery), or act as a centrally acting muscle r. exerting its effects within the brain and spinal cord to diminish muscle tone (and thus useful in muscle spasm or spasticity).

re

neuromuscular r., an agent, e.g., curare or succinylcholine, that produces relaxation of striated muscle by interruption of transmission of nervous impulses at the myoneural junction.

nondepolarizing r., an agent, e.g., tubocurarine, that paralyzes skeletal muscle without depolarization of the motor endplate, as in phase II block.

smooth muscle r., an agent, such as an antispasmodic, bronchodilator, or vasodilator, that reduces the tension or tone of smooth (involuntary) muscle.

re·lax·a·tion (rē-lak-sā′shŭn). **1.** Loosening, lengthening, or lessening of tension in a muscle. **2.** In nuclear magnetic resonance, r. is the decay in magnetization of protons after the direction of the surrounding magnetic field is changed; the different rates of r. for individual nuclei and tissues are used to provide contrast in imaging. [L. *relaxatio* (see relax)]

cardioesophageal r., r. of the lower esophageal sphincter, which can allow reflux of acidic gastric contents into the lower esophagus, producing esophagitis.

isometric r., decrease in tension of a muscle while the length remains constant because of fixation of the ends.

isovolumetric r., SYN isovolumic r.

isovolumic r., that part of the cardiac cycle between the time of aortic valve closure and mitral opening, during which the ventricular muscle decreases its tension without lengthening so that ventricular volume remains unaltered; the heart is never precisely isovolumetric (vs. isovolumic) except during long diastoles with a midiastolic period of diastasis. SYN isovolumetric r.

longitudinal r., in nuclear magnetic resonance, the return of the magnetic dipoles of the hydrogen nuclei (magnetization vector) to equilibrium parallel to the magnetic field, after they have been flipped 90°; varies in rate in different tissues, taking up to 15 s for water. SEE TI. SYN spin-lattice r., spin-spin r.

spin-lattice r., SYN longitudinal r.

spin-spin r., SYN longitudinal r.

transverse r., in nuclear magnetic resonance, the decay of the nuclear magnetization vector at right angles to the magnetic field after the 90° pulse is turned off; the signal is called free induction decay. SEE T2; Cf. longitudinal r.

re·lax·in (rē-lak′sin). A polypeptide hormone secreted by the corpora lutea of mammalian species during pregnancy. Facilitates the birth process by causing a softening and lengthening of the pubic symphysis and cervix; it also inhibits contraction of the uterus and may play a role in timing of parturition. SYN cervilaxin, ovarian hormone, releasin. [relax + -in]

re·learn·ing (rē-lern′ing). The process of regaining a skill or ability that has been partially or entirely lost; savings involved in r., as compared with original learning, give an index of the degree of retention.

re·leas·in. SYN relaxin.

re·li·a·bil·i·ty (rē-lī-ă-bil′i-tē). The degree of stability exhibited when a measurement is repeated under identical conditions. SEE correlation *coefficient*, reliability *coefficient*. [M.E. *relien*, fr. O.Fr. *relier*, fr. L. *religo*, to bind]

equivalent form r., in psychology, the consistency of measurement based on the correlation between scores on two similar forms of the same test taken by the same individual. SEE ALSO reliability *coefficient*.

interjudge r., in psychology, the consistency of measurement obtained when different judges or examiners independently administer the same test to the same individual. SYN interrater r.

interrater r., SYN interjudge r.

test-retest r., in psychology, the consistency of measurement based on the correlation between test and retest scores for the same individual. SEE ALSO coefficient, reliability.

re·lief (rē-lēf′). **1.** Removal of pain or distress, physical or mental. **2.** In dentistry, reduction or elimination of pressure from a specific area under a denture base. SEE ALSO relief *area*, relief *chamber*. [see relieve]

re·lieve (rē-lēv′). To free wholly or partly from pain or discomfort, either physical or mental. [through O. Fr. fr. L. *re-levo*, to lift up, lighten]

re·line (rē′līn′). In dentistry, to resurface the tissue side of a denture with new base material to make it fit more accurately. SEE ALSO rebase.

REM 1. Acronym for rapid eye *movements*, under *movement*. **2.** Acronym for reticular erythematous *mucinosis*. SEE REM *syndrome*.

rem Abbreviation for *roentgen*-equivalent-man.

Remak, Robert, Polish-German anatomist and histologist, 1815–1865. SEE R. nuclear *division*, *fibers*, under *fiber*, *ganglia*, under *ganglion*, *plexus*.

Remak, Ernst J., German neurologist, 1848–1911. SEE R. *reflex*, *sign*.

re·me·di·a·ble (rĕ-mē′dē-ă-bl). Curable. [L. *remediabilis*, fr. *remedio*, to cure]

re·me·di·al (rĕ-mē′dē-ăl). Curative or acting as a remedy.

rem·e·dy (rem′ĕ-dē). An agent that cures disease or alleviates its symptoms. [L. *remedium*, fr. *re-*, again, + *medeor*, cure]

re·min·er·al·i·za·tion (rē′min′er-ăl-i-zā′shŭn). **1.** The return to the body or a local area of necessary mineral constituents lost through disease or dietary deficiencies; commonly used in referring to the content of calcium salts in bone. **2.** In dentistry, a process enhanced by the presence of fluoride whereby partially decalcified enamel, dentin, and cementum become recalcified by mineral replacement.

rem·i·nis·cence (rem-i-nis′sens). In the psychology of learning, an improvement in recall, over that shown on the last trial, of incompletely learned material after an interval without practice. [L. *reminiscentiae*, from *reminiscor*, to remember]

re·mis·sion (rē-mish′ŭn). **1.** Abatement or lessening in severity of the symptoms of a disease. **2.** The period during which such abatement occurs. [L. *remissio*, fr. *re-mitto*, pp. *-missus*, to send back, slacken, relax]

spontaneous r., disappearance of symptoms without formal treatment.

re·mit (rē-mit′). To become less severe for a time without absolutely ceasing. [see remission]

re·mit·tence (rē-mit′ens). A temporary amelioration, without actual cessation, of symptoms.

re·mit·tent (rē-mit′ent). Characterized by temporary periods of abatement of the symptoms of a disease.

rem·nant (rem′nant). Something remaining, a residue or vestige. [O. Fr., fr. *remaindre*, to remain, fr. L. *remaneo*]

re·mod·el·ing (rē-mod′el-ing). **1.** A cyclic process by which bone maintains a dynamic steady state through sequential resorption and formation of a small amount of bone at the same site; unlike the process of modeling, the size and shape of remodeled bone remain unchanged. **2.** Any process of reshaping or reorganizing.

heart chamber r., an architectural change in any cardiac chamber (usually one or both ventricles) due to a pathologic or normal (neonatal) stimulus.

ren, gen. **re·nis,** pl. **re·nes** (ren, rē′nis, rē′nēz). SYN kidney. [L.]

re·nal (rē′năl). SYN nephric.

re·nat·ur·a·tion (rē-nā-tū-rā′shŭn). The conversion of a denatured and inactive macromolecule back to its natured and bioactive configuration.

ren·cu·lus (ren′koo-lŭs). **1.** SYN cortical *lobules* of kidney, under *lobule*. **2.** SYN reniculus (2).

Rendu, Henri J.L.M., French physician, 1844–1902. SEE R.-Osler-Weber *syndrome*.

△**reni-.** SEE reno-.

ren·i·cap·sule (ren′i-kap′sool). The capsule of the kidney. [reni- + L. *capsula*, capsule]

ren·i·car·di·ac (ren′i-kar′dē-ak). SYN cardiorenal. [reni- + G. *kardia*, heart]

re·nic·u·lus, pl. **re·nic·u·li** (rĕ-nik′ū-lŭs, -lī). **1.** SYN cortical *lobules* of kidney, under *lobule*. **2.** A lobe of the human fetal kidney and that of some lower animals in which fibrous septa subdivide the organ. SYN renculus (2), renunculus (2). [L. dim. of *ren*, kidney]

ren·i·form (ren′i-fōrm). SYN nephroid.

re·nin (rē′nin). A term originally used for a pressor substance obtained from rabbits' kidneys, now an enzyme that converts angiotensinogen to angiotensin I. SYN angiotensinogenase.

ren·i·por·tal (ren′i-pōr′tăl). **1.** Relating to the hilum of the kidney. **2.** Relating to the portal, or venous capillary circulation in the kidney. [reni- + L. *porta,* gate]

ren·nase (ren′ās). SYN chymosin.

ren·net (ren′et). SYN chymosin.

ren·nin (ren′in). SYN chymosin.

ren·nin·o·gen, ren·no·gen (rĕ-nin′ō-jen, ren′ō-jen). SYN prochymosin. [rennin + G. *-gen,* producing]

♻**reno-, reni-.** The kidney. SEE ALSO nephro-. [L. *ren*]

re·no·cu·ta·ne·ous (rē′nō-kū-tā′nē-ŭs). Relating to the kidneys and the skin. [reno- + L. *cutis,* skin]

re·no·gas·tric (rē′nō-gas′trik). Relating to the kidneys and the stomach. [reno- + G. *gastēr,* stomach]

re·no·gen·ic (rē-nō-jen′ik). Originating in or from the kidney.

re·no·gram (rē′nō-gram). The assessment of renal function by external radiation detectors after the administration of a radiopharmaceutical that is filtered and excreted by the kidney. [reno- + G. *gramma,* something written]

re·nog·ra·phy (rē-nog′ră-fē). Radiography of the kidney.

re·no·in·tes·ti·nal (rē′nō-in-tes′ti-năl). Relating to the kidneys and the intestine.

re·no·meg·a·ly (rē′nō-meg′ă-lē). Enlargement of the kidney.

re·nop·a·thy (rē-nop′ă-thē). A rarely used term for nephropathy.

re·no·pri·val (rē-nō-prī′văl). Relating to, characterized by, or resulting from total loss of kidney function or from removal of all functioning renal tissue. [reno- + L. *privus,* deprived of]

re·no·pul·mo·nary (rē′nō-pŭl′mo-nār-ē). Relating to the kidneys and the lungs.

re·no·tro·phic (rē-nō-trof′ik). Relating to any agent influencing the growth or nutrition of the kidney or to the action of such an agent. SYN nephrotrophic, nephrotropic, renotropic. [reno- + G. *trophē,* nourishment]

re·no·tro·phin (rē-nō-trō′fin). An agent affecting the growth or nutrition of the kidney. SYN renotropin.

re·no·tro·pic (rē-nō-trop′ik). SYN renotrophic. [reno- + G. *tropē,* a turning]

re·no·tro·pin (rē-nō-trō′pin). SYN renotrophin.

re·no·vas·cu·lar (rē-nō-vas′kū-ler). Pertaining to the blood vessels of the kidney, denoting especially disease of these vessels.

Renpenning, H., 20th century Canadian physician. SEE R. *syndrome.*

ren. sem. Abbreviation for [L.] renovetur semel, shall be renewed (only) once.

Renshaw, B., 20th century U.S. neurophysiologist. SEE R. *cells,* under *cell.*

re·nun·cu·lus (rē-nŭng′kū-lŭs). **1.** SYN cortical *lobules* of kidney, under *lobule.* **2.** SYN reniculus (2). [L. dim. of *ren*]

Re·o·vir·i·dae (rē-ō-vir′i-dē). A family of double-stranded RNA viruses, some of which (Reovirus) previously were included with ECHO viruses, and others (Orbivirus), with arboviruses. Virions are 60–80 nm in diameter, usually naked, and ether-resistant; genomes contain double-stranded, segmented RNA (MW $10–16 \times 10^6$); capsids are of icosohedral symmetry with two layers of capsomeres. The family comprises nine genera: Orthoreovirus, Orbivirus, Rotavirus, Coltivirus, Aquareovirus, cytoplasmic polyhedrosis virus group (Cypovirus), and three plant reovirus groups (Phytoreovirus, Fijivirus, and Oryzavirus). [*R*espiratory *E*nteric *O*rphan + viridae]

Re·o·vi·rus (rē′ō-vī′rŭs). A genus of viruses currently called Orthoreovirus (family Reoviridae) that are 80 nm in diameter, with distinct double layers of capsomeres, and have vertebrates as hosts; they have been recovered from children with upper respiratory tract infections, mild fever, and sometimes diarrhea, and from children with no apparent infection; from chimpanzees with coryza; monkeys and mice; and cattle feces. There are three antigenically distinct human types related by a common complement-fixing antigen and at least 12 avian orthoreoviruses.

re·pair (rē-pār′). Restoration of diseased or damaged tissues naturally by healing processes or artificially, as by surgical means. [M.E., fr. O.Fr., fr. L. *re-paro,* fr. re-, back, again, + *paro,* prepare, put in order]

chemical r., conversion of a free radical to a stable molecule.

error-prone r., SYN SOS r.

excision r., the use of a complementary DNA strand as a template to replace a damaged segment of DNA.

mismatch r., replacement of mismatched base pairs by removal of the incorrect base and replacement with the correct base by DNA polymerase.

recombinatorial r., the incorporation of corresponding DNA of a DNA segment from an identical DNA molecule for the purpose of replacing a damaged segment of DNA.

SOS r., a system that repairs severely damaged bases in DNA by base excision and replacement, even if there is no template to guide base selection. This process is a last resort for repair and is often the cause of mutations. SYN error-prone r.

re·pand (rē-pand′). Denoting a bacterial colony with edges marked by a series of slightly concave segments with angular projections at their points of union. [L. *repandus,* bent or turned back, fr. re-, back, + *pandus,* curved]

re·pel·lent (rē-pel′ent). **1.** Capable of driving off or repelling; repulsive. **2.** An agent that drives away or prevents annoyance or irritation by insect pests. **3.** An astringent or other agent that reduces swelling. [L. *re-pello,* pp. *-pulsus,* to drive back]

rep·e·ti·tion-com·pul·sion (rep-e-tish′ŭn-kŏm-pŭl′shŭn). In psychoanalysis, the tendency to repeat earlier experiences or actions, in an unconscious effort to achieve belated mastery over them; a morbid need to repeat a particular behavior such as handwashing or repeated checking to see if the door is locked.

re·place·ment (rē-plās′ment). **1.** Restoration. **2.** Substitution.

cephalic r., in cases of shoulder dystocia when vaginal delivery cannot be effected, the fetal head is flexed and reinserted into the vagina to re-establish umbilical cord blood flow and delivery performed through cesarean section. SYN Zavanelli maneuver.

re·plant (rē′plant). **1.** To perform replantation. **2.** A part or organ so replaced or about to be so replaced.

re·plan·ta·tion (rē-plan-tā′shŭn). Replacement of an organ or part in its original site and reestablishing its circulation. SYN reimplantation. [L. re-, again, + *planto,* pp. -atus, to plant, fr. *planta,* a sprout, slip]

intentional r., elective extraction of a tooth, obturation of the root canal(s), and replacement of the tooth into the alveolus.

re·ple·tion (rē-plē′shŭn). SYN hypervolemia. [L. *repletio,* fr. re-pleo, pp. -pletus, to fill up]

rep·li·ca (rep′li-kă). A specimen for electron microscopic examination obtained by coating a crystalline array or other virus material with carbon; the mold (the r.) obtained after the viral material has been dissolved provides details of structure and arrangement. [It., fr. L.L. *re-plico,* to fold back]

rep·li·case (rep′li-kās). **1.** Descriptive term for RNA-directed RNA polymerase associated with replication of RNA viruses. **2.** An enzyme that replicates nucleic acids.

rep·li·cate (rep′li-kāt). **1.** One of several identical processes or observations. **2.** To repeat; to produce an exact copy.

rep·li·ca·tion (rep-li-kā′shŭn). **1.** The execution of an experiment or study more than once so as to confirm the original findings, increase precision, and obtain a closer estimate of sampling error. **2.** Autoreproduction or duplication, as in mitosis or cellular biology. SEE autoreproduction. **3.** DNA-directed DNA synthesis. [L. *replicatio,* a reply, fr. replico, pp. -atus, to fold back]

bidirectional r., a situation in which DNA r. proceeds with two r. forks moving in opposite directions around a circle or D-loop-type structure.

conservative r., a hypothetical form of r. in which a double-stranded DNA (dsDNA) produces two daughter dsDNAs, one of which consists of the two original strands while the other daughter DNA consists of two newly synthesized chains.

semiconservative r., r. in which a double-stranded DNA

(dsDNA) produces two daughter dsDNAs, each of which contains one of the original chains and one newly synthesized strand.

unidirectional r., r. in which there is movement by a single r. fork.

rep·li·ca·tor (rep′li-kā-ter). The specific site of a bacterial genome (chromosome) at which replication begins.

rep·li·con (rep′li-kon). **1.** A segment of a chromosome (or of the DNA of a chromosome or similar entity) that can replicate, with its own initiation and termination codons, independently of the chromosome in which it may be located. **2.** The replication unit; several are found per DNA in eukaryotic systems. [*replic*ation + -on]

re·po·lar·i·za·tion (rē′pō-lăr-i-zā′shŭn). The process whereby the membrane, cell, or fiber, after depolarization, is polarized again, with positive charges on the outer and negative charges on the inner surface.

re·po·si·ti·o. SYN reposition.

re·po·si·tion. Movement returning palm and fingers from opposed position; opposite of opposition. SYN repositio.

re·po·si·tion·ing (rē′pō-zish′ŭn-ing). **1.** To place in another position as during an operation. **2.** SYN reduction (1).

gingival r., surgical relocation of the attached gingiva to eliminate pathosis or to establish more acceptable form and function.

jaw r., the changing of any relative position of the mandible to the maxillae, by altering the occlusion of the natural or artificial teeth or by surgical means.

muscle r., the surgical replacement of a muscle attachment into a more functional position.

re·pos·i·tor (rē-poz′i-ter, -tōr). An instrument used to reposition a displaced organ.

representation.

internal r., term used by neurolinguistic programming to denote the way people use mental imagery (visual, auditory, or kinesthetic) to encode experience, the composite of which comprises their internal and external reality.

re·pressed (rē-prest′). Subjected to repression.

re·pres·sion (rē-presh′ŭn). **1.** In psychotherapy, the active process or defense mechanism of keeping out and ejecting and banishing from consciousness those ideas or impulses that are unacceptable to the ego or superego. **2.** Decreased expression of some gene product. [L. *re-primo,* pp. *-pressus,* to press back, repress]

catabolite r., the decreased expression of an operon because of elevated levels of a catabolite of a biochemical pathway.

end product r., catabolite r. in which the catabolite is an end product of a particular pathway.

enzyme r., inhibition of enzyme synthesis by some metabolite.

primal r., r. of material never in conscious thought.

re·pres·sor (rē-pres′er). The product of a regulator or r. gene.

active r., a r. that combines directly with an operator gene to repress the operator and its structural genes, thus repressing protein synthesis; an active r. may be repressed by an inducer, with resulting protein synthesis; a homeostatic mechanism for regulation of inducible enzyme systems.

inactive r., a r. that cannot combine with an operator gene until it has combined with a corepressor (usually a product of a protein pathway); after activation, the r. arrests production of the proteins controlled by the operator gene; a homeostatic mechanism for regulation of repressible enzyme systems.

re·pro·duc·i·bil·i·ty (rē-prō-dus′i-bil′i-tē). **1.** Ability to cause to exist again or to present again. **2.** Ability to duplicate measurements over long periods of time by different laboratories.

re·pro·duc·tion (rē-prō-dŭk′shŭn). **1.** The total process by which organisms produce offspring. SYN generation (1), procreation. **2.** The recall and presentation in the mind of the elements of a former impression. [L. *re-,* again, + *pro-duco,* pp. *-ductus,* to lead forth, produce]

asexual r., r. other than by union of male and female sex cells. SYN agamogenesis, agamogony.

cytogenic r., r. by means of unicellular germ cells; includes both sexual r. and asexual r. by means of spores.

sexual r., r. by union of male and female gametes to form a zygote. SYN gamogenesis, syngenesis.

somatic r., asexual r. by fission or budding of somatic cells.

vegetative r., SEE asexual r.

re·pro·duc·tive (rē′prō-dŭk′tiv). Relating to reproduction.

rep·ti·lase (rep′til-as). An enzyme found in the venom of *Bothrops atrox* that clots fibrinogen by splitting off its fibrinopeptide. [reptile + -ase]

Rep·til·ia (rep-til′ē-ă). A class of vertebrates comprising the alligators, crocodiles, lizards, turtles, tortoises, and snakes. [L. *reptilis,* ntr. *-e,* creeping; ntr. as n., reptile]

re·pul·lu·la·tion (rē-pul-ū-lā′shŭn). Renewed germination; return of a morbid process or growth. [L. *re-,* again, + *pullulo,* pp. *-atus,* to sprout]

re·pul·sion (rē-pŭl′shŭn). **1.** The act of repelling or driving apart, in contrast to attraction. **2.** Strong dislike; aversion; repugnance. **3.** Coupling phase of genes at linked loci that are borne on opposite chromosomes. SEE coupling *phase.* [L. *re-pello,* pp. *-pulsus,* to drive back]

re·quire·ment (rē-kwīr′ment). **1.** Something needed. **2.** A condition.

minimum protein r., the age-dependent amount of protein required daily in the diet.

quantum r., the number of quanta of light absorbed required for the transformation of one molecule; the inverse of the quantum yield.

RES Abbreviation for reticuloendothelial *system.*

res·a·zu·rin (rē-saz′ū-rin). A blue compound used as a redox indicator in the reductase test of milk and also as a pH indicator (orange at 3.8, violet at 6.5).

res·cin·na·mine (rē-sin′ă-mēn, -min). 3,4,5-Trimethoxycinnamic acid ester of methyl reserpate; a purified ester alkaloid of the alseroxylon fraction of species of *Rauwolfia;* chemically and pharmacologically related to reserpine, with similar uses.

research (rē-surch′, rē′surch). **1.** (n) The organized quest for new knowledge and better understanding, e.g., of the natural world, determinants of health and disease. Several types of r. are recognized: observational (empiric); analytic; experimental; theoretical; applied. **2.** (v) To conduct such scientific inquiry. [O.Fr. *re-cerche,* fr. *cerchier,* to search, fr. L. *circare,* to go around, fr. *circus,* circle]

re·sect (rē-sekt′). **1.** To cut off or remove, especially to cut off the articular ends of one or both bones forming a joint. **2.** To excise a segment of a part. [L. *re-seco,* pp. *sectus,* to cut off]

re·sect·a·ble (rē-sek′tă-bl). Amenable to resection.

re·sec·tion (rē-sek′shŭn). **1.** A procedure performed for the specific purpose of removal, as in removal of articular ends of one or both bones forming a joint. **2.** To remove a part. **3.** SYN excision (1).

abdominoperineal r. (APR), a surgical cancer treatment involving r. of the lower sigmoid colon, rectum, anus, and surrounding skin, and formation of a sigmoid colostomy; performed as a synchronous or sequential transabdominal and perineal procedure.

gum r., SYN gingivectomy.

loop r., SYN loop *excision.*

muscle r., shortening of the tendon of the ocular muscle in strabismus.

root r., SYN apicoectomy.

scleral r., shortening of the outer coat of the eye in retinal separation.

transurethral r., endoscopic removal of the prostate gland or bladder lesions, usually for relief of prostatic obstruction or treatment of bladder malignancies.

wedge r., removal of a wedge-shaped portion of the ovary; used in the treatment of virilizing disorders of ovarian origin, such as the polycystic ovarian syndrome.

re·sec·to·scope (rē-sek′tō-skōp). A special endoscopic instrument for the transurethral electrosurgical removal of lesions involving the bladder, prostate gland, or urethra.

re·ser·pine (rē-ser′pēn, -pin). An ester alkaloid isolated from the root of certain species of *Rauwolfia;* it decreases the 5-hydroxytryptamine and catecholamine concentrations in the central nervous system and in peripheral tissues; used in conjunction with other hypotensive agents in the management of essential hypertension and useful as a tranquilizer in psychotic states.

re·serve (rē-zerv′). Something available but held back for later use, as strength or carbohydrates. [L. *re-servo,* to keep back, reserve]

alkali r., the sum total of the basic ions (mainly bicarbonates) of the blood and other body fluids that, acting as buffers, maintain the normal pH of the blood.

breathing r., the difference between the pulmonary ventilation (i.e., the volume of air breathed under ordinary resting conditions) and the maximum breathing capacity.

cardiac r., the work that the heart is able to perform beyond that required under the ordinary circumstances of daily life, depending upon the state of the myocardium and the degree to which, within physiologic limits, the cardiac muscle fibers can be stretched by the volume of blood reaching the heart during diastole.

res·er·voir (rez′ĕv-wor). SYN receptaculum. [Fr.]

r. of infection, living or nonliving material in or on which an infectious agent multiplies and/or develops and is dependent for its survival in nature.

Ommaya r., a plastic container placed in the subgaleal space that is connected to the lateral ventricle or tumor cyst by tubing; it is used to instill medication into, or remove fluid from, the ventricle or tumor cyst.

Pecquet r., SYN *cisterna* chyli.

r. of spermatozoa, the site where spermatozoa are stored; the distal portion of the tail of the epididymis and the beginning of the ductus deferens.

vitelline r., SYN vitellarium.

re·set no·dus si·nu·a·tri·a·lis (rē′set nō′dŭs sī′noo-ā-trē-ā′lis). Reset of the sinoatrial node produced by premature depolarization (usually atrial) when the sum of the duration of the premature cycle and the return cycle is less than twice the spontaneous cycle length. Cf. nonreset nodus sinuatrialis. SYN sinus node reset.

res·i·dent (rez′i-dent). A house officer attached to a hospital for clinical training; formerly, one who actually resided in the hospital. SYN resident physician. [L. *resideo,* to reside]

re·sid·ua (rē-zid′ū-ă). Plural of residuum.

re·sid·u·al (rē-zid′ū-ăl). Relating to or of the nature of a residue.

res·i·due (rez′i-doo). That which remains after removal of one or more substances. SYN residuum. [L. *residuum*]

day r., psychoanalytic term for a dream related to an experience of the previous day.

re·sid·u·um, pl. **re·sid·ua** (rē-zid′ū-ŭm, -ū-ă). SYN residue. [L. ntr. of *residuus,* left behind, remaining, fr. *re- sideo,* to sit back, remain behind]

re·sil·ience (rē-zil′yens). **1.** Energy (per unit of volume) released upon unloading. **2.** Springiness or elasticity. [L. *resilio,* to spring back, rebound]

res·in (rez′in, roz′in). **1.** An amorphous brittle substance consisting of the hardened secretion of a number of plants, probably derived from a volatile oil and similar to a stearoptene. **2.** SYN rosin. **3.** A precipitate formed by the addition of water to certain tinctures. **4.** A broad term used to indicate organic substances insoluble in water; these monomers are named according to their chemical composition, physical structure, and means for activation or curing, e.g., acrylic r., autopolymer r. [L. *resina*]

acrylic r., a general term applied to a resinous material of the various esters of acrylic acid; used as a denture base material, for other dental restorations, and for trays.

activated r., SYN autopolymer r.

anion-exchange r., SEE anion exchange, anion exchanger.

autopolymer r., autopolymerizing r., any r. that can be polymerized by chemical catalysis rather than by the application of heat or light; used in dentistry for dental restoration, denture repair, and impression trays. SYN activated r., cold cure r., cold-curing r., quick cure r., self-curing r.

carbacrylamine r.'s, a mixture of the cation-exchange r.'s, carbacrylic r. and potassium carbacrylic r. (87.5%), and of the anion-exchange r., polyamine-methylene r. (12.5%), used to increase the fecal excretion of sodium in edema associated with excessive sodium retention by the kidneys, e.g., in congestive heart failure, cirrhosis of the liver, and nephrosis.

cation-exchange r., SEE cation exchange, cation exchanger.

chemically cured r., a r. that contains an initiator, usually benzoyl peroxide, and an activator, usually a tertiary amine, in separate pastes. When mixed, the amine reacts with the benzoyl peroxide to form free radicals and polymerization occurs.

cholestyramine r., a strongly basic anion-exchange r. in the chloride form, consisting of a copolymer of styrene and divinylbenzene with quaternary ammonium functional groups; it lowers the blood cholesterol by binding the bile acids in the intestine, thus promoting their excretion in the feces instead of reabsorption from the bowel; used in the treatment of hypercholesterolemia, xanthomatous biliary cirrhosis, and other forms of xanthomatosis; also will bind numerous drugs in the intestine, reducing their bioavailability.

cold cure r., cold-curing r., SYN autopolymer r.

composite r., a synthetic r. usually acrylic based, to which a glass or natural silica filter has been added. Used mainly in dental restorative procedures. [L. *compositus,* put together, fr. *compono,* to put together]

copolymer r., synthetic r. produced by joint polymerization of two or more different monomers or polymers.

cross-linked r., SYN cross-linked *polymer.*

direct filling r., an autopolymerizing r. especially designed as a dental restorative material.

dual-cure r., a r. that utilizes both light and chemical initiation to activate polymerization.

epoxy r., any thermosetting r. based on the reactivity of epoxy; used as adhesives, protective coatings, and embedding media for electron microscopy.

gum r., the dry exudate from a number of plants, consisting of a mixture of a gum and a r., the former soluble in water but not alcohol, the latter soluble in alcohol but not water.

heat-curing r., r. that requires heat to initiate polymerization.

Indian podophyllum r., r. obtained from *Podophyllum emodi;* a cathartic and cholagogue.

ion-exchange r., SEE ion exchange, ion exchanger.

ipomea r., r. obtained from the dried root of *Ipomoea orizabensis;* a cathartic. SEE ALSO scammony.

jalap r., r. extracted from the dried tuberous root of *Exogonium purga;* a purgative.

light-activated r., SYN light-cured r.

light-cured r., a r. that uses visible or ultraviolet light to excite a photoinitiator, which interacts with an amine to form free radicals and initiate polymerization; used mainly in restorative dentistry. SYN light-activated r.

melamine r., a plastic material mixed with plaster of Paris for casts. Such a cast is lighter and stronger than one made with plaster of Paris alone. SYN melamine formaldehyde.

methacrylate r., a translucent plastic material, used for the manufacture of various medical appliances, surgical instruments, and seating components used in total joint replacement; it possesses the optical properties of fused quartz and is readily molded when heated; formerly used in electron microscopy for embedding tissues, now superseded by epoxy r.'s.

podophyllum r., a r. extracted from the dried roots and rhizomes of *Podophyllum peltatum,* a perennial herb common in moist, shady situations in the eastern parts of Canada and the United States. The drug has been used by American Indians as a vermifuge and emetic. The chief constituents of the r. belong to the group of lignins, which are C_{118} compounds related biosynthetically to the flavonoids and derived by dimerization of two C_6-C_3 units. The most important ones present in podophyllum r. are podophyllotoxin (about 20%), β-peltatin (about 10%), and α-peltatin (about 5%). All three occur both free and as glucosides. The r. has been used as a purgative but has been replaced by milder agents. It is cytotoxic and used as a paint in the treatment

re

of soft venereal and other warts. SYN May apple root, podophyllin, wild mandrake.

polyamine-methylene r., a synthetic acid-binding r. used as a gastric antacid.

polyester r., r. in which the polymers are insoluble in most organic solvents and are polymerized by light, heat, or oxygen; used in electron microscopy as a tissue-embedding medium.

quick cure r., SYN autopolymer r.

quinine carbacrylic r., SYN azuresin.

self-curing r., SYN autopolymer r.

res·in ac·ids. A class of organic compounds derived from various natural plant resins; diterpenes containing a phenanthrene ring system; e.g., abietic acid, pimaric acid, ester gums. SYN resinic acids.

res·in·ates (rez′in-āts). Salts or esters of resin acids.

res·ines (rez′ēns). Esters of resin acids.

res·in·ic ac·ids. SYN resin acids.

res·in·oid (rez′i-noyd). **1.** A substance containing a resin or resembling one. **2.** An extract obtained by evaporating a tincture. **3.** Resembling rosin.

res·in·ols (rez′in-ols). Resin alcohols.

res·in·ous (rez′i-nŭs). Relating to or derived from a resin.

re·sis·tance (rē-zis′tans). **1.** A force exerted in opposition to an active force. **2.** The opposition in a conductor to the passage of a current of electricity, whereby there is a loss of energy and a production of heat; specifically, the potential difference in volts across the conductor per ampere of current flow; unit: ohm. Cf. impedance (1). **3.** The opposition to flow of a fluid through one or more passageways (e.g., blood flow, respiratory gases in the tracheobronchial tree), analogous to (2); units are usually those of pressure difference per unit flow. Cf. impedance (2). **4.** In psychoanalysis, an individual's unconscious defense against bringing repressed thoughts to consciousness. **5.** The ability of red blood cells to resist hemolysis and to preserve their shape under varying degrees of osmotic pressure in the blood plasma. **6.** The natural or acquired ability of an organism to maintain its immunity to or to resist the effects of an antagonistic agent, e.g., pathogenic microorganism, toxin, drug. [L. *re-sisto,* to stand back, withstand]

airway r., in physiology, the r. to flow of gases during ventilation due to obstruction or turbulent flow in the upper and lower airways; to be differentiated during inhalation from r. to inflation due to decreases in pulmonary or thoracic compliance.

bacteriophage r., r. of a bacterial mutant to infection by a bacteriophage to which the parent (wild-type) strain is susceptible.

dicumarol r. [MIM*122700], an autosomal dominant disorder characterized by r. to dicumarol, over and above general variability in tolerance to the drug; caused by mutation in the coumarin 7-hydroxylase gene (CYP2A6) on chromosome 19p.

drug r., the capacity of disease-causing microorganisms to withstand drugs previously toxic to them; achieved by spontaneous mutation or through selective pressure after exposure to the drug in question. Pathogenic microorganisms resist antibiotics by various mechanisms, including the production of enzymes (e.g., β-lactamases) that chemically inactivate antibiotic molecules. In mixed infections of the respiratory tract, a β-lactamase (penicillinase) produced by one organism (e.g., *Haemophilus influenzae*) can inactivate penicillin and so block its effectiveness against other organisms in the mixture that possess no resistance of their own (e.g., group A β-hemolytic streptococci). Usually an organism that has acquired resistance to a given antibiotic is resistant to others in the same chemical class. Some bacteria transmit antibiotic r. to their offspring not chromosomally but via plasmids, which lie outside the bacterial nucleus but perform certain genetic functions. Bacteria of one species can develop r. to certain antibiotics by acquiring plasmids from bacteria of another species.

Drug resistance is a growing problem worldwide. Many strains of bacteria, fungi, and parasites have developed resistance, including pneumococci, gonococci, salmonellae, *Mycobacterium tuberculosis, Tinea tonsurans,* and *Plasmodium falciparum.* In some parts of the U.S., 40% of

pneumococcal isolates and 90% of staphylococci are resistant to penicillin. The prevalence of both vancomycin-resistant enterococci and methicillin-resistant *Staphylococcus aureus* has increased 20-fold since 1989. Factors favoring development of antibiotic resistance include inappropriate prescribing of antibiotics (e.g., to treat viral infections); indiscriminate use of newly developed, extended-spectrum agents; empiric and broad-spectrum treatment of infections in certain populations (e.g., children, the elderly, and residents of long-term care facilities); prescribing of sublethal doses; and failure of patients to complete courses of antibiotic treatment. The Centers for Disease Control and Prevention estimates that U.S. physicians write 50 million unnecessary antibiotic prescriptions annually, including 17 million to treat the common cold. Infectious disease experts and public health authorities have called for restraint by primary care physicians in prescribing antibiotics, particularly for children and for uncomplicated upper respiratory infections, acute bronchitis (nearly always viral), and acute sinusitis and otitis media (in neither of which have reliable diagnostic criteria for bacterial infection been established). They have also stressed the importance of public education, since inappropriate expectations of patients or their parents have been a driving factor in antibiotic overuse by physicians. Administration of antibiotics to livestock animals, chiefly for disease prophylaxis and growth promotion, has also contributed to the emergence of resistant strains of bacteria.

expiratory r., r. to flow of gas out of the lungs or the total r. to flow of gas during the expiratory phase of the respiratory cycle.

impact r., the ability of a lens for eyewear to withstand impact without shattering or breaking, i.e., of a ⅜-inch steel ball dropped 50 ft; criteria for determination of impact r. are specified by U.S. regulations.

inductive r., SYN reactance.

insulin r., diminished effectiveness of insulin in lowering plasma glucose levels, arbitrarily defined as a daily requirement of at least 200 units of insulin to prevent hyperglycemia or ketosis; usually due to binding of insulin or insulin receptor sites by antibodies; associated with obesity, ketoacidosis, and infection.

Impairment of the normal response of muscle and other cells to endogenous or exogenous insulin often complicates the deficiency of endogenous insulin that is characteristic of type 2 diabetes mellitus. It is a peripheral phenomenon and can occur even when the quality and quantity of insulin produced by the pancreas are normal. It apparently results from a decrease in the number of insulin receptor sites on cells, a malfunction of the biochemical glucose transport system, or both. Insulin resistance is often associated with high levels of circulating antibody to insulin receptors. The phenomenon of insulin resistance explains why some people with type 2 diabetes have hyperinsulinemia in the fasting state, often coexisting with elevated plasma glucose levels. Insulin resistance correlates closely with obesity in diabetes. It occurs less frequently in lean diabetics, whose principal problem is usually primary failure of insulin production. Insulin resistance is often seen in persons with or without frank diabetes who have other endocrine or systemic disorders, including dyslipidemias, hypertension, hyperuricemia, and chronic infection. Some women with polycystic ovaries, hirsutism, and anovulation also have insulin resistance and hyperinsulinemia. Troglitazone, a newer agent used in the treatment of type 2 diabetes mellitus, improves insulin sensitivity.

multidrug r., the insensitivity of various tumors to a variety of chemically related anticancer drugs; mediated by a process of inactivating the drug or removing it from the target tumor cells.

mutual r., SYN antagonism.

peripheral r., SYN total peripheral r.

synaptic r., the ease or difficulty with which a nerve impulse can cross a synapse.

systemic vascular r., an index of arteriolar compliance or constriction throughout the body; proportional to the blood pressure divided by the cardiac output.

thyrotropin r., an autosomal recessive disorder in which the thyrocytes are unresponsive to thyrotropin. Cf. pseudohypoparathyroidism.

total peripheral r. (TPR), the total r. to flow of blood in the systemic circuit; the quotient produced by dividing the mean arterial pressure by the cardiac minute-volume. SYN peripheral r.

re·sis·tiv·i·ty (rē′zis-tiv′ĭ-tē). A measure of a material's resistance to the passage of electrical current; the reciprocal of conductivity. [L. *re-sito,* to withstand]

re·sis·tor (rē-zis′ter, -tōr). An element included in an electric circuit to provide resistance to the flow of current.

res·o·lu·tion (rez-ō-loo′shŭn). **1.** The arrest of an inflammatory process without suppuration; the absorption or breaking down and removal of the products of inflammation or of a new growth. SEE line *pairs,* under *pair.* **2.** The optical ability to distinguish detail such as the separation of closely adjacent objects. SYN resolving power (3). [L. *resolutio,* a slackening, fr. *re-solvo,* pp. *-solutus,* to loosen, relax]

re·sol·vase (rē-sol′vāz). A gene encoded by a transposon that can catalyze a second stage of transposition as well as participate in the regulation of its own expression. [resolve + -ase]

re·solve (rē-zolv′). To return or cause to return to the normal, particularly without suppuration, said of a phlegmon or other form of inflammation. [L. *resolvo,* to loosen]

re·sol·vent (rē-zol′vent). **1.** Causing resolution. **2.** An agent that arrests an inflammatory process or causes the absorption of a neoplasm.

res·o·nance (rez′ō-nans). **1.** Sympathetic or forced vibration of air in the cavities above, below, in front of, or behind a source of sound; in speech, modification of the quality (e.g., harmonics) of a tone by the passage of air through the chambers of the nose, pharynx, and head, without increasing the intensity of the sound. **2.** The sound obtained on percussing a part that can vibrate freely. **3.** The intensification and hollow character of the voice sound obtained on auscultating over a cavity. **4.** In chemistry, the manner in which electrons or electric charges are distributed among the atoms in compounds that are planar and symmetric, particularly those with conjugated (alternating) double bonds; the existence of r. in the latter case lowers the energy content and increases the stability of a compound. **5.** The natural or inherent frequency of any oscillating system. **6.** SYN resonant *frequency.* [L. *resonantia,* echo, fr. *re-sono,* to resound, to echo]

amphoric r., a percussion sound, like that produced by striking a large empty bottle, obtained by percussing over a pulmonary cavity. SYN cavernous r.

bandbox r., SYN vesiculotympanitic r.

bellmetal r., in cases of a large pulmonary cavity or of pneumothorax, a clear metallic sound obtained by striking a coin, held against the chest, by another coin, or by flicking the chest wall with one's fingernail; the sound is heard on auscultating the chest wall on the same side anteroposteriorly. SYN anvil sound, bell sound, coin test.

cavernous r., SYN amphoric r.

cracked-pot r., a peculiar sound, resembling that heard on striking a cracked pot, elicited on percussing over a pulmonary cavity that communicates with a bronchial tube, when the patient's mouth is open. SYN cracked-pot sound.

electron paramagnetic r. (EPR), SYN electron spin r.

electron spin r. (ESR), a spectrometric method, based on measurement of electron spins and magnetic moments, for detecting and estimating free radicals in reactions and in biologic systems. SYN electron paramagnetic r.

hydatid r., a peculiar vibratile r. heard on auscultatory percussion over a hydatid cyst.

nuclear magnetic r. (NMR), the phenomenon in which certain atomic nuclei possessing a magnetic moment will precess around the axis of a strong external magnetic field, the frequency of precession (Larmor frequency) being specific for each nucleus and the strength of the magnetic field; spinning nuclei induce their own oscillating magnetic fields and therefore emit electromagnetic radiation that can produce a detectable signal at the Larmor frequency. NMR is used as a method of identifying covalent bonds and is applied clinically in magnetic resonance *imaging.*

skodaic r., a peculiar, high-pitched sound, less musical than that obtained over a cavity, elicited by percussion just above the level of a pleuritic effusion. SYN Skoda sign, Skoda tympany.

tympanitic r., SYN tympany.

vesicular r., the sound obtained on percussing over the normal lungs.

vesiculotympanitic r., a peculiar, partly tympanitic, partly vesicular sound, obtained on percussion in cases of pulmonary emphysema. SYN bandbox r., wooden r.

vocal r. (VR), the voice sounds as heard on auscultation of the chest.

wooden r., SYN vesiculotympanitic r.

res·o·na·tor (rez′ō-nā-ter). A device for employing inductance to create an electric current of very high potential and small volume.

re·sorb (rē-sōrb′). To reabsorb; to absorb what has been excreted, as an exudate or pus. [L. *re-sorbeo,* to suck back]

res·or·cin (rē-zōr′sin). SYN resorcinol.

res·or·cin·ol (rē-zōr′si-nol). An external antiseptic in psoriasis, eczema, seborrhea, and ringworm; pyrocatechol and hydroquinone are isomers of r. SYN resorcin.

r. monoacetate, used externally in the treatment of acne, sycosis, and seborrhea.

r. phthalic anhydride, SYN fluorescein.

res·or·cin·ol·phtha·lein (rē-zōr′si-nol-thal′ē-in). SYN fluorescein.

r. sodium, SYN *fluorescein* sodium.

re·sorp·tion (rē-sōrp′shŭn). **1.** The act of resorbing. **2.** A loss of substance by lysis, or by physiologic or pathologic means.

bone r., the removal of osseous tissue.

gingival r., SYN gingival *recession.*

horizontal r., SYN horizontal *atrophy.*

internal r., a loss of tooth structure originating within the pulp cavity.

ridge r., a loss in the volume and size of the alveolar portion of the mandible or maxilla.

root r., dissolution of the root of a tooth; either external, with loss or blunting of the apical portion, or internal, with loss of dentin from the inside (pulpal) part of the root area.

res·pi·ra·ble (re-spīr′ă-bl, res′pĭ-ră-bl). Capable of being breathed.

res·pi·ra·tion (res-pi-rā′shŭn). **1.** A fundamental process of life, characteristic of both plants and animals, in which oxygen is used to oxidize organic fuel molecules, providing a source of energy as well as carbon dioxide and water. In green plants, photosynthesis is not considered r. **2.** SYN ventilation (2). [L. *respiratio,* fr. *respiro,* pp. *-atus,* to exhale, breathe]

abdominal r., breathing effected mainly by the action of the diaphragm.

aerobic r., a form of r. in which molecular oxygen is consumed and carbon dioxide and water are produced.

amphoric r., a sound like that made by blowing across the mouth of a bottle, heard on auscultation in some cases in which a large pulmonary cavity exists, or occasionally in pneumothorax.

anaerobic r., a form of r. in which molecular oxygen is not consumed; e.g., nitrate r., sulfate r.

artificial r., SYN artificial *ventilation.*

assisted r., SYN assisted *ventilation.*

Biot r., completely irregular breathing pattern, with continually variable rate and depth of breathing; results from lesions in the respiratory centers in the brainstem, extending from the dorsomedial medulla caudally to the obex. SYN ataxic breathing, Biot breathing, respiratory ataxia.

re

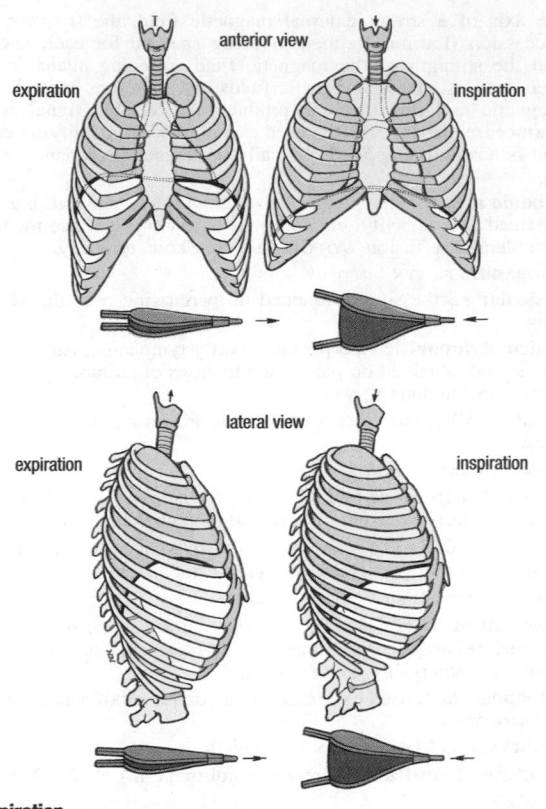

anterior view

expiration — inspiration

lateral view

expiration — inspiration

respiration

bronchial r., a tubular blowing sound caused by the passage of air through a bronchus in an area of consolidated lung tissue.

bronchovesicular r., combined bronchial and vesicular r.

cavernous r., a hollow reverberating sound heard on auscultation over a cavity in the lung.

Cheyne-Stokes r., the pattern of breathing with gradual increase in depth and sometimes in rate to a maximum, followed by a decrease resulting in apnea; the cycles ordinarily are 30 seconds to 2 minutes in duration, with 5–30 seconds of apnea; seen with bilateral deep cerebral hemispheric lesions, with metabolic encephalopathy, and, characteristically, in coma from affection of the nervous centers of respiration.

cogwheel r., the inspiratory sound interrupted by one or two by silent intervals. SYN interrupted r., jerky r.

controlled r., SYN controlled *ventilation*.

costal r., SYN thoracic r.

diffusion r., maintenance of oxygenation during apnea by intratracheal insufflation of oxygen at high flow rates. SYN apneic oxygenation.

electrophrenic r., the rhythmic electric stimulation of the phrenic nerve by an electrode applied to the skin at the motor points of the phrenic nerve; it is used in paralysis of the respiratory center resulting from acute bulbar poliomyelitis.

external r., the exchange of respiratory gases in the lungs as distinguished from internal or tissue r.

forced r., voluntary hyperventilation.

internal r., SYN tissue r.

interrupted r., SYN cogwheel r.

jerky r., SYN cogwheel r.

Kussmaul r., deep, rapid r. characteristic of diabetic or other causes of acidosis. SYN Kussmaul-Kien r.

Kussmaul-Kien r., SYN Kussmaul r.

labored r., difficult, usually deep, breathing in patients with cardiac or pulmonary disease or disease affecting nervous system control of ventilation.

mouth-to-mouth r., a method of artificial ventilation involving an overlap of the patient's mouth (and nose in small children) with the operator's mouth to inflate the patient's lungs by blowing, followed by an unassisted expiratory phase brought about by elastic recoil of the patient's chest and lungs; repeated 12–16 times a minute; where the nose is not covered by the operator's mouth, the nostrils must be closed by pinching.

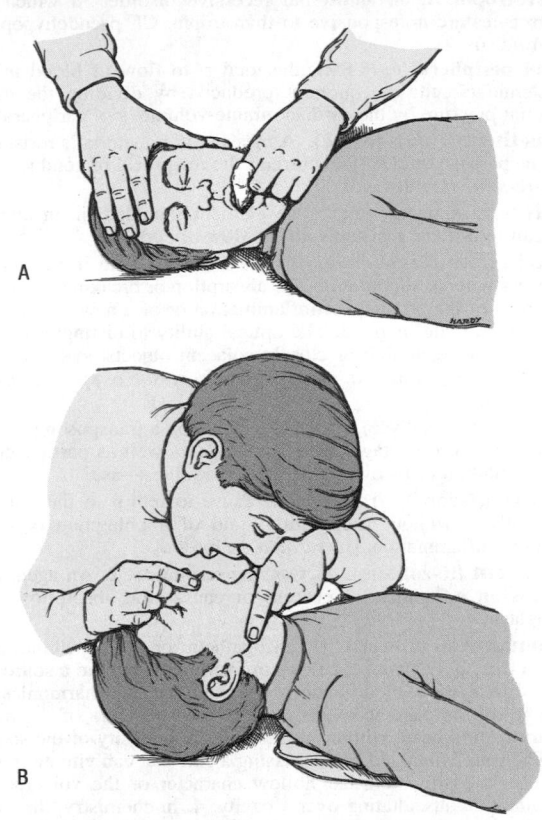

A

B

mouth-to-mouth-respiration: (A) attempt to remove any foreign matter in mouth with index finger wrapped in cloth or a handkerchief; (B) tilting head back and pinching nose, give two slow breaths into the victim's mouth with lips making a tight seal; breath into victim until chest gently rises

nitrate r., the process of r. used by some anaerobic organisms, in which nitrate rather than molecular oxygen is used to oxidize organic molecules to obtain energy.

paradoxical r., deflation of the lung during inspiration and inflation of the lung during the phase of expiration; seen in the lung on the side of an open pneumothorax.

puerile r., an exaggeration of the normal respiratory sounds, heard in children and in adults after exertion.

stertorous r., harsh, noisy breathing usually heard in a comatose patient. SYN stertorous breathing.

sulfate r., the process of r. used by some anaerobic organisms, in which sulfate rather than molecular oxygen is used to oxidize organic molecules to obtain energy.

thoracic r., r. effected chiefly by the action of the intercostal and other muscles that raise the ribs, causing expansion of the chest. SYN costal r.

tissue r., the interchange of gases between the blood and the tissues. SYN internal r.

tubular r., high-pitched bronchial r.

vesicular r., the respiratory murmur heard on auscultating over the normal lung. SYN respiratory murmur, vesicular murmur.

vesiculocavernous r., cavernous r., due to the presence of a cavity, mingled with the vesicular murmur of the surrounding normal lung tissue.

res·pi·ra·tor (res′pi-rā-ter, -tōr). **1.** An apparatus for administering artificial respiration in cases of respiratory failure. **2.** An appliance fitting over the mouth and nose, used for the purpose of excluding dust, smoke, or other irritants, or of otherwise altering the air before it enters the respiratory passages. SYN inhaler (1). SYN ventilator.

cuirass r., one of several types of r.'s producing alternating negative pressure about the thoracic cage; now rarely used.

Drinker r., a mechanical r. in which the body (except the head) is encased within a metal tank, which is sealed at the neck with an airtight gasket; artificial respiration is induced by making the air pressure inside negative. SYN iron lung, tank r.

pressure-controlled r., a r. that provides a predetermined pressure to gases during inhalation, the volume of gas moved being variable, depending upon resistance.

tank r., SYN Drinker r.

volume-controlled r., a r. that provides a predetermined volume of gases during inhalation, with the pressure required to move that volume remaining variable, depending upon resistance.

res·pi·ra·to·ry (res′pi-ră-tōr-ē, rĕ-spīr′ă-tōr-ē). Relating to respiration.

re·spire (rĕ-spīr′). **1.** To breathe. **2.** To consume oxygen and produce carbon dioxide by metabolism. [L. *respiro,* to breathe]

res·pi·rom·e·ter (res-pĭ-rom′ĕ-ter). **1.** An instrument for measuring the extent of the respiratory movements. **2.** An instrument for measuring oxygen consumption or carbon dioxide production, usually of an isolated tissue. [L. *respiro,* to breathe, + G. *metron,* measure]

Dräger r., an inferential meter to measure tidal and minute volume from the number of revolutions of a vane rotated by the gas stream as the latter passes through two lightweight lozenge-shaped meshing rotors.

Wright r., an inferential meter to measure tidal and minute volume from the number of revolutions of a vane rotated by the gas stream as the latter passes through 10 tangential slots in a cylindric stator ring to turn a flat two-bladed rotor; also called Wright spirometer.

re·sponse (rĕ-spons′). **1.** The reaction of a muscle, nerve, gland, or other excitable tissue to a stimulus. **2.** Any act or behavior, or its constituents, that a living organism is capable of emitting. Reflexes are usually excluded because they are typically elicited by a specifiable (unconditioned or natural) stimulus rather than emitted under circumstances in which the stimulus was not specifiable. [L. *responsus,* an answer]

acute phase r., SYN acute phase *reaction.*

anamnestic r. (an′am-nes-tik), SYN secondary immune r; SEE immune r.

auditory brainstem r. (ABR), an electrophysiologic measure of auditory function utilizing computer-averaged responses produced by the auditory nerve and the central auditory pathways principally in the brainstem to repetitive acoustic stimuli. ABR is also used to locate the lesion and determine the type of hearing impairment (sensory versus neural). SYN brainstem evoked r.

automatic auditory brainstem r., a technique of ABR in which the stimulus modification is programmed on the basis of the electrical responses recorded. The device determines automatically if predetermined thresholds have been achieved. It is useful in newborn hearing screening.

biphasic r., (1) two separate and distinct responses that are separated in time; **(2)** immediate reaction to an antigenic challenge followed by a recurrence of symptoms after an interval of quiescence.

blink r., a r. elicited during nerve conduction studies, consisting of muscle action potentials evoked from orbicularis oculi muscles after brief electric or mechanical stimuli to the cutaneous area supplied by the ophthalmic branch of the trigeminal nerve. Characteristically, there is an early r. (approximately 10 ms after stimulus) ipsilateral to the stimulation site (labeled R1) and bilateral late r.'s (approximately 30 ms after stimulus; labeled R2); the latter are responsible for the visible twitch of the orbicularis oculi muscles.

booster r., SYN secondary immune r; SEE immune r.

brainstem evoked r. (BSER), SYN auditory brainstem r.

conditioned r., a r. already in an individual's repertoire but which, through repeated pairings with its natural stimulus, has been acquired or conditioned anew to a previously neutral or conditioned stimulus. SEE conditioning; Cf. unconditioned r.

Cushing r., SYN Cushing *phenomenon.*

depletion r., subnormal metabolic r. to trauma in a person whose physiologic processes are already depressed by disease.

early-phase r., prompt onset of symptoms following an antigenic stimulus.

evoked r., an alteration in the electrical activity of a region of the nervous system through which an incoming sensory stimulus is passing; may be somatosensory (SER), brainstem auditory (BAER), or visual (VER). SEE ALSO evoked *potential.*

flight or fight r., SEE emergency *theory.*

galvanic skin r. (GSR), a measure of changes in emotional arousal recorded by attaching electrodes to any part of the skin and recording changes in moment-to-moment perspiration and related autonomic nervous system activity. SYN galvanic skin reaction, galvanic skin reflex, psychogalvanic reaction, psychogalvanic skin reaction, psychogalvanic reflex, psychogalvanic skin reflex, psychogalvanic r., psychogalvanic skin r.

Henry-Gauer r., inhibition of antidiuretic hormone secretion due to a rise in atrial pressure that stimulates atrial stretch receptors.

immune r., (1) any r. of the immune system to an antigen including antibody production and/or cell-mediated immunity; **(2)** the r. of the immune system to an antigen (immunogen) that leads to the condition of induced sensitivity; the immune r. to the initial antigenic exposure (primary immune r.) is detectable, as a rule, only after a lag period of from several days to 2 weeks; the immune r. to a subsequent stimulus (secondary immune r.) by the same antigen is more rapid than in the case of the primary immune r.

isomorphic r., a r. to trauma at sites of injury in previously uninvolved areas of patients with skin diseases such as psoriasis and lichen planus, typically with linear lesions at sites of scratching or a scar. SYN Köbner phenomenon.

late auditory-evoked r., r. of the auditory cortex to acoustic stimulation.

late-phase r., recurrence of symptoms after an appreciable interval following challenge with an antigen; preceded by an initial early-phase r.

level-dependent frequency r., one of several strategies used in hearing aids to alter the balance in amplification between high- and low-frequency sounds.

middle latency r., a r. to acoustic stimulation recorded from the auditory cortex of the brain.

myotonic r., failure of muscle relaxation caused by repetitive discharge of muscle fiber action potentials.

oculomotor r., widespread myogenic potential evoked by visual stimuli.

orienting r., SYN orienting *reflex.*

postural sway r., the body sway induced by vestibular stimulation.

primary immune r., SEE immune r.

psychogalvanic r. (PGR), psychogalvanic skin r., SYN galvanic skin r.

recruiting r., SYN recruitment (2).

relaxation r., an integrated hypothalamic reaction resulting in decreased sympathetic nervous system activity which, physiologically and psychologically, is almost a mirror image of the body's r.'s to Cannon emergency theory (flight or fight r.); can be self-induced through the use of techniques associated with transcendental meditation, yoga, and biofeedback. SEE ALSO emergency *theory.*

secondary immune r., SYN anamnestic r., booster r. SEE immune r.

sonomotor r., widespread myogenic potential evoked by click stimulation.

stringent r., the cellular response to amino acid starvation that reduces the amount of ribosomes to what can be employed under the nutrient conditions.

re

target r., SYN operant.

triple r., the triphasic r. to the firm stroking of the skin. Phase 1 is the sharply demarcated erythema that follows a momentary blanching of the skin and is the result of release of histamine from the mast cells. Phase 2 is the intense red flare extending beyond the margins of the line of pressure but in the same configuration, and is the result of arteriolar dilation; also called axon flare because it is mediated by axon reflex. Phase 3 is the appearance of a line wheal in the configuration of the original stroking.

unconditioned r., a r., such as salivation, which is a part of the animal or human repertoire. Cf. conditioned r.

rest. 1. Quiet; repose. [A.S. *raest*] 2. To repose; to cease from work. [A.S. *raestan*] 3. A group of cells or a portion of fetal tissue that has become displaced and lies embedded in tissue of another character. [L. *restare*, to remain] 4. In dentistry, an extension from a prosthesis that affords vertical support for a restoration.

adrenal r., SYN accessory *adrenal*.

bed r., maintenance of the recumbent position, in bed, to minimize activity and help recovery from disease; formerly used extensively in treatment of tuberculosis, myocardial infarction, and other diseases.

cingulum r., the rigid part of a removable partial denture supported by a prepared r. area on the cingulum of an anterior tooth or crown.

incisal r., the portion of a removable partial denture supported by an incisal edge.

lingual r., a metallic extension onto the lingual surface of a tooth to provide support or indirect retention for a removable partial denture.

Malassez epithelial r.'s, epithelial remains of Hertwig root sheath in the periodontal ligament.

Marchand r., SYN Marchand *adrenals*, under *adrenal*.

mesonephric r., SYN wolffian r.

occlusal r., a rigid extension of a removable partial denture onto the occlusal surface of a posterior tooth for support of the prosthesis.

precision r., a r. consisting of closely interlocking parts.

r.'s of Serres, remnants of dental lamina epithelium entrapped within the gingiva.

Walthard cell r., a nest of epithelial cells occurring in the peritoneum of the uterine tubes or ovary; when neoplastic, possibly comprising one of the components of the Brenner tumor.

wolffian r., remnants of the wolffian duct in the female genital tract that give rise to cysts; e.g., Gartner cyst. SYN mesonephric r.

re·ste·no·sis (rē'sten-ō-sis). Recurrence of stenosis after corrective surgery on the heart valve; narrowing of a structure (usually a coronary artery) following the removal or reduction of a previous narrowing. [re-, + G. *stenōsis*, a narrowing]

res·ti·form (res'ti-fōrm). Ropelike; rope-shaped; referring to the restiform body, the larger (lateral) part of the inferior cerebellar peduncle; contains fibers from the spinal cord (spinocerebellar) and medulla (cuneo-, olivo-, reticulocerebellar, etc.) to cerebellum. [L. *restis*, rope, + *forma*, form]

rest·i·tope (res'ti-tōp). The part of the T cell receptor that associates with the class II major histocompatibility molecule. [*restriction* + -tope]

res·ti·tu·tion (res-ti-too'shŭn). In obstetrics, the return of the rotated head of the fetus to its natural relation with the shoulders after its emergence from the vulva. [L. *restitutio*, act of restoring]

res·to·ra·tion (res-tō-rā'shŭn). In dentistry: 1. A prosthetic r. or appliance; a broad term applied to any inlay, crown, bridge, partial denture, or complete denture that restores or replaces lost tooth structure, teeth, or oral tissues. 2. A plug or stopping; any substance such as gold, amalgam, etc., used for restoring the portion missing from a tooth as a result of removing decay in the tooth. [L. *restauro*, pp. *-atus*, to restore, to repair]

acid-etched r., the r. of tooth structure with a resin after the surface of the tooth has been treated with an acid solution that etches the tooth surface, thereby increasing retention of the r.

combination r., a tooth r. of two or more materials applied in layers.

compound r., a r. of more than one surface of a tooth.

direct acrylic r., a direct resin r. of autopolymerizing acrylic.

direct composite resin r., SYN direct resin r.

direct resin r., a direct r. made by inserting a plastic mix of auto- or light-polymerized resins in a cavity prepared in a tooth. SYN direct composite resin r.

overhanging r., a r. with excessive material at the junction of the r. margin and the tooth.

permanent r., a definitive r., in contradistinction to a temporary or provisional r.

provisional r., SYN temporary r.

root canal r., a gutta-percha, silver, or plastic cone that has been carried into a root canal, either alone or in conjunction with a cement, paste, or solvent, for the purpose of obturating the canal space.

silicate r., restoration of lost tooth structure made with silicate cement.

temporary r., a r. to be used for a limited period of time, in contradistinction to a permanent r. SYN provisional r.

re·stor·a·tive (re-stōr'ă-tiv). 1. Renewing health and strength. 2. An agent that promotes a renewal of health or strength. [L. *restauro*, to restore]

re·straint (rē-strānt'). In hospital psychiatry, intervention to prevent an excited or violent patient from doing harm to self or others; may involve the use of a camisole (straightjacket). [O. Fr. *restrainte*]

re·stric·tion (rē-strik'shŭn). 1. The process with which foreign DNA that has been introduced into a prokaryotic cell becomes ineffective. 2. A limitation.

asymmetric fetal growth r., normal fetal head size as a result of preferential shunting of blood to brain, and decreased abdominal circumference from decreased adipose tissue and liver size; probably caused by placental insufficiency.

fetal growth r., fetal weight ≤5th percentile for gestational age. SYN intrauterine growth retardation.

lactase r., an inherited trait in which there is low lactase activity and thus there is defective lactose intestinal metabolism. Cf. lactase *persistence*.

MHC r., T helper cells only recognize an antigen that is presented with class II major histocompatibility antigens whereas T cytotoxic cells usually only recognize a processed antigen in conjunction with class I major histocompatibility antigens.

symmetric fetal growth r., proportional reduction in fetal head and body size, commonly constitutional or caused by an early intrauterine insult such as infection.

re·sus·ci·tate (rē-sŭs'i-tāt). To perform resuscitation. [L. *resuscito*, to raise up again, revive]

re·sus·ci·ta·tion (rē-sŭs'i-tā'shŭn). Revival from potential or apparent death. [L. *resuscitatio*]

cardiopulmonary r. (CPR), restoration of cardiac output and pulmonary ventilation following cardiac arrest and apnea, using artificial respiration and manual closed-chest compression or open-chest cardiac massage.

mouth-to-mouth r., mouth-to-mouth respiration (q.v.) employed as part of emergency cardiopulmonary r.

re·tain·er (rē-tān'er). Any type of clasp, attachment, or device used for the fixation or stabilization of a prosthesis; an appliance used to prevent the shifting of teeth following orthodontic treatment.

continuous bar r., a metal bar, usually resting on lingual surfaces of teeth, to aid in their stabilization and to act as indirect r.'s. SYN continuous clasp.

direct r., a clasp or attachment applied to an abutment tooth for the purpose of maintaining a removable appliance in position.

extracoronal r., a r. that depends upon contact with the outer circumference of the crown of a tooth for its retentive qualities.

Hawley r., a removable wire and acrylic palatal appliance used to retain or stabilize the teeth in their new position following orthodontic tooth movement; with modifications it can be used to move teeth as an active orthodontic appliance. SYN Hawley appliance.

indirect r., a part of a removable partial denture that assists the direct r.'s in preventing occlusal displacement of the distal extension bases by functioning through lever action on the opposite side of the fulcrum line.

intracoronal r., a r. that depends upon components placed within the crown portion of a tooth for its retentive qualities.

matrix r., a mechanical device designed to hold a matrix around a tooth during restorative procedures, usually by engaging the ends of the matrix band and drawing the band tight.

space r., SYN space *maintainer*.

re·tard·ate (rē-tahr′dāt). A mildly pejorative term, which is decreasing in usage, for a person who has mental retardation. [L. *retardo*, to delay, hinder]

re·tar·da·tion (rē-tahr-dā′shŭn). Slowness or limitation of development.

intrauterine growth r., SYN fetal growth *restriction*.

mental r., subaverage general intellectual functioning that originates during the developmental period and is associated with impairment in adaptive behavior. The American Association on Mental Deficiency lists eight medical classifications and five psychologic classifications; the latter five replace the three former classifications of moron, imbecile, and idiot. Mental r. classification requires assignment of an index for performance relative to a person's peers on two interrelated criteria: measured intelligence (IQ) and overall socioadaptive behavior (a judgmental rating of the individual's relative level of performance in school, at work, at home, and in the community). In general an IQ of 70 or below indicates mental retardation (mild = 50/55–70; moderate = 35/40–50/55; severe = 20/25–35/40; profound = below 20/25); an IQ of 70–85 signifies borderline intellectual functioning. SYN amentia (1), mental deficiency, oligophrenia.

psychomotor r., slowed psychic activity or motor activity, or both.

viscoelastic r., a technique for the measurement of the molecular weight of large DNA molecules; the DNA is stretched by hydrodynamic shear forces and, when the molecules relax, the relaxation time is measured.

re·tard·er (rē-tar′der). An agent used to slow the chemical hardening of gypsum, resins, or impression materials used in dentistry.

retch. To make an involuntary effort to vomit. [A.S. *hraecan*, to hawk]

retch·ing. Gastric and esophageal movements of vomiting without expulsion of vomitus. SYN dry vomiting, vomiturition.

re·te, pl. **re·tia** (rē′tē; rē′shē-ă, -tē-ă). **1.** SYN network (1). **2.** A structure composed of a fibrous network or mesh. [L. a net]

r. acromia′le arteriae thoracoacromialis [TA], SYN acromial *anastomosis* of the thoracoacromial artery.

r. arterio′sum [TA], SYN arterial *plexus*.

r. articula′re cu′biti [TA], SYN cubital *anastomosis*.

r. articula′re ge′nus [TA], SYN genicular *anastomosis*.

r. calca′neum [TA], SYN calcaneal *anastomosis*.

r. cana′lis hypoglos′si, SYN venous *plexus* of canal of hypoglossal nerve.

r. car′pale dorsa′le [TA], SYN dorsal carpal arterial *arch*.

r. car′pi poste′rius, SYN dorsal carpal arterial *arch*.

r. cuta′neum co′rii, the network of vessels parallel to the surface between the corium and the tela subcutanea.

r. foram′inis ova′lis, SYN venous *plexus* of foramen ovale.

Haller r., SYN r. testis.

r. halleri, SYN r. testis.

r. malleola′re latera′le [TA], SYN lateral malleolar *network*.

r. malleola′re media′le [TA], SYN medial malleolar *network*.

malpighian r., SYN malpighian *stratum*.

r. mirab′ile [TA], a vascular network interrupting the continuity of an artery or vein, such as occurs in the glomeruli of the kidney (arterial) or in the liver (venous).

r. ova′rii, a transient network of cells in the developing ovary; homologous to the r. testis.

r. patella′re [TA], SYN patellar *anastomosis*.

r. subpapilla′re, the network of vessels between the papillary and reticular strata of the corium.

r. tes′tis [TA], the network of canals at the termination of the straight tubules in the mediastinum testis. SYN Haller r., r. halleri.

r. vasculosum articula′re [TA], SYN articular vascular *plexus*.

r. veno′sum dorsa′le ma′nus [TA], SYN dorsal venous *network* of hand.

r. veno′sum dorsa′le pe′dis [TA], SYN dorsal venous *network* of foot.

r. veno′sum planta′re [TA], SYN plantar venous *network*.

re·ten·tion (rē-ten′shŭn). **1.** The keeping in the body of what normally belongs there, especially the retaining of food and drink in the stomach. **2.** The keeping in the body of what normally should be discharged, as urine or feces. **3.** Retaining that which has been learned so that it can be utilized later as in recall, recognition, or, if r. is partial, relearning. SEE ALSO memory. **4.** Resistance to dislodgement. **5.** In dentistry, a passive period following treatment when a patient is wearing an appliance or appliances to maintain or stabilize the teeth in the new position into which they have been moved. [L. *retentio*, a holding back]

denture r., the means by which dentures are held in position in the mouth.

direct r., r. obtained in a removable partial denture by the use of attachments or clasps that resist their removal from the abutment teeth.

indirect r., r. obtained in a removable partial denture through the use of indirect retainers.

partial denture r., the fixation of a removable partial denture by the use of clasps, indirect retainers, or precision attachments.

re·tia (rē′shē-ă, -tē-ă). Plural of rete. [L.]

re·ti·al (rē′shē-ăl). Relating to a rete.

reticul-. SEE reticulo-.

re·tic·u·la (re-tik′ū-lă). Plural of reticulum. [L.]

re·tic·u·lar, re·tic·u·lated (re-tik′ū-lăr, -lāt-ed). Relating to a reticulum.

re·tic·u·la·tion (re-tik-ū-lā′shŭn). The presence or formation of a reticulum or network, such as that observed in the red blood cells during active regeneration of blood. Also used to describe a chest radiographic pattern. SEE reticulonodular *pattern*.

re·tic·u·lin (re-tik′ū-lin). Name given to the chemical substance of reticular fibers, which once were thought to be distinct from collagen by reason of their distinctive structure and staining properties but are now regarded as type III collagen (with its associated proteoglygans and structural glycoproteins).

reticulo-, reticul-. Reticulum; reticular. [L. *reticulum*, a small net, dim. of *rete*, a net]

re·tic·u·lo·cyte (re-tik′ū-lō-sīt). A young red blood cell containing a basophilic cytoplasmic network precipitated by brilliant cresyl blue representing residual polyribosomes; such cells become more numerous during the process of active blood regeneration. SEE ALSO erythroblast. SYN reticulated corpuscle, skein cell. [reticulo- + G. *kytos*, cell]

re·tic·u·lo·cy·to·pe·nia (re-tik′ū-lō-sī-tō-pē′nē-ă). Paucity of reticulocytes in the blood. SYN reticulopenia. [reticulocyte + G. *penia*, poverty]

re·tic·u·lo·cy·to·sis (re-tik′ū-lō-sī-tō′sis). An increase in the number of circulating reticulocytes above the normal, which is less than 1% of the total number of red blood cells; it occurs during active blood regeneration (stimulation of red bone marrow) and in certain anemias, especially congenital hemolytic anemia. [reticulocyte + G. *osis*, condition]

re·tic·u·lo·en·do·the·li·al (re-tik′ū-lō-en-dō-thē′lē-ăl). Denoting or referring to reticuloendothelium. SEE reticuloendothelial *system*.

re·tic·u·lo·en·do·the·li·o·ma (re-tik′ū-lō-en′dō-thē-lē-ō′mă). Obsolete term for a localized reticulosis, or neoplasm derived from reticuloendothelial tissue. [reticuloendothelium + G. *-oma*, tumor]

re·tic·u·lo·en·do·the·li·um (re-tik′ū-lō-en-dō-thē′lē-ŭm). The cells making up the reticuloendothelial system. [reticulo- + endothelium]

re·tic·u·lo·his·ti·o·cy·to·ma (re-tik′ū-lō-his′tē-ō-sī-tō′mă). A solitary skin nodule composed of glycolipid-containing multinu-

re

cleated large histiocytes; multiple lesions sometimes occur in association with arthritis. [reticulo- + histiocytoma]

re·tic·u·lo·his·ti·o·cy·to·sis (re-tik′u-lō-his′tē-ō-sī-tō′sis). SEE reticulosis.

multicentric r., a rare disease in which cutaneous papules composed of histiocytes containing glycolipids are associated with polyarthritis, often leading to shortening of the fingers.

re·tic·u·loid (re-tik′u-loyd). **1.** Resembling a reticulosis. **2.** A condition resembling reticulosis.

actinic r., chronic pruritic erythema beginning on sun-exposed areas in elderly males, with marked thickening and ridging of exposed skin simulating lymphoma; there is infiltration by atypical CD8-positive T lymphocytes.

re·tic·u·lo·pe·nia (re-tik′u-lō-pē′nē-ă). SYN reticulocytopenia.

re·tic·u·lo·sis (re-tik-u-lō′sis). An increase in histiocytes, monocytes, or other reticuloendothelial elements. [reticulo- + G. -osis, condition]

benign inoculation r., SYN catscratch *disease*.

leukemic r., obsolete term for monocytic leukemia.

malignant midline r., obsolete term for polymorphic r.

midline malignant reticulosis r., SYN lethal midline *granuloma*.

pagetoid r., a usually solitary verrucous plaque on the extremities characterized histologically by predominantly epidermal infiltration of mononuclear cells resembling those found in mycosis fungoides; prognosis is good. SYN Woringer-Kolopp disease.

polymorphic r., a necrotizing lymphoproliferative lesion with a predilection for the upper respiratory tract; previously called lethal midline granuloma or malignant midline reticulosis; treatment is irradiation.

re·tic·u·lo·spi·nal (re-tik-u-lō-spī′năl). Pertaining to the reticulospinal *tract*.

re·tic·u·lot·o·my (rē-tik-u-lot′ō-mē). Production of lesions in the reticular formation. [reticulo- + G. *tomē,* incision]

re·tic·u·lum, pl. **re·tic·u·la** (re-tik′u-lŭm, -lă) [TA]. **1.** A fine network formed by cells, or formed of certain structures within cells or of connective tissue fibers between cells. **2.** SYN neuroglia. **3.** The second compartment of the stomach of a ruminant, a comparatively small chamber communicating with the rumen; sometimes called the honeycomb because of the characteristic structure of its wall. [L. dim of *rete,* a net]

agranular endoplasmic r., endoplasmic r. that is lacking in ribosomal granules; involved in synthesis of complex lipids and fatty acids, detoxification of drugs, carbohydrate synthesis, and sequestering of Ca^{++}. SYN smooth-surfaced endoplasmic r.

Ebner r., a network of nucleated cells in the seminiferous tubules.

endoplasmic r. (ER), the network of cytoplasmic tubules or flattened sacs (cisternae) with (rough ER) or without (smooth ER) ribosomes on the surface of their membranes in eukaryotes. SYN endomembrane system.

Golgi internal r., SYN Golgi *apparatus.*

granular endoplasmic r., endoplasmic r. in which ribosomal granules are applied to the cytoplasmic surface of the cisternae; involved in the synthesis and secretion of protein via membrane-bound vesicles to the extracellular space. SYN chromidial substance, ergastoplasm, rough-surfaced endoplasmic r.

Kölliker r., SYN neuroglia.

rough-surfaced endoplasmic r., SYN granular endoplasmic r.

sarcoplasmic r., the endoplasmic r. of skeletal and cardiac muscle; the complex of vesicles, tubules, and cisternae forming a continuous structure around striated myofibrils, with a repetition of structure within each sarcomere.

smooth-surfaced endoplasmic r., SYN agranular endoplasmic r.

stellate r., a network of epithelial cells disposed in a fluid-filled compartment in the center of the enamel organ between the outer and inner enamel epithelium.

trabecular r., SYN trabecular *tissue* of sclera.

r. trabecula′re sclerae [TA], SYN trabecular *tissue* of sclera.

trans-Golgi r., that part of the Golgi apparatus that takes newly processed proteins and delivers them to secretory vesicles that will fuse with other biomembranes (e.g., the plasma membrane).

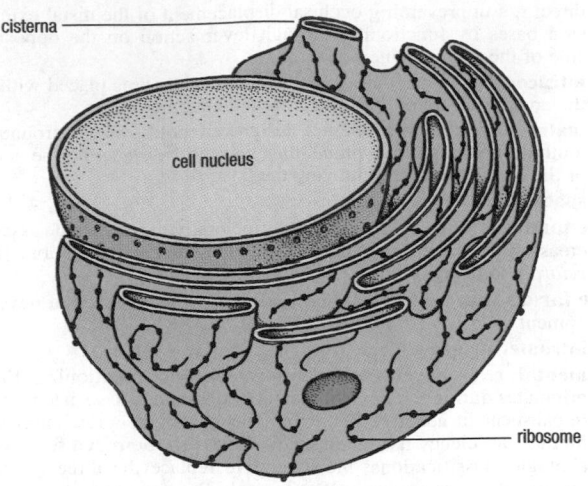

cisterna

cell nucleus

ribosome

granular endoplasmic reticulum

ret·i·form (ret′i-fōrm). Resembling a net or network. [L. *rete,* network]

retin-. SEE retino-.

ret·i·na (ret′i-nă) [TA]. Grossly, the r. consists of three parts: optic part of retina, ciliary part of retina, and iridial part of retina. The optic part, the physiologic portion that receives the visual light rays, is further divided into two parts, the pigmented part (pigment epithelium) and the nervous part, which are arranged in the following layers: 1) pigmented layer; 2) layer of inner and outer segments (of rods and cones); 3) outer limiting layer (actually a row of junctional complexes); 4) outer nuclear layer; 5) outer plexiform layer; 6) inner nuclear layer; 7) inner plexiform layer; 8) ganglionic (cell) layer; 9) layer of nerve fibers; and 10) inner limiting layer. Layers 2–10 compose the neural layer. At the posterior pole of the visual axis is the macula, in the center of which is the fovea, the area of acute vision. Here layers 6–9 and blood vessels are absent, and only elongated cones are present. About 3 mm medial to the fovea is the optic disk, where axons of the ganglionic cells converge to form the optic nerve. The ciliary and iridial parts of the r. are forward prolongations of the pigmented layer and a layer of supporting columnar or epithelial cells over the ciliary body and the posterior surface of the iris, respectively. SYN optomeninx. [Mediev. L. prob. fr. L. *rete,* a net]

detached r., SYN retinal *detachment.*

flecked r., an r. exhibiting fundus flavimaculatus, hereditary drusen, or fundus albipunctatus.

fleck r. of Kandori [MIM*228990], an autosomal recessive disorder of the retinal pigment epithelium characterized by retinal flecks and night blindness, occurring among Japanese.

leopard r., SYN tessellated *fundus.*

shot-silk r., the appearance of numerous wavelike, glistening reflexes, like the shimmer of silk, observed sometimes in the r. of a young person. SYN shot-silk phenomenon, shot-silk reflex.

tigroid r., SYN tessellated *fundus.*

ret·i·nac·u·lum, gen. **ret·i·nac·u·li,** pl. **ret·i·nac·u·la** (ret-i-nak′u-lŭm, -lī, -lă) [TA]. A frenum, or a retaining band or ligament. [L. a band, a halter, fr. *retineo,* to hold back]

antebrachial flexor r., thickening of distal antebrachial fascia just proximal to radiocarpal (wrist) joint. Continuous with extensor r. at margins of forearm. This structure is distinct from the transverse carpal *ligament,* commonly called "the flexor retinaculum," which forms the roof of the carpal tunnel. SYN flexor r. of forearm, palmar carpal ligament.

r. of articular capsule of hip, one of several longitudinal folds of the articular capsule of the hip joint reflected onto the femoral neck deep to which the retinacular branches of the medial femoral circumflex artery pass to reach the femoral head. SYN r. capsulae articularis coxae, Weitbrecht fibers.

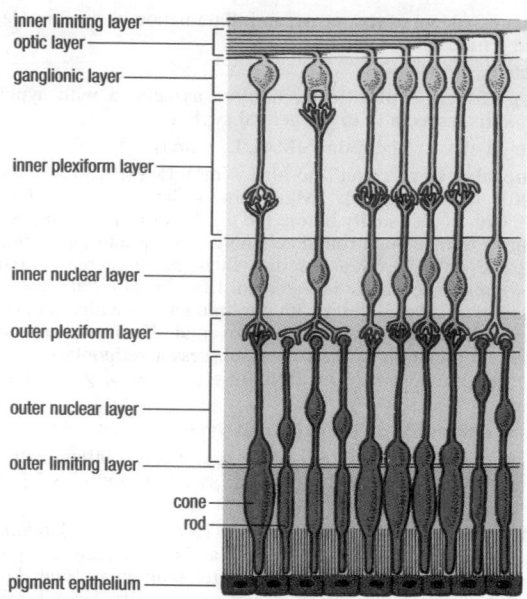

inner limiting layer
optic layer
ganglionic layer
inner plexiform layer
inner nuclear layer
outer plexiform layer
outer nuclear layer
outer limiting layer
cone
rod
pigment epithelium

layers of the retina

r. cap'sulae articula'ris cox'ae, SYN r. of articular capsule of hip.

caudal r., SYN r. caudale.

r. cauda'le [TA], fibrous bands, remnants of the notochord, that extend from the skin to the coccyx, forming the coccygeal foveola. SYN caudal ligament, caudal r., ligamentum caudale.

r. cu'tis [TA], SYN skin ligaments, under ligament.

r. cutis mammae, ✭official alternate term for suspensory ligaments of breast, under ligament.

extensor r. [TA], a strong fibrous band formed as a thickening of the antebrachial deep fascia, stretching obliquely across the back of the wrist, attaching deeply to ridges on the dorsal aspect of the radius, triquetral, and pisiform bones, and binding down the extensor tendons of the fingers and thumb. SYN r. musculorum extensorum [TA], dorsal carpal ligament, ligamentum carpi dorsale.

retinacula of extensor muscles, SEE inferior extensor r., superior extensor r.

flexor r. [TA], a strong fibrous band crossing the front of the carpus and binding down the flexor tendons of the digits and the flexor carpi radialis tendon and the median nerve; in so doing it creates the carpal tunnel. SYN r. musculorum flexorum [TA], deep part of flexor retinaculum, ligamentum carpi transversum, ligamentum carpi volare, transverse carpal ligament, volar carpal ligament.

flexor r. of forearm, SYN antebrachial flexor r.

flexor r. of lower limb [TA], a wide band passing from the medial malleolus to the medial and upper border of the calcaneus and to the plantar surface as far as the navicular bone; it holds in place the tendons of the tibialis posterior, flexor digitorum longus, and flexor hallucis longus. SYN r. musculorum flexorum membri inferioris [TA], laciniate ligament, ligamentum laciniatum, r. of flexor muscles.

r. of flexor muscles, SYN flexor r. of lower limb.

inferior extensor r. [TA], a Y-shaped ligament restraining the extensor tendons of the foot distal to the ankle joint. SYN r. musculorum extensorum inferius [TA], cruciate ligament of leg, inferior r. of extensor muscles, ligamentum cruciatum cruris.

inferior r. of extensor muscles, SYN inferior extensor r.

inferior fibular r. [TA], broad thickened band of deep fascia overlying fibularis longus and brevis tendons as they pass along the lateral margin of the foot, anchoring the tendons and their associated bursae in place; it is a lateral continuation of the stem of the Y-shaped inferior extensor retinaculum which attaches to

the fibular trochlea of the calcaneus (which intervenes between the two tendons) and then continues to attach to the inferolateral aspect of the calcaneous. SYN r. musculorum fibularium inferius [TA], inferior peroneal r.✭, r. musculorum peroneorum inferius✭.

inferior peroneal r., ✭official alternate term for inferior fibular r.

lateral patellar r. [TA], part of the aponeurosis of the vastus lateralis muscle passing lateral to the patella to attach to the tibial tuberosity. SYN r. patellae laterale [TA].

medial patellar r. [TA], part of the aponeurosis of the vastus medialis muscle passing medial to the patella to attach to the medial condyle of the tibia, forming the anteromedial aspect of the fibrous capsule of the knee joint. SYN r. patellae mediale [TA].

Morgagni r., SYN frenulum of ileal orifice.

r. musculorum extenso'rum [TA], SYN extensor r.

r. musculo'rum extenso'rum infe'rius [TA], SYN inferior extensor r.

r. musculo'rum extenso'rum supe'rius [TA], SYN superior extensor r.

r. musculo'rum fibula'rium, SYN peroneal r.

r. musculorum fibularium inferius [TA], SYN inferior fibular r.

r. musculorum fibularium superius [TA], SYN superior fibular r.

r. musculorum flexo'rum [TA], SYN flexor r.

r. musculo'rum flexo'rum membri inferioris [TA], SYN flexor r. of lower limb.

r. musculo'rum peroneo'rum, SYN peroneal r.

retinacula of nail, fibrous attachments of the nail-bed to the underlying phalanx. SYN retinacula unguis.

r. patel'lae latera'le [TA], SYN lateral patellar r.

r. patel'lae media'le [TA], SYN medial patellar r.

patellar r., extensions of the aponeuroses of the vasti medialis and lateralis muscles that pass on each side of the patella, attaching to the margins of the patella and patellar ligament anteriorly, the collateral ligaments posteriorly, and the tibial condyles distally; form the anteromedial and (with the fibrous expansion of the iliotibial tract) the anteromedial portions of the fibrous capsule of the knee. SEE lateral patellar r., medial patellar r.

peroneal r., superior and inferior fibrous bands retaining the tendons of the peroneus longus and brevis in position as they cross the lateral side of the ankle. SYN retinacula of peroneal muscles, r. musculorum fibularium, r. musculorum peroneorum.

r. musculorum peroneorum inferius, ✭official alternate term for inferior fibular r.

r. musculorum peroneorum superius, ✭official alternate term for superior fibular r.

retinacula of peroneal muscles, SYN peroneal r.

r. of skin, SYN skin ligaments, under ligament.

superior extensor r. [TA], the ligament that binds down the extensor tendons proximal to the ankle joint; it is continuous with (a thickening of) the deep fascia of the leg. SYN r. musculorum extensorum superius [TA], ligamentum transversum cruris, superior r. of extensor muscles, transverse crural ligament, transverse ligament of leg.

superior r. of extensor muscles, SYN superior extensor r.

superior fibular r. [TA], SYN r. musculorum fibularium superius [TA], r. musculorum peroneorum superius✭, superior peroneal r.✭.

superior peroneal r., ✭official alternate term for superior fibular r.

suspensory r. of breast, ✭official alternate term for suspensory ligaments of breast, under ligament.

r. ten'dinum, a ligamentous structure to restrain tendons, such as the flexor or extensor retinacula, or the annular parts of the digital fibrous sheaths.

retinac'ula un'guis, SYN retinacula of nail.

ret·i·nal (ret'i-nal). **1.** Relating to the retina. **2.** Retinaldehyde; most commonly referring to the all-trans form.

r. dehydrogenase, an oxidoreductase catalyzing the interconversion of retinaldehyde and NAD⁺ to retinoic acid and NADH, thus affecting growth and differentiation. SYN retinaldehyde dehydrogenase.

r. isomerase, an isomerase that catalyzes the *cis-trans*-interconversion of all-*trans*-retinal to 11-*cis*-retinal(dehyde); a part of the vision cycle. SYN retinaldehyde isomerase.

r. reductase, alcohol dehydrogenase (NAD(P)⁺).

11-*cis*-ret·i·nal. The isomer of retinaldehyde that can combine with opsin to form rhodopsin; it is formed from 11-*trans*-retinal by retinal isomerase. SYN neoretinal b.

***trans*-ret·i·nal.** SYN all-*trans*-retinal.

ret·i·nal·de·hyde (ret-i-nal'dĕ-hīd). Retinol oxidized to a terminal aldehyde; retinal; a carotene released (as all-*trans*-retinal) in the bleaching of rhodopsin by light and the dissociation of opsin in the vision cycle. SYN retinene-1, retinene, vitamin A aldehyde.

r. dehydrogenase, SYN *retinal* dehydrogenase.

r. isomerase, SYN *retinal* isomerase.

r. reductase, alcohol dehydrogenase (NAD(P)⁺).

ret·i·nec·to·my (ret'in-ek'tō-mē). A surgical excision of a piece of the retina.

ret·i·nene (ret'i-nēn). SYN retinaldehyde.

ret·i·nene-1. SYN retinaldehyde.

ret·i·nene-2. SYN dehydroretinaldehyde.

ret·i·ni·tis (ret-i-nī'tis). Inflammation of the retina. [retina + G. -*itis,* inflammation]

albuminuric r., SEE hypertensive *retinopathy.*

circinate r., SEE circinate *retinopathy.*

diabetic r., SEE diabetic *retinopathy.*

exudative r., r. exudati'va, a chronic abnormality characterized by deposition of cholesterol and cholesterol esters in outer retinal layers and subretinal space. In adults, often preceded by uveitis; in children, often preceded by retinal vascular abnormalities. SYN Coats disease.

leukemic r., SEE leukemic *retinopathy.*

metastatic r., purulent or septic r. resulting from the arrest of septic emboli in the retinal vessels. SYN purulent r., septic r.

r. pigmento'sa, a progressive retinal degeneration characterized by bilateral nyctalopia, constricted visual fields, electroretinogram abnormalities, and pigmentary infiltration of the inner retinal layers; may be sporadic or demonstrate autosomal dominant [MIM*180100], autosomal recessive, or X-linked inheritance [MIM*268000, *312600, *312610]. SYN pigmentary retinopathy.

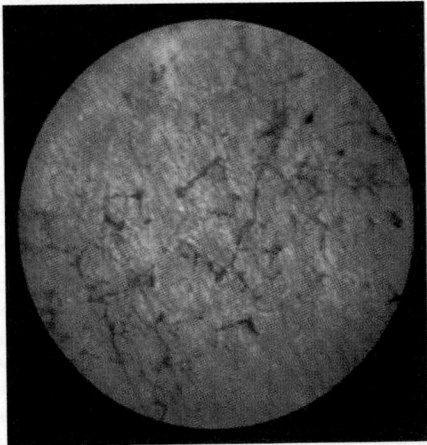

retinitis pigmentosa (advanced stage)

r. prolif'erans, SYN proliferative *retinopathy.*

punctate r., SEE *retinopathy* punctata albescens.

purulent r., SYN metastatic r.

r. sclopeta'ria, a severe contusion lesion of the retina, as from a shot pellet or BB. [from *sclopetum,* a medieval handgun]

secondary r., r. that follows uveal inflammation.

septic r., SYN metastatic r.

serous r., edema of the retina; an inflammation of the inner layers of the retina. SYN simple r.

simple r., SYN serous r.

r. syphilit'ica, syphilitic r., r. often associated with syphilitic choroiditis, especially in congenital syphilis.

△**retino-, retin-.** The retina. [Med. L. *retina*]

ret·i·no·blas·to·ma (ret'i-nō-blas-tō'mǎ) [MIM*180200, MIM* 180201, MIM*180202]. Malignant ocular neoplasm of childhood, with onset usually before the third year of life, composed of primitive retinal small round cells with deeply staining nuclei and elongated cells forming rosettes; there is an increased risk of developing osteosarcoma later in life. In familial cases, the disease is usually bilateral with multiple lesions within an eye, but in sporadic cases rarely so. Autosomal dominant inheritance caused by mutation in the tumor-suppressor retinoblastoma gene (RB) on chromosome 13q. [retino- + G. *blastos,* germ, + -*oma,* tumor]

ret·i·no·cho·roid (ret'i-nō-kō'royd). SYN chorioretinal.

ret·i·no·cho·roid·i·tis (ret'i-nō-kō-roy-dī'tis). Inflammation of the retina extending to the choroid. SYN chorioretinitis. [retinochoroid + G. -*itis,* inflammation]

bird shot r., bilateral diffuse retinal vasculitis with depigmentation of multiple areas of the choroid and retinal pigment epithelium posterior to the ocular equator, often with an associated papillitis or optic atrophy; vitiligo occurs occasionally. SYN vitiliginous choroiditis.

r. juxtapapilla'ris, r. close to the optic disk. SYN Jensen disease.

ret·i·no·di·al·y·sis (ret'i-nō-dī-al'i-sis). SYN *dialysis* retinae. [retino- + G. *dialysis,* separation]

ret·i·no·ic ac·id (ret-i-nō'ik). Vitamin A₁ acid; retinal in which the terminal –CHO has been oxidized to a –COOH; used topically in the treatment of acne; plays an important role in growth and differentiation. SYN vitamin A₁ acid.

13-*cis*-r. a., the retinoid most used in the U.S. to treat acne; it works by reducing sebum secretion. Use in pregnancy is contraindicated because of teratogenicity.

ret·i·noid (ret'i-noyd). **1.** Resembling a resin; resinous. [G. *rētinē,* resin, + *eidos,* resemblance] **2.** Resembling the retina. [Mediev. L. *retina*] **3.** In plural form, term used to describe the natural forms and synthetic analogs of retinol.

ret·i·noids (ret'i-noydz). A class of keratolytic drugs derived from retinoic acid and used for treatment of severe acne and psoriasis.

ret·i·nol (ret'i-nol). A half-carotene bearing the β (or β-ionone) form of the cyclic end group and a CH₂OH at the C-15 position (numbering as in carotenoids) or 9′-position (numbering as a nonyl side chain on a cyclohexene ring); an intermediate in the vision cycle, it also plays a role in growth and differentiation. SEE ALSO dehydroretinol. SYN vitamin A₁ alcohol, vitamin A₁.

r. dehydrogenase, an oxidoreductase catalyzing interconversion of retinal and NADH to retinol and NAD⁺.

11-*cis*-ret·i·nol. Retinol with *cis* configuration at the 11-position (carotenoid numbering) or 5′-position (retinol numbering) of the side chain; an intermediate in the vision cycle. SYN neoretinene B.

ret·i·no·pap·il·li·tis (ret'i-nō-pap-i-lī'tis). Inflammation of the retina extending to the optic disk.

r. of premature infants, SYN *retinopathy* of prematurity.

ret·i·nop·a·thy (ret-i-nop'ă-thē). Noninflammatory degenerative disease of the retina. [retino- + G. *pathos,* suffering]

arteriosclerotic r., r. distinguished by attenuated retinal arterioles with increased tortuosity, copper- or silver-wire appearance, perivascular sheathing, irregularity of lumen and scattered small hemorrhages, and small, sharp-edged deposits without surrounding edema.

central angiospastic r., SYN central serous *choroidopathy.*

central serous r., SYN central serous *choroidopathy.*

circinate r., a retinal degeneration marked by a girdle of sharply defined white exudates around an edematous macula; usually bilateral and typically affects the aged.

compression r., (1) SEE Berlin *edema.* SEE traumatic r.

diabetic r., retinal changes occurring in diabetes mellitus, marked by microaneurysms, exudates, and hemorrhages, and sometimes by neovascularization. SYN fundus diabeticus.

> Diabetic eye disease is responsible for approximately 25% of all newly reported cases of blindness in the U.S. The principal form is nonproliferative retinopathy, which results directly from degenerative changes in retinal capillaries. Features of this disorder, as observed on funduscopic examination, include microaneurysms; soft or cotton-wool exudates, which are actually areas of microinfarction; hard or waxy exudates, which are deposits of lipid and protein from leaking capillaries; and flame hemorrhages. A few patients, principally those with type 1 diabetes, develop a proliferative retinopathy characterized by neovascularization (proliferation of new capillary loops on the retinal surface). Either type of retinopathy can impair vision by destroying retinal tissue directly and by predisposing to retinal edema, retinal detachment, and vitreous hemorrhage. Controlled clinical studies have shown that maintaining blood glucose levels as near as possible to normal at all times in persons with diabetes mellitus substantially retards the onset and rate of progression of retinopathy. Laser photocoagulation is effective in arresting neovascularization in proliferative diabetic retinopathy.

dysproteinemic r., retinal venous congestion due to increased blood viscosity in dysproteinemia.

electric r., SYN photoretinopathy.

external exudative r., SEE exudative *retinitis.*

hypertensive r., a retinal condition occurring in accelerated vascular hypertension, marked by arteriolar constriction, flame-shaped hemorrhages, cotton-wool patches, star-figure edema at the macula, and papilledema.

Leber idiopathic stellate r., SEE neuroretinitis.

leukemic r., appearance of the retina in all types of leukemia, characterized by engorgement and tortuosity of veins, scattered hemorrhages, and edema of the retina and disk.

lipemic r., a milkiness of the retinal vessels (lipemia retinalis) combined with hard-edged fatty exudates, seen in patients with diabetic acidosis and hyperlipemia.

macular r., SYN maculopathy.

pigmentary r., SYN *retinitis* pigmentosa.

r. of prematurity, abnormal replacement of the sensory retina by fibrous tissue and blood vessels, occurring mainly in premature infants having a birth weight of less than 1500 g who are placed in a high-oxygen environment. SYN retinopapillitis of premature infants, retrolental fibroplasia, Terry syndrome.

proliferative r., neovascularization of the retina extending into the vitreous humor. SYN retinitis proliferans.

r. puncta′ta al′bescens [MIM*136880], a disease in which both fundi show numerous white dots or flecks through the retinae, causing night blindness; autosomal dominant inheritance, caused by mutation in the "retinal degeneration, slow" gene (RDS) encoding peripherin on chromosome 6p. There is also a recessive form [MIM*210370].

Purtscher r., transient traumatic retinal angiopathy due to a sudden rise in venous pressure, as in compression of the body from seat belt injury; ocular fundi show large white patches associated with the retinal veins about the disk or macula, hemorrhages, and retinal edema; thought to be due to fat embolism from bone marrow. SYN Purtscher disease, transient r., traumatic r.

renal r., hypertensive r. associated with chronic glomerulonephritis or nephrosclerosis.

rubella r., peripheral pigmentary retinal changes in congenital rubella, not affecting visual function.

sickle cell r., a condition marked by dilation and tortuosity of retinal veins and by microaneurysms and retinal hemorrhages; advanced stages may show neovascularization, vitreous hemorrhage, or retinal detachment.

solar r., SYN photoretinopathy.

toxemic r. of pregnancy, sudden angiospasm of retinal arterioles, later followed by retinal vascular signs of advanced hypertensive

r.; vascular changes disappear rapidly after termination of the pregnancy.

toxic r., retinal changes due to prolonged administration of various drugs.

transient r., SYN Purtscher r.

traumatic r., SYN Purtscher r.

venous-stasis r., a uniocular retinopathy associated with occlusion of the central retinal vein; a nonischemic central retinal vein occlusion.

whiplash r., an injury to the retina caused by a sudden acceleration/deceleration injury.

ret·i·no·pexy (ret′i-nō-pek′sē). A procedure to repair a detached retina by holding it in place; e.g., by producing chorioretinal adhesions by freezing ("retinal cryopexy"). [retino- + G. *pēxis,* fixation]

fluid r., a procedure to repair a detached retina by holding it in place with a fluid that is heavier than vitreous fluid.

gas r., a retinal detachment repair in which the retina is held in place by an expandable gas. SYN pneumatic r.

pneumatic r., SYN gas r.

ret·i·no·pi·e·sis (ret′i-nō-pī-ē′sis). Repositioning a detached retina by pressing it into position by gas or fluid. SEE retinopexy. [retino- + G. *piesis,* pressure]

ret·i·nos·chi·sis (ret-i-nos′ki-sis). Degenerative splitting of the retina, with cyst formation between the two layers. [retino- + G. *schisis,* division]

juvenile r. [MIM*268100], r. occurring before 10 years of age and within the nerve-fiber layer, with frequent macular involvement; at first, the inner wall is a translucent veil-like membrane, but it becomes more dense and may render the retina white; autosomal recessive inheritance. There is a form of this condition in middle age that is X-linked [MIM*312700] and a rare autosomal dominant form [MIM*180270].

senile r., r. occurring most often in the elderly and affecting the outer plexiform layer; it begins in the extreme inferotemporal periphery and is not significantly progressive; vision usually is good.

ret·i·no·scope (ret′i-nō-skōp). An optical device used to illuminate a subject's retina during retinoscopy. [retino- + G. *skopeō,* to view]

luminous r., a portable optical device providing either a circular or linear (streak) beam of light.

reflecting r., a plane or concave mirror with a central perforation that allows the observer to see rays emerge from the subject's eye.

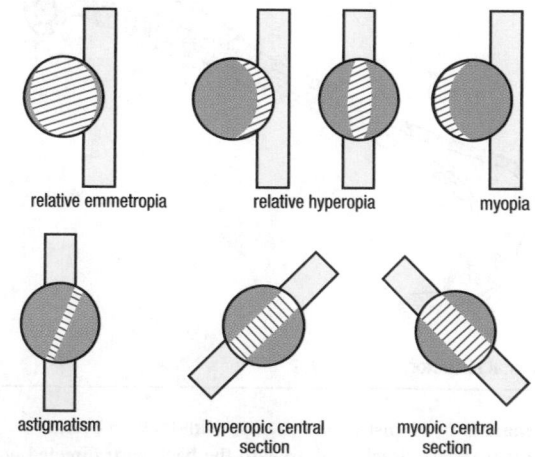

retinoscopy: characteristic appearances of light in pupil (*bars* represent light bands of retinoscope)

ret·i·nos·co·py (ret′i-nos′kŏ-pē). A method of determining errors of refraction by illuminating the retina and observing the rays of

re

light emerging from the eye. SYN scotoscopy, shadow test, skiascopy. [retino- + G. *skopeō,* to view]

cylinder r., determination of spherical, astigmatic, and refractive error using cylindric lenses.

fogging r., the method of reducing vision with convex lenses until accommodation is suspended; a static, noncycloplegic technique.

ret·i·not·o·my (ret′in-ot′ō-mē). A surgical incision through the retina.

ret·i·nyl phos·phate (ret′i-nil fos′fāt). The phosphoester of all-*trans*-retinol; essential for the biosynthesis of certain glycoproteins needed for growth regulation and for mucous secretion.

ret·o·per·i·the·li·um (rē′to-per-i-thē′lē-ŭm). The reticular cells related to the reticular fiber network, as in the stroma of lymphatic tissue. [L. *rete,* net, + G. *peri,* around, + Mod. L. *thelium,* fr. G. *thēlē,* nipple]

re·tort (rē-tōrt′). **1.** A flasklike vessel with a long neck passing outward, once used in distilling. **2.** A small furnace. [Mediev. L. *retorta,* fem. pp. of *retorqueo,* pp. *-tortus,* to twist or bend back]

Re·tor·tam·o·nas (rē-tōr-tam′ō-nas). A genus of protozoan flagellates, one species of which, *R. intestinalis,* is found occasionally in the human intestine, although it is nonpathogenic and infrequently reported. [L. *re-torqueo,* to twist back, + G. *monas,* single, a unit]

re·tract (rē-trakt′). To shrink, draw back, or pull apart. [L. *re-traho,* pp. *-tractus,* a drawing back]

re·trac·tile (rē-trak′til). Retractable; capable of being drawn back.

re·trac·tion (rē-trak′shŭn). **1.** A shrinking, drawing back, or pulling apart. **2.** Posterior movement of teeth, usually with the aid of an orthodontic appliance. [L. *retractio,* a drawing back]

gingival r., (1) lateral movement of the gingival margin away from the tooth surface; may be indicative of underlying inflammation or pocket formation; (2) displacement of the marginal gingivae away from the tooth by mechanical, chemical, or surgical means.

mandibular r., a type of facial anomaly in which the gnathion lies posterior to the orbital plane.

re·trac·tor (rē-trak′ter, -tōr). **1.** An instrument for drawing aside the edges of a wound or for holding back structures adjacent to the operative field. **2.** A muscle that draws a part backward, e.g., the middle part of the trapezius muscle is a r. of the scapula; the horizontal fibers of the temporalis muscle serve to retract the mandible.

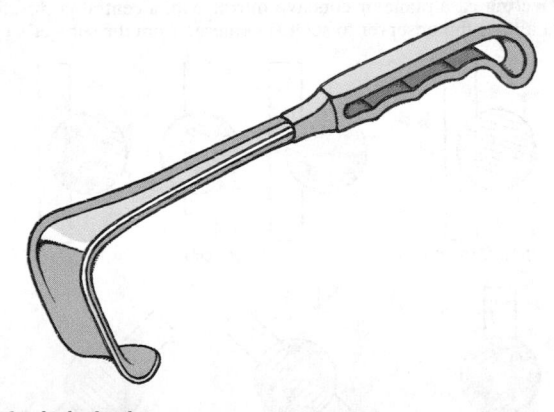

abdominal retractor

Desmarres r., an instrument used to withdraw an eyelid.

re·trad (rē′trad). Backward; toward the back part; directed posteriorly. [L. *retro,* backward, + *ad,* to]

re·tra·hens au·rem, re·tra·hens au·ric·u·lam (rēt′rǎ-henz aw′rem, aw-rik′ū-lam). SEE auricularis posterior (*muscle*). [L. drawing back the ear, or auricle]

re·treat from re·al·i·ty. Substitution of imaginary satisfactions or fantasy for relations with the real world.

re·trench·ment (rē-trench′-ment). The cutting away of superfluous tissue. [F. *re-,* back, + *trancher,* to cut]

re·triev·al (rē-trē′văl). The third stage in the memory process, after encoding and storage, involving mental processes associated with bringing stored information back into consciousness. SEE ALSO memory.

retro-. Backward or behind. [L. back, backward]

ret·ro·au·ric·u·lar (re′trō-aw-rik′ū-lăr). Behind the auricle.

ret·ro·buc·cal (re′trō-bŭk′ăl). Relating to the back part of, or behind, the cheek.

ret·ro·bul·bar (re′trō-bŭl′bar). Behind the eyeball. SYN retroocular.

ret·ro·cal·ca·ne·o·bur·si·tis (re′trō-kal-kā′nē-ō-ber-sī′tis). SYN achillobursitis. [retro- + L. *calcaneum* heel, + bursitis]

ret·ro·ce·cal (re′trō-sē′kăl). Posterior to the cecum.

ret·ro·cer·vi·cal (re′trō-ser′vi-kăl). Posterior to the cervix uteri.

ret·ro·ces·sion (re-trō-sesh′ŭn). **1.** A going back; a relapse. **2.** Cessation of the external symptoms of a disease followed by signs of involvement of some internal organ or part. **3.** Denoting a position of the uterus or other organ farther back than is normal. [L. *retro-cedo,* pp. *-cessus,* to go back, retire]

ret·ro·clu·sion (re-trō-kloo′zhŭn). A form of acupressure for the arrest of bleeding; the needle is passed through the tissues above the cut end of the artery, is turned around, and then is passed backward beneath the vessel to come out near the point of entrance. [retro- + L. *claudo* (*cludo*) to close]

ret·ro·col·ic (re′trō-kol′ik). Posterior to the colon. [retro- + G. *kolon,* colon]

ret·ro·col·lic (re′trō-kol′ik). Relating to the back of the neck; drawing back the head. [retro- + L. *collum,* neck]

ret·ro·con·duc·tion (re-trō-kon-dŭk′shŭn). SYN retrograde VA conduction.

ret·ro·cur·sive (re′trō-ker′siv). Running backward. [retro- + L. *cursus,* a running]

ret·ro·de·vi·a·tion (re′trō-dē-vē-ā′shŭn). A backward bending or inclining.

ret·ro·dis·place·ment (re′trō-dis-plās′ment). Any backward displacement, such as retroversion or retroflexion of the uterus.

ret·ro·e·soph·a·ge·al (re′trō-ē-sof′ă-jē′ăl). Posterior to the esophagus.

ret·ro·fil·ling (re-trō-fil′ing). Placement of a sealing material into the apical foramen of a dental root from the apical end.

ret·ro·flect·ed (re′trō-flek-ted). SYN retroflexed.

ret·ro·flec·tion (re-trō-flek′shŭn). SYN retroflexion.

ret·ro·flexed (re′trō-flekst). Bent backward or posteriorly. SYN retroflected. [retro- + L. *flecto,* pp. *flexus,* to bend]

ret·ro·flex·ion (re-trō-flek′shŭn). Backward bending, as of the uterus when the corpus is bent back, forming an angle with the cervix. SYN retroflection.

r. of iris, abnormal position of the iris on the ciliary body after severe concussion.

ret·ro·gnath·ic (re-trō-nath′ik). Denoting a state in which the mandible is located posterior to its normal position in relation to the maxillae.

ret·ro·gnath·ism (re-trō-nath′izm). A condition of facial disharmony in which one or both jaws are posterior to normal in their craniofacial relationships; usually used in reference to the mandible. [retro- + G. *gnathos,* jaw]

ret·ro·grade (ret′rō-grād). **1.** Moving backward. **2.** Degenerating; reversing the normal order of growth and development. [L. *retrogradus,* fr. retro- + *gradior,* to go]

ret·rog·ra·phy (re-trog′rǎ-fē). SYN mirror-writing. [retro- + G. *graphō,* to write]

ret·ro·gres·sion (re-trō-gresh′ŭn). SYN cataplasia. [L. *retrogressus* fr. *retrogradior,* to go backwards]

ret·ro·in·hi·bi·tion (re′trō-in-hi-bish′ŭn). SYN feedback inhibition.

ret·ro·i·rid·i·an (re′trō-i-rid′ē-an). Posterior to the iris.

ret·ro·jec·tion (re-trō-jek′shŭn). The washing out of a cavity by

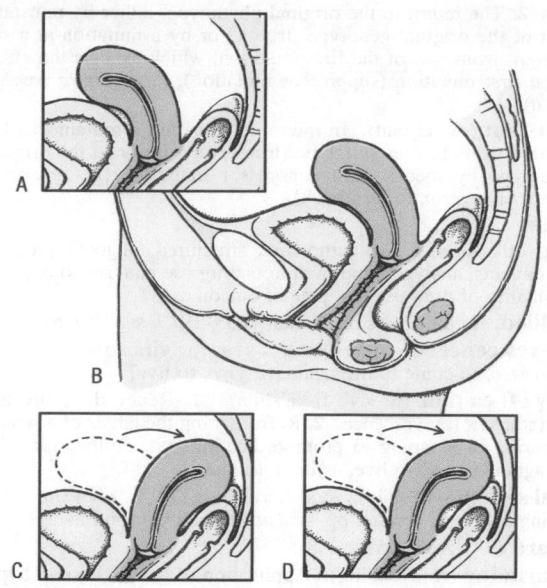

position of the uterus: (A) anteflexion, (B) anteversion (normal), (C) retroversion, (D) retroflexion

the backward flow of an injected fluid. [L. *retro,* backward, + *jacio,* to throw]

ret·ro·jec·tor (re′trō-jek-ter, -tōr). A form of syringe with long tubular attachment to the nozzle, used in retrojection.

ret·ro·len·tal (re′trō-len′tăl). Posterior to the lens of the eye. SYN retrolenticular (1).

ret·ro·len·tic·u·lar (re′trō-len-tik′ū-lăr). **1.** SYN retrolental. **2.** Behind the lentiform nucleus of the brain.

ret·ro·lin·gual (re′trō-ling′gwăl). Relating to the back part of the tongue; posterior to the tongue. [retro- + L. *lingua,* tongue]

ret·ro·mam·ma·ry (re′trō-mam′ă-rē). Posterior to the mamma.

ret·ro·man·dib·u·lar (re′trō-man-dib′ū-lăr). Posterior to the lower jaw. [retro- + L. *mandibula,* lower jaw]

ret·ro·mas·toid (re′trō-mas′toyd). Posterior to the mastoid process; relating to the posterior mastoid cells.

ret·ro·mo·lar (re-trō-mō′lăr). Distal (or posterior) to the last erupted (or present) molar tooth.

ret·ro·mor·pho·sis (re-trō-mōr′fō-sis, -mōr-fō′sis). SYN cataplasia. [retro- + G. *morphōsis,* process of forming]

ret·ro·na·sal (re′trō-nā′zăl). Posterior nasal; relating to the posterior nares.

ret·ro-oc·u·lar (re′trō-ok′ū-lăr). SYN retrobulbar.

ret·ro·per·i·to·ne·al (re′trō-per′i-tō-nē′ăl). External or posterior to the peritoneum.

ret·ro·per·i·to·ne·um (re′trō-per′i-tō-nē′ŭm). SYN retroperitoneal *space.* [retro- + peritoneum]

ret·ro·per·i·to·ni·tis (ret′rō-per-i-tō-nī′tis). Inflammation of the cellular tissue behind the peritoneum.

idiopathic fibrous r., SYN retroperitoneal *fibrosis.*

ret·ro·pha·ryn·ge·al (re′trō-fă-rin′jē-ăl). Posterior to the pharynx.

ret·ro·phar·ynx (re′trō-făr′ingks). The posterior part of the pharynx.

ret·ro·pla·cen·tal (re′trō-pla-sen′tăl). Behind the placenta.

ret·ro·pla·sia (ret-rō-plā′zē-ă). That state of cell or tissue in which activity is decreased below that considered normal; associated with retrogressive changes (e.g., injury, degeneration, death, necrosis). [retro- + G. *plasis,* a molding]

ret·ro·posed (re′trō-pōzd). Denoting retroposition. [retro- + L. *pono,* pp. *positus,* to place]

ret·ro·po·si·tion (re′trō-pō-zish′ŭn). Simple backward displacement of a structure or organ, as the uterus, without inclination, bending, retroversion, or retroflexion. [retro- + L. *positio,* a placing]

ret·ro·pos·on (re-trō-pōs′on). A transposition of sequences in a DNA that does not originate in the DNA but rather in an mRNA that is transcribed back into the genomic DNA by reverse transcription. [retro- + L. *pono,* pp. *positum,* to place, + -on]

ret·ro·pu·bic (re-trō-pū′bik). Posterior to the pubic bone.

ret·ro·pul·sion (re-trō-pŭl′shŭn). **1.** An involuntary backward walking or running, occurring in patients with the parkinsonian syndrome. **2.** A pushing back of any part. [retro- + L. *pulsio,* a pushing, fr. *pello,* pp. *pulsus,* beat, drive]

ret·ro·spec·tion (re-trō-spek′shŭn). The act or process of surveying and reviewing the past. [retro- + L. *specto,* pp. *spectatus,* to look at]

ret·ro·spec·tive (re-trō-spek′tiv). Relating to retrospection.

ret·ro·spon·dy·lo·lis·the·sis (re′trō-spon′di-lō-lis-thē′sis). Slipping posteriorly of the body of a vertebra, bringing it out of line with the adjacent vertebrae. [retro- + G. *spondylos,* vertebra, + *olisthēsis,* a slipping]

ret·ro·ster·nal (re′trō-ster′năl). Posterior to the sternum.

ret·ro·ste·roid (re-trō-stēr′oyd, -ster′oyd). A term sometimes used to designate a steroid in which the orientations of the substituents at carbons-9 and -10 are the opposite of those of the reference or "parent" compound.

ret·ro·tar·sal (re′trō-tar′săl). Posterior to the tarsus, or edge of the eyelid.

ret·ro·u·ter·ine (re′trō-ū′ter-in). Posterior to the uterus.

ret·ro·ver·si·o·flex·ion (re-trō-ver′sē-ō-flek′shŭn, -ver′zhō-). Combined retroversion and retroflexion of the uterus.

ret·ro·ver·sion (re-trō-ver′zhŭn). **1.** A turning backward, as of the uterus. **2.** Condition in which the teeth are located in a more posterior position than is normal. [retro- + L. *verto,* pp. *versus,* to turn]

ret·ro·vert·ed (re′trō-ver-ted). Denoting retroversion.

Ret·ro·vir·i·dae (re-trō-vir′i-dē). A family of RNA viruses 80–100 nm in diameter, enveloped, and containing two identical molecules of positive sense, single-stranded RNA, molecular weight 3–6 × 10⁶; genomic RNA serves as a template for the synthesis of a complementary DNA, which may be integrated into the host DNA. There are currently 7 genera: Mammalian type B retroviruses, Mammalian type C retroviruses, Avian type C retroviruses, Type D retroviruses, BLV-HTLV retroviruses, Lentivirus, and Spumovirus.

ret·ro·vi·rus (re′trō-vī′rŭs). Any virus of the family Retroviridae.

> Retroviruses are potent disease agents, but they have also served as invaluable research tools in molecular biology. In 1979, the molecular biologist Richard Mulligan used a genetically altered retrovirus to trigger the production of hemoglobin in vitro by monkey kidney cells. His technique for using retroviruses to import alien genes into cells has been widely adopted. Medical researchers have also explored retroviral transport as a means of gene therapy. However, evidence suggesting that retroviruses may play a role in carcinogenesis raises questions as to the safety of their use in gene therapy. See oncogene.

re·tru·sion (rē-troo′zhŭn). **1.** Retraction of the mandible from any given point. **2.** The backward movement of the mandible. [L. *retrudo,* pp. *-trusus,* to push back]

Rett, Andreas, 20th century Austrian pediatrician. SEE R. *syndrome.*

return.

total anomalous pulmonary venous r. (TAPVR), SEE anomalous pulmonary venous *connections,* total or partial, under *connection.*

venous r., the blood returning to the heart via the great veins and coronary sinus.

re

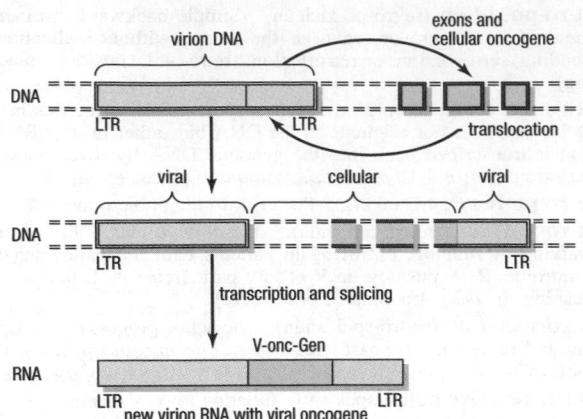

retrovirus: incorporation of cellular oncogene into a retrovirus, whereby it becomes a viral oncogene (LTR, long terminal repeats)

Retzius, Magnus G., Swedish anatomist and anthropologist, 1842–1919. SEE R. *striae*, under *stria; lines* of R., under *line; foramen* of R.; calcification *lines* of R., under *line; foramen* of Key-R.; *sheath* of Key and R.

Retzius, Anders A., Swedish anatomist and anthropologist, 1796–1860. SEE R. *cavity; cavum retzii;* R. *fibers*, under *fiber, gyrus, ligament, space;* retroperitoneal *veins*, under *vein.*

re·u·ni·ent (rē-ū′nē-ent). Connecting; denoting the ductus reuniens. [L. *re-,* again, + *unio,* pp. *unitus,* to unite]

Reuss, August von, Austrian ophthalmologist, 1841–1924. SEE R. *formula, test.*

re·vac·ci·na·tion (rē′vak-si-nā′shŭn). Vaccination of an individual previously successfully vaccinated.

re·vas·cu·lar·i·za·tion (rē-vas′kū-lăr-i-zā′shŭn). Reestablishment of blood supply to a part.

re·ver·ber·a·tion (rē′vĕr-bĕ-rā′shŭn). Multiple echoes or reflections; in ultrasonography, an artifactual image caused by delay of an echo that has been reflected back and forward again before returning to the transducer.

Reverdin, Jacques L., Swiss surgeon, 1842–1929. SEE R. *graft.*

re·ver·sal (rē-ver′săl). **1.** A turning or changing to the opposite direction, as of a process, disease, symptom, or state. **2.** The changing of a dark line or a bright one of the spectrum into its opposite. **3.** Denoting the difficulty of some persons in distinguishing the lowercase printed or written letter *p* from *q* or *g, b* from *d,* or *s* from *z.* **4.** In psychoanalysis, the change of an instinct or affect into its opposite, as from love into hate. [L. *reverto,* pp. *-versus,* to turn back or about]

adrenaline r., SYN epinephrine r.

epinephrine r., the fall in blood pressure produced by epinephrine when given following blockage of α-adrenergic receptors by an appropriate drug such as phenoxybenzamine; the vasodilation reflects the ability of epinephrine to activate β-adrenergic receptors that, in vascular smooth muscle, are inhibitory; in the absence of α-receptor blockade, the β-receptor activation by epinephrine is masked by its predominant action on vascular α-receptors, which causes vasoconstriction. SYN adrenaline r.

narcotic r., the use of narcotic antagonists, such as naloxone, to terminate the action of narcotics.

pressure r., cessation of anesthesia by hyperbaric pressure; of major importance in understanding the mode of action of anesthetics.

sex r., SYN sex *reassignment.*

re·vers·i·ble (rē-ver′si-bl). Capable of reversal; said of diseases or chemical reactions.

re·ver·sion (rē-ver′zhŭn). **1.** The manifestation in an individual of certain characteristics, peculiar to a remote ancestor, which have been suppressed during one or more of the intermediate genera-

tions. **2.** The return to the original phenotype, either by reinstatement of the original genotype (true r.) or by a mutation at a site different from that of the first mutation, which cancels the effect of the first mutation (suppressor mutation). [L. *reversio* (see reversal)]

re·ver·tant (rē-ver′tant). In microbial genetics, a mutant that has reverted to its former genotype (true reversion) or to the original phenotype by means of a suppressor mutation. [L. *revertans,* pros.p. of *reverto,* to turn back]

review.

   drug utilization r., an authorized, structured, ongoing program that collects, analyzes, and interprets drug use patterns to improve the quality of drug use and patient outcomes.

Revilliod, Léon, Swiss physician, 1835–1919. SEE R. *sign.*

rev·i·ves·cence (re-vi-ves′ens). SYN revivification (1). [L. *re-vivesco,* to come to life again, fr. *vivo,* to live]

re·viv·i·fi·ca·tion (rē-viv′i-fi-kā′shŭn). **1.** Renewal of life and strength. SYN revivescence. **2.** Refreshening the edges of a wound by paring or scraping to promote healing. SYN vivification. [L. *re-,* again, + *vivo,* to live, + *facio,* to make]

re·vul·sion (rē-vŭl′shŭn). SYN derivation (1). [L. *revulsio,* act of pulling away, fr. *revello,* pp. *-vulsus,* to pluck or pull away]

re·ward (rē-ward′). SYN reinforcer.

re·warm·ing (rē-warm′ing). Application of heat to correct hypothermia.

Rexed. Bror A., Swedish physician, scientist, and public servant, *1914. SEE *lamina* of Rexed.

Reye, Ralph Douglas Kenneth, 20th century Australian pathologist. SEE R. *syndrome.*

Reymond. SEE Du Bois-Reymond.

Reynolds, Osborne, English physicist, 1842–1912. SEE Reynolds *number.*

RF Abbreviation for releasing *factors;* rheumatoid *factors,* under *factor;* replicative *form;* reticular *formation.*

RFA Abbreviation for right frontoanterior position.

RFLP Abbreviation for restriction fragment length *polymorphism.*

RFP Abbreviation for right frontoposterior position.

RFT Abbreviation for right frontotransverse position.

RH Abbreviation for releasing *hormone.*

Rh 1. Symbol for rhodium. **2.** See Rh blood group, Blood Groups appendix.

Rha Abbreviation for L-rhamnose.

rha·bar·ber·one (ra-bar′ber-ōn). SYN aloe-emodin.

△**rhabd-.** SEE rhabdo-.

rhabditiform. SEE rhabditiform *larva.*

Rhab·di·tis-like. SEE rhabditiform *larva.*

△**rhabdo-, rhabd-.** Rod; rod-shaped (rhabdoid). [G. *rhabdos*]

rhab·do·cyte (rab′dō-sīt). Rarely used term for band cell or metamyelocyte. [rhabdo- + G. *kytos,* cell]

rhab·doid (rab′doyd). Rod-shaped. [rhabdo- + G. *eidos,* resemblance]

rhab·do·my·o·blast (rab-dō-mī′ō-blast). Large round, spindle-shaped, or strap-shaped cells with deeply eosinophilic fibrillar cytoplasm that may show cross striations; found in some rhabdomyosarcomas. [rhabdo- + G. *mys,* muscle, + *blastos,* germ]

rhab·do·my·ol·y·sis (rab′dō-mī-ol′i-sis). An acute, fulminating, potentially fatal disease of skeletal muscle that entails destruction of muscle, as evidenced by myoglobinemia and myoglobinuria. [rhabdo- + G. *mys,* muscle, + *lysis,* loosening]

   acute recurrent r. [MIM*268200], repeated paroxysmal attacks of muscle pain and weakness followed by passage of dark red-brown urine, often precipitated by intercurrent illness and diagnosed by demonstration of myoglobin in the urine; it is attributed to abnormal phosphorylase activity in skeletal muscle, but there may be more than one biologic type; probably autosomal recessive inheritance. In some cases, at least, there is deficiency of carnitine palmitoyl transferase. SYN familial paroxysmal r.

   exertional r., r. produced in susceptible individuals by muscular exercise.

familial paroxysmal r., SYN acute recurrent r.

idiopathic paroxysmal r., SYN myoglobinuria.

rhab·do·my·o·ma (rab′dō-mī-ō′mă). A benign neoplasm derived from striated muscle, occurring in the heart in children, probably as a hamartomatous process. [rhabdo- + G. *mys*, muscle, + *-oma*, tumor]

rhab·do·my·o·sar·co·ma (rab′dō-mī-ō-sar-kō′mă). A malignant neoplasm derived from skeletal (striated) muscle, occurring in children or, less commonly, in adults; classified as embryonal alveolar (composed of loose aggregates of small round cells) or pleomorphic (containing rhabdomyoblasts). SYN rhabdosarcoma. [rhabdo- + G. *mys*, muscle, + *sarkōma*, sarcoma]

embryonal r., malignant neoplasm occurring in children, consisting of loose, spindle-celled tissue with rare cross-striations, and arising in many parts of the body in addition to skeletal muscles.

rhab·do·pho·bia (rab-dō-fō′bē-ă). Morbid fear of a rod (or switch) as an instrument of punishment. [rhabdo- + G. *phobos*, fear]

rhab·do·sar·co·ma (rab′dō-sar-kō′mă). SYN rhabdomyosarcoma.

rhab·do·sphinc·ter (rab′dō-sfingk′ter). A sphincter made up of striated musculature. SYN striated muscular sphincter. [rhabdo- + G. *sphinktēr*, sphincter]

Rhab·do·vir·i·dae (rab′dō-vir′i-dē). A family of rod- or bullet-shaped viruses of vertebrates, insects, and plants, including rabiesvirus and vesicular stomatitis virus (of cattle). Virions (100–430 by 45–100 nm), formed by budding from surface membranes of cells, are enveloped and ether sensitive, with surface spikes 5–10 nm long; nucleocapsids contain negative sense single-stranded RNA (MW ~4.4 × 10⁶) and are of helical symmetry. There are five genera: Vesiculovirus, Lyssavirus, Ephemerovirus, Nucleorhabdovirus, and Cytorhabdovirus.

rhab·do·vi·rus (rab′dō-vī′rŭs). Any virus of the family Rhabdoviridae.

rhachi-. For words so beginning, see rachi-.

Rhad·in·o·vi·rus (rad-ēn′ō-vī-rus). A herpesvirus genus, subfamily Gammaherpesvirinae, associated with Kaposi sarcoma.

rhag·a·des (rag′ă-dēz). Chaps, cracks, or fissures occurring at mucocutaneous junctions; seen in vitamin deficiency diseases and in congenital syphilis. [G. *rhagas*, pl. *rhagades*, a crack]

rha·gad·i·form (ră-gad′i-fōrm). Resembling or characterized by rhagades. [G. *rhagas* (*rhagad*-), crack, + L. *forma*, shape]

-rhagia. SEE -rrhagia.

L-rham·nose (Rha) (ram′nōs). A methylpentose present in a number of plant glycosides, found in free form in poison sumac, in lipopolysaccharides of *Enterobacteriaceae*, and in rutinose (a disaccharide). SYN isodulcit.

rham·no·side (ram′nō-sīd). A glycoside of rhamnose.

rham·no·xan·thin (ram-nō-zan′thin). SYN frangulin.

Rhamnus (ram′nŭs). A genus of shrubs and trees (family Rhamnaceae). The bark and berries of *R. cathartica* are cathartic; *R. frangula* is the source of frangula; *R. purshiana* is the source of cascara sagrada. SYN buckthorn. [G. *rhamnos*]

rha·pha·nia (ră-fā′nē-ă). SYN raphania.

rha·phe (rā′fē). SYN raphe.

-rhaphy. SEE -rrhaphy.

rhe (rē). The absolute unit of fluidity, the reciprocal of the unit of viscosity. [G. *rheos*, a stream]

-rhea. SEE -rrhea.

rheg·ma (reg′mă). A rent or fissure. [G. breakage]

rheg·ma·tog·e·nous (reg-mă-toj′ĕ-nŭs). Arising from a bursting or fractioning of an organ. SEE rhegmatogenous retinal *detachment*. [G. *rhēgma*, breakage, + *-gen*, producing]

rhe·ic (rē′ik). Relating to *Rheum* (rhubarb).

Rheinberg mi·cro·scope. See under microscope.

rhe·ni·um (Re) (rē′nē-ŭm). A metallic element of the platinum group; atomic wt. 186.207, atomic no. 75. [Mod. L., fr. L. *Rhenus*, Rhine river]

rheo-. Blood flow; electrical current. [G. *rheos*, stream, current, flow]

rhe·o·base (rē′ō-bās). The minimal strength of an electrical stimulus of indefinite duration that is able to cause excitation of a tissue, e.g., muscle or nerve. SEE ALSO chronaxie. SYN galvanic threshold. [rheo- + G. *basis*, a base]

rhe·o·ba·sic (rē-ō-bā′sik). Pertaining to or having the characteristics of a rheobase.

rhe·o·car·di·og·ra·phy (rē′ō-kar-dē-og′ră-phē). Impedance plethysmography applied to the heart. [rheo- + cardiography]

rhe·o·chrys·i·din (rē-ō-kris′i-din). The 3-methyl ether of emodin.

rhe·o·en·ceph·a·lo·gram (rē′ō-en-sef′ă-lō-gram). Graphic registration of the changes in conductivity of tissue of the head caused by vascular factors.

rhe·o·en·ceph·a·log·ra·phy (rē′ō-en-sef-ă-log′ră-fē). The technique of measuring blood flow of the brain; commonly used to denote impedance r., which uses changes in electrical impedance and resistance as a measure of flow. [rheo- + encephalography]

rhe·o·gram (rē′ō-gram). A plot of the shear stress versus the shear rate for a fluid. [rheo- + G. *gramma*, something written]

rhe·ol·o·gist (rē-ol′ō-jist). A specialist in rheology.

rhe·ol·o·gy (rē-ol′ō-jē). The study of the deformation and flow of materials. [rheo- + G. *logos*, study]

rhe·om·e·ter (rē-om′ĕ-ter). **1.** An instrument for measurement of the rheologic properties of materials, e.g., of blood. **2.** A galvanometer. [rheo- + G. *metron*, measure]

rhe·om·e·try (rē-om′ĕ-trē). Measurement of electrical current or blood flow.

rhe·o·pexy (rē′ō-pek-sē). A property of certain materials in which an increased rate of shear favors an increase in viscosity. [rheo- + G. *pēxis*, fixation]

rhe·o·stat (rē′ō-stat). A variable resistor used to adjust the current in an electrical circuit. [rheo- + G. *statos*, stationary]

rhe·os·to·sis (rē-os-tō′sis). A hypertrophying and condensing osteitis that tends to run in longitudinal streaks or columns, like wax drippings on a candle, and that involves a number of the long bones. SYN flowing hyperostosis, streak hyperostosis. [rheo- + G. *osteon*, bone, + *-osis*, condition]

rhe·o·tax·is (rē-ō-tak′sis). A form of positive barotaxis, in which a microorganism in a fluid is impelled to move against the current flow of its medium. [rheo- + G. *taxis*, orderly arrangement]

rhe·ot·ro·pism (rē-ot′rō-pizm). A movement contrary to the motion of a current, involving part of an organism, rather than the organism as a whole, as in rheotaxis. [rheo- + G. *tropos*, a turning]

rhes·to·cy·the·mia (res′tō-sī-thē′mē-ă). An obsolete term for the presence of broken-down red blood cells in the peripheral circulation. [G. *rhaiō*, to destroy, + *kytos*, a hollow (a cell), + *haima*, blood]

rhe·sus (rē′sŭs). Generic name for *Macaca mulatta*. [Mod. L., fr. L. *Rhesus*, G. *Rhesos*, a mythical king of Thrace]

rheum (room). A mucous or watery discharge. [G. *rheuma*, a flux]

rheu·ma·tal·gia (roo-mă-tal′jē-ă). Obsolete term for rheumatic pain. [G. *rheuma*, flux, + *algos*, pain]

rheu·mat·ic (roo-mat′ik). Relating to or characterized by rheumatism. SYN rheumatismal. [G. *rheumatikos*, subject to flux, fr. *rheuma*, flux]

rheu·ma·tid (roo′mă-tid). Rheumatic nodules or other eruptions that may accompany rheumatism. [G. *rheum*, flux, + *-id* (1)]

rheu·ma·tism (roo′mă-tizm). **1.** Obsolete term for rheumatic *fever*. **2.** Indefinite term applied to various conditions with pain or other symptoms of articular origin or related to other elements of the musculoskeletal system. [G. *rheumatismos*, rheuma, a flux]

articular r., SYN arthritis.

cerebral r., central nervous system symptoms resulting from a rheumatic disease. Formerly seen primarily as a manifestation of rheumatic *fever*, now seen less frequently as a part of other diseases such as systemic *lupus* erythematosus. SEE ALSO Sydenham *chorea*.

chronic r., a nonspecific disorder of the joints, slow in progress, producing a painful thickening and contraction of the fibrous structures, interfering with motion, and causing deformity.

gonorrheal r., an arthritis, usually initially a polyarthritis, but often localizing in one joint as a pyarthrosis caused by systemic infection with the gonococcus.

r. of the heart, rheumatic cardiac valvular disease, most often of the mitral and aortic valves.

inflammatory r., rheumatoid arthritis or other cause of joint inflammation.

Macleod r., rheumatoid arthritis with abundant serous effusion in the affected joints.

muscular r., SYN fibrositis (2).

nodose r., (1) SYN rheumatoid *arthritis*; (2) an acute or subacute articular r., accompanied by the formation of nodules on the tendons, ligaments, and periosteum in the neighborhood of the affected joints.

subacute r., a mild but usually protracted form of acute rheumatic fever, often resistant to treatment.

tuberculous r., an inflammatory condition of the joints or fibrous tissues during the course of tuberculosis.

rheu·ma·tis·mal (roo-mă-tiz′măl). SYN rheumatic.

rheu·ma·toid (roo′mă-toyd). Resembling r. arthritis in one or more features. [G. *rheuma*, flux, + *eidos*, resemblance]

rheu·ma·tol·o·gist (roo-mă-tol′ō-jist). A specialist in rheumatology.

rheu·ma·tol·o·gy (roo-mă-tol′ō-jē). The medical specialty concerned with the study, diagnosis, and treatment of rheumatic conditions. [G. *rheuma*, flux, + *logos*, study]

rhig·ot·ic (ri-got′ik). Pertaining to rhigosis.

rhIL-11. SYN recombinant human *interleukin* 11.

△**rhin-, rhino-.** The nose. [G. *rhis*]

rhi·nal (rī′năl). SYN nasal.

rhi·nal·gia (rī-nal′jē-ă). Pain in the nose. SYN rhinodynia. [rhin- + G. *algos*, pain]

rhin·e·de·ma (rī′ne-dē′mă). Swelling of the nasal mucous membrane. [rhin- + G. *oidēma*, swelling]

rhin·en·ce·phal·ic (rī′nen-se-fal′ik). Relating to the rhinencephalon.

rhin·en·ceph·a·lon (rī′nen-sef′ă-lon). A largely archaic collective term denoting the parts of the cerebral hemisphere directly related to the sense of smell: the olfactory bulb, olfactory peduncle (together still listed as the first cranial nerve or olfactory nerve despite the fact that they form part of the central nervous system), olfactory tubercle, and olfactory or piriform cortex including the cortical nucleus of the amygdala. The term originally also encompassed the hippocampus, the entire amygdala, and the fornicate gyrus, all of which are no longer believed to be specifically related to the sense of smell. SEE ALSO limbic *system*. SYN smell-brain. [rhin- + G. *enkephalos*, brain]

rhin·en·chy·sis (rī-nen′kī-sis). A nasal douche; washing out the nasal cavities. [rhin- + G. *enchysis*, a pouring in]

rhin·i·on (rin′ē-on). A craniometric point: the lower end of the internal suture. [G. *rhinion*, nostril, dim. of *rhis* (*rhin-*), nose]

rhi·nism (rī′nizm). SYN rhinolalia.

rhi·ni·tis (rī-nī′tis). Inflammation of the nasal mucous membrane. SYN nasal catarrh. [rhin- + G. *-itis*, inflammation]

acute r., an acute catarrhal inflammation of the mucous membrane of the nose, marked by sneezing, lacrimation, and a profuse secretion of watery mucus; usually associated with infection by one of the common cold viruses. SYN coryza, head cold.

🔲**allergic r.,** r. associated with hay fever.

atrophic r., chronic r. with thinning of the mucous membrane; often associated with crusts and foul-smelling discharge. SYN ozena.

r. caseo′sa, caseous r., a form of chronic r. in which the nasal cavities are more or less completely filled with an ill-smelling cheesy material.

chronic r., a protracted sluggish inflammation of the nasal mucous membrane; in the later stages the mucous membrane with its glands may be thickened (hypertrophic r.) or thinned (atrophic r.).

gangrenous r., SEE *cancrum* nasi.

hypertrophic r., chronic r. with permanent thickening of the mucous membrane.

r. medicamento′sa, inflammation of the nasal mucous membrane secondary to excessive or improper topical medication.

scrofulous r., tuberculous infection of the nasal mucous membrane.

r. sic′ca, a form of chronic r. with little or no secretion.

vasomotor r., congestion of nasal mucous membrane and rhinorrhea without infection or allergy.

△**rhino-.** SEE rhin-.

rhi·no·an·e·mom·e·ter (rī′nō-an-ĕ-mom′ĕ-ter). SYN rhinomanometer. [rhino- + G. *anemos*, wind, + *metron*, measure]

rhi·no·cele (rī′nō-sēl). Cavity (ventricle) of the rhinencephalon, the primitive olfactory part of the telencephalon. [rhino- + G. *koilia*, a hollow]

rhi·no·ceph·a·ly, rhi·no·ce·pha·lia (rī′nō-sef′ă-lē, -se-fā′lē-ă). Rhinencephaly; a form of cyclopia in which the nose is represented by a fleshy proboscis-like protuberance arising above the slit-like orbits, and the rhinencephalic lobes of the telencephalon are poorly developed with some tendency to become fused together. [rhino- + G. *kephalē*, head]

Rhi·no·clad·i·el·la (rī′nō-klad-ē-el′ă). A genus of dematiaceous (dark colored) fungi, characterized by acrotheca, that cause chromoblastomycosis. SEE ALSO *Phialophora*.

rhi·no·clei·sis (rī-nō-klī′sis). SYN rhinostenosis. [rhino- + G. *kleisis*, a closure]

rhi·no·dym·ia (rī-nō-dim′ē-ă). Duplication of the nose on an otherwise normal face. [rhino- + G. *-dymos*, fold]

rhi·no·dyn·ia (rī-nō-din′ē-ă). SYN rhinalgia. [rhino- + G. *odynē*, pain]

rhi·no·es·tro·sis (rī′nō-es-trō′sis). Infection of horses and donkeys, rarely humans, with larvae of the fly *Rhinoestrus purpureus;* human infection is usually benign and of short duration, limited to the first stage of the larva and resulting in a mild ophthalmomyiasis.

Rhi·no·es·trus pur·pu·re·us (rī-nō-es′trŭs pŭr-poo′rē-ŭs). A species of fly of the family Oestridae, the nasal botflies, that causes rhinoestrosis.

rhi·nog·e·nous (rī-noj′ĕ-nŭs). Originating in the nose. [rhino- + G. *-gen*, producing]

rhi·no·ky·pho·sis (rī′nō-kī-fō′sis). A hump deformity of the nose. [rhino- + G. *kyphōsis*, humped condition]

rhi·no·la·lia (rī′nō-lā′lē-ă). Nasalized speech. SYN rhinism, rhinophonia. [rhino- + G. *lalia*, talking]

r. aper′ta, abnormal speech attributable to inadequate velopharyngeal closure.

r. clau′sa, abnormal speech attributable to nasal obstruction.

rhi·no·lite (rī′nō-līt). SYN rhinolith.

rhi·no·lith (rī′nō-lith). A calcareous concretion in the nasal cavity often around a foreign body. SYN nasal calculus, rhinolite. [rhino- + G. *lithos*, stone]

rhi·no·li·thi·a·sis (rī′nō-li-thī′ă-sis). The presence of a nasal calculus. [rhinolith + G. *-iasis*, condition]

rhi·no·log·ic (rī-nō-loj′ik). Relating to rhinology.

rhi·nol·o·gist (rī-nol′ō-jist). A specialist in diseases of the nose.

rhi·nol·o·gy (rī-nol′ō-jē). The branch of medical science concerned with the nose and paranasal sinuses and their diseases. [rhino- + G. *logos*, study]

rhi·no·ma·nom·e·ter (rī′nō-mă-nom′ĕ-ter). A manometer used to determine the presence and amount of nasal obstruction, and the nasal air pressure and flow relationships. SYN rhinoanemometer. [rhino- + manometer]

rhi·no·ma·nom·e·try (rī′nō-mă-nom′ĕ-trē). 1. The use of a rhinomanometer. 2. The study and measurement of nasal air flow and pressures.

rhi·no·ne·cro·sis (rī′nō-ne-krō′sis). Necrosis of the bones of the nose. [rhino- + necrosis]

rhi·nop·a·thy (rī-nop′ă-thē). Disease of the nose. [rhino- + G. *pathos*, suffering]

rhi·no·pha·ryn·ge·al (rī′nō-fă-rin′jē-ăl). **1.** SYN nasopharyngeal. **2.** Relating to the rhinopharynx.

rhi·no·pha·ryn·go·lith (rī′nō-fă-ring′gō-lith). A concretion in the nasopharynx. [rhinopharynx + G. *lithos,* stone]

rhi·no·phar·ynx (rī′nō-far′ingks). SYN nasopharynx. [rhino- + pharynx]

rhi·no·pho·nia (rī′nō-fō′nē-ă). SYN rhinolalia. [rhino- + G. *phōnē,* voice]

rhi·no·phy·ma (rī′nō-fī′mă). Hypertrophy of the nose with follicular dilation, resulting from hyperplasia of sebaceous glands with fibrosis and increased vascularity; a form of acne rosacea. SYN brandy nose, copper nose, hammer nose, hypertrophic rosacea, potato nose, rum nose, rum-blossom, toper's nose. [rhino- + G. *phyma,* tumor, growth]

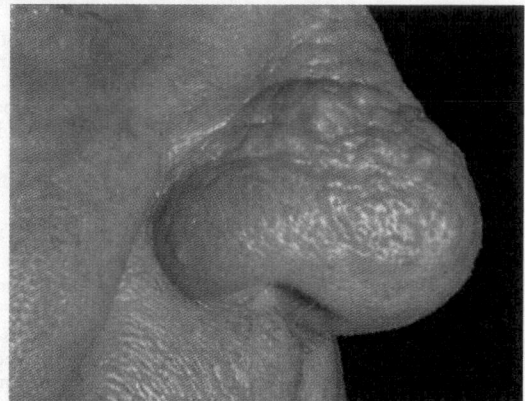

rhinophyma

rhi·no·plas·ty (rī′nō-plas-tē). **1.** Repair of a defect of the nose. **2.** Plastic surgery to change the shape or size of the nose. [rhino- + G. *plastos,* formed]

rhi·no·pneu·mo·ni·tis (rī′nō-noo-mō-nī′tis). Inflammation of the mucous membranes of the nose and lung. [rhino- + G. *pneumōn,* lung, + *-itis,* inflammation]

rhi·nor·rhea (rī-nō-rē′ă). A discharge from the nose. [rhino- + G. *rhoia,* flow]

cerebrospinal fluid r., a discharge of cerebrospinal fluid from the nose.

gustatory r., watery nasal discharge associated with eating.

rhi·no·sal·pin·gi·tis (rī′nō-sal-pin-jī′tis). Inflammation of the mucous membrane of the nose and eustachian tube. [rhino- + G. *salpinx,* tube, + *-itis,* inflammation]

rhi·no·scle·ro·ma (rī′nō-sklē-rō′mă). A chronic granulomatous process involving the nose, upper lip, mouth, and upper air passages; starts usually as a growth of hard smooth nodules in the anterior nares that spreads backward into the pharynx, larynx, trachea, and even into the bronchi; it may involve the external auditory meatus and is believed to be due to a specific bacterium, *Klebsiella rhinoscleromatis.* [rhino- + G. *sklērōma,* an induration]

rhi·no·scope (rī′nō-skōp). A small mirror attached at a suitable angle to a rodlike handle, used in posterior rhinoscopy and nasopharyngoscopy.

rhi·no·scop·ic (rī′nō-skop′ik). Relating to the rhinoscope or to rhinoscopy.

rhi·nos·co·py (rī-nos′kŏ-pē). Inspection of the nasal cavity. [rhino- + G. *skopeō,* to view]

anterior r., inspection of the anterior portion of the nasal cavity with or without the aid of a nasal speculum.

median r., inspection of the roof of the nasal cavity and openings of the posterior ethmoid cells and sphenoidal sinus by means of a long-bladed nasal speculum or nasopharyngoscope.

posterior r., inspection of the nasopharynx and posterior portion of the nasal cavity by means of the rhinoscope, or with a nasopharyngoscope. SEE ALSO nasopharyngoscopy.

rhi·no·si·nus·i·tis (rī-nō-sī-noo-sī′tis). Inflammation of the mucous membrane of the nose and paranasal sinuses.

rhi·no·spo·rid·i·o·sis (rī′nō-spō-rid-ē-ō′sis). Invasion of the nasal cavity or, occasionally, the conjunctiva, or other superficial structures by *Rhinosporidium seeberi,* resulting in a chronic granulomatous disease producing polyps or other forms of hyperplasia on mucous membranes; it is found principally in India and Sri Lanka.

Rhi·no·spo·rid·i·um see·beri (rī′nōspō-rid′ē-ŭm sē-bē′rī). A funguslike organism, of worldwide distribution and uncertain taxonomic position, found in certain vascular raspberry-like nasal polyps (rhinosporidiosis). [rhino- + G. *sporidion,* dim. of *sporos,* seed]

rhi·no·ste·no·sis (rī′nō-ste-nō′sis). Nasal obstruction. SYN rhinocleisis. [rhino- + G. *stenōsis,* a narrowing]

rhi·not·o·my (rī-not′ō-mē). **1.** Any cutting operation on the nose. **2.** Operative procedure in which the nose is incised along one side so that it may be turned away to provide full vision of the nasal passages for radical sinus operations. [rhino- + G. *tomē,* incision, cutting]

rhi·no·tra·che·i·tis (rī′nō-trā-kē-ī′tis). Inflammation of the nasal cavities and trachea. [rhino- + trachea + *-itis,* inflammation]

Rhi·no·vi·rus (rī′nō-vī′rŭs). A genus of acid-labile viruses (family Picornaviridae) of worldwide distribution, with a single-stranded positive sense RNA genome, associated with the common cold in humans. There are more than 110 antigenic types, formerly classified as M strains (culturable in rhesus monkey kidney and human cells) and H strains (growing only in cultures of human cells).

rhi·no·vi·rus. Any virus of the genus Rhinovirus.

bovine r.'s, viruses that cause widespread subclinical and occasionally mild clinical respiratory diseases of calves in the United States and Europe.

equine r.'s, viruses that cause inapparent as well as mild to relatively severe upper respiratory tract disease in the United States and Europe; most prevalent in breeding stables, and associated with high morbidity but negligible mortality; all equine isolates are related serologically to the original isolate.

Rhi·pi·ceph·a·lus (rī-pi-sef′ă-lŭs). A genus of inornate hard ticks (family Ixodidae) consisting of about 50 species, all of which are Old World except *R. sanguineus.* Eyes and festoons are present in both sexes; short palpi and ventral plates are present only in the male. The genus includes important vectors of disease in humans and domestic animals. [G. *rhipis,* fan, + *kephalē,* head]

R. sanguin′eus, the brown dog tick, probably the most common and cosmopolitan species found on dogs in the U.S.; it may attack other animals but rarely attacks humans; it is a vector of Rocky Mountain spotted fever in Mexico and is a vector of the rickettsia of boutonneuse fever.

rhizo-. Combining form denoting root. [G. *rhiza*]

rhi·zoid (rī′zoyd). **1.** Rootlike. **2.** Irregularly branching, like a root; denoting a form of bacterial growth. **3.** In fungi, the rootlike hyphae that arise at the nodes of the hyphae of *Rhizopus* species. [rhizo- + G. *eidos,* resemblance]

rhi·zome (rī′zōm). The creeping underground stem of plants such as iris, calamus, and sanguinaria. [G. *rhizōma,* mass of roots, fr. *rhiza,* root, + *-oma,* mass]

rhi·zo·me·lia (rī-zō-mē′lē-ă). **1.** Disproportion in the length of the most proximal segment of the limbs (upper arms and thighs). **2.** A disorder involving the shoulder and hip joint. [rhizo- + G. *melos,* limb]

rhi·zo·melic (rī-zō-mel′ik). Of or relating to the hip joint or the shoulder joint.

rhi·zo·me·nin·go·my·e·li·tis (rī′zō-mĕ-ning′gō-mī-ĕ-lī′tis). Inflammation of the nerve roots, the meninges, and the spinal cord. SYN radiculomeningomyelitis. [rhizo- + G. *mēninx,* membrane, + *myelon,* marrow, + *-itis,* inflammation]

Rhizomucor (rī-zō-moo-kōr). A genus of fungi in the family Mucoraceae; a cause of mucormycosis.

rhi·zo·plast (rī′zō-plast). A fine connection between the flagellum or blepharoplast and the nucleus of a protozoan. [rhizo- + G. *plastos,* formed]

Rhi·zop·o·da (rī-zō-pō'dă). A superclass in the subphylum Sarcodina that includes the amebae of humans, having pseudopodia of various forms but without axial filaments. SYN Rhizopodasida, Rhizopodea. [rhizo + G. *pous (pod-),* foot]

Rhi·zo·po·das·i·da (rī'zō-pō-das'i-dă). SYN Rhizopoda.

Rhi·zo·po·dea (rī-zō-pō'dē-ă). SYN Rhizopoda. [rhizo- + G. *pous (pod-),* foot]

rhi·zop·ter·in (rī-zop'ter-in). A folic acid factor for certain bacteria. SYN SLR factor, *Streptococcus lactis* R factor.

Rhi·zo·pus (rī-zō'pŭs). A genus of fungi (class Zygomycetes, family Mucoraceae); some species cause mucormycosis in humans.

rhi·zot·o·my (rī-zot'ō-mē). Section of the spinal nerve roots for the relief of pain or spastic paralysis. SYN radicotomy, radiculectomy. [G. *rhiza,* root, + *tomē,* section]

anterior r., section of anterior spinal root.

facet r., a percutaneous radiofrequency lysis of the innervation of a facet.

posterior r., section of posterior spinal root. SYN Dana operation.

trigeminal r., division or section of a sensory root of the fifth cranial nerve, accomplished through a subtemporal (Frazier-Spiller operation), suboccipital (Dandy operation), or transtentorial approach. SYN retrogasserian neurectomy, retrogasserian neurotomy.

rho (ρ) (rō). **1.** The 17th letter of the Greek alphabet. **2.** Symbol for density. **3.** SEE rho *factor.*

△**rhod-.** SEE rhodo-.

rho·da·mine B (rō'dă-mēn, -min) [C.I. 45170]. A fluorescent red basic xanthene dye, tetraethylrhodamine chloride, used in histology as a contrasting stain to methylene blue and methyl green, and as a vital fluorochrome.

rho·da·nate (rō'dă-nāt). SYN thiocyanate.

rho·da·nese (rō'dă-nēz). SYN *thiosulfate* sulfurtransferase.

rho·dan·ic ac·id (rō-dan'ik). SYN thiocyanic acid.

rho·da·nile blue (rō'dă-nīl). A dye mixture, considered by some to be a salt of rhodamine B and Nile blue, used to stain keratinized epithelium (red) and fibroblasts (blue), as well as spermatozoa and normal and pathologic acidophilic, basophilic, and certain neutrophilic elements of cells and tissues; used as a substitute for hematoxylin and eosin.

rho·de·ose (rō'dē-ōs). SYN fucose.

rho·din (rō'din). A dihydroporphyrin derivative (the two additional hydrogens being at positions 17 and 18) of the type found in chlorophyll *b* and with a formyl group on position 7 rather than a methyl group.

rho·di·um (Rh) (rō'dē-ŭm). A metallic element, atomic no. 45, atomic wt. 102.90550. [Mod. L. fr. G. *rhodon,* a rose]

Rhod·ni·us (rod'nē-us). Genus of reduvid bug that is the principal vector of *Trypanosoma cruzi* in Venezuela, Colombia, French Guiana, Guyana, and Surinam.

R. prolixus, a reduvid bug, an important cause of South American trypanosomiasis.

△**rhodo-, rhod-.** Rosy, red color. [G. *rhodon,* rose]

Rho·do·coc·cus (rō-dō-kok'us). A genus of rod-shaped, Gram-positive, partially acid-fast, aerobic bacteria found in soil and in the feces of herbivores. Some species are pathogenic for animals and humans. The type species is *Rhodococcus rhodochrous.*

R. equi, a bacterial species causing bronchopneumonia and the formation of abscesses in the lungs of foals. It can cause bronchopneumonia in immunodeficient humans, especially those with AIDS. SYN *Corynebacterium equi.*

rho·do·gen·e·sis (rō'dō-jen'ĕ-sis). The production of rhodopsin by the combination of 11-*cis*-retinal and opsin in the dark. [rhodopsin + G. *genesis,* production]

rho·do·phy·lac·tic (rō'dō-fī-lak'tik). Relating to rhodophylaxis.

rho·do·phy·lax·is (rō'dō-fī-lak'sis). The action of the pigment cells of the choroid in preserving or facilitating the reproduction of rhodopsin. [rhodopsin + G. *phylaxis,* a guarding]

rho·dop·sin (rō-dop'sin). A purplish-red thermolabile protein, MW about 40,000, found in the external segments of the rods of the retina; it is bleached by the action of light, which converts it to opsin and all-*trans*-retinal, and is restored in the dark by rhodogenesis; the dominant protein in the plasma membrane of rod cells. SYN visual purple.

r. kinase, an enzyme that regulates r. function by phosphorylating activated r. at a number of sites; phosphorylated photoactivated r. binds to arrestin.

meta-**rho·dop·sin I,** *meta*-**rho·dop·sin II,** *meta*-**rho·dop·sin III.** Precursors of opsin and all-*trans*-retinal, formed from lumirhodopsin in the visual cycle.

Rho·do·tor·u·la (rō-dō-tōr'ū-lă). A genus of yeasts, usually pink to red and of questionable pathogenicity, which are generally introduced iatrogenically in prosthetic implants and into immunocompromised patients via intravenous catheters.

rhomb·en·ceph·a·lon (rom-ben-sef'ă-lon) [TA]. That part of the developing brain that is the most caudal of the three primary vesicles of the embryonic neural tube; secondarily divided into metencephalon and myelencephalon; the r. includes the pons, cerebellum, and medulla oblongata. SYN hindbrain [TA], hindbrain vesicle*. [rhombo- + G. *enkephalos,* brain]

rhom·bic (rom'bik). **1.** SYN rhomboid. **2.** Relating to the rhombencephalon.

△**rhombo-.** Rhombic, rhomboid. [G. *rhombos*]

rhom·bo·at·loi·de·us. SEE musculus rhomboatloideus.

rhom·bo·cele (rom'bō-sēl). SYN rhomboidal *sinus.* [rhombo- + G. *koilia,* a hollow]

rhom·boid, rhom·boi·dal (rom'boyd, rom-boy'dăl). Resembling a rhomb; i.e., an oblique parallelogram, but having unequal sides; in anatomy, denoting especially a ligament and two muscles. SYN rhombic (1). [rhombo- + G. *eidos,* appearance]

rhom·boi·de·us (rom-bō-id'ē-ŭs). SEE rhomboid minor (*muscle*).

rhom·bo·mere. Segments of the developing neural tube in the rhombencephalon; nine rhombomeres appear in the developing human. [rhombencephalon + G. *meros,* part]

rhon·chal, rhon·chi·al (rong'kăl, rong'kē-ăl). Relating to or characteristic of a rhonchus.

rhon·chus, pl. **rhon·chi** (rong'kŭs, -kī). An added sound with a musical pitch occurring during inspiration or expiration, heard on auscultation of the chest and caused by air passing through bronchi that are narrowed by inflammation, spasm of smooth muscle, or presence of mucus in the lumen; if low-pitched, it is called **sonorous r.;** if high-pitched, with a whistling or squeaky quality, **sibilant r..** [L. fr. G. *rhenchos,* a snoring]

cavernous r., SYN cavernous *rale.*

rho·phe·o·cy·to·sis (rō'fē-ō-sī-tō'sis). Formation of vacuoles at a cell surface without prior formation of cytoplasmic projections, by which the cell appears to aspirate surrounding material. SEE ALSO pinocytosis. [G. *rhopheō,* to gulp down, or aspirate, + *kytos,* cell, + *-osis,* condition]

rhop·try, pl. **rhop·tries** (rōp'trē, -trēs). Electron-dense club-shaped, tubular or saccular organelles, extending back from the anterior end of sporozoites and other stages of certain sporozoans in the subphylum Apicomplexa. SYN paired organelles, toxoneme. [G. *rhopalon,* club]

rho·ta·cism (rō'tă-sizm). Mispronunciation of the "r" sound. [G. *rhō,* the letter r]

rhu·barb (roo'barb). Any plant of the genus *Rheum* (family Polygonaceae), especially *R. rhaponticum,* garden rhubarb, and *R. officinale* or *R. palmatum;* the last two species or their hybrids, deprived of periderm tissues, dried, and powdered, are used for their astringent, tonic and laxative effects.

Rhus (roos, rŭs). A genus of vines and shrubs (family Anacardiaceae) containing various species that are used for their ornamental foliage; formerly used in tanning. Certain poisonous species are classified as *Toxicodendron.* [L., fr. G. *rhous,* sumac]

rhy·po·pho·bia (rī-pō-fō'bē-ă). SYN mysophobia. [G. *rhypos,* filth, + *phobos,* fear]

■**rhythm** (rith'ŭm). **1.** Measured time or motion; the regular alternation of two or more different or opposite states. **2.** SYN rhythm *method.* **3.** Regular or irregular occurrence of an electrical event in the electrocardiogram or electroencephalogram. SEE ALSO wave. **4.** Sequential beating of the heart generated by a single beat or sequence of beats. [G. *rhythmos*]

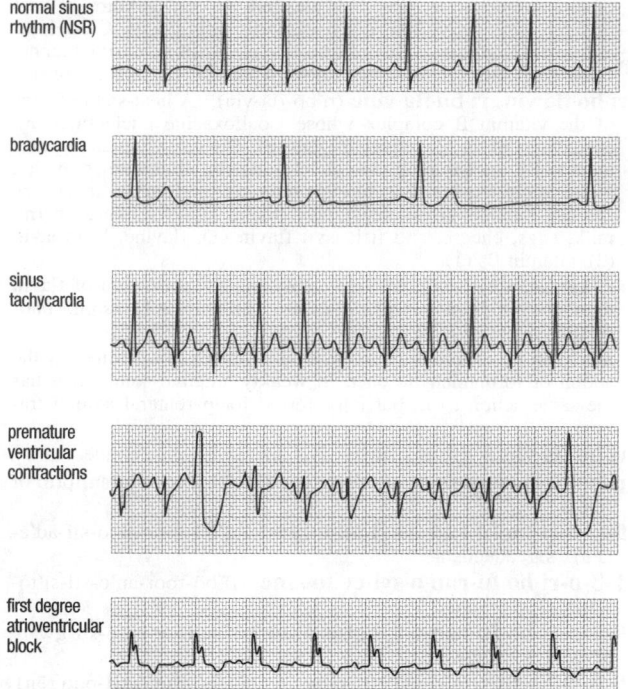

normal sinus rhythm (NSR)

bradycardia

sinus tachycardia

premature ventricular contractions

first degree atrioventricular block

atrial flutter

ventricular fibrillation

rhythm: electrocardiogram tracings showing common types of arrhythmia

agonal r., an idioventricular r., characterized by unusually wide and bizarre ventricular complexes, often seen in moribund patients.

alpha r., (1) a wave pattern in the encephalogram in the frequency band of 8–13 Hz; (2) the posterior dominant 8–13 Hz r. in the awake, relaxed person with closed eyes, that attenuates with eye opening. SYN alpha wave, Berger r.

atrioventricular junctional r., the cardiac r. when the heart is controlled by the AV junction (including node); arising in the AV junction, the impulse ascends to the atria and descends to the ventricles, each at varying speeds depending on the site of the pacemaker; only descends to the ventricles in the common form of atrioventricular dissociation and in idiojunctional rhythm. SYN AV junctional r., nodal bradycardia, nodal r.

AV junctional r., SYN atrioventricular junctional r.

basic electrical r. (BER), a slow wave of depolarization of smooth muscle from the fundus to the pylorus that coordinates gastric peristalsis and emptying.

Berger r., SYN alpha r.

beta r., a wave pattern in the electroencephalogram in the frequency band of 18–30 Hz. SYN beta wave.

bigeminal r., that cardiac r. when each beat of the dominant

rhythm (sinus or other) is followed by a premature beat, with the result that the heartbeats occur in pairs (bigeminy). SYN coupled r.

cantering r., SYN gallop.

chaotic r., completely irregular cardiac r. at varying rates. SEE ALSO arrhythmia.

circadian r., SEE circadian.

circus r., SYN circus *movement.*

coronary nodal r., formerly applied by some authorities to the electrocardiographic pattern of normal upright P waves in leads I and II with a short P-R interval.

coronary sinus r., an ectopic atrial r. supposedly originating from a pacemaker at the mouth of the coronary sinus; recognized in the electrocardiogram by P-waves that are inverted in leads II, III, and aVF with a normal or prolonged P-R interval; an ectopic ("lower") atrial rhythm.

coupled r., SYN bigeminal r.

delta r., a wave pattern in the electroencephalogram in the frequency band of 1.5–4.0 Hz.

diurnal r., SEE diurnal.

ectopic r., any cardiac r. arising from a center other than the normal pacemaker, the sinus node.

escape r., three or more consecutive impulses at a rate not exceeding the upper limit of the inherent pacemaker; extreme range of impulse formation at the sinoatrial node is between 40 and 180 impulses per minute, that of the atrioventricular junction is normally 40–60 impulses per min, and the normal rate of the ventricular myocardium (idioventricular rhythm) is 20–40 impulses per min.

gallop r., SYN gallop.

idiojunctional r., SYN idionodal r.

idionodal r., an independent r., the ventricles being under control of the AV node (AV junction). SYN idiojunctional r.

idioventricular r., a slow independent ventricular r. under control of a ventricular center (which is, by definition, ectopic). SYN ventricular r.

junctional r., r.'s originating anywhere within the AV junction. Formerly, "AV nodal" or simply "nodal" r.'s.

nodal r., SYN atrioventricular junctional r.

pendulum r., SYN embryocardia.

quadrigeminal r., a cardiac arrhythmia in which the heartbeats are grouped in fours, each usually composed of one sinus beat followed by three extrasystoles, but a repetitive group of four of any composition is quadrigeminal. SYN quadrigeminy.

quadruple r., a quadruple cadence to the heart sounds due to the easy audibility of both third and fourth heart sounds, indicative of serious myocardial disease. SYN trainwheel r.

reciprocal r., a cardiac arrhythmia in which the impulse arising in the AV junction descends to and activates the ventricles on one intrajunctional pathway and simultaneously ascends toward the atria in parallel pathways; before reaching the atria, however, the impulse is reflected downward and again activates the ventricles, producing an echo or reciprocal beat; recognized in the electrocardiogram by the presence of an inverted P wave in lead aVF and usually II sandwiched between two ventricular complexes aberrantly, both of which may be normal or one of which may be conducted.

reciprocating r., a cardiac arrhythmia initiated by an AV junctional beat followed in turn by a reciprocal beat; the descending impulse of the reciprocal beat, before reaching the ventricles, is also reflected backward to the atria, but before reaching the atria is reflected downward again to the ventricles, so that there is both retrograde atrial activation and orthograde ventricular activation.

reversed reciprocal r., a cardiac arrhythmia in which a normal sinus impulse, before reaching the ventricles, is reflected backward to the atria; thus in the electrocardiogram a ventricular complex is sandwiched between a normal sinus P wave and a retrograde P wave; if the dysrhythmia continues, subsequent cycles are similar to those of reciprocating r.

sinus r., normal cardiac r. proceeding from the sinoatrial node; in healthy adults its rate is 60–90 beats/min.

systolic gallop r., obsolete term for extra sounds, usually clicks, heard during systole.

rh

theta r., a wave pattern in the electroencephalogram in the frequency band of 4–7 Hz. SYN theta wave.

tic·tac r., SYN embryocardia.

trainwheel r., SYN quadruple r.

trigeminal r., a cardiac arrhythmia in which the beats are grouped in trios, usually composed of a sinus beat followed by two extrasystoles. SYN trigeminy.

triple r., a triple cadence to the heart sounds at any heart rate, due to the easy audibility of a third (S_3) (usually) or fourth (S_4) heart sound, or at faster rates a summation sound due to coincidence of the third and fourth heart sounds ("S_7" = S_3 + S_4).

ultradian r., SEE ultradian.

ventricular r., SYN idioventricular r.

rhytide (rī′tīd). A skin wrinkle. [[G. *rhytis, -idos,* wrinkle]]

rhyt·i·dec·tomy (rit-i-dek′tō-mē). Elimination of wrinkles from, or reshaping of, the face by excising any excess skin and tightening the remainder; the so-called face-lift. SYN face-lift, rhytidoplasty. [G. *rhytis* (*rhytid-*), a wrinkle]

rhyt·i·do·plas·ty (rit′i-dō-plas-tē). SYN rhytidectomy. [G. *rhytis,* a wrinkle, + *plastos,* formed]

rhyt·i·do·sis (rit-i-dō′sis). **1.** Wrinkling of the face to a degree disproportionate to age. **2.** Laxity and wrinkling of the cornea, an indication of approaching death. SYN rutidosis. [G. a wrinkling, fr. *rhytis,* a wrinkle, + *-osis,* condition]

r. retinae, retinal wrinkling.

RIA Abbreviation for radioimmunoassay.

Rib Symbol for ribose. SYN os costale.

△**rib-.** SEE ribo-.

ri·ba·vi·rin (rī′bă-vī-rin). A synthetic nucleoside antiviral agent that, by its inhibitory effect on the synthesis of guanosine 5′-phosphate, inhibits both DNA and RNA synthesis; used for treatment of viral pneumonia caused by respiratory syncytial virus.

α-ri·ba·zole (rī′bă-zōl). The benzimidazole nucleoside in vitamin B_{12}.

rib·bon (rib′ŏn). A ribbon-shaped structure. [M. E. *riban*]

Reil r., SYN medial *lemniscus.*

Ribes, François, French physician, 1765–1845. SEE R. *ganglion.*

ri·bi·tol (rī′bi-tol). Reduction product of ribose (–CHO at position 1 of ribose reduced to –CH_2OH). SYN adonitol.

ri·bi·tyl (rī′bi-til). The radical of ribitol; a constituent of riboflavin.

rib [I–XII]. One of the 24 elongated curved bones forming the main portion of the bony wall of the chest. SYN costa (1). [A.S. *ribb*]

bicipital r., fusion of first thoracic r. with cervical vertebra.

bifid r., one in which the body bifurcates.

cervical r. [TA], a supernumerary rib articulating with a cervical vertebra, usually the seventh, but not reaching the sternum anteriorly. SEE ALSO cervical rib *syndrome.* SYN costa cervicalis [TA].

false r.'s, five lower ribs on either side that do not articulate with the sternum directly. SYN costae spuriae [VII–XII] [TA], vertebrochondral r.'s.

first r. [I] [TA], atypical rib having a single facet on its head, for articulation with the T1 vertebra, and the broadest, shortest and most sharply curved shaft; it also bears two transverse grooves on its superior surface for the subclavian vessels, separated by the scalene tubercle and ridge. SYN costa prima [I] [TA].

floating r.'s [XI–XII], the two lower ribs on either side that are not attached anteriorly. SYN costae fluctuantes [XI–XII], costae fluitantes, vertebral r.'s.

lumbar r. [TA], an occasional r. articulating with the transverse process of the first lumbar vertebra.

r. notching, a smooth defect in the lower border of one or more upper r.'s caused by enlarged intercostal collateral vessels, most often a sign of coarctation of the aorta.

slipping r., subluxation of a r. cartilage, with costochondral separation.

true r.'s [I–VII], seven upper ribs on either side whose cartilages articulate directly with the sternum. SYN costae verae [I–VII] [TA], vertebrosternal r.'s.

vertebral r.'s, SYN floating r.'s [XI–XII].

vertebrochondral r.'s, SYN false r.'s.

vertebrosternal r.'s, SYN true r.'s [I–VII].

△**ribo-.** **1.** Ribose. **2.** As an italicized prefix to the systematic name of a monosaccharide, *ribo-* indicates that the configuration of a set of three consecutive, but not necessarily contiguous, CHOH (or asymmetric) groups is that of ribose; e.g., D-ribose, a trivial name, is D-*ribo*-pentose in systematic nomenclature. [German *Ribose*]

ri·bo·fla·vin, ri·bo·fla·vine (rī′bō-flā-vin). A heat-stable factor of the vitamin B complex whose isoalloxazine nucleotides are coenzymes of the flavodehydrogenases. The daily human requirement is 1.7 mg for adult men and 1.3 mg for adult women, with a higher daily requirement during pregnancy and lactation; dietary sources include green vegetables, liver, kidneys, wheat germ, milk, eggs, cheese, and fish. SYN flavin (1), flavine, lactoflavin (2), vitamin B_2 (1).

r. kinase, a cytosolic enzyme catalyzing the formation of flavin mononucleotide (r. phosphate) from r., utilizing ATP as phosphorylating agent. SYN flavokinase.

methylol r., a mixture of methylol derivatives of r. formed by the action of formaldehyde on r. in weakly alkaline solution; it has the same action as r., but is preferred for parenteral administration.

ri·bo·fla·vin 5′-phos·phate. SYN *flavin* mononucleotide.

ri·bo·fu·ra·nose (rī-bō-foor′ă-nōs). The 1,4 cyclic furan form of ribose.

9-β-D-ri·bo·fu·ran·o·syl·ad·e·nine (rī′bō-foor-an′o-sil-ad′ĕ-nēn). SYN adenosine.

1-β-D-ri·bo·fu·ran·o·syl·cy·to·sine (rī′bō-foor-an′o-sil-sī′tō-sēn). SYN cytidine.

9-β-D-ri·bo·fu·ran·o·syl·gua·nine (rī′bō-foor-an′ō-sil-gwah′nēn). SYN guanosine.

9-β-ri·bo·fu·ran·o·syl·pu·rine (rī′bō-foo-ran′ō-sil-poo′rēn). SYN nebularine.

ri·bo·fu·ran·o·syl·thy·mine (rī′bō-foor-an′ō-sil-thī′mēn). SYN ribothymidine.

1-β-D-ri·bo·fu·ran·o·syl·u·ra·cil (rī′bō-foor-an′ō-sil-ūr′ă-sil). SYN uridine.

ri·bo-2-hex·u·lose. SYN psicose.

ri·bo·nu·cle·ase (RNase) (rī-bō-noo′klē-ās). A transferase or phosphodiesterase that catalyzes the hydrolysis of ribonucleic acid. SEE ALSO ribonuclease (pancreatic), ribonuclease (*Bacillus subtilis*). SYN ribonucleinase.

RNase A, ribonuclease (pancreatic).

alkaline RNase, ribonuclease (pancreatic).

RNase α, an enzyme catalyzing endonucleolytic cleavage of *O*-methylated RNA yielding 5′-phosphomonoesters.

r. D (RNase D), an enzyme (endonuclease) that trims the extra 3′ nucleotides from immature tRNA.

Escherichia coli **RNase I,** SYN RNase T_2.

RNase I, ribonuclease (pancreatic).

RNase II, an enzyme cleaving RNA exonucleolytically in the 3′ to 5′ direction, yielding 5′-phosphomononucleotides. SEE ALSO microbial RNase II.

RNase III, an enzyme catalyzing endonucleolytic cleavage of double-stranded RNA, yielding 5′-phosphomonoesters.

microbial RNase II, SYN RNase T_2.

RNase N_1, SYN RNase T_1.

RNase N_2, SYN RNase T_2.

RNase P, an enzyme catalyzing the endonucleolytic cleavage tRNA precursors to yield 5′-phosphomonoesters.

pancreatic RNase, SEE ribonuclease (pancreatic).

plant RNase, SYN RNase T_2.

RNase T_1, an enzyme endonucleolytically cleaving ribonucleic acids at the 3′-5′ link of a guanosine 3′-phosphate residue, producing oligonucleotides terminating in this nucleotide; a transferase (endonuclease) in the first (cyclizing) step, a phosphodiesterase on the second (hydrolyzing) step. SYN guanyloribonuclease, RNase N_1.

RNase T_2, an enzyme endonucleolytically cleaving RNA to 3′-

nucleotides with 2′,3′-cyclic nucleotides as intermediates. SYN *Escherichia coli* RNase I, microbial RNase II, plant RNase, RNase N_2.

RNase U_2, an enzyme endonucleolytically cleaving RNA to 3′-phosphomono- and 3′-phosphooligonucleotides ending in adenylate or guanylate residues with 2′,3′-cyclic phosphate intermediates.

RNase U_4, SYN yeast RNase.

yeast RNase, an enzyme catalyzing the exonucleolytic cleavage of RNA to yield 3′-phosphomononucleotides. SYN RNase U_4.

ri·bo·nu·cle·ase (*Ba·cil·lus sub·ti·lis*). 1. Ribonuclease (*Azotobacter agilis*); ribonuclease (*Proteus mirabilis*); an enzyme catalyzing the endonucleolytic cleavage of RNA to yield 2′,3′-cyclic nucleotides. **2.** Ribonuclease T_1.

ri·bo·nu·cle·ase (pan·cre·at·ic). An enzyme isolated from the pancreas of ruminants that transfers the 3′-phosphate of a pyrimidine ribonucleotide residue in a polynucleotide from the 5′-position of the adjoining nucleotide to the 2′-position of the pyrimidine nucleotide itself (a transferase, endonuclease action), thus breaking the chain and forming a pyrimidine 2′,3′-cyclic phosphate, then (or independently) hydrolyzing this phosphodiester to leave a pyrimidine nucleoside 3′-phosphate residue (phosphodiesterase action); used in cytochemistry to selectively degrade and remove RNA as a control for staining of RNA.

ri·bo·nu·cle·ic ac·id (RNA) (rī′bō-noo-klē′ik). A macromolecule consisting of ribonucleoside residues connected by phosphate from the 3′-hydroxyl of one to the 5′-hydroxyl of the next nucleoside. RNA is found in all cells, in both nuclei and cytoplasm and in particulate and nonparticulate form, and also in many viruses; polynucleotides made in vitro are generally called such. Various RNA fractions are identified by location, form, or function.

acceptor RNA, SYN transfer RNA.

antisense RNA, the transcription product of the DNA antisense strand; it can play a role in the inhibition of translation. SEE ALSO antisense DNA.

chromosomal RNA, RNA associated with the chromosome (not mRNA, tRNA, or rRNA) that may have a role in transcription.

heterogeneous nuclear RNA (hnRNA), an ill-defined form of RNA, of high molecular weight, that never leaves the nucleus and is thought to be the precursor of messenger RNA.

informational RNA, SYN messenger RNA.

initiation tRNA, tRNA in prokaryotes containing a formyl-methionyl residue that initiates translation. SYN formyl-methionyl-tRNA, starter tRNA.

messenger RNA (mRNA), the RNA reflecting the exact nucleoside sequence of the genetically active DNA and carrying the "message" of the latter, coded in its sequence, to the cytoplasmic areas where protein is made in amino acid sequences specified by the mRNA, and hence primarily by the DNA; viral RNAs are considered to be natural messenger RNAs. SYN informational RNA, template RNA.

messengerlike RNA (mlRNA), SEE heterogeneous nuclear RNA.

nuclear RNA (nRNA), rNA found in nuclei, or associated with DNA, or with nuclear structures (nucleoli).

RNA polymerase, SEE nucleotidyltransferases.

ribosomal RNA, the RNA of ribosomes and polyribosomes.

small nuclear RNA (snRNA), small RNA (i.e., about 90–300 nucleotides long) in the nucleus believed to have a role in RNA processing and cellular architecture.

soluble RNA (sRNA), SYN transfer RNA. [soluble in molar salt]

starter tRNA, SYN initiation tRNA.

suppressor tRNA, the tRNA associated with a suppressor mutation.

template RNA, SYN messenger RNA.

transfer RNA (tRNA), short-chain RNA molecules present in cells in at least 20 varieties, each variety capable of combining with a specific amino acid (see aminoacyl-tRNA). By joining (through their anticodons) with particular spots (codons) along the messenger RNA molecule and carrying their amino acyl residues along, they lead to the formation of protein molecules with a specific amino acid arrangement—the one ultimately dictated by a segment of DNA in the chromosomes. Each tRNA has about 80

nucleotides (MW about 25,000); most of the 20 varieties occur in multiple "isoacceptor" forms, separable by chromatography. Further subvarieties exist in, e.g., different strains of an organism, in subcellular organelles, and in different metabolic states. Cognate tRNAs are the tRNAs recognized by the specific amino acyl-tRNA synthetases. SYN acceptor RNA, soluble RNA.

ri·bo·nu·cle·i·nase (rī-bō-noo′klē-i-nās). SYN ribonuclease.

ri·bo·nu·cle·o·pro·tein (RNP) (rī′bō-noo′klē-ō-prō′tēn). A combination of ribonucleic acid and protein.

ri·bo·nu·cle·o·side (rī-bō-noo′klē-ō-sīd). A nucleoside in which the sugar component is ribose; the common r.'s of RNA are adenosine, cytidine, guanosine, and uridine.

ri·bo·nu·cle·o·tide (rī-bō-noo′klē-ō-tīd). A nucleotide (nucleoside phosphate) in which the sugar component is ribose; the major r.'s of RNA are adenylic acid, cytidylic acid, guanylic acid, and uridylic acid.

r. reductase, a protein complex that converts ribonucleotide diphosphates (NDPs) such as ADP and CDP to 2′-deoxyribonucleotide diphosphates (dNDPs) such as dADP and dCDP. This complex requires thioredoxin, thioredoxin reductase, and NADPH. It is crucial for DNA synthesis.

ri·bo·pho·rins (rī′-bō-for′inz). Ribosome receptor proteins that interact specifically with the large ribosomal subunit and aid in translocation of newly synthesized proteins across the endoplasmic reticulum. [*ribo*nucleic acid + G. *phoros,* carrying, + -in]

ri·bo·pyr·a·nose (rī-bō-pir′ă-nōs). The 1,5-cyclic form of ribose.

ri·bose (Rib) (rī′bōs). The pentose that, as the D-isomer, is present in ribonucleic acid; epimers of D-r. are D-arabinose, D-xylose, and L-lyxose.

ri·bose-5-phos·phate. Ribose phosphorylated on carbon-5; an intermediate in the pentose phosphate pathway.

r.-5-p. isomerase, an enzyme catalyzing interconversion of D-ribose 5-phosphate and D-ribulose 5-phosphate; of importance in ribose metabolism and in the pentose phosphate pathway. SYN phosphopentose isomerase, phosphoriboisomerase.

ri·bo·side (rī′bō-sīd). The product formed by replacement of the H of the C-1 OH of ribose by an alcohol residue (which may be another sugar); differs from ribosyl compounds and does not occur in ribonucleic acids, where the radical is a ribosyl (1-OH missing entirely). See structure for methyl β-D-ribofuranoside below.

ri·bo·some (rī′bō-sōm). A granule of ribonucleoprotein, 120–150 Å in diameter, that is the site of protein synthesis from aminoacyl-tRNAs as directed by mRNAs. SYN Palade granule.

ri·bo·su·ria (rī-bō-soo′rē-ă). The enhanced urinary excretion of D-ribose; commonly one manifestation of muscular dystrophy. [ribose + G. *ouron,* urine]

ri·bo·syl (rī′bō-sil). The radical formed by loss of the hemiacetal OH group from either of the two cyclic forms of ribose (yielding ribofuranosyl and ribopyranosyl compounds), by combination with an H of an –NH– or a –CH– group; the natural nucleosides are ribosyl compounds, not riboside, as the bond between ribose and aglycon is C–N or C–C, not –C–O–X–.

ri·bo·syl·a·tion (rī-bō-sil-ā-shŭn). The covalent attachment of one or more ribosyl groups to a molecule (usually a macromolecule).

ADP r., covalent attachment of an ADP-ribosyl moiety to a macromolecule; e.g., the action of diphtheria toxin.

1-ri·bo·syl·or·o·tate (rī′bō-sil-ōr′ō-tāt). SYN orotidine.

ri·bo·syl·pur·ine (rī′bō-sil-pūr′ēn). SYN nebularine.

ri·bo·syl·thy·mi·dine. SYN ribothymidine.

ri·bo·thy·mi·dine (T, Thd) (rī-bō-thī′mi-dēn). 5-Methyluridine; the ribosyl analog of thymidine (deoxyribosylthymine); a nucleoside found in small amounts in ribonucleic acids. SYN ribofuranosylthymine, ribosylthymidine.

ri·bo·thy·mi·dyl·ic ac·id (rTMP, TMP) (rī′bō-thī-mi-dil′ik). Ribothymidine 5′-phosphate; the ribose analog of thymidylic acid; a rare component of transfer RNAs.

ri·bo·tide (rī′bō-tīd). A corruption of riboside, by analogy with nucleoside-nucleotide, to mean ribonucleotide.

ri·bo·vi·rus (rī′bō-vī′rŭs). SYN RNA *virus*.

ri

ri·bo·zyme (rī'bō-zīm). A nonprotein biocatalyst; several cleave precursors of tRNA to yield functional tRNAs; others act on rRNA; plays a key role in intron splicing events. SYN organic catalyst (1), RNA enzyme. [ribonucleic acid + -zyme]

ri·bu·lose (rī'bū-lōs). The 2-keto isomer of ribose. As the 5-phosphate, it participates in the pentose monophosphate shunt; as the 1,5-bisphosphate, it combines with CO_2 at the start of the photosynthetic process in green plants ("carbon dioxide trap"); D-r. is the epimer of D-xylulose.

ri·bu·lose-1,5-bis·phos·phate car·box·yl·ase. A dimerizing carboxy-lyase; an enzyme that catalyzes the addition of carbon dioxide to D-ribulose 1,5-bisphosphate and the hydrolysis of the addition product to two molecules of 3-D-phosphoglyceric acid, a key reaction in the fixation of CO_2 in photosynthesis. SYN carboxydismutase.

ri·bu·lose-phos·phate 3-ep·i·mer·ase. An enzyme catalyzing the reversible interconversion of D-xylulose 5-phosphate and its epimer, D-ribulose 5-phosphate; a step in the nonoxidative phase of the pentose phosphate pathway. SYN phosphoribulose epimerase.

Ricco, Annibale, Italian astrophysicist, 1844–1919. SEE R. *law.*

rice (rīs). The grain of *Oryza sativa* (family Gramineae), the rice plant; a food; also used, finely pulverized, as a dusting powder. [G. *oryza*]

Rich, Arnold R., U.S. pathologist, 1893–1968. SEE Hamman-R. *syndrome.*

Richards, Barry Wyndham, 20th century English physician. SEE Richards-Rundle *syndrome.*

Richardson, John Clifford, Canadian neurologist, *1909. SEE Steele-R.-Olszewski *disease, syndrome.*

Richter, August G., German surgeon, 1742–1812. SEE R. *hernia;* R.-Monro *line;* Monro-R. *line.*

Richter, Maurice N., U.S. pathologist, *1897. SEE R. *syndrome.*

ri·cin (rī'sin, ris'in). A highly toxic lectin and hemagglutin occurring in the seeds (castor beans) of the castor oil plant, *Ricinus communis;* if eaten, acts as a violent irritant and may be fatal; an *N*-glycosidase that acts on the GOS subunit of rRNA.

ric·i·nism (ris'i-nizm). Poisoning by ingestion of toxic principles from seeds (castor beans) or leaves of the castor oil plant, *Ricinus communis.*

ri·cin·o·le·ate (ris-i-nō'lē-āt). A salt of ricinoleic acid.

ri·cin·o·le·ic ac·id (ris-i-nō-lē'ik, rī-si-). An unsaturated hydroxy acid present in castor oil.

Ric·i·nus (ris'i-nŭs). A genus of plants (family Euphorbiaceae) with one species, *R. communis,* the castor oil plant, the source of castor oil; the leaves are said to be a galactagogue. SYN castor bean. [L.]

rick·ets (rik'ets). A disease due to vitamin D deficiency and characterized by overproduction and deficient calcification of osteoid tissue, with associated skeletal deformities, disturbances in growth, hypocalcemia, and sometimes tetany; usually accompanied by irritability, listlessness, and generalized muscular weakness; fractures are frequent. SYN infantile osteomalacia, juvenile osteomalacia, rachitis. [E. *wrick,* to twist]

acute r., SYN hemorrhagic r.

adult r., SYN osteomalacia.

celiac r., arrested growth and osseous deformities associated with defective absorption of fat and calcium in celiac disease.

familial hypophosphatemic r., SYN vitamin D-resistant r.

hemorrhagic r., bone changes seen in infantile scurvy, consisting of subperiosteal hemorrhage and deficient osteoid tissue formation; often used to indicate simultaneous occurrence of r. and scurvy. SYN acute r.

hereditary hypophosphatemic r., with hypercalciuria, an inherited disorder in which there is a defect in renal tubular reabsorption.

late r., SYN osteomalacia.

refractory r., r. that does not respond to treatment with usual doses of vitamin D and adequate dietary calcium and phosphorus; most often due to inherited renal tubular disorder, e.g., Fanconi syndrome.

renal r., a form of r. occurring in children in association with and apparently caused by renal disease with hyperphosphatemia. SYN pseudorickets, renal fibrocystic osteosis, renal infantilism, renal osteitis fibrosa.

scurvy r., SYN infantile *scurvy.*

vitamin D-resistant r., a group of metabolic disorders characterized by renal tubular defect in phosphate transport and bone abnormalities resulting in hypophosphatemic r. or osteomalacia; hypocalcemia and tetany are not features. There is an autosomal dominant form [MIM*193100] and an X-linked dominant form [MIM*307800], the latter caused by mutation in the phosphate-regulating gene with homologies to endopeptidases (PHEX) on chromosome Xp. Both forms are not responsive to standard therapeutic doses of vitamin D but they may respond to very large doses of phosphate and/or vitamin D. There is also an autosomal recessive form [MIM*277440] caused by mutation in the vitamin D receptor gene (VDR) on 12q. SYN familial hypophosphatemic r.

Ricketts, Howard T., U.S. pathologist, 1871–1910. SEE *Rickettsia.*

Rick·ett·sia (ri-ket'sē-ă). A genus of bacteria (order Rickettsiales) containing small (nonfilterable), often pleomorphic, coccoid to rod-shaped, Gram-negative organisms that usually occur intracytoplasmically in lice, fleas, ticks, and mites but do not grow in cell-free media; pathogenic species infect humans and other animals, causing epidemic typhus, murine, or endemic typhus, Rocky Mountain spotted fever, tsutsugamushi disease, rickettsialpox, and other diseases; type species is *R. prowazekii.* [Howard T. *Ricketts*]

R. africae, a species of R. studied principally in Zimbabwe that appears to be carried by the tick *Amblyomma hebraeum;* a cause of spotted fever.

R. ak'ari, a bacterial species causing human rickettsialpox; transmitted by the house mouse mite, *Liponyssoides sanguineus;* a mild febrile disease of 7–10 days is produced with an urban distribution in the northeastern U.S. and in wild or commensal rodents in the countries of the former USSR and Africa.

R. austral'is, a bacterial species causing a spotted fever, North Queensland tick typhus, clinically and serologically similar to the disease caused by the agent of rickettsialpox; *Ixodes holocyclus* and *I. tasmani* are probable vectors. Small marsupials are suspected reservoirs of this agent, which is found over much of coastal Queensland, especially in secondary scrub and savannah.

R. burnet'ii, former name for *Coxiella burnetii.*

R. canis, former name for *Ehrlichia canis.*

R. conorii, a species of bacteria causing boutonneuse fever in southern Europe, Africa, and the Middle East; transmitted by various ticks, such as the dog tick *Rhipicephalis sanguineus.*

R. honei, a bacterial species causing Flinders Island spotted fever in Australia.

R. japonica, a bacterial species causing Japanese spotted fever.

R. mooseri, a species similar to *R. prowazekii* but with less variation in appearance; the resultant endemic typhus is milder and has a somewhat slower onset.

R. prowazek'ii, a bacterial species causing epidemic and recrudescent typhus, transmitted by body lice; type species of the genus R.

R. psi'ttaci, former name for *Chlamydia psittaci.*

R. ricketts'ii, a bacterial species, the agent of Rocky Mountain spotted fever, South African tick-bite fever, São Paulo exanthematic typhus of Brazil, Tobia fever of Colombia, and spotted fevers of Minas Gerais and Mexico; transmitted by infected ixodid ticks, especially *Dermacentor andersoni* and *D. variabilis.*

R. sennet'su, SYN *Ehrlichia sennetsu.*

R. sibir'ica, a bacterial species, the agent of Siberian or North Asian tick typhus, transmitted by various ixodid ticks, which also serve as reservoirs, possibly aided by rodents and hares; the disease resembles Rocky Mountain spotted fever.

R. slovaca, a bacterial species causing a newly recognized rickettsiosis associated with local erythema and possibly meningoencephalitis; transmitted by the tick *Dermacentor marginatus.*

R. tsutsugamu'shi, former name for *Orientia tsutsugamushi.*

R. ty'phi, a bacterial species causing murine or endemic typhus fever, transmitted by the rat flea.

rick·ett·si·al (ri-ket′sē-ăl). Pertaining to or caused by rickettsiae.

rick·ett·si·al·pox (ri-ket′sē-ăl-poks′). Infection with *Rickettsia akari*, which is spread by mites from reservoir in house mice; a benign, self-limited process first recognized in 1946 in the Kew Gardens area of New York City; a few limited outbreaks have been observed elsewhere since then. SYN Kew Gardens fever, mite-born typhus, vesicular rickettsiosis.

rick·ett·si·o·sis (ri-ket-sē-ō′sis). Infection with rickettsiae.
vesicular r., SYN rickettsialpox.

rick·ett·si·o·stat·ic (ri-ket′sē-ō-stat′ik). An agent inhibitory to the growth of *Rickettsia*. [*Rickettsia* + G. *statikos,* bringing to a standstill]

rick·e·ty (rik′ĕ-tē). SYN rachitic.

Rickles, Norman H., U.S. oral pathologist, *1920. SEE R. *test.*

RID Abbreviation for radial *immunodiffusion.*

Riddoch, George, British physician, 1888–1947. SEE Riddoch *phenomenon.* SEE ALSO Riddoch *phenomenon.*

Rideal, Samuel, English chemist and bacteriologist, 1863–1929. SEE R.-Walker *coefficient, method.*

ridge (rij). **1.** A (usually rough) linear elevation. SEE ALSO crest. **2.** In dentistry, any linear elevation on the surface of a tooth. **3.** The remainder of the alveolar process and its soft tissue covering after the teeth are removed. [A. S. *hrycg,* back, spine]
alveolar r., SYN alveolar *process* of maxilla.
apical ectodermal r., the layer of surface ectodermal cells at the apex of the embryonic limb bud; thought to exert an inductive influence on the condensation of underlying mesenchyme and be necessary for continued outgrowth of the limb.
basal r., (1) SYN alveolar *process* of maxilla; **(2)** SYN *cingulum* of tooth.
bicipital r.'s, SYN *crest* of greater tubercle, *crest* of lesser tubercle.
buccocervical r., a convexity within the cervical third of the buccal surface of molars.
buccogingival r., a distinct r. on the buccal surface of a deciduous molar tooth, approximately 1.5 mm from the crown-root junction.
bulbar r., one of two spiral subendocardial thickenings in the embryonic bulbus cordis; when they fuse, they divide the bulbus into the aorta and pulmonary artery.
bulboventricular r., an elevation on the inner surface of the embryonic heart at 4–5 weeks; it indicates the division between the developing ventricles and the bulbus cordis.
dental r., the prominent border of a cusp or margin of a tooth.
dermal r.'s [TA], surface ridges of the epidermis of the palms and soles, where the sweat pores open. SYN cristae cutis [TA], epidermal r.'s, papillary r.'s, skin r.'s.
epidermal r.'s, SYN dermal r.'s.
epipericardial r., an elevation separating the developing pharyngeal region from the embryonic pericardium.
external oblique r., SYN oblique *line* of mandible.
ganglion r., SYN neural *crest.*
genital r., SYN gonadal r.
gluteal r., SYN gluteal *tuberosity.*
gonadal r., an elevation of thickened mesothelium and underlying mesenchyme on the ventromedial border of the embryonic mesonephros; the primordial germ cells become embedded in it, establishing it as the primordium of the testis or ovary. SYN genital r.
interpapillary r.'s, SYN rete r.
key r., SYN zygomaxillare.
lateral epicondylar r., SYN lateral supraepicondylar r.
lateral supracondylar r., ✭official alternate term for lateral supraepicondylar r.
lateral supraepicondylar r. [TA], the distal sharp portion of the lateral margin of the humerus. SYN crista supraepicondylaris lateralis [TA], crista supracondylaris lateralis✭, lateral supracondylar r.✭, lateral epicondylar crest, lateral epicondylar r., lateral supracondylar crest.
linguocervical r., SYN linguogingival r.

linguogingival r., a r. occurring on the lingual surface, near the cervix, of the incisor and cuspid teeth. SYN linguocervical r.
Mall r.'s, rarely used eponym for pulmonary r.'s.
mammary r., bandlike thickening of ectoderm in the embryo extending on either side from just below the axilla to the inguinal region; in human embryos, the mammary glands arise from primordia in the thoracic part of the r., the balance of the r. disappearing; in some lower mammals that give birth to a litter of young, several milk glands develop along these lines. SYN mammary fold, milk line, milk r.
marginal r., SYN marginal *crest* of tooth.
medial epicondylar r., SYN medial supraepicondylar r.
medial supracondylar r., ✭official alternate term for medial supraepicondylar r.
medial supraepicondylar r. [TA], the distal sharp portion of the medial margin of the humerus. SYN crista supraepicondylaris medialis [TA], crista supracondylaris medialis✭, medial supracondylar r.✭, medial epicondylar crest, medial epicondylar r., medial supracondylar crest.
mesonephric r., a r. that, in early human embryos, composes the entire urogenital r.; however, later in development a more medial genital r., the potential gonad, is demarcated from it. SEE ALSO urogenital r. SYN mesonephric fold.
milk r., SYN mammary r.
mylohyoid r., SYN mylohyoid *line.*
nasal r., SYN *agger* nasi.
oblique r., a r. on the masticatory surface of an upper molar tooth from the mesiolingual to the distobuccal cusp.
oblique r. of trapezium, SYN *tuberculum* of trapezium bone.
palatine r., SYN palatine *raphe.*
papillary r.'s, SYN dermal r.'s.
Passavant r., a prominence on the posterior wall of the nasopharynx formed by contraction of the superior constrictor muscle of the pharynx during swallowing. SYN Passavant bar, Passavant cushion, Passavant pad.
pectoral r., SYN *crest* of greater tubercle.
pharyngeal r., SYN posterior *fascicle* of palatopharyngeus muscle.
primitive r., one of the paired r.'s on either side of the primitive groove.
pronator r., an oblique r. on the anterior surface of the ulna, giving attachment to the pronator quadratus muscle.
pterygoid r. of sphenoid bone, SYN infratemporal *crest* of greater wing of sphenoid.
pulmonary r.'s, a pair of r.'s overlying the common cardinal veins and bulging from the lateral body wall into the embryonic celom; so called because they give early indication of where the pleuropericardial folds will develop.
residual r., that portion of the processus alveolaris remaining in the edentulous mouth following resorption of the section containing the alveoli.
rete r., downward thickening of the epidermis between the dermal papillae; peg is a misnomer because the dermal papillae are cylindric but the epidermal thickening between papillae is not. SYN interpapillary r.'s, rete pegs.
skin r.'s, SYN dermal r.'s.
sphenoidal r.'s, sharp posterior margins of the lesser wings of the sphenoid bone that end medially in the anterior clinoid process; the sphenoidal r.'s demarcate the anterior cranial fossa from the lateral part of the middle cranial fossa.
superciliary r., SYN superciliary *arch.*
supplemental r., a r. on the surface of a tooth that is not normally present.
supraorbital r., SYN supraorbital *margin.*
taste r., one of the r.'s surrounding the vallate papillae of the tongue.
temporal r., SYN inferior temporal *line* of parietal bone, superior temporal *line* of parietal bone.
transverse r. [TA], SYN *crista* transversalis.
transverse palatine r., SYN transverse palatine *fold.*
transverse r.'s of sacrum [TA], one of four ridges that cross the pelvic surface of the sacrum; these mark the positions of the

ri

intervertebral disks between the bodies of the five sacral vertebrae in the immature bone. SYN lineae transversae ossis sacri [TA].

trapezoid r., SYN trapezoid *line.*

triangular r. [TA], SYN *crista triangularis.*

urogenital r., one of the paired longitudinal r.'s developing in the dorsal body wall of the embryo on either side of the dorsal mesentery; the r. is formed at first by the growing mesonephros and later by the mesonephros and the gonad. SYN genital fold, wolffian r.

wolffian r., SYN urogenital r.

Ridley, Humphrey, English anatomist, 1653–1708. SEE R. *circle, sinus; circulus* venosus ridleyi.

Riedel, Bernhard M.C.L., German surgeon, 1846–1916. SEE R. *disease, lobe, struma, thyroiditis.*

Rieder, Hermann, German pathologist, 1858–1932. SEE R. *cells,* under *cell,* cell *leukemia, lymphocyte.*

Riegel, Franz, German physician, 1843–1904. SEE R. *pulse.*

Rieger, Herwigh, German ophthalmologist. SEE R. *anomaly, syndrome.*

Riehl, Gustav, Austrian dermatologist, 1855–1943. SEE R. *melanosis.*

RIF Abbreviation for resistance-inducing *factor.*

ri·fam·pi·cin (rif′am-pi-sin). SYN rifampin.

rif·am·pin (rif′am-pin). A first-line antituberculosis drug; a bactericidal agent used in the treatment of tuberculosis and other infections, that, like all antituberculosis drugs, must not be used alone in the treatment of active tuberculosis; a powerful inducer of hepatic microsomal enzymes. SYN rifampicin.

rif·a·my·cin, rif·o·my·cin (rif-ă-mī′sin, rif-ō-). A complex antibiotic, isolated from *Nocardia mediterranei,* that is active against *Mycobacterium tuberculosis* and *Staphylococcus aureus;* it is poorly absorbed from the gastrointestinal tract and often causes irritation and severe pain at the sites of injection.

Riga, Antonio, Italian physician, 1832–1919. SEE R.-Fede *disease.*

right-eyed (rīt-īd). SYN dextrocular.

right-foot·ed (rīt′fŭt-ed). SYN dextropedal.

right-hand·ed (rīt′hand-ed). Denoting the habitual or more skillful use of the right hand for writing and most manual operations. SYN dextral, dextromanual.

ri·gid·i·ty (ri-jid′i-tē). **1.** Stiffness or inflexibility. SYN rigor (1). **2.** In psychiatry and clinical psychology, an aspect of personality characterized by an individual's resistance to change. **3.** In neurology, one type of increase in muscle tone at rest; characterized by increased resistance to passive stretch, independent of velocity and symmetric about joints; increases with activation of corresponding muscles in the contralateral limb. Two basic types are cogwheel r. and lead-pipe r. SEE ALSO nuchal r. [L. *rigidus,* rigid, inflexible]

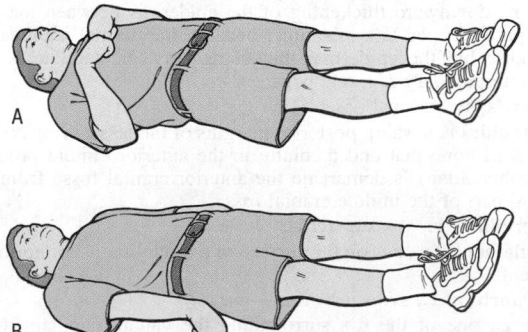

rigidity: (A) decorticate, (B) decerebrate

cadaveric r., SYN *rigor* mortis.

catatonic r., r. associated with catatonic psychotic states in which all muscles exhibit flexibilitas cerea.

cerebellar r., increased tone of the extensor muscles, related to injury of the vermis of the cerebellum.

clasp-knife r., SYN clasp-knife *spasticity.*

cogwheel r., a type of r. seen in parkinsonism in which the muscles respond with cogwheel-like jerks to the use of constant force in bending the limb.

decerebrate r., a postural change that occurs in some comatose patients, consisting of episodes of opisthotonos, rigid extension of the limbs, internal rotation of the upper extremities, and marked plantar flexion of the feet; produced by a variety of metabolic and structural brain disorders. SYN decerebrate state.

decorticate r., a unilateral or bilateral postural change, consisting of the upper extremities flexed and adducted and the lower extremities in rigid extension; due to structural lesions of the thalamus, internal capsule, or cerebral white matter. SYN decorticate state.

lead-pipe r., the plastic type of r. resembling that of a pipe of lead seen in certain forms of parkinsonism.

nuchal r., impaired neck flexion resulting from muscle spasm (not actual r.) of the extensor muscles of the neck; usually attributed to meningeal irritation.

ocular r., the resistance offered by the eyeball to a change in intraocular volume; manifested as a change in intraocular pressure.

postmortem r., SYN *rigor* mortis.

scleral r., the resistance of the eye to changes in shape with changes in intraocular pressure.

rig·or (rig′er). **1.** SYN rigidity (1). **2.** SYN chill (2). [L. stiffness]

acid r., coagulation of muscle protein induced by acids.

calcium r., arrest of the heart in the fully contracted state as a result of poisoning with calcium.

heat r., coagulation of muscle protein induced by heat.

r. mor′tis, stiffening of the body, 1–7 hours after death, from hardening of the muscular tissues as a consequence of the coagulation of the myosinogen and paramyosinogen; it disappears after 1–6 days or when decomposition begins. SYN cadaveric rigidity, postmortem rigidity.

myocardial r. mortis, SYN ischemic *contracture* of the left ventricle.

Riley, Conrad M., U.S. pediatrician, *1913. SEE R.-Day *syndrome.*

Riley, Harris D., Jr., 20th century U.S. physician. SEE Smith-R. *syndrome.*

riluzole (ril′oo-zōl). A drug used to treat amyotrophic lateral sclerosis; mechanism of action not known.

rim. A margin, border, or edge, usually circular in form.

bite r., SYN occlusion r.

occlusal r., SYN occlusion r.

occlusion r., occluding surfaces built on temporary or permanent denture bases for the purpose of making maxillomandibular relation records and for arranging teeth. SYN bite r., occlusal r., record r.

orbital r., SYN orbital *margin.*

record r., SYN occlusion r.

ri·ma, gen. and pl. **ri·mae** (rī′mă, rī′mē) [TA]. A slit or fissure, or narrow elongated opening between two symmetric parts. [L. a slit]

r. glot′tidis [TA], the interval between the true vocal cords. SYN r. vocalis☆, glottis vera, true glottis.

r. o′ris [TA], SYN oral *fissure.*

r. palpebra′rum [TA], SYN palpebral *fissure.*

r. puden′di [TA], SYN pudendal *cleft.*

r. respirato′ria, SYN r. vestibuli.

r. vestib′uli [TA], the interval between the false vocal cords or vestibular folds. SYN false glottis, glottis spuria, r. respiratoria.

r. voca′lis, ☆official alternate term for r. glottidis.

r. vul′vae, SYN pudendal *cleft.*

ri·man·ta·dine (rĭ-man′tă-dēn). An antiviral agent resembling amantadine in its activity but seemingly with fewer central nervous system adverse reactions.

Rimini test. See under test.

ri·mose (rī'mōs). Fissured; marked by cracks in all directions, like the crackle of porcelain. [L. *rimosus,* fr. *rima,* a fissure]

rim·u·la (rim'ū-lă). A minute slit or fissure. [L. dim. of *rima*]

Rindfleisch, Georg E., German physician, 1836–1908. SEE R. *folds,* under *fold.*

ring (rĭng) [TA]. **1.** A circular band surrounding a wide central opening; a ring-shaped or circular structure surrounding an opening or level area. SYN anulus [TA]. **2.** The closed (i.e., endless) chain of atoms in a cyclic compound; commonly used for "cyclic" or "cycle." **3.** A marginal growth on the upper surface of a broth culture of bacteria, adhering to the sides of the test tube in the form of a circle. SYN annulus. [A.S. *hring*]

abdominal r., SYN deep inguinal r.

amnion r., the r. formed by the attachment of the amnion to the umbilical cord at its point of emergence from the umbilicus.

annuloplasty r., the dilated annulus is sutured, often to a prosthetic r., thereby reducing it to its normal systolic size.

anterior limiting r., SYN anterior limiting *lamina.*

Balbani r., an extremely large puff at a band of a polytene chromosome.

benzene r., the closed-chain arrangement of the carbon and hydrogen atoms in the benzene molecule. SEE ALSO cyclic *compound.*

Bickel r., SYN pharyngeal lymphatic r.

Cannon r., SYN Cannon *point.*

cardiac lymphatic r., SYN *lymph nodes* around cardia of stomach, under *lymph node.*

casting r., SYN refractory *flask.*

choroidal r., a lightly pigmented crescent or r. adjacent to the optic disk.

ciliary r., SYN orbiculus ciliaris.

common tendinous r. of extraocular muscles [TA], a fibrous ring that surrounds the optic canal and the medial part of the superior orbital fissure; it gives origin to the four rectus muscles of the eye and is partially fused with the sheath of the optic nerve. SYN anulus of Zinn, anulus tendineus communis, Zinn ligament, Zinn r., Zinn tendon.

conjunctival r. [TA], a narrow ring at the junction of the periphery of the cornea with the conjunctiva. SYN anulus conjunctivae [TA].

constriction r., **(1)** true spastic stricture of the uterine cavity resulting when a zone of muscle goes into local tetanic contraction and forms a tight constriction about some part of the fetus; **(2)** SYN amnionic *band.*

crural r., SYN femoral r.

deep inguinal r. [TA], the opening in the transversalis fascia through which the ductus deferens and gonadal vessels (or round ligament in the female) enter the inguinal canal. Located midway between anterior superior iliac spine and pubic tubercle, it is bounded medially by the lateral umbilical fold (inferior epigastric vessels) and inferiorly by the iliopubic tract. Indirect inguinal hernias exit the abdominal cavity via the deep inguinal r. SYN anulus inguinalis profundus [TA], abdominal r., anulus abdominalis, internal inguinal r.

external inguinal r., SYN superficial inguinal r.

femoral r. [TA], the superior opening of the femoral canal, bounded anteriorly by the inguinal ligament, posteriorly by the pectineus muscle, medially by the lacunar ligament, and laterally by the femoral vein. Passageway by which many lymphatics from lower limb pass to abdomen. Accommodates enlargement of femoral vein in Valsalva maneuver. Often occupied by a lymph node (Cloquet) and is the site of femoral hernias. SYN anulus femoralis [TA], crural r.

fibrocartilaginous r. of tympanic membrane [TA], the thickened portion of the circumference of the tympanic membrane that is fixed in the tympanic sulcus. SYN anulus fibrocartilagineus membranae tympani [TA], Gerlach annular tendon.

fibrous r., **(1)** SYN (right and left) fibrous r.'s of heart; **(2)** SYN *anulus* fibrosus of intervertebral disk.

fibrous r. of intervertebral disk, SYN *anulus* fibrosus of intervertebral disk.

Fleischer r., an incomplete ring often present at the base of the keratoconus cone; it may be yellow or greenish from deposition of hemosiderin.

Fleischer-Strümpell r., SYN Kayser-Fleischer r.

Flieringa r., a stainless steel r. sutured to the sclera to prevent collapse of the globe in difficult intraocular operations.

gestational r., the white r. identified by pulse echosonography that signals an early stage of pregnancy.

glaucomatous r., SYN glaucomatous *halo* (1).

Graefenberg r., obsolete term for a silver or silkworm gut r. designed for insertion into the uterine cavity as a means of contraception.

greater r. of iris, SYN outer *border* of iris.

internal inguinal r., SYN deep inguinal r.

r. of iris, SYN *border* of iris.

Kayser-Fleischer r., a greenish yellow pigmented r. encircling the cornea just within the corneoscleral margin, seen in hepatolenticular degeneration, due to copper deposited in Descemet *membrane.* SYN Fleischer-Strümpell r.

lesser r. of iris, SYN inner *border* of iris.

Liesegang r.'s, colored r.'s of precipitated silver chromate formed when a drop of concentrated silver nitrate is added to the surface of a gel (such as gelatin, agar, or silica gel) containing potassium dichromate.

Lower r., SYN (right and left) fibrous r.'s of heart.

lymphatic r. of cardiac part of stomach, SYN *lymph nodes* around cardia of stomach, under *lymph node.*

neonatal r., SYN neonatal *line.*

pathologic retraction r., a constriction located at the junction of the thinned lower uterine segment with the thick retracted upper uterine segment, resulting from obstructed labor; this is one of the classic signs of threatened rupture of the uterus.

pharyngeal lymphatic r. [TA], the broken r. of lymphoid tissue, formed of the lingual, faucial, and pharyngeal tonsils. SYN anulus lymphoideus pharyngis [TA], Bickel r., tonsillar r., Waldeyer throat r.

physiologic retraction r., a ridge on the inner uterine surface at the boundary line between the upper and lower uterine segment that occurs in the course of normal labor.

polar r., a thickened, electron-dense ring at the anterior end of certain stages of the Apicomplexa; part of the apical complex characteristic of these sporozoans.

(right and left) fibrous r.'s of heart [TA], two fibrous r.'s that surround atrioventricular orifices of the heart, providing attachment for the atrioventricular valve leaflets and maintaining patency of the orifices. As part of the fibrous skeleton of the heart, the fibrous r.'s also provide origin and insertion for the myocardium. SYN anulus fibrosus (1) [TA], anulus fibrosus dexter/sinister cordis, coronary tendon, fibrous r. (1), Lower r.

Schatzki r., a contraction r. or incomplete mucosal diaphragm in the lower third of the esophagus, which is occasionally symptomatic.

Schwalbe r., SYN anterior limiting *lamina.*

scleral r., the appearance of the sclera adjacent to the optic disk when the retinal pigment epithelium does not extend to the optic nerve.

signet r., the early stage of trophozoite development of the malaria parasite in the red blood cell; the parasite cytoplasm stains blue around its circular margin, and the nucleus stains red in Romanowsky stains, while the central vacuole is clear, giving the ring-like appearance.

r. of Soemmerring, a mass of lenticular fibers enclosed between the anterior and posterior portion of the lenticular capsule, leaving the pupillary area relatively free.

subcutaneous r., SYN superficial inguinal r.

superficial inguinal r. [TA], the slitlike opening in the aponeurosis of the external oblique muscle of the abdominal wall through which the spermatic cord (round ligament in the female) and inguinal hernias emerge from the inguinal canal. SEE ALSO *apo-*

ri

neurosis of external oblique muscle. SYN anulus inguinalis superficialis, external inguinal r., subcutaneous r.

tonsillar r., SYN pharyngeal lymphatic r.

tracheal r., SYN tracheal *cartilages,* under *cartilage.*

tympanic r. [TA], in the fetus, a more or less complete bony ring at the medial end of the cartilaginous external acoustic meatus, to which is attached the tympanic membrane. SYN anulus tympanicus, tympanic bone.

umbilical r. [TA], an opening in the linea alba through which pass the umbilical vessels in the fetus; in young embryos it is relatively nearer to the pubis, but gradually ascends to the center of the abdomen; it is closed in the adult, its site being indicated by the umbilicus or navel. SYN anulus umbilicalis, canalis umbilicalis.

vascular r., anomalous arteries (aortic arches) congenitally encircling the trachea and esophagus, at times producing pressure symptoms.

Vieussens r., SYN *limbus* fossae ovalis.

Vossius lenticular r., a ring-shaped opacity found on the anterior lens capsule after contusion of the eye, due to pigment and blood.

Waldeyer throat r., SYN pharyngeal lymphatic r.

Zinn r., SYN common tendinous r. of extraocular muscles.

Ringer, Sydney, English physiologist, 1835–1910. SEE R. *injection, solution;* lactated R. *injection;* Krebs-R. *solution;* Locke-R. *solution;* Ringer *lactate.*

ring-knife (ring-nīf). A circular or oval ring with internal cutting edge, on the model of the carpenter's spoke-shave, for shaving off tumors in the nasal and other cavities. SYN spoke-shave.

ring·worm (ring′werm). SYN tinea.

r. of beard, SYN *tinea* barbae.

black-dot r., tinea capitis due most commonly to *Trichophyton tonsurans* or *T. violaceum.*

r. of body, SYN *tinea* corporis.

crusted r., SYN favus.

r. of foot, SYN *tinea* pedis.

honeycomb r., SYN favus.

r. of nails, SYN onychomycosis.

Oriental r., SYN *tinea* imbricata.

r. of scalp, SYN *tinea* capitis.

scaly r., SYN *tinea* imbricata.

Tokelau r., SYN *tinea* imbricata. [*Tokelau* Islands in S. Pacific Ocean]

Rinne, Friedrich Heinrich A., German otologist, 1819–1868. SEE R. *test.*

Riolan, Jean, French anatomist and botanist, 1577–1657. SEE R. *anastomosis, arc, arcades,* under *arcade, bones,* under *bone, bouquet, muscle.*

RIP. Abbreviation for radioimmunoprecipitation.

ri·par·i·an (ri-pār′ē-an, rī-). Relating to a ripa; marginal.

Ripault, Louis H.A., French physician, 1807–1856. SEE R. *sign.*

rip·en·ing (rī′pen-ing). Denoting progressive oxidation of dye solutions, as in the r. of hematoxylin solutions to hematein or of methylene blue to azure dyes.

Ripstein, Charles B., 20th century U.S. surgeon. SEE Ripstein *operation.*

RISA Abbreviation for radioiodinated serum *albumin.*

risk. The probability that an event will occur.

attributable r., the rate of a disease or other outcome in exposed individuals that can be attributed to the exposure.

competing r., an event that removes a subject from being at r. for an outcome under investigation.

empiric r., r. that is based on empiric evidence alone, without any appeal to formal theory or surmise.

radiation r.'s, the r.'s to health posed by exposure to radiation. Sources of exposure are both natural and artificial (e.g., medical and occupational). SEE background *radiation.*

Excessive exposure to ionizing radiation is associated with increased risk of malignant diseases, particularly of the skin and blood-forming organs; increased risk of abnormal variation in reproductive cells, with the possibility of abnormality in offspring; and increased risk of fetal abnormality from maternal exposure during early pregnancy. For most people, natural sources account for the bulk of received radiation, with artificial sources adding only a small percentage to the average annual dose. Public perception of the hazards of radiation is often at odds with scientific positions on the subject. Equivocal research results (as in attempts to assess the added cancer risk posed by mammograms) have contributed to public fears. Some studies have concluded that, whether or not public fears of nuclear power plants are justified, the added stress caused by such fears in itself constitutes a threat to health.

recurrence r., r. that a disease will occur elsewhere in a pedigree, given that at least one member of the pedigree (the proband) exhibits the disease.

relative r., the ratio of the r. of disease among those exposed to a r. factor to the r. among those not exposed.

Risley, Samuel D., U.S. ophthalmologist, 1845–1920. SEE R. rotary *prism.*

ri·so·ri·us (ri-sōr′ē-ŭs). SEE risorius (*muscle*). [L. *risor,* a laughter, fr. *rideo,* pp. *risus,* to laugh]

RIST Abbreviation for radioimmunosorbent *test.*

ris·to·ce·tin (ris-tō-sē′tin). An antibiotic produced by the fermentation of *Amycolatopsis orientalis* subsp. *lurida,* comprising two substances; r. A and r. B; it is useful against staphylococcic and enterococcic infections refractory to other antibiotics.

ri·sus (rī′sŭs). Laughter. [laughter]

r. caninus (rī′sŭs kā-nī′nŭs), the semblance of a grin caused by facial spasm, seen especially in tetanus but also in some kinds of poisoning. SYN canine spasm, r. sardonicus, sardonic grin, trismus sardonicus. [L. *risus,* laugh + *caninus,* doglike]

r. sardonicus (sar-don′i-kŭs), SYN r. caninus. [L. *risus,* laughter, + *sardonicus,* fr. G. *sardanios,* scornful, infl. by *sardonios,* Sardinian, ref. to effects of *Strychnos nux-vomica,* poisonous herb fr. Sardinia]

Ritgen, Ferdinand A.M.F. von, German obstetrician, 1787–1867. SEE R. *maneuver.*

ri·to·drine (rī′tō-drēn). A sympathomimetic agent with β_2-adrenergic stimulant actions, used as a uterine relaxant.

Ritter, Johann W., German physicist, 1776–1810. SEE R. opening *tetanus;* R.-Rollet *phenomenon.*

rit·u·al (rich′oo-ăl). In psychiatry and psychology, any psychomotor activity (e.g., morbid handwashing) performed by a person to relieve anxiety or forestall its development; typically seen in obsessive-compulsive disorder. [L. *ritualis,* fr. *ritus,* rite]

rituximab (rit-ŭks′im-ab). Monoclonal antibody used in the treatment of non-Hodgkin lymphoma.

ri·val·ry (rī′văl-rē). Competition between two or more individuals or entities for the same object or goal. [L. *rivalis,* competitor, rival]

binocular r., alteration in perception of portions of the visual field when the two eyes are simultaneously and rapidly exposed to targets containing dissimilar colors or borders.

r. of retina, simultaneous excitation of corresponding retinal areas of each eye by stimuli that differ in size, color, shape, or luminance, making fusion impossible.

sibling r., jealous competition among children, especially for the attention, affection, and esteem of their parents; by extension, a factor in both normal and abnormal competitiveness throughout life.

Riv·ea co·rym·bo·sa (riv′ē-ă kō-rim-bō′să). Mexican bindweed, a plant of the family Convolvulaceae, the seeds of which were used in ceremonies by Aztec Indians in Mexico and contain lysergic acid amide, isolysergic acid, lysergic acid monoethylamide, chanoclavine, and other indole alkaloids; several hundred seeds must be ingested to produce hallucinatory and euphoric effects. SYN morning glory (2).

Riverius. SEE Rivière.

Rivero-Carvallo, José Manuel, Mexican cardiologist, *1905. SEE Carvallo *sign;* Rivero-Carvallo *effect.*

Rivers, William H., English physician, 1864–1922. SEE R. *cocktail.*

Rivière (Riverius), Lazare (Lazarus), French physician, 1589–1655. SEE R. *salt.*

Rivinus (Latin form of Bachmann). August Q., German anatomist, 1652–1723. SEE Rivinus *canals,* under *canal,* Rivinus *ducts,* under *duct,* Rivinus *gland,* Rivinus *incisure,* Rivinus *membrane,* Rivinus *notch.*

ri·vus la·cri·ma·lis (rī'vŭs lak-ri-mā'lis) [TA]. SYN lacrimal *pathway.* [L. *rivus,* stream, + Mediev. L. *lacrimalis,* fr. L. *lacrima,* a tear]

riz·i·form (riz'i-fōrm). Resembling rice grains. [Fr. *riz,* rice]

RLL Abbreviation for right lower lobe (of lung).

RLQ Abbreviation for right lower quadrant (of abdomen).

RMA Abbreviation for right mentoanterior position.

RML Abbreviation for right middle lobe (of lung).

RMP Abbreviation for right mentoposterior position.

RMT Abbreviation for right mentotransverse position.

RMV Abbreviation for respiratory minute *volume.*

R.N. Abbreviation for registered *nurse.*

Rn Symbol for radon.

RNA Abbreviation for ribonucleic acid. For terms bearing this abbreviation, see subentries under ribonucleic acid.

RNase Abbreviation for ribonuclease. For terms bearing this abbreviation, see subentries under ribonuclease.

RNase D Abbreviation for *ribonuclease* D.

RNA splic·ing. SYN splicing (2).

RNP Abbreviation for ribonucleoprotein.

ROA Abbreviation for right occipitoanterior position.

Roach, F. Ewing, U.S. prosthodontist, 1868–1960. SEE R. *clasp.*

Roaf, R. SEE R. *syndrome.*

Robert, Heinrich, L.F., German gynecologist, 1814–1878. SEE R. *pelvis.*

Roberts, J.B., 20th century U.S. physician. SEE R. *syndrome.*

Robertshaw, Frank L., 20th century English anesthesiologist. SEE R. *tube.*

Robertson, SEE Argyll R.

Robin, Pierre, French pediatrician, 1867–1950. SEE Pierre R. *syndrome.*

Robin, Charles P., French physician, 1821–1885. SEE Virchow-R. *space.*

Robinow, Meinhard, U.S. physician, *1909. SEE Robinow *dwarfism,* Robinow *syndrome.*

Robinson, Brian F., 20th century British cardiologist. SEE R. *index.*

Robison, Robert, English chemist, 1884–1941. SEE R. *ester,* ester *dehydrogenase;* R.-Embden *ester.*

Robles, Rudolfo (Valverde), Guatemalan dermatologist, 1878–1939.

ro·bot·ic (rō-bot'ik). Pertaining to or characteristic of a robot, an automatic mechanical device designed to duplicate a human function without direct human operation. [Czech *robot,* robot, fr. *robota,* drudgery, + -ic]

Robson. SEE Mayo-Robson.

ro·bust·ness (rō-bust'ness). In statistics, the degree to which the probability of drawing a wrong conclusion from the test result is not seriously affected by moderate departures from the assumptions implicit in the model on which the test is based. [L. *robustus,* hale, strong, fr. *robur,* oak, hard, strong]

ROC Acronym for receiver operating *characteristic,* an analytic expression of diagnostic accuracy. SEE ROC *curve.*

roc·cel·lin (rok'sel-in) [C.I. 15620]. SYN archil.

Ro·cha·li·maea (rō-chă-lī'mā-ă). Former name for *Bartonella.* [H. da *Rocha-Lima,* Brazilian microbiologist]

  Rochalimaea henselae, SEE *Bartonella henselae.*

  Rochalimaea quintana, SEE *Bartonella quintana.*

rod (rŏd). **1.** A slender cylindric structure or device. **2.** The photosensitive, outward-directed process of a rhodopsin-containing r. cell in the external granular layer of the retina; many millions of such r.'s, together with the cones, form the photoreceptive layer of r.'s and cones. SYN rod cell of retina. [A.S. *rōd*]

analyzing r., a device used with a surveyor to determine the relative positions of parallel surfaces and undercuts when designing removable partial dentures.

Auer r.'s, SYN Auer *bodies,* under *body.*

basal r., SYN costa (2).

Corti r.'s, SYN pillar *cells,* under *cell.*

enamel r.'s, SYN *prismata* adamantina, under *prisma.*

germinal r., SYN sporozoite.

Maddox r., a glass r., or a series of parallel glass r.'s, that converts the image of a light source into a streak of light perpendicular to the axis of the r. The position of this streak in relation to the image of the light source seen by the fellow eye indicates the presence and amount of heterophoria.

surgical r., a cylindric implant, usually composed of metal, used to align and internally fix fractures of long bones. SEE ALSO nail, pin.

Ro·den·tia (rō-den'shē-ă). The rodents; the largest order of placental mammals (class Eutheria), all possessing one pair of chisel-like upper incisors for gnawing and flat-crowned premolars and molars for grinding; it includes the mice, rats, guinea pigs, squirrels, beavers, and many more. [Mod. L., fr. L. *rodo,* pres. p. *rodens,* to gnaw]

ro·den·ti·cide (rō-den'ti-sīd). An agent lethal to rodents. [rodent + L. *caedo,* to kill]

Roentgen, Wilhelm K., German physicist and Nobel laureate, 1845–1923. Discovered x-rays in November, 1895; awarded Nobel Prize in Physics in 1901 for his discovery. SEE roentgen; roentgen *ray.*

roent·gen (R, r) (rent'gen, rent'chen). The international unit of exposure dose for x-rays or gamma rays; that quantity of radiation that will produce in 1 cc or 0.001293 g of air at STP, 2.08×10^9 ions of both signs, each totaling 1 electrostatic unit (e.s.u.) of charge; in the MKS system this is 2.58×10^{-4} coulombs per kg of air. [W. K. *Roentgen*]

r.-equivalent-man (rem), a unit of dose equivalent to that quantity of ionizing radiation of any type that produces in humans the same biologic effect as 1 rad of x-rays or gamma rays; the number of rems is equal to the absorbed dose, measured in rads, multiplied by the quality factor of the radiation in question. 100 rem = 1 Sv.

r.-equivalent-physical, obsolete unit of measurement; that quantity of ionizing radiation of any kind that, upon absorption by living tissue, produces an energy gain per gram of tissue equivalent to that produced by 1 rad of x-rays or gamma-rays. SEE rad.

roent·gen·ky·mo·gram (rent'gen-kī'mō-gram). A record of the heart's movements taken with the roentgenkymograph.

roent·gen·ky·mo·graph (rent'gen-kī'mō-graf). An apparatus for recording the movements of the heart and great vessels or of the diaphragm on a single film. It consists of a lead sheet called the grid in which are cut horizontal or vertical slits, typically less than 1 mm wide, spaced 1–2 cm apart. During an x-ray exposure lasting as long as several cardiac or respiratory cycles, the grid or the film is moved vertically to record cardiac motion or horizontally for diaphragm motion.

roent·gen·ky·mog·ra·phy (rent'gen-kī-mog'ră-fē). An obsolete technique involving the recording of movements of the heart by means of the roentgenkymograph.

roent·gen·o·gram (rent'gen-ō-gram). SYN radiograph.

roent·gen·o·graph (rent'gen-ō-graf). SYN radiograph.

roent·gen·og·ra·phy (rent'ge-nog'ră-fē). SYN radiography.

roent·gen·ol·o·gist (rent'ge-nol'ō-jist). A person skilled in the diagnostic or therapeutic application of roentgen rays; a radiologist.

roent·gen·ol·o·gy (rent'gen-ol'ō-jē). The study of roentgen rays in all their applications. Radiology is the preferred term in the context of medical imaging.

ro

roent·gen·om·e·ter (rent'ge-nom'ĕ-ter). SYN radiometer.

roent·gen·om·e·try (rent-ge-nom'ĕ-trē). Measurement of an administered therapeutic or diagnostic dose and the penetrating power of x-rays. SYN x-ray dosimetry.

roent·gen·o·scope (rent'gen-ō-scōp). Obsolete term for fluoroscope.

roent·gen·os·co·py (rent-gen-os'kŏ-pē). Obsolete term for fluoroscopy.

roent·gen·o·ther·a·py (rent'gen-ō-thār'ă-pē). Obsolete term for radiotherapy.

roeth·eln. SEE röteln.

Roger, Georges Henri, French physiologist, 1860–1946. SEE R. *reflex.*

Roger, Henri L., French physician, 1809–1891. SEE R. *disease, murmur; bruit* de R.; *maladie* de R.

Rogers, Oscar H., U.S. physician, 1857–1941. SEE R. *sphygmomanometer.*

Rohr, Karl, Swiss embryologist and gynecologist, *1863. SEE R. *stria.*

Röhrer in·dex. See under index.

Rokitansky, Karl Freiherr von, Austrian pathologist, 1804–1878. SEE R. *disease, hernia;* R.-Aschoff *sinuses,* under *sinus;* Mayer-R.-Küster-Hauser *syndrome.*

ro·lan·dic (rō-lan'dik). Relating to or described by Luigi Rolando.

Rolando, Luigi, Italian anatomist, 1773–1831. SEE R. *angle, area, cells,* under *cell, column;* rolandic *epilepsy;* R. gelatinous *substance, tubercle; fissure* of R.

role (rōl). The pattern of behavior that a person exhibits in relationship to significant persons in his or her life; it has its roots in childhood and is influenced by significant people with whom the person has or had primary relationships. [Fr.]

complementary r., a r. in which the behavior pattern conforms with the expectations and demands of other people.

gender r., the public presentation of gender identity; specifically, everything a person says and does that signals to others or to the self that one is male or female (or androgynous). SEE sex r., gender *identity.*

noncomplementary r., a r. that does not conform with the expectations and demands of other people.

sex r., specifically, the pattern of behavior and thought related to sex organs and procreation; but more generally, behavior and thought that is stereotypically classified as belonging to either one sex or the other. SEE gender r.

sick r., in medical sociology, the familially or culturally accepted behavior pattern or r. which one is permitted to exhibit during illness or disability, including sanctioned absence from school or work and a submissive, dependent relationship to family, health care personnel, and significant others.

role-play·ing. A psychotherapeutic method used in psychodrama to understand and treat emotional conflicts through the enactment or reenactment of stressful interpersonal events. SEE psychodrama.

ro·li·tet·ra·cy·cline (rō'li-tet-ră-sī'klēn). A more soluble and less irritating derivative of tetracycline; uses and effectiveness are similar to those of tetracycline, and it may be administered intravenously or intramuscularly, which makes it useful when oral administration of a tetracycline is impossible or impractical.

roll (rōl). **1.** A mass or structure in the shape of a roll. **2.** The process by which a round entity is moved by a pressure gradient, as a leukocyte moves along a blood vessel wall.

iliac r., a sausage-shaped, often painful, nonfluctuating mass, with convexity to the right, palpable in the left iliac fossa, due to induration of the walls of the sigmoid flexure.

scleral r., SYN scleral *spur.*

Roller, Christian F.W., German neurologist and psychiatrist, 1844–1978. SEE R. *nucleus.*

roll·er (rō'ler). SEE roller *bandage.*

Rolleston, Sir Humphry D., British physician, 1862–1944. SEE R. *rule.*

Rollet, Alexander, Austrian physiologist, 1834–1903. SEE R. *stroma;* Ritter-R. *phenomenon.*

Romaña, Cecilio, Argentinian physician in Brazil, *1899. SEE R. *sign.*

Romano, C., 20th century Italian physician. SEE Romano-Ward *syndrome.*

Romanowsky, Dimitri L., Russian physician, 1861–1921. SEE R. blood *stain.*

Romberg, Moritz H., German physician, 1795–1873. SEE R. *test, disease;* facial *hemiatrophy* of R.; R. *syndrome, sign.*

rom·berg·ism (rom'berg-izm). SYN Romberg *sign.*

Römer, Paul H., German bacteriologist, 1876–1916. SEE R. *test.*

ron·geur (rawn-zhĕr'). A strong biting forceps for nipping away bone. [Fr. *ronger,* to gnaw]

Rønne, Henning K.T., Danish ophthalmologist, 1878–1947. SEE R. nasal *step.*

roof (roof). A covering or rooflike structure; e.g., a tectorium, tectum, tegmen, tegmentum, integument. [A.S. *hróf*]

r. of fourth ventricle [TA], SYN *tegmen* ventriculi quarti.

r. of mouth, SYN palate.

r. of orbit [TA], formed by the orbital plate of the frontal bone and the lesser wing of the sphenoid bone, the optic canal opens at its posterior limit; an indentation, the fossa for the lacrimal gland, is located in the anterolateral part of the roof. SYN paries superior orbitae [TA], superior wall of orbit.

r. of skull, SYN calvaria.

r. of tympanic cavity, SYN tegmental *wall* of tympanic cavity.

r. of tympanum, SYN *tegmen* tympani.

roof·plate (roof'plāt). SEE roof *plate.*

room·ing-in (room'ing-in). Placement of newborn with mother, rather than in nursery, during the postpartum hospital stay.

root (rōōt) [TA]. **1.** The primary or beginning portion of any part, as of a nerve at its origin from the brainstem or spinal cord. SYN radix (1) [TA]. **2.** SYN r. of tooth. **3.** The descending underground portion of a plant; it absorbs water and nutrients, provides support, and stores nutrients. For r.'s of pharmacologic significance not listed below, see specific names. [A.S. *rot*]

accessory r. of tooth [TA], an anomalous additional tooth root. SYN radix accessoria [TA].

anatomical r., that portion of a tooth extending from the cervical line to its apical extremity.

anterior r. of spinal nerve [TA], the motor root of a spinal nerve. SYN radix anterior nervi spinalis [TA], motor r. of spinal nerve⋆, radix motoria nervi spinalis⋆, ventral r. of spinal nerve⋆, radix ventralis nervi spinalis.

buccal r. of tooth [TA], root of a multirooted tooth which is located toward the buccal side of the alveolar ridge. SYN radix buccalis [TA].

clinical r. of tooth [TA], that portion of a tooth embedded in the investing structures; the portion of a tooth not visible in the oral cavity. SYN radix clinica dentis [TA].

cochlear r. of VIII nerve, one of the components of the vestibulocochlear nerve; it is made up of the central processes of the bipolar neurons that compose the spiral (cochlear) ganglion in the spiral canal of the modiolus of the bony cochlea; the cochlear r. enters the cranial cavity by passing in fascicles through the spiral foraminous tract at the bottom of the internal auditory meatus; it enters the brainstem through the pontomedullary groove, closely adhering to the caudoventral aspect of the vestibular r., and distributes its fibers to the ventral and dorsal cochlear nuclei in the floor of the lateral recess of the fourth ventricle. SYN radix inferior nervi vestibulocochlearis.

cranial r. of accessory nerve [TA], the r.'s of the accessory nerve that arise from the medulla; the nerve fibers of the cranial r. join the intracranial portion of the vagus nerve and are distributed to the pharyngeal plexus, providing the motor innervation of the soft palate (except the tensor veli palati) and the pharynx. SEE ALSO accessory *nerve* [CN XI]. SYN radix cranialis nervi accessorii [TA], pars vagalis nervi accessorii⋆, vagal part of accessory nerve⋆, accessory portion of spinal accessory nerve.

Culver r., SYN leptandra.

dorsal r. of spinal nerve, ✫official alternate term for posterior r. of spinal nerve.

facial r., SYN *nerve* of pterygoid canal.

r. of facial nerve, fibers running from the facial motor nucleus upward to the facial colliculus where they curve around the abducens nucleus and then pass peripherally between the superior olive and sensory nucleus of the trigeminal, to emerge as the facial nerve from the pontomedullary groove. SYN radix nervi facialis.

r. of foot, SYN tarsus (1).

hair r., the part of a hair that is embedded in the hair follicle, its lower succulent extremity capping the dermal papilla pili in the deep bulbous portion of the follicle. SYN radix pili.

inferior r. of ansa cervicalis [TA], fibers from the second and third cervical nerves that pass forward and downward along the internal jugular vein; they contribute to the ansa cervicalis and innervate the infrahyoid muscles. SYN radix inferior ansae cervicalis [TA], inferior limb of ansa cervicalis✫, descendens cervicalis.

lateral r. of median nerve [TA], the part of the median nerve arising from the lateral cord of the brachial plexus. SYN radix lateralis nervi mediani [TA].

lateral r. of optic tract [TA], the larger division of the posterior end of the optic tract that terminates in the lateral geniculate body. SYN radix lateralis tractus optici [TA].

long r. of ciliary ganglion, SYN sensory r. of ciliary ganglion.

r. of lung [TA], all the structures entering or leaving the lung at the hilum, forming a pedicle invested with the pleura; includes the bronchi, pulmonary artery and veins, bronchial arteries and veins, lymphatics, and nerves. SYN radix pulmonis [TA].

May apple r., SYN podophyllum *resin*.

medial r. of median nerve [TA], the part of the median nerve coming from the medial cord of the brachial plexus. SYN radix medialis nervi mediani [TA].

medial r. of optic tract [TA], the smaller division of the posterior end of the optic tract that disappears under the medial geniculate body. SYN radix medialis tractus optici [TA].

r. of mesentery [TA], the origin of the mesentery of the small intestine (jejunum and ileum) from the posterior parietal peritoneum; about 9 inches (23 cm) in length, it extends from the duodenojejunal flexure (just to the left of the midline at the L2 vertebral level) to the ileocecal junction (iliac fossa). SYN radix mesenterii [TA].

motor r. of ciliary ganglion, SYN parasympathetic r. of ciliary ganglion.

motor r. of spinal nerve, ✫official alternate term for anterior r. of spinal nerve.

motor r. of trigeminal nerve [TA], the smaller root of the trigeminal nerve, composed of fibers originating from the trigeminal motor nucleus and emerging from the pons medial to the much larger sensory root, to join the mandibular nerve; it carries motor and proprioceptive fibers to the muscles derived from the first bronchial (mandibular) arch, including the four muscles of mastication, plus the mylohyoid, anterior belly of the digastric, and the tensores tympani and veli palati. SYN radix motoria nervi trigemini [TA], masticator nerve, portio minor nervi trigemini.

r. of nail, the proximal end of the nail, concealed under a fold of skin. SYN radix unguis.

nasociliary r. of ciliary ganglion, ✫official alternate term for sensory r. of ciliary ganglion.

nerve r., one of the two bundles of nerve fibers (posterior and anterior r.'s) emerging from the spinal cord that join to form a single segmental (mixed) spinal nerve; some of the cranial nerves are similarly formed by the union of two r.'s, in particular the fifth or trigeminal nerve.

r. of nose [TA], the upper least protruding portion of the external nose situated between the two orbits. SYN radix nasi [TA].

oculomotor r. of ciliary ganglion, ✫official alternate term for parasympathetic r. of ciliary ganglion.

olfactory r.'s, SYN olfactory *striae*, under *stria*.

r.'s of olfactory tract, lateral and medial, the two fiber bands that form the caudal continuation of the olfactory tract that, upon diverging, enclose the olfactory tubercle.

parasympathetic r. of ciliary ganglion [TA], a branch of the oculomotor nerve supplying parasympathetic preganglionic nerve fibers to the ciliary ganglion. SYN radix parasympathica ganglii ciliaris [TA], oculomotor r. of ciliary ganglion✫, radix nervi oculomotorii ad ganglion ciliare✫, radix oculomotoria ganglii ciliaris✫, branch of oculomotor nerve to ciliary ganglion, motor r. of ciliary ganglion, radix brevis ganglii ciliaris, short r. of ciliary ganglion.

parasympathetic r. of otic ganglion, ✫official alternate term for lesser petrosal *nerve*.

parasympathetic r. of pelvic ganglia, ✫official alternate term for pelvic splanchnic *nerves*, under *nerve*.

parasympathetic r. of pterygopalatine ganglion, ✫official alternate term for greater petrosal *nerve*.

parasympathetic r. of submandibular ganglion, SYN *chorda* tympani.

r. of penis [TA], the proximal attached part of the penis, including the two crura and the bulb. SYN radix penis [TA].

posterior r. of spinal nerve [TA], the sensory root of a spinal nerve, having a dorsal r. ganglion containing the nerve cell bodies of the fibers conveyed by the root in its distal end. SYN radix posterior nervi spinalis [TA], dorsal r. of spinal nerve✫, radix sensoria nervi spinalis✫, sensory r. of spinal nerve✫, radix dorsalis nervi spinalis.

sensory r. of ciliary ganglion [TA], sensory fibers passing from the eyeball through the ciliary ganglion to their cell bodies in the trigeminal ganglion via the nasociliary nerve. SYN radix sensoria ganglii ciliaris [TA], nasociliary r. of ciliary ganglion✫, radix nasociliaris ganglii ciliaris✫, ramus communicans nervi nasociliaris cum ganglio ciliari✫, communicating branch of nasociliary nerve with ciliary ganglion, long r. of ciliary ganglion, radix longa ganglii ciliaris.

sensory r. of pterygopalatine ganglion [TA], the ganglionic branches, two short sensory branches of the maxillary nerve in the pterygopalatine fossa, the fibers of which pass through the pterygopalatine ganglion without synapse. SYN radix sensoria ganglii pterygopalatini [TA], ganglionic branches of maxillary nerve to pterygopalatine ganglion✫, rami ganglionici nervi maxillaris✫, ganglionic branches of maxillary nerve, nervi pterygopalatini, nervi sphenopalatini, pterygopalatine nerves, rami ganglionares.

sensory r. of spinal nerve, ✫official alternate term for posterior r. of spinal nerve.

sensory r. of sublingual ganglion [TA], branch or branches of the lingual nerve conveying sensory fibers to the sublingual ganglion that traverse the ganglion without synapse for distribution to the floor of the mouth. SYN radix sensoria ganglii sublingualis [TA], ganglionic branches of lingual nerve to sublingual ganglion✫, ganglionic branches of lingual nerve to submandibular ganglion✫, rami communicantes ganglii sublingualis cum nervo linguali✫.

sensory r. of submandibular ganglion [TA], motor roots of submandibular ganglion; communicating r.'s between submandibular ganglion and lingual nerve. SYN radix sensoria ganglii submandibularis [TA], rami communicantes ganglii submandibularis cum nervo linguali✫, ganglionic branches of lingual nerve.

sensory r. of trigeminal nerve [TA], the large sensory root of the trigeminal (or fifth cranial) nerve, extending from the semilunar ganglion into the pons through the middle cerebellar peduncle or brachium pontis, immediately lateral to the small motor r. SYN radix sensoria nervi trigemini [TA], portio major nervi trigemini.

short r. of ciliary ganglion, SYN parasympathetic r. of ciliary ganglion.

spinal r. of accessory nerve [TA], originates from the upper five or six cervical spinal segments, emerges from the lateral surface of the spinal cord and ascends through the foramen magnum to join the cranial root. SYN radix spinalis nervi accessorii [TA], pars spinalis nervi accessorii✫, spinal part of accessory nerve✫.

superior r. of ansa cervicalis [TA], the fibers that arise from the first and second cervical nerves, accompany the hypoglossal nerve, then branch off to meet the inferior root in the ansa cervicalis; they innervate the infrahyoid muscles. SYN radix superior ansae cervicalis [TA], superior limb of ansa cervicalis✫, descendens hypoglossi, descending branch of hypoglossal nerve.

ro

sympathetic r. of ciliary ganglion [TA], postganglionic fibers, having cell bodies in the superior cervical ganglion, branching from the carotid plexus passing through the ciliary ganglion without synapse to reach the eyeball. SYN radix sympathica ganglii ciliaris [TA].

sympathetic r. of otic ganglion [TA], branch arising from the periarterial plexus of the middle meningeal artery, bringing postsynaptic sympathetic fibers from the superior cervical sympathetic ganglion that traverse the ganglion without synapse for distribution to blood vessels within the parotid gland. SYN radix sympathica ganglii otici [TA].

sympathetic r. of pterygopalatine ganglion, ☆official alternate term for deep petrosal *nerve*.

sympathetic r. of sublingual ganglion [TA], branch arising from the periarterial plexus of the facial artery, bringing postsynaptic sympathetic fibers from the superior cervical sympathetic ganglion that traverse the ganglion without synapse for distribution to blood vessels of the sublingual gland. SYN radix sympathica ganglii sublingualis [TA].

sympathetic r. of submandibular ganglion [TA], branch to the submandibular ganglion composed of postsynaptic sympathetic fibers from the internal carotid plexus conveyed largely by a periarterial plexus of the facial artery. SYN radix sympathica ganglii submandibularis [TA], ramus sympathicus (sympatheticus) ad ganglion submandibulare, sympathetic branch to submandibular ganglion.

tegmental r. of tympanic cavity, ☆official alternate term for tegmental *wall* of tympanic cavity.

r. of tongue [TA], the posterior attached portion of the tongue. SYN radix linguae [TA], base of tongue.

r. of tooth [TA], that part of a tooth below the neck, covered by cementum rather than enamel, and attached by the periodontal ligament to the alveolar bone. SYN radix dentis [TA], radix (2) [TA], root (2) [TA].

r.'s of trigeminal nerve, collective term for the sensory r. of trigeminal nerve and motor r. of trigeminal nerve. SYN radices nervi trigemini.

tuberous r., a r. that is swollen for food storage; tuberous primary r.'s occur in aconite, beet, and carrot; tuberous secondary r.'s occur in plants of the Umbelliferae; and tuberous adventitious roots occur in jalap and sweet potato.

ventral r. of spinal nerve, ☆official alternate term for anterior r. of spinal nerve.

vestibular r., vestibular r. of VIII nerve, a collective term for those sensory fibers of the 8th cranial nerve (vestibulocochlear) that originate from the vestibular labyrinth, have their cell bodies of origin in the vestibular ganglion, and function in the sphere of balance and equilibrium; centrally these fibers end primarily in the vestibular nuclei of the brainstem and in the cerebellum. SYN radix superior nervi vestibulocochlearis, radix vestibularis, vestibular r. of vestibulocochlear nerve.

vestibular r. of vestibulocochlear nerve, SYN vestibular r.

root·lets (root′lets). In neuroanatomy, nerve rootlets (radicular fila). SEE filum. SEE ALSO radicular *fila*, under *filum*.

root plan·ing (plān′ing). In dentistry, abrading of rough root surfaces to achieve a smooth surface.

ROP Abbreviation for right occipitoposterior position.

ro·pal·o·cy·to·sis (rō-pal′ō-sī-tō′sis). Formation of numerous processes of erythroid cells, which in ultrathin sections appear club-shaped, associated with cytoplasmic vesicles and found in some diseases of the blood. [G. *ropalon,* club, + *kytos,* cell, + *-osis,* condition]

Ropes test. See under test.

Rorschach, Hermann, Swiss psychiatrist, 1884–1922. SEE R. *test.*

Ro·sa (rō′ză). A genus of plants including the roses (family Rosaceae); several varieties are the sources of rose oil: *R. alba,* cottage rose; *R. centifolia,* the pale rose or cabbage rose (source of official rose oil); *R. damascena,* damask rose; and *R. gallica,* red rose or French rose. [L. rose]

ro·sa·cea (rō-zā′shē-ă). Chronic vascular and follicular dilation involving the nose and contiguous portions of the cheeks; may vary from mild but persistent erythema to extensive hyperplasia of the sebaceous glands, seen especially in men as rhinophyma and by deep-seated papules and pustules; accompanied by telangiectasia at the affected erythematous sites. SYN acne rosacea. [L. *rosaceus,* rosy]

granulomatous r., papular lesions in r., characterized microscopically by perifollicular granulomas with central necrosis and scattered giant cells. Lupus miliaris disseminatus faciei is probably a form of granulomatous r. SYN rosacea-like tuberculid, tuberculoid r.

hypertrophic r., SYN rhinophyma.

tuberculoid r., SYN granulomatous r.

Rosai, Juan, U.S. pathologist, b. 1941. SEE Rosai-Dorfman *disease.*

ros·an·i·lin (rō-zan′i-lin) [C.I. 42510]. A tris(aminophenyl)-methyl compound; together with pararosanilin it is a component of basic fuchsin; also used as an antifungal agent.

ro·sap·ros·tol (rō′să-prost-ol). A prostaglandin analog with protective properties for the gastric mucosa; similar to misoprostol and also used as an antiulcerative drug.

ro·sa·ry (rō′zer-ē). A beadlike arrangement or structure.

rachitic r., a row of beading at the junction of the ribs with their cartilages, often seen in rachitic children. SYN beading of the ribs.

Roscoe, Sir Henry E., British chemist, 1833–1915. SEE Bunsen-R. *law.*

Rose, Edmund, German physician, 1836–1914. SEE R. *position.*

Rose, Harry M., U.S. microbiologist, *1906. SEE R.-Waaler *test.*

rose (rōz). 1. Any shrub of the genus *Rosa.* 2. The petals of *Rosa gallica,* collected before expanding; used for its agreeable odor. [L. *rosa*]

r. hips, the fruit or berries from wild rose bushes and in particular *Rosa canina, R. gallica, R. condita,* and *R. Rugosa,* (family Rosaceae). A rich source of vitamin C (ascorbic acid). SYN hipberries.

r. oil, a volatile oil from *Rosa centifolia;* used in perfumery and in ointments. SYN attar of rose.

rose ben·gal (rōz′ ben′gal) [C.I. 45440]. The sodium salt of tetraiodotetra-chlorfluorescein, used as a stain for bacteria, as a stain in the diagnosis of keratitis sicca, and in liver function tests.

Rose-Bradford kid·ney. See under kidney.

rose·mary oil (rōz′mār-ē). The volatile oil distilled with steam from the fresh flowering tops of *Rosmarinus officinalis* (family Labiatae); used as a flavoring and in perfumery.

Rosenbach, Ottomar, German physician, 1851–1907. SEE R. *law, sign, test;* R.-Gmelin *test.*

Rosenmüller, Johann C., German anatomist, 1771–1820. SEE R. *fossa, gland, node, recess, valve; organ* of R.

Rosenthal, Curt, 20th century German psychiatrist. SEE Melkersson-R. *syndrome.*

Rosenthal, Friedrich C., German anatomist, 1780–1829. SEE R. *canal, vein;* basal *vein* of R.

Rosenthaler-Turk re·a·gent. See under reagent.

Rosenthal fi·ber. See under fiber.

ro·se·o·la (rō-zē′ō′lă). A symmetrical eruption of small, closely aggregated patches of rose-red color. It is believed to be caused by human herpesvirus type 6. SEE ALSO *exanthema* subitum. SYN macular erythema. [Mod. L. dim. of L. *roseus,* rosy]

epidemic r., SYN rubella.

idiopathic r., r. not occurring as a symptom of a recognized general disease.

r. infan′tilis, r. infan′tum, SYN *exanthema* subitum.

syphilitic r., usually the first eruption of syphilis, occurring 6 to 12 weeks after the initial lesion.

Roser, Wilhelm, German surgeon, 1817–1888. SEE R.-Nélaton *line.*

ro·sette (rō-zet′). 1. The quartan malarial parasite *Plasmodium malariae* in its segmented or mature phase. 2. A grouping of cells characteristic of neoplasms of neuroblastic, neuroectodermal, or ependymal origin; a number of nuclei form a ring from which neurofibrils, which can be demonstrated by silver impregnation, extend to interlace in the center (Homer-Wright rosette). 3. Rose-like coiling of the uterus among certain pseudophyllidean tapeworms, such as *Diphyllobothrium latum*. **4.** Cells of one type surrounding a cell of another type. [Fr. a little rose]

E r. (ro-zet′), the adherence of erythrocytes to cells. Sheep erythrocytes will adhere spontaneously to human T cells, forming rosettes.

EAC r., indicates the presence of complement receptors. Erythrocytes (E) coated with antibody (A) and complement (C) are incubated with test cells; if the test cells have complement receptors, the EAC will adhere to these cells, forming rosettes.

Homer-Wright r.'s, pseudorosettes formed by the arrangement of tumor cells around an area of fibrillarity, evidence of neuroblastic differentiation in a medulloblastoma or primitive neuroectodermal tumor.

Wintersteiner r.'s, r.'s found only in retinal embryonic tumors, formed by a group of columnar cells with a peripheral basement membrane arranged in a radial manner around a central cavity, the spokes corresponding to the photoreceptors.

ros·in (roz′in). The solid resin obtained after steam distillation of crude balsam from *Pinus palustris* and from other species of *Pinus* (family Pinaceae); used in plasters to render them adhesive and also in ointments to render them locally stimulating. SYN colophony, resin (2).

p-ro·so·lic ac·id (rō-sol′ik). SYN aurin.

Ross, Sir George W., Canadian physician, 1841–1931. SEE R.-Jones *test*.

Ross, Donald N., Br. cardiac surgeon, * 1922; introduced aortic valve replacement using a pulmonic valve autograft. SEE R. *procedure*.

Ross, Sir Ronald, English physician and Nobel laureate, 1857–1932. SEE R. *cycle*.

Rossolimo, Grigoriy I., Russian neurologist, 1860–1928. SEE R. *reflex*, *sign*.

ros·tel·lum (ros-tel′ŭm). The anterior fixed or invertible portion of the scolex of a tapeworm, frequently provided with a row (or several rows) of hooks. [L. dim. of *rostrum*, a beak]

armed r., r. with one or more rows of hooks.

unarmed r., r. lacking hooks.

ros·trad (ros′trăd). **1.** In a direction toward any rostrum. **2.** Situated nearer a rostrum or the snout end of an organism in relation to a specific reference point; opposite of caudad (2). [L. *rostrum*, beak, + *-ad*, toward]

ros·tral (ros′trăl) [TA]. **1.** Relating to any rostrum or anatomic structure resembling a beak. **2.** At the head end. SYN rostralis [TA]. [L. *rostralis*, fr. *rostrum*, beak]

ros·tra·lis (ros′trā′lis) [TA]. SYN rostral. [L. fr. *rostrum*, beak]

ros·trate (ros′trāt). Having a beak or hook. [L. *rostratus*]

ros·tri·form (ros′tri-fōrm). Beak-shaped. [L. *rostrum*, beak]

ros·trum, pl. **ros·tra**, **ros·trums** (ros′trŭm, -tră) [TA]. Any beak-shaped structure. [L. a beak]

r. cor′poris callo′si [TA], SYN r. of corpus callosum.

r. of corpus callosum [TA], beak of the corpus callosum, the recurved portion of the corpus callosum passing backward from the genu to the anterior commissure. SYN r. corporis callosi [TA].

sphenoidal r. [TA], the anterior projecting part of the body of the sphenoid bone that articulates with the vomer. SYN r. sphenoidale [TA], r. of the sphenoid bone.

r. sphenoida′le [TA], SYN sphenoidal r.

r. of the sphenoid bone, SYN sphenoidal r.

ROT Abbreviation for right occipitotransverse position.

rot. To decay or putrify. [A.S. *rotian*]

ro·ta·mase (rō′ta-māz). Enzyme capable of altering the rotational conformation of a molecule.

ro·ta·mer (rō′ta-mer). An isomer differing from other conformation(s) only in rotational positioning of its parts, such as *cis*- and *trans*- forms.

ro·tam·e·ter (rō-tam′ĕ-ter). A device for measuring the flow of gas or liquid; the fluid flowing up through a slightly tapered tube elevates a ball or other weight that partially obstructs the flow,

until the wider cross-section allows that flow to pass around the floating obstruction. [L. *rota*, wheel, + G. *metron*, measure]

ro·ta·tion (rō-tā′shŭn). **1.** Turning or movement of a body around its axis. **2.** A recurrence in regular order of certain events, such as the symptoms of a periodic disease. **3.** In medical education, a period of time on a particular service or specialty. [L. *rotatio*, fr. *roto*, pp. *rotatus*, to revolve, rotate]

intestinal r., r. of the primitive intestinal loop around an axis formed by the superior mesenteric artery. SEE malrotation.

molecular r., one-hundredth of the product of the specific r. of an optically active compound and its molecular weight.

off-vertical r., r. about an axis eccentric to the body.

optic r., the change in the plane of polarization of polarized light of a given wavelength upon passing through optically active substances; measured in terms of specific rotation by polarimetry, an important tool in chemical structural work, especially on carbohydrates.

specific optic r. ([α]), the arc through which the plane of polarized light is rotated by 1 g of a substance per milliliter of water when the length of the light path through the solution is 1 decimeter, typically using light corresponding to the D line of sodium.

ro·ta·tor (rō-tā′ter, -tōr). SYN rotator *muscle*. SEE rotatores (*muscles*), under *muscle*. [L. See rotation]

medial r., a muscle that turns a part medialward. SEE ALSO invertor. SYN intortor.

ro·ta·vi·rus (rō′tă-vī′rŭs). A group of RNA viruses (family Reoviridae) wheel-like in appearance that form a genus, Rota virus, which includes the human gastroenteritis viruses (a major cause of infant diarrhea throughout the world). Separated into groups A through F, rotaviruses can infect a number of vertebrates. They are fastidious, and in vitro culture is difficult. SYN duovirus, gastroenteritis virus type B, infantile gastroenteritis virus, reoviruslike agent. [L. *rota*, wheel, + virus]

Rotch, Thomas M., U.S. physician, 1849–1914. SEE R. *sign*.

röt·eln, roeth·eln (ruht′eln). SYN rubella. [Ger. little red spots, fr. *rot*, red, + *-el*, dim. suffix]

ro·te·none (rō′te-nōn). The principal insecticidal component of derris root, *Derris elliptica*, *D. malaccensis*, and other species of *D.*, and from *Lonchocarpus nicou* (family Leguminosae); used externally for the treatment of scabies and infestation with chiggers, and in veterinary medicine for follicular mange and infestation with lice, fleas, and ticks; an inhibitor of the respiratory chain.

Roth, Vladimir K., Russian neurologist, 1848–1916. SEE Bernhardt-R. *syndrome*.

Roth, Moritz, Swiss physician and pathologist, 1839–1914. SEE R. *spots*, under *spot*; *vas* aberrans of R.

Roth. SEE Benedict-Roth *apparatus*.

Rothera, Arthur C.H., English biochemist, 1880–1915. SEE Rothera nitroprusside *test*.

Roth·ia (roth′ē-ă). A genus of nonmotile, non–spore-forming, non–acid-fast, aerobic to facultatively anaerobic bacteria (family Actinomycetaceae) containing Gram-positive, coccoid, diphtheroid, or filamentous cells; metabolism is fermentative, and glucose fermentation yields primarily lactic acid but no propionic acid. These organisms are normal inhabitants of the human oral cavity and are opportunistic pathogens. The type species is *R. dentocariosa*. [G. D. *Roth*]

R. dentocariosa, rare cause of infective endocarditis in humans.

Rothmund, August von, German physician, 1830–1906. SEE R. *syndrome*; R.-Thomson *syndrome*.

Rotor, Arturo B., 20th century Philippine internist. SEE R. *syndrome*.

ro·to·sco·li·o·sis (rō′tō-skō-lē-ō′sis). Combined lateral and rotational deviation of the vertebral column. [L. *roto*, to rotate, + G. *skoliōsis*, crookedness]

ro·to·tome (rō′tō-tōm). A rotating cutting instrument used in arthroscopic surgery.

ro·tox·a·mine (rō-tok′să-mēn). Active isomer of carbinoxamine; an antihistaminic.

ro

Rouget, Charles M.B., French physiologist, 1824–1904. SEE R. *muscle;* R.-Neumann *sheath.*

Rouget, Antoine D., 19th century French physiologist. SEE R. *bulb.*

rough (rŭf). Not smooth; denoting the irregular, coarsely granular surface of a certain bacterial colony type.

rough·age (rŭf´ij). Anything in the diet, e.g., bran, serving as a bulk stimulant of intestinal peristalsis.

Roughton, Francis J.W., British scientist, 1899–1972. SEE R.-Scholander *apparatus, syringe.*

Rougnon de Magny, Nicholas F., French physician, 1727–1799. SEE Rougnon-Heberden *disease.*

▣**rou·leau,** pl. **rou·leaux** (roo-lō´). An aggregate of erythrocytes stacked like a pile of coins. R. formation commonly indicates an increase in plasma immunoglobulin. [Fr. spool, cylinder, fr. *rouler,* to roll, fr. L.L. *rotulo,* fr. *rota,* wheel]

round·worm (rownd´werm). A nematode member of the phylum Nematoda, commonly confined to the parasitic forms.

Rous, F. Peyton, U.S. pathologist and Nobel laureate, 1879–1970. SEE R. *sarcoma,* sarcoma *virus, tumor;* R.-associated *virus.*

Roussy, Gustave, French pathologist, 1874–1948. SEE R.-Lévy *disease, syndrome;* Dejerine-R. *syndrome.*

Rouviere, Henri, French anatomist and embryologist, *1875. SEE *node* of R.

Roux, César, Swiss surgeon, 1857–1934. SEE R.-en-Y *anastomosis, operation.*

Roux, Philibert J., French surgeon, 1780–1854. SEE R. *method.*

Roux, Pierre P.E., French bacteriologist, 1853–1933. SEE Ro *spatula;* R. *stain.*

Rovsing, Niels T., Danish surgeon, 1862–1927. SEE R. *sign.*

RPF Abbreviation for renal plasma flow. SEE effective renal plasma *flow.*

R.Ph. Abbreviation for Registered Pharmacist.

rpm Abbreviation for revolutions per minute.

▣**RPO 1.** Abbreviation for right posterior oblique, a radiographic projection. **2.** Abbreviation for radiation protection officer.

R.Q. Abbreviation for respiratory *quotient.*

△**-rrhagia.** Excessive or unusual discharge; hemorrhage. [G. *rhēgnymi,* to burst forth]

△**-rrhaphy.** Surgical suturing. [G. *rhaphē,* suture]

△**-rrhea.** A flowing; a flux. [G. *rhoia,* a flow]

△**-rrhoea.** SEE -rrhea.

rRNA Abbreviation for ribosomal ribonucleic acid.

RSA Abbreviation for right sacroanterior position.

RSD Abbreviation for reflex sympathetic *dystrophy.*

RSP Abbreviation for right sacroposterior position.

RST Abbreviation for right sacrotransverse position.

RSV Abbreviation for Rous sarcoma *virus;* respiratory syncytial *virus.*

RT, rt Abbreviation for room *temperature.*

RT₃ Symbol for reverse triiodothyronine.

rTMP Abbreviation for ribothymidylic acid.

RT-PCR Abbreviation for reverse transcriptase polymerase chain *reaction.*

RU-486. SYN mifepristone.

Ru Symbol for ruthenium.

rub (rŭb). Friction encountered in moving one body in contact with another.

friction r., SYN friction *sound.*

pericardial r., pericardial friction r., SYN pericardial friction *sound.*

pleural r., friction rub sound caused by inflammation of the pleura. SYN pleural friction r., pleural rale.

pleural friction r., SYN pleural r.

pleuritic r., a friction sound produced by the rubbing together of the roughened surfaces of the costal and visceral pleurae.

Rubarth, Sven, Swedish veterinarian, *1905. SEE R. disease *virus.*

rub·ber (rŭb´er). The prepared inspissated milky juice of *Hevea brasiliensis* and other species of *Hevea* (family Euphorbiaceae), known in commerce as pure Para r.; used in the manufacture of various plasters, tissues, bandages, etc.

rub·ber po·lice·man. SEE policeman.

ru·be·an·ic ac·id (roo´bē-an-ik). Dithiooxamide, which forms complete dark greenish-black complexes with copper in alkaline ethanolic solution; used histochemically for demonstrating pathologic copper deposits, as in Wilson disease; also reacts with cobalt and nickel.

ru·be·do (roo-bē´dō). A temporary redness of the skin. [L. redness, fr. *ruber,* red]

ru·be·fa·cient (roo-bē-fā´shent). **1.** Causing a reddening of the skin. **2.** A counterirritant that produces erythema when applied to the skin surface. [L. *rubi-facio,* fr. *ruber,* red, + *facio,* to make]

ru·be·fac·tion (roo-bē-fak´shŭn). Erythema of the skin caused by local application of a counterirritant. [see rubefacient]

ru·bel·la (roo-bel´ă). An acute but mild exanthematous disease caused by rubella virus (Rubivirus family Togaviridae), with enlargement of lymph nodes, but usually with little fever or constitutional reaction; a high incidence of birth defects in children results from maternal infection during the first trimester of fetal life (congenital rubella syndrome). SYN epidemic roseola, German measles, röteln, roetheln, third disease, three-day measles. [L. *rubellus,* fem. *-a,* reddish, dim. of *ruber,* red]

ru·bel·lin (roo-bel´in). A cardiac glycoside with a digitalis-like action, obtained from *Urginia rubella* (family Liliaceae).

ru·be·o·la (roo-bē´ō-lă, -bē-ō´lă). A term used for measles; not to be confused with rubella. [Mod. L. dim. of *ruber,* red, reddish]

ru·be·o·sis (roo-bē-ō´sis). Reddish discoloration, as of the skin. [L. *ruber,* red, + G. *-osis,* condition]

r. i´ridis diabet´ica, neovascularization of the anterior surface of the iris in diabetes mellitus.

ru·bes·cent (roo-bes´ent). Reddening. [L. *rubesco,* pr. p. *rubescens,* to become red]

ru·bid·i·um (Rb) (roo-bid´ē-ŭm). An alkali element, atomic no. 37, atomic wt. 85.4678; its salts have been used in medicine for the same purposes as the corresponding sodium or potassium salts. [L. *rubidus,* reddish, dark red, fr. *rubeo,* to be red]

ru·bid·o·my·cin (dau·no·ru·bi·cin) (roo-bid´ō-mī-sin). An antibiotic used as an antineoplastic particularly in acute leukemias; similar to doxorubicin in antitumor activity and in exhibiting cumulative cardiotoxicity.

Rubin, Isidor C., U.S. gynecologist, 1883–1958. SEE R. *test.*

ru·bin S, ru·bine (roo´bin, bēn) [C.I. 42685]. SYN acid *fuchsin.*

Rubinstein, Jack H., U.S. child psychiatrist and pediatrician, *1925. SEE R.-Taybi *syndrome.*

Ru·bi·vi·rus (roo´bi-vī´rŭs). A genus of viruses (family Togaviridae) that includes the rubella virus. [*rubella* + virus]

Rubner, Max, German hygienist and biochemist, 1854–1932. SEE R. *laws* of growth, under *law, test.*

ru·bor (roo´bōr). Redness, as one of the four signs of inflammation (r., calor, dolor, tumor) enunciated by Celsus. [L.]

ru·bra·tox·in (roo-bră-tok´sin). A mycotoxin produced by *Penicillium rubrum* and *P. purpurogenum,* which form readily on cereal grains; responsible for outbreaks of toxicosis in the U.S.

ru·bre·dox·ins (roo-brē-dok´sinz). Ferredoxins without acid-labile sulfur and with the iron in a typical mercaptide coordination.

ru·bri·blast (roo´bri-blast). SYN pronormoblast. [L. *ruber,* red, + G. *blastos,* germ]

pernicious anemia type r., SYN promegaloblast; SEE erythroblast.

rub·ric. Section or chapter heading, used with reference to groups of diseases, as in ICD. [M.E. *rubrike,* title or heading in red, fr. *ruber,* red]

ru·bri·cyte (roo´bri-sīt). Polychromatic normoblast. SEE erythroblast. [L. *ruber,* red, + *kytos,* cell]

ru·bro·spi·nal (roo´brō-spī´năl). Relating to the nerve fibers passing from the red nucleus to the spinal cord: the rubrospinal *tract* [TA].

Ru·bu·la·vi·rus (roo-boo′la-vī-rus). A genus in the family Paramyxoviridae; causes mumps. SYN mumpvirus.

ruc·tus (rŭk′tŭs). SYN eructation. [L. fr. *ructo*, pp. -*atus*, to belch]

Rud, Einar, Danish physician, *1892. SEE R. *syndrome*.

ru·di·ment (roo′di-ment). **1.** An organ or structure that is incompletely developed. **2.** The first indication of a structure in the course of ontogeny. SYN rudimentum. [L. *rudimentum*, a beginning, fr. *rudis*, unformed]

ru·di·men·ta·ry (roo-di-men′tār-ē). Relating to a rudiment. SYN abortive (2).

ru·di·men·tum, pl. **ru·di·men·ta** (roo′di-men′tŭm, -tă). SYN rudiment, rudiment. [L.]

  r. hippocam′pi, SEE *indusium* griseum.

ruff (rŭf). A collar or ruffle.

  pupillary r., the dark-brown, wrinkled rim of the normal pupil, which is the posterior pigment epithelium of the iris showing itself at the pupillary margin.

Ruffini, Angelo, Italian histologist, 1864–1929. SEE R. *corpuscles*, under *corpuscle;* flower-spray *organ* of R.

ru·fous (roo′fŭs). Having a reddish complexion and red hair. SYN erythristic. [L. *rufus*, reddish]

ru·ga, pl. **ru·gae** (roo′gă, roo′gē) [TA]. A fold, ridge, or crease; a wrinkle. [L. a wrinkle]

  rugae of gallbladder, ☆official alternate term for mucosal *folds* of gallbladder, under *fold*.

  gastric rugae, ☆official alternate term for gastric *folds*, under *fold*.

  r. gas′trica, SYN gastric *folds*, under *fold*.

  r. palati′na, SYN transverse palatine *fold*.

  rugae of stomach, SYN gastric *folds*, under *fold*.

  rugae of vagina, SYN vaginal rugae.

  vaginal rugae [TA], a number of transverse ridges in the mucous membrane of the vagina. SYN rugae vaginales [TA], rugae of vagina.

  ru′gae vagina′les [TA], SYN vaginal rugae.

  rugae vesicae biliaris, ☆official alternate term for mucosal *folds* of gallbladder, under *fold*.

ru·gine (roo-zhēn′). **1.** SYN periosteal *elevator*. **2.** A raspatory. [Fr.]

ru·gi·tus (roo′ji-tŭs). A rumbling sound in the intestines. SEE ALSO borborygmus. [L. a roaring, fr. *rugio*, to roar]

ru·gose (roo′gōs). Marked by rugae; wrinkled. SYN rugous. [L. *rugosus*]

ru·gos·i·ty (roo-gos′i-tē). **1.** The state of being thrown into folds or wrinkles. **2.** A ruga.

ru·gous (roo′gŭs). SYN rugose.

Ruhemann pur·ple. a blue-violet dye formed in the reaction of ninhydrin with amino acids.

RUL Abbreviation for right upper lobe (of lung).

rule (rool). A criterion, standard, or guide governing a procedure, arrangement, action, etc. SEE ALSO law, principle, theorem. [O. Fr. *reule*, fr. L. *regula*, a guide, pattern]

  Abegg r., the tendency of the sum of the maximum positive and maximum negative valence of a particular element to equal 8; e.g., C may have a valence of +4 and −4, O of +6 and −2. Sometimes loosely stated as all atoms have the same number of valences, a consequence of the tendency of valence electron shells to be filled to 8.

  American Law Institute r., a test of criminal responsibility (1962): "a person is not responsible for criminal conduct if at the time of such conduct as a result of mental disease or defect he or she lacks substantial capacity either to appreciate the wrongfulness of the conduct or to conform the conduct to the requirements of law."

  r. of bigeminy, r. that a ventricular premature beat will follow the beat terminating a long cycle. Sudden prolongation of the ventricular cycle, by changing the refractoriness in the conduction system, causes a peripheral region of bidirectional block to become

transiently unidirectional and thus opens potential pathways for reentry to occur.

  Chargaff r., in DNA the number of adenine units equals the number of thymine units; likewise, the number of guanine units equals the number of cytosine units.

  Clark weight r., an obsolete r. for an approximate child's dose, obtained by dividing the child's weight in pounds by 150 and multiplying the result by the adult dose.

  Cowling r., an obsolete r. for a child's dose: that fraction of the adult dose obtained by dividing the age of the child at the nearest birthday by 24.

  Durham r., an American test of criminal responsibility (1954) under which an accused person is not held criminally responsible if the unlawful act was the product of mental disease or mental defect.

  Gibb phase r., SYN phase r.

  Goriaew r., rarely used term for a r. of a blood counting field by which it is marked off in a series of squares, some of which are again subdivided into 16 smaller ones.

  Haase r., the length of the fetus in centimeters, divided by 5, is the duration of pregnancy in months, i.e., the age of the fetus.

  Hückel r., the number of depolarized electrons in an aromatic ring is equal to $4n + 2$ where n is 0 or any positive integer; L-tyrosine, L-phenylalanine, L-tryptophan, and L-histidine (when the imidazole ring is deprotonated) obey this rule.

  Ingelfinger r., a principle developed by Franz Ingelfinger for use in the editorial offices of the *New England Journal of Medicine*, stating that original articles submitted for publication will be reviewed on the understanding that the same information will not be submitted for publication elsewhere during the period of review; has been adopted by many other peer-reviewed medical journals.

  isoprene r., the classical, outmoded statement that naturally occurring terpenes are built up by condensation of isoprene units by either a 1-4 linkage ("head to tail") or a 4-4 linkage ("tail to tail").

  Jackson r., after an epileptic attack, simple and quasiautomatic functions are less affected and more rapidly recovered than the more complex ones.

  Le Bel-van't Hoff r., the number of stereoisomers of an organic compound is 2^n, where n represents the number of asymmetric carbon atoms (unless there is an internal plane of symmetry); a corollary of their simultaneously announced conclusions, in 1874, that the most probable orientation of the bonds of a carbon atom linked to four groups or atoms is toward the apexes of a tetrahedron, and that this accounted for all then-known phenomena of molecular asymmetry (which involved a carbon atom bearing four different atoms or groups). SEE ALSO stereoisomerism.

  Liebermeister r., in adult febrile tachycardia, about eight pulse beats correspond to an increase of 1°C.

  Meyer-Overton r., because inhalation agents act via the lipid-rich CNS cells, anesthetic potency increases with lipid solubility.

  M'Naghten r., the classic English test of criminal responsibility (1843): "to establish a defense on the ground of insanity, it must be clearly proved that, at the time of committing the act, the party accused was laboring under such a defect of reasoning, from disease of the mind, as not to know the nature and quality of the act he was doing, or if he did know it, that he did not know he was doing what was wrong."

  Nägele r., determination of the estimated delivery date by adding 7 days to the first day of the last normal menstrual period, counting back 3 months, and adding 1 year.

  New Hampshire r., pioneering American test of criminal responsibility (1871): "if the [criminal] act was the offspring of insanity, a criminal intent did not produce it."

  r. of nines, method used in calculating body surface area involved in burns whereby values of 9% or 18% of surface area are assigned to specific regions as follows: Head and neck, 9%; anterior thorax, 18%; posterior thorax, 18%; arms, 9% each; legs, 18% each; and perineum, 1%.

  Ogino-Knaus r., the time in the menstrual period when conception is most likely to occur is at about midway between two menstrual periods; fertilization of the ovum is least likely just before or just after menstruation; the basis for the rhythm method of contraception.

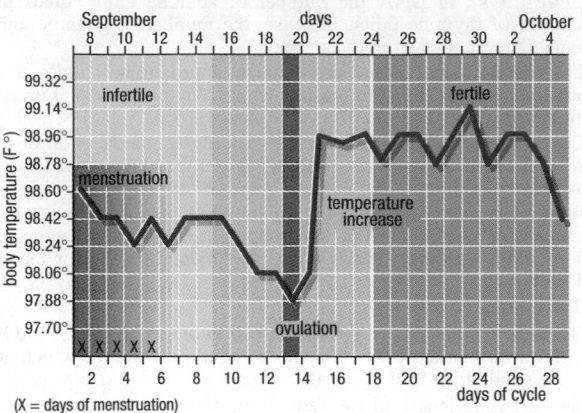

Ogino-Knaus rule

r. of outlet, an obstetric r. for determining whether the pelvic outlet will permit the passage of a fetus; the sum of the posterior sagittal diameter and the transverse diameter of the outlet must equal at least 15 cm if a normal-sized baby is to pass.

phase r., an expression of the relationships existing between systems in equilibrium: $P + V = C + 2$, where P is the number of phases, V the variance or degrees of freedom, and C the number of components; it also follows that the variance is $V = C + 2 - P$. For H_2O at its triple point, $V = 1 + 2 - 3 = 0$, i.e., both temperature and pressure are fixed. SYN Gibb phase r.

Prentice r., each centimeter of decentration of a lens results in 1 prism diopter of deviation of light for each diopter of lens power.

Rolleston r., the ideal adult systolic blood pressure is 100 plus half the age, whereas the maximal physiologic pressure is 100 plus the age; of historical interest.

Schütz r., the rate of an enzyme reaction is proportional to the square root of the enzyme concentration; applied specifically to pepsin within a limited range. SYN Schütz law.

stopping r.'s, in randomized controlled trials and other systematic experiments on human subjects, r.'s laid down in advance that specify conditions under which the experiment will be terminated, e.g., unequivocal demonstration that one regimen in a randomized controlled trial is clearly superior to the other, or that one is clearly harmful.

Trusler r. for pulmonary artery banding, a method that gives guidance as to the correct tightness of the band; the degree of banding for a complex congenital cardiac anomaly with bidirectional shunting less than that for simple ones.

Young r., an obsolete r. to determine a child's dose: 12 is added to the child's age and the sum is divided by the age; the adult dose divided by the figure so obtained gives the proper dose.

rul·er (roo′ler). A calibrated strip for measuring plane surfaces.

isometric r., a calibrated scale for eliminating distortion in the measurement of plane surfaces.

rum (rŭm). A spirit distilled from the fermented juice of the sugar cane.

rum-blos·som (rŭm-blos′ŭm). SYN rhinophyma.

ru·mi·nant (roo′mi-nănt). An animal that chews the cud, material regurgitated from the rumen for rechewing; e.g., the sheep, cow, deer, or antelope.

ru·mi·na·tion (roo-mi-nā′shŭn). **1.** The physiologic process in ruminant animals in which coarse, hastily eaten food is regurgitated from the rumen, thoroughly rechewed, reduced to finer particles, mixed with saliva, and reswallowed. **2.** A disorder of infancy characterized by repeated regurgitation of food, with weight loss or failure to thrive, developing after a period of normal functioning. **3.** Periodic reconsideration of the same subject. [L. *ruminatio,* fr. *rumino,* to chew the cud, think over, fr. *rumen,* throat]

ru·mi·na·tive (roo′min-ă-tiv). Characterized by a preoccupation with certain thoughts and ideas.

Ru·mi·no·coc·cus (room′ē-nō-kok′us). A genus of anaerobic, Gram-positive coccobacilli isolated from the repiratory tract of humans and the intestinal tract of humans and animals. The type species is *Ruminococcus productus,* formerly *Peptostreptococcus productus.*

Rumpel, Theodor, German physician, 1862–1923. SEE R.-Leede *sign, test, phenomenon.*

run (rŭn). A group of successive measurements in an analytic process or during a period of time within which the accuracy and precision of the measuring system are expected to be stable. [ME *runnen,* fr. A. S. *rinnan,* fr. O.N. *rinna*]

Rundle. A.T., British physician. SEE Richards-Rundle *syndrome.*

Runeberg, Johan W., Finnish physician, 1843–1918. SEE R. *formula.*

run·off (rŭn′awf). Delayed part of the angiographic examination of a vascular bed, to show small artery patency.

runt (rŭnt). A stunted animal, occurring most frequently in species that give birth to large litters. [A.S.]

ru·pia (roo′pē-ă). **1.** Ulcers of late secondary syphilis, covered with yellowish or brown crusts that have been compared in their appearance to oyster shells. **2.** Term occasionally used to designate a very scaly, heaped-up, and secondarily infected psoriatic lesion. [G. *rhypos,* filth]

ru·pi·oid (roo′pē-oyd). Resembling rupia. [G. *rhypos,* filth (rupia), + *eidos,* resemblance]

rup·ture (rŭp′choor). **1.** SYN hernia. **2.** A solution of continuity or a tear; a break of any organ or other of the soft parts. [L. *ruptura,* a fracture (of limb or vein), fr. *rumpo,* pp. *ruptus,* to break]

artificial membrane r., r. of the membranes induced by use of an amniohook or similar device.

membrane r., r. of the amnionic sac allowing the amnionic fluid to escape through the vagina.

premature membrane r., r. of the membranes before the onset of labor.

preterm membrane r., r. of membranes before term (<37 weeks gestation).

spontaneous membrane r., spontaneous r. of membranes, with or without associated labor.

RUQ Abbreviation for right upper quadrant (of abdomen).

Rushton, Martin A., British pathologist, 1903–1970. SEE R. *bodies.*

Russell, Albert L., U.S. dentist, 1905–1985. SEE R. Periodontal Index.

Russell, Alexander, 20th century British pediatrician. SEE R. *syndrome;* Silver-R. *dwarfism, syndrome.*

Russell, Gerald F.M., 20th century English physician. SEE R. *sign.*

Russell, Hamilton, 20th century Australian surgeon. SEE R. *traction.*

Russell, James S. Risien, British physician, 1863–1939. SEE hooked *bundle* of R.; uncinate *bundle* of R.

Russell, Patrick, Irish physician in India, 1727–1805. SEE R.'s viper *venom, viper.*

Russell, William James, English chemist, 1830–1909. SEE R. *effect.*

Russell, William, Scottish physician, 1852–1940. SEE R. *bodies,* under *body.*

Russell Per·i·o·don·tal In·dex. An index that estimates the degree of periodontal disease present in the mouth by measuring both bone loss around the teeth and gingival inflammation; used frequently in the epidemiologic investigation of periodontal disease.

Rust, Johann N., German surgeon, 1775–1840. SEE R. *phenomenon.*

rusts (rŭsts). Species of *Puccinia* and other microbes constituting important pathogens of plants, especially cereal grains; they are important allergens for humans when inhaled in large numbers, as in harvesting processes.

ru·the·ni·um (Ru) (roo-thē′nē-ŭm). A metallic element of the platinum group; atomic no. 44, atomic wt. 101.07; ^{106}Ru, with a half-life of 1.020 years, has been used in the treatment of certain eye problems. [Mediev. L. *Ruthenia,* Russia, where first obtained]

ru·the·ni·um red. Ammoniated r. r. oxychloride, used in histology and electron microscopy as a stain for certain complex polysaccharides.

ruth·er·ford (rŭth′er-ferd). Obsolete term for a unit of radioactivity, representing that quantity of radioactive material in which a million disintegrations are taking place per second; 37 r. = 1 mCi. SEE Becquerel. [Ernest *Rutherford,* British physicist and Nobel laureate, 1871–1937]

ru·ti·do·sis (roo-ti-dō′sis). SYN rhytidosis.

ru·tin (roo′tin). A flavonoid obtained from buckwheat, which causes decreased capillary fragility. SYN rutoside.

ru·tin·ose (roo′ti-nōs). A disaccharide of D-glucose and L-rhamnose, and a component of rutin.

ru·to·side (roo′tō-sīd). SYN rutin.

Ruysch, Frederik, Dutch anatomist, 1638–1731. SEE R. *membrane, muscle, tube, veins,* under *vein.*

RV Abbreviation for residual *volume.*

Ryan, Norbert J., 20th century Australian pathologist. SEE R. *stain.*

ry·an·o·dine (rī-an′ō-dēn). An alkaloid obtained from *Ryania speciosa* (family Flacourtiaceae); has a disruptive effect on calcium storage in cardiac and skeletal muscle, where it produces sustained contractions; used as an insecticide.

rye smut (rī′ smŭt′). SYN ergot.

Ryle, John A., English physician, 1889–1950. SEE R. *tube.*

Ry

σ, Σ 1. The 18th letter of the Greek alphabet, sigma. **2.** (σ) Symbol for reflection *coefficient*; standard *deviation*; a factor in prokaryotic RNA initiation; wavenumber; surface *tension*. **3.** (Σ) Summation of a series.

S 1. Abbreviation for sacral vertebra (S1–S5); spherical, spherical *lens*; Svedberg *unit*. **2.** Symbol for siemens; sulfur; entropy in thermodynamics; substrate in the Michaelis-Menton mechanism; percentage saturation of hemoglobin (when followed by subscript O_2 or CO); serine; one of the two stereochemical designations (in italics) in the Cahn-Ingold-Prelog system. **3.** Designation of a rare human antigen (hemagglutinogen) related genetically to the MNSs blood group. See Blood Groups appendix.

S100. An acidic, calcium-binding protein characterized by its partial solubility in saturated ammonium sulfate; stains for S100 are used in the differential diagnosis of melanomas, which are commonly positive for S100.

^{35}S Symbol for sulfur-35.

S_1 Symbol for first heart *sound*.

S Symbol for entropy.

S_2 Symbol for second heart *sound*.

S_3 Symbol for third heart *sound*.

S_4 Symbol for fourth heart *sound*.

S_7 SYN summation *gallop*.

S_f Symbol for flotation *constant*.

s Abbreviation of L. *sinister*, left; L. *semis*, half; second; as a subscript, denotes steady *state*.

s̄ Abbreviation for L. *sine*, without.

s Symbol for selection *coefficient*; sedimentation *coefficient*.

S-A Abbreviation for sinuatrial.

SA Abbreviation for sacroanterior *position*.

sab·a·dil·la (sab-ă-dil′ă). The seed of *Schoenocaulon officinale* (family Liliaceae), a plant of the shores of the Gulf of Mexico and Caribbean Sea; it yields cevadine, veratridine, and several other alkaloids; has been used externally as a parasiticide. SYN cevadilla. [Sp. *cevadilla,* ult. fr. L. *cibus,* food]

Sabin, Albert B., Polish-U.S. virologist, 1906–1993. SEE S. *vaccine;* S.-Feldman dye *test.*

Sabouraud, Raymond J.A., French dermatologist, 1864–1938. SEE S. *agar, pastils,* under *pastil;* S.-Noiré *instrument.*

sab·u·lous (sab′ū-lŭs). Sandy; gritty. [L. *sabulosus,* fr. *sabulum,* coarse sand]

sa·bur·ra (să-bŭr′ă). Foulness of the stomach or mouth resulting from decomposed food. [L. sand]

sa·bur·ral (să-bŭr′ăl). Relating to saburra.

sac (sak) [TA]. **1.** A pouch or bursa. SYN saccus [TA]. SEE ALSO sacculus. **2.** An encysted abscess at the root of a tooth. **3.** The capsule of a tumor, or envelope of a cyst. [L. *saccus,* a bag]

abdominal s., the part of the embryonic celom that becomes the abdominal cavity.

air s., SYN alveolar s.

allantoic s., the dilated distal portion of the allantois; it forms part of the placenta in many mammals.

alveolar s., (1) terminal dilation of the alveolar ducts that give rise to alveoli in the lung; a small air chamber in the pulmonary tissue from which the pulmonary alveoli project like bays and into which an alveolar duct opens; SYN sacculus alveolaris [TA]. **(2)** in birds, air-containing extensions of bronchi that connect with bone cavities. SYN air s.

amnionic s., SYN amnion.

aneurysmal s., the dilated wall of an artery in a saccular aneurysm.

aortic s., in mammalian embryos, the endothelially lined dilation just distal to the truncus arteriosus; it is the primordial vascular channel from which the aortic arch/arteries arise and is homologous to the ventral aorta of gill-bearing vertebrates.

chorionic s., SYN chorion.

conjunctival s. [TA], the space bound by the conjunctival membrane between the palpebral and bulbar conjunctiva, into which the lacrimal fluid is secreted; it is a closed space when eye is

closed; when eye is open, the sac is open anteriorly via the palpebral fissure (between the eyelids). SYN saccus conjunctivalis [TA].

cupular blind s., SYN cupular *cecum* of the cochlear duct.

dental s., the outer investment of mesenchymal tissue surrounding a developing tooth; involved in formation of the root and periodontal ligament. SEE ALSO dental *follicle.*

endolymphatic s. [TA], the dilated blind extremity of the endolymphatic duct, which lies external to the dura on the posterior aspect of the petrous part of the temporal bone. SYN saccus endolymphaticus [TA], Böttcher space, Cotunnius space, sacculus endolymphaticus.

gestational s., cystic structure of early pregnancy that represents the amnionic s., fluid, and placenta.

heart s., SYN pericardium.

hernial s., the protruding envelope of peritoneum in a hernia.

Hilton s., SYN laryngeal *saccule.*

lacrimal s. [TA], the dilated upper portion of the nasolacrimal duct into which the two lacrimal canaliculi empty. SYN saccus lacrimalis [TA], dacryocyst, sacculus lacrimalis, tear s.

lesser peritoneal s., SYN omental *bursa.*

lymph s.'s, the earliest lymphatic vessels formed in the embryo.

nasal s.'s, the deepened nasal pits that develop into the definitive nasal cavities.

omental s., SYN omental *bursa.*

preputial s., the space between the prepuce and the glans penis.

pudendal s., a pear-shaped encapsulated collection of connective tissue and fat in each labium majus. SYN Broca pouch.

tear s., SYN lacrimal s.

tooth s., a capsule that encloses the developing tooth.

vestibular blind s., SYN vestibular *cecum* of the cochlear duct.

vitelline s., SYN yolk s.

yolk s., (1) in vertebrates with telolecithal eggs; the highly vascular layer of splanchnopleure surrounding the yolk of an embryo; **(2)** in humans and other mammals, the s. of extraembryonic membrane that is located ventral to the embryonic disk and, after formation of the gut tube, is connected to the midgut; by the second month of development, this connection has become the narrow yolk stalk; the yolk s. is the first hematopoietic organ of the embryo, and its vitelline circulation plays an important role in the early embryonic circulation; the s. is also the site of origin of the primordial germ cells. SYN umbilical vesicle, vesicula umbilicalis, vitelline s.

sac·cade (să-kād′). Rapid eye movement to redirect the line of sight. [Fr. *saccade,* sudden check of a horse]

sac·cad·ic (să-kad′ik). Jerky. SEE saccadic *movement.*

sac·cate (sak′āt). Relating to a sac. [L. *saccus,* sac]

△**sacchar-.** SEE saccharo-.

sac·cha·rase (sak′ă-rās). SYN β-fructofuranosidase.

sac·cha·rate (sak′ă-rāt). A salt or ester of saccharic acid.

sac·char·eph·i·dro·sis (sak-ar-ef-i-drō′sis). The presence of sugar in the sweat. [sacchar- + G. *ephidrōsis,* a slight perspiration]

△**sacchari-.** SEE saccharo-.

sac·char·ic (să-kar′ik). Relating to sugar.

sac·char·ic ac·id (sak′ă-rik). Term used to denote the class of dicarboxy sugar acids.

△ **Combining Forms**

🄸 **Indicates term is illustrated,** see Illustration Index

SYN Synonym

Cf. Compare

[NA] Nomina Anatomica

[TA] Terminologia Anatomica

☆ **Official alternate Terminologia Anatomica term**

[MIM] Mendelian Inheritance in Man

C.I. Colour Index

High Profile Term

sac·cha·rides (sak′ă-rīdz). S.'s are classified as mono-, di-, tri-, and polysaccharides according to the number of monosaccharide groups composing them. SEE carbohydrates.

sac·cha·rif·er·ous (sak′ă-rif′er-ŭs). Producing sugar.

sac·char·i·fi·ca·tion (să-kar′i-fi-kā′shŭn). The process of saccharifying.

sac·char·i·fy (să-kar′i-fī). To convert starch or cellulose or other polysaccharides into sugar. [facchari- + L. *facio*, to make]

sac·cha·rim·e·ter (sak-ă-rim′ĕ-ter). An instrument for determining the amount of sugar in a solution; it may be a polarimeter, a hygrometer, or a container in which the solution is fermented and the amount estimated by the volume of CO_2 produced. SYN saccharometer. [(facchari- + G. *metron*, measure]

sac·cha·rin (sak′ă-rin). In dilute aqueous solution it is 300–500 times sweeter than sucrose; used as a noncaloric sweetening agent (sugar substitute); s. sodium and s. calcium have the same use. SYN benzosulfimide.

sac·cha·rine (sak′ă-rēn, -rin, -rīn). Relating to sugar; sweet.

♺**saccharo-, facchar-, facchari-.** Combining forms denoting sugar (faccharide). [G. *fakcharon*, sugar]

sac·cha·ro·gen am·y·lase (sak′ă-rō-jen). SYN β-amylase.

sac·cha·ro·lyt·ic (sak′ă-rō-lit′ik). Capable of hydrolyzing or otherwise breaking down a sugar molecule. [faccharo- + G. *lysis*, loosening]

sac·cha·ro·met·a·bol·ic (sak′ă-rō-met′ă-bol′ik). Relating to saccharometabolism.

sac·cha·ro·me·tab·o·lism (sak-ă-rō-mĕ-tab′ō-lizm). Metabolism of sugar; the process of utilization of sugar in cells.

sac·cha·rom·e·ter (sak-ă-rom′ĕ-ter). SYN saccharimeter.

Sac·cha·ro·my·ces (sak′ă-rō-mī′sēz). A genus of budding yeasts (family Saccharomycetaceae); an ascomycete. *S. cerevisiae* is used to produce brewer's yeast and ethanol. *S. cerevisiae* is a very rare pathogen in humans. [faccharo- + G. *mykēs*, fungus]

Sac·cha·ro·my·ce·ta·ce·ae (sak′ă-rō-mī-sē-tā′sē-ē). The family of yeasts; that group of fungi comprising the ascomycetes which possess a predominantly unicellular thallus, reproduce asexually by budding, transverse division, or both, and produce ascospores in an ascus, originating from a zygote or pathogenetically from a single somatic cell. The term yeastlike fungus is often applied to fungi that are not known to form ascospores, but otherwise possess the characteristics of yeasts; such forms are properly placed with the Fungi Imperfecti unless methods of sexual reproduction are known; e.g., *Cryptococcus neoformans.*

Sac·cha·ro·my·ce·ta·les (sak′ă-rō-mī′sē-tā′lēz). SYN Endomycetales.

sac·cha·ro·pine (sak-ar′ō-pēn). A derivative of α-ketoglutarate and L-lysine that is an intermediate in L-lysine catabolism; elevated in cases of saccharopinuria.

s. dehydrogenase, two enzymes that are used in the pathway of L-lysine catabolism; the first isoform catalyzes the reversible conversion of L-lysine, α-ketoglutarate, and NADH to s. and NAD$^+$; the other isoform reversibly catalyzes to conversion of s. and NAD$^+$ to L-glutamate, NADH, and L-α-aminoadipate δ-semialdehyde. A deficiency of one of these isoforms is associated with familial hyperlysinemia and saccharopinuria.

sac·cha·ro·pi·nu·ria (sak-ar′ō-pēn-oor-ē-ă). Elevated levels of saccharopine in the urine; associated with a variant of familial hyperlysinuria.

sac·cha·rose (sak′ă-rōs). SYN sucrose.

sac·cha·rum (sak′ă-rŭm). SYN sucrose. [Mod. L. fr. G. *fakcharon*]

s. canaden′se, SYN maple *sugar.*

s. lac′tis, SYN lactose.

sac·ci·form (sak′si-fōrm). Pouched; sac-shaped. SYN saccular, sacculated. [L. *saccus*, sack, + *forma*, form]

sac·cu·lar (sak′ū-lăr). SYN sacciform.

sac·cu·lat·ed (sak′ū-lā′ted). SYN sacciform.

sac·cu·la·tion (sak′ū-lā′shŭn). **1.** A structure formed by a group of sacs. **2.** The formation of a sac or pouch.

s.'s of colon, SYN *haustra* of colon, under *haustrum.*

sac·cule (sak′ūl) [TA]. **1** [TA]. The smaller of the two membranous sacs in the vestibule of the labyrinth, lying in the spherical recess; it is connected with the cochlear duct by a very short tube, the ductus reuniens, and with the utriculus by the beginning of the ductus endolymphaticus and the ductus utriculosaccularis that joins it. **2.** The immense bag-shaped structure formed by peptidoglycans as part of the cell wall of certain microorganisms. SYN sacculus [TA], sacculus proprius, sacculus vestibuli. [L. *sacculus*]

laryngeal s. [TA], a small diverticulum provided with mucous glands extending upward from the ventricle of the larynx between the vestibular fold and the lamina of the thyroid cartilage; it is a vestigial structure, being a much larger structure interdigitating with the neck musculature in some of the great apes, where it serves as a resonating chamber. SYN sacculus laryngis [TA], appendix ventriculi laryngis, Hilton sac, laryngeal pouch, s. of larynx.

s. of larynx, SYN laryngeal s.

sac·cu·lo·co·chle·ar (sak′ū-lō-kok′lē-ăr). Relating to the sacculus and the membranous cochlea.

sac·cu·lus, pl. **sac·cu·li** (sak′ū-lŭs, -lī) [TA]. SYN saccule. [L. dim. of *saccus*, sac]

s. alveola′ris, pl. **sacculi alveola′res** [TA], SYN alveolar *sac* (1).

s. commu′nis, SYN utricle.

s. endolymphat′icus, SYN endolymphatic *sac.*

s. lacrima′lis, SYN lacrimal *sac.*

s. laryn′gis [TA], SYN laryngeal *saccule.*

s. pro′prius, SYN saccule.

s. vestib′uli, SYN saccule.

sac·cus, pl. **sac·ci** (sak′ŭs, sak′sī) [TA]. SYN sac (1). [L. a bag, sack]

s. conjunctiva′lis [TA], SYN conjunctival *sac.*

s. endolymphat′icus [TA], SYN endolymphatic *sac.*

s. lacrima′lis [TA], SYN lacrimal *sac.*

s. reu′niens, SYN *sinus* venosus.

s. vagina′lis, an embryonic peritoneal fossa indicating the site where the processus vaginalis peritonei extends through the anterior abdominal wall during descent of the testis.

Sachs, Bernard, U.S. neurologist, 1858–1944. SEE Tay-S. *disease.*

Sachs, Hans, German bacteriologist, 1877–1945. SEE S.-Georgi *test.*

Sachs, Maurice D., U.S. radiologist, *1909. SEE Hill-S. *lesion.*

Sacks, Benjamin, U.S. physician, 1896–1939. SEE Libman-S. *endocarditis, syndrome.*

♺**sacr-.** SEE sacro-.

sa·crad (sā′krad). In the direction of the sacrum. [sacr- + L. *ad,* to]

sa·cral (sā′krăl). Relating to or in the neighborhood of the sacrum.

sa·cral·gia (sā-kral′jē-ă). Pain in the sacral region. SYN sacrodynia. [sacr- + G. *algos,* pain]

sa·cral·i·za·tion (sā′kral-i-zā′shŭn). Lumbar development and appearance of the first sacral vertebra.

sa·crec·to·my (sā-krek′tō-mē). Resection of a portion of the sacrum to facilitate an operation. SYN sacrotomy. [sacr- + G. *ektomē,* excision]

♺**sacro-, sacr-.** The sacrum. [L. *os sacrum,* sacred bone]

sa·cro·coc·cyg·e·al (sā-krō-kok-sij′ē-ăl). Relating to both sacrum and coccyx.

sa·cro·coc·cyg·e·us (sā′krō-kok-si-jē′ŭs). SEE muscle.

sa·cro·dyn·ia (sā′krō-din′ē-ă). SYN sacralgia. [sacro- + G. *odynē,* pain]

sa·cro·il·i·ac (sā-krō-il′ē-ak). Relating to the sacrum and the ilium.

sa·cro·il·i·i·tis (sā′krō-il-ē-ī′tis). Inflammation of the sacroiliac joint.

sa·cro·lum·ba·lis (sā′krō-lŭm-bā′lis). The iliocostalis lumborum muscle.

sa·cro·lum·bar (sā′krō-lŭm′băr). SYN lumbosacral.

sa

sa·cro·sci·at·ic (sā'krō-sī-at'ik). Relating to both sacrum and ischium.

sa·cro·spi·nal (sā'krō-spī'năl). Relating to the sacrum and the vertebral column above.

sa·crot·o·my (sā-krot'ō-mē). SYN sacrectomy. [sacro- + G. *tomē*, incision]

sa·cro·ver·te·bral (sā'krō-ver'tē-brăl). Relating to the sacrum and the vertebrae above.

sa·crum, pl. **sa·cra** (sā'krŭm, sā'kră) [TA]. The segment of the vertebral column forming part of the pelvis; a broad, slightly curved, spade-shaped bone, thick above, thinner below, closing in the pelvic girdle posteriorly; it is formed by the fusion of five originally separate sacral vertebrae; it articulates with the last lumbar vertebra, the coccyx, and the hip bone on either side. SYN os sacrum [TA], sacred bone, vertebra magna. [L. (lit. sacred bone), neuter of *sacer* (*sacr-*), sacred]

assimilation s., one which is composed of six segments, the last lumbar vertebra assuming the appearance of a sacral segment; or one which is composed of but four segments, the first sacral being free and having the characteristics of a lumbar vertebra.

SACT Abbreviation for sinoatrial conduction *time*.

SAD Abbreviation for seasonal affective *disorder*.

sad·dle (sad'l). **1.** A structure shaped like, or suggestive of, a seat or s. used in horseback riding. SYN sella. **2.** SYN denture *base*.

 Turkish s., SYN *sella* turcica.

sa·dism (sā'dizm, sad'izm). A form of perversion, often sexual in nature, in which a person finds pleasure in inflicting abuse and maltreatment. Cf. masochism. [Marquis de *Sade*, 1740–1814, confessedly addicted to the practice]

sa·dist (sā'dist, sad'ist). One who practices sadism.

sa·dis·tic (să-dis'tik). Pertaining to or characterized by sadism.

sa·do·mas·och·ism (sā-dō-mas'ō-kizm, sad-o-). A form of perversion marked by enjoyment of cruelty and/or humiliation in its received or active and/or dispensed and passive form. [sadism + masochism]

Saemisch, Edwin T., German ophthalmologist, 1833-1909. SEE S. *section, ulcer*.

Saenger, M., Prague obstetrician, 1853–1903. SEE S. *operation*.

saf·flow·er (saf'low-er). SYN carthamus. [Ar. *safrā*, yellow]

saf·flow·er oil. An oil extracted from the seeds of *Carthamus tinctorius*, containing 74.5% linoleic acid and 6.6% saturated fatty acids; recommended for use in hypercholesteremia, myocardial infarction, and coronary insufficiency.

saf·fron (saf'ron). SYN crocus. [Ar. *zafarān*, fr. *safrā*, yellow]

saf·ra·nin O (saf'ră-nin) [C.I. 50240]. A mixture of dimethyl- and trimethylphenosafranin chloride, a basic red dye that exhibits orange metachromasia; used in histology as a nuclear stain, in microbiology as a counterstain in the Gram method, and to demonstrate enterochromaffin.

saf·ra·no·phil, saf·ra·no·phile (saf'ră-nō-fil, -fīl). Staining readily with safranin; denoting certain cells and tissues.

saf·role (saf'rōl). The methylene ether of allyl pyrocatechol; contained in oil of sassafras, oil of camphor, and various other volatile oils; it is obtained chiefly from oil of camphor by fractional distillation; used as a tonic and carminative; prolonged administration causes fatty degeneration.

sage (sāj). SYN salvia. [L. *salvia*, the sage plant, fr. *salvus*, safe]

sa·git·ta (saj'i-tă). SYN otoliths.

sag·it·tal (saj'i-tăl) [TA]. Resembling an arrow; in the line of an arrow shot from a bow, i.e., in an anteroposterior direction; referring to a sagittal plane or direction. SYN sagittalis [TA]. [L. *sagitta*, an arrow]

sa·git·ta·lis (saj-i-tā'lis) [TA]. SYN sagittal. [L.]

Saint, Charles F.M., African surgeon, *1886. SEE S. *triad*.

Saint Anthony fire (sānt anth-ō-nē). **1.** SYN ergotism. **2.** Any of several inflammations or gangrenous conditions of the skin (e.g., erysipelas). [St. Anthony, Egyptian monk, about 250–350 AD]

Sakaguchi re·ac·tion. See under reaction.

Saksenaea vasiformis. one of the fungal species that cause mucormycosis. This species is notable for the proportion of cases with subcutaneous infection, rather than pulmonary or paranasal sinus disease, more typical manifestations of mucormycosis.

Sakurai. Japanese ophthalmologist. SEE Sakurai-Lisch *nodule*.

sal, pl. **sales** (sal, sal'ēz). SYN salt. [L.]

 s. alem'broth, the product obtained by crystallization from a solution of equal parts of ammonium chloride and mercuric chloride. SYN salt of wisdom. [an alchemist's term of unknown origin]

 s. ammo'niac, SYN *ammonium* chloride.

 s. diuret'icum, SYN *potassium* acetate.

 s. soda, SYN *sodium* carbonate.

 s. vol'atile, SYN aromatic ammonia *spirit*.

Salah, M., 20th century Egyptian surgeon. SEE S. sternal puncture *needle*.

sal·bu·ta·mol (sal-bū'tă-mol). SYN albuterol.

Saldino, Ronald M., American radiologist.

sal·i·cin (sal'i-sin). A glucoside of *o*-hydroxybenzylalcohol, obtained from the bark of several species of *Salix* (willow) and *Populus* (poplar); s. is hydrolyzed to glucose and saligenin (salicyl alcohol); formerly used in rheumatoid arthritis.

sal·i·cyl (sal'i-sil). The acyl radical of salicylic acid.

 s. aldehyde, obtained from *Spirea ulmaria* (meadow sweet), and made synthetically; used as a diuretic and antiseptic, and in perfumery. SYN salicylic aldehyde.

sal·i·cyl·am·ide (sal-i-sil'ă-mīd). The amide of salicylic acid, *o*-hydroxybenzamide; an analgesic, antipyretic and antiarthritic, similar in action to aspirin.

sal·i·cyl·an·i·lide (sal'i-sil-an'i-līd). An antifungal agent especially useful in the treatment of tinea capitis caused by *Microsporum audouinii*.

sa·lic·y·late (să-lis'i-lāt). **1.** A salt or ester of salicylic acid. **2.** To treat foodstuffs with salicylic acid as a preservative. SYN salicylize.

sa·lic·y·lat·ed (să-lis'i-lāt-ĕd). Treated by the addition of salicylic acid as a preservative.

sal·i·cyl·az·o·sul·fa·pyr·i·dine (sal'i-sil-az'ō-sool-fă-pir'i-dēn). SYN sulfasalazine.

sal·i·cyl·ic ac·id (sal-i-sil'ik). A component of aspirin (acetylsalicylic acid), derived from salicin and made synthetically; used externally as a keratolytic agent, antiseptic, and fungicide.

sal·i·cyl·ic al·de·hyde (sal-i-sil'ik). SYN *salicyl* aldehyde.

sal·i·cyl·ism (sal'i-sil-izm). Poisoning by salicylic acid or any of its compounds.

sal·i·cyl·ize (sal'i-sil-īz). SYN salicylate (2).

sal·i·cyl·sal·i·cyl·ic ac·id (sal'i-sil-sal-i-sil'ik). SYN salsalate.

sal·i·cyl·sul·fon·ic ac·id (sal'i-sil-sŭl-fon'ik). SYN sulfosalicylic acid.

sal·i·cyl·u·ric ac·id (sal'i-sil-ūr'ik). The conjugation product of glycine with salicylic acid; excreted in urine after the administration of salicylic acid or some of its compounds.

sa·lient (sā'lē-ent, sāl'yent). **1.** SYN projection. **2.** In radiology, an obsolete term for projection. [L. *salio,* to leap or spring up]

sal·i·fi·a·ble (sal-i-fī'ă-bl). Capable of being made into salts; said of a base that combines with acids to make salts.

sal·i·fy (sal'i-fī). To convert into a salt.

sal·i·gen·in, sal·i·gen·ol (sal-i-jen'in, sal'i-jen-ol). Obtained by the hydrolysis of salicin; a local anesthetic.

sa·lim·e·ter (să-lim'ĕ-ter). A hydrometer used to determine the specific gravity, or the concentration, of a saline solution.

sa·line (sā'lēn, -līn). **1.** Relating to, of the nature of, or containing salt; salty. **2.** A salt solution, usually sodium chloride. [L. *salinus*, salty, fr. *sal*, salt]

 physiologic s., an isotonic aqueous solution of salts, containing 0.9% sodium chloride.

sa·li·nom·e·ter (sal-i-nom'ĕ-ter). A hydrometer so calibrated as to give a direct reading of the percentage of a particular salt present in solution.

sa·li·va (să-lī'vă). A clear, tasteless, odorless, slightly acid (pH

6.8) viscid fluid, consisting of the secretion from the parotid, sublingual, and submandibular salivary glands and the mucous glands of the oral cavity; its function is to keep the mucous membrane of the mouth moist, to lubricate the food during mastication, and, in a measure, to convert starch into maltose, the latter action being effected by a diastatic enzyme, ptyalin. SYN spittle. [L. akin to G. *sialon*]

chorda s., the secretion of the submaxillary gland obtained by stimulation of the chorda tympani nerve.

ganglionic s., submaxillary s. obtained by direct irritation of the gland.

resting s., the s. found in the mouth in the intervals of food taking and mastication.

sympathetic s., submaxillary s. obtained by stimulation of the sympathetic fibers innervating the gland.

sal·i·vant (sal′i-vant). **1.** Causing a flow of saliva. **2.** An agent that increases the flow of saliva. SYN salivator.

sal·i·vary (sal′i-vār-ē). Relating to saliva. SYN sialic, sialine. [L. *salivarius*]

sal·i·vate (sal′i-vāt). To cause an excessive flow of saliva.

sal·i·va·tion (sal′i-vā′shŭn). SYN sialorrhea.

sal·i·va·tor (sal′i-vā-ter). SYN salivant (2).

sa·li·vo·li·thi·a·sis (sa-lī′vō-li-thī′ă-sis). SYN sialolithiasis.

Salk, Jonas, U.S. immunologist, 1914–1995. SEE S. *vaccine*.

Sal·mo·nel·la (sal′mō-nel′ă). A genus of aerobic to facultatively anaerobic bacteria (family Enterobacteriaceae) containing Gram-negative rods that are either motile or nonmotile; motile cells are peritrichous. These organisms do not liquefy gelatin or produce indole and vary in their production of hydrogen sulfide; they utilize citrate as a sole source of carbon; their metabolism is fermentative, producing acid and usually gas from glucose, but they do not attack lactose; most are aerogenic, but *S. typhi* never produces gas; they are pathogenic for humans and other animals. The type species is *S. choleraesuis.* [Daniel E. *Salmon,* U.S. pathologist, 1850–1914]

S. enterica subsp. *enterit′idis,* a widely distributed bacterial species that occurs in humans and in domestic and wild animals, especially rodents; it causes human gastroenteritis.

S. enterica subsp. *paratyphi A,* a bacterial species that is an important etiologic agent of enteric fever in developing countries.

S. enterica subsp. *paratyphi B,* (formerly known as *S. schottmülleri*), consists of two distinct types of strains, those that produce enteric fever, found primarily in humans, and those producing gastroenteritis in humans, also found in animal species. This species includes 56 strains distinguishable by phage typing and/or biotyping, features of epidemiologic value.

S. enterica subsp. *typhi,* SYN *S. typhi.*

S. enterica subsp. *typhimu′rium,* a bacterial species causing food poisoning in humans; it is a natural pathogen of all warm-blooded animals and is also found in snakes and pet turtles; worldwide, it is the most frequent cause of gastroenteritis due to *S. enterica* species.

S. enterica subsp. *choleraesuis,* a bacterial species that occurs in pigs, where it is an important secondary invader in the virus disease hog cholera, but does not occur as a natural pathogen in other animals; occasionally causes acute gastroenteritis and enteric fever in humans; it is the type species of the genus *S.*

S. ty′phi, the bacterial species that causes typhoid fever in humans; transmitted through ingestion of contaminated water or food. SYN Eberth bacillus, *S. enterica* subsp. *typhi,* typhoid bacillus.

S. typho′sa, former name for *S. typhi.*

sal·mo·nel·lo·sis (sal′mō-nel-ō′sis). Infection with bacteria of the genus *Salmonella.* Patients with sickle cell anemia and compromised immune systems are particularly susceptible. [*Salmonella* + G. *-osis,* condition]

sal·ol (sal′ol). SYN *phenyl* salicylate.

△**salping-.** SEE salpingo-.

sal·pin·gec·to·my (sal-pin-jek′tō-mē). Removal of the fallopian tube. SYN tubectomy. [salping- + G. *ektomē,* excision]

abdominal s., removal of one or both fallopian tubes through an abdominal incision.

sal·pin·ges (sal-pin′jēz). Plural of salpinx.

sal·pin·gi·an (sal-pin′jē-ăn). Relating to the fallopian tube or to the auditory tube.

sal·pin·gi·o·ma (sal-pin-jē-ō′mă). Any tumor arising in the tissues of a uterine tube. [salping- + G. *-oma,* tumor]

sal·pin·git·ic (sal-pin-jit′ik). Relating to salpingitis.

sal·pin·gi·tis (sal-pin-jī′tis). Inflammation of the uterine or the eustachian tube. [salping- + G. *-itis,* inflammation]

chronic interstitial s., s. in which fibrosis or mononuclear cell infiltration involves all layers of the uterine or eustachian tube.

foreign body s., s. in which giant cells form in the tissue, as a result of introduction of foreign material into the uterine tube.

gonorrheal s., inflammation of the uterine tube following acute gonorrheal infection.

s. isth′mica nodo′sa, a condition of the fallopian tube characterized by nodular thickening of the tunica muscularis of the isthmic portion of the tube enclosing glandlike or cystic duplications of the lumen. SYN adenosalpingitis.

pyogenic s., a form of acute s. usually occurring with puerperal infection.

△**salpingo-, salping-.** A tube (usually the uterine or auditory tube). SEE ALSO tubo-. [G. *salpinx,* trumpet (tube)]

sal·pin·go·cele (sal-ping′gō-sēl). Hernia of a fallopian tube. [salpingo- + G. *kēlē,* hernia]

sal·pin·go·cy·e·sis (sal-ping′gō-sī-ē′sis). SYN tubal *pregnancy.* [salpingo- + G. *kyēsis,* pregnancy]

sal·pin·gog·ra·phy (sal-ping-gog′ră-fē). Radiography of the fallopian tubes after the injection of radiopaque contrast medium. [salpingo- + G. *graphō,* to write]

sal·pin·gol·y·sis (sal-ping-gol′i-sis). Freeing the fallopian tube from adhesions. [salpingo- + G. *lysis,* loosening]

sal·pin·go·ne·os·to·my (sal-ping′ō-nē-os′tō-mē). Surgical reopening of a uterine tube clubbed because of fimbrial adhesions. [salpingo- + neostomy]

△**salpingo-oophor-, salpingo-oophoro-.** The uterine tube and ovary. [salpingo- + Mod. L. *oophoron,* ovary, fr. G. *ōophoros,* egg-bearing]

sal·pin·go-o·o·pho·rec·to·my (sal-ping′gō-ō-of-ō-rek′tō-mē). Removal of the ovary and its fallopian tube. SYN salpingo-ovariectomy, tubo-ovariectomy.

sal·pin·go-o·o·pho·ri·tis (sal-ping′gō-ō-of-ō-rī′tis). Inflammation of both fallopian tube and ovary. SYN tubo-ovaritis.

sal·pin·go-o·oph·ro·cele (sal-ping′gō-ō-of′ō-rō-sēl). Hernia of both ovary and fallopian tube.

sal·pin·go-o·var·i·ec·to·my (sal-ping′gō-ō-var-ē-ek′tō-mē). SYN salpingo-oophorectomy.

sal·pin·go·per·i·to·ni·tis (sal-ping′gō-per-i-tō-nī′tis). Inflammation of the fallopian tube, perisalpinx, and peritoneum. [salpingo- + peritonitis]

sal·pin·go·pexy (sal-ping′gō-pek-sē). Operative fixation of an oviduct. [salpingo- + G. *pēxis,* fixation]

sal·pin·go·pha·ryn·ge·al (sal-ping′gō-fă-rin′jē-ăl). Relating to the auditory tube and pharynx.

sal·pin·go·pha·ryn·ge·us. SEE salpingopharyngeus (*muscle*).

sal·pin·go·plas·ty (sal-ping′gō-plas-tē). Plastic surgery of the fallopian tubes. SYN tuboplasty. [salpingo- + G. *plastos,* formed]

sal·pin·gor·rha·gia (sal-ping-gō-rā′jē-ă). Hemorrhage from a fallopian tube. [salpingo- + G. *rhēgnymi,* to burst forth]

sal·pin·gor·rha·phy (sal-ping-gōr′ă-fē). Suture of the fallopian tube. [salpingo- + G. *rhaphē,* stitching]

sal·pin·gos·co·py (sal-ping-gos′kō-pē). Visualization of the intraluminal portion of the fallopian tubes, usually by x-ray or by means of an endoscope. [salpingo- + G. *skopeō,* to view]

sal·pin·gos·to·my (sal-ping-gos′tō-mē). Establishment of an artificial opening in a fallopian tube primarily as surgical treatment for an ectopic pregnancy. [salpingo- + G. *stoma,* mouth]

sa

sal·pin·got·o·my (sal-ping-got′ō-mē). Incision into a fallopian tube. [salpingo- + G. *tomē,* incision]

    abdominal s., incision into the fallopian tube through an opening in the abdominal wall.

sal·pinx, pl. **sal·pin·ges** (sal′pingks, sal-pin′jēz). ⋆official alternate term for uterine *tube.* [G. a trumpet (tube)]

    s. uteri′na, SYN uterine *tube.*

sal·sa·late (sal′să-lāt). A combination of 2 molecules of salicylic acid in ester linkage. The compound is hydrolyzed during and after absorption to salicylic acid which, like other salicylates, exerts analgesic and anti-inflammatory effects. SYN salicylsalicylic acid.

salt. **1.** A compound formed by the interaction of an acid and a base, the ionizable hydrogen atoms of the acid being replaced by the positive ion of the base. **2.** Sodium chloride, the prototypical s. **3.** A saline cathartic, especially magnesium sulfate, sodium sulfate, or Rochelle s.; often denoted by the plural, salts. SYN sal. [L. *sal*]

    acid s., a s. in which not all of the ionizable hydrogen of the acid is replaced by the electropositive element; e.g., $NaHSO_4$, KH_2PO_4. SYN protosalt.

    artificial Carlsbad s., a mixture of potassium sulfate, sodium chloride, sodium bicarbonate, and dried sodium sulfate; a laxative.

    artificial Kissingen s., a mixture of potassium chloride, sodium chloride, anhydrous magnesium sulfate, and sodium bicarbonate; an antacid and laxative.

    artificial Vichy s., a mixture of sodium bicarbonate, anhydrous magnesium sulfate, potassium carbonate, and sodium chloride; an antacid.

    basic s., a s. in which there are one or more hydroxyl ions not replaced by the electronegative element of an acid; e.g., Fe(OH)$_2$Cl.

    bile s.'s, the s. forms of bile acids; e.g., taurocholate, glycocholate.

    bone s., SEE bone-salt.

    common s., SYN *sodium* chloride.

    diazonium s.'s, s.'s of a theoretical base, R–$\overset{+}{N}$=N or R–N=NOH, useful in histochemistry to demonstrate tissue phenols and aryl amines or with enzymatically released naphthols and naphthylamines to form the chromophore azo group –N=N–; diazonium s.'s contain only one R–N=N group, tetrazonium s.'s contain two, and hexazonium s.'s contain three; examples include fast garnet GBC base and naphthol AS.

    double s., a s. in which two different positive ions are bonded to the same negative ion, or vice versa; e.g., $NaKSO_4$.

    effervescent s.'s, preparations made by adding sodium bicarbonate and tartaric and citric acids to the active s.; when thrown into water the acids break up the sodium bicarbonate, setting free the carbonic acid gas.

    Epsom s.'s, SYN *magnesium* sulfate.

    Glauber s., SYN *sodium* sulfate.

    hexazonium s.'s, diazonium s.'s that contain three azo groups.

    Reinecke s., an ammonium salt prepared by fusing ammonium thiocyanate with ammonium dichromate; dark red crystals; used in the detection and analysis of primary and secondary amines, including amino acids; also used as a reagent for mercury.

    Rivière s., SYN *potassium* citrate.

    Rochelle s., SYN *potassium* sodium tartrate.

    Seignette s., SYN *potassium* sodium tartrate.

    smelling s.'s, SYN aromatic ammonia *spirit.*

    s. substitute, A low-sodium food additive that tastes like salt, such as potassium chloride; useful as a dietary alternative to salt.

    table s., SYN *sodium* chloride.

    tetrazonium s.'s, diazonium s.'s that contain two azo groups.

    s. of wisdom, SYN *sal* alembroth.

sal·ta·tion (sal-tā′shŭn). A dancing or leaping, as in a disease (e.g., chorea) or physiologic function (e.g., saltatory conduction). [L. *saltatio,* fr. *salto,* pp. -*atus,* to dance, fr. *salio,* to leap]

sal·ta·to·ry (sal′tă-tōr-ē). Pertaining to, or characterized by, saltation.

Salter, Sir Samuel J.A., English dentist, 1825–1897. SEE S. incremental *lines,* under *line.*

Salter, Robert B., 20th century Canadian orthopedist. SEE S.-Harris *classification* of epiphysial plate injuries.

salt·ing in (salt′ing). The increase in solubility (as observed for some proteins) by dilute salt solutions (as compared to pure water).

salt·ing out. The precipitation of a protein from its solution by saturation or partial saturation with such neutral salts as sodium chloride, magnesium sulfate, or ammonium sulfate.

salt·pe·ter (salt′pē-ter). SYN *potassium* nitrate.

    Chilean s., SYN *sodium* nitrate.

sa·lu·bri·ous (să-loo′brē-ŭs). Healthful, usually in reference to climate. [L. *salubris,* healthy, fr. *salus,* health]

sal·u·re·sis (sal-ū-rē′sis). Excretion of sodium in the urine. [L. *sal,* salt, + G. *ourēsis,* uresis (urination)]

sal·u·ret·ic (sal-ū-ret′ik). Facilitating the renal excretion of sodium.

Salus, Robert, Bohemian ophthalmologist, *1877. SEE Koerber-Salus-Elschnig *syndrome.*

sal·u·ta·ri·um (sal-ū-tār′ē-ŭm). SYN sanitarium. [L. *salutaris,* healthful, fr. *salus* (*salut*-), health]

sal·u·tary (sal′ū-tār-ē). Healthful; wholesome. [L. *salutaris*]

Sal·var·san (sal′var-san). Historic proprietary name for arsphenamine. [L. *salvare,* to preserve, + *sanitas,* health]

salve (sav). SYN ointment. [A.S. *sealf*]

sal·via (sal′vē-ă). The dried leaves of *Salvia officinalis* (family Labiatae), garden or meadow sage; it inhibits secretory activity, especially of the sweat glands, and was also used in bronchitis and inflammation of the throat. SYN sage. [L.]

Salzmann, Maximilian, German ophthalmologist, 1862–1954. SEE S. nodular corneal *degeneration.*

SAM Abbreviation for *S*-adenosyl-L-methionine.

sam·an·da·rine (sa-măn′da-rēn). A toxic alkaloid from salamanders; causes hemolysis.

sa·mar·i·um (Sm) (să-mār′ē-ŭm). A metallic element of the lanthanide group, atomic no. 62, atomic wt. 150.36. [bands indicating its presence first found in the spectrum of *samarskite,* a mineral named after Col. von Samarski, 19th century Russian mine official]

sam·bu·cus (sam-bū′kŭs). The dried flowers of *Sambucus canadensis* or *S. nigra* (family Caprifoliaceae), the common elder or black elder; slightly laxative. SYN elder, elder flowers. [L. an elder-tree]

sAMP Abbreviation for adenylosuccinic acid.

sam·ple (sam′pel). **1.** A specimen of a whole entity small enough to involve no threat or damage to the whole; an aliquot. **2.** A selected subset of a population; a sample may be random or nonrandom (haphazard), representative or nonrepresentative. [M.E. *ensample,* fr. L. *exemplum,* example]

    cluster s., each sampling unit is a group of individuals.

    end-tidal s., a s. of the last gas expired in a normal expiration, ideally consisting only of alveolar gas.

    Haldane-Priestley s., an approximation of alveolar gas obtained from the end of a sudden maximal expiration into a Haldane tube.

    probability s., each individual in the s. has a known, generally equal, chance of being selected.

    proficiency s.'s, s.'s sent to a laboratory as unknowns to allow an external assessment of laboratory performance, a frequent practice as part of proficiency testing programs to ensure the laboratory is generating correct results. SEE ALSO proficiency *testing.*

    Rahn-Otis s., an approximation of alveolar gas continuously provided by a simple device that admits just the latter part of each expiration.

    random s., a selection on the basis of chance of individuals or items in a population for research; selection is made in such a way that all members presumably have the same chance of being selected.

    stratified s., a subset of a total population, defined by some objective criterion such as age or occupation, is sampled.

sam·pling. The policy of inferring the behavior of a whole batch by studying a fraction of it. [MF essample, fr. L. exemplum, taking out]

biological s., denotes s. that can be taken without jeopardy to the whole organism (e.g., for hematological or biochemical study). Because of the complexity of biological samples it is usually supposed that the source of the sample is thoroughly mixed and hence representative; this assumption is often not true, e.g., in genetic studies in mosaic patients.

chemical s., a sample that is obtained by whatever means is convenient and then purified of irrelevant elements before analysis; the assumption of thorough mixing is not necessary.

continuous interleaved s., a strategy in speech processing for cochlear implants in which brief pulses are presented to each electrode in a nonoverlapping sequence.

haphazard s., the assembly of data in an unprescribed and undefined fashion that allows no sound scientific inferences other than establishing the existence of types. (Finding even one unicorn in such a set would establish that unicorns can exist, but no inference about their prevalence could be made from it.) Cf. random *sample.*

random s., a selection of elements from a population such that each possible outcome is independent of other possible outcomes and the probability of each member of the population being chosen is equal.

snowball s., a method whereby the names of prospective interview subjects for a statistical study are obtained from subjects already interviewed for the study.

Sanarelli, Giuseppe, Italian bacteriologist, 1865–1940. SEE S. *phenomenon;* S.-Shwartzman *phenomenon.*

san·a·tive (san´ă-tiv). Having a tendency to heal. [L. *sano,* to cure, heal]

san·a·to·ri·um (san´ă-tōr´ē-ŭm). An institution for the treatment of chronic disorders and a place for recuperation under medical supervision. Cf. sanitarium. [Mod. L. neuter of *sanatorius,* curative, fr. *sano,* to cure, heal]

san·a·to·ry (san´ă-tōr-ē). Health-giving; conducive to health. [Mod. L. *sanatorius*]

Sanchez Salorio, Manuel, Spanish ophthalmologist, *1930. SEE Sanchez Salorio *syndrome.*

sand. The fine granular particles of quartz and other crystalline rocks, or a gritty material resembling s. [A.S.]

brain s., SYN *corpora* arenacea, under *corpus.*

hydatid s., the scoleces, daughter cysts, hooks, and calcareous corpuscles of *Echinococcus* tapeworms in the fluid within a primary or daughter hydatid cyst.

intestinal s., minute calculi or gritty material occurring in feces, composed of soaps, bile pigment, cholesterol, magnesium salts, succinic acid, etc.

urinary s., multiple small calculous particles passed in the urine of patients with nephrolithiasis; each particle is usually too small to cause significant symptoms or to be identified as a true calculus.

san·dal·wood oil (san´dăl-wood). SYN santal oil.

sand·fly (sand´flī). A small, biting, dipterous midge of the genus *Phlebotomus* or *Lutzomyia;* a vector of leishmaniasis.

Sandhoff, K., contemporary German biochemist. SEE S. *disease.*

Sandison, J. Calvin, U.S. surgeon, *1899. SEE S.-Clark *chamber.*

Sandström, I., Swedish anatomist, 1852–1889. SEE S. *bodies,* under *body.*

sand·worm (sand´werm). Any of the various dog and cat hookworms whose larvae cause cutaneous larva migrans.

sane (sān). Denoting sanity. [L. *sanus*]

Sanfilippo, Sylvester J., 20th century U.S. pediatrician. SEE S. *syndrome.*

Sanger, Frederick, English biochemist and twice Nobel laureate, *1918. SEE S. *reagent, method.*

⟁**sangui-, sanguin-, sanguino-.** Blood, bloody. [G. *sanguis*]

san·gui·fa·ci·ent (sang-gwi-fā´shent). SYN hemopoietic. [sangui- + L. *facio,* to make]

san·guif·er·ous (sang-gwif´er-ŭs). Conveying blood. SYN circulatory (2). [sangui- + L. *fero,* to carry]

san·gui·fi·ca·tion (sang´gwi-fi-kā´shŭn). SYN hemopoiesis. [sangui- + L. *facio,* to make]

san·guin·a·rine (sang-gwi-nă´rēn). An alkaloid obtained from the bloodroot plant, *Sanguinaria canadensis,* used to treat and remove dental plaque.

san·guine (sang´gwin). **1.** SYN plethoric. **2.** Formerly, denoting a temperament characterized by a light, fair complexion, full pulse, good digestion, optimistic outlook, and a quick but not lasting temper. SYN sanguineous (3). [L. *sanguineus*]

san·guin·e·ous (sang-gwin´ē-ŭs). **1.** Relating to blood; bloody. **2.** SYN plethoric. **3.** SYN sanguine (2). [L. *sanguineus*]

san·guin·o·lent (sang-gwin´ō-lent). Bloody; tinged with blood. [L. *sanguinolentus*]

san·gui·no·pu·ru·lent (sang´gwi-nō-poo´roo-lent). Denoting exudate or matter containing blood and pus. [sanguino- + L. *purulentus,* festering (suppurative), fr. *pus,* pus]

San·gui·su·ga (sang-gwi-soo´gă). Former name for *Hirudo.* [L. a leech, fr. *sanguis,* blood, + *sugo,* pp. *suctus,* to suck]

san·guiv·or·ous (sang-gwiv´er-ŭs). Bloodsucking, as applied to certain bats, leeches, insects, etc. [sangui- + L. *voro,* to devour]

sa·ni·es (sā´nē-ēz). A thin, blood-stained, purulent discharge. [L.]

sa·ni·o·pu·ru·lent (sā´nē-ō-poo´roo-lent). Characterized by bloody pus. [L. *sanies,* thin, bloody matter, + *purulentus,* festering (suppurative), fr. *pus,* pus]

sa·ni·o·se·rous (sā´nē-ō-sēr´ŭs). Characterized by blood-tinged serum.

sa·ni·ous (sā´nē-ŭs). Relating to sanies; ichorous and blood-stained.

san·i·tar·i·an (san-i-tār´ē-ăn). One who is skilled in sanitation and public health. [L. *sanitas,* health, fr. *sanus,* sound]

san·i·tar·i·um (san-i-tār´ē-ŭm). A health resort. Cf. sanatorium. SYN salutarium. [L. *sanitas,* health]

san·i·tary (san´i-tār-ē). Healthful; conducive to health; usually in reference to a clean environment. [L. *sanitas,* health]

san·i·ta·tion (san-i-tā´shŭn). Use of measures designed to promote health and prevent disease; development and establishment of conditions in the environment favorable to health. [L. *sanitas,* health]

san·i·ti·za·tion (san´i-ti-zā´shŭn). The process of making something sanitary.

san·i·ty (san´i-tē). Soundness of mind, emotions, and behavior; of a sound degree of mental health. [L. *sanitas,* health]

San Jose, Hermenia, 20th century Chilean pathologist. SEE Maldonado-San Jose *stain.*

Sansom, Arthur E., English physician, 1839–1907. SEE S. *sign.*

Sanson, Louis J., French physician, 1790–1841. SEE S. *images,* under *image;* Purkinje-S. *images,* under *image.*

san·tal oil (san´tăl). A volatile oil distilled from the wood of *Santalum album* (family Santalaceae), a tree of India; formerly used in subacute bronchitis and in gonorrhea. SYN sandalwood oil.

san·to·nin (san´tō-nin). The inner anhydride or lactone of santoninic acid, obtained from santonica, the unexpanded flower heads of *Artemisia cina* and other species of *Artemisia* (family Compositae); has been used to effect expulsion of roundworms (*Ascaris lumbricoides*), and in the treatment of urinary incontinence. [G. *santonikon,* wormwood]

Santorini, Giandomenico (Giovanni Domenico), Italian anatomist, 1681–1737. SEE S. *canal, cartilage,* major *caruncle,* minor *caruncle, concha, duct, fissures,* under *fissure, incisure, incisures,* under *incisure, labyrinth, muscle, tubercle, vein; incisura* santorini.

sap. The juice or tissue fluid of a living organism.

cell s., contents of vacuoles.

nuclear s., SYN karyolymph.

sa·phe·na (să-fē´nă). SEE vein. [Med. L. attributed by some as derived fr. Ar. *safin,* standing; by others, fr. G. *saphēnēs,* manifest, clearly visible]

saph·e·nec·to·my (saf-ĕ-nek'tō-mē). Excision of a saphenous vein. [saphena + G. *ektomē*, excision]

sa·phe·nous (să-fē'nŭs). Relating to or associated with a saphenous vein; denoting a number of structures in the leg. [see saphena]

⌂**sapo-, sapon-.** Soap. [L. *sapo*]

sap·o·gen·in (să-poj'ĕ-nin). The aglycon of a saponin; one of a family of steroids of the spirostan type (a 16,22:22,26-diepoxycholestane).

sap·o·na·ceous (sap-ō-nā'shŭs). Soapy; relating to or resembling soap.

sap·o·na·tus (sap-ŏ-nā'tŭs). Mixed with soap. [L.]

sa·pon·i·fi·ca·tion (să-pon'i-fi-kā'shŭn). Conversion into soap, denoting the hydrolytic action of an alkali on fat, especially on triacylglycerols; in histochemistry, s. is used to demethylate or reverse blockage of carboxylic acid groups, thus permitting basophilia to occur. [sapo- (sapon-) + L. *facio*, to make]

sa·pon·i·fy (să-pon'i-fī). To perform or undergo saponification.

sap·o·nins (sap'ō-ninz). Glycosides of plant origin characterized by properties of foaming in water and of lysing cells (as in hemolysis of erythrocytes when s. are injected into the bloodstream); powerful surfactants; many have antibiotic activities.

Sappey, Marie P.C., French anatomist, 1810–1896. SEE S. *fibers,* under *fiber, plexus, veins,* under *vein.*

sap·phism (saf'izm). SYN lesbianism. [*Sapphō,* homosexual Greek poet, queen of the island of Lesbos]

⌂**sapr-.** SEE sapro-.

sa·pre·mia (să-prē'mē-ă). Obsolete term for septicemia. [sapr- + G. *haima,* blood]

⌂**sapro-, sapr-.** Rotten, putrid, decayed. [G. *sapros*]

sap·robe (sap'rōb). An organism that lives upon dead organic material. This term is preferable to saprophyte, since bacteria and fungi are no longer regarded as plants. [sapro- + G. *bios,* life]

sa·pro·bic (sap-rō'bik). Pertaining to a saprobe.

sap·ro·don·tia (sap-rō-don'shē-ă). SYN dental *caries.* [sapro- + G. *odous,* tooth]

sap·ro·gen (sap'rō-jen). An organism living on dead organic matter and causing the decay thereof. [sapro- + G. *-gen,* producing]

sap·ro·gen·ic, sa·prog·e·nous (sap-rō-jen'ik, să-proj'ĕ-nŭs). Causing or resulting from decay.

sa·proph·i·lous (să-prof'i-lŭs). Thriving on decaying organic matter. [sapro- + G. *philos,* fond]

sap·ro·phyte (sap'rō-fīt). An organism that grows on dead organic matter, plant or animal. SEE saprobe. SYN necroparasite. [sapro- + G. *phyton,* plant]

facultative s., an organism, usually parasitic, that occasionally may live and grow as a s.

sap·ro·phyt·ic (sap-rō-fit'ik). Relating to a saprophyte.

sap·ro·zo·ic (sap-rō-zō'ik). Living in decaying organic matter; especially denoting certain protozoa. [sapro- + G. *zōikos,* relating to animals]

sap·ro·zo·o·no·sis (sap'rō-zō-ō-nō'sis). A zoonosis, the agent of which requires both a vertebrate host and a nonanimal (food, soil, plant) reservoir or developmental site for completion of its life cycle. Combination terms may be used, such as saprometazoonoses for fluke infections, when metacercariae encyst on plants, or saprocyclozoonoses for tick infestations, whose agents complete part of their life cycles in soil. [sapro- + G. *zōon,* animal, + *nosos,* disease]

SAR Abbreviation for scaffold-associated *regions,* under *region.*

Sar Abbreviation for sarcosine.

sar·al·a·sin ac·e·tate (sar-al'ă-sin). An angiotensin II antagonist used in the treatment of essential hypertension.

α-sar·cin (sar'sin). A fungal toxin that acts on the large subunit of rRNA and inactivates the ribosome.

Sar·ci·na (sar'si-nă). A genus of nonmotile, strictly anaerobic bacteria (family Peptococcaceae) containing Gram-positive cocci, 1.8–3.0 μm in diameter, which divide in three perpendicular planes, producing regular packets of eight or more cells. The metabolism of these chemoorganotrophic organisms is fermentative. Saprophytic and facultatively parasitic species occur. The type species is *S. ventriculi.* [L. *sarcina,* a pack, bundle, fr. *sarcio,* to mend, patch]

S. ventric'uli, a bacterial species found in soil, mud, the contents of a diseased human stomach, rabbit and guinea pig stomach contents, and on the surfaces of cereal seeds; it is the type species of the genus *S.*

sar·cine (sar'sēn). Obsolete term for hypoxanthine.

⌂**sarco-.** Combining form denoting muscular substance or a resemblance to flesh. [G. *sarx (sark-),* flesh]

sar·co·blast (sar'kō-blast). SYN myoblast. [sarco- + G. *blastos,* germ]

Sar·co·cys·tis (sar-kō-sis'tis). A genus of protozoan parasites, related to the sporozoan genera *Eimeria, Isospora,* and *Toxoplasma,* and placed in a distinct family, Sarcocystidae, but with the above genera in the same suborder, Eimeriina, within the subclass Coccidia, class Sporozoea, and phylum Apicomplexa. Tissue stages of *S.* are usually seen as thick-walled cylindrical or (often extremely large (1 cm or more), fusiform cysts (Miescher tubes) in reptile, bird, or mammal striated muscles. Cysts are smooth in the house mouse form or with radial spines (cytophaneres) in sheep or rabbit; contents may be compartmentalized by septa. Variably shaped spores (Rainey corpuscles) probably are peripheral rounded cells (sporoblasts, cytomeres) that divide to form mature "spores" (bradyzoites), motile bodies when released from the cyst; sexual stages have been described in tissue cultures. These parasites are abundant but rarely of pathogenic significance. Humans who have ingested meat containing the mature sarcocysts serve as the definitive hosts; fever, severe diarrhea, abdominal pain, and weight loss have been reported in a small number of immunocompromised hosts. When humans accidentally ingest oocysts from other animal stool sources, the sarcocysts that develop in human muscle appear to cause no inflammatory response. [sarco- + G. *kystis,* bladder]

S. bovih'ominis, SYN *S. hominis.*

S. fusifor'mis, a species found in the striated and heart muscle of cattle and water buffalo.

S. hom'inis, a species now recognized as a two-host infection, with beef serving as the intermediate host source of infective tissue cysts to humans, who serve as the final host. Gamogony and sporogony occur in mucosal cells of the human small intestine; cattle become infected from human feces contaminated with *S. hominis* sporocysts. SYN *S. bovih'ominis.*

S. lindeman'ni, a protozoan species described on rare occasions from the striated and heart muscles of humans, probably as an infection due to various species, possibly from domestic dogs or other final hosts from which infective oocysts or sporocysts were passed to humans via water or direct exposure; in these instances humans serve as an intermediate rather than a final host.

S. miescheria'na, a common species of worldwide distribution that is found in the striated and heart muscle of pigs; it is the type species of the genus *S.*

S. suihom'inis, a form of *S.* in which humans serve as the final host, with the pig serving as intermediate host, the source of infected tissues to humans. The life cycle and moderate disease induced follow the pattern of *S. hominis,* though the disease appears to be somewhat more pathogenic. Human infection is widespread, having been reported in Europe, the Mediterranean, West Africa, Indonesia, and South America.

S. tenel'la, an extremely common species of worldwide distribution that is found in the striated and heart muscle of sheep and goats.

sar·co·cys·to·sis (sar'kō-sis-tō'sis). Infection with protozoan parasites of the genus *Sarcocystis.*

sar·code (sar'kōd). A term of historical interest (1835), applied to the protoplasm of protozoa before the term protoplasm was coined. [sarco- + G. *eidos,* resemblance]

Sar·co·di·na (sar'kō-dī'nă, -dē'nă). The amebae; a subphylum of protozoa in the phylum Sarcomastigophora, possessing pseudopodia or locomotive protoplasmic flow for movement. Includes forms that possess flagella during development and forms with an internal or external test or skeleton and others lacking such a structure; asexual reproduction occurs by fission, and sexual reproduction, if present, by flagellate or ameboid gametes; most species are free-living. [Mod. L. fr. G. *sarx*, flesh]

sar·cog·lia (sar-kog′lē-ă). The accumulation of neurolemma cells at the motor endplate. [sarco- + G. *glia*, glue]

sar·coid (sar′koyd). SYN sarcoidosis. [sarco- + G. *eidos*, resemblance]

Boeck s., SYN sarcoidosis.

Spiegler-Fendt s., SYN benign *lymphocytoma* cutis.

sar·coid·o·sis (sar-koy-dō′sis). A systemic granulomatous disease of unknown cause, especially involving the lungs with resulting interstitial fibrosis, but also involving lymph nodes, skin, liver, spleen, eyes, phalangeal bones, and parotid glands; granulomas are composed of epithelioid and multinucleated giant cells with little or no necrosis. SYN Besnier-Boeck-Schaumann disease, Besnier-Boeck-Schaumann syndrome, Boeck disease, Boeck sarcoid, sarcoid, Schaumann syndrome. [sarcoid + G. *-osis*, condition]

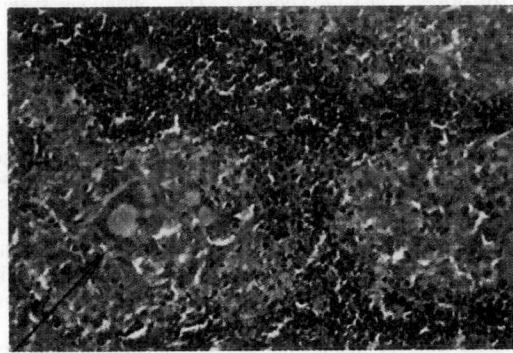

sarcoidosis: microscopic section of lymph node showing epithelioid cell clusters and a solitary giant cell (arrow)

hypercalcemic s., s. with hypercalcemia of unknown cause, not necessarily associated with detectable bone involvement by s.

sar·co·lem·ma (sar′kō-lem′ă). The plasma membrane of a muscle fiber; formerly, the delicate connective tissue of the endomysium was included under this term by some. SYN myolemma. [sarco- + G. *lemma*, husk]

sar·co·lem·mal, sar·co·lem·mic, sar·co·lem·mous (sar′kō-lem′ăl, -lem′ik, -lem′ŭs). Relating to the sarcolemma.

sar·col·o·gy (sar-kol′ō-jē). **1.** SYN myology. **2.** The anatomy of the soft parts, as distinguished from osteology. [sarco- + G. *logos*, study]

sar·co·ly·sine (sar-kō-lī′sēn). SYN merphalan.

sar·co·ma (sar-kō′mă). A connective tissue neoplasm, usually highly malignant, formed by proliferation of mesodermal cells. [G. *sarkōma*, a fleshy excrescence, fr. *sarx*, flesh, + *-oma*, tumor]

alveolar soft part s., a malignant tumor formed of a reticular stroma of connective tissue enclosing aggregates of large round or polygonal cells; occurs in subcutaneous and fibromuscular tissues.

ameloblastic s., SYN ameloblastic *fibrosarcoma*.

angiolithic s., obsolete term for psammomatous *meningioma*.

avian s., SYN Rous s.

botryoid s., a polypoid form of embryonal rhabdomyosarcoma that occurs in children, most frequently in the urogenital tract, characterized by the formation of grossly apparent grapelike clusters of neoplastic tissue that consist of rhabdomyoblasts and spindle and stellate cells in a myxomatous stroma; neoplasms of this type grow relatively rapidly and are highly malignant.

endometrial stromal s., a term sometimes used for a relatively rare s. believed to be a form of endometriosis in which the lesions form multiple foci in the myometrium and in vascular spaces in other sites, and which consist of histologic and cytologic elements that resemble those of the endometrial stroma.

Ewing s., SYN Ewing *tumor*.

fascicular s., SYN spindle cell s.

giant cell s., a malignant giant cell tumor of bone.

giant cell monstrocellular s. of Zülch, SYN giant cell *glioblastoma multiforme*.

granulocytic s., a malignant tumor of immature myeloid cells, frequently subperiosteal, associated with or preceding granulocytic leukemia. SEE ALSO chloroma. SYN myeloid s.

immunoblastic s., obsolete term for immunoblastic *lymphoma*.

Jensen s., a mouse tumor transmissible by inoculation.

juxtacortical osteogenic s., a form of osteogenic s. of relatively low malignancy, probably arising from the periosteum and initially involving cortical bone and adjacent connective tissue, which occurs in middle-aged as well as young adults and most commonly affects the lower part of the femoral shaft. SYN periosteal s.

Kaposi s., a multifocal malignant neoplasm of primitive vasoformative tissue, occurring in the skin and sometimes in lymph nodes or viscera, consisting of spindle cells and irregular small vascular spaces frequently infiltrated by hemosiderin-pigmented macrophages and extravasated red cells; clinically manifested by cutaneous lesions consisting of reddish-purple to dark-blue macules, plaques, or nodules; seen most commonly in men over 60 years of age and, in AIDS patients, as an opportunistic disease associated with human herpes virus 8 infection. SYN multiple idiopathic hemorrhagic s.

leukocytic s., SYN leukemia.

lymphatic s., obsolete term for lymphosarcoma.

medullary s., a soft, extremely vascular s.

multiple idiopathic hemorrhagic s., SYN Kaposi s.

myelogenic s., s. originating in the bone marrow.

myeloid s., SYN granulocytic s.

osteogenic s., the most common and malignant of bone s.'s, which arises from bone-forming cells and affects chiefly the ends of long bones; its greatest incidence is in the age group between 10 and 25 years. SYN osteosarcoma.

periosteal s., SYN juxtacortical osteogenic s.

reticulum cell s., obsolete term for histiocytic *lymphoma*.

round cell s., obsolete term for an undifferentiated malignant neoplasm, believed to be of mesenchymal origin, composed chiefly of closely packed round cells.

Rous s., a fibrosarcoma, originally observed in a Plymouth Rock hen, now thought to be an expression of infection by certain viruses of the avian leukosis-sarcoma complex in the family Retroviridae. SYN avian s., Rous tumor.

spindle cell s., a malignant neoplasm of mesenchymal origin composed of elongated, spindle-shaped cells. SYN fascicular s.

synovial s., a rare malignant tumor of synovial origin, most commonly involving the knee joint and composed of spindle cells usually enclosing slits or pseudoglandular spaces that may be lined by radially disposed epithelial-like cells.

telangiectatic osteogenic s., a lytic cystic variant of osteogenic s. composed of aneurysmal blood-filled spaces lined by sarcoma cells producing osteoid.

Sar·co·mas·ti·goph·o·ra (sar′kō-mas-ti-gof′ŏ-ră). A phylum of the subkingdom Protozoa characterized by flagellae, pseudopodia, or both types of locomotory organelles; includes both the flagellates (subphylum Mastigophora) and the amebae (subphylum Sarcodina) in a single large assemblage. [sarco- + G. *mastix* (*mastig*-), whip, + *phoros*, to bear]

sar·co·ma·toid (sar-kō′mă-toyd). Resembling a sarcoma. [sarcoma + G. *eidos*, resemblance]

sar·co·ma·to·sis (sar′kō-mă-tō′sis). Occurrence of several sarcomatous growths on different parts of the body. [sarcoma + G. *-osis*, condition]

sar·com·a·tous (sar-kō′mă-tŭs). Relating to or of the nature of sarcoma.

sar·co·mere (sar′kō-mēr). The segment of a myofibril between two adjacent Z lines, representing the functional unit of striated muscle. [sarco- + G. *meros*, part]

sa

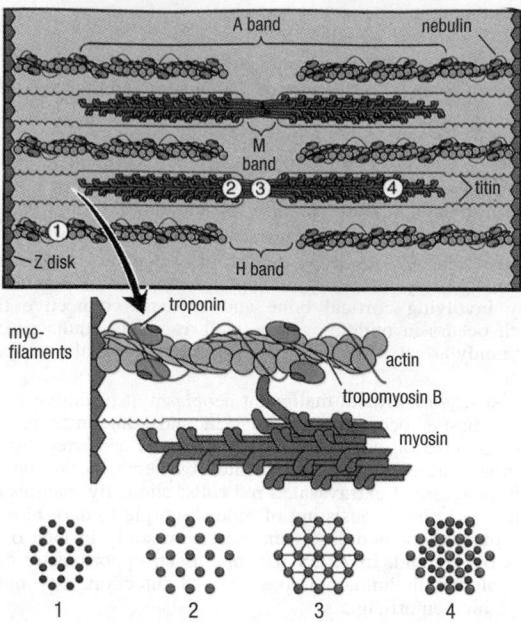

sarcomere: molecular structure; each thick filament is surrounded by a hexagonal array of thin filaments

sar·co·neme (sar'kō-nēm). SYN microneme. [sarco- + G. *nēma*, thread]

sar·co·plasm (sar'kō-plazm). The nonfibrillar cytoplasm of a muscle fiber. [sarco- + G. *plasma*, a thing formed]

sar·co·plas·mic (sar-kō-plaz'mik). Relating to sarcoplasm.

sar·co·plast (sar'kō-plast). SYN satellite *cell* of skeletal muscle. [sarco- + G. *plastos*, formed]

sar·co·poi·et·ic (sar'kō-poy-et'ik). Forming muscle. [sarco- + G. *poiēsis*, a making]

Sar·cop·syl·la pen·e·trans (sar-kō-sil'ă pen'ĕ-tranz). SYN *Tunga penetrans.*

Sar·cop·syl·li·dae (sar-kop-sil'li-dē). Older name for Tungidae. [sarco- + G. *psylla*, flea]

Sar·cop·tes sca·biei (sar-kop'tēz skā'bē-ī). Formerly *Acarus scabiei*, the itch mite, varieties of which are distributed worldwide and affect humans, horses, cattle, swine, sheep, dogs, cats, and many wild animals; serious and fatal infections are not uncommon in untreated animals. Although considered to belong to a single species, they do not readily pass from one host to another of a different animal species; transitory infections of this type do occur, however, especially from various animals to humans, and are spread by direct contact. The mite burrows into the skin and lays eggs within the burrow; intense itching and rash develop near the burrow in about a month. SEE scabies, mange. [sarco- + G. *koptō*, to cut; L. *scabies*, scurf]

sar·cop·tic (sar-kop'tik). Of, relating to, or caused by mites of the genus *Sarcoptes* or other members of the family Sarcoptidae.

sar·cop·tid (sar-kop'tid). Common name for members of the Sarcoptidae, a family of mites that includes the genera *Sarcoptes, Knemidokoptes,* and *Notoedres.*

sar·co·sine (Sar) (sar'kō-sēn). *N*-Methylglycine; an intermediate in the metabolism of choline; it can donate a methyl group to tetrahydrofolate, yielding N^5,N^{10}-methylenetetrahydrofolate; demethylation by s. dehydrogenase yields formaldehyde, glycine, and a reduced acceptor; elevated in certain inherited disorders.

s. dehydrogenase, an enzyme that cleaves s. using some acceptor to produce glycine, formaldehyde, and a reduced acceptor molecule; a deficiency of this enzyme will result in sarcosinemia.

sar·co·si·ne·mia (sar'kō-si-nē'mē-ă) [MIM*268900]. A disorder of amino acid metabolism due to deficiency of sarcosine dehydro-

genase, causing the sarcosine level to rise in blood plasma and be excreted in the urine; some affected infants fail to thrive, are irritable, may have muscle tremors, and have retarded motor and mental development; autosomal recessive inheritance. SYN hypersarcosinemia.

sar·co·sis (sar-kō'sis). 1. An abnormal increase of flesh. 2. A multiple growth of fleshy tumors. 3. A diffuse sarcoma involving the whole of an organ. [G. *sarkōsis*, the growth of flesh, fr. *sarx*, flesh]

sar·co·some (sar'kō-sōm). 1. Formerly, any granule in a muscle fiber. 2. Now, sometimes used synonymously with myomitochondrion. [sarco- + G. *soma*, body]

sar·cos·to·sis (sar-kos-tō'sis). Ossification of muscular tissue. [sarco- + G. *osteon*, bone, + -*osis*, condition]

sar·cot·ic (sar-kot'ik). 1. Relating to sarcosis. 2. Causing an increase of flesh.

sar·co·trip·sy (sar'kō-trip-sē). Rarely used term for use of a crushing forceps to stop hemorrhage. [sarco- + G. *tripsis*, a rubbing]

sar·co·tu·bules (sar-kō-too'boolz). The continuous system of membranous tubules in striated muscle that corresponds to the smooth endoplasmic reticulum of other cells.

sar·cous (sar'kŭs). Relating to muscular tissue; fleshy. [G. *sarx*, flesh]

sar·don·ic grin (sar-don'ik). SYN *risus* caninus.

sargramostim (sar-gra-mos'tim). A recombinant human granulocyte-macrophage colony-stimulating factor (GM-CSF); used to protect against infection in the presence of acute myelogenous leukemia and in bone marrow transplants.

sa·rin (zah-rēn'). A nerve poison similar to diisopropyl fluorophosphate and tetraethyl pyrophosphate; a very potent irreversible cholinesterase inhibitor and a more toxic nerve gas than tabun or soman. [Ger.]

sar·mas·sa·tion (sar-mă-sā'shŭn). Erotic squeezing, kneading, or caressing of female tissues and organs. [G. *sarx*, flesh, + *massō*, to knead]

sar·sa·pa·ril·la (sar'sā-per-il'ă, sas-per-il'ă). The dried root of *Smilax aristolochiaefolia* (Mexican s.), *S. regelii* (Honduras s.), *S. febrifuga* (Ecuadorian s.), or of undetermined species of *Smilax* (family Liliaceae), a thorny vine widely distributed throughout the tropical and semitropical world; it has been used in treatments of psoriasis, gout, rheumatism, and syphilis, and popularly as a "blood purifier." [Sp. *zarza*, a bramble]

SART Abbreviation for sinoatrial recovery *time.*

sar·to·ri·us (sar-tōr'ē-ŭs). SEE sartorius (*muscle*). [L. *sartor*, a tailor, the muscle being used in crossing the legs in the tailor's position, fr. *sarcio* pp. *sartus*, to patch, mend]

Sartwell, Philip, U.S. epidemiologist, *1908. SEE S. incubation *model.*

sas·sa·fras (sas'ă-fras). The dried bark of the root of *Sassafras albidum* (family Lauraceae), a tree of the eastern U.S.; a flavoring agent, diuretic, and diaphoretic; s. oil, a volatile oil obtained by distillation from the bark of *S. albidum* and *S. variifolium*, is used as a carminative, topical antiseptic, pediculicide, and flavoring agent.

sat. Abbreviation for saturated or saturation, as in O_2 sat.

sat·el·lite (sat'ĕ-līt). 1. A minor structure accompanying a more important or larger one; e.g., a vein accompanying an artery, or a small or secondary lesion adjacent to a larger one. 2. The posterior member of a pair of gregarine gamonts in syzygy, several of which may be found in some species. SEE ALSO primite. [L. *satelles* (*satellit-*), attendant]

chromosome s., a small chromosomal segment separated from the main body of the chromosome by a secondary constriction; in humans it is usually associated with the short arm of an acrocentric chromosome.

perineuronal s., an oligodendroglia cell surrounding the neuron.

sat·el·lit·o·sis (sat'ĕ-lī-tō'sis). 1. A condition marked by an accumulation of neuroglia cells around the neurons of the central nervous system. 2. The presence of satellite, smaller structures, or lesions, e.g., metastatic melanoma in the skin adjacent to the primary tumor, or lymphocytes in contact with a damaged keratinocyte in acute cutaneous graft versus host reaction. [L. *satelles* (*satellit-*), an attendant, + G. *-ōsis,* condition]

sa·ti·a·tion (sā-shē-ā′shŭn). The state produced by fulfillment of a specific need, such as hunger or thirst. [L. *satio,* pp. *-atus,* to fill, satisfy]

sat. sol., sat. soln. Abbreviation for saturated *solution.*

Sattler, Hubert, Austrian ophthalmologist, 1844–1928. SEE S. elastic *layer, veil.*

sat·u·rate (satch′ŭ-rāt). **1.** To impregnate to the greatest possible extent. **2.** To neutralize; to satisfy all the chemical affinities of a substance (as by converting all double bonds to single bonds). **3.** To dissolve a substance up to that concentration beyond which the addition of more results in two phases. [L. *saturo,* pp. *-atus,* to fill, fr. *satur,* sated]

sat·u·ra·tion (satch-ŭ-rā′shŭn). **1.** Impregnation of one substance by another to the greatest possible extent. **2.** Neutralization, as of an acid by an alkali. **3.** That concentration of a dissolved substance that cannot be exceeded. **4.** In optics, see saturated *color.* **5.** Filling of all the available sites on an enzyme molecule by its substrate, or on a hemoglobin molecule by oxygen (symbol S_{O_2}) or carbon monoxide (symbol S_{CO}). [L. *saturatio,* fr. *saturo,* to fill, fr. *satis,* enough]

secondary s., a technique of nitrous oxide anesthesia consisting of an abrupt curtailment of the oxygen in the inhaled mixture to produce a deep plane of anesthesia, following which oxygen is administered to correct hypoxia.

sat·ur·nine (sat′er-nīn). **1.** Relating to lead. **2.** Due to or symptomatic of lead poisoning. [Mediev. L. *saturninus,* fr. *saturnus,* lead, fr. L. *saturnus,* the god and planet Saturn]

sat·urn·ism (sat′er-nizm). SYN lead *poisoning.* [Mediev. L. *saturnus,* alchemical term for lead]

sat·y·ri·a·sis (sat-i-rī′ă-sis). Satyromania; excessive sexual excitement and behavior in the male; the counterpart of nymphomania in the female. SYN satyrism. [G. *satyros,* a satyr]

sat·y·rism (sat′i-rizm). SYN satyriasis.

sau·cer·i·za·tion (saw′ser-i-zā′shŭn). Excavation of tissue to form a shallow depression, performed in wound treatment to facilitate drainage from infected areas. SYN craterization.

Saundby, Robert, English physician, 1849–1918. SEE S. *test.*

sau·ri·a·sis (saw-rī′ă-sis). SYN ichthyosis. [G. *sauros,* lizard, + *-iasis,* condition]

Savage, Henry, English anatomist and gynecologist, 1810–1900. SEE S. perineal *body.*

saw. A metal operating instrument having an edge of sharp, toothlike projections, for dividing bone, cartilage, or plaster; edges may be attached to a rigid band, a flexible wire or chain, or a motorized oscillator. [A.S. *saga*]

Gigli s., a hand-held wire s. for use in craniotomy.

Stryker s., a rapidly oscillating s. used for cutting bone or plaster casts; it cuts hard matter, but soft tissues give and thus are not injured.

sax·i·tox·in (sak-si-tok′sin). A potent neurotoxin found in shellfish, such as the mussel or the clam, produced by the dinoflagellate *Gonyaulax catenella,* which is ingested by the shellfish; the cause of cases of poisoning from eating California sea mussel (*Mytilus californianus*), the scallop, and the Alaskan butterclam (*Saxidomus giganteus*).

Sayre, George P., U.S. ophthalmologist, *1911. SEE Kearns-S. *syndrome.*

Sb Symbol for antimony.

SBE Abbreviation for subacute bacterial *endocarditis.*

SBS Abbreviation for shaken baby *syndrome.*

Sc Symbol for scandium.

s.c. Abbreviation for subcutaneous; subcutaneously.

scab (skab). A crust formed by coagulation of blood, pus, serum, or a combination of these, on the surface of an ulcer, erosion, or other type of wound. [A.S. *scaeb*]

scab·i·ci·dal (skā-bi-sī′dăl). Destructive to scabies mites.

scab·i·cide (skā′bi-sīd). An agent lethal to scabies mites.

sca·bies (skā′bēz). **1.** An eruption due to the mite *Sarcoptes scabiei* var. *hominis;* the female of the species burrows into the skin, producing a vesicular eruption with intense pruritus between the fingers, on the male or female genitalia, buttocks, and elsewhere on the trunk and extremities. **2.** In animals, s. or scab is usually applied to cutaneous acariasis in sheep, which may be caused by *Sarcoptes, Psoroptes,* or *Chorioptes.* [L. *scabo,* to scratch]

crusted s., SYN Norwegian s.

Norwegian s., a severe form of s. with innumerable mites in thickened stratum corneum; has been linked with cellular immune deficiencies, including AIDS. SYN crusted s., Norway itch.

sca·brit·i·es (skā-brish′i-ēz). Roughness of the skin. [L., fr. *scaber,* scurfy]

s. un′guium, thickening and distortion of the nails.

sca·la, pl. **sca·lae** (skā′lă, -lē). One of the cavities of the cochlea winding spirally around the modiolus. [L. a stairway]

Löwenberg s., SYN cochlear *duct.*

s. me′dia, SYN cochlear *duct.*

s. tym′pani [TA], the division of the spiral canal of the cochlea lying on the basal side of the spiral lamina.

s. vestib′uli [TA], the division of the spiral canal of the cochlea lying on the apical side of the spiral lamina and vestibular membrane. SYN vestibular canal.

scald (skawld). **1.** To burn by contact with a hot liquid or steam. **2.** The lesion resulting from such contact. [L. *excaldo,* to wash in hot water]

scald·ing (skawl′ding). A burning pain on urinating.

scale (skāl). **1.** A standardized test for measuring psychological, personality, or behavioral characteristics. SEE ALSO score, test. **2.** SYN squama. **3.** A small thin plate of horny epithelium, resembling a fish s., cast off from the skin. **4.** To desquamate. **5.** To remove tartar from the teeth. **6.** A device by which some property can be measured. [L. *scala,* a stairway]

absolute s., obsolete term for Kelvin s.

activities of daily living s., a s. to score physical activity and its limitations, based on answers to simple questions about mobility, self-care, grooming, etc; widely used in geriatrics, rheumatology, etc.

adaptive behavior s.'s, a behavioral assessment device to quantify the levels of skills of mentally retarded and developmentally delayed individuals in interacting with the environment; consists of three developmentally related factors: 1) personal self-sufficiency, e.g., eating, dressing; 2) community self-sufficiency, e.g., shopping, communicating; 3) personal and social responsibility, e.g., use of leisure time, job performance. SEE intelligence.

Ångström s., a table of wavelengths of a large number of light rays corresponding to as many Fraunhofer lines in the spectrum.

Baumé s., a hydrometer s. for determining the specific gravity of liquids heavier and lighter than water, respectively: for liquids lighter than water, divide 140 by 130 plus the Baumé degree; for liquids heavier than water, divide 145 by 145 minus the Baumé degree.

Bayley s.'s of Infant Development, a psychological test used to measure the developmental progress of infants over the first 2 1/2 of life; consists of three scales: mental, motor, and behavior record.

Binet s., a measure of intelligence designed for both children and adults.

Binet-Simon s., forerunner of individual intelligence tests, particularly the Stanford-Binet intelligence s., and sometimes referred to as the Binet s.

Brazelton Neonatal Behavioral Assessment s.'s, a s. used by obstetricians, pediatricians, and pediatric psychologists to assess the sensory, motor, emotional and physical development of the neonate, usually beginning at birth or in the first month of life.

Cattell Infant Intelligence S., a standardized s. for assessment of the cognitive development of infants between the ages of 3 and 30 months.

Celsius s., a temperature s. that is based upon the triple point of water (defined to be 273.16 K) and assigned the value of 0.01°C;

SC

this has replaced the centigrade scale because the triple point of water can be more accurately measured than the ice point, although, for most practical purposes, the two s.'s are equivalent.

centigrade s., a thermometer s. in which there are 100 degrees between the freezing point of water (assigned the value of 0.0°C) and the boiling point of water at sea level; technically, supplanted by the Celsius s. Cf. Celsius s.

Charrière s., SYN French s.

Columbia Mental Maturity S., an individually administered intelligence test that provides an estimate of the intellectual ability of children; provides mental ages ranging from 3–12 years and requires no verbal response and minimal motor response. [Columbia University, NY]

🛈**coma s.,** a clinical s. to assess impaired consciousness; assessment may include motor responsiveness, verbal performance, and eye opening, as in the Glasgow (Scotland) c.s., or the same three items and dysfunction of cranial nerves, as in the Maryland (U.S.) c.s.

Glasgow coma scale		
monitored performance	**reaction**	**score**
eye opening	spontaneous	4
	open when spoken to	3
	open at pain stimulus	2
	no reaction	1
verbal performance	coherent	5
	confused, disoriented	4
	disconnected words	3
	unintelligible sounds	2
	no verbal reaction	1
motor responsiveness	follows instructions	6
	intentional pain-avoidance	5
	large motor movement	4
	flexor synergism	3
	extensor synergism	2
	no reaction	1

digital gray s., SYN latitude.

expanded disability status s. (EDSS), a commonly used rating system for evaluating the degree of neurologic impairment in multiple sclerosis, based on neurologic findings, and not symptoms; there are 10 grades in all, in steps and half-steps (e.g., 4, 4.5, 5), with "1" being neurologically normal and "10" being death. SYN Kurtzke multiple sclerosis disability s.

Fahrenheit s., a thermometer s. in which the freezing point of water is 32°F and the boiling point of water 212°F; 0°F indicates the lowest temperature Fahrenheit could obtain by a mixture of ice and salt in 1724; $°C = \frac{5}{9}(°F - 32)$.

French s. (F), a s. for grading sizes of sounds, tubes, and catheters as based on a diameter of $\frac{1}{3}$ mm equaling 1 F on the scale (e.g., 3 F = 1 mm); grading to scale is carried out using a metal plate with holes ranging from $\frac{1}{3}$ mm to 1 cm in diameter. SYN Charrière s.

Gaffky s., SYN Gaffky table.

gray s., SYN latitude. SEE gray-scale ultrasonography.

Guttman s., a measurement s. that ranks response categories to a question with each unit representing an increasingly strong expression of an attribute such as pain or disability.

Hamilton anxiety rating s., a list of specific symptoms used as a measure of severity of anxiety.

Hamilton depression rating s., a list of specific symptoms used as a measure of severity of depression.

hardness s., a qualitative s. in which minerals are classified in order of their increasing hardness, based on the fact that the harder of two materials will scratch the softer and will not be scratched by it. The s. lists 15 substances: 1, talc; 2, gypsum; 3, calcite; 4, fluorite; 5, apatite; 6, orthoclase, periclase; 7, vitreous pure silica; 8, quartz, stellite; 9, topaz; 10, garnet; 11, tantalum carbide, fused zirconia; 12, fused alumina; 13, silicon carbide; 14, boron carbide; 15, diamond. SYN Mohs s.

homigrade s., a special thermometer s. in which 100° indicates the normal human temperature (98.6°F, 37°C), 0° the freezing point, and 270° the boiling point of water.

interval s., like a temperature s. in centigrade or Fahrenheit units, a s. on which the intervals are equal but which has an arbitrary zero point; e.g., intelligence quotient values are values along an interval s.

Karnofsky s., a performance s. for rating a person's usual activities; used to evaluate a patient's progress after a therapeutic procedure.

Kelvin s., temperature scale in which the triple point of water is assigned the value of 273.16 K; °C = K − 273.15.

Kurtzke multiple sclerosis disability s., SYN expanded disability status s.

Leiter International Performance S., a nonverbal (performance) test for measuring intelligence that contains norms for each age between 2 and 18; originally developed as a method of assessing the comparative intellectual abilities of Caucasian, Chinese, and Japanese children, but now occasionally used for assessing slow learners and those who are blind, deaf, or verbally handicapped.

Likert s., ordinal s. of responses to a question or statement, ordered in hierarchical sequence from strongly negative to strongly positive. Used mainly in behavioral sciences and psychiatry.

masculinity-femininity s., any s. on a psychological test that assesses the relative masculinity or femininity of an individual; s.'s vary and may focus, for example, on basic identification with either sex or preference for a particular sex role.

Mohs s., SYN hardness s.

ordinal s., a s. that is based on classification of persons or things into ordered qualitative categories, such as socioeconomic status.

pH s., SYN Sörensen s.

Rahe-Holmes social readjustment rating s., a widely used s. in the social and behavioral sciences that assigns values to significant life events such as marriage, birth of offspring, bereavement, loss of job; such events correlate with emotional states.

Rankine s., a thermometer s. in which each degree Rankine (°Rank) is equal to the Fahrenheit but applied to the absolute temperature s. with its zero point at absolute zero; °Rank = °F + 459.67.

ratio s., a s. that involves physical units and demonstrates their relations.

Réaumur s., a thermometer s. in which each degree Réaumur (°R) is $\frac{1}{80}$ of the temperature difference between the freezing point and boiling point of pure water at 1 atm, with 0°R set at the freezing point and 80°R set at the boiling point of water.

Shipley-Hartford s., a test of intellectual and conceptual aptitude. [Hartford Retreat, CT, where Shipley was employed]

Sörensen s., the negative logarithm of the hydrogen ion concentration, used as a s. for expressing acidity and alkalinity. SEE ALSO pH. SYN pH s.

Stanford-Binet intelligence s., a standardized test for the measurement of intelligence consisting of a series of questions, graded according to the intelligence of normal children at different ages, the answers to which indicate the mental age of the person tested; primarily used with children, but also contains norms for adults standardized against adult age levels rather than those of children, as formerly was the case. SYN Binet test.

Wechsler-Bellevue s., a measure of general intelligence superseded by the Wechsler adult intelligence s. and its subsequent revision. SEE ALSO Wechsler intelligence s.'s.

Wechsler intelligence s.'s, continuously revised and updated standardized s.'s for the measurement of general intelligence in preschool children (Wechsler preschool and primary s. of intelligence), in children (Wechsler intelligence s. for children), and in adults (Wechsler adult intelligence s., the successor to the Wechsler-Bellevue s.).

Zubrod s., a 5-point s. similar to the 10-point Karnofsky s.; both measure the performance status of a patient's ambulatory nature, from normal activity to total dependence on others for care. SEE ALSO Karnofsky s.

sca·lene (skā'lēn). **1.** Having sides of unequal length, said of a triangle so formed. **2.** One of several muscles so named. SEE scalenus anterior (*muscle*), musculus scalenus anticus, scalenus medius (*muscle*), scalenus minimus (*muscle*), scalenus posterior (*muscle*), musculus scalenus posticus. SYN scalenus. [G. *skalēnos*, uneven]

sca·le·nec·to·my (skā'lĕ-nek'tō-mē). Resection of the scalene muscles. [scalene + G. *ektomē*, excision]

sca·le·not·o·my (skā'lĕ-not'ō-mē). Division or section of the anterior scalene muscle. [scalene + G. *tomē*, incision]

sca·le·nus (skā-lē'nŭs). SYN scalene. [L.]

scal·er (skā'ler). **1.** An instrument for removing tartar from the teeth. **2.** A device for counting electrical impulses, as in the assay of radioactive materials.

hoe s., a hoe-shaped s. with a very short blade.

ultrasonic s., an ultrasonic instrument that uses high frequency vibration to remove adherent deposits from the teeth.

scal·ing (skā'ling). In dentistry, removal of accretions from the crowns and roots of teeth by use of special instruments.

scal·lop·ing (skal'ō-ping). A series of indentations or erosions on a normally smooth margin of a structure.

scalp (skalp). The skin and subcutaneous tissue, normally hair-bearing, covering the neurocranium. [M. E. fr. Scand. *skalpr*, sheath]

scal·pel (skal'pl). A knife used in surgical dissection. [L. *scalpellum;* dim. of *scalprum,* a knife]

plasma s., a s. that uses a fine high-temperature gas jet, instead of a blade, for cutting.

scal·pri·form (skal'pri-fōrm). Chisel-shaped. [L. *scalprum,* chisel, + *forma,* shape]

scal·prum (skal'prŭm). **1.** A large, strong scalpel. **2.** A raspatory. [L. chisel, penknife, fr. *scalpo,* pp. *scalptus,* to carve]

scaly (skā'lē). SYN squamous.

scam·mo·ny (skam'ō-nē). The plant, *Convolvulus scammonia* (family Convolvulaceae), the dried root of which contains a cathartic resin. SEE ALSO ipomea. [G. *skammōnia*]

⊞scan (skan). **1.** To survey by traversing with an active or passive sensing device. **2.** The image, record, or data obtained by scanning, usually identified by the technology or device employed; e.g., CT s., radionuclide s., ultrasound s., etc. **3.** Abbreviated form of scintiscan, usually identified by the organ or structure examined; e.g., brain s., bone s., etc.

CT s., SEE tomography.

duplex Doppler s., a method of visualizing and selectively assessing the flow patterns of peripheral arteries and veins using ultrasound imaging and pulsed Doppler.

EMI s., historically, the name commonly used for computed tomography of the head, the technique devised by Hounsfield, who was a scientist at EMI, an English electronics firm.

Meckel s., use of ⁹⁹ᵐtechnetium pertechnetate in a s. of the small bowel to detect ectopic gastric mucosa in Meckel diverticulum; the pertechnetate anion is secreted by epithelial cells in the gastric mucosa.

multiple-gated acquisition s. (MUGA), a nuclear medicine cardiac blood pool study collected by multiple-gated acquisition; used for ejection *fraction* and wall motion assessment. SEE ALSO radionuclide ejection *fraction.*

renal cortical s., an imaging technique wherein a renal cortex–localizing radiopharmaceutical (e.g., ⁹⁹ᵐTc-DMSA, ⁹⁹ᵐTc-glucohepatanate) is injected to image the renal cortex to find scarring or pyelonephritis.

sector s., in ultrasonography, a system in which the transducer or transmitted ultrasound beam is rotated through an angle, resulting in a pie-shaped image.

⊞ventilation-perfusion s., a lung function test, especially useful for pulmonary embolism, employing an inhaled radionuclide for ventilation and an intravenous radionuclide for perfusion; their respective distributions in the lung are recorded scintigraphically.

scan·di·um (Sc) (skan'dē-ŭm). A metallic element, atomic no.

21, atomic wt. 44.955910. [L. *Scandia,* Scandinavia, where discovered]

scan·ner (skan'er). A device or instrument that scans.

scan·ning (skan'ing). The act of imaging by traversing with an active or passive sensing device, often identified by the technology or device employed.

transvaginal s., ultrasonography of the female pelvis with the transducer placed inside the vagina.

scan·o·gram (skan'ō-gram). A radiographic technique for showing true dimensions by moving a narrow orthogonal beam of x-rays along the length of the structure being measured, e.g., the lower extremities. [scan- + G. *gramma,* something written]

Scanzoni, Friedrich W., German obstetrician, 1821–1891. SEE S. *maneuver.*

sca·pha (skaf'ă, skā'fă). **1** [TA]. The longitudinal furrow between the helix and the antihelix of the auricle. SYN fossa of helix. **2.** Obsolete term for scaphoid *fossa.* [L. fr. G. *skaphē,* skiff]

△**scapho-.** A scapha, scaphoid. [G. *skaphē,* skiff, boat]

scaph·o·ce·phal·ic (skaf-ō-se-fal'ik). Denoting or relating to scaphocephaly. SYN scaphocephalous, tectocephalic.

scaph·o·ceph·a·lism (skaf-ō-sef'ă-lizm). SYN scaphocephaly.

scaph·o·ceph·a·lous (skaf-ō-sef'ă-lŭs). SYN scaphocephalic.

scaph·o·ceph·a·ly (skaf-ō-sef'ă-lē). A form of craniosynostosis that results in a long, narrow head in which the parietal eminences are absent and frontal and occiptal protrusions are conspicuous; there may be a crest indicating the site of a prenatally closed sagittal suture; sometimes accompanied by mental retardation. SYN cymbocephaly, sagittal synostosis, scaphocephalism, tectocephaly. [scapho- + G. *kephalē,* head]

scaph·o·hy·dro·ceph·a·lus, scaph·o·hy·dro·ceph·a·ly (skaf'ō-hī'drō-sef'ă-lŭs, -lē). Occurrence of hydrocephalus in a scaphocephalic individual.

scaph·oid (skaf'oyd) [TA]. Boat-shaped; hollowed. SEE scaphoid (*bone*). [scapho- + G. *eidos,* resemblance]

scap·u·la, gen. and pl. **scap·u·lae** (skap'ū-lă, -lē) [TA]. A large triangular flattened bone lying over the ribs, posteriorly on either side, articulating laterally with the clavicle at the acromioclavicular joint and the humerus at the glenohumeral joint. It forms a functional articulation with the chest wall, the scapulothoracic articulation. SYN blade bone, shoulder blade. [L. *scapulae,* the shoulder blades]

s. ala'ta, SYN winged s.

s. eleva'ta, SYN Sprengel *deformity.*

winged s., condition wherein the medial border of the scapula protrudes away from the thorax; the protrusion is posterior and lateral, as the scapula rotates out; most commonly caused by paralysis of the serratus anterior muscle. SYN s. alata.

scap·u·lal·gia (skap'ū-lal'jē-ă). Rarely used term meaning pain in the shoulder blades. SYN scapulodynia. [scapula + G. *algos,* pain]

scap·u·lar (skap'ū-lăr). Relating to the scapula.

scap·u·lary (skap'ū-lăr-ē). A form of brace or suspender for keeping a belt or body bandage in place.

scap·u·lec·to·my (skap'ū-lek'tō-mē). Excision of the scapula. [scapula + G. *ektomē,* excision]

△**scapulo-.** Scapula, scapular. [L. *scapulae,* shoulder blades]

scap·u·lo·cla·vic·u·lar (skap'ū-lō-klă-vik'ū-lăr). **1.** SYN acromioclavicular. **2.** SYN coracoclavicular.

scap·u·lo·dyn·ia (skap'ū-lō-din'ē-ă). SYN scapulalgia. [scapulo- + G. *odynē,* pain]

scap·u·lo·hu·mer·al (skap'ū-lō-hū'mer-ăl). Relating to both scapula and humerus. SEE ALSO glenohumeral.

scap·u·lo·pexy (skap'ū-lō-pek-sē). Operative fixation of the scapula to the chest wall or to the spinous process of the vertebrae. [scapulo- + G. *pēxis,* fixation]

sca·pus, pl. **sca·pi** (skā'pŭs, -pī). A shaft or stem. [L. shaft, stalk]

s. pe'nis, SYN *body* of penis.

s. pi'li, SYN hair *shaft.*

scar (skar). Fibrous tissue replacing normal tissues destroyed by injury or disease. [G. *eschara,* scab]

cigarette-paper s.'s, atrophic s.'s in the skin at sites of minor

SC

lacerations over the knees, shins, and elbows of persons with Ehlers-Danlos syndrome. SYN papyraceous s.'s.

hypertrophic s., an elevated s. resembling a keloid but which does not spread into surrounding tissues, is rarely painful, and regresses spontaneously; collagen bundles run parallel to the skin surface.

papyraceous s.'s, SYN cigarette-paper s.'s.

radial s., SYN radial sclerosing *lesion.*

Scardino, Peter T., U.S. urologist, *1915. SEE S. vertical flap *pyeloplasty.*

Scarff, John E., U.S. neurosurgeon, 1898–1978. SEE Stookey-S. *operation.*

scar·i·fi·ca·tion (skar-i-fi-kā′shŭn). The making of a number of superficial incisions in the skin. [L. *scarifico,* to scratch, fr. G. *skariphos,* a style for sketching]

scar·i·fy (skar′i-fī). To produce scarification.

scar·la·ti·na (skar′lă-tē′nă). An acute exanthematous disease, caused by infection with streptococcal organisms producing erythrogenic toxin, marked by fever and other constitutional disturbances, and a generalized eruption of closely aggregated points or small macules of a bright red color followed by desquamation in large scales, shreds, or sheets; mucous membrane of the mouth and fauces is usually also involved. SYN scarlet fever. [through It. fr. Mediev. L. *scarlatum,* scarlet, a scarlet cloth]

anginose s., s. angino′sa, a form of s. in which the throat affection is unusually severe. SYN Fothergill disease (2).

s. hemorrhag′ica, a form of s. in which blood extravasates into the skin and mucous membranes, giving to the eruption a dusky hue; frequent bleeding from the nose and into the intestine also occurs.

s. la′tens, latent s., a form of s. in which the rash is absent, but other complications of streptococcal infection occur, such as acute nephritis.

s. malig′na, a severe scarlet fever in which the patient is quickly overcome with the intensity of the systemic intoxication.

s. rheumat′ica, SYN dengue.

s. sim′plex, a mild form of the disease.

scar·la·ti·nal (skar-lă-tē′năl). Relating to scarlatina.

scar·la·ti·nel·la (skar-lă-ti-nel′ă). SYN Filatov-Dukes *disease.* [dim. of *scarlatina*]

scar·la·ti·ni·form (skar-lă-tē′ni-fōrm, -tin′i-fōrm). Resembling scarlatina, denoting a rash. SYN scarlatinoid (1).

scar·la·ti·noid (skar-lă-tē′noyd, skar-lat′i-noyd). **1.** SYN scarlatiniform. **2.** SYN Filatov-Dukes *disease.* [scarlatina + G. *eidos,* resemblance]

scar·let (skar′let). Denoting a bright red color tending toward orange. [Mediev. L. *scarlatum,* scarlet cloth]

scar·let red [C.I. 26905]. An azo dye; a dark, brownish red powder, soluble in oils, fats, and chloroform, but insoluble in water; used in medicine as a vulnerary, in histology to stain fat in tissue sections and basic proteins at high pH, and in immunoelectrophoresis. SYN Biebrich scarlet red, medicinal scarlet red, scharlach red, Sudan IV.

scar·let red sul·fo·nate. An azo dye that has been used to stimulate healing of chronic superficial wounds and ulcers.

Scarpa, Antonio, Italian anatomist, orthopedist, and ophthalmologist, 1747–1832. SEE *canals* of S., under *canal;* membranous *layer* of subcutaneous tissue of abdomen; S. *fluid, foramina,* under *foramen; fossa* scarpae major; S. *ganglion, habenula, hiatus, liquor, membrane, method, sheath, staphyloma, triangle.*

Scatchard, George, U.S. chemist and biochemist, 1892–1973. SEE S. *plot.*

sca·te·mia (skă-tē′mē-ă). Intestinal autointoxication. [scato- + G. *haima,* blood]

⚠**scato-.** Feces. SEE ALSO copro-, sterco-. [G. *skōr (skat-),* excrement]

scat·o·log·ic (skat-ō-loj′ik). Pertaining to scatology.

sca·tol·o·gy (skă-tol′o-jē). **1.** The scientific study and analysis of feces, for physiologic and diagnostic purposes. SYN coprology. **2.**

The study relating to the psychiatric aspects of excrement or excremental (anal) function. [scato- + G. *logos,* study]

sca·to·ma (ska-tō′mă). SYN fecaloma. [scato- + G. *-oma,* tumor]

sca·toph·a·gy (skă-tof′ă-jē). SYN coprophagia. [scato- + G. *phagō,* to eat]

sca·tos·co·py (skă-tos′kŏ-pē). Examination of the feces for purposes of diagnosis. [scato- + G. *skopeō,* to view]

scat·ter (skat′er). **1.** A change in direction of a photon or subatomic particle, as the result of a collision or interaction. **2.** The secondary radiation resulting from the interaction of primary radiation with matter.

Compton s., the mechanism of s. called the Compton effect.

scat·ter·gram (skăt-er-gram). Graphical display of distribution of two variables in relation to each other. [scatter + G. *gramma,* something written]

scat·u·la (skat′ū-lă). A square pillbox. [Mediev. L. a rectangular figure whose width is one-tenth of its length]

Scedosporium (se-dō-spōr′ē-um). An imperfect fungus of the form-class Hyphomycetes; anamorph of *Pseudallescheria.*

S. apiosper′mum (sked-os-pōr′ē-ŭm), the imperfect state of the fungus *Pseudallescheria boydii,* one of the 16 species of true fungi that may cause mycetoma in humans or severe infection in immunosuppressed patients.

S. infla′tum, SEE S. prolificans.

S. proli′ficans, a mold; a rare cause of deep fungal infection. Formerly called *S. inflatum.*

sce·lal·gia (se-lal′jē-ă). Pain in the leg. [G. *skelos,* leg, + *algos,* pain]

scene.

primal s., in psychoanalysis, the actual or fantasied observation by a child of sexual intercourse, particularly between the parents.

scent (sent). SYN odor. [M.E., fr. O.Fr., fr. L. *sentio,* to feel]

Schacher, Polycarp G., German physician, 1674–1737. SEE S. *ganglion.*

Schaer re·a·gent. See under reagent.

Schäfer, Sir Edward A. Sharpey-, English physiologist and histologist, 1850–1935. SEE S. *method.*

Schäffer, Max, German neurologist, 1852–1923. SEE S. *reflex.*

Schaffer test. See under test.

Schamberg, Jay F., U.S. dermatologist, 1870–1934. SEE Schamberg *fever.*

Schapiro, Heinrich, Russian physician, 1852–1901. SEE S. *sign.*

Schardinger, Franz, Austrian scientist, 1853–1920. SEE S. *dextrins,* under *dextrin, enzyme, reaction.*

schar·lach red (shar′lak). SYN scarlet red.

Schatzki, Richard, U.S. radiologist, 1901–1992. SEE Schatzki *ring.*

Schaudinn, Fritz R., German bacteriologist, 1871–1906. SEE S. *fixative.*

Schaumann, Jörgen N., Swedish physician, 1879–1953. SEE S. *bodies,* under *body, lymphogranuloma, syndrome;* Besnier-Boeck-S. *disease, syndrome.*

Schaumberg, H.H., U.S. neuropathologist, *1912.

Schauta, Friedrich, Austrian gynecologist, 1849–1919. SEE S. vaginal *operation.*

Schede, Max, German surgeon, 1844–1902. SEE S. *method.*

sched·ule (sked′jool). A procedural plan for a proposed objective, especially the sequence and time allotted for each item or operation required for its completion. [L. *scheda,* fr. *scida,* a strip of papyrus, leaf of paper]

s.'s of reinforcement, in the psychology of conditioning, established procedures or sequences for reinforcing operant behavior; e.g., in a lever-pressing situation, every displacement of the lever will bring a pellet of food or comparable reinforcer (**continuous reinforcement s.**), or the reinforcer will come at every 5 seconds, regardless of how many displacements occur earlier (**fixed-interval reinforcement s.**), at every 10th displacement (**fixed-ratio reinforcement s.**), or on an average of every 5 seconds (**variable-interval reinforcement s.**), or the reinforcer will come in a noncontinuous fashion in which less than 100% of the displacements bring a reinforcer (**intermittent reinforcement s.**).

Scheele, Karl W., Swedish chemist, 1742–1786. SEE S. *green.*

Scheibe, A., U.S. physician, *1875. SEE Scheibe *hearing impairment.*

Scheibler re·a·gent. See under reagent.

Scheie, Harold G., U.S. ophthalmologist, *1909. SEE S. *syndrome.*

Scheiner, Christoph, German physicist, 1575–1650. SEE S. *experiment.*

Schellong, Fritz, German physician, 1891–1953. SEE S. *test;* S.-Strisower *phenomenon.*

sche·ma, pl. **sche·ma·ta** (skē′mă, skē-mah′tă). **1.** A plan, outline, or arrangement. SYN scheme. **2.** In sensorimotor theory, the organized unit of cognitive experience. [G. *schēma,* shape, form]

  body s., SYN body *image.*

sche·mat·ic (skē-mat′ik). Made after a definite type of formula; representing in general, but not with absolute exactness; denoting an anatomical drawing or model. [G. *schēmatikos,* in outward show, fr. *schēma,* shape, form]

sche·mat·o·graph (skē-mat′ō-graf). An instrument for making a tracing in reduced size of the outline of the body. [G. *schēma,* form, + *graphō,* to write]

scheme (skēm). SYN schema (1).

  occlusal s., SYN occlusal *system.*

sche·mo·chromes (skē-mō-krōmz). SYN structural *color.*

Schenck, Benjamin R., U.S. surgeon, 1873–1920. SEE S. *disease.*

Scheuermann, Holger W., Danish surgeon, 1877–1960. SEE S. *disease.*

Schick, Bela, Austrian pediatrician in U.S., 1877–1967. SEE S. *method, test,* test *toxin.*

Schiff, Hugo, German chemist in Florence, 1834–1915. SEE S. *base, reagent;* Kasten fluorescent S. *reagents,* under *reagent;* periodic acid-S. *stain;* ninhydrin-S. *stain* for proteins.

Schiff, Moritz, German physiologist, 1823–1896. SEE S.-Sherrington *phenomenon.*

Schilder, Paul Ferdinand, Austrian neurologist, 1886–1940.

Schiller, Walter, Austrian pathologist in U.S., 1887–1960. SEE S. *test.*

Schilling, Victor, German hematologist, 1883–1960. SEE S. *blood count,* band *cell, index, test,* type of monocytic *leukemia.*

schin·dy·le·sis (skin-dī-lē′sis) [TA]. A form of fibrous joint in which the sharp edge of one bone is received in a cleft in the edge of the other, as in the articulation of the vomer with the rostrum of the sphenoid. SYN schindyletic joint, wedge-and-groove joint, wedge-and-groove suture. [G. *schindylēsis,* splintering]

Schiötz, Hjalmar, Norwegian physician, 1850–1927. SEE S. *tonometer.*

Schirmer, Otto W.A., German ophthalmologist, 1864–1917. SEE S. *test.*

◇**schisto-.** Cleft, division. SEE ALSO schizo-. [G. *schistos,* split]

schis·to·ce·lia (skis-tō-sē′lē-ă). Congenital fissure of the abdominal wall. [schisto- + G. *koilia,* a hollow]

schis·to·cor·mia (skis-tō-kōr′mē-ă). Congenital clefting of the trunk, the lower extremities of the fetus usually being imperfectly developed. SYN schistosomia. [schisto- + G. *kormos,* trunk of a tree]

schis·to·cys·tis (skis-tō-sis′tis). Fissure of the bladder. [schisto- + G. *kystis,* bladder]

schis·to·cyte (skis′tō-sīt). A variety of poikilocyte that owes its abnormal shape to fragmentation occurring as the cell flows through damaged small vessels. SYN schizocyte. [schisto- + G. *kytos,* cell]

schis·to·cy·to·sis (skis′tō-sī-tō′sis). The occurrence of many schistocytes in the blood. SYN schizocytosis.

schis·to·glos·sia (skis-tō-glos′ē-ă). Congenital fissure or cleft of the tongue. [schisto- + G. *glōssa,* tongue]

schis·to·me·lia (skis′tō-mel′ē-ă). Congenital cleft of a limb.

schis·tor·rha·chis (skis-tōr′ă-kis). SYN *spina* bifida. [schisto- + G. *rhachis,* spine]

Schis·to·so·ma (skis-tō-sō′mă). A genus of digenetic trematodes, including the important blood flukes of humans and domestic animals, that cause schistosomiasis; characterized by elongate shape, by separate sexes with marked sexual dimorphism, by their unusual location in the smaller blood vessels of their host, and by utilization of water snails as intermediate hosts. [schisto- + G. *sōma,* body]

S. haemato′bium, the vesical blood fluke, a species with terminally spined eggs that occurs as a parasite in the portal system and mesenteric veins of the bladder (causing human schistosomiasis haematobium) and rectum; common in the Nile delta but is found along waterways, irrigation ditches, or streams throughout Africa and in parts of the Middle East; the intermediate host is *Bulinus truncatus* in Egypt; elsewhere, other snails of the subfamily Bulininae (*Bulinus, Physopsis, Pyrgophysa*) are involved.

S. intercala′tum, a blood fluke species related to *S. haematobium* locally distributed in Zaire and other areas of central Africa, causing mild dysentery and abdominal pains, with enlargement of the spleen and liver; a planorbid snail, *Bulinus (Physopsis) africanus,* serves as the intermediate host.

S. japon′icum, the Oriental or Japanese blood fluke, a species having eggs with small lateral spines, usually only a small knob; causes schistosomiasis japonica, with extensive pathology from encapsulation of the eggs, particularly in the liver, and is the most pathogenic of the three common schistosome species afflicting man, possibly owing to greater egg production per female worm; it is also the most intractable to treatment and the most difficult to control, as the intermediate hosts are amphibious snails (species of *Oncomelania,* family Hydrobiidae) that can leave the water to avoid molluscicides, and also because many other animals, such as pigs, oxen, cattle, and dogs, serve as reservoir hosts.

S. malayen′sis, a member of the *S. japonicum* complex described from the rodent *Rattus muelleri* in peninsular Malaysia. The aquatic snail *Robertsiella kaporensis* and two other species of this genus were found to be naturally infected. *S. malayensis* is considered most closely related to *S. mekongi.* Human infections, based on serologic evidence, were reported among the indigenous people of central peninsular Malaysia.

🔲*S. manso′ni,* a common species of trematode characterized by large eggs with a strong lateral spine and transmitted by planorbid snails of the genus *Biomphalaria;* causes schistosomiasis mansoni in humans in Africa, parts of the Middle East, South America, and certain Caribbean islands.

S. mat′theei, a species found in the portal and mesenteric veins of ruminants, primates (including humans), zebra, and rodents in Africa.

S. mekon′gi, the Mekong schistosome, a species described from the Mekong delta in southern Laos and northern Cambodia. Infection rates are highest for ages 7–15; dogs appear to be the chief reservoir host; the intermediate host snail is the operculid snail, *Tricula aperta.* Pathology is similar to but generally less severe than that of *S. japonicum.*

schis·to·some (skis′tō-sōm). Common name for a member of the genus *Schistosoma.*

schis·to·so·mia (skis-tō-sō′mē-ă). SYN schistocormia. [schisto- + G. *sōma,* body]

schis·to·so·mi·a·sis (skis′tō-sō-mī′ă-sis). Infection with a species of *Schistosoma;* manifestations of this often chronic and debilitating disease vary with the infecting species but depend in large measure upon tissue reaction (granulation and fibrosis) to the eggs deposited in venules and in the hepatic portals, the latter resulting in portal hypertension and esophageal varices, as well as liver damage leading to cirrhosis. SEE tropical *diseases,* under *disease.* SEE ALSO schistosomal *dermatitis,* Symmers clay pipestem *fibrosis.* SYN bilharziasis, bilharziosis, hemic distomiasis, snail fever.

Asiatic s., SYN s. japonica.

bladder s., SYN s. haematobium.

cutaneous s. japonica, SYN s. japonica.

ectopic s., a clinical form of s. that occurs outside of the normal site of parasitism (mesenteric vein or hepatic portals); may result from accidental blood-borne transport of schistosome eggs or, rarely, adult worms, to various unusual sites such as the skin, brain, or spinal cord.

SC

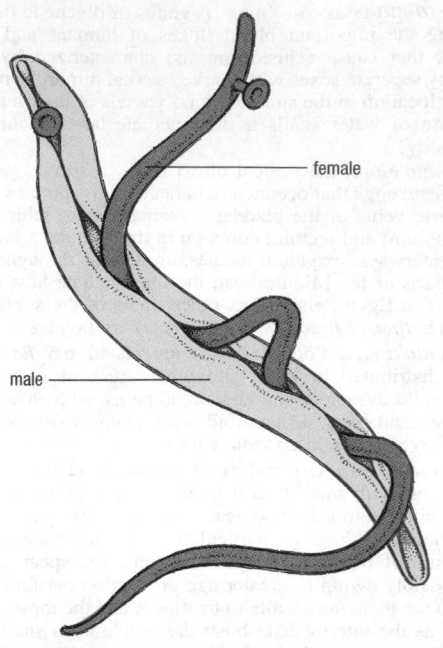

female

male

Schistosoma mansoni: copulating

s. haemato′bium, infection with *Schistosoma haematobium*, the eggs of which invade the urinary tract, causing cystitis and hematuria, and possibly an increased likelihood of bladder cancer. SYN bladder s., Egyptian hematuria, endemic hematuria, urinary s.

s. intercalatum, infection with *Schistosoma intercalatum;* occurs only in West Africa; few symptoms reported and no cases of hepatic fibrosis known.

intestinal s., SYN s. mansoni.

s. japon′ica, Japanese s., infection with *Schistosoma japonicum*, characterized by dysenteric symptoms, painful enlargement of the liver and spleen, dropsy, urticaria, and progressive anemia. SYN Asiatic s., cutaneous s. japonica, kabure itch, kabure, Katayama syndrome, Kinkiang fever, Oriental s., rice itch, urticarial fever, Yangtze Valley fever.

Manson s., SYN s. mansoni.

s. manso′ni, infection with *Schistosoma mansoni*, the eggs of which invade the wall of the large intestine and the liver, causing irritation, inflammation, and ultimately fibrosis. SYN intestinal s., Manson disease, Manson s.

s. mekon′gi, infection with *Schistosoma mekongi*, which chiefly afflicts children in the Mekong delta, where it was discovered; the disease is similar to s. japonica.

Oriental s., SYN s. japonica.

pulmonary s., pulmonary manifestations of infection with *Schistosoma*, usually *Schistosoma mansoni*, occurring when schistosomals, which form in the skin from the cercariae which have entered from infected water, migrate via the bloodstream to the lungs, en route to the gastrointestinal tract and the portal vein; symptoms are usually limited to cough.

urinary s., SYN s. haematobium.

schis·to·som·u·lum, pl. **schis·to·som·u·la** (skis-tō-sō′mū-lŭm, -lă). The stage in the life cycle of a blood fluke of the genus *Schistosoma* immediately after penetration of the skin as a cercaria; marked by loss of the tail and gaining of physiological modifications allowing it to survive in a mammalian bloodstream.

schis·to·ster·nia (skis-tō-ster′nē-ă). SYN schistothorax. [schisto- + G. *sternon*, sternum]

schis·to·tho·rax (skis-tō-thōr′aks). Congenital cleft of the chest wall. SYN schistosternia. [schisto- + G. *thōrax*, thorax]

△**schiz-.** SEE schizo-.

schiz·am·ni·on (skiz-am′nē-on). An amnion developing, as in the human embryo, by the formation of a cavity over or within the inner cell mass. [schiz- + amnion]

schiz·ax·on (skiz-ak′son). An axon divided into two branches. [schiz- + G. *axōn*, axis]

schiz·en·ceph·a·ly (skiz-en-sef′ă-lē). Abnormal divisions or clefts of the brain substance. [schiz- + G. *enkephalos*, brain]

△**schizo-, schiz-.** Split, cleft, division; schizophrenia. SEE ALSO schisto-. [G. *schizō*, to split or cleave]

schiz·o·af·fec·tive (skiz′ō-ă-fek′tiv). Having an admixture of symptoms suggestive of both schizophrenia and affective (mood) disorder.

schiz·o·cyte (skiz′ō-sīt). SYN schistocyte. [schizo- + G. *kytos*, cell]

schiz·o·cy·to·sis (skiz′ō-sī-tō′sis). SYN schistocytosis.

schiz·o·gen·e·sis (skiz-ō-jen′ĕ-sis). Reproduction by fission. SYN fissiparity, scissiparity. [schizo- + G. *genesis*, origin]

schi·zog·o·ny (ski-zog′ō-nē). Multiple fission in which the nucleus first divides and then the cell divides into as many parts as there are nuclei; called merogony if daughter cells are merozoites, sporogony if daughter cells are sporozoites, or gametogony if daughter cells are gametes. SYN agamocytogeny. [schizo- + G. *gonē*, generation]

schiz·o·gy·ria (skiz-ō-jī′rē-ă, -jir′ē-ă). Deformity of the cerebral convolutions marked by occasional interruptions of their continuity. [schizo- + G. *gyros*, circle (convolution)]

schiz·oid (skiz′oyd). Socially isolated, withdrawn, having few (if any) friends or social relationships; resembling the personality features characteristic of schizophrenia, but in a milder form. SEE ALSO schizoid *personality*. [schizo(phrenia), + G. *eidos*, resemblance]

schiz·oid·ism (skiz′oy-dizm). A schizoid state; the manifestation of schizoid tendencies.

schiz·o·my·cete (skiz′ō-mī-sēt). A member of the class Schizomycetes; a bacterium.

schiz·o·my·cet·ic (skiz-ō-mī-sē′tik). Relating to or caused by fission fungi (bacteria).

schiz·ont (skiz′ont). A sporozoan trophozoite (vegetative form) that reproduces by schizogony, producing a varied number of daughter trophozoites or merozoites. SEE ALSO meront, segmenter. SYN agamont, segmenting body. [schizo- + G. *ōn* (*ont-*), a being]

schi·zon·ti·cide (ski-zon′ti-sīd). An agent that kills schizonts. [schizont + L. *caedo*, to kill]

schiz·o·nych·ia (skiz-ō-nik′ē-ă). Splitting of the nails. [schizo- + G. *onyx*, nail]

schiz·o·pha·sia (skiz-ō-fā′zē-ă). A rarely used term for the disordered speech (word salad) of the schizophrenic individual. [schizo- + G. *phasis*, speech]

schiz·o·phre·nia (skiz-ō-frē′nē-ă, skit′sō-). A term coined by Bleuler, synonymous with and replacing *dementia praecox;* a common type of psychosis, characterized by abnormalities in perception, content of thought, and thought processes (hallucinations and delusions) and by extensive withdrawal of interest from other people and the outside world, with excessive focusing on one's own mental life; now considered a group or spectrum of disorders rather than a single entity, with distinction sometimes made between process s. and reactive s. The "split" personality of s., in which individual psychic components or functions split off and become autonomous, is popularly but erroneously identified with multiple personality, in which 2 or more relatively complete personalities dominate by turns the psychic life of an individual. [schizo- + G. *phrēn*, mind]

Schizophrenia is the most prevalent psychosis, affecting some 2 million Americans. The annual cost of the disease to the U.S. economy is estimated at $65 billion, of which $46 billion reflects lost productivity of patients and their caregivers. The lifetime incidence risk is about 1%. Onset is typically gradual, without an obvious precipitating cause. Early symptoms include shortened attention span, memory deficits, and diminished ability to make decisions. Most patients become ill before age 40. Psychotic symptoms persist for months or years, and there is a lifelong risk of relapse. Cognitive malfunctions are typically accompanied by reduced energy level, flat or depressed affect, anhedonia, and abulia. Virtually all patients display impoverished thought content, social withdrawal, and impairment of occupational functioning, and even with intensive psychotherapy and drug treatment about 25% require custodial or institutional care. Although some persons with schizophrenia become assassins or mass murderers, the vast majority pose no threat to society; about 10% commit suicide. Neurophysiologic studies have shown generalized limbic lobe and prefrontal cortical abnormalities, abnormal smallness of the thalamus, and changes in signal intensity in adjacent white matter. Brain imaging inconsistently demonstrates structural or physiologic abnormalities in the prefrontal cortex, cingulate cortex, temporal cortex, and hippocampal formation. The amelioration or exacerbation of schizophrenia by certain pharmacologic agents seems to indicate that it represents a malfunction of neuronal systems using dopamine, serotonin, glutamate, and γ-aminobutyric acid (GABA) as transmitters or modulators. Genetic studies suggest that susceptibility to schizophrenia is inherited as a complex of variations affecting several genes. According to the neurodevelopmental hypothesis, a brain lesion is present or acquired early in life but does not fully manifest itself until late adolescence or early adulthood, when it triggers abnormalities of neuronal proliferation, axonal outgrowth, cell migration, cell survival, synaptic regression, or myelination. Psychotherapy and behavioral therapy are inconsistently effective in the treatment of schizophrenia. Neuroleptic drugs shorten episodes of acute psychosis, limit the need for institutional care, and reduce the risk of relapse, but their long-term use is associated with serious side effects, particularly tardive dyskinesia. Newer agents such as clozapine, olanzipine, quetiapine, and risperidone are more effective in improving cognitive function and less likely to induce extrapyramidal side effects. Persons with schizophrenia frequently stop taking their medicine, and it is estimated that at any given time only one-half of them are receiving medical treatment or supervision.

---

acute s., a disorder in which the symptoms of s. occur abruptly; they may subside or become chronic over time. SYN acute schizophrenic episode.

ambulatory s., a milder form of s. in which the patient is capable of maintaining himself or herself in society and need not be hospitalized.

catatonic s., s. characterized by marked disturbance, which may involve stupor, negativism, rigidity, excitement, or posturing; sometimes there is rapid alternation between the extremes of excitement and stupor. Associated features include stereotypic behavior, mannerisms, and waxy flexibility; mutism is particularly common.

childhood s., SYN infantile *autism*.

disorganized s., a severe form of s. characterized by the predominance of incoherence, blunted, inappropriate or silly affect, and the absence of systematized delusions. SYN hebephrenic s.

hebephrenic s., SYN disorganized s.

latent s., a preexisting susceptibility for developing overt s. under strong emotional stress.

paranoid s., s. characterized predominantly by delusions of persecution and megalomania.

process s., an obsolete term for those forms of severe schizophrenic disorders in which chronic and progressive biologic conditions in the brain are considered to be the primary cause and in which prognosis is poor as well, with insidious onset at a young age, as contrasted with reactive s.

pseudoneurotic s., s. in which the underlying psychotic process is masked by complaints ordinarily regarded as neurotic.

reactive s., those forms of severe schizophrenic disorders which

are distinguished from process s. by their more acute onset, greater relation to environmental stress, and better prognosis.

residual s., blunted or inappropriate affect, social withdrawal, eccentric behavior, or loose associations, but without prominent psychotic symptoms, as the remains of former psychotic symptoms of s.

simple s., s. characterized by withdrawal, apathy, indifference, and impoverishment of human relationships without overt psychotic features.

schiz·o·phren·ic (skiz-ō-fren′ik, -frē′nik, skit-sō-). Relating to, characteristic of, or suffering from one of the schizophrenias.

schiz·o·to·nia (skiz-ō-tō′nē-ă). Division of the distribution of tone in the muscles. [schizo- + G. *tonos,* tension, tone]

schiz·o·trich·ia (skiz-ō-trik′ē-ă). A splitting of the hairs at their ends. SYN scissura pilorum. [schizo- + G. *thrix,* hair]

Schiz·o·tryp·a·num cru·zi (skiz-ō-trī′pan-ŭm kroo′zī). A distinct generic designation used for *Trypanosoma cruzi,* used frequently by workers in the endemic area of South American trypanosomiasis; also used as a subgeneric designation, i.e., *Trypanosoma (Schizotrypanum) cruzi.* [schizo- + G. *trypanon,* a borer, an auger]

schiz·o·zo·ite (skiz-ō-zō′īt). A merozoite prior to schizogony, as in the exoerythrocytic phase of the development of the *Plasmodium* agent after sporozoite invasion of the hepatocyte and before multiple division. [schizo- + G. *zōon,* animal]

schlamm·fie·ber (shlăm′fē-ber). Name given to an outbreak of leptospirosis near Breslau in Germany thought to have been due to infection with *Leptospira grippotyphosa.*

Schlatter, Carl B., Swiss surgeon, 1864–1934. SEE Osgood-S. *disease.*

Schlemm, Friedrich, German anatomist, 1795–1858. SEE S. *canal.*

Schlesinger, Hermann, Austrian physician, 1868–1934. SEE S. *sign;* Pool-S. *sign.*

schlieren (shlēr′en). SEE schlieren *optics.*

Schmid, Rudi, Swiss-U.S. internist and biochemist, *1922. SEE McArdle-S.-Pearson *disease.*

Schmid, W. SEE S.-Fraccaro *syndrome.*

Schmidel, Kasimir C., German anatomist, 1718–1792. SEE S. *anastomoses,* under *anastomosis.*

Schmidt, Gerhard, U.S. biochemist, *1900. SEE S.-Thannhauser *method.*

Schmidt, Henry D., U.S. anatomist and pathologist, 1823–1888. SEE S.-Lanterman *clefts,* under *cleft, incisures,* under *incisure.*

Schmidt, Johann F.M., German laryngologist, 1838–1907. SEE S. *syndrome.*

Schmidt, Martin Benno, German physician, 1863–1949. SEE S. *syndrome.*

Schmorl, Christian G., German pathologist, 1861–1932. SEE S. *nodule,* ferric-ferricyanide reduction *stain,* picrothionin *stain, jaundice.*

Schneider, C.V., German anatomist, 1614–1680. SEE schneiderian *membrane.*

Schneider, Franz C., German chemist, 1813–1897. SEE S. *carmine.*

Schneider, Kurt, German psychiatrist, 1887–1967.

Schnei·der·sitz (shnī′der-zitz). A typical sitting position with legs crossed in front, exhibited by severely defective patients with phenylketonuria and resembling the position which was commonly attributed to tailors. [Ger.]

Schnitzler, L., 20th century European physician. SEE S. *syndrome.*

Scholander, Per F., Norwegian physiologist, 1905–1980. SEE S. *apparatus;* Roughton-S. *apparatus, syringe.*

Scholz, Willibald, German neurologist, 1889–1971. SEE S. *disease.*

Schönbein, Christian F., German chemist, 1799–1868. SEE S. *test.*

Schönlein, Johann L., German physician, 1793–1864. SEE S. *purpura;* Henoch-S. *purpura.*

Sc

school (skool). A set of beliefs, teachings, methods, etc. [O. E. *scōl*]

biometrical s., a group of British geneticists, followers of Galton and Karl Pearson, whose approach to genetics was quantitative rather than enumerative.

dogmatic s., ancient Greek s. or tradition in medicine whose members were the successors to or followers of Hippocrates; they based their conceptions of disease upon the humoral theory and their practice upon experience and sound reasoning, and were comparatively free from fads, speculative theories, and dogma, which the term dogmatic falsely implies.

dynamic s., a group of theorists founded by G.E. Stahl, who professed the belief that all vital action is the result of an internal force independent of anything external to the body.

hippocratic s., the followers of the teachings of Hippocrates. SEE ALSO dogmatic s.

iatromathematical s., a group of academicians, of whom Descartes was one of the foremost proponents, who maintained that all physiologic processes were the result of physical laws. SYN mechanistic s.

mechanistic s., SYN iatromathematical s.

Schott, Theodor, 1850–1921, German physician in Bad Nauheim. SEE S. *treatment.*

schra·dan (schrā'dan). A potent irreversible organophosphate cholinesterase inhibitor used as an insecticide. It was prepared for potential use as a nerve gas. Poisoning produces a cholinergic crisis which can be fatal. SYN octamethyl pyrophosphoramide. [Gerhard *Schrader*, Ger. chemist, + -an]

Schreger, Christian H.T., German anatomist and chemist, 1768–1833. SEE S. *lines,* under *line;* Hunter-S. *bands,* under *band, lines,* under *line.*

Schridde, Hermann R.A., German pathologist, *1876. SEE S. cancer *hairs,* under *hair.*

Schroeder, Karl L.E., German gynecologist, 1838–1887. SEE S. *operation.*

Schuchardt, Karl A., German surgeon, 1856–1902. SEE S. *operation.*

Schüffner, Wilhelm, German pathologist in Sumatra, 1867–1949. SEE S. *granules,* under *granule, dots,* under *dot.*

Schüller, Karl H.L.A. Max, German surgeon, 1843–1907. SEE S. *ducts,* under *duct.*

Schüller, Artur, Austrian neurologist, *1874. SEE S. *disease, phenomenon, syndrome;* Hand-S.-Christian *disease.*

Schultes, Johann. SEE Scultetus.

Schultz, Arthur R.H., German physician, *1890. SEE S. *reaction, stain.*

Schultz, Werner, German internist, 1878–1947. SEE S.-Charlton *phenomenon, reaction;* S.-Dale *reaction.*

Schultze, Bernhard S., German obstetrician, 1827–1919. SEE S. *fold, mechanism, phantom, placenta.*

Schultze, Max J.S., German histologist and zoologist, 1825–1874. SEE S. *cells,* under *cell, membrane, sign;* comma *bundle* of S.; comma *tract* of S.

Schütz, Erich, German biochemist, *1902. SEE S. *law, rule.*

Schütz, Hugo, 19th century German anatomist. SEE S. *bundle.*

Schwabach, Dagobert, German otologist, 1846–1920. SEE S. *test.*

Schwalbe, Gustav A., German anatomist, 1844–1916. SEE S. *corpuscle, nucleus, ring, spaces,* under *space.*

Schwann, Theodor, German histologist and physiologist, 1810–1882. SEE S. *cells,* under *cell,* cell *unit,* white *substance; sheath* of S.

schwan·no·ma (shwah-nō'mă). A benign, encapsulated neoplasm in which the fundamental component is structurally identical to a syncytium of Schwann cells; the neoplastic cells proliferate within the endoneurium, and the perineurium forms the capsule. The neoplasm may originate from a peripheral or sympathetic nerve, or from various cranial nerves, particularly the eighth nerve; when the nerve is small, it is usually found (if at all) in the capsule of the neoplasm; if the nerve is large, the neurilemoma may develop within the sheath of the nerve, the fibers of which may then spread over the surface of the capsule as the neoplasm enlarges. Microscopically, neurilemoma is composed of combinations of two patterns, Antoni types A and B, either of which may be predominant in various examples of neurilemomas. SEE ALSO neurofibroma. SYN neurilemoma, neuroschwannoma. [Theodor *Schwann* + -oma]

acoustic s., SYN vestibular s.

vestibular s., a benign but life-threatening tumor arising from Schwann cells, usually of the vestibular division of the eighth cranial nerve; produces hearing loss, tinnitus, and vestibular disturbances, early and cerebellar, brainstem, and other cranial nerve signs and increased intracranial pressure in late stages. SYN acoustic neurinoma, acoustic neuroma, acoustic s., acoustic tumor, cerebellopontine angle tumor, eighth nerve tumor.

schwan·no·sis (shwan-nō'sis). A nonneoplastic proliferation of Schwann cells in the perivascular spaces of the spinal cord; seen particularly in older patients, especially those with diabetes mellitus.

Schwartz, Henry G., U.S. neurosurgeon, *1909. SEE S. *tractotomy.*

Schwartz, Oscar, U.S. pediatrician, *1919. SEE S. *syndrome.*

Schweigger-Seidel, Franz, German physiologist, 1834–1871. SEE *sheath* of Schweigger-Seidel.

Schweninger, Ernst, German dermatologist, 1850–1924. SEE S.-Buzzi *anetoderma;* S. *method.*

sci·age (sē-ahzh'). A to-and-fro, sawlike movement of the hand in massage. [Fr. *scie,* saw]

sci·at·ic (sī-at'ik). **1.** Relating to or situated in the neighborhood of the ischium or hip. Ischial or sciatic. SYN ischiadic, ischial, ischiatic. **2.** Relating to sciatica. SYN ischiadicus. [Mediev. L. *sciaticus,* a corruption of G. *ischiadikos,* fr. *ischion,* the hip joint]

sci·at·i·ca (sī-at'i-kă). Pain in the lower back and hip radiating down the back of the thigh into the leg, initially attributed to sciatic nerve dysfunction (hence the term), but now known to usually be due to herniated lumbar disk compromising a nerve root, most commonly the L5 or S1 root. SYN sciatic neuralgia, sciatic neuritis. [see sciatic]

SCID Abbreviation for severe combined *immunodeficiency.*

SCID mice Abbreviation for severe combined immunodeficient mice.

sci·ence (sī'ens). **1.** The branch of knowledge that produces theoretical explanations of natural phenomena based on experiments and observations. **2.** An area of such knowledge that is restricted to explaining a limited class of phenomena. [L. *scientia,* knowledge, fr. *scio,* to know]

scientometrics (sī-en-tō-met'riks). The measurement of scientific output, and the impact of scientific findings, e.g., on public policy. [L. *scientia,* science, knowledge, fr. *scio,* to know, + G. *metron,* measure, + -ics]

scil·la (sil'ă). SYN squill. [G.]

scil·la·ren (sil'lă-ren). A mixture of glycosides, possessing digitalis-like actions, present in squill.

s. A, a crystalline steroidal glycoside (*Scilla maritima*), present in squill that can be hydrolyzed to glucose and proscillaridin A; the latter can be hydrolyzed to rhamnose and the steroid aglycone scillaridin A; has the same actions and uses as digitalis glycosides. SYN transvaalin.

s. B, an amorphous glycosidal fraction obtained from squill, consisting of at least seven cardioactive glycosides: glucoscillaren A, scillipheoside, glucoscillipheoside, scillicryptoside, scilliglaucoside, scillicyanoside, and scillazuroside.

scil·lar·i·cide (sil'ar-ĭ-sīd). A toxic principle from squill used as a rodenticide.

scil·lir·o·side (sil'ir-ō-sīd). Glycoside from red squill, the red variety of *Urginea maritima* (family Liliaceae). Used as a rodenticide.

scin·ti·cis·tern·og·ra·phy (sin'ti-sis-tern-og'ră-fē). Cisternography performed with a radiopharmaceutical and recorded with a radionuclide imaging device.

scin·ti·gram (sin'ti-gram). SYN scintiscan. [L. *scintilla,* spark, + G. *gramma,* something written]

scin·ti·graph·ic (sin'ti-graf'ik). Relating to or obtained by scintigraphy.

scin·tig·ra·phy (sin-tig'ră-fē). A diagnostic procedure consisting of the administration of a radionuclide with an affinity for the organ or tissue of interest, followed by recording the distribution of the radioactivity with a stationary or scanning external scintillation camera. SEE gamma *camera*.

scin·til·la·scope (sin-til'ă-skōp). Obsolete term for scintillation *counter*. [L. *scintilla*, spark, + G. *skopeō*, to observe]

scin·til·la·tion (sin-til-lā'shŭn). **1.** Flashing or sparkling; a subjective sensation as of sparks or flashes of light. **2.** In radiation measurement, the light produced by an ionizing event in a phosphor, as in a crystal or liquid scintillator. SEE ALSO scintillation *counter*. [L. *scintilla*, a spark]

scin·til·la·tor (sin'ti-lā-ter, -tōr). A substance that emits visible light when hit by a subatomic particle or x- or gamma ray. SEE ALSO scintillation *counter*.

liquid s., a liquid with the properties of a scintillator, in which the substance whose radioactivity is to be measured can be dissolved, to be placed in a well counter.

scin·til·lom·e·ter (sin-til-lom'ĕ-ter). SYN scintillation *counter*. [L. *scintilla*, spark, + G. *metron*, measure]

scin·ti·mam·mog·ra·phy (sin'tē-mam-og'ră-fē). Breast imaging that uses a radionuclide for the detection of cancer.

scin·ti·pho·to·graph (sin-ti-fō'tō-graf). The image obtained by scintiphotography; obsolete. SEE ALSO scintiscan.

scin·ti·pho·tog·ra·phy (sin'ti-fō-tog'ră-fē). The process of obtaining a photographic recording of the distribution of an internally administered radiopharmaceutical with the use of a gamma camera; obsolete. SYN scintography.

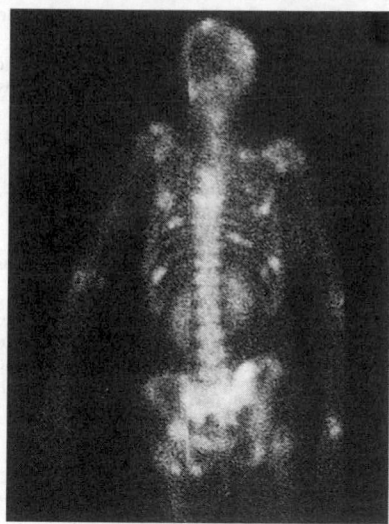

scintiphotography: widespread metastases in a patient with breast cancer

scin·ti·scan (sin'ti-skan). The record obtained by scintigraphy. SEE ALSO scan. SYN photoscan, scintigram.

scin·ti·scan·ner (sin'ti-skan'er). The apparatus used to make a scintiscan.

scint·og·ra·phy (sin-tog'ra-tē). SYN scintiphotography.

sci·on (sī'on). In experimental embryology, an embryonic tissue or part grafted to another embryo of the same or of another species. SEE ALSO chimera. [O. Fr. *sion*, shoot, sprig, fr. L. *seco*, to cut]

scir·rhos·i·ty (skir-os'i-tē, sir-). A scirrhous state or hardness of a tumor.

scir·rhous (skir'us, sir'). Hard; relating to a scirrhus.

scir·rhus (skir'ŭs, sir'). Obsolete term for any fibrous indurated area, especially an indurated carcinoma. [G. *skirrhos*, hard, a hard tumor]

scis·sion (sizh'ŭn). **1.** A separation, division, or splitting, as in fission. **2.** SYN cleavage (2). [L. *scissio*, fr. *scindo*, pp. *scissus*, to cleave]

scis·si·par·i·ty (sis-i-par'i-tē). SYN schizogenesis. [L. *scissio*, cleavage, + *pario*, to bring forth]

scis·sors (siz'erz). An instrument with two blades, moving on a pivot, that cut against each other. SYN shears. [L. *scindo*, pp. *scissus*, to cut]

de Wecker s., a small s. with sharp points for intraocular cutting of the iris and lens capsule.

Smellie s., obsolete term for lance-pointed shears, with external cutting edges, used for fetal craniotomy.

scis·sors-shad·ow. A distorted image seen in mixed astigmatism by retinoscopy.

scis·su·ra, pl. **scis·su·rae** (si-soo'ră, -rē). **1.** Cleft or fissure. **2.** A splitting. SYN scissure. [L.]

s. pilo'rum, SYN schizotrichia.

scis·sure (sish'oor). SYN scissura.

scler-. SEE sclero-.

scle·ra, pl. **scle·ras**, **scler·ae** (sklēr'ă, -ăz, -ē) [TA]. A portion of the fibrous layer forming the outer envelope of the eyeball, except for its anterior sixth, which is the cornea. SYN sclerotic coat, sclerotica, tunica albuginea oculi, tunica sclerotica. [Mod. L. fr. G. *sklēros*, hard]

blue s., appearance of the uveal tissue through a thin s. seen in a number of conditions including myopia, buphthalmos, scleral *staphyloma*, Ehlers-Danlos *syndrome*, Marfan *syndrome*, *osteogenesis* imperfecta, Paget *disease*, and Pierre Robin *syndrome*.

scler·ad·e·ni·tis (sklēr'ad-ĕ-nī'tis). Inflammatory induration of a gland. [scler- + G. *adēn*, gland, + *-itis*, inflammation]

scle·ral (sklēr'ăl). Relating to the sclera. SYN sclerotic (2).

scle·ra·tog·e·nous (sklēr-ă-toj'ĕ-nŭs). SYN sclerogenous.

scle·rec·ta·sia (sklēr-ek-tā'zē-ă). Localized bulging of the sclera. SYN scleral ectasia. [scler- + G. *ektasis*, an extension]

partial s., partial protrusion of a portion of the sclera, typically seen in severe myopia. SEE staphyloma.

total s., uniform stretching of the entire sclera, typically seen in buphthalmos.

scle·rec·to·my (sklĕ-rek'tō-mē). **1.** Excision of a portion of the sclera. **2.** Removal of the fibrous adhesions formed in chronic otitis media. [scler- + G. *ektomē*, excision]

scle·re·de·ma (sklēr-e-dē'mă). Hard nonpitting edema of the skin of the dorsal aspect of the upper body and extremities, giving a waxy appearance and no sharp demarcation; seen in diabetics and in s. adultorum. [scler- + G. *oidēma*, a swelling (edema)]

s. adulto'rum, a benign spreading induration of the skin and subcutaneous tissue, possibly streptoccocal in origin, that may follow a febrile illness, with nonpitting thickening and induration of the skin by collagen and mucin deposit appearing first on the head and neck and extending over the trunk; a misnomer, because the disease is not restricted to adults. SYN Buschke disease.

scle·re·ma (sklĕ-rē'mă). Induration of subcutaneous fat. [scler- + edema]

s. neonato'rum, s. appearing at birth or in early infancy, usually in premature and hypothermic infants, as sharply demarcated and yellowish white indurated plaques that usually involve the cheeks, buttocks, shoulders, and calves; subcutaneous fat has a high proportion of saturated fatty acids; microscopically, there is thickening of interlobular fibrous tissue and formation of triglyceride crystals and foreign body giant cells; prognosis is poor for widespread lesions, but localized lesions may resolve slowly over a period of many months.

scle·ren·ceph·a·ly, **scle·ren·ce·pha·lia** (sklēr-en-sef'ă-lē, -en-sĕ-fā'lē-ă). Sclerosis and shrinkage of the brain substance. [scler- + G. *enkephalos*, brain]

scle·ri·tis (sklĕ-rī'tis). Inflammation of the sclera.

anterior s., inflammation of the sclera adjacent to the cornea.

anular s., an often protracted inflammation of the anterior portion of the sclera, forming a ring around the corneoscleral limbus.

brawny s., a gelatinous-appearing swelling surrounding, and with a tendency to involve the periphery of, the cornea. SYN gelatinous s.

deep s., severe inflammation of the sclera, with involvement of the underlying uvea.

gelatinous s., SYN brawny s.

malignant s., progressive inflammation of the anterior sclera and adjacent choroid with associated uveitis.

necrotizing s., fibrinoid degeneration and necrosis of the sclera.

nodular s., firm, immobile, single or multiple areas of localized s.

posterior s., inflammation, often monocular, of the sclera adjacent to the optic nerve, with frequent extension to the retina and choroid.

⊘**sclero-, scler-.** Hardness (induration), sclerosis, relationship to sclera. [G. *skleros,* hard]

scle·ro·at·ro·phy (sklēr-ō-at′rō-fē). SYN sclerotylosis.

scle·ro·blas·te·ma (sklēr-ō-blas-tē′mă). The embryonic tissue entering into the formation of bone. [sclero- + G. *blastēma,* sprout]

scle·ro·cho·roi·dal (sklēr-ō-kō-roy′dăl). Relating to both the sclera and the choroid.

scle·ro·cho·roid·i·tis (sklēr-ō-kō-roy-dī′tis). Inflammation of the sclera and choroid.

s. ante′rior, a secondary inflammation of the sclera by an extension of a process from the uvea.

s. poste′rior, SYN posterior *staphyloma.*

scle·ro·con·junc·ti·val (sklēr′ō-kon-jŭngk-tī′văl). Relating to the sclera and the conjunctiva.

scle·ro·cor·nea (sklēr-ō-kōr′nē-ă). **1.** The cornea and sclera regarded as forming together the hard outer coat of the eye, the fibrous tunic of the eye. **2.** A congenital anomaly in which the whole or part of the cornea is opaque and resembles the sclera; other ocular abnormalities are frequently present.

scle·ro·dac·ty·ly, scle·ro·dac·tyl·ia (sklēr-ō-dak′ti-lē, -dak-til′ē-ă). SYN acrosclerosis. [sclero- + G. *daktylos,* finger or toe]

▣**scle·ro·der·ma** (sklēr-ō-der′mă). Thickening and induration of the skin caused by new collagen formation, with atrophy of pilosebaceous follicles; either a manifestation of progressive systemic sclerosis or localized (morphea). SEE systemic *sclerosis,* morphea. SYN systemic s., systemic sclerosis (2). [sclero- + G. *derma,* skin]

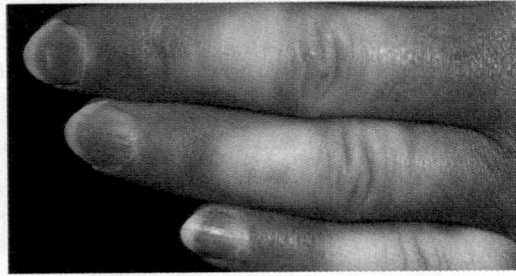

scleroderma: early stage

linear s., localized s. with band-like lesions of skin with induration, atrophy, hyper- or hypopigmentation, which may be disfiguring with extension into underlying tissues and joint contractures. Involvement of the forehead and scalp has been called coup de sabre (q.v.). SYN morphea linearis.

localized s., SYN morphea.

progressive familial s. [MIM*181750], a syndrome characterized by calcinosis cutis, Raynaud phenomenon, sclerodactyly, and telangiectasia; usually due to s.; autosomal dominant form of progressive systemic sclerosis.

systemic s., SYN scleroderma.

scle·ro·der·ma·tous (sklēr-ō-der′mă-tŭs). Marked by, or resembling, scleroderma.

scle·rog·e·nous, scle·ro·gen·ic (skle-roj′ĕ-nŭs, sklēr-ō-jen′ik). Producing hard or sclerotic tissue; causing sclerosis. SYN scleratogenous. [sclero- + G. *-gen,* producing]

scle·roid (sklēr′oyd). Indurated or sclerotic, of unusually firm texture, leathery, or of scarlike texture. SYN sclerosal, sclerous. [sclero- + G. *eidos,* resemblance]

scle·ro·i·ri·tis (sklēr′ō-ī-rī′tis). Inflammation of both sclera and iris.

scle·ro·ker·a·ti·tis (sklēr′ō-ker-ă-tī′tis). Inflammation of the sclera and cornea. [sclero- + G. *keras,* horn]

scle·ro·ker·a·to·i·ri·tis (sklēr-ō-ker′ă-tō-ī-rī′tis). Inflammation of sclera, cornea, and iris.

scle·ro·ma (skle-rō′mă). A circumscribed indurated focus of granulation tissue in the skin or mucous membrane. [G. *sklērōma,* an induration]

respiratory s., rhinoscleroma in which the lesion involves the mucous membrane of the greater part or all of the upper respiratory tract.

scle·ro·ma·la·cia (sklēr′ō-mă-lā′shē-ă). Degenerative thinning of the sclera, occurring in persons with rheumatoid arthritis and other collagen disorders. [sclero- + G. *malakia,* a softening]

scle·ro·mere (sklēr′ō-mēr). **1.** Any metamere of the skeleton, such as a vertebral segment. **2.** Caudal half of a sclerotome. [sclero- + G. *meros,* part]

scle·rom·e·ter (sklē-rom′ĕ-ter). A device for determining the density or hardness of any substance. [sclero- + G. *metron,* measure]

scle·ro·myx·e·de·ma (sklēr′ō-mik-se-dē′mă). Generalized lichen myxedematosus with diffuse thickening of the skin underlying the papules.

scle·ro·nych·ia (sklēr-ō-nik′ē-ă). Induration and thickening of the nails. [sclero- + G. *onyx,* nail, + *-ia,* condition]

scle·ro·o·o·pho·ri·tis (sklēr′ō-ō-of′ō-rī′tis). Inflammatory induration of the ovary. [sclero- + Mod. L. *oophoron,* ovary + G. *-itis,* inflammation]

scle·roph·thal·mia (sklēr-of-thal′mē-ă). An abnormality in which most of the normally transparent cornea resembles the opaque sclera. [sclero- + G. *ophthalmos,* eye]

scle·ro·plas·ty (sklēr′ō-plas-tē). Plastic surgery of the sclera. [sclero- + G. *plastos,* formed]

scle·ro·pro·tein (sklēr-ō-prō′tēn). SYN albuminoid (3). SEE ALSO fibrous *protein.*

scle·ro·sal (sklĕ-rō′săl). SYN scleroid.

scle·ro·sant (sklēr′ō-sant). An injectable irritant used to treat varices by producing thrombi in them.

scle·rose (sklĕ-rōz′). To harden; to undergo sclerosis.

scle·ro·sis, pl. **scle·ro·ses** (sklĕ-rō′sis, -sēz). **1.** SYN induration (2). **2.** In neuropathy, induration of nervous and other structures by a hyperplasia of the interstitial fibrous or glial connective tissue. [G. *sklērōsis,* hardness]

Alzheimer s., hyaline degeneration of the medium and smaller blood vessels of the brain.

amyotrophic lateral s. (ALS), a fatal degenerative disease involving the corticobulbar, corticospinal, and spinal motor neurons, manifested by progressive weakness and wasting of muscles innervated by the affected neurons; fasciculations and cramps commonly occur. The disorder is 90–95% sporadic in nature (although a number of cases are inherited as an autosomal dominant trait [MIM*105400]), affects adults (typically, older adults), and usually is fatal within 2–5 years of onset. It is the most common subgroup of motor neuron disease, and the only one manifested by a combination of upper and lower abnormalities. Variants include: 1) progressive bulbar palsy, in which isolated or predominant lower brainstem motor involvement occurs; 2) primary lateral sclerosis, in which only upper motor neuron abnormalities are seen; and 3) progressive spinal muscle atrophy, in which only lower motor neuron dysfunction is noted. SYN Aran-Duchenne disease, Charcot disease, Duchenne-Aran disease, Lou Gehrig disease, progressive muscular atrophy, progressive spinal amyotrophy.

arterial s., SYN arteriosclerosis.

arteriocapillary s., arteriosclerosis, especially of the finer vessels.

arteriolar s., SYN arteriolosclerosis.

bone s., SYN eburnation.

Canavan s., SYN Canavan *disease.*

central areolar choroidal s., SYN areolar *choroidopathy.*

combined s., SYN subacute combined *degeneration* of the spinal cord.

diffuse infantile familial s., SYN globoid cell *leukodystrophy.*

disseminated s., SYN multiple s.

endocardial s., SYN endocardial *fibrosis.*

glomerular s., SYN glomerulosclerosis.

hippocampal s., a loss of cortical neurons and a reactive astrocytosis in the hippocampal regions of some persons with epilepsy.

idiopathic hypercalcemic s. of infants, SEE idiopathic *hypercalcemia* of infants.

insular s., SYN multiple s.

laminar cortical s., a degeneration of nerve fibers in the corona radiata in a laminar pattern.

lateral spinal s., SYN primary lateral s.

lobar s., SYN Pick *atrophy.*

mantle s., a common cerebral lesion in the palsied states of early life characterized by nodular cortical atrophy.

menstrual s., SYN physiologic s.

Mönckeberg s., SYN Mönckeberg *arteriosclerosis.*

∎multiple s. (MS), common demyelinating disorder of the central nervous system, causing patches of sclerosis (plaques) in the brain and spinal cord; occurs primarily in young adults, and has protean clinical manifestations, depending upon the location and size of the plaque; typical symptoms include visual loss, diplopia, nystagmus, dysarthria, weakness, paresthesias, bladder abnormalities, and mood alterations; characteristically, the plaques are "separated in time and space" and clinically the symptoms show exacerbations and remissions. SYN disseminated s., insular s.

nodular s., SYN atherosclerosis.

nuclear s., increased refractivity of the central portion of the lens of the eye. SEE nuclear *cataract.*

ovulational s., SYN physiologic s.

physiologic s., a slowly progressive s. in the walls of the ovarian arteries that commences after puberty. SYN menstrual s., ovulational s.

posterior s., SYN tabetic *neurosyphilis.*

posterior spinal s., SYN tabetic *neurosyphilis.*

primary lateral s., considered by many to be a subgroup of motor neuron disease; a slowly progressive degenerative disorder of the motor neurons of the cerebral cortex, resulting in widespread weakness on an upper motor neuron basis; spasticity, hyperreflexia, and Babinski signs are present, but not fasciculation potentials, nor any electrodiagnostic evidence of a lower motor neuron lesion. SYN lateral spinal s.

systemic s., (1) a systemic disease characterized by formation of hyalinized and thickened collagenous fibrous tissue, with thickening of the skin and adhesion to underlying tissues (especially of the hands and face), dysphagia due to loss of peristalsis and submucosal fibrosis of the esophagus, dyspnea due to pulmonary fibrosis, myocardial fibrosis, and renal vascular changes resembling those of malignant hypertension; Raynaud phenomenon, atrophy of the soft tissues, and osteoporosis of the distal phalanges (acrosclerosis), sometimes with gangrene at the ends of the digits, are common findings. The term progressive systemic s. is commonly used and is appropriate for cases with initially widespread skin involvement including the trunk. However, when skin involvement is limited to the distal extremities and face, there is often prolonged delay in appearance of visceral manifestations. SEE ALSO CREST *syndrome;* **(2)** SYN scleroderma.

tuberous s. [MIM*191100], phacomatosis characterized by the formation of multisystem hamartomas producing seizures, mental retardation, and angiofibromas of the face; the cerebral and retinal lesions are glial nodules; other skin lesions are hypopigmented macules, shagreen patches, and periungual fibromas; autosomal dominant inheritance with variable expression, caused by mutation in either the tuberous sclerosis gene (TSC1) on chromosome 9q or TSC2 on 16p. SYN Bourneville disease, epiloia.

unicellular s., a growth of fibrous tissue between and isolating the individual cells of a part.

valvular s., fibrosis, often with calcification of valves, considered to be an aging change and not due to primary valvular disease.

vascular s., SYN arteriosclerosis.

s. of white matter, SYN leukodystrophy.

scle·ro·ste·no·sis (sklēr-ō-ste-nō′sis). Induration and contraction of the tissues. [sclero- + G. *stenōsis,* a narrowing]

Scle·ros·to·ma (sklĕ-ros′tō-mă). A former generic name for strongyle (hookworm) nematodes and for trichostrongyle worms of horses; now replaced by other genera but still used as a collective term for this group. Species include *S. duodenale (Ancylostoma duodenale)* and *S. syngamus (Syngamus trachea)* [sclero- + G. *stoma,* mouth]

scle·ros·to·my (sklĕ-ros′tō-mē). Surgical perforation of the sclera, as for the relief of glaucoma. [sclero- + G. *stoma,* mouth]

scle·ro·ther·a·py (sklēr-ō-thār′ă-pē). Treatment involving the injection of a sclerosing solution into vessels or tissues. SYN sclerosing therapy.

scle·ro·thrix (sklēr′ō-thriks). Induration and brittleness of the hair. SYN sclerotrichia. [sclero- + G. *thrix,* hair]

scle·rot·ic (sklĕ-rot′ik). **1.** Relating to or characterized by sclerosis. **2.** SYN scleral.

scle·rot·i·ca (sklĕ-rot′i-kă). SYN sclera. [Mod. L. *scleroticus,* hard]

scle·ro·ti·um, pl. **scle·ro·tia** (sklĕ-rō′shē-ŭm, -shē-ă). **1.** In fungi, a variably sized resting body composed of a hardened mass of hyphae with or without host tissue, usually with a darkened rind, from which fruit bodies, stromata, conidiophores, or mycelia may develop. **2.** The hardened resting condition of the plasmodium of Myxomycetes.

scle·ro·tome (sklēr′ō-tōm). **1.** A knife used in sclerotomy. **2.** The group of mesenchymal cells emerging from the ventromedial part of a somite and migrating toward the notochord. Sclerotomal cells from adjacent somites become merged in intersomitically located masses that are the primordia of the centra of the vertebrae. [sclero- + G. *tomē,* a cutting]

scle·rot·o·my (sklĕ-rot′ō-mē). An incision through the sclera. [sclero- + G. *tomē,* incision]

anterior s., incision into the anterior chamber of the eye.

posterior s., incision through the sclera into the vitreous humor.

scle·ro·trich·i·a (sklēr-ō-trik′ē-ă). SYN sclerothrix.

scle·ro·ty·lo·sis (sklēr′ō-tī-lō′sis) [MIM*181600]. Atrophic fibrosis of the skin, hypoplasia of the nails, and palmoplantar keratoderma; associated with skin and gastrointestinal cancers; autosomal dominant inheritance. SYN scleroatrophy. [sclero- + G. *tylōsis,* the process of becoming callous]

scle·rous (sklēr′ŭs). SYN scleroid. [G. *sklēros,* hard]

SCM Abbreviation for sternocleidomastoid *(muscle).*

scol·e·ces (skō′le-sez). Plural of scolex.

sco·le·ci·a·sis (skō-lē-sī′ă-sis). Infection of the intestine by larvae of lepidopterans (moths and butterflies). [G. *skōlēx,* worm, + *-iasis,* condition]

sco·le·ci·form (skō-lē′si-fōrm). SYN scolecoid.

sco·le·coid (skō′lē-koyd). **1.** Resembling a tapeworm scolex. **2.** Wormlike. SEE ALSO lumbricoid (1), vermiform. SYN scoleciform. [G. *skōlēkoeidēs,* fr. *skōlēx,* worm, + *eidos,* appearance]

sco·le·col·o·gy (skō-lē-kol′ŏ-jē). SYN helminthology. [G. *skōlēx,* worm, + *logos,* study]

sco·lex, pl. **scol·e·ces, scol·i·ces** (skō′leks, skō′le-sēz, skō′li-sēz). The head or anterior end of a tapeworm attached by suckers, and frequently by rostellar hooks, to the wall of the intestine; it is formed within the hydatid cyst in *Echinococcus,* within a cysticercus in *Taenia,* a cysticercoid in *Hymenolepis,* or by a plerocercoid, as in *Diphyllobothrium latum.* The form of the s. varies greatly, the most familiar being rounded or club-shaped with four circular muscular suckers and an armed or unarmed rostellum, or a spatulate flattened s. with a pair of slitlike suckers (bothria) and no rostellum, as in *Diphyllobothrium* and its allies. Other forms have complex leaflike, cup-shaped, or fimbriated shapes, or re-

SC

tractile, multiply spined proboscides. These varied forms characterize the orders of cestodes, which are particularly well developed as parasites of sharks and skates or rays. [G. *skōlēx*, a worm]

sco·li·o·ky·pho·sis (skō′lē-ō-kī-fō′sis). SYN kyphoscoliosis. [G. *scolios*, curved, + *kyphōsis*, kyphosis]

sco·li·om·e·ter (skō-lē-om′ĕ-ter). An instrument for measuring curves, especially those in lateral curvature of the spine. [G. *skolios*, curved, + *metron*, measure]

sco·li·o·sis (skō-lē-ō′sis) [TA]. Abnormal lateral and rotational curvature of the vertebral column. Depending on the etiology, there may be one curve, or primary and secondary compensatory curves; s. may be "fixed" as a result of muscle and/or bone deformity or "mobile" as a result of unequal muscle contraction. [G. *skoliōsis*, a crookedness]

   coxitic s., s. in the lumbar spine resulting from tilting of the pelvis in the presence of hip disease.

   empyemic s., s. due to retraction of one side of the chest following an empyema.

   habit s., s. supposedly due to habitual standing or sitting in an improper position.

   myopathic s., lateral curvature due to weakness of the spinal muscles, as in poliomyelitis.

   ocular s., ophthalmic s., s. supposed to be due to head tilting, caused by ophthalmological dysfunction.

   osteopathic s., lateral curvature of the spine due to vertebral disease.

   paralytic s., lateral curvature of the spine due to paralysis of spinal muscles.

   rachitic s., s. occurring as a result of rickets.

   sciatic s., s. caused by asymmetric spasm of spinal muscles usually associated with sciatica, usually presenting as a list toward one side.

   static s., lateral curvature of the spine due to inequality in length of the legs.

sco·li·ot·ic (skō′lē-ot′ik). Relating to or suffering from scoliosis.

sco·li·o·tone (skō′lē-ō-tōn). An apparatus for stretching the spine and reducing the curve in scoliosis. [G. *skolios*, crooked, + *tonos*, tension]

Scol·o·pen·dra (skō-lō-pen′dră). A genus of centipedes characterized by 21–23 pairs of legs. Common U.S. species are *S. heros* (the Western house centipede) and *S. morsitans*. [Mod. L., fr. G. *skōlopendra*, multipede]

s-cone. Short wavelength sensitive c. (blue c.).

scoop (skoop). A narrow, spoonlike instrument for extracting the contents of cavities or cysts. [A.S. *skopa*]

△**-scope.** Denoting an instrument for viewing, but extended to include other methods of examination (e.g., stethoscope). [G. *skopeō*, to view]

sco·pine (skō′pēn). Scopolamine less the tropic acid side chain, i.e., 6,7-epoxytropine, or 6,7-epoxy-3-hydroxytropane.

sco·pol·a·mine (skō-pol′ă-mēn, -min). An alkaloid found in the leaves and seeds of *Hyoscyamus niger*, *Duboisia myoproides*, *Scopolia japonica*, *Scopolia carniolica*, *Atropa belladonna*, and other solanaceous plants; the 6,7-epoxide of atropine, i.e., 6,7-epoxytropine tropate. Exerts anticholinergic actions similar to atropine; thought to have greater central nervous system effects; useful in preventing motion sickness. SYN hyoscine.

   s. hydrobromide, anticholinergic action is similar to that of atropine. SYN hyoscine hydrobromide.

   s. methylbromide, a quaternary ammonium derivative of s.; used when spasmolytic or antisecretory effects are desired.

sco·po·lia (skō-pō′lē-ă). The dried rhizome and roots of *Scopolia carniolica* (family Solanaceae), a herb of Austria and neighboring countries of Europe; it resembles belladonna in pharmacologic action. [G.A. *Scopoli*, Italian naturalist, 1723–1788]

   S. japon'ica, Japanese belladonna, the leaves, root, and seeds of which contain scopolamine.

sco·po·line (skō′pō-lēn). A decomposition product of scopolamine, and an isomer of scopine, in that the epoxy and hydroxyl groups are in different locations.

sco·pom·e·ter (skō-pom′ĕ-ter). A device for determining the

density of a precipitate by the degree of translucency of a fluid containing it. SEE ALSO nephelometer. [G. *skopeō*, to view, + *metron*, measure]

sco·po·phil·ia (skō-pō-fil′ē-ă). SYN voyeurism. [G. *skopeō*, to view, + *philos*, fond]

sco·po·pho·bia (skō-pō-fō′bē-ă). Morbid dread of being stared at. [G. *skopeō*, to view, + *phobos*, fear]

Scop·u·lar·i·op·sis (skō′pū-lar-ē-op′sis). A genus of filamentous fungi rarely pathogenic for humans; several species have been implicated in onychomycosis, ulcerating granuloma, and other "mycotic" entities. *Penicillium*-like, it is common in nature and generally a contaminant in laboratory cultures of human tissues. [Mod. L. *scopula*, a small broom, + G. *opsis*, appearance]

△**-scopy.** An action or activity involving the use of in instrument for viewing. [G. *skopeō*, to view]

scor·bu·tic (skōr-bū′tik). Relating to, suffering from, or resembling scurvy (scorbutus).

scor·bu·ti·gen·ic (skōr-bū-ti-jen′ik). Scurvy-producing.

scor·bu·tus (skōr-bū′tŭs). SYN scurvy. [Mediev. L. form of Teutonic *schorbuyck*, scurvy]

scor·di·ne·ma (skōr′di-nē′mă). Heaviness of the head with yawning and stretching, occurring as a prodrome of an infectious disease. [G. *skordinēma*, yawning]

score (skōr). An evaluation, usually expressed numerically, of status, achievement, or condition in a given set of circumstances. [M. E. *scor*, notch, tally]

   APACHE s., *A*cute *p*hysiology *a*nd *c*hronic *h*ealth *e*valuation. The most widely used method of assessing the severity of illness in acutely ill patients in intensive care units.

   Apgar s., evaluation of a newborn infant's physical status by assigning numerical values (0–2) to each of 5 criteria: 1) heart rate, 2) respiratory effort, 3) muscle tone, 4) response stimulation, and 5) skin color; a score of 8–10 indicates the best possible condition.

Apgar score				
after 60 seconds	**score**	**0**	**1**	**2**
heart rate	....	absent	under 100	over 100
respiratory effort	....	absent	slow, irregular	good (screams)
muscle tone	....	limp	good in limbs	active movement
reaction to nasal catheter	....	none	makes grimaces	coughing or sneezing
skin color	....	pale	rosy trunk, blue extremities	rosy
score	_____	(total points: 8–10 is normal)		

   Bishop s., system to determine the inducibility of the cervix in a pregnant patient, based on dilation, effacement, station, and cervical consistency and position.

   discrimination s., the percentage of words that a subject can repeat correctly from a list of phonetically balanced words presented at 25–40 dB above the speech reception threshold.

   Dubowitz s., a method of clinical assessment of gestational age in the newborn that includes neurological criteria for the infant's maturity and other physical criteria to determine the gestational age of the infant; useful from birth to 5 days of life.

   Gleason s., SEE Gleason tumor *grade*.

   Jarman s., index of social and medical deprivation, used mainly by family doctors, especially in the U.K.

   Logistic Organ Dysfunction S., an evaluation method used in intensive care that enumerates the level of dysfunction of each organ system and among organ systems; includes evaluation of degree of dysfunction of cardiovascular, hepatic, hematologic, pulmonary, renal, and nervous systems.

raw s., the actual s., measurement, or value obtained before any statistics are applied to it. Cf. standard s.

recovery s., a number expressing the condition of an infant at various stipulated intervals greater than 1 min after birth and based on the same features assessed by the Apgar s. at 60 seconds after birth.

standard s., a statistically referenced or derived s. representing the deviation of a raw s. from its mean in standard deviation units.

symptom s., American Urological Association's scoring system to evaluate prostatic obstruction.

scor·pi·on (skōr′pē-on). A member of the order Scorpionida; includes the devil s., *Vejovis*, and the hairy s., *Hadrurus*. [G. *skorpios*]

Scor·pi·on·i·da (skōr-pē-on′i-dă). The scorpions; an order of venomous, predaceous, arachnid arthropods characterized by a distinctly segmented bony abdomen terminating in a sharply recurved stinging spine equipped with a poison gland; causes a severely painful but rarely fatal sting. North American genera include *Centruroides*, *Hadrurus*, and *Vejovis*. [Mod. L.]

scoto-. Darkness. [G. *skotos*]

scot·o·chro·mo·gens (skō′tō-krō′mō-jenz). SYN Runyon group II *mycobacteria*. [scoto- + G. *chrōma*, color, + -gen, producing]

scot·o·graph (skō′tō-graf). An appliance for aiding one to write in straight lines in the dark or for aiding the blind to write, as used by the historian W.H. Prescott. SYN noctograph. [scoto- + G. *graphō*, to write]

sco·to·ma, pl. **sco·to·ma·ta** (skō-tō′mă, skō-tō′mă-tă). **1.** An isolated area of varying size and shape, within the visual field, in which vision is absent or depressed. **2.** A blind spot in psychological awareness. [G. *skotōma*, vertigo, fr. *skotos*, darkness]

absolute s., a s. in which there is no perception of light.

anular s., a circular s. surrounding the center of the field of vision. SEE ring s.

arcuate s., a s. extending from the blind spot and arching into the nasal field following the lines of retinal nerve fibers.

Bjerrum s., a comet-shaped s., occurring in glaucoma, attached at the temporal end to the blind spot or separated from it by a narrow gap; the defect widens as it extends above and nasally curves around the fixation spot, and then extends downward to end exactly at the nasal horizontal meridian. SYN Bjerrum sign, sickle s.

cecocentral s., a s. involving the optic disk area (blind spot) and the papillomacular fibers; there are three forms: 1) the cecocentral defect, which extends from the blind spot toward or into the fixation area; 2) angioscotoma; 3) glaucomatous nerve-fiber bundle s., due to involvement of nerve-fiber bundles at the edge of the optic disk. SEE ALSO Bjerrum s., Rønne nasal *step*.

central s., a s. involving the fixation point.

color s., an area of depressed color vision in the visual field.

flittering s., SYN scintillating s.

glaucomatous nerve-fiber bundle s., SEE cecocentral s.

hemianopic s., a s. involving half of the central field.

mental s., absence of insight into, or inability to comprehend, items relative to a subject whose content is highly emotional to the individual. SYN blind spot (2).

negative s., a s. that is not ordinarily perceived, but is detected only on examination of the visual field.

paracentral s., a s. adjacent to the fixation point.

pericentral s., a s. that surrounds the fixation point more or less symmetrically.

peripheral s., a s. outside of the central 30 degrees of the visual field.

physiologic s., the negative s. in the visual field, corresponding to the optic disk. SYN blind spot (1).

positive s., a s. that is perceived as a black spot within the field of vision.

quadrantic s., a s. involving a quarter segment of the central visual field.

relative s., a s. in which there is visual depression but not complete loss of light perception.

ring s., an annular area of blindness in the visual field surround-

ing the fixation point in pigmentary degeneration of the retina and in glaucoma.

scintillating s., a localized area of blindness edged by brilliantly colored shimmering lights (teichopsia); usually a prodromal symptom of migraine. SEE ALSO fortification *spectrum*. SYN flittering s.

Seidel s., a form of Bjerrum s. SEE ALSO Seidel *sign*.

sickle s., SYN Bjerrum s.

zonular s., a curved s. not corresponding to the path of retinal nerve fibers.

sco·to·ma·ta (skō-tō′mă-tă). Plural of scotoma.

sco·tom·a·tous (skō-tō′mă-tŭs). Relating to scotoma.

sco·tom·e·ter (skō-tom′ĕ-ter). An instrument for determining the size, shape, and intensity of a scotoma.

sco·tom·e·try (skō-tom′ĕ-trē). The plotting and measuring of a scotoma. [scoto- + G. *metron*, measure]

scot·o·phil·ia (skō-tō-fil′ē-ă). SYN nyctophilia. [scoto- + G. *philos*, fond]

scot·o·pho·bia (skō-tō-fō′bē-ă). SYN nyctophobia. [scoto- + G. *phobos*, fear]

sco·to·pia (skō-tō′pē-ă). SYN scotopic *vision*. [scoto- + G. *opsis*, vision]

sco·top·ic (skō-tō′pik, -top′ik). Referring to low illumination to which the eye is dark-adapted. SEE scotopic *vision*.

sco·top·sin (skō-top′sin). The protein moiety of the pigment in the rods of the retina.

sco·tos·co·py (skō-tos′kŏ-pē). SYN retinoscopy. [scoto- + G. *skopeō*, to view]

Scott, Charles I., Jr., U.S. pediatrician, *1934. SEE Aarskog-S. *syndrome*.

Scott, Henry William Jr., U.S. surgeon, *1916. SEE S. *operation*.

Scott-Wilson, H., English scientist. SEE Scott-Wilson *reagent*.

scot·ty dog (scot′tē dawg). The fancied appearance of the articular facets on oblique radiographs of the lumbar spine; the neck of the s. d. is the pars interarticularis, site of the most common defect in spondylolysis.

scrape. SYN scraping.

scrap·ie (skrap′ē, skrā′pē). A communicable spongiform encephalopathy of the central nervous system of sheep and goats caused by a prion and characterized by a very long incubation period followed by pruritus, abnormalities of gait, and invariably death; it resembles Creutzfeldt-Jakob disease and kuru in humans. [from scraping by affected animals against objects to relieve itching]

scrap·ing (skrāp′ing). A specimen scraped from a lesion or specific site, for cytologic examination. SEE ALSO smear. SYN scrape.

screen (skrēn). **1.** A sheet of any substance used to shield an object from any influence, such as heat, light, x-rays, etc. **2.** A sheet upon which an image is projected. **3.** Formerly, to make a fluoroscopic examination. **4.** In psychoanalysis, concealment, as one image or memory concealing another. SEE ALSO screen *memory*. **5.** To examine, evaluate; to process a group to select or separate certain individuals from it. **6.** A thin layer of crystals that converts x-rays to light photons to expose film; used in a cassette to produce radiographic images on film. [Fr. *écran*]

Bjerrum s., SYN tangent s.

s.-film contact, the closeness and uniformity with which the x-ray film in a cassette lies against the s. (6). Image resolution is dependent on this property.

fluorescent s., a s. coated with fluorescent crystals such as the calcium tungstate used in the fluoroscope.

Hess s., a s. used in the measurement of ocular deviation.

intensifying s., a s. (6) used in radiography.

multiple marker s., use of two or more markers in the maternal serum to determine the relative risk of an abnormal fetus. SEE ALSO triple s.

rare-earth s., an intensifying s. (6) made of a rare-earth oxide phosphor, more efficient than calcium tungstate, especially at the higher kilovoltages used in modern radiography.

tangent s., a flat, usually black surface used to measure the central 30 degrees of the field of vision. SYN Bjerrum s.

SC

triple s., test of maternal serum α-fetoprotein, chorionic gonadotropin, and unconjugated estrogen for indications of increased risk of fetal abnormality, especially trisomy 21.

vestibular s., a s. made of acrylic resin that covers the labial or buccal surfaces of one or both dental arches; used to treat oral habits and to stimulate tooth movement by using perioral muscle force.

screen·ing (skrēn′ing). **1.** To screen (5). **2.** Examination of a group of usually asymptomatic individuals to detect those with a high probability of having a given disease, typically by means of an inexpensive diagnostic test. **3.** In the mental health professions, initial patient evaluation that includes medical and psychiatric history, mental status evaluation, and diagnostic formulation to determine the patient's suitability for a particular treatment modality.

carrier s., indiscriminate examination of members of a population to detect heterozygotes for serious disorders and counsel about the risks of marriages with other carriers, and by antenatal diagnosis where a married couple are both carriers; often sacrifices specificity to sensitivity and is most effectively applied to populations known to be at high risk.

cytologic s., a s. for the detection of early disease, usually cancer, through microscopic examination of a cellular specimen by inspecting each cell and structure present, usually at ×100 magnification with a mechanical stage, so that all areas are screened; the findings are evaluated and significant abnormalities are flagged (e.g., by dotting the cover slip) for further evaluation by a cytopathologist. This s. is usually performed by a cytotechnologist, but at times is done by automated machine prescreening.

familial s., s. directed at close relatives of probands with diseases that may lie latent, as in age-dependent dominant traits, or that may involve risk to progeny, as X-linked traits.

mass s., examination of a large population to detect the manifestation of a disease in order to initiate treatment or prevent spread, as part of a public health campaign.

multiphasic s., the routine use of multiple tests, usually biochemical, for the purpose of detecting disease at a preventable or curable stage.

neonatal s., testing of newborns for the detection of preventable or curable disease or for diagnosis of genetic disease.

prenatal s., s. for the detection of fetal disease, usually by ultrasound examination or by testing amnionic fluid obtained by amniocentesis. Other s. techniques include testing maternal serum and placental biopsy.

screw (skroo). A helically grooved cylinder for fastening two objects together or for adjusting the position of an object resting on one end of the s.

afterloading s., a device for setting the length at which a contracting muscle encounters an afterload.

screw-worm (skroo′werm). The larva of the botfly, *Cochliomyia hominivorax,* and other similar forms that cause human and animal myiasis.

primary s.-w., an obligatory s.-w. that can penetrate normal tissues and feed as a primary invader. The important myiasis flies of humans that serve as p. s.-w.'s are *Cochliomyia hominivorax, Chrysomyia bezziana,* and *Wohlfahrtia magnifica.*

secondary s.-w., an accidental or facultative s.-w. that enters a prior wound or suppurated condition and feeds on infected rather than intact tissues. Many blowflies are included, such as *Calliphora vicina, Phaenicia sericata, Phormia regina, Cochliomyia macellaria, Chrysomyia* species, and other fleshflies.

scribe (skrīb). **1.** To write, trace, or mark by making a line with a marker or pointed instrument, as in surveying a dental cast for a removable prosthesis. **2.** To form, by instrumentation, negative areas within a master cast to provide a positive beading in the framework of a removable partial denture, or the posterior palatal seal area for a complete denture. [L. *scribo,* pp. *scripto,* to write]

Scribner, Belding H., U.S. nephrologist, *1921. SEE S. *shunt.*

scro·bic·u·late (skrō-bik′ū-lāt). Pitted; marked with minute depressions. [L. *scrobiculus;* dim. of *scrobis,* a trench]

scro·bic·u·lus cor·dis (skrō-bik′ū-lŭs kōr′dis). SYN epigastric *fossa.* [L. pit or fossa of the heart]

scrof·u·la (skrof′ū-lă). Historic term for cervical tuberculous lymphadenitis. [L. *scrofulae* (pl. only), a glandular swelling, scrofula, fr. *scrofa,* a breeding sow]

scrof·u·lo·der·ma (skrof′ū-lō-der′mă). Tuberculosis resulting from extension into the skin from underlying atypical mycobacterial infection, most commonly of cervical lymph nodes in children with tonsillar infection by bovine tubercle bacillus. [scrofula + G. *derma,* skin]

scrof·u·lous (skrof′ū-lŭs). Relating to or suffering from scrofula.

scro·tal (skrō′tăl). Relating to the scrotum. SYN oscheal.

scro·tec·to·my (skrō-tek′tō-mē). Removal of all or part of the scrotum. [scrotum, + G. *ektomē,* excision]

scro·ti·form (skrō′ti-fōrm). Having the shape or form of a scrotum.

scro·ti·tis (skrō-tī′tis). Inflammation of the scrotum.

scro·to·plas·ty (skrō′tō-plas-tē). Surgical reconstruction of the scrotum. SYN oscheoplasty. [scrotum + G. *plastos,* formed]

scro·tum, pl. **scro·ta, scro·tums** (skrō′tŭm, -tă, -tŭmz) [TA]. A musculocutaneous sac containing the testes; it is formed of skin, containing a network of nonstriated muscular fibers (the dartos or dartus fascia), which also forms the scrotal septum internally. SYN marsupium (1). [L.]

lymph s., SYN *elephantiasis* scroti.

watering-can s., urinary fistulas in scrotum and perineum, resulting from disease of the perineal urethra. SEE ALSO watering-can *perineum.*

scru·ple (skroo′pl). An apothecaries' weight of 20 grains or one-third of a dram. [L. *scrupulus,* a small sharp stone, a weight, the 24th part of an ounce, a scruple, dim. of *scrupus,* a sharp stone]

SCUBA Acronym for *s*elf-*c*ontained *u*nderwater *b*reathing *a*pparatus.

Scultetus (Scul·tet), Originally Schultes, Johann, German surgeon, 1595–1645. SEE S. *bandage, position.*

scum (skŭm). A film of insoluble material that rises to the surface of a liquid, as in epistasis. [M.E.]

scurf (skerf). SYN dandruff. [A.S.]

scur·vy (sker′vē). A disease marked by inanition, debility, anemia, and edema of the dependent parts; a spongy condition sometimes with ulceration of the gums and loss of teeth, hemorrhages into the skin from the mucous membranes and internal organs, and poor wound healing; due to a diet lacking vitamin C. SYN scorbutus, sea s. [fr. A.S. *scurf*]

Alpine s., SYN pellagra.

hemorrhagic s., s. with extensive hemorrhages in gums, skin, and other tissues, typical of severe stage of the disease.

infantile s., osteopathia hemorrhagia infantum; a cachectic condition in infants, resulting from malnutrition and marked by pallor, fetid breath, coated tongue, diarrhea, and subperiosteal hemorrhages; probably a combination of s. and rickets due to combined deficiency of vitamins C and D. SYN Barlow disease, Cheadle disease, osteopathia hemorrhagica infantum, scurvy rickets.

land s., formerly, s. occurring in people who had not been to sea.

sea s., SYN scurvy.

scu·tate (skoo′tāt). SYN scutiform.

scute (skoot). A thin lamina or plate. SYN scutum (1). [L. *scutum,* shield]

tympanic s., the thin bony plate separating the epitympanic recess from the mastoid cells.

scu·ti·form (skoo′ti-fōrm). Shield-shaped. SYN scutate. [L. *scutum,* shield, + *forma,* form]

Scu·tig·e·ra (skoo-tij′er-ă). A genus of centipedes commonly found in the eastern U.S.; the Eastern house centipede is a member of the species *S. cleopatra.* [L. *scutum,* an oblong shield]

scu·tu·lum, pl. **scu·tu·la** (skoo′tū-lŭm, -lă; skoo′choo-loom). A yellow, saucer-shaped crust, the characteristic lesion of favus, consisting of a mass of hyphae, pus, and scales. [L. dim. of *scutum,* shield]

scu·tum, pl. **scu·ta** (skoo′tŭm, -tă). **1.** SYN scute. **2.** In ixodid (hard) ticks, a plate that largely or entirely covers the dorsum of the male and forms an anterior shield behind the capitulum of the female or immature ticks. [L. shield]

scyb·a·la (sib'ă-lă). Plural of scybalum.

scyb·a·lous (sib'ă-lŭs). Relating to scybala.

scyb·a·lum, pl. **scyb·a·la** (sib'ă-lŭm, -lă). A hard, round mass of inspissated feces. [G. *skybalon,* excrement]

scy·phi·form (sī'fi-fōrm). SYN scyphoid. [G. *skyphos,* goblet, cup, + L. *forma,* form]

scy·phoid (sī'foyd). Cup-shaped. SYN scyphiform. [G. *skyphos,* cup, + *eidos,* resemblance]

SD Abbreviation for streptodornase; standard *deviation.*

SDA Abbreviation for specific dynamic *action.*

SDS Abbreviation for *sodium* dodecyl sulfate.

Se Symbol for selenium.

seal (sēl). 1. A tight closure. 2. To effect a tight closure.

    border s., the contact of the denture border with the underlying or adjacent tissues to prevent the passage of air or other substances. SYN peripheral s.

    palatal s., SYN posterior palatal s.

    peripheral s., SYN border s.

    posterior palatal s., the s. at the posterior border of a denture. SEE ALSO posterior palatal seal *area.* SYN palatal s., post dam, postdam, postpalatal s.

    postpalatal s., SYN posterior palatal s.

    velopharyngeal s., closure between the oral and nasopharyngeal cavities.

seal·ant (sē'lănt). A material used to effect an airtight closure.

    dental s., SYN fissure s.

    fissure s., a dental material usually made from interaction between bisphenol A and glycidyl methacrylate; such s.'s are used to seal nonfused, noncarious pits and fissures on surfaces of teeth. SYN dental s.

sea nettle (sē net'il). SYN *Chrysaora quinquecirrha.*

search·er (ser'cher). A form of sound used to determine the presence of a calculus in the bladder.

Seashore, Carl E., U.S. psychologist, 1866–1949. SEE S. *test.*

sea·sick·ness (sē'sik-nes). A form of motion sickness caused by the motion of a floating platform, such as a ship, boat, or raft. SYN mal de mer, naupathia, vomitus marinus.

sea·son (sē'zŏn). A particular phase of some slow cyclic phenomenon, especially the annual weather cycle.

seat (sēt). A surface against which an object may rest to gain support.

    basal s., SYN denture foundation *area.*

    rest s., SYN rest *area.*

seat·worm (sēt'werm). SYN pinworm.

sea wasp. SYN *Chiropsalmus quadrumanus.*

△**seb-.** SEE sebo-.

se·ba·ceous (sē-bā'shŭs). Relating to sebum; oily; fatty. SYN sebaceus. [L. *sebaceus*]

se·ba·ceus (sē-bā'shŭs). SYN sebaceous. [L.]

seb·i·a·gog·ic (seb'ē-ă-goj'ik). SYN sebiferous. [sebi- + G. *agōgos,* leading]

se·bif·er·ous (sē-bif'er-ŭs). Producing sebaceous matter. SYN sebiagogic, sebiparous. [sebi- + L. *fero,* to bear]

Sebileau, Pierre, French anatomist, 1860–1953. SEE S. *hollow, muscle.*

se·bip·a·rous (sē-bip'ă-rŭs). SYN sebiferous. [sebi- + L. *pario,* to produce]

△**sebo-, seb-, sebi-.** Sebum, sebaceous. [L. *sebum,* suet, tallow]

seb·or·rhea (seb-ō-rē'ă). Overactivity of the sebaceous glands, resulting in an excessive amount of sebum. [sebo- + G. *rhoia,* a flow]

    s. cap'itis, s. of the scalp.

    eczematoid s., seborrheic eczema in which lesions have lost definition and have become confluent, usually as a result of trauma and overzealous use of soap and medication.

    s. facie'i, s. of face, s. affecting especially the nose and forehead.

    s. furfura'cea, SYN s. sicca (1).

    s. oleo'sa, a greasy condition of the skin due to excessive secretion of the sebaceous glands.

    s. sic'ca, (1) an accumulation on the skin, especially the scalp, of dry scales; SYN s. furfuracea. **(2)** SYN dandruff.

    s. squamo'sa neonato'rum, seborrheic dermatitis in infants.

seb·or·rhe·ic (seb-ō-rē'ik). Relating to seborrhea.

se·bum (sē'bŭm). The secretion of the sebaceous glands. [L. tallow]

sec Abbreviation for second.

Se·cer·nen·tas·i·da (se-ser-nen-tas'i-dă). A class of nematodes possessing lateral canals opening into the excretory system and phasmids; it includes most of the familiar nematode parasites of humans and domestic animals, including the soil-borne nematodes, strongyles, and filiariae. SEE ALSO Adenophorasida. SYN Phasmidia, Secernentia. [L. *secerno,* to separate, hide]

Se·cer·nen·tia (se-ser-nen'shē-ă). SYN Secernentasida.

Seckel, Helmut P.G., German physician, *1900. SEE S. *dwarfism, syndrome.*

sec·o·bar·bi·tal (sē-kō-bar'bi-tahl). An obsolescent sedative and short-acting hypnotic; largely replaced by benzodiazepines.

sec·on·dar·ies (sek'ŏn-dār-ēz). 1. SYN metastasis. 2. The lesions of secondary syphilis.

se·cos·te·roid (sek'ō-stēr'oyd). A compound derived from a steroid in which there has been a ring cleavage. [L. *seco,* to cut, + steroid]

se·cre·ta (se-krē'tă). Secretions. [L. neuter pl. of *secretus,* pp. of *se-cerno,* to separate]

se·cre·ta·gogue (se-krē'tă-gog). An agent that promotes secretion; e.g., acetylcholine, gastrin, secretin. SYN secretogogue. [secreta + G. *agōgos,* drawing forth]

se·cre·tase (sē-krē'tās). A term used to describe a proteinase that acts on amyloid precursor protein to produce peptides that do not contain the entire amyloid β protein (a major constituent of the plaques found in Alzheimer disease), are soluble, and do not precipitate to produce amyloid.

se·crete (se-krēt'). To elaborate or produce some physiologically active substance (e.g., enzyme, hormone, metabolite) by a cell and to deliver it into blood, body cavity, or sap, either by direct diffusion, cellular exocytosis, or by means of a duct. [L. *se-cerno,* pp. -*cretus,* to separate]

se·cre·tin (se-krē'tin). A hormone, formed by the epithelial cells of the duodenum under the stimulus of acid contents from the stomach, that incites secretion of pancreatic juice; used as a diagnostic aid in the diagnosis of pancreatic exocrine disease and as an adjunct in obtaining desquamated pancreatic cells for cytological examination. SYN oxykrinin. [secrete + -in]

    s. family, a class of hormones that are structurally and functionally similar to s.; e.g., s., glucagon, gastric inhibitory polypeptide, vasoactive intestinal polypeptide, and glicentin.

se·cre·tion (se-krē'shŭn). 1. Production by a cell or aggregation of cells (a gland) of a physiologically active substance and its movement out of the cell or organ in which it is formed. 2. The solid, liquid, or gaseous product of cellular or glandular activity that is stored in or used by the organism in which it is produced. Cf. excretion. [L. *secerno,* pp. -*cretus,* to separate]

    cytocrine s., the transfer of secretory material from one cell to another, such as the transfer of melanin granules from melanocytes to epidermal cells.

    external s., a substance formed by a cell and transported outside the cell walls as a means of ridding the cell of the substance or as a messenger to affect the function of other cells.

    neurohumoral s., transmission of a nerve impulse across a synapse or to an end-organ by s. of a minute amount of a chemical transmitter such as acetylcholine.

se·cre·to·gogue (se-krē'tō-gog). SYN secretagogue.

se·cre·to·mo·tor, se·cre·to·mo·tory (se-krē'tō-mō'ter, -mō'ter-ē). Stimulating secretion. [secrete + *motor,* mover]

se·cre·tor (se-krē'ter, tōr). An individual whose bodily fluids (saliva, semen, vaginal secretions) contain a water-soluble form of the antigens of the ABO blood group. S.'s constitute 80% of

se

the population. In forensic medicine, the examination of fluids has enhanced the ability of law enforcement officials to develop identifying information about perpetrators and narrow a field of suspects.

se·cre·to·ry (se-krēt′ĕ-rē, sē′krĕ-tōr-ē). Relating to secretion or the secretions.

sec·tile (sek′til, tīl). **1.** Capable of being cut or divided. **2.** Having the appearance of being divided. [L. *sectilis,* fr. *seco,* to cut]

sec·tio, pl. **sec·ti·o·nes** (sek′shē-ō, sek-shē-ō′nēz) [TA]. In anatomy, a subdivision or segment. [L.]

sec·tion (sek′shŭn). **1.** The act of cutting. **2.** A cut or division. **3.** A segment or part of any organ or structure delimited from the remainder. **4.** A cut surface. **5.** A thin slice of tissue, cells, microorganisms, or any material for examination under the microscope. SYN microscopic s. [L. *sectio,* a cutting, fr. *seco,* to cut]

abdominal s., SYN celiotomy.

attached cranial s., SYN attached *craniotomy.*

axial s., SYN transverse s.

cesarean s., incision through the abdominal wall and the uterus (abdominal hysterotomy) for extraction of the fetus.

classical cesarean s., a cesarean s. in which the uterus is entered through a vertical fundal incision.

coronal s., a cross section attained by slicing, actually or through imaging techniques, the body or any part of the body or any anatomic structure in the coronal or frontal plane, i.e., in a vertical plane perpendicular to the median or sagittal plane. Since actual sectioning in the coronal plane results in an anterior and a posterior portion, an anatomic coronal section may be a two-dimensional view of the cut surface of the posterior aspect of the anterior portion, or of the anterior aspect of the posterior portion. SYN frontal s.

cross s., (1) a planar or two-dimensional view, diagram, or image of the internal structure of the body, part of the body, or any anatomic structure afforded by slicing, actually or through imaging (radiographic, magnetic resonance, or microscopic) techniques, the body or structure along a particular plane. Traditionally, "cross section" referred to views resulting from slicing at right angles to the longitudinal axis of the structure (axial or transaxial), but in contemporary use, the term is applied when the structure is sliced in any given plane; (2) the slice or section of a given thickness created by actual serial parallel cuts through a structure or by the application of imaging technique.

detached cranial s., SYN detached *craniotomy.*

diagonal s., SYN oblique s.

frontal s., SYN coronal s.

frozen s., a thin slice of tissue cut from a frozen specimen, often used for rapid microscopic diagnosis.

Latzko cesarean s., a cesarean s. in which the uterus is entered by paravesical blunt dissection without entering the peritoneal cavity.

longitudinal s., a cross s. attained by slicing in any plane parallel to the long or vertical axis, actually or through imaging techniques, the body or any part of the body or anatomic structure. Longitudinal sections include, but are not limited to, median, sagittal, and coronal sections.

lower uterine segment cesarean s., a cesarean s. in which the uterus is entered in its lower segment by a transperitoneal approach.

median s., a cross s. attained by slicing in the median plane, actually or through imaging techniques, the body or any part of the body which occupies or crosses the median plane or by slicing any generally symmetrical anatomic structure, such as a finger or a cell, in its midline. Since actual sectioning of the median plane results in a right and a left half, an anatomical median s. may be a two-dimensional view of the cut surface on the medial aspect of either half. SYN midsagittal s.

microscopic s., SYN section (5).

midsagittal s., SYN median s.

oblique s., a diagonal cross s. attained by slicing, actually or through imaging techniques, the body or any part of the body or anatomic structure, in any plane which does not parallel the longi-

tudinal axis or intersect it at a right angle, i.e., which is neither longitudinal (vertical) nor transverse (horizontal). SYN diagonal s.

parasagittal s., SYN sagittal s.

perineal s., any s. through the perineum, either lateral or median lithotomy (operations of historical importance) or external urethrotomy.

pituitary stalk s., transection of the neurovascular connection between the hypothalamus and the pituitary gland.

Saemisch s., procedure of transfixing the cornea beneath an ulcer and then cutting from within outward through the base.

sagittal s., a cross s. obtained by slicing, actually or through imaging techniques, the body or any part of the body, or any anatomic structure in the sagittal plane, i.e., in a vertical plane parallel to the median plane. Since actual sectioning in the sagittal plane results in a right and a left portion, an anatomical sagittal s. may be a two-dimensional view of the cut surface on the medial aspect of either portion. SYN parasagittal s.

serial s., one of a number of consecutive microscopic s.'s.

thin s., ultrathin s., a s. of tissue for electron microscopic examination; the specimen is fixed, typically in glutaraldehyde and/or in osmium tetroxide, embedded in a plastic resin, and sectioned at less than 0.1 μm in thickness with a glass or diamond knife in an ultramicrotome.

transverse s., a cross s. obtained by slicing, actually or through imaging techniques, the body or any part of the body structure, in a horizontal plane, i.e., a plane which intersects the longitudinal axis at a right angle. Since actual sectioning in the transverse plane results in an inferior and a superior portion, an anatomical transverse section may be a two-dimensional view of the cut surface on the inferior aspect of the superior portion, or of the superior aspect of the inferior portion. By convention, in medical imaging transverse sections demonstrate the former unless otherwise stated. SYN axial s.

sec·tor·an·o·pia (sek′tŏr-an-ō′pē-ă). Loss of vision in a sector of the visual field. [sector + G. *an-* priv. + *opsis,* vision]

sec·to·ri·al (sek-tōr′ē-ăl). **1.** Relating to a sector. **2.** Cutting or adapted for cutting; denoting the carnassial or shearing molar and premolar teeth of carnivores. [L. *sector,* cutter]

se·cun·di·grav·i·da (sek′ŭn-di-grav′i-dă). SEE gravida.

se·cun·di·na, pl. **se·cun·di·nae** (sek-ŭn-dī′nă, -nē). SYN afterbirth. [L. *secundinae,* the afterbirth, fr. *secundus,* second]

se·cun·dines (sek′ŭn-dēnz). SYN afterbirth. [L. *secundinae,* the afterbirth]

se·cun·dip·a·ra (sek′ŭn-dip′ă-ră). SEE para.

se·date (sĕ-dāt′). To bring under the influence of a sedative. [L. *sedatus;* see sedation]

se·da·tion (sĕ-dā′shŭn). **1.** The act of calming, especially by the administration of a sedative. **2.** The state of being calm. [L. *sedatio,* to calm, allay]

sed·a·tive (sed′ă-tiv). **1.** Calming; quieting. **2.** A drug that quiets nervous excitement; designated according to the organ or system upon which specific action is exerted; e.g., cardiac, cerebral, nervous, respiratory, spinal. [L. *sedativus;* see sedation]

SEDC Abbreviation for spondyloepiphyseal *dysplasia* congenita.

se·dig·i·tate (se-dij′i-tāt). SYN sexdigitate. [L. *sex,* six, + *digitus,* digit]

sed·i·ment (sed′i-ment). **1.** Insoluble material that tends to sink to the bottom of a liquid, as in hypostasis. SYN sedimentum. **2.** To cause or effect the formation of a sediment or deposit, as in the case of centrifugation or ultracentrifugation. SYN sedimentate. [L. *sedimentum,* a settling, fr. *sedeo,* to sit, settle down]

sed·i·men·tate (sed′i-men-tāt). SYN sediment (2).

sed·i·men·ta·tion (sed′i-men-tā′shŭn). Formation of a sediment.

sed·i·men·ta·tor (sed′i-men-tā′ter, tōr). A centrifuge.

sed·i·men·tom·e·ter (sed′ĭ-men-tom′ĕ-ter). A photographic apparatus for the automatic recording of the blood sedimentation rate. [sediment + G. *metron,* measure]

sed·i·men·tum (sed-i-men′tŭm). SYN sediment (1). [L.]

   s. laterit′ium, SYN brickdust *deposit.*

se·do·hep·tu·lose (sē-dō-hep′tū-lōs). A 2-ketoheptulose formed metabolically in the pentose monophosphate pathway as the 7-phosphate by condensation of D-xylulose 5-phosphate and D-ribose 5-phosphate, splitting out D-glyceraldehyde 3-phosphate; the unphosphorylated sugar is found in *Sedum* (stonecrop). SYN D-*altro*-2-heptulose.

sedoxantrone trihydrochloride (se-doks′an-trōn trī-hī-drō-klōr-īd). A topoisomerase II inhibitor in cancer chemotherapy.

seed (sēd). **1.** The reproductive body of a flowering plant; the mature ovule. SYN semen (2). **2.** In bacteriology, to inoculate a culture medium with microorganisms. [A.S. *soed*]

Seeligmüller, Otto L.G.A., German neurologist, 1837–1912. SEE S. *sign*.

Seessel, Albert, U.S. embryologist, 1850–1910. SEE S. *pocket, pouch*.

seg·ment (seg′ment) [TA]. **1.** A section; a part of an organ or other structure delimited naturally, artificially, or by invagination from the remainder. SYN segmentum [TA]. SEE ALSO metamere. **2.** A territory of an organ having independent function, supply, or drainage. **3.** To divide and redivide into minute equal parts. [L. *segmentum*, fr. *seco*, to cut]

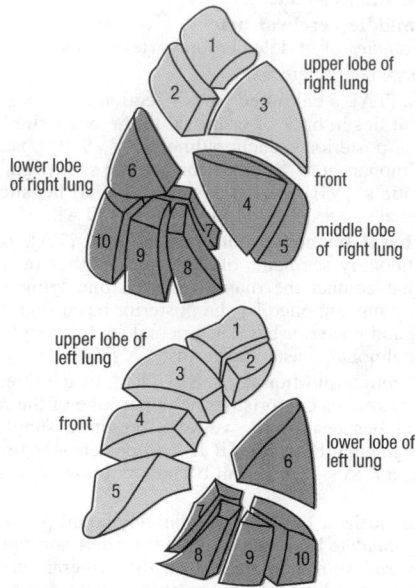

bronchopulmonary segments: lateral views; (1) apical segment (s.), (2) posterior s. (in left lung, 1+2 = apicoposterior s., formerly "apicobasal," (3) anterior s., (4) lateral s. of right lung (for left lung, superior lingular s.), (5) medial s. of right lung (for left lung, inferior lingular s.), (6) apical s. (or superior), (7) medial basal s. (or cardiac s. of right lung; inconstant in left lung), (8) anterior basal s., (9) lateral basal s., (10) posterior basal s.

A1 s. of anterior cerebral artery, ☆official alternate term for precommunicating *part* of anterior cerebral artery.

A2 s. of anterior cerebral artery, ☆official alternate term for postcommunicating *part* of anterior cerebral artery.

abnormal ST s., SYN isoelectric *period*.

anterior s. [TA], a delimited part or section of an organ or other structure that lies in front of or ventral to the other similar parts or sections. SEE anterior (bronchopulmonary) s. [S III], anterior basal (bronchopulmonary) s. [S VIII], anterior inferior renal s., anterior superior renal s., anterior ocular s. SYN segmentum anterius [TA].

anterior basal (bronchopulmonary) s. [S VIII], of the four bronchopulmonary segments of the inferior lobes of the right or left lung that contact the diaphragm, the one lying in front, i.e., nearest the costal cartilages; supplied by the anterior basal segmental bronchi [B VIII] and anterior basal segmental (pulmonary) artery. SYN segmentum (bronchopulmonale) basale anterius [S VIII].

anterior (bronchopulmonary) s. [S III] [TA], of the three bronchopulmonary segments comprising the upper lobe of the right or left lungs, the one that lies nearest the costal cartilages, supplied by the anterior segmental bronchis [B III] and anterior segmental (pulmonary) artery. SYN segmentum (bronchopulmonale) anterius S III [TA].

anterior inferior renal s., portion of the kidney exclusively supplied by the anterior inferior segmental (renal) artery. SYN segmentum renale anterius inferius.

anterior ocular s., portion of the eyeball comprised by the cornea, iris, and lens and the associated chambers (anterior and posterior), which are filled with aqueous humor. SYN segmentum oculare anterius [TA].

anterior superior renal s. [TA], portion of the kidney exclusively supplied by the anterior superior segmental (renal) artery. SYN segmentum renale anterius superius.

apical (bronchopulmonary) s. [S I], of the three bronchopulmonary segments comprising the superior lobe of the right lung, the one extending to the highest level (into the cervical parietal pleura) that is supplied by the apical segmental bronchus [B I] and the apical segmental (pulmonary) artery. SYN segmentum bronchopulmonale apicale S I.

apicoposterior (bronchopulmonary) s. [SI + SII], of the four bronchopulmonary segments typically comprising the superior lobe of the left lung, the most superior and posterior, supplied by the left apicoposterior segmental bronchus [B I + II]; they correspond approximately in position to the separate apical and posterior bronchopulmonary segments of the superior lobe of the right lung. SYN segmentum (bronchopulmonale) apicoposterius [SI + II].

arterial s.'s of kidney, SYN renal s.'s.

s. bronchopulmonale basale posterius S X [TA], SYN posterior basal bronchopulmonary s. S X.

bronchopulmonary s. [TA], smallest surgically resectable subdivision of the lobes of the lungs, supplied exclusively by a tertiary (segmental) bronchus and the corresponding tertiary branch of the pulmonary artery (segmental pulmonary artery); typically, the right lung has ten bronchopulmonary segments, and the left has eight or nine due to a merging of the apical and posterior segments of the upper lobe and of the anterior and medial basal segments of the lower lobe. SYN segmentum bronchopulmonale [TA].

cardiac s., SYN medial basal bronchopulmonary s. S VII.

cervical s.'s of spinal cord [C1–C8], ☆official alternate term for cervical *part* of spinal cord.

coccygeal s. of spinal cord [Co], inferiormost segment of spinal cord that gives rise to the coccygeal pair of spinal nerves and constitutes the coccygeal part of the spinal cord. SYN segmentum medullae spinalis coccygeum [Co] [TA].

hepatic s.'s [TA], surgically resectable portions of the liver supplied by independent branches of the portal vein and hepatic artery, and drained by independent lobular branches of the hepatic bile ducts; thus, the naming and numbering of the eight hepatic segments in TA is based on the portobilioarterial distribution: posterior [I], lateral [II], left lateral anterior [III], and medial [IV] segments of the left (part of) liver, and anterior medial [V], right anterior lateral [VI], posterior lateral [VII], and posterior medial [VIII] segments of the right (part of) liver; the hepatic segments are separated by the vertical planes of the three major (right, intermediate, and left) hepatic veins; those of the right (part of) liver are also separated by the horizontal plane of the right division of the portobilioarterial tree. SEE anterior s., lateral s., medial s., posterior s. SYN segmenta hepatis [TA], s.'s of liver.

s. I, ☆official alternate term for posterior hepatic s. I.

inferior s. [TA], a delimited part or section of an organ or other structure that lies at the lowest level (nearest the feet) compared with the other similar parts or sections. SYN segmentum inferius [TA].

inferior lingular (bronchopulmonary) s. [S V], of the four bronchopulmonary segments that typically comprise the superior lobe of the left lung, the most inferior, supplied by the inferior lingular bronchus [B V] and inferior lingular segmental (pulmonary) artery; corresponds approximately in position to the medial [S V] segment of the middle lobe of the right lung; the lingula is a feature of this part of the left lung. SYN segmentum lingulare bronchopulmonale inferius S V [TA].

inferior renal s., portion of the kidney exclusively supplied by the inferior segmental (renal) artery. SYN segmentum renale inferius [TA].

interannular s., SYN internodal s.

intermaxillary s., the primordial mass of tissue formed by the merging of the medial nasal prominences of the embryo; it contributes to the intermaxillary portion of the upper jaw, the prolabial portion of the upper lip, and the primary palate.

internodal s., the portion of a myelinated nerve fiber between two successive nodes. SYN interannular s., internode, Ranvier s., segmentum internodale.

Lanterman s.'s, the divisions of the nerve fiber between the Schmidt-Lanterman incisures.

lateral s. [TA], a delimited part or section of an organ or other structure that lies farthest to the left or right compared with the other similar parts or sections. SEE lateral bronchopulmonary s. S IV, lateral basal (bronchopulmonary) s. [S IX], (left anterior) lateral hepatic s. [III], (left posterior) lateral hepatic s. III, right anterior lateral hepatic s. [VI], (right) posterior lateral hepatic s. [VII]. SYN segmentum laterale [TA].

lateral basal (bronchopulmonary) s. [S IX], of the four bronchopulmonary segments of the inferior lobes of the right or left lung that contact the diaphragm, the one lying farthest to the right in the right lung, and farthest to the left in the left lung, supplied by the lateral basal segmental bronchi [B IX] and lateral basal segmental (pulmonary) artery. SYN segmentum (bronchopulmonale) basale laterale [S IX].

lateral bronchopulmonary s. S IV [TA], of the two bronchopulmonary segments comprising the middle lobe of the right lung, the one placed on the right side that is supplied by the lateral segmental bronchus [B IV] and the lateral segmental (pulmonary) artery. SYN segmentum bronchopulmonale laterale S IV [TA].

(left anterior) lateral hepatic s. [III] [TA], one of the three hepatic segments that constitute the left (part of) liver, the one which lies to the left of the inferior portion of the falciform ligament, typically overlapping the stomach anteriorly, supplied by the lower lateral branch from the umbilical part of the left branch of the hepatic portal vein. SYN lateral inferior hepatic area [TA], segmentum hepatis anterius laterale sinistrum [III] [TA], segmentum III⋆.

(left) medial hepatic s. [IV] [TA], of the three hepatic segments that constitute the left (part of) liver, the one that lies to the right of the falciform ligament; it lies between that ligament and the vertical plane of the right hepatic vein, that is demarcated on the diaphragmatic surface of the liver by a line extrapolated from the fossa for the gallbladder to the inferior vena cava; the quadrate lobe of the visceral surface of the liver is also part of the medial hepatic segment; the medial segment is supplied by medial branches of the umbilical part of the left branch of the portal vein. SYN segmentum hepatis mediale (sinistrum) [IV] [TA], segmentum IV⋆.

(left posterior) lateral hepatic s. III [TA], of the three hepatic segments that constitute the left (part of) liver, the one that lies to the left of the superior portion of the falciform ligament and the fissure for the ligamentum venosum; typically, it lies superior to the stomach and is supplied by the upper lateral branch from the umbilical part of the left branch of the hepatic portal vein. SYN lateral superior hepatic area [TA], segmentum hepatis posterius laterale sinistrum [II] [TA], segmentum II⋆.

s.'s of liver, SYN hepatic s.'s.

lower uterine s., the inferior portion or isthmus of the uterus, the lower extremity of which joins with the cervical canal and, during pregnancy, expands to become the lower part of the uterine cavity. This is not the active contracting portion of the uterus.

lumbar s.'s L1–L5 of spinal cord, SYN lumbar *part* of spinal cord.

lumbar s.'s of spinal cord L1–5, the five segments of the spinal cord that give rise to the five pairs of lumbar spinal nerves [L1–L5] and constitute the lumbar part of the spinal cord, that in the adult, lies within the portion of the vertebral canal formed by the

T11–L1 vertebrae. SYN segmenta medullae spinalis lumbaria L1–L5.

medial s. [TA], a delimited part or section of an organ or other structure that lies closest to the midline compared with the other similar parts or sections. SEE medial bronchopulmonary s. S V, medial basal bronchopulmonary s. S VII, (left) medial hepatic s. [IV], (right) posterior medial hepatic s. [VIII], (right) anterior medial hepatic segment [V]. SYN segmentum mediale [TA].

medial basal bronchopulmonary s. S VII [TA], of the four bronchopulmonary segments of the inferior lobes of the right or left lung that contact the diaphragm, the one lying directly inferior to the hilum of the lung in contact with the middle of the lateral aspect of the mediastinum, supplied by the medial basal segmental bronchis [B VII] and medial basal segmental (pulmonary) artery. SYN segmentum bronchopulmonale basale mediale S VII [TA], cardiac s., segmentum cardiacum.

medial bronchopulmonary s. S V [TA], of the two bronchopulmonary segments comprising the middle lobe of the right lung, the one placed on the left that is supplied by the medial segmental bronchus [B V] and the medial segmental (pulmonary artery). SYN segmentum bronchopulmonale mediale S V [TA].

mesoblastic s., SYN somite.

M2 s. of middle cerebral artery, ⋆official alternate term for terminal *branches* of middle cerebral artery, under *branch.*

neural s., SYN neuromere.

posterior s. [TA], a delimited part or section of an organ or other structure that lies in back of or dorsal to the other similar parts or sections. SEE posterior bronchopulmonary s. S II, posterior basal bronchopulmonary s. S X, posterior hepatic s. I, (right) posterior lateral hepatic s. [VII], (right) posterior medial hepatic s. [VIII], posterior renal s. SYN segmentum posterius [TA].

posterior basal bronchopulmonary s. S X [TA], of the four bronchopulmonary segments of the inferior lobes of the right or left lung that contact the diaphragm, the one lying nearest the vertebral column, supplied by the posterior basal segmental bronchus [B X] and posterior basal segmental (pulmonary) artery. SYN s. bronchopulmonale basale posterius S X [TA].

posterior bronchopulmonary s. S II [TA], of the three bronchopulmonary segments comprising the upper lobe of the right lungs, the one that lies nearest the vertebral column, supplied by the posterior segmental bronchus [B II] and posterior segmental (pulmonary) artery. SYN segmentum bronchopulmonale posterius S II [TA].

posterior hepatic s. I [TA], the relatively small part of the liver supplied by caudate branches of the left (or left and right) branches of the portal vein, demarcated on the visceral surface of the liver as the caudate lobe. SYN segmentum hepatis posterius I [TA], caudate lobe⋆, lobus caudatus⋆, posterior liver⋆, posterior part of liver⋆, s. I⋆, segmentum I⋆, Spigelius lobe.

posterior renal s. [TA], part of the kidney exclusively supplied by the posterior segmental (renal) artery. SYN segmentum renale posterius [TA].

P1 s. of posterior cerebral artery, SYN precommunicating *part* of posterior cerebral artery.

P2 s. of posterior cerebral artery, ⋆official alternate term for postcommunicating *part* of posterior cerebral artery.

P3 s. of posterior cerebral artery [TA], SYN lateral occipital *artery.*

P4 s. of posterior cerebral artery, ⋆official alternate term for medial occipital *artery.*

PR s., that part of the electrocardiographic curve between the end of the P wave and the beginning of the QRS complex.

precommunical s. of anterior cerebral artery, SYN precommunicating *part* of anterior cerebral artery.

precommunical s. of posterior cerebral artery, SYN precommunicating *part* of posterior cerebral artery.

Ranvier s., SYN internodal s.

renal s.'s [TA], regions of the kidney supplied by end arteries branching from the renal arteries; they are named anterior inferior s., anterior superior s., inferior s., posterior s., and superior s. SYN segmenta renalia [TA], arterial s.'s of kidney.

right anterior lateral hepatic s. [VI] [TA], of the four segments comprising the right (part of) liver (i.e., that lie to the right side of the plane of the middle hepatic vein), the one that also lies to the right of the plane of the right hepatic vein and inferior to the plane of the transverse portion of the right branch of the hepatic portal vein; it is supplied by the lateral anterior branch of the hepatic portal vein. SYN segmentum hepatis anterius laterale dextrum [VI] [TA].

(right) anterior medial hepatic segment [V] [TA], of the four segments comprising the right (part of) liver (i.e., that lie to the right side of the plane of the middle hepatic vein), the one that lies between that plane and the plane of the right hepatic vein and inferior to the plane of the transverse portion of the right branch of the hepatic portal vein; it is supplied by the medial anterior branch of the portal vein. SYN segmentum hepatis anterius mediale (dextrum) [V] [TA].

(right) posterior lateral hepatic s. [VII] [TA], of the four segments comprising the right (part of) liver (i.e., that lie to the right side of the plane of the middle hepatic vein), the one that also lies to the right of the plane of the right hepatic vein and superior to the plane of the transverse portion of the right branch of the hepatic portal vein; it is supplied by the lateral posterior branch of the portal vein. SYN segmentum hepatis posterius laterale (dextrum) [VII] [TA].

(right) posterior medial hepatic s. [VIII] [TA], of the four segments comprising the right (part of) liver (i.e., that lie to the right side of the plane of the middle hepatic vein), the one that lies between that plane and the plane of the right hepatic vein and superior to the plane of the transverse portion of the right branch of the hepatic portal vein; it is supplied by the medial posterior branch of the portal vein. SYN segmentum hepatis posterius mediale (dextrum) [VIII] [TA].

RST s., the part of the electrocardiogram between the QRS complex and the T wave. Virtually never distinct in normal hearts in which it forms the initial limb of the T wave without an agreed endpoint. SYN ST s.

s.'s of spinal cord [C1–Co] [TA], one of the 31 portions of the spinal cord, each of which gives rise to the anterior and posterior roots that combine to form a single pair of spinal nerves. These are the cervical spinal cord segments [C1–C8]; the thoracic spinal cord segments [T1–T12]; the lumbar spinal cord segments [L1–L5]; the sacral spinal cord segments [S1–S5], and the coccygeal spinal cord segment [Co]. SYN segmenta medullae spinalis C1–Co [TA].

s.'s of spleen, splenic territories receiving independent arterial supply or drained by independent roots of the splenic vein. SYN segmenta lienis.

ST s., SYN RST s.

subapical s., an inconstant segment of the inferior lobe of the right and left lungs. SYN segmentum subapicale, segmentum subsuperius, subsuperior s.

subsuperior s., SYN subapical s.

superior s., the uppermost segment of the kidney;

superior lingular bronchopulmonary s. S IV [TA], of the four bronchopulmonary segments that typically comprise the superior lobe of the left lung, the segment that lies centrally and posteriorly, supplied by the superior lingular bronchus [B IV] and superior lingular segmental (pulmonary) artery; corresponds approximately in position to the lateral [S IV] segment of the middle lobe of the right lung. SYN segmentum bronchopulmonale lingulare superius[S IV] [TA].

superior renal s. [TA], portion of the kidney exclusively supplied by the superior segmental (renal) artery. SYN segmentum renale superius [TA].

sympathetic s., a divison of the sympathetic trunks based on the origins of the gray communicating branches.

upper uterine s., the main portion of the body of the gravid uterus, the contraction of which furnishes the chief force of expulsion in labor.

venous s.'s of the kidney, anatomic s.'s of the kidney drained by tributaries of the renal vein; not a true segmental distribution, since cross communication exists between the various tributaries within the kidney.

seg·men·ta (seg-men′tă). Plural of segmentum.

seg·men·tal (seg-men′tăl). Relating to a segment.

seg·men·ta·tion (seg′men-tā′shŭn). **1.** The act of dividing into segments; the state of being divided into segments. **2.** SYN cleavage (1).

seg·men·tec·to·my (seg-men-tek′tō-mē). Excision of an anatomic segment of any organ or gland.

seg·ment·er (seg′men-ter). A schizont; usually applied to the malaria parasite developing in a red blood cell after having undergone nuclear and cytoplasmic division, just before cell rupture and release of the merozoites.

Seg·men·ti·na (seg-men-tī′nă). A genus of freshwater pulmonate snails (family Planorbidae, subfamily Segmentininae); includes the species *S. hemisphaerula*, an important intermediate host of *Fasciolopsis buski*. [L. segmentum, fr. seco, to cut]

seg·men·tum, pl. **seg·men·ta** (seg-men′tŭm, -tă) [TA]. SYN segment (1). [L. segment]

s. A1 arteriae cerebri anterioris, ✩official alternate term for precommunicating *part* of anterior cerebral artery.

s. A2 arteriae cerebri anterioris, ✩official alternate term for postcommunicating *part* of anterior cerebral artery.

s. ante′rius [TA], SYN anterior *segment*.

s. apica′le, apical segment of the inferior lobe of the right and left lungs.

s. bronchopulmona′le [TA], SYN bronchopulmonary *segment*.

s. (bronchopulmonale) anterius S III [TA], SYN anterior (bronchopulmonary) *segment* [S III].

s. bronchopulmonale apicale S I, SYN apical (bronchopulmonary) *segment* [S I].

s. (bronchopulmonale) basa′le latera′le [S IX], SYN lateral basal (bronchopulmonary) *segment* [S IX].

s. bronchopulmonale basale mediale S VII [TA], SYN medial basal bronchopulmonary *segment* S VII.

s. bronchopulmonale laterale S IV [TA], SYN lateral bronchopulmonary *segment* S IV.

s. bronchopulmonale lingulare superius[S IV] [TA], SYN superior lingular bronchopulmonary *segment* S IV.

s. bronchopulmonale mediale S V [TA], SYN medial bronchopulmonary *segment* S V.

s. bronchopulmonale posterius S II [TA], SYN posterior bronchopulmonary *segment* S II.

s. (bronchopulmonale) apicoposte′rius [SI + II], SYN apicoposterior (bronchopulmonary) *segment* [SI + SII].

s. cardi′acum, SYN medial basal bronchopulmonary *segment* S VII.

segmenta cervicalia C1–C5, SYN cervical *part* of spinal cord.

segmen′ta cervica′lia medul′lae spina′lis [TA], SYN cervical *part* of spinal cord.

segmen′ta coccyg′ea medul′lae spina′lis [TA], SYN coccygeal *part* of spinal cord.

segmen′ta hep′atis [TA], SYN hepatic *segments*, under *segment*.

s. hepatis anterius laterale dextrum [VI] [TA], SYN right anterior lateral hepatic *segment* [VI].

s. hepatis anterius laterale sinistrum [III] [TA], SYN (left anterior) lateral hepatic *segment* [III].

s. hepatis anterius mediale (dextrum) [V] [TA], SYN (right) anterior medial hepatic segment [V].

s. hepatis mediale (sinistrum) [IV] [TA], SYN (left) medial hepatic *segment* [IV].

s. hepatis posterius I [TA], SYN posterior hepatic *segment* I.

s. hepatis posterius laterale sinistrum [II] [TA], SYN (left posterior) lateral hepatic *segment* III.

s. hepatis posterius laterale (dextrum) [VII] [TA], SYN (right) posterior lateral hepatic *segment* [VII].

s. hepatis posterius mediale (dextrum) [VIII] [TA], SYN (right) posterior medial hepatic *segment* [VIII].

s. I, ✩official alternate term for posterior hepatic *segment* I.

s. II, ✩official alternate term for (left posterior) lateral hepatic *segment* III.

s. III, ✩official alternate term for (left anterior) lateral hepatic *segment* [III].

s. inferius [TA], SYN inferior *segment*.

se

s. internoda′le, SYN internodal *segment.*

s. IV, ⁺official alternate term for (left) medial hepatic *segment* [IV].

s. latera′le [TA], SYN lateral *segment.*

segmen′ta lien′is, SYN *segments* of spleen, under *segment.*

s. lingulare bronchopulmonale inferius S V [TA], SYN inferior lingular (bronchopulmonary) *segment* [S V].

segmenta lumbalia L1–L5, SYN lumbar *part* of spinal cord.

segmenta lumbalia medullae spinalis, SYN lumbar *part* of spinal cord.

s. media′le [TA], SYN medial *segment.*

segmenta medullae spinalis C1–Co [TA], SYN *segments* of spinal cord [C1–Co], under *segment.*

segmenta medullae spinalis cervicalia C1–C8 [TA], SYN cervical *part* of spinal cord.

s. medullae spinalis coccygeum [Co] [TA], SYN coccygeal *segment* of spinal cord [Co].

segmenta medullae spinalis lumbaria L1–L5, SYN lumbar *segments* of spinal cord L1–5, under *segment.*

s. oculare anterius [TA], SYN anterior ocular *segment.*

s. P4 arteriae cerebri posterioris, ⁺official alternate term for medial occipital *artery.*

s. P3 arteriae cerebri posterioris [TA], SYN lateral occipital *artery.*

s. P1 arteriae cerebri posterioris, ⁺official alternate term for medial occipital *artery.*

s. poste′rius [TA], SYN posterior *segment.*

s. renale ante′rius infe′rius, SYN anterior inferior renal *segment.*

s. renale ante′rius supe′rius, SYN anterior superior renal *segment.*

s. renale inferius [TA], SYN inferior renal *segment.*

segmen′ta rena′lia [TA], SYN renal *segments,* under *segment.*

s. renale posterius [TA], SYN posterior renal *segment.*

s. renale superius [TA], SYN superior renal *segment.*

segmen′ta sacra′lia medul′lae spina′lis [TA], SYN sacral *part* of spinal cord.

s. (bronchopulmonale) basale anterius [S VIII], SYN anterior basal (bronchopulmonary) *segment* [S VIII].

s. subapica′le, SYN subapical *segment.*

s. subsupe′rius, SYN subapical *segment.*

segmen′ta thora′cica medul′lae spina′lis [TA], SYN thoracic *part* of spinal cord.

seg·re·ga·tion (seg-rĕ-gā′shŭn). **1.** Removal of certain parts from a mass, e.g., those with infectious diseases. **2.** Separation of contrasting characters in the offspring of heterozygotes. **3.** Separation of the paired state of genes, which occurs at the reduction division of meiosis; only one member of each somatic gene pair is normally included in each sperm or ovum; e.g., an individual heterozygous for a gene pair, *Aa,* will form gametes half containing gene *A* and half containing gene *a.* **4.** Progressive restriction of potencies in the zygote to the following embryo. [L. *segrego,* pp. -*atus,* to set apart from the flock, separate]

seg·re·ga·tor (seg′re-gā-ter, tōr). SYN separator (2).

Seidel, Erich, German ophthalmologist, 1882–1946. SEE S. *scotoma, sign.*

Seignette, Pierre, French apothecary, 1660–1719. SEE S. *salt.*

Seiler, Carl, Swiss laryngologist and anatomist in U.S., 1849–1905. SEE S. *cartilage.*

Seip, Martin, 20th century Scandinavian physician. SEE Lawrence-S. *syndrome;* S. *syndrome.*

seis·mo·car·di·o·gram (sīz′mō-kar′dē-ō-gram). Recording of cardiac vibrations as they affect the entire body, by various techniques. [G. *seismos,* a shaking, + cardiogram]

seis·mo·ther·a·py (sīz-mō-thār′ă-pē). SYN vibratory *massage.* [G. *seismos,* a shaking, vibration]

sei·zure (sē′zher). **1.** An attack; the sudden onset of a disease or of certain symptoms. **2.** An epileptic attack. SYN convulsion (2). [O. Fr. *seisir,* to grasp, fr. Germanic]

absence s., a s. characterized by impaired awareness of interaction with, or memory of, ongoing events external or internal to the person; may comprise the following elements: mental confusion,

diminished awareness of environment, inability to respond to internal or external stimuli, and amnesia. (The term absence was first used by Louis-Florentin Calmeil (1798–1895) to introduce the concept of epileptic absence for the brief loss of consciousness or confusion seen in epileptic patients.)

akinetic s., SYN atonic s.

anosognosic s.'s, SYN anosognosic *epilepsy.*

astatic s., s. causing loss of erect posture.

atonic s., a s. characterized by sudden, brief (1–2 s.) loss of muscle tone, involving postural muscles; the term usually applies to bilaterally synchronous events. SYN akinetic s.

atypical absence s., an absence s. associated with an EEG pattern of irregular or slow spike and wave at less than 2.5 Hz or paroxysmal fast activity on an abnormally slow background EEG.

audiogenic s., a reflex s. precipitated by loud noises, rare in humans. Audiogenic seizures in rodents are an animal model of epilepsy.

automotor s., s. characterized by an automatism predominantly involving the distal limbs.

autonomic s., s. characterized by objectively documented dysfunction of the autonomic nervous system, usually involving cardiovascular, gastrointestinal, or sudomotor functions.

clonic s., a s. characterized by repetitive rhythmical jerking of all or part of the body.

complex motor s., s. characterized by muscles of each limb contracting asynchronously and sequentially to produce a movement that may resemble voluntary activity.

complex partial s., s. with impairment of consciousness, occurring in a patient with focal epilepsy.

convulsive s., s. with clonic or tonic-clonic motor activity.

dileptic s., s. characterized by impaired awareness of, interaction with, or memory of ongoing events.

early s., a s. occurring within one week after craniocerebral trauma.

electrographic s., SYN subclinical s.

epileptic s., clinical and/or laboratory manifestations of an epileptic attack.

febrile s., SYN febrile *convulsion.*

focal motor s., a simple partial s. with localized motor activity.

gelastic s., a s. characterized by bursts of involuntary laughter or giggling, usually without an appropriate affective tone; most often related to hypothalamic lesions, such as hamartomas.

generalized s., s.'s characterized by generalized clinical manifestations.

generalized tonic-clonic s., a generalized s. characterized by the sudden onset of tonic contraction of the muscles often associated with a cry or moan, and frequently resulting in a fall to the ground. The tonic phase of the s. gradually give way to clonic convulsive movements occurring bilaterally and synchronously before slowing and eventually stopping, followed by a variable period of unconsciousness and gradual recovery. SYN cryptogenic epilepsy, generalized tonic-clonic epilepsy, grand mal s., grand mal, idiopathic epilepsy (2), major epilepsy.

grand mal s., SYN generalized tonic-clonic s.

hypermotor s., s. characterized by automatisms involving predominantly proximal limb muscles and producing marked limb displacement.

hypomotor s., s. characterized by complete or partial arrest of ongoing motor activity in a patient whose level of consciousness cannot be determined accurately (e.g., newborns, infants, mentally retarded patients).

jacksonian s., a motor s. that initially involves one part of the body and then progressively spreads to other parts of the body on the same side; may become generalized; often originates in or near the contralateral rolandic neocortex. SYN jacksonian epilepsy.

late s., a s. that occurs greater than one week after a craniocerebral trauma or CNS insult.

major motor s., a grand mal s. or other convulsive s.

minor motor s., old term for nonconvulsive s. seen in patients with secondary generalized epilepsies.

myoclonic s., a s. characterized by sudden, brief (200-ms) contractions of muscle fibers, muscles, or groups of muscles of variable topography (axial, proximal, or distal limb).

negative myoclonic s., s. characterized by abrupt, brief cessation of muscular activity, occasionally preceded by a single myoclonic contraction; term usually is applied to unilateral, distal muscles.

nonconvulsive s., a s. without clonic or tonic activity or other convulsive motor activity. SEE ALSO complex partial s., absence s.

nonepileptic s., any behavior that resembles a s., but is not epileptic, i.e., not associated with abnormal cerebral EEG activity. SEE ALSO psychogenic s.

partial s., s. characterized by localized cerebral ictal onset. The symptoms experienced are dependent on the cortical area of ictal onset or seizure spread.

petit mal s., obsolescent term for a cerebral s. not manifested by tonic-clonic movements (i.e., grand mal); formerly thought to be the clinical manifestation solely of a 3-s. spike in wave pattern, as seen on electroencephalography, but now known to be associated with several different EEG patterns.

psychic s., a simple partial s. characterized by an attack of psychic phenomena such as a dreamy state, déjà vu, autonomic sensation or emotion; commonly, but not exclusively, associated with temporal lobe epilepsy.

psychogenic s., a clinical spell that resembles an epileptic s., but is not due to epilepsy. The EEG is normal during an attack, and the behavior is often related to psychiatric disturbance, such as a conversion disorder.

psychomotor s., a s. characterized by psychic manifestation, and a complex motor s. SEE psychic s.

secondarily generalized tonic-clonic s., a generalized tonic-clonic s. that begins with a partial s. and evolves into a generalized tonic-clonic s.

simple partial s., a partial s. that is not associated with impairment of consciousness; seen in patients with focal epilepsy.

subclinical s., a s. detected by EEG, which has no clinical correlate, i.e., an EEG seizure alone. SYN electrographic s.

tonic s., a s. characterized by a sustained increase in muscle tone, of abrupt or gradual onset and offset, lasting a few seconds to a minute, usually 10–20 s.; tonic s.'s affecting proximal muscles bilaterally frequently lead to the adoption of a posture.

tonic-clonic s., a s. characterized by a sequence consisting of a tonic-clonic phase; when generalized, constitutes what has been known as a "grand mal" s.

versive s., a s. characterized by sustained, forced conjugate ocular and cephalic and/or truncal deviation.

se·la·pho·bia (sē-lă-fō′bē-ă). Rarely used term for a morbid fear of a flash of light. [G. *selas*, light, + *phobos*, fear]

Sel·din·ger, Sven Ivar, Swedish radiologist, *1921. SEE Seldinger technique.

se·lec·tin (sel-ek′tin). A cell surface molecule involved in immune adhesion and cell trafficking. [L. *se-ligo*, pp. *se-lectum*, to sort, choose, + -in]

E selectin, cell surface receptor produced by endothelium.

L selectin, cell surface receptor produced by leukocytes.

P selectin, cell surface receptor present on endothelium that is involved with neutrophil migration into inflamed tissue.

se·lec·tion (sĕ-lek′shŭn). The combined effect of the causes and consequences of genetic factors that determine the average number of progeny of a species that attain sexual maturity; phenotypes that are lethal early in life (e.g., Tay-Sachs disease), that cause sterility (e.g., Turner syndrome), or that produce sterile progeny are selected against. When s. is used of individual pedigrees, other factors, notably variance of the number of progeny and number that survive to maturity, are important considerations; in large populations, these factors even out and the mean only is of importance. [L. *se-ligo*, to separate, select, fr. *se*, apart, + *lego*, to pick out]

artificial s., interference by humans with natural s. by purposeful breeding of animals or plants of specific genotype or phenotype to produce a strain with desired characteristics; e.g., breeding of dairy cattle for high milk production.

medical s., preservation, by medical care and treatment, of individuals of pathologic genotypes who would not otherwise reproduce, thus tending to increase the frequency of pathologic genes in the population; conversely, reduction of the frequency of pathologic genes by preventing reproduction of individuals of specified genotype by surgical sterilization or other means.

natural s., "survival of the fittest," the principle that in nature those individuals best able to adapt to their environment will survive and reproduce, while those less able will die without progeny, and the genes carried by the survivors will increase in frequency. This principle is heuristic rather than rigorous since it cannot be tested, the outcome being tautologous with the empirical definition of fitness.

sexual s., a form of natural s. in which, according to Darwin theory, the male or female is attracted by certain characteristics, form, color, behavior, etc., in the opposite sex; thus modifications of a special nature are brought about in the species.

se·leg·i·line (sē-lej′e-lēn). A monoamine oxidase enzyme inhibitor; inhibits only the type B isozyme so that consuming tyramine-containing foods or beverages is less likely to induce hypertensive crisis in persons treated with selegiline than in persons treated with nonselective monoamine oxidase inhibitors. The drug is used in the treatment of Parkinson disease. SYN deprenyl.

se·le·ne un·gui·um (sē-lē′nē ŭng′gwi-ŭm). SYN *lunule* of nail. [G. *selēnē*, moon; gen. pl. of L. *unguis*, nail]

se·le·ni·um (Se) (sĕ-lē′nē-ŭm). A metallic element chemically similar to sulfur, atomic no. 34, atomic wt. 78.96; an essential trace element toxic in large quantities; required for glutathione peroxidase and a few other enzymes; ^{75}Se (half-life equal to 119.78 days) is used in scintography of the pancreas and parathyroid glands. [G. *selēnē*, moon]

s. sulfide, a mixture of crystalline s. monosulfide and solid solutions of s. and sulfur in an amorphous form, containing 52–55.5% Se; used in the treatment of seborrhea of the scalp or dandruff; it is applied to the scalp as a suspension.

se·le·no·cys·teine (se-lē-nō-sis′tēn). Cysteine containing selenium in place of one sulfur atom.

se·len·o·dont (sĕ-lē′nō-dont). Denoting an animal, or humans, having teeth, as the human molars, with longitudinal crescent-shaped ridges. [G. *selēnē*, moon, + *odous* (*odont-*), tooth]

se·le·no·me·thi·o·nine (sĕ-lē′nō-me-thī′ō-nēn). Methionine containing selenium in place of sulfur.

Se·le·no·mo·nas (sĕ-lē′nō-mō′nas). A genus of bacteria of uncertain taxonomic affiliation, containing curved to crescentic or helical, Gram-negative, strictly anaerobic rods that are motile with an active tumbling motion. Several flagella are present in a tuft, often near the center of the concave side. The type species, *S. sputigena*, is found in the human buccal cavity. [G. *selēnē*, moon, + *monas*, single (unit)]

self. **1.** A sum of the attitudes, feelings, memories, traits, and behavioral predispositions that make up the personality. **2.** The individual as represented in his or her own awareness and in his or her environment. **3.** In immunology, an individual's autologous cell components as contrasted with non-s., or foreign, constituents; the basic mechanism underlying recognition of s. from non-s. is unknown, but serves to protect the host from an immunologic attack on the host's own antigenic constituents, as opposed to immune system destruction or elimination of foreign antigens.

subliminal s., the sum of the mental processes which take place without the conscious knowledge of the individual. SYN subconscious mind.

self-ac·cu·sa·tion. A common psychiatric symptom, encountered most characteristically in agitated depression.

self-a·naly·sis. SYN autoanalysis.

self-a·ware·ness. Realization of one's ongoing feeling and emotional experience; a major goal of all psychotherapy.

self-cen·tered·ness. SYN autosynnoia.

self-com·mit·ment. Voluntary mental hospitalization.

self-con·trol. **1.** Self-regulation of one's behavior in accordance with personal beliefs, goals, attitudes and societal expectations. **2.** Use by an individual of active coping strategies to deal with problem situations, in contrast to passive conditioning strategies which do things to the individual and require no action by the person.

se

self·dif·fer·en·ti·a·tion. Differentiation resulting from the action of intrinsic causes.

self·dis·cov·e·ry. In psychoanalysis, the freeing of the repressed ego in a person raised to be submissive to those around him.

self·ef·fi·ca·cy. An individual's estimate or personal judgment of his or her own ability to succeed in reaching a specific goal, e.g., quitting smoking or losing weight, or a more general goal, e.g., continuing to remain at a prescribed weight level.

self·fer·til·i·za·tion. Fecundation of the ovules by the pollen of the same flower, or of the ova by the spermatozoa of the same animal in hermaphrodite forms; denoting an extreme type of in-breeding seen in certain plants and animal forms which produce both male and female gametes.

self·in·fec·tion. SYN autoinfection.

self·knowl·edge. SYN autognosis.

self·lim·it·ed. Denoting a disease that tends to cease after a definite period; e.g., pneumonia.

self-love. SYN narcissism.

self·poi·son·ing. SYN autointoxication.

self·reg·u·la·tion. A three-stage strategy patients are taught to use in order to end risky health-associated behaviors such as smoking and overeating: 1. self-monitoring (self-observation), the first stage in self-regulation involves the individual's deliberately attending to and recording his or her own behavior; 2. self-evaluation, the second stage, in which the individual assesses what was learned by self-monitoring, such as how often and where one smokes, and uses those observational data to establish health goals or criteria; and 3. self-reinforcement, the third stage, in which the individual rewards him/herself for each behavioral success on the road to that goal, thereby enhancing the chance of reaching it.

self·stim·u·la·tion. A technique for electrical stimulation of peripheral nerves, spinal cord, or brain by the patient to relieve pain.

self-tolerance. SYN *horror* autotoxicus.

Selivanoff, Feodor, Russian chemist, *1859. SEE S. *test.*

sel·la (sel′ă). SYN saddle (1). [L. saddle]

  empty s., a sella turcica, often enlarged, that contains no discernible pituitary gland; may be primarily due to an incompetent sellar diaphragm with compression of the pituitary gland by herniating arachnoid or secondarily due to surgery or radiotherapy.

  s. tur′cica [TA], a saddlelike bony prominence on the upper surface of the body of the sphenoid bone, constituting the middle part of the butterfly-shaped middle cranial fossa; it includes the tuberculum sellae anteriorly and the dorsum sellae posteriorly; with its covering of dura mater it constitutes the hypophysial fossa that accommodates the hypophysis or pituitary gland. SYN pars sellaris, Turkish saddle.

sel·lar (sel′ăr). Relating to the sella turcica.

Sellick, Brian A., 20th century British anesthetist. SEE S. *maneuver.*

Selye, Hans, Austrian endocrinologist in Canada, 1907–1982. SEE adaptation *syndrome* of S.

SEM Abbreviation for standard error of the *mean.*

se·man·tics (se-man′tiks). A branch of semiotics: **1.** The study of the significance and development of the meaning of words. **2.** The study concerned with the relations between signs and their referents; the relations between the signs of a system; and human behavioral reaction to signs, including unconscious attitudes, influences of social institutions, and epistemological and linguistic assumptions. [G. *sēmainō,* to show]

Sémélaigne, Georges, 20th century French pediatrician. SEE Debré-S. *syndrome;* Kocher-Debré-S. *syndrome.*

sem·el·in·ci·dent (sem-el-in′si-dent). An obsolete term that means happening once only; said of an infectious disease, one attack of which confers permanent immunity. [L. *semel,* once, + *incido,* to happen, fr. *cado,* to fall]

se·men, pl. **sem·i·na, se·mens** (sē′men, sē-mi′nă, sē′menz). **1** [NA]. The penile ejaculate; a thick, yellowish-white, viscid fluid containing spermatozoa; a mixture produced by secretions of the testes, seminal vesicles, prostate, and bulbourethral glands. SYN

seminal fluid. **2.** SYN seed (1). [L. *semen* (*semin-*), seed (of plants, men, animals)]

se·me·nu·ria (sē-mĕ-noo′rē-ă). The excretion of urine containing semen. SYN seminuria, spermaturia.

△**semi-.** One-half; partly. Cf. hemi-. [L. *semis,* half]

sem·i·al·de·hyde (sem-ē-al′dĕ-hīd). The monoaldehyde of a dicarboxylic acid, so called because half the COOH groups of the original acid are reduced to the aldehyde while the other half are unchanged; e.g., glutamic acid γ-s., OHC–CH₂CH₂CH(NH₃)⁺–COO⁻. Many s.'s are intermediates in the biosynthesis and metabolic degradation of amino acids (e.g., L-proline, L-lysine, L-glutamate).

sem·i·ca·nal (sem-ē-kă-nal′). A half canal; a deep groove on the edge of a bone that, uniting with a similar groove or part of an adjoining bone, forms a complete canal. SYN semicanalis.

  s. of auditory tube, SYN *canal* for pharyngotympanic (auditory) tube.

  s. for tensor tympani muscle, SYN *canal* for tensor tympani muscle.

sem·i·ca·na·lis, pl. **sem·i·ca·na·les** (sem′ē-kă-nal′is, -ēz). SYN semicanal. [L.]

  s. mus′culi tensor′is tym′pani [TA], SYN *canal* for tensor tympani muscle.

  s. tu′bae auditi′vae [TA], SYN *canal* for pharyngotympanic (auditory) tube.

  s. t′ubae audito′riae, SYN *canal* for pharyngotympanic (auditory) tube.

sem·i·car·ti·lag·i·nous (sem′ē-kar-ti-laj′i-nŭs). Composed partly of cartilage.

sem·i·cir·cu·lar (sem′ē-sir′kū-lăr). Forming a half circle or an incomplete circle. SYN semiorbicular.

sem·i·co·ma (sem′ē-kō′ma). SEE semicomatose.

sem·i·com·a·tose (sem′ē-kō′ma-tōs). An imprecise term for a state of drowsiness and inaction, in which more than ordinary stimulation may be required to evoke a response, and the response may be delayed or incomplete. SYN semiconscious.

sem·i·con·duc·tor (sem′ē-kon-dŭk′ter). A metalloid, in one form or another, that conducts electricity more easily than a true non-metal but less easily than a metal; e.g., silicon, germanium.

sem·i·con·scious (sem′ē-kon′shŭs). SYN semicomatose.

sem·i·con·serv·a·tive. The process of replicating DNA in which the two strands remain intact, separate, and are copied and one parental strand goes to each daughter cell.

sem·i·cris·ta (sem′ē-kris′tă). A small or imperfect ridge or crest. [semi- + L. *crista,* crest, tuft]

  s. incisi′va, SYN nasal *crest.*

sem·i·de·cus·sa·tion (sem′ē-dē-kŭs-sā′shŭn). Incomplete decussation such as occurs in the human optic chiasm.

sem·i·flex·ion (sem-ē-flek′shŭn). The position of a joint or segment of a limb midway between extension and flexion.

sem·i·lu·nar (sem-ē-loo′năr). SYN lunar (2). [semi- + L. *luna,* moon]

sem·i·lu·na·re (sem-ē-loo-nā′rē). Obsolete term for lunate (*bone*).

sem·i·lux·a·tion (sem-ē-lŭk-sā′shŭn). SYN subluxation.

sem·i·mem·bra·no·sus (sem′ē-mem-bră-nō′sŭs). SEE semimembranosus (*muscle*).

sem·i·mem·bra·nous (sem′ē-mem′brā-nŭs). Consisting partly of membrane; denoting the semimembranosus muscle.

sem·i·nal (sem′i-năl). **1.** Relating to the semen. **2.** Original or influential of future developments.

sem·i·na·tion (sem-i-nā′shŭn). SYN insemination.

sem·i·nif·er·ous (sem′i-nif′er-ŭs). Carrying or conducting the semen; denoting the tubules of the testis. [L. *semen,* seed (semen) + *fero,* to carry]

sem·i·no·ma (sem-i-nō′mă). A radiosensitive malignant neoplasm usually arising from germ cells in the testis of young male adults which metastasizes to the paraortic lymph nodes; a counterpart of dysgerminoma of the ovary. [L. *semen,* seed (semen) + G. *-oma,* tumor]

spermacytic s., a relatively slow-growing, locally invasive type of testicular s. that does not metastasize and has no ovarian counterpart.

se·mi·no·ma·tous (sem-i-nō′mă-tŭs). Relating to a seminoma.

sem·i·nor·mal (N/2) (sem-ē-nōr′măl). Denoting a solution one-half the strength of a normal solution (0.5 N).

se·mi·nu·ria (sē-mi-noo′rē-ă). SYN semenuria.

se·mi·o·path·ic, se·mei·o·path·ic (sē′mē-ō-path′ik). Denoting the disordered use of symbols. [G. *sēmeion*, sign, + *pathos*, disease]

sem·i·or·bic·u·lar (sē-mē-ōr-bik′ū-lăr). SYN semicircular.

se·mi·o·sis, se·mei·o·sis (sē-mē-ō′sis) The mental or symbolic process in which something (e.g., word, symbol, nonverbal cue) functions as a sign for the organism. [G. *sēmeiōsis*, fr. *sēmeion*, sign]

se·mi·ot·ic, se·mei·ot·ic (sē-mē-ot′ik, sem-ē-). **1.** Relating to semiotics. **2.** Relating to signs, linguistic or bodily. [G. *sēmeiō-tikos*, fr. *sēmeion*, sign]

se·mi·ot·ics, se·mei·ot·ics (sē-mē-ot′iks, sem-e-). **1.** The general philosophic theory of signs and symbols in communication, having three branches: syntactics, semantics, and pragmatics. **2.** Obsolete term for symptomatology. [see semiotic]

se·mi·pen·nate (sem′ē-pen′āt) [TA]. **1.** Having a feather arrangement on one side; resembling one-half of a feather. **2.** Denoting certain muscles with fibers running at an acute angle from one side of a tendon. SYN unipennate✶, demipenniform.

sem·i·pen·ni·form (sem′ē-pen′i-fōrm). Penniform on one side. SEE semipennate *muscle*.

sem·i·per·me·a·ble (sem-ē-per′mē-ă-bl). Freely permeable to water (or other solvent) but relatively impermeable to solutes. Depending on the context, it has been used to imply impermeability to all solutes except very small uncharged molecules (e.g., a cell membrane), or merely impermeability to very large molecules such as proteins (e.g., a capillary membrane).

sem·i·pro·na·tion (sem′ē-prō-nā′shŭn). The attitude or assumption of a partly prone position, as in Sims position.

sem·i·prone (sem-ē-prōn′). Denoting semipronation.

sem·i·qui·none (sem-ē-kwin′ōn). A free radical resulting from the removal of one hydrogen atom with its electron during the process of dehydrogenation of a hydroquinone to quinone or similar compound (e.g., flavin mononucleotide).

sem·i·spi·nal (sem-ē-spī′năl). Half spinal; denoting muscles attached in part to the spinous processes of the vertebrae.

Sem·i·sul·co·spi·na (sem′ē-sŭl-kō-spī′nă). A genus of operculate snails (family Pleuroceriidae, subclass Prosobranchiata). An oriental form, *S. libertina*, is the first intermediate host of a number of trematodes, including *Paragonimus westermani*. [semi- + L. *sulcus*, a furrow + *spina*, thorn, spine]

sem·i·sul·cus (sem′ē-sŭl′kŭs). A slight groove on the edge of a bone or other structure, which, uniting with a similar groove on the corresponding adjoining structure, forms a complete sulcus.

sem·i·su·pi·na·tion (sem′ē-soo-pi-nā′shŭn). The attitude or assumption of a partly supine position.

sem·i·su·pine (sem-ē-soo-pīn′). Denoting semisupination.

sem·i·syn·thet·ic (sem′ē-sin-thet′ik). Describing the process of synthesizing a particular chemical utilizing a naturally occurring chemical as a starting material, thus obviating part of a total synthesis; e.g., the conversion of cholesterol (obtained from a natural source) into a corticosteroid.

sem·i·sys·tem·at·ic name (sem′ē-sis-tĕ-mat′ik). A name of a chemical of which at least one part is systematic and at least one part is not (i.e., is trivial). For example, calciferol includes the -ol suffix denoting an –OH radical, while calcifer-, which has no systematic meaning, is used only in this word. Cortisone contains the -one suffix, indicating a ketone group, but the rest of the term derives from cortex (adrenal). Hippuric acid (trivial) may be defined as *N*-benzoylglycine (semitrivial name); benzoyl is systematic for the C_6H_5–CO– radical, whereas glycine is the trivial name for α-aminoacetic (or 2-aminoethanoic, to be completely systematic) acid, and the *N* signifies that the benzoyl is attached to the nitrogen of glycine; from this, the structure C_6H_5–CO–NH–CH_2–

COOH is uniquely defined. Many generic or nonproprietary names of drugs, including USAN names, hormones, etc., are semitrivial in this chemical sense, although often termed trivial names; distinction between trivial and semitrivial is not often made. SYN semitrivial name.

sem·i·ten·di·no·sus (sem′ē-ten-di-nō′sŭs). SYN semitendinous. [L.]

sem·i·ten·di·nous (sem′ē-ten′di-nŭs). Composed in part of tendon; denoting the semitendinosus muscle. SYN semitendinosus. [L. *semitendinosus*]

sem·i·ter·tian (sem-ē-ter′shē-ăn, -ter′shŭn). Partly tertian, partly quotidian; denoting a malarial fever in which two paroxysms occur on one day and one on the succeeding day.

sem·i·triv·i·al name (sem-ē-triv′ē-ăl). SYN semisystematic name.

sem·i·va·lent (sem-ē-vā′lent). Denoting the ability to form a one-electron bond.

Semon, Richard W., German biologist, 1859–1918. SEE S.-Hering *theory*.

Semple, Sir David, English physician, 1856–1937. SEE S. *vaccine*.

se·mus·tine (se-mus′ten). SYN methyl-CCNU.

Senear, Francis E., U.S. dermatologist, 1889–1958. SEE S.-Usher *disease, syndrome*.

Se·ne·cio (sĕ-nē′sē-ō, -shē-ō). **1.** A large genus of plants (family Compositae), many species of which contain alkaloids that produce hepatic necrosis. **2.** A common weed of the eastern U.S., formerly used in the treatment of amenorrhea and other menstrual irregularities. [L. a plant, groundsel, fr. *senecio*, an old man]

se·ne·ci·o·ic ac·id (sĕ-nē′si-ō-ik). A polymer precursor and a precursor of isoprenoid and terpene compounds; the acid component of binapacryl in which it is esterified with 4,6-dinitro-2-(1-methylpropyl)phenol; the coenzyme A derivative is an intermediate in L-leucine degradation; used as a fungicide and miticide.

se·ne·ci·o·sis (sĕ-nē-sē-ō′sis). Liver degeneration and necrosis caused by ingestion of plants of the genus *Senecio*, such as ragwort and groundsel; similar hepatotoxic properties have been observed after ingestion of some kinds of *Crotalaria* and *Heliotropium*.

sen·e·ga (sen′ē-gă). The dried root of *Polygala senega* (family Polygalaceae), a herb of eastern and central North America; an expectorant. SYN Seneca snakeroot. [*Seneca*, an Indian tribe]

se·nes·cence (se-nes′ens). The state of being old. [L. *senesco*, to grow old, fr. *senex*, old]

dental s., that condition of the teeth and associated structures in which there is deterioration due to normal or premature aging processes.

se·nes·cent (sē-nes′ent). Growing old.

Sengstaken, Robert W., U.S. neurosurgeon, *1923. SEE S.-Blakemore *tube*.

se·nile (sē′nīl, sen′īl). Relating to or characteristic of old age. [L. *senilis*]

se·nil·i·ty (se-nil′i-tē). Old age; a general term for a variety of organic disorders, both physical and mental, occurring in old age. [see senile]

se·ni·um (sē′nē-ŭm). Rarely used term for old age; especially the debility of advanced age. [L. the feebleness of age, fr. *seneo*, to be old, feeble]

sen·na (sen′ă). The dried leaflets or legumes of *Cassia acutifolia* (Alexandrine s.) and *C. angustifolia* (Tinnevelly or Indian s.); a laxative. [Ar. *senā*]

sen·no·side A, sen·no·side B (sen′ō-sīd). Two anthraquinone glucosides that are the laxative principles of senna.

sen·sate (sen′sāt). Able to perceive touch and other sensations; used in reference to patients who have had partial nerve or spinal cord injuries.

■**sen·sa·tion** (sen-sā′shŭn). A feeling; the translation into consciousness of the effects of a stimulus exciting any of the organs of sense. [L. *sensatio*, perception, feeling, fr. *sentio*, to perceive, feel]

se

sensation			
modality of sensation	object of perception	nature of stimuli	receptor type
sense of sight	brightness, darkness, colors	electromagnetic radiation 4000–7000 Å	photo-receptors
sense of temperature	cold, heat	electromagnetic radiation 7000–9000 Å, convective heat transport	thermo-receptors
tactile sense of skin	pressure, touch		
sense of hearing	sound frequencies		
statokinetic sense	absolute body position, speed of body, relative body position and movement of body parts and joints, sense of strength	modification of mechano-receptors by solid objects or transmission of air-pressure changes	mechano-receptors
sense of smell	odors	chemical substances	
sense of taste	sour, salty, sweet, bitter	ions	chemo-receptors
sense of pain	pain	mechanical tissue injury	nociceptors

delayed s., a s. that is not perceived until the lapse of an appreciable interval following the application of the stimulus.

general s., a s. referred to the body as a whole rather than to any particular part.

girdle s., SYN zonesthesia.

primary s., a s. that is the direct result of a stimulus.

referred s., a s. felt in one place in response to a stimulus applied in another.

sense (sens). The faculty of perceiving any stimulus. [L. *sentio,* pp. *sensus,* to feel, to perceive]

chemical s.'s, the s.'s of smell and taste.

color s., the ability to perceive variations in hue, luminosity, and saturation of light.

s. of equilibrium, the s. that makes possible a normal physiologic posture. SYN static s.

geometric s., one or other of two directions along a curve in which something is moving, e.g., clockwise or counterclockwise.

joint s., SYN articular *sensibility.*

kinesthetic s., the sensation felt in muscle when it is contracting; awareness of movement or activity in muscles or joints; sense of position or movement mediated in large part by the posterior columns and medial lemniscus. SEE ALSO bathyesthesia. SYN deep sensibility, muscular s., myesthesia, myoesthesis, myoesthesia.

light s., the ability to perceive variations in the degree of light or brightness.

muscular s., SYN kinesthetic s.

obstacle s., the ability, often found in the blind, to avoid objects without visual warning.

position s., SYN posture s.

posture s., the ability to recognize the position in which a limb is passively placed, with the eyes closed. SYN position s.

pressure s., the faculty of discriminating various degrees of pressure on the surface. SYN baresthesia, weight s.

seventh s., SYN visceral s.

space s., the faculty of perceiving the relative positions of objects in the external world.

special s., one of the five senses related respectively to the organs of sight, hearing, smell, taste, and touch.

static s., SYN s. of equilibrium.

tactile s., SYN touch (1).

temperature s., SYN thermoesthesia.

thermal s., thermic s., SYN thermoesthesia.

time s., the faculty by which the passage of time is appreciated.

visceral s., the perception of the existence of the internal organs. SYN seventh s., splanchnesthesia, splanchnesthetic sensibility.

weight s., SYN pressure s.

sen·si·bil·i·ty (sen-si-bil′i-tē). The consciousness of sensation; the capability of perceiving sensible stimuli. [L. *sensibilitas*]

articular s., appreciation of sensation in joint surfaces. SYN arthresthesia, joint sense.

bone s., SYN pallesthesia.

cortical s., the integration of sensory stimuli by the cerebral cortex.

deep s., SYN bathyesthesia, kinesthetic *sense.*

dissociation s., the loss of the pain and the thermal senses with preservation of tactile sensibility or vice versa.

electromuscular s., s. of muscular tissue to stimulation by electricity.

epicritic s., SEE epicritic.

pallesthetic s., SYN pallesthesia.

proprioceptive s., SEE proprioceptive.

protopathic s., SEE protopathic.

splanchnesthetic s., SYN visceral *sense.*

vibratory s., SYN pallesthesia.

sen·si·ble (sen′si-bl). **1.** Perceptible to the senses. **2.** Capable of sensation. **3.** SYN sensitive. **4.** Having reason or judgment; intelligent. [L. *sensibilis,* fr. *sentio,* to feel, perceive]

sen·sif·er·ous (sen-sif′er-ŭs). Conducting a sensation. [L. *sensus,* sense, + *fero,* to carry]

sen·sig·e·nous (sen-sij′e-nŭs). Giving rise to sensation. [L. *sensus,* sense, + G. *-gen,* to produce]

sen·sim·e·ter (sen-sim′ĕ-ter). An instrument that measures degrees of cutaneous sensation. [L. *sensus,* sense, + G. *metron,* measure]

sensing.

quorum s., a phenomenon in bacteria that limits certain behaviors to occurring only above a certain population density.

sen·si·tive (sen′si-tiv). **1.** Capable of perceiving sensations. **2.** Responding to a stimulus. **3.** Acutely perceptive of interpersonal situations. **4.** One who is readily hypnotizable. **5.** Readily undergoing a chemical change, with but slight change in environmental conditions, as a s. reagent. **6.** In immunology, denoting: 1) a sensitized *antigen;* 2) a person (or animal) rendered susceptible to immunological reactions by previous exposure to the antigen concerned. SYN sensible (3).

sen·si·tiv·i·ty (sen-si-tiv′i-tē). **1.** The ability to appreciate by one or more of the senses. **2.** State of being sensitive. SYN esthesia (2). **3.** In clinical pathology and medical screening, the proportion of affected individuals who give a positive test result for the disease that the test is intended to reveal, i.e., true positive results divided by total true positive and false negative results, usually expressed as a percentage. Cf. specificity (2). [L. *sentio,* pp. *sensus,* to feel]

acquired s., SYN allergy (1).

analytical s., (1) the minimum detection limit; **(2)** the degree of response to a change in concentration of analyte being measured in an assay.

antibiotic s., microbial susceptibility to antibiotics. SEE ALSO antibiotic sensitivity *test,* minimal inhibitory *concentration.*

clinical s., test positivity in disease; ability of a test to correctly identify disease. SEE ALSO diagnostic s.

contrast s., in optics, the ability to discern the difference in brightness of adjacent areas; in radiology, allergic reaction to iodinated radiographic contrast medium.

diagnostic s., the probability (P) that, given the presence of disease (D), an abnormal test result (T) indicates the presence of disease; i.e., P(T/D). SEE ALSO clinical s.

idiosyncratic s., atopy, a type I allergic reaction.

induced s., SYN allergy (1).

multiple chemical s., a symptom array of variable presentation attributed to recurrent exposure to known environmental chemicals at dosages generally below levels established as harmful; complaints involve multiple organ systems. SYN environmental illness.

pacemaker s., the minimum cardiac activity required to consistently trigger a pulse generator.

photoallergic s., SEE photosensitization.

phototoxic s., SEE photosensitization.

primaquine s., nonimmunologic inborn s. to primaquine, causing hemolysis on exposure to the drug, due to deficiency of glucose 6-phosphate dehydrogenase in red cells.

relative s., the s. of a medical screening test as determined by comparison with the same type of test; e.g., s. of a new serologic test relative to s. of an established serologic test.

salt s., the tendency of certain bacterial suspensions to agglutinate spontaneously in physiologic saline solution.

spectral s., the reciprocal of the amount of monochromatic radiation that produces a fixed response.

sen·si·ti·za·tion (sen′si-ti-zā′shŭn). Immunization, especially with reference to antigens (immunogens) not associated with infection; the induction of acquired sensitivity or of allergy.

autoerythrocyte s., SEE autoerythrocyte sensitization *syndrome.*

covert s., aversive conditioning or training to rid oneself of an unwanted behavior during which the patient is taught to imagine unpleasant and related aversive consequences while engaging in the unwanted habit.

photodynamic s., the action by which certain substances, notably fluorescing dyes (acridine, eosin, methylene blue, rose bengal) absorb visible light and emit the energy at wavelengths that are deleterious to microbes or other organisms in the dye-containing suspension, or selectively destroy cancer cells sensitized by intravenous porphyrin and exposed to red laser light. SYN photosensitization (2).

sen·si·tize (sen′si-tīz). To render sensitive; to induce acquired sensitivity, to immunize. SEE ALSO sensitized *antigen.*

sen·si·tiz·er (sen′si-tīz-er). 1. A substance that causes allergy or dermatitis only after alteration (sensitization) of the skin by previous exposure to that substance. 2. SYN antibody.

sens·i·tom·e·try (sen-si-tom′ĕ-trē). In radiology, the procedure of measuring film response to radiation. [sensitivity + G. *metron,* measure]

sen·so·mo·bile (sen-sō-mō′bēl). Capable of movement in response to a stimulus.

sen·so·mo·bil·i·ty (sen-sō-mō-bil′i-tē). The state of being sensomobile.

sen·so·mo·tor (sen-sō-mō′ter). SYN sensorimotor.

sen·sor (sen′sŏr). A device designed to respond to physical stimuli such as temperature, light, magnetism, or movement, and to transmit resulting impulses for interpretation, recording, movement, or operating control. SEE sense.

⌂**sensori-.** Sensory. [L. *sensorius*]

sen·so·ri·al (sen-sōr′ē-ăl). Relating to the sensorium.

sen·so·ri·glan·du·lar (sen′sōr-i-glan′dū-lăr). Relating to glandular secretion excited by stimulation of the sensory nerves.

sen·so·ri·mo·tor (sen′sōr-i-mō′ter). Both sensory and motor; denoting a mixed nerve with afferent and efferent fibers. SYN sensomotor.

sen·so·ri·mus·cu·lar (sen′sōr-i-mŭs′kū-lăr). Denoting muscular contraction in response to a sensory stimulus.

sen·so·ri·um, pl. **sen·so·ria, sen·so·ri·ums** (sen-sōr′ē-ŭm, -ă, -ŭmz). 1. An organ of sensation. 2. The hypothetical "seat of sensation." SYN perceptorium. 3. In human biology and psychology, consciousness; sometimes used as a generic term for the intellectual and cognitive functions. [Late L.]

sen·so·ri·vas·cu·lar (sen′sōr-i-vas′kū-lăr). SYN sensorivasomotor.

sen·so·ri·vas·o·mo·tor (sen′sōr-i-vas-ō-mō′ter). Denoting con-

traction or dilation of the blood vessels occurring as a sensory reflex. SYN sensorivascular.

sen·so·ry (sen′sŏ-rē). Relating to sensation. [L. *sensorius,* fr. *sensus,* sense]

sen·su·al (sen′shoo-ăl). 1. Relating to the body and the senses, as distinguished from the intellect or spirit. 2. Denoting bodily or sensory pleasure, not necessarily sexual. [L. *sensualis,* endowed with feeling]

sen·su·al·ism (sen′shoo-ăl-izm). 1. Domination by the emotions. 2. Indulgence in sensory pleasures. [L. *sensualis,* endowed with feeling, fr. *sentio,* to feel]

sen·su·al·i·ty (sen-shŭ-al′i-tē). The state or quality of being sensual.

sen′su la′to. In a broad sense. [L.]

sen′su stri′cto. In a strict sense. [L.]

sen·tient (sen′shent, sen′shē-ent). Capable of, or characterized by, sensation. [L. *sentiens,* pres. p. of *sentio,* to feel, perceive]

sen·ti·ment (sen′ti-ment). 1. Feeling or emotion in relation to one idea. 2. A complex disposition or organization of a person with reference to a given object (a person, thing, or abstract idea) that makes the object what it is for him or her. [L. *sentio,* to feel]

sen·ti·sec·tion (sen-ti-sek′shŭn). Vivisection of an animal that is not anesthetized. [L. *sentio,* to feel, + *sectio,* a cutting]

sep·a·ra·tion (sep-ă-rā′shŭn). 1. The act of keeping apart or dividing, or the state of being held apart. 2. In dentistry, the process of gaining slight spaces between the teeth preparatory to treatment.

jaw s., the amount of space between the jaws at any degree of opening.

s. of retina, SYN retinal *detachment.*

sternochondral s., s. of the costal cartilage from the sternum, especially of the 2nd to 7th ribs, which are true joints lined with synovial membranes.

s. of teeth, (1) loss of proximal contact of teeth; (2) in orthodontics, the creation of interproximal spaces for the fitting of an appliance.

sep·a·ra·tor (sep′er-ā-ter). 1. That which divides or keeps apart two or more substances or prevents them from mingling. 2. In dentistry, an instrument for forcing two teeth apart, so as to gain access to adjacent proximal walls. SYN segregator. [L. *se-paro,* pp. *-atus,* to separate, fr. *se,* apart, + *paro,* to prepare]

Se·pha·dex (sef′a-deks). Trade name for certain polydextrans used in column chromatography.

sep·sis, pl. **sep·ses** (sep′sis, -sēz). The presence of various pathogenic organisms, or their toxins, in the blood or tissues; septicemia is a common type of s. [G. *sēpsis,* putrefaction]

intestinal s., s. associated with autointoxication of intestinal origin.

s. len′ta, a slowly developing and more or less localized infection.

puerperal s., SYN puerperal *fever.*

⌂**sept-.** SEE septi-, septico-, septo-.

sep·ta (sep′tă). Plural of septum. [L.]

intra-alveolar septa, SYN interradicular *septa* of maxilla and mandible, under *septum.*

sep·tal (sep′tăl). Relating to a septum.

sep·tan (sep′tăn). Denoting a malarial fever the paroxysms of which recur every seventh day, counting the day of the occurrence as the first day, i.e., with a five-day asymptomatic interval. [L. *septem,* seven]

Sep·ta·ta (sep-tă′tă). A recently described member of the protozoan phylum Microspora found in the intestine of an immunocompromised individual. The species described is *S. intestinalis.* This organism has been reclassified as *Encephalitozoon intestinalis.* SEE ALSO *Encephalitozoon intestinalis.*

sep·tate (sep′tāt). Having a septum; divided into compartments. [L. *saeptum,* septum]

sep·tec·to·my (sep-tek′tō-mē). Operative removal of the whole or a part of a septum, specifically of the nasal septum. [L. *saeptum,* septum, + G. *ektomē,* excision]

sep·te·mia (sep-tē′mē-ă). A rarely used term for septicemia.

se

⟳septi-, sept-. Seven. [L. *septem*]

sep·tic (sep′tik). Relating to or caused by sepsis.

sep·ti·ce·mia (sep-ti-sē′mē-ă). Systemic disease caused by the spread of microorganisms and their toxins via the circulating blood; formerly called "blood poisoning." SEE ALSO pyemia. SYN septic fever, septic intoxication. [G. *sēpsis,* putrefaction, + *haima,* blood]

acute fulminating meningococcal s., SYN Waterhouse-Friderichsen *syndrome.*

anthrax s., SYN anthracemia.

cryptogenic s., a form of s. in which no primary focus of infection can be found.

metastasizing s., sepsis, with entry of microorganisms into the bloodstream leading to abscess formation at a distance from the original site of infection.

morphine injector's s., bloodstream infection in an individual who injects him or herself with narcotics, usually intravenously, due to bacterial contamination of equipment used. Seen more often with heroin and narcotics other than morphine.

plague s., infection with the plague organism, *Yersinia pestis,* with bloodstream infection.

puerperal s., a severe bloodstream infection resulting from an obstetric delivery or procedure.

typhoid s., typhoid during the phase when the organism can be cultured from the blood. SYN typhosepsis.

sep·ti·ce·mic (sep-ti-sē′mik). Relating to, suffering from, or resulting from septicemia.

⟳septico-, septic-. Sepsis, septic. [G. *sēptikos,* putrifying, fr. *sēpsis,* putrefaction]

sep·ti·co·py·e·mia (sep′ti-kō-pī-ē′mē-ă). Pyemia and septicemia occurring together.

sep·ti·co·py·e·mic (sep′ti-kō-pī-ē′mik). Relating to septicopyemia.

sep·ti·va·lent (sep-ti-vā′lent, sep-tiv′ă-lent). Having a combining power (valency) of seven.

⟳septo-, sept-. Septum. [L. *saeptum*]

sep·to·der·mo·plas·ty (sep-tō-der′mō-plas-tē). Operation to graft squamous epithelium and dermis to replace the mucous membrane of the nasal septum, especially for patients with hereditary hemorrhagic telangiectasia. [septo- + dermo- + G. *plastos,* formed]

sep·to·mar·gi·nal (sep′tō-mar′ji-năl). Relating to the margin of a septum, or to both a septum and a margin.

sep·to·na·sal (sep′tō-nā′săl). Relating to the nasal septum.

sep·to·plas·ty (sep′tō-plas-tē). Operation to correct defects or deformities of the nasal septum, often by alteration or partial removal of skeletal structures. [septo- + G. *plastos,* formed]

sep·to·rhi·no·plas·ty (sep-tō-rī′nō-plas-tē). Combined operation to repair defects or deformities of the nasal septum and of the external nose. [septo- + G. *rhis,* nose, + *plastos,* formed]

sep·tos·to·my (sep-tos′tō-mē). Surgical creation of a septal defect. [septo- + G. *stoma,* mouth]

atrial s., establishment of a communication between the two atria of the heart. SYN atrioseptostomy.

balloon s., s. performed by cardiac catheterization with the use an of inflated balloon pulled across the interatrial septum through the foramen ovale; used in cases of transposition of the great vessels and tricuspid atresia.

sep·tu·lum, pl. **sep·tu·la** (sep′tū-lŭm, -lă). A minute septum. [Mod. L. dim. of *septum*]

s. tes′tis, SYN septula of testis.

septula of testis, one of the trabeculae of the testis; imperfect septa and fibrous cords radiating toward the surface of the gland from the mediastinum testis. SYN s. testis, trabecula testis.

SEPTUM

sep·tum, gen. **sep·ti,** pl. **sep·ta** (sep′tŭm, -tī, -tă). **1** [TA]. A thin wall dividing two cavities or masses of softer tissue. SEE septal *area,* transparent s. **2.** In fungi, a wall; usually a cross-wall in a hypha. [L. *saeptum,* a partition]

s. accesso′rium, an additional ridge forming the lower border of the limbus fossae ovalis.

alveolar s., SYN interalveolar s.

anteromedial intermuscular s. [TA], dense fascial triangle extending from the inferior medial border of the adductor magnus muscle to the vastus medialis muscle. Along with the sartorius muscle, this dense s. forms the roof of the lower half of the adductor canal and, as the femoral vessels pass deep to it, is often mistaken for the adductor hiatus. SYN s. intermusculare vastoadductorium [TA], subsartorial fascia, vastoadductor fascia.

aortopulmonary s., the spiral s. which, during development, separates the truncus arteriosus into a ventral pulmonary trunk and dorsal aorta. SEE ALSO bulbar *ridge.*

atrioventricular s. [TA], the small part of the membranous s. of the heart just above the septal cusp of the tricuspid valve that separates the right atrium from the left ventricle. SYN s. atrioventriculare [TA].

s. atrioventricula′re [TA], SYN atrioventricular s.

Bigelow s., SYN *calcar* femorale.

bony nasal s. [TA], the bones supporting the bony part of the nasal septum; these are the perpendicular plate of the ethmoid, the vomer, the sphenoidal rostrum, the crest of the nasal bones, the frontal spine, and the median crest formed by the apposition of the maxillary and palatine bones. SYN s. nasi osseum [TA].

bulbar s., obsolete term for spiral s.

s. bul′bi ure′thrae, a fibrous s. in the interior of the bulb of the penis which divides it into two hemispheres.

s. cana′lis musculotuba′rii, SYN s. of pharyngotympanic (auditory) tube.

cartilaginous s., SYN septal nasal *cartilage.*

s. cervica′le interme′dium [TA], SYN intermediate cervical s.

s. clitor′idis, SYN s. of corpora cavernosa of clitoris.

Cloquet s., SYN femoral s.

comblike s., SYN pectiniform s.

s. of corpora cavernosa of clitoris [TA], an incomplete fibrous s. between the corpora cavernosa of the clitoris. SYN s. corporum cavernosorum clitoridis [TA], s. clitoridis.

s. cor′porum cavernoso′rum clitor′idis [TA], SYN s. of corpora cavernosa of clitoris.

crural s., SYN femoral s.

distal spiral s., SEE spiral s.

endovenous s., s. endoveno′sum, a remnant of the primitive separation between veins that fused to form a definitive trunk, such as the trunk leading to the left common iliac and the left renal veins.

femoral s. [TA], mass of connective tissue that occupies the femoral canal, effectively closing the canal but permitting the passage of lymphatics draining the lower limb. SYN s. femorale [TA], Cloquet s., crural s.

s. femora′le [TA], SYN femoral s.

s. of frontal sinuses [TA], the bony partition between the right and left frontal sinuses; it is often deflected to one side of the middle line. SYN s. sinuum frontalium [TA].

gingival s., SYN gingival *papilla.*

s. glan′dis [TA], SYN s. of glans penis.

s. of glans penis [TA], a fibrous partition extending through the glans penis from the lower surface of the tunica albuginea to the urethra. SYN s. glandis [TA].

hanging s., the deformity caused by an abnormal width of the septal portion of the alar cartilages.

interalveolar s. [TA], **(1)** the tissue intervening between two adjacent pulmonary alveoli; it consists of a close-meshed capillary network covered on both surfaces by very thin alveolar epithelial cells; **(2)** one of the bony partitions between the tooth sockets of the mandible and maxilla (septa interalveolare mandibulae et maxillae). SYN s. interalveolare [TA], alveolar s., septal bone.

s. interalveola're, pl. **sep'ta interalveola'ria** [TA], SYN interalveolar s.

interatrial s. [TA], the wall between the atria of the heart. SEE ALSO s. primum, s. secundum. SYN s. interatriale [TA].

s. interatria'le [TA], SYN interatrial s.

interdental s., the bony portion separating two adjacent teeth in a dental arch.

interlobular s., the connective tissue between secondary pulmonary lobules, usually containing a vein and lymphatics; seen radiographically when thickened as a Kerley B or septal line.

intermediate cervical s. [TA], a thin s. composed of glia fiber and leptomeningeal connective tissue in the cervical spinal cord marking the border between the gracile fasciculi and cuneatus of the dorsal funiculus. SYN s. cervicale intermedium [TA].

s. interme'dium, old term for the s. of the atrioventricular canal of the embryonic heart formed by the fusion of the dorsal and ventral atrioventricular canal cushions.

intermuscular s. [TA], a term applied to aponeurotic sheets separating various muscles of the limbs; these are anterior and posterior crural intermuscular septa of leg (septa intermuscularis cruris anterius et posterius), lateral and medial femoral intermuscular septa (septa intermuscularis femoris laterale et mediale), lateral and medial intermuscular septa of arm (septa intermuscularis brachii laterale et mediale). SYN s. intermusculare [TA].

s. intermuscula're [TA], SYN intermuscular s.

s. intermuscula're va'stoadducto'rium [TA], SYN anteromedial intermuscular s.

interpulmonary s., SYN mediastinum (2).

sep'ta interradicula'ria mandi'bulae et ma'xillae [TA], SYN interradicular septa of maxilla and mandible.

interradicular septa of maxilla and mandible [TA], the bony partitions that project into the alveoli between the roots of the molar teeth. SYN septa interradicularia mandi'bulae et ma'xillae [TA], intra-alveolar septa.

interventricular s. [TA], the wall between the ventricles of the heart. SYN s. interventriculare [TA], ventricular s.

s. interventricula're [TA], SYN interventricular s.

s. lin'guae [TA], SYN lingual s.

lingual s. [TA], the median vertical fibrous partition of the tongue merging posteriorly into the aponeurosis of the tongue. SYN s. linguae [TA], s. of tongue.

s. lu'cidum, SYN s. pellucidum.

s. mediastina'le, SYN mediastinum (2).

s. membrana'ceum ventriculo'rum, SYN membranous *part* of interventricular septum.

membranous s., (1) SYN membranous *part* of nasal septum; **(2)** SYN membranous *part* of interventricular septum.

s. mo'bile na'si, SYN mobile *part* of nasal septum.

s. muscula're ventriculo'rum, SYN muscular *part* of interventricular septum (of heart).

s. of musculotubal canal, SYN s. of pharyngotympanic (auditory) tube.

nasal s. [TA], the wall dividing the nasal cavity into halves; it is composed of a central supporting skeleton covered on each side by a mucous membrane. SYN s. nasi [TA].

s. na'si [TA], SYN nasal s.

s. na'si oss'eum [TA], SYN bony nasal s.

orbital s. [TA], a fibrous membrane attached to the margin of the orbit and extending into the lids, containing the orbital fat and constituting in great part the posterior fascia of the orbicularis oculi muscle. SYN s. orbitale [TA].

s. orbita'le [TA], SYN orbital s.

pectiniform s., s. pectinifor'me, the anterior portion of the s. penis which is broken by a number of slitlike perforations. SYN comblike s.

s. pellu'cidum [TA], a thin plate of brain tissue, containing nerve cells and numerous nerve fibers, that is stretched like a flat, vertical sheet between the column and body of fornix below, and the corpus callosum above and anteriorly; it is usually fused in the median plane with its partner on the opposite side so as to form a thin, median partition between the left and right frontal horn of the lateral ventricles; in less than 10% of humans there is a blind, slitlike, fluid-filled space between the two transparent septa, the cavity of s. pellucidum. The transparent s. is continuous ventralward through the interval between the corpus callosum and the anterior commissure with the precommissural septum and subcallosal gyrus. SEE ALSO *cavity* of septum pellucidum, septal *area*. SYN s. lucidum, transparent s.

s. pe'nis [TA], the portion of the tunica albuginea incompletely separating the two corpora cavernosa of the penis.

s. of pharyngotympanic (auditory) tube [TA], a very thin horizontal plate of bone forming two semicanals, the upper, smaller, for the tensor tympani muscle, and the lower, larger for the pharyngotympanic (auditory) tube; its termination in the middle ear is the processus cochleariformis. SYN s. canalis musculotubarii, s. of musculotubal canal, s. tubae.

placental septa, incomplete partitions between placental cotyledons; they are covered with trophoblast and contain a core of maternal tissue.

precommissural s., SEE septal *area*.

s. pri'mum, a crescentic s. in the embryonic heart that develops on the dorsocephalic wall of the originally single atrium and initiates its partitioning into right and left chambers; the tips of the s. grow toward and fuse with the atrioventricular canal cushions.

proximal spiral s., SEE spiral s.

rectovaginal s. [TA], the fascial layer between the vagina and the lower part of the rectum. SYN s. rectovaginale [TA].

s. rectovagina'le [TA], SYN rectovaginal s.

rectovesical s. [TA], a fascial layer that extends superiorly from the central tendon of the perineum to the peritoneum between the prostate and rectum. SYN s. rectovesicale [TA], Denonvilliers aponeurosis, rectovesical fascia, Tyrrell fascia.

s. rectovesica'le [TA], SYN rectovesical s.

scrotal s. [TA], an incomplete wall of connective tissue and nonstriated muscle (dartos fascia) dividing the scrotum into two sacs, each containing a testis. SYN s. scroti [TA].

s. scro'ti [TA], SYN scrotal s.

s. secun'dum, the second of two major septal structures involved in the partitioning of the atrium, developing later than the s. primum and located to the right of it; like the s. primum, it is crescentic, but its tips are directed toward the sinus venosus, and it is more heavily muscular; it remains an incomplete partition until after birth, with its unclosed area constituting the foramen ovale.

sinus s., a small fold forming the medial end of the valve of the inferior vena cava; it is developed from the dorsal wall of the embryonic sinus venosus.

s. sin'uum fronta'lium [TA], SYN s. of frontal sinuses.

s. sin'uum sphenoida'lium [TA], SYN s. of sphenoidal sinuses.

s. of sphenoidal sinuses [TA], the bony partition between the two sphenoidal sinuses, often deflected to one side of the midline. SYN s. sinuum sphenoidalium [TA].

spiral s., a s. dividing the embryonic bulbus cordis into pulmonary and aortic outflow tracts from the developing heart; the distal spiral s. is derived from the right and left endocardial cushions and so separates the pulmonary and aortic orifices; the proximal spiral s. is the portion of the s. that is incorporated into the membranous part of the interventricular s.

spiral bulbar s., SEE spiral s.

s. spu'rium, a s. in the right atrium of the embryonic heart formed by the right venous valve and its continuation onto the dorsocephalic wall of the atrium; in human embryos, it reaches its fullest development during the third month and then undergoes regression, taking no part in atrial partitioning (hence its designation as false); reduced portions persist as the valve of the inferior vena cava and the valve of the coronary sinus.

s. of testis, SYN *mediastinum* of testis.

se

s. of tongue, SYN lingual s.

transparent s., SYN s. pellucidum.

transverse s., (1) SYN ampullary *crest*; (2) the mesodermal mass separating the pericardial and peritoneal cavities; it is covered with mesothelium except where intimately associated with the liver, which originally develops within it; the s. is definitively incorporated into the diaphragm as the central tendon.

s. tu′bae, SYN s. of pharyngotympanic (auditory) tube.

urogenital s., the coronally placed ridge formed by the caudal portion of the urogenital ridges meeting in the midline of the embryo; it lies between the hindgut dorsally and the bladder ventrally.

urorectal s., in embryos, a partition dividing the cloaca into a dorsal, rectal portion and a ventral portion called the urogenital sinus; reaching the cloacal membrane at about the time of its disintegration, the urorectal s. divides the cloacal exit into an anal and a urogenital orifice. SYN urorectal fold.

ventricular s., SYN interventricular s.

---

se·que·la, pl. **se·que·lae** (sē-kwel′ă, sē-kwel′ē). A condition following as a consequence of a disease. [L. *sequela,* a sequel, fr. *sequor,* to follow]

se·quence (sē′kwens). The succession, or following, of one thing or event after another. [L. *sequor,* to follow]

Alu s.′s, in the human genome a repeated, relatively conserved s. of about 300 bp that often contains a cleavage site for the restriction enzyme AluI near the center; about 1 million copies in the human genome.

chi s., an octameric s. of bases in DNA that participates in RecBC-mediated genetic recombination.

coding s., the portion of DNA that codes for transcription of messenger RNA. SEE exon.

insertion s., discrete DNA s.′s of nucleotides that are repeated at various sites on bacterial chromosomes, certain plasmids, and bacteriophages and that can move from one site to another on the chromosome, to another plasmid in the same bacterium, or to a bacteriophage.

intervening s., SYN intron.

s. ladder, The array of bands, made conspicuous by labeling, when DNA fragmented by endonucleases is subject to gel electrophoresis; corresponds to the nucleotide sequence.

leader s.′s, s.′s at the end of either nucleic acids (DNA and RNA) or proteins that must be processed off to allow for a specific function of the mature molecule.

long terminal repeat s.′s (LTR), regions of the RNA genome associated with regulation, integration, and expression of retroviruses.

monotonic s., a s. in which each value in a set is greater than the preceding value.

palindromic s., SEE palindrome.

pulse s., in magnetic resonance imaging, a series of changes in the induced magnetic field, which include the phase and frequency-encoding gradients and read-out functions.

regulatory s., any DNA s. that is responsible for the regulation of gene expression, such as promoters and operators.

Shine-Dalgarno s., a purine-rich, untranslated region of mRNA upstream from the initiation codon in prokaryotes; assists in aligning the mRNA on the ribosome.

termination s., SYN termination *codon.*

twin reversed arterial perfusion s. (TRAP), a circulatory anomaly in monozygotic twins wherein there are placental arterioarterial and venovenous anastomoses and umbilical anomalies, with one fetus being perfused with deoxygenated blood; the recipient fetus develops as an acardiac acephalic, and the pump or donor twin is at risk for cardiac failure.

se·quenc·ing (sē′kwens-ing). The determination of the sequence of subunits in a macromolecule.

dideoxy sequencing, a method of sequencing DNA using 2′,3′-dideoxyribonucleoside triphosphates.

Maxim-Gilbert sequencing, a method of sequencing DNA using dimethyl sulfate and hydrazinolysis.

se·quen·tial (sē-kwen′shăl). Occurring in sequence.

se·ques·tra (sē-kwes′tră). Plural of sequestrum.

se·ques·tral (sē-kwes′trăl). Relating to a sequestrum.

se·ques·tra·tion (sē-kwes-trā′shŭn). **1.** Formation of a sequestrum. **2.** Loss of blood or of its fluid content into spaces within the body so that it is withdrawn from the circulating volume, resulting in hemodynamic impairment, hypovolemia, hypotension, and reduced venous return to the heart. [L. *sequestratio,* fr. *sequestro,* pp. *-atus,* to lay aside]

bronchopulmonary s., a congenital anomaly in which a mass of lung tissue becomes isolated, during development, from the rest of the lung; the bronchi in the mass are usually dilated or cystic and are not connected with the bronchial tree; it is supplied by a branch of the aorta.

se·ques·trec·to·my (sē-kwes-trek′tō-mē). Operative removal of a sequestrum. SYN sequestrotomy. [sequestrum + G. *ektomē,* excision]

se·ques·trot·o·my (sē-kwes-trot′ō-mē). SYN sequestrectomy. [sequestrum + G. *tomē, incision*]

se·ques·trum, pl. **se·ques·tra** (sē-kwes′trŭm, -tră). A piece of necrotic tissue, usually bone, that has become separated from the surrounding healthy tissue. [Mod. L. use of Mediev. L. *sequestrum,* something laid aside, fr. L. *sequestro,* to lay aside, separate]

primary s., a completely detached s.

se·quoi·o·sis (sē-kwoy-ō′sis). Extrinsic allergic alveolitis caused by inhalation of redwood sawdust containing spores of *Graphium, Pullularia, Aureobasidium,* and other fungi. [*Sequoia* (genus name) for *Sequoah* (George Guess), Cherokee scholar, + G. *-osis,* condition]

SER Abbreviation for somatosensory evoked response. SEE ALSO evoked *response.*

Ser Symbol for serine and its radical.

se·ra (sēr′ă). Plural of serum.

ser·al·bu·min (sēr-al-bū′min). SYN serum *albumin.*

ser·en·dip·i·ty (ser-en-dip′i-tē). Accidental discovery; in science, finding one thing while looking for something else, as in Fleming's discovery of penicillin. [coined by Horace Walpole and relates to *The Three Princes of Serendip,* fr. alternate spelling of *Serendib,* ancient name for Sri Lanka]

Sergent, Emile, French physician, 1867–1943. SEE S. white *line;* Bernard-S. *syndrome.*

se·ries, pl. **se·ries** (sēr′ēz). **1.** A succession of similar objects following one another in space or time. **2.** In chemistry, a group of substances, either elements or compounds, having similar properties or differing from each other in composition by a constant ratio. [L. fr. *sero,* to join together]

aromatic s., all the compounds derived from benzene, or similar cyclic compounds that obey the Hückel rule, distinguished from those compounds that are acyclic or that contain rings that lack the conjugated double bond structure characteristic of benzene.

erythrocytic s., the cells in the various stages of development in the red bone marrow leading to the formation of the erythrocyte, e.g., erythroblasts, normoblasts, erythrocytes.

fatty s., the alkanes; all the acyclic compounds in the methane, ethane, propane, etc., group, as distinguished from the aromatic s.

granulocytic s., the cells in the several stages of development in the bone marrow leading to the mature granulocyte of the circulation, e.g., myeloblasts, different stages of the myelocyte, granulocytes.

Hofmeister s., the series of cations Mg^{2+}, Ca^{2+}, Sr^{2+}, Ba^{2+}, Li^+, Na^+, K^+, Rb^+, Cs^+, and of anions citrate^{3-}, tartrate^{2-}, SO_4^{2-}, acetate$^-$, NO_3^-, ClO_3^-, I^-, CNS^- (among others), each series arranged in order of decreasing ability to: 1) precipitate the dispersed substance of lyophilic sols; 2) "salt out" organic substances (e.g., aniline, ethyl acetate) from aqueous solutions; or 3) inhibit the swelling of gels. These effects, among other related ones, are ascribable to the abstraction and binding of water by these ions (i.e., hydration), which also decreases in the orders given, so that (in the monovalent cation series) Li^+, with the smallest crystal radius, has the largest hydrated radius, and vice versa for Cs^+. SYN lyotropic s.

homologous s., a s. of organic compounds, the succeeding members of which differ from each other by the radical CH_2 (as in the fatty series).

lymphocytic s., lymphoid s., the cells at various states in the development in lymphoid tissue of the mature lymphocytes, e.g., lymphoblasts, young lymphocytes, mature lymphocytes.

lyotropic s., SYN Hofmeister s.

myeloid s., the granulocytic and the erythrocytic s.

small bowel s., radiographic examination of the small intestine following the oral administration of contrast medium, usually barium sulfate. Cf. small bowel *enema*.

thrombocytic s., the cells of successive stages in thrombocytic (platelet) development in the bone marrow, e.g., thromboblasts, thrombocytes.

🔢**upper GI s.,** a radiographic contrast study of the esophagus, stomach, and duodenum.

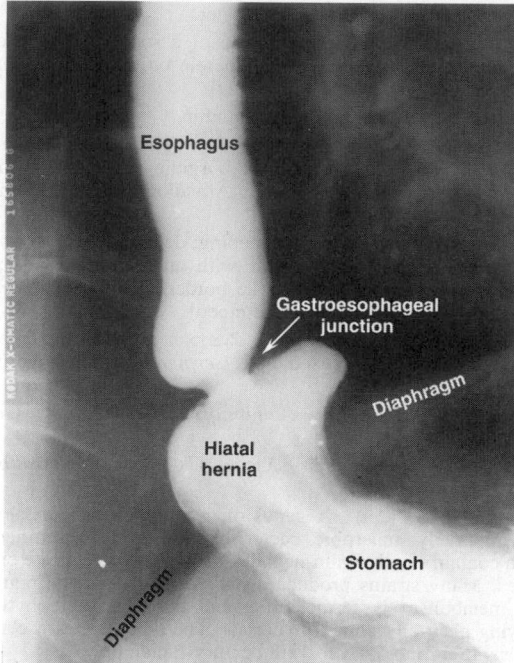

upper gastrointestinal series: radiograph showing hiatal hernia

---

ser·ine (S, Ser) (ser'ēn). 2-Amino-3-hydroxypropanoic acid; the L-isomer is one of the amino acids occurring in proteins.

s. deaminase, SYN *threonine* dehydratase.

s. dehydrase, SYN L-s. dehydratase.

L-s. dehydratase, L-hydroxyamino acid dehydratase; a deaminating hydro-lyase converting L-serine to pyruvate and NH_3; a part of amino acid catabolism. SEE ALSO *threonine* dehydratase. SYN s. dehydrase.

s. sulfhydrase, SYN cystathionine β-synthase.

se·ri·o·graph (sēr'ē-ō-graf). An instrument for making a series of radiographs; used, e.g., in cerebral angiography; an obsolete term for rapid film changer. [series + G. *graphō*, to write]

se·ri·og·ra·phy (sēr-ē-og'ră-fē). The making of a series of radiographs by means of the seriograph.

se·ri·os·co·py (sēr-ē-os'kŏ-pē). Formerly, a series of radiographs of a region taken from different directional points and later combined. [series + G. *skopeō*, to view]

ser·i·scis·sion (ser-i-sish'ŭn). Rarely used term denoting division of the pedicle of a tumor or other tissue by a silk ligature. [L. *sericum*, silk, + *scissio*, a cleaving]

SERM Abbreviation for selective estrogen receptor *modulator*.

sero-. Serum, serous. [L. *serum*, whey]

se·ro·co·li·tis (sēr'ō-kō-lī'tis). SYN pericolitis. [Mod. L. *serosa*, serous membrane, + colitis]

se·ro·con·ver·sion (sēr'ō-kon-ver'zhŭn). Development of detectable specific antibodies in the serum as a result of infection or immunization.

se·ro·cys·tic (sēr-ō-sis'tik). Relating to one or more serous cysts.

se·ro·di·ag·no·sis (sēr'ō-dī-ag-nō'sis). Diagnosis by means of serologic reactions using blood serum or other serous fluids in the body.

se·ro·en·ter·i·tis (sēr'ō-en-ter-ī'tis). SYN perienteritis. [Mod. L. *serosa*, serous membrane, + enteritis]

se·ro·ep·i·de·mi·ol·o·gy (sēr'ō-ep-i-dē-mē-ol'ō-jē). Epidemiologic study based on the detection of infection by serologic testing.

se·ro·fast (sēr'ō-fast). SYN serum-fast.

se·ro·fi·brin·ous (sēr-ō-fī'bri-nŭs). Denoting an exudate composed of serum and fibrin.

se·ro·fi·brous (sēr-ō-fī'brŭs). Relating to a serous membrane and a fibrous tissue.

serogroup (ser'ō-groop, sēr). **1.** A group of bacteria containing a common antigen, used in the classification of certain genera of bacteria. **2.** A group of viral species that are antigenically closely related.

se·ro·log·ic (sēr-ō-loj'ik). Relating to serology.

se·rol·o·gy (sĕ-rol'ō-jē). The branch of science concerned with serum, especially with specific immune or lytic serums; to measure either antigens or antibodies in sera. [sero- + G. *logos*, study]

se·ro·ma (sē-rō'mă). A mass or tumefaction caused by the localized accumulation of serum within a tissue or organ. [sero- + G. *-oma*, tumor]

se·ro·mem·bra·nous (sēr'ō-mem'bră-nŭs). Relating to a serous membrane.

se·ro·mu·coid (sēr-ō-mū'koyd). General term for a mucoprotein (glycoprotein) from serum.

acid s., SYN orosomucoid.

se·ro·mu·cous (sēr-ō-mū'kŭs). Pertaining to a mixture of watery and mucinous material, such as that of certain glands.

ser·o·my·ot·o·my (se'rō-mī-ot'ō-me). Incision in the wall of a hollow viscus that involves the serosa and muscularis but not the mucosa. [serosa (1) + G. *mys*, muscle, + *tomē*, a cutting]

se·ro·neg·a·tive (sēr-ō-neg'ă-tiv). Lacking an antibody of a specific type in serum; used to mean absence of prior infection with a specific agent (e.g., rubella virus), disappearance of antibodies after treatment of a disease (e.g., syphilis), or absence of antibody usually found in a given syndrome (e.g., rheumatoid arthritis without rheumatoid factor).

se·ro·pos·i·tive (sēr-ō-poz'i-tiv). Containing antibody of a specific type in serum; used to indicate presence of immunological evidence of a specific infection (e.g., Lyme disease, syphilis) or presence of a diagnostically useful antibody (e.g., rheumatoid arthritis with rheumatoid factor).

se·ro·pu·ru·lent (sēr'ō-poo'roo-lent). Composed of or containing both serum and pus; denoting a discharge of thin watery pus (seropus).

se·ro·pus (sēr'ō-pŭs). Purulent serum, i.e., pus largely diluted with serum.

se·ro·re·ver·sion (sir-ō-rē-vur'zhŭn). A loss in serological reactivity; may be spontaneous or in response to therapy.

se·ro·sa (se-rō'să) [TA]. **1.** The outermost coat or serous layer of a visceral structure that lies in the body cavities of the abdomen or thorax; it consists of a surface layer of mesothelium reinforced by irregular fibroelastic connective tissue. **2.** The outermost of the extraembryonic membranes that encloses the embryo and all its other membranes; it consists of somatopleure, i.e., ectoderm reinforced by somatic mesoderm; the serosa of mammalian embryos is frequently called the trophoderm. SYN membrana serosa (2). SEE ALSO chorion. SYN tunica serosa [TA], serous coat✱, membrana serosa (1), serous membrane, serous tunic. [fem. of Mod. L. *serosus*, serous]

s. of colon, SYN s. of large intestine.

s. of esophagus [TA], serous coat of the abdominal part of the esophagus. SYN tunica serosa esophagi [TA].

s. of gallbladder [TA], serous coat of the gallbladder; the visceral peritoneum covering the portions of the gallbladder not in direct contact with the liver. SYN tunica serosa vesicae biliaris [TA], tunica serosa vesicae felleae⭐.

s. of large intestine [TA], serous coat of the colon; the visceral peritoneum of the large intestine. SYN tunica serosa intestini crassi [TA], s. of colon, tunica serosa coli.

s. of liver [TA], serous coat of the liver; peritoneal covering of the liver, enclosing almost all except for a triangular area on its posterior surface (the "bare area of the liver") and a smaller area where the liver and gallbladder are in direct contact. SYN tunica serosa hepatis [TA].

s. of parietal pleura [TA], glistening inner surface of the parietal pleura. SYN tunica serosa pleurae perietalis [TA].

s. of peritoneum, simple squamous epithelium that forms the glistening surface of the parietal and visceral layers of peritoneum. SYN tunica serosa peritonei [TA], serous coat of peritoneum⭐, serous layer of peritoneum.

s. of serous pericardium [TA], single layer of flat cells that lines the pericardial sac and heart; this layer, plus the subserous layer, constitute the serous pericardium. SYN tunica serosa pericardii serosi [TA].

s. of small intestine [TA], serous coat of the small intestine; the peritoneal covering of the external surface of the small intestine. SYN tunica serosa intestini tenuis [TA].

s. of the spleen [TA], visceral peritoneum covering the spleen. SYN tunica serosa splenis [TA].

s. of stomach [TA], serous coat of the stomach; the visceral peritoneum covering the outer surface of the stomach. SYN tunica serosa gastricae [TA], tunica serosa ventriculi.

s. of (urinary) bladder [TA], serous coat of the urinary bladder; the visceral peritoneum covering the roof and lateral walls of the urinary bladder. SYN tunica serosa vesicae (urinariae) [TA].

s. of uterine tube [TA], serous coat of the uterine tube; the visceral peritoneum forming the outer surface of the uterine tubes. SYN tunica serosa tubae uterinae [TA].

s. of uterus [TA], serous coat of uterus; the visceral peritoneum covering the fundus and posterior body of the uterus. SYN tunica serosa uteri [TA].

s. of visceral pleura [TA], single layer of flat cells lining and thus forming the glistening outermost surface of the lungs. SYN tunica serosa pleurae visceralis [TA].

se·ro·sa·mu·cin (se-rō-să-mū′sin). Mucoid material found in serous fluids, e.g., in ascitic or synovial fluid.

se·ro·san·guin·e·ous (sēr′ō-sang-gwin′ē-ŭs). Denoting an exudate or a discharge composed of or containing serum and also blood.

se·ro·se·rous (sēr-ō-sēr′ŭs). **1.** Relating to two serous surfaces. **2.** Denoting a suture, as of the intestine, in which the edges of the wound are infolded so as to bring the two serous surfaces in apposition.

se·ro·si·tis (sēr-ō-sī′tis). Inflammation of a serous membrane.
multiple s., SYN polyserositis.

se·ros·i·ty (se-ros′i-tē). **1.** A serous fluid or a serum. **2.** The condition of being serous. **3.** The serous quality of a liquid.

se·ro·syn·o·vi·al (sēr′ō-si-nō′vē-ăl). Relating to serum and also synovia.

se·ro·syn·o·vi·tis (sēr′ō-sin-ō-vī′tis). Synovitis attended with a copious serous effusion.

se·ro·tax·is (sēr-ō-tak′sis). Edema of the skin induced by the application of a strong cutaneous irritant. [sero- + G. *taxis,* an arranging]

se·ro·ther·a·py (sēr-ō-thār′ă-pē). Treatment of an infectious disease by injection of an antitoxin or serum containing specific antibody. SYN serum therapy.

se·ro·ti·na (sēr′ō-tī′nă). SEE decidua. [L. fem. of *serotinus,* late]

se·ro·to·ner·gic (sēr-ō-tō-ner′jik, sěr-). Related to the action of serotonin or its precursor L-tryptophan. [serotonin + G. *ergon,* work]

se·ro·to·nin (sēr-ō-tō′nin). A vasoconstrictor, liberated by blood platelets, that inhibits gastric secretion and stimulates smooth muscle; present in relatively high concentrations in some areas of the central nervous system (hypothalamus, basal ganglia), and occurring in many peripheral tissues and cells and in carcinoid tumors. SYN 5-hydroxytryptamine, enteramine, thrombocytin, thrombotonin. [sero- + G. *tonos,* tone, tension, + -in]

se·ro·type (sēr′ō-tīp). SYN serovar.
heterologous s., an antibody that was induced by one antigen and reacts with another antigen.
homologous s., an antibody that was induced by a particular antigen and reacts with that antigen.

se·rous (sēr′ŭs). Relating to, containing, or producing serum or a substance having a watery consistency.

se·ro·vac·ci·na·tion (sēr′ō-vak-si-nā′shŭn). A process for producing mixed immunity by the injection of a serum to secure passive immunity, and by vaccination with a modified or killed culture to acquire active immunity later.

se·ro·var (sēr′ō-var). A subdivision of a species or subspecies distinguishable from other strains therein on the basis of antigenicity. SYN serotype. [sero- + *variant*]

se·ro·zyme (sēr′ō-zīm). SYN prothrombin.

ser·pen·tar·ia (ser-pen-tā′rē-ă, -tar′ē-ă). The dried rhizome and roots of *Aristolochia serpentaria,* Virginia snakeroot, or of *A. reticulata,* Texas snakeroot (family Aristolochiaceae); a stomachic. SYN snakeroot. [L. snakeweed]

ser·pig·i·nous (ser-pij′i-nŭs). Creeping; denoting an ulcer or other cutaneous lesion that extends with an arciform border; the margin has a wavy or serpent-like border. [Mediev. L. *serpigo-* (-gin-), ringworm, fr. L. *serpo,* to creep]

ser·pi·go (ser-pī′gō). **1.** SYN tinea. **2.** SYN herpes. **3.** Any creeping or serpiginous eruption. [Mediev. L. *serpigo* (-gin-), ringworm, fr. L. *serpo,* to creep]

ser·pins. SYN serine protease *inhibitors,* under *inhibitor.* [*ser*ine *protease inhibitors*]

ser·rate, ser·rat·ed (ser′āt, -ā′ted). Toothed. [L. *serratus,* fr. *serra,* a saw]

Ser·ra·tia (se-rā′shē-ă). A genus of motile, peritrichous, aerobic to facultatively anaerobic bacteria (family Enterobacteriaceae) which contain small, Gram-negative rods. Some strains are encapsulated. Many strains produce a pink, red, or magenta pigment; their metabolism is fermentative and they are saprophytic on decaying plant and animal materials. The type species is *S. marcescens.* [Serafino *Serrati,* 18th century Italian physicist]
S. marces′cens, a species found in water, soil, milk, foods, and silkworms and other insects; a significant cause of hospital-acquired infection, especially in patients with impaired immunity; it is the type species of the genus *S.*

ser·ra·tion (se-rā′shŭn). **1.** The state of being serrated or notched. **2.** Any one of the processes in a serrate or dentate formation. [L. *serra,* saw]

serre·fine (ser-e-fēn′). A small spring forceps used for approximating the edges of a wound or for temporarily closing an artery during an operation. [Fr.]

ser·re·no·eud (ser-e-no-ood′). An instrument for tightening a ligature. [Fr. *serrer,* to press, + *noeud,* knot]

Serres, Antoine E.R.A., French anatomist, 1786–1868. SEE S. *angle, glands,* under *gland; rests* of S., under *rest.*

ser·ru·late, ser·ru·lat·ed (ser′ū-lāt, -lā′ted). Finely serrate. [L. *serrula,* a small saw, dim. of *serra*]

Sertoli, Enrico, Italian histologist, 1842–1910. SEE *Sertoli cell tumor;* S. *cells,* under *cell, columns,* under *column;* S.-cell-only *syndrome;* Sertoli-Leydig cell *tumor;* Sertoli-stromal cell *tumor.*

ser·tra·line (ser′tră-lēn). An antidepressant which exhibits selectivity for the blockade of serotonin reuptake; similar to fluoxetine.

se·rum, pl. **se·rums, se·ra** (sēr′ŭm, -ŭmz, -ă). **1.** A clear, watery fluid, especially that moistening the surface of serous membranes, or exuded in inflammation of any of those membranes. **2.** The fluid portion of the blood obtained after removal of the fibrin clot and blood cells, distinguished from the plasma in circulating blood. Sometimes used as a synonym for antiserum or antitoxin. [L. whey]

anticomplementary s., s. that destroys or inactivates complement.

antiepithelial s., an antiserum (cytotoxin) for epithelial cells.

antilymphocyte s. (ALS), antiserum against lymphocytes, used to suppress rejection of grafts or organ transplants; when used in man, the globulin fraction of the heterologous s. (prepared in horse or other animals) is usually used in conjunction with other immunosuppressive agents (drugs or chemicals) and for a limited period of time. SYN antilymphocyte globulin.

antirabies s., a sterile solution containing antibodies obtained from the blood s. or plasma of a healthy animal, or human, that has been immunized against rabies by means of vaccine; administered immediately after severe or multiple bites by domestic animals suspected to be rabid and in all wild animal bites, to be followed by a regimen of rabies vaccine.

antireticular cytotoxic s., an antiserum specific for cells of the reticuloendothelial system.

antitoxic s., an antitoxin.

bacteriolytic s., an antiserum (bacteriolysin) that sensitizes a bacterium to the lytic action of complement.

blood s., SEE serum (2).

convalescent s., s. from patients recently recovered from a disease; useful for diagnosis by demonstrating a fourfold increase in specific antibodies or in preventing or modifying by passive immunization the same disease in exposed susceptible individuals.

Coombs s., SYN antihuman *globulin*.

dried human s., s. prepared by drying liquid human s. by freeze-drying or by any other method that will avoid denaturation of the proteins and will yield a product readily soluble in a quantity of water equal to the volume of liquid human s. from which it was prepared.

foreign s., a s. derived from an animal and injected into an animal of another species or into humans.

human s., SEE dried human s., normal human s.

human measles immune s., obtained from the blood of a healthy person who has survived an attack of measles. SYN measles convalescent s.

human pertussis immune s., the sterile s. prepared from the pooled blood of healthy adult human beings who have received repeated courses of phase I pertussis vaccine; administered intravenously or intramuscularly for the prophylaxis or treatment of whooping cough.

human scarlet fever immune s., scarlet fever convalescent s., obtained from healthy persons who have survived an attack of scarlet fever.

hyperimmune s., antisera with a high antibody titer produced by repeated injections of antigens.

immune s., SYN antiserum.

inactivated s., s. that has been heated to 56°C for 30 min to destroy the lytic activity of complement.

s. lactis, SYN whey.

liquid human s., the pool of fluids separated from blood withdrawn from human subjects and allowed to clot in the absence of any anticoagulant; not more than 10 separate donations are pooled; the contributions from donors of A, O, and either B or AB groups are represented in approximately the ratio 9:9:2.

measles convalescent s., SYN human measles immune s.

muscle s., the fluid remaining after the coagulation of muscle plasma and the separation of myosin.

nonimmune s., a s. from a subject that is not immune; a s. that is free of antibodies to a given antigen.

normal s., a nonimmune s., usually with reference to a s. obtained prior to immunization.

normal horse s., the sterile and filtered s. of a healthy, unvaccinated horse.

normal human s., sterile s. obtained by pooling approximately equal amounts of the liquid portion of coagulated whole blood

from eight or more persons who are free from any disease transmissible by transfusion.

polyvalent s., an antiserum obtained by inoculating an animal with several different antigens or species or strains of bacteria.

pooled s., pooled blood s., the mixed s. from a number of individuals.

salted s., SYN salted *plasma*.

specific s., a monovalent antiserum, i.e., one obtained by inoculating an animal with one antigen or species or strain of bacteria.

thyrotoxic s., an antiserum obtained by injecting into animals the nucleoproteins of the thyroid gland.

truth s., colloquialism for a drug, such as amobarbital sodium or thiopental sodium, intravenously injected with scopolamine for the purpose of eliciting information from the subject under its influence; a misnomer because the subject's revelations may or may not be factually true, and its legal status and use is questionable.

se·rum·al (sēr′ŭm-ăl). Relating to or derived from serum.

se·rum-fast (sēr′ŭm-fast). **1.** Pertaining to a serum in which there is little or no change in the titer of antibody, even under conditions of treatment or immunologic stimulation. **2.** Resistant to the destructive effect of sera. SYN serofast.

se·rum glu·tam·ic-ox·a·lo·ace·tic trans·am·i·nase (SGOT). SYN *aspartate* aminotransferase.

se·rum glu·tam·ic-py·ru·vic trans·am·i·nase (SGPT). SYN alanine aminotransferase.

ser·va·tion (ser-vā′shŭn). The use or function of an organ.

Servetus (Servet, Servide), Miguel, Spanish anatomist and theologian, 1511–1553. SEE S. *circulation.*

ser·vo·mech·a·nism (ser′vō-mek′ă-nizm). **1.** A control system using negative feedback to operate another system. **2.** A process that behaves as a self-regulatory device; e.g., the reaction of the pupil to light. [L. *servus,* servant, + G. *mēchanē,* contrivance]

ser·yl (ser′il). A radical of serine.

ses·a·me (ses′ă-mē). Benne plant, an herb, *Sesamum indicum* (family Pedaliaceae), the seeds of which are used as a food, and which are the source of sesame oil. [G. *sēsamē,* sesame, an Eastern leguminous plant]

s. oil, the refined fixed oil obtained from the seed of one or more cultivated varieties of *Sesamum indicum;* a solvent for intramuscular injections. SYN benne oil, gingili oil, teel oil.

ses·a·moid (ses′ă-moyd). **1.** Resembling in size or shape a grain of sesame. **2.** Denoting a sesamoid bone. [G. *sēsamoeidēs,* like sesame]

△**sesqui-.** Prefix denoting ³⁄₂; at one time used in chemistry to indicate a ratio of 3:2 between the two parts of a compound (e.g., sesquisulfide, sesquibasic), but presently used only for sesquihydrates and sesquiterpenes. [L.]

ses·qui·hy·drates (ses-kwi-hī′drāts). Compounds crystallizing with (nominally) 1.5 molecules of water.

ses·qui·ter·penes (ses-kwi-ter′pēnz). Compounds formed from three isoprene units; may be acyclic, mono-, di-, or tricyclic; synthesized from farnesylpyrophosphate (e.g., trichothecin, nicin).

ses·sile (ses′il). Having a broad base of attachment; not pedunculated. [L. *sessilis,* low-growing, fr. *sedeo,* pp. *sessus,* to sit]

ses·ter·ter·penes (ses′ter-ter-pēnz). Compounds formed from five isoprene units; often have a tricyclic structure; formed from geranylfarnesylpyrophosphate (e.g., cochliobolin B). [L. *sestertius,* two and one-half, fr. *semis,* half, + *tertius,* third, + terpene]

set. 1. A readiness to perceive or to respond in some way; an attitude which facilitates or predetermines an outcome; e.g., prejudice or bigotry as a s. to respond negatively, independently of the merits of the stimulus. **2.** To reduce a fracture; i.e., to bring the bones back into a normal position or alignment. **3.** Defined group of events, objects, data, distinguishable from other groups. [M.E. *sette,* fr. O.Fr., fr. Med. L. *secta,* course, fr. *sequor,* to follow]

haploid s., the genetic content of a normal gamete in which every autosomal locus is represented by a single allele and either one full set of X-linked genes or one full set of Y-linked genes; the normal adult somatic cell contains two haploid s.'s.

learning s., a readiness or predisposition to learn developed from previous learning experiences, as when an organism learns to solve each successive problem (of equal or increasing difficulty) in fewer trials.

postural s., an overall motor readiness to respond, as in a runner instructed to get set and on the mark.

se·ta, pl. **set·ae** (sē'tă, -tē). A bristle or a slender, stiff, bristle-like structure. SYN chaeta. [L. *saeta* or *seta,* a stiff hair or bristle]

se·ta·ceous (sē-tā'shŭs). **1.** Having bristles. **2.** Resembling a bristle. [L. *seta,* a bristle]

Se·tar·ia (sē-tā'rē-ă, -tar'ē-ă). A nematode genus of the family Stephanofilariidae (superfamily Filarioidea). Adults are long and thin, typically occur in the peritoneal cavity, and produce sheathed microfilariae in the blood that are transmitted to other hosts after cyclical development in appropriate mosquito hosts. They are parasitic in cattle or equines (wild or domestic) and generally are nonpathogenic, although occasionally young worms may wander into the anterior chamber of the eye. [L. *seta,* a bristle]

S. cer'vi, a species that occurs in the abdominal cavity of cattle, buffalo, bison, yak, and various deer, but rarely in sheep.

S. equi'na, a species that is a common parasite of horses and other equids in all parts of the world; they are slender whitish filaments, several inches in length, usually found free in the peritoneal cavity, but occasionally reported in the pleural cavity, lungs, scrotum, eye, and intestine.

set·back (set'bak). A surgical operation for treatment of a bilateral cleft of the palate in which the premaxilla is moved posteriorly; the procedure is often accompanied by bone grafting.

se·tif·er·ous (sĕ-tif'er-ŭs). Bristly or having bristles. SYN setigerous. [L. *seta,* bristle, + *fero,* to carry]

se·tig·er·ous (sĕ-tij'er-ŭs). SYN setiferous. [L. *seta,* bristle, + *gero,* to bear]

se·ton (sē'tŏn). A wisp of threads, a strip of gauze, a length of wire, or other foreign material passed through the subcutaneous tissues or a cyst to form a sinus or fistula. [L. *seta,* bristle]

set·ting. Hardening, as of amalgam.

set-up. 1. The arrangement of teeth on a trial denture base. **2.** A procedure in dental case analysis involving cutting off and repositioning of teeth in the desired positions on a plaster cast.

se·vere com·bined im·mu·no·de·fi·cient mice (SCID mice). Mice that lack both T and B lymphocytes and are used for transplantation and study of human lymphoid tissues resulting in a SCID-human mouse chimera. SEE ALSO severe combined *immunodeficiency.*

Severinghaus, John W., U.S. physiologist and anesthesiologist, *1922. SEE S. *electrode.*

se·vo·flu·rane (sev-ō-floor'ān). A halogenated ether for inhalation anesthesia.

se·vum (sē'vŭm). Suet or tallow. [L.]

sex (seks). **1.** The biologic character or quality that distinguishes male and female from one another as expressed by analysis of the individual's gonadal, morphologic (internal and external), chromosomal, and hormonal characteristics. Cf. gender. **2.** The physiologic and psychological processes within an individual which prompt behavior related to procreation or erotic pleasure. [L. *sexus*]

s. assignment, process whereby the sex of an intersex (hermaphroditic) newborn is initially assigned.

safe s., sexual practices that limit the risk of transmitting or acquiring an infectious disease via exchanges of semen, blood, and other bodily fluids, e.g., use of a condom, mutual masturbation, and avoidance of anal intercourse.

sex·dig·i·tate (seks-dij'i-tāt). Having six digits on one or both hands or feet. SYN sedigitate. [L. *sex,* six, + *digitus,* finger or toe]

sex-in·flu·enced. Denoting a class of genetic disorders in which the same genotype has differing manifestations in the two sexes; the variation may be rational (e.g., breast cancer occurs less frequently in males) or have only empirical support (e.g., pattern baldness behaves as a dominant trait in the male and as a recessive trait in the female). SEE ALSO sex-influenced *inheritance.*

sex·i·va·lent (sek-sĭ-vā'lent, sek-siv'ă-lent). Having a valence of six. [L. *sex,* six, + *valencia,* strength]

sex-lim·it·ed. Occurring in one sex only. SEE sex-limited *inheritance.*

sex-linked. SEE sex *linkage.*

sex·ol·o·gy (sek-sol'ō-jē). The scientific study of all aspects of sex, including differentiation and dimorphism, and, particularly, sexual behavior. [L. *sexus,* sex, + G. *logos,* study]

sex·tan (seks'tăn). Denoting a malarial fever the paroxysms of which recur every sixth day, counting the day of the episode as the first; i.e., with a four-day asymptomatic interval. [L. *sextus,* sixth]

sex·u·al (sek'shoo-ăl). Relating to sex, including stimulation, responsiveness, and functioning of the sex organs. [L. *sexualis,* fr. *sexus,* sex]

sex·u·al·i·ty (sek-shoo-al'i-tē). **1.** The sum of a person's sexual behaviors and tendencies, and the strength of such tendencies. **2.** One's degree of sexual attractiveness. **3.** The quality of having sexual functions or implications.

infantile s., in psychoanalytic personality theory, the concept concerning psychosexual development in infants and children; encompasses the overlapping oral, anal, and phallic phases during the first five years of life.

sex·u·al·i·za·tion (sek'shoo-ăl-i-zā'shŭn). **1.** The state characterized by the presence of sexual energy or drive. **2.** The act of acquiring sexual energy or drive. **3.** The act of imputing a sexual meaning or quality to persons or behaviors.

sex·u·al pref·er·ence. The gender sought in one's sexual partners. **2.** A particular mode of behavior leading to sexual satisfaction.

Sézary, Albert, French dermatologist, 1880–1956. SEE S. *cell, erythroderma, syndrome.*

SFO Abbreviation for subfornical *organ.*

S.G.O. Abbreviation for Surgeon General's Office.

SGOT Abbreviation for serum glutamic-oxaloacetic transaminase.

SGPT Abbreviation for serum glutamic-pyruvic transaminase.

SH 1. Abbreviation for serum *hepatitis.* **2.** Abbreviation for sulfhydryl.

shad·ow (shad'ō). **1.** A surface area defined by the interception of light or x-rays by a body. SEE ALSO density (3). **2.** In jungian psychology, the archetype consisting of collective animal instincts. **3.** SYN achromocyte.

acoustic s., sonographic appearance of reduced echo amplitude from regions lying beyond an attenuating object. Cf. acoustic *enhancement.*

Gumprecht s.'s, SYN smudge *cells,* under *cell.*

hilar s., radiographic hilum of the lung; a composite radiographic shadow of the central pulmonary arteries and veins, with associated bronchial walls and lymph nodes, within the right or left lung.

Ponfick s., SYN achromocyte.

radiographic parallel line s., SYN tram *lines,* under *line.*

shad·ow-cast·ing. Vacuum evaporation and deposition of a film of carbon or metals such as palladium, platinum, or chromium on a contoured microscopic object in order to allow the object to be seen in relief with the electron microscope or sometimes with the light microscope.

Shaffer, A., U.S. biochemist, 1881–1960. SEE S.-Hartmann *method.*

shaft [TA]. SYN diaphysis. [A.S. *sceaft*]

s. of clavicle [TA], the elongated, rodlike body of the clavicle. SYN corpus claviculae [TA], body of clavicle★.

s. of femur [TA], the cylindrical shaft of the thigh bone. SYN corpus ossis femoris [TA], body of femur★, body of thigh bone, corpus femoris.

s. of fibula [TA], the body of fibula; of the fibula elongated, rodlike portion which accounts for most of its length. SYN corpus fibulae [TA], body of fibula★.

hair s., the non-growing portion of a hair which protrudes from the skin, i.e., from the follicle. SYN scapus pili.

s. of humerus [TA], the elongated rodlike portion of the humerus between the surgical neck proximally and the emergence of the supracondylar ridges distally. SYN corpus humeri [TA], body of humerus⋆.

s. of metacarpal [TA], the elongated, rodlike portion of the metacarpal bone. SYN corpus metacarpale [TA], body of metacarpal⋆.

s. of metatarsal [TA], the elongated, rodlike portion of the metatarsal bone. SYN corpus metatarsale [TA], body of metatarsal⋆.

s. of phalanx [TA], the shaft of each phalanx of the hand or foot. SYN corpus phalangis [TA], body of phalanx⋆.

s. of radius [TA], the triangular body of the radius located between the expanded proximal and distal extremities of the bone. SYN corpus radii [TA], body of radius⋆.

s. of tibia [TA], the triangular body of tibia between its expanded proximal and distal ends. SYN corpus tibiae [TA], body of tibia⋆.

s. of ulna [TA], the s. of the ulna between the proximal extremity and the head. SYN corpus ulnae [TA], body of ulna⋆.

shakes. The vernacular term for a paroxysm associated with an intermittent fever.

smelter's shakes, SYN smelter's *fever.*

shank. **1.** The tibia; the shin; the leg. **2.** The portion of an instrument that connects the cutting or functional portion to a handle; with rotary tools, such as burrs and drills, the end that fits into the chuck. [A.S. *sceanca*]

shap·ing (shāp′ing). In operant conditioning, when the operant response is not in the organism's repertoire, a procedure in which the experimenter breaks down the response into those parts which appear most frequently, begins reinforcing them, and then slowly and successively withholds the reinforcer until more and more of the operant is emitted.

shark liv·er oil. Oil extracted from the livers of sharks, mainly of the species *Hypoprion brevirostris;* a rich source of vitamins A and D.

Sharpey, William, Scottish physiologist and histologist, 1802–1880. SEE S. *fibers,* under *fiber.*

Sharpey-Schäfer. SEE Schäfer.

Shaver, Cecil Gordon, Canadian physician, *1901. SEE S. *disease.*

SHBG Abbreviation for sex hormone-binding *globulin.*

shear (shēr). The distortion of a body by two oppositely directed parallel forces. The distortion consists of a sliding over one another of imaginary planes (within the body) parallel to the planes of the forces. [A.S.]

shears (shērz). SYN scissors.

Liston s., strong s. for cutting plaster of Paris bandages.

sheath (shēth). **1.** Any enveloping structure, such as the membranous covering of a muscle, nerve, or blood vessel. Any sheathlike structure. SYN vagina (1). **2.** The prepuce of male animals, especially of the horse. **3.** A specially designed tubular instrument through which special obturators or cutting instruments can be passed, or through which blood clots, tissue fragments, calculi, etc. can be evacuated. **4.** A tube used as an orthodontic appliance, usually on molars. [A.S. *scaeth*]

anterior tarsal tendinous s.'s [TA], synovial tendon s.'s that allow movement of tendons across the anterior aspect of the tarsal bones, deep to the extensor retinacula; included are the tendinous s.'s (vagina tendini musculi...) of: (1) the tibialis anterior (muscle) [TA] (...tibialis anterioris [TA]), (2) the extensor hallucis longus (muscle) [TA] (...extensoris hallucis longi [TA]), and (3) the extensor digitorum longus (muscle) [TA] (...extensoris digitorum longi [TA]). SYN vaginae tendinum tarsales anteriores [TA].

axillary s., fibrous neurovascular s., formed as an extension of the prevertebral layer of deep cervical fascia through the cervicoaxillary canal, which enclosed the first part of the axillary artery, the axillary vein, and the brachial plexus.

carotid s. [TA], the dense fibrous investment of the carotid artery, internal jugular vein, and vagus nerve on each side of the neck, deep to the sternocleidomastoid muscle; the layers of cervical fascia blend with it. SYN vagina carotica [TA].

carpal tendinous s.'s [TA], tendon s.'s occurring in relation to the wrist, allowing tendons to slide freely across the bones and

bony formations of the wrist as they are held in place by the flexor and extensor retinacula. SYN vaginae tendinum carpalium [TA].

caudal s., a group of microtubules arranged cylindrically around the caudal pole of the nucleus in a developing spermatozoon.

common flexor s. (of hand) [TA], the synovial palmar carpal tendinous s. that surrounds the eight tendons of the superficial and deep flexors of the digits of the hand as they pass through the carpal canal; it is commonly continuous with the synovial digital s. of the little finger. SYN vagina communis tendinum musculorum flexorum (manus) [TA], ulnar bursa.

common peroneal tendon s., the s. that surrounds the tendons of the fibularis (peroneus) longus and brevis muscles in their passage across the ankle. SYN vagina communis tendinum musculorum fibularium communis [TA], vagina tendinum musculorum fibularium communis, vagina tendinum musculorum peroneorum communis.

crural s., SYN femoral s.

dentinal s., a layer of tissue relatively resistant to the action of acids, which forms the walls of the dentinal tubules. SYN Neumann s.

dorsal carpal tendinous s.'s [TA], synovial tendon s.'s enabling tendon movement across the posterior aspect of the wrist deep to the extensor retinaculum; they are the following six tendinous s.'s (vaginae tendinum... [TA]): (1) of abductor longus and extensor pollicis brevis (muscles) [TA] (...musculorum abductoris longi et extensoris pollicis brevis [TA]); (2) of extensors carpi radiales (muscles) [TA] (...musculi extensorum carpi radialium [TA]); (3) of extensor pollicis longus (muscle) [TA] (...musculi extensoris pollicis longi [TA]); (4) of extensor digitorum and extensor indicis (muscles) [TA] (...musculorum extensoris digitorum et extensoris indicis [TA]); (5) of extensor digiti minimi (muscle) (...musculi extensoris digiti minimi [TA]); and (6) of extensor carpi ulnaris (muscle) [TA] (...musculi extensoris carpi ulnaris [TA]). SYN vaginae tendinum carpalium dorsalium [TA].

dural s., an extension of the dura mater that ensheathes the roots of spinal nerves or, more particularly, the vagina externa nervi optici.

dural s. of optic nerve, SYN outer s. of optic nerve.

enamel rod s., organic covering of the individual enamel rod.

external s. of optic nerve, SYN outer s. of optic nerve.

external root s., SEE root s.

s. of eyeball, SYN fascial s. of eyeball.

fascial s.'s of extraocular muscles, SYN muscular *fascia* of extraocular muscle.

fascial s. of eyeball [TA], a condensation of connective tissue on the outer aspect of the sclera from which it is separated by a narrow cleftlike episcleral space; the s. is attached to the sclera near the sclerocorneal junction and blends with the fascia of the extraocular muscles. SYN vagina bulbi [TA], capsula bulbi, eye capsule, fascia bulbi, s. of eyeball, Tenon capsule, vagina oculi.

femoral s., the fascia enclosing the femoral vessels, formed by the transversalis fascia anteriorly and the iliac fascia posteriorly; two septa divide the s. into three compartments, the lateral of which contains the femoral artery and the femoral branch of the genitofemoral nerve, the middle contains the femoral vein, and the medial is the femoral canal. SYN crural s., infundibuliform s.

fenestrated s., a s. with a window cut in the tip or lateral convexity, through which special cutting instruments can be passed.

fibrous s.'s, SEE fibrous tendon s., fibrous s.'s of digits of hand, fibrous digital s.'s of toes.

fibrous digital s.'s of foot, SYN fibrous digital s.'s of toes.

fibrous digital s.'s of hand, SYN fibrous digital s.'s of digits of hand.

fibrous digital s.'s of toes [TA], fibrous s.'s of the toes, the tubular fibrous layer enclosing the synovial s. and the tendons of the long and short flexors of the toes and the flexor hallucis longus in the digits; they are composed of annular and cruciform parts. SYN vaginae fibrosae digitorum pedis [TA], fibrous digital s.'s of foot.

fibrous s.'s of digits of hand [TA], fibrous s.'s of the digits of the hand, the tubular fibrous layers that enclose the synovial s.'s and the superficial and deep flexor tendons and the tendon of the

sh

flexor pollicis longus in their passage along their respective digits; they are composed of annular and cruciform parts. SYN vaginae fibrosae digitorum manus [TA], fibrous digital s.'s of hand.

fibrous tendon s. [TA], fibrous s. of a tendon. SYN stratum fibrosum vaginae tendinis⋆, vagina fibrosa tendinis.

fibular tarsal tendinous s.'s [TA], synovial tendon s.'s of flexor tendons enabling movement of tendons posterior to the lateral malleolus and across tarsal bones, passing deep to the fibular retinacula; includes (1) the common tendinous s. of fibulares (peronei) muscles [TA] (vagina communis tendineum musculorum fibularum (peroneum) [TA]); and (2) the plantar tendinous s. of fibularis (peroneus) (muscle) [TA]) (vagina plantaris tendinis musculi fibularis (peronei) longi [TA]). SYN vaginae tendinum tarsales fibulares [TA].

Henle s., SYN endoneurium.

Hertwig s., the merged outer and inner epithelial layers of the enamel organ which extends beyond the region of the anatomical crown and initiates formation of dentin in the root of a developing tooth; it atrophies as the root is formed, and any of the cells that persist are called Malassez epithelial rests.

Huxley s., SYN Huxley layer.

infundibuliform s., SYN femoral s.

inner s. of optic nerve [TA], the innermost s. around the optic nerve, continuous with the leptomeninges (pia-arachnoid) and including a cerebrospinal fluid-filled intervaginal space, continuous with the subarachnoid space. SYN vagina interna nervi optici [TA], internal s. of optic nerve.

internal s. of optic nerve, SYN inner s. of optic nerve.

internal root s., SEE root s.

intertubercular tendon s. [TA], the extension of the synovial membrane of the shoulder joint downward in the intertubercular groove to surround the tendon of the long head of the biceps. SYN vagina tendinis intertubercularis [TA].

s. of Key and Retzius, SYN endoneurium.

Mauthner s., SYN axolemma.

medullary s., SYN myelin s.

microfilarial s., the membrane surrounding the embryos of certain blood-borne microfilariae, such as *Wuchereria*, *Brugia*, and *Loa* of humans; thought to be derived from the vitelline membrane.

mitochondrial s., the spirally arranged mitochondria in the middle piece of a spermatozoon; provides energy for the movement of the tail.

mucous s. of tendon, SYN synovial tendon s.

myelin s., the lipoproteinaceous envelope in vertebrates surrounding most axons of more than 0.5-μm diameter; it consists of a double plasma membrane wound tightly around the axon in a variable number of turns, and supplied by oligodendroglia cells (in the brain and spinal cord) or Schwann cells (in peripheral nerves); unwound, the double membrane would appear as a sheetlike cell expansion that is empty of cytoplasm but for a few narrow cytoplasmic strands corresponding to apparent interruptions of the regular myelin structure, the incisures of Schmidt-Lanterman; the myelin s. of each axon is composed of a fairly regular longitudinal sequence of segments, each corresponding to the length of s. supplied by a single oligodendroglia or Schwann cell; in the short interval between each two neighboring segments, the nodes of Ranvier, the axon is unmyelinated even though enclosed by complex finger-like plasmatic expansions of the neighboring oligodendroglia or Schwann cells. SYN medullary s.

Neumann s., SYN dentinal s.

neurovascular s., fibrous tissue enveloping and binding together arteries, their accompanying veins (venae comitantes) and nerves that run together; often it is merely the adventitious tissue of the neurovascular structures, but may be highly developed as a distinct fascial layer (e.g., in the case of the carotid or axillary s.'s).

notochordal s., the fibrous outer covering of the notochord.

outer s. of optic nerve [TA], the outer s. around the optic nerve, continuous with the dura mater. SYN vagina externa nervi optici [TA], dural s. of optic nerve, external s. of optic nerve.

palmar carpal tendinous s.'s [TA], three synovial tendon s.'s that allow movement of tendons across the anterior aspect of the wrist, deep to or within the flexor retinaculum; they are the: (1) tendinous s. of flexor pollicis longus (muscle) [TA] (vagina tendinis musculi flexoris pollicis longi [TA]); (2) tendinous s. of flexor carpi radialis (muscle) [TA] (vagina tendinis musculi flexoris carpi radialis [TA]); and (3) common flexor s. [TA] (vagina communis tendineum musculorum flexorum [TA]). SYN vaginae tendinum carpales palmares [TA].

parotid s., SYN parotid *fascia.*

periarterial lymphatic s. (PALS), the accumulation of lymphocytes investing the central arteries of the spleen and comprising the white pulp.

plantar tendon s. of fibularis longus muscle [TA], the synovial s. surrounding the tendon of the peroneus longus in its course across the sole of the foot. SYN vagina tendinis musculi fibularis longi plantaris [TA], plantar tendon s. of peroneus longus muscle⋆, vagina tendinis musculi peronei longi plantaris⋆.

plantar tendon s. of peroneus longus muscle, ⋆official alternate term for plantar tendon s. of fibularis longus muscle.

prostatic s., loose fibrous, partly vascular enclosure of the prostate and its dense (true) fibrous capsule; it is continuous inferiorly with the superior fascia of the urogenital diaphragm and posteriorly becomes part of the rectovesical septum; it contains the prostatic venous plexus.

rectus s. [TA], s. of the rectus abdominis, formed by the aponeuroses of the three anterolateral muscles of the abdominal wall that split to enclose the rectus and fuse medially to form the linea alba; it consists of an anterior lamina and a posterior lamina, the latter being absent below the arcuate line. SEE ALSO *aponeurosis* of external oblique muscle, *aponeurosis* of internal oblique muscle. SYN vagina musculi recti abdominis [TA].

resectoscope s., an operative s. through which transurethral electroresection of bladder tumors or prostate gland can be performed.

root s., one of the epidermic layers of the hair follicle: external root s. is continuous with the stratum basale and stratum spinosum of the epidermis; internal root s. comprises the cuticle of the internal roots, Huxley layer, and Henle layer.

Rouget-Neumann s., the amorphous ground substance between an osteocyte and the lacunar or canalicular wall.

Scarpa s., SYN cremasteric *fascia.*

s. of Schwann, SYN neurilemma.

s. of Schweigger-Seidel, SYN ellipsoid.

s. of styloid process [TA], a crest of bone (edge of the tympanic portion of the temporal bone) running from the front and medial side of the mastoid process to the spine of the sphenoid; it splits to ensheath the base of the styloid process. SYN vagina processus styloidei [TA], vaginal process.

synovial s. [TA], SEE synovial tendon s., *vagina* synovialis trochleae, synovial s.'s of digits of hand, synovial s.'s of toes. SYN vagina synovialis [TA].

synovial s.'s of digits of foot, SYN synovial s.'s of toes.

synovial s.'s of digits of hand [TA], the synovial s.'s that enclose the flexor tendons of the fingers and line the inside of the fibrous tendon s.'s. SYN vaginae synoviales digitorum manus [TA].

synovial tendon s. [TA], a s. of synovial membrane enveloping certain of the tendons; it contains a small amount of synovial fluid. SYN vagina synovialis tendinis [TA], mucous s. of tendon, theca tendinis, vagina mucosa tendinis, vaginal synovial membrane.

synovial s.'s of toes [TA], similar in structure to the corresponding s.'s of the hand. SYN vaginae tendinum digitorum pedis [TA], synovial s.'s of digits of foot.

tail s., the fibrous envelope in the tail of a spermatozoon.

tendinous s. of abductor pollicis longus and extensor pollicis brevis muscles [TA], the dorsal carpal synovial tendinous s. lining the compartment of the extensor retinaculum that contains the abductor pollicis longus and extensor pollicis brevis tendons. SYN vagina tendinum musculorum abductoris longi et extensoris brevis pollicis [TA].

tendinous s. of extensor carpi radialis muscles [TA], the dorsal carpal synovial tendon s. lining the compartment of the extensor retinaculum containing the tendons of the extensor carpi radialis

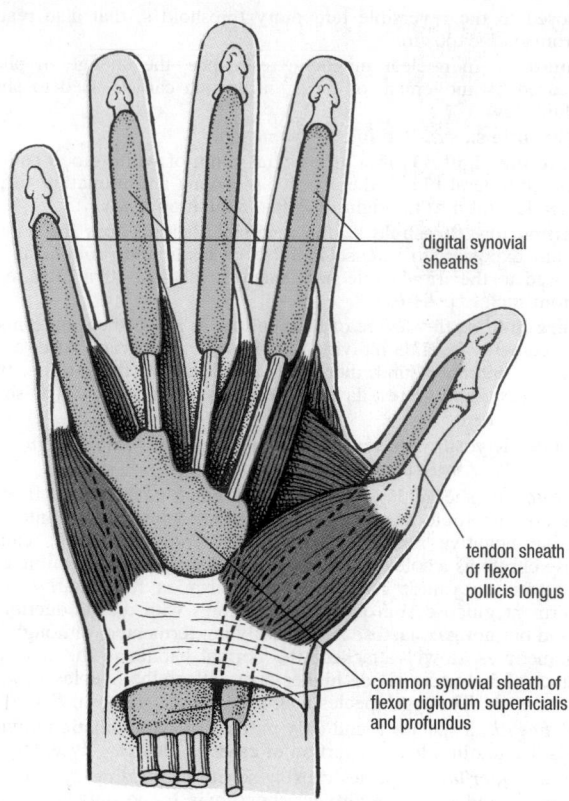

digital synovial
sheaths

tendon sheath
of flexor
pollicis longus

common synovial sheath of
flexor digitorum superficialis
and profundus

flexor tendon sheaths: the hand

longus and brevis muscles. SYN vagina tendinum musculorum extensorum carpi radialium [TA].

tendinous s. of extensor carpi ulnaris muscle [TA], the dorsal carpal synovial tendon s. surrounding the tendon of the extensor carpi ulnaris in its course deep to the extensor retinaculum. SYN vagina tendinis musculi extensoris carpi ulnaris [TA], peritenon.

tendinous s. of extensor digiti minimi muscle [TA], the dorsal carpal synovial tendon s. surrounding the tendon of the extensor digiti minimi in its passage deep to the extensor retinaculum. SYN vagina tendinis musculi extensoris digiti minimi [TA].

tendinous s. of extensor digitorum and extensor indicis muscles [TA], the dorsal carpal synovial tendon s. that surrounds the four tendons of the extensor digitorum muscle and the tendon of the extensor indicis deep to the extensor retinaculum. SYN vagina tendinum musculorum extensoris digitorum et extensoris indicis [TA].

tendinous s. of extensor digitorum longus muscle of foot [TA], the anterior tarsal synovial tendon s. that surrounds the tendons of the extensor digitorum longus muscle and the peroneus tertius in their passage across the ankle. SYN vagina tendinum musculi extensoris digitorum pedis longi [TA].

tendinous s. of extensor hallucis longus muscle [TA], the anterior tarsal synovial tendon s. that surrounds the tendon of the extensor hallucis longus in its passage across the ankle. SYN vagina tendinis musculi extensoris hallucis longi [TA].

tendinous s. of extensor pollicis longus muscle [TA], the dorsal carpal synovial tendon s. surrounding the extensor pollicis longus tendon in its passage deep to the extensor retinaculum. SYN vagina tendinis musculi extensoris pollicis longi [TA].

tendinous s. of flexor carpi radialis muscle [TA], the palmar carpal synovial tendon s. enclosing the tendon of the flexor carpi radialis as it crosses the wrist. SYN vagina tendinis musculi flexoris carpi radialis [TA].

tendinous s. of flexor digitorum longus muscle (of foot) [TA], the tibial tarsal synovial tendon s. that envelops the flexor digito-

rum longus tendons as they pass into the foot deep to the flexor retinaculum. SYN vagina tendinum musculi flexoris digitorum pedis longi [TA].

tendinous s. of flexor hallucis longus muscle [TA], the tibial tarsal synovial tendon s. that envelops the tendon of the flexor hallucis longus as it passes into the foot deep to the flexor retinaculum. SYN vagina tendinis musculi flexoris hallucis longi [TA].

tendinous s. of flexor pollicis longus muscle [TA], the palmar carpal synovial tendon s. that envelops the tendon of the flexor pollicis longus in its course through the carpal canal; it is continuous with the digital sheath of the thumb, the two generally being considered as one sheath. SYN vagina tendinis musculi flexoris pollicis longi [TA], radial bursa.

tendinous s. of superior oblique muscle [TA], the synovial s. enclosing the tendon of the superior oblique muscle as it passes through the trochlea. SYN vagina tendinis musculi obliqui superioris [TA], synovial trochlear bursa, trochlear synovial bursa, vagina synovialis trochleae.

tendinous s. of tibialis anterior muscle [TA], the anterior tarsal synovial tendon s., deep to the extensor retinaculum, that surrounds the tendon of the tibialis anterior as it crosses the ankle. SYN vagina tendinis musculi tibialis anterioris [TA].

tendinous s. of tibialis posterior muscle [TA], the tibial tarsal synovial tendon s. surrounding the tendon of the tibialis posterior as it passes into the foot deep to the flexor retinaculum. SYN vagina tendinis musculi tibialis posterioris [TA].

s. of thyroid gland, covering of the thyroid gland external to its capsule formed by a splitting of the pretracheal layer of deep cervical fascia at the gland's posterior border; the anterior lamina covers the gland anterolaterally, attaching to the arch of the cricoid cartilage superior to the isthmus of the gland (causing it to move with the trachea during elevation/depression of the larynx); the posterior lamina passes posterior to the esophagus to blend with the buccopharyngeal fascia; inferiorly, the s. extends along the inferior thyroid veins to open into the superior mediastinum (hence, expansion of the thyroid, as by goiter, can take this direction).

tibial tarsal tendinous s.'s [TA], synovial tendon s.'s that allow movement of tendons across the medial side of the tarsal bones, deep to flexor retinaculum; included are (1) the tendinous s. (vagina tendinis/tendinum musculi...) of flexor digitorum longus (muscle) [TA] (...flexoris digitorum longi [TA]); (2) the tibialis posterior (muscle) [TA] (...tibialis posterioris [TA]); and (3) the flexor hallucis longus (muscle) [TA] (...flexoris hallucis longi [TA]). SYN vaginae tendinum tarsales tibialis [TA].

vascular s.'s, fibrous envelopes ensheathing the arteries with their accompanying veins and sometimes nerves as well. SYN s.'s of vessels, vaginae vasorum.

s.'s of vessels, SYN vascular s.'s.

Waldeyer s., the tubular space between the bladder wall and the intramural portion of the ureter as it courses obliquely through this structure; actually a space and not a true s. SYN Waldeyer space.

Sheehan, Harold L., British pathologist, *1900. SEE S. *syndrome.*

Sheldon, J.H., English pediatrician, 1920–1964. SEE Freeman-S. *syndrome.*

shelf. In anatomy, a structure resembling a shelf.

Blumer s., SYN rectal s.

dental s., SYN dental *ledge.*

palatal s., a medially directed outgrowth of the embryonic maxilla; when fused with its opposite number it forms the secondary palate.

rectal s., a s. palpable by rectal examination, due to metastatic tumor cells gravitating from an abdominal cancer and growing in the rectovesical or rectouterine pouch. SYN Blumer s.

vocal s., SYN vocal *fold.*

shell. An outer covering.

cytotrophoblastic s., the external layer of fetally derived trophoblastic cells on the maternal surface of the placenta.

diffusion s., a small vessel made of a semipermeable membrane through which peptone, but not serum albumin, can pass; used in performing the Abderhalden test.

sh

K s., the innermost electron orbit or shell; it can hold two electrons.

L s., the next lowest energy level of electrons in the atom, after the K s. (q.v.).

M s., the lowest energy level at which electron transitions give rise to x-rays.

O s., the outermost s. of electrons, so called because displacement of electrons causes an emission in the visible or optical range.

shel·lac (shĕ-lak′). A resinous excretion of an insect, *Laccifer (Tachardia) lacca* (family Coccidae). The insects suck the juice of various resiniferous Asiatic (chiefly Indian) trees and excrete and deposit "stick-lac." S. softens at a low temperature. It has many nonmedicinal uses and is also used to coat confections and tablets and in dental materials, e.g., impression compound and denture base plates. SYN lacca.

Shemin, David, U.S. biochemist, *1911. SEE S. *cycle.*

Shenton, Edward W.H., English radiologist, 1872–1955. SEE S. *line.*

Shepherd, Francis J., Canadian surgeon, 1851–1929. SEE S. *fracture.*

Sherman, Henry C., U.S. biochemist, 1875–1955. SEE S. *unit;* S.-Bourquin *unit* of vitamin B$_2$; S.-Munsell *unit.*

Sherrington, Sir Charles S., English physiologist and Nobel laureate, 1857–1952. SEE S. *phenomenon, law;* Schiff-S. *phenomenon;* Liddell-S. *reflex.*

shield (shēld). A protecting screen; lead sheet for protecting the operator and patient from x-rays. [A.S. *scild*]

embryonic s., a thickened area of the embryonic blastoderm from which the embryo develops.

nipple s., a cap or dome placed over the nipple to protect it during nursing.

oral s.'s, removable appliances used in orthodontic treatment, usually placed between the labial and buccal mucosa and the teeth.

shift. SYN change. SEE ALSO deviation.

antigenic s., mutation, i.e., sudden change in molecular structure of RNA/DNA in microorganisms, especially viruses, which produces new strains; hosts previously exposed to other strains have little or no acquired immunity to the new strain; antigenic s. is believed to be the explanation for the occurrence of new strains of influenza virus, which occur by recombination or genetic reassortment of 2 different viral strains in a given host, and is associated with large-scale epidemics.

axis s., SYN axis *deviation.*

chemical s., dependence of the resonance frequency of a nucleus on the chemical binding of the atom or molecule in which it is contained. SEE chemical shift *artifact.*

chloride s., when CO$_2$ enters the blood from the tissues, it passes into the red blood cell and is converted by carbonate dehydratase to bicarbonate (HCO$_3^-$); HCO$_3^-$ ion passes out into the plasma while Cl$^-$ migrates into the red blood cell. Reverse changes occur in the lungs when CO$_2$ is eliminated from the blood. SYN Hamburger phenomenon.

Doppler s., the magnitude of the frequency change in hertz when sound and observer are in relative motion away from or toward each other. SEE ALSO Doppler *effect.*

s. to the left, (1) a marked increase in the percentage of immature cells in the circulating blood, based on the premise in hematology that the bone marrow with its immature myeloid cells is on the left, while the circulating blood with its mature neutrophils is on the right; SYN deviation to the left. **(2)** SEE maturation *index.*

luteoplacental s., the change in site of production of the estrogen and progesterone essential for human pregnancy from the corpus luteum to the placenta; ovariectomy always terminates pregnancy in most mammals because their placentas never produce enough estrogen and progesterone, but, after the sixth week of pregnancy, a human placenta can produce enough of these hormones to prevent abortion despite ovariectomy.

permanent threshold s., the irreversible hearing loss that results from exposure to intense impulse or continuous sound, as op-

posed to the reversible temporary threshold s. that also results from such exposure.

phase s., in nuclear magnetic resonance, the change in phase caused by movement of the spins, which can be used to show fluid flow.

Purkinje s., SYN Purkinje *phenomenon.*

s. to the right, (1) in a differential count of white blood cells in the peripheral blood, the absence of young and immature forms; SYN deviation to the right. **(2)** SEE maturation *index.*

temporary threshold s., the reversible hearing loss that results from exposure to intense impulse or continuous sound, as opposed to the irreversible permanent threshold s. that may result from such exposure.

threshold s., the degree of hearing loss or impairment in terms of a decibel s. from an individual's previous audiogram. After exposure to intense sound, there may be temporary threshold s. with recovery in hours or days or permanent threshold s. (noise-induced *hearing loss*).

Shiga, Kiyoshi, Japanese bacteriologist, 1870–1957. SEE *Shigella;* S. *bacillus;* S.-Kruse *bacillus.*

Shi·gel·la (shē-gel′lă). A genus of nonmotile, aerobic to facultatively anaerobic bacteria (family Enterobacteriaceae) containing Gram-negative nonencapsulated rods. These organisms cannot use citrate as a sole source of carbon; their growth is inhibited by potassium cyanide and their metabolism is fermentative; they ferment glucose and other carbohydrates with the production of acid but not gas; lactose is ordinarily not fermented, although it is sometimes slowly attacked; the normal habitat is the intestinal tract of humans and of higher apes; all of the species produce dysentery. The type species is *S. dysenteriae.* [Kiyoshi *Shiga*]

S. boy′dii, a species found only in feces of symptomatic individuals; occurs in a low proportion of cases of bacillary dysentery.

S. dysenter′iae, a species causing severe necrotizing dysentery in humans induced by a virulent shiga toxin found only in feces of symptomatic individuals; the type species of the genus *S.* SYN Shiga bacillus, Shiga-Kruse bacillus.

S. flexne′ri, a species found in the feces of symptomatic individuals and of convalescents or carriers; a common cause of dysentery epidemics, especially in Asia and the Middle East. Now known sometimes to be sexually transmitted through anal intercourse. SYN Flexner bacillus, paradysentery bacillus.

S. son′nei, a species causing dysentery, sometimes milder than that caused by other species. The most common S. species causing disease in the U.S.

shig·el·lo·sis (shig-ĕ-lō′sis). Bacillary dysentery caused by bacteria of the genus *Shigella,* often occurring in epidemic patterns; an opportunistic infection of persons with AIDS.

shi·kim·ate de·hy·dro·gen·ase (shi-kim′āt). An oxidoreductase reversibly reacting 3-dehydroshikimic acid with NADPH acid to produce shikimic acid and NADP$^+$ in L-phenylalanine and L-tyrosine biosynthesis.

Shiley, D. B., 20th century U.S. engineer. SEE Björk-Shiley *valve.*

shim (shim). In magnetic resonance imaging, fine adjustment of the magnetic field to improve uniformity.

shin. SYN anterior *border* of tibia. [A.S. *scina*]

saber s., the sharp-edged, anteriorly convex tibia in congenital syphilis.

toasted s.'s, SYN *erythema* ab igne.

Shine, J., contemporary Australian molecular biologist.

shin·gles (shing′glz). SYN *herpes* zoster. [L. *cingulum,* girdle]

shin-splints. Tenderness and pain with induration and swelling of pretibial muscles, following athletic overexertion by the untrained; it may be a mild form of anterior tibial compartment syndrome.

ship. A structure resembling the hull of a ship.

Fabricius s., the outlines of the sphenoid, occipital, and frontal bones, from their fancied resemblance to the hull of a s.

Shipley, Walter C., U.S. psychiatrist, *1903. SEE S.-Hartford *scale.*

Shirodkar, N.V., Indian obstetrician and gynecologist, 1900–1971. SEE S. *operation.*

shiv·er. **1.** To shake or tremble, especially from cold. **2.** A tremor; a slight chill.

shiv·er·ing. Trembling from cold or fear.

shock (shok). **1.** The condition in which the cells of the body receive inadequate amounts of oxygen secondary to changes in perfusion; most commonly secondary to blood loss or sepsis. **2.** A sudden physical or biochemical disturbance that results in inadequate blood flow and oxygenation of an animal's vital organs. **3.** A state of profound mental and physical depression consequent upon severe physical injury or an emotional disturbance. **4.** A state characterized by inadequacy of blood flow throughout the body to the extent that damage occurs to the cells of the tissues; if the s. is prolonged, the cardiovascular system itself becomes damaged and begins to deteriorate, resulting in a vicious cycle that leads to death. SEE diastolic s., systolic s. [Fr. *choc,* fr. Germanic]

anaphylactic s., a severe, often fatal form of s. characterized by smooth muscle contraction and capillary dilation initiated by cytotropic (IgE class) antibodies; typically an antibody-associated phenomenon (type I allergic reaction). SEE ALSO anaphylaxis, serum *sickness.*

anaphylactoid s., a reaction that is similar to anaphylactic s., but which does not require the incubation period characteristic of induced sensitivity (anaphylaxis); it is unrelated to antigen-antibody reactions. SYN anaphylactoid crisis (1), pseudoanaphylactic s.

anesthetic s., s. produced by the administration of anesthetic drug(s), usually in relative overdosage.

break s., the s. produced by breaking a constant current passing through the body.

cardiac s., SYN cardiogenic s.

cardiogenic s., s. resulting from decline in cardiac output secondary to serious heart disease, usually myocardial infarction. SYN cardiac s.

chronic s., the state of peripheral circulatory insufficiency developing in elderly patients with a debilitating disease, e.g., carcinoma; a subnormal blood volume makes the patient susceptible to hemorrhagic s. as a result of even a moderate blood loss such as may occur during an operation.

counter-s., SEE countershock.

cultural s., a form of stress associated with the beginning of a person's assimilation into a new culture vastly different from that in which he or she was raised.

declamping s., SYN declamping *phenomenon.*

deferred s., delayed s., a state of s. coming on at a considerable interval after the receipt of the injury.

diastolic s., the abnormally palpable impact, appreciated by a hand on the chest wall, of an accentuated third heart sound.

electric s., a sudden violent impression caused by the passage of a current of electricity through any portion of the body.

endotoxin s., s. induced by release of endotoxin from Gram-negative bacteria, especially by *Escherichia coli.*

hemorrhagic s., hypovolemic s. resulting from acute hemorrhage, characterized by hypotension, tachycardia, pale, cold, and clammy skin, and oliguria.

histamine s., the s. state produced in animals by the injection of histamine; characterized by bronchiolar spasm in the guinea pig and constriction of hepatic veins in the dog.

hypovolemic s., s. caused by a reduction in volume of blood, as from hemorrhage or dehydration.

insulin s., severe hypoglycemia produced by administration of insulin, manifested by sweating, tremor, anxiety, vertigo, and diplopia, followed by delirium, convulsions, and collapse. SYN wet s.

irreversible s., s. that has progressed because of cell injury beyond the stage where resuscitation is possible.

nitroid s., a syndrome resembling that produced by the administration of a large dose of a nitrite, sometimes caused by a too rapid intravenous injection of arsphenamine or some other drug; SEE nitritoid *reaction.*

oligemic s., s. associated with pronounced fall in blood volume, sometimes resulting from increased permeability of blood vessels.

osmotic s., a sudden change in the osmotic pressure to which a cell is subjected, usually in order to cause it to lyse.

primary s., s. mainly nervous in nature, from pain, anxiety, etc., which ensues almost immediately upon the receipt of a severe injury.

protein s., the systemic reaction following the parenteral administration of a protein.

pseudoanaphylactic s., SYN anaphylactoid s.

reversible s., s. that will respond to treatment and from which recovery is possible.

septic s., **(1)** s. associated with infection that has released large enough quantities of toxins or vasoactive substances including, cytokines, to be associated with hypotension; **(2)** s. associated with septicemia caused by Gram-negative bacteria.

serum s., anaphylactic or anaphylactoid s. caused by the injection of antitoxic or other foreign serum.

shell s., SYN battle *fatigue.*

spinal s., transient depression or abolition of reflex activity below the level of an acute spinal cord injury or transection.

systolic s., the abnormally palpable impact, appreciated by a hand on the chest wall, of an accentuated first heart sound.

toxic s., SEE toxic shock *syndrome.*

vasogenic s., s. resulting from depressed activity of the higher vasomotor centers in the brain stem and the medulla, producing vasodilation without loss of fluid so that the container is disproportionately large. In oligemic s., blood volume is reduced; in both, return of venous blood is inadequate.

wet s., SYN insulin s.

Shone, John D., 20th century English cardiologist. SEE S. *anomaly, complex, syndrome.*

shook jong (shuk-yong′). SYN koro.

Shope, Richard E., U.S. pathologist, 1902–1966. SEE S. *fibroma,* fibroma *virus, papilloma,* papilloma *virus.*

short-chain ac·yl-CoA de·hy·dro·gen·ase. SEE *acyl-CoA* dehydrogenase (NADPH).

short·sight·ed·ness (shōrt′sīt-ed-nes). SYN myopia.

shot-feel (shot′fēl). A peculiar sensation as of a nervous discharge or electric shock passing rapidly from the top of the head to the feet, sometimes described as a sensation of the rolling of shot down the body, occurring in acromegaly.

shoul·der (shōl′der). **1.** The lateral portion of the scapular region, where the scapula joins with the clavicle and humerus and is covered by the rounded mass of the deltoid muscle. **2.** In dentistry, the ledge formed by the junction of the gingival and axial walls in extracoronal restorative preparations. [A.S. *sculder*]

frozen s., SYN adhesive *capsulitis.*

shoul·der blade (shōl′der blād). SYN scapula.

show (shō). **1.** An appearance. **2.** First appearance of blood in beginning menstruation. **3.** Sign of impending labor, characterized by the discharge from the vagina of a small amount of blood-tinged mucus representing the extrusion of the mucous plug which has filled the cervical canal during pregnancy. [A.S. *sceáwe*]

Shprintzen, R.J. SEE Shprintzen *syndrome.*

Shrapnell, Henry J., English anatomist, 1761–1841. SEE S. *membrane.*

shud·der (shŭd′er). A convulsive or involuntary tremor. [M.E. *shodderen*]

carotid s., vibrations at the crest of the carotid pulse tracing, seen in aortic stenosis.

Shulman, Lawrence E., U.S. rheumatologist, *1919. SEE S. *syndrome.*

Shumway, Norman, U.S. surgeon, *1923, developed method for dealing with tissue rejection related to heart transplants.

shunt (shŭnt). **1.** To bypass or divert. **2.** A bypass or diversion of fluid to another fluid-containing system by fistulation or a prosthetic device. The nomenclature commonly includes origin and terminus, e.g., atriovenous, splenorenal, ventriculocisternal. SEE ALSO bypass. [M.E. *shunten,* to flinch]

arteriovenous s. (A-V s.), the passage of blood directly from arteries to veins, without going through the capillary network.

Blalock s., subclavian artery to pulmonary artery s. to increase pulmonary circulation in cyanotic heart disease with decreased pulmonary flow.

Blalock-Taussig s., a palliative subclavian artery to pulmonary artery anastomosis.

cavopulmonary s., SYN cavopulmonary *anastomosis.*

Denver s., a tube placed subcutaneously that connects the abdominal cavity in a patient with ascites to the low pressure superior vena cava. Not only does this s. have a one-way valve but also a manually compressible chamber to facilitate flow.

dialysis s., arteriovenous s. connecting the arterial and venous cannulas in arm or leg.

Dickens s., SYN pentose phosphate *pathway.*

distal splenorenal s., anastomosis of the splenic vein to the left renal vein, usually end-to-side, for control of portal hypertension. SYN renal-splenic venous s., Warren s.

Glenn s., SYN cavopulmonary *anastomosis.*

H s., a side-to-side s. between adjacent vessels that uses a connecting conduit; this s. is most commonly placed between the superior mesentary vein and the inferior vena cava in patients with portal hypertension. SYN H graft.

hexose monophosphate s., SYN pentose phosphate *pathway.*

jejunoileal s., SYN jejunoileal *bypass.*

left-to-right s., a diversion of blood from the left side of the heart to right (as through a septal defect), or from the systemic circulation to the pulmonary (as through a patent ductus arteriosus).

LeVeen s., a subcutaneously placed tube with an inline one-way valve used to transport ascitic fluid from the abdomen, via the jugular vein, to the superior vena cava.

mesocaval s., (1) anastomosis of the side of the superior mesenteric vein to the proximal end of the divided inferior vena cava, for control of portal hypertension; (2) H-shunt anastomosis of the inferior vena cava to the superior mesenteric vein, using a synthetic conduit or autologous vein.

pentose monophosphate s., SYN pentose phosphate *pathway.*

peritoneovenous s., a s., usually by a catheter, between the peritoneal cavity and the thoracic central venous system.

pleuroperitoneal s., a surgically implanted catheter for transport of fluid from a pleural space into the peritoneal *cavity,* where it is absorbed; used mainly for treatment of malignant pleural effusions.

pleurovenous s., a surgically implanted catheter for transport of fluid from a pleural space into the venous system; rarely used, mainly for treatment of malignant pleural effusions.

portacaval s., (1) surgical anastomosis between portal and systemic veins; (2) surgical anastomosis between the portal vein and the vena cava.

portasystemic s., a s. between any parts of the portal and systemic venous systems, including portacaval, mesocaval, splenorenal s.'s or spontaneously occurring s.'s.

proximal splenorenal s., anastomosis of the proximal end of the cut splenic vein to the side of the left renal vein for control of portal hypertension; this is considered a central or complete visceral venous s.

Rapoport-Luebering s., part of the glycolytic pathway characteristic of human erythrocytes in which 2,3-bisphosphoglycerate (2,3-P$_2$Gri) is formed as an intermediate between 1,3-P$_2$Gri and 3-phosphoglycerate; 2,3-P$_2$Gri is an important regulator of the affinity of hemoglobin for oxygen.

renal-splenic venous s., SYN distal splenorenal s.

reversed s., right-to-left s. that had previously been a left-to-right s.; rarely the opposite.

right-to-left s., the passage of blood from the right side of the heart into the left (as through a septal defect), or from the pulmonary artery into the aorta (as through a patent ductus arteriosus); such a shunt can occur only when the pressure on the right side exceeds that in the left, as in advanced pulmonic stenosis, or when the pulmonary artery pressure exceeds aortic pressure, as in one form of Eisenmenger syndrome or in tricuspid atresia.

Scribner s., connection of an artery, customarily the radial, to the cephalic vein via a short extracorporeal catheter.

Torkildsen s., a ventriculocisternal s. SEE shunt (2).

tracheoesophageal s., SEE tracheoesophageal *puncture.*

transjugular intrahepatic portosystemic s. (TIPS), an interventional radiology procedure to relieve portal hypertension.

Warburg-Dickens-Horecker s., SYN pentose phosphate *pathway.*

Warburg-Lipmann-Dickens-Horecker s., SYN pentose phosphate *pathway.*

Warren s., SYN distal splenorenal s.

Waterston s., creation of a narrow (about 3 mm) opening between the ascending aorta and the subjacent right pulmonary artery to increase pulmonary circulation in cyanotic heart disease with decreased pulmonary flow.

shut·tle (shut'il). A going back and forth regularly; used in respect to certain transport processes across a biomembrane.

glycerophosphate s., a mechanism for the transfer of reducing equivalents from the cytosol into the mitochondria; NADH is used to synthesize glycerol 3-phosphate in the cytosol; this compound is then transported into the mitochondria where it is converted to dihydroxyacetone phosphate (DHAP) using FAD; DHAP then returns to the cytosol to complete the cycle; found in brain tissue, brown adipose tissue, and white muscle.

malate-aspartate s., a mechanism for the transfer of NADH, reducing equivalents from the cytosol into the mitochondria using two isozymes of malate dehydrogenase and aspartate transaminase.

Shwachman, Harry, U.S. pediatrician, 1910–1986. SEE Shwachman *syndrome,* Shwachman-Diamond *syndrome.*

Shwartzman, Gregory, Russian bacteriologist in U.S., 1896–1965. SEE S. *phenomenon, reaction;* generalized S. *phenomenon;* Sanarelli-S. *phenomenon.*

Shy, George Milton, U.S. neurologist, 1919–1967. SEE S.-Drager *syndrome.*

Shy Abbreviation for 6-mercaptopurine.

SI Abbreviation for International System of Units (Système International d'Unités).

Si Symbol for silicon.

sI Abbreviation for 6-mercaptopurine ribonucleoside (or 6-thioinosine).

Sia Abbreviation for sialic acids.

SIADH Abbreviation for *syndrome* of inappropriate secretion of antidiuretic hormone.

△**sial-.** SEE sialo-.

si·al·a·den (sī-al'ă-den). A salivary gland. [sial- + G. *adēn,* gland]

si·al·ad·e·ni·tis (sī'al-ad-ĕ-nī'tis). Inflammation of a salivary gland. SYN sialoadenitis. [sial- + G. *adēn,* gland, + *-itis,* inflammation]

si·al·ad·e·no·tro·pic (sī'al-ad'ĕ-nō-trop'ik). Having an influence on the salivary glands. [sial- + G. *adēn,* gland, + *tropē,* a turning]

si·al·a·gogue (sī-al'ă-gog). 1. Promoting the flow of saliva. 2. An agent having this action (e.g., anticholinesterase agents). SYN ptyalagogue, sialogogue. [sial- + G. *agōgos,* drawing forth]

si·al·ec·ta·sis (sī'al-ek'tă-sis). Dilation of a salivary duct. SYN ptyalectasis. [sial- + G. *ektasis,* a stretching]

si·al·em·e·sis, si·al·e·me·sia (sī'al-em'ē-sis, -ĕ-mē'zē-ă). Vomiting of saliva, or vomiting caused by or accompanying an excessive secretion of saliva. [sial- + G. *emesis,* vomiting]

si·al·ic (sī-al'ik). SYN salivary.

si·al·ic ac·ids (Sia) (sī-al'ik). Esters and other *N*- and *O*-acyl derivatives of neuraminic acid; radicals of s. a. are sialoyl, if the OH of the COOH is removed, and sialosyl, if the OH comes from the anomeric carbon (C-2) of the cyclic structure; e.g., *N*-acetylneuraminic acid.

si·al·i·dase (sī-al'i-dās). An enzyme that cleaves terminal acetylneuraminic residues from oligosaccharides, glycoproteins, or glycolipids; present on the surface antigen in myxoviruses; used in histochemistry to selectively remove sialomucins, as from bronchial mucous glands and the small intestine; a deficiency of this enzyme will result in sialidosis. SYN neuraminidase.

si·al·i·do·sis (sī-al-i-dō'sis). SYN cherry-red spot myoclonus *syndrome*.

si·a·line (sī'ă-lēn). SYN salivary.

si·a·lism, si·a·lis·mus (sī'ă-lizm, sī'ă-liz'mŭs). SYN sialorrhea. [G. *sialismos*]

△**sialo-, sial-.** Saliva, salivary glands. SEE ALSO ptyal-. Cf. ptyal-. [G. *sialon*]

si·a·lo·ad·e·nec·to·my (sī'ă-lō-ad-ĕ-nek'tō-mē). Excision of a salivary gland. [sialo- + G. *adēn*, gland, + *ektomē*, excision]

si·a·lo·ad·e·ni·tis (sī'ă-lō-ad-ĕ-nī'tis). SYN sialadenitis.

si·a·lo·ad·e·not·o·my (sī'ă-lō-ad-ĕ-not'ŏ-mē). Incision of a salivary gland. [sialo- + G. *adēn*, gland, + *tomē*, incision]

si·a·lo·aer·oph·a·gy (sī'ă-lō-ār-of'ă-jē). A habit of frequent swallowing whereby quantities of saliva and air are taken into the stomach. SYN aerosialophagy. [sialo- + G. *aēr*, air, + *phagō*, to eat]

si·a·lo·an·gi·ec·ta·sis (sī'ă-lō-an-jē-ek'tă-sis). Dilation of salivary ducts. [sialo- + G. *angeion*, vessel, + *ektasis*, a stretching]

si·a·lo·an·gi·i·tis (sī'ă-lō-an-jē-ī'tis). Inflammation of a salivary duct. [sialo- + G. *angeion*, vessel, + -*itis*, inflammation]

si·a·lo·cele (sī'ă-lō-sēl). SYN ranula (2). [sialo- + G. *kēlē*, tumor]

si·a·lo·do·chi·tis (sī'ă-lō-dō-kī'tis). Inflammation of the duct of a salivary gland. [sialo- + G. *dochē*, receptacle, + -*itis*, inflammation]

si·a·lo·do·cho·plas·ty (sī'ă-lō-dō'kō-plas'tē). Repair of a salivary duct. [sialo- + G. *dochē*, receptacle, + *plassō*, to fashion]

si·a·log·e·nous (sī'ă-loj'ĕ-nŭs). Producing saliva. SEE ALSO sialagogue. [sialo- + G. -*gen*, producing]

si·a·lo·glyc·o·sphin·go·lip·id (sī'ă-lō-glī-kō-sfin-gō-lip'id). SYN ganglioside.

si·a·lo·gogue (sī-al'ă-gog). SYN sialagogue.

si·a·lo·gram (sī-al'ō-gram). A radiograph of sialography. [sialo- + G. *gramma*, a writing]

si·a·log·ra·phy (sī-ă-log'ră-fē). Radiography of the salivary glands and ducts after the introduction of contrast medium into the ducts. SYN ptyalography. [sialo- + G. *graphō*, to write]

si·a·lo·lith (sī'ă-lō-lith). A salivary calculus. SYN ptyalolith. [sialo- + G. *lithos*, stone]

si·a·lo·li·thi·a·sis (sī'ă-lō-li-thī'ă-sis). The formation or presence of a salivary calculus. SYN ptyalolithiasis, salivolithiasis. [sialolith + G. -*iasis*, condition]

si·a·lo·li·thot·o·my (sī'ă-lō-li-thot'ō-mē). Incision of a salivary duct or gland to remove a calculus. SYN ptyalolithotomy. [sialolith + G. *tomē*, incision]

si·al·o·met·a·pla·sia (sī'ă-lō-met-ă-plā'zē-ă). Squamous cell metaplasia in the salivary ducts. [sialo- + metaplasia]

necrotizing s., squamous cell metaplasia of the salivary gland ducts and lobules, with necrosis of the salivary gland lobules; seen most frequently in the hard palate.

si·a·lom·e·try (sī-ă-lom'ĕ-trē). A measurement of salivary secretion, generally for a comparison of a denervated or diseased gland with its healthy counterpart. [sialo- + G. *metron*, measure]

si·a·lor·rhea (sī'ă-lō-rē'ă). Excessive flow of saliva. SYN hygrostomia, ptyalism, salivation, sialism, sialismus, sialosis. [sialo- + G. *rhoia*, a flow]

si·a·los·che·sis (sī'ă-los'kĕ-sis). Suppression of the secretion of saliva. [sialo- + G. *schesis*, retention]

si·a·lo·se·mi·ol·o·gy, si·a·lo·se·mei·ol·o·gy (sī-ă-lō-sē-mē-ol'ō-jē). The study and analysis of saliva as an aid to diagnosis. [sialo- + G. *sēmeion*, sign, + *logos*, study]

si·a·lo·sis (sī'ă-lō'sis). SYN sialorrhea.

si·a·lo·ste·no·sis (sī'ă-lō-ste-nō'sis). Stricture of a salivary duct. [sialo- + G. *stenōsis*, a narrowing]

sib. A member of a sibship. SYN sibling.

sib·i·lant (sib'i-lănt). Hissing or whistling in character; denoting a form of rhonchus. [L. *sibilans* (-*ant*-), pres. p. of *sibilo*, to hiss]

sib·i·lus (sib'i-lŭs). A sibilant rale. [L. a hissing]

sib·ling. SYN sib. [A. S. *sib*, relation, + -*ling*, diminutive]

sib·ship. **1.** The reciprocal state between individuals who have the same pair of parents. **2.** All progeny of one pair of parents. [A.S. *sib*, relationship]

Sibson, Francis, English anatomist, 1814–1876. SEE S. *aponeurosis, fascia, groove, muscle,* aortic *vestibule*.

Sicard, Jean A., French physician, 1872-1929. SEE Collet-S. *syndrome*.

sic·cant (sik'ant). **1.** Drying; removing moisture from surrounding substances. **2.** A substance with such properties. SYN siccative. [L. *siccans* (-*ant*-), pres. p. of *sicco*, pp. -*atus*, to dry]

sic·ca·tive (sik'ă-tiv). SYN siccant.

sic·cha·sia (sĭ-kā'zē-ă). **1.** SYN nausea. **2.** Loathing for food. [G. *sikchasia*, loathing, fr. *sikchos*, squeamish]

sic·co·la·bile (sik-ō-lā'bil, -bīl). Subject to alteration or destruction on drying. [L. *siccus*, dry, + *labilis*, perishable]

sic·co·sta·bile, sic·co·sta·ble (sik-ō-stā'bil; -bīl, -bl). Not subject to alteration or destruction on drying. [L. *siccus*, dry, + *stabilis*, stable]

sick (sik). **1.** Unwell; suffering from disease. **2.** SYN nauseated. [A.S. *seóc*]

sick·le·mia (sik-lē'mē-ă). Presence of sickle- or crescent-shaped erythrocytes in peripheral blood; seen in sickle cell anemia and sickle cell trait.

sick·ling (sik'ling). Production of sickle-shaped erythrocytes in the circulation, as in sickle cell anemia.

sick·ness (sik'nes). SYN disease (1).

acute African sleeping s., SYN Rhodesian *trypanosomiasis*.

aerial s., SYN altitude s.

African sleeping s., SEE Gambian *trypanosomiasis*, Rhodesian *trypanosomiasis*.

air s., a form of motion s. caused by flying in an airplane.

altitude s., a syndrome caused by low inspired oxygen pressure (as at high altitude) and characterized by nausea, headache, dyspnea, malaise, and insomnia; in severe instances, pulmonary edema and adult respiratory distress syndrome can occur; SYN Acosta disease, mountain s., puna, soroche. SYN aerial s., altitude disease.

balloon s., a form of altitude s. occurring in someone as a result of ascent in a balloon.

black s., SYN visceral *leishmaniasis*.

caisson s., disease caused by rapid decompression; so named since it appeared in workers building tunnels or supports for bridges working in enclosed units under high atmospheric pressure to keep out surrounding water, called caissons. SEE decompression s.

car s., a form of motion s. caused by riding on a train or in an automobile or bus.

cave s., histoplasmosis acquired by inhalation of organism *Histoplasma capulatum* in caves (while spelunking) or mine shafts containing bird roosts or bats, prime conditions for growth of the organisms.

chronic African sleeping s., SYN Gambian *trypanosomiasis*.

chronic mountain s., loss of high altitude tolerance after prolonged exposure (e.g., by residence), characterized by extreme polycythemia, exaggerated hypoxemia, and reduced mental and physical capacity; relieved by descent. SYN altitude erythremia, chronic soroche, Monge disease.

decompression s., a symptom complex caused by the escape from solution in the body fluids of nitrogen bubbles absorbed originally at high atmospheric pressure, as a result of abrupt reduction in atmospheric pressure (either rapid ascent to high altitude or return from a compressed-air environment); it is characterized by headache, pain in the arms, legs, joints, and epigastrium, itching of the skin, vertigo, dyspnea, coughing, choking, vomiting, weakness and sometimes paralysis, and severe peripheral circulatory collapse; bone infarcts can occur from bubbles in nutrient vessels leading to long-term consequences. SEE ALSO caisson s. SYN caisson disease, decompression disease, diver's palsy.

East African sleeping s., SYN Rhodesian *trypanosomiasis*.

falling s., SYN epilepsy.

green s., SYN chlorosis.

green tobacco s., an illness of tobacco harvest workers characterized by headache, dizziness, and vomiting.

si

Indian s., SYN epidemic gangrenous *proctitis.*

Jamaican vomiting s., SYN ackee *poisoning.*

milk s., a disease of humans caused by ingesting contaminated milk from cows suffering from trembles; clinical manifestations include severe vomiting, labored breathing, delirium, convulsions, coma, and death; recovery from nonlethal illness is slow. SYN lactimorbus.

morning s., the nausea and vomiting of early pregnancy. SYN morning vomiting, nausea gravidarum.

motion s., the syndrome of pallor, nausea, weakness, and malaise, which may progress to vomiting and incapacitation, caused by stimulation of the semicircular canals during travel or motion as on a boat, plane, train, car, swing, or rotating amusement ride. SYN kinesia.

mountain s., SYN altitude s.

radiation s., a systemic condition caused by substantial whole-body irradiation, seen after nuclear explosions or accidents, rarely after radiotherapy. Manifestations depend on dose, ranging from anorexia, nausea, vomiting, and mild leukopenia, to thrombocytopenia with hemorrhage, severe leukopenia with infection, anemia, central nervous system damage, and death. SYN radiation poisoning.

sea s., motion s. occurring in boat travelers.

serum s., an immune complex disease appearing some days (usually 1–2 weeks) after injection of a foreign serum or serum protein, with local and systemic reactions such as urticaria, fever, general lymphadenopathy, edema, arthritis, and occasionally albuminuria or severe nephritis; originally described in patients receiving serotherapy. The term is sometimes used for clinically similar allergic reactions to drugs. SYN serum disease, serum reaction.

sleeping s., SEE Gambian *trypanosomiasis,* Rhodesian *trypanosomiasis.*

space s., dizziness as result of changes in inner ear resulting from absence of gravity. SYN physiologic vertigo.

West African sleeping s., SYN Gambian *trypanosomiasis.*

side (sīd). One of the two lateral margins or surfaces of a body, midway between the front and back. [A.S. *side*]

balancing s., in dentistry, the nonfunctioning s. from which the mandible moves during the working bite.

working s., in dentistry, the lateral segment of a dentition toward which the mandible is moved during occlusal function.

side ef·fect. A result of drug or other therapy in addition to or in extension of the desired therapeutic effect; usually but not necessarily, connoting an undesirable effect. Although technically the therapeutic effect carried beyond the desired limit (e.g., a hemorrhage from an anticoagulant) is a s. e., the term more often refers to pharmacologic results of therapy unrelated to the usual objective (e.g., a development of signs of Cushing syndrome with steroid therapy).

sid·er·a·tion (sid-er-ā′shŭn). Any sudden attack, as of apoplexy. [L. *sideror,* pp. *sideratus,* to be blasted or palsied by a constellation, fr. *sidus* (*sider-*), a constellation, the heavens]

△**sidero-.** Iron. [G. *sideros*]

sid·er·o·blast (sid′er-ō-blast). An erythroblast containing granules of ferritin stained by the Prussian blue reaction. [sidero- + G. *blastos,* germ]

sid·er·o·cyte (sid′er-ō-sīt). An erythrocyte containing granules of free iron, as detected by the Prussian blue reaction, in the blood of normal fetuses, where they constitute from 0.10–4.5% of the erythrocytes. [sidero- + G. *kytos,* cell]

sid·er·o·fi·bro·sis (sid′er-ō-fī-brō′sis). Fibrosis associated with small foci in which iron is deposited.

sid·er·og·en·ous (sid-er-oj′ĕ-nŭs). Iron forming. [sidero- + G. *-gen,* producing]

sid·er·o·pe·nia (sid′er-ō-pē′nē-ă). An abnormally low level of serum iron. [sidero- + G. *penia,* poverty]

sid·er·o·pe·nic (sid′er-ō-pē′nik). Characterized by sideropenia.

sid·er·o·phage (sid′er-ō-fāj). SYN siderophore. [sidero- + G. *phagō,* to eat]

sid·er·o·phil, sid·er·o·phile (sid′er-ō-fil, -fīl). **1.** Absorbing

iron. SYN siderophilous. **2.** A cell or tissue that contains iron. [sidero- + G. *philos,* fond]

sid·er·oph·i·lins (sid-er-ō-fil′in, -of′ĭ-lin). Nonheme, iron-binding proteins; there are three central classes of s.: transferrin (1) (in vertebrate blood), lactoferrin (in mammalian milk and other secretions), and conalbumin or ovotransferrin (avian blood and avian egg white).

sid·er·oph·i·lous (sid-er-of′i-lŭs). SYN siderophil (1).

sid·er·o·phore (sid′er-ō-fōr). A large extravasated mononuclear phagocyte containing granules of hemosiderin, found in the sputum or in the lungs of individuals with longstanding pulmonary congestion from left ventricular failure. SEE ALSO heart failure *cell.* SYN siderophage. [sidero- + G. *phoros,* bearing]

sid·er·o·sil·i·co·sis (sid′er-ō-sil′i-kō′sis). Silicosis due to inhalation of dust containing iron and silica. SYN silicosiderosis. [sidero- + silicosis]

sid·er·o·sis (sid-er-ō′sis). **1.** A form of pneumoconiosis due to the presence of iron dust. **2.** Discoloration of any part by disposition of a pigment containing iron; usually called hemosiderosis. **3.** An excess of iron in the circulating blood. **4.** Degeneration of the retina, lens, and uvea as a result of the deposition of intraocular iron. [sidero- + G. *-osis,* condition]

pulmonary s., SYN *pneumoconiosis* siderotica.

sid·er·ot·ic (sid-er-ot′ik). Related to siderosis; pigmented by iron or containing an excess of iron.

SIDS Acronym for sudden infant death *syndrome.*

Siegert, Ferdinand, German pediatrician, 1865–1946. SEE S. *sign.*

Siegle, Emil, German otologist, 1833–1900. SEE S. *otoscope.*

sie·mens (S) (sē′menz). The SI unit of electrical conductance; the conductance of a body with an electrical resistance of 1 ohm, allowing 1 ampere of current to flow per volt applied; equal to 1 mho. SYN mho. [Sir William *Siemens,* Ger. born British engineer, 1823–1883]

Siemerling, Ernst, German physician, 1857–1931.

sieve (siv). A meshed or perforated device for separating fine particles from coarser ones. [O.E. *sive*]

molecular s., a gel-like material with pore sizes of such ranges as to exclude molecules above certain sizes; used in fractionating or purifying macromolecules.

sie·vert (Sv) (sē′vert). The SI unit of ionizing radiation effective dose, equal to the absorbed dose in gray, weighted for both the quality of radiation in question and the tissue response to that radiation. The unit is the joule per kilogram and 1 Sv = 100 rem. SEE effective *dose,* equivalent *dose.*

SIF Abbreviation for somatotropin release-inhibiting *factor.*

Sig. Abbreviation for L. *signa,* label, write, or *signetur,* let it be labeled.

Siggaard-Andersen, Ole, Danish clinical biochemist, *1932. SEE Siggaard-Andersen *nomogram.*

sigh (sī). **1.** An audible inspiration and expiration under the influence of some emotion. **2.** To perform such an act. [A.S. *sican*]

sight (sīt). The ability or faculty of seeing. SEE ALSO vision. [A.S. *gesihth*]

day s., SYN nyctalopia.

far s., SYN hyperopia.

long s., SYN hyperopia.

near s., SYN myopia.

night s., SYN hemeralopia.

second s., improved near vision in the aged as a result of increased refractivity of the nucleus of the lens causing myopia. SYN senile lenticular myopia.

short s., SYN myopia.

sig·ma (sig′mă). The 18th letter of the Greek alphabet, σ.

sig·ma·tism (sig′mă-tizm). SYN lisping. [G. *sigma,* the letter S]

sig·moid (sig′moyd). Resembling in outline the letter S or one of the forms of the Greek sigma. [G. *sigma,* the letter S, + *eidos,* resemblance]

△**sigmoid-.** SEE sigmoido-.

sig·moi·dec·to·my (sig-moy-dek′tō-mē). Excision of the sigmoid colon. [sigmoid- + G. *ektomē*, excision]

sig·moid·ic·i·ty (sig′moyd-i-sa-tē). Describing an S-shaped curve; e.g., shape of enzyme-kinetic curves for enzymes displaying positive homotropic cooperativity.

sig·moid·i·tis (sig-moy-dī′tis). Inflammation of the sigmoid colon. [sigmoid- + G. *-itis*, inflammation]

⌂**sigmoido-, sigmoid-.** Sigmoid, usually the sigmoid colon. [G. *sigma*, the letter σ, + *eidos*, resemblance]

sig·moi·do·pexy (sig-moy′dō-pek-sē). Operative attachment of the sigmoid colon to a firm structure to correct rectal prolapse. [sigmoido- + G. *pēxis*, fixation]

sig·moi·do·proc·tos·to·my (sig-moy′dō-prok-tos′tō-mē). Anastomosis between the sigmoid colon and the rectum. SYN sigmoidorectostomy. [sigmoido- + G. *prōktos*, anus, + *stoma*, mouth]

sig·moi·do·rec·tos·to·my (sig-moy′dō-rek-tos′tō-mē). SYN sigmoidoproctostomy.

sig·moi·do·scope (sig-moy′dō-skōp). An endoscope for viewing the lumen of the sigmoid colon. SYN sigmoscope. [sigmoido- + G. *skopeō*, to view]

sig·moi·dos·co·py (sig′moy-dos′kŏ-pē). Inspection, through an endoscope, of the interior of the sigmoid colon.

sig·moi·dos·to·my (sig′moy-dos′tō-mē). Establishment of an artificial anus by opening into the sigmoid colon. [sigmoido- + G. *stoma*, mouth]

sig·moi·dot·o·my (sig′moy-dot′ō-mē). Surgical opening of the sigmoid. [sigmoido- + G. *tomē*, incision]

sig·mo·scope (sig′mō-skōp). SYN sigmoidoscope.

SIGN

sign (sīn). **1.** Any abnormality indicative of disease, discoverable on examination of the patient; an objective indication of disease, in contrast to a symptom, which is a subjective indication of disease. **2.** An abbreviation or symbol. **3.** In psychology, any object or artifact (stimulus) that represents a specific thing or conveys a specific idea to the person who perceives it. [L. *signum*, mark]

Aaron s., in acute appendicitis, a referred pain or feeling of distress in the epigastrium or precordial region on continuous firm pressure over the McBurney point.

Abadie s. of tabes dorsalis, insensibility to pressure over the tendo achillis.

Abrahams s., an obsolete sign. **(1)** rales and other adventitious sounds, changes in the respiratory murmurs, and increase in the whispered sound can be heard on auscultation over the acromial end of the clavicle some time before they become audible at the apex; heard primarily in pulmonary tuberculosis affecting the apical portion of the lung; **(2)** a dull-flat note, i.e., one between the normal dullness at the right apex and absolute flatness, heard on percussion in that region, indicating progress from incipient to advanced tuberculosis.

accessory s., a finding frequently but not consistently present in a disease. SYN assident s.

antecedent s., SYN prodromic s.

assident s., SYN accessory s.

Auenbrugger s., an epigastric prominence seen in cases of marked pericardial effusion.

Aufrecht s., diminished or noisy breath sounds in the trachea just above the jugular notch, in cases of stenosis.

Auspitz s., a finding typical of psoriasis in which removal of a scale leads to pinpoint bleeding.

Babinski s., (1) extension of the great toe and abduction of the other toes instead of the normal flexion reflex to plantar stimulation, considered indicative of pyramidal tract involvement ("positive" Babinski); SYN Babinski phenomenon, Babinski reflex, great-toe reflex, paradoxical extensor reflex, toe phenomenon. **(2)**

in hemiplegia, weakness of the platysma muscle on the affected side, as is evident in such actions as blowing or opening the mouth; **(3)** when the patient is lying supine, with arms crossed on the front of the chest, and attempts to assume the sitting posture, the thigh on the side of an *organic* paralysis is flexed and the heel raised, whereas the limb on the sound side remains flat; **(4)** in hemiplegia, the forearm on the affected side turns to a pronated position when placed in a position of supination.

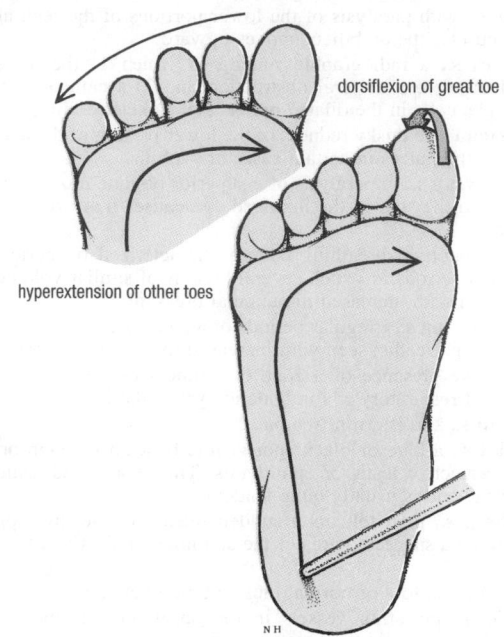

dorsiflexion of great toe

hyperextension of other toes

N H

Babinski sign: on stimulation of sole of foot, extension of the great toe with fanning of the other toes is a normal response up to six months of age, but abnormal thereafter; a positive response is considered indicative of pyramidal tract involvement

Baccelli s., an obsolete s.: good conduction of the whisper in nonpurulent pleural effusions. SYN aphonic pectoriloquy.

Ballance s., the presence of a dull percussion note in both flanks, constant on the left side but shifting with change of position on the right, said to indicate ruptured spleen; the dullness is due to the presence of fluid blood on the right side but coagulated blood on the left.

Bamberger s., (1) jugular pulse in tricuspid insufficiency; **(2)** SYN allochiria; **(3)** dullness on percussion at the angle of the scapula, clearing up as the patient leans forward, indicating pericarditis with effusion. SYN Bamberger-Pins-Ewart s.

Bamberger-Pins-Ewart s., SYN Bamberger s.

banana s., the abnormal curvature of the cerebellum noted on ultrasound imaging in a fetus with Arnold-Chiari *malformation*.

Bárány s., in cases of ear disease, in which the vestibule is healthy, injection into the external auditory canal of water below the body temperature will cause rotatory nystagmus toward the opposite side; when the injected fluid is above the body temperature the nystagmus will be toward the injected side; if the labyrinth is diseased or nonfunctional there may be diminished or absent nystagmus.

Barré s., a hemiplegic placed in the prone position with the limbs flexed at the knees is unable to maintain the flexed position on the side of the lesion but extends the leg.

Bassler s., in chronic appendicitis, pinching the appendix between the thumb and the iliacus muscle causes sharp pain.

Bastedo s., an obsolete s.: in chronic appendicitis, pain and tenderness in the right iliac fossa on inflation of the colon with air.

Battle s., postauricular ecchymosis in cases of fracture of the base of the skull.

B6 bronchus s., in lung radiology, appearance of an air bronchogram of the superior segmental bronchus of the lower lobe because of segmental atelectasis or consolidation.

beak s., appearance of the distal esophagus, on a contrast esophagram, in achalasia; also used to describe the proximal pyloric canal on upper GI series in congenital pyloric stenosis.

Bechterew s., paralysis of automatic facial movements, the power of voluntary movement being retained.

Beevor s., with paralysis of the lower portions of the recti abdominis muscles the umbilicus moves upward.

Bergman s., a radiographic finding in which 1) the ureter is dilated distal to a ureteral obstruction and 2) a catheter, passed retrograde, coils in the dilated ureter. SYN catheter coiling s.

Biederman s., a dusky redness of the lower portion of the anterior pillars of the fauces in certain cases of syphilis.

Bielschowsky s., in paralysis of a superior oblique muscle, tilting the head to the side of the involved eye causes that eye to rotate upward.

Biot s., abnormal breathing pattern characterized by periods of apnea and periods in which several breaths of similar volume are taken; seen with increased intracranial pressure.

Biot breathing s., irregular periods of apnea alternating with four or five deep breaths; seen with increased intracranial pressure.

Bird s., the presence of a zone of dullness on percussion with absence of respiratory s.'s in hydatid cyst of the lung.

Bjerrum s., SYN Bjerrum *scotoma*.

blue dot s., a blue or black spot visible beneath the skin on the cranial aspect of testis or epididymis. This is a torsed testicular appendage and is usually quite tender.

Blumberg s., pain felt upon sudden release of steadily applied pressure on a suspected area of the abdomen, indicative of peritonitis.

Bonhoeffer s., loss of normal muscle tone in chorea.

Bozzolo s., pulsating vessels in the nasal mucous membrane, noted occasionally in thoracic aneurysm.

Branham s., bradycardia following compression or excision of an arteriovenous fistula.

Braxton Hicks s., irregular uterine contractions occurring after the third month of pregnancy.

Broadbent s., a retraction of the thoracic wall, synchronous with cardiac systole, visible anywhere, but particularly in the left posterior axillary line; a s. of adherent pericardium.

Brockenbrough s., absolute decrease in pulse pressure of the beat immediately following a premature beat; a s. of idiopathic hypertrophic subaortic stenosis.

Brudzinski s., (1) in meningitis, on passive flexion of the leg on one side, a similar movement occurs in the opposite leg. SYN contralateral reflex, contralateral s. **(2)** in meningitis, involuntary flexion of the knees and hips following flexion of the neck while supine. SYN neck s.

burning drops s., in certain cases of perforated gastric ulcer, a sensation as of drops of hot liquid falling into the abdominal cavity or as of a stream of intensely hot liquid being poured into the cavity.

calcium s., in chest radiography, displacement of the line of the calcified intima of the aorta away from its outer wall, a finding in a small percentage of cases of dissection of blood in the aortic media; the expression "displaced intimal calcification" is preferred to the listed term. SEE aortic *dissection*.

Calkins s., the change of shape of the uterus from discoid to ovoid, indicating placental separation from the uterine wall.

Cantelli s., SEE doll's eye s.

Carman s., in gastric radiology, the appearance of a contrast-filled malignant ulcer, which does not extend beyond the line of the gastric wall as a benign ulcer would; also has a thick overhanging rim of tumor tissue.

Carnett s., disappearance of abdominal tenderness to palpation when the anterior abdominal muscles are contracted, indicating pain of intra-abdominal origin; its persistence suggests a source in the abdominal wall, which is also indicated when tenderness is caused by gently pinching a fold of skin and fat between the thumb and forefinger.

Carvallo s., an increase in the intensity of the pansystolic murmur of tricuspid regurgitation during or at the end of inspiration that distinguishes tricuspid from mitral involvement.

catheter coiling s., SYN Bergman s.

Chaddock s., when the external malleolar skin area is irritated, extension of the great toe occurs in cases of organic disease of the corticospinal reflex paths. SYN Chaddock reflex.

Chadwick s., a bluish discoloration of the cervix and vagina, a s. of pregnancy.

chandelier s., colloquial term referring to severe pain elicited during pelvic examination of patients with pelvic inflammatory disease in which the patient responds by reaching upwards towards the ceiling for relief.

Chaussier s., severe pain in the epigastrium, a prodrome of eclampsia; may be of central origin or caused by distention of the capsule of liver by hemorrhage.

Chvostek s., facial irritability in tetany, unilateral spasm of the orbicularis oculi or oris muscle being excited by a slight tap over the facial nerve just anterior to the external auditory meatus. SYN Weiss s.

Claybrook s., in rupture of abdominal viscus, transmission of breath and heart sounds through the abdominal wall.

clenched fist s., in angina pectoris, pressing of the clenched fist against the chest to indicate the constricting, pressing quality of the pain.

Collier s., unilateral or bilateral lid retraction due to midbrain lesion; occurring at any age. SEE setting sun s., Epstein s. SYN Collier tucked lid s.

Collier tucked lid s., SYN Collier s.

colon cutoff s., radiographic s. of (usually) inflammatory disease preventing distention of the distal transverse colon.

Comby s., an early s. of measles, consisting of thin, whitish patches on the gums and buccal mucous membrane, formed of desquamating epithelial cells.

comet s., SYN comet tail s.

comet tail s., in chest radiology, the curved appearance of pulmonary arteries and veins associated with rounded atelectasis, fibrosis associated with organizing pleurisy. SYN comet s.

commemorative s., a phenomenon pointing to the previous existence of some disease other than the one present at the time.

contralateral s., SYN Brudzinski s. (1).

conventional s.'s, s.'s that acquire their function through social (linguistic) custom; e.g., words, mathematical symbols. SEE ALSO symbol (4).

Corrigan s., a full, hard pulse followed by a sudden collapse easily palpated and occurring in aortic regurgitation. SYN Corrigan pulse.

Courvoisier s., SYN Courvoisier *law*.

crescent s., (1) in radiography of the lung, a crescent of gas near the top of a mass lesion, signifying cavitation with a space above the debris; seen in aspergilloma, hydatidoma; **(2)** in computed *tomography*, a high attenuating layer of new blood in an aneurysm; indicates a ruptured abdominal aortic aneurysm; **(3)** in diagnostic *ultrasound*, a sonolucent crescentic layer in a tumor mass, typically necrosis in stromal tumors of the small bowel; **(4)** in diagnostic ultrasound, a hyperechoic crescent, representing the entering limb of an intussusception; also known as crescent-in-a-doughnut; **(5)** in osteoradiology, a subcortical lucent crescent in the femoral head, signifying osteonecrosis. SYN meniscus s.

Cruveilhier-Baumgarten s., a murmur over the umbilicus often in the presence of caput medusae, resulting from portal hypertension, usually with hepatic cirrhosis; recanalization of the umbilical vein with reverse blood flow from the liver into the abdominal wall veins creates the murmur.

Cullen s., periumbilical darkening of the skin from blood, a s. of intraperitoneal hemorrhage, especially in ruptured ectopic pregnancy.

Dalrymple s., retraction of the upper eyelid in Graves disease, causing abnormal wideness of the palpebral fissure.

Dance s., a slight retraction in the neighborhood of the right iliac fossa in some cases of intussusception.

Danforth s., shoulder pain on inspiration, due to irritation of the diaphragm by a hemoperitoneum in ruptured ectopic pregnancy.

Darier s., urtication on stroking of cutaneous lesions of urticaria pigmentosa (mastocytosis).

Dejerine s., aggravation of symptoms of root irritation by the acts of coughing, sneezing, or straining to defecate.

Delbet s., in a case of aneurysm of a main artery, efficient collateral circulation if the nutrition of the part below is well maintained, despite the fact that the pulse has disappeared.

de Musset s., SYN Musset s.

D'Éspine s., an obsolete sign (1) bronchophony over the spinous processes heard, at a lower level than in health, in pulmonary tuberculosis; (2) an echoed whisper following a spoken word, heard in the stethoscope placed over the seventh cervical or first or second dorsal spine, in cases of tuberculosis of the mediastinal glands.

dimple s., in dermatofibroma, dimpling elicited when the lesion is squeezed.

doll's eye s., reflex movement of the eyes in the opposite direction to that which the head is moved, e.g., the eyes being lowered as the head is raised, and the reverse (Cantelli sign); an indication of functional integrity of the brainstem tegmental pathways and cranial nerves involved in eye movement.

Dorendorf s., fullness of one supraclavicular groove in aneurysm of the aortic arch.

double bubble s., in pediatric radiology, appearance of the dilated air-filled stomach and duodenal bulb, associated with duodenal atresia or web, less often midgut volvulus.

double ring s., two concentric rings around the optic nerve characteristic of optic nerve hypoplasia.

double track s., in pediatric radiology, a less common s. of congenital pyloric stenosis, when barium is caught between mucosal folds in the hypertrophied pylorus.

drawer s., in a knee examination, the forward or backward sliding of the tibia under applied stress, which indicates laxity or tear of the anterior (forward slide) or posterior (backward slide) cruciate ligaments of the knee. SYN drawer test.

drooping lily s., in urography, a s. of a double renal collecting system with an obstruction of the upper system depressing the opacified calyces of the lower system so they appear to droop.

Drummond s., in certain cases of aortic aneurysm, a puffing sound, synchronous with cardiac systole, heard from the nostrils, when the mouth is closed.

Duchenne s., falling in of the epigastrium during inspiration in paralysis of the diaphragm.

Dupuytren s., (1) in congenital dislocation, free up and down movement of the head of the femur occurs upon intermittent traction; (2) a crackling sensation on pressure over the bone in certain cases of sarcoma.

Duroziez s., SYN Duroziez *murmur.*

Ebstein s., in pericardial effusion, obtuseness of the cardiohepatic angle on percussion.

s. of edema of lower eyelid, swelling of the lower lid found in congestive failure, myxedema, or nephrosis.

Epstein s., lid retraction in an infant giving it a frightened expression and a "wild glance." SEE setting sun s., Collier s.

Ewart s., in large pericardial effusions, an area of dullness with bronchial breathing and bronchophony below the angle of the left scapula. SYN Pins s.

Ewing s., tenderness at the upper inner angle of the orbit at the point of attachment of the pulley of the superior oblique muscle, denoting closure of the outlet of the frontal sinus.

Faget s., a slow pulse with an elevated temperature, often seen in yellow fever.

fan s., the spreading apart of the toes in the complete Babinski sign.

Fischer s., an obsolete s.: in tuberculosis of the mediastinal or peribronchial glands, after bending the patient's head as far back as possible, auscultation over the manubrium sterni will sometimes reveal a continuous loud murmur caused by the pressure of the enlarged glands on the large mediastinal vessels. SYN Fischer symptom.

fissure s., in perfusion scintigraphy of the lungs, decreased uptake of radionuclide in the periphery of each lobe, making the fissures visible; caused by a variety of diseases and artifacts.

flag s., bands of discoloration of hair (reddish, blond, or gray, depending on original color) resulting from fluctuations in nutrition characteristic of kwashiorkor and in diseases with protein depletion such as ulcerative colitis.

Forchheimer s., the presence, in German measles, of a reddish maculopapular eruption on the soft palate.

Fothergill s., in rectus sheath hematoma, the hematoma produces a mass that does not cross the midline and remains palpable when the rectus muscle is tense.

Friedreich s., in adherent pericardium, sudden collapse of the previously distended veins of the neck at each diastole of the heart.

Froment s., flexion of the distal phalanx of the thumb when a sheet of paper is held between the thumb and index finger in ulnar nerve palsy.

Gaenslen s., pain on hyperextension of the hip with pelvis fixed by flexion of opposite hip; causes a torsion stress at the sacroiliac and lumbosacral joints.

Gauss s., marked mobility of the uterus in the early weeks of pregnancy.

Glasgow s., a systolic murmur heard over the brachial artery in aneurysm of the aorta.

gloved-finger s., in chest radiology, the appearance of mucoid impaction of branching bronchi.

Goggia s., the fibrillation of the biceps muscle, when pinched and tapped, is confined to a limited area in cases of debilitating disease, whereas in health it is general.

Goldstein toe s., increased space between the great toe and its neighbor, seen in Down syndrome, occasionally in cretinism, and as a normal variant.

Goodell s., softening of the cervix and vagina as being usually indicative of pregnancy.

Gordon s., SYN finger *phenomenon.*

Gorlin s., unusual ease in touching the tip of the nose with the tongue; seen in Ehlers-Danlos syndrome.

Gower s., use of limb muscles to assume an upright sitting position, with the patient using the hands to "walk" up the legs; seen in conditions of weak pelvic girdle and proximal leg muscles.

Graefe s., in Graves disease, lag of the upper eyelid as it follows the rotation of the eyeball downward. SYN von Graefe s.

Grasset s., normal contraction of the sternocleidomastoid muscle on the paralyzed side in cases of hemiplegia.

Grey Turner s., local areas of discoloration about the umbilicus and in the region of the loins, in acute hemorrhagic pancreatitis and other causes of retroperitoneal hemorrhage.

Griesinger s., erythema and edema over the posterior part of the mastoid process due to septic thrombosis of the mastoid emissary vein and indicating thrombophlebitis of the sigmoid sinus.

Grocco s., (1) acute dilation of the heart following a muscular effort, described in Graves disease; also occurring in various forms of myocardiopathy; (2) extension of the liver dullness several centimeters to the left of the midspinal line in cases of enlargement of that organ.

groove s., large, hard, fixed, and extremely tender lymph nodes in the groin above and below the inguinal ligament, with a groove along the ligament; characteristic of lymphogranuloma venereum.

Gunn s., (1) compression of the underlying vein at arteriovenous crossings seen ophthalmoscopically in arteriolar sclerosis; (2) on alternate stimulation with light, the pupil of an eye with optic nerve transmission defect constricts poorly or even dilates when stimulated (a relative afferent pupillary defect). SYN Marcus Gunn s.

Gunn crossing s., retinal arteriovenous crossing with venous compression in hypertensive disease.

Guyon s., (1) ballottement of the kidney in cases of nephroptosis, especially when there is also a renal tumor; (2) the hypoglossal nerve lies directly upon the external carotid artery, whereby this vessel may be distinguished from the internal carotid when ligation is necessary.

si

halo s., elevation of the subcutaneous fat layer over the fetal skull in a dead or dying fetus; said to be the most common radiologic sign of fetal death.

halo s. of hydrops, a discredited radiographic s. of fetal hydrops caused by scalp edema so that a definite corona surrounds the skull.

Hamman s., a crunching, rasping sound, synchronous with heart beat, heard over the precordium and sometimes at a distance from the chest in mediastinal *emphysema*.

Hawkins impingement s., pain produced by forced internal rotation of the humerus in 90° of abduction.

Hegar s., softening and compressibility of the lower segment of the uterus in early pregnancy (about the seventh week) which, on bimanual examination, is felt by the finger in the vagina as though the neck and body of the uterus were separated, or connected by only a thin band of tissue.

Heim-Kreysig s., in adherent pericardium, an indrawing of the intercostal spaces, synchronous with the cardiac systole. SYN Kreysig s.

Hennebert s., nystagmus produced by pressure applied to a sealed external auditory canal; may be seen in labyrinthine fistula or with intact tympanic membrane in syphilitic involvement of the otic capsule.

Higoumenakia s., sternoclavicular swelling in late congenital syphilis.

Hill s., in aortic insufficiency, greater systolic blood pressure in the legs than in the arms; normal arterial systolic pressure in the leg is 10–20 mm of Hg above that in the arm, whereas in aortic insufficiency the difference may be 60–100 mm of Hg. SYN Hill phenomenon.

Hoagland s., eyelid edema in infectious mononucleosis.

Hoffmann s., (1) in latent tetany mild mechanical stimulation of the trigeminal nerve causes severe pain; (2) flexion of the terminal phalanx of the thumb and of the second and third phalanges of one or more of the fingers when the volar surface of the terminal phalanx of the fingers is flicked. SYN digital reflex, Hoffmann reflex, snapping reflex.

Homans s., pain in the calf when the ankle is slowly and gently dorsiflexed (with the knee bent), indicative of incipient or established thrombosis in the veins of the leg.

Hoover s.'s, (1) when a subject lying supine is asked to raise one leg, he or she involuntarily creates counterpressure with the heel of the other leg; if this leg is paralyzed, whatever muscular power is preserved in it will be exerted in this way; or if the patient attempts to lift a paralyzed leg, counterpressure will be made with the other heel, whether any movement occurs in the paralyzed limb or not; not present in hysteria or malingering; (2) a modification in the movement of the costal margins during respiration, caused by a flattening of the diaphragm; suggestive of empyema or other intrathoracic condition causing a change in the contour of the diaphragm.

iconic s.'s, s.'s that acquire their function through similarity to what they signify; e.g., a photograph as a s. of the person in the picture.

impingement s., pain in patients with rotator cuff tendinitis or tears within the subacromial space elicited by provocative physical examination maneuvers.

indexical s.'s, s.'s that acquire their function through a causal connection with what they signify; e.g., smoke as a s. of fire.

inferior triangle s., in chest radiology, lateral displacement of the mediastinal pleura near the diaphragm, associated with collapse of the upper lobe, usually on the right side. Cf. superior triangle s.

Jackson s., during quiet respiration the movement of the paralyzed side of the chest may be greater than that of the opposite side, while in forced respiration the paralyzed side moves less than the other.

Joffroy s., disorder of the arithmetical faculty (the person being unable to do simple sums in addition or multiplication) in the early stages of organic brain disease.

Kehr s., violent pain in the left shoulder in a case of rupture of the spleen.

Kerandel s., delayed sensation to pain indicative of African trypanosomiasis.

Kernig s., when a subject is supine and the thigh is flexed to a right angle with the axis of the trunk, complete extension of the leg on the thigh is impossible; present in various forms of meningitis.

Kestenbaum s., a decrease in the number of arterioles crossing optic disk margins as a s. of optic neuritis.

knuckle s., in chest radiography, an abrupt tapering of a large pulmonary artery caused by pulmonary embolism.

Kocher s., in Graves disease, on upward gaze, the globe lags behind the movement of the upper eyelid.

Kreysig s., SYN Heim-Kreysig s.

Kussmaul s., in constrictive pericarditis, a paradoxical increase in venous distention and pressure or failure to collapse during inspiration; seen occasionally in effusive-constrictive pericarditis when tamponading pericardial fluid overlies a constricting epicarditis.

Lancisi s., a large systolic jugular venous wave caused by tricuspid regurgitation replacing the normal negative systolic trough ("x" descent).

Landolfi s., in aortic insufficiency, systolic contraction and diastolic dilation of the pupil.

Lasègue s., when a subject is supine with hip flexed and knee extended, dorsiflexion of the ankle causing pain or muscle spasm in the posterior thigh indicates lumbar root or sciatic nerve irritation.

Legendre s., in facial hemiplegia of central origin, when the examiner raises the lids of the actively closed eyes the resistance is less on the affected side.

lemon s., the ultrasound finding of frontal bone scalloping associated with Arnold-Chiari *malformation*.

Leri s., voluntary flexion of the elbow is impossible in a case of hemiplegia when the wrist on that side is passively flexed.

Leser-Trélat s., the sudden appearance and rapid increase in the number and size of seborrheic keratoses with pruritus; associated with internal malignancy.

Lhermitte s., sudden electric-like shocks extending down the spine on flexing the head.

local s., the characteristic of a sensation that permits distinguishing it from another sensation by locating its position in space.

Lorenz s., an obsolete s.: stiffness of the thoracic spine in early pulmonary tuberculosis.

Lovibond profile s., SYN Lovibond *angle*.

Macewen s., percussion of the skull gives a cracked-pot sound in cases of hydrocephalus. SYN Macewen symptom.

Magendie-Hertwig s., skew deviation of the eyes in acute cerebellar lesions. SYN Magendie-Hertwig syndrome.

Magnan s., paresthesia in the psychosis of cocaine addicts, who imagine they have a foreign body, in the shape of a powder or fine sand, under the skin, and that it is constantly changing its position.

Magnus s., an obsolete s.: after death, constriction of a limb or one of its segments is followed by venous congestion of the distal part.

Mannkopf s., acceleration of the pulse when a painful point is pressed upon.

Marañón s., in Graves disease, a vasomotor reaction following stimulation of the skin over the throat.

Marcus Gunn s., SYN Gunn s.

McBurney s., tenderness at site two-thirds of the distance between the umbilicus and the anterior-superior iliac spine; seen in appendicitis.

meniscus s., SYN crescent s.

Metenier s., easy eversion of the upper eyelid in Ehlers-Danlos syndrome.

Mirchamp s., a premonitory symptom of mumps; if a strongly flavored substance is placed on the tongue, a painful reflex secretion of saliva occurs in the gland that is the seat of the incipient infection.

Möbius s., impairment of ocular convergence in Graves disease.

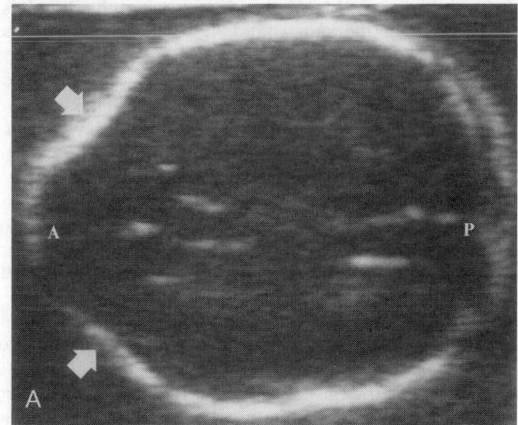

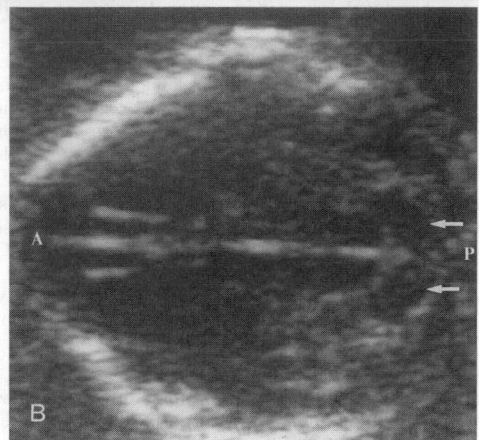

lemon and banana signs: (A) lemon sign, concavity of frontal bones (arrows) causes a "lemon" shape to fetal skull in axial plane images; this appearance suggests a possible spina bifida defect; (B) banana sign, compression of cerebellar hemispheres associated with downward herniation of brainstem and the Chiari II malformation results in a hypoechoic "banana" (arrows) in the posterior aspect of the fetal skull in axial plane (small A indicates anterior, P indicates posterior)

Mosler s., tenderness over the sternum in a patient with acute myeloblastic anemia.

Muehrcke s., SYN Muehrcke *bands*, under *band*.

Müller s., in aortic insufficiency, rhythmical pulsatory movements of the uvula, synchronous with the heart's action; accompanied by swelling and redness of the velum palati and tonsils.

Munson s., in keratoconus, the extra bowing of the lower eyelid caused by the misshapen cornea as the eye rotates downward.

Murphy s., pain on palpation of the right subcostal area during inspiration frequently associated with acute cholecystitis.

Musset s., in incompetence of the aortic valve, rhythmical nodding of the head, synchronous with the heart beat. SYN de Musset s.

neck s., SYN Brudzinski s. (2).

Neer impingement s., pain produced by forceful maximum forward elevation of the upper extremity.

Néri s., in hemiplegia, the knee bends spontaneously when the leg is passively extended.

Nikolsky s., a peculiar vulnerability of the skin in pemphigus vulgaris; the apparently normal epidermis may be separated at the basal layer and rubbed off when pressed with a sliding motion.

objective s., a s. that is evident to the examiner.

s. of the orbicularis, in hemiplegia, inability to voluntarily close the eye on the paralyzed side except in conjunction with closure of the other eye. SYN Revilliod s.

Osler s., SYN Osler *node*.

painful arc s., pain elicited during active abduction of the upper extremity between 60° and 120°.

Pastia s., the presence of pink or red transverse lines at the bend of the elbow in the preeruptive stage of scarlatina; they persist through the eruptive stage and remain as pigmented lines after desquamation. SYN Thomson s.

patellar apprehension s., a physical finding in which forced lateral displacement of the patella produces anxiety and resistance in patients with a history of lateral patellar instability.

Payr s., pain on pressure over the sole of the foot; a s. of thrombophlebitis.

Perez s., rales audible over the upper part of the chest when the arms are alternately raised and lowered; common in cases of fibrous mediastinitis and also of aneurysm of the aortic arch.

Pfuhl s., the pressure of pus within a subphrenic abscess rises during inspiration and falls during expiration, the reverse of what happens in the case of a purulent collection above the diaphragm; when the diaphragm is paralyzed this distinction is lost.

physical s., a s. that is observed or elicited by inspection, palpation, percussion, or auscultation.

Piltz s., SYN eye-closure pupil *reaction*.

Pins s., SYN Ewart s.

Pitres s., (1) SYN haphalgesia; (2) diminished sensation in the testes and scrotum in tabes dorsalis.

placental s., slight endometrial oozing of blood which occurs in certain animals and sometimes in women at the time of implantation of the fertilized ovum; in women, if the blood appears externally it may be mistaken for a scanty menstrual period.

Pool-Schlesinger s., SYN Pool *phenomenon* (1).

Potain s., in dilation of the aorta, dullness on percussion extending from the manubrium sterni toward the second intercostal space and the third costal cartilage on the right, the upper limit extending from the base of the sternum in the segment of a circle to the right.

prodromic s., a s. that appears during the prodrome of a disease. SYN antecedent s.

pseudo-Graefe s., a lid retraction phenomenon similar to Graefe s., but due to aberrant regeneration of fibers of the oculomotor nerve into the levator of the upper lid.

puddle s., a s. of free abdominal fluid: the patient assumes a position on all fours; one flank is percussed by repeated light flicking of constant intensity while a Bowles-type stethoscope is placed over the most dependent portion of the abdomen and gradually moved toward the flank opposite the percussion; a sharp increase in the intensity of the sound picked up by the stethoscope indicates the level of fluid.

pyramid s., any symptoms or signs indicative of damage of the pyramidal tracts, such as the Babinski or Gordon s., spastic spinal paralysis, foot clonus, etc.

Quant s., a T-shaped depression in the occipital bone occurring in many cases of rickets, especially in infants lying constantly in bed with pressure on the occiput.

Quénu-Muret s., in aneurysm, well-maintained collateral circulation indicated by issue of blood when the main artery of the limb is compressed and a puncture is made at the periphery.

Quincke s., SYN Quincke *pulse*.

Ransohoff s., yellow pigmentation in the umbilical region in rupture of the common bile duct.

Raynaud s., SYN acrocyanosis.

red, white, and blue s., the contemporaneous occurrence of erythema, ischemia, and necrosis in a wound, as in loxoscelism.

Remak s., dissociation of the sensations of touch and of pain in tabes dorsalis and polyneuritis.

reversed-three s., on an esophagram of a patient with coarctation of the aorta, the shape of the contrast-filled esophagus caused by the aortic arch (upper convexity) and post-stenotic dilatation (lower convexity); the cusp of the backwards 3 is at the level of the coarctation itself.

Revilliod s., SYN s. of the orbicularis.

si

Ripault s., a s. of death, consisting in a permanent change in the shape of the pupil produced by unilateral pressure on the eyeball.

Romaña s., marked edema of one or both eyelids, usually a unilateral palpebral edema, thought to be a sensitization response to the bite of a triatomine bug infected with *Trypanosoma cruzi*, and a strong suggestion of acute Chagas disease.

Romberg s., with feet approximated, the subject stands with eyes open and then closed; if closing the eyes increases the unsteadiness, a loss of proprioceptive control is indicated, and the sign is positive. SYN Romberg test, rombergism, station test.

Rosenbach s., loss of the abdominal reflex in cases of acute inflammation of the viscera.

Rossolimo s., SYN Rossolimo *reflex.*

Rotch s., in pericardial effusion, percussion dullness in the fifth intercostal space on the right.

Rovsing s., pain at McBurney point induced in cases of appendicitis, by pressure exerted over the descending colon.

Rumpel-Leede s., SYN capillary fragility *test.*

Russell s., abrasions and scars on the back of the hands of individuals with bulimia, usually due to manual attempts at self-induced vomiting.

Sansom s., in mitral stenosis, apparent duplication of the second heart sound.

scarf s., s. used in Dubowitz scoring (q.v.) to assess developmental age and muscle tone in neonates. The infant's arm is pulled laterally across the chest; in the hypotonic infant, the elbow will cross the midline; in a term infant with normal tone, the elbow will not reach the midline.

Schapiro s., in myocardial weakness, no slowing of the pulse occurs when the patient lies down.

Schlesinger s., SYN Pool *phenomenon* (1).

Schultze s., in latent tetany, tapping the tongue causes its depression with a concave dorsum. SYN tongue phenomenon.

scimitar s., a curvilinear structure seen radiographically in the lung and associated with anomalous pulmonary venous drainage, suggesting the sickle shape of a saber; also used to refer to the scalloped shape of the sacrum in spinal dysraphism with anterior meningocele.

Seeligmüller s., contraction of the pupil on the affected side in facial neuralgia.

Seidel s., a sickle-shaped scotoma appearing as an upward or downward extension of the blind spot.

sentinel loop s., in gastrointestinal radiology, dilation of a segment of large or small intestine, indicative of localized ileus from nearby inflammation.

setting sun s., retraction of the upper lid without upgaze so that the iris seems to "set" below the lower lid; suggestive of neurologic damage in the newborn, but usually clears up without sequelae. SEE Collier s., Epstein s.

S s. of Golden, in pulmonary radiology, the combination of an atelectatic lobe and a central obstructing mass produces a concavity and a convexity, like the letter "S."

Shibley s., on auscultation of the chest, the spoken sound "e" is heard as "ah" over an area of pulmonary consolidation or immediately above a pleural effusion.

shoulder apprehension s., a physical finding in which placement of the humerus in the position of abduction to 90° and maximum external rotation produces anxiety and resistance in patients with a history of anterior glenohumeral instability. SYN anterior apprehension test (1).

Siegert s., shortness and inward curvature of the terminal phalanges of the fifth fingers in Down syndrome.

silhouette s. of Felson, in pulmonary radiology, the obliteration of a normal air-soft tissue interface, such as the cardiac silhouette, when fluid fills the adjacent part of the lung.

Skoda s., SYN skodaic *resonance.*

Snellen s., bruit heard on auscultation over the eye in a patient with Graves *disease,* due to the hyperdynamic circulation.

spinal s., in pleurisy, the spinal muscles are in a state of tonic contraction on the affected side.

spine s., resistance to flexion of the spine in cases of meningitis.

Steinberg thumb s., in Marfan syndrome, when the thumb is held across the palm of the same hand, it projects well beyond the ulnar surface of the hand.

Stellwag s., infrequent and incomplete blinking in Graves disease.

Sternberg s., unilateral tenderness or discomfort on palpation of the shoulder girdle muscles in a patient with pleurisy on that side.

Stewart-Holmes s., in cerebellar disease, the inability to check a movement when passive resistance is suddenly released. SYN rebound phenomenon (1).

Stierlin s., repeated emptying of the cecum, seen radiographically, with barium remaining in the terminal part of the ileum and in the transverse colon; due to irritation of the cecum, sometimes caused by tuberculous cecitis (typhlitis).

Straus s., in facial paralysis, if an injection of pilocarpine is followed by sweating on the affected side later than on the other, the lesion is peripheral.

string s., in pediatric gastrointestinal radiology, the narrowed pyloric canal seen with congenital pyloric stenosis; also used to describe a narrowed segment in regional ileitis on small bowel series.

subjective s., a s. that is perceived only by the patient.

Sumner s., a slight increase in tonus of the abdominal muscles, an early indication of inflammation of the appendix, stone in the kidney or ureter, or a twisted pedicle of an ovarian cyst; it is detected by exceedingly gentle palpation of the right or left iliac fossa.

superior triangle s., in chest radiology, widening of the superior mediastinum, usually on the right, associated with collapse of the lower lobe producing traction on the mediastinal pleura. Cf. inferior triangle s.

ten Horn s., pain caused by gentle traction on the right spermatic cord, indicative of appendicitis.

Thomson s., SYN Pastia s.

Tinel s., a sensation of tingling, or of "pins and needles," felt at the lesion site or more distally along the course of a nerve when the latter is percussed; indicates a partial lesion or early regeneration in the nerve. SYN distal tingling on percussion.

Toma s., to distinguish between inflammatory and noninflammatory ascites: in inflammatory conditions of the peritoneum, the mesentery contracts, drawing the intestines over to the right side; consequently, with the patient supine, tympany is elicited on the right side, dullness on the left.

Topolanski s., congestion of the pericorneal region of the eye in Graves disease.

Tournay s., SYN Tournay *phenomenon.*

Traube s., a double sound or murmur heard in auscultation over arteries (particularly the femoral arteries) in significant aortic regurgitation.

Trendelenburg s., a physical examination finding associated with various hip abnormalities (e.g., congenital dislocation, hip abductor weakness, rheumatic arthritis, osteoarthritis) in which the pelvis sags on the side opposite the affected side during single leg stance on the affected side; during gait, compensation occurs by leaning the torso toward the involved side during stance phase on the affected extremity. SYN Trendelenburg gait.

Tresilian s., a reddish prominence at the orifice of Stenson duct, noted in mumps.

trough s., an anteromedial glenoid defect resultant from posterior shoulder dislocation.

Trousseau s., in latent tetany, the occurrence of carpopedal spasm accompanied by paresthesia elicited when the upper arm is compressed, as by a tourniquet or a blood pressure cuff.

Trunecek s., palpable impulse of the subclavian artery near the point of origin of the sternomastoid muscle in cases of aortic sclerosis.

Uhthoff s., SEE Uhthoff *symptom.*

Vierra s., yellowing and canalization of the nail in fogo selvagem.

Vipond s., a generalized adenopathy occurring during the period of incubation of various of the exanthemas of childhood, affording an early diagnostic s. in a case of known exposure.

vital s.'s, determination of temperature, rate of breathing, and level of blood pressure.

von Graefe s., SYN Graefe s.

Weber s., SYN Weber *syndrome.*

Weiss s., SYN Chvostek s.

Wernicke s., SYN Wernicke *reaction.*

Westermark s., in chest radiography, decreased lung markings from oligemia caused by pulmonary embolism.

Wilder s., a slight twitch of the eyeball when changing its movement from abduction to adduction or the reverse, noted in Graves disease.

Winterbottom s., swelling of the posterior cervical lymph nodes, characteristic of early stages of African trypanosomiasis; useful for surveys or control of migrations from endemic areas of persons with preclinical infections.

wrist s., in Marfan syndrome, when the wrist is gripped with the opposite hand, the thumb and fifth finger overlap appreciably.

---

sig·nal (sig′nal). **1.** Something that causes an action. **2.** A DNA template sequence that alters RNA polymerase transcription. **3.** The end product observed when a specific sequence of DNA or RNA is deleted by some method.

arrest s., a DNA sequence that causes arrest of RNA polymerase transcription.

contralateral routing of s.'s, a hearing aid configuration for greater hearing loss in one ear than the other in which sound is picked up by the microphone at the worse hearing ear and delivered to the better hearing ear.

pause s., a DNA sequence that causes pausing of RNA polymerase transcription.

termination s., SYN termination *codon.*

sig·na·ture (sig′nă-choor, -toor). The part of a prescription containing the directions to the patient. [Mediev. L. *signatura,* fr. L. *signum,* a sign, mark]

Signed English. A system of communication that is a semantic representation of English in which American Sign Language signs are used in English word order and additional signs are used for inflection; used principally in the education of children younger than 6 years.

sig·nif·i·cant (sig-nif′i-kant). In statistics, denoting the reliability of a finding or, conversely, the probability of the finding being the result of chance (generally less than 5%). [L. *significo,* to make known, signify, fr. *signum,* sign, + *facio,* to make]

sig·u·a·tera (sēg-wă-tā′ă). SEE ciguatera.

SIH Abbreviation for somatotropin release-inhibiting *hormone.*

Silber, Robert H., U.S. biochemist, *1915. SEE Porter-S. *chromogens,* under *chromogen, reaction,* chromogens *test.*

sil·den·a·fil (sil-den′ă-fil). A selective inhibitor of cGMP-specific phosphodiesterase type 5 (PDE5); relaxes the muscle in the penis, resulting in greater blood flow and erection; used to treat male impotence; potentiates the hypotensive effects of nitrates.

si·lent (sī′lent). Producing no detectable signs or symptoms, said of certain diseases or morbid processes.

sil·i·ca (sil′ĭ-kă). The chief constituent of sand, hence of glass. SYN silicic anhydride, silicon dioxide. [Mod. L. fr. L. *silex* (*silic-*), flint]

s. gel, a precipitated form of silicic acid, used for adsorption of various gases.

sil·i·cate (sil′i-kāt). **1.** A salt of silicic acid. **2.** The term sometimes applied to dental restorations of synthetic porcelain.

sil·i·ca·to·sis (sil′i-kă-tō′sis). SYN silicosis.

si·li·ceous (si-lish′ŭs). Containing silica. SYN silicious.

si·lic·ic (si-lis′ik). Relating to silica or silicon.

si·lic·ic ac·id. Obtained in water as a colloid by treating silicates; precipitated s. a. is silica gel.

si·lic·ic an·hy·dride. SYN silica.

si·li·cious (si-lish′ŭs). SYN siliceous.

sil·i·co·an·thra·co·sis (sil′ĭ-kō-an′thră-kō- sis). A pneumoconio-

sis consisting of a combination of silicosis and anthracosis, seen in hard coal miners.

sil·i·co·flu·o·ride (sil′i-kō-flōr′īd). A compound of silicon and fluorine with another element.

sil·i·con (Si) (sil′i-kon). A very abundant nonmetallic element, atomic no. 14, atomic wt. 28.0855, occurring in nature as silica and silicates; in pure form, used as a semiconductor and in solar batteries; also found in certain polysaccharide structures in mammary tissue. [L. *silex,* flint]

amorphous s., light-sensitive material used in digital *radiography* (q.v.) and fluoroscopy (q.v.).

sil·i·con di·ox·ide. SYN silica.

colloidal s. d., a submicroscopic fumed silica prepared by the vapor-phase hydrolysis of a silicon compound; used as a tablet diluent and as a suspending and thickening agent.

sil·i·cone (sil′i-kōn). A polymer of organic silicon oxides, which may be a liquid, gel, or solid, depending on the extent of polymerization; formerly widely used in surgical implants, in intracorporeal tubes to conduct fluids, as dental impression material, as a grease or sealing substance, as a coating on the inside of glass vessels for blood collection, and in various ophthalmological procedures.

s.-related disease problems, disease allegedly resulting from release of silicone into the body.

sil·i·co·pro·te·i·no·sis (sil′i-kō-prō′tē-i-nō′sis). An acute pulmonary disorder, radiographically and histologically similar to pulmonary alveolar proteinosis, resulting from relatively short exposure to high concentrations of silica dust; pulmonary symptoms are of rapid onset and the condition is invariably fatal.

sil·i·co·sid·er·o·sis (sil′i-kō-sid′er-ō′sis). SYN siderosilicosis.

ⅰ sil·i·co·sis (sil-i-kō′sis). A form of pneumoconiosis resulting from occupational exposure to and inhalation of silica dust over a period of years; characterized by a slowly progressive fibrosis of the lungs, which may result in impairment of lung function; s. predisposes to pulmonary tuberculosis. SYN pneumosilicosis, silicatosis, stone-mason's disease. [L. *silex,* flint, + *-osis,* condition]

sil·i·co·tu·ber·cu·lo·sis (sil′i-kō-too-ber-kū-lō′sis). Silicosis associated with tuberculous pulmonary lesions.

si·li·qua oli·vae (sil′i-kwă ō-lī′vē). The arcuate fibers, which appear to encircle the inferior olive in the medulla oblongata. [L. the husk of the olive]

silk. The fibers or filaments obtained from the cocoon of the silkworm.

floss s., SYN dental *floss.*

surgical s., thread prepared from the cocoon filaments of glutinous gum that are spun by the mulberry silkworm *Bombyx mori;* can be obtained in various sizes and used as suture material.

virgin s., an extremely fine ophthalmic suture material consisting of two to seven natural s. filaments bonded together by sericin, a natural adhesive.

Silver, Henry K., U.S. pediatrician, *1918. SEE S.-Russell *dwarfism, syndrome.*

sil·ver (Ag). L. argentum; a metallic element, atomic no. 47, atomic wt. 107.8682. Many salts have clinical applications. SYN argentum. [A.S. *seolfor*]

s. chloride, used in the preparation of antiseptic silver preparations.

colloidal s. iodide, an antiseptic used for treatment of inflammation of the mucous membranes.

s. fluoride, $AgF_2 \cdot H_2O$; an antiseptic.

fused s. nitrate, SYN toughened s. nitrate.

s. iodate, a reagent for the determination of chloride.

s. lactate, has been used as an astringent and antiseptic.

mild s. protein, a complex prepared by the reaction of s. oxide with either gelatin or serum albumin. Black shiny crystals liberate s. and it was formerly widely used as a topical anti-infective on mucous membranes. Contains 19–25% s., only a small fraction of which is ionizable. Can produce black or brown pigmentation due to deposition of reduced s. in the tissues. SYN argyrol, silvol.

s. nitrate, an antiseptic and astringent; used externally, in solution, in the prevention of ophthalmia neonatorum (currently penicillin is often used); also used in the special staining of the nervous system, spirochetes, reticular fibers, Golgi apparatus, nucleolar organizer region, and calcium.

s. oxide, has been used in epilepsy and chorea; it is explosive when mixed with readily combustible substances.

s. picrate, an ionizable salt of s.; has been used in the treatment of trichomoniasis and moniliasis of the vagina.

strong s. protein, a compound of s. and protein containing not less than 7.5 and not more than 8.5% of s.; used externally as an antiseptic, devoid of astringent and nearly so of irritant properties.

s. sulfadiazine, the s. derivative of sulfadiazine, used externally as a topical antibacterial agent in preventing and treating infections in burns.

toughened s. nitrate, s. nitrate mixed with s. chloride and allowed to dry. Usually applied to the ends of small wooden applicator sticks or made available as pencils. These are used after wetting as a caustic chemical for the removal of warts. SYN fused s. nitrate, lunar caustic.

sil·ver im·preg·na·tion. Silver complexes employed to demonstrate reticulin in normal and diseased tissues, as well as neuroglia, neurofibrillae, argentaffin cells, and Golgi apparatus.

Silverman, Leslie, U.S. engineer, 1914–1966. SEE S.-Lilly *pneumotachograph.*

Silverman, William A., 20th century U.S. pediatrician. SEE Caffey-S. *syndrome.*

Silverskiöld, Nils G., Swedish orthopedist, 1888–1957. SEE S. *syndrome.*

sil·vol (sil'vŏl). SYN mild *silver* protein.

si·meth·i·cone (si-meth'i-kōn). A mixture of dimethyl polysiloxanes and silica gel; an antiflatulent.

si·mi·lia si·mi·li·bus cur·an·tur (si-mil'ē-ă si-mil'i-bŭs ker-an'ter). The homeopathic concept expressing the law of similars (literally, "likes are cured by likes"), the doctrine that any drug capable of producing morbid symptoms in the healthy will remove similar symptoms occurring as an expression of disease. Another reading of the concept, employed by Hahnemann, the founder of homeopathy, is *similia similibus curentur,* "let likes be cured by likes." [L. likes are cured by likes]

si·mil·i·mum, si·mil·li·mum (si-mil'i-mŭm). In homeopathy, the remedy indicated in a certain case because the same drug, when given to a healthy person, will produce the symptom complex most nearly approaching that of the disease in question. [L. *simillimus,* most like, superl. of *similis,* like]

Simmonds, Morris, German physician, 1855–1925. SEE S. *disease.*

Simmons, James S., U.S. bacteriologist, 1890–1954. SEE S. *citrate medium.*

Simon, Gustav, German surgeon, 1824–1876. SEE S. *position.*

Simon, Richard, 20th century U.S. oncologist. SEE Norton-S. *hypothesis.*

Simon, Théodore, French physician, 1873–1961. SEE Binet-S. *scale.*

Simonart, Pierre J.C., Belgian obstetrician, 1816–1846. SEE S. *bands,* under band, *ligaments,* under *ligament.*

Simons, Arthur, German physician, *1877. SEE S. *disease.*

Simonsiella (sī'mon-sē-el'ah). Genus of nonphotosynthetic, nonfruiting, Gram-negative, chemoorganotrophic, gliding bacteria that exist as multicellular filaments with the long axis of individual cells perpendicular to the long axis of the filament. The cells are flattened and curved to yield a convex-concave, crescent shaped symmetry. Isolated from the oral cavity of mammals. Type species is *Simonsiella muelleri.*

sim·ple (sim'pl). **1.** Not complex or compound. **2.** In anatomy, composed of a minimum number of parts. **3.** A medicinal herb. [L. *simplex*]

Sim·plex·vi·rus (sim'pleks-vi'rŭs). SYN *herpes* simplex.

Sim·pli·fied Oral Hy·giene In·dex (OHI-S). An index that measures the current oral hygiene status based upon the amount of debris and calculus occurring on six representative tooth surfaces in the mouth; often used in field surveys of periodontal disease.

Simpson, William, British civil engineer, †1917.

Simpson, Sir James Y., Scottish obstetrician, 1811–1870. SEE S. uterine *sound, forceps.*

Sims, James Marion, U.S. gynecologist, 1813–1883. SEE S. *position,* uterine *sound.*

sim·u·la·tion (sim-ū-lā'shŭn). **1.** Imitation; said of a disease or symptom that resembles another, or of the feigning of illness as in factitious illness or malingering. **2.** In radiation therapy, use of a geometrically similar radiographic system or computer to plan the location of therapy ports. [L. *simulatio,* fr. *simulo,* pp. -*atus,* to imitate, fr. *similis,* like]

computer s., SYN computer *model.*

sim·u·la·tor (sim'ū-lā-ter, tōr). An apparatus designed to produce effects simulating those of specific environmental conditions; used in experimentation and training.

Sim·u·lium (si-mū'lē-ŭm). A genus of biting gnats or midges, the black flies, humpbacked flies, or buffalo gnats in the dipteran family Simuliidae. The aquatic larvae require swift-flowing streams or highly oxygenated waters for their development, a critical epidemiologic factor in the role of these flies as disease vectors. In Central and South America, Mexico, and across central Africa, various species transmit *Onchocerca volvulus,* agent of human onchocerciasis. SYN *Eusimulium.* [L. *simulo,* to simulate]

S. damno'sum, species that is an important vector of onchocerciasis in central Africa.

S. neav'ei, species that is an important vector of onchocerciasis in eastern Africa where its larvae and pupae are attached to the shells of crabs of the genus *Potamonantes.*

S. ochra'ceum, species that is a vector of human onchocerciasis in Central America.

S. ruggle'si, species that is a vector of *Leucocytozoon simondi* in Canada and the northern U.S.

simultagnosia (sī-mul-tag-nō'sē-ă). SYN simultanagnosia.

si·mul·tan·ag·no·sia (sī-mŭl-tan-ag-nō'sē-ă). Inability to recognize multiple elements in a visual presentation, i.e., one object or some elements of a scene can be appreciated but not the display as a whole. SYN simultagnosia. [simultaneous + agnosia]

SIMV Abbreviation for synchronized intermittent mandatory *ventilation.*

sim·va·sta·tin (sim'vă-sta-tin). A potent HMG-CoA reductase (the rate-limiting enzyme for cholesterol biosynthesis) inhibitor. Used for the treatment of hyperlipidemia; similar to lovastatin.

sin·ca·lide (sin'kă-līd). The C-terminal octapeptide of cholecystokinin; it causes smooth muscle contraction of the gallbladder and small intestine, relaxation of the choledoduodenal junction, and stimulates pancreatic and gastric secretions; also used as a diagnostic aid to retrieve bile for analysis.

sin·cip·i·tal (sin-sip'i-tăl). Relating to the sinciput.

sin·ci·put, pl. **sin·cip·i·ta, sin·ci·puts** (sin'si-put, sin-sip'i-tă). ☆official alternate term for forehead. [L. half of the head]

SINES Abbreviation for short interspersed *elements,* under *element.*

sin·ew (sin'oo). SYN tendon. [A.S. *sinu*]

Singer, Mark I., U.S. laryngologist, *1945. SEE Blom-S. *valve.*

sin·gle·ton (sing'gel-tun). **1.** A fetus that develops alone. **2.** SYN sport. [unknown]

sin·gul·ta·tion (sing'gŭl-tā'shŭn). Hiccupping. SEE hiccup. [L. *singulto,* pp. -*atus,* to hiccup]

sin·gul·tous (sing-gŭl'tŭs). Relating to hiccups.

sin·gul·tus (sing-gŭl'tŭs). SYN hiccup. [L.]

sin·i·grase, sin·i·gri·nase (sin'i-grās, -gri-nās). SYN thioglucosidase.

sin·is·ter (si-nis'ter) [TA]. Left. [L.]

sin·is·trad (sin'is-trad, si-nis'trad). Toward the left side. [L. *sinister,* left, + *ad,* to]

sin·is·tral (sin'is-trăl, sĭ-nis'trăl). **1.** Relating to the left side. SYN sinistrous. **2.** Denoting a left-handed person.

sin·is·tral·i·ty (sin-is-tral'i-tē). The condition of being left-handed.

△**sinistro-.** Left, toward the left. [L. *sinister*]

sin·is·tro·car·dia (sin'is-trō-kar'dē-ă). Displacement of the heart beyond the normal position on the left side. [sinistro- + G. *kardia*, heart]

sin·is·tro·ce·re·bral (sin'is-trō-ser'ĕ-brăl). Relating to the left cerebral hemisphere. [sinistro- + L. *cerebrum*, brain]

sin·is·troc·u·lar (sin-is-trok'ū-lăr). Seldom-used term denoting one who prefers the left eye in monocular work, such as in the use of a microscope. Cf. dominant *eye*. [sinistro- + L. *oculus*, eye]

sin·is·tro·gy·ra·tion (sin'is-trō-jī-rā'shŭn). SYN sinistrotorsion. [sinistro- + L. *gyratio*, a turning around (gyration)]

sin·is·tro·man·u·al (sin'is-trō-man'ū-ăl). SYN left-handed. [sinistro- + L. *manus*, hand]

sin·is·trop·e·dal (sin-is-trop'ĕ-dăl). Denoting one who uses the left leg by preference. SYN left-footed. [sinistro- + L. *pes (ped-)*, foot]

sin·is·tro·ro·ta·tion (sin'is-trō-rō-tā'shŭn). SYN sinistrotorsion.

sin·is·trorse (sin'is-trors). Turned or twisted to the left. [L. *sinistrorsus*, on the left side, fr. *sinister*, left, + *verto*, pp. *versus*, to turn]

sin·is·tro·tor·sion (sin'is-trō-tōr'shŭn). A turning or twisting to the left. SYN levocycleduction, levorotation (2), levotorsion (1), sinistrogyration, sinistrorotation. [sinistro- + L. *torsio*, a twisting (torsion)]

sin·is·trous (sin'is-trŭs, si-nis'trŭs). SYN sinistral (1).

si·no·a·tri·al (sī'nō-ā'trē-ăl). SYN sinuatrial.

si·nog·ra·phy (sī-nog'ră-fē). Radiologic use of a contrast medium to opacify a sinus tract. [sinus + G. *graphō*, to write]

si·no·pul·mo·nary (sī'nō-pŭl'mŏ-nār-ē). Relating to the paranasal sinuses and the pulmonary airway.

si·no·vag·i·nal (sī-nō-vaj'i-năl). Relating to that part of the vagina derived from the urogenital sinus.

sin·ter (sin'ter). To heat a powdered substance without thoroughly melting it, causing it to fuse into a solid but porous mass. [Ger. dross, slag]

si·nu·a·tri·al (S-A) (sin'ū-ā'trē-ăl, sī'noo-). Relating to the sinus venosus and the right atrium of the heart. SYN sinoatrial.

SINUS

si·nus, pl. **si·nus**, **si·nus·es** (sī'nŭs, -ĕz). **1** [TA]. A channel for the passage of blood or lymph, without the coats of an ordinary vessel; e.g., blood passages in the gravid uterus or those in the cerebral meninges. **2** [TA]. A cavity or hollow space in bone or other tissue. **3** [TA]. A dilation in a blood vessel. **4.** A fistula or tract leading to a suppurating cavity. [L. *sinus*, cavity, channel, hollow]

s. a′lae par′vae, SYN sphenoparietal s.

anal sinuses [TA], **(1)** the grooves between the anal columns; SYN Morgagni s. (1). **(2)** pockets or crypts in the columnar zone of the anal canal between the anocutaneous line and the anorectal line; the sinuses give the mucosa a scalloped appearance. SYN s. anales [TA], anal crypts, Morgagni crypts, rectal sinuses.

s. ana′les [TA], SYN anal sinuses.

anterior sinuses, SYN anterior ethmoidal *cells*, under *cell*.

s. aor′tae [TA], SYN aortic s.

aortic s. [TA], the space between the superior aspect of each cusp of the aortic valve and the dilated portion of the wall of the ascending aorta, immediately above each cusp. SYN s. aortae [TA], Petit s., Valsalva s.

Arlt s., an inconstant depression on the lower portion of the internal surface of the lacrimal sac.

barber pilonidal s., pilonidal s. occurring in barbers, usually in the web between the fingers, due to the burying of exogenous hairs by the alternate loosening and tightening of tissues of the hand by the manipulation of scissors.

basilar s., SYN basilar venous *plexus*.

Breschet s., SYN sphenoparietal s.

s. carot′icus [TA], SYN carotid s.

carotid s. [TA], a slight dilation of the common carotid artery at its bifurcation into external and internal carotids; it contains baroreceptors that, when stimulated, cause slowing of the heart, vasodilation, and a fall in blood pressure and is innervated primarily by the glossopharyngeal nerve. SYN s. caroticus [TA], carotid bulb.

s. caverno′sus [TA], SYN cavernous s.

cavernous s. [TA], a paired dural venous s. on either side of the sella turcica, the two being connected by anastomoses, the anterior intercavernosus s. (sinus intercavernosus anterior [TA]) and posterior intercavernosus sinus [TA] (sinus intercavernosus posterior [TA]), in front of and behind the hypophysis, respectively, making thus the circular s.; the cavernous s. is unique among dural venous sinuses in being trabeculated; coursing within the s. are the internal carotid artery and the abducent nerve. SYN s. cavernosus [TA].

cerebral sinuses, SYN dural venous sinuses.

cervical s., in young mammalian embryos a depression in the nuchal region caudal to the hyoid arch, with the third and fourth branchial arches and ectodermal grooves in its floor; normally it is obliterated after the second month, but occasionally cervical fistulae persist as vestiges of it. SYN precervical s.

circular s., (1) dural venous formation that surrounds the hypophysis, composed of right and left cavernous sinuses and the intercavernous sinuses; SYN circulus venosus ridleyi, Ridley circle. **(2)** a venous s. at the periphery of the placenta; **(3)** SYN scleral venous s.

s. circula′ris, SYN scleral venous s.

coccygeal s., a fistula opening in the region of the coccyx. SEE ALSO pilonidal s.

s. corona′rius [TA], SYN coronary s.

coronary s. [TA], a short trunk receiving most of the cardiac veins, beginning at the junction of the great cardiac vein and the oblique vein of the left atrium, running in the posterior part of the coronary sulcus and emptying into the right atrium between the inferior vena cava and the atrioventricular orifice. SYN s. coronarius [TA].

costomediastinal s., SYN costomediastinal *recess*.

cranial sinuses, SYN dural venous sinuses.

dermal s., a s. lined with epidermis and skin appendages extending from the skin to some deeper-lying structure, most frequently the spinal cord.

s. du′rae ma′tris [TA], SYN dural venous sinuses.

dural venous sinuses [TA], endothelium-lined venous channels in the dura mater. SYN s. durae matris [TA], cerebral sinuses, cranial sinuses, sinuses of dura mater, venous sinuses.

sinuses of dura mater, SYN dural venous sinuses.

Englisch s., SYN inferior petrosal s.

s. epididym′idis [TA], SYN s. of epididymis.

s. of epididymis [TA], a narrow space between the body of the epididymis and the testis. SYN s. epididymidis [TA].

ethmoidal sinuses, SYN ethmoid *cells*, under *cell*.

s. ethmoida′les, SYN ethmoid *cells*, under *cell*.

s. ethmoidales anterio′res, SYN anterior ethmoidal *cells*, under *cell*.

s. ethmoidales me′diae, SYN middle ethmoidal *cells*, under *cell*.

s. ethmoidales posterio′res, SYN posterior ethmoidal *cells*, under *cell*.

frontal s. [TA], a hollow paranasal sinus formed on either side in the lower part of the squama of the frontal bone; it communicates by the ethmoidal infundibulum with the middle meatus of the nasal cavity of the same side. SYN s. frontalis [TA].

s. fronta′lis [TA], SYN frontal s.

Guérin s., a cul-de-sac or diverticulum behind the valve of the navicular fossa.

Huguier s., SYN *fossa* of oval window.

inferior longitudinal s., SYN inferior sagittal s.

inferior petrosal s. [TA], a paired dural venous s. running in the

si

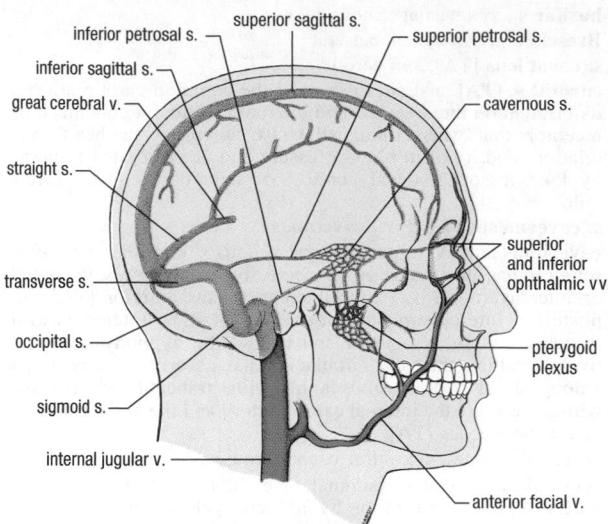

the cranial venous sinuses

groove on the petrooccipital fissure connecting the cavernous s. with the superior bulb of the internal jugular vein. SYN s. petrosus inferior [TA], Englisch s.

inferior sagittal s. [TA], an unpaired dural venous s. in the lower margin of the falx cerebri, running parallel to the superior sagittal s. and merging with the great cerebral vein to form the straight s. SYN s. sagittalis inferior [TA], inferior longitudinal s.

s. intercaverno'si anterior et posterior [TA], SYN intercavernous sinuses.

intercavernous sinuses, the anterior and posterior anastomoses between the cavernous sinuses, passing anterior and posterior to the hypophysis and forming, with the cavernous sinuses, the circular sinus. SEE ALSO cavernous s. SYN s. intercavernosi anterior et posterior [TA], Ridley s.

jugular s., s. jugula'ris, one of three enlargements of the jugular veins; the external jugular s. is between the two sets of valves; the internal jugular sinuses are at the origin (superior bulb) and near the termination (inferior bulb).

s. lactif'eri [TA], SYN lactiferous s.

lactiferous s. [TA], a circumscribed spindle-shaped dilation of the lactiferous duct just before it enters the nipple. In nursing mothers, this dilation stores a droplet of milk that is expressed by compression as the infant begins to suckle; this is thought to encourage continual suckling while the let-down reflex ensues. SYN s. lactiferi [TA], ampulla lactifera, ampulla of lactiferous duct, ampulla of milk duct, lactiferous ampulla.

laryngeal s., SYN laryngeal *ventricle.*

s. laryn'geus, SYN laryngeal *ventricle.*

lateral s., SYN transverse s.

s. lie'nis, SYN splenic s.

longitudinal s., SEE inferior sagittal s., superior sagittal s.

longitudinal vertebral venous s., large, plexiform veins forming portions of the anterior internal vertebral venous plexus lying on the posterior surfaces of the vertebral bodies on either side of the posterior longitudinal ligament. SYN s. vertebrales longitudinales.

Luschka s., venous s. in the petrosquamous suture.

lymph s., SYN lymphatic s.

lymphatic s., the channels in a lymph node crossed by a reticulum of cells and fibers and bounded by littoral cells; there are subcapsular, trabecular, and medullary sinuses. SYN lymph s.

Maier s., an infundibuliform depression on the internal surface of the lacrimal sac which receives the lacrimal canaliculi.

marginal sinuses of placenta, discontinuous venous lakes at the margin of the placenta.

mastoid sinuses, SYN mastoid *cells,* under *cell.*

s. maxilla'ris [TA], SYN maxillary s.

maxillary s. [TA], the largest of the paranasal sinuses occupying the body of the maxilla, communicating with the middle meatus of the nose. SYN s. maxillaris [TA], antrum of Highmore, genyantrum, maxillary antrum.

Meyer s., a small concavity in the floor of the external auditory canal near the membrana tympani.

middle ethmoidal sinuses, SYN middle ethmoidal *cells,* under *cell.*

Morgagni s., (1) SYN anal sinuses (1); **(2)** SYN prostatic *utricle*; **(3)** SYN laryngeal *ventricle.*

s. of nail, SYN s. unguis.

oblique pericardial s. [TA], the recess in the pericardial cavity posterior to the base of the heart bounded laterally by the pericardial reflections on the pulmonary veins and inferior vena cava, and posteriorly by the pericardium overlying the anterior aspect of the esophagus. SYN s. obliquus pericardii [TA], oblique s. of pericardium.

oblique s. of pericardium, SYN oblique pericardial s.

s. obli'quus pericar'dii [TA], SYN oblique pericardial s.

occipital s. [TA], an unpaired dural venous s. commencing at the confluence of the sinuses and passing downward in the base of the falx cerebelli to the foramen magnum. SYN s. occipitalis [TA].

s. occipita'lis [TA], SYN occipital s.

Palfyn s., a space within the crista galli of the ethmoid described as communicating with the ethmoidal and frontal sinuses.

paranasal sinuses [TA], the paired air-filled cavities in the bones of the face lined by mucous membrane continuous with that of the nasal cavity; these sinuses are the frontal, sphenoidal, maxillary, and ethmoidal. SYN s. paranasales [TA].

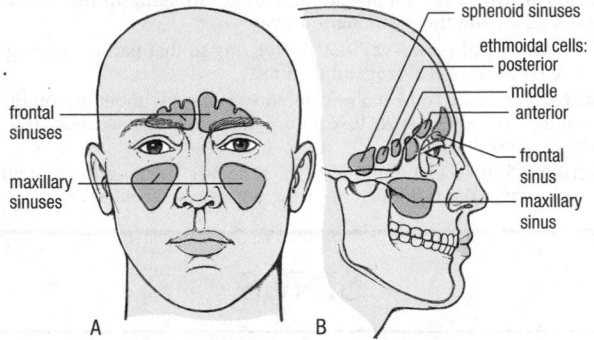

paranasal sinuses: (A) anterior and (B) lateral views of head

s. paranasa'les [TA], SYN paranasal sinuses.

parasinoidal sinuses, SYN lateral *lacunae* of superior sagittal sinus, under *lacuna.*

Petit s., SYN aortic s.

petrosal s., SEE inferior petrosal s., superior petrosal s.

s. petro'sus infe'rior [TA], SYN inferior petrosal s.

s. petro'sus supe'rior [TA], SYN superior petrosal s.

phrenicocostal s., SYN costodiaphragmatic *recess.*

pilonidal s., a fistula or pit in the sacral region, communicating with the exterior, containing hair which may act as a foreign body producing chronic inflammation. SYN pilonidal fistula.

piriform s., SYN piriform *fossa.*

pleural sinuses, SYN pleural *recesses,* under *recess.*

s. pocula'ris, SYN prostatic *utricle.*

s. poste'rior cavi tympani [TA], SYN posterior s. of tympanic cavity.

posterior s. of tympanic cavity [TA], a deep groove above the pyramidal eminence extending to the incudal fossa in the posterior wall of the tympanic cavity. SYN s. posterior cavi tympani [TA].

preauricular s., s. tract or pit in preauricular skin, resulting from developmental defect of the first and second branchial arches. SYN preauricular pit.

precervical s., SYN cervical s.

prostatic s. [TA], the groove on either side of the urethral crest in the prostatic part of the urethra into which the prostatic ducts open. SYN s. prostaticus [TA].

s. prostat′icus [TA], SYN prostatic s.

pulmonary sinuses, SYN s. of pulmonary trunk.

s. of pulmonary trunk [TA], the space at the origin of the pulmonary trunk between the dilated wall of the vessel and each cusp of the pulmonic valve. SYN s. trunci pulmonalis [TA], pulmonary sinuses.

rectal sinuses, SYN anal sinuses.

s. rec′tus [TA], SYN straight s.

renal s. [TA], the cavity of the kidney, containing the calices and pelvis of the ureter and the segmental vesels embedded within a fatty matrix. The renal sinuses cause the kidneys to appear hollow or C-shaped on cross section or medical imaging. SYN s. renalis [TA].

s. rena′lis [TA], SYN renal s.

s. reu′niens, obsolete term for s. venosus.

rhomboidal s., s. rhomboidalis, a dilation of the central canal of the spinal cord in the lumbar region. SYN rhombocele.

Ridley s., SYN intercavernous sinuses.

Rokitansky-Aschoff sinuses, small outpocketings of the mucosa of the gallbladder which extend through the muscular layer; they may be congenital.

s. sagitta′lis infe′rior [TA], SYN inferior sagittal s.

s. sagitta′lis supe′rior [TA], SYN superior sagittal s.

scleral venous s. [TA], the vascular structure encircling the anterior chamber of the eye and through which the aqueous is returned to the blood circulation. SYN s. venosus sclerae [TA], circular s. (3), Fontana canal, Lauth canal, Schlemm canal, s. circularis, venous s. of sclera.

sigmoid s. [TA], the S-shaped dural venous s. lying deep to the mastoid process of the temporal bone and immediately posterior to the petrous temporal bone; it is continuous with the transverse s. and empties into the internal jugular vein as it passes through the jugular foramen. SYN s. sigmoideus [TA].

s. sigmoi′deus [TA], SYN sigmoid s.

sphenoidal s. [TA], one of a pair of paranasal sinuses in the body of the sphenoid bone communicating with the upper posterior nasal cavity or sphenoethmoidal recess. SYN s. sphenoidalis [TA].

s. sphenoida′lis [TA], SYN sphenoidal s.

sphenoparietal s. [TA], a paired dural venous s. beginning on the parietal bone, running along the sphenoidal ridges and emptying into the cavernous s. SYN s. sphenoparietalis [TA], Breschet s., s. alae parvae.

s. sphenoparieta′lis [TA], SYN sphenoparietal s.

splenic s., an elongated venous channel, 12–40 μm wide, lined by rod-shaped cells. SYN s. lienis.

straight s. [TA], an unpaired dural venous s. in the posterior part of the falx cerebri where it is attached to the tentorium cerebelli; it is formed anteriorly by the merging of the great cerebral vein with the inferior sagittal sinus, and passes horizontally and posteriorly to the confluence of sinuses. SYN s. rectus [TA], tentorial s.

superior longitudinal s., SYN superior sagittal s.

superior petrosal s. [TA], a paired dural venous s. in the groove along the crest of the petrous temporal bone, connecting the cavernous s. with the termination of the transverse s. or beginning of the sigmoid sinus. SYN s. petrosus superior [TA].

superior sagittal s. [TA], an unpaired dural venous s. in the sagittal groove, beginning at the foramen caecum and terminating at the confluence of sinuses where it merges with the straight sinus; receives the superior cerebral veins and has lateral extensions, the lateral venous lacunae. SYN s. sagittalis superior [TA], superior longitudinal s.

tarsal s. [TA], a hollow or canal formed by the groove of the talus and the interosseous groove of the calcaneus that is occupied by the interosseous talocalcaneal ligament. SYN s. tarsi [TA], tarsal canal.

s. tar′si [TA], SYN tarsal s.

tentorial s., SYN straight s.

terminal s., s. termina′lis, the vein bounding the area vasculosa in the blastoderm.

s. tonsilla′ris, SYN tonsillar *fossa*.

Tourtual s., SYN supratonsillar *fossa*.

transverse s. [TA], a paired dural venous s. that drains the confluence of sinuses, running along the occipital attachment of the tentorium cerebelli and terminating in the sigmoid s. SYN s. transversus [TA], lateral s.

transverse pericardial s. [TA], a passage in the pericardial sac between the origins of the great vessels, i.e., posterior to the intrapericardial portions of the pulmonary trunk and ascending aorta and anterior to the superior vena cava and superior to the atria; it is formed as a result of the flexure of the heart tube, partially approximating the great venous and arterial vessels. SYN s. transversus pericardii [TA], Theile canal, transverse s. of pericardium.

transverse s. of pericardium, SYN transverse pericardial s.

s. transver′sus [TA], SYN transverse s.

s. transver′sus pericar′dii [TA], SYN transverse pericardial s.

s. trun′ci pulmona′lis [TA], SYN s. of pulmonary trunk.

s. tym′pani [TA], SYN tympanic s.

tympanic s. [TA], a depression in the tympanic cavity posterior to the tympanic promontory. SYN s. tympani [TA].

s. un′guis, the deep cleft housing the root of the nail. SYN s. of nail.

urogenital s., (1) the ventral part of the cloaca after its separation from the rectum by the growth of the urorectal septum; from it develops the lower part of the bladder in both sexes, the prostatic portion of the male urethra, and the urethra and vestibule in the female; (2) SYN persistent *cloaca*.

s. urogenita′lis, SYN persistent *cloaca*.

uterine s., a small irregular vascular channel in the endometrium, of a type that forms during pregnancy. SYN uterine sinusoid.

uteroplacental sinuses, irregular vascular spaces in the zone of the chorionic attachment to the decidua basalis.

Valsalva s., SYN aortic s.

s. of the vena cava [TA], the portion of the cavity of the right atrium of the heart that receives the blood from the venae cavae; it is separated from the rest of the atrium by the crista terminalis. SYN s. venarum cavarum [TA].

s. vena′rum cava′rum [TA], SYN s. of the vena cava.

s. veno′sus [TA], a cavity at the caudal end of the embryonic cardiac tube in which the veins from the intra- and extraembryonic circulatory arcs unite; in the course of development it forms the portion of the right atrium known in adult anatomy as the sinus of the vena cava. SYN saccus reuniens.

s. veno′sus scle′rae [TA], SYN scleral venous s.

venous sinuses, SYN dural venous sinuses.

venous s. of sclera, SYN scleral venous s.

s. vertebra′les longitudina′les, SYN longitudinal vertebral venous s.

---

si·nus·i·tis (sī-nŭ-sī′tis). Inflammation of the mucous membrane of any sinus, especially of one of the paranasal sinuses. [sinus + G. -itis, inflammation]

si·nus·oid (si′nŭ-soyd). **1.** Resembling a sinus. **2.** Sinusoidal capillary; a thin-walled terminal blood vessel having an irregular and larger caliber than an ordinary capillary; its endothelial cells have large gaps and the basal lamina is either discontinuous or absent. SYN sinusoidal capillary. [sinus + G. *eidos,* resemblance]

uterine s., SYN uterine *sinus*.

si·nus·oi·dal (sī-nŭ-soy′dăl). Relating to a sinusoid.

si·nus·ot·o·my (sin-ŭ-sot′ŏ-mē). Incision into a sinus. [sinus + G. *tomē,* incision]

si op. sit Abbreviation for L. *si opus sit,* if needed.

si·phon (sī′fŏn). A tube bent into two unequal lengths, used to remove fluid from a cavity or vessel by atmospheric pressure. [G. *siphōn,* tube]

si·phon·age (sī′fŏn-ij). Emptying of the stomach or other cavity by means of a siphon.

si

Si·pho·na ir·ri·tans (sī-fō'nă ir'i-tanz). The horn fly, a blood-sucking muscoid fly that causes great irritation and annoyance to cattle, and transmits *Stephanofilaria stilesi*. [G. *siphōn*, tube]

Si·pho·nap·tera (sī-fō-nap'tĕ-ră). The fleas, an order of wingless insect ectoparasites highly adapted for survival in mammalian fur; they are flattened laterally, spined, and equipped with well-developed metathoracic legs for jumping. [G. *siphōn*, tube, + G. *a*-priv. + *pteron*, wing]

Sipho·vir·i·dae (sif'ō-vī'ră-dā). A family of bacterial viruses with long, noncontractile tails and isometric or elongated heads, containing double-stranded DNA (MW $25–79 \times 10^6$); includes the λ temperate phage group and probably other genera. [L. *sipho*, little tube, pipe, fr. G. *siphōn*, + virus]

Sipple, John H., U.S. physician, *1930. SEE S. *syndrome*.

Sippy, Bertram W., U.S. physician, 1866–1924. SEE S. *diet*.

si·ren·i·form (sī-ren'i-fōrm). Denoting a malformation with the appearance of sirenomelia.

si·re·no·me·lia (sī'rĕ-nō-mē'lē-ă). Union of the legs with partial or complete union of the feet. SEE ALSO sympus. SYN mermaid malformation, symmelia. [L. *siren*, G. *seirēn*, a siren]

si·ri·a·sis (si-rī'ă-sis). SYN sunstroke. [G. *seiriasis*, from *seiriaō*, to be hot]

Siris, Evelyn, U.S. radiologist, *1914. SEE Coffin-S. *syndrome*.

sir·up (sir'ŭp). SYN syrup.

sis·mo·ther·a·py (sis-mō-thār'ă-pē). SYN vibratory *massage*. [G. *seismos*, a shaking, fr. *seiō*, fut. *seisō*, to shake]

sis·o·mi·cin sul·fate (sis-ō-mī'sin). An antibiotic produced by *Micromonospora inyoensis* that has a spectrum of activity and application similar to that of gentamicin.

sis·ter. In Great Britain and its Commonwealth countries: **1.** The title of a head nurse in a public hospital or in a ward or the operating room of a hospital. **2.** Any registered nurse in private practice.

Sistrunk, Walter Ellis, U.S. surgeon, 1880–1933. SEE S. *operation*.

site (sīt). A place or location or locus. SYN situs. [L. *situs*]

acceptor s., the ribosomal binding s. for the aminoacyl-tRNA during protein synthesis.

acceptor splicing s., SYN right splicing *junction*.

active s., that portion of an enzyme molecule at which the actual reaction proceeds; considered to consist of one or more residues or atoms in a spatial arrangement that permits interaction with the substrate to effect the reaction of the latter.

allosteric s., postulated as the place on an enzyme, other than the active s., where a compound, which may be the ultimate product of the biosynthetic pathway involving the enzyme, may bind and influence the activity of the enzyme by changing the enzyme's conformation; the influence of CTP on aspartate carbamoyltransferase activity exemplifies the concept of an allosteric site on an allosteric protein.

antibody-combining s., SYN paratope.

antigen-binding s., SYN paratope.

cleavage s., SYN restriction s.

fragile s. [MIM*136540, MIM*136670], a nonstaining gap at a specific point on a chromosome, usually involving both chromatids, always at the same point on chromosomes of different cells from an individual or kindred; it results in in vitro production of acentric fragments, deleted chromosomes, or other chromosome anomalies; inherited as a dominant chromosome marker.

immunologically privileged s.'s, s.'s where allografts are not readily rejected or tumors escape immune surveillance probably because these particular areas have poor lymphatic drainage and are not readily accessible to effector cells of the immune system.

ligand-binding s., the s. on a protein's surface that binds a ligand; equivalent to the active s. if the ligand is the substrate of an enzyme.

privileged s., an anatomic area lacking lymphatic drainage, such as the brain, cornea, and hamster cheek pouch, in which heterologous tumors may grow because the host does not become sensitized.

▪ receptor s., point of attachment for viruses, hormones, or other activators to cell membranes.

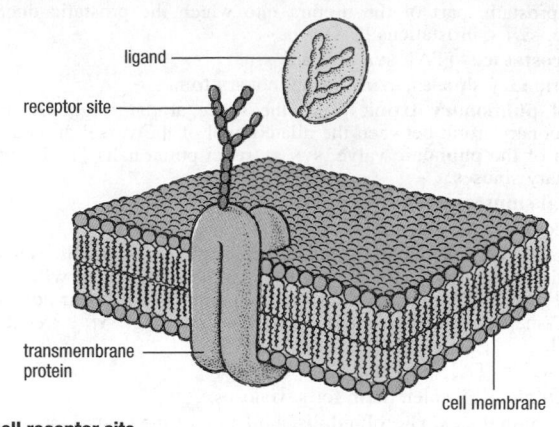

cell receptor site

replication s., the in vivo s. on DNA of DNA replication.

restriction s., a s. in nucleic acid in which the bordering bases are of such a type as to leave them vulnerable to the cleaving action of an endonuclease. SYN cleavage s.

sequence-tagged s.'s (STSs), short stretches of DNA sequences that can be detected by use of the polymerase chain reaction.

switching s., the break point in a DNA sequence at which a gene segment unites with another gene segment, as in the production of the immunoglobulins.

△**sito-.** Food, grain. [G. *sitos, sition*]

si·to·stane (sī'tō-stān). SYN stigmastane.

β-**si·tos·ter·ol** (sī-tō-stēr'ol). A phytosterol and anticholesteremic. SYN cinchol.

sitosterolemia (sī-tō-stēr-ō-lē-mē-ă). SYN phytosterolemia.

si·to·tax·is (sī-tō-tak'sis). SYN sitotropism. [sito- + G. *taxis*, orderly arrangement]

si·to·tox·in (sī-tō-tok'sin). Any food poison, especially one developing in grain. [sito- + G. *toxikon*, poison]

si·to·tox·ism (sī-tō-tok'sizm). **1.** Poisoning by spoiled or fungous grain. **2.** Food poisoning in general. [sito- + G. *toxikon*, poison]

si·tot·ro·pism (sī-tot'rō-pizm). Turning of living cells to or away from food. SYN sitotaxis. [sito- + G. *tropē*, a turning]

sit·u·a·tion (sich-ū-ā'shŭn). The aggregate of biological, psychological, and sociological factors that affect an individual's behavioral pattern.

psychoanalytic s., the relationship, characteristically restricted to the therapist's office, between patient and therapist.

si·tus (sī'tŭs). SYN site. [L.]

s. inver'sus, reversal of position or location. SYN s. transversus.

s. inversus viscerum, a transposition of the viscera, e.g., the liver developing on the left side or the heart on the right. SYN visceral inversion.

s. perver'sus, malposition of any viscus.

s. sol'itus, the normal visceral arrangement.

s. transver'sus, SYN s. inversus.

Siwe, Sture A., Swedish pediatrician, 1897–1966. SEE Letterer-S. *disease*.

siz·er (sī'zer). A cylinder of variable diameter, with rounded ends, used to measure the internal diameter of the bowel in preparation for stapling.

Sjögren, Henrik C., Swedish ophthalmologist, 1899–1986. SEE S. *disease, syndrome;* Gougerot-S. *disease*.

Sjögren, Torsten, Swedish physician, 1859–1939. SEE S.-Larsson *syndrome;* Torsten S. *syndrome;* Marinesco-Sjögren *syndrome*.

Sjöqvist, O., Swedish neurosurgeon, 1901–1954. SEE S. *tractotomy*.

SK Abbreviation for streptokinase.

△**skato-.** Obsolete spelling of scato-.

skat·ole (skat′ōl). 3-Methyl-1*H*-indole, formed in the intestine by the bacterial decomposition of ʟ-tryptophan and found in fecal matter, to which it imparts its characteristic odor.

skat·ox·yl (skă-tok′sil). 3-Hydroxymethylindole, formed in the intestine by the oxidation of skatole; some undergoes conjugation in the body with sulfuric or gluronic acids and is excreted in the urine in conjugated form.

skein (skān). The coiled threads of chromatin seen in the prophase of mitosis. [Gael. *sgeinnidh,* hempen thread]

    choroid s., SYN choroid *enlargement.*

skel·e·tal (skel′ĕ-tăl). Relating to the skeleton.

skel·e·tol·o·gy (skel-ĕ-tol′ō-jē). The branch of anatomy and of mechanics dealing with the skeleton.

skel·e·ton (skel′ĕ-tŏn). **1.** The bony framework of the body in vertebrates (endoskeleton) or the hard outer envelope of insects (exoskeleton or dermoskeleton). **2.** All the dry parts remaining after the destruction and removal of the soft parts; this includes ligaments and cartilages as well as bones. **3.** All the bones of the body taken collectively. **4.** A rigid or semirigid nonosseous structure which functions as the supporting framework of a particular structure. [G. *skeletos,* dried, ntr. *skeleton,* a mummy, a skeleton]

    appendicular s. [TA], the bones of the limbs including the shoulder and pelvic girdles. SYN s. appendiculare [TA].

    s. appendicula′re [TA], SYN appendicular s.

    articulated s., mounted s., one with the various parts connected in such a way as to demonstrate normal relationships and allow motion between components as in the living body.

    axial s. [TA], articulated bones of head and vertebral column, i.e., head and trunk, as opposed to the appendicular skeleton, the articulated bones of the upper and lower limbs. SYN s. axiale [TA].

    s. axia′le [TA], SYN axial s.

    cardiac s., SYN fibrous s. of heart.

    cardiac fibrous s., SYN fibrous s. of heart.

    s. of eyelid, SYN tarsus (2).

    facial s., ✩official alternate term for viscerocranium.

    fibrous s. of heart, a complex framework of dense collagen forming four fibrous rings (annuli fibrosi), which surround the ostia of the valves, a right and left fibrous trigone, formed by connecting the rings, and the membranous portions of the interatrial and interventricular septa; it is found in association with the base of the ventricles, i.e., at the level of the coronary sulcus; its functions include: 1) contributing reinforcement of the valvular ostia while providing attachment for the leaflets and cusps of the valves; 2) providing origin and insertion for the myocardium; and 3) serving as a sort of electrical "insulator," separating the electrically conducted impulses of the atria and ventricles and providing passage for the common atrioventricular bundle of conductive tissue through the right fibrous trigone and membranous interventricular septum. SYN cardiac fibrous s., cardiac s., s. of heart.

    s. of free inferior limb, the bones of the lower limb except the hip bones, i.e., all lower limb bones including and distal to the femur.

    s. of free superior limb, the bones of the upper limb except the scapula and clavicle, i.e., all upper limb bones including and distal to the humerus.

    gill arch s., cartilages associated with the visceral portion of the embryonic mammalian chondrocranium, representing the gill arch (branchial) skeletons as seen in shark-type fishes; they are the primordia of Meckel cartilage, the styloid, hyoid, cricoid, thyroid, and arytenoid cartilages, and the auditory ossicles. SEE ALSO branchial *arches,* under *arch.*

    s. of heart, SYN fibrous s. of heart.

    jaw s., SYN viscerocranium.

    thoracic s. [TA], the bones and cartilage that comprise the thoracic cage. SYN s. thoracis [TA], s. thoracicus.

    s. thoracicus, SYN thoracic s.

    s. thoracis [TA], SYN thoracic s.

    visceral s., SYN visceroskeleton (2).

Skene, Alexander J.C., U.S. gynecologist, 1837–1900. SEE S.

glands, under *gland, tubules,* under *tubule; ducts* of S. glands, under *duct.*

ske·nei·tis, ske·ni·tis (skē-nī′tis). Inflammation of Skene glands.

skene·o·scope (skēn′ō-skōp). A form of endoscope for inspecting Skene glands.

skew (skū). In statistics, departure from symmetry of a frequency distribution.

△**skia-.** Shadow; superseded by radio-. [G. *skia*]

ski·as·co·py (skī-as′kŏ-pē). SYN retinoscopy.

Skillern, Penn Gaskell Jr., U.S. surgeon, *1882. SEE S. *fracture.*

⬛**skin** [TA]. The membranous protective covering of the body, consisting of the epidermis and corium (dermis). SYN cutis [TA]. [A.S. *scinn*]

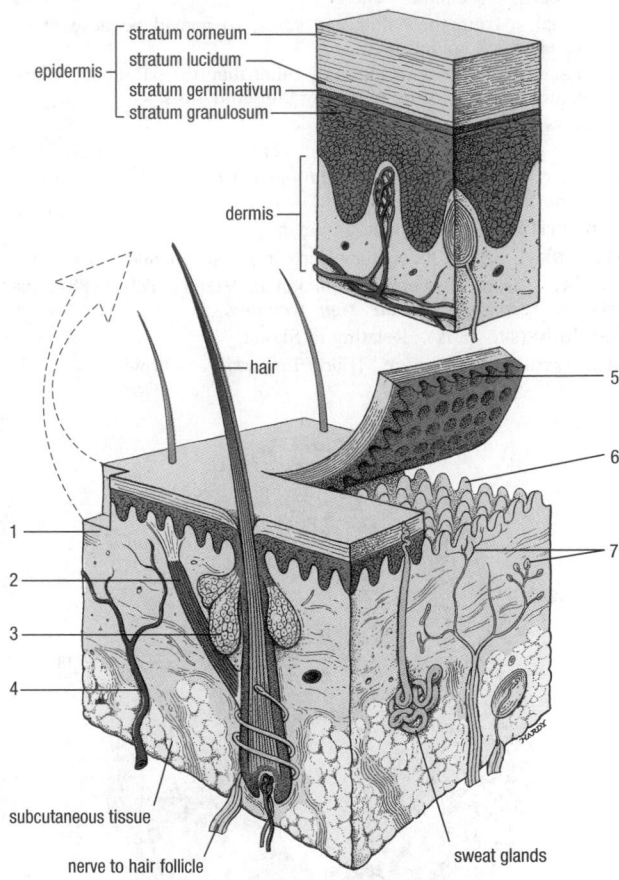

skin components and layers: (1) dermis, (2) arrector muscle of hair, (3) sebaceous gland, (4) blood vessel, (5) epidermis lifted to reveal papillae of the dermis, (6) papillae, (7) nerve endings

alligator s., SYN ichthyosis.

bronzed s., the dark s. in Addison disease.

deciduous s., SYN keratolysis (2).

elastic s., SEE Ehlers-Danlos *syndrome.*

farmer's s., dry, wrinkled s. with presence of dry premalignant keratoses; observed most commonly in fair-skinned, blue-eyed persons who are exposed by occupation or sport to sunshine for prolonged periods and over many years. SYN golfer's s., sailor's s.

fish s., SYN ichthyosis.

glabrous s., s. that is normally devoid of hair.

glossy s., shiny atrophy of the s., usually of the hands, following nerve injury; a type of neurotrophic atrophy. SYN atrophoderma neuriticum.

golfer's s., SYN farmer's s.

hidden nail s., SYN eponychium (2).

loose s., SYN dermatochalasis.

parchment s., parchmentlike appearance of the s. caused by loss of underlying connective and elastic tissue, or by the relatively rapid and persistent loss of water from the horny layer.

piebald s., SYN piebaldism.

pig s., soft s. in which follicles are widely dilated; seen in pretibial myxedema.

porcupine s., SYN epidermolytic *hyperkeratosis.*

sailor's s., SYN farmer's s.

shagreen s., an oval-shaped, elevated nevoid plaque, skin-colored or occasionally pigmented, smooth or crinkled, appearing on the trunk or lower back in early childhood; sometimes seen with other signs of tuberous sclerosis. SYN shagreen patch.

s. of teeth, SYN enamel *cuticle.*

thick s., s. from the palms and soles, so named because of its relatively thick epidermis.

thin s., s. from areas of the body other than the palms and soles, so named because of its relatively thin epidermis.

toad s., SYN phrynoderma.

yellow s., (1) SYN xanthochromia; **(2)** SYN xanthoderma (2).

Skinner, Burrhus F., U.S. psychologist, 1904–1990. SEE skinnerian *conditioning;* S. *box.*

skin writ·ing. SYN dermatographism.

Sklowsky, E.L., 20th century German physician. SEE S. *symptom.*

Skoda, Joseph, Bohemian clinician in Vienna, 1805–1881. SEE skodaic *resonance;* S. *rale, sign, tympany.*

sko·da·ic (skō-dā′ik). Relating to Skoda.

skull (skŭl). SYN cranium. [Early Eng. *skulle,* a bowl]

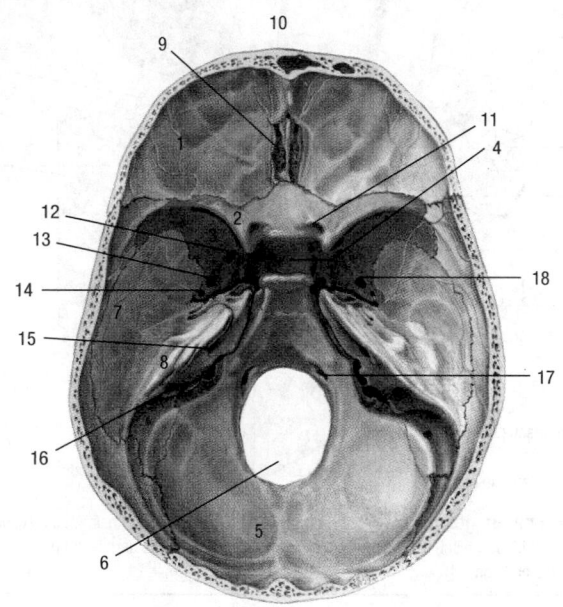

skull: internal view of base

1 frontal bone	10 frontal sinus
2 lesser wing of sphenoid bone	11 optic canal
3 greater wing of sphenoid bone	12 foramen rotundum
4 sella turcica	13 foramen ovale
5 occipital bone	14 foramen spinosum
6 foramen magnum	15 internal acoustic meatus
7 temporal bone	16 jugular foramen
8 petrous portion of temporal bone	17 hypoglossal canal
9 cribriform plate of ethmoid bone	18 carotid canal

cloverleaf s., SEE cloverleaf skull *syndrome.*

maplike s., various defects in the s., especially in the temporal bone, the anterior fossa, and orbits, forming irregular outlines resembling the national boundaries in an atlas.

natiform s., palpable bony nodules on the surface of the skull in infants with congenital *syphilis.*

steeple s., tower s., SYN oxycephaly.

skull·cap (skŭl′kap). SYN calvaria.

sky blue (skī′ bloo′). A pigment mixture of cobaltous stannate and calcium sulfate; used biologically as an injection mass.

SL Abbreviation for spinal *length.*

sl Symbol for slyke.

slab-off. A process by which prism base-up is produced in the reading field of a spectacle lens through bicentric grinding.

SLE Abbreviation for systemic *lupus* erythematosus.

sleep (slēp). A physiologic state of relative unconsciousness and inaction of the voluntary muscles, the need for which recurs periodically. The stages of sleep have been variously defined in terms of depth (light, deep), EEG characteristics (delta waves, synchronization), physiologic characteristics (REM, NREM), and presumed anatomic level (pontine, mesencephalic, rhombencephalic, Rolandic, etc.). [A.S. *slaep*]

electric s., a condition of convulsions and unconsciousness induced by the passage of an electric current through the brain.

electrotherapeutic s., SEE electrotherapeutic sleep *therapy.*

hypnotic s., SYN hypnosis.

light s., SYN dysnystaxis.

paroxysmal s., SYN narcolepsy.

rapid eye movement s., REM s., that state of deep s. in which rapid eye movements, alert EEG pattern, and dreaming occur; several central and autonomic functions are distinctive during this state.

s. terror, SYN night terrors.

winter s., SYN hibernation.

sleep·i·ness (slēp′i-nes). SYN somnolence (1).

sleep·less·ness (slēp′les-nes). SYN insomnia.

sleep·talk·ing. 1. SYN somniloquence (1). **2.** SYN somniloquy.

sleep·walk·er. SYN somnambulist.

sleep·walk·ing. SYN somnambulism (1).

slide (slīd). A rectangular glass plate on which is placed an object to be examined under the microscope.

sling. A supporting bandage or suspensory device; especially a loop suspended from the neck and supporting the flexed forearm.

slit. A long, narrow opening, incision, or aperture.

Cheatle s., a longitudinal incision into the antimesenteric border of the small intestine, which when closed transversely creates a larger lumen than would be possible by simple end-to-end anastomosis; currently modified to include longitudinal incisions into the cut ends of the transected small intestine or other tubular structures, allowing a wide caliber elliptical anastomosis to be performed.

filtration s.'s, SYN slit *pores,* under *pore.*

pudendal s., SYN pudendal *cleft.*

vulvar s., SYN pudendal *cleft.*

slit·lamp. In ophthalmology, an instrument consisting of a microscope combined with a rectangular light source that can be narrowed into a slit. SYN biomicroscope, Gullstrand s.

Gullstrand s., SYN slitlamp.

slope (slōp). An inclination or slant.

lower ridge s., the s. of the mandibular residual ridge in the second and third molar as seen from the buccal side.

slough (slŭf). **1.** Necrosed tissue separated from the living structure. **2.** To separate from the living tissue, said of a dead or necrosed part. [M.E. *slughe*]

Sluder, Greenfield, U.S. laryngologist, 1865–1928.

Sluder neu·ral·gia. See under neuralgia.

sludge (slŭdj). A muddy sediment. SEE ALSO sludged *blood.*

activated s., SEE activated sludge *method.*

sluice (sloos). SYN waterfall.

sluice·way (sloos′wā). SYN spillway.

slur·ry (sler′ē). A thin semifluid suspension of a solid in a liquid.

slyke (sl) (slīk). A unit of buffer value, the slope of the acid-base titration curve of a solution; the millimoles of strong acid or base that must be added per unit of change in pH. [D.D. Van *Slyke,* U.S. physician and chemist, 1883–1971]

Sm Symbol for samarium.

SMA Abbreviation for sequential multichannel *autoanalyzer*; spinal muscular *atrophy.*

small·pox (smawl'poks). An acute eruptive contagious disease caused by a poxvirus (Orthopoxvirus, a member of the family Poxviridae) and marked at the onset by chills, high fever, backache, and headache; in 2–5 days the constitutional symptoms subside and an eruption appears as papules, which become umbilicated vesicles, develop into pustules, dry, and form scabs that, on falling off, leave a permanent marking of the skin (pock marks); average incubation period is 8–14 days. As a result of increasingly aggressive vaccination programs carried out over a period of about 200 years, smallpox is now extinct. SYN variola major, variola. [E. *small pocks,* or pustules]

> Smallpox was a universally dreaded scourge for more than 3 millennia, with case fatality rates sometimes exceeding 20%. In many ways a unique disease, it had no nonhuman reservoir species and no human carriers. First subjected to some control by variolation in the 10th century in India and China, it was gradually suppressed in the industrialized world after Edward Jenner's 1776 landmark discovery that infection with the harmless cowpox (vaccinia) virus renders humans immune to the smallpox virus. A global eradication program was initiated by the World Health Organization in 1966, and the last naturally occurring case of the disease was reported in Somalia in 1977. The disease is now of mainly historical interest.

confluent s., a severe form in which the lesions run into each other, forming large suppurating areas.

discrete s., the usual form in which the lesions are separate and distinct from each other.

fulminating s., SYN hemorrhagic s.

hemorrhagic s., a severe and frequently fatal form of s. accompanied by extravasation of blood into the skin in the early stage, or into the pustules at a later stage, accompanied often by nosebleed and hemorrhage from other orifices of the body. SYN fulminating s., variola hemorrhagica.

malignant s., SYN *variola* maligna.

modified s., varicelloid s., SYN varioloid (2).

West Indian s., SYN alastrim.

smear (smēr). A thin specimen for examination; it is usually prepared by spreading material uniformly onto a glass slide, fixing it, and staining it before examination.

alimentary tract s., a group of cytologic specimens containing material from the mouth (oral s.), esophagus and stomach (gastric s.), duodenum (paraduodenal s.), and colon, obtained by specialized lavage techniques; used principally for the diagnosis of cancer of those areas.

bronchoscopic s., SYN lower respiratory tract s.

buccal s., a cytologic s. containing material obtained by scraping the lateral buccal mucosa above the dentate line, smearing, and fixing immediately; used principally for determining somatic sex as indicated by the presence of the sex chromocenter (Barr body).

cervical s., a generic name for different types of s.'s of the cervix uteri, e.g., ectocervical, endocervical, pancervical; used principally for cervical screening.

colonic s., SEE alimentary tract s.

cul-de-sac s., a cytologic specimen of material obtained by aspirating the pouch of Douglas from the posterior vaginal fornix and prepared by smearing, centrifuging, or filtering; used principally for ovarian cancer.

cytologic s., a type of cytologic specimen made by smearing a sample (obtained by a variety of methods from a number of sites), then fixing it and staining it, usually with 95% ethyl alcohol and Papanicolaou stain. SYN cytosmear.

duodenal s., SEE alimentary tract s.

ectocervical s., a cytologic s. of material obtained from the ectocervix, usually by scraping; used principally for the diagnosis of late cervical cancers involving the ectocervix.

endocervical s., a cytologic s. of material obtained from the endocervical canal by swab, aspiration, or scraping; used principally for the detection of early cervical cancer.

endometrial s., a group of cytologic s.'s containing material obtained directly from the endometrium by aspiration, lavage, or brushing of the uterine cavity.

esophageal s., SEE alimentary tract s.

fast s., a cytologic smear containing material from the vaginal pool and pancervical scrapings, mixed and prepared on one microscopic slide, smeared, and fixed immediately; used principally for routine screening of ovaries, endometrium, cervix, vagina, and hormonal states.

gastric s., SEE alimentary tract s.

lateral vaginal wall s., a cytologic s. containing material obtained by scraping the lateral wall of the vagina near the junction of its upper and middle third; used for cytohormonal evaluation.

lower respiratory tract s., a group of cytologic specimens containing material from the lower respiratory tract and consisting mainly of sputum (spontaneous, induced) and material obtained at bronchoscopy (aspirated, lavaged, brushed); used for cytologic study of cancer and other diseases of the lungs. SYN bronchoscopic s., sputum s.

oral s., SEE alimentary tract s.

pancervical s., a cytologic s. of material obtained from the endocervical canal, external os, and ectocervix by scraping these areas with a properly designed cervical spatula; used principally for early cervical cancer detection.

Pap s., a s. of vaginal or cervical cells obtained for cytological study. SYN Papanicolaou s.

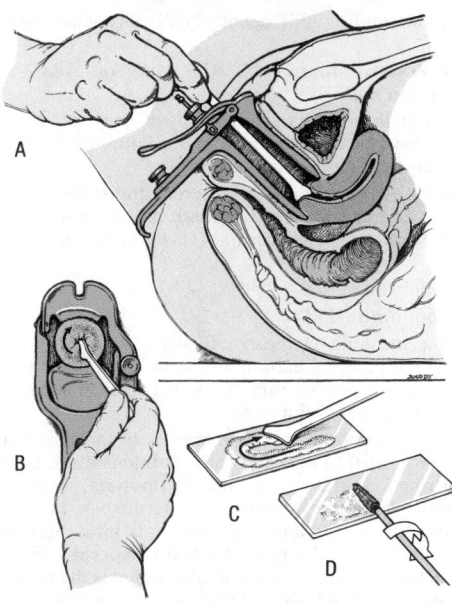

Pap smear: (A) speculum in place and Ayre spatula in position at cervical os, (B) tip of spatula placed in the cervical os and rotated 360 degrees, (C) cellular material clinging to spatula is then smeared smoothly on glass slide, which is promptly placed in fixative solution, (D) Cytobrush is rotated in cervical os and rolled onto glass slide

Papanicolaou s., SYN Pap s.

sputum s., SYN lower respiratory tract s.

urinary s., a group of cytologic specimens containing processed urine obtained from bladder, ureters, or renal pelvis; used for cytologic study of cancer and other diseases of the urinary tract.

vaginal s., a s. of debris from the vaginal lumen of mammals, used to determine the stage of their reproductive cycle. It is most

sm

useful in subprimate mammals having short estrous cycles; nucleated epithelial cells and leukocytes prevail in the s. during diestrus and proestrus, and cornified cells during estrus.

VCE s., a cytologic s. of material obtained from the vagina, ectocervix, and endocervix, smeared separately (in that order) on one slide, and fixed immediately; used principally for the detection of cervical cancer and identification of the sites of diseases of those areas, and for hormonal evaluation.

smeg·ma (smeg′mă). A foul-smelling, pasty accumulation of desquamated epidermal cells and sebum that has collected in moist areas of the genitalia. [G. unguent]

s. clitor′idis, the secretion of the apocrine glands of the clitoris, in combination with desquamating epithelial cells.

s. prepu′tii, whitish secretion that collects under the prepuce of the foreskin of the penis or of the clitoris; it is comprised chiefly of desquamating epithelial cells.

smeg·ma·lith (smeg′mă-lith). A calcareous concretion in the smegma. [smegma + G. *lithos,* stone]

smell. **1.** To scent; to perceive an odor by means of the olfactory apparatus. **2.** SYN olfaction (1). **3.** SYN odor.

smell-brain (smel′brān). SYN rhinencephalon.

Smellie, William, English obstetrician, 1698–1763. SEE S. *scissors.*

Smith, David W., U.S. pediatrician, 1926–1981. SEE S.-Lemli-Opitz *syndrome.*

Smith, Henry, Irish-born British military surgeon in India, 1862–1948. SEE S. *operation;* S.-Indian *operation.*

Smith, M.J.V., 20th century U.S. urologist.

Smith, Robert W., Irish surgeon, 1807–1873. SEE S. *fracture.*

Smith, Theobald, U.S. pathologist, 1859–1934. SEE Theobald S. *phenomenon.*

Smith, William R., 20th century U.S. physician. SEE S.-Riley *syndrome.*

Smith-Petersen, Marius N., U.S. surgeon, 1886–1953. SEE Smith-Petersen *nail.*

smog. Air pollution characterized by a hazy and often highly irritating atmosphere resulting from a mixture of fog with smoke and other air pollutants. [smoke + fog]

smut (smŭt). A fungal disease of cereal grains caused by species of *Ustilago* and characterized by dark brown or black masses of spores on the plants; e.g., corn s. (*U. maydis*); loose s. of wheat (*U. nuda*)

Sn Symbol for tin.

113Sn Symbol for tin-113.

⌂sn-. Prefix meaning stereospecifically numbered; a system of numbering the glycerol carbon atoms in lipids, so that the locant numbers remain constant regardless of chemical substitutions, as opposed to systematic numbering.

snail (snāl). Common name for members of the class Gastropoda (phylum Mollusca). The freshwater pulmonate (nonoperculated, air-breathing) snails (subclass Pulmonata, order Basommatophora) include the majority of intermediate hosts of trematodes parasitic in humans and domestic birds and mammals, chiefly in the families Lymnaeidae and Planorbidae. The subclass Prosobranchiata, the operculate snails, includes the order Neogastropoda, which includes the venomous stinging cone snails (genus *Conus*), and the order Mesogastropoda, of which the family Hydrobiidae includes most of the medically important host snails. [M.E. *snaile*]

snake (snāk). An elongated, limbless, scaly reptile of the suborder Ophidia.

snake·root (snāk′root). SYN serpentaria.

Canada s., SYN *Asarum* canadense.

European s., SYN *Asarum* europaeum.

Seneca s., SYN senega.

Texas s., botanical source of serpentaria.

Virginia s., *Aristolochia serpentaria;* botanical source of serpentaria.

snap. A click; a short sharp sound; said especially of cardiac sounds.

closing s., the accentuated first heart sound of mitral stenosis, related to closure of the abnormal valve.

opening s., a sharp, high-pitched click in early diastole, usually best heard between the cardiac apex and the lower left sternal border, related to opening of the abnormal valve in cases of mitral stenosis.

snare (snār). An instrument for removing polyps and other projections from a surface, especially within a cavity; it consists of a wire loop passed around the base of the tumor and gradually tightened. [A.S. *snear,* a cord]

cold s., an unheated s.

galvanocaustic s., hot s., a s. the wire of which is heated to a high temperature by an electric current.

SNE Abbreviation for subacute necrotizing *encephalomyelopathy.*

Sneddon, Ian B., 20th century English dermatologist. SEE S. *syndrome;* S.-Wilkinson *disease.*

sneeze (snēz). **1.** To expel air from the nose and mouth by an involuntary spasmodic contraction of the muscles of expiration. **2.** An act of sneezing; a reflex excited by an irritation of the mucous membrane of the nose or, sometimes, by a bright light striking the eye. [A.S. *fneōsan*]

Snell, Simeon, English ophthalmologist, 1851–1909. SEE S. *law.*

Snellen, Hermann, Dutch ophthalmologist, 1834–1908. SEE S. *sign, test types.*

snore (snōr). **1.** A rough, rattling, inspiratory noise produced by vibration of the pendulous palate, or sometimes of the vocal cords, during sleep or coma. SEE ALSO stertor, rhonchus. **2.** To breathe noisily, or with a s. [A.S. *snora*]

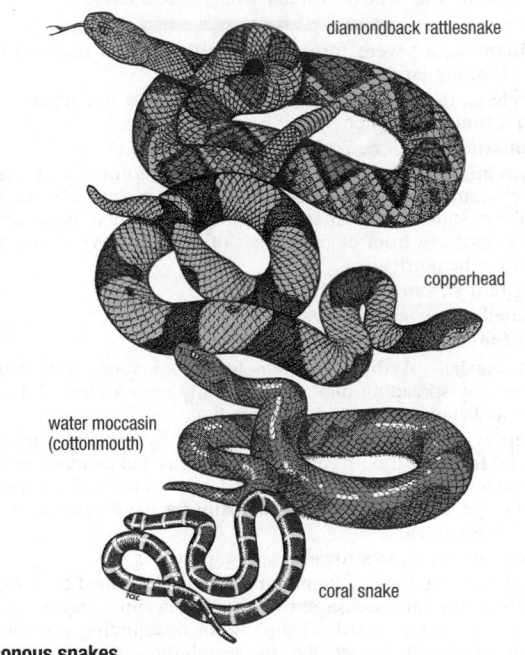

poisonous snakes

snow (snō). SEE *carbon* dioxide snow.

snRNA Abbreviation for small nuclear RNA.

snuff (snŭf). **1.** To inhale forcibly through the nose. **2.** Finely powdered tobacco used by inhalation through the nose or applied to the gums. **3.** Any medicated powder applied by insufflation to the nasal mucous membrane. [echoic]

snuff·box (snŭf′boks). SEE anatomic snuffbox.

snuf·fles (snŭf′lz). Obstructed nasal respiration, especially in the newborn infant, sometimes due to congenital syphilis.

Snyder, Marshall L., U.S. microbiologist, 1907–1969. SEE S. *test.*

SOAP Acronym for *s*ubjective, *o*bjective, *a*ssessment, and *p*lan;

used in problem-oriented records for organizing follow-up data, evaluation, and planning.

soap (sōp). The sodium or potassium salts of long-chain fatty acids (e.g., sodium stearate); used as an emulsifier for cleansing purposes and as an excipient in the making of pills and suppositories. [A.S. *sape*, L. *sapo*, G. *sapōn*]

animal s., s. made with sodium hydroxide and a purified animal fat consisting chiefly of stearin; used in pharmacy in the preparation of certain liniments. SYN curd s., domestic s., tallow s.

Castile s., SYN hard s.

curd s., domestic s., SYN animal s.

green s., SYN medicinal soft s.

hard s., a s. made with olive oil, or some other suitable oil or fat, and sodium hydroxide; used as a detergent, and in the form of a suppository or soapsuds enema for constipation; used also as an excipient in pills. SYN Castile s.

insoluble s., s. made with a fatty acid and an earthy or metallic base (iron or calcium salts of fatty acids).

marine s., a s. made of palm or coconut oil for use with sea water in which it is soluble. SYN salt water s.

medicinal soft s., a s. made with vegetable oils, potassium hydroxide, oleic acid, glycerin, and purified water; used as a cleansing agent and stimulant in chronic skin diseases. SYN green s., soft s.

salt water s., SYN marine s.

soft s., SYN medicinal soft s.

soluble s., any s. made with potassium, sodium, or ammonium hydroxide: ordinary animal s., Castile s., green s., etc.

superfatted s., a s. containing an excess (3–5%) of fat above that necessary to completely neutralize all the alkali; used in the manufacture of medicated s., and in the treatment of skin diseases.

tallow s., SYN animal s.

soap·stone (sōp′stōn). SYN talc.

Soave, F., 20th century Italian pediatric surgeon. SEE S. *operation.*

so·cal·o·in (sō-kal′ō-in). An aloin obtained from aloes of the island of Socotra.

so·cia (sō′shē-ă). An ectopic, supernumerary, or accessory portion of an organ.

socia parotidis (sō′shē-ă pa-rot′i-dis), SYN accessory parotid *gland.* [L. companion of the parotid]

so·cial·i·za·tion (sō′shăl-i-zā′shŭn). **1.** The process of learning attitudes and interpersonal and interactional skills which are in conformity with the values of one's society. **2.** In a group therapy setting, a way of learning to participate effectively in the group. [L. *socius,* partner, companion]

♻**socio-.** Social, society. [L. *socius,* companion]

so·ci·o·ac·u·sis (sō-sē-ō-ak-ū′sis). The hearing loss produced by exposure to nonoccupational noise such as small arms fire in hunting and target practice. [socio- + G. *akousis,* hearing]

so·ci·o·cen·tric (sō′sē-ō-sen′trik). Outgoing; reactive to the social or cultural milieu. [socio- + L. *centrum,* center]

so·ci·o·cen·trism (sō′sē-ō-sen′trizm). Taking one's own social group as the standard by which others are measured.

so·ci·o·cosm (sō′sē-ō-kozm). The totality that includes human society, human thought, and the relationship of humans to nature. [socio- + G. *kosmos,* universe]

so·ci·o·gen·e·sis (sō′sē-ō-jen′ĕ-sis). The origin of social behavior from past interpersonal experiences. [socio- + G. *genesis,* origin]

so·ci·o·gram (sō′sē-ō-gram). A diagrammatic representation of the valences and degrees of attractiveness and acceptance of each individual rated according to the interpersonal interactions between and among members of a group; a diagram in which group interactions are analyzed on the basis of mutual attractions or antipathies between group members. [socio- + G. *gramma,* something written]

so·ci·o·med·i·cal (sō′sē-ō-med′i-kăl). Pertaining to the relation of the practice of medicine to society.

so·ci·om·e·try (sō-sē-om′ĕ-trē). The study of interpersonal relationships in a group. [socio- + G. *metron,* measure]

so·ci·o·path (sō′sē-ō-path). A designation for a person with an antisocial personality disorder. SEE ALSO antisocial *personality,* psychopath.

so·ci·op·a·thy (sō-sē-op′ă-thē). A term for the behavioral pattern exhibited by persons with an antisocial personality disorder. SEE ALSO personality *disorder.* [socio- + G. *pathos,* suffering]

sock·et (sok′et). SYN gomphosis. **1.** The hollow part of a joint; the excavation in one bone of a joint which receives the articular end of the other bone. **2.** Any hollow or concavity into which another part fits, as the eye s. [thr. O. Fr. fr. L. *soccus,* a shoe, a sock]

dry s., SYN alveoalgia.

eye s., generally the orbit, although the true "socket" for the eyeball, into which a prosthetic eye would be inserted, is formed by the fascial sheath of the eyeball. SYN orbit.

tooth s. [TA], a socket in the alveolar process of the maxilla or mandible, into which each tooth fits and is attached by means of the periodontal ligament. SYN alveolus dentalis [TA], alveolus (4) [NA].

SOD Abbreviation for *superoxide* dismutase.

so·da (sō′dă). SYN *sodium* carbonate. [It., possibly fr. Mediev. L. barilla plant]

baking s., SYN *sodium* bicarbonate.

caustic s., SYN *sodium* hydroxide.

s. lime, a mixture of calcium and sodium hydroxides used to absorb carbon dioxide in situations in which rebreathing occurs; e.g., in basal determinations or in certain types of anesthesia circuits.

washing s., SYN *sodium* carbonate.

so·dic (sō′dik). Relating to or containing soda or sodium.

♻**sodio-.** A compound containing sodium; as sodiocitrate, sodiotartrate, a citrate or tartrate of some element containing sodium in addition.

SODIUM

so·di·um (Na) (sō′dē-ŭm). A metallic element, atomic no. 11, atomic wt. 22.989768; an alkali metal oxidizing readily in air or water; its salts are found in natural biologic systems and are extensively used in medicine and industry. The s. ion is the most plentiful extracellular ion in the body. For organic s. salts not listed below, see under the name of the organic acid portion. SYN natrium. [Mod. L. fr. *soda*]

s. acetate, a systemic and urinary alkalizer, expectorant, and diuretic.

s. acid carbonate, SYN s. bicarbonate.

s. acid citrate, SYN s. citrate.

s. acid phosphate, SYN s. biphosphate.

s. alginate, SYN algin.

s. *p*-aminohippurate, used intravenously in renal function tests, to determine the renal plasma flow and the tubular excretion.

s. *p*-aminophenylarsonate, a compound that was one of the first modern pentavalent arsenicals. SYN s. arsanilate.

s. aminosalicylate, used for the same purposes as aminosalicylic acid.

s. antimonylgluconate, SYN stibogluconate *sodium* (2).

s. antimonyl tartrate, SYN *antimony* sodium tartrate.

s. arsanilate, SYN s. *p*-aminophenylarsonate.

s. ascorbate, same actions and uses as ascorbic acid; it is preferred for intramuscular administration.

s. aurothiomalate, SYN *gold* sodium thiomalate.

s. aurothiosulfate, SYN *gold* sodium thiosulfate.

s. benzoate, used in chronic and acute rheumatism, as a liver function test, and as a preservative.

s. bicarbonate, $NaHCO_3$; used as a gastric and systemic antacid, to alkalize urine, and for washes of body cavities. SYN baking soda, s. acid carbonate, s. hydrogen carbonate.

SO

s. biphosphate, used to increase urinary acidity. SYN primary s. phosphate, s. acid phosphate, s. dihydrogen phosphate.

s. bisulfite, $NaHSO_3$; acid s. sulfite, used in gastric and intestinal fermentation, externally in the treatment of parasitic diseases, and as an antioxidant in certain injections (s. metabisulfite). SYN s. hydrogen sulfite, s. pyrosulfite.

s. borate, used in lotions, gargles, mouthwashes, and as a detergent. SYN borax, s. pyroborate, s. tetraborate.

s. bromide, NaBr; an obsolete hypnotic and sedative; occasionally used in epilepsy and other functional disorders of the nervous system.

s. cacodylate, used in anemia, leukemia, and malaria. SYN s. dimethylarsenate.

s. carbonate, used in the treatment of scaly skin diseases; otherwise rarely used in medicine because of its irritant action. SYN sal soda, soda, washing soda.

s. carboxymethyl cellulose, the s. salt of a polycarboxymethyl ether of cellulose; used as a laxative due to its indigestibility and binding of water within the gastrointestinal tract.

s. chloride, NaCl; the chief component of blood and other body fluids, and urine; used to make isotonic and physiological saline solutions, in the treatment of salt depletion, and topically for inflammatory lesions. SYN common salt, table salt.

s. citrate, used as diuretic, antilithic, systemic and urinary alkalizer, expectorant, and anticoagulant (in vitro). SYN s. acid citrate.

s. citrate, acid, same actions and uses as s. citrate; in addition, it may be used in solutions of glucose without producing caramelization of the latter during autoclaving.

s. cromoglycate, SYN cromolyn sodium.

s. dehydrocholate, a cholagogue; also used to determine circulation time.

s. diatrizoate, a water-soluble organic iodine compound formerly used for intravenous excretory urography and angiography.

dibasic s. phosphate, SYN s. phosphate.

s. dihydrogen phosphate, SYN s. biphosphate.

s. dimethylarsenate, SYN s. cacodylate.

s. dodecyl sulfate (SDS), SYN s. lauryl sulfate.

effervescent s. phosphate, exsiccated s. phosphate 200, s. bicarbonate 477, tartaric acid 252, and citric acid 162, mixed and passed through a sieve to make a granular salt.

exsiccated s. sulfite, anhydrous s. sulfite, used as a preservative in pharmaceutical preparations.

s. fluoride, used as a dental prophylactic against caries in drinking water, and topically as a 2% solution applied on the teeth.

s. fluosilicate, SYN s. hexafluorosilicate.

s. folate, the s. salt of folic acid; action and uses are the same as those of folic acid, but it is preferred for parenteral administration. SYN s. pteroylglutamate.

s. fusidate, SYN fusidate sodium.

s. glycerophosphate, has been used as a tonic.

s. hexafluorosilicate, Na_2SiF_6; used (in dilute solutions) as an antiseptic and deodorant, and for fluoridation of drinking water. SYN s. fluosilicate, s. silicofluoride.

s. hydrogen carbonate, SYN s. bicarbonate.

s. hydrogen sulfite, SYN s. bisulfite.

s. hydroxide, NaOH; used externally as a caustic. SYN caustic soda.

s. hypochlorite, strong oxidizer; explosive when anhydrous. Decomposes by absorbing carbon dioxide from the air. Liberates chlorine and oxygen; used in aqueous solution as a bleach and disinfectant. The active constituent of many household bleaches, e.g., Clorox.

s. hypophosphite, formerly used as a nerve tonic.

s. hyposulfite, SYN s. thiosulfate.

s. ichthyolsulfonate, an alterative and antiseptic.

s. indigotin disulfonate, SYN indigo carmine.

s. iodide, NaI; used as a source of iodine.

s. lactate, a systemic and urinary alkalizer.

s. lauryl sulfate, a surface-active agent of the anionic type used in toothpastes. SYN s. dodecyl sulfate.

s. levothyroxine, s. salt of the natural isomer of thyroxine, a thyroid hormone. It is twice as effective as the racemic form. Used in the treatment of hypothyroidism in humans and animals, to treat lowered fertility in bulls, and to stimulate lactation in animals.

s. liothyronine, s. L-triiodothyronine, the physiologically active isomer of triiodothyronine, twice as active as the racemic form; used in the treatment of thyroid deficiency syndromes. A metabolite of thyroxine.

s. metabisulfite, used as an antioxidant in injectable solutions.

s. methicillin, SYN methicillin sodium.

s. methylarsonate, formerly used in tuberculosis, chorea, and other affections in which the cacodylates were used.

s. nitrate, $NaNO_3$; formerly used for dysentery and as a diuretic. SYN Chilean saltpeter, cubic niter.

s. nitrite, $NaNO_2$; used to lower systemic blood pressure, to relieve local vasomotor spasms, especially in angina pectoris and Raynaud disease, to relax bronchial and intestinal spasms, and as an antidote for cyanide poisoning.

s. nitroferricyanide, SYN s. nitroprusside.

s. nitroprusside, a rapidly acting and potent arterial and venous vasodilator used in hypertensive emergencies and administered intravenously. Acts in a manner similar to vasodilator nitrates and nitrites by donating nitric oxide which produces vasodilation; also used as a reagent for detection of organic compounds in the urine. SYN s. nitroferricyanide.

s. orthophosphate, SYN s. phosphate.

s. perborate, used in the extemporaneous preparation of hydrogen peroxide; a 2% solution is equivalent in germicidal action to 0.4% of hydrogen peroxide.

s. peroxide, Na_2O_2; used externally as a paste or soap in the treatment of comedones and acne.

s. pertechnetate, $Na^{99m}TcO_4$; a radiopharmaceutical used for brain, thyroid, and salivary gland scanning.

s. phosphate, a laxative. SYN dibasic s. phosphate, s. orthophosphate.

s. phosphate ^{32}P, anionic radioactive phosphorus in the form of a solution of s. acid phosphate and s. basic phosphate; a beta emitter with a half-life of 14.3 days; after administration, highest concentrations are found in rapidly proliferating tissues; it is used in the treatment of polycythemia vera, chronic myelogenous leukemia, and osseous metastases. SEE ALSO chromic phosphate ^{32}P colloidal *suspension.*

s. polyanhydromannuronic acid sulfate, an anticoagulant drug prepared from alginic acid and having an action similar to that of heparin.

s. polystyrene sulfonate, a cationic exchange resin used in hyperpotassemia.

s. potassium tartrate, SYN *potassium* sodium tartrate.

pravastatin s., antihyperlipoproteinemic. An HMG-Co reductase inhibitor resembling lovastatin and simvastatin, which inhibits cholesterol formation.

primary s. phosphate, SYN s. biphosphate.

s. propionate, the s. salt of propionic acid; used for fungus infections of the skin, usually in combination with calcium propionate; used as a preservative.

s. psylliate, the s. salt of the liquid fatty acids of psyllium oil, prepared by dissolving the fatty acid in dilute s. hydroxide solution; used like morrhuate s. as a sclerosing agent in the treatment of varicose veins.

s. pteroylglutamate, SYN s. folate.

s. pyroborate, SYN s. borate.

s. pyrosulfite, SYN s. bisulfite.

s. rhodanate, SYN s. thiocyanate.

s. ricinoleate, s. ricinate, the s. salt of ricinoleic acid; a sclerosing agent similar in action to morrhuate s.

s. salicylate, an analgesic, antipyretic, and antirheumatic.

s. silicofluoride, SYN s. hexafluorosilicate.

s. stearate, stearic acid sodium salt, used as a pharmaceutical adjuvant in ointments, creams, and suppositories.

s. sulfate, an ingredient of many of the natural laxative waters, and also used as a hydragogue cathartic primarily in large animals. SYN Glauber salt.

s. sulfite, has been used for the relief of intestinal fermentation, and externally for aphthous stomatitis.

s. sulfocyanate, SYN s. thiocyanate.

s. sulforicinate, s. sulforicinoleate, made by combining castor oil, sulfuric acid, and s. hydroxide and chloride; used as a solvent for iodine, iodoform, resorcinol, pyrogallol, and a number of other substances for external use.

s. tartrate, a laxative.

s. taurocholate, the s. salt of taurocholic acid, extracted from the bile of carnivora; a cholagogue.

s. tetraborate, SYN s. borate.

s. tetradecyl sulfate, an anionic surface-active agent used for its wetting properties to enhance the surface action of certain antiseptic solutions; also used as a sclerosing agent similar to morrhuate s. in the treatment of varicose veins.

s. thiocyanate, formerly used in the management of essential hypertension. SYN s. rhodanate, s. sulfocyanate.

s. thiosulfate, an antidote in cyanide poisoning in conjunction with s. nitrite; used as a prophylactic agent against ringworm infections in swimming pools and baths, and to measure the extracellular fluid volume of the body. SYN s. hyposulfite.

s. tungstoborate, used in electron microscopy as a negative stain.

so·di·um-24 (^{24}**Na**). The isotope of sodium with an atomic weight of 24, and a half-life of 14.96 hr; it emits beta and gamma rays, and is more easily prepared than the longer-lived, positron-emitting ^{22}Na (half-life, 2.605 yr). It is used to measure extracellular fluid by indicator dilution.

so·di·um group. The alkali metals: cesium, lithium, potassium, rubidium, and sodium.

so·do·ku (sō-dō'koo). SYN rat-bite *fever.* [Jap. rat poison]

sod·om·ist, sod·om·ite (sod'ŏ-mist, -mīt). One who practices sodomy. [G. *sodomitēs,* an inhabitant city of Sodom, said in the Bible to have been destroyed by fire because of the wickedness of its people]

sod·o·my (sod'ŏm-ē). A term denoting a number of sexual practices variously proscribed by law, especially bestiality, oral-genital contact, and anal intercourse. SYN buggery. [see sodomist]

Soemmerring, Samuel Thomas von, German anatomist, 1755–1830. SEE S. *ganglion, ligament, muscle, spot; ring* of S.

Soffer, Louis J., U.S. internist, *1904. SEE Sohval-S. *syndrome.*

soft·ware. The program or instructions for a computer.

Sohval, Arthur R., U.S. internist, *1904. SEE S.-Soffer *syndrome.*

soil (soyl). Dirt.

night s., human feces used for fertilizer.

so·ja (sō'yah). SYN soybean.

so·ko·sho (sō-kō'shō). SYN rat-bite *fever.* [Jap. *so,* rat, + *ko,* bite, + *sho,* malady]

sol. 1. A colloidal dispersion of a solid in a liquid. Cf. gel. **2.** Abbreviation for solution.

So·la·na·ce·ae (sō-lă-nā'sē-ē). A family of plants that includes the genus *Solanum* (nightshade) and some 84 other genera comprising 1,800 species, including belladonna, the tomato, and potato plants.

so·la·na·ceous (sō-lă-nā'shŭs, sol'ă-). Pertaining to plants of the family Solanaceae, or to drugs derived from them.

sol·a·no·chro·mene (sol'ă-nō-krō'mēn). SYN plastochromenol-8.

so·lap·sone (sō-lap'sōn). SYN solasulfone.

sol·a·sul·fone (sol-ă-sŭlf'ōn). A leprostatic agent. SYN solapsone.

sol·a·tion (sol-ā'shŭn). In colloidal chemistry, the transformation of a gel into a sol, as by melting gelatin.

sol·der (sod'er). **1.** A fusible alloy used to unite edges or surfaces of two pieces of metal of higher melting point; hard s.'s, usually containing gold or silver as their main constituent, are usually used in dentistry to connect noble metal alloys. **2.** To join two pieces of metal with such an alloy. [L. *solido,* to make solid, through Fr., various forms]

sol·der·ing (sod'er-ing). A laser technique to make one tissue adhere to another.

sole (sōl) [TA]. The plantar surface or under part of the foot. SYN planta [TA], pelma. [A.S.]

s. of foot [TA], the inferior aspect or bottom of the foot, much of which is in contact with the ground when standing; it is covered with hairless, usually nonpigmented skin that is especially thickened and provided with epidermal ridges over the weightbearing areas. SYN planta pedis [TA], plantar region⋆, regio plantaris⋆, plantar surface of foot.

So·le·nog·ly·pha (sō-lĕ-nog'li-fă). A major category of snakes that includes the viper and rattlesnake families. [L., fr. G. *sōlēn,* pipe channel, + *glyphō,* to carve]

so·le·noid (sol'ĕ-noyd). A helical coil of wire energized electrically to produce a magnetic field, which induces a current in any conductor placed within or near the coil.

So·le·no·po·tes cap·il·la·tus (sō-lĕ-nop'ŏ-tēz kap-i-lā'tŭs). A sucking louse of cattle, called the little blue cattle louse in the U.S. and the tubercle-bearing louse in Australia. [G. *solen,* pipe, + *potos,* a drinking]

so·le·nop·sin A (sō-lĕ-nop'sin). One of several, probably five, alkaloidal constituents present in the venom of the imported fire ant, *Solenopsis saevissima;* the venom has necrotoxic, hemolytic, insecticidal, and antibiotic properties.

Solenopsis (sōl-ĕ-nop'sis). A genus of ants known as fire ants, which can inflict painful burning stings that cause local and occasionally systemic reactions.

S. invicta, the red imported fire ant, a species imported from South America which has spread extensively within the southeastern United States where it has become a major pest of humans and animals; it readily stings humans, producing local swelling and pruritus with development of a pustule at the site of the sting and, in rare cases, it can cause anaphylactic shock with death from respiratory or cardiac arrest. SEE ALSO *S. richteri.* SYN red imported fire ant.

S. richteri, the black imported fire ant, a species imported from South America but less extensively established in the United States than *S. invicta.* SEE ALSO *S. invicta.* SYN black imported fire ant.

so·le·us (sō-lē'ŭs). SEE soleus *(muscle).* [Mod. L. fr. L. *solea,* a sandal, sole of the foot (of animals), fr. *solum,* bottom, floor, ground]

sol·id. 1. Firm; compact; not fluid; without interstices or cavities; not cancellous. **2.** A body that retains its form when not confined; one that is not fluid, neither liquid nor gaseous. [L. *solidus*]

sol·id·ism (sol'i-dizm). The theory propounded by Asclepiades and his followers that disease was due to an imbalance between solid particles (atoms) of the body and the spaces (pores) between them, a doctrine that opposed the humoral conception of Hippocrates. SYN methodism.

sol·id·ist (sol'i-dist). An adherent of the doctrine of solidism.

sol·id·is·tic (sol'i-dis'tik). Relating to solidism.

sol·i·dus (sol'i-dŭs). That line on a constitution diagram indicating the temperature below which all metal is solid.

sol·i·ped (sol'i-ped). A solid-hoofed animal such as the horse. [L. *solidus,* solid, + *pes,* foot]

sol·ip·sism (sō'lip-sizm, sol'ip-). A philosophical concept that whatever exists is a product of will and the ideas of the perceiving individual. [L. *solus,* alone, + *ipse,* self]

soln. Abbreviation for solution.

sol·u·bil·i·ty (sol-ū-bil'i-tē). The property of being soluble.

sol·u·ble (sol'ū-bl). Capable of being dissolved. [L. *solubilis,* fr. *solvo,* to dissolve]

so·lum (sō'lŭm). Bottom; the lowest part. [L.]

sol·ute (sol'ūt, sō'loot). The dissolved substance in a solution. [L. *solutus,* dissolved, pp. of *solvo,* to dissolve]

so·lu·tio (sō-loo'shē-ō). SYN solution. [L.]

so·lu·tion (sol., soln.) (sō-loo'shŭn). **1.** The incorporation of a solid, a liquid, or a gas in a liquid or noncrystalline solid resulting in a homogeneous single phase. SEE dispersion, suspension. **2.**

Generally, an aqueous s. of a nonvolatile substance. **3.** In the language of the Pharmacopeia, an aqueous s. of a nonvolatile substance is called a s. or liquor; an aqueous s. of a volatile substance is a water (aqua); an alcoholic s. of a nonvolatile substance is a tincture (tinctura); an alcoholic s. of a volatile substance is a spirit (spiritus); a s. in vinegar is a vinegar (acetum); a s. in glycerin is a glycerol (glyceritum); a s. in wine is a wine (vinum); a s. of sugar in water is a syrup (syrupus); a s. of a mucilaginous substance is a mucilage (mucilago); a s. of an alkaloid or metallic oxide in oleic acid is an oleate (oleatum). **4.** The termination of a disease by crisis. **5.** A break, cut, or laceration of the solid tissues. SEE s. of contiguity, s. of continuity. SYN solutio. [L. *solutio*]

acetic s., a vinegar.

amaranth s., a 1% s. of amaranth (trisodium naphthol sulfonic acid), a synthetic vivid red dye, stable in acid and intensified in sodium hydroxide s.; used as a red or pink colorant in liquid pharmaceuticals.

aqueous s., a s. containing water as the solvent; examples include lime water, rose water, saline s., and a large number of s.'s intended for intravenous administration.

Benedict s., an aqueous solution of sodium citrate, sodium carbonate, and copper sulfate which changes from its normal blue color to orange, red, or yellow in the presence of a reducing sugar such as glucose. SEE ALSO Benedict *test* for glucose.

Burow s., a preparation of aluminium subacetate and glacial acetic acid, used for its antiseptic and astringent action on the skin.

chemical s., SEE solution (1).

colloidal s., a dispersoid, emulsoid, or suspensoid. SYN colloidal dispersion.

s. of contiguity, the breaking of contiguity; a dislocation or displacement of two normally contiguous parts.

s. of continuity, division of bones or soft parts that are normally continuous, as by a fracture, a laceration, or an incision. SYN dieresis.

Dakin s., a bactericidal wound irrigant. SYN Dakin fluid.

disclosing s., a s. that selectively stains all soft debris, pellicle, and bacterial plaque on teeth; used as an aid in identifying bacterial plaque after rinsing with water.

Earle s., a tissue culture medium containing $CaCl_2$, $MgSO_4$, KCl, $NaHCO_3$, NaCl, $NaH_2PO_4 \cdot H_2O$, and glucose.

ethereal s., a s. of any substance in ether.

Fehling s., an alkaline copper tartrate s. formerly used for detection of reducing sugars. SYN Fehling reagent.

ferric and ammonium acetate s., a clear, aromatic, reddish-brown liquid which has been used in iron-deficiency anemia in animals and man; a source of iron. SYN Basham mixture.

Fonio s., a diluent with magnesium sulfate, used for stained smears of blood platelets.

Gallego differentiating s., a dilute s. of formaldehyde and acetic acid used in a modified Gram stain to differentiate and enhance the basic fuchsin binding to Gram-negative microorganisms.

Gey s., a salt s. usually used in combination with naturally occurring body substances (e.g., blood serum, tissue extracts) and/or more complex chemically defined nutritive s.'s for culturing animal cells.

Hanks s., a salt s. usually used in combination with naturally occurring body substances (e.g., blood serum, tissue extracts) and/or more complex chemically defined nutritive s.'s for culturing animal cells; two variations contain $CaCl_2$, $MgSO_4 \cdot 7H_2O$, KCl, KH_2PO_4, $NaHCO_3$, NaCl, $Na_2HPO_4 \cdot 2H_2O$, and D-glucose.

Hartman s., a s. used to desensitize dentin in dental operations; contains thymol, ethyl alcohol, and sulfuric ether.

Hartmann s., SYN lactated Ringer s.

Hayem s., a blood diluent used prior to counting red blood cells.

Krebs-Ringer s., a modification of Ringer s., prepared by mixing NaCl, KCl, $CaCl_2$, $MgSO_4$, and phosphate buffer, pH 7.4.

lactated Ringer s., a s. containing NaCl, sodium lactate, $CaCl_2$(dihydrate), and KCl in distilled water; used for the same purposes as Ringer s. SYN Hartmann s.

Lange s., a colloidal gold s. used to demonstrate protein abnormalities in spinal fluid. SEE Lange *test*.

Locke s.'s, s.'s containing, in varying amounts, NaCl, $CaCl_2$, KCl, $NaHCO_3$, and D-glucose; used for irrigating mammalian heart and other tissues, in laboratory experiments; also used in combination with naturally occurring body substances (e.g., blood serum, tissue extracts) and/or more complex chemically defined nutritive s.'s for culturing animal cells.

Locke-Ringer s., a s. containing NaCl, $CaCl_2$, KCl, $MgCl_2$, $NaHCO_3$, D-glucose, and water; used in the laboratory for physiological and pharmacological experiments.

Lugol iodine s., an iodine-potassium iodide s. used as an oxidizing agent, for removal of mercurial fixation artifacts, and also in histochemistry and to stain amebas.

molecular dispersed s., SYN dispersoid.

Monsel s., ferric subsulfate s. used to coagulate superficial bleeding such as that following skin biopsy.

normal s., SEE normal (3).

ophthalmic s.'s, sterile s.'s, free from foreign particles and suitably compounded and dispensed for instillation into the eye.

Ringer s., (1) a s. resembling the blood serum in its salt constituents; it contains 8.6 g of NaCl, 0.3 g of KCl, and 0.33 g of $CaCl_2$ in each 1000 mL of distilled water; used as a fluid and electrolyte replenisher by intravenous infusion. (2) a salt s. usually used in combination with naturally occurring body substances (e.g., blood serum, tissue extracts) and/or more complex chemically defined nutritive s.'s for culturing animal cells. SYN Ringer lactate. SEE Ringer *injection*.

saline s., (1) a s. of any salt; SYN salt s. (2) specifically, an isotonic sodium chloride s.; 0.85–0.9 per 100 mL of water.

salt s., SYN saline s. (1).

saturated s. (sat. sol., sat. soln.), a s. that contains all of a substance capable of dissolving; a solution of a substance in equilibrium with an excess undissolved substance.

standard s., standardized s., a s. of known concentration, used as a standard of comparison or analysis.

supersaturated s., a s. containing more of the solid than the liquid would ordinarily dissolve; it is made by heating the solvent when the substance is added, and on cooling the latter is retained without precipitation; addition of a crystal or solid of any kind usually results in precipitation of the excess solute, leaving a saturated s.

test s., a s. of some reagent, in definite strength, used in chemical analysis or testing.

Tyrode s., a modified Locke s.; it contains 8 g of NaCl, 0.2 g of KCl, 0.2 g of $CaCl_2$, 0.1 g of $MgCl_2$, 0.05 g of NaH_2PO_4, 1 g of $NaHCO_3$, 1 g of D-glucose, and water to make 1000 mL; used to irrigate the peritoneal cavity, and in laboratory work.

volumetric s. (VS), a s. made by mixing measured volumes of the components.

Weigert iodine s., an iodine-potassium iodide mixture used as a reagent to alter crystal and methyl violet so that they are retained by certain bacteria and fungi.

sol·vate (sol′vāt). A nonaqueous solution or dispersoid in which there is a noncovalent or easily reversible combination between solvent and solute, or dispersion means and disperse phase; when water is the solvent or dispersion medium, it is called a hydrate.

sol·va·tion (sol-vā′shŭn). Noncovalent or easily reversible combination of a solvent with solute, or of a dispersion means with the disperse phase; if the solvent is water, s. is called hydration. S. affects the size of ions in solution, thus Na^+ is much larger in H_2O than in solid NaCl.

sol·vent. A liquid that holds another substance in solution, i.e., dissolves it. [L. *solvens,* pres. p. of *solvo,* to dissolve]

amphiprotic s., a s. capable of acting as an acid or a base; e.g., H_2O. SEE solvolysis.

fat s.'s, organic liquids notable for their ability to dissolve lipids; usually, but not always, immiscible in water; e.g., diethyl ether, carbon tetrachloride. SYN nonpolar s.'s.

nonpolar s.'s, SYN fat s.'s.

polar s.'s, s.'s that exhibit polar forces on solutes, due to high dipole moment, wide separation of charges, or tight association; e.g., water, alcohols, acids.

universal s., a substance sought by the alchemists, and claimed by some to have been found, supposedly capable of dissolving all substances; sometimes, in a physiological sense, applied to water.

sol·vol·y·sis (sol-vol′ĭ-sis). The reaction of a dissolved salt with the solvent to form an acid and a base; the (partial) reverse of neutralization. If the solvent is water, an amphiprotic solvent, s. is called hydrolysis.

so·ma (sō′mă). **1.** The axial part of the body, i.e., head, neck, trunk, and tail, excluding the limbs. **2.** All of an organism with the exception of the germ cells. SEE ALSO body. **3.** The body of a nerve cell, from which axons, dendrites, etc. project. [G. *sōma,* body]

so·man (sō′man). An extremely potent cholinesterase inhibitor. SEE ALSO sarin, tabun.

so·mas·the·nia (sō-mas-thē′nē-ă). SYN somatasthenia.

△**somat-.** SEE somato-.

so·ma·tag·no·sia (sō′mă-tag-nō′sē-ă). SYN somatotopagnosis. [somat- + G. *a-* priv. + *gnōsis,* recognition]

so·ma·tal·gia (sō-mă-tal′jē-ă). **1.** Pain in the body. **2.** Pain due to organic causes, as opposed to psychogenic pain. [somat- + G. *algos,* pain]

so·ma·tas·the·nia (sō′mă-tas-thē′nē-ă). A condition of chronic physical weakness and fatigability. SYN somasthenia. [somat- + G. *astheneia,* weakness]

so·ma·tes·the·sia (sō′mă-tes-thē′zē-ă). Bodily sensation, the conscious awareness of the body. SYN somesthesia. [somat- + G. *aisthēsis,* sensation]

so·mat·es·the·tic (sō′mat-es-thet′ik). Relating to somatesthesia.

so·mat·ic (sō-mat′ik). **1.** Relating to the soma or trunk, the wall of the body cavity, or the body in general. SYN parietal (2). **2.** Relating to or involving the skeleton or skeletal (voluntary) muscle and the innervation of the latter, as distinct from the viscera or visceral (involuntary) muscle and its (autonomic) innervation. SYN parietal (3). **3.** Relating to the vegetative, as distinguished from the generative, functions. [G. *sōmatikos,* bodily]

so·mat·i·co·splanch·nic (sō-mat-i-kō-splangk′nik). Relating to the body and the viscera. SYN somaticovisceral. [G. *sōmatikos,* relating to the body, + *splanchnikos,* relating to the viscera]

so·mat·i·co·vis·cer·al (sō-mat-i-kō-vis′er-ăl). SYN somaticosplanchnic.

so·ma·tist (sō′mă-tist). An older term for one who considers that neuroses and psychoses are manifestations of organic disease.

so·ma·ti·za·tion (sō′mat-i-zā′shŭn). The process by which psychological needs are expressed in physical symptoms; e.g., the expression or conversion into physical symptoms of anxiety, or a wish for material gain associated with a legal action following an injury, or a related psychological need. SEE ALSO somatization *disorder.*

△**somato-, somat-, somatico-.** The body, bodily. [G. *sōma,* body]

so·ma·to·chrome (sō-mat′ō-krōm). Denoting the group of neurons or nerve cells in which there is an abundance of cytoplasm completely surrounding the nucleus. [somato- + G. *chrōma,* color]

so·ma·to·crin·in (sō′mă-tō-crin′in). Hypothalamic growth releasing hormone, GHRH. [somato- + G. *krinō,* to secrete, + -in]

so·ma·to·gen·ic (sō′mă-tō-jen′ik). **1.** Originating in the soma or body under the influence of external forces. **2.** Having origin in body cells. [somato- + G. *genesis,* origin]

so·ma·to·lib·er·in (sō′mă-tō-lib′er-in). A decapeptide released by the hypothalamus, which induces the release of human growth hormone (somatotropin). SYN growth hormone-releasing factor, growth hormone-releasing hormone, somatotropin-releasing factor, somatotropin-releasing hormone. [somatotropin + L. *libero,* to free, + -in]

so·ma·tol·o·gy (sō-mă-tol′ŏ-jē). The science concerned with the study of the body; includes both anatomy and physiology. [somato- + G. *logos,* study]

so·ma·to·mam·mo·tro·pin (sō′mă-tō-mam′ō-trō-pin). A peptide hormone, closely related to somatotropin in its biologic proper-

ties, produced by the normal placenta and by certain neoplasms. [somato- + L. *mamma,* breast, + G. *tropē,* a turning, + -in]

human chorionic s. (HCS), SYN human placental *lactogen.*

so·ma·to·me·din (sō′mă-tō-mē′din). S. A is a peptide (MW about 4,000), synthesized in the liver and probably in the kidney, that is capable of stimulating certain anabolic processes in bone and cartilage, such as synthesis of DNA, RNA, and protein (including chondromucoprotein), and the sulfation of mucopolysaccharides; secretion and/or biological activity of s. is known to be dependent on somatotropin. SEE ALSO insulinlike growth *factor.* [*somato,* tropin + *med*iator + -in]

so·ma·to·me·dins. SYN insulinlike growth *factor.*

so·ma·tom·e·try (sō-mă-tom′ĕ-trē). Classification of persons according to body form, and relation of the types to physiologic and psychologic characteristics. [somato- + G. *metron,* measure]

so·ma·top·a·gus (sō-mă-top′ă-gŭs). Conjoined twins united in their body regions. SEE conjoined *twins,* under twin. [somato- + G. *pagos,* something fixed]

so·ma·to·path·ic (sō′mă-tō-path′ik). Relating to bodily or organic illness, as distinguished from mental (psychologic) disorder. [somato- + G. *pathos,* suffering]

so·ma·top·a·thy (sō-mă-top′ă-thē). Obsolete term for any disease of the body. [somato- + G. *pathos,* suffering]

somatopause. Decrease in growth hormone–insulinlike growth factor axis activities associated with aging.

so·ma·to·phre·nia (sō′mă-tō-frē′nē-ă). An older term for a tendency to imagine or exaggerate body ills. [somato- + G. *phrēn,* mind]

so·ma·to·plasm (sō-mat′ō-plazm). Aggregate of all the forms of specialized protoplasm entering into the composition of the body, other than germ plasm. [somato- + G. *plasma,* something formed]

so·ma·to·pleure (sō′mă-tō-ploor). Embryonic layer formed by association of the parietal layer of the lateral plate mesoderm with the ectoderm. [somato- + G. *pleura,* side]

so·ma·to·pros·thet·ics (sō′ma-tō-pros-thet′iks). The art and science of prosthetically replacing external parts of the body that are missing or deformed. [somato- + G. *prosthesis,* an addition]

so·ma·to·psy·chic (sō′mă-tō-sī′kik). Relating to the body-mind relationship; the study of the effects of the body upon the mind, as opposed to psychosomatic, which is mind on body. [somato- + G. *psychē,* soul]

so·ma·to·psy·cho·sis (sō′mă-tō-sī-kō′sis). An emotional disorder associated with an organic disease. [somato- + G. *psychōsis,* an animating]

so·ma·tos·co·py (sō-mă-tos′kŏ-pē). Examination of the body. [somato- + G. *skopeō,* to view]

so·ma·to·sen·so·ry (sō-mă-tō-sen′sō-rē). Sensation relating to the body's superficial and deep parts as contrasted to specialized senses such as sight.

so·ma·to·sex·u·al (sō′mă-tō-sek′shoo-ăl). Denoting the somatic aspects of sexuality as distinguished from its psychosexual aspects.

so·ma·to·stat·in (sō′mă-tō-stat′in). A tetradecapeptide capable of inhibiting the release of somatotropin by the anterior lobe of the pituitary gland; s. has a short half-life; it also inhibits the release of insulin and gastrin. SYN growth hormone-inhibiting hormone, somatotropin release-inhibiting factor, somatotropin release-inhibiting hormone. [somatotropin + G. *stasis,* a standing still, + -in]

so·ma·to·stat·i·no·ma (sō′mă-tō-stat-i-nō′mă). A somatostatin-secreting tumor of the pancreatic islets.

so·ma·to·ther·a·py (sō′mă-tō-thār′ă-pē). **1.** Therapy directed at physical disorders. **2.** In psychiatry, a variety of therapeutic interventions employing chemical or physical, as opposed to psychological, methods.

so·ma·to·top·ag·no·sis (sō′mă-tō-top′ag-nō′sis). The inability to identify any part of the body, either one's own or another's body. Cf. autotopagnosia. SYN somatagnosia. [somato- + top- + G. *a-* priv. + G. *gnōsis,* knowledge]

so·ma·to·top·ic (sō-mă-tō-top′ik). Relating to somatotopy.

so·ma·tot·o·py (sō-mă-tot′ō-pē). The topographic association of

SO

positional relationships of receptors in the body via respective nerve fibers to their terminal distribution in specific functional areas of the cerebral cortex; the continuation of these positional relationships in all stages of the ascent of nerve fibers through the central nervous system enables the brain and spinal cord to function on a basis of spatially designated units. [somato- + G. *topos*, place]

so·ma·to·tropes (sō-mă′tō-trōps). A subclass of pituitary acidophilic cells; site of synthesis of growth hormone.

so·ma·to·troph (sō′mat′ō-trof). A cell of the adenohypophysis that produces somatotropin.

so·ma·to·tro·phic (sō′mă-tō-trof′ik). SYN somatotropic. [somato- + G. *trophē*, nourishment]

so·ma·to·tro·pic (sō′mă-tō-trop′ik). Having a stimulating effect on body growth. SYN somatotrophic. [somato- + G. *tropē*, a turning]

so·ma·to·tro·pin (sō′mă-tō-trō′pin). A protein hormone of the anterior lobe of the pituitary, produced by the acidophil cells, that promotes body growth, fat mobilization, and inhibition of glucose utilization; diabetogenic when present in excess; a deficiency of s. is associated with a number of types of dwarfism (type III is an X-linked disorder). SYN growth hormone, pituitary growth hormone, somatotropic hormone. [for *somatotrophin*, fr. somato- + G. *trophē* nourishment; corrupted to *-tropin* and reanalyzed as fr. G. *tropē*, a turning]

so·ma·to·type (sō′mă-tō-tīp). **1.** The constitutional or body type of an individual. **2.** The particular constitutional or body type associated with a particular personality type.

so·ma·to·ty·pol·o·gy (sō′mă-tō-tī-pol′ō-jē). The study of somatotypes. [somato- + G. *typos*, form, + *logos*, study]

so·ma·trem (sō′mă-trem). *N*-L-Methionyl growth hormone (human); a purified polypeptide hormone, made by recombinant DNA techniques, that contains the identical sequence of 191 amino acids constituting naturally occurring somatotropin, plus an additional amino acid, methionine; used in long-term treatment of children deficient in somatotropin.

somatropin (so-ma-trō′pin). A drug identical with human growth hormone; used in the treatment of growth disturbances due to insufficient secretion of growth hormone in children or adults or associated with gonadal dysgenesis (Turner syndrome) and of growth disturbance in prepubertal children with chronic renal insufficiency.

som·es·the·sia (sō-mes-thē′zē-ă). SYN somatesthesia.

so·mite (sō′mīt). One of the paired, metamerically arranged cell masses formed in the early embryonic paraxial mesoderm; commencing in the third or early fourth week in the region of the hindbrain, they develop in a caudal direction typically until 42 pairs are formed. SYN mesoblastic segment. [G. *sōma*, body, + *-ite*]

occipital s., one of the four most rostral s.'s; these become incorporated into the occipital region of the embryonic skull.

som·nam·bu·lance (som-nam′bū-lans). SYN somnambulism (1).

som·nam·bu·lism (som-nam′bū-lizm). **1.** A disorder of sleep involving complex motor acts which occurs primarily during the first third of the night but not during rapid eye movement sleep. SYN oneirodynia activa, sleepwalking, somnambulance. **2.** A form of hysteria in which purposeful behavior is forgotten. [L. *somnus*, sleep, + *ambulo*, to walk]

som·nam·bu·list (som-nam′bū-list). One who is subject to somnambulism (1). SYN sleepwalker.

som·ni·fa·cient (som-ni-fā′shent). SYN soporific (1). [L. *somnus*, sleep, + *facio*, to make]

som·nif·er·ous (som-nif′er-ŭs). SYN soporific (1). [L. *somnus*, sleep, + *fero*, to bring]

som·nif·ic (som-nif′ik). SYN soporific (1).

som·nil·o·quence, som·nil·o·quism (som-nil′ō-kwens, -kwizm). **1.** Talking or muttering in one's sleep. SYN sleeptalking (1). **2.** SYN somniloquy. [L. *somnus*, sleep, + *loquor*, to talk]

som·nil·o·quist (som-nil′ō-kwist). A habitual sleep-talker.

som·nil·o·quy (som-nil′ō-kwē). Talking under the influence of

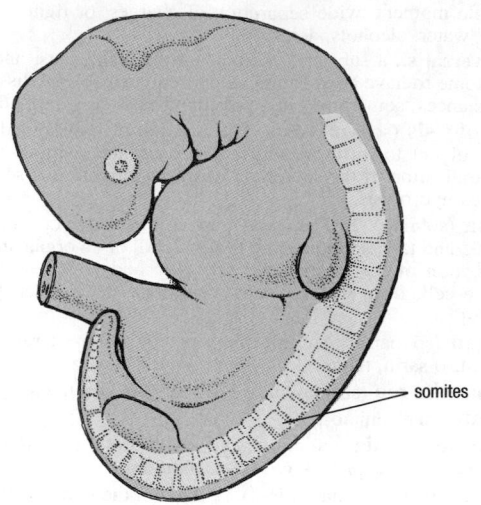

somites: in a 29-day human embryo

hypnotic suggestion. SYN sleeptalking (2), somniloquence (2), somniloquism. [L. *somnus*, sleep, + *loquor*, to speak]

som·no·lence, som·no·len·cy (som′nō-lens, -len-sē). **1.** An inclination to sleep. SYN sleepiness. **2.** A condition of obtusion. SYN somnolentia (1). [L. *somnolentia*]

som·no·lent (som′nō-lent). **1.** Drowsy; sleepy; having an inclination to sleep. **2.** In a condition of incomplete sleep; semicomatose. [L. *somnus*, sleep]

som·no·len·tia (som-nō-len′shē-ă). **1.** SYN somnolence. **2.** SYN sleep *drunkenness*. [L.]

som·no·les·cent (som-nō-les′ent). Inclined to sleep; drowsy.

som·no·lism (som′nō-lizm). SYN hypnotism (1).

Somogyi, Michael, U.S. biochemist, 1883–1971. SEE S. *effect, method, unit.*

Sondermann, R., 20th century German ophthalmologist. SEE S. *canal.*

sone (sōn). A unit of loudness; a pure tone of 1000 Hz at 40 dB above the normal threshold of audibility has a loudness of 1 s. [L. *sonus*, sound]

son·ic (son′ik). Of, pertaining to, or determined by sound; e.g., s. vibration. [L. *sonus*, sound]

son·i·cate (son′i-kāt). To expose a suspension of cells or microbes to the disruptive effect of the energy of high frequency sound waves.

son·i·ca·tion (son-i-kā′shŭn). The process of disrupting biologic materials by use of sound wave energy.

son·i·fi·ca·tion (son′i-fi-kā′shŭn). The production of sound, or of sound waves.

son·i·fi·er (son′i-fī-er). An instrument which produces sound waves, especially those of the frequencies used in sonification procedures.

son·i·fy (son′i-fī). To produce sound.

Sonne, Carl, Danish bacteriologist, 1882–1948.

son·o·chem·is·try (son-ō-kem′is-trē). The branch of chemistry concerned with chemical changes caused by, or involving, sound, particularly ultrasound.

son·o·gram (son′ō-gram). SYN ultrasonogram. [L. *sonus*, sound, + G. *gramma*, a drawing]

son·o·graph (son′ō-graf). SYN ultrasonograph. [L. *sonus*, sound, + G. *graphō*, to write]

so·nog·ra·pher (sŏ-nog′ră-fer). SYN ultrasonographer.

so·nog·ra·phy (sŏ-nog′ră-fī). SYN ultrasonography. [L. *sonus*, sound. + G. *graphō*, to write]

son·o·lu·cent (son-o-lu′sent). In ultrasonography, containing few or no echoes; a misnomer for transonic or anechoic. SEE anechoic. [L. *sonus*, sound + L. *luceo*, to shine]

son·o·mic·rom·e·ter (son'ō-mī-krom'e-ter). An operatively implanted ultrasonic dimension gauge to measure the wall thickening and motion of the heart.

son·o·mo·tor (son-ō-mō'ter). Related to movements caused by sound. SEE sonomotor *response*.

so·phis·ti·cate (sō-fis'ti-kāt). To adulterate. [Mod. L. *sophisticare*, pp. *sophisticatus*, to alter deceptively, fr. G. *sophistikos*, deceitful]

soph·o·re·tin (sof-ŏ-rē'tin). SYN quercetin.

so·por (sō'pōr). An unnaturally deep sleep. [L.]

so·po·rif·er·ous (sō-pōr-if'er-ŭs, sop'ōr-). SYN soporific (1). [L. *soporifer*, fr. *sopor*, deep sleep, + *fero*, to bring]

so·po·rif·ic (sō-pōr-if'ik, sop'ōr-). **1.** Causing sleep. SYN somnifacient, somniferous, somnific, soporiferous. **2.** SYN hypnotic (2). [L. *sopor*, deep sleep, + *facio*, to make]

sop·o·rose, so·po·rous (sō'pŏ-rōs, -rŭs). Relating to or causing an unnaturally deep sleep. [L. *sopor*, deep sleep]

sor·be·fa·cient (sōr-bĕ-fā'shent). **1.** Causing absorption. **2.** An agent that causes or facilitates absorption. [L. *sorbeo*, to suck up, + *facio*, to make]

sor·bic ac·id (sōr'bik). Obtained from berries of the mountain ash, *Sorbus aucuparia* (family Rosaceae), or prepared synthetically; it inhibits growth of yeast and mold and is nearly nontoxic to humans; used as a preservative.

sor·bin (sōr'bin). SYN L-sorbose.

sor·bin·ose (sōr-bin-ōs). SYN L-sorbose.

sor·bi·tan (sōr'bi-tan). Sorbitol or sorbose and related compounds in ester combination with fatty acids and with short oligo (ethylene oxide) side chains and an oleate terminus to form detergents such as polysorbate 80.

sor·bite (sōr'bīt). SYN sorbitol.

sor·bi·tol (sōr'bi-tol). A reduction product of glucose and sorbose found in the berries of the mountain ash, *Sorbus aucuparia* (family Rosaceae), and in many fruits and seaweeds. It has many industrial and pharmaceutical uses; medicinally, it is used as a laxative and as a sweetening agent, and is almost completely metabolized (to CO_2 and H_2O); accumulates in type I diabetes mellitus; elevated levels can cause osmotic damage. SYN sorbite.

D-sor·bi·tol-6-phos·phate de·hy·dro·gen·ase. An oxidoreductase that catalyzes the interconversion of D-sorbitol 6-phosphate and NAD^+ to D-fructose 6-phosphate and NADH. A key step in fructose metabolism in the lens. SYN ketose reductase.

sor·bi·tose (sōr'bi-tōs). SYN L-sorbose.

L-sor·bose (sōr'bōs). A very sweet reducing, but not fermentable, 2-ketohexose obtained from the berries of the mountain ash, *Sorbus aucuparia* (family Rosaceae), and from sorbitol by fermentation with *Acetobacter suboxydans;* L-sorbose is epimeric with D-fructose and is used in the manufacture of vitamin C. SYN sorbin, sorbinose, sorbitose.

sor·des (sōr'dēz). A dark brown or blackish crustlike collection on the lips, teeth, and gums of a person with dehydration associated with a chronic debilitating disease. [L. filth, fr. *sordeo*, to be foul]

sore (sōr). **1.** A wound, ulcer, or any open skin lesion. **2.** Painful; aching; tender. [A.S. *sār*]

bed s., SEE bedsore.

canker s.'s, SYN aphtha (2).

cold s., colloquialism for *herpes* simplex.

Delhi s., SYN Oriental s.

desert s., any of a variety of chronic nonspecific cutaneous ulcers, most commonly on the shins, knees, hands, and forearms, and probably a variant of ecthyma, that occur in tropical and desert areas. SYN veldt s.

hard s., SYN chancre.

Lahore s., SYN Oriental s.

Natal s., lesion of cutaneous leishmaniasis.

Oriental s., SEE cutaneous *leishmaniasis.* SYN Delhi s., Lahore s.

pressure s., SYN decubitus *ulcer.*

soft s., SYN chancroid.

tropical s., SYN tropical *ulcer* (1); SEE cutaneous *leishmaniasis.*

veldt s., SYN desert s.

venereal s., SYN chancroid.

sore·mouth (sōr'mowth). SYN orf.

Sörensen, Sören P.L., Danish chemist, 1868–1939. SEE S. *scale.*

Soret, C., French radiologist, †1931. SEE S. *band, phenomenon.*

so·ro·che (sō-rō'chē). SYN altitude *sickness.* [Sp. (orig. ore, formerly attributed to toxic emanations of ores in mountains)]

chronic s., SYN chronic mountain *sickness.*

sorp·tion (sōrp'shŭn). Adsorption or absorption.

Sorsby, Arnold, British ophthalmologist, 1900–1980. SEE S. macular *degeneration, syndrome.*

s.o.s. Abbreviation for L. *si opus sit,* if needed.

so·ta·lol hy·dro·chlo·ride (sō'tă-lol). A β-receptor blocking agent with uses similar to those of propranolol; also possesses potassium channel blocking properties.

Sotos, J.F., U.S. pediatrician, *1927. SEE S. *syndrome.*

Sottas, Jules, French neurologist, 1866–1943. SEE Dejerine-S. *disease.*

souf·fle (soo'fl). A soft blowing sound heard on auscultation. [Fr. *souffler,* to blow]

cardiac s., a soft puffing heart murmur.

fetal s., a blowing murmur, synchronous with the fetal heart beat, sometimes only systolic and sometimes continuous, heard on auscultation over the pregnant uterus. SYN funic s., funicular s., umbilical s.

funic s., funicular s., SYN fetal s.

mammary s., a blowing murmur heard late in pregnancy and during lactation at the medial border of the breast, sometimes only systolic and sometimes continuous.

placental s., SYN uterine s.

umbilical s., SYN fetal s.

uterine s., a blowing sound, synchronous with the cardiac systole of the mother, heard on auscultation of the pregnant uterus. SYN placental s.

Soulier, Jean Pierre, French hematologist, 1915–1985. SEE Bernard-S. *disease, syndrome.*

sound (sownd). **1.** The vibrations produced by a sounding body, transmitted by the air or other medium, and perceived by the internal ear. **2.** An elongated cylindrical, usually curved, instrument of metal, used for exploring the bladder or other cavities of the body, for dilating strictures of the urethra, esophagus, or other canal, for calibrating the lumen of a body cavity, or for detecting the presence of a foreign body in a body cavity. **3.** To explore or calibrate a cavity with a s. **4.** Whole; healthy; not diseased or injured.

adventitious breath s.'s, s.'s heard by auscultation of abnormal lungs. SEE ALSO rale, rhonchus, crackle, crepitation, wheeze, rub, crunch.

after-s., SEE aftersound.

amphoric voice s., SEE amphoric *voice.*

anvil s., SYN bellmetal *resonance.*

atrial s., SYN fourth heart s.

auscultatory s., a rale, murmur, bruit, fremitus, or other s. heard on auscultation of the chest or abdomen.

bell s., SYN bellmetal *resonance.*

bowel s.'s, relatively high-pitched abdominal s.'s caused by propulsion of intestinal contents through the lower alimentary tract.

breath s.'s, a murmur, bruit, fremitus, rhonchus, or rale heard on auscultation over the lungs or any part of the respiratory tract. SYN respiratory s.'s.

bronchial breath s.'s, loud, high-pitched, hollow-toned breath s.'s heard by auscultation mainly over the sternum; when heard elsewhere in the chest they may indicate consolidated lung or another pathologic condition.

bronchovesicular breath s.'s, s.'s intermediate between bronchial and vesicular breath s.'s; they can be abnormal, but are normal when heard between the 1st and 2nd intercostal spaces anteriorly and posteriorly between scapulae.

SO

Campbell s., a miniature s. with a short round-tipped beak, especially curved for the deep urethra of the young male.

cannon s., SYN *bruit* de canon.

cardiac s., SYN heart s.'s.

cavernous voice s., SEE cavernous *voice*.

coconut s., a s. like that produced when a cracked coconut is tapped; it is elicited by percussing the skull of a patient with osteitis deformans.

complex s., a s. composed of a number of sounds of different frequencies.

cracked-pot s., SYN cracked-pot *resonance*.

Davis interlocking s., a s. comprised of two instruments with curved male and female tips, used to introduce a catheter into the bladder in the treatment of ruptured urethra; the male s. is introduced into the distal urethra via the meatus and the female s. is passed downward through the bladder neck into the proximal urethra via an open cystotomy; the ends of the two instruments are engaged, with the female s. guiding the male s. upward into the bladder; a catheter is then sutured to the tip of the male s. and withdrawn through the urethra to restore continuity of its lumen.

double-shock s., SYN *bruit* de rappel.

eddy s.'s, s.'s that punctuate the continuous murmur of patent ductus arteriosus, imparting to it a characteristically "uneven" quality.

ejection s.'s, click-like s.'s during ejection from a hypertensive aorta or pulmonary artery or associated with stenosis (particularly congenital) of the aortic or pulmonic valve.

first heart s. (S_1), occurs with ventricular systole and is mainly produced by closure of the atrioventricular valves.

fourth heart s. (S_4), the s. produced in late diastole in association with ventricular filling due to atrial systole and related to reduced ventricular compliance. It is a low frequency oscillation that may be normal at older ages owing to a physiologic decline in ventricular compliance but is nearly always abnormal at younger ages if it is of high intensity or palpable. It is common in ventricular hypertrophy, particularly with hypertension, and is almost invariable during acute myocardial infarction. Fourth heart s.'s may arise from the right or left ventricle or both. SYN atrial s.

friction s., the s., heard on auscultation, made by the rubbing of two opposed serous surfaces roughened by an inflammatory exudate, or, if chronic, by nonadhesive fibrosis. SYN friction murmur, friction rub.

gallop s., the abnormal third or fourth heart s. which, when added to the first and second s.'s, produces the triple cadence of gallop rhythm. SEE ALSO gallop.

heart s.'s, the noise made by muscle contraction and the closure of the heart valves during the cardiac cycle. SEE first heart s., second heart s., third heart s., fourth heart s. SYN cardiac s., heart tones.

hippocratic succussion s., a splashing s. elicited by shaking a patient with hydro- or pyopneumothorax, the physician's ear being applied to the chest.

Jewett s., a short straight s. for dilating the anterior urethra.

Korotkoff s.'s, s.'s heard over an artery when pressure over it is reduced below systolic arterial pressure, as when blood pressure is determined by the auscultatory method.

Le Fort s., a curved s. threaded for a filiform bougie, used for dilation of urethral strictures in the male when small caliber or presence of false passages prevents safe passage of a standard s. or catheter.

McCrea s., a gently curved s. used to dilate the urethra in infants or children.

Mercier s., a catheter the beak of which is short and bent almost at a right angle.

muscle s., a noise heard on auscultation over the belly of a contracting muscle.

percussion s., any s. elicited on percussing over one of the cavities of the body.

pericardial friction s., a to-and-fro grating, rasping, or, rarely, creaking s. heard over the heart in some cases of pericarditis, due to rubbing of the inflamed pericardial surfaces as the heart contracts and relaxes; during normal sinus rhythm it is usually triphasic; during any rhythm it may be biphasic or uniphasic. SYN pericardial rub, pericardial friction rub.

pistol-shot s., s. created by lightly compressing an artery during aortic regurgitation; sometimes is audible without compression.

pistol-shot femoral s., a shotlike systolic s. heard over the femoral artery in high output states, especially aortic insufficiency; presumably due to sudden stretching of the elastic wall of the artery; pistol-shot s.'s may also be heard over other relatively large arteries, e.g., brachial, radial.

posttussis suction s., a s. produced by the falling back of a drop of mucus or pus into a pulmonary cavity after the latter has been emptied by coughing.

respiratory s.'s, SYN breath s.'s.

sail s., a s., likened to the snapping of a sail; the abnormal first heart s. in some patients with Ebstein anomaly.

Santini booming s., a sonorous booming s. heard on auscultatory percussion of a hydatid cyst.

second s., SYN second heart s.

second heart s. (S_2), the second s. heard on auscultation of the heart; signifies the beginning of diastole and is due to closure of the semilunar valves. SYN second s.

Simpson uterine s., a slender flexible metal rod used to calibrate or dilate the cervical canal, or to hold the uterus in various positions during gynecologic surgery.

Sims uterine s., a slender flexible s. with a small projection about 7 cm from its tip, used to estimate the size and caliber of the uterine cavity.

splitting of heart s.'s, the production of major components of the first and second heart s.'s (rarely the third and fourth) due to contribution by the left-sided and right-sided valves; thus, the first heart s. would have a mitral and a tricuspid component and the second heart s. an aortic and pulmonic component. The latter are best appreciated during respiration, with inspiration delaying the pulmonic component and producing an earlier aortic component.

succussion s., the noise made by fluid with overlying air when shaken, such as occurs with gastric dilation or with fluid and air in a pleural cavity (hydropneumothorax).

tambour s., SYN *bruit* de tambour.

third s., SYN third heart s.

third heart s. (S_3), occurs in early diastole and corresponds with the end of the first phase of rapid ventricular filling; normal in children and younger people but abnormal in others. SYN third s.

tic-tac s.'s, SYN embryocardia.

to-and-fro s., doubling of an abnormal murmur usually in systole and diastole and formerly applied to pericardial rubs.

tracheal breath s.'s, loud, harsh, hollow breath s.'s usually heard only over the neck.

van Buren s., a standard s., available in several calibers, with a gently curved tip designed to follow the contour of the bulbous urethra in the male; used for urethral calibration or dilation.

vesicular breath s.'s, the gentle rustling s.'s of normal breathing heard by auscultation over most of the lung fields; the inspiratory phase is usually longer than the expiratory.

waterwheel s., s. made by cardiac motion inducing splashes in the presence of fluid and air within the pericardial sac.

water-whistle s., a bubbling whistle heard on auscultation over a bronchial or pulmonary fistula.

Winternitz s., a double-current catheter in which water at any desired temperature circulates.

xiphisternal crunching s., SEE Hamman *sign*.

Southern, M.E., 20th century British biologist. SEE Southern blot *analysis*.

Southey, Reginald, English physician, 1835–1899. SEE S. *tubes*, under *tube*.

soy·a (soy′ă). SYN soybean. [Hind. *soyā*, fennel]

soy·bean (soy′bēn). The bean of the climbing herb *Glycine soja* or *G. hispida* (family Leguminosae); a bean rich in protein and containing little starch; it is the source of s. oil; s. flour is used in preparing a bread for diabetics, in feeding formulas for infants who are unable to tolerate cow's milk, and for adults allergic to cow's milk. SYN soja, soya. [Hind. *soyā*, fennel]

s. oil, obtained from s.'s by expression or solvent extraction; contains triglycerides of linoleic acid, oleic acid, linolenic acid, and saturated fatty acids; used as a food and in the manufacture of margarine and other food products.

SP Abbreviation for sacroposterior *position*.

SP1 Abbreviation for stimulatory *protein* 1.

sp. Abbreviation for species; pl. form is spp. [*L. spiritus, spirit.*]

spa (spah). A health resort, especially one where there are one or more mineral springs whose waters possess therapeutic properties. [*Spa,* a mineral spring health resort in Belgium]

SPACE

space (spās) [TA]. Any demarcated portion of the body, either an area of the surface, a segment of the tissues, or a cavity. SEE ALSO area, region, zone. SYN spatium [TA]. [*L. spatium,* room, space]

alveolar dead s., the difference between physiologic dead s. and anatomic dead s.; it represents that part of the physiologic dead s. resulting from ventilation of relatively underperfused or nonperfused alveoli; it differs specifically in being placed so as to fill and empty in parallel with functional alveoli, rather than being interposed in the conducting tubes between functional alveoli and the external environment.

anatomic dead s., the volume of the conducting airways from the external environment (at the nose and mouth) down to the level at which inspired gas exchanges oxygen and carbon dioxide with pulmonary capillary blood; formerly presumed to extend down to the beginning of alveolar epithelium in the respiratory bronchioles, but more recent evidence indicates that effective gas exchange extends some distance up the thicker-walled conducting airways because of rapid longitudinal mixing. Cf. alveolar dead s., physiologic dead s. SYN anatomic airway.

antecubital s., SYN cubital *fossa.*

anterior clear s., SYN retrosternal s.

apical s., the s. between the alveolar wall and the apex of the root of a tooth where an alveolar abscess usually has its origin.

axillary s., SYN axilla.

Berger s., the s. between the patellar fossa of the vitreous and the lens.

Bogros s., SYN retroinguinal s.

Böttcher s., SYN endolymphatic *sac.*

Bowman s., SYN capsular s.

Burns s., SYN suprasternal s.

capsular s., the slitlike s. between the visceral and parietal layers of the capsule of the renal corpuscle; it opens into the proximal tubule of the nephron at the neck of the tubule. SYN Bowman s., filtration s.

cartilage s., SYN cartilage *lacuna.*

cavernous s. [TA], an anatomic cavity with many interconnecting chambers. SYN cavern, caverna.

cavernous s.'s of corpora cavernosa [TA], the vascular s.'s of the corpora cavernosa that, together with the intervening fibrous trabeculae, form the erectile tissue of the penis or clitoris. SYN cavernae corporum cavernosorum [TA], caverns of corpora cavernosa, cavities of corpora cavernosa.

cavernous s.'s of corporus spongiosum [TA], the vascular s.'s forming the erectile tissue of the corpus spongiosum penis in the male and the bulb of the vestibule in the female. SYN cavernae corporis spongiosi [TA], caverns of corpus spongiosum, cavities of corpus spongiosum.

central palmar s., the more medial of the central palmar s.'s, bounded medially by the hypothenar compartment; related distally to the synovial tendon sheaths of digits 3 and 4 and proximally to the common flexor sheath. SYN medial midpalmar s., middle palmar s.

Chassaignac s., potential s. between the pectoralis major and the mammary gland.

Cloquet s., a s. between the ciliary zonule and the vitreous body.

Colles s., SYN superficial perineal s.

corneal s., one of the stellate s.'s between the lamellae of the cornea, each of which contains a cell or corneal corpuscle. SYN lacuna (4).

Cotunnius s., SYN endolymphatic *sac.*

(cranial) extradural s. [TA], s. between the cranial bones and the external periosteal layer of the dura; it becomes an actual s. only pathologically, as when as extra- or epidural hemorrhage occurs forming a hematoma.

dead s., (1) a cavity, potential or real, remaining after the closure of a wound that is not obliterated by the operative technique; (2) SEE anatomic dead s., physiologic dead s.

deep perineal s., the region immediately superior to the perineal membrane, occupied by the membranous part of the urethra, the bulbourethral gland (in the male), the deep transverse perineal and sphincter urethrae muscles, and the dorsal nerve and artery of the penis or clitoris. SYN deep perineal pouch, spatium perinei profundum.

denture s., (1) that portion of the oral cavity which is, or may be, occupied by maxillary and/or mandibular denture(s); (2) the s. between the residual ridges which is available for dentures. SEE ALSO interarch *distance.*

disk s., on radiographs of the spine, the radiolucent region between each pair of vertebral bodies.

Disse s., SYN perisinusoidal s.

s. of Donders, the s. between the dorsum of the tongue and the hard palate when the mandible is in rest position following the expiratory cycle of respiration.

endolymphatic s. [TA], endolymph-filled space contained by the membranous labyrinth. SYN spatium endolympha'ticum [TA].

epidural s., the space between the walls of the vertebral canal and the dura mater of the spinal cord. SYN extradural s. [TA], spatium extradurale [TA], spatium extradura'le*, cavum epidurale, epidural cavity.

episcleral s. [TA], the s. between the fascial sheath of the eyeball and the sclera. SYN spatium episclerale [TA], interfascial s., spatium interfasciale, spatium intervaginale bulbi oculi, Tenon s.

epitympanic s., SYN epitympanic *recess.*

extradural s. [TA], SYN epidural s.

extraperitoneal s. [TA], loose areolar s. (potential only in many places) or plane immediately external to the peritoneum; in surgery, this plane enables dissection within the body wall but external to the peritoneum. SEE ALSO retroperitoneal s. SYN spatium extraperitonea'le [TA].

filtration s., SYN capsular s.

Fontana s.'s, SYN s.'s of iridocorneal angle.

freeway s., the s. between the occluding surfaces of the maxillary and mandibular teeth when the mandible is in physiologic resting position. SYN interocclusal clearance, interocclusal distance (2), interocclusal gap, interocclusal rest s. (2).

gingival s., SYN gingival *sulcus.*

haversian s.'s, s.'s in bone formed by the enlargement of haversian canals.

Henke s., SYN retropharyngeal s.

His perivascular s., SYN Virchow-Robin s.

infraglottic s., SYN infraglottic *cavity.*

interalveolar s., SYN interarch *distance.*

intercostal s. [TA], an interval between the ribs, occupied by intercostal muscles, veins, arteries, and nerves. SYN spatium intercostale [TA].

interfascial s., SYN episcleral s.

interglobular s., one of a number of irregularly branched spaces near the periphery of the dentin of the crown of a tooth, through which pass the ramifications of the tubules; they are caused by failure of calcification of the dentin. SYN interglobular s. of Owen, spatium interglobulare.

interglobular s. of Owen, SYN interglobular s.

intermembrane s., the s. between the two membranes in a cell or organelle enclosed by a double biomembrane; e.g., the space

sp

between the inner and outer membranes of the mitochondria; sometimes referred to as the external matrix.

interocclusal rest s., (1) SYN interocclusal *distance* (1); (2) SYN freeway s.

interosseous metacarpal s.'s [TA], the s.'s between the metacarpal bones in the hand. SYN spatia interossea metacarpi [TA].

interosseous metatarsal s.'s [TA], the s.'s between the metatarsal bones in the foot. SYN spatia interossea metatarsi [TA].

interpleural s., SYN mediastinum (2).

interproximal s., the s. between adjacent teeth in a dental arch; it is divided into the embrasure occlusal to the contact area, and the septal s. gingival to the contact area.

interradicular s., the s. between the roots of multirooted teeth.

interseptovalvular s., the interval in the developing embryonic heart between the septum primum and the left valve of the sinus venosus.

intersheath s.'s of optic nerve, SYN intervaginal subarachnoid s. of optic nerve.

intervaginal subarachnoid s. of optic nerve [TA], the s.'s within the internal sheath of the optic nerve, between the arachnoidal and pial layers, filled with cerebrospinal fluid and continuous with the subarachnoid s. SYN spatium intervaginale subarachnoidale nervi optici [TA], intersheath s.'s of optic nerve, Schwalbe s.'s.

intervillous s.'s, the s.'s containing maternal blood, located between placental villi; they are lined with syncytiotrophoblast.

intraretinal s., the potential cleft between the pigmented and neural layers of the retina; it represents the cavity of the embryonic optic vesicle; retinal detachment occurs by the opening of this s.

s.'s of iridocorneal angle [TA], irregularly shaped endothelium-lined s.'s within the trabecular reticulum, through which the aqueous filters to reach the sinus venosus sclerae. SYN spatia anguli iridocornealis [TA], ciliary canals, Fontana s.'s.

Kiernan s., interlobular s. in the liver.

Kretschmann s., a slight depression in the epitympanic recess below the superior recess of the tympanic membrane.

Kuhnt s.'s, shallow diverticula or recesses between the ciliary body and ciliary zonule that open into the posterior chamber of the eye.

lateral central palmar s., the more lateral (radial) of the central palmar s.'s, bounded laterally by the thenar compartment; related distally to the synovial tendon sheath of the index finger and proximally to the common flexor sheath. SYN lateral midpalmar s., thenar s.

lateral midpalmar s., SYN lateral central palmar s.

lateral pharyngeal s. [TA], that part of the peripharyngeal space located at the sides of the pharynx. SYN spatium lateropharyngeum [TA], spatium pharyngeum laterale [TA].

leeway s., the difference between the combined mesiodistal widths of the deciduous cuspids and molars and their successors.

leptomeningeal s., SYN subarachnoid s. SYN spatium leptomeningeum [TA].

lymph s., a s., in tissue or a vessel, filled with lymph.

Magendie s.'s, s.'s between the pia and arachnoid at the level of the fissures of the brain.

Malacarne s., SYN posterior perforated *substance*.

masticator s., a s. subtended by the superficial layer of the deep cervical fascia that splits into lateral and medial slings at the inferior border of the mandible to enclose the masseter muscle, part of the temporalis muscle, and the medial and pterygoid muscles before attaching to the zygomatic arch and base of the skull.

Meckel s., SYN trigeminal *cave*.

medial midpalmar s., SYN central palmar s.

mediastinal s., SYN mediastinum (2).

medullary s., the central cavity and the cellular intervals between the trabeculae of bone, filled with marrow.

middle palmar s., SYN central palmar s.

midpalmar s., either of the two central palmar s.'s (medial or lateral).

Mohrenheim s., SYN infraclavicular *fossa*.

muscular s. of retroinguinal compartment [TA], the lateral compartment beneath the inguinal (Poupart) ligament, for the passage of the iliopsoas muscle and femoral nerve; it is separated by the iliopectineal arch from the vascular lacuna. SYN lacuna musculorum retroinguinalis, lacuna musculorum, muscular lacuna.

Nuel s., an interval in the spiral organ (of Corti) between the outer pillar cells on one side and the phalangeal cells and hair cells on the other.

paraglottic s., the s. on each side of the glottis bounded laterally by the perichondrium of the thyroid cartilage and the cricothyroid membrane and posteriorly by the mucous membrane of the pyriform sinus; anterosuperiorly it extends into the preepiglottic space. It is an important route of transglottic and extralaryngeal spread of carcinoma of the larynx.

parapharyngeal s. [TA], SYN pharyngomaxillary s. SYN spatium parapharyngeum.

Parona s., a s. between the pronator quadratus deep and the overlying flexor tendons of the forearm which is continuous through the carpal tunnel with the medial central palmar space.

parotid s., a deep hollow on the side of the face flanking the posterior aspect of the ramus of the mandible with its attached muscles that is occupied by the parotid gland; it is lined with fascial laminae (the parotid sheath) derived from the investing layer of deep cervical fascia; the structures bounding the s. collectively constitute the parotid bed. Surgeons operating in the area take advantage of the fact that the anteroposterior dimensions of the parotid s. increase with protrusion of the mandible. SYN bed of parotid gland, parotid recess, recessus parotideus.

perforated s., SEE anterior perforated *substance*, posterior perforated *substance*.

perichoroid s., SYN perichoroidal s.

perichoroidal s. [TA], the interval between the choroid and the sclera filled by the loose meshes of the lamina fusca of sclera and the suprachoroid lamina. SYN spatium perichoroideum [TA], perichoroid s.

perilymphatic s. [TA], space between the bony and membranous portions of the labyrinth. SYN spatium perilymphaticum [TA], cisterna perilymphatica.

perineal s.'s, SEE deep perineal s., superficial perineal s.

perinuclear s., SYN cisterna caryothecae.

peripharyngeal s. [TA], the s., filled with loose areolar tissue, around the pharynx; it is divided into two portions, parapharyngeal (lateral pharyngeal) s. and retropharyngeal s. SYN spatium peripharyngeum [TA].

periportal s. of Mall, a tissue s. between the limiting lamina and the portal canal in the liver.

perisinusoidal s., the potential extravascular s. between the liver sinusoids and liver parenchymal cells. SYN Disse s.

perivitelline s., the s. between the vitelline membrane and the zona pellucida, appearing in an ovum immediately following fertilization.

personal s., a term used in the behavioral sciences to denote the physical area immediately surrounding an individual who is in proximity to one or more others, whether known or unknown, and which serves as a body buffer zone in such interpersonal transactions.

pharyngeal s., the area occupied by the pharynx (naso-, oro-, and laryngopharynx). Not to be confused with the retropharyngeal s.

pharyngomaxillary s., the s. limited by the lateral wall of the pharynx, the cervical vertebrae, and the medial pterygoid muscle. SYN parapharyngeal s. [TA].

physiologic dead s. (V_D), unthe sum of anatomic and alveolar dead s.; the dead s. calculated when the carbon dioxide pressure in systemic arterial blood is used instead of that of alveolar gas in the Bohr equation; it is a virtual or apparent volume that takes into account the impairment of gas exchange because of uneven distributions of lung ventilation and perfusion.

plantar s., one of four areas between fascial layers in the foot, where pus may be confined when the foot is infected.

pleural s., SYN pleural *cavity*.

pneumatic s., any one of the paranasal sinuses.

Poiseuille s., SYN still *layer*.

popliteal s., SYN popliteal *fossa*.

postpharyngeal s., SYN retropharyngeal s.

preepiglottic s., the s. anterior to the epiglottis that is bounded anteriorly by the thyrohyoid membrane and the superior parts of the lamina of the thyroid cartilage, superiorly by the hyoepiglottic ligament and inferiorly by the thyroepiglottic ligament; laterally it extends into the paraglottic s.'s. Carcinoma of the infrahyoid portion of the epiglottis often extends into the preepiglottic s.

Proust s., SYN rectovesical *pouch*.

Prussak s., SYN superior *recess* of tympanic membrane.

pterygomandibular s., the area between the mandibular ramus and the pterygoid process of the sphenoid bone.

quadrangular s., musculotendinous formation providing passageway for the axillary nerve, posterior humeral circumflex artery, and accompanying veins as they run from the axilla to the superior posterior arm; as the neurovascular structures enter the formation anteriorly, it is bounded superiorly by the shoulder joint, medially by the lateral border of subscapularis, laterally by the surgical neck of the humerus, and inferiorly by the tendon of latissimus dorsi; where the vessels exit the formation posteriorly, it is bounded superiorly by the teres minor, medially by the long head of the triceps, laterally by the lateral head of the triceps and inferiorly by the teres major muscle or tendon; as they emerge, most of the neurovascular structures run on the deep surface of the deltoid muscle, which they supply. SYN quadrilateral s.

quadrilateral s., SYN quadrangular s.

Reinke s., a potential s. between the lamina propria and the external elastic lamina of the vocal fold. Edema in this s. produces hoarseness in chronic inflammation.

respiratory dead s., that part of the respiratory tract or of a single breath which fails to exchange oxygen and carbon dioxide with pulmonary capillary blood; a nonspecific term which fails to distinguish between anatomical dead s. and physiologic dead s.

retroadductor s., potential s. between the adductor pollicis and first dorsal interosseous muscles.

retroinguinal s. [TA], a triangular s. between the peritoneum and the transversalis fascia, at the lower angle of which is the inguinal ligament; it contains the lower portion of the external iliac artery. SYN spatium retroinguinale [TA], Bogros s.

retromylohyoid s., the sulcus at the posterior end of the mylohyoid line.

retroperitoneal s. [TA], the s. between the parietal peritoneum and the muscles and bones of the posterior abdominal wall. SYN spatium retroperitoneale [TA], retroperitoneum.

retropharyngeal s. [TA], that part of the peripharyngeal s. located posterior to the pharynx. SYN spatium retropharyngeum [TA], Henke s., postpharyngeal s.

retropubic s. [TA], the area of loose connective tissue between the bladder with its related fascia and the pubis and anterior abdominal wall. SYN spatium retropubicum [TA], cavum retzii, Retzius cavity, Retzius s.

retrosternal s., on lateral chest radiographs, the region dorsal to the sternum and ventral to the ascending aorta. SYN anterior clear s.

retrozonular s. [TA], potential s. of the chamber of the eyeball immediately posterior to the zonule and anterior to the vitreous body. SYN spatium retrozonulare [TA].

Retzius s., SYN retropubic s.

Schwalbe s.'s, SYN intervaginal subarachnoid s. of optic nerve.

(spinal) epidural space [TA], fat-filled s. immediately external to the dura mater ensheathing the spinal cord; contains the internal vertebral (epidural) venous plexus, and is the target site for epidural anesthesia. SYN spatium peridurale★.

subarachnoid s. [TA], the s. between the arachnoidea and pia mater, traversed by delicate fibrous trabeculae and filled with cerebrospinal fluid. Since the pia mater immediately adheres to the surface of the brain and spinal cord, the s. is greatly widened wherever the brain surface exhibits a deep depression (e.g., between the cerebellum and medulla); such widenings are called cisternae. The large blood vessels supplying the brain and spinal cord lie in the subarachnoid s. SYN spatium subarachnoideum

[TA], cavum subarachnoideum, leptomeningeal s., subarachnoid cavity.

subchorial s., the part of the placenta adjacently beneath the chorionic plate; it joins with irregular channels to form the marginal lakes. SYN subchorial lake.

subdural s. [TA], originally thought to be a narrow fluid-filled interval between the dural and arachnoid; now known to be an artificial s. created by the separation of the arachnoid from the dura as the result of trauma or some ongoing pathologic process; in the healthy state, the arachnoid is lightly attached to the dura (maintained in that position by the pressure of the cerebrospinal fluid) and a naturally occurring subdural s. is not present. SYN spatium subdurale [TA], cavum subdurale, subdural cavity, subdural cleavage, subdural cleft.

subgingival s., SYN gingival *sulcus*.

subhepatic s. [TA], the part of the peritoneal cavity between the visceral surface of the liver and the transverse colon. SYN recessus subhepaticus [TA], subhepatic recess.

subphrenic s. [TA], the recesses in the peritoneal cavity between the anterior part of the liver and the diaphragm, separated into right and left by the falciform ligament. SYN recessus subphrenicus [TA], subphrenic recesses, suprahepatic s.'s.

superficial perineal s. [TA], the superficial compartment of the perineum; the s. bounded superiorly by the perineal membrane (formerly the now obsolete inferior fascia of the urogenital diaphragm) and inferiorly by the superficial perineal (Colles) fascia; it contains the root structure of the penis or clitoris and associated musculature, plus the superficial transverse perineal muscle and, in the female only, the greater vestibular glands. SYN spatium perinei superficiale [TA], Colles s., superficial perineal pouch.

suprahepatic s.'s, SYN subphrenic s.

suprasternal s. [TA], a narrow interval between the deep and superficial layers of the cervical fascia above the manubrium of the sternum through which pass the anterior jugular veins. SYN spatium supraspinale [TA], Burns s.

Tarin s., SYN interpeduncular *cistern*.

Tenon s., SYN episcleral s.

thenar s., SYN lateral central palmar s.

Traube semilunar s., a crescentic s. about 12 cm wide, bounded medially by the left border of the sternum, above by an oblique line from the sixth costal cartilage to the lower border of the eighth or ninth rib in the midaxillary line and below by the costal margin; the percussion tone here is normally tympanitic, because of the underlying stomach, but is modified by pulmonary emphysema, a pleural effusion, or an enlarged spleen.

Trautmann triangular s., the area of the temporal bone bounded by the sigmoid sinus, the superior petrosal sinus, and a tangent to the posterior semicircular canal.

vascular s. of retroinguinal compartment [TA], the medial compartment beneath the inguinal ligament, for the passage to the femoral vessels; it is separated from the muscular s. by the iliopectineal arch. SYN lacuna vasorum retroinguinalis [TA], lacuna vasorum, vascular lacuna.

vertebral epidural s., SEE spinal *dura mater*.

Virchow-Robin s., a tunnel-like extension of the subarachnoid s. surrounding blood vessels that pass into the brain or spinal cord from the subarachnoid s.; the lining of the channel is composed of pia and glial feet of astrocytes; a continuation of the s. around capillaries and nerve cells probably does not occur. SYN His perivascular s.

Waldeyer s., SYN Waldeyer *sheath*.

Westberg s., the s. surrounding the origin of the aorta which is invested with the pericardium.

zonular s.'s [TA], the s.'s between the fibers of the ciliary zonule at the equator of the lens of the eye. SYN spatia zonularia [TA], Petit canals.

---

spacing (spā′sing). Making or arranging spaces, especially at intervals.

third spacing, loss of extracellular fluid from the vascular to other body compartments.

spa·gyr·ic (spă-jir′ik). Relating to the paracelsian or alchemical system of medicine, which stressed the treatment of disease by various types of chemical substances. [G. *spaō,* to tear open, + *ageirō,* to collect]

spag·y·rist (spaj′ĭ-rist). A physician of the 16th century, a follower of the teachings of Paracelsus who believed in the essential importance of chemical or alchemical knowledge in the understanding and treatment of disease.

spall (spawl). 1. A fragment. 2. To break up into fragments.

Spallanzani, Lazaro, Italian priest and scientist, 1729–1799. SEE S. *law.*

spall·a·tion (spaw-lā′shŭn). 1. SYN fragmentation. 2. Nuclear reaction in which nuclei, on being bombarded by high energy particles, liberate a number of protons and alpha particles. [M.E. *spalle,* fragment]

span. The amount, distance, or length between two points; the full extent or reach of anything.

   attention s., the length of time a person can concentrate on a subject.

   memory s., the maximum number of items recalled after a single presentation (auditory or visual).

spar·ga·no·ma (spar-gă-nō′mă). A localized mass resulting from sparganosis.

spar·ga·no·sis (spar-gă-nō′sis). Infection with the plerocercoid or sparganum of a pseudophyllidean tapeworm, usually in a dermal sore resulting from application of infected flesh as a poultice; infection may also occur from ingestion of uncooked frog, snake, mammal, or bird intermediate or transport host bearing the spargana, but not from fish with *Diphyllobothrium* larvae, since s. is an infection with nonhuman pseudophyllidean tapeworms, usually species of *Spirometra.* S. may also develop from ingestion of water containing procercoid-infected *Cyclops.*

   ocular s., infestation of the orbits with the sparganum of *Spirometra mansoni;* characterized by redness and edema of the eyelids, lacrimation, and blepharoptosis; acquired by application of infected raw frog flesh against the eye as a poultice.

spar·ga·num (spar′gă-nŭm). Originally described as a genus, but now restricted to the plerocercoid stage of certain tapeworms. [G. *sparganon,* a swathing band, fr. *spargō,* to swathe]

spar·te·ine (spar′tē-ēn, -tē-in). An alkaloid obtained from scoparius, *Cytisus scoparius* and *Lupinus luteus;* s. sulfate was used as an oxytocic drug. SYN lupinidine.

spasm (spazm). A sudden involuntary contraction of one or more muscles; includes cramps, contractures. SYN muscle s., spasmus. [G. *spasmos*]

   s. of accommodation, excessive contraction of the ciliary muscle.

   affect s.'s, rarely used term for spasmodic attacks of laughing, weeping, and screaming, accompanied by marked tachypnea.

   anorectal s., SYN *proctalgia* fugax.

   Bell s., SYN facial *tic.*

   cadaveric s., rigor mortis occurring irregularly in the different muscles, causing movements of the limbs.

   canine s., SYN *risus* caninus.

   carpopedal s., s. of the feet and hands observed in hyperventilation, calcium deprivation, and tetany: flexion of the hands at the wrists and of the fingers at the metacarpophalangeal joints and extension of the fingers at the phalangeal joints; the feet are dorsiflexed at the ankles and the toes plantar flexed.

   diffuse esophageal s., abnormal contraction of the muscular wall of the esophagus causing pain and dysphagia, often in response to regurgitation of acid gastric contents.

   epidemic transient diaphragmatic s., SYN epidemic *pleurodynia.*

   epileptic s., s. characterized by a sudden flexion-extension, or mixed extension-flexion, predominantly proximal (including truncal muscles), which is usually more sustained than a myoclonic movement but not as sustained as a tonic seizure. Occurs frequently in clusters, with the individual events ranging in duration from myoclonic to tonic seizure components.

   esophageal s., a disorder of the motility of the esophagus characterized by pain or forceful eructations after swallowing food. Esophageal muscle contractions are of excessive force and dura-

tion. Chest pain can be confused with symptoms of cardiac or other origin.

   facial s., SYN facial *tic.*

   habit s., SYN tic.

   hemifacial s., a facial nerve disorder, with onset in late adult life, characterized by episodes of irregular, sometimes painful, myoclonic contractions of various facial muscles; triggered by voluntary or reflex movements of the face, s. typically begins in the orbicularis oculi muscle and then spreads; occasionally a sequela of Bell palsy, but more often the result of proximal compression of the facial nerve by an aberrant blood vessel or neoplasm.

   infantile s., brief (1–3 seconds) muscular s.'s in infants with West syndrome, which often appear as nodding or salaam s.'s. SYN salaam convulsions.

   intention s., a spasmodic contraction of the muscles occurring when a voluntary movement is attempted.

   masticatory s., involuntary convulsive muscular contraction affecting the muscles of mastication.

   mobile s., a tonic s. occurring in spastic infantile hemiplegia on attempted movement.

   muscle s., SYN spasm.

   nictitating s., involuntary spasmodic winking. SYN spasmus nictitans, winking s.

   nodding s., (1) in infants, a drop of the head on the chest due to loss of tone in the neck muscles as in epilepsia nutans, or to tonic spasm of anterior neck muscles as in West syndrome; (2) in adults, a nodding of the head from clonic s.'s of the sternomastoid muscles. SYN salaam attack, salaam s., spasmus nutans (1).

   salaam s., SYN nodding s.

   saltatory s., a spasmodic affection of the muscles of the lower extremities. SYN Bamberger disease (1), Gowers disease (1).

   winking s., SYN nictitating s.

△spasmo-. Spasm. [G. *spasmos*]

spas·mod·ic (spaz-mod′ik). Relating to or marked by spasm. [G. *spasmōdes,* convulsive, fr. *spasmos,* + *eidos,* form]

spas·mo·gen (spaz′mō-jen). A substance causing contraction of smooth muscle; e.g., histamine.

spas·mo·gen·ic (spaz-mō-jen′ik). Causing spasms. [spasmo- + G. *-gen,* producing]

spas·mol·y·sis (spaz-mol′i-sis). The arrest of a spasm or convulsion. [spasmo- + G. *lysis,* dissolution]

spas·mo·lyt·ic (spaz′mō-lit′ik). 1. Relating to spasmolysis. 2. Denoting a chemical agent that relieves smooth muscle spasms.

spas·mo·phil·ic (spaz-mō-fil′ik). Relating to spasmophilia.

spas·mus (spaz′mŭs). SYN spasm. [L. fr. G. *spasmos,* spasm]

   s. coordina′tus, compulsive movements, such as imitative or mimic tics, festinatio.

   s. glot′tidis, SYN *laryngismus* stridulus.

   s. nic′titans, SYN nictitating *spasm.*

   s. nu′tans, (1) SYN nodding *spasm;* (2) a fine nystagmus, sometimes rotary, sometimes monocular, associated with head-nodding movements.

spas·tic (spas′tik). 1. SYN hypertonic (1). 2. Relating to spasm or to spasticity. [L. *spasticus,* fr. G. *spastikos,* drawing in]

spas·tic·i·ty (spas-tis′i-tē). One type of increase in muscle tone at rest; characterized by increased resistance to passive stretch, velocity dependent and asymmetric about joints (i.e., greater in the flexor muscles at the elbow and the extensor muscles at the knee). Exaggerated deep tendon reflexes and clonus are additional manifestations. SEE ALSO clasp-knife s.

   clasp-knife s., initial increased resistance to stretch of the extensor muscles of a joint that give way rather suddenly allowing the joint then to be easily flexed; the rigidity is due to an exaggeration of the stretch reflex. SEE ALSO lengthening *reaction.* SYN clasp-knife effect, clasp-knife rigidity.

spa·tia (spā′shē-ă). Plural of spatium. [L.]

spa·tial (spā′shăl). Relating to space or a space.

spa·ti·um, pl. spa·tia (spā′shē-ŭm, -shē-ă) [TA]. SYN space. [L.]

   spa′tia an′guli iridocornea′lis [TA], SYN *spaces* of iridocorneal angle, under *space.*

s. endolympha′ticum [TA], SYN endolymphatic *space.*

s. episclera′le [TA], SYN episcleral *space.*

s. extradura′le, ☆official alternate term for epidural *space.*

s. extradurale [TA], SYN epidural *space.*

s. extraperitonea′le [TA], SYN extraperitoneal *space.*

s. intercosta′le [TA], SYN intercostal *space.*

s. interfascia′le, SYN episcleral *space.*

s. interglobula′re, pl. **spa′tia interglobula′ria**, SYN interglobular *space.*

spa′tia interos′sea metacar′pi [TA], SYN interosseous metacarpal *spaces,* under *space.*

spa′tia interos′sea metatar′si [TA], SYN interosseous metatarsal *spaces,* under *space.*

s. intervagina′le bulb′i oc′uli, SYN episcleral *space.*

s. intervagina′le subarachnoidale ner′vi op′tici [TA], SYN intervaginal subarachnoid *space* of optic nerve.

s. lateropharyn′geum [TA], SYN lateral pharyngeal *space;* SEE ALSO retropharyngeal *space.*

s. leptomeningeum [TA], SYN leptomeningeal *space.*

s. parapharyngeum, SYN parapharyngeal *space.*

s. perichoroideum [TA], SYN perichoroidal *space.*

s. peridurale, ☆official alternate term for (spinal) epidural space.

s. perilymphat′icum [TA], SYN perilymphatic *space.*

s. perine′i profun′dum, SYN deep perineal *space.*

s. perine′i superficia′le [TA], SYN superficial perineal *space.*

s. peripharyn′geum [TA], SYN peripharyngeal *space.*

s. pharyngeum laterale [TA], SYN lateral pharyngeal *space.*

s. retroinguina′le [TA], SYN retroinguinal *space.*

s. retroperitonea′le [TA], SYN retroperitoneal *space.*

s. retropharyn′geum [TA], SYN retropharyngeal *space;* SEE ALSO lateral pharyngeal *space.*

s. retropu′bicum [TA], SYN retropubic *space.*

s. retrozonulare [TA], SYN retrozonular *space.*

s. subarachnoideum [TA], SYN subarachnoid *space.*

s. subdura′le [TA], SYN subdural *space.*

s. supraspinale [TA], SYN suprasternal *space.*

spa′tia zonula′ria [TA], SYN zonular *spaces,* under *space.*

spat·u·la (spach′ŭ-lă). A flat blade, like a knife blade but without a sharp edge, used in pharmacy for spreading plasters and ointments and as an aid to mixing ingredients with a mortar and pestle. [L. dim. of *spatha,* a broad, flat wooden instrument, fr. G. *spathē*]

iris s., a flat surgical instrument used for repositioning an iris that has prolapsed through a wound.

Ro s., a very small nickeled steel s. used to transfer bits of infected material, such as diphtheritic membrane, to culture tubes.

spat·u·late (spach′ŭ-lāt). **1.** Shaped like a spatula. **2.** To manipulate or mix with a spatula. **3.** To incise the cut end of a tubular structure longitudinally and splay it open, to allow creation of an elliptical anastomosis of greater circumference than would be possible with conventional transverse or oblique (bevelled) end-to-end anastomoses. SYN spatulated.

spat·u·lat·ed (spach′ŭ-lāt-ed). SYN spatulate.

spat·u·la·tion (spach′ŭ-lā′shŭn). Manipulation of material with a spatula.

Spatz, Hugo, German neurologist and psychiatrist, 1888–1969. SEE Hallervorden-S. *disease, syndrome.*

spay (spā). To remove the ovaries of an animal. [Gael. *spoth,* castrate, or G. *spadōn,* eunuch]

SPCA Abbreviation for serum prothrombin conversion *accelerator.*

spear·mint (spēr′mint). The leaves and flowering tops of *Mentha viridis* (green garden or lamb mint) or *M. cardiaca* (family Labiatae); a carminative and flavoring agent.

s. oil, the volatile oil, distilled with steam from the fresh overground parts of the flowering plant of *Mentha viridis* or *M. cardiaca,* a flavoring agent.

spe·cial·ist (spesh′ă-list). One who has developed professional expertise in a particular specialty or subject area.

spe·cial·i·za·tion (spesh′ă-li-zā′shŭn). **1.** Professional attention limited to a particular specialty or subject area for study, research, and/or treatment. **2.** SYN differentiation (1).

spe·cial·ize (spesh′ă-līz). To engage in specialization (1).

spe·cial·ty (spesh′al-tē). The particular subject area or branch of medical science to which one devotes professional attention. [L. *specialitas* fr. *specialis,* special]

spe·ci·a·tion (spē-shē-ā′shŭn). The evolutionary process by which diverse species of animals or plants are formed from a common ancestral stock.

spe·cies, pl. **spe·cies** (spē′shēz). **1.** A biologic division between the genus and a variety or the individual; a group of organisms that generally bear a close resemblance to one another in the more essential features of their organization, and breed effectively producing fertile progeny. **2.** A class of pharmaceutical preparations consisting of a mixture of dried plants, not pulverized, but in sufficiently fine division to be conveniently used in the making of extemporaneous decoctions or infusions, as a tea. [L. appearance, form, kind, fr. *specio,* to look at]

type s., the name of the single s. or of one of the s. of a genus or subgenus when the name of the genus or subgenus was originally validly published.

spe·cies-spe·cif·ic. Characteristic of a given species; serum that is produced by the injection of immunogens into an animal, and that acts only upon the cells, protein, etc., of a member of the same species as that from which the original antigen was obtained.

spe·cif·ic (spĕ-sif′ik). **1.** Relating to a species. SEE ALSO specific *epithet.* **2.** Relating to an individual infectious disease, one caused by a special microorganism. **3.** A remedy having a definite therapeutic action in relation to a particular disease or symptom, as quinine in relation to malaria. [L. *specificus* fr. *species + facio,* to make]

spec·i·fic·i·ty (spes-i-fis′i-tē). **1.** The condition or state of being specific, of having a fixed relation to a single cause or to a definite result; manifested in the relation of a disease to its pathogenic microorganism, of a reaction to a certain chemical union, or of an antibody to its antigen or the reverse. **2.** In clinical pathology and medical screening, the proportion of individuals with negative test results for the disease that the test is intended to reveal, i.e., true negative results as a proportion of the total of true negative and false-positive results. Cf. sensitivity (2).

analytical s., freedom from interference by any element or compound other than the analyte.

diagnostic s., the probability (P) that, given the absence of disease (D), a normal test result (T) excludes disease; i.e., P(T/D).

relative s., the s. of a medical screening test as determined by comparison with the same type of test (e.g., s. of a new serological test relative to s. of an established serological test).

substrate s., the ability of an enzyme to recognize and bind its substrates, typically measured by the V_{max}/K_m or k_{cat}/K_m ratios.

spe·cil·lum, pl. **spe·cil·la** (spe-sil′ŭm, -lă). A probe or small sound. [L. a probe, fr. *specio,* to look at]

spec·i·men (spes′ĭ-men). A small part, or sample, of any substance or material obtained for testing. [L. fr. *specio,* to look at]

cytologic s., a s. obtainable by a variety of methods from many areas of the body, including the female genital tract, respiratory tract, urinary tract, alimentary tract, and body cavities; used for cytologic examination and diagnosis (e.g., cytologic smears, filter preparations, centrifuged buttons).

SPECT Abbreviation for single photon emission computed *tomography.*

spec·ta·cles (spek′tĭ-klz). Lenses set in a frame that holds them in front of the eyes, used to correct errors of refraction or to protect the eyes. The parts of the s. are the *lenses;* the *bridge* between the lenses, resting on the nose; the *rims* or *frames,* encircling the lenses; the *sides* or *temples* that pass on either side of the head to the ears; the *bows,* the curved extremities of the temples; the *shoulders,* short bars attached to the rims or the lenses and jointed with the sides. SYN eyeglasses, glasses (1). [L. *specto,* pp. *-atus,* to watch, observe]

bifocal s., s. with bifocal lenses. SEE lens.

sp

clerical s., SYN half-glass s.

divers' s., strongly convex lenses for clear vision underwater.

divided s., SYN Franklin s.

Franklin s., an early form of bifocal s. in which the lower half of the lens is for near vision, the upper half for distant vision. SYN divided s.

half-glass s., s., used for reading, in which the upper portion of the lenses are removed. SYN clerical s., pantoscopic s., pulpit s.

hemianopic s., s. with a prism or mirror to allow the person with homonymous hemianopia to see objects in the blind half field.

lid crutch s., s. with little offsets of metal with smooth edges which engage above the upper eyelid and keep it raised above the pupil in cases of paralytic blepharoptosis. SYN Masselon s.

Masselon s., SYN lid crutch s.

orthoscopic s., convex lenses with base-in prisms for close work.

pantoscopic s., SYN half-glass s.

photochromic s., s. with lenses that darken on exposure to ultraviolet light.

protective s., s. which protect against ultraviolet or infrared rays or against mechanical injuries. SYN safety s.

pulpit s., SYN half-glass s.

safety s., SYN protective s.

stenopeic s., stenopaic s., (1) opaque disks with narrow slits in the center allowing only a minimum amount of light to enter; used as a protection against snow blindness; **(2)** s. having opaque disks with multiple perforations used to aid vision in incipient cataract and in discrete opacities of the cornea; occasionally used as a substitute for corrective lenses or sunglasses.

telescopic s., magnifying s. obtained by using a convex objective lens and a concave eyepiece separated by the difference in their focal lengths.

spec·ti·no·my·cin hy·dro·chlo·ride (spek'ti-nō-mī'sin). An antibiotic antibacterial agent.

spec·tra (spek'tră). Plural of spectrum. [L.]

spec·tral (spek'trăl). Relating to a spectrum.

spec·trin (spek'trin). A filamentous contractile protein that together with actin and other cytoskeleton proteins forms a network that gives the red blood cell membrane its shape and flexibility; a defect or deficiency of s. is associated with hereditary spherocytosis and hereditary elliptocytosis; the principal component of the membrane skeleton of red cells. It comprises two units, an alpha unit of MW 240,000 [MIM*182860] and a beta unit of MW 225,000 [MIM*182870].

spectro-. A spectrum. [L. *spectrum,* an image]

spec·tro·chem·is·try (spek'trō-kem'is-trē). The study of chemical substances and their identification by means of spectroscopy, i.e., by light emitted or absorbed.

spec·tro·col·or·im·e·ter (spek'trō-kŏl-er-im'ĕ-ter). A colorimeter using a source of light from a selected portion of the spectrum, i.e., of a selected wavelength.

spec·tro·flu·o·rom·e·ter (spek-trō-flōr-om'ĕ-ter). An instrument for measuring the intensity and quality of fluorescence.

spec·tro·gram (spek'trō-gram). A graphic representation of a spectrum. [spectro- + G. *gramma,* something written]

spec·tro·graph (spek'trō-graf). An instrument used in spectography.

mass s., an instrument that subjects charged and accelerated ions (atomic or molecular) to a magnetic field that imparts a curved path that differs for each mass-to-charge ratio, thus separating individual species; used in detecting and assaying isotopic ratios and in molecular structure determinations.

spec·trog·ra·phy (spek-trog'ră-fē). The procedure of photographing or tracing a spectrum. [spectro- + G. *graphō,* to write]

spec·trom·e·ter (spek-trom'ĕ-ter). An instrument for determining the wavelength or energy of light or other electromagnetic emission. [spectro- + G. *metron,* measure]

spec·trom·e·try (spek-trom'ĕ-trē). The procedure of observing and measuring the wavelengths of light or other electromagnetic emissions.

clinical s., SYN biospectrometry.

spec·tro·pho·bia (spek-trō-fō'bē-ă). Morbid fear of mirrors or of one's mirrored image. [spectro- + G. *phobos,* fear]

spec·tro·pho·to·flu·o·rim·e·try (spek'trō-fō'tō-flōr-im'ĕ- trē). Measurement of the intensity and quality of fluorescence by means of a spectrophotometer.

spec·tro·pho·tom·e·ter (spek'trō-fō-tom'ĕ-ter). An instrument for measuring the intensity of light of a definite wavelength transmitted by a substance or a solution, giving a quantitative measure of the amount of material in the solution absorbing the light; a colorimeter with a choice of wavelength and photometric measurement. [spectro- + photometer]

spec·tro·pho·tom·e·try (spek'trō-fō-tom'ĕ-trē). Analysis by means of a spectrophotometer.

atomic absorption s., determination of concentration by the ability of atoms to absorb radiant energy of specific wavelengths.

flame emission s., determination of the concentration of an element by measurement of light emitted when the element is excited by energy in the form of heat.

spec·tro·po·lar·im·e·ter (spek'trō-pō-lar-im'ĕ-ter). An instrument for measuring the rotation of the plane of polarized light of specific wavelength upon passage through a solution or translucent solid. [spectro- + polarimeter]

spec·tro·scope (spek'trō-skōp). An instrument for resolving light from any luminous body into its spectrum, and for the analysis of the spectrum so formed. It consists of a prism that refracts the light or a grating for diffraction of the light, an arrangement for rendering the rays parallel, and a telescope that magnifies the spectrum. [spectro- + G. *skopeō,* to view]

direct vision s., a s. consisting of a single tube containing a series of prisms; one end of the tube is placed in as close contact as possible with the substance to be examined while the observer's eye is at the opposite end; it can be used to make a spectroscopic examination of the blood in vivo, as in the ear lobe or web of the thumb.

spec·tro·scop·ic (spek-trō-skop'ik). Relating to or performed by means of a spectroscope.

spec·tros·co·py (spek-tros'kŏ-pē). Observation and study of spectra of absorbed or emitted light by means of a spectroscope.

clinical s., SYN biospectroscopy.

infrared s., the study of the specific absorption in the infrared region of the electromagnetic spectrum; used in the study of the chemical bonds within molecules.

magnetic resonance s., detection and measurement of the resonant spectra of molecular species in a tissue or sample.

s., pl. spec·tra, spec·trums (spek'trŭm, -ă, -ŭmz). **1.** The range of colors presented when white light is resolved into its constituent colors by being passed through a prism or through a diffraction grating: red, orange, yellow, green, blue, indigo, and violet, arranged in increasing frequency of vibration or decreasing wavelength. **2.** Figuratively, the range of pathogenic microorganisms against which an antibiotic or other antibacterial agent is active. **3.** The plot of intensity vs. wavelength of light emitted or absorbed by a substance, usually characteristic of the substance and used in qualitative and quantitative analysis. **4.** The range of wavelengths presented when a beam of radiant energy is subjected to dispersion and focused. [L. an image, fr. *specio,* to look at]

absorption s., the s. observed after light has passed through, and been partially absorbed by, a solution or translucent substance; many molecular groupings have characteristic light absorption patterns, which can be used for detection and quantitative assay.

antimicrobial s., SEE *spectrum* (2).

broad s., a term indicating a broad range of activity of an antibiotic against a wide variety of microorganisms.

chromatic s., the continuum of colors that white light forms on passing through a prism or diffraction grating. SYN color s.

color s., SYN chromatic s.

continuous s., a s. in which there are no absorption bands or lines.

excitation s., fluorescence produced over a range of wavelengths of the exciting light.

fluorescence s., fluorescence evoked over a range of wavelengths when the excitation wavelength is at a maximum.

fortification s., the zigzag banding of light, resembling the walls of fortified medieval towns, that marks the margin of the scintillating scotoma of migraine. SYN fortification figures, telehopsias.

frequency s., the range of frequencies in a signal, used to describe the resolving power of an imaging system in radiology.

infrared s., the part of the invisible s. of wavelengths just longer than that of visible red light. SYN thermal s.

invisible s., the radiation lying on either side of visible light, i.e., infrared and ultraviolet light.

Raman s., the characteristic array of light produced by the Raman effect.

thermal s., SYN infrared s.

ultraviolet s., the electromagnetic s. at wavelengths shorter than the violet end of the visible s.

visible s., that part of electromagnetic radiation that is visible to the human eye; it extends from extreme red, 7606 Å (760.6 nm), to extreme violet, 3934 Å (393.4 nm).

vocal s., the frequency and intensity ranges of the voice.

wide s., SEE *spectrum* (3).

spec·u·lum, pl. **spec·u·la** (spek′ū-lŭm, -lă). An instrument for exposing the opening of any canal or cavity in order to facilitate inspection of its interior. [L. a mirror, fr. *specio,* to look at]

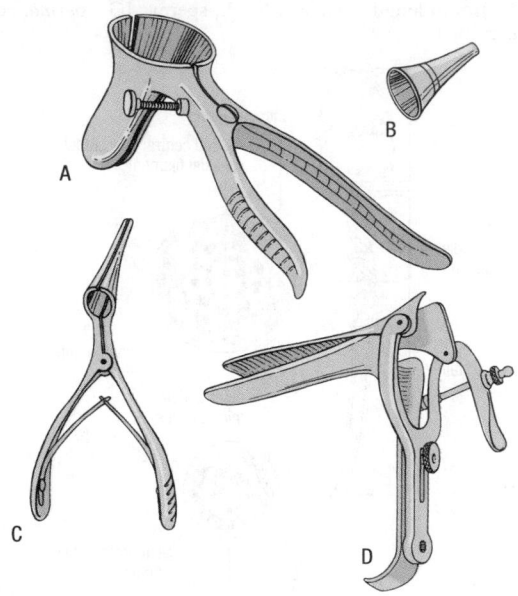

speculum: (A) rectal, (B) ear, (C) nasal, (D) vaginal duckbill

bivalve s., a s. with two adjustable blades.

Cooke s., a three-pronged s. for rectal examinations and operations.

duckbill s., a bivalve s., the blades of which are broad and flattened, resembling a duck's bill, used in inspection of the vagina and cervix.

eye s., an instrument for keeping the eyelids apart during inspection of or operation on the eye. SYN blepharostat.

Kelly rectal s., a tubular s. with obturator for rectal examination.

Pedersen s., a narrow flat s. used in vaginas with a narrow introitus.

stop-s., a dilating s., as a s. of the eyelids, which is provided with a catch to prevent its being opened too wide.

Spee, Ferdinand Graf von, German embryologist, 1855–1937. SEE *curve* of S.

SPEECH1. Gene that when mutated is responsible for motor dyspraxia.

speech. Talk; the use of the voice in conveying ideas. [A.S. *spaec*]

alaryngeal s., a form of s. achieved after laryngectomy by using either an external vibratory source or the pharyngoesophageal segment as an internal vibratory source. SEE ALSO esophageal s. Tracheoesophageal s. may be produced after laryngectomy by surgically diverting exhaled air to the pharynx by a permanently constructed tracheoesophageal fistula.

cerebellar s., an explosive type of utterance, with slurring of words.

clipped s., SYN scamping s.

cued s., a system of communication with a person with profound hearing impairment in which handshapes are used to cue sounds to supplement spoken language.

echo s., SYN echolalia.

esophageal s., a technique for speaking following total laryngectomy; consists of drawing air into the esophagus and regurgitating it, producing a vibration in the hypopharynx.

explosive s., loud, sudden s. related to injury of the nervous system. SYN logospasm (2).

helium s., the peculiar high-pitched, often unintelligible speech sounds produced when one breathes a mixture of up to 80° per cent helium and 20° per cent oxygen.

mirror s., a reversal of the order of syllables in a word, analogous to mirror writing.

scamping s., a form of lalling in which consonants or syllables that are difficult to pronounce are omitted. SYN clipped s.

scanning s., measured or metered, often slow s. with interruptions.

slurring s., slovenly articulation of the more difficult letter sounds.

spastic s., labored s. related to increased tone of muscles.

staccato s., an abrupt utterance, each syllable being enunciated separately; noted especially in multiple sclerosis. SYN syllabic s.

subvocal s., slight movements of the muscles of s. related to thinking but producing no sound.

syllabic s., SYN staccato s.

tracheoesophageal s., a form of alaryngeal s. obtained by a surgical technique which creates a shunt between trachea and esophagus, allowing pulmonary air to generate upper esophageal and pharyngeal mucosal vibrations as a substitute for vocal cord vibrations when the larynx is surgically removed.

speed (spēd). The magnitude of velocity without regard to direction. Cf. velocity.

spe·len·ceph·a·ly (spē-len-sef′ă-lē). SYN porencephaly. [*spēlaion,* cave, + *enkephalos,* brain]

Spens, Thomas, Scottish physician, 1769–1842. SEE S. *syndrome.*

sperm. SYN spermatozoon. [G. *sperma,* seed]

sperma-, spermato-, spermo-. Semen, spermatozoa. [G. *sperma,* seed]

sper·ma·ce·ti (sper-mă-set′ē). A peculiar fatty, waxy substance, chiefly cetin (cetyl palmitate), obtained from the head of the sperm whale, *Physeter macrocephalus;* used to impart firmness to ointment bases. SYN cetaceum. [sperma- + G. *ketos,* whale]

sperm·ag·glu·ti·na·tion (sperm′ă-gloo-ti-nā′shŭn). Agglutination of spermatozoa.

sperm-as·ter (sperm′-as-ter). Cytocentrum with astral rays in the cytoplasm of an inseminated ovum; it is brought in by the penetrating spermatozoon and evolves into the mitotic spindle of the first cleavage division. [sperm + G. *astēr,* a star (aster)]

sper·mat·ic (sper-mat′ik). Relating to the sperm or semen.

sper·ma·tid (sper′mă-tid). A cell in a late stage of the development of the spermatozoon; it is a haploid cell derived from the secondary spermatocyte and evolves by spermiogenesis into a spermatozoon. SYN nematoblast. [spermat- + *-id* (2)]

sper·ma·tin (sper′mă-tin). Name proposed for an albuminoid in the seminal fluid.

spermato-. SEE sperma-.

sper·ma·to·blast (sper′mă-tō-blast). SYN spermatogonium. [spermato- + G. *blastos,* germ]

sp

sper·ma·to·cele (sper′mă-tō-sēl). Cyst of the epididymis containing spermatozoa. SYN spermatocyst. [spermato- + G. *kēlē*, tumor]

sper·ma·to·ci·dal (sper′mă-tō-sī′dăl). Destructive to spermatozoa. SYN spermicidal.

sper·ma·to·cide (sper′mă-tō-sīd). An agent destructive to spermatozoa. SYN spermicide. [spermato- + L. *caedo*, to kill]

sper·ma·to·cyst. SYN spermatocele.

sper·ma·to·cy·tal (sper-mă-tō-sī′tăl). Relating to spermatocytes.

sper·ma·to·cyte (sper′mă-tō-sīt). Parent cell of a spermatid, derived by mitotic division from a spermatogonium. [spermato- + G. *kytos*, cell]

    primary s., the s. derived by a growth phase from a spermatogonium, and that undergoes the first division of meiosis.

    secondary s., the s. derived from a primary s. by the first meiotic division; each secondary s. produces two spermatids by the second meiotic division.

sper·ma·to·cy·to·gen·e·sis (sper′mă-tō-sī′tō-jen′ĕ-sis). SYN spermatogenesis.

◼**sper·ma·to·gen·e·sis** (sper′mă-tō-jen′ĕ-sis). The entire process by which spermatogonial stem cells divide and differentiate into spermatozoa. SEE ALSO spermiogenesis. SYN spermatocytogenesis, spermatogeny. [spermato- + G. *genesis*, origin]

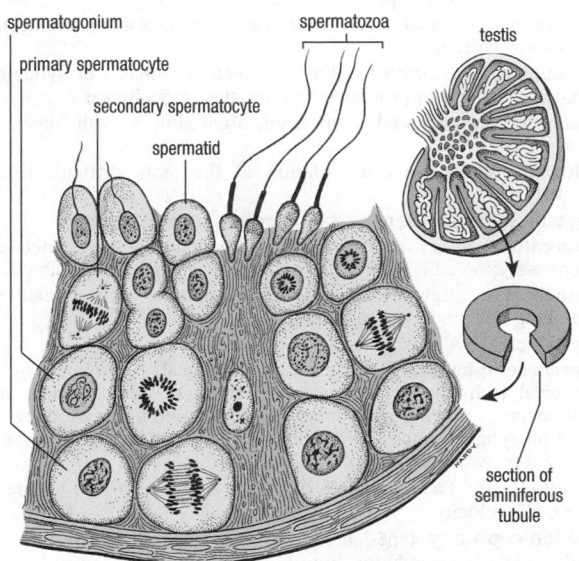

spermatogenesis: various stages seen in a section of a seminiferous tubule

sper·ma·to·ge·net·ic (sper′mă-tō-jĕ-net′ik). SYN spermatogenic.

sper·ma·to·gen·ic (sper′mă-tō-jen′ik). Relating to spermatogenesis; sperm-producing. SYN spermatogenetic, spermatogenous, spermatopoietic (1).

sper·ma·tog·e·nous (sper-mă-toj′ĕ-nŭs). SYN spermatogenic.

sper·ma·tog·e·ny (sper-mă-toj′ĕ-nē). SYN spermatogenesis.

sper·ma·to·gone (sper′mă-tō-gōn). SYN spermatogonium.

sper·ma·to·go·ni·um (sper′mă-tō-gō′nē-ŭm). The primitive sperm cell derived by mitotic division from the germ cell; increasing several times in size, it becomes a primary spermatocyte. SEE ALSO spermatid. SYN spermatoblast, spermatogone. [spermato- + G. *gonē*, generation]

sper·ma·toid (sper′mă-tōid). **1.** Resembling a sperm, a sperm tail, or semen. **2.** A male or flagellated form of the malarial microparasite. [spermato + G. *eidos*, form]

sper·ma·tol·o·gy (sper-mă-tol′ō-jē). The branch of histology, physiology, and embryology concerned with sperm and/or seminal secretion. [spermato- + G. *logos*, study]

sper·ma·tol·y·sin (sper-mă-tol′i-sin). A specific lysin (antibody) formed in response to the repeated injection of spermatozoa.

sper·ma·tol·y·sis (sper-mă-tol′i-sis). Destruction, with dissolu-tion, of the spermatozoa. SYN spermolysis. [spermato- + G. *lysis*, dissolution]

sper·ma·to·lyt·ic (sper′mă-tō-lit′ik). Relating to spermatolysis.

sper·ma·to·pho·bia (sper′mă-tō-fō′bē-ă). Morbid fear of spermatorrhea or loss of semen. [spermato- + G. *phobos*, fear]

sper·ma·to·phore (sper′mă-tō-fōr). A capsule containing spermatozoa; found in a number of invertebrates. [spermato- + G. *phoros*, bearing]

sper·ma·to·poi·et·ic (sper′mă-tō-poy-et′ik). **1.** SYN spermatogenic. **2.** Secreting semen. [spermato- + G. *poieō*, to make]

sper·ma·tor·rhea (sper′mă-tō-rē′ă). An involuntary discharge of semen, without orgasm. [spermato- + G. *rhoia*, a flow]

sper·ma·tox·in (sper-mă-tok′sin). A cytotoxic antibody specific for spermatozoa. SYN spermotoxin.

sper·ma·to·zoa (sper′mă-tō-zō′ă). Plural of spermatozoon.

sper·ma·to·zo·al, sper·ma·to·zo·an (sper′ma-tō-zō′ăl, -zō′ăn). Relating to spermatozoa.

◼**sper·ma·to·zo·on,** pl. **sper·ma·to·zoa** (sper′mă-tō-zō′on, -zō′ă). The male gamete or sex cell that contains the genetic information to be transmitted by the male, exhibits autokinesis, and is able to effect zygosis with an ovum. The human s. is composed of a head and a tail, the tail being divisible into a neck, a middle piece, a principal piece, and an end piece; the head, 4–6 μm in length, is a broadly oval, flattened body containing the nucleus; the tail is about 55 μm in length. SYN sperm cell, sperm. [G. *sperma*, seed, + *zōon*, animal]

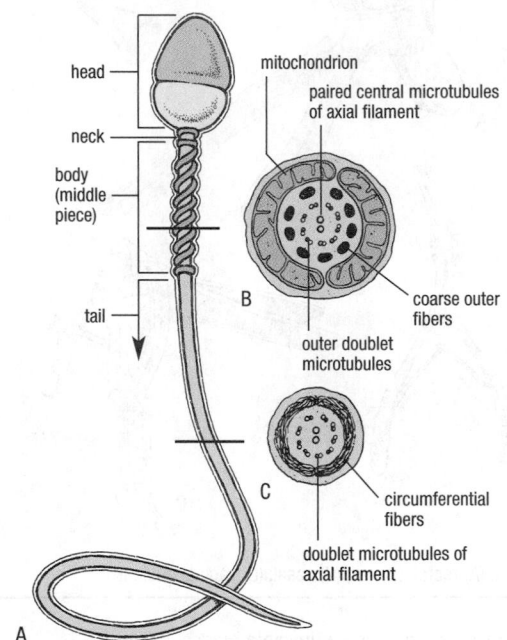

human spermatozoon: longitudinal section (A); transverse sections of body (B) and tail (C)

sper·ma·tu·ria (sper-mă-too′rē-ă). SYN semenuria.

sper·mia (sper′mē-ă). Plural of spermium.

sper·mi·ci·dal (sper-mi-sī′dăl). SYN spermatocidal.

sper·mi·cide (sper′mi-sīd). SYN spermatocide.

sper·mi·dine (sper′mi-dēn). A polyamine found with spermine in a wide variety of organisms and tissues; found in human sperm; important in cell and tissue growth.

sper·mi·duct (sper′mi-dŭkt). **1.** SYN *ductus* deferens. **2.** SYN ejaculatory *duct*.

sperm·ine (sper′mēn). A polyamine found in some bacteria; associated with nucleic acids in some viruses; found in human sperm; important in cell and tissue growth. SYN gerontine, musculamine, neuridine.

sper·mi·o·gen·e·sis (sper′mē-ō-jen′ĕ-sis). That segment of spermatogenesis during which immature spermatids become spermatozoa. [sperm- + G. *genesis,* origin]

sperm·ism (sper′mizm). The belief by preformationists that the male sex cell (sperm) contains a miniature preformed body called the homunculus.

sperm·ist. A preformationist who believed in the concept of spermism. Cf. ovist.

sper·mi·um, pl. **sper·mia** (sper′mē-ŭm, -ă). H.W.G. Waldeyer term for the mature male germ cell or spermatozoon.

⌂**spermo-.** SEE sperma-.

sper·mo·lith (sper′mō-lith). A concretion in the ductus deferens. [spermo- + G. *lithos,* stone]

sper·mol·y·sis (sper-mol′i-sis). SYN spermatolysis.

Sper·moph·il·us (sper-mot′il-us). A genus of ground squirrel. *S. beecheyi, S. grammurus, S. pygmaeus, S. townsendi,* and several other species act as an important reservoir of *Yersinia pestis.*

sper·mo·tox·in (sper-mō-tok′sin). SYN spermatoxin.

SPF Abbreviation for sun protection *factor.*

sp. gr. Abbreviation for specific *gravity.*

sph. Abbreviation for spherical, or spherical *lens.*

sphac·e·late (sfas′ĕ-lāt). To become gangrenous or necrotic. [G. *sphakelos,* gangrene]

sphac·e·la·tion (sfas-ĕ-lā′shŭn). 1. The process of becoming gangrenous or necrotic. 2. Gangrene or necrosis. [G. *sphakelos,* gangrene]

sphac·el·ism (sfas′ĕ-lizm). The condition manifested by a sphacelus.

sphac·e·lous (sfas′ĕ-lŭs). Sloughing, gangrenous, or necrotic.

sphac·e·lus (sfas′ĕ-lŭs). A mass of sloughing, gangrenous, or necrotic matter. [G. *sphakelos,* gangrene]

Sphaer·ol·tilus (sfēr-ol′til-us). A genus of bacteria closely related to *Leptothrix* found in fresh water; *S. natans* grows a thick biofilm mat in sulfite-containing water, especially as drained from paper mills.

sphen·eth·moid (sfē-neth′moyd). SYN sphenoethmoid.

sphe·ni·on (sfē′nē-on). The tip of the sphenoidal angle of the parietal bone; a craniometric point. [Mod. L. fr. G. *sphēn,* wedge, + dim. *-iŏn*]

⌂**spheno-.** Wedge, wedge-shaped; the sphenoid bone. [G. *sphēn,* wedge]

sphe·no·bas·i·lar (sfē′nō-bas′i-lăr). Relating to the sphenoid bone and the basilar process of the occipital bone. SYN sphenoccipital, sphenooccipital.

sphe·noc·cip·i·tal (sfē′nok-sip′i-tăl). SYN sphenobasilar.

sphe·no·ceph·a·ly (sfē′nō-sef′ă-lē). Condition characterized by a deformation of the skull giving it a wedge-shaped appearance. [spheno- + G. *kephalē,* head]

sphe·no·eth·moid (sfē-nō-eth′moyd). Relating to the sphenoid and ethmoid bones. SYN sphenethmoid.

sphen·o·eth·moi·dec·to·my (sfē′nō-eth-moy-dek′tō-mē). An operation to remove diseased tissue from the sphenoid and ethmoid sinuses.

sphe·no·fron·tal (sfē′nō-fron′tăl). Relating to the sphenoid and frontal bones.

sphe·noid (sfē′noyd) [TA]. 1. SYN sphenoidal. 2. SYN sphenoid (*bone*). [G. *sphēnoeidēs,* fr. *sphēn,* wedge, + *eidos,* resemblance]

sphe·noi·dal (sfē-noy′dăl). 1. Relating to the sphenoid bone. 2. Wedge-shaped. SYN sphenoid (1) [TA].

sphe·noi·da·le (sfē-noy-dā′lē). The point of greatest convexity between the anterior contour of the sella turcica and the jugum sphenoidale.

sphe·noid·i·tis (sfē-noy-dī′tis). 1. Inflammation of the sphenoid sinus. 2. Necrosis of the sphenoid bone. [sphenoid + G. *-itis,* inflammation]

sphe·noi·dos·to·my (sfe-noy-dos′tō-mē). An operative opening

made in the anterior wall of the sphenoid sinus. [sphenoid + G. *stoma,* mouth]

sphe·noi·dot·o·my (sfē′noy-dot′ō-mē). Any operation on the sphenoid bone or sinus. [sphenoid + G. *tomē,* a cutting]

sphe·no·ma·lar (sfē′nō-mā′lăr). SYN sphenozygomatic.

sphe·no·max·il·lary (sfē′nō-mak′si-lār-ē). Relating to the sphenoid bone and the maxilla.

sphe·no·oc·cip·i·tal (sfē′nō-ok-sip′i-tăl). SYN sphenobasilar.

sphe·no·pal·a·tine (sfē-nō-pal′ă-tīn). Relating to the sphenoid and the palatine bones.

sphe·no·pa·ri·e·tal (sfē′nō-pă-rī′ă-tăl). Relating to the sphenoid and the parietal bones.

sphe·no·pe·tro·sal (sfē′nō-pe-trō′săl). Relating to the sphenoid bone and the petrous portion of the temporal bone.

sphe·nor·bit·al (sfē-nōr′bit-ăl). Denoting the portions of the sphenoid bone contributing to the orbits.

sphe·no·sal·pin·go·staph·y·li·nus (sfē′nō-sal-ping′gō-staf-i-lī′nŭs). SEE tensor veli palati (*muscle*). [L.]

sphe·no·squa·mo·sal (sfē′nō-skwā-mō′săl). SYN squamosphenoid.

sphe·no·tem·po·ral (sfē′nō-tem′pŏ-răl). Relating to the sphenoid and the temporal bones.

sphe·not·ic (sfē-nō′tik). Relating to the sphenoid bone and the bony case of the ear. [spheno- + G. *ous,* ear]

sphe·no·tur·bi·nal (sfē′nō-ter′bi-năl). Denoting the concha sphenoidalis.

sphe·no·vo·mer·ine (sfē′nō-vō′mer-ēn, -īn). Relating to the sphenoid bone and the vomer.

sphe·no·zy·go·mat·ic (sfē′nō-zī-gō-mat′ik). Relating to the sphenoid and the zygomatic bones. SYN sphenomalar.

sphere (sfēr). A ball or globular body. [G. *sphaira*]
   attraction s., SYN astrosphere.
   Morgagni s.'s, SYN Morgagni *globules,* under *globule.*

spher·i·cal (sph.) (sfēr′i-kăl). Pertaining to, or shaped like, a sphere.

⌂**sphero-.** Spherical, a sphere. [G. *sphaira,* globe]

sphe·ro·cyl·in·der (sfēr′ō-sil′in-der). SYN spherocylindrical *lens.*

sphe·ro·cyte (sfēr′ō-sīt). A small, spherical red blood cell. [sphero- + G. *kytos,* cell]

⬛**sphe·ro·cy·to·sis** (sfēr′ō-sī-tō′sis). Presence of sphere-shaped red blood cells in the blood. SYN microspherocytosis. [spherocyte + G. *-osis,* condition]
   hereditary s. [MIM*182900], a congenital defect of spectrin [MIM*182860], the main component of the erythrocyte cell membrane, which becomes abnormally permeable to sodium, resulting in thickened and almost spherical erythrocytes that are fragile and susceptible to spontaneous hemolysis, with decreased survival in the circulation; results in chronic anemia with reticulocytosis, episodes of mild jaundice due to hemolysis, and acute crises with gallstones, fever, and abdominal pain; symptomatology is highly variable; autosomal dominant inheritance, caused by mutation in the ankyrin gene (ANK1) on 8p. However, as with elliptocytosis, there is an autosomal recessive form [MIM*270970], caused by mutation in the alpha-spectrin 1 gene (SPTA1) on chromosome 1q. SYN chronic acholuric jaundice, chronic familial icterus, chronic familial jaundice, congenital hemolytic icterus, congenital hemolytic jaundice, spherocytic anemia.

sphe·roid, sphe·roi·dal (sfēr′oyd, sfir-; sfē-royd′ăl). Shaped like a sphere. [L. *spheroideus*]

sphe·rom·e·ter (sfēr-om′ĕ-ter). An instrument to determine the curvature of a sphere or a spherical lens. SEE Geneva lens *measure.* [sphero- + G. *metron,* measure]

sphe·ro·pha·ki·a (sfēr-ō-fā′kē-ă). A congenital bilateral aberration in which the lenses are small, spherical, and subject to subluxation; may occur as an independent anomaly or may be associated with the Weill-Marchesani syndrome. [sphero- + G. *phakos,* lens]

sphe·ro·plast (sfēr′ō-plast). A bacterial cell from which the rigid cell wall has been incompletely removed. The bacterium loses its characteristic shape and becomes round. [sphero- + G. *plastos,* formed]

sphe·ro·prism (sfēr′ō-prizm). A spherical lens decentered to produce a prismatic effect, or a combined spherical lens and prism.

sphe·ro·sper·mia (sfēr′ō-sper′mē-ă). Spheroid spermatozoa lacking an elongated tail, in contrast to the threadlike, tailed sperm of humans and other mammals (nematospermia). [sphero- + G. *sperma,* seed]

spher·ule (sfer′ool). **1.** A small spherical structure. **2.** A sporangiallike structure filled with endospores at maturity, produced within tissue and in vitro by *Coccidioides immitis*. [LL. *sphaerula,* dim. of L. *sphaera,* sphere, ball]

sphinc·ter (sfingk′ter) [TA]. A muscle that encircles a duct, tube, or orifice in such a way that its contraction constricts the lumen or orifice. SYN musculus sphincter [TA], sphincter muscle [TA]. [G. *sphinktēr,* a band or lace]

s. of ampulla, ^{�star}official alternate term for s. of hepatopancreatic ampulla.

anatomic s., an accumulation of muscular circular fibers or specially arranged oblique fibers the function of which is to reduce partially or totally the lumen of a tube, the orifice of an organ, or the cavity of a viscus; the closing component of a pylorus.

s. angula′ris, angular s., thickening of the circular muscular layer forming a proposed intermediate s. at the level of the angular notch of the stomach. While the thickening of the circular muscle may indicate the commencement of the pyloric antrum, true functional sphincteric activity distinct from the other peristaltic contractions of the stomach is not observed although some of these may in fact temporarily close off the antrum from the remainder of the stomach lumen. SYN antral s., midgastric transverse s., s. antri, s. intermedius, s. of antrum, s. of gastric antrum.

s. a′ni, anal s., SEE external anal s., internal anal s.

s. a′ni ter′tius, the third s. of the anorectum, a physiological s. at the sigmoidorectal junction.

antral s., SYN s. angularis.

s. an′tri, SYN s. angularis.

s. of antrum, SYN s. angularis.

anular s., a short thickening of circular muscular fibers, similar to a ring; a ring-shaped s. as opposed to a segmental s.

artificial s., a s. produced by surgical procedures to reduce speed of flow in the digestive system or to maintain continence of the intestine.

basal s., the thickening of the circular muscular coat at the base of the ileal papilla at the terminal ileum. SYN sphincteroid tract of ileum.

bicanalicular s., a s. encircling two canals, such as the terminal portions of the common bile duct and the main pancreatic duct.

s. of biliaropancreatic ampulla, [✫]official alternate term for s. of hepatopancreatic ampulla.

Boyden s., SYN s. of (common) bile duct.

canalicular s., a s. located somewhere along the course of an organ, a tube, or a duct, as opposed to ostial s.

choledochal s., SYN s. of (common) bile duct.

colic s., one of the physiological s.'s of the colon.

s. of (common) bile duct [TA], smooth muscle s. of the common bile duct immediately proximal to the hepatopancreatic ampulla and organized into a superior and inferior s.; it is this s. that controls the flow of bile in the duodenum. SYN musculus sphincter ductus choledochi [TA], musculus sphincter ductus biliaris[✫], Boyden s., choledochal s., sphincter muscle of common bile duct.

s. constric′tor car′diae, SYN inferior esophageal s.

duodenal s., one of the physiologic s.'s described in the duodenum.

duodenojejunal s., the s. supposedly present at the duodenojejunal flexure.

external anal s. [TA], a fusiform ring of striated muscular fibers surrounding the anus, attached posteriorly to the coccyx and anteriorly to the central tendon of the perineum; it is subdivided, often indistinctly, into a subcutaneous part, a superficial part, and a deep part for descriptive purposes. SYN musculus sphincter ani externus [TA], external sphincter muscle of anus.

external urethral s. [TA], muscle that constricts membranous urethra to retain urine in bladder; nerve supply, pudendal. SYN s. urethrae externus [TA], Guthrie muscle, musculus constrictor urethrae, musculus sphincter urethrae externus, sphincter muscle of urethra, Wilson muscle (1).

external urethral s. of female [TA], composed of striated (voluntary) muscle and more properly a urogenital s., part forms a true anular s. around the urethra, part extends superiorly to the neck of the bladder, part passing anterior to the urethra that attaches to the ischial rami (compressor urethrae muscle) and a bandlike part that encircles both the urethra and the vagina (urethrovaginal s.). SYN musculus sphincter urethrae externus femininae [TA].

external urethral s. of male [TA], composed of striated (voluntary) muscle, includes a tubelike portion that encircles the membranous urethra, but also has a large, troughlike portion that ascends the anterior aspect of the prostatic urethra to the neck of the bladder and a part that passes anteriorly to the membranous urethra and attaches to the ischial rami on each side (compressor urethrae muscle). SYN musculus sphincter urethrae externus masculinae [TA].

extrinsic s., a s. provided by circular muscular fibers extraneous to the organ.

first duodenal s., the s. supposedly located at the level of the aboral extremity of the duodenal bulb.

functional s., SYN physiologic s.

s. of gastric antrum, SYN s. angularis.

Glisson s., SYN s. of hepatopancreatic ampulla.

s. of hepatic flexure of colon, physiological s. at the level of the right colic flexure.

hepatopancreatic s., SYN s. of hepatopancreatic ampulla.

s. of hepatopancreatic ampulla [TA], the smooth muscle s. of the hepatopancreatic ampulla within the duodenal papilla. SYN musculus sphincter ampullae hepatopancreaticae [TA], musculus sphincter ampullae biliaropancreaticae[✫], musculus sphincter ampullae[✫], s. of ampulla[✫], s. of biliaropancreatic ampulla[✫], Glisson s., hepatopancreatic s., Oddi s.

hypertensive upper esophageal s., SYN cricopharyngeal *achalasia*.

Hyrtl s., a band, generally incomplete, of circular muscular fibers in the rectum about 10 cm above the anus (upper rectal ampulla).

ileal s., a thickening of circular musculature at the free margin of the ileal papilla. SYN ileocecocolic s., marginal s., operculum ilei, Varolius s.

ileocecocolic s., SYN ileal s.

iliopelvic s., SYN midsigmoid s.

inferior esophageal s., a physiologic s. at the level of the esophagogastric junction; this is in fact an extrinsic sphincter formed by the surrounding musculature of the esophageal hiagus of the right crus of the diaphragm; causes a normally occurring constriction at the esophagogastric junction observable with a barium swallow. SYN s. constrictor cardiae.

s. intermedius, SYN s. angularis.

internal anal s. [TA], a smooth muscle ring, formed by an increase of the circular fibers of the rectum, situated at the upper end of the anal canal, internal to the outer voluntary external anal s. This s. is maximally contracted when the rectal ampulla is "at rest"—empty or relaxed to accommodate a distending fecal mass. It is inhibited with filling of the ampulla, increased distension, and peristalsis. SYN musculus sphincter ani internus [TA], internal sphincter muscle of anus.

internal urethral s. [TA], the complete collar of smooth muscle cells of the neck of the urinary bladder that extends distally to surround the preprostatic portion of the male urethra. There is not comparable structure in the neck of the female bladder; the internal urethral s. may exist to prevent reflux of semen into the bladder. SYN musculus sphincter urethrae internus[✫], preprostatic s.[✫], supracollicular s.[✫], anulus urethralis, muscular s. supracollicularis, musculus sphincter vesicae, preprostate urethral s., proximal urethral s., sphincter muscle of urinary bladder, s. vesicae.

intrinsic s., a thickening of the circular fibers of the muscular coat of an organ.

lower esophageal s. (LES), musculature of the gastroesophageal junction that is tonically active except during swallowing.

macroscopic s., a s. visible to the naked eye.

marginal s., SYN ileal s.

mediocolic s., a physiological s. located midway in the ascending colon.

microscopic s., a s. visible only under the microscope.

midgastric transverse s., SYN s. angularis.

midsigmoid s., the physiologic s. midway in the sigmoid colon. SYN iliopelvic s.

muscular s. supracollicularis, SYN internal urethral s.

myovascular s., a s. having a muscular and a vascular (usually venous) component. SEE myovenous s.

myovenous s., a s. having a muscular and a venous component, e.g., at the pharyngoesophageal junction and anal canal.

Nélaton s., SEE transverse *folds* of rectum, under *fold.* SYN Nélaton fibers.

O'Beirne s., SYN rectosigmoid s.

s. oc'uli, SYN orbicularis oculi (*muscle*).

Oddi s., SYN s. of hepatopancreatic ampulla.

s. o'ris, SYN orbicularis oris (*muscle*).

ostial s., a thickening of circular muscular fibers at the level of an orifice.

palatopharyngeal s., ☆official alternate term for posterior *fascicle* of palatopharyngeus muscle.

pancreatic s., SYN s. of pancreatic duct.

s. of pancreatic duct [TA], smooth muscle s. of the main pancreatic duct immediately proximal to the hepatoduodenal ampulla. SYN musculus sphincter ductus pancreatici, pancreatic s., sphincter muscle of pancreatic duct.

pathologic s., a thickening of circular musculature caused by disease.

pelvirectal s., SYN rectosigmoid s.

s. of the pharyngeal isthmus, SYN posterior *fascicle* of palatopharyngeus muscle.

physiologic s., a section of a tubular structure that acts as if it has a band of circular muscle to constrict it, although no such specialized structure can be found on morphologic examination. SYN functional s., radiologic s.

postpyloric s., the duodenal portion of the s. or closing mechanism of the gastroduodenal pylorus.

prepapillary s., a s. of duodenum described in the location oral to the major duodenal papilla.

preprostate urethral s., SYN internal urethral s.

preprostatic s., ☆official alternate term for internal urethral s.

prepyloric s., a band of circular muscular fibers in the wall of the stomach near the gastroduodenal pylorus.

proximal urethral s., SYN internal urethral s.

s. pupil'lae [TA], a ring of smooth muscle fibers surrounding the pupillary border of the iris. SYN musculus sphincter pupillae [TA], sphincter muscle of pupil.

pyloric s. [TA], a thickening of the circular layer of the gastric musculature encircling the gastroduodenal junction. SYN musculus sphincter pylori [TA], sphincter muscle of pylorus.

radiologic s., SYN physiologic s.

rectosigmoid s., a circular band of muscular fibers at the rectosigmoid junction. SYN O'Beirne s., O'Beirne valve, pelvirectal s.

segmental s., a s. of a segment of an organ, a tube, or a canal, and longer than an annular s.

smooth muscular s., SYN lissosphincter.

striated muscular s., SYN rhabdosphincter.

superior esophageal s., SYN inferior constrictor (*muscle*) of pharynx; SEE inferior constrictor (*muscle*) of pharynx.

supracollicular s., ☆official alternate term for internal urethral s.

s. of third portion of duodenum, a physiologic s. supposedly located at the horizontal (inferior) portion of the duodenum.

unicanalicular s., a s. limited to one visceral canal or tube.

s. ure'thrae externus [TA], SYN external urethral s.

urethrovaginal s. [TA], voluntary, bandlike part of external urethral s. of female that encircles both urethra and vagina superior to the perineal membrane. SYN musculus sphincter urethrovaginalis [TA].

s. vagi'nae, SYN bulbospongiosus (*muscle*).

Varolius s., SYN ileal s.

velopharyngeal s., SYN posterior *fascicle* of palatopharyngeus muscle.

s. vesi'cae, SYN internal urethral s.

s. vesi'cae biliaris, the s. of the gallbladder, at the transition between the neck of the gallbladder and the cystic duct.

sphinc·ter·al (sfingk'ter-ăl). Relating to a sphincter. SYN sphincterial, sphincteric.

sphinc·ter·al·gia (sfingk-ter-al'jē-ă). Pain in the sphincter ani muscles. [sphincter + G. *algos,* pain]

sphinc·ter·ec·to·my (sfingk-ter-ek'tō-mē). **1.** Excision of a portion of the pupillary border of the iris. **2.** Dissecting away any sphincter muscle. [sphincter + G. *ektomē,* excision]

sphinc·te·ri·al, sphinc·ter·ic (sfingk-tēr'ē-ăl, -ter-ik). SYN sphincteral.

sphinc·ter·is·mus (sfingk-ter-iz'mŭs). Spasmodic contraction of the sphincter ani muscles.

sphinc·ter·i·tis (sfingk'ter-ī'tis). Inflammation of any sphincter.

sphinc·ter·oid (sfingk'ter-oyd). Denoting similarity to a musculus sphincter. [sphincter + G. *eidos,* resemblance]

sphinc·ter·ol·y·sis (sfingk-ter-ol'i-sis). An operation for freeing the iris from the cornea in anterior synechia involving only the pupillary border. [sphincter, + G. *lysis,* loosening]

sphinc·ter·o·plas·ty (sfingk'ter-ō-plas-tē). Operation on any sphincteric muscle. [sphincter + G. *plastos,* formed]

sphinc·ter·o·scope (sfingk'ter-ō-skōp). A speculum to facilitate inspection of the internal sphincter ani muscle. [sphincter + G. *skopeō,* to view]

sphinc·ter·os·co·py (sfingk'ter-os'kŏ-pē). Visual examination of a sphincter.

sphinc·ter·o·tome (sfingk'ter-ō-tōm). An instrument for incising a sphincter.

sphinc·ter·ot·o·my (sfingk'tĕ-rot'ō-mē). Incision or division of a sphincter muscle. [sphincter + G. *tomē,* incision]

external s., transurethral incision of external urethral sphincter.

transduodenal s., division of Oddi sphincter; an operation to open the lower end of the common duct to remove impacted stones or to relieve spasm or stricture of the terminal bile and pancreatic ducts.

sphin·ga·nine (sfing'gă-nēn). Dihydrosphingosine; a constituent of the sphingolipids.

(4E)-sphin·gen·ine (sfing'gen-ēn). SYN sphingosine.

sphing·ol (sfing'gol). SYN sphingosine.

sphin·go·lip·id (sfing'gō-lip-id). Any lipid containing a long-chain base like that of sphingosine (e.g., ceramides, cerebrosides, gangliosides, sphingomyelins); a constituent of nerve tissue.

◼sphin·go·lip·i·do·sis (sfing'gō-lip-i-dō'sis). Collective designation for a variety of diseases characterized by abnormal sphingolipid metabolism, e.g., gangliosidosis, Gaucher disease, Niemann-Pick disease. SYN sphingolipodystrophy.

cerebral s., any one of a group of inherited diseases characterized by failure to thrive, hypertonicity, progressive spastic paralysis, loss of vision and occurrence of blindness, usually with macular degeneration and optic atrophy, convulsions, and mental deterioration; associated with abnormal storage of sphingomyelin and related lipids in the brain. Four types are recognized as clinically and enzymatically distinct: 1) **infantile type** (Tay-Sachs disease, G_{M2} gangliosidosis) due to a deficiency of hexosaminidase A; 2) **early juvenile type** (Jansky-Bielschowsky or Bielschowsky disease); 3) **late juvenile type** (Spielmeyer-Vogt disease; Spielmeyer-Sjögren disease; Batten-Mayou disease; ceroid lipofuscinosis); and 4) **adult type** (Kufs disease). SYN cerebral lipidosis.

sphin·go·lip·o·dys·tro·phy (sfing'gō-lip-ō-dis'trō-fē). SYN sphingolipidosis.

sp

sphingolipidoses		
classified according to storage substance and corresponding enzyme defect (not all variants included)		
disease	storage substance	deficient enzyme
Niemann-Pick disease (sphingomyelinosis, type A)	sphingomyelin	sphingo-myelinase
Gaucher disease	glucocerebroside	β-glucosidase
globoid cell leukodystrophy	galactocerebroside	cerebroside-β-galactosidase
metachromatic leukodystrophy	sulfatide	cerebroside sulfatase, arylsulfatase A
Fabry disease	ceramide trihexoside	α-galactosidase
gangliosidoses	gangliosides	β-galactosidase hexosaminidase N-acetylgalactosaminyl transferase

sphin·go·my·e·li·nase (sfing'gō-mi'ĕ-li-nās). SYN sphingomyelin phosphodiesterase.

sphin·go·my·e·lin phos·pho·di·es·ter·ase (sfing'gō-mī'ĕ-lin). An enzyme catalyzing hydrolysis of sphingomyelin to *N*-acyl-sphingosine (a ceramide) and phosphocholine; a deficiency of this enzyme is associated with type I Niemann-Pick disease. SYN sphingomyelinase.

sphin·go·my·e·lins (sfing'gō-mī'ĕ-linz). A group of phospholipids, found in brain, spinal cord, kidney, and egg yolk, containing 1-phosphocholine (choline *O*-phosphate) combined with a ceramide (a long-chain fatty acid linked to the nitrogen of a long-chain base, such as sphingosine). SYN ceramide 1-phosphorylcholine, phosphosphingosides.

sphin·go·sine (sfing'gō-sēn). The principal long-chain base found in sphingolipids. SYN (4*E*)-sphingenine, sphingol.

△**sphygm-.** SEE sphygmo-.

sphyg·mic (sfig'mik). Relating to the pulse.

△**sphygmo-, sphygm-.** Pulse. [G. *sphygmos*]

sphyg·mo·car·di·o·graph (sfig'mō-kar'dē-ō-graf). A polygraph recording both the heartbeat and the radial pulse. SYN sphygmocardioscope. [sphygmo- + G. *kardia*, heart, + *graphō*, to write]

sphyg·mo·car·di·o·scope (sfig'mō-kar'dē-ō-skōp). SYN sphygmocardiograph. [sphygmo- + G. *skopeō*, to view]

sphyg·mo·chron·o·graph (sfig'mō-kron'ō-graf). A modified sphygmograph that represents graphically the time relations between the beat of the heart and the pulse; one recording the character of the pulse as well as its rapidity. [sphygmo- + G. *chronos*, time, + *graphō*, to write]

sphyg·mo·gram (sfig'mō-gram). The graphic curve made by a sphygmograph. SYN pulse curve. [sphygmo- + G. *gramma*, something written]

sphyg·mo·graph (sfig'mō-graf). An instrument consisting of a lever, the short end of which rests on the radial artery at the wrist, its long end being provided with a stylet which records on a moving ribbon of smoked paper the excursions of the pulse. [sphygmo- + G. *graphō*, to write]

sphyg·mo·graph·ic (sfig-mō-graf'ik). Relating to or made by a sphygmograph; denoting the s. tracing, or sphygmogram.

sphyg·mog·ra·phy (sfig-mog'ră-fē). Use of the sphygmograph in recording the character of the pulse.

sphyg·moid (sfig'moyd). Pulselike; resembling the pulse. [sphygmo- + G. *eidos*, resemblance]

sphyg·mo·ma·nom·e·ter (sfig'mō-mă-nom'ĕ-ter). An instrument for measuring arterial blood pressure consisting of an inflatable cuff, inflating bulb, and a gauge showing the blood pressure. SYN sphygmometer. [sphygmo- + G. *manos*, thin, scanty, + *metron*, measure]

Mosso s., an apparatus for measuring the blood pressure in the digital arteries.

Riva-Rocci s., the original blood pressure apparatus first used to noninvasively measure arterial pressure.

Rogers s., an s. with an aneroid barometer gauge.

sphyg·mo·ma·nom·e·try (sfig'mō-mă-nom'ĕ-trē). Determination of the blood pressure by means of a sphygmomanometer.

sphyg·mom·e·ter (sfig-mom'ĕ-ter). SYN sphygmomanometer.

sphyg·mo·met·ro·scope (sfig-mō-met'rō-skōp). An instrument for auscultating the pulse, used especially in the auscultatory method of reading the blood pressure, particularly the diastolic pressure. [sphygmo- + G. *metron*, measure, + *skopeō*, to view]

sphyg·mo·os·cil·lom·e·ter (sfig'mō-os'i-lom'ĕ-ter). An instrument resembling an aneroid sphygmomanometer used in the measurement of the systolic and diastolic blood pressure. [sphygmo- + L. *oscillo*, to swing, + G. *metron*, measure]

sphyg·mo·pal·pa·tion (sfig'mō-pal-pa'shŭn). Feeling the pulse. [sphygmo- + L. *palpatio*, palpation]

sphyg·mo·phone (sfig'mō-fōn). An instrument by which a sound is produced with each beat of the pulse. [sphygmo- + G. *phōnē*, sound]

sphyg·mo·scope (sfig'mō-skōp). An instrument by which the pulse beats are made visible by causing fluid to rise in a glass tube, by means of a mirror projecting a beam of light, or simply by a moving lever as in the sphygmograph. [sphygmo- + G. *skopeō*, to view]

Bishop s., an instrument for measuring the blood pressure, with special reference to diastolic pressure; the tube is filled with a solution of cadmium borotungstate, and the scale is the reverse of that of a mercurial manometer, the pressure being made directly by the weight of the liquid and not by compressed air.

sphyg·mos·co·py (sfig-mos'kŏ-pē). Examination of the pulse. [sphygmo- + G. *skopeō*, to view]

sphyg·mo·sys·to·le (sfig-mō-sis'tō-lē). Obsolete term for that segment of the pulse wave corresponding to the cardiac systole. [sphygmo- + G. *systolē*, a contracting]

sphyg·mo·ton·o·graph (sfig-mō-tō'nō-graf). An instrument for recording graphically both the pulse and the blood pressure. [sphygmo- + G. *tonos*, tension, + *graphō*, to write]

sphyg·mo·to·nom·e·ter (sfig-mō-tō-nom'ĕ-ter). An instrument, like the sphygmotonograph, for determining the degree of blood pressure. [sphygmo- + G. *tonos*, tension, + *metron*, measure]

sphyg·mo·vis·co·sim·e·try (sfig-mō-vis-kō-sim'ĕ-trē). Measurement of the pressure and the viscosity of the blood.

spi·ca, pl. **spi·cae** (spī'kă, spī'kē). SEE bandage. [L. a point, an ear of grain]

spic·u·la (spik'ū-lă). Plural of spiculum. [L.]

spic·u·lar (spik'ū-lăr). Relating to or having spicules.

spic·ule (spik'ūl). **1.** A small needle-shaped body. **2.** Accessory reproductive structure in male nematodes; useful in identification of species. [L. *spiculum*, dim. of *spica*, or *spicum*, a point]

spic·u·lum, pl. **spic·u·la** (spik'ū-lŭm, -lă). A spicule or small spike. [L.]

spi·der (spī'der). **1.** An arthropod of the order Araneida (subclass Arachnida) characterized by four pairs of legs; a cephalothorax; a globose, smooth abdomen; and a complex of web-spinning spinnerets. Among the venomous s.'s found in the New World are the black widow s., *Latrodectus mactans;* red-legged widow s., *Latrodectus bishopi;* pruning s., or Peruvian tarantula, *Glyptocranium gasteracanthoides;* Chilean brown s., *Loxosceles laeta;* Peruvian brown s., *Loxosceles rufiper;* brown recluse s. of North America, *Loxosceles reclusus.* **2.** An obstructive growth in the teat of a cow. [O. E. *spinnan*, to spin]

arterial s., SYN spider *angioma.*

vascular s., SYN spider *angioma.*

spi·der-burst (spī'der-berst). Radiating dull red capillary lines on the skin of the leg, usually without any visible or palpable varicose veins, but nevertheless due to deep-seated venous dilation. [*spider*web + sun*burst*]

Spiegelberg, Otto, German gynecologist, 1830–1881. SEE S. *criteria,* under *criterion.*

Spieghel, Adrian van der. SEE Spigelius.

Spiegler, Eduard, Austrian dermatologist, 1860–1908. SEE cutaneous *pseudolymphoma;* S.-Fendt *sarcoid.*

Spielmeyer, Walter, Munich neurologist, 1879–1935. SEE S. acute *swelling;* S.-Stock *disease;* S.-Vogt *disease.*

spi·ge·li·an (spī-jē'lē-an). Relating to or described by Spigelius.

Spigelius, Adrian (van der Spieghel), Flemish anatomist in Padua, 1578–1625. SEE spigelian *hernia;* S. *line, lobe.*

spike. **1.** A brief electrical event of 3–25 ms that gives the appearance in the electroencephalogram of a rising and falling vertical line. **2.** In electrophoresis, a sharply angled upward deflection on a densitometric tracing.

ponto-geniculo-occipital s., EEG spikes during REM sleep that arise in the pons and pass to the lateral geniculate body and occipital cortex.

spill. An overflow; a scattering of fluid or finely divided matter.

cellular s., a dissemination of cells through the lymph or blood, thereby resulting in metastases or implantation of foreign tissue in any part or organ.

Spiller, William G., U. S. neurologist, 1863–1940. SEE Frazier-S. *operation.*

spill·way. A groove or channel through which food may pass from the occlusal surfaces of teeth during the masticatory process. SYN sluiceway.

spi·lus (spī'lŭs). SYN *nevus* spilus. [Mod. L. fr. G. *spilos,* a spot]

△**spin-.** SEE spino-.

spi·na, gen. and pl. **spi·nae** (spī'nă, -nē) [TA]. SYN spine (1). [L. a thorn, the backbone, spine]

s. angula'ris, SYN *spine* of sphenoid bone.

▣**s. bif'ida,** embryologic failure of fusion of one or more vertebral arches; subtypes of s. bifida are based on degree and pattern of malformation associated with neuroectoderm involvement. SYN hydrocele spinalis, schistorrhachis.

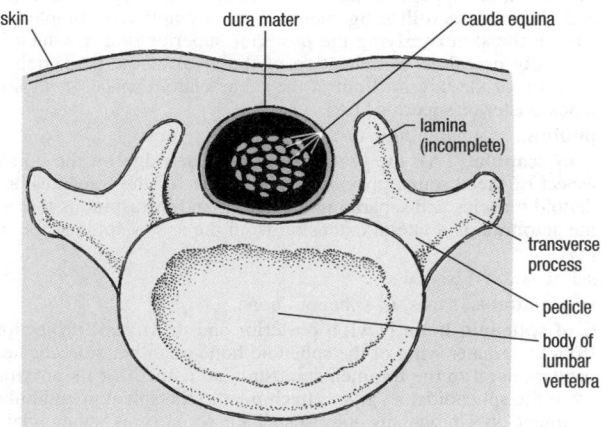

skin · dura mater · cauda equina · lamina (incomplete) · transverse process · pedicle · body of lumbar vertebra

spina bifida occulta

s. bif'ida aper'ta, SYN s. bifida cystica.

s. bif'ida cys'tica, s. bifida associated with a meningeal cyst (meningocele) or a cyst containing both meninges and spinal cord (meningomyelocele) or only spinal cord (myelocele). SYN s. bifida aperta, s. bifida manifesta.

s. bif'ida manifes'ta, SYN s. bifida cystica.

s. bif'ida occul'ta, s. bifida in which there is a spinal defect, but no protrusion of the cord or its membrane, although there is often some abnormality in their development.

s. dorsa'lis, SYN vertebral *column.*

s. fronta'lis, s, nasalis ossis frontalis.

spinae geniorum inferior et superior, SYN mental *spine.*

s. hel'icis [TA], SYN *spine* of helix.

s. ili'aca ante'rior infe'rior, SYN anterior inferior iliac *spine.*

s. ili'aca ante'rior supe'rior, SYN anterior superior iliac *spine.*

s. ili'aca poste'rior infe'rior [TA], SYN posterior inferior iliac *spine.*

s. ili'aca poste'rior supe'rior [TA], SYN posterior superior iliac *spine.*

s. ischiad'ica [TA], SYN ischial *spine.*

s. mea'tus, SYN suprameatal *spine.*

s. menta'lis (inferior et superior) [TA], SYN mental *spine.*

s. nasa'lis ante'rior corporis maxillae [TA], SYN anterior nasal *spine* of maxilla.

s. nasa'lis os'sis fronta'lis [TA], SYN nasal *spine* of frontal bone.

s. nasa'lis poste'rior laminae horizontalis ossis palatini [TA], SYN posterior nasal *spine* of horizontal plate of palatine bone.

s. os'sis sphenoida'lis [TA], SYN *spine* of sphenoid bone.

spi'nae palati'nae [TA], SYN palatine *spines,* under *spine.*

s. peronea'lis, SYN fibular *trochlea* of calcaneus.

s. pu'bis, SYN pubic *tubercle.*

s. scap'ulae [TA], SYN *spine* of scapula.

s. suprameatalis, ✕official alternate term for suprameatal *spine.*

s. supramea'tica, SYN suprameatal *spine.*

s. trochlea'ris [TA], SYN trochlear *spine.*

s. tympan'ica ma'jor [TA], SYN greater tympanic *spine.*

s. tympan'ica mi'nor [TA], SYN lesser tympanic *spine.*

spi·nal (spī'năl). **1.** Relating to any spine or spinous process. **2.** Relating to the vertebral column. SYN rachial, rachidial, rachidian, spinalis. [L. *spinalis*]

spi·na·lis (spī-nā'lis). SYN spinal. [L.]

spi·nate (spī'nāt). Spined; having spines.

spin·dle (spin'dl). In anatomy and pathology, any fusiform cell or structure. [A.S.]

aortic s., a fusiform dilation of the aorta immediately beyond the isthmus. SYN His s.

central s., a central group of microtubules (continuous fibers) that course uninterrupted, between the asters, in contrast to the microtubules attached to the individual chromosomes (s. fibers).

cleavage s., the s. formed during the cleavage of a zygote or its blastomeres.

His s., SYN aortic s.

Krukenberg s., a vertical fusiform area of melanin pigmentation on the posterior surface of the central cornea.

Kühne s., SYN neuromuscular s.

mitotic s., the fusiform figure characteristic of a dividing cell; it consists of microtubules (s. fibers), some of which become attached to each chromosome at its centromere and are involved in chromosomal movement; other microtubules (continuous fibers) pass from pole to pole. SYN nuclear s.

muscle s., SYN neuromuscular s.

neuromuscular s., a fusiform end organ in skeletal muscle in which afferent and a few efferent nerve fibers terminate; it contains from 3–10 striated muscle fibers (intrafusal fibers) that are much smaller than the ordinary muscle fibers, are separated from them by a capsule that encloses the organ, and are innervated by the thin axon of a gamma motoneuron (gamma motor fiber); the sensory endings that occur on the intrafusal fibers are either annulospiral or flower spray endings; this sensory end organ is particularly sensitive to passive stretch of the muscle in which it is enclosed. SYN Kühne s., muscle s.

neurotendinous s., SYN Golgi tendon *organ.*

nuclear s., SYN mitotic s.

▣**sleep s.,** the electroencephalographic record of 14-per-second bursts of wave frequency seen on EEG examination.

spine (spīn) [TA]. **1.** A short, sharp, thornlike process of bone; a spinous process. SYN spina [TA]. **2.** SYN vertebral *column.* [L. *spina*]

alar s., SYN s. of sphenoid bone.

angular s., SYN s. of sphenoid bone.

anterior inferior iliac s. [TA], spine on the anterior border of the ilium between the anterior superior iliac s. and the acetabulum; site of origin for the direct head of the rectus femoris muscle. SYN spina iliaca anterior inferior [TA].

anterior nasal s. (ANS), SYN anterior nasal s. of maxilla.

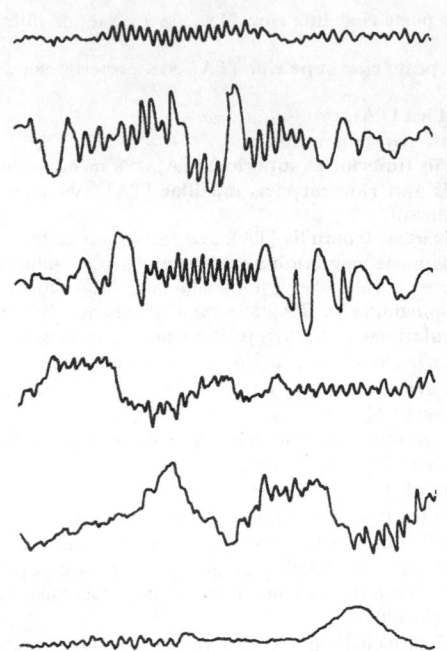

sleep spindle: EEG showing spindle-shaped runs of alpha rhythm (9–14 Hz) in first and third tracing

anterior nasal s. of maxilla [TA], a pointed projection at the anterior extremity of the intermaxillary suture; the tip, as seen on a lateral cephalometric radiograph, is used as a cephalometric landmark. SYN spina nasalis anterior corporis maxillae [TA], anterior nasal s.

anterior superior iliac s. [TA], the anterior extremity of the iliac crest, which provides attachment for the inguinal ligament and the sartorius muscle. SYN spina iliaca anterior superior [TA].

bamboo s., in radiology, the appearance of the thoracic or lumbar spine with ankylosing spondylitis.

cleft s., SEE *spina* bifida.

dendritic s.'s, variably long excrescences of nerve cell dendrites, varying in shape from small knobs to thornlike or filamentous processes, usually more numerous on distal dendrite arborizations than on the proximal part of dendritic trunks; they are a preferential site of synaptic axodendritic contact; sparse or absent in some types of nerve cells (motor neurons, the large cells of the globus pallidus, stellate cells of the cerebral cortex), exceedingly numerous in others such as the pyramidal cells of the cerebral cortex and the Purkinje cells of the cerebellar cortex. SYN dendritic thorns, gemmule (2).

dorsal s., SYN vertebral *column.*

greater tympanic s. [TA], the anterior edge of the tympanic notch (of Rivinus). SYN spina tympanica major [TA].

s. of helix [TA], an anteriorly directed s. at the extremity of the crus of the helix of the auricle. SYN spina helicis [TA], apophysis helicis.

hemal s., the middle point on the underside of the hemal arch of a vertebra in lower vertebrates; considered by some to be represented by the sternum in humans.

Henle s., SYN suprameatal s.

iliac s., SEE anterior inferior iliac s., anterior superior iliac s., posterior inferior iliac s., posterior superior iliac s.

ischiadic s., SYN ischial s.

ischial s. [TA], a pointed process from the posterior border of the ischium on a level with the lower border of the acetabulum; gives attachment to the coccygeus muscle and sacrospinous ligament; the pudendal nerve passes dorsal to the ischial s., which is palpable per vagina or rectum, and thus is used as a target for the

needle tip in administering a pudendal nerve block. SYN spina ischiadica [TA], ischiadic s., sciatic s.

lesser tympanic s. [TA], the posterior edge of the tympanic notch (of Rivinus). SYN spina tympanica minor [TA].

meatal s., SYN suprameatal s.

mental s. [TA], a slight projection, sometimes two (superior and inferior), in the middle line of the posterior surface of the body of the mandible, giving attachment to the geniohyoid muscle (below) and the genioglossus (above). SYN spina mentalis (inferior et superior) [TA], genial tubercle, spinae geniorum inferior et superior.

nasal s. of frontal bone [TA], a projection from the center of the nasal part of the frontal bone, which lies between and articulates with the nasal bones and the perpendicular plate of the ethmoid. SYN spina nasalis ossis frontalis [TA].

neural s., the middle point of the neural arch of the typical vertebra, represented by the spinous process.

palatine s.'s [TA], the longitudinal ridges along the palatine grooves on the inferior surface of the palatine process of the maxilla. SYN spinae palatinae [TA].

poker s., stiff s. resulting from widespread joint immobility or overwhelming muscle spasm as might be evoked by an osteomyelitis of a vertebra or a rheumatoid spondylitis.

posterior inferior iliac s. [TA], s. at the inferior end of the posterior border of the ilium between the posterior superior iliac s. and the greater sciatic notch; it forms the upper margin of the latter. SYN spina iliaca posterior inferior [TA].

posterior nasal s. of horizontal plate of palatine bone [TA], the sharp posterior extremity of the nasal crest of the hard palate. SYN spina nasalis posterior laminae horizontalis ossis palatini [TA], posterior palatine s.

posterior palatine s., SYN posterior nasal s. of horizontal plate of palatine bone.

posterior superior iliac s. [TA], the posterior extremity of the iliac crest, the uppermost point of attachment of the sacrotuberous and posterior sacroiliac ligaments; a readily apparent dimple occurs in the skin overlying the posterior superior iliac s. which is clinically useful as an indication of the level of the S2 vertebra, the level of the inferior limit of the subarachnoid space. SYN spina iliaca posterior superior [TA].

pubic s., SYN pubic *tubercle.*

s. of scapula [TA], the prominent triangular ridge on the dorsal aspect of the scapula, providing attachment for the trapezius and deltoid muscles and separating the supra- and infraspinous fossae; the acromion is a lateral extension from the s. SYN spina scapulae [TA].

sciatic s., SYN ischial s.

sphenoidal s., SYN s. of sphenoid bone.

s. of sphenoid bone [TA], a posterior and downward projection from the greater wing of the sphenoid bone on either side, located posterolateral to the foramen spinosum, so named for its proximity to the sphenoidal s.; gives attachment to the sphenomandibular ligament. SYN processus spinosus [TA], spina ossis sphenoidalis [TA], alar s., angular s., sphenoidal s., spina angularis, spinous process of sphenoid.

Spix s., SYN *lingula* of mandible.

suprameatal s. [TA], small bony prominence anterior to the supramastoid pit at the posterosuperior margin of the bony external acoustic meatus. SYN spina suprameatalis ☆, Henle s., meatal s., spina meatus, spina suprameatica.

thoracic s., the thoracic region of the vertebral column; the thoracic vertebrae [T1–T12] as a whole; that part of the vertebral column which enters into the formation of the thorax.

trochlear s. [TA], a spicule of bone arising from the edge of the trochlear fovea, giving attachment to the pulley of the superior oblique muscle of the eyeball. SYN spina trochlearis [TA].

Spinelli, Pier G., Italian gynecologist, 1862–1929. SEE S. *operation.*

spinn·bar·keit (spin′bahr-kīt). The stringy, elastic character of cervical mucus during the ovulatory period; in contrast to other times in the menstrual cycle, cervical secretions at midcycle are clear, abundant, and of low viscosity. [Ger. *Spinnbarkeit,* viscosity, ability to form a thread]

⚠️**spino-, spin-. 1.** The spine. **2.** Spinous. [L. *spina*]

spi·no·bul·bar (spī′nō-bŭl′bar). SYN bulbospinal.

spi·no·cer·e·bel·lum (spī′nō-sār-ĕ-bel′ŭm) [TA]. SYN paleocerebellum.

spi·no·col·lic·u·lar (spī′nō-col-ik′ū-lar). SYN spinotectal.

spi·no·cos·ta·lis (spī′nō-kos-tā′lis). The superior and inferior serratus posterior muscles regarded as one. [L.]

spi·no·gle·noid (spī′nō-glē′noyd). Relating to the spine and the glenoid cavity of the scapula.

spi·no·mus·cu·lar (spī′nō-mŭs′kū-lăr). Relating to the spinal cord and the muscles supplied by the spinal nerves.

spi·no·neu·ral (spī′nō-noo′răl). Relating to the spinal cord and the nerves given off from it.

spi·nose (spī′nōs). SYN spinous.

spi·no·tec·tal (spī′nō-tek′tăl). Passing upward from the spinal cord to the tectum. SYN spinocollicular.

spi·no·trans·ver·sar·i·us (spī′nō-trans-ver-sār′ē-ŭs). The splenius and obliquus capitis major muscles regarded as one.

spi·nous (spī′nŭs). Relating to, shaped like, or having a spine or spines. SYN spinose.

spin·thar·i·con (spin-thăr′i-kon). A spark chamber device used to record the distribution of low energy emissions from radiopharmaceuticals administered internally, especially for thyroid scans using iodine-125. [G. *spinthēr*, spark]

spin·thar·i·scope (spin-thăr′i-skōp). SYN scintillation *counter*. [G. *spinthēr*, spark, + *skopeō*, to view]

spip·e·rone (spip′ĕ-rōn). An antipsychotic.

⚠️**spir-.** SEE spiro-.

spi·ra·cle (spī′ră-kl, spir-). An aperture for breathing in arthropods and in sharks and related fishes. [L. *spiraculum*, fr. *spiro*, to breathe]

spi·rad·e·no·ma (spī-rad-ĕ-nō′mă). A benign tumor of sweat glands. [G. *speira*, coil, + adenoma]

eccrine s., a typically painful benign skin tumor composed of two cell types derived from the secretory part of eccrine sweat glands.

spi·ral (spī′răl). **1.** Coiled; winding around a center like a watch spring; winding and ascending like a wire spring. **2.** A structure in the shape of a coil. [Mediev. L. *spiralis*, fr. G. *speira*, a coil]

Curschmann s.'s, spirally twisted masses of mucus occurring in the sputum in bronchial asthma.

s. of Tillaux, an imaginary line connecting the insertions of the recti muscles of the eye.

spir·a·my·cin (spir-ă-mī′sin). An antibiotic substance (almost identical to leucomycin) produced by *Streptomyces ambofaciens;* an antimicrobial agent.

spi·rem, spi·reme (spī′rem, spī′rēm). Term formerly applied to the first stage of mitosis or meiosis (prophase) when extended chromosome filaments have the appearance of a loose ball of yarn, on the incorrect supposition that the filaments were continuous and later broke apart to form individual chromosomes. [G. *speirēma*, a coil 1]

spi·ril·la (spī-ril′ă). Plural of spirillum.

Spi·ril·la·ce·ae (spī-ri-lā′sē-ē). A family of usually motile, aerobic to facultatively anaerobic bacteria (order Pseudomonadales) containing Gram-negative, rod-shaped cells which are curved or spirally twisted. Motile cells contain a single polar flagellum or a tuft of polar flagella. These organisms are primarily water forms, although some are parasitic or pathogenic on humans and other higher animals. The type genus is *Spirillum.* SEE *Spirillum.*

spi·ril·lar (spī-ril′ăr). S-shaped; referring to a bacterial cell with an S shape.

spi·ril·li·ci·dal (spī-ril-i-sī′dăl). Destructive to spirilla or spirochetes. [spirilla + L. *caedo*, to kill]

spi·ril·lo·sis (spī′ri-lō′sis). Any disease caused by the presence of spirilla in the blood or tissues.

Spi·ril·lum (spī-ril′ŭm). A genus of large (1.4–1.7 μm in diameter), rigid, helical, Gram-negative bacteria (family Spirillaceae) that are motile by means of bipolar fascicles of flagella. These freshwater organisms are obligately microaerophilic and chemoorganotrophic, possessing a strictly respiratory metabolism; they

neither oxidize nor ferment carbohydrates. The type species is *S. volutans.* [Mod. L. dim. of L. *spira*, coil, fr. G. *speira*]

S. mi′nus, a species of uncertain taxonomic classification that causes a form of rat-bite fever (sodoku). This species has never been cultured.

S. volu′tans, a species found in fresh water; it is the type species of *S.*

spi·ril·lum, pl. **spi·ril·la** (spī-ril′ŭm, -ă). A member of the genus *Spirillum.*

Obermeier s., SYN *Borrelia recurrentis.*

Vincent s., the s. or spirochete found in association with Vincent bacillus. *Fusobacterium nucleatum* is frequently the only bacillus isolated.

spir·it (spir′it). **1.** An alcoholic liquor stronger than wine, obtained by distillation. **2.** Any distilled liquid. **3.** An alcoholic or hydroalcoholic solution of volatile substances; some s.'s are used as flavoring agents, others have medicinal value. SYN spiritus. [L. *spiritus,* a breathing, life soul, fr. *spiro,* to breathe]

ardent s.'s, brandy, whiskey, and other forms of distilled alcoholic liquors.

aromatic ammonia s., a hydroalcoholic solution containing approximately 2% ammonia and 4% ammonium carbonate and the aromatics: lemon oil, lavender oil, and myristica oil. Used mainly by inhalation to produce reflex stimulation in persons who have fainted or are at risk of syncope. SYN sal volatile, smelling salts.

industrial methylated s., methylated s., SYN denatured *alcohol.*

neutral s.'s, s.'s distilled from suitable raw materials, are 95% ethanol (v/v), that is, at least 190 proof when distilled. Used for blending with straight whiskey and for making gin, cordials, liqueurs, and vodka. SEE ALSO alcohol.

proof s., dilute alcohol, specific gravity 0.920, containing 49.5% by weight (57.27% by volume) of C_2H_5OH at 15.56°C. Originally in Great Britain it was the weakest alcohol that would permit ignition of gunpowder moistened with it. British proof s. has a specific gravity of 0.9198 and contains 49.2% C_2H_5OH by weight, or 57.1% by volume at the temperature of 10.56°C.

pyroligneous s., pyroxylic s., SYN methyl *alcohol.*

rectified s., SYN alcohol (2).

vital s.'s, in the galenic teachings, a vital essence or principle supposed to be generated from the air or pneuma in the left ventricle of the heart; carried in the blood to the brain and converted to animal s.'s which then flowed along the nerves to all parts of the body.

wine s., SYN alcohol (2).

wood s., SYN methyl *alcohol.*

spir·i·tu·ous (spir′i-choo-ŭs). Containing alcohol in large amount, denoting liquors.

spir·i·tus, gen. and pl. **spir·i·tus** (spir′i-tŭs). SYN spirit. [L.]

⚠️**spiro-, spir-. 1.** Coil, coil-shaped. [G. *speira*] **2.** Breathing. [L. *spiro,* to breathe]

Spi·ro·cer·ca lu·pi (spi-rō-ser′kă loo′pī). The esophageal worm of dogs and other carnivores, a red spiruroid nematode that occurs in nodules in the wall of the esophagus, stomach, and aorta of dogs, foxes, and wolves; intermediate hosts are various coprophagic beetles. Clinical symptoms occur only in very heavy infections, which are associated with esophageal carcinomata in dogs and with hypertrophic pulmonary osteoarthropathy. [L., fr. G. *speira*, coil, + G. *kerkos*, tail; L. *lupus*, wolf]

🔲***Spi·ro·chae·ta*** (spī′rō-kē′tă). A genus of motile bacteria (order Spirochaetales) containing presumably Gram-negative, flexible, undulating, spiral-shaped rods that may or may not possess flagelliform, tapering ends. The protoplast is spirally wound around an axial filament. No obvious periplast membrane or cross-striations occur. These organisms are motile by means of a creeping motion over the surfaces of supporting objects. They are not parasitic but are found free-living in fresh or sea water slime; they are commonly found in sewage and foul waters. At present the genus contains five species. The type species is *S. plicatilis.* [Mod. L. fr. G. *speira*, a coil, + *chaitē,* hair]

S. obermei′eri, SYN *Borrelia recurrentis.*

S. plicat′ilis, a very large species (sometimes as long as 200 μm)

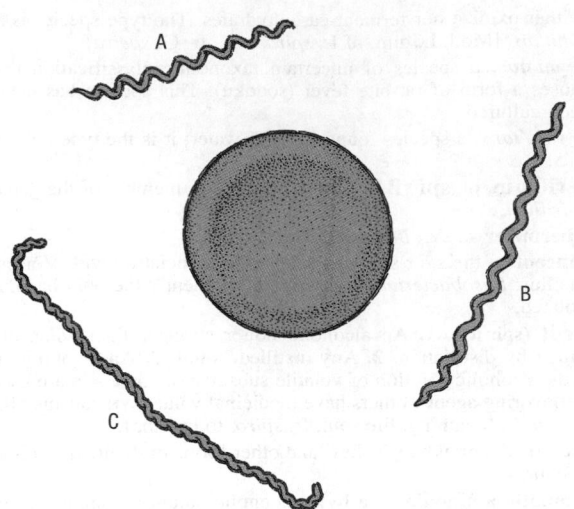

spirochetes: (shown for size comparison with red blood cell) (A) *Treponema*; (B) *Borrelia*; (C) *Leptospira*

---

of bacteria; it is nonparasitic, so far as known; it is the type species of the genus *S.*

Spi·ro·chae·ta·ce·ae (spī-rō-kē-tā'sē-ē). A family of bacteria (order Spirochaetales) consisting of coarse, spiral cells, 30–50 μm in length and possessing definite protoplasmic structures. These organisms occur in stagnant, fresh, or salt water and in the intestinal tracts of bivalve molluscs. The type genus is *Spirochaeta*. SEE *Spirochaeta*.

Spi·ro·chae·ta·les (spī-rō-kē-tā'lēz). An order of bacteria containing slender, flexuous cells, 6–500 μm in length, in the form of spirals with at least one complete turn. Some species may have an axial filament, a lateral crista, or ridge, or transverse striations. All of these organisms are motile, whirling or spinning about the long axis, thus driving the organism forward or backward. Free-living, saprophytic, and parasitic forms occur. The type family is Spirochaetaceae.

spi·ro·chet·al (spī-rō-kē'tăl). Relating to spirochetes, especially to infection with such organisms.

spi·ro·chete (spī'rō-kēt). A vernacular term used to refer to any organism resembling a *Leptospira*, *Spirochaeta*, or *Treponema* cell.

spi·ro·chet·e·mia (spī'rō-kē-tē'mē-ă). Presence of spirochetes in the blood. [spirochete + G. *haima*, blood]

spi·ro·che·ti·cide (spī-rō-kē'tĭ-sīd). An agent destructive to spirochetes. [spirochete + L. *caedo*, to kill]

spi·ro·che·tol·y·sis (spī'rō-kē-tol'i-sis). Destruction of spirochetes, as by chemotherapy or by specific antibodies. [spirochete + G. *lysis*, a loosening]

spi·ro·che·to·sis (spī'rō-kē-tō'sis). Any disease caused by a spirochete.

bronchopulmonary s., SYN hemorrhagic *bronchitis*.

spi·ro·che·tot·ic (spī'rō-kē-tot'ik). Relating to or marked by spirochetosis.

spi·ro·gram (spī'rō-gram). The tracing made by the spirograph.

spi·ro·graph (spī'rō-graf). A device for representing graphically the depth and rapidity of respiratory movements. [L. *spiro*, to breathe, + G. *graphō*, to write]

spi·ro·in·dex (spī'rō-in-deks). Vital capacity divided by the height of the individual.

spi·rom·e·ter (spī-rom'ĕ-ter). In clinical practice and research, any device used for measuring flows and volumes, inspired and expired by the lungs, thus assessing pulmonary function. Considered the most basic measurement device of pulmonary function. [L. *spiro*, to breathe, + G. *metron*, measure]

chain-compensated s., a Tissot s. in which compensation for

change in bell buoyancy is accomplished automatically by a suspending chain of correct mass per unit length.

Krogh s., a water-sealed s. in which the bell is a large, shallow, rectangular box rotating slightly around a horizontal axis extending along one edge, with an arm extending beyond that axis to a counterbalancing weight; comparable with a wedge s.

Tissot s., a very large water-sealed s. designed for accumulating expired gas over a long period of time; the counterbalancing of the bell (almost frictionless) is compensated for by the bell's change in buoyancy as it emerges from the water, keeping the contained gas precisely at ambient atmospheric pressure.

wedge s., a waterless s. constructed of two large rectangular plates with edges connected by accordion-pleated rubber so that large changes in volume are accommodated by small changes in the acute angle of the wedge-shaped interior, sensed by an electrical transducer; designed for rapid response by reducing the acceleration of the moving parts.

Spi·ro·me·tra (spī-rō-mē'tră). A genus of pseudophyllid tapeworms. [G. *speira*, coil, + *mētra*, womb (uterus)]

S. manso'ni, a species of pseudophyllid tapeworms of wild and feral cats, the larval form of which (sparganum) may survive in human tissues; it has been commonly found in humans in the Orient, but is also reported from widely scattered areas elsewhere; infection of humans with the sparganum occurs from active migration of the larva from freshly split infected frogs used as a poultice for wounds, sore eyes (as in ocular sparganosis), bruises, or ulcerations; it is also likely that humans may be infected with sparganum larvae from eating any vertebrate harboring these plerocercoids. SYN *Diphyllobothrium linguloides, Diphyllobothrium mansoni*.

S. mansonoi'des, a species of pseudophyllid tapeworms from North America, whose larva (sparganum) may be a cause of sparganosis of humans in Florida and the Gulf of Mexico states. SYN *Diphyllobothrium mansonoides*.

spi·rom·e·try (spī-rom'ĕ-trē). Making pulmonary measurements with a spirometer.

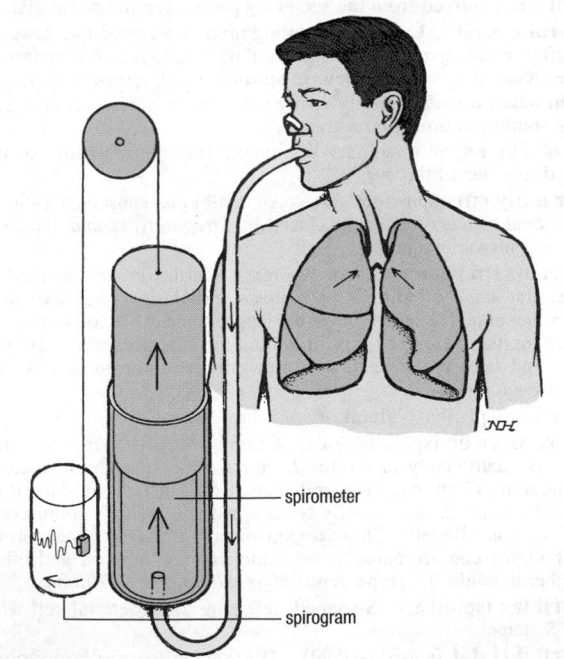

spirometry: principle of closed-circuit spirometry

---

forced s., inspiration and more particularly expiration in which volume is plotted against time, giving a measure of pulmonary function. The amount of air expelled in one second (FEV) is often considered the single most important measurement in clinical respiratory physiology.

spi·ro·no·lac·tone (spī'rō-nō-lak'tōn). A diuretic agent that blocks the renal tubular actions of aldosterone. It increases the urinary excretion of sodium and chloride, decreases the excretion of potassium and ammonium, and reduces the titratable acidity of the urine; most effectively used to potentiate the natriuretic action and reduce the potassium excretion produced by other diuretics.

spi·ro·scope (spī'rō-skōp). A device for measuring the air capacity of the lungs. [L. *spiro*, to breathe, + G. *skopeo*, to view]

spi·ro·stan (spī'rō-stan). A 16,22:22,26-diepoxycholestane.

spi·ru·roid (spī'roo-royd). Common name for a member of the superfamily Spiruroidea.

Spi·ru·roi·dea (spī-roo-roy'dē-ă). A superfamily of arthropod-borne nematode parasites of the alimentary tract, respiratory system, or orbital, nasal, or oral cavities of vertebrates. They are common and frequently pathogenic parasites of domestic mammals and birds, producing ulcerations from penetration of the anterior end of these spiny worms through the alimentary lining; includes the families Acuariidae, Gnathostomatidae, Rictulariidae, Seuratidae, Physalopteridae, Spiruridae, and Thelaziidae. [G. *speiroeidēs*, spiral]

spis·si·tude (spis'i-tood). The state of being inspissated; the condition of a fluid thickened almost to a solid by evaporation or inspissation. [L. *spissitudo*, fr. *spissus*, thick]

spit·ting. SYN expectoration (2).

spit·tle (spit'l). SYN saliva. [A.S. *spātl*]

Spitz, Sophie, 20th century U.S. pathologist. SEE S. *nevus*.

Spitzer, Alexander, Austrian anatomist, 1868–1943. SEE S. *theory*.

Spitzka, Edward C., U.S. neurologist, 1852–1914. SEE S. *nucleus*, marginal *tract*, marginal *zone; column* of S.-Lissauer.

Spix, Johann B., German anatomist, 1781–1826. SEE S. *spine*.

SPL Abbreviation for sound pressure *level*.

△**splanchn-.** SEE splanchno-.

splanch·nap·o·phys·i·al, splanch·nap·o·phys·e·al (splangk'nă-pō-fiz'ē-ăl). Relating to a splanchnapophysis.

splanch·na·poph·y·sis (splangk'nă-pof'i-sis). An apophysis of the typical vertebra, on the side opposite to the neural apophysis, or any bony process, giving attachment to a viscus or part of the alimentary tract. [splanchn- + G. *apophysis*, offshoot]

splanch·nec·to·pia (splangk-nek-tō'pē-ă). Displacement of any of the viscera. [splanchn- + G. *ektopos*, out of place]

splanch·nes·the·sia (splangk-nes-thē'zē-ă). SYN visceral *sense*. [splanch- + G. *aisthēsis*, sensation]

splanch·nic (splangk'nik). SYN visceral.

splanch·ni·cec·to·my (splangk-ni-sek'tō-mē). Resection of the splanchnic nerves and usually of the celiac ganglion as well. [splanchni- + G. *ektomē*, excision]

splanch·ni·cot·o·my (splangk-ni-kot'ō-mē). Section of a splanchnic nerve or nerves, a surgical procedure formerly used in the treatment of hypertension. [splanchni- + G. *tomē*, incision]

△**splanchno-, splanchn-, splanchni-.** The viscera. SEE ALSO viscero-. [G. *splanchnon*, viscus]

splanch·no·cele (splangk'nō-sēl). **1.** The primitive body cavity or celom in the embryo. [G. *koilos*, hollow] **2.** Hernia of any of the abdominal viscera. [G. *kēlē*, hernia]

splanch·no·cra·ni·um (splangk-nō-krā'nē-ŭm). SYN viscerocranium.

splanch·nog·ra·phy (splangk-nog'ră-fē). A treatise on or description of the viscera. [splanchno- + G. *graphō*, to write]

splanch·no·lith (splangk'nō-lith). An intestinal calculus. [splanchno- + G. *lithos*, stone]

splanch·no·lo·gia (splangk'nō-lō'jē-ă). SYN splanchnology, splanchnology.

splanch·nol·o·gy (splangk-nol'ŏ-jē). The branch of medical science dealing with the viscera. SYN splanchnologia. [splanchno- + G. *logos*, study]

splanch·no·meg·a·ly (splangk-nō-meg'ă-lē). SYN visceromegaly. [splanchno- + G. *megas*, large]

splanch·no·mic·ria (splangk-nō-mik'rē-ă). Condition in which the splanchnic organs are of smaller than normal size. [splanchno- + G. *mikros*, small]

splanch·nop·a·thy (splangk-nop'ă-thē). Any disease of the abdominal viscera. [splanchno- + G. *pathos*, disease]

splanch·no·pleu·ral (splangk-nō-ploor'ăl). SYN splanchnopleuric.

splanch·no·pleure (splangk'nō-ploor). The embryonic layer formed by association of the visceral layer of the lateral plate mesoderm with the endoderm. [splanchno- + G. *pleura*, side]

splanch·no·pleu·ric (splangk-nō-ploor'ik). Relating to the splanchnopleure. SYN splanchnopleural.

splanch·nop·to·sis, splanch·nop·to·sia (splangk'nō-tō'sis, -tō'sē-ă). SYN visceroptosis. [splanchno- + G. *ptōsis* a falling]

splanch·no·scle·ro·sis (splangk'nō-skle-rō'sis). Hardening, through connective tissue overgrowth, of any of the viscera. [splanchno- + G. *sklērōsis*, hardening]

splanch·no·skel·e·tal (splangk-nō-skel'ĕ-tăl). SYN visceroskeletal.

splanch·no·skel·e·ton (splangk-nō-skel'ĕ-tŏn). SYN visceroskeleton (2).

splanch·no·so·mat·ic (splangk'nō-sō-mat'ik). SYN viscerosomatic. [splanchno- + G. *sōma*, body]

splanch·not·o·my (splangk-not'ō-mē). Dissection of the viscera by incision. [splanchno- + G. *tomē*, incision]

splanch·no·tribe (splangk'nō-trīb). An instrument resembling a large angiotribe used for occluding the intestine temporarily, prior to resection. [splanchno- + G. *tribō*, to rub, bruise]

splay (splā). **1.** To lay open the end of a tubular structure by making a longitudinal incision to increase its potential diameter. SEE ALSO spatulate. **2.** The rounding of the corner on the graph relating rate of renal tubular secretion or reabsorption of a substance to its arterial plasma concentration, due primarily to the fact that some nephrons reach their tubular maximum before others do.

spleen (splēn) [TA]. A large vascular lymphatic organ lying in the upper part of the abdominal cavity on the left side, between the stomach and diaphragm, composed of white and red pulp; the white consists of lymphatic nodules and diffuse lymphatic tissue; the red consists of venous sinusoids between which are splenic cords; the stroma of both red and white pulp is reticular fibers and cells. A framework of fibroelastic trabeculae extending from the capsule subdivides the structure into poorly defined lobules. It is a blood-forming organ in early life and later a storage organ for red corpuscles and platelets; because of the large number of macrophages, it also acts as a blood filter, both identifying and destroying effete erythrocytes. SYN splen [TA], lien ☆. [G. *splēn*]

accessory s. [TA], one of the small globular masses of splenic tissue occasionally found in the region of the s., in one of the peritoneal folds or elsewhere. SYN splen accessorius [TA], lien accessorius ☆, lien succenturiatus, lienculus, lienunculus, spleneolus, spleniculus, splenule, splenulus, splenunculus.

diffuse waxy s., a condition of amyloid degeneration of the s., affecting chiefly the extrasinusoidal tissue spaces of the pulp.

floating s., a s. that is palpable because of excessive mobility from a relaxed or lengthened pedicle rather than because of enlargement. SYN lien mobilis, movable s.

lardaceous s., SYN waxy s.

movable s., SYN floating s.

sago s., amyloidosis in the s. affecting chiefly the malpighian bodies.

sugar-coated s., hyaloserositis involving the s.

waxy s., amyloidosis of the s. SYN lardaceous s.

splen [TA]. SYN spleen. [G. *splen*, spleen]

s. accessorius [TA], SYN accessory *spleen*.

△**splen-.** SEE spleno-.

sple·nal·gia (splē-nal'jē-ă). A rarely used term for a painful condition of the spleen. SYN splenodynia. [splen- + G. *algos*, pain]

Splendore, Alfonso, 20th century Italian physician. SEE S.-Hoeppli *phenomenon;* Lutz-S.-Almeida *disease*.

Sp

sple·nec·to·my (splē-nek'tō-mē). Removal of the spleen. [splen- + G. *ektomē*, excision]

sple·nec·to·pia, sple·nec·to·py (splen'ek-tō'pē-ă, splē-nek'tō-pē). **1.** Displacement of the spleen, as in a floating spleen. **2.** The presence of rests of splenic tissue, usually in the region of the spleen. [splen- + G. *ektopos*, out of place]

sple·nel·co·sis (splen-el-kō'sis). Abscess of the spleen. [splen- + G. *helkōsis*, ulceration]

sple·ne·o·lus (splē-nē'ō-lŭs). SYN accessory *spleen*. [Mod. L. dim. of G. *splēn*]

sple·net·ic (splē-net'ik). **1.** SYN splenic. **2.** Fretfully surly.

sple·ni·al (splē'nē-ăl). **1.** Relating to the splenium. **2.** Relating to a splenius muscle. [G. *splēnion*, bandage]

splen·ic (splen'ik). Relating to the spleen. SYN lienal, splenetic (1).

sple·ni·cu·lus (splen-ik'ū-lŭs). SYN accessory *spleen*. [Mod. L.]

splen·i·form (splen'i-fōrm, splē'ni-). SYN splenoid.

splen·i·ser·rate (splen'i-ser'āt). Relating to the splenius and serratus muscles.

sple·ni·tis (splē-nī'tis). Inflammation of the spleen. [splen- + G. *-itis*, inflammation]

sple·ni·um, pl. **sple·nia** (splē'nē-ŭm, -ă). **1.** A compress or bandage. **2** [TA]. A structure resembling a bandaged part. [Mod. L. fr. G. *splēnion*, bandage]
s. cor'poris callo'si [TA], SYN s. of corpus callosum.
s. of corpus callosum [TA], the thickened posterior extremity of the corpus callosum. SYN s. corporis callosi [TA], tuber corporis callosi.

sple·ni·us (splē'nē-ŭs). SEE splenius *muscle* of head, splenius *muscle* of neck. [Mod. L. fr. G. *splēnion*, a bandage]

△**spleno-, splen-.** The spleen. [G. *splēn*]

sple·no·cele (splē'nō-sēl). A splenic hernia. [spleno- + G. *kēlē*, tumor, hernia]

sple·no·clei·sis (splē-nō-klī'sis). Inducing the formation of new fibrous tissue on the surface of the spleen by friction or wrapping with gauze. [spleno- + G. *kleisis*, closure]

sple·no·co·lic (splē'nō-kol'ik). Relating to the spleen and the colon; denoting a ligament or fold of peritoneum passing between the two viscera.

sple·no·dyn·ia (splē'nō-din'ē-ă). SYN splenalgia. [spleno- + G. *odynē*, pain]

sple·no·he·pa·to·meg·a·ly, sple·no·he·pa·to·me·ga·lia (splē'-nō-hep'ă-tō-meg'ă-lē, -mě-gā'ē-ă). Enlargement of both spleen and liver. [spleno- + G. *hēpar*, liver, + *megas*, large]

sple·noid (splē'noyd). Resembling the spleen. SYN spleniform. [spleno- + G. *eidos*, resemblance]

sple·no·lym·phat·ic (splē'nō-lim-fat'ik). Relating to the spleen and the lymph nodes.

sple·no·ma (splē-nō'mă). General nonspecific term for an enlarged spleen. [spleno- + G. *-oma*, tumor]

sple·no·ma·la·cia (splē'nō-mă-lā'shē-ă). Softening of the spleen. [spleno- + G. *malakia*, softness]

sple·no·med·ul·lary (splē-nō-med'ŭ-lār-ē). SYN splenomyelogenous. [spleno- + L. *medulla*, marrow]

▣ **sple·no·meg·a·ly, sple·no·me·ga·lia** (splē-nō-meg'ă-lē, -mě-gā'lē-ă). Enlargement of the spleen. SYN megalosplenia. [spleno- + G. *megas* (*megal-*), large]
  congestive s., enlargement of the spleen due to passive congestion; sometimes used as a synonym for Banti syndrome.
  Egyptian s., term sometimes used as a synonym for schistosomiasis mansoni, although hepatomegaly and fibrosis are more consistently found than is an enlarged spleen.
  hemolytic s., s. associated with hemolytic jaundice.
  hyperreactive malarious s., a syndrome characterized by persistent splenomegaly, exceptionally high serum IgM and malaria antibody levels, and hepatic sinusoidal lymphocytosis; believed to be a disturbance in the T-lymphocyte control of the humoral response to recurrent malaria. SYN tropical splenomegaly syndrome.
  Niemann s., enlargement of spleen occurring in Niemann-Pick disease.
  tropical s., SYN visceral *leishmaniasis*.

sple·no·my·e·log·e·nous (splē'nō-mī-ě-loj'ě-nŭs). Originating in the spleen and bone marrow, denoting a form of leukemia. SYN lienomedullary, lienomyelogenous, splenomedullary. [spleno- + G. *myelos*, marrow, + *-gen*, producing]

sple·no·my·e·lo·ma·la·cia (splē'nō-mī'ě-lō-mă-lā'shē-ă). Pathologic softening of the spleen and bone marrow. [spleno- + G. *myelos*, marrow, + *malakia*, softness]

sple·no·neph·ric (splē'nō-nef'rik). SYN splenorenal. [spleno- + G. *nephros*, kidney]

sple·no·pan·cre·at·ic (splē'nō-pan-krē-at'ik). Relating to the spleen and the pancreas. SYN lienopancreatic.

sple·nop·a·thy (splē-nop'ă-thē). Any disease of the spleen. [spleno- + G. *pathos*, suffering]

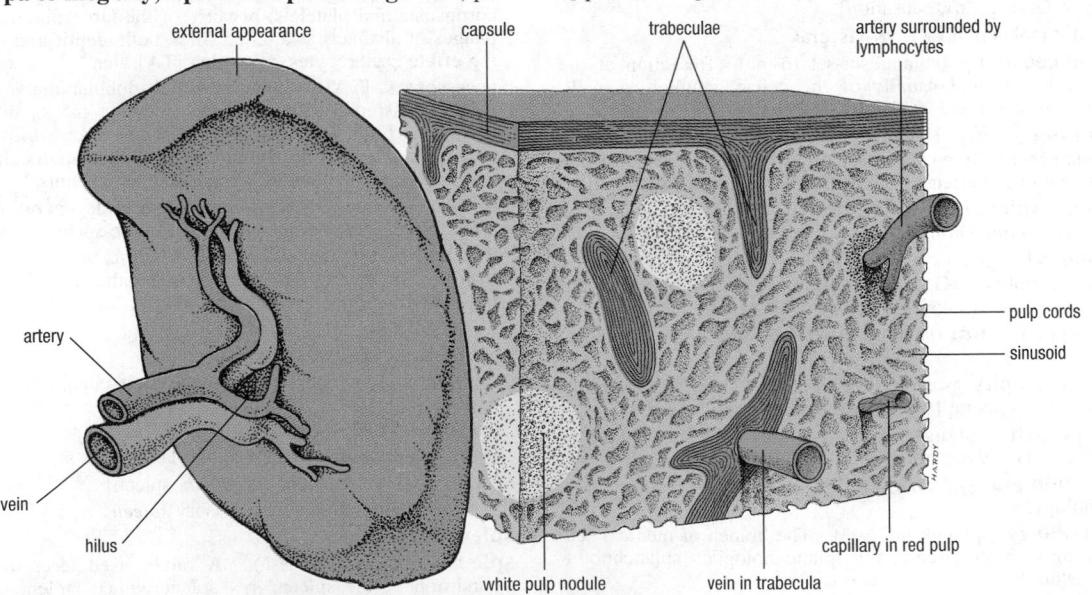

external appearance   capsule   trabeculae   artery surrounded by lymphocytes

artery

vein

hilus

pulp cords

sinusoid

white pulp nodule   vein in trabecula   capillary in red pulp

spleen section: showing general arrangement of splenic tissue

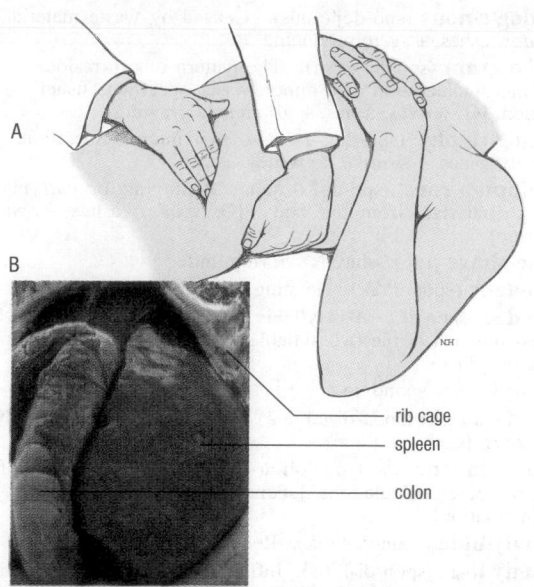

splenomegaly: (A) palpation technique used in diagnosis; (B) splenomegaly due to granulocytic leukemia as seen at autopsy (weight of spleen: 4200g)

sple·no·pexy, sple·no·pex·ia (splē′nō-pek-sē, splē-nō-pek′sē-ă). Suturing in place an ectopic or floating spleen. SYN splenorrhaphy (2). [spleno- + G. *pēxis*, fixation]

sple·no·phren·ic (splē′nō-fren′ik). Relating to the spleen and the diaphragm; denoting a ligament or fold of peritoneum extending between the two structures. [spleno- + G. *phrēn*, diaphragm]

sple·no·por·to·gram (splē-nō-pōr′tō-gram). Radiographic record of the splenic and portal veins and their collaterals following direct injection of water-soluble contrast material into the spleen.

sple·no·por·tog·ra·phy (splē′nō-pōr-tog′ră-fē). Introduction of radiopaque material into the spleen to obtain radiographic visualization of the splenic and main portal veins of the portal circulation. SYN splenic portal venography. [spleno- + portography]

sple·nop·to·sis, sple·nop·to·sia (splē-nop-tō′sis, -tō′sē-ă). Downward displacement of the spleen, as in a floating spleen. [spleno- + G. *ptōsis*, falling]

sple·no·re·nal (splē′nō-rē′năl). Relating to the spleen and the kidney; denoting a ligament or fold of peritoneum extending between the two structures. SYN lienorenal, splenonephric.

sple·nor·rha·gia (splē′nō-rā′jē-ă). Hemorrhage from a ruptured spleen. [spleno- + G. *rhēgnymi*, to burst forth]

sple·nor·rha·phy (splē-nōr′ă-fē). **1.** Suturing a ruptured spleen. **2.** SYN splenopexy. [spleno- + G. *rhaphē*, suture]

sple·no·sis (splē-nō′sis). Implantation and subsequent growth of splenic tissue within the abdomen as a result of disruption of the spleen.

thoracic s., presense of splenic tissue in the thorax, resultant from combined thoracic and abdominal trauma followed by splenectomy.

sple·not·o·my (splē-not′ō-mē). **1.** Anatomy or dissection of the spleen. **2.** Surgical incision of the spleen. [spleno- + G. *tomē*, incision]

sple·no·tox·in (splē-nō-tok′sin). A cytotoxin specific for cells of the spleen. [spleno- + G. *toxikon*, poison]

splen·ule (splen′ūl). SYN accessory *spleen*. [Mod. L. *splenulus*]

splen·u·lus, pl. **splen·u·li** (splen′ū-loos, -lī). SYN accessory *spleen*. [Mod. L. dim. of L. *splen*, spleen]

sple·nun·cu·lus, pl. **sple·nun·cu·li** (splē-nŭng′kū-lŭs, -lī). SYN accessory *spleen*. [Mod. L. dim. of L. *splen*, spleen]

splice·o·some (splī′sē-ō-sōm). A specialized structure that participates in the removal of introns and resplicing of remaining exons of mRNA; in addition to the mRNA primary transcript, at least four small nuclear RNAs (snRNAs) and some proteins are involved. [splice + -some]

splic·ing (splīs′ing). **1.** Attachment of one DNA molecule to another. SYN gene splicing. **2.** Removal of introns from mRNA precursors and the reattachment or annealing of exons. SYN RNA splicing.

alternative s., different ways of assembling exons to produce different mature mRNAs.

splint. 1. An appliance for preventing movement of a joint or for the fixation of displaced or movable parts. **2.** The s. bone, or fibula. [Middle Dutch *splinte*]

acid etch cemented s., a s. of heavy wire which is cemented to the labial surfaces of teeth with any of the acid etch cement techniques; used to stabilize traumatically displaced or periodontally diseased teeth.

active s., SYN dynamic s.

air s., a plastic s. inflated by air used to immobilize part or all of an extremity. SYN inflatable s.

airplane s., a complicated s. that holds the arm in abduction at about shoulder level with the forearm midway in flexion, generally with an axillary strut for support.

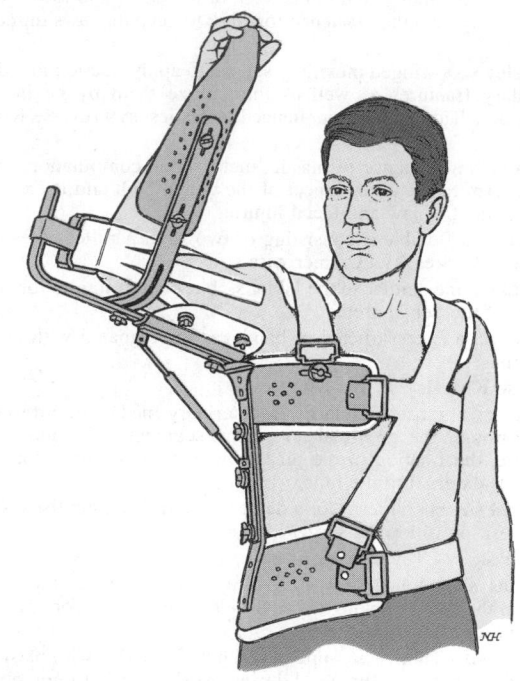

airplane splint

anchor s., a s. used for fracture of the jaw, with wires around the teeth and a rod to hold it in place.

Anderson s., a contained skeletal traction s. with pins inserted into proximal and distal ends of a fracture; reduction is obtained by an external rod attached to the pins; also referred to as external fixation.

backboard s., a board s. with slots for fixation of the body by straps; shorter ones are used for neck injuries, longer ones for back injuries.

Balkan s., SYN Balkan *frame*.

cap s., a plastic or metallic fracture appliance designed to cover the crowns of the teeth and usually cemented to them.

coaptation s., a short s. designed to prevent overriding of the ends of a fractured bone, usually supplemented by a longer s. to fix the entire limb. Most commonly used for repair of fractures of the humeral shaft.

Cramer wire s., SYN ladder s.

Denis Browne s., a light aluminum s. applied to the lateral aspect

sp

of the leg and foot; used for torsional deformities of the leg, ankle, or foot in children.

dynamic s., a s. utilizing springs or elastic bands that aids in movements initiated by the patient by controlling the plane and range of motion. SYN active s., functional s. (1).

Essig s., a stainless steel wire passed labially and lingually around a segment of the dental arch and held in position by individual ligature wires around the contact areas of the teeth; used to stabilize fractured or repositioned teeth and the involved alveolar bone.

Frejka pillow s., a pillow s. used for abduction and flexion of the femurs in treatment of congenital hip dysplasia or dislocation in infants.

functional s., (1) SYN dynamic s; **(2)** the joining of two or more teeth into a rigid unit by means of fixed restorations that cover all or part of the abutment teeth.

Gunning s., a prosthesis fabricated from models of endentulous maxillary and mandibular arches in order to aid in reduction and fixation of a fracture.

inflatable s., SYN air s.

interdental s., a s. for a fractured jaw, consisting of two metal or acrylic resin bands wired to the teeth of the upper and lower jaws, respectively, and then fastened together to keep the jaws immovable.

Kingsley s., a winged maxillary s. used to apply traction to reduce maxillary fractures as well as immobilize them by having the wings attached to a head appliance by elastics. SYN reverse Kingsley s.

labial s., an appliance of plastic, metal, or in combination, made to conform to the outer aspect of the dental arch and used in the management of jaw and facial injuries.

ladder s., a flexible s. consisting of two stout parallel wires with finer cross wires. SYN Cramer wire s.

lingual s., one similar to the labial s., but conforming to the inner aspect of the dental arch.

plaster s., a s. constructed of bandages impregnated with plaster of Paris.

reverse Kingsley s., SYN Kingsley s.

Stader s., a s. used primarily in veterinary medicine; with metal pins through the proximal and distal segments of a long bone fracture, the fixation of the pins is maintained by the apparatus, which is external to the limb.

surgical s., general term for a device used to maintain tissues in a new position following surgery.

Taylor s., SYN Taylor back *brace*.

Thomas s., a long leg s. extending from a ring at the hip to beyond the foot, allowing traction to a fractured leg, for emergencies and transportation.

Tobruk s., a Thomas s., applied and held in plaster with plaster of Paris dressings; a s. first used during World War II to immobilize the limb during hazardous conditions such as transport from small to large boats. [port of *Tobruk*, Libya]

wire s., a device to stabilize teeth loosened by accident or by a periodontal condition in the maxilla or mandible; a device to reduce and stabilize maxillary or mandibular fractures by applying it to both jaws and connecting it by intermaxillary wires or rubber bands.

splint·ing. 1. Application of a splint or treatment using a splint. **2.** In dentistry, the joining of two or more teeth into a rigid unit by means of fixed or removable restorations or appliances. **3.** Stiffening of a body part to avoid pain caused by movement of the part, as from a fracture or other injury. **4.** In psychiatry, the exercise by family, friends, or coworkers of the various strategies designed to minimize the impairment and increase the function of a person with diminished higher cortical function.

splints. Exostoses occurring along the course of the small metacarpal and metatarsal bones of the horse. SEE splint.

split·ting. In chemistry, the cleavage of a covalent bond, fragmenting the molecule involved.

spm Abbreviation for a gene that leads to *s*uppression and *m*utation of alleles that are unstable.

spo·dog·e·nous (spŏ-doj′ĕ-nŭs). Caused by waste material. [G. *spodos*, ashes, + -*gen*, producing]

spod·o·gram (spŏ′dō-gram). The pattern of ash residue formed by microincineration of a minute tissue specimen, usually a thin section. [G. *spodos*, ashes, + *gramma*, a drawing]

spo·dog·ra·phy (spŏ-dog′-ră-fē). SYN microincineration. [G. *spodos*, ashes, + *graphō*, to write]

spo·doph·o·rous (spŏ-dof′ō-rŭs). Removing or carrying off waste materials from the body. [G. *spodos*, ashes, + *phoros*, bearing]

spoke-shave (spōk′-shāv). SYN ring-knife.

spon·da·ic (spon-dā′ik). Relating to spondee.

spon·dee (spon′dē). A bisyllabic word with generally equivalent stress on each of the two syllables; used in the testing of speech hearing. [Fr.]

⬨**spondyl-.** SEE spondylo-.

spon·dy·lal·gia (spon-di-lal′jē-ă). Pain in the spine. [spondyl- + G. *algos*, pain]

spon·dy·lar·thri·tis (spon′dil-ar-thrī′tis). Inflammation of the intervertebral articulations. [spondyl- + G. *arthron*, joint, + -*itis*, inflammation]

spon·dy·lit·ic (spon-di-lit′ik). Relating to spondylitis.

spon·dy·li·tis (spon-di-lī′tis). Inflammation of one or more of the vertebrae. [spondyl- + G. -*itis*, inflammation]

ankylosing s., arthritis of the spine, resembling rheumatoid arthritis, that may progress to bony ankylosis with lipping of vertebral margins; the disease is more common in the male, often with the rheumatoid factor absent and the HLA antigen present. There is a striking association with the B27 tissue type and the strong familial aggregation suggest an important genetic factor, perhaps inherited as an autosomal dominant [MIM*106300]; the mechanism, however, remains obscure. SYN Marie-Strümpell disease, rheumatoid s., Strümpell-Marie disease.

s. defor′mans, arthritis and osteitis deformans involving the spinal column; marked by nodular deposits at the edges of the intervertebral disks with ossification of the ligaments and bony ankylosis of the intervertebral articulations, it results in a rounded kyphosis with rigidity. SYN Bechterew disease, poker back, Strümpell disease (1).

rheumatoid s., SYN ankylosing s.

tuberculous s., tuberculous infection of the spine associated with a sharp angulation of the spine at the point of disease. SYN Pott disease.

⬨**spondylo-, spondyl-.** The vertebrae. [G. *spondylos*, vertebra]

🅱**spon·dy·lo·lis·the·sis** (spon′di-lō-lis-thē′sis). Forward movement of the body of one of the lower lumbar vertebrae on the vertebra below it, or upon the sacrum. SYN spondyloptosis. [spondylo- + G. *olisthēsis*, a slipping and falling]

spon·dy·lo·lis·thet·ic (spon′di-lō-lis-thet′ik). Relating to or marked by spondylolisthesis.

spon·dy·lol·y·sis (spon-di-lol′i-sis). Degeneration or deficient development of a portion of the vertebra; commonly involves the pars interarticularis, which can result in a spondylolithesis. [spondylo- + G. *lysis*, loosening]

spon·dy·lo·ma·la·cia (spon′di-lō-mă-lā′shē-ă). Softening of vertebrae with multiple collapsed vertebral bodies. [spondylo- + G. *malakia*, softness]

spon·dy·lop·a·thy (spon-di-lop′ă-thē). Any disease of the vertebrae or spinal column. [spondylo- + G. *pathos*, suffering]

spon·dy·lop·to·sis (spon′di-lō-tō′sis). SYN spondylolisthesis. [spondylo- + G. *ptōsis*, a falling]

spon·dy·lo·py·o·sis (spon′di-lō-pī-ō′sis). Suppurative inflammation of one or more of the vertebral bodies. [spondylo- + G. *pyōsis*, suppuration]

spon·dy·los·chi·sis (spon-di-los′ki-sis). Embryologic failure of fusion of the vertebral arch. SEE *spina* bifida. [spondylo- + G. *schisis*, fissure]

spon·dy·lo·sis (spon-di-lō′sis). Ankylosis of the vertebra; often applied nonspecifically to any lesion of the spine of a degenerative nature. [G. *spondylos*, vertebra]

cervical s., s. affecting the cervical vertebrae, intervertebral discs, and surrounding soft tissue.

hyperostotic s., SYN diffuse idiopathic skeletal *hyperostosis.*

spon·dy·lo·syn·de·sis (spon′di-lō-sin-dē′sis). SYN spinal *fusion.* [spondylo- + G. *syndesis,* binding together]

spon·dy·lo·tho·rac·ic (spon′di-lō-thō-ras′ik). Relating to the vertebra and the thorax.

spon·dyl·ous (spon′di-lŭs). Relating to a vertebra.

sponge (spŭnj). **1.** Absorbent material, such as gauze or prepared cotton, used to absorb fluids. **2.** A member of the phylum Porifera, the cellular endoskeleton of which is a source of commercial s.'s. SYN spongia. [G. *spongia*]

absorbable gelatin s., a sterile, absorbable, water-insoluble gelatin base s., used to control capillary bleeding in surgical operations; it is left in situ and is absorbed in from 4 to 6 weeks.

Bernays s., a compressed disk of aseptic cotton that swells when moistened; used in packing cavities.

compressed s., a s. that is impregnated with a thin mucilage of acacia, wrapped with twine to the desired shape, and then dried; used to dilate sinuses, the os uteri, etc. by absorbing moisture after insertion. SYN sponge tent.

contraceptive s., a resilient, hydrophilic s. of polyurethane foam impregnated with a spermicide; contraception is achieved by action of the spermicide; no longer manufactured in the U.S.

spon·gia (spŭn′jē-ă). SYN sponge. [G.]

spon·gi·form (spŭn′ji-fŏrm). SYN spongy.

△**spongio-.** Sponge, spongelike, spongy. [G. *spongia*]

spon·gi·o·blast (spŭn′jē-ō-blast). A neuroepithelial, filiform ependymal cell extending across the entire thickness of the wall of the brain or spinal cord, i.e., from the internal to the external limiting membrane; s.'s become neuroglial and ependymal cells. SEE ALSO glioblast. [spongio- + G. *blastos,* germ]

spon·gi·o·blas·to·ma (spŭn′jē-ō-blas-tō′mă). **1.** A glioma consisting of cells (elongated, spindle-shaped, and sometimes pleomorphic, with one or two fibrillary processes) that resemble the embryonic spongioblasts, occurring normally around the neural canal of the human embryo; it grows relatively slowly, usually originating in the brainstem, optic chiasm, or infundibulum, and infiltrates adjacent structures or causes compression of the third and fourth ventricles. S.'s were formerly subclassified as s. polare and s. unipolare. **2.** Obsolete term for glioblastoma multiforme. [spongioblast + G. *-oma* tumor]

spon·gi·o·cyte (spŭn′jē-ō-sīt). **1.** A neuroglial cell. **2.** A cell in the zona fasciculata of the adrenal containing many droplets of lipid material which, after staining with hematoxylin and eosin, show pronounced vacuolization. [spongio- + G. *kytos,* cell]

spon·gi·oid (spŭn′jē-oyd). SYN spongy. [spongio- + G. *eidos,* resemblance]

spon·gi·ose (spŭn′jē-ōs). Resembling or characteristic of a sponge. [L. *spongiosus*]

spon·gi·o·sis (spŭn-jē-ō′sis). Inflammatory intercellular edema of the epidermis.

spon·gi·o·si·tis (spŭn-jē-ō-sī′tis). Inflammation of the corpus spongiosum, or corpus cavernosum urethrae.

spongy (spŭn′jē). Of spongelike texture or appearance. SYN spongiform, spongioid.

spon·ta·ne·ous (spon-tā′nē-ŭs). Without apparent cause; said of disease processes or remissions. [L. *spontaneus,* voluntary, capricious]

spoon (spoon). An instrument with a handle and a small bowl- or cup-shaped extremity. [A.S. *spōn,* chip]

cataract s., a small concave instrument for removing a cataractous lens.

Daviel s., a small ovoid instrument for removing the remains of a cataract after discission.

sharp s., an instrument with a small cup-shaped extremity having sharpened edges, used for scraping skin lesions.

Volkmann s., a sharp s. for scraping away carious bone or other diseased tissue.

△**spor-.** SEE sporo-.

spo·rad·ic (spō-rad′ik). **1.** Denoting a temporal pattern of disease occurrence in an animal or human population in which the disease occurs only rarely and without regularity. SEE endemic, epidemic, enzootic, epizootic. **2.** In the genetic context denotes a singleton or sport. Several quite different and disparate phenomena are covered by this term, including a new mutation; occult nonpaternity; the chance outcome for a recessive trait in two carrier parents with a small family; extreme variability in the expression of a gene; an environmental phenocopy; a multilocal genocopy, etc. No useful properties can be predicated of all members of this class; and the term is notionally useless. **3.** Occurring irregularly, haphazardly. [G. *sporadikos,* scattered]

spo·ra·din (spōr′ă-din). Gamont stage of a gregarine parasite after it has lost its epimerite or mucron.

spo·ran·gi·o·phore (spō-ran′jē-ō-fōr). In fungi, a specialized hypha that bears a sporangium at its tip. [sporangium + G. *phoros,* bearing]

spo·ran·gi·um (spō-ran′jē-ŭm). A saclike structure (a cell) within a fungus, in which asexual spores are borne by progressive cleavage. [L. fr. G. *sporos,* seed, + *angeion,* vessel]

spore (spōr). **1.** The asexual or sexual reproductive body of fungi or sporozoan protozoa. **2.** A cell of a plant lower in organization than the seed-bearing spermatophytic plants. **3.** A resistant form of certain species of bacteria. **4.** The highly modified reproductive body of certain protozoa, as in the phyla Microspora and Myxozoa. [G. *sporos,* seed]

black s., a degenerating malarial or other blood parasite in the body of the mosquito.

spo·ri·ci·dal (spōr-i-sī′dăl). Lethal to spores. [spori- + L. *caedo,* to kill]

spo·ri·cide (spōr′i-sīd). An agent that kills spores.

spo·rid·i·um, pl. **spo·rid·ia** (spō-rid′ē-ŭm, -ă). A protozoan spore; an embryonic protozoan organism. [Mod. L. dim., fr. G. *sporos,* seed]

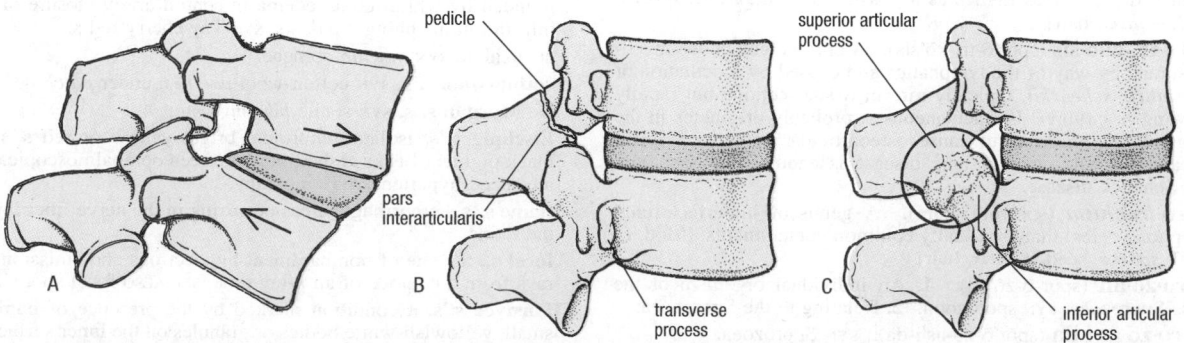

spondylolisthesis: (A) showing forward slippage of lumbar vertebrae; **spondylolysis:** (B) showing fracture of pars interarticularis; **spondylosis:** (C) showing fixation of the articular processes

⌂**sporo-, spori-, spor-.** Seed, spore. [G. *sporos*]

spo·ro·ag·glu·ti·na·tion (spōr'ō-ă-gloo-ti-nā'shŭn). A diagnostic method in relation to the mycoses, based upon the fact that the blood of patients with diseases caused by fungi contains specific agglutinins that cause clumping of the spores of these organisms.

spo·ro·blast (spōr'ō-blast). An early stage in the development of a sporocyst prior to differentiation of the sporozoites. SEE ALSO oocyst, sporocyst (2), pansporoblast. SYN zygotomere. [sporo- + G. *blastos*, germ]

spo·ro·cyst (spōr'ō-sist). **1.** A larval form of digenetic trematode (fluke) that develops in the body of its molluscan intermediate host, usually a snail; the s. forms a simple saclike structure with germinal cells that bud off internally and develop into other larval types that continue this process of larval multiplication (considered to be a form of polyembryony). SEE ALSO miracidium, redia, cercaria. **2.** A secondary cyst that develops within the oocyst of Coccidia, a group of sporozoans that includes many of the most important disease agents of domestic animals and fowl; the s. develops from a sporoblast and produces within itself one or several sporozoites, the infective agents for infection and multiplication in the next host. [sporo- + G. *kystis*, bladder]

Spo·ro·cys·tin·ea (spōr'ō-sis-tin'ē-ă). In older classification schemes, a suborder of Coccidia in which the sporoblasts develop sporocysts. [sporo + G. *kystis*, bladder]

spo·ro·do·chi·um (spō-rō-dō'kē-ŭm). In fungi, a cushion-shaped stroma covered with conidiophores.

spo·ro·gen·e·sis (spōr-ō-jen'ē-sis). SYN sporogony. [sporo- + G. *genesis*, production]

spo·rog·e·nous (spŏ-roj'ĕ-nŭs). Relating to or involved in sporogony.

spo·rog·e·ny (spŏ-roj'ĕ-nē). SYN sporogony.

spo·rog·o·ny (spŏ-rog'ŏ-nē). The formation of sporozoites in sporozoan protozoa, a process of asexual division within the sporoblast, which becomes the sporocyst within an oocyst; follows fusion of gametes (gametogony) and zygote (sporont) formation. SYN sporogenesis, sporogeny. [sporo- + G. *goneia*, generation]

spo·ront (spōr'ont). The zygote stage within the oocyst wall in the life cycle of coccidia; gives rise to sporoblasts, which form sporocysts, within which the infective sporozoites are produced. [sporo- + G. *ōn* (*ont-*), being]

spo·ro·phore (spōr'ō-fōr). Any specialized hyphas in fungi that give rise to spores. [sporo- + G. *phoros*, bearing]

spo·ro·plasm (spōr'ō-plazm). The protoplasm of a spore. [sporo- + G. *plasma*, thing formed]

spo·ro·the·ca (spōr'o-the'ka). The envelope enclosing the minute needle-like spores of certain Sporozoea. [sporo- + G. *thēkē*, case]

Spo·ro·thrix (spōr'ō-thriks). A genus of dimorphic imperfect fungi, including the species *S. schenckii*, an organism of worldwide distribution and the causative agent of sporotrichosis in humans and animals, which grows in soil or vegetation, especially in thorny bushes, and is acquired by humans when infected thorns are introduced into subcutaneous tissues; at 37°C it grows as a yeast and parasitizes tissues as a yeast. [Mod. L., fr. G. *sporos*, seed, + *thrix*, hair]

spo·ro·tri·cho·sis (spōr'ō-tri-kō'sis). A chronic cutaneous mycosis spread by way of the lymphatics and caused by inoculation of *Sporothrix schenckii*, typically rare in tissue sections but rapidly growing in cultures. Extracutaneous s. probably originates in the lung but disseminates to cause osteoarticular or other visceral disease. Chronic cavitary lung disease is another manifestation. SYN Schenck disease.

Spo·ro·tri·chum (spŏ-rot'ri-kŭm). A genus of imperfect fungi (Hyphomycetes) that are usually common contaminants. [Mod. L. fr. G. *sporos*, seed, + *thrix*, hair]

spo·ro·zo·an (spōr-ō-zō'an). **1.** An individual organism of the class Sporozoea. SYN sporozoon. **2.** Relating to the Sporozoea.

Spo·ro·zo·as·i·da (spōr'ō-zō-as'i-dă). SYN Sporozoea.

Spor·o·zo·ea (spōr-ō-zō'ē-ă). A large class of protozoans (phylum Apicomplexa, subkingdom Protozoa) consisting of obligatory parasites with simple spores lacking polar filaments; cilia and flagella are absent (except for microgametes, found in some

groups), and locomotion is by undulation, gliding, or body flexion; sexuality, when present, is by syngamy, forming oocysts with infective sporozoites from sporogony. The class includes the gregarines and coccidia, the latter including many agents of human and animal disease, such as the plasmodia of malaria. SYN Sporozoasida, Telosporea. [Mod. L., fr. G. *sporos*, seed, + *zōon*, animal]

spo·ro·zo·ite (spōr-ō-zō'īt). One of the minute elongated bodies resulting from the repeated division of the oocyst during sporogony. In the case of the malarial parasite, it is the form that is concentrated in the salivary glands and introduced into the blood by the bite of a mosquito; it enters the liver cells (exoerythrocytic cycle), whose progeny, the merozoites, infect the red blood cells to initiate clinical malaria. SYN germinal rod, zoite, zygotoblast. [sporo- + G. *zōon*, animal]

spo·ro·zo·on (spōr-ō-zō'on). SYN sporozoan (1).

sport (spōrt). An organism varying in whole or in part, without apparent reason, from others of its type; this variation may be transmitted to the descendants or the latter may revert to the original type. SYN singleton (2). [M.E. *disporte*, fr. O.Fr. *desport*, diversion]

spor·u·lar (spōr'ū-lăr). Relating to a spore or sporule.

spor·u·la·tion (spor'oo-lā'shŭn). The process by which yeasts undergo meiosis, and the meiotic products are encased in spore coats.

spor·ule (spōr'ool). A spore; a small spore. [Mod. L. *sporula*; dim. of G. *sporos*, seed]

spot. **1.** SYN macula. **2.** To lose a slight amount of blood through the vagina.

acoustic s.'s, SEE *macula* of utricle, *macula* of saccule.

Bitot s.'s, small, circumscribed, lusterless, grayish white, foamy, greasy, triangular deposits on the bulbar conjunctiva adjacent to the cornea in the area of the palpebral fissure of both eyes; occurs in vitamin A deficiency.

blind s., **(1)** SYN physiologic *scotoma*; **(2)** SYN mental *scotoma*; **(3)** SYN optic *disk*.

blood s.'s, hemorrhagic graafian follicles seen in ovaries of mice, caused by injection of urine of pregnant women; a positive result in the now obsolete Aschheim-Zondek test for pregnancy.

blue s., **(1)** SYN *macula* cerulea; **(2)** SYN mongolian s.

❚**Brushfield s.'s,** light-colored condensations of the surface of the mid-iris; seen in Down syndrome.

café au lait s.'s, pigmented cutaneous lesions, ranging from light to dark brown, and due to an excess of melanosomes in the malpighian cells, rather than to an excess of melanocytes; café au lait s.'s are one of the major cutaneous manifestations of neurofibromatosis (von Recklinghausen disease), with type 1 (peripheral) neurofibromatosis, almost always 6 or more café-au-lait s.'s can be found with at least some exceeding 1.5 cm in diameter. These are often accompanied by frecklelike s.'s in the axilla.

cherry-red s., the ophthalmoscopic appearance of the normal choroid beneath the fovea centralis, appearing as a red s. surrounded by white retinal edema in central artery closure or lipid infiltration in sphingolipidosis. SYN Tay cherry-red s.

corneal s., SYN *macula* corneae.

cotton-wool s.'s, SYN cotton-wool *patches*, under *patch*.

De Morgan s.'s, SYN senile *hemangioma*.

Elschnig s.'s, isolated choroidal bright yellow or red s.'s with black pigment flecks at their borders, seen ophthalmoscopically in advanced hypertensive retinopathy.

flame s.'s, hemorrhagic areas occurring in the nerve fiber layer of the retina.

focal s., the site of bombardment by electrons and emission of x-rays from the anode of an x-ray tube. SEE ALSO focal spot size.

❚**Fordyce s.'s,** a condition marked by the presence of numerous small, yellowish-white bodies or granules on the inner surface and vermilion border of the lips; histologically the lesions are ectopic sebaceous glands. SYN Fordyce disease, Fordyce granules.

Fuchs black s., an area of pigment proliferation in the macular region in degenerative myopia.

hot s., a region in a gene in which there is a putatively high rate of mutation or recombination.

hypnogenic s., a pressure-sensitive point on the body of certain susceptible persons, which, when pressed, causes the induction of sleep.

Koplik s.'s, small red s.'s on the buccal mucous membrane, in the center of each of which may be seen, in a strong light, a minute bluish white speck; they occur early in measles (morbilli), before the skin eruption, and are regarded as a pathognomonic sign of the disease.

liver s., SYN senile *lentigo*.

Mariotte blind s., SYN optic *disk*.

milk s.'s, (1) white plaques of hyalinized fibrous tissue situated in the epicardium overlying the right ventricle of the heart where it is not covered by lung; SYN soldier's patches. **(2)** white macroscopic areas in the omentum, due to accumulation of macrophages and lymphocytes. SYN tache laiteuse (1).

mongolian s., any of a number of dark-bluish or mulberry-colored rounded or oval s.'s on the sacral region due to the ectopic presence of scattered melanocytes in the dermis. These congenital lesions are frequent in black, native American, and Asian children from 2 to 12 years, after which time they gradually recede; they do not disappear on pressure and are sometimes mistaken for bruises from child abuse. SYN blue s. (2).

mulberry s.'s, the abdominal eruption in typhus fever.

rose s.'s, characteristic exanthema of typhoid fever; 10–20 small pink papules on the lower trunk lasting a few days and leaving hyperpigmentation.

Roth s.'s, a round white retina s. surrounded by hemorrhage in bacterial endocarditis, and in other retinal hemorrhagic conditions.

saccular s., SYN *macula* of saccule.

Soemmerring s., SYN *macula* of retina.

spongy s., SYN vascular *zone*.

Tardieu s.'s, SYN Tardieu *ecchymoses*, under *ecchymosis*.

Tay cherry-red s., SYN cherry-red s.

temperature s., one of a number of definitely arranged s.'s on the skin sensitive to heat and cold, but not to ordinary pressure or pain stimuli.

tendinous s., SYN *macula* albida.

Trousseau s., SYN meningitic *streak*.

utricular s., SYN *macula* of utricle.

white s., SYN *macula* albida.

yellow s., SYN *macula* of retina.

spp. Abbreviation for plural of species.

sprain (sprān). **1.** An injury to a ligament as a result of abnormal or excessive forces applied to a joint, but without dislocation or fracture. **2.** To cause a s. of a joint.

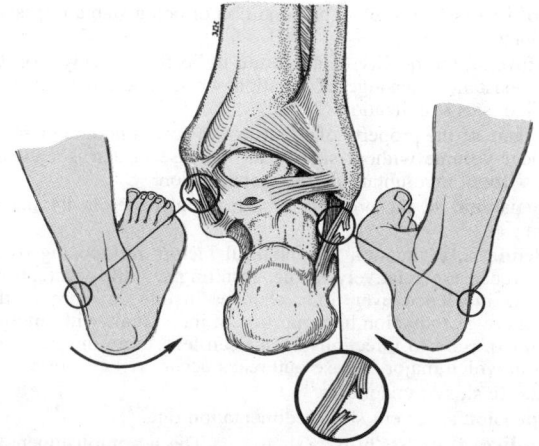

sprain: involving ankle ligaments

spray (sprā). A jet of liquid in fine drops, coarser than a vapor; it is produced by forcing the liquid from the minute opening of an atomizer, mixing it with air.

spread·er (spred'er). **1.** An instrument used to distribute a substance over a surface or area. **2.** A device for spacing or parting structures.

gutta-percha s., an instrument used in dentistry for condensing gutta-percha laterally in a root canal.

rib s., a retractor for widening the space between ribs in intrathoracic operations.

root canal s., a tapered instrument utilized for condensing root filling materials laterally.

Sprengel, Otto G.K., German surgeon, 1852–1915. SEE S. *deformity*.

sprout (sprowt). A structure resembling the s. of a plant.

syncytial s., SYN syncytial *knot*.

sprue (sproo). **1.** Primary intestinal malabsorption with steatorrhea. SYN cachexia aphthosa. **2.** In dentistry, wax or metal used to form the aperture(s) for molten metal to flow into a mold to make a casting; also, the metal that later fills the s. hole(s). [D. *spruw*]

celiac s., SYN celiac *disease*.

nontropical s., s. occurring in persons away from the tropics; usually called celiac disease; due to gluten-induced enteropathy.

tropical s., s. occurring in the tropics, often associated with enteric infection and nutritional deficiency, and frequently complicated by folate deficiency with macrocytic anemia. SYN tropical diarrhea.

sprue-form·er (sproo-fōr'mer). The base to which the sprue (2) is attached while the wax pattern is being invested in a refractory investment in a casting flask; it is sometimes referred to as a crucible-former.

spud (spŭd). A triangular knife used for removing foreign bodies from the cornea.

Spu·ma·vir·i·nae (spoo'mă-vir'i-nē). Formerly a subfamily of viruses (family Retroviridae) that includes the foamy viruses (agents) of primates and other mammals; they are now placed in the genus Spumavirus. In common with other retroviruses, they possess RNA-dependent DNA polymerases (reverse transcriptase). [L. *spuma*, foam]

Spu·ma·vi·rus (spoo'mă-vī'rŭs). A virus genus encompassing a poorly characterized group of retroviruses that cause vacuolation (foaming) of cultured cells; usually cause persistent but silent infections in their natural hosts and no diseases caused by these agents have been identified.

spur (sper) [TA]. SYN calcar. [A.S. *spora*]

calcarine s. [TA], the lower of two elevations on the medial wall of the posterior horn of the lateral ventricle of the brain, caused by the depth of the calcarine sulcus. SYN calcar avis [TA], Haller unguis, hippocampus minor, minor hippocampus, Morand s., unguis avis.

Fuchs s., epithelial outgrowth of the dilator muscle of the pupil about midway in the breadth of the sphincter; part of the insertion of the dilator muscle onto the iris sphincter.

Grunert s., epithelial outgrowth of the dilator muscle of the pupil at the junction of the iris and the ciliary body; part of the origin of the iris dilator muscle.

heel s., bony thickening of the flexor surface of the calcaneus associated with severe pain on standing.

Michel s., epithelial outgrowth of the dilator muscle of the pupil at the peripheral border of the sphincter; part of the insertion of the dilator muscle onto the iris sphincter.

Morand s., SYN calcarine s.

scleral s. [TA], circular ridge of sclera on the internal aspect of the corneoscleral junction; on cross-section, it appears as a hook-like process deep to the scleral venous sinus; relatively rigid, it provides attachment (origin) of the meridional fibers of the ciliary body. SYN calcar sclerae [TA], scleral roll.

vascular s., partial septum between vessels (arteries and veins) at the level of fusion or branching at acute angle. SEE ALSO calcar (1).

spu·ri·ous (spoo'rē-ŭs). False; not genuine. [L. *spurius*]

spu·tum, pl. **spu·ta** (spū'tŭm, -tă). **1.** Expectorated matter, espe-

sp

cially mucus or mucopurulent matter expectorated in diseases of the air passages. SEE ALSO expectoration (1). **2.** An individual mass of such matter. [L. *sputum*, fr. *spuo*, pp. *sputus*, to spit]

s. aerogeno′sum, a green expectoration seen occasionally in jaundice, due to staining of the s. by bile pigments. SYN green s.

globular s., SYN nummular s.

green s., SYN s. aerogenosum.

nummular s., a thick, coherent mass expectorated in globular shape which does not run at the bottom of the cup but forms a discoid mass resembling a coin. SYN globular s.

prune-juice s., a thin reddish expectoration, characteristic of necrosis of lung tissue, usually by infection; due to hemorrhage caused by destruction of the lung parenchyma; sometimes seen with lung tumors. SYN prune-juice expectoration.

rusty s., a reddish brown, blood-stained expectoration characteristic of lobar pneumonococcal pneumonia.

SQ Abbreviation for subcutaneous.

squalamine lactate (skwal′ă-mēn lak′tāt). An antiangiogenic, noncytotoxic drug used to treat solid tumors.

squa·lene (skwā′lēn). A hexaisoprenoid (triterpenoid) hydrocarbon found in shark oil and in some plants; intermediate in the biosynthesis of cholesterol and other sterols and triterpenes.

s. epoxidase, an enzyme that catalyzes the conversion of s. to s. 2,3-oxide in the endoplasmic reticulum; a required step in order for cyclization to occur, resulting in the synthesis of the first sterol, lanosterol, in steroidogenesis; uses NADPH.

s. synthase, an enzyme that catalyzes the formation of s. from two molecules of farnesylpyrophosphate using NADPH and concomitant production of two molecules of pyrophosphate.

squa·ma, pl. **squa·mae** (skwā′mă, skwā′mē). **1.** A thin plate of bone. **2.** An epidermal scale. SYN squame. SYN scale (2). [L. a scale]

frontal s., SYN squamous *part* of occipital bone.

s. fronta′lis [TA], SYN squamous *part* of frontal bone.

s. occipita′lis, occipital s. [TA], SYN squamous *part* of occipital bone.

temporal s., SYN squamous *part* of temporal bone.

s. tempora′lis, SYN squamous *part* of temporal bone.

squa·ma·ti·za·tion (skwā′mă-ti-zā′shŭn). Transformation of other types of cells into squamous cells.

squame (skwām). SYN squama (2).

△**squamo-.** Squama, squamous. [L. *squama*, a scale]

squa·mo·cel·lu·lar (skwā-mō-sel′ū-lăr). Relating to or having squamous epithelium.

squa·mo·co·lum·nar (skwā-mō-kol′ŭm-nar). Pertaining to the junction between a stratified squamous epithelial surface and one lined by columnar epithelium; e.g., the cardia of the stomach or anus.

squa·mo·fron·tal (skwā′mō-frŏn′tăl). Relating to the squamous part of the frontal bone.

squa·mo·mas·toid (skwā′mō-mas′toyd). Relating to the squamous and petrous portions of the temporal bone.

squa·mo·oc·cip·i·tal (skwā′mō-ok-sip′i-tăl). Relating to the squamous portion of the occipital bone, developing partly in membrane and partly in cartilage.

squa·mo·pa·ri·e·tal (skwā′mō-pă-rī′e-tăl). Relating to the parietal bone and the squamous portion of the temporal bone.

squa·mo·pe·tro·sal (skwā′mō-pĕ-trō′săl). SYN petrosquamosal.

squa·mo·sa, pl. **squa·mo·sae** (skwā-mō′să, -sē). The squamous parts of the frontal, occipital, or temporal bone, especially the latter. [L. *squamosus*, scaly, fr. *squama*, scale]

squa·mo·sal (skwā-mō′săl). Relating especially to the squamous part of the temporal bone.

squa·mo·sphe·noid (skwā′mō-sfē′noyd). Relating to the sphenoid bone and the squamous part of the temporal bone. SYN sphenosquamosal.

squa·mo·tem·po·ral (skwā′mō-tem′pŏ-răl). Relating to the squamous part of the temporal bone.

squa·mo·tym·pan·ic (skwa′mō-tim-man′ik). SYN tympanosquamosal.

squa·mous (skwā′mŭs). Relating to or covered with scales. SYN scaly. [L. *squamosus*]

squa·mo·zy·go·mat·ic (skwā′mō-zī-gō-mat′ik). Relating to the squamous part of the temporal bone and the zygomatic process of the temporal bone.

squill (skwil). The cut and dried fleshy inner scales of the bulb of the white variety of *Urginea maritima* (Mediterranean s.), or of *U. indica* (Indian s.) (family Liliaceae); the central portion of the bulb is excluded during its processing; s. contains cardiac glycosides (scillaren-A and scillaren-B) and scillaricide, a rodenticide. SYN scilla. [L. *squilla* or *scilla*]

squint (skwint). **1.** SYN strabismus. **2.** To suffer from strabismus.

convergent s., SYN esotropia.

divergent s., SYN exotropia.

external s., SYN exotropia.

internal s., SYN esotropia.

87mSr Abbreviation for strontium-87m.

Sr Symbol for strontium.

sr. Abbreviation for steradian.

85Sr Abbreviation for strontium-85.

89Sr Symbol for strontium-89.

90Sr Symbol for strontium-90.

SRF Abbreviation for somatotropin-releasing *factor*.

SRF-A Abbreviation for slow-reacting *factor* of anaphylaxis.

SRH Abbreviation for somatotropin-releasing *hormone*.

SRIF Abbreviation for somatotropin release-inhibiting *factor*.

sRNA Abbreviation for soluble RNA. See entries under ribonucleic acid.

S ro·ma·num (rō-mā′nŭm). Archaic term for sigmoid *colon.*

SRP Abbreviation for signal recognition *particle*.

SRS Abbreviation for slow-reacting *substance*.

SRS-A Abbreviation for slow-reacting *substance* of anaphylaxis.

ss Abbreviation for single-stranded, steady *state*.

SSPE Abbreviation for subacute sclerosing *panencephalitis*.

SSPL Abbreviation for saturation sound pressure *level*.

SSS Abbreviation for soluble specific *substance*.

stab. To pierce with a pointed instrument, as a knife or dagger. [Gael. *stob*]

sta·bi·late (stā′bi-lāt). A sample of organisms preserved alive on a single occasion, i.e., by freezing.

sta·bile (stā′bīl, -bil). Steady; fixed; denoting: 1) certain constituents of serum unaffected by ordinary degrees of heat; 2) an electrode held steadily on a part during the passage of an electric current. Cf. labile. [L. *stabilis*]

stab·i·lim·e·ter (stā-bi-lim′ĕ-ter). An instrument to measure the sway of the body when standing with feet together and usually with eyes closed. [L. *stabilitas*, firmness, + G. *metron*, measure]

sta·bil·i·ty (stă-bil′i-tē). The condition of being stable or resistant to change.

denture s., the quality of a denture to be firm, steady, constant, and resistant to change of position when functional forces are applied. SYN stabilization (2).

detrusor s., the property of a detrusor to accommodate increasing bladder volume without significant increase in detrusor pressure and without involuntary detrusor contraction.

dimensional s., the property of a material to retain its size and form.

endemic s., a situation in which all factors influencing disease occurrence are relatively stable, resulting in little fluctuation in disease incidence over time; changes in one or more of these factors (e.g., reduction in proportion of individuals with immunity from exposure to infectious agent) can lead to an unstable situation in which major disease outbreaks occur. SYN enzootic s.

enzootic s., SYN endemic s.

suspension s., a very slow sedimentation rate.

sta·bi·li·za·tion (stā′bĭ-li-zā′shŭn). **1.** The accomplishment of a stable state. **2.** SYN denture *stability*.

sta·bi·liz·er (stā′bĭ-lī-zer). **1.** That which renders something else more stable. **2.** An agent that retards the effect of an accelerator, thus preserving a chemical equilibrium. **3.** A part possessing the quality of rigidity or creating rigidity when added to another part.

endodontic s., a pin implant passing through the apex of a tooth from its root canal and extending well into the underlying bone to provide immobilization of periodontally involved teeth.

sta·ble (stā′bl). Steady; not varying; resistant to change. SEE ALSO stabile.

stach·y·bot·ry·o·tox·i·co·sis (stak-ē-bot′rē-ō-tok-si-kō′sis). A type of mycotoxicosis seen in horses and cattle following ingestion of hay and fodder overgrown by the fungus *Stachybotrys atra;* may also occur in humans exposed to hay either by inhalation or by absorbing the toxin through the skin, and is manifested by skin rash, pharyngitis, and mild leukopenia.

stach·y·drine (stak′i-drēn). The betaine of L-proline found in alfalfa, chrysanthemum, and citrus plants.

stach·y·ose (stak′ē-ōs). A raffinosegalactopyranoside; a tetrasaccharide that yields D-glucose, D-fructose, and 2 mol of D-galactose upon hydrolysis; present in certain tubers and other plant tissues.

stac·tom·e·ter (stak-tom′ĕ-ter). SYN stalagmometer. [G. *staktos,* dropping, fr. *stazō,* to let fall by drops, + *metron,* measure]

Stader, Otto, U.S. veterinary surgeon, *1894. SEE S. *splint.*

Staderini, Rutilio, 19th century Italian neuroanatomist. SEE S. *nucleus.*

sta·di·om·e·ter (stā-dē-om′ĕ-ter). An instrument for measuring standing or sitting height. [L. *stadium,* fr. G. *stadion,* a fixed length, + G. *metron,* measure]

sta·di·um, pl. **sta·dia** (stā′dē-ŭm, -dē-ă). Obsolete term for a stage in the course of a disease, especially of an acute pyretic disease. [L. fr. G. *stadion,* a fixed standard length]

staff. 1. A specific group of workers. **2.** SYN director (1). [A.S. *staef*]

attending s., physicians and surgeons who are members of a hospital s. and regularly attend their patients at the hospital; may also supervise and teach house s., fellows, and medical students.

consulting s., specialists affiliated with a hospital who serve in an advisory capacity to the attending s.

house s., physicians and surgeons in specialty training at a hospital who care for the patients under the direction and supervision of the attending s.

staff of Aes·cu·la·pi·us. A rod encircled by a serpent; symbol of medicine and emblem of the American Medical Association, Royal Army Medical Corps (Britain), and Royal Canadian Medical Corps. SEE ALSO caduceus. [L. *Aesculapius,* G. *Asklēpios,* god of medicine]

Stafne, Edward C., U.S. oral pathologist, 1894–1981. SEE S. bone *cyst.*

stage (stāj). **1.** A period in the course of a disease; a description of the extent of involvement of a disease process or the status of a patient with a specific disease, as of the distribution and extent of dissemination of a malignant neoplastic disease; also, the act of determining the s. of a disease, especially cancer. SEE ALSO period. **2.** The part of a microscope on which the microslide bears the object to be examined. **3.** A particular step, phase, or position in a developmental process. For psychosexual stages, see entries under phase. [M.E. thr. O. Fr. *estage,* standing-place, fr. L. *sto,* pp. *status,* to stand]

algid s., the s. of collapse in cholera.

Arneth s.'s, a differential grouping of polymorphonuclear neutrophils in accordance with the number of lobes in their nuclei, i.e., cells with 1, 2, 3, 4, or 5 (or more) lobes are designated, respectively, as class I, II, and so on. SEE ALSO Arneth *formula.*

bell s., third s. of tooth development, wherein the cells form the inner enamel epithelium, the stratum intermedium, the stellate reticulum, and the outer enamel epithelium; the enamel organ assumes a bell shape.

bud s., first s. of tooth development; development of the primordia of the enamel organs, the tooth buds.

cap s., second s. of tooth development wherein there is development of the inner and outer enamel epithelium.

cold s., the s. of chill in a malarial paroxysm.

defervescent s., SEE defervescence.

end s., the late, fully developed phase of a disease; e.g., in end-stage renal disease, a shrunken and scarred kidney that may result from a variety of chronic diseases that have become indistinguishable in their effect on the kidney.

eruptive s., the stage of an exanthematous illness in which the rash appears.

exoerythrocytic s., developmental s. of the malaria parasite (*Plasmodium*) in liver parenchyma cells of the vertebrate host before erythrocytes are invaded. The initial generation produces cryptozoites, the next generation metacryptozoites; reinfection of liver cells from blood cells apparently does not occur. Delayed development of the sporozoite (hypnozoite) of *Plasmodium vivax* and *P. ovale* appears to be responsible for malarial relapse that may occur with these disease agents.

genital s., referring to the psychic organization derived from, and which is characteristic of, the Freudian genital period of the infant's psychosocial organization. SEE genitality; SEE ALSO anality, orality.

imperfect s., a mycologic term used to describe the asexual life cycle phase of a fungus. SEE anamorph.

incubative s., SYN incubation *period* (1).

intuitive s., in psychology, a s. of development, usually occurring between 4 and 7 years of age, in which a child's thought processes are determined by the most prominent aspects of the stimuli to which the child is exposed, rather than by some form of logical thought.

s. of invasion, SYN incubation *period* (1).

s.'s of labor, SEE labor.

latent s., SYN incubation *period* (1).

perfect s., a mycologic term used to describe the sexual life cycle phase of a fungus in which spores are formed after nuclear fusion. SYN teleomorph.

preconceptual s., in psychology, the s. of development in an infant's life, prior to actual conceptual thinking, in which sensorimotor activity predominates.

prodromal s., early stage/symptoms of disease prior to the appearance of characteristic symptoms.

resting s., the quiescent s. of a cell or its nucleus in which no karyokinetic changes are taking place. SYN vegetative s.

Tanner s., a s. of puberty in the Tanner growth chart, based on pubic hair growth, development of genitalia in boys, and breast development in girls.

trypanosome s., SEE trypomastigote.

tumor s., the extent of the spread of a malignant neoplasm from its site of origin. SEE ALSO TNM *staging.*

vegetative s., SYN resting s.

stag·ger (stag′er). To walk unsteadily; to reel.

stag·gers (stag′erz). A form of decompression sickness in which vertigo, mental confusion, and muscular weakness are the chief symptoms.

stag·ing (stāj′ing). **1.** The determination or classification of distinct phases or periods in the course of a disease or pathological process. **2.** The determination of the specific extent of a disease process in an individual patient.

Jewett and Strong s., obsolete term for s. of bladder carcinoma: O, noninvasive; A, with submucosal invasion; B, with muscle invasion; C, with invasion of perivascular fat; D, with lymph node metastasis.

TNM s., a system of clinicopathologic evaluation of tumors based on the extent of tumor involvement at the primary site (T, followed by a number indicating size and depth of invasion), and lymph node involvement (N) and metastasis (M) each followed by a number starting at 0 for no evident metastasis; numbers used depend on the organ involved and influence the prognosis and choice of treatment.

stag·na·tion (stag-nā′shŭn). Retardation or cessation of flow of blood in the vessels, as in passive congestion; marked slowing or accumulation in any part of a normally circulating fluid. [L. *stagnum,* a pool]

st

Ann Arbor staging system

stage I	involvement in single lymph node region or single extralymphatic site
stage II	involvement of two or more lymph node regions on the same side of diaphragm
	localized contiguous involvement of only one extralymphatic site and lymph node region (stage IIE)
stage III	involvement of lymph node regions on both sides of diaphragm; may include spleen
stage IV	disseminated involvement of one or more extralymphatic organs with or without lymph node involvement

TNM staging

T — primary tumor
TX primary tumor cannot be judged
T0 no basis for primary tumor
Tis carcinoma/tumor in situ
T1, T2, T3, T4 increasing sizes and/or extent of primary tumor invasion

N — regional lymph nodes
NX regional lymph nodes cannot be judged
N0 no regional lymph node metastases
N1, N2, N3 increasing invasion of regional lymph nodes

M — metastasis
MX existence of metastases cannot be judged
M0 no metastases
M1 metastases present

the category M1 can be subdivided as follows:

lung	PUL	marrow	MAR
bone	OSS	rib	PLE
liver	HEP	peritoneum	PER
brain	BRA	skin	SKI
lymph nodes	LYM	other organs	OTH

R — residual tumor (postoperative)
R0 no residual tumor
R1 microscopic residual tumor
R2 macroscopic residual tumor

G — histopathologic differentiation grade (grading)
GX differentiation grade cannot be determined
G1 well-differentiated
G2 moderately differentiated
G3 poorly differentiated
G4 undifferentiated

Stahl, George E., German physician and chemist, 1660–1734. He promulgated the phlogiston theory. SEE phlogiston.

Stahl, Friedrich K., German physician, 1811–1873. SEE S. *ear*.

Stähli, Jean, Swiss ophthalmologist, *1890. SEE Hudson-S. *line*.

STAIN

stain (stān). **1.** To discolor. **2.** To color; to dye. **3.** A discoloration. **4.** A dye used in histologic and bacteriologic technique. **5.** A procedure in which a dye or combination of dyes and reagents is used to color the constituents of cells and tissues. For individual dyes or staining substances, see the specific names. [M.E. *steinen*]

Abbott s. for spores, spores are stained blue with alkaline methylene blue; bodies of the bacilli become pink with eosin counterstain.

aceto-orcein s., a s. used for chromosomes in air-dried or squashed cytologic material.

acid s., a dye in which the anion is the colored component of the dye molecule, e.g., sodium eosinate (eosin).

Ag-AS s., SYN silver-ammoniac silver s.

Albert s., a s. for diphtheria bacilli and their metachromatic granules; contains toluidine blue, methyl green, glacial acetic acid, alcohol, and distilled water.

Altmann anilin-acid fuchsin s., a mixture of picric acid, anilin, and acid fuchsin which stains mitochondria crimson against a yellow background.

auramine O fluorescent s., a rapid and accurate technique for *Mycobacterium tuberculosis*, using auramine O-phenol and a methylene blue counterstain.

basic s., a dye in which the cation is the colored component of the dye molecule that binds to anionic groups of nucleic acids ($PO_4^=$) or acidic mucopolysaccharides (e.g., chondroitin sulfate).

basic fuchsin-methylene blue s., a s. for intact epoxy sections; semithick sections of plastic-embedded tissues have nuclei stained purple; collagen, elastic lamina, and connective tissue are stained blue; mitochondria, myelin, and lipid droplets are stained red; cytoplasm, smooth muscle cells, axoplasm, and chrondroblasts are stained pink.

Bauer chromic acid leucofuchsin s., a s. for glycogen and fungi utilizing chromic acid as an oxidizing agent of polysaccharides, followed by Schiff reagent; glycogen and fungi cell walls appear deep red.

Becker s. for spirochetes, a s. applied to thin films fixed in formaldehyde-acetic acid; preparations are treated successively with tannin, carbolic acid, and carbol fuchsin.

Bennhold Congo red s., an amyloid s. useful for amyloid detection in pathologic tissue; gives red staining of amyloid; also induces green birefringence to amyloid under polarized light.

Berg s., a method for staining spermatozoa, utilizing a carbol-fuchsin solution followed by dilute acetic acid and methylene blue; spermatozoa are stained a brilliant red and most other structures appear blue to purple.

Best carmine s., a method for the demonstration of glycogen in tissues.

Bielschowsky s., a method of treating tissues with silver nitrate to demonstrate reticular fibers, neurofibrils, axons, and dendrites.

Biondi-Heidenhain s., an obsolete s. for spirochetes, using acid fuchsin and orange G.

Birch-Hirschfeld s., an obsolete s. for demonstrating amyloid, using Bismarck brown and crystal violet; amyloid is usually stained a bright ruby red, whereas the cytoplasm of cells is not stained and nuclei are brown.

Bodian copper-PROTARGOL s., a s. employing a silver proteinate complex (PROTARGOL) to demonstrate axis cylinders and neurofibrils.

Borrel blue s., a s. for demonstrating spirochetes, treponemes, and Borrelia organisms, using silver oxide (prepared by means of mixing solutions of silver nitrate and sodium bicarbonate) and methylene blue.

Bowie s., a s. for juxtaglomerular granules in which the kidney sections are stained in a mixture of Biebrich scarlet red and ethyl violet; juxtaglomerular granules and elastic fibers are stained a deep purple, erythrocytes are amber, and background tissue appears in shades of red.

Brown-Brenn s., a method for differential staining of Gram-positive and Gram-negative bacteria in tissue sections; it utilizes a modified Gram s. of crystal violet, Gram iodine, and basic fuchsin.

Cajal astrocyte s., a method for demonstrating astrocytes by impregnation in a solution containing gold chloride and mercuric chloride.

carbol-thionin s., a s. useful for demonstrating typhoid bacilli in films and sections, and for Nissl substance.

C-banding s., a selective chromosome banding s. used in human cytogenetics, employing Giemsa s. after most of the DNA is denatured or extracted by treatment with alkali, acid, salt, or heat; only heterochromatic regions close to the centromeres and rich in satellite DNA stain, with the exception of the Y chromosome, whose long arm usually stains throughout. SYN centromere banding s.

centromere banding s., SYN C-banding s.

chromate s. for lead, a method in which tissues preserved in chromate-containing fixatives, such as Regaud or Orth fixatives, precipitate lead as yellow lead chromate crystals; formalin-fixed sections are treated with potassium chromate acidified with acetic acid.

chrome alum hematoxylin-phloxine s., a s. used to demonstrate pancreatic islet cells; alpha cells appear red, beta cells blue or unstained.

Ciaccio s., a method for demonstrating complex insoluble intracellular lipids using fixation in a formalin-dichromate solution, embedding in paraffin, staining with Sudan III or IV, and examination in aqueous mountant.

contrast s., a dye used to color one portion of a tissue or cell which remained unaffected when the other part was stained by a dye of different color. SYN differential s.

Cresylecht violet s., a s. used for identification of *Pneumocystis carinii*.

Da Fano s., a silver s. that produces a blackening of Golgi elements after tissues are fixed in a mixture of nitrate and formalin.

Dane s., a s. for prekeratin, keratin, and mucin that employs hemalum, phloxine, Alcian blue, and orange G; nuclei appear orange to brown, acid mucopolysaccharides pale blue, and keratins orange to red-orange.

DAPI s., a sensitive fluorescent probe for DNA, 4′6-diamidino-2-phenylindole·2HCl, used in fluorescence microscopy to detect DNA in yeast mitochondria, chloroplasts, viruses, mycoplasma, and chromosomes; DNA is visualized in vitally stained living cells and after cells are fixed in formaldehyde.

diazo s. for argentaffin granules, in enterochromaffin cells, a variety of diazonium salts are used to blacken the cells.

Dieterle s., s. used to demonstrate spirochetes and Leishman-Donovan bodies; employs silver nitrate and uranium nitrate.

differential s., SYN contrast s.

double s., a mixture of two dyes, each of which stains different portions of a tissue or cell.

Ehrlich acid hematoxylin s., an alum type of hematoxylin s. used as a regressive staining method for nuclei, followed by differentiation to required staining intensity; the solution may be allowed to ripen naturally in sunlight or partially oxidized with sodium iodate.

Ehrlich aniline crystal violet s., a s. for Gram-positive bacteria.

Ehrlich triacid s., a differential leukocytic s. comprised of saturated solutions of orange G, acid fuchsin, and methyl green.

Ehrlich triple s., a mixture of indulin, eosin Y, and aurantia.

Einarson gallocyanin-chrome alum s., a method for staining both RNA and DNA a deep blue; with proper controls, nucleic acid content of stained cells and nuclei may be estimated by cytophotometry; also used for Nissl substance.

Eranko fluorescence s., exposure of frozen sections to formaldehyde that produces a strong yellow-green fluorescence from cells containing norepinephrine.

Feulgen s., a selective cytochemical reaction for DNA in which sections or cells are first hydrolyzed with hydrochloric acid to produce apurinic acid and then are stained with Schiff reagent to produce magenta-stained nuclei; generally the concentration of DNA in nucleoli and mitochondria is too low to permit detection by this s. SEE ALSO Kasten fluorescent Feulgen s.

Field rapid s., a s. to permit rapid positive diagnosis of malaria in endemic areas by using thick films; it employs methylene blue and azure B in a phosphate buffer, with the preparation counterstained by eosin in a phosphate buffer.

Fink-Heimer s., a method used for histologic demonstration of degenerating nerve fibers and terminals of the central nervous system (black on a yellow background).

Flemming triple s., a s. composed of safranin, methyl violet, and orange G.

fluorescence plus Giemsa s., a s. used to demonstrate sister chromatid exchange; cells are grown in 5-bromodeoxyuridine,

followed by chromosome preparation, staining in HOECHST 33258, exposure to light, and staining in Giemsa; chromosomes exhibit a "harlequin" appearance.

fluorescent s., a s. or staining procedure using a fluorescent dye or substance that will combine selectively with certain tissue components and that will then fluoresce upon irradiation with ultraviolet or violet-blue light.

Fontana s., a traditional method for silver impregnation of treponemes and other spirochetal forms.

Fontana-Masson silver s., SYN Masson-Fontana ammoniac silver s.

Foot reticulin impregnation s., a silver s. in which reticulin stains black and collagen stains golden brown; sections are floated on the surface of solutions to avoid contamination with silver debris.

Fouchet s., Fouchet reagent employed to demonstrate bile pigments; paraffin sections are used for conjugated bile pigments, frozen sections for unconjugated ones.

Fraser-Lendrum s. for fibrin, a multistaining procedure after Zenker fixative in which fibrin, keratin, and some cytoplasmic granules appear red, erythrocytes appear orange, and collagen appears green.

Friedländer s. for capsules, an obsolete s. employing gentian violet.

G-banding s., a chromosome-staining technique used in human cytogenetics to identify individual chromosomes which produces characteristic bands; it utilizes acetic acid fixation, air drying, denaturing chromosomes mildly with proteolytic enzymes, salts, heat, detergents, or urea, and finally Giemsa s.; chromosome bands appear similar to those fluorochromed by Q-banding s. SYN Giemsa chromosome banding s.

Giemsa s., compound of methylene blue-eosin and methylene blue used for demonstrating Negri bodies, *Tunga* species, spirochetes and protozoans, and differential staining of blood smears; also used for chromosomes, sometimes after hydrolyzing the cytologic preparation in hot hydrochloric acid, and for showing chromosome G bands; often used in glycerol-methanol buffer solution.

Giemsa chromosome banding s., SYN G-banding s.

Glenner-Lillie s. for pituitary, a modification of Mann methyl blue-eosin s. that changes the dye proportions, buffering the dye mixture, and staining at 60°C; basophils are stained blue to black, acidophils are dark red, chromophobe granules are gray to pink, and erythrocytes are orange; with modification, the method is also useful for enterochromaffin cells, goblet cells, Paneth cells, and pancreatic islet cells.

Golgi s., any of several methods for staining nerve cells, nerve fibers, and neuroglia using fixation and hardening in formalin-osmic-dichromate combinations for various times, followed by impregnation in silver nitrate.

Gomori aldehyde fuchsin s., a s. used to demonstrate beta cells of the pancreas, storage form of thyrotrophic hormone in beta cells of the anterior pituitary, hypophyseal neurosecretory substance, mast cells, granules, elastic fibers, sulfated mucins, and gastric chief cells.

Gomori chrome alum hematoxylin-phloxine s., a technique used to demonstrate cytoplasmic granules, after Bouin or formalin-Zenker fixatives, using oxidized hematoxylin plus phloxine; in the pancreas, beta cells are blue, alpha and delta cells are red, and zymogen granules are red to unstained; in the pituitary, alpha cells are pink, beta cells and chromophobes are gray-blue, and nuclei are purple to blue.

Gomori-Jones periodic acid-methenamine-silver s., a staining method using methenamine silver, periodic acid, gold chloride, hematoxylin, and eosin to delineate basement membrane, reticulin, collagen, and nuclei; used in renal histopathology. SEE ALSO Rambourg periodic acid-chromic methenamine-silver s.

Gomori methenamine-silver s.'s (GMS), techniques for 1) *argentaffin cells:* a method using a methenamine-silver solution in combination with gold chloride, sodium thiosulfate, and safranin O; argentaffin granules appear brown-black against a green background; 2) *urates:* warm sections are treated directly with a hot methenamine-silver solution to produce a blackening of urates; 3)

st

fungi: see Grocott-Gomori methenamine-silver s.; 4) *melanin,* which reduces silver nitrate.

Gomori nonspecific acid phosphatase s., a method in which formalin-fixed frozen sections are incubated in a substrate containing sodium β-glycerophosphate and lead nitrate at pH 5.0; the insoluble lead phosphate produced is treated with ammonium sulfide to give a black lead sulfide.

Gomori nonspecific alkaline phosphatase s., a calcium-cobalt sulfide method using frozen sections or cold acetone- or formalin-fixed paraffin sections, plus sodium β-glycerophosphate as a substrate at pH 9.0–9.5 with Mg^{2+} as activator; calcium ions precipitate the liberated phosphate, cobalt salt replaces the calcium phosphate, and ammonium sulfide converts the product to a black cobalt sulfide.

Gomori one-step trichrome s., a connective tissue s. that uses hematoxylin and a dye mixture containing chromotrope 2R and light green or aniline blue; muscle fibers appear red, collagen is green (or blue if aniline blue is used), and nuclei are blue to black.

Gomori silver impregnation s., a reliable method for reticulin, as an aid in the diagnosis of neoplasm and early cirrhosis of the liver; the staining solution employs silver nitrate, potassium hydroxide, and ammonia water carefully prepared to avoid having silver precipitate.

Goodpasture s., a s. for Gram-negative bacteria, using aniline fuchsin.

Gordon and Sweet s., a s. for reticulin, using acidified potassium permanganate, oxalic acid, iron alum, silver nitrate, formaldehyde, gold chloride, and sodium thiosulfate.

Gram s., a method for differential staining of bacteria; smears are fixed by flaming, stained in a solution of crystal violet, treated with iodine solution, rinsed, decolorized, and then counterstained with safranin O; Gram-positive organisms stain purple-black and Gram-negative organisms stain pink; useful in bacterial taxonomy and identification, and also in indicating fundamental differences in cell wall structure.

Gram-chromotrope s., a modified trichrome s. for microsporidian spores that combines Gram-stain reagents in the procedure.

green s., a deposit, produced by chromogenic bacteria, found on the cervicolabial portions of the teeth, usually in children. SEE ALSO acquired *pellicle.*

Gridley s., a silver staining method for reticulum.

Gridley s. for fungi, a method for fixed tissue sections based on Bauer chromic acid leucofuchsin s. with the addition of Gomori aldehyde fuchsin s. and metanil yellow as counterstains; against a yellow background, hyphae, conidia, yeast capsules, elastin, and mucin appear in different shades of blue to purple.

Grocott-Gomori methenamine-silver s., a modification of Gomori methenamine-silver s. for fungi in which sections are pretreated with chromic acid before addition of the methenamine-silver solution and then counterstained with light green to demonstrate black-brown fungi against a pale green background.

Hale colloidal iron s., a s. used to distinguish acid mucopolysaccharides such as hyaluronic acid; may be combined with PAS to also visualize carbohydrate-containing proteins and glycoproteins.

Heidenhain azan s., a technique using azocarmine B or G followed by aniline blue to stain nuclei and erythrocytes red, muscle orange, glia fibrils reddish, mucin blue, and collagen and reticulum dark blue. [*az*ocarmine + *ani*line blue]

Heidenhain iron hematoxylin s., an iron alum hematoxylin s. used for staining muscle striations and mitotic structures blue-black.

hematoxylin and eosin s., probably the most generally useful of all staining methods for tissues; nuclei are stained a deep blue with hematoxylin, and cytoplasm is stained pink after counterstaining with eosin, usually in water.

hematoxylin-malachite green-basic fuchsin s., a s. for epoxy resin-extracted sections; semithick sections have their plastic dissolved out and the residual tissue is stained sequentially with the various dyes; nuclei and astrocytes are purplish-pink and myelin, lipid droplets, nucleoli, and oligodendrocytes are bright blue-green.

hematoxylin-phloxine B s., a s. for intact epoxy sections; semithick sections of plastic-embedded tissues have the following

structures stained blue to black: chromatin, nucleoli, basophilic cytoplasm, mitochondria, plasma and nuclear membranes, anisotropic myofibrils, mast cell granules, and elastic membranes of blood vessels; appearing pink to red are collagen fibrils, reticulum, goblet cell mucins, hyalin cartilage matrix, stereocilia, cytoplasm, and erythrocytes; fat droplets and perichondrocyte matrix are green.

Hirsch-Peiffer s., a s. used for cytologic demonstration staining of metachromatic leukodystrophy; excess sulfatides stain metachromatically (golden brown) with cresyl violet in acetic acid.

Hiss s., a s. for demonstrating the capsules of microorganisms, using gentian violet or basic fuchsin followed by a copper sulfate wash.

Holmes s., a silver nitrate staining method for nerve fibers.

Hortega neuroglia s., one of several silver carbonate methods to demonstrate astrocytes, oligodendroglia, and microglia.

Hucker-Conn s., a crystal violet-ammonium oxalate mixture used in Gram stain.

immunofluorescent s., s. resulting from combination of fluorescent antibody with antigen specific for that antibody.

India ink capsule s., a negative s. for crystal bacteria in which cells appear purple (Gram crystal violet) and the capsules appear clear against a dark background.

intravital s., a s. which is taken up by living cells after parenteral administration, e.g., intravenously or subcutaneously.

iodine s., a s. to detect amyloid, cellulose, chitin, starch, carotenes, and glycogen, and to stain amebas by virtue of their glycogen; feces and other wet preparations are stained directly with Lugol iodine solution; smears are treated with Schaudinn fixative and then stained with alcoholic iodine, followed by Heidenhain iron hematoxylin.

Jenner s., a methylene blue eosinate similar to Wright s. but differing in not using polychromed methylene blue; used for staining of blood smears.

Kasten fluorescent Feulgen s., a fluorescent modification of the Feulgen s., utilizing any one of a variety of fluorescent basic dyes to which SO_2 is added; the brilliant fluorescence makes this method unusually sensitive and adaptable to cytofluorometric quantification of DNA.

Kasten fluorescent PAS s., a fluorescent modification of the periodic acid-Schiff s. for polysaccharides which uses one of Kasten fluorescent Schiff reagents.

Kinyoun s., a method for demonstrating acid-fast microorganisms, using carbol fuchsin, acid alcohol, and methylene blue; acid-fast microorganisms appear red against a blue background.

Kleihauer s., a combination of aniline blue and Biebrich scarlet red used for detection of fetal cells in the maternal blood.

Klinger-Ludwig acid-thionin s. for sex chromatin, a method using a preliminary acid treatment on buccal smears, prior to staining with buffered thionin, to differentiate Barr body.

Klüver-Barrera Luxol fast blue s., in combination with cresyl violet, a s. useful for demonstrating myelin and Nissl substance.

Kokoskin s., a modified trichrome s. for microsporidian spores in which heat is used to shorten the staining times.

Kossa s., SYN von Kossa s.

Kronecker s., a 5% sodium chloride s. rendered faintly alkaline with sodium carbonate, used in the examination of fresh tissues under the microscope.

lactophenol cotton blue s., a solution consisting of phenol crystals, glycerol, lactic acid, and distilled water to which cotton blue or crystal violet is added; used as a s. in mycology.

Laquer s. for alcoholic hyalin, a combination of Altmann aniline-acid fuchsin s. with a Masson trichrome s. which, on a gray-brown background, stains alcoholic hyalin red, collagen green, and nuclei brown.

lead hydroxide s., a s. for electron microscopy; after aldehyde fixation, alkaline lead hydroxide preferentially stains RNA, but after OsO_4 fixation, it reacts largely with osmium in tissues to give a general s.; in addition to binding to cytomembranes, it also stains carbohydrates (e.g., glycogen).

Leishman s., a polychromed eosin-methylene blue s. used in the examination of blood films.

Lendrum phloxine-tartrazine s., a s. for demonstrating acidophilic inclusion bodies, which appear red on a yellow background; nuclei stain blue, but Negri bodies do not stain.

Lepehne-Pickworth s., a staining technique for hemoglobin and other heme-containing substances in cryostat or frozen sections, which utilizes the presence of tissue peroxidase to oxidize benzidine to a blue quinhydrone.

Levaditi s., a silver nitrate s. for blackening spirochetes in tissue sections.

Lillie allochrome connective tissue s., a procedure using PAS, hematoxylin, picric acid, and methyl blue; used for distinction between basement membrane and reticulin, and for demonstration of arteriosclerotic lesions.

Lillie azure-eosin s., a s. in which an azure eosinate solution is used to s. bacteria and rickettsiae in tissues.

Lillie ferrous iron s., a method using potassium ferrocyanide in acetic acid that demonstrates melanins as a deep green color; lipofuscins and heme pigments are unreactive.

Lillie sulfuric acid Nile blue s., a technique for showing fatty acids when present in high concentrations.

Lison-Dunn s., a technique using leuco patent blue V and hydrogen peroxidase to demonstrate hemoglobin peroxidase on time sections and smears.

Loeffler s., a s. for flagella; the specimen is treated with a mixture of ferrous sulfate, tannic acid, and alcoholic fuchsin, then stained with aniline-water fuchsin or gentian violet made alkaline with sodium hydroxide solution.

Loeffler caustic s., a s. for flagella, utilizing an aqueous solution of tannin and ferrous sulfate with the addition of an alcoholic fuchsin s.

Luna-Ishak s., a staining method using celestine blue and acid fuchsin in which bile canaliculi stain pink to red.

Macchiavello s., a basic fuchsin-citric acid-methylene blue sequence in smears which produces red staining of rickettsiae and inclusion bodies, with nuclei staining blue.

MacNeal tetrachrome blood s., a s. for blood smears composed of a mixture of methylene blue, azure A, methylene violet, and eosin Y.

malarial pigment s., a s. using phloxine-toluidine blue O sequence; malarial pigment and nuclei are bluish, erythrocytes and cytoplasm are red to orange; found in phagocytic cells of the reticuloendothelial system.

Maldonado-San Jose s., a staining method for staining pancreatic islet cells, using a phloxine-azure B-hematoxylin sequence; alpha cells are purple, beta cells are violet-blue, delta cells are light blue, and exocrine cells are grayish blue with red secretion granules.

Mallory s. for actinomyces, a s. using alum hematoxylin, followed by eosin; immersion in Ehrlich aniline crystal violet s., and Weigert iodine solution; mycelia stain blue and clubs stain red.

Mallory aniline blue s., SYN Mallory trichrome s.

Mallory collagen s., one of a number of staining methods using phosphomolybdic or phosphotungstic acid with an acid s., such as aniline blue, or with hematoxylin for connective tissue staining.

Mallory s. for hemofuchsin, sections are stained sequentially in alum hematoxylin and basic fuchsin; the lipofuchsin-like pigment and ceroid stain bright red, nuclei stain blue, while melanin and hemosiderin appear unstained in their natural browns.

Mallory iodine s., amyloid appears red-brown after Gram iodine, then violet and blue after flooding with dilute sulfuric acid.

Mallory phloxine s., a technique based on retention of phloxine by hyaline after overstaining and then decolorizing with lithium carbonate, used in combination with alum hematoxylin to give nuclear staining; hyaline appears red, older hyaline is pink to colorless, amyloid is pale pink, and nuclei are blue-black.

Mallory phosphotungstic acid hematoxylin s., SYN phosphotungstic acid *hematoxylin*.

Mallory trichrome s., a method especially suitable for studying connective tissue; sections are stained in acid fuchsin, aniline blue-orange G solution, and phosphotungstic acid; fibrils of collagen are blue, fibroglia, neuroglia, and muscle fibers are red, and fibrils of elastin are pink or yellow. SYN Mallory aniline blue s., Mallory triple s.

Mallory triple s., SYN Mallory trichrome s.

Mann methyl blue-eosin s., a s. useful for anterior pituitary and viral inclusion bodies; a mixture of the two dyes stains alpha cell granules red, beta cell granules dark blue, chromophobes gray to pink, colloid red, erythrocytes orange-red, and collagen fibers blue; this method is also useful for enterochromaffin, goblet, Paneth, and pancreatic islet cells; Negri bodies appear red while their nuclei and central granules are blue.

Marchi s., a staining method in which the specimen is hardened for 8–10 days in a modified Müller fixative, followed by immersion for 1–3 weeks in the same with the addition of osmic acid; fat and degenerating nerve fibers stain black.

Masson argentaffin s., a s. used to stain enterochromaffin granules brown-black.

Masson-Fontana ammoniac silver s., a s. used to demonstrate melanin and argentaffin granules. SYN Fontana-Masson silver s.

Masson trichrome s., original composition for multicolored tissue preparations including ponceau de xylidine, acid fuchsin, iron alum hematoxylin, and either aniline blue or fast green FCF; chromatin stains black, cytoplasm is in shades of red, granules of eosinophils and mast cells are deep red, erythrocytes are black, elastic fibers are red, and collagen fibers and mucus are dark blue (aniline blue) or green (fast green FCF); modifications substitute other dyes, such as Biebrich scarlet red and wool green s.

Maximow s. for bone marrow, an alum-hematoxylin and azure II-eosin s. used to distinguish granulated leukocytes, mast cells, and cartilage.

Mayer hemalum s., a progressive nuclear s. also used as a counterstain.

Mayer mucicarmine s., SEE mucicarmine.

Mayer mucihematein s., SEE mucihematein.

May-Grünwald s., a German equivalent of Jenner s., used for blood staining and in cytology; often used in combination with Giemsa s.; valuable in demonstrating parasitic flagellates.

metachromatic s., a s., such as methylene blue, thionin, or azure A, that has the ability to produce different colors with various histologic or cytologic structures.

methenamine silver s., a s. used for cysts of *Pneumocystis carinii*.

methyl green-pyronin s., a staining method useful for identification of plasma cells which are intensely pyroninophilic; a mixture of a green and a red dye that has the property of staining highly polymerized nucleic acid (DNA) green and low molecular weight nucleic acids (RNA) red. SEE Unna-Pappenheim s.

modified acid-fast s., a s. for coccidia (*Cryptosporidium, Cyclospora, Isospora*) in which the decolorizer is a very dilute acid (1–3% sulfuric acid); less likely to remove too much dye.

modified trichrome s., a s. developed from the Wheatley modification of the Gomori trichrome s. using 10 times the amount of chromotrope 2R dye for microsporidian spores, which stain pink to red.

Mowry colloidal iron s., a s. used for demonstrating acid mucopolysaccharides.

MSB trichrome s., a s. for fibrin using martius yellow, brilliant crystal scarlet 6R, and soluble blue; fibrin is selectively stained red and connective tissue appears blue.

multiple s., a mixture of several dyes each having an independent selective action on one or more portions of the tissue.

Nair buffered methylene blue s., s. used to show nuclear detail of protozoan trophozoites when used at low pH (3.6–4.8).

Nakanishi s., a method for vital staining of bacteria in which a slide is treated with hot methylene blue solution until it acquires a sky-blue color, after which a drop of an emulsion of the bacteria is put on the cover glass and the latter laid on the slide; the bacteria are stained differentially, some parts more intensely than others.

Nauta s., a s. for degenerating axons in which they stain with silver and appear as fragmented and swollen fibers.

negative s., s. forming an opaque or colored background against

st

which the object to be demonstrated appears as a translucent or colorless area; in electron microscopy, an electron opaque material, such as phosphotungstic acid or sodium phosphotungstate, is used to give detail as to surface structure.

Neisser s., a s. for the polar nuclei of the diphtheria bacillus which uses a mixture of methylene blue and crystal violet.

neutral s., a compound of an acid s. and a basic s., such as the eosinate of methylene blue, in which the anion and cation each contains a chromophore group. SYN salt dye.

Nicolle s. for capsules, s. in a mixture of a saturated solution of gentian violet in alcohol-phenol.

ninhydrin-Schiff s. for proteins, proteins are revealed by using ninhydrin or alloxan to produce aldehydes from primary aliphatic amines by oxidative deamination; the aldehydes are shown by reaction with Schiff reagent.

Nissl s., (1) a method for staining nerve cells with basic fuchsin; (2) a method for staining aggregates of rough endoplasmic reticulum and ribosomes in neuronal cell bodies and dendrites with basic dyes such as cresyl violet (or cresyl echt violet), thionine, toluidin blue O, or methylene blue.

Noble s., a basic fuchsin-orange G staining technique for detection of viral inclusion bodies in fixed tissues.

nuclear s., a s. for cell nuclei, usually based on the binding of a basic dye to DNA or nucleohistone.

Orth s., a lithium carmine s. for nerve cells and their processes.

Padykula-Herman s. for myosin ATPase, a technique similar to that of Gomori nonspecific alkaline phosphatase s., except that incubation is carried out with ATP as the substrate at pH 9.4 in the absence of Mg^{2+}; enzyme activity is demonstrated as blackened deposits in the A band of striated muscle sarcomeres; control tissue sections lacking substrate and containing sulfhydryl inhibitors are necessary.

Paget-Eccleston s., an aldehyde-thionin-PAS-orange G staining technique modified to identify seven different cell types in the anterior pituitary gland.

panoptic s., a s. in which a Romanowsky-type s. is combined with another s.; such a combination improves the staining of cytoplasmic granules and other bodies.

Papanicolaou s., a multichromatic s. used principally on exfoliated cytologic specimens and based on aqueous hematoxylin with multiple counterstaining dyes in 95% ethyl alcohol, giving great transparency and delicacy of detail; important in cancer screening, especially of gynecologic smears.

Pappenheim s., a methyl green-pyronin stain, originally used as a stain for lymphocytes.

paracarmine s., a staining fluid consisting of a solution of calcium chloride and carminic acid in 75% alcohol.

PAS s., SYN periodic acid-Schiff s.

periodic acid-Schiff s. (PAS), a tissue-staining procedure in which 1,2-glycol groupings are first oxidized with periodic acid to aldehydes, which then react with the sulfite leucofuchsin reagent of Schiff, and become colored red-violet; strong staining occurs with polysaccharides, such as glycogen, and mucopolysaccharides of epithelial mucins, basement membranes, and connective tissue. SYN PAS s.

Perls Prussian blue s., a s. for ferric iron as in hemosiderins, using potassium ferrocyanide in acetic acid or dilute hydrochloric acid followed by a red counterstain such as safranin O or neutral red; various hemosiderins and most mineral irons give a blue-green reaction, while nuclei stain red.

peroxidase s., a method for demonstrating peroxidase granules in some neutrophils and in eosinophils; the enzyme promotes the oxidation of benzidine by hydrogen peroxide; tissues treated with horseradish peroxidase can also have the enzyme detected in the electron microscope.

phosphotungstic acid s., the first general s. used for electron microscopy; a selective s. for extracellular components such as elastin, collagen, and basement membrane mucopolysaccharides; it can be followed by uranyl acetate or lead. SYN PTA s.

picrocarmine s., a red crystalline powder derived from a solution of carmine, ammonia, and picric acid, which is evaporated, leav-

ing the powder (soluble in water); it produces excellent staining of keratohyaline granules.

picro-Mallory trichrome s., a modification of Mallory trichrome s. that involves the addition of picric acid.

picronigrosin s., a solution of nigrosin in picric acid, used for staining connective tissue.

plasma s., plasmatic s., plasmic s., a s. whose principal affinity is for the cytoplasm of cells.

plastic section s., (1) for electron microscopy, a s. (e.g., osmic acid, PTA, potassium permanganate) used on thin sections of plastic-embedded tissues, utilizing differential attachment of heavy atoms to various cellular and tissue structures so that electrons will be absorbed and scattered by these structures to produce an image; to achieve differential staining, the s. must penetrate nonwettable plastic embedments; (2) for light microscopy, a s. (e.g., alkaline toluidine blue, silver methenamine) used on plastic-embedded tissues to attain higher resolution and more detail than normally possible; semi-thick (0.5-1.5 μm) sections are particularly useful in renal pathology, especially in combination with the phase microscope.

port-wine s., SYN *nevus* flammeus.

positive s., direct binding of a dye with a tissue component to produce contrast; in electron microscopy, heavy metals like uranyl and lead salts are used to bind to selective cell constituents to produce increased density to the electron beam, i.e., contrast.

Prussian blue s., a s. employing acid potassium ferrocyanide to demonstrate iron, as in siderocytes.

PTA s., SYN phosphotungstic acid s.

Puchtler-Sweat s. for basement membranes, a staining method using resorcin-fuchsin and nuclear fast red solutions after Carnoy fixative; basement membranes are gray to black and nuclei pink to red.

Puchtler-Sweat s. for hemoglobin and hemosiderin, a complex staining method in which, on a yellow background, hemoglobin is stained red, hemosiderin blue to green, and elastic fibers pink.

Q-banding s., a fluorescent s. for chromosomes which produces specific banding patterns for each pair of homologous chromosomes; the acridine dye derivative, quinacrine hydrochloride, or other derivatives like quinacrine mustard dihydrochloride produces a green-yellow fluorescence at pH 4.5 in chromosome segments rich in constitutive heterochromatin with deoxyadenylate-deoxythymidilate (A-T) bases of DNA; centromeric regions of human chromosomes 3, 4, and 13 are specifically stained, as are satellites of some acrocentric chromosomes and the end of the long arm of the Y chromosome; banding patterns are similar to those obtained with G-banding stain; similar fluorescent s. results are seen with the antibiotics adriamycin and daunomycin, as well as the tertiary dyes butyl proflavine and DAPI, and the bis-benzimidazole dye HOECHST 33258. SYN quinacrine chromosome banding s.

quinacrine chromosome banding s., SYN Q-banding s.

Rambourg chromic acid-phosphotungstic acid s., a s. for glycoproteins, used with an electron microscope, with which ultra-thin tissue sections reveal complex carbohydrates in the same locations as shown by Rambourg periodic acid-chromic methenamine-silver s.

Rambourg periodic acid-chromic methenamine-silver s., a s. for glycoproteins, used with an electron microscope, adapted from the Gomori-Jones periodic acid-methenamine-silver s.; it produces silver deposits in mature saccules of the Golgi apparatus, lysosomal vesicles, cell coat, and basement membranes.

R-banding s., a reverse Giemsa chromosome banding method that produces bands complementary to G-bands; induced by treatment with high temperature, low pH, or acridine orange staining; often used together with G-banding on human karyotype to determine whether there are deletions.

Romanowsky blood s., prototype of the eosin-methylene blue s.'s for blood smears, using aqueous solutions made of a mixture of methylene blue (saturated) and eosin. Romanowsky-type s.'s depend for their action on compounds formed by interaction of methylene blue and eosin; most are of no value if water is present in the alcohol because neutral dyes become precipitated.

Roux s., a double s. for diphtheria bacilli which employs crystal violet or dahlia and methyl green.

Ryan s., a modified trichrome s. for microsporidian spores in which the chromotrope 2R is 10 times the normal concentration used in trichrome s.'s for stool specimens and the counterstain is aniline blue.

Schaeffer-Fulton s., a s. for bacterial spores using malachite green and safranin so that bacterial bodies are red to pink and spores are green.

Schmorl ferric-ferricyanide reduction s., a s. to test for reducing substances in tissues, including melanin, argentaffin granules, thyroid colloid, keratin, keratohyalin, and lipofuscin pigments; ferricyanide is converted into ferrocyanide which is converted to insoluble Prussian blue in the presence of ferric ions.

Schmorl picrothionin s., a s. for compact bone which employs thionin and picric acid solutions to produce blue to blue-black staining of bone canaliculi and cells; bone matrix is yellowish and cartilage ground substance is purple.

Schultz s., a s. for cholesterol; a relatively specific but insensitive histochemical test for cholesterol and cholesterol esters in which frozen sections of formalin-fixed tissues are oxidized in iron alum, hydrogen peroxide, or sodium iodate, then treated with sulfuric acid to give a blue-green to red color in a positive reaction; the presence of glycerol inhibits the reaction.

selective s., a s. that colors one portion of a tissue or cell exclusively or more deeply than the remaining portions.

Semichon acid carmine s., s. for adult trematodes.

silver s., any of a variety of s.'s (e.g., Bielschowsky, Gomori silver, impregnation s.'s) which employ alkaline silver nitrate solutions to stain connective tissue fibers (reticulin, collagen), calcium salt deposits, spirochaetes, neurological tissue, and nucleolar organizer regions.

silver-ammoniac silver s., a s. for the acid protein component of nucleolar regions that are active or that were transcriptionally active in the preceding interphase; uses silver nitrate, ammoniacal silver, and formalin. SYN Ag-AS s.

silver protein s., a silver proteinate complex used in staining nerve fibers, nerve endings, and flagellate protozoa; also used to demonstrate phagocytosis in living animals by the cells of the reticuloendothelial system.

Stirling modification of Gram s., a stable aniline-crystal violet s.

supravital s., a procedure in which living tissue is removed from the body and cells are placed in a nontoxic dye solution so that their vital processes may be studied.

Taenzer s., an orcein solution used for staining elastic tissue. SYN Unna-Taenzer s.

Takayama s., a s. containing pyridine, sodium hydrate, and dextrose; used for identification of blood stains; a drop added to a suspected blood stain results in the formation of hemochromogen crystals.

telomeric R-banding s., a modified R-banding s. in which the telomeres become strongly stained and faint R-banding still occurs over the rest of the chromosomes; uses air-dried slides, aging for several days, and staining in hot phosphate-buffered Giemsa s.

thioflavine T s., a s. employed to detect amyloid, which induces specific yellow fluorescence; tissue sections are first put in alum-hematoxylin to quench nuclear fluorescence and then stained in thioflavine T.

Tizzoni s., a s. used as a test for iron in tissue; the tissue is treated with a solution of potassium ferrocyanide and then with dilute hydrochloric acid; a blue coloration indicates the presence of iron.

Toison s., a blood diluent and leukocyte stain containing methyl violet, sodium chloride, sodium sulfate, and glycerin; also used for erythrocyte counts.

toluidine blue s., a s. used for *Pneumocystis carinii* trophozoites.

trichrome s., staining combinations that usually contain three dyes of contrasting colors selected to stain connective tissue, muscle, cytoplasm, and nuclei in bright colors; generally, tissue sections are first dyed in iron hematoxylin before being treated with the other dyes.

trypsin G-banding s., SEE G-banding s.

ultrafast Pap s., a modified Papanicolaou s. suitable for use in

situations in which rapid decisions are essential and frozen sections may not be sufficiently reliable or practical. SEE ALSO Papanicolaou s.

Unna s., (1) an alkaline methylene blue s. for plasma cells; **(2)** a polychrome methylene blue s. with which mast cells are stained red (metachromatic).

Unna-Pappenheim s., a contrast s. consisting of a methyl green-pyronin solution; originally used for gonococci, but later used to detect RNA and DNA in tissue sections; RNA is stained red and DNA appears green; used to demonstrate plasma cells during chronic inflammation. SEE methyl green-pyronin s.

Unna-Taenzer s., SYN Taenzer s.

uranyl acetate s., a s. used in electron microscopy; uranyl acetate binds specifically to nucleic acids but selectively tends to be abolished by osmium fixation; proteins are well-stained, but cytomembranes are poorly stained.

urate crystals s., a s. using silver methenamine to detect crystals, which polarize light in contrast with calcium crystals; useful in diagnosing gout and kidney infarcts resulting from uric acid build-up.

van Ermengen s., a method for staining flagella that uses glacial acetic acid, osmic acid, tannic acid, silver nitrate, gallic acid, and potassium acetate.

van Gieson s., a mixture of acid fuchsin in saturated picric acid solution, used in collagen staining.

Verhoeff elastic tissue s., a s. for tissue sections in which a mixture of hematoxylin, ferric chloride, and Lugol iodine solution is used; tissue may be counterstained, if desired, with eosin or van Gieson s.; elastic fibers and nuclei appear blue-black to black while collagen and other components are shades of pink to red.

vital s., a s. applied to cells or parts of cells while they are still living.

von Kossa s., a s. for calcium in mineralized tissue, utilizing a silver nitrate solution followed by sodium thiosulfate; calcified bone but not osteoid is stained brown to black. SYN Kossa s.

Wachstein-Meissel s. for calcium-magnesium-ATPase, a method similar to that of Gomori nonspecific acid phosphatase s., except that incubation is carried out with ATP as substrate at neutral pH; enzyme activity is generally demonstrated at cell membranes.

Warthin-Starry silver s., a s. for spirochetes in which preparations are incubated in 1% silver nitrate solution followed by a developer.

Weber s., a modified trichrome s. for microsporidian spores in which the chromotrope 2R is 10 times the normal concentration used in trichrome s.'s for stool specimens and the counterstain is fast green.

Weigert s. for actinomyces, a staining method using immersion in a dark red orsellin solution in alcohol, then staining in crystal-violet solution. SEE ALSO iron *hematoxylin*.

Weigert s. for elastin, a staining solution of fuchsin, resorcin, and ferric chloride; elastic fibers stain blue-black.

Weigert s. for fibrin, a staining method using solutions of aniline-crystal violet and iodine-potassium iodide, then decolorizing in aniline oil and xylol; the fibrin is stained dark blue.

Weigert-Gram s., a s. for bacteria in tissues in which sections are stained in alum-hematoxylin, then in eosin, aniline methyl violet, and Lugol solution.

Weigert iron hematoxylin s., a nuclear staining solution containing hematoxylin, ferric chloride, and hydrochloric acid; useful in combination with van Gieson s., especially for demonstrating connective tissue elements or *Entamoeba histolytica* in sections.

Weigert s. for myelin, a staining method using ferric chloride and hematoxylin; myelin stains deep blue, degenerated portions a light yellowish color.

Weigert s. for neuroglia, a complicated process in which the final treatment is like that for staining fibrin; neuroglia and nuclei stain blue.

Wilder s. for reticulum, a silver impregnation technique in which reticulum appears as black, well-defined fibers without beading and with a relatively clear background.

Williams s., a s. for Negri bodies that uses picric acid, fuchsin, and methylene blue; Negri bodies are magenta, granules and nerve cells blue, and erythrocytes yellowish.

ℹ️**Wright s.,** a staining mixture of eosinates of polychromed methylene blue used in staining of blood smears.

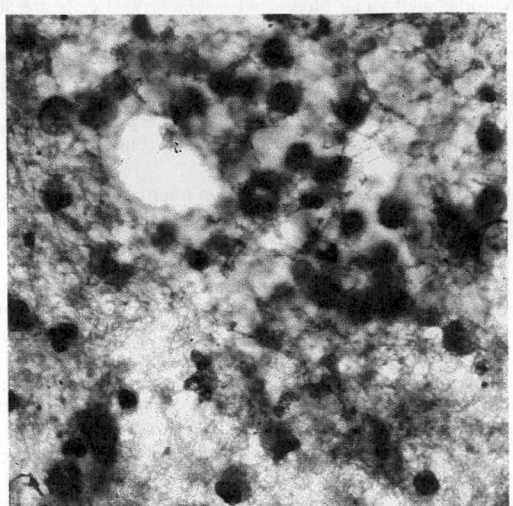

Ziehl-Neelsen stain: used here to show granulomatous inflammation in a liver aspirate

Ziehl s., a carbol-fuchsin solution of phenol and basic fuchsin used to demonstrate bacteria and cell nuclei.

ℹ️**Ziehl-Neelsen s.,** a method for staining acid-fast bacteria using Ziehl s., decolorizing in acid alcohol, and counterstaining with methylene blue; acid-fast organisms appear red, other tissue elements light blue; a modification of this s. is also used for *Actinomycetes* and *Brucella*.

stain·ing (stān′ing). **1.** The act of applying a stain. SEE ALSO stain. **2.** In dentistry, modification of the color of the tooth or denture base.

progressive s., a procedure in which s. is continued until the desired intensity of coloring of tissue elements is attained.

regressive s., a type of s. in which tissues are overstained and the excess dye is then removed selectively until the desired intensity is obtained.

stains-all (stainz′awl). A dye that stains phosphoproteins blue, proteins red, nucleic acids purple, and mucoproteins and mucopolysaccharides various colors on acrylamide gels; also used on tissue sections.

stair·case (stār′kās). A series of reactions that follow one another in progressively increasing or decreasing intensity, so that a chart shows a continuous rise or fall. SEE treppe.

stal·ag·mom·e·ter (stal-ă-gom′ĕ-ter). An instrument for determining exactly the number of drops in a given quantity of liquid; used as a measure of the surface tension of a fluid (the lower the tension, the smaller the drops and, consequently, the more numerous in a given quantity of the fluid). SYN stactometer. [G. *stalagma*, a drop, + *metron*, measure]

stalk (stawk). A narrowed connection with a structure or organ.

allantoic s., the narrow connection between the intraembryonic portion of the allantois and the extraembryonic allantoic vesicle.

body s., the extraembryonic precursor of the connecting s. or umbilical cord by which the embryo is attached to its trophoblastic chorion. SYN connecting s.

connecting s., SYN body s.

s. of epiglottis, the lower end or pedicle of the cartilage of the epiglottis, attached to the superior notch of the thyroid cartilage. SYN petiolus epiglottidis.

infundibular s., SYN infundibular *stem*.

optic s., the constricted proximal portion of the optic vesicle in the embryo; it contributes to the optic nerve.

pineal s., the attachment of the pineal body to the roof of the third ventricle; it contains the pineal recess of the third ventricle.

pituitary s., a process comprising the tuberal part investing the infundibular stem that attaches the hypophysis to the tuber cinereum at the base of the brain.

yolk s., the narrowed connection between the intraembryonic gut and the yolk sac; its walls are splanchnopleure. SYN umbilical duct, vitelline duct, vitellointestinal duct.

stam·mer (stam′er). **1.** To hesitate in speech, halt, repeat, and mispronounce, by reason of embarrassment, agitation, unfamiliarity with the subject, or as yet unidentified physiologic causes. Cf. stutter. **2.** To mispronounce or transpose certain consonants in speech. [A.S. *stamur*]

stam·mer·ing (stam′er-ing). **1.** A speech disorder characterized by hesitation and repetition of words, or by mispronunciation or transposition of certain consonants, especially *l*, *r*, and *s*. **2.** Sounds other than speech, that are similar to stammering. SYN paralalia literalis, psellism.

s. of the bladder, SYN urinary *stuttering*.

Stam·no·so·ma (stam-nō-sō′mă). A genus of flukes of the family Heterophyidae, identical with *Centrocestus*. Two species, *S. armatum* and *S. formosanum*, have been described as sometimes infecting humans. [G. *stamnos*, a jar, + *sōma*, body]

stan·dard (stan′dard). **1.** Something that serves as a basis for comparison; a technical specification or written report by experts. **2.** SEE standard *substance*. [M.E., fr. O.Fr. *estandard*, rallying place, fr. Frankish *standan*, to stand, + *hard*, hard, fast]

stan·dard·i·za·tion (stan′dard-i-zā′shŭn). **1.** The making of a solution of definite strength so that it may be used for comparison and in tests. **2.** Making any drug or preparation conform to the type or standard. **3.** A set of techniques used to remove as far as possible the effects of differences in the age or other confounding variables when comparing two or more populations.

s. of a test, in psychology, the following of definite procedures for administering, scoring, evaluating, and reporting the results of a new test which is under development.

stand·still. Cessation of activity.

atrial s., cessation of atrial contractions, marked by absence of atrial waves in the electrocardiogram. SYN auricular s.

auricular s., SYN atrial s.

cardiac s., SYN asystole.

sinus s., cessation of sinus node activity, marked by absence of normal P waves in the electrocardiogram.

ventricular s., cessation of ventricular contractions, marked by absence of ventricular complexes in the electrocardiogram.

Stanley, Edward, English surgeon, 1793–1862. SEE S. cervical *ligaments*, under *ligament*.

stan·nic (stan′ik). Relating to tin, especially when in combination in its higher valency. [L. *stannum*, tin]

stan·nic chlo·ride. $SnCl_4$; a fuming liquid (fuming spirit of Libavius), specific gravity 2.23, boiling point 115°C, that forms several hydrates; the pentahydrate (butter of tin) is used for mordanting and "loading" or "weighting" silk.

stan·nic ox·ide. SnO_2; used in industry; it is a cause of pneumoconiosis. SYN tin oxide.

Stannius, Herman F., German biologist, 1808–1883. SEE S. *ligature*.

stan·nous (stan′ŭs). Relating to tin, especially when in combination in its lower valency. [L. *stannum*, tin]

stan·nous flu·o·ride. A preparation containing not less than 71.2% of stannous tin and not less than 22.3% nor more than 25.5% of fluoride; used as a prophylactic against caries in dentistry.

stan·num (stan′ŭm). SYN tin. [L.]

stan·o·lone (stan′ŏ-lōn). An androgen with the same actions and uses as testosterone; used for its anabolic and tumor-suppressing effects, specifically, in carcinoma of the breast. SYN dihydrotestosterone.

stan·o·zo·lol (stan-ō′zō-lol, -lōl). Stanozol, 17α-methyl-5α-androstan-17β-ol carrying a pyrazole ring (=CH–NH–N=) attached to C-2 and C-3 (see steroids for androstane structure). A semisynthetic, orally effective anabolic agent.

sta·pe·dec·to·my (stă-pĕ-dek′tō-mē). Operation to remove the stapes in whole or part with replacement of the stapes by a metal or plastic prosthesis; used for otosclerosis with stapes fixation to overcome a conductive hearing loss. [stapes + G. *ektomē,* excision]

sta·pe·di·al (stā-pē′dē-ăl). Relating to the stapes.

sta·pe·di·o·te·not·o·my (stā-pē′dē-ō-tĕ-not′ŏ-mē). Division of the tendon of the stapedius muscle. [stapedius + G. *tenōn,* tendon, + *tomē,* incision]

sta·pe·di·o·ves·tib·u·lar (stā-pē′dē-ō-ves-tib′ū-lăr). Relating to the stapes and the vestibule of the ear.

sta·pe·di·us, pl. **sta·pe·dii** (stā-pē′dē-ŭs, stā-pē′dē-ī). SYN stapedius (*muscle*). [Mod. L.]

sta·pe·dot·o·my (stā-pē-dot′ō-mē). A surgical technique for the improvement of hearing in otosclerosis: a hole is made in the footplate of the stapes bone through which is placed the piston-shaped end of a prosthesis, the other end of which is attached to the long process of the incus bone.

sta·pes, pl. **sta·pes, sta·pe·des** (stā′pēz, stā′pē-dēz) [TA]. The smallest of the three auditory ossicles; its base, or footpiece, fits into the vestibular (oval) window, while its head is articulated with the lenticular process of the long limb of the incus. SYN stirrup. [Mod. L. stirrup]

staphyl-. SEE staphylo-.

staph·y·lec·to·my (staf-i-lek′tō-mē). SYN uvulectomy. [staphyl- + G. *ektomē,* excision]

staph·yl·e·de·ma (staf′il-e-dē′mă). Edema of the uvula. [staphyl- + G. *oidēma,* swelling (edema)]

staph·y·line (staf′i-līn, -lēn). SYN botryoid.

sta·phyl·i·on (stă-fil′ē-on). The midpoint of the posterior edge of the hard palate; a craniometric point. SEE ALSO posterior nasal *spine* of horizontal plate of palatine bone. [G. dim. of *staphylē,* a bunch of grapes]

staphylo-, staphyl-. Resemblance to a grape or a bunch of grapes, hence relating usually to staphylococci or, in obsolescent image, to the uvula palatina. SEE ALSO uvulo-. [G. *staphylē,* a bunch of grapes]

staph·y·lo·coc·cal (staf′i-lō-kok′ăl). Relating to or caused by any organism of the genus *Staphylococcus.*

staph·y·lo·coc·ce·mia (staf′i-lō-kok-sē′mē-ă). The presence of staphylococci in the circulating blood. [staphylo- + G. *haima,* blood]

staph·y·lo·coc·ci (staf′i-lō-kok′sī). Plural of staphylococcus.

staph·y·lo·coc·cic (staf′i-lō-kok′sik). Relating to or caused by any species of *Staphylococcus.*

staph·y·lo·coc·col·y·sin (staf′i-lō-kŏ-kol′i-sin). SYN staphylolysin.

staph·y·lo·coc·col·y·sis (staf′i-lō-kŏ-kol′i-sis). Lysis or destruction of staphylococci. [staphylo- + G. *lysis,* dissolution]

staph·y·lo·coc·co·sis, pl. **staph·y·lo·coc·co·ses** (staf′i-lō-kok-ō′sis, -sēz). Infection by species of the bacterium *Staphylococcus.*

Sta·phy·lo·coc·cus (staf′i-lō-kok′ŭs). A genus of nonmotile, nonspore-forming, aerobic to facultatively anaerobic bacteria (family Micrococcaceae) containing Gram-positive, spherical cells, 0.5–1.5 μm in diameter, which divide in more than one plane to form irregular clusters. These organisms are chemoorganotrophic, and their metabolism is respiratory and fermentative. Under anaerobic conditions, lactic acid is produced from glucose; under aerobic conditions, acetic acid and small amounts of CO_2 are produced. Coagulase-positive strains produce a variety of toxins and are therefore potentially pathogenic and may cause food poisoning. These organisms are usually susceptible to antibiotics such as the β-lactam and macrolide antibiotics, tetracyclines, novobiocin, and chloramphenicol but are resistant to polymyxin and polyenes. They are susceptible to antibacterials such as phenols and their derivatives, surface-active compounds, salicylanilides, carbanilides, and halogens (chlorine and iodine) and their derivatives, such as chloramines and iodophors. They are found on the skin, in skin glands, on the nasal and other mucous membranes of warm-blooded animals, and in various food products. The type species is *S. aureus.* [staphylo- + G. *kokkos,* a berry]

S. au′reus, a common species found especially on nasal mucous membrane and skin (hair follicles); bacterial species that produces exotoxins including those that cause toxic shock syndrome, with resulting skin rash, and renal, hepatic, and central nervous system disease, and an enterotoxin associated with food poisoning; it causes furunculosis, cellulitis, pyemia, pneumonia, osteomyelitis, endocarditis, suppuration of wounds, other infections; also a cause of infection in burn patients; humans are the chief reservoir. The type species of the genus *S.* SYN *S. pyogenes aureus.*

S. epider′midis, a species of bacteria, the most common of the coagulase-negative *S.* group.

S. haemoly′ticus, coagulase-negative staphylococcus indigenous to human and mammalian hosts.

S. hominis, coagulase-negative staphylococcus indigenous to human and mammalian hosts.

S. pyog′enes al′bus, a name formerly applied to the organisms that are now regarded as the mutants of *S. aureus* that form white colonies.

S. pyog′enes au′reus, SYN *S. aureus.*

S. saprophyticus, a coagulase negative species that causes urinary tract infections.

S. simulans, coagulase-negative staphylococcus indigenous to human and mammalian hosts.

S. species, coagulase-negative, includes a group of species present as normal flora of human skin, respiratory, and mucous membrane surfaces. Although a normal commensal, strains are prominent causes of nosocomial infections, especially in patients with implanted intravenous access devices; some strains are abscess forming and cause diverse infections including sinusitis, wound infections, and osteomyelitis.

staph·y·lo·coc·cus, pl. **staph·y·lo·coc·ci** (staf′i-lō-kok′ŭs, kok′sī). A vernacular term used to refer to any member of the genus *Staphylococcus.*

staph·y·lo·di·al·y·sis (staf′i-lō-dī-al′i-sis). SYN uvuloptosis. [staphylo- + G. *dialysis,* a separation]

staph·y·lo·he·mia (staf′i-lō-hē′mē-ă). Obsolete term for staphylococcemia.

staph·y·lo·he·mo·ly·sin (staf′i-lō-hē-mol′i-sin). A mixture of hemolysins (alpha, beta, gamma, and delta), included in staphylococcal exotoxin; the α hemolysin has a marked effect on vascular muscle.

staph·y·lo·ki·nase (staf′i-lō-kī′nās). A microbial metalloenzyme from *Staphylococcus aureus,* with action similar to that of urokinase and streptokinase, that can convert plasminogen to plasmin but requires Ca^{2+}; separated in forms A, B, and C.

staph·y·lol·y·sin (staf-i-lol′i-sin). **1.** A hemolysin elaborated by a staphylococcus. **2.** An antibody causing lysis of staphylococci. SYN staphylococcolysin.

staph·y·lo·ma (staf-i-lō′mă). A bulging of the cornea or sclera containing uveal tissue. [staphylo- + G. *-ōma,* tumor]

anterior s., a bulging near the anterior pole of the eyeball. SYN corneal s.

anular s., a s. extending around the periphery of the cornea.

ciliary s., scleral s. occurring in the region of the ciliary body.

corneal s., SYN anterior s.

equatorial s., a s. occurring in the area of exit of the vortex veins. SYN scleral s.

intercalary s., a scleral s. occurring between the insertion of the ciliary body and the root of the iris.

posterior s., a bulging near the posterior pole of the eyeball due to degenerative changes in severe myopia. SYN Scarpa s., sclerochoroiditis posterior.

Scarpa s., SYN posterior s.

scleral s., SYN equatorial s.

uveal s., seldom-used term for protrusion of the iris through a rupture of the sclera.

staph·y·lom·a·tous (staf-i-lō′mă-tŭs). Relating to or marked by staphyloma.

st

staph·y·lo·phar·yn·gor·rha·phy (staf'i-lō-far-in-gōr'ă-fē). Surgical repair of defects in the uvula or soft palate and the pharynx. SYN palatopharyngorrhaphy. [staphylo- + pharynx + G. *rhaphē*, suture]

staph·y·lo·plas·ty (staf'i-lō-plas-tē). SYN palatoplasty. [staphylo- + G. *plassō*, to form]

staph·y·lop·to·sis (staf'i-lop-tō'sis). SYN uvuloptosis. [staphylo- + G. *ptōsis*, a falling]

staph·y·lor·rha·phy (staf-i-lōr'ă-fē). SYN palatorrhaphy. [staphylo- + G. *rhaphē*, suture]

staph·y·lo·tox·in (staf'i-lō-tok'sin). The toxin elaborated by any species of *Staphylococcus*. SEE ALSO staphylohemolysin. [staphylo- + G. *toxikon*, poison]

sta·pling (stăp'ling). Use of a stapling device that unites two tissues, such as the two ends of bowel, by applying a row or circle of staples.

gastric s., partitioning of the stomach by rows of staples; used to treat severe obesity.

star (stăr). Any star-shaped structure. SEE ALSO aster, astrosphere, stella, stellula. [A.S. *steorra*]

daughter s., one of the figures forming the diaster. SYN polar s.

lens s.'s, (1) SYN *radii* of lens, under *radius;* **(2)** congenital cataracts with opacities along the suture lines of the lens; may be anterior or posterior, or both.

mother s., SYN monaster.

polar s., SYN daughter s.

venous s., a small, red nodule formed by a dilated vein in the skin; caused by increased venous pressure.

Verheyen s.'s, SYN *venulae* stellatae, under *venula.*

Winslow s.'s, SYN *stellulae* winslowii, under *stellula.*

starch. A high molecular weight polysaccharide built up of D-glucose residues in α-1,4 linkage, differing from cellulose in the presence of α- rather than β-glucoside linkages, that exists in most plant tissues; converted into dextrin when subjected to the action of dry heat, and into dextrin and D-glucose by amylases and glucoamylases in saliva and pancreatic juice; used as a dusting powder, an emollient, and an ingredient in medicinal tablets, and is an important raw material for the manufacture of alcohol, acetone, *n*-butanol, lactic acid, citric acid, glycerine, and gluconic acid by fermentation; chief storage carbohydrate in most higher plants. SYN amylum. [A.S. *stearc*, strong]

animal s., SYN glycogen.

liver s., SYN glycogen.

moss s., SYN lichenin.

rice s., rice product used as a supplement in many media formulations used for the culture of intestinal protozoa (e.g., *Entamoeba histolytica*).

soluble s., a high molecular weight, water-soluble dextrin produced by the partial acid hydrolysis of s.; useful in iodimetry, as it gives an easily visible purple-black end point in the presence of free iodine.

starch·eat·ing. SYN amylophagia.

stare (stăr). **1.** To look intently or fixedly. **2.** An intent gaze. [A.S. *starian*]

Stargardt, Karl, German ophthalmologist, 1875–1927. SEE S. *disease.*

Starling, Ernest H., English physiologist, 1866–1927. SEE S. *curve, hypothesis, law, reflex;* Frank-S. *curve.*

Starr, Albert, U.S. physician, *1926. SEE Starr-Edwards *valve.*

Starry. SEE Warthin-Starry silver *stain.*

start·er (start'er). SYN primer (1).

star·va·tion (star-vā'shŭn). Lengthy and continuous deprivation of food.

starve. 1. To suffer from lack of food. **2.** To deprive of food so as to cause suffering or death. **3.** Formerly, to die of cold. [A.S. *steorfan*, to die]

Stas, Jean-Servais, Belgian chemist, 1813–1891. SEE S.-Otto *method.*

stas·i·mor·phia (stas-i-mōr'fē-ă). Dysmorphogenesis due to arrested development. [G. *stasis*, a standing still, + *morphē*, shape]

sta·sis, pl. **sta·ses** (stā'sis, stas'is; -ēz). Stagnation of the blood or other fluids. [G. a standing still]

intestinal s., SYN enterostasis.

papillary s., obsolete term for papilledema.

pressure s., SYN traumatic *asphyxia.*

venous s., congestion and slowing of circulation in veins due to blockage by either obstruction or high pressure in the venous system, usually best seen in the feet and legs.

stat. Abbreviation for L. *statim*, at once, immediately.

△**stat-.** Prefix applied to electrical units in the CGS-electrostatic system to distinguish them from units in the CGS-electromagnetic system (prefix ab-) and those in the metric system or SI (no prefix).

△**-stat.** An agent intended to keep something from changing, flowing, or moving. [G. *statēs*, stationary]

stat·am·pere (stat-am'pēr). The electrostatic unit of current; the flow of 1 electrostatic unit of charge (1 statcoulomb) per second; equal to 3.335641×10^{-10} ampere. [G. *statos*, standing (stationary), + ampere]

stat·cou·lomb (stat-koo'lom). The electrostatic unit of charge, such that two objects, each carrying such a charge and separated (center to center) by 1 cm in a vacuum, will repel each other with a force of 1 dyne (or 10^{-5} newton); equal to 3.335641×10^{-10} coulomb. [G. *statos*, standing (stationary), + coulomb]

state (stāt). A condition, situation, or status. [L. *status*, condition, state]

absent s., SYN dreamy s.

activated s., SYN excited s.

anxiety tension s., a milder form of an anxiety disorder. SEE anxiety *disorders*, under *disorder.*

apallic s., (1) diffuse, bilateral cerebral cortical degeneration caused by head injury, anoxia, or encephalitis; **(2)** a state of persistent unresponsiveness, such as akinetic mutism, caused by brain damage. SEE ALSO vegetative. SYN apallic syndrome, apallic.

carrier s., the s. of being a carrier of pathogenic organisms; i.e., one who is infected but free of disease.

central excitatory s., the building up of excitatory influences produced by individual impulses finally causes firing of the next neuron.

convulsive s., SYN epilepsy.

decerebrate s., SYN decerebrate *rigidity.*

decorticate s., SYN decorticate *rigidity.*

dreamy s., the semiconscious s. associated with an epileptic attack. SYN absent s.

eunuchoid s., an imprecisely delineated condition of a male manifesting signs of inadequate androgen secretion during adolescent growth, regardless of the cause; usually referring to long legs, short trunk, and boyish beardless faces.

excited s., the condition of an atom or molecule after absorbing energy, which may be the result of exposure to light, electricity, elevated temperature, or a chemical reaction; such activation may be a necessary prelude to a chemical reaction or to the emission of light. SYN activated s.

ground s., the normal, inactivated s. of an atom from which, on activation, the singlet, triplet, and other excited s.'s are derived.

hypnoid s., a drowsy or sleeplike s. artificially induced by a hypnotist in individuals of higher than average levels of suggestibility. SEE hypnosis.

hypnotic s., SYN hypnosis.

hypometabolic s., a rare s. of reduced metabolism with symptoms resembling hypothyroidism but with some tests for thyroid gland function normal; also used to describe the reduced metabolic activity seen in true hypothyroidism.

imperfect s., in fungi, the s. or stage at which only asexual spores such as conidia are formed; most such species are classified as Deuteromycetes (Fungi Imperfecti).

lacunar s., the presence of lacunes in the brain. One of the major factors underlying cerebrovascular disease; high correlation with hypertension and atherosclerosis. Symptomatic forms include pure motor hemiplegia and pure hemisensory syndrome; multiple lacunar infarcts are the most common cause of pseudobulbar palsy.

local excitatory s., increased irritability of a nerve fiber or muscle fiber which is produced by a subthreshold electrical stimulus; summation of the stimuli may occur, resulting in a propagated impulse if two or more subliminal stimuli are applied in rapid succession.

multiple ego s.'s, various psychological organizational s.'s reflecting different personas or life experiences.

perfect s., in fungi, that portion of the life cycle in which spores are formed after nuclear fusion.

persistent vegetative s. (PVS), vegetative s. (q.v.) of prolonged duration (defined in different sources as duration of greater than 1 month, 1 year, or 2 years); usually permanent. SEE ALSO vegetative.

post–steady s., any period of time, particularly in an enzyme-catalyzed reaction, after the steady-state interval; e.g., when the rate of product formation is declining in an enzyme-catalyzed reaction.

pre–steady s., those conditions and the time interval prior to establishment of steady s.

refractory s., subnormal excitability immediately following a response to previous excitation; the s. is divided into absolute and relative phases.

singlet s., a transient, excited s. of a molecule (e.g., of chlorophyll, upon absorbing light) that can release energy as heat or light (fluorescence) and thus return to the initial (ground) s.; it may alternatively assume a slightly more stable, but still excited s. (triplet s.), with an electron still dislocated as before but with reversed spin.

steady s. (ss, s), (1) a s. obtained in moderate muscular exercise, when the removal of lactic acid by oxidation keeps pace with its production, the oxygen supply being adequate, and the muscles do not go into debt for oxygen; **(2)** any condition in which the formation or introduction of substances just keeps pace with their destruction or removal so that all volumes, concentrations, pressures, and flows remain constant; **(3)** in enzyme kinetics, conditions such that the rate of change in the concentration of any enzyme species (e.g., free enzyme or the enzyme-substrate binary complex) is zero or much less than the rate of formation of product. [often subscript s or ss]

triplet s., a second excited s. of a molecule (e.g., chlorophyll) produced by absorption of light to produce the singlet s., then loss of some energy (fluorescence) to arrive at the longer-lived triplet s. The molecule may remain sufficiently long in the triplet s. for a second activating light quantum to be effective in producing a "second triplet" s., obviously at still a higher level of excitation, hence reactivity. Alternatively, it may lose the triplet s. energy directly and return to the ground s.

twilight s., a condition of disordered consciousness during which actions may be performed without the conscious volition of the individual and with no memory of such actions. Cf. somnambulic *epilepsy.*

vegetative s., a clinical condition in which there is complete absence of awareness of the self and the environment, accompanied by sleep-wake cycles, but with either partial or complete preservation of hypothalamic and brainstem autonomic functions; may be transient or permanent. There are multiple causes, all involving the brain, including traumatic and nontraumatic injuries, metabolic and degenerative disorders, and congenital malformations.

stat·far·ad (stat-fa'rad). An electrostatic unit of capacitance, equal to 1.112650×10^{-12} farad.

stat·hen·ry (stat-hen'rē). An electrostatic unit of inductance, equal to 8.987552×10^{11} henry.

stath·mo·ki·ne·sis (stath'mō-ki-nē'sis). Condition of arrested mitosis after treatment with an agent, such as colchicine, which effectively alters the mitotic spindle to prevent typical rearrangement of the chromosomes preceding cell division. [G. *stathmos,* standing place, + *kinēsis,* motion]

sta·tim (stā'tim). At once; immediately. [L.]

stat·ins (stat'ins). SYN releasing *factors.*

sta·tion. The degree of descent of the presenting part of the fetus through the maternal pelvis, as measured in relation to the ischial spines of the maternal pelvis.

sta·tis·ti·cal sig·nif·i·cance. Statistical methods allow an estimate to be made of the probability of the observed degree of association between variables, and from this the statistical significance can be expressed, commonly in terms of the P value.

sta·tis·tics (stă-tis'tiks). **1.** A collection of numerical values, items of information, or other facts which are numerically grouped into definite classes and subject to analysis, particularly analysis of the probability that the resulting empirical findings are due to chance. **2.** The science and art of collecting, summarizing, and analyzing data that are subject to random variation.

descriptive s., numerical values such as mean, median, and mode which describe the chief features of a group of scores, without regard to a larger population.

inferential s., s. from which an inference is made about the nature of a population; the purpose is to generalize about the population, based upon data from the sample selected from the population.

vital s., systematically tabulated information concerning births, marriages, divorces, separations, and deaths, based on the numbers of official registrations of these vital events; the branch of s. concerned with such data.

stat·o·a·cou·stic (stat'ō-ă-koo'stik). Relating to equilibrium and hearing. SYN vestibulocochlear (2). [G. *statos,* standing, + *akoustikos,* acoustic]

stat·o·co·nia, sing. **stat·o·co·ni·um** (stat'ō-kō'nē-ă, -nē-ŭm) [TA]. SYN otoliths. [L. fr. G. *statos,* standing, *konis,* dust]

stat·o·ki·net·ic (stat'ō-ki-net'ik). Pertaining to statokinetics.

stat·o·ki·net·ics (stat'ō-ki-net'iks). The adjustment made by the body in motion to maintain stable equilibrium. [G. *statos,* standing, + *kinēsis,* movement]

stat·o·liths (stat'ŏ-liths). SYN otoliths. [G. *statos,* standing, + *lithos,* stone]

sta·tom·e·ter (stă-tom'ě-ter). SYN exophthalmometer. [G. *statos,* standing, + *metron,* measure]

stat·o·sphere (stat'ō-sfēr). SYN centrosphere.

stat·ure (statch'er). The height of a person. [L. *statura,* fr. *statuo,* pp. *statutus,* to cause to stand]

sta·tus (stā'tŭs, stat'ŭs). A state or condition. [L. a way of standing]

s. angino'sus, prolonged angina pectoris refractory to treatment.

s. arthrit'icus, obsolete term for gouty diathesis or predisposition.

s. asthmat'icus, a condition of severe, prolonged asthma.

s. cholera'icus, the cold stage of shock and depression in cholera, due to fluid and electrolyte loss and resulting hypovolemia; characterized by weak pulse, cold clammy skin, confusion, and depression.

s. chore'icus, a very severe form of chorea in which the persistence of the movements prevents sleep and the patient may die of exhaustion.

s. cribro'sus, a condition marked by dilations of the perivascular spaces in the brain.

s. crit'icus, a very severe and persistent form of crisis in tabes dorsalis.

s. dysmyelinisa'tus, SYN Hallervorden-Spatz *syndrome.*

s. dysra'phicus, a condition in which there is failure of fusion of midline structures, especially failure of neural tube closure. SYN arrhaphia.

s. epilep'ticus, repeated seizure or a seizure prolonged for at least 30 min; may be convulsive (tonic-clonic), nonconvulsive (absence or complex partial), partial (epilepsia partialis continuans), or subclinical (electrographic status epilepticus).

s. hemicra'nicus, a condition in which attacks of migraine succeed each other with such short intervals as to be almost continuous.

s. hypnot'icus, rarely used term for hypnosis.

s. lacuna'ris, a condition, occurring in cerebral arteriosclerosis, in which there are numerous small areas of degeneration in the brain.

s. lymphat'icus, SYN s. thymicolymphaticus.

st

s. marmora′tus, a congenital condition due to maldevelopment of the corpus striatum associated with choreoathetosis, in which the striate nuclei have a marblelike appearance caused by altered myelination.

nonreassuring fetal s., abnormal fetal heart rate or rhythm on electronic monitoring, suggesting fetal ischemia. SYN fetal distress.

performance s., a measure of a patient's well-being defined as the amount of normal activity the patient can maintain.

s. prae′sens, obsolete term for the part of the history of a case describing the condition of the patient at initial observation.

s. spongio′sus, multiple fluid-filled spaces of microscopic size in the cerebral white matter; seen in certain hypoxic, toxic, and metabolic diseases.

s. ster′nuens, a state of continual sneezing.

s. thymicolymphat′icus, obsolete term for a syndrome of supposed enlargement of the thymus and lymph nodes in infants and young children, formerly believed to be associated with unexplained sudden death; it was also erroneously believed that pressure of the thymus on the trachea might cause death during anesthesia. Prominence of these structures is now considered normal in young children, including those who have died suddenly without preceding illnesses that might lead to atrophy of lymphoid tissue. SEE ALSO sudden infant death *syndrome.* SYN s. lymphaticus, s. thymicus.

s. thy′micus, SYN s. thymicolymphaticus.

s. vertigino′sus, a condition in which attacks of vertigo occur in rapid succession. SYN chronic vertigo.

stat·volt (stat′vōlt). An electrostatic unit of potential or electromotive force, equal to 299.7925 V. [G. *statos,* standing (stationary), + volt]

Staub, Hans, Swiss internist, 1890–1967. SEE S.-Traugott *effect, phenomenon.*

stau·ri·on (staw′rē-on). A craniometric point at the intersection of the median and transverse palatine sutures. [G. dim. of *stauros,* cross]

STD Abbreviation for sexually transmitted *disease.*

steal (stēl). Diversion of blood via alternate routes or reversed flow, from one vascular bed to another, often causing symptoms in the organ from which blood flow has been diverted. [M.E. *stelen,* fr. A.S. *stelan*]

coronary s., a s. caused by anomalous origin of the coronary artery from the pulmonary artery.

iliac s., the decrease in flow in one common iliac artery when an occlusion of the other common iliac artery is released.

renal-splanchnic s., diversion of blood from the right renal artery via the inferior adrenal branch into splanchnic collaterals distal to a stenosis of the celiac axis.

subclavian s., obstruction of the subclavian artery proximal to the origin of the vertebral artery; blood flow through the vertebral artery is reversed and the subclavian artery thus "steals" cerebral blood, causing symptoms of vertebrobasilar insufficiency (subclavian s. syndrome); manifest during vigorous use of an upper extremity.

ste·ap·sin (stē-ap′sin). SYN *triacylglycerol* lipase.

⌂**stear-.** SEE stearo-.

ste·a·ral (stē′ă-răl). Octadecanal(dehyde); the aldehyde of stearic acid. SYN stearaldehyde.

ste·a·ral·de·hyde (stē-ă-ral′dĕ-hīd). SYN stearal.

ste·a·rate (stē′ă-rāt). A salt of stearic acid.

ste·ar·ic ac·id (stē′ă-rik). *n*-Octadecanoic acid; one of the most abundant fatty acids found in animal lipids; used in pharmaceutical preparations, ointments, soaps, and suppositories.

ste·a·rin (stē′ă-rin). Tristearoylglycerol; the "triglyceride" of stearic acid present in solid animal fats and in some vegetable fats; source of stearic acid; commercial s. also contains some palmitic acid. SYN tristearin.

Stearns, A. Warren, U.S. physician, 1885–1959.

⌂**stearo-, stear-.** Combining form denoting fat. SEE ALSO steato-. [G. *stear,* tallow]

ste·ar·rhea (stē-ă-rē′ă). SYN steatorrhea.

ste·a·ryl al·co·hol (stē′ă-ril). An ingredient of hydrophilic ointment and hydrophilic petrolatum; also used in the preparation of creams.

ste·a·ryl-CoA, ste·a·ryl-co·en·zyme A. The coenzyme A thioester of stearic acid; precursor to oleic acid and, in the brain, the C_{22} and C_{24} fatty acids present in sphingomyelins; in the brain, use of s.-CoA increases during myelination.

s.-CoA desaturase, a protein complex that is key in the synthesis of unsaturated fatty acids; it introduces a double bond at Δ^9; high dietary levels of unsaturated fatty acids decrease this enzyme's activity in the liver; a number of agents will induce this enzyme (e.g., insulin, hydrocortisone, and triiodothyronine).

ste·a·tite (stē′ă-tīt). Talc in the form of a mass.

ste·a·ti·tis (stē-ă-tī′tis). Inflammation of adipose tissue. [G. *stear* (*steat-*), tallow, + *-itis,* inflammation]

⌂**steato-.** Combining form denoting fat. SEE stearo-. [G. *stear* (*steat-*), tallow]

ste·a·to·cys·to·ma (stē′ă-tō-sis-tō′mă). A cyst with sebaceous gland cells in its wall.

s. mul′tiplex, widespread, multiple, thin-walled cysts of the skin that are lined by squamous epithelium, including lobules of sebaceous cells.

ste·a·to·gen·e·sis (stē′ă-tō-jen′ĕ-sis). Biosynthesis of lipids. The term is used specifically to designate lipid accumulation in the testes of nonmammalian vertebrates on completion of spermatogenesis in the breeding period. [steato- + G. *genesis,* production]

ste·a·tol·y·sis (stē-ă-tol′i-sis). The hydrolysis or emulsion of fat in the process of digestion. [steato- + G. *lysis,* dissolution]

ste·a·to·ly·tic (stē-ă-tō-lit′ik). Relating to steatolysis.

ste·a·to·ne·cro·sis (stē′ă-tō-ne-krō′sis). SYN fat *necrosis.* [steato- + G. *nekrōsis,* death]

ste·a·to·py·ga, ste·a·to·py·gia (stē′ă-tō-pī′gă, -pij′ē-ă). Excessive accumulation of fat on the buttocks. [steato- + G. *pygē,* buttocks]

ste·a·to·py·gous (stē-ă-top′ă-gŭs). Having excessively fat buttocks.

ste·a·tor·rhea (stē′ă-tō-rē′ă). Passage of fat in large amounts in the feces, due to failure to digest and absorb it; occurs in pancreatic disease and the malabsorption syndromes. SYN stearrhea. [steato- + G. *rhoia,* a flow]

biliary s., s. due to the absence of bile from the intestine; usually accompanied by jaundice.

intestinal s., s. due to malabsorption resulting from intestinal disease. SEE ALSO sprue, celiac *disease.*

pancreatic s., s. due to the absence of pancreatic juice from the intestine.

ste·a·to·sis (stē-ă-tō′sis). **1.** SYN adiposis. **2.** SYN fatty *degeneration.* [steato- + G. *-osis,* condition]

s. cardiaca, excessive fat on the pericardium and invading the cardiac muscle.

s. cor′dis, fatty degeneration of the heart.

hepatic s., SYN fatty *liver.*

ste·a·to·zo·on (stē′ă-tō-zō′on). Common name for *Demodex folliculorum.* [steato- + G. *zōon,* animal]

Steele, John C., Canadian neurologist, fl. 1951–1968. SEE S.-Richardson-Olszewski *disease, syndrome.*

Steell, Graham, British physician, 1851–1942. SEE Graham Steell *murmur.*

Steenbock, Harry, U.S. physiologist and chemist, 1886–1967. SEE S. *unit.*

ste·ge (stē′gē). The internal pillar of Corti organ. [G. *stegos,* roof, a house]

steg·no·sis (steg-nō′sis). **1.** A stoppage of any of the secretions or excretions. **2.** A constriction or stenosis. [G. stoppage]

steg·not·ic (steg-not′ik). **1.** Astringent or constipating. **2.** An astringent or constipating agent.

Stein, Stanislav A.F. von, Russian otologist, *1855. SEE S. *test.*

Stein, Irving F., U.S. gynecologist, *1887. SEE S.-Leventhal *syndrome*.

Steinberg, I. SEE S. thumb *sign*.

Steinbrinck, W., 20th century Germany physician. SEE Chédiak-S.-Higashi *anomaly*, *syndrome*.

Steinert, Hans, German physician, *1875. SEE S. *disease*.

Steinmann, Fritz, Swiss surgeon, 1872–1932. SEE S. *pin*.

stein·stras·se (stīn′stra-se). A complication of extracorporeal shock wave lithotripsy for urinary tract calculi in which stone fragments block the ureter to form a "stone street." [Ger. *Stein,* stone, + *Strasse,* street]

STEL Abbreviation for short-term exposure *limit*.

stel·la, pl. **stel·lae** (stel′ă, -ē). A star or star-shaped figure. [Mod. L.]

  s. len′tis hyaloi′dea, the posterior pole of the lens. SEE *radii* lentis, under *radius*.

  s. len′tis irid′ica, the anterior pole of the lens. SEE *radii* lentis, under *radius*.

stel·late (stel′āt). Star-shaped. [L. *stella,* a star]

stel·lec·to·my (stel-ek′tō-mē). Stellate ganglionectomy.

stel·lu·la, pl. **stel·lu·lae** (stel′ū-lă, -lē). A small star or star-shaped figure. [L. dim. of *stella,* star]

stel′lulae vasculo′sae, SYN stellulae winslowii.

stel′lulae verheyen′ii, SYN *venulae* stellatae, under *venula*.

stel′lulae winslo′wii, capillary whorls in the lamina choroidocapillaris from which arise the venae vorticosae. SYN stellulae vasculosae, Winslow stars.

Stellwag, Carl von C., Austrian ophthalmologist, 1823–1904. SEE S. *sign*.

stem. A supporting structure similar to the stalk of a plant.

  brain s., SEE brainstem.

  infundibular s., the neural component of the pituitary stalk that contains nerve tracts passing from the hypothalamus to the pars nervosa. SYN infundibular stalk.

sten. A statistical term which uses the standard deviation to convert data into standardized scores which define 10 steps along a normal distribution, with five steps on either side of the mean.

Stender, Wilhelm P., 19th century Leipzig manufacturer of scientific apparatus. SEE S. *dish*.

Stenger test. See under test.

ste·ni·on (sten′ē-on). The termination in either temporal fossa of the shortest transverse diameter of the skull; a craniometric point. [G. *stenos,* narrow, + dim. *-iōn*]

Steno. SEE Stensen.

steno-. Narrowness, constriction; opposite of eury-. [G. *stenos,* narrow]

sten·o·breg·mat·ic (sten′ō-breg-mat′ik). Denoting a skull narrow anteriorly, at the part where the bregma is. [steno- + G. *bregma*]

sten·o·car·dia (sten-ō-kar′dē-ă). SYN *angina* pectoris. [steno- + G. *kardia,* heart]

sten·o·ce·pha·lia (sten-ō-se-fā′lē-ă). SYN stenocephaly.

sten·o·ceph·a·lous, sten·o·ce·phal·ic (sten-ō-sef′ă-lŭs, -se-fal′ik). Pertaining to, or characterized by, stenocephaly.

sten·o·ceph·a·ly (sten-ō-sef′ă-lē). Marked narrowness of the head. SYN stenocephalia. [steno- + G. *kephalē,* head]

sten·o·cho·ria (sten-ō-kō′rē-ă). Abnormal contraction of any canal or orifice, especially of the lacrimal ducts. [G. *stenochōria,* narrowness, fr. steno- + *chōra,* place, room]

sten·o·com·pres·sor (sten′ō-kom-pres′er, ōr). An instrument for compressing the ducts of the parotid glands (Stensen duct) in order to keep back the saliva during dental operations.

sten·o·crot·a·phy, sten·o·cro·ta·phia (sten′ō-krot′ă-fē, -krō-tā′fē-ă). Narrowness of the skull in the temporal region; the condition of a stenobregmate skull. [steno- + G. *krotaphos,* temple]

Stenon. SEE Stensen. [*Stenonius,* Latin form of Stensen]

sten·o·pe·ic, sten·o·pa·ic (stĕn-ō-pē′ik, sten-ō-pā′ik). Provided with a narrow opening or slit, as in s. spectacles. [steno- + G. *opē,* opening]

ste·no·sal (ste-nō′săl). SYN stenotic.

ste·nosed (sten′ōzd). Narrowed; contracted; strictured.

ste·no·sis, pl. **ste·no·ses** (ste-nō′sis, -sēz). A stricture of any canal or orifice. [G. *stenōsis,* a narrowing]

  aortic s., pathologic narrowing of the aortic valve orifice.

  bronchial s., narrowing of the lumen of a bronchial tube. SYN bronchiostenosis.

  buttonhole s., extreme narrowing, usually of the mitral valve.

  calcific nodular aortic s., most common type of aortic s., occurring usually in elderly men, in which the cusps contain calcified fibrous nodules on both surfaces; the causes include rheumatic fever, atherosclerosis, age-related degeneration, and congenitally bicuspid aortic valve.

  congenital pyloric s., SYN hypertrophic pyloric s.

  coronary ostial s., narrowing of the mouths of the coronary arteries as a result of syphilitic aortitis or atherosclerosis.

  Dittrich s., SYN infundibular s.

  double aortic s., subaortic s. associated with s. of the valve itself, both lesions being congenital.

  fish-mouth mitral s., extreme mitral s.

  hypertrophic pyloric s., muscular hypertrophy of the pyloric sphincter, associated with projectile vomiting appearing in the first few weeks of life, more commonly seen in males. SYN congenital pyloric s.

  idiopathic hypertrophic subaortic s., left ventricular outflow obstruction due to hypertrophy, usually congenital, of the ventricular septum. SYN muscular subaortic s.

  idiopathic subglottic s., narrowing of the infraglottic lumen, of unknown cause; apparently occurring only in women.

  infundibular s., narrowing of the outflow tract of the right ventricle below the pulmonic valve; may be due to a localized fibrous diaphragm just below the valve or, more commonly, to a long narrow fibromuscular channel. SYN Dittrich s.

  laryngeal s., narrowing or stricture of any or all areas of the larynx; may be congenital or acquired.

  mitral s. (MS), pathologic narrowing of the orifice of the mitral valve.

  muscular subaortic s., SYN idiopathic hypertrophic subaortic s.

  pulmonary s., narrowing of the opening into the pulmonary artery from the right ventricle.

  pyloric s., narrowing of the gastric pylorus, especially by congenital muscular hypertrophy or scarring resulting from a peptic ulcer. SEE ALSO hypertrophic pyloric s.

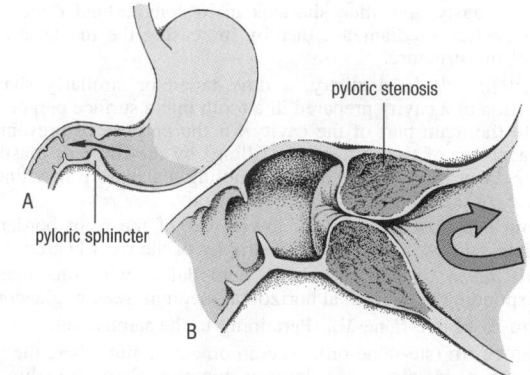

pyloric stenosis: (A) normal passage through pyloric sphincter, (B) stoppage of flow due to stenotic sphincter

  subaortic s., congenital narrowing of the outflow tract of the left ventricle by a ring of fibrous tissue or by hypertrophy of the muscular septum below the aortic valve. SYN subvalvar s.

  subvalvar s., SYN subaortic s.

  subvalvular aortic s., congenital narrowing below the aortic valves due to a membrane or to a muscular hypertrophy frequently confused with valvular aortic stenosis.

  supravalvar s., narrowing of the aorta above the aortic valve by a

st

constricting ring or shelf, or by coarctation or hypoplasia of the ascending aorta.

supravalvular s., s. distal to the aortic valve due usually to a congenital membrane. Patients usually have a kind of elfin facies and resemble each other more than they do members of their family.

tricuspid s., pathologic narrowing of the orifice of the tricuspid valve.

sten·o·ste·no·sis (sten′ō-stĕ-nō′sis). Stricture of the parotid duct (Steno or Stensen duct).

sten·o·sto·mia (sten-ō-stō′mē-ă). Narrowness of the oral cavity. [steno- + G. *stoma*, mouth]

sten·o·ther·mal (sten-ō-ther′măl). Thermostable through a narrow temperature range; able to withstand only slight changes in temperature. [steno- + G. *thermē*, heat]

sten·o·tho·rax (sten′ō-thōr′aks). A narrow contracted chest. [steno- + thorax]

ste·not·ic (ste-not′ik). Narrowed; affected with stenosis. SYN stenosal.

Sten·o·tro·pho·mo·nas (sten′ō-trō-fō-mōn′as). A genus of Gram-negative bacilli that typically reside in soil and water and are not a part of normal human flora.

S. maltophilia, an opportunistic ocular bacterial pathogen producing keratitis, keratopathy, and conjunctivitis; a Gram-negative non-sporebearing rod, a major emerging nosocomial pathogen, it is of especial importance in intensive care units in part because of its resistance to most penicillins and to cephalosporins and aminoglycosides. Formerly called *Xanthomonas maltophilia* and *Pseudomonas maltophilia.*

sten·ox·e·nous (sten-ok′sě-nŭs). Denoting a parasite with a narrow host range; e.g., *Eimeria* (among the Coccidia), hookworm, biting and sucking lice. [steno- + G. *xenos,* a stranger, foreigner]

Stensen (Steno, Stenon, Stenonius). Niels (Nicholaus), Danish anatomist, 1638–1686. SEE Stensen *duct,* Stensen *foramen,* Stensen *plexus,* Stensen *veins,* under *vein.*

Stent, Charles R., English dentist, †1901. SEE stent; S. *graft.*

stent. 1. A thread, rod, or catheter, lying within the lumen of tubular structures, used to provide support during or after their anastomosis, or to assure patency of an intact but contracted lumen. 2. The process of placing a stent. 3. Device used to maintain a bodily orifice or cavity during skin grafting. 4. To immobilize a skin graft after placement. [Charles R. *Stent*]

expandable s., s. placed within the lumen of a structure, often percutaneously, that then shortens in its longitudinal dimension and increases its diameter, thereby increasing the inside dimension of the structure.

step (stĕp). 1. In dentistry, a dove-tailed or similarly shaped projection of a cavity prepared in a tooth into a surface perpendicular to the main part of the cavity for the purpose of preventing displacement of the restoration (filling) by the force of mastication. 2. A change in direction resembling a stair-step in a line, a surface, or the construction of a solid body.

Krönig s.'s, extension of the lower part of the right border of absolute cardiac dullness in hypertrophy of the right heart.

Rónne nasal s., a nasal visual field defect with one margin corresponding to the retinal horizontal medium; seen in glaucoma.

ste·pha·ni·al (ste-fā′nē-ăl). Pertaining to the stephanion.

ste·pha·ni·on (ste-fā′nē-on). A craniometric point where the coronal suture intersects the inferior temporal line. [G. dim. of *stephanos,* crown]

Steph·a·no·fi·lar·ia (stef′ă-fī-lār′ē-ă). A genus of Filaroid nematodes in the family Stephanofilariidae, subcutaneous parasites of large mammals, especially cattle.

S. stilesi, a skin-infecting species of filaria parasitic in cattle and transmitted by the horn fly, *Haematobia irritans;* the only species known to occur in the U.S.; characterized by a row of spines behind the mouth of the adult worm, which is 6–8 mm in the female, 2–3 mm in the male. Both adults and larvae are found in granulomatous skin lesions in cattle, usually on the underside of the abdomen. [G. *stephanos,* crown, + filaria]

Steph·a·nu·rus den·ta·tus (stef-ă-noo′rŭs). The kidney worm or

lard worm of swine, a strongyle nematode parasite species that also occurs, though rarely, in the liver of cattle. Adult worms in swine live in the perirenal fat, the kidney pelvis, or as erratic forms in many other locations. Eggs are passed through the urine and infection is direct, by ingestion of infective larvae or by skin infection, or indirect, by ingestion of earthworms in which the larvae can survive. [G. *stephanos,* crown, + *oura,* tail]

step·page (step′aj). SYN steppage *gait.* [Fr.]

ste·ra·di·an (sr) (stě-rā′dē-ăn). The unit of solid angle; the solid angle that encloses an area on the surface of a sphere equivalent to the square of the radius of the sphere. [G. *stereos,* solid, + *radion,* radius]

ster·ane (ster′ān, stēr′ān). The hypothetical parent molecule for any steroid hormone; a saturated hydrocarbon compound that contains no oxygen. The name was originally conceived to achieve forms of systematic nomenclature, but is now supplanted by the fundamental variants: gonane, estrane, androstane, norandrostane (etiane), cholane, cholestane, ergostane, and stigmastane. SEE ALSO steroids.

sterco-. Feces. SEE ALSO copro-, scato-. [L. *stercus,* excrement]

ster·co·bi·lin (ster′kō-bī′lin, -bil′in). A brown degradation product of hemoglobin, present in the feces. SEE ALSO bilirubinoids.

l-ster·co·bi·lin·o·gen (ster′kō-bī-lin′ō-jen). Reduction product of *l*-urobilinogen, precursor of *l*-stercobilin in the final stages of bilirubin metabolism; excreted in feces, wherein it is oxidized to stercobilin. SEE ALSO bilirubinoids.

ster·co·lith (ster′kō-lith). SYN fecalith. [sterco- + G. *lithos,* stone]

ster·co·ra·ceous (ster-kō-rā′shŭs). Relating to or containing feces. SYN stercoral, stercorous.

ster·co·ral (ster′kō-răl). SYN stercoraceous.

ster·co·rin (ster′kō-rin). SYN coprosterol.

ster·co·ro·ma (ster-kō-rō′mă). SYN fecaloma. [sterco- + G. *-oma,* tumor]

ster·co·rous (ster′kō-rŭs). SYN stercoraceous.

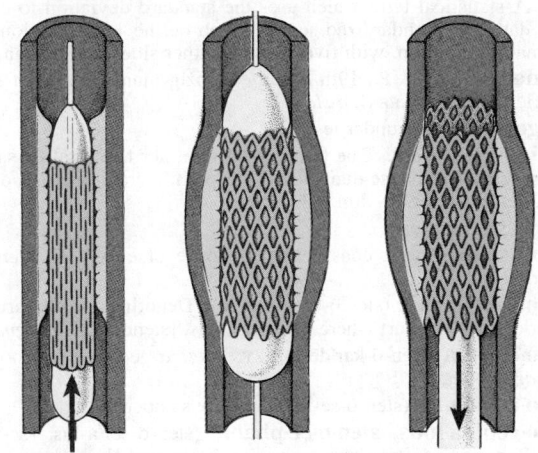

vascular stent

ster·cus (ster′kŭs). SYN feces. [L. feces, excrement]

stere (stēr, stār). A measure of capacity; equivalent to a cubic meter or a kiloliter; equal to 1.307951 cubic yards. [Fr. fr. G. *stereos,* solid]

stereo-. 1. A solid; a solid condition or state. 2. Spatial qualities, three-dimensionality. [G. *stereos,* solid]

ster·e·o·ag·no·sis (ster′ē-ō-ag-nō′sis). SYN tactile *agnosia.*

ster·e·o·an·es·the·sia (ster′ē-ō-an-es-thē′zē-ă). SYN tactile *agnosia.* [stereo- + G. *an-* priv. + *aisthēsis,* sensation]

ster·e·o·ar·throl·y·sis (ster′ē-ō-ar-throl′i-sis). Production of a new joint with mobility in cases of bony ankylosis. [stereo- + G. *arthron,* joint, + *lysis,* loosening]

ster·e·o·cam·pim·e·ter (ster′ē-ō-kam-pim′ě-ter). An apparatus for studying the central visual fields while the fellow eye holds fixation. [stereo- + L. *campus,* field, + G. *metron,* measure]

ster·e·o·chem·i·cal (ster′ē-ō-kem′i-kăl). Relating to stereochemistry.

ster·e·o·chem·is·try (ster-ē-ō-kem′is-trē). The branch of chemistry concerned with the spatial three-dimensional relations of atoms in molecules, i.e., the positions the atoms in a compound bear in relation to one another in space.

ster·e·o·cil·i·um, pl. **ster·e·o·cil·ia** (ster′ē-ō-sil′ē-ŭm, -ă). A nonmotile long microvillus. [stereo- + L. *cilium,* eyelid]

ster·e·o·cin·e·flu·o·rog·ra·phy (ster′ē-ō-sin′ē-flōr-og′ră-fē). Obsolete practice of recording on motion picture film the images obtained by stereoscopic fluoroscopy; three-dimensional views are obtained.

ster·e·o·col·po·gram (ster′ē-ō-kol′pō-gram). Picture taken with the stereocolposcope.

ster·e·o·col·po·scope (ster′ē-ō-kol′pō-skōp). Instrument that provides the observer with a magnified three-dimensional gross inspection of the vagina and cervix. [stereo- + G. *kolpos,* a hollow (vagina), *skopeō,* to view]

ster·e·o·e·lec·tro·en·ceph·a·log·ra·phy (ster-ē-ō-ē-lek′trō-en-sef-ă-log′ră-fē). Recording of electrical activity in three planes of the brain, i.e., with surface and depth electrodes.

ster·e·o·en·ceph·a·lom·e·try (ster′ē-ō-en-sef′ă-lom′ĕ-trē). The localization of brain structures by use of three-dimensional coordinates.

ster·e·og·no·sis (ster′ē-og′nō′sis). The appreciation of the form of an object by means of touch. [stereo- + G. *gnōsis,* knowledge]

ster·e·og·nos·tic (ster′ē-og-nos′tik). Relating to stereognosis.

ster·e·o·gram (ster′ē-ō-gram). A stereoscopic radiographic image of a pair.

ster·e·o·graph (ster′ē-ō-graf). A stereoscopic x-ray apparatus.

ster·e·og·ra·phy (ster-ē-og′ră-fē). SYN stereoradiography.

ster·e·o·i·so·mer (ster′ē-ō-ī′sō-mer). A molecule containing the same number and kind of atom groupings as another but in a different arrangement in space; the stereoisomers are not interconvertible unless bonds are broken and reformed, by virtue of which it exhibits different optic properties, e.g., as between D- and L-amino acids, 5α- and 5β-steroids. Cf. isomer. [stereo- + G. *isos,* equal, + *meros,* part]

ster·e·o·i·so·mer·ic (ster′ē-ō-ī-sō-mer′ik). Relating to stereoisomerism.

ster·e·o·i·som·er·ism (ster′ē-ō-ī-som′er-izm). Molecular asymmetry, isomerism involving different spatial arrangements of the same groups (e.g., androsterone and isoandrosterone, differing only in that one has a 3α-OH, the other a 3β-OH). SEE ALSO stereoisomer, Le Bel-van't Hoff *rule.* SYN stereochemical isomerism.

ster·e·ol·o·gy (ster′ē-ol′ō-jē). A study of the three-dimensional aspects of a cell or microscopic structure. [stereo- + G. *logos,* study]

ster·e·om·e·ter (ster-ē-om′ĕ-ter). An instrument used in stereometry. [stereo- + G. *metron,* measure]

ster·e·om·e·try (ster-ē-om′ĕ-trē). **1.** Measurement of a solid object or the cubic capacity of a vessel. **2.** Determination of the specific gravity of a liquid.

ster·e·o·or·thop·ter (ster′ē-ō-ōr-thop′ter). A type of stereoscope used in visual training. [stereo- + G. *orthos,* straight, + *optikos,* optical]

ster·e·op·a·thy (ster-ē-op′ă-thē). Persistent stereotyped thinking.

ster·e·o·pho·rom·e·ter (ster′ē-ō-fō-rom′ĕ-ter). A phorometer with a stereoscopic attachment.

ster·e·o·pho·to·mi·cro·graph (ster′ē-ō-fō′tō-mī′krō-graf). A stereoscopic photomicrograph that, when viewed with a stereoscope, appears three dimensional.

ster·e·op·sis (ster-ē-op′sis). SYN stereoscopic *vision.* [stereo- + G. *opsis,* vision]

ster·e·o·ra·di·og·ra·phy (ster′ē-ō-rā-dē-og′ră-fē). Preparation of a pair of radiographs with appropriate shift of the x-ray tube or film so that the images can be viewed stereoscopically to give a three-dimensional appearance. SYN stereography, stereoroentgenography.

ster·e·o·roent·gen·og·ra·phy (ster′ē-ō-rent′gen-og′ră-fē). SYN stereoradiography.

ster·e·o·scope (ster′ē-ō-skōp). An instrument producing two horizontally separated images of the same object, providing a single image with an appearance of depth. [stereo- + G. *skopeō,* to view]

ster·e·o·scop·ic (ster′ē-ō-skop′ik). Relating to a stereoscope, or giving the appearance of three dimensions.

ster·e·os·co·py (ster-ē-os′kŏ-pē). **1.** An optic technique by which two images of the same object are blended into one, giving a three-dimensional appearance to the single image. **2.** SEE radiostereoscopy.

ster·e·o·se·lec·tive (ster′ē-ō-sĕ-lek′tiv). As applied to a reaction, denoting a process in which of two or more possible stereoisomeric products only one predominates; a s. process is not necessarily stereospecific.

ster·e·o·spe·cif·ic (ster′ē-ō-spĕ-sif′ik). As applied to a reaction, denoting a process in which stereoisomerically different starting materials give rise to stereoisomerically different products; a s. process is thus necessarily stereoselective, but not all stereoselective processes are s.

ster·e·o·tac·tic, ster·e·o·tax·ic (ster′ē-ō-tak′tik, -tak′sik). Relating to stereotaxis or stereotaxy.

ster·e·o·tax·is (ster′ē-ō-tak′sis). **1.** Three-dimensional arrangement. **2.** Stereotropism, but applied more exactly where the organism as a whole, rather than a part only, reacts. **3.** SYN stereotaxy. [stereo- + G. *taxis,* orderly arrangement]

ster·e·o·taxy (ster′ē-ō-tak′sē). A precise method of identifying nonvisualized anatomic structures by use of three-dimensional coordinates; more frequently used for brain and spinal surgery. SYN stereotactic surgery, stereotaxic surgery, stereotaxis (3).

ster·e·o·tro·pic (ster′ē-ō-trop′ik). Relating to or exhibiting stereotropism.

ster·e·ot·ro·pism (ster′ē-ot′rō-pizm). Growth or movement of a plant or animal toward (**positive s.**) or away from (**negative s.**) a solid body, usually applied where a part of the organism rather than the whole reacts. [stereo- + G. *tropos,* a turning]

ster·e·o·typy (ster′ē-ō-tī′-pē). **1.** Maintenance of one attitude for a long period. **2.** Constant repetition of certain meaningless gestures or movements, as in certain forms of schizophrenia. [stereo- + G. *typos,* impression, type]

oral s., SYN verbigeration.

ste·ric (ster′ik, stēr-). Pertaining to stereochemistry.

s. hindrance, interference with or inhibition of a seemingly feasible reaction (usually synthetic) because the size of one or another reactant prevents approach to the required interatomic distance.

ster·id (ster′id, stēr-). SYN steroid (2).

ste·rig·ma, pl. **ste·rig·ma·ta** (ste-rig′mă, -mă-tă). A slender, pointed structure arising from a basidium upon which a basidiospore will develop. [G. *stērigma,* a support]

ster·ile (ster′il). Relating to or characterized by sterility. [L. *sterilis,* barren]

ste·ril·i·ty (stĕ-ril′i-tē). **1.** In general, the incapability of fertilization or reproduction. SEE female s., male s. **2.** Condition of being aseptic, or free from all living microorganisms. [L. *sterilitas*]

aspermatogenic s., s. due to a failure to produce living spermatozoa.

dysspermatogenic s., male s. due to some abnormality in production of spermatozoa.

female s., the inability of the female to conceive, due to inadequacy in structure or function of the genital organs. SYN infecundity.

male s., the inability of the male to fertilize the ovum; it may or may not be associated with impotence.

normospermatogenic s., male s. due to some cause other than failure to produce live, normal spermatozoa, e.g., blockage of the seminiferous passages.

ster·i·li·za·tion (ster′ĭ-li-zā′shŭn). **1.** The act or process by which an individual is rendered incapable of fertilization or reproduction, as by vasectomy, partial salpingectomy, or castration. **2.** The

st

destruction of all microorganisms in or about an object, as by steam (flowing or pressurized), chemical agents (alcohol, phenol, heavy metals, ethylene oxide gas), high-velocity electron bombardment, heat, or ultraviolet light radiation.

discontinuous s., SYN fractional s.

fractional s., exposure to a temperature of 100°C (flowing steam) for a definite period, usually an hour, on each of several days; at each heating the developed bacteria are destroyed; spores, which are unaffected, germinate during the intervening periods and are subsequently destroyed. SYN discontinuous s., intermittent s., tyndallization.

intermittent s., SYN fractional s.

ster·il·ize (ster'ĭ-līz). To produce sterility.

ster·il·iz·er (ster'i-lī-zer). An apparatus for rendering objects sterile.

glass bead s., a s. for endodontic equipment; the heat is transmitted to the instruments, absorbent points, or cotton pellets by means of glass beads.

hot salt s., a s. for endodontic equipment in which table salt is heated in a container at 218–246°C; the dry heat is transmitted to root canal instruments, absorbent points, or cotton pellets for their rapid (5–10 seconds) sterilization.

Stern, Heinrich, U.S. physician, 1868–1918. SEE S. *posture.*

⌂**stern-.** SEE sterno-.

ster·na (ster'nă). Plural of sternum.

ster·nad (ster'nad). In a direction toward the sternum.

ster·nal (ster'năl). Relating to the sternum.

ster·nal·gia (ster-nal'jē-ă). Pain in the sternum or the sternal region. SYN sternodynia. [stern- + G. *algos,* pain]

ster·na·lis (ster-nā'lis). SEE sternalis *(muscle).*

Sternberg, George M., U.S. bacteriologist, 1838–1915. SEE S. *cell;* S.-Reed *cell;* Reed-S. *cell.*

ster·ne·bra, pl. **ster·ne·brae** (ster'nē-bră, -brē). One of the four segments of the primordial sternum of the embryo by the fusion of which the body of the adult sternum is formed. [Mod. L. fr. stern(um) + (vert)ebra]

ster·nen. Relating to the sternum independent of any other structures. [stern- + G. *en,* in]

⌂**sterno-, stern-.** The sternum, sternal. [G. *sternon,* chest]

ster·no·chon·dro·sca·pu·la·ris (ster'nō-kon'drō-skap-ū-lā'ris). SEE sternochondroscapular *muscle.* [Mod. L.]

ster·no·cla·vic·u·lar (ster'nō-kla-vik'ū-lăr). Relating to the sternum and the clavicle.

ster·no·cla·vi·cu·la·ris (ster'nō-kla-vik'ū-lā'ris). SEE sternoclavicular *muscle.*

ster·no·clei·dal (ster'nō-klī'dăl). Relating to the sternum and the clavicle. [sterno- + G. *kleis,* key (clavicle)]

ster·no·clei·do·mas·toid (ster'nō-klī'dō-mas'toyd). Relating to sternum, clavicle, and mastoid process.

ster·no·clei·do·mas·toi·de·us (ster'nō-klī'dō-mas-tō-id'-ē-ŭs). SEE sternocleidomastoid *(muscle).* [Mod. L.]

ster·no·cos·tal (ster'nō-kos'tăl). Relating to the sternum and the ribs. [L. *costa,* rib]

ster·no·dyn·ia (ster-nō-din'ē-ă). SYN sternalgia. [sterno- + G. *odynē,* pain]

ster·no·fas·ci·a·lis (ster'nō-fash-ē-ā'lis). SEE *musculus* sternofascialis.

ster·no·glos·sal (ster-nō-glos'ăl). Denoting muscular fibers that occasionally pass from the sternohyoid muscle to join the hyoglossal muscle.

ster·no·hy·oi·de·us (ster'nō-hī-oyd'ē-ŭs). SEE sternohyoid *(muscle).* [Mod. L.]

ster·noid (ster'noyd). Resembling the sternum. [sterno- + G. *eidos,* resemblance]

ster·no·mas·toid (ster'nō-mas'toyd). Relating to the sternum and the mastoid process of the temporal bone; applied to the sternocleidomastoid muscle.

ster·no·pa·gia (ster-nō-pā'jē-ă). Condition shown by conjoined twins united at the sterna or more extensively at the ventral walls

of the chest. SEE conjoined *twins,* under twin. [sterno- + G. *pagos,* something fixed]

ster·no·per·i·car·di·al (ster'nō-per'i-kar'dē-ăl). Relating to the sternum and the pericardium.

ster·nos·chi·sis (ster-nos'ki-sis). Congenital cleft of the sternum. [sterno- + G. *schisis,* a cleaving]

ster·no·thy·roi·de·us (ster'nō-thī-royd'ē-ŭs). SEE sternothyroid *(muscle).* [Mod. L.]

ster·not·o·my (ster-not'ō-mē). Incision into or through the sternum. [sterno- + G. *tomē,* incision]

median s., incision through the midline of the sternum usually used to gain access to the heart, mediastinal structures, and great vessels.

ster·no·tra·che·al (ster'nō-trā'kē-ăl). Relating to the sternum and the trachea.

ster·no·try·pe·sis (ster'nō-trī-pē'sis). Trephining of the sternum. [sterno- + G. *trypēsis,* a boring]

ster·no·ver·te·bral (ster'nō-ver'tĕ-brăl). Relating to the sternum and the vertebrae; denoting the true ribs, or the seven upper ribs on either side, which articulate with the vertebrae and with the sternum. SYN vertebrosternal.

ⓘ**ster·num,** gen. **ster·ni,** pl. **ster·na** (ster'nŭm, -nī, -nă) [TA]. A long flat bone, articulating with the cartilages of the first seven ribs and with the clavicle, forming the middle part of the anterior wall of the thorax; it consists of three portions: the corpus or body, the manubrium, and the xiphoid process. SYN breast bone. [Mod. L. fr. G. *sternon,* the chest]

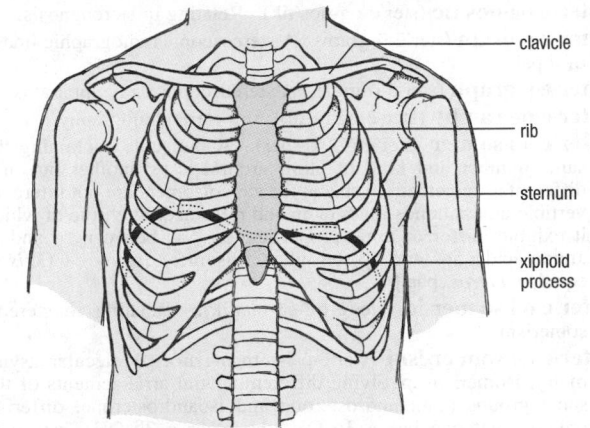

clavicle

rib

sternum

xiphoid process

sternum and surrounding structures

ster·nu·ta·tion (ster'noo-tā'shŭn). The act of sneezing. [L. *sternutatio,* fr. *sternuo (sternuto),* pp. *sternutatus,* to sneeze]

ster·nu·ta·tor (ster'noo-tā-ter, -tōr). A substance, such as a gas, that induces sneezing. SYN sneezing gas.

ster·nu·ta·to·ry (ster-noo'tă-tōr-ē). 1. Causing sneezing. 2. An agent that provokes sneezing. SYN ptarmic.

ste·roid (stēr'oyd, ster'oyd). 1. Pertaining to the steroids. SYN steroidal. Cf. steroids. 2. One of the steroids. SYN sterid. 3. Generic designation for compounds closely related in structure to the steroids, such as sterols, bile acids, cardiac glycosides, androgens, estrogens, corticosteroids, and precursors of the D vitamins.

anabolic s., a s. compound with the capacity to increase muscle mass; compounds with androgenic properties which increase muscle mass and are used in the treatment of emaciation. Sometimes used by athletes in an effort to increase muscle size, strength, and endurance. Examples include methyltestosterone, nandrolone, methandrostenolone, and stanozolol.

s. hydroxylases, SYN s. monooxygenases.

s. 21-monooxygenase, an enzyme catalyzing the reaction of a steroid, O_2, and some reduced compound to produce water, the oxidized compound, and a 21-hydroxysteroid; a deficiency of this

st

enzyme results in decreased cortisol synthesis, of which there are three types (salt-wasting, simple virilizing, and nonclassical).

s. monooxygenases, enzymes catalyzing addition of hydroxyl groups to the s. rings utilizing O_2; differentiated into, for example, s. 11β-monooxygenase, s. 17α-monooxygenase, and s. 21-monooxygenase, in accordance with the position of the catalytically introduced hydroxyl group. SYN s. hydroxylases.

s. 5α-reductase, an enzyme that uses NADPH to reduce certain steroids (e.g., the conversion of testosterone to dihydrotestosterone); a deficiency of this enzyme is associated with a form of male pseudohermaphroditism in which genetic males have male genitals as well as female external genitalia.

s. sulfatase deficiency, SYN X-linked *ichthyosis.*

ste·roi·dal (stēr′oy-dăl, ster′). SYN steroid (1).

ste·roi·do·gen·e·sis (stēr′oy-dō-jen′ĕ-sis, ster′). The formation of steroids; commonly referring to the biological synthesis of steroid hormones, but not to the production of such compounds in a chemical laboratory. [steroid + G. *genesis,* production]

ste·roids (stēr′oydz, ster-). A large family of chemical substances, comprising many hormones, body constituents, and drugs, each containing the tetracyclic cyclopenta[*a*]phenanthrene skeleton. Stereoisomerism among s. is not only common but of critical biologic significance. The nomenclature conventions are that the nucleus is presented as if projected onto the plane of the paper, with groups then lying above that plane being denoted by thickened bonds and called β and those then lying below that plane being denoted by broken bonds and called α; the letter ξ indicates unknown or unspecified orientation. The principal classes of steroids, with the names for the unsubstituted, saturated hydrocarbon forms that are clearly related to physiologic functions or sources are: 1) gonanes (in which the methyl groups C-18 and C-19, have been replaced by H), 2) estranes (in which the C-19 methyl groups have been replaced by H), 3) androstanes (equivalent to Formula II), 4) norandrostanes (in which one of the methyl groups, typically C-18, has been replaced by H), 5) cholanes (with $-CH(CH_3)(CH_2)_2CH_3$ bonded to C-17), 6) cholestanes (with $-CH(CH_3)(CH_2)_3CH(CH_3)_2$ at C-17, 7) ergostanes (with $-CH(CH_3)(CH_2)_2CH(CH_3)CH(CH_3)_2$ at C-17), and 8) stigmastanes (with $-CH(CH_3)(CH_2)_2CH(CH_2CHCH_3)CH(CH_3)_2$ at C-17). In addition, each of the classes can be in a 5α or 5β series.

The steroid derivatives known as cardanolides are androstanes with a 5-membered lactone linked to C-17. The squill-toad poisons known as the bufanolides are androstanes with a 6-membered lactone linked to C-17. Spirostans and furostans (the basic structures of many "genins," including the sapogenins) are androstanes having certain cyclic ether moieties.

The natural and synthetic derivatives are named by adding conventional chemical prefixes and suffixes for substituents; e.g., -ol for a hydroxyl group, -on(e) for a keto group, -al for an aldehyde group. "Nor" indicates loss of a $-CH_2-$ group; "homo," the addition of a $-CH_2-$ group; each is preceded by the letter indicating which ring is contracted or expanded, respectively, or, in the case where the $-CH_2-$ is lost from a methyl group, the number of the carbon atom lost. "Seco" indicates fission of a ring with the addition of hydrogen atoms at the positions indicated by numerals preceding the term. Unsaturation is denoted, as usual, by substituting appropriate terms, e.g., -en(e), -yn(e), -adien(e), for the -ane or -an parts of the hydrocarbon or parent class names, with numerals indicating locations of the unsaturated bonds. The locations of double bonds are specified by the lower of the two (consecutive) numbers of the carbon atoms involved. When a double bond is formed between two nonconsecutive carbon atoms, the second is indicated in parentheses after the first; e.g., estriol and the estradiols possess three double bonds, between C-1 and C-2, between C-3 and C-4, and between C-5 and C-10, respectively.

Steroid alkaloids may be named from the steroid parent, as above, or from trivial family names usually ending in -anine if the steroid is saturated or in -enine, -adienine, etc., if it is not saturated (e.g., conanine, tomatanine).

ste·rol (stēr′ol). A steroid with one OH (alcohol) group; the systematic names contain either the prefix hydroxy- or the suffix -ol, e.g., cholesterol, ergosterol.

ster·tor (ster′tōr). A noisy inspiration occurring in coma or deep sleep, sometimes due to obstruction of the larynx or upper airways. [L. *sterto,* to snore]

hen-cluck s., a breath sound like the clucking of a hen, sometimes heard in cases of retropharyngeal abscess.

ster·to·rous (ster′tōr-ŭs). Relating to or characterized by stertor or snoring.

△**steth-.** SEE stetho-.

ste·thal·gia (ste-thal′jē-ă). Pain in the chest. [steth- + G. *algos,* pain]

steth·ar·te·ri·tis (steth′ar-ter-ī′tis). Inflammation of the aorta or other arteries in the chest. [steth- + L. *arteria,* artery, + G. -*itis,* inflammation]

△**stetho-, steth-.** Combining forms denoting the chest. [G. *stēthos*]

steth·o·graph (steth′ō-graf). An apparatus for recording the respiratory movements of the chest. [stetho- + G. *graphō,* to write]

steth·o·my·i·tis (steth′ō-mī-ī′tis). Inflammation of the muscles of the chest wall. SYN stethomyositis. [stetho- + G. *mys,* muscle, + -*itis,* inflammation]

steth·o·my·o·si·tis (steth′ō-mī-ō-sī′tis). SYN stethomyitis.

steth·o·pa·ral·y·sis (steth′ō-pă-ral′i-sis). Paralysis of the respiratory muscles.

steth·o·scope (steth′ō-skōp). An instrument originally devised by Laennec for aid in hearing the respiratory and cardiac sounds in the chest, but now modified in various ways and used in auscultation of any of vascular or other sounds anywhere in the body. [stetho- + G. *skopeō,* to view]

binaural s., a s. in which the two ear pieces connect with a single bell.

Bowles type s., a s. in which the chest piece is a shallow metal cup about 4.5 cm in diameter, the mouth of which is covered by a hard rubber or celluloid diaphragm.

differential s., a s. having two chest pieces so that two sounds in different parts of the chest may be heard simultaneously and compared.

steth·o·scop·ic (steth-ō-skop′ik). **1.** Relating to or effected by means of a stethoscope. **2.** Relating to an examination of the chest.

ste·thos·co·py (stĕ-thos′kŏ-pē). **1.** Examination of the chest by means of auscultation, either mediate or immediate, and percussion. **2.** Mediate auscultation with the stethoscope.

Stevens, Albert M., U.S. pediatrician, 1884–1945. SEE S.-Johnson *syndrome.*

Stewart, Fred Waldorf, U.S. physician, 1894–1991. SEE S.-Treves *syndrome.*

Stewart, George N., Canadian-U.S. scientist, 1860–1930. SEE S. *test;* Stewart-Hamilton *method.*

Stewart, R.M., 20th century English neurologist. SEE S.-Morel *syndrome.*

Stewart, Thomas Grainger, 20th century English neurologist, 1877–1957. SEE S.-Holmes *sign.*

STH Abbreviation for somatotropic *hormone.*

sthe·nia (sthē′nē-ă). A condition of activity and apparent force, as in an acute sthenic fever. [G. *sthenos,* strength, + -*ia,* condition]

sthen·ic (sthen′ik). Active; marked by sthenia; said of a fever with strong bounding pulse, high temperature, and active delirium.

△**stheno-.** Strength, force, power. [G. *sthenos*]

sthe·nom·e·ter (sthĕ-nom′ĕ-ter). An instrument for measuring muscular strength. [stheno- + G. *metron,* measure]

sthe·nom·e·try (sthĕ-nom′ĕ-trē). The measurement of muscular strength. [stheno- + G. *metrin,* to measure]

stib·a·mine glu·co·side (stib′ă-mēn). A nitrogen glycoside of sodium *p*-aminobenzenestibonate; a pentavalent antimony compound; has been used in leishmaniasis (kala azar) and certain other tropical diseases, but is no longer marketed.

stib·e·nyl (stib′ĕ-nil). The first pentavalent antimonial used in the treatment of leishmaniasis (kala azar).

stib·i·al·ism (stib′ē-ă-lizm). Chronic antimonial poisoning. [L. *stibium,* antimony]

stib·i·a·ted (stib′ē-ā-ted). Impregnated with or containing antimony.

stib·i·a·tion (stib-ē-ā′shŭn). Impregnation with antimony.

stib·i·um (stib′ē-ŭm). SYN antimony. [L. fr. G. *stibi*]

stib·o·cap·tate (stib-ō-kap′tāt). SYN *antimony* dimercaptosuccinate.

stib·o·glu·co·nate s. s. (stib-ō-gloo′kŏ-nāt). **1.** Pentavalent sodium stibogluconate, used in the treatment of all types of leishmaniasis; toxic effects are frequent. SYN antimony sodium gluconate. **2.** Trivalent antimony sodium gluconate, used in the treatment of schistosomiasis; toxic effects are frequent. SYN sodium antimonylgluconate.

sti·bo·ni·um (sti-bō′nē-ŭm). The hypothetical radical, SbH_4^+, analogous to ammonium.

stib·o·phen (stib′ō-fen). An organic trivalent antimony compound, used in the treatment of schistosomiasis, filariasis, leishmaniasis, and lymphogranuloma inguinale.

stich·o·chrome (stik′ō-krōm). Denoting a nerve cell in which the chromophil substance, or stainable material, is arranged in roughly parallel rows or lines. [G. *stichos,* a row, + *chrōma,* color]

Stickler, Gunnar B., U.S. physician, *1925. SEE S. *syndrome.*

Stieda, Ludwig, German anatomist, 1837–1918. SEE S. *process.*

Stieda, Alfred, German surgeon, 1869–1945. SEE Pellegrini-S. *disease.*

Stierlin, Eduard, German surgeon, 1878–1919. SEE S. *sign.*

stig·ma, pl. **stig·mas, stig·ma·ta** (stig′mă, -mă-tă). **1.** Visible evidence of a disease. **2.** SYN follicular s. **3.** Any spot or blemish on the skin. **4.** A bleeding spot on the skin, which is considered a manifestation of conversion hysteria. **5.** The orange-pigmented eyespot of certain chlorophyll-bearing protozoa, such as *Euglena viridis,* which serves as a light filter by absorbing certain wavelengths. **6.** A mark of shame or discredit. [G. a mark. fr. *stizō,* to prick]

follicular s., the point where the graafian follicle is about to rupture on the surface of the ovary. SYN macula pellucida, stigma (2).

malpighian stigmas, the points of entrance of the smaller veins into the larger veins of the spleen.

s. ventric′uli, one of a number of miliary ecchymoses of the gastric mucosa.

stig·mas·tane (stig-mas′tān). The parent substance of sitosterol. SYN sitostane.

stig·ma·ta (stig′mă-tă). Alternative plural of stigma.

stig·mat·ic (stig-mat′ik). Relating to or marked by a stigma.

stig·ma·tism (stig′mă-tizm). The condition of having a stigma. SYN stigmatization (1).

stig·ma·ti·za·tion (stig′mă-ti-zā′shŭn). **1.** SYN stigmatism. **2.** Production of stigmas, especially of a hysterical nature. **3.** Debasement of a person by attributing a negatively toned characteristic or other stigma to him or her.

stil·bam·i·dine (stil-bam′i-dēn). A compound used in the treatment of leishmaniasis (kala azar), in infections due to *Blastomyces dermatitidis,* and in actinomycosis; also used in multiple myeloma for the relief of bone pain.

stil·baz·i·um io·dide (stil-baz′ē-ŭm). An anthelmintic.

stil·bene (stil′bēn). **1.** $C_6H_5CH=CHC_6H_5$; α,β-diphenylethylene; an unsaturated hydrocarbon, the nucleus of stilbestrol and other synthetic estrogenic compounds. **2.** A class of compounds based on s. (1).

stil·bes·trol (stil-bes′trol). SYN diethylstilbestrol.

Stiles, Walter S., English physicist, 1901–1985. SEE S.-Crawford *effect.*

sti·let, sti·lette (stī′let, stī-let′). SEE stylet.

Still, Sir George F., English physician, 1868–1941. SEE S. *disease, murmur;* S.-Chauffard *syndrome.*

still·birth (stil′berth). The birth of an infant who has died prior to delivery.

still·born (stil′bōrn). Born dead; denoting an infant dead at birth.

Stilling, Benedict, German anatomist, 1810–1879. SEE S. *canal, column, nucleus, raphe,* gelatinous *substance.*

sti·lus (stī′lŭs). SEE stylus.

stim·u·lant (stim′ū-lănt). **1.** Stimulating; exciting to action. **2.** An agent that arouses organic activity, strengthens the action of the heart, increases vitality, and promotes a sense of well-being; classified according to the parts upon which they chiefly act: cardiac, respiratory, gastric, hepatic, cerebral, spinal, vascular, genital. SYN excitor, stimulator. SEE ALSO stimulus. SYN excitant. [L. *stimulans,* pres. p. of *stimulo,* pp. -*atus,* to goad, incite, fr. *stimulus,* a goad]

diffusible s., a s. that produces a rapid but temporary effect.

general s., a s. that affects the entire body.

local s., a s. whose action is confined to the part to which it is applied.

stim·u·la·tion (stim-ū-lā′shŭn). **1.** Arousal of the body or any of its parts or organs to increased functional activity. **2.** The condition of being stimulated. **3.** In neurophysiology, the application of a stimulus to a responsive structure, such as a nerve or muscle, regardless of whether the strength of the stimulus is sufficient to produce excitation. [see stimulant]

dorsal column s., electrical s., either percutaneously or by direct application of electrodes to the dorsal columns of the spinal cord.

fetal scalp s., intrapartum test for fetal well-being; acceleration of the fetal heart rate in response to digital or forceps stimulation of scalp is associated with a normal scalp blood pH.

Ganzfeld s., illumination of the entire retina in the electroretinogram. [Ger. *Ganzfeld,* whole field]

percutaneous s., electrical s. of the peripheral nerves or spinal cord by the application of electrodes to the skin.

photic s., the use of a flickering light at various frequencies to influence the pattern of the occipital electroencephalogram and also to activate latent abnormalities.

vagal nerve s., an adjunctive treatment for patients with intractable epilepsy, particularly complex partial or secondarily generalized seizures; stimulation is delivered to the left vagus nerve in the neck, usually in 30-s bursts every 5½ min by a stimulator implanted in the anterior chest wall.

stim·u·la·tor (stim′ū-lā-ter, -tōr). SYN stimulant (2).

long-acting thyroid s. (LATS), a substance, found in the blood of some hyperthyroid patients, that exerts a prolonged stimulatory effect on the thyroid gland; associated in plasma with the IgG (7 S γ-globulin) fraction and seems to be an antibody or, perhaps, an immune complex.

stim·u·lus, pl. **stim·u·li** (stim′ū-lŭs, -lī). **1.** A stimulant. **2.** That which can elicit or evoke action (response) in a muscle, nerve, gland or other excitable tissue, or cause an augmenting action upon any function or metabolic process. [L. a goad]

adequate s., a s. to which a particular receptor responds effectively and that gives rise to a characteristic sensation; e.g., light and sound waves that stimulate, respectively, visual and auditory receptors.

aversive s., a noxious stimulus such as an electric shock used in aversive *training* or conditioning. SEE ALSO aversive *training.*

conditioned s., (1) a s. applied to one of the sense organs (e.g., receptors of vision, hearing, touch) which are an essential and integral part of the neural mechanism underlying a conditioned reflex; SEE classical *conditioning,* higher order *conditioning;* **(2)** a neutral s., when paired with the unconditioned s. in simultaneous presentation to an organism, capable of eliciting a given response.

discriminant s., a s. which can be differentiated from all other stimuli in the environment because it has been, and continues to serve as, an indicator of a potential reinforcer.

heterologous s., a s. that acts upon any part of the sensory apparatus or nerve tract.

heterotopic s., any electrical activation from an abnormal locus.

homologous s., a s. that acts only on the nerve terminations in a special sense organ.

inadequate s., SYN subthreshold s.

liminal s., SYN threshold s.

maximal s., a s. strong enough to evoke a maximal response.

square wave stimuli, electrical stimulation in which the intensity of the current is brought suddenly to a given level and maintained at that level until it suddenly is cut off; this type of s. is particularly useful in obtaining a strength-duration curve.

subliminal s., SYN subthreshold s.

subthreshold s., a s. too weak to evoke a response. SYN inadequate s., subliminal s.

supramaximal s., a s. having strength significantly above that required to activate all of the nerve or muscle fibers in contact with the electrode; used when response of all the fibers is desired.

threshold s., a s. of threshold strength, i.e., one just strong enough to excite. SEE ALSO adequate s. SYN liminal s.

train-of-four s., a method for measuring magnitude and type of neuromuscular blockade, based upon the ratio of the amplitude of the fourth evoked mechanical response to the first one, when four supramaximal 2-Hz electrical currents are applied for 2 s to a peripheral motor nerve.

unconditioned s., a s. that elicits an unconditioned response; e.g., food is an unconditioned s. for salivation, which in turn is an unconditioned response in a hungry animal. SEE classical *conditioning*.

stim·u·lus word. The word used in association tests to evoke a response.

sting. 1. Sharp momentary pain, most commonly produced by the puncture of the skin by many species of arthropods, including hexapods, myriapods, and arachnids; can also be produced by jellyfish, sea urchins, sponges, mollusks, and several species of venomous fish, such as the stingray, toadfish, rabbitfish, and catfish. **2.** The venom apparatus of a stinging animal, consisting of a chitinous spicule or bony spine and a venom gland or sac. **3.** To introduce (or the process of introducing) a venom by stinging. [O.E. *stingan*]

sting·ers (sting′erz). SYN burners.

stink weed. SYN *Datura stramonium.*

stip·pling (stip′ling). **1.** A speckling of a blood cell or other structure with fine dots when exposed to the action of a basic stain, due to the presence of free basophil granules in the cell protoplasm. SYN punctate basophilia. **2.** An orange peel appearance of the attached gingiva. **3.** A roughening of the surfaces of a denture base to stimulate natural gingival s.

geographic s. of nails, regularly arranged longitudinal s. found commonly in psoriasis and occasionally in alopecia areata. SEE ALSO nail *pits*, under *pit*.

Ziemann s., SYN Ziemann *dots*, under *dot*.

STIR Acronym for short TI inversion *recovery*.

Stirling, William, British histologist and physiologist, 1851–1932. SEE S. modification of Gram *stain*.

stir·rup (ster′ŭp, stir′ŭp). SYN stapes. [A.S. *stīrāp*]

stitch. 1. A sharp sticking pain of momentary duration. **2.** A single suture. **3.** SYN suture (2). [A.S. *stice*, a pricking]

lock s., SYN locking *suture.*

STM Abbreviation for short-term *memory*.

Stock, Wolfgang, German ophthalmologist, 1874–1956. SEE Spielmeyer-S. *disease.*

stock (stok). All the populations of organisms derived from an isolate without any implication of homogeneity or characterization. [A.S. *stoc*]

Stocker, Frederick William, U.S. ophthalmologist, 1893–1974. SEE S. *line.*

Stoffel, Adolf, German orthopedic surgeon, 1880–1937. SEE S. *operation.*

stoi·chi·ol·o·gy (stoy-kē-ol′-ō-jē). The science concerned with the elements or principles in any branch of knowledge, especially in chemistry, cytology, or histology. [G. *stoicheion,* element (lit. one of a row), fr. *stoichos,* a row, + *logos,* study]

stoi·chi·o·met·ric (stoy′kē-ō-met′rik). Pertaining to stoichiometry.

stoi·chi·om·e·try (stoy-kē-om′ĕ-trē). Determination of the relative quantities of the substances concerned in any chemical reaction; e.g., with the laws of definite proportions in chemistry, as in the molar proportions in a reaction. [G. *stoicheion,* element, + *metron,* measure]

stoke (stōk). A unit of kinematic viscosity, that of a fluid with a viscosity of 1 poise and a density of 1 g/ml; equal to 10^{-4} m²/s. [Sir George Gabriel *Stokes*]

Stokes, Sir George Gabriel, British physicist and mathematician, 1819–1903. SEE stoke; S. *law* (2), *law* (3).

Stokes, William, Irish physician, 1804–1878. SEE S. *law* (1); Cheyne-S. *psychosis, respiration;* S.-Adams *disease;* Adams-S. *disease;* Morgagni-Adams-S. *syndrome.*

Stokes, Sir William, Irish surgeon, 1839–1900. SEE S. *amputation;* Gritti-S. *amputation.*

sto·lon (stō′lon). A runner or connective aerial hypha that forms a cluster of rhizoids when it touches the substrate, and then sends out other runners to produce the aerial mycelium and sporangiosphores typical of *Rhizopus.* [L. *stolō,* branch, shoot, twig]

△**stom-.** SEE stomato-.

sto·ma, pl. **sto·mas, sto·ma·ta** (stō′mă, stō′maz, stō′mă-tă). **1.** A minute opening or pore. **2.** An artificial opening between two cavities or canals, or between such and the surface of the body. [G. a mouth]

Fuchs stomas, small depression on the surface of the iris near the margin of the pupil.

loop s., a specialized s. of intestine or ureter by which a loop of the hollow viscus is brought through an opening in the abdominal wall, with an opening created in the apex of the viscus to allow egress of its contents.

stom·ach (stŭm′ŭk) [TA]. A large irregularly piriform sac between the esophagus and the small intestine, lying just beneath the diaphragm; when distended it is 25–28 cm in length and 10–10.5 cm in its greatest diameter, and has a capacity of about 1 L. Its wall has four coats or tunics: mucous, submucous, muscular, and peritoneal; the muscular coat is composed of three layers, the fibers running longitudinally in the outer, circularly in the middle, and obliquely in the inner layer. SYN gaster (1) [TA], ventriculus (1) [TA]. [G. *stomachos,* L. *stomachus*]

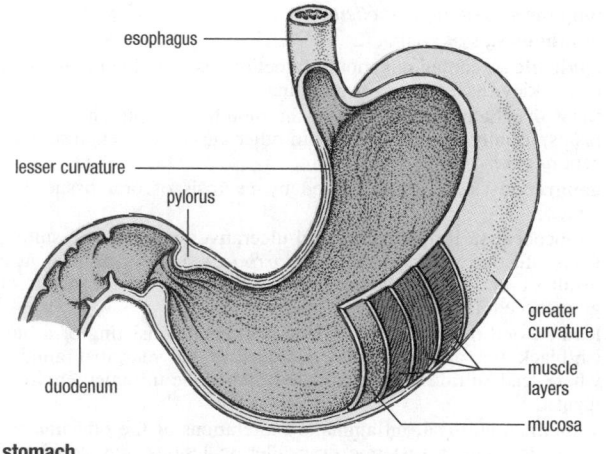

esophagus

lesser curvature

pylorus

greater curvature

muscle layers

mucosa

duodenum

stomach

bilocular s., SYN hourglass s.

s. bubble, the gas in the fundus of the s. seen on an upright radiograph.

cascade s., a radiographic description: when contrast material is swallowed while the patient is in the upright position, the gastric fundus acts as a reservoir until contrast overflows (cascades) into the antrum; a normal variant in a horizontal s.

drain-trap s., SYN water-trap s.

hourglass s., a condition in which there is a central constriction of the wall of the s. dividing it into two cavities, cardiac and pyloric. SYN bilocular s., ectasia ventriculi paradoxa.

leather-bottle s., marked thickening and rigidity of the s. wall,

st

with reduced capacity of the lumen although often without obstruction; nearly always due to scirrhous carcinoma, as in linitis plastica. SYN sclerotic s.

miniature s., SYN Pavlov *pouch.*

Pavlov s., SYN Pavlov *pouch.*

powdered s., the dried and powdered defatted wall of the s. of the hog, *Sus scrofa;* it contains thermolabile factors including native vitamin B_{12} and intrinsic factor; has been used in the treatment of pernicious anemia.

sclerotic s., SYN leather-bottle s.

thoracic s., a condition in which part or all of the s. is contained within the thorax because of a paraesophageal hiatus hernia.

trifid s., a condition in which the s. is divided by two constrictions into three pouches.

wallet s., a form of dilated s. in which there is a general baglike distention, the antrum and fundus being indistinguishable.

water-trap s., a ptotic and dilated s., having a relatively high (though normally placed) pyloric outlet which is held up by the gastrohepatic ligament. SYN drain-trap s.

stom·ach·al (stŭm′ă-kăl). Relating to the stomach. SYN stomachic (1).

stom·a·chal·gia (stŭm-ă-kal′jē-ă). Obsolete term for stomach *ache.* [stomach + G. *algos,* pain]

sto·mach·ic (sto′mak′ik). **1.** SYN stomachal. **2.** An agent that improves appetite and digestion.

stom·a·cho·dyn·ia (stŭm′ă-kō-din′ē-ă). Obsolete term for stomach *ache.* [stomach + G. *odynē,* pain]

sto·mal (stō′măl). Relating to a stoma.

△**stomat-.** SEE stomato-.

sto·ma·ta (stō′mă-tă). Alternate plural of stoma.

sto·ma·tal (stō′mă-tăl). Relating to a stoma.

sto·ma·tal·gia (stō-mă-tal′jē-ă). Pain in the mouth. SYN stomatodynia. [stomat- + G. *algos,* pain]

sto·mat·ic (stō-mat′ik). Relating to the mouth; oral.

sto·ma·ti·tis (stō-mă-tī′tis). Inflammation of the mucous membrane of the mouth. [stomat- + G. *-itis,* inflammation]

angular s., SYN angular *cheilitis.*

aphthous s., SYN aphtha (2).

epidemic s., contagious mouth infection, usually due to Group A coxsackievirus. SEE ALSO herpangina.

fusospirochetal s., infection of the mouth with spirochetal organisms, usually in association with other anaerobes. SEE ALSO Vincent *angina.*

gangrenous s., s. characterized by necrosis of oral tissue. SEE noma.

gonococcal s., inflammatory and ulcerative oral lesions resulting from infection with *Neisseria gonorrhoeae;* usually primary as a result of oral-genital contact, but occasionally is the result of gonococcemia.

lead s., oral manifestation of lead poisoning consisting of a bluish-black line following the contours of the marginal gingiva where lead sulfide has precipitated due to the inflamed environment.

s. medicamento′sa, inflammatory alterations of the oral mucosa associated with a systemic drug allergy; lesions may consist of erythema, vesicles, bullae, ulcerations, or angioneurotic edema.

mercurial s., alterations of the oral mucosa arising from chronic mercury poisoning; may consist of mucosal erythema and edema, ulceration, and deposition of mercurial sulfide in inflamed tissues, resulting in oral pigmentation resembling that of lead s.

nicotine s., heat-stimulated lesions, usually on the palate, that begin with erythema and progress to multiple white papules with a red dot in the center. The red dot represents a dilated, inflamed salivary duct orifice.

primary herpetic s., first infection of oral tissues with herpes simplex virus; characterized by gingival inflammation, vesicles, and ulcers. SYN primary herpetic gingivostomatitis.

recurrent aphthous s., SYN aphtha (2).

recurrent herpetic s., reactivation of herpes simplex virus infec-

tion, characterized by vesicles and ulceration limited to the hard palate and attached gingiva.

recurrent ulcerative s., SYN aphtha (2).

ulcerative s., SYN aphtha (2).

vesicular s., a vesicular disease of horses, cattle, swine, and occasionally humans caused by a Vesiculovirus (vesicular stomatitis virus) in the family Rhabdoviridae; in horses and cattle the disease usually causes mouth vesicles which, in cattle, cannot be differentiated clinically from those of foot-and-mouth disease.

△**stomato-, stom-, stomat-.** Mouth. [G. *stoma*]

sto·ma·to·cyte (stō′mă-tō-sīt). A red blood cell that exhibits a slit or mouth-shaped pallor rather than a central one on air-dried smears; e.g., Rh null cells. [stomato- + G. *kytos,* cell]

sto·ma·to·cy·to·sis (stō′mă-tō-sī-tō′sis). A hereditary deformation of red blood cells, which are swollen and cup-shaped, causing congenital hemolytic anemia. SEE ALSO Rh null *syndrome.*

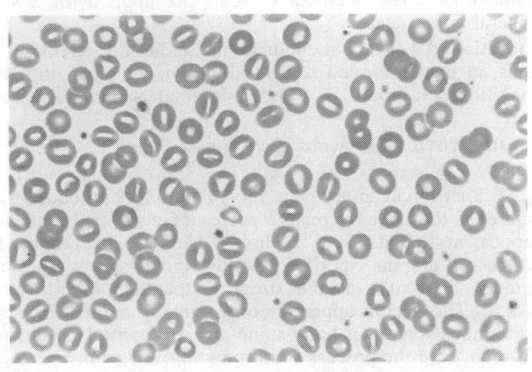

stomatocytosis: peripheral blood picture from patient with hereditary stomatocytosis reveals erythrocytes with slitlike or mouthlike (stoma = mouth) areas of pallor (250 2 original magnification)

sto·ma·to·de·um (stō′mă-tō-dē′ŭm). SYN stomodeum (1).

sto·ma·to·dyn·ia (stō′mă-tō-din′ē-ă). SYN stomatalgia. [stomato- + G. *odynē,* pain]

sto·ma·to·dys·o·dia (stō′mă-tō-di-sō′dē-ă). SYN halitosis. [stomato- + G. *dysōdia,* bad odor]

sto·ma·to·gnath·ic (stō′mă-tog-nath′ik). Pertaining to the mouth and jaw. [stomato- + G. *gnathos,* jaw]

sto·ma·to·log·ic (stō′mă-tō-loj′ik). Relating to stomatology.

sto·ma·tol·o·gist (stō-mă-tol′ŏ-jist). A specialist in diseases of the oral cavity.

sto·ma·tol·o·gy (stō-mă-tol′ō-jē). The study of the structure, function, and diseases of the mouth. [stomato- + G. *logos,* study]

sto·ma·to·ma·la·cia (stō′mă-tō-mă-lā′shē-ă). Pathologic softening of any of the structures of the mouth. [stomato- + G. *malakia,* softness]

sto·ma·to·my·co·sis (stō′mă-tō-mī-kō′sis). Disease of the mouth due to a fungus. [stomato- + G. *mykēs,* fungus, + *-osis,* condition]

sto·ma·to·ne·cro·sis (stō′mă-tō-ně-krō′sis). SYN noma. [stomato- + G. *nekrōsis,* death]

sto·ma·top·a·thy (stō-mă-top′ă-thē). Any disease of the oral cavity. SYN stomatosis. [stomato- + G. *pathos,* suffering]

sto·ma·to·plas·ty (stō′mă-tō-plas-tē). Old term for corrective operation of the mouth. [stomato- + G. *plastos,* formed]

sto·ma·tor·rha·gia (stō′mă-tō-rā′jē-ă). Bleeding from the gums or other part of the oral cavity. [stomato- + G. *rhēgnymi,* to burst forth]

sto·ma·to·scope (stō′mă-tō-skōp). An apparatus for illuminating the interior of the mouth to facilitate examination. [stomato- + G. *skopeō,* to view]

sto·ma·to·sis (stō-mă-tō′sis). SYN stomatopathy. [stomato- + G. *-osis,* condition]

sto·mi·on (stō′mē-on). The median point of the oral slit when the lips are closed.

sto·mo·ceph·a·lus (stō′mō-sef′ă-lŭs). Malformed individual with an undeveloped jaw and a snoutlike mouth; likely to be combined with an ethmocephalic type of cyclopia. [G. *stoma*, mouth, + *kephalē*, head]

sto·mo·de·al (stō′mō-dē′ăl). Relating to a stomodeum.

sto·mo·de·um (stō-mō-dē′ŭm). **1.** A midline ectodermal depression ventral to the embryonic brain and surrounded by the mandibular arch; when the buccopharyngeal membrane disappears, it becomes continuous with the foregut and forms the mouth. SYN stomatodeum. **2.** The anterior portion of the insect alimentary canal, consisting of mouth, buccal cavity, pharynx, esophagus, crop (frequently a diverticulum), and the proventriculus. [Mod. L. fr. G. *stoma*, mouth, + *hodaios*, on the way, fr. *hodos*, a way]

Sto·mox·ys cal·ci·trans (stō-mok′sis kal′si-tranz). The stable fly, a species of biting fly, resembling in size and general appearance the common housefly, which is an annoying pest of humans and domestic animals worldwide and is implicated in the mechanical transmission of diseases. [Mod. L., fr. C. *stoma*, mouth, + *oxys*, sharp; L. pres. p. of *calcitro*, to kick, fr. *calx*, the heel]

-stomy. Artificial or surgical opening. SEE stomato-. [G. *stoma*, mouth]

stone (stōn). **1.** SYN calculus. **2.** An English unit of weight of the human body, equal to 14 pounds. [A.S. *stān*]

    artificial s., a specially calcined gypsum derivative similar to plaster of Paris, but stronger, because the grains are nonporous.

    bladder s.'s, urinary tract calculi in the bladder. Throughout most of the history of humans, this was the predominant form of urinary tract stone disease, mentioned in the Hippocratic oath, and giving rise to the common ancient surgical procedure, lithotomy. In much of the world, bladder s. disease has become uncommon and renal and ureteral s.'s (which are usually of different origins) have become more common. Bladder s.'s are now typically seen in patients with neurogenic bladders, urinary tract reconstruction, or infravesical obstruction. SYN bladder calculus.

    philosopher's s., a s. sought by the alchemists of the Middle Ages that was supposedly able to transmute base metals into gold, to make precious s.'s, and to cure all ills, and thus confer longevity; it was also believed to be a universal solvent.

    pulp s., SYN endolith.

    tear s., SYN dacryolith.

    vein s., SYN phlebolith.

Stookey, Byron P., U.S. neurosurgeon, 1887–1966. SEE S.-Scarff *operation;* Queckenstedt-S. *test.*

stool (stool). **1.** A discharging of the bowels. **2.** The matter discharged at one movement of the bowels. SYN evacuation (2). SYN motion (3), movement (2). [A.S. *stōl*, seat]

    butter s.'s, fatty s.'s, occurring especially in steatorrhea.

    currant jelly s., feces that contain blood and products of inflammation, which cause it to resemble currant jelly in appearance; considered a sign of intussusception.

    fatty s., a s. containing excessive amounts of fat.

    rice-water s., a watery fluid containing whitish flocculi, discharged from the bowel in cholera and occasionally in other cases of serous diarrhea.

    spinach s.'s, dark greenish porridge-like s.'s, resembling chopped spinach.

    Trélat s.'s, glairy s.'s streaked with blood, occurring in proctitis.

stops. Bends in, or wires soldered to, an archwire to limit passage through a bracket or tube.

stor·age (stōr′ij). The second stage in the memory process, following encoding and preceding retrieval, involving mental processes associated with retention of stimuli that have been registered and modified by encoding. SEE memory.

sto·rax (stōr′aks). A liquid balsam obtained from the wood and inner bark of *Liquidamber orientalis,* a tree of Asia Minor, or *L. styraciflua* (family Hamamelidaceae); has been used in the treatment of chronic inflammation of the mucous membranes, and externally for scabies. SYN styrax. [G. *styrax,* a sweet-smelling gum]

STORCH A revision of the TORCH acronym (q.v.) to include syphilis as a cause of congenital infections.

sto·ri·form (stōr′i-fōrm). Having a cartwheel pattern, as of spindle cells with elongated nuclei radiating from a center. [L. *storea,* woven mat, + *-formis,* form]

storm (stōrm). An exacerbation of symptoms or a crisis in the course of a disease.

    thyroid s., SYN thyrotoxic *crisis.*

Stout wir·ing. See under wiring.

STPD Abbreviation indicating that a gas volume has been expressed as if it were at standard temperature (0°C), standard pressure (760 mm Hg absolute), and dry; under these conditions a mole of gas occupies 22.4 L.

stra·bis·mal (stra-biz′măl). Relating to or affected with strabismus. SYN strabismic.

stra·bis·mic (stra-biz′-mik). SYN strabismal.

stra·bis·mol·o·gist (stra-biz-mol′ah-jist). A physician subspecializing in pediatric ophthalmology with an emphasis on the management of strabismus and amblyopia.

stra·bis·mus (stra-biz′mŭs). A manifest lack of parallelism of the visual axes of the eyes. SYN crossed eyes, heterotropia, heterotropy, squint (1). [Mod. L., fr. G. *strabismos,* a squinting]

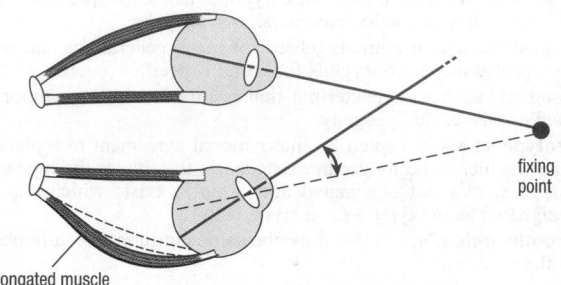

fixing point

elongated muscle

convergent strabismus (esotropia): in this case, right eye deviates inward because of an elongated lateral rectus muscle

    A-s., (1) s. in which esotropia is more marked in looking upward than downward; **(2)** s. in which exotropia is more marked on looking downward than upward. SYN A-pattern s.

    accommodative s., s. in which the severity of deviation varies with accommodation.

    alternate day s., SYN cyclic *esotropia.*

    alternating s., a form of s. in which either eye fixes.

    A-pattern s., SYN A-s.

    comitant s., a condition in which the degree of s. is the same in all directions of gaze. SYN concomitant s.

    concomitant s., SYN comitant s.

    convergent s., SYN esotropia.

    cyclic s., a s. that appears and disappears in rhythm, most frequently at 48-hour intervals.

    divergent s., SYN exotropia.

    incomitant s., SYN paralytic s.

    kinetic s., s. due to spasm of an extraocular muscle.

    manifest s., evident deviation of one eye or the other; may be alternating or monocular.

    mechanical s., s. due to restriction of action of the ocular muscle within the orbit.

    paralytic s., s. due to weakness of an ocular muscle or muscles. SYN incomitant s.

    vertical s., a form of s. in which the visual axis of one eye deviates upward (s. sursum vergens) or downward (s. deorsum vergens).

    X-s., s. in which exotropia is more marked when looking upward or downward than when looking straight ahead.

strain (strān). **1.** A population of homogeneous organisms possessing a set of defined characteristics; in bacteriology, the set of descendants that retains the characteristics of the ancestor; members of a s. that subsequently differ from the original isolate are regarded as belonging either to a substrain of the original s., or to

st

a new s. **2.** Specific host cell(s) designed or selected to optimize production of recombinant products. [A.S. *strēon,* progeny] **3.** To make an effort to the limit of one's strength. **4.** To injure by overuse or improper use (usually refers to a muscle tear). **5.** An act of straining. **6.** Injury resulting from s. or overuse. [L. *stringere, to draw tight]* **7.** The change in shape that a body undergoes when acted upon by an external force. **8.** To filter; to percolate.

auxotrophic s.'s, s.'s which are derived from the prototrophic s. but which require extra growth factors.

carrier s., a bacterial s. that is contaminated with a bacteriophage of low infectivity. SYN pseudolysogenic s.

cell s., in tissue culture, cells derived from a primary culture or a single cell (clone) and possessing a specific feature such as a marker chromosome, antigen, or resistance to a virus.

congenic s., an inbred s. of animals produced by continued crossing of a gene of one line onto another inbred (isogenic) line.

HFR s., Hfr s., a s., or clone, in which a conjugative plasmid (such as an F′), integrated in the bacterial genome, is instrumental in the transfer (along with plasmid DNA) of integrated bacterial DNA in a sequential manner to a suitable recipient. [*h*igh *f*requency of *r*ecombination]

hypothetical mean s. (HMS), a hypothetical s. that possesses the characteristics of a calculated mean organism.

isogenic s., a s. of animals inbred for many generations and with high probability homozygous for certain specified genes.

lysogenic s., a s. of bacterium that is infected with a temperate bacteriophage. SEE lysogeny.

neotype s., a s. accepted by international agreement to replace a type s. which is no longer in existence or to serve as the type s. if a type s. was not designated and if no s. exists which can be designated as the type. SYN neotype culture.

prototrophic s.'s, s.'s that have the same nutritional requirements as the wild-type s.

pseudolysogenic s., SYN carrier s.

recombinant s., SEE recombinant (1).

stock s., a bacterial or other microbial s. that has been maintained under laboratory conditions as representative of its type.

type s., the nomenclatural type of a species or subspecies.

wild-type s., a s. found in nature or a standard s. SEE ALSO auxotrophic s.'s, prototrophic s.'s.

strait (strāt). A narrow passageway. **inferior s.,** *apertura* pelvis inferior; **superior s.,** *apertura* pelvis superior. [M.E. *streit* thr. O. Fr. fr. L. *strictus,* drawn together, tight]

strait·jack·et (strāt′jak-et). A garmentlike device with long sleeves that can be secured to restrain a violently disturbed person. SYN camisole.

stra·mo·ni·um (stra-mō′nē-ŭm). The dried leaves and flowering or fruiting tops with branches of *Datura stramonium* or *D. tatula* (family Solanaceae), a herb abounding in temperate and subtropical countries; it contains an alkaloid, daturine, identical with hyoscyamine. It is an antispasmodic and has been used in the treatment of asthma and parkinsonism; when abused or taken inadvertently, it may cause an atropine-like toxic psychosis. [Mod. L.]

strand. In microbiology, a filamentous or threadlike structure.

anticoding s., the s. of duplex DNA which is used as a template for the synthesis of mRNA. SYN antisense s.

antiparallel s., a macromolecular s. that is oriented in the opposite direction of a neighboring s.

antisense s., SYN anticoding s.

coding s., the s. of duplex DNA that has the same sequence as the mRNA (except that mRNA contains ribonucleotides instead of deoxyribonucleotides). SYN sense s.

complementary s., SEE replicative *form.*

minus s., SEE replicative *form.*

plus s., SEE replicative *form.*

sense s., SYN coding s.

viral s., SEE replicative *form.*

Strandberg, James Victor., Swedish dermatologist, *1883. SEE Grönblad-S. *syndrome.*

stran·gal·es·the·sia (strang′gal-es-thē′zē-ă). SYN zonesthesia. [G. *strangalē,* halter, + *aisthēsis,* sensation]

stran·gle (strang′gl). To suffocate; to choke; to compress the trachea so as to prevent sufficient passage of air. [G. *strangaloō,* to choke, fr. *strangalē,* a halter]

stran·gu·lat·ed (strang′gū-lā-ted). Constricted so as to prevent sufficient passage of air, as through the trachea, or to cut off venous return and/or arterial flow so as to compromise viability, as in the case of a hernia. [L. *strangulo,* pp. *-atus,* to choke, fr. G. *strangaloō,* to choke (strangle)]

stran·gu·la·tion (strang′gū-lā′shŭn). The act of strangulating or the condition of being strangulated, in any sense: compression, constriction, herniation.

stran·gu·ry (strang′gū-rē). Difficulty in micturition, with straining to void; urine may be passed intermittently with pain and tenesmus. [G. *stranx* (*strang-*), something squeezed out, a drop, + *ouron,* urine]

strap. **1.** A strip of adhesive plaster. **2.** To apply overlapping strips of adhesive plaster. [A.S. *stropp*]

Strassburg, Gustav A., German physiologist, *1848. SEE S. *test.*

strat·i·fi·ca·tion (strat′i-fi-kā′shŭn). The process or result of separating a sample into subsamples according to specified criteria such as age or occupational groups. [L. *stratum,* layer, + *facio,* to make]

strat·i·fied (strat′i-fīd). Arranged in the form of layers or strata.

stra·tig·ra·phy (stra-tig′ră-fē). SYN tomography. [L. *stratum,* layer, + G. *graphē,* a writing]

STRATUM

stra·tum, gen. **stra·ti,** pl. **stra·ta** (strat′ŭm, tă; strā′tŭm; tī). One of the layers of differentiated tissue, the aggregate of which forms any given structure, such as the retina or the skin. SEE ALSO lamina, layer. [L. *sterno,* pp. *stratus,* to spread out, strew, ntr. of pp. as noun, *stratum,* a bed cover, layer]

s. aculea′tum, obsolete term for s. spinosum.

s. basa′le, (1) the outermost layer of the endometrium which undergoes only minimal changes during the menstrual cycle; SYN basal layer. **(2)** SYN s. basale epidermidis.

s. basa′le epider′midis, the deepest layer of the epidermis, composed of dividing stem cells and anchoring cells. SYN basal cell layer, columnar layer, germinative layer, palisade layer, s. basale (2), s. cylindricum, s. germinativum.

s. cerebra′le ret′inae, SYN cerebral *layer* of retina.

s. cine′reum collic′uli superio′ris, SYN gray *layers* of superior colliculus, under *layer.*

s. circula′re membra′nae tym′pani, circular fibers deep to the radiate layer of the membrane that are more abundant near the periphery; not present in the pars flaccida. SYN circular layer of tympanic membrane.

s. circulare musculi detrusoris vesicae [TA], SYN circular *layer* of detrusor (muscle) of urinary bladder.

s. circula′re tu′nicae muscula′ris [TA], SYN circular *layer* of muscular coat.

s. circula′re tu′nicae muscula′ris co′li, circular layer of muscular coat of colon.

s. circulare tunicae muscularis intestini tenuis [TA], SYN circular *layer* of muscle coat of small intestine.

s. circula′re tu′nicae muscula′ris rec′ti, circular layer of muscular coat of rectum.

s. circula′re tu′nicae muscula′ris ventric′uli, circular layer of muscular coat of stomach.

s. compac′tum, the superficial layer of decidual tissue in the pregnant uterus, in which the interglandular tissue preponderates. SYN compacta.

s. cor′neum epider′midis, the outer layer of the epidermis, consisting of several layers of flat keratinized non-nucleated cells. SYN corneal layer of epidermis, horny layer of epidermis.

st

s. cor′neum un′guis, the outer, horny layer of the nail. SYN cornified layer of nail, horny layer of nail.

s. cuta′neum membra′nae tym′pani, the thin layer of skin on the external surface of the tympanic membrane. SYN cutaneous layer of tympanic membrane.

s. cylin′dricum, SYN s. basale epidermidis.

s. disjunc′tum, the layer of partly detached cells on the free surface of the s. corneum, as seen in sections under the microscope; likely an artifact of fixation.

s. fibrosum vaginae tendinis, ⭐official alternate term for fibrous tendon *sheath*.

s. fibrosum [TA], SYN fibrous *capsule*.

s. fibro′sum capsulae articularis, SYN fibrous *layer* of joint capsule, fibrous *capsule*.

s. fibrosum panniculi adiposi telae subcutaneae [TA], SYN fibrous *layer* in or on deep aspect of fatty layer of subcutaneous tissue.

s. functiona′le, the endometrium except for the s. basale; formerly believed to be lost during menstruation but now considered to be only partially disrupted.

s. gangliona′re ner′vi op′tici, SYN ganglionic *layer* of optic nerve.

s. ganglionicum [TA], SYN ganglionic *layer*.

s. germinati′vum, SYN s. basale epidermidis.

s. germinati′vum un′guis, the deeper layer of the nail that is continuous with the s. germinativum of the surrounding skin and from which the nail plate is continuously formed. SYN germinative layer of nail.

s. granulare [TA], SYN granular *layer*; SEE *layers* of dentate gyrus, under *layer*.

s. granulo′sum corticis cerebel′li [TA], SYN granular *layer* of cerebellum.

s. granulo′sum epider′midis, SYN granular *layer* of epidermis.

s. granulo′sum follic′uli ova′rici vesiculo′si, the layer of small cells that forms the wall of an ovarian follicle. SYN granular layer of a vesicular ovarian follicle, granulosa, membrana granulosa, s. granulosum ovarii.

s. granulo′sum ova′rii, SYN s. granulosum folliculi ovarici vesiculosi.

s. gris′eum collic′uli superio′ris, SYN gray *layers* of superior colliculus, under *layer*.

s. gris′eum interme′dium [TA], SEE gray *layers* of superior colliculus, under *layer*.

s. gris′eum profun′dum [TA], SEE gray *layers* of superior colliculus, under *layer*.

s. griseum profundum colliculis superioris [TA], SYN deep gray *layer* of superior colliculus.

s. gris′eum superficia′le [TA], SEE gray *layers* of superior colliculus, under *layer*.

strata gyri dentati [TA], SYN *layers* of dentate gyrus, under *layer*.

s. helicoidale brevis gradus, ⭐official alternate term for circular *layer* of muscle coat of small intestine.

s. helicoidale longi gradus, ⭐official alternate term for longitudinal *layer* of muscle coat of small intestine.

strata hippocampi [TA], SYN *layers* of hippocampus, under *layer*.

s. interoliva′re lemnis′ci, the medial region of the medulla oblongata between the left and right olivary nucleus, traversed longitudinally by the left and right medial lemniscus, and transversely by the decussating olivocerebellar fibers.

s. lemnis′ci, a largely fibrous (hence whitish) layer of the superior colliculus separating the middle gray layer of superior colliculus from the deep gray layer of superior colliculus and containing, among others, fibers from the spinal and trigeminal lemnisci. SYN fillet layer.

s. limitans externum [TA], SYN outer limiting *layer*.

s. limitans internum [TA], SYN inner limiting *layer*.

s. longitudina′le tu′nicae muscula′ris [TA], SYN longitudinal *layer* of muscular coat.

s. longitudina′le tu′nicae muscula′ris co′li, longitudinal layer of the muscular tunic of the colon.

s. longitudina′le tu′nicae muscula′ris intesti′ni ten′uis [TA], SYN longitudinal *layer* of muscle coat of small intestine.

s. longitudina′le tu′nicae muscula′ris rec′ti, longitudinal layer of muscular coat of rectum.

s. longitudina′le tu′nicae muscula′ris ventric′uli, longitudinal layer of muscular coat of stomach.

s. lu′cidum, a layer of lightly staining corneocytes in the deepest level of the s. corneum; found primarily in the thick epidermis of the palmar and plantar skin. SYN clear layer of epidermis.

strata magnocellularia [TA], SEE lateral geniculate *body*.

malpighian s., the living layer of the epidermis comprising the s. basale, s. spinosum, and s. granulosum. SYN malpighian layer, malpighian rete.

s. medullare intermedium [TA], SYN intermediate white *layer* [TA] of superior colliculus.

s. medullare profundum [TA], SYN deep white *layer* of superior colliculus.

s. molecula′re, SYN molecular *layer*.

s. molecula′re corticis cerebel′li [TA], SYN molecular *layer* of cerebellar cortex.

s. moleculare et substratum lacunosum [TA], SYN lacunar-molecular *layer*; SEE *layers* of hippocampus, under *layer*.

s. molecula′re ret′inae, SYN molecular *layer* of retina.

s. multiforme [TA], SYN multiform *layer*; SEE *layers* of dentate gyrus, under *layer*.

s. musculosum panniculi adiposi telae subcutaneae [TA], SYN muscle *layer* in fatty layer of subcutaneous tissue.

s. neuroepithelia′le ret′inae, SYN neuroepithelial *layer* of retina.

s. neurofibrarum [TA], SYN *layer* of nerve fibers.

s. neurono′rum pirifor′mium, obsolete term for Purkinje cell *layer*.

s. nucleare externum [TA], SYN outer nuclear *layer*.

s. nucleare internum [TA], SYN inner nuclear *layer*.

strata nuclea′ria exter′na et inter′na ret′inae, SYN nuclear *layers* of retina, under *layer*.

s. op′ticum [TA], SYN optic *layer*.

s. oriens [TA], SYN oriens *layer*; SEE *layers* of hippocampus, under *layer*.

s. papilla′re cor′ii, the more superficial layer of the corium whose papillae interdigitate with the epidermis. SYN corpus papillare, papillary layer.

strata parvocellularia [TA], SEE lateral geniculate *body*.

s. pigmen′ti bul′bi, SYN pigmented *layer* of retina.

s. pigmen′ti cor′poris cilia′ris, the continuation of the pigment layer of the retina onto the posterior aspect of the ciliary body. SYN pigmented layer of ciliary body.

s. pigmen′ti i′ridis, the double layer of pigmented epithelium on the posterior surface of the iris. SYN pigmented layer of iris.

s. pigmen′ti ret′inae, SYN pigmented *layer* of retina.

s. plexiforme externum, SYN plexiform *layers* of retina, under *layer*.

s. plexiforme externum [TA], SYN outer plexiform *layer*.

s. plexiforme internum [TA], SYN plexiform *layers* of retina, under *layer*.

s. plexiforme internum [TA], SYN inner plexiform *layer*.

s. purkinjense corticis cerebelli [TA], SYN Purkinje cell *layer*.

s. pyramidale [TA], SYN pyramidal *layer*; SEE *layers* of hippocampus, under *layer*.

s. radiatum [TA], SYN radiant *layer*; SEE *layers* of hippocampus, under *layer*.

s. radia′tum membra′nae tym′pani, the connective tissue layer of the tympanic membrane beneath the stratum cutaneum, the fibers of which radiate from the manubrium of the malleus to the peripheral fibrocartilaginous ring of the membrane; absent from the pars flaccida. SYN radiate layer of tympanic membrane.

s. reticula′re co′rii, the thicker deep layer of the corium consisting of dense irregularly arranged connective tissue. SYN reticular layer of corium, s. reticulare cutis, tunica propria corii.

s. reticula′re cu′tis, SYN s. reticulare corii.

s. segmentorum externorum et internorum [TA], SYN *layer* of inner and outer segments.

s. spino'sum epider'midis, the layer of polyhedral cells in the epidermis; shrinkage artifacts and adhesion of these cells at their desmosomal junctions gives a spiny or prickly appearance. SYN prickle cell layer, spinous layer.

s. spongio'sum, the middle layer of the endometrium formed chiefly of dilated glandular structures; it is flanked by the compacta on the luminal side and the basalis on the myometrial side.

s. subcuta'neum, SYN subcutaneous *tissue.*

s. synovia'le, SYN synovial *membrane,* synovial *membrane.*

s. zona'le [TA], SYN zonular *layer.*

Straus, Isidore, French physician, 1845–1896. SEE S. *reaction, sign.*

Strauss, Lotte, U.S. pathologist, *1913. SEE Churg-S. *syndrome.*

Straüssler. SEE Gerstmann-Sträussler-Scheinker *syndrome.*

streak (strēk). A line, stria, or stripe, especially one that is indistinct or evanescent. [A.S. *strica*]

angioid s.'s, calcification of lamina basalis choroideae visible in the peripapillary fundus oculi; associated with pseudoexanthoma elasticum, sickle cell disease, and Paget disease; predisposing to choroidal neovascularization. SYN elastosis dystrophica, Knapp s.'s, Knapp striae.

germinal s., SYN primitive s.

gonadal s., a form of aplasia in which the ovary is replaced by a functionless tissue, as found in Turner syndrome. SYN streak gonad.

Knapp s.'s, SYN angioid s.'s.

meningitic s., a line of redness resulting from drawing a point across the skin, especially notable in cases of meningitis. SYN Trousseau spot.

Moore lightning s.'s, photopsia manifested by vertical flashes of light, seen usually on the temporal side of the affected eye, caused by the involutional shrinkage of vitreous humor.

primitive s., ridge of epiblast in the midline at the caudal end of the embryonic disk from which arises the intraembryonic mesoderm and definitive endoderm; achieved by inward and then lateral migration of cells; in human embryos, it appears on day 15 and provides visual evidence of the cephalocaudal axis. SYN germinal s.

stream (strēm). SYN flumen.

hair s.'s, the curved lines along which the hairs are arranged on the head and various parts of the body, especially noticeable in the fetus. SYN flumina pilorum.

stream·ing (strēm'ing). SEE ameboid *movement.*

streb·lo·dac·ty·ly (streb-lō-dak'ti-lē). SYN camptodactyly. [G. *streblos,* twisted, + *daktylos,* finger]

Streeter, George L., U.S. embryologist, 1873–1948. SEE S. developmental horizon(s).

Streeter de·vel·op·men·tal ho·ri·zon(s). A term borrowed from geology and archeology by Streeter to define 23 developmental stages in young human embryos, from fertilization through the first 2 months; each horizon spanned 2–3 days and emphasized specific anatomic characteristics, to avoid discrepancies in the determination of age and body dimensions. [G.L. Streeter]

Streiff, Enrico Bernard, Swiss ophthalmologist, *1908. SEE Hallermann-S. *syndrome;* Hallermann-S.-François *syndrome.*

strength. 1. The quality of being strong or powerful. **2.** The degree of intensity. **3.** The property of materials by which they endure the application of force without yielding or breaking.

associative s., in psychology, the s. of a stimulus response linkage as measured by the frequency with which a stimulus elicits a particular response. SEE conditioning.

biting s., SYN *force* of mastication.

compressive s., tensile s., except that the stress is in compression.

fatigue s., the stress level below which a particular component will survive an indefinite number of load cycles (typically about 50% of the ultimate s. of the component).

ionic s. (I), symbolized as $\Gamma/2$ or I and set equal to $0.5\Sigma m_i z_i^2$,

where m_i equals the molar concentration and z_i the charge of each ion present in solution; if molar concentrations (c_i) are used instead of molality (and the solution is dilute), then I = $0.5(1/\rho_o)\Sigma c_i z_i^2$ where ρ_o is the density of the solvent; a number of biochemically important events (e.g., protein solubility and rates of enzyme action) vary with the ionic s. of a solution.

tensile s., the maximum tensile stress or load that a material is capable of sustaining; usually expressed in pounds per square inch.

ultimate s., the maximum stress achieved prior to failure of a component on a single application of the load.

yield s., the amount of stress at which a permanent (plastic) deformation in a component becomes measurable (usually taken as 0.2% permanent strain).

streph·o·sym·bo·lia (stref'ō-sim-bō'lē-ă). **1.** Generally, the perception of objects reversed as if in a mirror. **2.** Specifically, difficulty in distinguishing written or printed letters that extend in opposite directions but are otherwise similar, such as *p* and *d,* or related kinds of mirror reversal. [G. *strephō,* to turn, + *symbolon,* a mark or sign]

stre·pi·tus (strep'i-tŭs). Rarely used term for a noise, usually an auscultatory sound. [L.]

streptavidin (strep-ta-vī'din). A bacterial protein used as a probe in immunologic assays because of its strong affinity and specificity for biotin; s. is used as a bridge to link a chromogen to a biotinylated substrate specific for the substance of interest. [*streptococcus* + *avidin*]

strep·ti·ce·mia (strep-ti-sē'mē-ă). Obsolete term for streptococcemia.

strep·ti·dine (strep'ti-dēn). An aglycone component of streptomycin.

△strepto-. Curved or twisted (usually relating to organisms thus described). [G. *streptos,* twisted, fr. *strephō,* to twist]

Strep·to·ba·cil·lus (strep-tō-ba-sil'ŭs). A genus of nonmotile, non–spore-forming, aerobic to facultatively anaerobic bacteria (family Bacteroidaceae) containing Gram-negative, pleomorphic cells that vary from short rods to long, interwoven filaments that have a tendency to fragment into chains of bacillary and coccobacillary elements. These organisms can be pathogenic for rats, mice, and other mammals. The type species is *S. moniliformis.* [strepto- + bacillus]

S. monilifor'mis, a bacterial species commonly found as an inhabitant of the nasopharynx of rats; it occurs as the etiologic agent of an epizootic septic polyarthritis in mice and of one type of rat-bite fever; it is the type species of the genus *S.*

strep·to·bi·o·sa·mine (strep'tō-bī-ō'să-mēn). A methylamino disaccharide (streptose + *N*-methyl-L-glucosamine), with the oxygen link between C-2 of streptose and C-1 of the glucosamine; with streptidine, it forms streptomycin.

strep·to·bi·ose (strep-tō-bī'ōs). Old term for streptose.

strep·to·cer·ci·a·sis (strep'tō-ser-kī'ă-sis). Infection of humans and higher primates with the nematode *Mansonella streptocerca.*

strep·to·coc·cal (strep'tō-kok'ăl). Relating to or caused by any organism of the genus *Streptococcus.*

strep·to·coc·ce·mia (strep'tō-kok-sē'-mē-ă). The presence of streptococci in the blood. SYN streptosepticemia. [streptococcus + G. *haima,* blood]

strep·to·coc·ci (strep'tō-kok'sī). Plural of streptococcus.

strep·to·coc·cic (strep'tō-kok'sik). Relating to or caused by any organism of the genus *Streptococcus.*

strep·to·coc·co·sis (strep'tō-kŏ-kō'sis). Any streptococcal infection.

Strep·to·coc·cus (strep-tō-kok'ŭs). A genus of nonmotile (with few exceptions), nonsporeforming, aerobic to facultatively anaerobic bacteria (family Lactobacillaceae) containing Gram-positive, spherical or ovoid cells that occur in pairs or short or long chains. Dextrorotatory lactic acid is the main product of carbohydrate fermentation. These organisms occur regularly in the mouth and intestines of humans and other animals, in dairy and other food products, and in fermenting plant juices. Some species are pathogenic. The type species is *S. pyogenes*. [strepto- + G. *kokkos*, berry (coccus)]

S. agalac'tiae, a species found in the milk and tissues from udders of cows with mastitis; also reported to be associated with a variety of human infections, especially those of the urogenital tract.

S. angino'sus, an α-hemolytic species of bacteria found in the human throat, sinuses, abscesses, vagina, skin, and feces; this organism is a common cause of isolated liver abscesses.

S. bo'vis, a bacterial species found in the bovine alimentary tract; this organism may also be found in blood and heart lesions in cases of subacute endocarditis.

S. constella'tus, an α-hemolytic species of bacteria found in tonsils, purulent pleurisy, appendix, the nose, throat, and gums, and infrequently on the skin and in the vagina.

S. dur'ans, a bacterial species found in dried milk powder and in the intestines of humans and other animals.

S. faeca'lis, SYN *Enterococcus faecalis.*

S. intermedius, one of a heterogenous collection of streptococci, generally found in the mouth or upper respiratory tract; classification is generally established by fermentation patterns, analysis of the sugar composition of the cell wall, and use of sugar production patterns. SYN *Peptostreptococcus intermedius.*

S. lac'tis, a bacterial species found commonly as a contaminant in milk and dairy products; a common cause of the souring and coagulation of milk; some strains produce nisin, a powerful antibiotic that inhibits the growth of many other Gram-positive organisms.

S. milleri, a term used to refer to the *S. intermedius* group, which contains three distinct streptococcal species including *S. intermedius,* *S. constellatus,* and *S. anginosus.* These bacteria are found in the human oral cavity and have been associated with a variety of infections including bacteremia; endocarditis; and CNS, oral, and thoracic infections.

S. mi'tis, a bacterial species found in the human mouth, throat, and nasopharynx; ordinarily, it is not considered to be pathogenic, but this organism may be recovered from ulcerated teeth and sinuses and from blood and heart lesions in cases of subacute endocarditis.

S. morbillorum, SYN *Peptostreptococcus morbillorum.*

S. mu'tans, a bacterial species associated with the production of dental caries in humans and in some other animals and with subacute endocarditis.

S. pneumo'niae, a species of Gram-positive, lancet-shaped cocci and diplococci frequently occurring in chains; cells are readily lysed by bile salts. Virulent forms are enclosed in type-specific polysaccharide capsules, the basis for an effective vaccine. Normal inhabitants of the respiratory tract, and the most common cause of lobar pneumonia, they are the most common causative agents of meningitis, and pneumonia worldwide, and also cause sinusitis, and other infections. It is the type species of the former genus *Diplococcus.* SYN Fraenkel pneumococcus, pneumococcus, pneumonococcus.

S. pyog'enes, a bacterial species found in the human mouth, throat, and respiratory tract and in inflammatory exudates, the bloodstream, and cellulitic lesions in human diseases; it is sometimes found in the udders of cows and in dust from sickrooms, hospital wards, schools, theaters, and other public places; it causes the formation of pus, fatal septicemia, and necrotizing fascitis and myositis. There is also a specific somatic antigen (M protein) for each of the approximately 85 types. It is the type species of the genus *S.*

S. saliva'rius, a bacterial species found in the human mouth, throat, and nasopharynx, and associated with dental disease.

S. san'guis, a bacterial species originally found in the so-called vegetation on heart valves from cases of subacute bacterial endocarditis; occasionally found in infected sinuses and teeth and in house dust.

S. vir'idans, a name applied not to a distinct species but rather to the group of α-hemolytic streptococci as a whole; viridans streptococci have been isolated from the mouth and intestines of humans, the intestines of horses, the milk and feces of cows, and milk products. SYN viridans streptococci.

strep·to·coc·cus, pl. **strep·to·coc·ci** (strep'tō-kok'ŭs, -kok'sī). A term used to refer to any member of the genus *Streptococcus.*

group A streptococci (GAS), a common bacteria that is the cause of strep throat, scarlet fever, impetigo, cellulitis-erysipelas, rheumatic fever, acute glomerular nephritis, endocarditis, and group A streptococcal necrotizing fasciitis. The prototype is *Streptococcus pyogenes.*

group B streptococci, a leading cause of a form of neonatal sepsis that has a 10–20% mortality rate and leaves a large number of survivors with brain damage; also a leading cause of meningitis.

hemolytic streptococci, SYN β-hemolytic streptococci.

α-hemolytic streptococci, streptococci that form a green variety of reduced hemoglobin in the area of the colony on a blood agar medium. SEE ALSO *Streptococcus viridans.*

β-hemolytic streptococci, those that produce active hemolysins (O and S) which cause a zone of clear hemolysis on the blood agar medium in the area of the colony; β-hemolytic streptococci are divided into groups (A to O) on the basis of cell wall C carbohydrate (see Lancefield *classification*); Group A (in the strains pathogenic for man) comprises more than 50 types (designated by Arabic numerals) determined by cell wall M protein, which seems to be associated closely with virulence and is produced chiefly by strains with matt or mucoid colonies, in contrast to nonvirulent, glossy colony-producing strains; other surface protein antigens such as R and T (T substance), and the nucleoprotein fraction (P substance) seem to be of less importance. The more than 20 extracellular substances elaborated by strains of β-hemolytic streptococci include erythrogenic toxin (elaborated only by lysogenic strains), deoxyribonuclease (streptodornase), hemolysins (streptolysins O and S), hyaluronidase, and streptokinase. SYN hemolytic streptococci.

viridans streptococci, SYN *Streptococcus viridans.*

strep·to·dor·nase (SD) (strep-tō-dōr'nās). A "dornase" (deoxyribonuclease) obtained from streptococci; used with streptokinase to facilitate drainage in septic surgical conditions.

strep·to·fu·ra·nose (strep-tō-foor'ă-nōs). SYN streptose.

strep·to·ki·nase (SK) (strep-tō-kī'nās). An extracellular metalloenzyme from hemolytic streptococci that cleaves plasminogen, producing plasmin, which causes the liquefaction of fibrin (same activity as staphylokinase and urokinase); thus, used in the removal of clots. SYN plasminokinase, streptococcal fibrinolysin.

strep·to·ki·nase-strep·to·dor·nase. A purified mixture containing streptokinase, streptodornase, and other proteolytic enzymes; used by topical application or by injection into body cavities to remove clotted blood and fibrinous and purulent accumulations of exudate; thus, used in the removal of clots.

strep·to·ly·sin (strep-tol'i-sin). A hemolysin produced by streptococci.

s. O, a hemolysin that is produced by β-hemolytic streptococci and is hemolytically active only in the reduced state; anti-s. O produced during infection is of diagnostic significance.

Strep·to·my·ces (strep-tō-mī'sēz). A genus of nonmotile, aerobic, Gram-positive bacteria (family Streptomycetaceae) that grow in the form of a many-branched mycelium; conidia are produced in chains on aerial hyphae. These organisms (several hundred species in the genus) are predominantly saprophytic soil forms; some are parasitic on plants or animals; many produce antibiotics. The type species is *S. albus.* [strepto- + G. *mykēs*, fungus]

S. al'bus, a bacterial species found in dust, soil, grains, and straw; some strains produce actinomycetin; others produce thiolutin or endomycin; it is the type species of the genus *S.*

S. gibso'nii, a bacterial species found in human infections. SYN *Nocardia gibsonii.*

S. somalien'sis, a bacterial species that causes Bouffardi white mycetoma.

Strep·to·my·ce·ta·ce·ae (strep'tō-mī-sĕ-tā'sē-ē). A family of aerobic Gram-positive bacteria (order Actinomycetales) that produce a vegetative mycelium which does not fragment into bacillary or coccoid forms; they produce conidia which are borne on sporophores. These organisms occur primarily in the soil; some

St

are thermophiles found in rotting manure, a few are parasitic, and many produce antibiotics. The type genus is *Streptomyces*.

strep·to·my·cete (strep'tō-mī'sēt). A term used to refer to a member of the genus *Streptomyces;* it is sometimes improperly used to refer to any member of the family Streptomycetaceae.

strep·to·my·cin (strep-tō-mī'sin). An antibiotic agent obtained from *Streptomyces griseus* that is active against the tubercle bacillus and a large number of Gram-positive and Gram-negative bacteria; also used in the form of dihydrostreptomycin (aldehyde of s. reduced to CH_2OH). It is a glucoside and contains streptidine and streptobiosamine linked by an oxygen bridge between C-4 of the inositol residue and C-1 of the streptose residue; s. B has a mannose residue attached to the glucosamine and is a natural product, with less activity than s. A. It is used virtually exclusively in the treatment of tuberculosis; toxicity includes eighth cranial nerve damage leading to deafness and/or vestibular dysfunction. SYN streptomycin A.

strep·to·my·cin A. SYN streptomycin.

strep·to·my·co·sis (strep'tō-mī-kō'sis). Old term for streptococcemia. [strepto- + G. *mykēs,* fungus, + *-osis,* condition]

strep·to·ni·vi·cin (strep'tō-ni-vī'sin). SYN novobiocin.

strep·tose (strep'tōs). An unusual L-pentose that is a component of streptobiosamine, hence of streptomycin. SYN streptofuranose.

strep·to·sep·ti·ce·mia (strep'tō-sep-ti-sē'mē-ă). SYN streptococcemia.

strep·to·thri·cho·sis (strep'tō-thri-kō'sis). SYN dermatophilosis.

strep·to·tri·chi·a·sis (strep'tō-tri-kī'ă-sis). SYN dermatophilosis.

strep·to·tri·cho·sis (strep'tō-tri-kō'sis). SYN dermatophilosis.

strep·to·zo·cin (strep-tō-zō'sin). An antineoplastic agent used in the treatment of metastatic islet-cell carcinoma of the pancreas. SYN streptozotocin.

streptozotocin (strep'tō-zō-toks'in). SYN streptozocin.

ℹ **stress** (stres). **1.** Reactions of the body to forces of a deleterious nature, infections, and various abnormal states that tend to disturb its normal physiologic equilibrium (homeostasis). **2.** In dentistry, the forces set up in teeth, their supporting structures, and structures restoring or replacing teeth as a result of the force of mastication. **3.** The force or pressure applied or exerted between portions of a body or bodies, generally expressed in pounds per square inch. **4.** In rheology, the force in a material transmitted per unit area to adjacent layers. **5.** In psychology, a physical or psychological stimulus such as very high heat, public criticism, or another noxious agent or experience which, when impinging upon certain individuals, produces psychological strain or disequilibrium. [L. *strictus,* tight, fr. *stringo,* to draw together]

life s., events or experiences that produce severe strain, e.g., failure on the job, marital separation, loss of a love object.

shear s., the force acting in shear flow expressed per unit area; units in the CGS system: dynes/cm².

tensile s., a s. acting on a body per unit cross-sectional area so as to elongate the body.

yield s., the critical s. that must be applied to a material before it begins to flow, as in a Bingham plastic.

stress break·er. A device that relieves the abutment teeth, to which a fixed or removable partial denture is attached, of all or part of the forces generated by occlusal function.

stress ris·er. A mechanical defect, such as a hole, in bone or other materials, that concentrates stress in the area and increases the risk of failure of the bone or material at that site.

stress shield·ing. Osteopenia occurring in bone as the result of removal of normal stress from the bone by an implant.

stretch·er (stre'cher). **1.** A litter, usually a sheet of canvas stretched to a frame with four handles, used for transporting the sick or injured. **2.** A cart with four wheels and a flat top for the transportation of patients, usually within hospitals. [A.S. *streccan,* to stretch]

stri·a, gen. and pl. **stri·ae** (strī'ă, strī'ē). **1.** A stripe, band, streak, or line, distinguished by color, texture, depression, or elevation from the tissue in which it is found. SYN striation (1). **2.** SYN striae cutis distensae. [L. channel, furrow]

acoustic striae, SYN medullary striae of fourth ventricle.

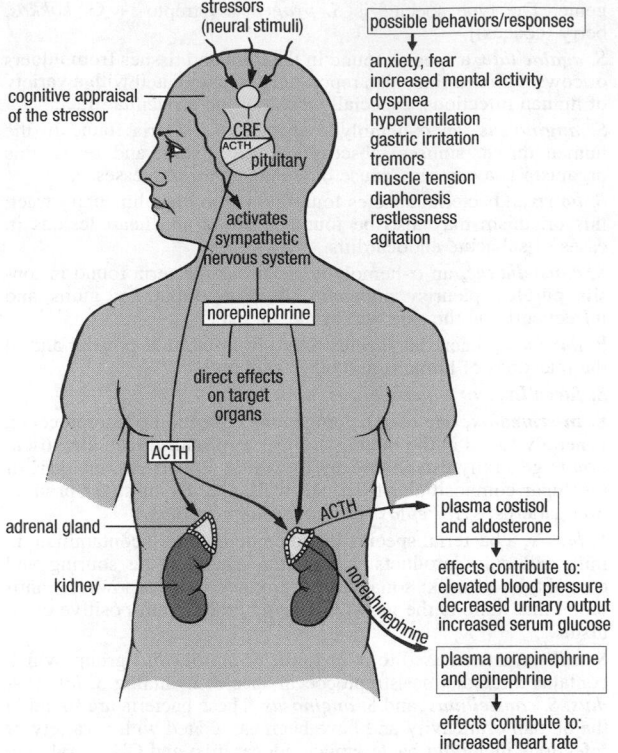

stress response: CRF, corticotropin releasing factor; ACTH, adrenocorticotropic hormone

anterior acoustic s. [TA], these axons originate in the ventral cochlear nucleus, cross the midline as part of the trapezoid body, join the lateral lemniscus, and terminate largely in the superior olivary complex. SYN s. cochlearis anterior [TA], ventral acoustic s. [TA].

stri'ae atroph'icae, SYN striae cutis distensae.

auditory striae, SYN medullary striae of fourth ventricle.

brown striae, SYN Retzius striae.

stri'ae cilia'res, shallow radial grooves on the surface of the orbiculus ciliaris extending from the teeth of the ora serrata and leading into the valleys between the ciliary processes.

s. cochlearis anterior [TA], SYN anterior acoustic s.

s. cochlearis intermedia [TA], SYN intermediate acoustic s.

s. cochlearis posterior [TA], SYN posterior acoustic s.

stri'ae cu'tis disten'sae, bands of thin wrinkled skin, initially red but becoming purple and white, which occur commonly on the abdomen, buttocks, and thighs at puberty and/or during and following pregnancy, and result from atrophy of the dermis and overextension of the skin; also associated with ascites and Cushing syndrome. SYN atrophoderma striatum, lineae atrophicae, linear atrophy, stretch marks, stria (2), striae atrophicae, striate atrophy of skin, traction atrophy.

diagonalis s., SEE Broca diagonal *band.*

s. diagonalis [TA], SYN Broca diagonal *band.*

s. externa medullae renalis [TA], SYN outer *stripes* of renal medulla, under *stripe.*

s. for'nicis, SYN medullary s. of thalamus.

Gennari s., SYN *line* of Gennari.

stri'ae gravida'rum, striae cutis distensae related to pregnancy.

intermediate acoustic s. [TA], these axons arise in the cochlear nuclei; some fibers cross adjacent to the trapezoid body, others ascend on the ipsilateral side; they terminate in periolivary nuclei and nuclei of the lateral lemniscus; may function to modulate activity in the olivocochlear tract. SYN s. cochlearis intermedia [TA].

s. of internal granular layer [TA], SEE Baillarger *lines*, under *line*.

s. of internal pyramidal layer [TA], SEE Baillarger *lines*, under *line*.

s. interna medullae renalis [TA], SYN inner *stripes* of renal medulla, under *stripe*.

Knapp striae, SYN angioid *streaks*, under *streak*.

s. laminae granularis internae [TA], SYN Baillarger *lines*, under *line*.

s. laminae molecularis [TA], SYN *band* of Kaes-Bechterew.

s. laminae pyramidalis internae [TA], SYN Baillarger *lines*, under *line*.

stri′ae lanci′si, the lateral longitudinal s. and the medial longitudinal s.

Langhans s., fibrinoid that accumulates on the chorionic plate between the bases of placental villi during the first half of pregnancy.

lateral longitudinal s. [TA], a thin longitudinal band of nerve fibers accompanied by gray matter, near each outer edge of the upper surface of the corpus callosum under cover of the cingulate gyrus. SYN s. longitudinalis lateralis [TA], s. tecta, tectal s.

s. longitudina′lis latera′lis [TA], SYN lateral longitudinal s.

s. longitudina′lis media′lis [TA], SYN medial longitudinal s.

s. mallea′ris [TA], SYN malleolar s.

malleolar s. [TA], a bright line seen through the membrana tympani, produced by the attachment of the manubrium of the malleus. SYN s. mallearis [TA], mallear stripe.

medial longitudinal s., a thin longitudinal band of nerve fibers accompanied by gray matter, running along the surface of the corpus callosum on either side of the median line. Together with the lateral longitudinal s. it forms part of a thin layer of gray matter on the dorsal surface of the corpus callosum, the indusium griseum, a rudimentary component of the hippocampus. SYN s. longitudinalis medialis [TA].

stri′ae medulla′res ventric′uli quar′ti [TA], SYN medullary striae of fourth ventricle.

s. medulla′ris thal′ami [TA], SYN medullary s. of thalamus.

medullary striae of fourth ventricle [TA], slender fascicles of fibers extending transversely below the ependymal floor of the ventricle from the median sulcus to enter the inferior cerebellar peduncle. They arise from the arcuate nuclei on the ventral surface of the medullary pyramid. SYN striae medullares ventriculi quarti [TA], acoustic striae, auditory striae, Bergmann cords, medullary teniae, taeniae acusticae.

medullary s. of thalamus [TA], a narrow, compact fiber bundle that extends along the line of attachment of the roof of the third ventricle to the thalamus on each side and terminates posteriorly in the habenular nucleus. It is composed of fibers originating in the septal area, the anterior perforated substance, the lateral preoptic nucleus, and the medial segment of the globus pallidus. SYN s. medullaris thalami [TA], s. fornicis, s. ventriculi tertii.

s. of molecular layer [TA], SYN *band* of Kaes-Bechterew.

s. na′si transver′sa, a single deep horizontal groove at the level of the alae, with no associated defects. SYN transverse nasal groove.

Nitabuch s., SYN Nitabuch *membrane*.

s. occipitalis [TA], SYN *line* of Gennari.

stri′ae olfacto′riae [TA], SYN olfactory striae.

olfactory striae [TA], three distinct fiber bands (s. medialis, s. intermedia, s. lateralis) that caudally extend the olfactory tract beyond its attachment to the olfactory trigone. The medial olfactory s. [TA] (s. olfactoria medialis [TA]) curves dorsally into the tenia tecta; the intermediate, often barely visible, extends straight back and terminates in the olfactory tubercle; the lateral olfactory s. [TA] (s. olfactoria lateralis [TA], the largest of the three, passes along the lateral side of the olfactory tubercle, curving laterally as far as the limen insulae, then sharply medially to reach the uncus of the parahippocampal gyrus where it terminates in the plexiform

layer of the olfactory cortex. SEE ALSO medial longitudinal s. SYN striae olfactoriae [TA], olfactory roots.

stri′ae paral′lelae, SYN Retzius striae.

posterior acoustic s. [TA], these axons originate from the dorsal cochlear nucleus, cross the midline dorsal to the trapezoid body, and join the lateral lemniscus; some fibers may terminate in the superior olivary nucleus but most pass directly to the inferior colliculus or synapse in the nuclei of the lateral lemniscus enroute. SYN s. cochlearis posterior [TA].

striae ret′inae, concentric lines on the surface of an abnormal retina. SYN Paton lines.

Retzius striae, dark concentric lines crossing the enamel prisms of the teeth, seen in axial cross sections of the enamel. SYN brown striae, striae parallelae.

Rohr s., layer of fibrinoid in the intervillous spaces of the placenta.

s. spino′sa, a faint groove occasionally caused by the chorda tympani nerve on the spine of the sphenoid. SYN Lucas groove, sulcus spinosus.

s. tec′ta, SYN lateral longitudinal s.

tectal s., SYN lateral longitudinal s.

terminal s. [TA], a slender, compact fiber bundle that connects the amygdala (amygdaloid body) with the hypothalamus and other basal forebrain regions. Originating from the amygdala, the bundle passes first caudalward in the roof of the temporal horn of the lateral ventricle; it follows the medial side of the caudate nucleus forward in the floor of the ventricle's central part (or body) until it reaches the interventricular foramen, in the posterior wall of which it curves steeply down to enter the hypothalamus, with fibers passing both rostral and caudal to the anterior commissure. Coursing caudalward in the medial part of the hypothalamus, the bundle terminates in the anterior and ventromedial hypothalamic nuclei. SYN s. terminalis [TA], Foville fasciculus, Tarin tenia, tenia semicircularis.

s. termina′lis [TA], SYN terminal s.

s. vascularis of cochlear duct [TA], the stratified epithelium lining the upper part of the ligamentum spirale cochleae; it is penetrated by capillaries and is believed to be the site of production of endolymph. SYN s. vascularis ductus cochlearis [TA], psalterial cord, vascular stripe.

s. vascula′ris duc′tus cochlea′ris [TA], SYN s. vascularis of cochlear duct.

ventral acoustic s. [TA], SYN anterior acoustic s.

s. ventric′uli ter′tii, SYN medullary s. of thalamus.

Wickham striae, fine whitish lines, having a network arrangement, on the surface of lichen planus papules.

striae of Zahn, SYN *lines* of Zahn, under *line*.

stri·a·tal (strī′ā-tăl). Relating to the corpus striatum.

stri·ate (strī′āt). Striped; marked by striae. [L. *striatus*, furrowed]

stri·a·tion (strī-ā′shŭn). 1. SYN stria (1). 2. A striate appearance. 3. The act of streaking or making striae.

basal s.'s, the vertical infranuclear s.'s due to the infolded plasma membrane and mitochondria; they are seen in kidney tubules and certain intralobular salivary ducts.

tabby cat s., SYN tigroid s.

tigroid s., linear whitish or yellowish markings on the fatty degenerated heart muscle. SYN tabby cat s.

stri·a·to·ni·gral (strī-ā-tō-nī′grăl). Referring to the efferent connection of the striatum with the *substantia* nigra.

stri·a·tum (strī-ā′tŭm) [TA]. Collective name for the caudate nucleus and putamen which together with the globus pallidus or pallidum form the striate body. SYN neostriatum*. [L. neut. of *striatus*, furrowed]

dorsal s. [TA], those portions of the caudate nucleus and especially the putamen located generally dorsal to a plane representing the anterior commissure; also called the dorsal basal ganglia; may function in motor activities with cognitive origins. SYN s. dorsale [TA].

s. dorsale [TA], SYN dorsal s.

ventral s. [TA], those portions of the striatum located generally ventral to a plane representing the anterior commissure; includes the nucleus accumbens and some nuclei of the olfactory tubercle; may function in motor activities with emotional or motivational origins. SYN s. ventrale [TA].

s. ventrale [TA], SYN ventral s.

stric·ture (strik'choor). A circumscribed narrowing or stenosis of a hollow structure, usually consisting of cicatricial contracture or deposition of abnormal tissue. [L. *strictura,* fr. *stringo,* pp. *strictus,* to draw tight, bind]

anastomotic s., narrowing, usually by scarring, of an anastomotic suture line.

anular s., a ringlike constriction encircling the wall of a canal.

bridle s., narrowing of a canal by a band of tissue stretching across part of its lumen.

contractile s., SYN recurrent s.

functional s., SYN spasmodic s.

organic s., a s. due to the presence of cicatricial or other new tissue, not spasmodic. SYN permanent s.

permanent s., SYN organic s.

recurrent s., a s. due to the presence of contractile tissue which may be dilated but soon returns. SYN contractile s.

spasmodic s., a s. due to localized spasm of muscular fibers in the wall of the canal. SYN functional s., temporary s.

temporary s., SYN spasmodic s.

urethral s., a stenosing lesion of the urethra, due usually to inflammation or to iatrogenic instrumentation and resulting in reduction of urethral caliber which may be focal or may involve virtually the entire length of the urethra.

stric·tur·o·plas·ty (strik'chur-plas'tē). Surgical procedure for widening a structured segment of intestine that involves incision and closure in opposing directions. [stricture + G. *plastos,* formed]

stric·tur·o·tome (strik'choor-ō-tōm). An instrument for use in dividing a stricture.

stric·tur·ot·o·my (strik-choor-ot'ō-mē). Surgical opening or division of a stricture. [stricture + G. *tomē,* incision]

stri·dent (strī'dent). Creaking; grating; harsh-sounding; denoting an auscultatory sound or rale. [L. *stridens,* pres. p. of *strideo,* to creak]

stri·dor (strī'dōr). A high-pitched, noisy respiration, like the blowing of the wind; a sign of respiratory obstruction, especially in the trachea or larynx. [L. a harsh, creaking sound]

congenital s., crowing inspiration occurring at birth or within the first few months of life; sometimes without apparent cause and sometimes due to abnormal flaccidity of epiglottis or arytenoids. SYN laryngeal s.

s. den'tium, grinding of the teeth.

expiratory s., a singing sound due to the semiapproximated vocal folds offering resistance to the escape of air or to tracheal or bronchial obstruction.

inspiratory s., a crowing sound during the inspiratory phase of respiration due to pathology involving the upper respiratory tract especially at the epiglottis or larynx.

laryngeal s., SYN congenital s.

s. serrat'icus, a rough grating like the sound of a saw.

strid·u·lous (strid'ū-lŭs). Having a shrill or creaking sound. [L. *stridulus,* fr. *strideo,* to creak, to hiss]

string. A slender cord or cordlike structure.

auditory s.'s, bundles of parallel filaments in the zona pectinata of the lamina basilaris of the cochlea; the length of the s.'s varies from 64 μm in the basal coil to 480 μm in the apex.

stri·o·la (strī'ō-la). The narrow central area of the utricular macula where the orientations of the tallest stereocilia and kinocilia change. [L. *stria,* stripe, + *-ola,* dim. suffix]

strip. **1.** To express the contents from a collapsible tube or canal, such as the urethra, by running the finger along it. SYN milk (4). **2.** Subcutaneous excision of a vein in its longitudinal axis, performed with a stripper. **3.** Any narrow piece, relatively long and of uniform width. [A.S. *strypan,* to rob]

abrasive s., a ribbon-like piece of linen on one side of which is bonded abrasive particles; used in dentistry for contouring and polishing proximal surfaces of restorations.

amalgam s., a linen s. without abrasive used to smooth proximal contours of newly placed amalgam restorations.

celluloid s., a clear plastic s. used as a matrix when inserting a cement or resin in proximal cavity preparations of anterior teeth.

lightning s., a s. of metal with abrasive on one side, used to open rough or improper contacts of proximal restorations.

stripe (strīp). **1.** In anatomy, a streak, line, band, or stria. **2.** In radiography, a linear opacity differing in density from the adjacent parts of the image; usually represents the tangential image of a planar structure such as the pleura or peritoneum. SEE ALSO psoas *margin.* [M.E.]

s. of Gennari, SYN *line* of Gennari.

Hensen s., a band on the undersurface of the membrana tectoria of the cochlear duct.

inner s.'s of renal medulla [TA], the deeper or more central portion of the outer medulla of the kidney, recognizable on sagittal section through the pyramid of a fresh specimen; it is structurally distinct from the outer stripe in that it is traversed by thin as well as thick portions (limbs) of nephron tubules. SYN stria interna medullae renalis [TA].

mallear s., SYN malleolar *stria.*

Mees s.'s, SYN Mees *lines,* under *line.*

occipital s. [TA], SYN *line* of Gennari.

outer s.'s of renal medulla [TA], the more superficial or more peripheral portion of the outer medulla of the kidney, recognizable on sagittal section through the pyramid of a fresh specimen; it is structurally distinct from the outer stripe in that it is traversed by only thick portions (limbs) of nephron tubules. SYN stria externa medullae renalis [TA].

pleural s., SYN pleural *lines,* under *line.*

tracheal wall s., on a chest radiograph, the linear opacity between air in the trachea and in the right upper lobe.

vascular s., SYN *stria* vascularis of cochlear duct.

strip·per.

vein s., an instrument used to remove a vein by tying the vein at one end and pulling it, tearing its branches, and thus, stripping it out of the body.

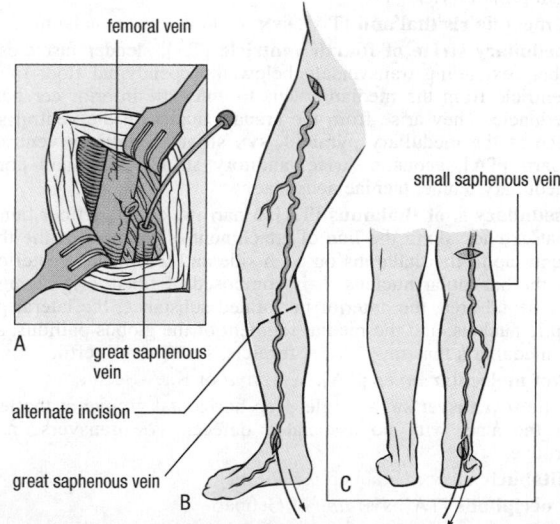

stripping of the saphenous veins: (A) tributaries of saphenous vein ligated, and saphenous vein ligated at the saphenofemoral junction; (B) vein stripper inserted from ankle superiorly to groin, vein is stripped from above downward; (C) small saphenous vein stripped from its junction with popliteal vein to a point posterior to lateral malleolus

strip·ping. Removal, often of a covering.

membrane s., separation of gestational membranes from the lower uterine segment by insertion of a finger through the cervical os, to initiate the Ferguson reflex or prostaglandin release from the decidua and hasten labor.

Strisower. SEE Schellong-Strisower *phenomenon.*

stro·bi·la, pl. **stro·bi·lae** (strō′bi-lă, -lē). A chain of segments, less the scolex and unsegmented neck portion, of a tapeworm; in the monozoic tapeworms (subclass Cestodaria and some members of the subclass Cestoda), it may consist of a single proglottid. [G. *stobilē,* a twist of lint]

stro·bi·lo·cer·cus (strō′bi-lō-ser′kŭs). A taenioid tapeworm larva of the cysticercus type, but with a conspicuous segmented neck, small terminal bladder, and everted scolex; the larval form of *Taenia taeniaeformis,* called *Cysticercus fasciolaris.* [G. *strobilē,* a twist of lint, + *kerkos,* tail]

stro·bi·loid (strō′bi-loyd). Resembling a chain of segments of a tapeworm. [G. *strobilē,* strobile, + *eidos,* resemblance]

stro·bo·scope (strō′bō-skōp). An electronic instrument that produces intermittent light flashes of controlled frequency; used to influence electrical activity of the cerebral cortex.

stro·bo·scop·ic (strō-bō-skop′ik). Pertaining to the illusion of motion, retarded or accelerated, produced by visual images observed intermittently in rapid succession. [G. *strobos,* a twisting around, fr. *strephō,* to twist, + *skopeō,* to view]

stro·bos·co·py (strō-bos′kō-pē). Endoscopy performed with an intermittent light at a frequency that approximates the frequency of movement of the object visualized so that it appears to be motionless; useful in analyzing vocal cord structure and motion.

stroke (strōk). **1.** Any acute clinical event, related to impairment of cerebral circulation, that lasts more than 24 hours. SYN apoplexy, brain attack. **2.** A harmful discharge of lightning, particularly one that affects a human being. **3.** A pulsation. **4.** To pass the hand or any instrument gently over a surface. SEE ALSO stroking. **5.** A gliding movement over a surface. [A.S. *strāc*]

Acute neurologic deficits resulting from circulatory impairment that resolve within 24 hours are called transient ischemic attacks (TIAs); most TIAs last only 15–20 minutes. In contrast, a stroke involves irreversible brain damage, the type and severity of symptoms depending on the location and extent of brain tissue whose circulation has been compromised. The outcome of a stroke varies from minimal impairment to rapid onset of coma followed quickly by death. Stroke ranks third as a cause of death in adults in the U.S., after ischemic heart disease and cancer. About 700,000 people a year experience strokes in this country, and at any given time the population includes about 3 million stroke survivors. The incidence of stroke has gradually declined during the past generation. Risk factors for stroke include hypertension, valvular heart disease, atrial fibrillation, hyperlipidemia, diabetes mellitus, cigarette smoking, and a family history of stroke. In addition, recent studies have shown that elevation of plasma homocysteine, low circulating levels of folic acid and pyridoxine (vitamin B_6), periodontal disease, and chronic bronchitis are all independent risk factors.

Ischemic stroke, which accounts for about 85% of all strokes, is generally caused by atherothrombosis or embolism of a major cerebral artery. Less common causes of ischemic stroke include nonatheromatous vascular disease and coagulation disorders. Severe, acute ischemia in nerve tissue triggers cellular changes (calcium influx, protease activation) that can swiftly cause irreversible damage (infarction). Around the infarct zone lies a so-called penumbra of ischemic, electrically silent tissue that may be salvageable by prompt reperfusion. The mortality of ischemic stroke is 15–30% within the first 30 days. Hemorrhagic stroke, which makes up the other 15%, has a graver prognosis, with a 30-day mortality rate of 40–80%. The diagnostic evaluation of the patient with stroke includes history, physical examination, blood count, blood chemistries, coagulation profile, electrocardiogram, and imaging studies. While cranial CT is the procedure of choice to identify subarachnoid hemorrhage, MRI is a more sensitive indicator of parenchyal hemorrhage as well as of ischemia and infarction. About 20% of persons initially thought to have had a stroke prove to have some other disorder, and as many as 20% of strokes

are missed on initial evaluation by emergency department physicians. Early and aggressive treatment is crucial in limiting damage to brain tissue and achieving an optimal outcome. In ischemic stroke, intravenous administration of tissue plasminogen activator (TPA) within the first 3 hours, with the purpose of dissolving an obstructing thrombus, has been shown to improve overall outcome at 90 days. Limiting factors in the use of thrombolytic therapy are the need to rule out hemorrhagic stroke (sometimes difficult with available imaging methods) and the fact that the therapy itself may induce hemorrhage. Intravenous thrombolytic agents other than TPA are not only less effective but also more likely to cause hemorrhage. In limited studies, intraarterial injection of prourokinase up to 6 hours after stoke onset has favorably influenced outcome. During the acute phase of a stroke, respiratory and circulatory support and attention to fluid and electrolyte balance and nutrition are vitally important. Hypothermia and intravenous administration of heparin and magnesium also improve outcome in selected cases. Long-term consequences may depend on the aggressiveness and persistence of physical therapy and rehabilitation.

Effective measures for the prevention of stroke include aggressive management of hypertension, hyperlipidemia, and diabetes mellitus, cessation of smoking, and chemoprophylaxis in persons at high risk. Administration of aspirin (acetylsalicylic acid) prophylactically inhibits platelet aggregation by suppressing thromboxane A_2. A meta-analysis of randomized controlled trials involving a total of more than 50,000 people indicated that low-dosage aspirin (80–325 mg/day) reduces the risk of ischemic stroke by 39 events per 10,000 persons but increases the risk of hemorrhagic stroke by 12 events per 10,000 persons. Other studies suggest that aspirin at higher dosage (1.3 g/day in divided doses) protects men but not women from ischemic stroke because in women aspirin also suppresses prostacyclin, a natural inhibitor of platelet aggregation. Prophylaxis with other antiplatelet agents (clopidogrel, ticlopidine) is equally effective in men and women and at least as protective as aspirin. In nonvalvular atrial fibrillation, warfarin prophylaxis reduces stroke risk by two-thirds. Most studies show that, in persons with carotid artery stenosis of at least 60%, carotid endarterectomy reduces the risk of stroke. The National Stroke Association has recommended adoption of the term *brain attack* for stroke, by analogy with the familiar *heart attack,* to emphasize to the public both the location of the lesion and the urgency of the need for assessment and treatment. See Also tissue plasminogen activator.

effective s., the rapid forward movement of cilia.

heart s., impact of the apex of the heart against the wall of the chest.

heat s., SEE heatstroke.

recovery s., the slow return movement of cilia.

spinal s., abrupt onset of focal spinal cord dysfunction caused by a disturbance in its blood supply.

sun s., SEE sunstroke.

strok·ing (strōk′ing). The nonverbal fondling and nurturance accorded infants or the nonverbal and verbal forms of acceptance, reassurance, and positive reinforcement accorded to children and adults either by an individual to himself or herself or to another person in order to satisfy a basic biopsychological need of all developing humans; various psychopathologic conditions are believed to result when such s. is absent or faulty.

stro·ma, pl. **stro·ma·ta** (strō′mă, strō′mă-tă). **1.** The framework, usually of connective tissue, of an organ, gland, or other structure, as distinguished from the parenchyma or specific substance of the part. **2.** Aqueous phase of chloroplasts; i.e., chloroplast matrix. **3.** Archaic term for mitochondrial matrix. [G. *strōma,* bed]

s. glan′dulae thyroi′deae, SYN s. of thyroid gland.

s. i′ridis, SYN s. of iris.

s. of iris, the delicate vascular connective tissue that lies between the anterior surface of the iris and the pars iridica retinae. SYN s. iridis.

lymphatic s., the network of reticular fibers and associated reticular cells of lymphatic tissue.

nerve s., the connective tissue supporting structures of peripheral

st

nerve fibers, consisting of endoneurium, perineurium, and epineurium.

s. ova′rii, SYN s. of ovary.

s. of ovary, the fibrous tissue of the medulla of the ovary. SYN s. ovarii.

Rollet s., the colorless s. of the red blood cells.

s. of thyroid gland, the connective tissue that supports the lobules and follicles of the thyroid gland. SYN s. glandulae thyroideae.

s. of vitreous, the delicate framework of the vitreous body embedded in or enclosing the vitrous humor. SYN s. vitreum.

s. vit′reum, SYN s. of vitreous.

stro·mal (strō′măl). Stromatic; relating to the stroma of an organ or other structure. SYN stromic.

stro·ma·tin (strō′mă-tin). An insoluble protein in the stroma of erythrocytes.

stro·ma·tol·y·sis (strō-mă-tol′i-sis). Destruction of the enveloping membrane of a cell, such as a red blood cell. [stroma + G. lysis, dissolution]

strom·ic (strō′mik). SYN stromal.

stro·muhr (strōm′oor). An instrument for measuring the quantity of blood that flows per unit of time through a blood vessel. [Ger. Strom, stream, + Uhr, clock]

Ludwig s., one of the first devices for measuring flow in blood vessels.

thermo-s., SEE thermostromuhr.

Strong, Edward K., Jr., U.S. psychologist, *1884. SEE S. vocational interest *test*.

stron·gyle (stron′jil). Common name for members of the family Strongylidae. [G. strongylos, round]

Stron·gyl·i·dae (stron-jil′i-dē). A family of parasitic nematode worms (order Strongyloidea) including the genera *Strongylus* and *Oesophagostomum*. [see *Strongyloides*]

Stron·gy·loi·dea (stron-ji-loy′dē-ă). A superfamily of strongyle nematode parasites including the genera *Ancyclostoma*, *Necator*, *Ostertagia*, *Haemonchus*, and *Strongylus*, as well as the tapeworms of fowl, the lungworms of carnivores, and some of the most important helminth pathogens of humans and domestic animals. [see *Strongyloides*]

Stron·gy·loi·des (stron-ji-loy′dēz). The threadworm, a genus of small nematode parasites (superfamily Rhabditoidea), commonly found in the small intestine of mammals (particularly ruminants), that are characterized by an unusual life cycle that involves one or several generations of free-living adult worms. Human infection is chiefly by *S. stercoralis*, the small roundworm of man, widespread in all tropical regions, or by *S. fuelleborni*, a parasite of non-human primates in African and Asian tropics and of humans in African tropics. The subspecies *S. fuelleborni kellyi* occurs in New Guinea where it causes widespread infection. Fatal infection in 2-month-old infants, possibly infected by transmammary transmission, produces the condition known locally as swollen belly disease or swollen belly syndrome, which causes grossly distended abdomens, invariably fatal in these infants. Other species include *S. papillosus* in cattle, sheep, and goats, and *S. ransomi* in swine. [G. strongylos, round, + eidos, resemblance]

stron·gy·loi·di·a·sis (stron′ji-loy-dī′ă-sis). Infection with soil-borne nematodes of the genus *Strongyloides*, considered to be a parthenogenetic parasitic female. Larvae passed to the soil develop through four larval instars to form free-living adults or develop from first and second free-living stages into infective third-stage strongyliform or filariform larvae, which penetrate the skin or enter the buccal mucosa via drinking water. Infection can occur by larvae of a new generation developed in the soil (indirect cycle), by infective larvae developed without an intervening adult stage (direct cycle), or by larvae that develop directly in the feces within the intestine of the host, penetrate the mucosa, and pass by blood/lung sputum migration back to the intestine (autoreinfection); most serious human infections and nearly all fatalities result from autoreinfection and subsequent disseminated infection, which commonly follow immunosuppression by steroids, ACTH, or other immunosuppressive agents. Autoreinfection also may develop in patients with AIDS. SYN strongyloidosis.

stron·gy·loi·do·sis (-dō′sis). SYN strongyloidiasis.

stron·gy·lo·sis (stron-ji-lō′sis). Disease caused by infection with a species of the nematode *Strongylus*; effects may be extreme from worm-caused lesions, nodules, and aneurysms.

Stron·gy·lus (stron′ji-loos). The palisade worm, a genus of large strongyle nematodes (subfamily Strongylinae, family Strongylidae) parasitic in horses and other equids, and the cause of strongylosis. [G. strongylos, round]

S. asi′ni, a species that occurs in the large intestine of the ass and other wild equids.

S. edenta′tus, a bloodsucking species occurring in the cecum and colon of the horse, ass, mule, and zebra.

S. equi′nus, a cosmopolitan bloodsucking species found in the cecum and (rarely) colon of horses and other equids.

S. radia′tus, SYN *Cooperia oncophora*.

S. ventrico′sus, SYN *Cooperia oncophora*.

S. vulga′ris, a bloodsucking species found chiefly in the cecum of horses and other equids; in the course of their migration, larvae commonly lodge in the wall of the posterior aorta, causing wall damage and the development of verminous aneurysms in this vessel, especially in the anterior mesenteric arteries.

stron·ti·um (Sr) (stron′shē-ŭm). A metallic element, atomic no. 38, atomic wt. 87.62; one of the alkaline earth series and similar to calcium in chemical and biological properties. Various salts of s. are used therapeutically for their anions; e.g., s. bromide, iodide, lactate. [*Strontian*, a town in Scotland]

stron·ti·um-85 (^{85}Sr). A radioactive strontium isotope with a half-life of 64.84 days; used in bone imaging.

stron·ti·um-87m (^{87m}Sr). A radioactive strontium isotope with a half-life of 2.80 h; used in bone imaging.

stron·ti·um-89 (^{89}Sr). A radioactive strontium isotope; a β emitter with a half-life of 50.52 days; used as a tracer in studies of strontium absorption by the body, strontium incorporation in bone, etc.

stron·ti·um-90 (^{90}Sr). A radioactive strontium isotope; a β emitter with a half-life of 29.1 years; a major component (about 5%) of the uranium fission products; it is incorporated into bone tissue where turnover is slow; used in the therapy of certain eye conditions (e.g., pterygia).

stro·phan·thin (strō-fan′thin). A glycoside or mixture of glycosides from *Strophanthus kombé*; a cardiac tonic, like ouabain (G-s.); extremely toxic.

Stro·phan·thus (strō-fan′thŭs). A genus of vines of east Africa (family Apocynaceae); the dried ripe seeds of *S. kombé* or *S. hispidus* contain the cardiac glycoside strophanthin and were used as an arrow poison; the seeds of *S. gratus* are the botanical source of ouabain. [G. strophos, a twisted cord, + anthos, flower]

stroph·o·ceph·a·ly (strof-ō-sef′ă-lē). Condition characterized by a congenitally distorted head and face, in which there is a tendency toward cyclopia and malformation of the oral region. [G. strophē, a twist, + kephalē, head]

stroph·o·so·mia (strof-ō-sō′mē-ă). Severe form of a congenital ventral fissure, extremely rare in humans. [G. strophē, a twist, + sōma, body]

struc·tura (strook-too′ra). SYN structure.

structurae oculi accessoriae [TA], SYN accessory visual structures, under structure.

struc·tur·al (strŭk′choor-ăl). Relating to the structure of a part; having a structure. SYN anatomical (2).

struc·tur·al·ism (strŭk′choor-ăl-izm). A branch of psychology interested in the basic structure and elements of consciousness.

struc·ture (strŭk′choor). **1.** The arrangement of the details of a part; the manner of formation of a part. **2.** A tissue or formation made up of different but related parts. **3.** In chemistry, the specific connections of the atoms in a given molecule. SYN structura. [L. structura, fr. struo, pp. structus, to build]

accessory s.'s [TA], parts accessory to the main organ or structure. SYN accessory organs (1), adnexa, annexa.

accessory visual s.'s [TA], the eyelids, with lashes and eyebrows, lacrimal apparatus, conjunctival sac, and extrinsic muscles of the eyeball. SYN structurae oculi accessoriae [TA], accessory organs of the eye, accessory visual apparatus, adnexa oculi, appendages of eye, organa oculi accessoria.

brush heap s., haphazard interlocking of fibrils in a gel or hydrocolloid impression material.

chi s., a joint between two DNA duplex molecules. SEE ALSO chi *sequence.*

cointegrate s., a s. of DNA produced by the fusion of two replicons, one possessing a transposon.

complementary s.'s, s.'s that define one another; e.g., the two strands of duplex DNA.

crystal s., the arrangement in space and the interatomic distances and angles of the atoms in crystals, usually determined by x-ray diffraction measurements.

denture-supporting s.'s, the tissues, teeth, and/or residual ridges, which serve as the foundation for removable partial or complete dentures.

fine s., SYN ultrastructure.

gel s., brush heap s. of fibrils giving firmness to hydrocolloids.

Holliday s., SYN Holliday *junction.*

primary s., in a macromolecule, the sequence of subunits that make up that macromolecule; e.g., the amino acid sequence of a protein.

quaternary s., the three-dimensional arrangement and constitution of a multimeric (i.e., a substance containing more than one biopolymer) macromolecule; e.g., the $\alpha_2\beta_2$ tetramer of hemoglobin A.

secondary s., the localized arrangement in space of regions of a biopolymer; often these types of s.'s are regular and recurring along one dimension; e.g., the α-helix often found in proteins.

tertiary s., the three-dimensional configuration of a biopolymer.

tuboreticular s., tubules 20–30 nm in length that lie within cisterns of smooth endoplasmic reticulum; observed in connective tissue diseases such as SLE, and in various cancers and virus infections.

stru·ma, pl. **stru·mae** (stroo′mă, -mē). **1.** SYN goiter. **2.** Formerly, any enlargement of a tissue. [L. a scrofulous tumor, fr. *struo,* to pile up, build]

s. aberra′ta, SYN aberrant *goiter.*

s. colloi′des, SYN colloid *goiter.*

Hashimoto s., SYN Hashimoto *thyroiditis.*

ligneous s., SYN Riedel *thyroiditis.*

s. lymphomato′sa, SYN Hashimoto *thyroiditis.*

s. malig′na, obsolete term for cancer of the thyroid gland.

s. medicamento′sa, goiter due to the use of some therapeutic agent.

s. ova′rii, a rare ovarian tumor, regarded as teratomatous, in which thyroid tissue has surpassed the other elements; occasionally associated with hyperthyroidism.

Riedel s., SYN Riedel *thyroiditis.*

stru·mi·form (stroo′mi-fōrm). Resembling a goiter. [struma + L. *forma,* form]

stru·mi·tis (stroo-mī′tis). Inflammation, with swelling, of the thyroid gland. SEE ALSO thyroiditis. [struma + G. *-itis,* inflammation]

stru·mous (stroo′mŭs). Denoting or characteristic of a struma.

Strümpell, Ernst Adolf von, German physician, 1853–1925. SEE S. *disease, phenomenon, reflex;* Fleischer-Strümpell *ring;* S.-Marie *disease;* Marie-S. *disease.*

Strutt, SEE Rayleigh.

stru·vite (stroo′vīt). The hexahydrate of magnesium ammonium phosphate; found in some renal calculi. Cf. bobierrite, newberyite. [H.C.G. von Struve, Russian diplomat + -ite]

strych·nine (strik′nin, -nēn, -nīn). An alkaloid from *Strychnos nux-vomica;* colorless crystals of intensely bitter taste, nearly insoluble in water. It stimulates all parts of the central nervous system, and was used as a stomachic, an antidote for depressant poisons, and in the treatment of myocarditis. S. blocks the inhibitory neurotransmitter glycine, and thus can cause convulsions. The formerly used salts of s. are s. hydrochloride, s. phosphate, and s. sulfate. It is a potent chemical capable of producing acute or chronic poisoning of humans or animals.

strych·nin·ism (strik′nin-izm). Chronic strychnine poisoning, the symptoms being those that arise from central nervous system stimulation; the first signs are tremors and twitching, progressing to severe convulsions and respiratory arrest.

Strych·nos (strik′nos). A genus of tropical shrubs or trees (family Loganiaceae); most South American species contain chiefly quaternary neuromuscular blocking alkaloids, e.g., curare; the African, Asiatic, and Australian species contain tertiary strychnine-like alkaloids (e.g., strychnine, brucine, and yohimbine-type alkaloids). [G. nightshade]

Stryker, Garold V., U.S. pathologist, *1896. SEE S.-Halbeisen *syndrome.*

Stryker, Homer H., U.S. orthopedic surgeon. SEE S. *frame, saw.*

STSs Abbreviation for sequence-tagged *sites,* under *site.*

Stuart. Surname of a patient in whom the S. or Stuart-Prower *factor* was first discovered.

Stu·dent. Pseudonym for William Sealy Gosset, British statistician, and chemist, 1876–1937. SEE Student's *t test.*

study (stŭd′ē). Research, detailed examination, and/or analysis of an organism, object, or phenomena. [L. *studium,* study, inquiry]

analytic s., in epidemiology, a s. designed to examine associations, commonly putative or hypothesized causal relationships; usually concerned with identifying or measuring the effects of risk factors or with the health effects of specific exposures.

blind s., a s. in which the experimenter is unaware of which group is subject to which procedure.

case control s., an epidemiologic method that begins by identifying persons with the disease or condition of interest (the cases) and compares their past history of exposure to identified or suspected risk factors with the past history of similar exposures among persons who resemble the cases but do not have the disease or condition of interest (the controls).

cohort s., a s. using epidemiologic methods, such as a clinical trial, in which a cohort with a particular attribute (e.g., smokers, recipients of a drug) is followed prospectively and compared for some outcome (e.g., disease, cure) with another cohort not possessing the attribute. SYN follow-up s. (1).

cross-over s., a s. in which the subject is switched from the experimental to the control procedure (or vice versa).

cross-sectional s., a s. in which groups of individuals of different types are composed into one large sample and studied at only a single point in time (e.g., a survey in which all members of a given population, regardless of age, religion, gender, or geographic location, are sampled for a given characteristic or finding in one day). SYN synchronic s.

diachronic s., SYN longitudinal s.

double blind s., a s. in which neither the patients, the experimenter, nor any other assessor of the results, knows which individuals are subject to which procedure, thus helping to ensure that the biases or expectations of either will not influence the results.

ecologic s., epidemiologic s. in which the units of analysis are populations or groups of people rather than individuals.

flow-volume loop s.'s, diagnostic methods in which inspiratory and expiratory flow-volume curves are used to determine the location of an obstruction in the tracheobronchial tree.

follow-up s., (1) SYN cohort s; **(2)** study in which persons exposed to risk or given a designated preventive or therapeutic regimen are observed over a period or at intervals to determine the outcome of the exposure or regimen.

Framingham Heart S., the first major U.S. s. of the epidemiology of cardiovascular disease, begun in Framingham, Massachusetts, in 1948 under the auspices of the National Heart Institute (now the National Heart, Lung, and Blood Institute) and still in operation. Initially the Framingham researchers enrolled over 5000 people between the ages of 30 and 60 to s. the evolution of heart disease and identify risk factors for heart attack. In 1971, offspring of the original study participants began to be enrolled for a second generation of observations.

The Framingham study has had a major impact on the modern understanding of cardiovascular disease and on the prevention and treatment not only of heart attack but also of stroke. During the 1960s, cigarette smoking, elevated cholesterol, hypertension, obesity, and lack of exercise were all statistically confirmed to be risk factors for heart attack. In the succeeding years, the study has provided invaluable information on triglycerides, LDL cholesterol, mitral valve prolapse, heart failure, atrial fibrillation, stroke, diabetes, cardiovascular risk factors in ethnic minorities, and the role of estrogen in preventing heart attack in postmenopausal women. After a half-century, the study continues to provide new clues to the causation and prevention of heart disease and other cardiovascular disorders.

longitudinal s., a s. of the natural course of life or disorder in which a cohort of subjects is serially observed over a period of time and no assumptions need be made about the stability of the system. SYN diachronic s.

multivariate s.'s, the use of statistical techniques for the simultaneous investigations of the influence of several variables.

synchronic s., SYN cross-sectional s.

stump (stŭmp). **1.** The extremity of a limb left after amputation. **2.** The pedicle remaining after removal of the tumor attached to it. [M.e. *stumpe*]

stun (stŭn). To stupefy; to render unconscious by cerebral trauma. [A.S. *stunian,* to make a loud noise]

stupe (stoop). A compress or cloth wrung out of hot water, usually impregnated with turpentine or other irritant, applied to the surface to produce counterirritation. [L. stupa, oakum, tow]

stu·por (stoo′per). A state of impaired consciousness in which the individual shows a marked diminution in reactivity to environmental stimuli and can be aroused only by continual stimulation. [L. fr. *stupeo,* to be stunned]

benign s., a stuporous syndrome from which recovery is the rule, as opposed to malignant s. SYN depressive s.

catatonic s., s. associated with catatonia.

depressive s., SYN benign s.

malignant s., a stuporous condition from which recovery is infrequent, as opposed to benign s.

stu·por·ous (stoo′per-ŭs). Relating to or marked by stupor. SYN carotic.

Sturge, William A., English physician, 1850–1919. SEE S.-Weber *syndrome, disease.*

Sturm, Johann C., 1635–1703. SEE S. *conoid, interval.*

Sturmdorf, Arnold, U.S. gynecologist, 1861–1934. SEE S. *operation.*

stut·ter (stŭt′er). To speak dysfluently; to enunciate certain words with difficulty and with frequent halting and repetition of the initial consonant of a word or syllable. [frequentative of *stut,* from Goth. *stautan,* to strike]

stut·ter·ing (stŭt′er-ing). A phonatory or articulatory disorder, characteristically beginning in childhood, with intense anxiety about the efficiency of oral communications, and characterized by dysfluency: hesitations, repetitions, and prolongations of sounds and syllables, interjections, broken words, circumlocutions, and words produced with excess tension. SYN logospasm (1).

urinary s., frequent involuntary interruption occurring during the act of urination. SYN stammering of the bladder.

sty, stye, pl. **sties, styes** (stī, stīz). SYN *hordeolum* externum.

meibomian s., SYN *hordeolum* internum.

zeisian s., inflammation of one of Zeis glands.

style (stīl). SYN stylet.

sty·let, sty·lette (stī′let, stī-let′). **1.** A flexible metallic rod inserted in the lumen of a flexible catheter to stiffen it and give it form during its passage. **2.** A slender probe. SYN style, stylus (3), stilus. [It. *stilletto,* a dagger; dim. of L. *stilus* or *stylus,* a stake, a pen]

endotracheal s., a rod of malleable metal used to maintain the desired curve of a tube for its insertion into the trachea.

sty·li·form (stī′li-fōrm). SYN styloid. [L. *stilus (stylus)*, a stake, + *forma,* form]

△**stylo-.** Styloid (specifically the styloid process of the temporal bone). [G. *stylos,* pillar, post]

sty·lo·au·ri·cu·la·ris (stī′lō-aw-rik-ū-lā′ris). SEE styloauricular *(muscle)*.

sty·lo·glos·sus (stī′lō-glos′ŭs). Relating to the styloid process and the tongue. SEE styloglossus *(muscle)*.

sty·lo·hy·al (stī-lō-hī′ăl). Relating to the styloid process of the temporal bone and to the hyoid bone. SYN stylohyoid (1).

sty·lo·hy·oid (stī-lō-hī′oyd). **1.** SYN stylohyal. **2.** Relating to the stylohyoid muscle.

sty·loid (stī′loyd). Peg-shaped; denoting one of several slender bony processes. SEE styloid *process* of third metacarpal bone, styloid *process* of temporal bone, styloid *process* of radius, styloid *process* of ulna. SYN styliform. [stylo- + G. *eidos,* resemblance]

sty·loi·di·tis (stī-loy-dī′tis). Inflammation of a styloid process.

sty·lo·la·ryn·ge·us (stī′lō-lar-in-jē′ŭs). SEE *musculus* stylolaryngeus.

sty·lo·man·dib·u·lar (stī′lō-man-dib′ū-lăr). Relating to the styloid process of the temporal bone and the mandible; denoting the stylomandibular ligament. SYN stylomaxillary.

sty·lo·mas·toid (stī′lō-mas′toyd). Relating to the styloid and the mastoid processes of the temporal bone; denoting especially a small artery and a foramen.

sty·lo·max·il·lary (stī′lō-mak′si-lăr-ē). SYN stylomandibular.

sty·lo·pha·ryn·ge·us (stī′lō-far-in-jē′ŭs). SEE stylopharyngeus *(muscle)*.

sty·lo·po·di·um (stī-lō-pō′dē-ŭm). The proximal intermediate segment of the limb skeleton, the humerus and the femur, in the embryo. [stylo- + G. *podion,* small foot]

sty·lo·staph·y·line (stī-lō-staf′i-līn). Relating to the styloid process of the temporal bone and the uvula.

sty·los·te·o·phyte (stī-los′tē-ō-fīt). A peg-shaped bony outgrowth. [G. *stylos,* post, + *osteon,* bone, + *phyton,* growth]

sty·lus, sti·lus (stī′lŭs, stī′lŭs). **1.** Any pencil-shaped structure. **2.** A pencil-shaped medicinal preparation for external application; e.g., a medicated bougie, or a pencil or stick of silver nitrate or other caustic. **3.** SYN stylet. [L. *stilus* or *stylus,* a stake or pen]

stype (stīp). A tampon. [G. *stypē,* tow]

styp·tic (stip′tik). **1.** Having an astringent or hemostatic effect. **2.** An astringent agent used topically to stop bleeding. SYN hemostyptic. [G. *styptikos,* astringent]

styr·a·mate (stī′ră-māt). An orally effective skeletal muscle relaxant with a relatively long duration of action.

sty·rax (stī′raks). SYN storax.

sty·rene (stī′rēn). Phenylethylene; the monomer from which polystyrenes, plastics, and synthetic rubber are made; together with divinylbenzene (for cross-linking), it is the basis of many synthetic ion exchangers. SYN cinnamene, ethenylbenzene, styrol, vinylbenzene.

sty·rol (stī′rol). SYN styrene.

sty·rone (stī′rōn). $C_9H_{10}O$; obtained from storax by distillation with potassium hydroxide; used as a deodorant in 12% glycerin solution, and as a decolorizing agent in histology. SYN cinnamic alcohol.

△**sub-.** Beneath, less than the normal or typical, inferior. Cf. hypo-. [L. *sub,* under]

sub·ab·dom·i·nal (sŭb-ab-dom′i-năl). Below the abdomen.

sub·ab·dom·i·no·per·i·to·ne·al (sŭb-ab-dom′i-nō-per-i-tō-nē′-ăl). Beneath the abdominal, as distinguished from the pelvic, peritoneum. SYN subperitoneoabdominal.

sub·ac·e·tate (sŭb-as′ĕ-tāt). A mixture or complex of a base and its acetate.

sub·a·cro·mi·al (sŭb-ă-krō′mē-ăl). Beneath the acromion process.

sub·a·cute (sŭb-ă-kūt′). Between acute and chronic; denoting the course of a disease of moderate duration or severity.

sub·al·i·men·ta·tion (sŭb′al-i-men-tā′shŭn). A condition of insufficient nourishment. SYN hypoalimentation.

sub·a·nal (sŭb-ā′năl). Below the anus.

sub·a·or·tic (sŭb′ā-ōr′tik). Below the aorta.

sub·ap·i·cal (sŭb-ap'i-kăl). Below the apex of any part.

sub·ap·o·neu·rot·ic (sŭb-ap-ō-noo-rot'ik). Beneath an aponeurosis.

sub·a·rach·noid (sŭb-ă-rak'noyd). Underneath the arachnoid membrane.

sub·ar·cu·ate (sŭb-ar'kū-āt). Slightly arcuate or bowed.

sub·a·re·o·lar (sŭb-ā-rē'ō-lăr). Beneath an areola; especially the areola of the mamma.

sub·as·trag·a·lar (sŭb-as-trag'ă-lăr). Beneath the calcaneus (astragalus).

sub·a·tom·ic (sŭb-ă-tom'ik). Pertaining to particles making up the intraatomic structure; e.g., protons, electrons, neutrons.

sub·au·ral (sŭb-aw'răl). Below the ear.

sub·au·ric·u·lar (sŭb-aw-rik'ū-lăr). Below an auricle; especially the concha or pinna of the ear.

sub·ax·i·al (sŭb-ak'sē-ăl). Below the axis of the body or any part.

sub·ax·il·lary (sŭb-ak'si-lār-ē). Below the axillary fossa. SYN infraaxillary.

sub·bas·al (sŭb-bā'săl). Beneath any base or basal membrane.

sub·brach·y·ce·phal·ic (sŭb-brak-ē-se-fal'ik). Slightly brachycephalic; having a cephalic index of 80.01–83.33.

sub·cal·ca·rine (sŭb-kal'kă-rīn). Below the calcarine fissure; denoting the lingual gyrus.

sub·cal·lo·sal (sŭb-ka-lō'săl). Below the corpus callosum; denoting either the subcallosal gyrus or the fasciculus.

sub·cap·su·lar (sŭb-kap'soo-lăr). Beneath any capsule.

sub·car·bon·ate (sŭb-kar'bon-āt). A mixture or complex of a base and its carbonate.

sub·car·di·nal (sŭb-kar'di-năl). Lying ventral to the anterior or posterior cardinal veins in the embryo.

sub·car·ti·lag·i·nous (sŭb'kar-ti-laj'i-nŭs). 1. Partly cartilaginous. 2. Beneath a cartilage.

sub·ce·cal (sŭb-sē'kăl). Below the cecum; denoting a fossa.

sub·cel·lu·lar (sŭb-sel'ū-lăr). SYN noncellular (1).

sub·cep·tion (sŭb-sep'shŭn). Subliminal perception as in the reaction to a stimulus not fully perceived. SEE subliminal. [sub- + L. -ceptum, perceived]

sub·chlo·ride (sŭb-klōr'īd). The chloride of a series that contains proportionally the greatest amount of the other element in the compound; e.g., s. of mercury is Hg_2Cl_2, whereas chloride or perchloride of mercury is $HgCl_2$.

sub·chon·dral (sŭb-kon'drăl). Beneath or below the cartilages of the ribs.

sub·cho·ri·on·ic (sŭb'kō-rē-on'ik). Beneath the chorion.

sub·cho·roi·dal (sŭb-kō-roy'dăl). Beneath the choroid coat of the eye.

sub·class (sŭb'klas). In biologic classification, a division between class and order.

sub·cla·vi·an (sŭb-klā'vē-an). 1. Beneath the clavicle. SYN infraclavicular. 2. Pertaining to the s. artery or vein.

sub·cla·vic·u·lar (sŭb-kla-vik'ū-lăr). Pertaining to the region beneath the clavicle.

sub·cla·vi·us (sŭb-klā'vē-ŭs). SEE subclavius (muscle).

sub·clin·i·cal (sŭb-klin'i-kăl). Denoting the presence of a disease without manifest symptoms; may be an early stage in the evolution of a disease.

sub·clon·ing (sŭb'klōn-ing). The process by which a DNA clone is cleaved into smaller pieces and recloned; analysis of overlapping regions of these smaller DNA fragments can confirm the entire sequence of the original DNA clone.

sub·col·lat·er·al (sŭb-kŏ-lat'er-ăl). Below the collateral fissure; denoting a cerebral convolution, or gyrus.

sub·con·junc·ti·val (sŭb-kon-jŭnk-tī'văl). Beneath the conjunctiva.

sub·con·junc·ti·vi·tis (sŭb'kon-jŭnk-ti-vī'tis). SYN episcleritis periodica fugax.

sub·con·scious (sŭb-kon'shŭs). 1. Not wholly conscious. 2. Denoting an idea or impression which is present in the mind, but of which there is at the time no conscious knowledge or realization. 3. That part of the mind that is outside conscious awareness.

sub·con·scious·ness (sŭb-kon'shŭs-nes). 1. Partial unconsciousness. 2. The state in which mental processes take place without the conscious perception of the individual.

sub·cor·a·coid (sŭb-kōr'ă-koyd). Beneath the coracoid process.

sub·cor·tex (sŭb-kōr'teks). Any part of the brain lying below the cerebral cortex, and not itself organized as cortex.

sub·cor·ti·cal (sŭb-kōr'ti-kăl). Relating to the subcortex; beneath the cerebral cortex.

sub·cos·tal (sŭb-kos'tăl). 1. Beneath a rib or the ribs. SYN infracostal. 2. Denoting certain arteries, veins, and nerves.

sub·cos·tal·gia (sŭb-kos-tal'jē-ă). Pain in the subcostal region. [subcostal + G. algos, pain]

sub·cos·to·ster·nal (sŭb-kos'tō-ster'năl). Below or beneath the ribs and sternum.

sub·cra·ni·al (sŭb-krā'nē-ăl). Beneath or below the cranium.

sub·crep·i·tant (sub-krep'i-tănt). Nearly, but not frankly, crepitant; denoting a rale.

sub·crep·i·ta·tion (sŭb'krep-i-tā'shŭn). 1. The presence of subcrepitant rales. 2. A sound approaching crepitation in character.

sub·cru·ra·lis (sŭb-kroo-rā'lis). SYN articularis genus (muscle).

sub·cru·re·us (sŭb-kroo-rē-ŭs). SYN articularis genus (muscle). [sub- + L. crus, leg]

sub·cul·ture (sŭb-kŭl'choor). 1. A culture made by transferring to a fresh medium microorganisms from a previous culture; a method used to prolong the life of a particular strain where there is a tendency to degeneration in older cultures. 2. To make a fresh culture with material obtained from a previous one.

sub·cu·ra·tive (sŭb-kūr'ă-tiv). Denoting a dose less than that necessary for a curative effect.

sub·cu·ta·ne·ous (s.c., SQ) (sŭb-koo-tā'nē-ŭs). Beneath the skin. SYN hypodermic (1). [sub- + L. cutis, skin]

sub·cu·tic·u·lar (sŭb-koo-tik'ū-lăr). Beneath the cuticle or epidermis. SYN subepidermal, subepidermic.

sub·cu·tis (sŭb-kū'tis). SYN subcutaneous tissue.

sub·de·lir·i·um (sŭb-dē-lir'ē-ŭm). A rarely used term for a slight or discontinuous delirium.

sub·del·toid (sŭb-del'toyd). Beneath the deltoid muscle; denoting a bursa.

sub·den·tal (sŭb-den'tăl). Beneath the roots of the teeth.

sub·di·a·phrag·mat·ic (sŭb'dī-ă-frag-mat'ik). Beneath the diaphragm. SYN infradiaphragmatic, subphrenic.

sub·dor·sal (sŭb-dōr'săl). Below the dorsal region.

sub·duce, sub·duct (sŭb-doos', sŭb-dŭkt'). To pull or draw downward. [L. sub-duco, pp. -ductus, to lead away]

sub·du·ral (sŭb-doo'răl). Beneath the dura mater or between it and the arachnoid. SEE spatium subdurale.

sub·en·do·car·di·al (sŭb-en-dō-kar'dē-ăl). Beneath the endocardium.

sub·en·do·the·li·al (sŭb'en-dō-thē'lē-ăl). Beneath the endothelium.

sub·en·do·the·li·um (sŭb'en-dō-thē'lē-ŭm). The connective tissue between the endothelium and inner elastic membrane in the intima of arteries.

sub·en·dy·mal (sŭb-en'di-măl). Beneath the endyma, or ependyma. SYN subependymal.

sub·ep·en·dy·mal (sŭb-ep-en'di-mal). SYN subendymal.

sub·ep·en·dy·mo·ma (sŭb-ep-en-di-mō'mă). Discrete lobulated ependymal nodules in the walls of the anterior third or posterior fourth ventricles commonly found at autopsy.

sub·ep·i·der·mal, sub·ep·i·der·mic (sŭb'ep-i-der'măl, -der'mik). SYN subcuticular.

sub·ep·i·the·li·al (sŭb'ep-i-thē'lē-ăl). Beneath the epithelium.

sub·ep·i·the·li·um (sŭb'ep-i-thē'lē-ŭm). Any structure beneath the epithelium.

sub·e·ric ac·id (soo-ber'ik). Used in plastics and in the crosslinking of biopolymers; found in the urine as a product of ω-oxidation of fatty acids. SYN octandioic acid. [L. *suber*, cork oak, + -ic]

su·ber·o·sis (soo-ber-ō'sis). Extrinsic allergic alveolitis caused by inhalation of mold spores from contaminated cork. [L. *suber*, cork, + G. *-osis*, condition]

sub·fam·i·ly (sŭb-fam'i-lē). In biologic classification, a division between family and tribe or between family and genus.

sub·fas·cial (sŭb-fash'ē-ăl). Beneath a fascia.

sub·fer·til·i·ty (sŭb-fer-til'i-tē). Less than normal capacity for reproduction.

sub·fis·sure (sŭb-fish'er). A cerebral fissure beneath the surface, concealed by overlapping convolutions.

sub·fo·li·um (sŭb-fō'lē-ŭm). A secondary division of a cerebellar folium.

sub·gal·late (sŭb-gal'āt). Partially neutralized gallic acid; a basic gallate, such as bismuth s.

sub·gem·mal (sŭb-jem'ăl). Below a gemma or bud (e.g., a taste bud).

sub·ge·nus (sŭb-jē'nŭs). In biologic classification, a division between genus and species.

sub·gin·gi·val (sŭb-jin'ji-văl). Below the gingival margin.

sub·gle·noid (sŭb-glē'noyd). SYN infraglenoid.

sub·glos·sal (sŭb-glos'ăl). Below or beneath the tongue. SYN sublingual.

sub·glot·tic (sŭb-glot'ik). SYN infraglottic.

sub·gran·u·lar (sŭb-gran'oo-lăr). Slightly granular.

sub·grun·da·tion (sŭb-grŭn-dā'shŭn). The depression of one fragment of a broken cranial bone below the other. [sub- + A.S. *grund*, bottom, foundation]

sub·he·pat·ic (sŭb-he-pat'ik). Below the liver. SYN infrahepatic.

sub·hy·a·loid (sŭb-hī'ă-loyd). Beneath, on the vitreous side of, the hyaloid (vitreous) membrane.

sub·hy·oid, sub·hy·oid·e·an (sŭb-hī'oyd, sŭb-hī-oyd'ē-an). SYN infrahyoid.

sub·ic·ter·ic (sŭb-ik'ter-ik). Slightly elevated serum bilirubin without clinical evidence of jaundice. [sub- + G. *ikterikos*, jaundiced]

su·bic·u·lar (soo-bik'ū-lăr, sŭ-bik'). Relating to the subiculum.

su·bic·u·lum, pl. **su·bic·u·la** (soo-bik'ū-lŭm, sŭ-bik'; -lă) [TA]. 1. A support or prop. 2 [TA]. The zone of transition between the parahippocampal gyrus and Ammon horn of the hippocampus. [L. dim. of *subex*, support]

s. promonto'rii [TA], support of the promontory; a bony ridge bounding the fossula fenestrae cochleae posteriorly. SYN ponticulus promontorii.

sub·il·i·ac (sŭb-il'ē-ak). 1. Below the ilium. 2. Relating to the subilium.

sub·il·i·um (sŭb-il'ē-ŭm). The portion of the ilium contributing to the acetabulum.

sub·in·fec·tion (sŭb-in-fek'shŭn). A secondary infection occurring in one exposed to and successfully resisting an epidemic of another infectious disease.

sub·in·flam·ma·to·ry (sŭb-in-flam'ă-tō-rē). Denoting a slightly inflammatory irritation of the tissues.

sub·in·ti·mal (sŭb-in'ti-măl). Beneath the intima.

sub·in·trant (sŭb-in'trant). SYN proleptic. [L. *sub-intro*, pres. p. *-ans*, to enter by stealth]

sub·in·vo·lu·tion (sŭb-in-vō-loo'shŭn). Arrest of the normal involution of the uterus following childbirth with the organ remaining abnormally large.

sub·i·o·dide (sŭb-ī'ō-dīd). That one of a series of iodine compounds with a given cation containing the least iodine; analogous to subchloride.

sub·ja·cent (sŭb-jā'sent). Below or beneath another part. [L. *sub-jaceo*, to lie under]

sub·ject (sŭb'jekt). A person or organism that is the object of research, treatment, experimentation, or dissection. [L. *subjectus*, lying beneath]

sub·jec·tive (sŭb-jek'tiv). 1. Perceived by the individual only and not evident to the examiner; said of certain symptoms, such as pain. 2. Colored by one's personal beliefs and attitudes. Cf. objective (2). [L. *subjectivus*, fr. *subjicio*, to throw under]

sub·jec·tive as·sess·ment da·ta. Those facts presented by the client that show his/her perception, understanding, and interpretation of what is happening.

sub·ju·gal (sŭb-joo'găl). Below the zygomatic (jugal) bone.

sub·king·dom (sŭb-king'dom). In biologic classification, a division between kingdom and phylum.

sub·la·tion (sŭb-lā'shŭn). Detachment, elevation, or removal of a part. [L. *sublatio*, a lifting up]

sub·le·thal (sŭb-lē'thăl). Not quite lethal.

sub·leu·ke·mia (sŭb-loo-kē'mē-ă). SYN subleukemic *leukemia*.

sub·li·mate (sŭb'lim-āt). 1. To perform or accomplish sublimation. 2. Any substance that has been submitted to sublimation. [L. *sublimo*, pp. *-atus*, to raise on high, fr. *sublimis*, high]

corrosive s., SYN mercuric chloride.

sub·li·ma·tion (sŭb-lim-ā'shŭn). 1. The process of converting a solid into a gas without passing through a liquid state; analogous to distillation. 2. In psychoanalysis, an unconscious defense mechanism in which unacceptable instinctual drives and wishes are modified into more personally and socially acceptable channels.

sub·lime (sŭb-līm'). 1. To sublimate. 2. To undergo a process of sublimation.

sub·lim·i·nal (sŭb-lim'i-năl). Below the threshold of perception or excitation; below the limit or threshold of consciousness. [sub- + L. *limen* (*limin-*), threshold]

sub·li·mis (sŭb-lī'mis). 1. At the top. 2. SYN superficialis. [L.]

sub·lin·gual (sŭb-ling'gwăl). SYN subglossal.

sub·lob·u·lar (sŭb-lob'ū-lăr). Beneath a lobule, as of the liver.

sub·lum·bar (sŭb-lŭm'băr). Below the lumbar region.

sub·lu·mi·nal (sŭb-loo'mi-năl). Below or beneath the structure facing the lumen of an organ.

sub·lux·a·tion (sŭb-lŭk-sā'shŭn). An incomplete luxation or dislocation; though a relationship is altered, contact between joint surfaces remains. SYN semiluxation. [sub- + L. *locatio*, luxation (dislocation)]

arytenoid s., SYN arytenoid *dislocation*.

sub·lym·phe·mia (sŭb-lim-fē'mē-ă). An obsolete term for a blood state in which there is a great increase in the proportion of lymphocytes although the total number of white cells is normal. [sub- + L. *lympha*, lymph, + G. *haima*, blood]

sub·mam·ma·ry (sŭb-mam'ă-rē). 1. Deep to the mammary gland. 2. SYN inframammary.

sub·man·dib·u·lar (sŭb-man-dib'ū-lăr). Beneath the mandible or lower jaw. SYN inframandibular, submaxillary (2).

sub·mar·gin·al (sŭb-mar'ji-năl). Near the margin of any part.

sub·max·il·la (sŭb-mak-sil'ă). SYN mandible.

sub·max·il·lary (sŭb-mak'si-lār-ē). 1. SYN mandibular. 2. SYN submandibular.

sub·me·di·al, sub·me·di·an (sŭb-mē'dē-ăl, sŭb-mē'dē-an). Almost, but not exactly in the middle.

sub·mem·bra·nous (sŭb-mem'bră-nŭs). Partly or nearly membranous.

sub·men·tal (sŭb-men'tăl). Beneath the chin.

sub·merged (sŭb-merjd'). In dentistry, describing a field of operation covered by saliva.

sub·met·a·cen·tric (sŭb'met-ă-sen'trik). SEE submetacentric *chromosome*.

sub·mi·cron·ic (sŭb-mī-kron'ik). Smaller than 1 micron in size.

sub·mi·cro·scop·ic (sŭb'mī-krō-skop'ik). Too minute to be visible with a light microscope. SYN amicroscopic, ultramicroscopic.

sub·mor·phous (sŭb-mōr'fŭs). Neither definitely amorphous nor definitely crystalline, denoting the structure of certain calculi.

sub·mu·co·sa (sŭb-moo-kō'să). A layer of tissue beneath a mucous membrane; the layer of connective tissue beneath the tunica mucosa. SYN tela submucosa, tunica submucosa.

sub·mu·cous (sŭb-moo'kŭs). Beneath a mucous membrane.

sub·nar·co·tic (sŭb-nar-kot′ik). Slightly narcotic.

sub·na·sal (sŭb-nā′săl). Under the nose.

sub·na·si·on (sŭb-nā′zē-on). The point of the angle between the septum of the nose and the surface of the upper lip.

sub·neu·ral (sŭb-noo′răl). Below the neural axis.

sub·ni·trate (sŭb-nī′trāt). A basic nitrate; a salt of nitric acid having one or more atoms of the base still capable of combining with the acid.

sub·nor·mal (sub-nōr′măl). Below the normal standard of some quality.

sub·nor·mal·i·ty (sŭb-nōr-mal′i-tē). A subnormal state or condition.

sub·no·to·chor·dal. Lying beneath the notochord.

sub·nu·cle·us (sŭb-noo′klē-ŭs). A secondary nucleus.

sub·oc·cip·i·tal (sŭb-ok-sip′i-tăl). Below the occiput or the occipital bone.

sub·op·ti·mal (sŭb-op′ti-măl). Below or less than the optimum.

sub·or·bit·al (sŭb-ōr′bi-tăl). SYN infraorbital.

sub·or·der (sŭb-ōr′der). In biologic classification, a division between order and family.

sub·ox·i·da·tion (sŭb′oks-i-dā′shŭn). Deficient oxidation.

sub·ox·ide (sŭb-ok′sīd). That one of a series of oxides containing the least oxygen. SYN protoxide.

sub·pa·ri·e·tal (sŭb-pa-rī′ĕ-tăl). Below or beneath any structure called parietal: bone, lobe, layer of a serous membrane, etc.

sub·pa·tel·lar (sŭb-pa-tel′ăr). 1. Deep to the patella. 2. SYN infrapatellar.

sub·pec·to·ral (sŭb-pek′tŏ-răl). Beneath the pectoralis muscle.

sub·pel·vi·per·i·to·ne·al (sŭb-pel′vi-per-i-tō-nē′ăl). Beneath the pelvic, as distinguished from the abdominal, peritoneum. SYN subperitoneopelvic.

sub·per·i·car·di·al (sŭb-per-i-kar′dē-ăl). Beneath the pericardium.

sub·per·i·os·te·al (sŭb-per-ē-os′tē-ăl). Beneath the periosteum.

sub·per·i·to·ne·al (sŭb-per-i-tō-nē′ăl). Beneath the peritoneum.

sub·per·i·to·ne·o·ab·dom·i·nal (sŭb-per-i-tō-nē′ō-ab-dom′i-năl). SYN subabdominoperitoneal.

sub·per·i·to·ne·o·pel·vic (sŭb-per-i-tō-nē′ō-pel′vik). SYN subpelviperitoneal.

sub·pe·tro·sal (sŭb-pe-trō′săl). 1. Denoting the inferior petrosal. 2. Denoting a dural venous sinus.

sub·pha·ryn·ge·al (sŭb-fă-rin′jē-ăl). Below the pharynx.

sub·phren·ic (sŭb-fren′ik). SYN subdiaphragmatic.

sub·phy·lum (sŭb-fī′lŭm). In biologic classification, a division between phylum and class.

sub·pi·al (sŭb-pī′ăl). Beneath the pia mater.

sub·pla·cen·tal (sŭb-pla-sen′tăl). Beneath the placenta; denoting the decidua basalis.

sub·pleu·ral (sŭb-plu′răl). Beneath the pleura.

sub·plex·al (sŭb-plek′săl). Below or beneath any plexus.

sub·pre·pu·tial (sŭb-prē-pū′shē-ăl). Beneath the prepuce.

sub·pu·bic (sŭb-pū′bik). Beneath the pubic arch; denoting a ligament, the arcuate pubic ligament, connecting the two pubic bones below the arch.

sub·pul·mo·nary (sŭb-pŭl′mŏ-nār-ē). Below the lungs.

sub·py·ram·i·dal (sŭb-pi-ram′i-dăl). 1. Below any pyramid; denoting especially the tympanic sinus. 2. Nearly pyramidal in shape.

sub·ret·i·nal (sŭb-ret′i-năl). 1. Between the sensory retina and the retinal pigment epithelium. 2. Between the retinal pigment epithelium and the choroid.

sub·salt (sŭb′salt). A basic salt; a salt in which the base has not been completely neutralized by the acid.

sub·sar·to·ri·al (sŭb-sar-tō′rē-ăl). Beneath the sartorius muscle; denoting a nerve plexus and a fascia.

sub·scap·u·lar (sŭb-skap′ū-lăr). 1. Deep to the scapula. 2. SYN infrascapular.

sub·scap·u·la·ris (sŭb-skap-ū-lā′ris). SEE subscapularis (*muscle*).

sub·scle·ral (sŭb-sklē′răl). Beneath the sclera of the eye, i.e., on the choroidal side of this layer. SYN subsclerotic (1).

sub·scle·rot·ic (sŭb-skle-rot′ik). 1. SYN subscleral. 2. Partly or slightly sclerotic or sclerosed.

sub·scrip·tion (sŭb-skrip′shŭn). The part of a prescription preceding the signature, in which are the directions for compounding. [L. *subscriptio,* fr. *subscribo,* pp. *-scriptus,* to write under, subscribe]

sub·ser·osa [TA]. The layer of connective tissue beneath a serous membrane such as that of the periconeum or pericardium. SYN tela subserosa [TA], subserous layer✶.

sub·se·rous, sub·se·ro·sal (sŭb-sē′rŭs, sŭb-se-rō′săl). Beneath a serous membrane.

sub·sib·i·lant (sŭb-sib′i-länt). Rarely used term denoting a rale with a quality between blowing and whistling.

sub·si·dence (sŭb-sī′dens). Sinking or settling in bone, as of a prosthetic component of a total joint implant.

sub·spi·na·le (sŭb-spi-nā′lē). In cephalometrics, the most posterior midline point on the premaxilla between the anterior nasal spine and the prosthion. SYN point A.

sub·spi·nous (sŭb-spī′nŭs). 1. SYN infraspinous. 2. Tendency to spininess.

sub·stage (sŭb′stāj). An attachment to a microscope, below the stage, supporting the condenser or other accessory.

sub·stance (sŭb′stans). Stuff; material. SYN substantia [TA], matter. [L. *substantia,* essence, material, fr. *sub- sto,* to stand under, be present]

alpha s., SYN reticular s. (1).

anterior perforated s. [TA], a region at the base of the brain through which numerous small branches of the anterior and middle cerebral arteries (lenticulostriate arteries) enter the depth of the cerebral hemisphere; it is bordered medially by the optic chasm and anterior half of the optic tract, rostrally and laterally by the lateral olfactory stria; its anteromedial part corresponds to the olfactory tubercle. SYN substantia perforata anterior [TA], locus perforatus anticus, olfactory area, substantia perforata rostralis.

autacoid s., SYN autocoid.

bacteriotropic s., opsonin or other s. that alters bacterial cells in such a manner that they are more susceptible to phagocytic action.

basophil s., SYN Nissl s.

basophilic s., SYN Nissl s.

blood group s., SYN blood group *antigen.*

blood group-specific s.'s A and B, solution of complexes of polysaccharides and amino acids that reduces the titer of anti-A and anti-B isoagglutinins in serum from group O persons; used to render group O blood reasonably safe for transfusion into persons of group A, B, or AB, but does not affect any incompatibility that results from various other factors, such as Rh.

cementing s., a deposit of amorphous mineralized matrix surrounding the osteons of compact bone.

central gray s., (1) in general: the predominantly small-celled gray matter adjoining or surrounding the central canal of the spinal cord and the third and fourth ventricles of the brainstem; (2) in particular: the thick sleeve of gray matter surrounding the cerebral sylvian aqueduct in the midbrain, rostrally continuous with the posterior nucleus of the hypothalamus; in sections stained for myelin it stands out from the adjoining tectum and tegmentum by the poverty of its myelinated fibers. SYN substantia grisea centralis [TA], periaqueductal gray s.

central and lateral intermediate s.'s, the central gray matter of the spinal cord surrounding the central canal. SYN anterior gray column, Stilling gelatinous s., substantia gelatinosa centralis.

chromidial s., SYN granular endoplasmic *reticulum.*

chromophil s., SYN Nissl s.

compact s., SYN compact *bone.*

controlled s., a s. subject to the Controlled Substances Act (1970), which regulates the prescribing and dispensing, as well as the manufacturing, storage, sale, or distribution of s.'s assigned to five schedules according to their 1) potential for or evidence of abuse, 2) potential for psychic or physiologic dependence, 3)

su

contribution to a public health risk, 4) harmful pharmacologic effect, or 5) role as a precursor of other controlled s.'s.

cortical s., SYN cortical *bone*.

exophthalmos-producing s. (EPS), a factor found in crude extract of pituitary tissue that produced exophthalmos in laboratory animals (especially fish). Its existence and role in producing exophthalmopathy in Graves *disease* is questioned.

filar s., SYN reticular s. (1).

gelatinous s. [TA], the apical part of the posterior horn (dorsal horn; posterior gray column) of the spinal cord's gray matter, composed largely of very small nerve cells; its gelatinous appearance is due to its very low content of myelinated nerve fibers; spinal lamina II (of Rexed). SYN substantia gelatinosa [TA], lamina spinalis II⋆, spinal lamina II⋆, Rolando gelatinous s., Rolando s.

glandular s. of prostate, the glandular tissue of the prostate as distinct from the stroma and capsule. SYN substantia glandularis prostatae.

gray s. [TA], SYN gray *matter*.

ground s., the amorphous material in which structural elements occur; in connective tissue, it is composed of proteoglycans, plasma constituents, metabolites, water, and ions present between cells and fibers. SYN substantia fundamentalis.

H s., designation given by Sir Thomas Lewis to a diffusible s. in skin, indistinguishable in action from histamine, that is liberated by injury and causes the triple response. SYN released s.

innominate s. [TA], the region of the forebrain that lies ventral to the anterior half or so of the lentiform nucleus, extending in the frontal plane from the lateral preopticohypothalamic zone laterally over the optic tract to the amygdala (amygdaloid body); rostrally it tapers off over the dorsal border of the olfactory tubercle, caudally it ends where the internal capsule reaches the surface to form the cerebral peduncle or pes pedunculi. Notable among its polymorphic cell population is the large-celled basal nucleus of Meynert. These magnocellular elements within the i. s. are present in the medial septum and the diagonal band of Broca, but occur in largest numbers ventral to the globus pallidus. Histochemical evidence indicates that magnocellular elements distribute cholinergic fibers widely in the cerebral cortex and that these cells undergo selective degeneration in Alzheimer disease. SYN substantia innominata [TA].

Kendall s., SYN Kendall *compounds*, under *compound*.

s. of lens of eye [TA], that which constitutes the lens of the eye, composed of a nucleus and a cortex and covered by an epithelium. SYN substantia lentis [TA].

medullary s., (1) the lipid material present in the myelin sheath of nerve fibers; SYN Schwann white s. **(2)** medulla of bones and other organs. SYN substantia medullaris (2).

müllerian inhibiting s. (MIS), a 535-amino acid glycoprotein secreted by the Sertoli cells of the testis. It is related to inhibin. SYN anti-müllerian hormone, müllerian inhibiting factor.

muscular s. of prostate, the smooth muscle in the stroma of the prostate. SYN musculus prostaticus, substantia muscularis prostatae.

neurosecretory s., the secretion of nerve cell bodies located in the hypothalamus; the s. is transported by way of hypothalamo-hypophysial tract fibers into the neurohypophysis where the terminals of the nerve fibers contain the secretion. As seen in the fibers and terminals with a light microscope, the s. appears as Herring bodies or hyaline bodies of the pituitary. SEE hyaline *bodies* of pituitary, under *body*.

Nissl s., the material consisting of granular endoplasmic reticulum and ribosomes that occurs in nerve cell bodies and dendrites. SYN basophil s., basophilic s., chromophil s., Nissl bodies, Nissl granules, substantia basophilia, tigroid bodies, tigroid s.

s. P, a peptide neurotransmitter composed of 11 amino acid residues (with the carboxyl group amidated), normally present in minute quantities in the nervous system and intestines of humans and various animals and found in inflamed tissue, that is primarily involved in pain transmission and is one of the most potent compounds affecting smooth muscle (dilation of blood vessels and contraction of intestine) and thus presumed to play a role in inflammation.

periaqueductal gray s., SYN central gray s.

P s. of Lewis, SYN *factor* P.

posterior perforated s. [TA], the bottom of the interpeduncular fossa at the base of the midbrain, extending from the anterior border of the pons forward to the mamillary bodies, and containing numerous openings for the passage of perforating branches of the posterior cerebral arteries. SYN substantia perforata posterior [TA], locus perforatus posticus, Malacarne space.

pressor s., SYN pressor *base*.

proper s., SEE *substantia* propria of cornea, *substantia* propria membranae tympani, *substantia* propria of sclera.

Reichstein s., one of several steroids; e.g., Reichstein s. F (cortisone), Reichstein s. H (corticosterone), Reichstein s. M (cortisol), Reichstein s. Q (cortexone), and Reichstein s. S (cortexolone). SYN Reichstein compound.

released s., SYN H s.

reticular s., (1) a filamentous plasmatic material, beaded with granules, demonstrable by means of vital staining in the immature red blood cells; SYN alpha s., filar mass, filar s., substantia reticularis (1), substantia reticulofilamentosa. **(2)** SYN reticular *formation*.

Rolando gelatinous s., Rolando s., SYN gelatinous s.

Schwann white s., SYN medullary s. (1).

slow-reacting s. (SRS), slow-reacting s. of anaphylaxis (SRS-A), a liproprotein of low molecular weight composed of leucotrienes that is released in anaphylactic shock and produces slower and more prolonged contraction of muscle than does histamine; it is active in the presence of antihistamines (but not epinephrine) and seems not to occur preformed in mast cells, but as a result of an antigen-antibody reaction on the granules; it induces the effect observed in anaphylactic reactions. Cf. peptidyl *leukotrienes*. SYN slow-reacting factor of anaphylaxis.

soluble specific s. (SSS), SYN specific capsular s.

specific capsular s., a soluble type-specific polysaccharide produced during active growth of virulent pneumococci comprising a large part of the capsule. SYN pneumococcal polysaccharide, soluble specific s., specific soluble polysaccharide, specific soluble sugar.

spongy s., SYN *substantia* spongiosa.

standard s., a pure, authentic s. used for identification purposes.

Stilling gelatinous s., SYN central and lateral intermediate s.'s.

threshold s., any material (e.g., glucose) that is excreted in the urine only when its plasma concentration exceeds a certain value, termed its threshold. SYN threshold body.

tigroid s., SYN Nissl s.

vasodepressor s., an incompletely characterized chemical, apparently produced during liver damage, that tends to decrease vascular pressures and relax arterial walls.

white s., SYN white *matter*.

zymoplastic s., SYN thromboplastin.

sub·stan·tia, pl. **sub·stan·ti·ae** (sŭb-stan′shē-ă, -shē-ē) [TA]. SYN substance. [L.]

s. adamanti′na, SYN enamel.

s. al′ba, SYN white *matter*.

basal s. [TA], basal structures associated with the amygdaloid complex and its connections; includes the basal nucleus [TA] (nucleus basalis [TA]) also called the nucleus of Ganser, the sublenticular extended nucleus [TA] (pars sublenticularis amygdalae [TA]), and bed nucleus of the stria terminalis [TA] (nucleus stria terminalis [TA]). SYN s. basalis [TA].

s. basalis [TA], SYN basal s.

s. basophi′lia, SYN Nissl *substance*.

s. cine′rea, SYN gray *matter*.

s. compac′ta [TA], SYN compact *bone*.

s. compac′ta os′sium, SYN compact *bone*.

s. cortica′lis [TA], SYN cortical *bone*.

s. ebur′nea, SYN dentine.

s. ferrugin′ea, SYN *locus* caeruleus.

s. fundamenta′lis, SYN ground *substance*.

s. gelatino′sa [TA], SYN gelatinous *substance*.

s. gelatino′sa centra′lis, SYN central and lateral intermediate *substances,* under *substance.*

s. glandula′ris pros′tatae, SYN glandular *substance* of prostate.

s. gris′ea [TA], SYN gray *matter.*

s. gris′ea centra′lis [TA], SYN central gray *substance.*

s. innomina′ta [TA], SYN innominate *substance.*

s. interme′dia centra′lis [TA], SEE central and lateral intermediate *substances,* under *substance.*

s. intermedia lateralis [TA], SYN lateral intermediate *substance;* SEE central and lateral intermediate *substances,* under *substance.*

s. len′tis [TA], SYN *substance* of lens of eye.

s. medulla′ris, (1) SYN medulla; (2) SYN medullary *substance.*

s. muscula′ris prosta′tae, SYN muscular *substance* of prostate.

s. ni′gra [TA], a large cell mass, crescentic on transverse section, extending forward over the dorsal surface of the crus cerebri from the rostral border of the pons into the subthalamic region; it is composed of a dorsal stratum of closely spaced pigmented (i.e., melanin-containing) cells, the pars compacta [TA], a larger ventral region of widely scattered cells, the pars reticulata [TA], and smaller less distinct regions, the pars lateralis [TA] and pars retrorubralis [TA], the pars compacta in particular includes numerous cells that project forward to the striatum (caudate nucleus and putamen) and contain dopamine, which acts as the transmitter at their synaptic endings; other, apparently nondopaminergic cells of the s. nigra project to a rostral part of the ventral nucleus of thalamus, to the middle layers of the superior colliculus, and to restricted parts of the reticular formation of the midbrain; the nigrostriatal projection is reciprocated by a massive striatonigral fiber system with multiple neurotransmitters, chief among which is γ-aminobutyric acid (GABA); s. n. receives smaller afferent projections from the subthalamic nucleus, the lateral segment of the globus pallidus, the dorsal nucleus of the raphe, and the pedunculopontine nucleus of the midbrain. The pars reticulata forms part of the output system for the striate body. The s. n. is involved in the metabolic disturbances associated with Parkinson disease and Huntington disease. SYN locus niger, nucleus niger, Soemmerring ganglion.

s. os′sea den′tis, SYN cement (1).

s. perfora′ta ante′rior [TA], SYN anterior perforated *substance.*

s. perforata rostralis, SYN anterior perforated *substance.*

s. perfora′ta poste′rior [TA], SYN posterior perforated *substance.*

s. propria of cornea, proper substance of cornea, modified transparent connective tissue, between the layers of which are open spaces or lacunae nearly filled with the corneal cells or corpuscles. SYN s. propria corneae.

s. pro′pria cor′neae, SYN s. propria of cornea.

s. pro′pria membra′nae tym′pani, proper substance of tympanic membrane, the layer of radial and circular collagenous fibers of the tympanic membrane.

s. propria of sclera [TA], proper substance of the sclera, the dense white fibrous tissue arranged in interlacing bundles that forms the main mass of the sclera, continuous anteriorly with the substantia propria of the cornea. SYN s. propria sclerae [TA].

s. pro′pria scle′rae [TA], SYN s. propria of sclera.

s. reticula′ris, (1) SYN reticular *substance* (1); (2) SYN reticular *formation.*

s. reticulofilamento′sa, SYN reticular *substance* (1).

s. spongio′sa [TA], bone in which the spicules or trabeculae form a three-dimensional latticework (cancellus) with the interstices filled with embryonal connective tissue or bone marrow. SYN spongy bone (1) [TA], s. trabecularis✶, trabecular bone✶, cancellous bone, spongy substance.

s. trabecula′ris, ✶official alternate term for s. spongiosa.

s. vit′rea, SYN enamel.

sub·ster·nal (sŭb-ster′năl). 1. Deep to the sternum. 2. SYN infrasternal.

sub·ster·no·mas·toid (sŭb-ster′nō-mas′toyd). Beneath the sternomastoid muscle; denoting a group of deep cervical lymph nodes.

sub·sti·tute (sŭb′sti-toot). 1. Anything that takes the place of another. 2. In psychology, a surrogate.

blood s., any material (e.g., human plasma, serum albumin, or a solution of such substances as dextran) used for transfusion in hemorrhage and shock.

plasma s., a solution of a substance (e.g., dextran) used for transfusion in hemorrhage or shock as a s. for plasma. SYN plasma expander.

volume s., infusion of cell-free or volume-expanding fluids such as dextran for replacement of fluid lost from the circulation as part of the prevention or treatment of circulatory shock.

sub·sti·tu·tion (sŭb-sti-too′shŭn). 1. In chemistry, the replacement of an atom or group in a compound by another atom or group (e.g., s. of H by Cl in CH_4 to give CH_3Cl). 2. In psychoanalysis, an unconscious defense mechanism by which an unacceptable or unattainable goal, object, or emotion is replaced by one that is more acceptable or attainable; the process is more acute and direct, and less subtle, than sublimation. [L. *substitutio,* to put in place of another]

generic s., the dispensing of a chemically equivalent, less expensive drug in place of a brand-name product that has an expired patent.

stimulus s., SYN classical *conditioning.*

symptom s., an unconscious psychological process by which a repressed impulse is indirectly manifested through a particular symptom, e.g., anxiety, compulsion, depression, hallucination, obsession. SYN symptom formation.

sub·strate (**S**) (sŭb′strāt). 1. The substance acted upon and changed by an enzyme; the reactant considered to be attacked in a chemical reaction. 2. The base on which an organism lives or grows; e.g., the s. on which microorganisms and cells grow in cell culture. [L. *sub-sterno,* pp. *-stratus,* to spread under]

insulin receptor s.-1, a cytoplasmic protein that is a direct substrate of the activated insulin receptor kinase. Insulin exposure results in its rapid phosphorylation at multiple tyrosine residues. Its phosphorylated sites associate with high affinity to certain cellular proteins. IRS-1 thus acts as an adaptor molecule that links the receptor kinase to various cellular activities regulated by insulin. IRS-1 is also phosphorylated after stimulation by insulinlike growth factor-1 and several interleukins.

suicide s., a competitive inhibitor that is converted to an irreversible inhibitor at the active site of the enzyme. SYN mechanism-based inhibitor, suicide inhibitor.

sub·stra·tum (sŭb-strā′tŭm). Any layer or stratum lying beneath another. [L. see substrate]

sub·struc·ture (sŭb-strŭk′choor). A tissue or structure wholly or partly beneath the surface.

implant denture s., the metal framework which is placed beneath the soft tissues in contact with, or embedded into, bone for the purpose of supporting an implant denture superstructure.

sub·sul·fate (sŭb-sŭl′fāt). A basic sulfate; a sulfate that contains some base unneutralized and still capable of combining with the acid.

sub·tar·sal (sŭb-tar′săl). Below the tarsus.

sub·ten·to·ri·al (sŭb-ten-tō′rē-ăl). Beneath the tentorium cerebelli.

sub·ter·mi·nal (sŭb-ter′mi-năl). Situated near the end or extremity of an oval or rod-shaped body.

sub·te·tan·ic (sŭb-te-tan′ik). Denoting tonic muscular spasms or convulsions that are not entirely sustained but have brief remissions.

sub·tha·lam·ic (sŭb-thă-lam′ik). Related to the subthalamus region or to the subthalamic nucleus.

sub·thal·a·mus (sŭb-thal′ă-mŭs) [TA]. That part of the diencephalon that lies wedged between the thalamus on the dorsal side and the cerebral peduncle ventrally, lateral to the dorsal half of the hypothalamus from which it cannot be sharply delineated. It is composed of the subthalamic nucleus (corpus luysi), the zona incerta, and the fields of Forel; laterally it expands in a winglike fashion into the reticular nucleus of the thalamus; caudally it is continuous with the midbrain tegmentum. SYN ventral thalamus.

sub·thy·roid·e·us (sŭb-thī-royd′ē-ŭs). A muscular bundle formed of fibers derived from the thyroarytenoid and vocalis muscles.

su

sub·til·i·sin (sŭb-ti-lī′sin). A proteinase formed by *Bacillus subtilis* and other species, similar to the serine proteinases of other molds and bacteria; it catalyzes the hydrolysis of a few specific peptide bonds in certain proteins, converting chymotrypsinogen to chymotrypsin and ovalbumin to plakalbumin in this manner, and cleaves pancreatic ribonuclease into S-peptide and S-protein. SYN subtilopeptidase.

sub·ti·lo·pep·ti·dase (sŭb′ti-lō-pep′ti-dās). SYN subtilisin.

sub·trac·tion (sŭb-trak′shŭn). A technique used to enhance detectability of opacified anatomic structures on radiographic or scintigraphic images; a negative of an image made before introduction of contrast medium or radionuclide is photographically or electronically removed from a later image; commonly used in cerebral angiography. SEE ALSO digital subtraction *angiography*, mask.

energy s., digital radiography using higher- and lower-energy exposures, either by double exposure at 2-kV levels or by interposing a copper filter that absorbs the lower-energy photons between two phosphor plates, with computer calculation of high-Z and low-Z images (bone and soft tissues, respectively); makes use of the fact that lower-energy x-rays are absorbed by more high-Z substances, such as calcium and copper, because of the photoelectric *effect*. SEE ALSO Z, photoelectric *effect*, phosphor *plate*.

sub·tra·pe·zi·al (sŭb-tra-pē′zē-ăl). Beneath the trapezius muscle; denoting a nerve plexus.

sub·tribe (sŭb-trīb). In biologic classification, a division between tribe and genus.

sub·tro·chan·ter·ic (sŭb-trō-kan-ter′ik). Below any trochanter.

sub·troch·le·ar (sŭb-trok′lē-ar). Below any trochlea.

sub·tu·ber·al (sŭb-too′ber-ăl). Lying below any tuber.

sub·tym·pan·ic (sŭb-tim-pan′ik). Below the tympanic cavity.

sub·um·bil·i·cal (sŭb-ŭm-bil′i-kăl). SYN infraumbilical.

sub·un·gual, sub·un·gui·al (sŭb-ŭng′gwăl, sŭb-ŭng′gwi-ăl). Beneath the finger or toe nail. SYN hyponychial (1). [L. *unguis*, nail]

sub·u·nit (sŭb′oo-nit). 1. A unit that forms a distinct part of a larger structure. SEE ALSO monomer. 2. The single protein or polypeptide chain that can be separated from an oligomer protein without cleaving covalent bonds other than disulfide bridges between cysteinyl residues. 3. A single biopolymer separated from a larger multimeric structure.

sub·u·re·thral (sŭb-ū-rē′thrăl). Beneath the male or female urethra.

sub·vag·i·nal (sŭb-vaj′i-năl). 1. Below the vagina. 2. On the inner side of any tubular membrane serving as a sheath.

sub·val·var, sub·val·vu·lar (sŭb-val′văr, sŭb-val′vū-lăr). Below any valve.

sub·ver·te·bral (sŭb-ver′tĕ-brăl). Beneath, or on the ventral side, of a vertebra or the vertebral column.

sub·vir·ile (sŭb-vir′il). Deficient in virility.

sub·vir·ion (sub-vir′ē-on). An incomplete viral particle. [sub- + virion]

sub·vit·ri·nal (sŭb-vit′ri-năl). Beneath the vitreous body.

sub·wak·ing (sŭb-wāk′ing). Denoting the mental state between sleeping and waking.

sub·zon·al (sŭb-zō′năl). Below or beneath any zona or zone, such as the zona radiata or zona pellucida.

sub·zy·go·mat·ic (sŭb-zī-gō-mat′ik). Below or beneath the zygomatic bone or arch.

suc·ca·gogue (sŭk′ă-gog). 1. Stimulating the flow of juice. 2. An agent having such an effect. [L. *succus*, juice, + G. *agōgos*, leading]

suc·ce·da·ne·ous (sŭk-sē-dā′nē-ŭs). 1. Relating to a succedaneum. 2. Relating to the permanent or second teeth that replace the deciduous or primary teeth. [see succedaneum]

suc·ce·da·ne·um (sŭk-sē-dā′nē-ŭm). A substitute; a drug or any therapeutic agent that has the properties of and can be used in place of another. [L. *succedaneus*, following after, substituting, fr. *suc-cedo*, to follow, to take the place of, fr. *sub*, under, + *cedo*, to go]

suc·cen·tu·ri·ate (sŭk-sen-tū′rē-āt). In anatomy, substituting for, or accessory to, some organ. [L. *suc-centurio*, pp. -*atus*, to substitute]

suc·ci·nate (sŭk′si-nāt). A salt of succinic acid.

active s., SYN succinyl-coenzyme A.

s. dehydrogenase, a flavoenzyme that catalyzes the removal of hydrogen from succinic acid and converts it into fumaric acid; e.g., s. + FAD ↔ fumarate + FADH$_2$; this complex is a part of the tricarboxylic acid cycle. SYN fumarate reductase (NADH), fumaric hydrogenase.

suc·ci·nate sem·i·al·de·hyde (sŭk′sin-āt sem-ē-ăl-dē -hīd). An intermediate in the catabolism of γ-aminobutyrate.

s. s. dehydrogenase, an enzyme that catalyzes the reaction of s. s. and either NAD$^+$ or NADP$^+$ to form succinate and NADH (or NADPH); a deficiency of this enzyme is associated with 4-hydroxybutyric aciduria.

suc·cin·ic ac·id (sŭk-sin′ik). An intermediate in the tricarboxylic acid cycle; several of its salts have been variously used in medicine.

suc·cin·ic thi·o·ki·nase. SYN *succinyl-CoA* synthetase.

suc·cin·i·mide (suk′sin-ă-mīd). Chemical class of drugs from which the antiepileptic agents ethosuximide, methsuximide, and phensuximide are derived. Unsubstituted s. has been used as an antiurolithic.

suc·ci·nyl·ac·e·tone (sŭk′sin-il-ăs′e-tōn). A minor metabolite that is elevated in individuals with tyrosinemia IA.

***N*-suc·cin·yl·ad·en·yl·ic ac·id** (sŭk-sin-il-ăd-ē-nil′ik). SYN adenylosuccinic acid.

suc·ci·nyl·cho·line (sŭk′si-nil-kō′lēn). A neuromuscular relaxant with short duration of action which characteristically first depolarizes the motor endplate (phase I block) but which is often later associated with a curare-like, nondepolarizing neuromuscular block (phase II block); used to produce relaxation for tracheal intubation and during surgical anesthesia. SYN diacetylcholine, suxamethonium.

suc·ci·nyl-CoA (sŭk′sin-il). SYN succinyl-coenzyme A.

s.-CoA synthetase, (1) a ligase reversibly reacting succinate and CoA with ATP to produce ADP, inorganic phosphate, and s.-CoA; **(2)** a similar synthetase, but one able to use itaconate as well as succinate and GTP (or ITP) in place of ATP; a part of the tricarboxylic acid cycle. SYN succinic thiokinase, succinyl-CoA ligase.

suc·ci·nyl-CoA li·gase. SYN *succinyl-CoA* synthetase.

suc·ci·nyl-co·en·zyme A (sŭk′si-nil-kō-en′zīm). The condensation product of succinic acid and CoA; one of the intermediates of the tricarboxylic acid cycle and a precursor in the synthesis of heme. SYN active succinate, succinyl-CoA.

suc·ci·nyl·di·cho·line (sŭk′si-nil-dī-kō′lēn). Succinylcholine chloride.

***O*-suc·ci·nyl·ho·mo·ser·ine (thi·ol)-ly·ase** (sŭk′si-nil-hō′mō-ser′ēn). An enzyme catalyzing the reaction between cystathionine and succinate to form L-cysteine and *O*-succinyl-L-homoserine. SYN cystathionine γ-synthase.

suc·ci·nyl·sul·fa·thi·a·zole (sŭk′si-nil-sŭl′fă-thī′ă-zōl). The most effective of the poorly absorbed bacteriostatic sulfonamides used for sterilization of the intestinal tract.

suc·ci·sul·fone im·i·no·di·eth·a·nol (sŭk-si-sŭl′fōn). An antimicrobial agent.

suc·cor·rhea (sŭk-ō-rē′ă). An abnormal increase in the secretion of a digestive fluid. [L. *succus*, juice, + G. *rhoia*, a flow]

suc·cu·bus (sŭk′ū-bŭs). A demon, in female form, believed to have sexual intercourse with a man during sleep. Cf. incubus. [L. *succubo*, to lie under]

suc·cuss (sŭ-kŭs′). To make succussion.

suc·cus·sion (sŭ-kŭsh′ŭn). A diagnostic procedure that consists in shaking the body so as to elicit a splashing sound in a cavity containing both gas and fluid. [L. *sucussio*, fr. *suc-cutio* (*subc*-), pp. -*cussus*, to shake up, fr. *quatio*, to shake]

hippocratic s., a splashing noise produced by shaking the body when there is gas or air and fluid in the stomach or intestine, or free in the peritoneum, thorax, and, rarely, the pericardium.

suck (sŭk). **1.** To draw a fluid through a tube by exhausting the air in front. **2.** To draw a fluid into the mouth; specifically, to draw milk from the breast. [A.S. *sūcan*]

suck·le (sŭk′l). **1.** To nurse; to feed by milk from the breast. **2.** To suck; to draw sustenance from the breast.

Sucquet, J.P., French anatomist, 1840–1870. SEE S. *anastomoses,* under *anastomosis, canals,* under *canal;* S.-Hoyer *anastomoses,* under *anastomosis, canals,* under *canal.*

su·cral·fate (soo-kral′fāt). Sucrose octakis (hydrogen sulfate) aluminum complex; a polysaccharide with antipeptic activity, used to treat duodenal ulcers by providing a protective coating to allow healing.

su·crase (soo′krās). SYN sucrose α-D-glucohydrolase.

su·crate (soo′krāt). A compound of sucrose.

su·crose (soo′krōs). A nonreducing disaccharide made up of D-glucose and D-fructose obtained from sugar cane, *Saccharum officinarum* (family Gramineae), from several species of sorghum, and from the sugar beet, *Beta vulgaris* (family Chenopodiaceae); the common sweetener, used in pharmacy in the manufacture of syrup, confections, etc. SYN saccharose, saccharum.

s. octaacetate, an alcohol denaturant.

su·crose α-D-glu·co·hy·dro·lase. An enzyme hydrolyzing sucrose and maltose in a complex with isomaltase; hence, it hydrolyzes both sucrose and isomaltose; found in the intestinal mucosa; a deficiency of this enzyme results in defective digestion of sucrose and linear α1,4-glucans. SYN sucrase.

su·cro·se·mia (soo-krō-sē′mē-ă). The presence of sucrose in the blood. [sucrose + G. *haima,* blood]

su·cro·su·ria (soo-krō-soo′rē-ă). The excretion of sucrose in the urine. [sucrose + G. *ouron,* urine]

suc·tion (sŭk′shŭn). The act or process of sucking. SEE ALSO aspiration (1), aspiration (2). [L. *sugo,* pp. *suctus,* to suck]

posttussive s., a s. sound heard on auscultation over a pulmonary cavity at the end of a cough.

Wangensteen s., a modified siphon that maintains constant negative pressure, used with a duodenal tube for the relief of gastric and intestinal distention. SYN Wangensteen tube.

suc·to·ri·al (sŭk-tō′rē-ăl). Relating to suction, or the act of sucking; adapted for sucking.

su·da·men, pl. **su·dam·i·na** (soo-dā′men, -dam′i-nă). A minute vesicle due to retention of fluid in a sweat follicle, or in the epidermis. [Mod. L., fr. L. *sudo,* to sweat]

su·dam·i·na (soo-dam′i-nă). **1.** Plural of sudamen. **2.** SYN *miliaria crystallina.*

Su·dan III [C.I. 26100]. A red stain, used for neutral fat in histologic technique; it also stains the fatty envelope of the tubercle bacillus. SYN Sudan red III.

Su·dan IV [C.I. 26105]. SYN scarlet red.

Su·dan black B [C.I. 26150]. A diazo dye, used as a stain for fats.

Su·dan brown [C.I. 12020]. A brown stain, derived from α-naphthylamine and used as a stain for fats.

su·dan·o·phil·ia (soo-dan-ō-fil′ē-ă). **1.** Affinity for an oil-soluble or Sudan dye. **2.** A condition in which leukocytes contain minute fat droplets that take a brilliant red stain when treated with 0.2% Sudan III and 0.1% cresyl blue in absolute alcohol.

su·dan·o·phil·ic (soo-dan-ō-fil′ik). Staining easily with Sudan dyes, usually referring to lipids in tissues.

su·dan·o·pho·bic (soo-dan-ō-fō′bik). Denoting tissue that fails to stain with a Sudan or fat-soluble dye.

Su·dan red III. SYN Sudan III.

Su·dan yel·low. Metadioxyazobenzene; a yellow stain for fats.

su·da·tion (soo-dā′shŭn). SYN perspiration (1). [L. *sudatio,* fr. *sudo,* pp. *-atus,* to sweat]

Sudeck, Paul H.M., German surgeon, 1866–1938. SEE S. *atrophy,* critical *point, syndrome.*

su·do·mo·tor (soo-dō-mō′ter). Denoting the autonomic (sympathetic) nerves that stimulate the sweat glands to activity. [L. *sudor,* sweat, + *motor,* mover]

su·dor (soo′dōr). SYN perspiration (3). [L.]

s. anglicus, SYN English sweating *disease.*

△**sudor-.** Sweat, perspiration. [L. *sudor*]

su·do·re·sis (soo-dō-rē′sis). Profuse sweating. [sudor- + G. *-ēsis,* condition]

su·do·rif·er·ous (soo-dō-rif′er-ŭs). Carrying or producing sweat. [sudor- + L. *fero,* to bear]

su·do·rif·ic (soo-dō-rif′ik). Causing sweat. [sudor- + L. *facio,* to make]

su·do·rom·e·ter (soo-dō-rom′ĕ-ter). An instrument for measuring the amount of perspiration. [sudor- + G. *metron,* measure]

su·dor·rhea (soo-dō-rē′ă). SYN hyperhidrosis. [sudor- + G. *rhoia,* a flow]

su·et (soo′et). The hard fat around the kidneys of cattle and sheep; when rendered it yields tallow.

prepared s., the internal fat of the abdomen of the sheep, *Ovis aries,* purified by melting and straining; formerly used in pharmacy in making ointments. SYN prepared mutton tallow.

su·fen·ta·nil cit·rate (soo-fen′tă-nil). An injectable narcotic with short duration of effect resembling fentanil; used in "balanced anesthesia."

suf·fo·cate (sŭf′ō-kāt). **1.** To impede respiration; to asphyxiate. **2.** To be unable to breathe; to suffer from asphyxiation. [L. *suffoco (subf-),* pp. *-atus,* to choke, strangle]

suf·fo·ca·tion (sŭf-ō-kā′shŭn). The act or condition of suffocating or of asphyxiation.

suf·fu·sion (sŭ-fū′zhŭn). **1.** The act of pouring a fluid over the body. **2.** A reddening of the surface. **3.** The condition of being wet with a fluid. **4.** SYN extravasate (2). [L. *suffusio,* fr. *suffundo (subf-),* to pour out]

sug·ar (shu-ger). One of the sugars, q.v., pharmaceutical forms are compressible s. and confectioner's s. SEE ALSO sugars. [G. *sakcharon;* L. *saccharum*]

amino s.'s, s.'s in which a hydroxyl group has been replaced with an amino group; e.g., D-glucosamine.

beechwood s., D-xylose. SEE xylose.

beet s., D-sucrose. SEE sucrose.

blood s., SEE D-glucose.

brain s., D-galactose. SEE galactose.

cane s., D-sucrose. SEE sucrose.

corn s., SEE D-glucose.

deoxy s., a s. containing fewer oxygen atoms than carbon atoms and in which, consequently, one or more carbons in the molecule lack an attached hydroxyl group. SYN desoxy s.

desoxy s., SYN deoxy s.

fruit s., D-fructose. SEE fructose.

gelatin s., SYN glycine.

grape s., SEE D-glucose.

invert s., a mixture of equal parts of D-glucose and D-fructose produced by hydrolysis of sucrose (inversion).

s. of lead, SYN lead acetate.

malt s., SYN maltose.

manna s., SYN mannitol.

maple s., sucrose extracted from the sap of the sugar maple, *Acer saccharinum.* SYN saccharum canadense.

milk s., SYN lactose.

oil s., SYN oleosaccharum.

pectin s., D-arabinose. SEE arabinose.

reducing s., a s., such as glucose in the urine, that has the property of reducing various inorganic ions, notably cupric ion to cuprous ion.

specific soluble s., SYN specific capsular *substance.*

starch s., SEE D-glucose.

wood s., D-xylose. SEE xylose.

sug·ar ac·ids. Acids, such as gluconic, glycuronic, and saccharic acid, produced by the oxidation of glucose.

sug·ar al·co·hol. The polyalcohol resulting from the reduction of the carbonyl group in a monosaccharide to a hydroxyl group.

sug·ar al·de·hyde. A sugar that contains an internal acetal.

sug·ars (shug′erz). Those carbohydrates (saccharides) having the

su

general composition $(CH_2O)_n$ and simple derivatives thereof. Although the simple monomeric s. (glycoses) are often written as polyhydroxy aldehydes or ketones, e.g., $HOCH_2$–$(CHOH)_4$–CHO for aldohexoses (e.g., glucose) or $HOCH_2$–$(CHOH)_3$–CO–CH_2OH for 2-ketoses (e.g., fructose), cyclization can give rise to varied structures as described below. S.'s are generally identifiable by the ending -ose or, if in combination with a nonsugar (aglycon), -oside or -osyl. S. especially D-glucose, are the chief source of energy by oxidation in nature, and they and their derivatives (e.g., D-glucosamine, D-glucuronic acid), in polymeric form, are major constituents of mucoproteins, bacterial cell walls, and plant structural material (e.g., cellulose). S. are often found in combination with steroids (steroid glycosides) and other aglycons.

Fischer projection formulas of s., representations, by projection, of cyclic s., or derivatives thereof, in which the carbon chain is depicted vertically. The lowest-numbered asymmetric carbon atom (C-1 in aldoses; C-2 in 2-ketoses, e.g., fructose) is drawn at the top, and the rest of the carbon atoms of the chain are drawn in sequence below the top carbon atom. For each carbon atom, depicted in projection as lying in the plane of the paper, the carbon-to-carbon bond(s), which actually point away from the viewer, are drawn as vertical lines. The left-hand and right-hand bonds of each carbon atom, which actually point toward the viewer, are, in projection, depicted as horizontal lines.

The conventions for the Fischer formulas of cyclic s. are as follows: 1) if the highest-numbered asymmetric carbon atom has its OH (or its replacement) lying to the right, as is the 2-OH of D-glyceraldehyde, the sugar has the D configuration; if the OH is to the left, the sugar has the L configuration; 2) on the anomeric carbon atom (C-1 in the aldoses; C-2 in the 2-ketoses), an OH or substituted OH that lies to the right, with the OH of the highest-numbered asymmetric carbon atom also to the right, is defined to be α; if it is to the left, with the OH of the highest-numbered carbon atom still to the right, it is β; the reverse applies if the latter OH is to the left; 3) the orientation of a terminal CH_2OH group in the aldoses carries no configurational significance, as it contains no asymmetric carbon atom.

Haworth conformational formulas of cyclic s., for the pyranoses, these depict those shapes (conformations) on which none, one, or two ring-atoms lie outside the plane of the ring. If there are two such atoms *para* to each other, they can lie 1) on opposite sides of the plane (*trans*), giving chair forms, or 2) on the same side of the plane (*cis*), giving boat forms.

Similarly, there are six boat conformations. If the two (*trans*) exoplanar atoms are *meta* to each other, the conformation is a skew form; if the two atoms are *ortho* to each other, the conformation is a half-chair form.

For the furanoses, the envelope conformations have one ring-atom exoplanar. If there are three adjacent, coplanar ring-atoms (the two exoplanar ring-atoms on opposite sides of the plane), the conformations are twist forms.

Haworth perspective formulas of cyclic s., perspective representations of furanose or pyranose structures as pentagons or hexagons, respectively, with the connecting bonds so shaded as to make them appear as though the plane of the ring is at an angle of 30° to the plane of the paper, and the bonds to H and OH at right angles to the plane of the ring. These formulas depict the planar conformation, a situation not usually met. Other conformational formulas, e.g., Haworth conformational formulas of cyclic s., attempt to depict the many deviations from planarity.

The basic conventions in Haworth formulas of cyclic s. (cyclic glycoses) are as follows: 1) the lowest-numbered asymmetric ring-carbon atom is depicted at the right; 2) if the highest-numbered asymmetric carbon atom is D, the sugar is D; the formula of an L-glycose may be derived from that of its D-isomer by reversing the up or down direction of all groups attached to the ring-carbon atoms; 3) if the hydroxyl group attached to the anomeric carbon (C-1 in aldoses, C-2 in 2-ketoses) is below the plane of the ring of a D-glycose, it is α; if above, it is β; the reverse applies if the sugar is L. SEE ALSO Fischer projection formulas of s.

sug·gest·i·bil·i·ty (sŭg-jes'tĭ-bil'i-tē). Responsiveness or susceptibility to a psychological process such as a hypnotic command whereby an idea is induced into, or adopted by, an individual without argument, command, or coercion. SYN sympathism.

sug·gest·i·ble (sŭg-jes'tĭ-bl). Susceptible to suggestion.

sug·ges·tion (sŭg-jes'chŭn). The implanting of an idea in the mind of another by some word or act on one's part, the subject's conduct or physical condition being influenced to some degree by the implanted idea. SEE ALSO autosuggestion. [L. *sug-gero* (*subg-*), pp. *-gestus,* to bring under, supply]

hypnotic s., a directive to a subject in trance, which is carried out either during or after the trance. SEE ALSO minor *hypnosis.*

posthypnotic s., s. given to a subject under hypnosis for certain actions to be performed after the subject is "awakened" from the hypnotic trance.

sug·ges·tive (sŭg-jes'tiv). Relating to suggestion.

sug·gil·la·tion (sŭg-ji-lā'shŭn, sŭj-i-). Obsolete term for a bruise or livedo. SEE ALSO contusion. [L. *sugillo,* pp. *-atus,* to beat black and blue]

postmortem s., SYN postmortem *livedo.*

Sugiura, M., 20th century Japanese surgeon. SEE S. *procedure.*

SUI Abbreviation for stress urinary *incontinence.*

su·i·cide (soo'i-sīd). **1.** The act of taking one's own life. **2.** A person who commits such an act. [L. *sui,* self, + *caedo,* to kill]

physician-assisted s., voluntary termination of one's own life by administration of a lethal substance with the direct or indirect assistance of a physician. Physician-assisted s. is to be distinguished from the withholding or discontinuance of life-support measures in terminal or vegetative states so that the patient dies of the underlying illness, and from administration of narcotic analgesics in terminal cancer, which may indirectly hasten death. SEE ALSO end-of-life *care,* advance *directive.*

Questions and controversies about assisted suicide have become widespread within the health care community and society at large. The U.S. Supreme Court, in a 9–0 decision, has ruled that citizens have no constitutional right to physician-assisted suicide, but has placed no obstacles to legalization of the practice by state legislatures. Under Oregon law any mentally competent resident of the state who has reached the age of 18, and who has a terminal illness that is expected to cause death within 6 months, may make a voluntary and informed decision to terminate life by taking a lethal overdose of oral medicine prescribed for that purpose by a physician. The physician is immune from civil or criminal prosecution. Despite the legalization of physician-assisted suicide in at least one state, and the highly publicized activities of "death doctors" in other states, the American Medical Association and the American Nurses Association have issued official position statements opposing assisted suicide in all circumstances. Among objections voiced by opponents of the legalization of physician-assisted suicide and its integration into medical practice are the erosion of public trust in the health care professions; the radical change in the traditional physician-patient relationship; the concern that if physician-assisted suicide were to become an accepted option for the "treatment" of certain illnesses, physicians might be required to present it to patients as an alternative, and managed-care or other third-party payers might favor it as least expensive; and the fear that, once legal, physician-assisted suicide would be permitted for conditions not terminal, and that people other than the patient would eventually be empowered to make the decision. The debate over physician-assisted suicide has drawn attention to shortcomings in the care of dying persons and to the preeminent obligation of health care professionals to provide responsible, respectful, appropriate, and ethically sound care.

sui·cid·ol·o·gy (soo'i-sī-dol'ō-jē). A branch of the behavioral sciences devoted to the study of the nature, causes, and prevention of suicide. [suicide + G. *logos,* study]

su·int (swint). The natural grease in sheep's wool, from which the official wool fat (anhydrous lanolin) is extracted. [Fr. wool-grease]

suit (soot). An outer garment designed for protection against specific environmental conditions.

anti-G s., a garment with bladders that expand to apply external pressure to the abdomen and lower extremities during positive G maneuvers in flight or on a human centrifuge; the anti-G s. is worn to prevent the pooling of blood and serves to increase the wearer's ability to withstand exposure to higher G forces.

sul·bac·tam (sŭl-bak′tam). A β-lactamase inhibitor with weak antibacterial action; when used in conjunction with penicillins (e.g., ampicillin) with little β-lactamase-inhibiting action, it greatly increases their effectiveness against organisms which would ordinarily not be susceptible.

sul·ben·tine (sŭl-ben′tēn). SYN dibenzthione.

sul·cal (sŭl′kăl). Relating to a sulcus.

sul·cate (sŭl′kāt). Grooved; furrowed; marked by a sulcus or sulci.

sul·ci·form (sŭl′si-fōm). Having the form of a groove or sulcus.

sul·cu·lus, pl. **sul·cu·li** (sŭl′kŭ-lŭs, -lī). A small sulcus. [Mod. L. dim. of L. *sulcus,* furrow]

SULCUS

---

sul·cus, gen. and pl. **sul·ci** (sool′kŭs, sŭl′sī). **1** [TA]. One of the grooves or furrows on the surface of the brain, bounding the several convolutions or gyri; a fissure. SEE ALSO fissure. **2** [NA]. Any long narrow groove, furrow, or slight depression. SEE ALSO groove. **3.** A groove or depression in the oral cavity or on the surface of a tooth. [L. a furrow or ditch]

alveolobuccal s., SYN alveolobuccal *groove.*

alveololabial s., SYN alveololabial *groove.*

alveololingual s., SYN alveololingual *groove.*

s. ampulla′ris [TA], SYN ampullary *groove.*

ampullary s., SYN ampullary *groove.*

s. angula′ris, SYN angular *incisure.*

anterior intermediate s., a furrow occasionally seen in the adult between the anterior median fissure and the anterior lateral s. of the spinal cord but usually present only in the fetus. It indicates the lateral border of the anterior corticospinal fasciculus. SYN anterior intermediate groove, s. intermedius anterior.

anterior interventricular s. [TA], a groove on the anterosuperior surface of the heart, marking the location of the septum between the two ventricles. SYN s. interventricularis anterior [TA], anterior interventricular groove, crena cordis (1).

anterior parolfactory s., a fissure marking the anterior border of the parolfactory area. SYN s. parolfactorius anterior.

anterolateral s., an indistinct furrow on the ventral surface of the spinal cord and medulla oblongata, on either side marking the line of exit of the anterior nerve roots. SYN s. anterolateralis [TA], ventrolateral s.[✗], anterolateral groove.

s. anterolatera′lis [TA], SYN anterolateral s.

s. anthel′icis transver′sus, SYN transverse anthelicine *groove.*

aortic s., SYN aortic *impression* of left lung.

s. aor′ticus, SYN aortic *impression* of left lung.

s. arte′riae occipita′lis [TA], SYN occipital *groove.*

s. arteriae subclaviae costae primae [TA], SYN *groove* of first rib for subclavian artery.

s. arte′riae tempora′lis me′diae [TA], SYN *groove* for middle temporal artery.

s. arte′riae vertebra′lis [TA], SYN *groove* for vertebral artery.

sul′ci arterio′si [TA], SYN arterial *grooves,* under *groove.*

atrioventricular s., SYN coronary s.

s. for auditory tube, SYN s. for pharyngotympanic tube.

s. auric′ulae ante′rior, SYN anterior *notch* of auricle.

basilar s. [TA], SYN basilar pontine s.

s. basila′ris [TA], SYN basilar pontine s.

basilar pontine s., a median groove on the ventral surface of the

pons varolii in which lies the basilar artery. SYN basilar s. [TA], s. basilaris [TA].

s. bicipita′lis latera′lis [TA], SYN lateral bicipital *groove.*

s. bicipita′lis media′lis [TA], SYN medial bicipital *groove.*

s. bicipitalis radialis, [✗]official alternate term for lateral bicipital *groove.*

s. bicipitalis ulnaris, [✗]official alternate term for medial bicipital *groove.*

s. bulbopontis [TA], SYN medullopontine s.

calcaneal s. [TA], the groove on the upper part of the calcaneus, which with a corresponding groove on the talus forms the sinus tarsi. SYN s. calcanei [TA], interosseous groove of calcaneus, interosseous groove (1).

s. calca′nei [TA], SYN calcaneal s.

calcarine s. [TA], a deep fissure on the medial aspect of the cerebral cortex, extending on an arched line from the isthmus of the fornicate gyrus back to the occipital pole, marking the border between the lingual gyrus below and the cuneus above it. The cortex in the depth of the sulcus corresponds to the horizontal meridian of the contralateral half of the visual field. SYN s. calcarinus [TA], calcarine fissure, fissura calcarina, posthippocampal fissure.

s. calcari′nus [TA], SYN calcarine s.

callosal s., SYN s. of corpus callosum.

callosomarginal s., SYN cingulate s.

s. callosomargina′lis, SYN cingulate s.

s. carot′icus [TA], SYN cavernous *groove.*

carotid s., SYN cavernous *groove.*

s. car′pi [TA], SYN carpal *groove.*

central s. [TA], a double-S-shaped fissure extending obliquely upward and backward on the lateral surface of each cerebral hemisphere at the boundary between frontal and parietal lobes. SYN s. centralis [TA], fissure of Rolando.

central s. of insula [TA], a s. traversing the insular cortex and dividing it into an anterior part, the gyri brevi and a posterior part, the gyri longi. SYN s. centralis insulae [TA].

s. centra′lis [TA], SYN central s.

s. centralis insulae [TA], SYN central s. of insula.

cerebellar sulci, grooves between the folia cerebelli; commonly called fissures in cerebellum.

cerebral sulci [TA], the grooves between the cerebral gyri or convolutions. SYN sulci cerebri [TA].

sul′ci cer′ebri [TA], SYN cerebral sulci.

chiasmatic s., SYN prechiasmatic s.

cingulate s. [TA], a fissure on the mesial surface of the cerebral hemisphere, bounding the upper surface of the cingulate gyrus (callosal convolution); the anterior portion is called the pars subfrontalis; the posterior portion which curves up to the superomedial margin of the hemisphere and borders the paracentral lobule posteriorly is the ramus marginalis. SYN s. cinguli [TA], callosomarginal fissure, callosomarginal s., s. callosomarginalis, s. of cingulum.

s. cin′guli [TA], SYN cingulate s.

s. of cingulum, SYN cingulate s.

circular s. of insula [TA], a semicircular fissure demarcating the insula from the opercula above, below, and behind. SYN s. circularis insulae [TA], circular s. of Reil, limiting s. of Reil.

s. circula′ris in′sulae [TA], SYN circular s. of insula.

circular s. of Reil, SYN circular s. of insula.

collateral s. [TA], a long, deep sagittal fissure on the undersurface of the temporal lobe, marking the border between the fusiform gyrus laterally and the hippocampal and lingual gyri medially; the great depth of the collateral s. results in a bulging of the floor of the occipital and temporal horn of the lateral ventricle, the collateral eminence. SYN occipitotemporal s. [TA], s. collateralis [TA], s. occipitotemporalis [TA], collateral fissure, fissura collateralis.

s. collatera′lis [TA], SYN collateral s.

s. corona′rius [TA], SYN coronary s.

coronary s. [TA], a groove on the outer surface of the heart marking the division between the atria and the ventricles. SYN s.

coronarius [TA], atrioventricular groove, atrioventricular s., auriculoventricular groove, coronary groove.

s. cor'poris callo'si [TA], SYN s. of corpus callosum.

s. of corpus callosum [TA], the fissure between the corpus callosum and the cingulate gyrus. SYN s. corporis callosi [TA], callosal s.

s. cos'tae [TA], SYN costal *groove*.

s. costae arte'riae subcla'viae, SYN *groove* of first rib for subclavian artery.

costophrenic s., the recess between the ribs and the lateral-most portion of the diaphragm, partially occupied by the most caudal part of the lung; seen on radiographs as the costophrenic angle.

s. cru'ris heli'cis [TA], SYN *groove* of crus of helix.

sul'ci cu'tis [TA], SYN skin sulci.

dorsal intermediate s., SYN posterior intermediate s.

dorsal median s., ⋆official alternate term for posterior median s. of medulla oblongata.

dorsolateral s., ⋆official alternate term for posterolateral s.

s. ethmoida'lis [TA], SYN ethmoidal *groove*.

external spiral s., SYN outer spiral s.

fimbriodentate s. [TA], a shallow groove between the fimbria and the dentate gyrus of the hippocampus. SYN s. fimbriodentatus [TA].

s. fimbriodenta'tus [TA], SYN fimbriodentate s.

s. fronta'lis infe'rior [TA], SYN inferior frontal s.

s. fronta'lis me'dius, SYN middle frontal s.

s. fronta'lis supe'rior [TA], SYN superior frontal s.

s. frontomargina'lis, SEE middle frontal s.

gingival s. [TA], the space between the surface of the tooth and the free gingiva. SYN s. gingivalis [TA], gingival crevice, gingival groove, gingival space, subgingival space.

s. gingiva'lis [TA], SYN gingival s.

gingivobuccal s., SYN alveolobuccal *groove*.

gingivolabial s., SYN alveololabial *groove*.

gingivolingual s., SYN alveololingual *groove*.

s. glu'teus [TA], SYN gluteal *fold*.

s. for greater palatine nerve, SYN greater palatine *groove*.

habenular s. [TA], a small groove located between the habenular trigone and the adjacent dorsal thalamus. SYN s. habenularis.

s. habenularis, SYN habenular s.

s. ham'uli pterygoi'dei [TA], SYN *groove* for pterygoid hamulus.

hippocampal s. [TA], a shallow groove between the dentate gyrus and the parahippocampal gyrus; the remains of a fissure extending deep into the hippocampus between the Ammon horn and the dentate gyrus which becomes obliterated during fetal development. SYN s. hippocampalis [TA], dentate fissure, fissura dentata, fissura hippocampi, hippocampal fissure.

s. hippocam'palis [TA], SYN hippocampal s.

hypothalamic s. [TA], a groove in the lateral wall of the third ventricle on either side leading from the interventricular foramen to the apertura aqueductus mesencephali; the s.-demarcated boundary between dorsal thalamus and hypothalamus. SYN s. hypothalamicus [TA], Monro s.

s. hypothalam'icus [TA], SYN hypothalamic s.

inferior frontal s. [TA], a sagittal fissure on the lateral convex surface of each frontal lobe of the cerebrum demarcating the middle from the inferior frontal gyrus. SYN s. frontalis inferior [TA].

inferior petrosal s., SYN *groove* for inferior petrosal sinus.

inferior temporal s. [TA], the s. on the basal aspect of the temporal lobe that separates the fusiform gyrus from the inferior temporal gyrus on its lateral side. SYN s. temporalis inferior [TA], Clevenger fissure.

s. infraorbita'lis [TA], SYN infraorbital *groove*.

infrapalpebral s., the hollow or furrow below the lower eyelid. SYN s. infrapalpebralis.

s. infrapalpebra'lis, SYN infrapalpebral s.

inner spiral s. [TA], a concavity in the floor of the cochlear duct formed by the overhanging vestibular lip. SYN s. spiralis internus [TA], internal spiral s.

s. interme'dius ante'rior, SYN anterior intermediate s.

s. interme'dius poste'rior [TA], SYN posterior intermediate s.

internal spiral s., SYN inner spiral s.

interparietal s., SYN intraparietal s.

intertubercular s. [TA], a furrow running down the shaft of the humerus between the two tubercles, lodging the tendon of the long head of the biceps, and giving attachment in its floor to the latissimus dorsi muscle. SYN intertubercular groove [TA], s. intertubercularis [TA], bicipital groove⋆.

s. intertubercula'ris [TA], SYN intertubercular s.

s. interventricula'ris ante'rior [TA], SYN anterior interventricular s.

s. interventricula'ris cor'dis, SEE anterior interventricular s., posterior interventricular s.

s. interventricula'ris poste'rior [TA], SYN posterior interventricular s.

intragracile s., a fissure between the gracilis minor and gracilis posterior lobuli of the cerebellum. SYN s. intragracilis.

s. intragra'cilis, SYN intragracile s.

intraparietal s. [TA], a horizontal s. extending back from the postcentral s. over some distance, then dividing perpendicularly into two branches so as to form, with the postcentral s., a figure H. It divides the parietal lobe into superior and inferior parietal lobules. SYN s. intraparietalis [TA], interparietal s., intraparietal s. of Turner, Turner s.

s. intraparieta'lis [TA], SYN intraparietal s.

intraparietal s. of Turner, SYN intraparietal s.

labial s., a furrow between the developing lip and gum. SYN labiodental s., lip s., primary labial groove.

labiodental s., SYN labial s.

s. lacrima'lis [TA], SYN lacrimal *groove*.

lateral s., the deepest and most prominent of the cortical sulci, extending from the anterior perforated substance first laterally at the deep incisure between the frontal and temporal lobes, then caudal and slightly dorsal over the lateral aspect of the cerebral hemisphere; the superior temporal gyrus forms its lower bank, the insula its greatly expanded floor, and the frontal and parietal opervula its upper bank. The s. is composed of three portions, a large posterior ramus [TA] (ramus posterior [TA]) that is commonly called the lateral s., a short anterior ramus [TA] (ramus posterior [TA]) located between the pars orbitalis and pars triangularis of the inferior frontal gyrus, and a short ascending ramus [TA] (ramus ascendens [TA]) located between the pars triangularis and pars opercularis. SYN s. lateralis [TA], fissura cerebri lateralis, lateral cerebral fissure, sylvian fissure, fissure of Sylvius.

s. latera'lis [TA], SYN lateral s.

lateral occipital s., one of several variable sulci on the lateral aspect of the occipital lobe of each cerebral hemisphere, bounding the lateral occipital convolutions. SYN s. occipitalis lateralis.

s. lim'itans [TA], SYN limiting s.

s. lim'itans ventriculi quarti [TA], SYN limiting s. of fourth ventricle.

limiting s., the medial longitudinal groove on the inner surface of the neural tube separating the alar and basal plates. SYN s. limitans [TA].

limiting s. of fourth ventricle [TA], a lateral groove running the whole length of the floor of the rhomboid fossa on either side of the midline, representing the remains of the s. demarcating the alar (dorsal) from the basal (ventral) plate of the embryonic rhombencephalon; position of s. indicates the general separation of motor nuclei of cranial nerves (located medially) from sensory nuclei of cranial nerves (located laterally). SYN s. limitans ventriculi quarti [TA].

limiting s. of Reil, SYN circular s. of insula.

lip s., SYN labial s.

longitudinal s. of heart, SEE anterior interventricular s., posterior interventricular s.

lunate s., a small, inconstant semilunar groove on the cortical convexity near the occipital pole, marking the anterior border of the striate cortex (area 17) and considered homologous with the major s. of the same name that is a more constant feature of the cerebral cortex in monkeys and apes. SYN lunate fissure [TA], s. lunatus [TA], simian fissure.

s. luna′tus [TA], SYN lunate s.

malleolar s., SYN malleolar *groove*.

s. malleola′ris [TA], SYN malleolar *groove*.

marginal s. [TA], the s. located immediately caudal to the posterior paracentral gyrus: the posterior ascending portion of the cingulate s.; may also be considered the marginal ramus of the cingulate s. SYN ramus marginalis [TA], s. marginalis [TA], marginal branch [TA] of cingulate sulcus.

s. marginalis [TA], SYN marginal s.

s. ma′tricis un′guis, the cutaneous furrow in which the lateral border of the nail is situated. SYN groove of nail matrix, vallecula unguis.

medial s. of crus cerebri, SYN oculomotor s. of mesencephalon.

s. media′lis cru′ris cer′ebri, SYN oculomotor s. of mesencephalon.

median s. of fourth ventricle [TA], the shallow midline groove in the floor of the ventricle. SYN s. medianus ventriculi quarti [TA].

median s. of tongue [TA], a slight longitudinal depression running forward on the dorsal surface of the tongue from the foramen cecum dividing the dorsum into right and left halves. SYN s. medianus linguae [TA], median groove of tongue, median longitudinal raphe of tongue, raphe linguae.

s. media′nus lin′guae [TA], SYN median s. of tongue.

s. media′nus poste′rior medul′lae oblonga′tae [TA], SYN posterior median s. of medulla oblongata.

s. media′nus poste′rior medul′lae spina′lis [TA], SYN posterior median s. of spinal cord.

s. media′nus ventric′uli quar′ti [TA], SYN median s. of fourth ventricle.

medullopontine s. [TA], the transverse groove on the ventral aspect of the brainstem that demarcates the medulla from the pons and contains the emerging roots of the 6th, 7th, and 8th cranial nerves. SYN s. bulbopontis [TA].

mentolabial s., the indistinct line separating the lower lip from the chin. SYN mentolabial furrow, s. mentolabialis.

s. mentolabia′lis, SYN mentolabial s.

middle frontal s., a relatively shallow sagittal fissure of the brain dividing the middle frontal convolution into an upper and lower part; this s. is found only in humans and anthropoid apes; at its anterior extremity it bifurcates, the two branches spreading out laterally and constituting the frontomarginal s. SYN s. frontalis medius.

middle temporal s., the s. between the middle temporal gyrus and inferior temporal gyrus. SYN s. temporalis medius.

s. for middle temporal artery, SYN *groove* for middle temporal artery.

Monro s., SYN hypothalamic s.

s. mus′culi subcla′vii [TA], SYN subclavian *groove*.

s. mylohyoi′deus [TA], SYN mylohyoid *groove*.

nasolabial s. [TA], a furrow between the wing of the nose and the lip. SYN s. nasolabialis [TA], nasolabial groove.

s. nasolabia′lis [TA], SYN nasolabial s.

s. nervi oculomotorii [TA], SYN oculomotor s. of mesencephalon.

s. ner′vi petro′si majo′ris [TA], SYN *groove* for greater petrosal nerve.

s. ner′vi petro′si mino′ris [TA], SYN *groove* of lesser petrosal nerve.

s. ner′vi radia′lis [TA], SYN radial *groove*.

s. ner′vi spina′lis [TA], SYN *groove* for spinal nerve.

s. ner′vi ulna′ris [TA], SYN *groove* for ulnar nerve.

nymphocaruncular s., a groove between the labium minor and the border of the remains of the hymen, in which is the opening of the duct of the greater vestibular gland on either side. SYN nymphohymenal s., s. nymphocaruncularis.

s. nymphocaruncula′ris, SYN nymphocaruncular s.

nymphohymenal s., SYN nymphocaruncular s.

s. obturato′rius [TA], SYN obturator *groove*.

s. of occipital artery, SYN occipital *groove*.

s. occipita′lis latera′lis, SYN lateral occipital s.

s. occipita′lis supe′rior, SYN superior occipital s.

s. occipita′lis transver′sus [TA], SYN transverse occipital s.

occipitotemporal s. [TA], SYN collateral s.

s. occipitotempora′lis [TA], SYN collateral s.

oculomotor s. of mesencephalon [TA], a groove in the lateral wall of the interpeduncular fossa of the midbrain from which the rootlets of the oculomotor nerve emerge. SYN s. nervi oculomotorii [TA], medial s. of crus cerebri, s. medialis cruris cerebri, s. of the oculomotor nerve.

s. of the oculomotor nerve, SYN oculomotor s. of mesencephalon.

s. olfacto′rius [TA], SYN olfactory s.

s. olfacto′rius cavi na′si [TA], SYN olfactory *groove* of nasal cavity.

olfactory s. [TA], the sagittal s. on the inferior or orbital surface of each frontal lobe of the cerebrum, demarcating the straight gyrus from the orbital gyri, and covered on the orbital surface by the olfactory bulb and tract. SYN s. olfactorius [TA], olfactory groove.

olfactory s. of nasal cavity, SYN olfactory *groove* of nasal cavity.

orbital sulci [TA], a number of irregularly disposed, variable sulci dividing the inferior or orbital surface of each frontal lobe of the cerebrum into the orbital gyri. SYN sulci orbitales [TA].

sul′ci orbita′les [TA], SYN orbital sulci.

outer spiral s. [TA], a concavity in the outer wall of the cochlear duct between the spiral prominence and the spiral organ. SYN s. spiralis externus [TA], external spiral s.

sulci palati′ni [TA], SYN palatine *grooves*, under *groove*.

s. palati′nus ma′jor [TA], SYN greater palatine *groove*.

s. palatovagina′lis [TA], SYN palatovaginal *groove*.

paracentral s. [TA], a s. on the medial surface of the hemisphere, sometimes regarded as a branch of the cingulate sulcus, located between the anterior portions of the paracentral lobule and the medial portions of the superior frontal gyrus. SYN s. paracentralis [TA].

s. paracentralis [TA], SYN paracentral s.

sul′ci paraco′lici [TA], SYN paracolic *gutters*, under *gutter*.

paraglenoid s., SYN preauricular *groove*.

s. paraglenoida′lis, SYN preauricular *groove*.

sulci paraolfactorii [TA], SYN parolfactory sulci.

parietooccipital s. [TA], a very deep, almost vertically oriented fissure on the medial surface of the cerebral cortex, marking the border between the precuneus portion of the parietal lobe and the cuneus of the occipital lobe; its lower part curves forward and fuses with the anterior extent of the calcarine fissure (sulcus calcarinus); the great depth of this combined fissure causes a bulge in the medial wall of the occipital horn of the lateral ventricle, the calcar avis. SYN s. parieto-occipitalis [TA], fissura parietooccipitalis, parietooccipital fissure.

s. parieto-occipita′lis [TA], SYN parietooccipital s.

s. parolfacto′rius ante′rior, SYN anterior parolfactory s.

s. parolfacto′rius poste′rior, SYN posterior parolfactory s.

parolfactory sulci [TA], small sulci found in the parolfactory area, which is located immediately rostral to the lamina terminalis; they frequently consist of anterior and posterior sulci. SEE ALSO anterior parolfactory s. SYN sulci paraolfactorii [TA].

periconchal s., SYN *fossa* antihelica.

s. for pharyngotympanic tube [TA], a furrow on the inner surface of the posterior border of the greater wing of the sphenoid bone, for the cartilaginous auditory tube. SYN s. tubae auditoriae [TA], groove for auditory tube, pharyngotympanic groove, s. for auditory tube.

s. poplit′eus [TA], SYN *groove* for popliteus.

postcentral s. [TA], the s. that demarcates the postcentral gyrus from the superior and inferior parietal lobules. SYN s. postcentralis [TA].

s. postcentra′lis [TA], SYN postcentral s.

s. poste′rior auric′ulae [TA], SYN posterior auricular *groove*.

posterior intermediate s. [TA], a longitudinal furrow between

su

the posterior median and the posterolateral sulci of the spinal cord in the cervical region, marking the gracile fasciculus from the cuneate fasciculus. SYN s. intermedius posterior [TA], dorsal intermediate s., posterior intermediate groove.

posterior interventricular s. [TA], a groove on the diaphragmatic surface of the heart, marking the location of the septum between the two ventricles. SYN s. interventricularis posterior [TA], crena cordis (2), posterior interventricular groove.

posterior median s. of medulla oblongata [TA], the longitudinal groove marking the posterior midline of the medulla oblongata; continuous below with the posterior median s. of the spinal cord. SYN s. medianus posterior medullae oblongatae [TA], dorsal median s.✩, posterior median fissure of the medulla oblongata.

posterior median s. of spinal cord [TA], a shallow furrow in the median line of the posterior surface of the spinal cord. SYN s. medianus posterior medullae spinalis [TA], posterior median fissure of spinal cord.

posterior parolfactory s. [TA], a shallow groove on the medial surface of the hemisphere demarcating the subcallosal gyrus or precommissural septum from the parolfactory area. SYN s. parolfactorius posterior.

posterolateral s. [TA], a longitudinal furrow on either side of the posterior median s. of the spinal cord marking the line of entrance of the posterior nerve roots. SYN s. posterolateralis [TA], dorsolateral s.✩, posterolateral groove.

s. posterolatera'lis [TA], SYN posterolateral s.

preauricular s., SYN preauricular *groove.*

precentral s. [TA], an interrupted fissure anterior to and in general parallel with the central s., marking the anterior border of the precentral gyrus. SYN s. precentralis [TA], s. verticalis.

s. precentra'lis [TA], SYN precentral s.

prechiasmatic s. [TA], the groove on the upper surface of the sphenoid bone running transversely between the optic canals bounded anteriorly by the sphenoidal limbus and posteriorly by the tuberculum sellae; forms in relationship to the optic chiasm. SYN s. prechiasmaticus [TA], chiasmatic groove, chiasmatic s., optic groove.

s. prechiasma'ticus [TA], SYN prechiasmatic s.

s. promonto'rii cavitatis tympanicae [TA], SYN *groove* of promontory of labyrinthine wall of tympanic cavity.

s. of promontory of tympanic cavity, SYN *groove* of promontory of labyrinthine wall of tympanic cavity.

s. of pterygoid hamulus, SYN *groove* for pterygoid hamulus.

s. pterygopalati'nus, SYN greater palatine *groove.*

s. pulmona'lis [TA], SYN pulmonary *groove.*

pulmonary s., SYN pulmonary *groove.*

rhinal s. [TA], the shallow rostral continuation of the collateral s. that delimits the rostral part of the parahippocampal gyrus from the fusiform or lateral occipitotemporal gyrus. One of the oldest sulci of the pallium, it marks the border between the neocortex and the allocortical (olfactory). SYN s. rhinalis [TA], rhinal fissure.

s. rhina'lis [TA], SYN rhinal s.

sagittal s., SYN *groove* for superior sagittal sinus.

s. of sclera, SYN s. sclerae.

s. scle'rae [TA], a slight groove on the external surface of the eyeball indicating the line of union of the sclera and cornea (corneoscleral junction or limbus of cornea). SYN scleral s., s. of sclera.

scleral s., SYN s. sclerae.

sigmoid s., SYN *groove* for sigmoid sinus.

s. si'nus petro'si inferio'ris [TA], SYN *groove* for inferior petrosal sinus.

s. si'nus petro'si superio'ris [TA], SYN *groove* for superior petrosal sinus.

s. si'nus sagitta'lis superio'ris, SYN *groove* for superior sagittal sinus.

s. si'nus sigmoi'dei [TA], SYN *groove* for sigmoid sinus.

s. si'nus transver'si [TA], SYN *groove* for transverse sinus.

skin sulci [TA], the numerous grooves of variable depth on the surface of the epidermis. SYN sulci cutis [TA], skin furrows, skin grooves.

s. spino'sus, SYN *stria* spinosa.

s. spira'lis exter'nus [TA], SYN outer spiral s.

s. spira'lis inter'nus [TA], SYN inner spiral s.

subclavian s., SYN subclavian *groove.*

s. subclavia'nus, SYN subclavian *groove.*

s. subcla'vius, SYN *groove* of lung for subclavian artery.

subparietal s. [TA], a s. continuing the direction of the cingulate s. from where the marginal part of that fissure bends upward; it forms the upper boundary of the posterior portion of the cingulate gyrus. SYN s. subparietalis [TA].

s. subparieta'lis [TA], SYN subparietal s.

superior frontal s. [TA], a sagittal fissure on the superior surface of each frontal lobe of the cerebrum starting from the precentral s.; it forms the lateral boundary of the superior frontal convolution. SYN s. frontalis superior [TA].

superior longitudinal s., SYN *groove* for superior sagittal sinus.

superior occipital s., one of several small and variable sulci bordering the superior occipital gyri on the upper aspect of the occipital lobe of the cerebrum. SYN s. occipitalis superior.

superior petrosal s., SYN *groove* for superior petrosal sinus.

superior temporal s. [TA], the longitudinal s. that separates the superior and middle temporal gyri. SYN s. temporalis superior [TA], superior temporal fissure.

supraacetabular s., SYN supra-acetabular *groove.*

s. supraacetabula'ris [TA], SYN supra-acetabular *groove.*

talar s., SYN s. tali.

s. ta'li [TA], the groove on the inferior surface of the talus, which with a corresponding groove on the calcaneus forms the sinus tarsi. SYN interosseous groove of talus, interosseous groove (2), talar s.

sul'ci tempora'les transver'si, SYN transverse temporal s.

s. tempora'lis infe'rior [TA], SYN inferior temporal s.

s. tempora'lis me'dius, SYN middle temporal s.

s. tempora'lis supe'rior [TA], SYN superior temporal s.

s. temporalis transversus [TA], SYN transverse temporal s.

s. ten'dinis mus'culi fibula'ris lon'gi [TA], SYN *groove* for tendon of fibularis longus.

s. ten'dinis mus'culi flexo'ris hal'lucis lon'gi [TA], SYN *groove* for tendon of flexor hallucis longus.

s. ten'dinis mus'culi perone'i lon'gi, (1) ✩official alternate term for *groove* for tendon of fibularis longus; **(2)** the groove distal to the tuberosity of the cuboid bone.

terminal s. [TA], SYN s. terminalis.

s. terminalis cordis [TA], a groove on the surface of the right atrium of the heart, marking the junction of the primitive sinus venosus with the atrium. SYN s. terminalis atrii dextri [TA].

s. termina'lis [TA], groove demarcating the end of a structure (and usually the beginning of another). SYN terminal s. [TA].

s. terminalis atrii dextri [TA], SYN s. terminalis cordis.

s. terminalis linguae [TA], SYN terminal s. of tongue.

terminal s. of tongue [TA], a V-shaped groove, with apex pointing backward, on the surface of the tongue, marking the separation between the anterior (oral or horizontal) and the posterior (pharyngeal or vertical) parts. SYN s. terminalis linguae [TA].

tonsillolingual s., the space between the palatine tonsil and the tongue.

transverse occipital s., the posterior, vertical limb of the intraparietal s. SYN s. occipitalis transversus [TA].

s. for transverse sinus, SYN *groove* for transverse sinus.

transverse temporal s. [TA], the shallow s. that demarcates the transverse temporal gyri on the opercular surface of the superior temporal gyrus. This s. frequently consists of more than a single s., depending on the exact configuration of the transverse temporal gyrus (gyri). SYN s. temporalis transversus [TA], sulci temporales transversi.

s. tu'bae auditoriae [TA], SYN s. for pharyngotympanic tube.

Turner s., SYN intraparietal s.

tympanic s. [TA], the groove on the inner aspect of the tympanic part of the temporal bone in which the tympanic membrane is fixed. SYN s. tympanicus [TA], tympanic groove.

s. tympan′icus [TA], SYN tympanic s.

s. of umbilical vein, the s. on the fetal liver occupied by the umbilical vein. SYN s. venae umbilicalis.

s. for vena cava [TA], a groove on the posterior surface of the liver between the caudate lobe and the right lobe which gives passage to the inferior vena cava. SYN s. venae cavae [TA], fossa venae cavae, groove for inferior venae cava.

s. ve′nae ca′vae [TA], SYN s. for vena cava.

s. ve′nae ca′vae crania′lis, SYN *groove* for superior vena cava.

s. ve′nae subcla′viae [TA], SYN *groove* for subclavian vein.

s. ve′nae umbilica′lis, SYN s. of umbilical vein.

sul′ci veno′si [TA], SYN venous *grooves,* under *groove.*

s. ventra′lis, SYN anterior median *fissure* of spinal cord.

ventrolateral s., ☆official alternate term for anterolateral s.

s. for vertebral artery, SYN *groove* for vertebral artery.

s. vertica′lis, SYN precentral s.

vomeral s., SYN vomerine *groove.*

s. vomera′lis, SYN vomerine *groove,* vomerine *groove.*

s. vo′meris [TA], SYN vomerine *groove.*

s. vomerovagina′lis [TA], SYN vomerovaginal *groove.*

♻**sulf-, sulfo-.** **1.** Prefix denoting that the compound to the name of which it is attached contains a sulfur atom. This spelling (rather than sulph-, sulpho-) is preferred by the American Chemical Society and has been adopted by the USP and NF, but not by the BP. **2.** Prefix form of sulfonic acid or sulfonate.

sul·fa (sŭl′fă). Denoting the sulfa drugs, or sulfonamides.

sul·fa·benz·am·ide (sŭl-fă-ben′ză-mīd). An antimicrobial of the sulfonamide group. SYN *N*-sulfanilylbenzamide.

sul·fa·cet·a·mide (sŭl-fă-set′ă-mīd). An antibacterial agent of the sulfonamide group, primarily used topically; s. sodium has the same uses as s. and also is used locally for eye infections and for prevention of gonorrheal ophthalmia in newborn infants. SYN *N*-sulfanilylacetamide.

sulf·ac·id (sŭlf-as′id). SYN thioacid.

sul·fa·cy·tine (sŭl-fă-sī′tēn). A sulfonamide used as an oral antibiotic in the treatment of urinary tract infections.

sul·fa·di·a·zine (sŭl-fă-dī′ă-zēn). One of a group of diazine derivatives of sulfanilamide, the pyrimidine analog of sulfapyridine and sulfathiazole; one of the components of the triple sulfonamide mixture. It is an inhibitor of bacterial folic acid synthesis, which has been highly effective against pneumococcal, staphylococcal, and streptococcal infections, against infections with *Escherichia coli* and *Klebsiella pneumoniae,* and in acute gonococcal arthritis; s. sodium has the same uses.

sul·fa·di·me·thox·ine (sŭl′fă-dī-mě-thok′sēn). A long-acting sulfonamide that is rapidly absorbed after oral administration and is slowly excreted by the kidney; it accumulates in the tissue and requires lower doses to attain effective tissue concentrations than do the other sulfonamides.

sul·fa·dim·i·dine (sŭl-fă-dim′i-dēn). SYN sulfamethazine.

sul·fa·dox·ine (sŭl-fă-dok′sēn). A long-acting sulfonamide, used with quinine and pyrimethamine to reduce the relapse rate of malaria. SYN sulformethoxine.

sul·fa·eth·i·dole (sŭl-fă-eth′i-dōl). A sulfonamide used in the treatment of systemic and urinary tract infections.

sul·fa·fur·a·zole (sŭl-fă-fūr′ă-zōl). SYN sulfisoxazole.

sul·fa·gua·ni·dine (sŭl-fă-gwahn′i-dēn). The guanidine derivative of sulfanilamide. It is poorly absorbed from the gastroenteric tract; useful for bacterial infections of the lower intestinal tract and for preoperative sterilization of the intestinal tract; a goitrogen. SYN sulfaguine.

sul·fa·guine (sul′fa-guīn). SYN sulfaguanidine.

sul·fa·lene (sŭl′fă-lēn). A very long-acting sulfonamide that enhances, as do other sulfonamides and sulfones, the effectiveness of antimalarial agents such as pyrimethamine, chloroguanide, or cycloguanil.

sul·fa·mer·a·zine (sŭl-fă-mer′ă-zēn). One of the components of the triple sulfonamide mixtures.

sul·fa·me·ter (sŭlf′ă-mē-ter). A slowly excreted sulfonamide once used in the treatment of acute and chronic urinary tract infections. SYN sulfamethoxydiazine.

sul·fa·meth·a·zine (sŭl-fă-meth′ă-zēn). One of the components of the triple sulfonamide mixture. SYN sulfadimidine.

sul·fa·meth·i·zole (sŭl-fă-meth′i-zōl). A sulfonamide useful for the treatment of urinary tract infection, because of its high solubility.

sul·fa·meth·ox·a·zole (sŭl′fă-meth-ok′să-zōl). A sulfonamide related chemically to sulfisoxazole, with a similar antibacterial spectrum, but a slower rate of absorption from the gastrointestinal tract and urinary excretion.

sul·fa·me·thox·y·di·a·zine (sŭl′fă-me-thok′si-dī′ă-zēn). SYN sulfameter.

sul·fa·me·thox·y·py·rid·a·zine (sŭl′fă-me-thok′si-pi-rid′ă-zēn). A long-acting sulfonamide that requires a single daily dose for maintaining effective tissue concentrations. S. acetyl is a preparation well suited for pediatric use because it is tasteless; it is also used to enhance the actions of quinine and other suppressants in the chemoprophylaxis of malaria.

sul·fa·mox·ole (sŭl-fă-mok′sōl). An antimicrobial agent of the sulfonamide group.

p-**sul·fa·myl·ac·e·tan·il·ide** (sŭl′fă-mil-as-e-tan′il-īd). SYN N^4-acetylsulfanilamide.

sul·fa·nil·a·mide (sŭl-fă-nil′ă-mīd). The first sulfonamide used for its chemotherapeutic effect in infections caused by some β-hemolytic streptococci, meningococci, gonococci, *Clostridium welchii,* and in certain infections of the urinary tract, especially those due to *Escherichia coli* and *Proteus vulgaris;* less effective than sulfapyridine in the treatment of pneumococcic, staphylococcic, and *Klebsiella pneumoniae* infections. Toxic manifestations include acidosis, cyanosis, hemolytic anemia, and agranulocytosis.

N-**sul·fan·i·lyl·a·cet·a·mide** (sŭl-fan′i-lil-ă-set′ă-mīd). SYN sulfacetamide.

N-**sul·fan·i·lyl·benz·a·mide** (sŭl-fan′i-lil-ben′ză-mīd). SYN sulfabenzamide.

sul·fa·phen·a·zole (sŭl-fă-fen′ă-zōl). A long-acting sulfonamide that is rapidly absorbed after oral administration; one dose is sufficient to maintain effective tissue concentration for 24 hours.

sul·fa·pyr·a·zine (sŭl-fă-pir′ă-zēn). An antibacterial agent of the sulfonamide group.

sul·fa·pyr·i·dine (sŭl-fă-pir′i-dēn). An antibacterial agent of the sulfonamide group.

sul·fa·sal·a·zine (sŭl-fă-sal′ă-zēn). A sulfonamide (acid-azosulfa compound) with a marked affinity for connective tissues, especially for those rich in elastin, used in chronic ulcerative colitis; it is broken down in the body to aminosalicylic acid and sulfapyridine. SYN salicylazosulfapyridine.

sul·fa·tase (sŭl′fă-tās). **1.** Trivial name for enzymes in EC group 3.1.6, the sulfuric ester hydrolases, which catalyze the hydrolysis of sulfuric esters (sulfates) to the corresponding alcohols plus inorganic sulfate; includes aryl-, sterol, glycol-, chondroitin, choline-, cellulose, cerebroside, and chondro- s.'s. **2.** SYN arylsulfatase.

multiple s. deficiency, an inherited disorder (autosomal recessive) in which there is a failure to hydrolyze sulfatides and sulfated mucopolysaccharides; this failure leads to their accumulation in neural and extraneural tissues, causing demyelination, sulfatiduria, facial and skeletal dysmorphism, etc.

sul·fate (sŭl′fāt). A salt or ester of sulfuric acid.

acid s., SYN bisulfate.

active s., SYN adenosine 3′-phosphate 5′-phosphosulfate.

s. adenylyltransferase, an enzyme that catalyzes a step in the pathway for the synthesis of active s.; the enzyme reacts ATP with s. to produce pyrophosphate and adenosine 5′-phosphosulfate (APS). SYN ATP sulfurylase.

codeine s., a water-soluble salt of codeine, often used in solid pharmaceutical dosage forms. Also used in cough preparations, where the drug suppresses the cough reflex.

dermatan s., an anticoagulant with properties similar to heparin and sharing with heparin a sulfated mucopolysaccharide structure; a repeating polymer of L-iduronic acid and N-acetyl-D-galactosamine. O-Sulfation of iduronic acid residues at the C-2 position and of galactosamine residues at the C-4 and C-6 positions occurs to a variable extent. SYN chondroitin sulfate B.

iron s., a soluble iron salt frequently used as an iron supplement in tablets and liquid preparations as a hematinic. SYN ferrous sulfate.

polysaccharide s. esters, s. esters of polysaccharides often found in cell walls.

sul·fa·thi·a·zole (sŭl-fă-thī′ă-zōl). An antibacterial agent of the sulfonamide group.

sul·fa·ti·dates (sŭl′fă-ti-dāts). SYN sulfatides.

sul·fa·tides (sŭl′fă-tīdz). Cerebroside sulfuric esters containing one or more sulfate groups in the sugar portion of the molecule. SYN sulfatidates.

sul·fa·ti·do·sis (sŭl′fă-ti-dō′sis) [MIM*272200]. A combination of metachromatic leukodystrophy and mucopolysaccharidosis caused by deficiency of sulfatase enzymes such as arylsulfatases A, B, and C, and steroid sulfatases; characterized by coarse facial features, ichthyosis, hepatosplenomegaly, and skeletal abnormalities, with increased urinary excretion of dermatan and heparan sulfates; autosomal recessive inheritance. SEE ALSO metachromatic *leukodystrophy*.

sul·fa·tion (sŭl-fā′shŭn). Addition of sulfate groups as esters to preexisting molecules.

sulf·he·mo·glo·bin (sŭlf-hē′mō-glō-bin). SYN sulfmethemoglobin.

sulf·he·mo·glo·bi·ne·mia (sŭlf-hē′mō-glō-bi-nē′mē-ă). A morbid condition due to the presence of sulfhemoglobin in the blood; it is marked by a persistent cyanosis, but the blood count does not reveal any special abnormality in that fluid; it is thought to be caused by the action of hydrogen sulfide absorbed from the intestine.

sulf·hy·drate (sŭlf-hī′drāt). A compound (hydrosulfide) containing the ion HS⁻. SYN sulfohydrate.

sulf·hy·dryl (SH) (sŭlf-hī′dril). The radical –SH; contained in glutathione, cysteine, coenzyme A, lipoamide (all in the reduced state), and in mercaptans (R–SH). SYN thiel.

sul·fide (sŭl′fīd). A compound of sulfur in which the sulfur has a valence of −2; e.g., Na_2S, HgS; also, a thioether (i.e., R–S–R′, such as lanthionine). SYN sulfuret.

sul·fi·ki·nase (sŭl′fō-kīn′ās). SYN sulfotransferase.

sul·fin·di·got·ic ac·id (sŭl′fin-dī-got′ik). Formed by the action of sulfuric acid on indigo, a reaction that also yields indigo carmine.

sul·fin·py·ra·zone (sŭl-fin-pir′ă-zōn). An analgesic and uricosuric agent, useful in gout, that promotes the excretion of uric acid, probably by interfering with the tubular reabsorption of uric acid.

β-sul·fi·nyl·py·ru·vic ac·id (sŭl′fi-nil-pī-roo′vik). An intermediate product of L-cysteine catabolism in mammalian tissue.

sul·fi·so·mi·dine (sŭl-fi-sō′mi-dēn). The structural isomer of sulfamethazine, used in the treatment of systemic and urinary tract infections.

sul·fi·sox·a·zole (sŭl-fi-sok′să-zōl). A sulfonamide used chiefly in bacterial infections of the urinary tract. SYN sulfafurazole.

s. diolamine, the 2,2′-iminodiethanol salt of s.; used for intravenous, subcutaneous, or intramuscular administration.

sul·fite (sŭl′fīt). A salt of sulfurous acid; elevated in cases of molybdenum cofactor deficiency.

s. dehydrogenase, an oxidoreductase catalyzing the reaction of s. with 2ferricytochrome *c* and water to sulfate and 2ferrocytochrome *c*.

s. oxidase, a liver oxidoreductase (hemoprotein) catalyzing the reaction of inorganic s. ion with O_2 and water to produce sulfate ion and H_2O_2; a lower activity of this enzyme is observed in cases of molybdenum cofactor deficiency.

s. reductase, oxidoreductase catalyzing reduction of s. to H_2S using some reduced acceptor.

sul·fi·tu·ria (sŭlf′īt-oor-ē-ă). Elevated levels of sulfites in the urine.

sulf·met·he·mo·glo·bin (sŭlf-met-hē′mō-glō-bin). The complex

formed by H_2S (or sulfides) and ferric ion in methemoglobin. SYN sulfhemoglobin.

△**sulfo-.** SEE sulf-.

sul·fo·ac·id (sŭl′fō-as-id). **1.** SYN thioacid. **2.** SYN sulfonic acid.

3-sul·fo·al·a·nine (sŭl-fō-al′ă-nēn). SYN cysteic acid.

sul·fo·bro·mo·phtha·lein so·di·um (sŭl′fō-brō-mō-thal′ē-in). A triphenylmethane derivative excreted by the liver, used in testing hepatic function, particularly of the reticuloendothelial cells. SYN bromosulfophthalein, bromsulfophthalein.

sul·fo·cy·a·nate (sŭl-fō-sī′ă-nāt). SYN thiocyanate.

sul·fo·cy·an·ic ac·id (sŭl-fō-sī-an′ik). SYN thiocyanic acid.

S-sul·fo·cys·teine (sŭl-fō-sis′tē-ēn). A sulfated derivative of cysteine that is elevated in individuals with a molybdenum cofactor deficiency.

3-sul·fo·ga·lac·to·syl·cer·a·mide. A sulfatide that accumulates in individuals with metachromatic leukodystrophy.

sul·fo·gel (sŭl′fō-jel). A hydrogel with sulfuric acid instead of water as the dispersion means.

sul·fo·hy·drate (sŭl-fō-hī′drāt). SYN sulfhydrate.

sul·fo·ki·nase (sŭl′fō-kīn-ās). SYN sulfotransferase.

sul·fol·y·sis (sul-fol′i-sis). Lysis brought on or accelerated by sulfuric acid.

sul·fo·mu·cin (sŭl-fō-mū′sin). A mucin containing sulfuric esters in its mucopolysaccharides or glycoproteins.

sul·fo·myx·in so·di·um (sŭl-fō-mik′sin). A mixture of sulfomethylated polymyxin B and sodium bisulfite; an antibacterial agent.

sul·fon·a·mides (sŭl-fon′ă-mīdz). The sulfa drugs, a group of bacteriostatic drugs containing the sulfanilamide group (sulfanilamide, sulfapyridine, sulfathiazole, sulfadiazine, and other sulfanilamide derivatives).

sul·fo·nate (sŭl′fō-nāt). A salt or ester of sulfonic acid.

sul·fone (sŭl-fōn). A compound of the general structure R′–SO₂–R″.

sul·fon·ic ac·id (sŭl-fon′ik). Any of the compounds in which a hydrogen atom of a CH group is replaced by the s. a. group, –SO₃H; general formula: R–SO₃H. SYN sulfoacid (2).

sul·fo·ni·um salts (sŭl-fō′nē-um). Compounds containing sulfur covalently linked to three moieties; e.g., RS⁺(R′)R‴, such as S-adenosyl-L-methionine.

sul·fo·nyl·u·re·as (sŭl′fō-nil-ū-rē′ăz). Derivatives of isopropylthiodiazylsulfanilamide, chemically related to the sulfonamides, which possess hypoglycemic action. Belonging to this series are acetohexamide, azepinamide, chlorpropamide, fluphenmepramide, glymidine, hydroxyhexamide, heptolamide, indylamide, thiohexamide, tolazamide, and tolbutamide.

sul·fo·pro·tein (sŭl-fō-prō′tēn). A protein molecule containing sulfate groups.

6-sul·fo·qui·no·vo·syl di·ac·yl·glyc·er·ol (sŭl′fō-kwī′nō-vō-sil, -kwin′ō). Quinovose containing an SO₃H on C-6 and a doubly substituted glycerol on C-1; the sulfolipid occurring in all photosynthetic tissues.

sul·fo·rho·da·mine B (sŭl-fō-rō′dă-mēn) [C.I. 45100]. A xanthene dye derivative, a fluorochrome used for tagging proteins by a sulfamido condensation; employed in immunofluorescence alone or in combination with fluorescein isothiocyanate for the simultaneous microscopic detection of two antigens in contrasting red and green colors. SYN lissamine rhodamine B 200.

sul·for·me·thox·ine (sŭl′fōr-me-thok′sēn). SYN sulfadoxine.

sul·fo·sal·i·cyl·ic ac·id (sŭl′fō-sal-i-sil′ik). Used as a test for albumin and ferric ion. SYN salicylsulfonic acid.

sul·fo·sol (sŭl′fō-sol). A hydrosol with sulfuric acid instead of water as the dispersion means.

sul·fo·trans·fer·ase (sŭl-fō-trans′fer-ās). Generic term for enzymes in EC sub-subclass 2.8.2 catalyzing the transfer of a sulfate group from 3′-phosphoadenylyl sulfate (active sulfate) to the hydroxyl group of an acceptor, producing the sulfated derivative and 3′-phosphoadenosine 5′-phosphate. SYN sulfikinase, sulfokinase.

sulf·ox·ide (sŭl-fok′sīd). The sulfur analog of a ketone, R′–SO–R″.

sulf·ox·one so·di·um (sŭl-fok′sōn). An antileprotic.

sul·fur (S) (sŭl′fer). An element, atomic no. 16, atomic wt. 32.066, that combines with oxygen to form s. dioxide (SO_2) and s. trioxide (SO_3), and these with water to make strong acids, and with many metals and nonmetallic elements to form sulfides; mildly laxative; has been used to treat rheumatism, gout, and bronchitis, and externally in the treatment of skin diseases. SYN brimstone. [L. *sulfur,* brimstone, sulfur]

s. dioxide, SO_2; a colorless, nonflammable gas with a strong, suffocating odor; a powerful reducing agent used to prevent oxidative deterioration of food and medicinal products. SEE ALSO sulfurous acid. SYN sulfurous oxide.

s. iodide, has been used in the treatment of certain skin diseases.

liver of s., SYN sulfurated *potash.*

precipitated s., sublimed s. boiled with lime water, the lime being removed from the precipitate by washing with diluted hydrochloric acid; used in preparing s. ointment and in the treatment of various skin disorders. SYN lac sulfuris, milk of sulfur.

roll s., sublimed s. melted and cast in cylindrical molds; sometimes called brimstone.

soft s., an allotropic form obtained by dropping very hot melted s. into water; it is then temporarily of a viscid or waxy consistency.

sublimed s., used in preparing s. ointment and in the treatment of various skin disorders. SYN flowers of sulfur.

s. trioxide, SO_3; forms sulfuric acid, H_2SO_4, by its reaction with water. SYN sulfuric oxide.

vegetable s., SYN lycopodium.

washed s., sublimed s. macerated in diluted ammonia water to remove the free acid; same therapeutic uses as sublimed s.

wettable s., s. prepared from calcium polysulfide solution containing a protective colloid such as casein; it is easily dispersed and suspended in water.

sul·fur-35 (^{35}S). A radioactive sulfur isotope; a beta emitter with a half-life of 87.2 days; used as a tracer in the study of metabolism of cysteine, cystine, methionine, etc.; also used to estimate, with labeled sulfate, extracellular fluid volumes.

sul·fu·ret (sŭl′fer-et). SYN sulfide.

sul·fur group. The elements sulfur, selenium, and tellurium; they form dibasic acids with hydrogen, and their oxyacids are also dibasic.

sul·fur·ic (sŭl-fū′rik). Related to sulfuric acid.

sul·fu·ric ac·id (sŭl-fūr′ik). H_2SO_4; a colorless, nearly odorless, heavy, oily, corrosive liquid containing 96% of the absolute acid; used occasionally as a caustic. SYN oil of vitriol.

fuming s. a., SYN Nordhausen s. a.

Nordhausen s. a., s. a. containing sulfurous acid gas in solution. SYN fuming s. a. [named for *Nordhausen,* a town in Saxony where it was first prepared]

sul·fu·ric ether. SYN diethyl ether.

sul·fu·ric ox·ide. SYN sulfur trioxide.

sul·fu·rous (sŭl′fŭr-ŭs). Designating a sulfur compound in which sulfur has a valence of +4 as contrasted to sulfuric compounds in which sulfur has a valence of +6, or sulfides (−2).

sul·fu·rous ac·id. A solution of about 6% sulfur dioxide in water; used chiefly as a disinfectant and bleaching agent; it has been used externally for its parasiticidal effect in various skin diseases.

sul·fu·rous ox·ide. SYN sulfur dioxide.

sul·fur·yl (sŭl′fŭr-il). The bivalent radical, $-SO_2-$.

sul·fy·drate (sŭl-fī′drăt). A compound of SH^-.

sul·in·dac (sŭl-in′dak). A nonsteroidal anti-inflammatory agent with analgesic and antipyretic actions. S. is a prodrug which is reduced to an active drug.

sul·i·so·ben·zone (soo-lī′sō-ben′zōn). A sunscreen agent.

Sulkowitch, Hirsh W., U.S. physician, *1906. SEE S. *reagent.*

△**sulph-, sulpho-.** SEE sulf-.

sul·pir·ide (sŭl′pir-īd). An antidepressant.

sul·thi·ame (sŭl-thi′ām). Inhibits carbonic anhydrase; an anticonvulsant used in the treatment of temporal lobe epilepsy and grand mal with psychomotor seizures; may cause ataxia, paresthesias, and psychotic episodes.

Sulzberger, Marion B., U.S. dermatologist, 1895–1983. SEE Bloch-S. *disease;* syndrome; S.-Garbe *disease, syndrome.*

sum·ma·tion (sŭm-ā′shŭn). The aggregation of a number of similar neural impulses or stimuli. [Mediev. L. *summatio,* fr. *summo,* pp. *-atus,* to sum up, fr. L. *summa,* sum]

s. of stimuli, cumulative muscular or neural effects produced by the frequent repetition of stimuli.

Sumner, F.W., 20th century British surgeon. SEE S. *sign.*

sun·burn (sŭn′bern). Erythema with or without blistering caused by exposure to critical amounts of ultraviolet light, usually within the range of 260–320 nm in sunlight (UVB). SYN erythema solare.

sun·down·ing (sŭn′down-ing). The onset or exacerbation of delirium during the evening or night with improvement or disappearance during the day; most often seen in mid and later stages of dementing disorders, such as Alzheimer disease.

sun·flow·er seed oil (sŭn′flow-er). Oil from the seeds of *Helianthus annuus* (family Compositae); the glycerides consist mainly of the mixed triglycerides, each containing one or two linoleic acid radicals; used as a food, and in dietary supplements.

sun·screen (sŭn′skrēn). A topical product that protects the skin from ultraviolet-induced erythema and resists washing off; its use also reduces formation of solar keratoses and reduces ultraviolet-B-induced melanoma and nonmelanoma skin cancers and wrinkling.

sun·stroke (sŭn′strōk). A form of heatstroke resulting from undue exposure to the sun's rays, probably caused by the action of actinic rays combined with high temperature; symptoms are those of heatstroke, but often without fever. SYN heliosis, ictus solis, insolation (2), siriasis, solar fever (2).

△**super-.** In excess, above, superior, or in the upper part of; often the same usage as L. supra-. Cf. hyper-. [L. *super,* above, beyond]

su·per·ab·duc·tion (soo-per-ab-dŭk′shŭn). Abduction of a limb beyond the normal limit. SYN hyperabduction.

su·per·a·cid·i·ty (soo′per-a-sid′i-tē). An excess of acid; excessive acidity.

su·per·a·cro·mi·al (soo-per-ă-krō′mē-ăl). Above the acromion process. SYN supra-acromial.

su·per·ac·tiv·i·ty (soo-per-ak-tiv′i-tē). Abnormally great activity. SYN hyperactivity (1).

su·per·a·cute (soo′per-ă-kūt′). Extremely acute; marked by extreme severity of symptoms and rapid progress, as of the course of a disease.

su·per·al·i·men·ta·tion (soo′per-al′i-men-tā′shŭn). SYN hyperalimentation.

su·per·a·nal (soo-per-ā′năl). SYN supra-anal.

su·per·an·ti·gen. An antigen that interacts with the T-cell receptor in a domain outside the antigen recognition site. This interaction induces the activation of larger numbers of T cells than are induced by antigens that are presented in the antigen recognition site leading to the release of numerous cytokines. SEE ALSO antigen.

su·per·cil·i·ary (soo-per-sil′ē-ār-ē). Relating to or in the region of the eyebrow. SYN supraciliary.

su·per·cil·i·um, pl. **su·per·cil·i·a** (soo′per-sil′ē-ŭm, -ă). SYN eyebrow. [L. fr. *super,* above, + *cilium,* eyelid]

su·per·coil·ing. SYN superhelicity.

su·per·di·crot·ic (soo-per-dī-krot′ik). SYN hyperdicrotic.

su·per·dis·ten·tion (soo′per-dis-ten′shŭn). SYN hyperdistention.

su·per·duct (sooper-dŭkt). To elevate or draw upward. [L. *super-duco,* pp. *-ductus,* to lead over]

su·per·e·go (soo-per-ē′gō). In psychoanalysis, one of the three components of the psychic apparatus in the freudian structural framework, the other two being the ego and the id. It is an outgrowth of the ego that has identified itself unconsciously with important persons, such as parents, from early life, and which results from incorporating the values and wishes of these persons and subsequently societal norms as part of one's own standards to form the "conscience."

su·per·e·rup·tion. Movement of a tooth beyond the normal plane of occlusion due to the loss of its antagonist(s).

su·per·ex·ci·ta·tion (soo'per-ek-sī-tā'shŭn). **1.** The act of exciting or stimulating unduly. **2.** A condition of extreme excitement or stimulation.

su·per·ex·ten·sion (soo-per-eks-ten'shŭn). SYN hyperextension.

su·per·fat·ted (soo'per-fat'ed). With additional fat added, as in the case of soap.

su·per·fe·ta·tion (soo'per-fe-tā'shŭn). The presence of two fetuses of different ages, not twins, in the uterus, due to the impregnation of two ova liberated at successive periods of ovulation; an obsolete concept. SYN hypercyesis, hypercyesia, multifetation, superimpregnation.

su·per·fi·cial (soo-per-fish'ăl) [TA]. **1.** Cursory; not thorough. **2.** Pertaining to or situated near the surface. **3.** SYN superficialis. [L. *superficialis,* fr. *superficies,* surface]

su·per·fi·ci·a·lis (soo'per-fish-ē-ā'lis) [TA]. Situated nearer the surface of the body in relation to a specific reference point. Cf. profundus. SYN superficial (3) [TA], sublimis (2). [L.]

s. vo'lae, SYN superficial palmar *branch* of radial artery.

su·per·fi·cies (su-per-fish'ĭ-ēz). Outer surface; facies. [L. the top surface, fr. *super,* above, + *facies,* figure, form]

su·per·flex·ion (soo-per-flek'shŭn). SYN hyperflexion.

su·per·fuse (soo-per-fūs'). To flush a fluid over the top of a tissue. Cf. perfuse, perifuse.

su·per·fu·sion (soo-per-fū'zhŭn). The act of superfusing.

su·per·gen·u·al (soo-per-jen'ū-ăl). Above the knee or any genu.

su·per·hel·ic·i·ty (soo'per-hē-li'si-tē). Referring to native duplex DNA structure in which there is further twisting or coiling of the double helix. SYN supercoiling.

su·per·im·preg·na·tion (soo'per-im-preg-nā'shŭn). SYN superfetation.

su·per·in·duce (soo'per-in-doos). To induce or bring on in addition to something already existing.

su·per·in·fec·tion (soo'per-in-fek'shŭn). A new infection in addition to one already present.

su·per·in·vo·lu·tion (soo'per-in-vō-loo'shŭn). An extreme reduction in size of the uterus, after childbirth, below the normal size of the nongravid organ. SYN hyperinvolution.

su·pe·ri·or (soo-pēr'ē-ōr). **1.** Situated above or directed upward. **2** [NA]. In human anatomy, situated nearer the vertex of the head in relation to a specific reference point; opposite of inferior. SYN cranial (2). [L. comparative of *superus,* above]

su·per·lac·ta·tion (soo'per-lak-tā'shŭn). The continuance of lactation beyond the normal period. SYN hyperlactation.

su·per·lig·a·men (soo-per-lig'ă-men). A retentive dressing; a bandage retaining a surgical dressing in place. [L. *ligamen,* bandage]

su·per·me·di·al (soo-per-mē'dē-ăl). Above the middle of any part.

su·per·mo·til·i·ty (soo'per-mō-til'i-tē). SYN hyperkinesis.

su·per·na·tant (soo-per-nā'tănt). SEE supernatant *fluid.* [super- + L. *natare,* to swim]

su·per·nu·mer·ary (soo-per-noo'mer-ār-ē). Exceeding the normal number. SYN epactal. [super- + L. *numerus,* number]

su·per·nu·tri·tion (soo'per-noo-trish'ŭn). Overeating leading to obesity. SYN hypernutrition.

su·per·o·lat·er·al (soo'per-ō-lat'er-ăl). At the side and above.

su·per·ov·u·la·tion (soo'per-ō-vū-lā'shŭn). Ovulation of a greater than normal number of ova; usually the result of the administration of exogenous gonadotropins.

su·per·ox·ide (soo-per-oks'īd). An oxygen free radical, O_2^-, which is toxic to cells.

s. dismutase (SOD), an enzyme that catalyzes the dismutation reaction, $2O_2 \cdot^- + 2H^+ \rightarrow H_2O_2 + O_2$; there are three isozymes of SOD: an extracellular form (ECSOD) that contains copper and zinc, a cytoplasmic form that also contains copper and zinc, and a

mitochondrial form that contains manganese; a deficiency of SOD is associated with amyotrophic lateral sclerosis.

su·per·par·a·site (soo-per-par'ă-sīt). A member of a large population of parasites living on a host, usually a parasitic hymenopteran larva in its insect host. SEE ALSO parasitoid.

su·per·par·a·sit·ism (soo-per-par'ă-si-tizm). **1.** Association between parasitic Hymenoptera and their insect hosts. **2.** An excess of parasites of the same species in a host, overtaxing the defense mechanism to the degree that disease or death results, in contrast to multiple parasitism.

su·per·pe·tro·sal (soo-per-pe-trō'săl). Above or at the upper part of the petrous portion of the temporal bone.

su·per·sat·u·rate (soo-per-sach'ŭ-rāt). To make a solution hold more of a salt or other substance in solution than it will dissolve when in equilibrium with that salt in the solid phase; such solutions are usually unstable with respect to precipitating the excess salt or substance and becoming saturated.

su·per·scrip·tion (soo'per-skrip'shŭn). The beginning of a prescription, consisting of the injunction, *recipe,* take, usually denoted by the sign ℞. [L. *super-scribo,* pp. *-scriptus,* to write upon or over]

su·per·son·ic (soo'per-son'ik). **1.** Pertaining to or characterized by a speed greater than the speed of sound. SEE ALSO hypersonic. **2.** Pertaining to sound vibrations of high frequency, above the level of human audibility. SEE ALSO ultrasonic. [super- + L. *sonus,* sound]

su·per·struc·ture (soo-per-strŭk'choor). A structure above the surface.

implant denture s., the denture which is retained and stabilized by the implant denture substructure.

su·per·ten·sion (soo-per-ten'shŭn). Extreme tension; incorrectly used as a synonym of high blood pressure, or hyperpiesis.

su·per·volt·age (soo'per-vol'tij). In radiation therapy, a descriptor for high-energy radiation above 1000 V.

su·pi·nate (soo'pi-nāt). **1.** To assume, or to be placed in, a supine (face upward) position. **2.** To perform supination of the forearm or of the foot. [L. *supino,* pp. *-atus,* to bend backwards, place on back, fr. *supinus,* supine]

su·pi·na·tion (soo'pi-nā'shŭn) [TA]. The condition of being supine; the act of assuming or of being placed in a supine position.

s. of the foot, inversion and abduction of the foot, causing an elevation of the medial edge.

s. of the forearm, rotation of the forearm in such a way that the palm of the hand faces foreward when the arm is in the anatomical position, or upward when the arm is extended at a right angle to the body.

su·pi·na·tor (soo'pi-nā-ter, -tōr) [TA]. SYN supinator (*muscle*). SEE supinator (*muscle*), biceps brachii (*muscle*).

su·pine (soo-pīn'). **1.** Denoting the body when lying face upward. **2.** Supination of the forearm or of the foot. [L. *supinus*]

sup·port (sŭ-pōrt'). **1.** To add to in an attempt to give greater strength. **2.** SYN supporter. **3.** In dentistry, a term used to denote resistance to vertical components of masticatory force. [L. *supporto,* to carry]

sup·port·er (sŭ-pōrt'er). An apparatus intended to hold in place a dependent or pendulous part, prolapsed organ, or joint. SYN support (2). [see support]

sup·pos·i·to·ry (sŭ-poz'i-tōr-ē). A small solid body shaped for ready introduction into one of the orifices of the body other than the oral cavity (e.g., rectum, urethra, vagina), made of a substance, usually medicated, which is solid at ordinary temperatures but melts at body temperature. S. bases usually used are theobroma oil, glycerinated gelatin, hydrogenated vegetable oils, mixtures of polyethylene glycols of various molecular weights, and fatty acid esters of polyethylene glycol. [L. *suppositorium,* fr. *suppositorius,* placed underneath]

glycerin s., a conical translucent dosage form for rectal administration intended for the relief of constipation; frequently used in young children. Contains glycerin and a stiffening agent such as sodium stearate (a soap). Action is produced by lubrication, water retention, and local irritation.

sup·pres·sion (sŭ-presh′ŭn). **1.** Deliberately excluding from conscious thought. Cf. repression. **2.** Arrest of the secretion of a fluid, such as urine or bile. Cf. retention (2). **3.** Checking of an abnormal flow or discharge, as in s. of a hemorrhage. **4.** The effect of a second mutation which overwrites a phenotypic change caused by a previous mutation at a different point on the chromosome. SEE epistasis. **5.** Inhibition of vision in one eye when dissimilar images fall on corresponding retinal points. [L. *sub-primo* (*subp-*), pp. *-pressus,* to press down]

    fixation s., the reduction in induced or spontaneous nystagmus that occurs with visual fixation.

    immune s., s. of the immune response by some compound or agent.

    intergenic s., SEE suppressor *mutation* (2).

    intragenic s., SEE suppressor *mutation* (2).

sup·pres·sor (soo-pres′ōr). A compound that suppresses the effects of mutation or suppresses what would be a normal course of events.

    amber s., a mutant gene that codes for a tRNA whose anticodon has been altered so that the altered tRNA responds to UAG codons as well.

sup·pu·rant (sŭp′ūr-ant). **1.** Causing or inducing suppuration. **2.** An agent with this action. [L. *suppurans,* causing suppuration]

sup·pu·rate (sŭp′yŭr-āt). To form pus. [L. *sup-puro* (*subp-*), pp. *-atus,* to form *pus* (*pur*), pus]

sup·pu·ra·tion (sŭp′yŭ-rā′shŭn). The formation of pus. SYN pyesis, pyogenesis, pyopoiesis, pyosis. [L. *suppuratio* (see suppurate)]

sup·pu·ra·tive (sŭp′yŭr-ă-tiv). Forming pus.

⏷**supra-.** A position above the part indicated by the word to which it is joined; in this sense, the same as super-; opposite of infra-. [L. *supra,* on the upper side]

su·pra·a·cro·mi·al (soo-pră-ă-krō′mē-ăl). SYN superacromial.

su·pra·a·nal (soo-pră-ā′năl). Above the anus. SYN superanal.

su·pra·au·ric·u·lar (soo-pră-aw-rik′ū-lăr). Above the auricle or pinna of the ear.

su·pra·ax·il·lary (soo′pră-ak′si-lār′ē). Above the axilla.

su·pra·buc·cal (soo-pră-bŭk′ăl). Above the cheek.

su·pra·bulge (soo′pră-bŭlj). The portion of the crown of a tooth that converges toward the occlusal surface of the tooth.

su·pra·car·di·nal (soo-pră-kar′di-năl). Lying dorsal to the anterior or posterior cardinal veins in the embryo.

su·pra·cer·e·bel·lar (soo-pră-ser-ĕ-bel′ar). On or above the surface of the cerebellum.

su·pra·ce·re·bral (soo-pră-ser′ĕ-brăl, -sĕ-rē′brăl). On or above the surface of the cerebrum.

su·pra·cho·roid (soo-pră-kō′royd). On the outer side of the choroid of the eye.

suprachoroidea. SYN suprachoroid *lamina* of sclera.

su·pra·cil·i·ary (soo-pră-sil′ē-ār-ē). SYN superciliary.

su·pra·cla·vic·u·lar (soo-pră-kla-vik′ū-lăr). Above the clavicle, denoting some cutaneous nerves.

su·pra·cla·vic·u·lar·is (soo′pră-kla-vik′ū-lār′is). SEE supraclavicular *muscle.*

su·pra·con·dy·lar (soo-pră-kon′di-lăr). Above a condyle. SYN supracondyloid.

su·pra·con·dy·loid (soo′-pra-kon′di-loyd). SYN supracondylar.

su·pra·cos·tal (soo-pră-kos′tăl). Above the ribs.

su·pra·cot·y·loid (soo-pră-kot′i-loyd). Above the cotyloid cavity, or acetabulum.

su·pra·cris·tal (soo-pră-kris′tăl). Above a crest or ridge; specifically used to denote a line or plane across the summits of the iliac crests.

su·pra·di·a·phrag·mat·ic (soo-pră-dī-ă-frag-mat′ik). Above the diaphragm.

su·pra·duc·tion (soo-pră-dŭk′shŭn). The upward rotation of one eye. SYN sursumduction.

su·pra·ep·i·con·dy·lar (soo-pră-ep′i-kon′di-lăr). Above an epicondyle.

su·pra·gle·noid (soo-pră-glē′noyd). Above the glenoid cavity or fossa.

su·pra·glot·tic (soo-pră-glot′ik). Above the glottis.

sup·ra·glot·ti·tis (soop′ra-gla-tī′tis). An infectious inflammation and swelling of the laryngeal tissue above the glottis, especially of the epiglottis, which becomes red and spherical leading to upper airway obstruction.

su·pra·he·pat·ic (soo-pră-he-pat′ik). Above the liver.

su·pra·hy·oid (soo-pră-hī′oyd). Above the hyoid bone, denoting, among other things, a group of muscles.

su·pra·in·gui·nal (soo-pră-ing′gwin-ăl). Above the inguinal region, or groin.

su·pra·in·tes·ti·nal (soo-pră-in-tes′ti-năl). Above the intestine.

su·pra·lim·i·nal (soo-pră-lim′i-năl). More than just perceptible; above the threshhold for conscious awareness. Cf. subliminal. [supra- + L. *limen,* threshold]

su·pra·lum·bar (soo-pră-lŭm′bar). Above the lumbar region.

su·pra·mal·le·o·lar (soo-pră-mal-ē-ō-lăr). Above a malleolus.

su·pra·mam·ma·ry (soo-pră-mam′ă-rē). Above the mammary gland.

su·pra·man·dib·u·lar (soo-pră-man-dib′ū-lăr). Above the mandible.

su·pra·mar·gin·al (soo-pră-mar′jin-ăl). Above any margin; denoting especially the s. gyrus.

su·pra·mas·toid (soo-pră-mas′toyd). Above the mastoid process of the temporal bone.

su·pra·max·il·la (soo′pră-mak-sil′ă). Obsolete term for maxilla.

su·pra·max·il·lary (soo-pră-mak′si-lār-ē). Above the maxilla.

su·pra·men·tal (soo-pră-men′tăl). Above the chin.

su·pra·men·ta·le (soo′pră-men-tā′lē). In cephalometrics, the most posterior midline point, above the chin, on the mandibula between the infradentate and the pogonion. SYN point B. [supra- + L. *mentum,* chin]

su·pra·na·sal (soo-pră-nā′săl). Above the nose.

su·pra·neu·ral (soo-pră-noo′răl). Above the neural axis.

su·pra·nu·cle·ar (soo-pră-noo′klē-er). Above (cranial to) the level of the motor neurons of the spinal or cranial nerves; the pathways the suprasegmental nerve fibers follow to reach the motor cell bodies in the brainstem; as used in clinical neurology, s. indicates disorders of movement caused by destruction or functional impairment of brain structures other than the motor neurons, such as the motor cortex, pyramidal tract, or striate body; e.g., supranuclear palsy, as distinguished from the nuclear (or flaccid, or "lower motor neuron") paralysis that results from destruction or functional impairment of the motor neurons or their axons in a peripheral nerve.

su·pra·oc·clu·sion (soo′pră-ō-kloo′zhŭn). An occlusal relationship in which a tooth extends beyond the occlusal plane.

su·pra·or·bit·al (soo-pră-ōr′bi-tăl). Above the orbit, either on the face or within the cranium; denoting numerous structures. SEE canal, foramen, notch, nerve.

su·pra·or·bi·to·me·a·tal (soo′pra-or-bit-ō-mē-at′al). Above or at the top of both the orbit and the external acoustic meatus; denotes a line or plane.

su·pra·pa·tel·lar (soo-pră-pă-tel′ăr). Above the patella, denoting especially a bursa.

su·pra·pel·vic (soo-pră-pel′vik). Above the pelvis.

su·pra·phys·i·o·log·ic, su·pra·phys·i·o·log·i·cal (soo′pră-fiz-ē-ō-loj′ik, -loj′i-kăl). Denoting any dose (of a chemical agent that either is or mimics a hormone, neurotransmitter, or other naturally occurring agent) that is larger or more potent than would occur naturally, or the effects of such a dose. Cf. homeopathic (2), pharmacologic (2), physiologic (4).

su·pra·pu·bic (soo-pră-pū′bik). Above the pubic bone.

su·pra·re·nal (soo′pră-rē′năl). **1.** Above the kidney. SYN surrenal. **2.** Pertaining to the suprarenal glands. [supra- + L. *ren,* kidney]

su·pra·scap·u·lar (soo-pră-skap′ū-lăr). Above the scapula, denoting especially an artery, vein, and nerve.

su·pra·scle·ral (soo-pră-sklēr′ăl). On the outer side of the sclera, denoting the s. or perisclerotic space between the sclera and the fascia bulbi.

su·pra·sel·lar (soo-pră-sel'ăr). Above or over the sella turcica.

su·pra·spi·nal (soo-pră-spī'năl). Above the vertebral column or any spine.

su·pra·spi·na·lis (soo-pră-spi-nā'lis). SEE supraspinalis (*muscle*).

su·pra·spi·na·tus (soo-pră-spī-nā'tŭs). SEE supraspinatus (*muscle*).

su·pra·spi·nous (soo-pră-spī'nŭs). Above any spine; especially above one or more of the vertebral spines (e.g., supraspinous ligament) or the spine of the scapula.

su·pra·sta·pe·di·al (soo-pră-sta-pēd'ē-ăl). Above the stapes.

su·pra·ster·nal (soo-pră-ster'năl). Above the sternum.

su·pra·syl·vi·an (soop-ră-sil'vē-an). Above the fissure of Sylvius or lateral sulcus.

su·pra·sym·phys·ary (soo-pră-sim-phiz'ă-rē). Above the pubic symphysis.

su·pra·tem·po·ral (soo-pră-tem'pŏ-răl). Above the temporal region.

su·pra·ten·to·ri·al (soo'pră-ten-tōr'ē-ăl). Denoting cranial contents located above the tentorium cerebelli; often used to describe functional symptoms.

su·pra·tho·rac·ic (soo-pră-thō-ras'ik). Above or in the upper part of the thorax.

su·pra·ton·sil·lar (soo-pră-ton'si-lăr). Above the tonsil; denoting a recess above and slightly back of the tonsil.

su·pra·troch·le·ar (soo-pră-trok'lē-ăr). Above a trochlea, denoting a nerve.

su·pra·tur·bi·nal (soo-pră-ter'bi-năl). SYN supreme nasal *concha*.

su·pra·tym·pan·ic (soo-pră-tim-pan'ik). Above the tympanic cavity.

su·pra·vag·i·nal (soo-pră-vaj'i-năl). Above the vagina, or above any sheath.

su·pra·val·var (soo-pră-val'văr). Above the valves, either pulmonary or aortic. SYN supravalvular.

su·pra·val·vu·lar (soo-pră-val'vū-lăr). SYN supravalvar.

su·pra·ven·tric·u·lar (soo-pră-ven-trik'ū-lăr). Above the ventricles; especially applied to rhythms originating from centers proximal to the ventricles, namely in the atrium, AV node, or AV junction, in contrast to rhythms arising in the ventricles themselves.

su·pra·ver·sion (soo-pră-ver'zhŭn). **1.** A turning (version) upward. **2.** In dentistry, the position of a tooth when it is out of the line of occlusion in an occlusal direction; a deep overbite. **3.** In ophthalmology, binocular conjugate rotation upward. [supra- + L. *verto*, pp. *versus*, to turn]

su·pro·fen (soo-prō'fen). A nonsteroidal anti-inflammatory agent with antipyretic and analgesic properties; similar to ibuprofen.

su·ral (soo'răl). Relating to the calf of the leg.

sur·al·i·men·ta·tion (ser-al'i-men-tā'shŭn). SYN hyperalimentation. [Fr. *sur*, fr. L. *super*, above]

sur·a·min so·di·um (soo'ră-min). A complex derivative of urea; used in the treatment of trypanosomiasis, onchocerciasis, and pemphigus.

sur·face (ser'făs) [TA]. The outer part of any solid. SYN face (2) [TA], facies (2) [TA]. [F. fr. L. *superficius*, see superficial]

acromial articular s. of clavicle, SYN acromial *facet* of clavicle.

anterior s. [TA], the surface of a structure or part of the body that faces forward. TA recognizes an anterior surface (facies anterior ...) of the following structures: heart (... cordis [TA]); cornea (... corneae [TA]); body of maxilla (... corporis maxillae [TA]); lens (... lentis [TA]); eyelids (... palpebrae [TA]); petrous part of temporal bone (... pars petrosi ossis temporalis [TA]); kidney (... renis [TA]); iris (... iridis [TA]); patella (... patellae [TA]); prostate (... prostatae [TA]); radius (... radii [TA]); suprarenal gland (... glandulae suprarenalis [TA]); ulna (... ulnae [TA]); uterus (... uteri [TA]). SYN facies anterior [TA].

anterior s. of arm, SYN anterior *region* of arm.

anterior articular s. of dens [TA], the curved articular facet on the anterior aspect of the dens of the axis that articulates with the facet for the dens of the axis anterior arch of the atlas. SYN facies articularis anterior dentis [TA].

anterior s. of cornea [TA], the external s. of the cornea. SYN facies anterior corneae [TA].

anterior s. of elbow, SYN anterior *region* of elbow.

anterior s. of eyelids, SYN *facies* anterior palpebrarum.

anterior s. of forearm, SYN anterior *region* of forearm.

anterior s. of iris [TA], the aspect of the iris of the eyeball visible through the cornea. SYN facies anterior iridis [TA].

anterior s. of kidney [TA], the aspect of the kidney facing th abdominal cavity. SYN facies anterior renis [TA].

anterior s. of leg, SYN anterior *region* of leg.

anterior s. of lens [TA], the aspect of the lens of the eyeball that forms the posterior boundary of the aqueous-filled anterior segment. SYN facies anterior lentis [TA].

anterior s. of lower limb [TA], the ventral or flexor aspect of the inferior limb. SYN facies anterior membri inferioris [TA].

anterior s. of maxilla [TA], the s. of the maxilla below the orbit and lateral to the nasal aperture. SYN facies anterior corporis maxillae [TA].

anterior s. of patella [TA], the subcutaneous aspect of the patella. SYN facies anterior patellae [TA].

anterior s. of petrous part of temporal bone [TA], the s. of the petrous part of the temporal bone contributing to the floor of the middle cranial fossa. SYN facies anterior partis petrosae ossis temporalis [TA].

anterior s. of prostate [TA], the aspect of the prostate facing the pubic symphysis. SYN facies anterior prostatae [TA].

anterior s. of radius [TA], the ventral aspect of the radius, much of which provides attachment for the flexor pollicis longus muscle. SYN facies anterior radii [TA].

anterior s. of suprarenal gland [TA], the aspect of the suprarenal gland facing the abdominal cavity. SYN facies anterior glandulae suprarenalis [TA].

anterior talar articular s. of calcaneus [TA], underlies the head of the talus and contributes to the talocalcaneonavicular joint. SYN facies articularis talaris anterior calcanei [TA].

anterior s. of thigh, SYN anterior *region* of thigh.

anterior s. of ulna [TA], the anterior s. of the ulna. SYN facies anterior ulnae [TA].

anterior s. of uterus [TA], ventral s. of uterus; in its normal position (anteverted and anteflexed) this is actually a mostly inferior s. SYN facies anterior uteri [TA].

anteroinferior s. of pancreas [TA], the s. of the body of the pancreas that faces forward and downward. SYN facies anteroinferior corporis pancreatis [TA].

anterolateral s. of arytenoid cartilage [TA], of the three nonarticular surfaces of the pyramidal arytenoid cartilage, the convex, rougher one that bears the oblong and triangular foveae, the former giving attachment to the vocalis and lateral cricoarytenoid muscles, the latter to the vestibular ligament. SYN facies anterolateralis cartilaginis arytenoideae [TA].

anterolateral s. of (shaft of) humerus [TA], the s. of the humerus lateral to the intertubercular groove. SYN facies anterolateralis corporis humeri [TA], facies anterior lateralis corporis humeri.

anteromedial s. of shaft of humerus [TA], the s. of the humerus between the anterior and medial borders of the bone. SYN facies anteromedialis corporis humeri [TA], facies anterior medialis corporis humeri.

anterosuperior s. of body of pancreas [TA], of the three s.'s of the prism-shaped body of the pancreas, the one which faces (contacts) the stomach, being separated from it by the potential space of the omental bursa. SYN facies anterosuperioris corporis pancreatis [TA].

approximal s. of tooth [TA], the s. of a tooth that faces an adjacent tooth in the dental arch; the contact s. that is closest to the anterior midline of the dental arch is the mesial s.; that farthest is the distal s. SYN interproximal s. of tooth⁎, contact s. of tooth, facies approximalis dentis, facies contactus dentis.

articular s. [TA], any articular s. SYN facies articularis [TA].

articular s. of acromion, SYN clavicular articular *facet* of acromion.

articular s. of arytenoid cartilage [TA], the oval s. on the undersurface of the muscular process of the arytenoid for articulation with the cricoid cartilage. SYN facies articularis cartilaginis arytenoideae [TA].

articular s. of mandibular fossa of temporal bone [TA], the smooth portion of the mandibular articular fossa and eminence of the temporal bone that articulates with the disk of the temporomandibular joint. SYN facies articularis fossae mandibularis ossis temporalis [TA].

articular s. on calcaneus for cuboid bone [TA], the saddle-shaped s. on the anterior end of the calcaneus for articulation with the cuboid (bone). SYN facies articularis cuboidea ossis calcanei [TA], cuboidal articular s. of calcaneus.

articular s. of patella [TA], the posterior s. of the patella, covered with hyaline cartilage and subdivided by a vertical ridge into a larger lateral and a smaller medial s. for articulation with the corresponding condyles of the femur. SYN facies articularis patellae [TA].

arytenoidal articular s. of cricoid [TA], one of two oval facets on the superolateral margin of the cricoid lamina for articulation with the arytenoid cartilages. SYN facies articularis arytenoidea cricoideae [TA].

auricular s. of ilium [TA], the irregular, L-shaped articular s. on the medial aspect of the ilium that articulates with the sacrum. SYN facies auricularis ossis ilii [TA].

auricular s. of sacrum [TA], the rough articular s. on the lateral aspect of the sacrum that articulates with the ilium on each side. SYN facies auricularis ossis sacri [TA].

axial s.'s, s.'s of a tooth parallel to its long axis; the axial s.'s are the vestibular (labial or buccal), lingual, and contact (mesial or distal).

balancing occlusal s., SYN balancing *contact*.

basal s., the s. of the denture of which the detail is determined by the impression and which rests upon the basal seat.

buccal s., (1) cheek portion of vestibular s. of tooth. (2) the mucosa of the cheek; (3) in prosthodontics, the side of a denture adjacent to the cheek.

calcaneal articular s. of talus [TA], one of three articular facets on the talus for union with the calcaneus: anterior facet on talus for calcaneus (facies articularis calcanea anterior tali [TA]), middle facet on talus for calcaneus (facies articularis calcanea media tali [TA]), and posterior facet on talus for calcaneus (facies articularis calcanea posterior tali [TA]). SYN facies articularis calcanea tali [TA].

carpal articular s. of radius [TA], the biconcave distal s. of the radius for articulation with the scaphoid bone laterally and the lunate medially. SYN facies articularis carpi radii [TA].

cerebral s., the internal s. of certain cranial bones; they are (the greater wing of) the sphenoid (facies cerebralis alae majoris ossis sphenoidale [TA]) and (the squamous part of) the temporal bone (facies cerebralis partis squamosae ossis temporale [TA]). SYN facies cerebralis.

colic s. of spleen, SYN colic *impression* of spleen.

contact s. of tooth, SYN approximal s. of tooth.

costal s. [TA], the s. of certain structures that face the ribs; they are the costal s.'s of the lungs (facies costalis pulmonis [TA]) and the scapula (facies costalis scapulae [TA]). SYN facies costalis [TA].

costal s. of lung [TA], the s. of each lung that lies in contact with the costal pleura. SYN facies costalis pulmonis [TA].

costal s. of scapula [TA], the concave aspect of the body of the scapula that faces the thorax and that principally lodges and gives origin to the subscapularis muscle. SYN facies costalis scapulae [TA].

cuboidal articular s. of calcaneus, SYN articular s. on calcaneus for cuboid bone.

denture basal s., SYN denture foundation s.

denture foundation s., that portion of the s. of a denture which has its contour determined by the impression and bears the greater part of the occlusal load. SYN denture basal s.

denture impression s., that portion of the s. of a denture which has its contour determined by the impression; it includes the borders of the denture and extends to the polished s.

denture occlusal s., that portion of the s. of a denture that makes contact or near contact with the corresponding s. of an opposing denture or tooth. SYN facies occlusalis dentis [TA], occlusal s. of tooth (2) [TA], facies masticatoria, grinding s., masticating s., masticatory s.

denture polished s., that portion of the denture which extends in an occlusal direction from the border of the denture and includes the palatal s.; it is the part of the denture base which is usually polished and includes the buccal and lingual s.'s of the teeth.

diaphragmatic s. [TA], the s. of an organ in contact with the diaphragm (facies diaphragmatica...) as of the heart (... cordis [TA]); liver (... hepatis [TA]); lungs (... pulmonis [TA]); and spleen (... splenica [TA]). SYN facies diaphragmatica [TA].

distal s. of tooth [TA], the contact s. of a tooth that is directed away from the median plane of the dental arch; opposite to the mesial s. of a tooth. SYN facies distalis dentis [TA].

dorsal s. [TA], the dorsal s. of a structure such as the sacrum, the finges, or the toes. SYN facies dorsalis [TA].

dorsal s. of digit (of hand or foot) [TA], the dorsal s. of a finger or toe. SYN facies digitalis dorsalis (manus et pedis) [TA].

dorsal s. of sacrum [TA], the posterosuperior aspect of the sacrum marked by a median and two lateral sacral crests between which four dorsal sacral foramina are located on each side. SYN facies dorsalis ossis sacri [TA].

dorsal s. of scapula, SYN posterior s. of scapula.

external s. [TA], the outer convex s. of either the frontal or the parietal bone. SYN facies externa [TA].

external s. of cochlear duct [TA], the aspect of the duct that faces the outer (spiral ligament) side of the cochlea. SYN paries externus ductus cochlearis [TA], external wall of cochlear duct.

external s. of cranial base [TA], external aspect of the base of skull. SYN basis cranii externa [TA], external base of skull, norma basilaris, norma inferior, norma ventralis.

external s. of frontal bone [TA], the convex outer s. of the frontal bone. SYN facies externa ossis frontalis [TA].

external s. of parietal bone [TA], the convex outer s. of the parietal bone. SYN facies externa ossis parietalis [TA].

facial s. of tooth, SYN vestibular s. of tooth.

fibular articular s. of tibia, SYN fibular articular *facet* of tibia.

gastric s. of spleen, SYN gastric *impression* on spleen.

glenoid s., SYN mandibular *fossa*.

gluteal s. of ilium [TA], the external s. of the wing of the ilium marked by the anterior, posterior, and inferior gluteal lines that separate the origins of the gluteal muscles. SYN facies glutea ossis ilii [TA].

grinding s., SYN denture occlusal s.

incisal s., SYN incisal *margin*.

inferior articular s. of atlas [TA], one of two concave s.'s on the lateral masses of the atlas that articulate with corresponding s.'s on the axis. SYN facies articularis inferior atlantis [TA], fovea articularis inferior atlantis, inferior articular facet of atlas, inferior articular pit of atlas.

inferior articular s. of tibia [TA], the quadrilateral s. on the distal end of the tibia for articulation with the talus; it is concave anteroposteriorly and broader anteriorly. SYN facies articularis inferior tibiae [TA].

inferior s. of cerebellar hemisphere, it rests in the posterior cranial fossa and overlies the medulla; it includes the semilunaris inferior, biventer lobule, cerebellar tonsil, and flocculus. SYN facies inferior hemispherii cerebri [TA].

inferior cerebral s., SYN base of brain.

inferior s. of petrous part of temporal bone [TA], the portion of the petrous part of the temporal bone that contributes to the external base of the skull. SYN facies inferior partis petrosae ossis temporalis [TA].

inferior s. of tongue [TA], the s. of the tongue that faces the floor of the oral cavity, its mucosa being thin, smooth, and devoid of papillae. SYN facies inferior linguae [TA].

su

inferolateral s. of prostate [TA], the s. of the prostate facing the body of the pubis and the pelvic diaphragm. SYN facies inferolateralis prostatae [TA].

infratemporal s. of (body of) maxilla [TA], the convex posterolateral s. of the body of the maxilla that form the anterior wall of the infratemporal fossa. SYN facies infratemporalis corporis maxillae [TA].

infratemporal s. of greater wing of sphenoid [TA], inferiorly directed s. of greater wing of sphenoid that forms a roof for the infratemporal fossa. SYN facies infratemporalis alaris majoris ossis sphenoidalis [TA].

interlobar s.'s of lung [TA], s. of a lobe of the lung that lies adjacent to (in contact with) the s. of another lobe; the two s.'s are separated by an interlobar fissure in the interlobar fissures of the lung. SYN facies interlobares pulmonis.

internal s. [TA], the internal concave s. of either the frontal or the parietal bone. SYN facies interna [TA].

internal s. of cranial base [TA], the interior aspect of the skull base on which the brain rests; the floor of the cranial cavity. SYN basis cranii interna [TA], internal base of skull.

internal s. of frontal bone [TA], the s. of the frontal bone that contributes to the wall of the cranial cavity. SYN facies interna ossis frontalis [TA].

internal s. of parietal bone [TA], the concave s. of the parietal bone forming part of the wall of the cranial cavity. SYN facies interna ossis parietalis [TA].

interproximal s. of tooth, ✱official alternate term for approximal s. of tooth.

intestinal s. of uterus [TA], the posterosuperior s. of the uterus with which loops of intestine come in contact. SYN facies intestinalis uteri [TA].

lateral s. [TA], the s. of a part of the body that faces away from the midline; TA recognizes a lateral s. on the following structures: fibula, ovary, radius, testis, tibia, zygomatic bone. SYN facies lateralis [TA].

lateral s. of arm, the lateral s. of the arm. SYN facies lateralis brachii.

lateral s. of fibula [TA], the lateral s. of the fibula. SYN facies lateralis fibulae [TA].

lateral s. of finger, the lateral s. of a finger. SYN facies lateralis digiti manus.

lateral s. of leg, the lateral s. of the part of the inferior limb between the knee and the ankle. SYN facies lateralis cruris.

lateral s. of lower limb, the lateral s. of the inferior limb. SYN facies lateralis membri inferioris.

lateral malleolar s. of talus, SYN lateral malleolar facet of talus.

lateral s. of ovary [TA], the s. of the ovary facing the pelvic wall. SYN facies lateralis ovarii [TA].

lateral s. of testis [TA], the laterally directed s. of the testis. SYN facies lateralis testis [TA].

lateral s. of tibia [TA], the laterally directed s. of the tibia. SYN facies lateralis tibiae [TA].

lateral s. of toe, the lateral s. of a toe. SYN facies lateralis digiti pedis.

lateral s. of zygomatic bone [TA], the lateral s. of the zygomatic bone. SYN facies lateralis ossis zygomatici [TA].

lingual s. of tooth [TA], the s. of a tooth that faces the tongue; opposite to the s. vestibulum dentis. SYN facies lingualis dentis [TA].

lunate s. of acetabulum [TA], the curved articular s. that surrounds the acetabular fossa and articulates with the head of the femur. SYN facies lunata acetabuli [TA].

malleolar articular s. of fibula, SYN articular facet of lateral malleolus.

malleolar articular s. of tibia, SYN articular facet of medial malleolus.

masticating s., SYN denture occlusal s.

masticatory s., SYN denture occlusal s.

maxillary s. of greater wing of sphenoid bone [TA], the part of the anterior s. of the greater wing of the sphenoid bone that is perforated by the foramen rotundum and forms the posterior boundary of the pterygopalatine fossa. SYN facies maxillaris alaris majoris ossis sphenoidalis [TA].

maxillary s. of palatine bone, the lateral s. of the perpendicular plate of the palatine bone; SYN facies maxillaris ossis palatini.

medial s. [TA], the surface of a part of the body that faces toward the midline. TA recognizes a medial surface on the following structures: arytenoid cartilage, cerebral hemisphere, fibula, ovary, testis, tibia, ulna. SYN facies medialis [TA].

medial s. of arytenoid cartilage [TA], the s. of the arytenoid cartilage that faces its contralateral partner. SYN facies medialis cartilaginis arytenoideae [TA].

medial cerebral s., SYN medial s. of cerebral hemisphere.

medial s. of cerebral hemisphere [TA], it faces, above as well as anterior and posterior to the corpus callosum, the falx cerebri; below it are the mesencephalon and the dura-covered medial wall of the middle cranial fossa. SYN facies medialis hemispherii cerebri [TA], medial cerebral s.

medial s. of fibula [TA], the s. of the fibula directed toward the midline. SYN facies medialis fibulae [TA].

medial s. of lung, SYN mediastinal s. of lung.

medial s. of ovary [TA], the s. of the ovary that faces the pelvic cavity. SYN facies medialis ovarii [TA].

medial s. of testis, SYN facies medialis testis.

medial s. of tibia, SYN facies medialis tibiae.

medial s. of toes [TA], the medial s. of a toe. SYN facies medialis digiti pedis [TA].

medial s. of ulna, SYN facies medialis ulnae.

mediastinal s. of lung [TA], the part of the medial s. of a lung in contact with the mediastinum. SYN facies mediastinalis pulmonis [TA], facies medialis pulmonis, medial s. of lung, mediastinal part of lung, pars mediastinalis pulmonis.

mesial s. of tooth [TA], the contact s. of a tooth that is directed toward the median plane of the dental arch; opposite to the s. distalis dentis. SYN facies mesialis dentis [TA].

middle talar articular s. of calcaneus [TA], underlies the head of the talus and contributes to the talocalcaneonavicular joint. SYN facies articularis talaris media calcanei [TA].

nasal s. of maxilla [TA], the s. of the maxilla that forms part of the lateral nasal wall with a large defect (maxillary hiatus) posteriorly and the lacrimal sulcus in its midportion. SYN facies nasalis maxillae [TA].

nasal s. of palatine bone [TA], (1) the nasal s. of the perpendicular lamina of the palatine bone that forms part of the lateral wall of the nasal cavity (facies nasalis lamina perpendicularis ossis palatini [TA]); (2) the nasal s. of the horizontal lamina of the palatine bone that forms part of the floor of the nasal cavity (facies nasalis lamina horizontalis ossis palatini [TA]). SYN facies nasalis ossis palatini [TA].

navicular articular s. of talus [TA], the large convex s. on the head of the talus for articulation with the navicular bone. SYN facies articularis navicularis tali [TA].

occlusal s. of tooth [TA], (1) the s. of a tooth that occludes with or contacts an opposing surface of a tooth in the opposing jaw; (2) SYN denture occlusal s.

orbital s. [TA], the s. of a bone that contributes to the walls of the orbit. TA recognizes an orbital s. (facies orbitalis... [TA]) on the following bones: greater wing of the sphenoid bone (... alaris majoris ossis sphenoidale [TA]); the body of the maxilla (... corporis maxillae [TA]); the frontal bone (... ossis frontalis [TA]); the zygomatic bone (... ossis zygomatici [TA]). SYN facies orbitalis [TA].

palatine s. of horizontal plate of palatine bone [TA], the inferior s. of the horizontal plate of the palatine bone. SYN facies palatina laminae horizontalis ossis palatini [TA].

palmar s.'s of fingers [TA], the flat of the fingers; the flexor or anterior s. of the fingers. SYN facies palmares digitorum [TA], facies digitalis palmaris, facies digitalis ventralis, ventral s. of digit.

patellar s. of femur [TA], the groove formed anteriorly between the anterosuperior portions of the femoral condyles that accommodates the patella. SYN facies patellaris femoris [TA], trochlea femoris.

pelvic s. of sacrum [TA], the s. of the sacrum that faces downward and forward forming the roof and part of the posterior wall of the pelvic cavity. SYN facies pelvica ossis sacri [TA].

Petzval s., the curved image plane upon which any extended linear object is focused by a lens; it is curved toward the edges of a convex *lens* and away from the edges of a concave *lens*. SEE barrel *distortion*, pincushion *distortion*.

plantar s. of foot, SYN *sole* of foot.

plantar s. of toe, SYN facies digitalis plantaris.

popliteal s. of femur [TA], the posterior s. of the lower end of the femur between the diverging lips of the linea aspera. SYN facies poplitea femoris [TA], planum popliteum, popliteal plane of femur.

posterior s. [TA], the surface of a part of the body that faces toward the posterior part of the body. TA recognizes a posterior surface of the following structures: arytenoid cartilage, cornea, eyelid, fibula, humerus, iris, kidney, lens, pancreas, petrous part of temporal bone, prostate, radius, scapula, suprarenal gland, tibia, ulna, uterus. SYN facies posterior [TA].

posterior s. of arm, SYN posterior *region* of arm.

posterior articular s. of dens, SYN posterior articular *facet* of dens.

posterior s. of arytenoid cartilage [TA], concave aspect of arytenoid cartilage that gives attachment to the arytenoid muscle and is directed toward the laryngopharynx. SYN facies posterior cartilaginis arytenoideae [TA].

posterior s. of cornea [TA], the deep or internal s. of the cornea in contact with the aqueous humor. SYN facies posterior corneae [TA].

posterior s. of elbow, SYN posterior *region* of elbow.

posterior s. of eyelids [TA], the internal s. of the eyelids, covered with conjunctiva. SYN facies posterior palpebrarum [TA].

posterior s. of fibula [TA], the aspect of the fibula that forms, with the tibia and interosseous membrane, the anterior boundary of the posterior compartment of the leg. SYN facies posterior fibulae [TA].

posterior s. of forearm, SYN posterior *region* of forearm.

posterior s. of iris [TA], the aspect of the iris covered with nonvisual retina, forming the anterior boundary of the posterior chamber of the eyeball. SYN facies posterior iridis [TA].

posterior s. of kidney [TA], the aspect of the kidney directed toward the posterior abdominal wall. SYN facies posterior renis [TA].

posterior s. of leg, SYN posterior *region* of leg.

posterior s. of lens [TA], the aspect of the lens of the eye that forms the anterior boundary of the postremal chamber and is adjacent to the vitreous body. SYN facies posterior lentis [TA].

posterior s. of lower limb, the posterior surface of the inferior limb. SYN facies posterior membri inferioris.

posterior s. of pancreas [TA], the aspect of the pancreas facing the posterior abdominal wall. SYN facies posterior pancreatis [TA].

posterior s. of petrous part of temporal bone [TA], the s. of the petrous part of the temporal bone that contributes to the posterior cranial fossa. SYN facies posterior partis petrosae ossis temporalis [TA].

posterior s. of prostate [TA], the aspect of the prostate that faces the rectum, separated from it by the retroprostatic fascia. SYN facies posterior prostatae [TA].

posterior s. of radius [TA], the dorsal aspect of the radius. SYN facies posterior radii [TA].

posterior s. of scapula [TA], the outer aspect of the body of the scapula, subdivided by the prominent spine of the scapula into a smaller supraspinous fossa and a larger infraspinous fossa. SYN dorsal s. of scapula, facies dorsalis scapulae.

posterior s. of shaft of humerus [TA], the portion of the humerus that features the linea aspera, and to which the intermuscular septa of the thigh attach. SYN facies posterior corporis humeri [TA].

posterior s. of suprarenal gland [TA], the posteromedial s. of the suprarenal gland that contacts the diaphragmatic crura. SYN facies posterior glandulae suprarenalis [TA].

posterior talar articular s. (of calcaneus) [TA], articulates with talus (subtalar joint) posterior to sinus tarsi. SYN facies articularis talaris posterior calcanei [TA].

posterior s. of thigh, SYN posterior *region* of thigh.

posterior s. of tibia [TA], the aspect of the tibia that, with the posterior s. of the fibula and the interosseous membrane, forms the anterior boundary of the posterior compartment of the leg. SYN facies posterior tibiae [TA].

posterior s. of ulna [TA], the dorsal aspect of the ulna. SYN facies posterior ulnae [TA].

renal s. of spleen, SYN renal *impression* of spleen.

renal s. of suprarenal gland [TA], s. of suprarenal gland in contact with the kidney. SYN facies renalis glandulae suprarenalis [TA].

right/left pulmonary s.'s of heart, the lateral s.'s of the heart, directed toward the lungs; on the left it is principally the left ventricular wall; on the right it is the right atrial wall and the upper part of the right ventricular wall. SYN facies pulmonales cordis dextra/sinistra.

sacropelvic s. of ilium [TA], the medial s. of the ilium behind and below the iliac fossa; it includes the iliac tuberosity, the auricular s. and the smooth pelvic s. below and in front of the auricular s. SYN facies sacropelvina ossis ilii [TA].

sternal articular s. of clavicle, SYN sternal *facet* of clavicle.

sternocostal s. of heart [TA], the anterior aspect of the heart, formed mostly by the right ventricle and to a lesser extent the left ventricle. SYN facies sternocostalis cordis [TA].

subocclusal s., a portion of the occlusal s. of a tooth which is below the level of the occluding portion of the tooth.

superior articular s. of atlas [TA], one of two concave articular s.'s on the superior aspect of the lateral masses of the atlas that articulate with the occipital condyles. SYN facies articularis superior atlantis [TA], fovea articularis superior atlantis, superior articular facet of atlas, superior articular pit of atlas.

superior articular s. of tibia [TA], the articular s. on the proximal end of the tibia that is divided into medial and lateral portions for articulation with the condyles of the femur. SYN facies articularis superior tibiae [TA].

superior s. of cerebellar hemisphere, it lies against the under s. of the tentorium and includes the ala lobuli centralis, quadrangular lobule, simple lobule, and superior semilunar lobule. SYN facies superior hemispherii cerebelli [TA].

superior s. of talus, SYN superior *facet* of trochlear of talus.

superolateral cerebral s., SYN superolateral s. of cerebrum.

superolateral s. of cerebrum [TA], the aspect of the cerebral hemisphere that lies in contact with the flat bones of the skull; it includes parts of the frontal, parietal, temporal, and occipital lobes. SYN facies superolateralis hemispherii cerebri [TA], superolateral face of cerebral hemisphere [TA], cortical convexity, superolateral cerebral s.

symphysial s. of pubis [TA], the medial, elongated oval s. of the pubis that faces and articulates with its contralateral partner by means of the interpubic disc, forming the pubic symphysis. SYN facies symphysialis [TA].

talar articular s.'s of calcaneus [TA], the three facets of the calcaneus that articulate with the overlying talus; the anterior and middle talar articular s. contribute to the talocalcaneonavicular joint and are separated by the tarsal sinus from the posterior talar articular s. which enters into the subtalar joint. SYN facies articularis talaris calcanei [TA].

temporal s. [TA], the s. of a bone that contributes to the temporal fossa, namely, the greater wing of the sphenoid, the squamous part of the temporal, frontal, and zygomatic bones. SYN facies temporalis [TA].

tentorial s., those areas of the occipital lobe (inferior aspect) and the cerebellum (superior aspect) that are apposed to the superior and inferior s.'s, respectively, of the tentorium cerebelli.

thyroid articular s. of cricoid (cartilage) [TA], one of two small circular facets on the lateral s. of the cricoid cartilage near the inferior margin of the junction of the arch and lamina for articulation with the inferior horns of the thyroid cartilage. SYN facies articularis thyroidea cricoideae [TA].

su

tympanic s. of cochlear duct [TA], the wall that separates the cochlear duct from the scala tympani; it consists of the osseous spiral lamina and the basilar membrane. SYN paries tympanicus ductus cochlearis [TA], membrana spiralis✲, spiral membrane✲, tympanic wall of cochlear duct.

urethral s. of penis [TA], the s. of the penis opposite to the dorsum penis. SYN facies urethralis penis [TA].

ventral s. of digit, SYN palmar s.'s of fingers.

vesical s. of uterus [TA], the s. of the uterus facing the bladder and separated from it by the uterovesical pouch of peritoneum. SYN facies vesicalis uteri [TA].

vestibular s. of cochlear duct [TA], the membrane separating the cochlear duct from the vestibular canal; it consists of squamous epithelial cells with microvilli toward the ductus, a basement membrane, and a thin layer of connective tissue toward the scala. SYN paries vestibularis ductus cochlearis [TA], membrana vestibularis ductus cochlearis✲, vestibular membrane✲, Reissner membrane, vestibular wall of cochlear duct.

vestibular s. of tooth [TA], the s. of a tooth that faces the buccal or labial mucosa of vestibule of the mouth; opposite to the lingual s. of tooth. SYN facies vestibularis dentis [TA], facial s. of tooth, facies facialis dentis.

visceral s. of liver [TA], the posteroinferior s. of the liver that faces adjacent abdominal organs; the porta hepatis and gallbladder are located on this s. SYN facies visceralis hepatis [TA].

visceral s. of the spleen [TA], the s. of the spleen in contact with adjacent viscera. SYN facies visceralis splenis [TA].

working occlusal s.'s, the s.'s of teeth upon which mastication can occur.

sur·face-ac·tive (ser'făs-ak'tiv). Indicating the property of certain agents of altering the physicochemical nature of surfaces and interfaces, bringing about lowering of interfacial tension; they usually possess both lipophilic and hydrophilic groups. SEE ALSO surfactant.

sur·fac·tant (ser-fak'tănt). **1.** A surface-active agent, including substances commonly referred to as wetting agents, surface tension depressants, detergents, dispersing agents, emulsifiers, quaternary ammonium antiseptics, etc. **2.** Those surface-active agents forming a monomolecular layer over pulmonary alveolar surfaces; lipoproteins that include lecithins and sphygomyelins that stabilize alveolar volume by reducing surface tension and altering the relationship between surface tension and surface area. [*surface active agent*]

nonionic s., a s. without a charged moiety.

zwitterionic s., a dipolar s.

sur·geon (ser'jŭn). A physician who treats disease, injury, and deformity by operation or manipulation. [G. *cheirougos;* L. *chirurgus*]

attending s., a surgical member of the attending staff of a hospital.

dental s., a general practitioner of dentistry; a dentist with the D.D.S. or D.M.D. degree.

genitourinary s., SYN urologist.

oral s., a dentist who specializes in oral surgery.

sur·geon gen·er·al. The chief medical officer in the U.S. Army, Navy, Air Force, or Public Health Service. In some foreign military services any member of the medical corps who has the rank of general, not necessarily the chief medical officer.

sur·gery (ser'jer-ē). **1.** The branch of medicine concerned with the treatment of disease, injury, and deformity by physical operation or manipulation. **2.** The performance or procedures of an operation. [L. *chirurgia;* G. *cheir,* hand, + *ergon,* work]

ambulatory s., operative procedures performed on patients who are admitted to and discharged from a hospital on the same day.

aseptic s., the performance of an operation with sterilized hands, instruments, etc., and utilizing precautions against the introduction of infectious microorganisms from without.

closed s., s. without incision into skin, e.g., reduction of a fracture or dislocation.

cosmetic s., s. in which the principal purpose is to improve the appearance. SYN esthetic s.

craniofacial s., simultaneous procedure on the cranium and facial bones.

endolymphatic sac s., a generic term for several operations performed on the endolymphatic sac for the treatment of Ménière disease.

esthetic s., SYN cosmetic s.

functional endoscopic sinus s. (FESS), a group of operations performed on the paranasal sinuses, with illumination and magnification through an endoscope.

keratorefractive s., SYN refractive *keratoplasty.*

laparoscopic s., operative procedure performed using minimally invasive surgical technique for exposure that avoids traditional incision; visualization is achieved using a fiber optic instrument, attached to a video camera.

laparoscopically assisted s., operative procedure performed using combined laparoscopic and open techniques.

left ventricular volume reduction s., operation in which the volume of a dilated, nonaneurysmal left ventricle is reduced by myocardial resection to improve ventricular geometry and mechanical function and thereby treat end-stage congestive heart *failure.* SYN Battista operation, partial left ventriculectomy, reduction left ventriculoplasty.

lung volume reduction s., procedure whereby nonfunctional lung tissue in emphysema patients is removed, allowing more room in the thoracic cavity for good relatively healthy tissue and thus theoretically improving lung function. SEE ALSO emphysema.

major s., SEE major *operation.*

microscopically controlled s., SYN Mohs *chemosurgery.*

minimally invasive s., operative procedure performed in a manner derived to result in the smallest possible incision or no incision at all; includes laparoscopic, laparoscopically assisted, thoracoscopic, and endoscopic surgical procedures.

minor s., SEE minor *operation.*

Mohs s., SYN Mohs *chemosurgery.*

Mohs micrographic s., SYN Mohs *chemosurgery.*

open heart s., operative procedure(s) performed on or within the exposed heart, usually with cardiopulmonary bypass.

oral s., the branch of dentistry concerned with the diagnosis and surgical and adjunctive treatment of diseases, injuries, and deformities of the oral and maxillofacial region.

orthognathic s., SYN surgical *orthodontics.*

orthopedic s., the branch of s. that embraces the treatment of acute and chronic disorders of the musculoskeletal system, including injuries, diseases, dysfunction, and deformities (orig. deformities in children) in the extremities and spine. SEE ALSO orthopaedics.

plastic s., the surgical specialty or procedure concerned with the restoration, construction, reconstruction, or improvement in the shape and appearance of body structures that are missing, defective, damaged, or misshapen.

reconstructive s., SEE plastic s.

skull base s., generic term to denote a specialty of s. and a group of operations, techniques, and approaches to lesions at or involving the base of the skull or its contents.

stereotactic s., SYN stereotaxy.

stereotaxic s., SYN stereotaxy.

thoracoscopic s., operation on the chest using a thoracoscope; formerly, a direct-view instrument used mainly for simple procedures such as collapse therapy and pleural biopsy; currently, employs video-endoscopic minimally invasive techniques and instruments and is applied to more complex procedures. Cf. video-assisted thoracic s.

transsexual s., procedures designed to alter a patient's external sexual characteristics so that they resemble those of the other sex.

ventricular reduction s., SYN Battista *procedure.*

video-assisted thoracic s. (VATS), thoracic s. performed using endoscopic cameras, optical systems, and display screens, as well as specially designed surgical instruments and staplers; the ability to make small incisions without spreading of the ribs is an advantage over standard thoracotomy; has been applied to most thoracic procedures.

sur·gi·cal (ser′ji-kăl). Relating to surgery.

sur·re·nal (ser-rē′năl). SYN suprarenal (1).

sur·ro·gate (ser′ŏ-gāt). **1.** A person who functions in another's life as a substitute for some third person such as a relative who assumes the nurturing and other responsibilities of the absent parent. **2.** A person who reminds one of another person so that one uses the first as an emotional substitute for the second. [L. *surrogo*, to put in another's place]

mother s., one who substitutes for or takes the place of the mother.

sur·round (ser-ownd′). Milieu; environment.

acoustical s., SYN sound *field*.

sur·sum·duc·tion (ser-sŭm-dŭk′shŭn). SYN supraduction. [L. *sursum*, upward, + *duco*, pp. *-ductus*, to draw]

sur·sum·ver·sion (ser-sŭm-ver′zhŭn). The act of rotating the eyes upward. [L. *sursum*, upward, + *verto*, pp. *versus*, to turn]

sur·veil·lance (ser-vā′lans). **1.** The collection, collation, analysis, and dissemination of data; a type of observational study that involves continuous monitoring of disease occurrence within a population. **2.** Ongoing scrutiny, generally using methods distinguished by practicability, uniformity, or rapidity, rather than complete accuracy. [Fr. *surveiller*, to watch over, fr. L. *super-* + *vigilo*, to watch]

immune s., a theory that the immune system recognizes and destroys tumor cells which are constantly arising during the life of the individual. SYN immunological s.

immunological s., SYN immune s.

post-marketing s., procedure implemented after a drug has been licensed for public use, designed to provide information on use and on occurrence of side effects, adverse effects, etc.

sur·vey (ser′vā). **1.** An investigation in which information is systematically collected but in which the experimental method is not used. **2.** A comprehensive examination or group of examinations to screen for one or more findings. **3.** A series of questions administered to a sample of individuals in a population. [O.Fr. *surveeir*, fr. Mediev.L. *supervideo*, fr. *super*, over, + *video*, to see]

field s., the planned collection of data among noninstitutionalized persons in the general population.

skeletal s., radiographic examination of all or selected parts of the skeleton, as for occult fractures, metastases, etc.

sur·vey·ing (ser-vā′ing). In dentistry, the procedure of locating and delineating the contour and position of the abutment teeth and associated structures before designing a removable partial denture.

sur·vey·or (ser-vā′er, ōr). In dentistry, the instrument used in surveying.

sur·viv·al (ser-vī′văl). Continued existence; persistence of life.

sus·cep·ti·bil·i·ty (su-sep-ti-bil′i-tē). **1.** Likelihood of an individual to develop ill effects from an external agent, such as *Mycobacterium tuberculosis*, high altitude, or ambient temperature. **2.** In magnetic resonance imaging, the loss of magnetization signal caused by rapid phase dispersion because of marked local inhomogeneity of the magnetic field, as with the multiple air–soft tissue interfaces in the lung.

sus·pen·sion (sŭs-pen′shŭn). **1.** A temporary interruption of any function. **2.** A hanging from a support, as used in the treatment of spinal curvatures or during the application of a plaster jacket. **3.** Fixation of an organ, such as the uterus, to other tissue for support. **4.** The dispersion through a liquid of a solid in finely divided particles of a size large enough to be detected by purely optical means; if the particles are too small to be seen by microscope but still large enough to scatter light (Tyndall phenomenon), they will remain dispersed indefinitely and are then called a colloidal s. SYN coarse dispersion. **5.** A class of pharmacopoeial preparations of finely divided, undissolved drugs (e.g., powders for s.) dispersed in liquid vehicles for oral or parenteral use. [L. *suspensio*, fr. *suspendo*, pp. *-pensus*, to hang up, suspend]

amorphous insulin zinc s., SYN prompt insulin zinc s.

chromic phosphate ^{32}**P colloidal s.,** a pure β-emitting colloidal, nonabsorbable radiopharmaceutical administered into body cavi-

ties such as the pleural or peritoneal spaces to control malignant effusions. SEE ALSO *sodium* phosphate ^{32}P.

Coffey s., an operative technique following partial excision of the cornu, as in salpingectomy, whereby the broad and the round ligaments are sutured over the cornual wound to restore continuity of the peritoneum and to suspend the uterus on the operated side.

crystalline insulin zinc s., SYN extended insulin zinc s.

extended insulin zinc s., a long-acting insulin s., obtained from beef, with an approximate time of onset of 7 hours and a duration of action of 36 hours. SYN crystalline insulin zinc s.

insulin zinc s., a sterile buffered s. with zinc chloride, usually containing 100 units per ml; the solid phase of the s. consists of a mixture of 7 parts of crystalline insulin and 3 parts of amorphous insulin. SYN lente insulin.

magnesia and alumina oral s., a mixture of magnesium hydroxide and variable amounts of aluminum oxide; used as an antacid.

prompt insulin zinc s., sterile s. of insulin in buffered water for injection, modified by the addition of zinc chloride such that the solid phase of the s. is amorphous; it usually contains 100 units per ml; the duration of action is equivalent to that of insulin injection. SYN amorphous insulin zinc s., semilente insulin.

sus·pen·soid (sŭs-pen′soyd). A colloidal solution in which the dispersed particles are solid and lyophobe or hydrophobe and are therefore sharply demarcated from the fluid in which they are suspended. SYN hydrophobic colloid, lyophobic colloid, suspension colloid. [suspension + G. *eidos*, resemblance]

sus·pen·so·ry (sŭs-pen′sŏ-rē). **1.** Suspending; supporting; denoting a ligament, a muscle, or other structure that keeps an organ or other part in place. **2.** A supporter applied to uplift a dependent part, such as the scrotum or a pendulous breast.

sus·ten·tac·u·lar (sŭs-ten-tak′ū-lăr). Relating to a sustentaculum; supporting.

sus·ten·tac·u·lum, pl. **sus·ten·tac·u·la** (sŭs′ten-tak′ū-lŭm, -lă). A structure that serves as a stay or support to another. [L. a prop, fr. *sustento*, to hold upright]

s. lienis, SYN phrenicosplenic *ligament*.

s. ta′li, support of the talus, a bracket-like lateral projection from the medial surface of the calcaneus, the upper surface of which presents a facet for articulation with the talus.

su·sur·rus (sŭ-ser′ŭs). SYN murmur (1). [L.]

s. au′rium, murmur in the ear.

Sutter blood group. See Blood Groups appendix.

Sutton, Richard L., Jr., U.S. dermatologist, *1908. SEE S. *disease*, ulcer.

Sutton, Richard L., U.S. dermatologist, 1878–1952. SEE S. *nevus*.

SUTURA

su·tu·ra, pl. **su·tu·rae** (soo′too′ră, -rē) [TA]. SYN suture (1). [L. a sewing, a suture, fr. *suo*, pp. *sutus*, to sew]

s. corona′lis [TA], SYN coronal *suture*.

sutu′rae cra′nii [TA], SYN cranial *sutures*, under *suture*.

s. ethmoidolacrima′lis [TA], SYN ethmoidolacrimal *suture*.

s. ethmoidomaxilla′ris [TA], SYN ethmoidomaxillary *suture*.

s. fronta′lis, SYN frontal *suture*.

s. frontalis persistens, *official alternate term for metopic *suture*.

s. frontoethmoida′lis [TA], SYN frontoethmoidal *suture*.

s. frontolacrima′lis [TA], SYN frontolacrimal *suture*.

s. frontomaxilla′ris [TA], SYN frontomaxillary *suture*.

s. frontonasa′lis [TA], SYN frontonasal *suture*.

s. frontozygomat′ica [TA], SYN frontozygomatic *suture*.

s. incisi′va [TA], SYN incisive *suture*.

s. infraorbita′lis [TA], SYN infraorbital *suture*.

s. intermaxilla′ris [TA], SYN intermaxillary *suture*.

s. internasa′lis [TA], SYN internasal *suture*.

su

s. interparieta′lis, SYN sagittal *suture*.

s. lacrimoconcha′lis [TA], SYN lacrimoconchal *suture*.

s. lacrimomaxilla′ris [TA], SYN lacrimomaxillary *suture*.

s. lambdoi′dea [TA], SYN lambdoid *suture*.

s. meto′pica [TA], SYN metopic *suture*.

s. nasofronta′lis, SYN frontonasal *suture*.

s. nasomaxilla′ris [TA], SYN nasomaxillary *suture*.

s. no′tha (nō′tă), SYN false *suture*. [G. fem. of *nothos*, spurious]

s. occipitomastoi′dea [TA], SYN occipitomastoid *suture*.

s. palati′na media′na [TA], SYN median palatine *suture*.

s. palati′na transver′sa [TA], SYN transverse palatine *suture*.

s. palatoethmoida′lis [TA], SYN palatoethmoidal *suture*.

s. palatomaxilla′ris [TA], SYN palatomaxillary *suture*.

s. parietomastoi′dea [TA], SYN parietomastoid *suture*.

s. pla′na [TA], SYN plane *suture*.

s. sagitta′lis [TA], SYN sagittal *suture*.

s. serra′ta [TA], SYN serrate *suture*.

s. sphenoethmoida′lis [TA], SYN sphenoethmoidal *suture*.

s. sphenofronta′lis [TA], SYN sphenofrontal *suture*.

s. sphenomaxilla′ris [TA], SYN sphenomaxillary *suture*.

s. spheno-orbita′lis, SYN spheno-orbital *suture*.

s. sphenoparieta′lis [TA], SYN sphenoparietal *suture*.

s. sphenosquamo′sa [TA], SYN sphenosquamous *suture*.

s. sphenovomeria′na [TA], SYN sphenovomerine *suture*.

s. sphenozygoma′tica [TA], SYN sphenozygomatic *suture*.

s. squamoparietalis, (1) SYN squamous *suture*; **(2)** SYN squamo-parietal *suture*.

s. squamosomastoi′dea [TA], SYN squamomastoid *suture*.

s. temporozygomat′ica [TA], SYN temporozygomatic *suture*.

s. zygomaticofronta′lis, SYN frontozygomatic *suture*.

s. zygomaticomaxilla′ris [TA], SYN zygomaticomaxillary *suture*.

s. zygomaticotempora′lis, SYN temporozygomatic *suture*.

---

su·tur·al (soo′choor-ăl). Relating to a suture in any sense.

SUTURE

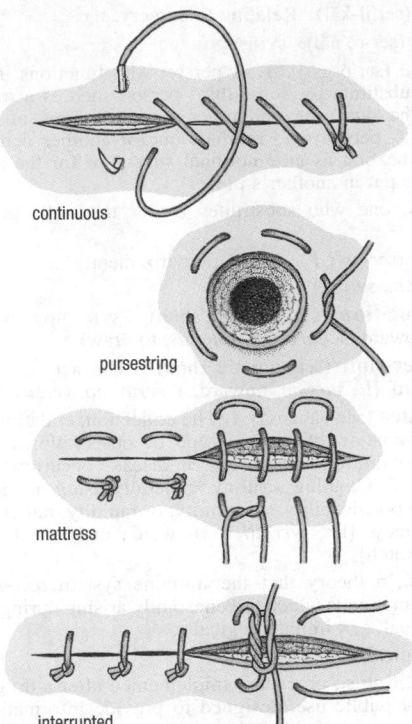

surgical sutures

su·ture (soo′choor) [TA]. **1.** A form of fibrous joint in which two bones formed in membrane are united by a fibrous membrane continuous with the periosteum. SYN sutura [TA], suture joint. **2.** To unite two surfaces by sewing. SYN stitch (3). **3.** The material (silk thread, wire, synthetic material, etc.) with which two surfaces are kept in apposition. **4.** The seam so formed, a surgical s. [L. *sutura*, a seam]

absorbable surgical s., a surgical s. material prepared from a substance that can be dissolved by body tissues and is therefore not permanent; it is available in various diameters and tensile strengths; the rate of disappearance of strength depends on the characteristics of the suture material.

Albert s., a modified Czerny s., the first row of stitches passing through the entire thickness of the wall of the gut.

apposition s., a s. of the skin only. SYN coaptation s.

approximation s., a s. that pulls together the deep tissues.

atraumatic s., a s. swaged onto the end of an eyeless needle.

blanket s., a continuous lock-stitch used to approximate the skin of a wound.

bridle s., a s. passed beneath the superior rectus muscle to rotate the globe downward in eye surgery.

Bunnell s., a method of tenorrhaphy using a pull-out wire affixed to buttons.

buried s., any s. placed entirely below the surface of the skin.

button s., a s. in which the threads are passed through the holes of a button and then tied; used to reduce the danger of the threads cutting through the flesh.

catgut s., SEE catgut.

coaptation s., SYN apposition s.

cobbler's s., SYN doubly armed s.

Connell s., a continuous s. used for inverting the gastric or intestinal walls in performing an anastomosis.

continuous s., an uninterrupted series of stitches using one s.; the stitching is fastened at each end by a knot. SYN spiral s., uninterrupted s.

control release s., eyeless s. with thread attached to a needle such that the two separate when tension is applied to the thread.

coronal s. [TA], the line of junction of the frontal with the two parietal bones of the skull. SYN sutura coronalis [TA].

cranial s.'s [TA], the s.'s between the bones of the skull. SYN suturae cranii [TA].

Cushing s., a running horizontal mattress s. used to approximate two adjacent surfaces.

Czerny s., the first row of the Czerny-Lembert intestinal s.; the needle enters the serosa and passes out through the submucosa or muscularis, and then enters the submucosa or muscularis of the opposite side and emerges from the serosa.

Czerny-Lembert s., an intestinal s. in two rows combining the Czerny s. (first) and the Lembert s. (second).

delayed s., a suturing of a wound after an interval of days.

dentate s., SYN serrate s.

doubly armed s., a s. with a needle attached at both ends. SYN cobbler's s.

Dupuytren s., a continuous Lembert s.

end-on mattress s., a vertical mattress s. used for exact skin approximation.

ethmoidolacrimal s. [TA], the line of union of the orbital plate of the ethmoid and the posterior margin of the lacrimal bone. SYN sutura ethmoidolacrimalis [TA].

ethmoidomaxillary s. [TA], line of apposition of the orbital surface of the body of the maxilla with the orbital plate of the ethmoid bone. SYN sutura ethmoidomaxillaris [TA].

Faden s., a s. placed between an ocular rectus muscle and the posterior sclera to limit excessive action of the eyeball. [Ger. *Faden*, thread, twine]

false s., one whose opposing margins are smooth or present only a few ill-defined projections. SYN sutura notha.

far-and-near s., an interrupted s. using alternate near and far stitches, used to approximate fascial edges.

figure-of-8 s., a s. using criss-cross stitches to approximate fascial edges or the musculofascial and outer layers of an abdominal wound.

frontal s., the suture between the two halves of the frontal bone, usually obliterated by about the sixth year; if persistent it is called a metopic s. or sutura frontalis persistens. SYN sutura frontalis.

frontoethmoidal s. [TA], line of union between the cribriform plate of the ethmoid and the orbital plate and posterior margin of the nasal process of the frontal bone. SYN sutura frontoethmoidalis [TA].

frontolacrimal s. [TA], line of union between the upper margin of the lacrimal and the orbital plate of the frontal bone. SYN sutura frontolacrimalis [TA].

frontomaxillary s. [TA], articulation of the frontal process of the maxilla with the frontal bone. SYN sutura frontomaxillaris [TA].

frontonasal s. [TA], line of union of the frontal and of the two nasal bones. SYN sutura frontonasalis [TA], sutura nasofrontalis.

frontozygomatic s. [TA], line of union between the zygomatic process of the frontal and the frontal process of the zygomatic bone. SYN sutura frontozygomatica [TA], sutura zygomaticofrontalis.

Frost s., intermarginal s. between the eyelids to protect the cornea.

Gély s., a cobbler's s. used in closing intestinal wounds.

glover s., a continuous s. in which each stitch is passed through the loop of the preceding one.

Gould s., an intestinal mattress s. in which each loop is invaginated in such a way that the tissue at the loop is bulged out, becoming convex instead of concave.

Gussenbauer s., a figure-of-8 s. for the intestine, resembling the Czerny-Lembert s. but not including the mucous membrane.

Halsted s., a s. placed through the subcuticular fascia; used for exact skin approximation.

harmonic s., SYN plane s.

implanted s., passage of a pin through each lip of the wound parallel to the line of incision, the pins then being looped together with s.'s.

incisive s. [TA], line of union of the two portions of the maxilla (pre- and postmaxilla); it is present at birth but may persist into old age. SYN sutura incisiva [TA], premaxillary s.

infraorbital s. [TA], an inconstant suture running from the infraorbital foramen to the infraorbital groove. SYN sutura infraorbitalis [TA].

intermaxillary s. [TA], the line of union of the two maxillae. SYN sutura intermaxillaris [TA].

internasal s. [TA], line of union between the two nasal bones. SYN sutura internasalis [TA].

interparietal s., SYN sagittal s.

interrupted s., a series of single stitches, the ends of each s. tied together.

Jobert de Lamballe s., an interrupted intestinal s., used for invaginating the margins of the intestines in circular enterorrhaphy.

lacrimoconchal s. [TA], line of union of the lacrimal bone with the inferior nasal concha. SYN sutura lacrimoconchalis [TA].

lacrimomaxillary s. [TA], line of union, on the medial wall of the orbit, between the anterior and inferior margin of the lacrimal bone and the maxilla. SYN sutura lacrimomaxillaris [TA].

lambdoid s. [TA], the inverted λ-shaped line of union between the occipital and the parietal bones. SYN sutura lambdoidea [TA].

Lembert s., the second row of the Czerny-Lembert intestinal s.; an inverting s. for intestinal surgery, used either as a continuous s. or interrupted s., producing serosal apposition and including the collagenous submucosal layer but not entering the lumen of the intestine.

lens s.'s, SYN *radii* of lens, under *radius*.

locking s., a running s. in which the s. material is made to pass through the loop made from the previous stitch. SYN lock stitch.

mattress s., a s. utilizing a double stitch that forms a loop about the tissue on both sides of a wound, producing eversion of the edges when tied. SYN quilted s.

median palatine s. [TA], line of union between the horizontal plates of the palatine bones, continuing the intermaxillary s. posteriorly. SYN sutura palatina mediana [TA].

metopic s. [TA], a persistent frontal s., sometimes discernible a short distance above s. frontonasalis. SEE ALSO frontal s. SYN sutura metopica [TA], persistent frontal s.✩, sutura frontalis persistens✩.

nasomaxillary s. [TA], line of union of the lateral margin of the nasal bone with the frontal process of the maxilla. SYN sutura nasomaxillaris [TA].

nerve s., SYN neurorrhaphy.

neurocentral s., SYN neurocentral *synchondrosis*.

nonabsorbable surgical s., surgical s. material that is relatively unaffected by the biologic activities of the body tissues and is therefore permanent unless removed; e.g., stainless steel, silk, cotton, nylon, and other synthetic materials.

occipitomastoid s. [TA], continuation of the lambdoid s. between the posterior border of the petrous portion of the temporal bone and the occipital. SYN sutura occipitomastoidea [TA].

palatoethmoidal s. [TA], line of junction of the orbital process of the palatine bone and the orbital plate of the ethmoid. SYN sutura palatoethmoidalis [TA].

palatomaxillary s. [TA], line of union, in the floor of the orbit, between the orbital process of the palatine bone and the orbital surface of the maxilla. SYN sutura palatomaxillaris [TA].

Paré s., the approximation of the edges of a wound by pasting strips of cloth to the surface and stitching them instead of the skin.

parietomastoid s. [TA], articulation of the posterior inferior angle of the parietal with the mastoid process of the temporal bone. SYN sutura parietomastoidea [TA].

Parker-Kerr s., a continuous inverting s. used to close an open end of intestine.

persistent frontal s., ✩official alternate term for metopic s.

petrosquamous s., SEE petrosquamous *fissure*.

plane s. [TA], a simple firm apposition of two smooth surfaces of bones, without overlap, as seen in the lacrimomaxillary s. SYN sutura plana [TA], harmonia, harmonic s.

pledgetted s., a s. supported by a small piece of fabric or tissue so that the s. will not tear through the tissue.

premaxillary s., SYN incisive s.

purse-string s., a continuous s. placed in a circular manner either for inversion (as for an appendiceal stump) or closure (as for a hernia).

quilted s., SYN mattress s.

relaxation s., a s. so arranged that it may be loosened if the tension of the wound becomes excessive.

retention s., a heavy reinforcing s. placed deep within the muscles and fasciae of the abdominal wall to relieve tension on the primary s. line. SYN tension s.

sagittal s. [TA], midline union between the two parietal bones. SYN sutura sagittalis [TA], interparietal s., sutura interparietalis.

secondary s., delayed closure of a wound.

serrate s. [TA], one whose opposing margins present deep sawlike indentations, as most of the sagittal s. SYN sutura serrata [TA], dentate s.

shotted s., a s. in which the ends are fastened by passing through a split shot (a partially divided lead pellet) which is then compressed.

sphenoethmoidal s. [TA], line of union between the crest of the sphenoid bone and the perpendicular and cribriform plates of the ethmoid. SYN sutura sphenoethmoidalis [TA].

sphenofrontal s. [TA], line of union between the orbital plate of the frontal and the lesser wings of the sphenoid on either side. SYN sutura sphenofrontalis [TA].

sphenomaxillary s. [TA], an inconstant s. between the pterygoid process of the sphenoid bone and the body of the maxilla. SYN sutura sphenomaxillaris [TA].

sphenooccipital s., SYN sphenooccipital *synchondrosis*.

spheno-orbital s., articulation between the orbital process of the palatine bone and the outer surface of the body of the sphenoid. SYN sutura spheno-orbitalis.

sphenoparietal s. [TA], line of union of the lower border of the parietal with the upper edge of the greater wing of the sphenoid. SYN sutura sphenoparietalis [TA].

sphenosquamous s. [TA], articulation of the greater wing of the sphenoid with the squamous portion of the temporal bone. SYN sutura sphenosquamosa [TA].

sphenovomerine s. [TA], the line of union of the vaginal process of the sphenoid with the wing of the vomer. SYN sutura sphenovomeriana [TA].

sphenozygomatic s. [TA], junction of the zygomatic bone and greater wing of the sphenoid. SYN sutura sphenozygomatica [TA].

spiral s., SYN continuous s.

squamomastoid s. [TA], line of union of the squamous and petrous portions of the temporal bone during development; it sometimes persists in the region of the mastoid process. SYN sutura squamosomastoidea [TA].

squamoparietal s., the articulation of the parietal with the squamous portion of the temporal bone. SYN sutura squamoparietalis (2).

squamous s. [TA], a scalelike s., one whose opposing margins are scalelike and overlapping; SYN sutura squamoparietalis (1).

subcuticular s., SEE Halsted s.

temporozygomatic s., line of junction of the zygomatic process of the temporal and the temporal process of the zygomatic bone. SYN sutura temporozygomatica [TA], sutura zygomaticotemporalis, zygomaticotemporal s.

tendon s., SYN tenorrhaphy.

tension s., SYN retention s.

transfixion s., (1) a criss-cross stitch so placed as to control bleeding from a tissue surface or small vessel when tied; (2) a s. used to fix the columella to the nasal septum.

transverse palatine s. [TA], line of union of the palatine processes of the maxillae with the horizontal plates of the palatine bones. SYN sutura palatina transversa [TA].

tympanomastoid s., SYN tympanomastoid *fissure.*

uninterrupted s., SYN continuous s.

wedge-and-groove s., SYN schindylesis.

zygomaticomaxillary s. [TA], articulation of the zygomatic bone with the zygomatic process of the maxilla. SYN sutura zygomaticomaxillaris [TA].

zygomaticotemporal s., SYN temporozygomatic s.

---

su·tur·ec·to·my (soo-choor-ek′tō-mē). Removal of cranial suture.

suxamethonium. SYN succinylcholine.

Suzanne, Jean G., French physician, *1859. SEE S. *gland.*

SV Abbreviation for simian *virus,* numbered serially; e.g., SV1.

SV40 Symbol for simian vacuolating *virus* No. 40.

Sv Abbreviation for sievert.

Svedberg, Theodor, Swedish chemist and Nobel laureate, 1884–1971. SEE S. *equation,* of flotation, *unit.*

Svedberg of flo·ta·tion. SYN flotation *constant.*

swab (swob). A wad of cotton, gauze, or other absorbent material attached to the end of a stick or clamp, used for applying or removing a substance from a surface.

swage (swāj). **1.** To fuse suture thread to suture needles. **2.** To shape metal by hammering or adapting it onto a die, often by using a counterdie. [Old F. *souage*]

▮swal·low (swawl′ō). To pass anything through the fauces, pharynx, and esophagus into the stomach; to perform deglutition. [A.S. *swelgan*]

Gastrografin s., esophagram or upper GI series using water-soluble iodinated contrast medium. SYN hypaque s.

hypaque s., SYN Gastrografin s.

somatic s., a swallowing pattern with muscular contractions which appear to be under control of the person at a subconscious level; distinguished from visceral s.

visceral s., the immature swallowing pattern of an infant or a person with tongue thrust, resembling peristaltic wavelike muscular contractions observed in the gut; adult or mature swallowing is more volitional and therefore somatic.

Swan, Harold James C., U.S. cardiologist, *1922. SEE S.-Ganz *catheter.*

swarm·ing (swŏrm′ing). A progressive spreading by motile bacteria over the surface of a solid medium. [A.S. *swearm*]

Sweat, Faye, 20th century pathologist. SEE Puchtler-S. stains. SEE Puchtler-S. stains.

sweat (swet). **1.** Perspiration (3), especially sensible perspiration. **2.** To perspire. [A.S. *swāt*]

night s.'s, profuse sweating at night, occurring in pulmonary tuberculosis and other chronic debilitating affections with low-grade fever.

red s., reddening of s., especially in the axilla, due to pigment produced by *Streptomyces roseofulvis.* SEE ALSO chromidrosis.

sweat·ing (swet′ing). SYN perspiration (1).

sweep (swēp). The travel of the beam of a cathode ray oscilloscope from left to right, representing the time axis, produced by an artificially generated sawtooth voltage.

Sweet, Robert Douglas, 20th century English dermatologist. SEE S. *disease.*

Sweet. SEE Gordon and Sweet *stain.*

swell·ing (swel′ing). **1.** An enlargement, e.g., a protuberance or tumor. **2.** In embryology, a primordial elevation that develops into a fold, ridge, or prominence.

albuminous s., SYN cloudy s.

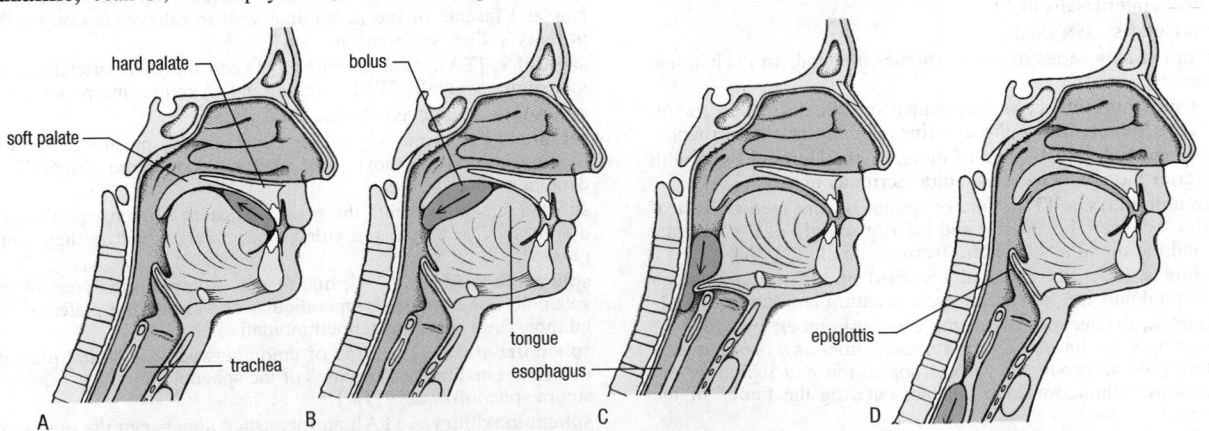

swallowing: (A) bolus is pushed back; (B) nasopharynx closes; (C) epiglottis closes the trachea; (D) bolus is moved down the esophagus

arytenoid s., paired primordial elevations, on either side of the embryonic larynx, within which the arytenoid cartilages are formed.

brain s., a pathologic entity, localized or generalized, characterized by an increase in bulk of brain tissue, due to expansion of the intravascular (congestion) or extravascular (edema) compartments that may coexist or may occur separately and be clinically indistinguishable; clinical manifestations depend on disturbed neuronal function due to local s., shifting of intracranial structures, and the effects of intracranial hypertension or circulatory disturbance.

Calabar s., SYN loiasis.

cloudy s., s. of cells due to injury to the membranes affecting ionic transfer; causes an accumulation of intracellular water. SYN albuminous s., granular degeneration, hydropic degeneration, parenchymatous degeneration.

fugitive s., SYN loiasis.

genital s.'s, paired primordial elevations flanking the genital tubercle and the urogenital orifice of the embryo; they develop into the labioscrotal folds, which become the labia majora in the female and unite to form the scrotal pouch of the male. SYN labioscrotal s.'s.

hunger s., starvation edema caused by many factors, primarily reduced serum albumin.

labial s., the female embryonic genital s. which elongates to become the definitive labium majus. SEE ALSO genital s.'s.

labioscrotal s.'s, SYN genital s.'s.

lateral lingual s.'s, in the embryo, paired oval elevations that appear in the floor of the mouth at the mandibular arch level; the primordial elevations, composed of mesenchyme covered by ectoderm of stomodeal origin, merge to form the greater part of the anterior two-thirds of the tongue.

levator s., SYN *torus* levatorius.

Neufeld capsular s., increase in opacity and visibility of the capsule of capsulated organisms exposed to specific agglutinating anticapsular antibodies. SYN Neufeld reaction, quellung phenomenon, quellung reaction (1), quellung test.

scrotal s., the s. formed after the embryonic genital s.'s have fused together, become spherical, and positioned at the base of the penis; just before birth the testis comes to lie within it.

Spielmeyer acute s., a form of degeneration of nerve cells in which the cell body and its processes swell and stain palely and diffusely.

switch·ing (swich'ing). **1.** Making a shift or exchange. **2.** The movement of a defined region of DNA within a genome.

class s., a change in the expression of the C region of an immunoglobulin heavy chain.

Swyer, Paul R., U.S. pediatrician, *1921. SEE Swyer-James *syndrome;* S.-James-MacLeod *syndrome.*

sy·co·sis (sī-kō'sis). A pustular folliculitis, particularly of the bearded area. [G. *sykōsis,* fr. *sykōn,* fig, + *-osis,* condition]

Sydenham, Thomas, English physician, 1624–1689. SEE S. *chorea, disease.*

Sydney crease. See under crease.

Sydney line. See under line.

syl·la·ble-stum·bling (sil'ă-bl-stŭm'bling). A form of stuttering in which halting occurs at certain syllables that are difficult for the individual to enunciate. SYN dyssyllabia. [L. *syllabē,* several letters or sounds taken together]

syl·vat·ic (sil-vat'ik). Occurring in or affecting wild animals. [L. *silva,* woods]

Sylvest, Ejnar, Norwegian physician, 1880–1931. SEE S. *disease.*

syl·vi·an (sil'vē-an). Relating to Franciscus or Jacobus Sylvius or to any of the structures described by either of them.

Sylvius, Le Böe, Franciscus (François), Dutch physician, anatomist, and physiologist, 1614–1672. SEE sylvian *angle;* sylvian *aqueduct;* sylvian *fissure;* sylvian *line;* sylvian *point;* sylvian *valve;* sylvian *ventricle; fossa* of S.; *vallecula* sylvii.

Sylvius, Jacobus (Jacques), French anatomist, 1478–1555. SEE *caro* quadrata sylvii; *os* sylvii.

△**sym-.** SEE syn-.

sym·bal·lo·phone (sim-bal'ō-fōn). A stethoscope having two chest pieces, designed to lateralize sound and produce a stereophonic effect. [G. *symballō,* to throw together, + *phōnē,* sound]

sym·bi·on, sym·bi·ont (sim'bē-on, -ont). An organism associated with another in symbiosis. SYN mutualist, symbiote. [G. *symbion,* neut. of *symbiōs,* living together]

sym·bi·o·sis (sim-bē-ō'sis). **1.** The biological association of two or more species to their mutual benefit. Cf. commensalism, mutualistic s., parasitism. **2.** The mutual cooperation or interdependence of two persons, as mother and infant, or husband and wife; sometimes used to denote excessive or pathological interdependence of two persons. [G. *symbiōsis,* state of living together, fr. sym- + *bios,* life, + *-osis,* condition]

dyadic s., s. between a child and one parent.

mutualistic s., s. in which all partners obtain an advantage.

triadic s., s. between a child and both parents.

sym·bi·ote (sim'bē-ōt). SYN symbion.

sym·bi·ot·ic (sim-bē-ot'ik). Relating to symbiosis.

sym·bleph·a·ron (sim-blef'ă-ron). Adhesion of one or both eyelids to the eyeball, partial or complete, resulting from burns or other trauma but rarely congenital. SYN atretoblepharia. [sym- + G. *blepharon,* eyelid]

anterior s., union between the lid and eyeball by a fibrous band not involving the fornix.

posterior s., adhesion between the eyeball and eyelid involving the fornix.

sym·bol (sim'bŏl). **1.** A conventional sign serving as an abbreviation. **2.** In chemistry, an abbreviation of the name of an element, radical, or compound, expressing in chemical formulas one atom or molecule of that element (e.g., H and O in H_2O); in biochemistry, an abbreviation of trivial names of molecules used primarily in combination with other similar s.'s to construct larger assemblies (e.g., Gly for glycine, Ado for adenosine, Glc for glucose). **3.** In psychoanalysis, an object or action that is interpreted to represent some repressed or unconscious desire, often sexual. **4.** A philosophical-linguistic sign. SEE ALSO conventional *signs,* under *sign.* [G. *symbolon,* a mark or sign, fr. *sym-ballō,* to throw together]

sym·bo·lia (sim-bō'lē-ă). The capability of recognizing the form and nature of an object by touch. [G. *symbolon,* a mark or sign]

sym·bol·ism (sim'bō-lizm). **1.** In psychoanalysis, the process involved in the disguised representation in consciousness of unconscious or repressed contents or events. **2.** A mental state in which a person regards everything that happens as symbolic of the person's own thoughts. **3.** The description of the emotional life and experiences in abstract terms.

sym·bol·i·za·tion (sim'bō-li-zā'shŭn). An unconscious mental mechanism whereby one object or idea is represented by another.

sym·brach·y·dac·ty·ly (sim-brak'i-dak'ti-lē). Condition in which abnormally short fingers are joined or webbed in their proximal portions. [sym- + G. *brachys,* short, + *daktylos,* finger]

Syme, James, Scottish surgeon, 1799–1870. SEE S. *amputation, operation.*

Symington, Johnson, Scottish anatomist, 1851–1924. SEE S. anococcygeal *body.*

sym·me·lia (si-mē'lē-ă). SYN sirenomelia. [sym- + G. *melos,* limb]

Symmers, W. St. C., British pathologist, 1863–1937. SEE S. clay pipestem *fibrosis.*

sym·me·try (sim'ĕ-trē). Equality or correspondence in form of parts distributed around a center or an axis, at the extremities or poles, or on the opposite sides of any body. [G. *symmetria,* fr. sym- + *metron,* measure]

inverse s., correspondence of the right or left side of an asymmetrical individual to the left or right side of another.

△**sympath-, sympatheto-, sympathico-, sympatho-.** The sympathetic part of the autonomic nervous system. [see sympathetic]

sym·pa·thec·to·my (sim-pă-thek'tō-mē). Excision of a segment of a sympathetic nerve or of one or more sympathetic ganglia. SYN

sy

sympathetectomy, sympathicectomy. [sympath- + G. *ektomē,* excision]

chemical s., destruction of the periareterial sympathetic nerves, as in Doppler operation, by a corrosive such as phenol.

periarterial s., sympathetic denervation by arterial decortication. SYN histonectomy, Leriche operation.

sym·pa·the·tec·to·my (sim-pă-thĕ-tek′tō-mē). SYN sympathectomy.

sym·pa·thet·ic (sim-pă-thet′ik). **1.** Relating to or exhibiting sympathy. **2.** Denoting the sympathetic part of the autonomic nervous system. SYN sympathic. [G. *sympathētikos,* fr. *sympatheō,* to feel with, sympathize, fr. *syn,* with, + *pathos,* suffering]

sym·pa·thet·o·blast (sim-pă-thet′ō-blast). SYN sympathoblast.

sym·pa·thic (sim-path′ik). SYN sympathetic.

sym·path·i·cec·to·my (sim-path′i-sek′tō-mē). SYN sympathectomy.

△**sympathico-.** SEE sympath-.

sym·path·i·co·blast (sim-path′i-kō-blast). SYN sympathoblast.

sym·path·i·co·neu·ri·tis (sim-path′i-kō-noo-rī′tis). Inflammation of the autonomic nerves.

sym·path·i·cop·a·thy (sim-path-i-kop′ă-thē). A disease resulting from a disorder of the autonomic nervous system. [sympathico- + G. *pathos,* suffering]

sym·path·i·co·to·nia (sim-path′i-kō-tō′nē-ă). A condition in which there is increased tonus of the sympathetic system and a marked tendency to vascular spasm and high blood pressure; opposed to vagotonia. [sympathico- + G. *tonos,* tone, tension]

sym·path·i·co·ton·ic (sim-path′i-kō-ton′ik). Relating to or characterized by sympathicotonia.

sym·path·i·co·trip·sy (sim-path′i-kō-trip′sē). Operation of crushing the sympathetic ganglion. [sympathico- + G. *tripsis,* a rubbing]

sym·pa·thin (sim′pă-thin). The substance diffusing into circulation from sympathetic nerve terminals when they are active. The term was introduced by W.B. Cannon, who thought that this substance differed from the mediator produced by the nerve ending (now known to be incorrect); the mediator itself (norepinephrine) diffuses into circulation. SYN sympathetic hormone.

sym·pa·thism (sim′pă-thizm). SYN suggestibility. [G. *sympatheia,* sympathy]

sym·pa·thiz·er (sim′pă-thī-zer). **1.** An eye affected with sympathetic ophthalmia. **2.** One who exhibits sympathy.

△**sympatho-.** SEE sympath-.

sym·pa·tho·ad·re·nal (sim′pă-thō-ă-drē′năl). Relating to the sympathetic part of the autonomic nervous system and the medulla of the adrenal gland, as the postganglionic neurons.

sym·pa·tho·blast (sim′pă-thō-blast). A primitive cell derived from the neural crest glia; with the pheochromoblasts, s.'s enter into the formation of the adrenal medulla and sympathetic ganglia. SYN sympathetoblast, sympathicoblast. [sympatho- + G. *blastos,* germ]

sym·pa·tho·go·nia (sim′pă-thō-gō′nē-ă). The completely undifferentiated cells of the sympathetic nervous system. [sympatho- + G. *gonē,* seed]

sym·pa·tho·lyt·ic (sim′pă-thō-lit′ik). Denoting antagonism to or inhibition of adrenergic nerve activity. SEE ALSO adrenergic blocking *agent,* antiadrenergic. [sympatho- + G. *lysis,* a loosening]

sym·pa·tho·mi·met·ic (sim′pă-thō-mi-met′ik). Denoting mimicking of action of the sympathetic system. SEE ALSO adrenomimetic. [sympatho- + G. *mimikos,* imitating]

sym·pa·thy (sim′pă-thē). **1.** The mutual relation, physiologic or pathologic, between two organs, systems, or parts of the body. **2.** Mental contagion, as seen in mass hysteria or in the yawning induced by seeing another person yawn. **3.** An expressed sensitive appreciation or emotional concern for and sharing of the mental and emotional state of another person. Cf. empathy (1). [G. *sympatheia,* fr. sym- + *pathos,* suffering]

sym·per·i·to·ne·al (sim′per-i-tō-nē′ăl). Relating to the surgical induction of adhesion between two portions of the peritoneum.

sym·pha·lan·gism, sym·pha·lan·gy (sim-fal′an-jizm, sim-fal′an-jē). **1.** SYN syndactyly. **2.** Ankylosis of the finger or toe joints. [sym- + phalanx]

sym·phys·i·al, sym·phys·e·al (sim-fiz′ē-ăl). Grown together; relating to a symphysis; fused. SYN symphysic.

sym·phys·ic (sim-fiz′ik). SYN symphysial.

sym·phys·i·on (sim-fiz′ē-on). A craniometric point, the most anterior point of the alveolar process of the mandible.

sym·phys·i·o·tome, sym·phys·e·o·tome (sim-fiz′ē-ō-tōm). Instrument for use in symphysiotomy.

sym·phys·i·ot·o·my, sym·phys·e·ot·o·my (sim-fiz-ē-ot′ō-mē). Division of the pubic joint to increase the capacity of a contracted pelvis sufficiently to permit passage of a living child. SYN synchondrotomy. [symphysis + G. *tome,* incision]

sym·phy·sis, gen. **sym·phy·ses** (sim′fi-sis, -sēz) [TA]. **1** [NA]. Form of cartilaginous joint in which union between two bones is effected by means of fibrocartilage. SYN amphiarthrosis. **2.** A union, meeting point, or commissure of any two structures. **3.** A pathologic adhesion or growing together. SYN secondary cartilaginous joint [TA]. [G. a growing together]

intervertebral s. [TA], the union between adjacent vertebral bodies composed of the nucleus pulposus, annular ligament, and the anterior and posterior longitudinal ligaments. SYN s. intervertebralis [TA].

s. intervertebra′lis [TA], SYN intervertebral s.

s. mandib′ulae [TA], SYN mandibular s.

mandibular s. [TA], the fibrocartilaginous union of the two halves of the mandible in the fetus; it becomes an osseous union during the first year. SYN s. mandibulae [TA], mental s., s. mentalis, s. menti.

manubriosternal s. [TA], the later union, by fibrocartilage, of the manubrium and the body of the sternum; it begins as a synchondrosis and becomes a symphysis, occasionally fusing to become a synostosis. SYN s. manubriosternalis [TA], sternomanubrial junction.

s. manubriosterna′lis [TA], SYN manubriosternal s.

mental s., SYN mandibular s.

s. menta′lis, SYN mandibular s.

s. men′ti, SYN mandibular s.

pericardial s., adhesion between the parietal and visceral layers of the pericardium.

pubic s. [TA], the firm fibrocartilaginous joint between the two pubic bones. SYN s. pubica [TA], s. pubis.

s. pu′bica [TA], SYN pubic s.

s. pu′bis, SYN pubic s.

s. sacrococcyg′ea, SYN sacrococcygeal *joint.*

s. xiphosternalis [TA], SYN xiphisternal *joint.*

sym·plas·mat·ic (sim-plaz-mat′ik). Relating to the union of protoplasm as in giant cell formation. [G. sym- *plassō,* to mold together]

sym·plast (sim′plast). A multinucleated cell that has formed by fusion of separate cells. [sym- + G. *plastos,* formed]

sym·po·dia (sim-pō′dē-ă). Condition characterized by union of the feet. SEE ALSO sirenomelia, sympus. [sym- + G. *pous,* foot]

sym·port (sim′pōrt). Coupled transport of two different molecules or ions through a membrane in the same direction by a common carrier mechanism (symporter). Cf. antiport, uniport. [sym- + L. *porto,* to carry]

sym·port·er (sim-pōrt′er). The protein responsible for mediating symport.

symp·tom (simp′tŏm). Any morbid phenomenon or departure from the normal in structure, function, or sensation, experienced by the patient and indicative of disease. SEE ALSO phenomenon (1), reflex (1), sign (1), syndrome. [G. *symptōma*]

abstinence s.'s, SYN withdrawal s.'s.

accessory s., a s. that usually but not always accompanies a certain disease, as distinguished from a pathognomonic s. SYN assident s., concomitant s.

accidental s., any morbid phenomenon coincidentally occurring in the course of a disease, but having no relation with it.

assident s., SYN accessory s.

Baumès s., pain behind the sternum in angina pectoris.

Bolognini s., a feeling of crepitation on gradually increasing pressure on the abdomen in cases of measles.

cardinal s., the primary or major s. of diagnostic importance.

concomitant s., SYN accessory s.

constitutional s., a s. indicating a systemic effect of a disease; e.g., weight loss.

deficiency s., manifestation of a lack, in varying degrees, of some substance (e.g., hormone, enzyme, vitamin) necessary for normal structure and/or function of an organism.

Demarquay s., absence of elevation of the larynx during deglutition, said to indicate syphilitic induration of the trachea.

Epstein s., SEE Epstein *sign*.

equivocal s., a s. that points definitely to no special disease, being associated with any one of a number of morbid states, or whose presence is uncertain or indefinite.

first rank s.'s (FRS), SYN Schneider first rank s.'s.

Fischer s., SYN Fischer *sign*.

Gordon s., SYN tonic *reflex*.

incarceration s., SYN Dietl *crisis*.

induced s., a s. excited by a drug, exercise, or other means, often intentionally for diagnostic purposes.

local s., a s. of limited extent, caused by disease of a particular organ or part.

localizing s., a s. indicating clearly the seat of the morbid process.

Macewen s., SYN Macewen *sign*.

negative s., one of the deficit s.'s of schizophrenia that follow from diminished volition and executive function including inertia, anergia, lack of involvement with the environment, poverty of thought, social withdrawal, and blunted affect.

objective s., a s. that is evident to the observer.

pathognomonic s., a s. that, when present, definitely points to the presence of a certain disease.

positive s., one of the acute or florid s.'s of schizophrenia, including hallucinations, delusions, thought disorder, loose associations, ambivalence, or affective lability.

Pratt s., rarely used term for rigidity in the muscles of an injured limb, which precedes the occurrence of gangrene.

presenting s., the complaint offered by the patient as the main reason for seeking medical care; usually synonymous with chief *complaint*.

rainbow s., SYN glaucomatous *halo* (2).

reflex s., a disturbance of sensation or function in an organ or part more or less remote from the morbid condition giving rise to it; e.g., muscle spasm due to joint inflammation. SYN sympathetic s.

Schneider first rank s.'s, those s.'s that, when present, indicate that the diagnosis of schizophrenia is likely, provided that organic or toxic etiology is ruled out: delusion of control, thought broadcasting, thought withdrawal, thought insertion, hearing one's thoughts spoken aloud, auditory hallucinations that comment on one's behavior, and auditory hallucinations in which two voices carry on a conversation. SYN first rank s.'s, schneiderian first rank s.'s.

schneiderian first rank s.'s, SYN Schneider first rank s.'s.

Sklowsky s., the rupture of a varicella vesicle on very slight pressure with the finger, greater pressure being necessary to break the vesicles of smallpox, herpes, or other affections.

subjective s., a s. apparent only to the patient.

sympathetic s., SYN reflex s.

Trendelenburg s., a waddling gait in paresis of the gluteal muscles, as in progressive muscular dystrophy.

Uhthoff s., a transient temperature-dependent numbness, weakness, or loss of vision. Conduction stops in any nerve if the temperature gets too high. In a damaged nerve, e.g., by demyelinization, this shutdown temperature is lowered, and may approach normal body temperature. Transient neurological dysfunction may then appear with a hot shower, exercise, or fever. SYN Uhthoff syndrome.

Wartenberg s., (1) flexion of the thumb when the patient attempts to flex the four fingers against resistance, a "pyramid sign". **(2)** intense pruritus of the tip of the nose and nostrils in cases of cerebral tumor;

withdrawal s.'s, a group of morbid s.'s, including excitability and irritability, occurring in an addict who is deprived of the accustomed dose of the addicting agent. SYN abstinence s.'s.

symp·to·mat·ic (simp-tō-mat'ik). Indicative; relating to or constituting the aggregate of symptoms of a disease.

symp·tom·a·tol·o·gy (simp'tō-mă-tol'ō-jē). **1.** The science of the symptoms of disease, their production, and the indications they furnish. **2.** The aggregate of symptoms of a disease. [symptom + G. *logos,* study]

symp·to·mat·o·lyt·ic (simp'tō-mat-ō-lit'ik). Removing symptoms. SYN symptomolytic. [symptom + G. *lytikos,* dissolving]

symp·to·mo·lyt·ic (sim-tō-mō-lit'ik). SYN symptomatolytic.

symp·to·sis (sim-tō'sis). A localized or general wasting of the body. [G. a falling together, collapse, fr. *syn,* together, + *ptōsis,* a falling]

sym·pus (sim'pŭs). An individual in which the legs and feet are united in the midline. [G. *sympous,* fr. sym- + *pous,* foot]

  s. a'pus, a sirenomelus without feet.

  s. di'pus, a sirenomelus with both feet more or less distinct.

  s. mo'nopus, a sirenomelus with but one foot externally visible.

Syms, Parker, U.S. surgeon, 1860–1933. SEE S. *tractor.*

syn-. Together, with, joined; appears as sym- before b, p, ph, or m; corresponds to L. con-. [G. *syn,* with, together]

syn·a·del·phus (sin-ă-del'fŭs). Conjoined twins with single head, partially united trunk, and four upper and four lower limbs. SEE conjoined *twins,* under *twin.* [syn- + G. *adelphos,* brother]

synanamorph (sin-an'ă-morf). The same fungal species growing in a different form.

syn·a·nas·to·mo·sis (sin'an-as-tō-mō'sis). An anastomosis between several blood vessels.

syn·an·dro·gen·ic (sin'an-drō-jen'ik). Relating to any agent or condition that enhances the effects of androgens.

sy·nan·them, syn·an·the·ma (si-nan'them, sin'an-thē'mă). An exanthem consisting of several different forms of eruption. [G. *syn- antheō,* to blossom together]

sy·naph·o·cep·tors (si-naf-ō-sep'terz). Receptors stimulated by direct contact. [G. *synaphe,* contact, + L. *recipio,* to receive]

syn·apse, pl. **syn·aps·es** (sin'aps, sĭ-naps'; sĭ-nap'sēz). The functional membrane-to-membrane contact of the nerve cell with another nerve cell, an effector (muscle, gland) cell, or a sensory receptor cell. The s. subserves the transmission of nerve impulses, commonly from a variably large (1–12 μm), generally knob-shaped or club-shaped axon terminal (the presynaptic element) to the circumscript patch of the receiving cell's plasma membrane (the postsynaptic element) on which the s. occurs. In most cases the impulse is transmitted by means of a chemical transmitter substance (such as acetylcholine, γ-aminobutyric acid, dopamine, norepinephrine) released into a synaptic cleft (15–50 μm wide) that separates the presynaptic from the postsynaptic membrane; the transmitter is stored in quantal form in synaptic vesicles: round or ellipsoid, membrane-bound vacuoles (10–50 nm in diameter) in the presynaptic element. In other synapses transmission takes place by direct propagation of the bioelectrical potential from the presynaptic to the postsynaptic membrane; in such electrotonic synapses ("gap junctions"), the synaptic cleft is no more than about 2 nm wide. In most cases, synaptic transmission takes place in only one direction ("dynamic polarity" of the s.), but in some synapses synaptic vesicles occur on both sides of the synaptic cleft, suggesting the possibility of reciprocal chemical transmission. [syn- + G. *hapto,* to clasp]

axoaxonic s., the synaptic junction between an axon terminal of one neuron and either the initial axon segment or an axon terminal of another nerve cell.

axodendritic s., the synaptic contact between an axon terminal of one nerve cell and a dendrite of another nerve cell.

axosomatic s., the synaptic junction of an axon terminal of one nerve cell to the cell body of another nerve cell. SYN pericorpuscular s.

electrotonic s., SYN gap *junction*; SEE ALSO synapse.

pericorpuscular s., SYN axosomatic s.

syn·ap·sin I (si-nap′sin). A fibrous phosphoprotein that links synaptic vesicles together in the axon terminal; s. I is a substrate for certain kinases; phosphorylation of s. I allows release of neurotransmitters.

syn·ap·sis (si-nap′sis). The point-for-point pairing of homologous chromosomes during the prophase of meiosis. SYN synaptic phase. [G. a connection, junction]

syn·ap·tic (si-nap′tik). **1.** Relating to a synapse. **2.** Relating to synapsis.

syn·ap·tol·o·gy (sin′ap-tol′ō-jē). Study of the synapse.

syn·ap·to·phys·in (si-nap′tō-fī′sin). An integral membrane protein found in many types of active neurons; believed to form a hexamer that forms an ion channel and is involved in the uptake of neurotransmitters; s. is found in the membrane only after stimulation of the neurons.

syn·ap·to·some (si-nap′tō-sōm). Membrane-bound sac containing synaptic vesicles that breaks away from axon terminals when brain tissue is homogenized under controlled conditions; such particles can be separated from other subcellular particles by differential and density gradient centrifugation. [synapse + G. *sōma*, body]

syn·ar·thro·dia (sin′ar-thrō′dē-ă). SYN fibrous *joint*.

syn·ar·thro·di·al (sin-ar-thrō′dē-ăl). Relating to synarthrosis; denoting an articulation without a joint cavity.

syn·ar·thro·phy·sis (sin-ar-thrō-fī′sis). The process of ankylosis. [syn- + G. *arthron*, joint, + *physis*, growth]

syn·ar·thro·sis, pl. **syn·ar·thro·ses** (sin′ar-thrō′sis, -sēz) [TA]. An immovable or nearly immovable union of rigid components of the skeletal system, including fibrous joints, cartilaginous joints, and bony unions (synostoses). SEE articulation. [G. fr. *syn*, together, + *arthrōsis*, articulation]

syn·can·thus (sin-kan′thŭs). Adhesion of the eyeball to orbital structures. [syn- + L. *canthus*, wheel]

syn·car·y·on (sin-kar′ē-on). SYN synkaryon.

syn·ceph·a·lus (sin-sef′ă-lŭs). Conjoined twins having a single head with two bodies. SEE conjoined *twins*, under *twin*. Cf. craniopagus, janiceps. SYN monocephalus, monocranius. [syn- + G. *kephalē*, head]

s. asymmet′ros, SYN *janiceps* asymmetrus.

syn·ceph·a·ly (sin-sef′ă-lē). The condition exhibited by a syncephalus. SYN prozygosis.

syn·chei·lia (sin-kī′lē-ă). A more or less complete adhesion of the lips; atresia of the mouth. SYN synchilia. [syn- + G. *cheilos*, lip]

syn·chei·ria (sin-kī′rē-ă). A form of dyscheiria in which the subject refers a stimulus applied to one side of the body to both sides. SYN synchiria. [syn- + G. *cheir*, hand]

syn·chi·lia. SYN syncheilia.

syn·chi·ria. SYN syncheiria.

syn·chon·dro·se·ot·o·my (sin-kon′drō-sē-ot′ō-mē). Operation of cutting through a synchondrosis; specifically, cutting through the sacroiliac ligaments and forcibly closing the arch of the pubes; used in the treatment of exstrophy of the bladder. [synchondrosis + G. *tomē*, cutting]

syn·chon·dro·sis, pl. **syn·chon·dro·ses** (sin′kon-drō′sis, -sēz) [TA]. Cartilaginous joint in which two bones are united either by hyaline cartilage or fibrocartilage. SYN synchondrodial joint [TA]. [Mod. L. fr. G. *syn*, together, + *chondros*, cartilage, + *-osis*, condition]

anterior intraoccipital s. [TA], cartilaginous union in the newborn between the lateral and the basilar portions of the occipital bone. SYN s. intraoccipitalis anterior [TA], anterior intraoccipital joint.

s. arycornicula′ta, SYN arycorniculate s.

arycorniculate s., the junction of the corniculate cartilage (of Santorini) with the arytenoid. SYN s. arycorniculata.

cranial synchondroses [TA], the cartilaginous joints of the skull; these include sphenoethmoidal s., sphenooccipital s., sphenope-

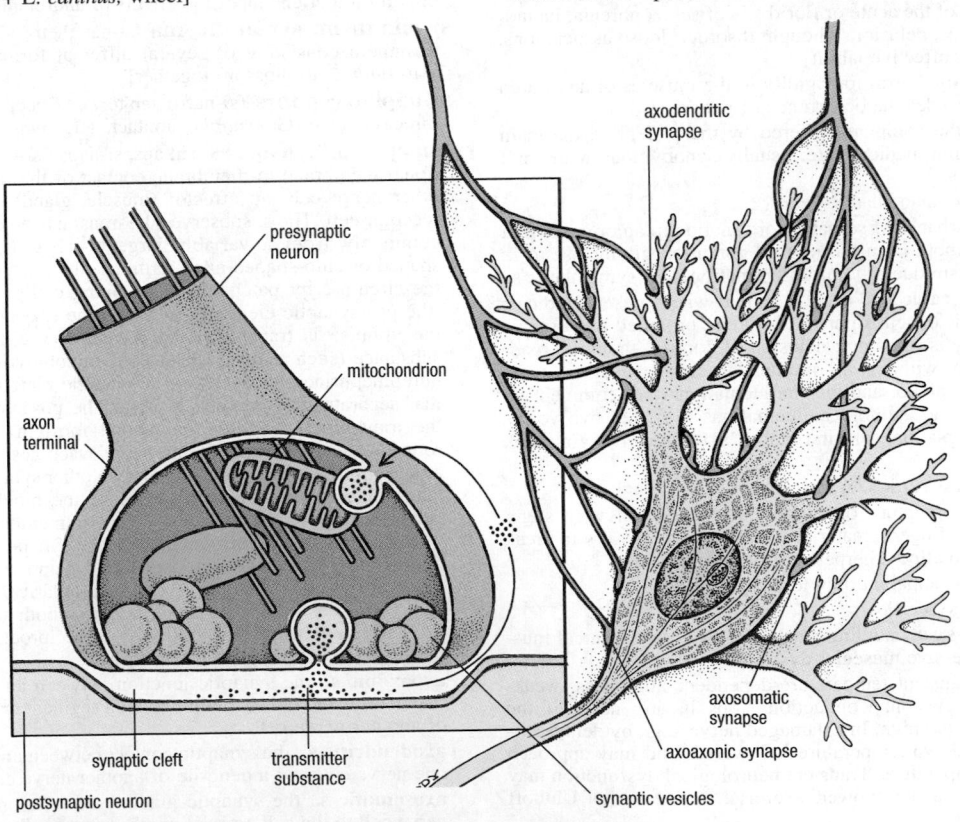

presynaptic neuron

axodendritic synapse

mitochondrion

axon terminal

synaptic cleft

transmitter substance

postsynaptic neuron

axosomatic synapse

axoaxonic synapse

synaptic vesicles

synapses

trosal s., petrooccipital s., anterior intraoccipital and posterior intraoccipital s. SYN synchondroses cranii [TA].

synchondro′ses cra′nii [TA], SYN cranial synchondroses.

s. epiphy′seos, SYN epiphysial line.

synchondroses intersternebra′les, persisting cartilages uniting the bony elements of the sternum, as in some domestic animals such as the dog. SYN intersternebral joints.

s. intraoccipita′lis ante′rior [TA], SYN anterior intraoccipital s.

s. intraoccipita′lis poste′rior [TA], SYN posterior intraoccipital s.

s. manubriosterna′lis [TA], SYN manubriosternal joint.

neurocentral s., the cartilaginous union on either side between the body and arch of a vertebra in the young child. SYN neurocentral joint, neurocentral suture.

petrooccipital s. [TA], fibrocartilage filling the petrooccipital fissure. SYN s. petro-occipitalis [TA], petrooccipital joint.

s. petro-occipita′lis [TA], SYN petrooccipital s.

posterior intraoccipital s. [TA], cartilaginous union between the squamous and lateral parts of the occipital bone in the newborn. SYN s. intraoccipitalis posterior [TA], Budin obstetrical joint, posterior intraoccipital joint.

sphenoethmoidal s. [TA], cartilaginous union between the body of the sphenoid and the posterior part of the ethmoidal labyrinth. SYN s. sphenoethmoidalis [TA].

s. sphenoethmoida′lis [TA], SYN sphenoethmoidal s.

sphenooccipital s. [TA], cartilaginous union between the body of the sphenoid and the basilar portion of the occipital; it fuses by the twentieth year and thus has particular importance in forensic anthropology; incorrectly called sphenooccipital suture. SYN s. spheno-occipitalis [TA], sphenooccipital joint, sphenooccipital suture.

s. spheno-occipita′lis [TA], SYN sphenooccipital s.

s. sphenopetro′sa [TA], SYN sphenopetrosal s.

sphenopetrosal s., sphenopetrous s. [TA], fibrocartilage filling the sphenopetrosal fissure. SYN s. sphenopetrosa [TA].

sternal synchondroses [TA], the cartilaginous junctions between the body of the sternum and the manubrium (manubriosternal joint or symphysis), and between the body of the sternum and the xiphoid process (xiphisternal joint or symphysis); in domestic animals, there may be several, e.g., the manubriosternal, intersternebral, and the xiphisternal joints. SYN synchondroses sternales [TA], sternal joints.

synchondro′ses sterna′les [TA], SYN sternal synchondroses.

s. xiphosterna′lis, SYN xiphisternal joint.

syn·chon·dro·to·my (sin-kon-drot′ō-mē). SYN symphysiotomy.

syn·cho·ri·al (sin-kōr′ē-ăl). Relating to fused chorions as are found in multiple-fetus pregnancies. [syn- + chorion]

syn·chro·nia (sin-krō′nē-ă). **1.** SYN synchronism. **2.** Origin, development, involution, or functioning of tissues or organs at the usual time for such an event. Cf. heterochronia. [syn- + G. chronos, time]

syn·chron·ic (sin′krŏn-ik). Referring to the study of the natural history of a disease by its state and distribution in a population at one time. The inferences about longitudinal course from such a study are warranted only under special conditions, notably that the longitudinal course of the disease is itself unchanging and that subjects in the sample are a representative sample of the survivors.

syn·chro·nism (sin′krō-nizm). Occurrence of two or more events at the same time; the condition of being simultaneous. SYN synchronia (1). [syn- + G. chronos, time]

syn·chro·nous (sin′krō-nŭs). Occurring simultaneously. SYN homochronous (1). [G. synchronos]

syn·chro·ny (sin′krō-nē). The simultaneous appearance of two separate events. [syn- + G. chronos, time]

bilateral s., electroencephalographic activity that is recorded over both hemispheres simultaneously; usually used in reference to spike and wave activity.

syn·chro·tron (sin′krō-tron). A machine for generating high speed electrons or protons, as for nuclear studies.

syn·chy·sis (sin′kĭ-sis). Collapse of the collagenous framework of the vitreous humor, with liquefaction of the vitreous body. [G. a mixing together, fr. syn- + chysis, a pouring]

s. scintil′lans, an appearance of glistening spots in the eye, due to cholesterol crystals floating in a fluid vitreous.

syn·ci·ne·sis (sin-si-nē′sis). SYN synkinesis.

syn·cli·nal (sin′klĭ-năl). Denoting two structures inclined one toward the other. [G. syn- klinō, to incline together]

syn·clit·ic (sin-klit′ik). Relating to or marked by synclitism.

syn·cli·tism (sin′kli-tizm). Condition of parallelism between the planes of the fetal head and of the pelvis, respectively. [G. syn-klinō, to incline together]

syn·co·pal (sin′kō-păl). Relating to syncope. SYN syncopic.

syn·co·pe (sin′kŏ-pē). Loss of consciousness and postural tone caused by diminished cerebral blood flow. [G. synkopē, a cutting short, a swoon]

Adams-Stokes s., s. due to complete AV block. SYN Morgagni-Adams-Stokes s.

cardiac s., fainting with unconsciousness of any cardiac cause.

carotid sinus s., s. resulting from overactivity of the carotid sinus; attacks may be spontaneous or produced by pressure on a sensitive carotid sinus.

deglutition s., faintness or unconsciousness upon swallowing. This is nearly always due to excessive vagal effect on a heart that may already have bradycardia or atrioventricular block. SYN swallow s.

hysterical s., fainting due to, or to avoid, emotional stress.

laryngeal s., a paroxysmal neurosis characterized by attacks of coughing, with unusual sensations, as of tickling, in the throat, followed by a brief period of unconsciousness.

local s., limited numbness in a part, especially of the fingers; one of the symptoms, usually associated with local asphyxia, of Raynaud disease.

micturition s., s. occurring in association with the act of emptying the bladder.

Morgagni-Adams-Stokes s., SYN Adams-Stokes s.

postural s., s. upon assuming an upright position; caused by failure of normal vasoconstrictive mechanisms.

swallow s., SYN deglutition s.

tussive s., fainting as a result of a coughing spell, caused by persistent increased intrathoracic pressure diminishing venous return to the heart, thus lowering cardiac output; most often occurs in heavy-set male smokers who have chronic bronchitis. SYN Charcot vertigo, laryngeal vertigo.

vasodepressor s., faintness or loss of consciousness due to reflex reduction in blood pressure. SYN vasovagal s.

vasovagal s., SYN vasodepressor s.

syn·cop·ic (sin-kop′ik). SYN syncopal.

syn·cre·tio (sin-krē′shē-ō). Development of adhesion between inflamed opposing surfaces. [Mod. L., fr. G. synkrētizō, to unite the Cretan cities, reanalyzed as fr. syn- + L. cresco, pp. cretum, to grow]

syn·cy·a·nin (sin-sī′ă-nin). A blue pigment produced by Pseudomonas syncyanea.

syn·cy·tial (sin-sish′ăl, -sish′ē-ăl, -sit′ē-ăl). Relating to a syncytium.

syn·cy·ti·o·tro·pho·blast (sin-sish′ē-ō-trō′fō-blast). The syncytial outer layer of the trophoblast; site of synthesis of human chorionic gonadotropin. SEE ALSO trophoblast. SYN placental plasmodium, plasmodial trophoblast, plasmodiotrophoblast, syncytial trophoblast, syntrophoblast. [syncytium + trophoblast]

syn·cy·ti·um, pl. **syn·cy·tia** (sin-sish′ē-ŭm, -ă; -sit′ē-ŭm). A multinucleated protoplasmic mass formed by the secondary union of originally separate cells. [Mod. L. fr. syn- + G. kytos, cell]

syn·dac·tyl, syn·dac·tyle (sin-dak′til, -dak′tīl). SYN syndactylous.

syn·dac·tyl·ia, syn·dac·ty·lism (sin-dak-til′ē-ă, -dak′ti-lizm). SYN syndactyly.

syn·dac·ty·lous (sin-dak′ti-lŭs). Having fused or webbed fingers or toes. SYN syndactyl, syndactyle.

syn·dac·ty·ly (sin-dak′ti-lē). Any degree of webbing or fusion of fingers or toes, involving soft parts only or including bone structure; usually autosomal dominant inheritance. SYN symphalangism (1), symphalangy, syndactylia, syndactylism. [syn- + G. *daktylos,* finger or toe]

syn·dein (sin-dē'in). SYN ankyrin. [G. *syndeō,* to bind together, + -in]

△**syndesm-.** SEE syndesmo-.

syn·des·mec·to·my (sin-dez-mek'tō-mē). Cutting away a section of a ligament. [syndesm- + G. *ektomē,* excision]

syn·des·mi·tis (sin-dez-mī'tis). Inflammation of a ligament. [syndesm- + G. *-itis,* inflammation]
   s. metatar'sea, inflammation of the metatarsal ligaments.

△**syndesmo-, syndesm-.** Ligament, ligamentous. [G. *syndesmos,* a fastening, fr. *syndeō,* to bind]

syn·des·mo·cho·ri·al (sin-dez-mō-kōr'ē-ăl). Relating to the placenta in ruminant animals. [syndesmo- + G. *chorion,* membrane]

syn·des·mo·di·al (sin-des-mō'dē-ăl). SYN syndesmotic.

syn·des·mog·ra·phy (sin-dez-mog'ră-fē). A treatise on or description of the ligaments. [syndesmo- + G. *graphō,* to write]

syn·des·mo·lo·gia (sin-dez'mō-lō'jē-ă). SYN arthrology.

syn·des·mol·o·gy (sin-dez-mol'ŏ-jē). SYN arthrology. [syndesmo- + G. *logos,* study]

syn·des·mo·phyte (sin-dez'mō-fīt). An osseous excrescence attached to a ligament. [syndesmo- + G. *phyton,* plant]

syn·des·mo·sis, pl. **syn·des·mo·ses** (sin'dez-mo'sis, -sēz) [TA]. A form of fibrous joint in which opposing surfaces that are relatively far apart are united by ligaments; e.g., the union of the styloid process of the temporal bone and the hyoid bone via the stylohyoid ligament, and the fibrous union between the radius and ulna (radioulnar syndesmoses) and the tibia and fibula (tibiofibular syndesmoses). SYN syndesmodial joint, syndesmotic joint. [syndesmo- + G. *-osis,* condition]
   radioulnar s. [TA], the fibrous union of the radius and ulna consisting of the oblique cord and the interosseous membrane. SYN s. radioulnaris [TA], middle radioulnar joint.
   s. radioulna'ris [TA], SYN radioulnar s.
   tibiofibular s. [TA], the fibrous union of the tibia and fibula consisting of the interosseous membrane and the anterior, interosseous and posterior tibiofibular ligaments at the distal extremities of the bones. SYN s. tibiofibularis [TA], distal tibiofibular joint, inferior tibiofibular joint, tibiofibular articulation (2).
   s. tibiofibula'ris [TA], SYN tibiofibular s.
   tympanostapedial s. [TA], the connection of the base or footplate of the stapes with the vestibular (oval) window. SYN s. tympanostapedialis [TA], tympanostapedial junction.
   s. tympanostapedia'lis [TA], SYN tympanostapedial s., tympanostapedial s.

syn·des·mot·ic (sin-des-mot'ik). Relating to syndesmosis. SYN syndesmodial.

SYNDROME

■**syn·drome** (sin'drōm). The aggregate of symptoms and signs associated with any morbid process, and constituting together the picture of the disease. SEE ALSO disease. [G. *syndromē,* a running together, tumultuous concourse; (in med.) a concurrence of symptoms, fr. *syn,* together, + *dromos,* a running]

Aagenaes s., an idiopathic form of familial intrahepatic cholestasis associated with lymphedema of the lower extremities.

Aarskog-Scott s., SYN faciodigitogenital *dysplasia.*

abdominal muscle deficiency s. [MIM*100100, MIM*264140], congenital absence (partial or complete) of abdominal muscles, in which the outline of the intestines is visible through the protruding abdominal wall; in males, genitourinary anomalies (urinary tract dilation and cryptorchidism) are also found; genetics unclear. SEE ALSO prune belly s. SYN prune belly.

abstinence s., a constellation of physiologic changes undergone by persons or animals who have become physically dependent on a drug or chemical due to prolonged use at elevated doses, but who are abruptly deprived of that substance. The abstinence s. varies with the drug to which dependence has developed. Generally the effects observed are in an opposite direction from those produced by the drug; e.g., the withdrawal s. from central nervous system depressants such as barbiturates and benzodiazepines consists of insomnia, restlessness, tremulousness, hallucinations, and, in the extreme, tonic-clonic convulsions which may prove fatal. The onset time and severity of the abstinence s. depend upon how rapidly the drug disappears from the body.

Achard s. [MIM*100700], arachnodactyly with small receding mandible, broad skull, and joint laxity limited to the hands and feet; genetics unclear.

Achard-Thiers s., one form of a virilizing disorder of adrenocortical origin in women, characterized by masculinization and menstrual disorders in association with manifestations of diabetes mellitus, such as glucosuria.

Achenbach s., hematoma of the finger pad with accompanying edema; of unknown cause in the absence of disturbances in blood coagulation mechanisms.

acquired immunodeficiency s., SYN AIDS.

acrofacial s., SYN acrofacial *dysostosis.*

acroparesthesia s., abnormal sensation such as numbness and tingling in the hands, usually in middle-aged women; now known to be a classic symptom of carpal tunnel syndrome.

acute organic brain s., SYN organic brain s.

acute radiation s., a s. caused by exposure of the body to large amounts of radiation, (e.g., from certain forms of therapy, accidents, and nuclear explosions; it is divided into three major forms which are, in ascending order of severity, the hematogic, gastrointestinal, and central nervous system-cardiovascular forms; its clinical manifestations are divided into prodromal, latent, overt, and recovery stages.

acute respiratory distress s., SYN adult respiratory distress s.

Adams-Stokes s., a s. characterized by slow or absent pulse, vertigo, syncope, convulsions, and sometimes Cheyne-Stokes respiration; usually as a result of advanced AV block or sick sinus syndrome. SYN Adams-Stokes disease, Morgagni disease, Morgagni-Adams-Stokes s., Spens s., Stokes-Adams disease, Stokes-Adams s.

adaptation s. of Selye, general nonspecific adaptation of the organism in response to specific stimuli which trigger a cycle of extensive physiological changes in the endocrine and other organ systems due to prolonged and intense stress. SEE general adaptation s.

addisonian s., SYN chronic adrenocortical *insufficiency.*

adherence s., restriction action of an ocular muscle owing to adhesions between the muscle and its fascial sheath.

Adie s. [MIM*100300], an idiopathic postganglionic denervation of the parasympathetically innervated intraocular muscles, usually complicated by signs of aberrant regeneration of these nerves: a weak light reaction with segmental palsy of iris sphincter, a strong, slow near response. Deep tendon reflexes are often asymmetrically reduced. SEE ALSO tonic *pupil.* SYN Adie pupil, Holmes-Adie pupil, Holmes-Adie s., pupillotonic pseudotabes.

adiposogenital s., SYN adiposogenital *dystrophy.*

adrenal cortical s., an inexact (and obsolete) term that has been applied to Cushing s., Addison disease, or the adrenogenital s.

adrenal virilizing s., SYN adrenal *virilism.*

adrenogenital s., generic designation for a group of disorders caused by adrenocortical hyperplasia or malignant tumors and characterized by masculinization of women, feminization of men, or precocious sexual development of children; representative of excessive or abnormal secretory patterns of adrenocortical steroids, especially those with androgenic or estrogenic effects.

adult respiratory distress s. (ARDS), acute lung injury from a variety of causes, characterized by interstitial and/or alveolar edema and hemorrhage as well as perivascular pulmonary edema associated with hyaline membrane formation, proliferation of collagen fibers, and swollen epithelium with increased pinocytosis.

SYN acute respiratory distress s., diffuse alveolar damage, wet lung (2), white lung.

afferent loop s., chronic obstruction of the duodenum and jejunum proximal to the gastrojejunostomy performed in a Billroth II-type gastrectomy; the distended afferent loop of jejenum and duodenum causes symptoms of pain and fullness associated with food injestion; weight loss is common. SYN gastrojejunal loop obstruction s.

aglossia-adactylia s. [MIM*103300], congenital absence or hypoplasia of the tongue, associated with absence of the digits.

Aicardi s. [MIM*304050], an X-linked dominant disorder with lethality in hemizygous males; characterized by agenesis of corpus collosum, chorioretinal abnormality with "holes," cleft lip with or without cleft palate, seizures, and characteristic EEG changes.

Alagille s. [MIM 118450], an autosomal dominant syndrome that becomes apparent in childhood and is associated with jaundice due to a paucity of intrahepatic bile ducts; characteristics include a narrow face and pointed chin, broad forehead, long, straight nose, deep-set eyes, posterior embryotoxon in the eye, cardiovascular abnormalities, vertebral defects, and nephropathy.

Albright s., (1) SYN McCune-Albright s; (2) SYN Albright hereditary *osteodystrophy.*

alcohol amnestic s., an amnestic s. resulting from alcoholism; alcoholic "blackouts." Cf. Korsakoff s.

Aldrich s., SYN Wiskott-Aldrich s.

Alice in Wonderland s., the illusion of dreams, feelings of levitation, and alteration in the sense of the passage of time, sometimes associated with migraine, epilepsy, and various diseases of the parietal lobe of the brain.

Allen-Masters s., pelvic pain resulting from an old laceration of the broad ligament received during delivery.

Allgrove s., SYN triple A s.

Alport s., a genetically heterogeneous disorder characterized by nephritis associated with microscopic hematuria and slow progression of renal failure, sensorineural hearing loss, and ocular abnormalities such as lenticonus and maculopathy; autosomal dominant [MIM*104200, MIM*153640, and MIM*153650], autosomal recessive [MIM*203780], and X-linked recessive [MIM*301050 and MIM*303630] forms exist. The X-linked form is caused by mutation in the collagen type IV alpha-5 gene (COL4A5) on chromosome Xq; the autosomal recessive form is due to mutation in the collagen type IV alpha-3 gene (COL4A3) or alpha-4 gene (COL4A4) on 2q.

Alström s. [MIM*203800], retinal degeneration with nystagmus and loss of central vision, associated with obesity in childhood; sensorineural hearing loss and diabetes mellitus usually occur after age 10; autosomal recessive inheritance.

amenorrhea-galactorrhea s., unphysiologic lactation from endocrinological causes or from a pituitary tumor.

amnestic s., (1) SYN Korsakoff s; (2) an organic brain s. with short-term (but not immediate) memory disturbance, regardless of the etiology.

amnionic band syndrome, SYN amnionic *band.*

amnionic fluid s., pulmonary embolic phenomena thought to be due to infusion of amniotic fluid containing epithelial squames into maternal blood vessels; shock ensues and sudden death may occur. SEE amnionic fluid *embolism.*

Amsterdam s., SYN de Lange s. [*Amsterdam,* the Netherlands]

androgen insensitivity s., SYN androgen resistance s.'s.

androgen resistance s.'s, a class of disorders associated with 5α-steroid reductase deficiency, testicular feminization, and related disorders. Cf. *steroid* 5α-reductase, Reifenstein s., infertile male s., testicular feminization s. SYN androgen insensitivity s.

Angelman s., microdeletion of 15q-13, of maternal origin, resulting in mental retardation, ataxia, paroxysms of laughter, seizures, characteristic facies, and minimal speech. SEE Prader-Willi s.

Angelucci s., extreme excitability, vasomotor disturbances, and palpitation associated with vernal conjunctivitis.

angioosteohypertrophy s., SYN Klippel-Trenaunay-Weber s.

ankyloglossia superior s., a congenital condition in which the tongue adheres to the hard palate; no evidence of genetic factors.

anorectal s., soreness, burning, itching, or other irritation of the rectum together with redness about the anus, and sometimes accompanied by diarrhea, occurring as a toxic effect of the oral administration of certain broad spectrum antibiotics.

anterior chamber cleavage s. [MIM*261540], a congenital disorder originating from faulty separation of embryonic structures; it results in bilateral central corneal opacities, with an anterior ring attachment of the iridic pupillary border and anterior polar cataracts; associated with short-limbed dwarfism; autosomal dominant inheritance. SEE iridocorneal endothelial s. SYN Peters anomaly.

anterior tibial compartment s., ischemia of the muscles of the anterior tibial compartment of the leg, presumably caused by transient compression of arterial blood flow from muscle swelling within a closed fascial compartment, following strenuous physical activity.

antibody deficiency s., any of a group of disorders associated with a defective antibody production due to defects in the B-type lymphocyte system or in T-type lymphocytes; chief manifestation is an increased susceptibility to infection by various microorganisms. SEE agammaglobulinemia, hypogammaglobulinemia, immunodeficiency. SYN antibody deficiency disease.

Anton s., in cortical blindness, lack of awareness of being blind.

anxiety s., the constellation of autonomic nervous system signs and symptoms accompanying the apprehension of danger and dread. SEE anxiety.

aortic arch s., atheromatous and/or thrombotic obliteration of the branches of the arch of the aorta leading to diminished or absent pulses in the neck and arms. SEE ALSO Takayasu *arteritis,* reversed *coarctation.* SYN Martorell s.

apallic s., SYN apallic *state.*

Apert s. [MIM*101200], disorder characterized by craniosynostosis and syndactyly of all the fingers and usually the toes as well; the thumbs are free; mental retardation is a variable feature. Autosomal dominant mutation with most cases sporadic, caused by mutation in the fibroblast growth factor receptor 2 gene (FGFR2) on 10q. SEE ALSO acrocephalosyndactyly. SYN type I acrocephalosyndactyly.

s. of approximate relevant answers, SYN Ganser s.

Arnold-Chiari s., SYN Arnold-Chiari *malformation.*

arterial thoracic outlet s., a rare disorder due to compression of the subclavian artery (with resultant poststenotic dilation) by a fully formed cervical rib or an abnormal first thoracic rib; thrombi form in the dilated distal arterial segment, and distal limb ischemia may occur due to thromboembolic events.

Ascher s. [MIM*109900], a condition in which a congenital double lip is associated with blepharochalasis and nontoxic thyroid gland enlargement.

Asherman s., SYN traumatic *amenorrhea.*

asplenia s., s. seen in patients who have no functional spleen, either because of surgical removal or disease (e.g., sickle cell anemia); includes increased susceptibility to bacterial infection, especially pneumococcal infection.

ataxia telangiectasia s., SYN *ataxia* telangiectasia.

auriculotemporal nerve s., localized flushing and sweating of the ear and cheek in response to eating. SYN Frey s., gustatory sweating s.

autoerythrocyte sensitization s., a condition, usually occurring in women, in which the individual bruises easily (purpura simplex) and the ecchymoses tend to enlarge and involve adjacent tissues, resulting in pain in the affected parts; so called because similar lesions are produced by inoculation of the individual's blood or various components of red blood cells and it is thought to be a form of localized autosensitization, although no specific antibodies have been demonstrable. SYN Gardner-Diamond s.

Avellis s., unilateral paralysis of the larynx and velum palati, with contralateral loss of pain and temperature sensibility in the parts below. SYN jugular foramen s.

A-V strabismus s., strabismus in which the angle of deviation is more marked on looking upward or downward. SEE ALSO A-pattern *esotropia,* V-pattern *esotropia,* A-pattern *exotropia,* V-pattern *exotropia.*

sy

Ayerza s., sclerosis of the pulmonary arteries in chronic cor pulmonale; associated with severe cyanosis, it is a condition resembling polycythemia vera but resulting from primary pulmonary arteriosclerosis or primary pulmonary hypertension and characterized by plexiform lesions of arterioles. SYN Ayerza disease, cardiopathia nigra, plexogenic pulmonary arteriopathy.

Babinski s., the combination of cardiac, arterial, and central nervous system manifestations of late *syphilis*.

baby bottle s., SYN nursing bottle *caries*.

Balint s., an entity characterized by optic *ataxia* and simultanagnosia. This difficulty in applying the visual system to a visual task is usually due to damage to the superior temporal-occipital areas in both hemispheres.

Bamberger-Marie s., SYN hypertrophic pulmonary *osteoarthropathy*.

Bannwarth s., neurologic manifestations of Lyme disease, also called chronic lymphocytic meningitis and tick-borne meningopolyneuritis.

Banti s., chronic congestive splenomegaly that occurs primarily in children as a sequel to hypertension in the portal or splenic veins, usually as a result of thrombosis in those veins; anemia, splenomegaly, and irregular episodes of gastrointestinal bleeding are usually observed, with ascites, jaundice, leukopenia, and thrombocytopenia developing in various conbinations. SYN Banti disease, splenic anemia.

Bardet-Biedl s. [MIM*209900], mental retardation, pigmentary retinopathy, polydactyly, obesity, and hypogenitalism; autosomal recessive inheritance. SEE ALSO Laurence-Moon s.

bare lymphocyte s., absence of HLA antigens on peripheral mononuclear cells, which may result in immunodeficiency.

Barlow s. [MIM*157700], late apical systolic murmur or (so-called "mid-late") systolic click, or both, due to billowing of the anterior and/or posterior (mural) mitral valvular leaflet into the left atrial cavity (also, floppy valve s.); electrocardiographically, ST-T changes in a posteroinferior distribution resembling those of myocardial ischemia often coexist for unknown reasons; rhythm disturbances may coexist with this s. without demonstrable pathogenetic relationship.

Barrett s., chronic peptic ulceration of the lower esophagus, which is lined by columnar epithelium, resembling the mucosa of the gastric cardia, acquired as a result of long-standing chronic esophagitis; esophageal stricture with reflux, and adenocarcinoma, also have been reported. SYN Barrett esophagus, Barrett metaplasia.

Bart s. [MIM*132000], a form of epidermolysis bullosa with blistering of the extremities and intertriginous areas, congenital localized absence of skin, erosions of the mouth, and dystrophic nails; there is often spontaneous improvement with no residual scarring; autosomal dominant inheritance, caused by mutation in the collagen type VII gene (COL7A1) on chromosome 3p.

Barth s., an X-linked s. characterized by poor growth, neutropenia, cardiomyopathy, and excess excretion of 3-methylglutaconic acid in the urine; some patients also show skeletal muscle weakness.

Bartter s. [MIM*241200], a disorder due to a defect in active chloride reabsorption in the loop of Henle; characterized by primary juxtaglomerular cell hyperplasia with secondary hyperaldosteronism, hypokalemic alkalosis, hypercalciuria, elevated renin or angiotensin levels, normal or low blood pressure, and growth retardation; edema is absent. Autosomal recessive inheritance, caused by mutation in either the Na-K-2Cl cotransporter gene (SLC12A1) on chromosome 15q or the K(+) channel gene (KCNJ1) on 11q.

basal cell nevus s. [MIM*109400], a s. of myriad basal cell nevi with development of basal cell carcinomas in adult life, odontogenic keratocysts, erythematous pitting of the palms and soles, calcification of the cerebral falx, and frequently skeletal anomalies, particularly ribs that are bifid or broadened anteriorly; autosomal dominant inheritance, caused by mutation in the PTCH gene, the human homolog of the "patched" gene of *Drosophila* on 9q. SYN Gorlin s.

Bassen-Kornzweig s., SYN abetalipoproteinemia.

battered child s., the clinical presentation of child abuse: various injuries to the skeleton, soft tissues, or organs of a child sustained as a result of repeated mistreatment or beating, usually by an individual responsible for the child's care.

battered spouse s., physical, psychological, and emotional injuries in a person subjected to abuse by a spouse or domestic partner; usually associated with alcoholism in the abusing spouse.

Bauer s., aortitis and aortic endocarditis as a little-recognized manifestation of rheumatoid arthritis.

Bazex s., SYN paraneoplastic *acrokeratosis*.

Beckwith-Wiedemann s. [MIM*130650], an overgrowth s. characterized by exomphalos, macroglossia, and gigantism, often with neonatal hypoglycemia; there is an association with hemihypertrophy and Wilms tumor. Autosomal dominant inheritance, with most cases sporadic; influenced by genomic imprinting and uniparental disomy; caused by mutation in the P57 (KIP2) gene on chromosome 11p. SYN EMG s.

Behçet s. [MIM*109650], a s. characterized by simultaneously or successively occurring recurrent attacks of genital and oral ulcerations (aphthae) and uveitis or iridocyclitis with hypopyon, often with arthritis; a phase of a generalized disorder, occurring more often in men than in women, with variable manifestations, including dermatitis, erythema nodosum, thrombophlebitis, and cerebral involvement. SYN Behçet disease, cutaneomucouveal s., iridocyclitis septica, oculobuccogenital s., recurrent hypopyon, triple symptom complex, uveoencephalitic s.

Behr s. [MIM*210000], characterized by bilateral optic atrophy with temporal field defects, nystagmus, ataxia, spasticity, and mental retardation; probably autosomal recessive inheritance. SYN Behr disease.

Benedikt s., hemiplegia with clonic spasm or tremor and oculomotor paralysis on the opposite side.

Beradinelli s., accelerated growth, lipodystrophy with muscular hypertrophy, hepatomegaly, and lipemia.

Berardinelli s., SYN congenital total *lipodystrophy*.

Bernard-Horner s., SYN Horner s.

Bernard-Sergent s., SYN acute adrenocortical *insufficiency*.

Bernard-Soulier s., a coagulation disorder characterized by thrombocytopenia, giant platelets, and a bleeding tendency.

Bernhardt-Roth s., SYN *meralgia* paresthetica.

Bernheim s., systemic congestion resembling the consequences of right heart failure (enlarged liver, distended neck veins, and edema) without pulmonary congestion in subjects with left ventricular enlargement from any cause; reduction in the size of the right ventricular cavity is found by contrast imaging or echocardiography or at postmortem due to encroachment by the hypertrophied or aneurysmal ventricular septum.

Besnier-Boeck-Schaumann s., SYN sarcoidosis.

Beuren s., supravalvular aortic stenosis with multiple areas of peripheral pulmonary arterial stenosis, mental retardation, and dental anomalies.

Biemond s. [MIM*210350], iris coloboma, mental retardation, obesity, hypogenitalism, and postaxial polydactyly; probably an autosomal recessive inheritance disorder resembling Laurence-Moon and Bardet-Biedel s.'s.

billowing mitral valve s., SYN mitral valve prolapse s.

Björnstad s. [MIM*262000], pili torti associated with sensorineural hearing loss, the severity of distortion and brittleness of the hair correlated with the degree of hearing impairment; autosomal dominant inheritance.

Blatin s., SYN hydatid *thrill*.

blind loop s., stagnation of intestinal contents with bacterial overgrowth producing substances that interfere with absorption of fat, vitamins, and other nutrients, usually occurs in a portion of small intestine that has been excluded from the flow of chyme.

Bloch-Sulzberger s., SYN *incontinentia* pigmenti.

Bloom s. [MIM*210900], congenital telangiectatic erythema, primarily in butterfly distribution, of the face and occasionally of the hands and forearms, with sun sensitivity of skin lesions and dwarfism with normal body proportions except for a narrow face and dolichocephalic skull; chromosomes are excessively unstable and there is a predisposition to malignancy; autosomal recessive inheritance, caused by mutation in the Bloom syndrome gene (BLM) on chromosome 15q.

blue diaper s., a disorder of tryptophan absorption; excess unabsorbed tryptophan in the intestine is metabolized to indoles and indicans, which are absorbed and lead to excretion of indican in the urine, which is oxidized in the diaper to indigo; patients also have hypercalcemia and nephrocalcinosis.

blue toe s., progressive tissue injury or gangrene from microthromboembolism in the presence of palpable pedal pulses.

Boerhaave s., rupture of the esophagus caused by increased intraluminal pressure during retching or vomiting with a closed glottis; results in mediastinitis and sometimes ruptures into the left pleural space.

Bonnet-Dechaume-Blanc s., SYN Wyburn-Mason s.

Bonnier s., a s. due to a lesion of Deiters nucleus and its connection; the symptoms include ocular disturbances (e.g., paralysis of accommodation, nystagmus, diplopia), as well as deafness, nausea, thirst, anorexia, and symptoms referable to the involvement of the vagus centers.

Böök s. [MIM*112300], premolar aplasia, hyperhidrosis, and premature canities; autosomal dominant trait.

BOR s., SYN branchiootorenal *dysplasia*.

Börjeson-Forssman-Lehmann s. [MIM*301900], a condition characterized by mental deficiency, epilepsy, hypogonadism, hypometabolism, obesity, large ears, and narrow palpebral fissures; X-linked recessive inheritance.

bowel bypass s., recurrent fever, chills, malaise, and inflammatory cutaneous papules and pustules on the extremities and upper trunk with diffuse neutrophil infiltration, sometimes with polyarthralgia or polyarthritis following bowel bypass surgery.

Bradbury-Eggleston s., SYN pure autonomic *failure*.

bradytachycardia s. (brā′dē-tă-kē-car′dē′ă), alternate rapid and slow cardiac rates that may represent any rhythm disturbances in any combination usually related to sinus node disease. SYN tachybradycardia s.

branchiootorenal s., an autosomal dominant disorder characterized by anomalies of the branchial arch derivatives, sensory hearing impairment, and renal abnormalities.

Briquet s., a chronic but fluctuating mental disorder, usually of young women, characterized by frequent complaints of physical illness involving multiple organ systems simultaneously.

Brissaud-Marie s., unilateral spasm of the tongue and lips, of hysterical nature.

Brock s., SYN middle lobe s.

bronze baby s., a brown or bronze discoloration of the skin that may occur in children with hyperbilirubinemia who have received phototherapy.

Brown s., SYN tendon sheath s.

Brown-Séquard s., s. with unilateral spinal cord lesions, proprioception loss and weakness occur ipsilateral to the lesion, while pain and temperature loss occur contralateral. SYN Brown-Séquard paralysis.

Budd s., SYN Chiari s.

Budd-Chiari s., SYN Chiari s.

Bürger-Grütz s., SYN type I familial *hyperlipoproteinemia*.

burner s., multiple episodes of upper extremity burning pain, sometimes accompanied by shoulder girdle weakness, experienced during contact sports, especially football, with each forceful blow to the head or shoulder; attributed to an upper trunk brachial plexopathy.

Burnett s., SYN milk-alkali s.

burning foot s., a disorder observed in prisoners-of-war in World War II, now believed to be due to a pantothenate deficiency.

burning mouth s., a clinical condition in which the patient complains of a burning sensation in the oral cavity although the appearance of the oral mucosa is normal; the cause has not been determined.

burning tongue s., a s. of pain in the tongue without apparent lesions, often associated with ageusia; more common in elderly women.

burning vulva s., persistent vulvodynia in which a physical cause has not been identified.

Buschke-Ollendorf s., SYN osteodermatopoikilosis.

Caffey s., SYN infantile cortical *hyperostosis*.

Caffey-Kempe s., SEE battered child s.

Caffey-Silverman s., SYN infantile cortical *hyperostosis*.

camptomelic s., also associated with flat facies, short vertebrae, hypoplastic scapula, and bowed tibia. SYN osteochondrodysplasia.

Capgras s., the delusional belief that a person (or persons) close to the schizophrenic patient has been substituted for by one or more impostors; may have an organic etiology. SYN Capgras phenomenon, illusion of doubles.

Caplan s., intrapulmonary nodules, histologically similar to subcutaneous rheumatoid nodules, associated with rheumatoid arthritis and pneumoconiosis in coal workers. SYN Caplan nodules.

carbonic anhydrase II deficiency s., an inherited deficiency of carbonic anhydrase II that results in osteopetrosis and metabolic acidosis. SYN osteopetrosis with renal tubular acidosis.

carcinoid s., a combination of symptoms and lesions mostly produced by the release of serotonin from carcinoid tumors of the gastrointestinal tract that have metastasized to the liver; consists of irregular mottled blushing, flat angiomas of the skin, acquired tricuspid and pulmonary stenosis often with regurgitation, occasionally with some minor involvement of valves on the left side of the heart, diarrhea, bronchial spasm, mental aberration, and excretion of large quantities of 5-hydroxyindoleacetic acid. SYN malignant carcinoid s., metastatic carcinoid s.

cardiofacial s., (1) transient or persistent unilateral partial lower facial paresis accompanying some congenital heart disease. (2) a group of syndromes characterized by congenital cardiovascular, bone, soft tissue, and facial abnormalities. Examples include Rubinstein-Taybi s., Noonan s. and Williams s.

Caroli s., congenital malformation of the bile ducts within the liver leading to formation of multifocal cystic dilatations.

carotid sinus s., stimulation of a hyperactive carotid sinus, causing a marked fall in blood pressure due to vasodilation, cardiac slowing, or both; syncope with or without convulsions or AV block may occur. SYN Charcot-Weiss-Baker s.

carpal tunnel s., the most common nerve entrapment s., characterized by nocturnal hand paresthesia and pain, and sometimes sensory loss and wasting in the median hand distribution; affects women more than men and is often bilateral; caused by chronic entrapment of the median nerve at the wrist, within the carpal tunnel.

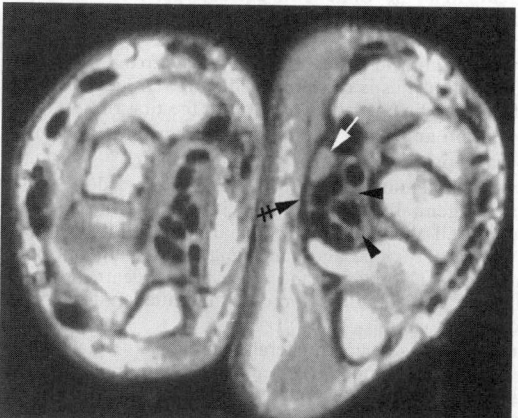

carpel tunnel syndrome: MRI of both wrists; swelling of right median nerve (white arrow), increased fluid between flexor tendons within tunnel (black arrowheads) and slight bowing of the flexor retinaculum (crossed arrow)

Carpenter s., the association of primary hypothyroidism, primary adrenocortical insufficiency, and diabetes mellitus. [C.C.J. Carpenter]

cataract-oligophrenia s., SYN Marinesco-Garland s.

cat's cry s., SYN cri-du-chat s.

cat's-eye s. [MIM*115470], a chromosomal disorder characterized by iris colobomas (resembling the vertical pupils of a cat), downslanting palpebral fissures, anal atresia, preauricular tags and/or pits, heart and renal malformations, and, occasionally, mild mental retardation; associated with chromosome partial tetrasomy 22. SYN Schmid-Fraccaro s.

cauda equina s., involvement, often asymmetric, of multiple roots making up the cauda equina (i.e., L2–S3 roots), manifested by pain, paresthesia, and weakness; often bladder and bowel sphincter function is unaffected because of sacral sparing (lack of compromise of the S2, S3, and S4 roots).

cavernous sinus s., a s. caused by thrombosis of the cavernous intracranial sinus characterized by edema of eyelids and conjunctivae, and paralysis of the third, fourth and sixth nerves.

Ceelen-Gellerstedt s., SYN idiopathic pulmonary *hemosiderosis.*

celiac s., SYN celiac *disease.*

cellular immunity deficiency s., a s. marked by increased susceptibility to infection, especially to viral infection, associated with defective functioning of the mechanism responsible for acquired immunity of the cell-mediated kind. SEE ALSO immunodeficiency.

central cord s., quadriparesis most severely involving the distal upper extremities, with or without sensory loss and bladder dysfunction, usually due to ischemia from osteophytic or traumatic compression of the central part of the cervical spinal cord and/or artery.

cerebellar s., the signs and symptoms of cerebellar dysfunction: dysmetria, dysarthria, asynergia, nystagmus, ataxia, staggering gait, and adiadochokinesia.

cerebellomedullary malformation s., SYN Arnold-Chiari *malformation.*

cerebellopontine angle s., a s. due most commonly to a lesion in the region between the cerebellum and pons that can affect multiple cranial nerves; may be marked by hearing loss, tinnitus, vertigo, ataxia, or facial weakness.

cerebrohepatorenal s. [MIM*214100, MIM*211410], SYN Zellweger s.

cervical compression s., SYN cervical disk s.

cervical disk s., pain, paresthesias, and sometimes weakness in the area of the distribution of one or more cervical roots, due to pressure of a protruded cervical intervertebral disk. SYN cervical compression s.

cervical fusion s., SYN Klippel-Feil s.

cervical rib s., indefinite term, equally applicable to two different syndromes: 1) arterial thoracic outlet s. in which the subclavian artery is compromised by a fully formed cervical rib, and 2) true neurogenic thoracic outlet s. in which the proximal lower trunk of the brachial plexus is compromised by a translucent band extending from a rudimentary cervical rib to the first rib.

cervical rib and band s., SYN true neurogenic thoracic outlet s.

cervical tension s., SYN posttraumatic neck s.

cervicooculoacoustic s. [MIM*314600], a disorder characterized by a congenitally short neck with fused cervical vertebrae (Klippel-Feil anomaly), sixth cranial nerve paralysis with retraction of the eye globe and narrowing of the palpebral fissure on adduction (Duane palsy), and sensorineural deafness; inheritance is thought to be multifactorial with limitation to females. SYN Wildervanck s.

Cestan-Chenais s., contralateral hemiplegia, hemianesthesia, and loss of pain and temperature sensibility, with ipsilateral hemiasynergia and lateropulsion, paralysis of the larynx and soft palate, enophthalmia, miosis, and ptosis, due to lesions of the brainstem.

chancriform s., an ulcerative lesion at the site of primary infection by microorganisms, with regional lymph node enlargement; it occurs not only in chancroid infections but also in various bacterial and fungal infections.

Chandler s., iris atrophy with corneal edema. SYN iridocorneal syndrome.

Charcot s., SYN intermittent *claudication.*

Charcot-Weiss-Baker s., SYN carotid sinus s.

CHARGE s., SYN CHARGE *association.*

Chauffard s., the symptoms of Still disease in one suffering from bovine or other nonhuman form of tuberculosis. SYN Still-Chauffard s.

Chédiak-Higashi s. [MIM*214500 and MIM*214450], a genetic disorder associated with abnormalities of granulation and nuclear structure of all types of leukocytes and with the presence of peroxidase-positive granules, cytoplasmic inclusions, and Dohle bodies; characterized by hepatosplenomegaly, lymphadenopathy, anemia, neutropenia, partial albinism, nystagmus, photophobia, and susceptibilities to infection and lymphoma; death usually occurs in childhood; occurs in mink, cattle, mice, killer whales, and humans; autosomal recessive inheritance, caused by mutation in the Chediak-Higashi gene (CHS) on chromosome 1q. SYN Béguez César disease, Chédiak-Higashi disease, Chédiak-Steinbrinck-Higashi anomaly, Chédiak-Steinbrinck-Higashi s.

Chédiak-Steinbrinck-Higashi s. [MIM*214500, MIM*214450], SYN Chédiak-Higashi s.

Cheney s., acroosteolysis with osteoporosis and changes in the skull and mandible.

cherry-red spot myoclonus s., a neuronal storage disorder in children characterized by a cherry-red spot at the macula, progressive myoclonus, and easily controlled seizures; the result of sialidase deficiency. Type 1 is characterized by normal body habitus, cherry-red macula, myoclonus, and normal β-galactosidase levels; type 2 by short stature, bony abnormalities, and deficient β-galactosidase. SYN sialidosis.

Chiari s., thrombosis of the hepatic vein with great enlargement of the liver and extensive development of collateral vessels, intractable ascites, and severe portal hypertension. SYN Budd s., Budd-Chiari s., Chiari disease, Chiari-Budd s., Rokitansky disease (2).

Chiari-Budd s., SYN Chiari s.

Chiari-Frommel s., unphysiological lactation and amenorrhea following pregnancy, but not caused by infant's nursing; characterized by hyperprolactinemia and a pituitary adenoma.

Chiari II s., displacement of the medulla and cerebellar tonsils and vermis through the foramen magnum into the upper spinal canal; often associated with other cerebral anomalies.

chiasma s., a s. characterized by a bitemporal visual field defect and optic nerve atrophy due to a lesion in or about the chiasm.

Chilaiditi s., interposition of the colon between the liver and the diaphragm.

CHILD s., *c*ongenital *h*emidysplasia with *i*chthyosiform erythroderma and *l*imb *d*efects.

Chinese restaurant s., development of chest pain, feelings of facial pressure, and sensation of burning over variable portions of the body surface after ingestion of food containing monosodium L-glutamate (MSG) by persons sensitive to this food additive.

Chotzen s. [MIM*101400], SYN Saethre-Chotzen s.

Christian s., SYN Hand-Schüller-Christian *disease.*

chromosomal s., general designation for s.'s due to chromosomal aberrations; typically associated with mental retardation and multiple congenital anomalies.

chromosomal instability s.'s, chromosomal breakage s.'s, a group of mendelian conditions associated with chromosomal instability and breakage in vitro, they often manifest an increased tendency to certain types of malignancies. SEE Bloom s., *xeroderma* pigmentosum.

chronic hyperventilation s., reduced CO_2 content of the blood (hypocapnia) as a result of hyperventilation of prolonged duration; may occur in anxiety states and in some chronic organic, usually cardiovascular, disease; alkalemia, paresthesia, and tetany may occur.

Churg-Strauss s., asthma, fever, eosinophilia, and varied symptoms and signs of vasculitis, primarily affecting small arteries, with vascular and extravascular granulomas. SYN allergic granulomatosis, allergic granulomatous angiitis.

Cianca s., a severe form of infantile esotropia characterized by cross-fixation and tight medial rectus muscles.

Clarke-Hadfield s., SYN cystic *fibrosis.*

classic cervical rib s., SYN true neurogenic thoracic outlet s.

Claude s., midbrain s. with oculomotor palsy on the side of the lesion and incoordination on the opposite side.

click s., a s., particularly of the atrioventricular valves, in which systole causes a sudden tensing of a scallop of a valve or an entire cusp producing the auscultatory click.

climacteric s., SYN menopausal s.

cloverleaf skull s. [MIM*148800], intrauterine bone dysplasia and synostosis of the coronal and lambdoid sutures producing a trilobar head shape, sometimes associated with exophthalmos, and various craniofacial and long-bone anomalies; the condition is sporadic.

Cobb s., cutaneous capillary malformation, usually in a dermatomal distribution on the trunk, associated with vascular abnormality of the spinal cord and resulting neurologic symptoms. SYN cutaneomeningospinal angiomatosis.

Cockayne s. [MIM*216400 and MIM*216411], dwarfism, precociously senile appearance, pigmentary degeneration of the retina, optic atrophy, deafness, sensitivity to sunlight, microcephaly, and mental retardation; autosomal recessive inheritance associated with defective excision repair of DNA. There are various complementation groups. SYN Cockayne disease.

Coffin-Lowry s. [MIM*303600], characterized by coarse facial features with bulbous nose, large ears, and thick lips; short stature; tapered fingers; skeletal anomalies and mental retardation. X-linked recessive inheritance, caused by mutation in the ribosomal S6 kinase gene (RSK) on chromosome Xp.

Coffin-Siris s. [MIM*135900], characterized by mental retardation, bulbous nose, flat nasal bridge, moderate hirsutism, and digital anomalies with absence or hypoplasia of the nail and terminal phalanx of the fifth finger and/or the fifth toe; probably autosomal dominant inheritance. SYN fifth digit s.

Cogan s., SYN oculovestibulo-auditory s.

Cogan-Reese s., SYN iridocorneal endothelial s.

cold agglutinin s., SYN cold hemagglutinin *disease.*

Collet-Sicard s., unilateral lesions of the ninth, tenth, eleventh, and twelfth cranial nerves producing Vernet syndrome and paralysis of the tongue on the same side.

combined immunodeficiency s., a serious primary immunodeficiency affecting both T and B cells.

compartment s., a condition in which increased pressure in a confined anatomical space adversely affects the circulation and threatens the function and viability of the tissues therein.

complete androgen insensitivity s., SYN testicular *feminization.*

compression s., SYN crush s.

congenital rubella s., fetal infection with rubella virus during the first trimester of pregnancy resulting in a series of congenital abnormalities including heart disease, deafness, and blindness.

Conn s., SYN primary *aldosteronism.*

Conradi-Hünermann s., one of the s.'s of chondrodysplasia punctata (q.v.), autosomal dominant, with variable skin keratinization disorders and facial, cardiac, optic, and central nervous system abnormalities; epiphyseal stippling is also present.

Cornelia de Lange s., SYN de Lange s.

corpus luteum deficiency s., functional disturbances caused by insufficient ovarian luteinization; reflected by inadequate luteal phase endometrial response.

Costen s., a symptom complex of loss of hearing, otalgia, tinnitus, dizziness, headache, and burning sensation of the throat, tongue, and side of the nose; originally attributed to temporomandibular joint dysfunction resulting from occlusal disharmony, but currently recognized as not being well founded on anatomic and physiologic principles.

costochondral s., pain in the chest with tenderness over one or more costochondral junctions.

costoclavicular s., one of the forerunners of thoracic outlet s., in which the subclavian artery and vein and, on later reports, the brachial plexus, were thought to be compressed between the clavicle and normal first rib, with the assumption of certain body postures, e.g., the military brace position.

Cotard s., psychotic depression involving delusion of the existence of one's body, along with ideas of negation and suicidal impulses.

Crandall s. [MIM*262000], characterized by pili torti, sensorineural deafness, and hypogonadism; a familial trait in which there is a deficiency of luteinizing and of growth hormone. SEE ALSO Björnstad s.

CREST s., a variant of systemic *sclerosis* characterized by *c*alcinosis, *R*aynaud phenomenon, *e*sophageal motility disorders, *s*clerodactyly, and *t*elangiectasia.

cri-du-chat s., cri du chat s., cat-cry s., a disorder due to deletion of the short arm of chromosome 5, characterized by microcephaly, hypertelorism, antimongoloid palpebral fissures, epicanthal folds, micrognathia, strabismus, mental and physical retardation, and a characteristic high-pitched catlike whine. SYN cat's cry s., Lejeune s.

Crigler-Najjar s. [MIM*218800], a rare defect in ability to form bilirubin glucuronide due to deficiency of bilirubin-glucuronide glucuronosyltransferase; characterized by familial nonhemolytic jaundice and, in its severe form, by irreversible brain damage in infancy that resembles kernicterus and may be fatal; autosomal recessive inheritance, caused by mutation in the uridine diphosphate glycosyltransferase 1 gene (UGT1) on chromosome 1q. There is an autosomal dominant form called Gilbert s., also caused by mutation in the UGT1 gene. SYN Crigler-Najjar disease.

crocodile tears s., a flow of tears, usually unilateral, upon eating or the anticipation of eating; this happens when nerve fibers originally destined for a salivary gland are damaged and regrow, aberrantly, into the lacrimal gland.

Cronkhite-Canada s. [MIM*175500], a sporadically occurring s. of gastrointestinal polyps with diffuse alopecia and nail dystrophy; probably not genetic.

Crouzon s. [MIM*123500], craniosynostosis with broad forehead, ocular hypertelorism, exophthalmos, beaked nose, and hypoplasia of the maxilla; autosomal dominant inheritance, caused by mutation in the fibroblast growth factor receptor 2 gene (FGFR2) on chromosome 10q. Crouzon s. with acanthosis nigricans is due to mutation in the fibroblast growth factor receptor 3 gene (FGFR3) on 4p. SYN craniofacial dysostosis, Crouzon disease.

Crow-Fukase s., SYN POEMS.

crush s., the shocklike state that follows release of a limb or limbs or the trunk and pelvis after a prolonged period of compression, as by a heavy weight; characterized by suppression of renal function, probably the result of damage to the renal tubules by myoglobin from the damaged muscles. SYN compression s.

Cruveilhier-Baumgarten s., cirrhosis of the liver with patent umbilical or paraumbilical veins and varicose periumbilical veins (caput medusae). SYN Cruveilhier-Baumgarten disease.

cryptophthalmus s., SYN Fraser s.

cubital tunnel s., a group of symptoms that develop from compression of the ulnar nerve within the cubital tunnel at the elbow; can include paresthesia into the 4th and 5th digits and weakness of the intrinsic muscles of the hand.

Cushing s., a disorder resulting from increased adrenocortical secretion of cortisol (giving clinical picture of Cushing *disease*), due to any one of several sources: ACTH-dependent adrenocortical hyperplasia or tumor, ectopic ACTH-secreting tumor, or excessive administrations of steroids; characterized by trunkal obesity, moon face, acne, abdominal striae, hypertension, decreased carbohydrate tolerance, protein catabolism, psychiatric disturbances, and osteoporosis, amenorrhea, and hirsutism in females; when associated with an ACTH-producing adenoma, called Cushing disease. SYN Cushing basophilism.

Cushing s. medicamentosus, a variable number of the signs and symptoms of Cushing s.; produced by the chronic administration of large doses of any steroid that is a potent glucocorticoid.

cutaneomucouveal s., SYN Behçet s.

Dandy-Walker s. [MIM*304340], developmental anomaly of the fourth ventricle associated with atresia of the foramina of Luschka and Magendie that results in cerebellar hypoplasia, hydrocephalus, and posterior fossa cyst formation.

dead arm s., sensory diminution or loss in the arm after anterior shoulder dislocation or subluxation.

dead fetus s., s. characterized by lengthy intrauterine retention of a dead fetus usually greater than 4 weeks with development of

sy

hypofibrinogenemia and occasionally disseminated intravascular coagulopathy.

dead-in-bed s., the finding of young, insulin-dependent diabetics without previous illness or abnormal glucose control dead in bed in the morning. Assumed to be due to hypoglycemia but it has been difficult to establish that fact postmortem. Usually occurs in diabetics taking three daily doses of insulin, suggesting inadvertent administration of erroneous dose, with lack of awareness of hypoglycemia during sleep.

Debré-Sémélaigne s., SYN Kocher-Debré-Sémélaigne s.

de Clerambault s., erotomania accompanied by the delusional belief that a certain person is in love with you.

Degos s., SYN malignant atrophic *papulosis.*

Dejerine-Klumpke s., SYN Klumpke *palsy.*

Dejerine-Roussy s., SYN thalamic s.

de Lange s. [MIM 122470], a multiple congenital anomaly s. characterized by mental retardation, distinctive facies with microcephaly, synophrys, low anterior hairline, depressed nasal bridge, anteverted nares, long philtrum, carp mouth, thin upper lip and low-set ears, prenatal and postnatal growth retardation, hirsutism, and frequently, limb anomalies. Genetics unclear, though some instances appear to be autosomal dominantly inherited. SYN Amsterdam s., Cornelia de Lange s.

Del Castillo s., SYN Sertoli-cell-only s.

de Morsier s., SYN septooptic *dysplasia.*

dengue shock s., dengue fever of grade III or IV severity.

Denys-Drash s., s. comprising nephropathy, Wilms tumor, and genital abnormalities.

depersonalization s., SYN depersonalization.

depressive s., SYN depression (4).

dermatitis-arthritis-tenosynovitis s., disseminated infection with *Neisseria gonorrhoeae*, causing skin lesions (often pustular or necrotic), plus synovitis of major joints (such as knee, ankle, elbow) and tendon sheaths.

De Sanctis-Cacchione s. [MIM*278800], xeroderma pigmentosum with mental deficiency, dwarfism, and gonadal hypoplasia; autosomal recessive inheritance associated with defective DNA repair following damage by ultraviolet irradiation.

s. of deviously relevant answers, SYN Ganser s.

dialysis disequilibrium s., nausea, vomiting, and hypertension, occasionally with convulsions, developing within several hours after starting hemodialysis for renal failure; apparently caused by too rapid removal of urea from the extracellular fluid compartment, with movement of water into cells, and cerebral edema.

dialysis encephalopathy s., a progressive, often fatal, diffuse encephalopathy occurring in a few patients on chronic hemodialysis; to be differentiated from the relatively acute, self-limited dialysis disequilibrium s. SYN dialysis dementia.

Diamond-Blackfan s., SYN congenital hypoplastic *anemia.*

diencephalic s. of infancy, profound emaciation after initial normal growth, locomotor hyperactivity and euphoria, usually with skin pallor, hypotension, and hypoglycemia; usually due to neoplasm involving the anterior hypothalamus.

Di Ferrante s. [MIM*253230], associated with a deficiency of *N*-acetylglucosamine 6-sulfatase and urinary excretion of heparan sulfate and keratan sulfate. SYN type VII mucopolysaccharidosis (2).

DiGeorge s. [MIM*188400], a condition arising from developmental failure of the third and fourth pharyngeal pouches, resulting in the absence or underdevelopment of the thymus and parathyroid gland, associated with abnormalities of the outflow tract of the heart, distinctive facies, hypoparathyroidism, hypocalcemia with tetany, and deficiency in T-cell immunity; this is a contiguous gene deletion s. involving chromosome 22q11; autosomal dominant inheritance. SYN congenital aplasia of thymus, immunodeficiency with hypoparathyroidism, pharyngeal pouch s., third and fourth pharyngeal pouch s., thymic hypoplasia.

Di Guglielmo s. [MIM*133180], SYN Di Guglielmo *disease.*

disconnection s., general term for various neurological disorders due to interruption of fiber pathways of the cerebrum.

disk s., a constellation of symptoms and signs, including pain, paresthesias, sensory loss, weakness, and impaired reflexes, due to a compressive radiculopathy caused by intervertebral disk pressure.

disputed neurogenic thoracic outlet s., a highly controversial disorder in which the brachial plexus is reputedly repressed at one or more sites along its course, particularly within the interscalene triangle, and between the normal first thoracic rib and some other structures; frequently attributed to trauma (particularly automobile accidents), and most often diagnosed in young to middle-aged women; no characteristic clinical presentation, although forequarter pain is characteristic; no definite objective findings are present, and no undisputed ancillary diagnostic studies are available.

distal intestinal obstructive s., a s. seen in cystic fibrosis secondary to impaction with feces and inspissated mucus.

Donohue s., SYN leprechaunism.

Doose s., a rare familial type of primary, generalized myoclonic astatic epilepsy characterized by a 2–3- or 4–6-Hz spike and wave complexes in the EEG; the condition usually responds to medication.

Dorfman-Chanarin s. [MIM*275630], congenital ichthyosis, leukocyte vacuoles, and variable involvement of other organ systems. SYN neutral lipid storage disease.

dorsal midbrain s., SYN Parinaud s.

Down s., a chromosomal dysgenesis s. consisting of a variable constellation of abnormalities caused by triplication or translocation of chromosome 21. The abnormalities include mental retardation, retarded growth, flat hypoplastic face with short nose, prominent epicanthic skin folds, small low-set ears with prominent antihelix, fissured and thickened tongue, laxness of joint ligaments, pelvic dysplasia, broad hands and feet, stubby fingers, and transverse palmar crease. Lenticular opacities and heart disease are common. The incidence of leukemia is increased and Alzheimer disease is almost inevitable by age 40. SYN trisomy 21 s.

Down syndrome		
frequency of some bodily symptoms		
order of relative frequency	**feature**	**percentage of cases with feature**
1	retarded development	99%
2	mongoloid face	90%
3	palpebral fissure	86.5%
4	brachycephaly	75%
5	clinodactyly V	50–70%
6	epicanthus	67%
7	open mouth	65%
8	transverse palmar crease	59%
9	gap between 1st and 2nd toes	53%
10	flat, short nose	53%
11	lingua scrotalis	51%
12	Brushfield spots	50%
13	deformity of external ear	50%
14	macroglossia	41%
15	congenital cardiac defects	40–60%
16	muscular hypotonia	31%
17	brachydactyly	29%
18	strabismus	14–23%

Dressler s., recurrent pericarditis following acute myocardial infarction.

dry eye s., SYN *keratoconjunctivitis* sicca.

Duane s., SYN retraction s.

Dubin-Johnson s. [MIM*237500], an inherited defect in hepatic excretory function characterized by jaundice with levels of serum bilirubin up to about 6 mg/dL, over half of which is conjugated, and excretion of abnormal proportions of coproporphyrin I in urine. There is also retention of a dark pigment in the hepatocytes that is derived either from melanin or catecholamines, but otherwise liver histology is normal. Oral cholecystogram fails to visualize the gallbladder, and excretion of test substances (e.g., bromosulfothalein) by the liver is abnormal. The basic defect is apparently in canalicular transport. No therapy is necessary; autosomal recessive inheritance caused by mutation in the canalicular multispecific organic anion transporter gene (CMOAT) on 10q. SYN chronic idiopathic jaundice.

Dubreuil-Chambardel s., simultaneous caries of the upper incisor teeth occurring in either sex between the ages of 14 and 17; after an interval of varying length the other teeth also become involved.

dumping s., the s. that occurs after eating, most often seen in patients with shunts of the upper alimentary canal; characterized by flushing, sweating, dizziness, weakness, and vasomotor collapse, resulting from rapid passage of large amounts of food into the small intestine, with an osmotic effect removing fluid from plasma and causing hypovolemia. SYN early dumping s., postgastrectomy s.

Duncan s., SYN X-linked lymphoproliferative s.

Dyggve-Melchior-Clausen s. [MIM*223800], a skeletal dysplasia that has some clinical resemblance to Morquio s. but without mucopolysacchariduria; characterized by mental retardation, short-trunk dwarfism, progressive sternal bulging, restricted joint mobility, waddling gait, and radiographic findings of irregular iliac crests and flattening of vertebral bodies; autosomal recessive inheritance. There is an X-linked form [MIM*304950].

dysarthria–clumsy hand s., a disorder characterized by dysarthria and a clumsiness of one hand, caused by a lacunar stroke in the basis pontis.

dyskinesia s. [MIM*242650], clearance of mucus is sluggish and bronchiectasis is prevalent and intractable. There is evidence that the defect lies in dynein, a protein in the cilia. The pattern of inheritance is apparently autosomal recessive.

dysmnesic s., SYN Korsakoff s.

dysplastic nevus s., SEE dysplastic *nevus*.

Eagle-Barrett s., SYN prune belly s.

early dumping s., SYN dumping s.

Eaton-Lambert s., SYN Lambert-Eaton s.

ectopic ACTH s., the association of Cushing s. with a nonpituitary neoplasm, usually a lung carcinoma that produces ACTH.

ectrodactyly–ectodermal dysplasia–clefting s., an autosomal recessive disorder resulting in defects of hands and feet; the ectodermal dysplasia causes fair skin, anodontia, and cleft palate.

Edwards s., SYN trisomy 18 s.

egg-white s., dermatitis, loss of hair, and loss of muscle coordination, produced in rats by diets containing large amounts of raw egg white, the avidin of which combines with biotin producing a deficiency of the latter. SYN egg-white injury.

Ehlers-Danlos s. (EDS), a group of connective tissue disorders characterized by hyperelasticity and fragility of the skin, hypermobility of the joints, and fragility of the cutaneous blood vessels and sometimes large arteries due to deficient quality or quantity of collagen; the most common types are inherited as autosomal dominant, caused by mutation in one of the following genes: the collagen V alpha-1 gene (COL5A1) on chromosome 9q or the collagen V alpha-2 gene (COL5A2) on 2q or COL3A1 gene on 2q.

Eisenmenger s., cardiac failure with significant right-to-left shunt producing cyanosis due to higher pressure on the right side of the shunt. Usually due to the Eisenmenger complex, a ventricular septal defect with right ventricular hypertrophy and dilatation, severe pulmonary hypertension, and frequent straddling of the defect by a misplaced aortic root.

Ekbom s., SYN restless legs s.

elfin facies s., SYN Williams s.

Ellis-van Creveld s., SYN chondroectodermal *dysplasia*.

E-M s., SYN eosinophilia-myalgia s.

EMG s., SYN Beckwith-Wiedemann s.

encephalotrigeminal vascular s., angiomatosis of the brain accompanied by nevi in the trigeminal area. SEE ALSO Sturge-Weber s.

eosinophilia-myalgia s., a probable autoimmune disorder precipitated by contaminated L-tryptophan tablets, and characterized by fatigue, low-grade fever, myalgias, muscle tenderness and cramps, weakness, paresthesias of the extremities, and skin indurations; marked eosinophilia is noted on peripheral blood studies, serum aldolase is increased, and biopsies of peripheral nerve, muscle, skin, and fascia show microangiopathy and inflammation in connective tissue. SYN E-M s.

episodic dyscontrol s., SYN intermittent explosive *disorder*.

erythrodysesthesia s., tingling sensation of the palms and soles, progressing to severe pain and tenderness with erythema and edema; caused by continuous infusion therapy.

euthyroid sick s., abnormalities in levels of hormones and function tests related to the thyroid gland occurring in patients with severe systemic disease. Thyroid function is actually normal in these patients, and it is uncertain whether treatment of these abnormalities would be beneficial. SYN sick euthyroid s.

Evans s., acquired hemolytic anemia and thrombocytopenia.

exfoliation s., SYN pseudoexfoliation s.

extrapyramidal s., abnormalities of movement related to injury of motor pathways other than the pyramidal tract.

Faber s., SYN achlorhydric *anemia*.

false memory s., an apparent memory of an imagined event, usually traumatic and remote in time; generally used pejoratively to imply that the memory was engendered by the therapist facilitating its recovery; a controversial concept.

familial aortic ectasia s., the concurrence as an autosomal dominant trait of bicuspid aortic valve often with premature calcification, ectasia, and dissection of the aorta and, rarely, coarctation of the aorta. Superficially resembles the Marfan s. SYN familial aortic ectasia.

familial chylomicronemia s., an inherited disorder resulting in accumulation of chylomicrons as well as triacylglycerols. SEE ALSO chylomicronemia.

Fanconi s. [MIM*227650–227660], **(1)** SYN Fanconi *anemia*; **(2)** a group of conditions with characteristic disorders of renal tubular function, which may be classified as: 1) cystinosis, an autosomal recessive disease of early childhood; 2) adult Fanconi s., a rare hereditary form, probably due to a recessive gene different from that found in cystinosis, characterized by the tubular malfunction seen in cystinosis and by osteomalacia, but without cystine deposit in tissues; 3) acquired Fanconi s., which may be associated with multiple myeloma or may result from chemical poisoning, injury, or persisting damage of proximal tubular epithelium due to various causes, leading to multiple defects of tubular function.

FAPA s., a syndrome of unknown etiology that causes periodic bouts of *f*ever, *a*denitis, *p*haryngitis, and *a*phthous ulcers.

Farber s. [MIM*228000], SYN disseminated *lipogranulomatosis*.

Favre-Racouchot s., SYN Favre-Racouchot *disease*.

Felty s., rheumatoid arthritis with splenomegaly and leukopenia.

fetal alcohol s., a pattern of malformation with growth deficiency, craniofacial anomalies, and functional deficits including mental retardation found among offspring of mothers who abuse alcohol.

fetal aspiration s., a s. resulting from uterine aspiration of amniotic fluid and meconium by the fetus, usually caused by hypoxia and often leading to aspiration pneumonia. SYN meconium aspiration s.

fetal face s., a s. of facies resembling an early fetus with short forearms, and genital hypoplasia at birth, but without evidence of achondroplasia; leads to dwarfism without mental retardation.

fetal hydantoin s., a s. resulting from maternal ingestion of hydantoin analog (e.g., phenytoin), characterized by growth deficiency, mental deficiency, dysmorphic facies, cleft palate and/or lip, cardiac defects, and abnormal genitalia.

fetal trimethadione s., a s. resulting from maternal ingestion of trimethadione during the early weeks of pregnancy and characterized by developmental delay, V-shaped eyebrows, epicanthus,

sy

low-set ears with anteriorly folded helix, palatal anomaly, and irregular teeth.

fetal warfarin s., fetal bleeding, nasal hypoplasia, optic atrophy, and death resulting from ingestion of warfarin by the pregnant patient.

fibrinogen-fibrin conversion s., a s. characterized by hypofibrinogenemia with incoagulable blood; it may be seen in abruptio placentae, prolonged retention of a dead fetus in an Rh-isosensitized mother, hemolytic blood reactions, bilateral renal cortical necrosis, and cases of trauma.

fibromyalgia s., SYN fibromyalgia.

Fiessinger-Leroy-Reiter s., SYN Reiter s.

fifth digit s., SYN Coffin-Siris s.

first arch s., generic term including s.'s of malformations involving derivatives of the first branchial arch, with or without associated malformations; includes mandibulofacial dysostosis, micrognathia with peromelia, otomandibular dystosis, acrofacial dysostosis, and others.

Fisher s., a s. characterized by ophthalmoplegia, ataxia, and areflexia; a form of polyneuroradiculitis.

Fitz-Hugh and Curtis s., perihepatitis in women with a history of gonococcal or chlamydial salpingitis.

flashing pain s. [MIM*190400], sudden, intermittent, and severe brief episodes of pain, without apparent cause, in the distribution of a spinal dermatome; resembles in character the pain of tic douloureux. Cf. *tic* douloureux.

flecked retina s. [MIM*228980], hereditary retinal disorder with abnormal transmission of fluorescence through the retinal pigment epithelium on angiography.

floppy valve s., retrograde slippage of degenerating mitral or tricuspid valve leaflets into the valve's orifice beyond the point of closure during systole of the left ventricle; a feature of Barlow s.

Flynn-Aird s. [MIM*136300], a familial s. characterized by muscle wasting, ataxia, dementia, skin atrophy, dental caries, joint stiffness, retinitis pigmentosa, and progressive sensorineural hearing loss; autosomal dominant inheritance.

Foix-Alajouanine s., thrombophlebitis of spinal veins resulting in a subacute ascending painful flaccid paralysis from necrotic myelitis.

Foix-Cavany-Marie s., constellation of faciopharyngoglossomasticatory diplegia with automatic voluntary dissociation without associated dementia or forced laughing or crying usually caused by bilateral large artery infarcts of the opercular cortex.

folded-lung s., SYN rounded *atelectasis.*

Forbes-Albright s., pituitary tumor in a patient without acromegaly, which secretes excessive amounts of prolactin (LTH) and produces persistent lactation.

Foster Kennedy s., SYN Kennedy s.

Foville s., a form of alternating hemiplegia characterized by abducens paralysis on one side, paralysis of the extremities on the other.

fragile X s., an X-linked recessive s. [MIM*309550] consisting of mental retardation, a characteristic facies, and macroorchidism; DNA analysis shows abnormal trinucleotide repeats on the X chromosome near the end of its long arm, at Xq27.3; a constriction is demonstrable at this site on karyotyping after culture in folate-deficient medium. SYN FMR1, marker X s., Martin-Bell s.

> The incidence of fragile X syndrome (about 1:2000 in males) is second only to that of Down syndrome among genetically identifiable sources of mental retardation. Phenotypic expression is variable, but mental retardation is the most commonly observed feature. The face is long and narrow, with large ears, a prominent mandibular symphysis, and a high-arched palate. Absolute or relative macrocephaly is common. Macroorchidism appears at puberty or before; histologic study shows only edema of the testis. Connective tissue abnormality may be manifested by hypermobility of fingers and other joints, pes planus, dilation of the aorta, and mitral valve prolapse. Besides intellectual impairment, neuropsychiatric findings include hyperactivity, short attention span, poor eye contact, autistic-like be-

havior, jocular speech, echolalia, and motor incoordination. The IQ may deteriorate with advancing age. A few males with this genetic defect, and about two-thirds of females, are phenotypically normal. Expression depends on a mutation that occurs in two or more steps and that is both meiotically and mitotically unstable. Transmission is complex and varies with the gender of both the proband and the transmitting parent. The fragile chromosomal locus represents a site of abnormal amplification with a variable number of CGG repeats. These block transcription of the FMR1 (familial mental retardation) gene, which normally encodes FMR1 protein; clinical expression is due to failure to synthesize FMR1 protein and to abnormal methylation of DNA sequences distal to the fragile site.

Fraley s., dilation of the upper pole renal calices due to stenosis of the upper infundibulum, usually caused by compression from vessels supplying the upper and middle segments of the kidney.

Franceschetti s., mandibulofacial *dysostosis,* when complete or nearly complete.

Franceschetti-Jadassohn s., SYN Naegeli s.

Fraser s. [MIM*219000], an association of cryptophthalmus with multiple anomalies, including middle and outer ear malformations, cleft palate, laryngeal deformity, displacement of umbilicus and nipples, digital malformations, separation of symphysis pubis, maldevelopment of kidneys, and masculinization of genitalia in females; autosomal recessive inheritance. SYN cryptophthalmus s.

Freeman-Sheldon s., SYN craniocarpotarsal *dystrophy.*

Frey s., SYN auriculotemporal nerve s.

Friderichsen-Waterhouse s., SYN Waterhouse-Friderichsen s.

Fröhlich s., SYN adiposogenital *dystrophy.*

Froin s., an alteration in the cerebrospinal fluid, which is yellowish and coagulates spontaneously in a few seconds after withdrawal, owing to its greatly increased protein (albumin and globulin) content; noted in loculated portions of the subarachnoid space isolated from spinal fluid circulation by an inflammatory or neoplastic obstruction. SYN loculation s.

Fuchs s. [MIM*136800], a s. characterized by corneal degeneration, heterochromia of the iris, iridocyclitis, keratic precipitates, and cataract; probably autosomal dominant inheritance. SYN Fuchs heterochromic cyclitis.

functional prepubertal castration s., a s. characterized by the absence of testes from the scrotum but in their place mesonephric duct derivatives, pronounced gynecomastia and eunuchoid habitus, and increased plasma levels and urinary excretion of gonadotrophins.

G s. [MIM*145410], a s. of characteristic facies associated with hypospadias, ventral curvature of the penis, and dysphagia. Apparently the same as the BBB syndrome of Opritz et al. Autosomal dominant inheritance. [first letter of surname of affected person reported]

Gaisböck s., SYN *polycythemia* hypertonica.

Ganser s., a psychoticlike condition, without the symptoms and signs of a traditional psychosis, occurring typically in prisoners who feign insanity; e.g., such a person, when asked to multiply 6 by 4, will give 23 as the answer, or will call a key a lock. SEE malingering, factitious *disorder.* SYN nonsense s., s. of approximate relevant answers, s. of deviously relevant answers.

Gardner s. [MIM*175100-0006], multiple polyposis predisposing to carcinoma of the colon; also multiple tumors, osteomas of the skull, epidermoid cysts, and fibromas; autosomal dominant inheritance, caused by mutation in the adenomatous polyposis coli gene (APC) on chromosome 5q. This disorder is allelic to familial adenomatous *polyposis* (FAP).

Gardner-Diamond s., SYN autoerythrocyte sensitization s.

gastrocardiac s., disturbances of the heart's action due to faulty action of the digestive system, especially of the stomach.

gastrojejunal loop obstruction s., SYN afferent loop s.

gay bowel s., gastrointestinal discomfort experienced by homosexual males; includes abdominal pain, cramps, bloating, flatulence, nausea, vomiting, or diarrhea caused by enteric bacteria, viruses, fungi, zooparasites, or trauma.

Gélineau s., SYN narcolepsy.

gender dysphoria s., a s. in which an individual experiences marked personal stress due to feelings that despite having the genitalia and secondary sexual characteristics of one gender there is a sense of compatibility and greater belonging to the other gender class; one may undergo surgery to reconstruct anatomy to that of the other gender.

general adaptation s., a s. introduced by Hans Selye to describe marked physiological changes in various organ systems of the body, especially the pituitary-endocrine system, as a result of exposure to prolonged physical or psychological stress, with the bodily changes progressing through three stages that the author described as the alarm reaction, resistance, and finally exhaustion.

Gerstmann s., finger agnosia, agraphia, confusion of laterality of body, and acalculia; caused by lesions between the occipital area and the angular gyrus.

Gerstmann-Sträussler-Scheinker s., a chronic cerebellar form of spongiform encephalopathy.

Gianotti-Crosti s., a cutaneous manifestation of hepatitis B infection occurring in young children; an exanthem comprising non-pruritic dusky papules on the legs, buttocks, and extensors of the arms; Gianotti-Crosti s. lasts 2–8 weeks and is associated with adenopathy, anicteric hepatomegaly, and malaise. SYN papular acrodermatitis of childhood.

Gilbert s., SYN familial nonhemolytic *jaundice*.

Gilles de la Tourette s. [MIM*137580], SYN Tourette s.

Gillespie s., s. of congenital absence of the iris, mental retardation, and cerebellar ataxia; etiology unknown.

Gitelman s., a disorder seen in older children and young adults characterized by hypokalemia, hypomagnesemia, hypocalciuria, and sometimes tetany.

glucagonoma s., necrolytic migratory erythema or intertriginous and periorofacial dermatitis, stomatitis, anemia, weight loss, and hyperglycemia resulting from glucagon-secreting pancreatic islet cell tumors.

Goldenhar s. [MIM*257700], SYN oculoauriculovertebral *dysplasia*.

Goldmann-Favre s., an autosomal recessive, progressive vitreo-tapetoretinal degeneration.

gold-myokymia s., the symptom complex of widespread myokymia, muscle aching, and autonomic disturbances (excess sweating, orthostatic hypotension) that can result from gold therapy.

Goltz s., SYN focal dermal *hypoplasia*.

Goodpasture s. [MIM*233450], glomerulonephritis of the anti-basement membrane type associated with or preceded by hemoptysis; the nephritis usually progresses rapidly to produce death from renal failure, and the lungs at autopsy show extensive hemosiderosis or recent hemorrhage.

Gopalan s., severe discomfort of the feet associated with elevated skin temperature and excessive sweating.

Gorham s., SYN disappearing bone *disease*.

Gorlin s., SYN basal cell nevus s.

Gorlin-Chaudhry-Moss s. [MIM*233500], craniofacial dysostosis, patent ductus arteriosus, hypertrichosis, hypoplasia of labia majora, and dental and ocular abnormalities. SEE ALSO Weill-Marchesani s.

Gougerot-Carteaud s., SYN confluent and reticulate *papillomatosis*.

Gowers s., s. consisting of palpitation, chest pain, respiratory difficulties, and disturbances in gastric motility; once attributed to vagal stimulation, now considered psychogenic (anxiety neurosis). SYN vagal attack, vasovagal attack, vasovagal s.

gracilis s., osteonecrosis of the pubic bone following trauma.

Gradenigo s., a s. consisting of otorrhea, headache, diplopia, and retroorbital pain in petrositis due to an epidural abscess at the apex of the anterior surface of the petrous pyramid causing compression of the abducens nerve in Dorello canal and irritation of the trigeminal ganglion.

gray s., gray baby s., gray appearance of an infant at birth and during the neonatal period which can be caused by transplacental

toxic effects of the drug chloramphenicol taken by the mother during late pregnancy; the s. may be fatal.

Greig s., SYN ocular *hypertelorism*.

Greig cephalopolysyndactyly s. [MIM*175700], an autosomal dominant disorder characterized by polysyndactyly of the hands and feet, macrocephaly, frontal bossing, hypertelorism, and flat nasal bridge, caused by mutation in the GLI3 gene on chromosome 7p13.

Grönblad-Strandberg s., angioid streaks of the retina together with pseudoxanthoma elasticum of the skin.

Gubler s., a form of alternating hemiplegia characterized by contralateral hemiplegia and ipsilateral facial paralysis. SYN Gubler paralysis, Millard-Gubler s.

Guillain-Barré s., an acute, immune-mediated disorder of peripheral nerves, spinal roots, and cranial nerves, commonly presenting as a rapidly progressive, areflexive, relatively symmetric ascending weakness of the limb, truncal, respiratory, pharyngeal, and facial musculature, with variable sensory and autonomic dysfunction; typically reaches its nadir within 2–3 weeks, followed initially by a plateau period of similar duration, and then subsequently by gradual but complete recovery in the majority of cases. Guillain-Barré s. is often preceded by a respiratory or gastrointestinal infection and is associated with albuminocytologic dissociation of the cerebral spinal fluid. Although classically considered pathologically to be an acute, inflammatory demyelinating polyradiculoneuropathy (q.v.), pure axon degeneration forms recently have been recognized. SYN acute idiopathic polyneuritis, acute inflammatory polyneuropathy, infectious polyneuritis, Landry paralysis, Landry s., Landry-Guillain-Barré s., myeloradiculopolyneuritis, postinfectious polyneuritis.

Gulf War s., a term often but inappropriately applied to various health problems experienced by U.S. military personnel after serving in the Persian Gulf conflict of 1991; symptoms of fatigue, musculoskeletal pain, headaches, dyspnea, memory loss, and diarrhea have been reported, but an NIH panel has concluded that evidence of a specific disease is lacking. SYN Persian Gulf s.

Gunn s., SYN jaw-winking s.

gustatory sweating s., SYN auriculotemporal nerve s.

Guyon tunnel s., entrapment or compression of the ulnar nerve within Guyon canal as the ulnar nerve passes into the wrist.

Haber s., a permanent flushing and telangiectasia of the cheeks, nose, forehead, and chin, with prominent follicular openings, small papules with scaling, and minute pitted areas; occasionally accompanied by scaly and keratotic lesions of the trunk.

HAIR-AN s., hyperandrogenism, insulin resistance, and *acanthosis* nigricans; virilization in pubertal girls associated with markedly elevated insulin levels and normal levels of luteinizing *hormone* and follicle-stimulating *hormone*. [hyperandrogenism, insulin resistance, *a*canthosis *n*igricans]

Hallermann-Streiff s., SYN *dyscephalia* mandibulo-oculofacialis.

Hallermann-Streiff-François s., SYN *dyscephalia* mandibulo-oculofacialis.

Hallervorden s., SYN Hallervorden-Spatz s.

Hallervorden-Spatz s., a disorder characterized by dystonia with other extrapyramidal dysfunctions appearing in the first two decades of life; associated with large amounts of iron in the globus pallidus and substantia nigra. SYN Hallervorden s., Hallervorden-Spatz disease, status dysmyelinisatus.

Hallgren s., vestibulocerebellar ataxia, pigmentary retinal dystrophy, congenital deafness, and cataract.

Hamman s., spontaneous mediastinal emphysema, resulting from rupture of alveoli. SYN Hamman disease.

Hamman-Rich s., SYN idiopathic pulmonary *fibrosis*.

hand-and-foot s., recurrent painful swelling of the hands and feet occurring in infants and young children with sickle cell anemia. SYN sickle cell dactylitis.

hand-foot s., a painful desquamative s. associated with 5-fluorouracil, especially if given in a continuous administration and with cytarabine.

Hanhart s., SYN *micrognathia* with peromelia.

hantavirus pulmonary s., a febrile disease caused by several species of Hantavirus (Andes, Bayou, Black Creek Canal, New

York, and Sin Nombre viruses) in North and South America and characterized by thrombocytopenia, leukocytosis, and capillary leakage in the lungs, with death due to shock and cardiac complications.

happy puppet s. [MIM*234400], a s. characterized by mental retardation, ataxia, hypotonia, epileptic seizures, easily provoked and prolonged spasms of laughter, prognathism, and an open-mouthed expression.

Harada s., bilateral retinal edema, uveitis, choroiditis, and retinal detachment, with temporary or permanent deafness, graying of the hair (poliosis), and alopecia; related to the Vogt-Koyanagi s. and sympathetic ophthalmia. SYN Harada disease, uveoencephalitis, uveomeningitis s.

Harris s., excessive insulin production with hypoglycemia, hunger, jitteriness, tachycardia, and flushing occurring in conditions such as functional disorders of the pancreas, hyperplasia of the islets of Langerhans, or insulinoma.

Hartnup s., SYN Hartnup *disease.*

Hayem-Widal s., obsolete term for acquired hemolytic *icterus.* SYN Widal s.

head-bobbing doll s., bobbing motion of the head usually due to cysts in or about the third ventricle.

Hegglin s., dissociation between electromechanical systole (QSII interval) and electrical systole (QT interval) so that the second heart tone (SII) is recorded before the end of the T wave; described by Hegglin as an energy-dynamic cardiac insufficiency during diabetic coma and other metabolic disorders.

HELLP s., type of severe preeclampsia involving *h*emolysis, *e*levated *l*iver function, and *l*ow *p*latelets.

Helweg-Larssen s. [MIM*125050], an autosomal dominant disorder characterized by anhidrotic ectodermal dysplasia and hearing loss, the latter developing in the fourth or fifth decade.

hemolytic uremic s., hemolytic anemia and thrombocytopenia occurring with acute renal failure; in children, characterized by sudden onset of gastrointestinal bleeding, hematuria, oliguria, and microangiopathic hemolytic anemia; in adults, associated with complications of pregnancy following normal delivery, or associated with oral contraceptive use or with infection; often caused by infection with *Escherichia coli.*

Henoch-Schönlein s., SYN Henoch-Schönlein *purpura.*

hepatorenal s., hepatonephric s., the occurrence of acute renal failure in patients with disease of the liver or biliary tract, apparently due to decreased renal blood flow and conditions that damage both organs, such as carbon tetrachloride poisoning and leptospirosis.

Herlitz s., SYN *epidermolysis* bullosa lethalis.

Hermansky-Pudlak s., a form of oculocutaneous albinism (autosomal recessive) with accumulation of ceroid in lysosomes with restrictive lung disease, granulomatous colitis, kidney failure, cardiomyopathy, and storage pool-deficient platelets. SEE oculocutaneous *albinism.*

heroin overdose s., SYN opiate intoxication s.

Herrmann s. [MIM*172500], a multisystem disorder beginning in late childhood or early adolescence, with photomyoclonus and hearing loss followed by diabetes mellitus, progressive dementia, pyelonephritis, and glomerulonephritis; progressive sensorineural hearing loss is of later onset; probably autosomal dominant inheritance with incomplete penetrance.

Hinman s., SYN nonneurogenic neurogenic *bladder.*

HIV wasting s., SYN wasting s. (2).

holiday s., regression, development of diffuse anxiety, feelings of helplessness, irritability, and depression; said to occur in certain psychoanalytic patients before Thanksgiving and continuing into the Christmas holiday season, ending a few days after January 1.

holiday heart s., arrhythmias of the heart, sometimes apparent after a vacation or weekend away from work, following excessive alcohol consumption; usually transient.

Holmes-Adie s., SYN Adie s.

Holt-Oram s. [MIM*142900], atrial septal defect in association with finger-like or absent thumb and other deformities of the forearm; autosomal dominant inheritance, caused by mutation in the T-box5 gene (TBX5) on chromosome 12q.

Horner s., ptosis, miosis, and anhidrosis on the side of asympathetic palsy. The enophthalmos is more apparent than real. The affected pupil is visibly slow to dilate in dim light; due to a lesion of the cervical sympathetic chain or its central pathways. SYN Bernard-Horner s., ptosis sympathetica.

Houssay s., the amelioration of diabetes mellitus by a destructive lesion in, or surgical removal of, the pituitary gland.

Houston-Harris s., SYN Type IA *achondrogenesis.*

Hughes-Stovin s., s. characterized by aneurysms of the large and small pulmonary arteries and thrombosis of peripheral veins and dural sinuses.

Hunt s. [MIM*159700], (1) an intention tremor beginning in one extremity, gradually increasing in intensity, and subsequently involving other parts of the body; SYN progressive cerebellar tremor. (2) facial paralysis, otalgia, and herpes zoster resulting from viral infection of the seventh cranial nerve and geniculate ganglion; (3) a form of juvenile paralysis agitans associated with primary atrophy of the pallidal system. SYN paleostriatal s., pallidal s. SYN Ramsay Hunt s. (1).

Hunter s. [MIM*309900], an error of mucopolysaccharide metabolism characterized by deficiency of iduronate sulfatase, with excretion of dermatan sulfate and heparan sulfate in the urine; clinically similar to Hurler s. but distinguished by less severe skeletal changes, no corneal clouding, and X-linked recessive inheritance; caused by mutation in the iduronate sulfatase gene (IDS) on chromosome Xq. SYN type II mucopolysaccharidosis.

Hurler s. [MIM*252800], mucopolysaccharidosis in which there is a deficiency of α-L-iduronidase, an accumulation of an abnormal intracellular material, and excretion of dermatan sulfate and heparan sulfate in the urine; with severe abnormality in development of skeletal cartilage and bone, with dwarfism, kyphosis, deformed limbs, limitation of joint motion, spadelike hand, corneal clouding, hepatosplenomegaly, mental retardation, and gargoyle-like facies; autosomal recessive inheritance, caused by mutation in the alpha-L-iduronidase gene (IDUA) on 4p. SEE ALSO mucolipidosis. SYN Hurler disease, lipochondrodystrophy, Pfaundler-Hurler s., type IH mucopolysaccharidosis.

Hurler-Scheie s., a phenotypic intermediate between Hurler s. and Scheie s.; a deficiency of α-L-iduronidase. SYN type I H/S mucopolysaccharidosis.

Hutchinson-Gilford s., SYN progeria.

Hutchison s., adrenal neuroblastoma of infants with metastasis to the orbit; at one time erroneously believed to arise predominantly from the left adrenal gland. SEE ALSO Pepper s.

hyaline membrane s., SYN hyaline membrane *disease* of the newborn.

hydralazine s., SYN drug-induced *lupus.*

17-hydroxylase deficiency s. [MIM*202110], congenital deficiency of adrenocortical, and possibly ovarian, steroid C-17α-hydroxylase; the resulting excessive secretion of corticosterone and deoxycorticosterone produces amenorrhea, ambiguous genitalia, hypertension, and hypokalemic alkalosis; autosomal recessive inheritance caused by mutation in one of the cytochrome P450 genes (CYP17) on chromosome 10q.

hyperabduction s., (1) diminution or loss of distal upper extremity pulses on hyperabduction of the limb; (2) one of the forerunners of thoracic outlet s., in which the subclavian or axillary artery in the brachial plexus was thought to be compressed, either in the costoclavicular space or beneath the pectoralis minor tendon, during hyperabduction of the limb. SYN subcoracoid-pectoralis minor tendon s., Wright s.

hyperactive child s., SYN attention deficit hyperactivity *disorder.*

hypereosinophilic s., persistent peripheral eosinophilia with eosinophilic infiltration into bone marrow, heart, and other organ systems; accompanied by nocturnal sweating, coughing, anorexia and weight loss, itching and various skin lesions, and symptoms of Löffler endocarditis.

hyper-IgM s., an X-linked immunodeficiency disorder with very low serum concentrations of IgG and IgA with a normal or a markedly elevated concentration of polyclonal IgM; affected boys develop recurrent bacterial infections in the 1st or 2nd year of life.

hyperimmunoglobulin E s., an immunodeficiency disorder characterized by high levels of plasma IgE concentrations, a leukocyte chemotactic defect, and recurrent staphylococcal infections of the skin, upper respiratory tract, and other sites. SYN Job s.

hyperkinetic s., a condition marked by pathologically excessive energy seen sometimes in young children with brain injury, mental illness, and attention deficit disorder, and in epileptics; hypermotility and emotional instability are the chief characteristics; distractibility, inattention, and lack of shyness and of fear are common accompaniments.

hyperkinetic heart s., loosely, a syndrome in which the heart appears to be "overworking", i.e., beating excessively fast and/or causing subjective awareness of continual cardiac activity.

hyperornithinemia-hyperammonemia-hypercitrullinuria s., a rare inherited disorder in which there is impaired ornithine transport into the mitochondria. SEE ALSO lysinuric protein *intolerance.*

hypersensitive xiphoid s., abnormal tenderness of the xiphoid, often associated with spontaneous pains in the chest, upper abdomen, and shoulders.

hyperventilation s., SEE chronic hyperventilation s.

hyperviscosity s., a s. resulting from increased viscosity of the blood; an increase in serum proteins may be associated with bleeding from mucous membranes, retinopathy, and neurological symptoms, and is sometimes seen in Waldenström macroglobulinemia and in multiple myeloma; an increased viscosity secondary to polycythemia may be associated with organ congestion and decreased capillary perfusion.

hypometabolic s., a clinical situation suggesting hypothyroidism or myxedema, in which some tests of thyroid function may be normal and the gland is not obviously atrophic or diseased; indicative of a lack of sensitivity of peripheral tissues to thyroid hormone.

hypoparathyroidism s., a s. characterized by fatigue, muscular weakness, paresthesia and cramps of the extremities, tetany, and laryngeal stridor; due to hypocalcemia resulting from a lack of parathyroid hormone; may be idiopathic, postoperative, or caused by organic lesions of the parathyroids.

hypophysial s., SYN adiposogenital *dystrophy.*

hypophysiosphenoidal s., neoplastic invasion of the base of the skull in the region of the sphenoidal sinus, often with destruction of the dorsum sellae.

hypoplastic left heart s. [MIM*241550], association of underdevelopment of the left heart chambers with atresia or stenosis of the aortic and/or mitral valve and hypoplasia of the ascending aorta.

iliotibial band s., a s. of knee pain that may result from inflammation due to mechanical friction of the iliotibial band and the lateral femoral epicondyle.

iliotibial band friction s., a painful condition affecting the hip, thigh, or knee; produced by irritation of the iliotibial tract as it glides over the greater trochanter, anterior superior iliac spine, Gerdy tubercle, or the lateral femoral condyle; sometimes associated with a snapping or grating sensation.

Imerslünd-Grasbeck s., enterocyte cobalamin malabsorption.

immotile cilia s. [MIM*242650], an inherited disorder characterized by recurrent sinopulmonary infections, reduced fertility in women, and sterility in men due to the inability of ciliated structures to beat effectively because of the absence of one or both dynein arms; autosomal recessive inheritance. Cf. Kartagener s.

immunodeficiency s., an immunologic deficiency or disorder, of which the chief symptom is an increased susceptibility to infection, the pattern of susceptibility being dependent upon the kind of deficiency. SEE ALSO immunodeficiency.

impingement s., SYN supraspinatus s.

s. of inappropriate secretion of antidiuretic hormone (SIADH), continued secretion of antidiuretic hormone despite low serum osmolality and expanded extracellular volume.

indifference to pain s., congenital insensitivity to pain, possibly due to an absence of organized nerve endings in the skin.

infertile male s., an inherited disorder of the androgen receptor protein resulting in defective androgen activity. SEE ALSO Reifenstein s.

inspissated bile s., persistent jaundice in newborns with hemolytic anemia, with elevations of both direct and indirect bilirubin.

internal capsule s., hemianopsia with contralateral hemianesthesia of the face.

inversed jaw-winking s., when there are supranuclear lesions of the trigeminal nerve, touching the cornea may produce a brisk movement of the mandible to the opposite side.

iridocorneal endothelial s., s. of glaucoma, iris atrophy, decreased corneal endothelium, anterior peripheral synechia, and multiple iris nodules. SYN Cogan-Reese s., iris-nevus s.

iridocorneal syndrome, SYN Chandler s.

iris-nevus s., SYN iridocorneal endothelial s.

Irvine-Gass s., macular edema, aphakia, and vitreous humor adherent to incision for cataract extraction.

Isaac s., a rare disorder resulting from abnormal, spontaneous muscle activity of neural origin, manifested as continuous muscle stiffness and delayed relaxation after exercise, often accompanied by pain, cramps, fasciculations, hyperhydrosis, and muscle hypertrophy (on EMG, manifests as myokymia). Isacc s. usually begins in the lower extremities but can affect abdominal, upper extremity, vocal, and respiratory muscles; it is most often sporadic, although autosomal dominant inheritance has been reported. Probably an autoimmune disease, with antibodies against the potassium channels of peripheral nerves. SYN Isaac-Merton s.

Isaac-Merton s., SYN Isaac s.

Ivemark s. [MIM*208530], SYN polysplenia.

Jadassohn-Lewandowski s., SYN pachyonychia congenita.

Jahnke s., sturge-Weber s. without glaucoma.

jaw-winking s. [MIM*154600], an increase in the width of the palpebral fissures during chewing, sometimes with a rhythmic elevation of the upper lid when the mouth is open and ptosis when the mouth is closed. SYN Gunn phenomenon, Gunn s., jaw-winking phenomenon, jaw-working reflex, Marcus Gunn phenomenon, Marcus Gunn s.

Jeghers-Peutz s., SYN Peutz-Jeghers s.

Jervell and Lange-Nielsen s. [MIM*220440 and MIM*176261], a prolonged Q-T interval recorded in the electrocardiogram of certain congenitally deaf children subject to attacks of unconsciousness resulting from Adams-Stokes seizures and ventricular fibrillation; autosomal recessive inheritance, caused by homozygosity for a mutation in the potassium channel gene (KVLQT1) on chromosome 11 or minimal potassium ion channel gene (KCNE1) on 21. SYN surdocardiac s.

Jeune s., SYN asphyxiating thoracic dystrophy.

Job s., SYN hyperimmunoglobulin E s. [Job, biblical char.]

Johanson-Blizzard s., a clinical s. manifested by pancreatic insufficiency, scalp defects, aplasia of the alae nasi, deafness, low birthweight, microcephaly, psychomotor delay, hypothyroidism, dwarfism, and missing permanent teeth.

Joubert s. [MIM*213300], agenesis of the cerebellar vermis, characterized clinically by attacks of tachypnea or prolonged apnea, abnormal eye movements, ataxia, and mental retardation.

jugular foramen s., SYN Avellis s.

Kallmann s., SYN hypogonadism with anosmia.

Kanner s., SYN infantile autism.

Kartagener s. [MIM*244400], complete situs inversus associated with bronchiectasis and chronic sinusitis associated with ciliary dysmotility and impaired ciliary mucous transport in the respiratory epithelium; autosomal recessive inheritance with variable penetrance. The mechanism of the reversal of laterality remains an enigma, but it appears to be strictly an abolition (indifference) of laterality rather than a true reversal. SEE ALSO immotile cilia s. SYN Kartagener triad, Zivert s.

Kasabach-Merritt s., in which platelets become trapped; associated with thrombocytopenic purpura.

Kast s., SYN Maffucci s.

Katayama s., SYN schistosomiasis japonica.

Kawasaki s., SYN Kawasaki disease.

Kearns-Sayre s. [MIM*165100], a form of chronic progressive external ophthalmoplegia with associated cardiac conduction defects, short stature, and hearing loss; a sporadically occurring mitochondrial myopathy presenting in childhood.

Kennedy s., ipsilateral optic atrophy with central scotoma and

sy

contralateral choked disk or papilledema, caused by a meningioma of the ipsilateral optic nerve. SYN Foster Kennedy s.

Kenny-Caffey s., a disorder characterized by intermittent hypocalcemia (associated with abnormalities in parathyroid hormone secretion) and bone and eye abnormalities; autosomal dominant and autosomal recessive forms exist.

Kimmelstiel-Wilson s., nephrotic syndrome and hypertension in diabetics, associated with diabetic glomerulosclerosis. SYN Kimmelstiel-Wilson disease.

Kleine-Levin s. [MIM*148840], a rare form of periodic hypersomnia associated with bulimia, occurring in males aged 10–25 years, characterized by periods of ravenous appetite alternating with prolonged sleep (as long as 18 hours), along with behavioral disturbances, impaired thought processes, and hallucinations; acute illness or fatigue may precede an episode, which may occur as often as several times a year.

Klinefelter s., a chromosomal anomaly with chromosome count 47, XXY sex chromosome constitution; buccal and other cells are usually sex chromatin positive; patients are male in development but have seminiferous tubule dysgenesis, elevated plasma and urinary gonadotropins, variable gynecomastia, and eunuchoid habitus; some patients are chromosomal mosaics, with two or more cell lines of different chromosome constitution; the male tortoise-shell cat (calico cat) is an animal model. SYN XXY s.

Klippel-Feil s. [MIM*148900], a congenital defect manifested as a short neck, fusion of cervical vertebrae, and abnormalities of the brainstem and cerebellum; autosomal dominant inheritance, with most cases sporadic. SYN cervical fusion s.

Klippel-Trenaunay-Weber s. [MIM*149000], an anomaly of the extremity in which there is a combination of angiomatosis and anomalous development of the underlying bone and muscle, sometimes associated with localized gigantism; probably autosomal dominant inheritance, with most cases sporadic. SYN angioosteohypertrophy s., congenital dysplastic angiectasia, hemangiectatic hypertrophy.

Klüver-Bucy s., a s. characterized by psychic blindness or hyperreactivity to visual stimuli, increased oral and sexual activity, and depressed drive and emotional reactions; reported in monkeys after bilateral temporal lobe ablation, but rarely reported in humans.

Kniest s. [MIM*156550 and MIM*120140], a chondrodysplasia characterized by round flat facies, enlargement and stiffness of joints, joint contractures, scoliosis, myopia with retinal detachment, cleft palate, deafness, and characteristic radiographic findings of metaphyseal flaring of long bones, flattening, and coronal clefting of vertebrae; autosomal dominant inheritance, caused by mutation in the type II collagen gene (COL2A1) on chromosome 12q.

Kobberling-Dunnigan s., SYN familial partial *lipodystrophy*.

Kocher-Debré-Sémélaigne s., autosomal recessive inherited athyrotic cretinism associated with muscular pseudohypertrophy. SYN Debré-Sémélaigne s.

Koenig s., alternating attacks of constipation and diarrhea, with colic, meteorism, and gurgling in the right iliac fossa, said to be symptomatic of cecal tuberculosis.

Koerber-Salus-Elschnig s., SYN convergence-retraction *nystagmus*.

Kohlmeier-Degos s., vascular occlusive disorder predominantly involving the small arteries of the skin and bowel with about one-fifth of patients having central nervous system symptoms secondary to arterial fibrosis and thrombosis.

Korsakoff s., an alcohol amnestic s. characterized by confusion and severe impairment of memory, especially for recent events, for which the patient compensates by confabulation; typically encountered in chronic alcoholics; delirium tremens may precede the s., and Wernicke s. often coexists; the precise pathogenesis is uncertain, but direct toxic effects of alcohol are probably less important than severe nutritional deficiencies often associated with chronic alcoholism. SYN amnestic s. (1), dysmnesic s., Korsakoff psychosis.

Kostmann s., severe infantile agranulocytosis, an inherited disorder of infancy characterized by severe, recurrent infections and neutropenia.

Kuskokwim s., congenital joint contractures resembling arthrogryposis, found in Inuits of the Kuskokwim River delta in Alaska.

Laband s. [MIM*135500 and 135300], fibromatosis of the gingivae associated with hypoplasia of the distal phalanges, nail dysplasia, joint hypermotility, and sometimes hepatosplenomegaly; autosomal dominant inheritance.

Lady Windemere's syndrome, nontuberculous mycobacterial pulmonary disease in a frail, elderly woman, often with pectus excavatum or scoliosis. [named for the main character in Oscar Wilde's play, *Lady Windemere's Fan*]

LAMB s. [MIM*160980], the concurrence of lentigines, atrial myxoma, mucocutaneous myxomas, and blue nevi. SEE ALSO NAME s.

Lambert s., SYN Lambert-Eaton s.

Lambert-Eaton s. (LES), a generalized disorder of neuromuscular transmission caused by a defect in the release of acetylcholine quanta from the presynaptic nerve terminals; often associated with small cell carcinoma of the lung, particularly in elderly men with a long history of cigarette smoking. In contrast to myasthenia gravis, weakness tends to affect solely axial muscles, girdle muscles, and less often the limb muscles; autonomic disturbances, e.g., dry mouth and impotence, are common; the deep tendon reflexes are unelicitable; on motor conduction studies, responses on initial stimulation are quite low in amplitude, but they show marked post-tetanic facilitation after a few seconds of exercise. Lambert-Eaton s. is due to loss of voltage-sensitive calcium channels located on the presynaptic motor nerve terminal. SEE myasthenic s. SYN carcinomatous myopathy, Eaton-Lambert s., Lambert s., myasthenic s.

Landau-Kleffner s., childhood disorder characterized by generalized and psychomotor seizures associated with acquired aphasia; multifocal spikes and spike and wave discharges in the electroencephalogram. SYN acquired epileptic aphasia.

Landry s., SYN Guillain-Barré s.

Landry-Guillain-Barré s., SYN Guillain-Barré s.

Langer-Saldino s., SYN Type II *achondrogenesis*.

Larsen s., a s. characterized by multiple congenital dislocations with osseous anomalies, including characteristic flattened facies and cleft soft palate.

Lasègue s., in conversion hysteria, inability to move an anesthetic limb, except under control of the sight.

late dumping s., a s. in patients who have had ablation of the pyloric sphincter mechanism; associated with flushing, sweating, dizziness, weakness, and vasomotor collapse 2–3 hours after a meal and caused by hypoglycemia resulting from the rapid absorption of a large carbohydrate load, which then stimulates insulin release. SEE ALSO dumping s.

lateral medullary s., SYN posterior inferior cerebellar artery s.

Launois-Bensaude s., SYN multiple symmetric *lipomatosis*.

Launois-Cléret s., SYN adiposogenital *dystrophy*.

Laurence-Moon s. [MIM*245800], disorder characterized by mental retardation, pigmentary retinopathy, hypogenitalism, and spastic paraplegia; autosomal recessive inheritance. This s. is to be distinguished from Bardet-Biedl [MIM*209900]: in the past, the two syndromes have been lumped together under the designation of Laurence-Moon-Bardet-Biedl s.

Lawrence-Seip s., SYN lipoatrophy.

Lejeune s., SYN cri-du-chat s.

Lenègre s., isolated damage of the cardiac conduction system as a result of a sclerodegenerative lesion; characterized ordinarily as idiopathic fibrosis of the atrioventricular nodal, His bundle, or bundle branches with corresponding conduction block(s). SYN Lenègre disease.

Lennox s., SYN Lennox-Gastaut s.

Lennox-Gastaut s., a generalized myoclonic astatic epilepsy in children, with mental retardation, resulting from various cerebral afflictions such as perinatal hypoxia, cerebral hemorrhage, encephalitides, maldevelopment or metabolic disorders of the brain; characterized by multiple seizure types (generalized tonic, atonic, myoclonic, tonic-clonic, and atypical absence) and background slowing and slow spike and wave pattern on EEG. SYN Lennox s.

LEOPARD s., s. consisting of *l*entigines (multiple), *e*lectrocardiographic abnormalities, *o*cular hypertelorism, *p*ulmonary stenosis, *a*bnormalities of genitalia, *r*etardation of growth, and *d*eafness (sensorineural). An autosomal dominant hereditary disorder. SYN multiple lentigines s.

Leriche s., aortoiliac occlusive *disease* producing distal ischemic symptoms and signs.

Leri-Weill s., SYN dyschondrosteosis.

Lermoyez s., increasing hearing loss and tinnitus preceding an attack of vertigo, after which the hearing improves. Variant of Ménière *disease*.

Lesch-Nyhan s. [MIM*308000 several kinds], a disorder of purine metabolism due to deficiency of hypoxanthine-guanine phosphoribosyltransferase (HPRT); characterized by hyperuricemia, uric acid renal stones, mental retardation, spasticity, choreoathetosis, and self-mutilation of fingers and lips by biting; X-linked inheritance, caused by mutation in the HPRT gene on Xq.

Lev s., bundle branch block in a patient with normal myocardium and normal coronary arteries resulting from fibrosis or calcification including the conducting system; affects the membranous septum, the apex of the muscular septum, and often the mitral and aortic valve rings. SYN Lev disease.

Libman-Sacks s., SYN Libman-Sacks *endocarditis*.

Li-Fraumeni cancer s. [MIM*151623 and 191170], familial breast cancer in young women, with soft-tissue sarcomas in children, brain tumors and other cancers in close relatives; autosomal dominant inheritance, caused by mutation in the P53 gene on chromosome 17p.

liver kidney s., severe loss of both liver and kidney function, seen in a variety of diseases, often with fatal outcome. Seen particularly in late-stage liver failure due to cirrhosis or hepatitis, and in several viral infections.

locked-in s., basis pontis infarct resulting in tetraplegia, horizontal ophthalmoplegia, dysphagia, and facial diplegia with preserved consciousness; caused by basilar artery occlusion. SYN pseudocoma.

loculation s., SYN Froin s.

Loeffler s. I, eosinophilic pulmonary infiltrates, often associated with parasitic migration; also associated with reactions to some antibiotics, to L-tryptophan, or to crack cocaine. SYN eosinophilic pneumonia.

Loeffler s. II, eosinophilic endocarditis/myocarditis.

Löffler s., (1) SYN simple pulmonary *eosinophilia*; **(2)** SYN Löffler *endocarditis*.

long QT s.'s, a group of congenital and acquired diseases in which the electrocardiographic QT interval is longer than established measurements for age and sex; the presence of long QT intervals presages arrhythmias and sudden death. SEE ALSO QT *interval*.

Lorain-Lévi s., SYN pituitary *dwarfism*.

Louis-Bar s., SYN *ataxia* telangiectasia.

Lowe s., SYN oculocerebrorenal s.

Lowe-Terrey-MacLachlan s., SYN oculocerebrorenal s.

Lown-Ganong-Levine s., electrocardiographic s. of a short PR interval with normal duration of the QRS complex; it lacks the slurred delta wave of the Wolff-Parkinson-White s., but resembles it in its frequent (controversial) association with paroxysmal tachycardia which qualifies it as a s.; otherwise short PR may occur in otherwise normal individuals.

low salt s., low sodium s., a s. resulting from salt restriction and use of diuretics in treatment of congestive heart failure and hypertension, characterized by weakness, drowsiness, muscle cramps, and a reduction in glomerular filtration with consequent nitrogen retention, renal failure, and sometimes death; occurs also in cirrhosis of the liver with ascites and in adrenal insufficiency. SYN salt depletion s.

lupus-like s., a clinical s. resembling that of systemic *lupus* erythematosus, but due to some other cause.

Lutembacher s., a congenital cardiac abnormality consisting of a defect of the interatrial septum, mitral stenosis, and enlarged right atrium.

Lyell s., SYN toxic epidermal *necrolysis*.

lymphoproliferative s., SYN Duncan *disease*.

Lynch s., type I, familial colorectal cancer, generally occurring at an early age; type II, familial colorectal cancer occurring at an early age in conjunction with female genital cancer or cancers at other sites proximal to the bowel.

Macleod s., SYN unilateral lobar *emphysema*.

Mad Hatter s., gastrointestinal and central nervous system manifestations of chronic mercury poisoning, including stomatitis, diarrhea, ataxia, tremor, hyperreflexia, sensorineural impairment, and emotional instability; previously seen in workers in felt hat manufacturing who put mercury-containing material in their mouths to make it more pliable. [fr. char. in *Alice in Wonderland*]

Maffucci s. [MIM*166000], enchondromas of the limbs in association with venous and lymphaticovenous malformation; propensity to develop other benign or malignant tumors. SYN dyschondroplasia with hemangiomas, Kast s.

Magendie-Hertwig s., SYN Magendie-Hertwig *sign*.

malabsorption s., a state characterized by diverse features such as diarrhea, weakness, edema, lassitude, weight loss, poor appetite, protuberant abdomen, pallor, bleeding tendencies, paresthesias, muscle cramps, and steatorrhea; caused by any of several conditions in which there is ineffective absorption of nutrients, e.g., sprue, gluten-induced enteropathy, gastroileostomy, tuberculosis, and certain fistulas.

malignant carcinoid s., SYN carcinoid s.

malignant mole s. [MIM*155600], irregularly shaped, variously colored, distinctively melanocytic, 5–10-mm nevi occurring in large numbers (to over 100) primarily on the trunk and extremities, with a high risk of malignancy; probably autosomal dominant inheritance. SEE ALSO dysplastic *nevus*.

Mallory-Weiss s., upper gastrointestinal hemorrhage resulting from a laceration in the mucosa at the gastroesophageal junction usually induced by retching or vomiting. SYN Mallory-Weiss lesion, Mallory-Weiss tear.

mandibulofacial dysotosis s., SYN mandibulofacial *dysostosis*.

mandibulo-oculofacial s., SYN *dyscephalia* mandibulo-oculofacialis.

Marchiafava-Micheli s., SYN paroxysmal nocturnal *hemoglobinuria*.

Marcus Gunn s., SYN jaw-winking s.

Marfan s. [MIM*154700], a connective tissue multisystemic disorder characterized by skeletal changes (arachnodactyly, long limbs, joint laxity, pectus), cardiovascular defects (aortic aneurysm which may dissect, mitral valve prolapse), and ectopia lentis; autosomal dominant inheritance, caused by mutation in the fibrillin-1 gene (FBN1) on chromosome 15q. SYN Marfan disease.

Marie-Robinson s., insomnia and mild melancholia associated with alimentary levulosuria.

Marine-Lenhart s., toxic multinodular goiter.

Marinesco-Garland s. [MIM*248800], a rare neurologic disorder characterized by cerebellar ataxia, congenital cataracts, and growth and mental retardation; autosomal recessive inheritance. SYN cataract-oligophrenia s., Marinesco-Sjögren s., Torsten Sjögren s.

Marinesco-Sjögren s., SYN Marinesco-Garland s.

marker X s., SYN fragile X s.

Maroteaux-Lamy s. [MIM*253200], an error of mucopolysaccharide metabolism characterized by excretion of dermatan sulfate in the urine, growth retardation, lumbar kyphosis, sternal protrusion, genu valgum, usually hepatosplenomegaly, and no mental retardation; onset occurs after 2 years of age; autosomal recessive inheritance, caused by mutation in the arylsulfatase B gene (ARSB) on chromosome 5q. SYN arylsulfatase B deficiency, type VI mucopolysaccharidosis.

Marshall s. [MIM*154780], s. of midface hypoplasia, cataract, sensorineural hearing loss, and hypohidrosis. It is disputed whether this s. is distinct from Stickler s.

Martin-Bell s., SYN fragile X s.

Martorell s., SYN aortic arch s.

opiate intoxication s., the triad of miosis with depressed consciousness and respiratory rate; the s. is often named for the specific opiate responsible, e.g., heroin intoxication s. SYN heroin overdose s.

sy

systemic capillary leak s., a rare disorder of unknown cause presenting with episodic hypotension, hemoconcentration, and hypoalbuminemia; monoclonal gammopathy is often associated.

MASS s., a s. closely resembling both Marfan s. and Barlow s. However, no dislocation of the lenses or aneurysmal changes occur in the aorta, and the mitral valve prolapse is by no means invariable. At present it has been assigned no separate MIM number, but shares that of the Barlow s. [MIM*157700]. [*m*itral valve prolapse, *a*ortic anomalies, *s*keletal changes, and *s*kin changes.]

massive bowel resection s., malabsorption following extensive resection of the bowel, particularly the small intestine, characterized by diarrhea, steatorrhea, hypoproteinemia, and malnutrition.

maternal deprivation s., a failure to thrive seen in infants and young children and exhibited as a constellation of physical signs, symptoms, and behaviors, usually associated with maternal loss, absence or neglect, and characterized by lack of responsiveness to the environment and often depression.

Mauriac s., dwarfism with obesity and hepatosplenomegaly in children with poorly controlled diabetes mellitus.

Mayer-Rokitansky-Küster-Hauser s., primary amenorrhea due to müllerian duct agenesis, resulting in absence of the vagina, or presence of a short vaginal pouch, and absence of the uterus with normal karyotype and ovaries. SYN müllerian agenesis, Rokitansky-Küster-Hauser s.

May-White s., progressive myoclonus epilepsy with lipomas, deafness, and ataxia; probably a familial form of mitochondrial encephalomyopathy.

McArdle s., SYN type 5 *glycogenosis.*

McCune-Albright s., polyostotic fibrous dysplasia with irregular brown patches of cutaneous pigmentation and endocrine dysfunction, especially precocious puberty in girls. SEE ALSO pseudohypoparathyroidism. SYN Albright disease, Albright s. (1).

Meadows s., cardiomyopathy developing during pregnancy or the puerperium.

Meckel s., SYN dysencephalia splanchnocystica.

Meckel-Gruber s., SYN dysencephalia splanchnocystica.

meconium aspiration s., SYN fetal aspiration s.

meconium blockage s., low intestinal obstruction in newborn infants resulting from blockage of meconium.

megacystic s., a combination of a large, smooth, thin-walled bladder, vesicoureteral reflux, and dilated ureters.

megacystitis-megaureter s., radiologic findings of a large capacity, thin-walled bladder and massive vesicoureteral reflux, without obstruction or underlying neuropathy or dysfunctional voiding.

megacystitis-microcolon-intestinal hypoperistalsis s., a rare condition characterized by abdominal distention, lax abdominal musculature, incomplete intestinal rotation, and deficient intestinal peristalsis. A large bladder and often vesicoureteral reflux are seen. Typically affects female neonates and usually fatal in first year of life.

Meigs s., fibromyoma of the ovary associated with hydroperitoneum and hydrothorax.

Meischer s., SYN *cheilitis* granulomatosa.

Melkersson-Rosenthal s. [MIM*155900], cheilitis granulomatosa, fissured tongue, and recurrent facial nerve paralysis.

Melnick-Needles s., SYN osteodysplasty.

Ménétrier s., SYN Ménétrier *disease.*

Ménière s., SYN Ménière *disease.*

Menkes s., SYN kinky-hair *disease.*

menopausal s., recurring symptoms experienced by some women during the climacteric period; they include hot flashes, chills, headache, irritability, and depression. SYN climacteric s.

Meretoja s., a familial form of systemic amyloidosis with lattice, corneal *dystrophy,* cranial and peripheral nerve palsies, protruding lips, masklike facies, and floppy ears.

metastatic carcinoid s., SYN carcinoid s.

methionine malabsorption s., an inherited disorder in which there is an inability to absorb L-methionine from the gut.

Meyenburg-Altherr-Uehlinger s., SYN relapsing *polychondritis.*

Meyer-Betz s., SYN myoglobinuria.

middle lobe s., atelectasis with chronic pneumonitis of the middle lobe of the (right) lung, due to compression of the middle lobe bronchus, usually by enlarged lymph nodes, which may be tuberculous; chief symptoms are chronic cough, wheezing, recurrent respiratory infections, hemoptysis, chest pain, malaise, easy fatigability, and loss of weight; sometimes confused with interlobar accumulation of fluid in the lateral x-ray view. SYN Brock s.

Mikulicz s., the symptoms characteristic of Mikulicz disease occurring as a complication of some other disease, such as lymphoma, leukemia, or uveoparotid fever.

milk-alkali s., a chronic disorder characterized by pathologic deposition of calcium in many sites, especially in the kidneys, reversible in its early stages, induced by ingestion of large amounts of calcium and alkali, which were formerly used in the therapy of peptic ulcer; can progress to renal failure. SYN Burnett s.

Milkman s., osteomalacia with multiple pseudofractures, usually bilateral and symmetrical, may develop true pathologic fractures.

Millard-Gubler s., SYN Gubler s.

minimal-change nephrotic s., nephrotic s. with minimal glomerular changes by light or electron microscopy, occurring most frequently in children, marked by edema, albuminuria, and an increase in cholesterol in the blood, but otherwise with fairly good renal function; tubular epithelium is vacuolated by cholesterol droplets, but the glomeruli show only that the foot processes of the glomerular epithelial cells are fused, probably secondary to the proteinuria; the cause of the increased glomerular permeability to plasma protein is unknown.

Mirizzi s., benign obstruction of the hepatic ducts due to spasm and/or fibrous scarring of surrounding connective tissue; often associated with a stone in the cystic duct and chronic cholecystitis.

mitral valve prolapse s., the clinical constellation of findings with or without symptoms due to prolapse of the mitral valve: a nonejection systolic click accentuated in the standing posture, sometimes multiple, sometimes with mitral regurgitation occurring relatively late in systole, and accompanied by echocardiographic evidence of the mitral valve prolapse, usually with thickened leaflets of the valve. Symptoms are nonspecific and may include vague chest pains and dyspnea on exertion. SYN billowing mitral valve s.

Möbius s. [MIM*157900], a developmental bilateral facial paralysis usually associated with oculomotor or other neurological disorders. SYN congenital facial diplegia.

Mohr s., autosomal recessive oral-facial-digital s.

Monakow s., contralateral hemiplegia, hemianesthesia, and homonomous hemianopsia due to occlusion of the anterior choroidal artery.

monofixation s., a small-angle strabismus (fewer than 10 prism diopters) with central fixation by the preferred eye, central suppression of the deviating eye, and binocular fusion of peripheral vision

Morgagni s. [MIM*144800], hyperostosis frontalis interna in elderly women, with obesity and neuropsychiatric disorders of uncertain cause; at least sometimes familial. SYN metabolic craniopathy, Stewart-Morel s.

Morgagni-Adams-Stokes s., SYN Adams-Stokes s.

morning glory s. [MIM*120330], a funnel-shaped hypoplastic optic nerve with a dot of white tissue at its center; surrounded by an elevated anulus of chorioretinal pigment.

Morquio s. [MIM*253000, MIM*253010, MIM*230500], an error of mucopolysaccharide metabolism with excretion of keratan sulfate in urine; characterized by severe skeletal defects with short stature, severe deformity of spine and thorax, long bones with irregular epiphyses but with shafts of normal length, enlarged joints, flaccid ligaments, and waddling gait; autosomal recessive inheritance; type IVA mucopolysaccharidosis is due to an absence of galactose-1-sulfatase and is caused by mutation in the *N*-acetylgalactosamine-6-sulfate sulfatase gene (GALNS) on 16q, while type IVB is due to a deficiency of a β-galactosidase, and is caused by mutation in β-galactosidase gene (GLB1) on 3p. SYN Brailsford-Morquio disease, Morquio disease, Morquio-Ullrich disease, type IVA, B mucopolysaccharidosis.

Morton s., congenital shortening of the first metatarsal causing metatarsalgia.

Mounier-Kuhn s., SYN tracheobronchomegaly.

Muckle-Wells s. [MIM*191900], a s. characterized by amyloidosis, notably involving the kidneys, progressive sensorineural hearing loss, and periods of febrile urticaria associated with pain in joints and muscles of the extremities; autosomal dominant inheritance.

mucocutaneous lymph node s., SYN Kawasaki *disease.*

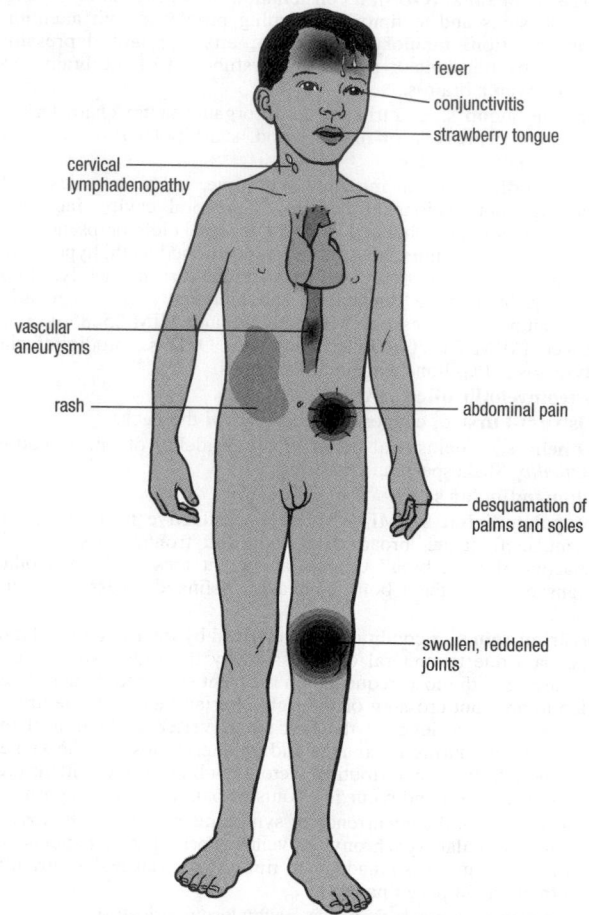

fever
conjunctivitis
strawberry tongue
cervical lymphadenopathy
vascular aneurysms
rash
abdominal pain
desquamation of palms and soles
swollen, reddened joints

mucocutaneous lymph node syndrome (Kawasaki disease): common signs and symptoms

Muir-Torre s., SYN Torre s.

multiple endocrine deficiency s., acquired deficiency of the function of several endocrine glands, usually on an autoimmune basis, as in Schmidt s. (2). SYN multiple glandular deficiency s., polyendocrine deficiency s., polyglandular deficiency s.

multiple endocrine neoplasia s., type 1, an autosomal-dominant predisposition to tumors of parathyroid glands, anterior pituitary, endocrine pancreas, and less commonly, other organs. SYN multiple endocrine neoplasia, type 1, Wermer s.

multiple endocrine neoplasia s., type 2A, an autosomal-dominant predisposition to tumors of thyroid C cells (medullary carcinoma), adrenal medulla (pheochromocytoma), and nodular hyperplasia of parathyroid glands. SYN multiple endocrine neoplasia, type 2A.

multiple endocrine neoplasia s., type 2B, an autosomal-dominant predisposition to tumors of thyroid C cells (medullary carcinoma), adrenal medulla (pheochromocytoma), peripheral nerves (mucosal neurinoma), and intestinal ganglioneuromatosis; associated with a tall, thin habitus.

multiple glandular deficiency s., SYN multiple endocrine deficiency s.

multiple hamartoma s., SYN Cowden *disease.*

multiple lentigines s., SYN LEOPARD s.

multiple mucosal neuroma s., multiple submucosal neuromas or neurofibromas of the tongue, lips, and eyelids in young persons; sometimes associated with tumors of the thyroid or adrenal medulla, or with subcutaneous neurofibromatosis.

Munchausen s., repeated fabrication of clinically convincing simulations of disease for the purpose of gaining medical attention; a term referring to patients who wander from hospital to hospital feigning acute medical or surgical illness and giving false and fanciful information about their medical and social background for no apparent reason other than to gain attention. SEE factitious *disorder.*

Munchausen s. by proxy, a form of child maltreatment or abuse inflicted by a caretaker (usually the mother) with fabrications of symptoms and/or induction of signs of disease, leading to unnecessary investigations and interventions, with occasional serious health consequences, including death of the child. SYN factitious illness by proxy.

Münchhausen s., SEE Munchausen s.

myasthenic s. (MS), SYN Lambert-Eaton s.

myelodysplastic s., SYN preleukemia.

myeloproliferative s.'s, a group of conditions that result from a disorder in the rate of formation of cells of the bone marrow, including chronic granulocytic leukemia, erythremia, myelosclerosis, panmyelosis, and erythremic myelosis and erythroleukemia.

myofascial s., irritation of the muscles and fascia of the back and neck causing acute and chronic pain not associated with any neurologic or bony evidence of disease; presumed to arise primarily from poorly understood changes in the muscle and fascia themselves.

myofascial pain-dysfunction s., dysfunction of the masticatory apparatus related to spasm of the muscles of mastication precipitated by occlusal dysharmony or alteration in vertical dimension of the jaws, and exacerbated by emotional stress; characterized by pain in the preauricular region, muscle tenderness, popping noise in the temporomandibular joint, and limitation of jaw motion. SYN temporomandibular joint pain-dysfunction s.

Naegeli s. [MIM*161000], reticular skin pigmentation, diminished sweating, hypodontia, hyperkeratosis of the palms and soles, and blistering; may be confused with *incontinentia* pigmenti but is as common in males as in females; autosomal dominant inheritance. SYN Franceschetti-Jadassohn s.

Naffziger s., scalenus-anticus s.

nail-patella s. [MIM*161200], a skeletal disorder characterized by absence or hypoplasia of the patella, iliac horns, dysplasia of the fingernails and toenails, and thickening of the glomerular lamina densa; the lower ends of the femur have a shape very similar to Erlenmeyer flask deformity; autosomal dominant inheritance, caused by mutation in the gene encoding LIM-homeodomain protein (LMX1B) onchromosome 9q.

NAME s., the concurrence of nevi, atrial myxoma, myxoid neurofibromas, and ephilides.

Nance-Insley s., SYN *chondrodystrophy* with sensorineural deafness.

Nelson s., a s. of hyperpigmentation, third nerve damage, and enlarging sella turcica caused by pituitary adenomas presumably present before adrenalectomy for Cushing s. but enlarging and symptomatic afterward. SYN postadrenalectomy s.

nephritic s., the clinical symptoms of acute glomerulonephritis, particularly hematuria, hypertension, and renal failure.

nephrotic s., a clinical state characterized by edema, albuminuria, decreased plasma albumin, doubly refractile bodies in the urine, and usually increased blood cholesterol; lipid droplets may be present in the cells of the renal tubules, but the basic lesion is increased permeability of the glomerular capillary basement membranes, of unknown cause or resulting from glomerulonephritis, diabetic glomerulosclerosis, systemic lupus erythematosus, amyloidosis, renal vein thrombosis, or hypersensitivity to various toxic agents. SYN nephrosis (3).

sy

Netherton s. [MIM*256500], congenital ichthyosiform erythroderma or ichthyosis linearis circumscripta associated with bamboo hair, atopy, urticaria, intermittent aminoaciduria, and mental retardation; probably an autosomal recessive trait that frequently resolves or improves in adolescence.

neural crest s., s. consisting of loss of pain sensibility, autonomic dysfunction, pupillary abnormalities, neurogenic anhidrosis, vasomotor instability, aplasia of dental enamel, meningeal thickening, hyperflexion, and a degree of albinism; may reflect developmental abnormalities of the neural crest.

neurocutaneous s., the occurrence of nevi and sometimes various skeletal deformities with symptoms pointing to gliosis or abiotrophy of the central nervous system.

neuroleptic malignant s., hyperthermia with extrapyramidal and autonomic disturbances which may result in death, following the use of neuroleptic agents.

Nezelof s., SYN cellular *immunodeficiency* with abnormal immunoglobulin synthesis.

Noack s., SYN Pfeiffer s.

nonsense s., SYN Ganser s.

Noonan s. [MIM*163950, MIM*163955], a s. found in both males and females, with a phenotype reminiscent of Turner s.; characterized by hypertelorism, downslanting of palpebral fissures, webbing of the neck, short stature, and congenital heart disease, especially pulmonary stenosis; normal chromosomal karyotype; autosomal dominant inheritance.

Nothnagel s., dizziness, staggering, and rolling gait, with irregular forms of oculomotor paralysis and often nystagmus, seen in cases of tumor of the midbrain.

numb chin s., paresthesia and sensory loss affecting one side of the chin and lower lip, resulting from neoplastic infiltration of the ipsilateral mental nerve; common causes include multiple myeloma and breast or prostate carcinoma.

nystagmus blockage s., strabismus with eyes and head in a position to minimize associated nystagmus.

OAV s., SYN oculoauriculovertebral *dysplasia*.

occipital horn s., an X-linked recessive disorder in which there is defective biliary excretion of copper, resulting in a deficiency of lysyl oxidase causing skin and joint laxity.

ocular-mucous membrane s., Stevens-Johnson s. with associated ocular lesions (conjunctivitis, panophthalmitis, iritis), oral lesions (bullae, erosions, superficial ulcers), and genital lesions (urethritis, balanitis circinata, blebs).

oculobuccogenital s., SYN Behçet s.

oculocerebrorenal s. [MIM*309000], a congenital s. with hydrophthalmia, cataracts, mental retardation, aminoaciduria, reduced ammonia production by the kidney, and vitamin D–resistant rickets; X-linked recessive inheritance, caused by mutation in the oculocerebrorenal gene (OCRL) on Xq. SYN Lowe s., Lowe-Terrey-MacLachlan s.

oculocutaneous s., SYN Vogt-Koyanagi s.

oculomandibulofacial s., SYN *dyscephalia* mandibulo-oculofacialis.

oculopharyngeal s. [MIM*164300], a myopathic disorder with a slowly progressive blepharoptosis and dysphagia, beginning late in life; autosomal dominant inheritance, caused by mutation in the gene encoding poly(A)-binding protein-2 (PABP2) on chromosome 14q.

oculovertebral s., SYN oculovertebral *dysplasia*.

oculovestibulo-auditory s., a nonsyphilitic interstitial keratitis characterized by an abrupt onset with vertigo and tinnitus followed by hearing impairment; about 50% of patients have an associated systemic disease, most commonly polyarteritis nodosa. SYN Cogan s.

OFD s., SYN orofaciodigital s.

Ogilvie s., pseudoobstruction, predominantly of the colon, believed to be the result of motility disturbance; without physical obstruction.

Oldfield s., familial polyposis of the colon.

Olmsted s., congenital palmar, plantar, and periorificial keratoderma leading to flexion contractures and digital spontaneous amputation.

Omenn s. [MIM*603554], a rapidly fatal immunodeficiency disease characterized by erythroderma, diarrhea, repeated infections, hepatosplenomegaly, and leukocytosis with eosinophilia; autosomal recessive inheritance, caused by mutation in either the recombination activating gene 1 (RAG1) or the adjacent RAG2 gene on chromosome 11p.

Opitz BBB s., SYN ocular *hypertelorism*.

Opitz G s., SYN ocular *hypertelorism*.

Oppenheim s., SYN *amyotonia* congenita.

organic brain s. (OBS), a constellation of behavioral or psychological signs and symptoms including problems with attention, concentration, memory, confusion, anxiety, and depression caused by transient or permanent dysfunction of the brain. SYN acute organic brain s.

organic mood s., s. attributed to an organic factor characterized by either depressive or manic mood. SEE bipolar *disorder*; SEE ALSO bipolar *disorder*.

orofaciodigital s., an inherited syndrome, lethal in males, with varying combinations of defects of the oral cavity, face, and hands, including lobulated or bifid tongue, cleft or pseudocleft palate, tongue tumors, missing or malpositioned teeth, hypoplastic nasal alar cartilage, depressed nasal bridge, brachydactyly, clinodactyly, incomplete syndactyly, and, frequently, mental retardation; autosomal recessive [MIM 252100 and MIM 258850] or X-linked [MIM 311200] inheritance. SYN OFD s., orodigitofacial dysostosis, Papillon-Léage and Psaume s.

osteomyelofibrotic s., SYN myelofibrosis.

Ostrum-Furst s., congenital synostosis of the neck.

Othello s., a delusional belief in the infidelity of one's spouse. [*Othello*, Shakespearean character]

otomandibular s., SYN otomandibular *dysostosis*.

otopalatodigital s. [MIM*311300], conductive hearing impairment, cleft palate, broad nasal root, and frontal bossing, wide spacing of toes, broad thumbs and great toes, and often other signs of generalized bone dysplasia; X-linked recessive inheritance.

ovarian vein s., a condition characterized by intermittent abdominal pain due to ureteral compression by the right ovarian vein, occurring with most frequency on the right side, and thought to be due to aberrant crossing of the right ovarian vein over the ureter, generally at the level of the first sacral vertebra; dilation of the ovarian vein during pregnancy and unilateral ptosis of the kidney are thought to be contributing factors leading to intermittent ureteral obstruction and recurring bouts of pain and pyelonephritis.

pacemaker s., the occurrence of symptoms relating to the loss of atrial-ventricular synchrony in ventricularly paced patients, or symptoms caused by inadequate timing of atrial and ventricular contractions in paced patients.

pachydermoperiostosis s., SEE pachydermoperiostosis.

Paget-von Schrötter s., stress thrombosis or spontaneous thrombosis of the subclavian or axillary vein; a thoracic outlet s. SYN effort-induced thrombosis.

painful arc s., SYN supraspinatus s.

painful-bruising s., an intense inflammatory reaction to slight extravasation of blood, due to an allergic sensitivity to red blood cells; more commonly seen in adult women.

paleostriatal s., SYN Hunt s. (3).

pallidal s., SYN Hunt s. (3).

Pancoast s., lower trunk brachial plexopathy and Horner s. due to malignant tumor in the region of the superior pulmonary sulcus.

pancreatorenal s., acute renal failure occurring in a patient with severe acute pancreatitis; the mortality rate is high.

papillary muscle s., SYN papillary muscle *dysfunction*.

Papillon-Léage and Psaume s., SYN orofaciodigital s.

Papillon-Lefèvre s. [MIM*245000], a congenital hyperkeratosis of the palms and soles, with progessive destruction of alveolar bone about the deciduous and permanent teeth beginning as early as 2 years of age, and also with premature exfoliation of teeth and calcification of the falx cerebri; autosomal recessive inheritance.

paraneoplastic s., a s. directly resulting from a malignant neoplasm, but not resulting from the presence of tumor cells in the affected parts.

Parenti-Fraccaro s., SYN Type IB *achondrogenesis.*

Parinaud s., paralysis of conjugate upward gaze with a lesion at the level of the superior colliculi; Bell phenomenon is present. SYN dorsal midbrain s., Parinaud ophthalmoplegia.

Parinaud oculoglandular s., unilateral conjunctival granuloma with preauricular adenopathy in tularemia, chancre, tuberculosis, and cat-scratch disease.

Parkes Weber s., concurrence of multiple congenital arteriovenous fistulae or arteriovenous malformations with capillary stain and lymphaticovenous anomalies in an enlarged limb.

Parsonage-Turner s., SYN neuralgic *amyotrophy.*

Patau s., SYN trisomy 13 s.

patellofemoral s., anterior knee pain due to a structural or functional disturbance in the relation between the patella and distal femur.

patellofemoral stress s., SYN runner's *knee.*

Paterson-Brown-Kelly s., SYN tendon sheath s.

Paterson-Kelly s., SYN Plummer-Vinson s.

pathologic startle s.'s, a group of disorders characterized by markedly exaggerated startle reflex and other exaggerated stimulus-induced responses. Includes hyperexplexia and probably latah and the jumping Frenchman of Maine s.

Pellizzi s., SYN *macrogenitosomia* praecox.

Pendred s. [MIM*274600], characterized by congenital sensorineural hearing impairment with goiter (usually small) due to defective organic binding of iodine in the thyroid; afflicted individuals are usually euthyroid; autosomal recessive inheritance, caused by mutation in the Pendred syndrome gene (PDS) encoding pendrin on chromosome 7q.

Pepper s., obsolete eponym for neuroblastoma of the adrenal gland with metastases in the liver; formerly believed to occur more frequently when the primary tumor was in the right adrenal, whereas tumors of the left adrenal tended to metastasize to the skull (Hutchison syndrome).

pericolic membrane s., a symptom complex simulating chronic appendicitis, caused by congenital constricting pericolic membranes.

Perrault s., XX gonadal dysgenesis associated with sensorineural deafness.

Persian Gulf s., SYN Gulf War s.

persistent müllerian duct s., familial disorder with presence of fallopian tube, uterus, and testis in a male. Deficient müllerian inhibitory substance secondary to Sertoli cell defect. SYN hernia uteri inguinale.

pertussis s., SYN pertussis.

pertussis-like s., a syndrome characterized by severe episodes of coughing resembling whooping *cough* (pertussis).

petrosphenoidal s., neoplastic infiltration of the apex of the petrous bone and the anterior part of the foramen lacerum.

Peutz s., SYN Peutz-Jeghers s.

Peutz-Jeghers s. [MIM*175200], generalized hamartomatous multiple polyposis of the intestinal tract, consistently involving the jejunum, associated with melanin spots of the lips, buccal mucosa, and fingers; autosomal dominant inheritance, caused by mutation in the serine/threonine kinase gene (STK11) on chromosome 19p. SYN Jeghers-Peutz s., Peutz s.

Pfaundler-Hurler s., SYN Hurler s.

Pfeiffer s. [MIM*101600], disorder characterized by broad, short thumbs and great toes, often with duplication of the great toes, and variable syndactyly of the digits; craniosynostosis is a variable feature. Autosomal dominant inheritance, caused by mutation in the fibroblast growth factor receptor 1 gene (FGFR1) on chromosome 8p or FGFR2 gene on 10q. SYN Noack s., type V acrocephalosyndactyly.

pharyngeal pouch s., SYN DiGeorge s.

phospholipid s., the combination of antiphospholipid antibodies and the presence of either arterial or venous occlusive events such as thrombosis.

Picchini s., a form of polyserositis involving the three great serosae in contact with the diaphragm, sometimes also the menin-

ges, tunica vaginalis testis, synovial sheaths, and bursae, caused by the presence of a trypanosome.

Pick s., SYN Pick *disease.*

pickwickian s., a combination of severe, grotesque obesity, somnolence, and general debility, theoretically resulting from hypoventilation induced by the obesity; hypercapnia, pulmonary hypertension, and cor pulmonale can result. [after the "fat boy" in Dickens' *Pickwick Papers*]

Pierre Robin s. [MIM*261800], micrognathia and U-shaped cleft palate, glossoptosis, often associated with upper airway obstruction and feeding difficulties; weak evidence of autosomal recessive inheritance. SYN Robin s.

pigment dispersion s., increased resistance to flow of aqueous humor through the pupil from the anterior chamber to the posterior chamber, leading to posterior bowing of the peripheral iris against the zonules; a possible mechanism for pigmentary glaucoma.

Pins s., dullness, diminution of vocal fremitus and of the vesicular murmur, and a slight distant blowing sound, heard in the posteroinferior region of the chest on the left side, in cases of pericardial effusion; there is sometimes also a fine rale in this region, but all the adventitious auscultatory signs disappear when the patient assumes the genupectoral position.

placental dysfunction s., fetal malnutrition and hypoxia resulting from impaired transfer of oxygen and various nutritive materials from mother to fetus.

placental transfusion s., in utero transfusion of blood from one twin to the other such that the donor becomes anemic and growth retarded and the recipient becomes polycythemic and develops hydrops. SEE ALSO twin-twin *transfusion.*

Plummer-Vinson s., iron deficiency anemia, dysphagia, esophageal stenosis, and atrophic glossitis. SYN Paterson-Kelly s., sideropenic dysphagia.

POEMS s., a condition characterized by *p*olyneuropathy, *o*rganomegaly, *e*ndocrinopathy, *m*onoclonal gammopathy, and *s*kin changes.

Poland s., an anomaly consisting of absence of the pectoralis major and minor muscles, ipsilateral breast hypoplasia, and absence of two to four rib segments.

polycystic ovary s. [MIM*184700], a condition commonly characterized by hirsutism, obesity, menstrual abnormalities, infertility, and enlarged ovaries; thought to reflect excessive androgen secretion of ovarian origin. SYN sclerocystic disease of the ovary, Stein-Leventhal s.

polyendocrine deficiency s., polyglandular deficiency s., SYN multiple endocrine deficiency s.

polysplenia s., SYN bilateral *left-sidedness.*

popliteal entrapment s., a crush s. resulting from compression of the popliteal artery and impairment of its blood flow by structures of the popliteal space.

postadrenalectomy s., SYN Nelson s.

postcardiotomy s., SYN postpericardiotomy s.

postcholecystectomy s., the recurrence or persistence of signs and symptoms that led to removal of the gallbladder, but after cholecystectomy.

postcommissurotomy s., SYN postpericardiotomy s.

postconcussion s., SEE posttraumatic s.

posterior inferior cerebellar artery s., a s. due usually to thrombosis, characterized by dysarthria, dysphagia, staggering gait, and vertigo, and marked by hypotonia, incoordination of voluntary movement, nystagmus, Horner s. on the ipsilateral side, and loss of pain and temperature senses on the side of the body opposite to the lesion. SYN lateral medullary s., Wallenberg s.

posterior leukoencephalopathy s., a reversible clinicoradiologic s. characterized by confusion, headaches, seizures, cortical blindness and other visual abnormalities, emesis, and motor signs, associated with MRI or CT evidence of bilateral white matter edema involving the parietal-occipital cerebral regions.

postgastrectomy s., SYN dumping s.

post–lumbar puncture s., SYN spinal *headache.*

postmalaria neurologic s., a self-limited central nervous system disorder that develops soon after recovery from a severe bout of falciparum malaria, characterized principally by an acute state of confusion or psychosis, generalized convulsions, or both, lasting 1–10 days and associated with negative blood smears for malaria parasite; linked to preceding mefloquine therapy.

postmaturity s., gestation extending 43 weeks or longer; sometimes associated with fetal dysmaturity.

postmyocardial infarction s. (PMIS), a complication developing several days to several weeks after myocardial infarction; its clinical features are fever, leukocytosis, chest pain, and evidence of pericarditis, sometimes with pleurisy and pneumonitis, with a strong tendency to recurrence; probably of immunopathogenetic origin.

postpartum pituitary necrosis s., SYN Sheehan s.

postpericardiotomy s., pericarditis, with or without fever and often in repeated episodes, weeks to months after cardiac surgery. SYN postcardiotomy s., postcommissurotomy s.

postphlebitic s., a state characterized by edema, pain, stasis dermatitis, cellulitis, and varicose veins, and in the late stages associated with ulceration of the lower leg, most often as a sequel to deep venous thrombosis of the lower extremity.

postrubella s., a group of congenital defects resulting from maternal rubella during the first trimester of pregnancy and including microphthalmos, cataracts, deafness, mental retardation, patent ductus arteriosus, and pulmonary artery stenosis.

postthrombotic s., a s. that follows a vascular thrombosis. Term is usually used to indicate difficulties, such as persistent edema, following venous thrombosis.

posttraumatic s., a clinical disorder that often follows head injury, characterized by headache, dizziness, neurasthenia, hypersensitivity to stimuli, and diminished concentration.

posttraumatic neck s., a clinical complex of pain, tenderness, tight neck musculature, vasomotor instability, and ill-defined symptoms such as dizziness and blurred vision as the result of trauma to the neck. Also variously termed occipital or suboccipital neuralgia or neuritis; cervical tension s.; cervical myospasm, myositis, or fibrositis. SYN cervical fibrositis, cervical tension s.

posttraumatic stress s., a disorder appearing after a physically or psychologically traumatic event outside the range of usual human experience, (e.g., a serious threat to one's life or seeing a loved one killed), characterized by symptoms of re-experiencing the event, numbing of responsiveness to the environment, exaggerated startle response, guilt feelings, impairment of memory, and difficulties in concentration and sleep.

Potter s., renal agenesis with hypoplastic lungs and associated neonatal respiratory distress, hemodynamic instability, acidosis, cyanosis, edema, and characteristic (Potter) facies; death usually occurs from respiratory insufficiency, which develops before uremia.

Prader-Willi s. [MIM*176270], a congenital s. characterized by short stature, mental retardation, polyphagia with marked obesity, and sexual infantilism; severe muscular hypotonia and poor responsiveness to external stimuli decrease with age; a small deletion is demonstrable in the paternal-derived chromosome 15q11–13 in many cases; some cases are due to maternal uniparental disomy (i.e., both chromosomes 15 are derived from the mother).

precordial catch s., a benign s. of uncertain origin, characterized by sharp, sudden pain in the region of the cardiac apex on inspiration, yet usually relieved by forcing a deeper breath; tenderness is absent.

preexcitation s., SYN Wolff-Parkinson-White s.

preinfarction s., abrupt development of angina pectoris or worsening of existing angina by increases in its frequency or severity; sometimes heralds myocardial infarction.

premature senility s., SYN progeria.

premenstrual s. (PMS), in women of reproductive age, a constellation of emotional, behavioral, and physical symptoms that occur in the luteal (premenstrual) phase of the menstrual cycle and subside with the onset of menstruation; characterized by swelling and weight gain due to fluid retention, breast tenderness, irritability, mood swings, anxiety, depression, drowsiness, fatigue, difficulty concentrating, and changes in appetite and libido. SYN late luteal phase dysphoria, late luteal phase dysphoric disorder, menstrual molimina, premenstrual tension s., premenstrual tension.

About 80% of menstruating women aged 25–40 experience some symptoms of PMS with at least some menstrual cycles, and about 5% have severe and disabling symptoms. A specific biologic cause has not been identified. Reported abnormalities in serotonin metabolism have led to the hypothesis that in women with PMS the normal hormonal fluctuations of the menstrual cycle interact with a neurotransmitter dysregulation to trigger mood and anxiety symptoms. No drug therapy has been approved by the FDA for the treatment of PMS. However, oral contraceptives and serotonergic antidepressants are widely used for this indication. Reducing caffeine and salt intake may lessen associated malaise and depression, and regular exercise and a diet high in complex carbohydrates may help to minimize the severity of episodes. In a large study, daily consumption of 1.2 g of calcium in a chewable supplement reduced symptoms to a greater extent than placebo. After its inclusion in the 1987 edition of the *Diagnostic and Statistical Manual of Mental Disorders* (*DSM-III*), PMS became a subject of debate among feminists, who doubted that it qualifies as a true disorder. PMS was used as a successful defense in a murder trial in the U.K.

premenstrual salivary s., glandular abnormalities occurring prior to the onset of menses, including swelling of the breast tissues and enlargement of the salivary glands.

premenstrual tension s., SYN premenstrual s.

premotor s., hemiplegia with spasticity, Rossolimo reflex, but not the Babinski sign, together with forced grasping and vasomotor disturbances.

pronator teres s., entrapment or compression of the median nerve in the proximal forearm usually where the nerve passes between the two heads of the pronator teres muscle.

Proteus s., a sporadic disorder of possible genetic origin, having a variable and changing phenotype; characterized by grossly enlarged hands and feet, distorted abnormal growth, and gigantism of the head; often confused with neurofibromatosis type I. SYN elephant man's disease (1).

prune belly s., a s. of deficient abdominal muscle, undescended testes, large hypotonic bladder and dilated, tortuous ureters. SYN Eagle-Barrett s.

pseudoexfoliation s., a condition, often leading to glaucoma, in which deposits on the surface of the lens resemble exfoliation of the lens *capsule*. SEE ALSO *pseudoexfoliation* of lens capsule. SYN exfoliation s.

psychogenic nocturnal polydipsia s., PNP s., emotionally induced excessive water drinking at night.

pterygium s. [MIM*178110, MIM*265000, MIM*312150], webbing of the neck, antecubital fossae, and popliteal fossae with flexion deformities of the limbs and anomalies of the vertebrae; autosomal dominant, autosomal recessive, and X-linked recessive inheritance have all been described.

pulmonary dysmaturity s., a respiratory disorder occurring in small, premature infants who are incapable of normal pulmonary ventilation and who often die of hypoxia after an illness of 6–8 weeks; the lungs contain widespread focal emphysematous blebs and the parenchyma has thickened alveolar walls; diagnosed principally on the basis of the clinical history, chest radiographic findings, and the findings at autopsy, which must include the absence of pathological changes characteristic of other pulmonary disorders commonly encountered in this age group. SYN Wilson-Mikity s.

punchdrunk s., a condition seen in boxers, often years after their retirement, and presumably caused by repeated cerebral injury; characterized by weakness in the lower limbs, unsteadiness of gait, slowness of muscular movements, tremors of hands, dysarthria, and slow cerebration.

Putnam-Dana s., SYN subacute combined *degeneration* of the spinal cord.

radial aplasia-thrombocytopenia s., thrombocytopenia-absent radius s.

radial tunnel s., pain in the lateral aspect of the elbow and forearm without motor or sensory deficits, resulting from compression of the radial nerve, at any of various sites along its course, as it passes the elbow and the proximal forearm.

radicular s., a group of symptoms resulting from any interference with the intradural portion of one or more spinal nerve roots; the chief symptoms are pain, paresthesia, hypesthesia, or hyperesthesia, motor, trophic, and reflex disturbances.

Raeder paratrigeminal s., a postganglionic Horner s. associated with trigeminal nerve dysfunction caused by involvement of the carotid sympathetic plexus, near Mechel cave.

Ramsay Hunt s., (1) SYN Hunt s; (2) SYN *herpes* zoster oticus.

Rasmussen s., SYN rasmussen *encephalitis.*

Raynaud s., idiopathic paroxysmal bilateral cyanosis of the digits due to arterial and arteriolar contraction; caused by cold or emotion. SEE ALSO Raynaud *phenomenon.* SYN Raynaud disease, symmetric asphyxia.

Refetoff s., a condition characterized by goiter and elevated serum level of thyroid hormones without manifestations of thyrotoxicosis, due to target organ unresponsiveness to thyroid hormones.

Refsum s., SYN Refsum *disease.*

Reifenstein s. [MIM*312300 and MIM*313700], partial androgen sensitivity; a familial form of male pseudohermaphroditism characterized by varying degrees of ambiguous genitalia or hypospadias, postpubertal development of gynecomastia, and infertility associated with seminiferous tubular sclerosis; cryptorchidism may be present, and Leydig cell hypofunction may lead to impotence in later years; chromosomal studies show 46,XY karyotype; X-linked recessive inheritance, caused by mutation in the androgen receptor gene (AR) on Xq.

Reiter s., the association of urethritis, iridocyclitis, mucocutaneous lesions, and arthritis, sometimes with diarrhea; one or more of these conditions may recur at intervals of months or years, but the arthritis may be persistent. SYN Fiessinger-Leroy-Reiter s., Reiter disease.

REM s., a reticular erythematous dermatitis of the upper trunk, more common in women, in which there is perivascular infiltrate of lymphocytes, few plasma cells, and upper dermal deposits of mucin; worsens on exposure to ultraviolet light. SYN reticular erythematous mucinosis.

Rendu-Osler-Weber s., SYN hereditary hemorrhagic *telangiectasia.*

Renpenning s. [MIM*309500], X-linked mental retardation with short stature and microcephaly not associated with the fragile X chromosome; occurs more frequently in males, although some females may also be affected.

residual ovary s., the development of a pelvic mass, pelvic pain, and occasionally dyspareunia following hysterectomy without removal of both ovaries.

resistant ovary s. [MIM*176440], amenorrhea associated with hypergonadotrophism and usually normal ovarian follicles; may be autosomal dominant in inheritance.

respiratory distress s. of the newborn, SYN hyaline membrane *disease* of the newborn.

respiratory distress s. type II, SYN transient *tachypnea* of the newborn.

restless legs s., a sense of indescribable uneasiness, twitching, or restlessness that occurs in the legs after going to bed, frequently leading to insomnia, which may be relieved temporarily by walking about; thought to be caused by inadequate circulation or as a side effect of antipsychotic medication. SEE ALSO akathisia. SYN Ekbom s., restless legs.

retraction s., a retraction of the globe and pseudoptosis on attempted adduction; due to co-innervation of the horizontal recti. Sometimes there is an inability to abduct the affected eye (type 1), or adduct the affected eye (type 2), or both (type 3). SYN Duane s.

Rett s. [MIM*312750], (1) a pervasive developmetnal disorder characterized by the development of several specific deficits after an apparently normal prenatal and perinatal period, including

deceleration in head growth, loss of purposeful hand skills with deterioration into stereotypical hand movements, impairment in expressive and receptive language, and significant psychomotor retardation; (2) a DSM diagnosis that is established when the specified criteria are met.

Reye s., an acquired encephalopathy of young children that follows an acute febrile illness, usually influenza or varicella infection; characterized by recurrent vomiting, agitation, and lethargy, which may lead to coma with intracranial hypertension; ammonia and serum transaminases are elevated; death may result from edema of the brain and resulting cerebral herniation.

Rh null s. [MIM*268150], a condition characterized by lack of all Rh antigens, compensated hemolytic anemia, and stomatocytosis; autosomal recessive inheritance, caused by mutation in the Rhesus-associated polypeptide 50-kD gene (RH50A) on chromosome 6p.

Richards-Rundle s. [MIM*245100], a neurologic disorder beginning in early childhood with severe, progressive sensorineural hearing loss, ataxia, muscle wasting nystagmus, absent deep tendon reflexes, mental retardation, failure to develop secondary sexual characteristics, and ketoaciduria; autosomal recessive inheritance.

Richter s., a high-grade lymphoma developing during the course of chronic lymphocytic leukemia; associated with cachexia, pyrexia, dysproteinemia, and lymphomas with multinucleated tumor cells.

Rieger s. [MIM*180500], iridocorneal mesenchymal dysgenesis combined with hypodontia or anodontia and maxillary hypoplasia; autosomal dominant; there is a delayed sexual development and hypothyroidism.

Riley-Day s., SYN familial *dysautonomia.*

Roaf s., a nonhereditary craniofacial-skeletal disorder characterized by congenital or early retinal detachment, cataracts, myopia, shortened long bones, and mental retardation; progressive sensorineural hearing loss is of later onset.

Roberts s. [MIM*268300], phocomelia or lesser degrees of hypomelia, microbrachycephaly, midfacial defect, prenatal growth deficiency, and cryptorchidism; associated with chromosomal centromeric abnormalities; autosomal recessive inheritance.

Robin s., SYN Pierre Robin s.

Robinow s. [MIM*180700], a skeletal dysplasia characterized by bulging forehead, hypertelorism, depressed nasal bridge (so-called fetal face), wide mouth, acromesomelic shortening of limbs, hemivertebrae, and hypoplastic genitalia; there is also an autosomal recessive form [MIM*268310]. SEE ALSO fetal face s. SYN Robinow dwarfism.

Rokitansky-Küster-Hauser s., SYN Mayer-Rokitansky-Küster-Hauser s.

Romano-Ward s. [MIM*192500], a prolonged Q-T interval in the electrocardiogram in children subject to attacks of unconsciousness that result from ventricular arrhythmias including ventricular fibrillation; autosomal dominant inheritance, with one form caused by mutation in the potassium channel gene (KVLQT1) on chromosome 11p. Cf. Jervell and Lange-Nielsen s. SYN Ward-Romano s.

Romberg s., SYN facial *hemiatrophy.*

Rothmund s. [MIM*268400], atrophy, pigmentation, and telangiectasia of the skin, usually with juvenile cataract, saddle nose, congenital bone defects, disturbance of hair growth, hypogonadism; autosomal recessive inheritance. SYN poikiloderma atrophicans and cataract, poikiloderma congenitale, Rothmund-Thomson s.

Rothmund-Thomson s., SYN Rothmund s.

Rotor s., jaundice appearing in childhood due to impaired biliary excretion; most of the plasma bilirubin is conjugated, liver function tests are usually normal, and there is no hepatic pigmentation.

Roussy-Lévy s., SYN Roussy-Lévy *disease.*

Rubinstein-Taybi s. [MIM*180849], mental retardation, broad thumb and great toe, antimongoloid slant to the eyes, thin and beaked nose, microcephaly, prominent forehead, low-set ears, high arched palate, and cardiac anomaly; there may be a submicroscopic chromosomal defect, but there is evidence that this s. is

sy

due to mutation in the gene encoding transcriptional coactivator CREB-binding protein (CREB) on chromosome 16p.

Rud s. [MIM*308200], ichthyosiform erythroderma associated with acanthosis nigricans, dwarfism, hypogonadism, and epilepsy; mostly sporadic, but may be an X-linked recessive trait.

runting s., if newborn mice are thymectomized, they do not gain weight and their lymphoid tissue atrophies. SYN wasting s. (1).

Russell s., failure of infants and young children to thrive due to suprasellar lesions, commonly astrocytomas of the anterior third ventricle; although the growth hormone may be elevated, the child is emaciated and has loss of body fat. SEE ALSO pseudohydrocephaly.

Saethre-Chotzen s., condition characterized by craniosynostosis, asymmetry of skull (plagiocephaly), ptosis, prominent ear crus, and cutaneous syndactyly of fingers 2–3 and toes 3–4; autosomal dominant inheritance, caused by mutation in the TWIST transcription factor gene on chromosome 7p. SYN Chotzen s., type III acrocephalosyndactyly.

salt depletion s., SYN low salt s.

salt-losing s., SYN salt-losing *nephritis*.

Samter s., a triad of asthma, nasal polyps, and aspirin intolerance.

Sanchez Salorio s., a s. characterized by retinal pigmentary dystrophy, cataract, hypotrichosis of the lashes, mental deficiencies, and retarded somatic development.

Sandifer s., torticollis (q.v.) in infants, associated with gastroesophageal reflux; may be a mechanism to protect the airway or reduce acid reflux–associated pain.

Sanfilippo s. [MIM*252900, MIM*252920, MIM*252930,], an error of the mucopolysaccharide metabolism, with excretion of large amounts of heparan sulfate in the urine; characterized by severe mental retardation with hepatomegaly; skeleton may be normal or may present mild changes similar to those in Hurler s.; several different types (A, B, C, and D) have been identified according to the enzyme deficiency; autosomal recessive inheritance. SYN type III mucopolysaccharidosis.

Savage s., obsolete term for resistant ovary s. [from surname of first reported patient]

scalded mouth s., a s. in which the patient complains of a burning sensation of the tongue, lips, throat, or palate, likened to scalding caused by hot liquids; clinically the tissues appear normal; it has been associated with angiotensin-converting enzyme (ACE) inhibitors.

scalded skin s., SEE staphylococcal scalded skin s.

scalenus anterior s., one of the precursors of disputed neurogenic thoracic outlet s.; a popular cause for upper extremity discomfort in the late 1930s and 1940s, based on the unproven concept that the lower trunk of the brachial plexus and the subclavian artery could be compressed in the intrascalene triangle by a hypertrophic scalenus anticus muscle, the compression in turn affecting the nerves to it and setting up a vicious circle; this concept was essentially abandoned in the 1950s, when actual causes, such as cervical radiculopathy and carpal tunnel syndrome, for upper extremity symptoms were appreciated, but resurrected in the 1980s, without attribution, as etiology for upper plexus type of disputed neurologic thoracic outlet syndrome.

scapulocostal s., pain of insidious development in the upper or posterior part of the shoulder radiating into the neck and occiput, down the arm, or around the chest; there may be numbness or tingling in the fingers; attributed to an alteration from the normal relationship between the scapula and posterior wall of the thorax.

Schaumann s., SYN sarcoidosis.

Scheie s. [MIM*252800], allelic to Hurler s. but with a much milder phenotype; characterized by α-L-iduronidase deficiency, corneal clouding, deformity of the hands, aortic valve involvement, and normal intelligence; autosomal recessive inheritance, caused by mutation in the alpha-L-iduronidase gene (IUDA) on chromosome 4p. SYN type IS mucopolysaccharidosis.

Schmid-Fraccaro s., SYN cat's-eye s.

Schmidt s., (1) unilateral paralysis of a vocal cord, the velum palati, trapezius, and sternocleidomastoid. [J.F.M. Schmidt] (2) the association of primary hypothyroidism, primary adrenocorti-

cal insufficiency, and insulin-dependent diabetes mellitus. [M.B. Schmidt]

Schnitzler s., tense, generalized chronic urticaria, joint or bone pain, and monoclonal gammopathy of kappa type.

Schönlein-Henoch s., SYN Henoch-Schönlein *purpura*.

Schüller s., SYN Hand-Schüller-Christian *disease*.

Schwartz s. [MIM*255800], a congenital disorder characterized by myotonic myopathy, dystrophy of epiphyseal cartilages resulting in dwarfism, joint contractures, blepharophimosis, and characteristic facies; autosomal recessive inheritance.

Seckel s. [MIM*210600], an autosomal recessive disorder characterized by low birth weight, dwarfism, microcephaly, large eyes, beaked nose, receding mandible, and moderate mental retardation. SYN Seckel dwarfism.

Seip s., SYN congenital total *lipodystrophy*.

Senear-Usher s., SYN *pemphigus* erythematosus.

sepsis s., clinical evidence of acute infection with hyperthermia or hypothermia, tachycardia, tachypnea and evidence of inadequate organ function or perfusion manifested by at least one of the following: altered mental status, hypoxemia, acidosis, oliguria, or disseminated intravascular coagulation.

Sertoli-cell-only s. [MIM*305700], the absence from the seminiferous tubules of the testes of germinal epithelium, Sertoli cells alone being present; there is sterility due to azoospermia but no other sexual abnormality, Leydig cells are normal, and the level of gonadotrophins in the plasma and urine is increased; probably represents one form of seminiferous tubule dysgenesis. SYN Del Castillo s.

Sézary s., exfoliative dermatitis with intense pruritus, resulting from cutaneous infiltration by atypical mononuclear cells (T lymphocytes with markedly convoluted or cerebriform nuclei) also found in the peripheral blood, and associated with alopecia, edema, and nail and pigmentary changes; a variant of mycosis fungoides. SYN Sézary erythroderma.

---

shaken baby s. (SBS), a s. of neurologic and other injuries, of variable presentation, induced by the violent shaking of an infant.

> Shaken baby syndrome is an increasingly recognized form of child abuse. Vigorous shaking of an infant, with or without direct violence to the head, can result in spinal cord injury or intracranial bleeding, with irreversible brain damage, blindness, hearing loss, seizures, learning disabilities, paralysis, or death. SBS occurs most often before the age of 1 and seldom after age 2. Infants under 6 months are particularly vulnerable because of their disproportionately heavy heads, weak neck muscles, and thin skulls. About 1000 babies are hospitalized annually in the U.S. with this diagnosis; about 25% of them die and about 25% of the survivors suffer irreversible brain damage. Men are more likely than women to inflict injury by shaking. Boys are more likely than girls to be victims, and twins are at higher risk than singletons. Most cases occur as an impulsive response of the caregiver to a child's persistent crying. In the typical incident, no one is present but the caregiver and the victim. There may be a prior history of abuse, or evidence of previous injury. The guilty person may invent a story of accidental injury to explain the findings. Signs of SBS vary widely, from a flulike presentation or lethargy to unexplained vomiting, seizures, or coma. The classical triad of subdural hematoma, cerebral edema, and retinal or subhyaloid hemorrhage is often absent. Finger marks may be found on the chest wall or around the shoulders, but often there are no external signs of injury. One-half of patients with subdural hematoma have no skull fracture. Prevention of shaken baby syndrome requires education of parents and others entrusted with the care of small children as to the grave danger of shaking a baby. New parents should be informed that all babies cry and that shaking is never an appropriate response. Alternative modes of coping with the stress of a crying baby should be planned. Parents must also exercise caution in selecting babysitters, day-care centers, or childcare agencies. All caregivers should be enjoined never to

touch a child in anger. Health professionals must be alert for subtle signs of SBS and other forms of child abuse.

Sheehan s., hypopituitarism developing postpartum as a result of pituitary necrosis; caused by ischemia resulting from a hypotensive episode during delivery. SYN pituitary cachexia, postpartum pituitary necrosis s., Simmonds disease, thyrohypophysial s.

Shone s., the association of obstructive lesions of the mitral valve complex, including supravalvar ring and parachute mitral valve, with left ventricular outflow obstruction and coarctation of the aorta.

short-bowel s., malabsorption and maldigestion resulting from disease or resection of large portions of the small intestine.

shoulder-girdle s., SYN neuralgic *amyotrophy.*

shoulder-hand s., SYN reflex sympathetic *dystrophy.*

Shprintzen s., SYN velocardiofacial s.

Shulman s., SYN eosinophilic *fasciitis.*

Shwachman s. [MIM*260400], an autosomal recessive disorder characterized by sinusitis, bronchiectasis, pancreatic insufficiency resulting in malabsorption, neutropenia with defect in neutrophile chemotaxis, short stature, and skeletal changes with radiographic findings of metaphyseal flaring of long bones. SYN Shwachman-Diamond s.

Shwachman-Diamond s., SYN Shwachman s.

Shy-Drager s. [MIM*146500], a now-obsolete term for multiple system atrophy in which autonomic nervous system failure predominates.

sicca s., SYN Sjögren s.

sick building s., old term for building-related illness.

sick euthyroid s., SYN euthyroid sick s.

▮**sick sinus s.** [MIM*182190], symptoms ranging from dizziness to unconsciousness due to chaotic or absent atrial activity often with bradycardia alternating with tachycardia, recurring ectopic beats including escape beats, runs of supraventricular and ventricular arrhythmias, sinus arrest, and sinoatrial block.

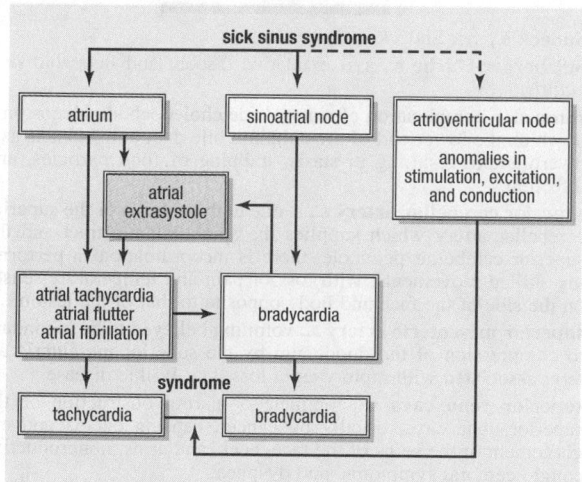

sick sinus syndrome: schematic diagram of pathogenesis of sick sinus syndrome showing tachycardial and bradycardial anomalies

Silver-Russell s. [MIM*270050], a disorder characterized by low birth weight, late closure of the anterior fontanel, bilateral bodily asymmetry, clinodactyly of the fifth fingers, triangular facies, and carp mouth; little useful genetic evidence. SYN Silver-Russell dwarfism.

Silverskiöld s., a type of osteochondrodystrophy with only slight vertebral changes but with shortened and curved long bones of the extremities.

Sinding-Larsen-Johansson s., apophysitis of the distal pole of the patella.

sinus venosus s., the association of partial anomalous, pulmonary-venous connection, and a small venosus ASD.

Sipple s. [MIM*171400], pheochromocytoma, medullary carcinoma of the thyroid, and parathyroid adenomas; autosomal dominant inheritance, caused by mutation in the RET oncogene on chromosome 10q.

Sjögren s., keratoconjunctivitis sicca, dryness of mucous membranes, telangiectasias or purpuric spots on the face, and bilateral parotid enlargement; seen in menopausal women and often associated with rheumatoid arthritis, Raynaud phenomenon, and dental caries; there are changes in the lacrimal and salivary glands resembling those of Mikulicz disease. SYN Gougerot-Sjögren disease, sicca s., Sjögren disease. [H.S.C. Sjögren]

Sjögren-Larsson s. [MIM*270200], congenital ichthyosis in association with oligophrenia and spastic paraplegia; autosomal recessive inheritance, caused by mutation in the fatty aldehyde dehydrogenase gene (FALDH) on chromosome 17p.

sleep apnea s., a disorder characterized by multiple episodes of partial or complete cessation of respiration during sleep.

sleep phase delay s., a disorder in which the circadian rhythm of sleep and waking falls into a delayed but stable relationship with external time cues of day and night.

SLE-like s., a disease with manifestations suggestive of systemic lupus erythematosus, without meeting diagnostic criteria for that disease; sometimes used for drug-induced lupus.

slit ventricle s., in shunt-dependent patients, a state characterized by intermittent or chronic headaches, small ventricles, and slow reflux of the valve mechanism.

Sly s., an autosomal recessive disorder due to a deficiency of a β-glucuronidase; defective lysosomal degradation of dermatan sulfate, heparan sulfate, and chondroitin sulfate; cellular function disrupted in most tissues. SYN type VII mucopolysaccharidosis (1).

Smith-Lemli-Opitz s. [MIM*270400], mental retardation, small stature, anteverted nostrils, ptosis, male genital anomalies, and syndactyly of the second and third toes, often in breech-born babies with delayed fetal activity; inherited as an autosomal recessive trait.

Smith-Riley s., multiple hemangiomas, macrocephaly, and blurred optic disks; angiomas appear at birth or later, and enlarge and multiply.

Sneddon s., a cerebral arteriopathy of unknown etiology, characterized by noninflammatory intimal hyperplasia of medium-sized vessels associated with diffuse cutaneous livedo reticularis.

Sohval-Soffer s. [MIM 307500], hypogonadism, gynecomastia, skeletal anomalies, and mental retardation; probably X-linked inheritance.

Sorsby s., congenital macular coloboma and apical dystrophy of the extremities.

Sotos s. [MIM*117550], cerebral gigantism and generalized large muscles in childhood, with mental retardation and defective coordination; of unknown etiology. Most cases have been sporadic, perhaps new dominant mutations with low fitness, but there is one set of concordant identical twins on record.

space adaptation s., alterations in normal physiology that occur during prolonged exposure to weightlessness, unless preventive measures are taken. Characterized by muscle atrophy, loss of mineral from bones, cardiovascular changes, etc.

Spens s., SYN Adams-Stokes s.

splenic flexure s., symptoms of pain, gas, bloating, a sense of fullness experienced in the left upper abdominal quadrant, sometimes beneath the ribs, in some instances radiating upward, and in some instances producing anterior chest pain central or predominantly on the left. It may be induced experimentally by the introduction and trapping of air in the splenic flexure.

staphylococcal scalded skin s., a disease affecting infants in which large areas of skin peel off, as in a second-degree burn, as a result of upper respiratory staphylococcal infection even though the skin lesions are sterile; the level of skin separation is subcorneal, unlike a burn or the clinically similar toxic epidermal necrolysis which occurs in children and adults and which involves subepidermal cleavage. SYN Lyell disease.

sy

Stauffer s., elevation of liver function tests, in the absence of metastatic disease, due to cholestasis in renal cell cancer patients.

Steele-Richardson-Olszewski s., SYN progressive supranuclear *palsy.*

Stein-Leventhal s., SYN polycystic ovary s.

steroid withdrawal s., a condition exhibited by persons who previously had been receiving large therapeutic doses of glucocorticoid hormones for long periods of time; pituitary-adrenocortical insufficiency is manifested, particularly during stress, for as long as a year or more thereafter and varying degrees of emotional disturbance may be exhibited.

Stevens-Johnson s., a bullous form of erythema multiforme which may be extensive, involving the mucous membranes and large areas of the body; it may produce serious subjective symptoms and may have a fatal termination. SEE ALSO ocular-mucous membrane s. SYN erythema multiforme bullosum, erythema multiforme exudativum, erythema multiforme major.

Stewart-Morel s., SYN Morgagni s.

Stewart-Treves s., angiosarcoma arising in arms affected by postmastectomy lymphedema.

Stickler s., SYN hereditary progressive *arthroophthalmopathy.*

stiff heart s., any condition, usually acute, that causes the heart to be restricted in diastole mainly affecting the ventricles and at one time a complication of cardiac surgery.

stiff man s., a rare disorder manifested clinically by the continuous isometric contraction of many of the somatic muscles; contractions are usually forceful and painful and most frequently involve the trunk musculature, although limb muscles may be involved. This is an autoimmune disease, with circulating antibodies against the GABA-synthesizing enzyme and glutamic acid decarboxylase, among other types of antibodies present.

Still-Chauffard s., SYN Chauffard s.

Stockholm s., a form of bonding between a captive and captor in which the captive begins to identify with, and may even sympathize with, the captor. [*Stockholm,* Sweden, where early case reported]

Stokes-Adams s., SYN Adams-Stokes s.

straight back s., loss of the normal concavity of the thoracolumbar spine with a narrowed anteroposterior chest dimension, resulting compression of the heart between spine and sternum, and consequent prominent precordial pulsations, an ejection murmur, and radiologic evidence of a widened cardiac silhouette (pancaked heart).

streptococcal toxic shock s., a toxic s. characterized by hypotension and a variety of signs and symptoms indicative of multiorgan failure including cerebral dysfunction, renal failure, acute respiratory distress s., toxic cardiomyopathy, and hepatic dysfunction. The s. is usually precipitated by local infections of skin or soft tissue by streptococci; mortality of 30% has been reported.

Stryker-Halbeisen s., reddish, scaling, macular eruption on the head and upper trunk due to vitamin B complex deficiency; associated with macrocytic anemia.

Sturge-Kalischer-Weber s., SYN Sturge-Weber s.

Sturge-Weber s. [MIM*185300], in its complete form, a triad of unilateral occurrence of 1) congenital capillary malformation (flame nevus) in the distribution of the trigeminal nerve; 2) leptomeningeal vascular malformations with intracranial calcification and neurologic signs; and 3) vascular malformation of the choroid, often with secondary glaucoma. Inheritance is unclear with most cases sporadic. SEE ALSO encephalotrigeminal vascular s. SYN cephalotrigeminal angiomatosis, encephalotrigeminal angiomatosis, Sturge-Kalischer-Weber s., Sturge-Weber disease.

subclavian steal s., symptoms of vertebrobasilar insufficiency resulting from subclavian steal.

subcoracoid-pectoralis minor tendon s., SYN hyperabduction s.

sudden infant death s. (SIDS), the sudden death of an apparently healthy infant that remains unexplained after all known possible causes have been ruled out through autopsy, death scene investigation, and review of the medical history. SYN cot death, crib death.

SIDS is the leading cause of death in infants between 1

week and 1 year of age, with an approximate rate of 2 per 1000 live births; 6000–7000 babies die of SIDS every year in the U.S. The peak age is 2–4 months and most deaths occur during the winter months (October to April in the northern hemisphere). The case definition specifically excludes death due to drugs or poisons, apnea, respiratory infection, suffocation, aspiration of vomitus, choking, accidental strangulation, and child abuse. Most victims appear healthy before death, which occurs rapidly, usually during sleep. SIDS strikes families of all races and socioeconomic levels. It is slightly more common in males, and the second child is more susceptible than the first. Some theories suggest a congenital or developmental defect, but the phenomenon does not show familial clustering. In the present state of knowledge, SIDS cannot be predicted, prevented, or reversed. However, statistical studies have identified certain risk factors, among them maternal smoking before and after birth, inadequate prenatal care, low birth weight, young maternal age, and maternal hard drug use. Some but not all studies have suggested that breastfeeding slightly reduces the risk. Gastric infection with *Helicobacter pylori* has been speculatively implicated in some cases. The most important risk factor identified to date is sleeping in the prone position. Sleeping on the side is less dangerous than sleeping prone, but more dangerous than sleeping supine. The reason for these differences is unknown, but the incidence of SIDS has markedly declined since 1992, when the American Academy of Pediatrics first recommended that healthy infants be placed on their backs for sleep. For infants with gastroesophageal reflux, swallowing dysfunction, or unilateral vocal cord paralysis, the prone position may be preferred. For healthy infants, the supine position does not increase the risk of vomiting and aspiration. Current medical practice emphasizes reduction of risk through avoidance of the prone sleeping position and of maternal smoking, and education, counseling, and emotional support of the parents of victims.

Sudeck s., SYN Sudeck *atrophy.*

Sulzberger-Garbe s., SYN exudative discoid and lichenoid *dermatitis.*

sump s., a complication of side-to-side choledochoduodenostomy in which the lower end of the common bile duct at times acts as a diverticulum, resulting in stasis, trapping of food particles, and infection.

superior cerebellar artery s., s. due to thrombosis of the superior cerebellar artery which supplies the spinothalamic tract and the superior cerebellar peduncle; there is incoordination in performing skilled movements, with loss of pain and temperature senses on the side of the face and body opposite to that of the lesion.

superior mesenteric artery s., vomiting believed to be secondary to compression of the duodenum by the superior mesenteric artery; associated with rapid weight loss. SYN Wilkie disease.

superior vena cava s., complete or partial obstruction of the superior vena cava, usually by cancer, causing edema and engorgement of the veins of the face, neck, and arms, nonproductive cough, cerebral symptoms, and dyspnea.

supine hypotensive s., in the supine pregnant woman at or near term, maternal hypotension; maternal hypotension is due to obstruction by the gravid uterus of the inferior vena cava with resulting decrease in venous return to the heart; fetal hypoxia is due to maternal hypotension and obstruction of the maternal aorta by the gravid uterus with resulting decrease in placental perfusion.

supraspinatus s., pain on elevation of the shoulder and tenderness on deep pressure over the supraspinatus tendon; due to pressure of an injured or inflamed tendon or inflamed subacromial bursa coming into contact or pressing on the overlying acromial process when the arm is elevated over the shoulder level. SYN impingement s., painful arc s.

supravalvar aortic stenosis s. [MIM*185500], supravalvar aortic stenosis (usually membranous) sometimes associated with pulmonary valvar or peripheral arterial stenosis but with normal facies and mentality; autosomal dominant inheritance, caused by mutation in the elastin gene (ELN) on chromosome 7q. Cf. Williams s.

supravalvar aortic stenosis-infantile hypercalcemia s. [MIM* 194050], SYN Williams s.

surdocardiac s., SYN Jervell and Lange-Nielsen s.

sweaty feet s., SYN isovaleric acidemia.

swollen belly s., SYN swollen belly *disease*.

Swyer s., gonadal dysgenesis in phenotypic females with XY genotype.

Swyer-James s., (1) SYN unilateral lobar *emphysema*; **(2)** hyperlucency of one lung from obliterating bronchiolitis, usually caused by adenovirus infection in childhood, with decreased size and vascularity of the lung; distinguished from other causes of unilateral hyperlucency by demonstration of air trapping without central obstruction.

Swyer-James-MacLeod s., SYN unilateral lobar *emphysema*.

tachybradycardia s., SYN bradytachycardia s.

tachycardia-bradycardia s., alternating periods of slow and rapid heart beat; often associated with disturbances of both sinoatrial and atrioventricular conduction. SEE ALSO sick sinus s.

Takayasu s., SYN Takayasu *arteritis*.

Tapia s., unilateral paralysis of the larynx, the velum palati, and the tongue, with atrophy of the latter.

tarsal tunnel s., s. produced by entrapment neuropathy of terminal branches of posterior tibial nerve (medial plantar, lateral plantar, and calcanial nerves) at the ankle.

Taussig-Bing s., complete transposition of the aorta, which arises from the right ventricle, with a left-sided pulmonary artery overriding the left ventricle, and with high ventricular septal defect, right ventricular hypertrophy, anteriorly situated aorta, and posteriorly situated pulmonary artery. SYN Taussig-Bing disease.

tegmental s., a s. usually caused by a vascular lesion in the tegmentum; marked by contralateral hemiplegia and ipsilateral ocular paresis.

temporomandibular s., symptoms of discomfort and pain caused by loss of vertical dimension, lack of posterior occlusion, or other malocclusion, trismus, muscle tremor, arthritis, or direct trauma to the temporomandibular joint.

temporomandibular joint pain-dysfunction s., SYN myofascial pain-dysfunction s.

tendon sheath s., limited elevation of the eye in adduction, appearing clinically as a paresis of the inferior oblique muscle, due to fascia contracting the superior oblique muscle on the same side. SYN Brown s., Paterson-Brown-Kelly s.

Terry s., SYN *retinopathy* of prematurity.

Terson s., vitreous, retinal, and subhyaloid hemorrhages associated with subarachnoid hemorrhage.

testicular feminization s. [MIM*313700], a type of male pseudohermaphroditism characterized by female external genitalia (may be ambiguous if the s. is incomplete), incompletely developed vagina often with rudimentary uterus and fallopian tubes, female habitus at puberty but with scanty or absent axillary and pubic hair and amenorrhea, and testes present within the abdomen or in the inguinal canals or labia majora; epididymis and vas deferens are usually present; androgens and estrogens are formed, but target tissues are largely unresponsive to androgens; individuals have a normal male karyotype; X-linked recessive inheritance, caused by mutation in the androgen receptor gene (AR) on chromosome Xq.

tethered cord s., abnormal low positioning (below the L_2 vertebrae) of the distal spinal cord (conus medullaris) by the filum terminale. May be associated with incontinence, progressive motor and sensory impairment in the legs, pain, and scoliosis.

thalamic s., a s. produced by infarction of the posteroinferior thalamus causing transient hemiparesis, severe loss of superficial and deep sensation with preservation of crude pain in the hypalgic limbs which frequently have vasomotor or trophic disturbances. SYN Dejerine-Roussy s.

Thiemann s., avascular necrosis of the epiphyses of phalanges of fingers or toes, usually familial, beginning in childhood or adolescence, leading to deformity of fingers; also called familial arthropathy of the fingers or toes. SYN Thiemann disease.

third and fourth pharyngeal pouch s., SYN DiGeorge s.

thoracic outlet s. (TOS), collective title for a number of conditions attributed to compromise of blood vessels or nerve fibers (brachial plexus) at any point between the base of the neck and the axilla; formerly classified on the basis of presumed injurious structure or mechanism, i.e., scalenus anticus syndrome, hyperabduction syndrome, costoclavicular syndrome; currently classified on the basis of the structure known or presumed to be compromised, and divided into two main groups: vascular and neurologic (simultaneous compromise of both neural and vascular structures is rare); vascular subdivisions include arterial and venous.

Thorn s., SYN salt-losing *nephritis*.

thrombocytopenia-absent radius s., TAR s. [MIM*274000], congenital absence of the radius associated with thrombocytopenia that is symptomatic in infancy but later improves; congenital heart disease and renal anomalies occur in some cases; autosomal recessive inheritance.

thrombopathic s., a nondescript term to describe any of a number of bleeding diseases in which clot formation is deficient rather than those in which there is an organic fault of the blood vessels.

thyrohypophysial s., SYN Sheehan s.

Tietz s., autosomal dominant inheritance of albinism and deafness caused at least in some subsets of families by a mutation of the microophthalmia transcription factor gene.

Tietze s., inflammation and painful, tender nonsuppurative swelling of a costochondral junction. SYN peristernal perichondritis.

Tolosa-Hunt s., cavernous sinus s. produced by an idiopathic granuloma.

tooth-and-nail s. [MIM*189500], hypodontia associated with absent or very small nails at birth. Common among Dutch Mennonites in Canada.

TORCH s., a group of infections seen in neonates that have crossed the placental barrier with similar clinical manifestations, although symptoms may vary in degree and time of appearance: *t*oxoplasmosis, *o*ther infections, *r*ubella, *c*ytomegalovirus infection, and *h*erpes simplex.

Tornwaldt s., nasopharyngeal discharge, occipital headache, and stiffness of posterior cervical muscles, with halitosis due to chronic infection of the pharyngeal bursa.

Torre s., multiple sebaceous gland adenomas associated with multiple visceral malignancies, often colorectal carcinoma. SYN Muir-Torre s.

Torsten Sjögren s., SYN Marinesco-Garland s.

Tourette s., a tic disorder appearing in childhood, characterized by multiple motor tics and vocal tics present for more than 1 year. Obsessive-compulsive behavior, attention-deficit disorder, and other psychiatric disorders may be associated; coprolalia and echolalia rarely occur; autosomal dominant inheritance. SYN Gilles de la Tourette disease, Gilles de la Tourette s., Tourette disease.

toxic shock s. (TSS), infection with toxin-producing staphylococci, occurring most often in the vagina of menstruating women using superabsorbent tampons but also prevalent in many soft tissue infections and characterized by high fever, vomiting, diarrhea, a scarlatiniform rash followed by desquamation, and decreasing blood pressure and shock, which can result in death; hyperemia of the conjunctival, oropharyngeal, and vaginal mucous membranes also occurs.

transplant lung s., a s. associated with fever and diffuse bilateral pulmonary infiltration mainly at the base or at the hilum of the lung; can accompany rejection of an organ (kidney, liver, etc.) transplant or follow a reduction in dosage of an immunosuppressive drug.

transurethral resection s., absorption of glycine from irrigation solution during TUR that the liver cannot metabolize, resulting in increased serum ammonia. SYN TUR s.

Treacher Collins s. [MIM*154500], mandibulofacial *dysostosis*, when limited to the orbit and malar region.

trichorhinophalangeal s., a condition characterized by sparse fine hair, broad nose with a long philtrum, swollen middle phalanges with cone-shaped epiphyses, and growth retardation. There

sy

seem to be at least three similar disorders, two dominant [MIM*150230 and MIM 190350] and one recessive [MIM*275500].

triple A s. [MIM*231550], autosomal recessive syndrome associated with *a*chalasia of the cardia, and *a*lacrima; associated problems include abnormalities of the nervous system such as mental retardation and autonomic dysfunction. SYN Allgrove s.

triple X s., trisomy of the X chromosome; original observations (made in mental institutions) were seriously biased and the phenotypic changes spurious. Intelligence may be at the lower range of normal, stature is usually tall, there may be speech and behavioral problems. The outstanding feature of the s. is the occurrence of twin Barr bodies in a typical cell.

trisomy 8 s., the full trisomy 8 is usually associated with early lethality, but most affected individuals are mosaic with craniofacial dysmorphism; short, wide neck; narrow cylindrical trunk; multiple joint and digital abnormalities; and deep creases of the palms and soles.

trisomy 13 s., a chromosomal disorder that is usually fatal within 2 years; characterized by mental retardation, malformed ears, cleft lip or palate, microphthalmia or coloboma, small mandible, polydactyly, cardiac defects, convulsions, renal anomalies, umbilical hernia, malrotation of intestines, and dermatoglyphic anomalies. SYN Patau s., trisomy D s.

trisomy 18 s., a chromosomal disorder that is usually fatal within 2–3 years; characterized by mental retardation, abnormal skull shape, lowset and malformed ears, small mandible, cardiac defects, short sternum, diaphragmatic or inguinal hernia, Meckel diverticulum, abnormal flexion of fingers, and dermatoglyphic anomalies. SYN Edwards s.

trisomy 20 s., a chromosomal disorder characterized by profound mental retardation, coarse facies, macrostomia and macroglossia, minor anomalies of the ears, pigmentary dysplasia of the skin, dorsal kyphoscoliosis, and other skeletal defects.

trisomy 21 s., SYN Down s.

trisomy C s., trisomy for any chromosome of group C, numbers 6–12, most often number 8.

trisomy D s., SYN trisomy 13 s.

trochanteric s., tendonitis and bursitis around the greater trochanter.

trophic s., ulceration of a denervated area, frequently secondary to picking at the anesthetic surface.

tropical splenomegaly s., SYN hyperreactive malarious splenomegaly.

Trousseau s., thrombophlebitis migrans associated with visceral cancer.

true neurogenic thoracic outlet s., very chronic axon loss brachial plexopathy, caused by compromise of the lower trunk fibers by a congenital band extending from a rudimentary cervical rib to the first thoracic rib; rare disorder, found mostly in young to middle-aged women, that presents with unilateral hand wasting and weakness, particularly involving the lateral thenar eminence; sometimes accompanied by intermittent discomfort along the medial forearm and hand. SYN cervical rib and band s., classic cervical rib s.

tumor lysis s., hyperphosphatemia, hypocalcemia, hyperkalemia, and hyperuricemia following induction chemotherapy of malignant neoplasms; believed to be due to the release of intracellular products by cell lysis.

TUR s., SYN transurethral resection s.

Turcot s. [MIM*276300], a rare and distinctive form of multiple intestinal polyposis associated with brain tumors; autosomal recessive inheritance, caused by mutation in one of the mismatch repair genes: either MLH1 on chromosome 3p, PMS2 on chromosome 7p, or the adenomatous polyposis coli gene (APC) on 5q.

Turner s., a s. with chromosome count 45 and only one X chromosome; buccal and other cells are usually sex chromatin-negative; anomalies include dwarfism, webbed neck, valgus of elbows, pigeon chest, infantile sexual development, and amenorrhea; the ovary has no primordial follicles and may be represented only by a fibrous streak; some individuals are chromosomal mosaic, with two or more cell lines of different chromosome constitution; seen in many animal species, in the meadow vole it is the normal female state. SYN XO s.

twiddler's s., condition in which a cardiac pacemaker wire is pulled out of position in the heart with rotation of the subcutaneous pacemaker by the patient's "twiddling."

Uhthoff s., SYN Uhthoff symptom.

Ullmann s., a systemic angiomatosis due to multiple arteriovenous malformations.

Ulysses s., the ill effects of extensive diagnostic investigations conducted because of a false-positive result in the course of routine laboratory screening. [L. Ulysses, fr. G. Odysseus, myth. char.]

uncombable hair s., a genetic syndrome in which the hair, which is often silvery blond, is unruly and resists lying flat because of irregularly shaped hair shafts. SYN spun glass hair.

Unna-Thost s., SYN diffuse hyperkeratosis of palms and soles.

unroofed coronary sinus s., a spectrum of cardiac anomalies in which part or all of the common wall between the coronary sinus and the left atrium is absent.

urethral s., a condition of no certain etiology, characterized by urinary frequency, urgency, dysuria in the absence of specific infection, obstruction, or dysfunction. Suprapubic pain, hesitancy, and back pain may also occur. Usually seen in females.

Usher s. [MIM*276900, MIM*276901], autosomal recessive inheritance with genetic heterogeneity; the three forms are distinguishable by linkage data: type 1 causes sensorineural hearing loss, loss of vestibular function, and retinitis pigmentosa; types 2 and 3 are characterized by hearing loss and retinitis pigmentosa.

uveocutaneous s., SYN Vogt-Koyanagi s.

uveoencephalitic s., SYN Behçet s.

uveomeningitis s., SYN Harada s.

VACTERL s., abnormalities of *v*ertebrae, *a*nus, *c*ardiovascular tree, *t*rachea, *e*sophagus, *r*enal system, and *l*imb buds reportedly associated with administration of sex steroids during early pregnancy.

van Buchem s. [MIM*239100], an osteosclerosing skeletal dysplasia, characterized by mandibular enlargement, thickening of the diaphyses and calvaria, and increased serum alkaline phosphatase; autosomal recessive inheritance. SYN generalized cortical hyperostosis.

van der Hoeve s., a subtype of osteogenesis imperfecta in which progressive conductive hearing loss begins in childhood because of stapedial fixation.

vanished testis s., absence of both testes in a male with normal chromosomes (XY) and otherwise normal genitalia at birth and during childhood. Testes were present in at least the first trimester of gestation, but vanished sometime thereafter.

vanishing lung s., progressive decrease of radiographic opacity of the lung caused by accelerated development of emphysema or rapid cystic destruction of the lung from infection.

Van Lohuizen s., SYN cutis marmorata telangiectatica congenita.

vasculocardiac s. of hyperserotonemia, obsolete term for carcinoid s.

vasovagal s., SYN Gowers s.

velocardiofacial s. [MIM*192430], a s. with hypernasal speech, dysmorphic facial features (long midface, cylindrical nose, downward turned corners of mouth), and cardiac abnormalities; same chromosomal abnormality as seen in DiGeorge s. (a microdeletion in chromosome 22q11); dominant inheritance. SYN Shprintzen s.

Verner-Morrison s., watery diarrhea, hypokalemia, and achlorhydria associated with secretion of vasoactive intestinal polypeptide by a pancreatic islet-cell tumor in the absence of gastric hypersecretion. SYN WDHA s.

Vernet s., a s. characterized by paralysis of the motor components of the glossopharyngeal, vagus, and accessory cranial nerves as they lie in the posterior fossa; it is most commonly the result of head injury.

vertical retraction s., SEE retraction s.

vibration s., tingling, numbness, and blanching of the fingers resulting from use of hand-held vibration tools; may persist without further exposure to vibration.

virus-associated hemophagocytic s., a s. closely resembling malignant histiocytosis but potentially reversible, following a herpes group virus infection such as by the Epstein-Barr virus.

vitreoretinal choroidopathy s. [MIM*193220], an ocular condition characterized by peripheral pigmentary retinopathy, retinal vascular abnormalities, vitreous opacities, choroidal atrophy, and presenile cataracts; autosomal dominant inheritance.

vitreoretinal traction s., traction on the internal limiting membrane of the retina by adherent vitreous fibrils in vitreous humor detachment.

Vogt s., SYN double *athetosis*. [Cècile and Oscar Vogt]

Vogt-Koyanagi s., bilateral uveitis with iritis and glaucoma, premature graying of the hair, and alopecia, vitiligo, and dysacusia; related to Harada s. and sympathetic ophthalmia. SYN oculocutaneous s., uveocutaneous s.

Vohwinkel s., SYN mutilating *keratoderma*.

voice fatigue s., weakness and loss of the voice usually toward the end of the day because of abuse by using it too long and too loudly.

von Hippel-Lindau s. [MIM*193300], a type of phacomatosis, consisting of retinal vascular malformations, which may be multiple and bilateral, associated with hemangioblastomas primarily of the cerebellum and walls of the fourth ventricle, occasionally involving the spinal cord; sometimes associated with renal cell carcinomas or cysts or hamartomas of kidney, adrenal, or other organs; autosomal dominant inheritance due to mutation in the von Hippel-Lindau gene (VHL) on 3p. SYN cerebroretinal angiomatosis, Lindau disease.

vulnerable child s., a reaction characterized by disturbance in psychosocial development, often occurring in children whose parents expect them to die prematurely.

Waardenburg s. [MIM*193500, MIM*193510], disorder characterized by lateral displacement of inner canthi (dystopia canthorum), broad nasal root, heterochromia iridis, cochlear deafness, white forelock, and synophrys; autosomal dominant inheritance with type I distinguished from type II by the presence of dystopia canthorum. Type I is caused by mutation in the PAX3 gene on chromosome 2q while some cases of type II are caused by mutation in the microphthalmia-associated transcription factor gene (MITF) on chromosome 3p.

Wagner s., SYN hyaloideoretinal *degeneration*.

WAGR s., acronym for *W*ilms tumor, *a*niridia, *g*enitourinary malformations, and mental *r*etardation.

Waldenström s., SYN Waldenström *macroglobulinemia*.

Wallenberg s., SYN posterior inferior cerebellar artery s.

Ward-Romano s., SYN Romano-Ward s.

wasting s., (1) SYN runting s; (2) progressive involuntary weight loss seen in patients with HIV infection; may be due to a number of factors acting alone or in combination, including inadequate oral intake of food, altered metabolic state and/or malabsorption. Does not respond to increased caloric intake. Defined as profound involuntary weight loss of greater than 10% of baseline body weight, plus either chronic diarrhea (at least 2 loose stools per day for >30 days or chronic weakness and documented fever (for >30 days, intermittent or constant) in the absence of concurrent illness or condition other than HIV infection that could explain the findings (such as cancer, tuberculosis, cryptosporidiosis, or other specific enteritis). SYN HIV wasting s.

Waterhouse-Friderichsen s., a condition occurring mainly in children under 10 years of age, characterized by vomiting, diarrhea, extensive purpura, cyanosis, tonic-clonic convulsions, and circulatory collapse, usually with meningitis and hemorrhage into the adrenal glands. SYN acute fulminating meningococcal septicemia, Friderichsen-Waterhouse s.

WDHA s., SYN Verner-Morrison s. [*w*atery *d*iarrhea, *h*ypokalemia, *a*chlorhydria]

Weber s., midbrain tegmentum lesion characterized by ipsilateral oculomotor nerve paresis and contralateral paralysis of the extremities, face, and tongue. SYN Weber sign.

Weber-Cockayne s. [MIM*131800], *epidermolysis* bullosa of the hands and feet; autosomal dominant inheritance, caused by

mutation in the keratin 5 gene (KRT5) on chromosome 12q or keratin 14 gene (KRT14) on 17q.

Weill-Marchesani s. [MIM*277600], ectopia lentis (lens abnormally round and small), short stature, and brachydactyly; autosomal recessive inheritance.

Wells s., SYN eosinophilic *cellulitis*.

Wermer s., SYN multiple endocrine neoplasia s., type 1.

Werner s. [MIM*277700], a prematurely aging disorder consisting of scleroderma-like skin changes, bilateral juvenile cataracts, progeria, hypogonadism, and diabetes mellitus; autosomal recessive inheritance, caused by mutation in the WRN gene, which encodes a helicase protein on chromosome 8p.

Wernicke s., a condition frequently encountered in chronic alcoholics, largely due to thiamin deficiency and characterized by disturbances in ocular motility, pupillary alterations, nystagmus, and ataxia with tremors; an organic-toxic psychosis is often an associated finding, and Korsakoff s. often coexists; characteristic cellular pathology found in several areas of the brain. SYN superior hemorrhagic polioencephalitis, Wernicke disease, Wernicke encephalopathy.

Wernicke-Korsakoff s., the coexistence of Wernicke and Korsakoff s.'s.

West s., an encephalopathy in infancy characterized by infantile spasms, arrest of psychomotor development, and hypsarrhythmia.

Weyers-Thier s., SYN oculovertebral *dysplasia*.

whistling face s., SYN craniocarpotarsal *dystrophy*.

white-out s., a psychosis which occurs in Arctic explorers or others similarly exposed to the stimulus deprivation of a snow-clad environment. SEE ALSO sensory *deprivation*.

Widal s., SYN Hayem-Widal s.

Wildervanck s., SYN cervicooculoacoustic s.

Williams s. [MIM*194050], disorder characterized by distinctive facies with shallow supraorbital ridges, medial eyebrow flare, stellate patterning of the irises, small nose with anteverted nares, malar hypoplasia with droopy cheeks, full lips, supravalvar aortic stenosis, neonatal hypocalcemia, mild mental retardation, and loquacious personality. Autosomal dominant inheritance; this is a contiguous gene deletion s. and one of the genes mutated is the elastin gene (ELN) on chromosome 7q. SYN elfin facies s., supravalvar aortic stenosis-infantile hypercalcemia s., Williams-Beuren s.

Williams-Beuren s., SYN Williams s.

Wilson-Mikity s., SYN pulmonary dysmaturity s.

Wiskott-Aldrich s. [MIM*301000], an immunodeficiency disorder occurring in male children and characterized by thrombocytopenia, eczema, melena, and susceptibility to recurrent bacterial infections; death occurs from severe hemorrhage or overwhelming infection; X-linked recessive inheritance, caused by mutation in the Wiskott-Aldrich syndrome gene (WASP) on chromosome Xp. SYN Aldrich s.

Wissler s., high intermittent fever, irregularly recurring macular and maculopapular eruption of the face, chest and limbs, leukocytosis, arthralgia, occasionally eosinophilia, and raised erythrocyte sedimentation rate; occurs in children and adolescents, with varying duration.

withdrawal s., the development of a substance-specific s. that follows the cessation of, or reduction in, intake of a psychoactive substance that the person previously used regularly; e.g., clinical syndrome of disorientation, perceptual disturbance, and psychomotor agitation following the cessation of chronic use of excessive quantities of alcohol is termed alcohol withdrawal syndrome. The s. that develops varies according to the psychoactive substance used. Common symptoms include anxiety, restlessness, irritability, insomnia, and impaired attention. SEE ALSO abstinence s.

Wolff-Parkinson-White s. [MIM*194200], an electrocardiographic pattern sometimes associated with paroxysmal tachycardia; it consists of short PR interval (usually 0.1 second or less; occasionally normal) together with a prolonged QRS complex with a slurred initial component (delta wave). SYN preexcitation s.

Wolfram s. (DIDMOD), a s. consisting of diabetes insipidus, diabetes mellitus, optic atrophy, and deafness; the genetic abnormality is located on chromosome 4p; autosomal recessive inheritance.

Wright s., SYN hyperabduction s.

Wyburn-Mason s., arteriovenous malformation on the cerebral cortex, retinal arteriovenous malformation, and facial nevus, usually occurring in mentally retarded individuals. SYN Bonnet-Dechaume-Blanc s.

X-linked lymphoproliferative s., an X-linked recessive immunodeficiency and lymphoproliferative disease caused by mutation in the SH2 domain protein 1A gene (SH2D1A) on Xq; characterized by defective cellular or humoral immune response to Epstein-Barr virus; manifestations include fulminant infectious mononucleosis, B-cell malignancies, and hypogammaglobulinemia. SYN Duncan disease, Duncan s., X-linked lymphoproliferative disease.

XO s., SYN Turner s.

XXY s., SYN Klinefelter s.

XYY s., a chromosomal anomaly with chromosome count 47, with a supernumerary Y chromosome; controversial evidence associates tallness, aggressiveness, and acne with this condition.

yellow nail s., SYN yellow *nail.*

Young s., obstructive azoospermia and chronic sinopulmonary infections.

Zellweger s., a metabolic disorder with neonatal onset, characterized by distinctive facies, muscular hypotonia, hepatomegaly with jaundice, renal cysts, epiphyseal stippling of the patellae, cerebral dysmyelination, and neuronal migration defects and psychomotor retardation; there is a perturbation in peroxisomal biogenesis; autosomal recessive inheritance, caused by mutation in any one of several peroxin (PEX) genes on chromosome 6, 7, 8, or 12. SYN cerebrohepatorenal s.

Zieve s., transient jaundice, hemolytic anemia, and hyperlipemia associated with acute alcoholism in patients with cirrhosis or a fatty liver.

Zivert s., SYN Kartagener s.

Zollinger-Ellison s. [MIM*131100], peptic ulceration with gastric hypersecretion and gastrinoma of the pancreas or duodenum, sometimes associated with familial multiple endocrine adenomatosis type 1.

---

syn·drom·ic (sin-drom′ik, -drō′mik). Relating to a syndrome.

syn·ech·ia, pl. **syn·ech·i·ae** (si-nek′ē-ă, -kē-ē; si-nē′kē-ă). Any adhesion; specifically, anterior or posterior s. [G. *synecheia,* continuity, fr. *syn,* together, + *echō,* to have, hold]

anterior s., adhesion of the iris to the cornea.

anular s., adhesion of the entire pupillary margin of the iris to the capsule of the lens.

peripheral anterior s., SYN goniosynechia.

posterior s., adhesion of the iris to the capsule of the lens.

total s., adhesion of the entire surface of the iris to the lens capsule.

syn·ech·i·ot·o·my (si-nek′ē-ot′ō-mē). Division of the adhesions in synechia. [synechia + G. *tomē,* incision]

syn·ech·o·tome (si-nek′ō-tōm). A small knife for use in synechiotomy.

syn·ec·ten·ter·ot·o·my (si-nek′ten-ter-ot′ō-mē). Division of intestinal adhesions. [G. *synektos,* held together (see synechia), + *enteron,* intestine, + *tomē,* incision]

syn·en·ceph·a·lo·cele (sin-en-sef′ă-lō-sēl). Protrusion of brain substance through a defect in the skull, with adhesions preventing reduction. [syn- + G. *enkephalos,* brain, + *kēlē,* hernia]

syn·er·e·sis (si-ner′ĕ-sis). **1.** The contraction of a gel, e.g., a blood clot, by which part of the dispersion medium is squeezed out. **2.** Degeneration of the vitreous humor with loss of gel consistency to become partially or completely fluid. [G. *synairesis,* a taking or drawing together]

syn·er·get·ic (sin-er-jet′ik). SYN synergistic.

syn·er·gia (si-ner′jē-ă). SYN synergism.

syn·er·gic (si-ner′jik). SYN synergistic.

syn·er·gism (sin′er-jizm). Coordinated or correlated action of two or more structures, agents, or physiologic processes so that the combined action is greater than the sum of each acting separately. Cf. antagonism. SYN synergia, synergistic effect, synergy. [G. *synergia,* fr. *syn,* together, + *ergon,* work]

syn·er·gist (sin′er-jist). A structure, agent, or physiologic process that aids the action of another. Cf. antagonist.

syn·er·gis·tic (sin-er-jis′tik). **1.** Pertaining to synergism. **2.** Denoting a synergist. SYN synergetic, synergic.

syn·er·gy (sin′er-jē). SYN synergism.

syn·es·the·sia (sin-es-thē′zē-ă). **1.** A condition in which a stimulus, in addition to exciting the usual and normally located sensation, gives rise to a subjective sensation of different character or localization; e.g., color hearing, color taste. **2.** From a neurolinguistic perspective, stimulus-response conditioning such as seen in a phobia. [syn- + G. *aisthēsis,* sensation]

s. al′gica, SYN synesthesialgia.

syn·es·the·si·al·gia (sin′es-thē-zē-al′jē-ă). Painful synesthesia. SYN synesthesia algica.

Syn·gam·i·dae (sin-gam′i-dē). A family of nematodes (order Strongyloidea) parasitic in the respiratory system of birds and mammals. [see *Syngamus*]

Syn·gamus (sin′ga-mŭs). A genus of bloodsucking, strongyle gapeworms of the family Syngamidae.

S. laryngeus, infestation of the larynx with nematodes of the *Syngamus* genus causing cough, hemoptysis, foreign body sensation, and shortness of breath.

syn·ga·my (sin′gă-mē). Conjugation of the gametes in fertilization. [syn- + G. *gamos,* marriage]

syn·ge·ne·ic (sin′jĕ-nē′ik). Relating to genetically identical individuals. SYN isogeneic, isogenic, isologous, isoplastic, syngenic. [G. *syngenēs,* congenital]

syn·gen·e·sis (sin-jen′ĕ-sis). SYN sexual *reproduction.* [syn- + G. *genesis,* origin]

syn·ge·net·ic (sin-jĕ-net′ik). Relating to syngenesis.

syn·gen·ic (sin-jen′ik). SYN syngeneic.

syn·gna·thia (sin-nath′ē-ă). Congenital adhesion of the maxilla and mandible by fibrous bands. [syn- + G. *gnathos,* jaw]

syn·graft (sin′graft). A tissue or organ transplanted between genetically identical individuals. SYN isogeneic graft, isograft, isologous graft, isoplastic graft, syngeneic graft.

syn·i·dro·sis (sin-i-drō′sis). A condition in which excessive sweating is part of the clinical manifestation. [syn- + G. *hidrosis,* sweating]

syn·i·ze·sis (sin-i-zē′sis). **1.** Closure or obliteration of the pupil. **2.** The massing of chromatin at one side of the nucleus that occurs usually at the beginning of synapsis. [G. collapse]

syn·kar·y·on (sin-kar′ē-on). The nucleus formed by the fusion of the two pronuclei in karyogamy. SYN syncaryon. [syn- + G. *karyon,* kernel (nucleus)]

syn·ki·ne·sis (sin-ki-nē′sis). Involuntary movement accompanying a voluntary one, as the movement of a closed eye following that of the uncovered one, or the movement occurring in a paralyzed muscle accompanying motion in another part. SYN syncinesis. [syn- + G. *kinēsis,* movement]

syn·ki·net·ic (sin-ki-net′ik). Relating to or marked by synkinesis.

syn·ne·ma·tin B (sin-ĕ-mā′tin, si-nē′mă-tin). SYN *cephalosporin N.*

syn·o·nych·ia (sin-ō-nik′ē-ă). Fusion of two or more nails of the digits, as in syndactyly. [sin- + G. *onyx* (*onych-*), nail]

syn·o·nym (sin′ō-nim). In biologic nomenclature, a term used to denote one of two or more names for the same species or taxonomic group (taxon).

objective s.'s, different names for the same organism, based on one and the same nomenclatural type, as when a species is transferred from one genus to another (e.g., the transfer of *Diplococcus pneumoniae* to the genus *Streptococcus* as *Streptococcus pneumoniae*), in contrast to subjective s.'s.

senior s., the earliest published of two or more available names for the same organism, usually used as the correct name (law of priority).

subjective s.'s, different names, based on different nomenclatural types, for organisms that were originally regarded as different but were later considered to be identical, or nearly so, as a matter of personal opinion, in contrast to objective s.'s.

syn·oph·rys (sin-of'ris). Hypertrophy and fusion of the eyebrows. [syn- + G. *ophrys*, eyebrow]

syn·oph·thal·mia (sin-of-thal'mē-ă). SYN cyclopia. [syn- + G. *ophthalmos*, eye]

syn·oph·thal·mus (-mŭs). SYN cyclopia.

syn·op·to·phore (sin-op'tō-fōr). A modified form of Wheatstone stereoscope used in orthoptic training. [syn- + G. *ōps*, eye, + *phoros*, bearing]

syn·or·chi·dism, syn·or·chism (sin-ōr'ki-dizm, sin-ōr'kizm). Congenital fusion of the testes in the abdomen or scrotum. [syn- + G. *orchis*, testis]

syn·os·che·os (sin-os'kē-os). Partial or complete adhesion of the penis and scrotum, a malformation in hermaphroditism. [syn- + G. *osche*, scrotum]

syn·os·te·ol·o·gy (sin-os-tē-ol'ō-jē). SYN arthrology. [syn- + G. *osteon*, bone, + *logos*, study]

syn·os·te·o·sis (sin-os-tē-ō'sis). SYN synostosis.

syn·os·to·sis (sin-os-tō'sis) [TA]. Osseous union between two bones that are not supposed to be united; commonly refers to formation of a bony bundle between the radius and ulna following fracture of these two bones. SYN bony ankylosis, synosteosis, true ankylosis. [syn- + G. *osteon*, bone, + *-osis*, condition]

sagittal s., SYN scaphocephaly.

tribasilar s., fusion in early life of the three bones at the base of the skull, resulting in interference with the development of the brain.

syn·os·tot·ic (sin-os-tot'ik). Relating to synostosis.

sy·no·tia (si-nō'shē-ă). Fusion or abnormal approximation of the lobes of the ears in otocephaly. [syn- + G. *ous*, ear]

syn·o·vec·to·my (sin-ō-vek'tō-mē). Excision of a portion or all of the synovial membrane of a joint. [synovia + G. *ektomē*, excision]

radiopharmaceutical s., the treatment of abnormal synovial membranes by radiation derived from the instillation in the joint of a radiopharmaceutical, such as radiogold.

syn·o·via (si-nō'vē-ă) [TA]. SYN synovial *fluid*. [Mod. L., a word coined by Paracelsus, fr. G. *syn*, together, + *ōon* (L. *ovum*), egg]

syn·o·vi·al (si-nō'vē-ăl). 1. Relating to, containing, or consisting of synovia. 2. Relating to the membrana synovialis.

syn·o·vip·a·rous (sin'ō-vip'ă-rŭs). Producing synovia. [synovia + L. *pario*, to produce]

syn·o·vi·tis (sin-ō-vī'tis). Inflammation of a synovial membrane, especially that of a joint; in general, when unqualified, the same as arthritis. [synovia + G. *-itis*, inflammation]

bursal s., SYN bursitis.

chronic hemorrhagic villous s., SYN pigmented villonodular s.

dry s., s. with little serous or purulent effusion. SYN s. sicca.

filarial s., synovial inflammation often followed by fibrotic ankylosis due to microfilariae in the joint.

pigmented villonodular s., diffuse outgrowths of synovial membrane of a joint, usually the knee, composed of synovial villi and fibrous nodules infiltrated by hemosiderin- and lipid-containing macrophages and multinucleated giant cells; the condition may be inflammatory, although recurrence is likely to follow incomplete removal. SYN chronic hemorrhagic villous s.

purulent s., SYN suppurative *arthritis*.

serous s., s. with a large effusion of nonpurulent fluid.

s. sic′ca, SYN dry s.

suppurative s., SYN suppurative *arthritis*.

tendinous s., SYN tenosynovitis.

syn·o·vi·um (si-nō'vē-ŭm). SYN synovial *membrane*.

syn·pol·y·dac·ty·ly (sin'pol-ē-dak'ti-lē). Associated syndactyly and polydactyly.

syn·tac·tics (sin-tak'tiks). A branch of semiotics concerned with the formal relations between signs, in abstraction from their meaning and their interpreters. [syn- + G. *taxis*, order]

syn·tal·i·ty (sin-tal'i-tē). The consistent and predictable behavior of a social group. [prob. telescoped from syn- + mentality]

syn·tec·tic (sin-tek'tik). Pertaining to or marked by syntexis.

syn·ten·ic (sin-ten'ik). Pertaining to synteny.

syn·te·ny (sin'ten-ē). The relationship between two genetic loci (not genes) represented on the same chromosomal pair or (for haploid chromosomes) on the same chromosome; an anatomic rather than a segregational relationship. [syn- + G. *tainia*, ribbon]

syn·tex·is (sin-tek'sis). Emaciation or wasting. [G. *syn-tēxis*, a melting together]

syn·thase (sin'thās). Trivial name used in the Enzyme Commission Report for a lyase reaction going in the reverse direction (NTP-independent). For individual s.'s, see the specific names. SEE ALSO synthetase.

syn·ther·mal (sin-ther'măl). Having the same temperature. [syn- + G. *thermē*, heat]

syn·the·sis, pl. **syn·the·ses** (sin'thĕ-sis, -sēz). 1. A building up, putting together, composition. 2. In chemistry, the formation of compounds by the union of simpler compounds or elements. 3. Stage in the cell *cycle* in which DNA is synthesized as a preliminary to cell division. [G. fr. *syn*, together, + *thesis*, a placing, arranging]

s. of continuity, healing of the edges of a wound or fracture.

enzymatic s., s. by enzymes. SEE biosynthesis.

Kiliani-Fischer s., a synthetic procedure for the extension of the carbon atom chain of aldoses by treatment with cyanide; hydrolysis of the cyanohydrins followed by reduction of the lactone yields the homologous aldose; with this method, D-glucose and D-mannose can be synthesized from D-arabinose.

Merrifield s., the s. of peptides and proteins via an automated system on carrier polymers.

protein s., the process in which individual amino acids, whether of exogenous or endogenous origin, are connected to each other in peptide linkage in a specific order dictated by the sequence of nucleotides in DNA; this governing sequence is conveyed to the synthesizing apparatus in the ribosomes by mRNA, formed by base-pairing on the DNA template.

syn·the·size (sin'thĕ-sīz). To make something by synthesis, i.e., synthetically.

syn·the·tase (sin'thĕ-tās). An enzyme catalyzing the synthesis of a specific substance. S. is limited, in the Enzyme Commission Report, to use as a trivial name for the ligases (EC class 6), which in turn are those synthesizing enzymes that require the cleavage of a pyrophosphate linkage in ATP or a similar compound. Reversal of lyase (EC class 4) reactions, producing a synthesis, is indicated (in trivial names) by synthase; such reactions do not involve pyrophosphate cleavage. For individual s.'s, see the specific names.

syn·thet·ic (sin-thet'ik). Relating to or made by synthesis.

syn·tho·rax (sin-thōr'aks). SYN thoracopagus.

syn·ton·ic (sin-ton'ik). Having even tone or temperament; a personality trait characterized by a high degree of emotional responsiveness to the environment. [G. *syntonos*, in harmony, fr. *syn*, together, + *tonos*, tone]

syn·tro·phism (sin'trō-fizm). State of mutual dependence, with reference to food supply, of organs or cells of a plant or an animal. [syn- + G. *trophē*, nourishment]

syn·tro·pho·blast (sin-trō'fō-blast, -trof'ō-). SYN syncytiotrophoblast.

syn·tro·pic (sin-trop'ik). Relating to syntropy.

syn·tro·py (sin'trō-pē). 1. The tendency sometimes seen in two diseases to coalesce into one. 2. The state of harmonious association with others. 3. In anatomy, a number of similar structures inclined in one general direction; e.g., the spinous processes of a series of vertebrae, the ribs. [syn- + G. *tropē*, a turning]

inverse s., a situation in which the presence of one disease tends to decrease the possibility of another.

syn·zyme (sin'zīm). A synthetic macromolecule having enzymatic activity. SYN enzyme analog.

Sy·pha·cia (si-fā'shē-ă). Genus of oxyurid nematode pinworms of rodents; *S. obvelata* is the common cecal pinworm of mice, and *S. muris*, of rats. SEE ALSO *Aspiculuris tetraptera*. [fr. L. *siphon*, tube]

sy

△**syphil-.** SEE syphilo-.

syph·i·le·mia (sif-i-lē′mē-ă). A state in which the specific organism, *Treponema pallidum*, is present in the bloodstream. [syphilis + G. *haima*, blood]

syph·i·lid (sif′i-lid). Historic term for any of the several kinds of cutaneous and mucous membrane lesions of secondary and tertiary syphilis. SYN syphiloderm, syphiloderma. [syphilis + *-id* (1)]

syph·i·lim·e·try (sif-i-lim′ĕ-trē). A test designed to determine intensity of syphilitic infection, e.g., titered serologic test. [syphilis + G. *metron*, measure]

🔲**syph·i·lis** (sif′i-lis). An acute and chronic infectious disease caused by the bacterium *Treponema pallidum* and transmitted by direct contact, usually through sexual intercourse. After an incubation period of 12–30 days, the first symptom is a chancre, followed by slight fever and other constitutional symptoms (*primary s.*), followed by a skin eruption of various appearances with mucous patches and generalized lymphadenopathy (*secondary s.*), and subsequently by the formation of gummas, cellular infiltration, and functional abnormalities usually resulting from cardiovascular and central nervous system lesions (*tertiary s.*). SYN lues venerea, malum venereum. [Mod. L. *syphilis* (*syphilid-*), (?) fr. a poem, *Syphilis sive Morbus Gallicus,* by Fracastorius, *Syphilus* being a shepherd and principal character]

cardiovascular s., involvement of the cardiovascular system seen in late s., usually resulting in aortitis, aneurysm formation, and aortic valvular insufficiency.

congenital s., s. acquired by the fetus in utero, thus present at birth. SYN hereditary s., s. hereditaria.

s. d'emblée, s. occurring without an initial sore. [Fr. right away]

early s., primary, secondary, or early latent s., before any tertiary manifestations have appeared.

early latent s., infection with *Treponema pallidum*, the organism of s., after the primary and secondary phases have subsided, during the first year after infection, before any manifestations of tertiary s. have appeared.

endemic s., SYN nonvenereal s.

s. heredita′ria, SYN congenital s.

s. heredita′ria tar′da, s., believed to be congenital, but not manifesting itself until several years after birth.

hereditary s., SYN congenital s.

late s., involvement of the cardiovascular or central nervous system, or the development of a gumma in any organ, due to infection with *Treponema pallidum;* usually several years to 2–3 decades after the initial infection. SYN tertiary s.

late benign s., late s., manifested by serologic evidence of infection, but without any clinical manifestations.

late latent s., usually infectious in pregnant women only, who may pass the infection on to the fetus.

latent s., infection with *Treponema pallidum*, after the manifestations of primary and secondary s. have subsided (or were never noticed), before any manifestations of tertiary s. have appeared.

meningovascular s., a rare manifestation of secondary or tertiary s. characterized by mild, nonsuppurative, chronic inflammation of the leptomeninges and an intracranial or spinal angiitis.

nonvenereal s., s. caused by organisms closely related to *Treponema pallidum;* spread by personal, but not necessarily venereal, contact; usually acquired in childhood, most common in areas of poverty and overcrowding; rare in the United States; includes yaws, pinta and bejel. SYN endemic s.

primary s., the first stage of s. SEE syphilis.

quaternary s., SYN parasyphilis.

secondary s., the second stage of s. SEE syphilis.

tertiary s., SYN late s.

syph·i·lit·ic (sif-i-lit′ik). Relating to, caused by, or suffering from syphilis. SYN luetic.

△**syphilo-, syph-, syphili-.** Syphilis. [see syphilis]

syph·i·lo·derm, syph·i·lo·der·ma (sif′i-lō-derm, -der′mă). SYN syphilid. [syphilo- + G. *derma*, skin]

syph·i·loid (sif′i-loyd). Resembling syphilis. [syphilo- + G. *eidos*, resemblance]

syph·i·lol·o·gist (sif-i-lol′o-jist). One who specializes in the study, diagnosis, and treatment of syphilis.

syph·i·lol·o·gy (sif-i-lol′ō-jē). The branch of medical science concerned with the origin, prevention, and treatment of syphilis. [syphilo- + G. *logos*, study]

syph·i·lo·ma (sif-i-lō′mă). SYN gumma. [syphilo- + G. *-oma*, tumor]

s. of Fournier, SYN Fournier *disease*.

syr Abbreviation of Mod. L. *syrupus*, syrup.

sy·rig·mus (sĭ-rig′mŭs). SYN *tinnitus* aurium. [L. fr. G. *syrigmos*, a hissing]

△**syring-.** SEE syringo-.

syr·ing·ad·e·no·ma (sir′ing-ad-ĕ-nō′mă). A benign sweat gland tumor showing glandular differentiation typical of secretory cells. SYN syringoadenoma. [syring- + G. *aden*, gland, + *-oma*, tumor]

syr·ing·ad·e·no·sus (sir′ing-ad-ĕ-nō′sŭs). Relating to the sweat glands. [L. fr. syring- + G. *aden*, gland]

sy·ringe (sĭ-rinj′, sir′inj). An instrument used for injecting or withdrawing fluids, consisting of a barrel and plunger. [G. *syrinx*, pipe or tube]

air s., SYN chip s.

chip s., a tapered metal tube through which air is forced from a rubber bulb or pressure tank to blow debris from, or to dry, a cavity in preparing teeth for restoration. SYN air s.

control s., a type of Luer-Lok s. with thumb and finger rings attached to the proximal end of the barrel and to the tip of the plunger, allowing operation of the s. with one hand. SYN ring s.

Davidson s., a rubber tube, armed with an appropriate nozzle, intersected with a compressible bulb, with valves so arranged that compression forces the fluid, into which one end of the tube is inserted, forward to the nozzle end.

dental s., a breech-loading metal cartridge s. into which fits a hermetically sealed glass cartridge containing the anesthetic solution.

fountain s., an apparatus consisting of a reservoir for holding fluid, to the bottom of which is attached a tube with a suitable nozzle; used for vaginal or rectal injections, irrigating wounds, etc., the force of the flow being regulated by the height of the reservoir above the point of discharge.

hypodermic s., a small s. with a barrel (which may be calibrated), perfectly matched plunger, and tip; used with a hollow needle for subcutaneous injections and for aspiration. SYN hypodermic (3).

Luer s., a glass s. with a metal tip and locking device to secure the needle; used for hypodermic and intravenous purposes. SYN Luer-Lok s.

Luer-Lok s., SYN Luer s.

Neisser s., a urethral s. used in treatment of gonococcal urethritis.

probe s., a s. with an olive-shaped tip, used in treatment of diseases of the lacrimal passages.

ring s., SYN control s.

Roughton-Scholander s., SYN Roughton-Scholander *apparatus*.

rubber-bulb s., a s. with a hollow rubber bulb and cannula provided with a check valve, used to obtain a jet of air or water.

sy·rin·ge·al (sĭ-rin′jē-ăl). Relating to a syrinx.

sy·rin·gec·to·my (si-rin-jek′tō-mē). SYN fistulectomy. [syring- + G. *ektomē*, excision]

sy·rin·gi·tis (si-rin-jī′tis). Inflammation of the eustachian tube. [syring- + G. *-itis,* inflammation]

△**syringo-, syring-.** A syrinx; syringeal. [G. *syrinx*, pipe or tube]

sy·rin·go·ad·e·no·ma (sĭ-ring′gō-ad-ĕ-nō′mă). SYN syringadenoma.

sy·rin·go·bul·bia (sĭ-ring′gō-bŭl′bē-ă). A fluid-filled cavity of the brainstem, analogous to syringomyelia. [syringo- + L. *bulbus*, bulb (medulla oblongata)]

sy·rin·go·car·ci·no·ma (sĭ-ring′gō-kar-si-nō′mă). Obsolete term for a malignant epithelial neoplasm which has undergone cystic change (cystic carcinoma). [syringo- + carcinoma]

sy·rin·go·cele (sĭ-ring′gō-sēl). **1.** SYN central *canal*. **2.** A meningomyelocele in which there is a cavity in the ectopic spinal cord. [syringo- + G. *koilia,* a hollow]

sy·rin·go·cys·tad·e·no·ma (sĭ-ring'gō-sis-tad-ĕ-nō'mă). A cystic benign sweat gland tumor. [syringo- + cystadenoma]

s. papillif'erum, a s. characterized by numerous fingerlike projections of proliferated neoplastic epithelial cells in two layers on a stromal core of fibrous connective tissue infiltrated by plasma cells occurring singly or as part of a nevus sebaceus.

sy·rin·go·cys·to·ma (sĭ-ring'gō-sis-tō'mă). SYN hidrocystoma. [syringo- + cystoma]

sy·rin·go·en·ceph·a·lo·my·e·lia (sĭ-ring'gō-en-sef'ă-lō-mī-ē'lē-ă). A tubular cavity involving both brain and spinal cord and etiologically unrelated to vascular insufficiency. [syringo- + G. *enkephalos,* brain, + *myelos,* marrow]

sy·rin·goid (sĭ-ring'goyd). Resembling a tube or fistula. [syringo- + G. *eidos,* resemblance]

sy·rin·go·ma (si-ring-gō'mă). A benign, often multiple, sometimes eruptive neoplasm of the sweat gland ducts composed of very small round cysts. [syringo- + G. *-ōma,* tumor]

chondroid s., a benign tumor of sweat glands with a mucoid stroma showing cartilaginous metaplasia. SYN mixed tumor of skin.

sy·rin·go·me·nin·go·cele (sĭ-ring'gō-mĕ-ning'gō-sēl). A form of spina bifida in which the dorsal sac consists chiefly of membranes, with very little spinal cord substance, enclosing a cavity that communicates with a syringomyelic cavity. [syringo- + meningocele]

sy·rin·go·my·e·lia (sĭ-ring'gō-mī-ē'lē-ă). The presence in the spinal cord of longitudinal cavities lined by dense, gliogenous tissue, which are not caused by vascular insufficiency. S. is marked clinically by pain and paresthesia, followed by muscular atrophy of the hands and analgesia with thermoanesthesia of the hands and arms, but with the tactile sense preserved; later marked by painless whitlows, spastic paralysis in the lower extremities, and scoliosis of the lumbar spine. Some cases are associated with low grade astrocytomas or vascular malformations of the spinal cord. SYN hydrosyringomyelia, Morvan disease, syringomyelus. [syringo- + G. *myelos,* marrow]

sy·rin·go·my·e·lo·cele (sĭ-ring'gō-mī'ĕ-lō-sēl). A form of spina bifida, consisting of a protrusion of the membranes and spinal cord through a dorsal defect in the vertebral column, the fluid of the syrinx of the cord being increased and expanding the cord tissue into a thin-walled sac which then expands through the vertebral defect. [syringo- + myelocele]

sy·rin·go·my·e·lus (sĭ-ring'gō-mī'ĕ-lŭs). SYN syringomyelia. [syringo- + G. *myelos,* marrow]

sy·rin·go·pon·tia (sĭ-ring'gō-pon'shē-ă). A condition of cavity formation in the pons, of the same nature as syringomyelia. [syringo- + L. *pons,* bridge]

sy·rin·go·tome (sĭ-rin'gō-tōm). SYN fistulatome.

sy·rin·got·o·my (si-rin-got'ō-mē). SYN fistulotomy.

syr·inx, pl. **sy·rin·ges** (sir'ingks, sĭ-rin'jēz). **1.** A rarely used synonym for fistula. **2.** A pathologic tubular cavity in the brain or spinal cord. [G. a tube, pipe]

sy·ro·sing·o·pine (sir-ō-sin'gō-pēn). Prepared from reserpine by hydrolysis and reesterification; an antihypertensive agent with actions similar to those of reserpine.

syr·up (ser'ŭp, sir'ŭp). **1.** Refined molasses; the uncrystallizable saccharine solution left after the refining of sugar. **2.** Any sweet fluid; a solution of sugar in water in any proportion. **3.** A liquid preparation of medicinal or flavoring substances in a concentrated aqueous solution of a sugar, usually sucrose; other polyols, such as glycerin or sorbitol, may be present to retard crystallization of sucrose or to increase the solubility of added ingredients. When the s. contains a medicinal substance, it is termed a medicated s.; although a s. tends (due to its very high [approximately 85%] sucrose content) to resist mold or bacterial contamination, a s. may contain antimicrobial agents to prevent bacterial and mold growth. SYN sirup, syrupus. [Mod. L. *syrupus,* fr. Ar. *sharāb*]

ipecac s., a sweetened liquid medicinal preparation containing powdered ipecac extract, which contains the alkaloids emetine and cephaline; used as an emetic in certain cases of poisoning and (at lower doses) as an expectorant.

syr·u·pus (syr) (sir'ŭ-pŭs). SYN syrup. [Mod. L.]

syr·upy (ser'ŭ-pē, sir'). Relating to syrup; of the consistency of syrup.

sys·sar·co·sic (sis'ar-kō'sik). SYN syssarcotic.

sys·sar·co·sis (sis'ar-kō'sis). A muscular articulation; union of bones by muscle; e.g., in man, the muscular connections of the patella. [G. *syssarkōsis,* a being overgrown with flesh, fr. *syn,* with, + *sarx,* flesh]

sys·sar·cot·ic (sis'ar-kot'ik). Relating to or characterized by syssarcosis. SYN syssarcosic.

SYSTEM

---

sys·tem (sis'tĕm). **1** [TA]. A consistent and complex whole made up of correlated and semiindependent parts. A complex of functionally related anatomic structures. **2.** The entire organism seen as a complex organization of parts. **3.** Any complex of structures anatomically related (e.g., vascular s.) or functionally related (e.g., digestive s.). **4.** A scheme of medical theory. SEE ALSO apparatus, classification. **5.** S. followed by one or more letters denotes specific amino acid transporters; s. N is a sodium-dependent transporter specific for amino acids such as L-glutamine, L-asparagine, and L-histidine; s. y⁺ is a sodium-independent transporter of cationic amino acids. SYN systema [TA]. [G. *systēma,* an organized whole]

absolute s. of units, a s. based on absolute units accepted as being fundamental (length, mass, time) and from which other units (force, energy or work, power) are derived; such s.'s in common use are the foot-pound-second, centimeter-gram-second, and meter-kilogram-second s.'s.

absorbent s., SYN lymphoid s.

alimentary s. [TA], the digestive tract from the mouth to the anus with all its associated glands and organs. SYN systema digestorium [TA], alimentary apparatus, apparatus digestorius, digestive apparatus, digestive s., systema alimentarium.

anterolateral s., a composite bundle of fibers, located in the ventrolateral part of the lateral funiculus, containing spinothalamic, spinohypothalamic, spinoreticular, and spinomesencephalic (spinotectal, spinal to periaqueductal grey, etc.) fibers; occupies the combined areas of the spinal white matter historically divided into anterior and lateral spinothalamic tracts; located in white matter ventral to the denticulate ligament, hence the anatomical basis for the anterolateral cordotomy; concerned with the transmission of nociceptive and thermal information and with crude (nondiscriminative) touch. SEE ALSO spinothalamic *tract.* SYN anterolateral tract, tractus anterolaterales.

arch-loop-whorl s. (ALW), SEE Galton system of classification of *fingerprints,* under *fingerprint.*

association s., groups or tracts of nerve fibers interconnecting different regions of one and the same major subdivision of the central nervous system, such as the various areas of the cerebral cortex or the various segments of the spinal cord.

autonomic nervous s. (ANS), SYN autonomic *division* of nervous system.

Bethesda s., a s. for reporting cervical or vaginal cytologic findings and diagnoses. SYN Bethesda classification. [*Bethesda,* Maryland, site of NIH]

George Papanicolaou divided cytologic findings on stained cervical smears into five classes, ranging from I (normal) to V (carcinoma). Classes II–IV represented increasing degrees of premalignant squamous cellular atypia. Later workers modified the system by introducing the terms *dysplasia* (mild, moderate, severe) and *cervical intraepithelial neoplasia (CIN)* (grades 1–3). Pap smear findings reported according to this nomenclature showed poor reproducibility between observers and even between separate readings by the same observer. In addition, there was little correlation between diagnostic categories and treatment options. In 1988 the National Cancer Institute sponsored a workshop in Bethesda, Maryland, to establish a more useful system. The Bethesda system was first used in 1991 and has now become standard throughout the world. This recording system replaces numerical designations with descriptive diagnoses of cellular changes. The accompanying table compares the Bethesda system with earlier classifications. The standard format for reporting cervical cytology findings according to the Bethesda system comprises three elements: 1) a statement of the adequacy of the specimen (satisfactory, unsatisfactory, or satisfactory but limited by, e.g., absence of endocervical cells); 2) general categorization (within normal limits, benign cellular changes, or epithelial cell abnormality); and 3) descriptive diagnosis, elaborating on the general categorization and including mention of all significant abnormalities, as well as of the patient's hormonal status (when vaginal cells are present in the smear). Benign cellular changes include those due to infection (*Candida*, *Trichomonas*, herpes simplex), atrophy, radiation therapy, or the presence of an IUD. Epithelial cell abnormalities may involve either squamous or glandular cells. Abnormal squamous cells of undetermined significance (ASCUS) show cellular atypia but not clear evidence of premalignant change. About 20% of women with ASCUS eventually develop squamous intraepithelial lesions or invasive carcinoma. Squamous cell changes formerly called mild dysplasia or CIN 1 (including cellular atypia characteristic of human papillomavirus infection) are now designated low-grade squamous intraepithelial lesion. The category of high-grade squamous intraepithelial lesion encompasses what were formerly called moderate and severe dysplasia or CIN 2 and CIN 3. Abnormalities of glandular cells are similarly categorized.

blood group s.'s, see Blood Groups appendix.

blood-vascular s., SYN cardiovascular s.

bulbosacral s., SYN parasympathetic *part* of autonomic division of peripheral nervous system.

cardiovascular s. [TA], the heart and blood vessels considered as a whole. SYN systema cardiovasculare [TA], blood-vascular s.

caudal neurosecretory s., urohypophysis.

centimeter-gram-second s. (CGS, cgs), the scientific s. of expressing the fundamental physical units of length, mass, and time,

autonomic nervous system				
organ	function of sympathetic nervous system	sympathetic nerve(s)	function of parasympathetic nervous system	parasympathetic nerve(s)
eye	pupil dilation, contraction of ciliary muscle for accommodation	postganglionic fibers from superior cervical ganglion (internal carotid nr.)	constriction of pupil	postganglionic fibers from ciliary ganglion via short ciliary nerves
lacrimal gland	slight or no effect	postganglionic fibers from superior cervical ganglion (external carotid nr.)	secretion	postganglionic fibers from pterygopalatine ganglion via zygomaticotemporal nerve
salivary glands	thick, viscous secretion	external carotid nerve	abundant, watery secretion	postganglionic fibers from submandibular ganglion and from otic ganglion
heart	increase of rate and strength of heartbeats, dilation of coronary vessels (indirectly?), reduction of conduction time	cervical cardiac and thoracic cardiac nerves	contraction of coronary vessels (indirectly?), increase of conduction time	postganglionic fibers from terminal/intermural ganglia via vagus nerve
lungs	bronchodilation, inhibition of secretion	pulmonary nerves	bronchial constriction, stimulation of secretion	postganglionic fibers from terminal/intramural ganglia via vagus nerve
digestive tract	peristaltic inhibition, vasoconstriction	greater, lesser, least splanchnic nerves and branches from celiac, superior mesenteric, and inferior mesenteric ganglia	stimulation of peristalsis and secretion	postganglionic fibers from terminal/intermural ganglia via vagus and pelvic nerves
liver and gallbladder	release of glucose	branches from celiac ganglion	excretion of bile	postganglionic fibers from terminal/intramural ganglia via vagus nerve
adrenal medulla	secretion of epinephrine	lesser splanchnic nerve	no connection	no nerves
kidney	vasoconstriction, inhibition of urine formation	branches from corticorenal ganglion	no effect (?)	no nerves
bladder	retention of urine	branches from inferior mesenteric ganglion (via hypogastric plexus)	release of urine	postganglionic fibers from terminal/intramural ganglia via pelvic nerves
genitalia	ejaculation	branches from inferior mesenteric ganglion (via hypogastric plexus)	penile and clitoral erections	postganglionic fibers from terminal/intramural ganglia via pelvic nerves
sweat glands	secretion	postganglionic fibers from sympathetic chain ganglia	no connection	no nerves
peripheral blood vessels	constriction of smooth muscle	postganglionic fibers from sympathetic chain ganglia	no connection, apart from dilation in the genital area	no nerves
skeletal muscle	constriction of smooth muscles in blood vessels	postganglionic fibers from sympathetic chain ganglia	dilation	no nerves

Bethesda system			
Papanicolaou class	dysplasia	CIN	Bethesda category
I–II	negative	negative	within normal limits
III	—	—	ASCUS
III	mild	1	LGSIL
III	moderate	2	HGSIL
IV	severe	3	HGSIL
IV	carcinoma in situ	3	HGSIL
V	carcinoma	carcinoma	carcinoma

and those units derived from them, in centimeters, grams, and seconds; currently being replaced by the International S. of Units based on the meter, kilogram, and second.

central nervous s. (CNS) [TA], the brain and the spinal cord. SYN pars centralis systematis nervosi [TA], systema nervosum centrale☆.

cerebrospinal s., the combined central nervous s. and peripheral nervous s.

charge transfer s., SYN charge transfer *complex.*

chromaffin s., the cells of the body that stain with chromium salts and occur in the medullary portion of the adrenal body, paraganglia, and in relation to certain sympathetic nerves.

circulatory s., SYN vascular s.

closed s., a s. in which there is no exchange of material, energy, or information with the environment.

colloid s., a combination of the two phases, internal and external, of a colloid solution; the various s.'s are: gas + liquid (foam); gas + solid (meerschaum); liquid + gas (fog); solid + gas (smoke); solid + liquid (sol); liquid + solid (gel); liquid + liquid (emulsion); solid + solid (colored glass).

complement s., a group of more than 20 serum proteins, some of which can be serially activated and participate in a cascade resulting in cell lysis; the complement s. also functions in chemotaxis, opsonization, and phagocytosis.

conducting s. of heart [TA], the s. of atypical modified muscle fibers comprising the sinoatrial node, atrioventricular node and bundle, the right and left bundles, and their terminal subendocardial branches (the Purkinje network). SYN complexus stimulans cordis [TA], systema conducens cordis☆.

craniosacral nervous s., SYN parasympathetic *part* of autonomic division of peripheral nervous system.

cytochrome s., SYN respiratory *chain.*

cytochrome P-450 s., a heterogeneous group of enzymes that catalyze various oxidative reactions in the human liver, intestine, kidney, lung, and central nervous system; these enzymes are involved in the metabolism of many endogenous and exogenous substrates, including drugs, toxins, hormones, and natural plant products. Cytochrome P-450 enzymes are classified on the basis of chemical structure (amino acid sequencing). The designation of each enzyme is CYP followed by a numeral for the family to which it has been assigned, a letter for its subfamily, and sometimes a second numeral for the individual enzyme.

The steady increase in the number and variety of pharmaceutical agents available for the treatment of infections, degenerative and malignant conditions, mental disorders, and other diseases has led to polypharmacy, with attendant risks of undesirable drug interactions. Disturbances in the function of the cytochrome P-450 system are increasingly recognized as important causes of such interactions. When a drug increases the formation of a P-450 enzyme, other drugs metabolized by that enzyme are eliminated more rapidly and may fail to produce the desired therapeutic effects. In contrast, a drug that inhibits P-450 enzyme activity can retard the metabolism of substrate drugs, with resultant increases in serum and tissue levels and in drug effects, including side effects. Inhibition usually involves competition between drugs for the same binding site on an enzyme molecule. Reversible inhibition is the most common mechanism of drug interactions involving the P-450 system. In general, drugs compete for a specific P-450 isoenzyme. Examples of agents that cause interactions through reversible inhibition are fluoroquinolone antibiotics, cimetidine, ketoconazole, and protease inhibitors used in the treatment of AIDS. CYP3A, the most abundant of human cytochrome P-450 enzymes, accounts for 30% of those found in the liver. Its substrates include many psychoactive medicines, ketoconazole, erythromycin, and protease inhibitors. This enzyme is inhibited by some antidepressants, azole antifungals, cimetidine, erythromycin, and other drugs. Increased formation of CYP3A is induced by carbamazepine, phenobarbital, phenytoin, and rifampin. Ethnic differences in the expression of CYP2D6 explain why whites are more likely than blacks and Asians to experience toxicity from accumulation and excessive serum levels of drugs metabolized by this enzyme, such as tricyclic antidepressants, SSRIs, antipsychotics, and beta-blockers.

digestive s., SYN alimentary s.

ecological s., SYN ecosystem.

electron-transport s., SYN respiratory *chain.*

endocrine s., SYN endocrine *glands,* under *gland.*

endomembrane s., SYN endoplasmic *reticulum.*

esthesiodic s., a s. of neurons and fiber tracts in the spinal cord and brain subserving sensation.

exterofective s., name applied by Cannon to the somatic nervous s. as opposed to the interofective or autonomic s.

extrapyramidal motor s., literally: all of the brain structures affecting bodily (somatic) movement, excluding the motor neurons, the motor cortex, and the pyramidal (corticobulbar and corticospinal) tract. Despite its very wide literal connotation, the term is more often used to denote in particular the striate body (basal ganglia), its associated structures (substantia nigra, subthalamic nucleus), and its descending connections with the midbrain.

feedback s., (1) a complex of neuronal circuits whereby a part of the efferent path returns to the input to modulate its activity, thus acting as a governor on the s.; **(2)** SEE feedback.

foot-pound-second s. (FPS, fps), a s. of absolute units based on the foot, pound, and second.

gamma motor s., SYN gamma *loop.*

genital s. [TA], the complex s. consisting of the male or female gonads, associated ducts, and external genitalia dedicated to the function of reproducing the species. SYN systema genitalia [TA], reproductive s.

genitourinary s., SYN urogenital s.

geographic information s., a computer-based s. that combines cartographic capabilities with electronic data processing to rapidly produce customized maps for use in epidemiologic studies.

glandular s., all the glands of the body collectively.

haversian s., SYN osteon.

health information s., combination of vital and health statistical data from multiple sources, used to derive information about the health needs, health resources, use of health services, and outcomes of use by the people in a defined region or jurisdiction.

hematopoietic s., the blood-making organs; in the embryo at different ages these are the yolk sac, liver, thymus, spleen, lymph nodes, and bone marrow; after birth they are principally the bone marrow, spleen, thymus, and lymph nodes.

hepatic portal s., a venous portal s. in which the portal vein receives blood via its tributaries from the capillaries of most of the abdominal viscera and drains it into the hepatic sinusoids.

heterogeneous s., in chemistry, a s. that contains various distinct and mechanically separable parts or phases; e.g., a suspension or an emulsion.

hexaxial reference s., the figure resulting if the lines of derivation of the unipolar limb leads of the electrocardiogram are added to the triaxial reference s.

His-Tawara s., the complex s. of interlacing Purkinje fibers

sy

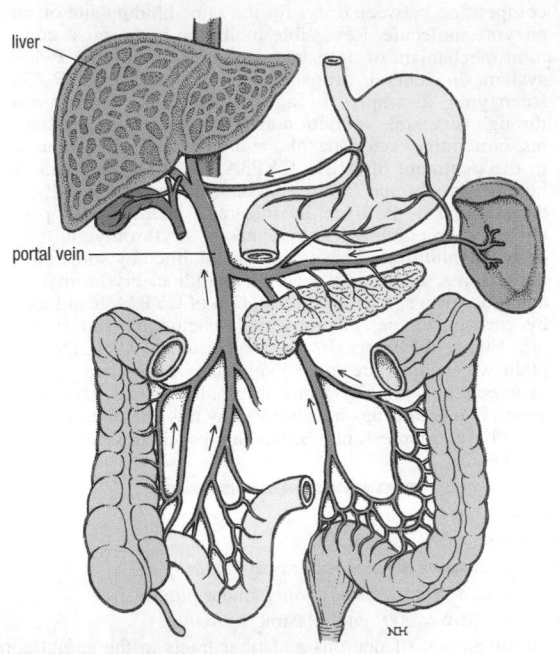

liver

portal vein

hepatic portal system

within the ventricular myocardium. SEE ALSO conducting s. of heart.

homogeneous s., in chemistry, a s. whose parts cannot be mechanically separated and is therefore uniform throughout and possesses in every part identically physical properties; e.g., a solution of sodium chloride in water.

hypophyseoportal s., SYN portal hypophysial *circulation.*

hypophysial portal s., SYN portal hypophysial *circulation.*

hypophysioportal s., SYN portal hypophysial *circulation.*

hypothalamohypophysial portal s., (1) SYN portal hypophysial *circulation;* **(2)** SYN renal portal s.

hypoxia warning s., a device designed to produce an audio or visual signal at a predetermined level of oxygen partial pressure; ideally, the system would warn of impending hypoxia in time for corrective action to be taken.

immune s., an intricate complex of interrelated cellular, molecular, and genetic components which provides a defense (immune response) against foreign organisms or substances and aberrant native cells.

indicator s., in in vitro immunological tests, a combination of reagents used to determine the degree to which immunologic reagents have combined (e.g., sensitized erythrocytes in complement-fixation tests; enzyme and substrate in enzyme-linked immunosorbent assays).

information s., combination of vital and health statistical data from multiple sources, used to derive information and make decisions about the health needs, health resources, costs, use, and outcome of health care.

integumentary s., SYN integument.

intermediary s., SYN interstitial *lamella.*

International S. of Units, SEE International System of Units.

interofective s., term applied by W. Cannon to the autonomic nervous s. as opposed to the somatic nervous s. or exterofective s.

involuntary nervous s., SYN autonomic *division* of nervous system.

kallikrein s., a blood serum s., the activity of which is initiated by factor XII (Hageman factor) leading to the production of prekallikrein activator and then to kallikrein which, after activation by plasmin, splits bradykinin from kininogen.

kinetic s., (1) a term proposed by G.W. Crile to denote the chain of organs through which latent energy is transformed into motion

and heat: it includes the brain, the thyroid, the adrenals, the liver, the pancreas, and the muscles; **(2)** that part of the neuromuscular s. whereby active movements are effected; distinguished from the static s.

limbic s., collective term denoting a heterogeneous array of brain structures at or near the edge (limbus) of the medial wall of the cerebral hemisphere, in particular the hippocampus, amygdala, and fornicate gyrus; the term is often used so as to include also the interconnections of these structures, as well as their connections with the septal area, the hypothalamus, and a medial zone of mesencephalic tegmentum. By way of the latter connections, the limbic s. exerts an important influence upon the endocrine and autonomic motor s.'s; its functions also appear to affect motivational and mood states. SYN visceral brain.

linnaean s. of nomenclature, the s. of nomenclature in which the names of species are composed of two parts, a generic name and a specific epithet (species name, in botany). SYN binary nomenclature, binomial nomenclature. [Carl von *Linné*]

lymphatic s., SYN lymphoid s.

lymphoid s. [TA], it consists of lymphatic vessels, nodes, and lymphoid tissue; it empties into the veins at the level of the superior aperture of the thorax. SYN systema lymphoideum [TA], absorbent s., lymphatic s., systema lymphaticum.

s. of macrophages, SYN mononuclear phagocyte s.

masticatory s., the organs and structures primarily functioning in mastication: the jaws, teeth with their supporting structures, temporomandibular joint, muscles of mastication, tongue, lips, cheeks, and oral mucosa. SYN dental apparatus, masticatory apparatus (1).

metameric nervous s., that part of the nervous s. which innervates body structures developed in ontogeny from the segmentally arranged somites or, in the head region, branchial arches. The term implies reference to the neural mechanisms intrinsic to the spinal cord and brainstem (represented by the sensory nuclei, motoneuronal cell groups, and their associated interneurons in the reticular formation); by strict definition it should exclude the autonomic nervous system.

meter-kilogram-second s., an absolute s. based on the meter, kilogram, and second; the basis of the International S. of Units.

metric s., a s. of weights and measures, universal for scientific use, based upon the meter, which was originally intended to be one ten-millionth of a quadrant of the earth's meridian and now is based on the length that light travels in a vacuum in a given period of time (see meter). Prefixes of the meter (and other standards) reflect either fractions or multiples of the meter and are identical to the International S. of Units (q.v.). The unit of weight is the gram, which is the weight of one cubic centimeter of water, equivalent to 15.432358 grains. The unit of volume is the liter or one cubic decimeter, equal to 1.056688 U.S. liquid quarts; a cubic centimeter is about 16.23073 U.S. minims.

mononuclear phagocyte s. (MPS), a widely distributed collection of both free and fixed macrophages derived from bone marrow precursor cells by way of monocytes; their substantial phagocytic activity is mediated by immunoglobulin and the serum complement s. In both connective and lymphoid tissue, they may occur as free and fixed macrophages; in the sinusoids of the liver, as Kupffer cells; in the lung, as alveolar macrophages; and in the nervous system, as microglia. SYN s. of macrophages.

muscular s., all the muscles of the body collectively.

nervous s. [TA], the entire nerve apparatus, composed of a central part, the brain and spinal cord, and a peripheral part, the cranial and spinal nerves, autonomic ganglia, and plexuses. SYN systema nervosum [TA].

neuromuscular s., the muscles of the body collectively and the nerves supplying them.

nonspecific s., SYN reticular activating s.

occlusal s., the form or design and arrangement of the occlusal and incisal units of a dentition or the teeth on a denture. SYN occlusal scheme.

oculomotor s., that part of the central nervous s. having to do with eye movements; it is composed of pathways connecting various regions of the cerebrum, brainstem, and ocular nuclei, utilizing multisynaptic articulations.

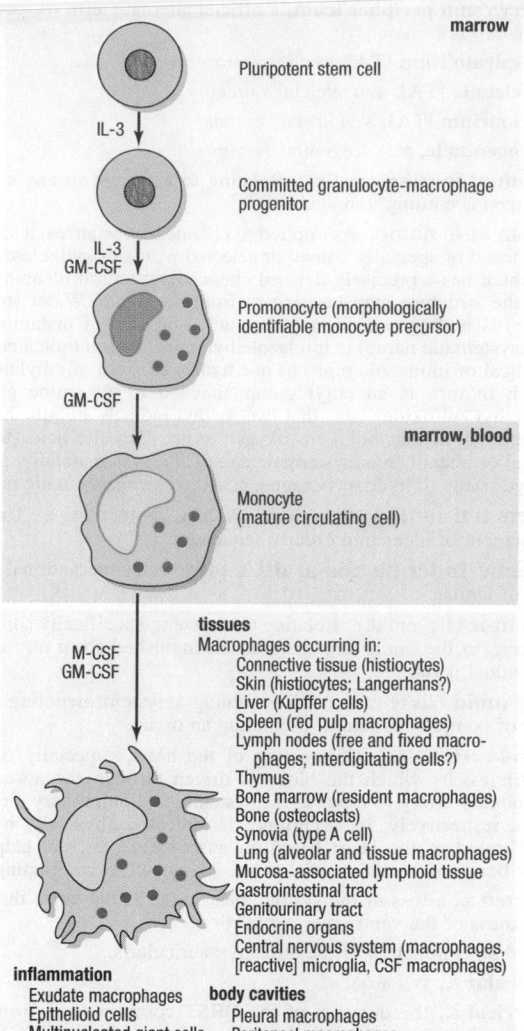

cells belonging to the **mononuclear phagocytic system**: IL=interleukin; GM-CSF=granulocyte-macrophage colony-stimulating factor

Labels within figure:
marrow
Pluripotent stem cell
IL-3
Committed granulocyte-macrophage progenitor
IL-3
GM-CSF
Promonocyte (morphologically identifiable monocyte precursor)
GM-CSF
marrow, blood
Monocyte (mature circulating cell)
tissues
M-CSF
GM-CSF
Macrophages occurring in:
Connective tissue (histiocytes)
Skin (histiocytes; Langerhans?)
Liver (Kupffer cells)
Spleen (red pulp macrophages)
Lymph nodes (free and fixed macrophages; interdigitating cells?)
Thymus
Bone marrow (resident macrophages)
Bone (osteoclasts)
Synovia (type A cell)
Lung (alveolar and tissue macrophages)
Mucosa-associated lymphoid tissue
Gastrointestinal tract
Genitourinary tract
Endocrine organs
Central nervous system (macrophages, [reactive] microglia, CSF macrophages)
inflammation
Exudate macrophages
Epithelioid cells
Multinucleated giant cells
body cavities
Pleural macrophages
Peritoneal macrophages

open s., a s. in which there is a continual exchange of material, energy, and information with the environment.

O-R s., abbreviation for oxidation-reduction s.

oxidation-reduction s. (O-R s.), an enzyme s. in the tissues by which oxidation and reduction proceed simultaneously through the transference of hydrogen or of one or more electrons from one metabolite to another. SEE ALSO oxidation-reduction. SYN redox s.

parasympathetic nervous s., SEE parasympathetic *part* of autonomic division of peripheral nervous system, autonomic *division* of nervous system.

pedal s., efferent fibers connecting the forebrain with more caudal structures.

periodic s., the arrangement of the chemical elements in a definite order as indicated by their respective atomic numbers in such a way that groups of elements with similar chemical properties (similar valence shell electron number) are grouped together. SEE Mendeléeff *law*.

peripheral nervous s. [TA], the peripheral part of the nervous system external to the brain and spinal cord from their roots to their peripheral terminations. This includes the ganglia, both sensory and autonomic, and any plexuses through which the nerve fibers run. SEE ALSO autonomic *division* of nervous system. SYN pars peripherica systematis nervosi [TA], systema nervosum periphericum ☆, peripheral part of nervous system.

Pinel s., the abolition of forcible restraint in the treatment of the mental hospital patient.

portal s., a s. of vessels in which blood, after passing through one capillary bed, is conveyed through a second capillary network, as in the hepatic portal system in which blood from the intestines passes through the liver sinusoids.

pressoreceptor s., the pressoreceptive areas which with their afferent fibers and connections with the autonomic system react to a rise in arterial blood pressure and serve to buffer it by inhibiting the heart rate and vascular tone. SEE ALSO baroreceptor.

projection s., the s. of axons carrying stimuli from one portion of the nervous system to other portions.

properdin s., an immunologic s. that is the alternative pathway for complement, composed of several distinct proteins that react in a serial manner and activate C3 (third component of complement), seemingly without utilizing components C1, C4, and C2; in addition to properdin, the s. includes Factors B, D, H, and I. The s. can be activated, in the absence of specific antibody, by bacterial endotoxins, by a variety of polysaccharides and lipopolysaccharides, and by a component of cobra venom.

Purkinje s., SYN subendocardial conducting s. of heart.

redox s., SYN oxidation-reduction s.

renal portal s., an arterial portal s., in which efferent glomerular arterioles receive blood from the capillaries of the renal glomeruli and carry it to the peritubular capillary plexus surrounding the proximal and distal convoluted tubules. SYN hypothalamohypophysial portal s. (2).

renin-angiotensin s., a selective regulator of the aldosterone biosynthetic pathway that acts by increasing aldosterone production and sodium retention as a result of volume depletion, with resulting increased renin production in the kidney and conversion of angiotensin I in the plasma to angiotensin II.

renin-angiotensin-aldosterone s., the hormones, renin, angiotensin, and aldosterone work together to regulate blood pressure. A sustained fall in blood pressure causes the kidney to release renin. This is converted to angiotensin in the circulation. Angiotensin then raises blood pressure directly by arteriolar constriction and stimulates the adrenal gland to produce aldosterone which promotes sodium and water retention by the kidney, such that blood volume and blood pressure increase.

reproductive s., SYN genital s.

respiratory s. [TA], all the air passages from the nose to the pulmonary alveoli. SYN systema respiratorium [TA], apparatus respiratorius, respiratory apparatus.

reticular activating s. (RAS), a physiologic term denoting that part of the brainstem reticular formation that plays a central role in the organism's bodily and behavioral alertness; it extends as a diffusely organized neural apparatus through the central region of the brainstem into the subthalamus and the intralaminar nuclei of the thalamus; by its ascending connections it affects the function of the cerebral cortex in the sense of behavioral responsiveness; its descending (reticulospinal) connections transmit its activating influence upon bodily posture and reflex mechanisms (e.g., muscle tonus), in part by way of the gamma motor neurons. SEE ALSO reticular *formation*. SYN nonspecific s.

reticuloendothelial s. (RES), a collection of putative macrophages, first described by Aschoff, which included most of the true macrophages (now classified under the mononuclear phagocytic s.) as well as cells lining the sinusoids of the spleen, lymph nodes, and bone marrow, and the fibroblastic reticular cells of hematopoietic tissues; all of these latter cells are only weakly phagocytic and are not true macrophages. The term persists in the literature and is often equated with the mononuclear phagocytic s.

second signaling s., pavlovian term for speech in which words are considered to be the "second signals" capable of producing conditioned responses.

skeletal s. [TA], the bones and cartilages of the body. SYN systema skeletale [TA].

somesthetic s., sensory data derived from skin, muscles, and body organs in contrast to that derived from the five special senses.

static s., that part of the neuromuscular s. whereby the animal

sy

organism is maintained in posture and equilibrium and counteracts the forces of gravity and atmospheric pressure; distinguished from the kinetic s. (2).

stomatognathic s., all of the structures involved in speech and in the reception, mastication, and deglutition of food. SEE ALSO masticatory s. SYN masticatory apparatus (2).

subendocardial conducting s. of heart, terminal ramifications in the ventricles of the specialized conducting s. of the heart. SYN Purkinje s.

sympathetic nervous s., SYN sympathetic *part* of autonomic division of peripheral nervous system.

T s., the transverse tubules that are continuous with the sarcolemma in skeletal and cardiac muscle fibers.

thoracolumbar s., SEE autonomic *division* of nervous system, sympathetic *part* of autonomic division of peripheral nervous system.

thoracolumbar nervous s., SYN sympathetic *part* of autonomic division of peripheral nervous system.

triaxial reference s., the figure resulting from rearranging the lines of derivation of the three standard limb leads of the electrocardiogram (as represented in the Einthoven triangle) so that, instead of forming the sides of an equilateral triangle, they bisect one another. SYN Dieuaide diagram.

urinary s. [TA], all organs concerned with the formation, storage, and voidance of urine including kidneys, ureters, bladder, and urethra. SYN systema urinarium [TA], urinary apparatus, uropoietic s.

urogenital s., includes all the organs concerned in reproduction and in the formation and voidance of urine. SYN apparatus urogenitalis, genitourinary apparatus, genitourinary s., systema urogenitale, urogenital apparatus.

uropoietic s., SYN urinary s.

vascular s., the cardiovascular and lymphatic s.'s collectively. SYN circulatory s.

vegetative nervous s., SYN autonomic *division* of nervous system.

vertebral-basilar s., the arterial complex comprising the two vertebral arteries joining to form the basilar artery, and their immediate branches.

vertebral venous s., any of four interconnected venous networks surrounding the vertebral column; anterior external vertebral venous plexus [TA] (plexus vertebralis externus anterior [TA]), the small s. around the vertebral bodies; posterior external vertebral venous plexus [TA] (plexus vertebralis internus anterior [TA]), the extensive s. around the vertebral processes; anterior internal vertebral venous plexus [TA] (plexus vertebralis internus posterior [TA]), the s. running the length of the vertebral canal anterior to the dura; posterior internal vertebral venous plexus, the s. running the length of the vertebral canal posterior to the dura; the latter two constitute the epidural venous plexus. SYN Batson plexus, plexus venosus vertebralis, vertebral venous plexus.

visceral motor s., SYN autonomic *division* of nervous system.

visceral nervous s., SYN autonomic *division* of nervous system.

Zaffaroni s., a chromatographic s. for the separation of steroids.

---

sys·te·ma (sis'tē'mă) [TA]. SYN system. SEE ALSO system, apparatus. [L. fr. G. *systēma*]

s. alimenta'rium, SYN alimentary *system*.

s. cardiovasculare [TA], SYN cardiovascular *system*.

s. conducens cordis, ✩official alternate term for conducting *system* of heart.

s. digesto'rium [TA], SYN alimentary *system*.

s. genitalia [TA], SYN genital *system*.

s. lymphat'icum, SYN lymphoid *system*.

s. lymphoideum [TA], SYN lymphoid *system*.

s. nervo'sum [TA], SYN nervous *system*.

s. nervo'sum autonom'icum, SYN autonomic *division* of nervous system.

s. nervo'sum centra'le, ✩official alternate term for central nervous *system*, central nervous *system*.

s. nervo'sum peripher'icum, ✩official alternate term for peripheral nervous *system*.

s. respirato'rium [TA], SYN respiratory *system*.

s. skeleta'le [TA], SYN skeletal *system*.

s. urinarium [TA], SYN urinary *system*.

s. urogenita'le, SYN urogenital *system*.

sys·tem·at·ic (sis'tĕ·mat'ik). Relating to a system in any sense; arranged according to a system.

sys·tem·at·ic name. As applied to chemical substances, a s. n. is composed of specially coined or selected words or syllables, each of which has a precisely defined chemical structural meaning, so that the structure may be derived from the name. Water (trivial name) is hydrogen oxide (systematic). The s. n. of histamine (a semisystematic name) is imidazolethylamine, which indicates that a radical of imidazole replaces one hydrogen atom of ethylamine, which in turn is an ethyl group attached to an amine group. Dimethyl sulfoxide states that two methyl radicals are attached to a sulfur atom that holds an oxygen atom. Carbolic acid (trivial name) or phenol (semisystematic name) are, systematically, phenyl hydroxide or hydroxybenzene. SEE ALSO semisystematic name.

sys·tem·a·ti·za·tion (sis·tĕ·mat'i·zā'shŭn, sis·tem'ă·ti·). The arrangement of ideas into orderly sequence.

Sys·tème In·ter·na·tion·al d'Un·i·tés. SEE International System of Units.

sys·tem·ic (sis·tem'ik). Relating to a system; specifically somatic, relating to the entire organism as distinguished from any of its individual parts.

sys·te·moid (sis'tĕ·moyd). Resembling a system; denoting a tumor of complex structure resembling an organ.

sys·to·le (sis'tō·lē). Contraction of the heart, especially of the ventricles, by which the blood is driven through the aorta and pulmonary artery to traverse the systemic and pulmonary circulations, respectively; its occurrence is indicated physically by the first sound of the heart heard on auscultation, by the palpable apex beat, and by the arterial pulse. [G. *systolē*, a contracting]

aborted s., a loss of the systolic beat in the radial pulse through weakness of the ventricular contraction.

atrial s., contraction of the atria. SYN auricular s.

auricular s., SYN atrial s.

electrical s., the duration of the QRST complex (i.e., from the earliest Q wave to the end of the latest T wave on the ECG).

electromechanical s., the period from the beginning of the QRS complex to the first (aortic) vibration of the second heart sound. SYN QS$_2$ interval.

extra-s., SEE extrasystole.

late s., SYN prediastole.

premature s., SYN extrasystole.

ventricular s., contraction of the ventricles.

sys·tol·ic (sis·tol'ik). Relating to, or occurring during cardiac systole.

sys·to·lom·e·ter (sis'tō·lom'ĕ·ter). **1.** An apparatus for determining the force of the cardiac contraction. **2.** An instrument for analyzing the sounds of the heart. [systole + G. *metron*, measure]

sys·trem·ma (sis·trem'ă). A muscular cramp in the calf of the leg, the contracted muscles forming a hard ball. [G. anything twisted]

sy·zyg·i·al (si·zij'ē·ăl). Relating to syzygy.

sy·zyg·i·ol·o·gy (si·zij'ē·ol'ō·jē). The study of interrelationships, or interdependencies, especially of the whole, as opposed to the study of separate parts or isolated functions. [G. *syzygios*, yoked (see syzygy), + *logos*, study]

sy·zyg·i·um (si·zij'ē·ŭm). SYN syzygy.

syz·y·gy (siz'i·jē). **1.** The association of gregarine protozoans end-to-end or in lateral pairing (without sexual fusion). **2.** Pairing of chromosomes in meiosis. SYN syzygium. [G. *syzygios*, yoked, bound together, fr. *syn*, together, + *zygon*, a yoke]

τ The 19th letter of the Greek alphabet, tau; symbol for relaxation *time*.

θ, Θ The eighth letter in the Greek alphabet, theta; symbol for angle.

T 1. Symbol for ribothymidine; tension (T+, increased tension; T–, diminished tension); tera-; tesla, the unit of magnetic field strength; tritium; threonine; torque; transmittance. **2.** As a subscript, refers to tidal *volume*. **3.** Abbreviation for thoracic vertebra (T1–T12); tocopherol.

α**-T** Symbol for α-tocopherol.

β**-T** Symbol for β-tocopherol.

γ**-T** Symbol for γ-tocopherol.

T1. In magnetic resonance, the time for 63% of longitudinal relaxation to occur; the value is a function of magnetic field strength and the chemical environment of the hydrogen nucleus; for protons in fat and in water, in a 1.5T magnet, about 250 msec and 3000 msec, respectively. A T1-weighted image will have a bright fat signal.

T2. In magnetic resonance, the time for 63% of transverse relaxation to occur; the value is a function of magnetic field strength and the chemical environment of the hydrogen nucleus; for protons in fat and in water, in a 1.5T magnet, about 60 msec and 250 msec respectively. A T2-weighted image will have a bright water signal.

2,4,5-T Abbreviation for (2,4,5-trichlorophenoxy)acetic acid.

T Symbol for absolute *temperature* (kelvin).

T_m Symbol for *temperature* midpoint (kelvin); melting *point*.

T_3 Symbol for 3,5,3'-triiodothyronine.

T_4 Symbol for thyroxine.

t Abbreviation for metric ton; time.

t Symbol for temperature (Celsius); tritium.

t_m Symbol for *temperature* midpoint (Celsius).

TA Abbreviation for *Terminologia Anatomica*.

Ta Symbol for tantalum.

tab·a·nid (tab′ă-nid). Common name for flies of the family Tabanidae. [L. *tabanus,* gadfly]

Ta·ban·i·dae (tă-ban′i-dē). A family of bloodsucking flies that includes the genera *Tabanus* (horsefly) and *Chrysops* (deerfly and mango fly), which are involved in transmission of several blood-borne parasites. [L. *tabanus,* gadfly]

Ta·ba·nus (tă-bā′nŭs). The gadflies and horseflies; a genus of biting flies, some species of which transmit surra, infectious equine anemia, anthrax, and other diseases. [L. a gadfly]

ta·bar·dil·lo (tah-bar-dē′yō). Mexican term for typhus. [Sp., fr. L.L. *tabardilii,* pustules]

ta·ba·tière an·a·to·mique (tab-ah-tē-ār′ an-ah-to-mēk′). SYN anatomic snuffbox. [Fr. snuffbox]

ta·bel·la, pl. **ta·bel·lae** (tă-bel′lă, -lē). A medicated tablet or lozenge. [L. dim. of *tabula,* tablet]

ta·bes (tā′bēz). Progressive wasting or emaciation. [L. a wasting away]

t. infan′tum, t. in infants with congenital syphilis.

t. mesenter′ica, tuberculosis of the mesenteric and retroperitoneal lymph nodes.

ta·bes·cence (ta-bes′ens). The state of progressive wasting away.

ta·bes·cent (ta-bes′ent). Characteristic of tabes. [L. *tabesco,* to waste away, fr. *tabes,* a wasting away]

ta·bet·ic (ta-bet′ik). Relating to or suffering from tabes, especially tabes dorsalis. SYN tabic, tabid.

ta·bet·i·form (ta-bet′i-fōrm). Resembling tabes, especially tabes dorsalis. [irreg. formed fr. L. *tabes,* a wasting, + *forma,* form]

tab·ic (tab′ik). SYN tabetic.

tab·id (tab′id). SYN tabetic. [L. *tabidus,* wasting away]

tab·la·ture (tab-lă-choor). The state of division of the cranial bones into two plates separated by the diploë. [L. *tabula,* tablet]

ta·ble (tā′bl). **1.** One of the two plates or laminae, separated by the diploë, into which the cranial bones are divided. **2.** An arrangement of data in parallel columns, showing the essential facts in a readily appreciable form. **3.** A platform upon which items can be placed. [L. *tabula*]

Aub-DuBois t., t. of basal metabolic rates in calories per square meter of body surface per hour or day for different ages.

contingency t., a tabular cross-classification of data such that subcategories of one characteristic are indicated in rows (horizontally) and subcategories of another are indicated in columns (vertically).

examining t., a t. on which the patient lies during a medical examination.

external t. of calvaria [TA], the outer compact layer of the cranial bones. SYN lamina externa calvaria [TA], lamina externa cranii, outer t. of skull.

Gaffky t., a numerical rating for the classification of tuberculosis according to the number of tubercle bacilli in the sputum, ranging from 1 (one to four organisms in the whole preparation) to 9 (an average of 100 per field). SYN Gaffky scale.

inner t. of skull, SYN internal t. of calvaria.

internal t. of calvaria [TA], the inner compact layer of the cranial bones. SYN lamina interna calvariae [TA], inner t. of skull, lamina interna cranii.

life t., a representation of the probable years of survivorship of a defined population of subjects; since survivorship is changed by new methods of prevention or treatment, a diachronic study is commonly used because the main interest lies in the composite structure of the current population. (In the summarizing technique used to describe the pattern of mortality and survival in a population, survivors to age *x* are denoted by the symbol l*x* and the expectation of life at age *x* is denoted by the symbol *x*.)

occlusal t., the occlusal or grinding surfaces of the bicuspid and molar teeth.

operating t., a t. on which the patient lies during a surgical operation.

outer t. of skull, SYN external t. of calvaria.

tilt t., a t. with a top capable of being rotated on its transverse axis so that a patient lying upon it can be brought to the erect position as desired; used in experimental investigation and in physical therapy.

vitreous t., the inner t. of one of the cranial bones; it is more compact and harder than the outer t. SYN lamina interna ossium cranii.

ta·ble·spoon (tā′bl-spoon). A large spoon, used as a measure of the dose of a medicine, equivalent to about 4 fluidrams or ½ fluidounce or 15 ml.

tab·let. A solid dosage form containing medicinal substances with or without suitable diluents; it may vary in shape, size, and weight, and may be classed according to the method of manufacture, as compressed t. SYN tabule. [Fr. *tablette,* L. *tabula*]

buccal t., usually a small, flat t. intended to be inserted in the buccal pouch, where the active ingredient is absorbed directly through the oral mucosa; such a t. dissolves or erodes slowly.

compressed t., a t. prepared, usually as a large-scale production, by means of great pressure; most compressed t.'s consist of the active ingredient and a diluent, binder, disintegrator, and lubricant.

dispensing t., a t. prepared by molding or by compression; used by the dispensing pharmacist to obtain certain potent substances in a convenient form for accurate compounding. Formerly used to

△ **Combining Forms**	☆ **Official alternate Terminologia Anatomica term**
▉ **Indicates term is illustrated, see Illustration Index**	
SYN **Synonym**	**[MIM] Mendelian Inheritance in Man**
Cf. **Compare**	C.I. **Colour Index**
[NA] **Nomina Anatomica**	
[TA] **Terminologia Anatomica**	**High Profile Term**

ta

prepare bulk solutions of germicidal chemicals, e.g., bichloride of mercury. Not intended for internal use.

enteric coated t., an oral dosage form in which a t. is coated with a material to prevent or minimize dissolution in the stomach but allow dissolution in the small intestine. This type of formulation either protects the stomach from a potentially irritating drug (e.g., aspirin) or protects the drug (e.g., erythromycin) from partial degradation in the acidic environment of the stomach.

hypodermic t., a compressed or molded t. that dissolves completely in water to form an injectable solution.

prolonged action t., repeat action t., SYN sustained action t.

sublingual t., usually a small, flat t. intended to be inserted beneath the tongue, where the active ingredient is absorbed directly through the oral mucosa; such a t. (e.g., nitroglycerine) dissolves very promptly.

sustained action t., sustained release t., a drug product formulation that provides the required dosage initially and then maintains or repeats it at desired intervals. SYN prolonged action t., repeat action t.

t. triturate, a small, usually cylindrical, molded or compressed disk of varying size, containing a diluent usually consisting of dextrose (glucose) or of a mixture of lactose and powdered sucrose and a moistening agent or excipient, such as dilute alcohol.

ta·boo, ta·bu (tă-boo′). Restricted, prohibited, or forbidden; set apart for religious or ceremonial purposes. [Tongan, set apart]

tab·u·lar (tab′ū-lăr). **1.** Tablelike. **2.** Arranged in the form of a table (2). [L. *tabularis,* fr. *tabula,* table]

tab·ule (tab′ūl). SYN tablet. [L. *tabula*]

ta·bun (tä′bŭn). An extremely potent cholinesterase inhibitor; the lethal dose for humans is believed to be as low as 0.01 mg/kg; median lethal dosage (respiratory) is about 40 mg/min/m³ for resting persons.

Tac (tak) A 55-kD polypeptide that is the one of the two chains that comprise the IL-2 receptor.

tache (tash). A circumscribed discoloration of the skin or mucous membrane, such as a macule or freckle. [Fr. spot]

t. blanche, SYN *macula* albida.

t. laiteuse, (1) SYN milk *spots,* under *spot*; **(2)** SYN *macula* albida. [Fr., milky spot]

ta·chis·to·scope (tă-kis′tō-skōp). An instrument to determine the shortest time an object must be exposed in order to be perceived. [G. *tachistos,* very rapid, fr. *tachys,* rapid, + *skopeō,* to view]

tach·o·gram (tak′ō-gram). Record made by a tachometer. [G. *tachos,* speed, + *gramma,* mark]

tach·o·graph (tak′ō-graf). A tachometer designed to provide a continuous record of speed or rate. [G. *tachos,* speed, + *graphō,* to write]

ta·chog·ra·phy (tă-kog′ră-fē). The recording of speed or rate. [G. *tachos,* speed, + *graphō,* to write]

ta·chom·e·ter (tă-kom′ĕ-ter). An instrument for measuring speed or rate; e.g., revolutions of a shaft, heart rate (cardiotachometer), arterial blood flow (hemotachometer), respiratory gas flow (pneumotachometer). [G. *tachos,* speed, + *metron,* measure]

△**tachy-.** Rapid. [G. *tachys,* quick]

tach·y·ar·rhyth·mia (tak′ē-ă-ridh′mē-ă). Any disturbance of the heart's rhythm, regular or irregular, resulting by convention in a rate over 100 beats/min during physical examination. [tachy- + G. *a-* priv. + *rhythmos,* rhythm]

tach·y·aux·e·sis (tak′ē-awk-sē′sis). Type of growth in which a part grows more rapidly than the whole. [tachy- + G. *auxō,* to increase]

tach·y·car·dia (tak′i-kar′dē-ă). Rapid beating of the heart, conventionally applied to rates over 90 beats/min. SYN polycardia, tachyrhythmia, tachysystole. [tachy- + G. *kardia,* heart]

atrial t., paroxysmal t. originating in an ectopic focus in the atrium. SYN auricular t.

atrial chaotic t., multifocal origin of tachycardia within the atrium; often confused with atrial fibrillation during physical examination. SYN multifocal atrial t.

atrioventricular junctional t., t. originating in the AV junction. SYN AV junctional t., nodal t.

auricular t., SYN atrial t.

AV junctional t., SYN atrioventricular junctional t.

bidirectional ventricular t., ventricular t. in which the QRS complexes in the electrocardiogram are alternately mainly positive and mainly negative; many such cases may represent ventricular t. with alternating forms of aberrant ventricular conduction.

Coumel t., a persistent junctional reciprocating t. that usually uses a slowly conducting posteroseptal pathway for the retrograde journey.

double t., the simultaneous t. of two ectopic pacemakers, e.g., atrial and junctional t.

ectopic t., a t. originating in a focus other than the sinus node, e.g., atrial, AV junctional, or ventricular t.

t. en salves, short runs of paroxysmal t. of the Gallavardin type. Cf. Gallavardin *phenomenon.* [Fr. *tachycardia in salvos*]

essential t., obsolete term for persistent rapid action of the heart due to no discoverable organic lesion.

t. exophthal′mica, rapid heart action occurring as one of the symptoms of exophthalmic goiter.

fetal t., a fetal heart rate of 160 or more beats/min.

junctional t., supraventricular t. arising from the atrioventricular junction (formerly called nodal t.).

multifocal atrial t. (MAT), SYN atrial chaotic t.

nodal t., SYN atrioventricular junctional t.

orthostatic t., increased heart rate on assuming the erect posture.

paroxysmal t., recurrent attacks of t., usually with abrupt onset and often also abrupt termination, originating from an ectopic focus which may be atrial, AV junctional, or ventricular.

reflex t., increased heart rate in response to some stimulus conveyed through the cardiac nerves.

sinus t., t. originating in the sinus node.

supraventricular t., rapid heart rate due to a pacemaker anywhere above the ventricular level, i.e., sinus node, atrium, atrioventricular junction. The QRS complexes are always narrow unless there is rate-related aberrancy or preexisting intraventricular conduction delay.

ventricular t., paroxysmal t. originating in an ectopic focus in the ventricle. SEE ALSO torsade de pointes.

tach·y·car·di·ac (tak-i-kar′dē-ak). Relating to or suffering from excessively rapid action of the heart.

tach·y·car·dic (tar-i-kar′dik). Relating to rapid heart rate.

tach·y·crot·ic (tak′i-krot′ik). Relating to, causing, or characterized by a rapid pulse. [tachy- + G. *krotos,* a striking]

tach·y·ki·nin (tak-ē-kī′nin). Any member of a group of polypeptides, widely scattered in vertebrate and invertebrate tissues, that have in common four of the five terminal amino acids: Phe–Xaa–Gly–Leu–Met–NH$_2$; pharmacologically, they all cause hypotension in mammals, contraction of gut and bladder smooth muscle, and secretion of saliva. [G. *tachys,* swift, + *kineō,* to move, + *-in*]

tach·y·pac·ing (tak′ĭ-pā′sing). Rapid pacing of the heart by an artificial electronic pacemaker operating faster than the basic cardiac rate.

tach·y·phy·lax·is (tak′i-fī-lak′sis). Rapid appearance of progressive decrease in response to a given dose following repetitive administration of a pharmacologically or physiologically active substance. [tachy- + G. *phylaxis,* protection]

tach·yp·nea (tak-ip-nē′ă). Rapid breathing. SYN polypnea. [tachy- + G. *pnoē (pnoiē),* breathing]

transient t. of the newborn, a syndrome of generally mild t. in otherwise healthy newborns, lasting usually only about 3 days. SYN respiratory distress syndrome type II.

tach·y·rhyth·mia (tak-i-ridh′mē-ă). SYN tachycardia. [tachy- + G. *rhythmos,* rhythm]

ta·chys·ter·ol (tă-kis′ter-ōl). Sterol(s) formed by ultraviolet irradiation of any 5,7-diene-3β-sterol, which breaks the 9,10 bond, but usually from either or both of ergosterol and lumisterol to produce t.$_2$ (ertacalciol, (6*E*,22*E*)-9,10-secoergosta-5(10),6,8,22-tetraen-3β-ol) and from 7-dehydrocholesterol to produce t.$_3$ (tacalciol, (6*E*,3*S*)-9,10-secocholesta-5(10),6,8-trien-3β-ol). When reduced to the 5,7-diene (or 5,7,22-triene) form, dihydrotachysterol$_3$ (10,19-dihydrocalciol) or dihydrotachysterol$_2$ (10,19-

dihydrotachisterol), antirachitic action appears. This property has been of therapeutic interest, but t. is being replaced by the true vitamin D hormone (calcitriol) and its derivatives.

tach·y·sys·to·le (tak-i-sis′tō-lē). SYN tachycardia. [tachy- + G. *systolē,* contracting]

tach·y·zo·ite (tak-ĭ-zō′īt). A rapidly multiplying stage in the development of the tissue phase of certain coccidial infections, as in *Toxoplasma gondii* development in acute infections of toxoplasmosis. [tachy- + G. *zōon,* animal]

tac·rine (tak′rēn). An anticholinesterase agent with nonspecific central nervous system stimulatory effects; used in early stages of Alzheimer disease.

tac·tile (tak′til). Relating to touch or to the sense of touch. [L. *tactilis,* fr. *tango,* pp. *tactus,* to touch]

tac·tion (tak′shŭn). **1.** The sense of touch. **2.** The act of touching. [L. *tactio,* fr. *tango,* pp. *tactus,* to touch]

tac·tom·e·ter (tak-tom′ĕ-ter). SYN esthesiometer. [L. *tactus,* touch, + G. *metron,* measure]

tac·tor (tak′tăr, -tōr). A tactile end organ. [L. one who or that which touches]

tac·tu·al (tak′chool). Relating to or caused by touch.

TAD Acronym for transient acantholytic *dermatosis.*

Tae·nia (tē′nē-ă). A genus of cestodes that formerly included most of the tapeworms, but is now restricted to those species infecting carnivores with cysticerci found in tissues of various herbivores, rodents, and other animals of prey. SEE ALSO tapeworm. [see taenia]

  T. africa′na, a tapeworm found in native Africans, the cysticercus of which is unknown.

  T. arma′ta, SYN *T. solium.*

  T. crassic′ollis, SYN *T. taeniaeformis.*

  T. demerarien′sis, former name for *Davainea madagascariensis.*

  T. denta′ta, SYN *T. solium.*

  T. equi′na, SYN *Anoplocephala perfoliata.*

  T. hom′inis, unusual form of *T. saginata.*

  T. hydatig′ena, a tapeworm of dogs, cats, wolves, foxes, and other carnivores; the larva is known as *Cysticercus tenuicollis.*

  T. madagascarien′sis, former name for *Davainea madagascariensis.*

  T. min′ima, former name for *Hymenolepis nana.*

  T. o′vis, a tapeworm of dogs and foxes whose larval form is found in the muscles of sheep; heavy larval infections in sheep can have severe economic consequences due to condemnation of carcasses at meat inspection.

  T. philippi′na, atypical form of *T. saginata.*

  T. pisifor′mis, a common tapeworm of dogs, foxes, and other carnivores; the larval form is *Cysticercus pisiformis.*

  T. quadriloba′ta, SYN *Anoplocephala perfoliata.*

  T. sagina′ta, the beef, hookless, or unarmed tapeworm of humans, acquired by eating insufficiently cooked flesh of cattle infected with *Cysticercus bovis.*

  T. so′lium, the pork, armed, or solitary tapeworm of humans, acquired by eating insufficiently cooked pork infected with *Cysticercus cellulosae;* hatching of ova within the human intestine may result in establishment of cysticerci in human tissues, resulting in cysticercosis. SYN *T. armata, T. dentata.*

  T. taeniaefor′mis, one of the common tapeworms of household cats; the larval form is called *Cysticercus fasciolaris.* SYN *Hydatigera taeniaeformis, T. crassicollis.*

tae·nia (tē′nē-ă). **1.** A coiled bandlike anatomic structure. SEE tenia (1). **2.** Common name for a tapeworm, especially of the genus *Taenia.* SYN tenia (2). [L., fr. G. *tainia,* band, tape, a tapeworm]

Tae·ni·a·rhyn·chus (tē′nē-ă-ring′kŭs). A genus established for the *Taenia* species having a rudimentary rostellum but lacking the rostellar hooklets typical of *Taenia.* The best known example is *Taeniarhynchus saginatus,* but the older name, *Taenia saginata,* is more commonly used. [G. *tainia,* band, + *rhynchos,* snout]

tae·ni·a·sis (tē-nē-ī′ă-sis). Infection with cestodes of the genus *Taenia.*

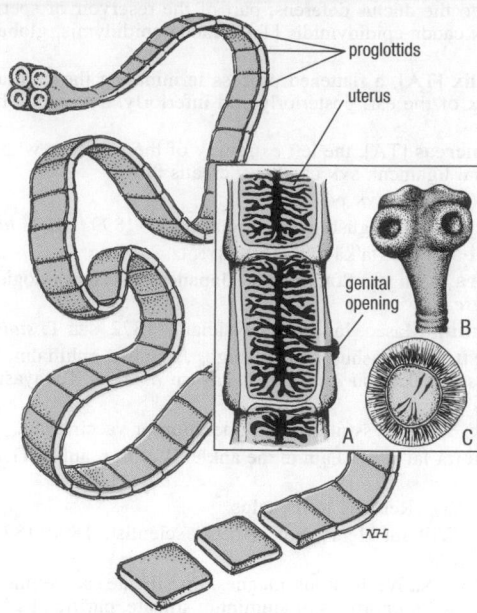

Taenia saginata (beef tapeworm): (A) body segment showing reproductive organs (x1.7), (B) scolex (x12), (C) egg (x550)

tae·ni·id (tē-nē′id). Common name for a member of the family Taeniidae.

Tae·ni·i·dae (tē-nē′i-dē). A family of parasitic cestodes (order Cyclophyllidea) that includes the genera *Taenia, Taeniarhynchus, Multiceps,* and *Echinococcus.*

tae·ni·oid (tē′nē-oyd). Denoting members of the genus *Taenia.*

Tae·ni·o·rhyn·chus (tē-nē-ō-ring′kŭs). A genus and subgenus of mosquitoes now considered synonymous with *Mansonia.* [G. *tainia,* band, + *rhynchos,* snout]

Taenzer, Paul R., German dermatologist, 1858–1919. SEE T. *stain;* Unna-T. *stain.*

TAF Abbreviation for tumor angiogenic *factor.*

tag. 1. SEE label, tracer. **2.** A small outgrowth or polyp. **3.** In magnetic resonance imaging, a band of saturation that can be followed to detect tissue motion.

  anal skin t., a fibrous polyp of the skin just outside the anus.

  epiploic t.'s, SYN omental *appendices,* under *appendix.*

  sentinel t., projecting edematous skin at the lower end of an anal fissure.

  skin t., (1) a polypoid outgrowth of both epidermis and dermal fibrovascular tissue; **(2)** in embryology, skin-covered projection that may or may not contain cartilage; typically located in a line between the tragus and corner of the mouth and associated with external ear anomalies. SYN acrochordon, fibroepithelial polyp, fibroma molle, papilloma molle, soft papilloma.

tag·a·tose (tag′ă-tōs). A ketohexose; D-t. is epimeric with D-fructose.

tag·li·a·co·ti·an (tal-yah-cō′shē-an). Pertaining to or described by Tagliacozzi.

Tagliacozzi, Gaspare, Italian surgeon, 1546–1599.

tail (tāl) [TA]. **1.** Any tail, or taillike structure, or tapering or elongated extremity of an organ or other part. SYN cauda [TA]. **2.** In veterinary anatomy, a free appendage representing the caudal end of the vertebral column; covered by skin and hair, feathers, or scales. [A.S. *taegl*]

  t. of caudate nucleus [TA], the elongated posterior extension of the caudate nucleus that parallels the body and inferior horn of the lateral ventricle. SYN cauda nuclei caudati [TA], cauda striati.

  t. of dentate gyrus, SYN uncus *band* of Giacomini.

  t. of epididymis [TA], the inferior part of the epididymis that leads into the ductus deferens; part of the reservoir of spermatozoa. SYN cauda epididymidis [TA], cauda epididymis, globus minor.

t. of helix [TA], a flattened process terminating the cartilage of the helix of the ear, posteriorly and inferiorly. SYN cauda helicis [TA].

t. of pancreas [TA], the left extremity of the pancreas within the lienorenal ligament. SYN cauda pancreatis [TA].

tail·gut (tāl′gŭt). SYN postanal *gut*.

Tait, Robert L., English gynecologist, 1845–1899. SEE T. *law*.

Ta·ka·di·as·tase (tă′kă-dī′as-tās). SYN α-amylase.

Takahara, Shigeo, 20th century Japanese otolaryngologist. SEE T. *disease*.

Takayama, Masao, Japanese physician, *1872. SEE T. *stain*.

Takayasu (Takayashu). Michishige, Japanese ophthalmologist, *1872. SEE Takayasu *arteritis*, Takayasu *disease*, Takayasu *syndrome*.

take (tāk). A successful grafting operation or vaccination.

ta·lal·gia (tă-lal′jē-ă). Pain in the ankle. [L. *talus,* ankle, G. *algos,* pain]

ta·lar (tā′lăr). Relating to the talus.

Talbot, William Henry Fox, British scientist, 1800–1877. SEE Plateau-T. *law*.

talc (tălk). Native hydrous magnesium silicate, sometimes containing small proportions of aluminum silicate, purified by boiling powdered t. with hydrochloric acid in water; used in pharmacy as a filter aid, as a dusting powder, and in cosmetic preparations. SYN French chalk, soapstone, talcum. [Ar. *talq*]

tal·co·sis (tal-kō′sis). A pulmonary disorder related to silicosis, occurring in workers exposed to talc mixed with silicates; characterized by restrictive or obstructive disorders of breathing or the two in combination. [talc + G. -osis, condition]

pulmonary t., pneumoconiosis from inhaling talc dusts.

tal·cum (tal′kŭm). SYN talc. [L.]

tal·i·on (tal′ē-on, tal′yŭn). The principle of retribution in intrapsychic behavior. [Welsh *tal,* compensation]

t. dread, The symbolic anxieties that represent the unconscious dread of penalties for an act.

tal·i·ped·ic (tal-i-ped′ik). Clubfooted.

tal·i·pes (tal′i-pēz). Any deformity of the foot involving the talus. [L. *talus,* ankle, + *pes,* foot]

t. calcaneoval′gus, t. calcaneus and t. valgus combined; the foot is dorsiflexed, everted, and abducted.

t. calcaneova′rus, t. calcaneus and t. varus combined; the foot is dorsiflexed, inverted, and adducted.

t. calca′neus, a deformity due to weakness or absence of the calf muscles, in which the axis of the calcaneus becomes vertically oriented; commonly seen in poliomyelitis. SYN calcaneus (2).

t. ca′vus, an exaggeration of the normal arch of the foot. SYN contracted foot, pes cavus, t. plantaris.

t. equinoval′gus, t. equinus and t. valgus combined; the foot is plantarflexed, everted, and abducted. SYN equinovalgus, pes equinovalgus.

t. equinova′rus, t. equinus and t. varus combined; the foot is plantarflexed, inverted, and adducted. SYN clubfoot, equinovarus, pes equinovarus.

t. equi′nus, permanent plantar flexion of the foot so that only the ball rests on the ground; it is commonly combined with t. varus.

t. planta′ris, SYN t. cavus.

t. pla′nus, SYN *pes* planus.

t. transversopla′nus, SYN *metatarsus* latus.

t. val′gus, permanent eversion of the foot, the inner side alone of the sole resting on the ground; it is usually combined with a breaking down of the plantar arch. SYN pes abductus, pes pronatus, pes valgus.

t. va′rus, inversion of the foot, the outer side of the sole only touching the ground; usually some degree of t. equinus is associated with it, and often t. cavus. SYN pes adductus, pes varus.

tal·low (tal′ō). The rendered fat from mutton suet.

prepared mutton t., SYN prepared *suet*.

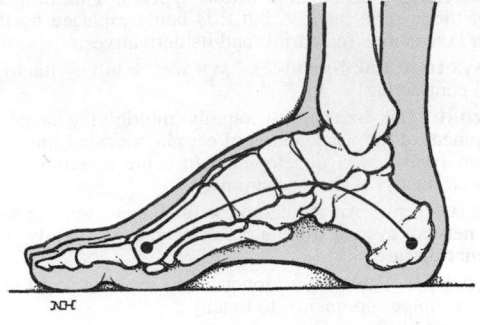

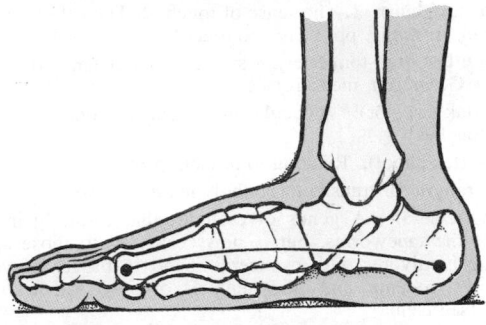

talipes cavus (top) and **talipes planus** (bottom)

talo-. The talus. [L. *talus,* ankle, ankle bone]

ta·lo·cal·ca·ne·al, ta·lo·cal·ca·ne·an (tā-lō-kal-kā′nē-ăl, tā-lō-kal-kā′nē-an). Relating to the talus and the calcaneus.

ta·lo·cru·ral (tā′lō-kroo′răl). Relating to the talus and the bones of the leg; denoting the ankle joint.

ta·lo·fib·u·lar (tă′lō-fib′ū-lăr). Relating to the talus and the fibula.

ta·lo·na·vic·u·lar (tā′lō-nă-vik′ū-lăr). Relating to the talus and the navicular bone. SYN astragaloscaphoid, taloscaphoid.

ta·lo·scaph·oid (tā′lō-skaf′oyd). SYN talonavicular.

tal·ose (tal′ōs). An aldohexose, isomeric with glucose; D-t. is epimeric with D-galactose.

ta·lo·tib·i·al (tā′lō-tib′ē-ăl). Relating to the talus and the tibia.

ta·lus, gen. **ta·li** (tā′lŭs, -lī) [TA]. The bone of the foot that articulates with the tibia and fibula to form the ankle joint. SYN ankle bone, ankle (3). [L. ankle bone, heel]

tam·a·rind (tam′ă-rind). The pulp of the fruit of *Tamarindus indica* (family Leguminosae), a large tree of India; mildly laxative. [Mediev. L. fr. Ar. *tamr*]

tam·bour (tahm-bur′). The recording part of a graphic apparatus, such as a sphygmograph, consisting of a membrane stretched across the open end of a cylinder and the recording stylus attached to it. [Fr. drum]

Tamm, Igor, U.S. virologist, *1922. SEE T.-Horsfall *mucoprotein, protein*.

ta·mox·i·fen cit·rate (tă-mok′sĭ-fen). A synthetic nonsteroidal estrogen antagonist used in the prevention and treatment of breast cancer.

By competing with naturally occurring estrogen for binding sites on tissue cells, tamoxifen inhibits the stimulant effect of estrogen on breast cancers. Tumors that have been shown by biochemical assay to be rich in estrogen receptors are most likely to respond to treatment. Since 1985, tamoxifen has been used in patients who have undergone surgery or irradiation for breast cancer, to delay or prevent relapse. The drug has been found effective in reducing the risk of cancer recurrence or disease progression in women with or without axillary node metastasis. In women with extensive disease, tamoxifen therapy has been as effective as oophorectomy in retarding progression. In 1992, the National Cancer Institute's Breast Cancer Prevention Trial (BCPT) enrolled more than 13,000 women in the U.S. and Canada to study the preventive value of tamoxifen. All participants were considered at high risk of breast cancer because of age (>60), strong family history, or a prior diagnosis of lobular carcinoma in situ. By March 1998 the difference in incidence of breast cancer between treated and placebo groups was so great that researchers concluded that the ethical need to inform participants of the clear benefits of active drug prophylaxis outweighed any possible benefits of further controlled study. Women in the highest risk categories showed 45% reduction in breast cancer. However, this study demonstrated no effect on mortality, and in two similar trials in Europe, tamoxifen failed to show a statistically significant protective effect. Women taking tamoxifen are at increased risk of endometrial carcinoma, deep venous thrombosis, pulmonary embolism, and cataracts. The danger of these adverse consequences is greatest in women over 50. Long-term use of the drug is associated with recurrent vaginal candidiasis. It is contraindicated during pregnancy because of the risk of fetal harm.

---

tam·pon. **1.** A cylinder or ball of cotton-wool, gauze, or other loose substance; used as a plug or pack in a canal or cavity to restrain hemorrhage, absorb secretions, or maintain a displaced organ in position. **2.** To insert such a plug or pack. [O. Fr.]

Corner t., a plug of omentum stuffed into a wound of the stomach or intestine as a temporary t.

tam·pon·ade, tam·pon·age (tam-pŏ-nād′, tam′pŏ-nij). **1.** Pathologic compression of an organ. **2.** SYN tamponing.

⬛**cardiac t.,** compression of the heart due to critically increased volume of fluid in the pericardium. SYN heart t.

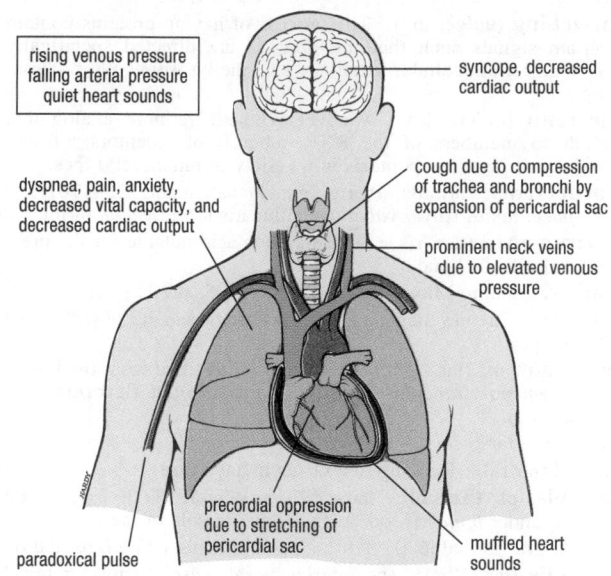

rising venous pressure falling arterial pressure quiet heart sounds

syncope, decreased cardiac output

dyspnea, pain, anxiety, decreased vital capacity, and decreased cardiac output

cough due to compression of trachea and bronchi by expansion of pericardial sac

prominent neck veins due to elevated venous pressure

precordial oppression due to stretching of pericardial sac

muffled heart sounds

paradoxical pulse

assessment for **cardiac tamponade** due to pericardial effusion

---

chronic t., cardiac compression over long periods due to pathologically increased fluid in the pericardial sac.

heart t., SYN cardiac t.

tam·pon·ing, tam·pon·ment (tam′pon-ing, tam-pon′ment). The act of inserting a tampon. SYN tamponade (2), tamponage.

ta·nace·tol, tan·a·ce·tone (ta-nās′tol, tan-ă-sē′tōn). SYN thujone.

tan·dem (tan′dem). Term used to describe multiple copies of the same sequence in a polynucleic acid that lie adjacent to one another.

tan·gen·ti·al·i·ty (tan-jen′shē-al′i-tē). A disturbance in the asso-

ciative thought process in which one tends to digress readily from one topic under discussion to other topics which arise in the course of associations; observed in bipolar disorder and schizophrenia and certain types of organic brain disorders. Cf. circumstantiality. [off on a tangent, fr. L. *tango,* to touch]

tan·gle (tang′l). A small irregular knot.

neurofibrillary t., intraneuronal accumulations of helical filaments that assume twisted contorted patterns; found in cells of the hippocampus and cerebral cortex in individuals with Alzheimer disease.

tank. A device made to receive and/or hold liquids.

Hubbard t., a large t., usually filled with warm water, used for therapeutic exercises in a program of physiotherapy.

tan·nase (tan′ās). Tannin acylhydrolase, an enzyme produced in cultures of *Penicillium glaucum* and found in certain tannin-forming plants; it hydrolyzes digallate to gallate, and also acts on ester links in other tannins.

tan·nate (tan′āt). A salt of tannic acid.

Tanner growth chart. See under chart.

Tanner stage. See under stage.

tan·nic (tan′ik). Relating to tan (tan-bark) or to tannin.

tan·nic ac·id. A tannin, $C_{76}H_{52}O_{46}$, that occurs in many plants, particularly in the bark of oaks and other members of the Fagaceae; used as a styptic and astringent, and in the treatment of diarrhea; available also as tannic acid glycerite. Sometimes used synonymously with tannin.

tan·nin (tan′in). Any one of a group of complex nonuniform plant constituents that can be classified into hydrolyzable t.'s (esters of a sugar, usually glucose, and one or several trihydroxybenzenecarboxylic acids) and condensed t.'s (derivatives of flavonols). T.'s are used in tanning, dyeing, photography, and as clarifying agents for beer and wine. Sometimes used synonymously with tannic acid. T.'s form black stains in the presence of iron.

tan·nyl·ac·e·tate (tan-il-as′ĕ-tāt). SYN acetyltannic acid.

tan·ta·lum (Ta) (tan′tă-lŭm). A heavy metal of the vanadium group, atomic no. 73, atomic wt. 180.9479; used in surgical prostheses because of its noncorrosive properties. [G. mythical king of Lydia, *Tantalus*]

tan·trum (tan′trŭm). A fit of bad temper, especially in children.

tan·y·cyte (tan′i-sīt). A variety of ependymal cell found principally in the walls of the third ventricle of the brain; the t.'s may have branched or unbranched processes, some of which end on capillaries or neurons.

tan·y·pho·nia (tan-i-fō′nē-ă). A thin, weak voice resulting from tension of vocal muscles. [G. *tanyō,* to stretch, + *phonē,* sound]

TAP. A protein that transports a peptide from the cytoplasm into the lumen of the endoplasmic reticulum.

tap. **1.** To withdraw fluid from a cavity by means of a trocar and cannula, hollow needle, or catheter. **2.** To strike lightly with the finger or a hammerlike instrument in percussion or to elicit a tendon reflex. **3.** A light blow. **4.** An East Indian fever of undetermined nature. **5.** An instrument to cut threads in a hole in bone prior to inserting a screw. [M.E. *tappe,* fr. A.S. *taeppa*]

heel t., a reflex movement of the toes when the heel is tapped, present in multiple sclerosis and other diseases of the pyramidal tract.

mitral t., **(1)** the palpable equivalent of the opening snap of the mitral valve; **(2)** the palpable accentuated first heart sound of mitral stenosis; often mistaken for the apex beat.

pericardial t., SYN pericardiocentesis.

pleural t., SYN thoracentesis.

spinal t., SYN lumbar *puncture.*

tape (tāp). A thin flat strip of fascia or tendon, or of synthetic material, used as a tie or suture. [A.S. *taeppe*]

adhesive t., fabric or film evenly coated on one side with a pressure-sensitive adhesive mixture.

ta·pe·to·cho·roi·dal (tă-pē′tō-kō-roy′dăl). Relating to the tapetum and the choroid.

ta·pe·to·ret·i·nal (tă-pē′tō-ret′i-năl). Relating to the retinal pigment epithelium and the sensory retina.

ta

ta·pe·to·ret·in·op·a·thy (tă-pē'tō-ret-in-op'ă-thē). Hereditary degeneration of the sensory retina and pigmentary epithelium; seen in pigmentary retinopathy, choroideremia, gyrate atrophy, congenital nyctalopia, congenital amaurosis, and heredomacular degeneration. [tapetum + retinopathy]

ta·pe·tum, pl. **ta·pe·ta** (tă-pē'tŭm, -tă). 1. In general, any membranous layer or covering. 2 [TA]. In neuroanatomy, a thin sheet of fibers in the lateral wall of the temporal and occipital horns of the lateral ventricle, continuous with the corpus callosum. SYN Fielding membrane, membrana versicolor. 3. A dense layer in the choroidea of the eye of many mammalian species, including the cat and dog but not humans, that forms a discrete or diffuse area of reflective cells, rodlets, and fibers; its strong light-reflecting properties cause the metallic hue and light-glow of such eyes in the dark. [L. tapeta, a carpet]

t. alve'oli, SYN periodontium.

t. ni'grum, SYN pigmented *layer* of retina.

t. oc'uli, SYN pigmented *layer* of retina.

tape·worm (tāp'werm). An intestinal parasitic worm, adults of which are found in the intestine of vertebrates; the term is commonly restricted to members of the class Cestoidea. T.'s consist of a scolex, variously equipped with spined or sucking structures by which the worm is attached to the intestinal wall of the host, and strobila having several to many proglottids that lack a digestive tract at any stage of development. The ovum, entering the intestine of an appropriate intermediate host, hatches and the hexacanth penetrates the gut wall and develops into a specific larval form (e.g., cysticercoid, cysticercus, hydatid, strobilocercus), which develops into an adult when the intermediate host is ingested by the proper final host. A three-host cycle with a swimming coracidium, procercoid and plerocercoid (sparganum) larva, and adult intestinal worm is found in aquatic life cycles, as in *Diphyllobothrium latum* (broad fish t.) and other pseudophyllid cestodes. Other important species of t. are *Echinococcus granulosus* (hydatid t.), *Hymenolepis nana* or *H. nana* var. *fraterna* (dwarf or dwarf mouse t.), *Taenia saginata* (beef, hookless, or unarmed t.), *T. solium* (armed, pork, or solitary t.), and *Thysanosoma actinoides* (fringed t. of sheep).

taph·o·phil·ia (taf-ō-fil'ē-ă). Morbid attraction for graves. [G. *taphos*, grave, + *phileō*, to love]

taph·o·pho·bia (taf-ō-fō'bē-ă). Morbid fear of being buried alive. [G. *taphos*, the grave, + *phobos*, fear]

Tapia, Antonio G., Spanish otolaryngologist, 1875–1950. SEE T. *syndrome*.

tap·i·no·ce·phal·ic (tap'i-nō-sĕ-fal'ik, tă-pī'nō-). Having a low flat head; relating to tapinocephaly.

tap·i·no·ceph·a·ly (tă-pi-nō-sef'ă-lē). A condition of flat head in which the skull has a vertical index below 72; similar to chamecephaly. [G. *tapeinos*, low, + *kephalē*, head]

tap·i·o·ca (tap'ē-ō'kă). A starch from the root of *Janipha manihot* and other species of *J.* (family Euphorbiaceae), plants of tropical America; an easily digested starch, free of irritant properties. SYN cassava starch. [Braz. *tipioca*]

ta·pote·ment (tă-pot-mawn'). A massage movement consisting in striking with the side of the hand, usually with partly flexed fingers. SYN tapping (1). [Fr. fr. *tapoter*, to tap]

tap·ping (tap'ing). 1. SYN tapotement. 2. SYN paracentesis.

TAPVC Abbreviation for total anomalous pulmonary venous connection. SEE anomalous pulmonary venous *connections*, total or partial, under *connection*.

TAPVR Abbreviation for total anomalous pulmonary venous *return*. SEE anomalous pulmonary venous *connections*, total or partial, under *connection*.

TAR Acronym for *t*hrombocytopenia and *a*bsent *r*adius. SEE thrombocytopenia-absent radius *syndrome*.

tar. A thick, semisolid, blackish brown mass, of complex hydrocarbon composition, obtained by the destructive distillation of carbonaceous materials. For individual t.'s, see specific names.

rectified t. oil, a volatile oil distilled from pine t.; used externally in the treatment of skin diseases such as eczema and psoriasis.

tar·an·tism (tar'an-tizm). A form of mass hysteria which origi-

nated in Taranto, Italy, in the late Middle Ages as a dancing mania to cure the madness allegedly caused by the bite of a tarantula.

ta·ran·tu·la (tă-ran'choo-lă). A very large, hairy spider, considered highly venomous and often greatly feared; the bite, however, is usually no more harmful than a bee sting, and the creature is relatively inoffensive. SEE tarantism.

American t., *Eurypelma hentzii*, the Arkansas t.; although greatly feared, its bite is relatively uncommon and harmless to humans.

black t., *Sericopelma communis*, a large black t. of Panama and the Canal Zone, whose bite is poisonous, although the effect is localized.

European t., *Lycosa tarentula*, the large European wolf spider or true t. Its bite was once believed to cause madness, which inspired frenzied contortions and dancing to rid the body of the venom, though the bite is, in fact, harmless, as is that of most of the large, hairy "tarantula spiders" of the tropics.

Peruvian t., pruning spider, *Glyptocranium gasteracanthoides*, a poisonous Peruvian spider whose bite causes local gangrene, hematuria, and neurotoxic symptoms.

ta·rax·a·cum (tă-rak'să-kŭm). The dried rhizome and root of *Taraxacum officinale* (family Compositae), the dandelion, a wild plant of wide distribution throughout the temperate regions of the northern hemisphere; alleged to be a tonic and hepatic stimulant. [Mod. L. fr. Ar. *tarakshagūn*, wild chicory]

Tardieu, Ambroise A., French physician, 1818–1879. SEE T. *ecchymoses*, under *ecchymosis*, *petechiae*, under *petechiae*, *spots*, under *spot*.

tar·dive (tar'div). Late; tardy.

cyanose t., SYN late *cyanosis*.

tar·get (tar'get). 1. An object fixed as goal or point of examination. 2. In the ophthalmometer, the mire. 3. SYN target *organ*. 4. Anode of an x-ray tube. SEE ALSO x-ray. [It. *targhetta*, a small shield]

tar·get·ing (tar'get-ing). The process of having proteins contain certain signals such that the proteins are directed specifically towards certain cellular locations, e.g., the lysosome. Cf. processing.

targretin (tar'gre-tin). A novel synthetic retinoid analog that binds to members of the RXR subclass of receptors; of low toxicity, it induces apoptosis in a variety of tumor cell types.

Tarin (Tarini, Tarinus), Pierre, French anatomist, 1725–1761. SEE T. *space*, *tenia*, *valve*; *valvula* semilunaris tarini; *velum* tarini.

ta·rir·ic ac·id (tă-rī'rik). An 18-carbon acid notable for the presence of a triple bond.

Tarlov, Isadore Max, U. S. surgeon, *1905. SEE T. *cyst*.

Tarnier, Étienne Stephane, French obstetrician, 1828–1897. SEE T. *forceps*.

tar·ra·gon oil (tar'ă-gon). A volatile oil distilled from the leaves of *Artemisia dranculus* (family Compositae); a flavoring. SYN estragon oil.

△**tars-.** SEE tarso-.

tar·sal (tar'săl). Relating to a tarsus in any sense.

tar·sa·le, pl. **tar·sa·lia** (tar-sā'lē, tar-sā'lē-ă) [TA]. SYN tarsal *bones*, under *bone*. [Mod. L. fr. G. *tarsos*, sole of the foot]

tars·al·gia (tar-sal'jē-ă). SYN podalgia. [tarsus + G. *algos*, pain]

tar·sa·lis (tar-sā'lis). SEE inferior tarsal *muscle*, superior tarsal *muscle*.

tars·ec·to·my (tar-sek'tō-mē). Excision of the tarsus of the foot or of a segment of the tarsus of an eyelid. [tarsus + G. *ektomē*, excision]

tar·sec·to·pia, tar·sec·to·py (tar-sek-tō'pē-ă, -sek'tō-pē). Subluxation of one or more tarsal bones. [tarsus + G. *ektopos*, out of place]

tar·sen. Within the tarsus; relating to the tarsus independent of other structures. [tarsus + G. *en*, in]

tar·si·tis (tar-sī'tis). 1. Inflammation of the tarsus of the foot. 2. Inflammation of the tarsal border of an eyelid.

△**tarso-, tars-.** A tarsus. [See tarsus]

tar·so·cla·sia, tar·soc·la·sis (tar-sō-klā'zē-ă, tar-sok'lă-sis). Instrumental fracture of the tarsus, for the correction of talipes equinovarus. [tarso- + G. *klasis*, a breaking]

tar·so·la·cia (tar′sō-mă-lā′shē-ă). Softening of the tarsal cartilages of the eyelids. [tarso- + G. *malakia*, softness]

tar·so·meg·a·ly (tar-sō-meg′ă-lē). A congenital maldevelopment and overgrowth of a tarsal or carpal bone. SYN dysplasia epiphysialis hemimelia. [tarso- + G. *megas*, large]

tar·so·met·a·tar·sal (tar-sō-met′ă-tar′săl). Relating to the tarsal and metatarsal bones; denoting the articulations between the two sets of bones, and the ligaments in relation thereto.

tar·so·or·bit·al (tar′sō-ōr′bi-tăl). Relating to the eyelids and the orbit.

tar·so·pha·lan·ge·al (tar-sō-fă-lan′jē-ăl). Relating to the tarsus and the phalanges.

tar·sor·rha·phy (tar-sōr′ă-fē). The suturing together of the eyelid margins, partially or completely, to shorten the palpebral fissure or to protect the cornea in keratitis or in paralysis of the orbicularis oculi muscle. [tarso- + G. *rhaphē*, suture]

tar·so·tar·sal (tar′sō-tar′săl). SYN intertarsal.

tar·so·tib·i·al (tar′sō-tib′ē-al). SYN tibiotarsal.

tar·sot·o·my (tar-sot′ō-mē). **1.** Incision of the tarsal cartilage of an eyelid. **2.** Rarely used term for any operation on the tarsus of the foot. [tarso- + G. *tomē*, incision]

tar·sus, gen. and pl. **tar·si** (tar′sŭs, -sī). **1.** As a division of the skeleton, the seven tarsal bones of the instep. SYN root of foot. SEE tarsal *bones*, under *bone*. [G. *tarsos*, a flat surface, sole of the foot, edge of eyelid] **2.** The fibrous plates giving solidity and form to the edges of the eyelids; often erroneously called tarsal or ciliary cartilages. SYN skeleton of eyelid. SEE ALSO inferior t., superior t.

   t. infe′rior [TA], SYN inferior t.

   inferior t. [TA], the fibrous plate in the lower eyelid. SYN t. inferior [TA].

   t. supe′rior [TA], SYN superior t.

   superior t. [TA], the fibrous plate in the upper eyelid. SYN t. superior [TA].

tar·tar (tar′tăr). **1.** A crust on the interior of wine casks, consisting essentially of potassium bitartrate. **2.** A white, brown, or yellow-brown deposit at or below the gingival margin of teeth, chiefly hydroxyapatite in an organic matrix. SYN dental calculus (2). [Mediev. L. *tartarum*, ult. etym. unknown]

   cream of t., SYN *potassium* bitartrate.

   t. emetic, SYN *antimony* potassium tartrate.

   soluble t., SYN *potassium* tartrate.

tar·tar·ic ac·id (tar-tar′ik). Made from crude tartar; a laxative and refrigerant; used in the manufacture of various effervescing powders, tablets, and granules.

tar·trate (tar′trāt). A salt of tartaric acid.

   acid t., a salt of tartaric acid which contains an acid group still capable of combining with a base; e.g., bitartrate.

   normal t., t. that contains no uncombined acid groups.

tar·trat·ed (tar′trāt-ed). Combined with or containing tartar or tartaric acid.

tar·tra·zine (tar′tră-zēn) [C.I. 19140]. A yellow acid dye used in place of orange G in a variant of Mallory aniline blue stain for collagen and cellular inclusion bodies. SYN hydrazine yellow.

tas·tant (tās′tant). Any chemical that stimulates the sensory cells in a taste bud.

taste (tāst). **1.** To perceive through the gustatory system. **2.** The sensation produced by a suitable stimulus applied to the taste buds. [It. *tastare*; L. *tango*, to touch]

   after-t., SEE aftertaste.

   color t., a form of synesthesia in which the color sense and t. are associated, with stimulation of either sense inducing a subjective sensation in the associated sense. SYN pseudogeusesthesia.

   franklinic t., a metallic or sour t. produced by the application of static electricity to the tongue. SYN voltaic t.

   voltaic t., SYN franklinic t.

TAT Abbreviation for thematic apperception *test*.

tat·too (tă-too′). **1.** A deliberate decorative implanting or injecting of indelible pigments into the skin or the tinctorial effect of accidental implantation. **2.** To produce such an effect. The procedure, historically and geographically widespread, is associated with risks of infection. Removal is difficult, with pulsed laser treatment offering low risks of scarring. [Tahiti, *tatu*]

   amalgam t., a bluish-black or gray macular lesion of the oral mucous membrane caused by accidental implantation of silver amalgam into the tissue during tooth restoration or extraction.

tau (τ). **1.** The 19th letter of the Greek alphabet. **2.** Symbol for tele; relaxation time. **3.** A protein that associates with microtubules and other elements of the cytoskeleton; t. accelerates tubulin polymerization and stabilizes microtubules; t. is also found in the plaque observed in individuals with Alzheimer disease and in cerebral neurons in other neurodegenerative disorders.

tau·rine (taw′rin, -rēn). **1.** An aminosulfonic acid, synthesized from L-cysteine and used in a number of roles, including in the synthesis of certain bile salts. **2.** Of or pertaining to a bull. [L. *taurinus*, of bulls, fr. *taurus*, bull, + suffix *-inus*, pertaining to]

tau·ro·cho·late (taw-rō-kō′lāt). A salt of taurocholic acid.

tau·ro·cho·lic ac·id (taw-rō-kō′lik). Choloyltaurine; *N*-choloyltaurine; a compound of cholic acid and taurine, involving the carboxyl group of the former and the amino of the latter; a common bile salt in carnivores. SYN cholaic acid.

tau·ro·don·tism (taw-rō-don′tizm). A developmental anomaly involving molar teeth in which the bifurcation or trifurcation of the roots is very near the apex, resulting in an abnormally large and long pulp chamber with exceedingly short pulp canals. [L. *taurus*, bull, + G. *odous*, tooth]

Taussig, Helen B., U.S. pediatrician, 1898–1986. SEE T.-Bing *disease, syndrome;* Blalock-T. *operation, shunt.*

tau·to·mer·ic (taw-tō-mer′ik). **1.** Relating to the same part. **2.** Relating to or marked by tautomerism. [G. *tautos*, the same, + *meros*, part]

tau·tom·er·ism (taw-tom′er-izm). A phenomenon in which a chemical compound exists in two forms of different structure (isomers) in equilibrium, the two forms differing, usually, in the position of a hydrogen atom; e.g., keto-enol t., $R–CH_2–C(O)–R'$ $\leftrightarrow R–CH=C(OH)–R'$. [G. *tautos*, the same, + *meros*, part]

Tawara, K. Sunao, Japanese pathologist, 1873–1952. SEE T. *node;* His-T. *system; node* of Aschoff and T.

taxa (tak′să). Plural of taxon.

taxanes (taks′ānz). A class of antitumor agents derived directly or semisynthetically from *Taxus brevifolius*, the Pacific yew; examples include paclitaxel and docetaxel.

tax·is (tak′sis). **1.** Reduction of a hernia or of a dislocation of any part by means of manipulation. **2.** Systematic classification or orderly arrangement. **3.** The reaction of protoplasm to a stimulus, by virtue of which animals and plants are led to move or act in certain definite ways in relation to their environment; the various kinds of t. are designated by a prefix denoting the stimulus governing them; e.g., chemotaxis, electrotaxis, thermotaxis. [G. orderly arrangement]

   negative t., the repulsion of protoplasm away from a stimulus.

   positive t., the attraction of protoplasm toward a stimulus.

tax·on, pl. **taxa** (tak′son, tak′să). The name given to a particular level or grouping in a systematic classification of living things or organisms (taxonomy). [G. *taxis*, order, arrangement, + -on]

tax·o·nom·ic (tak-sō-nom′ik). Relating to taxonomy.

tax·on·o·my (tak-săn′ŏ-mē). The systematic classification of living things or organisms. Kingdoms of living organisms are divided into groups (taxa) to show degrees of similarity or presumed evolutionary relationships, with the higher categories being larger, more inclusive, and more broadly defined, and the lower categories being more restricted, with fewer species more closely related. The divisions below kingdom are, in descending order: phylum, class, order, family, genus, species, and subspecies (variety). Infra- and supra- or sub- and super- categories can be used when needed; additional categories, such as tribe, section, level, group, etc., are also used. [G. *taxis*, orderly arrangement, + *nomos*, law]

   chemical t., an approach to the classification of organisms based on the distribution of natural products.

ta

taxonomy	
sample taxonomic classification of *Leptospira interrogans*	
kingdom	Procaryotae
phylum	Gracilicutes
class	Scotobacteria
order	Spirochaetales
family	Leptospiraceae
genus	*Leptospira*
species	*Leptospira interrogans*
subspecies serovar	e.g., *Leptospira interrogans* icterohemorrhagiae

numerical t., an approach to the classification of organisms that strives for objectivity, wherein characteristics of organisms are given equal weight (adansonian classification) and the relationships of the organisms are numerically determined, usually by computer.

Taxus (taks′us). Genus of plants including the Pacific yew (*Taxus brevifolius*); its bark yields antitumor agents of the taxane group.

Tay, Warren, English physician, 1843–1927. SEE T. cherry-red spot; T.-Sachs *disease*.

Taybi, Hooshang, U.S. pediatrician and radiologist, *1919. SEE Rubinstein-T. *syndrome*.

Taylor, Charles F., U.S. orthopedic surgeon, 1827–1899. SEE T. back *brace, apparatus, splint*.

Taylor, Robert W., U.S. dermatologist, 1842–1908. SEE T. *disease*.

TB Colloquial abbreviation for tuberculosis.

Tb Symbol for terbium.

TBG Abbreviation for thyroxine-binding *globulin*.

tBoc Abbreviation for *tert*-butyloxycarbonyl.

TBP Abbreviation for thyroxine-binding *protein*.

TBPA Abbreviation for thyroxine-binding *prealbumin*.

TBV Abbreviation for total blood volume.

TBW Abbreviation for total body *water*.

Tc Symbol for technetium.

Tc Abbreviation for T cytotoxic *cells*, under *cell*.

^{99m}Tc Symbol for technetium-99m.

^{99}Tc Symbol for technetium-99.

2,3,7,8-TCDD. Abbreviation for 2,3,7,8-tetrachlorodibenzo[b,e]-[1,4]dioxin. SEE dioxin (3).

^{99m}Tc-dimercaptosuccinic acid. Radiopharmaceutical that localizes to the renal cortex for imaging to determine scarring or pyelonephritis.

^{99m}Tc-DMSA Abbreviation for ^{99m}Tc-dimercaptosuccinic acid.

TCG Abbreviation for time compensation *gain*.

^{99m}Tc-glucoheptanate. Radiopharmaceutical possessing renal cortical-localizing and excretion-handling properties; may be used either for renal cortical imaging to determine scarring or for renal function imaging by renography.

TCID$_{50}$, TCD$_{50}$ Abbreviation for tissue culture infectious *dose*.

TDF Abbreviation for testis-determining *factor*.

TDP Abbreviation for ribothymidine 5′-diphosphate. The thymidine analog is dTDP.

TdT Abbreviation for terminal deoxynucleotidyl *transferase*.

TE In magnetic resonance spin echo pulse sequences, the time to echo, when the magnetization signal is sampled.

Te Symbol for tellurium.

tea (tē). **1.** The dried leaves of various genera of the family Theaceae, including *Thea* (*T. senensis*), *Camellia*, and *Gordonia*, a shrub indigenous to China, southern and southeastern Asia, and Japan. Its chief constituent, upon which its stimulating action largely depends, is the alkaloid caffeine, which is present in the

amount of 1–4%; theophylline, a chemically related alkaloid, is also present. **2.** The infusion made by pouring boiling water upon t. leaves. **3.** Any infusion or decoction made extemporaneously. SEE ALSO species (2). SYN thea. [Chinese (Amoy dial.) *t'e*, Mod. L. *thea*]

Hottentot t., SYN buchu.

Jesuit t., Mexican t., SYN chenopodium.

Paraguay t., SYN maté.

Teale, Thomas P., English surgeon, 1801–1868.

tear (tār). A discontinuity in substance of a structure. Cf. laceration.

bucket-handle t., a t. and separation in the central part of a semilunar cartilage with the ends intact that produces a resemblance to the handle of a bucket.

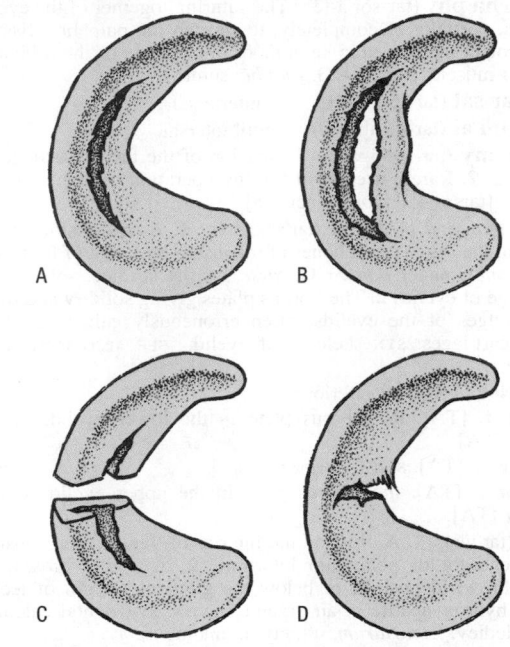

meniscal tears: (A) longitudinal, (B) bucket-handle, (C) horizontal, (D) parrot beak

Mallory-Weiss t., SYN Mallory-Weiss *syndrome*.

tear (tēr). The fluid secreted by the lacrimal glands by means of which the conjunctiva and cornea are kept moist. [A.S. *teár*]

artificial t.'s, mixtures of fluid compounds to substitute for naturally produced t's.

crocodile t.'s, SEE crocodile tears *syndrome*.

tear·ing (tēr′ing). SYN epiphora.

tease (tēz). To separate the structural parts of a tissue by means of a needle, in order to prepare it for microscopic examination. [A.S. *taesan*]

tea·spoon (tē′spoon). A small spoon, holding about 1 dram (or about 5 mL) of liquid; used as a measure in the dosage of fluid medicines.

teat (tēt). **1.** SYN nipple. **2.** SYN breast. **3.** SYN papilla. [A.S. *tit*]

teb·u·tate (teb′ū-tāt). USAN-approved contraction for tertiary butylacetate, $(CH_3)_3C–CH_2–CO_2^-$.

tech·ne·ti·um (Tc) (tek-nē′shē-um). An artificial radioactive element, atomic no. 43, atomic wt. 99, produced in 1937 by bombardment of molybdenum by deuterons; also a product of the fission of ^{235}U; used extensively as a radiographic tracer in imaging studies of internal organs. [G. *technetos*, artificial]

tech·ne·ti·um-99 (^{99}Tc). A radioisotope of technetium which is the decay product of technetium-99m and has a weak beta emission and a physical half-life of 213,000 years.

tech·ne·ti·um-99m (^{99m}Tc). A radioisotope of technetium that decays by isomeric transition, emitting an essentially monoenergetic gamma ray of 142 keV with a half-life of 6.01 hr. It is usually obtained from a radionuclide generator of molybdenum-99 and is used to prepare radiopharmaceuticals for scanning the brain, parotid, thyroid, lungs, blood pool, liver, heart, spleen, kidney, lacrimal drainage apparatus, bone, and bone marrow.

^{99m}Tc diphosphonate, a radionuclide complex used for bone scans.

^{99m}Tc-DTPA, a radionuclide chelate complex used for renal imaging and function testing; also known as ^{99m}Tc pentatate. [*d*iethylene *t*riamine *p*enta*a*cetic *a*cid]

^{99m}Tc sestamibi, a lipophilic cationic complex of a ^{99m}Tc-labeled isonitrite, used as a radionuclide in several organs (e.g., brain, bone, thyroid, breast) for the detection of cancer, or in the heart for identifying coronary artery occlusion. It has superseded Tl-201 in cardiac imaging and in experimental breast imaging.

^{99m}Tc sulfur colloid, a particulate radionuclide complex taken up by the reticuloendothelial system; used for imaging the liver and spleen.

tech·nic (tek-nik′). SYN technique.

tech·ni·cal (tek′ni-kăl). **1.** Relating to technique. **2.** Pertaining to some particular art, science, or trade. **3.** In connection with a chemical substance, denoting that the substance contains appreciable quantities of impurities.

tech·ni·cian (tek-nish′ŭn). SYN technologist. [G. *technē,* an art]

tech·nique (tek-nēk′). The manner of performance, or the details, of any surgical operation, experiment, or mechanical act. SEE ALSO method, operation, procedure. SYN technic. [Fr., fr. G. *technikos,* relating to *technē,* art, skill]

airbrasive t., a method of grinding, cutting tooth structure, or roughening the natural tooth surface or the surface of a restoration, by means of a device utilizing a gas-impelled jet of fine Al_2O_3 particles which, after striking the tooth, are removed by an aspirator. SEE ALSO microetching t.

air-gap t., chest radiography performed using a space between the subject and film instead of a grid to absorb scattered radiation; usually requires a target-film distance of 10 feet.

atrial-well t., an obsolete semiclosed surgical t. for repairing atrial septal defects and other cardiac abnormalities.

ballpoint pen t., a t. to measure the induration of intradermal tuberculin tests; a ballpoint pen is used to draw two opposing lines on the skin beginning 1–2 cm away from the dermal reaction site on opposite sides, stopping as the induration edge is felt. The distance between the proximal ends of the lines is the reported extent of induration.

Barcroft-Warburg t., SEE Warburg *apparatus.*

Begg light wire differential force t., SEE light wire *appliance.*

cellulose tape t., use of a piece of transparent cellulose tape applied to a glass slide to obtain perianal samples for identification of pinworm eggs.

direct t., SYN direct *method* for making inlays.

Ficoll-Hypaque t., a density-gradient centrifugation t. for separating lymphocytes from other formed elements in the blood; the sample is layered onto a Ficoll-sodium metrizoate gradient of specific density; following centrifugation, lymphocytes are collected from the plasma-Ficoll interface.

flicker fusion frequency t., SYN flicker *perimetry.*

fluorescent antibody t., a t. used to test for antigen with a fluorescent antibody, usually performed by one of two methods: *direct,* in which immunoglobulin (antibody) conjugated with a fluorescent dye is added to tissue and combines with specific antigen (microbe, or other), the resulting antigen-antibody complex being located by fluorescence microscopy; or *indirect,* in which unlabeled immunoglobulin (antibody) is added to tissue and combines with specific antigen, after which the antigen-antibody complex may be labeled with fluorescein-conjugated anti-immunoglobulin antibody, the resulting triple complex then being located by fluorescence microscopy.

flush t., a t. for determining the systolic blood pressure in infants; the elevated limb is "milked" of blood from the hand or foot proximally; the blood pressure cuff is then inflated above the

likely systolic pressure and the limb lowered; the cuff pressure is then gradually released until the blanched limb flushes.

Hampton t., obsolete term for atraumatic, nonpalpation, fluoroscopic examination of the upper gastrointestinal tract in peptic ulcer disease with acute hemorrhage.

Hartel t., a method of reaching the gasserian ganglion by passing a needle from the mouth, inserting it about the level of the upper midmolar tooth, and passing it inward until the point reaches the bone in front and to the outer side of the foramen ovale, allowing an alcohol injection to be made for the relief of trigeminal neuralgia.

high-kV t., chest radiography using a kilovoltage of at least 125 kVp, usually 140–150 kVp, to reduce patient dose and increase latitude.

Ilizarov t., a method of promoting controlled osteogenesis to lengthen bone and correct angular and rotational deformities, in which gradually increasing force is applied to the apposed fragments of a surgically divided bone by an external fixation frame (Ilizarov device).

immunoperoxidase t., an immunologic test that utilizes antibodies chemically conjugated to the enzyme peroxidase.

indirect t., SYN indirect *method* for making inlays.

Jerne t., a t. for measuring immunocompetence by quantitating the number of splenic antibody-forming cells found in a mouse that has been sensitized to sheep erythrocytes. The number of plaques formed correlates with the number of splenic antibody-forming cells.

Judkins t., a method of selective coronary artery catheterization utilizing the standard Seldinger t. through a percutaneous femoral artery puncture.

Knott t., concentration procedure using blood and dilute formalin; designed to detect microfilaria.

long cone t., the use of a cone distance of 14 inches or more in making oral roentgenographs.

McGoon t., plastic reconstruction of an incompetent mitral valve, when the incompetence is due to rupture of chordae to the posterior leaflet, by plication of the redundant leaflet.

Merendino t., plastic reconstruction of an incompetent mitral valve using heavy sutures to narrow the annulus in the region of the medial commissure.

microetching t., a method of roughening the surface of a natural tooth or a dental restoration utilizing a gas-impelled jet of fine abrasive. It enhances the attachment of resin cements or restorative materials to the surface. SEE ALSO airbrasive t.

Mohs fresh tissue chemosurgery t., chemosurgery in which superficial cancers are excised after fixation in vivo.

Ouchterlony t., a t. in which both reaction partners (antigen and antibody) are allowed to diffuse to each other in a gel in a precipitation reaction.

PAP t., an unlabeled antibody peroxidase method that reacts both with the rabbit antihorseradish peroxidase antibody and free horseradish peroxidase to form a soluble complex of peroxidase antiperoxidase or PAP; a uniquely sensitive immunohistochemical method that is applicable to paraffin-embedded tissues.

rebreathing t., use of a breathing or anesthesia circuit in which exhaled air is subsequently inhaled either with or without absorption of CO_2 from the exhaled air.

Rebuck skin window t., an in vivo test of the inflammatory response in which the skin is abraded and a slide applied to the abraded area to permit visualization of leukocyte mobilization.

sealed jar t., a t. for producing suspended animation in small experimental animals, consisting of sealing the animal in a jar which is then refrigerated.

Seldinger t., a method of percutaneous insertion of a catheter into a blood vessel or space: a needle is used to puncture the structure and a guide wire is threaded through the needle; when the needle is withdrawn, a catheter is threaded over the wire; the wire is then withdrawn, leaving the catheter in place.

sterile insect t., a t. used to control or eradicate insect pests or vectors, utilizing induction by irradiation of dominant lethality in the chromosomes of the released insects.

vacuum pack t., a temporary closing of the abdomen by using a fenestrated plastic sheet over the intestine but under the anterior abdominal wall followed by the placement of moistened pads with a suction catheter within the wound. The entire defect is then covered by a nonporous plastic sheet; permits drainage of the abdominal cavity by suction while maintaining anterior abdominal wall rigidity.

washed field t., the cutting of cavity preparations in teeth utilizing a constant irrigant which is immediately removed from the mouth by means of a vacuum device.

tech·no·cau·sis (tek-nō-kaw'sis). SYN actual *cautery*. [G. *technē*, art, + *kausis*, a burning]

tech·nol·o·gist (tek-nol'ŏ-jist). One trained in and using the techniques of a profession, art, or science. SYN technician.

tech·nol·o·gy (tek-nol'ŏ-jē). The knowledge and use of the techniques of a profession, art, or science. [G. *technē*, an art, + *logos*, study]

assisted reproductive t., originally, a range of techniques for manipulating eggs and sperm in order to overcome infertility. Encompasses drug treatments to stimulate ovulation; surgical methods for removing eggs (e.g., laparoscopy and ultrasound-guided transvaginal aspiration) and for reimplanting embryos (e.g., zygote intrafallopian transfer (or ZIFT); in vitro and in vivo fertilization (e.g., artificial insemination and gamete intrafallopian transfer (or GIFT); ex utero and in utero fetal surgery; as well as laboratory regimes for freezing and screening sperm and embryos, and micromanipulating and cloning embryos. SEE eugenics.

tec·lo·thi·a·zide (tek-lō-thī'ă-zīd). SYN tetrachlormethiazide.

tec·tal (tek'tăl). Relating to a tectum.

tec·ti·form (tek'ti-fōrm). Roof-shaped.

Tec·ti·vi·ri·dae (tek'tē-vī'rā-dā). A name for a family of icosahedral nonenveloped double-stranded DNA bacteriophages that have double capsids. [L. *tectum*, roof, covering, + virus]

tec·to·ce·phal·ic (tek'tō-sĕ-fal'ik). SYN scaphocephalic. [L. *tectum*, roof, + G. *kephalē*, head]

tec·to·ceph·a·ly (tek'tō-sef'ă-lē). SYN scaphocephaly.

tec·tol·o·gy (tek-tol'ŏ-jē). Structural morphology. [G. *tektōn*, builder, + *-logia*]

tec·ton·ic (tek-ton'ik). Relating to variations in structure in the eye, particularly the cornea. [G. *tektonikos*, relating to building]

tec·to·ri·al (tek-tōr'ē-ăl). Relating to or characteristic of a tectorium.

tec·to·ri·um (tek-tōr'ē-ŭm). **1.** An overlaying structure. **2.** SYN tectorial *membrane* of cochlear duct. [L. an overlaying surface (plaster, stucco), fr. *tego*, pp. *tectus*, to cover]

tec·to·spi·nal (tek-tō-spī'năl). Denoting nerve fibers passing from the mesencephalic tectum to the spinal cord.

tec·tum, pl. **tec·ta** (tek'tŭm, tek'tă). Any rooflike covering or structure. [L. roof, roofed structure, fr. *tego*, pp. *tectus*, to cover]

t. mesenceph'ali [TA], SYN *lamina* of mesencephalic tectum.

t. of midbrain, SYN *lamina* of mesencephalic tectum.

TEDD Abbreviation for total end-diastolic *diameter*.

teel oil (tēl). SYN *sesame* oil.

teeth (tēth). Plural of tooth.

acoustic teeth [TA], tooth-shaped formations or ridges occurring on the vestibular lip of the limbus lamina spiralis of the cochlear duct. SYN dentes acustici [TA], auditory teeth, Corti auditory teeth, Huschke auditory teeth.

teeth·ing (tē'thing). Eruption or "cutting" of the teeth, especially of the deciduous teeth. SYN odontiasis.

tef·lu·rane (tef'loo-rān). A nonexplosive and nonflammable inhalation anesthetic of moderate potency.

teg·men, gen. **teg·mi·nis,** pl. **teg·mi·na** (teg'men, -mi-nis, -mi-nă). A structure that covers or roofs over a part. [L. a covering, fr. *tego*, to cover]

t. cru'ris, old term for *tegmentum* mesencephali.

t. mastoi'deum, the lamina of bone roofing over the mastoid cells.

t. tym'pani [TA], the roof of the middle ear, formed by the thinned anterior surface of the petrous portion of the temporal bone. Its anterior edge is inserted into the petrosquamous fissure

so that it can be seen as a wedge of bone subdividing that fissure into a squamotympanic and a petrotympanic fissure. SYN roof of tympanum.

t. ventric'uli quar'ti [TA], roof of fourth ventricle, formed in its upper part by the superior medullary velum stretching between the two brachia conjunctiva (superior cerebellar peduncles) and in its lower part by the inferior medullary velum composed of the choroid membrane and choroid plexus of the fourth ventricle. SYN roof of fourth ventricle [TA].

teg·men·tal (teg-men'tăl). Relating to, characteristic of, or placed or oriented toward a tegmentum or tegmen.

teg·men·tot·o·my (teg-men-tot'ŏ-mē). Production of lesions in the reticular formation of the midbrain tegmentum. [tegmentum + G. *tomē*, incision]

teg·men·tum, pl. **teg·men·ta** (teg-men'tŭm, -tă). **1.** A covering structure. **2.** SYN mesencephalic t. [L. covering structure, fr. *tego*, to cover]

t. mesenceph'ali [TA], SYN mesencephalic t.

mesencephalic t., that major part of the substance of the mesencephalon or midbrain that extends from the substantia nigra to the level of the cerebral aqueduct. SYN t. mesencephali [TA], t. of midbrain [TA], midbrain t., tegmentum (2).

midbrain t., SYN mesencephalic t.

t. of midbrain [TA], SYN mesencephalic t.

t. of pons [TA], SYN dorsal *part* of pons.

t. pontis [TA], SYN dorsal *part* of pons.

t. rhombenceph'ali, SYN rhombencephalic t.

rhombencephalic t., the portion of the pons continuous with the mesencephalic t.; it consists of reticular formation, tracts, and cranial nerve nuclei, and forms the dorsal part of the pons (pars dorsalis pontis). SYN t. of rhombencephalon, t. rhombencephali.

t. of rhombencephalon, SYN rhombencephalic t.

teg·u·ment (teg'ū-ment). **1.** SYN integument. **2.** SYN integument (2). [L. *tegumentum*, a collat. form of *tegmentum*]

teg·u·men·tal, teg·u·men·ta·ry (teg-ū-men'tăl, teg-ū-men'tă-rē). Relating to the integument.

Teichmann, Ludwig, German histologist, 1823–1895. SEE T. *crystals*, under *crystal*.

tei·cho·ic ac·ids (tī-kō'ik). One of two classes (the other being the muramic acids or mucopeptides) of polymers constituting the cell walls of Gram-positive bacteria, but also found intracellularly; linear polymers of a polyol (ribitol phosphate or glycerol phosphate) carrying D-alanyl residues esterified to OH groups and glycosidically linked sugars.

tei·chop·sia (tī-kop'sē-ă). The jagged, shimmering visual sensation resembling the fortifications of a walled medieval town; the scintillating scotoma of migraine. [G. *teichos*, wall, + *opsis*, vision]

◁tel-, tele-, telo-. Distance, end, other end. [G. *tēle*, distant, *telos*, end]

te·la, gen. and pl. **te·lae** (tē'lă, tē'lē). **1.** Any thin weblike structure. **2.** A tissue; especially one of delicate formation. [L. a web]

t. choroi'dea [TA], that portion of the pia mater that covers the ependymal roof or, in the case of the lateral ventricle, medial wall of a cerebral ventricle. SYN choroid membrane [TA].

t. choroi'dea of fourth ventricle [TA], the sheet of pia mater covering the lower part of the ependymal roof of the fourth ventricle. SYN t. choroidea ventriculi quarti [TA], t. choroidea inferior.

t. choroi'dea infe'rior, SYN t. choroidea of fourth ventricle.

t. choroi'dea supe'rior, SYN t. choroidea of third ventricle.

t. choroi'dea of third ventricle, a double fold of pia mater, enclosing subarachnoid trabeculae, between the fornix above and the epithelial roof of the third ventricle and the thalami below; at each lateral margin is a vascular fringe projecting into the choroidal fissure of the lateral ventricle; on its undersurface are several small vascular projections filling the folds of the ependymal roof of the third ventricle. SYN t. choroidea ventriculi tertii [TA], t. choroidea superior, triangular lamella, velum interpositum, velum triangulare.

t. choroi′dea ventric′uli quar′ti [TA], SYN t. choroidea of fourth ventricle.

t. choroi′dea ventric′uli ter′tii [TA], SYN t. choroidea of third ventricle.

t. conjuncti′va, SYN connective *tissue.*

t. elas′tica, SYN elastic *tissue.*

t. subcuta′nea [TA], SYN subcutaneous *tissue.*

t. subcuta′nea penis [TA],

t. subcuta′nea perinei [TA],

t. submuco′sa, SYN submucosa.

t. submuco′sa pharyn′gis, SYN pharyngobasilar *fascia.*

t. subsero′sa [TA], SYN subserosa.

t. vasculo′sa, SYN choroid *plexus.*

Te·la·dor·sa·gia dav·ti·ani (tē′lă-dōr-sā′jē-ă dav-shē-ān′ī). One of the medium stomach worm species (family Trichostrongylidae) of sheep, goats, and deer occurring in the abomasum; it is similar to *Ostertagia trifurcata.* [tele- + L. *dorsum,* back]

tel·al·gia (tel-al′jē-ă). SYN referred *pain.* [G. *tēle,* distant, + *algos,* pain]

🔲 **tel·an·gi·ec·ta·sia** (tel-an′jē-ek-tā′zē-ă). Dilation of the previously existing small or terminal vessels of a part. SYN angiotelectasis, angiotelectasia. [G. *telos,* end, + *angeion,* vessel, + *ektasis,* a stretching out]

cephalo-oculocutaneous t., an angioma involving the skin of the face, orbit, meninges, and brain. SEE ALSO Sturge-Weber *syndrome.*

essential t., (1) localized capillary dilation of undetermined origin; **(2)** SYN *angioma* serpiginosum.

hereditary benign t., an autosomal dominant disorder in which the face, upper trunk, and arms develop telangiectasias.

hereditary hemorrhagic t. [MIM*187300], a disease with onset usually after puberty, marked by multiple small telangiectases and dilated venules that develop slowly on the skin and mucous membranes; the face, lips, tongue, nasopharynx, and intestinal mucosa are frequent sites, and recurrent bleeding may occur; autosomal dominant inheritance, caused by mutation in the gene (ENG) encoding endoglin on chromosome 9q. SYN Rendu-Osler-Weber syndrome.

t. lymphat′ica, SYN lymphangiectasis.

t. macula′ris erupti′va per′stans, a disseminated eruption of telangiectases associated with erythematous and edematous macules.

primary t., SYN *angioma* serpiginosum.

secondary t., t. related to a known cause of prolonged dermal vascular dilation such as sunlight, varicose veins, and connective tissue diseases; often associated with atrophy of the skin.

spider t., SYN spider *angioma.*

t. verruco′sa, SYN angiokeratoma.

tel·an·gi·ec·ta·sis, pl. **tel·an·gi·ec·ta·ses** (tel-an′jē-ek′tă-sis, -sēz). A lesion formed by a dilated capillary or terminal artery, most commonly on the skin. SEE telangiectasia.

tel·an·gi·ec·tat·ic (tel-an′jē-ek-tat′ik). Relating to or marked by telangiectasia.

tel·an·gi·ec·to·des (tel-an′jē-ek-tō′dēz). A term used to qualify highly vascular tumors. [telangiectasis + G. *-ōdēs,* fr. *eidos,* resemblance]

tel·an·gi·o·ma (tel-an′jē-ō′mă). Angioma due to dilation of the capillaries or terminal arterioles.

tel·an·gi·on (tel-an′jē-on). One of the terminal arterioles or a capillary vessel. SYN trichangion. [G. *telos,* end, + *angeion,* vessel]

tel·an·gi·o·sis (tel′an-jē-ō′sis). Any disease of the capillaries and terminal arterioles.

tele (tel′ē). Referring to the nitrogen atom of the imidazole ring of histidine that is the farthest from the β-carbon. Cf. *pros.* [G. far]

△**tele-.** SEE tel-.

tel·e·can·thus (tel-ĕ-kan′thŭs). Increased distance between the medial canthi of the eyelids. SYN canthal hypertelorism. [G. *tēle,* distant, + *kanthos,* canthus]

tel·e·car·di·o·gram (tel-ĕ-kar′dē-ō-gram). SYN telelectrocardiogram.

tel·e·car·di·o·phone (tel-ĕ-kar′dē-ō-fōn). A specially constructed stethoscope by means of which heart sounds can be heard by listeners at a distance from the patient. [G. *tēle,* distant, + *kardia,* heart, + *phōnē,* sound]

tel·e·co·balt (tel′ĕ-kō′bawlt). Teletherapy using radioactive cobalt as the source.

tel·e·di·ag·no·sis (tel′ĕ-dī-ag-nō′sis). Detection of a disease by evaluation of data transmitted to a receiving station, a process normally involving patient-monitoring instruments and a transfer link to a diagnostic center at some distance from the patient.

tel·e·di·a·stol·ic (tel′ĕ-dī-ă-stol′ik). Pertaining to or occurring toward the end of ventricular diastole. [G. *telos,* end, + *diastolē,* dilation]

telehopsias. SYN fortification *spectrum.*

tel·e·lec·tro·car·di·o·gram (tel′ē-lek-trō-kar′dē-ō-gram). An electrocardiogram recorded at a distance from the subject being tested; e.g., the electrocardiogram obtained through telemetry, or, as with a galvanometer in the laboratory, being connected by a wire with the patient in another room. SYN telecardiogram. [G. *tēle,* distant, + electrocardiogram]

te·lem·e·ter (tĕ-lem′ĕ-ter). An electronic instrument that senses and measures a quantity, then transmits radio signals to a distant station for recording and interpretation. [G. *tēle,* distant, + *metron,* measure]

te·lem·e·try (tĕ-lem′ĕ-trē). The science of measuring a quantity, transmitting the results by radio signals to a distant station, and there interpreting, indicating, and/or recording the results. SEE ALSO biotelemetry.

cardiac t., transmission of cardiac signals (electric or pressure derived) to a receiving location where they are displayed for monitoring.

tel·en·ce·phal·ic (tel′en-se-fal′ik). Relating to the telencephalon or endbrain.

tel·en·ceph·al·i·za·tion (tel-en-sef′ăl-i-zā′shŭn). SYN corticalization.

tel·en·ceph·a·lon (tel-en-sef′ă-lon) [TA]. The anterior division of the prosencephalon, which develops into the olfactory lobes, the cortex of the cerebral hemispheres, and the subcortical telencephalic nuclei, and the basal ganglia (nuclei), particularly the striatum and the amygdala. SYN endbrain. [G. *telos,* end, + *enkephalos,* brain]

te·le·ol·o·gy (tel-ē-ol′ō-jē). The philosophical doctrine according to which events, especially in biology, are explained in part by reference to final causes or end goals; the doctrine that goals or end states have a causal influence on present events and that the future as well as the past affect the present. [G. *telos,* end, + *logos,* study]

te·le·o·mi·to·sis (tel′ē-ō-mī-tō′sis). A completed mitosis. [G. *teleos,* complete, + mitosis]

tel·e·o·morph (tel′ē-ō-morf). A reproductive structure of a fungus that is a result of plasmogamy and nuclear recombination; sexual state (sexual reproduction). SYN perfect stage.

tel·e·o·nom·ic (tel′ē-ō-nom′ik). **1.** Pertaining to teleonomy. **2.** In psychology, pertaining to those patterns of behavior that are a function of an inferred purpose or motive; e.g., a child's behavior pattern may be classified teleonomically by an observer as attention-getting.

tel·e·on·o·my (tel-ē-on′ō-mē). The doctrine that life is characterized by endowment with a project or purpose; i.e., the existence in an organism of a structure or function implies that it has had evolutionary survival value. [G. *telos,* end, + *nomos,* law]

tel·e·op·sia (tel-ē-op′sē-ă). An error in judging the distance of objects arising from lesions in the parietal temporal region. [G. *tēle,* distant, + *opsis,* vision]

tel·e·or·gan·ic (tel′ē-ōr-gan′ik). Manifesting life. [G. *teleos,* complete, + *organikos,* organic]

tel·e·path·ine (tel-ĕ-path′ēn). SYN harmine.

te·lep·a·thy (tĕ-lep′ă-thē). Transmittal and reception of thoughts by means other than through the normal senses, as a form of

te

extrasensory perception. SYN extrasensory thought transference, mind-reading. [G. *tēle*, distant, + *pathos*, feeling]

tel·e·ra·di·og·ra·phy (tel-ĕ-rā-dē-og'ră-fē). Radiography with the x-ray tube positioned about 2 m from the film thereby securing practical parallelism of the x-rays to minimize geometric distortion; the standard configuration for chest radiography. Cf. air-gap *technique*. SYN teleroentgenography. [G. *tēle*, distant, + radiography]

tel·e·ra·di·ol·o·gy (tel-ĕ-rā-dē-ol'ō-jē). The interpretation of digitized diagnostic images transmitted by modem over telephone lines. [tele- + radiology]

tel·e·ra·di·um (tel'ĕ-rā'dē-ŭm). SEE teleradium *therapy*.

tel·e·re·cep·tor (tel'ĕ-rē-sep'ter, -tōr). An organ, such as the eye, that can receive sense stimuli from a distance.

tel·er·gy (tel'er-jē). SYN automatism. [G. *tēle*, far off, + *ergon*, work]

tel·e·roent·gen·og·ra·phy (tel'ĕ-rent-gen-og'ră-fē). SYN teleradiography.

tel·e·roent·gen·ther·a·py (tel'ĕ-rent'gen-thār'ă-pē). SYN teletherapy.

telescope.

    Hopkins rod-lens t., an endoscopic t. in which the air-containing spaces between the conventional series of lenses are replaced with glass rods with polished ends separated by small "air-lenses." This system transmits more light, yields greater magnification and provides greater depth and breadth of field than conventional lens systems.

tel·e·sis (tel-ē'sis). A goal to be attained by planned conduct. [G. *telos*, end, + *-osis*, condition]

tel·e·sys·tol·ic (tel'ĕ-sis-tol'ik). Relating to the end of ventricular systole. [G. *telos*, end, + *systolē*, a contracting]

tel·e·ther·a·py (tel-ĕ-thār'ă-pē). Radiation therapy administered with the source at a distance from the body. Cf. interstitial *therapy*. SYN teleroentgentherapy. [G. *tēle*, distant, + *therapeia*, treatment]

TeLinde, Richard W., U.S. gynecologist, *1894. SEE T. *operation*.

tel·lu·ric (tĕ-loor'ik). **1.** Relating to or originating in the earth. **2.** Relating to the element tellurium, especially in its 6+ valence state. [L. *tellus* (*tellur-*), the earth]

tel·lu·rism (tel'oo-rizm). The alleged influence of soil emanations in producing disease. [L. *tellus* (*tellur-*), the earth]

tel·lu·ri·um (Te) (tel-oo'rē-ŭm). A rare semimetallic element, atomic no. 52, atomic wt. 127.60, belonging to the sulfur group. [L. *tellus* (*tellur-*), the earth]

△**telo-.** SEE tel-.

tel·o·den·dron (tel-ō-den'dron). An anomalous term that refers to the terminal arborization of an axon. SYN end-brush. [G. *telos*, end, + *dendron*, tree]

tel·o·gen (tel'ō-jen). Resting phase of hair cycle. [G. *telos*, end, + *-gen*, producing]

te·log·lia (tĕ-log'lē-ă). Accumulation of neurolemmal cells at the myoneural junction. [G. *telos*, end, + *glia*, glue]

tel·og·no·sis (tel-og-nō'sis). Obsolete term denoting diagnosis by means of radiographs or other diagnostic tests transmitted by telephone or radio. SEE teleradiology. [G. *tēle*, distant, + *gnōsis*, a knowing]

tel·o·ki·ne·sia (tel'ō-ki-nē'zē-ă). SYN telophase. [G. *telos*, end, + *kinēsis*, movement]

tel·o·lec·i·thal (tel-ō-les'i-thăl). Denoting an ovum in which a large amount of deuteroplasm or yolk accumulates at the vegetative pole, as in the eggs of birds and reptiles. [G. *telos*, end, + G. *lekithos*, yolk]

tel·o·me·rase (tel-ō'mer-ās). A reverse transcriptase comprising an RNA template, which acts as a die for the TTAGGG sequence, and a catalytic protein component that is not found in normal, aging somatic cells. Telomerase mediates the repair or preservation of telomere regions (terminal sequences) of chromosomes.

    The aging process that takes place in normal somatic cells, and the natural limit on the number of times such cells can undergo mitosis, involves a sequential shortening of telomeres due to failure of terminal sequences to be replicated during mitosis. Cells in which this shortening does not occur (cancer cells, germ cells, hematopoietic stem cells, and others) display a transient expression of telomerase, which not only delays the erosion of telomeres but actually adds DNA bases to telomeres. Experimental transfection of a gene for the catalytic component of telomerase into normal, aging cells results in extension of telomeres. Restoring telomere length appears to reset gene expression, cell morphology, and the replicative life span. It has therefore been suggested that such procedures may permit therapeutic modification of the cellular mechanisms underlying age-related diseases such as atherosclerosis, osteoarthritis, macular degeneration, and Alzheimer dementia. Cellular aging is but one element of clinical aging, however, others being heredity and environment. Although telomerase expression is an important marker of malignancy, it is not itself the cause of cancer. Telomerase expression and telomere lengthening apparently do not alter normal cell cycle control, chromosome complement, or cell morphology.

tel·o·mere (tel'ō-mēr). The distal end of a chromosome arm. [G. *telos*, end, + *meros*, part]

tel·o·pep·tide (tel-ō-pep'tīd). A peptide covalently bound in or on a protein, protruding therefrom and therefore subject to enzyme attack and maturation modification or cross-linking, and conferring immunogenic specificity.

tel·o·phase (tel'ō-fāz). The final stage of mitosis or meiosis that begins when migration of chromosomes to the poles of the cell has been completed; the chromosomes progressively lengthen while the nuclear membranes of the two daughter nuclei are reconstructed and a cell membrane at the equator complete the separation of the two daughter cells. SYN telokinesia. [G. *telos*, end, + *phasis*, appearance]

Te·lo·spo·rea (tel-ō-spō'rē-ă). SYN Sporozoea.

Te·lo·spo·rid·ia (tel'ō-spō-rid'ē-ă). A former order of Sporozoea. [G. *telos*, end, + *sporos*, seed]

tel·o·tism (tel'ō-tizm). The perfect performance of a function, as that of sight or hearing. [G. *telos*, end]

TEM Abbreviation for triethylenemelamine.

te·maz·e·pam (te-maz'ĕ-pam). A benzodiazepine sedative-hypnotic primarily used to relieve insomnia.

tem·per. **1.** Disposition; in general, any characteristic or particular state of mind. SYN temperament (2). **2.** A display of irritation or anger. SEE tantrum. **3.** To treat metal by application of heat, as in annealing or quenching.

tem·per·a·ment (tem'per-ă-ment). **1.** The psychological and biological organization peculiar to the individual, including one's character or personality predispositions, that influence the manner of thought and action and general views of life. **2.** SYN temper (1). [L. *temperamentum*, proper measure, moderation, disposition]

tem·per·ance (tem'per-ans). Moderation in all things; especially, abstinence from the use of alcoholic beverages. [L. *temperantia*, moderation]

tem·per·ate (tem'per-ăt). Moderate; restrained in the indulgence of any appetite or activity.

tem·per·a·ture (tem'per-ă-chŭr). The sensible intensity of heat of any substance; the manifestation of the average kinetic energy of the molecules making up a substance due to heat agitation. SEE ALSO scale. [L. *temperatura*, due measure, temperature, fr. *tempero*, to proportion duly]

    absolute t. (T), t. reckoned in Kelvins from absolute zero.

    basal body t., the t. at rest, usually obtained on arising in the morning, without any influences that might increase it; can give indirect evidence of ovulation.

    critical t., the t. of a gas above which it is no longer possible by use of any pressure, however great, to convert it into a liquid.

    denaturation t. of DNA, that t. at which, under a given set of conditions, double-stranded DNA is changed (50%) to single-stranded DNA; under standard conditions, the base composition of the DNA can be estimated from the denaturation t., since the greater the denaturation t., the greater the guanine-plus-cytosine content (i.e., GC content) of the DNA. SYN melting t. of DNA.

effective t., a comfort index or scale which takes into account the t. of air, its moisture content, and movement.

equivalent t., the t. of a thermally uniform enclosure in which, under still air conditions, a "sizable" black body loses heat at the same rate as in the nonuniform environment.

eutectic t., the t. at which a eutectic mixture becomes fluid (melts).

fusion t. (wire method), (1) the recorded t. at which a 20-gauge metal wire will collapse under a 3-ounce load. **(2)** the recorded t. at which porcelain becomes glazed.

maximum t., in bacteriology, denoting a t. above which growth will not take place.

mean t., the average atmospheric t. in any locality for a designated period of time, as a month or a year.

melting t., SYN t. midpoint.

melting t. of DNA, SYN denaturation t. of DNA.

t. midpoint (T_m, t_m), the midpoint in the change in optical properties (absorbance, rotation) of a structured polymer (e.g., DNA) with increasing t. SYN melting t.

minimum t., in bacteriology, denoting a t. below which growth will not take place.

optimum t., the t. at which any operation, such as the culture of any special microorganism, is best carried on.

room t. (RT, rt), the ordinary t. (65°F to slightly less than 80°F, 18.3°C–26.7°C) of the atmosphere in the laboratory; a culture kept at room t. is one kept in the laboratory, not in an incubator.

sensible t., the atmospheric t. as felt by the individual, supposed to be that recorded by the wet-bulb thermometer.

standard t., a t. of 0°C or 273.15° absolute (Kelvin).

tem·plate (tem′plăt). **1.** A pattern or guide that determines the shape of a substance. **2.** Metaphorically, the specifying nature of a macromolecule, usually a nucleic acid or polynucleotide, with respect to the primary structure of the nucleic acid or polynucleotide or protein made from it in vivo or in vitro. **3.** In dentistry, a curved or flat plate utilized as an aid in setting teeth. **4.** An outline used to trace teeth, bones, or soft tissue in order to standardize their form. **5.** A pattern or guide that determines the specificity of antibody globulins. [Fr. *templet,* temple of a loom, fr. L. *templum,* small timber]

surgical t., (1) a thin, transparent, resin base shaped to duplicate the form of the impression surface of an immediate denture, used as a guide for surgically shaping the alveolar process to fit an immediate denture; **(2)** a guide for various osteotomy procedures; **(3)** a guide for duplicating size and shape for an autogenic (free) gingival graft.

tem·ple (tem′pl). **1** [TA]. The area of the temporal fossa on the side of the head above the zygomatic arch. **2.** The part of a spectacle frame passing from the rim backward over the ear. [L. *tempus* (*tempor-*), time, temple]

tem·po·la·bile (tem-pō-lā′bil, -bīl). Undergoing spontaneous change or destruction during the passage of time. [L. *tempus,* time, + *labilis,* perishable]

tem·po·ra (tem′pŏ-ră). The temples. [L. pl. of *tempus*]

tem·po·ral (tem′pŏ-răl). **1.** Relating to time; limited in time; temporary. **2.** Relating to the temple. SEE temporal *region* of head. [L. *temporalis,* fr. *tempus* (*tempor-*), time, temple]

tem·po·ra·lis (tem-pŏ-rā′lis). SYN temporalis (*muscle*). [L.]

⌂**temporo-.** Temporal (2). [L. *temporalis,* temporal]

tem·po·ro·au·ric·u·lar (tem′pŏ-rō-aw-rik′ū-lăr). Relating to the temporal region and the auricle.

tem·po·ro·hy·oid (tem′pŏ-rō-hī′oyd). Relating to the temporal and the hyoid bones or regions.

tem·po·ro·ma·lar (tem′pŏ-rō-mā′lăr). SYN temporozygomatic.

tem·po·ro·man·dib·u·lar (tem′pŏ-rō-man-dib′ū-lăr). Relating to the temporal bone and the mandible; denoting the joint of the lower jaw. SYN temporomaxillary (2).

tem·po·ro·max·il·lary (tem′pŏ-rō-mak′si-lār′ē). **1.** Relating to

the regions of the temporal and maxillary bones. **2.** SYN temporomandibular.

tem·po·ro·oc·cip·i·tal (tem′pŏ-rō-ok-sip′i-tăl). Relating to the temporal and the occipital bones or regions.

tem·po·ro·pa·ri·e·tal (tem′pŏ-rō-pă-rī′ĕ-tăl). Relating to the temporal and the parietal bones or regions.

tem·po·ro·pon·tine (tem-pŏ-rō-pon′tīn). Referring to the projection fibers from the temporal lobe of the cerebral cortex to the basilar part of the pons.

tem·po·ro·sphe·noid (tem′pŏ-rō-sfē′noyd). Relating to the temporal and sphenoid bones.

tem·po·ro·zy·go·mat·ic (tem′pŏ-rō-zī′gō-mat′ik). Relating to the temporal and zygomatic bones or regions. SYN temporomalar.

tem·po·sta·bile, tem·po·sta·ble (tem-pō-stā′bil, -stā′bl). Not subject to spontaneous alteration or destruction. [L. *tempus,* time + *stabilis,* stable]

temps utile (temp′ oo-tēl′). SYN utilization *time.* [Fr. service or utilization time]

tem·pus, gen. **tem·po·ris,** pl. **tem·po·ra** (tem′pŭs, -pŏ-ris, -pŏ-ră). **1.** The temple. **2.** SYN time. [L. time]

TEN Abbreviation for toxic epidermal *necrolysis.*

te·na·cious (tĕ-nā′shŭs). Sticky; denoting tenacity. [L. *tenax* (*tenac-*), fr. *teneo,* to hold]

te·nac·i·ty (tĕ-nas′i-tē). Adhesiveness; the character or property of holding fast. [L. *tenacitas,* fr. *teneo,* to hold]

cellular t., the inherent property of all cells to persist in a given form or direction of activity.

te·nac·u·lum, pl. **te·nac·u·la** (tĕ-nak′ū-lŭm, -lă). A surgical clamp designed to hold or grasp tissue during dissection, commonly used to grasp the cervix. [L. a holder, fr. *teneo,* to hold]

tenac′ula ten′dinum, a tendinous restraining structure, such an extensor or flexor retinaculum; historically applied to the vincula of tendon which are not however, restraining structures.

te·nal·gia (te-nal′jē-ă). Obsolete term for pain referred to a tendon. SYN tenodynia. [G. *tenōn,* tendon, + *algos,* pain]

t. crep′itans, SYN *tenosynovitis* crepitans.

ten·as·cin (ten-as′sin). A protein that is present in the mesenchyme that surrounds epithelia in organs undergoing development in embryos; believed to participate in inducing differentiation of epithelia.

ten·der. Sensitive or painful as a result of pressure or contact that is not sufficent to cause discomfort in normal tissues. [L. *tener,* soft, delicate]

ten·der·ness (ten′der-nes). The condition of being tender.

pencil t., strictly localized t., elicited by pressure with the rubber tip of a pencil, e.g., in cases of incomplete or subperiosteal fracture.

rebound t., t. felt when pressure, particularly pressure on the abdomen, is suddenly released.

ten·di·ni·tis (ten-di-nī′tis). SYN tendonitis.

ten·di·no·plas·ty (ten′din-ō-plas-tē). Reparative or plastic surgery of the tendons. SYN tenontoplasty, tenoplasty. [Mediev. L. *tendo* (*tendin-*), tendon, + G. *plastos,* formed]

ten·di·no·su·ture (ten′di-nō-soo′choor). SYN tenorrhaphy.

ten·di·nous (ten′di-nŭs). Relating to, composed of, or resembling a tendon.

ten·do, gen. **ten·di·nis,** pl. **ten·di·nes** (ten′dō, -di-nis, -di-nēz) [TA]. SYN tendon. For histologic description, see tendon. [Mediev. L., fr. L. *tendo,* to stretch out, extend]

t. Achil′lis, SYN calcaneal *tendon,* calcaneal *tendon.*

t. calca′neus [TA], SYN calcaneal *tendon.*

t. calca′neus commu′nis, SEE hamstring (2).

t. conjuncti′vus, ✩official alternate term for inguinal *falx.*

t. cricoesopha′geus [TA], SYN cricoesophageal *tendon.*

t. oc′uli, SYN medial palpebral *ligament.*

t. palpebra′rum, SYN medial palpebral *ligament.*

⌂**tendo-.** A tendon. SEE ALSO teno-. [L. *tendo*]

ten·dol·y·sis (ten-dol′i-sis). SYN tenolysis. [tendo- + G. *lysis,* dissolution]

te

ten·do·mu·cin, ten·do·mu·coid (ten-dō-mū'sin, -mū'koyd). A form of mucin found in tendons.

⊞ **ten·don** (ten'dŏn) [TA]. A nondistensible fibrous cord or band of variable length that is the part of the muscle that connects the fleshy (contractile) part of muscle with its bony attachment or other structure; it may unite with the fleshy part of the muscle at its extremity or may run along the side or in the center of the fleshy part for a longer or shorter distance, receiving the muscular fibers along its border; when determining the length of a muscle, the tendon length is included as well as the fleshy part; it consists of fascicles of very densely arranged, almost parallel collagenous fibers, rows of elongated fibrocytes, and a minimum of ground substance. SYN tendo [TA], sinew. [L. *tendo*]

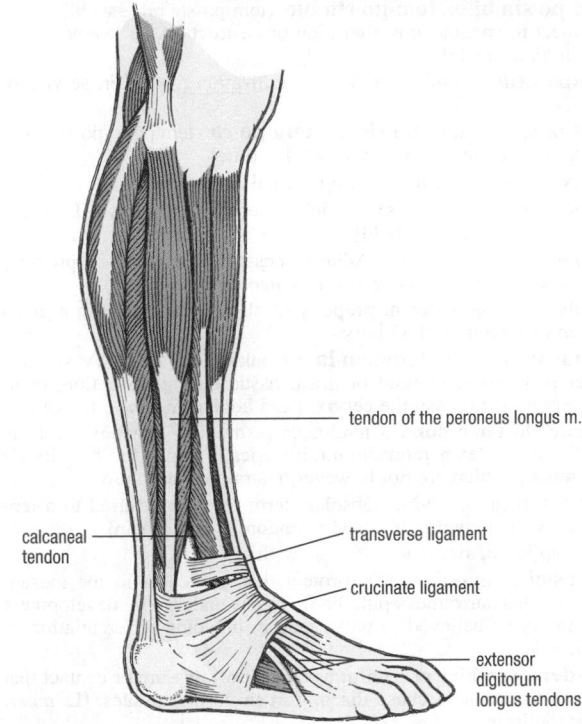

tendon of the peroneus longus m.

calcaneal tendon

transverse ligament

crucinate ligament

extensor digitorum longus tendons

tendons and ligaments of the lower leg

Achilles t., SYN calcaneal t.

calcaneal t. [TA], the thick tendon of insertion of the triceps surae (gastrocnemius and soleus) into the tuberosity of the calcaneus. SYN tendo calcaneus [TA], Achilles t., chorda magna, heel t., tendo Achillis.

central t. of diaphragm [TA], a three-lobed fibrous sheet comprising the center of the diaphragm; superiorly it is fused with the fibrous pericardium that provides attachment (insertion) for the moving end of the muscle fibers. SYN centrum tendineum diaphragmatis [TA], trefoil t.

central t. of perineum [TA], the fibromuscular mass between the anal canal and the urogenital diaphragm in the median plane onto which several perineal muscles insert (bulbospongiosus, external anal sphincter, superficial, and deep transverse perineal muscles); midline episiotomies extend into this structure. SYN centrum tendineum perinei [TA], perineal body, Savage perineal body.

conjoined t., SYN inguinal *falx.*

conjoint t., ☆official alternate term for inguinal *falx*; SEE ALSO *aponeurosis* of internal oblique muscle.

coronary t., SYN (right and left) fibrous *rings* of heart, under *ring.*

cricoesophageal t. [TA], longitudinal fiber of the esophagus that attaches to the posterior aspect of the cricoid cartilage of the larynx. SYN tendo cricoesophageus [TA], Gillette suspensory ligament, suspensory ligament of esophagus.

Gerlach annular t., SYN fibrocartilaginous *ring* of tympanic membrane.

hamstring t., SEE hamstring.

heel t., SYN calcaneal t.

Todaro t., an inconstant tendinous structure that extends from the right fibrous trigone of the heart toward the valve of the inferior vena cava.

trefoil t., SYN central t. of diaphragm.

Zinn t., SYN common tendinous *ring* of extraocular muscles.

ten·don·i·tis (ten-dō-nī'tis). Inflammation of a tendon. SYN tendinitis, tenonitis (2), tenontitis.

ten·doph·o·ny (ten-dof'ō-nē). SYN tenophony.

ten·do·syn·o·vi·tis (ten'dō-si-nō-vī'tis). SYN tenosynovitis.

ten·dot·o·my (ten-dot'ō-mē). SYN tenotomy.

ten·do·vag·i·nal (ten-dō-vaj'i-năl). Relating to a tendon and its sheath. [tendo- + L. *vagina,* sheath]

ten·do·vag·i·ni·tis (ten'dō-vaj-i-nī'tis). SYN tenosynovitis. [tendo- + L. *vagina,* sheath, + G. *-itis,* inflammation]

radial styloid t., SYN de Quervain *disease.*

te·nec·to·my (tĕ-nek'tō-mē). Resection of part of a tendon. SYN tenonectomy. [G. *tenōn,* tendon, + *ektomē,* excision]

te·nes·mic (tĕ-nez'mik). Relating to or marked by tenesmus.

te·nes·mus (te-nez'mŭs). A painful spasm of the urogenital diaphragm with an urgent desire to evacuate the bowel or bladder, involuntary straining, and the passage of little fecal matter or urine. [G. *teinesmos,* ineffectual effort to defecate, fr. *teinō,* to stretch]

ten Horn, C., Dutch surgeon. SEE t. H. *sign.*

te·nia, pl. **te·ni·ae** (tē'nē-ă, tē'nē-ē). **1.** Any anatomic bandlike structure. **2.** SYN taenia (2). [L. fr. G. *tainia,* band, tape, a tapeworm]

tae'niae acus'ticae, SYN medullary *striae* of fourth ventricle, under *stria.*

t. choroi'dea [TA], the somewhat thickened line along which a choroid membrane or plexus is attached to the rim of a brain ventricle. SYN choroid line [TA], t. telae.

te'niae co'li [TA], the three bands in which the longitudinal muscular fibers of the large intestine, except the rectum, are collected; these are the mesocolic t. (t. mesocolica [TA]), situated at the place corresponding to the mesenteric attachment; the free t. (t. libera [TA]), opposite the mesocolic t.; and the omental t. (t. omentalis [TA]), at the place corresponding to the site of adhesion of the greater omentum to the transverse colon. SYN bands of colon, colic teniae, teniae of Valsalva.

colic teniae, SYN teniae coli.

t. fim'briae, SYN t. fornicis.

t. for'nicis [TA], the line of attachment of the choroid plexus of the lateral ventricle to the fornix. SYN t. fimbriae, t. of the fornix.

t. of the fornix, SYN t. fornicis.

t. of fourth ventricle, SYN t. ventriculi quarti.

free t. [TA], SYN teniae coli. SYN t. libera [TA].

t. hippocam'pi, SYN *fimbria* hippocampi.

t. lib'era [TA], SYN free t. SEE teniae coli.

medullary teniae, SYN medullary *striae* of fourth ventricle, under *stria.*

mesocolic t., SEE teniae coli. SYN t. mesocolica [TA].

t. mesocol'ica [TA], SYN mesocolic t.

omental t. [TA], SEE teniae coli. SYN t. omentalis [TA].

t. omenta'lis [TA], SYN omental t. SEE teniae coli.

t. semicircula'ris, SYN terminal *stria.*

Tarin t., SYN terminal *stria.*

t. tec'ta, SEE *indusium* griseum.

t. te'lae, SYN t. choroidea.

t. termina'lis, SYN *crista* terminalis of right atrium.

t. thal'ami [TA], the sharp edge or angle between the superior and medial surfaces of the thalamus on either side; to it is attached the epithelial lamina forming the roof of the third ventricle. SYN t. ventriculi tertii, thalamic t.

thalamic t., SYN t. thalami.

teniae of Valsalva, SYN teniae coli.

t. ventric′uli quar′ti, the line of attachment of the choroid roof to the rim of the fourth ventricle. SYN t. of fourth ventricle.

t. ventric′uli ter′tii, SYN t. thalami.

te·ni·a·cide (tē′nē-ă-sīd). An agent destructive to tapeworms. SYN tenicide. [L. *taenia*, tapeworm, + *caedo*, to kill]

te·ni·a·fuge (tē′nē-ă-fooj). An agent that causes the expulsion of tapeworms. SYN tenifuge. [L. *taenia*, tapeworm, + *fugo*, to put to flight]

ten·i·al (ten′ē-ăl). **1.** Relating to a tapeworm. **2.** Relating to one of the structures called tenia.

te·ni·a·sis (tē-nī′ă-sis). Presence of a tapeworm in the intestine.

somatic t., invasion of the body by the cysticercus of a tenioid worm.

ten·i·cide (ten′i-sīd). SYN teniacide.

ten·i·form (ten′i-fōrm). SYN tenioid.

te·nif·u·gal (te-nif′ū-găl). Having the power to expel tapeworms.

ten·i·fuge (ten′i-fūj). SYN teniafuge.

te·ni·oid (tē′nē-oyd). **1.** Band-shaped; ribbon-shaped. **2.** Resembling a tapeworm. SYN teniform. [G. *tainia*, a tape, + *eidos*, resemblance]

te·ni·o·la (tē-nī′ō-lă). A slender tenia or bandlike structure. [L. dim. of *taenia*, ribbon]

t. cor′poris callo′si, SYN rostral *lamina.*

♲**teno-, tenon-, tenont-, tenonto-.** Tendon. SEE ALSO tendo-. [G. *tenōn*]

te·no·de·sis (tĕ-nod′ē-sis, ten′ō-dē′sis). Stabilizing a joint by anchoring the tendons which move that joint and thereby preventing any further excursion of the tendons. [teno- + G. *desis*, a binding]

ten·o·dyn·ia (ten-ō-din′ēă). SYN tenalgia. [teno- + G. *odynē*, pain]

ten·o·fi·bril (ten-ō-fī′bril). SYN tonofibril. [teno- + Mod. L. *fibrilla*, a small fiber]

ten·ol·y·sis (ten-ol′i-sis). Release of a tendon from adhesions. SYN tendolysis.

ten·o·my·o·plas·ty (ten-ō-mī′ō-plas-tē). SYN tenontomyoplasty.

ten·o·my·ot·o·my (ten-ō-mī-ot′ō-me). SYN myotenotomy.

Tenon, Jacques R., French pathologist and oculist, 1724–1816. SEE T. *capsule, space.*

♲**tenon-.** SEE teno-.

ten·o·nec·to·my (ten-ō-nek′tō-me). SYN tenectomy. [tenon- + G. *ektomē*, excision]

ten·o·ni·tis (ten-ō-nī′tis). **1.** Inflammation of Tenon capsule or the connective tissue within Tenon space. **2.** SYN tendonitis. [tenont- + G. *-itis*, inflammation]

ten·on·ti·tis (ten′on-tī′tis). SYN tendonitis. [tenont- + G. *-itis*, inflammation]

♲**tenonto-.** SEE teno-.

te·non·tog·ra·phy (ten′on-tog′ră-fē). A treatise on or description of the tendons. [tenonto- + G. *graphē*, description]

te·non·tol·o·gy (ten′on-tol′ŏ-jē). The branch of science that has to do with the tendons. [tenonto- + G. *logos*, study]

te·non·to·my·o·plas·ty (te-non′tō-mī′ō-plas-tē). Obsolete term for a combined tenontoplasty and myoplasty, used in the radical correction of a hernia. SYN tenomyoplasty. [tenonto- + G. *mys*, muscle, + *plastos*, formed]

te·non·to·my·ot·o·my (te-non′tō-mī-ot′ō-me). SYN myotenotomy.

te·non·to·plas·tic (te-non′tō-plas-tik). Relating to tenontoplasty.

te·non·to·plas·ty (te-non′tō-plas-tē). SYN tendinoplasty. [tenonto- + G. *plastos*, formed]

te·noph·o·ny (te-nof′ō-nē). A heart murmur assumed to be due to an abnormal condition of the chordae tendineae. SYN tendophony. [teno- + G. *phōnē*, sound]

ten·o·phyte (ten′ō-fīt). Bony or cartilaginous growth in or on a tendon. [teno- + G. *phyton*, plant]

ten·o·plas·tic (ten-ō-plas′tik). Relating to tenoplasty.

ten·o·plas·ty (ten′ō-plas-tē). SYN tendinoplasty.

ten·o·re·cep·tor (ten′ō-rē-sep′ter, -tōr). A receptor in a tendon, activated by increased tension.

te·nor·rha·phy (te-nōr′ă-fē). Suture of the divided ends of a tendon. SYN tendinosuture, tendon suture, tenosuture. [teno- + G. *rhaphē*, suture]

ten·os·to·sis (ten-os-tō′sis). Ossification of a tendon. [teno- + G. *osteon*, bone, + *-osis*, condition]

ten·o·sus·pen·sion (ten′ō-sŭs-pen′shŭn). Using a tendon as a suspensory ligament, sometimes as a free graft or in continuity.

ten·o·su·ture (ten-ō-soo′choor). SYN tenorrhaphy.

ten·o·syn·o·vec·to·my (ten′ō-sin-ō-vek′tō-me). Excision of a tendon sheath. [teno- + synovia + G. *ektomē*, excision]

ten·o·syn·o·vi·tis (ten′ō-sin-ō-vī′tis). Inflammation of a tendon and its enveloping sheath. SYN tendinous synovitis, tendosynovitis, tendovaginitis, tenovaginitis. [teno- + synovia + G. *-itis*, inflammation]

t. crep′itans, inflammation of a tendon sheath in which movement of the tendon is accompanied by a cracking sound. SYN tenalgia crepitans.

de Quervain t., inflammation of the tendons of the first dorsal compartment of the wrist, which includes the abductor pollicis longus and extensor pollicis brevis; diagnosed by a specific provocative test (Finkelstein test).

localized nodular t., SYN giant cell *tumor* of tendon sheath.

pigmented villonodular t., SYN villous t.

stenosing t., inflammation of a tendon and its sheath resulting in contracture of the sheath causing an obstruction of tendon gliding; can be a cause of trigger finger conditions.

villous t., a condition resembling pigmented villonodular synovitis but arising in periarticular soft tissue rather than in joint synovia; occurs most commonly in the hands. SYN pigmented villonodular t.

te·not·o·my (te-not′ō-me). The surgical division of a tendon for relief of a deformity caused by congenital or acquired shortening of a muscle, as in clubfoot or strabismus. SYN tendotomy. [teno- + G. *tomē*, incision]

curb t., SYN tendon *recession.*

graduated t., partial incisions of the tendon of an eye muscle for correction of strabismus.

subcutaneous t., division of a tendon by means of a small pointed knife introduced through skin and subcutaneous tissue without an open operation.

ten·o·vag·i·ni·tis (ten′ō-vaj-i-nī′tis). SYN tenosynovitis. [teno- + L. *vagina*, sheath, + G. *-itis*, inflammation]

tense (tens). Tight, rigid, or strained; characterized by anxiety and psychological strain. [L. *tensus*, pp. of *tendo*, to stretch]

ten·si·om·e·ter (ten-sē-om′ĕ-ter). A device for measuring tension. [L. *tensio*, tension, + G. *metron*, measure]

ten·sion (ten′shŭn). **1.** The act of stretching. **2.** The condition of being tense, or a stretching or pulling force. **3.** The partial pressure of a gas, especially that of a gas dissolved in a liquid such as blood. **4.** Mental, emotional, or nervous strain; strained relations or barely controlled hostility between persons or groups. [L. *tensio*, fr. *tendo*, pp. *tensus*, to stretch]

arterial t., the blood pressure within an artery.

interfacial surface t., the t. or resistance to separation possessed by the film of liquid between two well-adapted surfaces, as of the thin film of saliva between the denture base and the tissues.

ocular t. (Tn), resistance of the tunics of the eye to deformation; it can be estimated digitally or measured by means of a tonometer.

premenstrual t., SYN premenstrual *syndrome.*

surface t. (γ, σ), the expression of intermolecular attraction at the surface of a liquid, in contact with air or another gas, a solid, or another immiscible liquid, tending to pull the molecules of the liquid inward from the surface; dimensional formula: mt^{-2}.

tissue t., a theoretical condition of equilibrium or balance between the tissues and cells whereby overaction of any part is restrained by the pull of the mass.

ten·sor, pl. **ten·so·res** (ten′sōr, ten-sō′rēz). A muscle the function

te

of which is to render a part firm and tense. [Mod. L. fr. L. *tendo,* pp. *tensus,* to stretch]

tent. 1. Canopy used in various types of inhalation therapy to control humidity and concentration of oxygen in inspired air. **2.** Cylinder of some material, usually absorbent, introduced into a canal or sinus to maintain its patency or to dilate it. **3.** To elevate or pick up a segment of skin, fascia, or tissue at a given point, giving it the appearance of a t. [L. *tendo,* pp. *tensus,* to stretch]

oxygen t., a transparent enclosure, suspended over the bed and enclosing the patient, used to supply a high concentration of oxygen.

sponge t., SYN compressed *sponge.*

ten·ta·cle (ten'tă-kl). A slender process for feeling, prehension, or locomotion in invertebrates. [Mod. L. *tentaculum,* a feeler, fr. *tento,* to feel]

ten·to·ri·al (ten-tō'rē-ăl). Relating to a tentorium.

ten·to·ri·um, pl. **ten·to·ria** (ten-tō'rē-ŭm, -rē-ă) [TA]. A membranous cover or horizontal partition. [L. tent, fr. *tendo,* to stretch]

t. cerebel'li [TA], a strong fold of dura mater roofing over the posterior cranial fossa with an anterior median opening, the tentorial notch, through which the midbrain passes; the t. cerebelli is attached along the midline to the falx cerebri and separates the cerebellum from the basal surface of the occipital and temporal lobes of the cerebral hemisphere. SYN cerebellar t. [TA].

cerebellar t. [TA], SYN t. cerebelli.

t. of hypophysis, SYN *diaphragma* sellae.

TEPA Abbreviation for triethylenephosphoramide.

teph·ro·ma·la·cia (tef'rō-mă-lā'shē-ă). Softening of the gray matter of the brain or spinal cord. [G. *tephros,* ashen-gray, + *malakia,* softness]

teph·ry·lom·e·ter (tef-ri-lom'ĕ-ter). An instrument for measuring the thickness of the cerebral cortex; it consists of a graduated tube of thin glass which is inserted into the brain substance, so the depth of the gray matter can be read off on the scale. [G. *tephros,* ashen, + *hylē,* stuff, + *metron,* measure]

TEPP Abbreviation for tetraethyl pyrophosphate.

tep·ro·tide (tē'prō-tīd). A nonapeptide in which glycine is replaced by tryptophan, leucine and the first proline are missing, and lysine is replaced by glutamine; an angiotensin-converting enzyme inhibitor. SYN bradykinin-potentiating peptide.

△**tera- (T). 1.** Prefix used in the SI and metric system to signify one trillion. **2.** Combining form denoting a teras. SEE ALSO terato-. [G. *teras,* monster]

ter·as, pl. **ter·a·ta** (ter'as, ter'ă-tă). Conceptus with deficient, redundant, misplaced, or grossly misshapen parts. [G.]

ter·at·ic (ter-at'ik). Relating to a teras.

ter·a·tism (ter'ă-tizm). SYN teratosis. [G. *teratisma,* fr. *teras*]

△**terato-.** A teras. SEE ALSO tera- (2). [G. *teras,* monster]

ter·a·to·blas·to·ma. A tumor containing embryonic tissue differing from a teratoma in that not all germ layers are present.

ter·a·to·car·ci·no·ma (ter'ă-tō-kar-si-nō'mă). **1.** A malignant teratoma, occurring most commonly in the testis in association with embryonal carcinoma. **2.** A malignant epithelial tumor arising in a teratoma.

te·rat·o·gen (ter'ă-tō-jen). A drug or other agent that causes abnormal prenatal development. [terato- + G. *-gen,* producing]

ter·a·to·gen·e·sis (ter'ă-tō-jen'ĕ-sis). The origin or mode of production of a malformed conceptus; the disturbed growth processes involved in the production of a malformed neonate. [terato- + G. *genesis,* origin]

ter·a·to·gen·ic, ter·a·to·ge·net·ic (ter'ă-tō-jen'ik, -jĕ-net'ik). **1.** Relating to teratogenesis. **2.** Causing abnormal prenatal development.

ter·a·to·ge·nic·i·ty (ter'ă-tō-jĕ-nis'i-tē). The property or capability of producing malformation. [terato- + G. *genesis,* generation]

ter·a·toid (ter'ă-toyd). Resembling a teras. [G. *teratōdēs,* fr. *teras* (*terat-*), monster, + *eidos,* resemblance]

ter·a·to·log·ic (ter'ă-tō-loj'ik). Relating to teratology.

ter·a·tol·o·gy (ter-ă-tol'ō-jē). The branch of science concerned with the production, development, anatomy, and classification of

malformed conceptuses. SEE ALSO dysmorphology. [terato- + G. *logos,* study]

⬛**ter·a·to·ma** (ter-ă-tō'mă). A neoplasm composed of multiple tissues, including tissues not normally found in the organ in which it arises. T.'s occur most frequently in the ovary, where they are usually benign and form dermoid cysts; in the testis, where they are usually malignant; and, uncommonly, in other sites, especially the midline of the body. SYN teratoid tumor. [terato- + G. *-oma,* tumor]

t. or'bitae, SYN orbitopagus.

sacrococcygeal t., found in the region of the tailbud. Most common tumor in the newborn period.

triphyllomatous t., a t. composed of tissues derived from all three germ layers. SYN tridermoma.

ter·a·tom·a·tous (ter'ă-tō'mă-tŭs). Relating to or of the nature of a teratoma.

ter·a·to·pho·bia (ter'ă-tō-fō'bē-ă). Morbid fear of carrying and giving birth to a malformed infant. [terato- + G. *phobos,* fear]

ter·a·to·sis (ter'ă-tō'sis). An anomaly producing a teras. SYN teratism. [terato- + G. *-osis,* condition]

atresic t., a t. in which any of the normal orifices, such as the nares, mouth, anus, or vagina, is imperforate.

ceasmic t., a t. in which there is a failure of the lateral halves of a part to unite, as in cleft palate.

ectogenic t., a t. in which there is a deficiency of parts.

ectopic t., a t. in which the organs or other parts are misplaced.

hypergenic t., a t. in which there is a redundancy of parts.

symphysic t., a t. in which there is a fusion of normally separated parts.

ter·a·to·sper·mia (ter'ă-tō-sper'mē-ă). SYN teratozoospermia. [terato- + G. *sperma,* seed]

teratozoospermia (ter'ă-tō-zō-ō-sperm'ē-ă). Condition characterized by the presence of malformed spermatozoa in the semen. SYN teratospermia. [terato- + G. *zōos,* living, + *sperma,* seed, semen, + *-ia*]

te·ra·zo·sin hy·dro·chlo·ride (tĕ-rā'zō-sin). A peripherally acting antiadrenergic used to treat benign prostatic hypertrophy and hypertension.

ter·bi·um (Tb) (ter'bē-ŭm). A metallic element of the lanthanide or rare earth series, atomic no. 65, atomic wt. 158.92534. [fr. *Ytterby,* a village in Sweden]

ter·bu·ta·line sul·fate (ter-bū'tă-lēn). A sympathomimetic drug with relatively selective B_2 agonistic activity, used principally as a bronchodilator or tocolytic agent.

ter·e·bene (ter'ĕ-bēn). A thin colorless liquid of an aromatic odor and taste, a mixture of terpene hydrocarbons, chiefly dipentene and terpinene, obtained from oil of turpentine; used as an expectorant and in cystitis and urethritis.

ter·e·bin·thi·nate (ter-ĕ-bin'thĭ-nāt). **1.** Containing or impregnated with turpentine. **2.** A preparation containing turpentine. SYN terebinthine. [G. *terebinthos,* the terebinth or turpentine-tree]

ter·e·bin·thine (ter-ĕ-bin'thin). SYN terebinthinate.

ter·e·bin·thin·ism (ter-ĕ-bin'thin-izm). SYN turpentine *poisoning.*

ter·e·brant, ter·e·brat·ing (ter'ĕ-brant, -brā-ting). Boring; piercing; used figuratively, as in the term t. pain. [L. *terebro,* pp. *-atus,* to bore, fr. *terebra,* an auger]

ter·e·bra·tion (ter-ĕ-brā'shŭn). **1.** The act of boring, or of trephining. **2.** A boring, piercing pain. [L. *terebro,* to bore, fr. *terebra,* an auger]

te·res, gen. **ter·e·tis,** pl. **ter·e·tes** (ter'ēz, -tēr-; ter'ĕ-tis; ter'ĕ-tēz). Round and long; denoting certain muscles and ligaments. SEE teres minor (*muscle*), teres major (*muscle*), round *ligament* of uterus, round *ligament* of liver, pronator teres (*muscle*). [L. round, smooth, fr. *tero,* to rub]

ter·fen·a·dine (ter-fen'ă-dēn). An H_1 antihistamine used to treat a variety of allergic conditions; has fewer sedative effects than other antihistamines, but in combination with several other drugs may cause serious cardiac arrhythmias.

ter·gal (ter'găl). SYN dorsal (1). [L. *tergum,* back]

ter·gum (ter'gŭm). SYN dorsum. [L.]

term. **1.** A definite or limited period. **2.** A name or descriptive word or phrase. SEE ALSO terminus, term *infant*. [L. *terminus*, a limit, an end]

ter·mi·nad (ter′mi-nad). Toward the terminus.

ter·mi·nal (ter′mi-năl). **1.** Relating to the end; final. **2.** Relating to the extremity or end of any body; e.g., the end of a biopolymer. **3.** A termination, extremity, end, or ending. [L. *terminus,* a boundary, limit]

amino-t., SEE amino-terminal.

axon t.'s, the somewhat enlarged, often club-shaped endings by which axons make synaptic contacts with other nerve cells or with effector cells (muscle or gland cells). As isolated, by homogenizing brain or spinal cord, they contain acetylcholine and the related enzymes. Axon t.'s contain neurotransmitters of various kinds, sometimes more than one. These can be demonstrated by chemical analysis and immunocytochemical methods. SEE ALSO synapse. SYN axonal terminal boutons, end-feet, neuropodia, pieds terminaux, synaptic boutons, synaptic endings, synaptic t.'s, terminal boutons, bouton terminaux.

carboxy t., SEE C *terminus.*

synaptic t.'s, SYN axon t.'s.

ter·mi·nal de·ox·y·nu·cle·o·ti·dyl·trans·fer·ase (dē-ok′sē-noo′klē-ō-tī-dil-trans′fer-ās). SYN DNA nucleotidylexotransferase.

ter·mi·na·tio, pl. **ter·mi·na·ti·o·nes** (ter′mi-nā′shē-ō, -ō′nēz) [TA]. SYN termination. SEE ALSO ending. [L.]

terminatio′nes nervo′rum li′berae, SYN free nerve *endings*, under *ending.*

ter·mi·na·tion (ter′mi-nā′shŭn). An end or ending. A termination or ending, particularly a nerve ending. SEE ending. SYN terminatio [TA]. [L. *terminatio*]

selective t., SYN selective *reduction.*

ter·mi·na·ti·o·nes (ter-mi-nā-shē-ō′nēz). Plural of terminatio. [L.]

Terminologia Anatomica (TA). A system of anatomic nomenclature, consisting of about 7500 terms, devised and approved by the International Federation of Associations of Anatomists (IFAA) and promulgated in August, 1997, at São Paulo, Brazil.

Since its foundation in 1903 the IFAA has held periodic conventions for the standardization of anatomic concepts and terminology. In 1989 the federation elected a 12-member Federative Committee on Anatomical Terminology (FCAT), consisting of experts from 11 countries, to undertake a wholesale revision of the last (sixth) edition of Nomina Anatomica (NA VI). With the election of additional members in 1994, the FCAT had representatives from 16 countries and 5 continents. The committee solicited suggestions from anatomists and others around the world, and from more than 10,000 terms proposed for introduction or retention, they formulated and published a list of those deemed worthy of consideration. During 8 years of deliberations they chose the simplest and most exact terms, preferring those that are descriptive of form or function over semantically opaque ones. Some 10% of formerly accepted terms were rejected or altered because they were considered inaccurate, ambiguous, or otherwise unsuitable. About 1000 new terms were introduced, including some for structures not officially named in earlier nomenclatural systems. Many of these terms had already been adopted informally in various countries. Adoption of the new terminology is expected to be widespread. Because English is spoken in many countries and serves as a common language for scientific and medical communication, English equivalents of Latin terms are given in the published version of TA. However, only the Latin terms have official status. The FCAT is currently working on complementary formulations of histologic, cytologic, embryologic, dental, and anthropologic terminology.

ter·mi·nus, pl. **ter·mi·ni** (ter′mi-nŭs, -nī). A boundary or limit. [L.]

C t., the end of a peptide or protein having a free carboxyl (–COOH) group.

ter′mini genera′les, general terms; words that are of general use in descriptive anatomy.

N t., SEE amino-terminal.

ter·mo·lec·u·lar (ter-mō-lek′oo-lar). Denoting three molecules; e.g., a termolecular reaction requires three molecules to come together in order for the reaction to occur. [L. *ter,* thrice, + molecular]

ter·mone (ter′mōn). A type of ectohormone, secreted by some invertebrate organisms, that stimulates gametogenesis. [L. *ter,* thrice, threefold, + hormone]

ter·na·ry (ter′nār-ē). Denoting or comprised of three compounds, elements, molecules, etc. [L. *ternarius,* of three]

Ter·ni·dens (Ter′nē-denz). Nematode genus found in the intestine of several simian species in Africa, India, and Indonesia, and in humans in parts of Africa; differentiated from hookworms by the anteriorly directed buccal capsule guarded by a double crown of stout bristles; ternidens inhabit the wall of the large bowel, where they may produce cystic nodules.

T. deminutus, nematode species whose larvae develop in soil; probably infective for humans; life cycle not known.

ter·ox·ide (ter-ok′sīd). SYN trioxide.

ter·pene (ter′pēn). One of a class of hydrocarbons with an empirical formula of $C_{10}H_{16}$, occurring in essential oils and resins. Acyclic t.'s may be regarded as isomers and polymers of isoprene units; cyclic forms include menthane, bornane, and camphene. T.'s containing 15, 20, 30, 40, etc., carbon atoms are called sesquiterpenes, diterpenes, triterpenes, tetraterpenes, etc.

***p*-ter·phen·yl** (ter-fen′il). $C_6H_5-C_6H_4-C_6H_5$; useful as a primary scintillator in liquid scintillation counting.

ter·pin. A cyclic terpene alcohol, $C_{10}H_{18}(OH)_2$, obtained by the action of nitric acid and dilute sulfuric acid on pine oil.

t. hydrate, monohydrate of terpin; alleged to be an expectorant. SYN terpinol.

ter·pin·e·ol (ter-pin′ē-ol). An unsaturated alcoholic terpene obtained by heating terpin hydrate with diluted phosphoric acid; an active antiseptic and a perfume.

ter·pi·nol (ter′pin-ol). SYN *terpin* hydrate.

ter·race (ter′as). To suture in several rows, in closing a wound through a considerable thickness of tissue. [thr. O. Fr. fr. L. *terra,* earth]

ter·ra ja·pon·i·ca (ter′rǎ jǎ-pon′i-kǎ). SEE gambir.

Terrey, Mary, 20th century U.S. physician. SEE Lowe-T.-MacLachlan *syndrome*.

Terrien, Louis-Felix, French surgeon, 1837–1908. SEE T. *valve,* marginal *degeneration.*

ter·ri·to·ri·al·i·ty (ter′i-tōr-ē-al′i-tē). **1.** The tendency of individuals or groups to defend a particular domain or sphere of interest or influence. **2.** The tendency of an individual animal to define a finite space as its own habitat from which it will fight off trespassing animals of its own species.

Terry, Theodore L., U.S. ophthalmologist, 1899–1946. SEE T. *syndrome.*

Terson, Albert, French ophthalmologist, 1867–1935. SEE T. *glands,* under *gland.*

ter·tian (ter′shǎn). Recurring every third day, counting the day of an episode as the first; actually, occurring every 48 hours or every other day. [L. *tertianus,* fr. *tertius,* third]

double t., denoting malarial infections with two different sets of organisms producing daily paroxysms. SEE ALSO quotidian *malaria.*

ter·ti·a·rism, ter·ti·a·ris·mus (ter′shē-ă-rizm, -riz′mŭs). All the symptoms of the tertiary stage of syphilis taken collectively.

TESD Abbreviation for total end-systolic *diameter.*

Tesla, Nikola, Serbian-American electrical engineer, 1856–1943. SEE tesla; T. *current.*

tesla (T) (tes′lǎ). In the SI system, the unit of magnetic flux density expressed as $kg\ s^{-2}\ A^{-1}$; equal to 1 Wb/m^2. [N. *Tesla*]

tes·sel·lat·ed (tes'ĕ-lāt-ed). Made up of small squares; checkered. [L. *tessella,* a small square stone]

Tessier, Paul, 20th century French physician. SEE Tessier *classification.*

TEST

test. 1. To prove; to try a substance; to determine the chemical nature of a substance by means of reagents. **2.** A method of examination, as to determine the presence or absence of a definite disease or of some substance in any of the fluids, tissues, or excretions of the body, or to determine the presence or degree of a psychologic or behavioral trait. **3.** A reagent used in making a t. **4.** SEE testa (1). SEE ALSO assay, reaction, reagent, scale, stain. [L. *testum,* an earthen vessel]

acetone t., a t. for ketonuria; the suspected urine is shaken up with a few drops of sodium nitroprusside, and strong ammonia water is then gently poured over the mixture; if acetone is present, a magenta ring forms at the line of contact; tablets containing sodium nitroprusside and alkali are now more commonly used.

achievement t., a standardized t. used to measure acquired learning, e.g., competence in a specific subject area such as reading or arithmetic, in contrast to an intelligence t., which is a useful index of potential ability or learning.

acidified serum t., lysis of the patient's red blood cells in acidified fresh serum, specific for paroxysmal nocturnal hemoglobinuria. SYN Ham t.

acid perfusion t., SYN Bernstein t.

acid phosphatase t. for semen, a screening t. for semen by determining acid phosphatase content; because seminal fluid contains high concentrations of acid phosphatase, while other body fluids and extraneous foreign materials have very low concentrations, high values of acid phosphatase on vaginal aspirate or lavage, or on wash fluid from stains, render positive identification of semen, even if the male is aspermic.

acid reflux t., a t. to detect gastroesophageal reflux by monitoring esophageal pH by an electrode in the distal esophagus either basally or after acid is instilled into the stomach.

acoustic stimulation t., a t. for fetal well-being through use of an acoustic device to stimulate the fetus and cause accelerated fetal heart rate.

ACTH stimulation t., a t. for adrenal cortical function; ACTH administered by continuous intravenous infusion, or intramuscularly, evokes an increase in plasma cortisol in normal persons; in adrenal cortical insufficiency, the expected increase in plasma cortisol is limited or nonexistent.

Addis t., SEE Addis *count.*

adhesion t., the diagnostic application of the immune adhesion phenomenon. SYN erythrocyte adherence t., immune adhesion t., red cell adherence t.

Adler t., SYN benzidine t.

Adson t., a t. for thoracic outlet syndrome; the patient is seated, with head extended and turned to the side of the lesion; with deep inspiration there is a diminution or total loss of radial pulse on the affected side. Not all patients with a positive Adson t. have thoracic outlet syndrome. SYN Adson maneuver.

agglutination t., any of a variety of t.'s that are dependent on the clumping of cells, microorganisms, or particles when mixed with specific antiserum.

Albarran t., a t. for renal insufficiency wherein the drinking of large quantities of water will cause a proportionate increase in the volume of urine if the kidneys are sound, but not if the epithelium of the secreting tubules is damaged. SYN polyuria t.

alkali denaturation t., a t. for hemoglobin F (Hb F), based on the fact that hemoglobins, with the exception of Hb F, are denatured by alkali to alkaline hematin; the t. is sensitive to 2% or more Hb F.

Allen t., (1) for phenol: upon the addition of 5 or 6 drops of hydrochloric acid and then 1 of nitric acid to the suspected fluid, a red color develops; [A.H. Allen] **(2)** for strychnine: fluid is extracted with ether, which is then evaporated by means of "drop-by-drop" pipetting into a warmed porcelain dish or crucible; the residue is treated with a small bit of manganese dioxide and dilute sulfuric acid; a red-blue or violet color develops if strychnine is present. [A.H. Allen] **(3)** a t. for radial or ulnar patency; either the radial or ulnar artery is digitally compressed by the examiner after blood has been forced out of the hand by clenching it into a fist; failure of the blood to diffuse into the hand when opened indicates that the artery not compressed is occluded. [Edgar Van Nuys Allen]

Allen-Doisy t., a t. for estrogenic activity; the material to be investigated is injected repeatedly into immature or spayed rats or mice; the disappearance of leukocytes from the vaginal smear and the appearance of cornified cells constitutes a positive reaction.

Almén t. for blood, an obsolete t. in which glacial acetic acid, gum guaiac solution, and hydrogen peroxide are added to an aqueous suspension of the suspected stain; if occult blood or blood pigment is present, a blue color develops. SYN guaiac t., Schönbein t., van Deen t.

Alpha t.'s, a set of paper and pencil-administered mental t.'s first used in the United States Army in 1917–1918 to determine the mental ability of literate recruits; the set includes 8 different types of t.'s: i.e., directions, arithmetical problems, practical judgement, synonyms and antonyms, disarrayed sentences, number series completions, analogies, and information; they are designed especially for testing large groups of individuals simultaneously, and for rapid machine scoring; distinguished from the Army Beta t.'s, a complementary set for administration to recruits who could not read or write English, in which the instructions are given in signs and the t. material is pictorial. SEE Beta t.'s. SYN Army Alpha t.

alternate binaural loudness balance t., ABLB t., a t. for recruitment in one ear; the comparison of relative loudness of a series of intensities presented alternately to either ear.

alternate cover t., a t. to detect phoria or strabismus; attention is directed to a small fixation object, and one eye is covered for several seconds; then the cover is moved quickly to the other eye; if the eye moves when it is uncovered, a strabismus or phoria is present. SYN cover-uncover t.

alternating light t., t. to detect a relative afferent defect in one eye by watching pupillary movements. With the patient fixing in the distance, the light is held on each eye for about a second, and quickly moved to the other eye. Assuming no defect of the innervation to the iris sphincter in one eye (which would produce an anisocoria in light), the eye with the weaker light response has a relative afferent pupillary defect. This asymmetry of pupillomotor input can be estimated by holding neutral density filters in front of the better eye until the pupillary responses of the two eyes are balanced. SYN swinging light t.

Ames t., a screening t. for possible carcinogens using strains of *Salmonella typhimurium* that are unable to synthesize histidine; if the t. substance produces mutations that regain the ability to synthesize histidine, the substance is carcinogenic. SYN Ames assay.

Amsler t., projection of a visual field defect onto an Amsler chart.

Anderson-Collip t., an obsolete procedure for evaluating the thyrotropic activity of an extract of the anterior lobe of the pituitary gland, as indicated by an increased basal metabolic rate or histologic evidence of stimulation of the thyroid gland in a hypophysectomized rat injected with the t. extract.

Anderson and Goldberger t., an obsolete t. for typhus in which the patient's blood is injected into a guinea pig's peritoneal cavity. In typhus a typical temperature curve will be observed.

anoxemia t., an obsolete t. for coronary insufficiency; the patient breathes a mixture of 10% oxygen and 90% nitrogen; if anginal pain or electrocardiographic abnormalities are induced, the t. is positive. SYN hypoxemia t.

anterior apprehension t., (1) SYN shoulder apprehension *sign*; **(2)** a t. of shoulder stability; apprehension with abduction and external rotation of the joint suggests anterior instability. SYN crank test.

antibiotic sensitivity t., the in vitro testing of bacterial cultures with antibiotics to determine susceptibility of bacteria to antibiotic therapy. SEE ALSO Bauer-Kirby t.

antiglobulin t., SYN Coombs t.

antihuman globulin t., SEE Coombs t.

antithrombin t., a procedure for estimating the inhibitory effect of a defibrinated specimen of plasma on the action of thrombin in converting fibrinogen to fibrin.

Apt t., a t. for identifying fetal blood by the addition of sodium hydroxide and water to a specimen.

aptitude t., an occupation-oriented intelligence t. used to evaluate a person's abilities, talents, and skills; particularly valuable in vocational counseling.

Army Alpha t., SYN Alpha t.'s.

Army Beta t.'s, SYN Beta t.'s.

Army General Classification T., a selection screening t. of overall intellectual ability administered to entering army recruits for use in determining qualifications for entry into one of the wide range of positions to which each individual is assigned at the end of basic training.

Ascoli t., a precipitin t. for anthrax using a tissue extract and anthrax antiserum.

ascorbate-cyanide t., a t. for glucose 6-phosphate-deficient red blood cells; blood is incubated with sodium cyanide and ascorbate; the hydrogen peroxide generated is free to oxidize hemoglobin to methemoglobin, since cyanide inhibits catalase; a brown color is produced more rapidly in glucose 6-phosphate-deficient cells.

association t., a word (stimulus word) is spoken to the subject, who is to reply immediately with another word (reaction word) suggested by the first; used as a diagnostic aid in psychiatry and psychology, clues being given by the length of time (association time) between the stimulus and reaction words, and also by the nature of the reaction words.

Astwood t., SYN metrotrophic t.

atropine t., SYN Dehio t.

augmented histamine t., SYN histamine t.

aussage t., a t. of ability to reproduce correctly something that has been seen for a brief interval. [Ger. *Aussage*, a declaration]

autohemolysis t., when sterile defibrinated blood is incubated at 37°C, normal red blood cells hemolyze slowly; cells with membrane or metabolic defects do so to a greater extent.

Bachman t., a skin t. for trichinosis in which an extract of *Trichinella* larvae is suspended in saline and injected intradermally. An immediate wheal-and-flare reaction or a delayed response indicates infection.

Bachman-Pettit t., a modification of the Kober t. for the detection of estradiol and similar estrogenic hormones in the urine.

Bagolini t., a t. for retinal correspondence with the subject observing a figure through two striated lenses.

Bárány caloric t., a t. for vestibular function, made by irrigating the external auditory meatus with either hot or cold water; this normally causes stimulation of the vestibular apparatus, resulting in nystagmus and past-pointing; in vestibular disease, the response may be reduced or absent. SYN caloric t., nystagmus t.

Barlow t., SYN Barlow *maneuver.*

Bauer-Kirby t., a standardized t. for microbiologic susceptibility performed by transferring a standardized pure culture of the organism of interest onto a sensitivity plate (Petri dish with Mueller-Hinton *agar*) and observing growth in the presence of disks containing antibiotics.

BEI t., SYN butanol-extractable iodine t.

belt t., an obsolete t.: firm upward pressure on the lower part of the abdomen will remove the feeling of discomfort in cases of enteroptosis.

Bender gestalt t., a psychological t. used by neurologists and clinical psychologists to measure a person's ability to visually copy a set of geometric designs; useful for measuring visuospatial and visuomotor coordination to detect brain damage. SYN Bender Visual Motor Gestalt t.

Bender Visual Motor Gestalt t., SYN Bender gestalt t.

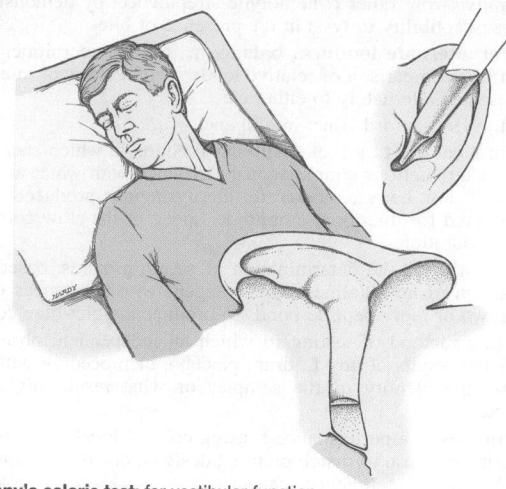

Bárány's caloric test: for vestibular function

Benedict t. for glucose, a copper-reduction t. for glucose in the urine, which involves thiocyanate in addition to copper sulfate for qualitative or quantitative use.

bentiromide t., a t. of pancreatic exocrine function that does not require duodenal intubation: orally administered bentiromide is cleaved by chymotrypsin within the lumen of the small intestine, releasing *p*-aminobenzoic acid which is absorbed and excreted in the urine; diminished urinary excretion of *p*-aminobenzoic acid suggests pancreatic insufficiency.

bentonite flocculation t., an obsolete flocculation t. for rheumatoid arthritis in which sensitized bentonite particles are added to inactivated serum; the t. is positive if half of the particles are clumped while the other half remain in suspension.

benzidine t., a t. for blood; the suspected fluid is treated with glacial acetic acid and ether, and the latter is then decanted and treated with hydrogen peroxide and a solution of benzidine in acetic acid; the presence of blood is indicated by a bluish color turning to purple. SYN Adler t.

Bernstein t., a t. to establish that substernal pain is due to reflux esophagitis, performed by instillation of a weak hydrochloric acid solution directly into the lower esophagus by means of a tube; symptoms disappear when the acid solution is replaced by normal saline solution. SYN acid perfusion t.

Berson t., a t. of thyroid clearance of ^{131}I from the plasma by the thyroid gland.

Beta t.'s, a set of pictorially administered mental t.'s first used in the United States Army in 1917–1918 to determine the relative mental ability of recruits who were illiterate or deficient in reading and writing English, the instructions being given in signs and the t. material is pictorial in character; distinguished from the Alpha t.'s, which were administered at the same time to literate recruits. SYN Army Beta t.'s.

Betke-Kleihauer t., a slide t. for the presence of fetal red blood cells among those of the mother; hemoglobins other than Hb F are eluted from the red blood cells on an air-dried blood film by a buffer of pH 3.3.

Bettendorff t., a t. for arsenic; after mixing the suspected fluid with hydrochloric acid a solution of stannous chloride is added; when a piece of tin foil is then added, a brown precipitate forms.

Bial t., an obsolete t. for pentose with orcinol. SYN orcinol t.

bile acid tolerance t., a sensitive t. of hepatic dysfunction; following oral administration of labeled or unlabeled bile acid, the measured fractional disappearance rate or 10-minute retention is measured.

bile esculin t., a biochemical t. used in characterizing group O streptococci, based on the ability of organisms to grow in a medium containing bile and to hydrolyze esculin.

bile solubility t., a procedure that differentiates *Streptococcus*

te

pneumoniae from other α-hemolytic streptococci by demonstrating its susceptibility to lysis in the presence of bile.

binaural alternate loudness balance t., a t. for recruitment in one ear; the comparison of relative loudness of a series of intensities presented alternately to either ear.

Binet t., SYN Stanford-Binet intelligence *scale.*

bithermal caloric t., a t. of vestibular function in which each ear canal is alternately or simultaneously irrigated with water at 7°C above or below body temperature; the nystagmus produced may be monitored for direction, amplitude, speed of the slow component, and duration.

biuret t., a t. for the determination of serum proteins, based on the reaction of an alkaline copper reagent with substances containing two or more peptide bonds to produce a violet-blue color.

blind t., a method of testing in which an independent observer records the results of any t., drug, placebo, or procedure without knowing the identity of the samples or what result might be expected.

block design t., a performance t. using colored blocks which the individual must use to match pictured designs; one of the subtests of the Wechsler intelligence scales.

Bonney t., SYN Marshall t.

breath t., any diagnostic test in which endogenous or exogenous materials are measured in samples of breath as a means of identifying pathologic processes; examples include hydrogen breath testing for lactose intolerance or urea breath testing to detect gastric colonization with *Helicobacter pylori.* SYN breath analysis.

breath-holding t., a rough index of cardiopulmonary reserve measured by the length of time that a subject can voluntarily stop breathing; normal duration is 30 sec or more; diminished cardiac or pulmonary reserve is indicated by a duration of 20 sec or less.

Brigg t., a t. using the reduction of molybdate to follow the excretion of homogentisic acid.

bromphenol t., a colorimetric t. for measurement of protein, albumin, and globulin in the urine by use of reagent strips.

bromsulphalein t., obsolete t. for liver function (hepatic excretory capacity) in which a known amount of dye, usually 5 mg/kg of body weight, is injected intravenously; subsequently (usually after 45 minutes elapsed time), the amount of dye remaining in the serum is measured; a concentration of 0.4 mg or less of bromsulphalein per 100 ml of serum or less than 4% of the injected dye is considered normal; bromsulphalein retention may follow decreased hepatic blood flow or biliary obstruction as well as hepatic cell damage. SYN BSP t.

BSP t., SYN bromsulphalein t.

butanol-extractable iodine t., an obsolete t. for thyroid function, applicable in patients who have received large amounts of iodine or iodized products. SYN BEI t.

California psychological inventory t., a personality inventory, used with normal persons, in which emphasis is upon social interaction variables.

Calmette t., conjunctival reaction to tuberculin.

caloric t., SYN Bárány caloric t.

CAMP t., a t. to identify Group B β-streptococci based on their formation of a substance (CAMP factor) that enlarges the area of hemolysis formed by streptococcal β-hemolysin. [*C*hristie, *A*tkins, and *M*unch-*P*etersen, developers of the t.]

cancer antigen 125 t. (CA125), t. for cell-surface antigen found on derivatives of coelomic epithelium. Elevated levels of this antigen are associated with ovarian malignancy and benign pelvic disease such as endometriosis.

capillary fragility t., a tourniquet t. used to determine the presence of vitamin C deficiency or thrombocytopenia; a circle 2.5 cm in diameter, the upper edge of which is 4 cm below the crease of the elbow, is drawn on the inner aspect of the forearm, pressure midway between the systolic and diastolic blood pressure is applied above the elbow for 15 minutes, and a count of petechiae within the circle is made: 10, normal; 10–20, marginal; more than 20, abnormal. SYN capillary resistance t., Rumpel-Leede sign, Rumpel-Leede t., vitamin C t.

capillary resistance t., SYN capillary fragility t.

carbohydrate utilization t., a t. for the definitive identification of clinically important yeasts and yeastlike organisms.

carotid sinus t., stimulation of one carotid sinus (never both) to produce reflex effects that may slow the heart, reduce the systolic blood pressure or both for diagnostic or, in the case of certain arrhythmias, therapeutic purposes.

Carr-Price t., a quantitative t. for vitamin A based on the reaction with antimony trichloride in chloroform.

Casoni intradermal t., a t. for hydatid disease in which hydatid fluid is injected intracutaneously; immediate or delayed wheal-and-flare reaction is positive. SYN Casoni skin t.

Casoni skin t., SYN Casoni intradermal t.

CF t., SYN complement *fixation.*

Chick-Martin t., a method of testing the in vitro efficiency of a bactericidal agent; a standard culture of *Salmonella typhi* which has been added to a fixed amount of sterilized feces or yeast is tested for a fixed period (30 minutes), against various concentrations of phenol solution and various concentrations of the disinfectant; the result is expressed as a ratio: the phenol coefficient, which is the highest dilution of the disinfectant under t. at which the bacteria are killed, divided by the highest dilution of phenol which sterilizes the solution in the same length of time.

chi-square t., a statistical method of assessing the significance of a difference, as when the data from two or more samples, such as the numbers of females and males attending each of two colleges, are represented by a discrete number. SYN χ^2 t.

cis/trans t., a t. on the relative configuration on expression of two mutations.

Clauberg t., a t. for progestational activity; immature rabbits are treated with 8 daily injections of estrogen and then given 5 daily injections of the t. substance; the amount required to produce definite progestational changes in the endometrium is taken as the unit; it is equivalent to 0.75 mg of progesterone.

clomiphene t., a t. of pituitary gonadotropin reserve using clomiphene.

clonidine growth hormone stimulation t., administration of the α-2 adrenoreceptor agonist clonidine fails to raise growth hormone levels in patients with multiple system atrophy; levels in normal patients increase.

coccidioidin t., an intracutaneous t. for determining the presence of infection with the fungus *Coccidioides immitis;* a reaction of delayed hypersensitivity indicates a positive t. and is interpreted as meaning past or present infection with the fungus.

coin t., SYN bellmetal *resonance.*

cold bend t., a t. of the ability of a wire to be shaped; performed by counting the number of times a wire can be bent to a right angle and reversed at the same point before breaking; important in establishing specifications for orthodontic wires.

cold pressor t., a cardiocirculatory challenge conventionally performed by immersing one hand in ice-cold water for two or more minutes (as tolerated) to acutely raise the blood pressure, thus imposing resistance to ejection of blood from the left ventricle into the systemic arterial system and consequently acutely increased afterload (afterload = increased left ventricular wall stress). SYN Hines-Brown t.

colloidal gold t., SEE Lange t.

colorimetric caries susceptibility t., SYN Snyder t.

complement-fixation t., an immunologic t. for determining the presence of a particular antigen or antibody when one of the two is known to be present, based on the fact that complement is "fixed" in the presence of antigen and its specific antibody. SEE ALSO Bordet-Gengou *phenomenon.*

contraction stress t., SYN oxytocin challenge t.

Coombs t., a t. for antibodies, the so-called anti–human globulin t. using either the direct or indirect Coombs t.'s. SYN antiglobulin t.

Corner-Allen t., a t. for progestational activity; adult female rabbits are mated during estrus and spayed 18 hours later; the t. substance is injected subcutaneously on 5 successive days; the minimal amount required to produce complete progestational proliferation of the endometrium is taken as a unit, equivalent to 1.25 mg of progesterone.

cover t., a t. used for objective demonstration of ocular deviation in strabismus; may be performed by two methods: the cover-uncover t. and the alternate cover t.

cover-uncover t., SYN alternate cover t.

CO₂-withdrawal seizure t., utilization of hyperventilation to demonstrate abnormalities in the brain waves or even to precipitate a convulsion.

Crampton t., a test for physical condition and resistance; a record is made of the pulse and the blood pressure in the recumbent and standing positions, and the difference is graded from the theoretical perfection of 100 (seldom attained) downward (a reading of 75 is considered excellent, 65 poor); high values indicate a good physical resistance but low ones indicate a nonconditioned state.

t.'s of criminal responsibility, in forensic psychiatry, legal precedents upon which are based decisions concerning insanity in criminals. SEE ALSO American Law Institute *rule,* Durham *rule,* M'Naghten *rule,* New Hampshire *rule.*

cutaneous t., SYN skin t.

cutaneous tuberculin t., SEE tuberculin t.

cyanide-nitroprusside t., a qualitative t. for diagnosis of cystinuria; the addition of fresh sodium cyanide formed by sodium nitroprusside to a sample of urine gives rise to a stable red-purple color in the presence of cystine.

cytotropic antibody t., a rosette t. for macrophage cytotropic antibody: monolayers of macrophages are exposed first to antibody cytotropic for macrophages, then to the antigen (for which the antibody is specific), and indicator sheep erythrocytes; if the antibody is specific for sheep erythrocytes, the latter will form a rosette around the macrophages directly, but if not, and the antigen is soluble, the antigen must be coupled to the sheep erythrocytes by an agent such as bis-diazotized benzidine.

DA pregnancy t., direct agglutination latex t. for pregnancy. SEE immunologic pregnancy t.

Day t., a t. for blood by the addition of the suspected fluid or the washing of a suspected stain with tincture of guaiac and then hydrogen peroxide; the presence of blood results in a blue color.

D-dimer t., t. that detects the cross-linked fibrin degradation fragment, D-dimer. Elevations in this fragment are seen in primary and secondary fibrinolysis; during thrombolytic or defibrination therapy with tissue plasminogen activator; as a result of thrombotic disease, such as deep-vein thrombosis, pulmonary embolism or DIC; in vasoocclusive crisis of sickle cell anemia; in malignancies; and in surgery.

Dehio t., if an injection of atropine relieves bradycardia, the condition is due to action of the vagus; if it does not, the condition may be due to an affection of the heart itself. SYN atropine t.

dehydrocholate t., a method of determining the speed of the blood circulation; a solution of sodium dehydrocholate is injected intravenously, and the time that elapses before a bitter taste is noted in the mouth is recorded; the average of this time is normally about 13 sec.

Denver Developmental Screening T., a scale used by psychologists and pediatricians to assess the developmental, intellectual, motor, and social maturity of children at any age level from birth to adolescence.

dexamethasone suppression t., a t. for the detection and diagnosis of Cushing syndrome; following administration of 1.0 mg of dexamethasone at 11 p.m., normal persons suppress plasma cortisol to low levels; patients with Cushing syndrome do not. Higher dose regimens distinguish between Cushing syndrome due to tumor and due to hyperplasia.

Dick t., an intracutaneous t. of susceptibility to the erythrogenic toxin of *Streptococcus pyogenes* responsible for the rash and other manifestations of scarlet fever. SYN Dick method.

differential renal function t., SYN differential ureteral catheterization t.

differential ureteral catheterization t., a study performed to determine various functional parameters of one kidney compared to the contralateral kidney; ureteral catheters are inserted at cystoscopy into the ureter or renal pelvis bilaterally, and simultaneous measurements are made of urine flow rate, insulin, or PAH (if

infused), endogenous creatinine, or various urinary solutes. SYN differential renal function t., split renal function t.

dinitrophenylhydrazine t., a screening t. for maple syrup urine disease; the addition of 2,4-dinitrophenylhydrazine in HCl to urine gives a chalky white precipitate in the presence of ketoacids.

direct Coombs t., a t. for detecting sensitized erythrocytes in erythroblastosis fetalis and in cases of acquired immune hemolytic anemia: the patient's erythrocytes are washed with saline to remove serum and unattached antibody protein, then incubated with Coombs anti-human globulin (usually serum from a rabbit or goat previously immunized with human globulin); after incubation, the system is centrifuged and examined for agglutination, which indicates the presence of so-called incomplete or univalent antibodies on the surface of the erythrocytes.

direct fluorescent antibody t., SEE fluorescent antibody *technique.*

discontinuation t., a t. to determine whether a certain drug is responsible for a reaction by observation of a remission of symptoms following cessation of its use.

Doerfler-Stewart t., examination of the patient's ability to respond to spondee words in the presence of a masking noise of the saw-tooth type; used especially in differentiating between functional and organic hearing loss. SYN D-S t.

double (gel) diffusion precipitin t. in one dimension, SEE gel diffusion precipitin t.'s in one dimension.

double (gel) diffusion precipitin t. in two dimensions, SEE gel diffusion precipitin t.'s in two dimensions.

Dragendorff t., an obsolete qualitative t. for bile; a play of colors is produced by adding a drop of nitric acid to white filter paper or unglazed porcelain, moistened with a fluid containing bile pigments. The t. is essentially the same as Gmelin t. for bile in urine.

drawer t., SYN drawer *sign.*

D-S t., SYN Doerfler-Stewart t.

Ducrey t., an intradermal t., using inactivated *Haemophilus ducreyi,* for diagnosis of chancroid; a positive delayed reaction is indicative of present or past infection; false-positive results.

Duke bleeding time t., a bleeding time t. in which an incision is made in the earlobe and the time until bleeding stops is measured.

dye disappearance t., SYN fluorescein instillation t.

dye exclusion t., a t. to determine cell viability in which a dilute solution of certain dyes (e.g., trypan blue, eosin Y, nigrosin, Alcian blue) is mixed with a suspension of live cells; cells that exclude dye are considered to be alive while cells that stain are considered dead; it is not always an accurate t. because it indicates only the structural integrity of the cell membrane.

Ebbinghaus t., a psychological t. in which the patient is asked to complete certain sentences from which several words have been left out.

Ellsworth-Howard t., measurement of serum and urinary phosphorus after intravenous administration of parathyroid extract; used in the diagnosis of pseudohypoparathyroidism.

E-rosette t., a t. to identify T lymphocytes by mixing purified blood lymphocytes with serum and sheep erythrocytes; rosettes of erythrocytes form around human T lymphocytes on incubation.

erythrocyte adherence t., SYN adhesion t.

erythrocyte fragility t., SYN fragility t.

exercise t., any t. using exercise to determine the patient's solidus responses and/or physical condition.

Farnsworth-Munsell color t., a t. for color perception; the task is to arrange 84 color disks (in four separate racks of 20–22 disks) in a sequence with minimal separation of hue between adjacent disks.

fern t., (1) a t. for estrogenic activity; cervical mucus smears form a fern pattern at those times when estrogen secretion is elevated, as at the time of ovulation; similar changes have been reported to occur in saliva; (2) a t. to detect ruptured amniotic membranes.

ferric chloride t., a qualitative t. for the detection of phenylketonuria; the addition of ferric chloride to urine gives rise to a blue-green color in the presence of phenylketonuria.

Finckh t., a psychological t. in which the patient is asked to explain certain proverbial expressions, such as "burn the candle at both ends," "the early bird catches the worm," etc.

finger-nose t., a t. of upper limb coordination and position sense; the subject is asked to slowly touch the tip of his or her nose with an extended index finger; assesses cerebellar function.

finger-to-finger t., a t. for coordination and position sense of the upper limbs; the subject is asked to approximate the ends of the index fingers; assesses cerebellar function.

Finkelstein t., t. to detect de Quervain tenosynovitis in which the thumb is flexed into the palm and is covered by the remaining four digits; the wrist is then bent toward the ulna; positive result of t. produces pain and crepitus along the path of the involved tendon.

Fishberg concentration t., a t. of renal water conservation; after overnight fluid deprivation, morning urine samples are collected and specific gravity is measured.

Fisher exact t., the t. for association in a two-by-two table that is based on the exact distribution of the frequencies within the table.

fistula t., compression or rarefaction of the air in the external auditory canal excites nystagmus when there is an erosion of the otic capsule, so long as the labyrinth is still capable of functioning.

FIT t., SYN fusion-inferred threshold t.

Fleitmann t., an obsolete t. for arsenic; hydrogen is generated in a t. tube containing the suspected fluid; the fluid is heated and a piece of filter paper moistened with silver nitrate solution is held over the top; if arsenic is present, the moistened paper is blackened.

flocculation t., SEE flocculation *reaction*.

fluorescein instillation t., a t. for patency of the lacrimal system; fluorescein instilled in the conjunctival sac can be recovered from the inferior nasal meatus. SYN dye disappearance t., Jones t.

fluorescein string t., an infrequently used t. in which a patient with gastrointestinal bleeding swallows a string; fluorescein is given intravenously; if the string fluoresces after removal, it has been contaminated by blood that has appeared since injection of the fluorescein; used to determine location of bleeding lesion.

fluorescent antinuclear antibody t., FANA t., a t. for antinuclear antibody components; used, in particular, for the diagnosis of collagen-vascular diseases.

fluorescent treponemal antibody-absorption t., a sensitive and specific serologic t. for syphilis using a suspension of the Nichols strain of *Treponema pallidum* as antigen; the presence or absence of antibody in the patient's serum is indicated by an indirect fluorescent antibody technique. SYN FTA-ABS t.

foam stability t., a t. for fetal pulmonary maturity, determined by the ability of pulmonary surfactant in amniotic fluid to generate stable foam in the presence of ethanol after mechanical agitation. SYN shake t.

Folin t., (1) a quantitative t. for uric acid by means of the color produced with phosphotungstic acid and a base; **(2)** a quantitative t. for urea; the urea is decomposed by boiling with magnesium chloride, and the freed ammonia is measured.

Folin-Looney t., an obsolete t. for tyrosine that gives a blue color in alkaline solution with a reagent consisting of sodium tungstate, phosphomolybdic acid, and phosphoric acid.

formol-gel t., a t. to detect the greatly increased serum proteins in visceral leishmaniasis; one drop of full-strength formalin is added to 1 mL of serum, with rapid and complete coagulation indicating the positive reaction.

Fosdick-Hansen-Epple t., a t. for determining dental caries activity based on a solution of powdered human enamel in a saliva-glucose-enamel mixture.

Foshay t., an intradermal t. for cat-scratch disease or tularemia, using material prepared from suppurative lymph nodes of persons known to have had the disease (not commercially available).

fragility t., a t. that measures the resistance of erythrocytes to hemolysis in hypotonic saline solutions; erythrocytes to be tested are added to varying concentrations of saline (usually ranging from 0.85–0.10% sodium chloride with 0.05% increments), and beginning and complete hemolysis are measured; normal erythrocytes show initial hemolysis at concentrations of 0.45–0.39% and complete hemolysis at 0.33–0.30%; in hereditary spherocytosis, the fragility of the erythrocytes is markedly increased, whereas in thalassemia, sickle cell anemia, and obstructive jaundice the fragility of the erythrocytes is usually reduced. SYN erythrocyte fragility t.

Frei t., an intracutaneous diagnostic t. for lymphogranuloma venereum: the Frei antigen is usually a sterile preparation of inactivated chlamydiae from domestic fowl; a positive delayed type reaction is not diagnostically specific for lymphogranuloma venereum and is rarely used. SYN Frei-Hoffmann reaction.

FTA-ABS t., SYN fluorescent treponemal antibody-absorption t.

fusion-inferred threshold t., employment of the phenomenon of cerebral fusion of binaural sounds to substitute for conventional masking in hearing testing. SYN FIT t.

Gaddum and Schild t., a sensitive method for identification of epinephrine in tissue or other material, based on the fluorescence of epinephrine exposed to ultraviolet light in the presence of alkali and oxygen; sensitivity ranges from 1:50 to 1:100 million.

galactose tolerance t., a liver function t., based on the ability of the liver to convert galactose to glycogen, measured by the rate of excretion of galactose following ingestion or intravenous injection of a known amount; normally, less than 3 g appear in the urine within 5 hours after the ingestion of 40 g.

gel diffusion precipitin t.'s, precipitin t.'s in which the immune precipitate forms in a gel medium (usually agar) into which one or both reactants have diffused; generally classified in two types, in one dimension and in two dimensions. SYN gel diffusion reactions.

gel diffusion precipitin t.'s in one dimension, precipitin t.'s in which antigen solution and antibody incorporated in agar are layered in tubes, permitting effective diffusion in the vertical dimension; the antibody-containing agar may be overlaid directly with antigen solution (single (gel) diffusion in one dimension).

gel diffusion precipitin t.'s in two dimensions, precipitin t.'s made in a layer of agar that permits radial diffusion, in both of the horizontal dimensions, of one or both reactants. Double (gel) diffusionin two dimensions (Ouchterlony test, technique, or method) incorporates antigen and antibody solutions placed in separate wells in a sheet of plain agar, permitting radial diffusion of both reactants; this method is widely used to determine antigenic relationships; the bands of precipitate that form where the reactants meet in optimal concentration are of three patterns, referred to as reaction of identity, reaction of partial identity (cross-reaction), and reaction of nonidentity.

Gellé t., a vibrating tuning fork is applied over the mastoid process; if it is heard, the air in the external auditory canal is compressed, by means of a rubber tube inserted into the canal and a hand bulb, thereby fixing the stapes in the oval window, and the sound ceases to be heard, but is again perceived if the air pressure is removed; a t. of the mobility of the ossicles.

Gerhardt t. for acetoacetic acid, in fresh urine a red color develops upon addition of $FeCl_3$; no color develops if the urine has first been boiled; this t. has low specificity and sensitivity. SYN Gerhardt reaction.

Gerhardt t. for urobilin in the urine, the urobilin is extracted with chloroform and then treated with iodine and potassium hydrate, a fluorescent green color being produced.

germ tube t., a t. for the identification of *Candida albicans;* after a 3-hour incubation in serum, an inoculum of *Candida* develops tubelike appendages.

glucose oxidase paper strip t., a qualitative t. for glucose in the urine, in which glucose is oxidized to gluconic acid by glucose oxidase; a specific t., unless ascorbic acid is present.

glucose tolerance t., a t. for diabetes, or for hypoglycemic states such as may be seen rarely in patients with insulinomas. Following ingestion of 75 g of glucose while the patient is fasting, the blood sugar promptly rises and then falls to normal within 2 hours; in diabetics, the increase is greater and the return to normal unusually prolonged; in hypoglycemic patients, depressed glucose levels may be observed in 3-, 4-, or 5-hour measurements.

glycerol dehydration t., transient hearing improvement in some persons with Ménière disease after an oral glycerol dose resulting in an osmotic diuresis.

Gmelin t., an obsolete t. for bile in the urine or other body fluid; nitric acid, with a little nitrous acid, is carefully added to a few milliliters of the material to be tested; if bile (bilirubin) is present, it is oxidized to varying degrees, thereby resulting in disklike zones that are (from the interface outward) yellow, red, violet, blue, and green; development of green and violet layers is essential to the validity of the t. SYN Rosenbach-Gmelin t.

Gofman t., a t. for various serum lipoproteins that contain cholesterol, as an index of the tendency to the development of atheromatous lesions and arteriosclerosis; the t. is based on the differential flotation of molecules of various sizes when the serum is treated in an ultracentrifuge.

Goldscheider t., determination of the temperature sense by touching the skin with a sharp-pointed metallic rod heated to varying degrees.

gold sol t., SYN Lange t.

Goodenough draw-a-man t., a brief t. for assessing an individual's level of intelligence based on how accurately drawn and how many elements are included when a child or adult is given a pencil and sheet of white paper and asked to draw a man, the best man he or she is able to draw. Also called the Goodenough draw-a-person t. and, in its current form, the Goodenough-Harris drawing t.

goodness of fit t., a statistical t. of the hypothesis that data have been randomly sampled or generated from a population that follows a particular theoretical distribution.

Göthlin t., a capillary fragility t. to determine the presence or absence of scurvy.

Graham-Cole t., SYN cholecystography.

group t., in psychology, a t. designed to be administered to more than one individual at a time; e.g., scholastic achievement t., medical college admissions t.

guaiac t., SYN Almén t. for blood.

Günzberg t., a t. for hydrochloric acid utilizing phloroglucin vanillin (Günzberg reagent), with which a bright red color is produced in the presence of the acid.

Guthrie t., bacterial inhibition assay for direct measurement of serum phenylalanine; in widespread use for detection of phenylketonuria in the newborn.

Gutzeit t., an obsolete t. for arsenic; a piece of zinc and a little sulfuric acid are added to the suspected liquid which is then boiled; a bit of filter paper with a silver nitrate solution is held in the vapor and will turn yellow if arsenic is present.

Ham t., SYN acidified serum t.

Hardy-Rand-Ritter t., a t. for color vision deficiency using pseudoisochromatic cards.

Harrington-Flocks t., a rapid screening t. for visual field defects; patterns are viewed tachistoscopically, and the patterns are visible only when illuminated by a flash of ultraviolet light.

Harris t., SYN Harris and Ray t.

Harris and Ray t., an obsolete t. for vitamin C in the urine; a microtitration t. of the urine against a known amount of 0.05% aqueous solution of the dye 2,6-dichloroindophenol in 10% acetic acid (usually 0.05 mL of dye is used, roughly equivalent to 0.025 mg of ascorbic acid). SYN Harris t.

head-dropping t., a t. used in the diagnosis of disease of the extrapyramidal or striatal system (e.g., parkinsonism, Wilson disease); with the patient supine and relaxed with attention diverted, the examiner briskly lifts the patient's head with the right hand and then allows it to drop upon the palm of the examiner's left hand; the head of a normal person drops suddenly like a dead weight; in striatal disease the head falls slowly, gently, and almost hesitantly.

heat coagulation t., a t. for measurement of protein in urine; albumin and globulin are coagulated by heat at an acid pH, and the amount of turbidity present provides a qualitative estimation of the degree of proteinuria.

heat instability t., a t. for the presence of unstable hemoglobins; fresh red blood cells lysed in distilled water develop a precipitate within 1 hour at 50°C if unstable hemoglobin is present.

heel-tap t., SEE heel *tap*.

heel-to-knee-to-toe t., SYN heel-to-shin t.

heel-to-shin t., a test of lower limb coordination and position sense; the subject places the heel of one foot on the opposite knee and then slides it distally along the shin to the opposite ankle. SYN heel-to-knee-to-toe t.

Heinz body t., a t. for glucose-6-phosphate dehydrogenase-deficient red blood cells; an oxidant (acetylphenylhydrazine) is added to blood; after incubation at 37°C, glucose-6-phosphate dehydrogenase-deficient samples exhibit more than 30% Heinz bodies.

hemadsorption virus t., a method for detecting hemagglutinating viruses that is based on adherence of erythrocytes to infected cells.

hemagglutination t., a sensitive t. to measure certain antigens, antibodies, or viruses, using their ability to agglutinate certain erythrocytes.

Hemoccult t., trade name for a qualitative t. for occult blood in stool based on detecting the peroxidase activity of hemoglobin; a t. kit can be used at home and the specimens (usually 3 collected on sequential days) mailed to a laboratory for evaluation.

Hering t., a t. of binocular vision; the subject looks through an apparatus having at its far end a thread near which a small sphere is dropped; with binocular vision the observer recognizes the location of the sphere in front of or behind the thread; with monocular vision this is not possible.

Hershberg t., a t. for anabolic steroids in which castrated male rats are treated with the substance being tested.

Hines-Brown t., SYN cold pressor t.

Hinton t., a formerly widely used precipitin (flocculation) t. for syphilis in which the "antigen" consisted of glycerol, cholesterol, and beef heart extract.

Hirschberg t., a t. of binocular motor alignment by which a penlight is shone at the eyes and the position of the light reflex on the cornea observed, allowing an estimate of the amount of deviation, if present.

Histalog t., a t. for measurement of maximal production of gastric acidity or anacidity; it is similar to the histamine t., but uses Histalog (betazole hydrochloride), an analog of histamine. SYN maximal Histalog t.

histamine t., a t. for maximal production of gastric acidity or anacidity; after preliminary administration of an antihistamine, histamine acid phosphate is injected subcutaneously in a dose of 0.04 mg/kg of body weight, followed by analysis of gastric contents. SEE ALSO Histalog t. SYN augmented histamine t.

histoplasmin-latex t., a passive agglutination t. for histoplasmosis; latex particles, sensitized with antigen extracted from *Histoplasma capsulatum*, are used in a flocculation reaction with the patient's serum.

Hollander t., SYN insulin hypoglycemia t.

Holmgren wool t., a t. for color blindness, in which the subject matches variously colored skeins of wool.

homovanillic acid t., a t. for homovanillic acid based upon the fact that dopamine is present in sympathetic nervous tissue as precursor of norepinephrine; since norepinephrine has a metabolic pathway which yields homovanillic acid, tumors such as neuroblastomas and ganglioneuromas may cause elevations of urinary dopamine and homovanillic acid. SYN HVA t.

Howard t., an obsolete t. in which a differential ureteral catheterization is performed by the insertion of bilateral ureteral catheters to measure simultaneous urinary volume and sodium concentration in patients with suspected renovascular hypertension.

Huhner t., SYN postcoital t.

HVA t., SYN homovanillic acid t.

17-hydroxycorticosteroid t., a t., dependent on the Porter-Silber reaction, that is used as a measure of adrenocortical function and is performed on urine. Low values are seen in Addison disease and hypopituitarism; high values are seen in Cushing syndrome and extreme stress. SYN 17-OH-corticoids t., Porter-Silber chromogens t.

hyperventilation t., producing respiratory alkalosis by overbreathing to 1) produce clinical abnormalities, e.g., tetany seizures; 2) cause EEG abnormalities; 3) cause EMG abnormalities.

hypoxemia t., SYN anoxemia t.

immune adhesion t., SYN adhesion t.

immunologic pregnancy t., a general term for t.'s for detection of increased human chorionic gonadotropin in plasma or urine by immunologic techniques including latex particle agglutination, hemagglutination inhibition, radioimmunoassay, radioreceptor assays, and enzyme immunoassays.

impingement t., diagnostic t. in which local anesthetic is injected into the subacromial space of a patient with impingement signs; relief of pain following the injection during provocative maneuvers is helpful in confirming the subacromial space as the source of the symptoms.

indirect t., SEE Prausnitz-Küstner *reaction*.

indirect Coombs t., a t. routinely performed in cross-matching blood or in the investigation of transfusion reaction: t. for patient's serum is incubated with a suspension of donor erythrocytes; if specific antibodies are present, they become attached to the antigen in the donor cells; after a washing with saline, Coombs antihuman globulin is added; agglutination at this point indicates that antibodies present in the original t. serum had indeed become attached to donor erythrocytes.

indirect fluorescent antibody t., SEE fluorescent antibody *technique*.

indirect hemagglutination t., SYN passive *hemagglutination*.

indole t., a t. used to identify members of the *Enterobacteriaceae* family and other Gram-negative bacilli, based on the ability of the organisms to produce indole from tryptophan.

inkblot t., SYN Rorschach t.

insulin hypoglycemia t., an infrequently used t. to determine the completeness of vagotomy; after the surgery, insulin is administered to cause hypoglycemia; if vagotomy is complete, the acid output from the stomach following administration of insulin is substantially less than that before insulin administration; if the level is unchanged, incomplete vagotomy is likely. Complications of hypoglycemia are such that the t. largely has been abandoned. SYN Hollander t.

intelligence t., a t., using well-researched items and involving a systematic method of administration and scoring, used to assess an individual's general aptitude or level of potential competence, in contrast to an achievement t.

intradermal t., SYN skin t.

iodine t., a t. for detecting the presence of starch based on its reaction with iodine.

Ishihara t., a t. for color vision deficiency that utilizes a series of pseudoisochromatic plates on which numbers or letters are printed in dots of primary colors surrounded by dots of other colors; the figures are discernible by individuals with normal color vision.

isopropanol precipitation t., a t. using the principle that the internal bonds of hemoglobin are weakened by nonpolar solvents; thus, unstable hemoglobins will precipitate more rapidly than other hemoglobins in isopropanol.

^{131}I uptake t., a t. of thyroid function in which ^{131}I-iodide is given orally; after 24 hours, the amount present in the thyroid gland is measured and compared with normal values. SYN radioactive iodide uptake t., RAI t.

Ivy bleeding time t., a bleeding time t. in which a sphygmomanometer is inflated to 40 mm Hg around the upper arm, a 5-mm deep incision is made on the flexor surface of the forearm, and the time is measured to cessation of bleeding.

Jacquemin t., a t. for phenol; to the suspected fluid an equal amount of aniline is added, and, after thorough admixture, a little solution of sodium hypochlorite; if phenol is present the fluid becomes blue.

Jaffe t., **(1)** a quantitative t. for creatinine based on its reaction with alkaline picrate; **(2)** a qualitative t. for the presence of indicanuria; after an equal amount of HCl is added to the urine, the further addition of chloroform and CaCl$_2$ gives rise to blue or purple chloroform droplets that sink to the bottom if indican is present.

Janet t., a t. for functional or organic anesthesia; the patient (with eyes closed) is told to say "yes" or "no" on feeling (or not) the touch of the examiner's finger; in the case of functional anesthesia the patient may say "no" when an anesthetic area is touched, but will say nothing, being unaware that he is touched, in cases of organic anesthesia.

Jolles t., a t. for bile; a precipitate is obtained by agitation with chloroform, a solution of barium chloride, and hydrochloric acid; the precipitate is removed, and the addition of a drop or two of sulfuric acid will produce a play of color if bile pigments are present.

Jones t., SYN fluorescein instillation t.

Jones I t., SYN primary dye t.

Jones II t., SYN secondary dye t.

Katayama t., a qualitative colorimetric t. for the presence of carboxyhemoglobin in the blood.

ketogenic corticoids t., SYN 17-ketogenic steroid assay t.

17-ketogenic steroid assay t., a colorimetric t., based on the Zimmermann reaction, which indicates metabolites or adrenal and testicular steroids excreted as 17-ketones in the urine; increased values are most striking in adrenocortical tumors, decreased values in Addison disease or in panhypopituitarism. SYN ketogenic corticoids t.

Knoop hardness t., SEE Knoop hardness *number*.

Kober t., a t. for naturally occurring estrogens, based upon the production of a pink color (absorption maximum: 520 μm) when an estrogen is heated in a mixture of phenol and sulfuric acid.

Kolmer t., a former standard quantitative method for the Wassermann t., with numerous modifications (especially as to antigen).

Korotkoff t., a t. of collateral circulation; while the artery above an aneurysm is compressed, the blood pressure in the distal circulation is estimated; if it is fairly high, the collateral circulation is good.

Krimsky t., a t. of binocular motor alignment by which a penlight is shone at the eyes and the position of the light reflex centered with a prism, thus indicating the amount of deviation.

Kurzrok-Ratner t., a t. for estrogens in the urine; the urine is extracted with ethyl acetate and, after purification, the extract is subjected to bioassay as in the Allen-Doisy t.

Kveim t., an intradermal t. for the detection of sarcoidosis, done by injecting Kveim antigen (obtained from spleens of persons with sarcoidosis) and examining skin biopsies after 3 and 6 weeks; a positive t. is indicated by typical nodules showing evidence of sarcoid tissue. SYN Kveim-Siltzbach t., Nickerson-Kveim t.

Kveim-Siltzbach t., SYN Kveim t.

Lachman t., a maneuver to detect deficiency of the anterior cruciate ligament; with the knee flexed 20–30°, the tibia is displaced anteriorly relative to the femur; a soft endpoint or greater than 4 mm of displacement is positive (abnormal).

Lancaster red green t., t. to measure ocular deviations in various fields of gaze in adult patients with acquired strabismus and diplopia by placing a red filter over the right eye and a green filter over the left eye followed by alignment by the patient of a red or green light with light of opposite color projected by the examiner.

Landsteiner-Donath t., SEE Donath-Landsteiner *phenomenon*.

Lange t., an obsolete, nonspecific t. for altered proteins in spinal fluid. As originally used by Lange in 1912, the t. was thought to be specific for neurosyphilis; however, this proved to be incorrect. Dilutions of spinal fluid are made in saline and to these a colloidal gold solution is added; if altered proteins are present, there is a color change or precipitate formed. SYN gold sol t., Zsigmondy t.

latex agglutination t., a passive agglutination t. in which antigen is adsorbed onto latex particles which then clump in the presence of antibody specific for the adsorbed antigen. SYN latex fixation t.

latex fixation t., SYN latex agglutination t.

LE cell t., in vitro incubation of blood or bone marrow of patients with systemic lupus erythematosus, or action of their serum on normal leukocytes, causes formation of characteristic LE cells. SYN lupus erythematosus cell t.

Legal t., a t. for acetone; the urine is rendered alkaline by a few drops of a solution of potassium hydroxide, and to this are added 2 or 3 drops of a freshly prepared 10% solution of sodium nitroprusside; it is colored red, then yellow; then a few drops of acetic acid are trickled down the side of the t. tube and at the line of junction of the two fluids is formed a carmine or purple ring.

leishmanin t., a delayed hypersensitivity t. for cutaneous leishmaniasis; a positive t. when granulomatous induration exceeds 5 min after 2–3 days at the intradermal injection site of a suspension of leishmanias in phenol. SYN Montenegro t. [leishmania + suffix -*in*, component, derivative]

lepromin t., a t. utilizing an intradermal injection of a lepromin, such as the Dharmendra antigen or Mitsuda antigen, to classify the stage of leprosy based on the lepromin reaction, such as the Fernandez reaction or Mitsuda reaction; it differentiates tuberculoid leprosy, in which there is a positive delayed reaction at the injection site, from lepromatous leprosy, in which there is no reaction (i.e., a negative t. result) despite the active malignant *Mycobacterium leprae* infection; the t. is not diagnostic, since normal uninfected persons may react.

leukocyte adherence assay t., a t. to detect the ability of leukocytes to adhere to bacteria, performed in vitro using nylon fibers to measure adherence.

leukocyte bactericidal assay t., a t. of leukocytes to determine their ability to kill a culture of live bacteria.

Liebermann-Burchard t., a colorimetric t. for unsaturated sterols, notably cholesterol; a blue-green color develops when such substances are added to acetic anhydride and sulfuric acid in chloroform.

limulus lysate t., a t. for the rapid detection of Gram-negative bacterial meningitis; Gram-negative endotoxin induces gel formation of *Limulus polyphemus* (horseshoe crab) lysates.

line t., a t. for rickets, based on observation of the lines of calcification in the growing ends of rachitic long bones in rats given vitamin D preparations under standard t. conditions; used in biological assay of vitamin D by the USP.

lipase t., a diagnostic t. based on the measurement of lipase in blood and urine as an indicator of pancreatic disease.

Lombard voice-reflex t., the observation of fluctuations in the intensity of a patient's voice when a masking noise is increased or decreased; a t. useful in assessing functional hearing loss.

Lücke t., a t. for hippuric acid; hot nitric acid is added to the urine and evaporated to dryness; the presence of hippuric acid is indicated by an odor of nitrobenzol upon further heating.

lupus band t., a direct immunofluorescent technique for demonstrating a band of immunoglobulins at the dermal-epidermal junction of the skin of patients with lupus erythematosus.

lupus erythematosus cell t., SYN LE cell t.

Machado-Guerreiro t., a complement-fixation t. for infection with *Trypanosoma cruzi*.

Maclagan t., SYN thymol turbidity t.

Maclagan thymol turbidity t., SYN thymol turbidity t.

macrophage migration inhibition t., SYN migration inhibitory factor t.

Mantel-Haenszel t., a summary chi-square t. developed by Mantel and Haenszel for stratified data.

Mantoux t., SEE tuberculin t.

Marshall t., manual deviation of bladder neck during strain or cough to ascertain presence of stress urinary incontinence. SYN Bonney t., Marshall-Marchetti t.

Marshall-Marchetti t., SYN Marshall t.

Master t., an early and long-used exercise challenge to identify ischemic heart disease using a pair of 9-inch steps with a platform on top, the number of trips by the patient arbitrarily chosen and related to age and body weight. SEE ALSO two-step exercise t. SYN Master two-step exercise t.

Master two-step exercise t., SYN Master t.

maximal Histalog t., SYN Histalog t.

Mazzotti t., a t. for onchocerciasis using an oral t. dose of diethylcarbamazine (50 or 100 mg), resulting in the appearance of an acute rash in 2–24 hours from death of microfilariae in the skin. SYN Mazzotti reaction.

McMurray t., rotation of the tibia on the femur to determine injury to meniscal structures.

McNemar t., a form of chi-square t. for matched paired data.

McPhail t., an obsolete t. for progesterone and like substances; immature female rabbits are treated with 150 IU of estrone over a period of 6 days; the t. material is then given in five daily subcutaneous doses; progestational proliferation of the endometrium is noted and the results estimated according to a scale from 0 to ++++; the amount required to produce an average (++) response is taken as a unit, equivalent to 0.25 mg of progesterone.

Meinicke t., the first successful application (1917–1918) of immune precipitation to diagnose syphilis, now obsolete.

Meltzer-Lyon t., a t. used in diagnosis of gallbladder conditions: 25 ml of a 25% solution of magnesium sulfate are delivered into the region of the sphincter of Oddi through a duodenal tube, causing contraction of the gallbladder, relaxation of the sphincter, and the expulsion of bile from the common duct and gallbladder; bile from the common duct is relatively pale and is expelled first, that from the gallbladder follows; samples aspirated from the tube are examined for pus cells, pigment granules, epithelial cells, cholesterol, etc.

metabisulfite t., a t. for sickle cell hemoglobin (Hb S); deoxygenation of cells containing Hb S is enhanced by addition of sodium metabisulfite to the blood, causing sickling visible on a slide; certain other abnormal hemoglobins (Hb C$_{Harlem}$ and Hb I) also sickle in this t.

methacholine challenge t., a t. that involves the inhalation of increasing concentrations of methacholine, a potent bronchoconstrictor, in patients with possible bronchial hyperreactivity; usually performed when a diagnosis of asthma or bronchospastic lung disease is not clinically obvious.

3-methoxy-4-hydroxymandelic acid t., SYN vanillylmandelic acid t.

metrotrophic t., an obsolete t. for the assay of estrogenic substances; immature female rats (25–49 g) are injected subcutaneously with the hormone and killed after 6 hours, when the increase in uterine weight (due largely to imbibation of water) is taken as the criterion of estrogenic activity. SYN Astwood t.

MHA-TP t., SYN microhemagglutination-Treponema pallidum t.

microhemagglutination-Treponema pallidum t., a microtiter version of the *Treponema pallidum* hemagglutination t. SYN MHA-TP t.

microprecipitation t., a precipitation t. in which reduced quantities of t. reagents are used.

migration inhibition t., SYN migration inhibitory factor t.

migration inhibitory factor t., a t. which measures the presence of migration inhibitory factor, a 25-kD lymphokine. Usually peritoneal macrophages are placed in a capillary tube in the presence or absence of supernatants from activated T cells in response to immunogenic challenge. If MIF is present, the migration of monocyte/macrophages is reduced. SYN macrophage migration inhibition t., migration inhibition t.

milk-ring t., a special form of agglutination t. done on the pooled milk of many cows, usually entire herds, for the detection of herds containing individuals infected with bovine brucellosis.

Millon Clinical Multiaxial Inventory t., a paper and pencil test, consisting of 20 clinical scales derived from 175 self-descriptive statements, and developed in 1977 for use in the assessment of psychopathology and the more enduring patterns of personality; specifically designed to correspond with some of the disorders of personality included in the Diagnostic and Statistical Manual of Mental Disorders used in diagnosis by mental health professionals. SYN Millon clinical multiaxial inventory.

Millon-Nasse t., a t. for protein, the tyrosine of which reacts with nitrite after a brief treatment with mercuric ion in acid to give a color.

Minnesota Multiphasic Personality Inventory t. (MMPI), a questionnaire type of psychological test for ages 16 and over, with 550 true-false statements coded in 4 validity and 10 personality scales which may be administered in both an individual or group format. SYN Minnesota Multiphasic Personality Inventory.

mixed agglutination t., SEE mixed agglutination *reaction*.

mixed lymphocyte culture t., a t. for histocompatibility of HL-A antigens in which donor and recipient lymphocytes are mixed in culture; the degree of incompatibility is indicated by the number of cells that have undergone transformation and mitosis, or by the uptake of radioactive isotope-labeled thymidine. SYN MLC t.

MLC t., SYN mixed lymphocyte culture t.

Molisch t., a color t. for sugar, which condenses with α-naphthol

te

or thymol in the presence of strong sulfuric acid, which converts the sugar to furfural derivatives.

Moloney t., a t. to detect a high degree of sensitivity to diphtheria toxoid; more than a minimal local reaction to diluted (1:20) toxoid given intradermally indicates that prophylactic toxoid should be inoculated in fractional doses at suitable intervals.

Montenegro t., SYN leishmanin t.

Mörner t., (1) for cysteine, which gives a brilliant purple color with sodium nitroprusside; (2) for tyrosine, which gives a green color on boiling with sulfuric acid containing formaldehyde.

Moschcowitz t., demonstration of lower limb ischemia by occlusion of the arterial circulation for 5 min with a tourniquet or Esmarch bandage. Following release, skin color normally will return in a few seconds; with arterial obstruction (e.g., arteriosclerotic) color returns more slowly.

Mosenthal t., an infrequently used t. to evaluate renal concentrating ability by measuring the density of urine every 2 hours during the ingestion of a controlled diet.

motility t., a t. based on microscopic observation or on the spread of growth in soft agar, used to determine if a microorganism is motile.

Motulsky dye reduction t., a t. for glucose-6-phosphate dehydrogenase deficiency in the blood, using a mixture of brilliant cresyl blue, glucose 6-phosphate, and NADP.

mucin clot t., a t. that reflects the polymerization of synovial fluid hyaluronate; a few drops of synovial fluid added to acetic acid form a clot; poor clot formation occurs in a variety of inflammatory conditions including septic arthritis, gouty arthritis, and rheumatoid arthritis. SYN Ropes t.

Mulder t., SEE xanthoprotein *reaction*.

multiple puncture tuberculin t., a kind of tine t. SEE tuberculin t.

multiple sleep latency t., a t. of the propensity to fall asleep, done by performing polysomnography during multiple brief opportunities to sleep.

mumps sensitivity t., a skin t. for sensitivity to mumps, in which inactivated mumps virus is used as antigen.

Nagel t., a t. for color vision in which the observer determines the relative amounts of red and green necessary to match spectral yellow; an instrument called Nagel anomaloscope is used.

NBT t., abbreviation for nitroblue tetrazolium t.

neutralization t., SYN protection t.

niacin t., a t. of the ability of mycobacteria to elaborate niacin; used to distinguish *Mycobacterium tuberculosis* from other strains.

Nickerson-Kveim t., SYN Kveim t.

nitroblue tetrazolium t. (NBT t.), a t. to detect the phagocytic ability of polymorphonuclear leukocytes by measuring the capacity of the oxygen-dependent leukocytic bactericidal system.

nitroprusside t., a qualitative t. for cystinuria; following the addition of sodium cyanide to the urine, the further addition of nitroprusside produces a red-purple color if the cyanide has reduced any cystine present to cysteine.

nonstress t., a t. to evaluate fetal well-being by evaluating fetal heart rate response to fetal movement; a reactive nonstress t. is fetal heart rate acceleration in response to fetal movement.

nystagmus t., SYN Bárány caloric t.

Ober t., t. to evaluate a tight, contracted, or inflamed iliotibial tract; the patient lies on the uninvolved side and the involved hip is abducted by the examiner as the knee is flexed to 90°; the hip is allowed to adduct passively; the degree of abduction or the production of pain along the iliotibial tract can assist in identifying the location of the inflammation or contracture.

Obermayer t., a t. for indican; solids in the urine are precipitated by means of a 20% solution of acetate of lead and then filtered, and to the filtrate is added fuming hydrochloric acid containing a small amount of ferric chloride solution; if indican is present, the addition of chloroform causes the formation of indigo, indicated by the blue color.

17-OH-corticoids t., SYN 17-hydroxycorticosteroid t.

oral lactose tolerance t., a t. for lactose deficiency; the plasma glucose response to an oral lactose load is measured as in the (oral) glucose tolerance t.

orcinol t., SYN Bial t.

Ortolani t., SYN Ortolani *maneuver*.

Ouchterlony t., double (gel) diffusion t. in two dimensions. SEE gel diffusion precipitin t.'s in two dimensions. SYN Ouchterlony method.

oxidase t., a t. for the presence of intracellular cytochrome oxidase based on the reaction with *p*-phenylenediamine; aids in the identification of *Neisseria* species and Pseudomonadaceae.

oxytocin challenge t., a contraction stress t. accomplished by administration of intravenous dilute oxytocin solution to stimulate contractions. SYN contraction stress t.

Pachon t., in a case of aneurysm, determination of the collateral circulation by estimation of the blood pressure.

Palmer acid t. for peptic ulcer, in duodenal ulcer, the administration of acid by duodenal tube causes severe pain.

palmin t., palmitin t., a t. of pancreatic efficiency, based upon the fact that the presence of fat in the stomach causes the pylorus to open and admit the pancreatic juice; this splits the palmin so that an examination of the stomach contents, after a t. meal containing palmin, will reveal the presence of fatty acids.

pancreozymin-secretin t., SEE secretin t.

Pandy t., SYN Pandy *reaction*.

Pap t., microscopic examination of cells exfoliated or scraped from a mucosal surface after staining with Papanicolaou stain; used especially for detection of cancer of the uterine cervix. SYN Papanicolaou smear t.

Papanicolaou smear t., SYN Pap t.

parallax t., measurement of the deviation in strabismus by the alternate cover t. combined with neutralization of the deviation using prisms.

parametric t., a statistical t. that depends on an assumption about the distribution of the data, e.g., that the data are normally distributed.

passive cutaneous anaphylaxis t., an animal is injected intradermally with antibody (usually IgE) and subsequently challenged intravenously with a mixture of antigen and Evans blue dye 24–48 hours later. A dark blue area indicates a positive reaction due to the leakage of the dye at the site of antigen-antibody reactions.

patch t., a t. of skin sensitiveness: a small piece of paper, tape, or a cup, wet with nonirritating diluted t. fluid, is applied to skin of the upper back or upper outer arm and after 48 hours the covered is compared with the uncovered surface; an erythematous reaction with vesicles occurs if the substance causes contact allergy. SEE ALSO photo-patch t.

Patrick t., a t. to determine the presence or absence of sacroiliac disease; with the patient supine, the hip and knee are flexed and the external malleolus is placed above the patella of the opposite leg; this can ordinarily be done without pain, but, on depressing the knee, pain is promptly elicited in sacroiliac disease.

Paul t., SYN Paul *reaction*.

Paul-Bunnell t., a t. for detection of heterophil antibodies in infectious mononucleosis. SEE Forssman *antigen*.

PBI t., SYN protein-bound iodine t.

pentagastrin t., an alternative to histamine for stimulation of acid secretion in gastric analysis.

performance t., a t., such as five of the eleven Wechsler adult intelligence scale subtests, requiring little or no verbal instruction from the examiner and virtually no verbal response by the examinee.

Perls t., a t. for hemosiderin, utilizing Perls Prussian blue *stain*.

personality t., any of the category of psychological t.'s designed to t. the characteristics of the personality, emotional status, mental disorder, etc., in contrast to an intelligence t.

Perthes t., a t. for patency of the deep femoral vein; with the patient standing, a tourniquet is applied above the knee; after walking, if the deep circulation is competent, the superficial varicosities remain unchanged; if the deep circulation is occluded, the legs become painful.

phentolamine t., a t. for pheochromocytoma; intravenous administration of phentolamine (5 mg) reduces hypertension due to a pheochromocytoma but not that due to other causes, e.g., essential hypertension; the blood pressure is raised by the drug in the latter form of hypertension.

photo-patch t., a t. of contact photosensitization: after application of a patch with the suspected sensitizer for 48 hours to two sites, if there is no reaction, one area is exposed to a weak erythema dose of sunlight or ultraviolet light; if positive, a more severe reaction with vesiculation develops at the exposed patch area than the nonexposed skin patch site.

photostress t., measurement of visual acuity before and after exposure of the eyes to intense light.

phrenic pressure t., pressure is applied on the phrenic nerve on each side, above the clavicles where the nerve passes over the scalenus anticus muscle; if pain is felt and the patient inclines the head to the painful side, the problem is in the pleural space; if the head does not incline to one side, the problem is in the abdominal cavity.

Pirquet t., a cutaneous tuberculin t. SEE tuberculin t. SYN dermotuberculin reaction, Pirquet reaction.

pivot shift t., a maneuver to detect a deficiency of the anterior cruciate ligament of the knee; when the knee is extended, a sudden subluxation of the lateral tibial condyle upon the distal femur is positive.

P-K t., SYN Prausnitz-Küstner *reaction.*

plasmacrit t., a serologic screening method used as an aid in the diagnosis of syphilis; after only a few drops of heparinized blood (obtained from a pricked finger) are collected in a special capillary tube, the capillary tube is centrifuged in order to collect plasma, which is then mixed with a 0.01-ml drop of antigen (cardiolipin previously treated with choline chloride as an antiinhibitor, in order to avoid falsely negative results that may occur with nonheated plasma or serum). After mechanically agitating the antigen-plasma mixture for 4 min, the presence or absence of flocculation is observed. A positive result should not be regarded as conclusively diagnostic, but a negative result excludes the likelihood of syphilis.

platelet aggregation t., a t. of the ability of platelets to adhere to each other and hence form a hemostatic plug to prevent bleeding; failure to aggregate occurs in several conditions, e.g., thrombasthenia, Von Willebrand disease, and following administration of aspirin, phenylbutazone, and indomethacin; the t. is conducted by quantitating the decrease in turbidity that occurs in platelet-rich plasma following the in vitro addition of one or several plateletaggregating agents (e.g., ADP, epinephrine, or serotonin).

polyuria t., SYN Albarran t.

Porges-Meier t., an early flocculation t. for syphilis; of significance in having introduced as antigens acetone-insoluble, alcohol-soluble fractions of tissue, and lecithin.

Porter-Silber chromogens t., SYN 17-hydroxycorticosteroid t.

postcoital t., a t. on cervical mucus about time of ovulation to evaluate its receptivity to sperm. SYN Huhner t.

precipitation t., SYN precipitin t.

precipitin t., an in vitro t. in which antigen is in soluble form and precipitates when it combines with added specific antibody in the presence of an electrolyte. SEE ALSO gel diffusion precipitin t.'s, ring precipitin t. SYN precipitation t.

primary dye t., assessment of lacrimal drainage following the fluorescein instillation t. by attempting to recover fluorescein dye beneath the inferior turbinate using a swab. SYN Jones I t.

prism cover t., measurement of the deviation in strabismus by the alternate cover t. combined with neutralization for the deviation using prisms.

prism vergence t., measurement of the amplitude of fusion by placing prisms of gradually increasing power in the direction tested until diplopia occurs.

progesterone challenge t., administration of a progestational agent in case of amenorrhea to detect the presence of an estrogen-primed endometrium.

projective t., a loosely structured psychological t. containing many ambiguous stimuli that require the subject to reveal feelings, personality, or psychopathology in response to them; e.g., Rorschach t., thematic apperception t.

protection t., a t. to determine the antimicrobial activity of a

serum or to identify a given organism by inoculating a susceptible animal or cell culture with a mixture of the serum and the virus or other microbe being tested. SYN neutralization t.

protein-bound iodine t., a formerly used t. of thyroid function in which serum protein-bound iodine is measured to provide an estimate of hormone bound to protein in peripheral blood. SYN PBI t.

prothrombin t., a quantitative t. for prothrombin in the blood based on the clotting time of blood plasma in the presence of thromboplastin and calcium chloride; measures the integrity of the extrinsic and common pathways of coagulation. SEE ALSO prothrombin *time.* SYN Quick method, Quick t.

prothrombin and proconvertin t., a t. formerly used by some to control anticoagulant therapy with bishydroxycoumarin and indandione drugs.

provocative t., any procedure in which a suspected pathophysiological abnormality is deliberately induced by manipulating conditions known to provoke the abnormality.

provocative Wassermann t., an obsolete t. of historical interest only; the use of the Wassermann t. from one or two days to one or two weeks after the administration of arsphenamine or neoarsphenamine; the result may then be positive when before the giving of arsphenamine it was negative.

psychological t.'s, t.'s designed to measure a person's achievements, intelligence, neuropsychological functions, skills, personality, or individual and occupational characteristics or potentialities. SEE ALSO scale.

psychomotor t.'s, psychological t.'s which, although based on other psychological processes (e.g., sensory, perceptual), require a motor reaction such as copying designs, building with blocks, or manipulating controls.

pulp t., SYN vitality t.

Q tip t., a t. for determining the mobility of the urethra.

Queckenstedt-Stookey t., compression of the jugular vein in a healthy person causes an increase in the pressure of the spinal fluid in the lumbar region within 10–12 sec, and an equally rapid fall to normal on release of the pressure on the vein; when there is a block of subarachnoid channels, compression of the vein causes little or no increase of pressure in the cerebrospinal fluid.

quellung t., SYN Neufeld capsular *swelling.*

Quick t., SYN prothrombin t.

quinine carbacrylic resin t., a t. for gastric anacidity. SEE azuresin.

Quinlan t., a t. for bile; when a thin layer of bile is examined through a spectroscope, absorption lines appear in the violet.

radioactive iodide uptake t., SYN ^{131}I uptake t.

radioallergosorbent t. (RAST), a radioimmunoassay t. to detect specific IgE antibodies responsible for hypersensitivity: the allergen is bound to insoluble material and the patient's serum is reacted with this conjugate; if the serum contains antibody to the allergen, it will be complexed to the allergen. Radiolabeled antihuman IgE antibody is added where it reacts with the bound IgE. The amount of radioactivity is proportional to the serum IgE.

radioimmunosorbent t. (RIST), a competition t., performed in vitro, used to measure IgE specific for a particular antigen. Known amounts of radiolabeled IgE compete with the patient's unlabeled IgE to bind to a surface coated with anti-IgE. The reduction in radiolabeled IgE due to the presence of IgE in the patient's serum can be determined by comparison to known IgE standards; thus, the amount of the patient's total serum IgE can be determined.

RAI t., SYN ^{131}I uptake t.

rapid plasma reagin t., a group of serologic t.'s for syphilis in which unheated serum or plasma is reacted with a standard t. antigen containing charcoal particles; positive t.'s yield a flocculation. A modification, called the RPR (circle) card t., is widely used as a screening t. SYN RPR t.

Rapoport t., a differential ureteral catheterization t. used to evaluate suspected renovascular hypertension; urine specimens from each kidney are obtained by bilateral ureteral catheterization, and the tubular rejection fraction ratio is determined by

te

measuring concentrations of sodium and creatinine in the urine from each kidney.

Rayleigh t., SYN Rayleigh *equation.*

red cell adherence t., SYN adhesion t.

Reinsch t., a t. for arsenic in which a strip of copper is placed in the suspected fluid, which is then acidulated with hydrochloric acid and boiled; if arsenic is present a gray deposit occurs on the copper, and this deposit on heating is sublimated and deposited as a crystalline layer on a piece of glass held above the copper strip.

Reiter t., a complement-fixation t. for syphilis using as antigen material prepared from the Reiter strain of *Treponema pallidum;* the t. has been largely replaced in laboratory medicine by the fluorescent treponemal antibody-absorption (FTA-ABS) t.

relocation t., a t. for anterior shoulder instability; the supine patient's humerus is abducted and rotated externally against the table edge as a fulcrum; patients with anterior stability loss become apprehensive with pressure.

resorcinol t., a t. for fructosuria; fresh urine treated with resorcinol in acid gives a red precipitate in the presence of fructose; the precipitate should form a red solution in ethanol. SYN Selivanoff t.

Reuss t., a t. for atropine; the addition of oxidizing agents and sulfuric acid to a liquid containing atropine produces an odor of orange-flowers and roses.

Rh blocking t., a t. for nonagglutinating Rh antibodies: an Rh agglutination t. is first carried out; if the t. for Rh agglutinins is negative, then 1 drop of anti-Rh_o agglutinating serum of moderate titer is mixed with the patient's serum containing Rh-positive t. cells; if after incubating for from 1–2 hr at 37°C no agglutination occurs, Rh_o-blocking antibodies are assumed to be present in the patient's serum.

Rickles t., a colorimetric t. for predicting dental caries activity by incubating saliva in sucrose and determining pH changes.

Rimini t., an obsolete t. for formaldehyde in urine, milk, and other fluids, by the use of dilute solution of phenylhydrazine hydrochloride, sodium nitroprusside, and sodium hydroxide.

ring t., SYN ring precipitin t.

ring precipitin t., a precipitin t. in which antigen solution is carefully layered over antibody solution in a tube; as diffusion proceeds, a disk of precipitate forms where the antibody ratio is optimal. SYN ring t.

Rinne t., (1) a vibrating tuning fork is held in contact with the skull (usually the mastoid process) until the sound is lost, its prongs are then brought close to the auditory orifice when, if the hearing is normal, a faint sound will again be heard; expressed as air conduction greater than bone conduction and indicative of a normal sound conducting mechanism through the middle ear; (2) a vibrating tuning fork is heard longer and louder when in contact with the skull than when held near the auditory orifice, expressed as bone conduction greater than air conduction, indicating some disorder of the sound conducting mechanism.

Romberg t., SYN Romberg *sign.*

Römer t., a t. of historical interest: tuberculin, either pure or diluted, is injected intracutaneously into a guinea pig; if the animal is tuberculous, a large papule with a necrotic hemorrhagic center appears in about 24 hours (cocarde or cockade reaction).

Ropes t., SYN mucin clot t.

Rorschach t., a projective psychological t. in which the subject reveals his or her attitudes, emotions, and personality by reporting what is seen in each of 10 inkblot pictures. SYN inkblot t.

rose bengal radioactive (^{131}I) t., a t. of liver function used as a means of measuring hepatic blood flow and for scintillation scanning of the liver to determine size and contour of the liver, or the presence of space-occupying masses in the liver.

Rosenbach t., an obsolete t. for bile in the urine; the suspected urine is passed several times through the same filter paper, which is then dried and touched with a drop of slightly fuming nitric acid; the presence of bile is indicated by the resulting play of colors characteristic of the bile pigments (a yellow spot surrounded by rings of red, violet, blue, and green).

Rosenbach-Gmelin t., SYN Gmelin t.

rosette t., a t. for rosette-forming cells (T lymphocytes) in which these cells and sheep erythrocytes are incubated and centrifuged

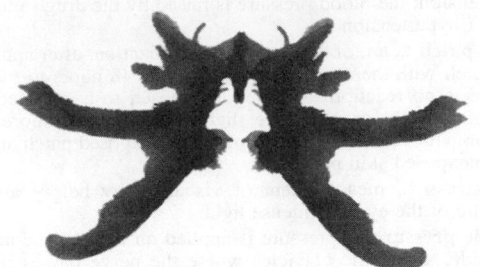

Rorschach test: example of picture used in testing

lightly, then examined under a microscope for rosette formation or adherence of erythrocytes to T lymphocytes.

Rose-Waaler t., a t. of historical interest: when sheep red cells are coated with a concentration of antiserum to sheep red cells which is too low to cause agglutination, the addition of serum from a patient with rheumatoid arthritis will cause agglutination.

Ross-Jones t., an obsolete t. for an excess of globulin in the cerebrospinal fluid; 1 ml of cerebrospinal fluid is carefully floated over 2 ml of a concentrated ammonium sulfate solution; if globulin is present in excess, a fine white ring appears at the line of junction in about 3 min.

Rothera nitroprusside t., a t. for ketone bodies; 5 ml of fresh urine are saturated with solid ammonium sulfate and mixed with 10 drops of freshly prepared 2% sodium nitroprusside solution, which is then mixed with 10 drops of concentrated ammonia water and allowed to stand for 15 min; the presence of acetoacetic acid, or of larger concentrations of acetone, is indicated by the development of a blue-purple color.

RPR t., SYN rapid plasma reagin t.

rubella HI t., a hemagglutination inhibition (HI) t. for rubella, often performed routinely as part of a prenatal workup of the pregnant woman; the presence of a detectable HI titer in the absence of disease indicates previous infection and immunity to reinfection; if HI antibody is undetected, the patient is considered potentially susceptible and is followed accordingly. SEE ALSO hemagglutination *inhibition.*

Rubin t., an obsolete t. of patency of the fallopian tubes; a cannula is introduced into the cervix uteri, and carbon dioxide gas is passed through the cannula by means of a syringe with manometer attachment; if the tubes are patent, the escape of gas into the abdominal cavity is evidenced by a high-pitched bubbling sound heard on auscultation over the lower abdomen, or free gas under the diaphragm can be demonstrated by x-ray.

Rubner t., an obsolete t. for lactose or glucose in the urine; lead acetate is added to the suspected urine which is then filtered; ammonia is added until a permanent precipitate is formed; if lactose is present, the precipitate will take on a pink to red color when the fluid is heated; if there is glucose, the color will be yellow to brown.

Rumpel-Leede t., SYN capillary fragility t.

Sabin-Feldman dye t., a method for the detection of antitoxoplasma antibody in serum, based on the fact that *Toxoplasma gondii* cells (from peritoneal exudate in mice) are fairly well stained with alkaline methylene blue, whereas organisms in a serum that contains specific antibody have no affinity for the dye; furthermore, normal toxoplasma cells become rounded, and the nucleus and cytoplasm deeply stained, when treated with methylene blue; on the other hand, when dye is mixed with organisms and antibody, the cells retain their crescent shape and only the shrunken nuclear endosome is stained.

Sachs-Georgi t., the first precipitin t. for syphilis of diagnostic practicality, the significant innovation having been the addition of cholesterol to the lipoidal antigen (alcoholic tissue extract) used in the earlier Meinicke t.

Saundby t., a t. for blood in the stool; on the addition of 30 drops of a 20-volume hydrogen peroxide solution to a mixture of 10 drops of a saturated benzidine solution and a small quantity of feces in a test tube, a persistent dark blue color denotes the presence of blood.

scarification t., a t., e.g., Pirquet t., in which a material is pricked or scratched into the skin.

Schaffer t., a t. for nitrites in the urine; urine is decolorized with animal charcoal and then 4 ml of a 10% solution of acetic acid and 3 drops of a 5% solution of potassium ferrocyanide are added; if nitrites are present, an intense yellow color will be produced.

Schellong t., a t. for circulatory function; the subject is required to stand for 10–20 min, during which time the blood pressure is measured continuously; a fall of systolic pressure of 20 mm Hg or more indicates poor circulatory function.

Schick t., a t. for susceptibility to *Corynebacterium diphtheriae* toxin: 0.1 ml of Schick test toxin is injected into the skin of one forearm (test site) and the same quantity of the same, but heat-inactivated, material into the skin of the other forearm (control site); individuals with toxin-neutralizing antibodies either will have no reaction at either injection site (negative test) or may have a pseudoreaction due to antibodies for substances (antigens) in the test materials other than diphtheria toxin; individuals lacking toxin-neutralizing antibodies may have a positive reaction, which consists of an area of redness appearing 24–36 hours at the test site only and persisting for 4–5 days. SYN Schick method.

Schiller t., a t. for nonglycogen-containing areas of the portio vaginalis of the cervix, which may be the site of early carcinoma; such areas fail to stain dark brown with iodine solution; loss of glycogen due to erosion and other benign conditions may also give a positive result.

Schilling t., a procedure for determining the amount of vitamin B_{12} excreted in the urine using cyanocobalamin tagged with a radioisotope of cobalt.

Schirmer t., a t. for tear production using a strip of filter paper; a measurement of basal and reflex lacrimal gland function.

Schober t., a measure of lumbar spine motion in which parallel horizontal lines are drawn 10 cm above and 5 cm below the lumbosacral junction in the erect subject; with maximum forward flexion, the distance between the lines increases at least 5 cm in normal patients but far less in patients with anklylosing spondylitis.

Schönbein t., SYN Almén t. for blood.

Schwabach t., a series of five tuning forks of different tones is used and the number of seconds is noted in which the patient can hear each by air and bone conduction.

scratch t., a form of skin t. in which antigen is applied through a scratch in the skin.

screening t., any testing procedure designed to separate people or objects according to a fixed characteristic or property, with the intention of detecting early evidence of disease.

Seashore t., a t. in which the individual must discriminate between two sounds; or in which the sense of pitch, intensity, rhythm, and other components of innate musical ability can be measured. SEE Halstead-Reitan *battery*.

secondary dye t., localization of lacrimal drainage obstruction following the fluorescein instillation and primary dye tests by intubating the lower punctum and canaliculus and irrigating with saline. SYN Jones II t.

secretin t., a t. of pancreatic exocrine function, variably performed and standardized, in which the bicarbonate, amylase, and volume of the duodenal aspirate are measured after intravenous administration of secretin.

Selivanoff t., SYN resorcinol t.

shadow t., SYN retinoscopy.

shake t., SYN foam stability t.

sickle cell t., in an anaerobic wet preparation containing equal amounts of blood and 2% sodium bisulfite, erythrocytes containing hemoglobin S undergo a change in shape to a sickle cell form; the number of sickled red cells per 1000 red blood cells is determined and expressed as a percentage.

single (gel) diffusion precipitin t. in one dimension, SEE gel diffusion precipitin t.'s in one dimension.

single (gel) diffusion precipitin t. in two dimensions, SEE gel diffusion precipitin t.'s in two dimensions.

SISI t., abbreviation for small increment sensitivity index t.

situational t., in psychology and psychiatry, a t. situation in which a subject is observed as he or she performs a task or an actual sample of the job or role to be performed; e.g., a test used to select people for the Office of Strategic Services during the Second World War and for managerial positions today.

skin t., a method for determining induced sensitivity (allergy) by applying an antigen (allergen) to, or inoculating it into, the skin; induced sensitivity (allergy) to the specific antigen is indicated by an inflammatory reaction of one of two general kinds: 1) immediate, appears in minutes and is dependent upon circulating immunoglobulins (antibodies); 2) delayed, appears in 12–48 hours and is not dependent upon these soluble substances but upon cellular response and infiltration. SYN cutaneous t., intradermal t., skin reaction.

skin-puncture t., t. for Behçet syndrome; after pricking the skin with a sterile needle, pustulation follows within 24 hours, owing to the dermal sensitivity in this disease.

small increment sensitivity index t. (SISI t.), the sounding of a tone 20 dB above threshold, followed by a series of 200–msec tones 1 dB louder; perception of these is indicative of cochlear damage; the percentage of small increments detected by the subject is the small increment sensitivity index. In sensory hearing losses, it will be high, and in normal hearing and neural hearing losses, it will be low.

sniff t., at fluoroscopy, a t. for diaphragmatic function; paradoxic motion of a hemidiaphragm when a patient sniffs vigorously shows phrenic nerve paralysis or paresis of the hemidiaphragm.

Snyder t., a colorimetric t. for determining dental caries activity or susceptibility based on the rate of acid production by acidogenic oral microorganisms (e.g., lactobacillus) in a glucose medium, using bromcresol green as the indicator, and producing a color change from green to yellow. SYN colorimetric caries susceptibility t.

solubility t., a screening t. for sickle cell hemoglobin (Hb S), which is reduced by dithionite and is insoluble in concentrated inorganic buffer; addition of blood showing Hb S to buffer and dithionite causes opacity of the solution.

spironolactone t., administration of spironolactone (400 mg orally) for 4 consecutive days: an increase in serum potassium during the t. and a decrease afterward strongly suggest primary aldosteronism.

split renal function t., SYN differential ureteral catheterization t.

spot t. for infectious mononucleosis, a slide t. widely used for the diagnosis of infectious mononucleosis, based on the principle that the heterophil antibodies that occur in the serum of patients with infectious mononucleosis are absorbed by beef red cells but not by guinea pig kidney cells; thus, when horse red cells (which provoke heterophil antibodies) are mixed with patient serum and agglutination occurs in the presence of beef red cells, the presumptive diagnosis is infectious mononucleosis.

Spurling t., evaluation for cervical nerve root impingement in which the patient extends the neck and rotates and laterally bends the head toward the symptomatic side; an axial compression force is then applied by the examiner through the top of the patient's head; the t. is considered positive when the maneuver elicits the typical radicular arm pain.

staggered spondaic word t., a t. of central auditory pathway integrity in which spondaic words are presented dichotically.

standard serologic t.'s for syphilis, STS for syphilis, nontreponemal antigen t.'s giving presumptive but not conclusive evidence of syphilis, including the Wassermann and VDRL t.'s.

standing t., a t. for the effect of a hypotensive drug, carried out by the patient: after taking the drug, the patient stands perfectly still for 1 min commencing from the time that the maximal action of the drug should be manifested; if the dose is adequate, the patient should experience a slight hypotensive reaction.

standing plasma t., if plasma is stored at 4°C upright in a t. tube, chylomicrons will float to the top and form a creamy layer.

starch-iodine t., a t. for sweating in which iodine in oil is painted on the skin, followed by dusting with a starch powder which turns blue-black in the presence of iodine and moisture.

station t., SYN Romberg *sign*.

Stein t., in cases of labyrinthine disease the patient is unable to stand or to hop on one foot with eyes shut.

Stenger t., a test for detecting simulation of unilateral hearing impairment, in which a tone below the admitted threshold is presented to the test ear and a tone of lesser intensity is presented to the other ear. If the subject is feigning a hearing loss, the lesser tone cannot be appreciated.

Stewart t., estimation of the amount of collateral circulation, in case of an aneurysm of the main artery of a limb, by means of a calorimeter.

Strassburg t., an obsolete t. for bile in the urine; albumin, if present, is precipitated, then cane sugar is added and filter paper is dipped in the fluid and dried; if bile pigments are present in the urine, sulfuric acid will turn the filter paper a reddish violet.

stress t., any standardized procedure for assessing the effect of stress on cardiac function and myocardial perfusion; stress may be induced by physical exercise or simulated by administration of a coronary vasodilator; heart rate, blood pressure, and electrocardiogram are monitored before, during, and after the challenge; other observations sometimes made are measurement of oxygen consumption, echocardiography, impedance cardiography, appraisal of both myocardial perfusion and cardiac wall motion by radionuclide tracer, and cardiac catheterization.

Although neither as sensitive nor as specific as invasive procedures, exercise stress testing has become a standard means of identifying and grading coronary artery disease in people with typical and atypical angina pectoris as well as in those in certain critical occupations (airline pilots, firefighters). It has been found useful for risk stratification in survivors of myocardial infarction (MI) and in planning and monitoring rehabilitation after MI, coronary bypass surgery, or balloon angioplasty. It is also used to assess the safety of exercise programs for people at risk of coronary artery disease because of age or personal or family history. The Masters two-step test, based on repeated ascent and descent of a step-stool, has been superseded by more sophisticated and reproducible methods. Standard exercise testing employs graded physical exertion on an electrically driven treadmill with variable inclination and speed. Alternative methods include a mechanical stair-climbing machine, a stationary bicycle ergometer, and (for those with certain physical disabilities) an arm-exercising (hand-crank) machine. Various protocols and end points are used to measure the outcome of stress testing. Workloads are measured in metabolic equivalents (MET), 1 MET being the amount of oxygen consumed at bedrest (3.5 mL/kg/min). In maximal (symptom-limited) stress testing, the subject continues to exercise at increasing levels of challenge until chest distress, significant hypertension or hypotension, certain arrhythmias, fatigue, gait problems, or severe dyspnea occurs. The Bruce protocol, a standard maximal exercise treadmill protocol, begins with a treadmill speed of 1.7 mph and a grade of 10°, designed to achieve a workload of 4.6 MET, and increases both speed and grade every 3 min. In submaximal (pulse-limited) stress testing, the subject continues exercising until reaching a target heart rate based on age, health history, and physical condition (unless the test must be stopped earlier because of symptoms). A stress test session usually lasts 6–10 min. Elevation or depression of ST segments by more than 1 mm during exercise is strongly suggestive of coronary artery disease. Other suggestive changes are T-wave inversion, arrhythmia, a fall in systolic blood pressure, and a marked rise in diastolic blood pressure. Exercise stress-testing protocols achieve 85–90% accuracy in identifying people without coronary artery disease. About 5% of asymptomatic adults have positive stress tests, but only one-third of these have angiographically demonstrable coronary artery disease. False-positive tests occur more frequently in women. Exercise stress testing is contraindicated in acute myocardial infarction, severe congestive heart failure, severe hypertension, hemodynamically significant valvular disease or arrhythmia, active

thromboembolic disease, and extreme obesity. As an alternative to exercise, pharmacologic challenge by intravenous infusion of dipyridamole or dobutamine may be performed. In addition to continuous ECG monitoring, the cardiac effects of stress or pharmacologic challenge can be assessed by myocardial scintigraphy after intravenous injection of thallium-201; cineangiography after injection of technetium-99m, with or without multiple-gated acquisition (MUGA) bloodpool imaging; or single-photon emission computed tomography (SPECT).

string t., (1) an infrequently used t. to locate gastrointestinal hemorrhage; a weighted string is repeatedly swallowed and removed, each time allowing the string to go further down the intestine until blood is encountered; (2) a similar procedure to obtain a specimen from the bowel lumen.

Strong vocational interest t., a t. that matches an individual's specific likes, dislikes, and interests to those characteristic of persons working in each of a number of vocations.

Student's *t* t., a statistical significance t. for assessing the difference between, or the equality of, two or more population means.

Stypven time t., a t. measuring the clotting time of plasma after addition of Russell's viper *venom*, useful in evaluating patients with deficiencies in factor X. [Trade name *styp*tic + *venom*]

sucrose hemolysis t., isotonic sucrose promotes binding of complement to red blood cells; in paroxysmal nocturnal hemoglobinuria a proportion of the cells is sensitive to complement-mediated lysis, and hemolysis ensues.

sulcus t., a t. for multidirectional shoulder instability; the seated patient's humerus is pulled caudally, with inferior mobility indicating positive result.

sulfosalicylic acid turbidity t., a t. for measurement of protein in the urine; sulfosalicylic acid precipitates protein in the urine with a turbidity that is approximately proportional to the concentration of protein in a solution.

sweat t., a t. for cystic fibrosis of the pancreas in which electrolytes are measured in collected sweat; sodium chloride concentration above 50 mEq/L (children) or 60 mEq/L (adults) is positive.

sweating t., a t. for locating the level of a lesion in the spinal cord; when the body is heated or the patient is given a diaphoretic, sweat secretion is absent below the level of the lesion.

swinging light t., SYN alternating light t.

t **t.,** a t. that uses a statistic which under the null hypothesis has the *t* distribution, to test whether two means differ significantly.

Tactual Performance T., SYN Halstead-Reitan *battery*.

thematic apperception t. (TAT), a projective psychological t. in which the subject is asked to tell a story about standard ambiguous pictures depicting life situations to reveal his or her own attitudes and feelings.

thermostable opsonin t., a t. for opsonic activity of antibody in the absence of effect of heat-labile complement.

Thompson t., (1) t. to detect Achilles tendon disruption; with the patient kneeling on a chair or platform with the feet unsupported, each calf is squeezed; if the Achilles tendon is disrupted, plantar-flexion of the foot will not occur. (2) an obsolete t. for gonorrhea in urine; urine is passed into two glasses; if the gonococci and gonorrheal threads are found only in the first glass, the probability is that the process is limited to the anterior urethra. SYN two-glass t.

Thormählen t., a t. for melanin; the suspected liquid is treated with sodium nitroprusside, caustic potash, and acetic acid; if melanin is present, the solution takes on a deep blue color.

Thorn t., a putative t. of adrenal cortical function; stimulation of a normally functioning adrenal cortex by the adrenocorticotrophic hormone is followed by a reduction in the number of circulating eosinophils and lymphocytes and an increase in the excretion of uric acid. The t. lacks sufficient specificity and is rarely used.

three-glass t., the bladder is emptied by passing urine into a series of 3-ounce test tubes, and the contents of the first and the last are examined; the first tube contains the washings from the anterior urethra, the second, material from the bladder, and the last, material from the posterior urethra, prostate, and seminal vesicles. SYN Valentine t.

thymol turbidity t., precipitation of abnormal proportions of albumin and globulin from the serum of patients with liver disease by addition of thymol. Although popular in the past it has been superseded by quantitative determination of specific proteins and direct measurement of liver enzymes. SYN Maclagan t., Maclagan thymol turbidity t.

thyroid-stimulating hormone stimulation t., TSH-stimulating t., a t. that measures the uptake of ^{131}I in the thyroid gland before and after administration of thyroid-stimulating hormone; useful in distinguishing primary hyperthyroidism (increased TSH serum concentration) from secondary or tertiary hyperthyroidism (low TSH serum concentrations).

thyroid suppression t., a thyroid function t. used to diagnose difficult cases of hyperthyroidism, now largely replaced by the thyrotropin-releasing hormone stimulation t.; triiodothyronine is administered for a week to 10 days, and a reduction of its uptake by the thyroid gland to less than half of the initial uptake is a normal response. SYN Werner t.

thyrotropin-releasing hormone stimulation t., TRH-stimulation t., a t. of pituitary response to injection of thyrotropin-releasing hormone, which normally stimulates pituitary secretion of thyroid-stimulating hormone (TSH, thyrotropin), used primarily to distinguish pituitary from hypothalamic causes of thyroid disorders; TSH does not rise in cases of pituitary dysfunction, but does rise in cases of hypothalamic disorders.

tilt t., any measurement of response during tilting of the body, usually head up but also head down. The t. may be monitored by catheterization, echocardiography, electrophysiologic measurements, electrocardiography, or mechanocardiography.

tine t., SEE tuberculin t.

titratable acidity t., the number of milliliters of 0.1 N NaOH required to neutralize a 24-hr specimen of urine.

tolbutamide t., a t. to detect insulin-producing tumors; after a 1-g intravenous dose of tolbutamide, plasma insulin and glucose are measured at intervals up to 3 hr; higher insulin responses and lower glucose values characterize patients with such tumors.

tone decay t., the sounding of a continuous tone at threshold for 1 min; if the intensity must be increased by more than 5 dB for continued perception, it is indicative of a neural hearing loss.

total catecholamine t., a determination of catecholamines in 24-hour urine specimens; elevated values are seen in patients with pheochromocytoma and neuroblastoma.

tourniquet t., SEE capillary fragility t.

TPHA t., SYN *Treponema pallidum* hemagglutination t.

TPI t., SYN *Treponema pallidum* immobilization t.

Trendelenburg t., a t. of the valves of the leg veins; the leg is raised above the level of the heart until the veins are empty and is then rapidly lowered; in varicosity and incompetence of the valves the veins will at once become distended, but placement of a tourniquet around the leg will prevent distention of veins below the incompetent perforators or valves below the tourniquet.

Treponema pallidum hemagglutination t., a highly sensitive and specific t. for the serologic diagnosis of syphilis; tanned sheep red blood cells are coated with the antigen of *Treponema pallidum* and, following absorption of nonspecific patient serum antibody, a positive reaction with tanned sheep red blood cells and patient serum indicates the presence of specific antibody for *Treponema pallidum* in patient serum. SYN TPHA t.

Treponema pallidum immobilization t., TPH t., a t. for syphilis in which an antibody other than Wassermann antibody is present in the serum of a syphilitic patient, which in the presence of complement causes the immobilization of actively motile *Treponema pallidum* obtained from testes of a rabbit infected with syphilis. SYN TPI t., *Treponema pallidum* immobilization reaction.

triiodothyronine uptake t., a t. of thyroid function in which triiodothyronine (T_3) is added to a patient's serum in vitro to measure the relative affinities of serum proteins and of an added competitive substance for T_3; higher T_3 uptakes are associated with hyperthyroidism. SYN T_3 uptake t.

tuberculin t., application of the skin t. to the diagnosis of infection by *Mycobacterium tuberculosis* in which tuberculin or its

"purified" protein derivative serves as an antigen (allergen); injection of graduated doses of tuberculin or of purified protein derivative into the skin, most often by means of a needle and syringe (Mantoux t.) or by means of tines (tine t.); t. material may also be applied by means of a "patch" in which it is absorbed but this method (patch t.) is viewed as being less reliable; the t. is read on the basis of induration and erythema, the former being considered the more diagnostic of infection with the tubercle bacillus (*M. tuberculosis*); the t. does not distinguish between infection in a resistant person without disease and an individual with clinical manifestations of disease.

T₃ uptake t., SYN triiodothyronine uptake t.

two-glass t., SYN Thompson t.

two-step exercise t., a t. used mainly for coronary insufficiency; significant depression of RST in the electrocardiogram is considered abnormal and suggests coronary insufficiency.

two-tail t., a statistical t. based on the assumption that the data are distributed in both directions from some central value.

Tzanck t., the examination of fluid from a bullous lesion for Tzanck cells (altered epithelial cells, rounded and devoid of intercellular attachments). The periphery of these cells is basophilic and the nucleus is spherical and enlarged with prominent nucleoli; they are characteristic of lesions due to varicella, herpes zoster, herpes simplex, and pemphigus vulgaris.

urea clearance t., a t. of renal function based on urea clearance.

urease t., (1) a t. for urea based on the conversion of urea into ammonium carbonate by the enzyme urease; **(2)** a t. for the production of urease, used for identification of *cryptococci* and *Helicobacter pylori*.

urecholine supersensitivity t., urodynamic t. that tries to elicit an abnormal cystometrogram after subcutaneous injection of a drug, urecholine. Urecholine may increase detrusor pressure response during filling in patients with some types of neuropathic bladder.

urinary concentration t., a t. of renal tubular function whereby the patient is dehydrated for a measured period of time and the specific gravity of the urine is subsequently determined.

vaginal cornification t., a t. for estrogenic activity, in which the appearance of cornified epithelial cells in a vaginal smear of a test animal is an indication of the action of an estrogen.

vaginal mucification t., a t. for progestational activity; stimulation of mucus production by the vaginal epithelium in rats, guinea pigs, or mice by progestogens.

Valentine t., SYN three-glass t.

Valsalva t., the heart is monitored by ECG, pressure recording, or other methods while the patient performs the Valsalva maneuver; the heart becomes smaller in normal persons but may dilate in the patient with impaired myocardial reserve; there is a characteristic complex sequence of cardiocirculatory events, departure from which indicates disease or malfunction.

van Deen t., SYN Almén t. for blood.

van den Bergh t., a t. for bile pigments (bilirubin) by reaction with diazotized sulfanilic acid (diazo reaction).

van der Velden t., a t. for free hydrochloric acid, the presence of which turns an added solution of methylene blue from violet to green.

vanillylmandelic acid t., a t. for catecholamine-secreting tumors (pheochromocytoma and neuroblastoma) performed on a 24-hour urine specimen; it is based on the fact that vanillylmandelic acid is the major urinary metabolite of norepinephrine and epinephrine. SYN 3-methoxy-4-hydroxymandelic acid t., VMA t.

VDRL t., a flocculation t. for syphilis, using cardiolipin-lecithin-cholesterol antigen as developed by the Venereal Disease Research Laboratory of the United States Public Health Service.

vitality t., a group of thermal and electrical t.'s used to aid in assessment of dental pulp health. SYN pulp t.

vitamin C t., SYN capillary fragility t.

VMA t., SYN vanillylmandelic acid t.

Volhard t., a t. for renal function: the patient drinks 1500 ml of water on an empty stomach; if the patient was not dehydrated beforehand and the kidneys are normal, this fluid will be excreted by the end of 4 hours with specific gravity of the urine being from 1.001 to 1.004.

Vollmer t., a tuberculin patch t.

Wada t., unilateral internal carotid injection of amobarbital to determine the laterality of speech; injection on the dominant side causes transient aphasia or mutism; used prior to surgical treatment of epilepsy.

Waldenström t., a t. for porphobilinogen or urobilinogen in urine that uses Ehrlich's aldehyde reagent to produce a red color if either of the two substances is present in the urine.

Wang t., a quantitative t. for indican, which is transformed into indigo-sulfuric acid and then titrated by a solution of potassium permanganate.

washout t., a means of estimating renal obstruction by the rate of disappearance of excreted radioactive material from the kidney.

Wassermann t., a complement-fixation t. used in the diagnosis of syphilis; originally the "antigen" was an extract of liver from a syphilitic fetus, but later the active substance, referred to as cardiolipin, was found to be present in normal tissues, including heart, and has been identified as a diphosphatidylglycerol. SYN Wassermann reaction.

water-drinking t., a t. of the assessment of open-angle glaucoma, measuring intraocular pressure after drinking a quart of water in 5 min.

Watson-Schwartz t., a qualitative screening t. for diagnosis of acute intermittent porphyria by the addition of Ehrlich reagent and saturated sodium acetate to the urine; a pink or red color indicates the presence of porphobilinogen or urobilinogen; the former indicates porphyria, the latter does not; therefore, positive results require further differential extraction with butanol and chloroform to eliminate false-positive results due to urobilinogen.

Weber t. for hearing, the application of a vibrating tuning fork to one of several points in the midline of the head or face, to ascertain in which ear the sound is heard by bone conduction, that ear being the affected one if the sound-conducting mechanism of the middle ear is at fault, but the normal one if there is a sensorineural hearing loss in the other ear.

Webster t., a t. for trinitrotoluene in the urine.

Weil-Felix t., a t. for the presence and type of rickettsial disease based on the agglutination of X-strains of *Proteus vulgaris* with suspected rickettsia in a patient's blood serum. SYN Weil-Felix reaction.

Werner t., SYN thyroid suppression t.

Wheeler-Johnson t., cystosine or uracil when treated with bromine yields dialuric acid which gives a green color with excess of barium hydroxide.

whiff t., t. for the fishy odor detectable when KOH is applied to a sample of vaginal discharge in case of bacterial vaginosis.

Whitaker t., a pressure-perfusion t. in the upper urinary tract to demonstrate impediment of flow.

Wormley t., a t. for alkaloids, by treating the solution with picric acid or a dilute iodine-potassium-iodide solution, the presence of alkaloids being shown by a color reaction.

Wurster t., an obsolete t. for tyrosine; the substance is dissolved in boiling water and quinone is added; if tyrosine is present a ruby-colored reaction takes place, the solution changing to brown after a few hours.

χ^2 **t.,** SYN chi-square t.

xylose t., a laboratory aid in diagnosing alimentary or essential pentosuria, conditions in which xylose (a pentose) is excreted; the xylose may be identified by rapid reduction of Benedict solution, by nonfermentation by yeasts, or by a positive Bial t. for pentose.

Yvon t., (1) for alkaloids; to the suspected solution is added a mixture of bismuth subnitrate, potassium iodide, and hydrochloric acid in water; a positive reaction is indicated by the appearance of a red color; **(2)** for acetanilid in the urine; the suspected fluid is extracted with chloroform and heated with yellow nitrate of mercury; if acetanilid is present, the fluid will be green.

Zimmermann t., SYN Zimmermann *reaction.*

Zsigmondy t., SYN Lange t.

tes·ta (tes′tă). **1.** In protozoology, usually termed test; an envelope of certain forms of ameboid protozoa, consisting of various earthy

materials cemented to a chitinous base (as in the testate rhizopods of the subclass Testacealobosia) or the calcareous, siliceous, organic, or strontium sulfate skeletons in the rhizopod subclass Foraminifera. **2.** In botany, the outer, sometimes the only, coat of a seed. [L. shell]

Tes·ta·ce·a·lo·bo·sia (tes-tā′shē-ă-lō-bō′zē-ă). A subclass of the subphylum Sarcodina (amebae), in which the cells are provided with a firm chitinous envelope, often containing earthy material, with an opening through which the pseudopodia are protruded. [L. *testa,* shell]

tes·tal·gia (tes-tal′jē-ă). SYN orchialgia. [testis + G. *algos,* pain]

test·cross (test′kros). Crossing of an unknown genotype to a recessive homozygote so that the phenotype of the progeny corresponds directly to the chromosomes carried by the parents of unknown genotype. SYN backcross (2).

tes·tec·to·my (tes-tek′tō-mē). SYN orchiectomy. [testis + G. G. *ektomē,* excision]

tes·tes (tes′tēz). Plural of testis. [L.]

tes·ti·cle (tes′tĭ-kl). SYN testis. [L. *testiculus,* dim. of *testis*]

tes·tic·u·lar (tes-tik′ū-lăr). Relating to the testes.

tes·tic·u·lus (tes-tik′ū-lŭs). SYN testis. [L.]

test·ing. SEE test.

bench t., t. of a device against specifications in a simulated (nonliving) environment.

contrast sensitivity t., examination of the visual recognition of the variation in brightness of an object.

genetic t., laboratory studies of human blood or other tissue for the purpose of identifying genetic disorders. Relatively large chromosomal abnormalities such as deletion or transposition are identified by microscopic examination of chromosomes from a cell undergoing mitosis (karyotyping). More subtle aberrations can be detected by DNA probes (fabricated lengths of single-stranded DNA that match parts of the known gene). Genetic testing in the broadest sense includes biochemical testing for abnormal substances, or abnormally high or low concentrations of normal substances, that serve as markers of genetic deficiency or abnormality. SYN DNA diagnostics.

Genetic testing has become a standard procedure in a number of settings: screening for genetic diseases such as hemochromatosis, screening of couples planning to have children for the cystic fibrosis carrier state, and screening for genetic mutations known to increase the risk of certain cancers such as retinoblastoma and early-onset breast cancer. In addition, genetic profiling ("genetic fingerprinting") can establish or rule out identity of source for 2 specimens of human material, or parent-child relationship between 2 persons, with a probability of 99.9%. The availability of tests to diagnose or predict untreatable disorders such as Huntington chorea and to identify persons at increased risk of malignant disease has raised many social, psychological, therapeutic, and legal questions. Authorities recommend that people about to undergo genetic testing receive advance counseling about the implications of positive or negative test results. Lay persons often misunderstand the concept of predisposition or risk, particularly with respect to oncogenes. The majority of people who develop cancer do so because of spontaneous genetic mutation, not because of inherited risk; and of those who inherit the risk, not all develop cancer. The discovery that certain populations, such as Ashkenazic Jews, Mormons, and Amish, have a much higher incidence of certain genetic disorders has threatened to reactivate or reinforce ethnic, racial, and religious prejudices. Social groups most likely to harbor easily identified genetic mutations are by definition those whose gene pools are most distinct, because they have tended to intermarry rather than to mix with outside populations. The 1.3% of Ashkenazic Jews who share a mutation on the BRCA2 tumor suppressor gene may all be descendants of a single person (founder effect). The possibility of identifying a person's genetic predisposition to severe, chronic, or disabling diseases raises the possibility of discrimination by employers and by health, life, and disability insurers. State governments and the federal government have established rules that limit the access of employers and insurers, actual and potential, to a person's genetic profile, and that forbid stigmatization, job discrimination, and refusal to issue insurance or to insure at standard rates, because of genetic profile.

histocompatibility t., a t. system for HLA antigens, of major importance in transplantation.

proficiency t., a program in which specimens of quality control material are periodically sent to members of a group of laboratories for analysis, with each laboratory's results compared with those of its peers. SEE ALSO proficiency *samples*, under *sample*.

reality t., in psychiatry and psychology, the ego function by which the objective or real world and one's subjectively sensed relationship to it are evaluated and appreciated; the ability to distinguish internal from external events.

susceptibility t., the determination of the ability of an antibiotic to kill or inhibit the growth of bacteria.

tes·tis, pl. **tes·tes** (tes′tis, -tēz) [TA]. One of the two male reproductive glands, located in the cavity of the scrotum. SEE ALSO *appendix* testis. SYN didymus, genital gland (1), male gonad, orchis, testicle, testiculus. [L.]

abdominal t., an undescended t. that has never descended from the retroperineal/abdominal origin through the internal inguinal ring.

cryptorchid t., SYN undescended t.

ectopic t., a variant of undescended t. wherein testicular position is outside the usual pathway of descent. SEE ALSO testis *ectopia*.

movable t., SYN retractile t.

peeping t., an undescended t. that migrates back and forth at the internal inguinal ring.

retractile t., a condition in which there is a tendency of the t. to ascend to the upper part of the scrotum or into the inguinal canal, as contrasted with an undescended t. SYN movable t., pseudocryptorchism.

undescended t., a t. that has failed to descend into the scrotum; there are palpable and nonpalpable (impalpable) variants. SYN cryptorchid t.

tes·ti·tis (tes-tī′tis). SYN orchitis.

test let·ter. SEE test types.

tes·toid (tes′toyd). **1.** SYN androgenic. **2.** SYN androgen. [testis + G. *eidos,* resemblance]

tes·to·lac·tone (tes-tō-lak′tōn). An androgenic agent used as an antineoplastic agent for treatment of mammary carcinoma.

tes·tos·ter·one (tes-tos′tĕ-rōn). The most potent naturally occurring androgen, formed in greatest quantities by the interstitial cells of the testes, and possibly secreted also by the ovary and adrenal cortex; may be produced in nonglandular tissues from precursors such as androstenedione; used in the treatment of hypogonadism, cryptorchism, certain carcinomas, and menorrhagia.

t. cypionate, a preparation with the same actions and uses as t. propionate, but with a prolonged duration of action.

t. enanthate, a preparation with the same actions and uses as t., but with a prolonged duration of action, being administered in oil.

t. phenylpropionate, an alternate preparation for the propionate.

t. propionate, a preparation that has an action similar to but more pronounced and prolonged than that of t.; used in the treatment of undescended testes and in menorrhagia.

tes·to·tox·i·co·sis (tes′tō-toks-ē-kō′sis). A G protein mutation disease resulting in autonomous testosterone overproduction, with precocious puberty.

test sym·bols. SEE test types.

test types. Letters of various sizes used to test visual acuity.

Jaeger t. t., type of different sizes used for testing the acuity of near vision.

point system t. t., a near-vision test chart in which the various t. t. are multiples of a point (¹⁄₇₂ inch), lower-case letters being

one-half the designated point size; reading 4-point at 16 inches is normal, and is designated N-4.

Snellen t. t., square black symbols employed in testing the acuity of distant vision; the letters vary in size in such a way that each one subtends a visual angle of 5′ at a particular distance.

⚠**tetan-.** SEE tetano-.

te·tan·ic (te-tan′ik). Relating to or marked by a sustained muscular contraction, as in tetanus. [G. *tetanikos*]

te·tan·i·form (te-tan′i-fōrm). SYN tetanoid (1).

tet·a·nig·e·nous (tet-ă-nij′ĕ-nŭs). Causing tetanus or tetaniform spasms. [tetanus + G. *-gen,* producing]

tet·a·nism (tet′ă-nizm). SYN neonatal *tetany.*

tet·a·ni·za·tion (tet′ă-ni-zā′shŭn). **1.** The act of tetanizing the muscles. **2.** A condition of tetaniform spasm.

tet·a·nize (tet′ă-nīz). To stimulate a muscle by a rapid series of stimuli so that the individual muscular responses (contractions) are fused into a sustained contraction; to cause tetanus (2) in a muscle.

⚠**tetano-, tetan-.** Combining forms denoting tetanus, tetany. [G. *tetanos,* convulsive tension]

tet·a·noid (tet′ă-noyd). **1.** Resembling or of the nature of tetanus. SYN tetaniform. **2.** Resembling tetany. [tetano- + G. *eidos,* resemblance]

tet·a·no·ly·sin (tet-ă-nol′i-sin). A hemolytic principle, elaborated by *Clostridium tetani,* which seems to have no role in the etiology of tetanus.

tet·a·nom·e·ter (tet-ă-nom′ĕ-ter). An instrument for measuring the force of tonic muscular spasms. [tetano- + G. *metron,* measure]

tet·a·no·mo·tor (tet′ă-nō-mō′ter). An instrument by means of which tonic spasms are produced by the mechanical irritation of a hammer striking the motor nerve of the muscle affected. [tetano- + L. *motor,* a mover]

tet·a·no·spas·min (tet′ă-nō-spaz′min). The neurotoxin of *Clostridium tetani,* which causes the characteristic signs and symptoms of tetanus; chief action is on the anterior horn cells, and the spasms seem to be due to action at inhibitory synapses.

tet·a·no·toxin (tet′ă-nō-tok′sin). SYN tetanus *toxin.* [tetano- + G. *toxikon,* poison]

tet·a·nus (tet′ă-nŭs). **1.** A disease marked by painful tonic muscular contractions, caused by the neurotropic toxin (tetanospasmin) of *Clostridium tetani* acting upon the central nervous system. Cf. lockjaw, trismus. **2.** A sustained muscular contraction caused by a series of nerve stimuli repeated so rapidly that the individual muscular responses are fused, producing a sustained tetanic contraction. SEE emprosthotonos, opisthotonos. [L. fr. G. *tetanos,* convulsive tension]

acoustic t., experimental t. induced by a faradic current, the speed of which is estimated by the pitch of the vibrations.

cephalic t., a type of local tetanus that follows wounds to the face and head; after a brief incubation (1–2 days) the facial and ocular muscles become paretic yet undergo repeated tetanic spasms. The throat and tongue muscles may also be affected. SYN cerebral t.

cerebral t., SYN cephalic t.

complete t., t. in which stimuli to a particular muscle are repeated so rapidly that decrease of tension between stimuli cannot be detected.

drug t., tonic spasms caused by strychnine or other tetanic. SYN toxic t.

generalized t., the most common type of t., often with trismus as its initial manifestation; the muscles of the head, neck, trunk and limbs become persistently contracted, and then painful paroxysmal tonic contractions (tetanic seizures) are superimposed; the high mortality rate (50%) is due to asphyxia or cardiac failure.

incomplete t., t. (2) in which each stimulus causes a contraction to be initiated when the muscle has only partly relaxed from the previous contraction.

local t., the most benign type of t.; the muscles in close proximity to an infected wound develop persistent involuntary contractions, often with transient, intense superimposed spasms triggered by

te

various stimuli. The more distal upper extremity muscles are most often affected; gradual but complete recovery is typical.

neonatal t., SYN t. neonatorum.

t. neonatorum, t. occurring in newborn infants, usually due to infection of umbilical area with *Clostridium tetani*, often a result of ritualistic practices; has high fatality rate (about 60%). SYN neonatal t.

postpartum t., SYN puerperal t.

puerperal t., t. occurring during the puerperium from infection of the obstetric wound. SYN postpartum t., uterine t.

Ritter opening t., the tetanic contraction that occasionally occurs when a strong current, passing through a long stretch of nerve, is suddenly interrupted.

toxic t., SYN drug t.

traumatic t., t. following infection of a wound.

uterine t., SYN puerperal t.

tet·a·ny (tet′ă-nē). A clinical neurologic syndrome characterized by muscle twitches, cramps, and carpopedal spasm, and when severe, laryngospasm and seizures; these findings reflect irritability of the central and peripheral nervous systems, usually resulting from low serum levels of ionized calcium or, less commonly, magnesium. Causes include hyperventilation, hypoparathyroidism, rickets, and uremia. SYN intermittent cramp. [G. *tetanos,* tetanus]

t. of alkalosis, t. due to a loss of acid from the body or an increase in alkali, resulting in a reduction of ionized calcium in plasma and body fluids, e.g., hyperventilation t. (loss of CO_2), gastric t. (loss of HCl by vomiting), or injection or ingestion of excessive amounts of sodium bicarbonate.

gastric t., t. associated with a gastric disorder, especially with loss of HCl by vomiting.

hyperventilation t., t. caused by forced overbreathing, due to a reduction in CO_2 in the blood.

hypoparathyroid t., SYN parathyroid t.

infantile t., t. of infants occurring usually in association with rickets, due to dietary deficiency of vitamin D.

manifest t., t. from any cause in which neuromuscular hyperexcitability is clearly evident, as opposed to latent t. SYN symptomatic t.

neonatal t., hypocalcemic t. occurring in neonates or young infants, due to transient functional hypoparathyroidism in consumption of cow's milk (high phosphorus content). SYN myotonia neonatorum, tetanism.

parathyroid t., t. due to lack of parathyroid function, spontaneous or following excision of the parathyroid glands. SYN hypoparathyroid t., parathyroprival t.

parathyroprival t., SYN parathyroid t.

phosphate t., t. due to the ingestion of an excess of alkaline phosphates (Na_2HPO_4 or K_2HPO_4); most commonly produced experimentally in animals by the injection of alkaline phosphate, which reduces the ionized calcium of the blood.

postoperative t., parathyroid t. caused by injury to or excision of the parathyroids during procedures in the neck.

symptomatic t., SYN manifest t.

△**tetra-.** Four. [G. *tetra-,* four]

tet·ra·a·me·lia (tet′ră-ă-mē′lē-ă). Absence of upper and lower limbs. [tetra- + G. *a-* priv. + *melos,* limb]

tet·ra·ba·sic (tet-ră-bā′sik). Denoting an acid having four acid groups and thereby being able to neutralize 4 Eq of base.

tet·ra·ben·a·zine (tet′ră-ben′ă-zen). Formerly used as a tranquilizer; resembles reserpine in its actions but duration of effect is shorter.

tet·ra·bo·ric ac·id (tet′ră-bōr′ik). Perboric or pyroboric acid. SYN pyroboric acid.

tet·ra·bra·chi·us (tet′ră-brā′kē-ŭs). An individual with four arms. [tetra- + G. *brachiōn,* arm]

tet·ra·bro·mo·phe·nol·phthal·ein so·di·um (tet′ră-brō′mō-fē′nol-thal′ēn, -ē-in). The sodium salt of a brominated dye; it was used early in the development of cholecystography.

tet·ra·caine hy·dro·chlo·ride (tet′ră-kān). A highly potent local anesthetic used for spinal, nerve block, and topical anesthesia.

tet·ra·chi·rus (tet′ră-kī′rŭs). An individual with four hands. [tetra- + G. *cheir,* hand]

tet·ra·chlor·eth·y·lene (tet′ră-klōr-eth′i-lēn). An anthelmintic against hookworm and other nematodes. SYN carbon dichloride, ethylene tetrachloride, tetrachloroethylene.

tet·ra·chlor·me·thi·a·zide (tet′ră-klōr-me-thī′ă-zīd). A diuretic of the thiazide type. SYN teclothiazide.

tet·ra·chlo·ro·eth·ane (tet′ră-klōr-ō-eth′ān). Acetylene tetrachloride; a nonflammable solvent for fats, oils, waxes, resins, etc.; used in the manufacture of paint and varnish removers, photographic films, lacquers, and insecticides. Its toxicity exceeds that of chloroform and carbon tetrachloride, and produces narcosis, liver damage, kidney damage, and gastroenteritis. SYN cellon.

tet·ra·chlo·ro·eth·yl·ene (tet′ră-klōr-ō-eth′i-lēn). SYN tetrachlorethylene.

tet·ra·chlo·ro·meth·ane (tet′tră-klōr-ō-meth′ān). SYN *carbon tetrachloride.*

tet·ra·coc·cus, pl. **tet·ra·coc·ci** (tet′ră-kok′ŭs, -kok′sī). An old term describing a spherical bacterium that divides in two planes and characteristically forms groups of four cells. [tetra- + G. *kokkos,* berry]

tet·ra·co·sac·tide, tet·ra·co·sac·tin (tet′ră-kō-sak′tid, -tin). SYN cosyntropin.

n-**tet·ra·co·sa·no·ic ac·id** (tet′ră-kō-să-nō′ik). SYN lignoceric acid.

tet·ra·crot·ic (tet′ră-krot′ik). Denoting a pulse curve with four upstrokes in the cycle. [tetra- + G. *krotos,* a striking]

tet·ra·cus·pid (tet-ră-kŭs′pid). Having four cusps. SYN quadricuspid.

∎tet·ra·cy·cline (tet-ră-sī′klēn, -klin). A broad spectrum antibiotic (a naphthacene derivative), the parent of oxytetracycline, prepared from chlortetracycline and also obtained from the culture filtrate of several species of *Streptomyces;* also available as t. hydrochloride and t. phosphate complex. T. fluorescence has been used in studies of growing tumors and calcium deposition in developing bone and teeth.

tet·rad (tet′rod). **1.** A collection of four things having something in common such as a deformity with four features, e.g., Fallot tetralogy. SYN tetralogy. **2.** In chemistry, a quadrivalent element. **3.** In heredity, a bivalent chromosome that divides into four chromatids during meiosis. [G. *tetras (tetrad-),* the number four]

Fallot t., SYN *tetralogy* of Fallot.

narcoleptic t., the clinical syndrome of narcolepsy, cataplexy, sleep paralysis, and hypnagogic hallucinations.

tet·ra·dac·tyl (tet-ră-dak′til). Having only four fingers or toes on a hand or foot. SYN quadridigitate. [tetra- + G. *daktylos,* finger or toe]

tet·ra·dec·a·no·ic ac·id (tet′ră-dek-ă-nō′ik). SYN myristic acid.

12-*O*-tet·ra·dec·a·no·yl·phor·bol 13-ac·e·tate (TPA, tPA) (tet′ră-dek′ă-nō-il-fōr′bol). A double ester of phorbol found in croton oil; a cocarcinogen or tumor promoter.

te·trad·ic (te-trad′ik). Relating to a tetrad.

tet·ra·eth·yl·am·mo·ni·um chlo·ride (tet-ră-eth′il-ă-mō′nē-ŭm). A quaternary ammonium compound that partially blocks transmission of impulses through parasympathetic and sympathetic ganglia and is used in pharmacologic studies to block ganglionic transmission; its clinical usefulness is limited; formerly used as an antihypertensive drug.

tet·ra·eth·yl·lead (tet′ră-eth′i-led). An anti-knock compound added to motor fuel; has a toxic action causing anorexia, nausea, vomiting, diarrhea, tremors, muscular weakness, insomnia, irritability, nervousness, and anxiety; death may occur. SYN lead tetraethyl.

tet·ra·eth·yl·mon·o·thi·o·no·py·ro·phos·phate (tet-ră-eth′il-mon-ō-thī′ō-nō-pī-rō-fos′făt). An anticholinesterase agent used in the treatment of glaucoma by local instillation in the eye.

tet·ra·eth·yl py·ro·phos·phate (TEPP) (tet′ră-eth′il). An organic phosphoric compound used as an insecticide; a potent irreversible cholinesterase inhibitor.

tet·ra·eth·yl·thi·u·ram di·sul·fide (tet′ră-eth-il-thī′ū-ram). SYN disulfiram.

tet·ra·gast·rin (tet-ră-gas′trin). **1.** A tetrapeptide (Trp–Met–Asp–Phe–NH$_2$) used to test the secretion of digestive juice. **2.** A pterin derivative that is a required cofactor for a number of enzymes; e.g., in the conversion of L-phenylalanine to L-tyrosine; the inability to synthesize tetrahydrobiopterin is associated with forms of malignant hyperphenylalaninemia.

tet·ra·gly·cine hy·dro·per·i·o·dide (tet-ră-glī′sēn). Dissolves in water to the extent of 380 g/L; used for the emergency disinfection of drinking water in amounts to yield 8 ppm of active iodine.

tet·ra·gon, tet·ra·go·num (tet′ră-gon, tet′ră-gō′nŭm). Quadrangle; a figure having four sides. [tetra- + G. *gōnia*, angle]

t. lumba′le, a quadrangular space bounded laterally by the obliquus externus abdominis muscle, medially by the erector spinae, above by the serratus posterior inferior, and below by the internal abdominal oblique muscle.

tet·ra·go·nus (tet′ră-gō′nŭs). Obsolete term for platysma (*muscle*).

tet·ra·hy·dric (tet-ră-hī′drik). Denoting a compound containing four ionizable hydrogen atoms (four acid groups).

⌂**tetrahydro-.** Prefix denoting attachment of four hydrogen atoms; e.g., tetrahydrofolate (H$_4$folate).

tet·ra·hy·dro·can·nab·i·nol (THC) (tet′ră-hī′drō-kă-nab′i-nol). The Δ^1-3,4-*trans* isomer and the Δ^6-3,4-*trans* isomer are believed to be the active isomers present in *Cannabis*, having been isolated from marijuana. SEE ALSO cannabis, dronabinol.

5,6,7,8-tet·ra·hy·dro·fo·late de·hy·dro·gen·ase (tet′ră-hī-drō-fō′lāt). SYN dihydrofolate reductase.

tet·ra·hy·dro·fo·late meth·yl·trans·fer·ase (tet′ră-hī-drō-fōl′āt). SYN *methionine* synthase.

tet·ra·hy·dro·fo·lic ac·id (FH$_4$) (tet′ră-hī-drō-fōl′ik). The active coenzyme form of folic acid; participates in one-carbon metabolism. SYN coenzyme F.

tet·ra·hy·droz·o·line hy·dro·chlo·ride (tet-ră-hī-droz′ō-lēn). A sympathomimetic agent related to ephedrine, used as a topical nasal and conjunctival decongestant; chronic excessive use may convert an acute congestion into a chronic reactive hyperemia.

Tet·ra·hy·me·na pyr·i·for·mis (tet-ră-hī′mē-nă pir-i-fōr′mis). A ciliate belonging to a large group characterized by three membranes on one side of the buccal cavity and one on the other; it somewhat resembles the paramecium and, like it, is readily cultured and used extensively for experimental studies. [tetra- + G. *hymēn*, membrane]

tet·ra·i·o·do·phe·nol·phthal·ein so·di·um (tet′ră-ī-ō′dō-fē′nol-thal′ēn, -thal′ē-in). SYN iodophthalein.

te·tral·o·gy (te-tral′ō-jē). SYN tetrad (1). [G. *tetralogia*]

Eisenmenger t., SYN Eisenmenger *complex.*

t. of Fallot, a set of congenital cardiac defects including ventricular septal defect, pulmonic valve stenosis or infundibular stenosis, and dextroposition of the aorta so that it overrides the ventricular septum and receives venous as well as arterial blood. Right ventricular hypertrophy is considered part of the tetralogy although it is reactive to the other defects. SYN Fallot tetrad.

tet·ra·mas·tia (tet′ră-mas′tē-ă). Presence of four breasts on an individual. [tetra- + G. *mastos*, breast]

tet·ra·mas·ti·gote (tet-ră-mas′ti-gōt). A protozoan or other microorganism possessing four flagella. [tetra- + G. *mastix*, whip]

tet·ra·mas·tous (tet′ră-mas′tŭs). Having four breasts.

te·tram·e·lus (tĕ-tram′e-lŭs). Conjoined twins possessing four arms (tetrabrachius), or four legs (tetrascelus). SEE conjoined *twins,* under *twin.* [tetra- + G. *melos*, limb]

Tet·ra·me·res (tet-ram′e-rēz). A genus of stomach-infecting parasitic nematodes (family Spiruridae) of birds. When filled with eggs, the female worm is enormously enlarged and has a globular, blood-red appearance. Species include *T. americana,* found in the proventriculus of chickens (sometimes severely pathogenic in young chicks), turkeys, grouse, and quail, and transmitted by infected cockroaches and grasshoppers, and *T. fissispina,* found in the proventriculum of ducks, geese, wild waterfowl, pigeons, and doves but rarely in gallinaceous birds. [see tetrameric]

tet·ra·mer·ic, te·tram·er·ous (tet′ră-mer′ik, tĕ-tram′ĕ-rŭs).

Having four parts, or parts arranged in groups of four, or capable of existing in four forms. [tetra- + G. *meros,* part]

tet·ra·meth·yl·am·mo·ni·um io·dide (tet-ră-meth′il-ă-mō′nē-ŭm). Dissolves in water to the extent of 0.25 g/L; used for the emergency disinfection of drinking water.

tet·ra·meth·yl·di·ar·sine (tet′ră-meth′il-dī-ar′sēn). SYN cacodyl.

tet·ra·meth·yl·pu·tres·cine (tet-ră-meth′il-pū-tres′ēn). A derivative of putrescine, C$_8$H$_{20}$N$_2$, similar in its action to muscarine.

tet·ra·ni·trol (tet-ră-nī′trol). SYN erythrityl tetranitrate.

tet·ra·nu·cle·o·tide (tet-ră-noo′klē-ō-tīd). A compound of four nucleotides; once thought to represent the actual structure of nucleic acid (tetranucleotide theory).

tet·ra·ot·us (tet′ră-ō′tus). SYN tetrotus.

tet·ra·pa·re·sis (tet′ră-pă-rē′sis). Weakness of all four extremities. SYN quadriparesis.

tet·ra·pep·tide (tet′ră-pep′tīd). A compound of four amino acids in peptide linkage.

tet·ra·pe·ro·me·lia (tet′ră-pē-rō-mē′lē-ă). Peromelia involving all four extremities. [tetra- + G. *peros,* maimed, + *melos,* limb]

tet·ra·pho·co·me·lia (tet′ră-fō-kō-mē′lē-ă). Phocomelia involving all four limbs.

tet·ra·ple·gia (tet′ră-plē′jē-ă). SYN quadriplegia. [tetra- + G. *plēgē,* stroke]

tet·ra·ple·gic (tet′ră-plē′jik). SYN quadriplegic.

tet·ra·ploid (tet′ră-ployd). SEE polyploidy. [G. *tetraploos,* fourfold, + *eidos,* form]

tet·ra·pus (tet′ră-pŭs). A malformed individual with four feet. [G. *tetrapous,* fr. tetra- + *pous,* foot]

tet·ra·pyr·role (tet′ră-pir′ol). A molecule containing four pyrrole nuclei; e.g., porphyrin.

tet·ra·sac·cha·ride (tet′ră-sak′ă-rīd). A sugar containing four molecules of a monosaccharide; e.g., stachyose.

te·tras·ce·lus (te-tras′e-lŭs). A malformed individual with four legs. [tetra- + G. *skelos,* leg]

tet·ra·so·mic (tet′ră-sō′mik). Relating to a cell nucleus in which one chromosome is represented four times while all others are present in the normal number. [tetra- + chromosome]

tet·ras·ter (tet-ras′ter). A figure exceptionally and abnormally occurring in mitosis, in which there are four asters. [tetra- +G. *astēr,* star]

tet·ra·sti·chi·a·sis (tet′ră-sti-kī′ă-sis). Duplication of the growth of the eyelashes (in four rows). [tetra- + G. *stichos,* row]

tet·ra·ter·penes (tet′ră-ter′pēnz). Hydrocarbons or their derivatives formed by the condensation of eight isoprene units (i.e., four terpenes) and therefore containing 40 carbon atoms; e.g., various carotenoids.

tet·ra·tom·ic (tet′ră-tom′ik). Denoting a quadrivalent element or radical. [tetra- + G. *atomos,* atom]

Tet·ra·trich·o·mo·nas (tet′ră-tri-kom′ŏ-nas). A genus of parasitic protozoan flagellates, formerly part of the genus *Trichomonas* but now separated into a distinct genus by the presence of four anterior and one trailing flagella, a pelta, and a disc-shaped parabasal body. SEE *Trichomonas.* [tetra- + *Trichomonas*]

T. o′vis, a species that occurs in the cecum or rumen of domestic sheep.

tet·ra·va·lent (tet′ră-vā′lent). SYN quadrivalent. [tetra- + L. *valentia,* strength]

tet·ra·zole (tet′ră-zōl). The compound CN$_4$H$_2$ with the structure of tetrazolium.

tet·ra·zo·li·um (tet′ră-zō′lē-ŭm). Any of a group of organic salts having the general structure that on reduction (cleaving the 2,3 bond) yields a colored insoluble formazan; used as a reagent in oxidative enzyme histochemistry.

nitroblue t. (NBT), a pale yellow dye that is converted on reduction to colored formazans in the histochemical demonstration of dehydrogenases; used in hematology for staining of neutrophils to help indicate the presence of bacterial infections.

tet·ro·do·tox·in (TTX) (tet′rō-dō-tok′sin). A potent neurotoxin found in the liver and ovaries of the Japanese pufferfish, *Sphoeroides rubripes,* other species of pufferfish, and certain newts;

te

produces axonal blocks of the preganglionic cholinergic fibers and the somatic motor nerves. T. blocks voltage-gated Na^+ channels in excitable tissues.

tet·rose (tet′rōs). A monosaccharide containing only four carbon atoms in the main chain; e.g., erythrose, threose, erythrulose.

te·tro·tus (te-trō′tŭs). A malformed individual with four ears, four eyes, two faces, and two almost separate heads. SYN tetraotus. [tetra- + G. *ous* (*ōt-*), ear]

te·trox·ide (te-trok′sīd). An oxide containing four oxygen atoms; e.g., OsO_4.

tet·ter (tet′er). An outmoded colloquial term, popularly applied to ringworm and eczema, and occasionally applied to other eruptions. [A.S. *teter*]

Teutleben, F.E.K. von, German anatomist, 1842–?. SEE T. *ligament*.

tex·ti·form (teks′tĭ-fōrm). Weblike. [L. *textum,* something woven]

tex·tur·al (teks′chŭr-ăl). Relating to the texture of the tissues.

tex·ture (teks′choor). The composition or structure of a tissue or organ. [L. *textura,* fr. *texo,* pp. *textus,* to weave]

tex·tus (teks′tŭs). A tissue. [L.]

TGC Abbreviation for time-varied gain *control;* time-gain *compensation.*

TGF Abbreviation for transforming growth *factors,* under *factor.*

TGFα Abbreviation for transforming growth *factor* α.

TGFβ Abbreviation for transforming growth *factor* β.

Th 1. Abbreviation for T helper *cells,* under *cell.* **2.** Symbol for thorium.

Thal, Alan P., U.S. surgeon, *1925. SEE T. *procedure.*

△**thalam-.** SEE thalamo-.

thal·a·mec·to·my (thal-ă-mek′tō-mē). SEE chemothalamectomy. [thalamus + G. *ektomē,* excision]

thal·a·men·ce·phal·ic (thal′ă-men-se-fal′ik). Relating to the thalamencephalon.

thal·a·men·ceph·a·lon (thal′ă-men-sef′ă-lon). That part of the diencephalon comprising the thalamus and its associated structures. [thalamus + G. *enkephalos,* brain]

tha·lam·ic (tha-lam′ik). Relating to the thalamus.

△**thalamo-, thalam-.** The thalamus. [G. *thalamos,* bedroom (thalamus)]

thal·a·mo·cor·ti·cal (thal′ă-mō-kōr′ti-kăl). Relating to the efferent connections of the thalamus with the cerebral cortex.

thal·a·mo·len·tic·u·lar (thal′ă-mō-len-tik′oo-lăr). Relating to the thalamus, usually the dorsal thalamus, and the lenticular nucleus (putamen and globus pallidus).

thal·a·mot·o·my (thal-ă-mot′ō-mē). Destruction of a selected portion of the thalamus by stereotaxy for the relief of pain, involuntary movements, epilepsy, and, rarely, emotional disturbances; produces few, if any, neurologic deficits or undesirable personality changes. [thalamus + G. *tomē,* incision]

thal·a·mus, pl. **thal·a·mi** (thal′ă-mŭs, -mī) [TA]. The large, ovoid mass of gray matter that forms the larger dorsal subdivision of the diencephalon; it is placed medial to the internal capsule and the body and tail of the caudate nucleus. Its medial aspect forms the dorsal half of the lateral wall of the third ventricle; its dorsal surface can be subdivided into a lateral triangle forming the floor of the body (central part) of the lateral ventricle, and a medial triangle covered by the velum interpositum; its tail-like caudal part curves ventralward around the posterolateral aspect of the cerebral peduncle and ends in the lateral geniculate body. The t. is composed of a large number of anatomically and functionally distinct cell groups or nuclei, usually classified as 1) sensory relay nuclei (ventral posterior nucleus, lateral and medial geniculate body) each receiving a modally specific sensory conduction system and in turn projecting each to the corresponding primary sensory area of the cortex; 2) "secondary" relay nuclei (ventral intermediate nucleus and ventral anterior nucleus) receiving fibers from the medial segment of the globus pallidus, the contralateral deep cerebellar nuclei (i.e., cerebellothalamic fibers), and the pars reticulata of the substantia nigra which project to various regions

of the motor cortex; 3) a nucleus associated with the limbic system: the composite anterior nucleus receiving the mamillothalamic tract and projecting to the fornicate gyrus; 4) association nuclei (medial dorsal nucleus, lateral nucleus including the large pulvinar) each projecting to a particular large expanse of association cortex; 5) the midline and intralaminar nuclei or "nonspecific" nuclei (centromedian nucleus, central lateral nucleus, paracentral nucleus, nucleus reuniens). SEE ALSO dorsal t. [G. *thalamos,* a bed, a bedroom]

dorsal t., the large part of the diencephalon located dorsal to the hypothalamus and excluding the subthalamus and the medial and lateral geniculate bodies (sometime the latter two are collectively called the metathalamus); the dorsal t. includes the major motor and somatosensory relay nuclei, nuclei that project to association areas, and the intralaminar nuclei. SEE ALSO thalamus.

ventral t., SYN subthalamus.

🔲 **thal·as·se·mia, thal·as·sa·ne·mia** (thal-ă-sē′mē-ă, thă-las-ă-nē′mē-ă). Any of a group of inherited disorders of hemoglobin metabolism in which there is impaired synthesis of one or more of the polypeptide chains of globin; several genetic types exist, and the corresponding clinical picture may vary from barely detectable hematologic abnormality to severe and fatal anemia. [G. *thalassa,* the sea, + *haima,* blood]

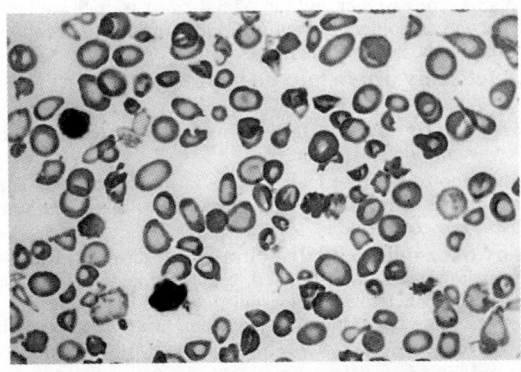

thalassemia: a blood film from a patient with homozygous β-thalassemia showing hypochromia, anisocytosis, and poikilocytosis (original magnification 250 x; Wright-Giemsa stain)

α **t.,** t. due to one of two or more genes that depress (severely or moderately) synthesis of α-globin chains by the chromosome with the abnormal gene. Heterozygous state: severe type, t. minor with 5–15% of Hb Barts at birth, only traces of Hb Barts in adult; mild type, 1–2% of Hb Barts at birth, not detectable in adult. Homozygous state: severe type, erythroblastosis fetalis and fetal death, only Hb Barts and Hb H present; mild type not clinically defined. SEE ALSO *hemoglobin* H.

A_2 **t.,** β **t.,** heterozygous state.

β **t.,** t. due to one of two or more genes that depress (partially or completely) synthesis of β-globin chains by the chromosome bearing the abnormal gene. Heterozygous state (A_2 t.): t. minor with Hb A_2 increased, Hb F normal or variably increased, Hb A normal or slightly reduced. Homozygous state: t. major with Hb A reduced to very low but variable levels, Hb F very high level.

β-δ **t.,** t. due to a gene that depresses synthesis of both β- and δ-globin chains by the chromosome bearing the abnormal gene. Heterozygous state: t. minor with Hb F comprising 5–30% of total hemoglobin but distributed unevenly among cells, Hb A_2 reduced or normal. Homozygous state: moderate anemia with only Hb F present, no Hb A or Hb A_2. SYN F t.

F t., SYN β-δ t.

t. interme′dia, a clinical variant of t. characterized by an intermediate degree of severity. These patients have severe anemia but usually do not require regular blood transfusions. Intermedia disorders represent a heterogeneous group of genetic disorders and may include cases with homozygous or heterozygous abnormalities in the β-globin chain gene.

α **t. interme′dia,** SEE *hemoglobin* H.

Lepore t. [MIM*142000.0020 and others], t. syndrome due to production of abnormally structured Lepore hemoglobin. Heterozygous state: t. minor with about 10% of Hb Lepore, Hb F moderately increased, Hb A$_2$ normal. Homozygous state: t. major with only Hb F and Hb Lepore produced, no Hb A or Hb A$_2$.

t. ma′jor [MIM*141800–142310 passim], the syndrome of severe anemia resulting from the homozygous state of one of the t. genes or one of the hemoglobin Lepore genes with onset, in infancy or childhood, of pallor, icterus, weakness, splenomegaly, cardiac enlargement, thinning of inner and outer tables of skull, microcytic hypochromic anemia with poikilocytosis, anisocytosis, stippled cells, target cells, and nucleated erythrocytes; types of hemoglobin are variable and depend on the gene involved. SYN Cooley anemia, primary erythroblastic anemia.

t. mi′nor [MIM*141800–142310 passim], the heterozygous state of a t. gene or a hemoglobin Lepore gene; usually asymptomatic and quite variable hematologically, with target cells, mild hypochromic microcytosis, and often slightly reduced hemoglobin level with slightly increased erythrocyte count; types of hemoglobin are variable and depend on the gene involved.

tha·las·so·pho·bia (thal′ă-sō-fō′bē-ă, thă-las′ō-). Morbid fear of the sea. [G. *thalassa,* the sea, + *phobos,* fear]

tha·las·so·po·sia (thal′ă-sō-pō′zē-ă, thă-las′ō-). SYN mariposia. [G. *thalassa,* the sea, + *posis,* drinking]

tha·las·so·ther·a·py (thal′ă-sō-ther′ă-pē). Treatment of disease by exposure to sea air, by sea bathing, or by a sea voyage. [G. *thalassa,* the sea]

tha·lid·o·mide (thă-lid′ō-mīd). A hypnotic drug which, if taken in early pregnancy, may cause the birth of infants with phocomelia and other defects; under investigational use for treatment of leprosy and as an immunomodulator in HIV infections and graft vs. host reactions.

thal·lic (thal′lik). Denoting conidia produced with no enlargement or growth after delimitation by septa in the hypha (thallus); the entire parent cell becomes an arthroconidium.

thal·li·um (Tl) (thal′ē-ŭm). A white metallic element, atomic no. 81, atomic wt. 204.3833; ^{201}Tl (half-life equal to 3.038 days) is used to scan the myocardium. [G. *thallos,* a green shoot (it gives a green line in the spectrum)]

t.-201 (^{201}Tl), the radioisotope of t. used widely for myocardial nuclear imaging; it is also taken up by certain tumors.

Thal·lo·phy·ta (thă-lof′i-tă). In older classification systems, a primary division of the plant kingdom whose members, with a few exceptions, were devoid of true roots, stems, and leaves; it included bacteria, fungi, and algae. [G. *thallos,* a green shoot, + *phyton,* plant]

thal·lo·phyte (thal′ō-fīt). A member of the division Thallophyta.

thal·lo·tox·i·co·sis (thal′ō-tok-si-kō′sis). Poisoning by thallium; marked by stomatitis, gastroenteritis, peripheral and retrobulbar neuritis, endocrine disorders, and alopecia. [thallium + G. *toxikon,* poison, + *-osis,* condition]

thal·lus (thal′ŭs). A simple plant or fungus body that is devoid of roots, stems, and leaves. The vegetative growth of a fungus. [G. *thallos,* a young shoot]

△**thanato-.** Death. SEE ALSO necro-. [G. *thanatos,* death]

than·a·to·bi·o·log·ic (than′ă-tō-bī-ō-loj′ik). Relating to the processes involved in life and death. [thanato- + G. *bios,* life, + *logos,* study]

than·a·to·gno·mon·ic (than′ă-tō-nō-mon′ik). Of fatal prognosis, indicating the approach of death. [thanato- + G. *gnōmē,* a sign]

than·a·tog·ra·phy (than-ă-tog′ră-fē). **1.** A description of one's symptoms and thoughts while dying. **2.** A treatise on death. [thanato- + G. *graphē,* a writing]

than·a·toid (than′ă-toyd). **1.** Resembling death. **2.** Deadly. [thanato- + G. *eidos,* resemblance]

than·a·tol·o·gy (than-ă-tol′ō-jē). The branch of science concerned with the study of death and dying. [thanato- + G. *logos,* study]

than·a·to·ma·nia (than′ă-tō-mā′nē-ă). Illness or death resulting from belief in the efficacy of magic; a phenomenon observed among those primitive societies or illiterate and superstitious peo-

ple who believe in the power of evil spirits, spells, curses, and individuals over one's bodily processes, with such belief and resulting fear manifesting itself as psychosomatic illness and even death. [thanato- + G. *mania,* frenzy]

than·a·to·phid·ia (than′ă-tō-fid′ē-ă). Venomous snakes. [thanato- + G. *ophidion,* dim. of *ophis,* a serpent]

than·a·to·pho·bia (than′ă-tō-fō′bē-ă). Morbid fear of death. [thanato- + G. *phobos,* fear]

than·a·to·phor·ic (than′ă-tō-fōr′ik). Leading to death. [thanato- + G. *phoros,* bearing]

than·a·tos (than′ă-tos). In psychoanalysis, the death principle, representing all instinctual tendencies toward senescence and death. See also entries under instinct. Cf. eros. [G. death]

Thane, Sir George D., English anatomist, 1850–1930. SEE T. *method.*

thau·mat·ro·py (thaw-mat′rō-pē). The transformation of one form of tissue into another. [G. *thauma (thaumat-),* a wonder, + *tropē,* a turning]

Thayer, James D. SEE T.-Martin *medium, agar.*

THC Abbreviation for tetrahydrocannabinol.

Thd Symbol for ribothymidine.

thea (thē-ă). SYN tea. [Mod. L.]

the·a·ism (thē′ă-izm). SYN theinism.

the·a·ter (thē′ă-ter). **1.** A large room for lectures and demonstrations; sometimes applied to an operating room equipped for observation by persons other than the surgical team. **2.** Any operating room or suite of such rooms. [G. *theatron,* a place for seeing, theater, fr. *theomai,* to look at]

the·ba·ic (thē-bā′ik). Relating to or derived from opium. [L. *Thebaicus,* relating to Thebes, whence opium was formerly obtained]

the·ba·ine (thē-bā′ēn, -in). An alkaloid obtained from opium (0.3–1.5%); it resembles strychnine in its action, causing tetanic convulsions. SYN paramorphine.

Thebesius, Adam C., German physician, 1686–1732. SEE thebesian *foramina,* under *foramen,* thebesian *valve,* thebesian *veins,* under *vein.*

the·ca, pl. **the·cae** (thē′kă, thē′sē). A sheath or capsule. [G. *thēkē,* a box]

t. cor′dis, SYN pericardium.

t. exter′na, SYN *tunica* externa thecae folliculi.

t. follic′uli, the wall of a vesicular ovarian follicle. SEE ALSO *tunica* externa, *tunica* interna thecae folliculi.

t. inter′na, SYN *tunica* interna thecae folliculi.

t. ten′dinis, SYN synovial tendon *sheath.*

t. vertebra′lis, SYN spinal *dura mater.*

the·cal (thē′kăl). Relating to a sheath, especially a tendon sheath. [see theca]

thec·o·dont (thē′kō-dont). Having the teeth inserted in alveoli. [G. *thēkē,* box, + *odous (odont-),* tooth]

the·co·ma (thē-kō′mă). A neoplasm derived from ovarian mesenchyme, consisting chiefly of spindle-shaped cells that frequently contain small droplets of fat; gross features generally resemble those of a granulosa cell tumor, i.e., firm, yellow, encapsulated mass, ordinarily about 10 cm or less in diameter, but it tends to be less malignant; it may form considerable quantities of estrogens, thereby resulting in precocious development of secondary sexual features in prepubertal girls, or hyperplasia of the endometrium in older patients. SYN theca cell tumor. [G. *thēkē,* box (theca), + *-oma,* tumor]

the·co·ma·to·sis (thē′kō-mă-tō′sis). A stromal hyperplasia or increase in the number of connective tissue elements of an ovary.

Theden, Johann C.A., German surgeon, 1714–1797. SEE T. *method.*

Theile, Friedrich W., German anatomist, 1801–1879. SEE T. *canal, glands,* under *gland, muscle.*

Theiler, Max, South African microbiologist in the U.S. and Nobel laureate, 1899–1972. SEE T. *virus.*

Thei·le·ri·i·dae (thī-lē′rē-i-dē). A family of sporozoan protozoa which, combined with the family Babesiidae, comprises the order

Th

Piroplasmida; it consists of one recognized genus, *Theileria*, transmitted by ixodid ticks.

the·in (thē'in, tē'in). SYN caffeine.

the·in·ism, the·ism (thē'i-nizm; thē'izm, tē'-). Chronic poisoning resulting from immoderate tea-drinking, marked by palpitation, insomnia, nervousness, headache, and dyspepsia. SYN theaism. [Mod. L. *thea,* tea]

thel-. SEE thelo-.

the·lar·che (thē-lar'kē). The beginning of development of the breasts in the female. [thel- + G. *archē,* beginning]

The·la·zia (thē-lā'zē-ă). The eye worms, a genus of spiruroid nematodes that inhabit the lacrimal ducts and surface of the eyes of various domestic and wild animals, but rarely humans; a number of species have been reported from wild birds. Cyclic development occurs in muscoid flies; infective larvae emerge from the fly mouthparts while the fly is feeding on or near the eyes of the host. [G. *thelazō,* to suck]

T. californien'sis, a nematode species occurring in the tear ducts, conjunctival sac, or under the nictitating membrane of dogs, coyotes, black bears, sheep, deer, jack rabbits, cats and, occasionally, humans in the western and southwestern U.S.; heavy infections cause photophobia, lacrimation, eyelid edema, conjunctivitis, and even blindness.

T. callipae'da, a species reported from humans in Southeast Asia and California; the worm, embedded in a subconjunctival tumor or swimming in the aqueous humor after penetrating the corneoscleral limbus, causes pain, photophobia, and tearing.

thel·a·zi·a·sis (thē-lă-zī'ă-sis, thel-ă-). Infection with nematodes of the genus *Thelazia.*

the·le (thē'lē). SYN nipple. [G.]

the·li·um, pl. **the·lia** (thē'lē-ŭm, -lē-ă). **1.** A nipplelike structure. **2.** A cellular layer. **3.** SYN nipple. [Mod. L., fr. G. *thēlē,* nipple]

thelo-, thel-. The nipples. Cf. mamil-. [G. *thēlē*]

the·lor·rha·gia (thē-lō-rā'jē-ă). Bleeding from the nipple. [thelo- + G. *rhēgnymi,* to burst forth]

the·nad (thē'nad). Toward the thenar or lateral side of the palm of the hand. [G. *thenar,* the palm of the hand, + L. *ad,* to]

the·nal (thē'năl). SYN thenar.

the·nal·dine (thē-nal'dēn). An antihistaminic and antipruritic agent (as the tartrate).

the·nar (thē'nar) [TA]. Term applied to any structure in relation with the base of the thumb or its underlying collective components. SYN thenal. SEE thenar *eminence.* [G. the palm of the hand]

the·nen (thē'nen). Relating only to the palm, specifically to the radial side. [G. *thenar,* palm, + *en, in*]

then·yl (then'il). The radical of 2-methylthiophene, (SC₄H₃)CH₂—. Cf. thienyl.

then·yl·di·a·mine hy·dro·chlo·ride (then-il-dī'ă-mēn). An antihistaminic.

Theobald Smith, SEE Smith.

the·o·bro·ma (thē-ō-brō'mă). SYN cacao. [G. *theos,* a god, + *brōma,* food]

t. oil, the fat obtained from the wasted seed of *Theobroma cacao* (family Sterculiaceae); it contains the glycerides of stearic, palmitic, oleic, arichidic, and linoleic acids; used as a base for suppositories and ointments and, in operative dentistry, as a lubricant and protective. SYN cacao butter, cocoa butter, cacao oil.

the·o·bro·mine (thē-ō-brō'mēn). An alkaloid resembling caffeine and theophylline in its action and chemical structure, prepared from the dried ripe seed of *Theobroma cacao* or made synthetically; formerly used widely as a diuretic, myocardial stimulant, dilator of coronary arteries, and smooth muscle relaxant. Compounds with calcium gluconate, calcium salicylate, sodium acetate, sodium lactate, and sodium salicylate have been listed.

the·o·ma·nia (thē-ō-mā'nē-ă). A delusion in which one believes that he or she is God. [G. *theos,* god, + *mania,* frenzy]

the·o·pho·bia (thē-ō-fō'bē-ă). Morbid fear of God. [G. *theos,* god, + *phobos,* fear]

the·o·phyl·line (thē-of'i-lēn, -lin). An alkaloid found with caffeine in tea leaves (commercial t. is prepared synthetically); a

smooth muscle relaxant, diuretic, cardiac stimulant, and vasodilator; used in bronchial asthma and other forms of chronic obstructive pulmonary disease as a bronchodilator and respiratory muscle stimulant. Also, thought to increase respiratory drive, so sometimes used in hypoventilation syndromes. Shares chemical and pharmacologic properties with caffeine and theobromine.

t. ethylenediamine, SYN aminophylline.

t. sodium glycinate, equilibrium mixture containing t. sodium and glycine in approximately molecular proportions, buffered with an additional mole of glycine; similar in action and uses to aminophylline but more stable in air, and less irritating to the gastric mucosa.

the·o·rem (thē'ō-rem). A proposition that can be tested, and can be established as a law or principle. SEE ALSO law, principle, rule.

Bayes t., the impacts of new data on the evidential merits of competing scientific hypotheses are compared by computing for each the product of the antecedent plausibility (the prior probability) and the likelihood of the current data given that hypothesis (the conditional probability) and rescaling them so that their total is unity (the rescaled values being posterior probabilities). SEE ALSO diagnostic *sensitivity,* diagnostic *specificity,* predictive *value.*

Bernoulli t., SYN Bernoulli *law.*

central limit t., the sum (or average) of *n* realizations of the same process, provided only that it has a finite variance, will approach the gaussian distribution as *n* becomes indefinitely large. This theory provides a broad warrant for the use of normal theory even for nongaussian data. In the form stated here, it constitutes the classical version; more general versions allow serious relaxation of the usual assumptions.

Gibbs t., substances that lower the surface tension of the pure dispersion medium tend to collect in its surface, whereas substances that raise the surface tension tend to remain out of the surface film.

THEORY

---

the·o·ry (thē'ōr-ē). A reasoned explanation of known facts or phenomena that serves as a basis of investigation by which to seek the truth. SEE ALSO hypothesis, postulate. [G. *theōria,* a beholding, speculation, theory, fr. *theōros,* a beholder]

adsorption t. of narcosis, that a drug becomes concentrated at the surface of the cell as a result of adsorption, and thus alters permeability and metabolism.

aerodynamic t., generally accepted t. that the vibration of the vocal folds in phonation is produced by the flow of exhaled air past lightly approximated vocal folds; opposed to the now untenable concept that vocal fold motion in phonation results from contraction of the intrinsic muscles of the larynx at the frequency of the vocal fold vibration.

Altmann t., a t. that protoplasm consists of granular particles (called bioblasts) that are clustered and enclosed in indifferent matter.

Arrhenius-Madsen t., that the reaction of an antigen with its antibody is a reversible reaction, the equilibrium being determined according to the law of mass action by the concentrations of the reacting substances.

atomic t., that chemical compounds are formed by the union of atoms in certain definite proportions; in its modern form, first advanced in 1803 by John Dalton.

Baeyer t., that carbon bonds are set at fixed angles (109° 28') and that those carbon rings are most stable that least distort those angles; for this reason, planar rings composed of 5 or 6 carbon atoms (e.g., cyclopentane, benzene) are more common than rings containing less than 5 or more than 6 carbon atoms.

balance t., in social psychology, a t. that assumes that steady and unsteady states can be specified for cognitive units (e.g., an individual and his or her attitudes or acts) and that such units tend to seek steady states (balance); e.g., balance exists when both parts of a unit are evaluated the same, but disequilibrium arises when both parts are not evaluated the same, which causes either cognitive reevaluation of the parts or their segregation. SEE ALSO cognitive dissonance t., consistency *principle*.

beta-oxidation-condensation t., that the two carbon fragments split from the fatty acid molecule by beta-oxidation are converted to acetic acid and then condensed to acetoacetic acid.

Bohr t., that spectrum lines are produced 1) by the quantized emission of radiant energy when electrons drop from an orbit of a higher to one of a lower energy level, or 2) by absorption of radiation when an electron rises from a lower to a higher energy level.

Brønsted t., that an acid is a substance, charged or uncharged, liberating hydrogen ions in solution, and that a base is a substance that removes them from solution (e.g., NH_4^+, CH_3COOH, and HSO_4^- are acids; NH_3, CH_3COO^-, and SO_4^- are bases); useful in the concept of weak electrolytes and buffers. Cf. Brønsted *acid*, Brønsted *base*.

Burn and Rand t., that stimulation of sympathetic fibers results first in the production of acetylcholine in the postganglionic nerve endings, which then release norepinephrine to act on the active site of the effector cell.

Cannon t., SYN emergency t.

Cannon-Bard t., the view that the feeling aspect of emotion and the pattern of emotional behavior are controlled by the hypothalamus.

catastrophe t., a branch of mathematics dealing with large changes in the total system that may result from a small change in a critical variable in the system; an example is the change in the physical properties of H_2O as the temperature reaches 0 or 100°C; many applications of catastrophe t. occur in clinical medicine and in epidemiology.

cellular immune t., a concept, put forth by Elie Metchnikoff, that cells, not antibodies, were responsible for the immune response of an organism.

celomic metaplasia t. of endometriosis, that endometrial tissue arises directly from the peritoneal mesothelium.

chaos t., a branch of mathematics dealing with events and processes that cannot be predicted precisely on the basis of conventional mathematical t.'s or laws; some biological processes, e.g., spread of malignant disease, appear to conform to chaos t., at least sometimes.

chemiosmotic t., a hypothesis proposing that cellular energy requiring processes such as ATP synthesis and ion pumping may be driven by a pH and membrane potential gradient; proposed by Peter Mitchell in 1961.

cloacal t., the belief sometimes held by neurotic adults or children that a child is born, as a stool is passed, from a common opening.

clonal deletion t., the elimination of certain T cell populations in the thymus that have receptors for self-antigens (forbidden clones). SEE immunologic *tolerance*.

clonal selection t., a t. which states that each lymphocyte has membrane-bound immunoglobulin receptors specific for a particular antigen and once the receptor is engaged, proliferation of the cell occurs such that a clone of antibody-producing cells (plasma cell) is produced.

cognitive dissonance t., a t. of attitude formation and behavior describing a motivational state that exists when an individual's cognitive elements (attitudes, perceived behaviors, etc.) are inconsistent with each other, such as the espousal of the Ten Commandments concurrent with the belief that it is all right to cheat on one's taxes; a t. which indicates that persons try to achieve consistency (consonance) and avoid dissonance which, when it arises, may be coped with by changing one's attitudes, rationalizing, selective perception, and other means. SEE ALSO balance t., consistency *principle*.

colloid t. of narcosis, that coagulation or flocculation of protein causes dehydration and reduction of metabolism.

darwinian t., the t. of the origin of species and of the development of higher organisms from lower forms through natural selection (survival of the fittest in the struggle for existence), and of the evolution of humans and apes from a common ancestor.

decay t., a t. of forgetting based on the premise that an engram or

memory trace dissipates progressively with time during the interval when it is not activated.

dipole t., a t. in which the activation current of the heart is conceived as a single net moving dipole, the positive pole leading.

duplicity t. of vision, that the cones of the retina function in bright light and the rods function in dim light.

Ehrlich t., SEE side-chain t.

t. of electrolytic dissociation, SEE Arrhenius *doctrine*.

emergency t., a t. of the emotions, advanced by W.B. Cannon, that animal and human organisms respond to emergency situations by increased sympathetic nervous system activity including an increased catecholamine production with associated increases in blood pressure, heart and respiratory rates, and skeletal muscle blood flow. SEE ALSO relaxation *response*. SYN Cannon t.

enzyme inhibition t. of narcosis, that narcotics inhibit respiratory enzymes by suppression of the formation of high-energy phosphate bonds within the cell.

Flourens t., an older t. that thought is a process depending upon the action of the entire cerebrum.

Frerichs t., that uremia represents a toxic condition caused by ammonium carbonate, which is formed as the result of the action of a plasma enzyme on the increased amounts of urea.

Freud t., a comprehensive t. of how personality is formed and develops in normal and emotionally disturbed individuals; e.g., that an attack of conversion hysteria is due to a psychic trauma which was not adequately reacted to at the time it was received, and persists as an affect memory. SEE ALSO psychoanalysis.

game t., the branch of mathematical logic concerned with the range of possible reactions to a particular strategy; each reaction can be assigned a probability and each reaction can lead to a counter-reaction by the "adversary" in the game. Used mainly in systems analysis, game t. has some applications in disease surveillance and control; it is one of the underlying t.'s in clinical decision analysis.

gastrea t., SYN Haeckel gastrea t.

gate-control t., a theory to explain the mechanism of pain; small-fiber afferent stimuli, particularly pain, entering the substantia gelatinosa can be modulated by large-fiber afferent stimuli and descending spinal pathways so that their transmission to ascending spinal pathways is blocked (gated). SYN gate-control hypothesis.

germ t., the t., now a doctrine, that infectious diseases are due to the presence and functional activity of microorganisms within the body.

germ layer t., the concept that young embryos differentiate three primary germ layers (ectoderm, mesoderm, and endoderm), each of which has the potentiality of forming different characteristic structures and organs in the developing body.

gestalt t., SEE gestaltism.

Haeckel gastrea t., that the two-layered gastrula is the ancestral form of all multicellular animals. SYN gastrea t.

Helmholtz t. of accommodation, that the ciliary muscle relaxes for near vision and allows the anterior aspect of the lens to become more convex.

Helmholtz t. of color vision, SYN Young-Helmholtz t. of color vision.

Helmholtz-Gibbs t., SEE Gibbs-Helmholtz *equation*.

Helmholtz t. of hearing, SYN resonance t. of hearing.

Hering t. of color vision, that there are three opponent visual processes: blue-yellow, red-green, and white-black.

humoral t., SEE humoral *doctrine*.

hydrate microcrystal t. of anesthesia, a t. of narcosis pertaining to nonhydrogen-bonding agents; postulates the interaction of the molecules of the anesthetic drug with water molecules in the brain. SYN Pauling t.

implantation t. of the production of endometriosis, that, at the time of menstruation, cells of the uterine mucosa pass through the fallopian tubes and escape into the pelvic cavity where they implant themselves on the peritoneum.

incasement t., SYN preformation t.

information t., in the behavioral sciences, a system for studying the communication process through the detailed analysis, often

th

mathematical, of all aspects of the process including the encoding, transmission, and decoding of signals; not concerned in any direct sense with the meaning of a message.

instructive t., a t. that states that an antibody learns or acquires its specificity after contact with a particular antigen.

kern-plasma relation t., a t. enunciated by Hertwig (1903) that a definite relation as to size normally exists in every cell between the mass of nuclear material and that of the protoplasm. [Ger. *kern,* kernel, nucleus]

Knoop t., that the catabolism of fatty acids occurs in stages in each of which there is a loss of two carbon atoms as a result of oxidation at the β-carbon atom, e.g.,

$$C_6H_5-\overset{\beta}{CH_2}-\overset{\alpha}{CH_2}-COOH \rightarrow C_6H_5-COOH.$$

Ladd-Franklin t., SYN molecular dissociation t.

lamarckian t., that acquired characteristics may be transmitted to the descendants and that experience, and not biology alone, can change and thereby influence genetic transmission.

learning t., any of several prominent theories designed to explain learning, especially those promulgated by Pavlov, Thorndike, Guthrie, Hull, Kohler, Spence, Miller, Skinner, and their modern followers. SEE ALSO conditioning.

libido t., Freud's t. that a person's psychic life results mainly from instinctual or libidinal needs and the attempts to satisfy them.

Liebig t., that the hydrocarbons that oxidize readily and burn are aliments that produce the greatest quantity of animal heat.

lipoid t. of narcosis, that narcotic efficiency parallels the coefficient of partition between oil and water, and that lipoids in the cell and on the cell membrane absorb the drug because of this affinity. SYN Meyer-Overton t. of narcosis.

mass action t., that large areas of brain tissue function as a whole in learned or intelligent action.

t. of medicine, the science, as distinguished from the art, or practice, of medicine.

membrane expansion t., that adsorption of anesthetics into membranes so alters membrane volume and/or configuration that membrane function is affected in such a way as to produce anesthesia.

Metchnikoff t., the phagocytic t., that the body is protected against infection by the leukocytes and other cells that engulf and destroy the invading microorganisms.

Meyer-Overton t. of narcosis, SYN lipoid t. of narcosis.

miasma t., an explanation of the origin of epidemics, based on the false notion that they were caused by air of bad quality, e.g., emanating from rotting vegetation in marshes or swamps.

Miller chemicoparasitic t., that dental caries is caused by microorganisms of the mouth fermenting dietary carbohydrates and producing acids that demineralize the teeth.

mnemic t., SYN mnemic *hypothesis.*

molecular dissociation t., a t., pertaining to color vision, that gray is the earliest of color sensations, from which are derived, by molecular change, two paired substances that, respectively, detect yellow and blue, and that the yellow gives rise to paired substances for detection of red and green. SYN Ladd-Franklin t.

monophyletic t., SYN monophyletism.

myoelastic t., a t. stating that sound of the human voice is produced by vibrations of the vocal cords resulting from folding upward due to air pressure below, and subsequent movement downward due to elastic tension of cords.

neurochronaxic t., t. stating that variations in the frequency of the human voice are produced by changes in the rate of contractions of the laryngeal muscles; no longer believed to be true.

Ollier t., a t. of compensatory growth; after resection of the articular extremity of a bone, the articular cartilage of the other bone entering into the structure of the joint takes on an increased growth.

omega-oxidation t., that the oxidation of fatty acids commences at the CH_3 group, i.e., the terminal or omega-group; beta-oxidation then proceeds at both ends of the fatty acid chain.

overproduction t., SYN Weigert *law.*

oxygen deprivation t. of narcosis, that narcotics inhibit oxidation, which causes the cell to be narcotized.

Pauling t., SYN hydrate microcrystal t. of anesthesia.

permeability t. of narcosis, that the permeability of the cell membrane is decreased by narcotic concentrations of aliphatic and other central nervous system depressants.

phlogiston t., SEE phlogiston.

pithecoid t., the t. of human's descent with the ape from a common ancestor. SEE ALSO darwinian t.

place t., a t. of pitch perception that states that the region of the basilar membrane of the cochlea that is set into vibration depends on the frequency of the sound. SEE ALSO resonance t. of hearing.

Planck t., SYN quantum t.

polyphyletic t., SYN polyphyletism.

preformation t., archaic t. that the embryo was fully formed in miniature within a gamete at the time of conception. SEE ALSO homunculus; Cf. epigenesis. SYN emboitement, incasement t.

quantum t., that energy can be emitted, transmitted, and absorbed only in discrete quantities (quanta), so that atoms and subatomic particles can exist only in certain energy states. SYN Planck t.

recapitulation t., the t. formulated by E.H. Haeckel that individuals in their embryonic development pass through stages similar in general structural plan to the stages their species passed through in its evolution; more technically phrased, the t. that ontogeny is an abbreviated recapitulation of phylogeny. SYN biogenetic law, law of biogenesis, Haeckel law, law of recapitulation.

Reed-Frost t. of epidemics, a mathematical t. to explain how epidemics originate and continue.

reed instrument t., a no longer tenable t. stating that in human voice production the larynx functions in a manner similar to a reed musical instrument.

reentry t., that extrasystoles are due to reentry of an impulse initiated by the sinus or AV junctional impulse, to which the extrasystole is coupled, into the ectopic focus.

resonance t. of hearing, that the basilar membrane of the cochlea acts as a resonating structure, with low frequency tones activating it in the apical turn and high frequency tones activating it in the basal turn. No longer considered correct; superseded by von Bekesy traveling wave theory. SYN Helmholtz t. of hearing.

scientific t., a t. that can be tested and potentially disproved; failure to disprove or refute it increases confidence in it, but it cannot be considered as proven.

Semon-Hering t., SYN mnemic *hypothesis.*

sensorimotor t., in the developmental t. of Piaget, the postulation that during the first 18 months of life there occurs a transformation of action into thought; at first there is a gradual shift from inborn to acquired behavior, then from body-centered to object-centered activity, ultimately permitting intentional behavior and inventive thinking.

side-chain t., Ehrlich postulated that cells contained surface extensions or side chains (haptophores) that bind to the antigenic determinants of a toxin (toxophores); after a cell is stimulated, the haptophores are released into the circulation and become the antibodies. SEE ALSO receptor. SYN Ehrlich postulate.

somatic mutation t. of cancer, that cancer is caused by a mutation or mutations in the body cells (as opposed to germ cells), especially nonlethal mutations associated with increased proliferation of the mutant cells.

Spitzer t., an interpretation of the partitioning of the heart of mammalian embryos primarily on the basis of recapitulations of the adult structural pattern of lower forms; most frequently cited in relation to the partitioning of the truncus arteriosus to form ascending aorta and pulmonary trunk, which is achieved by the phylogenetic development of the lungs.

stringed instrument t., a no longer tenable t. stating that in human voice production the vocal cords function in a manner similar to the strings in a stringed musical instrument.

surface tension t. of narcosis, that substances which lower the surface tension of water pass more readily into the cell and cause narcosis by decreasing metabolism.

telephone t., a t. of pitch perception that states that the cochlea possesses no faculty of sound analysis, but that the frequency of the impulses transmitted over the auditory nerve fibers corresponds to the frequency of the sound vibrations, and is the sole basis for pitch discrimination; a t. no longer tenable. SEE ALSO traveling wave t.

thermodynamic t. of narcosis, that the interposition of narcotic molecules in nonaqueous cellular phase causes changes that interfere with facilitation of ionic exchange.

traveling wave t., generally held t. that a wave travels from the base to the apex of the basilar membrane of the cochlea in response to acoustic stimulation, and that the site of maximal displacement of the basilar membrane depends on the frequency of the stimulating tone with higher frequencies causing maximal displacement near the base and lower frequencies causing maximal displacement near the apex.

van't Hoff t., that substances in dilute solution obey the gas laws. Cf. van't Hoff *law.*

Warburg t., that the development of cancer is due to irreversible damage to the respiratory mechanism of cells, leading to the selective multiplication of cells with increased glycolytic metabolism, both aerobic and anaerobic.

Wollaston t., a t. that the semidecussation of the optic nerves at the chiasm is proved by the homonymous hemianopia seen in brain lesions.

Young-Helmholtz t. of color vision, a t. that there are three color-perceiving elements in the retina: red, green, and blue. Perception of other colors arises from the combined stimulation of these elements; deficiency or absence of any one of these elements results in inability to perceive that color and a misperception of any other color of which it forms a part. SYN Helmholtz t. of color vision.

---

the·o·ther·a·py (thē-ō-thār′ă-pē). Treatment of disease by prayer or religious exercises. [G. *theos,* god, + *therapeia,* therapy]

thèque (tek). A nest or aggregation of nevocytes in the epidermis. [Fr. a small box]

ther·a·peu·sis (thār-ă-pū′sis). **1.** SYN therapeutics. **2.** SYN therapy.

ther·a·peu·tic (thār-ă-pū′tik). Relating to therapeutics or to the treatment, remediating, or curing of a disorder or disease. [G. *therapeutikos*]

ther·a·peu·tics (ther-ă-pū′tiks). The practical branch of medicine concerned with the treatment of disease or disorder. SYN therapeusis (1), therapia (2). [G. *therapeutikē,* medical practice]

ray t., obsolete term for radiotherapy.

suggestive t., treatment of disease or disorder by means of suggestion.

ther·a·peu·tist (thār-ă-pū′tist). An older term to denote one skilled in therapeutics.

the·ra·pia (thār-ă-pē′ă). **1.** SYN therapy. **2.** SYN therapeutics. [L. fr. G. *therapeia,* therapy]

t. mag′na sterili′sans, Ehrlich concept that an infectious disease, especially one of protozoal origin, can be cured by one large dose of a suitable remedy, large enough to sterilize all the tissues and to destroy the microorganism contained therein.

ther·a·pist (thār-ă-pist). One professionally trained and/or skilled in the practice of a particular type of therapy.

THERAPY

---

ther·a·py (ther-ă-pē). **1.** The treatment of disease or disorder by any method. SEE ALSO therapeutics. **2.** In psychiatry, and clinical psychology, a short term for psychotherapy. SEE ALSO psychotherapy, psychiatry, psychology, psychoanalysis. SYN therapeusis (2), therapia (1). [G. *therapeia,* medical treatment]

alkali t., SEE alkalitherapy.

analytic t., short term for psychoanalytic t.

anticoagulant t., the use of anticoagulant drugs to reduce or prevent intravascular or intracardiac clotting.

antisense t., use of antisense DNA for the inhibition of transcription or translation of a specific gene or gene product for therapeutic purposes.

autoserum t., t. with serum obtained from the patient's own blood.

aversion t., a form of behavior t. that pairs an unpleasant stimulus with undesirable behavior(s) so that the patient learns to avoid the latter. SEE ALSO aversive *training.*

behavior t., an offshoot of psychotherapy involving the use of procedures and techniques associated with research in the fields of conditioning and learning for the treatment of a variety of psychologic conditions; distinguished from psychotherapy because specific symptoms (e.g., phobia, enuresis, high blood pressure) are selected as the target for change, planned interventions or remedial steps to extinguish or modify these symptoms are then employed, and the progress of changes is continuously and quantitatively monitored. SEE systematic *desensitization.* SYN conditioning t.

client-centered t., a system of nondirective psychotherapy based on the assumption that the client (patient) both has the internal resources to improve and is in the best position to resolve his or her own personality dysfunction, provided that the therapist can establish a permissive, accepting, and genuine atmosphere in which the client feels free to discuss problems and to obtain insight into them in order to achieve self-actualization.

cognitive t., any of a variety of techniques in psychotherapy that utilizes guided self-discovery, imaging, self-instruction, symbolic modeling, and related forms of explicitly elicited cognitions as the principal mode of treatment.

collapse t., the surgical treatment of pulmonary tuberculosis whereby the diseased lung is placed, totally or partially, temporarily or permanently, in a nonfunctional respiratory state of retraction and immobilization. Now rarely performed.

conditioning t., SYN behavior t.

conjoint t., a type of t. in which a therapist sees the two spouses, or parent and child, or other partners together in joint sessions.

convulsive t., SYN electroshock t.

cytoreductive t., t. with the intention of reducing the number of cells in a lesion, usually a malignancy.

depot t., injection of a drug together with a substance that slows the release and prolongs the action of the drug.

diathermic t., treatment of various lesions by diathermy.

directly observed t., visual monitoring by a health care worker of ingestion of medications, to ensure compliance in difficult or long-term regimens, such as in oral treatment for tuberculosis; a contentious aspect of some WHO programs.

electroconvulsive t. (ECT), SYN electroshock t.

electroshock t. (ECT), a form of treatment of mental disorders in which convulsions are produced by the passage of an electric current through the brain. SYN convulsive t., electroconvulsive t.

electrotherapeutic sleep t., treatment by inducing sleep by means of nonconvulsive electric stimulation of the brain.

estrogen replacement t., administration of sex hormones to women after menopause or oophorectomy. SYN hormone replacement t.

> Administration of estrogen after natural or surgical menopause reverses atrophic vaginitis, relieves vasomotor instability ("hot flashes"), lowers LDL cholesterol, raises HDL cholesterol, reduces the risk of osteoporosis and colorectal cancer, and may retard onset and progression of parkinsonism, Alzheimer dementia, and type 2 diabetes mellitus. Observational studies have found lower rates of coronary artery disease (CAD) in postmenopausal women taking estrogen, but clinical trials have not confirmed this effect. A large randomized study of postmenopausal women with established CAD showed no difference between women taking estrogen-progestogen and controls in the incidence of fatal and nonfatal myocardial infarction, congestive heart failure, stroke, and in total mortality. In limited stud-

th

ies, estrogen has reduced left ventricular mass substantially more than placebo in hypertensive postmenopausal women using standard antihypertensive therapy. Medical opinion as to the safety of estrogen replacement therapy remains divided. Although some studies have indicated an increased incidence of breast cancer, the bulk of evidence does not support this conclusion. Administration of estrogen does, however, increase the risk of endometrial carcinoma. Combining cyclic progestogen administration with daily estrogen probably reduces this risk (besides restoring menstrual cycles), but the safety of long-term combined estrogen and progestogen treatment in postmenopausal women is unknown. Younger women who take this combination at higher dosages in oral contraceptives experience an increased risk of hypertension and thromboembolic disease. Some progestogens may negate the favorable effects of estrogen on lipoproteins. Raloxifene, a selective estrogen receptor modulator (SERM), probably does not increase the risk of endometrial cancer, but also does not relieve hot flashes, nor does it inhibit osteoclastic activity or control cholesterol as well as estrogen. As an alternative to the oral route, estrogen can be administered by transdermal patch, either alone or in combination with progestogen.

extended family t., a type of family t. that involves family members outside the nuclear family and who are closely associated with it and affect it.

family t., a type of group psychotherapy in which a family in conflict meets as a group with the therapist and explores its relationships and processes; focus is on the resolution of current interactions between members rather than on individual members.

fast-neutron radiation t., radiation t. using high-energy neutrons from cyclotrons or proton accelerators.

fever t., SEE pyrotherapy.

foreign protein t., SYN protein shock t.

functional orthodontic t., SYN functional jaw *orthopedics*.

gene t., alteration of somatic or germ-line DNA to correct or prevent disease; the process of inserting a gene artificially into the genome of an organism to correct a genetic defect or to add a new biologic property or function with therapeutic potential.

In somatic gene therapy, functional DNA sequences are inserted into cells that lack a specific gene or bear a faulty version of it. Vectors include replication-defective viruses, liposomes, and plasmids. For transfer of genetic material by viral infection (called transduction), retroviruses are particularly suitable as vectors because their RNA, converted to DNA by reverse transcriptase, becomes part of the genome of the infected cell. Adenovirus and herpesvirus are also used. Progress has been made in treating a number of inherited disorders, including severe combined immunodeficiency disease, cystic fibrosis, and hemophilia B. Gene therapy has several applications in oncology, including the transduction into malignant tumor cells of genes encoding cytokines or coactivation factors, in order to augment host antitumor responses, and the transfer of tumor suppressor genes, particularly p53 (the most commonly mutated gene found in human cancers), in order to enhance the sensitivity of malignant cells to chemotherapeutic agents. Germ-line therapy inserts specific genes directly into the DNA of sperm, egg, or embryo, producing heritable alterations of the genome. Chimeras have been created by insertion of human DNA into germ cells of pigs, mice, and other laboratory animals, but experiments with human germ cells are under federal ban.

geriatric t., SYN gerontotherapy.

gestalt t., a type of psychotherapy, used with individuals or groups, that emphasizes treatment of the person as a whole: the individual's biologic component parts and their organic functioning, perceptual configuration, and interrelationships with the external world; it focuses on the sensory awareness of the person's immediate experiences rather than on past recollections or future expectations, employing role-playing and other techniques to promote the person's growth and develop full potential.

heterovaccine t., t. with a vaccine obtained from organisms not directly concerned with the disorder being treated.

hormone replacement t. (HRT), SYN estrogen replacement t.

hyperbaric oxygen t., treatment in which oxygen is provided in a sealed chamber at an ambient pressure greater than 1 atmosphere. SEE ALSO hyperbaric *oxygenation*.

implosive t., a type of behavior t. using implosion.

individual t., SYN dyadic *psychotherapy*.

inhalation t., therapeutic use of gases or aerosols by inhalation.

insulin coma t., SEE insulin coma *treatment*.

interstitial t., radiation t. by means of radioactive seeds or needles implanted directly into the tissues to be irradiated.

intralesional t., t. by injection directly into a lesion, as in corticosteroid injections into skin lesions.

maintenance drug t., in chemotherapy, systematic dosage at a level that maintains protection against exacerbation.

marital t., SYN marriage t.

marriage t., a type of family t. that involves both husband and wife and focuses on the marital relationship as it affects the individual personalities, behaviors, and psychopathologies of the partners; the rationale for this method is the assumption that emotional or psychopathologic processes within the family structure and in the social matrix of the marriage perpetuate individual pathologic personality structures, which find expression in the disturbed marriage and are aggravated by the feedback between partners. SYN marital t.

microwave t., SYN microkymatotherapy.

milieu t., psychiatric treatment employing manipulation of the social environment for the benefit of the patient; e.g., using the day-to-day experiences of patients living in a ward as the stimuli for discussion and therapeutic change.

myofunctional t., t. of malocclusion and other dental and speech disorders utilizing muscular exercises of the tongue and lips; most often intended to alter a tongue thrust swallowing pattern.

nonspecific t., a t. that does not directly relate to the cause; e.g., the injection of a foreign protein, typhoid vaccine, etc., to induce fever in the treatment of certain diseases, especially those of a parasyphilitic nature. SYN phlogotherapy.

occupational t. (OT), therapeutic use of self-care, work, and recreational activities to increase independent function, enhance development, and prevent disability; may include adaptation of tasks or environment to achieve maximum independence and optimum quality of life.

orthodontic t., SEE orthodontics.

orthomolecular t., treatment designed to remedy deficiencies in any of the normal chemical constituents of the body.

oxygen t., treatment in which an increased concentration of oxygen is made available for breathing, through a nasal catheter, tent, chamber, or mask.

parenteral t., t. introduced usually by a needle through some other route than the alimentary canal.

photodynamic t., SYN photoradiation.

photoradiation t., SYN photoradiation.

physical t. (PT), (1) treatment of pain, disease, or injury by physical means; SYN physiotherapy. **(2)** the profession concerned with promotion of health, with prevention of physical disabilities, with evaluation and rehabilitation of persons disabled by pain, disease, or injury, and with treatment by physical therapeutic measures as opposed to medical, surgical, or radiologic measures.

plasma t., treatment with plasma.

play t., a type of t. used with children in which they can express or reveal their problems and fantasies by playing with dolls or other toys, drawing, etc.

proliferation t., rehabilitation of an incompetent structure (ligament or tendon) by the induced proliferation of new cells; accomplished by injecting an irritating substance into the loose ligament or tendon, the resulting scar formation and contracture serving to tighten up the ligament or tendon as scar tissue proliferates; rarely used.

protein shock t., the injection of a foreign protein to induce fever as a means of treating certain diseases. SYN foreign protein t.

psychedelic t., psychiatric t. utilizing psychedelic drugs.

psychoanalytic t., SYN psychoanalysis (1).

pulse t., a short, intensive course of pharmacotherapy, usually given at intervals such as weekly or monthly; often used in chemotherapy of malignancy.

quadrangular t., marriage t. involving the husband and wife and their respective therapists.

radiation t., treatment with x-rays or radionuclides. SEE radiation *oncology*.

radium beam t., SYN teleradium t.

rational t., therapeutic procedures introduced by Albert Ellis and based on the premise that lack of information or illogical thought patterns are basic causes of a patient's difficulties; it is assumed that the patient can be assisted in overcoming his or her problems by a direct, prescriptive, advice-giving approach by the therapist.

reflex t., treatment of some morbid condition by exciting a reflex action, as in the household treatment of nosebleed by a piece of ice applied to the cervical spine. SYN reflexotherapy.

replacement t., t. designed to compensate for a lack or deficiency arising from inadequate nutrition, from certain dysfunctions (e.g., glandular hyposecretion), or from losses (e.g., hemorrhage); replacement may be physiologic or may entail administration of a substitute (e.g., a synthetic estrogen in place of estradiol).

respiratory t., (1) treatment of various respiratory tract–related conditions, such as increased secretions and bronchospasm; (2) the profession charged with administering any of the therapies related to the respiratory system and breathing.

root canal t., dental t. for damaged pulp by removal of the pulp and sterilization and filling of the root canal.

rotation t., teletherapy in which a desirable radiation dose distribution is achieved by rotating the patient or machine about an axis passing through the center of the tumor.

salvage t., SYN salvage *chemotherapy*.

sclerosing t., SYN sclerotherapy.

serum t., SYN serotherapy.

shock t., SEE shock *treatment*.

social t., a psychiatric rehabilitative t. to improve a patient's social functioning.

social network t., a type of t. involving the assembling of all persons emotionally or functionally important to the patient for the purpose of affecting behavioral change in the patient.

solar t., treatment of disease by exposure to sunlight. SYN solar treatment.

specific t., t. aimed at the cause(s) of a disease process, as opposed to symptomatic therapy.

substitution t., replacement t., particularly when replacement is not physiologic but entails administration of a substitute.

substitutive t., SYN allopathy.

teleradium t., therapeutic use of radium rays, the source of which is a quantity of radium at a distance from the patient. SYN radium beam t.

thrombolytic t., intravenous administration of an agent intended to dissolve a clot causing acute ischemia, as in myocardial infarction, stroke, and peripheral arterial or venous thrombosis. Thrombolytic agents degrade fibrin clots by activating plasminogen, a naturally occurring modulator of hemostatic and thrombotic processes. Synthesized by the liver, plasminogen is present in circulating blood and binds to platelets, endothelium, and fibrin. At sites of vascular injury with thrombus formation, tissue plasminogen activator (TPA), produced by endothelial cells, also binds to fibrin and converts fibrin-bound plasminogen to plasmin by cleaving the arginine-valine bond in the 560–561 position of plasminogen. The resulting clot lysis is due to degradation of fibrin threads as well as of glycoproteins required for platelet adhesion and aggregation. Thrombolytic agents in current use mimic the effects of natural TPA. These include alteplase, a TPA produced by recombinant DNA technology; reteplase, a variant of the TPA molecule, also genetically engineered; urokinase, a tissue protein derived from human kidney cell cultures; streptokinase, a product of β-hemolytic streptococci that catalyzes the conversion of plasminogen to plasmin; and anistreplase, an inactive form of plasminogen that is bound to streptokinase and undergoes deacylation after administration, resulting in persistent activation of plasminogen. The latter 2 products are potentially antigenic and can cause systemic hypersensitivity reactions. SEE ALSO tissue plasminogen *activator*.

> Thrombolytic therapy reduces the in-hospital and 1-year mortality of acute myocardial infarction (MI) by 20–40% when administered promptly (within the first 100 minutes); some benefit may accrue even after a delay of 6–12 hours. About one-half of people treated for acute MI with a thrombolytic agent have patent coronary arteries after 90 minutes. Emergency percutaneous transluminal coronary angioplasty may provide better survival figures, but can only be undertaken in a setting where emergency coronary artery bypass graft is feasible in case of failure. Streptokinase has sometimes been preferred to TPA in acute MI because it is much less expensive. However, an exhaustive analysis has shown that the use of TPA is cost-effective, particularly in anterior MI. The fact that thrombolytic drugs activate platelets partially negates their effectiveness. In preliminary trials, combining heparin and the platelet inhibitor abciximab with TPA markedly enhanced its ability to restore arterial patency in acute MI. In ischemic stroke, administration of TPA within the first 3 hours has been shown to improve overall outcome at 90 days. The usefulness of thrombolytic therapy in stroke is limited by the difficulty of excluding hemorrhagic stroke and the risk of hemorrhage as a side effect of therapy. Of five clinical trials to evaluate the use of thrombolytics in stroke patients, four were stopped prematurely because of excess mortality in the treatment groups. Only TPA is currently recommended in the treatment of stroke. In addition to stroke and myocardial infarction, thrombolytic therapy has been used in pulmonary embolism, deep venous thrombosis, and peripheral arterial occlusion. Thrombolytic therapy in acute occlusion of a lower-limb artery (or arterial bypass graft) can obviate the need for surgery in many patients without increasing mortality or amputation rate. Recanalization occurs in as many as 80% of patients. The chief risk of thrombolytic therapy is major hemorrhage. It is contraindicated in the presence of active or recent hemorrhage, recent surgery, intracranial neoplasm or recent head trauma, aortic dissection, acute pericarditis, prolonged or traumatic cardiopulmonary resuscitation, pregnancy, or sensitivity to the specific agent.

thyroid t., the treatment of hypothyroidism.

Time-Line t., a technique, based on the principles of neurolinguistic programming, for releasing negative emotions and revising limiting decisions, that directs the client, in a dissociated state, to return to significant past events with new resources so that negative emotions can be released or limiting decisions revised. SEE ALSO dissociation (4).

total push t., the application of all available t.'s to the treatment of a psychiatric patient in a hospital setting.

ultrasonic t., t. for musculoskeletal disease using ultrasonic waves to produce heat.

viral t., the use of genetically altered virus particles for delivering genes to specific sites for the purpose of t.

x-ray t., radiation t. using x-rays; sometimes used ironically to refer to excessive use of diagnostic radiation.

ther·en·ceph·a·lous (thēr′en-sef′ă-lŭs, ther-). Denoting a skull in which the angle at the hormion, formed by lines converging from the inion and nasion, measures from 116°–129°. [G. *thēr*, wild beast, + *enkephalos*, brain]

the·ri·a·ca (thē-rī′ă-kă). A mixture containing a great number of ingredients, used in the Middle Ages and believed to possess antidotal and curative powers to an almost miraculous degree. [L. antidote to snake bite, fr. G. *thēriakos*, pertaining to wild beasts]

△**therio-.** Animals. [G. *thēr, thērion*, beast]

the·ri·o·mor·phism (thēr′ē-ō-mōr′fizm). Ascription of animal characteristics to human beings. Cf. anthropomorphism. [therio- + *morphē*, form]

therm. A unit of heat used indiscriminately for: 1) a small calorie, 2) a large calorie, 3) 1000 large calories, 4) 100,000 British thermal units. [G. *thermē*, heat]

△**therm-.** SEE thermo-.

ther·ma·co·gen·e·sis (ther′mă-kō-jen′ĕ-sis). The elevation of body temperature by drug action. [G. *thermē*, heat, + *pharmakon*, drug, + *genesis*, production]

ther·mal (ther′măl). Pertaining to heat.

ther·mal·ge·sia (ther-mal-jē′zē-ă). High sensibility to heat; pain caused by a slight degree of heat. SYN thermoalgesia. [therm- + G. *algēsis*, sense of pain]

ther·mal·gia (ther-mal′jē-ă). Burning pain. SEE ALSO causalgia. [therm- + G. *algos*, pain]

therm·an·al·ge·sia (therm′an-al-jē′zē-ă). SYN thermoanesthesia. [therm- + analgesia]

therm·an·es·the·sia (therm′an-es-thē′zē-ă). SYN thermoanesthesia.

ther·ma·tol·o·gy (ther-mă-tol′ō-jē). The branch of therapeutics concerned with the application of heat. SEE ALSO thermotherapy. [therm- + G. *logos*, study]

ther·me·lom·e·ter (ther-mĕ-lom′ĕ-ter). An electric thermometer, especially used for recording slight variations of temperature. [therm- + electric + G. *metron*, measure]

therm·es·the·sia (therm-es-thē′zē-ă). SYN thermoesthesia.

therm·es·the·si·om·e·ter (therm′es-the-zē-om′ĕ-ter). SYN thermoesthesiometer.

therm·is·tor (ther′mis-ter, -tōr). A device for determining temperature; also may be used to monitor control of temperature. [G. *thermē*, heat]

△**thermo-, therm-.** Heat. [G. *thermē*, heat; *thermos*, warm or hot]

ther·mo·ac·id·o·philes (ther′mō-as-id-ō-fīlz). Archaebacteria that grow in hot sulfur springs at low pH.

ther·mo·al·ge·sia (ther′mō-al-jē′zē-ă). SYN thermalgesia.

ther·mo·an·al·ge·sia (ther′mō-an′al-jē′zē-ă). SYN thermoanesthesia.

ther·mo·an·es·the·sia (ther′mō-an-es-thē′zē-ă). Loss of the temperature sense or of the ability to distinguish between heat and cold; insensibility to heat or to temperature changes. SYN thermanalgesia, thermanesthesia, thermoanalgesia. [thermo- + G. *an*-priv. + *aisthēsis*, sensation]

ther·mo·cau·ter·ec·to·my (ther′mō-kaw-ter-ek′tō-mē). Removal of tissue by thermocautery. [thermocautery + G. *ektomē*, excision]

ther·mo·cau·tery (ther′mō-kaw′ter-ē). The use of an actual cautery, such as an electrocautery. [thermo- + G. *kautērion*, branding iron (cautery)]

ther·mo·chem·is·try (ther′mō-kem′is-trē). The interrelation of chemical action and heat.

ther·mo·chro·ic (ther′mō-krō′ik). 1. Relating to thermochrose. 2. Exerting a selective action on heat rays.

ther·moch·ro·ism (ther-mok′rō-izm). SYN thermochrosis.

ther·mo·chrose (ther′mō-krōz). The property possessed by heat rays of reflection, refraction, and absorption, similar to that of light rays. SYN thermochrosy. [thermo- + G. *chrōsis*, coloring]

ther·mo·chro·sis (ther-mō-krō′sis). The selective action of certain substances on radiant heat, absorbing some of the rays, reflecting or transmitting others. SYN thermochroism. [thermo- + G. *chrōsis*, coloring]

ther·moch·ro·sy (ther-mok′rŏ-sē). SYN thermochrose.

ther·mo·co·ag·u·la·tion (ther′mō-kō-ag-ū-lā′shŭn). The process of converting tissue into a gel by heat. SYN endocoagulation.

ther·mo·cou·ple (ther-mō-kŭp′l). A device for measuring slight changes in temperature, consisting of two wires of different met-

als, one wire being kept at a certain low temperature, the other in the tissue or other material whose temperature is to be measured; a thermoelectric current is set up which is measured by a potentiometer. SYN thermojunction.

ther·mo·cur·rent (ther-mō-ker′ent). A current of thermoelectricity.

ther·mo·dif·fu·sion (ther′mō-di-fū′zhŭn). Diffusion of fluids, either gaseous or liquid, as influenced by the temperature of the fluid.

ther·mo·di·lu·tion (ther′mō-di-loo′shŭn). Reduction in temperature in a liquid that occurs when it is introduced into a colder liquid; the volume of the latter liquid can be calculated from the amount of rise in its temperature.

ther·mo·du·ric (ther-mō-doo′rik). Resistant to the effects of exposure to high temperature; used especially with reference to microorganisms. [thermo- + L. *durus*, hard, enduring]

ther·mo·dy·nam·ics (ther′mō-dī-nam′iks). 1. The branch of physicochemical science concerned with heat and energy and their conversions one into the other involving mechanical work. 2. The study of the flow of heat. [thermo- + G. *dynamis*, force]

ther·mo·e·lec·tric (ther′mō-ē-lek′trik). Relating to thermoelectricity.

ther·mo·e·lec·tric·i·ty (ther′mō-ē-lek-tris′i-tē). An electrical current generated in a thermopile.

ther·mo·es·the·sia (ther′mō-es-thē′zē-ă). The ability to distinguish differences of temperature. SYN temperature sense, thermal sense, thermic sense, thermesthesia. [thermo- + G. *aisthēsis*, sensation]

ther·mo·es·the·si·om·e·ter (ther′mō-es-thē′zē-om′ĕ-ter). An instrument for testing the temperature sense, consisting of a metal disk with thermometer attached, by which the exact temperature of the disk at the time of application may be known. SYN thermesthesiometer. [thermo- + G. *aisthēsis*, sensation, + *metron*, measure]

ther·mo·ex·ci·to·ry (ther′mō-ek-sī′tŏ-rē). Stimulating the production of heat.

ther·mo·gen·e·sis (ther′mō-jen′ĕ-sis). The production of heat; specifically the physiologic process of heat production in the body. [thermo- + G. *genesis*, production]

nonshivering t., t. resulting from the effects of the sympathetic nervous system neurotransmitters, epinephrine, and norepinephrine, acting to increase the cellular metabolic rate in skeletal muscle and other tissues, thereby increasing heat production. In a specialized form of adipose tissue, brown fat, the effect of the sympathetic neurotransmitters is to increase the rate of uncoupled oxidative phosphorylation by the mitochondria, which results in heat production without formation of ATP.

shivering t., t. resulting from the increase in metabolism of the skeletal muscles due to shivering.

ther·mo·ge·net·ic, ther·mo·gen·ic (ther′mō-je-net′ik, -jen′ik). 1. Relating to thermogenesis. SYN thermogenous. 2. SYN calorigenic (2).

ther·mo·gen·ics (ther-mō-jen′iks). The science of heat production.

ther·mo·gen·in (ther-mō-jen′in). A protein found in brown adipose tissue that acts as a thermogenic uncoupling protein of oxidative phosphorylation; it allows thermogenesis in this type of tissue.

ther·mog·e·nous (ther-moj′ĕ-nŭs). SYN thermogenetic (1).

ther·mo·gram (ther′mō-gram). 1. A regional temperature map of the surface of a part of the body, obtained by an infrared sensing device; it measures radiant heat, and thus subcutaneous blood flow, if the environment is constant. 2. The record made by a thermograph. [thermo- + G. *gramma*, a writing]

ther·mo·graph (ther′mō-graf). An instrument or device used in producing a thermogram. [thermo- + G. *graphō*, to write]

ther·mog·ra·phy (ther-mog′ră-fē). The technique for making a thermogram.

infrared t., measurement of the regional skin temperature with an infrared sensing device.

liquid crystal t., measurement of the regional skin temperature by contact with a flexible plate containing liquid crystals that change color with changes in temperature.

ther·mo·hy·per·al·ge·sia (ther'mō-hī'per-al-jē'zē-ă). Excessive thermalgesia. [thermo- + G. *hyper,* over, *algēsis,* sense of pain]

ther·mo·hy·per·es·the·sia (ther'mō-hī'per-es-thē'zē-ă). Very acute thermoesthesia or temperature sense; exaggerated perception of hot and cold. [thermo- + G. *hyper,* over, + *aisthēsis,* sensation]

ther·mo·hyp·es·the·sia (ther-mō-hip'es-thē'zē-ă, -hī'pes-thē'zē-ă). Diminished perception of temperature differences. SYN thermohypoesthesia. [thermo- + G. *hypo,* under, + *aisthēsis,* sensation]

ther·mo·hy·po·es·the·sia (ther-mō-hī'pō-es-thē'zē-ă). SYN thermohypesthesia.

ther·mo·in·hib·i·to·ry (ther'mō-in-hib'i-tōr-ē). Inhibiting or arresting thermogenesis.

ther·mo·in·te·gra·tor (ther-mō-in'tĕ-grā-ter, -tōr). Any device for assessing the effective warmth or coldness of an environment as it might be experienced by a living organism, taking into account radiation and convection as well as conduction. Conceived of as a thermal model of an organism, the device usually consists of a standard object (e.g., sphere, cylinder), the surface temperature of which is measured while it is being heated internally at a standard rate.

ther·mo·junc·tion (ther-mō-jŭngk'shŭn). SYN thermocouple.

ther·mo·ker·a·to·plas·ty (ther-mō-ker'ă-tō-plas-tē). A procedure in which the application of heat shrinks the collagen of the corneal stroma and flattens the cornea in the area of heat application. This tends to make the eye less myopic. SEE refractive *keratoplasty.* [thermo- + G. *keras,* horn, + *plassō,* to form]

ther·mo·la·bile (ther-mō-lā'bīl, -bil). Subject to alteration or destruction by heat. [thermo- + L. *labilis,* perishable]

ther·mol·o·gy (ther-mol'ō-jē). The science of heat. SYN thermotics. [thermo- + G. *logos,* study]

ther·mol·y·sis (ther-mol'i-sis). **1.** Loss of body heat by evaporation, radiation, etc. **2.** Chemical decomposition by heat. [thermo- + G. *lysis,* dissolution]

ther·mo·lyt·ic (ther-mō-lit'ik). **1.** Relating to thermolysis. **2.** An agent promoting heat dissipation.

ther·mo·mas·sage (ther'mō-mă-sahzh'). Combination of heat and massage in physical therapy.

ther·mom·e·ter (ther-mom'ĕ-ter). An instrument for indicating the temperature of any substance; often a sealed vacuum tube containing mercury, which expands with heat and contracts with cold, its level accordingly rising or falling in the tube, with the exact degree of variation of level being indicated by a scale, or, more recently, a device with an electronic sensor that displays the temperature without the use of mercury. SEE ALSO scale. [thermo- + G. *metron,* measure]

air t., SEE gas t.

axilla t., t. used by placing it in the armpit, with the arm held closely to the side. SYN axillary t.

axillary t., SYN axilla t.

clinical t., a small, self-registering t., consisting of a simple scaled glass tube containing mercury, used for taking the temperature of the body.

differential t., SYN thermoscope.

gas t., a t. filled with dry air or a gas, the expansion or increased pressure of which indicates the degree of heat; used to measure high temperatures.

resistance t., a device measuring temperature by the change of the electrical resistance of a metal wire. SYN resistance pyrometer.

self-registering t., a t. in which the maximum or minimum temperature, during the period of observation, is registered by means of a special appliance; in the clinical t. only the highest temperature is registered, usually by a steel bar above the column of mercury or by a segment of the mercury separated from the main column by a bubble of air; after the maximum temperature is registered, the bar or segment of mercury remains in place as the column of mercury contracts.

spirit t., a t. filled with alcohol, used to measure extreme degrees of cold.

surface t., a t. in the form of a disk or strip that indicates the temperature of the portion of the skin to which it is applied.

wet and dry bulb t., SYN psychrometer.

ther·mo·met·ric (ther-mō-met'rik). Relating to thermometry or to a thermometer reading.

ther·mom·e·try (ther-mom'ĕ-trē). The measurement of temperature. [thermo- + G. *metron,* measure]

ther·mo·neu·ro·sis (ther'mō-noo-rō'sis). Elevation of the temperature of the body due to an emotional influence.

ther·mo·nu·cle·ar (ther-mō-noo'klē-er). Pertaining to nuclear reactions brought about by nuclear fusion (e.g., the fusion of hydrogen to helium at temperatures of over 100,000,000°C; the reaction in the "hydrogen bomb").

ther·mo·pen·e·tra·tion (ther'mō-pen-ĕ-trā'shŭn). SYN medical *diathermy.*

ther·mo·phile, ther·mo·phil (ther'mō-fīl, -fil). An organism that thrives at a temperature of 50°C or higher. [thermo- + G. *phileō,* to love]

ther·mo·phil·ic (ther-mō-fil'ik). Pertaining to a thermophile.

ther·mo·pho·bia (ther-mō-fō'bē-ă). Morbid fear of heat. [thermo- + G. *phobos,* fear]

ther·mo·phore (ther'mō-fōr). **1.** An arrangement for applying heat to a part; consists of a water heater, a tube conveying hot water to a coil, and another tube conducting the water back to the heater. **2.** A flat bag containing certain salts that produce heat when moistened; used as a substitute for the hot-water bag. [thermo- + G. *phoros,* bearing]

ther·mo·phy·lic (ther-mō-fī'lik). Resistant to heat, denoting certain microorganisms. [thermo- + G. *phylaxis,* protection]

ther·mo·pile (ther'mō-pīl). A thermoelectric battery, consisting usually of a series of bars of antimony and bismuth joined together, that generates a thermoelectric current when the junctions are heated; used as a thermoscope. SYN thermoelectric pile. [thermo- + pile]

ther·mo·plac·en·tog·ra·phy (ther'mō-plă-sen-tog'ră-fē). Obsolete method for determination of placental position by detection of infrared rays from the large amounts of blood flowing through the placenta. [thermo- + L. *placenta,* placenta, + G. *graphō,* to write]

Ther·mo·plas·ma (ther'mō-plaz'mă). A genus of bacteria (order Mycoplasmatales) which possess the same characteristics as the organisms in the genus *Mycoplasma* except that the thermoplasmas do not require sterol for growth, have an optimal temperature of 55–59°C, have an optimal pH of 1.0–2.0, and reproduce by budding. The type species is *T. acidophilum.* [thermo- + G. *plasma,* something formed]

T. acidoph'ilum, a species found in a coal refuse pile which had undergone self-heating; it is also found in acid hot springs; it is the type species of the genus *T.*

ther·mo·plas·ma, pl. **ther·mo·plas·ma·ta** (ther'mō-plaz'mă, -plaz'mah-tă). A vernacular term used to refer to any member of the genus *Thermoplasma.*

ther·mo·plas·tic (ther-mō-plas'tik). A classification for materials that can be made soft by the application of heat and harden upon cooling.

ther·mo·ple·gia (ther-mō-plē'jē-ă). A rarely used term for sunstroke. [thermo- + G. *plēgē,* stroke]

ther·mo·re·cep·tor (ther'mō-rē-sep'ter, -tōr). A receptor that is sensitive to heat.

ther·mo·reg·u·la·tion (ther'mō-reg-ū-lā'shŭn). Temperature control, as by a thermostat.

ther·mo·reg·u·la·tor (ther-mō-reg'ū-lā-ter, -tōr). SYN thermostat.

ther·mo·scope (ther'mō-skōp). An instrument for indicating slight differences of temperature, without registering or recording them. SYN differential thermometer. [thermo- + G. *skopeō,* to view]

ther·mo·set (ther'mō-set). A classification for materials that become hardened or cured by the application of heat.

ther·mo·sta·bile, ther·mo·sta·ble (ther-mō-stā'bil, -stā'bl). Not

th

readily subject to alteration or destruction by heat. SYN heat-stable. [thermo- + L. *stabilis,* stable]

ther·mo·stat (ther′mō-stat). An apparatus for the automatic regulation of heat, as in an incubator. SYN thermoregulator. [thermo- + G. *statos,* standing]

ther·mo·ste·re·sis (ther′mō-stĕ-rē′sis). The abstraction or deprivation of heat. [thermo- + G. *sterēsis,* deprivation, loss]

ther·mo·stro·muhr (ther-mō-strom′oor). A stromuhr that consists of a heating element between two thermocouples, which are applied to the outside of a vessel; blood flow is calculated from the difference in temperatures recorded by the proximal and distal thermocouples.

ther·mo·sys·tal·tic (ther′mō-sis-tal′tik). Relating to thermosystaltism. [thermo- + G. *systaltikos,* contractile]

ther·mo·sys·tal·tism (ther-mō-sis′tal-tizm). Contraction, as of the muscles, under the influence of heat. [see thermosystaltic]

ther·mo·tac·tic, ther·mo·tax·ic (ther-mō-tak′tik, tak′sik). Relating to thermotaxis.

ther·mo·tax·is (ther-mō-tak′sis). **1.** Reaction of living protoplasm to the stimulus of heat. Cf. thermotropism. **2.** Regulation of the temperature of the body. [thermo- + G. *taxis,* orderly arrangement]

   negative t., repulsion of a plant or animal from heat.

   positive t., attraction of a plant or animal to heat.

ther·mo·ther·a·py (ther′mō-thār′ă-pē). Treatment of disease by therapeutic application of heat. [thermo- + G. *therapeia,* treatment]

ther·mot·ic (ther-mot′ik). Relating to thermotics.

ther·mot·ics (ther-mot′iks). SYN thermology. [G. *thermotēs,* heat]

ther·mo·to·nom·e·ter (ther′mō-tō-nom′ĕ-ter). An instrument for measuring the degree of thermosystaltism, or muscular contraction under the influence of heat. [thermo- + G. *tonos,* tone, tension, + *metron,* measure]

ther·mot·ro·pism (ther-mot′rō-pizm). The motion by a part of an organism (e.g., leaves or stems) toward or away from a source of heat. Cf. thermotaxis. [thermo- + G. *tropē,* a turning]

the·roid (thē′royd). Resembling an animal in instincts or propensities. [G. *thēr,* a wild beast, + *eidos,* resemblance]

the·rol·o·gy (thē-rol′ō-jē). The study of mammals. [G. *thēr,* a wild beast, + *logos,* study]

the·sau·ris·mo·sis (thē-saw-riz-mō′sis). Rarely used term for a metabolic disorder in which a substance accumulates or is stored in certain cells, usually in large amounts. [G. *thēsauros,* store, storehouse, + G. *-osis,* condition]

the·sau·ris·mot·ic (thē′saw-riz-mot′ik). Pertaining to thesaurismosis.

the·sau·ro·sis (thē-saw-rō′sis). Abnormal or excessive storage in the body of normal or foreign substances. [G. *thēsauros,* store, storehouse]

the·sis, pl. **the·ses** (thē′sis, -sēz). **1.** Any theory or hypothesis advanced as a basis for discussion. **2.** A proposition submitted by the candidate for a doctoral degree in some universities, which must be sustained by argument against any objections offered. **3.** An essay on a medical topic prepared by the graduating student. [G. a placing, a position, thesis]

the·ta (θ, Θ) (thā′ta). **1.** The 8th letter in the Greek alphabet, θ. **2.** The eighth in a series; denotes the position of a substituent located on the eighth atom from the carboxyl or other functional group. **3.** Symbol for angle.

the·tins (thē′tinz). Methyl sulfonium compounds, abundant in marine algae, in which the *S*-methyl group is "active," and that therefore act as methyl donors in some plants; e.g., dimethyl-propriothetin, $(CH_3)_2S^+–CH_2–CH_2–COO^-$.

THF Abbreviation for tetrahydrofolate. SEE 5,6,7,8-tetrahydrofolate dehydrogenase, tetrahydrofolate methyltransferase.

△**thia-.** The replacement of carbon by sulfur in a ring or chain. Cf. thio-. [G. *theion*]

thi·a·ben·da·zole (thī-ă-ben′dă-zōl). A broad spectrum anthel-

mintic especially useful against *Strongyloides stercoralis* and, with corticosteroids, against *Trichinella* infection (trichina worm).

thi·a·bu·ta·zide (thī-ă-bū′tă-zīd). SYN buthiazide.

thi·a·cet·a·zone (thī-ă-set′ă-zōn, -ă-se′tă-zōn). SYN amithiozone.

thi·al·bar·bi·tal (thī-al-bar′bi-tawl). An ultra-short-acting thiobarbiturate for induction of general anesthesia by intravenous injection; used as the sodium salt.

thi·am·bu·to·sine (thī-am-bū′tō-sēn). An antileprotic agent.

thi·a·min (thī′ă-min). A heat-labile and water-soluble vitamin contained in milk, yeast, and in the germ and husk of grains; also artificially synthesized; essential for growth; a deficiency of t. is associated with beriberi and Wernicke-Korsakoff syndrome. SYN aneurine, antiberiberi factor, antiberiberi vitamin, antineuritic factor, antineuritic vitamin, thiamine, vitamin B_1. [*thia-* + vitamin]

   t. hydrochloride, a coenzyme used in the prevention of beriberi and other conditions associated with a deficiency of t. in the diet. SYN aneurine hydrochloride.

   t. mononitrate, same action as t. hydrochloride.

   t. pyridinylase, an enzyme catalyzing transfer of a pyridine or other bases into the position of the pyrimidine in t.; e.g., t. reacting with pyridine produces heteropyrithiamin and 4-methyl-5-(2′-hydroxyethyl)thiazole. SYN pyrimidine transferase, thiaminase I.

   t. pyrophosphate (TPP), the diphosphoric ester of t., a coenzyme of several (de)carboxylases, transketolases, and α-oxoacid dehydrogenases. SYN aneurine pyrophosphate, cocarboxylase, diphosphothiamin.

thi·am·i·nase (thī-am′i-nās). **1.** An enzyme present in raw fish that destroys thiamin and may produce thiamin deficiency in animals on a diet largely composed of raw fish. **2.** A hydrolase cleaving thiamin into a pyrimidine moiety (i.e., 2-methyl-4-amino-5-hydroxymethylpyrimidine) and a thiazole moiety (i.e., 4-methyl-5-(2′-hydroxyethyl)thiazole); the pyrimidine moiety may appear in the urine as pyramin. SYN t. II.

   t. I, SYN *thiamin* pyridinylase.

   t. II, SYN thiaminase (2).

thi·a·mine (thī′ă-min, -mēn). SYN thiamin.

thi·am·phen·i·col (thī-am-fen′i-kol). An antibiotic with uses and toxicity similar to those of chloramphenicol. SYN thiophenicol.

thi·am·y·lal so·di·um (thī-am′i-lawl). A short-acting barbiturate, prepared as a mixture with sodium bicarbonate, used intravenously to produce anesthesia.

Thi·a·ra (thī-ah′ră). A widespread genus of operculate snails (family Thiaridae, subclass Prosobranchiata) found in fresh and brackish waters, chiefly in tropical and subtropical Africa and Asia. *T. tuberculata* is one of the initial intermediate hosts of the human lung fluke, *Paragonimus westermani,* and of several fishborne heterophyid flukes of humans and fish-eating mammals.

thi·a·zides (thī′ă-zīdz). Abbreviated form of benzothiadiazides.

thi·a·zin (thī′ă-zin). Parent substance of a family of biologic blue dyes; e.g., methylene blue, thionin, toluidine blue.

thiazolidinediones (thī′ă-zol′ĭ-dīn-dī-ōnz). SYN glitazones.

thi·a·zol·sul·fone (thī-ă-zol-sŭl′fōn). It has the same uses as glucosulfone sodium, but is less toxic and also less effective in the treatment of leprosy.

thick·ness (thik′nes). **1.** The measure of the depth of something, as opposed to its length or width. **2.** A layer or stratum.

   Breslow t., maximal t. of a primary cutaneous melanoma measured in tissue sections from the top of the epidermal granular layer, or from the ulcer base (if the tumor is ulcerated), to the bottom of the tumor; metastatic rates correlate closely with tumor t.

thi·el. SYN sulfhydryl.

thi·e·mia (thī-ē′mē-ă). The presence of sulfur in the circulating blood. [G. *theion,* sulfur, + *haima,* blood]

thi·e·na·my·cin (thī′en-ă-mī′sin). The first member of a family of des-thia-carbapenem nucleus antibiotics having a thioethylamine side chain on the enamine portion of the fused 5-membered ring.

thi·e·nyl (thī′en-il). The radical of thiophene, $SC_4H_3–$. Cf. thenyl.

thi·e·nyl·al·a·nine (thī′ĕ-nil-al′ă-nēn). A compound structurally similar to phenylalanine that inhibits the growth of *Escherichia* *coli*, presumably by competitive inhibition of enzymes for which L-phenylalanine is the substrate.

Thier, Carl Jörg, German physician. SEE Weyers-T. *syndrome.*

Thiers, Joseph, French physician, *1885. SEE Achard-T. *syndrome.*

Thiersch, Karl, German surgeon, 1822–1895. SEE T. *graft, canaliculi,* under *canaliculus;* Ollier-T. *graft.*

thi·eth·yl·per·a·zine ma·le·ate (thī-eth′il-per′ă-zēn). An antiemetic agent used to control nausea and vomiting associated with vertigo, the administration of general anesthetics, and with several other clinical conditions; also has weak hypotensive, spasmolytic, antihistaminic, and hypothermic actions.

thigh (thī) [TA]. The part of the inferior limb between the hip and the knee. SYN femur (1) [TA], os femoris⚹, thigh bone⚹.

Heilbronner t., in cases of organic paralysis, flattening and broadening of the t., when the patient lies supine on a hard mattress; absent in hysterical paralysis.

thig·mes·the·sia (thig-mes-thē′zē-ă). Sensibility to touch. [G. *thigma,* touch, + *aisthēsis,* sensation]

thig·mo·tax·is (thig-mō-tak′sis). A form of barotaxis; denoting the reaction of plant or animal protoplasm to contact with a solid body. Cf. thigmotropism. [G. *thigma,* touch, + *taxis,* orderly arrangement]

thig·mo·tro·pism (thig-mot′rō-pizm). A movement toward or away from a touch stimulus on the part of a portion of an organism, such as leaves or tendrils. Cf. thigmotaxis. [G. *thigma,* touch, + *tropē,* a turning]

thi·mer·o·sal (thī-mer′ō-săl). An antiseptic. SYN thiomersal, thiomersalate.

think·ing. The act of reasoning.

abstract t., t. in terms of concepts and general principles (e.g., perceiving a table and a chair as furniture), as contrasted with concrete t.

archaic-paralogical t., SYN prelogical t.

concrete t., t. of objects or ideas as specific items rather than as an abstract representation of a more general concept, as contrasted with abstract t. (e.g., perceiving a chair and a table as individual useful items and not as members of the general class, furniture).

creative t., productive t., with novel rather than routine elements and results.

magical t., the irrational equating of t. with doing.

prelogical t., a concrete type of t., characteristic of children and primitives, to which schizophrenic persons are sometimes said to regress. SYN archaic-paralogical t., prelogical mind.

t. through, the psychologic process of understanding, with insight, one's own behavior.

thin·ning (thin′ing). Causing a decrease in viscosity by dilution, including by chemical means, as by the addition of a solvent, or by mechanical means, as in shear t.

shear t., decreasing the viscosity of a polymer or macromolecule or gel by increasing the rate of shear; not ordinarily a function of time. SEE ALSO thixotropy.

♻**thio-.** Prefix denoting the replacement of oxygen by sulfur in a compound. Cf. thia-. [G. *theion,* sugar]

thi·o·ac·id (thī-ō-as′id). An organic acid in which one or more of the oxygen atoms have been replaced by sulfur atoms; e.g., thiosulfuric acid. SYN sulfacid, sulfoacid (1).

thi·o·al·co·hol (thī-ō-al′kō-hol). SYN mercaptan (1).

thi·o·am·ide (thī-ō-am′īd). An amide in which S replaces O.

thi·o·ate (thī′ō-āt). A salt or ester of a -thioic acid.

thi·o·bar·bi·tu·rates (thī′ō-bar-bich′ŭr-āts). Hypnotics of the barbiturate group, e.g., thiopental, in which the oxygen atom at carbon-2 is replaced by sulfur.

thi·o·car·bam·ide (thī-ō-kar′bă-mīd). SYN thiourea.

thi·o·car·lide (thī-ō-kar′līd). A synthetic compound whose molecule contains the three antituberculous groups *p*-aminosalicylic acid, *p*-aminobenzaldehyde thiosemicarbazone, and the thiocarbamide group; an antituberculous agent.

thi·o·chrome (thī′ō-krōm). A fluorescent compound, produced by the oxidation of thiamin; used in methods for detection and determination of thiamin.

thi·oc·tic ac·id (thī-ok′tik). SYN lipoic acid.

thi·o·cy·a·nate (thī-ō-sī′ă-nāt). A salt of thiocyanic acid. SYN rhodanate, sulfocyanate.

thi·o·cy·an·ic ac·id (thī-ō-sī-an′ik). HS–CN; hydrogen thiocyanate. SYN rhodanic acid, sulfocyanic acid.

thi·o·dep·si·pep·tide (thī-ō-dep′-sē-pep-tīd). Peptides that also contain one or more acylated thiol groups (e.g., of cysteine). [thio- + G. *depseō,* to knead, blend, + peptide]

thi·o·di·phen·yl·a·mine (thī′ō-dī-fen′il-am′ēn). SYN phenothiazine.

thi·o·es·ter (thī-ō-es′ter). An acylated thiol; RCOSR′; e.g., acetyl-CoA. SYN acylmercaptan.

thi·o·es·ter·ase (thī-ō-es-ter-ās). An enzyme that hydrolyzes thioesters; e.g., the deacylating activity at the end of fatty acid biosynthesis that releases palmitate. SYN thiolesterase.

thi·o·es·ters (thī′ō-es′-terz). In enzymology, an ester where the oxygen bridging the substrate or product carbonyl carbon and the enzyme is replaced by a sulfur (usually through a Cys residue); a high-energy intermediate in many enzymes.

thi·o·eth·a·nol·a·mine ace·tyl·trans·fer·ase (thī′ō-eth-ă-nol′ă-mēn). An enzyme transferring acetyl from acetyl-CoA to the sulfur atom of thioethanolamine, thus producing coenzyme A and *S*-acetylthioethanolamine. SYN thiotransacetylase B.

thi·o·e·ther (thī-ō-ē′ther). An organic sulfide; an ether in which the oxygen is replaced by sulfur; R–S–R′.

thi·o·fla·vine S (thī-ō-flā′vin) [C.I. 49010]. A methylated and sulfonated derivative of primulin; a yellowish dye used in fluorescence microscopy as a vital stain.

thi·o·fla·vin T (thī-ō-flā′vin) [C.I. 49005]. A yellow thiazole dye, used in histopathology as a fluorochrome for hyaline and amyloid.

thi·o·fu·ran (thī′ō-foor′an). SYN thiophene.

thi·o·glu·co·si·dase (thī-ō-gloo′kō-si-dās). An enzyme in mustard seed that converts thioglycosides into thiols plus sugars. SYN myrosinase, sinigrase, sinigrinase.

thi·o·glyc·er·ol (thī-ō-glis′er-ol). SYN monothioglycerol.

thi·o·gly·co·late, thi·o·gly·col·late (thī-ō-glī′kō-lāt). A salt or ester of thioglycolic acid; frequently used in bacterial media to reduce their oxygen content so as to create favorable conditions for the growth of anaerobes; the t. will also inactivate any mercurial that might be carried over with the inoculum.

thi·o·gly·col·ic ac·id (thī-ō-glī-kol′ik). Used as a reagent for the detection of metals such as iron, molybdenum, silver, and tin; the ammonium and sodium salts are used in home permanents; the calcium salt as a depilatory. SYN mercaptoacetic acid.

thi·o·gua·nine (thī-ō-gwah′nēn). An antineoplastic agent used for leukemias and nephrosis.

♻**-thioic ac·id.** Suffix denoting the radical, –C(S)OH or –C(O)SH, the sulfur analog of a carboxylic acid, i.e., a thiocarboxylic acid.

thi·o·ki·nase (thī-ō-kī′nās). Group term for enzymes that form acyl-CoA compounds from the corresponding fatty acids and CoA; the bond is through the sulfur atom of the CoA.

thi·ol (thī′ol). **1.** The monovalent radical –SH when attached to carbon; a hydrosulfide; a mercaptan. **2.** A mixture of sulfurated and sulfonated petroleum oils purified with ammonia; used in the treatment of skin diseases.

thi·o·lase (thī′ō-lās). SYN *acetyl-CoA* acetyltransferase.

thi·ole (thī′ōl). SYN thiophene.

thi·ol·es·ter·ase (thī′ōl-es′ter-āz). SYN thioesterase.

thi·ol·his·ti·dyl·be·ta·ine (thī′ol-his′ti-dil-bē′tă-ēn). SYN ergothioneine.

thi·ol·trans·a·cet·y·lase A (thī′ol-trans-ă-set′i-lās). SYN dihydrolipoamide *S*-acetyltransferase.

thi·ol·y·sis (thī-ol′i-sis). The cleavage of a chemical bond with the addition of coenzyme A to one part; analogous to hydrolysis and phosphorolysis.

thi·o·mer·sal (thī-ō-mer′săl). SYN thimerosal.

thi·o·mer·sa·late (thī-ō-mer′să-lāt). SYN thimerosal.

th

thi·o·meth·yl·a·den·o·sine (thī′ō-meth′il-ă-den′ō-sēn). SYN methylthioadenosine.

β-thi·o·nase (thī′ō-nās). SYN cystathionine β-synthase.

△**-thione.** Suffix denoting the radical =C=S, the sulfur analog of a ketone, i.e., a thiocarbonyl group.

thi·o·nein (thī′ō-nēn). The apoprotein of metallothionein.

thi·o·ne·ine (thī′ō-ne′in). SYN ergothioneine.

thi·on·ic (thī-on′ik). Relating to sulfur.

thi·o·nine (thī′ō-nin) [C.I. 52000]. Amidophenthiazine; a dark-green powder, giving a purple solution in water; useful as a basic stain in histology for chromatin and mucin because of its metachromatic properties. SYN Lauth violet.

△**thiono-.** Prefix sometimes used for thioxo-.

thi·o·pan·ic ac·id (thī-ō-pan′ik). SYN pantoyltaurine.

thi·o·pen·tal so·di·um (thī-ō-pen′tawl). An ultra–short-acting barbiturate administered intravenously or rectally for induction of anesthesia.

thi·o·phene (thī′ō-fēn). The fundamental ring compound. SYN thiofuran, thiole.

thi·o·phe·ni·col (thī-ō-fen′i-kol). SYN thiamphenicol.

thi·o·pro·pa·zate hy·dro·chlo·ride (thī-ō-prō′pă-zāt). A phenothiazine derivative related chemically and pharmacologically to prochlorperazine and perphenazine; an antipsychotic.

thi·o·pro·per·a·zine (thī′ō-prō-per′ă-zēn). An antiemetic and antianxiety agent.

thi·o·re·dox·in (thī-ō-rē-doks′in). A protein that participates in the oxidation-reduction reactions associated with the biosynthesis of deoxyribonucleotides.

t. reductase, a flavoprotein that uses NADPH to re-reduce t. in the formation of deoxyribonucleotides.

thi·o·rid·a·zine hy·dro·chlo·ride (thī-ō-rid′ă-zēn). An antipsychotic with action similar to that of chlorpromazine but with relatively stronger anticholinergic effects.

thi·o·sem·i·car·ba·zide (thī′ō-sem′ē-kar′bă-zīd). One of the group of thiosemicarbazones with a tuberculostatic action; used as a reagent in the detection of metals.

thi·o·sem·i·car·ba·zone (thī′ō-sem′ē-kar′bă-zōn). **1.** A compound containing the thiosemicarbazide radical, =N—NH—C(S)—NH$_2$. **2.** One of a group of tuberculostatic drugs that includes thiosemicarbazide, benzaldehyde thiosemicarbazone, and 4-aminoacetylbenzaldehyde thiosemicarbazone.

thi·o·sul·fate (thī-ō-sŭl′fāt). S$_2$O$_3^=$; the anion of thiosulfuric acid; elevated in individuals with a molybdenum cofactor deficiency.

t. cyanide transsulfurase, SYN t. sulfurtransferase.

t. sulfurtransferase, a transferase that catalyzes the formation of thiocyanate and sulfite from cyanide and t. SYN rhodanese, t. cyanide transsulfurase, t. thiotransferase.

t. thiotransferase, SYN t. sulfurtransferase.

thi·o·sul·fur·ic ac·id (thī′ō-sŭl-fūr′ik). H$_2$S$_2$O$_3$; sulfuric acid in which an atom of oxygen has been replaced by one of sulfur.

thi·o·te·pa (thī-ō-tep′ă). SYN triethylenethiophosphoramide.

thi·o·thix·ene (thī-ō-thik′sēn). An antipsychotic.

thi·o·trans·a·cet·y·lase B (thī′ō-trans-ă-set′i-lās). SYN thioethanolamine acetyltransferase.

2-thi·o·u·ra·cil (thī-ō-ūr′ă-sil). A rare component of transfer RNAs; a thioamide derivative that inhibits the synthesis of thyroid hormones; hence, a goitrogen; similar to propylthiouracil.

4-thi·o·u·ra·cil (thī-ō-ūr′ă-sil). Uracil with S replacing O in position 4, isomeric with 2-thiouracil; a rare component of transfer RNAs.

thi·o·u·rea (thī′ō-ū-rē′ă). An antithyroid compound of the thioamide group, with the same actions and uses as thiouracil. Several derivatives of t. are useful in the treatment of leprosy. SYN thiocarbamide.

thi·o·xan·thene (thī-ō-zan′thēn). A class of tricyclic compounds resembling phenothiazine, but with the central ring nitrogen replaced by a carbon atom; current use emphasizes the antipsychotic and antiemetic properties of this class.

△**thioxo-.** Prefix indicating =S in a thioketone.

thi·ox·o·lone (thī-ok′sō-lōn). An antiseborrheic.

THIP. An agonist at γ-aminobutyric acid (GABA) type A receptors. Unlike other agonists of this type, upon systemic administration THIP penetrates the blood-brain barrier and is used as a pharmacologic tool to explore GABA receptor function in the brain and spinal cord.

thi·phen·a·mil hy·dro·chlo·ride (thī-fen′ă-mil). An anticholinergic drug.

thirst (thurst). A desire to drink associated with uncomfortable sensations in the mouth and pharynx. [A.S. *thurst*]

false t., t. that is not satisfied by drinking or taking water; t. associated with a dry mouth but not with a bodily need for water. SYN pseudodipsia.

insensible t., SYN hypodipsia.

morbid t., SYN dipsesis.

subliminal t., SYN hypodipsia.

true t., t. that can be satisfied by drinking water.

Thiry, Ludwig, Austrian physiologist, 1817–1897. SEE T. *fistula*; T.-Vella *fistula*.

thix·o·la·bile (thik-sō-lā′bil, -bīl). Susceptible to thixotropy.

thix·o·tro·pic (thik-sō-trop′ik). Pertaining to, or characterized by, thixotropy.

thix·ot·ro·py (thik-sot′rō-pē). The property of certain gels of becoming less viscous when shaken or subjected to shearing forces and returning to the original viscosity upon standing (e.g., synovial fluid, ferrous hydroxide gel); a characteristic of a system exhibiting a decrease in viscosity with an increase in the rate of shear, usually a function of time. SYN reclotting phenomenon. [G. *thixis,* a touching, + *tropē,* turning]

Tho·go·to·vi·ruses (thō-gō-tō-vī-rus-ez). A group of unclassified viruses that are similar to the Orthoviruses and share some amino acid homology.

Thoma, Richard, German histologist, 1847–1923. SEE T. *ampulla, fixative, laws,* under law.

Thomas, Hugh Owen, British surgeon, 1834–1891. SEE T. *splint*.

Thompson, Sir Henry, English surgeon, 1820–1904. SEE T. *test*.

Thomsen, Asmus J., Danish physician, 1815–1896. SEE T. *disease*.

Thomson, Frederic H., English physician, 1867–1938. SEE T. *sign*.

Thomson, Matthew Sidney, English dermatologist, 1894–1969. SEE Rothmund-T. *syndrome*.

thon·zo·ni·um bro·mide (thon-zō′nē-ŭm). A surface-active agent used in ear drops and aerosols.

thon·zyl·a·mine hy·dro·chlo·ride (thon-zil′ă-mēn). An antihistamine at H$_1$ receptors.

△**thorac-.** SEE thoraco-.

tho·ra·cal (thor′ă-kăl). SYN thoracic.

tho·ra·cal·gia (thōr-ă-kal′jē-ă). Pain in the chest. SYN thoracodynia. [thoraco- + G. *algos,* pain]

tho·ra·cen·te·sis (thōr′ă-sen-tē′sis). Paracentesis of the pleural cavity. SYN pleuracentesis, pleural tap, pleurocentesis, thoracocentesis. [thoraco- + G. *kentēsis,* puncture]

tho·rac·ic (thō-ras′ik). Relating to the thorax. SYN thoracal.

△**thoracico-.** SEE thoraco-.

tho·rac·i·co·ab·dom·i·nal (thŏ-ras′i-kō-ab-dom′i-năl). SYN thoracoabdominal.

tho·rac·i·co·a·cro·mi·al (thor-as′i-kō-ă-krō′mē-al). SYN thoracoacromial.

tho·rac·i·co·hu·mer·al (thŏ-ras′i-kō-hū′mer-ăl). Relating to the thorax and the humerus.

△**thoraco-, thorac-, thoracico-.** The chest (thorax). [G. *thōrax*]

tho·ra·co·ab·dom·i·nal (thōr′ă-kō-ab-dom′i-năl). Relating to the thorax and the abdomen. SYN thoracicoabdominal.

tho·ra·co·a·cro·mi·al (thōr′ă-kō-ă-krō′mē-ăl). Relating to the acromion and the thorax; denoting especially the thoracoacromial *artery.* SYN acromiothoracic, thoracicoacromial.

tho·ra·co·ce·los·chi·sis (thōr′ă-kō-sē-los′ki-sis). A congenital fissure of the trunk involving both the thoracic and abdominal cavities. SYN thoracogastroschisis. [thoraco- + G. *koilia*, belly, + *schisis*, fissure]

tho·ra·co·cen·te·sis (thōr'ă-kō-sen-tē'sis). SYN thoracentesis.

tho·ra·co·cyl·lo·sis (thōr'ă-kō-si-lō'sis). A deformity of the chest. [thoraco- + G. *kyllōsis*, a crippling]

tho·ra·co·cyr·to·sis (thōr'ă-kō-ser-tō'sis). Abnormally wide curvature of the chest wall. [thoraco- + G. *kyrtōsis*, a being crooked]

tho·ra·co·del·phus (thōr'ă-kō-del'fŭs). SYN thoradelphus.

tho·ra·co·dor·sal (thor-ak-ō-dōr'sal). Relating to the external posterior chest wall, denoting especially an artery, vein, and nerve.

tho·ra·co·dyn·ia (thōr'ă-kō-din'ē-ă). SYN thoracalgia. [thoraco- + G. *odynē*, pain]

tho·ra·co·gas·tros·chi·sis (thōr'ă-kō-gas-tros'ki-sis). SYN thoracoceloschisis. [thoraco- + G. *gastēr*, belly, + *schisis*, fissure]

tho·ra·co·lap·a·rot·o·my (thōr'ă-kō-lap-ă-rot'ō-mē). Exposure of diaphragmatic region by an incision that opens both thorax and abdomen (thoracoabdominal incision). [thoraco- + laparotomy]

tho·ra·co·lum·bar (thōr'ă-kō-lŭm'bar). **1.** Relating to the thoracic and lumbar portions of the vertebral column. **2.** Relating to the origins of the sympathetic division of the autonomic nervous system. SEE autonomic *division* of nervous system.

tho·ra·col·y·sis (thōr-ă-kol'i-sis). Breaking up of pleural adhesions. [thoraco- + G. *lysis*, dissolution]

tho·ra·com·e·lus (thōr-ă-kom'ě-lŭs). Unequal conjoined twins in which the parasite, often only a single arm or leg, is attached to the thorax of the autosite. SEE conjoined *twins*, under *twin*. [thoraco- + G. *melos*, limb]

tho·ra·com·e·ter (thōr-ă-kom'ě-ter). An instrument for measuring the circumference of the chest or its variations in respiration. [thoraco- + G. *metron*, measure]

tho·ra·co·my·o·dyn·ia (thōr'ă-kō-mī-ō-din'ē-ă). Pain in the muscles of the chest wall. [thoraco- + G. *mys*, muscle, + *odynē*, pain]

tho·ra·cop·a·gus (thōr-ă-kop'ă-gŭs). Conjoined twins with union in the thoracic region. SEE conjoined *twins*, under *twin*. SYN synthorax. [thoraco- + G. *pagos*, something fastened]

tho·ra·co·par·a·ceph·a·lus (thōr'ă-kō-par-ă-sef'ă-lŭs). Unequal conjoined twins in which a rudimentary parasitic head is attached to the thorax of the autosite. SEE conjoined *twins*, under *twin*. [thoraco- + G. *para*, beside, + *kephalē*, head]

tho·ra·cop·a·thy (thōr-ă-kop'ă-thē). Rarely used term. Any disease of the thoracic organs or tissues. [thoraco- + G. *pathos*, suffering]

tho·ra·co·plas·ty (thōr'ă-kō-plas-tē). An operation that reduces intrathoracic space by removal of portions of the rigid chest wall. [thoraco- + G. *plastos*, formed]

  conventional t., resection of ribs to allow inward retraction of the chest wall to reduce size of the pleural space; may be used in the treatment of empyema.

tho·ra·co·pneu·mo·plas·ty (thōr'ă-kō-noo'mō-plas-tē). Plastic surgery of the chest in which the lung is also involved. [thoraco- + G. *pneumōn*, lung, + *plastos*, formed]

tho·ra·cos·chi·sis (thōr-ă-kos'ki-sis). Congenital fissure of the chest wall. [thoraco- + G. *schisis*, fissure]

tho·ra·co·scope (thō-rak'ō-skōp). An endoscope for viewing intrathoracic structures; may be video-assisted. [thoraco- + G. *skopeō*, to view]

tho·ra·cos·co·py (thōr-ă-kos'kŏ-pē). Examination of the pleural cavity with an endoscope. SYN pleuroscopy. [thoraco- + G. *skopeō*, to view]

tho·ra·co·ste·no·sis (thōr'ă-kō-stě-nō'sis). Narrowness of the chest. [thoraco- + G. *stenōsis*, narrowing]

thoracosternotomy. Chest incision combining an intercostal incision and transsection of the sternum.

  transverse t., chest incision combining an intercostal incision and transsection of the sternum.

tho·ra·cos·to·my (thōr-ă-kos'tō-mē). Establishment of an opening into the chest cavity, as for the drainage of an empyema. [thoraco- + G. *stoma*, mouth]

tho·ra·cot·o·my (thōr-ă-kot'ō-mē). Incision through the chest wall into the pleural space. SYN pleurotomy. [thoraco- + G. *tomē*, incision]

  anterior t., anterior incision into the chest, usually submammary.

  axillary t., lateral t. placed below the axillary hairline; may be transverse or vertical.

  clamshell t., SYN clamshell *incision*.

  minithoracotomy, any t. involving less muscle division than the classic posterolateral t. [colloquial]

  muscle-sparing t., any type of t. that does not involve significant division of the latissimus dorsi (*muscle*) and the serratus anterior (*muscle*).

  posterolateral t., t., involving division of the latissimus dorsi (*muscle*) and the serratus anterior (*muscle*).

tho·ra·del·phus (thōr-ă-del'fŭs). Duplicitas posterior in which the individual is duplicated from the navel downward. SEE conjoined *twins*, under *twin*. SYN thoracodelphus. [thoraco- + G. *adelphos*, brother]

tho·rax, gen. **tho·ra·cis,** pl. **tho·ra·ces** (thō'raks, thō'rā-sis, -rā'sēz) [TA]. The upper part of the trunk between the neck and the abdomen; it is formed by the 12 thoracic vertebrae, the 12 pairs of ribs, the sternum, and the muscles and fasciae attached to these; below, it is separated from the abdomen by the diaphragm; it contains the chief organs of the circulatory and respiratory systems. [L. fr. G. *thōrax*, breastplate, the chest, fr. *thōrēssō*, to arm]

  barrel-shaped t., increased anteroposterior dimension of the t., so that lateral and anteroposterior dimensions are about equal, due to hyperinflation of the lungs. Seen in patients with emphysema.

  Peyrot t., an obliquely oval deformity of the chest in cases of a very large pleural effusion.

tho·ri·um (Th) (thō'rē-ŭm). A radioactive metallic element; atomic no. 90, atomic wt. 232.0381. ^{232}Th, the only naturally occurring nuclide, with a half-life of 14×10^9 years, is used in colloidal form in electron microscopy as a stain for acid mucopolysaccharides. [*Thor*, Norse god of thunder]

Thormählen, Johann, 19th century German physician. SEE T. *test.*

Thorn, George W., U.S. physician, *1906. SEE T. *test, syndrome.*

thorn (thōrn). In anatomy, a thornlike or spinous structure.

  dendritic t.'s, SYN dendritic *spines*, under *spine.*

thorn ap·ple. SYN *Datura stramonium.*

Thornwaldt, Gustavus Ludwig. SEE Tornwaldt.

thought. 1. The faculty of reasoning. **2.** The process or act of thinking. **3.** The result of thinking.

  t. broadcasting, the delusion of experiencing one's thoughts, as they occur, as being broadcast from one's head to the external world where other people can hear them.

  t. insertion, the delusion that one's thoughts are not really one's own but are being placed into one's mind by an external force.

  trend of t., thinking with a tendency toward or centering on a particular idea with a particular affect.

  t. withdrawal, the delusion that one's thoughts have been removed from one's head resulting in a diminished number of thoughts remaining.

Thr Symbol for threonine or its radical forms.

thread (thred). **1.** A fine strand of suture material. **2.** A filamentous structure. [M.E., fr. A.S. *thraed*]

  terminal t., SYN terminal *filum.*

thread·worm (thred'werm). Common name for species of the genus *Strongyloides;* sometimes applied to any of the smaller parasitic nematodes.

thre·on·ic ac·id (thrē-on'ik). The acid derived by oxidation of the CHO group of threose to COOH; a product of the oxidation of ascorbic acid by hypoiodite.

thre·o·nine (T, Thr) (thrē'ō-nēn). 2-Amino-3-hydroxybutyric acid; the L-isomer is one of the naturally occurring amino acids, included in the structure of most proteins, and nutritionally essential in the diet of humans and other mammals.

  t. deaminase, SYN t. dehydratase.

  t. dehydratase, an enzyme catalyzing the anaerobic deamination of L-t. to 2-ketobutyric acid and ammonia; a central step in t. catabolism. SYN serine deaminase, t. deaminase.

thre·ose (thrē'ōs). An aldotetrose; one of the two aldoses (the other is erythrose) containing four carbon atoms.

thresh·old (thresh'ōld). **1.** The point at which a stimulus first produces a sensation. **2.** The lower limit of perception of a stimulus. **3.** The minimal stimulus that produces excitation of any structure; e.g., the minimal stimulus eliciting a motor response. SYN limen (2) [TA]. [A.S. *therxold*]

absolute t., the lowest limit of any perception whatever. Cf. differential t. SYN stimulus t.

achromatic t., SYN visual t.

auditory t., the intensity of any barely perceptible sound.

brightness difference t., the smallest difference that can be perceived as a difference in brightness. SYN light difference (2).

t. of consciousness, the lowest point at which a stimulus sensation can be perceived.

convulsant t., the smallest amount of stimulation, electric current, or drug required to induce a convulsion.

differential t., the lowest limit at which two stimuli can be differentiated. SYN threshold differential.

displacement t., the least distinguishable break in the contour of a line.

double-point t., the least degree of separation of two points applied to the body surface that permits their being felt as two.

erythema t., the dose at which erythema of the skin is produced by irradiation with ultraviolet, gamma, or x-rays.

fibrillation t., least intensity of an electrical stimulus that will initiate fibrillation.

galvanic t., SYN rheobase.

t. of island of Reil, SYN *limen* insulae.

light differential t., the smallest difference in light intensity that can be appreciated.

minimum light t., SYN visual t.

t. of nose, SYN *limen* nasi.

pain t., the smallest intensity of a painful stimulus at which the subject perceives pain.

phenotypic t., a quantitative genetic trait with a continuous distribution termed its liability; may generate two kinds of phenotype, according to whether the liability lies above or below some critical t. at about which a radical change in behavior occurs. For instance, blood uric acid level is a liability with an approximately gaussian distribution. At a critical point of chemical saturation (the t.), crystallization occurs and the resulting gout or nongout is a t. trait.

relational t., the smallest degree of difference between two stimuli that permits them to be perceived as different.

renal t., concentration of plasma substance above which the substance appears in the urine.

speech awareness t., the lowest sound intensity at which speech can be detected. SYN speech detection t.

speech detection t., SYN speech awareness t.

speech reception t., the intensity at which speech is recognized as meaningful symbols; in speech audiometry, it is the decibel level at which 50% of spondee words can be repeated correctly by the subject.

stimulus t., SYN absolute t.

swallowing t., (1) the moment that the act of swallowing begins after the mastication of food; **(2)** the critical moment of reflex action initiated by minimum stimulation, prior to the act of deglutition.

visual t., t. of visual sensation, the minimal light intensity evoking a visual sensation. SYN achromatic t., minimum light t.

thrill. A vibration accompanying a cardiac or vascular murmur that can be palpated. SEE ALSO fremitus.

diastolic t., a t. felt over the precordium or over a blood vessel during ventricular diastole.

hydatid t., the peculiar trembling or vibratory sensation felt on palpation of a hydatid cyst. SYN Blatin syndrome, hydatid fremitus.

presystolic t., a t. immediately preceding the ventricular contrac-

tion that is sometimes felt on palpation over the apex of the heart, as in mitral stenosis.

systolic t., a t. felt over the precordium or over a blood vessel during ventricular systole.

thrix (thriks) [TA]. SYN hair. [G.]

throat (thrōt). **1.** The fauces and pharynx. SYN gullet. **2.** The anterior aspect of the neck. SYN jugulum. **3.** Any narrowed entrance into a hollow part. [A.S. *throtu*]

sore t., a condition characterized by pain or discomfort on swallowing; it may be due to any of a variety of inflammations of the tonsils, pharynx, or larynx.

throb. 1. To pulsate. **2.** A beating or pulsation.

thromb-. SEE thrombo-.

throm·base (throm'bās). SYN thrombin.

throm·bas·the·nia (throm-bas-thē'nē-ă). An abnormality of platelets characteristic of Glanzmann t. SEE ALSO Bernard-Soulier *syndrome.* SYN thromboasthenia. [thromb- + G. *astheneia,* weakness]

Glanzmann t. [MIM*273800], a hemorrhagic diathesis characterized by normal or prolonged bleeding time, normal coagulation time, defective clot retraction, normal platelet count but morphologic or functional abnormality of platelets; several different kinds of platelet abnormalities have been described; caused by defect in platelet membrane glycoprotein IIb-IIIa complex; autosomal recessive inheritance, caused by mutation in the platelet-membrane glycoprotein IIb-IIIa complex gene (ITGA2B) on chromosome 17. SYN constitutional thrombopathy, Glanzmann disease, hereditary hemorrhagic t.

hereditary hemorrhagic t., SYN Glanzmann t.

throm·bec·to·my (throm-bek'tō-mē). The excision of a thrombus. [thromb- + G. *ektomē,* excision]

throm·bi (throm'bī). Plural of thrombus.

throm·bin. 1. An enzyme (proteinase), formed in shed blood, that converts fibrinogen into fibrin by hydrolyzing peptides (and amides and esters) of L-arginine; formed from prothrombin by the action of prothrombinase (factor Xa, another proteinase). **2.** A sterile protein substance prepared from prothrombin of bovine origin through interaction with thromboplastin in the presence of calcium; causes clotting of whole blood, plasma, or a fibrinogen solution; used as a topical hemostatic for capillary bleeding with or without fibrin foam in general and plastic surgical procedures. SYN factor IIa, fibrinogenase, thrombase, thrombosin.

human t., t. obtained from human plasma by precipitation with suitable salts and organic solvents; same uses as t.

throm·bin·o·gen (throm-bin'ō-jen). SYN prothrombin.

throm·bi·no·gen·e·sis (throm'bi-nō-jen'ě-sis). Thrombin production.

thrombo-, thromb-. Blood clot; coagulation; thrombin. [G. *thrombos,* clot (thrombus)]

throm·bo·an·gi·i·tis (throm'bō-an-ji-ī'tis). Inflammation of the intima of a blood vessel, with thrombosis. [thrombo- + G. *angeion,* vessel, + *-itis,* inflammation]

t. oblit'erans, inflammation of the entire wall and connective tissue surrounding medium-sized arteries and veins, especially of the legs of young and middle-aged men; associated with thrombotic occlusion and commonly resulting in gangrene. SYN Buerger disease, Winiwarter-Buerger disease.

throm·bo·ar·te·ri·tis (throm'bō-ar-ter-ī'tis). Arterial inflammation with thrombus formation.

throm·bo·as·the·nia (throm'bō-as-thē'nē-ă). SYN thrombasthenia.

throm·bo·blast (throm'bō-blast). SYN megakaryocyte. [thrombo- + G. *blastos,* germ]

throm·bo·clas·tic (throm-bō-klas'tik). SYN thrombolytic.

throm·bo·cyst, throm·bo·cys·tis (throm'bō-sist, -sis'tis). A membranous sac enclosing a thrombus. [thrombo- + G. *kystis,* a bladder]

throm·bo·cy·tas·the·nia (throm'bō-sī-tas-thē'nē-ă). A term for a group of hemorrhagic disorders in which the platelets may be only slightly reduced in number, or even within the normal range, but are morphologically abnormal, or are lacking in factors that are effective in the coagulation of blood. [thrombocyte + G. *astheneia*, weakness]

throm·bo·cyte (throm′bō-sīt). SYN platelet. [thrombo- + G. *kytos*, cell]

throm·bo·cy·the·mia (throm′bō-sī-thē′mē-ă). SYN thrombocytosis. [thrombocyte + G. *haima*, blood]

throm·bo·cy·tin (throm-bō-sī′tin). SYN serotonin.

throm·bo·cy·top·a·thy (throm′bō-sī-top′ă-thē). General term for any disorder of the coagulating mechanism that results from dysfunction of the blood platelets. [thrombocyte + G. *pathos*, suffering]

throm·bo·cy·to·pe·nia (throm′bō-sī-tō-pē′nē-ă). A condition in which there is an abnormally small number of platelets in the circulating blood. SYN thrombopenia. [thrombocyte + G. *penia*, poverty]

autoimmune neonatal t., SYN isoimmune neonatal t.

essential t., a primary form of t., in contrast to secondary forms that are associated with metastatic neoplasms, tuberculosis, and leukemia involving the bone marrow, or with direct suppression of bone marrow by the use of chemical agents, or with other conditions.

immune t., t. associated with antiplatelet antibodies. SEE isoimmune neonatal t.

isoimmune neonatal t., immune t. resulting from maternal-fetal platelet incompatibility. SYN autoimmune neonatal t.

throm·bo·cy·to·poi·e·sis (throm′bō-sī-tō-poy-ē′sis). The process of formation of thrombocytes or platelets. [thrombocyte + G. *poiēsis*, a making]

throm·bo·cy·to·sis (throm′bō-sī-tō′sis). An increase in the number of platelets in the circulating blood. SYN thrombocythemia. [thrombocyte + G. *-osis*, condition]

throm·bo·e·las·to·gram (throm′bō-ē-las′tō-gram). Registration of the coagulation process by a thromboelastograph.

throm·bo·e·las·to·graph (throm′bō-ē-las′tō-graf). Apparatus for registering elastic variations of a thrombus during the process of coagulation. [thromb- + G. *elastreō*, to push, + *graphō*, to write]

throm·bo·em·bo·lec·to·my (throm′bō-em-bō-lek′tō-mē). Extraction of an embolic thrombus. [thrombo- + G. *embolos*, embolus, + *ektomē*, excision]

throm·bo·em·bo·lism (throm′bō-em′bō-lizm). Embolism from a thrombus. [thrombo- + G. *embolismos*, embolism]

throm·bo·end·ar·ter·ec·to·my (throm′bō-end-ar-ter-ek′tō-mē). An operation that involves opening an artery, removing an occluding thrombus along with the intima and atheromatous material, and leaving a clean, fresh plane internal to the adventitia. [thrombo- + endarterectomy]

throm·bo·en·do·car·di·tis (throm′bō-en′dō-kar-dī′tis). SYN nonbacterial thrombotic *endocarditis*.

throm·bo·gen (throm′bō-jen). SYN prothrombin. [thrombo- + G. *-gen*, producing]

throm·bo·gene (throm′bō-jēn). SYN *factor* V.

throm·bo·gen·ic (throm-bō-jen′ik). **1.** Relating to thrombogen. **2.** Causing thrombosis or coagulation of the blood.

throm·boid (throm′boyd). Resembling a thrombus. [thrombo- + G. *eidos*, resemblance]

throm·bo·kat·i·ly·sin (throm′bō-kat-i-lī′sin). Obsolete term for factor VIII.

throm·bo·ki·nase (throm-bō-kī′nās). SYN thromboplastin.

throm·bol·ic (throm-bol′ik). Relating to a thrombolus.

throm·bo·lus (throm′bō-lŭs). An embolus composed mainly of agglutinated platelets. [thrombo- + G. *embolos*, embolus]

throm·bo·lym·phan·gi·tis (throm′bō-lim-fan-jī′tis). Inflammation of a lymphatic vessel with the formation of a lymph clot.

throm·bol·y·sis (throm-bol′i-sis). Fluidifying or dissolving of a thrombus. [thrombo- + G. *lysis*, a dissolving]

throm·bo·lyt·ic (throm-bō-lit′ik). Breaking up or dissolving a thrombus. SYN thromboclastic.

throm·bo·mod·u·lin (throm′bō-mo-doo-lin). A glycoprotein present in the plasma membrane of endothelial cells that binds

thrombin; participates in an additional regulatory mechanism in coagulation. [thrombo- + odulate + -in]

throm·bon. An all-inclusive term for circulating thrombocytes (blood platelets) and the cellular forms from which they arise (thromboblasts or megakaryocytes). It is analogous to erythron and leukon of the red and white blood cells, respectively.

throm·bo·ne·cro·sis (throm′bō-ne-krō′sis). Necrosis of the walls of a blood vessel, with thrombosis in the lumen.

throm·bop·a·thy (throm-bop′ă-thē). A nonspecific term applied to disorders of blood platelets resulting in defective thromboplastin, without obvious change in the appearance or number of platelets. [thrombo- + G. *pathos*, disease]

constitutional t., SYN Glanzmann *thrombasthenia*.

throm·bo·pe·nia (throm-bō-pē′nē-ă). SYN thrombocytopenia.

throm·bo·phil·ia (throm-bō-fil′ē-ă). A disorder of the hemopoietic system in which there is a tendency to the occurrence of thrombosis. [thrombo- + G. *philos*, fond]

throm·bo·phle·bi·tis (throm′bō-flĕ-bī′tis). Venous inflammation with thrombus formation. [thrombo- + G. *phleps*, vein, + *-itis*, inflammation]

t. mi′grans, creeping or slowly advancing t., appearing in first one vein and then another.

t. sal′tans, t. occurring in the same vein, but at a distance from the original lesion, or appearing suddenly in a distant vein.

throm·bo·plas·tid (throm-bō-plas′tid). **1.** SYN platelet. **2.** A nucleated spindle cell in submammalian blood. [thrombo- + G. *plastos*, formed]

throm·bo·plas·tin (throm-bō-plas′tin). A substance present in tissues, platelets, and leukocytes necessary for the coagulation of blood; in the presence of calcium ions t. is necessary for the conversion of prothrombin to thrombin, an important step in coagulation of blood. It is now generally believed that t. activity may be developed through blood (intrinsic) or tissue (extrinsic) systems. Tissue t. (factor III) interacts with factor VII and calcium to activate factor X; active factor X combines with factor V in the presence of calcium and phospholipid to produce t. activity (also commonly called t.). SYN platelet tissue factor, thrombokinase, thrombozyme, tissue factor, zymoplastic substance.

throm·bo·plas·tin·o·gen (throm′bō-plas-tin′ō-jen). Obsolete term for factor VIII.

throm·bo·poi·e·sis (throm′bō-poy-ē′sis). Precisely, the process of a clot forming in blood, but generally used with reference to the formation of blood platelets (thrombocytes). [thrombo- + G. *poiēsis*, a making]

thrombopoietin (throm′bō-poy′ĕ-tin). A cytokine that serves as a humoral regulator for the production of blood platelets through action on the receptor c-mp1. SYN megakaryocyte growth and development factor, megapoietin. [thrombo- + G. *poiētēs*, maker, + in]

throm·bosed (throm′bōsd). **1.** Clotted. **2.** Denoting a blood vessel that is the seat of thrombosis.

throm·bo·ses (throm-bō′sēz). Plural of thrombosis.

throm·bo·sin (throm′bō-sin). SYN thrombin.

throm·bo·sis, pl. **throm·bo·ses** (throm-bō′sis, -sēz). Formation or presence of a thrombus; clotting within a blood vessel which may cause infarction of tissues supplied by the vessel. [G. *thrombōsis*, a clotting, fr. *thrombos*, clot]

atrophic t., t. due to feebleness of the circulation, as in marasmus. SYN marantic t., marasmic t.

cerebral t., clotting of blood in a cerebral vessel.

compression t., t. due to arrest of the circulation in a vessel by compression, as from a tumor.

coronary t., coronary occlusion by thrombus formation, usually the result of atheromatous changes in the arterial wall and usually leading to myocardial infarction.

creeping t., a gradually increasing t. involving one section of a vein after another in continuity.

dilation t., t. due to slowed circulation consequent upon dilation of a vein.

effort-induced t., SYN Paget-von Schrötter *syndrome*.

marantic t., marasmic t., SYN atrophic t.

th

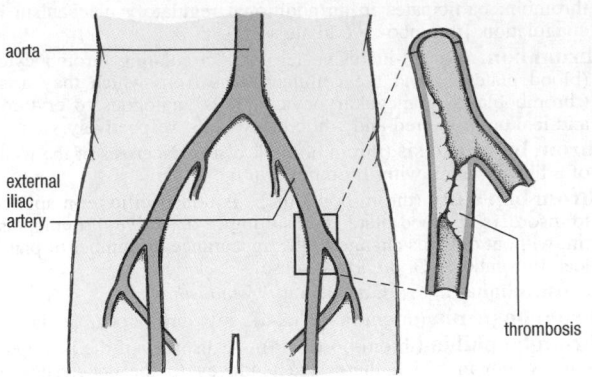

aorta

external
iliac
artery

thrombosis

thrombosis in the iliofemoral region

mural t., the formation of a thrombus in contact with the endocardial lining of a cardiac chamber, or a large blood vessel, if not occlusive.

placental t., t. of the veins of the uterus at the placental site.

plate t., platelet t., t. due to an abnormal accumulation of platelets.

posttraumatic arterial t., posttraumatic venous t., intravascular clotting due to injury to a vessel wall.

throm·bo·sta·sis (throm-bos′tă-sis). Local arrest of the circulation by thrombosis. [thrombo- + G. *stasis,* a standing]

throm·bo·sthe·nin (throm-bō-sthē′nin). SYN platelet *actomyosin.*

throm·bot·ic (throm-bot′ik). Relating to, caused by, or characterized by thrombosis.

throm·bo·to·nin (throm-bō-tō′nin). SYN serotonin.

throm·box·ane (throm-bok′sān). The formal parent of the thromboxanes; prostanoic acid in which the –COOH has been reduced to –CH₃ and an oxygen atom has been inserted between carbons 11 and 12.

throm·box·anes (throm′bok-zānz). A group of compounds, included in the eicosanoids, formally based on thromboxane, but with the terminal COOH group present; biochemically related to the prostaglandins and formed from them through a series of steps involving the formation of an endoperoxide (an O–O bridge between carbons 9 and 11 in the prostaglandins) by a cyclooxygenase, followed by a rearrangement (catalyzed by thromboxane synthase) that inserts one of the two oxygen atoms between carbons 11 and 12, leaving the other still bridging carbons 9 and 11. T. are so named from their influence on platelet aggregation and the formation of the oxygen-containing six-membered ring (pyran or oxane). Like the prostaglandins, individual t. (abbreviated TX) are designated by letters (A, B, C, etc.) and subscripts indicating structural features.

throm·bo·zyme (throm′bō-zīm). SYN thromboplastin.

throm·bus, pl. **throm·bi** (throm′bŭs, -bī). A clot in the cardiovascular systems formed during life from constituents of blood; it may be occlusive or attached to the vessel or heart wall without obstructing the lumen (mural t.). [L. fr. G. *thrombos,* a clot]

agglutinative t., SYN hyaline t.

agonal t., a heart clot formed during the act of dying after prolonged heart failure.

antemortem t., a clot formed in the circulation during life.

ball t., an unattached, spherical antemortem t. found in the left or right atrium usually in certain cases of mitral stenosis.

ball-valve t., ball t. intermittently occluding the mitral or tricuspid orifice.

bile t., an intracanalicular deposit of bile, usually a result of obstruction to bile drainage.

currant jelly t., SYN postmortem t.

fibrin t., a t. formed by repeated deposits of fibrin from the circulating blood; it usually does not completely occlude the vessel.

globular t., one of a number of thrombi of varying size, from a pea to a walnut, within the heart cavity, connected by a delicate fibrinous network.

hyaline t., a translucent colorless plug, partly or wholly filling a capillary or small artery or vein, formed by agglutination of red blood corpuscles. SYN agglutinative t.

infective t., a t. formed in septic phlebitis.

laminated t., a t. formed gradually by clotting of the blood in successive layers.

marantic t., marasmic t., a t. formed in cases of marasmus or general debility.

mixed t., a laminated t., the layers of different ages being of different color or consistency. SYN stratified t.

mural t., a t. formed on and attached to a diseased patch of endocardium, not on a valve or on one side of a large blood vessel. SEE ALSO parietal t.

obstructive t., a t. due to obstruction in the vessel from compression or other cause.

pale t., SYN white t.

parietal t., an arterial t. adhering to one side of the wall of the vessel. SEE ALSO mural t.

postmortem t., a clot formed within the heart or in a blood vessel after death, usually mainly red blood cells. SYN currant jelly t.

propagated t., SEE creeping *thrombosis.*

red t., a t. formed rapidly by the coagulation of stagnating blood, composed mainly of red blood cells rather than platelets.

secondary t., a t. formed about an embolus as a nucleus.

stratified t., SYN mixed t.

valvular t., a parietal t. that projects into the lumen of the vessel.

white t., an opaque dull white t. composed essentially of blood platelets. SYN pale t.

throughput (throo′put). A term applied to analytic instruments specifying the number of tests that can be performed in a given time.

thrush (thrŭsh). Infection of the oral tissues with *Candida albicans;* often an opportunistic infection in humans with AIDS or humans suffering from other conditions that depress the immune system; also common in normal infants who have been treated with antibiotics. [fr. the thrush fungus, *Candida albicans*]

thu·ja (thoo′jă, -yă). The fresh tops of *Thuja occidentalis* (family Pinaceae), an ornamental evergreen tree of eastern North America, a source of cedar leaf oil; has been used internally as an expectorant, emmenagogue, and anthelmintic, and externally as a mild counterirritant. SYN thuya. [G. *thyia,* an African tree with sweet-smelling wood]

t. oil, SYN cedar leaf oil.

thu·jol (thoo′jol). SYN thujone.

thu·jone (thoo′jōn). $C_{10}H_{16}O$; the chief constituent of cedar leaf oil; a stimulant and convulsant similar to camphor. SYN absinthol, tanacetol, tanacetone, thujol, thuyol, thuyone.

thu·li·um (Tm) (thoo′lē-ŭm). A metallic element of the lanthanide series, atomic no. 69, atomic wt. 168.93421. [L. *Thule,* the earliest name for Scandinavia]

thumb (thŭmb) [TA]. The first digit on the radial side of the hand. SYN pollex [TA], digitus (manus) primus✶, first finger. [A.S. *thuma*]

bifid t., a congenital malformed t. where the distal phalanx is divided.

gamekeeper's t., chronic radial subluxation of the metacarpophalangeal joint of the t.

hitchhiker t., malposition of the t., which, as a result of shortness of the first metacarpal, stands at right angles to the radial border of the hand and in the same place as it; a characteristic sign of diastrophic dwarfism.

tennis t., tendinitis with calcification in the tendon of the long flexor of the t. (flexor pollicis longus) caused by friction and strain as in tennis playing, but also occurring in other exercises in which the t. is subject to repeated pressure or strain.

thumb·print·ing (thŭm′print-ing). A radiographic sign of intestinal ischemia associated with hematoma formation and edema in the bowel wall; the thickened or edematous tissues encroach on the air- or contrast-filled lumen radiographically.

thumps (thŭmps). Spasmodic contractions of the diaphragm, or hiccups, occasionally seen in animals.

thus (thŭs, thoos). SYN olibanum. [L. incense]

thu·ya (thoo′yă). SYN thuja.

thu·yol, thu·yone (thoo′yol, thoo′yōn). SYN thujone.

Thy Abbreviation for thymine.

Thygeson, Phillips, U.S. ophthalmologist, *1903. SEE T. *disease*.

△**thym-.** SEE thymo-.

thyme (tīm). The dried leaves and flowering tops of *Thymus vulgaris* (family Labiatae), used as a condiment; it contains a volatile oil (t. oil) and is a source of thymol. [G. *thymon*, thyme]

t. oil, oil of t., a volatile oil distilled from the flowering plants of *Thymus vulgaris* or *T. zygis;* a flavoring agent.

thy·mec·to·my (thī-mek′tō-mē). Removal of the thymus gland. [thymus + G. *ektomē*, excision]

extended t., t. performed via combined sternotomy and a cervical incision to allow removal of all extraglandular thymic tissue. SYN maximal t.

maximal t., SYN extended t.

transcervical t., t. performed via a cervical incision only.

thy·mel·co·sis (thī-mel-kō′sis). Obsolete term for suppuration of the thymus gland. [thymus + G. *helkōsis*, ulceration]

△**thymi-.** SEE thymo-.

△**-thymia.** Mind, soul, emotions. SEE ALSO thymo- (2). [G. *thymos*, the mind or heart as the seat of strong feelings or passion]

thy·mic (thī′mik). Relating to the thymus gland.

thy·mic ac·id. SYN thymol. [see thyme]

thy·mi·co·lym·phat·ic (thī′mi-kō-lim-fat′ik). Relating to the thymus and the lymphatic system.

thy·mi·dine (dThd) (thī′mi-dēn). 1-(2-Deoxyribosyl)thymine; one of the four major nucleosides in DNA (the others being deoxyadenosine, deoxycytidine, and deoxyguanosine). SYN deoxythymidine, thymine deoxyribonucleoside.

t. phosphorylase, phosphorylase that catalyzes the phosphorolysis of t.; i.e., thymidine and P$_i$ react to form thymine and 2-deoxy-D-ribose 1-phosphate.

tritiated t., t. containing the hydrogen α-emitting radionuclide, tritium (^{3}H or hydrogen-3); used as a marker to measure and localize by radioautography the synthesis of DNA, into which it is incorporated.

thy·mi·dine 5′-di·phos·phate (dTDP). Thymidine esterified at its 5′ position with diphosphoric acid.

thy·mi·dine 5′-monophos·phate (dTMP). SYN thymidylic acid.

thy·mi·dine 5′-tri·phos·phate (dTTP). Thymidine esterified at its 5′ position with triphosphoric acid; the immediate precursor of thymidylic acid in DNA.

thy·mi·dyl·ate syn·thase (thī-mi-dil′āt). An enzyme catalyzing conversion of deoxyuridine 5′-monophosphate to thymidine 5′-monophosphate, the methyl group coming from N^5,N^{10}-methylenetetrahydrofolate.

thy·mi·dyl·ic ac·id (thī′mi-dil′ik). A major constituent of DNA. SYN thymidine 5′-monophosphate, thymine nucleotide.

thy·min (thī′min). SEE thymopoietin.

thy·mine (Thy) (thī′mēn, -min). 5-Methyluracil; a constituent of thymidylic acid and DNA; elevated in hyperuracil thyminuria.

t. deoxyribonucleoside, SYN thymidine.

t. deoxyribonucleotide, SYN deoxythymidylic acid.

t. nucleotide, SYN thymidylic acid.

thy·mi·nu·ria (thī-mēn-oor′ē-ă). SEE hyperuracil thyminuria.

thy·mi·tis (thī-mī′tis). Inflammation of the thymus gland.

△**thymo-, thym-, thymi-.** **1.** The thymus. [G. *thymos*] **2.** Mind, soul, emotions. [G. *thymos*, the mind or heart as the seat of strong feelings or passions] **3.** Wart, warty. [G. *thymos, thymion*]

thy·mo·cyte (thī′mō-sīt). A cell that develops in the thymus, seemingly from a stem cell of bone marrow and of fetal liver, and is the precursor of the thymus-derived lymphocyte (T lympho-

cyte) that effects cell-mediated (delayed type) sensitivity. [thymus + G. *kytos,* cell]

thy·mo·gen·ic (thī-mō-jen′ik). Of affective origin. [G. *thymos,* mind, + *genesis,* origin]

thy·mo·ki·net·ic (thī′mō-ki-net′ik). Activating the thymus gland. [thymus + G. *kinēsis,* movement]

thy·mol (thī′mol). A phenol present in the volatile oil of *Thymus vulgaris* (thyme), *Monarda punctata* (horsemint), and other volatile oils; used externally and internally as an antiseptic, as a deodorizer of offensive discharges, and as a specific for ancylostomiasis. SYN thyme camphor, thymic acid.

t. blue [C.I. 52025], a dye used as an acid-base indicator, with a pK value at 1.7 and another at 8.9; red at pH values below 1.2, yellow between 2.8 and 8.0, and blue above 9.6.

t. iodide, a dry powder antiseptic; has been used as a substitute for iodoform in skin diseases, wounds, ulcers, purulent rhinitis, otitis, etc.

thy·mo·ma (thī-mō′mă). A neoplasm in the anterior mediastinum, originating from thymic tissue, usually benign, and frequently encapsulated; occasionally invasive, but metastases are rare; histologically, consists of any type of thymic epithelial cell as well as lymphocytes that are usually abundant. Malignant lymphoma that involves the thymus, e.g., Hodgkin disease, should not be regarded as t. [thymus + G. *-oma,* tumor]

thy·mo·nu·cle·ase (thī-mō-noo′klē-ās). SYN *deoxyribonuclease* I.

thy·mo·poi·et·in (thī′mō-poy-ē′tin). Formerly called thymin; a polypeptide hormone that induces differentiation of lymphocytes to thymocytes. SEE ALSO thymic lymphopoietic *factor*.

thy·mo·pri·val, thy·mo·priv·ic, thy·mo·pri·vous (thī-mō-prī′văl, -priv′ik, -prī′vŭs). Relating to or marked by premature atrophy or removal of the thymus. [thymus + L. *privus,* deprived of]

thy·mo·sin (thī′mō-sin). A polypeptide hormone that restores T cell function in a thymectomized animal. SEE ALSO thymic lymphopoietic *factor*.

thy·mox·a·mine (thī-mok′să-mēn). SYN moxisylyte.

thy·mus, pl. **thy·mi, thy·mus·es** (thī′mŭs, thī′mī) [TA]. [NA] A primary lymphoid organ, located in the superior mediastinum and lower part of the neck, that is necessary in early life for the normal development of immunologic function. It reaches its greatest relative weight shortly after birth and its greatest absolute weight at puberty; it then begins to involute, and much of the lymphoid tissue is replaced by fat. The t. consists of two irregularly shaped parts united by a connective tissue capsule. Each part is partially subdivided by connective tissue septa into lobules, 0.5 to 2 mm in diameter, which consist of an inner medullary portion, continuous with the medullae of adjacent lobules, and an outer cortical portion. It is supplied by the inferior thyroid and internal thoracic arteries, and its nerves are derived from the vagus and sympathetic nerves. SYN thymus gland. [G. *thymos,* excrescence, sweetbread]

△**thyr-.** SEE thyro-.

△**thyreo-.** SEE thyro-.

△**thyro-, thyr-.** The thyroid gland. [see thyroid]

thy·ro·a·ce·tic ac·id (thī′rō-ă-sē′tik). A degradation product of thyronine (alanine side chain reduced to acetic acid), itself a degradation product (or precursor) of thyroxine.

thy·ro·ad·e·ni·tis (thī′rō-ad-ĕ-nī′tis). SYN thyroiditis. [thyro- + G. *adēn,* gland, + *-itis,* inflammation]

thy·ro·a·pla·sia (thī′rō-ă-plā′zē-ă). Anomalies observed in individuals with congenital defects of the thyroid gland and deficiency of its secretion. [thyro- + G. *a-* priv. + *plasis,* a molding]

thy·ro·ar·y·te·noid (thī′rō-ar′i-tē′noyd). Relating to the thyroid and arytenoid cartilages. SEE thyroarytenoid (*muscle*).

thy·ro·cal·ci·to·nin (thī′rō-kal-si-tō′nin). SYN calcitonin.

thy·ro·car·di·ac (thī-rō-kar′dē-ak). Affecting the heart as a result of hypo- or hyperthyroidism.

thy·ro·cele (thī′rō-sēl). A tumor of the thyroid gland, such as a goiter. [thyro- + G. *kēlē,* tumor]

thy·ro·cer·vi·cal (thī′rō-ser′vi-kăl). Relating to the thyroid gland and the neck, denoting an arterial trunk.

th

thy·ro·col·loid (thī-rō-kol′oyd). A colloid substance in the thyroid gland.

thy·ro·ep·i·glot·tic (thī′rō-ep-i-glot′ik). Relating to the thyroid cartilage and the epiglottis.

thy·ro·fis·sure (thī′rō-fish′er). SYN laryngofissure.

thy·ro·gen·ic, thy·rog·e·nous (thī-rō-jen′ik, -roj′ě-nŭs). Of thyroid gland origin. [thyroid + G. *-gen*, producing]

thy·ro·glob·u·lin (thī-rō-glob′ū-lin). **1.** A protein that contains precursors of thyroid hormone usually stored in the colloid within the thyroid follicles; biosynthesis of thyroid hormone entails iodination of the L-tyrosyl moieties of this protein and the combination of two iodotyrosines to form thyroxine, the fully iodinated thyronine; secretion of thyroid hormone requires proteolytic degradation of t., with the attendant release of free hormone; a defect in t. metabolism will lead to hypothyroidism. SYN iodoglobulin, thyroprotein (1). **2.** A substance obtained by the fractionation of thyroid glands from the hog, *Sus scrofa*, containing not less than 0.7% of total iodine; used as a thyroid hormone in the treatment of hypothyroidism.

thy·ro·glos·sal (thī-rō-glos′ăl). Relating to the thyroid gland and the tongue, denoting especially an embryologic duct. SYN thyrolingual.

thy·ro·hy·al (thī-rō-hī′ăl). The greater cornu of the hyoid bone.

thy·ro·hy·oid (thī-rō-hī′oyd). Relating to the thyroid cartilage and the hyoid bone. SEE thyrohyoid (*muscle*).

thy·roid (thī′royd). **1.** Resembling a shield; denoting a gland (t. gland) and a cartilage of the larynx (t. cartilage) having such a shape. **2.** The cleaned, dried, and powdered t. gland obtained from one of the domesticated animals used for food and containing 0.17–0.23% of iodine; formerly widely used in the treatment of hypothyroidism, cretinism, and myxedema, in certain cases of obesity, and in skin disorders. [G. *thyreoeidēs*, fr. *thyreos*, an oblong shield, + *eidos*, form]

accessory t., SYN accessory thyroid *gland*.

thy·roi·dea (thī-roy′dē-ă). SYN thyroid *gland*.

t. acces·so′ria, t. i′ma, SYN accessory thyroid *gland*.

thy·roid·ec·to·my (thī-roy-dek′tō-mē). Removal of the thyroid gland. [thyroid + G. *ektomē*, excision]

"chemical" t., jargon for the reduction of thyroid function produced by the administration of antithyroid drugs. SEE ALSO radiothyroidectomy.

near-total t., removal of nearly all of each thyroid lobe leaving unresected only a small portion of gland adjacent to the entrance of the recurrent laryngeal nerve into the larynx.

subtotal t., removal of at least one thyroid lobe and up to a near-total thyroidectomy.

thy·roid·ism (thī′roy-dizm). Obsolete designation for: **1.** SYN hyperthyroidism. **2.** Poisoning by overdoses of a thyroid extract.

thy·roid·i·tis (thī-roy-dī′tis). Inflammation of the thyroid gland. SYN thyroadenitis. [thyroid + G. *-itis*, inflammation]

autoimmune t., SYN Hashimoto t.

chronic atrophic t., replacement of the thyroid gland by fibrous tissue, the commonest cause of myxedema in older persons.

chronic fibrous t., SYN Riedel t.

chronic lymphadenoid t., SYN Hashimoto t.

chronic lymphocytic t., SYN Hashimoto t.

de Quervain t., SYN subacute granulomatous t.

focal lymphocytic t., focal infiltration of the thyroid by lymphocytes and plasma cells. SEE ALSO Hashimoto t.

giant cell t., SYN subacute granulomatous t.

giant follicular t., a variant of Hashimoto t. in which lymphocytic infiltrate in thyroid has formed into giant follicles.

Hashimoto t., diffuse infiltration of the thyroid gland with lymphocytes, resulting in diffuse goiter, progressive destruction of the parenchyma and hypothyroidism. SYN autoimmune t., chronic lymphadenoid t., chronic lymphocytic t., Hashimoto disease, Hashimoto struma, lymphocytic t., struma lymphomatosa.

ligneous t., SYN Riedel t.

lymphocytic t., SYN Hashimoto t.

parasitic t., chronic South American trypanosomiasis with involvement of the thyroid gland, causing myxedema.

Riedel t., a rare fibrous induration of the thyroid gland, with adhesion to adjacent structures, which may cause tracheal compression. SYN chronic fibrous t., ligneous struma, ligneous t., Riedel disease, Riedel struma.

subacute granulomatous t., t. with round cell (usually lymphocytes) infiltration, destruction of thyroid cells, epithelial giant cell proliferation, and evidence of regeneration; thought by some to be a reflection of a systemic infection and not an example of true chronic t. SYN de Quervain t., giant cell t.

subacute lymphocyte t., a subacute variant of Hashimoto t.

thy·roi·dol·o·gy (thī-roy-dol′ō-jē). The study of the thyroid gland, both normal and pathologic. [thyroid + G. *logos*, study]

thy·roid·o·to·my (thī′roy-dot′ō-mē). SYN laryngofissure. [thyroid + G. *tomē*, incision]

thy·ro·in·tox·i·ca·tion. SYN hyperthyroidism.

thy·ro·la·ryn·ge·al (thī′rō-lă-rin′jē-ăl). Relating to the thyroid gland or cartilage and the larynx.

thy·ro·lib·er·in (thī-rō-lib′er-in). A tripeptide hormone from the hypothalamus, which stimulates the anterior lobe of the hypophysis to release thyrotropin; L-pyroglutamyl-L-histidyl-L-prolinamide. SYN thyroid-stimulating hormone-releasing factor, thyrotropin-releasing hormone. [thyrotropin + L. libero, to free, + -in]

thy·ro·lin·gual (thī′rō-ling′gwăl). SYN thyroglossal. [thyro- + L. *lingua*, tongue]

thy·ro·lyt·ic (thī-rō-lit′ik). Causing destruction of thyroid gland cells. [thyro- + G. *lytikos*, dissolving]

thy·ro·meg·a·ly (thī-rō-meg′ă-lē). Enlargement of the thyroid gland. [thyro- + G. *megas*, large]

thy·ro·nine (thī′rō-nēn, -nin). An amino acid with a diphenyl ether group in the side chain; occurs in proteins only in the form of iodinated derivatives (iodothyronines), such as thyroxine.

thy·ro·pal·a·tine (thī-rō-pal′ă-tīn). Denoting the palatopharyngeus muscle.

thy·ro·par·a·thy·roid·ec·to·my (thī′rō-par-ă-thī′roy-dek′tō-mē). Excision of thyroid and parathyroid glands.

thy·rop·a·thy (thī-rop′ă-thē). A disorder of the thyroid gland. [thyro- + G. *pathos*, suffering]

thy·ro·per·ox·i·dase (thī-rō-per-oks′i-dās). A protein that participates in iodine metabolism in the thyroid follicle or in the follicular space; it utilized H_2O_2 to produce I^+.

thy·ro·pha·ryn·ge·al (thī-rō-fă-rin′jē-ăl). Denoting the thyropharyngeal portion of the inferior pharyngeal constrictor muscle.

thy·ro·plas·ty. A surgical method of restoring vocal quality by altering the geometry of the thyroid cartilage. [thyro- + G. *plastos*, formed]

thy·ro·pri·val (thī-rō-prī′văl). Relating to thyroprivia, denoting hypothyroidism produced by disease or thyroidectomy. SYN thyroprivic, thyroprivous. [thyro- + L. *privus*, deprived of]

thy·ro·priv·i·a (thī-rō-priv′ē-ă). A state characterized by reduced activity of the thyroid.

thy·ro·priv·ic, thy·ro·pri·vous (thī-rō-priv′ik, -priv′ŭs). SYN thyroprival.

thy·ro·pro·tein (thī-rō-prō′tēn). **1.** SYN thyroglobulin (1). **2.** An iodinated protein, usually casein, that has thyroxine activity.

thy·rop·to·sis (thī-rop-tō′sis). Downward dislocation of the thyroid gland. [thyro- + G. *ptōsis*, a falling]

thy·rot·o·my (thī′rot′ō-mē). **1.** Any cutting operation on the thyroid gland. **2.** SYN laryngofissure. [thyro- + G. *tomē*, a cutting]

thy·ro·tox·ic (thī-rō-tok′sik). Denoting thyrotoxicosis.

thy·ro·tox·i·co·sis (thī′rō-tok-si-kō′sis). The state produced by excessive quantities of endogenous or exogenous thyroid hormone. [thyro- + G. *toxikon*, poison, + *-osis*, condition]

apathetic t., chronic t., presenting as cardiac disease or as a wasting syndrome, with weakness of proximal muscles and depression but with few of the more typical clinical manifestations of t.

t. medicamento′sa, a hyperthyroid state resulting from excessive doses of thyroid hormone preparation.

thy·ro·tox·in (thī-rō-tok′sin). **1.** A hypothetical substance formerly believed to be an abnormal product of diffusely hyperplastic thyroid glands in persons with Graves disease, and presumed to be the cause of the distinctive signs and symptoms of that condition (in contrast to simple hyperthyroidism). **2.** A complement-fixing antigenic factor associated with certain diseases of the thyroid gland. **3.** Rarely used term referring to any material toxic to thyroidal tissue.

thy·ro·troph (thī′rō-trof). A cell in the anterior lobe of the pituitary that produces thyrotropin.

thy·ro·tro·phic (thī-rō-trof′ik). SYN thyrotropic. [thyro- + G. trophē, nourishment]

thy·rot·ro·phin (thī-rot′rō-fin, thī-rō-trō′fin). SYN thyrotropin.

thy·ro·tro·pic (thī-rō-trop′ik). Stimulating or nurturing the thyroid gland. SYN thyrotrophic. [thyro- + G. tropē, a turning]

thy·rot·ro·pin (thī-rot′rō-pin, thī-rō-trō′pin). A glycoprotein hormone produced by the anterior lobe of the hypophysis that stimulates the growth and function of the thyroid gland; it also is used as a diagnostic test to differentiate primary and secondary hypothyroidism. SYN thyroid-stimulating hormone, thyrotrophin, thyrotropic hormone. [for thyrotrophin, fr. thyro- + G. trophē, nourishment; corrupted to -tropin, and reanalyzed as fr. G. tropē, a turning]

thy·rox·ine (T_4), **thy·rox·in** (thī-rok′sēn, -sin). The L-isomer is the active iodine compound existing normally in the thyroid gland and extracted therefrom in crystalline form for therapeutic use; also prepared synthetically; used for the relief of hypothyroidism, cretinism, and myxedema.

labeled t., SYN radioactive t.

radioactive t., t. in which a radioisotope of iodine (^{125}I or ^{131}I) is incorporated into its molecule; used in experiments tracing the metabolism of t. SYN labeled t., radiolabeled t., radiothyroxin.

radiolabeled t., SYN radioactive t.

t. sodium, a preparation obtained by the action of a limited amount of sodium carbonate upon t.; it contains between 61 and 65% of iodine. SEE sodium levothyroxine, sodium liothyronine.

Thys·a·no·so·ma ac·ti·noi·des (this-ă-nō-sō′mă ak-ti-noyd′ēz). Fringed tapeworm of sheep, a relatively short, thick worm (family Anocephalidae) in which the posterior borders of the proglottids are fringed. It inhabits the small intestine, but often invades the bile ducts and causes many livers to be condemned for human food. It is essentially nonpathogenic and is common in stock-raising countries, where it infects a wide variety of ruminants; oribatid mites are probably the vectors.

TI The delay time between the inverting pulse and the "read" pulse in the inversion recovery experiment, in magnetic resonance imaging.

Ti Symbol for titanium.

TIA Abbreviation for transient ischemic *attack.*

tib·ia, gen. and pl. **tib·i·ae** (tib′ē-ă, tib′ē-ē) [TA]. The medial and larger of the two bones of the leg, articulating with the femur, fibula, and talus. SYN shin bone. [L. the large shinbone]

saber t., deformity of the t. occurring in tertiary syphilis or yaws, the bone having a marked forward convexity as a result of the formation of gummas and periostitis.

t. val′ga, SYN *genu* valgum.

t. va′ra, SYN *genu* varum.

tib·i·ad (tib′ē-ad). In a direction toward the tibia. [tibia + L. ad, to]

tib·i·al (tib′ē-ăl) [TA]. Relating to the tibia or to any structure named from it; also denoting the medial or tibial aspect of the lower limb. SYN tibialis [TA]. [L. tibialis]

tib·i·a·le pos·ti·cum (tib-ē-ā′lē pos-tī′kŭm). SYN os tibiale posterius.

tib·i·a·lis (tib-ē-ā′lis) [TA]. SYN tibial. [L.]

△**tibio-.** The tibia. [L. tibia, the shinbone]

tib·i·o·cal·ca·ne·an (tib′ē-ō-kal-kā′nē-an). Relating to the tibia and the calcaneus.

tib·i·o·fas·ci·a·lis (tib-ē-ō-fas-ē-ā′lis). See entries under musculus tibiofascialis.

tib·i·o·fem·o·ral (tib-ē-ō-fem′ō-răl). Relating to the tibia and the femur.

tib·i·o·fib·u·lar (tib-ē-ō-fib′ū-lăr). Relating to both tibia and fibula; denotes especially the joints and ligaments between the two bones. SYN peroneotibial, tibioperoneal.

tib·i·o·na·vic·u·lar (tib-ē-ō-na-vik′ū-lăr). Relating to the tibia and the navicular bone of the tarsus. SYN tibioscaphoid.

tib·i·o·per·o·ne·al (tib′ē-ō-per′ō-nē′ăl). SYN tibiofibular.

tib·i·o·scaph·oid (tib′ē-ō-skaf′oyd). SYN tibionavicular.

tib·i·o·tar·sal (tib-ē-ō-tar′săl). Relating to the tarsal bones and the tibia. SYN tarsotibial.

tic (tik). Habitual, repeated contraction of certain muscles, resulting in stereotyped individualized actions that can be voluntarily suppressed for only brief periods, e.g., clearing the throat, sniffing, pursing the lips, excessive blinking; especially prominent when the person is under stress; there is no known pathologic substrate. SEE ALSO spasm. SYN Brissaud disease, habit chorea, habit spasm. [Fr.]

convulsive t., SYN facial t.

t. de pensée, a rarely used term for the habit of involuntarily giving expression to any thought that comes to mind. [Fr. of thought]

t. douloureux, SYN trigeminal *neuralgia.* [Fr. painful]

facial t., involuntary twitching of the facial muscles, sometimes unilateral. SYN Bell spasm, convulsive t., facial spasm, palmus (1).

glossopharyngeal t., SYN glossopharyngeal *neuralgia.*

habit t., a habitual repetition of some grimace, shrug of the shoulder, twisting or jerking of the head, or the like.

local t., a t. of very limited extent, as the winking of an eye or a twitch of a finger.

psychic t., a gesture or exclamation made under the influence of an irresistible morbid impulse.

rotatory t., SYN spasmodic *torticollis.*

spasmodic t., a disorder in which sudden spasmodic coordinated movements of certain muscles or groups of physiologically related muscles occur at irregular intervals. SYN Henoch chorea.

ti·car·cil·lin di·so·di·um (tī-kar-sil′in). The disodium salt of 6-(α-carboxy-α-thien-3-ylacetamido)penicillanic acid; a bactericidal antibiotic useful in treating *Pseudomonas aeruginosa* infections and similar in effect to carbenicillin disodium.

tick (tik). An acarine of the families Ixodidae (hard t.'s) or Argasidae (soft t.'s), which contain many bloodsucking species that are important pests of humans and domestic birds and mammals, and that probably exceed all other arthropods in the number and variety of disease agents that they transmit. T.'s are differentiated from the much smaller true mites by possession of an armed hypostome and a pair of tracheal spiracular openings located behind the basal segment of the third or fourth pair of walking legs; the larva (seed t.) has six legs, and after molting appears as an eight-limbed nymph. Some important t.'s are *Amblyomma americanum* (Lone Star t.) and *A. hebraeum* (South African bont t.); *Argas persicus* (adobe, fowl, or Persian t.) and *A. reflexus* (pigeon t.); *Boophilus* (cattle t.'s); *Dermacentor albopictus* (horse or winter t.), *D. andersoni* (Rocky Mountain spotted fever or wood t.), *D. nitens* (tropical horse t.), *D. occidentalis* (Pacific or wood t.), and *D. variabilis* (American dog t.); *Haemaphysalis chordeilis* (bird t.) and *H. laporis-palustris* (rabbit t.); *Ixodes pacificus* (California black-legged t.), *I. pilosus* (paralysis t.), *I. ricinus* (castor bean t.), and *I. scapularis* (black-legged or shoulder t.); *Ornithodoros coriaceus* (pajaroello t.) and *O. moubata* (African relapsing fever or tampan t.); and *Rhipicephalus everti* (African red t.), *R. sanguineus* (brown dog t.), and *R. simus* (black-pitted t.).

tick·ling (tik′ling). Denoting a peculiar itching or tingling sensation caused by excitation of surface nerves, as of the skin by light stroking.

ticolubant (tī-kol′oo-bant). A leukotriene B_4 receptor antagonist used as an antipsoriatic.

t.i.d. Abbreviation for L. ter in die, three times a day.

ti

tid·al (tī′dăl). Relating to or resembling the tides, alternately rising and falling.

tide (tīd). An alternate rise and fall, ebb and flow, or an increase or a decrease. [A.S. *tīd*, time]

acid t., a temporary increase in the acidity of the urine occurring during fasting. SYN acid wave.

alkaline t., a period of urinary neutrality or even alkalinity after meals due to withdrawal of hydrogen ion for the purpose of secretion of the highly acid gastric juice. SYN alkaline wave.

fat t., an increase in the fat content of blood and lymph following a meal.

red t., a natural phenomenon resulting from higher than normal concentrations of the microscopic algae *Gymnodinium breve* in seawater. [when the causative organism is extremely concentrated, sea water can have a reddish-brown color.]

Tiedemann, Friedrich, German anatomist, 1781–1861. SEE T. *gland*, *nerve*.

Tietze, Alexander, German surgeon, 1864–1927. SEE T. *syndrome*.

tig·late (tig′lāt). A salt or ester of tiglic acid.

tig·li·an (tig′lē-ăn). Original trivial name for the saturated form of phorbol. [fr. *Croton tiglium* (Euphorbiaceae)]

tig·lic ac·id (tig′lik). An unsaturated fatty acid present in glycerides in croton oil.

ti·glyl-CoA (tig′lil). An intermediate in the degradation of L-isoleucine. SYN tiglyl-coenzyme A.

ti·glyl-coen·zyme A. SYN tiglyl-CoA.

ti·groid (tī′groyd). SEE chromophil *substance*. [G. *tigroeidēs*, fr. *tigris*, tiger, + *eidos*, appearance]

ti·grol·y·sis (tī-grol′i-sis). SYN chromatolysis. [tigroid + G. *lysis*, dissolution]

TIL. Abbreviation for tumor-infiltrating *lymphocytes*, under *lymphocyte*.

Tillaux, Paul Jules, French surgeon, 1834–1904. SEE *spiral* of T.

til·or·one (til′or-ōn). A small synthetic molecule used to induce interferon in mice.

TILS Abbreviation for tumor-infiltrating *lymphocytes*, under *lymphocyte*.

tilt (tilt). Slope.

pantoscopic t., an oblique astigmatism caused by slanting a spherical lens so that light rays strike the lens at a nonperpendicular angle, altering the spherical and cylindrical refractive power of the lens.

tim·bre (tam′br, tim′br). The distinguishing quality of a sound, by which one may determine its source, based principally on the distribution of overtones. SYN tone color. [Fr.]

time (t) (tīm). **1.** That relation of events which is expressed by the terms past, present, and future, and measured by units such as minutes, hours, days, months, or years. **2.** A certain period during which something definite or determined is done. SYN tempus (2). [A.S. *tima*]

activated clotting t. (ACT), the most common test used for coagulation t. in cardiovascular surgery.

activated partial thromboplastin t. (aPTT), the t. needed for plasma to form a fibrin clot following the addition of calcium and a phospholipid reagent; used to evaluate the intrinsic clotting system.

AH conduction t., SEE atrioventricular *conduction*.

association t., t. elasping between a stimulus and the verbalized response to it.

biologic t., the concept that our appreciation of t. varies with age and is governed by the neural organization of the individual; it obeys a logarithmic rather than an arithmetic law.

bleeding t., the t. interval between the appearance of the first drop of blood and the removal of the last drop following puncture of the ear lobe or the finger, usually 1–3 min; it provides a global but imprecise evaluation of platelet and capillary function.

circulation t., the t. taken for the blood to pass through a given circuit of the vascular system, e.g., the pulmonary or systemic circulation, from one arm to another, from arm to tongue, or from arm to lung; it is measured by the injection into an arm vein of a substance, such as sodium dehydrocholate, ether, fluorescein, histamine, or a radium salt, which can be detected when it arrives at another point in the vascular system.

clot retraction t., the t. required for a blood clot to separate from the tube wall and express serum, usually completed in 18–24 hours, but retarded or absent in persons with thrombocytopenic purpura.

clotting t., SYN coagulation t.

coagulation t., the t. required for blood to coagulate. SYN clotting t.

doubling t., the t. it takes for the number of cells in a neoplasm to double, with shorter doubling times implying more rapid growth.

euglobulin clot lysis t., a measure of the ability of plasminogen activators and plasmin to lyse a clot; normally, clot lysis is determined by the balance of factors which activate fibrinolysis (plasminogen activators and plasmin) and those which inhibit lysis; in certain conditions (e.g., carcinoma or hepatic insufficiency) activating factors predominate and can be measured by noting the t. it takes the euglobulin fraction of plasma (excluding inhibitors of fibrinolysis) to clot.

fading t., the t. required for a constant stimulus applied to a fixed area of the peripheral visual field to stop.

t. of flight, the t. for a photon created by annihilation of a positron-electron pair to reach a detector; since annihilation photons are created in pairs and travel in opposite directions at about 3×10^{10} cm/sec, measurement of the difference in arrival t. at detectors with subnanosecond resolution allows calculation of the location of the event; the basic physics of positron emission tomography.

forced expiratory t. (FET), the t. taken to expire a given volume or a given fraction of vital capacity during measurement of forced vital capacity; subscripts specify the exact parameters measured.

half-t., SEE half-time.

HR conduction t., SEE intraventricular *conduction*.

HV conduction t., SEE intraventricular *conduction*.

inertia t., the interval elapsing between the reception of the stimulus from a nerve and the contraction of the muscle.

interatrial conduction t., SYN intraatrial conduction t. (2).

intraatrial conduction t., (1) the total duration of electrical activity of the atria in one cardiac cycle; (2) the time between right atrial and left atrial activation. SYN interatrial conduction t.

left ventricular ejection t. (LVET), the t. measured clinically from onset to incisural notch of the carotid or other pulse; properly, the time of ejection of blood from the left ventricle beginning with aortic valve opening and ending with aortic valve closure.

PA conduction t., SEE atrioventricular *conduction*.

partial thromboplastin t. (PTT), SEE activated partial thromboplastin t.

PH conduction t., SEE atrioventricular *conduction*.

prothrombin t. (PT), the t. required for clotting after thromboplastin and calcium are added in optimal amounts to blood of normal fibrinogen content; if prothrombin is diminished, the clotting t. increases; used to evaluate the extrinsic clotting system. SEE ALSO prothrombin *test*.

reaction t., the interval between the presentation of a stimulus and the responsive reaction to it.

recognition t., the interval between the application of a stimulus and the recognition of its nature.

relaxation t. (τ), the time required for the substrate in an enzymatic or chemical reaction to fall to 1/e of its initial value.

repetition t. (TR), in magnetic resonance imaging, the t. between repetitions of the pulse sequence.

rise t., (1) the t. required for a pulse or echo to rise from onset to its peak amplitude; (2) the t. required for a pulse or echo to rise from 10–90% peak amplitude.

running t., the t. during which an activity (e.g., chromatography development) occurs.

Russell's viper venom clotting t., a clotting t. determination performed on citrated platelet-poor plasma using Russell's viper *venom* as an activating agent. This allows activation of factor X directly without the need for other coagulation factors and is used to confirm factor X defects. SEE ALSO Stypven time *test*.

sensation t., the minimal t. a visual image must be exposed in order to be perceived.

sinoatrial conduction t. (SACT), the t. required for an impulse to travel from sinus node to atrium; estimated indirectly during reset nodus sinuatrialis period by halving the average interval from the premature beat to the following normal sinus beat of the atrium.

sinoatrial recovery t. (SART), interval from the last paced P wave to the first succeeding spontaneous P wave (after 2–5 min of right atrial pacing at 120–140 beats/min, and when expressed as percentage of control cycle length, it normally ranges from 115–159%).

survival t., (1) the period elapsing between the completion or institution of any procedure and death; **(2)** the lifespan of biologically or physically marked erythrocytes or other cells.

thrombin t., the t. needed for a fibrin clot to form after the addition of thrombin to citrated plasma; prolonged thrombin t. is seen in patients receiving heparin therapy.

tissue thromboplastin inhibition t., a test used to identify lupus anticoagulant; the thromboplastin source used in the prothrombin test is diluted to increase sensitivity to inhibitors.

utilization t., the minimum duration of a stimulus of rheobasic strength that is just sufficient to produce excitation. SYN temps utile.

TIMI Acronym for *t*hrombolysis *i*n *m*yocardial *i*nfarction; a large multicenter controlled clinical trial.

tim·no·don·ic ac·id (tim-nō-don′ok).   A 20-carbon fatty acid with five *cis* double bonds located on carbons 5, 8, 11, 14, and 17; an important component of fish oils; a precursor to the 3-series prostaglandins, e.g., PGE$_3$.

ti·mo·lol ma·le·ate (tī′mō-lōl).   A β-adrenergic blocking agent used in the treatment of hypertension and used in eyedrops in the treatment of chronic open-angle glaucoma.

tin (Sn) (tin).   A metallic element, atomic no. 50, atomic wt. 118.710. SYN stannum. [AS, tin]

t. oxide, SYN stannic oxide.

tin-113 (¹¹³Sn).   A radioisotope of tin with a physical half-life of 115.1 days; used in the manufacture of radionuclide generators for the production of indium-113m.

tinct.   Abbreviation of L. *tinctura*, tincture.

tinc·ta·ble (tingk′tă-bl).   Stainable.

tinc·tion (tingk′shŭn).   **1.** A stain; a preparation for staining. **2.** The act of staining. [L. *tingo*, pp. *tinctus*, to dye]

tinc·to·ri·al (tingk-tōr′ē-ăl).   Relating to coloring or staining. [L. *tinctorius*, fr. *tingo*, to dye]

tinc·tu·ra, gen. and pl. **tinc·tu·rae** (tingk-too′ră, -rē).   SYN tincture. [L. a dyeing, fr. *tingo*, pp. *tinctus*, to dye]

tinc·ture (tingk′choor).   An alcoholic or hydroalcoholic solution prepared from vegetable materials or from chemical substances; most t.'s are prepared by percolation or by maceration. The proportions of drug represented in the different t.'s are not uniform, but vary according to the established standards for each. T.'s of potent drugs essentially represent the activity of 10 g of the drug in each 100 mL of t., the potency being adjusted after assay; most other t.'s represent 20 g of drug in each 100 mL of t. Compound t.'s are made according to long-established formulas. SYN tinctura.

alcoholic t., a t. made with undiluted alcohol.

ammoniated t., a t. made with ammoniated alcohol.

belladonna t., a green hydroalcoholic mobile liquid containing the alkaloids atropine and scopolamine and other substances extracted from the leaves of *Atropa belladonna*, the botanical source for these anticholinergic drugs. The t. allows for gradual titration of dose by counting drops of the preparation ingested. Formerly widely used in ulcer therapy or the symptomatic treatment of diarrhea, alone or in combination with antacids and insoluble clays.

digitalis t., an hydroalcoholic solution containing the glycosides of the leaves of the foxglove (digitalis) plant *Digitalis purpurea* or *D. lanata*. Although digitalis preparations are used extensively, they are currently used as the pure glycosides, digoxin and digi-

toxin. The t. was formerly widely used but was standardized by bioassay using frogs, cats, or pigeons.

ethereal t., a class of preparations consisting of 10% percolations of drugs in a menstruum of ether (1) and alcohol (2).

glycerinated t., a t. made with diluted alcohol to which glycerin is added to facilitate the extraction or to preserve the preparation.

green soap t., a liquid preparation containing potassium soaps and alcohol; frequently advocated in skin cleansing, particularly after exposure to plant toxins such as poison ivy.

hydroalcoholic t., a t. made with diluted alcohol in various proportions with water.

tine (tīn).   **1.** In dentistry, the slender, pointed end of an explorer. **2.** An instrument used to introduce antigen, such as tuberculin into the skin, and usually containing several individual t.'s. [A.S. *tind*, a prong]

tin·ea (tin′ē-ă).   A fungus infection (dermatophytosis) of the keratin component of hair, skin, or nails. Genera of fungi causing such infection are *Microsporum*, *Trichophyton*, and *Epidermophyton*. SYN ringworm, serpigo (1). [L. worm, moth]

t. bar′bae, a fungus infection of the beard, occurring as a follicular infection or as a granulomatous lesion; the primary lesions are papules and pustules. SYN barber itch, folliculitis barbae, ringworm of beard, t. sycosis.

t. cap′itis, a common form of fungus infection of the scalp caused by various species of *Microsporum* and *Trichophyton* on or within hair shafts, occurring most commonly in children and characterized by irregularly placed and variously sized patches of apparent baldness because of hairs breaking off at the surface of the scalp, scaling, black dots (see black-dot *ringworm*), and occasionally erythema and pyoderma. SYN ringworm of scalp.

t. circina′ta, SYN t. corporis.

t. cor′poris, a well-defined, scaling, macular eruption of dermatophytosis that frequently forms annular lesions and may appear on any part of the body. SYN ringworm of body, t. circinata.

t. favo′sa, SYN favus.

t. glabro′sa, ringworm or fungus infection of the hairless skin.

t. imbrica′ta, an eruption consisting of a number of concentric rings of overlapping scales forming papulosquamous patches scattered over the body; it occurs in tropical climates and is caused by the fungus *Trichophyton concentricum*. SYN Oriental ringworm, scaly ringworm, Tokelau ringworm.

t. ke′rion, an inflammatory fungus infection of the scalp and beard, marked by pustules and a boggy infiltration of the surrounding parts; most commonly caused by *Microsporum audouinii*.

t. ma′nus, ringworm of the hand, usually referring to infections of the palmar surface. SEE ALSO t. corporis.

t. ni′gra, a fungus infection due to *Exophiala werneckii*, marked by dark lesions giving a spattered appearance and occurring most commonly on the palms of the hands. SYN pityriasis nigra.

t. pe′dis, dermatophytosis of the feet, especially of the skin between the toes, caused by one of the dermatophytes, usually a species of *Trichophyton* or *Epidermophyton;* the disease consists of small vesicles, fissures, scaling, maceration, and eroded areas between the toes and on the plantar surface of the foot; other skin areas may be involved. SYN athlete's foot, dermatomycosis pedis, ringworm of foot.

t. profun′da, SYN Majocchi *granulomas*, under *granuloma*.

t. syco′sis, SYN t. barbae.

t. tonsu′rans, t. capitis or t. corporis caused by the fungus *Trichophyton tonsurans;* characterized by small plaques and fewer broken off hairs than in t. capitis caused by other species.

t. un′guium, ringworm of the nails due to a dermatophyte.

t. versic′olor, an eruption of tan or brown branny patches on the skin of the trunk, often appearing white, in contrast with hyperpigmented skin after exposure to the summer sun; caused by growth of the fungus *Malassezia furfur* in the stratum corneum with minimal inflammatory reaction. SYN pityriasis versicolor.

Tinel, Jules, French neurologist, 1879–1952. SEE T. *sign*.

tin·foil (tin′foyl).   **1.** Tin rolled into extremely thin sheets. **2.** A base metal foil used as a separating material, as between the cast and denture base material during flasking and curing procedures.

ti

tin·gi·bil·i·ty (tin′ji-bil′i-tē). The property of being tingible.

tin·gi·ble (tin′ji-bl). Capable of being stained. [L. *tingo,* to dye]

tin·gle (ting′gl). To feel a peculiar pricking sensation.

tin·gling (ting′ling). A pricking type of paresthesia.

distal t. on percussion (DTP), SYN Tinel *sign.*

ti·nid·a·zole (ti-nid′ă-zōl). An antiprotozoal agent.

tin·ni·tus (ti-nī′tŭs). Noises (ringing, whistling, hissing, roaring, booming, etc.) in the ears. [L. a jingling, fr. *tinnio,* pp. *tinnitus,* to jingle, clink]

t. au′rium, sensation of sound in one or both ears usually associated with disease in the middle ear, the inner ear, or the central auditory pathways. SYN syrigmus.

t. cere′bri, subjective sensation of noise in head rather than ears.

clicking t., an objective clicking sound in the ear in cases of chronic catarrhal otitis media; it may be audible to the bystander as well as to the patient and is supposed to be due to an opening and closing of the mouth of the eustachian tube, or to a rhythmical spasm of the velum palati.

Leudet t., a dry spasmodic click, audible also through the otoscope, heard in catarrhal inflammation of the eustachian tube; caused by reflex spasm of the tensor palati muscle.

tint. A shade of color varying according to the amount of white admixed with the pigment. [L. *tingo,* pp. *tinctus,* to dye]

ti·o·con·a·zole (tī-ō-kon′ă-zōl). An antifungal agent.

tip. 1. A point; a more or less sharp extremity. **2.** A separate, but attached, piece of the same or another structure, forming the extremity of a part.

t. of auricle, SYN *apex* of auricle.

t. of ear, ⋆official alternate term for *apex* of auricle.

t. of elbow, SYN olecranon.

t. of nose, ⋆official alternate term for *apex* of nose.

t. of posterior horn, SYN *apex* of posterior horn.

root t., SYN root *apex.*

t. of tongue, ⋆official alternate term for *apex* of tongue.

t. of tooth root, SYN root *apex.*

Woolner t., SYN *apex* of auricle.

tip·ping. A tooth movement in which the angulation of the long axis of the tooth is altered.

ti·pren·o·lol hy·dro·chlo·ride (tip-ren′ō-lol). A β-receptor blocking agent.

TIPS Acronym for transjugular intrahepatic portosystemic *shunt.*

Tiselius, Arne W.K., Swedish biochemist and Nobel laureate, 1902–1971. SEE T. *apparatus,* electrophoresis *cell.*

Tis·si·er·el·la prae·acuta. SYN *Bacteroides praeacutus.*

Tissot, Jules, early 20th century French physiologist. SEE T. *spirometer.*

tis·sue (tish′ū). A collection of similar cells and the intercellular substances surrounding them. There are four basic tissues in the body: 1) epithelium; 2) connective tissues, including blood, bone, and cartilage; 3) muscle tissue; and 4) nerve tissue. [Fr. *tissu,* woven, fr. L. *texo,* to weave]

adenoid t., SYN lymphatic t.

adipose t., a connective t. consisting chiefly of fat cells surrounded by reticular fibers and arranged in lobular groups or along the course of one of the smaller blood vessels. SYN fat (1), fatty t. (1), white fat (1).

areolar t., loose, irregularly arranged connective t. that consists of collagenous and elastic fibers, a protein polysaccharide ground substance, and connective t. cells (fibroblasts, macrophages, mast cells, and sometimes fat cells, plasma cells, leukocytes, and pigment cells).

bone t., SYN osseous t.

bronchus-associated lymphoid t. (BALT), patches of lymphoid t.'s composed mainly of B and T lymphocytes and extending throughout the bronchial airways of the lung.

brown adipose t., SYN brown *fat.*

cancellous t., latticelike or spongy osseous t.

cardiac muscle t., SEE cardiac *muscle.*

cartilaginous t., SEE cartilage.

cavernous t., SYN erectile t.

chondroid t., (1) in an adult, t. resembling cartilage; SYN fibrohyaline t., pseudocartilage. **(2)** in an embryo, an early stage in cartilage formation.

chromaffin t., a cellular t., vascular and well supplied with nerves, made up chiefly of chromaffin cells; it is found in the medulla of the suprarenal glands and, in smaller collections, in the paraganglia.

connective t., the supporting or framework t. of the animal body, formed of fibrous and ground substance with more or less numerous cells of various kinds; it is derived from the mesenchyme, and this in turn from the mesoderm; the varieties of connective t. are: areolar or loose; adipose; dense, regular or irregular, white fibrous; elastic; mucous; and lymphoid t.; cartilage; and bone; the blood and lymph may be regarded as connective t.'s the ground substance of which is a liquid. SYN interstitial t., tela conjunctiva.

dartoic t., t. resembling tunica dartos.

elastic t., a form of connective t. in which the elastic fibers predominate; it constitutes the ligamenta flava of the vertebrae and the ligamentum nuchae, especially of quadrupeds; it occurs also in the walls of the arteries and of the bronchial tree, and connects the cartilages of the larynx. SYN elastica (2), tela elastica.

epithelial t., SEE epithelium.

erectile t., a t. with numerous vascular spaces that may become engorged with blood. SYN cavernous t.

fatty t., (1) SYN adipose t; **(2)** in some animals, brown *fat.*

fibrohyaline t., SYN chondroid t. (1).

fibrous t., a t. composed of bundles of collagenous white fibers between which are rows of connective t. cells; the tendons, ligaments, aponeuroses, and some of the membranes, such as the dura mater.

Gamgee t., a thick layer of absorbent cotton between two layers of absorbent gauze, used in surgical dressings.

gelatinous t., SYN mucous connective t.

gingival t.'s, SEE gingiva.

granulation t., vascular connective t. forming granular projections on the surface of a healing wound, ulcer, or inflamed t. surface. SEE ALSO granulation.

gut-associated lymphoid t. (GALT), lymphoid t. of the gastrointestinal mucosa that contains both B and T cells. This t. is responsible for localized immunity to pathogens such as bacteria, viruses, and parasites.

Haller vascular t., SYN vascular *lamina* of choroid.

hard t., (1) t. that has become mineralized; **(2)** t. having a firm intercellular substance, e.g., cartilage and bone.

hemopoietic t., t. in which there is a development of blood cells or other formed elements.

indifferent t., undifferentiated, nonspecialized, embryonic t.

interstitial t., SYN connective t.

investing t.'s, the t.'s covering or enclosing a structure.

islet t., SYN *islets* of Langerhans, under *islet.*

lymphatic t., lymphoid t., a three-dimensional network of reticular fibers and cells the meshes of which are occupied in varying degrees of density with lymphocytes; there is nodular, diffuse, and loose lymphatic t. SYN adenoid t.

mesenchymal t., embryonic connective tissue. SEE mesenchyme.

mesonephric t., intermediate mesoderm situated in the thoracic and lumbar regions of the embryo or fetus; it develops into the mesonephros and associated structures.

metanephrogenic t., t. derived from the intermediate mesoderm caudal to mesonephric levels and concerned with the formation of the nephrons of the metanephros.

mucosa-associated lymphoid t. (MALT), a class of lymphoid t. comprising nodular aggregates found in association with the wet mucosal surfaces of the body such as those of the respiratory, digestive, and urinary systems.

mucous connective t., a type of connective t. little differentiated beyond the mesenchymal stage; its ground substance of glycoproteins is abundant and contains fine collagenous fibers and fibroblasts; in its most characteristic form, it appears in the umbilical cord as Wharton jelly. SYN gelatinous t.

multilocular adipose t., SYN brown *fat.*

muscular t., a t. characterized by the ability to contract upon stimulation; its three varieties are skeletal, cardiac, and smooth. SEE muscle. SYN flesh (2).

myeloid t., bone marrow consisting of the developmental and adult stages of erythrocytes, granulocytes, and megakaryocytes in a stroma of reticular cells and fibers, with sinusoidal vascular channels.

nasion soft t., the outer point of intersection between the nasion-sella line and the soft tissue profile.

nephrogenic t., the t. from which the pronephros, mesonephros, and metanephros develop.

nervous t., a highly differentiated t. composed of nerve cells, nerve fibers, dendrites, and a supporting t. (neuroglia).

nodal t., SEE atrioventricular *node*, sinuatrial *node*.

osseous t., a connective t., the matrix of which consists of collagen fibers and ground substance and in which are deposited calcium salts (phosphate, carbonate, and some fluoride) in the form of an apatite. SYN bone t.

osteogenic t., a connective t. with the property of forming osseous t.

osteoid t., osseous t. prior to calcification.

periapical t., the structures adjacent to a root apex, particularly the periodontal ligament and bone.

reticular t., retiform t., a t. in which the argyrophilic collagenous fibers form a network and that usually has a network of reticular cells associated with the fibers.

rubber t., a thin sheet of rubber used as a cover in surgical dressings.

skeletal muscle t., SEE skeletal *muscle*.

smooth muscle t., SEE smooth *muscle*.

subcutaneous t. [TA], an irregular layer of loose connective tissue immediately deep to the skin and superficial to the deep fascia, usually consisting primarily of a fatty layer [TA] (panniculus adiposus [TA]) which may also include a muscle layer [TA] (stratum musculosum [TA]) and/or a fibrous layer [TA] (stratum fibrosum [TA]}, or it may occur as a membranous layer [TA] (stratum membranosum [TA]) only, being nearly devoid of fat (as in the auricles, eyelids, scrotum, and penis); it is penetrated by, and gains support from, skin ligaments [TA] (retinacula cutis [TA]) extending between the dermis and the deep fascia; cutaneous nerves and superficial vessels course within the subcutaneous tissue, with only their terminal branches passing to the skin; of the body's coverings, this layer varies most between sexes and in different nutritional states. Terminologia Anatomica [TA] has recommended that the terms "superficial fascia" and "deep fascia" not be used generically in an unqualified way because of variation in their meanings internationally. The recommended terms are "subcutaneous tissue [TA] (tela subcutanea)" for the former superficial fascia, and "muscular fascia" or "visceral fasci viscera[is]) in place of deep fascia. SYN tela subcutanea [TA], hypodermis ☆, fascia superficialis, hypoderm, stratum subcutaneum, subcutis, superficial fascia.

subcutaneous t. of penis [TA], a superficial layer continuous with t. perinei superficialis. SYN fascia penis superficialis, superficial fascia of penis.

subcutaneous t. of perineum [TA], the membranous layer of the subcutaneous tissue in the urogenital region attaching posteriorly to the border of the urogenital diaphragm, at the sides to the ischiopubic rami, and continuing anteriorly onto the abdominal wall. SYN Colles fascia, Cruveilhier fascia, fascia perinei superficialis, membranous layer of superficial fascia of perineum (1), membranous layer of superficial fascia (1), superficial fascia of perineum.

trabecular t. of sclera [TA], the network of fibers (pectinate ligaments) at the iridocorneal angle between the anterior chamber of the eye and the venous sinus of the sclera; it contains spaces between the fibers that are involved in drainage of the aqueous humor, and is composed of two portions: the corneoscleral part (the part attached to the sclera) and the uveal part (the part attached to the iris). SYN reticulum trabeculare sclerae [TA], Gerlach valvula, Hueck ligament, ligamentum anulare bulbi, pectinate ligaments of iridocorneal angle, pillar of iris, trabecular meshwork, trabecular network, trabecular reticulum, trabecular zone.

tis·sue-trim·ming. SYN border *molding.*

tis·su·lar (tish'ū-lăr). Relating or pertaining to a tissue.

ti·ta·ni·um (Ti) (tī-tā'nē-ŭm). A metallic element, atomic no. 22, atomic wt. 47.88. [*Titans,* in G. myth., sons of Earth]

t. dioxide, TiO_2; contains not less than 99.0% and not more than 100.5% of TiO_2, calculated on the dry basis; used in creams and powders as a protectant against external irritations and solar rays.

ti·ter (tī'ter). The standard of strength of a volumetric test solution; the assay value of an unknown measure by volumetric means. [Fr. *titre,* standard]

TITh Abbreviation for 3,5,3'-triiodothyronine.

tit·il·la·tion (tit-i-lā'shŭn). The act or sensation of tickling. [L. *titillatio,* fr. *titillo,* pp. *-atus,* to tickle]

ti·tin (tī'tin). A very large fibrous protein that connects thick myosin filaments to Z discs in the sarcomere.

ti·trant (tī'trant). In chemistry, the solution that is added (titrated with) in a titration.

ti·trate (tī'trāt). To analyze volumetrically by a solution (the titrant) of known strength to an end point.

ti·tra·tion (tī-trā'shŭn). Volumetric analysis by means of the addition of definite amounts of a test solution to a solution of the substance being assayed. [Fr. *titre,* standard]

colorimetric t., a t. in which the end point is marked by a color change.

formol t., a method of titrating the amino groups of amino acids, by adding formaldehyde to the neutral solution; the formaldehyde reacts with the NH_3^+ group, liberating an equivalent quantity of H^+, which may then be estimated by t. with NaOH.

potentiometric t., a t. during which the pH is continually measured with some value of the pH serving as end point.

tit·u·ba·tion (tit-ū-bā'shŭn). **1.** A staggering or stumbling in trying to walk. **2.** A tremor or shaking of the head, of cerebellar origin. [L. *titubo,* pp. *-atus,* to stagger]

Tizzoni, Guido, Italian physician, 1853–1932. SEE Tizzoni *stain.*

Tl Symbol for thallium.

²⁰¹Tl Abbreviation for *thallium*-201.

TLC Abbreviation for thin-layer *chromatography*; total lung *capacity.*

TLE Abbreviation for thin-layer *electrophoresis.*

TLV Abbreviation for threshold limit *value.*

TM Abbreviation for transcendental meditation.

Tm Symbol for thulium; transport *maximum* or tubular *maximum.*

TMD Abbreviation for temporomandibular joint *dysfunction.*

TMJ Colloquial abbreviation for temporomandibular joint *dysfunction.*

TM-mode. SYN M-mode.

TMP Abbreviation for ribothymidylic acid; trimethoprim; sometimes for deoxyribothymidylic acid.

T-my·co·plas·ma. SYN *Ureaplasma.*

Tn Abbreviation for ocular *tension.*

TNF Abbreviation for tumor necrosis *factor.*

TNM Acronym for Tumor-Node-Metastasis. SEE TNM *staging.*

TNP-470. An angiogenesis inhibitor used in the treatment of cancer to reduce blood vessel formation in tumors.

TNT Abbreviation for trinitrotoluene.

to·bac·co (tō-bak'ō). A South American herb, *Nicotiana tabacum,* that has large ovate to lanceolate leaves and terminal clusters of tubular white or pink flowers. Tobacco leaves contain 2–8% of nicotine and are the source of smoking and chewing tobacco. Tobacco smoke contains nicotine, carbon monoxide (4%), nitric oxide, and numerous aromatic hydrocarbons and other substances known to be carcinogens, including benzo[*a*]pyrene, β-naphthylamine, and nitrosamines.

Cigarette smoking is the leading preventable cause of disease and death in the U.S., being responsible for ap-

to

proximately 434,000 deaths (20% of all deaths) each year. Smoking 2 packages of cigarettes a day reduces life span by 8.3 years. Smoking tobacco in any form (cigarettes, cigars, pipe) is a strong independent risk factor for atherosclerosis, acute myocardial infarction, unstable angina, stroke, and sudden death. It is responsible for 45% of all deaths due to coronary artery disease in men under 65 and more than 50% of all strokes in both sexes before age 65. Smoking lowers HDL cholesterol and raises LDL and VLDL cholesterol, and increases the risk of intermittent claudication and aortic aneurysm. It may cause as much as a 30-fold increase in the risk of thromboembolic disease in women taking oral contraceptives. Smoking is responsible for 100,000 deaths each year due to lung cancer, and markedly increases the risk of other cancers, particularly those of the oral cavity, larynx, esophagus, kidney, bladder, uterine cervix, and pancreas. Cigarette smoking is the principal cause of chronic bronchitis and emphysema. Passive smoking (inhalation by nonsmokers of second-hand or sidestream smoke) causes 53,000 deaths annually, 37,000 of them due to coronary artery disease. Maternal smoking during pregnancy is associated with increased risk of miscarriage, stillbirth, and low birth weight. Children of smokers are at increased risk of sudden infant death syndrome and meningococcal meningitis. Use of smokeless tobacco (chewing tobacco, snuff) greatly increases the risk of cancer and premalignant lesions of the oral cavity. Nicotine use is powerfully addictive, leading to habituation, tolerance, and dependency. In the U.S., 90% of smokers become habituated to tobacco before age 21; 3000 children begin smoking each day. The likelihood of becoming and remaining a smoker increases in inverse proportion to the number of years of education completed. Quitting smoking decreases the risk of death from all causes by 30%. Effective strategies for smoking cessation include behavior modification therapy, nicotine replacement (gum, skin patches, inhaler), hypnosis, and drug therapy (bupropion), but the relapse rate 3 months after smoking cessation is 60%.

---

wild t., SYN lobelia.

to·bra·my·cin (tō-bră-mī′sin). An aminoglycoside antibiotic produced by *Streptomyces tenebrarius*, having bactericidal effects and used mainly in the treatment of *Pseudomonas* infections.

to·cai·nide hy·dro·chlo·ride (tō-kā′nīd). An oral antiarrhythmic agent, similar in action to lidocaine, used in the treatment of ventricular arrhythmias.

△toco-. Childbirth. [G. *tokos,* birth]

to·co·chro·ma·nol-3 (tō′kō-krō′mă-nol). An α-tocotrienol. SEE tocotrienol.

toc·o·dy·na·graph (tō-kō-dī′nă-graf, tok-ō-). A recording of the force of uterine contractions. SYN tocograph. [toco- + G. *dynamis,* force, + *graphē,* a writing]

toc·o·dy·na·mom·e·ter (tō′kō-dī-nă-mom′ĕ-ter, tok′ō-). An instrument for measuring the force of uterine contractions. SYN tocometer. [toco- + G. *dynamis,* force, + *metron,* measure]

toc·o·graph (tō′kō-graf). SYN tocodynagraph.

to·cog·ra·phy (tō-kog′ră-fē). The process of recording uterine contractions. [toco- + G. *graphō,* to write]

to·col (tō′kol). Fundamental unit of the tocopherols; 6-phytylhydroquinone is in equilibrium with, in the chromanol form, 2-methyl-2-(4,8,12-trimethyltridecyl)chroman-6-ol.

to·col·o·gy (tō-kol′ō-jē). SYN obstetrics. [toco- + G. *logos,* study]

to·co·lyt·ic (tō-kō-lit′ik). Denoting any pharmacologic agent used to arrest uterine contractions; often used in an attempt to arrest premature labor contractions, e.g., ritodrine or terbutaline. [G. *tokos,* childbirth, labor, + *lysis,* loosening]

to·com·e·ter (tō-kom′ĕ-ter). SYN tocodynamometer.

to·coph·er·ol (T) (tō-kof′er-ōl). **1.** Name given to vitamin E by its discoverer, but now a generic term for vitamin E and compounds chemically related to it, with or without biological activi-

ty; similar in chemical structure and properties to vitamins K and coenzyme Q. **2.** A methylated tocol or methylated tocotrienol.

mixed t.'s concentrate, a source of vitamin E, obtained by vacuum distillation of edible vegetable oils or their by-products.

α-to·coph·er·ol (α-T). 5,7,8-Trimethyltocol; a light yellow, viscous, odorless, oily liquid that deteriorates on exposure to light, is obtained from wheat germ oil or by synthesis, biologically exhibits the most vitamin E activity of the α-T.'s, and is an antioxidant retarding rancidity by interfering with the autoxidation of fats. Prepared from natural phytol, it is called 2-*ambo*-α-t.; from synthetic phytol, *all-rac*-α-t. or *synt*-α-t.; also available are *d*-α-tocopheryl acetate, *dl*-α-tocopheryl acetate, *d*-α-tocopheryl acid succinate, and *d*-α-tocopheryl acetate concentrate. One of several forms of vitamin E. SYN vitamin E (1).

β-to·coph·er·ol (β-T). A lower homolog of α-tocopherol that contains one less methyl group in the aromatic nucleus and is less active biologically; accompanies α-tocopherol and γ-β-t.

γ-to·coph·er·ol (γ-T). A form biologically less active than α-γ-t.

to·coph·er·ol·qui·none (TQ) (tō-kof′er-ol-kwi′nōn). An oxidized tocopherol, formed from the isomeric 2-methyl-2-phytyl-6-chromenol with methyl groups in one or more of positions 5, 7, and 8, by migration of an H atom from 6-OH to C-4, which yields a 1,4-benzoquinone. Abbreviated TQ and preceded by α-, β-, etc., as in the tocopherols, to indicate degree of methylation. SYN tocopherylquinone.

to·coph·er·yl·qui·none (tō-kof′er-il-kwi′nōn). SYN tocopherolquinone.

toc·o·pho·bia (tō′kō-fō′bē-ă, tok′ō-). Morbid dread of childbirth. [toco- + G. *phobos,* fear]

to·co·qui·none (tō-kō-kwi′nōn). Class name for the 2,3,5-trimethyl-6-multiprenyl-1,4-benzoquinones.

to·co·tri·en·ol (tō-kō-trī′en-ol). A tocol with three double bonds in the side chain, i.e., with three additional double bonds in the phytyl chain. The natural products carry methyls at one or more of positions 5, 7, and 8 of the chromanol and are thus identical, except for the unsaturation in the phytyl-like side chain, to the tocopherols; also analogous is the cyclization to form a chromanol derivative and oxidation to form the tocotrienolquinones (or chromenols). Abbreviated T-*n* (hydroquinone form) or TQ-*n* (quinone form) and preceded by α-, β-, etc., as in the tocopherols, to indicate degree of methylation (the *n* indicates the number of intact isoprene or prenyl units remaining in the chromanol or chromenol form). T. terminology is used to indicate relationships to tocols and tocoenols (vitamin E-like), the chromanol terminology to indicate relationship to the isoprenoidal compounds of the vitamin K and coenzyme Q series.

to·co·tri·en·ol·qui·none (tō-kō-trī′en-ol-kwi′nōn). A tocotrienol in which the hydroquinone has been oxidized to a quinone (the chromanol has become a chromenol); the t.'s carry α, β, γ, and δ prefixes in accordance with the degree of methylation, as do the tocotrienols.

TOCP Abbreviation for triorthocresyl phosphate.

Tod, David, British surgeon, 1794–1856. SEE T. *muscle.*

Todaro, Francesco, Italian anatomist, 1839–1918. SEE T. *tendon.*

Todd, Robert B., English physician, 1809–1860. SEE T. *paralysis,* postepileptic *paralysis.*

toe (tō) [TA]. One of the digits of the feet. SYN digitus pedis [TA], digits of foot✩. [A.S. *ta*]

fourth t. [IV] [TA], fourth digit of foot. SYN digitus (pedis) quartus [IV] [TA].

great t. I [TA], the first digit of the foot. SYN hallux [TA], digitus pedis primus I✩, hallex, hallus, pollex pedis, primary digit of foot.

hammer t., permanent flexion at the midphalangeal joint of one or more of the t.'s.

little t. [V] [TA], fifth digit of the foot. SYN digitus (pedis) minimus [V] [TA], digitus (pedis) quintus [V]✩.

Morton t., a particular form of metatarsalgia caused by enlargement of the digital nerve. Cf. Morton *syndrome.*

painful t., SYN *hallux* dolorosus.

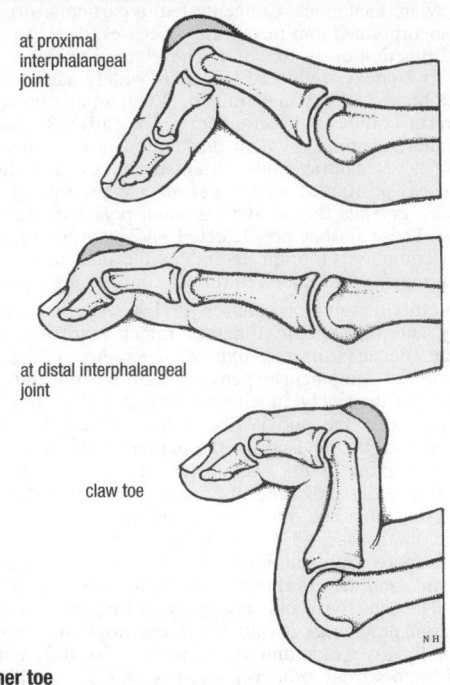

at proximal interphalangeal joint

at distal interphalangeal joint

claw toe

N H

hammer toe

---

second t. [II] [TA], second digit of foot. SYN digitus (pedis) secundus [II] [TA].

stiff t., SYN *hallux* rigidus.

third t. [III] [TA], third digit of foot. SYN digitus (pedis) tertius [III] [TA].

webbed t.'s, syndactyly involving the toes.

toe-drop (tō′drop). Inability to dorsiflex the toes, usually due to paralysis of the toe extensor muscles.

toe·nail (tō′nāl). SEE nail.

ingrowing t., SYN ingrown *nail.*

to·fen·a·cin hy·dro·chlo·ride (tō-fen′ă-sin). An anticholinergic drug.

To·ga·vir·i·dae (tō-gă-vir′i-dē). A family of viruses that includes two genera: Alphavirus, which includes eastern equine encephalitis, western equine encephalitis, and Venezuelan equine encephalitis virus, and Rubivirus, the rubella virus. Virions are 70 nm in diameter, enveloped, and ether-sensitive; the capsid is of icosahedral symmetry, containing single-stranded positive sense RNA.

to·ga·vi·rus (tō′gă-vi′rŭs). Any virus of the family Togaviridae. [L. *toga,* garment covering, + virus]

toi·let (toy-let′). **1.** Cleansing of the obstetric patient after childbirth. **2.** Cleansing of the surface of a wound after an operation preparatory to the application of the dressing. **3.** In dentistry, cavity debridement, the final step before placing a restoration in a tooth whereby the cavity is cleaned and all debris is removed. [Fr. *toilette*]

pulmonary t., attempts to clear mucus and secretions from the trachea and bronchial tree by deep breathing, insentive spiratomy, postural drainage, and percussion.

Toison, J., French histologist, 1858–1950. SEE T. *stain.*

Toker, Cyril, U.S. pathologist, *1930. SEE T. *cell.*

△**toko-.** SEE toco-.

to·laz·a·mide (tō-laz′ă-mīd). An oral hypoglycemic agent similar in use to tolbutamide.

to·laz·o·line hy·dro·chlo·ride (tō-laz′ō-lēn). An adrenergic α-receptor blocking agent used to augment blood flow in peripheral vascular disorders.

tol·bu·ta·mide (tol-bū′tă-mīd). An orally active hypoglycemic agent used in the management of adult-onset diabetes mellitus; it

appears to stimulate the synthesis and release of endogenous insulin from functional islets; available as t. sodium for injection.

tol·cy·cla·mide (tol-sī′klă-mīd). SYN glycyclamide.

Toldt, Karl, Austrian anatomist, 1840–1920. SEE T. *fascia, membrane;* white *line* of T.

tol·er·ance (tol′er-ăns). **1.** The ability to endure or be less responsive to a stimulus, especially over a period of continued exposure. **2.** The power of resisting the action of a poison or of taking a drug continuously or in large doses without injurious effects. [L. *tolero,* pp. *-atus,* to endure]

acoustic t., the maximum sound pressure level that can be experienced without producing pain or permanent hearing threshold shift in a normal individual.

cross t., the resistance to one or several effects of a compound as a result of t. developed to a pharmacologically similar compound.

frustration t., the level of an individual's ability to withstand frustration without developing inadequate modes of response, such as "going to pieces" emotionally.

high dose t., the induction of t. by exposure to high doses of antigen.

immunologic t., lack of immune response to antigen. Theories of t. induction include clonal deletion and clonal anergy. In clonal deletion, the actual clone of cells is eliminated whereas in clonal anergy the cells are present but nonfunctional. SYN immunotolerance, nonresponder t.

immunologic high dose t., induction of tolerance by exposure to large amounts of protein antigens.

impaired glucose t., excessive levels of blood glucose developing after a carbohydrate-rich meal or test dosage of glucose (usually 75 g). Not necessarily diagnostic of diabetes mellitus.

individual t., t. to a drug that the person has never received before.

nonresponder t., SYN immunologic t.

pain t., the greatest intensity of painful stimulation that an individual is able to tolerate.

species t., the insensitivity to a particular drug exhibited by a particular species.

split t., reaction to one (or more) antigen on a cell surface but no reaction to others. SYN immune deviation.

vibration t., the maximum vibratory or oscillatory movements that an individual can experience and bear without pain; the limit of t. is a function of amplitude and frequency of the vibration and varies with the direction of application.

tol·er·ant (tol′er-ănt). Having the property of tolerance.

tol·er·ize (tol′er-īz). To induce tolerance.

tol·er·o·gen (tol′er-ō-jen). A substance that produces immunological tolerance.

tol·er·o·gen·ic (tol′er-ō-jen′ik). Producing immunologic tolerance.

tol·hex·a·mide (tol-hek′să-mīd). SYN glycyclamide.

tol·met·in (tol′met-in). An anti-inflammatory drug used in the treatment of rheumatoid arthritis.

tol·naf·tate (tol-naf′tāt). A topical antifungal agent.

to·lo·ni·um chlo·ride (tō-lō′nē-ŭm). The medicinal grade of toluidine blue O, used as an antiheparin compound.

Tolosa, Eduardo, 20th century Spanish neurosurgeon. SEE T.-Hunt *syndrome.*

tol·pro·pa·mine (tol-prō′pă-mēn). A topical antipruritic agent.

tol·u·ene (tol′ū-ēn). A colorless liquid obtained by the dry distillation of tolu and other resinous bodies, and also derived from coal tar; its physical and chemical properties resemble those of benzene. Used in explosives and dyes, and as a solvent in the extraction of various principles from plants. SYN methylbenzene, toluol.

to·lu·ic ac·id (tō-loo′ik). Methylbenzoic acid; an oxidation product of xylene.

to·lu·i·dine (tō-loo′i-dēn, -din). Aminotoluene; one of three isomeric substances, derived from toluene.

alkaline t. blue O, t. blue O in borax solution, used with heat on semithick sections of epoxy embedded tissues.

to

t. blue O [C.I. 52040], a blue basic dye, used as an antibacterial agent, as a nuclear stain, and to stain metachromatically certain structures (e.g., the granules in mast cells which are believed to contain heparin and cartilage matrix which is rich in chondroitin sulfate), and in electrophoresis to stain RNA, RNase, and mucopolysaccharides; it also antagonizes the anticoagulant action of heparin. SEE ALSO tolonium chloride.

tol·u·ol (tol′oo-ol). SYN toluene.

tol·u·o·yl (tol-oo′ō-il). $CH_3C_6H_4CO-$; the radical of toluic acid.

tol·u·yl·ene red (tol-oo′i-lēn). SYN neutral red.

tol·yl (tol′il). $CH_3C_6H_4-$; the univalent radical of toluene.

Toma sign. See under sign.

△**-tome. 1.** A cutting instrument, the first element in the compound usually indicating the part that the instrument is designed to cut. **2.** Segment, part, section. **3.** Tomography. **4.** Surgery. [G. *tomos,* cutting, sharp; a cutting (section or segment)]

to·men·tum, to·men·tum ce·re·bri (tō-men′tŭm, tō-men′tŭm ser′ĕ-brī). The numerous small blood vessels passing between the cerebral surface of the pia mater and the cortex of the brain. [L. a stuffing for cushions]

Tomes, Sir Charles S., English dentist, 1846–1928. SEE T. *processes,* under *process.*

Tomes, Sir John, English dentist and anatomist, 1815–1895. SEE T. *fibers,* under *fiber,* granular *layer.*

Tommaselli, Salvatore, Italian physician, 1834–1906. SEE T. *disease.*

to·mo·gram (tō′mō-gram). A radiograph obtained by tomography. [G. *tomos,* a cutting (section) + *gramma,* a writing]

to·mo·graph (tō′mō-graf). The radiographic equipment used in tomography. [G. *tomos,* a cutting (section), + *graphō,* to write]

to·mog·ra·phy (tō-mog′ră-fē). Making of a radiographic image of a selected plane by means of reciprocal linear or curved motion of the x-ray tube and film cassette; images of all other planes are blurred ("out of focus") by being relatively displaced on the film. SYN conventional t., planigraphy, planography, sectional radiography, stratigraphy.

computed t. (CT), imaging anatomic information from a cross-sectional plane of the body, each image generated by a computer synthesis of x-ray transmission data obtained in many different directions in a given plane. SYN computerized axial t.

computerized axial t. (CAT), SYN computed t.

conventional t., SYN tomography.

dynamic computed t., computed t. with rapid injection of contrast medium, usually with sequential scans at only one or a few levels; used to enhance the vascular compartment. SYN dynamic CT.

electron beam t. (EBT), computed t. in which the circular motion of the x-ray tube is replaced by rapid electronic positioning of the cathode ray around a circular anode, allowing full scans in tens of milliseconds.

helical computed t., SYN spiral computed t.

high-resolution computed t. (HRCT), computed t. with narrow collimation to reduce volume-averaging and an edge-enhancing reconstruction algorithm to sharpen the image, sometimes with a restricted field of view to minimize the size of pixels in the region imaged; used particularly for lung imaging.

hypocycloidal t., body section radiography using a complex film and tube motion with a pattern resembling a three-leaf clover.

nuclear magnetic resonance t., SYN magnetic resonance *imaging.*

positron emission t. (PET), creation of tomographic images revealing certain biochemical properties of tissue by computer analysis of positrons emitted when radioactively tagged substances are incorporated into the tissue. Radiotracers used in PET are analogs of physiologic or pharmaceutical agents into which positron-emitting isotopes with short half-lives (2–110 min) have been incorporated. Radioisotopes are produced artificially by bombarding a stable compound with a proton beam generated by a cyclotron. The uptake and metabolism of these positron emitters mimic, at least in part, those of the radiostable natural substances to which they are analogous. Concentrated in particular organs or tissues and incorporated into metabolic processes, they can reflect biochemical function or dysfunction. The glucose analog 2-(fluorine-18)fluoro-2-deoxy-D-glucose (FDG) is widely used to locate zones of heightened energy metabolism. When a positron emitted by a radiotracer collides with an electron, the particles annihilate each other and 2 gamma rays are discharged in opposite directions (at 180°). After intravenous administration of the radiotracer, the subject is positioned within a scanner consisting of a ring of scintillation crystals that convert gamma rays into flashes of visible light. These flashes are detected and recorded electronically, and a computer program assembles the data into a three-dimensional image, color-coded to reflect concentration density.

Unlike other imaging procedures, PET assesses metabolic activity and physiologic function rather than anatomic structure. Because the half-lives of the radionuclides are short and the equipment expensive, PET has not thus far been used extensively in clinical settings. But since its development in the mid-1970s, it has proved the most important tool yet devised for the experimental investigation of the living brain, whether healthy, traumatized, or diseased. Besides providing important diagnostic information in Alzheimer and other dementias, parkinsonism, and Huntington disease, PET can localize epileptic foci in preparation for surgical intervention, assess intracranial neoplasms, and help to direct therapeutic choices in acute stroke. The sensitivity and specificity of PET in determining malignancy render it valuable in oncology in avoiding biopsies for low grade tumors, in noninvasive differentiation of tumors from radiation necrosis, in early modification of ineffective chemotherapy, and in avoiding unnecessary diagnostic and therapeutic surgery. PET has been employed in cardiology to screen for coronary artery disease, to assess flow rates and flow reserve, and to distinguish viable from nonviable myocardium in bypass and transplant candidates.

single photon emission computed t. (SPECT), tomographic imaging of metabolic and physiologic functions in tissues, the image being formed by computer synthesis of photons of a single energy emitted by radionuclides administered in suitable form to the patient.

spiral computed t., computed t. in which the x-ray tube continuously revolves around the patient, who is simultaneously moved longitudinally; computer interpolation allows reconstruction of standard transverse scans or images in any preferred plane. SYN helical computed t., helical CT, spiral CT.

trispiral t., hypocycloidal t. that allows a much thinner and more uniform plane of focus; formerly used especially for inner ear t.

to·mo·lev·el (tō′mō-lev-el). Obsolete term for the level at which tomography is performed.

to·mo·ma·nia (tō-mō-mā′nē-ă). An irrational desire to use operative procedures by a doctor or a patient. [G. *tomos,* cutting, + *mania,* frenzy]

△**-tomy.** A cutting operation. SEE ALSO -ectomy. [G. *tomē,* incision]

ton·a·pha·sia (tōn-ă-fā′zē-ă). Loss, through cerebral lesion, of the ability to remember tunes. [G. *tonos,* tone, + *a-* priv. + *phasis,* speech]

tone (tōn). **1.** A musical sound. **2.** The character of the voice expressing an emotion. **3.** The tension present in resting muscles. **4.** Firmness of the tissues; normal functioning of all the organs. **5.** To perform toning. [G. *tonos,* tone, or a tone]

affective t., emotional t., SYN feeling t.

feeling t., the mental state (pleasure, repugnance, etc.) that accompanies every act or thought. SYN affective t., emotional t., affectivity.

fundamental t., the component of lowest frequency in a complex sound.

heart t.'s, SYN heart *sounds,* under *sound.*

Traube double t., a double sound heard on auscultation over the femoral vessels in cases of aortic and tricuspid insufficiency.

ton·er (tō′ner). A solution used in toning.

tongue (tŭng) [TA]. **1.** A mobile mass of muscular tissue covered with mucous membrane, occupying the cavity of the mouth and forming part of its floor, constituting also by its posterior portion the anterior wall of the pharynx. It bears taste buds and assists in mastication, deglutition, and articulation. SYN glossa, lingua (1). **2.** A tonguelike structure. SYN lingua (2). [A.S. *tunge*]

coatings of the tongue

underlying illness	clinical symptoms	other findings
nonspecific mouth infection	whitish coating (scales)	connected with reduced nutrient intake in gastritis and enteritis and with fever
thrush	whitish, membranous plaques; difficult to remove, with red edges	evidence of *Candida albicans* in smear
scarlet fever	opaque white coating with redness at tip and edges of tongue	pharyngitis, exanthema, evidence of β-hemolytic streptococci in throat culture
diphtheria	grayish white membranous coating, sickly-sweet odor	coating difficult to remove, under-layer bleeds easily; general symptoms
typhoid fever	gray-white tongue with bright-red edges	infection by *Salmonella typhi*; general symptoms
uremia	lumpy brown coating on tongue	kidney failure

baked t., the dry blackish t. noted when patients with typhoid fever or other disorders are allowed to become dehydrated.

bald t., SYN atrophic *glossitis.*

beet-t., appearance of the t. in pellagra, where intense erythema appears, first at the tip, then along the edges, and finally over the dorsum; there may be pain and increased elevation; the shiny appearance results from edema, not atrophy, except in chronic pellagra.

bifid t., a structural defect of the t. in which the extremity is divided longitudinally for a greater or lesser distance. SEE diglossia. SYN cleft t.

black t., (1) in canines, a disorder associated with a deficency of nicotinic acid. (2) black to yellowish-brown discoloration of the dorsum of the t. due to staining by exogenous material such as the components of tobacco; usually superimposed on hairy t. SYN black hairy t., lingua nigra, melanoglossia, nigrities linguae.

black hairy t., SYN black t.

burning t., SYN glossodynia.

t. of cerebellum, SYN *lingula* of cerebellum.

cleft t., SYN bifid t.

coated t., a t. with a whitish layer on its upper surface, composed of epithelial debris, food particles, and bacteria; often an indication of indigestion or of fever. SYN furred t.

tongue crib, An appliance used to control visceral (infantile) swallowing and tongue thrusting and to encourage the mature or somatic tongue posture and function.

dotted t., one in which each separate papilla is capped with a whitish deposit. SYN stippled t.

fissured t., a painless condition of the t. characterized by numerous grooves or furrows on the dorsal surface. SYN grooved t., lingua fissurata, lingua plicata, scrotal t.

furred t., SYN coated t.

geographic t., idiopathic, asymptomatic erythematous circinate macules, often bounded peripherally by a white band, as a result of atrophy of the filiform papillae; with time the lesions resolve, coalesce, and change in distribution; frequently associated with fissured t.'s. SYN benign migratory glossitis, glossitis areata exfoliativa, pityriasis linguae.

grooved t., SYN fissured t.

hairy t., a t. with abnormal elongation of the filiform papillae, resulting in a thickened furry appearance. SYN glossotrichia, trichoglossia.

hobnail t., interstitial glossitis with hypertrophy and verrucous changes in papillae; seen in some cases of late acquired syphilis.

magenta t., purplish red coloration of the t., with edema and flattening of the filiform papillae, occurring in riboflavin deficiency. Cf. cyanosis.

mandibular t., SYN *lingula* of mandible.

raspberry t., strawberry t. that is a dark red color.

red strawberry t., clinical manifestation of Kawasaki *disease.*

scrotal t., SYN fissured t.

smoker's t., term for leukoplakia.

stippled t., SYN dotted t.

strawberry t., a t. with a whitish coat through which the enlarged fungiform papillae project as red points, characteristic of scarlet fever and of mucocutaneous lymph node syndrome.

tongue-swallowing, A slipping back of the tongue against the pharynx, causing choking.

tongue thrust, The infantile pattern of the suckle-swallow movement in which the tongue is placed between the incisor teeth or the alveolar ridges during the initial stage of swallowing, resulting sometimes in an anterior open bite.

tongue-tie. SYN ankyloglossia.

ton·ic (ton′ik). **1.** In a state of continuous unremitting action; denoting especially a prolonged muscular contraction. **2.** Invigorating; increasing physical or mental tone or strength. **3.** A remedy purported to restore enfeebled function and promote vigor and a sense of well-being; t.'s are qualified, according to the organ or system on which they are presumed to act, as cardiac, digestive, hematic, vascular, nerve, uterine, general, etc. [G. *tonikos,* fr. *tonos,* tone]

bitter t., a t. of bitter taste, such as quinine, gentian, quassia, etc., which acts chiefly by stimulating the appetite and improving digestion.

to·nic·i·ty (tō-nis′i-tē). **1.** A state of normal tension of the tissues by virtue of which the parts are kept in shape, alert, and ready to function in response to a suitable stimulus. In the case of muscle, it refers to a state of continuous activity or tension beyond that related to the physical properties; i.e., it is active resistance to stretch; in skeletal muscle it is dependent upon the efferent innervation. SYN tonus. **2.** The osmotic pressure or tension of a solution, usually relative to that of blood. SEE ALSO isotonicity. [G. *tonos,* tone]

ton·i·co·clon·ic (ton-i-kō-klon′ik). Both tonic and clonic, referring to repeated muscular contractions. SYN tonoclonic.

to·nin (tō′nin). An enzyme converting angiotensin I to angiotensin II, thus similar to or identical with angiotensin-converting enzyme.

ton·ing (tōn′ing). The replacing of a silver deposit with one of gold in an impregnated histologic section, by treatment with a solution of gold chloride.

ton·i·tro·pho·bia (tō′ni-trō-fō′bē-ă). SYN brontophobia. [L. *tonitrus,* thunder, + G. *phobos,* fear]

tono-. Tone, tension, pressure. [G. *tonos*]

ton·o·clon·ic (ton-ō-klon′ik). SYN tonicoclonic.

ton·o·fi·bril (ton-ō-fī′bril). One of a system of fibers found in the cytoplasm of epithelial cells. SEE cytoskeleton, tonofilament. SYN epitheliofibril, tenofibril.

ton·o·fil·a·ment (ton-ō-fil′ă-ment). A structural cytoplasmic protein, of a class known as intermediate filaments, bundles of which together form a tonofibril; a t. is made up of a variable number of related proteins, keratins, and is found in all epithelial cells, but is particularly well developed in the epidermis.

ton·o·graph (ton′ō-graf, tō′nō-). A recording tonometer. [tono- + G. *graphō,* to write]

to·nog·ra·phy (tō-nog′ră-fē). Continuous measurement of intraocular pressure by means of a recording tonometer, in order to determine the facility of aqueous outflow.

to·nom·e·ter (tō-nom′ĕ-ter). **1.** An instrument for determining pressure or tension, especially an instrument for determining ocular tension. **2.** A vessel for equilibrating a liquid (e.g., blood) with

to

a gas, usually at a controlled temperature; originally so named because it was used with a very small gas/blood ratio to allow the gas to approach blood oxygen tension and thus serve as a measure of it; now commonly used with a very large gas/blood ratio to adjust the blood to the oxygen pressure of the gas. SYN aerotonometer (2). [tono- + G. *metron,* measure]

applanation t., an instrument for determining ocular tension by application of a small, flat disk to the cornea.

Gärtner t., an apparatus for estimating the blood pressure by noting the force, expressed by the height of a column of mercury, needed to arrest pulsation in a finger encircled by a compressing ring.

Goldmann applanation t., an applanation t. that flattens only 3 mm² of cornea, used with a slitlamp.

Mackay-Marg t., a recording electronic applanation t.

Mueller electronic t., a Schiötz-type t. that electronically indicates the extent of corneal indentation; may also have an attached recorder for continuous pressure readings (tonography).

pneumatic t., a recording applanation t. operated by compressed gas.

Schiøtz t., an instrument that measures ocular tension by indicating the ease with which the cornea is indented.

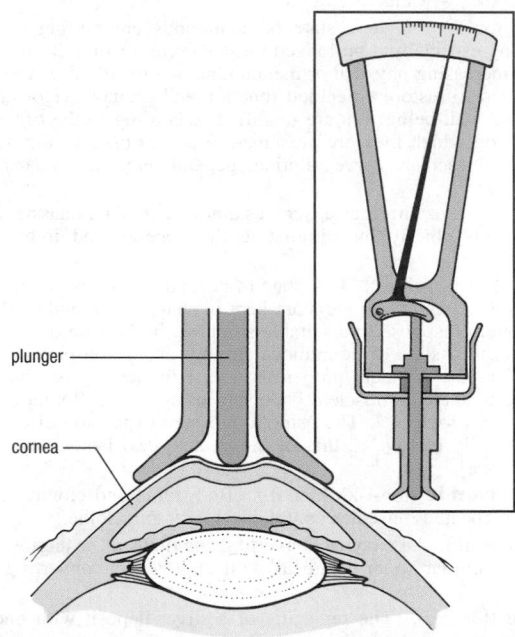

plunger

cornea

Schiøtz tonometer: indentation of the anesthetized cornea by the plunger (exaggerated here) measures ocular tension; (insert) entire tonometer

to·nom·e·try (tō-nom'ĕ-trē). **1.** Measurement of the tension of a part, e.g., intravascular tension or blood pressure. **2.** Measurement of ocular tension.

ton·o·phant (tō'nō-fant, ton'ō-). An instrument for visualizing sound waves. [tono- + G. *phainō,* to appear]

ton·o·plast (tō'nō-plast, ton'ō-). An intracellular structure or vacuole. [tono- + G. *plastos,* formed]

to·nos·cil·lo·graph (tō-nos'i-lō-graf). An instrument that produces graphic records of arterial and capillary pressures as well as of individual pulse characters. [tono- + L. *oscillo,* to swing, + G. *graphō,* to write]

to·no·top·ic (tō-nō-top'ik). Denoting a spatial arrangement of structures that subserve various frequencies, as in the auditory pathway. [tono- + G. *topos,* place]

to·no·tro·pic (tō-nō-trop'ik). Denoting the shortening of the resting length of a muscle. [G. *tonikos, tonos,* tone, + *tropos,* a turning]

ton·sil (ton'sil). **1.** Intraepithelial collection of lymphocytes forming a lymphoepithelial ring in the pharynx. **2.** SYN palatine t. [L. *tonsilla,* a stake, in pl. the tonsils]

cerebellar t., SYN t. of cerebellum.

t. of cerebellum [TA], a rounded lobule on the undersurface of each cerebellar hemisphere, continuous medially with the uvula of the cerebellar vermis. SYN tonsilla cerebelli [TA], cerebellar t.

eustachian t., SYN tubal t.

faucial t., SYN palatine t.

Gerlach t., SYN tubal t.

laryngeal t.'s, SYN laryngeal lymphoid *nodules,* under *nodule.*

lingual t. [TA], a collection of lymphoid follicles on the posterior or pharyngeal portion of the dorsum of the tongue. SYN tonsilla lingualis [TA].

Luschka t., SYN pharyngeal t.

palatine t. [TA], a large oval mass of lymphoid tissue embedded in the lateral wall of the oral pharynx on either side between the pillars of the fauces. SYN tonsilla palatina [TA], faucial t., tonsil (2), tonsilla.

pharyngeal t. [TA], a collection of more or less closely aggregated lymphoid nodules on the posterior wall and roof of the nasopharynx, the hypertrophy of which constitutes the morbid condition called adenoids. SYN tonsilla pharyngealis [TA], Luschka gland (1), Luschka t., third t., tonsilla adenoidea.

submerged t., a faucial t. that is flat and lying below the level of the pillars of the fauces.

third t., SYN pharyngeal t.

tubal t. [TA], a collection of lymphoid nodules near the pharyngeal opening of the auditory tube. SYN tonsilla tubaria [TA], eustachian t., Gerlach t.

ton·sil·la, pl. **ton·sil·lae** (ton-sil'ă, -ē). SYN palatine *tonsil.* [L. (see tonsil)]

t. adenoi'dea, SYN pharyngeal *tonsil.*

t. cerebel'li [TA], SYN *tonsil* of cerebellum.

t. intestina'lis, SEE aggregated lymphoid *nodules* of small intestine, under *nodule.*

t. lingua'lis [TA], SYN lingual *tonsil.*

t. palati'na [TA], SYN palatine *tonsil.*

t. pharyngea'lis [TA], SYN pharyngeal *tonsil.*

t. tuba'ria [TA], SYN tubal *tonsil.*

ton·sil·lar, ton·sil·lary (ton'si-lăr, ton'si-lă-rē). Relating to a tonsil, especially the palatine tonsil. SYN amygdaline (3).

ton·sil·lec·to·my (ton'si-lek'tō-mē). Removal of the entire tonsil. [tonsil + G. *ektomē,* excision]

ton·sil·li·tis (ton'si-lī'tis). Inflammation of a tonsil, especially of the palatine tonsil. [tonsil + G. *-itis,* inflammation]

lacunar t., inflammation of the mucous membrane lining the tonsillar crypts.

Vincent t., angina limited chiefly to the tonsils, caused by Vincent organisms (bacillus and spirillum).

tonsillo-. Tonsil. [L. *tonsilla*]

ton·sil·lo·lith (ton-sil'ō-lith). A calcareous concretion in a distended tonsillar crypt. SYN tonsillar calculus, tonsilolith. [tonsillo- + G. *lithos,* stone]

ton·sil·lop·a·thy (ton'si-lop'ă-the). Disease of the tonsil. [tonsillo- + G. *pathos,* suffering]

ton·sil·lo·tome (ton-sil'ō-tōm). An instrument, sometimes modelled after a guillotine, for use in tonsillectomy. [tonsillo- + G. *tomos,* cutting]

ton·sil·lot·o·my (ton'si-lot'ō-mē). The cutting away of a portion or all of a hypertrophied faucial tonsil. [tonsillo- + G. *tomē,* incision]

ton·sil·o·lith (ton'si-lith). SYN tonsillolith.

to·nus (tō'nŭs). SYN tonicity (1). [L., fr. G. *tonos*]

baseline t., intrauterine pressure between contractions during labor.

myogenic t., contraction of a muscle caused by intrinsic properties of the muscle or by its intrinsic innervation.

neurogenic t., contraction of a muscle caused by the influence of its extrinsic nerve supply.

Tooth, Howard H., English physician, 1856–1925. SEE Charcot-Marie-T. *disease.*

TOOTH

tooth, pl. **teeth** (tooth, tēth) [TA]. One of the hard conical structures set in the alveoli of the upper and lower jaws, used in mastication and assisting in articulation. A t. is a dermal structure composed of dentin and encased in cementum on the anatomic root and enamel on its anatomic crown. It consists of a root buried in the alveolus, a neck covered by the gum, and a crown, the exposed portion. In the center is the pulp cavity filled with a connective tissue reticulum containing a jellylike substance (dental pulp) and blood vessels and nerves that enter through an aperature or aperatures at the apex of the root. The 20 deciduous teeth or primary teeth appear between the sixth and ninth and the 24th month of life; these exfoliate and are replaced by the 32 permanent teeth appearing between the fifth and seventh year and the 17th to 23rd year. There are four kinds of teeth: incisor, canine, premolar, and molar. SYN dens (1) [TA]. [A.S. *tōth*]

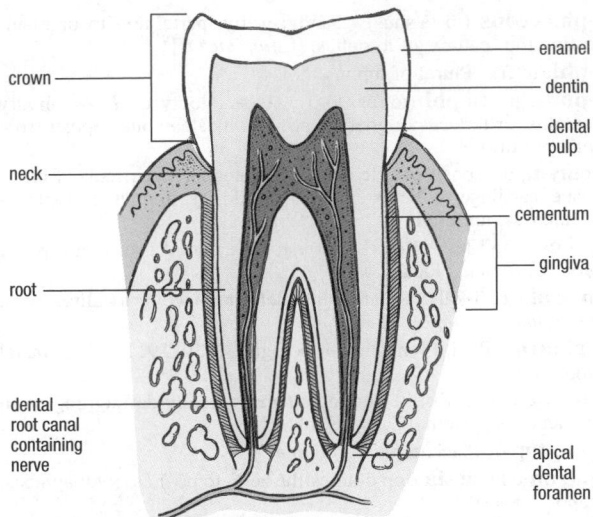

tooth and supporting tissues

Labels: crown, neck, root, dental root canal containing nerve, enamel, dentin, dental pulp, cementum, gingiva, apical dental foramen

acrylic resin t., a t. made of acrylic resin.

anatomic t., an artificial t. that duplicates the anatomic form of a natural t.

ankylosed t., SEE dental *ankylosis.*

anterior t., a central incisor, lateral incisor, or cuspid t. They comprise the organs for incision and are located in the front portion of the jaws. SYN oral teeth.

t. arrangement, (1) the placement of teeth on a denture base with definite objectives in mind; **(2)** the setting of teeth on temporary bases.

auditory teeth, SYN acoustic *teeth.*

baby t., SYN deciduous t.

back t., a t. posterior to the canines.

bicuspid t., SYN premolar t.

buck t., an anterior t. in labioversion.

canine t. [TA], a t. having a crown of thick conical shape and a long, slightly flattened conical root; there are two canine teeth in each jaw, one on either side adjacent to the distal surface of the lateral incisors, in both the deciduous and the permanent dentition. SYN dens caninus [TA], canine (3), cuspid t., cuspidate t., cuspid (2), dens angularis, dens cuspidatus, eye t.

carnassial t., (1) a t. adapted to shear flesh; **(2)** the last upper premolar or first lower molar t. of certain carnivores.

cheek t., SYN molar t.

Corti auditory teeth, SYN acoustic *teeth.*

crossbite t., a posterior t. designed to permit the modified cusp of the upper t. to be positioned in the fossae of the lower t.

cuspid t., cuspidate t., SYN canine t.

cuspless t., (1) a t. devoid of cusp formation; **(2)** severe abrasion of an occlusal surface; **(3)** a type of artificial denture t.

cutting teeth, the maxillary and mandibular anterior teeth.

dead t., a misnomer for pulpless t.

deciduous t. [TA], a t. of the first set of teeth, comprising 20 in all, that erupts between the mean ages of 6 and 24 months of life. SYN dens deciduus [TA], baby t., deciduous dentition, dens lacteus, first dentition, milk t., primary dentition, primary t., temporary t.

devitalized t., a misnomer for a pulpless t.

extruded teeth, SEE *extrusion* of a tooth.

eye t., SYN canine t.

fluoridated t., a t. exposed to fluorine salts during odontogenesis.

fused teeth, teeth joined by dentin as a result of embryologic fusion or juxtaposition of two adjacent tooth germs.

geminated teeth, a developmental anomaly arising from the attempted division of one t. bud, resulting in incomplete formation of two teeth and usually manifest as a bifid crown upon a single root.

ghost t., a t. with reduced radiodensity seen in regional odontodysplasia.

green t., green to brown discoloration of the primary teeth associated with erythroblastosis fetalis and caused by deposition of hemoglobin pigments in the developing teeth.

Horner teeth, incisor teeth having a horizontal, hypoplastic groove.

Huschke auditory teeth, SYN acoustic *teeth.*

Hutchinson teeth, the teeth of congenital syphilis in which the incisal edge is notched and narrower than the cervical area. SEE ALSO Hutchinson crescentic *notch.* SYN Hutchinson incisors, notched teeth, screwdriver teeth, syphilitic teeth.

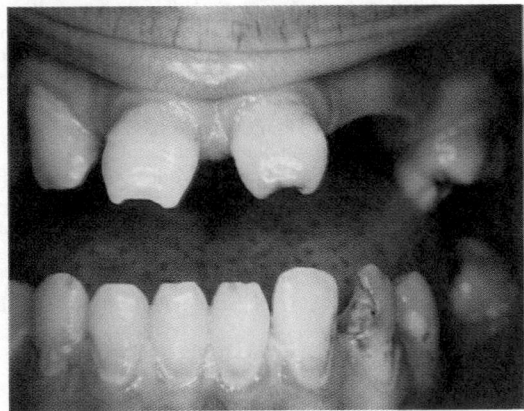

Hutchinson incisors: in congenital syphilis

impacted t., (1) a t. whose normal eruption is prevented by adjacent teeth or bone; **(2)** a t. that has been driven into the alveolar process or surrounding tissue as a result of trauma.

incisor t. [TA], a t. with a chisel-shaped crown and a single conical tapering root; there are four of these teeth in the anterior part of each jaw, in both the deciduous and the permanent dentitions. SYN dens incisivus [TA], incisor.

metal insert teeth, prosthetic teeth containing metal cutting surfaces in the occlusal surfaces.

migrating teeth, teeth which are changing position under natural forces.

milk t., SYN deciduous t.

to

molar t. [TA], a t. having a somewhat quadrangular crown with four or five cusps on the grinding surface; the root is bifid in the lower jaw, but there are three conical roots in the upper jaw; there are six molars in each jaw, three on either side behind the premolars in the permanent dentition; in the deciduous dentition there are but four molars in each jaw, two on either side behind the canines. SYN dens molaris [TA], cheek t., molar (2), multicuspid t.

mottled t., SEE mottled *enamel.*

multicuspid t., SYN molar t.

natal t., a predeciduous supernumerary t. present at birth.

neonatal t., a t. erupting up to 30 days after birth.

nonanatomic teeth, (1) teeth with occlusal surfaces not based on anatomic forms; **(2)** artificial teeth so designed that the occlusal surfaces are not copied from natural forms, but rather are given forms which in the opinion of the designer seem more nearly to fulfill the requirements of mastication, tissue tolerance, etc.

nonvital t., a t. with a nonvital pulp.

normally posed t., a t. in correct spatial relationship with its antagonist.

notched teeth, SYN Hutchinson teeth.

oral teeth, SYN anterior t.

pegged t., a conical t. whose sides converge from the cervical to the incisal region.

permanent t. [TA], 1 of 32 teeth belonging to the second, or permanent, dentition; eruption of the permanent teeth begins from the fifth to the seventh year, and is not completed until the 17th to the 23rd year, when the last of the third molars appears. SYN dens permanens [TA], dens succedaneus, second t., secondary dentition, succedaneous dentition, succedaneous t.

perpetually growing t., a physiologic phenomenon whereby the t. continually or constantly grows, calcifies, and erupts; e.g., the rat incisor t. SYN persistently growing t.

persistently growing t., SYN perpetually growing t.

plastic teeth, artificial teeth constructed of synthetic resins.

posterior t., a bicuspid or molar t.; these teeth comprise the organs of mastication and are located in the back part of the jaws.

premolar t. [TA], a t. usually having two tubercles or cusps on the grinding surface and a flattened root, single in the lower jaw and upper second premolar, and furrowed in the upper first premolar. There are four premolars in each jaw, two on either side between the canine and the molars; there are no premolars in the deciduous dentition. SYN dens premolaris [TA], bicuspid t., dens bicuspidus.

primary t., SYN deciduous t.

protruding teeth, teeth extending beyond the normal contour of the dental arches; usually in an anterior direction.

pulpless t., a t. with a nonvital or necrotic pulp, or one from which the pulp has been extirpated.

sclerotic teeth, teeth that are naturally hard and resistant to caries.

screwdriver teeth, SYN Hutchinson teeth.

second t., SYN permanent t.

spaced teeth, teeth which have separated and lost proximal contact with adjacent teeth.

stomach t., one of the lower canine teeth.

succedaneous t., SYN permanent t.

syphilitic teeth, SYN Hutchinson teeth.

temporary t., SYN deciduous t.

third-year molar t. [TA], eighth permanent t. in the maxilla and mandible on each side, making it the most posterior t. in human dentition; usually erupts between the 17th and 23rd years; the roots are often fused, the separation being marked only by grooves; because it tends to erupt in an anterosuperior direction, the lower third molar often becomes impacted against the lower second molar; it is common for one or more third molar to fail to develop. SYN dens molaris tertius [TA], dens serotinus ⭐, dens sapientiae, third molar, wisdom t.

tricuspid t., a t. having a crown with three cusps.

tube t., an artificial t. constructed with a vertical, cylindric aperture extending from the center of the base up into the body of the t. into which a pin may be placed or cast for the attachment of the t. to a denture base.

Turner t., enamel hypoplasia involving a solitary permanent t.; related to infection in the primary t. that preceded it or to trauma during odontogenesis.

unerupted t., (1) a t. prior to emergence; **(2)** a t. unable to break out or emerge from the dental alveolar tissues into the oral cavity.

vital t., a t. with a living pulp.

wisdom t., SYN third-year molar t.

zero degree teeth, prosthetic teeth having no cusp angles in relation to the horizontal.

---

tooth·ache (tooth'āk). Pain in a tooth due to the condition of the pulp or periodontal ligament resulting from caries, infection, or trauma. SYN dentalgia, odontalgia, odontodynia.

tooth-borne. A term used to describe a prosthesis or part of a prosthesis which depends entirely upon the abutment teeth for support.

△**top-.** SEE topo-.

top·ag·no·sis (top-ag-nō'sis). Inability to localize tactile sensations. SYN topoanesthesia. [top- + G. *a-* priv. + *gnōsis,* recognition]

top·es·the·sia (top'es-thē'zē-ă). The ability to localize a light touch applied to any part of the skin. [top- + G. *aisthēsis,* sensation]

to·pha·ceous (tō-fā'shŭs). Sandy; gritty; pertaining to or manifesting the features of a tophus. [L. *tophaceus*]

to·phi (tō'fī). Plural of tophus.

to·phus, pl. **to·phi** (tō'fŭs, tō'fī). **1.** SEE gouty t. **2.** A salivary calculus, or tartar. SYN gouty pearl. [L. a calcareous deposit from springs, tufa]

gouty t., a deposit of uric acid and urates in periarticular fibrous tissue, cartilage of the external ear, or kidney, in gout. SYN arthritic calculus, uratoma.

top·i·ca (top'i-kă). Remedies for local external use. [neut. pl. of Mod. L. *topicus,* local]

top·i·cal (top'i-kăl). Relating to a definite place or locality; local. [G. *topikos,* fr. *topos,* place]

Topinard, Paul, French anthropologist, 1830–1911. SEE T. facial *angle, line.*

to·pis·tic (tō-pis'tik). Denoting an anatomically defined region in the nervous system. [G. *topos,* place]

△**topo-, top-.** Place, topical. [G. *topos*]

top·o·an·es·the·sia (top'ō-an-es-thē'zē-ă, tō'pō-). SYN topagnosis. [topo- + anesthesia]

top·og·no·sis, top·og·no·sia (top-og-nō'sis, -nō'zē-ă). Recognition of the location of a sensation; in the case of touch, topesthesia. [topo- + G. *gnōsis,* knowledge]

top·o·gom·e·ter (top-ō-gom'ĕ-ter). A movable fixation target attached to the front of a keratometer, used in fitting contact lenses to measure the curvatures of the cornea in its peripheral zones. [topo- + G. *gonia,* angle, + *metron,* measure]

to·pog·ra·phy (tō-pog'ră-fē). In anatomy, the description of any part of the body, especially in relation to a definite and limited area of the surface. [topo- + G. *graphē,* a writing]

to·po·i·som·er·ase (tō'pō-i-som'er-ās). A type of enzyme converting (isomerizing) one topological version of DNA into another; acts by catalyzing the breakage and reformation of DNA phosphodiester linkages. [topo- + isomerase]

Topolanski, Alfred, Austrian ophthalmologist, 1861–1960. SEE T. *sign.*

to·pol·o·gy (tō-pol'ō-jē). **1.** SYN regional *anatomy.* **2.** The study of the dimensions of personality. [topo- + G. *logos,* study]

top·o·nar·co·sis (top'ō-nar-kō'sis). A localized cutaneous anesthesia. [topo- + narcosis]

top·o·nym (tō'pō-nim). A regional term; one designating a region as distinguished from the name of a structure, system, or organ. [topo- + G. *onyma,* name]

to·pon·y·my (tō-pon'i-mē). Topical or regional nomenclature, as distinguished from organonymy. [topo- + G. *onyma,* name]

top·o·path·o·gen·e·sis (tō'pō-path-ō-jen'ĕ-sis). Topography of lesions related to their pathogenesis. [topo- + pathogenesis]

top·o·pho·bia (tō-pō-fō'bē-ă). A neurotic dread of or related to a particular place or locality. [topo- + G. *phobos,* fear]

top·o·phy·lax·is (tō'pō-fī-lak'sis). Prevention of arsphenamine shock by a tourniquet applied to the limb above the site of injection and its slow release five or six minutes later. [topo- + G. *phylaxis,* protection]

topotecan (tō-pō-tek'an). A topoisomerase I inhibitor with antitumor activity used in the treatment of ovarian cancer.

TORCH Acronym for *to*xoplasmosis, *o*ther infections, *r*ubella, *c*ytomegalovirus infection, and *h*erpes simplex. SEE TORCH *syndrome.*

tor·cu·lar he·roph·i·li (tōr'kū-lăr hĕ-rof'i-lī). Archaic term for *confluence* of sinuses. [L. wine-press of *Herophilus,* fr. *torqueo,* to twist]

Torek, Franz J.A., U.S. surgeon, 1861–1938. SEE T. *operation.*

to·ric (tō'rik). Relating to, or having the curvature of, a torus.

Torkildsen, Arne, Norwegian neurosurgeon, 1899–1968 . SEE T. *shunt.*

Tornwaldt, Gustavus Ludwig, German physician, 1843–1910. SEE T. *abscess, cyst, disease, syndrome.*

to·rose, to·rous (tō'rōs, -rŭs). Bulging; knobby. [L. *torosus,* fleshy, fr. *torus,* a knot, bulge]

To·ro·vi·rus (tō-rō-vī'rus). A genus in the family Coronaviridae that causes enteric infections in animals.

tor·pent (tōr'pent). **1.** SYN torpid. **2.** A benumbing agent. [L. *torpeo,* pres. p. *-ens,* to be sluggish]

tor·pid (tōr'pid). Inactive; sluggish. SYN torpent (1). [L. *torpidus,* fr. *torpeo,* to be sluggish]

tor·pid·i·ty (tōr-pid'i-tē). SYN torpor.

tor·por (tōr'per, pōr). Inactivity, sluggishness. SYN torpidity. [L. sluggishness, numbness]

torque (T) (tōrk). **1.** A rotatory force. **2.** In dentistry, a torsion force applied to a tooth to produce or maintain crown or root movement. [L. *torqueo,* to twist]

torr (tōr). A unit of pressure sufficient to support a 1-mm column of mercury at 0°C against the standard acceleration of gravity at 45° north latitude (980.621 cm/s^2); equivalent to 1333.224 dynes/cm^2, 1.333224 millibars, 1.35951 cm of H_2O, 133.3224 newtons/m^2 (or Pa); 1 atm equals 760 Torr. [Evangelista *Torricelli*]

Torre, Douglas P., U.S. dermatologist, *1919. SEE T. *syndrome;* Muir-Torre *syndrome.*

tor·re·fac·tion (tōr-ē-fak'shŭn). Parching or drying by heat; a pharmaceutical operation for rendering drugs friable. [L. *tor-re-facio,* pp. *-factus,* to make dry by heat, fr. *torreo,* to parch]

tor·re·fy (tōr'ē-fī). To parch.

Torricelli, Evangelista, Italian scientist, 1608–1647. SEE torr.

tor·sade de pointes (tōr-săd dĕ pwant'). "Twisting of the points," a form of ventricular tachycardia nearly always due to medications and characterized by a long QT interval and a "short-long-short" sequence in the beat preceding its onset. The QRS complexes during this rhythm tend to show a series of complexes points up followed by complexes points down, often with a narrow waist between and no definite T waves; at one time referred to as "cardiac ballet." [Fr. *torsade,* fringe, twist, or coil, + *pointe,* point or tip (euphonious for "wave burst")]

tor·sion (tōr'shŭn). **1.** A twisting or rotation of a part upon its long axis or on its mesentery; often associated with compromise of the blood supply. **2.** Twisting of the cut end of an artery to arrest hemorrhage. **3.** Rotation of the eye around its anteroposterior axis. SEE ALSO intorsion, extorsion, dextrotorsion, levotorsion. [L. *torsio,* fr. *torqueo,* to twist]

  t. of appendage, t. of testicular or epididymal appendix.

  extravaginal t., high t. above insertion of tunica vaginalis; tends to occur in neonatal period.

  intravaginal t., t. below insertion of tunica vaginalis, the most common type of testicular t. SEE bell clapper *deformity.*

  perinatal t., tends to be extravaginal type.

◨t. of testis, rotation of spermatic cord producing ischemia of testis.

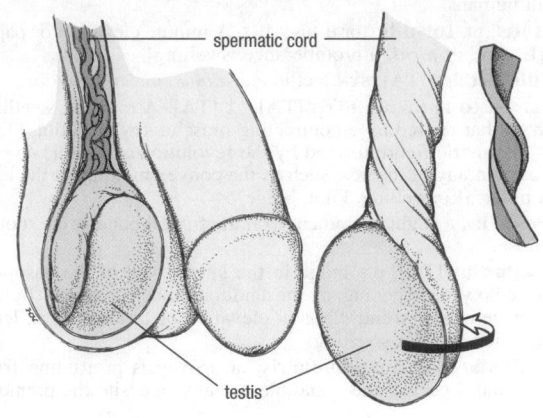

spermatic cord

testis

torsion of the spermatic cord

  t. of a tooth, rotation of a tooth in its socket.

tor·sion·om·e·ter (tōr-shŭn-om'ĕ-ter). A device for measuring the degree of rotation of the spinal column.

tor·si·ver·sion (tōr-si-ver'shŭn). A malposition of a tooth in which it is rotated on its long axis. SYN torsive occlusion, torsoclusion (2).

tor·so (tōr'sō). The trunk; the body without relation to head or extremities. [It.]

tor·so·clu·sion (tōr'sō-kloo-zhŭn). **1.** Obsolete term for acupressure performed by entering a needle in the tissues parallel with the artery, then turning it so that it crosses the artery transversely, and passing it into the tissues on the opposite side of the vessel. **2.** SYN torsiversion. [L. *torqueo,* to twist, + *claudo* or *cludo,* to close]

tor·ti·col·lar (tōr-ti-kol'ăr). Relating to or marked by torticollis.

tor·ti·col·lis (tōr-ti-kol'is). A contraction, or shortening, of the muscles of the neck, chiefly those supplied by the spinal accessory nerve; the head is drawn to one side and usually rotated so that the chin points to the other side. SEE ALSO dystonia. SYN wry neck, wryneck. [L. *tortus,* twisted, + *collum,* neck]

  benign paroxysmal t. of infancy, intermittent recurrent episodes of head tilt and t. usually associated with vomiting; the disorder usually appears between 2 and 8 months of age and resolves by age 3.

  congenital t., t. due to a unilateral fibrous tumor in the sternocleidomastoid muscle, present at birth as a swelling that may subside or may lead to t. by shortening of the muscle. SYN muscular t.

  dermatogenic t., painful stiff neck with limitation of motion due to extensive skin lesions in the area.

  dystonic t., SYN spasmodic t.

  fixed t., persistent contracture of cervical muscles on one side.

  hysterical t., t. believed to be psychosomatic in etiology. SEE hysteria.

  labyrinthine t., t. due to vestibular disorder.

  muscular t., SYN congenital t.

  ocular t., t. incident to paralysis of an extraocular muscle, especially an oblique muscle.

  psychogenic t., spasmodic contractions of the neck muscles, of psychosomatic origin. SEE ALSO spasmodic t.

  spasmodic t., a disorder of unknown cause, manifested as a restricted dystonia, localized to some of the neck muscles, especially the sternomastoid and trapezius; occurs in adults and tends to progress slowly; the head movements increase with standing and walking and decrease with contractual stimuli, e.g., touching the chin or neck. SYN dystonic t., rotatory tic.

tor·ti·pel·vis (tōr-ti-pel'vis). Twisted pelvis.

tor·tu·ous (tōr'choo-ŭs). Having many curves; full of turns and twists. [L. *tortuosus,* fr. *torqueo,* to twist]

Tor·u·lop·sis (tōr-oo-lop'sis). A genus of yeasts with smaller

to

blastoconidia (2–4 nm) with a wide attachment to the parent cell; *T. glabrata,* now called *Candida glabrata,* is a cause of candidiasis in humans.

tor·u·lus, pl. **tor·u·li** (tōr′ū-lŭs, -lī). A minute elevation or papilla. [L. dim. of *torus,* a protuberance, swelling]

　tor′uli tact′iles [TA], SYN tactile *elevations,* under *elevation.*

to·rus, pl. **to·ri** (tō′rŭs, tō′rī) [TA]. **1** [TA]. A rounded swelling, such as that caused by a contracting muscle. SYN elevation [TA]. **2.** A geometric figure formed by the revolution of a circle around the base of any of its arcs, such as the convex molding at the base of a pillar. [L. swelling, knot, bulge]

　t. fronta′lis, a slight prominence on the frontal bone at the root of the nose.

　t. levator′ius [TA], the bulge in the lateral wall of the nasopharynx, below the opening of the auditory tube, produced by the levator veli palatini muscle. SYN elevation of levator palati, levator cushion, levator swelling.

　mandibular t., t. mandibula′ris, an exostosis protruding from the lingual aspect of the mandible, usually opposite the premolar teeth.

　t. ma′nus, archaic term for the carpal bones.

　t. occipita′lis, an occasional ridge near the superior nuchal line of the occipital bone.

　⊡palatine t., t. palati′nus, an exostosis protruding from the midline of the hard palate.

　t. tuba′rius [TA], a ridge in the nasopharyngeal wall posterior to the opening of the pharyngotympanic (auditory) tube, caused by the projection of the cartilaginous portion of this tube. SYN eustachian cushion, tubal prominence.

　t. ureter′icus, SYN interureteric *crest.*

　t. uteri′nus, a transverse ridge on the back part of the cervix of the uterus, formed by the junction of the rectouterine folds.

TOS Abbreviation for thoracic outlet *syndrome.*

tos·yl (tō′sil). Toluenesulfonyl radical, widely used to block amino groups in the course of organic syntheses of drugs and other biologically active compounds.

tos·yl·ate (tō′si-lāt). USAN-approved contraction for *p*-toluenesulfonate.

to·tem (tō′tem). An object (usually an animal or plant) serving as the emblem of a family or clan and often as a reminder of its ancestry; something that serves as a revered symbol. [Amer. Indian]

to·tem·ism (tō′tem-izm). Belief in a kinship with, or a mystical relationship between, a group or individual and a totem.

to·tem·is·tic (tō-tem-is′tik). Relating to totemism.

to·tip·o·ten·cy, to·tip·o·tence (tō-ti-pō′ten-sē, tō-tip′ō-tens). The ability of a cell to differentiate into any type of cell and thus form a new organism or regenerate any part of an organism; e.g., a fertilized ovum, or a small excised portion of a *Planaria,* which is capable of regenerating a complete new organism. [L. *totus,* entire, + *potentia,* power]

to·tip·o·tent, to·ti·po·ten·tial (tō-tip′ŏ-tent, tō′ti-pō-ten′shăl). Relating to totipotency.

touch (tŭch). **1.** The sense by which slight contact with the skin or mucous membrane is appreciated. SYN tactile sense. **2.** Digital examination. [Fr. *toucher*]

　royal t., a touching of a patient by the king, which was thought to be curative; usually applied to patients with scrofula, but also done with patients with enlarged lymph glands (buboes) of plague.

Toupet, A., French surgeon. SEE T. *fundoplication.*

Tourette. SEE Gilles de la Tourette.

Tournay, Auguste, French ophthalmologist, 1878–1969. SEE T. *sign.*

tour·ni·quet (toor′ni-ket). An instrument for temporarily arresting the flow of blood to or from a distal part by pressure applied with an encircling device. [Fr. fr. *tourner,* to turn]

　Dupuytren t., an instrument for compression on the abdominal aorta.

　Esmarch t., a rubber t. that is wrapped around an extremity from distal to proximal before starting a surgical procedure to exsanguinate the limb before the inflation of a proximally placed pneumatic tourniquet. SYN Esmarch bandage.

　Rummel t., a t. fashioned by passing an umbilical tape around a vessel and bringing both ends through a short red rubber catheter. The t. can be tightened and secured with a perpendicularly placed hemostat at the end of the catheter farthest from the vessel.

Tourtual, Kaspar, Prussian anatomist, 1802–1865. SEE T. *membrane, sinus.*

Touton, Karl, German dermatologist, *1858. SEE T. giant *cell.*

Tovell, Ralph M., U.S. anesthesiologist, 1901–1967. SEE T. *tube.*

Towne, E.B., U.S. otolaryngologist, 1883–1957. SEE T. *projection,* projection *radiograph, view.*

△tox-. SEE toxico-.

tox·al·bu·mins (toks-al-bū′minz). Phytotoxins that inhibit protein synthesis.

tox·a·ne·mia (tok-să-nē′mē-ă). Anemia resulting from the effects of a hemolytic poison. [G. *toxikon,* poison, + anemia]

tox·a·phene (tok′să-fēn). A chlorinated hydrocarbon insecticide.

Tox·as·ca·ris le·o·ni·na (tok-sas′kă-ris lē-ō-nī′nă). An ascarid nematode of the dog that differs from *Toxocara* in that the larvae do not migrate through the lungs; the entire developmental cycle occurs in the gut. This parasite has been found in humans in a few instances and is a cause of visceral larva migrans in children, though less frequently implicated than is *Toxocara canis.* [G. *toxon,* bow, + *Ascaris*]

tox·e·mia (tok-sē′mē-ă). **1.** Clinical manifestations observed during certain infectious diseases, assumed to be caused by toxins and other noxious substances elaborated by the infectious agent; in certain infections by Gram-negative bacteria, endotoxins probably play a role when the bacterial cell wall breaks down, releasing a complex lipopolysaccharide; however, the role of other bacterial substances is unclear, except in the case of the specific exotoxins such as those of diphtheria and tetanus. **2.** The clinical syndrome caused by toxic substances in the blood. **3.** A lay term referring to the hypertensive disorders of pregnancy. SYN toxicemia. [G. *toxikon,* poison, + *haima,* blood]

tox·e·mic (tok-sē′mik). Pertaining to, affected by, or manifesting the features of toxemia.

△toxi-. SEE toxico-.

tox·ic (tok′sik). **1.** SYN poisonous. **2.** Pertaining to a toxin. [G. *toxikon,* an arrow-poison]

tox·i·cant (tok′si-kant). **1.** SYN poisonous. **2.** Any poisonous agent, specifically an alcoholic or other poison, causing symptoms of what is popularly called intoxication.

tox·i·ce·mia (tok-si-sē′mē-ă). SYN toxemia.

tox·ic·i·ty (tok-sis′i-tē). The state of being poisonous.

　oxygen t., **(1)** a body disturbance resulting from breathing high partial pressures of oxygen; characterized by visual and hearing abnormalities, unusual fatigue while breathing, muscular twitching, anxiety, confusion, incoordination, and convulsions; can occur when excessive quantities of oxygen are administered in patients (such as adult respiratory distress syndrome), resulting in worsening of pulmonary infiltrates and clinical deterioration; although the mechanism for development of the condition is obscure, a disruption of enzymatic activity is likely, perhaps as a result of free radical formation. Cf. retrolental *fibroplasia;* **(2)** exposure of the lungs to greater than 60% oxygen for periods exceeding 24–48 hours can lead to severe, irreversible pulmonary fibrosis. SYN oxygen poisoning.

△toxico-, tox-, toxi-, toxo-. Poison, toxin. [G. *toxikon,* bow, hence (arrow) poison]

Tox·i·co·den·dron (tok′si-kō-den′dron). A genus of poisonous plants (family Anacardiaceae), also known as *Rhus,* with smooth fruits and foliage that contain urushiol, which produces a contact dermatitis (rhus dermatitis); species include poison ivy (*T. radicans*), poison oak (*T. diversilobum*), and poison sumac (*T. vernix*) [toxico- + G. *dendron,* tree]

tox·i·co·gen·ic (tok′si-kō-jen′ik). **1.** Producing a poison. **2.** Caused by a poison. [toxico- + G. *-gen,* producing]

tox·i·coid (tok'si-koyd). Having an action like that of a poison; temporarily poisonous. [toxico- + G. *eidos,* resemblance]

tox·i·co·log·ic (tok'si-kō-loj'ik). Relating to toxicology.

tox·i·col·o·gist (tok-si-kol'ŏ-jist). A specialist or expert in toxicology.

tox·i·col·o·gy (tok-si-kol'ŏ-jē). The science of poisons, including their source, chemical composition, action, tests, and antidotes. [toxico- + G. *logos,* study]

tox·i·co·path·ic (tok'si-kō-path'ik). Denoting any morbid state caused by the action of a poison.

tox·i·co·pho·bia (tok'si-kō-fō'bē-ă). Morbid fear of being poisoned. SYN toxiphobia. [toxico- + G. *phobos,* fear]

tox·i·co·sis (tok-si-kō'sis). Any disease of toxic origin. SYN systemic poisoning. [toxico- + G. *-osis,* condition]

endogenic t., SYN autointoxication.

exogenic t., any disease caused by a poison introduced from without and not generated within the body.

thyroid t., SYN triiodothyronine t.

triiodothyronine t., T$_3$ **t.,** hyperthyroidism resulting from excessive circulating 3,5,3'-triiodothyronine. SYN thyroid t.

tox·if·er·ines (tok-sif'er-ēnz). The most potent group of the curare alkaloids; the principal source is *Strychnos toxifera.*

tox·if·er·ous (tok-sif'er-ŭs). SYN poisonous. [toxi- + L. *fero,* to bear]

tox·i·gen·ic (tok-si-jen'ik). SYN toxinogenic.

tox·i·ge·nic·i·ty (tok-si-jĕ-nis'i-tē). SYN toxinogenicity.

tox·il·ic ac·id (tok-sil'ik). SYN maleic acid.

tox·in (tok'sin). A noxious or poisonous substance that is formed or elaborated either as an integral part of the cell or tissue, as an extracellular product (exotoxin), or as a combination of the two, during the metabolism and growth of certain microorganisms and some higher plant and animal species. [G. *toxikon,* poison]

animal t., SYN zootoxin.

anthrax t., a culture filtrate of *Bacillus anthracis* containing an exotoxin with at least three different antigenically distinct components: edema factor, lethal factor, and protective antigen. SYN *Bacillus anthracis* t.

***Bacillus anthracis* t.,** SYN anthrax t.

bacterial t., any intracellular or extracellular t. formed in or elaborated by bacterial cells.

bee t., the t. delivered by a bee sting; contains three active principles: biogenic amines, active peptides, and certain hydrolytic enzymes.

botulinus t., a potent exotoxin that is highly neurotoxic from *Clostridium botulinum.* SYN botulin, botulismotoxin.

cholera t., SEE *Vibrio cholerae.*

***Clostridium perfringens* alpha t.,** a phospholipase produced by *Clostridium perfringens* that increases vascular permeability and produces necrosis.

***Clostridium perfringens* beta t.,** a substance produced by *Clostridium perfringens* that causes necrosis and induces hypertension by causing release of catecholamine.

***Clostridium perfringens* epsilon t.,** a t. produced by *Clostridium perfringens* that increases the permeability of the gastrointestinal wall.

***Clostridium perfringens* iota t.,** a binary t. produced by *Clostridium perfringens* responsible for necrosis and increased vascular permeability.

cobra t., SYN cobrotoxin.

Crotalus t., the t. of rattlesnake.

diagnostic diphtheria t., SYN Schick test t.

Dick test t., SYN streptococcus erythrogenic t.

dinoflagellate t., a potent neurotoxin that is thought to act similarly to botulinus t. by impairing the synthesis or the release of acetylcholine. Responsible for "red tide" loss of shellfish.

diphtheria t., SEE *Corynebacterium diphtheriae.*

erythrogenic t., SYN streptococcus erythrogenic t.

extracellular t., SYN exotoxin.

intracellular t., SYN endotoxin.

normal t., a t. solution holding exactly 100 lethal doses in 1 mL.

plant t., SYN phytotoxin.

scarlet fever erythrogenic t., SYN streptococcus erythrogenic t.

Schick test t., *Corynebacterium diphtheriae* t. diluted so that the inoculated dose (0.1 or 0.2 mL) will contain ⅟₅₀th of a guinea pig minimal lethal dose. SEE ALSO Schick *test.* SYN diagnostic diphtheria t.

Shiga t., the endotoxin formed by *Shigella dysenteriae* type 1.

Shigalike t., SYN vero *cytotoxin.*

streptococcus erythrogenic t., a culture filtrate of lysogenized group A strains of β-hemolytic streptococci, erythrogenic when inoculated into the skin of susceptible persons, and neutralized by antibodies that appear during scarlet fever convalescence; three immunologic types (A, B, and C) are recognized. SYN Dick test t., erythrogenic t., scarlet fever erythrogenic t.

tetanus t., the neurotropic, heat-labile exotoxin of *Clostridium tetani* and the cause of tetanus; it has been isolated as a crystalline protein (molecular weight 67,000), is one of the most poisonous substances known, and seems to function by blocking inhibitory synaptic impulses. SYN tetanotoxin.

tox·in·ic (tok-sin'ik). Relating to a toxin.

tox·i·no·gen·ic (tok'si-nō-jen'ik). Producing a toxin, said of an organism. SYN toxigenic. [toxin + G. *-gen,* producing]

tox·i·no·ge·nic·i·ty (tok'si-nō-jĕ-nis'i-tē). The capacity to produce toxin. SYN toxigenicity.

tox·i·nol·o·gy (tok'si-nol'ō-jē). The study of toxins, in a restricted sense, with reference to the relatively unstable proteinaceous substances of microbial, plant, or animal origins. [toxin + G. *logos,* study]

tox·i·no·sis (tok-si-nō'sis). Any disease or lesion caused by the action of a toxin. SYN toxonosis. [toxin + G. *-osis,* condition]

tox·i·pho·bia (tok-si-fō'bē-ă). SYN toxicophobia.

tox·is·ter·ol (tok-sis'ter-ol). A toxic substance formed by excessive irradiation of ergosterol or calciferol.

♻**toxo-.** SEE toxico-.

Tox·o·ca·ra (tok'sō-kar'ă). A genus of ascarid nematodes, chiefly found in carnivores, that cause toxocariasis. [G. *toxon,* bow, + *kara,* head]

T. ca'nis, the common ascarid species in the small intestine of the dog, where prenatal infection is a common mode of infection of pups; it is also reported in cats, wolves, foxes, coyotes, and badgers; the second-stage larva is the most frequent cause of visceral larva migrans in the liver of children.

T. mys'tax, a common ascarid species of cats, but not reported from dogs; prenatal infection of kittens does not occur, infection being by infective eggs, which hatch in the intestine, releasing second-stage larvae, which then undergo migration through the heart, lung, trachea, mouth, and gut, as with *Ascaris lumbricoides* in man; mice and other vertebrates, and also some invertebrates (e.g., earthworms, cockroaches) may serve as transport hosts, in which the migrating larvae encyst in the tissues.

tox·o·ca·ri·a·sis (tok'sō-kă-rī'ă-sis). Infection with nematodes of the genus *Toxocara;* parenterally migrating larvae, chiefly of *Toxocara canis,* may cause visceral larva migrans; ocular involvement results in either a solitary granuloma in the retina, peripheral inflammatory masses, or chronic endophthalmitis.

tox·oid (tok'soyd). A toxin that has been treated (commonly with formaldehyde) so as to destroy its toxic property but retain its antigenicity, i.e., its capability of stimulating the production of antitoxin antibodies and thus of producing an active immunity. For specific toxoids, see entries under vaccine. SYN anatoxin. [toxin + G. *eidos,* resemblance]

tox·on, tox·one (tok'sŏn, tok'sōn). A hypothetical bacterial product, of feeble toxicity and weak affinity for antitoxin.

tox·o·neme (tok'sō-nēm). SYN rhoptry. [G. *toxon,* bow, + *nema,* thread]

tox·o·no·sis (tok-sō-nō'sis). SYN toxinosis. [toxo- + G. *nosos,* disease]

tox·o·phil, tox·o·phile (tok'sō-fil, -fīl). Susceptible to the action of a poison; having an affinity for toxins. [toxo- + G. *philos,* fond]

tox·o·phore (tok'sō-fōr). Denoting the atomic group of the toxin

to

molecule which carries the poisonous principle. [toxo- + G. *phoros,* bearing]

tox·oph·o·rous (tok-sof′ăr-ŭs). Relating to the toxophore group of the toxin molecule.

Tox·o·plas·ma gon·dii (tok-sō-plaz′mă gon′dē-ī). An abundant, widespread sporozoan species (family Toxoplasmatidae) that is an intracellular, non–host-specific parasite in a great variety of vertebrates. It develops its sexual cycle, leading to oocyst production, exclusively in cats and other felids; proliferative stages (tachyzoites) and tissue cysts (containing bradyzoites) develop in a wide variety of animal species that acquire the infection from ingestion of oocysts, tissue cysts from infected meat, organ transplantation or by transplacental migration, leading to infection in utero. [G. *toxon,* bow or arc, + *plasma,* anything formed]

Tox·o·plas·mat·i·dae (tok′sō-plaz-mat′i-dē). A family of coccidian sporozoa including the genera *Toxoplasma* and *Frankelia,* characterized by endodyogeny and by the presence of cysts (sometimes termed pseudocysts) containing bradyzoites in parenteral cells of the host; schizonts and gamonts are produced in intestinal cells, and gamonts give rise to oocysts. Final hosts of *Toxoplasma* are cats and other felids; final hosts of *Frankelia* are unknown.

tox·o·plas·mo·sis (tok′sō-plaz-mō′sis). Disease caused by the protozoan parasite *Toxoplasma gondii,* which can produce abortion in sheep, encephalitis in mink, and a variety of syndromes in humans. Prenatally acquired human infection can result in the presence of abnormalities such as microcephalus or hydrocephalus at birth, the development of jaundice with hepatosplenomegaly or meningoencephalitis in early childhood, or the delayed appearance of ocular lesions such as chorioretinitis in later childhood. Postnatally acquired human infections typically remain subclinical; if clinical disease does occur, symptoms include fever, lymphadenopathy, headache, myalgia, and fatigue, with eventual recovery, except in the immunocompromised patient where fatal encephalitis often develops.

acquired t. in adults, a form of t. that may result in fever, encephalomyelitis, chorioretinopathy, maculopapular rash, arthralgia, myalgia, myocarditis, and pneumonitis; a lymphadenopathic form seems to be more prevalent in adults, and such persons may manifest fever, lymphadenopathy, malaise, and headache, a form frequently found in patients with AIDS.

congenital t., t. apparently resulting from parasites in an infected mother being transmitted in utero to the fetus, observed as three syndromes: 1) acute: most of the organs contain foci of necrosis in association with fever, jaundice, hydrocephaly, encephalomyelitis, pneumonitis, cutaneous rash, ophthalmic lesions, hepatomegaly, and splenomegaly; 2) subacute: most of the lesions are partly healed or calcified, but those in the brain and eye seem to remain active, inasmuch as chorioretinitis is observed in more than 80% of diseased infants; 3) chronic: usually not recognized during the newborn period, but chorioretinitis and cerebral lesions may be detected weeks to years later.

tox·o·py·rim·i·dine (toks′ō-pi-rim′i-dēn). One of the products resulting from the hydrolysis of thiamin by thiaminase and appearing in the urine; a competitive inhibitor of pyridoxal. SYN pyramin, pyramine.

Toynbee, Joseph, English otologist, 1815–1866. SEE T. *corpuscles,* under *corpuscle, muscle, tube.*

TPA, tPA Abbreviation for tissue plasminogen *activator.*

TPN Abbreviation for total parenteral *nutrition.*

TPP Abbreviation for *thiamin* pyrophosphate.

TPR Abbreviation for total peripheral *resistance.*

TQ Abbreviation for tocopherolquinone.

TR Abbreviation for repetition *time* in magnetic resonance imaging.

tr. Abbreviation for L. *tinctura,* or tincture.

tra·bec·u·la, gen. and pl. **tra·bec·u·lae** (tră-bek′ū-lă, -lē) [TA]. **1.** A meshwork; one of the supporting bundles of fibers traversing the substance of a structure, usually derived from the capsule or one of the fibrous septa. **2.** A small piece of the spongy substance of bone usually interconnected with other similar pieces. **3.** In

histopathology, a band of neoplastic tissue two or more cells wide. [L. dim. of *trabs,* a beam]

anterior chamber t., tissue at the angle of the anterior chamber through which aqueous humor exits from the eye.

arachnoid t. [TA], fine, delicate strands composed of fibroblast and extracellular collagen that traverse the subarachnoid space between the arachnoid mater, which is attached to the dura, and the pia mater, which is adherent to the surface of the brain. SYN trabeculae arachnoideae [TA].

trabeculae arachnoideae [TA], SYN arachnoid t.

trabec′ulae car′neae (of right and left ventricles) [TA], muscular bundles on the lining walls of the ventricles of the heart. SYN columnae carneae, Rathke bundles, trabeculae carneae ventriculorum dextri et sinistri.

trabeculae carneae ventriculorum dextri et sinistri, SYN trabeculae carneae (of right and left ventricles).

trabeculae of corpora cavernosa [TA], fibromuscular bands and cords given off from the fibrous envelopes and septum of the corpora cavernosa penis and that separate the cavernous veins. SYN trabeculae corporum cavernosorum [TA].

trabec′ulae cor′poris spongio′si pe′nis [TA], SYN trabeculae of corpus spongiosum.

trabec′ulae cor′porum cavernoso′rum [TA], SYN trabeculae of corpora cavernosa.

trabeculae of corpus spongiosum [TA], the fibrous bands interlacing between the vascular spaces of the corpus spongiosum and glans penis. SYN trabeculae corporis spongiosi penis [TA].

trabec′ulae cra′nii, a pair of chondrification centers in the base of the embryonic cartilaginous neurocranium, lying in front of the developing hypophysis; they become the sella turcica.

trabec′ulae lie′nis, ✫ official alternate term for splenic trabeculae.

trabeculae of lymph node [TA], supporting bundles of connective tissue traversing the substance of the spleen, derived from the capsule of the spleen. SYN trabeculae nodi lymphoidei [TA].

trabeculae nodi lymphoidei [TA], SYN trabeculae of lymph node.

septomarginal t. [TA], one of the trabeculae carneae in the right ventricle of the heart; it carries part of the right branch of the AV bundle from the septum to the anterior papillary muscle on the opposite wall of the ventricle. SYN t. septomarginalis [TA], moderator band, Reil band (1).

t. septomargina′lis [TA], SYN septomarginal t.

trabeculae of spleen, SYN splenic trabeculae.

splenic trabeculae [TA], small fibrous bands given off from the capsule of the spleen and constituting the framework of that organ. SYN trabeculae splenicae [TA], trabeculae lienis ✫, trabeculae of spleen.

trabec′ulae sple′nicae [TA], SYN splenic trabeculae.

t. tes′tis, SYN *septula* of testis, under *septulum.*

tra·bec·u·lar (tră-bek′ū-lăr). Relating to or containing trabeculae. SYN trabeculate.

tra·bec·u·late (tră-bek′ū-lāt). SYN trabecular.

tra·bec·u·la·tion (tră-bek′ū-lā′shŭn). **1.** The occurrence of trabeculae in the walls of an organ or part. **2.** The process of forming trabeculae, as in spongy bone.

tra·bec·u·lec·to·my (tră-bek′ū-lek′tō-mē). A filtering operation for glaucoma by creation of a fistula between the anterior chamber of the eye and the subconjunctival space, through a subscleral excision of a portion of the trabecular meshwork. [trabecula + G. *ektomē,* excision]

tra·bec·u·lo·plas·ty (tră-bek′ū-lō-plas-tē). Photocoagulation of the trabecular meshwork of the eye using the laser in the treatment of glaucoma.

laser t. (LTP), an operation for glaucoma in which laser energy is applied to the trabecular meshwork.

Investigations into laser treatments of open-angle glaucoma began in the early 1970s, but not until the late 1980s was LTP adopted as a standard treatment for the condition. In this procedure, a laser (usually argon) is used to create small openings in the trabecular meshwork at the ocular drainage angle, so as to improve the drainage of aqueous humor and relieve intraocular pressure. Laser iridotomy is sometimes performed at the same time. LTP lessens chances of postoperative infection and hemorrhage, and can be performed on an outpatient basis. This technique has achieved a 2-year success rate of over 70% (dropping to 59% after 5 years), but has been effective only in certain types of glaucoma (especially capsular and pigmentary glaucomas).

tra·bec·u·lot·o·my (tră-bek-ū-lot′ō-mē). Surgical opening of the sinus venosus sclerae (canal of Schlemm) to treat glaucoma. [trabekula + G. *tomē,* incision]

trace (trās). **1.** Evidence of the former existence, influence, or action of an object, phenomenon, or event. **2.** An extremely small amount or barely discernible indication of something.

trac·er (trā′ser). **1.** An element or compound containing atoms that can be distinguished from their normal counterparts by physical means (e.g., radioactivity assay or mass spectrography) and can thus be used to follow (trace) the metabolism of the normal substances. **2.** A colored or radioactive substance that can be injected in the region of a tumor (melanoma, breast, etc.) to map the flow of lymph from the tumor to its nearest nodal basin; used in sentinel node detection. **3.** A colored substance (e.g., a dye) used as a t. to follow the flow of water. **4.** An instrument used in dissecting out nerves and blood vessels. **5.** A mechanical device with a marking point attached to one jaw and a graph plate or tracing plate attached to the other jaw; used to record the direction and extent of movements of the mandible. SEE ALSO tracing (2). [M.E. track, fr. O. Fr. *tracier,* to make one's way, fr. L. *traho,* pp. *tractum,* to draw, + *-er,* agent suffix]

△**trache-.** SEE tracheo-.

▣**tra·chea**, pl. **tra·che·ae** (trā′kē-ă, -kē-ē) [TA]. The air tube extending from the larynx into the thorax (level of the fifth or sixth thoracic vertebra) where it bifurcates into the right and left main bronchi. The t. is composed of 16–20 rings of hyaline cartilage connected by a membrane (annular ligament); posteriorly, the rings are deficient for one-fifth to one-third of their circumference, the interval forming the membranous wall being closed by a fibrous membrane containing smooth muscular fibers. Internally, the mucosa is composed of a pseudostratified ciliated columnar epithelium with mucous goblet cells; numerous small mixed mucous and serous glands occur, the ducts of which open to the surface of the epithelium. SYN windpipe. [G. *tracheia artēria,* rough artery]

saber-sheath t., a type of tracheal collapse seen in chronic obstructive pulmonary disease in which there is an increase in the outer posterior tracheal dimension with side-to-side narrowing involving the lower two-thirds of the trachea.

scabbard t., a deformity of the t. caused by flattening and approximation of the lateral walls, producing more or less pronounced stenosis.

tra·che·al (trā′kē-ăl). Relating to the trachea.

tra·che·al·gia (trā-kē-al′jē-ă). Pain in the trachea. [trachea + G. *algos,* pain]

tra·che·a·lis. SEE trachealis (*muscle*).

tra·che·i·tis (trā-kē-ī′tis). Inflammation of the mucous membrane of the trachea. SYN trachitis. [trachea + G. *-itis,* inflammation]

△**trachel-.** SEE trachelo-.

trach·e·la·lis (trak-ĕ-lā′lis). Archaic term for longissimus capitis (*muscle*).

trach·e·lec·to·my (trak-ĕ-lek′tō-mē). SYN cervicectomy. [trachel- + G. *ektomē,* excision]

trach·e·le·ma·to·ma (trak′ĕ-lē-mă-tō′mă). A hematoma of the neck. [trachel- + hematoma]

trach·e·li·an (tră-kē′lē-an). Archaic term for cervical. [G. *trachēlos,* neck]

trach·e·lism, trach·e·lis·mus (trak′ĕ-lizm, -liz′mŭs). A bending backward of the neck, such as sometimes ushers in an epileptic attack. [G. *trachēlismos,* a seizing by the throat]

trach·e·li·tis (trak-ĕ-lī′tis). SYN cervicitis.

△**trachelo-, trachel-.** Neck. [G. *trachēlos*]

trach·e·lo·cele (trak′ĕ-lō-sēl). SYN tracheocele. [trachelo- + G. *kēlē,* tumor, hernia]

trach·e·lo·mas·toid (trak′ĕ-lō-mas′toyd). Archaic term for longissimus capitis (*muscle*).

trach·e·lo·oc·cip·i·ta·lis (trak′ĕ-lō-ok-sip′i-tā′lis). Archaic term for semispinalis capitis (*muscle*).

trach·e·lo·pa·nus (trak-ĕ-lō-pā′nŭs). **1.** Swelling of the lymphatic vessels of the neck. **2.** Lymphatic engorgement of the cervix uteri. [trachelo- + L. *panus,* tumor, swelling]

trach·e·lo·pex·ia, trach·e·lo·pexy (trak′ĕ-lō-pek′sē-ă, -pek-sē). Surgical fixation of the cervix uteri. [trachelo- + G. *pēxis,* fixation]

trach·e·lo·plas·ty (trak′ĕ-lō-plas-tē). Rarely used term for plastic surgery of the cervix uteri. [trachelo- + G. *plastos,* formed]

trach·e·lor·rha·phy (trak-ĕ-lōr′ă-fē). Repair by suture of a laceration of the cervix uteri. SYN Emmet operation. [trachelo- + G. *rhaphē,* suture]

trach·e·los (trak′ĕ-los). Archaic term for collum. [G. *trachēlos*]

trach·e·los·chi·sis (trak-ĕ-los′ki-sis). Congenital fissure in the neck. [trachelo- + G. *schisis,* fissure]

trach·e·lot·o·my (trak-ĕ-lot′ō-mē). SYN cervicotomy. [trachelo- + G. *tomē,* incision]

△**tracheo-, trache-.** The trachea. [see trachea]

tra·che·o·aer·o·cele (trā′kē-ō-ār′ō-sēl). An air cyst in the neck caused by distention of a tracheocele. [tracheo- + G. *aēr,* air, + *kēlē,* hernia]

tra·che·o·bil·i·ary (trā′kē-ō-bil′ē-ār-ē). Relating to the trachea or bronchi and the biliary duct system.

tra·che·o·bron·che·o·pa·thia os·te·o·plas·ti·ca. A benign submucoid tumor or series of tumors that ossify near the tracheal walls.

tra·che·o·bron·chi·al (trā′kē-ō-brong′kē-ăl). Relating to both trachea and bronchi, denoting especially a set of lymph nodes.

tra·che·o·bron·chi·tis (trā′kē-ō-brong-kī′tis). Inflammation of the mucous membrane of the trachea and bronchi.

tra·che·o·bron·cho·meg·a·ly (trā′kē-ō-brong′kō-meg′ă-lē). Gross widening of the trachea and main bronchi, usually congenital. SYN Mounier-Kuhn syndrome. [tracheo- + bronchus + G. *megas,* large]

tra·che·o·bron·chos·co·py (trā′kē-ō-brong-kos′kŏ-pē). Inspection of the interior of the trachea and bronchi. [tracheo- + bronchus, + G. *skopeō,* to view]

tra·che·o·cele (trā′kē-ō-sēl). A protrusion of the mucous membrane through a defect in the wall of the trachea. SYN trachelocele. [tracheo- + G. *kēlē,* hernia]

tra·che·o·e·soph·a·ge·al (trā′kē-ō-ē-sof′ă-jē′ăl). Relating to the trachea and the esophagus.

tra·che·o·la·ryn·ge·al (trā′kē-ō-lă-rin′jē-ăl). Relating to the trachea and the larynx.

tra·che·o·ma·la·cia (trā′kē-ō-mă-lā′shē-ă). Softening of the cartilages of the trachea. [tracheo- + G. *malakia,* softness]

tra·che·o·meg·a·ly (trā′kē-ō-meg′ă-lē). An abnormally dilated trachea which may, like bronchiectasis, result from infection or prolonged positive pressure ventilation. [tracheo- + G. *megas (megal-),* large]

tra·che·o·path·ia, tra·che·op·a·thy (trā′kē-ō-path′ē-ă, -op′ă-thē). Any disease of the trachea. [tracheo- + G. *pathos,* disease]

t. osteoplas′tica, a rare disease characterized by cartilaginous and bony growths in the trachea and bronchi that produce sessile polyps and plaques projecting into and partly obstructing the lumina.

tra·che·o·pha·ryn·ge·al (trā′kē-ō-fă-rin′jē-ăl). Relating to both trachea and pharynx; denoting an occasional band of muscular fibers passing from the inferior constrictor of the pharynx to the trachea.

tra·che·o·pho·ne·sis (trā′kē-ō-fō-nē′sis). Auscultation of the heart sounds at the sternal notch. [tracheo- + G. *phōnēsis,* a sounding]

tra·che·oph·o·ny (trā-kē-of′ō-nē). The hollow voice sound heard

tr

in auscultating over the trachea. SEE ALSO bronchophony. [tracheo- + G. *phōnē*, voice]

tra·che·o·plas·ty (trā′kē-ō-plas-tē). Plastic surgery of the trachea. [tracheo- + G. *plastos*, formed]

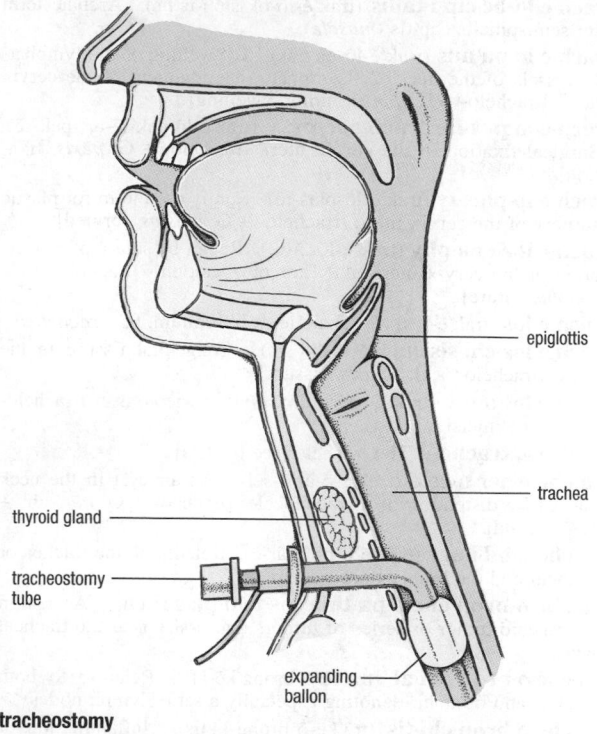

epiglottis

trachea

thyroid gland

tracheostomy tube

expanding ballon

tracheostomy

slide t., an operation for the repair of long tracheal stenosis in which anterior and posterior sliding flaps of tracheal wall are sutured together to reconstruct the tracheal lumen.

tra·che·or·rha·gia (trā-kē-ō-rā′jē-ă). Hemorrhage from the mucous membrane of the trachea. [tracheo- + G. *rhēgnymi*, to burst forth]

tra·che·os·chi·sis (trā-kē-os′ki-sis). A fissure into the trachea. [tracheo- + G. *schisis*, fissure]

tra·che·o·scope (trā′kē-ō-skōp). An instrument used in tracheoscopy.

tra·che·o·scop·ic (trā-kē-ō-skop′ik). Relating to tracheoscopy.

tra·che·os·co·py (trā-kē-os′kŏ-pē). Inspection of the interior of the trachea. [tracheo- + G. *skopeō*, to examine]

tra·che·o·ste·no·sis (trā′kē-ō-stĕ-nō′sis). Narrowing of the lumen of the trachea. [tracheo- + G. *stenōsis*, constriction]

tra·che·os·to·ma (trā′kē-os′tō-mă). Permanent opening into the trachea through the neck; also the opening after permanent laryngectomy. [tracheo- + G. *stoma*, mouth]

■**tra·che·os·to·my** (trā′kē-os′tō-mē). An operation to make an opening into the trachea. SEE ALSO tracheotomy. [tracheo- + G. *stoma*, mouth]

tra·che·o·tome (trā′kē-ō-tōm). A knife used in the operation of tracheotomy.

tra·che·ot·o·my (trā-kē-ot′ŏ-mē). The operation of incising the trachea, usually intended to be temporary. SEE ALSO tracheostomy. [tracheo- + G. *tomē*, incision]

Tra·chi·pleis·toph·ora (trā-kē-plī-stof′er-ă). A genus of microsporidia that can infect humans and cause myositis, keratoconjunctivitis, and sinusitis in the immunocompromised person.

tra·chi·tis (trā-kī′tis). SYN tracheitis.

■**tra·cho·ma** (tră-kō′mă). Chronic contagious microbial inflammation, with hypertrophy, of the conjunctiva, marked by the formation of minute grayish or yellowish translucent granules caused by

Chlamydia trachomatis. SYN Egyptian ophthalmia, granular lids, granular ophthalmia. [G. *trachōma*, fr. *trachys*, rough, harsh]

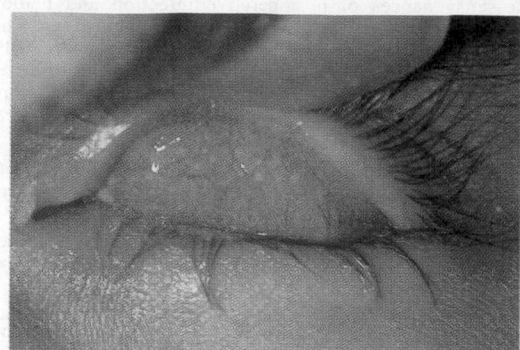

trachoma: note whitish follicles on the inner surface of the eyelid

follicular t., the ordinary form of t. marked by the presence of granulations on the conjunctiva. SYN granular t.

granular t., SYN follicular t.

tra·chom·a·tous (tră-kō′mă-tŭs). Relating to or suffering from trachoma.

tra·chy·chro·mat·ic (trak-i-krō-mat′ik). Denoting a nucleus with very deeply staining chromatin. [G. *trachys*, rough, + *chrōmatikos*, chromatic]

tra·chy·o·nych·ia (trak′ē-ō-nik′ē-ă). Rough-surfaced nails. [G. *trachys*, rough, + *onyx, onychos*, nail, + suffix *-ia*, condition]

tra·chy·pho·nia (trak′ē-fō′nē-ă). Roughness of voice. [G. *trachys*, rough, + *phōnē*, voice]

trac·ing (trās′ing). **1.** Any graphic display of electrical or mechanical cardiovascular events, e.g., electrocardiogram, phlebogram. SEE ALSO curve. **2.** In dentistry, a line or lines, scribed on a table or plate by a pointed instrument, representing a record of movements of the mandible; may be extraoral (made outside the oral cavity) or intraoral (made within the oral cavity).

arrow point t., SYN needle point t.

cephalometric t., an overlay drawing or t. of the teeth, facial bones, and anthropometric landmarks made directly from a cephalometric radiograph and used as a basis for cephalometric analysis.

Gothic arch t., SYN needle point t.

needle point t., a t. of mandibular movements made by means of a device attached to the opposing arches; its shape resembles that of an arrowhead or a Gothic arch, and when the instrument's marking point is at the apex of the arch, the jaws are considered to be in centric relation. SYN arrow point t., Gothic arch t., Gothic arch, stylus t.

stylus t., SYN needle point t.

TRACT

tract (trakt). An elongated area, e.g., path, track, way. SEE ALSO fascicle. SYN tractus. [L. *tractus*, a drawing out]

alimentary t., SYN digestive t.

anterior corticospinal t., uncrossed fibers forming a small bundle in the anterior funiculus of the spinal cord. SEE pyramidal t; SEE ALSO corticospinal t. SYN tractus corticospinalis anterior [TA], anterior pyramidal fasciculus, anterior pyramidal t., direct pyramidal t., fasciculus corticospinalis anterior, fasciculus pyramidalis anterior, tractus pyramidalis anterior, Türck bundle, Türck column, Türck t.

anterior pyramidal t., SYN anterior corticospinal t.

anterior raphespinal t. [TA], a group of axons that originate in the raphe nuclei, primarily of the medulla oblongata and caudal pons, and descend in the anterior funiculus. SYN tractus raphespinalis anterior [TA], ventral raphespinal t. [TA].

anterior spinocerebellar t. [TA], a bundle of fibers originating in the base of the posterior horn and zona intermedia throughout lumbosacral segments of the spinal cord, crossing to the opposite side and ascending in a peripheral position in the ventral half of the lateral funiculus. In its ascent through the rhombencephalon, the tract curves sharply dorsalward along the rostral border of the trigeminal motor nucleus, entering the cerebellum in a caudal direction over the dorsal surface of the superior cerebellar peduncle, and terminating as mossy fibers in the granular layer of the cortex of the cerebellar vermis. The bundle conveys proprioceptive and exteroceptive information largely from the opposite lower extremity, although some of its fibers recross in the cerebellum. SYN tractus spinocerebellaris anterior [TA], ventral spinocerebellar t.★, Gowers column, Gowers t.

anterior spinothalamic t. [TA], the more anterior or ventral part of the composite bundle, the anterolateral system, formed by the anterior and lateral spinothalamic tracts. These specific fibers are involved in tactile sensation. SEE spinothalamic t; SEE ALSO anterolateral *system*. SYN tractus spinothalamicus anterior [TA], ventral spinothalamic t.

anterior trigeminothalamic t. [TA], fibers that originate from the spinal trigeminal nucleus, cross the midline, and ascend on the contralateral side to terminate in the ventral posteromedial nucleus (VPM). This tract also contains, in the rostral pons and in the midbrain, fibers that originate in the contralateral principal sensory nucleus and that also terminate in the VPM. SYN tractus trigeminothalamicus anterior [TA], ventral trigeminothalamic t. [TA].

anterolateral t., SYN anterolateral *system*.

Arnold t., SYN temporopontine t.

association t., SEE association *system*.

auditory t., SYN lateral *lemniscus*.

bulboreticulospinal t. [TA], a t. that originates from the gigantocellular reticular nucleus of the medulla, descends primarily as an uncrossed t., and terminates mainly in spinal laminae VII and VIII. SYN lateral reticulospinal t. [TA], medullary reticulospinal t. [TA], tractus bulboreticulospinalis [TA].

Burdach t., SYN cuneate *fasciculus*.

caerulospinal t. [TA], a collection of axons that originate from the nucleus caeruleus and subcaeruleus area and project bilaterally to the gray matter of the spinal cord to all spinal levels; they are a major source of noradrenergic input to the spinal cord. SYN tractus caeruleospinalis [TA].

central tegmental t. [TA], a large fiber bundle passing longitudinally through the central mesencephalic and pontine tegmentum, distinguished from adjacent longitudinal groups of fiber-fascicles of the reticular formation by a more compact composition. In transverse sections of the mesencephalon the bundle occupies a large triangular area lateral to the medial longitudinal fasciculus; farther caudally it expands ventralward and finally passes over the lateral side of the (inferior) olivary nucleus, becoming part of the latter's fiber capsule. The bundle contains fibers from the mesencephalic tegmentum and regions surrounding the central gray substance descending to the olivary nucleus; it also includes numerous fibers ascending from the medullary, pontine, and mesencephalic reticular formation to the thalamus and subthalamus region. SYN tractus tegmentalis centralis [TA], central tegmental fasciculus.

cerebellorubral t., that component of the superior cerebellar peduncle (brachium conjunctivum) which distributes fibers within the red nucleus of the opposite side. SYN tractus cerebellorubralis.

cerebellothalamic t., that component of the superior cerebellar peduncle (brachium conjunctivum) which originates in the cerebellar nuclei, crosses completely in the decussation of the brachia conjunctiva, bypasses the red nucleus, and terminates in parts of the ventral anterior, ventral intermediate, ventral posterolateral, and central lateral nuclei of the thalamus. SYN dentatothalamic t., tractus cerebellothalamicus.

Collier t., SYN medial longitudinal *fasciculus*.

comma t. of Schultze, SYN semilunar *fasciculus*.

corticobulbar t., SEE corticonuclear *fibers*, under *fiber*. SYN tractus corticobulbaris.

corticopontine t., collective term for the multitude of fibers which, originating in all of the major subdivisions of the cerebral cortex, descend in the internal capsule and crus cerebri to terminate in the nuclei of the basilar part of the pons. Individual components of this massive fiber system are indicated, according to their origin in the cerebral cortex, as the frontopontine fibers [TA], parietopontine fibers [TA], occipitopontine fibers [TA], and temporopontine fibers [TA]. SYN tractus corticopontinus [TA].

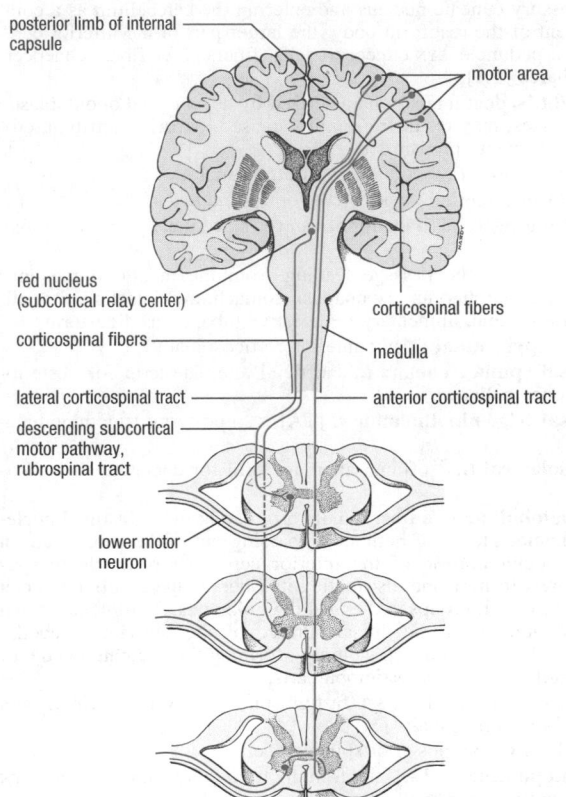

posterior limb of internal capsule

motor area

red nucleus (subcortical relay center)

corticospinal fibers

corticospinal fibers

medulla

lateral corticospinal tract

anterior corticospinal tract

descending subcortical motor pathway, rubrospinal tract

lower motor neuron

diagrammatic representation of motor pathways to the spinal cord via a direct route **(corticospinal tract)** and through a subcortical relay station (rubrospinal tract); the presence of a decussation means that one side of the brain controls skeletal muscle on the opposite side of the body

corticospinal t., a composite bundle of corticospinal fibers [TA] that descend into and through the medulla to form the lateral corticospinal tract [TA] and the anterior corticospinal tract [TA]. This massive bundle of fibers originates from pyramidal cells of various sizes in the fifth layer of the precentral motor (area 4), the premotor area (area 6), and to a lesser extent from the postcentral gyrus. Cells of origin in area 4 include the gigantopyramidal cells of Betz. Fibers from these cortical regions descend through the internal capsule, the middle third of the crus cerebri, and the ventral part of the pons to emerge on the ventral surface of the medulla oblongata as the pyramid. Continuing caudally, most of the fibers cross to the opposite side in the pyramidal decussation and descend in the dorsal half of the lateral funiculus of the spinal cord as the lateral corticospinal t., which distributes its fibers throughout the length of the spinal cord to interneurons of the zona intermedia of the spinal gray matter. In the (extremity-related) spinal cord enlargements, fibers also pass directly to motoneuronal groups that innervate distal extremity muscles subserving particular hand-and-finger or foot-and-toe movements. The uncrossed fibers form a small bundle, the anterior corticospinal t., which descends in the anterior funiculus of the spinal cord

tr

and terminates in synaptic contact with interneurons in the medial half of the anterior horn on both sides of the spinal cord. Interruption of corticospinal fibers at or below its cortical origin causes impairment of movement in the opposite body-half, especially severe in the arm and leg; characterized by muscular weakness, spasticity and hyperreflexia, and a loss of discrete finger and hand movements. Babinski sign is associated with this condition of hemiplegia. SYN pyramidal t. [TA], tractus pyramidalis [TA], tractus corticospinalis.

crossed pyramidal t., SYN lateral corticospinal t.

cuneocerebellar t., the nerve fiber system originating from the accessory cuneate nucleus and entering the cerebellum as a component of the restiform body, the larger part of the inferior cerebellar peduncle. SYN cuneocerebellar fibers [TA], fibrae cuneocerebellares [TA].

dead t.'s, dentin areas characterized by degenerated odontoblastic processes; may result from injury caused by caries, attrition, erosion, or cavity preparation.

deiterospinal t., SYN lateral vestibulospinal t.

dentatothalamic t., SYN cerebellothalamic t.

descending t. of trigeminal nerve, SYN spinal t. of trigeminal nerve.

digestive t., the passage leading from the mouth to the anus through the pharynx, esophagus, stomach, and intestine. SYN alimentary canal, alimentary t., digestive tube, tubus digestorius.

direct pyramidal t., SYN anterior corticospinal t.

dorsal spinocerebellar t., ✗official alternate term for posterior spinocerebellar t.

dorsal trigeminothalamic t. [TA], SYN posterior trigeminothalamic t.

dorsolateral t., ✗official alternate term for dorsolateral *fasciculus*.

fastigiobulbar t., a fiber bundle originating in the fastigial nucleus (nucleus tecti) of both sides, passing out of the cerebellum in the medial portion of the inferior cerebellar peduncle (corpus juxtarestiforme), and distributing its fibers to the vestibular nuclei and other cell groups in the medulla oblongata. Prominent crossed fibers loop over the dorsal surface of the superior cerebellar peduncle before turning ventrally, forming the uncinate bundle of Russell. SYN tractus fastigiobulbaris.

fastigiospinal t. [TA], SEE fastigiospinal *fibers*, under *fiber*. SYN tractus fastigiospinalis [TA].

Flechsig t., SYN posterior spinocerebellar t.

frontopontine t. [TA], SEE frontopontine *fibers*, under *fiber*. SYN tractus frontopontinus.

frontotemporal t., SYN unciform *fasciculus*.

gastrointestinal t., (G.I. t.) the stomach, small intestine, and large intestine; often used as a synonym of digestive t.

geniculocalcarine t., SYN optic *radiation*.

genital t., the genital passages of the urogenital apparatus. SYN genital duct.

t. of Goll, SYN gracile *fasciculus*.

Gowers t., SYN anterior spinocerebellar t.

habenulointerpeduncular t., habenulopeduncular t. [TA], SYN retroflex *fasciculus*.

Hoche t., SEE semilunar *fasciculus*.

hypothalamohypophysial t. [TA], SYN supraopticohypophysial t.

iliopubic t. [TA], thickened inferior margin of the transversalis fascia seen as a fibrous band running parallel and posterior (deep) to the inguinal ligament, contributing to the posterior wall of the inguinal canal as it bridges the external iliac-femoral vessels from the iliopectineal arch to the superior pubic ramus. It marks the inferior edge of the deep inguinal ring and the medial margin of the femoral canal. Seen only when the inguinal region is viewed from its internal aspect, it is a useful landmark in laparoscopy of this region, as for repair of inguinal herniae. SYN tractus iliopubicus [TA], deep crural arch, Thompson ligament.

iliotibial t. [TA], a fibrous reinforcement of the fascia lata on the lateral surface of the thigh, extending from the crest of the ilium (especially the tuberculum of the crest) to the anterolateral aspect of the lateral condyle of the tibia (Gerdy tubercle). SYN tractus iliotibialis [TA], iliotibial band, Maissiat band.

interpositospinal t. [TA], a group of axons that originate in the anterior and posterior interposed cerebellar nuclei, primarily the latter, and descend to the spinal cord. SYN tractus interpositospinalis [TA].

interstitiospinal t. [TA], a group of axons that originate in the interstitial nucleus of the midbrain, descend ipsilaterally, and terminate primarily in spinal laminae VII, VIII of Rexed. SYN tractus interstitiospinalis [TA].

James t.'s, SYN James *fibers*, under *fiber*.

lateral corticospinal t. [TA], those fibers that cross to the opposite side in the corticospinal (pyramidal) decussation and descend in the dorsal half of the lateral funiculus of the spinal cord; they are distributed throughout the length of the spinal cord to interneurons of the zona intermedia of the spinal gray matter, to some of the nuclei of the posterior horn, and to interneuron pools of the anterior horn. SEE ALSO corticospinal t. SYN tractus corticospinalis lateralis [TA], crossed pyramidal t., fasciculus corticospinalis lateralis, fasciculus pyramidalis lateralis, lateral pyramidal fasciculus, lateral pyramidal t., tractus pyramidalis lateralis.

lateral pyramidal t., SYN lateral corticospinal t.

lateral raphespinal t. [TA], a group of axons that arise in the nucleus raphe magnus, descend in the posterior portion of the lateral funiculus, and terminate primarily in the posterior (dorsal) horn. These serotoninergic fibers are involved in the inhibition of transmission of nociceptive information through the dorsal horn. SYN tractus raphespinalis lateralis [TA].

lateral reticulospinal t. [TA], SYN bulboreticulospinal t.

lateral spinothalamic t. [TA], the more dorsal or dorsolateral part of the composite bundle, the anterolateral system, formed by the lateral and anterior spinothalamic tracts; these specific fibers convey impulses associated with pain and temperature sensation. SEE spinothalamic t. SYN tractus spinothalamicus lateralis [TA].

lateral vestibulospinal t., a somatopically organized fiber bundle originating from the lateral vestibular nucleus (nucleus of Deiters) which descends uncrossed into the anterior funiculus of the spinal cord lateral to the anterior median fissure; the t. extends throughout the length of the cord, distributing fibers at all levels to the medial part of the anterior horn. Excitatory impulses conveyed by the vestibulospinal t. increase extensor muscle tone. SYN tractus vestibulospinalis lateralis [TA], deiterospinal t., tractus vestibulospinalis.

Lissauer t., SYN dorsolateral *fasciculus*.

Loewenthal t., SYN tectospinal t.

mamillothalamic t., SYN mammillothalamic *fasciculus*.

Marchi t., SYN tectospinal t.

medial reticulospinal t. [TA], SYN pontoreticulospinal t.

medial vestibulospinal t. [TA], fibers that originate from the medial vestibular nucleus and descend in the spinal cord as a component of the medial longitudinal fasciculus. SYN tractus vestibulospinalis medialis [TA], tractus vestibulospinalis medialis [TA].

medullary reticulospinal t. [TA], SYN bulboreticulospinal t.

mesencephalic t. of trigeminal nerve [TA], located alongside the central substance of the midbrain and composed of primary sensory fibers, the cells of origin of which compose the mesencephalic nucleus of the trigeminus. SYN tractus mesencephalicus nervi trigemini [TA].

Monakow t., SYN rubrospinal t.

t. of Münzer and Wiener, SYN tectopontine t.

nerve t., a bundle or group of nerve fibers in the brain or spinal cord.

occipitocollicular t., SYN occipitotectal t.

occipitopontine t., SEE occipitopontine *fibers*, under *fiber*. SYN tractus occipitopontinus.

occipitotectal t., SEE occipitotectal *fibers*, under *fiber*. SYN occipitocollicular t.

olfactory t. [TA], a nervelike, white band composed primarily of nerve fibers originating from the mitral cells and tufted cells of the olfactory bulb but also containing the scattered cells of the anterior olfactory nucleus. The t. is closely applied to the ventral surface of the frontal lobe, and attaches itself to the base of the cerebral hemisphere at the olfactory trigone, beyond which it extends in the form of the olfactory striae which distribute their fibers to the olfactory tubercle and, in largest number, to the olfactory cortex on and around the uncus of the parahippocampal gyrus. SEE ALSO olfactory *nerves* [CN I], under *nerve*. SYN tractus olfactorius [TA], olfactory peduncle.

olivocerebellar t. [TA], a large group of loosely arranged fiber fascicles emerging from the hilus of the olivary nucleus, crossing to the opposite side of the medulla oblongata through the stratum interolivare lemnisci and the contralateral olive, and joining the restiform body, the larger part of the contralateral inferior cerebellar peduncle; its fibers terminate in all parts of the cerebellar cortex as climbing fibers and in the cerebellar nuclei; all olivocerebellar projections are crossed. SYN tractus olivocerebellaris [TA].

olivocochlear t. [TA], fibers that originate from the periolivary nuclei bilaterally, exit the brianstem on the vestibular nerve, join the cochlear nerve in the inner ear, and terminate on outer hair cells. SYN tractus olivocochlearis [TA], bundle of Rasmussen.

olivospinal t., SEE olivospinal *fibers*, under *fiber*. SYN Helweg bundle.

optic t. [TA], the continuation of the optic nerve fibers beyond (behind) the latter's hemidecussation in the optic chiasm; each of the two symmetric optic t.'s is composed of fibers originating from the temporal half of the retina of the ipsilateral eye and a nearly equal number of fibers from the nasal half of the contralateral retina; it forms a compact, somewhat flattened fiber band passing caudolaterally alongside the base of the hypothalamus and over the basal surface of the crus cerebri; most of its fibers terminate in the lateral geniculate body; a smaller number of fibers enter the brachium of the superior colliculus, to terminate in the superior colliculus and the pretectal region. SYN tractus opticus.

parietopontine t., SEE parietopontine *fibers*, under *fiber*. SYN tractus parietopontinus.

pontoreticulospinal t. [TA], a t. that originates from oral and caudal pontine reticular nuclei, descends bilaterally but with an ipsilateral preponderance, and terminates mainly in spinal laminae VII and VIII. SYN medial reticulospinal t. [TA], tractus pontoreticulospinalis [TA].

posterior spinocerebellar t. [TA], a compact bundle of heavily myelinated, thick fibers at the periphery of the dorsal half of the lateral funiculus of the spinal cord, originating in the ipsilateral thoracic nucleus (column of Clarke) and ascending by way of the inferior cerebellar peduncle. Terminals end as mossy fibers in the granular layer of the cortex of the cerebellar vermis and, via collaterals, in the cerebellar nuclei. The bundle conveys largely proprioceptive information originating from the annulospiral nerve endings surrounding muscle spindles and from Golgi tendon organs. SYN tractus spinocerebellaris posterior [TA], dorsal spinocerebellar t.✶, Flechsig t.

posterior trigeminothalamic t. [TA], fibers that originate primarily in dorsomedial portion of the principal sensory nucleus and ascend on the ipsilateral side to terminate in the ventral posteromedial nucleus. SYN dorsal trigeminothalamic t. [TA], tractus trigeminothalamicus posterior [TA].

posterolateral t. [TA], SYN dorsolateral *fasciculus*.

prepyramidal t., SYN rubrospinal t.

pyramidal t. [TA], SYN corticospinal t.

respiratory t., the air passages from the nose to the pulmonary alveoli, through the pharynx, larynx, trachea, and bronchi.

reticulospinal t., collective term denoting a variety of fiber t.'s descending to the spinal cord from the reticular formation of the pons and medulla oblongata. Part of these fibers conduct impulses from the neural mechanisms regulating autonomic functions to the corresponding somatic and visceral motor neurons of the spinal cord; others form links in nonpyramidal motor mechanisms affecting muscle tonus, reflex activity, and somatic movement. SEE ALSO bulboreticulospinal t., pontoreticulospinal t. SYN tractus reticulospinalis.

rubrobulbar t. [TA], **(1)** that component of the rubrospinal t. which distributes its fibers to lateral parts of the rhombencephalic tegmentum rather than the spinal cord; **(2)** uncrossed rubro-olivary fibers. SYN tractus rubrobulbaris [TA], tractus rubrobulbaris.

rubropontine t. [TA], axons arising in cells of the red nucleus of the midbrain and terminating in the pontine nuclei of the basilar pons. SYN tractus rubropontinus [TA].

rubroreticular t., fibers that pass from the red nucleus to the reticular formation of the pons and medulla.

▣ **rubrospinal t.** [TA], a somatotopically organized fiber bundle, relatively small in humans, arising from the red nucleus, immediately crossing in the ventral tegmental decussation, descending near the lateral surface of the brainstem into the lateral funiculus of the spinal cord at the ventral border of the lateral pyramidal t. It terminates in the zona intermedia of the spinal cord where its distribution coincides with that of the lateral pyramidal t.; in contrast to the latter it appears not to have direct connections with spinal motor neurons. Impulses conveyed by this t. indirectly increase flexor muscle tone. SYN tractus rubrospinalis [TA], Monakow bundle, Monakow t., prepyramidal t.

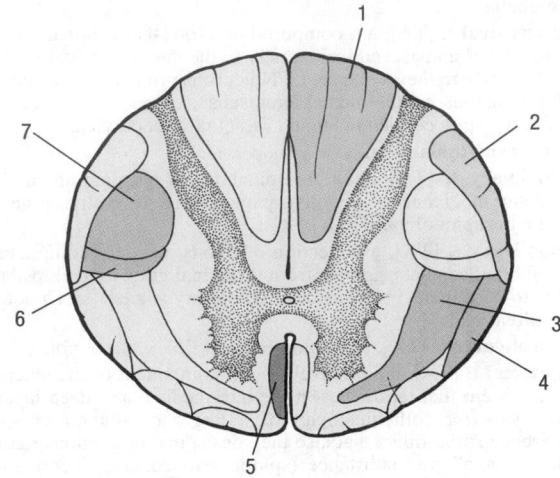

(1) posterior columns: conscious muscle sense, precise touch
(2) posterior spinocerebellar tract: unconscious muscle sense
(3) anterolateral system: pain, temperature, and light touch
(4) anterior spinocerebellar tract: unconscious muscle sense
(5) anterior corticospinal tract: voluntary control of skeletal muscle
(6) rubrospinal tract: control of skeletal muscle
(7) lateral corticospinal tract: voluntary control of skeletal muscle

diagrammatic cross-sectional representation of the spinal cord showing its principal pathways; all **tracts** are bilateral; ascending tracts are numbered on the right, descending ones on the left

t. of Schütz, SYN dorsal longitudinal *fasciculus*.

sensory t., SEE lemniscus.

septomarginal t., SEE semilunar *fasciculus*.

solitariospinal t. [TA], a group of axons that arise in the solitary nucleus and descend bilaterally, mainly in dorsal regions of the lateral funiculus. SYN tractus solitariospinalis [TA].

solitary t. [TA], a slender, compact fiber bundle extending longitudinally through the dorsolateral region of the medullary tegmentum, surrounded by the nucleus of the solitary t., below the obex decussating over the central canal, and descending over some distance into the upper cervical segments of the spinal cord. It is composed of primary sensory fibers that enter with the vagus, glossopharyngeal, and facial nerves, and in part convey information from stretch receptors and chemoreceptors in the walls of the cardiovascular, respiratory, and intestinal t.'s; in rostral parts of the t. impulses are generated by the receptor cells of the taste buds in the mucosa of the tongue. Its fibers are distributed to the nucleus of the solitary t. SYN tractus solitarius [TA], fasciculus rotundus, fasciculus solitarius, funiculus solitarius, Gierke respiratory bundle, Krause respiratory bundle, round fasciculus, solitary bundle, solitary fasciculus.

sphincteroid t. of ileum, SYN basal *sphincter*.

spinal t., any one of a multitude of fiber bundles ascending or descending in the spinal cord.

spinal t. of trigeminal nerve [TA], a compact fiber bundle, comma-shaped on transverse section, composed of primary sensory fibers of the portio major of the trigeminal nerve, descending from the level of the entrance of the trigeminus in the upper pons down through the dorsolateral region of the rhombencephalic tegmentum along the lateral side of the descending or spinal nucleus of the trigeminus, emerging on the dorsolateral surface of the lower medulla oblongata as the tuberculum cinereum, and continuing as far as the second cervical segment of the spinal cord. Its fibers are distributed to the descending or spinal nucleus of the trigeminus. SYN tractus spinalis nervi trigemini [TA], descending t. of trigeminal nerve, tractus descendens nervi trigemini.

spinocerebellar t.'s, SEE anterior spinocerebellar t., posterior spinocerebellar t.

spinocervical t. [TA], a t. composed of axons that originate from laminae III-V and ascend ipsilaterally to the lateral cervical nucleus (LCN) where they synapse, LCN neurons project to the contralateral thalamus via the medial lemniscus. SYN tractus spinocervicalis [TA], spinocervicothalamic t., tractus spinocervicalis.

spinocervicothalamic t., SYN spinocervical t.

spinoolivary t. [TA], multiple spinal tracts terminating in the dorsal and medial accessory olivary nuclei. SEE ALSO olivospinal t. SYN tractus spinoolivaris [NA].

spinoolivary t. [TA], a collection of axons, actually comprising several bundles, that originate from the spinal gray, ascend ipsilaterally to terminate in the accessory olivary nuclei. SYN tractus spinoolivaris [TA].

spinoreticular t. [TA], SYN spinoreticular *fibers*, under *fiber.*

spinotectal t. [TA], the relatively small component of the anterolateral system that terminates in the intermediate and deep layers of the superior colliculus; part of a larger population of spinomesencephalic fibers that also includes spinal projections to the periaqueductal gray substance (spinoperiaqueductal fibers). SYN tractus spinotectalis [TA].

spinothalamic t., a general term describing a large ascending fiber bundle in the ventral half of the lateral funiculus of the spinal cord, arising from cells in the posterior horn at all levels of the cord, which cross within their segments of origin in the white commissure. This t., part of a larger bundle commonly called the spinal lemniscus or anterolateral t. (anterolateral system), contains spinothalamic fibers, spinoreticular fibers, spinohypothalamic fibers, spinomesencephalic fibers (as spinotectal and spinoperiaqueductal fibers), and some projections from the spinal cord to the inferior olivary complex (spinoolivary). In their contralateral ascent, the bundle is intermingled with numerous intersegmental fibers. These fibers continue from the spinal cord into the brainstem, occupying a ventrolateral position and issuing numerous fibers to the rhombencephalic and mesencephalic reticular formation (spinoreticular fibers) to the accessory olivary nuclei (spinoolivary) fibers, to the lateral part of the central gray substance of the mesencephalon (spinoperiaqueductal fibers), and to the deep and intermediate layers of the superior colliculus (spinotectal fibers); the relatively few fibers (10–20%) that remain are the spinothalamic fibers which enter the diencephalon and ends in the nucleus ventralis posterior (caudal part) and intralaminar nuclei of the thalamus. In its ascent in the spinal cord this t. was originally described as being composed of a dorsal part, the lateral spinothalamic t., which conveys impulses associated with pain and temperature sensation, and a more ventral part, the anterior spinothalamic t., involved in tactile sensation. It is now known that this division is not as obvious as originally thought. SYN lemniscus spinalis [TA], spinal lemniscus [TA], tractus spinothalamicus.

spinovestibular t. [TA], a group of axons that originate from neurons primarily in lumbosacral levels, ascend ipsilaterally and in close apposition to the posterior spinocerebellar tract, and terminate in the lateral, medial and spinal vestibular nuclei. Some of these axons may be collaterals of posterior spinocerebellar fibers. SYN tractus spinovestibularis [TA].

spiral foraminous t., SYN *tractus* spiralis foraminosus.

Spitzka marginal t., SYN dorsolateral *fasciculus.*

sulcomarginal t., collective term for those fiber t.'s which descend in the anterior funiculus of the spinal cord along the wall of the anterior median fissure: tectospinal t., medial longitudinal fasciculus, and anterior pyramidal t.

supraopticohypophysial t. [TA], a bundle of unmyelinated fibers originating from all cells of the supraoptic nucleus and an estimated 20% of those of the paraventricular nucleus of the hypothalamus, which extend through the infundibulum and pituitary stalk to their endings in the posterior lobe of the hypophysis; the fibers convey neurosecretory substances, vasopressin and oxytocin, which are stored in (and can be released into the circulating blood from) their terminals. SEE ALSO pituitary *gland*, neurosecretion. SYN hypothalamohypophysial t. [TA], tractus supraopticohypophysialis [TA].

tectobulbar t. [TA], fibers originating in the deep layers of the superior colliculus and accompanying the tectospinal t. but, unlike the latter, terminating in medial regions of the pontine and medullary tegmentum. SYN tractus tectobulbaris [TA].

tectopontine t. [TA], a fiber bundle arising in the superior colliculus, passing caudoventrally on the same side along the medial side of the lateral lemniscus, issuing fibers terminating in the lateral zone of the mesencephalic tegmentum, and ending in the lateral part of the gray matter of the ventral part of the pons. SYN tractus tectopontinus [TA], t. of Münzer and Wiener.

tectospinal t. [TA], a bundle of thick, heavily myelinated fibers originating in the deep layers of the superior colliculus, crossing to the opposite side in the dorsal tegmental decussation, descending along the median plane, between the medial longitudinal fasciculus dorsally, the medial lemniscus ventrally, into the anterior funiculus of the spinal cord. The t. ends in the medial region of the anterior horn of the cervical spinal cord, and appears to be involved in head movements during visual and auditory tracking. Throughout its course in the brainstem it is accompanied by fibers of the tectobulbar t. SYN tractus tectospinalis [TA], Held bundle, Loewenthal bundle, Loewenthal t., Marchi t., predorsal bundle.

temporofrontal t., SYN unciform *fasciculus.*

temporopontine t., SEE temporopontine *fibers*, under *fiber.* SYN Arnold bundle, Arnold t., tractus temporopontinus.

trigeminospinal t. [TA], axons that originate from neurons in the spinal nucleus of the trigeminal nerve and descend to the spinal cord primarily on the ipsilateral side. SYN tractus trigeminospinalis [TA].

trigeminothalamic t., general term designating projections from the spinal trigeminal and principal sensory nuclei of the trigeminal nerve to the thalamus. SEE ALSO trigeminal *lemniscus.*

tuberoinfundibular t., a system of fine, unmyelinated fibers apparently originating from small-celled nuclei of the tuber cinereum, especially the arcuate nucleus, and terminating in the median eminence of the infundibulum, in contact with modified ependymal cells and the capillary tufts from which the hypothalamohypophysial portal veins originate. SEE ALSO pituitary *gland*, neurosecretion. SYN tractus tuberoinfundibularis.

Türck t., SYN anterior corticospinal t.

urinary t., the passage from the pelvis of the kidney to the urinary meatus through the ureters, bladder, and urethra.

uveal t., SYN vascular *layer* of eyeball.

ventral raphespinal t. [TA], SYN anterior raphespinal t.

ventral spinocerebellar t., ☆official alternate term for anterior spinocerebellar t.

ventral spinothalamic t., SYN anterior spinothalamic t.

ventral trigeminothalamic t. [TA], SYN anterior trigeminothalamic t.

vestibulospinal t.'s, SEE medial vestibulospinal t.

vocal t., the air passages above the glottis (including the pharynx, oral and nasal cavities, and the paranasal sinuses) that contribute to the quality of the voice.

Waldeyer t., SYN dorsolateral *fasciculus.*

---

trac·tel·lum, pl. **trac·tel·la** (trak-tel'ŭm, -ă). An anterior locomotor flagellum of a protozoon. [Mod. L. dim. of L. *tractus*]

trac·tion (trak'shŭn). **1.** The act of drawing or pulling, as by an

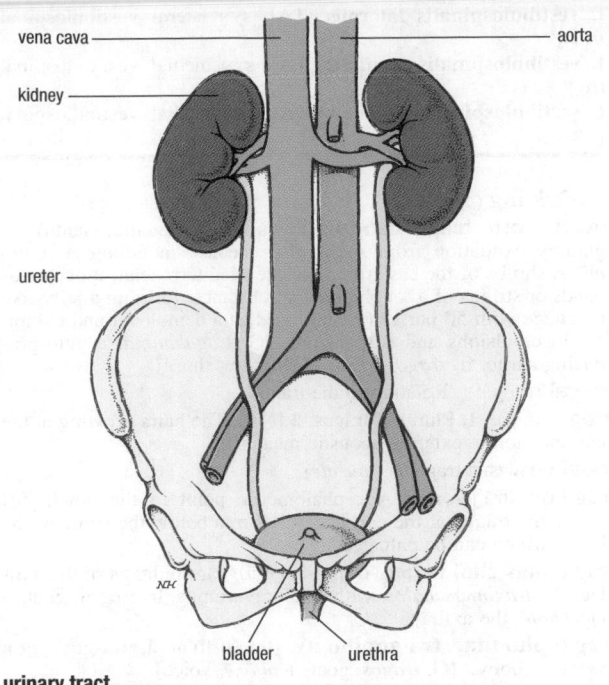

urinary tract

elastic or spring force. **2.** A pulling or dragging force exerted on a limb in a distal direction. [L. *tractio,* fr. *traho,* pp. *tractus,* to draw]

axis t., rarely used procedure to apply t. upon the fetal head in the line of the birth canal by means of axis t. forceps.

Bryant t., t. upon the lower limb placed vertically, employed especially in fractures of the femur in children.

Buck t., apparatus for applying longitudinal skin t. on the leg through contact between the skin and adhesive tape; friction between the tape and skin permits application of force, which is applied through a cord over a pulley, suspending a weight; elevation of the foot of the bed allows the body to act as a counterweight. SYN Buck extension.

external t., a pulling force created by using fixed anchorage (e.g., a headcap or bed frame) outside the oral cavity; principally used in the management of midfacial fractures.

halo t., application of skeletal t. to the head by means of a halo device.

intermaxillary t., SYN maxillomandibular t.

internal t., a pulling force created by using one of the cranial bones, above the point of fracture, for anchorage.

isometric t., t. in which the length of the limb does not change.

isotonic t., t. in which the amount of force does not change.

maxillomandibular t., a pulling force developed by using elastic or wire ligatures and interdental wiring or splints, or both. SYN intermaxillary t.

Russell t., an improvement of Buck extension that permits the resultant vector of the applied t. force to be changed; for fractures of the femur.

skeletal t., t. pull on a bone structure mediated through a pin or wire inserted into the bone to reduce a fracture of long bones. SYN skeletal extension.

skin t., t. on an extremity by means of adhesive tape or other types of strapping applied to the limb.

trac·tor (trak'ter, tōr). An instrument for exerting traction upon an organ or structure. [Mod. L. a drawer, see traction]

Lowsley t., a slender curved instrument with flexible blades at its tip, which can be opened or closed by rotation at the proximal end of the t.; it is passed through the urethra into the bladder and used to retract the prostate gland downward into the operative field in the initial stages of perineal prostatectomy.

Syms t., a collapsible rubber bag attached to the extremity of a tube; the tube is introduced into the bladder through the perineal wound and the bag is inflated; traction produced draws the enlarged prostate into the wound where it is more accessible.

Young prostatic t., a short, straight tubular instrument with blades at its tip, which can be rotated open and closed; it is passed into the prostatic urethra, through a prostatotomy incision made during the later stages of open perineal prostatectomy, with its tip into the bladder; direct traction on the instrument brings the prostate gland down into the operative field where enucleation can be more easily performed.

trac·tot·o·my (trak-tot'ō-mē). Interruption of a nerve tract in the brainstem or spinal cord. [L. *tractus,* tract, + G. *tomē,* incision]

anterolateral t., SYN anterolateral *cordotomy.*

intramedullary t., SYN trigeminal t.

pyramidal t., may be mesencephalic (pedunculotomy or crusotomy), medullary (medullary pyramidotomy), or spinal (spinal pyramidotomy).

Schwartz t., a medullary spinothalamic t.

Sjöqvist t., SYN trigeminal t.

spinal t., SYN anterolateral *cordotomy.*

spinothalamic t., may be spinal (cordotomy), medullary (Schwartz t.), or mesencephalic (Walker t.).

trigeminal t., division of the descending fibers of the trigeminal tract in the medulla. SYN intramedullary t., Sjöqvist t.

Walker t., a mesencephalic spinothalamic t.

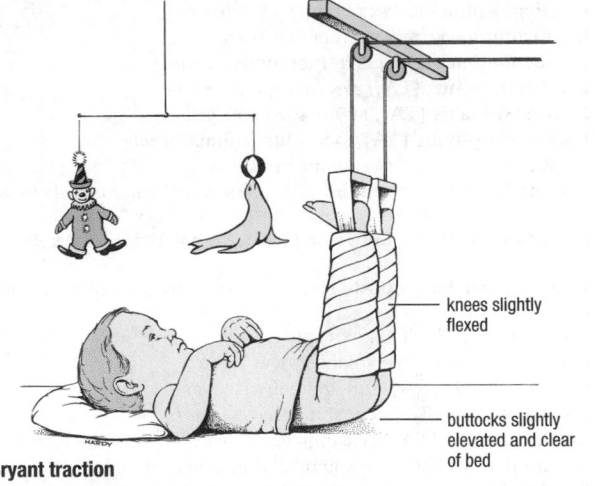

knees slightly flexed

buttocks slightly elevated and clear of bed

Bryant traction

TRACTUS

trac·tus (trak'tŭs). SYN tract. [L. a drawing, drawing out, extent, tract, fr. *traho,* pp. *tractus,* to draw]

t. anterolaterales, SYN anterolateral *system.*

t. bulboreticulospinalis [TA], SYN bulboreticulospinal *tract.*

t. caeruleospinalis [TA], SYN caerulospinal *tract.*

t. cerebellorubra'lis, SYN cerebellorubral *tract.*

t. cerebellothalam'icus, SYN cerebellothalamic *tract.*

t. corticobulba'ris, SYN corticobulbar *tract.*

t. corticoponti'nus [TA], SYN corticopontine *tract.*

t. corticospina'lis, SYN corticospinal *tract.*

t. corticospina'lis ante'rior [TA], SYN anterior corticospinal *tract.*

t. corticospina'lis latera'lis [TA], SYN lateral corticospinal *tract.*

t. descen'dens ner'vi trigem'ini, SYN spinal *tract* of trigeminal nerve.

tr

t. dorsolatera'lis [TA], SYN dorsolateral *fasciculus*.

t. fastigiobulba'ris, SYN fastigiobulbar *tract*.

t. fastigiospinalis [TA], SYN fastigiospinal *tract*; SEE fastigiospinal *fibers*, under *fiber*.

t. frontoponti'nus, SYN frontopontine *tract*.

t. habenulointerpeduncula'ris [TA], SYN retroflex *fasciculus*.

t. iliopubicus [TA], SYN iliopubic *tract*.

t. iliotibia'lis [TA], SYN iliotibial *tract*.

t. interpositospinalis [TA], SYN interpositospinal *tract*.

t. interstitiospinalis [TA], SYN interstitiospinal *tract*.

t. mesencephal'icus ner'vi trigem'ini [TA], SYN mesencephalic *tract* of trigeminal nerve.

t. occipitoponti'nus, SYN occipitopontine *tract*.

t. olfacto'rius [TA], SYN olfactory *tract*.

t. olivocerebella'ris [TA], SYN olivocerebellar *tract*.

t. olivocochlearis [TA], SYN olivocochlear *tract*; SEE olivocochlear *bundle*.

t. op'ticus, SYN optic *tract*.

t. parietoponti'nus, SYN parietopontine *tract*.

t. pontoreticulospinalis [TA], SYN pontoreticulospinal *tract*.

t. posterolateralis [TA], SYN dorsolateral *fasciculus*.

t. pyramida'lis [TA], SYN corticospinal *tract*.

t. pyramida'lis ante'rior, SYN anterior corticospinal *tract*.

t. pyramida'lis latera'lis, SYN lateral corticospinal *tract*.

t. raphespinalis anterior [TA], SYN anterior raphespinal *tract*.

t. raphespinalis lateralis [TA], SYN lateral raphespinal *tract*.

t. reticulospina'lis, SYN reticulospinal *tract*.

t. rubrobulbaris, SYN rubrobulbar *tract*.

t. rubrobulbaris [TA], SYN rubrobulbar *tract*.

t. rubropontinus [TA], SYN rubropontine *tract*.

t. rubrospina'lis [TA], SYN rubrospinal *tract*.

t. solitariospinalis [TA], SYN solitariospinal *tract*.

t. solita'rius [TA], SYN solitary *tract*.

t. spina'lis ner'vi trigem'ini [TA], SYN spinal *tract* of trigeminal nerve.

t. spinocerebella'ris ante'rior [TA], SYN anterior spinocerebellar *tract*.

t. spinocerebella'ris poste'rior [TA], SYN posterior spinocerebellar *tract*.

t. spinocervicalis [TA], SYN spinocervical *tract*.

t. spinocervicalis, SYN spinocervical *tract*.

t. spinoolivaris [NA], SYN spinoolivary *tract*.

t. spinoolivaris [TA], SYN spinoolivary *tract*.

t. spinotecta'lis [TA], SYN spinotectal *tract*.

t. spinothalam'icus, SYN spinothalamic *tract*.

t. spinothalam'icus ante'rior [TA], SYN anterior spinothalamic *tract*.

t. spinothalam'icus latera'lis [TA], SYN lateral spinothalamic *tract*.

t. spinovestibularis [TA], SYN spinovestibular *tract*.

t. spira'lis foramino'sus [TA], openings in the cochlear area of the bottom of the internal acoustic meatus through which the fibers of the cochlear nerve leave the bony labyrinth to enter the cranial cavity. SYN spiral foraminous tract.

t. supraopticohypophysia'lis [TA], SYN supraopticohypophysial *tract*.

t. tectobulba'ris [TA], SYN tectobulbar *tract*.

t. tectoponti'nus [TA], SYN tectopontine *tract*.

t. tectospina'lis [TA], SYN tectospinal *tract*.

t. tegmenta'lis centra'lis [TA], SYN central tegmental *tract*.

t. temporoponti'nus, SYN temporopontine *tract*.

t. trigeminospinalis [TA], SYN trigeminospinal *tract*.

t. trigeminothalamicus anterior [TA], SYN anterior trigeminothalamic *tract*.

t. trigeminothalamicus posterior [TA], SYN posterior trigeminothalamic *tract*.

t. tuberoinfundibula'ris, SYN tuberoinfundibular *tract*.

t. vestibulospina'lis, SYN lateral vestibulospinal *tract*.

t. vestibulospinalis lateralis [TA], SYN lateral vestibulospinal *tract*.

t. vestibulospinalis medialis [TA], SYN medial vestibulospinal *tract*.

t. vestibulospinalis medialis [TA], SYN medial vestibulospinal *tract*.

---

traf·fick·ing (traf'ik-ing). SYN processing (1). SEE targeting.

trag·a·canth, trag·a·can·tha (trag'ă-kanth, -kan'thă; -santh). A gummy exudation from *Astragalus* species, including *A. gummifer*, shrubs of the eastern end of the Mediterranean; it occurs as bands or strings of a tough gummy substance, forming a jelly-like mucilage with 50 parts of water; used as a demulcent and excipient in emulsions and suspensions. [G. *tragakantha,* a gum-producing shrub, fr. *tragos,* goat, + *akanthos,* thorn]

tra·gal (trā'găl). Relating to the tragus.

tra·gi (trā'jī). **1.** Plural of tragus. **2** [NA]. The hairs growing at the entrance to the external acoustic meatus.

tra·gi·cus. SEE tragicus (*muscle*).

trag·i·on (trā'jē-on). A cephalometric point in the notch just above the tragus of the ear; it lies 1–2 mm below the spine of the helix, which can be palpated.

trag·o·mas·chal·ia (trag-ō-mas-kal'ē-ă). Bromidrosis of the axillae. [G. *tragomaschalos,* with smelling armpits, fr. *tragos,* goat, + *maschalē,* the axilla]

trag·o·pho·nia, tra·goph·o·ny (trag'ō-fō'nē-ă, tră-gof'ō-nē). SYN egophony. [G. *tragos,* goat, + *phōnē,* voice]

tra·gus, pl. **tra·gi** (trā'gŭs, -jī). **1** [NA]. A tonguelike projection of the cartilage of the auricle in front of the opening of the external acoustic meatus and continuous with the cartilage of this canal. SYN antilobium, hircus (3). **2.** SEE tragi (2). [G. *tragos,* goat, in allusion to the hairs growing on the part, like a goatee]

accessory t., small nodules present at birth, anterior to the t., derived from first branchial arch remnants and often containing central cartilage.

TRAIL. A member of the tumor necrosis factor ligand family that rapidly induces apoptosis in a variety of transformed cell lines. SYN apo-2L.

train·ing (trān'ing). An organized system of education, instruction, or discipline.

assertive t., a form of behavior modification or therapy in which a client is taught to feel free to make legitimate demands and refusals in situations which previously elicited diffident responses. SYN assertive conditioning.

aversive t., a form of behavior t. or modification in which a noxious event is used to punish or extinguish undesirable behavior. SEE ALSO aversion *therapy.* SYN aversive conditioning.

avoidance t., SYN avoidance *conditioning.*

escape t., SYN escape *conditioning.*

toilet t., t. directed at teaching a child proper control of bladder and bowel functions; psychoanalytic personality theory believes that the attitudes of both parent and child concerning this t. may have important psychologic implications for the child's later development.

trait (trāt). A qualitative characteristic; a discrete attribute as contrasted with metric character. A t. is amenable to segregation rather than quantitative analysis; it is an attribute of phenotype, not of genotype. [Fr. from L. *tractus,* a drawing out, extension]

Bombay t., SEE Bombay *phenomenon.*

categorical t., in genetics, a feature that can conveniently and effectively be analyzed by sorting into classes either because there is no satisfactory way of measuring it (as with blood groups) or because it falls into natural classes so that the variation among classes far exceeds that within classes (e.g., the phenotypic effects of many enzyme polymorphisms); existence of categories suggests but does not prove the operation of a major, simple, underlying cause. SYN qualitative t.

chromosomal t., a t. dependent on a recurrent chromosomal aberration.

codominant t., SEE codominant.

dominant t., an outstanding mental or physical characteristic. SEE *dominance* of traits.

dominant lethal t., t., expressed in the phenotype if present in the genotype, that precludes having descendants. All such cases are necessarily sporadic and must represent new mutations as the usual methods of classical genetics provide no means of demonstrating any genetic component whatsoever, except for tenuous arguments such as advanced paternal age. Molecular biology may help although the methods may be tedious; if there is an epistatic gene that may mask the trait, the logic is more tractable, though complex.

galtonian t., a quantitative genetic t. due to contributions from many more of less equally important loci that resembles a continuous t.

intermediate t., a measurable t. in which there is some evidence of the operation of a simple major cause, but in which the variation within the putative categories is such as to cause overlap and hence ambiguity in classification of any particular reading.

liminal t., SYN threshold t.

marker t., a t. that may be of little importance in itself but which by association, linkage, or other means facilitates the detection, anticipation, or understanding of a disease or (for genetic diseases) the localization of the causative gene on the karyotype.

mendelian t., a categorical t. that segregates in accordance with a single-locus genetic system.

nonpenetrant t., a genetic t. that is not phenotypically manifest because of nongenetic factors; it therefore does not include recessivity, epistasis, hypostasis, or parastasis but does include environmental factors and pure random effects such as lyonization.

penetrant t., a t. that in the appropriate genotypes is phenotypically manifest; strictly, it is the t. that is penetrant, not the gene. SEE penetrance.

qualitative t., SYN categorical t.

recessive t., SEE *dominance* of traits.

sickle cell t., the heterozygous state of the gene for hemoglobin S in sickle cell anemia.

threshold t., a t. that falls into natural groups that originate not in categorically distinct causes but in whether or not the outcome attains critical values; e.g., gallstones may result from a categorical cause or from unusual levels of causal factors that themselves show no evidence of grouping. SYN liminal t.

tra·jec·tor (tră-jek′ter, -tōr). An infrequently used instrument for locating the course of a bullet in a wound. [L. fr. *tra-jicio,* pp. *-jectus,* to throw over or across]

tram·a·dol (tră′mă-dol). An analgesic drug whose mechanism of action is unusual in that one optical isomer exerts typical opioid-type effects and the other isomer interacts with the reuptake and/or release of norepinephrine and serotonin in nerve terminals.

tra·maz·o·line hy·dro·chlo·ride (tră-maz′ō-lēn). An adrenergic and sympathomimetic agent used for nasal decongestion.

trance (trans). An altered state of consciousness as in hypnosis, catalepsy, or ecstasy. [L. *transeo,* to go across]

death t., a condition of suspended animation, marked by unconsciousness and barely perceptible respiration and heart action.

induced t., the artificially induced state of hypnosis or of somnambulistic t.

somnambulistic t., a state of somnambulism, paralysis, anesthesia, or catalepsy induced by suggestion in major hypnosis.

tran·ex·am·ic ac·id (tran-eks-am′ik). A competitive inhibitor of plasminogen activation and of plasmin; used in hemophilia to reduce or prevent hemorrhage.

tran·quil·iz·er (trang′kwi-lī-zer). A drug that promotes tranquility by calming, soothing, quieting, or pacifying with minimal sedating or depressant effects.

major t., SYN antipsychotic *agent.*

minor t., SYN antianxiety *agent.*

△**trans-.** **1.** Prefix (in italics) denoting across, through, beyond; opposite of *cis-.* **2.** In genetics, a prefix denoting the location of two genes on opposite chromosomes of a homologous pair. **3.** In organic chemistry (in italics), a form of geometric isomerism in which the atoms attached to two carbon atoms, joined by double

bonds, are located on opposite sides of the molecule. **4.** In biochemistry, a prefix to a group name in an enzyme name or a reaction denoting transfer of that group from one compound to another; e.g., transformylase (transfers a formyl group), transpeptidation. [L. *trans,* through, across]

trans·a·cet·y·lase (trans-ă-set′i-lās). SYN acetyltransferase.

trans·a·cet·y·la·tion (trans′ă-set-i-lā′shŭn). Transfer of an acetyl group ($CH_3CO–$) from one compound to another; such reactions, usually involving formation of acetyl-CoA, occur notably in the initiation of the tricarboxylic acid cycle by the transfer of an acetyl group to oxaloacetate to form citrate.

trans·ac·tion (tranz-ak′shŭn). **1.** Interaction arising from the encounter of two or more persons. **2.** In transactional analysis, the unit of analysis involving a social stimulus and a response.

trans·ac·yl·as·es (trans-as′i-lā-sez). SYN acyltransferases.

trans·ac·yl·a·tion (trans-as′il-ā′shŭn). The reversible transfer of acyl groups.

trans·al·dol·ase (trans-al′dō-lās). Transferase interconverting sedoheptulose 7-phosphate and D-glyceraldehyde 3-phosphate to D-erythrose 4-phosphate and D-fructose 6-phosphate; part of the pentose phosphate pathway. SEE ALSO transketolase.

trans·al·do·la·tion (trans′al-dō-lā′shŭn). A reaction involving the transfer of an aldol group ($CH_2OH–CO–CHOH–$) from one compound to another; such reactions generally involve the sugar phosphates and occur in the phosphogluconate oxidation pathway of carbohydrate catabolism.

trans·a·mi·da·tion (trans-am′i-dā-shŭn). The transfer of NH_2 from an amide moiety (e.g., from glutamine) to another molecule.

trans·am·i·di·nas·es (trans-am′i-di-nās-ez). SYN amidinotransferases.

trans·am·i·di·na·tion (trans-am′i-di-nā′shŭn). A reaction involving the transfer of an amidine group ($NH_2C=NH$) from one compound to another; the amidine donor is generally L-arginine and the reaction is of significance in the biosynthesis of creatine.

trans·am·i·nas·es (trans-am′i-nās-ez). SYN aminotransferases.

trans·am·i·na·tion (trans-am′i-nā′shŭn). The reaction between an amino acid and an α-keto acid through which the amino group is transferred from the former to the latter; in certain cases the reaction may be between an amino acid and an aldehyde (e.g., glutamate with glutamate semialdehyde via ornithine transaminase).

trans·au·di·ent (trans-aw′dē-ent). Permeable to sound waves. [trans- + L. *audio,* pres. p. *audiens,* to hear]

trans·ca·lent (trans-kā′lent). SYN diathermanous. [trans- + L. *caleo,* to be warm]

trans·cap·si·da·tion (trans-kap-si-dā′shŭn). The phenomenon whereby the adenovirus capsid of the SV40 adenovirus "hybrid" is replaced by the capsid of another type of adenovirus; extended to include a similar phenomenon in other viruses.

trans·car·bam·o·y·las·es (trans-kar-bam′ō-i-lā-sez). SYN carbamoyltransferases.

trans·car·bam·o·yl·a·tion (trans-kar-bam′ō-il-ā′shŭn). The transfer of a carbamoyl moiety from one molecule to another; e.g., the reaction catalyzed by ornithine transcarbamoylase in the urea cycle.

trans·car·box·yl·as·es (trans-kar-boks′i-lās-ez). SYN carboxyltransferases.

tran·scen·den·tal med·i·ta·tion (TM) (tranz′en-den-tal med′ĭ-tă-shŭn). A form of meditation practiced over 2500 years ago in Eastern cultures and which was recently made popular in the West by Maharishi Mahesh Yogi as a means to help increase energy, reduce stress, and have a positive effect on mental and physical health; it involves the person sitting upright for 20 min, with eyes closed, and silently speaking a mantra (a key stimulus word used uniquely by each individual to return to the proper meditative state) whenever thought occurs.

trans·co·bal·a·mins (trans-kō-bal′ă-minz). Substances included in "R binder," the name given a family of cobalamin-binding proteins; deficiencies have been associated with low serum cobalamin levels, and can lead to megaloblastic anemia.

tr

trans·con·dy·lar (trans-kon′di-lăr). Across or through the condyles; denoting the line of bone incision in Carden amputation.

trans·cor·ti·cal (tranz-kōr′ti-kăl). **1.** Across or through the cortex of the brain, ovary, kidney, or other organ. **2.** From one part of the cerebral cortex to another; denoting the various association tracts.

trans·cor·tin (trans-kōr′tin). An α_2-globulin in blood that binds cortisol and corticosterone; the principal corticosteroid-binding protein in the plasma. SYN corticosteroid-binding globulin, corticosteroid-binding protein.

tran·scrip·tase (tran-skrip′tās). A polymerase associated with the process of transcription; may be RNA-dependent or DNA-dependent. [L. *transcribo*, pp. *transcriptum*, to copy, + -ase]

ℹ **reverse t.,** rNA-dependent DNA polymerase, present in virions of RNA tumor viruses (retroviruses).

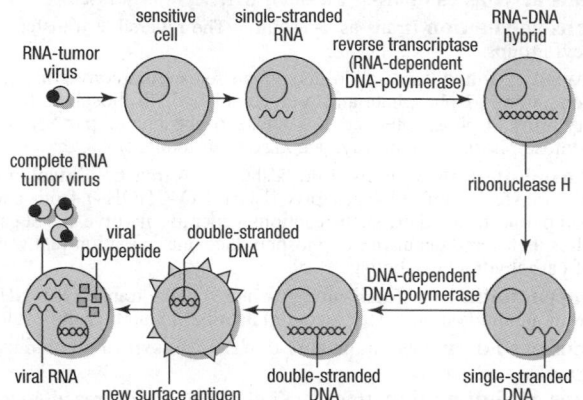

reverse transcriptase: integration of RNA tumor virus into cell DNA

ℹ **tran·scrip·tion** (tran-skrip′shŭn). Transfer of genetic code information from one kind of nucleic acid to another, especially with reference to the process by which a base sequence of messenger RNA is synthesized (by an RNA polymerase) on a template of complementary DNA.

   reverse t., reversal of the normal pattern of t. (from DNA to RNA); the effective means is the viral enzyme reverse transcriptase.

trans·cu·ta·ne·ous (trans-kū-tā′nē-ŭs). SYN percutaneous.

trans·cy·to·sis (trans-sī-tō′sis). A mechanism for transcellular transport in which a cell encloses extracellular material in an invagination of the cell membrane to form a vesicle (endocytosis), then moves the vesicle across the cell to eject the material through the opposite cell membrane by the reverse process (exocytosis). The transport mechanism by which most proteins reach the Golgi apparatus or the plasma membrane; the vesicles targeted toward lysosomes and secretory storage granules appear to be coated with clathrin. SYN cytopempsis, vesicular transport.

trans·der·mic (trans-der′mik). SYN percutaneous.

trans·duce (trans-doos′). To effect transduction.

trans·duc·er (trans-doo′ser). A device designed to convert energy from one form to another. SEE ALSO transduction.

   piezoelectric t., a t. that converts electric into mechanical energy and vice versa, used in ultrasound diagnosis or therapy.

   ultrasound t., a piezoelectric t. used in diagnostic ultrasound.

trans·duc·in (trans-doo′sin). A protein that binds guanine nucleotides (i.e., a G protein), found in retinal rods and cones, that plays a major role in signal transduction; in vertebrate rod cells it acts as a link of the photolysis of rhodopsin to the activation of cGMP phosphodiesterase.

trans·duc·tant (trans-dŭk′tănt). A cell that has acquired a new character by means of transduction; may be *complete*, with integration of the transferred genetic material into its genome, or *abortive*, in which case the genetic fragment is not integrated and passes to only one of the two daughter cells on division.

trans·duc·tion (trans-dŭk′shŭn). **1.** Transfer of genetic material (and its phenotypic expression) from one cell to another by viral infection. **2.** A form of genetic recombination in bacteria. **3.** Conversion of energy from one form to another. [trans- + L. *duco*, pp. *ductus*, to lead across]

   abortive t., t. in which the genetic fragment from the donor bacterium is not integrated in the genome of the recipient bacterium, and, when the latter divides, is transmitted to only one of the daughter cells.

   complete t., t. in which the transferred genetic fragment is fully integrated in the genome of the recipient bacterium.

   Davis battery model of t., a concept in which the positive endocochlear potential and the negative intracellular potential of the hair cells provide the electromotive force to pass current through the reticular lamina of the organ of Corti.

   general t., t. in which the transducing bacteriophage is able to transfer any gene of the donor bacterium.

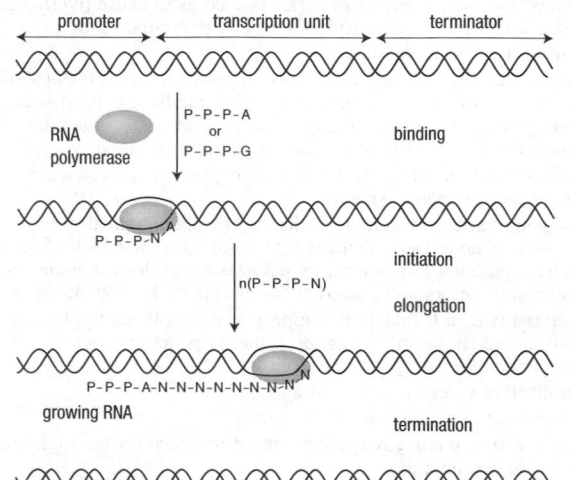

transcription; schematic representation: P-P-P-A = ATP; P-P-P-G = GTP; P-P-P-N = any nucleoside triphosphate

   high-frequency t., specialized t. in which the donor bacterium contains not only the transducing, defective probacteriophage but also nondefective prophage that serves as "helper" virus, enabling most of the defective prophage particles to develop sufficiently to function as transducing agents.

   low-frequency t., specialized t. in which only a small portion of the prophage particles, because of their defectiveness, are able to develop sufficiently to serve as effective transducing agents.

   mechanoelectric t., the conversion of mechanical energy to electric energy by sensory cells such as auditory and vestibular hair cells.

   specialized t., t. in which the bacteriophage strain is able to transfer only some, or only one, of the donor bacterium genes. SYN specific t.

   specific t., SYN specialized t.

tran·sec·tion (tran-sek′shŭn). **1.** A cross-section. **2.** Cutting across. SYN transsection. [trans- + L. *seco*, pp. *sectus*, to cut]

trans·eth·moi·dal (trans′eth-moy′dăl). Across or through the ethmoid bone.

trans·fec·tion (trans-fek′shŭn). A method of gene transfer utilizing infection of a cell with nucleic acid (as from a retrovirus) resulting in subsequent viral replication in the transfected cell. [trans- + in*fection*]

trans·fer. 1. Process of removal or transferral. **2.** A condition in which learning in one situation influences learning in another situation; a carry-over of learning that may be positive in effect, as when learning one behavior facilitates the learning of something else, or may be negative, as when one habit interferes with the acquisition of a later one. SYN transmission (1). [L. *trans-fero,* to bear across]

embryo t., after in vitro artificial insemination, the fertilized ovum is transferred at the blastocyst stage to the recipient's uterus or oviduct.

Fourier t., SYN Fourier *analysis.*

gamete intrafallopian t. (GIFT), placement of the oocyte and sperm into the ampulla of the fallopian tube; a form of assisted reproduction.

group t., the t. of a functional moiety from one molecule to another.

Jones t., surgical procedure to treat claw deformities of the great toe in which the extensor hallucis longus tendon is transferred to the neck of the metatarsal; can also be used to correct claw deformities of the lesser toes.

linear energy t. (LET), the amount of energy deposited by radiation per unit length of travel, expressed in keV per micron; protons, neutrons, and α particles have much higher LET than gamma or x-rays. A property of radiation considered in radiation protection. SEE relative biologic *effectiveness.*

trans·fer·as·es (trans′fer-ās-ez). Enzymes (EC class 2) transferring: one-carbon groups (2.1, including methyltransferases, 2.1.1; formyltransferases, 2.1.2; carboxyl- and carbamoyltransferases, 2.1.3; and amidinotransferases, 2.1.4); acyl residues (acyltransferases, 2.3); glycosyl residues (glycosyltransferases, 2.4, including hexosyltransferases, 2.4.1, and pentosyltransferases, 2.4.2); alkyl or aryl groups (2.5); nitrogenous groups (2.6); phosphorus-containing groups (2.7, phosphotransferases); and sulfur-containing groups (2.8, including sulfurtransferases, 2.8.1; sulfotransferases, 2.8.2; and CoA-transferases, 2.8.3). SYN transferring enzymes.

terminal t., enzymes that covalently add nucleotides to the 3′ end of polynucleic acids; e.g., DNA nucleotidylexotransferase.

terminal deoxynucleotidyl t. (TdT), a specialized DNA polymerase expressed in immature, pre-B, pre-T lymphoid cells, and acute lymphoblastic leukemia/lymphoma cells.

trans·fer·ence (trans-fer′ens). **1.** Conveyance of an object from one place to another. **2.** Shifting of symptoms from one side of the body to the other, as seen in certain cases of conversion hysteria. **3.** Displacement of affect from one person or one idea to another; in psychoanalysis, generally applied to the projection of feelings, thoughts, and wishes onto the analyst, who has come to represent some person from the patient's past.

counter t., SEE countertransference.

extrasensory thought t., SYN telepathy.

t. love, love expressed by the patient for the psychoanalyst as a manifestation of t. (3).

negative t., t. characterized by predominantly hostile feelings on the part of the patient toward the analyst.

passive t., the passage of an immunity or allergic susceptibility by the injection of serum of an animal or individual who has acquired an active immunity to the disease.

positive t., t. characterized by predominantly friendly, respectful, and positive feelings on the part of the patient toward the analyst.

trans·fer·rin (trans-fer′in). **1.** A nonheme β_1-globulin of the plasma, capable of associating reversibly with up to 1.25 μg of iron per gram, and acting therefore as an iron-transporting protein. **2.** A glycoprotein, found in mammalian milk (lactoferrin) and egg white (conalbumin, ovotransferrin), that binds and transports iron (Fe^{3+}). [trans- + L. *ferrum,* iron, + -ia]

trans·fer-RNA. See entries under ribonucleic acid.

trans·fix (trans′fiks). To pierce with a sharp instrument. [L. *trans-figo,* pp. *-fixus,* to pierce through, fr. *figo,* to fasten]

trans·fix·ion (trans-fik′shŭn). A maneuver in amputation in which the knife is passed from side to side through the soft parts, close to the bone, and the muscles are then divided from within outward. [L. *transfixio* (see transfix)]

transform.

Fourier t., SYN Fourier *analysis.*

trans·form·ant (trans-fōr′mănt). A bacterium that has received

genetic material (and its phenotypic expression) from another bacterium by means of transformation.

trans·for·ma·tion (trans-fōr-mā′shŭn). **1.** SYN metamorphosis. **2.** A change of one tissue into another, as cartilage into bone. **3.** In metals, a change in phase and physical properties in the solid state caused by heat treatment. **4.** In microbial genetics, transfer of genetic information between bacteria by means of "naked" intracellular DNA fragments derived from bacterial donor cells and incorporated into a competent recipient cell. [L. *trans-formo,* pp. *-atus,* to transform]

cavernous t. of portal vein, replacement of the portal vein by a number of collateral channels, a consequence of thrombosis.

cell t., morphologic and physiologic changes including loss of contact inhibition resulting from infection of an animal cell by an oncogenic virus.

Haldane t., the multiplication of inspired oxygen concentration by the ratio of expired to inspired nitrogen concentrations in the calculation of oxygen consumption or respiratory quotient by the open circuit method.

Lobry de Bruyn-van Ekenstein t., the conversion of glucose to fructose and mannose in dilute alkali by enolization adjacent to the carbonyl group to form an enediol, a reaction analogous to certain biochemical transformations.

logit t., a method of linearizing dose-response curves for radioimmunoassay techniques; i.e., logit B (bound)/B_0 (initial binding) = log (B/B_0/1 $-$ B/B_0).

lymphocyte t., the t. into large, blastlike forms (immunoblasts) that occurs when lymphocytes are exposed to histoincompatible antigens (mixed lymphocyte culture) or mitogens. SEE ALSO mixed lymphocyte culture *test.*

nodular t. of the liver, a rare condition in which nodules of hyperplastic hepatocytes develop without fibrosis or general loss of lobular architecture. SYN nodular regenerative hyperplasia.

trans·fuse (trans-fūz′). To perform transfusion.

trans·fu·sion (trans-fū′zhŭn). Transfer of blood or blood component from one individual (donor) to another individual (receptor). [L. *transfundo,* pp. *-fusus,* to pour from one vessel to another]

drip t., t. slow enough to measure by drops.

exchange t., removal of most of a patient's blood followed by introduction of an equal amount from donors. SYN exsanguination t., substitution t., total t.

exsanguination t., SYN exchange t.

fetomaternal t., passage of fetal blood into maternal circulation.

indirect t., t. into a patient of blood previously obtained from a donor and stored under suitable conditions. SYN mediate t.

intramedullary t., t., most commonly in infants, into the medullary cavity of a long bone, usually the femur or tibia.

intrauterine t., to treat erythroblastosis fetalis, Rh-negative blood is placed into the peritoneal cavity of the fetus.

mediate t., SYN indirect t.

placental t., return to the newborn via the umbilical vessels of some of the fetal placental blood.

reciprocal t., an attempt to confer immunity by transfusing blood taken from a donor into a receiver suffering from the same affection, the balance being maintained by transfusing an equal amount from the receiver to the donor.

subcutaneous t., an infusion of absorbable solutions beneath the skin.

substitution t., SYN exchange t.

total t., SYN exchange t.

twin-twin t., direct vascular anastomosis, arterial or venous, between the placental circulations of twins.

trans·gene (trans′gēn). A newly introduced gene.

transgenesis (tranz-jen′e-sis). Reproduction involving introduction of foreign species DNA into an ovum.

trans·gen·ic (trans-jen′ik). Referring to an organism in which new DNA has been introduced into the germ cells by injection into the nucleus of the ovum.

trans·glot·tic (trans-glot′ik). Vertical crossing of the glottis, as in the spread of carcinoma from the supraglottic to the infraglottic area.

tr

trans·glu·co·syl·ase (trans-gloo′kō-si-lās). SYN glucosyltransferase.

trans·glu·ta·min·ase (trans-gloo-ta′min-ās). A group of enzymes that catalyze the calcium-dependent acyl transfer reaction in which the amide moiety of peptide-bound glutaminyl residues serve as acyl donor; a specific t. covalently cross-links fibrin molecules between glutamine and the ε-amino group of a lysyl residue, thus producing a more stable fibrin clot; another t. participates in the formation of the chemically resistant envelope of the stratum corneum during terminal differentiation of keratinocytes.

trans·gly·co·si·da·tion (trans-glī-ko-sid′ā-shŭn). The transfer of a glycosidically bound sugar to another molecule.

trans·gly·co·syl·ase (trans-glī′kō-si-lās). SYN glycosyltransferase.

trans·hi·a·tal (trans-hī-ā′tăl). By way of a hiatus; e.g., transhiatal esophagectomy, performed partially through the esophageal hiatus.

tran·sient (trans′shĕnt, -sē-ĕnt). **1.** Short-lived; passing; not permanent; said of a disease or an attack. **2.** A short-lived cardiac sound having little duration (less than 0.12 s) as distinct from a murmur; e.g., first, second, third, and fourth heart sounds, clicks, and opening snaps. [L. *transeo,* pres. p. *transiens,* to cross over]

trans·il·i·ac (tran-sil′ē-ak). Extending from one ilium or iliac crest or spine to the other.

tran·sil·i·ent (tran-sil′yent, -zil-). Jumping across; passing over; pertaining to those cortical association fibers in the brain that pass from one convolution to another nonadjacent one. [L. *transilio,* to leap across, fr. *salio,* to leap]

trans·il·lu·mi·na·tion (trans-i-loo′mi-nā′shŭn). Method of examination by the passage of light through tissues or a body cavity. [trans- + L. *illumino,* pp. *-atus,* to light up]

trans·in·su·lar (tranz-in′soo-lăr). Across the insula or island of Reil.

trans·is·chi·ac (trans-is′kē-ak). Extending from one ischium to the other.

trans·isth·mi·an (trans-is′mē-an). Across any isthmus; specifically, across the isthmus of the fornicate gyrus, denoting the gyrus transitivus.

tran·si·tion (tran-sish′ŭn, -zish′ŭn). **1.** Passage from one condition or one part to another. **2.** In polynucleic acid, replacement of a purine base by another purine base or a pyrimidine base by a different pyrimidine. [L. *transitio,* fr. *transeo,* pp. *-itus,* to go across]

cervicothoracic t., the junction between the last cervical vertebra and first thoracic vertebra.

isomeric t., the t. of a nuclear isomer to a lower quantum state; e.g., $^{131m}Xe \rightarrow {}^{131}Xe + \gamma$.

tran·si·tion·al (tran-sish′ŭn-ăl, -zish-). Relating to or marked by a transition; transitory.

trans·ke·tol·ase (trans-kē′tō-lās). A transferase bringing about the reversible interconversion of sedoheptulose 7-phosphate and D-glyceraldehyde 3-phosphate to produce D-ribose 5-phosphate and D-xylulose 5-phosphate, and also other similar reactions, such as hydroxypyruvate and an aldehyde into CO_2 and an extended hydroxypyruvate; a part of the nonoxidative phase of the pentose phosphate pathway. SEE ALSO transaldolase. SYN glycolaldehyde-transferase.

trans·ke·to·la·tion (trans′kē-tō-lā′shŭn). A reaction involving the transfer of a ketole group ($HOCH_2CO-$) from one compound to another.

trans·la·tion (trans-lā′shŭn). **1.** A change or conversion into another form. **2.** The rather complex process by which messenger RNA, transfer RNA, and ribosomes effect the production of protein from amino acids, the specificity of synthesis being controlled by the base sequences of the messenger RNA. **3.** In dentistry, the movement of a tooth through alveolar bone without change in axial inclination. [L. *translatio,* a transferring, fr. *transfero* pp. *-latus,* to carry across]

nick t., a technique in which a bacterial DNA polymerase is used to degrade a single strand of DNA that has been nicked and then to resynthesize that strand, often with labeled nucleoside triphosphates.

⊞ trans·lo·ca·tion (trans-lō-kā′shŭn). **1.** Transposition of two segments between nonhomologous chromosomes as a result of abnormal breakage and refusion of reciprocal segments. **2.** Transport of a metabolite across a biomembrane. [trans- + L. *location,* placement, fr. *loco,* to place]

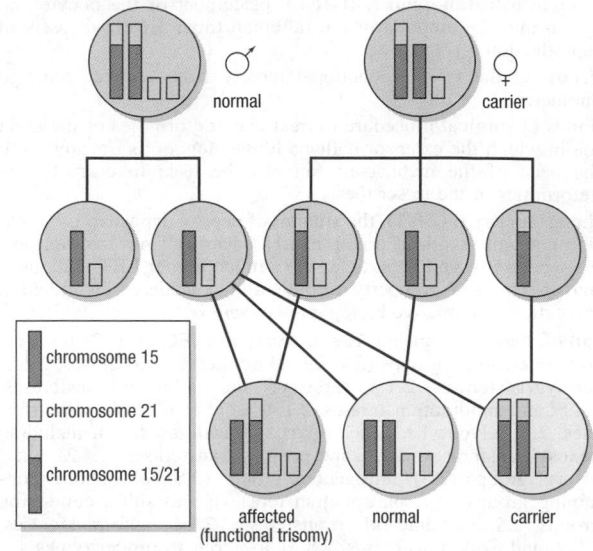

chromosome 15

chromosome 21

chromosome 15/21

normal

carrier

affected (functional trisomy)

normal

carrier

inheritance of translocation trisomy

bacterial t., the movement of bacteria or bacterial products across the intestinal membrane to emerge either in the lymphatics or the visceral circulation.

balanced t., t. of the long arm of an acrocentric chromosome to another chromosome; an individual with a balanced t. has a normal diploid genome and is clinically normal but has a chromosome count of 45 and as a result of asymmetric meiosis may have children lacking the genes on the translocated segment or have them in trisomy.

group t., a form of active transport across a biomembrane in which the transporting molecule is altered in the course of the transport.

reciprocal t., t. without demonstrable loss of genetic material.

robertsonian t., t. in which the centromeres of two acrocentric chromosomes appear to have fused, forming an abnormal chromosome consisting of the long arms of two different chromosomes with loss of the short arms. A carrier of a balanced robertsonian t. has only 45 chromosomes but near normal chromosomal complement and a clinically normal phenotype; however, he or she is at risk of having a child with unbalanced chromosomal complement. A person with an unbalanced robertsonian t. is trisomic for the long arm of the chromosome. SYN centric fusion. [W.R.B. *Robertson,* U.S. geneticist, *1881]

unbalanced t., condition resulting from fertilization of a gamete containing a t. chromosome by a normal gamete; if this abnormality is compatible with life, the individual would have 46 chromosomes but a segment of the t. chromosome would be represented three times in each cell and a partial or complete trisomic state would exist.

trans·lu·cent (trans-loo′sent). Partially transparent; permitting light to pass through diffusely. [L. *translucens,* fr. trans- + *luceo,* to shine through]

trans·mem·brane (trans-mem′brān). Through or across a membrane.

trans·meth·yl·ase (trans-meth′i-lās). SYN methyltransferase.

trans·meth·yl·a·tion (trans′meth-i-lā′shŭn). Transfer of a methyl group from one compound to another; e.g., L-homocysteine is converted to L-methionine by the transfer to the latter of a methyl group. SEE *methionine* synthase.

trans·mi·gra·tion (trans-mī-grā′shŭn). Movement from one site to another; may entail the crossing of some usually limiting barrier, as in the passage of blood cells through the walls of the vessels (diapedesis). [L. *transmigro,* pp. -*atus,* to remove from one place to another]

ovular t., the passage of an ovum from one ovary into the fallopian tube of the other side; **external ovular t., direct ovular t.** occurs when the ovum passes across the pelvic cavity; **internal ovular t., indirect ovular t.** occurs when the ovum crosses the uterine cavity and so enters the tube of the opposite side.

trans·mis·si·ble (trans-mis′i-bl). Capable of being transmitted (carried across) from one person to another, as a t. disease, an infectious or contagious disease.

trans·mis·sion (trans-mish′ŭn). **1.** SYN transfer. **2.** The conveyance of disease from one person to another. **3.** The passage of a nerve impulse across an anatomic cleft, as in autonomic or central nervous system synapses and at neuromuscular junctions, by activation of a specific chemical mediator that stimulates or inhibits the structure across the synapse. SEE neurohumoral t. **4.** In general, passage of energy through a material. [L. *transmissio,* a sending across]

duplex t., the passage of impulses in both directions through a nerve trunk.

horizontal t., t. of infectious agents from an infected individual to a susceptible contemporary, in contradistinction to vertical t.

iatrogenic t., t. of infectious agents due to medical interference (e.g., t. by contaminated needles).

neurohumoral t., a process by which a presynaptic cell, upon excitation, releases a specific chemical agent (a neurotransmitter) to cross a synapse to stimulate or inhibit the postsynaptic cell. SYN neurotransmission.

transovarial t., passage of parasites or infective agents from the maternal body to eggs within the ovaries; commonly used to describe certain arthropods, to explain the ability of larvae of the next generation to transmit disease pathogens, as with the infection of larval mites or ticks with rickettsiae or viruses.

transstadial t., passage of a microbial parasite, such as a virus or rickettsia, from one developmental stage (stadium) of the host to its subsequent stage or stages, particularly as seen in mites. SEE ALSO transovarial t.

vertical t., (1) t. of a virus (e.g., RNA tumor virus) by means of the genetic apparatus of a cell in which the viral genome is integrated; **(2)** for infectious agents in general, t. of an agent from an individual to its offspring, i.e., from one generation to the next. Cf. horizontal t.

trans·mu·ral (trans-mū′răl). Through any wall, as of the body or of a cyst or any hollow structure. [trans- + L. *murus,* wall]

trans·mu·ta·tion (trans-mū-tā′shŭn). A change; transformation. SYN conversion (1). [L. *transmuto,* pp. -*atus,* to change, transmute]

trans·oc·u·lar (trans-ok′ū-lăr). Across the eye.

tran·so·nance (trans′ō-nans). Transmission of a sound arising in one organ through another. [trans- + L. *sonans,* sounding]

tran·son·ic (tran-son′ik). In ultrasound, describes a region of a relatively unattenuating medium. A distinction should be made between a t. region and an acoustic echo. [trans- + sonic]

trans·pa·ri·e·tal (trans-pă-rī′ĕ-tăl). Through or across a parietal region, area, or structure.

trans·pep·ti·dase (trans-pep′ti-dās). An enzyme catalyzing a transpeptidation reaction; many proteolytic enzymes (e.g., trypsin, papain) act as t.'s in the course of proteolysis, forming an acylated enzyme as an intermediate in the process; e.g., γ-glutamyl transpeptidase.

trans·pep·ti·da·tion (trans′pep-ti-dā′shŭn). A reaction involving the transfer of one or more amino acids from one peptide chain to another, as by transpeptidase action, or of a peptide chain itself, as in bacterial cell wall synthesis.

trans·per·i·to·ne·al (trans′per-i-tō-nē′ăl). Through the peritoneum; e.g., denoting a nephrectomy performed by abdominal section.

trans·phos·pha·tas·es (trans-fos′fă-tās-ez). SYN phosphotransferases.

trans·phos·pho·ryl·as·es (trans-fos-fōr′i-lā-sez). SEE phosphotransferases, phosphorylases, kinase.

trans·phos·pho·ryl·a·tion (trans′fos-fōr-i-lā′shŭn). A reaction involving the transfer of a phosphoric group from one compound to another, often with the involvement of ATP, as by the action of a phosphotransferase or kinase.

tran·spir·a·ble (trans-pī′ră-bl). Capable of transpiring or being transpired.

tran·spi·ra·tion (trans-pi-rā′shŭn). Passage of watery vapor through the skin or any membrane. SEE ALSO insensible *perspiration.* [trans- + L. *spiro,* pp. -*atus,* to breathe]

pulmonary t., the passage of water vapor from the blood into the air via the respiratory tract.

tran·spire (trans-pīr′). To exhale vapor from the skin or respiratory mucous membrane. [trans- + L. *spiro,* to breathe]

trans·pla·cen·tal (tranz-pla-sen′tăl). Crossing the placenta.

trans·plant (tranz′plant). **1.** To transfer from one part to another, as in grafting and transplantation. **2.** The tissue or organ in grafting and transplantation. SEE ALSO graft. [trans- + L. *planto,* to plant]

Gallie t., narrow strips of the femoral fascia lata used for suture material.

hair t., autografts of punch biopsies of hair-bearing skin, such as occipital scalp, onto frontal scalp in male pattern alopecia.

trans·plan·tar (trans-plan′tar). Across the sole of the foot; denoting certain muscular fibers or ligamentous structures.

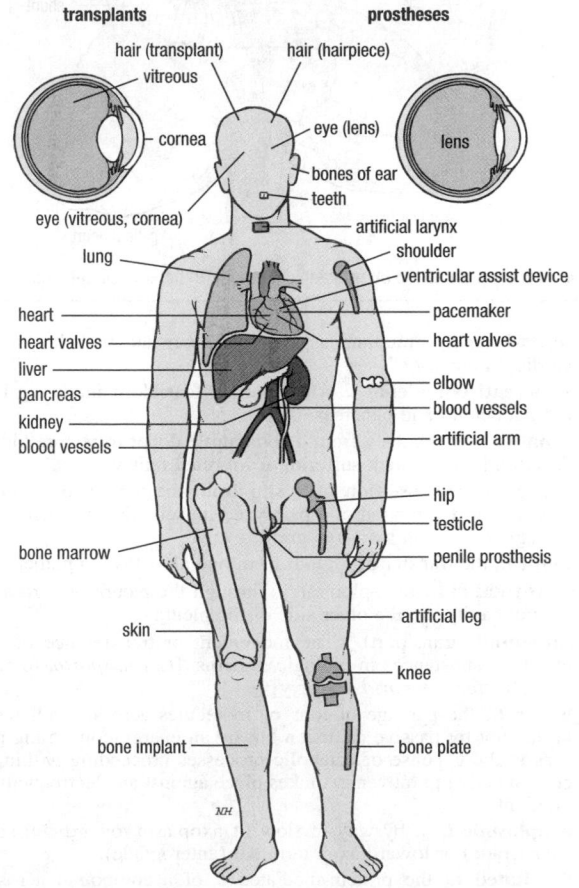

transplants and prostheses

---

trans·plan·ta·tion (tranz-plan-tā′shŭn). Implanting in one part a tissue or organ taken from another part or from another individual. SEE ALSO graft. [L. *transplanto,* pp. *-atus,* to transplant]

bone marrow t., grafting of bone marrow tissue; used in aplastic anemia, primary immunodeficiency, acute leukemia (following total body irradiation), and in patients with cancer (e.g., breast) who undergo extensive chemotherapy such that their bone marrow is destroyed.

cardiopulmonary t., SYN heart-lung t.

t. of cornea, SYN keratoplasty.

corneal t., SYN keratoplasty.

heart t., replacement of a severely damaged heart with a normal heart from a brain-dead donor.

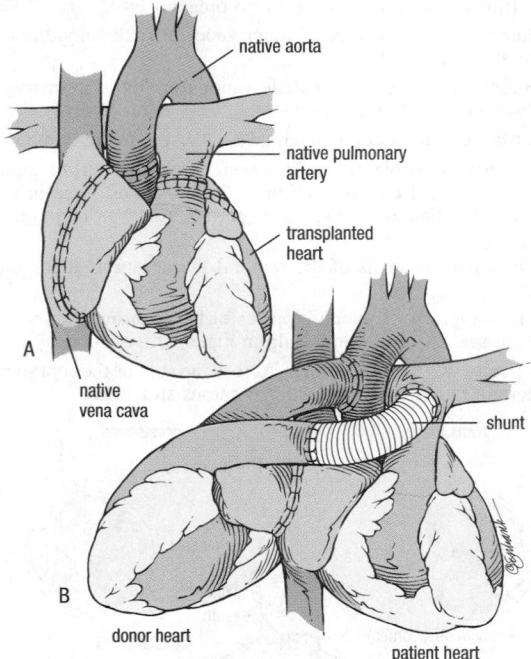

heart transplantation: (A) orthotopic method, (B) heterotopic method

heart-lung t., simultaneous t. of the heart and both lungs. SYN cardiopulmonary t.

pancreaticoduodenal t., a technically feasible t. including both the duodenum and pancreas.

renal t., t. of a kidney from a compatible donor to restore kidney function in a recipient suffering from renal failure.

tendon t., (1) insertion of a slip from the tendon of a sound muscle into the tendon of a paralyzed muscle; **(2)** replacement of a length of tendon by a free graft.

tooth t., the transfer of a tooth from one alveolus to another.

trans·pleu·ral (trans-ploo′răl). Through the pleura or across the pleural cavity; on the other side of the pleura.

trans·port (trans′pōrt). The movement or transference of biochemical substances in biologic systems. [L. *transporto,* to carry over, fr. trans- + *porto,* to carry]

active t., the passage of ions or molecules across a cell membrane, not by passive diffusion but by an energy-consuming process at the expense of catabolic processes proceeding within the cell; in active t., movement takes place against an electrochemical gradient.

axoplasmic t., t. by way of flow of axoplasm toward cell soma (retrograde) or toward axon terminal (anterograde).

facilitated t., the protein-mediated t. of a compound across a biomembrane that is not ion-driven; a saturable t. system. SYN passive t.

hydrogen t., the transfer of hydrogen from one metabolite (hydrogen donor) to another (hydrogen acceptor) through the action

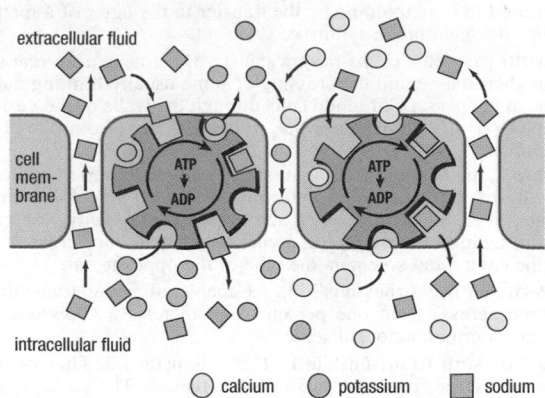

active transport: sodium diffuses into the cell through pores in cell membrane and is actively pumped out of cell by a carrier system; calcium and potassium diffuse out of cell and are actively pumped back into the cell; energy for this transport is obtained from ATP

of an enzyme system; the donor is thus oxidized and the acceptor reduced.

paracellular t., solvent movement across an epithelial cell layer through the tight junctions between cells. Cf. transcellular t.

passive t., SYN facilitated t.

transcellular t., solute movement across an epithelial cell layer through the cells. Cf. paracellular t.

vesicular t., SYN transcytosis.

trans·pos·ase (tranz-pōz′ās). An enzyme that is required for transposition of DNA segments. [L. *trans-pono,* pp. *transpositum,* to set across, transfer, + -ase]

trans·pose (tranz-pōz). To transfer one tissue or organ to the place of another and vice versa. [L. *trans-pono,* pp. *-positus,* to place across, transfer]

trans·po·si·tion (tranz-pō-zish′ŭn). **1.** Removal from one place to another; metathesis. **2.** The condition of being in the wrong place or on the wrong side of the body, as in t. of the viscera, in which the viscera are located opposite their normal position; e.g., the liver on the left, the apex of the heart on the right. **3.** Positioning of teeth out of their normal sequence in an arch.

t. of arterial stems, SYN t. of the great vessels.

corrected t. of the great vessels, anatomically or physiologically corrected malposition of the great arteries. In anatomically corrected t., they arise from the correct ventricles but have an abnormal relation to each other (actually a malposition rather than a t.) In physiologically or functionally corrected t., the aorta arises from a systemic ventricle that has the morphologic characteristics of a right ventricle, and the pulmonary artery arises from a "venous" ventricle that has the morphologic characteristics of a left ventricle.

t. of the great vessels, congenital malformation in which the aorta arises from the morphologic right ventricle and the pulmonary artery from the morphologic left ventricle resulting in two separate and parallel circulations. The condition is lethal unless some communication exists between the systemic and pulmonic circulation after birth; otherwise, unoxygenated venous blood inappropriately enters the systemic circulation, and oxygenated pulmonary venous blood is inappropriately directed to the pulmonary circulation. The life-sustaining communication may be an intraatrial passage or a patent ductus arteriosus. SYN t. of arterial stems.

penoscrotal t., a developmental error, seen with hypospadias, whereby hemiscrotal units are separated and lie lateral to the penile shaft or even cranial to it.

trans·po·son (trans-pō′son). A segment of DNA (e.g., an R-factor gene) which has a repeat of an insertion sequence element at each end that can migrate from one plasmid to another within the same bacterium, to a bacterial chromosome, or to a bacteriophage; the mechanism of transposition seems to be independent of the host's usual recombination mechanism. SEE jumping *gene*, transposable *element*. [L. *transpono*, pp. *transpositum*, to transfer, + -on]

trans·sec·tion (trans-sek'shŭn). SYN transection.

trans·seg·men·tal (trans-seg-men'tăl). Across or through a segment.

trans·sep·tal (trans-sep'tăl). Across or through a septum; on the other side of a septum.

trans·sex·u·al (trans-sek'shoo-ăl). **1.** A person with the external genitalia and secondary sexual characteristics of one sex, but whose personal identification and psychosocial configuration is that of the opposite sex; a study of morphologic, genetic, and gonadal structure may be genitally congruent or incongruent. **2.** Denoting or relating to such a person. **3.** Relating to medical and surgical procedures designed to alter a patient's external sexual characteristics so that they resemble those of the opposite sex.

trans·sex·u·al·ism (tranz-sek'shoo-ă-lizm). **1.** The state of being a transsexual. **2.** The desire to change anatomic sexual characteristics to conform physically with one's perception of oneself as a member of the opposite sex, coupled with a desire to live fulltime in the role of the opposite sex.

trans·sphe·noi·dal (trans-sfē-noy'dăl). Through or across the sphenoid bone.

trans·splic·ing (trans-splīs'ing). Formation of spliced products containing portions of two different transcripts.

trans·sul·fu·rase (trans-sŭl'fer-ās). Descriptive term applied to the enzymes catalyzing, among others, the following reactions involving sulfur-containing compounds: 1) cystathionine → cysteine + α-ketobutyrate + NH_3 (cystathionine γ-lyase); 2) cystathionine → homocysteine + pyruvate + NH_3 (cystathionine β-lyase); 3) cystine → thiocysteine + pyruvate + NH_3 (cystathionine γ-lyase); 4) cystathionine → serine + homocysteine (cystathionine synthase). SYN transulfurase.

trans·sul·fur·a·tion (trans-sŭl'fer-ā'shŭn). The exchange of sulfur, or sulfur-containing moiety, between two different compounds.

trans·syn·ap·tic (trans-si-nap'tik). Indicating transmission of a nerve impulse across a synapse.

trans·ten·to·ri·al (trans-ten-tōr'ē-ăl). Passing across or through either the tentorial notch or the tentorium cerebelli.

trans·tha·lam·ic (trans-tha-lam'ik). Passing across the thalamus.

trans·ther·mia (trans-ther'mē-ă). SYN diathermy. [trans- + G. *thermē*, heat]

trans·tho·rac·ic (trans-thōr-as'ik). Passing through the thoracic cavity.

trans·tho·ra·cot·o·my (trans-thōr'ă-kot'ō-mē). A surgical procedure carried out through an incision into the chest wall. [trans- + thorax + G. *tomē*, incision]

trans·thy·ret·in (trans-thī'rē-tin). SYN prealbumin (1).

tran·su·date (tran'soo-dāt). Any fluid (solvent and solute) that has passed through a presumably normal membrane, such as the capillary wall, as a result of imbalanced hydrostatic and osmotic forces; characteristically low in protein unless there has been secondary concentration. Cf. exudate. SYN transudation (2). [trans- + L. *sudo*, pp. *-atus*, to sweat]

tran·su·da·tion (tran-soo-dā'shŭn). **1.** Passage of a fluid or solute through a membrane by a hydrostatic or osmotic pressure gradient. SEE transudate. **2.** SYN transudate.

tran·sude (tran-sood'). In general, to ooze or to pass a liquid gradually through a membrane, more specifically, through a normal membrane, as a result of imbalanced hydrostatic and osmotic forces. [see transudate]

tran·sul·fu·rase (tran-sŭl'fer-ās). SYN transsulfurase.

trans·u·re·ter·o·u·re·ter·os·to·my (TUU) (tranz-ū-rē'ter-ō-ū-rē-ter-os'tō-mē). Anastomosis of the transected end of one ureter into the intact contralateral ureter, by direct or elliptical end-to-side technique. SEE ureteroureterostomy. SYN transureteroureteral anastomosis.

trans·u·re·thral (trans-ū-rē'thrăl). Through the urethra.

trans·vaa·lin. SYN *scillaren* A.

trans·vag·i·nal (trans-vaj'i-năl). Across or through the vagina.

trans·vec·tor (trans-vek'tŏr, tōr). An animal that transmits a toxic substance that it does not produce, but that may be accumulated from animal (dinoflagellate) or plant (algae) sources; e.g., filter-feeding mollusks.

trans·ver·sa·lis (trans-ver-sā'lis) [TA]. Transverse, denotes especially a fascia. SYN transverse, transverse. [L.]

trans·verse (trans-vers') [TA]. Crosswise; lying across the long axis of the body or of a part. SYN transversalis [TA], transversus [TA]. [L. *transversus*]

trans·ver·sec·to·my (trans-ver-sek'tō-mē). Resection of the transverse process of a vertebra. [transverse + G. *ektomē*, excision]

trans·ver·sion (trans-ver'zhŭn). **1.** Substitution in DNA and RNA of a pyrimidine for a purine, or vice versa, by mutation. **2.** In dentistry, the eruption of a tooth in a position normally occupied by another; transposition of a tooth.

trans·ver·so·cos·tal (trans-ver'sō-kos'tăl). SYN costotransverse.

transversospinales (tranz-ver-sō-spin-al'es). SYN transversospinales (*muscles*), under *muscle*.

trans·ver·so·u·re·thra·lis (trans-ver-sō-ū-rē-thrā'lis). Denoting the transverse fibers of the sphincter urethrae muscle, arising from the arch of the pubes.

trans·ver·sus (trans-ver'sŭs) [TA]. SYN transverse. [L. fr. *trans*, across, + *verto*, pp. *versus*, to turn]

trans·ves·tism (trans-ves'tizm). The practice of dressing or masquerading in the clothes of the opposite sex; especially the adoption of feminine mannerisms and costume by a male. SYN transvestitism. [trans- + L. *vestio*, to dress]

trans·ves·tite (trans-ves'tīt). A person who practices transvestism.

trans·ves·ti·tism (trans-ves'ti-tizm). SYN transvestism.

Trantas, Alexios, Greek ophthalmologist, 1867–1960. SEE T. *dots*, under *dot*; Horner-T. *dots*, under *dot*.

tran·yl·cyp·ro·mine sul·fate (tran-il-sip'rō-mēn). A monoamine oxidase inhibitor; an antidepressant used in the treatment of severe mental depression. Interacts with many foods and drugs to produce hypertensive crisis.

TRAP Abbreviation for twin reversed arterial perfusion.

tra·pe·zi·al (tra-pē'zē-ăl). Relating to any trapezium.

tra·pe·zi·form (tra-pē'zi-form). SYN trapezoid (1).

tra·pe·zi·o·met·a·car·pal (tra-pē'zē-ō-met'ă-kar'păl). Relating to the trapezium and the metacarpus.

tra·pe·zi·um, pl. **tra·pe·zia, tra·pe·zi·ums** (tra-pē'zē-ŭm, -ă). **1.** A four-sided geometrical figure having no two sides parallel. **2.** SYN trapezium *bone*. [G. *trapezion*, a table or counter, a trapezium, dim. of *trapeza*, a table, fr. *tra-* (= *tetra-*), four, + *pous* (*pod-*), foot]

tra·pe·zi·us (tra-pē'zē-ŭs). SYN trapezius (*muscle*).

trap·e·zoid (trap'ĕ-zoyd) [TA]. **1.** Resembling a trapezium. SYN trapeziform. **2.** A geometrical figure resembling a trapezium except that two of its opposite sides are parallel. **3.** SYN trapezoid (*bone*). **4.** SYN trapezoid *body*. [G. *trapeza*, table, + *eidos*, resemblance]

trap·i·dil (trap'ĭ-dil). An antagonist and selective synthesis inhibitor of thromboxane A_2; used to prevent cerebral vasospasm.

Trapp, Julius, Russian pharmacist, 1815–1908. SEE T. *formula*; T.-Häser *formula*.

Traube, Ludwig, German physician and pathologist, 1818–1876. SEE T. *bruit, corpuscle, dyspnea, plugs*, under *plug*, semilunar *space, sign*, double *tone*; T.-Hering *curves*, under *curve*, *waves*, under *wave*.

Traugott, Carl, German internist, *1885. SEE Staub-T. *effect*.

△**traum-.** SEE traumato-.

trau·ma, pl. **trau·ma·ta, trau·mas** (traw'mă, -mă-tă). An injury, physical or mental. SYN traumatism. [G. wound]

   birth t., (1) physical injury to an infant during its delivery; **(2)** the supposed emotional injury, inflicted by events incident to birth, upon an infant which allegedly appears in symbolic form in patients with mental illness.

tr

t. from occlusion, a reversible lesion in the periodontium caused by excessive movement of teeth.

occlusal t., abnormal occlusal stresses capable of producing or which have produced pathologic changes in the tooth and its surrounding structures.

psychic t., an upsetting experience precipitating or aggravating an emotional or mental disorder.

trau·ma·ta (traw′mă-tă). Plural of trauma.

trau·mat·ic (traw-mat′ik). Relating to or caused by trauma. [G. *traumatikos*]

trau·ma·tism (traw′mă-tizm). SYN trauma.

trau·ma·tize (traw′mă-tīz). To cause or inflict trauma. [G. *traumatizō*, to wound]

△**traumato-, traumat-, traum-.** Wound, injury. [G. *trauma*]

trau·ma·tol·o·gy (traw-mă-tol′ō-jē). The branch of surgery concerned with the injured. [traumato- + G. *logos,* study]

trau·ma·to·ne·sis (traw′mă-tō-nē′sis, -ton′ē-sis). Surgical repair of an accidental wound. [traumato- + G. *nēis,* a spinning]

trau·ma·top·a·thy (traw-mă-top′ă-thē). Any pathologic condition resulting from violence or wounds. [traumato- + G. *pathos,* suffering]

trau·ma·top·nea (traw′mă-top-nē′ă). Passage of air in and out through a wound of the chest wall. [traumato- + G. *pnoē,* breath]

trau·ma·to·py·ra (traw′mă-tō-pī′ră). Obsolete synonym of traumatic *fever.* [traumato- + G. *pyr,* fire, fever]

trau·ma·to·sep·sis (traw′mă-tō-sep′sis). Infection of a wound; septicemia following a wound. [traumato- + G. *sēpsis,* putrefaction]

trau·ma·to·ther·a·py (traw′mă-tō-thār′ă-pē). Treatment of trauma or the result of injury.

Trautmann, Moritz F., German otologist, 1832–1902. SEE T. triangular *space.*

tra·verse (trav′ers). In computed tomography, one complete linear movement of the gantry across the object being scanned, as occurred in the original translate and rotate CT machines. [M.E., fr. O.Fr., fr. L.L. *transverso,* fr. L. *trans-verto,* to turn across]

tray (trā). A flat receptacle with raised edges.

acrylic resin t., a plastic impression t. used in dentistry; usually fashioned for the individual patient from an autopolymerizing acrylic resin.

annealing t., an electrically heated, thermostatically controlled device used to drive off the protective NH_3 gas coating from the surface of cohesive gold foil.

impression t., a receptacle used to carry and confine plastic impression material when making an impression of oral structures.

traz·o·done hy·dro·chlo·ride (traz′ō-dōn). An antidepressant structurally unrelated to other antidepressants.

Trea·cher Collins, Edward, English ophthalmologist, 1862–1919. SEE Treacher Collins *syndrome.*

trea·cle (trē′kl). **1.** Molasses, a viscid syrup that drains from sugar-refining molds. **2.** A saccharine fluid. **3.** Formerly, a remedy for poison, hence any effective remedy. SEE ALSO theriaca. [M.E. *triacle,* antidote, fr. L. *theriaca,* antidote to snake bite, fr. G. *thēriakos,* pertaining to wild beasts]

treat (trēt). To manage a disease by medicinal, surgical, or other measures; to care for a patient medically or surgically. [Fr. *traiter,* fr. L. *tracto,* to drag, handle, perform]

treat·ment (trēt′ment). Medical or surgical management of a patient. SEE ALSO therapy, therapeutics. [Fr. *traitement* (see treat)]

active t., a therapeutic substance or course intended to ameliorate the basic disease problem, as opposed to supportive or palliative t. Cf. causal t.

Carrel t., t. of wound surfaces by intermittent flushing with Dakin solution. SYN Dakin-Carrel t.

causal t., t. aimed at reversing the causal factor in a disease.

conservative t., a course of therapeutic action designed to avoid harm, with less possibility of benefit than more risky actions.

Dakin-Carrel t., SYN Carrel t.

dietetic t., treatment of a clinical condition with a specific diet.

empiric t., a t. based on experience, usually without adequate data to support its use.

endodontic t., SYN root canal t.

Goeckerman t., a t. for psoriasis; the involved areas are painted with a solution of coal tar, or are covered with crude coal tar ointment and subsequently irradiated with ultraviolet (UVB).

heat t., in dentistry, a method of controlled temperature handling of metals so as to change the microscopic structure and thus the physical properties. SEE ALSO temper, anneal.

insulin coma t., formerly used t. of major mental illness by means of hypoglycemic coma induced by insulin. SYN insulin shock t.

insulin shock t., SYN insulin coma t.

isoserum t., therapeutic use of serum taken from a person having or having had the same disease as the patient under treatment.

Kenny t., an obsolete method for the t. of anterior poliomyelitis; the affected parts were wrapped in woolen cloth wrung out with hot water; after the acute stage of the disease had passed, the limbs were passively exercised to reeducate the paralyzed muscles.

light t., SYN phototherapy.

medical t., t. of disease by hygienic and pharmacologic remedies, as distinguished from invasive surgical procedures.

Mitchell t., t. of mental illness by rest, nourishing diet, and a change of environment. SYN Weir Mitchell t.

moral t., a type of milieu therapy utilized in the 19th century, emphasizing religious doctrine and benevolent guidance in activities of daily living; as such it was a form of psychotherapy as opposed to somatic t.'s such as bloodletting and purging.

Nauheim t., t. of certain cardiac affections by baths in water through which carbonic acid gas is bubbling, followed by resisting exercises. SYN Nauheim bath, Schott t. [*Bad Nauheim,* W. Germany]

palliative t., t. to alleviate symptoms without curing the disease.

preventive t., SYN prophylactic t.

prophylactic t., the institution of measures designed to protect a person from an attack of a disease to which the person has been or is liable to be exposed. SYN preventive t.

root canal t., **(1)** the means by which painful or diseased teeth, in which the pulp is involved, are restored to a healthy state; **(2)** removal of a normal, diseased, or dead pulp by biochemical and mechanical means, enlargement and sterilization of the root canal, followed by filling the canal, to effect healing of diseased periapical tissues; **(3)** the diagnosis and t. of diseases of the pulp and their sequelae. SYN endodontic t.

Schott t., SYN Nauheim t.

shock t., SEE electroshock *therapy.*

solar t., SYN solar *therapy.*

symptomatic t., therapy aimed at relieving symptoms without necessarily affecting the basic underlying cause(s) of the symptoms.

Tallerman t., use of special apparatus to administer dry heat to rheumatic disorders, traumatic sprains, etc.

thymus t., t. of disease by administration of extracts of thymus gland.

Tweed edgewise t., SEE edgewise *appliance.*

Weir Mitchell t., SYN Mitchell t.

tre·ha·la (trē-hah′lă). A saccharine substance containing trehalose and resembling manna, excreted by a parasitic beetle, *Larinus maculatus.* [Fr., fr. Turk. *tigala,* fr. Pers. *tīghāl*]

tre·ha·lase (trē-hă′lās). A glycosidase secreted in the duodenum that hydrolyzes α-glycosidic 1,1 bonds; an absence or deficiency of this enzyme will lead to deficient digestion of trehalose (autosomal recessive).

tre·ha·lose (trē′hă-lōs). A nonreducing disaccharide, (α-D-glucosido)-α-D-glucoside, contained in trehala; also found in fungi, such as *Amanita muscaria;* elevated in individuals with a trehalase deficiency. SYN mycose.

Treitz, Wenzel, Bohemian pathologist, 1819–1872. SEE T. *arch, fascia, fossa, hernia, ligament, muscle.*

Trélat, Ulysse, French surgeon, 1828–1890. SEE T. *stools,* under *stool;* Leser-T. *sign.*

tre·ma (trē′mă). **1.** SYN foramen. **2.** SYN vulva. [G. *trēma,* a hole]

tre·ma·camra (trē-ma-kam′ra). The extracellular part of the cell surface adhesion molecule ICAM-1 involved in rhinovirus attachments to mucosal cells.

Trem·a·to·da (trem′ă-tō′dă). A class in the phylum Platyhelminthes (the flatworms), consisting of flukes with a leaf-shaped body and two muscular suckers, and an acelomate parenchyma-filled body cavity. Circulatory system and sense organs are not present, but an incomplete alimentary canal is found (lacking an anus). Flukes of interest to human or veterinary medicine are members of the order Digenea, with complete life cycles involving embryonic multiplication in a mollusk as their first intermediate host. The other order, Monogenea, consists chiefly of parasites of fish that have a simpler pattern of direct development on a single host. [G. *trēmatōdēs,* full of holes, fr. *trēma,* a hole, + *eidos,* appearance]

trem·a·tode, trem·a·toid (trem′ă-tōd, trem′ă-toyd). **1.** Common name for a fluke of the class Trematoda. **2.** Relating to a fluke of the class Trematoda.

trem·bles (trem′blz). An intoxication of cattle, caused by eating white snakeroot, *Eupatorium urticaefolium,* or the rayless goldenrod; the active agent is a higher alcohol, tremetol, which intoxicated cows eliminate in their milk, causing milk *sickness* when ingested by humans. [L. *tremulus,* trembling, fr. *tremo,* to tremble]

trem·bling (trem′bling). The shaking or quaking of a tremor.

trem·el·loid, trem·el·lose (trem′ĕ-loyd, -lōs). Jelly-like. [L. *tremulus,* trembling]

trem·o·gram (trem′ō-gram). The graphic representation of a tremor taken by means of the tremograph or kymograph. SYN tremorgram.

trem·o·graph (trem′ō-graf). An apparatus for making a graphic record of a tremor. [L. *tremor,* a shaking, + G. *graphō,* to write]

trem·o·la·bile (trem-ō-lā′bil, -bīl). Inactivated or destroyed by shaking. [L. *tremor,* a shaking, + *labilis,* perishable]

trem·o·pho·bia (trem-ō-fō′bē-ă). Morbid fear of trembling. [L. *tremor,* trembling, + G. *phobos,* fear]

trem·or (trem′er, -ōr). **1.** Repetitive, often regular, oscillatory movements caused by alternate, or synchronous, but irregular contraction of opposing muscle groups; usually involuntary. **2.** Minute ocular movement occurring during fixation on an object. [L. a shaking]

action t., SYN intention t.

alcoholic withdrawal t., intention t. present in the withdrawal period of one of two types: 1) a t. of greater than 8 Hz, with continuous antagonistic muscle activity, and 2) a t. of less than 8 Hz, with intermittent spontaneous antagonistic muscle activity.

alternating t., a form of hyperkinesia characterized by regular, symmetric, to-and-fro movements (at about 4 per second) that are produced by patterned, alternating contraction of muscles and their antagonists.

alternative t., a coarse, low frequency (3–8 Hz) pathologic t. produced by alternating contraction of muscles and their antagonists; seen with Parkinson disease and kinetic predominant action t.

benign essential t., SYN heredofamilial t.

coarse t., a t. in which the amplitude is large and the oscillations are usually irregular and slow.

continuous t., SYN persistent t.

essential t., an action t. of 4–8 Hz frequency that usually begins in early adult life and is limited to the upper limbs and head; called familial when it appears in several family members.

familial t., SYN heredofamilial t.

fine t., a t. in which the amplitude is small and the frequency is usually greater than 12 Hz.

flapping t., SYN asterixis.

head t.'s, SYN head-nodding.

heredofamilial t. [MIM*190300], a benign t. inherited as a dominant character; it may be a rapid oscillation resembling that seen in thyrotoxicosis, a coarse t. during rest and inhibited by a voluntary effort, or one which appears only upon movement; of autosomal dominant inheritance. SYN benign essential t., familial t.

hysterical t., usually an intermittent, coarse, irregular t. limited to one limb. SYN psychogenic t.

intention t., a t. that occurs during the performance of precise voluntary movements, caused by disorders of the cerebellum or its connections. SYN action t., kinetic t., volitional t. (2).

kinetic t., SYN intention t.

passive t., SYN resting t.

persistent t., a t. that is constant, whether the subject is at rest or moving. SYN continuous t.

physiologic t., fine t., 8–13 Hz frequency, which is a normal phenomenon.

pill-rolling t., resting t. of the thumb and fingers seen in Parkinson disease.

postural t., t. present when the limbs or trunk are kept in certain positions and when they are moved actively, usually due to near-synchronous rhythmic bursts in opposing muscle groups. SYN static t.

progressive cerebellar t., SYN Hunt *syndrome* (1).

psychogenic t., SYN hysterical t.

resting t., a coarse, rhythmic t., 3–5 Hz frequency, usually confined to hands and forearms, that appears when the limbs are relaxed, and disappears with active limb movements; characteristic of Parkinson disease. SYN passive t.

senile t., an essential t. that becomes symptomatic in elderly adults.

static t., SYN postural t.

volitional t., (1) a t. that can be arrested by a strong effort of the will; **(2)** SYN intention t.

wing-beating t., a coarse, irregular t. that is most prominent when the limbs are held outstretched, reminiscent of a bird flapping its wings; due to up and down excursion of arm at abducted shoulder. Seen mainly with Wilson disease.

trem·or·gram (trem′ōr-gram). SYN tremogram.

trem·or·ine (trem′er-ēn). A chemical which in the laboratory produces a tremor resembling parkinsonian tremor and is used to produce experimental parkinsonism.

trem·o·sta·ble (trem-ō-stā′bl). Not subject to alteration or destruction by being shaken. [L. *tremor,* a shaking, + *stabilis,* stable]

trem·u·lor (trem′ū-ler, -lōr). An instrument for giving vibratory massage.

trem·u·lous (trem′ū-lŭs). Characterized by tremor.

Trenaunay, Paul, French physician, *1875. SEE Klippel-T.-Weber *syndrome.*

Trendelenburg, Friedrich, German surgeon, 1844–1924. SEE T. *operation, position;* reverse T. *position;* T. *sign, symptom, test;* Trendelenburg *gait.*

trep·a·na·tion (trep-ă-nā′shŭn). SYN trephination.

corneal t., t. of cornea, SYN keratoplasty.

treph·i·na·tion (tref-i-nā′shŭn). Removal of a circular piece ("button") of cranium by a trephine. SYN trepanation.

tre·phine (trē-fīn′, -fēn′). **1.** SYN perforator. **2.** To remove a disk of bone or other tissue by means of a t. [contrived fr. L. *tres fines,* three ends]

treph·o·cyte (tref′ō-sīt). SYN trophocyte. [G. *trephō,* to nourish, + *kytos,* cell]

trep·i·da·tio cor·dis (trep-i-dā′shē-ō kōr′dis). SYN palpitation.

trep·i·da·tion (trep-i-dā′shŭn). Anxious fear. [L. *trepidatio,* fr. *trepido,* to tremble, to be agitated]

Trep·o·ne·ma (trep-ō-nē′mă). A genus of anaerobic bacteria (order Spirochaetales) consisting of cells, 3–8 μm in length, with acute, regular, or irregular spirals and no obvious protoplasmic structure. A terminal filament may be present. They stain with difficulty except with Giemsa stain or silver impregnation. Some species are pathogenic and parasitic for humans and other animals, generally producing local lesions in tissues. The type species is *T. pallidum.* [G. *trepō,* to turn, + *nēma,* thread]

T. cara′teum, a bacterial species that causes pinta, or carate.

tr

T. cunic'uli, a bacterial species that causes spirochetosis in rabbits.

T. dentico'la, cultivatable bacterial species that does not ferment carbohydrates and can be isolated from the oral cavity of humans.

T. genita'lis, a nonpathogenic bacterial species found on the genitalia of humans.

T. hyodysente'riae, an enteropathogenic bacterial species that causes swine dysentery.

T. muco'sum, a bacterial species found in pyorrhea alveolaris; it possesses pyogenic properties.

T. pal'lidum, a bacterial species that causes syphilis in humans; this organism can be experimentally transmitted to anthropoid apes and to rabbits; it is the type species of the genus *T.*

T. perten'ue, a bacterial species that causes yaws; patients with this disease give positive results in serologic screening tests for syphilis.

trep·o·ne·ma·to·sis (trep'ō-nē-mă-tō'sis). SYN treponemiasis.

trep·o·neme (trep'ō-nēm). A vernacular term used to refer to any member of the genus *Treponema*.

trep·o·ne·mi·a·sis (trep'ō-nē-mī'ă-sis). Infection caused by *Treponema*. SYN treponematosis.

trep·o·ne·mi·ci·dal (trep'ō-nē'mi-sī'dăl). Destructive to any species of *Treponema*, but usually with reference to *T. pallidum*, the microorganisms responsible for syphillis. SYN antitreponemal. [*Treponema* + L. *caedo*, to kill]

trep·pe (trep'eh). A phenomenon in cardiac muscle first observed by H.P. Bowditch; if a number of stimuli of the same intensity are sent into the muscle after a quiescent period, the first few contractions of the series show a successive increase in amplitude (strength). SYN staircase phenomenon. [Ger. *Treppe*, staircase]

Tresilian, Frederick J., English physician, 1862–1926. SEE T. *sign.*

tre·sis (trē'sis). SYN perforation. [G. *trēsis*, a boring]

tret·i·noin (tret'i-nō-in). A keratolytic agent. SEE retinoic acid.

Treves, Sir Frederick, English surgeon, 1853–1923. SEE T. *fold.*

Treves, Norman, U.S. surgeon, 1894–1964. SEE Stewart-T. *syndrome.*

Trevor, David, 20th century British orthopedic surgeon. SEE T. *disease.*

TRF Abbreviation for thyrotropin-releasing *factor*.

TRH Abbreviation for thyrotropin-releasing *hormone*.

△**tri-.** Three. Cf. tris-. [L. and G.]

tri·a·ce·tic ac·id (trī-ă-sē'tik). Formed by condensation of acetyl and malonyl CoA's in the course of fatty acid synthesis.

tri·ac·e·tin (trī-as'ĕ-tin). Used as a solvent of basic dyes, as a fixative in perfumery, and as a topical antifungal agent. SYN glyceryl triacetate, triacetylglycerol.

tri·a·ce·tyl·glyc·er·ol (trī-as'i-til-glis'er-ol). SYN triacetin.

tri·a·ce·tyl·o·le·an·do·my·cin (trī-as'ĕ-til-ō'lē-an-dō-mī'sin). SYN troleandomycin.

tri·ac·yl·glyc·er·ol (trī-as'il-glis'er-ol). Glycerol esterified at each of its three hydroxyl groups by a fatty (aliphatic) acid; e.g., tristearoylglycerol. SYN triglyceride.

t. lipase, the fat-splitting enzyme in pancreatic juice; it hydrolyzes t. to produce a diacylglycerol and a fatty acid anion; a deficiency of the hepatic enzyme results in hypercholesterolemia and hypertriglyceridemia. SYN lipase (2), steapsin, tributyrase, tributyrinase.

tri·ad (trī'ad). **1.** A collection of three things having something in common. **2.** The transverse tubule and the terminal cisternae on each side of it in skeletal muscle fibers. **3.** SYN portal t. **4.** The father, mother, and child relationship projectively experienced in group psychotherapy. [G. *trias* (*triad-*), the number 3, fr. *treis,* three]

acute compression t., the rising venous pressure, falling arterial pressure, and decreased heart sounds of pericardial tamponade. SYN Beck t.

Beck t., SYN acute compression t.

Charcot t., (1) in multiple (disseminated) sclerosis, the three

symptoms: nystagmus, tremor, and scanning speech; **(2)** combination of jaundice, fever, and upper abdominal pain that occurs as a result of cholangitis.

Fallot t., SYN *trilogy* of Fallot.

hepatic t., SYN portal t.

Hull t., the association of diastolic gallop, anasarca, and small pulse pressure.

Hutchinson t., parenchymatous keratitis, labyrinthine disease, and Hutchinson teeth, significant of congenital syphilis.

Kartagener t., SYN Kartagener *syndrome.*

portal t., branches of the portal vein, hepatic artery, and the biliary ducts bound together in the perivascular fibrous capsule or portal tract as they ramify within the substance of the liver. SYN hepatic t., triad (3).

Saint t., the concurrence of hiatal hernia, diverticulosis, and cholelithiasis.

tri·age (trē'ahzh). **1.** Medical screening of patients to determine their relative priority for treatment. **2.** The separation of a large number of casualties, in military or civilian disaster medical care, into three groups: 1) those who cannot be expected to survive even with treatment; 2) those who will recover without treatment; and 3) the highest priority group, those who will not survive without treatment. [Fr. sorting]

tri·al. A test or experiment, usually conducted under specific conditions.

clinical t., a controlled experiment involving a defined set of human subjects, having a clinical event as an outcome measure, and intended to yield scientifically valid information about the efficacy or safety of a drug, vaccine, diagnostic test, surgical procedure, or other form of medical intervention.

> Four phases of clinical trial are distinguished. Phase I trials usually involve fewer than 100 healthy volunteers who are exposed to a new drug or vaccine. Such studies seek to establish optimal dosage and route of administration and to detect adverse reactions. Phase II trials generally involve 200–500 volunteers randomly assigned to control and study groups. These are pilot efficacy studies, with emphasis on immunogenicity in the case of vaccines, and on relative efficacy and safety in the case of drugs. Phase III trials, often multicenter, involve thousands of volunteers, randomly assigned to control and study groups. The aim is to generate statistically relevant data. Phase IV trials are conducted after a national drug registration authority (in the U.S., the Food and Drug Administration) has approved an agent for distribution or sale. They may explore specific pharmacologic effect, adverse reactions, or long-term effects.

randomized controlled t. (RCT), an epidemiologic experiment in which subjects in a population are allocated randomly into groups, called "experimental" or "study" and "control" groups to receive or not receive an experimental therapeutic or preventive regimen, procedure, maneuver, or intervention.

tri·al and er·ror. The apparently random, haphazard, hit-or-miss exploratory activity which often precedes the acquisition of new information or adjustments; it may be overt, as in a rat running in a maze, or covert (vicarious), as when one thinks of various ways of coping with a situation.

tri·am·cin·o·lone (trī-am-sin'ō-lōn). A glucocorticoid with actions and uses similar to those of prednisolone.

t. acetonide, a potent glucocorticoid for topical treatment of dermatoses.

t. diacetate, an anti-inflammatory and antiallergic agent for parenteral use.

tri·a·me·lia (trī'ă-mē'lē-ă). Absence of three limbs. [tri- + G. *a*-priv. + *melos*, limb]

tri·am·ter·ene (trī-am'ter-ēn). A potassium sparing diuretic agent, often used in combination with hydrochlorthiazide.

TRIANGLE

tri·an·gle (trī′ang-gl) [TA]. In anatomy and surgery, a three-sided area with arbitrary or natural boundaries. SEE ALSO trigonum, region. [L. *triangulum,* fr. *tri-,* three, + *angulus,* angle]

anal t. [TA], the posterior portion of the perineal region through which the anal canal opens; bounded by a line through both ischial tuberosities, the sacrotuberous ligaments, and the coccyx. SYN regio analis [TA], anal region.

anterior t. of neck, ☆official alternate term for anterior cervical *region.*

Assézat t., a t. formed by lines connecting the nasion with the alveolar and nasal point; used to indicate prognathism in comparative craniology.

auricular t., a t. formed by the base of the auricle and by lines drawn from the true tip of the auricle to the extremities of the base.

ausculatory t. [TA], space bounded by the lower border of the trapezius, the latissimus dorsi, and the medial margin of the scapula, where the absence of musculature allows respiratory sounds to be heard clearly with a stethoscope. SYN trigonum auscultationis [TA], t. of auscultation ☆.

t. of auscultation, ☆official alternate term for ausculatory t.

axillary t., a triangular area embracing the medial aspect of the arm, the axilla, and the pectoral region which is one of the seats of predilection for the petechial initial rash of smallpox. SEE ALSO axillary *region.*

Béclard t., area bounded by the posterior border of the hyoglossus muscle, the posterior belly of the digastric, and the greater horn of the hyoid bone.

Bonwill t., an equilateral t. formed by lines from the contact points of the lower central incisors, or the medial line of the residual ridge of the mandible, to the condyle on either side and from one condyle to the other.

Burger t., a scalene t. representing the frontal plane electrocardiographic leads comparable to, but more accurate than, the Einthoven t. SEE Einthoven t.

Burow t., a t. of skin and subcutaneous fat excised so that a flap can be advanced without buckling the adjacent tissue.

Calot t. [TA], SYN cystohepatic t.

cardiohepatic t., SYN cardiohepatic *angle.*

carotid t. [TA], a space bounded by the superior belly of the omohyoid muscle, anterior border of the sternocleidomastoid, and posterior belly of the digastric; it contains the bifurcation of the common carotid artery. SYN trigonum caroticum [TA], fossa carotica, Gerdy hyoid fossa, Malgaigne fossa, Malgaigne t., superior carotid t.

cephalic t., a t. on the cranium formed by lines connecting the metopion, the pogonion, and the occipital point.

cervical t., any of the t.'s of the neck.

clavipectoral t. [TA], area of anterior thoracic region bounded superiorly by the clavicle, inferomedially by the pectoral major (muscle) and superolaterally by the deltoid (muscle); the cephalic vein typically passes from superficial to deep here, and the pectoral branch of the thoracoacromial (arterial) trunk emerges here. SYN trigonum clavipectorale [TA], trigonum deltopectorale ☆, deltoideopectoral t., deltopectoral t., trigonum deltoideopectorale.

Codman t., in radiology, the interface between growing bone tumor and normal bone, presenting as an incomplete triangle formed by periosteum.

crural t., an area of predilection for the petechial initial rash of smallpox; it occupies the lower abdominal, inguinal, and genital regions and the inner aspects of the thighs, the base of the t. traversing the umbilicus.

cystohepatic t. [TA], area bounded by the cystic artery, cystic duct, and (common) hepatic duct—important structures to identify in performing a laparoscopic cholecystectomy. SYN Calot t. [TA], trigonum cystohepaticum [TA].

deltoideopectoral t., SYN clavipectoral t.

deltopectoral t., SYN clavipectoral t.

digastric t., SYN submandibular t.

Einthoven t., an imaginary equilateral t. with the heart at its center, its equal sides representing the three standard limb leads of the electrocardiogram.

Elaut t., t. formed by the iliac arteries and the promontory of the sacrum.

t. of elbow, SYN cubital *fossa.*

facial t., a t. formed by lines connecting the basion, the prosthion, and the nasion.

Farabeuf t., the t. formed by the internal jugular and facial veins and the hypoglossal nerve.

femoral t. [TA], a triangular space at the upper part of the thigh, bounded by the sartorius and adductor longus muscles and the inguinal ligament, with a floor formed laterally by the iliopsoas muscle and medially by the pectineus muscle; the branches of the femoral nerve are distributed within the femoral t.; it is bisected by the femoral vessels, which enter the adductor canal at the t.'s apex. SYN trigonum femorale [TA], trigonum femoris ☆, fossa scarpae major, Scarpa t., subinguinal t.

t. of fillet, SYN *trigone* of lateral lemniscus.

frontal t., a t. bounded above by the maximum frontal diameter and laterally by lines joining the extremities of this diameter with the glabella.

Garland t., a triangular area of relative resonance in the lower back near the spine, found on the same side as a pleural effusion.

Gombault t., SEE semilunar *fasciculus.*

Grocco t., a triangular patch of dullness at the base of the chest alongside the spinal column, on the side opposite a pleural effusion. SYN paravertebral t.

Grynfeltt t., a triangular space bounded above by the end of the last rib and the serratus posterior inferior muscle, anteriorly by the internal oblique, and posteriorly by the quadratus lumborum; lumbar hernia occurs in this space. SYN Lesshaft t.

Hesselbach t., SYN inguinal t.

inferior carotid t., SYN muscular t. (of neck).

inferior lumbar t. [TA], an area of the back (posterior abdominal wall) bounded by the edges of the latissimus dorsi and external oblique muscles and the iliac crest; herniations occasionally occur here. SYN trigonum lumbale inferius [TA], lumbar t., Petit lumbar t.

inferior occipital t., a t. with its apex at the external occipital protuberance; its base is formed by a line joining the two mastoid processes.

infraclavicular t., SYN infraclavicular *fossa.*

inguinal t. [TA], the triangular area in the lower abdominal wall bounded inferiorly by the inguinal ligament (externally) or iliopubic tract (internally), the border of the rectus abdominis medially and the inferior epigastric vessels (lateral umbilical fold) laterally. It is the site of direct inguinal hernia. SYN trigonum inguinale [TA], Hesselbach t., inguinal trigone.

interscalene t., SYN scalene *hiatus.*

Killian t., the triangular-shaped area of the cervical esophagus bordered by the oblique fibers of the inferior constrictor muscle of the pharynx and the transverse fibers of the cricopharyngeus muscle through which Zenker diverticulum occurs.

Koch t., a triangular area of the wall of the right atrium of the heart, that marks the approximate situation of the atrioventricular node.

Labbé t., an area bounded below by a horizontal line touching the lower edge of the cartilage of the left ninth rib, laterally by the line of the false ribs, and to the right side by the liver; here the stomach is normally in contact with the abdominal wall.

Langenbeck t., a t. formed by lines drawn from the anterior superior iliac spine to the surface of the great trochanter and to the surgical neck of the femur; a penetrating wound in this area probably involves the joint.

lateral pelvic wall t. [TA], area of lateral wall of pelvis covered by the portion of the obturator internus muscle and fascia superior to the tendinous arch of levator ani (muscle), anterior to the

tr

sciatic notch, and inferior to the arcuate line of the ilium. SYN trigonum parietale laterale pelvis [TA].

Lesser t., the space between the bellies of the digastric muscle and the hypoglossal nerve.

Lesshaft t., SYN Grynfeltt t.

Lieutaud t., SYN *trigone* of bladder.

lumbar t., SYN inferior lumbar t.

lumbocostal t. of diaphragm [TA], a triangular area in the diaphragm between its lumbar and costal parts and superior to the lateral arcuate ligament that is devoid of muscle fibers; it is covered by pleura superiorly and by peritoneum inferiorly; when it fails to form congenitally (a closure defect of the fetal pleuroperitoneal hiatus), the consequent foramen of Bochdalek is the most common site of diaphragmatic hernia of abdominal viscera. SYN trigonum lumbocostale diaphragmatis [TA], Bochdalek gap, vertebrocostal trigone.

lumbocostoabdominal t., an irregular area bounded by the serratus posterior inferior, obliquus externus, obliquus internus, and erector spinae muscles.

Macewen t., SYN suprameatal t.

Malgaigne t., SYN carotid t.

Marcille t., an area bounded by the medial border of the psoas major, the lateral margin of the vertebral column, and the iliolumbar ligament below; it is crossed by the obturator nerve.

muscular t. (of neck) [TA], the t. bounded by the sternocleidomastoid muscle, the superior belly of the omohyoid muscle, and the anterior midline of the neck; the infrahyoid muscles occupy most of it. SYN trigonum musculare (regionis cervicalis anterioris) [TA], omotracheal t.⋆, trigonum omotracheale⋆, inferior carotid t., tracheal t.

occipital t., a t. of the neck bounded by the trapezius, the sternocleidomastoid, and the omohyoid muscles. SEE ALSO inferior occipital t.

omoclavicular t. [TA], SYN supraclavicular t.

omotracheal t., ⋆official alternate term for muscular t. (of neck).

palatal t., a triangular area bounded by the greatest transverse diameter of the palate and by lines converging from its extremities to the alveolar point. SYN trigonum palati.

paravertebral t., SYN Grocco t.

Petit lumbar t., SYN inferior lumbar t.

Philippe t., SEE semilunar *fasciculus.*

Pirogoff t., a t. formed by the intermediate tendon of the digastric muscle, the posterior border of the mylohyoid muscle, and the hypoglossal nerve.

posterior t. of neck, ⋆official alternate term for lateral cervical region.

pubourethral t., a t. in the perineum bounded by the transversus perinei, the ischiocavernosus, and the bulbocavernosus muscles.

Reil t., SYN *trigone* of lateral lemniscus.

retromolar t. [TA], triangular area posterior to the third mandibular molar tooth. SYN trigonum retromolare [TA].

sacral t., the surface area over the sacrum.

t. of safety, the area at the lower left sternal border where the pericardium is not covered by lung (pericardial notch); preferred site for aspiration of pericardial fluid.

Scarpa t., SYN femoral t.

sternocostal t., SYN *trigonum* sternocostale.

sternocostal t. (of diaphragm) [TA], fibrous (nonmuscular) area of diaphragm between the muscular slips of the sternal part of the diaphragm and the costal part; when it fails to form congenitally, the consequent foramen of Morgagni may allow herniation of abdominal viscera into thorax. SYN trigonum sternocostale diaphragmatis [TA].

subclavian t., ⋆official alternate term for supraclavicular t.

subinguinal t., SYN femoral t.

submandibular t. [TA], the t. of the neck bounded by the mandible and the two bellies of the digastric muscle; it contains the submandibular gland. SYN trigonum submandibulare [TA], digastric t., submaxillary t.

submaxillary t., SYN submandibular t.

submental t. [TA], a t. bounded by the anterior belly of the digastric muscles, the hyoid bone, and the midline; the mylohyoid muscle forms its floor. SYN trigonum submentale [TA].

suboccipital t., a deep t. bounded by the obliquus capitis inferior, the obliquus capitis superior, and the rectus capitis posterior major muscles.

superior carotid t., SYN carotid t.

supraclavicular t. [TA], the t. bounded by the clavicle, the omohyoid muscle, and the sternocleidomastoid muscle; it contains the subclavian artery and vein. SYN omoclavicular t. [TA], trigonum omoclaviculare [TA], subclavian t.⋆.

suprameatal t. [TA], a t. formed by the root of the zygomatic arch, the posterior wall of the bony external acoustic meatus, and an imaginary line connecting the extremities of the first two lines; the suprameatal spine lies in its anterior margins; used as a guide in mastoid operations since it is the lateral wall of the mastoid antrum. SYN foveola suprameatica [TA], foveola suprameatalis, Macewen t., mastoid fossa, fossa mastoidea, supramastoid fossa, suprameatal pit.

tracheal t., SYN muscular t. (of neck).

Tweed t., a t. defined by facial and dental landmarks on a lateral cephalometric film, using the Frankfort horizontal plane as a base and intended for use as a guide in the evaluation and planning of orthodontic treatment.

umbilicomammillary t., a t. with its apex at the umbilicus and its base at the line joining the nipples.

urogenital t. [TA], the anterior portion of the perineal region containing the openings of the urethra and vagina in the female and the urethra and root structures of the penis in the male. SYN regio urogenitalis [TA], urogenital region.

t. of vertebral artery, triangular area in the root of the neck bounded laterally by the scalenus anterior and medially by the longus colli (muscles); the two muscles meet at the t.'s apex, formed by the anterior (carotid) tubercle of the transverse process of vertebra C6; the vertebral artery arises from the subclavian artery at the base of the t., bisecting the t. as it ascends to the apex to enter the transverse foramen of vertebra C6.

vesical t., SYN *trigone* of bladder.

Ward t., an area of diminished density in the trabecular pattern of the neck of the femur evident by x-ray as well as by direct inspection of a specimen.

Weber t., on the sole of the foot, an area indicated by the heads of the first and fifth metatarsal bone and the center of the plantar surface of the heel.

Wilde t., SYN light *reflex* (3).

---

tri·an·gu·la·ris. SEE triangular *muscle.* [L. triangular]

tri·an·gu·lum (trī-ang′goo-lŭm). SEE triangle. [L.]

Tri·at·o·ma (trī-ă-tō′mă). A genus of insects (subfamily Triatominae, family Reduviidae) that includes important vectors of *Trypanosoma cruzi,* such as *T. dimidiata, T. infestans,* and *T. maculata.*

Tri·a·tom·i·nae (trī-ă-tō′mi-nē). A subfamily of insects (family Reduviidae, suborder Heteroptera) that are vertebrate bloodsuckers and include such important disease vector species as *Panstrongylus, Rhodnius,* and *Triatoma;* they are commonly called conenose or kissing bugs.

tri·a·zo·lam (trī-ā′zō-lam). A short-acting benzodiazepine derivative used as a sedative and hypnotic.

tri·az·o·lo·gua·nine (trī′ă-zol-ō-gwah′nēn). SYN 8-azaguanine.

tri·ba·sic (trī-bā′sik). Having three titratable hydrogen atoms; denoting an acid with a basicity of 3.

tri·bas·i·lar (trī-bas′i-lăr). Having three bases.

tribe (trīb). In biologic classification, an occasionally used division between the family and the genus; often the same as the subfamily. [L. *tribus*]

tri·bol·o·gy (tri-bol′ō-jē). The study of friction and its effects in biologic systems, especially in regard to articulated surfaces of the skeleton. [G. *tribō,* to rub, + *logos,* study]

tri·bo·lu·mi·nes·cence (trib′ō-loo-mi-nes′ens). Luminosity produced by friction. [G. *tribō,* to rub, + luminescence]

tri·bra·chia (trī-brā′kē-ă). Condition seen in conjoined twins in which there are only three arms for the two bodies. SEE conjoined *twins*, under *twin*. [tri- + G. *brachiōn*, arm]

tri·bra·chi·us (trī-brā′kē-ŭs). Conjoined twins exhibiting tribrachia.

tri·brom·sa·lan (trī-brom′să-lan). A disinfectant used in soaps.

tri·bu·ty·rase (trī-bū′ti-rās). SYN *triacylglycerol* lipase.

tri·bu·tyr·in (trī-bū′ti-rin). A synthetic substrate for lipase assays. SYN glyceryl tributyrate, tributyrylglycerol.

tri·bu·tyr·in·ase (trī-bū′ti-ri-nās). SYN *triacylglycerol* lipase.

tri·bu·tyr·yl·glyc·er·ol (trī-bū′ti-ril-glis′er-ol). SYN tributyrin.

TRIC Acronym for *t*rachoma and *i*nclusion *c*onjunctivitis. SEE TRIC *agents*, under *agent*.

tri·cal·ci·um phos·phate (trī-kal′sē-ŭm). SYN tribasic *calcium* phosphate.

tri·ceph·a·lus (trī-sef′ă-lŭs). Fetus with three heads. [tri- + G. *kephalē*, head]

tri·ceps (trī′seps). Three-headed; denoting especially two muscles: t. brachii and t. surae. SEE muscle. [L. fr. *tri-*, three, + *caput*, head]

⟳**trich-.** SEE tricho-.

trich·al·gia (trik-al′jē-ă). Pain produced by touching the hair; painful hair, as can occur with atypical angina. SYN trichodynia. [trich- + G. *algos*, pain]

trich·an·gi·on (trik-an′jē-on). SYN telangion. [trich- + G. *angeion*, vessel]

trich·a·tro·phia (trik-ă-trō′fē-ă). Atrophy of the hair bulbs, with brittleness, splitting, and falling out of hair. [trich- + G. *atrophia*, atrophy]

trich·aux·is (trik-awk′sis). Excessive growth of hair in length and quantity. [trich- + G. *auxis*, increase]

⟳**trichi-.** SEE tricho-.

⟳**-trichia.** Condition or type of hair. [G. *thrix* (*trich-*), hair, + *-ia*, condition]

tri·chi·a·sis (trī-kī′ă-sis). A condition in which the hair adjacent to a natural orifice turns inward and causes irritation; e.g., in inversion of an eyelid (entropion), eyelashes irritate the eye. SYN trichoma, trichomatosis. [trich- + G. *-iasis*, condition]

trich·i·lem·mo·ma (trik′i-le-mō′mă). A benign tumor derived from outer root sheath epithelium of a hair follicle, consisting of cells with pale-staining cytoplasm containing glycogen; multiple t.'s are present on the face in Cowden disease. SYN tricholemmoma. [trichi- + G. *lemma*, husk, + *-ōma*, tumor]

Tri·chi·na (tri-kī′nă). Old name for a genus of nematode worms, correctly called *Trichinella*.

tri·chi·na, pl. **tri·chi·nae** (tri-kī′nă, -nē). A larval worm of the genus *Trichinella*; the infective form in pork. [Mod. L., fr. G. *thrix* (*trich-*), a hair]

▣*Trich·i·nel·la* (trik′i-nel′ă). A nematode genus in the aphasmid group that causes trichinosis in humans and carnivores. [Mod. L. fr. *trichina* + dim. suffix *ella*]

T. pseudospiralis., nematode species with normal life cycle in small predators; humans are an accidental host.

▣*T. spira′lis,* the pork or trichina worm, a species of parasites that cause trichinosis, found in most regions of the world but more frequently in the Northern Hemisphere; transmission occurs as a result of ingesting raw or inadequately cooked meat (especially pork) that contains encysted larvae which develop into adults that survive in the jejunum and ileum for approximately 6 weeks; the female worm is viviparous, and bears approximately 1500 embryonic larvae that are laid deep in the mucosa so that they are picked up in the submucosal capillaries and are transported via the liver to the heart, lungs, and systemic circulation; eventually the larvae break out of the body capillaries, penetrate a muscle fiber, coil, and encyst, thereby inducing the strong sensitization, pain, fever, edema, and eosinophilic reaction characteristic of trichinosis.

trich·i·nel·li·a·sis (trik′i-nel-ī′ă-sis). SYN trichinosis.

Trich·i·nel·li·cae (tri-ki-nel′i-kē). SYN Trichinelloidea.

Trich·i·nel·loi·dea (trik′i-nel-oy′dē-ă). A superfamily of nematodes, including the following roundworms that are parasitic in

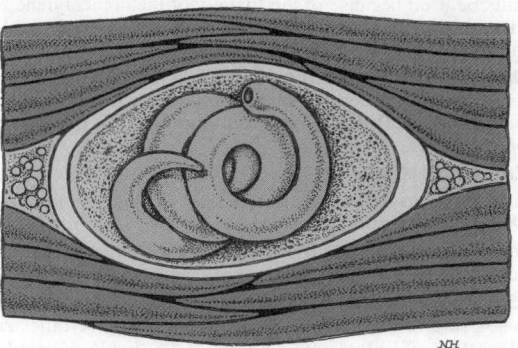

Trichinella spiralis: showing larva encysted in human muscle

man: *Trichinella spiralis*, the trichina worm (family Trichinellidae); *Trichuris trichiura*, the human whipworm; *Capillaria hepatica*, the capillary liver worm; and *C. philippinensis* (family Trichuridae). SYN Trichinellicae.

trich·i·nel·lo·sis (trik′i-nel-ō′sis). SYN trichinosis.

trich·i·ni·a·sis (trik-i-nī′ă-sis). SYN trichinosis.

trich·i·nif·er·ous (trik-i-nif′ĕ-rŭs). Containing trichina worms.

trich·i·ni·za·tion (trik′i-ni-zā′shŭn). Infection with trichina worms.

tri·chi·no·scope (trik′i-nō-skōp). A magnifying glass used in the examination of meat suspected of being trichinous. [trichina + G. *skopeō*, to view]

▣**trich·i·no·sis** (trik-i-nō′sis). The disease resulting from ingestion of raw or inadequately cooked pork (or bear or walrus meat) that contains encysted larvae of the nematode parasite *Trichinella spiralis*. The initial symptoms of human disease are abdominal pain, cramping, and diarrhea, associated with the development of the parasites in the small intestine. Once the resultant larval parasites migrate and invade muscular tissue, a second set of symptoms is manifest, including facial and periorbital edema, myalgia, fever, pruritus, urticaria, conjunctivitis, and signs of myocarditis. SYN trichinelliasis, trichinellosis, trichiniasis. [*Trichinella* (trichina) + G. *-osis*, condition]

tri·chi·nous (trik′i-nŭs). Infected with trichina worms.

trich·i·on (trik′ē-on). A cephalometric point at the midpoint of the hairline at the top of the forehead. [G. *thrix*, hair]

trich·ite (trik′īt). SYN trichocyst.

tri·chlo·ral (trī-klōr′ăl). SYN *m*-chloral.

tri·chlor·fon (trī-klōr′fon). An organophosphorus compound effective against immature and mature stages of *Schistosoma haematobium*, but ineffective against other species of *Schistosoma* in humans. SYN metrifonate.

tri·chlo·ride (trī-klōr′īd). A chloride having three chlorine atoms in the molecule; e.g., PCl_3.

tri·chlor·me·thi·a·zide (trī-klōr-me-thī′ă-zīd). An orally effective benzothiazide diuretic and antihypertensive agent.

tri·chlor·meth·ine (trī-klōr-meth′ēn). A nitrogen mustard used in the treatment of leukemia.

tri·chlo·ro·a·ce·tic ac·id (trī-klōr′ō-ă-sē′tik). Used as an astringent antiseptic in 1–5% solution or as an escharotic for venereal and other warts; a widely used protein precipitant.

tri·chlo·ro·eth·ane (trī-klōr-ō-eth′ān). An industrial solvent with pronounced inhalation anesthetic activity. SYN methylchloroform.

tri·chlo·ro·eth·a·nol (trī-klōr-ō-eth′ă-nol). A hypnotic and sedative; as a metabolite of chloral hydrate, it contributes to the depressant activity of chloral hydrate. SYN trichloroethyl alcohol.

tri·chlo·ro·eth·ene (trī-klōr-ō-eth′ēn). SYN trichloroethylene.

tri·chlo·ro·eth·yl al·co·hol (trī-klōr-ō-eth′il). SYN trichloroethanol.

tri·chlo·ro·eth·yl·ene (trī-klōr-ō-eth′i-lēn). An analgesic and inhalation anesthetic used in minor surgical operations and in obstetric practice; administration requires that only nonrebreathing

tr

circuits be used because of the toxicity of dichloracetylene resulting from interaction of t. with soda lime. SYN ethinyl trichloride, trichloroethene.

tri·chlo·ro·flu·o·ro·meth·ane (trī-klōr′ō-flōr-ō-meth′ān). A propellant used for aerosol sprays; has anesthetic and arrhythmogenic activity if inhaled in high concentration. SYN trichloromonofluoromethane.

tri·chlo·ro·meth·ane (trī-klōr-ō-meth′ān). SYN chloroform.

tri·chlo·ro·mon·o·flu·o·ro·meth·ane (trī-klōr-ō-mon′ō-flōr-ō-meth′ān). SYN trichlorofluoromethane.

tri·chlo·ro·phe·nol (trī-klōr-ō-fē′nol). Used as an antiseptic, disinfectant, and fungicide.

(2,4,5-tri·chlo·ro·phen·oxy)ace·tic ac·id (2,4,5-T) (trī-klōr-ō-fe-nok′sē-a-sē-tik). A herbicide and defoliant synthesized by condensation of chloracetic acid and 2,4,5-trichlorophenol, used as the principal constituent of Agent Orange.

⌂**tricho-, trich-, trichi-.** The hair; a hairlike structure. [G. *thrix* (*trich*-)]

Trich·o·ceph·a·lus (trik-ō-sef′ă-lŭs). Incorrect name for *Trichuris*. [tricho- + G. *kephalē*, head]

trich·o·chrome (trī′kō-krōm). Yellow-orange and violet natural pigments related to melanins; partly responsible for the red and auburn colors of human hair. [tricho- + G. *chrōma*, color]

trich·o·cyst (trik′ō-sist). One of a number of structures, in the form of minute elongated cysts, arranged radially around the periphery of a protozoan cell and containing fluid which when discharged serves for offense or defense; found in ciliates, such as *Paramecium* species. SYN trichite. [tricho- + G. *kystis*, bladder]

Trich·o·dec·tes (trik-ō-dek′tēz). A genus of biting lice that includes the species *T. canis* (*T. latus*), the biting louse of dogs that commonly serves as an intermediate host for the dog tapeworm, *Dipylidium caninum*, as well as the species *T. climax* (*Bovicola caprae*), *T. parumpilosus* (*B. equi*), *T. scalaris* (*B. bovis*), and *T. sphaerocephalus* (*B. ovis*). SEE ALSO *Bovicola, Damalinia*. [tricho- + G. *dektēs*, a beggar]

Trich·o·der·ma (trik-ō-der′mă). A genus of fungi in soil that furnishes the antibiotic gliotoxin. Has produced rare opportunistic infections. [tricho- + G. *derma*, skin]

trich·o·dis·co·ma (trik′ō-dis-kō′mă). Dominantly inherited or nonfamilial elliptical parafollicular mesenchymal hamartomas.

trich·o·dyn·ia (trik-ō-din′ē-ă). SYN trichalgia. [tricho- + G. *odynē*, pain]

trich·o·dys·tro·phy (trik′ō-dis-trō-fē). Defective nutrition or growth of hair, often culminating in alopecia. May be acquired or congenital; the latter often with metabolic or other birth defects. [tricho- + G. prefix *dys-*, abnormal, + *trophē*, growth]

trich·o·ep·i·the·li·o·ma (trik′ō-ep-i-thē-lē-ō′mă) [MIM*132700]. Multiple small benign nodules, occurring mostly on the skin of the face, derived from basal cells of hair follicles enclosing small keratin cysts; autosomal dominant inheritance. SYN Brooke tumor, epithelioma adenoides cysticum, hereditary multiple t. [tricho- + epithelioma]

desmoplastic t., a solitary, hard, annular, centrally depressed papule, occurring usually in women on the face, consisting of dermal strands of basaloid cells and small keratinous cysts within sclerotic desmoplastic stroma.

hereditary multiple t., SYN trichoepithelioma.

trich·o·es·the·sia (trik′ō-es-thē′zē-ă). 1. The sensation felt when a hair is touched. 2. A form of paresthesia in which there is a sensation as of a hair on the skin, on the mucous membrane of the mouth, or on the conjunctiva. [tricho- + G. *aisthēsis*, sensation]

trich·o·fol·lic·u·lo·ma (trik′ō-fol-ik-ū-lō′mă). A usually solitary tumor or hamartoma in which multiple abortive hair follicles open into a central cyst or space opening on the skin surface. [tricho- + L. *folliculus*, fountain, spring, + G. *-oma*, tumor]

trich·o·gen (trik′o-jen). An agent that promotes the growth of hair. [tricho- + G. *-gen*, producing]

trich·o·glos·sia (trik-ō-glos′ē-ă). SYN hairy tongue. [tricho- + G. *glōssa*, tongue]

trich·o·hy·a·lin (trik-ō-hī′ă-lin). A substance of the nature of keratohyalin found in the developing inner root sheath of the hair follicle.

trich·oid (trik′oyd). Hairlike. [tricho- + G. *eidos*, resemblance]

trich·o·lem·mo·ma (trik′ō-le-mō′mă). SYN trichilemmoma.

trich·o·lo·gia (trik-ō-lō′jē-ă). A nervous habit of plucking at the hair. SYN trichology (2). [G. *trichologeō*, to pluck hairs, fr. tricho- + *legō*, to pick out, gather]

tri·chol·o·gy (tri-kol′ō-jē). 1. The study of the anatomy, growth, and diseases of the hair. [tricho- + G. *logos*, study] 2. SYN trichologia. [G. *trichologeo*, fr. tricho- + *legō*, to pick out]

tri·cho·ma (tri-kō′mă). SYN trichiasis. [tricho- + G. *-oma*, tumor]

tri·cho·ma·to·sis (tri-kō′mă-tō′sis). SYN trichiasis.

trich·o·meg·a·ly (trik′ō-meg′ă-lē). Congenital condition characterized by abnormally long eyelashes; associated with dwarfism. [tricho- + G. *megas*, large]

trich·o·mo·na·cide (trik-ō-mō′nă-sīd). An agent that is destructive to *Trichomonas* organisms.

trich·o·mon·ad (trik-ō-mō′nad). Common name for members of the family Trichomonadidae.

Trich·o·mo·nad·i·dae (trik′ō-mō-nad′i-dē). A family of protozoan flagellates that includes the genus *Trichomonas*.

Trich·o·mon·as (trik-ō-mō′nas). A genus of parasitic protozoan flagellates (subfamily Trichomonidinae, family Trichomonadidae) causing trichomoniasis in humans, other primates, and birds. Specificity is more marked for its precise microhabitat than for host species. The genus has been divided into several genera: *Trichomonas, Pentatrichomonas, Tetratrichomonas,* and *Tritrichomonas*. [tricho- + G. *monas*, single (unit)]

T. bucca′lis, SYN *T. tenax*.

T. foe′tus, former name for *Tritrichomonas foetus*.

T. gallina′rum, former name for *Tetratrichomonas gallinarium*.

🔲 ***T. hom′inis,*** former name for *Pentatrichomonas hominis*.

T. o′vis, former name for *Tetratrichomonas ovis*.

T. su′is, former name for *Tritrichomonas suis*.

T. te′nax, a species that lives as a commensal in the mouth of humans and other primates, especially in the tartar around the teeth or in the defects of carious teeth; there is no evidence of direct pathogenesis, but it is frequently associated with pyogenic organisms in pus pockets or at the base of teeth. SYN *T. buccalis*.

T. vagina′lis, a species frequently found in the vagina and urethra of women (in whom it causes trichomoniasis vaginitis) and in the urethra and prostate gland of men (the only known natural hosts); considerable differences in pathogenicity exist among various strains of this species.

trich·o·mo·ni·a·sis (trik′ō-mō-nī′ă-sis). Disease caused by infection with a species of protozoon of the genus *Trichomonas* or related genera.

t. vagini′tis, acute vaginitis or urethritis caused by infection with *Trichomonas vaginalis*, which does not invade the mucosa or the tissue but provokes an inflammatory reaction; infection is venereal or by other forms of contact; widespread infection in human populations is usually asymptomatic but may produce vaginitis, with vaginal and vulvar pruritis, leukorrhea with frothy watery discharge, and (rarely) purulent urethritis in males.

trich·o·my·ce·to·sis (trik′ō-mī-sē-tō′sis). SYN trichomycosis.

trich·o·my·co·sis (trik′ō-mī-kō′sis). Term formerly used to mean any disease of the hair caused by a fungus; now synonymous with trichonocardiosis or t. axillaris. In present usage, t. is a misnomer because the causative agent of the disease is a nocardia (an entity intermediate between fungus and bacterium) or *Corynebacterium* and not a true fungus. SYN trichomycetosis. [tricho- + G. *mykēs*, fungus, + G. *-osis*, condition]

t. axilla′ris, *Corynebacterium* infection of axillary and pubic hairs with development of yellow (flava), black (nigra), or red (rubra) concretions around the hair shafts; frequently asymptomatic. SYN lepothrix, trichonodosis.

trich·o·no·do·sis (trik′ō-nō-dō′sis). SYN *trichomycosis* axillaris. [tricho- + L. *nodus*, node (swelling), + G. *-osis*, condition]

trich·o·no·sis (trik′ō-nō′sis). SYN trichopathy.

trich·o·path·ic (trik-ō-path'ik). Relating to any disease of the hair.

trich·o·path·o·pho·bia (trik'ō-path-ō-fō'bē-ă). Excessive worry regarding disease of the hair, its color, or abnormalities of its growth. [tricho- + G. *pathos,* suffering, + *phobos,* fear]

tri·chop·a·thy (tri-kop'ă-thē). Any disease of the hair. SYN trichonosis, trichosis. [tricho- + G. *pathos,* suffering]

trich·o·pha·gia (tri-kō-fāj'ē-a). The eating of hair or wool.

tri·choph·a·gy (tri-kof'ă-jē). Habitual biting of the hair. [tricho- + G. *phagein,* to eat]

trich·o·pho·bia (trik-ō-fō'bē-ă). Morbid disgust caused by the sight of loose hairs on clothing or elsewhere. [tricho- + G. *phobos,* fear]

trich·o·phyt·ic (trik-ō-fit'ik). Relating to trichophytosis.

trich·o·phy·to·be·zoar (trik'ō-fi'tō-bē'zōr). A mixed hair and food ball, consisting of vegetable fibers, seeds and skins of fruits, and animal hair matted together to form a ball in the stomach of humans or other animals, especially ruminants. SYN phytotrichobezoar. [tricho- + G. *phyton,* plant, + bezoar]

Trich·o·phy·ton (tri-kof'i-tŏn). A genus of pathogenic fungi causing dermatophytosis in humans and animals; species may be anthropophilic, zoophilic, or geophilic, and attack the hair, skin, and nails, and are characterized by their growth in hair. Endothrix species grow from the skin into the hair follicle, penetrate the shaft, and grow into it, producing rows of arthroconidia as the hyphae septate; there is no growth on the external surface of the shaft. Ectothrix species are of two kinds, large spored and small spored. In both, the fungus grows into the hair follicle, surrounds the hair shaft, and penetrates it, but continues to grow both within and outside the hair shaft, producing arthroconidia externally. [tricho- + G. *phyton,* plant]

T. concen'tricum, an anthropophilic fungal species that is the causative agent of tinea imbricata; it closely resembles the branching mycelium of *T. schoenleinii.*

T. equi'num, a zoophilic fungal species causing ectothrix infections of hair in horses, from which humans may also be infected; it requires nicotinic acid for growth.

T. megnin'ii, an anthropophilic ectothrix species of dermatophyte fungi with spores in chains, causing infection in humans; it requires histidine, which differentiates it from *Microsporum gallinae.*

T. mentagrophy'tes, a zoophilic small-spored ectothrix species of fungi that causes infection of the hair, skin, and nails; it is a cause of ringworm in dogs, horses, rabbits, mice, rats, chinchillas, foxes, and humans (especially tinea pedis with severe inflammation, and tinea cruris).

T. ru'brum, a widely distributed anthropophilic fungal species that causes persistent infections of the skin, especially tinea pedis and tinea cruris, and in the nails that are unusually resistant to therapy; it rarely invades the hair, where it is ectothrix in nature; occasional subcutaneous and systemic infections have been reported.

T. schoenlei'nii, an anthropophilic endothrix species of dermatophyte fungi causing favus in humans; it is endemic throughout Eurasia and Africa and, because of travel, is seen more frequently in the Western Hemisphere; it produces tunnels within the hair shaft that are filled with air bubbles after the hyphae disintegrate.

T. sim'ii, a zoophilic species of fungi that causes infection in rhesus monkeys, dogs, and humans; most infections have had their origin in India.

T. ton'surans, an anthropophilic endothrix species of fungi that causes epidemic dermatophytosis in Europe, South America, and the U.S.; it infects some animals and requires thiamin for growth. It is the most common cause of tinea capitis in the U.S., forming black dots where hair breaks off at the skin surface.

T. verrucos'um, a zoophilic species of fungi that causes ringworm in cattle, from which humans can become infected.

T. viola'ceum, an anthropophilic species of fungi that causes black-dot ringworm or favus infection of the scalp; hair infection is of the endothrix type; usually found in South America, Europe, Asia, and Africa.

trich·o·phyt·o·sis (trik'ō-fī-tō'sis). Superficial fungus infection caused by species of *Trichophyton.* [tricho- + G. *phyton,* plant, + -*osis,* condition]

Trich·o·pleu·ris (trik'ō-ploo'ris). A genus of biting lice that infest ruminants, e.g., *T. lipeuroides* and *T. parallelus* in American deer; considered by some to be a subgenus of *Damalinia.* [tricho- + G. *pleura,* rib, side]

tri·chop·o·li·o·dys·tro·phy. SYN kinky-hair *disease.*

trich·o·po·li·o·sis (trik'ō-pō-lē-ō'sis). SYN poliosis. [tricho- + G. *polios,* gray, + -*osis,* condition]

Tri·chop·tera (tri-kop'ter-ă). An order of insects in which the aquatic larvae (caddis flies) construct a protective case (caddis) of bits of submerged material in a highly specific form; commonly found attached under stones in freshwater streams. The adult caddis flies, having hairy wings, shed their hairs and epithelia, causing hay fever-like (allergic) symptoms in sensitive people. [tricho- + G. *pteron,* wing]

trich·o·pti·lo·sis (trik'ō-ti-lō'sis, tri-kop-ti-lō'sis). A condition of splitting of the shaft of the hair, giving it a feathery appearance. [tricho- + G. *ptilōsis,* plumage, + -*osis,* condition]

trich·or·rhex·is (trik-ō-rek'sis). A condition in which the hairs tend to readily break or split. [tricho- + G. *rhēxis,* a breaking]

t. invagina'ta, SYN bamboo *hair.*

t. nodo'sa, a congenital or acquired condition in which minute nodes are formed in the hair shafts; splitting and breaking, complete or incomplete, may occur at these points or nodes.

tri·chos·chi·sis (tri-kos'ki-sis). The presence of broken or split hairs. SEE ALSO trichorrhexis. [tricho- + G. *schisis,* a cleaving]

tri·cho·sis (tri-kō'sis). SYN trichopathy. [tricho- + G. -*osis,* condition]

t. carun'culae, a growth of hair on the lacrimal caruncle.

t. sensiti'va, hyperesthesia of the hairy parts.

t. seto'sa, coarseness of the hair.

trich·o·so·ma·tous (trik-ō-sō'mă-tŭs). Having flagella with a small body; denoting certain protozoan organisms. SEE *Trichomonas.* [tricho- + G. *sōma,* body]

Tri·cho·spo·ron (tri-kos'pō-ron, trik-ō-spōr'on). A genus of imperfect fungi that possess branching septate hyphae with arthroconidia and blastoconidia; these organisms are part of the normal flora of the intestinal tract of humans. *T. beigelii* is the causative agent of white piedra or trichosporonosis and fatal fungemia in immunocompromised patients. [tricho- + G. *sporos,* seed (spore)]

trich·o·spor·o·no·sis (trik'ō-spor-o-nō-sis). Systemic infection by *Trichosporan beigelii;* marked by fever or pneumonia with a high mortality; seen in neutropenic patients. Local infection with *T. beigelii* is white piedra, also known as trichosporosis.

trich·o·spo·ro·sis (trik'ō-spō-rō'sis). Infection with *Trichosporon beigelii.* [*Trichosporon* + G. -*osis,* condition]

trich·o·sta·sis spi·nu·lo·sa (tri-kos'tă-sis spī'noo-lō'să). A condition in which hair follicles are blocked with a keratin plug containing multiple vellus hairs forming pruritic papules. [tricho- + G. *stasis,* a standing; L. *spinulosus,* thorny]

trich·o·stron·gyle (trik-ō-stron'jil). Common name for members of the family Trichostrongylidae.

Trich·o·stron·gyl·i·dae (trik'ō-stron-jil'i-dē). A family of nematodes (order Strongylida or, in older terminology, Strongylata); includes the important genera *Cooperia, Ostertagia, Haemonchus, Trichostrongylus, Nematodirus,* and *Hippostrongylus.* SEE *Trichostrongylus.*

trich·o·stron·gy·lo·sis (trik'ō-stron-ji-lō'sis). Infection with nematodes of the genus *Trichostrongylus.*

Trich·o·stron·gy·lus (trik-ō-stron'ji-lŭs). The hairworm, or bankrupt or black scour worm; an economically important genus (about 30 species) of small slender nematodes (family Trichostrongylidae) that inhabit the small intestine, in some cases the stomach, of a variety of herbivorous animals and gallinaceous birds. They burrow into the mucosa and suck blood; in large numbers they do serious damage, especially to young hosts. [tricho- + G. *strongylos,* round]

T. ax'ei, the most common species in cattle, occurring also in the

tr

abomasum of sheep, horses, antelope, bison, llama, and deer, and in the stomach of pigs and horses.

T. capric'ola, a species that occurs in the small intestine and abomasum of sheep, goats, deer, and pronghorn.

T. colubrifor'mis, a species that occurs in anterior portions of the small intestine and sometimes in the abomasum of sheep, goats, cattle, camels, and some wild ruminants, and in the stomach of primates (including humans), rabbits, and squirrels; it is distributed worldwide and is common in the U.S., especially in sheep.

T. longispicula'ris, a species found in the small intestine of cattle, sheep, and goats; it is distributed worldwide but uncommon in the U.S.

T. ten'uis, a species that is a widespread pathogenic parasite of the ceca and small intestines of fowl, including ducks, geese, turkeys, pheasants, and partridges.

T. vitri'nus, a species that is an important pathogen of lambs, found chiefly in the duodenum of sheep, camels, rabbits, and goats but also reported from humans and pigs.

Trich·o·the·ci·um (tri-kō-thē'sē-ŭm). A genus of imperfect fungi generally considered a common saprophyte.

trich·o·thi·o·dys·tro·phy (trik'ō-thī'ō-dis'trō-fē) [MIM*234050]. Congenital brittle hair resulting from low sulfur-containing amino acid (cysteine) content sometimes associated with mental impairment and short stature; autosomal recessive inheritance. [tricho- + thio- + G. *dys,* bad, + *trophē,* nourishment]

trich·o·til·lo·ma·nia (trik'ō-til-ō-mā'nē-ă). A compulsion to pull out one's own hair. [tricho- + G. *tillo,* pull out, + *mania,* insanity]

tri·chot·o·my (tri-kot'ō-mē). A division into three parts. [G. *trichia,* threefold, + *tomē,* a cutting]

trich·o·tox·in (trik'ō-tok'sin). A cytotoxin having an injurious effect specifically for ciliated epithelium.

tri·chot·ro·phy (tri-kot'rō-fē). Nutrition of the hair. [tricho- + G. *trophē,* nourishment]

tri·chro·ic (trī-krō'ik). Relating to or marked by trichroism.

tri·chro·ism (trī'krō-izm). The property of some crystals of emitting different colors in three different directions. [G. *trichroos,* three-colored, fr. tri- + *chroa,* color]

tri·chro·mat (trī-krō'mat). A person who sees three primary colors; hence, one with normal color vision. [tri- + G. *chrōma,* color]

tri·chro·mat·ic (trī-krō-mat'ik). 1. Having, or relating to, the three primary colors: red, green, and blue. 2. Capable of perceiving the three primary colors; having normal color vision. SYN trichromic.

tri·chro·ma·tism (trī-krō'mă-tizm). The state of being trichromatic. [tri- + G. *chrōma,* color]

anomalous t., a defect in color perception in which there appears to be an abnormality or deficiency in one of the three primary pigments of the retinal cones. SEE protanomaly, deuteranomaly, tritanomaly.

tri·chro·ma·top·sia (trī-krō'mă-top'sē-ă). Normal color vision; the ability to perceive the three primary colors. [tri- + G. *chrōma,* color, + *opsis,* vision]

tri·chro·mic (trī-krō'mik). SYN trichromatic.

trich·ter·brust (tricht'er-broost). SYN *pectus* excavatum. [Ger. *Trichterbrust,* funnel chest]

trich·u·ri·a·sis (tri-koo-rī'ă-sis). Infection with nematodes of the genus *Trichuris.* In humans, intestinal parasitization by *T. trichiura* is usually asymptomatic and not associated with peripheral eosinophilia; in massive infections it frequently induces diarrhea or rectal prolapse.

Trich·u·ris (tri-koo'ris). A genus of aphasmid nematodes (sometimes improperly termed *Trichocephalus*) related to the trichina worm, *Trichinella spiralis,* and having a body with a slender, elongated, anterior portion threaded into the mucosa of the colon or large intestine of the host and a thick posterior portion bearing reproductive organs and their products. *T.* contains about 70 species, all in mammals. [tricho- + G. *oura,* tail]

T. suis, a nematode species found in the pig; adult worms have been found in humans.

T. trichiu'ra, the whipworm of humans, a species that causes

trichuriasis; the body is filiform and slender in the anterior three-fifths, and more robust posteriorly; females are 4 or 5 cm long, males are shorter (with coiled caudal extremity and a single eversible spicule); eggs are barrel-shaped, 50–56 μm by 20–22 μm, with double shell and translucent knobs at each of the two poles; humans are the only susceptible hosts and usually acquire infection by direct finger-to-mouth contact or by ingestion of soil, water, or food that contains larvated eggs (development in the soil takes 3–6 weeks under proper conditions of warmth and moisture, hence distribution is chiefly tropical); larvae escape from eggs in the ileum, mature in approximately a month, and then pass directly into the cecum without undergoing a parenteral migration as occurs with *Ascaris lumbricoides;* adults may persist for 2–7 years.

T. vulpis, a nematode species found in the dog; the sexually mature adult has been found in the human appendix.

tri·cip·i·tal (trī-sip'i-tăl). Having three heads; denoting a triceps muscle.

tri·clo·bi·so·ni·um chlo·ride (trī'klō-bi-sō'nē-ŭm). A bisquaternary ammonium compound used topically in the treatment of superficial infections of the skin and vagina; a cationic antiseptic effective against both Gram-negative and Gram-positive organisms. It is inactivated by soap and pH changes.

tri·clo·fen·ol pi·per·a·zine (trī-klō'fen-ol). An anthelmintic.

tri·clo·fos (trī'klō-fōs). A phosphorylated derivative of chloral hydrate, which is hydrolyzed to chloral hydrate in the body and produces characteristic sedative-hypnotic properties.

tri·corn (trī'kōrn). 1. One of the lateral ventricles of the brain. 2. SYN tricornute. [tri- + L. *cornu,* horn]

tri·cor·nute (trī-kōr'noot). Having three cornua or horns. SYN tricorn (2). [tri- + L. *cornutus,* horned, fr. *cornu,* a horn]

tri·cre·sol (trī-krē'sol). SYN cresol.

tri·crot·ic (trī-krot'ik). Thrice-beating; marked by three waves in the arterial pulse tracing. SYN tricrotous. [tri- + G. *krotos,* a beat]

tri·cro·tism (trī'krō-tizm). The condition of being tricrotic.

tri·cro·tous (trī'krō-tŭs). SYN tricrotic.

Tric·u·la (trik'ū-lă). A genus of operculate freshwater snails related to *Oncomelania* (the *Schistosoma japonicum* intermediate hosts) of the subfamily triculinae, family Hydrobiidae, subclass Prosobranchiata; it includes *T. aperta,* intermediate host of *Schistosoma mekongi.*

tri·cus·pid, tri·cus·pi·dal, tri·cus·pi·date (trī-kŭs'pid, -kŭs'pi-dăl, -kŭs'pi-dāt). 1. Having three points, prongs, or cusps, as the tricuspid valve of the heart. 2. Having three tubercles or cusps, as the second upper molar tooth (occasionally) and the upper third molar (usually). SYN tritubercular.

tri·cy·cla·mol chlo·ride (trī-sī'klă-mol). SYN procyclidine methochloride.

tri·dac·ty·lous (trī-dak'ti-lŭs). SYN tridigitate.

tri·dent (trī'dent). SYN tridentate.

tri·den·tate (trī-den'tāt). Three-toothed; three-pronged. SYN trident. [tri- + L. *dentatus,* toothed]

tri·der·mic (trī-der'mik). Relating to or derived from the three primary germ layers of the embryo: ectoderm, endoderm, and mesoderm. [tri- + G. *derma,* skin]

tri·der·mo·ma (trī-der-mō'mă). SYN triphyllomatous *teratoma.* [tri- + G. *derma,* skin, + *-oma,* tumor]

tri·dig·i·tate (trī-dij'i-tāt). Having three fingers or three toes on one hand or foot. SYN tridactylous. [tri- + L. *digitus,* digit]

tri·di·hex·eth·yl chlo·ride (trī'dī-heks-eth'il). An anticholinergic drug.

trid·y·mite (trid'i-mīt). A form of silica used in dental casting investment. [fr. G. *tridymos,* threefold]

trid·y·mus (trid'i-mŭs). SYN triplet (1). [L. fr. G. *tridymos,* threefold]

tri·el·con (trī-el'kon). A long, three-jawed forceps for the extraction of foreign bodies from wounds or canals. [tri- + G. *helkō,* to draw]

tri·en·tine hy·dro·chlo·ride (trī'en-tēn). A chelating agent used to remove excess copper from the body in Wilson disease. SYN triethylenetetramine dihydrochloride.

tri·eth·a·nol·a·mine (trī′eth-ă-nol′ă-mēn). A mixture of mono-, di-, and triethanolamine, used as an emulsifying agent in the preparation of medicated ointments and lotions and as an aid in the absorption of such medicaments through the skin.

tri·eth·yl·ene gly·col (trī-eth′i-lēn). Used in the vapor state as an air-sterilizing agent; toxic to bacteria, fungi, and viruses in very low concentrations in air; variations in the humidity of the air limit the germicidal effectiveness.

tri·eth·yl·ene·mel·a·mine (TEM) (trī-eth′i-lēn-mel′ă-mēn). An antineoplastic agent chemically related to the nitrogen mustards; used in the treatment of leukemia.

tri·eth·yl·ene·phos·phor·a·mide (TEPA) (trī-eth′i-lēn-fos-fōr′ă-mīd). A drug with the same actions and uses as triethylenemelamine in the treatment of leukemias.

tri·eth·yl·ene·tet·ra·mine di·hy·dro·chlo·ride (trī-eth′i-lēn-tet′ră-am′ēn). SYN trientine hydrochloride.

tri·eth·yl·ene·thi·o·phos·phor·a·mide (trī-eth′i-lēn-thī′ō-fos-fōr′ă-mīd). An alkylating agent used for the palliative treatment of malignant diseases such as leukemia, lymphoma, and carcinoma. SYN thiotepa.

tri·fa·cial (trī-fā′shăl). Denoting the fifth pair of cranial nerves, the trigeminal nerves. [tri- + L. *facies,* face]

tri·fid (trī′fid). Split into three. [L. *trifidus,* three-cleft]

tri·flu·o·per·a·zine hy·dro·chlo·ride (trī′floo-ō-per′ă-zēn). An antipsychotic of the phenothiazine type.

tri·flu·o·ro·ace·tyl (trī-flur′ō-as′ē-til). A group used to protect amino moieties of amino acid and peptides during peptide synthesis.

2,2,2-tri·flu·o·ro·ethyl vi·nyl (trī-flōr-ō-eth′il). SYN fluroxene.

5-tri·flu·o·ro·meth·yl·de·ox·y·u·ri·dine (trī-flōr′ō-meth′il-dē-ok-si-ū′ri-dēn). A pyrimidine analog used topically in the treatment of herpes simplex keratitis.

tri·flu·per·i·dol hy·dro·chlo·ride (trī-floo-per′i-dol). A tranquilizer.

tri·flu·pro·ma·zine hy·dro·chlo·ride (trī-floo-prō′mă-zēn). An antipsychotic closely related chemically and pharmacologically to chlorpromazine.

tri·flur·i·dine (trī-floor′i-dēn). An antiviral agent used in eye drops to treat herpes simplex infections of the eye.

tri·fo·cal (trī′fō-kăl). Having three foci. SEE trifocal *lens.*

tri·fur·ca·tion (trī-fŭr-kā′shŭn). **1.** A division into three branches. **2.** The area where the tooth roots divide into three distinct portions. [tri- + L. *furca,* fork]

tri·gas·tric (trī-gas′trik). Having three bellies; denoting a muscle with two tendinous interruptions. [tri- + G. *gastēr,* belly]

tri·gem·i·nal (trī-jem′i-năl). Relating to the fifth cranial or trigeminus nerve. SYN trigeminus. [L. *trigeminus,* threefold]

tri·gem·i·nus (trī-jem′i-nŭs). SYN trigeminal. [L. threefold, fr. tri- + *geminus,* twin]

tri·gem·i·ny (trī-jem′i-nē). SYN trigeminal *rhythm.* [L. *trigeminus,* threefold]

trig·e·nol·line (trig-ĕ-nol′ēn). SYN trigonelline.

trig·ger (trig′er). Term describing a system in which a relatively small input turns on a relatively large output, the magnitude of which is unrelated to the magnitude of the input.
    ECG t., use of the electrocardiogram, usually the R wave, to control electronically some recording or imaging apparatus. SEE cardiac *gating.* SYN EKG t.
    EKG t., SYN ECG t.

tri·glyc·er·ide (trī-glis′er-īd). SYN triacylglycerol.

tri·go·na (trī-gō′nă). Plural of trigonum. [L.]

trig·o·nal (trig′ō-năl). Triangular; relating to a trigonum.

tri·gone (trī′gōn) [TA]. **1.** SYN trigonum. **2.** The first three dominant cusps (protocone, paracone, and metacone), taken collectively, of an upper molar tooth. [L. *trigonum,* fr. G. *trigōnon,* triangle]
    t. of auditory nerve, the slight prominence of the floor of the lateral recess of the fourth ventricle, corresponding to the underly-

ing cochlear and vestibular nuclei. SYN acoustic tubercle, trigonum nervi acustici.
    t. of bladder [TA], a triangular smooth area at the base of the bladder between the openings of the two ureters and that of the urethra. SYN trigonum vesicae [TA], Lieutaud body, Lieutaud triangle, Lieutaud t., vesical triangle.
    cerebral t., SYN fornix.
    collateral t. [TA], a triangular prominence of the floor of the lateral ventricle at the transition between occipital and temporal horn, continuous rostrally with the collateral eminence and, like the latter, caused by the deep penetration of the collateral sulcus from the ventral surface of the temporal lobe. SYN trigonum collaterale [TA], t. of lateral ventricle, trigonum ventriculi, ventricular t.
    deltoideopectoral t., SYN infraclavicular *fossa.*
    fibrous t.'s of heart, SEE right fibrous t. (of heart), left fibrous t. (of heart).
    t. of fillet, SYN t. of lateral lemniscus.
    t. of habenula, SYN habenular t.
    habenular t. [TA], a small triangular area on the dorsomedial surface of the thalamus at the caudal end of the medullary stria, corresponding to the underlying habenula. SYN trigonum habenulae [TA], t. of habenula.
    hypoglossal t. [TA], a slight elevation in the floor of the inferior recess of the fourth ventricle, beneath which is the nucleus of origin of the twelfth cranial nerve. SYN trigonum nervi hypoglossi [TA], t. of hypoglossal nerve⋆, eminentia hypoglossi, hypoglossal eminence, trigonum hypoglossi, tuberculum hypoglossi.
    t. of hypoglossal nerve, ⋆official alternate term for hypoglossal t.
    inguinal t., SYN inguinal *triangle.*
    t. of lateral lemniscus [TA], a triangular area on the lateral surface of the caudal half of the mesencephalon, bordered caudally by the slight prominence of the lateral lemniscus, dorsally by the base of the inferior colliculus and the brachium of the superior colliculus, and ventrally by the crus cerebri. SYN lemniscal t., Reil triangle, triangle of fillet, t. of fillet.
    t. of lateral ventricle, SYN collateral t.
    left fibrous t. (of heart), the part of the fibrous skeleton of the heart located in the interval between the left side of the left atrioventricular ring and the aortic ring. SYN trigonum fibrosum sinistrum.
    lemniscal t., SYN t. of lateral lemniscus.
    Lieutaud t., SYN t. of bladder.
    Müller t., the floor of the supraoptic recess of the third ventricle.
    olfactory t. [TA], a grayish triangular area corresponding to the attachment of the olfactory peduncle ("olfactory nerve" or olfactory tract) to the base of the brain, at the anterior border of the anterior perforated substance. SYN trigonum olfactorium [TA].
    right fibrous t. (of heart) [TA], part of the fibrous skeleton of the heart located between the aortic fibrous ring and rings surrounding the right and left atrioventricular ostia. SYN trigonum fibrosum dextrum.
    vagal (nerve) t. [TA], a prominence in the floor of the inferior fovea of the fourth ventricle that overlies the dorsal motor nucleus of the vagus. SYN trigonum nervi vagi [TA], t. of vagus nerve⋆, trigonum vagale⋆, ala cinerea, ashen wing, gray wing, vagi eminentia.
    t. of vagus nerve, ⋆official alternate term for vagal (nerve) t.
    ventricular t., SYN collateral t.
    vertebrocostal t., SYN lumbocostal *triangle* of diaphragm.

trig·o·nel·line (trig-ō-nel′ēn). The methyl betaine of nicotinic acid; a product of the metabolism of nicotinic acid; excreted in the urine. SYN caffearine, trigenolline.

tri·go·nid (trī-gon′id, -gō′nid). The first three dominant cusps, taken collectively, of a lower molar tooth. SEE ALSO trigone.

tri·go·ni·tis (trī′gō-nī′tis). Inflammation of the urinary bladder, localized in the trigone. [trigone + G. *-itis,* inflammation]

trig·o·no·ce·phal·ic (trig′ō-nō-se-fal′ik). Pertaining to trigonocephaly.

trig·o·no·ceph·a·ly (trig′ō-nō-sef′ă-lē, trī′gō-nō-). Malformation

tr

characterized by a triangular configuration of the skull, due in part to premature synostosis of the cranial bones with compression of the cerebral hemispheres. [trigone + G. *kephalē*, head]

tri·go·num, pl. **tri·go·na** (trī-gō′nŭm, -nă) [TA]. Any triangular area. SEE triangle. SYN trigone (1) [TA]. [L., fr. G. *trigōnon*, a triangle]

t. auscultationis [TA], SYN ausculatory *triangle*.

t. carot′icum [TA], SYN carotid *triangle*.

t. cerebra′le, SYN fornix (2).

t. cervica′le, any one of the triangles of the neck. SYN t. colli.

t. cervica′le ante′rius, ✠official alternate term for anterior cervical *region*.

t. cervica′le poste′rius, ✠official alternate term for lateral cervical *region*.

t. clavipectorale [TA], SYN clavipectoral *triangle*.

t. collatera′le [TA], SYN collateral *trigone*.

t. col′li, SYN t. cervicale.

t. colli anterius, ✠official alternate term for anterior cervical region.

t. colli laterale, ✠official alternate term for lateral cervical region.

t. cystohepaticum [TA], SYN cystohepatic *triangle*.

t. deltoideopectora′le, SYN clavipectoral *triangle*.

t. deltopectorale, ✠official alternate term for clavipectoral *triangle*.

t. femora′le [TA], SYN femoral *triangle*.

t. femoris, ✠official alternate term for femoral *triangle*.

trigo′na fibro′sa cor′dis, SEE right fibrous *trigone* (of heart), left fibrous *trigone* (of heart).

t. fibro′sum dex′trum, SYN right fibrous *trigone* (of heart).

t. fibro′sum sinis′trum, SYN left fibrous *trigone* (of heart).

t. haben′ulae [TA], SYN habenular *trigone*.

t. hypoglos′si, SYN hypoglossal *trigone*.

t. inguina′le [TA], SYN inguinal *triangle*.

t. lemnis′ci lateralis [TA], SYN trigone of lateral lemniscus.

t. lumba′le inferius [TA], SYN inferior lumbar *triangle*.

t. lumbocosta′le diaphragmatis [TA], SYN lumbocostal *triangle* of diaphragm.

t. muscula′re (regionis cervicalis anterioris) [TA], SYN muscular *triangle* (of neck).

t. nervi acus′tici, SYN *trigone* of auditory nerve.

t. ner′vi hypoglos′si [TA], SYN hypoglossal *trigone*.

t. ner′vi va′gi [TA], SYN vagal (nerve) *trigone*.

t. olfacto′rium [TA], SYN olfactory *trigone*.

t. omoclavicula′re [TA], SYN supraclavicular *triangle*.

t. omotrachea′le, ✠official alternate term for muscular *triangle* (of neck).

t. pala′ti, SYN palatal *triangle*.

t. parietale laterale pelvis [TA], SYN lateral pelvic wall *triangle*.

t. retromolare [TA], SYN retromolar *triangle*.

t. sternocosta′le, a muscular defect in the diaphragm between the costal and the sternal portions. SYN Larrey cleft, sternocostal triangle.

t. sternocostale diaphragmatis [TA], SYN sternocostal *triangle* (of diaphragm).

t. submandibula′re [TA], SYN submandibular *triangle*.

t. submenta′le [TA], SYN submental *triangle*.

t. vagale, ✠official alternate term for vagal (nerve) *trigone*.

t. ventric′uli, SYN collateral *trigone*.

t. vesi′cae [TA], SYN *trigone* of bladder.

tri·hex·o·syl·cer·a·mide. SYN globotriaosylceramide.

tri·hex·y·phen·i·dyl hy·dro·chlo·ride (trī-heks′ē-fen′ĭ-dil). A synthetic anticholinergic agent reputed to exert a higher degree of anticholinergic activity in the brain as compared with peripheral parasympathetic neuroeffector junctions. Widely used in the treatment of parkinsonism secondary to idiopathic or neuroleptic-induced parkinsonism.

tri·hy·brid (trī-hī′brid). The offspring of parents that differ in three mendelian characters. [tri- + L. *hybrida*, hybrid]

tri·hy·dric (trī-hī′drik). Denoting a chemical compound containing three replaceable hydrogen atoms.

tri·hy·drox·y·es·trin (trī′hī-drok′sē-es′trin). SYN estriol.

tri·in·i·od·y·mus (trī-in′i-od′i-mŭs). A grossly malformed fetus with three heads, joined at the occiput, and a single body. [tri- + G. *inion*, nape of the neck, + *didymos*, twin]

tri·i·o·dide (trī-ī′ō-did, -dīd). An iodide with three atoms of iodine in the molecule; e.g., KI_3.

tri·i·o·do·meth·ane (trī-ī′ō-dō-meth′ān). SYN iodoform.

3,5,3′-tri·i·o·do·thy·ro·nine (TITh, T$_3$) (trī-ī′ō-dō-thī′rō-nēn). A thyroid hormone normally synthesized in smaller quantities than thyroxine; present in blood and thyroid gland and exerts the same biologic effects as thyroxine but, on a molecular basis, is more potent and the onset of its effect is more rapid.

tri·ke·to·hy·drin·dene hy·drate (trī-kē-tō-hī′drin-dēn). Former name for ninhydrin.

tri·ke·to·pu·rine (trī-kē-tō-pūr′ēn). SYN uric acid.

tri·labe (trī′lāb). A three-pronged forceps for removal of foreign bodies from the bladder. [tri- + G. *labē*, a handle, hold]

tri·lam·i·nar (trī-lam′i-nar). Having three laminae.

tri·lat·er·al (tri-lat′ĕ-răl). Having three sides.

tri·lo·bate, tri·lobed (trī-lō′bāt, trī′lobd). Having three lobes.

tri·loc·u·lar (trī-lok′ū-lăr). Having three cavities or cells.

tril·o·gy (tril′ō-jē). A triad of related entities. [G. *trilogia*, fr. tri- + *logos*, study, discourse]

t. of Fallot, a set of congenital defects including pulmonic stenosis, atrial septal defect, and right ventricular hypertrophy. SYN Fallot triad.

tri·lo·stane (trī′lō-stān). An adrenal steroid inhibitor used for amelioration of adrenal hyperfunction in Cushing syndrome.

tri·mas·ti·gote (trī-mas′ti-gōt). Having three flagella, as observed in certain protozoan organisms. [tri- + G. *mastix*, whip]

tri·mep·ra·zine tar·trate (trī-mep′ră-zēn). A phenothiazine compound related chemically and pharmacologically to promazine but with a more pronounced histamine-antagonizing action; used for the symptomatic relief of pruritus.

trim·er (trī′mer). A compound, complex, or structure made up of three components.

tri·mes·ter (trī′mes-ter, trī-mes′ter). A period of 3 months; one-third of the length of a pregnancy. [L. *trimestris*, of three-month duration]

tri·met·a·phan cam·sy·late (trī-met′ă-fan). SYN trimethaphan camsylate.

tri·me·taz·i·dine (trī-me-taz′i-dēn). A coronary vasodilator.

tri·meth·a·di·one (trī′meth-ă-dī′ōn). An obsolescent anticonvulsant used for the treatment of absence seizures (petit mal) and psychomotor epilepsy. SYN troxidone.

tri·meth·a·phan cam·sy·late (trī-meth′ă-fan). A ganglionic blocking agent that produces vasodilation of brief duration; used in surgery, particularly neurosurgery, to produce a relatively bloodless operative field (controlled hypotension). SYN trimetaphan camsylate.

tri·meth·i·di·um meth·o·sul·fate (trī-me-thid′ē-ŭm meth-ō-sŭl′fāt). Quaternary ammonium compound that blocks ganglionic transmission at sympathetic and parasympathetic ganglia; used in the treatment of severe hypertension.

tri·meth·o·benz·a·mide hy·dro·chlo·ride (trī′meth-ō-ben′ză-mīd). An antiemetic.

tri·meth·o·prim (trī-meth′ō-prim). An antimicrobial agent that potentiates the effect of sulfonamides and sulfones; usually used in combination with sulfamethoxazole.

tri·meth·o·prim-sul·fa·meth·ox·a·zole. A drug combination consisting of a dihydrofolate reductase inhibitor (trimethoprim) and a sulfonamide antibacterial drug (sulfamethoxazole). The drug combination is synergistic as the drugs interfere with two successive steps in the formation/utilization of folic acid by microorganisms. Used to treat many infectious diseases.

tri·meth·yl·a·mine (trī-meth′il-am′ēn). A degradation product, often by putrefaction, of nitrogenous plant and animal substances such as beet sugar residue or herring brine; in the body, it probably results from decomposition of choline.

tri·meth·yl·am·i·nur·ia (trī-meth'il-am-i-noor'ē-ă). Increased excretion of trimethylamine in urine and sweat, with characteristic offensive fishy body odor.

tri·meth·yl·car·bin·ol (trī-meth'il-kar'bin-ol). Tertiary butyl alcohol. SEE *butyl* alcohol.

tri·meth·yl·ene (trī-meth'il-ēn). SYN cyclopropane.

tri·meth·yl·eth·yl·ene (trī-meth-il-eth'il-ēn). SYN amylene.

N^e-tri·meth·yl·ly·sine (trī-meth-il-lī-sēn). An amino acid residue found in a number of proteins by the action of *S*-adenosyl-L-methionine on L-lysyl residues; upon release by proteolysis, *N^e*-trimethyllysine becomes the precursor of carnitine.

tri·meth·y·lo·mel·a·mine (trī'meth-i-lō-mel'ă-mēn). An antineoplastic agent.

tri·met·o·zine (trī-met'ō-zēn). An antianxiety agent.

tri·me·trex·ate (trī-me-treks'āt). An antineoplastic agent and antiprotozoal orphan drug used in the treatment of *Pneumocystis carinii* pneumonia in AIDS patients.

tri·mip·ra·mine (trī-mip'ră-mēn). An antidepressant.

tri·mor·phic (trī-mōr'fik). SYN trimorphous.

tri·mor·phism (trī-mōr'fizm). Existence under three forms, as in holometabolous insects that pass through larval, pupal, and imago stages. [tri- + G. *morphē*, form]

tri·mor·phous (trī-mōr'fŭs). Existing under three forms; marked by trimorphism. SYN trimorphic.

tri·ni·tro·cel·lu·lose (trī'nī-trō-sel'ū-lōs). A constituent of soluble guncotton; used in the preparation of collodion and of pyroxylin.

tri·ni·tro·glyc·er·in (trī'nī-trō-glis'ĕ-rin). SYN nitroglycerin.

tri·ni·tro·tol·u·ene (TNT) (trī'nī-trō-tol'ū-ēn). An explosive made by the nitrification of toluene; it causes gastric and intestinal disturbances and dermatitis in workers in munition factories. SYN trinitrotoluol.

tri·ni·tro·tol·u·ol (trī'nī-trō-tol'ū-ol). SYN trinitrotoluene.

tri·nu·cle·o·tide (trī-noo'klē-ō-tīd). A combination of three adjacent nucleotides, free or in a polynucleotide or nucleic acid molecule; often used with specific reference to the unit (codon or anticodon) specifying a particular amino acid in expression of the genetic code.

tri·o·ki·nase (trī-ō-kī'nās). A phosphotransferase catalyzing the phosphorylation of D-glyceraldehyde by ATP to produce D-glyceraldehyde 3-phosphate and ADP; participates in a step in D-fructose metabolism. SYN triosekinase.

tri·ol (trī-ol). A compound containing three hydroxyl groups; e.g., glycerol.

tri·o·le·in (trī-ō'lē-in). SYN olein.

tri·oph·thal·mos (trī-of-thal'mos). Conjoined twins with union in the facial region such that there is a common eye on the joined sides; a variety of opodidymus. SEE conjoined *twins*, under *twin*. [tri- + G. *ophthalmos*, eye]

tri·or·chism (trī-ōr'kizm). Condition of having three testes.

tri·orth·o·cres·yl phos·phate (TOCP) (trī'-ōr-thō-kres'il). A triaryl phosphate; produces a delayed neurotoxicity. An infamous incident occurred when it appeared as an adulterant in Jamaica ginger and was responsible for thousands of cases of paralysis during the Prohibition era.

tri·ose (trī'ōs). A three-carbon monosaccharide; e.g., glyceraldehyde and dihydroxyacetone.

tri·ose·ki·nase (trī'ōs-kī'nās). SYN triokinase.

tri·ose·phos·phate isom·er·ase (trī'ōs-fos'fāt). An isomerizing enzyme that catalyzes the reversible interconversion of D-glyceraldehyde 3-phosphate and dihydroxyacetone phosphate, a reaction of importance in glycolysis and gluconeogenesis; a deficiency of this enzyme will result in hemolytic anemia and severe neurologic deficits. SYN phosphotriose isomerase.

tri·o·tus (trī-ō'tŭs). Diprosopus in which three ears are present. [tri- + G. *ous*, ear]

tri·ox·ide (trī-oks'īd). A molecule containing three atoms of oxygen. SYN teroxide.

tri·ox·sa·len (trī-ok'să-len). An orally effective pigmenting, photosensitizing agent; used as a tanning agent and in the treatment of vitiligo.

tri·ox·y·meth·yl·ene (trī'ok-sē-meth'i-lēn). SYN paraformaldehyde.

tri·pal·mi·tin (trī-pal'mi-tin). SYN palmitin.

tri·par·a·nol (trī-par'ă-nol). Formerly used as inhibitor of cholesterol biosynthesis but withdrawn from the market because it promoted the formation of cataracts.

tri·pel·en·na·mine hy·dro·chlo·ride (trī-pĕ-len'ă-mēn). An antihistamine. Also available, with the same actions, is t. h. citrate; it is less bitter than the hydrochloride salt, and is therefore used in elixir.

tri·pep·tid·ases (trī-pep'ti-dās-es). A class of enzymes of different specificities that catalyzes the hydrolysis of tripeptides, producing a dipeptide and an amino acid.

tri·pep·tide (trī-pep'tīd). A compound containing three amino acids linked together by peptide bonds.

tri·pha·lan·gia (trī-fă-lan'jē-ă). Malformation in which three phalanges are present in the thumb or great toe. [tri- + phalanx]

Tripier, Léon, French surgeon, 1842–1891. SEE T. *amputation*.

tri·plant (trī'plant). SEE triplant *implant*.

tri·ple·gia (trī-plē'jē-ă). **1.** Paralysis of three limbs, both extremities on one side and one on the other. **2.** Paralysis of an upper and a lower extremity and of the face. [tri- + G. *plēgē*, stroke]

trip·let. 1. One of three children delivered at the same birth. SYN tridymus. **2.** A set of three similar objects, as a compound lens in a microscope, formed of three planoconvex lenses. **3.** SYN codon.

nonsense t., (1) a trinucleotide (codon) in which a base change to a termination codon results in premature termination of the growing polypeptide chain and, consequently, incomplete protein molecules; (2) a termination codon.

trip·lo·blas·tic (trip-lō-blas'tik). Formed of three primary germ layers (ectoderm, mesoderm, endoderm), or containing tissue derived from all three layers. [G. *triploos*, threefold, + *blastos*, germ]

trip·loid (trip'loyd). Pertaining to or characteristic of triploidy. [tri- + -ploid]

trip·loi·dy (trip'loy-dē). The presence of three haploid sets of chromosomes, instead of two, in all cells; results in fetal or neonatal death.

trip·lo·pia (trip-lō'pē-ă). Visual defect in which three images of the same object are seen. SYN triple vision. [G. *triploos*, triple, + *opsis*, sight]

tri·pod (trī'pod). **1.** Three-legged. **2.** A stand having three legs or supports. [G. *tripous*, fr. tri- + *pous*, foot]

Haller t., SYN celiac (arterial) *trunk*.

vital t., the brain, the heart, and the lungs, regarded as the three organs essential to life.

tri·po·dia (trī-pō'dē-ă). Condition in conjoined twins in which the lower extremities on the joined sides form a single foot, so that there are only three feet for the two bodies. SEE conjoined *twins*, under *twin*. [tri- + G. *pous*, foot]

tri·prol·i·dine hy·dro·chlo·ride (trī-prol'i-dēn). An H$_1$ antihistaminic used in the management of allergic and pruritic conditions.

tri·pro·so·pus (trī'prō-sō'pŭs). Fetus with three united heads, with only parts of three faces. [tri- + G. *prosōpon*, face]

trip·sis (trip'sis). **1.** SYN trituration (1). **2.** SYN massage. [G. a rubbing]

tri·que·trous (trī-kwē'trŭs, -kwet-). Triangular. [L. *triquetrus*, three-cornered]

tri·que·trum (trī-kwē'trŭm, -kwet-) [TA]. A bone on the medial (ulnar) side of the proximal row of the carpus, articulating with the lunate, pisiform, and hamate. SYN os triquetrum [TA], cubital bone, os pyramidale, os triangulare, pyramidal bone, pyramidale, three-cornered bone, triquetrum bone. [L. *triquetrus*, three-cornered]

tri·ra·di·al, tri·ra·di·ate (trī-rā'dē-ăl, trī-rā'dē-āt). Radiating in three directions.

tr

tri·ra·di·us (trī-rā'dē-ŭs). In dermatoglyphics, the figure at the base of each finger in the palm, produced by rows of papillae running in three directions so as to form a triangle. SYN Galton delta (2).

Tris Abbreviation for tris(hydroxymethyl)aminomethane and tris-(hydroxymethyl)methylamine; used as a trivial name.

⚠**tris-.** Chemical prefix indicating three of the substituents that follow, independently linked. Cf. tri-.

tri·sac·cha·ride (trī-sak'ă-rīd). A carbohydrate containing three monosaccharide residues, e.g., raffinose.

tris(hy·drox·y·meth·yl)a·mi·no·meth·ane (Tris). SYN tromethamine.

tris(hy·drox·y·meth·yl)meth·yl·a·mine (Tris). SYN tromethamine.

tris·kai·dek·a·pho·bia (tris'kī-dek-ă-fō'bē-ă). Superstitious dread of the number 13. [G. *triskaideka,* thirteen, + *phobos,* fear]

tris·mic (triz'mik). Relating to or marked by trismus.

tris·moid (triz'moyd). 1. Resembling trismus. 2. Trismus nascentium, formerly regarded as a distinct variety due to pressure on the occiput during birth. [trismus + G. *eidos,* resemblance]

tris·mus (triz'mŭs). Persistent contraction of the masseter muscles due to failure of central inhibition; often the initial manifestation of generalized tetanus. SYN *Ankylostoma* (2), lock-jaw, lockjaw. [L. fr. G. *trismos,* a creaking, rasping]

t. capistra'tus, congenital adhesion of the cheeks to the gums.

t. nascen'tium, stiffness of the jaw muscles in neonates, usually as the beginning of tetanus neonatorum. SYN t. neonatorum.

t. neonato'rum, SYN t. nascentium.

t. sardon'icus, SYN *risus* caninus.

tri·so·mic (trī-sō'mik). Relating to trisomy.

tri·so·my (trī'sō-mē). The state of an individual or cell with an extra chromosome instead of the normal pair of homologous chromosomes; in humans, the state of a cell containing 47 normal chromosomes. For various types of trisomy syndrome, see under syndrome. [tri- + (chromo)some]

tri·splanch·nic (trī-splangk'nik). Relating to the three visceral cavities: skull, thorax, and abdomen. [tri- + G. *splanchnon,* viscus]

tri·ste·a·rin (trī-stē'ă-rin). SYN stearin.

tri·stich·ia (trī-stik'i-ă). Presence of three rows of eyelashes. [G. *tristichos,* in three rows, fr. *tri-,* three, + *stichos,* row]

tri·sul·cate (trī-sŭl'kāt). Marked by three grooves.

tri·ta·nom·a·ly (trī'tă-nom'ă-lē). A type of partial color deficiency due to a deficiency or abnormality of blue-sensitive retinal cones. [G. *tritos,* third, + *anōmalia,* irregularity]

trit·an·o·pia (trī'tă-nō'pē-ă). Deficient color perception in which there is an absence of blue-sensitive pigment in the retinal cones. [G. *tritos,* third, + *an-* priv. + *ōps,* eye]

tri·ter·penes (trī-ter'pēnz). Hydrocarbons or their derivatives formed by the condensation of six isoprene units (equivalent to three terpene units) and containing, therefore, 30 carbon atoms; e.g., squalene, certain steroids, cardiac glycosides.

trit·i·at·ed (trit'ē-ā-ted). Containing atoms of tritium (hydrogen-3) in the molecule.

tri·ti·ce·o·glos·sus (tri-tish'ē-ō-glos'ŭs). SEE *musculus* triticeoglossus. [L. *triticeum,* + G. *glōssa,* tongue]

tri·ti·ceous (tri-tish'ŭs). Resembling or shaped like a grain of wheat. [L. *triticeus,* fr. *triticum,* a grain of wheat]

tri·tic·e·um (tri-tish'ē-ŭm). SYN triticeal *cartilage.* [L. *triticeus,* triticeous, like a grain of wheat]

trit·i·um (T, *t*) (trit'ē-ŭm, trish'-). SYN hydrogen-3.

Tri·trich·o·mon·as (trī'trīk-ō-mō'nas). A genus of parasitic protozoan flagellates, formerly part of the genus *Trichomonas* but now separated as a distinct genus by the absence of a pelta and the presence of three anterior flagella. Species include *T. foetus,* which causes bovine trichomoniasis, and *T. suis,* which occurs in the nasal passages, stomach, cecum, and colon of pigs. SEE ALSO *Trichomonas.* [G. *tri-,* three, + *Trichomonas*]

tri·tu·ber·cu·lar (trī-too-ber'kū-lăr). SYN tricuspid (2).

trit·u·ra·ble (trit'ū-ră-bl). Capable of being triturated.

trit·u·rate (trit'ū-rāt). 1. To accomplish trituration. 2. A triturated substance.

trit·u·ra·tion (trit-ū-rā'shŭn). 1. The act of reducing a drug to a fine powder and incorporating it thoroughly with sugar of milk by rubbing the two together in a mortar. SYN tripsis (1). 2. Mixing of dental amalgam in a mortar and pestle or with a mechanical device. [L. *trituratio,* fr. *trituro,* to thresh, fr. *tero,* pp. *tritus,* to rub]

tri·tyl (trī'til). The triphenylmethyl radical, Ph_3C-.

tri·va·lence, tri·va·len·cy (trī-vā'lens, -len-sē). The property of being trivalent.

tri·va·lent (trī-vā'lent). Having the combining power (valence) of 3.

tri·valve (trī'valv). Provided with three valves, as a speculum with three diverging blades.

triv·i·al name. A name of a chemical, no part of which is necessarily used in a systematic sense; i.e., it gives little or no indication as to chemical structure. Such names are common for drugs, hormones, proteins, and other biologicals, and are used by the general public. They may not be officially sanctioned, in contrast to nonproprietary names, but may be adopted as official nonproprietary names as a result of widespread usage. Examples are water, aspirin, chlorophyll, heme, methotrexate, folic acid, caffeine, thyroxine, epinephrine, barbital, etc.; also common abbreviations for chemically defined substances, such as ACTH, MSH, BAL, DDT, which are spoken as such and not in terms of the words they represent. The distinction between trivial and semitrivial names is seldom made; thus tetrahydrofolate, methylglycine, glucosamine, etc., are often termed trivial even though each contains a systematic part that is used in the correct systematic sense (tetrahydro for four hydrogen atoms, methyl for a $-CH_3$ group, amine for $-NH_2$ in the above examples). Trivial names are often assigned arbitrarily to chemical compounds, especially from natural sources, before the chemical structures, hence systematic names can be assigned. Also, they afford useful shortenings of long systematic names even when these can be stated (although most such shortenings turn out to be semisystematic, as they incorporate some portion of the systematic name).

tri·zon·al (trī-zō'năl). Having, or arranged in, three zones or layers.

tRNA Abbreviation for transfer RNA.

tro·car (trō'kar). An instrument for withdrawing fluid from a cavity, or for use in paracentesis; it consists of a metal tube (cannula) into which fits an obturator with a sharp three-cornered tip, which is withdrawn after the instrument has been pushed into the cavity; the name t. is usually applied to the obturator alone, the entire instrument being designated t. and cannula. [Fr. *trocart,* fr. *trois,* three, + *carre,* side (of a sword blade)]

Hasson t., a blunt t. inserted into the peritoneal cavity after making a small celiotomy; used for insufflation and introduction of a laparoscope.

troch Abbreviation for trochiscus.

tro·chan·ter (trō-kan'ter). One of the bony prominences developed from independent osseous centers near the upper extremity of the femur; there are two in humans, three in the horse. [G. *trochantēr,* a runner, fr. *trechō,* to run]

greater t. [TA], a strong process at the proximal and lateral part of the shaft of the femur, overhanging the root of the neck; it gives attachment to the gluteus medius and minimus, piriformis, obturator internus and externus, and gemelli muscles. SYN t. major [TA].

lesser t. [TA], a pyramidal process projecting from the medial and proximal part of the shaft of the femur at the line of junction of the shaft and the neck; it receives the insertion of the psoas major and iliacus (iliopsoas) muscles. SYN t. minor [TA], small t., trochantin.

t. ma'jor [TA], SYN greater t.

t. mi'nor [TA], SYN lesser t.

small t., SYN lesser t.

t. tertius [TA], SYN third t.

third t. [TA], an occasional process at the proximal end of the lateral lip of the linea aspera of the femur, about on a level with the lesser t., giving insertion to the greater part of the gluteus maximus muscle. SEE ALSO gluteal *tuberosity*. SYN t. tertius [TA].

tro·chan·ter·i·an, tro·chan·ter·ic (trō-kan-ter′ē-an, -ter′ik). Relating to a trochanter; especially the greater trochanter.

tro·chan·ter·plas·ty (trō-kan′ter-plas-tē). Plastic surgery of the trochanters and neck of the femur. [trochanter + G. *plastos*, formed]

tro·chan·tin (trō-kan′tin). SYN lesser *trochanter*.

tro·chan·tin·i·an (trō-kan-tin′ē-an). Relating to the trochanter minor.

tro·che (trōk, trō′kē). A small, disk-shaped or rhombic body composed of solidifying paste containing an astringent, antiseptic, or demulcent drug, used for local treatment of the mouth or throat, the t. being held in the mouth until dissolved. The vehicle or base of the t. is usually sugar, made adhesive by admixture with acacia or tragacanth, fruit paste, made from black or red currants, confection of rose, or balsam of tolu. SYN lozenge, morsulus, pastil (2), pastille, trochiscus. [L. *trochiscus* fr. G. *trochiskos*, a little wheel, fr. *trochos*, a wheel]

tro·chis·cus (troch), pl. **tro·chis·ci** (trō-kis′kŭs). SYN troche. [L., fr. G. *trochiskos*, a small wheel, a lozenge, fr. *trochos*, a wheel]

troch·lea, pl. **troch·le·ae** (trok′lē-ă, -lē-ē) [TA]. **1.** A structure serving as a pulley. **2.** A smooth articular surface of bone upon which another glides. [L. pulley, fr. G. *trochileia*, a pulley, fr. *trechō*, to run]

t. fem′oris, SYN patellar *surface* of femur.

fibular t. of calcaneus [TA], a projection from the lateral side of the calcaneus between the tendons of the peroneus longus and brevis. SYN t. fibularis calcanei [TA], peroneal t. of calcaneus✭, t. peronealis✭, peroneal pulley, processus trochlearis, spina peronealis, trochlear process.

t. fibula′ris calca′nei [TA], SYN fibular t. of calcaneus.

t. hu′meri [TA], SYN t. of humerus.

t. of humerus [TA], the grooved surface at the lower end of the humerus articulating with the trochlear notch of the ulna. SYN t. humeri [TA], pulley of humerus.

muscular t. [TA], a fibrous loop through which the tendon of a muscle passes; the intermediate tendon of the digastric and omohyoid muscles pass through such a t. SYN t. muscularis [TA], muscular pulley.

t. muscula′ris [TA], SYN muscular t.

t. musculi obliqui superioris bulbi, SYN t. of superior oblique (muscle).

peroneal t. of calcaneus, ✭official alternate term for fibular t. of calcaneus.

t. peronea′lis, ✭official alternate term for fibular t. of calcaneus.

trochleae of phalanges of hand and foot, palmar or plantar aspect of the intercondylar groove of the heads of the phalanges that accommodate the long flexor tendons. SYN t. phalangis (manus et pedis).

t. phalan′gis (manus et pedis), SYN trochleae of phalanges of hand and foot.

t. of superior oblique (muscle), a fibrous loop in the orbit, near the nasal process of the frontal bone, through which passes the tendon of the superior oblique muscle of the eye. SYN t. musculi obliqui superioris bulbi.

t. ta′li [TA], SYN t. of the talus.

t. of the talus [TA], the rounded superior articular surface of the talus that articulates with the distal ends of the tibia and fibula. SYN t. tali [TA], pulley of talus.

troch·le·ar (trok′lē-ar). **1.** Relating to a trochlea, especially the trochlea of the superior oblique muscle of the eye. SYN trochlearis (1). **2.** SYN trochleiform.

troch·le·ar·i·form (trok-lē-ar′i-fŏrm). SYN trochleiform.

troch·le·ar·is (trok-lē-ā′ris). **1.** SYN trochlear (1). **2.** SYN trochleiform. [L.]

troch·le·i·form (trok′lē-i-fŏrm). Pulley-shaped. SYN trochlear (2), trochleariform, trochlearis (2).

troch·o·car·dia (trok-ō-kar′dē-ă). Rotary displacement of the heart around its axis. [G. *trochos,* wheel, + *kardia,* heart]

tro·choid (trō′koyd). Revolving; rotating; denoting a revolving or wheel-like articulation. [G. *trochōdēs,* fr. *trochos,* wheel, + *eidos,* resemblance]

tro·chor·i·zo·car·dia (trō-kōr-ī′zō-kar′dē-ă). Combined trochocardia and horizocardia.

troglitazone (trō-glī′ta-zon). An insulin sensitizer used with a sulfonylurea or insulin to improve glycemic control.

Trog·lo·tre·ma sal·min·co·la (trog-lō-trē′mă sal-mingk′ō-lă). SYN *Nanophyetus salmincola.*

Troisier, Charles Émile, French physician, 1844–1919. SEE T. *ganglion, node.*

tro·la·mine (trō′lă-mēn). USAN-approved contraction for triethanolamine, $N(CH_2CH_2OH)_3$.

Troland, L.T., U.S. physicist, 1889–1932. SEE troland.

tro·land (trō′land). A unit of visual stimulation at the retina equal to the illumination per square millimeter of pupil received from a surface of 1 lux brightness.

Trolard, Paulin, French anatomist, 1842–1910. SEE T. *vein.*

tro·le·an·do·my·cin (trō′lē-an-dō-mī′sin). The triacetyl ester of oleandomycin, a macrolide antibiotic, with a potency of not less than 760 μg per mg; an orally effective antibiotic for infections produced by Gram-positive, penicillin-resistant bacteria. SYN triacetyloleandomycin.

trol·ni·trate phos·phate (trol-nī′trāt). An organic nitrate with mild but persistent vasodilator action on smooth muscle of the smaller vessels of postarteriolar vascular beds; used to prevent attacks of angina pectoris.

Tröltsch, Anton F. von, German otologist, 1829–1890. SEE T. *corpuscles,* under *corpuscle, pockets,* under *pocket, recesses,* under *recess.*

Trom·bic·u·la (trom-bik′ŭ-lă). The chigger mite, a genus of mites (family Trombiculidae) whose larvae (chiggers, red bugs) include pests of humans and other animals, and vectors of rickettsial diseases.

T. akamu′shi, SYN *Leptotrombidium akamushi.*

T. alfredduge′si, a mite species common in second growth and grassy brush areas of the Americas; the larvae attack humans (as well as reptiles, birds, and wild and domestic mammals), causing an intensely itching dermatitis.

T. delien′sis, SEE *Leptotrombidium akamushi.*

trom·bic·u·li·a·sis (trom-bik-ū-lī′ă-sis). Infestation by mites of the genus *Trombicula.*

trom·bic·u·lid (trom-bik′ŭ-lid). Common name for members of the family Trombiculidae.

Trom·bic·u·li·dae (trom-bik-oo-lī′dē). A family of mites whose larvae (redbugs, rougets, harvest mites, scrub mites, or chiggers) are parasitic on vertebrates and whose nymphs and adults are bright red and free-living, living on insect eggs or minute organisms in the soil. The six-legged larvae are barely visible red or orange parasites that attach to the skin for a few days to a month, producing an exceedingly irritating reaction. In the Orient, trombiculid chiggers of the genus *Leptotrombidium* transmit tsutsugamushi disease, caused by *Rickettsia tsutsugamushi,* which is transovarially transmitted in these mites.

Trom·bi·di·i·dae (trom-bi-dī′i-dē). A family of mites that formerly included the subfamily Trombiculinae, now raised to the family Trombiculidae (including the vectors of tsutsugamushi disease). T. larvae are characteristically parasitic on insects, not on vertebrates as with the larvae of Trombiculidae.

tro·meth·a·mine (trō-meth′ă-mēn). A weakly basic compound used as an alkalizing agent and as a buffer in enzymic reactions. SYN tris(hydroxymethyl)aminomethane, tris(hydroxymethyl)methylamine.

Trömner, Ernest L.O., German neurologist, *1868. SEE T. *reflex.*

tro·na (trō′nă). A native sodium carbonate.

tro·pa·ic ac·id (trō-pā′ik). SYN tropic acid.

tro·pane (trō′pān). **1.** A bicyclic hydrocarbon, the fundamental structure of tropine, atropine, and other physiologically active substances. **2.** In plural form, a class of alkaloids containing the t. (1) structure.

tro·pate (trō′pāt). A salt or ester of tropic acid.

tro·pe·ic ac·id (trō-pē′ik). SYN tropic acid.

tro·pe·ine (trō′pē-in). An ester of tropine; either a naturally occurring alkaloid or prepared synthetically.

tro·pen·tane (trō-pen′tān). An antispasmodic with anticholinergic properties.

tro·pe·o·lins (trō-pē′ō-linz). A group of azo dyes used as indicators; e.g., methyl orange. [G. *tropaios*, pertaining to a turning or change, fr. *trope*, a turn]

△**troph-.** SEE tropho-.

troph·ec·to·derm (trof-ek′tō-derm). Outermost layer of cells in the mammalian blastodermic vesicle, which will make contact with the endometrium and take part in establishing the embryo's means of receiving nutrition; the cell layer from which the trophoblast differentiates. [troph- + ectoderm]

Tropheryma whippelii. An unclassified, nonculturable organism, named in 1992, which has been identified by electron microscopy and defined by DNA amplification technologies; it has been proven to be the infectious agent responsible for Whipple disease.

tro·phic (trof′ik, trō′fik). **1.** Relating to or dependent upon nutrition. **2.** Resulting from interruption of nerve supply. [G. *trophe*, nourishment]

△**-trophic.** Nutrition. Cf. -tropic. [G. *trophe*, nourishment]

tro·phic·i·ty (trō-fis′i-tē). A trophic influence or condition. SYN trophism (1).

tro·phism (trof′izm). **1.** SYN trophicity. **2.** SYN nutrition (1). [G. *trophe*, nourishment]

△**tropho-, troph-.** Food, nutrition. [G. *trophe*, nourishment]

troph·o·blast (trof′ō-blast, trō′fō-blast). The mesectodermal cell layer covering the blastocyst that erodes the uterine mucosa and through which the embryo receives nourishment from the mother; the cells do not enter into the formation of the embryo itself, but contribute to the formation of the placenta. The t. develops processes that later receive a core of vascular mesoderm and are then known as the chorionic villi; the t. soon becomes two-layered, differentiating into the syncytiotrophoblast, an outer layer consisting of a multinucleated protoplasmic mass (syncytium), and the cytotrophoblast, the inner layer next to the mesoderm in which the cells retain their membranes. SYN chorionic ectoderm. [tropho- + G. *blastos*, germ]

plasmodial t., SYN syncytiotrophoblast.

syncytial t., SYN syncytiotrophoblast.

troph·o·blas·tic (trō-fō-blas′tik). Relating to the trophoblast.

tro·pho·blas·tin (trō-fō-blas′tin). SYN *interferon*-tau.

troph·o·chro·ma·tin (trof-ō-krō′mă-tin). SYN trophochromidia. [tropho- + G. *chroma*, color]

troph·o·chro·mid·ia (trof′ō-krō-mid′ē-ă). Nongerminal or vegetative extranuclear masses of chromatin, found in certain protozoan forms; e.g., the macronucleus of certain ciliates, such as *Paramecium*. SYN trophochromatin.

troph·o·cyte (trof′ō-sīt). A cell that supplies nourishment; e.g., Sertoli cells in the seminiferous tubules. SYN trephocyte. [tropho- + G. *kytos*, cell]

troph·o·derm (trof′ō-derm). The trophectoderm, or trophoblast, together with the vascular mesodermal layer underlying it. SEE ALSO serosa (2). [tropho- + G. *derma*, skin]

troph·o·der·ma·to·neu·ro·sis (trof′ō-der′mă-tō-noo-rō′sis). Cutaneous trophic changes due to neural involvement.

troph·o·dy·nam·ics (trof′ō-dī-nam′iks). The dynamics of nutrition or metabolism. SYN nutritional energy. [tropho- + G. *dynamis*, power]

troph·o·neu·ro·sis (trof′ō-noo-rō′sis). A trophic disorder, such as atrophy, hypertrophy, or a skin eruption, occurring as a consequence of disease or injury of the nerves of the part. [tropho- + G. *neuron*, nerve, + -osis, condition]

troph·o·neu·rot·ic (trof-ō-noo-rot′ik). Relating to a trophoneurosis.

troph·o·nu·cle·us (trof-ō-noo′klē-ŭs). SYN macronucleus (2).

troph·o·plast (trof′ō-plast). SYN plastid (1). [tropho- + G. *plastos*, formed]

troph·o·spon·gia (trof′ō-spon′jē-ă). **1.** Canalicular structures described by A.F. Holmgren in the protoplasm of certain cells. **2.** Vascular endometrium of the uterus between the myometrium and the trophoblast. [tropho- + G. *spongia*, a sponge]

troph·o·tax·is (trof-ō-tak′sis). SYN trophotropism. [tropho- + G. *taxis*, arrangement]

troph·o·tro·pic (trof-ō-trop′ik). Relating to trophotropism.

tro·phot·ro·pism (trō-fot′rō-pizm). Chemotaxis of living cells in relation to nutritive material; it may be positive (toward nutritive material) or negative (away from nutritive material). SYN trophotaxis. [tropho- + G. *trope*, a turning]

troph·o·zo·ite (trof-ō-zō′īt). The ameboid, vegetative, asexual form of certain Sporozoea, such as the schizont of the plasmodia of malaria and related parasites. [tropho- + G. *zoon*, animal]

△**-trophy.** Food, nutrition. [G. *trophe*, nourishment]

tro·pia (trō′pē-ă). Abnormal deviation of the eye. SEE strabismus. [G. trope, a turning]

△**-tropic.** A turning toward, having an affinity for. Cf. -trophic. [G. *trope*, a turning]

tro·pic ac·id (trop′ik). A constituent of atropine and of scopolamine, in which it is esterified through its COOH to the 3-CHOH of tropine. SYN tropaic acid, tropeic acid.

tro·pic·a·mide (trō-pik′ă-mīd). An anticholinergic agent used to effect a rapid and brief mydriasis for eye examinations.

tro·pine (trō′pēn). The major constituent of atropine and scopolamine, from which it is obtained on hydrolysis.

t. mandelate, SYN homatropine.

t. tropate, SYN atropine.

tro·pism (trō′pizm). The phenomenon, observed in living organisms, of moving toward (**positive t.**) or away from (**negative t.**) a focus of light, heat, or other stimulus; usually applied to the movement of a portion of the organism as opposed to taxis, the movement of an entire organism. [G. *trope*, a turning]

viral t., the specificity of a virus for a particular host tissue, determined in part by the interaction of viral surface structures with host cell-surface receptors.

tro·po·col·la·gen (trō-pō-kol′ă-jen, trop′ō-). The fundamental units of collagen fibrils, consisting of three helically arranged polypeptide chains.

trop·o·e·las·tin (trō-pō-ē-las′tin). The precursor to elastin; t. does not contain desmosine or isodesmosine cross-links.

tro·pom·e·ter (trō-pom′ĕ-ter). Any instrument for measuring the degree of rotation or torsion, as of the eyeball or the shaft of a long bone. [G. *trope*, a turning, + *metron*, measure]

tro·po·my·o·sin (trō-pō-mī′ō-sin). A fibrous protein extractable from muscle; sometimes specified as t. B to distinguish it from t. A (paramyosin) prominent in mollusks.

tro·po·nin (trō′pō-nin). A globular protein of muscle that binds to tropomyosin and has considerable affinity for calcium ions; a central regulatory protein of muscle contraction. T. T binds to tropomyosin; t. I inhibits F-actin-myosin interactions; t. C is a calcium-binding protein and has a key role in muscle contraction.

trough (trawf). A long, narrow, shallow channel or depression.

gingival t., the formation of a crater as a result of destruction of interdental tissues so that, in effect, there exists a labial and lingual curtain of gingiva with no interproximal connection at all.

Langmuir t., a t. with a movable surface barrier for studying the compression of surface films.

synaptic t., the depression of the surface of the striated muscle fiber that accommodates the motor endplate.

Trousseau, Armand, French physician, 1801–1867. SEE T. *point*, *sign*, *spot*, *syndrome*; T.-Lallemand *bodies*, under *body*.

trox·e·ru·tin (troks′ē-roo-tin). Used for treatment of venous disorders.

trox·i·done (trok′si-dōn). SYN trimethadione.

Trp Symbol for tryptophan and its radicals.

trun·cal (trŭng′kăl). Relating to the trunk of the body or to any arterial or nerve trunk, etc.

trun·cate (trŭng′kāt). Truncated; cut across at right angles to the long axis, or appearing to be so cut. [L. *trunco,* pp. *-atus,* to maim, cut off]

trun·cus, gen. and pl. **trun·ci** (trŭn′kŭs, -kī) [TA]. SYN trunk. [L. stem, trunk]

t. arterio′sus, the common arterial trunk opening out of both ventricles in early fetal life, later destined to be divided into aorta and pulmonary artery by development of the spiral septum.

t. arterio′sus commu′nis, SEE t. arteriosus.

t. brachiocepha′licus [TA], SYN brachiocephalic (arterial) *trunk.*

t. celi′acus [TA], SYN celiac (arterial) *trunk.*

t. cor′poris callo′si [TA], SYN *trunk* of corpus callosum.

t. costocervica′lis [TA], SYN costocervical (arterial) *trunk.*

t. encephali [TA], SYN brainstem.

t. fascicula′ris atrioventricula′ris, SYN atrioventricular *bundle;* SEE ALSO conducting *system* of heart.

t. infe′rior plex′us brachia′lis [TA], SYN inferior *trunk* of brachial plexus.

t. linguofacia′lis [TA], SYN linguofacial (arterial) *trunk.*

t. lum′bosacra′lis [TA], SYN lumbosacral (nerve) *trunk.*

trun′ci (lymphatici) intestina′les [TA], SYN intestinal (lymphatic) *trunks,* under *trunk.*

trun′ci (lymphatici) lumba′les [TA], SYN lumbar (lymphatic) *trunks,* under *trunk.*

t. (lymphaticus) bronchiomediastina′lis [TA], SYN bronchomediastinal (lymphatic) *trunk.*

t. (lymphaticus) jugula′ris [TA], SYN jugular lymphatic *trunk.*

t. me′dius plex′us brachia′lis [TA], SYN middle *trunk* of brachial plexus.

t. nervi accessorii [TA], SYN accessory nerve *trunk.*

persistent t. arterio′sus, a congenital cardiovascular anomaly resulting from failure of development of the spiral septum and consisting of a common arterial trunk opening out of both ventricles, the pulmonary arteries being given off from the ascending common trunk.

trun′ci plex′us brachia′lis [TA], SYN *trunks* of brachial plexus, under *trunk.*

t. pulmona′lis [TA], SYN pulmonary *trunk.*

t. subcla′vius [TA], SYN subclavian lymphatic *trunk.*

t. supe′rior plex′us brachia′lis [TA], SYN superior *trunk* of brachial plexus.

t. sympath′icus [TA], SYN sympathetic *trunk.*

t. thyrocervica′lis [TA], SYN thyrocervical (arterial) *trunk.*

t. vaga′lis, SYN vagal (nerve) *trunk.*

Trunecek, Karel, Czechoslovakian physician, *1865. SEE T. *sign.*

trunk (trŭnk) [TA]. **1.** The body (trunk or torso), excluding the head and extremities. **2.** A primary nerve, vessel, or collection of tissue before its division. **3.** A large collecting lymphatic vessel. SYN truncus [TA]. [L. *truncus*]

accessory nerve t. [TA], part of the accessory nerve formed within the cranial cavity by the union of the cranial and spinal roots, which then divides within the jugular foramen into internal and external branches, the former uniting with the vagus, the latter exiting the foramen as an independent branch which is commonly considered to be the accessory nerve. SYN truncus nervi accessorii [TA].

t. of atrioventricular bundle, SYN atrioventricular *bundle.*

t.'s of brachial plexus [TA], the superior, middle, and inferior trunks; they divide distally to form the cords (fasciculi) of the plexus. SYN trunci plexus brachialis [TA].

brachiocephalic (arterial) t. [TA], *origin,* arch of aorta; *branches,* right subclavian and right common carotid; occasionally it gives off the thyroidea ima. SYN truncus brachiocephalicus [TA].

bronchomediastinal (lymphatic) t. [TA], a lymphatic vessel arising from the union of the efferent lymphatics from the tracheo-bronchial and mediastinal nodes on either side. On the left side, it may be largely replaced by direct drainage into the thoracic duct. SYN truncus (lymphaticus) bronchiomediastinalis [TA].

celiac (arterial) t. [TA], *origin,* abdominal aorta just below diaphragm; *branches,* left gastric, common hepatic, splenic. SYN truncus celiacus [TA], arteria celiaca, celiac artery, celiac axis, Haller tripod.

t. of corpus callosum [TA], the main arched portion of the corpus callosum. SYN truncus corporis callosi [TA], body of corpus callosum☆.

costocervical (arterial) t. [TA], a short artery that arises from the subclavian artery on each side and divides into deep cervical and superior intercostal branches, the latter dividing usually to form the first and second posterior intercostal arteries. SYN truncus costocervicalis [TA], costocervical artery.

inferior t. of brachial plexus [TA], the nerve bundle formed by the union of the ventral rami of the eighth cervical and first thoracic nerves; it provides fibers to the posterior and medial cords (fasciculi) of the brachial plexus. SYN truncus inferior plexus brachialis [TA].

intestinal (lymphatic) t.'s [TA], the vessels conveying lymph from the lower part of the liver, the stomach, spleen, pancreas, and small intestine; they discharge into the cisterna chyli and are sometimes duplicated. SYN trunci (lymphatici) intestinales [TA].

jugular lymphatic t. [TA], lymphatic vessel on each side, conveying the lymph from the head and neck; that on the right side empties into the right lymphatic duct, that on the left into the thoracic duct. SYN truncus (lymphaticus) jugularis [TA], jugular duct.

linguofacial (arterial) t. [TA], the common t. by which the lingual and facial arteries frequently arise from the external carotid artery. SYN truncus linguofacialis [TA].

lumbar (lymphatic) t.'s [TA], two lymphatic ducts conveying lymph from the lower limbs, pelvic viscera and walls, large intestine, kidneys, and suprarenal glands; they discharge into the cisterna chyli. SYN trunci (lymphatici) lumbales [TA].

lumbosacral (nerve) t. [TA], a large nerve, formed by the union of the fifth lumbar and first sacral nerves, with a branch from the fourth lumbar nerve, which enters into the formation of the sacral plexus. SYN truncus lumbosacralis [TA].

middle t. of brachial plexus [TA], the continuation of the ventral ramus of the seventh cervical nerve; it contributes fibers to the posterior and lateral cords (fasciculi) of the brachial plexus. SYN truncus medius plexus brachialis [TA].

nerve t., a collection of funiculi or bundles of nerve fibers enclosed in a connective tissue sheath, the epineurium.

pulmonary t. [TA], *origin,* right ventricle of heart; *distribution,* it divides into the right pulmonary artery and the left pulmonary artery, which enter the corresponding lungs and branch along with the segmental bronchi. SYN truncus pulmonalis [TA], arteria pulmonalis, pulmonary artery, venous artery.

subclavian lymphatic t. [TA], it is formed by the union of the vessels draining the lymph nodes of either upper limb, emptying into the thoracic duct at the root of the neck on the left or into the right lymphatic duct. SYN truncus subclavius [TA], subclavian duct.

superior t. of brachial plexus [TA], the nerve bundle formed by the union of the ventral rami of the fifth and sixth cervical nerves and some fibers from the fourth; it contributes fibers to the posterior and lateral cords (fasciculi) of the brachial plexus. SYN truncus superior plexus brachialis [TA].

sympathetic t. [TA], one of the two long ganglionated nerve strands alongside the vertebral column that extend from the base of the skull to the coccyx; they are connected to each spinal nerve by gray rami and receive fibers from the spinal cord through white rami connecting with the thoracic and upper lumbar spinal nerves. SYN truncus sympathicus [TA], gangliated cord, ganglionic chain.

thoracoacromial t., SYN thoracoacromial *artery.*

thyrocervical (arterial) t. [TA], a short arterial t. arising from the subclavian artery, giving rise to the suprascapular (which may instead arise directly from the subclavian artery) and terminating by dividing into the ascending cervical and inferior thyroid arteries. SYN truncus thyrocervicalis [TA], thyroid axis.

tr

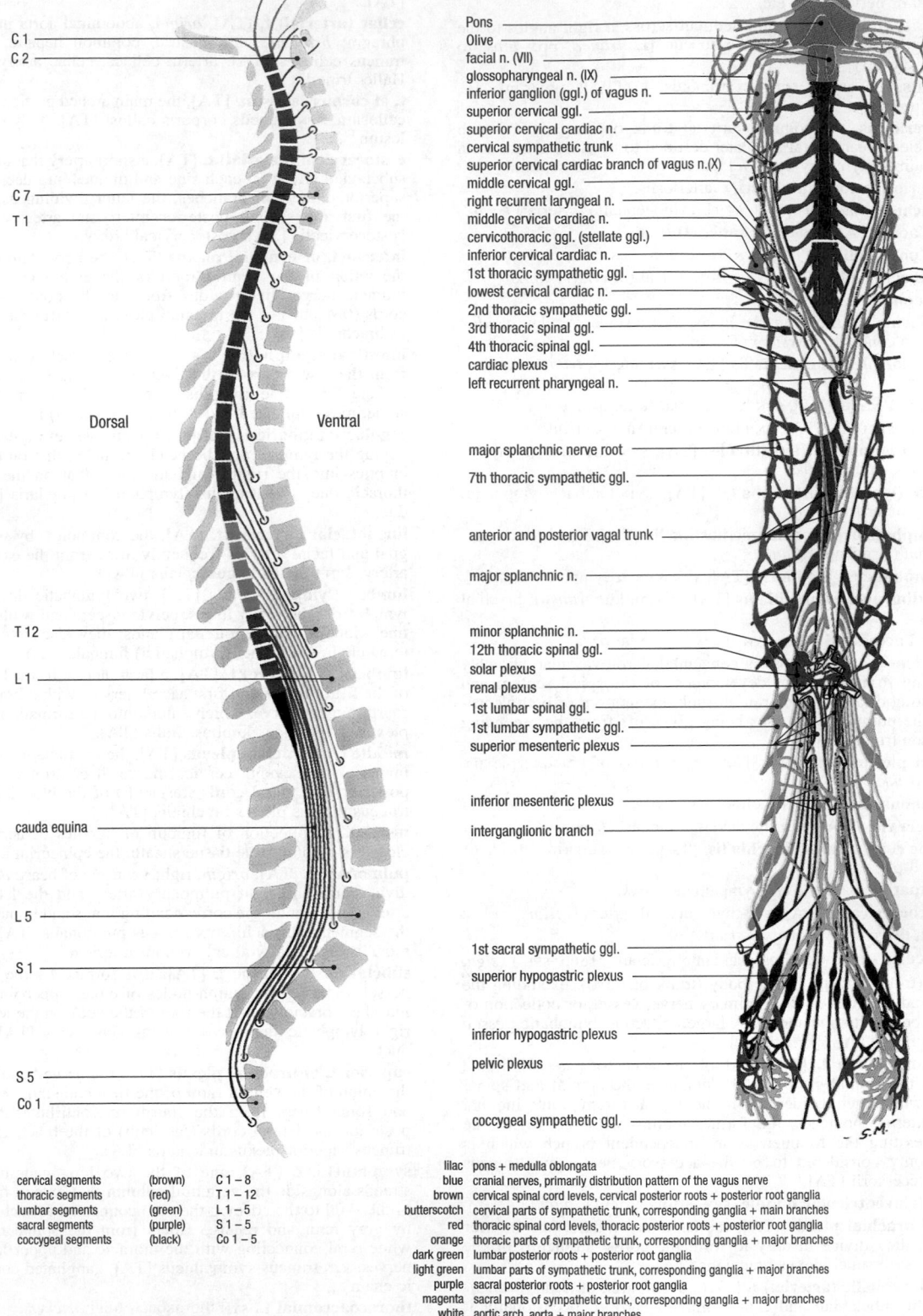

C 1
C 2

C 7
T 1

Dorsal   Ventral

T 12

L 1

cauda equina

L 5

S 1

S 5

Co 1

Pons
Olive
facial n. (VII)
glossopharyngeal n. (IX)
inferior ganglion (ggl.) of vagus n.
superior cervical ggl.
superior cervical cardiac n.
cervical sympathetic trunk
superior cervical cardiac branch of vagus n.(X)
middle cervical ggl.
right recurrent laryngeal n.
middle cervical cardiac n.
cervicothoracic ggl. (stellate ggl.)
inferior cervical cardiac n.
1st thoracic sympathetic ggl.
lowest cervical cardiac n.
2nd thoracic sympathetic ggl.
3rd thoracic spinal ggl.
4th thoracic spinal ggl.
cardiac plexus
left recurrent pharyngeal n.

major splanchnic nerve root

7th thoracic sympathetic ggl.

anterior and posterior vagal trunk

major splanchnic n.

minor splanchnic n.
12th thoracic spinal ggl.
solar plexus
renal plexus
1st lumbar spinal ggl.
1st lumbar sympathetic ggl.
superior mesenteric plexus

inferior mesenteric plexus

interganglionic branch

1st sacral sympathetic ggl.

superior hypogastric plexus

inferior hypogastric plexus

pelvic plexus

coccygeal sympathetic ggl.

– S.M. –

cervical segments	(brown)	C 1 – 8
thoracic segments	(red)	T 1 – 12
lumbar segments	(green)	L 1 – 5
sacral segments	(purple)	S 1 – 5
coccygeal segments	(black)	Co 1 – 5

lilac	pons + medulla oblongata
blue	cranial nerves, primarily distribution pattern of the vagus nerve
brown	cervical spinal cord levels, cervical posterior roots + posterior root ganglia
butterscotch	cervical parts of sympathetic trunk, corresponding ganglia + main branches
red	thoracic spinal cord levels, thoracic posterior roots + posterior root ganglia
orange	thoracic parts of sympathetic trunk, corresponding ganglia + major branches
dark green	lumbar posterior roots + posterior root ganglia
light green	lumbar parts of sympathetic trunk, corresponding ganglia + major branches
purple	sacral posterior roots + posterior root ganglia
magenta	sacral parts of sympathetic trunk, corresponding ganglia + major branches
white	aortic arch, aorta + major branches

spinal cord: left, spinal medulla in the vertebral column with color coding showing relation between neural segments and vertebrae; right, color coding shows relation of sympathetic trunk to spinal nerves and branches

vagal (nerve) t., one of the two nerve bundles, anterior and posterior, into which the esophageal plexus continues as it passes through the diaphragm. SYN truncus vagalis.

tru·sion (troo'zhŭn). Displacement of a body, e.g., a tooth, from an initial position. [L. *trudo,* pp. *trusus,* to thrust]

truss (trŭs). An appliance designed to prevent the return of a reduced hernia or the increase in size of a hernia; it consists of a pad attached to a belt and kept in place by a spring or straps. [Fr. *trousser,* to tie up, to pack]

Try Former abbreviation for tryptophan.

try-in (trī'in). Preliminary insertion of a complete denture wax-up (trial denture), of a partial denture casting, or of a finished restoration to determine the fit, esthetics, maxillomandibular relation, etc.

try·pan blue (trī'pan, trip') [C.I. 23850]. An acid azo dye, used for vital staining of the reticuloendothelial system, uriniferous tubules, and cells in tissue culture, and as an experimental teratogen; formerly used as a trypanocide.

try·pan·i·ci·dal (tri-pan-i-sī'dăl). SYN trypanocidal.

try·pan·i·cide (tri-pan'i-sīd). SYN trypanocide.

tryp·a·nid (trip'ă-nid). SYN trypanosomatid.

try·pan·o·ci·dal (tri-pan'ō-sī'dăl, trip'ă-nō-). Destructive to trypanosomes. SYN trypanicidal.

try·pan·o·cide (tri-pan'ō-sīd, trip'ă-nō-). An agent that kills trypanosomes. SYN trypanicide, trypanosomicide. [trypanosome + L. *caedo,* to kill]

Try·pan·o·plas·ma (tri-pan-ō-plaz'mă, trip'ă-nō-). A genus of flagellate Protozoa (family Cryptobiidae), the members of which have a body of varying shape, an undulating membrane, and a flagellum projecting from either extremity; parasitic in the blood of fishes. [G. *trypanon,* auger, + *plasma,* anything formed]

Try·pan·o·so·ma (tri-pan'ō-sō'mă, trip'ă-nō-). A genus of asexual digenetic protozoan flagellates (family Trypanosomatidae) that have a spindle-shaped body with an undulating membrane on one side, a single anterior flagellum, and a kinetoplast; they are parasitic in the blood plasma of many vertebrates (only a few being pathogenic) and as a rule have an intermediate host, a bloodsucking invertebrate, such as a leech, tick, or insect; pathogenic species cause trypanosomiasis in humans and a number of other diseases in domestic animals. [G. *trypanon,* an auger, + *sōma,* body]

T. a'vium, a species that occurs in owls, crows, and other birds; various bloodsucking arthropods are the vectors, including mosquitoes, black flies, and hippoboscids; this species was reported under a large number of names now considered to be physiologic strains of the species.

T. bru'cei, a protozoan species now divided into three subspecies: *T. brucei brucei, T. brucei rhodesiense,* and *T. brucei gambiense.*

T. bru'cei bru'cei, a protozoan subspecies causing nagana in Africa; it produces fatal disease in camels, acute disease in equines, dogs, and cats, and chronic disease in swine, cattle, sheep, and goats; it is transmitted primarily by tsetse flies of the genus *Glossina.* In wild African ungulates the infection is widespread but rarely fatal.

T. bru'cei gambien'se, a protozoan subspecies causing Gambian trypanosomiasis in humans; transmitted by tsetse flies, especially *Glossina palpalis.* SYN *T. gambiense, T. hominis, T. ugandense.*

T. bru'cei rhodesien'se, a protozoan subspecies causing Rhodesian trypanosomiasis; it is transmitted by tsetse flies, especially *Glossina morsitans* in humans; various game animals can act as reservoir hosts. SYN *T. rhodesiense.*

T. cru'zi, a species that causes South American trypanosomiasis and is endemic in Mexico and various countries of Central and South America; transmission and infection are common only where the triatomine bug vector defecates while taking blood, as the bug feces contains the infective agents that are scratched into the skin or brought in contact with mucosal surfaces. Trypomastigotes are found in the blood, and amastigotes occur intracellularly in clusters or colonies in the tissues; heart muscle fibers and cells of many other organs are attacked, the organisms not being restricted to macrophages as in visceral leishmaniasis; humans, dogs, cats, house rats, armadillos, bats, certain monkeys, and opossums are the usual vertebrate hosts; vectors are members of the family Triatominae. Also known as *Schizotrypanum cruzi,* a distinct generic designation widely used in the endemic regions. SYN *T. escomelis, T. triatomae.*

T. dimor'phon, an African species found in horses, cattle, sheep, goats, pigs, and dogs, formerly thought to be the same as *T. congolense* but now recognized as a distinct and more pathogenic species in cattle, sheep, and dogs; it is spread by tsetse flies across central Africa.

T. escome'lis, SYN *T. cruzi.*

T. gambien'se, SYN *T. brucei gambiense.*

T. hom'inis, SYN *T. brucei gambiense.*

T. igno'tum, old name for *T. simiae.*

T. lew'isi, species that is a worldwide nonpathogenic parasite in the blood of rats widely used for laboratory study; it is transmitted by the rat flea, *Nosopsyllus fasciatus.*

T. melopha'gium, a nonpathogenic species (related to *T. theileri*) found in sheep throughout the world, and probably in goats as well; the vector is *Melophagus ovinus.*

T. range'li, a species that parasitizes a wide variety of mammals, including humans, in South America and is transmitted by the triatomid bugs *Rhodnius prolixus* and *Tiratoma dimidiata,* and probably others; it is apparently nonpathogenic but may be pathogenic in the bug host.

T. rhodesien'se, SYN *T. brucei rhodesiense.*

T. thei'leri, a large, relatively nonpathogenic species found in African antelopes and in cattle in many parts of the world; the parasites are spread by bloodsucking tabanid horseflies.

T. triatom'ae, SYN *T. cruzi.*

T. uganden'se, SYN *T. brucei gambiense.*

try·pan·o·so·mat·id (trī-pan'ō-sō-mat'id). Common name for a member of the family Trypanosomatidae. SYN trypanid.

Try·pan·o·so·mat·i·dae (trī-pan'ō-sō-mat'i-dē). A protozoan family of hemoflagellates (order Kinetoplastida, class Zoomastigophorea, subphylum Mastigophora); asexual blood and/or tissue parasites of leeches, insects, and vertebrates and sap inhabitants of plants, characterized by a rounded or elongate form, a single nucleus, elongate mitochondrion (its position in relation to the nucleus is a characteristic of each genus), and an anteriorly directed single flagellum (in some genera, it borders an undulating membrane). T. includes the genera *Crithidia, Herpetomonas, Leptomonas,* and *Blastocrithidia,* all of which are monogenetic and found in insects, and *Phytomonas* (found in plants), *Endotrypanum, Leishmania,* and *Trypanosoma,* all of which are digenetic; *Leishmania* and *Trypanosoma* include important pathogens of humans and animals. Many trypanosomes pass through developmental or life cycle stages similar to the body forms characteristic of the genera; these forms include amastigote, choanomastigote, opisthomastigote, promastigote, epimastigote, and trypomastigote.

try·pan·o·some (tri-pan'ō-sōm, trip'ă-nō-). Common name for any member of the genus *Trypanosoma* or of the family Trypanosomatidae. [G. *trypanon,* an auger, + *sōma,* body]

try·pan·o·so·mi·a·sis (tri-pan'ō-sō-mī'ă-sis, trip'ă-nō-). Any disease caused by a trypanosome. SYN trypanosomosis.

acute t., SYN Rhodesian t.

African t., a serious endemic disease in tropical Africa, of two types: Gambian or West African t. and Rhodesian or East African t.

American t., SEE South American t.

chronic t., SYN Gambian t.

Cruz t., SYN South American t.

East African t., SYN Rhodesian t.

Gambian t., a chronic disease of humans caused by *Trypanosoma brucei gambiense* in northern and sub-Saharan Africa from Senegal east to Sudan and Uganda; characterized by splenomegaly, drowsiness, an uncontrollable urge to sleep, and the development of psychotic changes; basal ganglia and cerebellar involvement commonly lead to chorea and athetosis; the terminal phase of the disease is characterized by wasting, anorexia, and emaciation that gradually leads to coma and death, usually from intercurrent in-

tr

fection. SYN chronic African sleeping sickness, chronic t., West African sleeping sickness, West African t.

Rhodesian t., a disease of humans caused by *Trypanosoma brucei rhodesiense* in eastern Africa from Ethiopia and Uganda south to Zimbabwe; it is clinically similar to Gambian t. but of shorter duration and more acute in form; patients suffer repeated episodes of pyrexia, become anemic, and die commonly from cardiac failure. SYN acute African sleeping sickness, acute t., East African sleeping sickness, East African t.

South American t., t. caused by Trypanosoma (or *Schizotrypanum) cruzi* and transmitted by certain species of reduviid (triatomine) bugs. In its acute form, it is seen most frequently in young children, with swelling of the skin at the site of entry, most often the face, and regional lymph node enlargement; in its chronic form it can assume several aspects, commonly cardiomyopathy, but megacolon and megaesophagus also occur; natural reservoirs include dogs, armadillos, rodents, and other domestic, domiciliated, and wild mammals. SYN Chagas disease, Chagas-Cruz disease, Cruz t.

West African t., SYN Gambian t.

try·pan·o·so·mic (tri-pan-ō-sō′mik, trip′ă-nō-). Relating to trypanosomes, especially denoting infection by such organisms.

try·pan·o·so·mi·cide (tri-pan′ō-sō′mi-sīd). SYN trypanocide.

try·pan·o·so·mid (tri-pan′ō-sō-mid). A skin lesion resulting from immunologic changes from trypanosome disease. [trypanosome + G. *-id* (1)]

trypanosomosis (trip′an-ō-sō-mō′sis, tri-pan′). SYN trypanosomiasis.

try·pan red (trī′pan, trip′) [C.I. 22850]. An azo dye formerly used in the treatment of trypanosomiasis.

tryp·ar·sa·mide (trī-par′să-mīd). Used in the treatment of trypanosomic and spirochetal infections, especially neurosyphilis, and the late stages of African sleeping sickness.

tryp·o·mas·ti·gote (trip-ō-mas′ti-gōt). Term to replace the older term, "trypanosome stage," which was often confused with the flagellate genus *Trypanosoma.* It denotes the stage (infective stage for South American trypanosomiasis and African trypanosomiasis, and the only stage found in humans in the latter illness) in which the flagellum arises from a posteriorly located kinetoplast and emerges from the side of the body, with an undulating membrane running along the length of the body. [G. *trypanon,* auger, + *mastix,* whip]

tryp·sin (trip′sin). A proteolytic enzyme formed in the small intestine from trypsinogen by the action of enteropeptidase; a serine proteinase that hydrolyzes peptides, amides, esters, etc., at bonds of the carboxyl groups of L-arginyl or L-lysyl residues; it also produces the meromyosins.

crystallized t., a purified preparation of the pancreatic enzyme; used as an adjunct to surgery for débridement of necrotic wounds and ulcers.

tryp·sin·o·gen, tryp·so·gen (trip-sin′ō-jen, trip′sō-jen). An inactive protein secreted by the pancreas that is converted into trypsin by the action of enteropepsidase. SYN protrypsin.

trypt·a·mine (trip′tă-mēn, -min). A decarboxylation product of L-tryptophan that occurs in plants and certain foods (e.g., cheese). It raises the blood pressure through vasoconstrictor action, by the release of norepinephrine at postganglionic sympathetic nerve endings, and is believed to be one of the agents responsible for hypertensive episodes following therapy with monoamine oxidase inhibitors (e.g., pargyline hydrochloride).

trypt·a·mine-stro·phan·thi·din (trip′ta-mēn-strō-fan′thi-din). A semisynthetic cardiac glycoside that is a condensation product of strophanthidin and tryptamine; given orally, it has a rapid onset and short duration of cardiac action.

tryp·tic (trip′tik). Relating to trypsin, as t. digestion.

tryp·tone (trip′tōn). A peptone produced by proteolytic digestion with trypsin.

tryp·to·ne·mia (trip-tō-nē′mē-ă). The presence of tryptone in the circulating blood.

tryp·to·phan (Trp, W) (trip′tō-fan). 2-Amino-3-(3-indolyl)-propionic acid; the L-isomer is a component of proteins; a nutritionally essential amino acid.

t. decarboxylase, SYN aromatic D-amino acid decarboxylase.

t. desmolase, SYN t. synthase.

t. 2,3-dioxygenase, an oxidoreductase catalyzing the reaction of L-t. and O_2 to produce L-N-formylkynurenine; an adaptive enzyme, the level (in the liver) being controlled by adrenal hormones; a step in t. catabolism; also, a step in the synthesis of NAD^+ from t. SYN pyrrolase, t. oxygenase, t. pyrrolase, tryptophanase (1).

t. oxygenase, SYN t. 2,3-dioxygenase.

t. pyrrolase, SYN t. 2,3-dioxygenase.

t. synthase, a nonmammalian hydro-lyase condensing L-serine indole-3-glycerol phosphate to produce L-tryptophan and glyceraldehyde phosphate; pyridoxal phosphate is required; it will also react L-serine with indole. SYN t. desmolase, t. synthetase.

t. synthetase, SYN t. synthase.

tryp·to·pha·nase (trip′to-fă-nās). 1. SYN *tryptophan* 2,3-dioxygenase. 2. An enzyme found in bacteria that catalyzes the cleavage of L-tryptophan to indole, pyruvic acid, and ammonia; pyridoxal phosphate is a coenzyme.

tryp·to·pha·nu·ria (trip′tō-fă-noo′rē-ă). Enhanced urinary excretion of tryptophan.

t. with dwarfism [MIM*276100], a syndrome of dwarfism, mental defect, cutaneous photosensitivity, and gait disturbance associated with t.; autosomal recessive inheritance.

tset·se (tset′sē, tsē′tsē). SEE *Glossina.* [S. African native name]

TSH Abbreviation for thyroid-stimulating *hormone.*

TSH-RF Abbreviation for thyroid-stimulating hormone-releasing *factor.*

TSI Abbreviation for thyroid-stimulating *immunoglobulins,* under *immunoglobulin.*

TSS Abbreviation for toxic shock *syndrome.*

TSTA Abbreviation for tumor-specific transplantation *antigens,* under *antigen.*

TTP Abbreviation for ribothymidine 5′-triphosphate.

TTP-HUS Abbreviation for thrombotic thrombocytopenic purpura and hemolytic uremic syndrome. SEE thrombotic thrombocytopenic *purpura,* hemolytic uremic *syndrome.*

TTX Abbreviation for tetrodotoxin.

T.U. Abbreviation for toxic *unit* or toxin *unit.*

tu·a·mi·no·hep·tane (too′am-i-nō-hep′tān). A sympathomimetic volatile amine, used by inhalation as a nasal decongestant; available also as t. sulfate, with the same actions, and more potent as a vasoconstrictor than ephedrine.

tu·ba, gen. and pl. **tu·bae** (too′bă, too′bē) [TA]. SYN tube. [L. a straight trumpet]

t. acus′tica, SYN pharyngotympanic (auditory) *tube.*

t. auditi′va [TA], SYN pharyngotympanic (auditory) *tube.*

t. audito′ria, ✯official alternate term for pharyngotympanic (auditory) *tube,* pharyngotympanic (auditory) *tube.*

t. eustachia′na, t. eusta′chii, SYN pharyngotympanic (auditory) *tube.*

t. fallopia′na, t. fallo′pii, SYN uterine *tube.*

t. uteri′na [TA], SYN uterine *tube.*

tub·age (too′baj). Introduction of a tube into a canal. SEE ALSO intubation.

tub·al (too′băl). Relating to a tube, especially the uterine tube.

tu·ba·tor·sion (too-bă-tōr′shŭn). SYN tubotorsion.

TUBE

tube (toob) [TA]. 1. A hollow cylindrical structure or canal. 2. A hollow cylinder or pipe. SYN tuba [TA]. [L. *tubus*]

Abbott t., SYN Miller-Abbott t.

air t., the trachea, or a bronchus or any of its branches conveying air to the lungs.

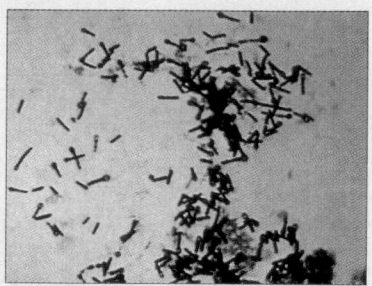

Gram stain: with spores characteristic of *Clostridium tetani*

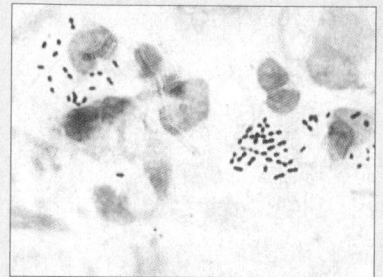

Gram stain: smear of purulent sputum demonstrating Gram-positive diplococci, characteristic of *Streptococcus pneumoniae*

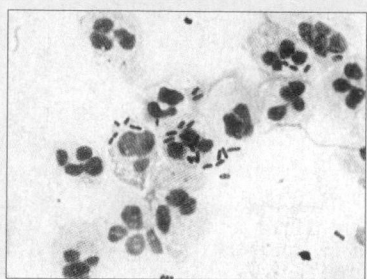

Gram stain: smear of urine sediment from a case of acute cystitis; note the several Gram-negative bacilli *(Escherichia coli)*

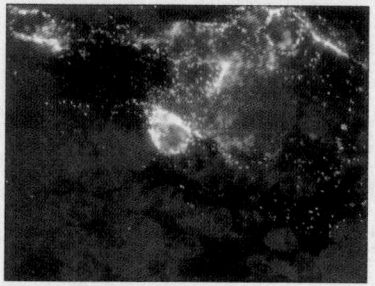

immunofluorescence: *Chlamydia trachomatis* cervicitis

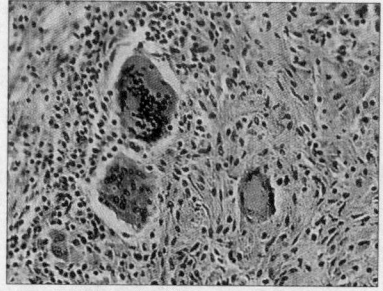

hematoxylin and eosin stain: liver section through a tuberculoma; note characteristic Langhans giant cells

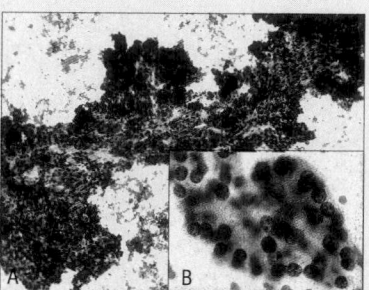

pancreatic acinar tissue: (A) low power, (B) high power showing acinar pattern

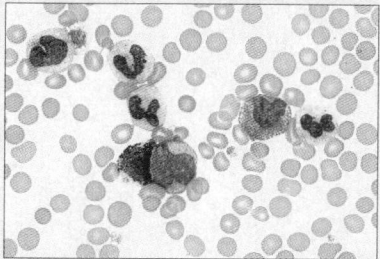

Wright-Giemsa stain: chronic myelocytic leukemia (CML) with leukocytosis; 250 ×

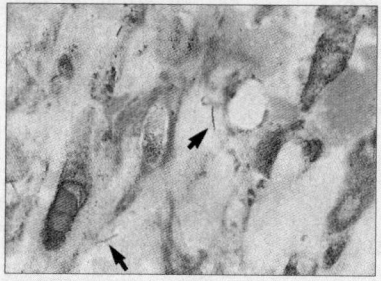

Warthin-Starry stain: *Treponema pallidum* in placenta from case of congenital syphilis, note tight spiral coils of spirochete (arrows); 1000 ×

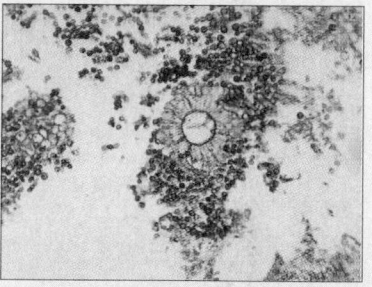

periodic acid-Schiff stain (PAS): fruiting body of *Aspergillus* in aspirate of fungus ball lesion of the lung

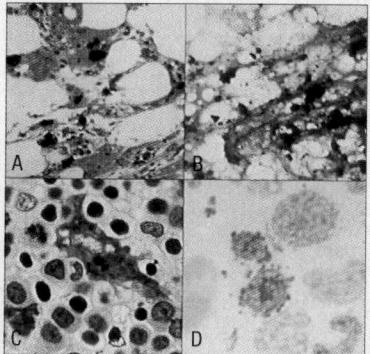

prussian blue stain: marrow clot sections (A,B) and smears (C,D) of a patient with refractory anemia; blue stain represents hemosiderin

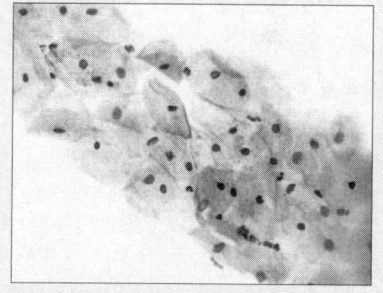

Papanicolaou stain: normal exfoliated cervical squamous epithelial cells in Pap smear

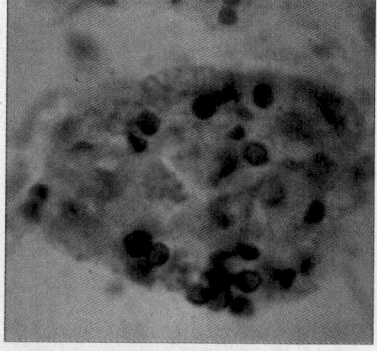

methenamine silver stain: *Pneumocystis carinii* in lung tissue; 1000 ×

Diseases/Abnormalities

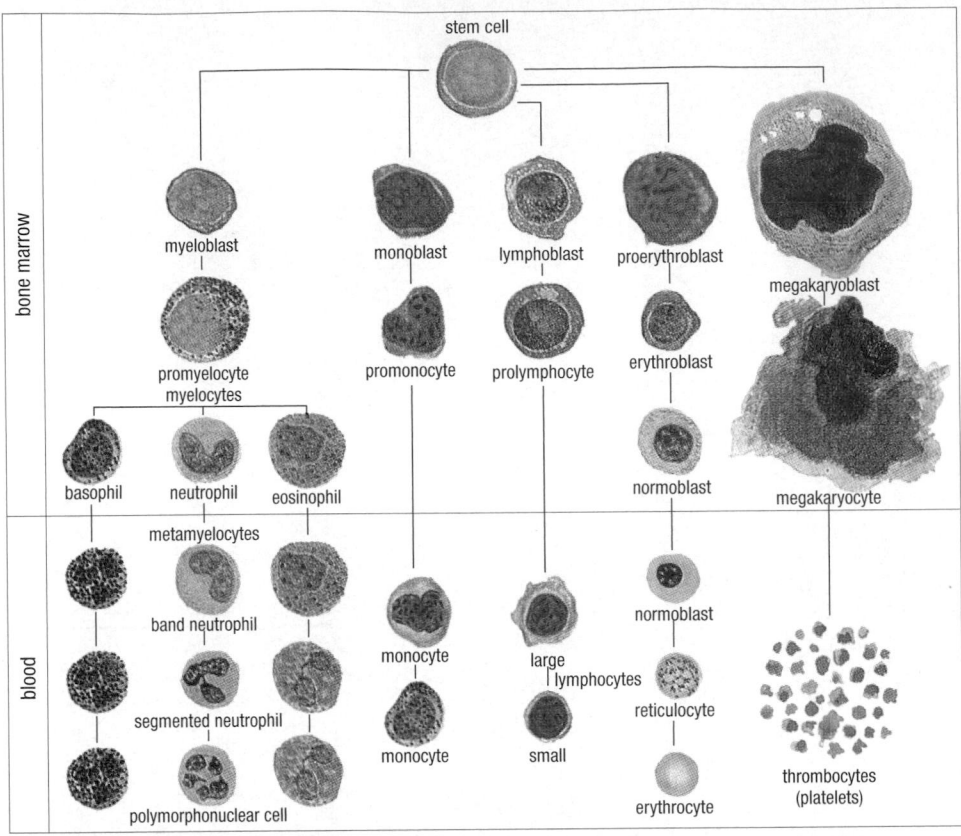

blood cells: developmental series (simplified scheme)

neutrophilic myelocyte: (peroxidase stain, 1325 ×); (ag) perioxidase-positive azurophils; (sg) specific granules; (is) immature specific granules; (G) Golgi region; (er) rough endoplasmic reticulum; (pn) perinuclear cisterna; (Gc) Golgi cisterna; (N) nucleus

red blood cells display a central clear region that represents the thinnest area of the biconcave disc; neutrophils display a somewhat granular cytoplasm and lobulated nuclei (arrows, right); eosinophils have large pink granules and sausage-shaped nuclei (arrow); basophils are characterized by their dense, dark, granules; monocytes are characterized by their large size, eccentric kidney-shaped nucleus, and lack of specific granules; lymphocytes are small cells that possess a single large, eccentrically located nucleus, and a narrow rim of light blue cytoplasm

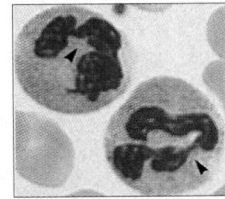

neutrophil, 1325 ×

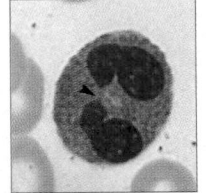

eosinophil, 1325 ×

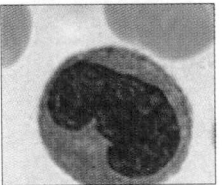

monocyte, 1325 ×

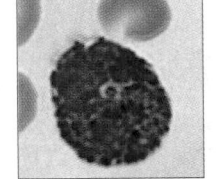

basophil, 1325 ×

erythroblasts: in iron-deficient blood

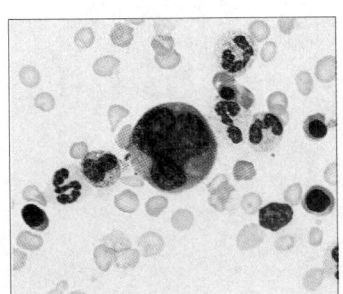

megakaryoblast

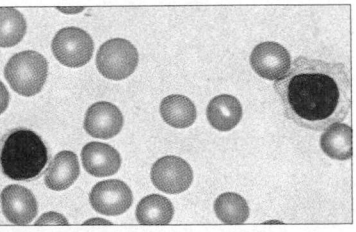

lymphocytes: small (left) and large (right) with erythrocytes in stained smear of normal blood

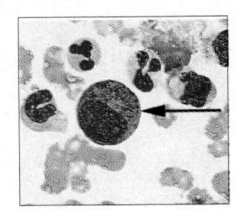

promyelocyte (arrow): bone marrow, 250 ×, Wright-Giemsa stain

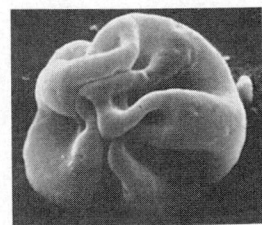

reticulocyte: as seen by scanning electron microscope

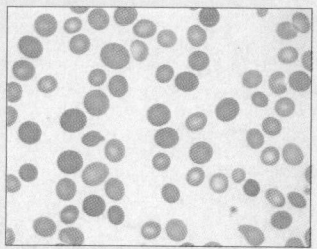

anisocytosis: PB; 250 ×, Wright-Giemsa stain

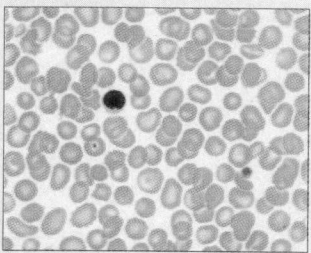

macrocytosis: peripheral blood from newborn; 250 ×, Wright-Giemsa stain

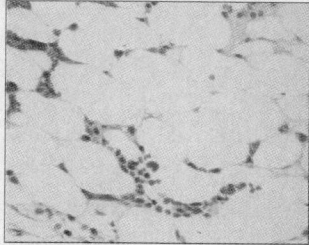

aplastic anemia: marrow smear showing lymphocytes and absence of red cell, white cell, and platelet precursors

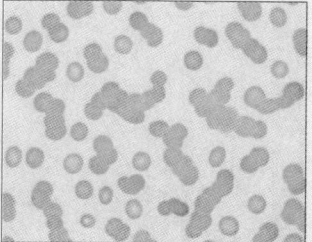

rouleaux: erythrocytes are stacked like coins; patient has multiple myeloma

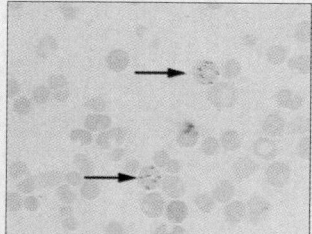

reticulocyte (arrows): supravital staining with brilliant cresyl blue; peripheral blood, 250 ×

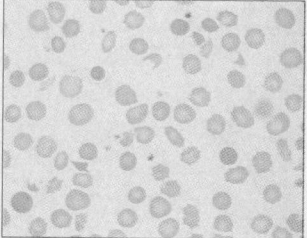

poikilocytosis: with various red blood cell types; 250 ×, Wright-Giemsa stain

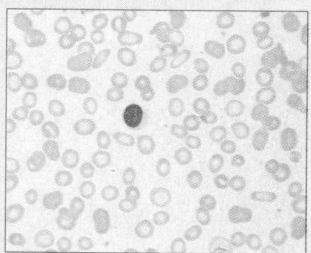

microcytic, hypochromic anemia: peripheral blood; 250 ×, Wright-Giemsa stain

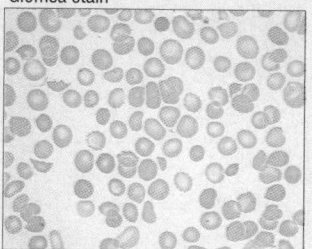

hemolytic anemia: showing poikilocytosis and absence of platelets, but no signs of hemolysis

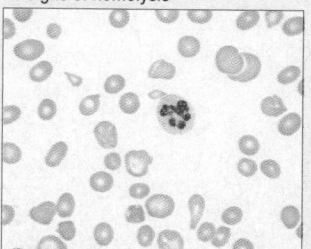

pernicious anemia: peripheral blood smear showing oval macrocytes and hypersegmented neutrophil nucleus

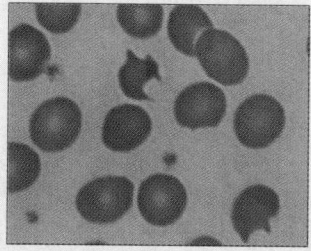

Heinz bodies: bite cells seen in Heinz-body-mediated hemolysis

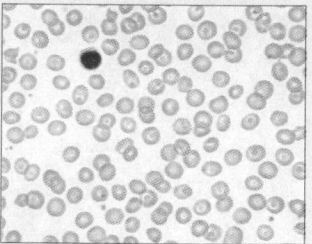

microcytosis: shown in heterozygous thalassemia (thalassemia minor)

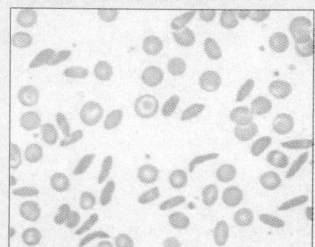

sickle cell anemia: showing poikilocytosis; peripheral blood; 250 ×, Wright-Giemsa stain

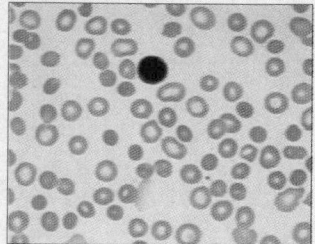

spherocytosis: blood smear; 250 ×, Wright-Giemsa stain

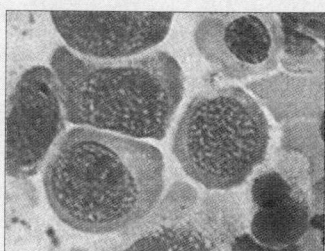

pernicious anemia: in bone marrow

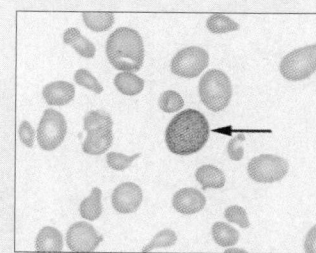

erythrocyte with **basophilic stippling:** 250 ×, Wright-Giemsa stain

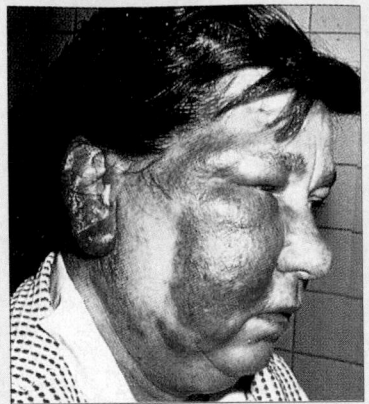

erysipelas

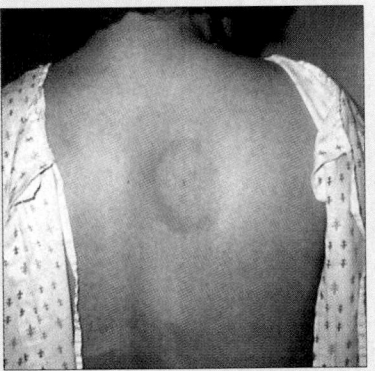

Lyme disease (erythema chronicum migrans)

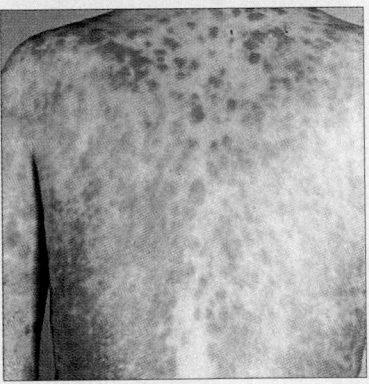

lepromatous leprosy

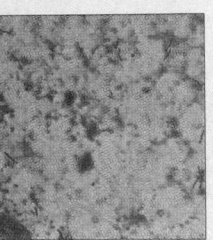

Mycobacterium tuberculosis

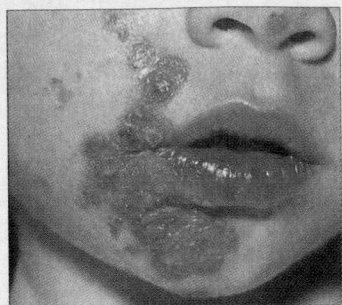

impetigo

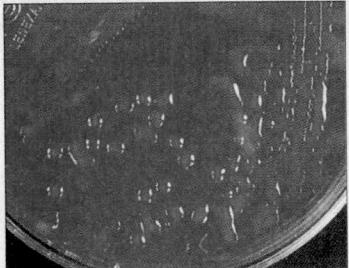

Pseudomonas: growing on blood agar

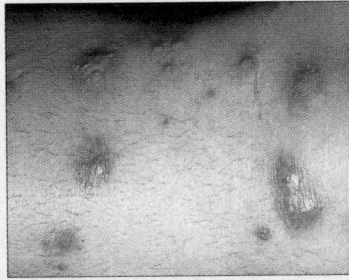

folliculitis: with multiple furuncles

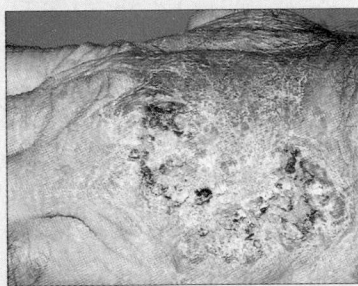

staphylococci: blastomycosis-like pyoderma

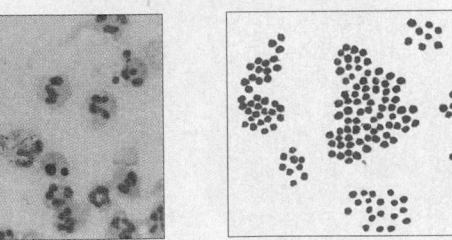

gonococci: Gram stain   **staphylococci**

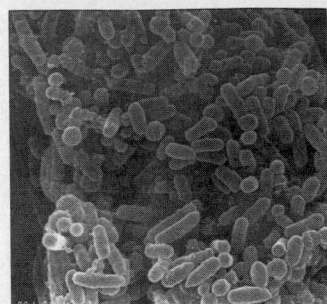

bacterial cell: scanning electron microscopy; 5000 ×

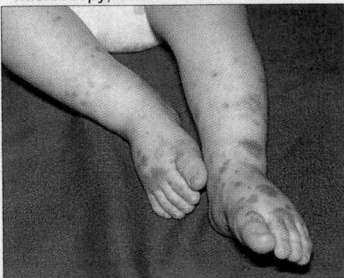

Henoch-Schönlein purpura

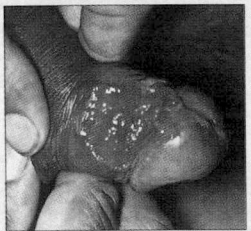

syphilis (primary chancre)

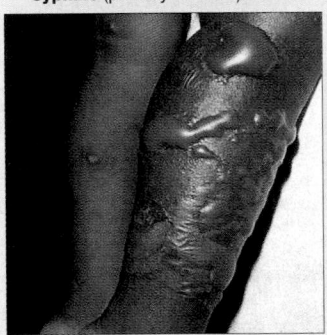

streptococci: cellulitis with bullous lesions

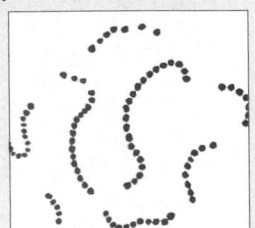

streptococci

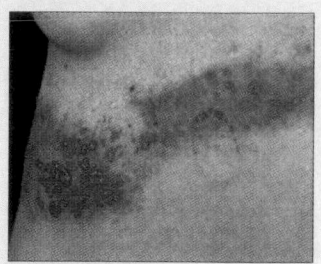

herpes zoster

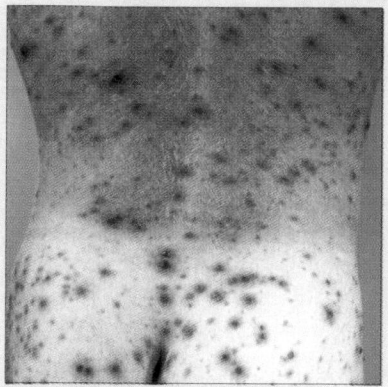

hemorrhagic varicella (chickenpox)

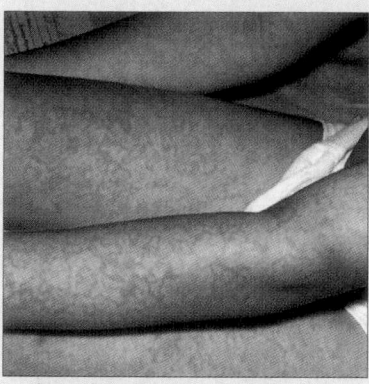

erythema infectiosum

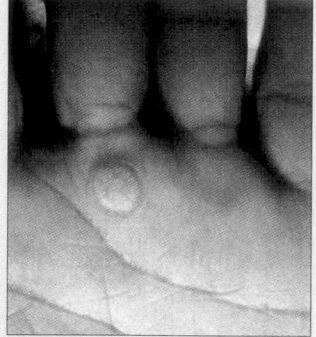

palmar wart

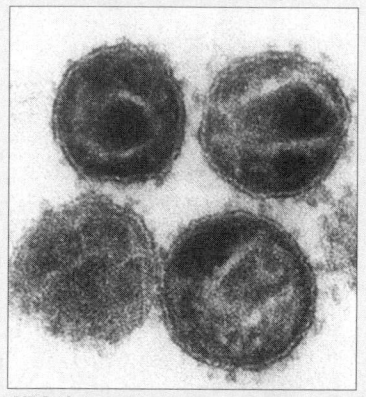

AIDS virus

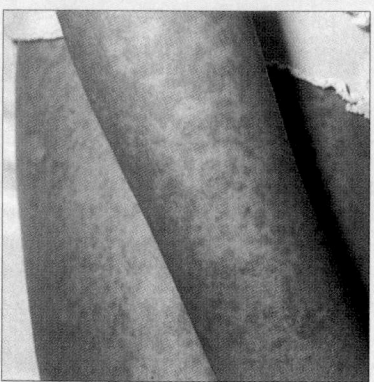

infectious mononucleosis

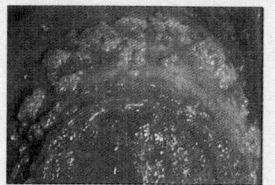

condyloma acuminatum (genital wart)

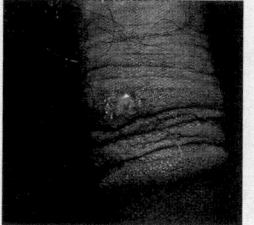

genital herpes (HSV-2)

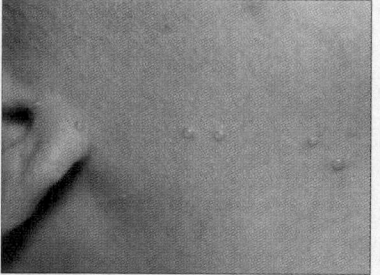

molluscum contagiosum

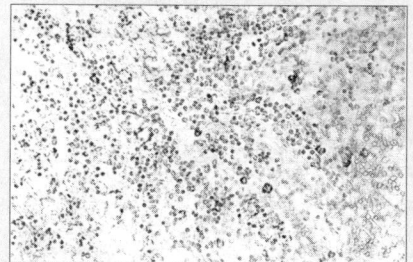

influenza A virus: Rhesus monkey kidney cells

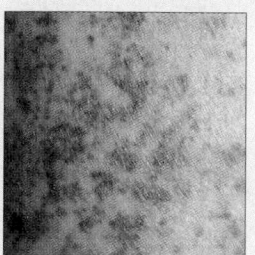

hepatitis C: showing petechial eruption

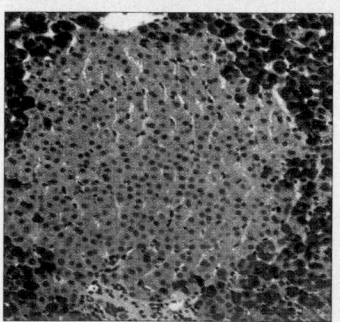

hepatitis B

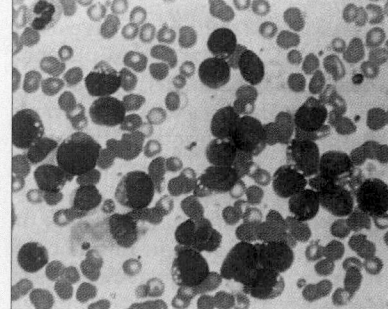

Burkitt's lymphoma

Diseases/Abnormalities

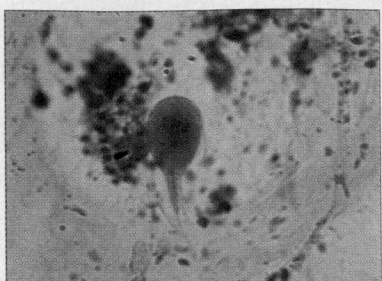

Giardia lamblia: trophozoite; trichrome, 400×

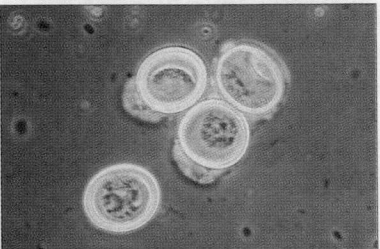

Taenia: phase contrast microscopy of four eggs

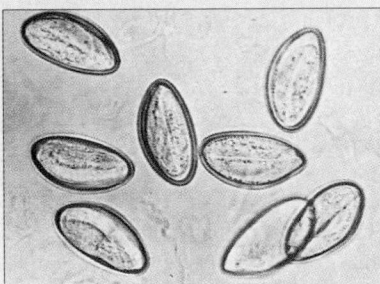

pinworm ova: transparent tape preparation

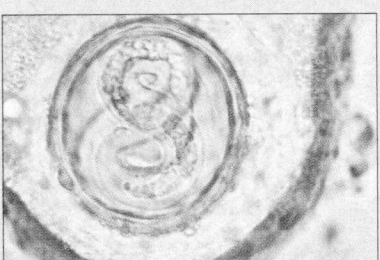

Ascaris lumbricoides: egg containing larvae

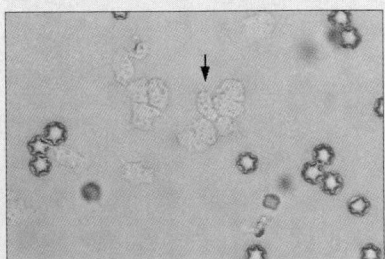

Acanthamoeba: trophozoites (arrow) and cysts; trypan blue; 40×

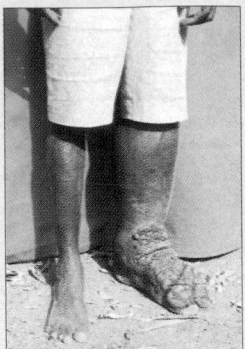

elephantiasis: with verrucous hyperplasia

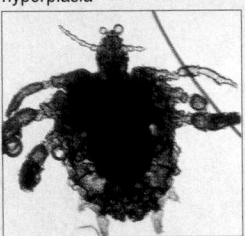

Pthirus pubis (adult female)

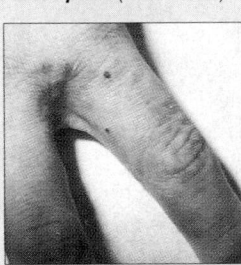

scabies: pruritic lesions

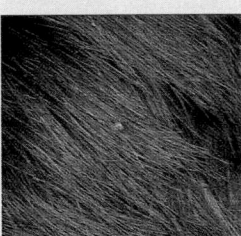

pediculosis capitis (head lice)

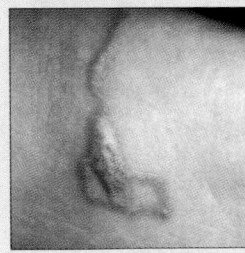

cutaneous larva migrans: serpiginous track with bulla formation on sole of foot

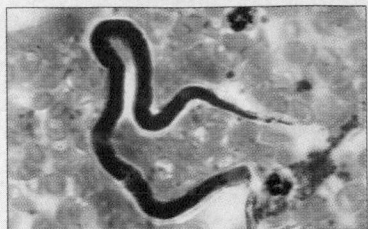

Brugia malayi: microfilaria; 300×

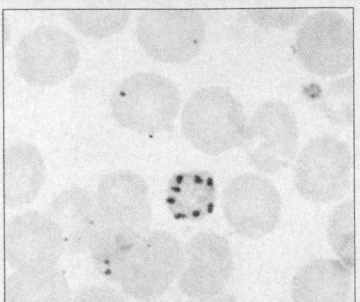

Plasmodium malariae: schizont with fewer than 13 segments in erythrocyte

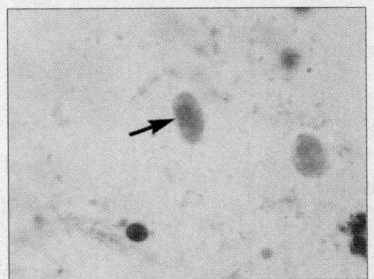

Trichomonas hominis: stool smear, trichrome, 400×

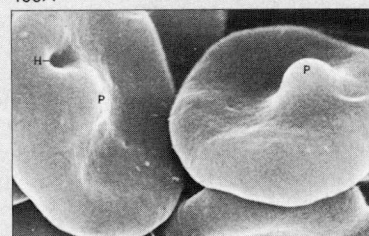

babesia: two infected erythrocytes; (H) perforation, (P) protrusion

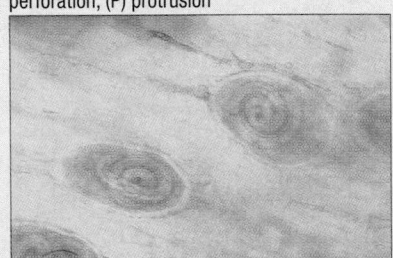

Trichinella: coiled larvae in laboratory mouse; unstained; 160×

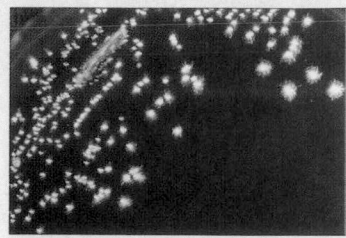

Candida albicans: showing footlike extensions of the colonies on the surface of 5% sheep blood agar

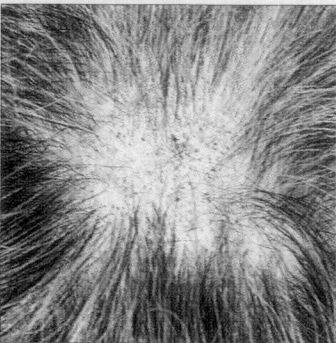

tinea capitis: black dot type; caused by *Trichophyton tonsurans*

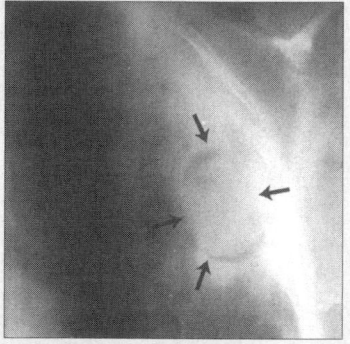

aspergilloma: tomogram of fungal infection in a tuberculous lung cavity

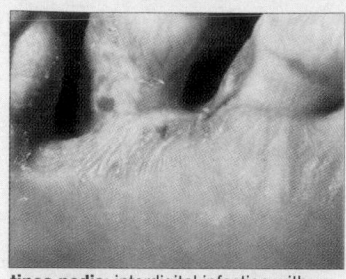

tinea pedis: interdigital infection with *Trichophyton mentagrophytes*

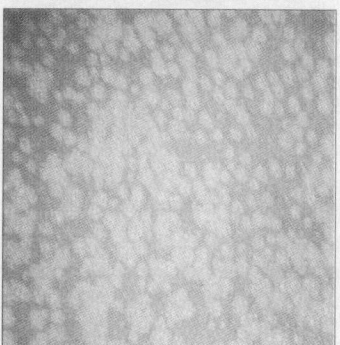

tinea versicolor: close-up view of hypopigmented macules on the back

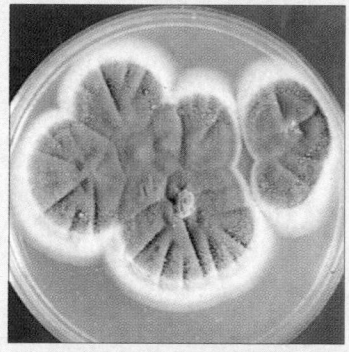

Alternaria *(Penicillium):* after 6 days' growth

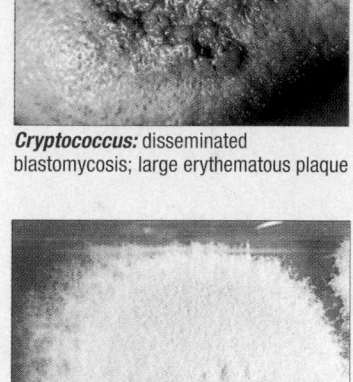

tinea corporis (ringworm)

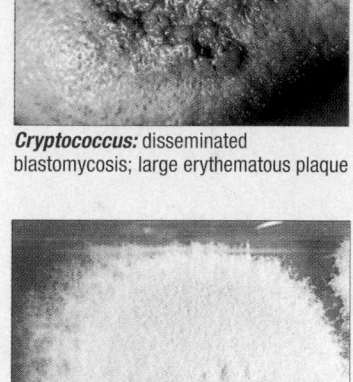

Cryptococcus: disseminated blastomycosis; large erythematous plaque

Microsporum gypseum: after 6 days' incubation

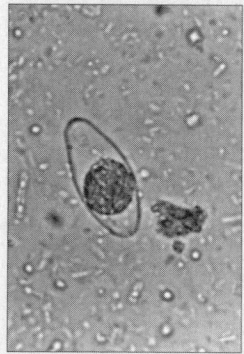

Isospora belli: immature oocyst

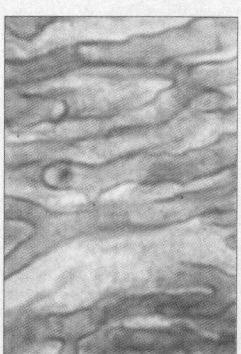

Aspergillus hyphae: in tissue; periodic acid-Schiff stain

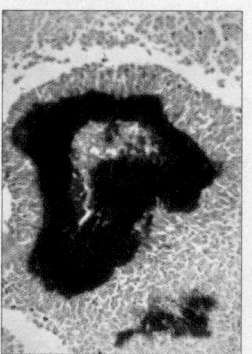

mycetoma granule: in tissue; Brown and Brenn stain

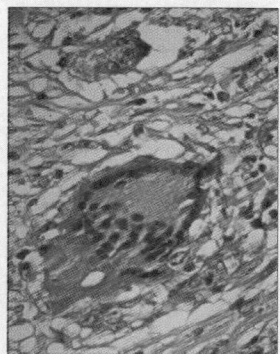

histoplasmosis: multinucleated giant cell in lung of patient with histoplasmosis

Diseases/Abnormalities

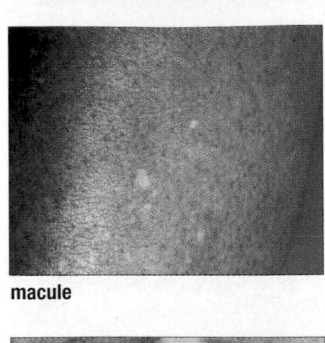

macule

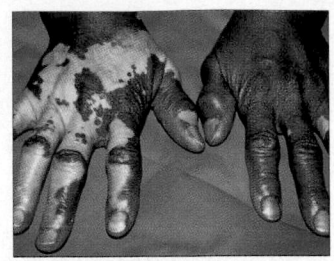

patch

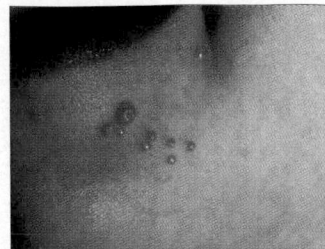

papule

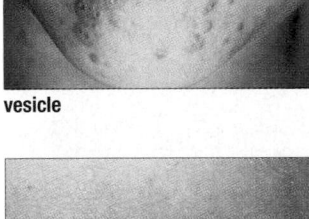
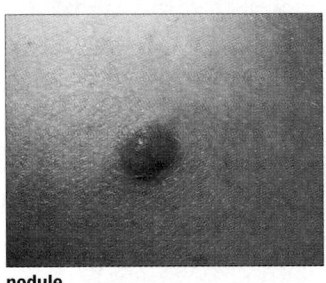

vesicle

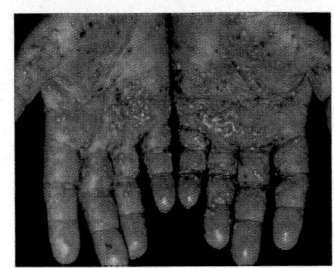

pustule

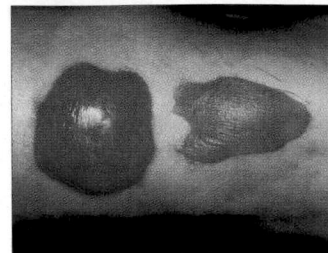

bulla

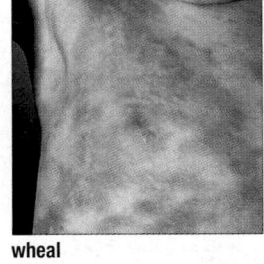

nodule

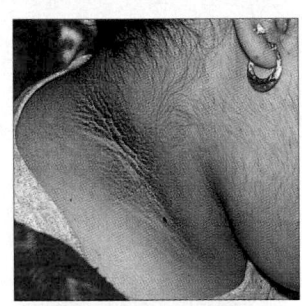

acanthosis nigricans (AN)

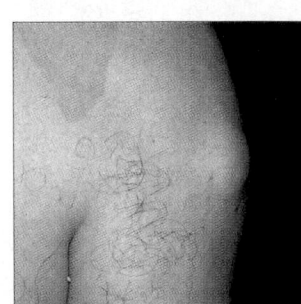

cyst: pilomatricoma

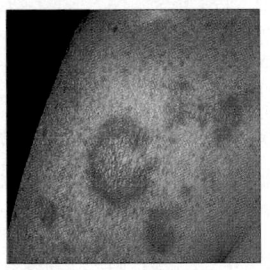

wheal

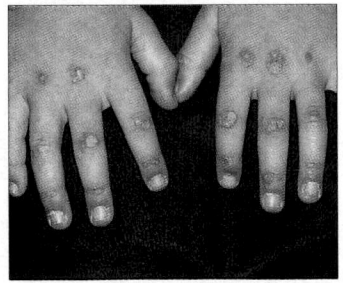

plaque

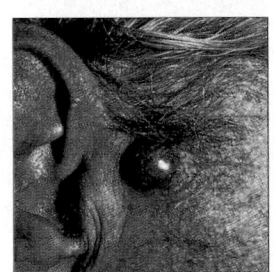

tumor

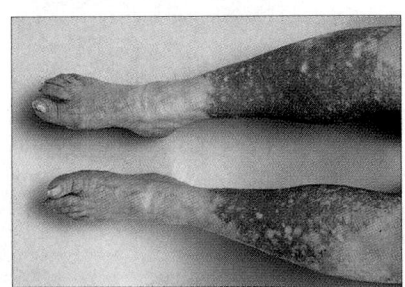

vitiligo: depigmented macules; (brown pigment on legs is patient's normal skin color)

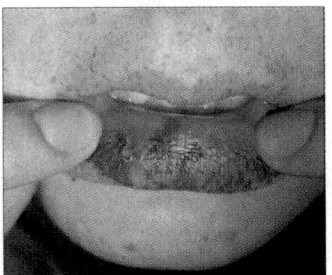

dermatomyositis: Gottron papules on joints of fingers

Peutz-Jeghers syndrome

secondary lesions

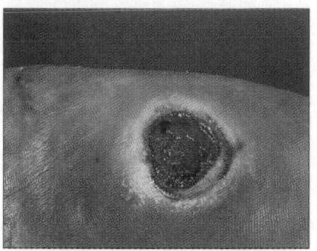

ulcer

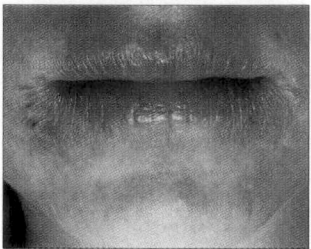

fissure

vascular lesions

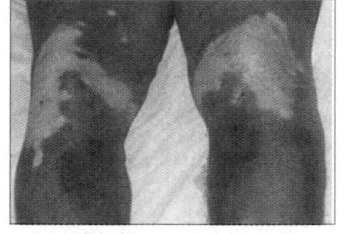

purpura fulminans

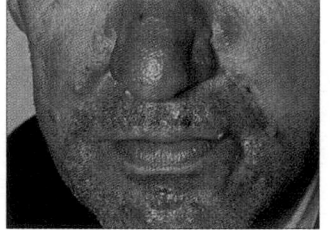

rosacea

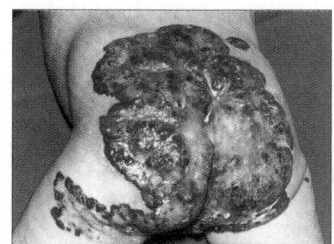

cavernous hemangioma

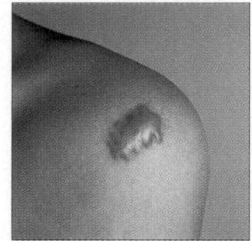

keloid

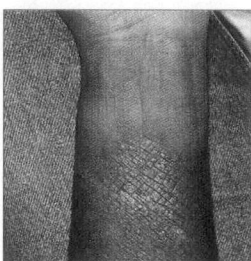

lichenification: chronic eczematous dermatitis (ED)

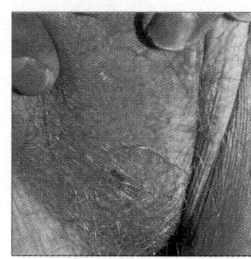

erosion

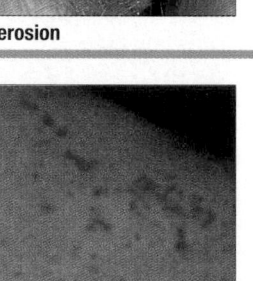

petechia

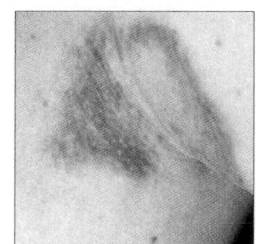

ecchymosis

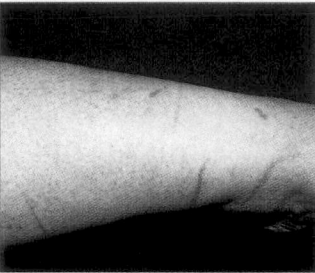

excoriation: cat scratches in patient with lichen planus

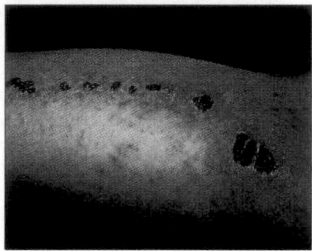

crust

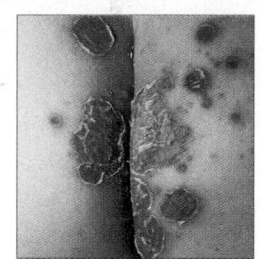

scale

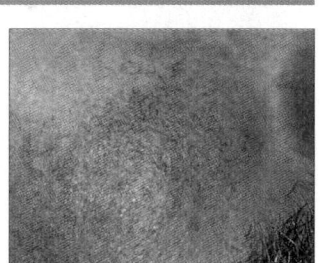

telangiectasia

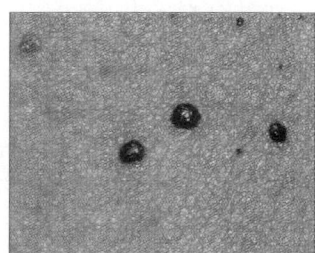

cherry angioma

Diseases/Abnormalities

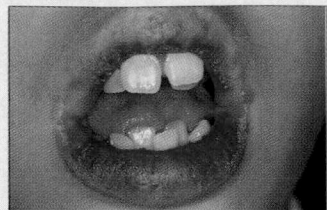

exfoliative cheilitis

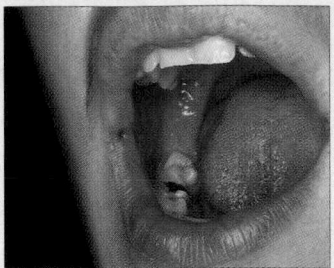

commissural lip pits

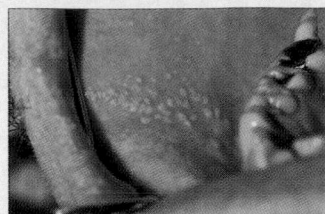

Fordyce granules

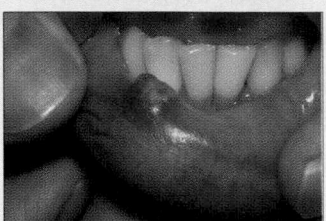

mucocele

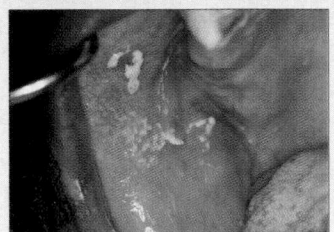

candidiasis

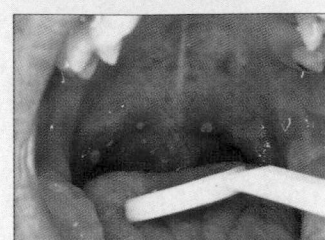

herpangina (coxsackievirus)

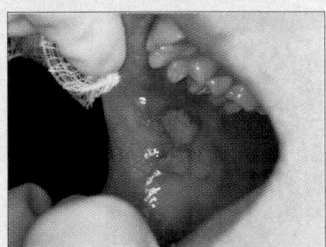

Behçet disease

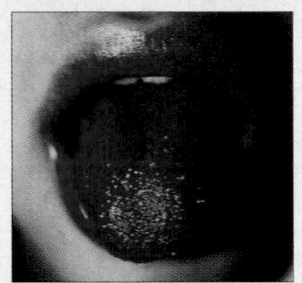

strawberry tongue: associated with Kawasaki disease

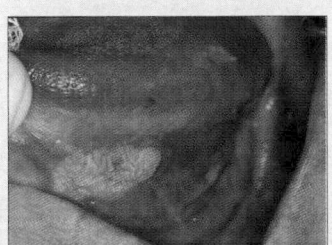

leukoplakia: with mild epithelial dysplasia

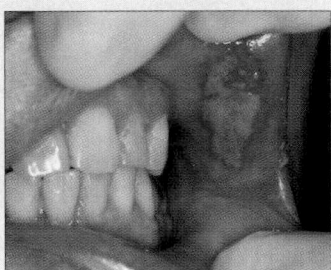

contact stomatitis: due to acrylic

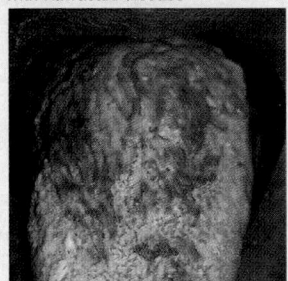

hairy tongue (glossotrichia)

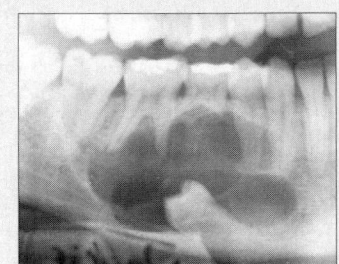

ameloblastoma: large multilocular ("soap bubble") lesion of the mandible

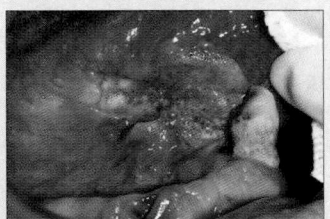

squamous cell carcinoma

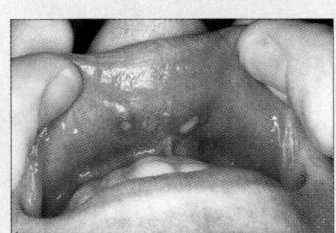

aphthous ulcerations (canker sores)

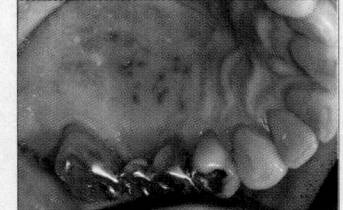

recurrent herpetic stomatitis

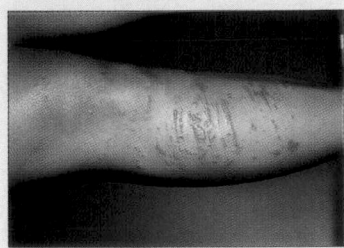

contact dermatitis (poison ivy)

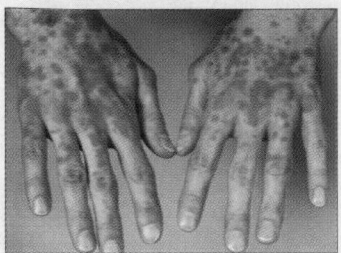

polymorphic light eruption

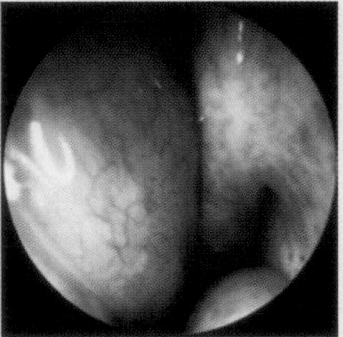

nasal polyps: associated with chronic nasal allergy; nasal illuminator view

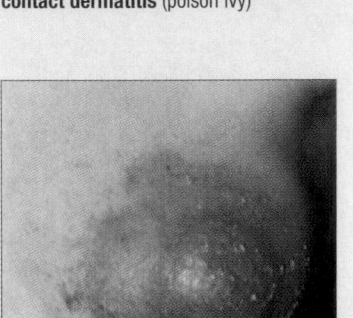

acute allergic contact dermatitis: Paget disease of nipple

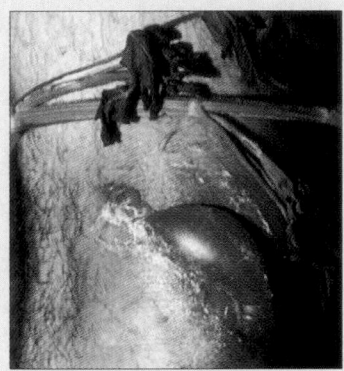

acute photodermatitis: (phototoxic type, phytophotodermatitis); bullous lesion formed after hogweed (plant shown) rubbed against skin, which was then exposed to sunlight

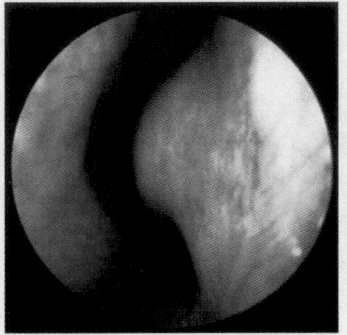

allergic rhinitis (rhinoscopic view)

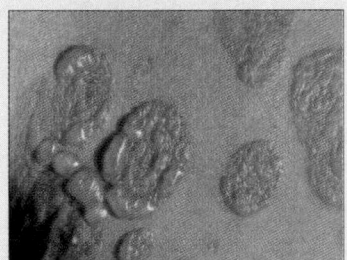

dermatitis herpetiformis

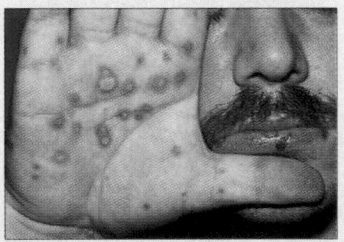

erythema multiforme minor: in patient with recurrent herpes simplex virus (HSV) infection

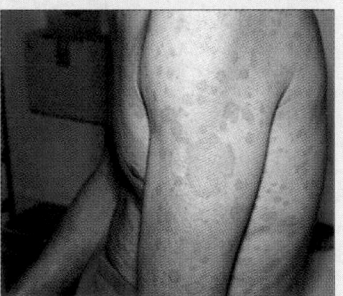

urticarial drug eruption

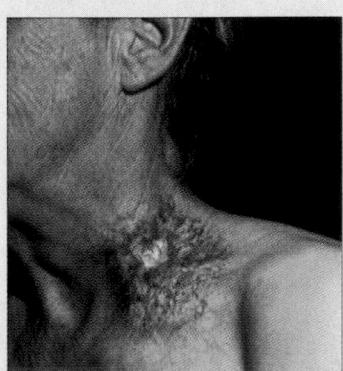

radiodermatitis: chronic ulceration

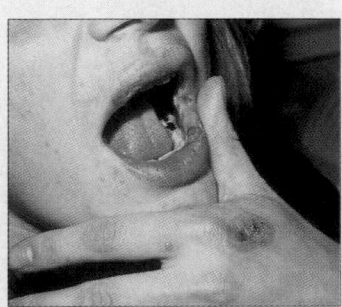

Stevens-Johnson syndrome (erythema multiforme major)

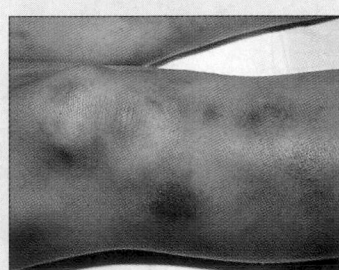

erythema nodosum (EN)

Diseases/Abnormalities

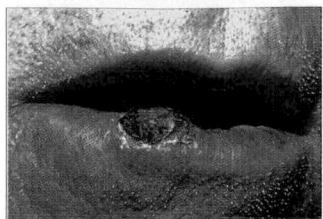

squamous cell carcinoma (lip)

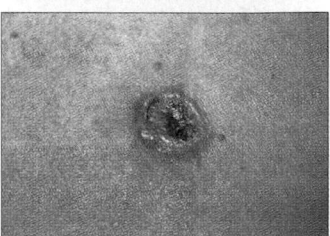

basal cell carcinoma

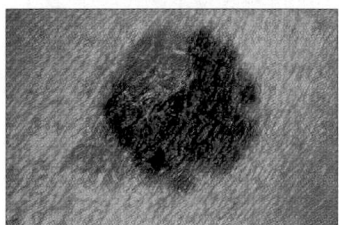

malignant melanoma

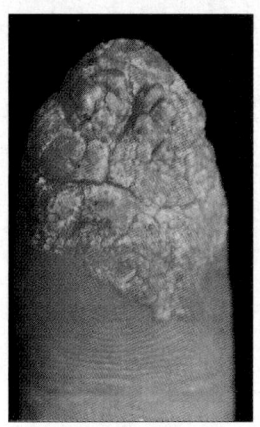

Bowen disease: squamous cell carcinoma in situ on fingertip

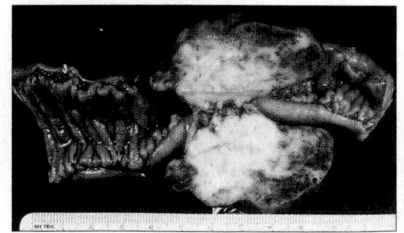

stromal tumor: malignant tumor of the bowel

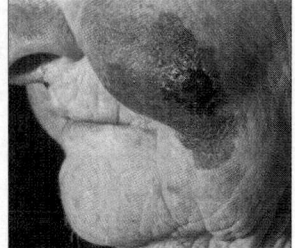

lentigo maligna melanoma

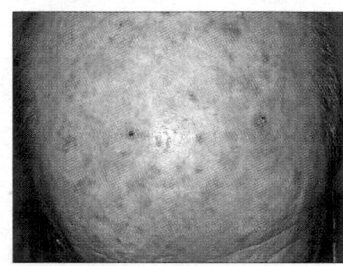

actinic keratosis: numerous keratoses over the scalp induced by chronic ultraviolet exposure

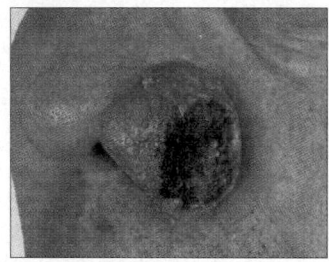

keratoacanthoma

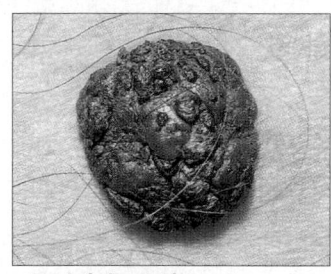

seborrheic keratosis

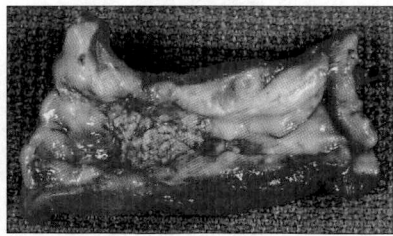

ulcerative squamous cell carcinoma: of the esophagus

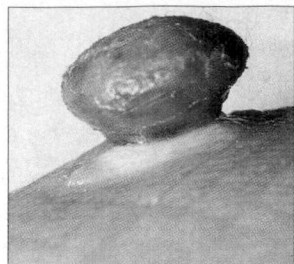

pyogenic granuloma

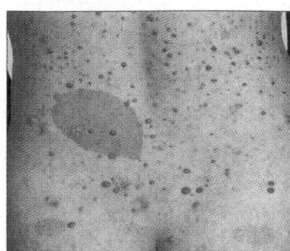

neurofibromatosis

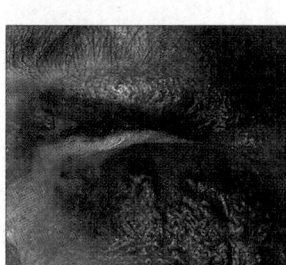

angiosarcoma: on left side of face

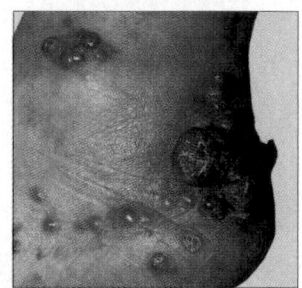

Kaposi sarcoma

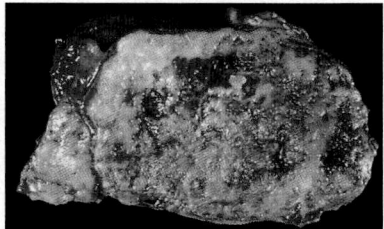

benign tumor of stomach

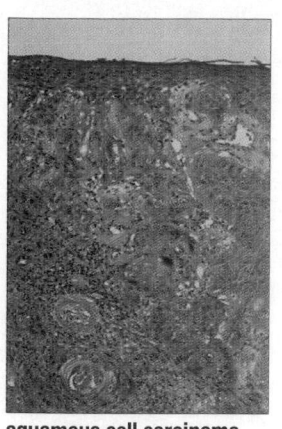

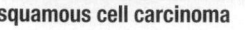

squamous cell carcinoma

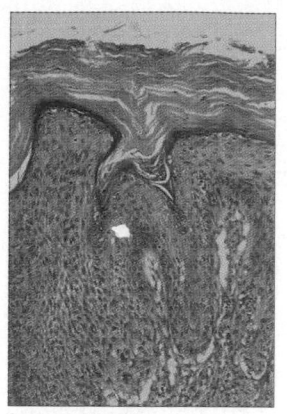

Bowen disease

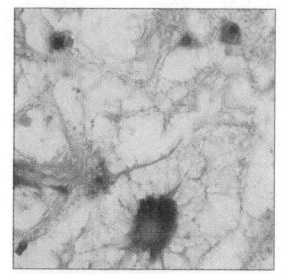

liposarcoma

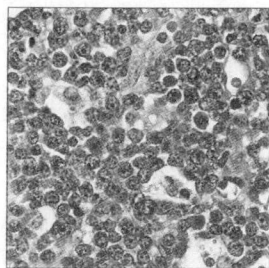

lymphoma

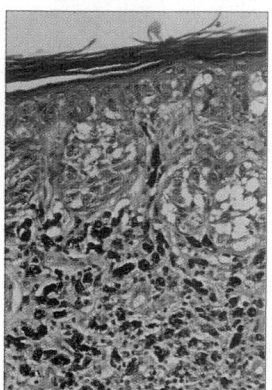

nodular melanoma

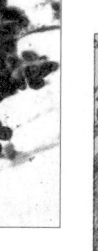

ependymoma: high power

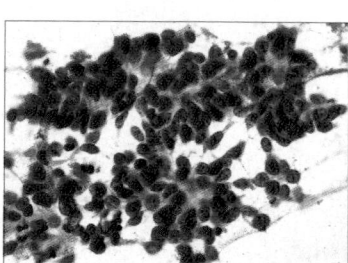

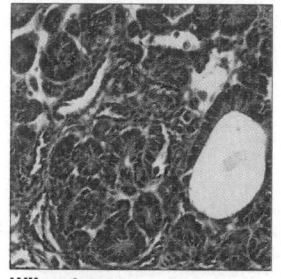

Wilms tumor

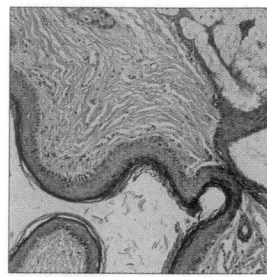

teratoma

actinic keratosis

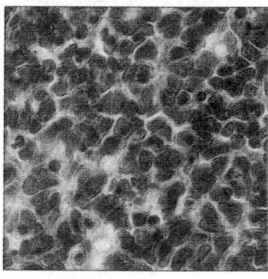

neuroblastoma

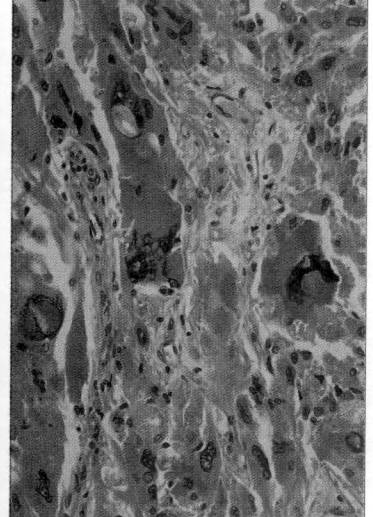

glioblastoma multiforme

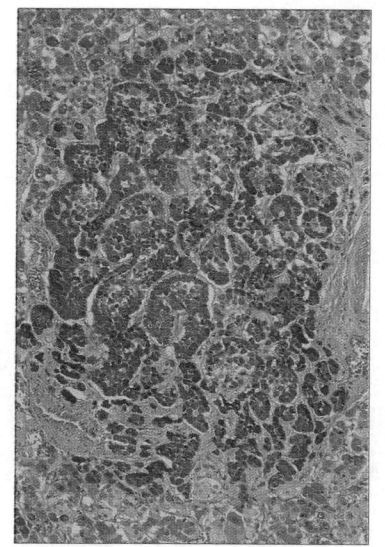

pituitary adenoma: microadenoma

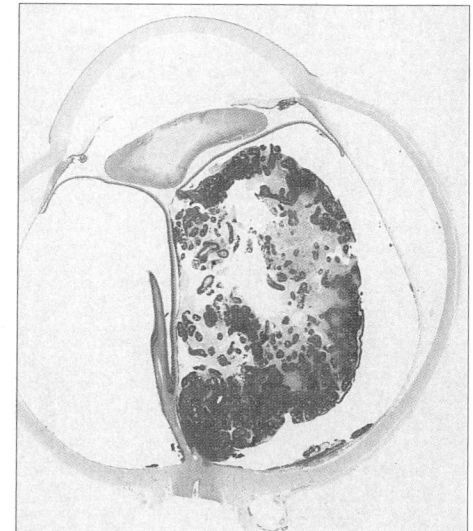

retinoblastoma

Diseases/Abnormalities

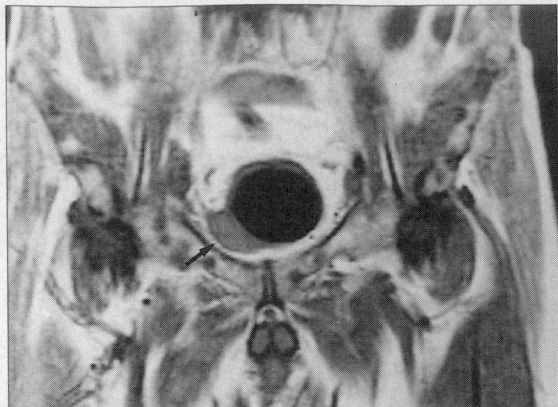

prostatic carcinoma: coronal T1-weighted MR image shows a mass (arrow) invading the floor of the bladder on the right side

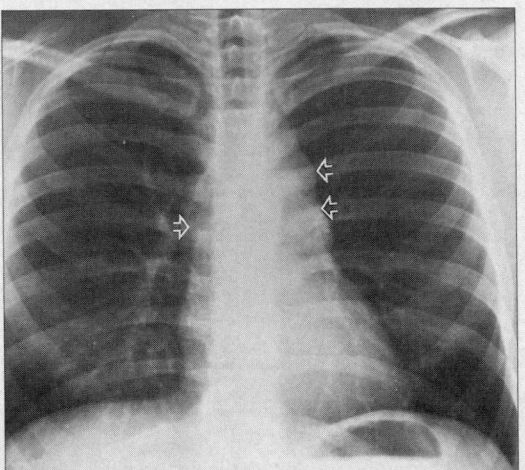

lymphoma: frontal radiograph shows a lobular mass in the mediastinum (arrows)

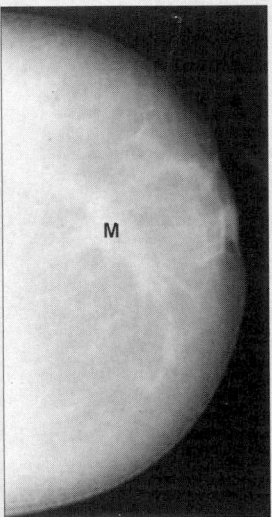

breast carinoma: mammogram revealing deep-seated carcinoma (M)

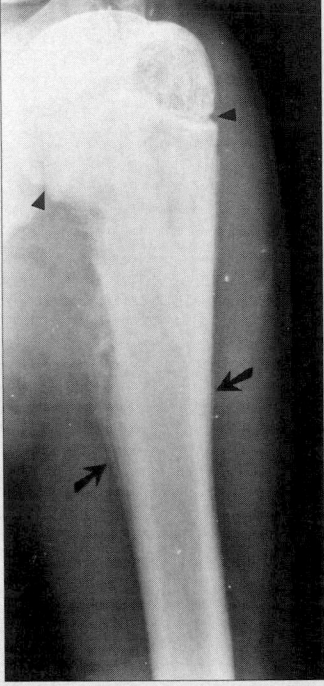

Ewing tumor: of the proximal humerus; note the interrupted laminated periosteal reaction (arrows)

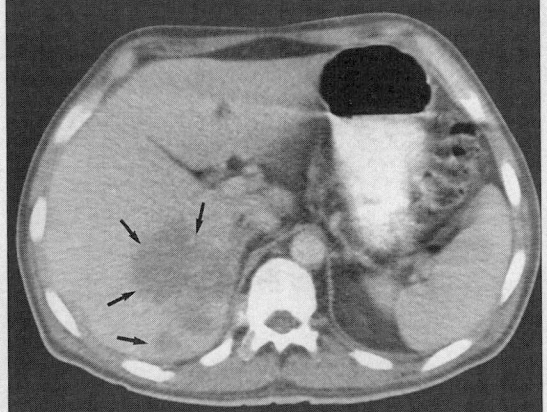

liver metastases: CT image of patient with renal carcinoma showing several lucent areas within the liver (arrows)

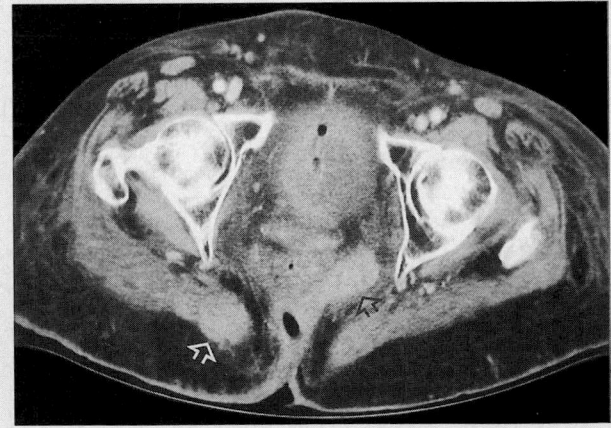

colon carcinoma: CT image of the pelvis shows recurrent perirectal masses (arrows)

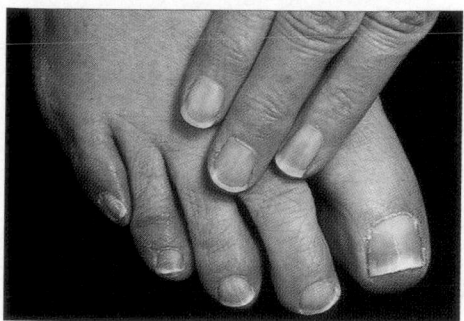

cyanosis: bluish color visible in nail beds

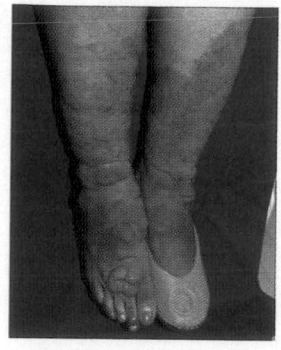

pretibial myxedema

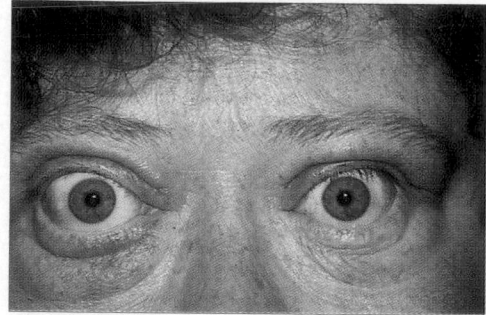

exophthalmos

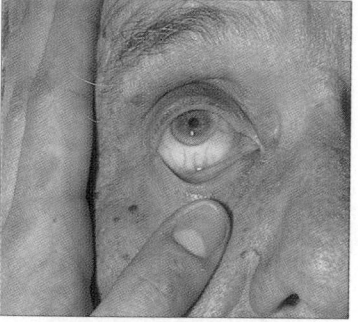

jaundice: note patient's yellow skin color in comparison to that of examiner's hand

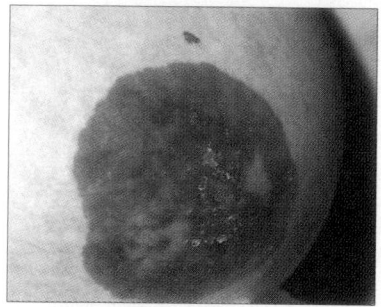

Paget disease: of the nipple

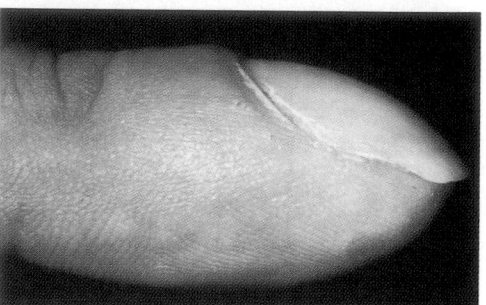

digital clubbing

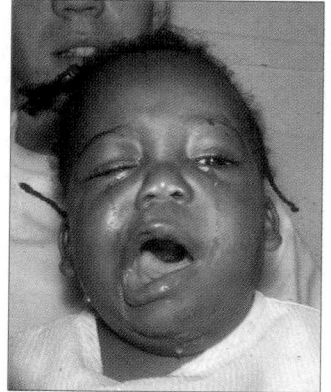

Bell palsy: peripheral (lower motor neuron) paralysis of the facial nerve

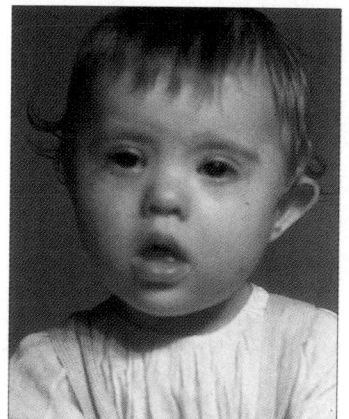

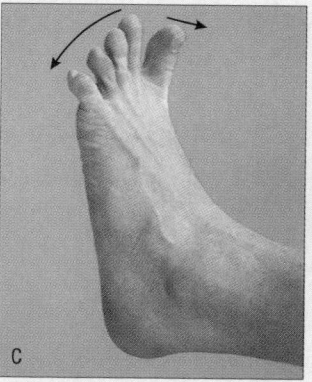

Down syndrome (Trisomy 21): (left) typical facial features including small rounded head, flattened nasal bridge, and relatively large tongue;
Brushfield spots: (above) strongly suggest Down syndrome

Diseases/Abnormalities

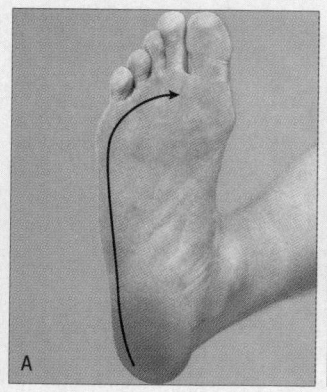

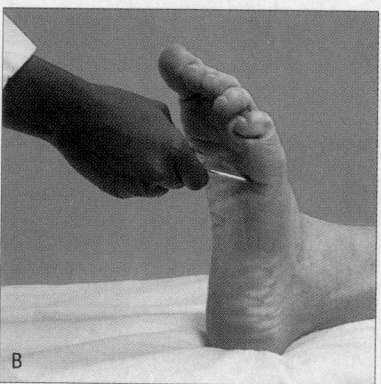

Babinski (extensor plantar) response: (A) lateral aspect of sole of foot is stroked from heel to ball of foot with a sharp object; (B) flexion of all toes is normal response; (C) extension of great toe, often with fanning of other toes, constitutes the Babinski sign; it often indicates a lesion of the motor cortex or of a pyramidal (corticospinal) tract.

microscopic unrinalysis

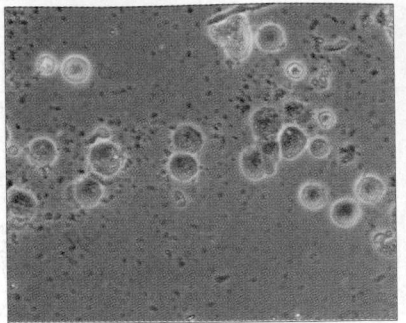

white blood cells (leukocytes)

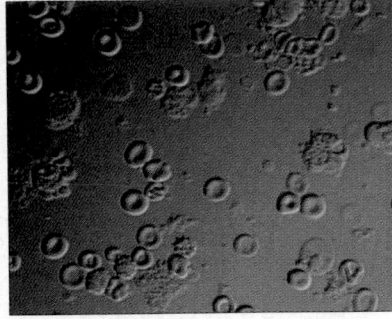

red blood cells

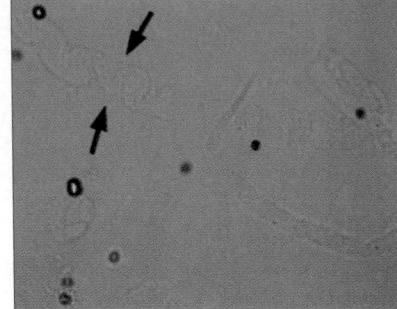

hyaline cast

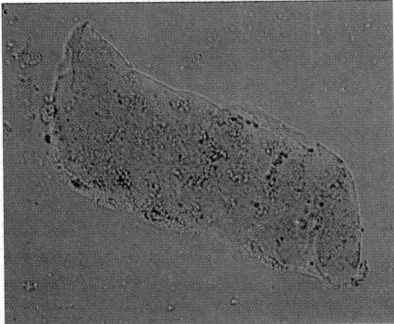

waxy cast

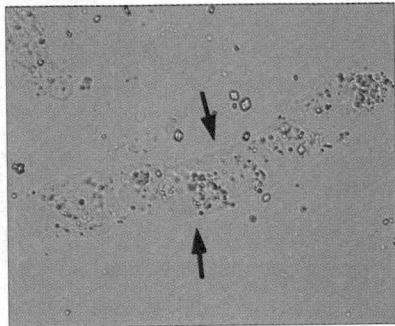

granular cast

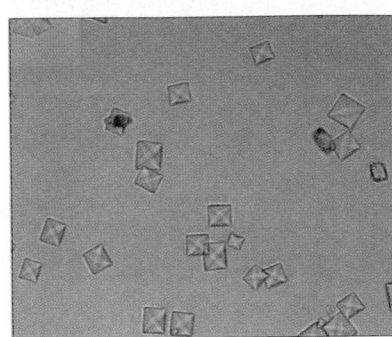

calcium oxalate crystals

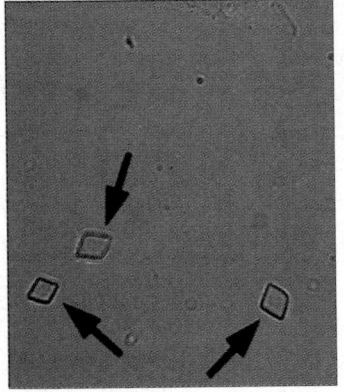

uric acid crystals

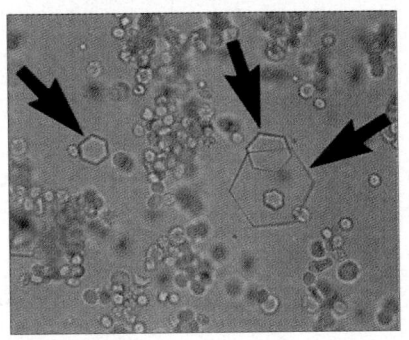

cystine crystals

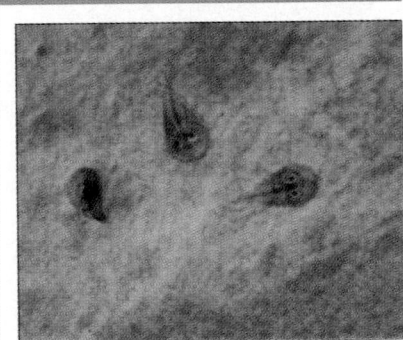

Giardia lamblia in fecal smear

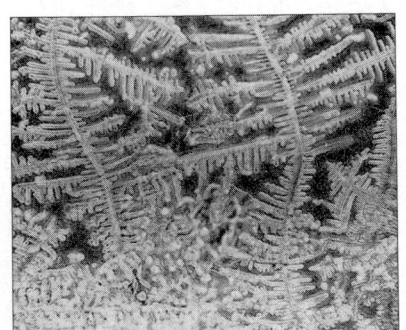

ferning of cervical mucus

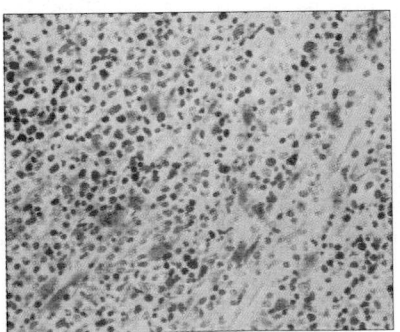

bone marrow aspirate showing iron stores

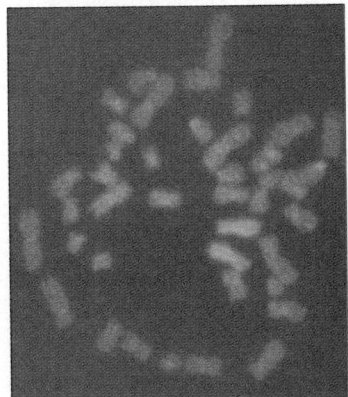

whole chromosome probe

auditory t., ☆official alternate term for pharyngotympanic (auditory) t.

Babcock t., a t. in which milk, after treatment with sulfuric acid, is centrifuged and its fat content then determined in a graduated neck.

Bouchut t., a short cylindrical t. used in intubation of the larynx.

bronchial t.'s, SYN bronchia.

Cantor t., a long, single-lumen intestinal t. with a sealed, mercury-filled rubber bag tip; used to decompress and/or stent the small intestine.

cardiac t., the primitive tubular heart in the embryo, before its division into chambers.

Carlen t., a double-lumen, flexible endobronchial t. used for bronchospirometry, for isolation of one lung to prevent contamination or secretions from the contralateral lung, or for ventilation of one lung.

cathode ray t. (CRT), an evacuated t. containing a beam of electrons which can be deflected to various parts of a fluorescent screen; used in the cathode ray oscilloscope.

Celestin t., a plastic t. introduced through a tumor in the esophagus; it permits swallowing of certain substances.

Coolidge t., an x-ray t., in which the cathode consists of a tungsten wire spiral surrounded by a focusing cup; the tungsten spiral is heated by an electric current; the quantity and quality of the x-rays so generated are regulated by varying the temperature of the cathode and the voltage between cathode and anode.

Crookes-Hittorf t., a simple evacuated t. containing a cathode, that emitted x-rays from the glass envelope when a current was passed through it; the type used by Roentgen to discover x-rays.

digestive t., SYN digestive *tract*.

drainage t., a t. introduced into a wound or cavity to facilitate removal of a fluid.

Durham t., a jointed tracheotomy t.

empyema t., a catheter used for drainage of an empyema.

endobronchial t., a single- or double-lumen t. with an inflatable cuff at the distal end that, after being passed through the larynx and trachea, is positioned so that ventilation is restricted to one lung; a single-lumen t. is placed in the mainstem bronchus of the lung; a double-lumen t. is positioned at the tracheal carina to permit ventilation of either or both lungs.

endotracheal t., a flexible t. inserted nasally, orally, or through a tracheotomy into the trachea to provide an airway, as in tracheal intubation SYN intratracheal t., tracheal t.

eustachian t., SYN pharyngotympanic (auditory) t.

fallopian t., SYN uterine t.

feeding t., a flexible t. passed through the nose and into the alimentary tract, through which liquid food is passed.

Ferrein t., SYN convoluted *tubule* of kidney.

field emission t., an x-ray t. that uses a cold cathode, relying on the t. voltage to pull electrons from it to the anode.

Geiger-Müller t., SEE Geiger-Müller *counter*.

germ t., a young hypha growing out of a yeast cell or spore, the beginning of a mycelium; also used as a rapid test for differentiating *Candida albicans* from other *Candida* species.

Haldane t., a t. for securing human alveolar air samples; consisting of a narrow hosepipe with a mouthpiece from which a t. is attached for the withdrawal of expired air at the end of a sudden, maximal expiration.

intratracheal t., SYN endotracheal t.

Levin t., a flexible t. introduced through the nose into the upper alimentary tract, to facilitate gastric decompression.

Martin t., a drainage t. with a cross piece near the extremity to keep it from slipping out of a cavity.

medullary t., SYN neural t.

Miescher t.'s, elongate fusiform or cylindrical bodies forming the encapsulated cystic intramuscular stage of the protozoan *Sarcocystis*.

Miller-Abbott t., a t. with two lumens, one ending in a small collapsible balloon and the other in a metallic tip with numerous perforations; used for decompression and stenting of the small intestine. SYN Abbott t.

molybdenum target t., an x-ray t. with an anode surface made of molybdenum instead of tungsten, used in mammography.

Moss t., (1) a triple-lumen, nasogastric, feeding-decompression t. that utilizes a gastric balloon to occlude the cardioesophageal junction, with simultaneous esophageal aspiration and intragastric feeding; **(2)** a double-lumen, gastric lavage t. that provides continuous delivery of saline via a small bore, with simultaneous aspiration of fluid and some particles via a large bore.

nasogastric t., a flexible t. passed through the nose and into the gastric pouch to decompress the stomach.

nasotracheal t., a tracheal t. inserted through the nasal passages.

nephrostomy t., a t. placed in the renal collecting system for drainage, diagnostic tests, or removal of calculi. May be placed through a percutaneous route or during an open surgical procedure.

neural t., the epithelial t. formed from the neuroectoderm of the early embryo by the closure of the neural groove; by complex processes of cell proliferation and organization the neural t. develops into the spinal cord and brain. SYN medullary t.

O'Dwyer t., a metal t. formerly used for intubation of the larynx in diphtheria.

orotracheal t., a tracheal t. inserted through the mouth.

otopharyngeal t., SYN pharyngotympanic (auditory) t.

pharyngotympanic (auditory) t. [TA], a t. leading from the tympanic cavity to the nasopharynx; it consists of an osseous (posterolateral) portion at the tympanic end, and a fibrocartilaginous (anteromedial) portion at the pharyngeal end; where the two portions join, in the region of the sphenopetrosal fissure, is the narrowest portion of the t. (isthmus); the auditory t. enables equalization of pressure within the tympanic cavity with ambient air pressure, referred to commonly as "popping of the ears." SYN tuba auditiva [TA], auditory t.☆, tuba auditoria☆, eustachian t., guttural duct, otopharyngeal t., otosalpinx, tuba acustica, tuba eustachiana, tuba eustachii.

photomultiplier t., a detector which amplifies a signal (by as much as 10^6) of electromagnetic radiation by an acceleration of electrons released from a photocathode through a series of dynodes; as each electron strikes a dynode stage, 3–4 electrons are liberated and accelerated to the subsequent dynode.

Pitot t., a stationary L-shaped t. inserted in a fluid stream, with its opening upstream, and used for measuring the velocity of fluid movement at that point in terms of the pressure developed in the t. by the fluid impinging on it, compared to a second t. opening laterally or downstream.

pus t., SYN pyosalpinx.

rectifier t., an electronic t., used in x-ray transformers, to convert alternating to direct current.

Rehfuss stomach t., a t. with a calibrated syringe, formerly used for aspiration of stomach contents in gastric analysis; replaced by plastic disposable stomach t.'s.

Robertshaw t., a variation of Carlen t. that eliminates some mechanical disadvantages of the latter.

roll t., a modification of the plate culture; a seeded medium containing agar is placed in a test t. which is rolled or spun horizontally until the medium solidifies evenly on the interior of the t.

rotating anode t., a modern x-ray t., in which heat buildup is distributed through a larger volume by rotating the target.

Ruysch t., a minute tubular cavity opening in the lower and anterior portion of each surface of the nasal septum; best seen in the early fetal period when it is associated with the vomeronasal organ (Jacobson organ).

Ryle t., a thin rubber t., with about the lumen of a no. 8 catheter, and an olive-tipped extremity, used in the giving of a test meal.

Sengstaken-Blakemore t., a t. with three lumens, one for drainage of the stomach and two for inflation of attached gastric and esophageal balloons; used for emergency treatment of bleeding esophageal varices.

Southey t.'s, obsolete cannulas of small, almost capillary, caliber, thrust by a trocar into the subcutaneous tissues to drain the fluid of anasarca.

tu

speaking t., a t. with an earpiece at one end and a cone at the other to amplify speech into the cone.

stomach t., a flexible t. passed into the stomach for lavage or feeding.

T t., a t. shaped like a T, the top of which is placed within a tubular structure such as the common bile duct and the stem placed through the skin; used for decompression.

test t., a t. of thin glass closed at one end, used in the examination of urine and other chemical operations, for bacterial cultures, etc.

thoracostomy t., a t. placed through the chest wall that drains the pleural space.

Tovell t., an endotracheal t. with a wire spiral embedded in the wall to prevent obstruction of the lumen when the t. is compressed and kinking or when the t. is bent at a sharp angle.

Toynbee t., a t. by which one can listen to the sounds in a patient's ear during politzerization.

tracheal t., SYN endotracheal t.

tracheostomy t., a curved t. used to keep the opening free after tracheotomy; may be metal or plastic. SYN tracheotomy t.

tracheotomy t., SYN tracheostomy t.

tympanostomy t., a small t. inserted through the tympanic membrane after myringotomy to ventilate the middle ear; often used for middle ear effusion.

uterine t. [TA], one of the t.'s leading on either side from the upper or outer extremity of the ovary, which is largely enveloped by its expanded infundibulum, to the fundus of the uterus; it provides the path by which the ovum travels from ovary to uterus where, if it is fertilized in the tube, it will implant as a zygote; it consists of infundibulum, ampulla, isthmus, and uterine parts. SYN tuba uterina [TA], salpinx☆, fallopian t., gonaduct (2), oviduct, salpinx uterina, tuba fallopiana, tuba fallopii.

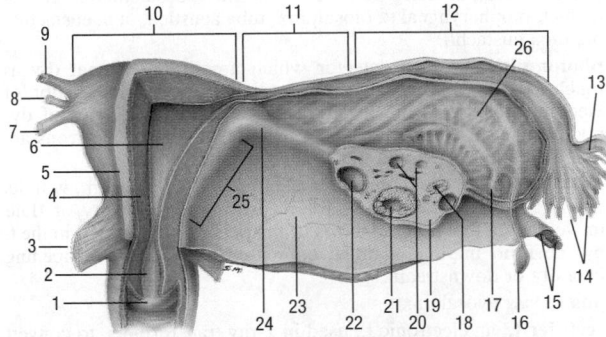

female genital tract: dorsal view with outstretched adnexa and opened uterus, vagina, and right uterine tube, right ovary is in frontal section;

1. cervix
2. cervical canal
3. sacrouterine ligament
4. myometrium
5. perimetrium
6. uterine cavity, endometrium
7. ovarian ligament
8. round ligament
9. uterine tube
10. fundus of uterus
11. isthmus of uterine tube
12. ampulla of uterine tube
13. infundibulum of uterine tube
14. fimbriae of uterine tube
15. ovarian vein and artery
16. stalked hydatid
17. ovarian fimbria
18. corpus albicans
19. stroma of ovary
20. primary ovarian follicles
21. corpus luteum
22. vesicular ovarian follicle
23. broad ligament
24. ovarian ligament
25. body of uterus
25. epoöphoron

vacuum t., a glass t. from which the air has been removed, containing two or more electrodes, between which passes an electrical current or spark; used in the production of x-rays, or to control circuits. Previously in wide use, the vacuum t. has been supplanted by transistors in electronic circuits.

Venturi t., a t. with a specially streamlined constriction to minimize energy losses in the fluid flowing through it while maximizing the fall in pressure in the constriction in accordance with Bernoulli law; the basis of the Venturi meter.

Wangensteen t., SYN Wangensteen *suction*.

x-ray t., SEE x-ray.

tu·bec·to·my (too-bek′tō-mē). SYN salpingectomy. [L. *tuba*, tube, + G. *ektomē*, excision]

tu·ber, pl. **tu·bera** (too′ber, too′ber-ă). **1** [TA]. A localized swelling; a knob. **2.** A short, fleshy, thick, underground stem of plants, such as the potato. [L. protuberance, swelling]

t. ante′rius, SYN t. cinereum.

ashen t., SYN t. cinereum.

calcaneal t., SYN calcaneal *tuberosity*.

t. calca′nei [TA], SYN calcaneal *tuberosity*.

t. cal′cis, SYN calcaneal *tuberosity*.

t. cine′reum [TA], a prominence of the base of the hypothalamus, bordered caudally by the mamillary bodies, rostrally by the optic chiasm, and laterally by the optic tract, extending ventrally into the infundibulum and hypophysial stalk. SYN ashen t., gray t., t. anterius.

t. coch′leae, SYN *promontory* of tympanic cavity.

t. cor′poris callo′si, SYN *splenium* of corpus callosum.

t. dorsa′le, SYN t. vermis.

eustachian t., a slight projection from the labyrinthine wall of the middle ear below the fenestra vestibuli (ovalis).

frontal t. [TA], the most prominent portion of the frontal bone on either side. SYN t. frontale [TA], eminentia frontalis☆, frontal eminence☆.

t. fronta′le [TA], SYN frontal t.

gray t., SYN t. cinereum.

t. ischiad′icum [TA], SYN ischial *tuberosity*.

t. of ischium, SYN ischial *tuberosity*.

t. maxil′lae [TA], SYN maxillary *tuberosity*.

omental t., SYN omental *eminence* of pancreas.

t. omentale hepatis [TA], SYN omental *tuberosity* of liver.

t. omentale pancreatis [TA], SYN omental *eminence* of pancreas.

parietal t. [TA], a prominent portion of the parietal bone, a little above the center of its external surface, usually corresponding to the point of maximum width of the head. SYN t. parietale [TA], eminentia parietalis☆, parietal eminence☆.

t. parieta′le [TA], SYN parietal t.

t. ra′dii, SYN radial *tuberosity*.

t. val′vulae, SYN t. vermis.

t. of vermis, SYN t. vermis.

t. ver′mis, the posterior division of the inferior vermis of the cerebellum located between the folium and the pyramis. SYN t. dorsale, t. of vermis, t. valvulae.

t. zygomat′icum, SYN articular *tubercle* of temporal bone.

tu·ber·cle (too′ber-kl). **1.** A nodule, especially in an anatomic, not pathologic, sense. **2.** A circumscribed, rounded, solid elevation on the skin, mucous membrane, or surface of an organ. **3.** A slight elevation from the surface of a bone giving attachment to a muscle or ligament. **4.** In dentistry, a small elevation arising on the surface of a tooth. **5.** A granulomatous lesion due to infection by *Mycobacterium tuberculosis*. Although somewhat variable in size (0.5–2 or 3 mm in diameter) and in the proportions of various histologic components, t.'s tend to be fairly well-circumscribed, spheroidal, firm lesions that usually consist of three irregularly outlined but moderately distinct zones: 1) an inner focus of necrosis, coagulative at first, and then becoming caseous; 2) a middle zone that consists of a fairly dense accumulation of large mononuclear phagocytes (macrophages), frequently arranged somewhat radially (with reference to the necrotic material) resembling an epithelium, and hence termed epithelioid cells; multinucleated giant cells of Langhans type may also be present; 3) an outer zone of numerous lymphocytes, and a few monocytes and plasma cells. In instances where healing has begun, a fourth zone of fibrous tissue may form at the periphery. Morphologically indistinguishable lesions may occur in diseases caused by other agents; many observers use the term nonspecifically, i.e., with reference to any such granuloma; others use "tubercle" only for tuberculous lesions, and then designate those of undetermined causes as epithelioid-cell granulomas. SYN tuberculum [TA]. [L. *tuberculum,* dim. of *tuber,* a knob, a swelling, a tumor]

accessory t., SYN accessory *process* of lumbar vertebra.

acoustic t., SYN *trigone* of auditory nerve.

adductor t. of femur [TA], the prominence above the medial epicondyle of the femur to which the tendon of the adductor magnus attaches. SYN tuberculum adductorium femoris [TA].

amygdaloid t., a projection from the roof of the anterior end-portion of the temporal horn of the lateral ventricle, marking the location of the amygdaloid nucleus.

anatomic t., SYN postmortem *wart.*

anterior t. of atlas [TA], a conical protuberance on the anterior surface of the arch of the atlas. SYN tuberculum anterius atlantis [TA].

anterior t. of cervical vertebrae [TA], the anterior projection from the transverse process. SYN tuberculum anterius vertebrarum cervicalium [TA].

t. of anterior scalene muscle, SYN scalene t.

anterior thalamic t. [TA], a prominence at the anterior extremity of the thalamus which corresponds to the nuclei anteriores. SYN tuberculum anterius thalami [TA], anterior t. of thalamus.

anterior t. of thalamus, SYN anterior thalamic t.

areolar t.'s [TA], small elevations on the areola of the female breast, especially prominent during pregnancy and lactation, that are a superficial manifestation of the underlying areolar glands. SYN tubercula areolae [TA].

articular t. of temporal bone [TA], articular eminence of the temporal bone which bounds the mandibular fossa anteriorly; it forms the anterior root of the zygomatic process; it is enclosed by the articular capsule of the temporomandibular joint with the articular fossa; the head of the mandible (and intervening articular disc) move onto the articular t. to allow full depression of the mandible (opening of the mouth). SYN tuberculum articulare ossis temporalis [TA], articular eminence of temporal bone, eminentia articularis ossis temporalis, tuber zygomaticum.

ashen t., SYN trigeminal t.

auricular t. [TA], a small inconstant projection from the upper end of the posterior portion of the incurved free margin of the helix of the auricle. SYN tuberculum auriculae [TA], darwinian t., tuberculum superius.

calcaneal t. [TA], the projection, often double, on the inferior aspect of the calcaneus at the anterior end of the area for attachment of the long plantar ligament. SYN tuberculum calcanei [TA].

Carabelli t., a small t., resembling a supernumerary cusp, found occasionally on the lingual surface of the mesiolingual cusp of a permanent maxillary first molar.

carotid t. [TA], the anterior t. of the transverse process of the sixth cervical vertebra, against which the carotid artery may be compressed by the finger. SYN tuberculum caroticum [TA], Chassaignac t.

caseous t., SYN soft t.

Chassaignac t., SYN carotid t.

conoid t. (of clavicle) [TA], the prominence near the lateral end of the inferior surface of the clavicle that gives attachment to the conoid ligament. SYN tuberculum conoideum (claviculare) [TA], conoid process.

corniculate t. [TA], the smaller and more medial of the two rounded eminences on the posterior part of the aryepiglottic fold, formed by the underlying corniculate cartilages. SYN tuberculum corniculatum [TA], Santorini t.

crown t., SYN dental t.

cuneate t., the bulbous rostral extremity of the fasciculus cuneatus corresponding to the position of the cunate nucleus, lying lateral to the clava and separated from the tuberculum cinereum on its lateral side by the posterior lateral sulcus. SYN tuberculum cuneatum, wedge-shaped t.

cuneiform t. [TA], the larger, more laterally placed of the two rounded eminences on the posterior part of the aryepiglottic fold, formed by the underlying cuneiform cartilage. SYN tuberculum cuneiforme [TA], Wrisberg t.

darwinian t., SYN auricular t.

deltoid t. (of spine of scapula) [TA], prominence on the dorsum of the scapular spine, lateral to the root of the spine, to which a flat, triangular tendon from the most inferior part of the middle part of the trapezius (muscle) is attached. SYN tuberculum deltoideum (spinae scapulae) [TA].

dental t. [TA], a small elevation on some portions of a crown produced by an extra formation of enamel. SYN tuberculum dentis [TA], crown t., t. of tooth, tuberculum coronae.

dorsal t. of radius [TA], a small prominence on the dorsal aspect of the distal end of the radius lateral to the groove for the extensor pollicis longus tendon; it serves as a trochlea or pulley for the tendon. SYN tuberculum dorsale radii [TA], Lister t.

epiglottic t. [TA], a convexity at the lower part of the epiglottis over the upper part of the thyroepiglottic ligament. SYN tuberculum epiglotticum [TA], cushion of epiglottis.

fibrous t., a t. in which fibroblasts proliferate about the periphery (and into the cellular zones), eventually resulting in a rim or wall of cellular fibrous tissue or collagenous material around the t.

genial t., SYN mental *spine.*

genital t., the median elevation just cephalic to the urogenital orifice of an embryo; it is the primordium of the penis of the male or the clitoris of the female. SYN phallic t.

Gerdy t., a t. on the anterolateral side of the upper end of the tibia giving attachment to the iliotibial tract and some fibers of the tibialis anterior muscle.

Ghon t., calcification seen in pulmonary parenchyma (usually midlung) resulting from earlier, usually childhood, infection with tuberculosis; sometimes confused with a combination of parenchymal lesion and calcified lymph node, which is properly termed a Ranke complex. SYN Ghon complex, Ghon focus, Ghon primary lesion.

gracile t., the somewhat expanded upper end of the gracile fasciculus, corresponding to the position of the gracile nucleus. SYN clava, tuberculum gracile.

gray t., SYN trigeminal t.

greater t. (of humerus) [TA], the larger of the two t.'s next to the head of the humerus; it gives attachment to the supraspinatus, infraspinatus, and teres minor muscles. SYN tuberculum majus (humeri) [TA], greater tuberosity of humerus.

hard t., a t. lacking necrosis.

hyaline t., a form of fibrous t. in which the cellular fibrous tissue and collagenous fibers become altered and merged into a fairly homogeneous, acellular, deeply acidophilic, firm mass.

iliac t., SYN t. of iliac crest.

t. of iliac crest [TA], a prominence on the outer lip of the iliac crest about 5 cm behind the anterior superior iliac spine. SYN tuberculum iliacum [TA], iliac t.

inferior thyroid t. [TA], a slight lateral projection from the lower margin of the lamina of the thyroid cartilage on either side, at the inferior end of the oblique line. SYN tuberculum thyroideum inferius [TA].

infraglenoid t. (of scapula) [TA], a rough surface below the glenoid cavity of the scapula, giving attachment to the long tendon of the triceps. SYN tuberculum infraglenoidale (scapulae) [TA], infraglenoid tuberosity.

intercolumnar t., SEE subfornical *organ.*

intercondylar t. [TA], one of two projections, medial and lateral, springing from the central lip of each articular surface of the tibia on either side of the intercondylar eminence. SYN tuberculum intercondylare (mediale et laterale) [TA].

intervenous t. (of right atrium) [TA], the slight projection on the wall of the right atrium between the orifices of the venae cavae. SYN tuberculum intervenosum (atrii dextri) [TA], Lower t.

jugular t. of occipital bone [TA], an oval elevation on the cerebral surface of the junction of the lateral and basal parts of the occipital bone, on either side of the foramen magnum medial to the lower border and anterosuperior to the opening of the hypoglossal canal. SYN tuberculum jugulare ossis occipitalis [TA].

labial t., SYN t. of upper lip.

lateral t. (of posterior process) of talus [TA], the prominence lateral to the groove for the flexor hallucis longus tendon. SYN tuberculum laterale (processus posterioris) tali [TA].

lesser t. (of humerus) [TA], the anterior of the two tubercles of

tu

the neck of the humerus on which the subscapularis is inserted. SYN tuberculum minus (humeri) [TA], lesser tuberosity of humerus.

Lisfranc t., SYN scalene t.

Lister t., SYN dorsal t. of radius.

Lower t., SYN intervenous t. (of right atrium).

mammillary t., SYN mammillary *process* of lumbar vertebra.

mammillary t. of hypothalamus, SYN mammillary *body*.

marginal t., SYN marginal t. (of zygomatic bone).

marginal t. (of zygomatic bone) [TA], an inconstant prominence on the temporal border of the zygomatic bone to which the temporal fascia is attached. SYN tuberculum marginale (ossis zygomatici) [TA], marginal t.

medial t. (of posterior process) of talus [TA], the eminence medial to the sulcus for the flexor hallucis longus tendon. SYN tuberculum mediale (processus posterioris) tali [TA].

mental t. (of mandible) [TA], a paired eminence on the mental protuberance of the mandible. SYN tuberculum mentale (mandibulae) [TA], eminentia symphysis.

molar t. [TA], occasional nonocclusive prominence of variable size on the crown of a molar tooth. SYN tuberculum molare [TA].

Montgomery t.'s, elevated reddened areolar glands, usually associated with pregnancy.

Morgagni t., SYN cuneiform *cartilage*.

Müller t., a median protuberance projecting into the embryonic urogenital sinus from its dorsal wall; it is formed from the fused caudal ends of the paramesonephric ducts and is the first evidence of the embryonic uterus and vagina. SYN sinus t.

nuchal t., SYN *vertebra* prominens.

obturator t. [TA], one of two processes, anterior and posterior, on the margin of the pubic portion of the obturator foramen, bounding the termination of the obturator groove; the posterior obturator t. is inconstant. SYN tuberculum obturatorium [TA].

olfactory t., a small, oval area at the base of the cerebral hemisphere, between the diverging medial and lateral olfactory striae, in the anteromedial part of the anterior perforated substance; it is formed by a small area of allocortex characterized by the presence of the islands of Calleja. Corresponding to a much more prominent structure in nonprimate mammals (especially rodents and insectivores), the olfactory tubercle receives fibers from the olfactory bulb by way of the intermediate olfactory stria; it has efferent connections with the hypothalamus and the mediodorsal nucleus of the thalamus. SYN tuberculum olfactorium [TA].

orbital t. (of zygomatic bone) [TA], a small elevation on the orbital surface of the zygomatic bone, just within the orbital margin, about 1 cm below the zygomaticofrontal suture; it gives attachment to the lateral check ligament, the lateral palpebral ligament, and the suspensory ligament of the eyeball. SYN tuberculum orbitale ossis zygomatici [TA], eminentia orbitalis (ossis zygomatici), orbital eminence of zygomatic bone, Whitnall t.

phallic t., SYN genital t.

pharyngeal t. (of basilar part of occipital bone) [TA], a projection from the undersurface of the basilar portion of the occipital bone, giving attachment to the fibrous raphe of the pharynx. SYN tuberculum pharyngeum (partis basilaris ossis occipitalis) [TA].

posterior t. of atlas [TA], a protuberance of the posterior extremity of the arch of the atlas, a rudiment of the spinous process giving attachment to the musculus rectus capitis posterior minor muscle. SYN tuberculum posterius atlantis [TA].

posterior t. of cervical vertebrae [TA], a posterior projection from the transverse processes. SYN tuberculum posterius vertebrarum cervicalium [TA].

Princeteau t., a slight prominence on the temporal bone near the apex of the petrous part where the superior petrosal sinus commences.

pterygoid t., a slight prominence on the posterior surface of the medial pterygoid plate, inferior and to the medial side of the pterygoid canal.

pubic t. [TA], a small palpable projection at the anterior extremity of the crest of the pubis about 2 cm from the symphysis; site of insertion of inguinal ligament. SYN tuberculum pubicum [TA], pubic spine, spina pubis.

t. of rib [TA], the knob on the posterior surface of a rib, at the junction of its neck and shaft, which articulates with the transverse process of the vertebra, whch corresponds in number to the rib, forming a costotransverse joint. SYN tuberculum costae [TA].

Rolando t., SYN trigeminal t.

t. of saddle, SYN *tuberculum* sellae.

Santorini t., SYN corniculate t.

scalene t. [TA], a small spine on the inner edge of the first rib, giving attachment to the scalenus anterior muscle, lying between and thus demarcating the grooves for the subclavian artery (anteriorly) and vein (posteriorly). SYN tuberculum musculi scaleni anterioris [TA], Lisfranc t., scalene t. of Lisfranc, t. of anterior scalene muscle.

scalene t. of Lisfranc, SYN scalene t.

t. of scaphoid (bone) [TA], a projection at the inferior lateral angle of the scaphoid bone; it can be felt at the root of the thumb; provides attachment for the transverse carpal ligament (flexor retinaculum). SYN tuberculum ossis scaphoidei [TA].

sinus t., SYN Müller t.

soft t., a t. showing caseous necrosis. SYN caseous t.

superior thyroid t. [TA], a blunt lateral projection on the external aspect lamina of the thyroid cartilage on either side at the superior end of the oblique line. SYN tuberculum thyroideum superius [TA].

supraglenoid t. (of scapula) [TA], a rough surface above the glenoid cavity of the scapula, giving attachment to the tendon of the long head of the biceps within the articular cavity of the shoulder joint. SYN tuberculum supraglenoidale (scapulae) [TA].

supratragic t. [TA], a small inconstant elevation often present on the edge of the upper tragus. SYN tuberculum supratragicum [TA].

t. of tooth, SYN dental t.

t. of trapezium (bone), SYN *tuberculum* of trapezium bone.

trigeminal t. [TA], a longitudinal prominence on the dorsolateral surface of the medulla oblongata along the lateral border of the cuneate t.; it is the surface profile of the spinal tract of trigeminal nerve, continuous caudally with the dorsolateral fasciculus (Lissauer's tract). SYN tuberculum trigeminale [TA], ashen t., gray t., Rolando t.

t. of upper lip [TA], the slight projection on the free edge of the center of the upper lip at the lower extent of the philtrum. SYN tuberculum labii superioris [TA], labial t., procheilon, prochilon.

wedge-shaped t., SYN cuneate t.

Whitnall t., SYN orbital t. (of zygomatic bone).

Wrisberg t., SYN cuneiform t.

⌂tubercul-. SEE tuberculo-.

tu·ber·cu·la (too-ber'kū-lă). Plural of tuberculum.

tu·ber·cu·lar, tu·ber·cu·lat·ed (too-ber'kū-lăr, -lāt-ed). Pertaining to or characterized by tubercles or small nodules. Cf. tuberculous.

tu·ber·cu·la·tion (too-ber-kū-lā'shŭn). The arrangement of tubercles or nodules in a part.

tu·ber·cu·lid (too-ber'kū-lid). A lesion of the skin or mucous membrane resulting from hypersensitivity to mycobacterial antigens disseminated from a distant site of active tuberculosis. [tubercul- + G. -id (1)]

nodular t., SYN erythema induratum.

papular t., SYN *lichen* scrofulosorum.

papulonecrotic t., dusky-red papules followed by crusting and ulceration with nongranulomatous vascular changes primarily on the extremities and predominantly in young adults with a deep focus of tuberculosis or with a history of preceding infection. SYN tuberculosis papulonecrotica.

rosacea-like t., SYN granulomatous *rosacea*.

tu·ber·cu·lin (too-ber'kū-lin). **1.** A glycerin-broth culture of *Mycobacterium tuberculosis* evaporated to $\frac{1}{10}$ volume at 100°C and filtered; introduced by Robert Koch for the treatment of tuberculosis but now used chiefly for diagnostic tests; originally known as Koch old t. (OT) or Koch original t. **2.** One or another of a relatively large number of extracts of *Mycobacterium tuberculosis* cultures, different from OT and now obsolete.

Koch old t. (OT), SEE tuberculin (1).

purified protein derivative of t. (PPD), purified t. containing the active protein fraction; the t. from which it is prepared differs from t. (1) chiefly in that the bacteria are grown in a synthetic rather than in a broth medium.

tu·ber·cu·li·tis (too-ber-kū-lī′tis). Inflammation of any tubercle. [tubercul- + G. -*itis*, inflammation]

tuberculo-, tubercul-. A tubercle, tuberculosis. [L. *tuberculum*, tubercle]

tu·ber·cu·lo·cele (too-ber′kū-lō-sēl). Tuberculosis of the testes. [tuberculo- + G. *kēlē*, tumor, hernia]

tu·ber·cu·lo·che·mo·ther·a·peu·tic (too-ber′kū-lō-kē′mō-ther-ă-pū′tik). Relating to the treatment of tuberculosis by tuberculostatic or tuberculocidal drugs.

tu·ber·cu·lo·ci·dal (too-ber′kū-lō-sī′dăl). Destructive to the tubercle bacillus.

tu·ber·cu·lo·der·ma (too-ber′kū-lō-der′mă). **1.** Any tubercular process of the skin. **2.** The cutaneous manifestation of tuberculosis.

tu·ber·cu·lo·fi·broid (too-ber′kū-lō-fī′broyd). A discrete, well-circumscribed, usually spheroidal, moderately to extremely firm, encapsulated nodule that is formed during the process of healing in a focus of tuberculous granulomatous inflammation.

tu·ber·cu·loid (too-ber′kū-loyd). Resembling tuberculosis or a tubercle. [tuberculo- + G. *eidos*, resemblance]

tu·ber·cu·lo·ma (too-ber-kū-lō′mă). A rounded tumorlike but nonneoplastic mass, usually in the lungs or brain, due to localized tuberculous infection. [tuberculo- + G. -*oma*, tumor]

tu·ber·cu·lo·pro·tein (too-ber′kū-lō-prō′tēn). Any one, or a mixture of any or all of the proteins present in the body of the tubercle bacillus, all of which have been found to possess certain properties of tuberculin.

tu·ber·cu·lo·sis (TB) (tū-ber′kyū-lō′sis). A specific disease caused by infection with *Mycobacterium tuberculosis*, the tubercle bacillus, which can affect almost any tissue or organ of the body, the most common seat of the disease being the lungs. Primary t. is typically a mild or asymptomatic local pulmonary infection. Regional lymph nodes may become involved, but in otherwise healthy people generalized disease does not immediately develop. A cell-mediated immune response arrests the spread of organisms and walls off the zone of infection. Infected tissues and lymph nodes may eventually calcify. The tuberculin skin test becomes positive within a few weeks, and remains positive throughout life. Organisms in a primary lesion remain viable and can become reactivated months or years later to initiate secondary t. Progression to the secondary stage eventually occurs in 10–15% of people who have had primary t. The risk of reactivation is increased by diabetes mellitus, HIV infection, silicosis, and various systemic or malignant conditions, as well as in alcoholics, IV drug abusers, nursing home residents, and those receiving adrenocortical steroid or immunosuppressive therapy. Secondary or reactivation t. usually results in a chronic, spreading lung infection, most often involving the upper lobes. Minute granulomas (tubercles), just visible to the naked eye, develop in involved lung tissue, each consisting of a zone of caseation necrosis surrounded by chronic inflammatory cells (epithelioid histiocytes and giant cells). These lesions, which give the disease its name, are also found in other tissues (lymph nodes, bowel, kidney, skin) to which the disease may spread. Rarely, reactivation results in widespread dissemination of tubercles throughout the body (miliary t.). The symptoms of active pulmonary t. are fatigue, anorexia, weight loss, low-grade fever, night sweats, chronic cough, and hemoptysis. Local symptoms depend on the parts affected. Active pulmonary t. is relentlessly chronic and, if untreated, leads to progressive destruction of lung tissue. Cavities form in the lungs, and erosion into pulmonary blood vessels can result in life-threatening hemorrhage. Gradual deterioration of nutritional status and general health culminates in death due to wasting, infection, or multiple organ failure. Variant syndromes (tuberculous lymphadenitis in children, severe systemic disease in persons with AIDS) are caused by organisms of the *Mycobacterium avium-intracellulare* complex. [tuberculo- + G. -*osis,* condition]

In 1993 the World Health Organization (WHO) declared tuberculosis a global emergency. Fully one-third of the world's population is infected with TB. On a global scale, TB ranks first among infectious diseases as a cause of death. Two-thirds of all the world's cases are in Asia, but the disease is also endemic in parts of Africa and other regions. War and social upheaval have played a role in the spread of tuberculosis beyond endemic zones; prevalence of infection is higher among refugees and immigrants. One-third of all persons with tuberculosis in the U.S. were born outside the country. From the 1950s, when antibiotics began to be used for the treatment of tuberculosis, until the 1980s, the incidence and mortality of the disease declined steadily in the U.S. During the 1980s the incidence began to rise because of many new cases in persons with AIDS and because of increasing prevalence of multidrug-resistant strains of *M. tuberculosis*. Since 1993 the figures have again declined, chiefly because of improvements in tuberculosis prevention and control programs in state and local health departments as a result of increased federal funding provided to states. At least one-third of persons with AIDS contract tuberculosis, and tuberculosis is the cause of death in one-third of persons who die of AIDS. Since antibiotic resistance in *M. tuberculosis* has been a growing problem for years, multidrug regimens, usually including isoniazid, rifampin, and pyrazinamide, are standard. Other drugs, such as ethambutol, streptomycin, kanamycin, and capreomycin, may be added or substituted. The success of treatment is limited not only by the resistance of organisms to several agents but also by the risk of severe toxic effects with all the standard agents. Unlike most infections treated with antibiotics, tuberculosis requires not days or weeks of treatment, but months and years. Long-term compliance tends to be poor among mobile, indigent, and uneducated persons. According to WHO, the principal reason for the spread of multidrug-resistant strains of *M. tuberculosis* is ineffectual management of tuberculosis control programs, particularly in third-world countries. An inappropriate or unfinished course of chemotherapy not only leaves the patient still sick and still contagious, but favors the selection of resistant bacteria. It is estimated that 50 million of the world's cases of tuberculosis involve multiply resistant tubercle bacilli. Currently WHO urges that tuberculosis programs worldwide adopt the practice of directly observed therapy (DOT), in which a health care worker observes each patient swallowing each dose of medicine. In a study performed at several U.S. centers, DOT for tuberculosis was found to be cost-effective when the cost of relapses and treatment failures was added to the cost of self-administered therapy, even though the raw cost of DOT was higher. U.S. public health authorities have established as a national goal the elimination of TB (defined as an incidence of <1 case per 1 million population) by 2010.

tu

adult t., SYN secondary t.

aerogenic t., infection with the *Mycobacterium tuberculosis* spread by inhalation of infected droplets.

anthracotic t., SYN pneumoconiosis.

arrested t., SYN inactive t.

attenuated t., a mild chronic form marked by caseous tubercles of the skin and the occurrence of cold abscesses.

basal t., t. of the basilar portions of the lungs.

cerebral t., (**1**) SYN tuberculous *meningitis*; (**2**) cerebral tuberculoma.

childhood t., initial (primary) infection with *Mycobacterium tuberculosis*, characterized by pneumonic lesions in the middle parts of the lungs, rarely cavitary, with rapid spread to lymph nodes in hilar and paratracheal areas; more often seen in childhood, but the pattern is not limited to children.

childhood type t., SYN primary t.

cutaneous t., pathologic lesions of the skin caused by *Mycobacterium tuberculosis*. SYN t. cutis.

t. cu′tis, SYN cutaneous t.

t. cu′tis orificia′lis, any tuberculous lesion in or about the mouth or anus.

t. cu′tis verruco′sa, a tuberculous skin lesion having a warty surface with a chronic inflammatory base seen on the hands in adults and lower extremities in children, with marked hypersensitivity to tuberculous antigens. SEE ALSO postmortem *wart.* SYN tuberculous wart.

disseminated t., SYN miliary t.

enteric t., a complication of cavitary pulmonary t. usually resulting from expectoration and swallowing of bacilli that then infect areas of the digestive tract where there is relative stasis or abundant lymphoid tissue; can be caused by ingestion of bovine tubercular organisms in infected milk, now rare. SEE ALSO tuberculous *enteritis.*

exudative t., a stage of infection with *Mycobacterium tuberculosis* causing severe edema and cellular inflammatory reaction without much necrosis or fibrosis.

generalized t., SYN miliary t.

healed t., a scar or a calcified, fibrous, or caseous nodule in the lung pleura, lymph node, or other organ, resulting from previous t. that has regressed. If truly healed, no organisms are present and reactivation is not possible.

inactive t., a fibrous or nodular area of previously active t. that has regressed, with the lesion having remained stable for a long period; can be calcified; reactivation is possible. SYN arrested t.

miliary t., general dissemination of tubercle bacilli in the blood, resulting in the formation of miliary tubercles in various organs and tissues, and occasionally producing symptoms of profound toxemia. SYN disseminated t., generalized t.

open t., pulmonary t., tuberculous ulceration, or other form in which the tubercle bacilli are present in the excretions or secretions; in the lung, usually the result of cavity formation.

t. papulonecrot′ica, SYN papulonecrotic *tuberculid.*

postprimary t., SYN secondary t.

primary t., first infection by *Mycobacterium tuberculosis,* typically seen in children but also occurs in adults, characterized in the lungs by the formation of a primary complex consisting of small peripheral pulmonary focus with spread to hilar or paratracheal lymph nodes; may proceed to cavitate or heal with scarring or may progress. SYN childhood type t.

pulmonary t., t. of the lungs.

reactivation t., SYN secondary t.

reinfection t., SYN secondary t.

secondary t., t. found in adults and characterized by lesions near the apex of an upper lobe, which may cavitate or heal with scarring without spreading to lymph nodes; theoretically, secondary t. may be due to exogenous reinfection or to reactivation of a dormant endogenous infection. SYN adult t., postprimary t., reactivation t., reinfection t.

tu·ber·cu·lo·stat (too-ber′kū-lō-stat). A tuberculostatic agent.

tu·ber·cu·lo·stat·ic (too-ber′kū-lō-stat′ik). Relating to an agent that inhibits the growth of tubercle bacilli. [tuberculo- + G. *statikos,* causing to stand]

tu·ber·cu·lous (too-ber′kū-lŭs). Relating to or affected by tuberculosis. Cf. tubercular.

TUBERCULUM

tu·ber·cu·lum, pl. **tu·ber·cu·la** (too-ber′kū-lŭm, -lă) [TA]. SYN tubercle. [L. dim. of *tuber,* a knob, swelling, tumor]

t. adducto′rium femoris [TA], SYN adductor *tubercle* of femur.

t. ante′rius atlan′tis [TA], SYN anterior *tubercle* of atlas.

t. ante′rius thal′ami [TA], SYN anterior thalamic *tubercle.*

t. ante′rius vertebra′rum cervica′lium [TA], SYN anterior *tubercle* of cervical vertebrae.

tubercula areolae [TA], SYN areolar *tubercles,* under *tubercle.*

t. arthrit′icum, (1) SYN Heberden *nodes,* under *node;* (2) any gouty concretion in or around a joint.

t. articula′re os′sis tempora′lis [TA], SYN articular *tubercle* of temporal bone.

t. auric′ulae [TA], SYN auricular *tubercle.*

t. calca′nei [TA], SYN calcaneal *tubercle.*

t. carot′icum [TA], SYN carotid *tubercle.*

t. cine′reum, a longitudinal prominence on the dorsolateral surface of the medulla oblongata along the lateral border of the t. cuneatum; it is the surface profile of the spinal tract of trigeminal nerve, continuous caudally with the dorsolateral fasciculus (Lissauer tract).

t. conoi′deum (claviculare) [TA], SYN conoid *tubercle* (of clavicle).

t. cornicula′tum [TA], SYN corniculate *tubercle.*

t. coro′nae, SYN dental *tubercle.*

t. cos′tae [TA], SYN *tubercle* of rib.

t. cunea′tum, SYN cuneate *tubercle.*

t. cuneifor′me [TA], SYN cuneiform *tubercle.*

t. deltoideum (spinae scapulae) [TA], SYN deltoid *tubercle* (of spine of scapula).

t. den′tis [TA], SYN dental *tubercle.*

t. dorsa′le radii [TA], SYN dorsal *tubercle* of radius.

t. epiglot′ticum [TA], SYN epiglottic *tubercle.*

t. grac′ile, SYN gracile *tubercle.*

t. hypoglos′si, SYN hypoglossal *trigone.*

t. ili′acum [TA], SYN *tubercle* of iliac crest.

t. im′par, a small median protuberance on the floor of the oral cavity of the embryo between the mandibular and hyoid arches, which plays a minor role in the development of the tongue. SYN median tongue bud.

t. infraglenoida′le (scapulae) [TA], SYN infraglenoid *tubercle* (of scapula).

t. intercondyla′re (mediale et laterale) [TA], SYN intercondylar *tubercle.*

t. interveno′sum (atrii dextri) [TA], SYN intervenous *tubercle* (of right atrium).

t. jugula′re ossis occipitalis [TA], SYN jugular *tubercle* of occipital bone.

t. la′bii superio′ris [TA], SYN *tubercle* of upper lip.

t. latera′le (proces′sus posterio′ris) ta′li [TA], SYN lateral *tubercle* (of posterior process) of talus.

t. ma′jus (hu′meri) [TA], SYN greater *tubercle* (of humerus).

t. mal′lei, SYN lateral *process* of malleus.

t. margina′le (os′sis zygomat′ici) [TA], SYN marginal *tubercle* (of zygomatic bone).

t. media′le (proces′sus posterio′ris) ta′li [TA], SYN medial *tubercle* (of posterior process) of talus.

t. menta′le (mandibulae) [TA], SYN mental *tubercle* (of mandible).

t. mi′nus (hu′meri) [TA], SYN lesser *tubercle* (of humerus).

t. molare [TA], SYN molar *tubercle.*

t. mus′culi scale′ni anterio′ris [TA], SYN scalene *tubercle.*

t. obturato′rium [TA], SYN obturator *tubercle.*

t. olfacto′rium [TA], SYN olfactory *tubercle.*

t. orbitale ossis zygomatici [TA], SYN orbital *tubercle* (of zygomatic bone).

t. os′sis scaphoi′dei [TA], SYN *tubercle* of scaphoid (bone).

t. os′sis trape′zii [TA], SYN t. of trapezium bone.

t. pharyn′geum (partis basilaris ossis occipitalis) [TA], SYN pharyngeal *tubercle* (of basilar part of occipital bone).

t. poste′rius atlan′tis [TA], SYN posterior *tubercle* of atlas.

t. poste′rius vertebra′rum cervica′lium [TA], SYN posterior *tubercle* of cervical vertebrae.

t. pu′bicum [TA], SYN pubic *tubercle.*

t. sel′lae [TA], the slight elevation in front of the pituitary fossa (sella turcica) on the body of the sphenoid bone. SYN tubercle of saddle.

t. sep′ti na′rium, a flat elevation on the septum in each naris opposite the anterior end of the middle concha; it is due to an aggregation of glands.

t. supe′rius, SYN auricular *tubercle*.

t. supraglenoida′le (scapulae) [TA], SYN supraglenoid *tubercle* (of scapula).

t. supratra′gicum [TA], SYN supratragic *tubercle*.

t. thyroi′deum infe′rius [TA], SYN inferior thyroid *tubercle*.

t. thyroi′deum supe′rius [TA], SYN superior thyroid *tubercle*.

t. of trapezium bone [TA], a prominent ridge on the trapezium forming the lateral border of the groove in which runs the tendon of the flexor carpi radialis and to which part of the transverse carpal ligament (flexor retinaculum) is attached. SYN t. ossis trapezii [TA], oblique ridge of trapezium, tubercle of trapezium (bone).

t. trigeminale [TA], SYN trigeminal *tubercle*.

tu·ber·if·er·ous (too-ber-if′er-ŭs). SYN tuberous. [tuber + L. *ferro,* to bear]

tu·ber·ose (too′ber-ōs). SYN tuberous.

tu·ber·os·i·tas (too′ber-os′i-tas) [TA]. SYN tuberosity. [LL., fr. L., *tuberosus,* full of lumps, fr. *tuber,* a knob]

t. coracoi′dea, SYN *tuberosity* for coracoclavicular ligament.

t. costa′lis, SYN *impression* for costoclavicular ligament.

t. deltoi′dea (humeri) [TA], SYN deltoid *tuberosity* (of humerus).

t. glu′tea [TA], SYN gluteal *tuberosity*.

t. ili′aca [TA], SYN iliac *tuberosity*.

t. ligamenti coracoclavicularis [TA], SYN *tuberosity* for coracoclavicular ligament.

t. masseter′ica [TA], SYN masseteric *tuberosity*.

t. mus′culi serra′ti anterio′ris [TA], SYN *tuberosity* for serratus anterior (muscle).

t. os′sis cuboi′dei [TA], SYN *tuberosity* of cuboid (bone).

t. os′sis metatarsa′lis pri′mi [I], SYN *tuberosity* of first metatarsal (bone) [I].

t. os′sis metatarsa′lis quin′ti [V] [TA], SYN *tuberosity* of fifth metatarsal (bone) [V].

t. os′sis navicula′ris [TA], SYN *tuberosity* of navicular bone.

t. phalan′gis dista′lis (manus et pedis) [TA], SYN *tuberosity* of distal phalanx (of hand and foot).

t. pronatoria [TA], SYN pronator *tuberosity*.

t. pterygoi′dea (mandibulae) [TA], SYN pterygoid *tuberosity* (of mandible).

t. ra′dii [TA], SYN radial *tuberosity*.

t. sacra′lis [TA], SYN sacral *tuberosity*.

t. tib′iae [TA], SYN tibial *tuberosity*.

t. ul′nae [TA], SYN *tuberosity* of ulna.

t. unguicula′ris, SYN *tuberosity* of distal phalanx (of hand and foot).

tu·ber·os·i·ty (too′ber-os′i-tē) [TA]. A large tubercle or rounded elevation, especially from the surface of a bone. SYN tuberositas [TA].

bicipital t., SYN radial t.

calcaneal t. [TA], the posterior extremity of the calcaneus, or os calcis, forming the projection of the heel. SYN tuber calcanei [TA], calcaneal tuber, tuber calcis.

t. for coracoclavicular ligament [TA], the conoid tubercle and trapezoid line of the coracoid process of the scapula, giving attachment to the two parts of the coracoclavicular ligament: the conoid and trapezoid ligaments. SYN tuberositas ligamenti coracoclavicularis [TA], coracoid t., tuberositas coracoidea.

coracoid t., SYN t. for coracoclavicular ligament.

costal t., SYN *impression* for costoclavicular ligament.

t. of cuboid (bone) [TA], a slight eminence on the lateral surface of the cuboid bone, capped with an articular facet for a sesamoid bone in the tendon of the peroneus longus muscle. SYN tuberositas ossis cuboidei [TA].

deltoid t. (of humerus) [TA], a rough elevation about the middle of the lateral side of the shaft of the humerus, providing attachment (insertion) for the deltoid muscle. SYN tuberositas deltoidea

(humeri) [TA], deltoid crest, deltoid eminence, deltoid impression.

t. of distal phalanx (of hand and foot) [TA], a roughened raised surface of horseshoe shape on the palmar surface of the distal end of the terminal or ungual phalanx of each finger and toe, which serves to support the pulp of the digit. SYN tuberositas phalangis distalis (manus et pedis) [TA], tuberositas unguicularis, ungual t.

t. of fifth metatarsal (bone) [V] [TA], a tubercle at the base of this bone to the posterior part of which is attached the tendon of the peroneus brevis muscle. SYN tuberositas ossis metatarsalis quinti [V] [TA].

t. of first metatarsal (bone) [I] [TA], a tubercle at the base of the bone to which is attached the tendon of the peroneus longus muscle. SYN tuberositas ossis metatarsalis primi [I].

gluteal t. [TA], the roughened area of insertion on the upper portion of the shaft of the femur of the deep, lesser part of the gluteus maximus muscle; when markedly developed this t. is called the third trochanter. SEE ALSO third *trochanter.* SYN tuberositas glutea [TA], crista glutea, gluteal crest, gluteal ridge.

greater t. of humerus, SYN greater *tubercle* (of humerus).

iliac t. [TA], a rough area above the auricular surface on the medial aspect of the ala of the ilium, giving attachment to the posterior sacroiliac ligament. SYN tuberositas iliaca [TA].

infraglenoid t., SYN infraglenoid *tubercle* (of scapula).

ischial t. [TA], the rough bony projection at the junction of the lower end of the body of the ischium and its ramus; this is a weight-bearing point in the sitting position; provides attachment for the sacrotuberous ligament and is the site of origin of the hamstring muscles. SYN tuber ischiadicum [TA], tuber of ischium.

lateral femoral t., SYN lateral *epicondyle* of femur.

lesser t. of humerus, SYN lesser *tubercle* (of humerus).

masseteric t. [TA], a roughened surface on the external aspect of the angle of the mandible, giving attachment to fibers of the masseter muscle. SYN tuberositas masseterica [TA].

maxillary t. [TA], the bulging lower extremity of the posterior surface of the body of the maxilla, behind the root of the last molar tooth. SYN tuber maxillae [TA], eminentia maxillae, maxillary eminence.

medial femoral t., SYN medial *epicondyle* of femur.

t. of navicular bone [TA], a rounded eminence on the medial surface of the navicular bone, giving attachment to a part of the tendon of the tibialis posterior muscle. SYN tuberositas ossis navicularis [TA], scaphoid t.

omental t. of liver [TA], an eminence on the visceral surface of the left hepatic lobe to the left of the fossa for the ductus venosus. SYN tuber omentale hepatis [TA].

pronator t. [TA], slight, roughened area on the middle of the convex lateal aspect of the shaft of the radius, to which the pronator teres (muscle) is attached (inserted). SYN tuberositas pronatoria [TA].

pterygoid t. (of mandible) [TA], a roughened area on the internal aspect of the mandible, giving attachment to fibers of the medial pterygoid muscle. SYN tuberositas pterygoidea (mandibulae) [TA].

radial t. [TA], an oval projection from the medial surface of the radius just distal to the neck, giving attachment (insertion) on its posterior half to the tendon of the biceps. SYN tuberositas radii [TA], bicipital t., tuber radii, t. of radius.

t. of radius, SYN radial t.

sacral t. [TA], a rough prominence on the lateral surface of the sacrum posterior to the auricular surface for attachment of posterior sacroiliac ligaments. SYN tuberositas sacralis [TA].

scaphoid t., SYN t. of navicular bone.

t. for serratus anterior (muscle) [TA], a rough oval area, about the middle of the outer surface and lower border of the second rib [II], for the attachment of the serratus anterior muscle. SYN tuberositas musculi serrati anterioris [TA].

tibial t. [TA], an oval elevation on the anterior surface of the tibia about 3 cm distal to the articular surface, giving attachment at its distal part to the patellar ligament. SYN tuberositas tibiae [TA].

t. of ulna [TA], a prominence at the lower border of the anterior surface of the coronoid process, giving attachment (insertion) to the brachialis muscle. SYN tuberositas ulnae [TA].

tu

ungual t., SYN t. of distal phalanx (of hand and foot).

tu·ber·ous (too′ber-ŭs). Knobby, lumpy, or nodular; presenting many tubers or tuberosities. SYN tuberiferous, tuberose. [L. *tuberosus*]

⌂**tubo-.** Tubular, a tube. SEE ALSO salpingo-. [L. *tubus, tuba,* tube]

tu·bo·ab·dom·i·nal (too′bō-ab-dom′i-năl). Relating to a uterine tube and the abdomen.

tu·bo·cu·ra·rine chlo·ride (too′bō-koor-ar′ēn). An alkaloid (obtained from the stems of *Chondodendron,* particularly *C. tomentosum*) that blocks the action of acetylcholine at the myoneural junction by occupying the receptors competitively; also blocks ganglionic transmission and releases histamine; used to produce muscular relaxation during surgical operations.

tu·bo·lig·a·men·tous (too′bō-lig-ă-men′tŭs). Relating to the uterine tube and the broad ligament of the uterus.

tu·bo·o·var·i·an (too′bō-ō-vā′rē-an). Relating to the uterine tube and the ovary.

tu·bo·o·var·i·ec·to·my (too′bō-ō-var-ē-ek′to-mǐ). SYN salpingo-oophorectomy.

tu·bo·o·va·ri·tis (too′bō-ō-va-rī′tis). SYN salpingo-oophoritis.

tu·bo·per·i·to·ne·al (too′bō-per-i-tō-nē′ăl). Relating to the uterine tubes and the peritoneum.

tu·bo·plas·ty (too′bō-plas-tē). SYN salpingoplasty.

tu·bo·tor·sion (too′bō-tōr-shŭn). Twisting of a tubular structure, such as an oviduct. SYN tubatorsion. [tubo- + L. *torsio,* torsion]

tu·bo·tym·pan·ic, tu·bo·tym·pa·nal (too′bō-tim-pan′ik, -tim′pă-năl). Relating to the pharyngotympanic (auditory) tube and the tympanic cavity of the ear.

tu·bo·u·ter·ine (too′bō-oo′ter-in). Relating to a uterine tube and the uterus.

tu·bo·vag·i·nal (too-bō-vaj′i-năl). Relating to a uterine tube and the vagina.

tu·bu·lar (too′bū-lăr). Relating to or of the form of a tube or tubule. SYN tubuliform.

tu·bu·la·ture (tu′bū-lă-choor). The short neck of a retort.

tu·bule (too′būl) [TA]. A small tube. SYN tubulus [TA]. [L. *tubulus,* dim. of *tubus,* tube]

Albarran y Dominguez t.'s, SYN Albarran *glands,* under *gland.*

connecting t., a narrow arching t. of the kidney joining the distal convoluted t. and the collecting t.

convoluted t. of kidney, the highly convoluted segments of the nephron in the renal labyrinth comprising the proximal convoluted tubule, which leads from Bowman capsule to the descending limb of Henle loop, and the distal convoluted t., which leads from the ascending limb of Henle loop to the collecting tube. SYN Ferrein tube, tubuli contorti (1), tubulus renalis contortus.

convoluted seminiferous t., SYN seminiferous t.'s.

dental t.'s, SYN *canaliculi* dentales, under *canaliculus.*

dentinal t.'s, SYN *canaliculi* dentales, under *canaliculus.*

discharging t., a urinary t. formed by the union of several collecting t.'s and terminating as a papillary duct.

Henle t.'s, the straight portions of the uriniferous t.'s that form the Henle loop, distinguished as the descending and ascending t.'s of Henle.

Kobelt t.'s, remnants of the mesonephric t.'s in the female, contained within the epoöphoron. SYN wolffian t.'s.

malpighian t.'s, in insects, slender tubular or hairlike excretory structures that emerge from the alimentary canal between the mesenteron (midgut) and proctodeum (hindgut) in a region frequently termed the pylorus; they vary in number from 1 to over 100, and may be assorted in equally sized bundles in some insects.

mesonephric t., an excretory t. of the mesonephros. SYN segmental t.

metanephric t., an excretory unit of the metanephros or permanent kidney.

paragenital t.'s, remnants of embryonic mesonephric t.'s, some of which form the paradidymis.

pronephric t., an excretory unit of the pronephros, present only in vestigial form in human embryos.

segmental t., SYN mesonephric t.

seminiferous t.'s, one of two or three twisted curved t.'s in each lobule of the testis, in which spermatogenesis occurs. SYN tubuli seminiferi recti [TA], convoluted seminiferous t., tubuli contorti (2).

Skene t.'s, the embryonic urethral glands which are the female homolog of the prostate.

spiral t., the segment of urinary t. coming next after the proximal convoluted t.

straight t., one of the straight t.'s of the kidney, present in the medulla and pars radiata of the cortex.

straight seminiferous t., ☆official alternate term for straight t. of testis.

straight t. of testis [TA], the continuation of the tubulus seminifer contortus which becomes straight just before entering the mediastinum to form the rete testis. SYN tubuli seminiferi recti testi [TA], straight seminiferous t.☆, tubulus rectus.

T t., SYN *tubulus* transversus.

uriniferous t., the functional unit of the kidney, composed of a long convoluted portion (nephron) and an intrarenal collecting duct.

wolffian t.'s, SYN Kobelt t.'s.

tu·bu·li (too′bū-lī). Plural of tubulus.

tu·bu·li·form (too′bū-li-fōrm). SYN tubular.

tu·bu·lin (too′bū-lin). A protein subunit of microtubules; it is a dimer composed of two globular polypeptides, α-tubulin and β-tubulin. SEE ALSO dynein.

t.-tyrosine ligase, an enzyme that covalently links a tyrosine to the C-terminal glutamyl residue of t., coupled with the hydrolysis of ATP to ADP and orthophosphate; this is a unique posttranslational modification that may have a significant role in cytoskeletal traffic, design, and stability.

tu·bu·li·za·tion (too′bū-li-zā′shŭn). Enclosing the joined ends of a divided nerve, after neurorrhaphy, in a cylinder of paraffin or of some slowly absorbable material to keep the surrounding tissues from pushing in and preventing union.

tu·bu·lo·cyst (too′bū-lō-sist). A cyst formed by the dilation of any occluded canal or tube. SYN tubular cyst.

tu·bu·lo·der·moid (too′bū-lō-der′moyd). A dermoid cyst arising from a persistent embryonal tubular structure.

tu·bu·lo·neo·gen·e·sis (too-bū-lō-nē′ō-jen′ĕ-sis). The formation of new tubules; usually refers to proliferation of tubules in renal tumors such as Wilms tumor or mesoblastic nephroma. [tubule + neogenesis]

tu·bu·lo·rac·e·mose (too′bū-lō-ras′ĕ-mōs). Denoting a gland of combined tubular and racemose structure.

tu·bu·lor·rhex·is (too′bū-lō-rek′sis). A pathologic process characterized by necrosis of the epithelial lining in localized segments of renal tubules, with focal rupture or loss of the basement membrane. [tubule + G. *rhēxis,* a breaking]

tu·bu·lose, tu·bu·lous (too′bū-lōs, -lŭs). Having many tubules.

tu·bu·lus, pl. **tu·bu·li** (too′bū-lŭs, -lī) [TA]. SYN tubule. [L. dim. of *tubus,* a pipe]

tu′buli bilif′eri, SYN biliary *ductules,* under *ductule.*

tubuli contor′ti, (1) SYN convoluted *tubule* of kidney; **(2)** SYN seminiferous *tubules,* under *tubule.*

tu′buli denta′les, SYN *canaliculi* dentales, under *canaliculus.*

tu′buli epoöph′ori, SYN transverse *ductules* of epoöphoron, under *ductule.*

tu′buli galactoph′ori, SYN lactiferous *ducts,* under *duct.*

tu′buli lactif′eri, SYN lactiferous *ducts,* under *duct.*

tu′buli paroöph′ori, SYN *ductuli* paroöphori, under *ductulus.*

t. rec′tus, SYN straight *tubule* of testis.

t. rena′lis contor′tus, SYN convoluted *tubule* of kidney.

tubuli semi′niferi recti [TA], SYN seminiferous *tubules,* under *tubule.*

tubuli semi′niferi rec′ti testi [TA], SYN straight *tubule* of testis.

t. transver′sus, a tubular invagination of the sarcolemma of skeletal or cardiac muscle fibers that surrounds myofibrils as the intermediate element of the triad; involved in transmitting the action potential from the sarcolemma to the interior of the myofibril. SYN T tubule.

tu·bus, pl. **tu·bi** (too′bŭs, -bī). A tube or canal. [L.]

    t. digesto′rius, SYN digestive *tract.*

    t. medulla′ris, SYN central *canal.*

    t. vertebra′lis, SYN vertebral *canal.*

Tucker, Ervin Alden, U.S. obstetrician, 1862–1902. SEE T.-McLean *forceps.*

tuft (tŭft). A cluster, clump, or bunch, as of hairs.

    enamel t., a group of structures representing defects in tooth mineralization that extend from the dentino-enamel junction into the enamel to about one-half its thickness.

    malpighian t., SYN glomerulus (2).

    synovial t.'s, SYN synovial *villi,* under *villus.*

tuft·sin (tuf′sin). A tetrapeptide derived from the Fc region of an immunoglobulin. Tuftsin enhances macrophage functions. [*Tufts* University + -in]

tug, tug·ging (tŭg, tŭg′ing). A pulling or dragging movement or sensation.

    tracheal t., (1) a downward pull of the trachea, manifested by a downward movement of the thyroid cartilage, synchronous with the action of the heart and symptomatic of an aneurysm of the aortic arch; the sign is elicited most easily by drawing the cricoid cartilage upward with the thumb and forefinger while the patient sits with head thrown back and mouth closed; **(2)** a jerky type of inspiration seen when the intercostal muscles and the sternocostal parts of the diaphragm are paralyzed by deep general anesthesia or muscle relaxants; due to the unopposed action of the crura pulling on the dome of the diaphragm and thence on the pericardium, lung roots, and tracheobronchial tree during each inspiration.

tu·la·re·mia (too-lă-rē′mē-ă). A disease caused by *Francisella tularensis* and transmitted to humans from rodents through the bite of a deer fly, *Chrysops discalis,* and other bloodsucking insects; can also be acquired directly through the bite of an infected animal or through handling of an infected animal carcass; symptoms, similar to those of undulant fever and plague, are a prolonged intermittent or remittent fever and often swelling and suppuration of the lymph nodes draining the site of infection; rabbits are an important reservoir host. SYN deer-fly disease, deer-fly fever, Pahvant Valley fever, Pahvant Valley plague, rabbit fever. [*Tulare,* Lake and County, CA, + G. *haima,* blood]

    glandular t., t. with predominant lymph node infection as the main manifestation.

    pulmonary t., t. affecting the lungs; tularemic *pneumonia.* SYN pulmonic t.

    pulmonic t., SYN pulmonary t.

tulle gras (tool grä′). A dressing for wounds, used chiefly in France, comprised of wide-mesh curtain net cut into squares and impregnated with soft paraffin (98 parts), balsam of Peru (1 part), and olive oil (1 part). [Fr. oily net]

Tulp (Tulpius), Nicholas (Nicolaus), Dutch anatomist, 1593–1674. SEE T. *valve.*

tu·me·fa·cient (too-mĕ-fā′shent). Causing or tending to cause swelling. [L. *tume-facio,* to cause to swell, fr. *tumeo,* to swell]

tu·me·fac·tion (too-mĕ-fak′shŭn). **1.** A swelling. SYN tumentia. **2.** SYN tumescence. [see tumefacient]

tu·me·fy (too′mĕ-fī). To swell or to cause to swell.

tu·men·tia (too-men′shē-ă). SYN tumefaction (1). [L. fr. *tumeo,* to swell]

tu·mes·cence (too-mes′ens). The condition of being or becoming tumid. SYN tumefaction (2), turgescence. [L. *tumesco,* to begin to swell]

tu·mes·cent (too-mes′ent). Denoting tumescence. SYN turgescent.

tu·mid (too′mid). Swollen, as by congestion, edema, hyperemia. SYN turgid. [L. *tumidus*]

TUMOR

◨ tu·mor (too′mŏr). **1.** Any swelling or tumefaction. **2.** SYN neoplasm. **3.** One of the four signs of inflammation (t., calor, dolor, rubor) enunciated by Celsus. [L. *tumor,* a swelling]

    acinar cell t., a solid and cystic t. of the pancreas, occurring in young women; t. cells contain zymogen granules.

    acoustic t., SYN vestibular *schwannoma.*

    acute splenic t., acute splenitis, enlargement, and softening of the spleen, usually due to bacteremia or severe bacterial toxemia.

    adenoid t., adenoma, or neoplasm with glandlike spaces.

    adenomatoid t., a small benign t. of the male epididymis and female genital tract, consisting of fibrous tissue or smooth muscle enclosing anastomosing glandlike spaces containing acid mucopolysaccharide lined by flattened cells that have ultra-structural characteristics of mesothelial cells. SYN benign mesothelioma of genital tract.

    adenomatoid odontogenic t., a benign epithelial odontogenic t. appearing radiographically as a well-circumscribed, radiolucent-radiopaque lesion usually surrounding the crown of an impacted tooth in an adolescent or young adult; characterized histologically by columnar cells organized in a ductlike configuration interspersed with spindle-shaped cells and amyloidlike deposition that gradually undergoes dystrophic calcification. SYN adenoameloblastoma, ameloblastic adenomatoid t.

    adipose t., SYN lipoma.

    ameloblastic adenomatoid t., SYN adenomatoid odontogenic t.

    amyloid t., SYN nodular *amyloidosis.*

    aortic body t., SYN chemodectoma.

    Bednar t., SYN pigmented *dermatofibrosarcoma protuberans.*

    ◨ benign t., a t. that does not form metastases and does not invade and destroy adjacent normal tissue. SYN innocent t.

    blood t., term sometimes used to denote an aneurysm, hemorrhagic cyst, or hematoma.

    borderline ovarian t., an ovarian surface epithelial t. in which the growth pattern is intermediate between benign and malignant; includes mucinous, serous, endometrioid, and Brenner t.'s of the ovary; highly curable but may recur after surgical removal. SYN low malignant potential t.

    Brenner t., a relatively infrequent benign neoplasm of the ovary, consisting chiefly of fibrous tissue that contains nests of cells resembling transitional type epithelium, as well as glandlike structures that contain mucin; origin is controversial, but it may arise from the Walthard cell rest; ordinarily found incidentally in ovaries removed for other reasons, especially in postmenopausal women.

    Brooke t., SYN trichoepithelioma.

    brown t., a mass of fibrous tissue containing hemosiderin-pigmented macrophages and multinucleated giant cells, replacing and expanding part of a bone in primary hyperparathyroidism.

    t. burden, the total mass of t. tissue carried by a patient with a malignancy.

    calcifying epithelial odontogenic t., a benign epithelial odontogenic neoplasm derived from the stratum intermedium of the enamel organ; a painless, slowly growing, mixed radiolucent-radiopaque lesion characterized histologically by cords of polyhedral epithelial cells, deposits of amyloid, and spherical calcifications. SYN Pindborg t.

    carcinoid t., a usually small, slow-growing neoplasm composed of islands of rounded, oxyphilic, or spindle-shaped cells of medium size, with moderately small vesicular nuclei, and covered by intact mucosa with a yellow cut surface; neoplastic cells are frequently palisaded at the periphery of the small groups, and the latter have a tendency to infiltrate surrounding tissue. Such neoplasms occur anywhere in the gastrointestinal tract (and in the lungs and other sites), with approximately 90% in the appendix and the remainder chiefly in the ileum, but also in the stomach, other parts of the small intestine, the colon, and the rectum; those

tu

of the appendix and small t.'s seldom metastasize, but reported incidences of metatases from other primary sites and from t.'s exceeding 2.0 cm in diameter vary from 25–75%; lymph nodes in the abdomen and the liver may be conspicuously involved, but metastases above the diaphragm are rare. SEE ALSO carcinoid *syndrome*.

carotid body t., SYN chemodectoma.

cellular t., a t. composed mainly of closely packed cells.

cerebellopontine angle t., SYN vestibular *schwannoma*.

chromaffin t., SYN chromaffinoma.

Codman t., chondroblastoma of the proximal humerus.

collision t., two originally separate t.'s, especially a carcinoma and a sarcoma, that appear to have developed by chance in close proximity, so that an area of mingling exists. SEE ALSO carcinosarcoma.

connective t., any t. of the connective tissue group, such as osteoma, fibroma, sarcoma.

dermal duct t., a benign small t. derived from the intradermal part of eccrine sweat gland ducts occurring often on the head and neck.

dermoid t., SYN dermoid *cyst*.

desmoid t., SYN desmoid (2).

desmoplastic small cell t., a high-grade malignant t. found most often in the abdomen of adolescent males; typically t. cells contain both desmin and keratin, i.e., show hybrid features like fetal mesothelial cells; the exact nature of these cells remains unknown.

dysembryoplastic neuroepithelial t., a rare low-grade neoplasm most frequently seen in children and associated with seizures and cortical dysplasia; the often multinodular, multicystic t. is composed of oligodendroglial-like cells with accompanying neurons.

eighth nerve t., SYN vestibular *schwannoma*.

embryonal t., embryonic t., a neoplasm, usually malignant, which arises during intrauterine or early postnatal development from an organ rudiment or immature tissue; it forms immature structures characteristic of the part from which it arises, and may form other tissues as well. The term includes neuroblastoma and Wilms t., and is also used to include certain neoplasms presenting in later life, this usage being based on the belief that such t.'s arise from embryonic rests. SEE ALSO teratoma. SYN embryoma.

embryonal t. of ciliary body, SYN embryonal *medulloepithelioma*.

endocervical sinus t., malignant germ cell t. commonly found in the ovary. The t. arises from primitive germ cells and develops into extra-embryonic tissue resembling the yolk sac. SYN yolk sac carcinoma.

endodermal sinus t., a malignant neoplasm occurring in the gonads, in sacrococcygeal teratomas, and in the mediastinum; produces α-fetoprotein and is thought to be derived from primitive endodermal cells. SYN yolk sac t.

endometrioid t., a t. of the ovary containing epithelial or stromal elements resembling t.'s of the endometrium.

Erdheim t., SYN craniopharyngioma.

▣**Ewing t.,** a malignant neoplasm which occurs usually before the age of 20 years, about twice as frequently in males, and in about 75% of patients involves bones of the extremities, including the shoulder girdle, with a predilection for the metaphysis; histologically, there are conspicuous foci of necrosis in association with irregular masses of small, regular, rounded, or ovoid cells (2–3 times the diameter of erythrocytes), with very scanty cytoplasm. SYN endothelial myeloma, Ewing sarcoma.

fecal t., SYN fecaloma.

fibroid t., old term for certain fibromas and leiomyomas.

gastrointestinal autonomic nerve t., benign or malignant t. of stomach and small intestine histogenetically related to myenteric plexus; may be familial and related to gastrointestinal neuronal dysplasia.

gastrointestinal stromal t., benign or malignant t. composed of unclassifiable spindle cells; immunohistochemically distinct from smooth muscle and Schwann cell t.'s.

giant cell t. of bone, a soft, reddish-brown, sometimes malignant, osteolytic t. composed of multinucleated giant cells and ovoid or spindle-shaped cells, occurring most frequently in an end of a long tubular bone of young adults. SYN giant cell myeloma, osteoclastoma.

giant cell t. of tendon sheath, a nodule, possibly inflammatory in nature, arising commonly from the flexor sheath of the fingers and thumb; composed of fibrous tissue, lipid- and hemosiderin-containing macrophages, and multinucleated giant cells. SYN localized nodular tenosynovitis.

glomus t. [MIM*138000], a vascular neoplasm composed of specialized pericytes (sometimes termed glomus cells), usually in single encapsulated nodular masses that may be several millimeters in diameter and occur almost exclusively in the skin, often subungually in the upper extremity; it is exquisitely tender and may be so painful that patients voluntarily immobilize an extremity, sometimes leading to atrophy of muscles; multiple glomus t.'s occur, sometimes with autosomal dominant inheritance. T.'s with cavernous spaces lined by glomus cells are called *glomangiomas*.

glomus jugulare t., a glomus t. arising from the jugular glomus and usually presenting initially in the hypotympanum.

glomus tympanicum t., a glomus t. arising on the medial wall of the middle ear.

Godwin t., SYN benign lymphoepithelial *lesion*.

granular cell t., a microscopically specific, generally benign t., often involving peripheral nerves in skin, mucosa, or connective tissue, derived from Schwann cells; the abundant cytoplasm contains lysosomal granules, the cells infiltrate between adjacent tissues although growth is slow, and adjacent surface epithelium may show hyperplasia.

granulosa cell t., a benign or malignant t. of the ovary arising from the membrana granulosa of the vesicular ovarian (graafian) follicle and frequently secreting estrogen; it is soft, solid, white or yellow, and consists of small round cells sometimes enclosing Call-Exner bodies; larger lipid-containing cells may be present. SYN folliculoma (1).

Grawitz t., old eponym for renal *adenocarcinoma*.

heterologous t., a t. composed of a tissue unlike that from which it springs.

hilar cell t. of ovary, SYN steroid cell t.

histoid t., old term for a t. composed of a single type of differentiated tissue.

homologous t., a t. composed of tissue of the same sort as that from which it springs.

innocent t., SYN benign t.

interstitial cell t. of testis, SYN Leydig cell t.

islet cell t., an endocrine t. composed of cells equivalent or related to those in the normal islet of Langerhans; may be benign or malignant; usually hormonally active; comprises insulinomas, glucagonomas, vipomas, somatostatinomas, gastrinomas, pancreatic polypeptide-secreting t., and multihormonal or hormonally inactive pancreatic islet cell t.'s.

juxtaglomerular cell t., a t. of juxtaglomerular cell origin usually presenting with symptoms of secondary aldosteronism, including severe diastolic hypertension, which appears to be due to t.-produced renin. The histologic appearance resembles that of a hemangiopericytoma.

Klatskin t., adenocarcinoma located at the bifurcation of the common hepatic duct.

Krukenberg t., a metastatic carcinoma of the ovary, usually bilateral and secondary to a mucous carcinoma of the stomach, which contains signet-ring cells filled with mucus.

Landschutz t., a transplantable, possibly isoantigenic, highly virulent neoplasm which can be grown in any strain of mice; the host is killed in a few days by what is apparently an anaplastic carcinoma.

Leydig cell t., a testicular and, less commonly, ovarian neoplasm composed of Leydig cells, usually benign but may be malignant; may secrete androgens or estrogens. SYN interstitial cell t. of testis.

Lindau t., SYN hemangioblastoma.

low malignant potential t., SYN borderline ovarian t.

▣**malignant t.,** a t. that invades surrounding tissues, is usually capable of producing metastases, may recur after attempted removal, and is likely to cause death of the host unless adequately treated. SEE ALSO cancer.

malignant mixed müllerian t. (MMMT), SYN mixed mesodermal t.

melanotic neuroectodermal t. of infancy, a benign neoplasm of neuroectodermal origin that most often involves the anterior maxilla of infants in the first year of life. It presents clinically as a rapidly growing blue-black lesion producing a destructive radiolucency; histologically, it is characterized by small, round, undifferentiated t. cells interspersed with larger polyhedral melanin-producing t. cells arranged in an alveolar configuration. SYN melanoameloblastoma, pigmented ameloblastoma, pigmented epulis, progonoma of jaw, retinal anlage t.

Merkel cell t., a rare malignant cutaneous t. seen in sun-exposed skin of elderly patients composed of dermal nodules of small round cells with scanty cytoplasm in a trabecular pattern; the t. cells contain cytoplasmic dense core granules resembling neurosecretory granules seen in Merkel cells. SYN primary neuroendocrine carcinoma of the skin, trabecular carcinoma.

mesonephroid t., SYN mesonephroma.

mixed t., a t. composed of two or more varieties of tissue.

mixed mesodermal t., a sarcoma of the body of the uterus arising in older women, composed of more than one mesenchymal tissue, especially including striated muscle cells. SYN malignant mixed müllerian t.

mixed t. of salivary gland, a t. composed of salivary gland epithelium and fibrous tissue with mucoid or cartilaginous areas. SYN pleomorphic adenoma.

mixed t. of skin, SYN chondroid *syringoma*.

mucoepidermoid t., SYN mucoepidermoid *carcinoma*.

Nelson t., a pituitary t. causing the symptoms of Nelson *syndrome*.

oil t., SYN lipogranuloma.

oncocytic hepatocellular t., SYN fibrolamellar liver cell *carcinoma*.

organoid t., a t. of complex structure, glandular in origin, containing epithelium, connective tissue, etc.

Pancoast t., any carcinoma of the lung apex causing the Pancoast syndrome by invasion or compression of the brachial plexus and stellate ganglion. SYN superior pulmonary sulcus t.

papillary t., SYN papilloma.

paraffin t., SYN paraffinoma.

phantom t., accumulation of fluid in the interlobar spaces of the lung, secondary to congestive heart failure, radiologically simulating a neoplasm.

phyllodes t., a spectrum of neoplasms consisting of a mixture of benign epithelium and stroma with variable cellularity and cytologic abnormalities, ranging from benign phyllodes t. to cytosarcoma phyllodes; most often involves the breast.

pilar t. of scalp, a solitary t. of the scalp in elderly women that may ulcerate; microscopically resembles squamous cell carcinoma composed of glycogen-rich clear cells, but is benign. SYN proliferating tricholemmal cyst.

Pindborg t., SYN calcifying epithelial odontogenic t.

Pinkus t., SYN fibroepithelioma.

placental site trophoblastic t., a t. usually arising in the uterus of parous women during reproductive years. Histologically, the t. consists of a predominance of intermediate trophoblastic cells with fibrinoid material and vascular invasion.

pontine angle t., a t. in the angle formed by the cerebellum and the lateral pons, often refers to an acoustic schwannoma.

potato t. of neck, a firm nodular mass in the neck, usually a carotid body t. (chemodectoma).

pregnancy t., SYN *granuloma* gravidarum.

primitive neuroectodermal t., a designation used to refer to a group of morphologically similar embryonal neoplasms that arise in intracranial and peripheral sites of the nervous system and which may show various degrees of cellular differentiation; includes medulloblastoma, pineoblastoma, etc.

ranine t., SYN ranula (2).

Rathke pouch t., SYN craniopharyngioma.

retinal anlage t., SYN melanotic neuroectodermal t. of infancy.

Rous t., SYN Rous *sarcoma*.

sand t., SYN psammomatous *meningioma*.

t. cell t., a t. of testis or ovary composed of Sertoli cells; most often benign but may be malignant.

Sertoli-Leydig cell t., an ovarian t. composed of Sertoli and Leydig cells; may secrete androgens. SYN arrhenoblastoma, gynandroblastoma (1).

Sertoli-stromal cell t., a generic term for ovarian sex-cord stromal t. composed of Sertoli cells, Leydig cells, and cells resembling rete epithelial cells, either in a pure form or as a mixture of these cell types.

solitary fibrous t., a benign t. of fibrous tissue which usually arises in the pleural space on other sites. SYN benign mesothelioma.

squamous odontogenic t., a benign epithelial odontogenic t. thought to arise from the epithelial cell rests of Malassez; appears clinically as a radiolucent lesion closely associated with the tooth root and histologically as islands of squamous epithelium enclosed by a peripheral layer of flattened cells.

steroid cell t., a collective term used for ovarian t.'s composed of cells resembling steroid-secreting lutein cells; comprises several t.'s such as stromal luteoma, Leydig cell t., steroid cell t. not otherwise specified; hormonally active; may be benign or malignant. SYN hilar cell t. of ovary.

sugar t., a benign clear cell t. of the lung containing abundant glycogen.

superior pulmonary sulcus t., SYN Pancoast t.

teratoid t., SYN teratoma.

theca cell t., SYN thecoma.

triton t., a peripheral nerve t. with striated muscle differentiation, seen most often in neurofibromatosis; named after the Masson theory of transformation of motor nerve fibers into muscle in triton salamanders.

turban t., multiple cylindromas the scalp which, when overgrown, may resemble a turban.

villous t., SYN villous *papilloma*.

Warthin t., SYN adenolymphoma.

Wilms t., a malignant renal t. of young children, composed of small spindle cells and various other types of tissue, including tubules and, in some cases, structures resembling fetal glomeruli, and striated muscle and cartilage. Often inherited as an autosomal dominant trait [MIM*194070, *194080, *194090]. SYN nephroblastoma.

yolk sac t., SYN endodermal sinus t.

Zollinger-Ellison t., a non–beta cell t. of pancreatic islets causing the Zollinger-Ellison syndrome.

---

tu·mor·i·ci·dal (too′mŏr-i-sī′dăl). Denoting an agent destructive to tumors. [tumor + L. *caedo,* to kill]

tu·mor·i·gen·e·sis (too′mŏr-i-jen′ĕ-sis). Production of a new growth or growths. [tumor + G. *genesis,* origin]

foreign body t., induction of malignant tumors in tissues by nonviable, nonabsorable solid material not known to contain a chemical carcinogen.

tu·mor·i·gen·ic (too′mŏr-i-jen′ik). Causing or producing tumors.

tu·mor·lets (too′mŏr-lets). Minute foci of atypical bronchiolar epithelial hyperplasia that are found multifocally; although now considered benign, they were once believed to be precursors of carcinoma.

tu·mor·ous (too′mŏr-ŭs). Swollen; tumorlike; protuberant.

tu·mul·tus cor·dis (too-mŭl′tŭs kōr′dis). Palpitation and irregular action of the heart.

TUNEL Abbreviation for terminal deoxynucleotidyl transferase-mediated dUTP-biotin end labeling of fragmented DNA; this method uses immunohistochemistry to identify DNA fragmentation in nuclei of cells undergoing apoptosis.

Tun·ga pen·e·trans (tŭng′ă pen′ĕ-tranz). A member of the flea family, Tungidae, commonly known as chigger flea, sand flea, chigoe, or jigger; the minute female penetrates the skin, fre-

TU

quently under the toenails; as she becomes distended with eggs to about pea size, a painful ulcer with inflammation develops at the site. SYN *Sarcopsylla penetrans.*

tun·gi·a·sis (tŭng-ī′ă-sis). Infestation with sand fleas (*Tunga penetrans*).

Tung·i·dae (tŭng′i-dē). A family of fleas containing the jigger or chigoe flea species, *Tunga penetrans.*

tung·state (tŭng′stāt). An anionic form of tungsten.

calcium t., a phosphor with a high stopping power for x-rays that was formerly used widely in fluoroscopic screens and intensifying screens for radiography.

tung·sten (W) (tŭng′sten). A metallic element, atomic no. 74, atomic wt. 183.85. SYN wolfram, wolframium. [Swed. *tung,* heavy, + *sten,* stone]

t. carbide, one of the hardest known materials, used as an abrasive and in the manufacture of dental cutting instruments.

tu·nic (too′nik). Coat or covering; one of the enveloping layers of a part, especially one of the coats of a blood vessel or other tubular structure. SEE ALSO layer. SYN tunica. [L. *tunica*]

Bichat t., the tunica intima of the blood vessels.

Brücke t., SYN *tunica* nervea.

fibrous t. of corpus spongiosum, SYN *tunica* albuginea of corpus spongiosum.

fibrous t. of eye, SYN fibrous *layer* of eyeball.

mucosal t.'s, mucous t.'s, SYN mucosa.

muscular t.'s, SEE muscular *layer.*

muscular t. of gallbladder, SYN muscular *layer* of gallbladder.

nervous t. of eyeball, SYN inner *layer* of eyeball.

serous t., SYN serosa.

vascular t. of eye, SYN vascular *layer* of eyeball.

TUNICA

tu·ni·ca, pl. **tu·ni·cae** (too′ni-kă, -kē). SYN tunic. [L. a coat]

t. adventi′tia, SYN adventitia.

t. albugin′ea, a dense white collagenous tunic surrounding a structure.

t. albuginea of corpora cavernosa [TA], a strong, fibrous membrane enveloping the corpora cavernosa penis. SYN t. albuginea corporum cavernosorum [TA].

t. albugin′ea cor′poris spongio′si [TA], SYN t. albuginea of corpus spongiosum.

t. albugin′ea cor′porum cavernoso′rum [TA], SYN t. albuginea of corpora cavernosa.

t. albuginea of corpus spongiosum [TA], the thick layer of fibrous tissue surrounding the corpus spongiosum penis; it is thinner than the corresponding layer around each corpus cavernosum. SYN t. albuginea corporis spongiosi [TA], fibrous tunic of corpus spongiosum.

t. albugin′ea oc′uli, SYN sclera.

t. albuginea ovarii [TA], SYN t. albuginea of ovary.

t. albuginea of ovary [TA], thin organ capsule of the ovary deep to the germinal epithelium. SYN t. albuginea ovarii [TA].

t. albugin′ea tes′tis [TA], SYN t. albuginea of testis.

t. albuginea of testis [TA], a thick white fibrous membrane forming the outer coat or capsule of the testis. SYN t. albuginea testis [TA], perididymis.

t. car′nea, SYN dartos *fascia.*

t. conjuncti′va [TA], SYN conjunctiva.

t. conjuncti′va bul′bi [TA], SYN bulbar *conjunctiva.*

t. conjuncti′va palpebra′rum [TA], SYN palpebral *conjunctiva.*

t. dar′tos [TA], SYN dartos *fascia;* SEE ALSO *dartos* muliebris.

t. elas′tica, t. media of large arteries.

t. exter′na [TA], **(1)** the outer of two or more enveloping layers of any structure; **(2)** specifically, the outer fibroelastic coat of a blood or lymph vessel. SYN t. extima [TA].

t. exter′na oc′uli, SYN fibrous *layer* of eyeball.

t. exter′na the′cae follic′uli, the external fibrous layer of the theca of a well-developed vesicular ovarian follicle; the cells and fibers are arranged in a concentric fashion. SYN theca externa.

t. ex′tima [TA], SYN t. externa.

t. fibromusculocartilaginea bronchi [TA], SYN fibromusculocartilagenous *layer* of bronchi.

t. fibro′sa [TA], SYN fibrous *capsule.*

t. fibro′sa bul′bi [TA], SYN fibrous *layer* of eyeball.

t. fibro′sa hep′atis [TA], SYN fibrous *capsule* of liver (2).

t. fibro′sa lie′nis, SYN fibrous *capsule* of spleen, fibrous *capsule* of spleen.

t. fibro′sa re′nis, SYN fibrous *capsule* of kidney.

t. fibro′sa sple′nis, ⋆official alternate term for fibrous *capsule* of spleen.

tu′nicae funic′uli spermat′ici, SYN *coverings* of spermatic cord, under *covering.*

Haller t. vasculosa, SYN vascular *layer* of eyeball.

t. interna bulbi [TA], SYN inner *layer* of eyeball.

t. inter′na the′cae follic′uli, the inner cellular and vascular layer of the vesicular ovarian follicle; there is evidence that the epithelioid cells produce estrogen and contribute to the formation of the corpus luteum after ovulation. SYN theca interna.

t. in′tima [TA], the innermost coat of a blood or lymphatic vessel; it consists of endothelium, usually a thin fibroelastic subendothelial layer, and an inner elastic membrane or longitudinal fibers.

t. me′dia [TA], the middle, usually muscular, coat of an artery or other tubular structure. SYN media (1).

t. muco′sa [TA], SYN mucosa.

t. muco′sa bronchi [TA], SYN *mucosa* of bronchi.

t. muco′sa cavita′tis tym′pani [TA], SYN *mucosa* of tympanic cavity.

t. muco′sa co′li, SYN *mucosa* of colon.

t. muco′sa duc′tus deferen′tis [TA], SYN *mucosa* of ductus deferens.

t. muco′sa esoph′agi [TA], SYN *mucosa* of esophagus.

t. muco′sa gas′trica [TA], SYN *mucosa* of stomach.

t. mucosa intestini crassi [TA], SYN *mucosa* of large intestine.

t. muco′sa intesti′ni ten′uis [TA], SYN *mucosa* of small intestine.

t. muco′sa laryn′gis [TA], SYN *mucosa* of larynx.

t. muco′sa lin′guae [TA], SYN *mucosa* of tongue.

t. muco′sa na′si [TA], SYN *mucosa* of nose.

t. muco′sa o′ris [TA], SYN *mucosa* of mouth.

t. mucosa pelvis renalis [TA], SYN *mucosa* of renal pelvis.

t. muco′sa pharyn′gis [TA], SYN *mucosa* of pharynx.

t. muco′sa tra′cheae [TA], SYN *mucosa* of trachea.

t. muco′sa tu′bae auditi′vae [TA], SYN *mucosa* of pharyngotympanic (auditory) tube.

t. mucosa tubae auditoriae, SYN *mucosa* of pharyngotympanic (auditory) tube.

t. muco′sa tu′bae uteri′nae [TA], SYN *mucosa* of uterine tube.

t. muco′sa ure′teris [TA], SYN *mucosa* of ureter.

t. muco′sa ure′thrae femini′nae [TA], SYN *mucosa* of female urethra.

t. muco′sa u′teri [TA], SYN endometrium.

t. muco′sa vagi′nae [TA], SYN *mucosa* of vagina.

t. muco′sa vesi′cae bilia′ris [TA], SYN *mucosa* of gallbladder.

t. muco′sa vesi′cae fel′leae, ⋆official alternate term for *mucosa* of gallbladder, *mucosa* of gallbladder.

t. muco′sa vesi′cae urina′riae [TA], SYN *mucosa* of (urinary) bladder.

t. muco′sa vesic′ulae semina′lis, ⋆official alternate term for *mucosa* of seminal gland.

t. muscula′ris [TA], SYN muscular *layer.*

t. muscula′ris bronchio′rum [TA], SYN muscular *layer* of bronchi.

t. muscula′ris co′li [TA], SYN muscular *layer* of colon.

t. muscula′ris duc′tus deferen′tis [TA], SYN muscular *layer* of ductus deferens.

t. muscula′ris esoph′agi [TA], SYN muscular *layer* of esophagus.

t. muscula′ris gas′trica [TA], SYN muscular *layer* of stomach.

t. muscularis glandulae vesiculosae [TA], SYN muscular *layer* of seminal gland.

t. muscularis intestini crassi [TA], SYN muscular *layer* of large intestine.

t. muscula′ris intesti′ni ten′uis [TA], SYN muscular *layer* of small intestine.

t. muscularis partis intermediae urethrae masculinae [TA], SYN muscular *layer* of intermediate part of (male) urethra.

t. muscularis partis prostaticae urethrae masculinae [TA], SYN muscular *layer* of prostatic urethra.

t. muscularis partis spongiosae urethrae masculinae [TA], SYN muscular *layer* of spongy (male) urethra.

t. muscularis pelvis renalis [TA], SYN muscular *layer* of renal pelvis.

t. muscula′ris pharyn′gis [TA], SYN muscular *layer* of pharynx.

t. muscula′ris rec′ti [TA], SYN muscular *layer* of rectum.

t. muscula′ris tra′cheae [TA], SYN muscular *layer* of trachea.

t. muscula′ris tu′bae uteri′nae [TA], SYN muscular *layer* of uterine tube.

t. muscula′ris ure′teris [TA], SYN muscular *layer* of ureter.

t. muscula′ris ure′thrae femini′nae [TA], SYN muscular *layer* of female urethra.

t. muscularis urethrae masculinae [TA], SYN muscular *layer* of male urethra.

t. muscula′ris u′teri [TA], SYN myometrium.

t. muscula′ris vagi′nae [TA], SYN muscular *layer* of vagina.

t. muscula′ris ventric′uli, SYN muscular *layer* of stomach.

t. muscula′ris vesi′cae bilia′ris [TA], SYN muscular *layer* of gallbladder.

t. muscula′ris vesi′cae fel′leae, ✫official alternate term for muscular *layer* of gallbladder.

t. muscula′ris vesi′cae urina′riae [TA], SYN muscular *layer* of urinary bladder.

t. ner′vea, an older term, formerly used to designate the retina exclusive of the layer of rods and cones. SYN Brücke tunic.

t. pro′pria, the special envelope of a part as distinguished from the peritoneal or other investment common to several parts.

t. pro′pria co′rii, SYN *stratum* reticulare corii.

t. pro′pria lie′nis, SYN fibrous *capsule* of spleen.

t. reflex′a, the reflected layer of the t. vasculosa testis that lines the scrotum.

t. sclerot′ica, SYN sclera.

t. sero′sa [TA], SYN serosa.

t. sero′sa co′li, SYN *serosa* of large intestine.

t. serosa esophagi [TA], SYN *serosa* of esophagus.

t. sero′sa gas′tricae [TA], SYN *serosa* of stomach.

t. sero′sa hep′atis [TA], SYN *serosa* of liver.

t. serosa intestini crassi [TA], SYN *serosa* of large intestine.

t. sero′sa intesti′ni ten′uis [TA], SYN *serosa* of small intestine.

t. serosa pericardii serosi [TA], SYN *serosa* of serous pericardium.

t. sero′sa peritone′i [TA], SYN *serosa* of peritoneum.

t. serosa pleurae parietalis [TA], SYN *serosa* of parietal pleura.

t. serosa pleurae visceralis [TA], SYN *serosa* of visceral pleura.

t. serosa splenis [TA], SYN *serosa* of the spleen.

t. sero′sa tu′bae uteri′nae [TA], SYN *serosa* of uterine tube.

t. sero′sa u′teri [TA], SYN perimetrium, *serosa* of uterus.

t. sero′sa ventric′uli, SYN *serosa* of stomach.

t. sero′sa vesi′cae bilia′ris [TA], SYN *serosa* of gallbladder.

t. sero′sa vesi′cae fel′leae, ✫official alternate term for *serosa* of gallbladder.

t. sero′sa vesi′cae (urina′riae) [TA], SYN *serosa* of (urinary) bladder.

t. spongiosa urethrae femininae [TA], SYN spongy *layer* of female urethra.

t. spongiosa vaginae [TA], SYN spongy *layer* of vagina.

t. submuco′sa, SYN submucosa.

t. urethrae masculinae [TA], SYN *mucosa* of male urethra.

t. vagina′lis commu′nis, SYN internal spermatic *fascia*.

t. vagina′lis tes′tis, the serous sheath of the testis and epididymis, derived from the peritoneum; it consists of outer parietal and inner visceral serous layers.

t. vasculo′sa, any vascular layer.

t. vasculo′sa bul′bi [TA], SYN vascular *layer* of eyeball.

t. vasculo′sa len′tis, a nutrient vascular layer enveloping the lens of the eye in the fetus.

t. vasculo′sa oc′uli, SYN vascular *layer* of eyeball.

t. vasculo′sa tes′tis, the vascular layer enveloping the testis beneath the t. albuginea.

t. vasculosa testis [TA], SYN vascular *layer* of testis.

t. vit′rea, SYN posterior limiting *lamina* of cornea.

tun·nel (tŭn′ĕl). An elongated passageway, usually open at both ends.

aortico-left ventricular t., congenital connection between the aorta above exit of coronary arteries and the left ventricle.

ⓘ**carpal t.** [TA], the passageway deep to the transverse carpal ligament between tubercles of the scaphoid and trapezoid bones on the radial side and the pisiform and hook of the hamate on the ulnar side, through which the median nerve and the flexor tendons of the fingers and thumb pass; compression of the median nerve may occur here (carpal t. syndrome). SYN canalis carpi [TA], carpal canal (1).

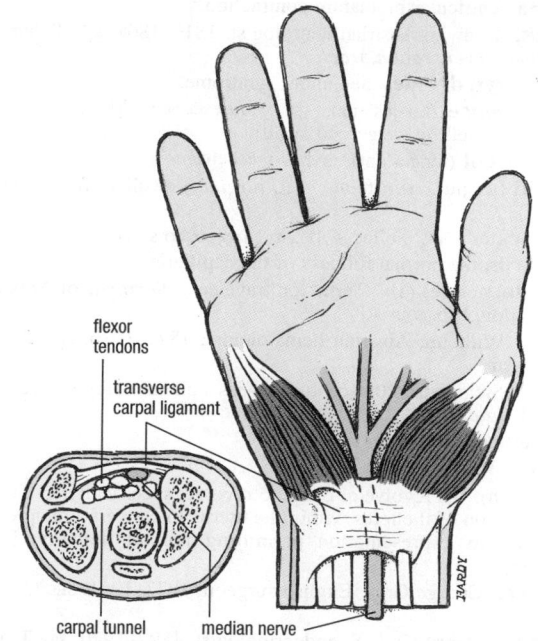

carpal tunnel: containing the median nerve and the flexor tendons of the fingers and thumb

Corti t., the spiral canal in the organ of Corti, formed by the outer and inner pillar cells or rods of Corti; it is filled with fluid and occasionally crossed by nonmedullated nerve fibers. SYN Corti canal.

Tuohy, Edward B., 20th century U.S. anesthesiologist. SEE T. *needle.*

tu·ran·ose (toor′ă-nōs). A reducing disaccharide.

Tur·ba·trix (ter-bā′triks). A genus of free-living nematodes in the family Cephalobidae. [L. *turbare,* to disturb]

T. aceti, a species found in old vinegar or in rotting fruits and vegetables and occasionally as a contaminant in laboratory solutions. SYN vinegar eel.

tur·bid (ter'bid). Cloudy, as by sediment or insoluble matter in a solution. [L. *turbidus,* confused, disordered]

tur·bi·dim·e·ter (ter-bi-dim'ĕ-ter). An instrument for measuring turbidity.

tur·bi·di·met·ric (ter'bid-i-met'rik). Pertaining to the measurement of turbidity.

tur·bi·dim·e·try (ter-bi-dim'ĕ-trē). A method for determining the concentration of a substance in a solution by the degree of cloudiness or turbidity it causes or by the degree of clarification it induces in a turbid solution. [turbidity + G. *metron,* measure]

tur·bid·i·ty (ter-bid'i-tē). The quality of being turbid, of losing transparency because of sediment or insoluble matter. [L. *turbiditas,* fr. *turbidus,* turbid]

tur·bi·nal (ter'bi-năl). SYN turbinated *body* (1).

tur·bi·nate (ter'bi-nāt). A bone shaped like a top, especially referring to turbinated bones. SEE inferior nasal *concha,* middle nasal *concha,* superior nasal *concha,* supreme nasal *concha.*

tur·bi·nat·ed (ter'bi-nāt-ed). Scroll-shaped. [L. *turbinatus,* shaped like a top]

tur·bi·nec·to·my (ter'bi-nek'tō-mē). Surgical removal of a turbinated bone. [turbinate + G. *ektomē,* excision]

tur·bi·no·tome (ter'bi-nō-tōm). An instrument for use in turbinotomy or turbinectomy.

tur·bi·not·o·my (ter'bi-not'ō-mē). Incision into or excision of a turbinated body. [turbinate + G. *tomē,* incision]

tur·bu·lence.

    heart rate t., fluctuations of electrocardiographic cycle length after a ventricular premature contraction.

Türck, Ludwig, Austrian neurologist, 1810–1868. SEE T. *bundle, column, degeneration, tract.*

Turcot syn·drome. See under syndrome.

tur·ges·cence (ter-jes'ens). SYN tumescence. [L. *turgesco,* to begin to swell, fr. *turgeo,* to swell]

tur·ges·cent (ter-jes'ent). SYN tumescent.

tur·gid (ter'jid). SYN tumid. [L. *turgidus,* swollen, fr. *turgeo,* to swell]

tur·gor (ter'gōr). Fullness. [L., fr. *turgeo,* to swell]
    t. vita'lis, the normal fullness of the capillaries.

tu·ris·ta (too-rēs'tă). Term for traveler's *diarrhea,* of Mexican derivation. [Sp. tourist]

Türk, Wilhelm, Austrian hematologist, 1871–1916. SEE T. *cell, leukocyte.*

Türk, Siegmund, 20th century Swiss ophthalmologist. SEE Ehrlich-T. *line.*

tur·key red (ter'kē). SYN madder.

tur·mer·ic (ter'mer-ik). Curcuma.

turn (tern). To revolve or cause to revolve; specifically, to change the position of the fetus within the uterus to convert a malpresentation into a presentation permitting normal delivery. [A.S. *tyrnan*]

Turner, George Grey, English surgeon, 1877–1951. SEE Grey T. *sign.*

Turner, Henry H., U.S. endocrinologist, 1892–1970. SEE T. *syndrome.*

Turner, Joseph G., English dentist, †1955. SEE T. *tooth.*

Turner, Sir William, English anatomist, 1832–1916. SEE intraparietal *sulcus* of Turner, Turner *sulcus.*

turn·o·ver (tern'ō-ver). The quantity of a material metabolized or processed, usually within a given length of time.

tur·pen·tine (ter'pen-tīn). An oleoresin from *Pinus palustris* and other species of *Pinus;* source of t. oil and a constituent of stimulating ointments. [G. *terebinthinos,* pertaining to *terebinthos,* the terebinth tree]

    Canada t., SYN Canada *balsam.*

    Chian t., an exudation from *Pistacia terebinthus,* a small tree of Chios and regions eastward; on exposure to air it thickens and forms translucent yellow masses similar to mastic.

    larch t., a transparent, yellowish, thick liquid, the oleoresin obtained from *Larix europaea* (family Pinaceae). SYN Venice t.

    Venice t., SYN larch t.

    white t., t. from *Pinus palustris.*

tur·pen·tine oil. A volatile oil, distilled from turpentine, that has been used as a diuretic, carminative, vermifuge, expectorant, rubefacient, and counterirritant. SYN oleum terebinthinae, turpentine spirit.

    rectified t. o., obtained by treating t. o. with sodium hydroxide, and redistilling; used externally as a counterirritant.

tur·pen·tine spir·it. SYN turpentine oil.

turps (terps). Popular name for turpentine oil.

tur·ri·ceph·a·ly (toor-i-sef'ă-lē). SYN oxycephaly. [L. *turris,* tower, + G. *kephalē,* head]

tu·run·da, pl. **tu·run·dae** (too-rŭn'dă, -dē). A surgical tent, gauze drain, or tampon. [L.]

tus·sal (tŭs'ăl). SYN tussive.

tus·sic·u·lar (tŭ-sik'ū-lăr). SYN tussive. [L. *tussicularis,* fr. *tussicula,* a slight cough, dim. of *tussis,* cough]

tus·sic·u·la·tion (tŭ-sik'ū-lā'shŭn). A hacking cough.

tus·sig·en·ic (tus'ĭ-jen'ik). Causing cough. [L. *tussis,* cough, + *-gen,* producing]

tus·sis (tŭs'is). A cough. [L.]

tus·sive (tŭs'siv). Relating to a cough. SYN tussal, tussicular. [L. *tussis,* a cough]

tu·ta·men, pl. **tu·ta·mi·na** (too-tā'men, -tā'mi-nă). Any defensive or protective structure. [L. protection]

    tuta'mina cer'ebri, the scalp, cranium, and cerebral meninges.

    tuta'mina oc'uli, the eyebrows, eyelids, and eyelashes.

Tuttle, James P., U.S. surgeon, 1857–1913. SEE T. *proctoscope.*

TUU Abbreviation for transureteroureterostomy.

TVG Abbreviation for time-varied *gain.*

TWAR SYN *Chlamydia pneumoniae.* [after the laboratory designations of the first two isolates, TW-83 and AR-39]

Tweed, Charles H., U.S. orthodontist, 1895–1970. SEE T. edgewise *treatment, triangle.*

tweez·ers (twē'zerz). An instrument with pincers that are squeezed together to grasp or extract fine structures. [A.S. *twisel,* fork]

twig. One of the finer terminal branches of an artery; a small branch or small ramus. [A.S.]

twi·light (twī'līt). **1.** Figuratively, a faint light. **2.** Pertaining to faint or indistinct mental perception, as in twilight *state.* [A.S. *twi-,* two]

twin. 1. One of two children born at one birth. **2.** Double; growing in pairs. [A.S. *getwin,* double]

    allantoidoangiopagous t.'s, unequal monochorial t.'s with fusion of their allantoic vessels within the placenta; the lesser t. is essentially a parasite on the placental circulation of the larger t.

    conjoined t.'s, monozygotic t.'s with varying extent of union and different degrees of residual duplication. The various types of union are named by the use of a prefix designating the region that is united and adding the suffix *-pagus,* meaning joined (e.g., craniopagus, thoracopagus); the various types of residual duplication are named by designating the parts duplicated and adding the suffix *-didymus,* or *-dymus,* meaning twin (e.g., cephalodidymus, cephalodymus).

    conjoined asymmetric t.'s, SYN conjoined unequal t.'s.

    conjoined equal t.'s, conjoined t.'s in which both members are approximately of the same size, and nearly normal except for the areas of union. SYN conjoined symmetric t.'s.

    conjoined symmetric t.'s, SYN conjoined equal t.'s.

    conjoined unequal t.'s, conjoined t.'s in which one member is nearly normal (host or autosite) and the other (parasite) is small, incomplete, and dependent for its nutrition upon the more nearly normal member. SYN conjoined asymmetric t.'s.

    dichorial t.'s, SYN dizygotic t.'s.

    diovular t.'s, SYN dizygotic t.'s.

dizygotic t.'s, t.'s derived from two separate zygotes. SYN dichorial t.'s, diovular t.'s, fraternal t.'s, heterologous t.'s.

enzygotic t.'s, SYN monozygotic t.'s.

fraternal t.'s, SYN dizygotic t.'s.

heterologous t.'s, SYN dizygotic t.'s.

identical t.'s, SYN monozygotic t.'s.

incomplete conjoined t.'s, conjoined t.'s, the two components of which equal one another but are less than entire individuals.

locked t.'s, a form of malpresentation in which a breech t. and a vertex t. become locked at the chin during labor and attempted delivery.

monoamniotic t.'s, t.'s within a common amnion; such t.'s are monovular in origin and may be conjoined.

monochorial t.'s, SYN monozygotic t.'s.

monovular t.'s, SYN monozygotic t.'s.

▣**monozygotic t.'s,** t.'s resulting from a single fertilized ovum that at an early stage of development becomes separated into independently growing cell aggregations giving rise to two individuals of the same sex and identical genetic constitution. SYN enzygotic t.'s, identical t.'s, monochorial t.'s, monovular t.'s, uniovular t.'s.

parasitic t., the smaller of unequal conjoined t.'s.

placental parasitic t., SYN omphalosite.

polyzygotic t.'s, t.'s resulting from fertilization of more than two ova discharged in a single ovulating cycle.

Siamese t.'s, originally, a much publicized conjoined pair of t.'s (xiphopagus) from Siam in the 19th century; this term has since come into general lay usage for any type of conjoined t.'s, but is incorrect.

uniovular t.'s, SYN monozygotic t.'s.

twinge (twinj). A sudden momentary sharp pain.

twin·ning. Production of equivalent structures by division; the tendency of divided parts to assume symmetric relations.

twitch. **1.** To jerk spasmodically. **2.** A momentary spasmodic contraction of a muscle fiber. [A.S. *twiccian*]

Twort, Frederick W., British bacteriologist, 1877–1950. SEE T. *phenomenon*; T.-d'Herelle *phenomenon*.

TX Abbreviation for individual thromboxanes, designated by capital letters with subscripts indicating structural features.

ty·ba·mate (tī'bă-māt). A tranquilizer related to meprobamate.

ty·lec·to·my (tī-lek'tō-mē). Surgical removal of a localized swelling or tumor. SEE ALSO lumpectomy. [G. *tylē*, lump, + *ektomē*, excision]

tyl·i·on, pl. **tyl·ia** (til'ē-on, -lē-ă; tī'lē-on). A craniometric point at the middle of the anterior edge of the chiasmatic groove. [G. a small pin, dim. of *tylē*, a lump]

ty·lo·ma (tī-lō'mă). SYN callosity. [G. a callus]

t. conjuncti'vae, localized keratinization of the conjunctiva, occurring in xerosis of the conjunctiva.

ty·lo·sis, pl. **ty·lo·ses** (tī-lō'sis, -sēz). Formation of a callus (tyloma). [G. a becoming callous]

t. cilia'ris, SYN pachyblepharon.

t. ling'uae, leukoplakia of the tongue.

t. palma'ris et planta'ris, SYN palmoplantar *keratoderma*.

ty·lox·a·pol (tī-lok'să-pol). A detergent and mucolytic agent used as an aerosol to liquify sputum.

ty·maz·o·line (tī-maz'ō-lēn). A nasal decongestant.

△**tympan-.** SEE tympano-.

tym·pa·nal (tim'pă-năl). **1.** SYN tympanic (1). **2.** Resonant. **3.** SYN tympanitic (2).

tym·pa·nec·to·my (tim'pă-nek'tō-mē). Excision of the tympanic membrane. [tympan- + G. *ektomē*, excision]

tym·pan·ia (tim-pan'ē-ă). SYN tympanites.

tym·pan·ic (tim-pan'ik). **1.** Relating to the t. cavity or membrane. SYN tympanal (1). **2.** Resonant. **3.** SYN tympanitic (2).

tym·pan·i·chord (tim-pan'i-kōrd). SYN *chorda* tympani.

tym·pan·i·chor·dal (tim-pan-i-kōr'dăl). Relating to the chorda tympani nerve.

tym·pa·nic·i·ty (tim'pă-nis'i-tē). The quality of being tympanic or drumlike in tone.

tym·pa·nism (tim'pă-nizm). SYN tympanites.

tym·pa·ni·tes (tim-pă-nī'tēz). Swelling of the abdomen from gas in the intestinal or peritoneal cavity. SYN meteorism, tympania, tympanism. [L. fr. G. *tympanitēs*, an edema in which the belly is stretched like a drum, *tympanon*]

uterine t., SYN physometra.

tym·pa·nit·ic (tim-pă-nit'ik). **1.** Referring to tympanites. SYN tympanous. **2.** Denoting the quality of sound elicited by percussing over the inflated intestine or a large pulmonary cavity. SYN tympanal (3), tympanic (3).

tym·pa·ni·tis (tim-pă-nī'tis). SYN myringitis.

△**tympano-, tympan-, tympani-.** Tympanum, tympanites. [G. *tympanon*, drum]

tym·pa·no·cen·te·sis (tim'pă-nō-sen-tē'sis). Puncture of the tympanic membrane with a needle to aspirate middle ear fluid. [tympano- + G. *kentēsis*, puncture]

tym·pa·no·eu·sta·chian (tim'pă-nō-oo-stā'shŭn, -stā'kē-an). Relating to the tympanic cavity and the auditory tube.

▣**tym·pan·o·gram** (tim'pah-nō-gram). The printout of an impedance bridge showing the stiffness or the compliance of the middle ear structures as it varies with changes in pressure within the external ear canal.

tym·pa·no·hy·al (tim'pă-nō-hī'ăl). Pertaining to the relationship between the tympanic cavity and the hyoid arch.

tym·pa·no·mal·le·al (tim'pă-nō-mal'ē-ăl). Relating to the tympanic membrane and the malleus.

tym·pa·no·man·dib·u·lar (tim'pă-nō-man-dib'ū-lăr). Relating to the tympanic cavity and the mandible.

tym·pa·no·mas·toid (tim'pă-nō-mas'toyd). Relating to the tympanic cavity and the mastoid process.

classification of conjoined twins		
terata catadidyma	**terata anadidyma**	**terata anacatadidyma**
joined by lower part of body, or twins single in lower body and double in upper body	single in upper body and double in lower body, or joined by some body part	united at midpoint of body
a) pygopagus back to back, coccyx and sacrum joined	a) cephalopagus fused in the cranial vault	a) thoracopagus attached along part of thoracic wall; thoracic and abdominal organs may be abnormal
b) ischiopagus inferior parts of coccyx and sacrum fused; separate vertebral columns lying in same axis	b) syncephalus united at the face; may also be joined by thorax (cephalothoracopagus)	b) omphalopagus attached from umbilicus to xiphoid cartilage
c) dicephalus two separate heads on one body	c) dipygus single head, thorax, and/or abdomen; pelvis, external genitalia, and limbs are duplicate	c) rachipagus attached at the vertebral column above the sacrum
d) diprosopus two faces with one head and one body		

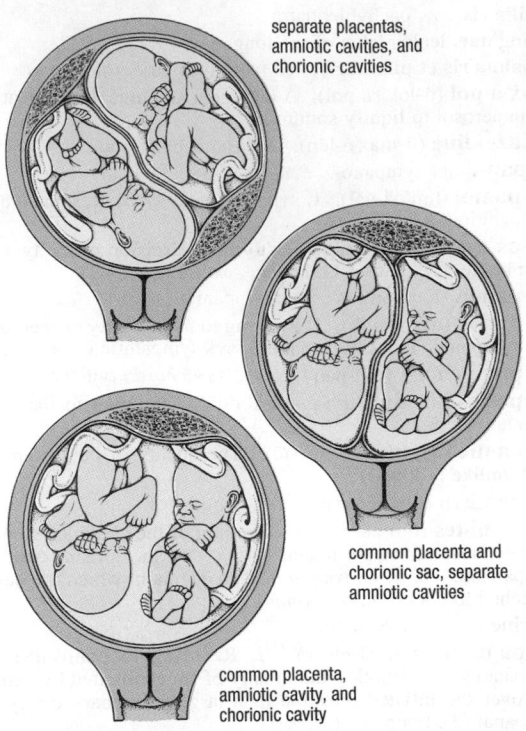

separate placentas, amniotic cavities, and chorionic cavities

common placenta and chorionic sac, separate amniotic cavities

common placenta, amniotic cavity, and chorionic cavity

twins: schematic diagrams showing the possible relations of the fetal membranes in monozygotic twins

tympanomastoidectomy. SYN radical *mastoidectomy.*

tym·pa·no·mas·toid·i·tis (tim′pă-nō-mas-toy-dī′tis). Inflammation of the middle ear and the mastoid cells.

tym·pan·om·et·ry (tim-pan-om′et-rē). A technique that measures compliance of the tympanic membrane at various levels of air pressure; helpful in diagnosing middle ear effusion, eustachian tube function, and otitis media.

tym·pa·no·pho·nia, tym·pa·noph·o·ny (tim′pă-nō-fō′nē-ă, tim′pă-nof′ō-nē). SYN autophony. [tympano- + G. *phōne,* sound]

tym·pa·no·plas·ty (tim′pă-nō-plas-tē). Operative correction of a damaged middle ear. [tympano- + G. *plassō,* to form]

■ tym·pan·o·scler·o·sis (tim′pan-ō-skler-ō′sis). The formation of dense connective tissue in the middle ear, often resulting in hearing loss when the ossicles are involved.

tym·pa·no·squa·mo·sal (tim′pă-nō-skwā-mō′săl). Relating to the tympanic and squamous parts of the temporal bone. SYN squamotympanic.

tym·pa·no·sta·pe·di·al (tim′pă-nō-stā-pē′dē-ăl). Relating to the tympanic cavity and the stapes.

tym·pan·os·to·my (tim-pan-os′tō-mē). An operation to make an opening in the tympanic membrane. SEE ALSO myringotomy. [tympano- + G. *ostium,* mouth]

tym·pa·no·tem·po·ral (tim′pă-nō-tem′pō-răl). Relating to the tympanic cavity and the temporal region or bone.

tym·pa·not·o·my (tim′pă-not′ō-mē). SYN myringotomy. [tympano- + G. *tomē,* incision]

tym·pa·nous (tim′pă-nŭs). SYN tympanitic (1).

tym·pa·num, pl. **tym·pa·na, tym·pa·nums** (tim′pă-nŭm, tim′pă-nă). SYN eardrum. [L., fr. G. *tympanon,* a drum]

tym·pa·ny (tim′pă-nē). A low-pitched, resonant, drumlike note obtained by percussing the surface of a large air-containing space, such as the distended abdomen or the thorax with or without pneumothorax. SYN tympanitic resonance.

Skoda t., SYN skodaic *resonance.*

Tyndall, John, English physicist, 1820–1893. SEE T. *effect;* tyndallization; T. *phenomenon.*

tyn·dal·li·za·tion (tin′dăl-i-zā′shŭn). SYN fractional *sterilization.* [John *Tyndall*]

type (tīp). **1.** The usual form, or a composite form, that all others of the class resemble more or less closely; a model, denoting especially a disease or a symptom complex giving the stamp or characteristic to a class. SEE ALSO constitution, habitus, personality. **2.** In chemistry, a substance in which the arrangement of the atoms in a molecule may be taken as representative of other substances in that class. **3.** A specific variation of a structure. SYN typus, variation (2). [G. *typos,* a mark, a model]

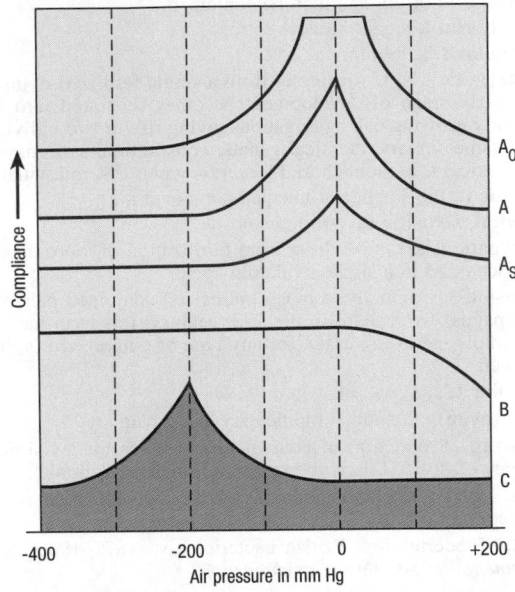

tympanogram: five tympanograms illustrating various conditions of the middle ear: type A is typical of normal middle ear; type A$_S$ is associated with stiffness of stapes; type A$_O$ is associated with interruptions in the chain of bones or flaccidity of the eardrum membrane; type B suggests fluid in the middle ear; type C suggests that the pressure within the middle ear is below atmospheric pressure

ampullary t. of renal pelvis [TA], saclike form of renal pelvis in which the calyces open onto a common dilated pelvis. SYN typus ampullaris pelvis renalis [TA].

basic personality t., (1) an individual's unique, covert, or underlying personality propensities, whether or not they are behaviorally manifest or overt; **(2)** personality characteristics of an individual which are also shared by a majority of the members of a social group.

blood t., SEE blood type.

branching t. of renal pelvis [TA], form of renal pelvis in which no common, expanded, saclike pelvis occurs; rather the major calyces merely merge to form the ureter. SYN typus dendriticus pelvis renalis [TA].

buffalo t., term used to describe the distribution of a fat deposit seen posteriorly over the upper thoracic spine; seen in hyperadrenocorticalism (Cushing *syndrome*). SYN buffalo hump.

nomenclatural t., the constituent element of a taxon to which the name of the taxon is permanently attached; the t. of a species is preferably a strain (in special cases it may be a description, a preserved specimen or preparation, or an illustration); the t. of a genus is a species; and the t. of an order, family, or tribe is the genus on whose name the name of the higher taxon is based.

test t., SEE test types.

wild t., a gene, phenotype, or genotype that is overwhelmingly common among those possible at a locus of interest that it represents the standard characteristic, and therefore presumably not harmful.

ty·phin·ia (tī-fin′ē-ă). SYN relapsing *fever*. [G. *typhos,* smoke, stupor arising from fever]

⚠**typhl-.** SEE typhlo-.

typh·lec·ta·sis (tif-lek′tă-sis). Dilation of the cecum. [G. *typhlon,* cecum, + *ektasis,* a stretching out]

typh·lec·to·my (tif-lek′tō-mē). SYN cecectomy.

typh·len·ter·i·tis (tif′len-ter-ī′tis). SYN cecitis.

typh·li·tis (tif′lī′tis). SYN cecitis.

⚠**typhlo-, typhl-.** 1. The cecum. SEE ALSO ceco-. [G. cecum] 2. Blindness. [G. *typhlos,* blind]

typh·lo·dic·li·di·tis (tif-lō-dik-li-dī′tis). Inflammation of the ileocecal valve. [G. *typhlon,* cecum, + *diklis (diklid-),* double-folding (of doors), + *-itis,* inflammation]

typh·lo·em·py·e·ma (tif′lō-em-pī-ē′mă). Presence of an abscess following typhlitis. [G. *typhlon,* cecum, + *empyēma,* abscess]

typh·lo·en·ter·i·tis (tif′lō-en-ter-ī′tis). SYN cecitis.

typh·lo·li·thi·a·sis (tif′lō-li-thī′ă-sis). Presence of fecal concretions in the cecum. [G. *typhlon,* cecum, + *lithos,* stone]

typh·lo·meg·a·ly (tif′lō-meg′ă-lē). Old term for enlargement of the cecum. [G. *typhlon,* cecum, + *megas (megal-),* large]

typh·lon (tif′lon). SYN cecum (1). [G.]

typh·lo·pexy, typh·lo·pex·ia (tif′lō-pek-sē, tif-lō-pek′sē-ă). SYN cecopexy.

typh·lor·rha·phy (tif-lōr′ă-fē). SYN cecorrhaphy.

typh·lo·sis (tif-lō′sis). SYN blindness. [G. *typhlos,* blind]

typh·los·to·my (tif-los′tō-mē). SYN cecostomy.

typh·lot·o·my (tif-lot′ō-mē). SYN cecotomy.

⚠**typho-.** Typhus, typhoid. [G. *typhos,* smoke, dullness]

ty·phoid (tī′foyd). 1. Typhus-like; stuporous from fever. 2. SYN typhoid *fever.* [typhus + G. *eidos,* resemblance]

   abdominal t., SYN typhoid *fever.*

   ambulatory t., SYN walking t.

   apyretic t., t. fever in which the temperature does not rise more than a degree or two.

   bilious t. of Griesinger, SYN relapsing *fever.*

   fowl t., a septicemic disease of chickens and turkeys, caused by *Salmonella gallinarum;* some human infections with this organism have been reported.

   latent t., SYN walking t.

   provocation t., an accelerated onset of t. fever, sometimes of unusual severity, resulting from typhoid-paratyphoid A and B (T.A.B.) vaccination late in the incubation period.

   walking t., t. fever without much prostration, the patient being up and around and sometimes working. SYN ambulatory t., latent t.

ty·phoi·dal (tī-foyd′ăl). Relating to or resembling typhoid fever.

ty·phol·y·sin (tī-fol′i-sin). A hemolysin formed by *Salmonella typhi.*

ty·pho·ma·nia (tī-fō-mā′nē-ă). A muttering delerium characteristic of that in typhoid fever and typhus. [typho- + G. *mania,* frenzy]

ty·pho·sep·sis (tī-fō-sep′sis). SYN typhoid *septicemia.*

ty·phous (tī′fŭs). Relating to typhus.

ty·phus (tī′foos). A group of acute infectious and contagious diseases, caused by rickettsiae that are transmitted by arthropods, and occurring in two principal forms: epidemic t. and endemic (murine) t.; typical symptoms include: severe headache, shivering and chills, high fever, malaise, and rash. Also called jail, camp, or ship fever. SYN jail fever, ship fever. [G. *typhos,* smoke, stupor]

   Australian tick t., rarely fatal form of t. caused by the *Rickettsia australis,* seen in eastern Australia, transmitted by tick bite, and characterized by severe headache and conjunctivitis. Reservoir is in rodents and marsupials. SYN Queensland tick t.

   endemic t., SYN murine t.

   epidemic t., t. caused by *Rickettsia prowazekii* and spread by body lice; marked by high fever, mental and physical depression, and a macular and papular eruption; lasts for about 2 weeks and occurs when large crowds are brought together and personal hy-

giene is at a low ebb; recrudescences can occur. SYN European t., hospital fever, louse-borne t., prison fever t.

   European t., SYN epidemic t.

   exanthematous t., t. fever with the usual petechial skin lesions seen in that disease.

   flea-borne t., SYN murine t.

   Indian tick t., SYN Mediterranean spotted *fever.*

   louse-borne t., SYN epidemic t.

   Manchurian t., tick transmitted infection with *Rickettsia sibirica.* SEE ALSO Korean hemorrhagic *fever.*

   Mexican t., infection with *Rickettsia typhi (mooseri)* causing a syndrome similar to epidemic t., but spread from rats to humans by the rat flea (*Xenopsylla (polyplax) cheopis*). Spread from rat to rat by the rat louse (*Polyplax spinulosa*). Most common form of t. in the U.S. It has various geographic names based on the region in which it was observed.

   mite t., SYN tsutsugamushi *disease.*

   mite-born t., SYN rickettsialpox.

   t. mit′ior, a mild or abortive t.

   murine t., a milder form of epidemic t. caused by *Rickettsia typhi* and transmitted to humans by rat or mouse fleas. SYN Congolian red fever, endemic t., flea-borne t., red fever, red fever of the Congo.

   North Queensland tick t., t. caused by *Rickettsia australis.*

   prison fever t., SYN epidemic t.

   Queensland tick t., SYN Australian tick t.

   recrudescent t., SYN Brill-Zinsser *disease.*

   Sao Paulo t., infection with *Rickettsia rickettsii;* spread by tick bite. SEE ALSO Rocky Mountain spotted *fever.*

   scrub t., SYN tsutsugamushi *disease.*

   shop t., a mild form of t. occurring in urban areas, reported in Mediterranean areas. SYN urban t.

   Siberian tick t., tick-borne rickettsiosis caused by infection with *Rickettsia sibirica.*

   tick t., SYN Mediterranean spotted *fever.*

   tropical t., SYN tsutsugamushi *disease.*

   urban t., SYN shop t.

typ·ing (tīp′ing). Classification according to type. [see type]

   bacteriophage t., a microbiological procedure, of epidemiologic importance, for distinguishing types within a seemingly homogeneous bacterial species or strain by the use of type-specific bacteriophage.

   HLA t., tests done in order to determine if a patient has antibodies against a potential donor's HLA antigens. The presence of antibodies means that a particular graft will be rapidly rejected. Also used to establish paternity and in forensic medicine.

typus. SYN type (3).

   typus ampullaris pelvis renalis [TA], SYN ampullary *type* of renal pelvis.

   typus dendriticus pelvis renalis [TA], SYN branching *type* of renal pelvis.

Tyr Symbol for tyrosine and tyrosyl.

ty·ra·mi·nase (tī′ră-mi-nās, tir′ă-). SYN *amine* oxidase (flavin-containing).

ty·ra·mine (tī′ră-mēn, tir′ă-). Decarboxylated tyrosine, a sympathomimetic amine having an action in some respects resembling that of epinephrine; present in ergot, mistletoe, ripe cheese, beers, red wines, and putrefied animal matter; elevated in individuals with tyrosinemia type II.

   t. oxidase, SYN *amine* oxidase (flavin-containing).

tyr·an·nism (tir′ă-nizm). A form of sadism characterized by a lust for domination and cruelty, with subsequent humiliation of the partner. [G. *tyrannos,* a tyrant]

ty·rem·e·sis (tī-rem′ĕ-sis). Vomiting of curdy material by infants. SYN tyrosis (1). [G. *tyros,* cheese, + *emesis,* vomiting]

ty·ro·ci·din, ty·ro·ci·dine (tī-rō-sī′din). An antibacterial cyclopeptide obtained from *Bacillus brevis.* SEE ALSO tyrothricin.

Tyrode, Maurice V., U.S. pharmacologist, 1878–1930. SEE T. *solution.*

ty·rog·e·nous (tī-roj′ĕ-nŭs). Produced by, or originating in, cheese. [G. *tyros,* cheese, + G. -gen, producing]

Ty·rog·ly·phus lon·gi·or (tī-rog′li-fŭs lon′gē-ōr, tī′rō-glif′ŭs). SYN *Tyrophagus putrescentiae.* [G. *tyros,* cheese, + *glyphē* carving]

ty·roid (tī′royd). Cheesy; caseous. [G. *tyrōdēs,* fr. *tyros,* cheese, + *eidos,* resemblance]

ty·ro·ke·to·nu·ria (tī′rō-kē-tō-noo′rē-ă). The urinary excretion of ketonic metabolites of tyrosine, such as *p*-hydroxyphenylpyruvic acid.

ty·ro·ma (tī-rō′mă). A caseous tumor. [G. *tyros,* cheese, + *-ōma,* tumor]

ty·ro·pa·no·ate so·di·um (tī′rō-pă-nō′āt). An oral contrast medium for cholecystography.

Ty·roph·a·gus pu·tres·cen·ti·ae (tī-rof′ă-gŭs pū′tre-sen′tē-ē). One of the grain mite species that cause various forms of dermatitis resulting from infestation by grain mites in food and produce, which sensitizes and causes dermatitis in storage and handling personnel. SYN *Tyroglyphus longior.* [G. *tyros,* cheese, + *phagō,* to eat]

ty·ro·sin·ase (tī′rō-si-nās, tir′ō-). SYN monophenol monooxygenase (1).

β-ty·ro·sin·ase. SYN *tyrosine* phenol-lyase.

ty·ro·sine (Tyr, Y) (tī′rō-sēn, -sin). 2-Amino-3-(4-hydroxyphenyl)propionic acid; 3-(4-hydroxyphenyl)alanine; the L-isomer is an α-amino acid present in most proteins.

t. aminotransferase, an enzyme that catalyzes the reversible reaction of L-t. and α-ketoglutarate producing *p*-hydroxyphenylpyruvate and L-glutamate; this enzyme catalyzes a step in L-phenylalanine and L-tyrosine catabolism; a deficiency of this enzyme is associated with tyrosinemia II. SYN t. transaminase.

t. iodinase, a postulated enzyme in the thyroid catalyzing iodination of t., a reaction important in the eventual biosynthesis of thyroxine. SEE ALSO peroxidases.

t. kinase, an enzyme that phosphorylates tyrosyl residues on certain proteins; many are products of viral oncogenes; a number of receptors (e.g., receptors for epidermal growth factor, insulin, etc.) have this enzymatic activity; a misnomer, since the physiologic substrate is not t. but tyrosyl residues in a protein.

t. phenol-lyase, an enzyme catalyzing the hydrolysis of L-tyrosine to phenol, pyruvate, and NH_3. SYN β-tyrosinase.

t. transaminase, SYN t. aminotransferase.

ty·ro·si·ne·mia (tī′rō-si-nē′mē-ă) [MIM*276600, *276700, and *276710]. A group of autosomal recessively inherited disorders of tyrosine metabolism associated with elevated blood concentration of tyrosine, and enhanced urinary excretion of tyrosine and tyrosyl compounds. Type I t., due to deficiency of fumarylacetoacetase (FAH), is characterized by hepatosplenomegaly, nodular liver cirrhosis, multiple renal tubular reabsorptive defects, and vitamin D–resistant rickets; caused by mutation in the FAH gene on chromosome 15q. Type II t., due to deficiency of tyrosine aminotransferase (TAT), is characterized by corneal ulcers and keratosis of digits, palms, and soles; caused by mutation in the TAT gene on 16q. Type III t. is associated with intermittent ataxia and drowsiness without liver dysfunction and is due to 4-hydroxyphenylpyruvate dioxygenase (4HPPD) deficiency. SYN hypertyrosinemia. [tyrosine + G. *haima,* blood]

ty·ro·si·no·sis (tī′rō-si-nō′sis) [MIM*276800]. A very rare, possibly heritable disorder of tyrosine metabolism that may be caused by defective formation of *p*-hydroxyphenylpyruvic acid oxidase or of tyrosine transaminase; characterized by enhanced urinary excretion of *p*-hydroxyphenylpyruvic acid and of other tyrosyl metabolites upon ingestion of tyrosine or proteins containing that amino acid; of autosomal recessive inheritance. [tyrosine + G. -*osis,* condition]

ty·ro·si·nu·ria (tī′rō-si-noo′rē-ă). The excretion of tyrosine in the urine. [tyrosine + G. *ouron,* urine]

ty·ro·sis (tī-rō′sis). 1. SYN tyremesis. 2. SYN caseation. [G. *tyros,* cheese]

ty·ro·sy·lu·ria (tī′rō-si-loo′rē-ă). Enhanced urinary excretion of certain metabolites of tyrosine, such as *p*-hydroxyphenylpyruvic acid; present in tyrosinosis, scurvy, pernicious anemia, and other diseases.

ty·ro·thri·cin (tī-rō-thrī′sin). An antibacterial mixture obtained from peptone cultures of *Bacillus brevis;* bactericidal and bacteriostatic, and active against Gram-positive bacteria. It yields the crystalline antibacterial agents gramicidin and tyrocidin; the gramicidin component is a polypeptide containing L-tryptophan, D-leucine, D-valine, L-valine, L-alanine, glycine, and an aminoethanol; the tyrocidin component is a cyclopolypeptide containing tyrosine, ornithine, and several other amino acids.

ty·ro·tox·ism (tī-rō-tok′sizm). Poisoning by cheese or any milk product. [G. *tyros,* cheese, + *toxikon,* poison]

Tyrrell, Frederick, English anatomist and surgeon, 1797–1843. SEE T. *fascia.*

Tyson, Edward, English anatomist, 1649–1708. SEE T. *glands,* under *gland.*

Tyz·ze·ria (tī-zē′rē-ă). A genus of coccidia (family Eimeriidae) in which the oocyst contains eight naked sporozoites. Important species are *T. anseris,* a relatively nonpathogenic species found in the small intestine of domestic and wild geese, whistling swans, and certain wild ducks, and *T. perniciosa,* which occurs in the small intestine of the domestic duck in North America and Europe, and is pathogenic in ducklings.

Tzanck, Arnault, Russian dermatologist, 1886–1954. SEE T. *cells,* under *cell, test.*

υ. 1. Upsilon, 20th letter of the Greek alphabet. **2.** Symbol for kinematic *viscosity*.

U 1. Abbreviation for unit. **2.** Symbol for kilurane; uranium; uridine in polymers; uracil; urinary concentration, followed by subscripts indicating location and chemical species.

U Symbol for internal *energy*.

ubi·hy·dro·qui·none (ū'bi-hī-drō-qui'nōn). SYN ubiquinol.

ubi·qui·nol (QH_2, H_2Q) (ū'bi-kwī'nol, ū-bik'wi-nol). The reduction product of a ubiquinone. SYN ubihydroquinone.

ubi·qui·none (ū'bi-kwī'nōn, ū-bik'wi-nōn). A 2,3-dimethoxy-5-methyl-1,4-benzoquinone with a multiprenyl side chain; a mobile component of electron transport. SEE ALSO coenzyme Q.

ubi·qui·none-6 (-Q_6). Ubiquinone-30; coenzyme Q_6; 2,3-dimethoxy-5-methyl-6-hexaprenyl-1,4 benzoquinone.

ubi·qui·none-10 (-Q_{10}). Ubiquinone-50; coenzyme Q_{10}; 2,3-dimethoxy-5-methyl-6-decaprenyl-1,4-benzoquinone.

ubiq·ui·tin (oo-bik'kwi-tin). A small (76 amino acyl residues) protein found in all cells of higher organisms and one whose structure has changed minimally during evolutionary history; involved in at least two processes; histone modification and intracellular protein breakdown.

UDP Abbreviation for *uridine* 5'-diphosphate.

UDP-*N*-ace·tyl·glu·co·sam·ine:ly·so·som·al en·zyme *N*-ace·tyl·glu·co·sam·in·yl-1-phos·pho·trans·fer·ase. An enzyme that participates in the posttranslational modification of a number of lysosomal proteins; a deficiency or defect in this enzyme results in two forms of mucolipidoses, I-cell disease, and pseudo-Hurler polydystrophy.

UDPG Abbreviation for uridine diphosphoglucose.

UDPGal Abbreviation for uridine diphosphogalactose.

UDPga·lac·tose. Uridine diphosphogalactose.

UDPga·lac·tose 4-ep·i·mer·ase. SYN UDPglucose 4-epimerase.

UDPGlc Abbreviation for uridine diphosphoglucose.

UDP-GlcUA Abbreviation for uridine diphosphoglucuronic acid.

UDPglu·cose. SYN uridine diphosphoglucose.

UDPglu·cose 4-ep·i·mer·ase. An enzyme that catalyzes the reversible Walden inversion of UDPglucose to UDPgalactose; a deficiency of this enzyme is associated with one type of galactosemia. SYN UDPgalactose 4-epimerase, uridine diphosphoglucose 4-epimerase.

UDPglu·cose-hex·ose-1-phos·phate uri·dyl·yl·trans·fer-·ase. An enzyme that catalyzes the reversible reaction of α-D-glucose 1-phosphate UDPgalactose to produce UDPglucose and α-D-galactose 1-phosphate. SEE ALSO UDPglucose 4-epimerase. SYN hexose-1-phosphate uridylyltransferase, phosphogalactoisomerase.

UDPglu·cur·o·nate-bil·i·ru·bin·glu·cu·ron·o·side glu·cu-·ron·o·syl·trans·fer·ase. SYN UDPglucuronate-bilirubin glucuronosyltransferase.

UDPglu·cur·o·nate-bil·i·ru·bin glu·cu·ron·o·syl·trans·fer-·ase. Hepatic transferases that catalyze the transfer of the glucuronic moiety of UDP-glucuronic acid to bilirubin or bilirubin glucuronide, thus producing UDP and either bilirubin-glucorono-side or bilirubin bisglucuronoside, respectively; these bile conjugates are then secreted into the bile. SYN UDPglucuronate-bilirubinglucuronoside glucuronosyltransferase.

UDP·xy·lose. A sugar derivative in which a pyrophosphate group links the 5' position of uridine and the 1-position of D-xylose; formed by the decarboxylation of UDPglucuronic acid; required for the synthesis of proteoglycans; inhibits UDPglucose dehydrogenase.

Uehlinger, E., Swiss pathologist, *1899. SEE Meyenburg-Altherr-U. *syndrome*.

UFA Abbreviation for unesterified free *fatty acid*.

Uffelmann, Jules A.C., German physician, 1837–1894. SEE U. *reagent*.

UGI Abbreviation for upper gastrointestinal series.

Uhl, Henry S.M., U.S. internist, *1921. SEE U. *anomaly*.

Uhthoff, Wilhelm, German ophthalmologist, 1853–1927. SEE U. *sign;* Uhthoff *symptom*.

UIP Abbreviation for usual interstitial *pneumonia* of Liebow.

ukam·bin (oo-kam'bin). An African arrow poison from plants of the family Apocynaceae; a heart poison resembling digitalis or strophanthus in its action.

ULCER

ul·cer (ŭl'ser). A lesion through the skin or a mucous membrane resulting from loss of tissue, usually with inflammation. SEE erosion. SYN ulcus. [L. *ulcus* (*ulcer*-), a sore, ulcer]

acute decubitus u., a severe form of bedsore, of neurotrophic origin, occurring in hemiplegia or paraplegia.

anastomotic u., an u. of jejunum, after gastroenterostomy.

Buruli u., an u. of the skin, with widespread necrosis of subcutaneous fat, due to infection with *Mycobacterium ulcerans;* occurs in Uganda in persons living on the Nile river banks. [*Buruli,* district in Uganda]

chrome u., an u. of the extremities or nasal septum produced by exposure to chromium compounds. SYN tanner's u.

chronic u., a longstanding u. with fibrous scar tissue in the floor of the u.

stress u., an u. of the duodenum in a patient with extensive superficial burns, intracranial lesions, or severe bodily injury. SYN Curling u.

decubitus u., a chronic u. that appears in pressure areas of skin overlying a bony prominence in debilitated patients confined to bed or otherwise immobilized, due to a circulatory defect. SYN bedsore, decubital gangrene, hospital gangrene, pressure gangrene, pressure sore, pressure u.

dendritic corneal u., keratitis caused by herpes simplex virus.

dental u., an u. on the oral mucuous membrane caused by biting or by rubbing against the edge of a broken tooth.

diphtheritic u., an u. covered with a gray adherent membrane, caused by *Corynebacterium diphtheriae*.

distention u., an u. of the intestine in the dilated part above a stricture.

elusive u., SYN Hunner u.

fascicular u., a localized vascularization of the cornea to the site of a corneal u.

Fenwick-Hunner u., SYN Hunner u.

Gaboon u., a form of tropical u. affecting the residents of this region; it resembles a syphilitic u., especially in the appearance of its scar. [*Gaboon,* a region in Africa]

gastric u., an u. of the stomach.

gravitational u., a chronic u. of the leg with impaired healing because of the dependent position of the extremity and the incompetence of the valves in the deep venous system of the leg and thigh; the venous return stagnates and creates hypoxemia. SEE ALSO varicose u.

gummatous u., lesion of the skin occurring in late syphilis.

hard u., SYN chancre.

△ Combining Forms	☆ Official alternate Terminologia Anatomica term
🔳 Indicates term is illustrated, see Illustration Index	
	[MIM] Mendelian Inheritance in Man
SYN Synonym	
Cf. Compare	C.I. Colour Index
[NA] Nomina Anatomica	
[TA] Terminologia Anatomica	**High Profile Term**

ul

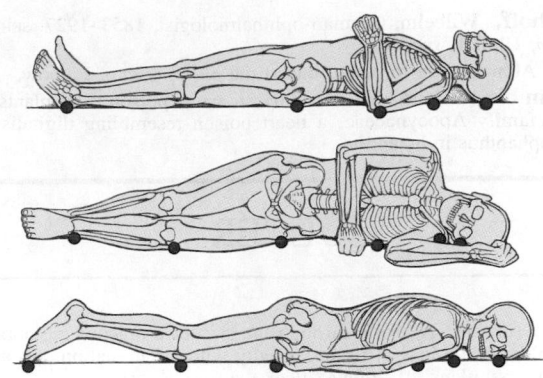

decubitus ulcer: most common sites due to proximity of bone to skin

healed u., an u. covered by epithelial regeneration, beneath which there may be scarring and absence of glands or appendages.

herpetic u., u. caused by herpes simplex virus.

Hunner u., a focal and often multiple lesion involving all layers of the bladder wall in chronic interstitial cystitis; the surface epithelium is destroyed by inflammation and the initially pale lesion cracks and bleeds with distention of the bladder. SYN elusive u., Fenwick-Hunner u.

hypopyon u., (1) an advancing central suppurative u. of the cornea; SEE ALSO hypopyon; **(2)** a corneal u. with pus in the anterior chamber;

indolent u., a chronic u., with hard elevated edges and few or no granulations, and showing no tendency to heal.

inflamed u., an u. with a purulent discharge and inflamed borders.

Mann-Williamson u., SEE Mann-Williamson *operation*.

marginal ring u. of cornea, a slowly advancing intermittent u. involving the circumference of the corneal margin.

Marjolin u., well-differentiated but aggressive squamous cell carcinoma occurring in cicatricial tissue at the epidermal edge of a sinus draining underlying osteomyelitis.

Meleney u., undermining u. of the skin and subcutaneous tissues caused by a synergistic infection by microaerophilic nonhemolytic streptococci and aerobic hemolytic staphylococci. SYN Meleney gangrene, progressive bacterial synergistic gangrene.

Mooren u., chronic inflammation of the peripheral cornea that slowly progresses centrally with corneal thinning and sometimes perforation.

Oriental u., the lesion occurring in cutaneous leishmaniasis.

penetrating u., an u. extending into deeper tissues of an organ.

peptic u., an u. of the alimentary mucosa, usually in the stomach or duodenum, exposed to acid gastric secretion.

perforated u., an u. extending through the wall of an organ.

perforating u. of foot, a round, deep, trophic u. of the sole of the foot, following disease or injury, in any part of its course from the center to the periphery of the nerve supplying the part.

phagedenic u., a rapidly spreading u. attended by the formation of extensive sloughing. SYN sloughing u.

phlegmonous u., a u. accompanied by inflammation of the neighboring tissues.

pressure u., SYN decubitus u.

recurrent aphthous u.'s, SYN aphtha (2).

ring u. of cornea, inflammation of the greater part or the whole of the corneal periphery.

rodent u., historic term for a slowly enlarging ulcerated basal cell carcinoma, usually on the face.

Saemisch u., a form of serpiginous keratitis, frequently accompanied by hypopyon.

serpent u. of cornea, SYN serpiginous *keratitis*.

serpiginous u., an u. extending on one side while healing at the opposite edge, forming an undulating margin.

serpiginous corneal u., serpentine ulceration of the cornea, due to infection, most often with *Streptococcus pneumoniae.*

simple u., a local, not constitutional, u. not accompanied by marked pain or inflammation.

sloughing u., SYN phagedenic u.

soft u., SYN chancroid.

stasis u., SYN varicose u.

stercoral u., an u. of the colon due to pressure and irritation of retained fecal masses.

stomal u., an intestinal u. occurring after gastrojejunostomy in the jejunal mucosa near the opening (stoma) between the stomach and the jejunum.

Curling u., SYN stress u.

Sutton u., a solitary, deep, painful u. of the buccal or genital mucous membrane.

syphilitic u., (1) SYN chancre; **(2)** any ulceration caused by a syphilitic infection.

Syriac u., Syrian u., old names for diphtheria.

tanner's u., SYN chrome u.

trophic u., u. resulting from cutaneous sensory denervation. SEE ALSO perforating u. of foot. SYN trophic gangrene.

tropical u., (1) the lesion occurring in cutaneous leishmaniasis; SYN tropical sore. SEE ALSO cutaneous *leishmaniasis*; **(2)** tropical phagedenic ulceration caused by a variety of microorganisms, including mycobacteria; common in northern Nigeria.

undermining u., a chronic cutaneous u. with overhanging margins; due to hemolytic streptococci, tubercle bacilli, or other bacteria.

varicose u., the loss of skin surface in the drainage area of a varicose vein, usually in the leg, resulting from stasis and infection. SEE ALSO gravitational u. SYN stasis u., venous u.

venereal u., SYN chancroid.

venous u., SYN varicose u.

Zambesi u., an u., usually single, about 3 cm in diameter, on the foot or leg, occurring in laborers in the Zambesi Delta; it has a sloughing surface, but does not spread and produces no constitutional symptoms or glandular enlargement; it is associated with the presence of a spirillum and a large fusiform bacillus; one attack seems to confer a partial immunity.

ul·cer·ate (ŭl′ser-āt). To form an ulcer.

ul·cer·at·ed (ŭl′ser-āt-ed). Having undergone ulceration.

ul·cer·a·tion (ŭl-ser-ā′shŭn). **1.** The formation of an ulcer. **2.** An ulcer or aggregation of ulcers.

tracheal u., erosion of the tracheal mucous membrane with, in some cases, exposure of the cartilaginous rings, at the site at which a cuffed tracheostomy tube has been present for some time.

ul·cer·a·tive (ŭl′ser-ă-tiv). Relating to, causing, or marked by an ulcer or ulcers.

ul·cer·o·gen·ic (ŭl′ser-ō-jen′ik). Ulcer-producing.

ul·cer·o·glan·du·lar (ŭl′ser-ō-gland′ū-lăr). Denoting a local ulceration at a site of infection followed by regional or generalized lymphadenopathy.

ul·cer·o·mem·bra·nous (ŭl′ser-ō-mem′bră-nŭs). Relating to or characterized by ulceration and the formation of a false membrane.

ul·cus, pl. **ul·ce·ra** (ŭl′kŭs, ŭl′ser-ă). SYN ulcer. [L.]

ule-. SEE ulo-.

ule·gy·ri·a (ū′lē-jī′rē-ă). A defect of the cerebral cortex characterized by narrow and distorted gyri; may be congenital or the result of scars. [G. *oulē,* scar, + *gyros,* ring]

uler·y·the·ma (oo′ler-i-thē′mă). Scarring with erythema. [G. *oulē,* scar, + *erythēma,* redness of the skin]

u. ophryog′enes, folliculitis of the eyebrows resulting in scarring and alopecia.

u·lex eu·ro·pae·us (oo-leks oor′o-pā-ŭs). A lectin that reacts specifically with α-L-fucose, used as a marker for endothelial cells in paraffin sections.

Ullmann, Emerich, Hungarian surgeon, 1861–1937. SEE U. *line, syndrome.*

Ullrich, Otto, German physician, 1894–1957. SEE Morquio-U. *disease.*

ul·na, gen. and pl. **ul·nae** (ŭl'nă, ŭl'nē) [TA]. The medial and larger of the two bones of the forearm. SYN cubitus (2) [TA]. [L. elbow, arm, fr. G. *ōlenē*]

ul·nad (ŭl'nad). In a direction toward the ulna. [ulna + L. *ad,* to]

ul·nar (ŭl'năr) [TA]. Relating to the ulna, or to any of the structures (e.g., artery, nerve) named from it; relating to the ulnar or medial aspect of the upper limb. SYN ulnaris [TA].

ul·na·ris (ŭl-nā'ris) [TA]. SYN ulnar. [Mod. L.]

ul·nen (ŭl'nen). Relating to the ulna independent of other structures. [ulna + G. *en,* in]

ul·no·car·pal (ŭl'nō-kar'păl). Relating to the ulna and the carpus, or to the ulnar side of the wrist.

ul·no·ra·di·al (ŭl'nō-rā'dē-ăl). Relating to both ulna and radius; denoting the two articulations, ligaments, etc., between them.

♲**ulo-, ule-.** **1.** Scar, scarring. [G. *oulē*] **2.** The gums. SEE ALSO gingivo-. [G. *oulon*] **3.** Curly. [G. *oulo-, ouli-,* woolly.]

uloid (ū'loyd). **1.** Resembling a scar. **2.** A scarlike lesion due to a degenerative process in deeper layers of skin. [G. *oulē,* scar + *eidos,* resemblance]

ulot·ri·chous (ū-lot'ri-kŭs). Having curly hair. Cf. leiotrichous. [G. *oulotrichos,* curly haired, fr. *oulos,* wooly, + *thrix* (trich-), hair]

ul·ti·mo·bran·chi·al (ŭl'ti-mō-brang'kē-ăl). In embryology, relating to the caudal-most pharyngeal pouch. [L. *ultimus,* last, + G. *branchia,* gills]

ul·ti·mum mo·ri·ens (ŭl'ti-mŭm mŏr'ĭ-enz). The right atrium of the heart, said to contract after the rest of the heart is still. [L. the last thing dying]

♲**ultra-.** Excess, exaggeration, beyond. [L. beyond]

ul·tra·brach·y·ce·phal·ic (ŭl-tră-brak-ē-se-fal'ik). Denoting an extremely short skull, one with an index of at least 90.

ul·tra·cen·tri·fu·ga·tion (ŭl-tră-sen'tri-fū-gā-shŭn). The process of subjecting to an ultracentrifuge.

ul·tra·cen·tri·fuge (ŭl'tră-sen'tri-fūj). A high-speed centrifuge (up to 100,000 rpm) by means of which large molecules, e.g., of protein or nucleic acids, are caused to sediment at practicable rates; used for determinations of molecular weights, separation of large molecules, criteria of homogeneity of large molecules, conformational studies, etc.

ul·tra·cy·to·stome (ŭl-tră-sī'tō-stōm). Former name for micropore. [ultra- + G. *kytos,* cell, + *stoma,* mouth]

ul·tra·di·an (ŭl-trā'dē-ăn). Relating to biologic variations or rhythms occurring in cycles more frequent than every 24 hours. Cf. circadian, infradian. [ultra- + L. *dies,* day]

ul·tra·dol·i·cho·ce·phal·ic (ŭl-tră-dol-i-kō-se-fal'ik). Denoting a very long skull, one with a cephalic index of less than 65.

ul·tra·fil·ter (ŭl'tră-fil-ter). A semipermeable membrane (collodion, fish bladder, or filter paper impregnated with gels) used as a filter to separate colloids and large molecules from water and small molecules, which pass through.

ul·tra·fil·tra·tion (ŭl'tră-fil-trā'shŭn). Filtration through a semipermeable membrane or any filter that separates colloid solutions from crystalloids or separates particles of different size in a colloid mixture.

ul·tra·li·ga·tion (ŭl-tră-lī-gā'shŭn). Ligation of a blood vessel beyond the point where a branch is given off.

ul·tra·mi·cro·scope (ŭl-tră-mī'krō-skōp). A microscope that utilizes refracted light for visualizing objects not visible with the ordinary microscope when direct light is used.

ul·tra·mi·cro·scop·ic (ŭl'tră-mī-krō-skop'ik). SYN submicroscopic.

ul·tra·mi·cro·tome (ŭl-tră-mī'krō-tōm). A microtome used in cutting sections 0.1 μm thick, or less, for electron microscopy.

ul·tra·mi·crot·o·my (ŭl'tră-mī-krot'ō-mē). The cutting of ultrathin sections for electron microscopy by use of an ultramicrotome.

ul·tra·son·ic (ŭl-tră-son'ik). Relating to energy waves similar to those of sound but of higher frequencies (above 30,000 Hz). [ultra- + L. *sonus,* sound]

ul·tra·son·ics (ŭl-tră-son'iks). The science and technology of ultrasound, its characteristics and phenomena.

ul·tra·son·o·gram (ŭl-tră-son'ō-gram). The image obtained by ultrasonography. SEE ALSO echogram. SYN sonogram.

ul·tra·son·o·graph (ŭl'tră-son'ō-graf). Computerized instrument used to create an image using ultrasound. SYN sonograph. [ultra- + L. *sonus,* sound, + G. *graphō,* to write]

ul·tra·so·nog·ra·pher (ŭl'tră-sŏ-nog'ră-fer). A person who performs and/or interprets ultrasonographic examinations. SYN echographer, sonographer.

ul·tra·so·nog·ra·phy (ŭl'tră-sŏ-nog'ră-fē). The location, measurement, or delineation of deep structures by measuring the reflection or transmission of high frequency or ultrasonic waves. Computer calculation of the distance to the sound-reflecting or absorbing surface plus the known orientation of the sound beam gives a two-dimensional image. SEE ALSO ultrasound. SYN echography, sonography. [ultra- + L. *sonus,* sound, + G. *graphō,* to write]

ⓘ**Doppler u.,** application of the Doppler effect in ultrasound to detect movement of scatterers (usually red blood cells) by the analysis of the change in frequency of the returning echoes.

> In many settings, ultrasound has supplanted x-radiography as the imaging method of choice, because it poses no known risk to patients and is noninvasive and of moderate cost. Doppler-created ultrasound makes possible real-time viewing of tissues, blood flow, and organs that cannot be observed by any other method. It is particularly valuable in cardiology and obstetrics.

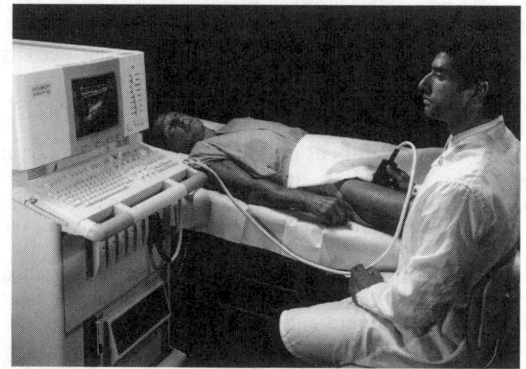

A

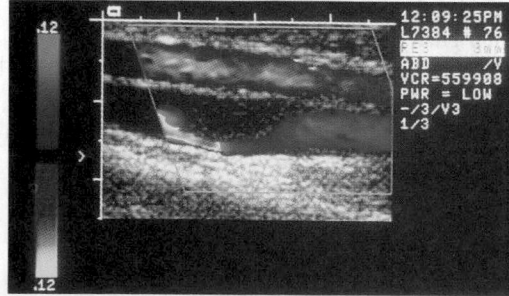

B

Doppler ultrasonography: (A) vascular imaging; (B) color flow Doppler showing femoral vein thrombus

duplex u., the combination of real-time and Doppler u.

endovaginal u., pelvic u. using a probe inserted into the vagina.

gray-scale u., the display of the ultrasound echo amplitude or

ul

signal intensity as different shades of gray, improving image quality compared to the obsolete black and white presentation.

real-time u., rapid serial ultrasound images produced using a phased array or scanning transducer; produces a video display of organ motion, such as heart valve or fetal motion.

ul·tra·son·o·sur·gery (ŭl′tră-son-ō-ser′jer-ē). Use of ultrasound techniques to disrupt cells, tissues, or tracts, particularly in the central nervous system.

ul·tra·sound (ŭl′tră-sownd). Sound having a frequency greater than 30,000 Hz.

diagnostic u., the use of u. to obtain images for medical diagnostic purposes, employing frequencies ranging from 1.6 to about 10 MHz.

▣obstetric u., use of diagnostic u. during pregnancy.

ul·tra·struc·ture (ŭl-tră-strŭk′choor). Structures or particles seen with the electron microscope. SYN fine structure.

ul·tra·therm (ŭl′tră-therm). A short-wave diathermy machine. [ultra- + G. *thermē,* heat]

ul·tra·vi·o·let (ŭl-tră-vī′ō-let). Denoting electromagnetic rays at higher frequency than the violet end of the visible spectrum.

u. A (UVA), u. radiation from 320 to 400 nm that causes skin tanning but is very weakly sunburn-producing and carcinogenic.

u. B (UVB), u. radiation from 290 to 320 nm that most effectively causes sunburning and tanning; excessive UVB exposure is a cause of cancer of fair skin.

u. C, u. radiation from 200 to 290 nm; UVC in sunlight does not reach the surface of the earth; germicidal and mercury arc lamps may cause sunburn and photokeratitis.

extravital u., having wavelengths of 2900 to 1850 Å.

intravital u., having wavelengths of 3900 to 3200 Å.

ul·tro·mo·tiv·i·ty (ŭl′trō-mō-tiv′i-tē). Power of spontaneous movement. [L. *ultro,* beyond, on one's own part + L. *motio,* movement]

ulu·la·tion (oo-loo-lā′shŭn). Rarely used term for the inarticulate crying of emotionally disturbed persons. [L. *ululo,* pp. -*atus,* to howl]

Ulysses, Latin form of Greek mythological character. SEE Ulysses *syndrome.*

um·bil·i·cal (ŭm-bil′i-kăl). Relating to the umbilicus. SYN omphalic.

um·bil·i·cate, um·bil·i·cat·ed (ŭm-bil′i-kāt, -kāt-ed). Of navel shape; pitlike; dimpled. [L. *umbilicatus*]

um·bil·i·ca·tion (ŭm-bil-i-kā′shŭn). **1.** A pit or navellike depression. **2.** Formation of a depression at the apex of a papule, vesicle, or pustule.

um·bil·i·cus, pl. **um·bil·i·ci** (ŭm-bil′i-kŭs, ŭm-bi-lī′kŭs; -i-sī, -lī′kī). The pit in the center of the abdominal wall marking the point where the umbilical cord entered in the fetus. SYN belly button, navel. [L. navel]

um·bo, gen. **um·bo·nis,** pl. **um·bo·nes** (ŭm′bō, -bō-nis, -bō-nēs) [TA]. **1** [NA]. A projecting point of a surface. **2.** SYN u. of tympanic membrane. [L. boss of a shield, a knob]

u. membra′nae tym′pani [TA], SYN u. of tympanic membrane.

u. of tympanic membrane [TA], the projection on the inner surface of the tympanic membrane at the end of the manubrium of the malleus; this corresponds to the most depressed point of the membrane, viewed laterally, that is commonly called the umbo. SYN u. membranae tympani [TA], umbo (2) [TA].

UMP Abbreviation for *uridine* 5′-monophosphate.

UMP syn·thase. SYN uridylic acid.

△un-. **1.** Not, akin to L. in- and G. a-, an-. **2.** Reversal, removal, release, deprivation. **3.** An intensive action. [M.E.]

un·cal (ŭng′kăl). Denoting or relating to the uncus.

un·ci (ŭn′sī). Plural of uncus.

un·cia (ŭn′sē-ă). An ounce. [L. a twelfth part, an ounce]

un·ci·form (ŭn′si-fōrm). SYN uncinate. [L. *uncus,* hook, + *forma,* form]

un·ci·for·me (ŭn-si-fōr′mē). SYN hamate (*bone*). [Mod. L. unciforme]

Un·ci·nar·ia (ŭn-si-nar′ē-ă). A genus of nematode hookworms that infect various mammals. Species include *U. stenocephala,* the European hookworm of dogs, cats, and various wild carnivores, also found in North America, where it is much less common than *Ancylostoma caninum,* though it has been implicated in human cutaneous larva migrans. [LL. *uncinus,* a hook]

un·ci·na·ri·a·sis (ŭn′si-nă-rī′ă-sis). SYN ancylostomiasis.

un·ci·nate (ŭn′si-nāt). **1.** Hooklike or hook-shaped. **2.** Relating to an uncus or, specifically, to the u. gyrus (2) or a process of the pancreas or of a vertebra. SYN unciform. [L. *uncinatus*]

un·ci·na·tum (ŭn-si-nā′tŭm). SYN hamate (*bone*).

un·ci·pres·sure (ŭn′si-presh-ŭr). Arrest of hemorrhage from a cut artery by pressure with a blunt hook. [L. *uncus,* hook]

un·com·ple·ment·ed (ŭn-kom′plĕ-men-ted). Not united with complement and therefore inactive.

un·con·scious (ŭn-kon′shŭs). **1.** Not conscious. **2.** In psychoanalysis, the psychic structure comprising the drives and feelings of which one is unaware. SYN insensible (1).

collective u., in jungian psychology, the combined engrams or memory potentials inherited from an individual's phylogenetic past.

un·con·scious·ness (ŭn-kon′shŭs-ness). An imprecise term for severely impaired awareness of self and the surrounding environment; most often used as a synonym for coma or unresponsiveness.

un·co·os·si·fied (ŭn-kō-os′i-fīd). Not co-ossified; not united into one bone.

un·cou·plers (ŭn-kŭp′lerz). Substances such as dinitrophenol that allow oxidation in mitochondria to proceed without the usual concomitant phosphorylation to produce ATP; these poisons thus "uncouple" oxidation and phosphorylation. SYN uncoupling factors.

un·co·ver·te·bral (ŭn-kō-ver′tĕ-brăl). Pertaining to or affecting the uncinate process of a vertebra.

unc·tion (ŭngk′shŭn). The action of anointing or rubbing with an ointment or oil. [L. *unctio,* fr. *ungo,* pp. *unctus,* to anoint]

unc·tu·ous (ŭngk′shoo-ŭs, -choo-ŭs). Greasy or oily. [L. *unctuosus,* fr. *unctio,* unction]

unc·ture (ŭnk′choor). SYN ointment.

un·cus, pl. **un·ci** (ŭn′kŭs, ŭn′sī) [TA]. **1.** Any hook-shaped process or structure. **2.** The anterior, hooked extremity of the parahippocampal gyrus on the basomedial surface of the temporal lobe; the anterior face of the u. corresponds to the olfactory cortex, its ventral surface to the entorhinal area; deep to the u. lies the amygdala (amygdaloid body). SYN uncinate gyrus, u. gyri parahippocampalis. [L. a hook, fr. G. *onkos*]

u. gy′ri parahippocampa′lis, SYN uncus (2).

un·dec·e·no·ic ac·id (ŭn′des-ĕ-nō′ik). SYN undecylenic acid.

un·de·co·yl·i·um chlo·ride (ŭn-de-kō-il′ē-ŭm). A topical antiseptic.

un·de·co·yl·i·um chlo·ride-io·dine. A complex of iodine with undecoylium chloride; a cationic detergent used topically as a germicidal agent.

un·dec·y·len·ate (ŭn-des′i-li-nāt). A salt of undecylenic acid.

un·dec·y·len·ic ac·id (ŭn-des-i-len′ik). An acid present in small amounts in sweat; used with its zinc salt in ointments, or as a powder in the treatment of fungus diseases of the skin, psoriasis, and certain other cutaneous affections. SYN undecenoic acid.

un·der·a·chieve·ment (ŭn′der-ă-chēv′ment). Failure to achieve as well as one's abilities would seem to allow.

un·der·a·chiev·er (ŭn′der-ă-chēv′er). One who manifests underachievement.

un·der·bite (ŭn′der-bīt). A nontechnical term applied to mandibular underdevelopment or to excessive maxillary development.

un·der·cut (ŭn′der-kŭt). **1.** That portion of a tooth that lies between the survey line (height of contour) and the gingivae. **2.** The contour of a cross-section of a residual ridge or dental arch which would prevent the insertion of a denture. **3.** The contour of a flasking stone which interlocks in such a way as to prevent the separation of the parts.

un·der·drive pac·ing (ŭn′der-drīv pās′ing). Electrical stimulation of the heart at a rate lower than that of an existing tachycardia; designed to capture the heart between beats, i.e., to interrupt a reentry pathway in order to terminate the tachycardia.

un·der·nu·tri·tion (ŭn′der-noo-tri′shŭn). A form of malnutrition resulting from a reduced supply of food or from inability to digest, assimilate, and utilize the necessary nutrients.

un·der·sens·ing (un′der-sen′sing). Non-sensing of the intracardiac atrial or ventricular depolarization signal by a pacemaker.

un·der·shoot (ŭn′der-shoot). A temporary decrease below the final steady-state value that may occur immediately following the removal of an influence that had been raising that value, i.e., overshoot in a negative direction.

un·der·stain (un′der-stān). To stain less deeply than usual.

un·der·ven·ti·la·tion (ŭn′der-ven-ti-lā′shŭn). SYN hypoventilation.

un·der·wind·ing (ŭn′der-wīnd′ing). The effect of negative supercoiling on a structure of DNA.

un·dif·fer·en·ti·at·ed (ŭn′dif-er-en′shē-ā-ted). Not differentiated; e.g., primitive, embryonic, immature, or having no special structure or function.

un·dine (ŭn′dēn, -dīn). A small glass flask that was used in irrigation of the conjunctiva. [Mod. L. *undina,* fr. L. *unda,* wave]

un·di·ver·sion (ŭn-di-ver′shŭn). Surgical restoration of continuity in any organ system, the flow through which had previously been diverted; e.g., between the upper urinary tract and bladder after supravesical urinary diversion.

un·do·ing (ŭn-doo′ing). In psychology and psychiatry, an unconscious defense mechanism by which one symbolically acts out in reverse some earlier unacceptable behavior.

un·du·late (ŭn′doo-lāt). Having an irregular, wavy border; denoting the shape of a bacterial colony. [Mod. L. *undula,* dim. of *unda,* wave]

un·du·li·po·di·um, pl. **un·du·li·po·dia** (ŭn′doo-li-pō′dē-um, -ă). A flexible whiplike intracellular extension of many eukaryotic cells, with a characteristic nine-fold symmetry, an arrangement of nine paired peripheral microtubules and one central pair, often termed 9 + 2 symmetry; it appears to grow out from a basal body (kinetosome) in the cell and is a fundamental component of the eukaryotic cell. Both the cilium and the eukaryotic flagellum (not the bacterial flagellum, which lacks the 9 + 2 pattern) are considered undulipodia. [LL. *undulo,* to move in waves, fr. L. *unda,* wave, + Mod.L. *podium,* fr. G. *podion,* dim. of *pous,* foot]

ung Abbreviation of L. *unguentum,* ointment.

un·gual (ŭng′gwăl). Relating to a nail or the nails. SYN unguinal. [L. *unguis,* nail]

un·guent (ŭng′gwent). SYN ointment. [L. *unguentum*]

un·gues (ŭng′gwēz). Plural of unguis.

Un·guic·u·la·ta (ŭng-gwik-ū-lā′tă). A division of Mammalia including all mammals having nails or claws, as distinguished from the Ungulata. [L. *unguiculus,* nail or claw]

un·guic·u·late (ŭng-gwik′ū-lāt). Having nails or claws, as distinguished from hooves.

un·guic·u·lus (ŭn-gwik′ū-lŭs). A small nail or claw. [L. dim. of *unguis,* nail]

un·gui·nal (ŭng′gwi-năl). SYN ungual.

un·guis, pl. **un·gues** (ŭng′gwis, -gwēz) [TA]. SYN nail (1). [L.]

   u. adun′cus, SYN ingrown *nail.*

   u. a′vis, SYN calcarine *spur.*

   Haller u., SYN calcarine *spur.*

   u. incarna′tus, SYN ingrown *nail.*

Un·gu·la·ta (ŭng-gū-lā′tă). A division of Mammalia containing the mammals with hooves, as distinguished from the Unguiculata.

un·gu·late (ŭng′gū-lāt). Having hooves. [L. *ungulatus,* fr. *ungula,* hoof]

un·gu·li·grade (ŭng′gū-li-grād). Walking on hooves, as by horses, pigs, and ruminants. [L. *ungula,* a hoof, + *gradus,* a step]

☊uni-. One, single, not paired; corresponds to G. mono-. [L. *unus*]

u·ni·ar·tic·u·lar (ū-nē-ar-tik′ū-lăr). SYN monarticular.

uni·ax·i·al (oo-nē-ak′sē-ăl). Having but one axis; growing chiefly in one direction.

uni·bas·al (ū-ni-bā′săl). Having but one base.

Un·i·blue A (ū′nē-bloo) [C.I. 14553]. A protein stain used in electrophoresis.

uni·cam·er·al, uni·cam·er·ate (oo-nē-kam′ĕ-răl, -kam′ĕ-rāt). SYN monolocular.

uni·cel·lu·lar (ū-ni-sel′ū-lăr). Composed of but one cell, as in the protozoons; for such u. organisms capable of undertaking life processes independently of other cells, the term acellular is also used.

u·ni·cen·tral (ū-ni-sen′trăl). Having a single center, as of growth or of ossification.

uni·corn (ū′nē-kōrn). SYN unicornous.

uni·cor·nous (ū′ni-kōr′nŭs). Having one horn, or cornu. SYN unicorn. [L. *unicornis,* fr. uni- + *cornu,* horn]

uni·cus·pid, uni·cus·pi·date (ū-ni-kŭs′pid, -kŭs′pi-dāt). Having only one cusp, as a canine tooth.

uni·fa·mil·i·al (ū′nē-fa-mil′ē-ăl). Relating to or occurring in a single family; denoting especially a nervous disease attacking several of the children in the same family in which no hereditary trait is apparent.

uni·fla·gel·late (ū-ni-flaj′ĕ-lāt). SYN monotrichous.

uni·fo·rate (oo-ni-fō′rāt). Having but one foramen, pore, or opening of any kind.

uni·form (oo′ni-fōrm). **1.** Having but one form; not variable in form. **2.** Of the same form or shape as another structure or object. [L. *uniformis,* fr. uni- + *forma,* form]

uni·ger·mi·nal (ū-ni-jer′mi-năl). Relating to a single germ or ovum, e.g., monozygotic. SYN monogerminal, monozygotic, monozygous.

uni·glan·du·lar (oo-ni-glan′doo-lăr). Involving, relating to, or containing but one gland.

uni·lam·i·nar, uni·lam·i·nate (oo-ni-lam′i-năr, -lam′i-nāt). Having but one layer or lamina.

uni·lat·e·ral (oo-ni-lat′ĕ-răl). Confined to one side only.

uni·lo·bar (oo-ni-lō′băr). Having but one lobe.

uni·lo·cal (ū-ni-lō′kăl). Strictly, denoting a trait in which the genetic component is contributed exclusively by one locus; in practice, any trait in which the contribution from one locus is so large that the data are readily interpreted as mendelian.

uni·loc·u·lar (oo-ni-lok′ū-lăr). Having but one compartment or cavity, as in a fat cell. [uni- + L. *loculus,* compartment]

uni·mo·lec·u·lar (ū′ni-mō-lek′ū-lăr). Denoting a single molecule. SEE ALSO molecularity. SYN monomolecular (1).

uni·nu·cle·ar, uni·nu·cle·ate (oo-ni-noo′klē-ăr, -noo′klē-āt). Having but one nucleus. Cf. mononuclear.

uni·oc·u·lar (ū-ni-ok′ū-lăr). **1.** Relating to one eye only. **2.** Having vision in only one eye.

un·ion (ŭn′yŭn). **1.** Joining or amalgamation of two or more bodies. **2.** Structural adhesion or growing together of the edges of a wound. **3.** Healing of a fracture represented by the development of continuity between fractured fragments. [L. *unus,* one]

   autogenous u., in dentistry, the u. of two pieces of metal without solder.

   faulty u., SYN fibrous u.

   fibrous u., u. of fracture by fibrous tissue. SEE nonunion. SYN faulty u.

   primary u., SYN *healing* by first intention.

   secondary u., SYN *healing* by second intention.

   vicious u., SYN malunion.

uni·o·val, uni·ov·u·lar (ū-nē-ō′văl, -ov′ū-lăr). Relating to or formed from a single ovum.

uni·pen·nate (ū-ni-pen′āt). ☆official alternate term for semipennate. [uni- + L. *penna,* feather]

uni·po·lar (oo-ni-pō′lăr). **1.** Having but one pole; denoting a nerve cell from which the branches project from one side only. **2.** Situated at one extremity only of a cell.

uni·port (ū′ni-pōrt). Transport of a molecule or ion through a

un

membrane by a carrier mechanism (uniporter), without known coupling to any other molecule or ion transport. Cf. antiport, symport. [uni- + L. *porto,* to carry]

uni·port·er (ū′ni-pōrt-er). A protein that mediates the transport of one molecule or ion through a membrane without known coupling to the transport of any other molecule or ion.

uni·po·tent (ū′ni-pō′tent). Referring to those cells that produce a single type of daughter cell; e.g., a u. stem cell. Cf. pluripotent *cells,* under *cell.*

uni·sep·tate (oo-ni-sep′tāt). Having but one septum or partition.

UNIT

---

unit (U) (ū′nit). **1.** One; a single person or thing. **2.** A standard of measure, weight, or any other quality, by multiplications or fractions of which a scale or system is formed. **3.** A group of persons or things considered as a whole because of mutual activities or functions. SEE ALSO international u. [L. *unus,* one]

absolute u., a u. whose value is constant regardless of place or time and not derived from or dependent on gravitation.

alexin u., SYN complement u.

Allen-Doisy u., the quantity of estrogen capable of producing in a spayed mouse a characteristic change in the vaginal epithelium, namely, disappearance of leukocytes and appearance of cornified cells, as determined by a vaginal smear; equal approximately to one-half of an estrone u. SYN mouse u.

alpha u.'s, cytoplasmic glycogen granules arranged in rosettes.

amboceptor u., SYN hemolysin u.

androgen u. (international), the androgenic activity of 100 μg (0.1 mg) of crystalline androsterone as assayed by the comb growth response in capons.

Ångström u. (Å), SEE Ångström.

antigen u., the smallest amount of antigen that, in the presence of specific antiserum, will fix 1 complement u.

antitoxin u., a u. expressing the strength or activity of an antitoxin; in general, determined with reference to a preserved standard preparation of antitoxin. SEE ALSO L *doses,* under *dose.*

antivenene u., the amount of antivenum which, injected in the ear vein, will protect 1 g weight of rabbit against a fatal dose of snake venom.

atomic mass u. (amu), a u. of mass by definition equal to $\frac{1}{12}$ of the mass of an atom of carbon-12, which equals $1.6605402 \times 10^{-27}$ kg; in terms of energy, 1 amu equals 931.49432 MeV. Cf. dalton.

base u.'s, the fundamental u.'s of length, mass, time, electric current, thermodynamic temperature, amount of substance, and luminous intensity in the International System of Units (SI); the names and symbols of the u.'s for these quantities are meter (m), kilogram (kg), second (s), ampere (A), kelvin (K), mole (mol), and candela (cd). SEE ALSO International System of Units.

Bethesda u., a measure of inhibitor activity: the amount of inhibitor that will inactivate 50% or 0.5 u. of a coagulation factor during the incubation period. [*Bethesda,* MD]

biological standard u., a specific quantity of biologically active reference material (antibiotic, antitoxin, enzyme, hormone, vitamin, etc.).

bird u., a u. of prolactin activity: the minimal quantity of the hormone which will cause a certain increase in weight of the crop gland of pigeons.

Bodansky u., that amount of phosphatase that liberates 1 mg of phosphorus as inorganic phosphate during the first hour of incubation with a buffered substrate containing sodium β-glycerophosphate.

British thermal u. (BTU), the quantity of heat required to raise 1 lb of water from 3.9°C to 4.4°C; equal to 251.996 calorie or 1055.056 J. SYN u. of heat (2).

capon u., amount of androgen needed to produce an increase in the capon comb surface of 20%. SYN capon-comb u.

capon-comb u., SYN capon u.

cat u., the dose of a drug (per kilogram of body weight of cat) which is just large enough to kill a cat when administered intravenously; was applied in the standardization of digitalis materials.

centimeter-gram-second u., CGS u., cgs u., an absolute u. of the centimeter-gram-second system.

chlorophyll u., the number of chlorophyll molecules required to reduce one molecule of carbon dioxide by photosynthesis.

chorionic gonadotropin u. (international), the specific gonadotropic activity of 0.1 mg of the standard preparation of chorionic gonadotropin originating from the urine or placentas of pregnant women.

Clauberg u., SEE Clauberg *test.*

colony-forming u., a u. of cells in bone marrow capable of generating or increasing the proliferation of new blood cells.

complement u., the smallest amount (highest dilution) of complement that will cause hemolysis of a u. of red blood cells in the presence of a hemolysin u. SYN alexin u.

Corner-Allen u., a u. of progestational activity, measured in rabbits; the minimum dose which, divided into five equal daily portions, produces on the sixth day the uterine changes characteristic of the eighth day of normal pregnancy; the u. has about the same potency as the international u.

coronary care u. (CCU), a group of beds within a hospital set aside for the care of patients having or suspected of having myocardial infarction.

corpus luteum hormone u., SYN progesterone u.

critical care u. (CCU), SYN intensive care u.

CT u., a u. of x-ray attenuation in each picture element of the CT image. SEE Hounsfield u.

Dam u., a u. of activity of vitamin K; the smallest amount of vitamin K, per gram of chick per day, capable of producing normal coagulability in the blood of K-avitaminotic chicks after 3 days of oral administration.

digitalis u. (international), the activity of 0.1 g of the international standard powdered digitalis.

diphtheria antitoxin u., the antitoxin activity of 0.0628 mg of standard diphtheria antitoxin.

dog u., the amount of adrenal cortical extract per kilogram of body weight which, given daily, will maintain an adrenalectomized dog in good condition for 7–10 days.

electromagnetic u. (emu), the u. in an absolute system (CGS) of u.'s utilizing the magnetic effects of current; e.g., abampere, abfarad, abhenry, abohm, abvolt.

electrostatic u. (esu), the u. in an absolute system (CGS) of u.'s utilizing static electricity; e.g., statampere, statcoulomb, statfarad, stathenry, statvolt.

u. of energy, (1) CGS system: erg, joule; **(2)** MKS system: newton-meter (joule); **(3)** FPS system: foot-poundal; **(4)** gravitational u.: gram-centimeter, gram-meter, kilogram-meter, footpound; **(5)** SI: joule.

epidermal-melanin u., an association of one melanocyte with several surrounding epidermal keratinocytes, presumably one that favors the transfer of melanin granules from the melanocyte to the keratinocytes.

equine gonadotropin u. (international), the specific gonadotropic activity of 0.25 mg of standard preparation of the gonadotropic principle of pregnant mares' serum.

estradiol benzoate u. (international), the estrogenic activity of 0.1 μg of a standard preparation of estradiol benzoate.

estrone u. (international), the estrogenic activity of 0.1 μg (0.0001 mg) of a standard preparation of crystalline estrone.

Fishman-Lerner u., a u. of serum acid phosphatase activity based upon measurement of the amount of phenol released from a phenylphosphate substrate.

Florey u., SYN Oxford u.

foot-pound-second u., FPS u., fps u., an absolute u. of the footpound-second system.

u. of force, (1) CGS system: dyne; **(2)** FPS system: poundal; **(3)** MKS system and SI: newton.

gravitational u.'s (G), of energy: gram-centimeter, gram-meter, kilogram-meter, and foot-pound.

G u. of streptomycin, SEE streptomycin u.'s.

u. of heat, (1) calorie (gram calorie; kilocalorie); **(2)** SYN British thermal u; **(3)** SYN joule.

hemolysin u., hemolytic u., the smallest quantity (highest dilution) of inactivated immune serum (hemolysin) that will sensitize the standard suspension of erythrocytes so that the standard complement will cause complete hemolysis. SYN amboceptor u.

heparin u., the quantity of heparin required to keep 1 ml of cat's blood fluid for 24 hours at 0°C; it is equivalent approximately to 0.002 mg of pure heparin. SYN Howell u.

Holzknecht u. (H), an obsolete u. of x-ray dosage equal to one-fifth of the erythema dose.

Hounsfield u., a normalized index of x-ray attenuation based on a scale of -1000 (air) to +1000 (bone), with water being 0; used in CT imaging.

Howell u., SYN heparin u.

insulin u. (international), the activity contained in $\frac{1}{22}$ mg of the international standard of zinc-insulin crystals.

intensive care u. (ICU), a hospital facility for provision of intensive nursing and medical care of critically ill patients, characterized by high quality and quantity of continuous nursing and medical supervision and by use of sophisticated monitoring and resuscitative equipment; may be organized for the care of specific patient groups, e.g., neonatal or newborn ICU, neurologic ICU, pulmonary ICU. SYN critical care u.

u. of intermedin, a u. based upon the action of the hormone in causing the expansion of the melanophores in a hypophysectomized frog; equal to 1 µg of alkali-treated USP Posterior-pituitary Reference Standard.

international u. (IU), the amount of a substance, such as a drug, hormone, vitamin, enzyme, etc., that produces a specific effect as defined by an international body and accepted internationally; e.g., for an enzyme it is micromoles of product formed (or substrate consumed) per minute.

International System of U.'s, SEE International System of Units.

Jenner-Kay u., that amount of phosphatase that liberates 1 mg of phosphorus; approximately 2 Bodansky u.'s or 1 King u.

Karmen u., a formerly used enzyme u. for aminotransferase activity; a change of 0.001 in the absorbance of NADH/min.

Kienböck u. (X), an obsolete u. of x-ray dosage equivalent to $\frac{1}{10}$ the erythema dose.

King u., the quantity of phosphatase that, acting upon disodium phenylphosphate in excess, at pH 9 for 30 min, liberates 1 mg of phenol. SYN King-Armstrong u.

King-Armstrong u., SYN King u.

u. of length, (1) metric system and SI: meter; **(2)** CGS system: centimeter; **(3)** variable in the English system: inch for short distances, foot for moderate distances and for elevation, mile for long distances.

u. of light, SEE candela, lux.

L u. of streptomycin, SEE streptomycin u.'s.

u. of luminous flux, SEE lumen.

u. of luminous intensity, SEE candela.

lung u., (1) a respiratory bronchiole together with the alveolar ducts and sacs and pulmonary alveoli into which the respiratory bronchiole leads; **(2)** considered by some to include the terminal bronchiole and its subdivisions, and called a pulmonary *acinus*.

u. of luteinizing activity (international), SYN progesterone u.

u. of magnetic field intensity, SEE gauss, tesla.

u. of magnetic flux intensity, SEE gauss, tesla.

u. of mass, (1) metric system: gram; **(2)** SI: kilogram; **(3)** English system: pound.

meter-kilogram-second u., MKS u., mks u., an absolute u. of the meter-kilogram-second system.

Montevideo u.'s, a measure of uterine contraction intensity in labor expressed as the sum of the intensity of each contraction within a 10-min period, with intensity defined as the peak pressure achieved by the contraction minus the baseline tone. [from Montevideo, Argentina, where developed]

motor u., a single somatic motor neuron and the group of muscle fibers innervated by it.

mouse u. (m.u.), SYN Allen-Doisy u.

u. of ocular convergence, SYN meter *angle*.

ostiomeatal u., SYN ostiomeatal *complex*.

Oxford u., the minimum amount of penicillin which will prevent the growth of *Staphylococcus aureus* over an area 26 mm in diameter in a standard culture medium; 1 u. equals 0.6 µg of crystalline sodium salt of penicillin. SYN Florey u.

u. of oxytocin, the oxytocic activity of 0.5 mg of the USP Posterior-pituitary Reference Standard; 1 mg of synthetic oxytocin corresponds to 500 IU.

u. of penicillin (international), the penicillin activity of 0.6 µg of penicillin G.

phosphatase u., SEE Bodansky u., King u.

physiologic u., (1) the ultimate (hypothetical) vital u. of protoplasm, as conceived by Spencer; **(2)** the smallest division of an organ that will perform its function; e.g., the uriniferous tubule.

practical u.'s, u.'s of magnitudes convenient for use in the practical applications of electricity; as originally defined they were absolute u.'s (multiples of CGS electromagnetic u.'s); they include the ampere, coulomb, farad, henry, joule, ohm, volt, and watt.

u. of progestational activity (international), SEE progesterone u.

progesterone u. (international), the progestational activity of 1 mg of u. of progestational activity (international); standard preparation of pure progesterone. SEE ALSO Clauberg *test*, Corner-Allen u. SYN corpus luteum hormone u., u. of luteinizing activity.

prolactin u. (international), the specific lactogenic activity contained in 0.1 mg of the standard preparation of the lactogenic substance of the anterior pituitary gland.

u. of radioactivity, SEE Becquerel.

riboflavin u., potency usually expressed in terms of weight of pure riboflavin. SEE ALSO Sherman-Bourquin u. of vitamin B₂. SYN vitamin B₂ u.

roentgen u., SEE Roentgen.

Schwann cell u., a single Schwann cell and all of the axons lying in troughs indenting its surface; this u. is regarded as an unmyelinated fiber in the peripheral nervous system.

Sherman u., u. of vitamin C, minimum protective dose; the minimum amount of vitamin C which, fed daily, will protect a 300-g guinea pig from scurvy for 90 days; equivalent to 0.5–0.6 mg of ascorbic acid.

Sherman-Bourquin u. of vitamin B₂, the amount of vitamin B₂ required in the diet daily to sustain an average weekly gain of 3 g for 8 weeks in standard test rats; one u. is equivalent to 1–7 µg (0.001–0.007 mg) of riboflavin, depending on the deficiency diet used in the above assay.

Sherman-Munsell u., a rat growth u.; the daily amount of vitamin A which sustains a rate of gain amounting to 3 g a week in standard test rats.

SI u.'s, SEE base u.'s, International System of Units.

Somogyi u., a measure of the level of activity of amylase in blood serum, as analyzed by means of the Somogyi method (the most frequently used procedure); one u. is equivalent to 1 mg of reducing sugar liberated as glucose per 100 ml of serum, when an aliquot of the latter is mixed with a standard starch substrate (plus sodium chloride for maximal activation) and incubated for a standard time; normal range is 80–150 u.'s, but values are usually not regarded as clinically significant unless they are greater than 200.

S u. of streptomycin, SEE streptomycin u.'s.

Steenbock u., a u. of vitamin D; the total amount of vitamin D which will produce within 10 days a narrow line of calcium deposit in the rachitic metaphyses of the distal ends of the radii and ulnae of standard rachitic rats.

streptomycin u.'s, (1) G u.: equals 1 g of the crystalline material or about 1,000,000 S u.'s; **(2)** L u.: equal to 1000 S u.'s; **(3)** S u.: the amount of streptomycin which will inhibit the growth of a standard strain of *Escherichia coli* in 1 mL of nutrient broth or other suitable medium.

Svedberg u. (S), a sedimentation constant of 1×10^{-13} s.

un

terminal respiratory u., all alveoli and alveolar ducts beyond the most proximal respiratory bronchiole; contains about 100 alveolar ducts and 2000 alveoli.

tetanus antitoxin u., the antitoxin activity of 0.3094 mg of standard tetanus antitoxin.

thiamin chloride u., thiamin hydrochloride u. (international).

thiamin hydrochloride u. (international), the antineuritic activity of 0.003 mg of the standard crystalline vitamin B_1 hydrochloride. SYN vitamin B_1 hydrochloride u.

u. of thyrotrophic activity, the activity of an amount of an extract of the anterior lobe of the hypophysis which, given daily for 5 days, will cause the thyroid of a guinea pig (weighing 200 g) to reach a weight of 600 mg.

Todd u., the u. in which the results of testing for antistreptolysin O (ASO) are expressed. It denotes the reciprocal of the highest dilution of test serum at which there continues to be neutralization of a standard preparation of the streptococcal enzyme streptolysin O.

toxic u. (T.U.), a u. formerly synonymous with minimal lethal dose in guinea pig but which, because of the instability of toxins, is now measured in terms of the quantity of standard antitoxin with which the toxin combines. SEE ALSO L *doses,* under *dose,* minimal lethal *dose.* SYN toxin u.

toxin u. (T.U.), SYN toxic u.

USP u., a u. as defined and adopted by the *United States Pharmacopeia.*

u. of vasopressin, the pressor activity of 0.5 mg of the USP Posterior-pituitary Reference Standard; 1 mg of synthetic vasopressin corresponds to 600 IU.

vitamin A u. (international), the specific biologic activity of 0.3 μg of vitamin A (alcohol form). SEE ALSO Sherman-Munsell u.

vitamin B_2 u., SYN riboflavin u.

vitamin B_6 u., potency expressed in terms of weight of pure crystalline pyridoxine.

vitamin B_1 hydrochloride u., SYN thiamin hydrochloride u.

vitamin C u. (international), the vitamin C activity of 0.05 mg of the standard crystalline levoascorbic acid; 1 mg of crystalline vitamin C provides 20 USP u.'s. SEE ALSO Sherman u.

vitamin D u. (international), the antirachitic activity contained in 0.025 μg of a preparation of crystalline vitamin D_3 (activated 7-dehydrocholesterol). SEE ALSO Steenbock u.

vitamin E u., potency usually expressed in terms of weight of pure α-tocopherol.

vitamin K u., SEE Dam u.

volume u. (VU), a u. of a logarithmic scale for expressing the power level of a complex audio frequency electrical signal, such as that transmitting music or speech; the power in volume u.'s equals the decibels of power above a reference level of one milliwatt, as measured with an appropriate meter.

u. of wavelength, SEE Ångström, nanometer.

u. of weight, SEE u. of mass.

Wood u.'s, a simplified measurement of pulmonary vascular resistance that uses pressures instead of more complicated u.'s measured by subtracting pulmonary capillary wedge pressure from the mean pulmonary arterial pressure and dividing by cardiac output in liters per minute.

u. of work, SEE u. of energy.

Uni·ted States Adopt·ed Names (USAN). Designation for nonproprietary names (for drugs) adopted by the USAN Council in cooperation with the manufacturers concerned; the designation USAN is applicable only to nonproprietary names coined since June 1961.

Uni·ted States Phar·ma·co·pe·ia (USP). SEE Pharmacopeia.

Uni·ted States Pub·lic Health Ser·vice (USPHS). A bureau of the Department of Health and Human Services, served by a corps of medical officers presided over by the Surgeon General, concerned with scientific research, domestic and insular quarantine, administration of government hospitals, publication of sanitary reports, and statistics; associated with it are the National Institutes of Health, Centers for Disease Control and Prevention, and other units.

uni·va·lence, uni·va·len·cy (ū-ni-vā′lens, -vā′len-sē). SYN monovalence.

uni·va·lent (ū-ni-vā′lent). SYN monovalent (1).

Universal Precautions. (in full, Universal Blood and Body Fluid Precautions). A set of procedural directives and guidelines published in August 1987 by the Centers for Disease Control and Prevention (CDC) (as *Recommendations for Prevention of HIV Transmission in Health-Care Settings*) to prevent parenteral, mucous membrane, and nonintact skin exposures of health care workers to bloodborne pathogens. In December 1991 the Occupational Safety and Health Administration (OSHA) promulgated its *Occupational Exposure to Bloodborne Pathogens Standard,* incorporating universal precautions and imposing detailed requirements on employers of health care workers, including engineering controls, provision of protective barrier devices, standardized labeling of biohazards, mandatory training of employees in Universal Precautions, management of accidental parenteral exposure incidents, and availability to employees of immunization against hepatitis B.

The principle underlying universal precautions is that the blood and certain other body fluids of all patients are to be considered potentially infected with human immunodeficiency virus (HIV), hepatitis B virus (HBV), and other bloodborne pathogens. Universal precautions apply to blood, unfixed tissues (except intact skin), cerebrospinal fluid, synovial fluid, pleural fluid, peritoneal fluid, pericardial fluid, amniotic fluid, semen, and vaginal secretions, but not to feces, nasal secretions, sputum, sweat, tears, urine, or vomitus unless these materials contain visible blood. Specific precautions are prescribed with respect to mouth-to-mouth resuscitation, surgery, invasive diagnostic procedures, obstetrics, renal dialysis, dentistry, clinical laboratories, morgues, and morticians' services. Barrier devices such as gloves, gowns, waterproof aprons, masks, and protective eyewear are required in certain settings, to prevent exposure to blood and other biologically hazardous materials. The OSHA standard requires glove wear for phlebotomy and intraoral examinations and manipulations. Standards are also imposed for laundry, cleaning of surfaces, and disposal of contaminated wastes. Special precautions are advised for handling needles, scalpels, and other sharp instruments or devices after use. Immunization with HBV vaccine is recommended as an important adjunct to universal precautions for health care workers exposed to blood. Universal precautions are intended to supplement, not replace, recommendations for routine infection control, such as handwashing and using gloves to prevent gross contamination of the hands. Implementation of universal precautions does not eliminate the need for other category- or disease-specific isolation precautions, such as enteric precautions for infectious diarrhea or isolation for pulmonary tuberculosis.

---

un·med·ul·lat·ed (ŭn-med′oo-lā-ted). SYN unmyelinated.

un·my·e·li·nat·ed (ŭn-mī′ĕ-li-nā-ted). Denoting nerve fibers (axons) lacking a myelin sheath. SYN amyelinated, amyelinic, nonmedullated, nonmyelinated, unmedullated.

Unna, Paul G., German dermatologist and staining expert, 1850–1929. SEE U. *disease;* Unna *nevus;* U. *stain;* U.-Pappenheim *stain;* U.-Taenzer *stain;* Unna-Thost *syndrome.*

un·of·fi·cial (ŭn-ŏ-fish′ăl). Denoting a drug that is not listed in the United States Pharmacopeia or the National Formulary.

un·phys·i·o·log·ic (ŭn-fis′ē-ō-loj′ik). Pertaining to conditions in the organism which are abnormal; can be used to refer to subjecting the body to abnormal amounts of substances normally present.

un·san·i·tary (ŭn-san′i-tār-ē). SYN insanitary.

un·sat·u·rat·ed (ŭn-sach′ŭr-āt-ed). **1.** Not saturated; denoting a solution in which the solvent is capable of dissolving more of the solute. **2.** Denoting a chemical compound in which all the affinities are not satisfied, so that still other atoms or radicals may be added to it. **3.** In organic chemistry, denoting compounds containing double and/or triple bonds or a ring structure.

un·sex (ŭn′seks). To castrate; to deprive of the gonads.

un·stri·at·ed (ŭn-strī′āt-ed). Without striations; not striped; denoting the structure of the smooth or involuntary muscles.

un·thrifty (ŭn-thrif′tē). In animals, denoting a failure to grow or develop normally as a result of disease.

Unverricht, Heinrich, German physician, 1853–1912. SEE U. *disease.*

UPJ Abbreviation for ureteropelvic *junction.*

up-reg·u·la·tion. Opposite of down-regulation.

up·si·loid (ŭp′si-loyd). SYN hypsiloid.

up·si·lon (up′si-lon). The 20th letter of the Greek alphabet, Ψ.

up·stream (ŭp′strēm). Refers to nucleic acid base sequences proceeding the opposite direction from expression.

up·take (ŭp′tāk). The absorption by a tissue of some substance, food material, mineral, etc., and its permanent or temporary retention.

Ura Abbreviation for uracil.

ura·chal (ūr′ă-kăl). Relating to the urachus.

ura·chus (ūr′ă-kŭs). That portion of the reduced allantoic stalk between the apex of the bladder and the umbilicus; postnatally, the u. is normally merely a fibrous cord, the median umbilical ligament, but occasionally the old allantoic lumen may persist as a vesicoumbilical fistula. [G. *ourachos,* the urinary canal of a fetus]

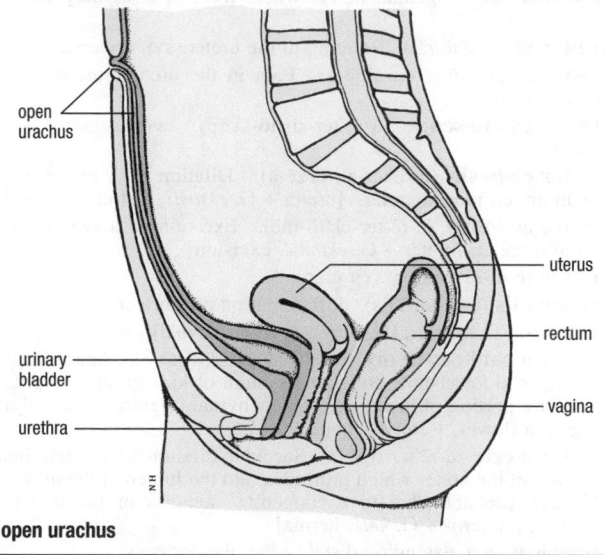

open urachus

uterus

rectum

urinary bladder

vagina

urethra

open urachus

ura·cil (Ura, U) (ūr′ă-sil). 2,4-Dioxopyrimidine; a pyrimidine (base) present in ribonucleic acid.

u. dehydrogenase, an oxidoreductase catalyzing oxidation of uracil to barbituric acid; also oxidizes thymine. SYN u. oxidase.

u. mustard, an alkylating antineoplastic agent. SYN uramustine.

u. oxidase, SYN u. dehydrogenase.

u. phosphoribosyltransferase, SEE phosphoribosyltransferase.

ura·cil-6-car·box·yl·ic ac·id. SYN orotic acid.

Ur·a·go·ga (ūr′ă-gō-gă). A genus of tropical plants (family Rubiaceae). *U. ipecacuanha* (*Cephaelis ipecacuanha*) is the source of Rio or Brazilian ipecac; *U. acuminata* (*C. acuminata*) is the source of Cartagena, Nicaragua, or Panama ipecac. SYN *Cephaelis.*

ur·a·mus·tine (ūr-ă-mŭs′tēn). SYN *uracil* mustard.

ura·nin (ū′ră-nin). SYN *fluorescein* sodium.

ura·ni·nite (ū-ran′i-nīt). SYN pitchblende.

uranisco-. SEE urano-.

ura·nis·co·chasm (ū-ră-nis′kō-kazm). SYN uranoschisis. [uranisco- + G. *chasma,* cleft]

ura·nis·co·ni·tis (ū′ră-nis-kō-nī′tis). SYN palatitis.

ura·nis·co·plas·ty (ū′ră-nis′kō-plas-tē). SYN palatoplasty. [uranisco- + G. *plassō,* to form]

ura·nis·cor·rha·phy (ū′ră-nis-kōr′ă-fē). SYN palatorrhaphy. [uranisco- + G. *rhaphē,* suture]

ura·nis·cus (ū′ră-nis′kŭs). SYN palate. [G. *ouraniskos,* roof of the mouth, dim. of *ouranos,* sky]

ura·ni·um (U) (ū-rā′nē-ŭm). A radioactive metallic element, atomic no. 92, atomic wt. 238.0289, occurring mainly in pitchblende and notable for its two isotopes: ^{238}U and ^{235}U (99.2745% and 0.720%, respectively, the rest being made up by ^{234}U), ^{235}U being the first substance ever shown capable of supporting a self-sustaining chain reaction. [G. myth. character, *Uranus*]

urano-, uranisco-. The hard palate. [G. *ouranos,* sky vault, *ouraniskos,* roof of mouth (palate)]

ura·no·plas·ty (ū′ră-nō-plas-tē). SYN palatoplasty.

ura·nor·rha·phy (ū′ră-nōr′ă-fē). SYN palatorrhaphy. [urano- + G. *rhaphē,* suture]

ura·nos·chi·sis (ū′ră-nos′ki-sis). Cleft of the hard palate. SYN uraniscochasm. [urano- + G. *schisis,* fissure]

ura·no·staph·y·lo·plas·ty (ū′ră-nō-staf′i-lō-plas-tē). Repair of a cleft of both hard and soft palates. SYN uranostaphylorrhaphy. [urano- + G. *staphylē,* uvula, + *plassō,* to form]

ura·no·staph·y·lor·rha·phy (ū′ră-nō-staf-i-lōr′ă-fē). SYN uranostaphyloplasty.

ura·no·staph·y·los·chi·sis (ū′ră-nō-staf′i-los′ki-sis). Cleft of the soft and hard palates. SYN uranoveloschisis. [urano- + G. *staphylē,* uvula, + *schisis,* fissure]

ura·no·ve·los·chi·sis (ū′ră-nō-vĕ-los′ki-sis). SYN uranostaphyloschisis.

ura·nyl (ūr′ă-nil). The ion, UO_2^{2+}, usually found in such salts as uranyl nitrate, $UO_2(NO_3)_2$; uranyl acetate, $UO_2(CH_3COO)_2$, is used in electron microscopy.

urap·i·dil (oo-ră′pĭ-dil). An antihypertensive agent which acts by influencing serotonin receptors.

ura·ro·ma (ū′ră-rō′mă). An obsolete term to describe a spicy, aromatic odor of the urine. [G. *ouron,* urine, + *arōma,* spice]

urar·thri·tis (ū-rar-thrī′tis). Gouty inflammation of a joint. [urate + arthritis]

urate (ūr′āt). A salt of uric acid.

u. oxidase, a copper-containing, oxygen-requiring oxidoreductase that oxidizes uric acid; used in the clinical diagnosis of increased uric acid levels. SYN uricase.

ura·te·mia (ū-ră-tē′mē-ă). The presence of urates, especially sodium urate, in the blood. [urate + G. *haima,* blood]

ur·ate·ri·bo·nu·cle·o·tide phos·pho·ryl·ase (ūr′āt-rī-bō-noo′klē-ō-tīd). A ribosyltransferase that reacts urate D-ribonucleotide with orthophosphate to produce urate plus D-ribose 1-phosphate.

urat·ic (ū-rat′ik). Pertaining to a urate or to urates.

ura·tol·y·sis (ū-ră-tol′i-sis). The decomposition or solution of urates. [urate + G. *lysis,* solution]

ura·to·ly·tic (ū′ră-tō-lit′ik). Causing the decomposition, or solution and removal of urates, from the tissues.

ura·to·ma (ū-ră-tō′mă). SYN gouty *tophus.* [urate + G. *-oma,* tumor]

ura·to·sis (ū-ră-tō′sis). Any morbid condition due to the presence of urates in the blood or tissues.

ura·tu·ria (ū-ră-too′rē-ă). The passage of an increased amount of urates in the urine. [urate + G. *ouron,* urine]

Urbach, Erich, U.S. dermatologist, 1893–1946. SEE U.-Wiethe *disease.*

Urban, Jerome A., U.S. surgeon, *1914. SEE U. *operation.*

ur·ce·i·form (ūr-sē′i-fōrm). Pitcher-shaped. SYN urceolate. [L. *urceus,* pitcher, + *forma,* form]

ur·ce·o·late (ūr′sē-ō-lāt). SYN urceiform. [L. *urceolus,* dim. of *urceus,* pitcher]

Urd Abbreviation for uridine.

Ur

ur·de·fens·es (oor′dē-fens-ez). A rarely used term for primitive defenses. [Ger. *ur-*, primitive, earliest, + defenses]

⚠**ure-, urea-, ureo-.** Urea; urine. SEE ALSO urin-, uro-. [G. *ouron*, urine]

urea (ū-rē′ă). The chief end product of nitrogen metabolism in mammals, formed in the liver by means of the Krebs-Henseleit cycle and excreted in normal adult human urine in the amount of about 32 g a day (about 6/7 of the nitrogen excreted from the body). It may be obtained artificially by heating a solution of ammonium cyanate. It occurs as colorless or white prismatic crystals, without odor but with a cooling saline taste, is soluble in water, and forms salts with acids; has been used as a diuretic in kidney function tests, and topically for various dermatitides. [G. *ouron*, urine]

u. peroxide, a white crystalline compound used in an aqueous solution as an oxidizing mouthwash.

u. stibamine, u. derivative of stibanilic acid, used in the treatment of kala azar and certain other tropical diseases.

ure·a·gen·e·sis (ū-rē-ă-jen′ĕ-sis). Formation of urea, usually referring to the metabolism of amino acids to urea. SYN ureapoiesis. [urea + G. *genesis*, production]

ure·al (ū-rē′ăl). Relating to or containing urea. SYN ureic.

Ure·a·plas·ma (ū-rē′ă-plaz′mă). A genus of microaerophilic to anaerobic, nonmotile bacteria (family Mycoplasmataceae) with no cell walls. Gram-negative, they are predominantly coccoidal to coccobacillary elements, approximately 0.3 μm in diameter, which frequently grow in short filaments; colonies are generally small, 20–30 μm in diameter, and may have no zones of surface growth. Ureaplasma hydrolyze urea with production of ammonia, and are found in the human genitourinary tract, occasionally in the pharynx and rectum. In males, they are associated with nongonococcal urethritis and prostatitis; in females, with genitourinary tract infections and reproductive failure; in neonates, they may cause pneumonia or meningitis. The type species is *U. urealyticum.* SYN T-mycoplasma.

U. urealy′ticum, a species that has been isolated from the respiratory tract and central nerve system of newborns. It causes infections of the genitourinary tract, particularly urethritis; thought to be sexually transmitted and transmitted from mother to infant. The laboratory diagnosis is simplified through the use of urea-containng agar, permitting detection of the tiny colonies.

ure·a·poi·e·sis (ū-rē′ă-poy-ē′sis). SYN ureagenesis. [urea + G. *poiēsis*, a making]

ure·ase (ūr′ē-ās). An enzyme that catalyzes the hydrolysis of urea to carbon dioxide and ammonia; used as an antitumor enzyme; it is present in intestinal bacteria and accounts for most of the ammonia generated from urea in mammals.

ure·de·ma (ū-re-dē′mă). Edema due to infiltration of urine into the subcutaneous tissues. [G. *ouron*, urine, + *oidēma*, swelling]

ure·ic (ū-rē′ik). SYN ureal.

ure·ide (ūr′ē-īd). Any compound of urea in which one or more of its hydrogen atoms have been substituted by acid radicals.

3-ure·i·do·hy·dan·to·in (u-rē′i-dō-hī′dan-tō-in). SYN allantoin.

3-ure·i·do·i·so·bu·tyr·ic ac·id (ū-rē′i-dō-ī′sō-bū-tir′ik). An intermediate in thymine catabolism.

3-ure·i·do·pro·pi·on·ic ac·id (ū-rē′i-dō-prō-pi-on′ik). An intermediate in uracil catabolism.

ure·i·do·suc·cin·ic ac·id (ū-rē′i-dō-sŭk-sin′ik). A precursor of the pyrimidines. SYN *N*-carbamoylaspartic acid.

urel·co·sis (ū-rel-kō′sis). Obsolete term for ulceration of any part of the urinary tract. [G. *ouron*, urine, + *helkōsis*, ulceration]

ure·mia (ū-rē′mē-ă). **1.** An excess of urea and other nitrogenous waste in the blood. **2.** The complex of symptoms due to severe persisting renal failure that can be relieved by dialysis. [G. *ouron*, urine, + *haima*, blood]

hypercalcemic u., u. due to renal failure caused by hypercalcemia with nephrocalcinosis.

ure·mic (ū-rē′mik). Relating to uremia.

ure·mi·gen·ic (ū-rē-mi-jen′ik). **1.** Of uremic origin or causation. **2.** Causing or resulting in uremia.

⚠**ureo-.** SEE ure-.

ure·o·tele (ū′rē-ō-tēl). An organism that is ureotelic; e.g., primates.

ure·o·tel·ia (ū′rē-ō-tēl′ē-a). The process or type of nitrogen excretion in which urea is the primary end product. [urea + G. *telos*, end, outcome, + -ia]

ure·o·tel·ic (ū′rē-ō-tel′ik). Excreting nitrogen primarily in the form of urea. [ureo- + G. *telos*, end]

ur·er·y·thrin (ūr-er′i-thrin). SYN uroerythrin.

ure·si·es·the·sia (ū-rē′si-es-thē′zē-ă). The desire to urinate. SYN uriesthesia. [G. *ourēsis*, a urinating, + *aisthēsis*, sensation]

ure·sis (ū-rē′sis). SYN urination. [G. *ourēsis*]

ure·ter (ū-rē′ter, ū′rē-ter) [TA]. The tube that conducts the urine from the renal pelvis to the bladder; it consists of an abdominal part and a pelvic part, is lined with transitional epithelium surrounded by smooth muscle, both circular and longitudinal, and is covered externally by a tunica adventitia. [G. *ourētēr*, urinary canal]

curlicue u., term given to the radiographic appearance of an opacified u., herniated through the sciatic foramen; a very rare condition.

ectopic u., opens somewhere other than the bladder wall.

ileal u., SYN ureteroileoneocystostomy.

postcaval u., congenital defect where the right u. passes deep to the inferior vena cava on its descent to the bladder.

retrocaval u., in urography, the medial deviation of the right u. in the rare circumstance in which it passes behind the inferior vena cava before entering the pelvis.

retroiliac u., congenital defect where the u. passes deep to the iliac artery.

ure·ter·al (ū-rē′tĕ-răl). Relating to the ureter. SYN ureteric.

ure·ter·al·gia (ū-rē-ter-al′jē-ă). Pain in the ureter. [ureter + G. *algos*, pain]

ure·ter·cys·to·scope (ū-rē′ter-sis′tō-skōp). SYN ureterocystoscope.

ure·ter·ec·ta·sia (ū-rē′ter-ek-tā′zē-ă). Dilation of a ureter. SYN hydroureter, megaloureter. [ureter + G. *ektasis*, a stretching out]

ure·ter·ec·to·my (ū-rē-ter-ek′tō-mē). Excision of a segment or all of a ureter. [ureter + G. *ektomē*, excision]

ure·ter·ic (ū-rē-ter′ik). SYN ureteral.

ure·ter·i·tis (ū-rē-ter-ī′tis). Inflammation of a ureter.

⚠**uretero-.** The ureter. [G. *ourētēr*, urinary canal]

ure·ter·o·cal·i·cos·to·my (ū-rē′ter-kal-ĭ-kos′-tō-ē). Anastomosis of ureter to lower-pole collecting system of kidney after amputation of a portion of lower-pole parenchyma. [uretero- + G. *kalyx*, cup of a flower, + *stoma*, mouth]

ure·ter·o·cele (ū-rē′ter-ō-sēl). Saccular dilation of the terminal portion of the ureter which protrudes into the lumen of the urinary bladder, probably due to a congenital stenosis of the ureteral meatus. [uretero- + G. *kēlē*, hernia]

ectopic u., a u. extending distal to the bladder neck.

orthotopic u., a u. entirely within the bladder.

ure·ter·o·cel·or·ra·phy (ū-rē′ter-ō-se-lōr′ă-fē). Excision and suturing of a ureterocele performed through an open cystotomy incision. [ureterocele + G. *raphē*, suture]

ure·ter·o·co·lic (ū-rē′ter-ō-kol′ik). Relating to the ureter and the colon, especially to an anastomosis for lesions of the lower urinary tract.

ure·ter·o·co·los·to·my (ū-rē′ter-ō-kō-los′tō-mē). Implantation of the ureter into the colon. SYN ureterosigmoidostomy. [uretero- + G. *kolon*, colon, + *stoma*, mouth]

ureterocystoplasty. Augmentation of the bladder using a native dilated ureter.

ure·ter·o·cys·to·scope (ū-rē′ter-ō-sis′tō-skōp). A cystoscope with an attachment for catheterization of the ureters; the catheter is passed into the ureter when its orifice is brought into view with the cystoscope. SYN uretercystoscope. [uretero- + G. *kystis*, bladder, + *skopeō*, to view]

ure·ter·o·cys·tos·to·my (ū-rē′ter-ō-sis-tos′tō-mē). SYN ureteroneocystostomy. [uretero- + G. *kystis*, bladder, + *stoma*, mouth]

ure·ter·o·en·ter·ic (ū-rē′ter-ō-en-ter′ik). Relating to a ureter and the intestine.

ure·ter·o·en·ter·os·to·my (ū-rē′ter-ō-en-ter-os′tō-mē). Formation of an opening between a ureter and the intestine. [uretero- + G. *enteron*, intestine, + *stoma*, mouth]

ure·ter·og·ra·phy (ū-rē′ter-og′ră-fē). Radiography of the ureter after the direct injection of contrast medium. [uretero- + G. *graphē*, a writing]

ure·ter·o·hy·dro·ne·phro·sis (ū-rē′ter-ō-hī′drō-nef-rō′sis). Hydronephrosis also involving the ureters. SYN hydroureteronephrosis, nephroureterectasis.

ure·ter·o·il·e·o·ne·o·cys·tos·to·my (ū-rē′ter-ō-il′ē-ō-nē′ō-sis-tos′tō-mē). Restoration of the continuity of the urinary tract by anastomosis of the upper segment of a partially destroyed ureter to a segment of ileum, the lower end of which is then implanted into the bladder. SYN ileal ureter. [uretero- + ileum + G. *neos*, new, + *hystis*, bladder, + *stoma*, mouth]

ure·ter·o·il·e·os·to·my (ū-rē′ter-ō-il-ē-os′tō-mē). Implantation of a ureter into an isolated segment of ileum which drains through an abdominal stoma. [uretero- + ileum + G. *stoma*, mouth]

ure·ter·o·li·thi·a·sis (ū-rē′ter-ō-li-thī′ă-sis). The formation or presence of a calculus or calculi in one or both ureters. [ureterolith + G. *-iasis*, condition]

ure·ter·o·li·thot·o·my (ū-rē′ter-ō-li-thot′ō-mē). Removal of a stone lodged in a ureter. [ureterolith + G. *tomē*, incision]

ure·ter·ol·y·sis (ū′rē-ter-ol′i-sis). Surgical freeing of the ureter from surrounding disease or adhesions. [uretero- + G. *lysis*, a loosening]

ure·ter·o·ne·o·cys·tos·to·my (ū-rē′ter-ō-nē′ō-sis-tos′tō-mē). An operation whereby a ureter is implanted into the bladder. SEE ALSO detrusorrhaphy. SYN neocystostomy, ureteral reimplantation, ureterocystostomy, ureterovesicostomy. [uretero- + G. *neos*, new, + *kystis*, bladder, + *stoma*, mouth]

ure·ter·o·ne·phrec·to·my (ū-rē′ter-ō-ně-frek′tō-mē). SYN nephroureterectomy. [uretero- + G. *nephros*, kidney, + *ektomē*, excision]

ure·ter·op·a·thy (ū-rē′ter-op′ă-thē). Disease of the ureter. [uretero- + G. *pathos*, suffering]

ure·ter·o·plas·ty (ū-rē′ter-ō-plas-tē). Surgical reconstruction of the ureters. [uretero- + G. *plastos*, formed]

ure·ter·o·proc·tos·to·my (ū-rē′ter-ō-prok-tos′tō-mē). Establishment of an opening between a ureter and the rectum. SYN ureterorectostomy. [uretero- + G. *prōktos*, rectum, + *stoma*, mouth]

ure·ter·o·py·e·li·tis (ū-rē′ter-ō-pī-ě-lī′tis). Inflammation of the pelvis of a kidney and its ureter. [uretero- + G. *pyelos*, pelvis, + *-itis*, inflammation]

ure·ter·o·py·e·log·ra·phy (ū-rē′ter-ō-pī′ě-log′ră-fē). SYN pyelography.

ure·ter·o·py·e·lo·plasty (ū-rē′ter-ō-pī′ě-lō-plas-tē). Surgical reconstruction of the ureter and of the pelvis of the kidney, usually for congenital ureteropelvic junction obstruction. [uretero- + G. *pyelos*, pelvis, + *plastos*, formed]

ure·ter·o·py·e·los·to·my (ū-rē′ter-ō-pī-ě-los′tō-mē). Formation of a junction of the ureter and the renal pelvis. [uretero- + pelvis, + *stoma*, mouth]

ure·ter·o·py·o·sis (ū-rē′ter-ō-pī-ō′sis). An accumulation of pus in the ureter. [uretero- + G. *pyōsis*, suppuration]

ure·ter·o·rec·tos·to·my (ū-rē′ter-ō-rek-tos′tō-mē). SYN ureteroproctostomy.

ure·ter·or·rha·gia (ū-rē′ter-ō-rā′jē-ă). Hemorrhage from a ureter. [uretero- + G. *rhēgnymi*, to burst forth]

ure·ter·or·rha·phy (ū-rē-ter-ōr′ă-fē). Suture of a ureter. [uretero- + G. *rhaphē*, suture]

ure·ter·o·scope (ū-rē′ter-o-skōp). An optical device passed in a retrograde fashion through the bladder up into the ureter to inspect the ureteral lumen and kidney collecting system.

ure·ter·o·sig·moid (ū-rē′ter-ō-sig′moyd). Relating to the ureter and the sigmoid colon, especially to an anastomosis between the two.

ure·ter·o·sig·moi·dos·to·my (ū-rē′ter-ō-sig-moy-dos′tō-mē). SYN ureterocolostomy.

ure·ter·o·sten·o·sis (ū-rē′ter-ō-ste-nō′sis). Stricture of a ureter. [uretero- + G. *stenōsis*, a narrowing]

ure·ter·os·to·my (ū-rē-ter-os′tō-mē). Establishment of an external opening into the ureter. [uretero- + G. *stoma*, mouth]

  cutaneous u., a stoma constructed of ureter at skin level for drainage of urine. This may be an end stoma or a loop stoma. Usually performed because of distal obstruction. SYN cutaneous loop u.

  cutaneous loop u., SYN cutaneous u.

ure·ter·ot·o·my (ū-rē-ter-ot′ō-mē). Incision into a ureter. [uretero- + G. *tomē*, incision]

ure·ter·o·tri·go·no·en·ter·os·to·my (ū-rē′ter-ō-tri-gō′nō-en-ter-os′tō-mē). Implantation of a ureter and its portion of the trigone of the bladder into the intestine. [uretero-, + trigone (of bladder), + enterostomy]

ure·ter·o·u·re·ter·al (ū-rē′ter-ō-ū-re′ter-ăl). Relating to two segments of the same ureter or to both ureters, especially an artificial anastomosis between them.

ure·ter·o·u·re·ter·os·to·my (ū-rē′ter-ō-ū-rē′ter-os′tō-mē). Establishment of an anastomosis between the two ureters or between two segments of the same ureter. SEE transureteroureterostomy.

ure·ter·o·ves·i·cal (ū-rē′ter-ō-ves′i-kăl). Relating to the ureter and the bladder, specifically the junction of ureter with bladder.

ure·ter·o·ves·i·cos·to·my (ū-rē′ter-ō-ves-i-kos′tō-mē). SYN ureteroneocystostomy. [uretero- + L. *vesica*, bladder, + *stoma*, mouth]

ure·than, ure·thane (ū′rě-than, -thān). Has antimitotic activity; formerly used medically as a hypnotic, but now more often used as an anesthetic for laboratory animals. SYN ethyl carbamate.

△**urethr-.** SEE urethro-.

ure·thra (ū-rē′thră) [TA]. The canal leading from the bladder, discharging the urine externally. [G. *ourēthra*]

  anterior u., the portion of u. distal to urogenital diaphragm (external sphincter).

  female u. [TA], a canal about 4 cm long passing from the bladder, in close relation with the anterior wall of the vagina and having a long axis that parallels that of the vagina, opening in the vestibule of the vagina posterior to the clitoris and anterior to the vaginal orifice. SYN u. feminina [TA], u. muliebris.

  u. femini′na [TA], SYN female u.

  male u. [TA], a canal about 20 cm in length that opens at the extremity of the glans penis; except for the intramural and upper prostatic parts, it gives passage to the spermatic fluid as well as urine; components include the intramural, prostatic, intermediate, and spongy urethrae. SYN u. masculina [TA], u. virilis.

  u. masculi′na [TA], SYN male u.

  membranous u., ☆official alternate term for intermediate *part* of male urethra.

  u. mulie′bris, SYN female u.

  penile u., SYN spongy u.

  posterior u., the portion of the u. posterior to the urogenital diaphragm (external sphincter).

  prostatic u. [TA], the prostatic part of the male u., about 2.5 cm in length, that traverses the prostate; it includes the seminal colliculus, and the ejaculatory and prostatic ducts open into it. SYN pars prostatica urethrae [TA].

  spongy u. [TA], the portion of the male u., about 15 cm in length, which traverses the corpus spongiosum. SYN pars spongiosa urethrae masculinae [TA], pars cavernosa, penile u., spongy part of the male urethra.

  u. viri′lis, SYN male u.

ure·thral (ū-rē′thrăl). Relating to the urethra.

ure·thral·gia (ū-rē-thral′jē-ă). Pain in the urethra. SYN urethrodynia. [urethr- + G. *algos*, pain]

ure·threc·to·my (ūr-ě-threk′tō-mē). Excision of a segment of or the entire urethra. [urethr- + G. *ektomē*, excision]

ure·threm·or·rha·gia (ū-rē′threm-ō-rā′jē-ă). SYN urethrorrhagia. [urethr- + G. *haima*, blood, + *rhēgnymi*, to burst forth]

ur

ure·thrism, ure·thris·mus (ū′rē-thrizm, -thriz′mŭs). Irritability or spasmodic stricture of the urethra. SYN urethrospasm.

ure·thri·tis (ū-rē-thrī′tis). Inflammation of the urethra. [ureth- + G. -*itis*, inflammation]

anterior u., inflammation of the portion of the urethra anterior to the triangular ligament.

follicular u., chronic u. with nodular lymphocytic infiltrations in the mucosa. SYN granular u.

gonorrheal u., infection of the urethra usually in association with a purulent discharge due to *Neisseria gonorrhoeae.*

granular u., SYN follicular u.

nongonococcal u., u. not resulting from gonococcal infection; venereally transmitted *Chlamydia trachomatis* is the most common cause.

nonspecific u., u. not resulting from gonococcal, chlamydial, or other specific infectious agents. SYN simple u.

u. petrif′icans, u., sometimes of gouty origin, in which there is a deposit of calcareous matter in the wall of the urethra.

posterior u., inflammation of the membranous and prostatic portions of the urethra.

simple u., SYN nonspecific u.

⚬**urethro-, urethr-.** The urethra. [G. *ourēthra*]

ure·thro·bul·bar (ū-rē′thrō-bŭl′băr). SYN bulbourethral.

ure·thro·cele (ū-rē′thrō-sēl). Prolapse of the female urethra. [urethro- + G. *kēlē,* tumor, hernia]

ure·thro·cys·to·me·trog·ra·phy (ū-rē′thrō-sis′tō-me-trog′ră-fē). SYN urethrocystometry. [urethro- + G. *kystis,* bladder, + *metron,* measure, + *skopeō,* to view]

ure·thro·cys·tom·e·try (ū-rē′thrō-sis-tom′ĕ-trē). A procedure that simultaneously measures pressures in the urinary bladder and urethra. SYN urethrocystometrography. [urethro- + G. *kystis,* bladder, + *metron,* measure]

ure·thro·cys·to·pexy (ū-rē′thrō-sis′tō-pek-sē). Fixation of urethra and bladder for stress incontinence. SYN urethropexy. [urethro- + G. *kystis,* bladder, + *pēxis,* fixation]

ure·thro·dyn·ia (ū-rē-thrō-din′ē-ă). SYN urethralgia. [urethro- + G. *odynē,* pain]

ure·throg·ra·phy (ū-rē-throg′ră-fē). Contrast radiography of the male or female urethra, by retrograde injection or during voiding of contrast medium in the bladder (cystourethrogram). [urethra + G. *graphō,* to write]

ure·throm·e·ter (ū-rē-throm′ĕ-ter). An instrument for measuring the caliber of the urethra. [urethro- + G. *metron,* measure]

ure·thro·pe·nile (ū-rē′thrō-pē′nīl). Relating to the urethra and the penis.

ure·thro·per·i·ne·al (ū-rē′thrō-pĕ-rī-nē′ăl). Relating to the urethra and the perineum.

ureth·ro·per·i·ne·o·scro·tal (ū-rē′thrō-pe-rī-nē-ō-skrō′tăl). Relating to the urethra, perineum, and scrotum.

ure·thro·pexy (ū-rē′thrō-pek-sē). SYN urethrocystopexy. [urethro- + G. *pēxis,* fixation]

ure·thro·plasty (ū-rē′thrō-plas-tē). Surgical reconstruction of the urethra. [urethro- + G. *plastos,* formed]

Cecil u., a staged urethral reconstructive procedure wherein the urethral portion of the penis is left buried in the scrotum after u. at the first stage because of inadequate ventral skin cover.

ure·thro·pros·ta·tic (ū-rē′thrō-pros-tat′ik). Relating to the urethra and the prostate.

ure·thro·rec·tal (ū-rē′thrō-rek′tăl). Relating to the urethra and the rectum.

ure·thror·rha·gia (ū-rē-thrō-rā′jē-ă). Bleeding from the urethra. SYN urethremorrhagia.

ure·thror·rha·phy (ū-rē-thrōr′ă-fē). Suture of the urethra. [urethro- + G. *rhaphē,* suture]

ure·thror·rhea (ū-rē-thrō-rē′ă). An abnormal discharge from the urethra. [urethro- + G. *rhoia,* a flow]

ure·thro·scope (ū-rē′thrō-skōp). An instrument for viewing the interior of the urethra. [urethro- + G. *skopeō,* to view]

ure·thro·scop·ic (ū-rē-thrō-skop′ik). Relating to the urethroscope or to urethroscopy.

ure·thros·co·py (ū-rē-thros′kŏ-pē). Inspection of the urethra with a urethroscope.

ure·thro·spasm (ū-rē′thrō-spazm). SYN urethrism.

ure·thro·stax·is (ū-rē′thrō-stak′sis). Oozing of blood from the urethra. [urethro- + G. *staxis,* trickling]

ure·thro·ste·no·sis (ū-rē′thrō-ste-nō′sis). Stricture of the urethra. [urethro- + G. *stenōsis,* a narrowing]

ure·thros·to·my (ū-rē-thros′tō-mē). Surgical formation of a permanent opening between the urethra and the skin. [urethro- + G. *stoma,* mouth]

perineal u., formation of a permanent opening into the bulbous portion of the urethra through a perineal skin incision.

ure·thro·tome (ū-rē′thrō-tōm). An instrument for dividing a stricture of the urethra. [urethro- + G. *tomos,* cutting]

ure·throt·o·my (ū-rē-throt′o-mē). Surgical incision of a stricture of the urethra. [urethro- + G. *tomē,* incision]

external u., u. via an external opening in the perineum or penile skin. SYN perineal u.

internal u., u. by means of an instrument passed through the urethra.

perineal u., SYN external u.

ure·thro·vag·i·nal (ū-rē′thrō-vaj′i-năl). Relating to the urethra and the vagina.

ure·thro·ves·i·cal (ū-rē′thrō-ves′i-kăl). Relating to the urethra and bladder.

ure·thro·ves·i·co·pexy (ū-rē′thrō-ves′i-kŏ-pek-sē). Surgical suspension of the urethra and the base of the bladder from the posterior surface of the pubic symphysis (or anterior abdominal wall or Cooper ligament) for correction of urinary stress incontinence. [urethro- + L. *vesica,* bladder, + G. *pexis,* fixation]

⚬**-uretic.** Urine. [G. *ourētikos,* relating to the urine]

URF Abbreviation for unidentified *reading frame.*

ur·gen·cy (er′jen-sē). A strong desire to void.

motor u., u. from overactive detrusor function.

sensory u., u. due to vesicourethral hypersensitivity.

ur·gi·nea (er-jin′ē-ă). The bulbs of *Urginea indica* (Indian squill) and *Urginea maritima* (white or Mediterranean squill); the source of squill. [L. *urgeo,* to press, referring to the shape of the seeds]

⚬**uri-, uric-, urico-.** Uric acid. [G. *ouron,* urine]

uri·an (ūr′ē-ăn). SYN urochrome.

uric (ūr′ik). Relating to urine.

▪**uric ac·id.** 2,6,8-Trioxypurine; white crystals, poorly soluble, contained in solution in the urine of mammals and in solid form in the urine of birds and reptiles; sometimes solidified in small masses as stones or crystals or in larger concretions as calculi; with sodium and other bases it forms urates; elevated levels associated with gout. SYN lithic acid, triketopurine.

u. a. oxidase, SEE *urate* oxidase.

uri·case (ūr′i-kās). SYN *urate* oxidase.

⚬**urico-.** SEE uri-.

uri·col·y·sis (ūr-i-kol′i-sis). Decomposition of uric acid. [urico- + G. *lysis,* a loosening]

uri·co·lyt·ic (ūr′i-kō-lit′ik). Relating to or effecting the hydrolysis of uric acid.

uri·cos·o·me (ūr-ik′ō-sōm). A microbody rich in urate oxidase.

uri·co·su·ria (ū′ri-kō-soo′rē-ă). Excessive amounts of uric acid in the urine. [urico- + G. *ouron,* urine]

uri·co·su·ric (ū′ri-kō-soo′rik). Tending to increase the excretion of uric acid.

uri·co·tele (oor′ik-ō-tēl). An organism that is uricotelic; e.g., birds and land-dwelling reptiles.

uri·co·tel·ia (ūr-ik′ō-tēl-ē-a). The process or type of nitrogen excretion in which uric acid is the chief excretion product. [uric (acid) + G. *telos,* end, outcome, + -ia]

uri·co·tel·ic (ūr′i-kō-tel′ik). Producing uric acid as the chief excretory product of nitrogen metabolism. [urico- + G. *telos,* end]

uri·dine (Urd) (ūr′i-dēn). Uracil ribonucleoside; one of the major nucleosides in RNAs; as the pyrophosphate (UDP, UDPG, etc.), u. is active in sugar metabolism. SYN 1-β-D-ribofuranosyluracil.

cyclic u. 3′,5′-monophosphate (cUMP), a cyclic nucleotide involved in metabolic regulation; inhibits the growth of some tumors.

u. 5′-diphosphate (UDP), uridine 5′-pyrophosphate; a condensation product of uridine and pyrophosphoric acid.

u. 5′-monophosphate (UMP), SYN uridylic acid.

u. phosphorylase, a ribosyltransferase that catalyzes the reaction of uridine with orthophosphate to produce uracil and α-D-ribose 1-phosphate.

u. 5′-triphosphate (UTP), u. esterified with triphosphoric acid at its 5′ position; the immediate precursor of uridylic acid residues in RNA.

uri·dine di·phos·pho·ga·lac·tose (UDPGal) (ūr′i-dēn-dī-fos′fō-gă-lak′tōs). A pyrophosphate group links the 5′ position of uridine and the 1 position of D-galactose.

u. d. 4-epimerase, SEE UDPglucose 4-epimerase.

uri·dine di·phos·pho·glu·cose (UDPG, UDPGlc) (ūr′i-dēn-dī-fos′fō-gloo′kōs). A pyrophosphate group links the 5′ position of uridine and the 1 position of D-glucose; an intermediate in glycogen biosynthesis. SYN UDPglucose.

u. d. 4-epimerase, SYN UDPglucose 4-epimerase.

uri·dine di·phos·pho·glu·cu·ron·ic ac·id (UDP-GlcUA) (ūr′i-dēn-dī-fos′fō-gloo-koo-ron′ik). Uridine diphosphoglucose in which the 6-CH₂OH of the glucose has been oxidized to COOH (thus, has become a glucuronyl residue); participates in the formation of conjugates of bilirubin or drugs such as aspirin.

uri·dine di·phos·pho·xylose. SYN xylose.

uri·dro·sis (ū-ri-drō′sis). The excretion of urea or uric acid in the sweat. [uri- + G. *hidrōs*, sweat]

u. crystalli′na, SYN urea *frost*.

uri·dyl·ic ac·id (ūr-i-dil′ik). Uridine esterified by phosphoric acid on one or more sugar hydroxyl groups; UMP is typically uridine 5′-monophosphate; 2′ and 3′ derivatives also occur; precursor for the biosynthesis of other pyrimidine nucleotides. SYN UMP synthase, uridine 5′-monophosphate.

u. a. synthase, a bifunctional enzyme that contains the activities of both orotate phosphoribosyltransferase and orotidine-5′-monophosphate decarboxylase; catalyzes a key step in pyrimidine biosynthesis; a deficiency of this enzyme leads to orotic aciduria.

uri·dyl·trans·fer·ase (ūr′i-dil-trans′fer-ās). UDPglucose-hexose 1-phosphate; uridylyltransferase.

uri·es·the·sia (ūri-es-thē′zē-ă). SYN uresiesthesia.

⚥**urin-, urino-.** Urine. SEE ALSO ure-, uro-. [G. *ouron*]

uri·nal (ū′rin-ăl). A vessel into which urine is passed.

⚑**uri·nal·y·sis** (ū-ri-nal′i-sis). Analysis of the urine.

uri·nary (ūr′i-nār-ē). Relating to urine.

uri·nate (ūr′i-nāt). To pass urine. SYN micturate.

uri·na·tion (ūr′i-nā′shŭn). The passing of urine. SYN miction, micturition (1), uresis.

stuttering u., the passage of urine in jets caused by intermittent spasmodic contraction of the bladder.

⚑**urine** (ūr′in). The fluid and dissolved substances excreted by the kidney. [L. *urina*; G. *ouron*]

ammoniacal u., SYN ammoniuria.

black u., the dark u. of melanuria or hemoglobinuria.

chylous u., u. of a milky appearance, containing chyle. SYN milky u.

cloudy u., u. with a cloudy appearance, usually due to pus, crystals, bacteria, blood, or free fat globules. SYN nebulous u.

crude u., pale u. of low specific gravity, with very little sediment.

febrile u., dark colored, concentrated u. of strong odor, passed by one suffering from fever. SYN feverish u.

urine

in general		organic components (in mg/24 hr., unless otherwise noted)	
quantity (in ml/24hr.)	500 − 2000	acetone bodies	10 − 100
specific gravity	1.010 − 1.025	amino acids, total (g/24 hr.)	1.3 − 3.2
solid matter (g/24hr., 100% dry residue)	40 − 60	amino acids, free (g/24 hr.)	0.35 − 1.20
freezing point depression (°C)	0.1 − 2.5	amino acid N	40 − 130
osmolality (mosm/l)	50 − 1400	creatine ♂	10 − 190
pH	4.8 − 7.5	creatine ♀	10 − 270
total acidity (mval/24 hr.)	50 − 60	creatinine	500 − 2500
acidity (by titration)	20 − 60	diazo bodies	traces
total nitrogen (g/24 hr.)	7 − 17	fatty acids	8 − 50
amino acid–N (% of total N)	< 2	bilirubin	0.02 − 1.9
ammonia (NH₄⁺)–N	4.6	urobilinogen	0.05 − 2.5
creatinine–N	3.7	bile acid (g/24 hr., as glyco and as taurocholic acid)	5 − 10
uric acid–N	1.6	glucuronic acid	200 − 600
urea–N	82.7	uric acid	80 − 1000
		urea (g/24 hr.)	12 − 30
inorganic components (in mg/24 hr., unless otherwise noted)		hippuric acid (g/24 hr.)	1.0 − 2.5
		hydroxyindoleacetic acid	1.0 − 14.7
ammonia	0.3 − 1.2	indican	4.0 − 20.0
calcium	130 − 330	indoxylsulfuric acid	15 − 100
chloride (g/24 hr.)	4.3 − 8.5	lactic acid	100 − 600
iron	0.4 − 0.15	oxal acid	10 − 25
iodine	0.02 − 0.5	aminolevulinic acid	1.5 − 7.0
potassium (g/24 hr.)	1.4 − 3.1	coproporphyrin	0.02 − 0.2
copper	0.03 − 0.07	porphobilinogen	0.4 − 2.4
magnesium	60.7 − 200	uroporphyrin	0.004 − 0.02
sodium (g/24 hr.)	2.8 − 5.0	proteins	10 − 100
phosphorus, total (g/24 hr.)	0.8 − 2.0	purine bases (g/24 hr.)	0.2 − 0.5
sulfur, total (g/24 hr.)	1.24 − 1.50	citric acid	150 − 1200
sulfur, inorganic (g/24 hr.)	1.07 − 1.30	sugar (reducing substances)	500 − 1500
sulfur, neutral (g/24 hr.)	0.05 − 0.08	galactose	3 − 25
sulfur, esterized (g/24 hr.)	0.08 − 0.10	glucose	15 − 130
zinc	0.14 − 0.70	lactose	0 − 90

feverish u., SYN febrile u.

gouty u., u. of a high color containing uric acid in excess.

honey u., obsolete term for *diabetes* mellitus.

maple syrup u., SEE maple syrup urine *disease.*

milky u., SYN chylous u.

nebulous u., SYN cloudy u.

residual u., u. remaining in the bladder at the end of micturition in cases of prostatic obstruction, bladder atony, etc.

uri·nif·er·ous (ūr-i-nif′ĕ-rŭs). Conveying urine; denoting the tubules of the kidney. [urine + L. *fero,* to carry]

uri·nif·ic (oor-i-nif′ik). SYN uriniparous. [urine + L. *facio,* to make]

uri·nip·a·rous (oor-i-nip′ă-rŭs). Producing or excreting urine; denoting the malpighian bodies and certain tubules in the renal cortex. SYN urinific. [urine + L. *pario,* to produce]

△**urino-.** SEE urin-.

uri·no·gen·i·tal (ūr′i-nō-jen′i-tăl). SYN genitourinary.

uri·nog·e·nous (ūr-i-noj′ĕ-nŭs). **1.** Producing or excreting urine. **2.** Of urinary origin. SYN urogenous.

uri·no·ma (ūr′i-nō′mă). A collection of extravasated urine. SYN urinary cyst.

uri·nom·e·ter (ūr-i-nom′ĕ-ter). A hydrometer for determining the specific gravity of the urine. SYN urogravimeter, urometer. [urine + G. *metron,* measure]

uri·nom·e·try (ūr-i-nom′ĕ-trē). The determination of the specific gravity of the urine.

uri·nos·co·py (ūr-i-nos′kŏ-pē). SYN uroscopy.

uri·no·sex·u·al (ūr-i-nō-sek′shoo-ăl). SYN genitourinary.

uri·nous (ūr′i-nŭs). Relating to or of the nature of urine.

uri·po·sia (ūr-i-pō′sē-ă). Urine-drinking. [urine + G. *posis,* drinking]

△**uro-.** Urine. SEE ALSO ure-, urin-. [G. *ouron*]

uro·am·mo·ni·ac (ū-rō-ă-mo′nē-ak). Relating to uric acid and ammonia; denoting a variety of urinary calculus.

uro·an·the·lone (ūr-ō-an′thĕ-lōn). SYN urogastrone.

uro·bi·lin (ūr-ō-bī′lin, -bil′in). A uroporphyrin; an acyclic tetrapyrrole that is one of the natural breakdown products of heme via choleglobin, verdohemochrome, biliverdin, bilirubin, and *d*-urobilinogen; a urinary pigment that gives a varying orange-red coloration to urine according to its degree of oxidation. SYN urohematin, urohematoporphyrin.

uro·bi·lin IXα. SYN mesobilene.

uro·bi·li·ne·mia (ū′rō-bil-i-nē′mē-ă). The presence of urobilins in the blood.

uro·bi·lin·o·gen (ūr-ō-bī-lin′ō-jen). Precursor of urobilin.

uro·bi·lin·o·gen IXα. SYN mesobilane.

uro·bi·lin·u·ria (ū′rō-bil-i-noo′rē-ă). The presence in the urine of urobilins in excessive amounts, formed mainly from hemoglobin.

uro·can·ase (ū′rō-kă-nās). SYN *urocanate* hydratase.

ur·o·can·ate (ūr′ō-kă-nāt). A salt or ester of urocanic acid.

u. hydratase, an enzyme catalyzing the reaction of water with urocanic acid to produce 4-imidazolone-5-propionic acid, a step in L-histidine catabolism; this enzyme is absent in cases of urocanic aciduria. SYN urocanase.

uro·can·ic ac·id (ūr-ō-kan′ik). 4-Imidazoleacrylic acid; an acid derived from the oxidative deamination of L-histidine; present in sweat and in dog's urine; elevated levels are observed in cases of urocanate hydratase deficiency. The *cis* form, resulting from exposure to UV radiation, activates suppressor T cells.

uro·can·ic ac·i·du·ria (oor′ō-kan′ik-as′id-ūr′ē-a). Elevated levels of urocanic acid in the urine.

uro·can·i·case (ūr-ō-kan′i-kās). One of a group of at least three enzymes that convert urocanic acid to glutamic acid.

uro·cele (ū′rō-sēl). Extravasation of urine into the scrotal sac. [uro- + G. *kēlē,* hernia]

uroch·er·as (ū-rok′er-as). **1.** SYN gravel. **2.** SYN uropsammus (2). [uro- + G. *cheras,* gravel (an incorrect form of *cherados,* gravel)]

uro·che·sia (ū-rō-kē′zē-ă). Passage of urine from the anus. [uro- + G. *chezō,* to defecate]

uro·chrome (ūr′ō-krōm). The principal pigment of urine, a compound of urobilin and a peptide of unknown structure. SYN urian.

uro·chro·mo·gen (ūr-ō-krō′mō-jen). Originally, a body in the urine that, on taking up oxygen, formed urochrome; now, probably urobilinogen.

uro·cris·ia (ū-rō-kris′ē-ă, -kriz′ē-ă). **1.** SYN urocrisis. **2.** Obsolete term for diagnosis based upon the results of a urinary examination. [uro- + G. *krinō,* to separate, judge]

uro·cri·sis (ū′rō-krī′sis). **1.** Obsolete term for the critical stage of a disease accompanied by a copious discharge of urine. **2.** Severe pain in any of the urinary organs or passages occurring in tabes dorsalis. SYN urocrisia (1). [uro- + G. *krisis,* crisis]

uro·cy·a·nin (ū′rō-sī′ă-nin). An indigo blue pigment sometimes observed in the urine in certain diseases, especially scarlet fever. SYN uroglaucin. [uro- + G. *kyanos,* a blue substance]

uro·cy·an·o·gen (ū-rō-sī-an′ō-jen). A blue pigment sometimes observed in the urine in cases of cholera.

uro·cy·a·no·sis (ū′rō-sī-ă-nō′sis). A bluish discoloration of the urine in indicanuria.

uro·cyst (ū′rō-sist). SYN urinary *bladder.* [uro- + G. *kystis,* bladder]

uro·cys·tic (ū′rō-sis′tik). Relating to the urinary bladder.

uro·cys·tis (ū′rō-sis′tis). SYN urinary *bladder.*

uro·dy·na·mics (ū′rō-dī-nam′iks). The study of the storage of urine within, and the flow of urine through and from, the urinary tract. [uro- + G. *dynamis,* force]

uro·dyn·ia (ūr-ō-din′ē-ă). Pain on urination. [uro- + G. *odynē,* pain]

uro·en·ter·one (ūr-ō-en′ter-ōn). SYN urogastrone.

uro·er·y·thrin (ū-rō-er′i-thrin). A urinary pigment that gives a pink color to deposits of urates; presumably derived from melanin. SYN purpurin (1), urerythrin.

uro·fla·vin (ūr-ō-flā′vin). A fluorescent product of riboflavin catabolism, or perhaps riboflavin itself, found in mammalian urine and feces.

uro·flow·me·ter (ū-rō′flō-mē-ter). A device that measures urine flow rates during micturition, including these parameters: peak flow rate, average flow rate, voided volume, and time of voiding.

ur·o·fol·li·tro·pin (ūr-ō-fol′i-trō-pin). A preparation of gonadotropin extracted from the urine of postmenopausal women, used in conjunction with human chorionic gonadotropin to induce ovulation. SEE ALSO menotropins.

uro·fus·co·hem·a·tin (ū-rō-fŭs-kō-hē′mă-tin). A brownish red pigment found in the urine in certain diseases such as leprosy.

uro·gas·trone (ūr-ō-gas′trōn). A fluorescent pigment extracted from urine; an inhibitor of gastric secretion and motility. Cf. enterogastrone. SYN anthelone U, anthelone, uroanthelone, uroenterone.

uro·gen·i·tal (ū′rō-jen′i-tăl). SYN genitourinary.

urog·e·nous (ū-roj′ĕ-nŭs). SYN urinogenous.

uro·glau·cin (ū-rō-glaw′sin). SYN urocyanin. [uro- + G. *glaukos,* bluish gray]

ur·o·go·nad·o·tro·pin (ūr′ō-gō-nad-ō-trō′pin). SEE human menopausal *gonadotropin.*

uro·graf·fin (ūr-ō-graf′fin). A mixture of salts of diatrizoic acid used to form density gradients.

uro·gram (ūr′ō-gram). The radiographic record obtained by urography.

urog·ra·phy (ū-rog′ră-fē). Radiography of any part (kidneys, ureters, or bladder) of the urinary tract. SEE ALSO pyelography. [uro- + G. *graphō,* to write]

antegrade u., radiography following intravenous or percutaneous injection of contrast agent with a needle or catheter into the renal calices or pelvis (antegrade pyelography), or into the urinary bladder (antegrade cystography).

cystoscopic u., SYN retrograde u.

■**intravenous u., excretory u.,** radiography of kidneys, ureters, and bladder following injection of contrast medium into a peripheral vein.

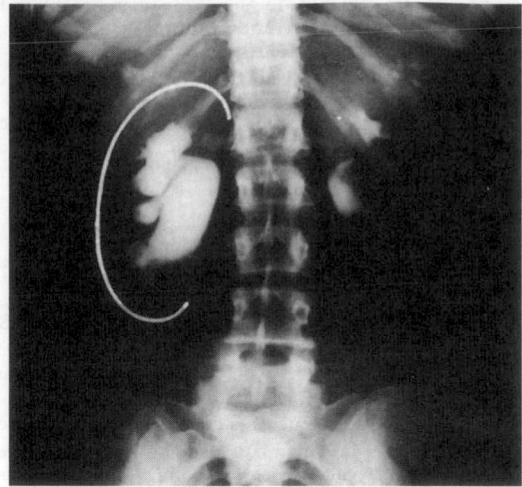

urography: intravenous urogram showing retention of a large amount of contrast medium in the right renal pelvis indicating hydronephrosis due to ureteral obstruction

retrograde u., radiography of the urinary tract following injection of contrast medium directly into the urethra, bladder, ureter, or renal pelvis. SYN cystoscopic u.

uro·gra·vim·e·ter (ū'rō-gră-vim'ĕ-ter). SYN urinometer. [uro- + L. *gravis,* heavy, + G. *metron,* measure]

uro·hem·a·tin (ūr-ō-hēm'ă-tin). SYN urobilin.

uro·hem·a·to·por·phy·rin (ūr'ō-hēm'ă-tō-pōr'fi-rin). SYN urobilin.

uro·hep·a·rin (ūr-ō-hep'ă-rin). An inactive form of heparin excreted in the urine.

uro·hy·per·ten·sin (ūr'ō-hī-per-ten'sin). A pressor substance derived from the urine.

uro·ki·nase (ūr-ō-kī'nās). SYN plasminogen *activator.*

uro·lag·nia (ūr-ō-lag'nē-ă). Sexual stimulation occasioned by the sight of a person urinating. [uro- + G. *lagneia,* lust]

uro·leu·cin·ic ac·id, uro·leu·cic ac·id (ū'rō-loo-sin'ik, ū-rō-loo'sik). An aromatic compound, excreted in the urine of persons with alcaptonuria.

uro·lith (ū'rō-lith). SYN urinary *calculus.* [uro- + G. *lithos,* stone]

uro·li·thi·a·sis (ū-rō-li-thī'ă-sis). Presence of calculi in the urinary system.

uro·lith·ic (ū-rō-lith'ik). Relating to urinary calculi.

uro·li·thol·o·gy (ū'rō-li-thol'ō-jē). The branch of medicine concerned with the formation, composition, effects, and removal of urinary calculi. [uro- + G. *lithos,* stone, + *logos,* study]

uro·log·ic, uro·log·i·cal (ū-rō-loj'ik, i-kăl). Relating to urology.

urol·o·gist (ū-rol'ō-jist). A specialist in urology. SYN genitourinary surgeon.

urol·o·gy (ū-rol'ō-jē). The medical specialty concerned with the study, diagnosis, and treatment of diseases of the genitourinary tract. [uro- + G. *logos,* study]

uro·lu·te·in (ū-rō-loo'tē-in). Name given to yellow pigment in the urine. SEE urochrome, uroporphyrin (1).

uro·mel·a·nin (ūr-ō-mel'ă-nin). A black pigment occasionally found in the urine, possibly a decomposition product of urochrome.

urom·e·ter (ū-rom'ĕ-ter). SYN urinometer.

uron·cus (ū-rong'kŭs). A urinary cyst; a circumscribed area of extravasation of urine. [uro- + G. *onkos,* mass (tumor)]

uron·ic ac·ids (ū-ron'ik). Acids derived from monosaccharides by oxidation of the primary alcohol group (–CH$_2$OH) farthest removed from the carbonyl group to a carboxyl group (–COOH); e.g., glucuronic acid.

uro·nos·co·py (ū-rō-nos'kŏ-pē). SYN uroscopy.

urop·a·thy (ū-rop'ă-thē). Any disorder involving the urinary tract. [uro- + G. *pathos,* suffering]

obstructive u., any pathologic condition, anatomic or functional, of the urinary tract caused by obstruction.

uro·phan·ic (ūr-ō-fan'ik). Appearing in the urine; denoting any constituent, normal or pathologic, of the urine. [uro- + G. *phainō,* to appear]

uro·phe·in (ū-rō-fē'in). A grayish pigment occasionally found in the urine, possibly identical with urobilin. [uro- + G. *phaios,* gray]

uro·poi·e·sis (ū'rō-poy-ē'sis). The production or secretion and excretion of urine. [uro- + G. *poiēsis,* a making]

uro·poi·e·tic (ū'rō-poy-et'ik). Relating or pertaining to uropoiesis.

uro·por·phy·rin (ūr-ō-pōr'fi-rin). **1.** Porphyrin excreted in the urine in porphyrinuria; e.g., urobilin. **2.** Class name for all porphyrins containing 4 acetic acid groups and 4 propionic acid groups in positions 1 through 8. SEE ALSO porphyrinogens.

u. I, porphin-1,3,5,7-tetraacetic acid-2,4,6,8-tetrapropionic acid; formed by the action of light on uroporphyrinogen I; elevated levels observed in certain porphyrias.

u. III, porphin-1,3,5,8-tetraacetic acid-2,4,6,7-tetrapropionic acid; formed by the action of light on uroporphyrinogen III; elevated levels observed in certain porphyrias.

ur·o·por·phy·rin·o·gen (ūr'ō-pōr-fi-rin'ō-jen). SEE porphyrinogens.

u. decarboxylase, an enzyme that participates in heme biosynthesis; it catalyzes the decarboxylation of uroporphyrin III to produce coproporphyrinogen III; it also acts on uroporphyrin I; a deficiency of this enzyme will result in either porphyria cutanea tarda or hepatoerythropoietic porphyria.

u. III cosynthase, an enzyme in heme biosynthesis that participates in the formation of u. III; a deficiency of this protein results in congenital erythropoietic porphyria.

uro·psam·mus (ū-rō-sam'ŭs). **1.** SYN gravel. **2.** Any inorganic or uratic urinary sediment. SYN urocheras (2). [uro- + G. *psammos,* sand]

urop·ter·in (ū-rop'ter-in). SYN urothion.

uro·pur·pur·in (ūr-ō-pŭr'poor-in). A purple pigment in the urine.

ur·o·ra·di·ol·o·gy (ū'rō-rā-dē-ol'ŏ-jē). The study of the radiology of the urinary tract.

uro·rec·tal (ū'rō-rek'tăl). Relating to the urinary tract and rectum.

uro·ro·se·in (ūr-ō-rō'zē-in). A chromogen in the urine that forms a red color on the addition of nitric acid; normally exists in very minute quantities but is increased in tuberculosis and other wasting diseases, and is related to ingestion of indole compounds.

uro·ru·bin (ūr-ō-roo'bin). A red pigment in urine made more visible by treatment with hydrochloric acid.

uro·ru·bro·hem·a·tin (ūr'ō-roo-brō-hē'mă-tin). A reddish pigment occasionally present in the urine in various chronic diseases.

uros·che·sis (ū-ros'kē-sis). **1.** Retention of urine. **2.** Suppression of urine. [uro- + G. *schesis,* a checking]

uro·scop·ic (ūr-ō-skop'ik). Relating to uroscopy.

uros·co·py (ū-ros'kŏ-pē). Examination of the urine, usually by means of a microscope. SYN urinoscopy, uronoscopy. [uro- + G. *skopeō,* to view]

uro·sem·i·ol·o·gy (ū'rō-sem-ē-ol'ō-jē). The study of the urine as an aid to diagnosis. [uro- + G. *sēmeion,* a sign, + *logos,* study]

uro·sep·sin (ūr-ō-sep'sin). An obsolete term for a substance formed by the decomposition of urine, supposed to be the cause of septic poisoning after urinary extravasation.

uro·sep·sis (ūr-ō-sep'sis). **1.** Sepsis resulting from the infection of extravasated urine. **2.** Sepsis from obstruction of infected urine. [uro- + G. *sēpsis,* decomposition]

uro·spec·trin (ūr-ō-spek'trin). A pigment found in the urine, possibly the same as urobilin.

ur

u·ro·the·li·um (ū-rō-thē′lē-ŭm). The epithelial lining of the urinary tract. [uro- + epithelium]

ur·o·thi·on (ūr-ō-thī′on). A sulfur-containing pteridine derivative isolated from urine. SYN uropterin.

ur·o·thor·ax (ūr-ō-thōr′aks). The presence of urine in the thoracic cavity, usually following complex multiple organ injuries.

uro·xan·thin (ūr-ō-zan′thin). SYN indican (2).

urox·in (ū-rok′sin). SYN alloxantin.

ursodeoxycholic acid. SYN ursodiol.

ursodiol (er-sō-dī′ōl). A bile acid used to facilitate the dissolution of gallstones in patients; a potential alternative to cholecystectomy. SYN ursodeoxycholic acid.

ur·ti·ca (er-tī′kă, er′ti-). The herb, *Urtica dioica* (family Urticaceae); a weed, the leaves of which produce a stinging sensation when touching the skin. It has been used as a diuretic and hemostatic in metrorrhagia, epistaxis, and hematemesis. SYN nettle. [L. a nettle, fr. *uro,* pp. *ustus,* to burn]

ur·ti·cant (er′ti-kant). Producing a wheal or other similar itching agent. [L. *urtica,* nettle; see urtica]

ur·ti·car·ia (er′ti-kar′i-ă). An eruption of itching wheals, usually of systemic origin; it may be due to a state of hypersensitivity to foods or drugs, foci of infection, physical agents (heat, cold, light, friction), or psychic stimuli. SYN hives (1), urtication (2). [L. *urtica*]

acute u., SYN febrile u.

u. bullo′sa, an eruption of wheals capped with subepidermal vesicles. SYN u. vesiculosa.

cholinergic u., a form of physical or nonallergic u. initiated by heat (e.g., hot baths, physical exercise, pyrexia, exposure to sun or to a warm room) or by excitement; the rather distinctive lesions consist of pruritic areas 1–2 mm in diameter surrounded by bright red macules. SYN heat u.

chronic u., a form of u. in which the wheals recur frequently, or persist. SYN u. chronica.

u. chron′ica, SYN chronic u.

cold u., wheal formation that develops after exposure to lowered temperatures, with or without demonstrable passive-transfer antibodies.

u. endem′ica, u. epidem′ica, u. caused by the nettling hairs of certain caterpillars.

factitious u., SYN dermatographism.

febrile u., u. accompanied by mild fever. SYN acute u.

giant u., SYN angioedema.

heat u., SYN cholinergic u.

u. hemorrhag′ica, u. bullosa in which the serous exudate contains blood.

u. maculo′sa, a chronic form of u. with lesions of a red color and little edema.

u. medicamento′sa, an urticarial form of drug eruption.

papular u., a sensitivity reaction to insect bites, especially human and pet fleas, seen mostly in young children as wheals followed by papules on exposed areas.

u. per′stans, a form of chronic u. in which the wheals persist unchanged for long periods; includes urticarial vasculitis.

u. pigmento′sa, cutaneous mastocytosis resulting from an excess of mast cells in the superficial dermis, producing a chronic eruption characterized by flat or slightly elevated brownish papules which urticate when stroked. The disease in children frequently involutes spontaneously whereas resolution is rare with adult onset and there may be systemic lesions. SEE ALSO diffuse cutaneous *mastocytosis.*

pressure u., u. of unknown etiology occurring after local pressure on the skin.

solar u., a form of u. resulting from exposure to sunlight; some patients have passive-transfer antibodies and others do not.

u. subcuta′nea, u. in which itching is present without the wheals.

u. vesiculo′sa, SYN u. bullosa.

vibratory u., a form of u. that occurs in response to vibratory stimuli.

ur·ti·car·i·al (er-ti-kar′ē-ăl). Relating to or marked by urticaria.

ur·ti·cate (er′ti-kāt). **1.** To perform urtication. **2.** Marked by the presence of wheals. [L. *urticatus*]

ur·ti·ca·tion (er-ti-kā′shŭn). **1.** A burning sensation resembling that produced by urticaria or resulting from nettle poisoning. **2.** SYN urticaria. [L. *urticatio*]

uru·shi·ol (oo′roo-shē-ōl). A mixture of nonvolatile hydrocarbons, derivatives of catechol with unsaturated C_{15} or C_{17} side chains, constituting the active allergen of the irritant oil of poison ivy, *Toxicodendron radicans,* poison oak, *T. diversilobum,* and the Asiatic laquer tree, *T. verniciferum.* [Jap. *urushi,* lac, + L. *oleum,* oil]

u. oxidase, SYN laccase.

USAN Abbreviation for United States Adopted Names.

Usher, Charles Howard, English ophthalmologist, 1865–1942. SEE U. *syndrome.*

Usher, Barney D., Canadian dermatologist, 1899–1978. SEE Senear-U. *disease, syndrome.*

USP Abbreviation for United States Pharmacopeia. SEE Pharmacopeia.

USPHS Abbreviation for United States Public Health Service.

us·ti·lag·i·nism (ŭs-ti-laj′i-nizm). Poisoning by *Ustilago maydis* (corn smut), which produces burning, itching, hyperemia, acrocyanosis, and edema of the extremities; resembles ergotism, pellagra, or infantile acrocynia.

Us·ti·la·go (ŭs-ti-lā′gō). A genus of smuts (order Ustilaginales). [L. a kind of thistle, fr. *ustio,* a burning]

U. may′dis, a smut species that resembles ergot of rye in its metabolic action; its black spores on the ears of corn are dispersed by wind and can cause contamination of laboratory cultures. SYN corn ergot, corn smut, *U. zeae.*

U. ze′ae, SYN *U. maydis.*

us·tu·la·tion (ŭs-tū-lā′shŭn). **1.** Separation of compounds by heat, as in the process of freeing ores from sulfur by roasting. **2.** Drying of a drug by heat to prepare it for pulverization. [L. *ustulo,* pp. *-atus,* to scorch]

usur·pa·tion (ū′ser-pā′shŭn). Assumption of pacemaker function of the heart by a subsidiary focus as a result of its own increased automaticity; e.g., accelerated junctional pacemaker takes command when it exceeds the sinus rate. [L. *usurpo,* pp. *-atus,* to seize]

uta (oo′tă). A mild form of New World or American cutaneous leishmaniasis caused by *Leishmania peruana,* occurring in the high Andean valleys of Peru and Bolivia, and characterized by numerous small dermal lesions occurring almost exclusively on exposed skin surfaces; the dog is an important reservoir. Unlike all other forms of American cutaneous leishmaniasis, this disease is found at high elevations (2000–2500 m) in barren open country, rather than in lowland tropical forests. [Sp.]

uter-. SEE utero-.

uter·ine (ū′ter-in, ū′ter-īn). Relating to the uterus.

in utero (in ū′ter-ō). Within the womb; not yet born. [L.]

utero-, uter-. The uterus. SEE ALSO hystero- (1), metr-. [L. *uterus*]

uter·o·ab·dom·i·nal (ū′ter-ō-ab-dom′i-năl). Relating to the uterus and the abdomen. SYN uteroventral.

uter·o·cer·vi·cal (ū′ter-ō-ser′vi-kăl). Relating to the cervix of the uterus.

uter·o·cys·tos·to·my (ū′ter-ō-sis-tos′tō-mē). Formation of a communication between the uterus (cervix) and the bladder. [utero- + G. *kystis,* bladder, + *stoma,* mouth]

uter·o·fix·a·tion (ū′ter-ō-fik-sā′shŭn). SYN hysteropexy.

uteroglobin. steroid-inducible, evolutionarily conserved, homodimeric secreted protein with many biological activities including a proinflammatory effect, inhibition of soluble lipoprotein-lipase A_2, and chemotaxis of neutrophils and monocytes. It binds to several putative receptors on several cell types and inhibits cellular invasion of the extracellular matrix. It is found in blood and urine, uterus and numerous other tissues but not kidneys. In mice uteroglobin has been shown to bind to fibronectin (Fn), preventing Fn self-aggregation and subsequent abnormal tissue deposition, especially in glomeruli. It is essential for maintaining normal renal function in mice. SYN bastokinin.

uteroglobin-adducin. An α/β heterodimeric protein found in renal tubule cells, thought to regulate ion transport through channels in the actin cytoskeleton. A mutant allele has been found in some patients with hypertension and it may be associated with the salt sensitive form of essential hypertension.

uter·o·lith (ū′ter-ō-lith). SYN uterine *calculus.* [utero- + G. *lithos,* stone]

uter·om·e·ter (ū-ter-om′ĕ-ter). SYN hysterometer.

uter·o·o·var·i·an (ū′ter-ō-ō-vār′ē-an). Relating to the uterus and an ovary.

uter·o·pa·ri·e·tal (ū′ter-ō-pa-rī′ĕ-tăl). Relating to the uterus and the abdominal wall.

uter·o·pel·vic (ū′ter-ō-pel′vik). Relating to the uterus and the pelvis.

uter·o·pexy (ū′ter-ō-pek-sē). SYN hysteropexy.

uter·o·pla·cen·tal (ū′ter-ō-pla-sen′tăl). Relating to the uterus and the placenta.

uter·o·plas·ty (ū′ter-ō-plas-tē). Plastic surgery of the uterus. SYN hysteroplasty, metroplasty. [utero- + G. *plastos,* formed]

uter·o·sa·cral (ū′ter-ō-sā′krăl). Relating to the uterus and the sacrum.

uter·o·sal·pin·gog·ra·phy (ū′ter-ō-sal-pin-gog′ră-fē). SYN hysterosalpingography.

uter·o·scope (ū′ter-ō-skōp). SYN hysteroscope.

uter·os·co·py (ū-ter-os′kŏ-pē). SYN hysteroscopy.

uter·ot·o·my (ū-ter-ot′ō-mē). SYN hysterotomy.

uter·o·ton·ic (ū′ter-ō-ton′ik). **1.** Giving tone to the uterine muscle. **2.** An agent that overcomes relaxation of the muscular wall of the uterus. [utero- + G. *tonos,* tone, tension]

uter·o·tro·pic (ū′ter-ō-trō′pik). Causing an effect on the uterus.

uter·o·tub·al (ū′ter-ō-too′băl). Pertaining to the uterus and the uterine tubes.

uter·o·tu·bog·ra·phy (ū′ter-ō-too-bog′ră-fē). SYN hysterosalpingography.

uter·o·vag·i·nal (ū-ter-ō-vaj′i-năl). Relating to the uterus and the vagina.

uter·o·ven·tral (ū′ter-ō-ven′trăl). SYN uteroabdominal. [utero- + L. *venter,* belly]

uter·o·ver·dine (ū′ter-ō-ver′din). Biliverdin from dog placenta.

uter·o·ves·i·cal (ū′ter-ō-ves′i-kăl). Relating to the uterus and the urinary bladder.

uter·us, pl. **uteri** (ū′ter-ŭs, ū′ter-ī) [TA]. The hollow muscular organ in which the impregnated ovum is developed into the child; it is about 7.5 cm in length in the nonpregnant woman, and consists of a main portion (body) with an elongated lower part (cervix), at the extremity of which is the opening (external os). The upper rounded portion of the u., opposite the os, is the fundus, at each extremity of which is the horn marking the part where the uterine tube joins the u. and through which the ovum reaches the uterine cavity after leaving the ovary. The organ is passively supported in the pelvic cavity by the cardinal ligaments and by the anteflexion and anteversion of the normal uterus, which places its mass superior to the bladder; it is actively supported by the tonic and phasic contraction of the muscles of the pelvic floor. SYN metra, womb. [L.]

u. acol′lis, a u. with atresia or absence of the cervix.

anomalous u., a malformed u. caused by abnormal development or fusion of the paramesonephric ducts.

arcuate u., a u. with a depression at the fundus; an incomplete u. bicornis. SYN u. arcuatus.

u. arcua′tus, SYN arcuate u.

bicornate u., a u. that is more or less completely divided into two lateral horns as a result of imperfect union of the paramesonephric ducts; it differs from septate u., in which there is no external mark of separation; in bicornate u., the cervix may be single (u. bicornis unicollis) or double (u. bicornis bicollis). SYN bifid u., u. bicornis, u. bifidus.

u. bicor′nis, SYN bicornate u.

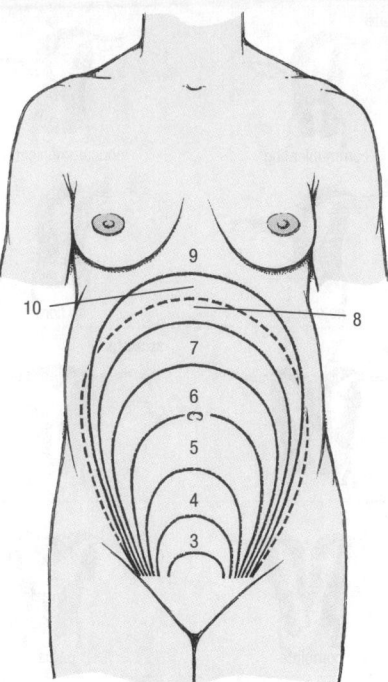

uterus: changes in size during pregnancy

u. bicornis bicollis, SEE bicornate u.

u. bicornis unicollis, SEE bicornate u.

bifid u., SYN bicornate u.

u. bi′fidus, SYN bicornate u.

biforate u., septate u. in which the cervix is divided into two by a septum. SYN double-mouthed u., u. biforis.

u. bifor′is, SYN biforate u.

u. bilocula′ris, SYN septate u.

bipartite u., SYN septate u.

u. biparti′tus, SYN septate u.

cordiform u., an incomplete u. bicornis with a wedge-shaped depression at the fundus. SYN heart-shaped u., u. cordiformis.

u. cordiform′is, SYN cordiform u.

Couvelaire u., extravasation of blood into the uterine musculature and beneath the uterine peritoneum in association with severe forms of abruptio placentae. SYN uteroplacental apoplexy.

u. didel′phys, double u. with double cervix and double vagina; due to failure of the paramesonephric ducts to unite. [G. *di-,* two, + *delphys,* womb]

double-mouthed u., SYN biforate u.

duplex u., any u. with double lumen (u. didelphys, u. bicornis bicollis, or septate u.). SYN u. duplex.

u. du′plex, SYN duplex u.

gravid u., the condition of the u. in pregnancy.

heart-shaped u., SYN cordiform u.

incudiform u., u. bicornis in which the fundus between the two cornua is broad and flat. SYN triangular u., u. incudiformis, u. triangularis.

u. incudiform′is, SYN incudiform u.

masculine u., SYN prostatic *utricle.*

u. masculi′nus, SYN prostatic *utricle.*

one-horned u., obsolete term for unicorn u.

u. parvicol′lis, a u. of normal size with an abnormal, disproportionately small cervix.

septate u., a u. divided into two cavities by an anteroposterior septum. SYN bipartite u., u. bilocularis, u. bipartitus, u. septus.

u. sep′tus, SYN septate u.

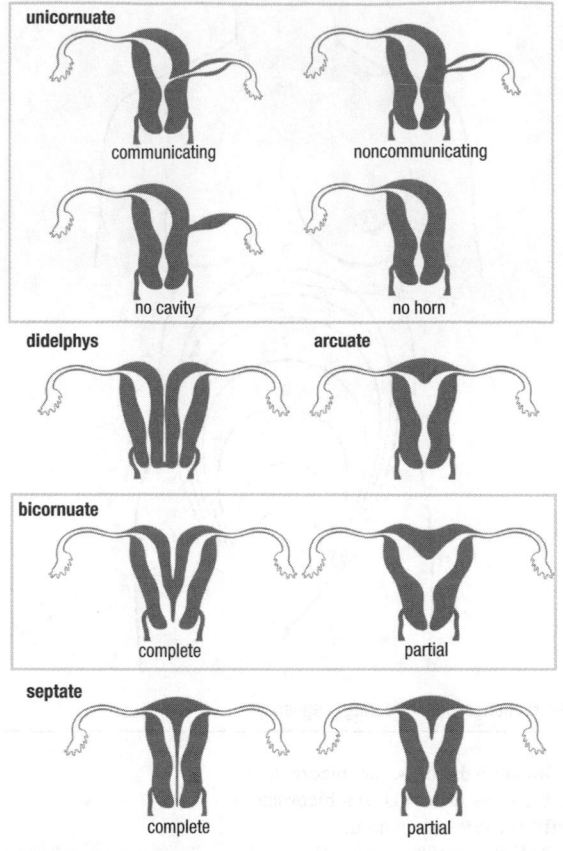

developmental anomalies of the uterus

---

subseptate u., an incomplete u. septus. SYN u. subseptus.

u. subsep'tus, SYN subseptate u.

triangular u., SYN incudiform u.

u. triangula'ris, SYN incudiform u.

unicorn u., a u. in which only one lateral half exists, the other half being undeveloped or absent. SYN u. unicornis.

u. unicor'nis, SYN unicorn u.

UTI Abbreviation for urinary tract *infection*.

util·i·ty. In biomedical ethics and clinical decision analysis, the satisfaction or economic advantage gained from the outcome that results from a particular decision.

UTP Abbreviation for *uridine* 5'-triphosphate.

utri·cle (oo'tri-kl) [TA]. SYN utriculus [TA], sacculus communis.

prostatic u. [TA], a minute pouch in the prostate that opens on the summit of the seminal colliculus, the analog of the uterus and vagina in the female, being the remains of the fused caudal ends of the paramesonephric ducts. SYN utriculus prostaticus [TA], masculine uterus, Morgagni sinus (2), sinus pocularis, uterus masculinus, vagina masculina, vesica prostatica, Weber organ.

u. of vestibular labyrinth [TA], the larger of the two membranous sacs in the vestibule of the labyrinth, lying in the elliptical recess; from it arise the semicircular ducts.

utric·u·lar (ū-trik'ū-lăr). Relating to or resembling a utricle.

utric·u·li (oo-trik'ū-lī). Plural of utriculus.

utric·u·li·tis (ū-trik-ū-lī'tis). Inflammation of the internal ear. [utriculus + G. *-itis,* inflammation]

utric·u·lo·sac·cu·lar (ū-trik'ū-lō-sak'ū-lăr). Relating to the utricle and the saccule of the labyrinth, denoting especially a duct connecting the two structures.

utric·u·lus, pl. **utric·u·li** (oo'trik'ū-lŭs, -lī) [TA]. SYN utricle. SEE ALSO vestibular *labyrinth*. [L. dim. of *uter,* leather bag]

u. prostat'icus [TA], SYN prostatic *utricle.*

utri·form (ū'tri-fōrm). Shaped like a leather bottle (wineskin). [L. *uter,* a skin bag, + *forma,* form]

UV, uv. Abbreviation for ultraviolet.

UVA Abbreviation for *ultraviolet* A.

uvae·for·mis (ū-vē-fōr'mis). SYN vascular *lamina* of choroid. [L. *uva,* grape, + *forma,* form]

uva ur·si (oo'vă er'sī). The dried leaves of *Arctostaphylos uva-ursi* (family Ericaceae), bearberry, mountain box, a common plant of the north temperate zone; contains antiseptic glycosides, arbutin, methylarbutin, and tannins; has been used in chronic inflammations of the urinary tract. [L. *uva,* grape + *ursus,* bear]

UVB Abbreviation for *ultraviolet* B.

uvea (oo'vē-ă). SYN vascular *layer* of eyeball. [L. *uva,* grape]

uve·al (oo'vē-ăl). Relating to the uvea.

uve·it·ic (ū-vē-it'ik). Relating to the uvea.

uve·i·ti·des (ū-vē-it'i-dēz). Plural of uveitis.

uve·i·tis, pl. **uve·i·ti·des** (ū-vē-ī'tis, -it'i-dēz). Inflammation of the uveal tract: iris, ciliary body, and choroid. [uvea + G. *-itis,* inflammation]

anterior u., inflammation involving the ciliary body and iris.

Förster u., syphilitic inflammation, with diffuse nodules involving the choroid and retinal vasculitis.

Fuchs u., SYN heterochromic u.

heterochromic u., anterior uveitis and depigmentation of the iris. SYN Fuchs u.

intermediate u., a u. that is neither anterior nor posterior but tends to involve the pars plana and the ciliary body.

lens-induced u., SYN phacoanaphylactic u.

phacoanaphylactic u., intraocular inflammation occurring after extracapsular cataract extraction; probably an immune reaction to the patient's liberated lenticular proteins. SYN lens-induced u.

phacogenic u., u. secondary to hypermature cataract.

posterior u., SYN choroiditis.

sympathetic u., a bilateral inflammation of the uveal tract caused by a perforating wound of one eye that injures the uvea.

uve·o·en·ceph·a·li·tis (ū'vē-ō-en-sef-ă-lī'tis). SYN Harada *syndrome.*

uve·o·scle·ri·tis (ū'vē-ō-sklē-rī'tis). Inflammation of the sclera involved by extension from the uvea.

uvi·form (oo'vi-fōrm). SYN botryoid. [L. uva, grape, + *forma,* form]

uvi·o·fast (ū'vē-ō-fast). Not weakened or destroyed by subjection to ultraviolet radiation. SYN uvioresistant. [uviol (*ultraviol*et), + fast]

uvi·ol (ū'vē-ol). A special kind of glass more than usually transparent to ultraviolet or actinic rays, e.g., crystalline quartz. [*ultraviol*et]

uvi·om·e·ter (ū-vē-om'ĕ-ter). An instrument for measuring ultraviolet radiation. [uviol (*ultraviol*et), + meter]

uvi·o·re·sis·tant (ū'vē-ō-rē-zis'tant). SYN uviofast.

uvi·o·sen·si·tive (ū'vē-ō-sen'si-tiv). Sensitive to ultraviolet rays. [uviol (*ultraviol*et) + sensitive]

uvitex 2B. A fluorescent stain that reacts with chitin; useful in the diagnosis of microsporidian or cryptosporidium infections.

uvo·mor·u·lin (ū-vō-mō'roo-lin). A transmembrane protein that links plasma membranes of adjacent cells together in a Ca^{2+}-dependent manner; aids in maintaining the rigidity of the cell layer. SYN E-cadherin. [L. *uva,* bunch of grapes, + Mod. L. *morula,* dim. of L. *morum,* fr. G. *moron,* mulberry, + -in]

uvul-. SEE uvulo-.

uvu·la, pl. **uvu·li** (ū'vū-lă, -lī) [TA]. An appendant fleshy mass; a structure bearing a fancied resemblance to the palatine u. [Mod. L. dim. of L. *uva,* a grape, the uvula]

bifid u., bifurcation of the u., constituting a partially cleft soft palate.

u. of bladder [TA], a slight projection into the cavity of the bladder, usually more prominent in old men, just behind the urethral opening, marking the location of the middle lobe of the prostate. SYN u. vesicae [TA], Lieutaud u.

u. cerebel′li, SYN uvula [TA] of cerebellum.

uvula [TA] of cerebellum, a triangular elevation on the vermis of the cerebellum, lying between the two tonsils anterior to the pyramis. SYN u. cerebelli, u. vermis.

Lieutaud u., SYN u. of bladder.

u. palati′na [TA], SYN u. of soft palate.

palatine u., SYN u. of soft palate.

u. of soft palate [TA], a conical projection from the posterior edge of the middle of the soft palate, composed of connective tissue containing a number of racemose glands, and some muscular fibers (uvulae muscle). SYN u. palatina [TA], palatine u., pendulous palate.

u. ver′mis, SYN uvula [TA] of cerebellum.

u. vesi′cae [TA], SYN u. of bladder.

uvu·lap·to·sis (ū′vū-lap-tō′sis). SYN uvuloptosis.

uvu·lar (ū′vū-lăr). Relating to the uvula.

uvu·la·ris (ū′vū-lā′ris). SYN *muscle* of uvula.

uvu·la·tome (ū′vū-lă-tōm). SYN uvulotome.

uvu·lec·to·my (ū-vū-lek′tō-mē). Excision of the uvula. SYN staphylectomy. [uvula + G. *ektomē,* excision]

uvu·li·tis (ū-vū-lī′tis). Inflammation of the uvula.

⌂**uvulo-, uvul-.** The uvula. SEE ALSO staphylo-. [L. *uvula*]

uvu·lo·pal·a·to·pha·ryn·go·plas·ty (ū′vū-lō-pal′ă-tō-fa-rin′gō-plas-tē). SYN palatopharyngoplasty.

uvu·lo·pal·a·to·plas·ty (ū′vū-lō-pal′ă-tō-plas-tē). SYN palatoplasty.

uvu·lop·to·sis (ū′vū-lop-tō′sis). Relaxation or elongation of the uvula. SYN falling palate, staphylodialysis, staphyloptosis, uvulaptosis. [uvulo- + G. *ptōsis,* a falling]

uvu·lo·tome (ū′vū-lō-tōm). An instrument for cutting the uvula. SYN uvulatome.

uvu·lot·o·my (ū-vū-lot′ō-mē). Any cutting operation on the uvula. [uvulo- + G. *tomē,* a cutting]

uv

V **1.** Abbreviation for vision or visual *acuity*; volt; with subscript 1, 2, 3, etc., the abbreviation for unipolar electrocardiogram leads. **2.** Symbol for vanadium; valine; valyl; volume, frequently with subscripts denoting location, chemical species, and/or conditions.

V̇ **1.** Symbol for gas flow, frequently with subscripts indicating location and chemical species. SEE flow (3). **2.** Symbol for ventilation (3), frequently with a subscript. See entries under ventilation (3). [volume + overdot denoting time derivative]

V$_D$. Symbol for physiologic dead *space*.

V$_T$. Symbol for tidal *volume*.

V̇$_{O2}$ Symbol for oxygen *consumption*.

V̇$_A$. Symbol for alveolar *ventilation*.

V̇$_{CO2}$ Symbol for carbon dioxide *elimination*.

V Abbreviation for volume.

V$_{max}$ Symbol for maximum *velocity*.

v **1.** Abbreviation for volt; initial rate velocity; velocity; vel [L. or]. **2.** As a subscript, refers to venous *blood*.

v̄. As a subscript, refers to mixed venous (pulmonary arterial) blood.

VA Abbreviation for ventriculoatrial.

VAC Abbreviation for ventriculoatrial *conduction*.

vac·cen·ic ac·id (vak-sen′ik). An unsaturated fatty acid of which both *cis* and *trans* isomers are found in butter and other animal fats.

vac·ci·na (vak-sin′ă). SYN vaccinia.

vac·ci·nal (vak′si-năl). Relating to vaccine or vaccination.

vac·ci·nate (vak′si-nāt). To administer a vaccine.

vac·ci·na·tion (vak′si-nā′shŭn). The act of administering a vaccine.

vac·ci·na·tor (vak′si-nā-tŏr). **1.** A person who vaccinates. SYN vaccinist. **2.** A scarifier or other instrument used in vaccination.

VACCINE

vac·cine (vak′sēn, vak-sēn′). Originally, the live v. (vaccinia, cowpox) virus inoculated in the skin as prophylaxis against smallpox and obtained from the skin of calves inoculated with seed virus. Usage has extended the meaning to include essentially any preparation intended for active immunologic prophylaxis; e.g., preparations of killed microbes of virulent strains or living microbes of attenuated (variant or mutant) strains; or microbial, fungal, plant, protozoal, or metazoan derivatives or products. Method of administration varies according to the v., inoculation being the most common, but ingestion is preferred in some instances and nasal spray is used occasionally. SYN vaccinum. [L. *vaccinus*, relating to a cow]

adjuvant v., a v. that contains an adjuvant; the antigen (immunogen) is included in a water-in-oil emulsion (Freund incomplete type adjuvant), or is adsorbed onto an inorganic gel (alum, aluminum hydroxide or phosphate) or mixed with another material to prevent rapid elimination by the host.

aqueous v., a v. having a liquid vehicle (e.g., physiologic salt solution) as distinguished from an emulsion.

attenuated v., live pathogens that have lost their virulence but are still capable of inducing a protective immune response to the virulent forms of the pathogen, e.g., Sabin polio v.

autogenous v., a v. made from a patient's own microorganisms.

bacillus Calmette-Guérin v., SYN BCG v.

BCG v., a suspension of an attenuated strain (bacillus Calmette-Guérin) of *Mycobacterium tuberculosis*, bovine type, which is inoculated into the skin for tuberculosis prophylaxis. SYN bacillus Calmette-Guérin v., Calmette-Guérin v., tuberculosis v.

brucella strain 19 v., a live bacterial v. prepared from an attenuated variant strain of *Brucella abortus* (strain 19); used for vaccinating cattle against brucellosis.

Calmette-Guérin v., SYN BCG v.

cholera v., an inactivated suspension of Inaba and Ogawa strains of *Vibrio cholerae* grown either on agar or in broth and preserved with phenol.

crystal violet v., SEE hog cholera v.'s.

diphtheria toxoid, tetanus toxoid, and pertussis v. (DTP), a v. available in three forms: 1) diphtheria and tetanus toxoids plus pertussis v. (DTP); 2) tetanus and diphtheria toxoids, adult type (Td); and 3) tetanus toxoid (T); used for active immunization against diphtheria, tetanus, and whooping cough.

duck embryo origin v. (DEV), SEE rabies v.

Flury strain v., SEE rabies v., Flury strain egg-passage.

foot-and-mouth disease virus v.'s, v.'s either of inactivated virus from infected cattle tongue epithelium or, more recently, of live virus attenuated by embryonated egg or mouse passage and propagated in tissue culture.

Haemophilus influenzae type B v., a conjugate of oligosaccharides of the capsular antigen of *H. influenzae* type B and diphtheria CRM protein. SYN Hib v.

Haffkine v., (1) a killed culture of *Vibrio cholerae* in two strengths, a weaker one for the initial inoculation and a stronger one for the second inoculation 7–10 days after the first; **(2)** a killed plague bacillus (*Yersinia pestis*) v.

hepatitis B v., originally a formalin-inactivated v. prepared from the surface antigen (HBsAg) of the hepatitis B virus; the antigen was formerly obtained from the plasma of human carriers of the virus; today in the U.S., purified HBsAg is now primarily prepared by recombinant DNA technology and is used almost exclusively for immunization.

heterogenous v., v. that is not autogenous, may be prepared from other species of bacterium.

Hib v., SYN *Haemophilus influenzae* type B v.

high-egg-passage v., HEP v., SEE rabies v., Flury strain egg-passage.

hog cholera v.'s, v.'s either of virus from blood of infected swine, inactivated with crystal violet, or live virus attenuated in rabbits or tissue culture and frequently used in conjunction with hog cholera virus antiserum.

human diploid cell v. (HDCV), an iodinated virus v. used for protection against rabies v. usually prepared in the human diploid cell WI-38. SYN human diploid cell rabies v.

human diploid cell rabies v. (HDCV), SYN human diploid cell v.

inactivated poliovirus v. (IPV), SEE poliovirus v.'s (2).

influenza virus v.'s, influenza virus grown in embryonated eggs and inactivated, usually by the addition of formalin; both whole virus and subunit preparations containing hemagglutinins and neuraminidase are used; because of the marked and progressive antigenic variation of the influenza viruses, the strains included are regularly changed following various outbreaks of influenza in order to include most recently isolated epidemic strains of both type A influenza and type B influenza.

live v., v. prepared from living, attenuated organisms.

live oral poliovirus v., SEE poliovirus v.'s (2).

low-egg-passage v., LEP v., SEE rabies v., Flury strain egg-passage.

measles, mumps, and rubella v. (MMR), a combination of live attenuated measles, mumps, and rubella viruses in an aqueous

△ **Combining Forms**	☆ **Official alternate Terminologia Anatomica term**
▣ **Indicates term is illustrated, see Illustration Index**	
	[MIM] Mendelian Inheritance in Man
SYN **Synonym**	
Cf. **Compare**	C.I. **Colour Index**
[NA] **Nomina Anatomica**	
[TA] **Terminologia Anatomica**	**High Profile Term**

suspension; used for immunization against the respective diseases.

measles virus v., v. containing live, attenuated strains of measles virus prepared in chick embryo cell culture. SEE measles, mumps, and rubella v.

multivalent v., SYN polyvalent v.

mumps virus v., v. containing live, attenuated mumps virus prepared in chick embryo cell cultures. SEE measles, mumps, and rubella v.

oil v., SEE adjuvant v.

oral poliovirus v. (OPV), SEE poliovirus v.'s (2).

Pasteur v., SEE rabies v.

pertussis v., SEE diphtheria toxoid, tetanus toxoid, and pertussis v.

plague v., v. (licensed for use in the U.S.) prepared from cultures of *Yersinia pestis,* inactivated with formaldehyde, and preserved with 0.5% phenol; injections are made intramuscularly, and booster inoculations are recommended every 6–12 months while individuals remain in an area of risk; live, attenuated bacterial and chemical fraction v.'s are also available.

pneumococcal v., v. comprised of purified capsular polysaccharide antigen from 23 types of *Streptococcus pneumoniae* (representing those types responsible for most of the reported pneumococcal diseases in the U.S.); some types have been conjugated with protein to make them antigenic for children under 2 years.

poliomyelitis v.'s, SYN poliovirus v.'s.

poliovirus v.'s, (1) inactivated poliovirus v. (IPV), an aqueous suspension of inactivated strains of poliomyelitis virus (types 1, 2, and 3) used by injection; has largely been replaced by the oral v.; SEE Salk v; **(2)** oral poliovirus v. (OPV), an aqueous suspension of live, attenuated strains of poliomyelitis virus (types 1, 2, and 3) given orally for active immunization against poliomyelitis. SEE Sabin v. SYN poliomyelitis v.'s.

polysaccharide conjugated v., a v. made from the capsular polysaccharide of the microorganism conjugated with a protein such as the *Haemophilus influenzae* type B vaccine against meningitis.

polyvalent v., a v. prepared from cultures of two or more strains of the same species or microorganism. SYN multivalent v.

rabies v., a v. introduced by Pasteur as a method of treatment for the bite of a rabid animal; daily (14–21) injections of virus that increased serially from noninfective to fully infective "fixed" virus were given to render the central nervous system refractory to infection by virulent virus; this v., with but slight modification (e.g., Semple v.), was used for many years but had the serious defect that the large quantity of heterologous nervous tissue inoculated along with the virus occasionally gave rise to an allergic (immunologic) demyelinization. It was replaced, in the case of humans, by rabies v. of duck embryo origin (DEV), prepared from embryonated duck eggs infected with "fixed" virus and inactivated with β-propiolactone. At the present time DEV has been replaced by either human diploid cell v. (HDCV), which is grown in WI-38 cells or rabies v. adsorbed (RVA), which is grown in fetal Rhesus monkey cells. They both are inactivated and have a low incidence of adverse reactions and require fewer injections.

rabies v., Flury strain egg-passage, (1) high-egg-passage (HEP) v.: living Flury strain rabies virus at the 180th to 190th level egg passage (embryonate eggs), used for vaccination of cattle and cats; **(2)** low-egg-passage (LEP) v.: at the 40th to 50th passage level, containing 10^3–10^4 mouse LD_{50}; nonpathogenic in dogs but retains some pathogenicity for cattle and cats.

rickettsia v., attenuated, SEE typhus v.

Rocky Mountain spotted fever v., suspension of inactivated *Rickettsia rickettsii* prepared by growing the rickettsiae in the embryonate yolk sac of fowl eggs.

rubella virus v., live, a live virus v. originally prepared from duck embryos (HPV77) but now prepared from human diploid cell cultures infected with rubella virus (RA27/3); administered as a single subcutaneous injection. SEE measles, mumps, and rubella v.

Sabin v., an orally administered v. containing live, attenuated strains of poliovirus. SEE poliovirus v.'s.

Salk v., the original poliovirus v., composed of virus propagated

in monkey kidney tissue culture and inactivated. SEE poliovirus v.'s.

Semple v., a modification of the original (Pasteur) rabies v., formerly widely used in the U.S., prepared from rabbit nerve tissue, inactivated with phenol and administered in 14–21 daily injections; has variable potency and is associated with a high incidence of postvaccinal demyelination.

smallpox v., v. of live vaccinia virus suspensions prepared from cutaneous vaccinial lesions of calves (calf lymph) or chick embryo origin; not currently used because of the worldwide elimination of smallpox.

split-virus v., SEE subunit v.

staphylococcus v., a suspension of organisms from cultures of one or more strains of *Staphylococcus;* used for furunculosis, acne, and other suppurative conditions.

stock v., a v. made from a stock microbial strain, in contradistinction to an autogenous v.

subunit v., a v. which, through chemical extraction, is free of viral nucleic acid and contains only specific protein subunits of a given virus; such v.'s are relatively free of the adverse reactions (e.g., influenza virus) associated with v.'s containing the whole virion.

T.A.B. v., SYN typhoid-paratyphoid A and B v.

tetanus v., SEE diphtheria toxoid, tetanus toxoid, and pertussis v.

tuberculosis v., SYN BCG v.

typhoid v., a suspension of *Salmonella typhi* inactivated either by heat or by chemical (acetone) with an added preservative; in the U.S., the combined typhoid and paratyphoid A and B v.'s have been largely replaced by the monovalent typhoid v. because of the lack of evidence of effectiveness of paratyphoid A and paratyphoid B ingredients.

typhoid-paratyphoid A and B v., a suspension of killed typhoid and paratyphoid A and B bacilli. SEE ALSO typhoid v. SYN T.A.B. v.

typhus v., a formaldehyde-inactivated suspension of *Rickettsia prowazekii* grown in embryonated eggs; effective against louse-borne (epidemic) typhus; primary immunization consists of two subcutaneous injections 4 or more weeks apart; booster doses are required every 6–12 months, as long as the possibility of exposure exists. A v. containing living rickettsiae of an attenuated strain of *R. prowazekii* has also been used.

whooping-cough v., SEE diphtheria toxoid, tetanus toxoid, and pertussis v.

yellow fever v., (1) a living, attenuated strain (17D) of yellow fever virus propagated in embryonated fowl eggs; **(2)** a suspension of dried mouse brain infected with French neurotropic (Dakar) strain of yellow fever virus, administered topically by the scratch method; not officially recommended in the United States because of meningoencephalitic reactions.

va

vac·cin·ia (vak-sin′ē-ă). An infection, primarily local and limited to the site of inoculation, induced in humans by inoculation with the v. virus, type species in the genus Orthopoxvirus (family Poxviridae) in order to confer resistance to smallpox. On about the third day after this vaccination, papules form at the site of inoculation which become transformed into umbilicated vesicles and later pustules; they then dry up, and the scab falls off on about the 21st day, leaving a pitted scar; in some cases there are more or less marked constitutional disturbances. Because of the global elimination of smallpox, routine vaccination is not now practiced. SYN primary reaction, vaccina, variola vaccine, variola vaccinia, variola vaccinia. [L. *vaccinus,* relating to a cow, fr. *vacca,* a cow]

v. gangreno′sa, SYN progressive v.

generalized v., secondary lesions of the skin following vaccination that may occur in subjects with previously healthy skin but are more common in the case of traumatized skin, especially in the case of eczema (eczema vaccinatum). In the latter instance, generalized v. may result from mere contact with a vaccinated person. Secondary vaccinial lesions may also occur following transfer of virus from the vaccination to another site by means of the fingers.

progressive v., a severe or even fatal form of v. occurring chiefly in subjects with an immunologic deficiency or dyscrasia and characterized by progressive enlargement of the initial and also of secondary lesions. SYN v. gangrenosa.

variola v., SYN vaccinia.

vac·cin·i·al (vak-sin′ē-ăl). Relating to vaccinia.

vac·cin·i·form (vak-sin′i-fōrm). Resembling vaccinia.

vac·ci·nist (vak′si-nist). SYN vaccinator (1).

vac·cin·i·za·tion (vak′sin-i-zā′shŭn). Vaccination repeated at short intervals until it will no longer take.

vac·cin·o·gen (vak-sin′-ō-jen). A source of vaccine, such as an inoculated heifer.

vac·ci·nog·e·nous (vak-si-noj′ĕ-nŭs). Producing vaccine, or relating to the production of vaccine.

vac·ci·noid (vak′si-noyd). Resembling vaccinia.

vac·ci·no·style (vak′si-nō-stīl). A pointed instrument used in vaccination.

vac·ci·num (vak′si-nŭm). SYN vaccine. [L.]

vac·u·o·lar (vak-oo-ō′lăr). Relating to or resembling a vacuole.

vac·u·o·late, vac·u·o·lat·ed (vak′oo-ō-lāt, -lāt′ed). Having vacuoles.

vac·u·o·la·tion (vak′oo-ō-lā′shŭn). 1. Formation of vacuoles. 2. The condition of having vacuoles. SYN vacuolization.

vac·u·ole (vak′oo-ōl). 1. A minute space in any tissue. 2. A clear space in the substance of a cell, sometimes degenerative in character, sometimes surrounding an englobed foreign body and serving as a temporary cell stomach for the digestion of the body. [Mod. L. *vacuolum,* dim. of L. *vacuum,* an empty space]

autophagic v., SYN cytolysosome.

contractile v., a cavity formed by the accumulation of fluid in the ectoplasm of a protozoan; after increasing for a time it empties itself externally by a sudden contraction; it functions as an osmoregulatory mechanism for water balance, especially in freshwater protozoans.

digestive v., SYN secondary *lysosomes,* under *lysosome.*

parasitophorous v., a v. formed by layers of endoplasmic reticulum around an intracellular parasite which may serve to isolate the parasite and enclose it for lysozymal attack.

vac·u·o·li·za·tion (vak′oo-ō-li-zā′shŭn). SYN vacuolation.

vac·u·ome (vak′oo-ōm). A system of vacuoles that can be stained with neutral red in the living cell. [vacuole + G. *-oma,* tumor]

vac·u·um (vak′oom). An empty space, one practically exhausted of air or gas. [L. ntr. of *vacuus,* empty]

va·dum (vā′dŭm). An occasional elevation from the bottom of a cerebral sulcus nearly obliterating it for a short distance. [L. a ford]

va·gal (vā′găl). Relating to the vagus nerve.

va·gec·to·my (vā-jek′tō-mē). Surgical removal of a segment of a vagus nerve.

va·gi (vā′gī, -jī). Plural of vagus.

△**vagin-.** SEE vagino-.

va·gi·na, gen. and pl. **va·gi·nae** (vă-jī′nă, -nē). 1. SYN sheath (1). 2 [TA]. The genital canal in the female, extending from the uterus to the vulva. [L. sheath, the vagina]

bipartite v., SYN septate v.

v. bul′bi [TA], SYN fascial *sheath* of eyeball.

v. carot′ica [TA], SYN carotid *sheath.*

v. cellulo′sa, the connective tissue sheath of a nerve or muscle (perineurium or perimysium, respectively).

v. commu′nis tendinum musculo′rum flexo′rum (manus) [TA], SYN common flexor *sheath* (of hand).

v. communis ten′dinum musculo′rum fibularium commu′nis [TA], SYN common peroneal tendon *sheath.*

v. exter′na ner′vi op′tici [TA], SYN outer *sheath* of optic nerve.

vagi′nae fibro′sae digito′rum ma′nus [TA], SYN fibrous *sheaths* of digits of hand, under *sheath;* SEE anular *part* of fibrous digital sheath of digits of hand and foot, cruciform *part* of fibrous digital sheath.

vagi′nae fibro′sae digito′rum pe′dis [TA], SYN fibrous digital

sheaths of toes, under *sheath;* SEE anular *part* of fibrous digital sheath of digits of hand and foot, cruciform *part* of fibrous digital sheath.

v. fibro′sa ten′dinis, SYN fibrous tendon *sheath.*

v. inter′na ner′vi op′tici [TA], SYN inner *sheath* of optic nerve.

v. masculi′na, SYN prostatic *utricle.*

v. muco′sa ten′dinis, SYN synovial tendon *sheath.*

v. mus′culi rec′ti abdo′minis [TA], SYN rectus *sheath.*

vagi′nae ner′vi op′tici, sheaths of the optic nerve, formed by extensions of the central meninges. SEE inner *sheath* of optic nerve, external *sheath* of optic nerve.

v. oc′uli, SYN fascial *sheath* of eyeball.

v. proces′sus styloi′dei [TA], SYN *sheath* of styloid process.

septate v., a bipartite v. caused by the presence of a more or less complete longitudinal septum. SYN bipartite v.

vagi′nae synovia′les digito′rum ma′nus [TA], SYN synovial *sheaths* of digits of hand, under *sheath.*

v. synovia′lis [TA], SYN synovial *sheath.*

v. synovia′lis ten′dinis [TA], SYN synovial tendon *sheath.*

v. synovia′lis troch′leae, SYN tendinous *sheath* of superior oblique muscle.

vaginae tendinum carpalium [TA], SYN carpal tendinous *sheaths,* under *sheath.*

vaginae tendinum carpalium dorsalium [TA], SYN dorsal carpal tendinous *sheaths,* under *sheath.*

v. ten′dinis intertubercula′ris [TA], SYN intertubercular tendon *sheath.*

v. ten′dinis mus′culi extenso′ris car′pi ulna′ris [TA], SYN tendinous *sheath* of extensor carpi ulnaris muscle.

v. ten′dinis mus′culi extenso′ris dig′iti min′imi [TA], SYN tendinous *sheath* of extensor digiti minimi muscle.

v. ten′dinis mus′culi extenso′ris hal′lucis lon′gi [TA], SYN tendinous *sheath* of extensor hallucis longus muscle.

v. ten′dinis mus′culi extenso′ris pol′licis lon′gi [TA], SYN tendinous *sheath* of extensor pollicis longus muscle.

v. tendinis musculi fibularis longi plantaris [TA], SYN plantar tendon *sheath* of fibularis longus muscle.

v. ten′dinis mus′culi flexo′ris car′pi radia′lis [TA], SYN tendinous *sheath* of flexor carpi radialis muscle.

v. ten′dinis mus′culi flexo′ris hal′lucis lon′gi [TA], SYN tendinous *sheath* of flexor hallucis longus muscle.

v. ten′dinis mus′culi flexo′ris pol′licis lon′gi [TA], SYN tendinous *sheath* of flexor pollicis longus muscle.

v. ten′dinis mus′culi obli′qui superio′ris [TA], SYN tendinous *sheath* of superior oblique muscle.

v. ten′dinis mus′culi perone′i lon′gi planta′ris, ⋆official alternate term for plantar tendon *sheath* of fibularis longus muscle.

v. ten′dinis mus′culi tibia′lis anterio′ris [TA], SYN tendinous *sheath* of tibialis anterior muscle.

v. ten′dinis mus′culi tibia′lis posterio′ris [TA], SYN tendinous *sheath* of tibialis posterior muscle.

vaginae tendinum carpales palmares [TA], SYN palmar carpal tendinous *sheaths,* under *sheath.*

vagi′nae tendinum digito′rum pe′dis [TA], SYN synovial *sheaths* of toes, under *sheath.*

v. ten′dinum mus′culi extenso′ris digito′rum pe′dis lon′gi [TA], SYN tendinous *sheath* of extensor digitorum longus muscle of foot.

v. ten′dinum mus′culi flexo′ris digito′rum pe′dis lon′gi [TA], SYN tendinous *sheath* of flexor digitorum longus muscle (of foot).

v. ten′dinum musculo′rum abducto′ris lon′gi et extenso′ris bre′vis pol′licis [TA], SYN tendinous *sheath* of abductor pollicis longus and extensor pollicis brevis muscles.

v. ten′dinum musculo′rum extenso′ris digitor′um et extenso′ris in′dicis [TA], SYN tendinous *sheath* of extensor digitorum and extensor indicis muscles.

v. ten′dinum musculo′rum extenso′rum car′pi radia′lium [TA], SYN tendinous *sheath* of extensor carpi radialis muscles.

v. ten′dinum musculo′rum fibula′rium commu′nis, SYN common peroneal tendon *sheath.*

v. tendinum musculo'rum peroneo'rum commu'nis, SYN common peroneal tendon *sheath.*

vaginae ten'dinum tarsa'les ante'riores [TA], SYN anterior tarsal tendinous *sheaths,* under *sheath.*

vaginae ten'dinum tarsa'les fibula'res [TA], SYN fibular tarsal tendinous *sheaths,* under *sheath.*

vaginae ten'dinum tarsa'les tibia'lis [TA], SYN tibial tarsal tendinous *sheaths,* under *sheath.*

vagi'nae vaso'rum, SYN vascular *sheaths,* under *sheath.*

vag·i·nal (vaj'i-năl). Relating to the vagina or to any sheath. [Mod. L. *vaginalis*]

va·gi·na·pexy (va-jī'nă-pek-sē). SYN vaginofixation.

vag·i·nate (vaj'i-nāt). **1.** To ensheathe; to enclose in a sheath. **2.** Ensheathed; provided with a sheath.

vag·i·nec·to·my (vaj-i-nek'tō-mē). Excision of the vagina or a segment thereof. SYN colpectomy. [vagina + G. *ektomē,* excision]

vag·i·nism (vaj'i-nizm). SYN vaginismus.

vag·i·nis·mus (vaj-i-niz'mŭs). Painful spasm of the vagina preventing intercourse. SYN vaginism, vulvismus. [vagina + L. *-ismus,* action, condition]

posterior v., spasmodic stenosis of the vagina caused by contraction of the levator ani muscle.

vag·i·ni·tis, pl. **vag·i·ni·ti·des** (vaj-i-nī'tis, -nī'ti-dēz). Inflammation of the vagina. [vagina + G. *-itis,* inflammation]

v. adhesi'va, SYN adhesive v.

adhesive v., inflammation of vaginal mucosa with adhesions of the vaginal walls to each other. SYN v. adhesiva.

amebic v., v. caused by *Entamoeba histolytica.*

atrophic v., thinning and atrophy of the vaginal epithelium usually resulting from diminished estrogen stimulation; a common occurrence in postmenopausal women.

v. cys'tica, SYN v. emphysematosa.

desquamative inflammatory v., an acute inflammation of the vagina of unknown cause, characterized by grayish pseudomembrane, free discharge, and easy bleeding on trauma; the discharge contains pus and immature epithelial cells, although estrogen levels are normal.

v. emphysemato'sa, v. characterized by accumulation of gas in small connective tissue spaces lined by foreign-body giant cells. SYN pachyvaginitis cystica, v. cystica.

Gardnerella v., SYN bacterial *vaginosis.*

nonspecific v., SYN bacterial *vaginosis.*

pinworm v., v. caused by *Enterobius vermicularis.*

senile v., atrophic v. resulting from withdrawal of estrogen stimulation of mucosa, often assuming the form of adhesive v. SYN v. senilis.

v. seni'lis, SYN senile v.

△**vagino-, vagin-.** The vagina. SEE ALSO colpo-. [L. *vagina,* sheath]

vag·i·no·ab·dom·i·nal (vaj'i-nō-ab-dom'i-năl). Relating to the vagina and the abdomen.

vag·i·no·cele (vaj'i-nō-sēl). SYN colpocele (1).

vag·i·no·dyn·ia (vaj'i-nō-din'ē-ă). Vaginal pain. SYN colpodynia.

vag·i·no·fix·a·tion (vaj'i-nō-fik-sā'shŭn). Suture of a relaxed and prolapsed vagina to the abdominal wall. SYN colpopexy, vaginapexy, vaginopexy.

vag·i·no·hys·ter·ec·to·my (vaj'i-nō-his-ter-ek'tō-mē). SYN vaginal *hysterectomy.*

vag·i·no·la·bi·al (vaj'i-nō-lā'bē-ăl). Relating to the vagina and the pudendal labia.

vag·i·no·my·co·sis (vaj'i-nō-mī-kō'sis). Vaginal infection due to a fungus. SYN colpomycosis.

vag·i·nop·a·thy (vaj-i-nop'ă-thē). Any diseased condition of the vagina. [vagino- + G. *pathos,* suffering]

vag·i·no·per·i·ne·al (vaj'i-nō-per-i-nē'ăl). Relating to or involving the vagina and perineum.

vag·i·no·per·i·ne·o·plas·ty (vaj'i-nō-per-i-nē'ō-plas-tē). Plastic surgery of the perineum involving the vagina. SYN colpoperineoplasty. [vagino- + perineum, + G. *plastos,* formed]

vag·i·no·per·i·ne·or·rha·phy (vaj'i-nō-per-i-nē-ōr'ă-fē). Repair of a lacerated vagina and perineum. SYN colpoperineorrhaphy. [vagino- + perineum, + G. *rhaphē,* suture]

vag·i·no·per·i·ne·ot·o·my (vaj'i-nō-per-i-nē-ot'ō-mē). SYN episiotomy. [vagino- + perineum, + G. *tomē,* incision]

vag·i·no·per·i·to·ne·al (vaj'i-nō-per-i-tō-nē'ăl). Relating to the vagina and the peritoneum.

vag·i·no·pexy (vaj'i-nō-pek-sē). SYN vaginofixation.

vag·i·no·plas·ty (vaj'i-nō-plas-tē). Plastic surgery of the vagina. SYN colpoplasty. [vagino- + G. *plastos,* formed]

vag·i·nos·co·py (vaj-i-nos'kŏ-pē). Inspection of the vagina, usually with an instrument.

vag·in·o·sis (vă'jin-ō'sis). Disease of the vagina.

bacterial v., infection of the human vagina that may be caused by anaerobic bacteria, especially by *Mobiluncus* species or by *Gardnerella vaginalis.* Characterized by excessive, sometimes malodorous, discharge. SYN *Gardnerella* vaginitis, nonspecific vaginitis.

vag·i·not·o·my (vaj-i-not'ō-mē). SYN colpotomy.

vag·i·no·ves·i·cal (vaj'i-nō-ves'i-kăl). Relating to the vagina and the urinary bladder.

vag·i·no·vul·var (vaj'i-nō-vŭl'văr). Relating to the vagina and the vulva.

Va·gin·u·lus **ple·be·i·us** (vaj-i-noo'lŭs plē'bē-ē-ŭs). The slug vector of *Angiostrongylus costaricensis.*

va·gi·tus uter·i·nus (va-jī'tŭs ū-ter-ī'nŭs). Crying of the fetus while still within the uterus, possible when the membranes have been ruptured and air has entered the uterine cavity. [L. fr. *vagio,* to squall; L. fr. *uterus,* womb]

△**vago-.** The vagus nerve. [L. *vagus*]

va·go·ac·ces·so·ri·us (vā-gō-ak-ses-sō'rē-ŭs). The vagus and the cranial root (accessory portion) of the accessory nerve, regarded as one nerve. SEE accessory *nerve* [CN XI].

va·go·glos·so·pha·ryn·ge·al (vā'gō-glos'ō-fă-rin'jē-ăl). Relating to the vagus and glossopharyngeal nerves; denoting their contiguous or common nuclei of origin and termination and regions innervated by both nerves such as the musculature of the pharynx.

va·gol·y·sis (vā-gol'i-sis). Surgical destruction of the vagus nerve. [vago- + G. *lysis,* a loosening]

va·go·lyt·ic (vā-gō-lit'ik). **1.** Pertaining to or causing vagolysis. **2.** A therapeutic or chemical agent that has inhibitory effects on the vagus nerve. **3.** Denoting an agent having such effects.

va·go·mi·met·ic (vā'gō-mi-met'ik). Mimicking the action of the efferent fibers of the vagus nerve.

🔳**va·got·o·my** (vā-got'ō-mē). Division of the vagus nerve. [vago- + G. *tomē,* incision]

va·go·to·nia (vā-gō-tō'nē-ă). Archaic designation for a condition in which the parasympathetic autonomic system is reputedly overactive. SYN parasympathotonia, sympathetic imbalance. [vago- + G. *tonos,* strain]

va·go·ton·ic (vā-gō-ton'ik). Relating to or marked by vagotonia.

va·go·tro·pic (vā-gō-trop'ik). Attracted by, hence acting upon, the vagus nerve. [vago- + G. *tropos,* turning]

va·go·va·gal (vā'gō-vā'găl). Pertaining to a process that utilizes both afferent and efferent vagal fibers.

va·gus, gen. and pl. **va·gi** (vā'gŭs; vā'gī, -jī). SYN vagus *nerve* [CN X]. [L. wandering, so-called because of the wide distribution of the nerve]

Val Symbol for valine and valyl.

va·lence, va·len·cy (vā'lens, -len-sē). The combining power of one atom of an element (or a radical), that of the hydrogen atom being the unit of comparison, determined by the number of electrons in the outer shell of the atom (v. electrons); e.g., in HCl, chlorine is monovalent; in H_2O, oxygen is bivalent; in NH_3, nitrogen is trivalent. [L. *valentia,* strength]

negative v., the number of v. electrons an atom can take up.

positive v., the number of v. electrons an atom can give up.

va·lent (vā'lent). Possessing valence.

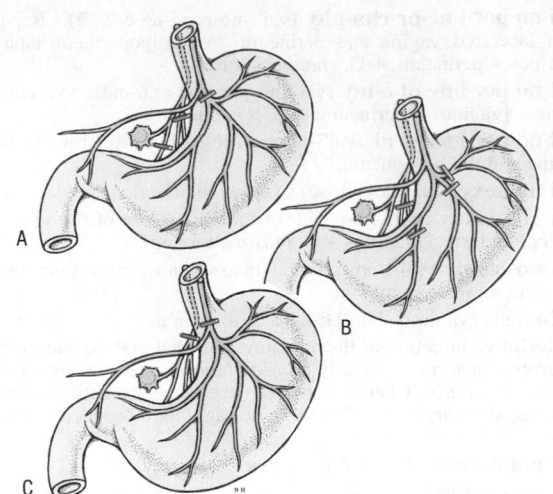

vagotomy: (A) selective gastric, (B) selective proximal, (C) truncal

Valentin, Gabriel G., German-Swiss physiologist, 1810–1883. SEE V. *corpuscles*, under *corpuscle, ganglion, nerve.*

Valentine, Ferdinand C., U.S. surgeon, 1851–1909. SEE V. *position, test.*

va·lep·o·tri·ates (val′ĕ-pō′trē-āts). A class of iridoid alkaloids from *Valeriana* sp. and *Kentranthus* sp.; e.g., the drug valtratum is a member of this class.

val·er·ate (val′ĕ-rāt). A salt of valeric acid; some are used in modern medicine. SYN valerianate.

va·le·ri·an (vă-lēr′ē-an). **1.** The rhizome and roots of *Valeriana officinalis* (family Valerianaceae), a herb native in southern Europe and northern Asia, cultivated also in Great Britain and the U.S.; has been used as a sedative in hysteria and at menopause. **2.** Referring to a class of terpene alkaloids obtained from v. (1). SYN vandal root.

va·le·ri·a·nate (va-lē′rē-ă-nāt). SYN valerate.

va·le·ric ac·id (vă-lēr′ik, vă-ler′ik). Normal aliphatic acid; distilled from valerian; some of its salts are used in medicine; found in human colon. SYN pentanoic acid.

va·leth·a·mate bro·mide (vă-leth′ă-māt). An anticholinergic agent.

val·e·tu·di·nar·i·an (val′ĕ-too-di-nār′ē-ăn). **1.** An invalid or person in chronically poor health. **2.** One whose chief concern is his/her invalidism or poor health. [L. *valetudinarius,* sickly]

val·e·tu·di·nar·i·an·ism (val′ĕ-too-di-nār′ē-ăn-izm). A weak or infirm state due to invalidism.

val·goid (val′goyd). Relating to valgus; knock-kneed; suffering from talipes valgus. [L. *valgus,* bowlegged, + G. *eidos,* resemblance]

val·gus (val′gŭs). Bent or twisted outward away from the midline or body; modern accepted usage, particularly in orthopedics, erroneously transposes the meaning of varus to v., as in *genu* valgum (knock-knee). [Mod. L. turned outward, fr. L. bowlegged]

val·id. Effective; producing the desired result; verifiably correct. [L. *valeo,* to be strong]

val·i·da·tion (val-i-dā′shŭn). The act or process of making valid.

consensual v., the confirmation of the experience or judgment of one person by another.

va·lid·i·ty (vă-lid′i-tē). An index of how well a test or procedure in fact measures what it purports to measure; an objective index by which to describe how valid a test or procedure is.

concurrent v., an index of criterion-related v. used to predict performance in a real-life situation given at about the same time as the test or procedure; the extent to which the index from one test correlates with that of a nonidentical test or index; e.g., how

well a score on an aptitude test correlates with the score on an intelligence test.

construct v., the extent to which a test or procedure appears to measure a higher order, inferred theoretical construct, or trait in contrast to measuring a more limited, specific dimension.

content v., the extent to which the items of a test or procedure are in fact a representative sample of that which is to be measured; e.g., items relating to ability in arithmetic and defining words are appropriate content for an intelligence test.

criterion-related v., the degree of effectiveness with which performance on a test or procedure predicts performance in a real-life situation; e.g., a good correlation between a score on an intelligence test such as the Scholastic Aptitude Test and one's 4-year college grade point average.

face v., the extent to which the items of a test or procedure appear superficially to sample that which is to be measured.

predictive v., criterion-related v. used to predict performance in a real-life task at a future time. SEE construct v., criterion-related v.

va·line (Val, V) (val′in). 2-Amino-3-methylbutanoic acid; the L-isomer is a constituent of most proteins; a nutritionally essential amino acid.

va·lin·o·my·cin (val′ĭ-nō-mī-sin). Cyclododecadepsipeptides ionophore antibiotic derived from *Streptomyces fulvissius;* a 36-membered ring structure consisting of 3 mol each of L-valine, D-α-hydroxyisovaleric acid, D-valine, and L-lactic acid linked alternately. The material is used as an insecticide and nematocide.

val·la (val′ă). Plural of vallum.

val·late (val′āt). Bordered with an elevation, as a cupped structure; denoting especially certain lingual papillae. SEE ALSO circumvallate. [L. *vallo,* pp. -*atus,* to surround with, fr. *vallum,* a rampart]

val·lec·u·la, pl. **val·lec·u·lae** (vă-lek′ū-lă, -lē) [TA]. A crevice or depression on any surface, particularly the spaces between the epiglottis and the base of the tongue, right and left. SYN valley. [L. dim. of *vallis,* valley]

v. cerebel′li [TA], a deep hollow on the inferior surface of the cerebellum, between the hemispheres, containing the medulla oblongata and the falx cerebelli. SYN v. of cerebellum [TA], vallis.

v. of cerebellum [TA], SYN v. cerebelli.

epiglottic v. [TA], a depression immediately posterior to the root of the tongue between the median and lateral glossoepiglottic folds on either side. SYN v. epiglottica [TA].

v. epiglot′tica [TA], SYN epiglottic v.

v. syl′vii, SYN lateral cerebral *fossa.*

v. un′guis, SYN *sulcus* matricis unguis.

Valleix, François L. I., French physician, 1807–1855. SEE V. *points,* under *point.*

val·ley (val′ē). SYN vallecula.

val·lis (val′is). SYN *vallecula* cerebelli. [L. valley]

val·lum, pl. **val·la** (val′ŭm, -ă). **1** [NA]. Any raised, more or less circular ridge. **2.** The slightly raised outer wall of the circular depression, or fossa, surrounding a vallate papilla of the tongue. [L. a rampart, fr. *vallus,* a stake]

v. un′guis [TA], SYN nail *wall.*

val·meth·a·mide (val-meth′ă-mīd). SYN valnoctamide.

val·noc·ta·mide (val-nok′tă-mīd). An antianxiety agent. SYN valmethamide.

val·oid (val′oyd). SYN equivalent *extract.* [L. *valeo,* to be strong]

val·pro·ic ac·id (val-prō′ik). An anticonvulsant used to treat seizure disorders; also used as the sodium salt, valproate sodium.

Valsalva, Antonio M., Italian anatomist, 1666–1723. SEE *aneurysm* of sinus of V.; V. *antrum, ligaments,* under *ligament, maneuver, muscle, sinus; teniae* of V., under *tenia;* V. *test.*

val·ue (val′ū). A particular quantitative determination. For v.'s not given below, see the specific name. SEE ALSO index, number. [M.E., fr. O.Fr., fr. L. *valeo,* to be of value]

acetyl v., the milligrams of KOH required to neutralize the acetic acid produced by the hydrolysis of 1 g of acetylated fat; a measure of the hydroxy acids present in glycerides; notably high in castor oil.

buffer v., the power of a substance in solution to absorb acid or alkali without change in pH; this is highest at a pH value equal to the pK_a value of the acid of the buffer pair. SEE ALSO buffer *capacity.* SYN buffer index.

buffer v. of the blood, the ability of the blood to compensate for additions of acid or alkali without disturbance of the pH.

C v., the total amount of DNA in a haploid genome.

caloric v., the heat evolved by a food when burnt or metabolized.

Hehner v., SYN Hehner *number.*

homing v., in a cybernetic system such as homeostasis, that v. of a trait of interest that the restorative forces are directed towards maintaining.

iodine v., SYN iodine *number.*

maturation v., an indicator of the level of maturation attained by vaginal epithelium and used as a factor in cytohormonal evaluation from the maturation index by valuing the parabasal cells at 0.0, the intermediate cells at 0.5, and the superficial cells at 1.0; for special investigations, subtypes of a major cell can be given different v.'s.

normal v.'s, a set of laboratory test v.'s used to characterize apparently healthy individuals; now replaced by reference v.'s.

pH v., SEE pH.

phenotypic v., in quantitative genetics, the metrical quantity of some trait associated with a particular phenotype.

predictive v., an expresion of the likelihood that a given test result correlates with the presence or absence of disease. A positive predictive v. is the ratio of patients with the disease who test positive to the entire population of individuals with a positive test result; a negative predictive v. is the ratio of patients without the disease who test negative to the entire population of individuals with a negative test.

R_f v., SEE R_f.

reference v.'s, a set of laboratory test v.'s obtained from an individual or group in a defined state of health; this term replaces normal v.'s, since it is based on a defined state of health rather than on apparent health.

thiocyanogen v., SYN thiocyanogen *number.*

threshold limit v. (TLV), the maximum concentration of a chemical recommended by the American Conference of Government Industrial Hygienists for repeated exposure without adverse health effects on workers.

val·va, pl. **val·vae** (val'vă, -vē) [TA]. SYN valve. [L. one leaf of a double door]

v. aor'tae [TA], SYN aortic *valve.*

v. atrioventricula'ris dex'tra [TA], SYN tricuspid *valve.*

v. atrioventricula'ris sinis'tra [TA], SYN mitral *valve.*

v. ileoceca'lis [TA], SYN ileal *papilla.*

v. mitra'lis, ✠official alternate term for mitral *valve.*

v. tricuspida'lis, ✠official alternate term for tricuspid *valve.*

v. trun'ci pulmona'lis [TA], SYN pulmonary *valve.*

val·val, val·var (val'văl, val'văr). Relating to a valve.

val·vate (val'văt). Relating to or provided with a valve. SYN valvular.

valve (valv) [TA]. **1.** A fold of the lining membrane of a canal or other hollow organ serving to retard or prevent a reflux of fluid. **2.** Any formation or reduplication of tissue, or flaplike structure, resembling or functioning as a v. SEE ALSO valvule, plica. SYN valva [TA]. [L. *valva*]

Amussat v., SYN spiral *fold* of cystic duct.

anal v.'s [TA], delicate crescent-shaped mucosal folds that pass between the lower ends of neighboring anal columns; the small pocket thus formed is an anal sinus. SYN valvulae anales [TA], Morgagni v.'s.

anterior urethral v., a crescentic horizontal fold in the proximal spongy urethra.

aortic v. [TA], the v. between the left ventricle and the ascending aorta, consisting of three fibrous semilunar cusps (valvules), located in the adult in anterior, right posterior, and left posterior positions; they are named, however, in accordance with their embryonic derivation in which the anteriorly located cusp is the right cusp (above which the right coronary artery arises), the left

posteriorly positioned cusp is designated as the left cusp (above which the left coronary artery arises), and the right posteriorly positioned cusp is designated as the posterior or noncoronary cusp. SYN valva aortae [TA].

⊞**atrioventricular v.'s,** SEE tricuspid v., mitral v.

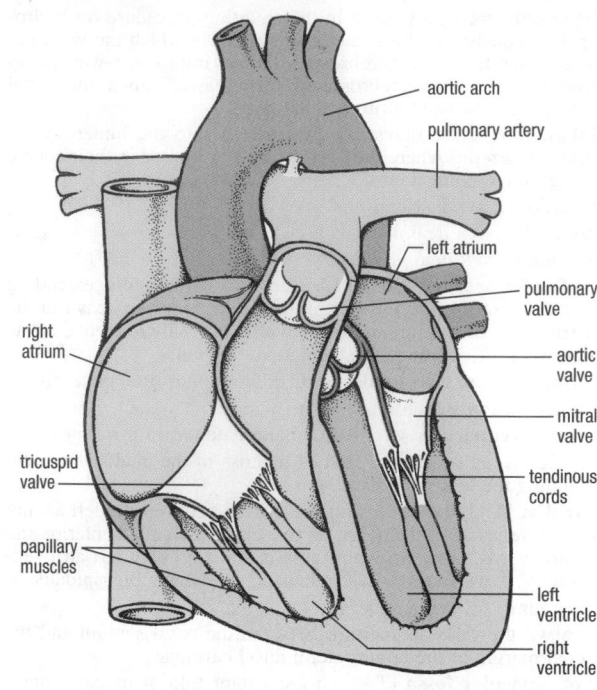

aortic arch
pulmonary artery
left atrium
pulmonary valve
aortic valve
mitral valve
tendinous cords
left ventricle
right ventricle
right atrium
tricuspid valve
papillary muscles

heart valves: aortic, pulmonary, tricuspid, and mitral valves

A-V v.'s, abbreviation for the cardiac atrioventricular valves; the mitral and tricuspid v.'s.

ball v., any of a variety of prosthetic cardiac v.'s comprising a ball within a retaining cage affixed to the orifice; when appropriately sized, used in aortic, mitral, or tricuspid position.

Bauhin v., SYN ileal *papilla.*

Béraud v., a small fold in the interior of the lacrimal sac at its junction with the lacrimal duct. SYN Krause v.

bicuspid v., SYN mitral v.

bi-leaflet v., a low profile mechanical heart v. that is less obstructive to outflow, especially in small size.

biologic v., SYN tissue v.

Björk-Shiley v., a low profile tilting disc mechanical heart v.

Blom-Singer v., a prosthesis for maintaining the patency of a tracheoesophageal puncture for vocal rehabilitation after laryngectomy.

Bochdalek v., a fold of mucous membrane in the lacrimal canaliculus at the lacrimal punctum. SYN Foltz valvule.

Braune v., a fold of mucous membrane at the junction of the esophagus with the stomach.

Carpentier-Edwards v., a bioprosthetic v. made from preserved porcine aortic v.'s.

caval v., SYN v. of inferior vena cava.

congenital v., an abnormal lining fold obstructing a passage; e.g., of a mucous membrane in the urethra.

coronary v., SYN v. of coronary sinus.

v. of coronary sinus [TA], a delicate fold of endocardium at the opening of the coronary sinus into the right atrium. SYN valvula sinus coronarii [TA], coronary v., thebesian v.

eustachian v., SYN v. of inferior vena cava.

v. of foramen ovale [TA], a fold projecting into the left atrium from the margin of the foramen ovale in the fetus; when, with beginning inspiration, the blood pressure within the left atrium increases, the v. closes and its edges become adherent to the

va

margin of the foramen ovale, occluding it. SYN valvula foraminis ovalis [TA], falx septi, v. of oval foramen.

Gerlach v., SYN v. of vermiform appendix.

Guérin v., SYN v. of navicular fossa.

Heister v., SYN spiral *fold* of cystic duct.

Heyer-Pudenz v., a v. used in the shunting procedure for hydrocephaly; consisting of a catheter-v. system in which the ventricular catheter leads the cerebrospinal fluid into a one-way pump through which the cerebrospinal fluid passes down the distal catheter into the right atrium of the heart.

Hoboken v.'s, the flangelike protrusions into the lumen of the umbilical arteries where they are twisted or kinked in their course through the umbilical cord.

Huschke v., SYN lacrimal *fold.*

ileocecal v., SYN ileal *papilla.*

ileocolic v., SYN ileal *papilla.*

v. of inferior vena cava [TA], an endocardial fold extending from the anterior inferior margin of the inferior vena cava to the anterior part of the limbus fossa ovalis. SYN valvula venae cavae inferioris [TA], caval v., eustachian v., sylvian v.

Kerckring v.'s, SYN circular *folds* of small intestine, under *fold.*

Krause v., SYN Béraud v.

left atrioventricular v., ⭐official alternate term for mitral v.

Mercier v., an occasional fold of mucosa of the bladder partially occluding the ureteral orifice.

mitral v. [TA], the v. closing the orifice between the left atrium and left ventricle of the heart; its two cusps are called anterior and posterior. SYN valva atrioventricularis sinistra [TA], left atrioventricular v.⭐, valva mitralis⭐, bicuspid v., valvula bicuspidalis.

Morgagni v.'s, SYN anal v.'s.

nasal v., the variable aperture between the nasal septum and the caudal margin of the upper lateral nasal cartilage.

v. of navicular fossa [TA], an inconstant fold of mucous membrane sometimes found in the root of the navicular fossa of the urethra. SYN valvula fossae navicularis [TA], Guérin fold, Guérin v.

nonrebreathing v., a type of v. that prevents mixture of inhaled and exhaled gases.

O'Beirne v., SYN rectosigmoid *sphincter.*

v. of oval foramen, SYN v. of foramen ovale.

parachute mitral v., congenital abnormality of the mitral v. characterized by the presence of a single papillary muscle from which the chordae of both v. leaflets divide; thus the resemblance to a parachute; the condition often produces a stenosis as the combined result of the tugging action of the chordae on, and the subsequent narrowing between, the leaflets. SYN parachute deformity.

porcine v., stented heterograft valve from pigs.

posterior urethral v.'s, anomalous folds occurring at the level of the seminal colliculus. SYN Amussat valvula.

prosthetic v.'s, v.'s used to replace human v.'s. They are divided into mechanical and tissue v.'s. The tissue is divided into homografts and heterografts.

pulmonary v. [TA], the v. at the entrance to the pulmonary trunk from the right ventricle; it consists of semilunar cusps (valvules), which are usually arranged in the adult in right anterior, left anterior, and posterior positions; however, they are named in accordance with their embryonic derivation; thus the posteriorly located cusp is designated as the left cusp, the right anteriorly located cusp is designated the right cusp, and the left anteriorly positioned cusp is called the anterior cusp. SYN valva trunci pulmonalis [TA], pulmonic v., v. of pulmonary trunk.

v. of pulmonary trunk, SYN pulmonary v.

pulmonic v., SYN pulmonary v.

rectal v.'s, SYN transverse *folds* of rectum, under *fold.*

reducing v., a v. designed to lower the pressure of a gas coming from a cylinder containing compressed gas under high pressure.

right atrioventricular v., ⭐official alternate term for tricuspid v.

Rosenmüller v., SYN lacrimal *fold.*

semilunar v. [TA], a heart v. comprised of a set of three semilu-

nar cusps (valvules); hence both the aortic and pulmonary valves are semilunar v.'s. SYN valvula semilunaris [TA].

spiral v. of cystic duct, SYN spiral *fold* of cystic duct.

Starr-Edwards v., a cage and ball artificial cardiac v. with high reliability and durability.

sylvian v., SYN v. of inferior vena cava.

Tarin v., SYN inferior medullary *velum.*

Terrien v., a valvelike fold between the gallbladder and the cystic duct; the first ridge of the spiral fold of the cystic duct.

thebesian v., SYN v. of coronary sinus.

tilting disk v., a variety of prosthetic cardiac v. composed of a caged disc.

tissue v., a prosthetic cardiac v. derived from the pig heart, bovine pericardium, or other biologic source. SEE ALSO prosthesis. SYN biologic v.

tricuspid v. [TA], the v. closing the orifice between the right atrium and right ventricle of the heart; its three cusps are called anterior, posterior, and septal. SYN valva atrioventricularis dextra [TA], right atrioventricular v.⭐, valva tricuspidalis⭐, valvula tricuspidalis.

Tulp v., Tulpius v., SYN ileal *papilla.*

urethral v.'s, folds in the urethral mucous membrane. SEE ALSO anterior urethral v., posterior urethral v.'s.

v. of Varolius, SYN ileal *papilla.*

ℹ **venous v.** [TA], a fold of the lining layer of a vein to prevent a reflux of blood. SYN valvula venosa (2) [TA].

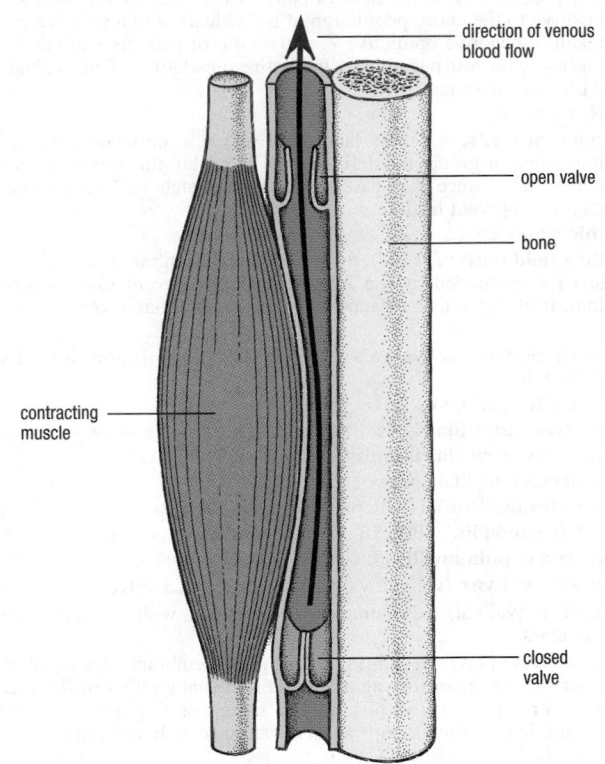

venous valves: principle of venous blood flow

v. of vermiform appendix, a fold of mucous membrane, simulating a v., sometimes found at the origin of the vermiform appendix. SYN Gerlach v., valvula processus vermiformis.

vesicoureteral v., a lock mechanism in the wall of the intravesical portion of the ureter that normally prevents urinary reflux.

v. of Vieussens, a prominent v. in the great cardiac vein where it turns around the obtuse margin to become the coronary sinus.

Vieussens v., SYN superior medullary *velum.*

valve·less (valv′les). Without valves; denoting certain veins, such as the portal, that are not provided with valves as are most of the veins.

val·vi·form (val'vi-fōrm). Valve-shaped.

val·vo·plas·ty (val'vō-plas-tē). Surgical reconstruction of a deformed cardiac valve, for the relief of stenosis or incompetence. SYN valvuloplasty. [valve + G. *plastos,* formed]

val·vot·o·my (val-vot'ō-mē). **1.** Cutting through a stenosed cardiac valve to relieve the obstruction. SYN valvulotomy. **2.** Incision of a valvular structure. [valve + G. *tomē,* incision]

mitral v., deliberate incision or enlargement by inserting a finger in the stenotic mitral valve.

rectal v., cutting through rectal folds that are too rigid or large.

val·vu·la, pl. **val·vu·lae** (val'vū-lă, -lē) [TA]. SYN valvule. [Mod. L. dim. of *valva*]

Amussat v., SYN posterior urethral *valves,* under *valve.*

val'vulae ana'les [TA], SYN anal *valves,* under *valve.*

v. bicuspida'lis, SYN mitral *valve.*

val'vulae conniven'tes, SYN circular *folds* of small intestine, under *fold.*

v. fora'minis ova'lis [TA], SYN *valve* of foramen ovale.

v. fos'sae navicula'ris [TA], SYN *valve* of navicular fossa.

Gerlach v., SYN trabecular *tissue* of sclera.

v. lymphat'ica [TA], SYN lymphatic *valvule.*

v. proces'sus vermifor'mis, SYN *valve* of vermiform appendix.

v. semiluna'ris [TA], SYN semilunar *valve.*

v. semiluna'ris ante'rior val'vae trun'ci pulmona'lis, anterior semilunar cusp of the pulmonary valve.

v. semiluna'ris dex'tra val'vae aor'tae, right semilunar cusp of the aortic valve.

v. semiluna'ris dex'tra val'vae trun'ci pulmona'lis, right semilunar cusp of the pulmonary valve.

v. semiluna'ris poste'rior val'vae aor'tae, posterior semilunar cusp of the aortic valve.

v. semiluna'ris sinis'tra val'vae aor'tae, left semilunar cusp of the aortic valve.

v. semiluna'ris sinis'tra val'vae trun'ci pulmona'lis, left semilunar cusp of the pulmonary valve.

v. semiluna'ris tari'ni, SYN inferior medullary *velum.*

v. si'nus corona'rii [TA], SYN *valve* of coronary sinus.

v. spiral'is, SYN spiral *fold* of cystic duct.

v. tricuspida'lis, SYN tricuspid *valve.*

v. ve'nae ca'vae inferio'ris [TA], SYN *valve* of inferior vena cava.

v. veno'sa [TA], **(1)** in the embryo, one of the pair of valves at the opening from the sinus venosus into the right atrium; **(2)** [NA], SYN venous *valve.*

v. vestib'uli, obsolete term for v. venosa (1).

val·vu·lar (val'vū-lăr). SYN valvate.

val·vule (val'vūl) [TA]. A valve, especially one of small size. SYN valvula [TA]. [L. *valvula*]

Foltz v., SYN Bochdalek *valve.*

lymphatic v. [TA], one of the delicate semilunar valves found in lymphatic vessels; they are usually paired and similar in structure to venous valves and occur at close intervals along the vessel wall. SYN valvula lymphatica [TA].

val·vu·li·tis (val-vū-lī'tis). Inflammation of a valve, especially a heart valve. [Mod. L. *valvula,* valve, + G. *-itis,* inflammation]

rheumatic v., v. characterized in the acute stage by small fibrin vegetations along the lines of closure and by Aschoff bodies in the cusps; in the chronic stage, it is characterized by scarring, commissural adhesion, and stenosis and/or regurgitation.

val·vu·lo·plas·ty (val'vū-lō-plas'tē). SYN valvoplasty.

val·vu·lo·tome (val'vū-lō-tōm). An instrument for sectioning a valve.

val·vu·lot·o·my (val-vū-lot'ō-mē). SYN valvotomy (1).

val·yl (Val, V) (val'il). The radical of valine.

Van, van. For some names with this prefix not found below, see the principal part of the name.

van·a·date (van'ă-dāt). A salt of vanadic acid.

va·na·dic ac·id (vă-nad'ik). An acid, H_3VO_4, derived from vanadium, forming salts with various bases.

va·na·di·um (V) (vă-nā'dē-ŭm). A metallic element, atomic no. 23, atomic wt. 50.9415; a bioelement, its deficiency can result in abnormal bone growth and a rise in cholesterol and triacylglycerol levels. [*Vanadis,* Scand. goddess]

v. group, those elements resembling vanadium in chemical and metallurgic properties; included with vanadium are niobium and tantalum.

van Bogaert, Ludo, 20th century Belgian neurologist. SEE Canavan-v. B.-Bertrand *disease;* v. B. *encephalitis.*

van Buchem, Francis Steven Peter, Dutch internist, *1897. SEE Van B. *syndrome.*

van Buren, William H., U.S. surgeon, 1819–1883. SEE van B. *sound, disease.*

van·co·my·cin (van-kō-mī'sin). An antibiotic isolated from cultures of *Nocardia orientalis,* bactericidal and bacteriostatic against Gram-positive organisms; available as the hydrochloride.

van Creveld, S., Dutch pediatrician, *1894. SEE Ellis-van C. *syndrome.*

van·dal root (van'dăl). SYN valerian.

van Deen, Izaak A., Dutch physiologist, 1804–1869. SEE van D. *test.*

van den Bergh, A.A.H., Dutch physician, 1869–1943. SEE van den B. *test.*

van der Kolk, Jacobus L.C.S., Dutch physician, 1797–1862.

van der Spieghel. SEE Spigelius.

van der Velden, Reinhardt, German physician, 1851–1903. SEE van der V.'s *test.*

van der Waals, Johannes D., Dutch physicist and Nobel laureate, 1837–1923. SEE van der W. *forces,* under *force.*

van Ekenstein, W.A., 19th century scientist. SEE Lobry de Bruyn-van E. *transformation.*

van Ermengen, Emile P., Belgian bacteriologist, 1851–1932. SEE van E. *stain.*

van Gieson, Ira, U.S. histologist and bacteriologist, 1865–1913. SEE van G. *stain.*

van Helmont, Jean B., Flemish physician and chemist, 1577–1644. SEE van H. *mirror.*

van Horne (Hoorne, Hoorn, Heurenius), Jan (Johannes), Dutch anatomist, 1621–1670. SEE van H. *canal.*

va·nil·la (vă-nil'ă). The cured, full-grown, unripe fruit of *Vanila planifolia* (Mexican or Bourbon v.) or of *V. tahitensis* (Tahiti v.), orchids (family Orchidaceae) native to Mexico and cultivated in other tropical countries; a flavoring agent. [Sp. *vainilla,* little pod]

va·nil·late (vă-nil'āt). A compound of vanillic acid; $C_8H_8O_4$.

va·nil·lic ac·id (vă-nil'ik). A flavoring agent.

va·nil·lin (vă-nil'in). Obtained from vanilla and also prepared synthetically; a flavoring agent; used to detect ornithine, sugar alcohols, phenols, and certain sterols.

va·nil·lism (vă-nil'izm). **1.** Symptoms of irritation of the skin, nasal mucous membrane, and conjunctiva from which workers with vanilla sometimes suffer. **2.** Infestation of the skin by sarcoptiform mites found in vanilla pods.

va·nil·lyl·man·del·ic ac·id (VMA) (van'i-lil-man-del'ik, vă-nil'il-). Misnomer for 4-hydroxy-3-methoxymandelic acid (α,3-dihydroxy-2-methoxybenzeneacetic acid); the major urinary metabolite of adrenal and sympathetic catecholamines (e.g., from both epinephrine and norepinephrine); elevated in most patients with pheochromocytoma.

Van Slyke, Donald D., U.S. biochemist, 1883–1971. SEE slyke; Van S. *apparatus, formula.*

van't Hoff, Jacobus H., Dutch chemist and Nobel laureate, 1852–1911. SEE van't H. *equation, law, theory;* Le Bel-van't H. *rule.*

va·por (vā'per). **1.** Molecules in the gaseous phase of a solid or liquid substance exposed to a gas. **2.** A visible emanation of fine particles of a liquid. **3.** A medicinal preparation to be administered by inhalation. [L. steam]

va

anesthetic v., the gaseous phase of a liquid anesthetic with sufficient partial pressure at room temperature to produce general anesthesia when inhaled.

va·por·i·za·tion (vā-pōr-i-zā'shŭn). **1.** The change of a solid or liquid to a state of vapor. **2.** The therapeutic application of a vapor.

va·por·ize (vā'-per-īz). **1.** To convert a solid or liquid into a vapor. **2.** To apply a vapor therapeutically.

va·por·iz·er (vā'per-īz-er). **1.** An apparatus for reducing medicated liquids to a state of vapor suitable for inhalation or application to accessible mucous membranes. SEE ALSO nebulizer, atomizer. **2.** A device for volatizing liquid anesthetics.

flow-over v., a device for vaporization of a liquid anesthetic by causing gases to pass over the anesthetic or over material saturated with the anesthetic.

temperature-compensated v., a v. of liquid anesthetics with graduated settings calibrated to deliver a known constant concentration of a specific anesthetic despite changes in inflow volume and despite cooling brought about by vaporization.

va·por·tho·rax (vāp-er-thō'raks). The existence of large water vapor bubbles in the pleural space between the lungs and the chest wall in an unprotected person exposed to altitudes above 63,000 ft., where the barometric pressure is less than 47 mm Hg and where water at body temperature vaporizes from the liquid state.

va·po·ther·a·py (vā'pō-thār'ă-pē). Treatment of disease by means of vapor or spray.

V̇a/Q̇ Abbreviation for ventilation/perfusion *ratio.*

Vaquez, Louis H., French physician, 1860–1936. SEE V. *disease.*

var·i·a·bil·i·ty (var'ē-ă-bil'i-tē). **1.** The capability of being variable. **2.** In genetics, the potential or actual differences, either quantitative or qualitative, in phenotype among individuals.

baseline v. of fetal heart rate, the beat-to-beat changes in fetal heart rate as recorded on a graph.

beat-to-beat v. of fetal heart rate, v. of fetal heart rate measured in changes in the QRS-QRS interval from heart beat to heart beat; measured with electronic internal fetal heart rate monitors.

var·i·a·ble (var'ē-ă-bl). **1.** That which is inconstant, which can or does change, as contrasted with a constant. **2.** Deviating from the type in structure, form, physiology, or behavior. [L. *vario,* to vary, change, differ]

continuous v., a v. that may take on any value in an interval or intervals (its domain).

continuous random v., continuous v. that may randomly assume any value in its domain but any particular value has no probability of occurring, only a probability density.

dependent v., in experiments, a v. that is influenced by or dependent upon changes in the independent v.; e.g., the amount of a written passage retained (dependent v.) as a function of the different numbers of minutes (independent v.) allowed to study the passage.

discrete v., a v. that may assume only a countable (usually finite) number of values.

discrete random v., a random v. that may assume a countable number of values, each with a probability strictly greater than zero.

independent v., a characteristic being measured or observed that is hypothesized to influence another event or manifestation (the dependent v.) within a defined area of relationships under study; that is, the independent v. is not influenced by the event or manifestation, but may cause it or contribute to its variation. SEE dependent v.

intermediate v., a v. in a causal pathway that causes variation in the dependent v. and is itself caused to vary by the independent v.

intervening v., an event, such as an attitude or emotion, inferred to occur within an organism between the stimulation and response in such a way as to influence or determine the response.

mixed discrete-continuous random v., a random v. that may assume some values with probabilities and others with probability densities. For example, in a 35-year-old man with familial polyposis of the colon, the distribution of time until malignant disease occurs consists of a probability that he already has cancer (which

would be assigned the waiting time 0), a probability density of developing it in the future, and a probability that he will die of some other cause before he develops cancer.

moderator v., a v. that interacts by virtue of being antecedent or intermediate in the causal pathway.

random v., a v. that may assume a set of values, each with fixed probabilities or probability densities (its distribution), in such a way that the total probability assigned to the distribution is unity; the random v. may be discrete, continuous, or mixed discrete-continuous.

var·i·ance (var'ē-ans). **1.** The state of being variable, different, divergent, or deviate; a degree of deviation. **2.** A measure of the variation shown by a set of observations, defined as the sum of squares of deviations from the mean, divided by the number of degrees of freedom in the set of observations.

ball v., swelling and changes in shape and consistency of the ball in a ball-valve prosthesis, especially in one replacing the aortic valve.

var·i·ant (var'ē-ant). **1.** That which, or one who, is variable. **2.** Having the tendency to alter or change, exhibit variety or diversity, not conform with, or differ from the type.

inherited albumin v.'s [MIM*103600], types of human serum albumin, distinguished by characteristic mobility patterns on electrophoresis; each type is due to a mutation of a gene controlling albumin synthesis; the mutant genes are codominant with the normal gene for albumin A, and the group forms a system of genetic polymorphism; types include: albumin b (slow), found occasionally in persons of European ancestry; albumin Ghent (fast), found first at Ghent, Belgium; albumin Mexico (slow), found in Indians of Mexico and the southwestern United States; albumin Naskapi (fast), found in the Naskapi and other Indians of northern North America; and albumin Reading (fast), found first at Reading, England.

L-phase v.'s, bacterial v.'s that do not have rigid cell walls but that may contain varying amounts of cell wall material; they are spherical to coccobacillary in shape and vary in size from small bodies that pass through filters which retain bacteria to bodies that are larger than the bacterial form; they are Gram-negative and resistant to penicillin. The v.'s differ greatly from the parent bacterial cells in mode of reproduction, physiology, growth requirements, and individual and colonial morphology; they are generally considered to be nonpathogenic, even if derived from a pathogenic bacterium. [L. fr. Lister Institute]

var·i·ate (var'ē-ăt). A measurable quantity capable of taking on a number of values; may be binary (i.e., capable of taking on two values in a certain interval of values), continuous (i.e., capable of taking on all values in a certain interval of real values), or discrete (i.e., capable of taking on a limited number of values in a certain interval of real values).

var·i·a·tion (var-ē-ā'shŭn). **1.** Deviation from the type, especially the parent type, in structure, form, physiology, or behavior. **2.** SYN type (3). [L. *variatio,* fr. *vario,* to change, vary]

continuous v., a series of very slight v.'s.

var·i·ca·tion (var-i-kā'shŭn). Formation or presence of varices.

var·i·ce·al (var-ĭ-sē'ăl, vă-ris'ē-ăl). Of or pertaining to a varix.

🔳 **var·i·cel·la** (var-i-sel'ă). An acute contagious disease, usually occurring in children, caused by the varicella-zoster virus genus, Varicellovirus, a member of the family Herpesviridae, and marked by a sparse eruption of papules, which become vesicles and then pustules, like that of smallpox although less severe and varying in stages, usually with mild constitutional symptoms; incubation period is about 14–17 days. SEE ALSO *herpes* zoster. SYN chickenpox. [Mod. L. dim. of *variola*]

v. gangreno'sa, gangrenous ulceration of v. lesions with or without secondary infection, occurring mainly in children with severe underlying disease.

var·i·cel·la·tion (var-i-sĕ-lā'shŭn). Inoculation with the virus of chickenpox as a means of protection against that disease.

var·i·cel·li·form (var-ĭ-sel'ĭ-fōrm). Resembling varicella. SYN varicelloid.

var·i·cel·loid (var-ĭ-sel'oyd). SYN varicelliform.

Var·i·cel·lo·vi·rus (var-ē-sel'ō-vi'rus). SYN varicella-zoster *virus.*

va·ri·ces (var′i-sēz). Plural of varix.

var·i·ci·form (var′ĭ-si-fōrm, vă-ris′ĭ-fōrm). Resembling a varix. SYN cirsoid, varicoid.

⟳**varico-.** A varix, varicose, varicosity. [L. *varix,* a dilated vein]

var·i·co·bleph·a·ron (var′i-kō-blef′a-ron). A varicosity of the eyelid. [varico- + G. *blepharon,* eyelid]

var·i·co·cele (var′i-kō-sēl). A condition manifested by abnormal dilation of the veins of the spermatic cord, caused by incompetent valves in the internal spermatic vein and resulting in impaired drainage of blood into the spermatic cord veins when the patient assumes the upright position. SYN pampinocele. [varico- + G. *kēlē,* tumor, hernia]

   ovarian v., a varicose condition of the pampiniform plexus in the broad ligament of the uterus. SYN tubo-ovarian v., utero-ovarian v.

   symptomatic v., a v. caused by obstruction of the internal spermatic vein, usually at the level of the renal vein and usually due to invasive renal cell carcinoma, characterized by failure of the dilated veins in the spermatic cord to empty when the patient assumes a recumbent position.

   tubo-ovarian v., SYN ovarian v.

   utero-ovarian v., SYN ovarian v.

var·i·co·ce·lec·to·my (var′i-kō-sē-lek′tō-mē). Operation for the correction of a varicocele by ligature and excision and by ligation alone of the dilated veins. [varicocele + G. *ektomē,* excision]

var·i·cog·ra·phy (var′ĭ-kog′ră-fē). Radiography of the veins after injection of contrast medium into varicose veins. [varico- + G. *graphō,* to write]

var·i·coid (var′i-koyd). SYN variciform.

var·i·com·pha·lus (var-i-kom′fă-lŭs). A swelling formed by varicose veins at the umbilicus. [varico- + G. *omphalos,* navel]

var·i·co·phle·bi·tis (var′i-kō-flě-bī′tis). Inflammation of varicose veins. [varico- + G. *phleps,* vein, + *-itis,* inflammation]

var·i·cose (var′i-kōs). Relating to, affected with, or characterized by varices or varicosis.

▤ **var·i·co·sis**, pl. **var·i·cos·es** (var-i-kō′sis, -sēz). A dilated or varicose state of a vein or veins. [varico- + G. *-osis,* condition]

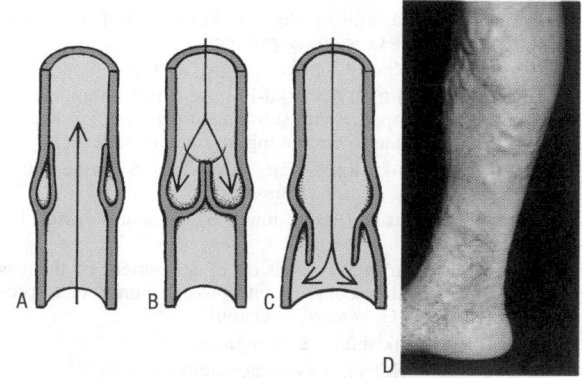

varicosis: in a healthy vein the valves allow blood to travel toward heart (A) while keeping blood from flowing back away from heart (B); valves in varicose veins (C) no longer function properly, thus allowing blood to travel back toward extremities, (D) photograph of leg with varicose veins

var·i·cos·i·ty (var-i-kos′i-tē). A varix or varicose condition.

var·i·cot·o·my (var-i-kot′ō-mē). An operation for varicose veins by subcutaneous incision. [varico- + G. *tomē,* a cutting]

va·ric·u·la (vă-rik′ū-lă). A varicose condition of the veins of the conjunctiva. SYN conjunctival varix. [L. dim. of *varix*]

var·i·cule (var′i-kūl). A small varicose vein ordinarily seen in the skin; may be associated with venous stars, venous lakes, or larger varicose veins. [L. *varicula,* dim. of *varix*]

va·ri·eg·a·tion (ver′ē-a-gā′shŭn). The diversification or alteration of a phenotype produced by a change in the genotype during somatic development.

va·ri·o·la (vă-rī′ō-lă). SYN smallpox. [Med. L. dim of L. *varius,* spotted]

   v. benig′na, SYN varioloid (2).

   v. hemorrha′gica, SYN hemorrhagic *smallpox.*

   v. ma′jor, SYN smallpox.

   v. malig′na, malignant smallpox, usually of the hemorrhagic form. SYN malignant smallpox.

   v. milia′ris, a form of varioloid in which the eruption consists of miliary vesicles without the formation of pustules.

   v. mi′nor, SYN alastrim.

   v. pemphigo′sa, a form of smallpox in which the eruption consists of pemphigus-like blebs.

   v. si′ne eruptio′ne, an abortive form of smallpox in which the disease subsides without the appearance of any eruption, or at most a few papules that never go on to pustulation.

   v. vaccine, variola v., SYN vaccinia.

   v. ve′ra, smallpox of ordinary severity in the unvaccinated.

   v. verruco′sa, a mild or abortive form of varioloid, the eruption of which consists mainly of papules, with occasionally minute vesicles at the apices, which persist for a time as wartlike lesions. SYN wartpox.

va·ri·o·lar (vă-rī′ō-lăr). Relating to smallpox. SYN variolic, variolous.

var·i·o·late (var′ē-ō-lāt). 1. To inoculate with smallpox. 2. Pitted or scarred, as if by smallpox.

var·i·o·la·tion (var′ē-ō-lā′shŭn). The obsolete process of inoculating a susceptible person with material from a vesicle of a patient with smallpox. SYN variolization.

var·i·ol·ic (var-ē-ol′ik). SYN variolar.

var·i·ol·i·form (vă-rī′ō-li-fōrm, var-ē-ō′li-fōrm). SYN varioloid (1). [variola + L. *forma,* form]

var·i·o·li·za·tion (var′ē-ō-li-zā′shŭn). SYN variolation.

va·ri·o·loid (var′ē-ō-loyd). 1. Resembling smallpox. SYN varioliform. 2. A mild form of smallpox occurring in persons who are relatively resistant, usually as a result of a previous vaccination. SYN modified smallpox, varicelloid smallpox, variola benigna. [variola + G. *eidos,* resemblance]

va·ri·o·lous (vă-rī′ō-lŭs). SYN variolar.

va·ri·o·lo·vac·cine (vă-rī′ō-lō-vak′sēn). A vaccine obtained from the eruption following inoculation of a heifer with smallpox from the human.

var·ix, pl. **va·ri·ces** (var′iks, var′i-sēz). 1. A dilated vein. 2. An enlarged and tortuous vein, artery, or lymphatic vessel. [L. *varix* (*varic-*), a dilated vein]

   v. anastomot′icus, SYN aneurysmal v.

   aneurysmal v., dilation and tortuosity of a vein resulting from an acquired communication with an adjacent artery. SYN Pott aneurysm, v. anastomoticus.

   cirsoid v., SYN cirsoid *aneurysm.*

   conjunctival v., SYN varicula.

   esophageal varices, longitudinal venous varices at the lower end of the esophagus as a result of portal hypertension; they are superficial and liable to ulceration and massive bleeding.

   gelatinous v., a lumpy or nodular condition of the umbilical cord.

   lymph v., the formation of varices or cysts in the lymph nodes in consequence of obstruction in the efferent lymphatics.

   turbinal v., a condition of permanent dilation of the veins of the turbinated bodies, especially of the inferior turbinate.

var·nish (den·tal). Solutions of natural resins and gums in a suitable solvent, of which a thin coating is applied over the surfaces of the cavity preparations before placement of restorations, used as a protective agent for the tooth against constituents of restorative materials. SYN cavity liner, vernix.

Varolius (Varolio), Constantius (Costanzio), Italian anatomist and physician, 1543–1575. SEE ileal *sphincter; valve* of V.; *pons varolii.*

var·us (va′rŭs). Bent or twisted inward toward the midline of the limb or body; modern accepted usage, particularly in orthopedics, erroneously transposes the meaning of valgus to v., as in *genu varum* (bow-leg). [Mod. L. bent inward, fr. L. knock-kneed]

va

vas, gen. **va·'sis**, pl. **va·sa**, gen. and pl. **va·so·rum** (vas, vā'sis, vā'să, vā-sō'rŭm) [TA]. A duct or canal conveying any liquid, such as blood, lymph, chyle, or semen. SEE ALSO vessel. [L. a vessel, dish]

v. aber'rans hep'atis, pl. **va'sa aberran'tia hep'atis**, blind and/or atrophic bile duct remnants in the fibrous appendix and in the capsule of the liver at the margins of the left lobe and the groove for the inferior vena cava.

v. aberrans of Roth, an occasional diverticulum of the rete testis or of the efferent ductules of the testis.

va'sa aberran'tia, SYN aberrant *ductules*, under *ductule*.

v. af'ferens, pl. **va'sa afferen'tia**, SYN afferent glomerular *arteriole*.

v. anastomot'icum [TA], SYN anastomotic *vessel*.

va'sa bre'via, SYN short gastric *arteries*, under *artery*.

v. capilla're [TA], SYN capillary (2); SEE blood *capillary*, lymph *capillary*.

va'sa chylif'era, chyle vessels. SEE lacteal (2).

v. collatera'le, SYN collateral *vessel*.

v. def'erens, pl. **va'sa deferen'tia**, SYN *ductus* deferens.

v. ef'ferens, pl. **va'sa efferen'tia**, (1) a vein carrying blood away from a part; SYN efferent lymphatic, v. lymphaticum efferens. (2) SYN efferent glomerular *arteriole*; (3) SYN efferent *ductules* of testis, under *ductule*.

Ferrein vasa aberrantia, biliary canaliculi that are not connected with hepatic lobules.

Haller v. aberrans, SYN inferior aberrant *ductule*.

va'sa lymphat'ica, SYN lymph *vessels*, under *vessel*.

v. lympha'ticum, SYN lymphatic (3).

v. lympha'ticum af'ferens, SYN afferent *lymphatic*.

v. lympha'ticum ef'ferens, SYN v. efferens (1).

v. lympha'ticum profun'dum [TA], SYN deep lymph *vessel*.

v. lympha'ticum superficia'le [TA], SYN superficial lymph *vessel*.

va'sa nervor'um, blood vessels supplying nerves.

va'sa pre'via, umbilical vessels presenting in advance of the fetal head, usually traversing the membranes and crossing the internal cervical os.

v. prom'inens duc'tus cochlea'ris, a blood vessel in the substance of the spiral prominence of the cochler duct.

va'sa rec'ta, straight vessels into which the efferent arteriole of the juxtamedullary glomeruli breaks up; they form a leash of vessels which, arising at the bases of the pyramids, run through the renal medulla toward the apex of each pyramid, then reverse direction in a hairpin turn, and run straight back again toward the base of the pyramid as venae rectae;

vasa recta renis [TA], arteries penetrating and supplying the renal medulla (pyramids). SYN arteriolae rectae [TA], straight arteries✩.

va'sa sanguinea aur'is inter'nae [TA], SYN *vessels* of internal ear, under *vessel*.

vasa sanguinea choroideae [TA], SYN choroid *blood vessels*, under *blood vessel*.

vasa sanguinea intrapulmonalia [TA], SYN intrapulmonary *blood vessels*, under *blood vessel*.

va'sa sanguin'ea ret'inae [TA], SYN retinal *blood vessels*, under *blood vessel*.

v. sanguineum [TA], SYN blood *vessel*.

v. spira'le, a blood vessel, larger than its fellows, running in the tympanic layer of the basilar membrane just beneath the tunnel of Corti.

va'sa vaso'rum [TA], small arteries distributed to the outer and middle coats of the larger blood vessels, and their corresponding veins. SYN vessels of vessels.

va'sa vortico'sa, SYN vorticose *veins*, under *vein*.

△**vas-**. A vas, blood vessel. SEE ALSO vasculo-, vaso-. [L. *vas*]

va·sa (vā'să). Plural of vas.

va·sal (vā'săl). Relating to a vas or to vasa.

vas·cu·lar (vas'kū-lăr). Relating to or containing blood vessels. [L. *vasculum*, a small vessel, dim. of *vas*]

vas·cu·lar·i·ty (vas-kū-lar'i-tē). The condition of being vascular.

vas·cu·lar·i·za·tion (vas'kū-lăr-i-zā'shŭn). The formation of new blood vessels in a part. SYN arterialization (3).

vas·cu·lar·ized (vas-kū-lăr-īzd). Rendered vascular by the formation of new vessels.

vas·cu·la·ture (vas'kū-lă-choor). The vascular network of an organ.

vas·cu·li·tis (vas-kū-lī'tis). SYN angiitis.

    cutaneous v., an acute form of v. that may affect the skin only, but also may involve other organs, with a polymorphonuclear infiltrate in the walls of and surrounding small (dermal) vessels. Nuclear fragments are formed by karyorrhexis of the neutrophils. SEE ALSO leukocytoclastic v. SYN hypersensitivity v.

    hypersensitivity v., SYN cutaneous v.

    hypocomplementemic v., SYN urticarial v.

    leukocytoclastic v., cutaneous acute v. characterized clinically by palpable purpura, especially of the legs, and histologically by exudation of the neutrophils and sometimes fibrin around dermal venules, with nuclear dust and extravasation of red cells; may be limited to the skin or involve other tissues as in Henoch-Schönlein purpura. SEE ALSO cutaneous v. [G. *leukos*, white, + *kytos*, cell, + *klastos*, broken, fr. *klao*, to break]

    livedo v., hyaline degeneration of the walls of small dermal blood vessels with thrombolic occlusion seen with cryoglobulinemia or in atrophie blanche. No necrosis is seen.

    nodular v., chronic or recurrent nodular lesions of subcutaneous tissue, especially of the legs of older women, with lobular panniculitis, granulomatous inflammation with multinucleated giant cells, focal necrosis, and obliterative inflammation of the small blood vessels, resembling erythema induratum but without evidence of associated tuberculosis.

    urticarial v., painful, purpuric cutaneous lesions resembling urticaria but lasting more than 24 hours, with biopsy findings of leukocytoclastic v. and variable systemic changes, often with hypocomplementemia. SYN hypocomplementemic v.

△**vasculo-**. A blood vessel. SEE ALSO vas-, vaso-. [L. *vasculum*, a small vessel, dim. of *vas*]

vas·cu·lo·car·di·ac (vas'kū-lō-kar'dē-ak). SYN cardiovascular.

vas·cu·lo·gen·e·sis (vas'kū-lō-jen'ĕ-sis). Formation of the vascular system. [vasculo- + G. *genesis*, production]

vas·cu·lo·mo·tor (vas'koo-lō-mō'ter). SYN vasomotor.

vas·cu·lo·my·e·li·nop·a·thy (vas'kū-lō-mī-ĕ-li-nop'ă-thē). Small cerebral vessel vasculopathy with subsequent perivascular demyelination, presumably due to circulating immune complexes.

vas·cu·lop·a·thy (vas-kū-lop'ă-thē). Any disease of the blood vessels. [vasculo- + G. *pathos*, disease]

vas·cu·lum, pl. **vas·cu·la** (vas'kū-lŭm, -lă). A small vessel. [L. dim of *vas*, a vessel]

▌**va·sec·to·my** (va-sek'tō-mē). Excision of a segment of the vas deferens, performed in association with prostatectomy, or to produce sterility. [vas- + G. *ektomē*, excision]

vas·i·fac·tion (vas-i-fak'shŭn). SYN angiopoiesis.

vas·i·fac·tive (vas-i-fak'tiv). SYN angiopoietic.

vas·i·form (vas'i-fōrm). Having the shape of a vas or tubular structure.

vas·i·tis (va-sī'tis). SYN deferentitis.

    v. nodo'sa (va-sī'tis nō-dō'sa), an inflammatory condition of the vas deferens characterized by the presence of numerous epithelium-lined spaces with the muscularis and adventitia, often containing spermatozoa; usually seen after vasectomy, and may clinically and microscopically mimic adenocarcinoma. SEE ALSO *vas* deferens.

△**vaso-**. Vas, blood vessel. SEE ALSO vas-, vasculo-. [L. *vas*, a vessel]

va·so·ac·tive (vā-sō-ak'tiv, vas-ō-). Influencing the tone and caliber of blood vessels.

va·so·con·stric·tion (vā'sō-kon-strik'shŭn, vas'ō-). Narrowing of the blood vessels.

    active v., reduced caliber of a vessel caused by increased tonus in the smooth muscle in its walls.

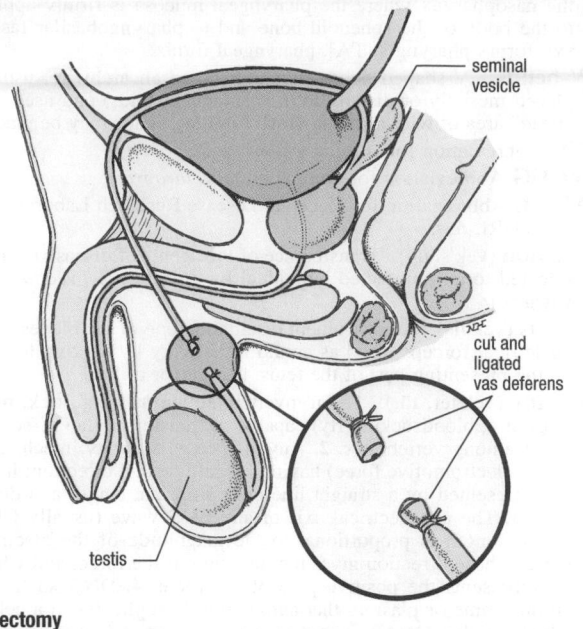

vasectomy

passive v., reduced caliber of a vessel caused by decreased intraluminal pressure.

va·so·con·stric·tive (vā′sō-kon-strik′tiv, vas′ō-). **1.** Causing narrowing of the blood vessels. **2.** SYN vasoconstrictor (1).

va·so·con·stric·tor (vā′sō-kon-strik′ter, vas′ō-). **1.** An agent that causes narrowing of the blood vessels. SYN vasoconstrictive (2). **2.** A nerve, stimulation of which causes vascular constriction.

va·so·den·tin (vā-sō-den′tin, vas-ō-). Dentin in which the primitive capillaries have remained uncalcified and so are wide enough to give passage to the formed elements of the blood. SYN vascular dentin.

va·so·de·pres·sion (vā′sō-dē-presh′ŭn, vas′ō). Reduction of tone in blood vessels with vasodilation and resulting in lowered blood pressure.

va·so·de·pres·sor (vā′sō-dē-pres′er, vas′ō). **1.** Producing vasodepression. **2.** SYN depressor (4).

va·so·di·la·ta·tion (vā′sō-dil-ă-tā′shŭn, vas′ō-). SYN vasodilation.

va·so·di·la·tion (vā′sō-dī-lā′shŭn, vas-ō-). Widening of the lumen of blood vessels. SYN vasodilatation.

active v., v. caused by a decrease in tonus of smooth muscle in the wall of a vessel.

passive v., v. related to increased pressure in lumen of a vessel.

va·so·di·la·tive (vā′sō-dī-lā′tiv, vas′ō-). **1.** Causing dilation of the blood vessels. **2.** SYN vasodilator (1).

va·so·di·la·tor (vā′sō-dī-lā′ter, vas′ō-). **1.** An agent that causes dilation of the blood vessels. SYN vasodilative (2). **2.** A nerve, stimulation of which results in dilation of the blood vessels.

va·so·ep·i·did·y·mos·to·my (vā′sō-ep-i-did-i-mos′tō-mē, vas′ō-). Surgical anastomosis of the vasa deferentia to the epididymis, to bypass an obstruction at the level of the mid to distal epididymis or proximal vas. [vaso- + epididymis + G. *stoma,* mouth]

va·so·fac·tive (vā-sō-fak′tiv, vas-ō-). SYN angiopoietic.

va·so·for·ma·tion (vā-sō-fōr-mā′shŭn, vas-ō-). SYN angiopoiesis.

va·so·for·ma·tive (vā-sō-fōr′mă-tiv, vas-ō-). SYN angiopoietic.

va·so·gan·gli·on (vā-sō-gang′glē-on, vas-ō-). A mass of blood vessels.

va·sog·ra·phy (vā-sog′ră-fē). Radiography of the vas deferens to determine patency, by injecting contrast medium into its lumen either transurethrally or by open vasotomy. [vas + G. *graphō,* to write]

va·so·in·hib·i·tor (vā′sō-in-hib′i-ter, vas′ō-). An agent that restricts or prevents the functioning of the vasomotor nerves.

va·so·in·hib·i·to·ry (vā′sō-in-hib′i-tōr-ē, vas′ō-). Restraining vasomotor action.

va·so·la·bile (vā-sō-lā′bil, -bīl, vas-ō-). Characterizing the condition in which there is lability or active vasomotion of blood vessels.

va·so·li·ga·tion (vā′sō-li-gā′shŭn, vas′ō-). Ligation of the vas deferens, usually after its division.

va·so·mo·tion (vā-sō-mō′shŭn, vas-ō-). Change in caliber of a blood vessel.

va·so·mo·tor (vā-sō-mō′ter, vas-ō-). **1.** Causing dilation or constriction of the blood vessels. **2.** Denoting the nerves which have this action. SYN vasculomotor.

va·so·neu·rop·a·thy (vā′sō-noo-rop′ă-thē, vas′ō-). Any disease involving both the nerves and blood vessels. [vaso- + G. *neuron,* nerve, + *pathos,* suffering]

va·so·or·chi·dos·to·my (vā′sō-ōr-ki-dos′tō-mē, vas′ō-). Reestablishment of the interrupted seminiferous channels by uniting the tubules of the epididymis or of the rete testis to the divided end of the vas deferens. [vaso- + G. *orchis,* testis, + *stoma,* mouth]

va·so·pa·ral·y·sis (vā′sō-pă-ral′i-sis, vas′ō-). Paralysis, atonia, or hypotonia of blood vessels. SYN angiohypotonia, angioparalysis.

va·so·pa·re·sis (vā′sō-pă-rē′sis, -par′ē-sis, vas′ō-). A mild degree of vasoparalysis. SYN angioparesis, vasomotor paralysis. [vaso- + G. *paresis,* weakness]

va·so·pres·sin (VP) (vā-sō-pres′in, vas-ō-). A nonapeptide neurohypophysial hormone related to oxytocin and vasotocin; synthetically prepared or obtained from the posterior lobe of the pituitary of healthy domestic animals. In pharmacological doses v. causes contraction of smooth muscle, notably that of all blood vessels; large doses may produce cerebral or coronary arterial spasm. SYN antidiuretic hormone, Pitressin. [vaso- + L. *premo,* pp. *pressum,* to press down, + -in]

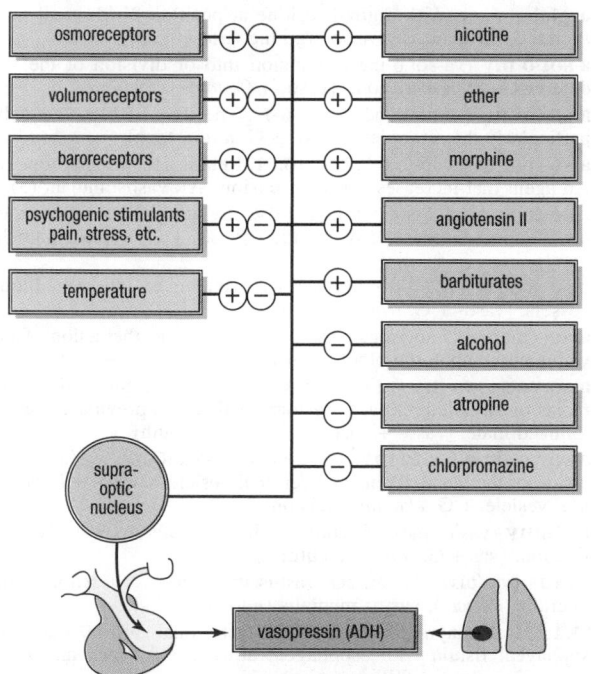

vasopressin: regulation of ADH secretion; effects of various neural and mechanical factors on the supraoptic nucleus (+ = stimulation, – = inhibition); note that some malignant neoplasms (e.g., bronchogenic carcinoma) may also secrete ADH

arginine v. (AVP), v. containing an arginyl residue in position 8 (as in chickens and most mammals, including humans); porcine v. has a lysyl residue at position 8. All are vasopressors. SYN argipressin.

va

va·so·pres·sor (vă-sō-pres´er, vas-ō-). **1.** Producing vasoconstriction and a rise in blood pressure, usually understood to be systemic arterial pressure unless otherwise specified. **2.** An agent that has this effect.

va·so·punc·ture (vă-sō-pŭnk´choor, vas-ō-). The act of puncturing a vessel with a needle.

va·so·re·flex (vă-sō-rē´fleks, vas´ō-). A reflex that influences the caliber of blood vessels.

va·so·re·lax·a·tion (vă´sō-rē-lak-sā´shŭn, vas-ō). Reduction in tension of the walls of the blood vessels.

va·so·sec·tion (vă-sō-sek´shŭn, vas-ō-). SYN vasotomy.

va·so·sen·so·ry (vă-sō-sen´ser-ē, vas-ō-). **1.** Relating to sensation in the blood vessels. **2.** Denoting sensory nerve fibers innervating blood vessels.

va·so·spasm (vā´sō-spazm, vas´ō-). Contraction or hypertonia of the muscular coats of the blood vessels. SYN angiohypertonia, angiospasm.

va·so·spas·tic (vă-sō-spas´tik, vas-ō-). Relating to or characterized by vasospasm. SYN angiospastic.

va·so·stim·u·lant (va-sō-stim´ū-lant). **1.** Exciting vasomotor action. **2.** An agent that excites the vasomotor nerves to action. **3.** SYN vasotonic (2).

va·sos·to·my (vă-sos´tō-mē). Establishment of an opening into the deferent duct. [vaso- + G. *stoma*, mouth]

va·so·throm·bin (vă-sō-throm´bin, vas-ō-). Thrombin derived from the lining cells of the blood vessels.

va·so·to·cin (vă-sō-tō´sin, vas-ō-). A nonapeptide hormone of the neurohypophysis of subvertebrates, with activities similar to that of vasopressin and oxytocin; chemically identical with human vasopressin except for an isoleucyl residue at position 3; thus [3-isoleucine]vasopressin or [Ile³]vasopressin. [*vaso*, pressin + *oxytocin*]

arginine v., v. with arginyl residue at position 8 (identical with arginine oxytocin). SEE ALSO arginine *vasopressin*.

va·sot·o·my (vă-sot´ō-mē). Incision into or division of the vas deferens. SYN vasosection. [vaso- + G. *tomē*, incision]

va·so·to·nia (vă-sō-tō´nē-ă, vas-ō-). The tone of blood vessels, particularly the arterioles. [vaso- + G. *tonos*, tone]

va·so·ton·ic (vă-sō-ton´ik, vas-ō-). **1.** Relating to vascular tone. **2.** An agent that increases vascular tension. SYN vasostimulant (3).

va·so·tro·phic (vă-sō-trof´ik, vas-ō-). Relating to the nutrition of the blood vessels or the lymphatics. [vaso- + G. *trophē*, nourishment]

va·so·tro·pic (vă-sō-trō´pik, vas-ō-). Tending to act on the blood vessels. [vaso- + G. *tropē*, a turning]

va·so·va·gal (vă-sō-vā´găl, vas-ō-). Relating to the action of the vagus nerve upon the blood vessels.

va·so·va·sos·to·my (vă´sō-vă-sos´tō-mē, vas´ō-). Surgical anastomosis of vasa deferentia, to restore fertility in a previously vasectomized male. [vaso- + vaso- + G. *stoma*, mouth]

va·so·ve·sic·u·lec·to·my (vă´sō-vĕ-sik-ū-lek´tō-mē, vas´ō-). Excision of the vas deferens and seminal vesicles. [vaso- + L. *vesicula*, vesicle, + G. *ektomē*, excision]

vas·tomy (vas´tō-mē). Section of the vas deferens, usually with ligation. [vas + G. *tomē*, a cutting]

vas·tus (vas´tŭs). Great. SEE vastus intermedius (*muscle*), vastus lateralis (*muscle*), vastus medialis (*muscle*). [L.]

VATER Acronym for *v*ertebral defects, *a*nal atresia, *t*racheoesophageal fistula with *e*sophageal atresia, and *r*adial and *r*enal anomalies. SEE VATER *complex*.

Vater, Abraham, German anatomist and botanist, 1684–1751. SEE *ampulla* of Vater; V. *corpuscles*, under *corpuscle*, *fold;* V.-Pacini *corpuscles*, under *corpuscle*.

VATS Abbreviation for video-assisted thoracic *surgery*.

vault (vawlt). A part resembling an arched roof or dome, e.g., the pharyngeal v. or fornix, the nonmuscular upper part of the nasopharynx; the palatine v., arch of the plate; v. of the vagina, fornix of vagina. [thr. O. Fr., fr. L. *volvo*, pp. *volutus*, to turn round]

cranial v., SYN neurocranium.

v. of pharynx [TA], the nonmuscular, noncollapsing upper end of the nasopharynx where the pharyngeal mucosa is firmly applied to the body of the sphenoid bone and to pharyngobasilar fascia. SYN fornix pharyngis [TA], pharyngeal fornix.

V-bends. V-shaped bends incorporated in an archwire, usually placed mesially or distally to the canines (cuspids) and used as a "dead" area of wire through which torquing bends may be placed.

VC Abbreviation for colored *vision*; vital *capacity*.

VCUG Abbreviation for voiding *cystourethrogram*.

VDRL Abbreviation for Venereal Disease Research Laboratories. SEE VDRL *test*.

vec·tion (vek´shŭn). Transference of the agents of disease from an infected to an uninfected individual by a vector. [L. *vectio*, conveyance]

vec·tis (vek´tis). An instrument resembling one of the blades of an obstetrical forceps, used as an aid in delivery by making leverge on the presenting part of the fetus. [L. a lever or bar]

vec·tor (vek´ter, tōr). **1.** An invertebrate animal (e.g., tick, mite, mosquito, bloodsucking fly) capable of transmitting an infectious agent among vertebrates. **2.** Anything (e.g., velocity, mechanical force, electromotive force) having magnitude and direction; it can be represented by a straight line of appropriate length and direction. **3.** The net electrical axis of any ECG wave (usually QRS) whose length is proportional to the magnitude of the electrical force, whose direction gives the direction of the force, and whose tip represents the positive pole of the force. **4.** DNA such as a chromosome or plasmid that autonomously replicates in a cell to which another DNA segment may be inserted and be itself replicated, as in cloning. **5.** SYN recombinant v. **6.** Recombinant DNA systems especially suited for production of large quantities of specific proteins in bacterial, yeast, insect, or mammalian cell systems. [L. *vector,* a carrier]

biologic v., a v., such as the *Anopheles* mosquito for malarial agents or the tsetse fly for agents of African sleeping sickness, in which the agent multiplies prior to being transmitted to another host.

cloning v., an autonomously replicating plasmid or phage with regions that are not essential for its propagation in bacteria and into which foreign DNA can be inserted; this foreign DNA is replicated and propagated as if it were a normal component of the v.

expression v., a v. (plasmid, yeast, or animal virus genome) used experimentally to introduce foreign genetic material into a propagatable host cell in order to replicate and amplify the foreign DNA sequences as a recombinant molecule (recombinant DNA cloning of sequences).

instantaneous v., the resultant v. of the heart's action currents at any given moment, usually represented as an arrow of appropriate direction and magnitude.

manifest v., projection of a spatial cardiac v. on a single plane.

mean v., a single cardiac v. representing the average of all v.'s present during a given time interval. SYN mean manifest v.

mean manifest v., SYN mean v.

mechanical v., a v. that conveys pathogens to a susceptible individual without essential biologic development of the pathogens in the v., as in the transfer of septic organisms on the feet or mouth parts of the housefly.

recombinant v., a v. into which a foreign DNA has been inserted. SYN vector (5).

retroviral v., a specially constructed retrovirus containing one or more genes to correct certain genetic disorders.

shuttle v., a v. (4) that contains both bacterial and eukaryotic replication signals; thus, replication can occur in both types of cells.

spatial v., a cardiac v. represented in more than one plane simultaneously; two- or three-dimensional orientation of a v.

vec·tor-borne (vek´ter-bōrn). Denoting a disease or infection that is transmitted by an invertebrate vector.

▣**vec·tor·car·di·o·gram** (vek´tōr-kar´dē-ō-gram). A graphic representation of the instant-to-instant magnitude and direction of the heart's action currents in the form of vector loops.

vec·tor·car·di·og·ra·phy. The integration of scalar electrocardi-

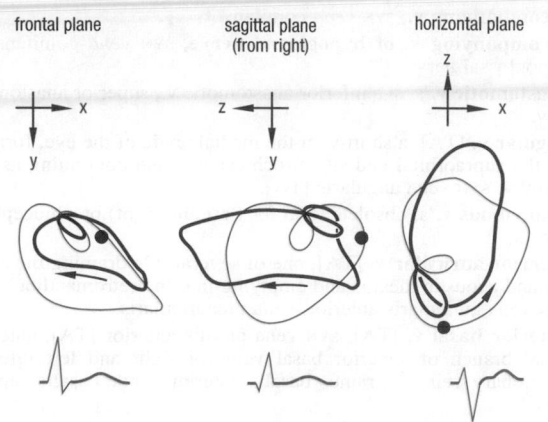

frontal plane

sagittal plane (from right)

horizontal plane

vectorcardiogram: normal scale ECG leads, as well as QRS and T vector loops in a vectorcardiogram (black line = adult; red line = child; thick dot = vector .02 s after beginning of ventricular stimulation)

ographic recordings on two or three planes to produce a vectorcardiogram consisting of loops divided by a timing mechanism for all the waves of the electrocardiogram.

spatial vectorcardiography, three-dimensional vectorcardiography in which vector loops are inscribed in frontal, sagittal, and horizontal planes.

vec·to·ri·al (vek-tōr′ē-ăl). Relating in any way to a vector.

ve·cu·ro·ni·um bro·mide (ve-kū-rō′nē-ŭm). A nondepolarizing neuromuscular relaxant with a relatively short duration of action; a monoquaternary homolog of pancuronium.

VEE Abbreviation for Venezuelan equine *encephalomyelitis*.

veg·an (veg′an). A strict vegetarian; i.e., one who consumes no animal or dairy products of any type. Cf. vegetarian.

veg·e·ta·ble (vej′tă-bl, vej′ĕ-tă-bl). **1.** A plant, specifically one used for food. **2.** Relating to plants, as distinguished from animals or minerals. SYN vegetal (1). [M.E., fr. L. *vegetabilis* (see vegetation)]

veg·e·tal (vej′ĕ-tăl). **1.** SYN vegetable (2). **2.** Denoting the vital functions common to plants and animals, such as respiration, metabolism, growth, generation, etc., distinguished from those peculiar to animals, such as conscious sensation and the mental faculties.

veg·e·tal·i·ty (vej-ĕ-tal′i-tē). The aggregate of the vital functions common to both plants and animals.

veg·e·tar·i·an (vej-ĕ-tār′ē-ăn). One whose diet is restricted to foods of vegetable origin, excluding primarily animal meats. Cf. vegan.

lacto-ovo-v., a v. who consumes dairy products and eggs but does not eat animal flesh.

ovo-v., a v. who consumes eggs but does not consume dairy products nor animal flesh.

semi-v., a v. who consumes dairy products, eggs, chicken, and fish, but does not consume other animal flesh.

veg·e·tar·i·an·ism (vej-ĕ-tār′ē-ăn-izm). The practice as to diet of a vegetarian.

veg·e·ta·tion (vej-ĕ-tā′shŭn). **1.** The process of growth in plants. **2.** A condition of sluggishness, comparable to the inactivity of plant life. **3.** A growth or excrescence of any sort. **4.** Specifically, a clot, composed largely of fused blood platelets, fibrin, and sometimes microorganisms, adherent to a diseased heart orifice or valve, and often initiated by infection of the structures involved. [Mod. L. *vegetatio,* growth]

bacterial v.'s, lesions of bacterial endocarditis that form anywhere on the endocardium but preferentially on higher pressure and injured areas and particularly valves. They may also appear on arterial intima and in a patent ductus arteriosus and other areas of shunt inside and outside the heart.

verrucous v.'s, wart-like v.'s sometimes due to endocarditis, also related to degenerative changes on the valves and amyloidosis.

veg·e·ta·tive (vej′ĕ-tā-tiv). **1.** Growing or functioning involuntarily or unconsciously, after the assumed manner of vegetable life; denoting especially a state of grossly impaired consciousness, as after severe head trauma or brain disease, in which an individual is incapable of voluntary or purposeful acts and only responds reflexively to painful stimuli. **2.** Resting; not active; denoting the stage of a cell or its nucleus in which the process of karyokinesis is quiescent. SEE ALSO vegetation.

veg·e·to·an·i·mal (vej′ĕ-tō-an′i-măl). Relating to both plants and animals.

ve·hi·cle (vē′hi-kl). **1.** An excipient or a menstruum; a substance, usually without therapeutic action, used as a medium to give bulk for the administration of medicines. **2.** An inanimate substance (e.g., food, milk, dust, clothing, instrument) by which or upon which an infectious agent passes from an infected to a susceptible host; v.'s consequently act as important sources of infection. [L. *vehiculum,* a conveyance, fr. *veho,* to carry]

veil (vāl). **1.** SYN velum (1). **2.** SYN caul (1). [L. *velum*]

aqueduct v., a membrane obstructing the sylvian aqueduct, causing a noncommunicating hydrocephalus.

Jackson v., SYN Jackson *membrane.*

Sattler v., a diffuse edema of the corneal epithelium that may develop after wearing contact lenses.

Veil·lo·nel·la (vā′yō-nel′ă). A genus of nonmotile, non–spore-forming, anaerobic bacteria (family Veillonellaceae) containing small (0.3–0.5 μm in diameter), Gram-negative cocci which occur as diplococci short chains and in masses. Carbon dioxide is required for growth, and carbohydrates are not fermented. These organisms are parasitic in the mouth and the intestinal and respiratory tracts of humans and other animals; they produce serologically specific endotoxins (lipopolysaccharides) that induce pyrogenicity and the Schwarzman phenomenon in rabbits; in humans, they have been associated with human bite infections and as a component of polymicrobial abscesses. The type species is *V. parvula.* [Adrien *Veillon,* French bacteriologist, 1864–1931]

V. alcales′cens subsp. *alcales′cens,* a bacterial subspecies found primarily in the mouth of humans but occasionally in the buccal cavity of rabbits and rats; it is the type subspecies of the species *V. alcalescens.*

V. alcales′cens subsp. *dis′par,* a subspecies found in the mouth and respiratory tract of humans.

V. alcales′ens, a bacterial species found in the saliva of humans and other animals.

V. aty′pica, SYN *V. parvula* subsp. *atypica.*

V. par′vula, a bacterial species found normally as a harmless parasite in the natural cavities, especially the mouth and digestive tract, of humans and other animals; it is the type species of the genus *V.*

V. par′vula subsp. *atyp′ica,* a bacterial subspecies found in the buccal cavity of rats and humans. SYN *V. atypica.*

V. par′vula subsp. *par′vula,* a bacterial subspecies found in the mouth or the intestinal or respiratory tract of humans; it is the type subspecies of the species *V. parvula.*

V. par′vula subsp. *roden′tium,* a bacterial subspecies found in the buccal cavity and intestinal tract of hamsters, rats, and rabbits. SYN *V. rodentium.*

V. roden′tium, SYN *V. parvula* subsp. *rodentium.*

Veil·lo·nel·la·ce·ae (vā′yō-nĕ-lā′sē-ē). A family of nonmotile, non–spore-forming, anaerobic bacteria (order Eubacteriales) containing Gram-negative (with a tendency to resist decolorization) cocci which vary in diameter from small (0.3–0.5 μm) to large (2.5 μm). Characteristically, they occur in pairs; single cells, masses, or chains may also occur, but the chains may show gaps illustrating the basic diplococcal arrangement. These organisms are chemoorganotrophic; they may or may not ferment carbohydrates; they are parasites of homothermic animals such as humans, ruminants, rodents, and pigs, and are primarily found in the alimentary tract. The type genus is *Veillonella.*

Ve

VEIN

⊞ vein (vān) [TA]. A blood vessel carrying blood toward the heart; postnatally, all v.'s except the pulmonary carry dark unoxygenated blood. SYN vena [TA]. [L. *vena*]

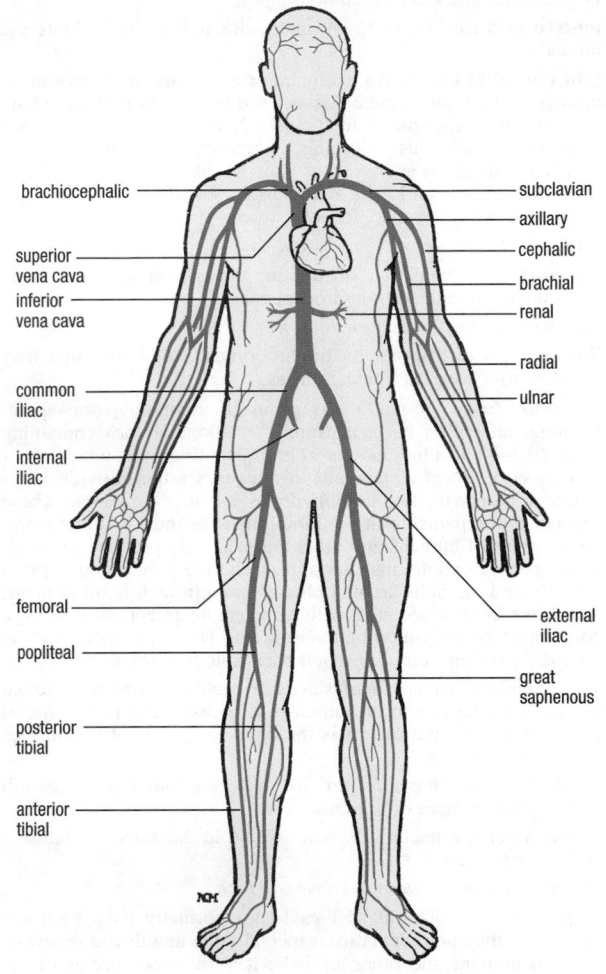

brachiocephalic

superior vena cava

inferior vena cava

common iliac

internal iliac

femoral

popliteal

posterior tibial

anterior tibial

subclavian

axillary

cephalic

brachial

renal

radial

ulnar

external iliac

great saphenous

major veins of the body

accessory cephalic v. [TA], a variable v. that passes along the radial border of the forearm to join the cephalic v. near the elbow. SYN vena cephalica accessoria [TA].

accessory hemiazygos v. [TA], formed by the union of the fourth to seventh left posterior intercostal v.'s, passes along the side of the bodies of the fifth, sixth, and seventh thoracic vertebrae, then crosses the midline behind the aorta, esophagus, and thoracic duct, and empties into the azygos v., sometimes in common with the hemiazygos v. SYN vena hemiazygos accessoria [TA], vena azygos minor superior.

accessory saphenous v. [TA], an occasional v. running in the thigh parallel to the great saphenous v. which it joins just before the latter empties into the femoral v. SYN vena saphena accessoria [TA].

accessory vertebral v. [TA], a v. that accompanies the vertebral v. but passes through the foramen of the transverse process of the seventh cervical vertebra and opens independently into the brachiocephalic v. SYN vena vertebralis accessoria [TA].

accompanying v., SYN *vena* comitans.

accompanying v. of hypoglossal nerve, SYN *vena* comitans of hypoglossal nerve.

anastomotic v.'s, SEE inferior anastomotic v., superior anastomotic v.

angular v. [TA], a short v. at the medial angle of the eye, formed by the supraorbital and supratrochlear v.'s and continuing as the facial v. SYN vena angularis [TA].

anonymous v.'s, obsolete term for (left and right) brachiocephalic v.'s.

anterior auricular v. [TA], one of several v.'s draining the auricle and acoustic meatus and emptying into the retromandibular v. SYN vena auricularis anterior, vena preauricularis.

anterior basal v. [TA], SYN vena basalis anterior [TA], anterior basal branch of superior basal vein (of right and left inferior pulmonary veins)✳, ramus basalis anterior venae basalis superioris✳.

anterior cardiac v.'s [TA], two or three small v.'s in the anterior wall of the right ventricle opening directly into the right atrium independently of the coronary sinus. SYN venae cardiacae anteriores [TA].

anterior cerebral v.'s [TA], small v.'s that parallel the anterior cerebral artery and drain into the basal v. SYN venae anteriores cerebri [TA].

anterior ciliary v.'s [TA], several small v.'s, anterior and posterior, coming from the ciliary body. SYN venae ciliares anteriores [TA].

anterior circumflex humeral v. [TA], vein accompanying the artery of the same name, passing anterior to the surgical neck of the humerus to enter the axillary vein. SYN vena circumflexa humeri anterior [TA].

anterior facial v., SYN facial v.

anterior intercostal v.'s [TA], tributaries to the musculophrenic or internal thoracic v.'s from the anterior portions of intercostal spaces. SYN venae intercostales anteriores [TA].

anterior jugular v. [TA], it arises below the chin from v.'s draining the lower lip and mental region, descends the anterior portion of the neck superficial or deep to the investing cervical fascia, and terminates in the external jugular v. at the lateral border of the scalenus anterior muscle. SYN vena jugularis anterior [TA].

anterior labial v.'s [TA], tributaries of the femoral or external pudendal v.'s draining the mons pubis and anterior labia majora. SYN venae labiales anteriores [TA].

anterior pontomesencephalic v., a v. in the midline of the interpeduncular fossa on the superior and anterior aspect of the pons; it communicates with the basal v. superiorly and the petrosal v. inferiorly. SYN vena pontomesencephalica anterior.

(anterior and posterior) vestibular v.'s [TA], v.'s draining the saccule and utricle; they are tributaries of both the labyrinthine v.'s and the v. of the vestibular aqueduct. SYN venae vestibulares (anterius et posterius) [TA].

anterior scrotal v.'s [TA], tributaries of the femoral or external pudendal v.'s draining the anterior aspect of the scrotum and the skin and dartos fascia of the shaft and base of the penis. SYN venae scrotales anteriores [TA].

anterior v. of septum pellucidum [TA], v. draining the anterior part of the transparent septum; it empties into the superior thalamostriate v. SYN vena anterior septi pellucidi [TA].

anterior tibial v.'s [TA], the venae comitantes of the anterior tibial artery that empty into the popliteal v. SYN venae tibiales anteriores [TA].

anterior vertebral v. [TA], the small v. that accompanies the ascending cervical artery; it opens below into the vertebral v. SYN vena vertebralis anterior [TA].

apical v. [TA], SYN vena apicalis [TA], apical branch of right superior pulmonary vein✳, ramus apicalis venae pulmonalis dextrae superioris✳.

apicoposterior v. [TA], drains the apicoposterior bronchopulmonary segment of the superior lobe of the left lung. SYN vena apicoposterior [TA], apicoposterior branch of left superior pulmonary vein★, ramus apicoposterior venae pulmonalis sinistrae superioris★.

appendicular v. [TA], the tributary of the ileocolic v. that accompanies the appendicular artery. SYN vena appendicularis [TA].

aqueous v., a tributary of the anterior ciliary v. that receives aqueous humor from the sinus venosus sclerae.

arciform v.'s of kidney, SYN arcuate v.'s of kidney.

arcuate v.'s of kidney, v.'s that parallel the arcuate arteries, receive blood from interlobular v.'s and straight venules, and terminate in interlobar v.'s. SYN arciform v.'s of kidney, venae arcuatae renis.

arterial v., so called because it ramifies like an artery (portal v.) or because, while proceeding from the heart like an artery, it contains unoxygenated blood, like a v. (pulmonary artery). SYN vena arteriosa.

ascending lumbar v. [TA], paired, vertical v. of the posterior abdominal wall, adjacent and parallel to the vertebral column, posterior to the origin of the psoas major muscle; it connects the common iliac, iliolumbar, and lumbar v.'s in the paravertebral line, the right v. joining the right subcostal v. to form the azygos v., the left v. uniting with the left subcostal v. to form the hemiazygos v. SYN vena lumbalis ascendens [TA].

auricular v.'s, SEE anterior auricular v., posterior auricular v.

axillary v. [TA], a continuation of the basilic and brachial v.'s running from the lower border of the teres major muscle to the outer border of the first rib where it becomes the subclavian v. SYN vena axillaris [TA].

azygos v. [TA], arises from the merger of the right ascending lumbar v. with the right subcostal v. and often a communication with the inferior vena cava; ascends through the aortic hiatus of the diaphragm or its right crus; it runs along the right side of the thoracic vertebral bodies in the posterior mediastinum, and terminates by arching anteriorly over the root of the right lung to enter the posterior aspect of the superior vena cava. SYN vena azygos [TA], azygos (2), vena azygos major.

basal v., a large v. originating from the confluence of v.'s from the orbital cortex (anterior cerebral veins [TA]) and the area of the insular cortex [deep middle cerebral vein [TA] (vena media profunda cerebri [TA]), insular veins [TA] (venae insulares [TA])], and passing caudally and dorsally along the medial surface of the temporal lobe, eventually emptying into the great cerebral vein. The basal v. receives tributaries from structures along its course; these include v. of olfactory gyrus [TA] (vena gyri olfactori [TA]), inferior thalamostriate v.'s [TA] (venae thalamostriatae inferiores [TA]), inferior ventricular v. [TA] (vena ventricularis inferior [TA]), inferior choroid v. [TA] (vena choroidea inferior [TA]), and peduncular v.'s [TA] (venae pedunculares [TA]). SEE ALSO common basal v., inferior basal v., superior basal v. SYN vena basalis [TA], basal v. of Rosenthal, Rosenthal v.

basal v. of Rosenthal, SYN basal v.

basilic v. [TA], arises from the ulnar side of the dorsal venous network of the hand; it curves around the medial side of the forearm (as the basilic vein of forearm), communicates with the cephalic v. via the median cubital v., and passes up the medial side of the arm to join the axillary v. SYN vena basilica [TA].

basivertebral v.'s [TA], v.'s in the spongy substance of the bodies of the vertebrae, emptying into the anterior internal vertebral venous plexus. SYN venae basivertebrales [TA].

Baumgarten v.'s, nonobliterated remnants of the vena umbilicalis.

Boyd communicating perforation v., a v. connecting the superficial and deep venous system in the anteromedial calf.

brachial v.'s [TA], venae comitantes of the brachial artery which empty into the axillary v. SYN venae brachiales [TA].

Breschet v., SYN diploic v.

bronchial v.'s [TA], many v.'s running in front of and behind the bronchi and uniting into two main trunks which empty on the right side into the azygos v., on the left into the accessory hemiazygos or the left superior intercostal v. SYN venae bronchiales [TA].

Browning v., SYN inferior anastomotic v.

v. of bulb of penis [TA], a tributary of the internal pudendal v. that drains the bulb of the penis. SYN vena bulbi penis [TA].

v. of bulb of vestibule [TA], the v. draining the bulb of the vestibule; a tributary of the internal pudendal v. SYN vena bulbi vestibuli [TA], v. of vestibular bulb.

Burow v., (1) an occasional v. passing from the inferior epigastric, sometimes receiving a tributary from the urinary bladder, which empties into the portal v.; (2) one of the renal v.'s.

capillary v., SYN venule.

cardiac v.'s, SEE anterior cardiac v.'s, great cardiac v., middle cardiac v., smallest cardiac v.'s.

cardinal v.'s, the major systemic venous channels in adult primitive vertebrates and in the embryos of higher vertebrates; the **anterior cardinal v.'s** are the major drainage channels from the cephalic part of the body, and the **posterior cardinal v.'s,** from the caudal part; the **common cardinal v.'s,** formed by the anastomosis of the anterior and posterior cardinal v.'s, are the main systemic return channels to the heart; in the older literature, sometimes called Cuvier ducts.

v.'s of caudate nucleus [TA], small v.'s from the caudate nucleus draining into the superior thalamostriate vein. SYN venae nuclei caudati [TA].

cavernous v.'s of penis [TA], the cavernous venous spaces in the erectile tissue of the penis. SYN venae cavernosae penis [TA].

central v.'s of liver [TA], initial v. of the hepatic venous system, located in the center of the conceptual hepatic lobule, receiving blood from sinuses and draining into collecting veins that become hepatic veins. SYN Krukenberg v.'s, venae centrales hepatis.

central retinal v. [TA], the v., formed by union of the retinal v.'s; accompanies the artery of the same name in the optic nerve. SYN vena centralis retinae [TA].

central v. of suprarenal gland [TA], the single draining v. of the gland; it receives a number of medullary v.'s; on the right side it empties directly into the inferior vena cava and on the left into the left renal v. SYN vena centralis glandulae suprarenalis [TA].

cephalic v. [TA], subcutaneous vein that arises at the radial border of the dorsal venous network of the hand, passes upward in front of the elbow and along the lateral side of the arm; it empties into the upper part of the axillary v. SYN vena cephalica [TA].

cephalic v. of forearm [TA], portion of cephalic vein between the dorsal venous network of the hand and the elbow (cubital) region. SYN vena cephalica antebrachii [TA].

cerebellar v.'s [TA], the v.'s draining the cerebellum. SEE inferior v.'s of cerebellar hemisphere, superior v.'s of cerebellar hemisphere, petrosal v., precentral cerebellar v., inferior v. of vermis, superior v. of vermis. SYN venae cerebelli [TA], v.'s of cerebellum.

v.'s of cerebellum, SYN cerebellar v.'s.

cerebral v.'s, SEE anterior cerebral v.'s, deep middle cerebral v., great cerebral v., superficial middle cerebral v.

cervical v., SEE deep cervical v.

choroid v., SEE inferior choroid v., superior choroid v.

choroid v.'s of eye, SYN vorticose v.'s.

circumflex v.'s, SEE anterior circumflex humeral v., circumflex scapular v., deep circumflex iliac v., lateral circumflex femoral v.'s, medial circumflex femoral v.'s, posterior circumflex humeral v., superficial circumflex iliac v.

circumflex scapular v. [TA], v. accompanying the artery of the same name draining the structures of infraspinous fossa around the lateral side of the scapula into the subscapular v.

v. of cochlear aqueduct, SYN v. of cochlear canaliculus.

v. of cochlear canaliculus, v. that drains the basal turn of the cochlea, the sacculus, and part of the utriculus, and empties into the superior bulb of the jugular v. by accompanying the perilymphatic duct (cochlear aqduduct) through the cochlear canaliculus. SYN v. of cochlear aqueduct, vena aqueductus cochleae, vena canaliculi cochleae.

v. of cochlear window [TA], v. of the internal ear draining the region of the round window; drains into the vestibulocochlear vein. SYN vena fenestrae cochleae [TA].

Cockett communicating perforating v.'s, mid-thigh perforation v.'s that connect the deep and superficial venous systems.

ve

colic v.'s, SEE right colic v., middle colic v., left colic v.

common basal v. [TA], the tributary to the inferior pulmonary v. (right and left) that receives blood from the superior and inferior basal v.'s. SYN vena basalis communis [TA].

common cardinal v.'s, SEE cardinal v.'s.

common facial v., a short vessel formed by the union of the facial v. and the retromandibular v., emptying into the jugular v.; considered to be a continuation of the facial v. in the NA. SYN vena facialis communis.

common iliac v. [TA], formed by the union of the external and internal iliac v.'s at the brim of the pelvis and passes upward behind the internal iliac artery to the right side of the body of the fifth lumbar vertebra where it unites with its fellow of the opposite side to form the inferior vena cava; the left common iliac v. is submitted to a pulsating compression by the right common iliac artery against the vertebral column which may result in partial obstruction of the v. SYN vena iliaca communis [TA].

common modiolar v. [TA], the v. running a spiral course in the modiolus of the cochlea; it is tributary to both the labyrinthine v. and the v. of the cochlear aqueduct. SYN vena modioli communis [TA], spiral v. of modiolus, vena spiralis modioli.

companion v.'s, SYN *venae* comitantes, under *vena*.

condylar emissary v. [TA], a v. that connects the sigmoid sinus and the external vertebral venous plexuses through the condylar canal of the occipital bone. SYN vena emissaria condylaris [TA], emissarium condyloideum.

conjunctival v.'s [TA], the v.'s of the conjunctiva that drain primarily to the ophthalmic v.'s. SYN venae conjunctivales [TA].

coronary v., SYN left gastric v.

v. of corpus striatum, SYN superior thalamostriate v.

costoaxillary v., one of a number of anastomotic v.'s connecting the intercostal v.'s of the first to seventh intercostal spaces with the lateral thoracic or the thoracoepigastric v.

cutaneous v., SYN superficial v.

Cuvier v.'s, the common cardinal v.'s of the embryo. SEE cardinal v.'s.

cystic v.'s [TA], v.'s, usually anterior and posterior, which drain the neck of the gallbladder and cystic duct, along which they pass to enter the right branch of the portal v.; they communicate extensively with surrounding v.'s of the stomach, duodenum, and pancreas. SYN vena cystica [TA].

deep cerebral v.'s [TA], the numerous v.'s draining the deep structures of the cerebral hemispheres; they empty into the tributaries of the great cerebral v. SYN venae profundae cerebri [TA].

deep cervical v. [TA], large v. running with the artery of the same name between the semispinalis capitis and semispinalis cervicis, draining the deep muscles at the back of the neck and emptying into the brachiocephalic or the vertebral v. SYN vena cervicalis profunda [TA], vena colli profunda ☆.

deep circumflex iliac v. [TA], corresponds to the artery of the same name, courses medially parallel to the inguinal ligament, and empties, near or in a common trunk with the inferior epigastric v., into the external iliac v. SYN vena circumflexa iliaca profunda [TA].

deep v.'s of clitoris [TA], the v.'s that pass from the dorsum of the clitoris to join the vesical plexus. SYN venae profundae clitoridis [TA].

deep dorsal v. of clitoris [TA], a tributary of the vesical venous plexus; it runs a course deep to the fascia on the dorsum of the clitoris. SYN vena dorsalis clitoridis profunda [TA].

deep dorsal v. of penis [TA], a vein on the dorsum of the penis deep to the fascia of the penis; it is a tributary to the prostatic venous plexus. SYN vena dorsalis penis profunda [TA].

deep epigastric v., SYN inferior epigastric v.

deep facial v. [TA], the communicating v. that passes from the pterygoid venous plexus of the infratemporal fossa to the facial v.; it is devoid of valves. SYN vena faciei profunda [TA].

deep femoral v., SYN profunda femoris v.

deep lingual v. [TA], the principal v. of the tongue that accompanies the deep lingual artery and joins the lingual v. It drains the body and apex of the tongue, running posteriorly near the median plane; often visible through the mucosa on the underside of the tongue, to each side of the frenulum. SYN vena profunda linguae [TA].

deep middle cerebral v. [TA], the v. that accompanies the middle cerebral artery in the depths of the lateral sulcus and empties into the basal v. of Rosenthal. SYN vena media profunda cerebri [TA].

deep v.'s of penis [TA], the veins deep to the fascia of the penis that drain via the internal pudendal vein to the internal iliac vein. SYN venae profundae penis.

deep temporal v.'s [TA], v.'s corresponding to the arteries of the same name; they empty into the pterygoid venous plexus. SYN venae temporales profundae [TA].

deep v. of thigh, ☆ official alternate term for profunda femoris v.

digital v.'s, SEE dorsal digital v.'s of foot, palmar digital v.'s, plantar digital v.'s.

diploic v. [TA], one of the v.'s in the diploë of the cranial bones, connected with the cerebral sinuses by emissary v.'s; the main diploic v.'s are the frontal, anterior temporal, posterior temporal, and occipital. SYN vena diploica [TA], Breschet v., Dupuytren canal.

direct lateral v.'s [TA], one or more veins running a subependymal course in a coronal plane over the thalamus, terminating in the internal cerebral vein. SYN venae directae laterales [TA], surface thalamic v.'s.

dorsal callosal v., SYN posterior v. of corpus callosum.

dorsal v.'s of clitoris, SEE deep dorsal v. of clitoris, superficial dorsal v.'s of clitoris.

dorsal v. of corpus callosum [TA], SYN posterior v. of corpus callosum.

dorsal digital v.'s of foot [TA], they receive intercapitular v.'s from the plantar venous arch, join to form four common dorsal digital v.'s, and terminate in the dorsal venous arch. SYN venae digitales dorsales pedis [TA], dorsal digital v.'s of toes.

dorsal digital v.'s of toes, SYN dorsal digital v.'s of foot.

dorsal lingual v. [TA], multiple tributaries of the lingual v. draining the dorsum of the tongue, becoming increasingly larger toward the root of the tongue. SYN venae dorsales linguae [TA].

dorsal metacarpal v.'s [TA], three v.'s on the dorsum of the hand draining blood from the four medial digits into the dorsal venous network of the hand. SYN venae metacarpeae dorsales [TA].

dorsal metatarsal v.'s [TA], v.'s arising from the dorsal digital v.'s forming the dorsal venous arch of the foot. SYN venae metatarseae dorsales [TA].

dorsal v.'s of penis, SEE deep dorsal v. of penis, superficial dorsal v.'s of penis.

dorsal scapular v. [TA], the vena comitans of the descending scapular artery; it is a tributary to the subclavian or the external jugular v. SYN vena scapularis dorsalis [TA].

dorsispinal v.'s, v.'s forming a plexus around the neural arches and processes of the vertebrae.

emissary v. [TA], one of the channels of communication between the venous sinuses of the dura mater and the v.'s of the diploë and the scalp. SEE ALSO condylar emissary v., mastoid emissary v., occipital emissary v., parietal emissary v. SYN vena emissaria [TA], emissarium, emissary (2).

epigastric v.'s, SEE inferior epigastric v., superficial epigastric v., superior epigastric v.'s.

episcleral v.'s [TA], a series of small venules in the sclera close to the corneal margin that empty into the anterior ciliary v.'s. SYN venae episclerales [TA].

esophageal v.'s [TA], series of v.'s draining the submucous venous plexus of the esophagus; proceeding inferiorly from the cervical portion of the esophagus, they drain to the inferior thyroid v., the superior intercostal v.'s, and the azygos, accessory hemiazygos, and hemiazygos v.'s, all of which are ultimately tributaries of the superior vena cava; the most inferior esophageal v.'s, from the cardiac portion of the esophagus, drain via the esophageal branches of the left gastric v., a tributary of the portal v. Thus, the submucosal v.'s of the inferior esophagus form a portocaval anastomoses, and are subject to the formation of varicosities in portal hypertension. SYN venae esophageae [TA].

ethmoidal v.'s [TA], v.'s that accompany the anterior and posterior ethmoidal arteries and pass into the superior ophthalmic v.; they drain the ethmoidal sinuses. SYN venae ethmoidales [TA].

external iliac v. [TA], a direct continuation of the femoral v. superior to the inguinal ligament, uniting with the internal iliac v. to form the common iliac v. SYN vena iliaca externa [TA].

external jugular v. [TA], superficial v. formed inferior to the parotid gland by the junction of the posterior auricular v. and the retromandibular v., and passing down the side of the neck crossing to the sternocleidomastoid muscle vertically to empty into the subclavian v. SYN vena jugularis externa [TA].

external nasal v.'s [TA], several vessels that drain the external nose, emptying into the angular or facial v. SYN venae nasales externae [TA].

external palatine v. [TA], drains the palatine regions and empties into the facial v. SYN vena palatina externa [TA].

external pudendal v.'s [TA], these correspond to the arteries of the same name; they empty into the great saphenous v. or directly into the femoral v., and receive the superficial dorsal v. of the penis (or clitoris) and the anterior scrotal (or labial) v.'s. SYN venae pudendae externae [TA].

v.'s of eyelids, SYN palpebral v.'s.

facial v. [TA], a continuation of the angular v. at the medial angle of the eye; it passes diagonally downward and outward, uniting with the retromandibular v. below the border of the lower jaw before emptying into the internal jugular v. SYN vena facialis [TA], anterior facial v., vena facialis anterior.

femoral v. [TA], a continuation of the popliteal v., it accompanies the femoral artery through the adductor canal and into the femoral triangle where it lies within the femoral sheath; it becomes the external iliac v. as it passes deep to the inguinal ligament. SYN vena femoralis [TA].

fibular v.'s [TA], venae comitantes of the peroneal artery; they join the posterior tibial v.'s to enter the popliteal v. SYN venae fibulares [TA], peroneal v.'s☆, venae peroneae☆.

frontal v.'s, (1) the superficial v.'s draining the frontal cortex and emptying into the superior sagittal sinus; **(2)** SYN supratrochlear v.'s.

v.'s of Galen, (1) SYN internal cerebral v.'s; **(2)** SEE great cerebral v.

gastric v.'s, SEE short gastric v.'s, right gastric v., left gastric v.

gastroepiploic v.'s, SEE right gastroomental v., left gastroomental v.

genicular v.'s [TA], the v.'s that accompany the genicular arteries; they drain blood from the structures around the knee, terminating in the popliteal v. SYN venae geniculares [TA], v.'s of knee.

gluteal v.'s, SEE inferior gluteal v.'s, superior gluteal v.'s.

great cardiac v. [TA], begins at the apex of the heart (where it anastomoses with the middle cardiac v.), runs first with the anterior interventricular artery as it ascends the anterior interventricular groove, then turns to the left as it approaches or reaches the coronary groove to run with the circumflex branch of the left coronary artery; it merges with the oblique v. of the left atrium to form the coronary sinus. SYN vena cordis magna [TA], left coronary v., vena cardiaca magna.

great cerebral v. [TA], SYN great cerebral v. of Galen.

great cerebral v. of Galen, a large, unpaired v. formed by the junction of the two internal cerebral v.'s in the caudal part of the tela choroidea of the third ventricle; it passes caudally between the splenium of the corpus callosum and the pineal gland, curving dorsally to merge with the inferior sagittal sinus to form the straight sinus. SYN great cerebral v. [TA], vena magna cerebri [TA], great v. of Galen.

great v. of Galen, SYN great cerebral v. of Galen.

great saphenous v. [TA], formed by the union of the dorsal v. of the great toe and the dorsal venous arch of the foot, ascends in front of the medial malleolus, behind the medial condyle of the femur, and traverses the saphenous hiatus in the fascia lata to empty into the femoral v. in the upper part of the femoral triangle. SYN vena saphena magna [TA], large saphenous v., long saphenous v.

v.'s of heart [TA], collective term for all venous structures of the heart, including the coronary sinus and all cardiac veins. SYN venae cordis [TA].

hemiazygos v. [TA], formed by the merger of the left ascending lumbar v. with the left subcostal v. or a communication from the inferior vena cava, it pierces the left crus of the diaphragm, ascends along the left side of the bodies of the lower thoracic vertebrae, opposite the eighth vertebra, crosses the midline behind the aorta, thoracic duct, and esophagus, and empties into the azygos v., sometimes in common with the accessory hemiazygos v. SYN vena hemiazygos [TA], inferior hemiazygos v., vena azygos minor inferior.

hemorrhoidal v.'s, obsolete term for rectal v.'s. SEE inferior rectal v.'s, middle rectal v.'s, superior rectal v.

hepatic v.'s [TA], the v.'s that drain the liver; they collect blood from the central v.'s and terminate in three large v.'s opening into the inferior vena cava below the diaphragm and several small inconstant v.'s entering the vena cava at more inferior levels. SYN venae hepaticae [TA].

hepatic portal v. [TA], a wide short v. formed by the confluence of the superior mesenteric and splenic v. posterior to the neck of the pancreas, ascending anterior to the inferior vena cava, and dividing at the right end of the porta hepatis into right and left branches, which ramify within the liver. SYN vena portae hepatis [TA], portal v., vena portalis.

highest intercostal v., SYN supreme intercostal v.

hypogastric v., obsolete term for internal iliac v.

ileal v.'s, SEE jejunal and ileal v.'s.

ileocolic v. [TA], a large tributary of the superior mesenteric v. that runs parallel to the ileocolic artery and drains the terminal ileum, appendix, cecum, and the lower part of the ascending colon. SYN vena ileocolica [TA].

iliac v.'s, SEE common iliac v., external iliac v., internal iliac v., deep circumflex iliac v., superficial circumflex iliac v.

iliolumbar v. [TA], accompanying the artery of the same name, anastomosing with the lumbar and deep circumflex iliac v.'s, and emptying into the internal iliac v. SYN vena iliolumbalis [TA].

inferior anastomotic v. [TA], an inconstant v. that passes from the superficial middle cerebral v. posteriorly over the lateral aspect of the temporal lobe to enter the transverse sinus. SYN vena anastomotica inferior [TA], Browning v., Labbé v.

inferior basal v. [TA], tributary to the common basal v. draining the medial and posterior part of the inferior lobe in each lung. SYN vena basalis inferior [TA].

inferior cardiac v., SYN middle cardiac v.

inferior v.'s of cerebellar hemisphere [TA], several v.'s draining the inferior portion of the cerebellar hemispheres; they terminate in the petrosal v. SYN venae inferiores cerebelli [TA].

inferior cerebral v.'s [TA], numerous cerebral v.'s that drain the undersurface of the cerebral hemispheres and empty into the cavernous and transverse sinuses. Included in these v.'s are named branches serving the uncus (vein of uncus [TA], vena uncalis [TA]), the orbital cortex (orbital veins [TA]), venae orbitae [TA], and the temporal lobe (temporal veins [TA], venae temporales [TA]). SYN venae inferiores cerebri [TA].

inferior choroid v. [TA], a small v. draining the lower part of the choroid plexus of the lateral ventricle into the basal v. SEE ALSO basal v. SYN vena choroidea inferior [TA], vena choroidea inferior [TA].

inferior epigastric v. [TA], corresponds to the artery of the same name and empties into the external iliac v. just proximal to the inguinal ligament. SYN vena epigastrica inferior [TA], deep epigastric v.

v.'s of inferior eyelid, SYN inferior palpebral v.'s.

inferior gluteal v.'s [TA], the venae comitantes of the inferior gluteal artery uniting at the sciatic foramen to form a common trunk which empties into the internal iliac v. SYN venae gluteae inferiores [TA].

inferior hemiazygos v., SYN hemiazygos v.

inferior hemorrhoidal v.'s, obsolete term for inferior rectal v.'s.

inferior labial v. [TA], a tributary of the facial v. draining the lower lip. SYN vena labialis inferior [TA].

inferior laryngeal v. [TA], the v. passing from the lower part of

ve

the larynx to the unpaired thyroid plexus. SYN vena laryngea inferior [TA].

inferior mesenteric v. [TA], a continuation of the superior rectal v. at the brim of the pelvis, ascending to the left of the aorta behind the peritoneum and emptying into the splenic v. or into the superior mesenteric v. or rarely in the angle between these v.'s. SYN vena mesenterica inferior [TA].

inferior ophthalmic v. [TA], arises from the inferior palpebral and lacrimal v.'s and divides into two terminal branches, one of which runs to the pterygoid plexus while the other joins the superior ophthalmic v. or empties into the cavernous sinus. SYN vena ophthalmica inferior [TA].

inferior palpebral v.'s [TA], v.'s of inferior eyelid; v.'s originating in the inferior eyelid and emptying into the angular v. SYN venae palpebrales inferiores [TA], v.'s of inferior eyelid.

inferior phrenic v. [TA], the v. that drains the substance of the diaphragm and empties on the right side into the inferior vena cava, on the left side into the left suprarenal v.; often a second v. on the left side passes transversely across the diaphragm anterior to the esophageal hiatus to enter the inferior vena cava. SYN vena phrenica inferior [TA].

inferior rectal v.'s [TA], v.'s that pass to the internal pudendal v. from the inferior rectal venous plexus around the anal canal. SYN venae rectales inferiores [TA].

inferior thalamostriate v.'s [TA], v.'s draining the thalamus and striate body exiting the anterior perforated substance; tributary to the basal v. SEE ALSO basal v. SYN venae thalamostriatae inferiores [TA], striate v.'s, venae striatae.

inferior thyroid v. [TA], unpaired v. formed by v.'s from the isthmus and lateral lobe of the thyroid gland and from the plexus thyroideus impar; it terminates in the left brachiocephalic v. SYN vena thyroidea inferior [TA], vena thyroidea ima.

inferior ventricular v. [TA], vein draining the deep white matter of the superior and lateral portions of the temporal lobe; it begins in the body of the lateral ventricle and exits from the choroid fissure of the inferior horn where it joins the basal vein. SEE ALSO basal v. SYN vena ventricularis inferior [TA].

inferior v. of vermis [TA], a v. draining part of the inferior part of the cerebellum; it courses on the inferior surface of the vermis and terminates in the straight sinus. SYN vena inferior vermis [TA].

infrasegmental v.'s, SEE intersegmental v.

innominate v.'s, obsolete term for (left and right) brachiocephalic v.'s.

innominate cardiac v.'s, the small superficial v.'s of the heart. SYN Vieussens v.'s.

insular v.'s [TA], SYN *venae* insulares, under *vena*.

intercapitular v.'s [TA], the v.'s connecting the dorsal and palmar v.'s in the hand, or the dorsal and plantar v.'s in the foot. SYN venae intercapitulares.

intercostal v.'s, SEE anterior intercostal v.'s, posterior intercostal v.'s, supreme intercostal v., left superior intercostal v.

interlobar v.'s of kidney [TA], the v.'s in the kidney that parallel the interlobar arteries, receiving blood from arcuate v.'s, and terminate in the renal v. SYN venae interlobares renis [TA].

interlobular v.'s of kidney [TA], v.'s that parallel the interlobular arteries and drain the peritubular capillary plexus, emptying into the arcuate v.'s. SYN venae interlobulares renis [TA].

interlobular v.'s of liver [TA], the terminal branches of the portal v. that course in the portal canals between the conceptual liver lobules and empty into the liver sinusoids. SYN venae interlobulares hepatis [TA].

intermediate antebrachial v., SYN median antebrachial v.

intermediate basilic v. [TA], the medial branch of the median antebrachial v. that joins the basilic v., often replacing a median cubital vein. SYN vena intermedia basilica [TA], median basilic v., vena mediana basilica.

intermediate cephalic v. [TA], the lateral branch of the median antebrachial v. that joins the cephalic v. near the elbow, often replacing a median cubital vein. SYN vena intermedia cephalica [TA], median cephalic v., vena mediana cephalica.

intermediate cubital v., SYN median cubital v.

intermediate v. of forearm, SYN median antebrachial v.

intermediate hepatic v.'s [TA], v.'s draining the central portion of the liver (the left sides of the superior anterior segment [VIII]) and the inferior anterior segment [V] of the right (part of the) liver and the right side of the medial segment [IV] of the left (part of the) liver, forming a trunk that merges with that of the left hepatic v.'s about 90% of the time prior to entering the left side of the inferior vena cava. SYN venae hepaticae intermediae [TA], venae hepaticae mediae [TA], middle hepatic v.'s.

internal auditory v.'s, SYN labyrinthine v.'s.

internal cerebral v.'s [TA], paired v.'s passing caudally near the midline in the tela choroidea of the third ventricle, formed by the union of the choroid v., thalamostriate (terminal) v., and v. of septum pellucidum, and uniting caudally so as to form the great cerebral v. SYN venae internae cerebri [TA], v.'s of Galen (1).

internal iliac v. [TA], v.'s that course in the lesser pelvis from the upper border of the greater sciatic notch to the brim of the pelvis where it joins the external iliac v. to form the common iliac v.; it drains most of the territory supplied by the internal iliac artery. SYN vena iliaca interna [TA].

internal jugular v. [TA], main venous structure of the neck, formed as a continuation of the sigmoid sinus of the dura mater, contained within the carotid sheath as it descends the neck uniting, behind the sternoclavicular joint, with the subclavian v. to form the brachiocephalic v. SYN vena jugularis interna [TA].

internal pudendal v. [TA], a tributary of the internal iliac v. that accompanies the internal pudendal artery as a single or double vessel. It drains the perineum. SYN vena pudenda interna [TA].

internal thoracic v. [TA], venae comitantes of each artery of the same name, fusing into one at the upper part of the thorax and emptying into the brachiocephalic v. of the same side; receive drainage of anterior chest wall. SYN vena thoracica interna [TA].

intersegmental v., a v. receiving blood from adjacent bronchopulmonary segments; it emerges from the inferior margin of a segment to become a tributary of a branch of a pulmonary v. SYN intersegmental part of pulmonary vein [TA], partes intersegmentales venarum pulmonum [TA], infrasegmental part.

intervertebral v. [TA], one of numerous v.'s accompanying the spinal nerves through the intervertebral foramina, draining the spinal cord and vertebral venous plexuses, and emptying in the neck into the vertebral v., in the thorax into the intercostal v.'s, in the lumbar and sacral regions into the lumbar and sacral v.'s. SYN vena intervertebralis [TA].

intrasegmental v.'s, SYN intrasegmental *part* of pulmonary veins.

jejunal and ileal v.'s [TA], the v.'s that drain the jejunum and ileum; they terminate in the superior mesenteric v. SYN venae jejunales et ilei [TA].

jugular v.'s, SEE anterior jugular v., external jugular v., internal jugular v; SEE ALSO posterior anterior jugular v., jugular venous *arch*.

key v., a deep-seated, dilated v. causing a "spider burst" on the surface.

v.'s of kidney [TA], the tributaries of the renal v. that drain the kidney; they parallel the arteries in the kidney and consist of interlobular, arcuate, and interlobar v.'s.

v.'s of knee, SYN genicular v.'s.

Krukenberg v.'s, SYN central v.'s of liver.

Labbé v., SYN inferior anastomotic v.

labial v.'s, SEE anterior labial v.'s, posterior labial v.'s, inferior labial v., superior labial v.

labyrinthine v.'s [TA], one or more v.'s accompanying the labyrinthine artery; they drain the internal ear, pass out through the internal acoustic meatus, and empty into the transverse sinus or the inferior petrosal sinus. SYN venae labyrinthi [TA], internal auditory v.'s.

lacrimal v. [TA], small v. that drains the lacrimal gland, passing posteriorly through the orbit with the lacrimal artery to empty into the superior ophthalmic v. SYN vena lacrimalis [TA].

large v., a v., such as the inferior vena cava, characterized by having a reduced or absent tunica media and an adventitia with large bundles of longitudinally disposed smooth muscle.

large saphenous v., SYN great saphenous v.

laryngeal v.'s, SEE inferior laryngeal v., superior laryngeal v.

Latarget v., SYN prepyloric v.

lateral atrial v., SYN lateral v. of lateral ventricle.

lateral circumflex femoral v.'s [TA], the v.'s that accompany the lateral circumflex femoral artery, usually terminating in the femoral v. SYN venae circumflexae femoris laterales [TA].

lateral direct v.'s [TA], one or more veins running a subependymal course in a coronal plane over the thalamus, terminating in the internal cerebral vein.

lateral v. of lateral ventricle [TA], a v. draining deep portions of the temporal and parietal lobes; it runs in the lateral wall of the lateral ventricle to terminate in the superior thalamostriate v. SYN vena lateralis ventriculi lateralis [TA], lateral atrial v., vena atrii lateralis.

v. of lateral recess of fourth ventricle [TA], a small vein originating in the cerebellar tonsil, coursing by the lateral recess of the fourth ventricle on its way to terminate in the petrosal vein. SYN vena recessus lateralis ventriculi quarti [TA].

lateral sacral v.'s [TA], several v.'s that receive the drainage of the sacral venous plexus and sacral intervertebral v.'s, then accompany the corresponding artery and empty into the internal iliac v. on each side. SYN venae sacrales laterales [TA].

lateral thoracic v. [TA], a tributary of the axillary v. that drains the lateral thoracic wall and communicates with the thoracoepigastric and intercostal v.'s. SYN vena thoracica lateralis [TA].

left colic v. [TA], a tributary of the inferior mesenteric v. that accompanies the left colic artery and drains the left flexure and descending colon. SYN vena colica sinistra [TA].

left coronary v., SYN great cardiac v.

left gastric v. [TA], arises from a union of v.'s from both surfaces of the cardia of the stomach and an esophageal tributary from the cardiac portion of the esophagus; it runs in the lesser omentum and empties into the portal v. SEE ALSO esophageal v.'s. SYN vena gastrica sinistra [TA], coronary v., vena coronaria ventriculi.

left gastroepiploic v., ✵official alternate term for left gastroomental v.

left gastroomental v. [TA], the v. that accompanies the left gastroepiploic artery along the greater curvature of the stomach; it empties into the splenic v. SYN left gastroepiploic v.✵, vena gastro-omentalis sinistra.

left hepatic v. [TA], vein draining the medial segment [IV] and the left lateral segments [II & III] of the liver, a single or paired trunk of variable size that usually (90% of the time) merges with the middle hepatic vein prior to entering the terminal portion of the superior vena cava. SYN venae hepaticae sinistrae [TA].

left inferior pulmonary v. [TA], the v. returning oxygenated blood from the inferior lobe of the left lung to the left atrium; tributaries include the superior and common basal veins (branches) from the inferior lobe. SYN vena pulmonalis inferior sinistra [TA].

left ovarian v. [TA], begins as the pampiniform plexus at the hilum of the ovary and empties into the left renal v. SYN vena ovarica sinistra [TA].

(left and right) brachiocephalic v.'s [TA], formed by the union of the internal jugular and subclavian v.'s; other tributaries of the right brachiocephalic v. are the right vertebral and internal thoracic v.'s, and the right lymphatic duct; other tributaries of the left brachiocephalic v. are the left vertebral, internal thoracic, superior intercostal, thyroidea ima, and various anterior pericardial, bronchial, mediastinal v.'s, and the thoracic duct. SYN venae brachiocephalicae (dextrae et sinistrae) [TA].

left superior intercostal v. [TA], the v. formed by the union of the left second, third, and fourth intercostal v.'s; it passes forward across the arch of the aorta to empty into the left brachiocephalic v. and frequently communicates also with the accessory hemiazygos v. SYN vena intercostalis superior sinistra [TA].

left superior pulmonary v. [TA], the v. returning oxygenated blood from the left superior lobe of the lung to the left atrium; tributaries include the apicoposterior, anterior, and lingular veins (branches) from the superior lobe. SYN vena pulmonalis superior sinistra [TA].

left suprarenal v. [TA], the v. from the hilum of the left suprare-

nal gland that passes downward to open into the left renal v.; it usually is joined by the left inferior phrenic v. SYN vena suprarenalis sinistra [TA].

left testicular v. [TA], v. conveying blood from the left testis, originating as the pampiniform plexus and entering the left renal v. SYN vena testicularis sinistra [TA].

left umbilical v., the v. that returns the blood from the placenta to the fetus; traversing the umbilical cord, it enters the fetal body at the umbilicus and passes thence into the liver, where it is joined by the portal v.; its blood then flows by way of the ductus venosus and the inferior vena cava to the right atrium. SYN vena umbilicalis [TA].

levoatrio-cardinal v., the communication of a systemic v. with the left atrium, other than a left superior vena cava or coronary sinus; may be the right superior vena cava.

lingual v. [TA], v. that receives blood from the tongue, sublingual and submandibular glands, and muscles of the floor of the mouth; empties into the internal jugular or the facial v. SYN vena lingualis.

lingular v. [TA], the lingular branch of the left superior pulmonary vein. SYN ramus lingularis venae pulmonis sinistrae superioris✵, vena lingularis.

long saphenous v., SYN great saphenous v.

long thoracic v., incorrect term for lateral thoracic v.

v.'s of lower limb [TA], all veins, superficial and deep, draining blood from the lower limb. SYN venae membri inferioris [TA].

lumbar v.'s [TA], five in number, these v.'s accompany the lumbar arteries, drain the posterior body wall and the lumbar vertebral venous plexuses, and terminate anteriorly as follows: the first and second in the ascending lumbar v., the third and fourth in the inferior vena cava, and the fifth in the iliolumbar v.; all communicate via the ascending lumbar v.'s. SYN venae lumbales [TA].

Marshall oblique v., SYN oblique v. of left atrium.

masseteric v.'s, plexiform v.'s accompanying the masseteric artery that empty into the pterygoid venous plexus.

mastoid emissary v. [TA], the vein that connects the sigmoid sinus with the occipital vein or one of the tributaries of the external jugular vein by way of the mastoid foramen. SYN vena emissaria mastoidea [TA], emissarium mastoideum.

maxillary v. [TA], the posterior continuation of the pterygoid plexus; it joins the superficial temporal vein to form the retromandibular vein. SYN vena maxillaris [TA].

Mayo v., SYN prepyloric v.

medial atrial v., SYN medial v. of lateral ventricle.

medial circumflex femoral v.'s [TA], the venae comitantes that parallel the medial circumflex femoral artery. SYN venae circumflexae femoris mediales [TA].

medial v. of lateral ventricle [TA], a v. that drains deep portions of the parietal and occipital lobes; it runs in the medial wall of the lateral ventricle to empty into the internal capsule v. or the great cerebral v. SYN vena medialis ventriculi lateralis [TA], medial atrial v., vena atrii medialis.

median antebrachial v. [TA], it begins at the base of the dorsum of the thumb, curves around the radial side, ascends the middle of the forearm, and just below the bend of the elbow divides into the intermediate basilic and intermediate cephalic v.'s; sometimes it divides lower down, one branch going to the basilic v., the other to the intermediate v. of the elbow. SYN vena mediana antebrachii [TA], median v. of forearm✵, intermediate antebrachial v., intermediate v. of forearm, vena intermedia antebrachii.

median basilic v., SYN intermediate basilic v.

median cephalic v., SYN intermediate cephalic v.

median cubital v. [TA], a v. which passes across the anterior aspect of the elbow from the cephalic v. to the basilic v.; commonly this v. is replaced by intermediate basilic and intermediate cephalic v.'s. The median cubital v. is often used for venipuncture. SYN vena mediana cubiti [TA], intermediate cubital v., vena intermedia cubiti.

median v. of forearm, ✵official alternate term for median antebrachial v.

ve

median v. of neck, a v. occasionally present due to fusion of the two anterior jugular v.'s.

median sacral v. [TA], an unpaired v. accompanying the middle sacral artery receiving blood from the sacral venous plexus and emptying into the left common iliac v. SYN vena sacralis mediana [TA].

mediastinal v.'s [TA], several small v.'s from the mediastinum emptying into the brachiocephalic v.'s or the superior vena cava. SYN venae mediastinales [TA].

medium v., a v. characterized by having a thinner wall and larger lumen than its corresponding artery, and a media with small bundles of circular muscle separated by considerable connective tissue; valves also occur.

v.'s of medulla oblongata, the several v.'s that drain the medulla oblongata; they are tributaries primarily of the anterior spinal and the petrosal veins. The veins of the medulla oblongata are the anteromedian medullary vein [TA] (vena medullaris anteromediana [TA]), anterolateral medullary vein [TA] (vena medullaris anteromedialis [TA]), transverse medullary veins [TA] (venae medullares transversae [TA]), dorsal medullary veins [TA] (venae medullares dorsales [TA]), and posteromedian medullary vein [TA] (vena medullaris posteromediana [TA]). SYN venae medullae oblongatae [TA].

meningeal v.'s [TA], v.'s that accompany the meningeal arteries; they communicate with venous sinuses and diploic v.'s and drain into regional v.'s outside the cranial vault. SYN venae meningeae [TA].

mesencephalic v.'s, the several veins that drain the mesencephalon; the posterior ones are tributaries to the great cerebral vein; the lateral ones are tributaries to the basal vein. The main veins are: pontomesencephalic vein [TA] (vena pontomesencephalica [TA]), interpeduncular veins [TA] (venae interpedunculares [TA]), intercollicular vein [TA] (vena intercollicularis [TA]), and the lateral mesencephalic vein [TA] (vena mesencephalica lateralis [TA]). SYN venae mesencephalicae.

mesenteric v.'s, SEE inferior mesenteric v., superior mesenteric v.

metacarpal v.'s, SEE dorsal metacarpal v.'s, palmar metacarpal v.'s.

middle cardiac v. [TA], v. that begins at the apex of the heart (where it anastomoses with the great cardiac v.), and ascends within the posterior interventricular sulcus to the coronary sinus. SYN vena cordis media [TA], inferior cardiac v.

middle colic v. [TA], the tributary of the superior mesenteric v. that carries drainage of the transverse colon and accompanies the middle colic artery. SYN vena colica media [TA].

middle hemorrhoidal v.'s, obsolete term for middle rectal v.'s.

middle hepatic v.'s, SYN intermediate hepatic v.'s.

middle lobe v. [TA], middle lobe branch of 1) the right pulmonary artery (arteriae pulmonalis dextrae [NA]); 2) the right superior pulmonary vein (venae pulmonalis dextrae superior [NA]). SYN vena lobi medii [TA], middle lobe branch of right superior pulmonary vein, ramus lobi medii venae pulmonalis dextrae superioris.

middle meningeal v.'s [TA], the venae comitantes of the middle meningeal artery that empty into the pterygoid plexus. SYN venae meningeae mediae [TA].

middle rectal v.'s [TA], several v.'s that pass from the rectal venous plexus (in which they anastomose with the superior rectal v.'s) to the internal iliac v., which ultimately drains into the inferior vena cava. Since the superior rectal v.'s ultimately drain into the portal v., the middle retal v.'s participate in a portocaval anastomosis, and the rectal venous plexus is subject to varicosities (hemorrhoids) although they commonly occur in the absence of portal hypertension. SYN venae rectales mediae [TA].

middle temporal v. [TA], v. that arises near the lateral angle of the eye and joins the superficial temporal v.'s to form the retromandibular v. SYN vena temporalis media [TA].

middle thyroid v. [TA], v. that passes from the thyroid gland across the common carotid artery (generally parallel with, but usually separate from) the inferior thyroid arteries to empty into the internal jugular v. SYN vena thyroidea media [TA].

musculophrenic v.'s [TA], the v.'s that accompany the musculophrenic artery and drain blood from the upper abdominal wall and anterior portions of the lower intercostal spaces and the diaphragm. SYN venae musculophrenicae [TA].

nasofrontal v. [TA], the v. located in the anterior medial part of the orbit that connects the superior ophthalmic v. with the angular v. SYN vena nasofrontalis [TA].

oblique v. of left atrium [TA], a small v. on the posterior wall of the left atrium which merges with the great cardiac v. to form the coronary sinus; it is developed from the left common cardinal v., and occasionally persists as a left superior vena cava. SYN vena obliqua atrii sinistri [TA], Marshall oblique v.

obturator v.'s [TA], formed by the union of tributaries draining the hip joint and the obturator and adductor muscles of the thigh; they enter the pelvis by the obturator canal as venae comitantes of the obturator artery and empty into the internal iliac v. SYN vena obturatoria [TA].

occipital v. [TA], v. that drains the occipital region and empties into the internal jugular v. or the suboccipital plexus. SYN vena occipitalis [TA].

occipital cerebral v.'s, the superior cerebral v.'s draining the occipital cortex and emptying into the superior sagittal sinus and the transverse sinus. SYN venae encephali occipitales [TA].

occipital emissary v. [TA], an inconstant vessel perforating the squama of the occipital bone to connect the occipital v.'s with the confluens sinuum. SYN vena emissaria occipitalis [TA], emissarium occipitale.

v. of olfactory gyrus [TA], a tributary of the basal v. which drains the medial olfactory stria. SEE ALSO basal v. SYN vena gyri olfactorii [TA].

ophthalmic v.'s, SEE inferior ophthalmic v., superior ophthalmic v.

ovarian v.'s, SEE right ovarian v., left ovarian v.

palmar digital v.'s [TA], paired venae comitantes of the proper and common digital arteries that empty into the superficial palmar venous arch. SYN venae digitales palmares [TA].

palmar metacarpal v.'s [TA], v.'s emptying into the deep venous arch from which the radial and ulnar v.'s arise. SYN venae metacarpeae palmares [TA].

palpebral v.'s [TA], v.'s draining the superior eyelid posteriorly as tributaries of the superior ophthalmic v. SYN venae palpebrales [TA], v.'s of eyelids.

pancreatic v.'s [TA], v.'s draining the pancreas, emptying into the splenic v. and the superior mesenteric v. SYN venae pancreaticae [TA].

pancreaticoduodenal v.'s [TA], v.'s that accompany the superior and inferior pancreaticoduodenal arteries, emptying into the superior mesenteric or portal v. SYN venae pancreaticoduodenales [TA].

paraumbilical v.'s [TA], several small v.'s arising from cutaneous v.'s about the umbilicus running along the round ligament of the liver, and terminating as accessory portal v.'s in the substance of this organ; they constitute a portocaval anastomosis and are subject to varicosity during portal hypertension; varicose paraumbilical v.'s form the "caput medussae." SYN venae paraumbilicales [TA], Sappey v.'s.

parietal v.'s [TA], the superficial v.'s draining the parietal cerebral cortex and emptying into the superior sagittal sinus. SYN venae parietales [TA].

parietal emissary v. [TA], the v. that connects the superior sagittal sinus with the tributaries of the superficial temporal v. and other v.'s of the scalp. SYN vena emissaria parietalis [TA], emissarium parietale, Santorini v.

parotid v.'s [TA], branches draining part of the parotid gland and emptying into the retromandibular v. SYN venae parotideae [TA], posterior parotid v.'s.

pectoral v.'s [TA], v.'s draining the pectoral muscles and emptying directly into the subclavian v. SYN venae pectorales [TA].

peduncular v.'s [TA], small tributaries of the basal vein from the cerebral peduncle. SEE ALSO basal v. SYN venae pedunculares [TA].

perforating v.'s [TA], **(1)** the v.'s that accompany the perforating arteries from the profunda femoris artery; they drain blood from the vastus lateralis and hamstring muscles and terminate in the profunda femoris v. **(2)** valved communicating veins that drain superficial veins—especially those of the lower limb—into deep (subfascial) veins so that the musculovenous pump can propel the venous blood to the heart against gravity. SYN venae perforantes [TA].

pericardiacophrenic v.'s [TA], the v.'s accompanying the pericardiacophrenic artery and emptying into the brachiocephalic v.'s or superior vena cava. SYN venae pericardiacophrenicae [TA].

pericardial v.'s [TA], several small v.'s from the pericardium emptying directly into the brachiocephalic v.'s or superior vena cava. SYN venae pericardiacae [TA].

peroneal v.'s, ☆official alternate term for fibular v.'s.

petrosal v. [TA], a tributary of the superior petrosal sinus that receives venous channels from the midbrain, pons, and the lateral portions of the anterior lobe of the cerebellum.

pharyngeal v.'s [TA], several v.'s from the pharyngeal venous plexus emptying into the internal jugular v. SYN venae pharyngeae [TA].

phrenic v.'s, SEE inferior phrenic v., superior phrenic v.'s.

plantar digital v.'s [TA], v.'s that drain the plantar and distal dorsal aspects (nail beds) of the toes and pass back to form four metatarsal v.'s that in turn empty into the plantar venous arch. SYN venae digitales plantares [TA].

plantar metatarsal v.'s [TA], v.'s receiving the plantar digital v.'s and draining in turn into the deep plantar venous arch, which empties into the medial and lateral plantar v.'s. SYN venae metatarseae plantares [TA].

v.'s of pons, SYN pontine v.'s.

pontine v.'s, several v.'s running transversely or obliquely on the pons to join the petrosal v.; the main pontine v.'s are: anteromedian pontine v. [TA] (vena pontis anteromediana [TA]), anterolateral pontine v. [TA] (vena pontis anterolateralis [TA]), transverse pontine v.'s [TA] (venae pontis transversae [TA]), and the lateral pontine vein [TA] (vena pontis lateralis [TA]). SYN venae pontis [TA], v.'s of pons.

pontomesencephalic v., SEE anterior pontomesencephalic v.

popliteal v. [TA], formed at the lower border of the popliteus muscle by the union of the anterior and posterior tibial v.'s, ascends through the popliteal space where it receives the lesser saphenous v. and passes through the adductor hiatus, entering the adductor canal as the femoral v. SYN vena poplitea [TA].

portal v., SYN hepatic portal v.

posterior anterior jugular v., a variable tributary of the external jugular v. arising in the upper posterior part of the neck.

posterior auricular v. [TA], v. that drains the region posterior to the ear and then merges with the retromandibular v. to form the external jugular v. SYN vena auricularis posterior [TA].

posterior cardinal v.'s, SEE cardinal v.'s.

posterior circumflex humeral v. [TA], vein accompanying the artery of the same name, passing posterior to the surgical neck of the humerus and through the quadrangular space to enter the axillary vein. SYN vena circumflexa humeri posterior [TA].

posterior v. of corpus callosum [TA], it originates on the superior surface of the corpus callosum and runs posteriorly to terminate in the great cerebral v. SYN dorsal v. of corpus callosum [TA], vena posterior corporis callosi [TA], vena dorsalis corporis callosi☆, dorsal callosal v., posterior marginal v., posterior pericallosal v.

posterior facial v., SYN retromandibular v.

v. of posterior horn, a small vein draining the surface region of the posterior horn of the lateral ventricle; it is a tributary to the great cerebral vein. SYN vena cornus posterioris [TA].

posterior intercostal v.'s [TA], v.'s draining the intercostal spaces posteriorly; those of the first 1-C space drain into the brachiocephalic v.'s; from spaces 2–3 they drain into right and left superior intercostal v.'s; from the 4th to the 11th spaces on the right they are tributaries of the azygos v.; on the left they empty into either the hemiazygos or accessory hemiazygos v.'s. SYN venae intercostales posteriores [TA].

posterior labial v.'s [TA], v.'s that pass posteriorly from the labia majora and minora to the internal pudendal v.'s. SYN venae labiales posteriores [TA].

posterior marginal v., SYN posterior v. of corpus callosum.

posterior parotid v.'s, SYN parotid v.'s.

posterior pericallosal v., SYN posterior v. of corpus callosum.

posterior scrotal v.'s [TA], v.'s from the posterior aspect of the scrotum to the internal pudendal v.'s. SYN venae scrotales posteriores [TA].

posterior v. of septum pellucidum [TA], v. draining the posterior part of the transparent septum; it empties into the superior thalamostriate v. SYN vena posterior septi pellucidi [TA].

posterior v.(s) of left ventricle [TA], arise(s) on the diaphragmatic surface of the heart near the apex, run(s) to the left and parallel to the posterior interventricular sulcus, and empties-(empty) in the coronary sinus. SYN vena(e) posterior(es) ventriculi sinistri.

posterior tibial v.'s [TA], venae comitantes of the posterior tibial artery that join those of the anterior tibial artery to form the popliteal v. SYN venae tibiales posteriores [TA].

precentral cerebellar v. [TA], an unpaired v. originating in the precentral cerebellar fissure passing anterior and superior to the culmen on its way to terminate in the great cerebral v. SYN vena precentralis cerebelli [TA].

prefrontal v.'s, the superficial veins draining the prefrontal cerebral cortex and emptying into the superior sagittal sinus. SYN venae prefrontales [TA].

prepyloric v. [TA], a tributary of the right gastric v. that passes anterior to the pylorus at its junction with the duodenum. SYN vena prepylorica [TA], Latarget v., Mayo v.

profunda femoris v. [TA], the v. that accompanies the deep femoral artery, receiving perforating v.'s from the lateral and posterior aspects of the thigh. It joins the femoral v. in the femoral triangle, usually in common with the medial and lateral circumflex femoral v.'s. SYN vena profunda femoris [TA], deep v. of thigh☆, deep femoral v.

v. of pterygoid canal [TA], a v. accompanying the nerve and artery through the pterygoid canal and emptying into the pharyngeal venous plexus. SYN vena canalis pterygoidei [TA], vidian v.

pudendal v.'s, SEE external pudendal v.'s, internal pudendal v.

pulmonary v.'s [TA], four v.'s, two on each side, conveying oxygenated blood from the lungs to the left atrium of the heart. Those from the left lung and the inferior v. from the right lung are lobar v.'s, each draining a single lobe with the corresponding name; the right superior pulmonary v. drains both the superior and middle lobes of the right lung. SEE ALSO left inferior pulmonary v., left superior pulmonary v., right inferior pulmonary v., right superior pulmonary v. SYN venae pulmonales [TA].

pyloric v., SYN right gastric v.

radial v.'s [TA], venae comitantes of the radial artery continuing from those of the radial aspect of the deep palmar arch, draining into the venae comitantes of the brachial artery in the cubital fossa. SYN venae radiales [TA].

renal v.'s [TA], large v.'s formed at the renal hilus by the merger of the segmental v.'s anterior to the corresponding arteries; they open at right angles into the inferior vena cava at the level of the second lumbar vertebra. The left renal v. receives the left suprarenal v. and the left gonadal v., and passes through the angle between the abdominal aorta and superior mesenteric artery where it may be compressed. SYN venae renales.

retromandibular v. [TA], v. formed by the union of the superficial temporal and maxillary v.'s in front of the ear; it runs posterior to the ramus of the mandible through the parotid gland, and unites with the posterior auricular v. to form the external jugular v.; it usually has a large communicating branch with the facial v. SYN vena retromandibularis [TA], posterior facial v., temporomaxillary v., vena facialis posterior.

retroperitoneal v.'s, portacaval anastomoses formed from v.'s in the walls of retroperitoneal viscera, such as the ascending and descending colon, passing to the tributaries of the inferior vena cava in the posterior body wall instead of those of the portal v. SYN Retzius v.'s, Ruysch v.'s, venae retroperitoneales.

Retzius v.'s, SYN retroperitoneal v.'s.

ve

right colic v. [TA], the v. that parallels the right colic artery and drains blood from the ascending colon and right colic flexure. SYN vena colica dextra [TA].

right gastric v. [TA], it receives v.'s from both surfaces of the upper portion of the stomach, runs to the right along the lesser curvature of the stomach, and empties into the portal v. SYN vena gastrica dextra [TA], pyloric v.

right gastroepiploic v., *official alternate term for right gastroomental v.

right gastroomental v. [TA], a tributary of the superior mesenteric v. that parallels the right gastroepiploic artery along the greater curvature of the stomach. SYN vena gastro-omentalis dextra [TA], right gastroepiploic v.*.

right hepatic v.'s [TA], v.'s draining much of the right lobe of the liver (posterior lateral segment [VI] and right anterior lateral segment [VI] and the lateral parts of the posterior and inferior anterior medial segments [V and VII]) that merge to form a single or sometimes double trunk, draining into the right side of the suprahepatic portion of the inferior vena cava (between the superior surface of the liver and the diaphragm); when single, it is the largest v. of the liver. SYN venae hepaticae dextrae [TA].

right inferior pulmonary v. [TA], the v. returning oxygenated blood from the inferior lobe of the right lung to the left atrium; tributaries include the superior vein and the common basal vein from the right inferior lobe. SYN vena pulmonalis inferior dextra [TA].

right ovarian v. [TA], begins as the pampiniform plexus at the hilum of the ovary and opens into the inferior vena cava. SYN vena ovarica dextra [TA].

right superior intercostal v. [TA], a tributary of the azygos v. formed by the union of the right second, third, and fourth posterior intercostal v.'s. SYN vena intercostalis superior dextra [TA].

right superior pulmonary v. [TA], the v. returning oxygenated blood from the superior and middle lobes of the right lung to the left atrium; tributaries include apical anterior and posterior veins (branches) from the right superior lobe and the middle lobe vein. SYN vena pulmonalis superior dextra [TA].

right suprarenal v. [TA], the short v. that passes from the hilum of the right suprarenal to the inferior vena cava. SYN vena suprarenalis dextra [TA].

right testicular v. [TA], begins as the pampiniform plexus and ascends to joint the inferior vena cava. SYN vena testicularis dextra [TA].

Rosenthal v., SYN basal v.

Ruysch v.'s, SYN retroperitoneal v.'s.

sacral v.'s, SEE lateral sacral v.'s, median sacral v.

Santorini v., SYN parietal emissary v.

saphenous v.'s, SEE accessory saphenous v., great saphenous v., small saphenous v.

Sappey v.'s, SYN paraumbilical v.'s.

v. of scala tympani [TA], tributary of common modiolar vein draining the scala tympani of the cochlea. SYN vena scalae tympani [TA].

v. of scala vestibuli [TA], tributary of the common modiolar vein draining the scala tympani of the cochlea. SYN vena scalae vestibuli [TA].

scleral v.'s [TA], small v.'s draining the sclera; they are tributaries of the anterior ciliary v.'s. SYN venae sclerales [TA].

scrotal v.'s, SEE anterior scrotal v.'s, posterior scrotal v.'s.

v.'s of semicircular ducts [TA], veins draining the semicircular ducts, especially the ampullary parts, into the vein of the vestibular aqueduct. SYN venae ductuum semicircularium [TA].

v. of septum pellucidum, SEE anterior v. of septum pellucidum, posterior v. of septum pellucidum.

short gastric v.'s [TA], small vessels that drain the fundus and left portion of the stomach wall and empty into the splenic v. SYN venae gastricae breves [TA].

short saphenous v., SYN small saphenous v.

sigmoid v.'s [TA], the several tributaries of the inferior mesenteric v. that drain the sigmoid colon. SYN venae sigmoideae [TA].

small v., a v. in which the three tunics are poorly defined and thin; longitudinal elastic networks occur and the smooth muscle of the media, which is circularly arranged, may be incomplete or in one or two layers.

small cardiac v. [TA], an inconstant vessel, accompanying the right coronary artery in the coronary sulcus, from the right margin of the right ventricle, and emptying into the coronary sinus or the middle cardiac v. SYN vena cordis parva [TA].

smallest cardiac v.'s [TA], numerous small valveless venous channels that open directly into the chambers of the heart from the capillary bed in the cardiac wall, enabling a form of collateral circulation unique to the heart. SYN venae cardiacae minimae [TA], venae cordis minimae*, thebesian v.'s.

small saphenous v. [TA], arises on the lateral side of the foot from a union of the dorsal v. of the little toe with the dorsal venous arch, ascends behind the lateral malleolus, along the lateral border of the calcanean tendon and then through the middle of the calf to the lower portion of the popliteal space where it empties into the popliteal v. SYN vena saphena parva [TA], short saphenous v.

spermatic v., SEE right testicular v., left testicular v.

spinal v.'s [TA], the v.'s that drain the spinal cord; they form a plexus on the surface of the cord from which v.'s pass along the spinal roots to the internal vertebral venous plexus and then to the regional segmental veins, e.g., the posterior intercostal veins in the thoracic region. SYN venae spinales [TA].

v.'s of spinal cord [TA], the anterior and posterior spinal veins that lie on the surface of the spinal cord. SYN venae medullae spinalis [TA].

spiral v. of modiolus, SYN common modiolar v.

splenic v. [TA], arises by the union of several small v.'s at the hilum on the anterior surface of the spleen with the short gastric and left gastroomental v.'s; passes backward through the splenorenal ligament to the left kidney, then runs behind the upper border of the pancreas to the neck of the pancreas where it joins the superior mesenteric v. to form the portal v. SYN vena splenica [TA], vena lienalis.

stellate v.'s, SYN *venulae* stellatae, under *venula.*

Stensen v.'s, SYN vorticose v.'s.

sternocleidomastoid v. [TA], arises in the sternocleidomastoid muscle and accompanies the sternocleidomastoid branch of the occipital artery; drains into the internal jugular or superior thyroid v. SYN vena sternocleidomastoidea [TA].

striate v.'s, SYN inferior thalamostriate v.'s.

stylomastoid v. [TA], drains the tympanic cavity, traverses the facial canal exiting via the stylomastoid foramen, and empties into the retromandibular v. SYN vena stylomastoidea [TA].

subclavian v. [TA], the direct continuation of the axillary v. at the lateral border of the first rib; it passes medially to join the internal jugular v. and form the brachiocephalic v. on each side. SYN vena subclavia [TA].

subcutaneous v.'s of abdomen, the network of superficial v.'s of the abdominal wall that empty into the thoracoepigastric, superficial epigastric, or superior epigastric v.'s and form portocaval anastomoses through their communications with the paraumbilical v.'s. SYN venae subcutaneae abdominis.

sublingual v. [TA], v. which accompanies the sublingual artery in the floor of the mouth, lateral to the hypoglossal nerve; it may join the deep lingual v. to form the lingual v., or join the vena comitans nerve hypoglossi. SYN vena sublingualis [TA].

submental v. [TA], a v. situated below the chin, anastomosing with the sublingual v., connecting with the anterior jugular v., and emptying into the facial v. SYN vena submentalis [TA].

⊞ superficial v. [TA], one of a number of v.'s that course in the subcutaneous tissue and empty into deep v.'s; they form prominent systems of vessels in the limbs and are usually not accompanied by arteries. SYN vena superficialis [TA], cutaneous v., vena cutanea.

superficial cerebral v.'s [TA], the v.'s on the superficial surface of the cerebral hemispheres; they comprise three groups: superior, middle, and inferior. SYN venae superficiales cerebri [TA].

superficial circumflex iliac v. [TA], corresponding to the artery

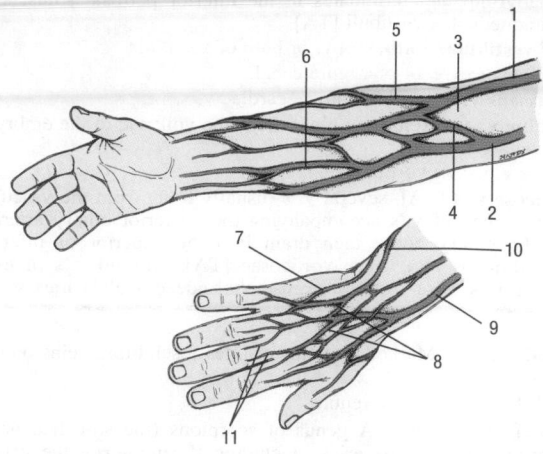

superficial veins of the hand and forearm: showing sites of selection for the insertion of intravenous needles or catheters for the parenteral administration of fluids, medications, or blood products; (1) cephalic vein, (2) basilic vein, (3) antecubital fossa, (4) median cubital vein, (5) accessory cephalic vein, (6) median antebrachial vein, (7) dorsal venous network, (8) metacarpal veins, (9) cephalic vein, (10) basilic vein, (11) digital veins

of the same name, emptying usually into the great saphenous v., or sometimes into the femoral v. SYN vena circumflexa iliaca superficialis [TA].

superficial dorsal v.'s of clitoris [TA], a pair of v.'s on the dorsum of the clitoris, tributary to the external pudendal v. on either side. SYN venae dorsales clitoridis superficiales [TA].

superficial dorsal v.'s of penis [TA], a pair of v.'s on the dorsum of the penis superficial to the fascia penis; they are tributaries of the external pudendal v.'s on each side. SYN venae dorsales penis superficiales [TA].

superficial epigastric v. [TA], drains the lower and medial part of the anterior abdominal wall and empties into the great saphenous v. SYN vena epigastrica superficialis [TA].

superficial middle cerebral v. [TA], a large v. passing along the line of the sylvian fissure to join the cavernous sinus; it communicates with the superior sagittal sinus and transverse sinus via the superior and inferior anastomotic v.'s, respectively. SYN vena media superficialis cerebri.

superficial temporal v.'s [TA], v.'s that pass from the temporal region to join the maxillary v. to form the retromandibular v. SYN venae temporales superficiales [TA].

superior anastomotic v. [TA], a large communicating v. between the superficial middle cerebral v. and the superior sagittal sinus; it passes upward from the lateral sulcus, often following the line of the central sulcus (Rolando fissure). SYN vena anastomotica superior [TA], Trolard v.

superior basal v. [TA], tributary to the common basal v. draining the lateral and anterior part of the inferior lobe of each lung. SYN vena basalis superior [TA].

superior v.'s of cerebellar hemisphere [TA], several v.'s draining the superior part of the cerebellar hemispheres; they terminate in the superior petrosal sinus or the petrosal v. SYN venae hemispherii cerebelli superiores [TA].

superior cerebral v.'s [TA], numerous (8–10) v.'s that drain the dorsal convexity of the cortical hemisphere and empty into the superior sagittal sinus, curving rostrally in passing through the subdural space so as to enter the sinus at an acute forward angle; can be divided into 5 general groups based on the area of cortex served: prefrontal veins [TA], frontal veins [TA] (venae frontales [TA]), parietal veins [TA], temporal veins [TA] (venae temporales [TA]), and occipital veins [TA] (venae occipitales [TA]). SYN venae superiores cerebri [TA].

superior choroid v. [TA], a tortuous v. that follows the choroid plexus of the lateral ventricle and unites with the superior thala-

mostriate v. and the anterior v. of the transparent septum to form the internal cerebral v. SYN vena choroidea superior [TA].

superior epigastric v.'s [TA], the venae comitantes of the artery of the same name, tributaries of the internal thoracic v. SYN venae epigastricae superiores [TA].

v.'s of superior eyelid, SYN superior palpebral v.'s.

superior gluteal v.'s [TA], the v.'s that accompany the superior gluteal artery, entering the pelvis as two v.'s which unite into one and empty into the internal iliac v. SYN venae gluteae superiores [TA].

superior hemorrhoidal v., outmoded term for superior rectal v.

superior intercostal v., SEE left superior intercostal v., right superior intercostal v.

superior labial v. [TA], v.'s taking blood from the upper lip and discharging into the facial v. SYN vena labialis superior [TA].

superior laryngeal v. [TA], vein which accompanies the superior laryngeal artery and empties into the superior thyroid vein. SYN vena laryngea superior [TA].

superior mesenteric v. [TA], begins at the ileum in the right iliac fossa, ascends in the root of the mesentery, and unites behind the pancreas with the splenic v. to form the hepatic portal v. SYN vena mesenterica superior [TA].

superior ophthalmic v. [TA], begins anteriorly from the nasofrontal v., passes along the upper part of the medial wall of the orbit, passes through the superior orbital fissure, to empty into the cavernous sinus. SYN vena ophthalmica superior [TA].

superior palpebral v.'s [TA], v.'s draining the superior eyelid anteriorly into the angular v. SYN venae palpebrales superiores [TA], v.'s of superior eyelid.

superior phrenic v.'s [TA], small v.'s that drain the upper surface of the diaphragm; they are tributaries of the azygos and hemiazygos v.'s. SYN venae phrenicae superiores [TA].

superior rectal v. [TA], it drains the greater part of the rectal venous plexus, and ascends between the layers of the mesorectum to the brim of the pelvis, where it becomes the inferior mesenteric v. As a tributary of the portal v., it forms a portocaval anastomosis with the middle and inferior rectal v.'s (caval tributaries) via the rectal venous plexus. SYN vena rectalis superior [TA].

superior thalamostriate v. [TA], a long v. passing forward in the groove between the thalamus and caudate nucleus, covered by the lamina affixa, receiving the transverse caudate v.'s along its lateral side, and joining at the caudal wall of Monro foramen with the choroidal v. and v. of septum pellucidum to form the internal cerebral v. SYN vena thalamostriata superior [TA], terminal v.☆, vena terminalis☆, v. of corpus striatum.

superior thyroid v. [TA], receives blood from the upper part of the thyroid gland and larynx, accompanies the artery of the same name, and empties into the internal jugular v. SYN vena thyroidea superior [TA].

superior v. of vermis [TA], a v. draining part of the superior part of the cerebellum; it runs on the superior surface of the vermis to terminate in the internal cerebral v. SYN vena superior vermis [TA].

supraorbital v. [TA], drains the front of the scalp and unites with the supratrochlear v.'s to form the angular v. SYN vena supraorbitalis [TA].

suprarenal v.'s, SEE right suprarenal v., left suprarenal v.

suprascapular v. [TA], v. that accompanies the suprascapular artery and empties into the external jugular v. SYN vena suprascapularis [TA], transverse v. of scapula, vena transversa scapulae.

supratrochlear v.'s [TA], several v.'s that drain the front part of the scalp and unite with the supraorbital v. to form the angular v. SYN venae supratrochleares [TA], frontal v.'s (2), venae frontales.

supreme intercostal v. [TA], the v. draining the first intercostal space into either the vertebral or the brachiocephalic v. SYN vena intercostalis suprema [TA], highest intercostal v.

surface thalamic v.'s, SYN direct lateral v.'s.

temporal v.'s, SEE middle temporal v., deep temporal v.'s, superficial temporal v.'s.

v.'s of temporomandibular joint, several small tributaries to the

ve

retromandibular v. from the temporomandibular joint. SYN venae articulares temporomandibulares.

temporomaxillary v., SYN retromandibular v.

terminal v., ☆official alternate term for superior thalamostriate v.

testicular v.'s, SEE right testicular v., left testicular v.

thalamostriate v.'s, SEE inferior thalamostriate v.'s, superior thalamostriate v.

thebesian v.'s, SYN smallest cardiac v.'s.

thoracic v.'s, SEE internal thoracic v., lateral thoracic v.

thoracoacromial v. [TA], v. corresponding to the artery of the same name, emptying into the axillary v., sometimes by a common trunk with the cephalic v. SYN vena thoracoacromialis [TA], thoracic axis (2).

thoracoepigastric v. [TA], one of two v.'s, sometimes a single v., arising from the region of the superficial epigastric v. and opening into the axillary or the lateral thoracic v., thus forming an anastomotic or collateral pathway between tributaries of the inferior and superior venae cavae. SYN vena thoracoepigastrica [TA].

thymic v.'s [TA], a number of small v.'s from the thymus emptying into the left brachiocephalic v. SYN venae thymicae [TA].

thyroid v.'s, SEE inferior thyroid v., middle thyroid v., superior thyroid v., *plexus* venosus thyroideus impar.

tracheal v.'s [TA], several small venous trunks from the trachea, emptying into the brachiocephalic v.'s or the superior vena cava. SYN venae tracheales [TA].

transverse cervical v.'s [TA], venae comitantes of the corresponding arteries, emptying into the external jugular v. or sometimes into the subclavian v. SYN venae transversae cervicis [TA], venae transversae colli☆, transverse v.'s of neck.

transverse v. of face, SYN transverse facial v.

transverse facial v. [TA], a tributary of the superficial temporal or retromandibular v.'s, anastomosing with the facial v. SYN vena transversa faciei [TA], transverse v. of face.

transverse v.'s of neck, SYN transverse cervical v.'s.

transverse v. of scapula, SYN suprascapular v.

Trolard v., SYN superior anastomotic v.

tympanic v.'s [TA], v.'s exiting from the tympanic cavity through the petrotympanic fissure with the chorda tympani and emptying into the retromandibular v. SYN venae tympanicae [TA].

ulnar v.'s [TA], venae comitantes of the ulnar artery, continuing from those of the superficial palmar arch and joining with those of the radial artery to form the brachial veins in the cubital fossa. SYN venae ulnares [TA].

umbilical v. [TA], SEE left umbilical v.

v. of uncus [TA], SYN *vena* uncalis.

v.'s of upper limb [TA], all veins, superficial and deep, that drain blood from the upper limb. SYN venae membri superioris [TA].

uterine v.'s [TA], two v.'s on each side that arise from the uterine venous plexus, pass through a part of the broad ligament and then through a peritoneal fold, and empty into the internal iliac v. SYN venae uterinae [TA].

varicose v.'s, permanent dilation and tortuosity of v.'s, most commonly seen in the legs, probably as a result of congenitally incomplete valves; there is a predisposition to varicose v.'s among persons in occupations requiring long periods of standing, and in pregnant women.

vertebral v. [TA], a v. derived from tributaries (venae comitantes) that run through the foramina in the transverse processes of the first six cervical vertebrae and form a plexus around the vertebral artery; it empties as a single trunk into the brachiocephalic v.'s. SYN vena vertebralis [TA].

v.'s of vertebral column [TA], includes the internal and external vertebral venous plexuses, the basivertebral v.'s, and the anterior and posterior spinal v.'s. SYN venae columnae vertebralis [TA].

Vesalius v., the emissary v. passing through the foramen venosum.

vesical v.'s [TA], v.'s that drain the vesical venous plexus; they join the internal iliac v.'s. SYN venae vesicales [TA].

v. of vestibular aqueduct [TA], a small v. accompanying the endolymphatic duct; it drains much of the vestibular portion of the labyrinth and terminates in the inferior petrosal sinus. SYN vena aqueductus vestibuli [TA].

v. of vestibular bulb, SYN v. of bulb of vestibule.

vidian v., SYN v. of pterygoid canal.

Vieussens v.'s, SYN innominate cardiac v.'s.

vitelline v., a v. returning blood from the yolk sac to the embryo. SYN vena vitellina.

vortex v.'s, SYN vorticose v.'s.

vorticose v.'s [TA], several v.'s (usually four) from the vascular tunic formed of v.'s accompanying the posterior ciliary arteries and the ciliary body; then drain into the superior or inferior ophthalmic v. SYN venae vorticosae [TA], choroid v.'s of eye, Stensen v.'s, vasa vorticosa, venae choroideae oculi, vortex v.'s.

veined (vānd). Marked by veins or lines resembling veins on the surface.

vein·let (vān'let). SYN venule.

Ve·jo·vis (vē-jō'vis). A genus of scorpions (the so-called devil scorpions of North America), including *V. spinigerus,* the striped-tailed devil scorpion; *V. carolinianus,* the southern devil scorpion; and *V. flavus,* the slender devil scorpion.

vel (vel). or [L. or]

ve·la (vē'lă). Plural of velum.

ve·la·men, pl. **ve·lam·i·na** (vĕ-lā'men, vĕ-lam'i-nă). SYN velum (1). [L. a veil]

v. vul'vae, obsolete term for hypertrophy of the labia minora.

vel·a·men·tous (vel-ă-men'tŭs). Expanded in the form of a sheet or veil. SYN veliform.

vel·a·men·tum, pl. **vel·a·men·ta** (vel'ă-men'tŭm, -tă). SYN velum (1). [L. a cover]

ve·lam·i·na (vĕ-lam'i-nă). Plural of velamen.

ve·lar (vē'lăr). Relating to any velum, especially the velum palati.

ve·li·form (vel'i-fōrm). SYN velamentous. [L. velum, veil, + forma, form]

Vella, Luigi, Italian physiologist, 1825–1886. SEE V. *fistula;* Thiry-V. *fistula.*

vel·li·cate (vel'i-kāt). To twitch or contract spasmodically; said especially of fibrillary muscular spasms. [L. vellico, pp. -atus, to pluck, to twitch, fr. vello, to deprive of hair, pluck]

vel·li·ca·tion (vel'i-kā'shŭn). A fibrillary muscular spasm.

vel·lus (vel'ŭs). 1. Fine nonpigmented hair covering most of the body. 2. A structure that is fleecy or soft and woolly in appearance. [L. fleece]

v. oli'vae inferio'ris, a stratum of nerve fibers surrounding the inferior olive.

ve·loc·i·ty (v) (vĕ-los'i-tē). Rate of movement; specifically, distance traveled or quantity converted per unit time in a given direction. Cf. speed. [L. velocitas, fr. velox (veloc-), quick, swift]

initial v., the rate of a reaction, e.g., an enzyme-catalyzed reaction, at the early stages of the reaction such that the product(s) concentrations have not risen to a level to significantly affect the observable rate; typically, initial v.'s are observed when less than 10% of the reaction's approach toward equilibrium has occurred. SYN initial rate.

maximum v. (V_{max}), (1) the maximum rate of an enzyme-catalyzed reaction that can be achieved by progressively increasing the substrate concentration at a given enzyme concentration; in cases of substrate inhibition, V_{max} is an extrapolated value in the absence of such inhibition; Cf. Michaelis-Menten *equation;* (2) the maximum initial rate of shortening of a myocardial fiber that can be obtained under zero load; used to evaluate the contractility of the fiber.

nerve conduction v., the rate of impulse conduction in a peripheral nerve or its various component fibers, generally expressed in meters per second.

PSA v., a measure of the rapidity of change in a person's PSA level.

sedimentation v., the rate of movement of a substance, typically a macromolecule, in centrifugation; these centrifugation studies provide data on the structure of the macromolecule.

steady-state v., the v. of an enzyme-catalyzed reaction in which, over the time course of the study, the concentration of any enzyme species is constant (i.e., for an enzyme-substrate binary complex, ES, $d[ES]/dt \cong 0$; for this to hold true, the total enzyme concentration must be much less than the initial substrate concentration. SYN steady-state rate.

vel·o·gen·ic (vel-ō-jen′ik). Denoting the virulence of a virus capable of inducing, after a brief incubation period, a fulminating and often lethal disease in embryonic, immature, and adult hosts; used in characterizing Newcastle disease virus. [L. *velox,* rapid, + G. -*gen,* producing]

vel·o·pha·ryn·ge·al (vē′lō-fă-rin′jē-ăl). Pertaining to the soft palate (velum palatinum) and the pharyngeal walls.

ve·lo·syn·the·sis (vē′lō-sin′thĕ-sis). SYN palatorrhaphy.

Velpeau, Alfred A.L.M., French surgeon, 1795–1867. SEE V. *bandage, canal, fossa, hernia.*

ve·lum, pl. **ve·la** (vē′lŭm, -lă). **1.** Any structure resembling a veil or curtain. SYN veil (1), velamen, velamentum. **2.** SYN caul (1). **3.** SYN greater *omentum.* **4.** Any serous membrane or membranous envelope or covering. [L. veil, sail]

anterior medullary v., SYN superior medullary v.

inferior medullary v. [TA], a thin sheet of white matter, hidden by the cerebellar tonsil, attached along the peduncle of the flocculus and, at or near the midline, to the nodulus of the vermis; it is continuous caudally with the epithelial lamina and choroid plexus of the fourth ventricle. SYN v. medullare inferius [TA], posterior medullary v., Tarin valve, valvula semilunaris tarini, v. semilunare, v. tarini.

v. interpos′itum, SYN *tela* choroidea of third ventricle.

v. medulla′re infe′rius [TA], SYN inferior medullary v.

v. medulla′re supe′rius [TA], SYN superior medullary v.

v. palati′num, ✕official alternate term for soft *palate.*

v. pen′dulum pala′ti, SYN soft *palate.*

posterior medullary v., SYN inferior medullary v.

v. semiluna′re, SYN inferior medullary v.

superior medullary v. [TA], the thin layer of white matter stretching between the two superior cerebellar peduncles, forming the roof of the superior recess of the fourth ventricle. SYN v. medullare superius [TA], anterior medullary v., Vieussens valve.

v. tari′ni, SYN inferior medullary v.

v. termina′le, SYN *lamina* terminalis of cerebrum.

transverse v., a fold in the dorsal wall of the embryonic brain at the boundary between the telencephalon and diencephalon. SYN v. transversum.

v. transver′sum, SYN transverse v.

v. triangula′re, SYN *tela* choroidea of third ventricle.

VENA

ve·na, gen. and pl. **ve·nae** (vē′nă, -nē) [TA]. SYN vein. [L.]

v. ad′vehens, pl. **ve′nae advehen′tes,** collective term for a series of branching channels in the early embryo receiving blood from the umbilical and/or vitelline venous systems and passing the mixed blood to the sinusoids of the liver; they become terminal branches of the hepatic portal vein. SYN v. afferens hepatis.

v. af′ferens hep′atis, SYN v. advehens.

v. anastomot′ica infe′rior [TA], SYN inferior anastomotic *vein.*

v. anastomot′ica supe′rior [TA], SYN superior anastomotic *vein.*

v. angula′ris [TA], SYN angular *vein.*

venae ante′riores cer′ebri [TA], SYN anterior cerebral *veins,* under *vein.*

v. ante′rior sep′ti pellu′cidi [TA], SYN anterior *vein* of septum pellucidum.

v. apicalis [TA], SYN apical *vein.*

v. apicoposterior [TA], SYN apicoposterior *vein.*

v. appendicula′ris [TA], SYN appendicular *vein.*

v. aqueduc′tus coch′leae, SYN *vein* of cochlear canaliculus.

v. aqueduc′tus vestib′uli [TA], SYN *vein* of vestibular aqueduct.

ve′nae arcua′tae re′nis, SYN arcuate *veins* of kidney, under *vein.*

v. arterio′sa, SYN arterial *vein.*

ve′nae articula′res temporomandibula′res, SYN *veins* of temporomandibular joint, under *vein.*

v. atrii lateralis, SYN lateral *vein* of lateral ventricle.

v. atrii medialis, SYN medial *vein* of lateral ventricle.

v. auricula′ris ante′rior, SYN anterior auricular *vein.*

v. auricula′ris poste′rior [TA], SYN posterior auricular *vein.*

v. axilla′ris [TA], SYN axillary *vein.*

v. az′ygos [TA], SYN azygos *vein.*

v. az′ygos ma′jor, SYN azygos *vein.*

v. az′ygos mi′nor infe′rior, SYN hemiazygos *vein.*

v. az′ygos mi′nor supe′rior, SYN accessory hemiazygos *vein.*

v. basa′lis [TA], SYN basal *vein.*

v. basalis anterior [TA], SYN anterior basal *vein.*

v. basa′lis commu′nis [TA], SYN common basal *vein.*

v. basa′lis infe′rior [TA], SYN inferior basal *vein.*

v. basa′lis supe′rior [TA], SYN superior basal *vein.*

v. basil′ica [TA], SYN basilic *vein.*

venae basivertebra′les [TA], SYN basivertebral *veins,* under *vein.*

Billroth venae cavernosae, SYN venae cavernosae of spleen.

ve′nae brachia′les [TA], SYN brachial *veins,* under *vein.*

ve′nae brachiocephal′icae (dextrae et sinistrae) [TA], SYN (left and right) brachiocephalic *veins,* under *vein.*

ve′nae bronchia′les [TA], SYN bronchial *veins,* under *vein.*

v. bul′bi pe′nis [TA], SYN *vein* of bulb of penis.

v. bul′bi vestib′uli [TA], SYN *vein* of bulb of vestibule.

v. canalic′uli coch′leae, SYN *vein* of cochlear canaliculus.

v. cana′lis pterygoi′dei [TA], SYN *vein* of pterygoid canal.

ve′nae cardiacae anterio′res [TA], SYN anterior cardiac *veins,* under *vein.*

venae cardiacae minimae [TA], SYN smallest cardiac *veins,* under *vein.*

v. cardi′aca mag′na, SYN great cardiac *vein.*

v. ca′va infe′rior [TA], SYN inferior v. cava.

v. ca′va supe′rior [TA], SYN superior v. cava.

ve′nae caverno′sae pe′nis [TA], SYN cavernous *veins* of penis, under *vein.*

ve′nae centra′les hep′atis, SYN central *veins* of liver, under *vein.*

v. centra′lis glan′dulae suprarena′lis [TA], SYN central *vein* of suprarenal gland.

v. centra′lis ret′inae [TA], SYN central retinal *vein.*

v. cephal′ica [TA], SYN cephalic *vein.*

v. cephal′ica accesso′ria [TA], SYN accessory cephalic *vein.*

v. cephalica antebrachii [TA], SYN cephalic *vein* of forearm.

ve′nae cerebel′li [TA], SYN cerebellar *veins,* under *vein.*

v. cervica′lis profun′da [TA], SYN deep cervical *vein.*

ve′nae choroi′deae oc′uli, SYN vorticose *veins,* under *vein.*

v. choroi′dea infe′rior, SYN inferior choroid *vein.*

v. choroidea inferior [TA], SYN inferior choroid *vein*; SEE basal *vein.*

v. choroi′dea supe′rior [TA], SYN superior choroid *vein.*

ve′nae cilia′res anteriores [TA], SYN anterior ciliary *veins,* under *vein.*

ve′nae circumflex′ae fem′oris latera′les [TA], SYN lateral circumflex femoral *veins,* under *vein.*

ve′nae circumflex′ae fem′oris media′les [TA], SYN medial circumflex femoral *veins,* under *vein.*

v. circumflexa humeri anterior [TA], SYN anterior circumflex humeral *vein.*

v. circumflexa humeri posterior [TA], SYN posterior circumflex humeral *vein.*

v. circumflex′a ili′aca profun′da [TA], SYN deep circumflex iliac *vein.*

v. circumflex′a ili′aca superficia′lis [TA], SYN superficial circumflex iliac *vein.*

ve

v. col′ica dex′tra [TA], SYN right colic *vein.*

v. col′ica me′dia [TA], SYN middle colic *vein.*

v. col′ica sinis′tra [TA], SYN left colic *vein.*

v. colli profunda, ✭official alternate term for deep cervical *vein.*

ve′nae colum′nae vertebra′lis [TA], SYN *veins* of vertebral column, under *vein.*

v. com′itans, a vein accompanying another structure. SYN accompanying vein.

v. comitans of hypoglossal nerve [TA], runs with the hypoglossal nerve below and lateral to the hyoglossus muscle, emptying usually into the lingual vein. SYN v. comitans nervi hypoglossi [TA], accompanying vein of hypoglossal nerve.

v. com′itans ner′vi hypoglos′si [TA], SYN v. comitans of hypoglossal nerve.

ve′nae comitan′tes [TA], a pair of veins, but occasionally more, that closely accompany an artery in such a manner that the pulsations of the artery aid venous return. SYN companion veins.

ve′nae conjunctiva′les [TA], SYN conjunctival *veins,* under *vein.*

venae cordis [TA], SYN *veins* of heart, under *vein.*

v. cor′dis mag′na [TA], SYN great cardiac *vein.*

v. cor′dis me′dia [TA], SYN middle cardiac *vein.*

ve′nae cor′dis min′imae, ✭official alternate term for smallest cardiac *veins,* under *vein.*

v. cor′dis par′va [TA], SYN small cardiac *vein.*

v. cor′nus posterio′ris [TA], SYN *vein* of posterior horn.

v. corona′ria ventric′uli, SYN left gastric *vein.*

v. cuta′nea, SYN superficial *vein.*

v. cys′tica [TA], SYN cystic *veins,* under *vein.*

ve′nae digita′les dorsa′les pe′dis [TA], SYN dorsal digital *veins* of foot, under *vein.*

ve′nae digita′les palma′res [TA], SYN palmar digital *veins,* under *vein.*

ve′nae digita′les planta′res [TA], SYN plantar digital *veins,* under *vein.*

v. diplo′ica [TA], SYN diploic *vein.*

ve′nae direc′tae latera′les [TA], SYN direct lateral *veins,* under *vein.*

ve′nae dorsa′les clitor′idis superficia′les [TA], SYN superficial dorsal *veins* of clitoris, under *vein.*

venae dorsa′les lin′guae [TA], SYN dorsal lingual *vein.*

ve′nae dorsa′les pe′nis superficia′les [TA], SYN superficial dorsal *veins* of penis, under *vein.*

v. dorsa′lis clitor′idis profun′da [TA], SYN deep dorsal *vein* of clitoris.

v. dorsa′lis cor′poris callo′si, ✭official alternate term for posterior *vein* of corpus callosum.

v. dorsa′lis pe′nis profun′da [TA], SYN deep dorsal *vein* of penis.

venae ductuum semicircularium [TA], SYN *veins* of semicircular ducts, under *vein.*

v. emissa′ria, pl. **ve′nae emissa′riae** [TA], SYN emissary *vein.*

v. emissa′ria condyla′ris [TA], SYN condylar emissary *vein.*

v. emissa′ria mastoi′dea [TA], SYN mastoid emissary *vein.*

v. emissa′ria occipita′lis [TA], SYN occipital emissary *vein.*

v. emissa′ria parieta′lis [TA], SYN parietal emissary *vein.*

ve′nae encephali occipita′les [TA], SYN occipital cerebral *veins,* under *vein.*

ve′nae epigas′tricae superio′res [TA], SYN superior epigastric *veins,* under *vein.*

v. epigas′trica infe′rior [TA], SYN inferior epigastric *vein.*

v. epigas′trica superficia′lis [TA], SYN superficial epigastric *vein.*

ve′nae episclera′les [TA], SYN episcleral *veins,* under *vein.*

ve′nae esopha′geae [TA], SYN esophageal *veins,* under *vein.*

ve′nae ethmoida′les [TA], SYN ethmoidal *veins,* under *vein.*

v. facia′lis [TA], SYN facial *vein.*

v. facia′lis ante′rior, SYN facial *vein.*

v. facia′lis commu′nis, SYN common facial *vein.*

v. facia′lis poste′rior, SYN retromandibular *vein.*

v. facie′i profun′da [TA], SYN deep facial *vein.*

v. femora′lis [TA], SYN femoral *vein.*

v. fenestrae cochleae [TA], SYN *vein* of cochlear window.

ve′nae fibula′res [TA], SYN fibular *veins,* under *vein,* fibular *veins,* under *vein.*

ve′nae fronta′les, [NA] SYN supratrochlear *veins,* under *vein.*

v. gas′trica dex′tra [TA], SYN right gastric *vein.*

ve′nae gas′tricae bre′ves [TA], SYN short gastric *veins,* under *vein.*

v. gas′trica sinis′tra [TA], SYN left gastric *vein.*

v. gastro-omenta′lis dex′tra [TA], SYN right gastroomental *vein.*

v. gastro-omenta′lis sinis′tra, SYN left gastroomental *vein.*

ve′nae geniculares [TA], SYN genicular *veins,* under *vein.*

ve′nae glu′teae inferio′res [TA], SYN inferior gluteal *veins,* under *vein.*

ve′nae glu′teae superio′res [TA], SYN superior gluteal *veins,* under *vein.*

v. gyri olfactorii [TA], SYN *vein* of olfactory gyrus; SEE basal *vein.*

v. hemiaz′ygos [TA], SYN hemiazygos *vein.*

v. hemiaz′ygos accesso′ria [TA], SYN accessory hemiazygos *vein.*

ve′nae hemisphe′rii cerebel′li superio′res [TA], SYN superior *veins* of cerebellar hemisphere, under *vein.*

ve′nae hemorrhoida′les inferio′res, outmoded term for inferior rectal *veins,* under *vein.*

ve′nae hemorrhoida′les me′diae, outmoded term for middle rectal *veins,* under *vein.*

v. hemorrhoida′lis supe′rior, outmoded term for superior rectal *vein.*

ve′nae hepat′icae [TA], SYN hepatic *veins,* under *vein.*

ve′nae hepat′icae dex′trae [TA], SYN right hepatic *veins,* under *vein.*

venae hepaticae intermediae [TA], SYN intermediate hepatic *veins,* under *vein.*

ve′nae hepat′icae me′diae [TA], SYN intermediate hepatic *veins,* under *vein.*

ve′nae hepat′icae sinis′trae [TA], SYN left hepatic *vein.*

v. hypogas′trica, obsolete term for internal iliac *vein.*

v. ileocol′ica [TA], SYN ileocolic *vein.*

v. ili′aca commu′nis [TA], SYN common iliac *vein.*

v. ili′aca exter′na [TA], SYN external iliac *vein.*

v. ili′aca inter′na [TA], SYN internal iliac *vein.*

v. iliolumba′lis [TA], SYN iliolumbar *vein.*

inferior v. cava (IVC) [TA], v. that receives the blood from the lower limbs and the greater part of the pelvic and abdominal organs; it begins at the level of the fifth lumbar vertebra on the right side by the merger of the right and left common iliac veins, pierces the diaphragm at the level of the eighth thoracic vertebra, and empties into the posteroinferior aspect of the right atrium of the heart. SYN v. cava inferior [TA], postcava.

ve′nae inferio′res cerebel′li [TA], SYN inferior *veins* of cerebellar hemisphere, under *vein.*

ve′nae inferio′res cer′ebri [TA], SYN inferior cerebral *veins,* under *vein.*

v. infe′rior ver′mis [TA], SYN inferior *vein* of vermis.

v. innomina′ta, archaic term for (left and right) brachiocephalic *veins,* under *vein.*

ve′nae insula′res [TA], veins draining the cortex of the insula, tributaries to the deep middle cerebral vein. SYN insular veins [TA].

ve′nae intercapitulares, SYN intercapitular *veins,* under *vein.*

ve′nae intercosta′les anterio′res [TA], SYN anterior intercostal *veins,* under *vein.*

ve′nae intercosta′les posterio′res [TA], SYN posterior intercostal *veins,* under *vein.*

v. intercosta′lis supe′rior dex′tra [TA], SYN right superior intercostal *vein.*

v. intercosta′lis supe′rior sinis′tra [TA], SYN left superior intercostal *vein.*

v. intercosta′lis supre′ma [TA], SYN supreme intercostal *vein.*

ve′nae interloba′res re′nis [TA], SYN interlobar *veins* of kidney, under *vein.*

ve′nae interlobula′res hep′atis [TA], SYN interlobular *veins* of liver, under *vein*.

ve′nae interlobula′res re′nis [TA], SYN interlobular *veins* of kidney, under *vein*.

v. interme′dia antebra′chii, SYN median antebrachial *vein*.

v. interme′dia basil′ica [TA], SYN intermediate basilic *vein*.

v. interme′dia cephal′ica [TA], SYN intermediate cephalic *vein*.

v. interme′dia cu′biti, SYN median cubital *vein*.

ve′nae inter′nae cer′ebri [TA], SYN internal cerebral *veins*, under *vein*.

v. intervertebra′lis [TA], SYN intervertebral *vein*.

ve′nae jejuna′les et il′ei [TA], SYN jejunal and ileal *veins*, under *vein*.

v. jugula′ris ante′rior [TA], SYN anterior jugular *vein*.

v. jugula′ris exter′na [TA], SYN external jugular *vein*.

v. jugula′ris inter′na [TA], SYN internal jugular *vein*.

ve′nae labia′les anterio′res [TA], SYN anterior labial *veins*, under *vein*.

ve′nae labia′les posterio′res [TA], SYN posterior labial *veins*, under *vein*.

v. labia′lis infe′rior [TA], SYN inferior labial *vein*.

v. labia′lis supe′rior [TA], SYN superior labial *vein*.

ve′nae labyrin′thi [TA], SYN labyrinthine *veins*, under *vein*.

v. lacrima′lis [TA], SYN lacrimal *vein*.

v. laryn′gea infe′rior [TA], SYN inferior laryngeal *vein*.

v. laryn′gea supe′rior [TA], SYN superior laryngeal *vein*.

v. latera′lis ventric′uli latera′lis [TA], SYN lateral *vein* of lateral ventricle.

v. liena′lis, SYN splenic *vein*.

v. lingualis, SYN lingual *vein*.

v. lingula′ris, SYN lingular *vein*.

v. lobi medii [TA], SYN middle lobe *vein*.

ve′nae lumba′les [TA], SYN lumbar *veins*, under *vein*.

v. lumba′lis ascen′dens [TA], SYN ascending lumbar *vein*.

v. mag′na cer′ebri [TA], SYN great cerebral *vein* of Galen.

v. mamma′ria inter′na, obsolete term for internal thoracic *vein*.

v. maxilla′ris, pl. ve′nae maxilla′res [TA], SYN maxillary *vein*.

v. media′lis ventric′uli latera′lis [TA], SYN medial *vein* of lateral ventricle.

v. media′na antebra′chii [TA], SYN median antebrachial *vein*.

v. media′na basil′ica, SYN intermediate basilic *vein*.

v. media′na cephal′ica, SYN intermediate cephalic *vein*.

v. media′na cu′biti [TA], SYN median cubital *vein*.

v. me′dia profun′da cer′ebri [TA], SYN deep middle cerebral *vein*.

ve′nae mediastina′les [TA], SYN mediastinal *veins*, under *vein*.

v. me′dia superficia′lis cer′ebri, SYN superficial middle cerebral *vein*.

ve′nae medul′lae oblonga′tae [TA], SYN *veins* of medulla oblongata, under *vein*.

venae medullae spinalis [TA], SYN *veins* of spinal cord, under *vein*.

venae membri inferioris [TA], SYN *veins* of lower limb, under *vein*.

venae membri superioris [TA], SYN *veins* of upper limb, under *vein*.

ve′nae menin′geae [TA], SYN meningeal *veins*, under *vein*.

ve′nae menin′geae me′diae [TA], SYN middle meningeal *veins*, under *vein*.

ve′nae mesencephal′icae, SYN mesencephalic *veins*, under *vein*.

v. mesenter′ica infe′rior [TA], SYN inferior mesenteric *vein*.

v. mesenter′ica supe′rior [TA], SYN superior mesenteric *vein*.

ve′nae metacar′peae dorsa′les [TA], SYN dorsal metacarpal *veins*, under *vein*.

ve′nae metacar′peae palma′res [TA], SYN palmar metacarpal *veins*, under *vein*.

ve′nae metatar′seae dorsa′les [TA], SYN dorsal metatarsal *veins*, under *vein*.

ve′nae metatar′seae planta′res [TA], SYN plantar metatarsal *veins*, under *vein*.

v. modioli communis [TA], SYN common modiolar *vein*.

ve′nae mus′culophren′icae [TA], SYN musculophrenic *veins*, under *vein*.

ve′nae nasa′les exter′nae [TA], SYN external nasal *veins*, under *vein*.

v. nasofronta′lis [TA], SYN nasofrontal *vein*.

ve′nae nu′clei cauda′ti [TA], SYN *veins* of caudate nucleus, under *vein*.

v. obli′qua a′trii sinis′tri [TA], SYN oblique *vein* of left atrium.

v. obturato′ria, pl. ve′nae obturato′riae [TA], SYN obturator *veins*, under *vein*.

v. occipita′lis [TA], SYN occipital *vein*.

v. ophthal′mica infe′rior [TA], SYN inferior ophthalmic *vein*.

v. ophthal′mica supe′rior [TA], SYN superior ophthalmic *vein*.

v. ova′rica dex′tra [TA], SYN right ovarian *vein*.

v. ova′rica sinis′tra [TA], SYN left ovarian *vein*.

v. palati′na externa [TA], SYN external palatine *vein*.

ve′nae palpebra′les [TA], SYN palpebral *veins*, under *vein*.

ve′nae palpebra′les inferio′res [TA], SYN inferior palpebral *veins*, under *vein*.

ve′nae palpebra′les superio′res [TA], SYN superior palpebral *veins*, under *vein*.

ve′nae pancreat′icae [TA], SYN pancreatic *veins*, under *vein*.

ve′nae pancreat′icoduodena′les [TA], SYN pancreaticoduodenal *veins*, under *vein*.

ve′nae paraumbilica′les [TA], SYN paraumbilical *veins*, under *vein*.

ve′nae parieta′les, SYN parietal *veins*, under *vein*.

ve′nae parotid′eae [TA], SYN parotid *veins*, under *vein*.

ve′nae pectora′les [TA], SYN pectoral *veins*, under *vein*.

venae pedunculares [TA], SYN peduncular *veins*, under *vein*; SEE basal *vein*.

ve′nae perforan′tes [TA], SYN perforating *veins*, under *vein*.

ve′nae pericardi′acae [TA], SYN pericardial *veins*, under *vein*.

ve′nae pericardiacophren′icae [TA], SYN pericardiacophrenic *veins*, under *vein*.

ve′nae perone′ae, ☆official alternate term for fibular *veins*, under *vein*.

v. petro′sa [TA], SEE petrosal *vein*.

ve′nae pharyn′geae [TA], SYN pharyngeal *veins*, under *vein*.

ve′nae phren′icae superio′res [TA], SYN superior phrenic *veins*, under *vein*.

v. phren′ica infe′rior [TA], SYN inferior phrenic *vein*.

ve′nae pon′tis [TA], SYN pontine *veins*, under *vein*.

v. pontomesencephalica [TA], SEE anterior pontomesencephalic *vein*.

v. pontomesencephal′ica ante′rior, SYN anterior pontomesencephalic *vein*.

v. poplit′ea [TA], SYN popliteal *vein*.

v. por′tae hep′atis [TA], SYN hepatic portal *vein*.

v. porta′lis, SYN hepatic portal *vein*.

v. posterior corporis callosi [TA], SYN posterior *vein* of corpus callosum.

v. poste′rior sep′ti pellu′cidi [TA], SYN posterior *vein* of septum pellucidum.

v.(e) poste′rior(es) ventric′uli sinis′tri, SYN posterior *vein*(s) of left ventricle.

v. preauricula′ris, SYN anterior auricular *vein*.

v. precentra′lis cerebel′li [TA], SYN precentral cerebellar *vein*.

ve′nae prefronta′les [TA], SYN prefrontal *veins*, under *vein*.

v. prepylo′rica [TA], SYN prepyloric *vein*.

ve′nae profun′dae cer′ebri [TA], SYN deep cerebral *veins*, under *vein*.

ve′nae profun′dae clitor′idis [TA], SYN deep *veins* of clitoris, under *vein*.

venae profun′dae pe′nis, SYN deep *veins* of penis, under *vein*.

v. profun′da fem′oris [TA], SYN profunda femoris *vein*.

v. profun'da lin'guae [TA], SYN deep lingual *vein.*

ve'nae puden'dae exter'nae [TA], SYN external pudendal *veins,* under *vein.*

v. puden'da inter'na [TA], SYN internal pudendal *vein.*

ve'nae pulmona'les [TA], SYN pulmonary *veins,* under *vein.*

v. pulmona'lis infe'rior dex'tra [TA], SYN right inferior pulmonary *vein.*

v. pulmona'lis infe'rior sinis'tra [TA], SYN left inferior pulmonary *vein.*

v. pulmona'lis supe'rior dex'tra [TA], SYN right superior pulmonary *vein.*

v. pulmona'lis supe'rior sinis'tra [TA], SYN left superior pulmonary *vein.*

ve'nae radia'les [TA], SYN radial *veins,* under *vein.*

v. reces'sus latera'lis ventric'uli quar'ti [TA], SYN *vein* of lateral recess of fourth ventricle.

ve'nae rec'tae, the ascending limbs of the vasa rectae in the renal medulla.

ve'nae recta'les inferio'res [TA], SYN inferior rectal *veins,* under *vein.*

ve'nae recta'les me'diae [TA], SYN middle rectal *veins,* under *vein.*

v. recta'lis supe'rior [TA], SYN superior rectal *vein.*

ve'nae rena'les, SYN renal *veins,* under *vein.*

v. retromandibula'ris [TA], SYN retromandibular *vein.*

venae retroperitoneales, SYN retroperitoneal *veins,* under *vein.*

v. re'vehens, pl. **ve'nae revehen'tes,** veins in the embryo, passing from the sinusoid vessels in the liver to the inferior v. cava, that develop into the hepatic veins.

ve'nae sacra'les latera'les [TA], SYN lateral sacral *veins,* under *vein.*

v. sacra'lis media'na [TA], SYN median sacral *vein.*

v. saphe'na accesso'ria [TA], SYN accessory saphenous *vein.*

v. saphe'na mag'na [TA], SYN great saphenous *vein.*

v. saphe'na par'va [TA], SYN small saphenous *vein.*

v. scalae tympani [TA], SYN *vein* of scala tympani.

v. scalae vestibuli [TA], SYN *vein* of scala vestibuli.

v. scapula'ris dorsa'lis [TA], SYN dorsal scapular *vein.*

ve'nae sclera'les [TA], SYN scleral *veins,* under *vein.*

ve'nae scrota'les anterio'res [TA], SYN anterior scrotal *veins,* under *vein.*

ve'nae scrota'les posterio'res [TA], SYN posterior scrotal *veins,* under *vein.*

ve'nae sigmoi'deae [TA], SYN sigmoid *veins,* under *vein.*

ve'nae spina'les [TA], SYN spinal *veins,* under *vein.*

v. spira'lis modi'oli, SYN common modiolar *vein.*

venae cavernosae of spleen, small tributaries of the splenic vein in the pulp of the spleen. SYN Billroth venae cavernosae.

v. sple'nica [TA], SYN splenic *vein.*

ve'nae stella'tae, SYN *venulae* stellatae, under *venula.*

v. sternocleidomastoi'dea [TA], SYN sternocleidomastoid *vein.*

ve'nae stria'tae, SYN inferior thalamostriate *veins,* under *vein.*

v. stylomastoi'dea [TA], SYN stylomastoid *vein.*

v. subcla'via [TA], SYN subclavian *vein.*

ve'nae subcuta'neae abdom'inis, SYN subcutaneous *veins* of abdomen, under *vein.*

v. sublingua'lis [TA], SYN sublingual *vein.*

v. submenta'lis [TA], SYN submental *vein.*

ve'nae superficia'les cer'ebri [TA], SYN superficial cerebral *veins,* under *vein.*

v. superficialis [TA], SYN superficial *vein.*

superior v. cava [TA], returns blood from the head and neck, upper limbs, and thorax to the posterosuperior aspect of the right atrium; formed in the superior mediastinum by union of the two brachiocephalic veins. SYN v. cava superior [TA], precava.

ve'nae superio'res cerebel'li [TA], SEE superior *veins* of cerebellar hemisphere, under *vein.*

ve'nae superio'res cer'ebri [TA], SYN superior cerebral *veins,* under *vein.*

v. supe'rior ver'mis [TA], SYN superior *vein* of vermis.

v. supraorbita'lis [TA], SYN supraorbital *vein.*

v. suprarena'lis dex'tra [TA], SYN right suprarenal *vein.*

v. suprarena'lis sinis'tra [TA], SYN left suprarenal *vein.*

v. suprascapula'ris [TA], SYN suprascapular *vein.*

ve'nae supratrochlea'res [TA], SYN supratrochlear *veins,* under *vein.*

ve'nae tempora'les profun'dae [TA], SYN deep temporal *veins,* under *vein.*

ve'nae tempora'les superficia'les [TA], SYN superficial temporal *veins,* under *vein.*

v. tempora'lis me'dia [TA], SYN middle temporal *vein.*

v. termina'lis, ☆official alternate term for superior thalamostriate *vein.*

v. testicula'ris dex'tra [TA], SYN right testicular *vein.*

v. testicula'ris sinis'tra [TA], SYN left testicular *vein.*

ve'nae thalamostria'tae inferio'res [TA], SYN inferior thalamostriate *veins,* under *vein.*

v. thalamostria'ta supe'rior [TA], SYN superior thalamostriate *vein.*

v. thora'cica inter'na [TA], SYN internal thoracic *vein.*

v. thora'cica latera'lis [TA], SYN lateral thoracic *vein.*

v. thoracoacromia'lis [TA], SYN thoracoacromial *vein.*

v. thoracoepigas'trica [TA], SYN thoracoepigastric *vein.*

ve'nae thy'micae [TA], SYN thymic *veins,* under *vein.*

v. thyroi'dea i'ma, SYN inferior thyroid *vein.*

v. thyroi'dea infe'rior [TA], SYN inferior thyroid *vein.*

v. thyroi'dea me'dia [TA], SYN middle thyroid *vein.*

v. thyroi'dea supe'rior [TA], SYN superior thyroid *vein.*

ve'nae tibia'les anterio'res [TA], SYN anterior tibial *veins,* under *vein.*

ve'nae tibia'les posterio'res [TA], SYN posterior tibial *veins,* under *vein.*

ve'nae trachea'les [TA], SYN tracheal *veins,* under *vein.*

venae transversae cervicis [TA], SYN transverse cervical *veins,* under *vein.*

ve'nae transver'sae col'li, ☆official alternate term for transverse cervical *veins,* under *vein.*

v. transver'sa facie'i [TA], SYN transverse facial *vein.*

v. transver'sa scap'ulae, SYN suprascapular *vein.*

ve'nae tympan'icae [TA], SYN tympanic *veins,* under *vein.*

ve'nae ulna'res [TA], SYN ulnar *veins,* under *vein.*

v. umbilica'lis [TA], SYN left umbilical *vein.*

v. un'calis [TA], a vein draining the uncus into the inferior cerebral vein of the same side. SYN vein of uncus [TA].

ve'nae uteri'nae [TA], SYN uterine *veins,* under *vein.*

v. ventricularis inferior [TA], SYN inferior ventricular *vein;* SEE basal *vein.*

v. vertebra'lis [TA], SYN vertebral *vein.*

v. vertebra'lis accesso'ria [TA], SYN accessory vertebral *vein.*

v. vertebra'lis ante'rior [TA], SYN anterior vertebral *vein.*

ve'nae vesica'les [TA], SYN vesical *veins,* under *vein.*

ve'nae vestibula'res (anterius et posterius) [TA], SYN (anterior and posterior) vestibular *veins,* under *vein.*

v. vitelli'na, SYN vitelline *vein.*

ve'nae vortico'sae [TA], SYN vorticose *veins,* under *vein.*

---

ve·na·ca·vog·ra·phy (vē'nă-kā-vog'ră-fē). Angiography of a vena cava. SYN cavography.

ve·na·tion (vē-nā'shŭn). The arrangement and distribution of veins. [L. *vena,* vein]

△**vene-.** **1.** The veins, venous. SEE ALSO veno-. [L. *vena,* vein] **2.** Combining form relating to venom. [L. *venenum,* poison]

ve·nec·ta·sia (ve-nek-tā'sē-ă). SYN phlebectasia.

ve·nec·to·my (ve-nek'tō-mē). SYN phlebectomy.

🔲 **ve·neer** (vĕ-nēr'). **1.** A thin surface layer laid over a base of common material. **2.** In dentistry, a layer of tooth-colored material, usually porcelain or composite resin, attached to and covering the surface of a metal crown or natural tooth structure. [Fr. *fournir,* to furnish]

ven·e·na·tion (ven-ĕ-nā'shŭn, vē-nĕ-). Poisoning, as from a sting or bite. [L. *veneno,* pp. -*atus,* to poison, fr. *venenum,* poison]

ven·e·nif·er·ous (ven-ĕ-nif'ĕ-rŭs). Conveying poison, as through a sting or bite. [L. *venenifer,* fr. *venenum,* poison, + *fero,* to carry]

ven·e·no·sal·i·vary (ven'ĕ-nō-sal'i-vār-ē). Secreting a poisonous saliva, said of venomous reptiles. SYN venomosalivary.

ven·e·nos·i·ty (ven-ĕ-nos'i-tē). The state of containing poison or being poisonous. [L. *venenosus,* poisonous]

ven·e·nous (ven'ĕ-nŭs). SYN poisonous. [L. *venenosus*]

ve·ne·re·al (ve-nēr'ē-ăl). Relating to or resulting from sexual intercourse. [L. *Venus* (*vener*-), goddess of love]

ve·ne·re·ol·o·gy (ve-nēr-ē-ol'ō-jē). The study of venereal disease. [venereal (disease) + G. *logos,* study]

ve·ne·re·o·pho·bia (ve-nēr'ē-ō-fō'bē-ă). Morbid fear of venereal disease. [venereal (disease) + G. *phobos,* fear]

ven·e·sec·tion (ven-ē-sek'shŭn). SYN phlebotomy. [L. *vena,* vein, + *sectio,* a cutting]

△**veni-.** SEE veno-.

ven·in (ven'in). Any poisonous substance found in snake venom. [see venom]

ven·i·punc·ture (ven'i-pŭnk-choor, vē'ni-). The puncture of a vein, usually to withdraw blood or inject a solution.

Venn, John, English logician and philosopher, 1834–1923. SEE Venn *diagram.*

△**veno-, veni-.** The veins. SEE ALSO vene- (1). [L. *vena*]

ve·no·cly·sis (vē-nok'li-sis). SYN phleboclysis. [veno- + G. *klysis,* a washing out]

ve·no·fi·bro·sis (vē'nō-fī-brō'sis). SYN phlebosclerosis.

ve·no·gram (vē'nō-gram). **1.** Radiograph of opacified veins. **2.** SYN phlebogram. [veno- + G. *gramma,* a writing]

ve·nog·ra·phy (vē-nog'ră-fē). Radiographic demonstration of a vein, after the injection of contrast medium. SYN phlebography (2). [veno- + G. *graphō,* to write]

splenic portal v., SYN splenoportography.

transosseous v., radiographic demonstration of veins that drain a bone's marrow, by injection of contrast medium into the marrow at an appropriate point, as in vertebral v. or azygography by rib injection.

vertebral v., radiographic demonstration of the epidural venous plexus by injection of contrast medium into the spinous process.

ven·om (ven'ŏm). A poisonous fluid secreted by snakes, spiders, scorpions, etc. [M. Eng. and O. Fr. *venim,* fr. L. *venenum,* poison]

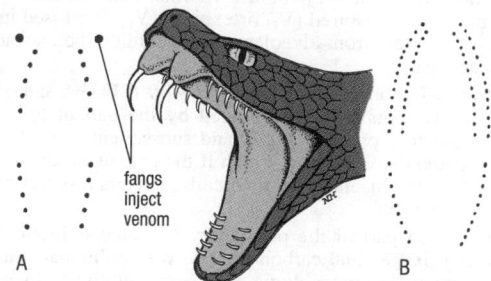

venom: teeth marks of a poisonous snake (A) as compared with that of a non-poisonous snake (B)

kokoi v., a potent neurotoxin found in the frog *Phyllobates bicolor;* it is a nonprotein compound with a molecular weight of approximately 400, and is lethal in microgram quantities.

Russell's viper v., a v. derived from Russell's viper (*Vipera russelli*), which acts as an intrinsic thromboplastin; used in the laboratory evaluation of deficiencies of factor X or topically to arrest local hemorrhage in hemophilia.

ven·o·mo·sal·i·vary (ven'ō-mō-sal'i-var-ē). SYN venenosalivary.

ve·no·mo·tor (vē'nō-mō'ter). Causing change in the caliber of a vein. [veno- + L. *motor,* a move]

ve·no·per·i·to·ne·os·to·my (vē'nō-per-i-tō-nē-os'tō-mē). An obsolete operation involving insertion of the cut end of the saphenous vein into the peritoneal cavity in cases of ascites; the vein is inverted so that the valves prevent regurgitation of blood into the cavity while the ascitic fluid flows into the vein. [veno- + peritoneum + G. *stoma,* mouth]

ve·no·pres·sor (vē-nō-pres'er). Relating to the venous blood pressure and consequently the volume of venous supply to the right side of the heart.

ve·no·scle·ro·sis (vē'nō-skle-rō'sis). SYN phlebosclerosis.

ve·nose (vē'nōs). Having veins; veiny. [L. *venosus*]

ve·no·si·nal (vē'nō-sī'năl). Pertaining to the vena cava and the atrial sinus of the heart.

ve·nos·i·ty (vē-nos'i-tē). **1.** A venous state; a condition in which the bulk of the blood is in the veins at the expense of the arteries. **2.** The unaerated condition of venous blood or of hypoxemic arterial blood.

ve·no·sta·sis (vē-nō-stā'sis, vē-nos'tă-sis). SYN phlebostasis. [veno- + G. *stasis,* a standing]

ve·no·stat (vē'nō-stat). Any instrument for arresting venous bleeding. [veno- + G. *statos,* standing, stationary]

ve·nos·to·my (vē-nos'tō-mē). SYN cutdown.

ve·not·o·my (vē-not'ō-mē). SYN phlebotomy.

ve·nous (vē'nŭs). Relating to a vein or to the veins. SYN phleboid (2). [L. *venosus*]

ve·no·ve·nos·to·my (vē'nō-vē-nos'tō-mē). The formation of an anastomosis between two veins. SYN phlebophlebostomy. [veno- + veno- + G. *stoma,* mouth]

vent. An opening into a cavity or canal, especially one through which the contents of such a cavity are discharged, as the anus. [O. Fr. *fente,* a chink, cleft]

ven·ter (ven'ter) [TA]. **1.** SYN abdomen. **2** [NA]. SYN belly (2). **3.** One of the great cavities of the body. **4.** The uterus. [L. *venter* (*ventr*-), belly]

v. ante'rior mus'culi digas'trici [TA], SYN anterior *belly* of digastric muscle.

v. fronta'lis mus'culi occipitofronta'lis [TA], SYN frontal *belly* of occipitofrontalis muscle.

v. infe'rior mus'culi omohyoi'dei [TA], SYN inferior *belly* of omohyoid *muscle.*

v. occipita'lis mus'culi occipitofron'talis [TA], SYN occipital *belly* of occipitofrontalis muscle.

v. poste'rior mus'culi digas'trici [TA], SYN posterior *belly* of digastric muscle.

v. supe'rior mus'culi omohyoi'dei [TA], SYN superior *belly* of omohyoid muscle.

ven·ti·late (ven'ti-lāt). To aerate, or oxygenate, the blood in the pulmonary capillaries. SYN air (2). [L. *ventilo,* pp. -*atus,* to fan, fr. *ventus,* the wind]

ven·ti·la·tion (ven-ti-lā'shŭn). **1.** Replacement of air or other gas in a space by fresh air or gas. **2.** Movement of gas(es) into and out of the lungs. SYN oxidative metabolism, respiration (2). **3 (V̇).** In physiology, the tidal exchange of air between the lungs and the atmosphere that occurs in breathing. SEE ALSO respiration. [see ventilate]

airway pressure release v., mechanical v. in which patients being treated with continuous positive airway pressure have intermittent decreases rather than increases in airway pressure and volume.

alveolar v. (V̇$_A$), the volume of gas expired from the alveoli to the outside of the body per minute; calculated as the respiratory frequency (f) multiplied by the difference between tidal volume and the dead space ($V_T - V_D$); units: ml/min BTPS.

artificial v., any means of producing gas exchange mechanically or manually between the lungs and the surrounding air, which is not performed entirely by the person's own respiratory system. SYN artificial respiration.

assist-control v., artificial positive-pressure v. by machine in

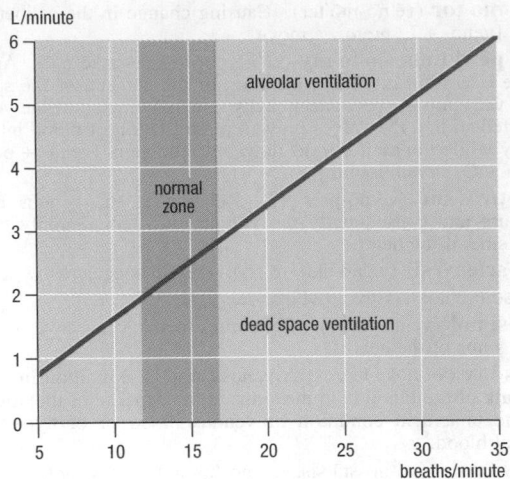

alveolar and dead space ventilation: depending on the number of breaths taken (respiratory frequency), with a constant tidal volume of 6 L

which a full breath is produced automatically, following a patient's natural inspiratory effort. In the event that the patient does not initiate such an effort, the machine will provide a baseline, or "backup" respiratory rate.

assisted v., application of mechanically or manually generated positive pressure to gas(es) in or about the airway during inhalation as a means of augmenting movement of gases into the lungs. SYN assisted respiration.

bag v., SYN manual v.

continuous positive pressure v. (CPPV), SYN controlled mechanical v.

controlled v., intermittent application of mechanically or manually generated positive pressure to gas(es) in or about the airway as a means of forcing gases into the lungs in the absence of spontaneous ventilatory efforts. SYN controlled respiration.

controlled mechanical v. (CMV), artificial v. in which all inspirations are provided by positive pressure applied to the airway, regardless of the patient's own efforts at breathing. In current clinical practice, this mode is almost never used. SYN continuous positive pressure v., intermittent positive pressure v.

high-frequency v., mechanical v. using "jet" administration of breaths at frequencies anywhere from 300–3000 breaths per minute to avoid some complications of more conventional v.

intermittent mandatory v. (IMV), mechanical application of positive pressure volume at a predetermined frequency to the airway, interspersed between the patient's own natural breathing through the ventilator circuit. No attempt is made to time the machine's breaths with the patient's own.

intermittent positive pressure v. (IPPV), SYN controlled mechanical v.

inverse-ratio v., mechanical v. in which the time allowed by the machine for inspiration exceeds that allowed for expiration, which is opposite the situation in more standard modes of v.

liquid v., an experimental means of ventilating lungs suffering from severe injury, through use of O_2 and CO_2 dissolved in perfluorocarbons in a liquid, thus (theoretically) decreasing the incidence of atelectasis and other problems.

mandatory minute v., mechanical v. in which the ventilator is configured to ensure a certain minute volume, but only if needed.

manual v., intermittent manual compression of a gas-filled reservoir bag to force gases into a patient's lungs and thus maintain oxygenation and carbon dioxide elimination during apnea or hypoventilation. SYN bag v.

maximum voluntary v. (MVV), the volume of air breathed when an individual breathes as deeply and as quickly as possible for a given time (e.g., 15 s.). Usually extrapolated to what could be breathed over 1 minute. SYN maximum breathing capacity.

mechanical v., any mechanically assisted breathing, employing either positive or negative pressure devices. Some positive-pressure devices require intubation of the trachea and some require only a mask applied to the mouth or nose. For the past several decades, the standard way of mechanicaly ventilating a patient with respiratory failure has involved intubation of the trachea and either pressure- or volume-limited application of positive pressure to the lungs through the endotracheal tube; currently, the need for intubation in all cases is coming into question and many chronic respiratory failure patients can be adequately ventilated by noninvasive devices.

negative pressure v., mechanical v. in which various devices that surround the thorax are used in such a way that the development of negative or subatmospheric pressure causes thoracic expansion and thus inhalation; the release of the negative pressure allows the thorax to relax and thus the lungs to exhale. This is the type of v. made famous by the "iron lung," used in so many patients with poliomyelitis. Other such ventilators include the cuirass and the body suit.

noninvasive positive pressure v., the application of positive pressure through a nasal or full-face mask encompassing the nose and mouth, which is cycled in a similar way to modes of v. in which more direct control of the patient's airway or trachea has been achieved. This type of v. is often used to temporize while treating the patient to avoid endotracheal intubation.

permissive hypercapnic v., mechanical v. in which the level of carbon dioxide in the blood is allowed to rise well above normal values, to minimize the amount of mechanical support given to the patient, and thus minimize complications of that support, such as barotrauma. This mode of v. is used commonly in severe asthmatic patients, who, if ventilated more traditionally, would generate huge pressures in their airways, with resultant pneumothorax.

pressure-controlled v., mechanical v. that is achieved regardless of the patient's spontaneous breathing, but that uses pressure as the major determining variable, along with rate and time, of how much air the patient receives.

pressure-support v., mechanical ventilatory assistance in which each breath triggers a pressure-limited amount of support. The ventilator only provides support of each breath to a preset amount of pressure, thus the volume breathed can differ from breath to breath taken.

proportional assist v., mechanical v. in which the ventilator, in synchrony with the patient's own breathing, gives support in proportion to the effort generated by the patient. This mode allows the patient to determine completely how much support is given by the machine.

pulmonary v., respiratory minute volume, i.e., the total volume of gas per minute inspired (V_I) or expired (V_E) expressed in liters per minute; differs from alveolar v. by including the exchange of dead space gas.

synchronized intermittent mandatory v. (SIMV), intermittent mandatory v. spontaneously initiated by the patient to increase tidal volume to a preset volume, and subsequently synchronized with the patient's respiratory cycle; if the patient makes no respiratory effort, the machine automatically delivers a preset number of breaths by itself.

wasted v., that part of the pulmonary v. which is ineffective in exchanging oxygen and carbon dioxide with pulmonary capillary blood; calculated as physiologic dead space multiplied by respiratory frequency.

ven·ti·la·tion/per·fu·sion mis·match. An imbalance between alveolar ventilation and pulmonary capillary blood flow.

ventilator (ven′til-ā-tōr). SYN respirator. [L. *ventilo,* to fan, fr. *ventus,* wind, + *-ator,* agent suffix]

cuirass v., rigid breast plate that fits over the anterior portion of the chest and by application and release of negative pressure moves the chest wall, thus "breathing" for the patient.

vent·plant. An endosteal implant, usually made of titanium, utilized to provide support and fixation for a dental prosthesis by means of projections through the mucosa; also used to designate a family of implants.

ven·trad (ven'trad). Toward the ventral aspect; opposed to dorsad. [L. *venter,* belly, + *ad,* to]

ven·tral (ven'trăl) [TA]. **1.** Pertaining to the belly or to any venter. **2.** SYN anterior (1). **3.** In veterinary anatomy, the undersurface of an animal; often used to indicate the position of one structure relative to another, i.e., situated nearer the undersurface of the body. [L. *ventralis*]

ven·tra·lis (ven-trā'lis) [TA]. SYN anterior (1). [L.]

ventral paraflocculus. A small hemisphere portion of the posterior lobe of the cerebellum (lobule IX) that is structurally associated with the tonsil of the cerebellum (also lobule HIX) and with the uvula (vermis lobule IX). SYN paraflocculus ventralis.

ven·tri·cle (ven'tri-kl) [TA]. A normal cavity, as of the brain or heart. SYN ventriculus (2) [TA]. [L. *ventriculus,* dim. of *venter,* belly]

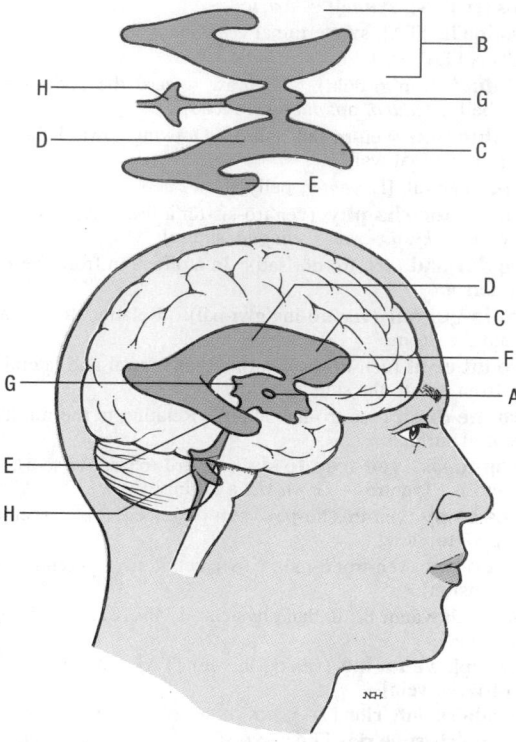

ventricles of the brain (superior and lateral views): (A) massa intermedia, (B) left ventricle, (C) anterior horn of right lateral ventricle, (D) central part of right lateral ventricle, (E) inferior horn of right lateral ventricle, (F) interventricular foramen, (G) third ventricle, (H) fourth ventricle

Arantius v., SYN *calamus* scriptorius.

cerebral v.'s, SEE lateral v., fourth v., third v., *cavity* of septum pellucidum.

v. of cerebral hemisphere, SYN lateral v.

v. of diencephalon, SYN third v.

double outlet right v., a heterogeneous category of congenital abnormalities as yet unclassified. Basically both great arteries arise in whole or in part from the right v. or an infundibular chamber. Ventricular septal defect is nearly always present.

Duncan v., SYN *cavity* of septum pellucidum.

fifth v., SYN *cavity* of septum pellucidum.

fourth v. [TA], a cavity of irregular tentlike shape extending from the obex rostralward to its communication with the sylvian aqueduct, enclosed between the cerebellum dorsally and the rhombencephalic tegmentum ventrally, having a rhomboid-shaped floor (rhomboid fossa) and a tentlike roof which in its caudal part is formed by the tela choroidea and the posterior medullary velum, in its middle part by the white matter of the cerebellum, and in its narrowing rostral part (recessus superior) by the anterior medullary velum. The fourth v. reaches its greatest width at the pontomedullary transition, where it expands laterally behind the cerebellar peduncles into the spoutlike lateral recess, and its greatest height at the fastigial recess, which reaches up into the cerebellar white matter. Direct communication of the brain's v. system and the subarachnoid space is established at the level of the fourth v. by a median opening in the tela choroidea, the medial aperture of Magendie's foramen, which opens into the cerebellomedullary cistern, and on both sides by the lateral aperture or foramen of Luschka, which connects the lateral recess with the interpeduncular cistern. SYN ventriculus quartus [TA], v. of rhombencephalon.

laryngeal v. [TA], the recess in each lateral wall of the larynx between the vestibular and vocal folds and into which the laryngeal sacculus opens. SYN ventriculus laryngis [TA], laryngeal sinus, Morgagni sinus (3), Morgagni v., sinus laryngeus.

lateral v. [TA], a cavity shaped somewhat like a horseshoe in conformity with the general shape of the hemisphere; each lateral v. communicates with the third v. through the interventricular foramen of Monro, and expands from there forward into the frontal lobe as the anterior horn as well as caudally over the thalamus as the central part (cella media) or body which, behind the thalamus, curves ventrally and laterally, then forward into the temporal lobe as the inferior horn; from the apex of the curve a variably sized posterior horn extends back into the white matter of the occipital lobe. The large choroid plexus of the lateral v. invades the cella media and the inferior horn (but not the anterior and posterior horn) from the medial side. SYN ventriculus lateralis [TA], v. of cerebral hemisphere.

left v. [TA], the lower chamber on the left side of the heart that receives the arterial blood from the left atrium and drives it by the contraction of its walls into the aorta. SYN ventriculus sinister [TA].

Morgagni v., SYN laryngeal v.

parchment right v., SYN Uhl *anomaly.*

v. of rhombencephalon, SYN fourth v.

right v. [TA], the lower chamber on the right side of the heart which receives the venous blood from the right atrium and drives it by the contraction of its walls into the pulmonary artery. SYN ventriculus dexter [TA].

(right/left) v.'s of heart, one of the two lower chambers of the heart. SYN ventriculus cordis dexter/sinister.

single v., congenital absence or near total absence of the ventricular septum.

sixth v., SYN Verga v.

sylvian v., SYN *cavity* of septum pellucidum.

v. of Sylvius, SYN *cavity* of septum pellucidum.

terminal v. [TA], a dilation of the central canal of the spinal cord at the tip of the medullary cone. SYN ventriculus terminalis [TA].

third v. [TA], a narrow, vertically oriented, irregularly quadrilateral cavity in the midplane, extending from the lamina terminalis to the rostral opening of the mesencephalic aqueduct. This v. communicates at its rostrodorsal corner with each of the two lateral v.'s through the left and right interventricular foramen of Monro. Its narrow roof is formed by the tela choroidea which is attached on either side to the tenia thalami; its lateral wall is formed by the medial surface of the thalamus and, below the hypothalamic sulcus, by the hypothalamus, which also forms its floor. In lateral profile, the third v. exhibits a number of recesses: in its floor, from before backward, 1) the preoptic recess in the acute angle between the base of the lamina terminalis and the dorsum of the optic chiasm, 2) the infundibular recess extending ventrally into the infundibulum but (in humans) not into the hypophysial stalk, and 3) the mamillary or inframamillary recess caused by the protrusion of the mamillary bodies into the v. From its dorsocaudal corner, the pineal recess extends caudally into the pineal stalk. SYN ventriculus tertius [TA], v. of diencephalon.

Verga v., an inconstant, horizontal, slitlike space between the posterior one-third of the corpus callosum and the underlying commissura fornicis (commissura hippocampi; psalterium) resulting from failure of these two commissural plates to fuse completely during fetal development; like the cavity of the septum pellucidum, the space is not a true v. in the sense that it did not develop from the central canal of the neural tube. SYN cavum psalterii, cavum vergae, sixth v.

Vieussens v., SYN *cavity* of septum pellucidum.

Wenzel v., SYN *cavity* of septum pellucidum.

ven·tri·cose (ven′tri-kōs). Bulging or swollen on one side or unequally.

ven·tric·u·lar (ven-trik′ū-lăr). Relating to a ventricle, in any sense. SYN ventricularis (1).

ven·tric·u·lar·is (ven-trik′ū-lā′ris). **1.** SYN ventricular. **2.** SYN thyroepiglottic *part* of thyroarytenoid (muscle). [Mod. L. fr. L. *ventriculus*]

ven·tric·u·lar·i·za·tion (ven-trik′ū-lar-i-zā′shŭn). Transformation of an atrial phenomenon to simulate a ventricular one, especially of the atrial (or venous) pulse tracing in tricuspid regurgitation.

ven·tric·u·lar pon·der·ance (ven-trik′7Macr;u-lăr pon′der-ans). A semiobsolete electrocardiographic term suggesting that one ventricle is either larger or thicker than the other.

ventriculectomy.

partial left v., SYN left ventricular volume reduction *surgery.*

ven·tric·u·li·tis (ven-trik-ū-lī′tis). Inflammation of the ventricles of the brain. [ventricle + G. *-itis,* inflammation]

△**ventriculo-.** A ventricle. [L. *ventriculus*]

ven·tric·u·lo·a·tri·al (VA) (ven-trik′ū-lō-ā′trē-ăl). Relating to both ventricles and atria, especially to the sequential passage of conduction in the retrograde direction from ventricle to atrium.

ven·tric·u·lo·cis·ter·nos·to·my (ven-trik′ū-lō-sis′ter-nos′tō-mē). An artificial opening between the ventricles of the brain and the cisterna magna. SEE ALSO shunt (2). [ventriculo- + L. *cisterna,* cistern, + G. *stoma,* mouth]

🔲 **ven·tric·u·log·ra·phy** (ven-trik-ū-log′ră-fē). **1.** Radiographic demonstration of the cerebral ventricles by direct injection of air or contrast medium; developed and described by Dandy in 1918. Cf. pneumoencephalography. **2.** Demonstration of the contractility of the cardiac ventricles by recording serially the distribution of intravenously injected radionuclide or that of radiographic contrast medium injected through an intracardiac catheter. [ventriculo- + G. *graphe,* a writing]

radionuclide v., SYN radionuclide *angiocardiography.*

ven·tric·u·lo·mas·toi·dos·to·my (ven-trik′ū-lō-mas′toy-dos′tō-mē). Operation for the establishment of a communication between the lateral cerebral ventricle and the mastoid antrum by means of a polythene tube for the relief of hydrocephalus. SEE ALSO shunt (2). [ventriculo- + mastoid, + G. *stoma,* mouth]

ven·tric·u·lo·nec·tor (ven-trik′oo-lō-nek′ter, -tōr). SYN atrioventricular *bundle.* [ventriculo- + L. *necto,* to join]

ven·tric·u·lo·pha·sic (ven-trik′ū-lō-fā′zik). Influenced by ventricular contraction; applied to the atrial rhythm when this is modified by ventricular contraction; in v. sinus arrhythmia in complete AV block the sinus impulse immediately following a ventricular contraction usually appears sooner than expected.

ven·tric·u·lo·plas·ty (ven-trik′ū-lō-plas-tē). Any surgical procedure to repair a defect of one of the ventricles of the heart. [ventriculo- + G. *plastos,* formed]

reduction left v., SYN left ventricular volume reduction *surgery.*

ven·tric·u·lo·punc·ture (ven-trik′ū-lō-pŭnk′choor). Insertion of a needle into a ventricle.

ven·tric·u·los·co·py (ven-trik-ū-los′kŏ-pē). Direct inspection of a ventricle with an endoscope. [ventriculo- + G. *skopeō,* to view]

ven·tric·u·los·to·my (ven-trik-ū-los′tō-mē). Establishment of an opening in a ventricle, usually through the floor of the third ventricle to the subarachnoid space to relieve hydrocephalus. SEE ALSO shunt (2). [ventriculo- + G. *stoma,* mouth]

third v., an operation to establish an opening from the third ventricle to the prechiasmal and interpeduncular cisterns (Stookey-Scarff operation) or from the third ventricle to the interpeduncular cistern (Dandy operation).

ven·tric·u·lo·sub·a·rach·noid (ven-trik′ū-lō-sŭb-ă-rak′noyd). Relating to the space occupied by the cerebrospinal fluid. [ventriculo- + subarachnoid]

ven·tric·u·lot·o·my (ven-trik-ū-lot′ō-mē). Incision into a ventricle; e.g., into the cerebral third ventricle for the relief of hydrocephalus or into a cardiac ventricle to surgically correct an abnormality. [ventriculo- + G. *tomē,* incision]

ven·tric·u·lus, pl. **ven·tric·u·li** (ven-trik′ū-lŭs, -lī) [TA]. **1.** stomach. **2.** SYN ventricle. **3.** The enlarged posterior portion of the mesenteron of the insect alimentary canal, in which digestion occurs. [L. dim. of *venter,* belly]

v. cor′dis dexter/sinister, SYN (right/left) *ventricles* of heart, under *ventricle.*

v. dex′ter [TA], SYN right *ventricle.*

v. laryn′gis [TA], SYN laryngeal *ventricle.*

v. latera′lis [TA], SYN lateral *ventricle.*

v. quar′tus [TA], SYN fourth *ventricle.*

v. quin′tus, SYN *cavity* of septum pellucidum.

v. sinis′ter [TA], SYN left *ventricle.*

v. termina′lis [TA], SYN terminal *ventricle.*

v. ter′tius [TA], SYN third *ventricle.*

ven·tri·duct (ven′tri-dŭkt). To draw toward the abdomen. [L. *venter,* belly, + *duco,* pp. *ductus,* to lead]

ven·tri·duc·tion (ven-tri-dŭk′shŭn). Drawing toward the abdomen or abdominal wall.

△**ventro-.** Ventral. [L. *venter,* belly]

ven·tro·cys·tor·rha·phy (ven′trō-sis-tōr′ă-fē). SYN cystopexy. [ventro- + G. *kystis,* cyst, + *rhaphē,* suture]

ven·tro·dor·sad (ven-trō-dōr′sad). In a direction from the venter to the dorsum.

ven·tro·in·gui·nal (ven′trō-ing′gwi-năl). Relating to the abdomen and the groin.

ven·tro·lat·er·al (ven-trō-lat′ĕ-răl). Both ventral and lateral, i.e., to the front and to the side.

ven·tro·me·di·an (ven-trō-mē′dē-an). Relating to the midline of the ventral surface.

ven·trop·to·sis, ven·trop·to·sia (ven-trō-tō′sis, -tō′sē-ă). SYN gastroptosis. [ventro- + G. *ptōsis,* a falling]

ven·tros·co·py (ven-tros′kŏ-pē). SYN peritoneoscopy. [ventro- + G. *skopeō,* to view]

ven·trot·o·my (ven-trot′ō-mē). SYN celiotomy. [ventro- + G. *tomē,* incision]

Venturi, Giovanni B., Italian physicist, 1746–1822. SEE V. *effect, meter, tube.*

ven·u·la, pl. **ven·u·lae** (ven′oo-lă, -lē) [TA]. SYN venule. [L. dim. of *vena,* vein]

v. macula′ris infe′rior [TA], SYN inferior macular *venule.*

v. macula′ris supe′rior [TA], SYN superior macular *venule.*

v. media′lis ret′inae [TA], SYN medial *venule* of retina.

v. nasa′lis ret′inae infe′rior [TA], SYN inferior nasal retinal *venule.*

v. nasa′lis ret′inae supe′rior [TA], SYN superior nasal retinal *venule.*

venulae rectae of kidney [TA], venules that drain the medullary pyramids of the kidney; they open into arcuate veins. SYN venulae rectae renis [TA], straight venules of kidney.

ven′ulae rec′tae re′nis [TA], SYN venulae rectae of kidney.

ven′ulae stella′tae, the star-shaped groups of venules in the renal cortex. SYN stellate veins, stellate venules, stellulae verheyenii, venae stellatae, Verheyen stars.

v. tempora′lis ret′inae infe′rior [TA], SYN inferior temporal retinal *venule.*

v. tempora′lis ret′inae supe′rior [TA], SYN superior temporal retinal *venule.*

ven·u·lar (ven′oo-lăr). Pertaining to venules. SYN venulous.

ven·ule (ven′ool, vē′nool) [TA]. A venous radicle continuous with a capillary. SYN venula [TA], capillary vein, veinlet.

high endothelial postcapillary v.'s, v.'s in the lymph nodes, tonsils, and Peyer patches that have a high-walled endothelium through which blood lymphocytes migrate from the blood into the lymphatic parenchyma.

inferior macular v. [TA], a small tributary of the central vein of the retina that drains the lower part of the macula. SYN venula macularis inferior [TA].

inferior nasal v. of retina, SYN inferior nasal retinal v.

inferior nasal retinal v. [TA], the small vein that passes from the inferior medial (nasal) part of the retina to join the central vein. SYN venula nasalis retinae inferior [TA], inferior nasal v. of retina.

inferior temporal v. of retina, SYN inferior temporal retinal v.

inferior temporal retinal v. [TA], the small vein that passes from the lower lateral (temporal) part of the retina to enter the central vein. SYN venula temporalis retinae inferior [TA], inferior temporal v. of retina.

medial v. of retina [TA], the small vein that passes from the part of the retina between the macula and the optic disk to join the central vein. SYN venula medialis retinae [TA].

nasal v.'s of retina, SEE inferior nasal retinal v., superior nasal retinal v.

pericytic v.'s, SYN postcapillary v.'s.

postcapillary v.'s, the microvasculature immediately following the capillaries, ranging in size from 10 to 50 μm, and characterized by investment of pericytes; they are the site of extravasation of blood cells, are particularly sensitive to histamine, and are believed to be important in blood-interstitial fluid exchanges. SYN pericytic v.'s.

stellate v.'s, SYN *venulae* stellatae, under *venula*.

straight v.'s of kidney, SYN *venulae* rectae of kidney, under *venula*.

superior macular v. [TA], a small tributary of the central vein of the retina that drains the upper part of the macula. SYN venula macularis superior [TA].

superior nasal v. of retina, SYN superior nasal retinal v.

superior nasal retinal v. [TA], the small vein that drains blood from the upper medial (nasal) part of the retina; it joins the central vein. SYN venula nasalis retinae superior [TA], superior nasal v. of retina.

superior temporal v. of retina, SYN superior temporal retinal v.

superior temporal retinal v. [TA], the v. that passes from the upper lateral (temporal) part of the retina to join the central vein. SYN venula temporalis retinae superior [TA], superior temporal v. of retina.

temporal v.'s of retina, SEE inferior temporal retinal v., superior temporal retinal v.

ven·u·lous (ven′oo-lŭs). SYN venular.

VER Abbreviation for visual evoked response. SEE evoked *response*.

ve·rap·a·mil (ver-ap′ă-mil). A calcium channel blocking agent used to treat cardiac arrhythmias and angina pectoris. SYN iproveratril.

ve·rat·ric ac·id (vĕ-rat′rik). Obtained by methylation and subsequent oxidation of protocatechuic acid; present in the seeds of *Schoenocaulon officinale* (*Sabadilla officinarum*).

ver·a·tri·dine (ver-ă-trī′dēn). An alkaloid derived from *Veratrum viridae* and *V. album*. Probably responsible for antihypertensive properties of this class of alkaloids.

ver·a·trine (ver′ă-trēn, -trin). A mixture of alkaloids from the seeds of *Schoenocaulon officinale* (*Sabadilla officinarum*) (family Liliaceae), including cevine, cevadine, cevadilline, sabadine, and veratridine; a powder of acrid taste, intensely irritating to the nasal mucous membrane, that has been used as an anodyne counterirritant in neuralgias and arthritis.

Ve·ra·trum (vĕ-rā′trŭm). A genus of toxic liliaceous plants. [L. hellebore]

V. al′bum, the rhizome has emetic and cathartic actions.

V. vir′ide, the dried rhizome and roots contain therapeutically important alkaloids (cevadine, veratridine, jervine, pseudojervine, rubijervine, and several ester alkaloids of the base germine) used in the treatment of hypertensive disorders.

ver·big·er·a·tion (ver-bij-er-ā′shŭn). Constant repetition of meaningless words or phrases; seen in schizophrenia. SYN oral stereotypy. [L. *verbum*, word, + *gero*, to carry about]

ver·bo·ma·nia (ver-bō-mā′nē-ă). A rarely used term for an ab-

normal talkativeness; a psychotic flow of speech. [L. *verbum*, word, + G. *mania*, frenzy]

ver·di·gris (ver′di-grēs, -gris, -grē). Cupric acetate (normal). [O. Fr. *verd*, green, *de*, of, *Gris*, Greeks]

ver·dine (ver′din). SYN biliverdin.

ver·do·glo·bin (ver-dō-glō-bin). Obsolete term for choleglobin.

ver·do·he·mo·chrome (ver-dō-hē′mō-krōm). An intermediate stage in hemoglobin degradation to yield the bile pigments, i.e., hemoglobin yields choleglobin (verdohemoglobin) and the loss of globin leaves v., the precursor of biliverdin.

ver·do·he·mo·glo·bin (ver′dō-hē-mō-glō′bin). SYN choleglobin.

ver·do·per·ox·i·dase (ver′dō-per-oks′i-dās). A peroxidase, occurring in leukocytes, that contains a greenish ferriheme; responsible for the peroxidase activity of pus.

Verga, Andrea, Italian neurologist, 1811–1895. SEE V. *ventricle; cavum* vergae.

verge (verj). An edge or margin.

anal v., the transitional zone between the moist, hairless, modified skin of the anal canal and the perianal skin.

ver·gence (ver′jens). A disjunctive movement of the eyes in which the fixation axes are not parallel, as in convergence or divergence. [L. *vergo*, to incline, to turn]

v. of lens, the reciprocal of the principal focal distance used as a measure of the divergence or convergence of parallel rays.

Verheyen, Philippe, Flemish anatomist, 1648–1710. SEE V. *stars*, under *star; stellulae* verheyenii, under *stellula*.

Verhoeff, Frederick H., U.S. ophthalmologist, 1874–1968. SEE V. elastic tissue *stain*.

Ver·mes (ver′mēz). Archaic term for a subkingdom of the animal kingdom containing worms and wormlike organisms; an unnatural division no longer in taxonomic use. [L. *vermis*, worm]

△**vermi-.** A worm; wormlike. [L. *vermis*]

ver·mi·ci·dal (ver′mi-sī′dăl). Destructive to worms; specifically, destructive to parasitic intestinal worms. [vermi- + L. *caedo*, to kill]

ver·mi·cide (ver′mi-sīd). An agent that kills intestinal parasitic worms. [vermi- + L. *caedo*, to kill]

ver·mic·u·lar (ver-mik′oo-lăr). Relating to, resembling, or moving like a worm. [L. *vermiculus*, dim. of *vermis*, worm]

ver·mic·u·la·tion (ver-mik-ū-lā′shŭn). A wormlike movement, as in peristalsis.

ver·mi·cule (ver′mi-kool). 1. A small worm or wormlike organism or structure. 2. SYN ookinete. [L. *vermiculus*, a small worm]

ver·mic·u·lose, ver·mic·u·lous (ver-mik′ū-lōs, -lŭs). 1. Wormy; infected with worms or larvae. 2. Wormlike. SEE ALSO vermiform.

ver·mic·u·lus (ver-mik′ū-lŭs). SEE vermicule. [L. dim. of *vermis*, worm]

ver·mi·form (ver′mi-fōrm). Worm-shaped; resembling a worm in form, denoting especially the appendix of the cecum. SEE ALSO lumbricoid, scolecoid (2). [vermi- + L. *forma*, form]

ver·mif·u·gal (ver-mif′ū-găl). SYN anthelmintic (2). [vermi- + L. *fugo*, to chase away]

ver·mi·fuge (ver′mi-fooj). SYN anthelmintic (1). [vermi- + L. *fugo*, to chase away]

ver·mil·ion (ver-mil′yon) [C.I. 77766]. A red pigment made from cinnabar or red mercuric sulfide.

ver·mil·ion·ec·to·my (ver-mil-yon-ek′tō-mē). Excision of the vermilion border of the lip. [vermilion border + G. *ektomē*, cutting out]

ver·min (ver′min). Parasitic insects, such as lice and bedbugs. [L. *vermis*, a worm]

ver·mi·nal (ver′mi-năl). SYN verminous.

ver·mi·na·tion (ver-mi-nā′shŭn). 1. The production or breeding of worms or larvae. 2. Infestation with vermin.

ver·min·ous (ver′mi-nŭs). Relating to, caused by, or infested with worms, larvae, or vermin. SYN verminal. [L. *verminosus*, wormy]

ver·mis, pl. **ver·mes** (ver′mis, -mēz). 1. A worm; any structure

ve

or part resembling a worm in shape. **2** [TA]. Vermis cerebelli, the narrow middle zone between the two hemispheres of the cerebellum; the portion projecting above the level of the hemispheres on the upper surface is called the superior v.; the lower portion, sunken between the two hemispheres and forming the floor of the vallecula, is the inferior v. [L. worm]

ver·mix (ver′miks). SYN appendix (2).

Verner, John, U.S. internist, *1927. SEE V.-Morrison *syndrome.*

Vernet, Maurice, French neurologist, 1887–1974. SEE V. *syndrome.*

Vernier, Pierre, French mathematician, 1580–1637. SEE V. *acuity.*

ver·nix (ver′niks). SYN varnish (dental). [Mod. L.]

v. caseo′sa, the fatty substance, consisting of desquamated epithelial cells, lanugo hairs, and sebaceous matter, which covers the skin of the fetus.

Verocay, José, Czechoslovakian pathologist, 1876–1927. SEE V. *bodies,* under *body.*

Ver·on·al (ver′ō-nal). SYN barbital.

ver·ru·ca, pl. **ver·ru·cae** (vĕ-roo′kă, -kē). A flesh-colored growth characterized by circumscribed hypertrophy of the papillae of the corium, with thickening of the malpighian, granular, and keratin layers of the epidermis, caused by human papilloma virus; also applied to epidermal verrucous tumors of nonviral etiology. SYN verruga, wart. [L.]

v. digita′ta, a wart in which the papillae project like fingers; they occur in groups, often on the scalp. SYN digitate wart.

v. filifor′mis, a wart composed of a single or many greatly elongated papillae; appears more commonly on the face and neck. SYN filiform wart.

v. perua′na, v. peruvia′na, SYN *verruga* peruana.

v. pla′na, a smooth, flat, flesh-colored wart of small size, occurring in groups, seen especially on the face of the young; often associated with common warts of the hands, due to human papilloma virus, commonly, types 3 and 10. SYN flat wart, plane wart, v. plana juvenilis.

v. pla′na juveni′lis, SYN v. plana.

v. pla′na seni′lis, SYN actinic *keratosis.*

v. planta′ris, SYN plantar *wart.*

seborrheic v., SYN seborrheic *keratosis.*

v. seni′lis, SYN actinic *keratosis.*

v. sim′plex, SYN v. vulgaris.

v. vulga′ris, a keratotic papilloma of the epidermis which occurs most frequently in young persons as a result of localized infection by human papilloma virus, usually types 2 and 4; the lesions are of variable duration, eventually undergoing spontaneous regression, and are both exophytic and endophytic, with hyperkeratosis, parakeratosis, hypergranulosis, koilocytosis, and papillomatosis. SYN common wart, infectious wart, v. simplex, viral wart.

ver·ru·ci·form (vĕ-roo′si-fōrm). Wart-shaped. [L. *verruca,* wart, + *forma,* form]

ver·ru·cose (vĕ-roo′kōs). Resembling a wart; denoting wartlike elevations. SYN verrucous. [L. *verrucosus*]

ver·ru·co·sis (ver-oo-kō′sis). A condition marked by the appearance of multiple warts. [L. *verruca,* wart, + G. *-osis,* condition]

lymphostatic v., SYN mossy *foot.*

ver·ru·cous (vĕ-roo′kŭs). SYN verrucose.

ver·ru·ga (vĕ-roo′gă). SYN verruca. [Sp.]

v. perua′na, a late, eruptive stage of bartonellosis; characterized by soft conical or pedunculated vascular papules anywhere on the skin or mucous membranes from miliary size to several centimeters, resolving without scars after a few months. SYN Peruvian wart, verruca peruana, verruca peruviana.

ver·si·col·or (ver-si-kŏl′ŏr). Variegated; marked by a variety of color. [L. particolored, fr. *verso,* to turn, twist, + *color,* color]

ver·sion (ver′zhŭn, -shŭn). **1.** Displacement of the uterus, with tilting of the entire organ without bending upon itself; such displacement may be anteversion, retroversion, or lateroversion. **2.** Change of position of the fetus in the uterus, occurring spontaneously or effected by manipulation. **3.** SYN inclination. **4.** Conju-

gate rotation of the eyes in the same direction; such rotation may be dextroversion, levoversion, supraversion, or infraversion. [L. *verto,* pp. *versus,* to turn]

bimanual v., turning of the baby in utero, performed by the hands acting upon both extremities of the fetus; it may be external v. or combined v. SYN bipolar v.

bipolar v., SYN bimanual v.

cephalic v., v. in which the fetus is turned so that the head presents; can be external cephalic v. or internal cephalic v. SEE ALSO external cephalic v., internal cephalic v.

combined v., bipolar v. by means of one hand in the vagina, the other on the abdominal wall.

external cephalic v., v. performed entirely by external manipulation. SEE ALSO cephalic v.

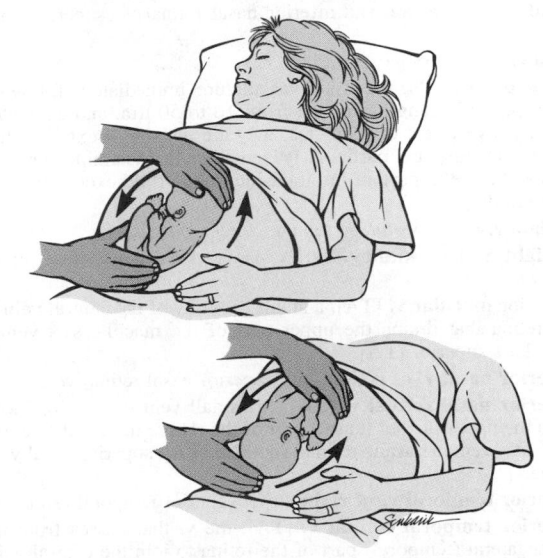

external cephalic version: the fetus is rotated by external pressure to a cephalic presentation

internal cephalic v., v. performed by means of one hand within the uterus. SEE ALSO cephalic v.

internal podalic v., maneuver to deliver the fetus by inserting a hand into the uterine cavity, grasping one or both feet, and drawing them through the cervix; rarely indicated today except for the delivery of a second twin. SYN podalic v.

pelvic v., v. by means of which a transverse or oblique presentation is converted into a pelvic presentation by manipulating the buttocks of the fetus.

podalic v., SYN internal podalic v.

postural v., nonmanual v. obtained by changing the position of the mother.

Potter v., obsolete term for a v. in which both feet are brought down until the buttocks are delivered, the back is then rotated to an anterior position, the arms and shoulders are delivered by twisting and downward movements.

spontaneous v., turning of the fetus effected by the unaided contraction of the uterine muscle.

Wright v., a cephalic v. employed in cases of shoulder presentation when the shoulders are pushed upward while the breech is moved toward the center of the uterus by the other hand; the head is then guided into the pelvis.

ver·te·bra, gen. and pl. **ver·te·brae** (ver′tĕ-bră, -brē) [TA]. One of the segments of the spinal column; in humans, there are usually 33 vertebrae: 7 cervical, 12 thoracic, 5 lumbar, 5 sacral (fused into one bone, the sacrum), and 4 coccygeal (fused into one bone, the coccyx). [L. joint, fr. *verto,* to turn]

basilar v., the lowest lumbar v.

block vertebrae, congenitally fused and hypoplastic vertebral

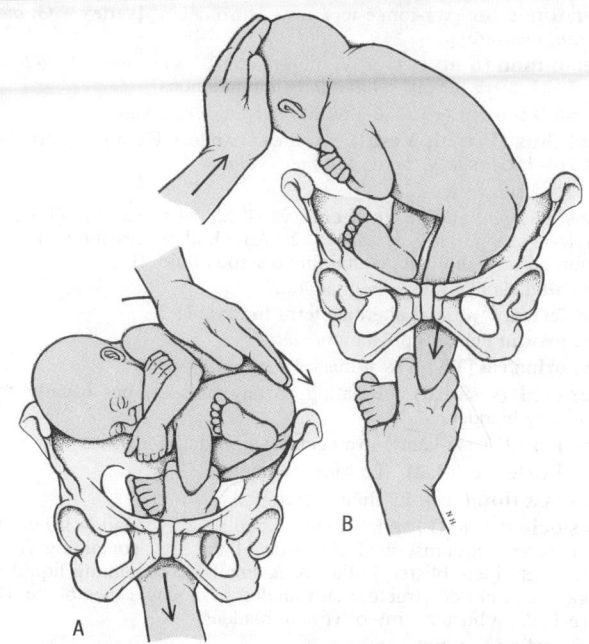

internal podalic version: conversion from dorsoposterior transverse lie to breech; (A) obstetrician's right hand grasps fetal foot within uterus while left hand applies pressure externally to rotate breech toward pelvic inlet; (B) obstetrician maneuvers fetus into longitudinal orientation by applying traction to foot while externally directing head into fundus, so that delivery can proceed as in breech presentation

bodies which, on radiographs, give the appearance of a more or less solid bony mass. SEE Klippel-Feil *syndrome*.

butterfly v., a hemivertebra or sagittally cleft v. that has a butterfly configuration on frontal radiographs; congenital in origin.

v. C1, ☆official alternate term for atlas.

v. C2, ☆official alternate term for axis (5).

caudal vertebrae, the vertebrae that form the skeleton of the tail.

cervical vertebrae [C1–C7] [TA], the seven segments of the vertebral column located in the neck. SYN vertebrae cervicales [C1–C7].

ver′tebrae cervica′les [C1–C7], SYN cervical vertebrae [C1–C7].

ver′tebrae coccyg′eae [Co1–Co4] [TA], SYN coccygeal vertebrae [Co1–Co4].

coccygeal vertebrae [Co1–Co4] [TA], the four terminal segments of the vertebral column, usually fused to form the coccyx. SYN vertebrae coccygeae [Co1–Co4] [TA], tail vertebrae.

codfish vertebrae, exaggeration of the concavity of the upper and lower end plates of the vertebrae, as demonstrated radiographically in various types of osteopenia.

cranial v., a segment of the skull regarded as homologous with a segment of the vertebral column.

v. denta′ta, SYN axis (5).

dorsal vertebrae, [L1–L4] an archaic term for thoracic vertebrae.

false vertebrae, the fused vertebral segments of the sacrum and coccyx. SYN vertebrae spuriae.

first cervical v., SYN atlas.

hourglass vertebrae, the radiographic appearance of some vertebrae in osteogenesis imperfecta tarda.

H-shape vertebrae, sharply delimited depression of the central portion of the endplates of the vertebrae, producing a stocky "H" shape on radiographs, as in sickle cell anemia.

ivory v., a radiographically dense v., usually from metastatic disease, especially lymphoma when solitary.

ver′tebrae lumba′les [L1–L5], SYN lumbar vertebrae [L1–L5].

lumbar vertebrae [L1–L5], the vertebrae, usually five in num-

ber, located in the lumbar region of the back. SYN vertebrae lumbales [L1–L5].

v. mag′na, SYN sacrum.

odontoid v., SYN axis (5).

picture frame v., radiographically diminished density of trabecular bone with relative preservation of the cortex, a sign of osteopenia.

v. pla′na, spondylitis with reduction of vertebral body to a thin disk.

v. prom′inens [TA], the v. in the cervicothoracic region which has the most prominent spinous process (seventh cervical v. in 70% of the cases, sixth in 20%, and first thoracic v. in 10%). SYN nuchal tubercle.

rugger jersey v., appearance of a vertebral body with horizontal sclerotic bands adjacent to the endplates; associated with renal osteodystrophy.

ver′tebrae sacra′les [S1–S5], SYN sacral vertebrae [S1–S5].

sacral vertebrae [S1–S5], the segments of the vertebral column, usually five in number, that fuse to form the sacrum. SYN vertebrae sacrales [S1–S5].

second cervical v., SYN axis (5).

ver′tebrae spu′riae, SYN false vertebrae.

tail vertebrae, SYN coccygeal vertebrae [Co1–Co4].

ver′tebrae thora′cicae [T1–T12], SYN thoracic vertebrae [T1–T12].

thoracic vertebrae [T1–T12] [TA], the segments of the vertebral column, usually 12, which articulate with ribs to form part of the thoracic cage. SYN vertebrae thoracicae [T1–T12].

toothed v., SYN axis (5).

true v., any one of the cervical, thoracic, or lumbar vertebrae. SYN v. vera.

v. ve′ra, SYN true v.

ver·te·bral (ver′tĕ-brăl). Relating to a vertebra or the vertebrae.

ver·te·bra·ri·um (ver-tĕ-brā′rē-ŭm). SYN vertebral *column*. [Mod. L.]

Ver·te·bra·ta (ver-tĕ-brah′tă, -brā′tă). The vertebrates, a major division of the phylum Chordata, consisting of those animals with a dorsal hollow nerve cord enclosed in a cartilaginous or bony spinal column; includes several classes of fishes, and the amphibians, reptiles, birds, and mammals. SYN Craniata. [L. *vertebratus*, jointed]

ver·te·brate (ver′tĕ-brāt). **1.** Having a vertebral column. **2.** An animal having vertebrae.

ver·te·brat·ed (ver′tĕ-brāt-ed). Jointed; composed of segments arranged longitudinally as in certain instruments.

ver·te·brec·to·my (ver′tĕ-brek′tō-mē). Resection of a vertebral body. [vertebra + G. *ektomē*, excision]

△**vertebro-.** A vertebra, vertebral. [L. *vertebra*]

ver·te·bro·ar·te·ri·al (ver′tĕ-brō-ar-tēr′ē-ăl). Relating to a vertebra and an artery, or to the vertebral artery.

ver·te·bro·chon·dral (ver′tĕ-brō-kon′drăl). Denoting the three false ribs (eighth, ninth, and tenth), which are connected with the vertebrae at one extremity and the costal cartilages at the other, these cartilages not articulating directly with the sternum. SYN vertebrocostal (2). [vertebro- + G. *chondros*, cartilage]

ver·te·bro·cos·tal (ver′tĕ-brō-kos′tăl). **1.** SYN costovertebral. **2.** SYN vertebrochondral. [vertebro- + L. *costa*, rib]

ver·te·bro·fem·o·ral (ver-tĕ-brō-fem′ŏ-răl). Relating to the vertebrae and the femur.

ver·te·bro·il·i·ac (ver′tĕ-brō-il′ē-ak). Relating to the vertebrae and the ilium.

ver·te·bro·sa·cral (ver-tĕ-brō-sā′krăl). Relating to the vertebrae and the sacrum.

ver·te·bro·ster·nal (ver′tĕ-brō-ster′năl). SYN sternovertebral.

ver·tex, pl. **ver·ti·ces** (ver′teks, ver′ti-sēz) [TA]. **1** [NA]. The topmost point of the vault of the skull, a landmark in craniometry. **2.** In obstetrics, the portion of the fetal head bounded by the planes of the trachelobregmatic and biparietal diameters, with the posterior fontanel at the apex. [L. whirl, whorl]

v. cor′dis, SYN *apex* of heart.

ve

v. of cornea, SYN corneal v.

v. cor′neae [TA], SYN corneal v.

corneal v. [TA], the central part of the cornea, slightly thinner than the peripheal part. SYN v. corneae [TA], v. of cornea.

ver·ti·cal (ver′ti-kăl) [TA]. **1.** Relating to the vertex, or crown of the head. **2.** Perpendicular. **3.** Denoting any plane or line that passes longitudinally through the body in the anatomic position. SYN verticalis [TA].

ver·ti·ca·lis (ver-ti-kā′lis) [TA]. SYN vertical. [L.]

ver·ti·ces (ver′ti-sēz). Plural of vertex.

ver·ti·cil (ver′ti-sil). A collection of similar parts radiating from a common axis. SYN vortex (1), whorl (4). [L. *verticillus,* the whirl of a spindle, dim. of *vertex,* a whirl]

ver·ti·cil·late (ver′ti-sil′āt). Disposed in the form of a verticil.

Ver·ti·cil·li·um (ver-ti-sil′ē-ŭm). A genus of hyphomycetous fungi often found in clinical specimens as contaminants. They are occasionally found in the meatus in cases of otitis externa, but are of doubtful pathogenicity. [L. *verticillus,* the whirl of a spindle]

ver·ti·co·men·tal (ver-ti-kō-men′tăl). Relating to the crown of the head and the chin; denoting a diameter in craniometry.

ver·tig·i·nous (ver-tij′i-nŭs). Relating to or suffering from vertigo.

ver·ti·go (ver′ti-gō, ver-tī′gō). **1.** A sensation of spinning or whirling motion. V. implies a definite sensation of rotation of the subject (subjective v.) or of objects about the subject (objective v.) in any plane. **2.** Imprecisely used as a general term to describe dizziness. [L. *vertigo* (*vertigin-*), dizziness, fr. *verto,* to turn]

aural v., (1) v. caused by disease of the internal ear or pressure of cerumen on the drum membrane; (2) nonspecific term for v. caused by labyrinthine disorders.

benign paroxysmal positional v., a recurrent, brief form of positional v. occurring in clusters; believed to result from displaced remnants of utricular otoconia. SYN cupulolithiasis.

benign positional v., brief attacks of paroxysmal v. and nystagmus that occur solely with certain head movements or positions, e.g., with neck extension; due to labyrinthine dysfunction. SYN positional v. of Bárány, postural v. (1).

Charcot v., SYN tussive *syncope.*

chronic v., SYN *status* vertiginosus.

endemic paralytic v., SYN vestibular *neuronitis.*

epidemic v., SYN vestibular *neuronitis.*

height v., dizziness experienced when looking down from a great height or in looking up at a high building or cliff. SYN vertical v. (1).

horizontal v., dizziness experienced on lying down.

hysterical v., a sensation of dizziness, as from a whirling motion, whose etiology is psychosomatic.

laryngeal v., SYN tussive *syncope.*

lateral v., dizziness caused by watching rows of vertical objects (e.g., telegraph poles, trees, and fences) from the window of a fast-moving vehicle.

mechanical v., v. caused by continued rotation or vibration of the body.

nocturnal v., a feeling of falling when dropping off to sleep.

ocular v., dizziness attributed to refractive errors or imbalance of the extrinsic muscles.

organic v., v. due to brain damage.

paralyzing v., SYN vestibular *neuronitis.*

physiologic v., SYN space *sickness.*

positional v., v. occurring with a change in body position.

positional v. of Bárány, SYN benign positional v.

postural v., (1) SYN benign positional v; (2) light-headedness that appears particularly in elderly people with change of position, usually from lying or sitting to standing; due to orthostatic hypotension.

sham-movement v., dizziness accompanied by an impression that the body is rotating or that objects are rotating about the body.

vertical v., (1) SYN height v; (2) dizziness experienced when standing upright.

visual v., v. induced by visual stimuli.

ver·tom·e·ter (ver-tom′ĕ-ter). SYN lensometer. [vertex + G. *metron,* measure]

ver·u·mon·ta·num (ver-oo-mon-tā′nŭm). SYN seminal *colliculus.* [L. *veru,* a spit, + *montanus,* mountainous]

ve·sa·li·a·num (ve-sā′lē-ā′nŭm). SYN os vesalianum.

Vesalius (Wesal, Vesal), Andreas (Andre), Flemish anatomist, 1514–1564. SEE V. *bone, foramen, vein.*

△**vesic-.** SEE vesico-.

ve·si·ca, gen. and pl. **ve·si·cae** (vĕ sī′ kă, vĕ sī′ sē; -kē) [TA]. **1** [NA]. SYN urinary *bladder.* **2.** Any hollow structure or sac, normal or pathologic, containing a serous fluid. [L.]

v. bilia′ris [TA], SYN gallbladder.

v. fel′lea, ✶official alternate term for gallbladder.

v. prostat′ica, SYN prostatic *utricle.*

v. urina′ria [TA], SYN urinary *bladder.*

ves·i·cal (ves′i-kăl). Relating to any bladder, but usually the urinary bladder.

ves·i·cant (ves′i-kănt). An agent that produces a vesicle.

ves·i·cate (ves′i-kāt). To form a vesicle.

ves·i·ca·tion (ves-i-kā′shŭn). SYN vesiculation (1).

ves·i·cle (ves′i-kl) [TA]. **1.** SYN vesicula. **2.** A small (<1.0 cm in diameter), circumscribed elevation of the skin containing fluid. SEE ALSO bleb, blister, bulla. **3.** A small sac containing liquid or gas. **4.** A closed structure surrounded by a single membrane. [L. *vesicula,* a blister, dim. of *vesica,* bladder]

acoustic v., SYN otic v.

acrosomal v., a v. derived from the Golgi apparatus during spermiogenesis whose limiting membrane adheres to the nuclear envelope; together with the acrosomal granule within, it spreads in a thin layer over the pole of the nucleus to form the acrosomal cap.

air v.'s, SYN pulmonary *alveolus.*

allantoic v., the hollow portion of the allantois.

amniocardiac v., the rostral portion of the most primitive intraembryonic celom.

auditory v., SYN otic v.

blastodermic v., SYN blastocyst.

cerebral v., each of the three divisions of the early embryonic brain (prosencephalon, mesencephalon, and rhombencephalon). SYN encephalic v., primary brain v.

cervical v., an abnormally persisting vestige of the cervical sinus or its associated branchial grooves.

coated v., a v. that has its biomembrane coated with the protein clathrin. It is involved in the transport of proteins from one membrane site to another.

encephalic v., SYN cerebral v.

forebrain v., ✶official alternate term for prosencephalon.

germinal v., archaic term for the nucleus of the ovum.

hindbrain v., ✶official alternate term for rhombencephalon.

lens v., in the embryo, the ectodermal invagination that forms opposite the optic cup; it is the primordium of the lens of the eye. SYN lenticular v.

lenticular v., SYN lens v.

malpighian v.'s, the minute air-filled v.'s on the surface of an expanded lung.

matrix v.'s, hydroxyapatite-containing, membrane-enclosed v.'s secreted by odontoblasts and some chondrocytes; believed to serve as nucleation centers for the mineralization process in dentin and calcified cartilage.

midbrain v., ✶official alternate term for mesencephalon.

ocular v., SYN optic v.

ophthalmic v., SYN optic v.

optic v., in the embryo, one of the paired evaginations from the ventrolateral walls of the forebrain from which the sensory and pigment layers of the retina develop. SYN ocular v., ophthalmic v., vesicula ophthalmica.

otic v., one of the paired sacs of invaginated ectoderm that develop into the membranous labyrinth of the internal ear. SYN acoustic v., auditory v.

pinocytotic v., a v., a fraction of a micrometer in diameter, containing fluid or solute being ingested into a cell by endocytosis. SEE ALSO pinocytosis.

primary brain v., SYN cerebral v.

seminal v., ⭐official alternate term for seminal *gland.*

synaptic v.'s, the small (average diameter 30 nm), intracellular, membrane-bound v.'s near the presynaptic membrane of a synaptic junction, containing the transmitter substance which, in chemical synapses, mediates the passage of nerve impulses across the junction. SEE ALSO synapse.

telencephalic v., paired diverticula arising from the prosencephalon, from which the forebrain develops.

umbilical v., SYN yolk *sac.*

△**vesico-, vesic-.** A vesica, vesicle. SEE ALSO vesiculo-. [L. *vesica,* bladder]

ves·i·co·ab·dom·i·nal (ves′i-kō-ab-dom′i-năl). Relating to the urinary bladder and the abdominal wall.

ves·i·co·bul·lous (ves′i-kō-bŭl′ŭs). Denoting an eruption of variously sized lesions containing fluid.

ves·i·co·cele (ves′i-kō-sēl). SYN cystocele.

ves·i·co·cer·vi·cal (ves′i-kō-ser′vi-kăl). Relating to the urinary bladder and the cervix of the uterus.

ves·i·coc·ly·sis (ves′i-kok′li-sis). Washing out, or lavage, of the urinary bladder. [vesico- + G. *klysis,* a washing out]

ves·i·co·in·tes·ti·nal (ves′i-kō-in-tes′ti-năl). Relating to the urinary bladder and the intestine; e.g., vesicointestinal fistula.

ves·i·co·li·thi·a·sis (ves′i-kō-li-thī′ă-sis). SYN cystolithiasis. [vesico- + G. *lithos,* stone, + -*iasis,* condition]

ves·i·co·pros·ta·tic (ves′i-kō-pros-tat′ik). Relating to the bladder and the prostate gland.

ves·i·co·pu·bic (ves′i-kō-pū′bik). Relating to the bladder and the os pubis.

ves·i·co·pus·tu·lar (ves′i-kō-pŭs′tū-lăr). Pertaining to a vesicopustule.

ves·i·co·pus·tule (ves′i-kō-pŭs′tūl). A vesicle which is developing pus formation.

ves·i·co·rec·tal (ves′i-kō-rek′tăl). Relating to the bladder and the rectum.

ves·i·co·rec·tos·to·my (ves′i-kō-rek-tos′tō-mē). Surgical urinary tract diversion by anastomosis of the posterior bladder wall to the rectum. [vesico- + rectum + G. *stoma,* mouth]

ves·i·co·sig·moid (ves′i-kō-sig′moyd). Relating to the bladder and the sigmoid colon.

ves·i·co·sig·moi·dos·to·my (ves′ĭ-kō-sig-moy-dos′tō-mē). Operative formation of a communication between the bladder and the sigmoid colon. [vesico- + sigmoid + G. *stoma,* mouth]

ves·i·co·spi·nal (ves′i-kō-spī′năl). Relating to the urinary bladder and the spinal cord; denoting the neural mechanisms that control retention and evacuation of urine by the bladder, located in the second lumbar and second sacral segment, respectively, of the spinal cord.

ves·i·cos·to·my (ves′i-kos′tō-mē). SYN cystostomy. [vesico- + G. *stoma,* mouth]

ves·i·cot·o·my (ves′i-kot′ō-mē). SYN cystotomy.

ves·i·co·um·bi·li·cal (ves′i-kō-ŭm-bil′i-kăl). Relating to the urinary bladder and the umbilicus. SYN omphalovesical.

ves·i·co·u·re·ter·al (ves′i-kō-ū-rē′ter-ăl). Relating to the bladder and the ureters.

ves·i·co·u·re·thral (ves′i-kō-ū-rē′thrăl). Relating to the bladder and the urethra.

ves·i·co·u·ter·ine (ves′i-kō-ū′ter-in). Relating to the bladder and the uterus.

ves·i·co·u·ter·o·vag·i·nal (ves′i-kō-ū′ter-ō-vaj′i-năl). Relating to the bladder, uterus, and vagina.

ves·i·co·vag·i·nal (ves-i-kō-vaj′i-năl). Relating to the bladder and vagina.

ves·i·co·vag·i·no·rec·tal (ves′i-kō-vaj′i-nō-rek′tăl). Relating to the bladder, vagina, and rectum.

ves·i·co·vis·cer·al (ves′i-kō-vis′er-ăl). Relating to the urinary bladder and any other adjacent organ or viscus.

ve·sic·u·la, gen. and pl. **ve·sic·u·lae** (vĕ-sik′ū-lă, -lē). A small bladder or bladder-like structure. SYN vesicle (1) [TA]. [L. blister, vesicle, dim. of *vesica,* bladder]

v. fel′lis, SYN gallbladder.

v. ophthal′mica, SYN optic *vesicle.*

v. semina′lis, ⭐official alternate term for seminal *gland.*

v. umbilica′lis, SYN yolk *sac.*

ve·sic·u·lar (vĕ-sik′ū-lăr). **1.** Relating to a vesicle. **2.** Characterized by or containing vesicles. SYN vesiculate (2).

ve·sic·u·late (vĕ-sik′ū-lāt). **1.** To become vesicular. **2.** SYN vesicular (2).

ve·sic·u·la·tion (vĕ-sik′ū-lā′shŭn). **1.** The formation of vesicles. SYN blistering, vesication. **2.** Presence of a number of vesicles.

ve·sic·u·lec·to·my (vĕ-sik′ū-lek′tō-mē). Resection of a portion or all of each of the seminal vesicles. [L. *vesicula,* vesicle, + G. *ektomē,* excision]

ve·sic·u·li·tis (vĕ-sik-ū-lī′tis). Inflammation of any vesicle; especially of a seminal vesicle. [L. *vesicula,* vesicle, + G. -*itis,* inflammation]

△**vesiculo-.** A vesicle. [L. *vesicula,* vesicle, dim. of *vesica,* bladder]

ve·sic·u·lo·bron·chi·al (vĕ-sik′ū-lō-brong′kē-ăl). Denoting an auscultatory sound having both a vesicular and a bronchial quality.

ve·sic·u·lo·cav·ern·ous (vĕ-sik′ū-lō-kav′er-nŭs). Both vesicular and cavernous; denoting: **1.** An auscultatory sound having both a vesicular and a cavernous quality; **2.** The structure of certain neoplasms.

ve·sic·u·log·ra·phy (vĕ-sik-ū-log′ră-fī). Radiographic contrast study of the seminal vesicles. [vesiculo- + G. *graphō,* to write]

ve·sic·u·lo·pap·u·lar (vĕ-sik′ū-lō-pap′ū-lăr). Pertaining to or consisting of a combination of vesicles and papules, or of papules becoming increasingly edematous with sufficient collection of fluid to form vesicles.

ve·sic·u·lo·pros·ta·ti·tis (vĕ-sik′ū-lō-pros′tă-tī′tis). Inflammation of the bladder and prostate. [vesiculo- + prostate + G. -*itis,* inflammation]

ve·sic·u·lot·o·my (vĕ-sik-ū-lot′ō-mē). Surgical incision of the seminal vesicles. [vesiculo- + G. *tomē,* incision]

ve·sic·u·lo·tu·bu·lar (vĕ-sik′ū-lō-too′bū-ler). Denoting an auscultatory sound having both a vesicular and a tubular quality.

ve·sic·u·lo·tym·pan·ic (vĕ-sik′ū-lō-tim-pan′ik). Denoting a percussion sound having both a vesicular and a tympanic quality.

Ve·si·cu·lo·vi·rus (vĕ-sik′ū-lō-vī′rŭs). A genus of viruses (family Rhabdoviridae) that includes the vesicular stomatitis virus (of cattle) and related viruses.

vesp. (ves′per). Abbreviation for L. vesper, evening. [L. evening]

ves·sel (ves′ĕl) [TA]. A structure conveying or containing a fluid, especially a liquid. SEE ALSO vas. [O. Fr. fr. L. *vascellum,* dim. of *vas*]

absorbent v.'s, SYN lymph v.'s.

afferent v., (1) any artery conveying blood to a part; **(2)** SYN afferent glomerular *arteriole;* **(3)** SYN afferent *lymphatic.*

anastomosing v., SYN anastomotic v.

anastomotic v. [TA], a v. that establishes a connection between arteries, between veins, or between lymph v.'s. SYN vas anastomoticum [TA], anastomosing v.

blood v., SEE blood vessel.

capillary v., SYN capillary (2); SEE blood *capillary,* lymph *capillary.*

chyle v., SYN lacteal (2).

collateral v., (1) a branch of an artery running parallel with the parent trunk; **(2)** a v. that runs in parallel with another v., nerve, or other long structure. SYN vas collaterale.

corkscrew v.'s, SYN hairpin v.'s.

deep lymph v. [TA], one of the v.'s that drain lymph from the deep structures of the body; they tend to follow the courses of blood v.'s to reach regional lymph nodes. SYN vas lymphaticum profundum [TA]

efferent v., SYN efferent glomerular *arteriole.*

ve

hairpin v.'s, atypical blood v.'s that double back on themselves, seen on colposcopy of the cervix; their presence indicates early invasive cervical cancer. SYN corkscrew v.'s.

v.'s of internal ear [TA], blood v.'s of the internal ear, consisting of the labyrinthine artery and its branches and the labyrinthine veins and their tributaries. SYN vasa sanguinea auris internae [TA].

lacteal v., SYN lacteal (2).

lymph v.'s [TA], the v.'s that convey the lymph; they anastomose freely with each other. SYN lymphatic v.'s [TA], absorbent v.'s, lymphatics, vasa lymphatica.

lymphatic v.'s [TA], SYN lymph v.'s.

nutrient v., SYN nutrient *artery*.

superficial lymph v. [TA], one of the lymphatic v.'s that lie in the skin and subcutaneous tissues; they join the deep lymphatic v.'s. SYN vas lymphaticum superficiale [TA].

v.'s of vessels, SYN *vasa* vasorum, under *vas*.

vitelline v.'s, SEE vitelline *artery*, vitelline *vein*.

ves·tib·u·la (ves-tib′ū-lă). Plural of vestibulum.

ves·tib·u·lar (ves-tib′ū-lăr). Relating to a vestibule, especially the vestibule of the ear. SYN vestibularis.

ves·ti·bu·la·ris (ves-tib-ū-lā′ris). SYN vestibular, vestibular. [L.]

ves·tib·u·late (ves-tib′ū-lăt). Possessing a vestibule.

ves·ti·bule (ves′ti-bool) [TA]. **1.** A small cavity or a space at the entrance of a canal. **2.** Specifically, the central, somewhat ovoid, cavity of the osseous labyrinth communicating with the semicircular canals posteriorly and the cochlea anteriorly. SYN vestibulum [TA]. [L. *vestibulum*]

aortic v. [TA], the anterosuperior portion of the left ventricle of the heart immediately below the aortic orifice, having fibrous walls and affording room for the segments of the closed aortic valve. SYN vestibulum aortae [TA], Sibson aortic v.

buccal v., that part of the oral vestibule related to the cheek.

esophagogastric v., SYN gastroesophageal v.

gastroesophageal v., the dilated aboral portion of the esophagus, just above the cardiac orifice; usually it corresponds to the lumen of abdominal part of the esophagus although its relation to diaphragm is variable. SYN esophagogastric v.

labial v., that part of the oval vestibule related to the lips.

v. of larynx [TA], the upper part of the laryngeal cavity from the superior aperture to the vestibular folds or rima vestibuli, bounded anteriorly by the epiglottis, laterally by the mucosa overlying the quadrangular membranes and posteriorly by the mucosa overlying the arytenoid cartilages and arytenoideus muscle. SYN vestibulum laryngis [TA], atrium glottidis, superior laryngeal cavity.

v. of mouth, SYN oral v.

nasal v. [TA], the anterior part of the nasal cavity, especially that enclosed by cartilage. SYN vestibulum nasi [TA], v. of nose.

v. of nose, SYN nasal v.

v. of omental bursa [TA], the upper part of the bursa omentalis, just within the epiploic foramen (of Winslow), behind the caudate lobe of the liver. SYN vestibulum bursae omentalis [TA].

oral v. [TA], that part of the mouth bounded anteriorly and laterally by the lips and the cheeks, posteriorly and medially by the teeth and/or gums, and above and below by the reflections of the mucosa from the lips and cheeks to the gums. SYN vestibulum oris [TA], buccal cavity, v. of mouth.

Sibson aortic v., SYN aortic v.

v. of vagina [TA], the space posterior to the glans clitoridis and between the labia minora, containing the openings of the vagina, urethra, and ducts of the greater vestibular glands. SYN vestibulum vaginae [TA], vaginal introitus, vestibulum pudendi.

ves·tib·u·li·tis. An inflammation of the vulvar vestibule and the periglandular and subepithelial stroma characterized by a burning sensation and painful coitus.

⏣**vestibulo-.** Vestibule, vestibulum. [L. *vestibulum*]

ves·tib·u·lo·cer·e·bel·lum (ves-tib′ū-lō-ser-ĕ-bel′ŭm) [TA]. Those regions of the cerebellar cortex whose predominant afferent fibers arise from the ganglion vestibulare and the vestibular nuclei; structures included under this term are nodulus, flocculus,

ventral parts of the uvula and small ventral parts of the lingula. SYN archeocerebellum. [vestibulo- + L. *cerebellum*]

ves·tib·u·lo·co·chle·ar (ves-tib′ū-lō-kok′lē-ăr). **1.** Relating to the vestibulum and cochlea of the ear. **2.** SYN statoacoustic.

ves·tib·u·lop·a·thy (ves-tib′ū-lop′a-thē). Any abnormality of the vestibular apparatus, e.g., Ménière disease.

idiopathic bilateral v., slowly progressive disorder affecting young to middle-aged adults, manifested as gait unsteadiness (especially when visual cues are absent) and oscillopsia, unaccompanied by vertigo and hearing loss.

migraine-related v., a disorder characterized by movement-associated disequilibrium, unsteadiness, space and motion discomfort, and vertigo before onset of headache.

ves·tib·u·lo·plas·ty (ves-tib′ū-lō-plas-tē). Any of a series of surgical procedures designed to restore alveolar ridge height by lowering muscles attaching to the buccal, labial, and lingual aspects of the jaws. [vestibulo- + G. *plassō*, to form]

ves·tib·u·lo·spi·nal (ves-tib′ū-lō-spī′năl). SEE lateral vestibulospinal *tract*.

ves·tib·u·lot·o·my (ves-tib′ū-lot′ō-mē). Operation for an opening into the vestibule of the labyrinth. [vestibulo- + G. *tomē*, incision]

ves·tib·u·lo·u·re·thral (ves-tib′ū-lō-oo-rē′thrăl). Relating to the vestibule of the vagina and urethra.

ves·tib·u·lum, pl. **ves·tib·u·la** (ves-tib′ū-lŭm, -lă) [TA]. SYN vestibule. [L. antechamber, entrance court]

v. aor′tae [TA], SYN aortic *vestibule*.

v. bur′sae omenta′lis [TA], SYN *vestibule* of omental bursa.

v. laryn′gis [TA], SYN *vestibule* of larynx.

v. na′si [TA], SYN nasal *vestibule*.

v. o′ris [TA], SYN oral *vestibule*.

v. puden′di, SYN *vestibule* of vagina.

v. vagi′nae [TA], SYN *vestibule* of vagina.

ves·tige (ves′tij) [TA]. A trace or a rudimentary structure; the degenerated remains of any structure which occurs as an entity in the embryo or fetus. SYN vestigium [TA]. [L. *vestigium*]

v. of ductus deferens [TA], remnant in a female of the portion of the embryonic mesonephric duct that develops into the ductus deferens in males.

v. of processus vaginalis [TA], incompletely obliterated remnants of the vaginal process of the peritoneum remaining in the spermatic cord. SYN vestigium processus vaginalis [TA], v. of vaginal process.

v. of vaginal process, SYN v. of processus vaginalis.

ves·tig·i·al (ves-tij′ē-ăl). Relating to a vestige.

ves·tig·i·um, pl. **ves·tig·ia** (ves-tij′ē-ŭm, -ă) [TA]. SYN vestige. [L. footprint (trace), fr. *vestigo*, to track, trace]

v. proces′sus vagina′lis [TA], SYN *vestige* of processus vaginalis.

ve·su·vin (vĕ-soo′vin) [C.I. 21000]. SYN Bismarck brown Y. [*Vesuvius*, volcano in Italy]

vet·er·i·nar·i·an (vet′ĕ-rin-ār′ē-ăn). A person who holds an academic degree in veterinary medicine; a licensed practitioner of veterinary medicine. [see veterinary]

vet·er·i·nary (vet′ĕ-rin-ār-ē). Relating to the diseases of animals. [L. *veterinarius*, fr. *veterina*, beast of burden]

via, pl. **vi·ae** (vī′ă, vī′ē; vē′ă). Any passage in the body, as the intestine, the vagina, etc. [L. way, road]

vi·a·bil·i·ty (vī-ă-bil′i-tē). Capability of living; the state of being viable; usually connotes a fetus that has reached 500 g in weight and 20 gestational weeks. [Fr. *viabilité* fr. L. *vita*, life]

vi·a·ble (vī′ă-bl). Capable of living; denoting a fetus sufficiently developed to live outside of the uterus. [Fr. fr. *vie*, life, fr. L. *vita*]

vi·al (vī′ăl). A small bottle or receptacle for holding liquids, including medicines. SYN phial. [G. *phialē*, a drinking cup]

vi·bes·ate (vī′bĕ-sāt). A mixture of polvinate and malrosinol in organic solvent and a propellant; a modified polyvinyl plastic used as a topical spray for wounds.

vi·bra·tion (vī-brā′shŭn). **1.** A shaking. **2.** A to-and-fro movement, as in oscillation. [L. *vibratio*, fr. *vibro*, pp. *-atus*, to quiver, shake]

vi·bra·tive (vī′bră-tiv). SYN vibratory.

vi·bra·tor (vī′brā-ter, tōr). An instrument used for imparting vibrations.

vi·bra·to·ry (vī′brā-tōr-ē). Marked by vibrations. SYN vibrative.

Vib·ri·o (vib′rē-ō). A genus of motile (occasionally nonmotile), nonsporeforming, aerobic to facultatively anaerobic, Gram-negative bacteria (family Spirillaceae) containing short (0.5–3.0 μm), curved or straight rods which occur singly or which are occasionally united into S-shapes or spirals. Motile cells contain a single polar flagellum; in some species, two or more flagella occur in one polar tuft. Some of these organisms are saprophytes in salt and fresh water and in soil; others are parasites or pathogens. The type species is *V. cholerae*. [L. *vibro*, to vibrate]

V. alginolyt′icus, a bacterial species associated with wound and ear infections, and with bacteremia in immunocompromised and in burn patients.

V. chol′erae, a bacterial species that produces a soluble exotoxin and is the cause of cholera in humans; it is the type species of the genus *V.* SYN cholera bacillus, comma bacillus.

V. fe′tus, former name for *Campylobacter fetus.*

V. fluvia′lis, a bacterial species similar to strains of *Aeromonas,* associated with diarrheal disease in humans.

V. furnis′sii, an aerogenic strain of bacteria, similar to *V. fluvialis,* associated with diarrheal disease and outbreaks of gastroenteritis.

V. hol′lisae, a bacterial species that can cause dysentery in humans.

V. metschniko′vii, a bacterial species causing acute enteric disease in chickens and other avian species; also isolated from human stool.

V. mim′icus, a sucrose-negative bacterial strain, similar to *V. cholerae,* isolated from human stool in diarrheal disease and from human ear infections.

V. parahaemolyt′icus, a marine bacterial species that causes gastroenteritis and bloody diarrhea, usually from eating contaminated shellfish.

V. sputo′rum, former name for *Campylobacter sputorum.*

V. vulnif′icus, a species capable of causing gastroenteritis and cutaneous lesions that may result in fatal septicemia, especially in a cirrhotic or immunocompromised patient; usually contracted from contaminated oysters; also a cause of wound infections, especially those associated with handling of shellfish.

vib·rio (vib′rē-ō). A member of the genus *Vibrio.*

El Tor v., a bacterium regarded as a biovar of *Vibrio cholerae.* It was originally isolated from six pilgrims who died of dysentery or gangrene of the colon at the Tor quarantine station on the Sinai Peninsula.

Nasik v., an organism differing from the cholera v., being shorter and stouter and less comma shaped; its cultures are very toxic to laboratory animals on intravenous injections.

Vib·ri·on sep·tique (vē-brē-on′ sep-tēk′). SYN *Clostridium septicum.* [Fr. septic vibrio]

vib·ri·o·sis, pl. **vib·ri·o·ses** (vib-rē-ō′sis). Infection caused by species of bacteria of the genus *Vibrio.*

vi·bris·sa, gen. and pl. **vi·bris·sae** (vī-bris′ă, vī-bris′ē) [TA]. SYN *hairs* of vestibule of nose, under *hair.* [L. found only in pl. *vibrissae,* fr. *vibro,* to quiver]

vi·bris·sal (vib-ris′ăl). Relating to the vibrissae.

vi·bro·car·di·o·gram (vī′brō-kar′dē-ō-gram). A graphic record of chest vibrations produced by hemodynamic events of the cardiac cycle; the record provides an indirect, externally recorded measurement of isovolumic contraction and ejection times. [L. *vibro,* to shake, + G. *kardia,* heart, + *gramma,* a drawing]

vi·bro·mas·seur (vī′brō-ma-ser′). A type of vibrator for giving vibratory massage.

vi·bro·ther·a·peu·tics (vī′brō-thār-ă-pū′tiks). SYN vibratory *massage.*

Vi·bur·num pru·ni·fo·li·um (vī-bur′num proo-′nī-fō′lē-ŭm). A medication derived from the root bark of *Viburnum prunifolium* (family Caprifoliaceae); contains viburnin; bitter resin; tannin; sugar; citric, malic, oxalic and valeric acids. Formerly used as a smooth muscle relaxant/antispasmodic (uterine).

vi·car·i·ous (vī-ker′ē-ŭs). Acting as a substitute; occurring in an abnormal situation. [L. *vicarius,* from *vicis,* supplying place of]

vi·cine (vī′sēn). A glucoside occurring in akta, a weed that contaminates *Lathyrus sativus,* and in the common vetch (*Vicia sativa*), a plant whose fruit is substituted for red lentils; thought by some to be responsible for the symptoms of lathyrism. [*Vicia* (genus name) + -ine]

Vicq d'Azyr, Félix, French anatomist, 1748–1794. SEE V. d' *bundle, centrum* semiovale, *foramen.*

Vic·to·ria blue. Any of several blue diphenylnaphthylmethane derivatives; used as a stain in histology. [Queen *Victoria*]

Vic·to·ria or·ange. An alkaline salt of dinitrocresol; a reddish yellow stain formerly used in histology.

vi·dar·a·bine (vī-der′ă-bēn). A purine nucleoside obtained from fermentation cultures of *Streptomyces antibioticus* and used to treat herpes simplex infections.

vid·e·o·en·do·scope (vid′ē-ō-end′ō-skōp). An endoscope fitted with a video camera.

vid·e·o·en·dos·co·py (vid′ē-ō-en-dos′ka-pē). Endoscopy performed with an endoscope fitted with a video camera.

vid·e·o·ker·a·to·scope (vid′ē-ō-ker′ah-tō-skōp). A keratoscope fitted with a video camera.

vid·i·an (vid′ē-an). Named after or described by Vidius.

Vidius (Vidus), Guidi (Guido), Italian anatomist and physician, 1500–1569. SEE vidian *artery,* vidian *canal,* vidian *nerve,* vidian *vein.*

Vierra, J.P., 20th century Brazilian dermatologist. SEE V. *sign.*

Vieussens, Raymond de, French anatomist, 1641–1715. SEE V. *anulus, ansa, centrum, foramina,* under *foramen, ganglia,* under *ganglion, isthmus, limbus, loop, ring; valve* of V.; V. *valve, veins,* under *vein, ventricle.*

view (vū). SYN projection.

axial v., SYN axial *projection.*

base v., SYN submentovertex *radiograph.*

Caldwell v., SYN Caldwell *projection.*

half axial v., SYN Towne *projection.*

Judet v., v. consisting of two oblique radiographic projections centered on the hip in question, tilted 45° medially or laterally from a true anteroposterior direction; useful for fractures or deformities of the acetabulum.

long axis v., in echocardiography or magnetic resonance imaging of the heart, a projection parallel to the ventricular axis and perpendicular to the interventricular septum of the heart; four-chamber view.

Stenvers v., SYN Stenvers *projection.*

Towne v., SYN Towne *projection.*

verticosubmental v., SYN axial *projection.*

Waters v., SYN Waters *projection.*

vig·a·bat·rin (vī-gă′bă-trin). An irreversible inhibitor of γ-aminobutyric acid transaminase, a degradative enzyme for γ-aminobutyric acid (GABA), the inhibitory neurotransmitter. The drug intensifies the effects of GABA and thus inhibition of the central nervous system; used as an antiepileptic agent.

vig·il (vij′il). A state of wakefulness or sleeplessness. [L. *vigilia,* wakefulness, alertness, fr. *vigeo,* to be active, to rouse]

coma v., SYN akinetic *mutism.*

vig·il·am·bu·lism (vij-i-lam′bū-lizm). An older term for a condition of unconsciously regarding one's surroundings, with automatism; resembling somnambulism but occurring in the waking state. [L. *vigil,* awake, alert, + *ambulo,* to walk about]

vig·i·lance (vij′i-lans). An attentiveness, alertness, or watchfulness for whatever may occur. [L. *vigilantia,* wakefulness]

vil·li (vil′ī). Plural of villus.

vil·lin (vil′in). An actin-binding protein that, at low calcium ion concentrations, nucleates polymerization of actin filaments; micromolar Ca^{2+} causes villin to sever actin filaments into short fragments.

vil·li·tis. SYN villositis.

vil·lose (vil′ōs). SYN villous (2).

vi

vil·lo·si·tis (vil-ō-sī'tis). Inflammation of the chorionic villi surface of the placenta. SYN villitis. [villous + G. -itis inflammation]

vil·los·i·ty (vi-los'i-tē). Shagginess; an aggregation of villi.

vil·lous (vil'ŭs). **1.** Relating to villi. **2.** Shaggy; covered with villi. SYN villose.

vil·lus, pl. **vil·li** (vil'ŭs, vil'ī). **1.** A projection from the surface, especially of a mucous membrane. If the projection is minute, as from a cell surface, it is termed a microvillus. **2.** An elongated dermal papilla projecting into an intraepidermal vesicle or cleft. SEE festooning. [L. shaggy hair (of beasts)]

anchoring v., a chorionic v. that is attached to the decidua basalis.

arachnoid villi, tufted prolongations of pia-arachnoid that protrude through the meningeal layer of the dura mater and have a thin limiting membrane; collections of arachnoid v. form arachnoid granulations that lie in venous lacunae at the margin of the superior sagittal sinus; the spongy tissue of the a. v. contains tubules that serve as one-way valves for transfer of cerebrospinal fluid from the subarachnoid space to the venous system. Both a. v. and the granulations formed from them are major sites of fluid transfer. SEE ALSO arachnoid *granulations*, under *granulation*.

chorionic villi, vascular processes of the chorion of the embryo entering into the formation of the placenta.

floating v., SYN free v.

free v., a chorionic v. that is not attached to the decidua basalis, but is "free" in the maternal blood of the intervillous spaces. SYN floating v.

intestinal villi [TA], projections (0.5–1.5 mm in length) of the mucous membrane of the small intestine; they are leaf-shaped in the duodenum and become shorter, more finger-shaped, and sparser in the ileum. SYN villi intestinales [TA].

vil'li intestina'les [TA], SYN intestinal villi.

vil'li pericardi'aci [TA], SYN pericardial villi.

pericardial villi [TA], minute filiform projections (synovial villi) from the surface of the serous pericardium. SYN villi pericardiaci [TA].

peritoneal villi [TA], synovial villi on the surface of the peritoneum. SYN villi peritoneales [TA].

vil'li peritonea'les [TA], SYN peritoneal villi.

pleural villi [TA], shaggy appendages (synovial villi) on the pleura in the neighborhood of the costomediastinal sinus. SYN villi pleurales [TA].

vil'li pleura'les [TA], SYN pleural villi.

primary v., the first stage of chorionic v. development, with columns of cytotrophoblastic cells covered by syncytiotrophoblast.

secondary v., an intermediate stage of chorionic v. development following invasion by a connective tissue core.

synovial villi [TA], small vascular processes given off from a synovial membrane. SYN villi synoviales [TA], synovial fringe, synovial tufts.

vil'li synovia'les [TA], SYN synovial villi.

tertiary v., the definitive chorionic v. with a vascular core separated from maternal blood by connective tissue, cytotrophoblast, and syncytiotrophoblast.

vi·men·tin (vī-men'tin). The major polypeptide that copolymerizes with other subunits to form the intermediate filament cytoskeleton of mesenchymal cells; they may have a role in maintaining the internal organization of certain cells. SEE ALSO desmin.

vin·blas·tine sul·fate (vin-blas'tēn). A dimeric alkaloid obtained from *Vinca rosea*. It arrests mitosis in metaphase (although vincristine is more active in this respect) and exhibits greater antimetabolic activity than does vincristine; used in the treatment of Hodgkin disease, choriocarcinoma, acute and chronic leukemias, and other neoplastic diseases; blocks microtubule assembly. SYN vincaleucoblastine.

vin·ca·leu·co·blas·tine (ving'kǎ-loo-kō-blas'tēn). SYN vinblastine sulfate.

Vin·ca ro·sea (ving'kǎ rō'zē-ǎ). A species of myrtle (family Myrtaceae) used in various parts of the world as a home remedy;

two active dimeric alkaloids obtained from this plant are vinblastine and vincristine. SYN periwinkle.

Vincent, Henri, French physician, 1862–1950. SEE V. *angina*, *bacillus*, *disease*, *infection*, *spirillum*, *tonsillitis*.

vin·cris·tine sul·fate (vin-kris'tēn). A dimeric alkaloid obtained from *Vinca rosea*; its antineoplastic activity is similar to that of vinblastine, but no cross-resistance develops between these two agents, and it is more useful than vinblastine in lymphocytic lymphosarcoma and acute leukemia. SYN leurocristine.

vin·cu·lin (ving'koo-lin). A protein associated with actin microfilaments; found in intercalated discs of cardiac muscle and focal adhesion plaques; may have a role in how a tumor virus causes pleiotropic effects of transformation. [L. *vinculum*, bond, fr. *vincio*, to bind + -in]

vin·cu·lum, pl. **vin·cu·la** (ving'koo-lŭm, -lǎ) [TA]. A frenum, frenulum, or ligament. [L. a fetter, fr. *vincio*, to bind]

v. bre've digitorum manus [TA], SYN v. breve of fingers; SEE ALSO vincula tendinea of digits of hand and foot.

v. breve of fingers [TA], a triangular band that extends from the dorsal surface of each of the flexor tendons of a digit to the capsule of the nearby interphalangeal joint and to the phalanx proximal to the insertion of the tendon. SYN v. breve digitorum manus [TA], short v.

v. lin'guae, SYN *frenulum* of tongue.

vin'cula lin'gulae cerebell'i, small lateral prolongations of the lingula of the vermis of the cerebellum resting on the dorsal surface of the superior cerebellar peduncle.

long v., SYN v. longum of fingers.

v. lon'gum digitorum manus [TA], SYN v. longum of fingers; SEE ALSO vincula tendinea of digits of hand and foot.

v. longum of fingers [TA], a long, threadlike band that extends from the dorsal surface of each of the flexor tendons of a digit to the proximal phalanx. SYN v. longum digitorum manus [TA], long v.

v. prepu'tii, SYN *frenulum* of prepuce.

short v., SYN v. breve of fingers.

vincula tendinea of digits of hand and foot [TA], fibrous bands that extend from the flexor tendons of the fingers and toes to the capsules of the interphalangeal joints and to the phalanges; they convey small vessels to the tendons. SYN synovial frena, synovial frenula, vincula of tendons, vincula tendinum digitorum manus et pedis.

vin'cula ten'dinum digitorum manus et pedis, SYN vincula tendinea of digits of hand and foot; SEE ALSO v. breve of fingers, v. longum of fingers.

vincula of tendons, SYN vincula tendinea of digits of hand and foot.

vin·de·sine (vin'dě-sēn). Synthetic derivative of vinblastine which shares antineoplastic properties with the latter agent. Used in the treatment of childhood lymphocytic leukemia.

Vineberg, Arthur M., Canadian thoracic surgeon, 1903–1988. SEE V. *procedure*.

vin·e·gar (vin'ě-găr). Impure dilute acetic acid, made from wine, cider, malt, etc. SYN acetum. [Fr. *vinaigre*, fr. *vin*, wine, + *aigre*, sour]

mother of v., in vinegar, the fungus of acetous fermentation appearing as a stringy sediment. [A.S. *modder*, mud]

pyroligneous v., SYN wood v.

wood v., impure acetic acid produced by the destructive distillation of pine tar and wood. SYN pyroligneous v.

vi·nic (vī'nik). Relating to or derived from wine. [L. *vinum*, wine]

vi·nous (vī'nŭs). Relating to, containing, or of the nature of wine.

Vinson, Porter P., U.S. surgeon, 1890–1959. SEE Plummer-V. *syndrome*.

vi·nyl (vī'nil). The hydrocarbon radical, $CH_2=CH-$. SYN ethenyl.

v. carbinol, SYN *allyl* alcohol.

v. chloride, a substance used in the plastics industry and suspected of being a potent carcinogen in humans. SYN chloroethylene.

vi·nyl·ben·zene (vī'nil-ben'zēn). SYN styrene.

vi·nyl·ene (vī′nil-ēn). The bivalent radical, –CH=CH–. SYN ethenylene.

vi·nyl·i·dene (vī-nil′i-dēn). The bivalent radical, $H_2C=C=$.

vi·o·la·ceous (vī-ō-lā′shŭs). Denoting a purple discoloration, usually of the skin. [L. *viola,* violet]

vi·o·let (vī′ō-let). The color evoked by wavelengths of the visible spectrum shorter than 450 nm. For individual violet dyes, see the specific name. [L. *viola*]

    Hoffman v., dahlia.

    visual v., SYN iodopsin.

vi·o·my·cin (vī-ō-mī′sin). An antibiotic agent obtained from *Streptomyces puniceus* var. *floridae;* active against acid-fast bacteria, including strains of tubercle bacilli resistant to streptomycin; may produce vestibular damage and deafness.

vi·os·ter·ol (vī-os′ter-ōl). SYN ergocalciferol.

VIP Abbreviation for vasoactive intestinal *polypeptide.*

vi·per (vī′per). A member of the snake family Viperidae. [L. *vipera,* serpent, snake]

    Russell's v., characteristically marked, highly venomous snake (*Vipera russellii*) of southeastern Asia. The venom is coagulant in action and is used locally in a 1:10,000 solution for the arrest of hemorrhage in hemophilia.

Vi·per·i·dae (vī-per′i-dē). A family of poisonous Old World snakes, the true vipers, composed of about 50 species and characterized by two relatively long caniculated fangs at the front of the upper jaw which are attached to movable bones, allowing them to be erect during the bite when the mouth is open, and folded into a palate skin fold when the jaws are shut. [L. *vipera,* viper]

VI·Po·ma (vi-pō′mă). An endocrine tumor, usually originating in the pancreas, which produces a vasoactive intestinal polypeptide believed to cause profound cardiovascular and electrolyte changes with vasodilatory hypotension, watery diarrhea, hypokalemia, and dehydration. [*v*asoactive *i*ntestinal *p*olypeptide + G. -*ōma,* tumor]

Vipond, French physician. SEE V. *sign.*

vip·ryn·i·um em·bo·nate (vip-rin′ē-ŭm em′bō-nāt). SYN pyrvinium pamoate.

vir·a·gin·i·ty (vir′ă-jin′i-tē). A rarely used term for the presence of pronounced masculine psychologic qualities in a woman. [L. *virago* (*viragin-*), a female warrior]

vi·ral (vī′răl). Of, pertaining to, or caused by a virus.

Virchow, Rudolf L.K., German pathologist and politician, 1821–1902. SEE V. *angle, cells,* under *cell, corpuscles,* under *corpuscle, crystals,* under *crystal, disease, node, psammoma;* V.-Holder *angle;* V.-Hassall *bodies,* under *body;* V.-Robin *space.*

vi·re·mia (vī-rē′mē-ă). The presence of a virus in the bloodstream. [virus + G. *haima,* blood]

vi·res (vī′rēz). Plural of vis.

vir·ga (vir′gă). SYN penis. [L. a rod]

vir·gin (ver′jin). **1.** A person who has never had sexual intercourse. **2.** Unused; uncontaminated. SYN virginal (2). [L. *virgo* (*virgin-*), maiden]

vir·gin·al (ver′ji-năl). **1.** Relating to a virgin. **2.** SYN virgin (2). [L. *virginalis*]

vir·gin·i·ty (ver-jin′i-tē). The virgin state. [L. *virginitas*]

vir·go·phre·nia (ver-gō-frē′nē-ă). A rarely used term for the receptive, capacious, and retentive mind of youth. [L. *virgo,* maiden, + G. *phrēn,* mind]

vir·i·ci·dal (vī-ri-sī′dă). SYN virucidal.

vir·i·cide (vī′ri-sīd). SYN virucide.

△**-viridae.** A virus family. [L. *virus,* venom]

vir·ile (vir′il). **1.** Relating to the male sex. **2.** Manly, strong, masculine. **3.** Possessing masculine traits. [L. *virilis,* masculine, fr. *vir,* a man]

vir·i·les·cence (vir-i-les′ens). A rarely used term for the assumption of male characteristics by the female.

vi·ril·ia (vi-ril′ē-ă). The male sexual organs. [L. ntr. pl. of *virilis,* virile]

vir·i·lism (vir′i-lizm). Possession of mature masculine somatic characteristics by a girl, woman, or prepubescent male; may be present at birth or may appear later, depending on its cause; may be relatively mild (e.g., hirsutism) or severe and is commonly the result of gonadal or adrenocortical dysfunction, or of androgenic therapy. [L. *virilis,* masculine]

    adrenal v., v. produced by excessive or abnormal secretory patterns of adrenocortical steroids. SYN adrenal virilizing syndrome.

vi·ril·i·ty (vi-ril′i-tē). The condition or quality of being virile. [L. *virilitas,* manhood, fr. *vir,* man]

vir·i·li·za·tion (vir′i-li-zā′shŭn). Production or acquisition of virilism.

vir·i·liz·ing (vir′i-līz-ing). Causing virilism.

△**-virinae.** A subfamily of viruses.

vi·ri·on (vī′rē-on, vir′ē-on). The complete virus particle that is structurally intact and infectious.

vi·rip·o·tent (vir-i-pō′tent, vĭ-rip′ō-tent). Obsolete term denoting a sexually mature male. [L. *viripotens,* fr. *vir,* man, + *potens,* having power]

vi·roid (vī′royd). An infectious pathogen of plants that is smaller than a virus (MW 75,000–100,000) and differs from one in that it consists only of single-stranded closed circular RNA, lacking a protein covering (capsid); replication does not depend on a helper virus, but is mediated by host cell enzymes. [virus + G. *eidos,* resemblance]

vi·rol·o·gist (vī-rol′ō-jist). A specialist in virology.

vi·rol·o·gy (vī-rol′ō-jē, vi-). The study of viruses and of viral disease. [virus + G. *logos,* study]

vi·ro·pex·is (vī-rō-pek′sis). Binding of virus to a cell and subsequent absorption (engulfment) of virus particles by that cell. [viro- + G. *pēxis,* fixation]

vi·ru·ci·dal (vī-rŭ-sī′dăl). Destructive to a virus. SYN viricidal.

vi·ru·cide (vī-rŭ-sīd). An agent active against virus infections. SYN viricide. [virus + L. *caedo,* to kill]

vi·ru·co·pria (vī-rŭ-kō′prē-ă). Presence of virus in feces. [virus + G. *kopros,* feces]

vir·u·lence (vir′oo-lens). The disease-evoking severity of a pathogen; numerically expressed as the ratio of the number of cases of overt infection to the total number infected, as determined by immunoassay. [L. *virulentia,* fr. *virulentus,* poisonous]

vir·u·lent (vir′oo-lent). Extremely toxic, denoting a markedly pathogenic microorganism. [L. *virulentus,* poisonous]

vir·u·lif·er·ous (vī-rŭ-lif′er-ŭs). Conveying virus.

vir·u·ria (vir-roo′rē-ă). Presence of viruses in the urine. [virus + G. *ouron,* urine]

VIRUS

▣**vi·rus,** pl. **vi·rus·es** (vī′rŭs). **1.** Formerly, the specific agent of an infectious disease. **2.** Specifically, a term for a group of infectious agents, which with few exceptions are capable of passing through fine filters that retain most bacteria, are usually not visible through the light microscope, lack independent metabolism, and are incapable of growth or reproduction apart from living cells. They have a prokaryotic genetic apparatus but differ sharply from bacteria in other respects. The complete particle usually contains either DNA or RNA, not both, and is usually covered by a protein shell or capsid that protects the nucleic acid. They range in size from 15 nanometers up to several hundred nanometers. Classification of viruses depends upon physiochemical characteristics of virions as well as upon mode of transmission, host range, symptomatology, and other factors. For viruses not listed below, see the specific name. SYN filtrable v. **3.** Relating to or caused by a v., as a virus disease. **4.** (Obsolete usage) Before the era of bacteriology, any agent causing disease, including a chemical substance such as an enzyme ("ferment") similar to snake venom; synonymous at that time with "poison." [L. poison]

    Abelson murine leukemia v., a retrovirus belonging to the Type C retrovirus group subfamily (family Retroviridae) that is associated with leukemia and induces in vitro transformation of certain mouse cells.

adeno-associated v. (AAV), SYN Dependovirus.

adenoidal-pharyngeal-conjunctival v., SYN adenovirus.

adenosatellite v., SYN Dependovirus.

AIDS-related v., obsolete term for human immunodeficiency v.

Akabane v., a v. of the genus Bunyavirus, family Bunyaviridae, causing abortion in cattle and congenital arthrogryposis and hydranencephaly in bovine fetuses in Israel, Japan, and Australia; it is transmitted by mosquitoes.

amphotropic v., a v. usually associated with retroviruses that may not produce disease in its natural host but does replicate in tissue culture cells of host species as well as in cells from other species.

Andes v., a species of Hantavirus in Argentina causing hantavirus pulmonary syndrome.

animal viruses, viruses occurring in humans and other animals, either causing inapparent infection or producing disease.

A-P-C v., SYN adenovirus.

Argentine hemorrhagic fever v., a member of the Arenaviridae.

attenuated v., a variant strain of a pathogenic v., so modified as to excite the production of protective antibodies, yet not producing the specific disease.

Aujeszky disease v., SYN pseudorabies v.

Australian X disease v., SYN Murray Valley encephalitis v.

avian encephalomyelitis v., a v. of the genus Enterovirus (family Picornaviridae) causing avian infectious encephalomyelitis in young chicks.

avian influenza v., a type A influenza v. (genus *Influenza* A virus) that causes fowl plague.

avian lymphomatosis v., SYN avian neurolymphomatosis v.

avian neurolymphomatosis v., the herpesvirus that causes avian lymphomatosis (Marek disease); is distinct from those causing other forms of leukosis. SYN avian lymphomatosis v., Marek disease v.

avian pneumoencephalitis v., SYN Newcastle disease v.

avian viral arthritis v., a v. of the genus Reovirus, family Reoviridae, causing tenosynovitis and arthritis in chickens.

B v., SYN cercopithecine *herpesvirus.* SYN monkey B v.

B19 v., a human parvovirus associated with arthritis and arthralgia and a number of specific clinical entities, including erythema infectiosum and aplastic crisis in the presence of hemolytic anemia.

bacterial v., a v. that "infects" bacteria; a bacteriophage.

Barmah Forest v., a species of Alphavirus that has caused outbreaks of polyarthritis in humans in Australia; transmitted by mosquitoes. [the virus was first isolated from mosquitoes collected at the Barmah Forest in southeastern Australia in 1974]

Bayou v., a species of Hantavirus in the U.S. causing hantavirus pulmonary syndrome; transmitted by the rice rat.

Bittner v. (bit'ner), SYN mammary tumor v. of mice.

BK v., a human polyomavirus, in the family Papovaviridae, of worldwide distribution, that produces kidney infections that are usually subclinical in immunocompetent persons. [initials of patient from whom first isolated]

Black Creek Canal v., a species of Hantavirus in the U.S. causing hantavirus pulmonary syndrome; transmitted by the cotton rat. [Black Creek Canal in Florida where the cotton rats were captured from which the virus was first isolated]

bluetongue v., a v. of the genus Orbivirus, in the family Reoviridae; the agent of bluetongue in sheep.

Bolivian hemorrhagic fever v., a member of the Arenavirus group of single-stranded RNA viruses also known as Machupo v.; primary reservoir in rodents; produces multiple abnormalities in the coagulation system including widespread capillary leak syndrome, which can be fatal.

Borna disease v., an unclassified negative sense single-stranded RNA v. that is the cause of Borna disease, a serious disease of horses that involves infection of the central nervous system. SYN enzootic encephalomyelitis v.

Bornholm disease v., SYN epidemic pleurodynia v.

bovine leukemia v. (BLV), a BLV-HTLV retrovirus in the family Retroviridae, commonly infecting cattle, especially dairy cows; in a small proportion of infected cattle, it will cause enzootic bovine leukosis. SYN bovine leukosis v.

bovine leukosis v., SYN bovine leukemia v.

bovine papular stomatitis v., a poxvirus of the genus Parapoxvirus, reported from North America, Africa and Europe, causing bovine papular stomatitis.

viral embryopathy

viral infections during pregnancy and the possible consequences for the child (embryopathy, fetopathy, perinatal infection)

virus	symptoms of infection during 1st to 14th week of pregnancy	symptoms of infection from 15th week to birth	symptoms of infection shortly before birth, or perinatal
cytomegalovirus	miscarriage, microcephaly	encephalitis, hepatosplenomegaly, chorioretinitis, premature birth, thrombocytopenia, minimal cerebral damage	cytomegaly
rubella	miscarriage, heart defects, cataract, microphthalmos, hearing deficiency, etc.	encephalitis, hepatosplenomegaly, thrombocytopenia, premature birth	—
measles	microcephaly, heart defects, anal atresia, etc.	fetal death, premature birth	measles
herpes simplex I and II	isolated cases: microphthalmos, microcephaly, chorioretinitis	—	generalized herpes infection, fatal encephalitis
varicella-zoster	isolated cases: eye deformity, cerebral damage	encephalitis, exanthema, premature birth	generalized varicella
coxsackie B	—	—	encephalitis, myocarditis, hepatitis
mumps	isolated cases: miscarriage	—	—
lymphocytic choriomeningitis	miscarriage (?)	isolated cases: encephalitis, chorioretinitis	—
hepatitis B	—	—	hepatitis (partly chronic)
hepatitis C	—	—	hepatitis
poliomyelitis	miscarriage	fetal death, premature birth	poliomyelitis

bovine virus diarrhea v., a v. of the genus Pestivirus, in the family Flaviviridae, causing bovine v. diarrhea; New York, Oregon, and Indiana strains of the v. are recognized. SYN mucosal disease v.

Bunyamwera v., a serologic group of the genus Bunyavirus, composed of over 150 v. types in the family Bunyaviridae. [*Bunyamwera,* Uganda, where first isolated]

Bwamba v., a species of Bunyavirus in the family Bunyaviridae; associated with cases of Bwamba fever in Uganda. [*Bwamba,* forest in Uganda where first isolated]

CA v., abbreviation for croup-associated v.

California v., a serologic group of the genus Bunyavirus, comprising about 14 strains including La Crosse and Tahyna v., and the type strain, California v., which causes encephalitis, chiefly in the age group 4–14 years.

canine distemper v., an RNA v. of the genus Morbillivirus, a member of the family Paramyxoviridae, that causes canine distemper. SYN dog distemper v.

Capim viruses, a serologic group of the genus Bunyavirus, the type species of which is Capim v.

Caraparu v., a species of C group Bunyavirus and an agent of bunyavirus encephalitis.

Catu v., an arbovirus of the genus Bunyavirus, of the family Bunyaviridae; an agent of bunyavirus encephalitis.

CELO v., a v. in the Aviadenovirus genus and similar to quail bronchitis v. SYN chicken embryo lethal orphan v.

Central European tick-borne encephalitis v., one of the viruses of the tick-borne encephalitis complex of group B arboviruses (genus Flavivirus); the causative agent of tick-borne encephalitis (Central European subtype).

C group viruses, a serologic group of the genus Bunyavirus (formerly called group C arboviruses), composed of about 14 species including Caraparu, Murutucu, and Oriboca v.

Chagres v., a v. in the genus Phlebovirus, family Bunyaviridae, an agent of bunyavirus encephalitis.

chicken embryo lethal orphan v., SYN CELO v.

chickenpox v., SYN varicella-zoster v.

chikungunya v., a mosquito-transmitted arbovirus of the genus Alphavirus (family Togaviridae) found in parts of Africa and in India, Thailand, and Malaysia; causes a febrile illness with joint pains. [named for the "bent up" position of persons so infected]

Coe v., obsolete name for the A-21 strain of coxsackievirus; the cause of a common-cold-like disease in military recruits.

cold v., SYN common cold v.

Colorado tick fever v., a v. of the genus Coltivirus, from the family Reoviridae, found in the Rocky Mountain region of the U.S. and transmitted by the tick, *Dermacentor andersoni;* it causes Colorado tick fever.

Columbia S. K. v., a strain of encephalomyocarditis v.

common cold v., any of the numerous strains of v. etiologically associated with the common cold, chiefly the rhinoviruses, but also strains of adenovirus, coxsackievirus, echovirus, and parainfluenza v. SYN cold v.

contagious ecthyma (pustular dermatitis) v. of sheep, the poxvirus of the genus Parapoxvirus causing contagious ecthyma (pustular dermatitis) of sheep. SYN soremouth v.

contagious pustular stomatitis v., (1) SYN horsepox v; **(2)** SYN orf v.

Côte-d'Ivoire virus, a variant of Ebola virus. SYN Ebola v. Côte-d'Ivoire.

cowpox v., a v. of the genus Orthopoxvirus that causes cowpox.

coxsackie v., SEE coxsackievirus.

Crimean-Congo hemorrhagic fever v., a v. of the genus Nairovirus (family Bunyaviridae) from Africa and carried by ticks (Hyalomma and Amblyomma) and found in human blood; the cause of Crimean-Congo hemorrhagic fever.

croup-associated v. (CA v.), parainfluenza v. types 1 and 2. SEE parainfluenza viruses.

cytopathogenic v., a v. whose multiplication leads to degenerative changes in the host cell. SEE ALSO cytopathic *effect*.

defective v., a v. particle that contains insufficient nucleic acid to

provide for production of all essential viral components; consequently, infectious v. is not produced except under certain conditions (e.g., when the host cell is infected with a "helper" v. also).

delta v., SYN hepatitis D v.

dengue v., a v. of the genus Flavivirus, about 50 nm in diameter; the etiologic agent of dengue in humans and also occurring in monkeys and chimpanzees, usually as inapparent infection; four serotypes are recognized; transmission is effected by mosquitoes of the genus *Aedes.*

distemper v., SEE canine distemper v.

🔲**DNA v.,** a major group of animal viruses in which the core consists of deoxyribonucleic acid (DNA); it includes parvoviruses, papovaviruses, adenoviruses, herpesviruses, poxviruses, and other unclassified DNA viruses. SYN deoxyribovirus.

representative DNA-containing tumor viruses		
virus	**host of origin**	**natural tumors (host of origin)**
papovaviruses		
polyoma	mouse	no
SV40	monkey	no
BK, JC	human	no
papilloma		
human	human	yes
rabbit	rabbit	yes
bovine	cow	yes
adenoviruses		
human (several types)	human	no
simian (some)	monkey	no
herpesviruses		
human		
herpes simplex type 2	human	
Ebstein-Barr virus	human	yes
cytomegalovirus	human	
monkey	monkey	no
avian (Marek)	chicken	yes
frog (Lucké)	frog	yes
Hepadnaviruses		
human hepatitis B	human	yes
woodchuck hepatitis	woodchuck	yes
poxviruses		
molluscum		
contagiosum	human	yes
Yaba	monkey	yes
fibroma-myxoma	rabbit, deer	yes

dog distemper v., SYN canine distemper v.

duck hepatitis v., a DNA v. of the genus Hepadnavirus, in the family Hepadnaviridae, causing v. hepatitis of ducks.

duck influenza v., an influenza A v., a member of the family Orthomyxoviridae, distinct from human influenza A strains on basis of hemagglutination inhibition.

duck plague v., a herpesvirus that causes duck plague.

Duvenhage v., a species of Lyssavirus causing a rabieslike disease in humans in Africa; transmitted by the bite of insectivorous bats. [the virus was named after its first victim, a man infected near Pretoria in South Africa]

eastern equine encephalomyelitis v., a v. of the genus Alphavirus (formerly group A arbovirus), in the family Togaviridae, occurring in the eastern U.S.; it is normally present in certain wild birds and small rodents as an inapparent infection, but is capable of causing eastern equine encephalomyelitis in horses and humans following transfer by the bites of culicine mosquitoes. SYN EEE v.

vi

EB v., SYN Epstein-Barr v.

Ebola v., a v. of the family Filoviridae, morphologically similar to but antigenically distinct from Marburg v.; the cause of Ebola fever (viral hemorrhagic fever). Transmission is parenteral, not oral, sexual, or by inhalation. After an incubation period of about 1 week, disease comes on acutely with fever, headache, vomiting and diarrhea, weakness, and a maculopapular rash. Gastrointestinal bleeding and other hemorrhagic manifestations, including disseminated intravascular coagulation, appear in a high percentage of cases and often prove fatal. The case fatality rate approximates 80%. Specific prevention and treatment are not available.

> Ebola virus made the headlines in 1995 when a sudden and devastating outbreak occurred in Kikwit, Zaire. In this cluster, which involved a number of health care workers, 315 persons became infected, of whom 243 (77%) died. Most cases in the Kikwit outbreak were blamed on the reuse, in clinics and hospitals, of unsterile medical and surgical equipment, contaminated with the blood, vomitus, stool, and urine of patients. In the following year, two large outbreaks occurred in Gabon. Serologic studies of patients in Gabon suggest that survival depends on early formation of IgG antibody directed against viral capsular protein. Despite sensational and exaggerated accounts by the news media, epidemics of Ebola virus disease and other viral hemorrhagic fevers do not occur when standard infection control measure is used. Further epidemics will occur in third-world countries as long as poverty and ignorance lead to unsound health care practices, but the disease poses no risk of epidemic spread in developed countries.

Ebola v. Côte-d'Ivoire, SYN Côte-d'Ivoire virus.
Ebola v. Reston, SYN Reston v.
Ebola v. Sudan, SYN Sudan v.
Ebola v. Zaire, SYN Zaire v.
ECHO v., an enterovirus from a large group of unrelated viruses belonging to the Picornaviridae, isolated from humans; while there are many inapparent infections, certain of the several serotypes are associated with fever and aseptic meningitis, and some appear to cause mild respiratory disease. SYN echovirus, enteric cytopathogenic human orphan v.
ECMO v., simian picornavirus recovered from monkey kidney cells and stools. SYN enteric cytopathogenic monkey orphan v.
ecotropic v., a retrovirus that does not produce disease in its natural host but does replicate in tissue culture cells derived from the host species.
ECSO v., a picornavirus isolated from outbreaks of enteritis in swine, but not known to be a natural pathogen. SYN enteric cytopathogenic swine orphan v.
ectromelia v., SYN infectious ectromelia v.
EEE v., SYN eastern equine encephalomyelitis v.
EMC v., SYN encephalomyocarditis v.
emerging viruses, in epidemiology, a class of viruses that have long infected humans or animals but now have the opportunity to attain epidemic proportions due to human encroachment on tropical rainforests, increased international travel, burgeoning populations in less developed countries, and, possibly, mutations. A number of viruses have been termed emergent, including hemorrhagic viruses such as Ebola, Marburg, and Hantaan; the rabies-like viruses Mokola and Duvenhage; rodent-borne Junin and Lassa virus; and mosquito-borne dengue. Virologists speculate that the strain of HIV that causes AIDS may also fall into this category, having entered humans through contact with monkeys in central Africa, possibly having existed among monkey populations for some 50,000 years.
encephalitis v., any one of a variety of viruses that cause encephalitis.
encephalomyocarditis v., a Cardiovirus in the family Picornaviridae, usually from rodents, isolated from blood and stools of humans, other primates, pigs, and rabbits; occasionally causes febrile illness with central nervous system involvement in humans, and an often fatal myocarditis in chimpanzees, monkeys

and pigs; strains of this v. include Columbia S. K. v. and Mengo v. SYN EMC v.
enteric viruses, viruses of the genus Enterovirus.
enteric cytopathogenic human orphan v., SYN ECHO v.
enteric cytopathogenic monkey orphan v., SYN ECMO v.
enteric cytopathogenic swine orphan v., SYN ECSO v.
enteric orphan viruses, enteroviruses isolated from humans and other animals, "orphan" implying lack of known association with disease when isolated; many viruses of the group are now known to be pathogenic; they include ECBO viruses, ECHO viruses, and ECSO viruses.
enzootic encephalomyelitis v., SYN Borna disease v.
ephemeral fever v., a rhabdovirus that causes ephemeral fever of cattle.
epidemic gastroenteritis v., a RNA v., about 27 nm in diameter, which has not been cultured in vitro; it is the cause of epidemic nonbacterial gastroenteritis; at least five antigenically distinct serotypes have been recognized, including the Norwalk agent. These viruses are classified with the Caliciviruses in the family Caliciviridae. SYN gastroenteritis v. type A.
epidemic keratoconjunctivitis v., an adenovirus (type 8) causing epidemic keratoconjunctivitis, especially among shipyard workers, and also associated with outbreaks of swimming pool conjunctivitis. SYN shipyard eye.
epidemic myalgia v., SYN epidemic pleurodynia v.
epidemic parotitis v., SYN mumps v.
epidemic pleurodynia v., a v. of Enterovirus coxsackievirus type B, in the family Picornaviridae, that causes epidemic pleurodynia. SYN Bornholm disease v., epidemic myalgia v.
Epstein-Barr v. (EBV), a herpesvirus in the genus Lymphocryptovirus that causes infectious mononucleosis and is also found in cell cultures of Burkitt lymphoma; associated with nasopharyngeal carcinoma. SYN EB v., human herpesvirus 4.
FA v., a strain of mouse encephalomyelitis v.
fibrous bacterial viruses, SYN filamentous bacterial viruses.
filamentous bacterial viruses, deoxyribonucleoproteins that "infect" and replicate in Gram-negative bacteria having sex pili and that, unlike bacteriophage, are released from infected bacteria without damage to the cell; they seem to be of two kinds, one of which has a specificity for F pili and the other for I pili. SYN fibrous bacterial viruses.
filtrable v., SYN virus (2).
fixed v., rabies v. whose virulence for rabbits has been stabilized by numerous passages through this experimental host. SEE ALSO street v.
Flury strain rabies v., SEE rabies v., Flury strain.
FMD v., SYN foot-and-mouth disease v.
foamy viruses, retroviruses of the genus Spumavirus, family Retroviridae, found in primates and other mammals; so named because of lacelike changes produced in monkey kidney cells; syncytia are also produced. SYN foamy agents.
foot-and-mouth disease v., a picornavirus of the genus Aphthovirus, family Picornaviridae, causing foot-and-mouth disease of cattle, swine, sheep, goats, and wild ruminants; it has wide distribution throughout Africa and Asia, causing serious economic losses; the v. is spread by contamination of the animal environment with infected saliva and excreta. SYN FMD v.
Four Corners v., SYN Sin Nombre v. [from the section of the U.S. where New Mexico, Colorado, Utah, and Arizona meet, site of a major occurrence]
Friend v., a strain of the splenic group of mouse leukemia viruses, related to Moloney and Rauscher viruses. SYN Friend leukemia v., Swiss mouse leukemia v.
Friend leukemia v., SYN Friend v.
GAL v., a v. with characteristics of adenovirus, not known to be associated with natural disease. SYN gallus adenolike v.
gallus adenolike v., SYN GAL v.
gastroenteritis v. type A, SYN epidemic gastroenteritis v.
gastroenteritis v. type B, SYN rotavirus.
GB viruses, members of the family Flaviviridae; GBV-A and GBV-B have been isolated from tamarins infected with human

viral agents; GBV-C is a human pathogen related to hepatitis G virus.

German measles v., SYN rubella v.

Germiston v., a virus in the genus Bunyavirus, family Bunyaviridae.

goatpox v., a v. of the genus Capripoxvirus; the cause of goatpox.

Graffi v., a type C mouse myeloleukemia v. from filtrates of transplantable tumors; possibly related to Gross v.

green monkey v., SYN Marburg v.

Gross v., the first strain of mouse leukemia v. isolated. SYN Gross leukemia v.

Gross leukemia v., SYN Gross v.

Guama v., a serologic group of the genus Bunyavirus, composed of 6 species including Catu v., and the type strain, Guama v.

Guanarito v., a species of Arenavirus causing Venezuelan hemorrhagic fever. [after municipality in Venezuela where all initial cases of Venezuelan hemorrhagic fever were confirmed]

Guaroa v., a v. of the Bunyamwera group of the genus Bunyavirus, and an agent of bunyavirus encephalitis.

HA1 v., SYN hemadsorption v. type 1; SEE parainfluenza viruses.

HA2 v., SYN hemadsorption v. type 2; SEE parainfluenza viruses.

hand-foot-and-mouth disease v., the v. causing hand-foot-and-mouth disease; chiefly type A16 but also types A4, A5, A7, A9, or A10 Entervirus coxsackievirus.

Hantaan v., a Hantavirus of the family Bunyaviridae that causes Korean hemorrhagic fever with renal syndrome.

helper v., a v. whose replication renders it possible for a defective v. or a virusoid (also present in the host cell) to develop into a fully infectious agent.

hemadsorption v. type 1, parainfluenza v. type 3. SEE parainfluenza viruses. SYN HA1 v.

hemadsorption v. type 2, parainfluenza v. type 1. SEE parainfluenza viruses. SYN HA2 v.

Hendra v., SYN equine *Morbillivirus*. [from Hendra, the suburb of Brisbane, Australia, where it was first isolated]

hepatitis A v. (HAV), an RNA virus, genus Hepatovirus, in the family Picornaviridae; the causative agent of viral hepatitis type A. SYN infectious hepatitis v.

hepatitis B v. (HBV), a DNA virus in the genus Orthohepadnavirus, family Hepadnaviridae; the causative agent of viral hepatitis type B. SYN serum hepatitis v.

hepatitis C v. (HCV), a non-A, non-B RNA v. causing posttransfusion hepatitis; it a member of the family Flaviviridae. There are now tests to detect hepatitis C infection.

hepatitis D v., a small "defective" RNA v., similar to viroids and virusoids, that requires the presence of hepatitis B v. for replication. The clinical course is variable but is usually more severe than other hepatitides. SYN delta agent, delta antigen, delta v., hepatitis delta v.

hepatitis delta v. (HDV), SYN hepatitis D v.

hepatitis E v. (HEV), a RNA v., possibly a Calicivirus, that is the principal cause of enterically transmitted, waterborne, or epidemic non-A, non-B hepatitis occurring primarily in Asia and Africa.

hepatitis G v. (HGV), an RNA v. related to the hepatitis C v., and which may cause co-infection with that agent.

herpes v., SEE herpesvirus.

herpes simplex v. (HSV), SEE *herpes* simplex.

herpes zoster v., SYN varicella-zoster v.

hog cholera v., an RNA virus of the genus Pestivirus, in the family Flaviviridae, that causes hog cholera. SYN swine fever v.

horsepox v., the poxvirus causing horsepox. SYN contagious pustular stomatitis v. (1).

human immunodeficiency v. (HIV), human T-cell lymphotropic v. type III; a cytopathic retrovirus (genus Lentvirus, family Retroviridae) that is 100–120 nm in diameter, has a lipid envelope, and has a characteristic dense cylindrical nucleoid containing core proteins and genomic RNA. There are currently two types: HIV-1 infects only human and chimpanzees and is more virulent than HIV-2, which is more closely related to Simian or monkey viruses. HIV-2 is found primarily in West Africa and is not as widespread as HIV-1. In addition to the usual gene associated with retroviruses, this virus has at least 6 genes that regulate its replication. It is the etiologic agent of acquired immunodeficiency syndrome (AIDS). Formerly or also known as the lymphadenopathy v. (LAV) or the human T-cell lymphotropic v. type III (HTLV-III). Identified in 1984 by Luc Montagnier and colleagues. SYN lymphadenopathy-associated v.

human immunodeficiency v.-2, a v., found primarily in West Africa, which causes a less virulent form of AIDS and is more closely related to Simian virus strains.

human T-cell lymphoma/leukemia v. (HTLV), a group of viruses (genus BLTV-HTLV retroviruses, family Retroviridae) that are lymphotropic with a selective affinity for the helper/inducer cell subset of T lymphocytes and that are associated with adult T-cell leukemia and tropical spastic paraparesis. SYN human T-cell lymphotropic v.

human T-cell lymphotropic v., SYN human T-cell lymphoma/leukemia v.

human T lymphotrophic v., a virus that has a predilection for human lymphoid cells.

v. III of rabbits, obsolete name for a latent herpesvirus infection of rabbits. [the third strain isolated, used for study]

Ilhéus v., a v. of the genus Flavivirus (group B arbovirus) first isolated in Brazil, later found in Colombia, Central America, and the Caribbean; the cause of Ilhéus encephalitis and Ilhéus fever.

inclusion conjunctivitis viruses, former name for *Chlamydia trachomatis*.

infantile gastroenteritis v., SYN rotavirus.

infectious ectromelia v., a virus belonging to the family Poxviridae morphologically similar to vaccinia v., which occurs as a latent infection in laboratory mice, but which may be activated by stresses such as irradiation and transport to cause disease; inoculation into the footpad results in edema and necrosis. SYN ectromelia v., mousepox v., pseudolymphocytic choriomeningitis v.

infectious hepatitis v., SYN hepatitis A v.

infectious papilloma v., SYN human papillomavirus.

infectious porcine encephalomyelitis v., SYN Teschen disease v.

vi

viruses associated with acute gastroenteritis in humans

virus	size (nm)	epidemiology
Rotavirus		
group A	70	single most important cause (viral or bacterial) of endemic severe diarrheal illness in infants and young children worldwide (in cooler months in temperate climates)
group B	70	outbreaks of diarrheal illness in adults and children in China
group C	70	sporadic cases and occasional outbreaks of diarrheal illness in children
Enteric adenovirus	70–80	second most important viral agent of endemic diarrheal illness of infants and young children worldwide
Norwalk virus and Norwalk-like viruses	27–32	important cause of outbreaks of vomiting and diarrheal illness in older children and adults in families, communities, and institutions, frequently associated with ingestion of food
Caliciviruses	28–40	sporadic cases and occasional outbreaks of diarrheal illness in infants, young children, and the elderly
Astroviruses	28	sporadic cases and occasional outbreaks of diarrheal illness in infants, young children, and the elderly

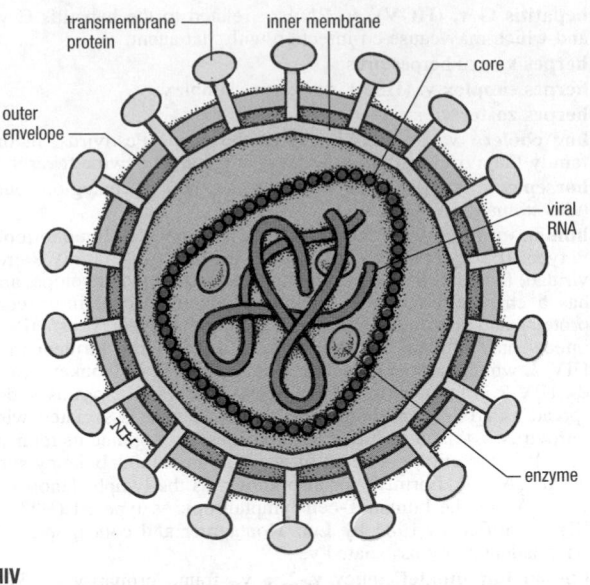

transmembrane protein

inner membrane

core

outer envelope

viral RNA

enzyme

HIV

influenza viruses, viruses of the family Orthomyxoviridae that cause influenza and influenzalike infections of humans and other animals. These viruses contain single-stranded RNA that is segmented, accounting in part, for their epidemic spread. Viruses included are influenza v. types A and B of the genus Influenzavirus, causing, respectively, influenza A and B, and Influenzavirus C, which belongs to a separate genus and causes influenza C.

insect viruses, viruses pathogenic for insects.

iridescent v., an insect virus in the family Iridoviridae.

Jamestown Canyon v., a member of the California group of arboviruses (family Bunyaviridae), which has been associated with a mild febrile illness in humans in North America.

Japanese B encephalitis v., a v. of the genus Flavivirus (group B arbovirus) occurring particularly in Japan but probably widespread throughout Southeast Asia; the v. is normally present in humans, especially in children, as an inapparent infection, but may cause febrile response and sometimes encephalitis; it may cause encephalitis in horses and abortion in pigs; wild birds are probably the natural hosts and culicine mosquitoes the vectors. SYN Russian autumn encephalitis v.

JC v., a human polyomavirus, family Papovaviridae, of worldwide distribution which produces infections that are usually subclinical in immunocompetent individuals, but is associated with progressive multifocal leukoencephalopathy in immunosuppressed individuals. [initials of patient from whom first isolated]

Junin v., a v. of the Tacaribe complex of arboviruses, genus Arenavirus, and the cause of Argentinian hemorrhagic fever; also isolated from mites and rodents.

K v., a polyomavirus, family Papovaviridae, that causes pneumonia in young mice by various routes of inoculation.

Kasokero v., a v. of the family Bunyaviridae causing a febrile disease in humans characterized by headache, abdominal pain, diarrhea, severe myalgia, and arthralgia. [after the Kasokero Cave in Uganda where the virus was first isolated from bats]

Kelev strain rabies v., SEE rabies v., Kelev strain.

Kilham rat v., a v. of the genus Parvovirus causing inapparent infection in rats; also recoverable from rat tumors. SYN latent rat v.

Koongol viruses, a serologic group of the genus Bunyavirus, comprising two species, Koongol (type species) and Wongal v.

Korean hemorrhagic fever v., SEE Hantavirus.

Kyasanur Forest disease v., a group B arbovirus, in the family Flaviviridae, isolated from monkeys in India and capable of causing Kyasanur Forest disease in humans; the v. is spread by monkeys and birds having mild infections; the vectors are probably species of the tick *Haemaphysalis*.

La Crosse v., a bunyavirus of the California group, family Bunyaviridae, and an agent of bunyavirus encephalitis.

lactate dehydrogenase v., an arterivirus present perhaps as a "passenger" in various transplantable mouse tumors; the v. may cause a life-long infection and be recognized by elevated plasma lactate dehydrogenose. SYN LDH agent.

Lassa v., an arenavirus, family Arenaviridae, that causes Lassa fever, an acute febrile disease with a high mortality.

latent rat v., SYN Kilham rat v.

LCM v., SYN lymphocytic choriomeningitis v.

louping-ill v., a v. of the genus Flavivirus that causes louping ill and is transmitted by the hard tick *Ixodes ricinus*.

Lucké v., a herpesvirus associated with Lucké carcinoma.

Lunyo v., an atypical strain of Rift Valley fever v.

lymphadenopathy-associated v. (LAV), SYN human immunodeficiency v.

lymphocytic choriomeningitis v., an RNA v. of the family Arenaviridae that infects mice, man, monkeys, dogs, and guinea pigs, and causes lymphocytic choriomeningitis; in man, infection may be inapparent, but sometimes the v. causes influenza-like disease, meningitis, or rarely meningoencephalomyelitis; in utero infections of mice establish a type of immunologic tolerance. SYN LCM v.

lymphogranuloma venereum v., former name for *Chlamydia trachomatis*.

Machupo v., a v. of the Tacaribe complex (genus Arenavirus, family Arenaviridae); the cause of Bolivian hemorrhagic fever.

malignant catarrhal fever v., a herpesvirus of wide distribution causing malignant catarrhal fever of cattle; sheep and wildebeests harbor inapparent infections and may transmit the v. to cattle.

mammary cancer v. of mice, SYN mammary tumor v. of mice.

mammary tumor v. of mice, one of the mammalian Type B retroviruses, antigenically distinct from the murine leukemia-sarcoma complex, that is associated with adenocarcinomatous tumors of the mammary gland, commonly latent in wild and laboratory mice and causing cancer only in genetically susceptible strains under certain hormonal influences. SYN Bittner agent, Bittner milk factor, Bittner v., mammary cancer v. of mice, milk factor, mouse mammary tumor v.

Marburg v., an RNA-containing v., genus Filovirus in the family Filoviridae, first recognized at Marburg University (Germany), where it was the cause of a highly fatal hemorrhagic fever among laboratory workers and handlers of green monkeys. SYN green monkey v.

Marek disease v., SYN avian neurolymphomatosis v.

marmoset v., a herpesvirus obtained repeatedly from throat swabs and tissues of New World monkeys.

masked v., a v. ordinarily occurring in the host in a noninfective state, but which may be activated and demonstrated by special procedures such as blind passage in experimental animals.

Mason-Pfizer v., a member of the genus D-type retroviruses in the family Retroviridae that was isolated from a mammary carcinoma of a rhesus monkey.

Mayaro v., a v. of the genus Alphavirus, family Togaviridae, causing epidemics of undifferentiated type fever in South America.

measles v., an RNA v. of the genus Morbillivirus, family Paramyxoviridae, that causes measles in humans and is transmitted via the respiratory tract; possesses hemagglutinating, hemadsorbing, and hemolyzing properties. SYN rubeola v.

Menangle v., a virus of the family Paramyxoviridae causing infection in pigs, humans, and fruit bats in Australia; human infection has resulted in an influenzalike illness with rash. [named after the location in Australia of the laboratory where it was first isolated]

Mengo v., a strain of encephalomyocarditis v.

milker's nodule v., a virus in the family Poxviridae.

mink enteritis v., a parvovirus that causes enteritis of mink.

MM v., a strain of encephalomyocarditis v.

Mokola v., a rabies related v. of the genus Lyssavirus, family Rhabdoviridae, first isolated from shrews (Crocidura spp.) in Nigeria, which has caused fatal neurologic disease in humans and cats in Africa.

molluscum contagiosum v., the poxvirus causing molluscum contagiosum of humans.

Moloney v., a lymphoid leukemia retrovirus of mice, in the family Retroviridae, isolated originally during propagation of S 37 mouse sarcoma.

monkey B v., SYN B v.

monkeypox v., a v. of the genus Orthopoxvirus causing monkeypox.

mouse encephalomyelitis v., a v. of the genus Enterovirus, family Picornaviridae, normally associated with inapparent infections and found in the intestinal tracts of infected mice, occasionally causing mouse encephalomyelitis in experimentally inoculated susceptible mice. SYN mouse poliomyelitis v., Theiler v.

mouse hepatitis v., a coronavirus, in the family Coronaviridae, that in the presence of *Eperythrozoon coccoides* causes fatal hepatitis in newly weaned mice; otherwise causes inapparent infection.

mouse leukemia viruses, retroviruses of the murine leukemia-sarcoma complex that produce leukemia and sometimes lymphosarcomas in mice, including the Abelson, Gross, Moloney, Friend, and Rauscher strains of v.; they have been isolated from inbred mice having a high incidence of spontaneous lymphoid leukemia.

mouse mammary tumor v., SYN mammary tumor v. of mice.

mouse parotid tumor v., SYN polyoma v.

mouse poliomyelitis v., SYN mouse encephalomyelitis v.

mousepox v., SYN infectious ectromelia v.

mouse thymic v., an ether-sensitive member of the herpesviridae family that causes necrosis of the thymus in young mice.

mucosal disease v., SYN bovine virus diarrhea v.

mumps v., a v. of the genus Rubulavirus, family Paramyxoviridae, causing parotitis in man, sometimes with complications of orchitis, oophoritis, pancreatitis, meningoencephalitis, and others, and transmitted by infectious salivary secretions. SYN epidemic parotitis v.

murine sarcoma v., a seemingly defective retrovirus that produces sarcomas in mice when growing in the presence of a "helper" v.; e.g., mouse leukemia v.

Murray Valley encephalitis v., a group B arbovirus of the genus Flavivirus that causes Murray Valley encephalitis; it is transmitted by *Culex* mosquitoes, and also infects birds and horses. SYN Australian X disease v., MVE v.

Murutucu v., a C group mosquito-borne v. of the genus Bunyavirus, which has caused undifferentiated type fever in Brazil and French Guiana.

MVE v., SYN Murray Valley encephalitis v.

myxomatosis v., SYN rabbit myxoma v.

naked v., a v. consisting only of a nucleocapsid; i.e., one that does not possess an enclosing envelope.

ND v., SYN Newcastle disease v.

negative strand v., a v. the genome of which is a strand of RNA that is complementary to messenger RNA; negative strand viruses also carry RNA polymerases necessary for the synthesis of messenger RNA.

Negishi v., one of the group B arboviruses (genus Flavivirus) of the tick-borne encephalitis complex, isolated from fatal infections in Japan.

neonatal calf diarrhea v., one of two viruses causing neonatal calf diarrhea; a rotovirus-like v. is associated with disease in newborn calves, and a coronavirus is associated with disease in calves over 5 days of age.

neurotropic v., a v. that has an affinity for nervous tissue, e.g., poliomyelitis v., neurotropic v. variant of yellow fever, and the "fixed" v. of rabies.

Newcastle disease v., a v. of the genus Rubulavirus, family Paranexoviridae, causing Newcastle disease in chickens and, to a lesser extent, in turkeys and other birds; it may occasionally infect laboratory and poultry workers, causing conjunctivitis and lymphadenitis. SYN avian pneumoencephalitis v., ND v.

New York v., a species of Hantavirus in the United States causing hantavirus pulmonary syndrome.

Nipah v., a paramyxovirus that can cause fatal disease in humans, with features of encephalitis and meningitis; the v. spreads from swine to humans. [Nipah, Malaysia, where first human case detected, 1999]

non-A, non-B hepatitis v., term used to group any of a number of viruses, other than A or B, that cause hepatitis in humans.

nonoccluded v., a v. not inclosed in an inclusion body, usually with reference to an insect v.

Norwalk v., a v. associated with acute viral gastroenteritis and belonging to the calicivirus group.

occluded v., a v. inclosed in an inclusion body, usually with reference to an insect v.

Omsk hemorrhagic fever v., a tick-borne v. of the genus Flavivirus causing Omsk hemorrhagic fever.

oncogenic v., any v. capable of inducing tumors. The RNA tumor viruses (family Retroviridae), which are well-defined and rather homogeneous, or the DNA viruses, which contain a number of viruses capable of inducing tumors, including poxviruses, herpesviruses, papillomaviruses, and polyomavirus. SYN tumor v.

o'nyong-nyong v., a v. of the genus Alphavirus, in the family Togaviridae, found in Uganda, Kenya, and Congo, which causes o'nyong-nyong fever.

orf v., a parapoxvirus causing orf in sheep and goats and sometimes humans. SYN contagious pustular dermatitis, contagious pustular stomatitis v. (2).

Oriboca v., a C group v. of the genus Bunyavirus, and an agent of bunyavirus encephalitis.

ornithosis v., former name for *Chlamydia psittaci*.

orphan viruses, viruses, such as the enteric orphan viruses, that when originally found were not specifically associated with disease; a number of these have since been shown to be pathogenic and subsequently reclassified.

Pacheco parrot disease v., a v. of the family Herpesviridae, possibly related to the v. of infectious laryngotracheitis. SYN parrot v. (2).

pantropic v., the ordinary strain of yellow fever v., as distinguished from the neurotropic strain; has an affinity for different tissues.

papilloma v., SYN Papillomavirus.

pappataci fever viruses, SYN phlebotomus fever viruses.

parainfluenza viruses, viruses of the genus Paramyxovirus, of four types: type 1 (hemadsorption v. type 2), which includes sendai v., causes acute laryngotracheitis in children and occasionally adults; type 2 (croup-associated v.) is associated especially with acute laryngotracheitis or croup in young children and minor upper respiratory infections in adults; type 3 (hemadsorption v. type 1; shipping fever v.) has been isolated from small children with pharyngitis, bronchiolitis, and pneumonia, and causes occasional respiratory infection in adults; bovine strains have been isolated from cattle with shipping fever, and the v. has also been isolated from sheep; type 4 has been isolated from a very few children with minor respiratory illness.

paravaccinia v., SYN pseudocowpox v.

parrot v., (1) obsolete term for *Chlamydia psittaci*; (2) SYN Pacheco parrot disease v.

Patois v., a serologic group of the genus Bunyavirus, comprising 4 species.

pharyngoconjunctival fever v., one of several types of adenoviruses associated with outbreaks of fever and pharyngitis, sometimes with conjunctivitis, especially in military recruits and people in boarding schools.

phlebotomus fever viruses, a group of at least 5 viruses in the family Bunyavirida but antigenically unrelated, transmitted by *Phlebotomus papatasi* (sandfly) and causing phlebotomus fever. SYN pappataci fever viruses, sandfly fever viruses.

plant viruses, viruses pathogenic to higher plants.

pneumonia v. of mice, an RNA v. of the genus Pneumovirus, a member of the family Paramyxoviridae, occurring normally as latent infection in laboratory mice, but capable of activation by serial intranasal passage and causing pneumonia. SYN PVM v.

vi

poliomyelitis v., a small single-stranded RNA v. of the genus Enterovirus, family Picornaviridae, causing poliomyelitis in humans; the route of infection is the alimentary tract, but the v. may enter the bloodstream and nervous system, sometimes causing paralysis of the limbs and, rarely, encephalitis; many infections are inapparent; serologic types 1, 2, and 3 are recognized, type 1 being responsible for most paralytic poliomyelitis and most epidemics. SYN poliovirus hominis.

polyoma v., a small naked v. with double-stranded circular DNA (genus Polyomavirus, family Papovaviridae) that normally occurs in inapparent infections in laboratory and wild mice, but after growth on tissue culture is capable of producing parotid tumors in mice and sarcomas in hamsters as well as tumors in other laboratory animals. SYN mouse parotid tumor v.

porcine hemagglutinating encephalomyelitis v., a Coronavirus causing vomiting, wasting, and encephalomyelitis in young pigs.

Powassan v., a v. of the genus Flavivirus (family Flaviviridae), transmitted by ixodid ticks and causing Powassan encephalitis in children; also capable of producing meningoencephalomyelitis in rabbits and children. [*Powassan,* Canada, where first isolated]

pseudocowpox v., a v. of the genus Parapoxvirus that causes pseudocowpox in humans and cattle; it is closely related to orf v. and papular stomatitis v. SYN paravaccinia v.

pseudolymphocytic choriomeningitis v., SYN infectious ectromelia v.

pseudorabies v., a herpesvirus, family Herpesviridae, causing pseudorabies in swine. SYN Aujeszky disease v.

psittacosis v., former name for *Chlamydia psittaci.*

Puumala v., a species of Hantavirus found in Europe causing hemorrhagic fever with renal syndrome.

PVM v., SYN pneumonia v. of mice.

quail bronchitis v., a v., in the genus Aviadenovirus, related antigenically to CELO v.

Quaranfil v., an ungrouped arbovirus isolated from human blood and from herons.

rabbit fibroma v., a poxvirus of the genus Leporipoxvirus, family Poxviridae, closely related to vaccinia and myxoma viruses, that causes Shope fibroma. SYN Shope fibroma v.

rabbit myxoma v., the poxvirus of the genus Leporipoxvirus causing myxomatosis of rabbits. SYN myxomatosis v.

rabbitpox v., an Orthopoxvirus that causes epidemics of pox in laboratory rabbits; immunologically, it is closely related to vaccinia v. but is more virulent in rabbits.

rabies v., a large bullet-shaped single-stranded RNA v. of the genus Lyssavirus, in the family Rhabdoviridae, that is the causative agent of rabies.

rabies v., Flury strain, a v. isolated from human brain, attenuated (fixed) by serial propagation in nonmammalian hosts, and subsequently established in chick embryo culture.

rabies v., Kelev strain, an attenuated, embryonate fowl egg-passaged strain.

Rauscher v., SYN Rauscher leukemia v.

Rauscher leukemia v., an RNA retrovirus associated with leukemia in rodents; similar to Friend v. SYN Rauscher v.

REO v., SYN respiratory enteric orphan v.

respiratory enteric orphan v., a nonenveloped icosahedral virus with a two-layered capsid whose genome consists of multiple segments of double-stranded RNA, belonging to the family Reoviridae, frequently found in both the respiratory and enteric tract. SYN REO v.

respiratory syncytial v. (RSV), an RNA v. of the genus Pneumovirus, in the family Paramyxoviridae, with a tendency to form syncytia in tissue culture, that causes minor respiratory infection with rhinitis and cough in adults, but is capable of causing severe bronchitis and bronchopneumonia in young children; first isolated from chimpanzees with respiratory disease. SYN chimpanzee coryza agent, Rs v.

Reston v., a variant of Ebola v. SYN Ebola v. Reston.

Rida v., a variant of the scrapie agent.

Rift Valley fever v., a v. of the genus Phlebovirus (family Bunyaviridae) that occurs in central and southern Africa in sheep, goats, and cattle, causing abortions and severe febrile disease, especially in young lambs; humans, especially herdsmen and veterinarians, may become infected through close contact with infected animals, developing a dengue-like disease; the v. also infects buffaloes, camels, and antelopes; it is mosquito-borne, but also probably infects by contact and respiratory tract.

RNA v., a group of viruses in which the core consists of RNA; a major group of animal viruses that includes the families Picornaviridae, Reoviridae, Togaviridae, Flaviviridae, Bunyaviridae, Arenaviridae, Paramyxoviridae, Retroviridae, Coronaviridae, Orthomyxoviridae, and Rhabdoviridae. SYN ribovirus.

RNA tumor viruses, RNA viruses of the family Retroviridae that cause tumors.

Ross River v., a mosquito-borne alphavirus, family Togaviridae, that causes epidemic polyarthritis.

Rous-associated v. (RAV), a leukemia v. of the Avian type C retroviruses (leukosis-sarcoma complex), family Retroviridae, that by phenotypic mixing with a defective (noninfectious) strain

oncogenic viruses			
virus family	virus	host of origin	associated tumors
Herpesviridae	frog, herpesvirus	leopard frog	adenocarcinomas
	Marek disease virus	fowl	neurolymphomatosis (T cell)
	herpesvirus	monkeys	lymphoma, leukemia
	Epstein-Barr virus (EBV)	human	Burkitt lymphoma, nasopharyngeal carcinoma
	herpes simplex (type 2)	human	cervical neoplasia
	herpes simplex type 8 (HHVS)	human	Kaposi sarcoma
Poxviridae	Shope fibroma	rabbit	fibroma
	Yaba virus	monkey	nodular fibromatous hyperplasia
	molluscum contagiosum	human	nodular epidermal hyperplasia
Hepadnaviridae	hepatitis B group	humans, apes, rodents, ducks	primary hepatocellular carcinoma
Papovaviridae	polyoma	mouse	various carcinomas and sarcomas
	SV40	monkey	sarcoma (in rodents)
	BK and JC	human	none in humans; neural tumors in rodents and monkeys
	papilloma	human	genital, laryngeal, and skin warts; may progress to cervical carcinoma, laryngeal carcinoma, skin carcinoma
		cattle	genital, alimentary, skin warts; may progress to alimentary carcinoma, skin carcinoma
		other mammals	papillomas: may progress to carcinomas

of Rous sarcoma v. effects production of infectious sarcoma v. with envelope antigenicity of the RAV.

Rous sarcoma v. (RSV), a sarcoma-producing v. of the Avian type C retroviruses (leukosis-sarcoma complex), family Retroviridae identified by Rous in 1911.

Rs v., SYN respiratory syncytial v.

Rubarth disease v., SYN canine *adenovirus* 1.

rubella v., an RNA v. of the genus Rubivirus in the family Togaviridae; the agent causing rubella (German measles) in humans. SYN German measles v.

rubeola v., SYN measles v.

Russian autumn encephalitis v., SYN Japanese B encephalitis v.

Russian spring-summer encephalitis v., SYN tick-borne encephalitis v.

Sabia v., an arenavirus associated with hemolytic fever.

Salisbury common cold viruses, strains of rhinovirus of historical interest because of early studies that established the viral etiology of common colds.

salivary v., SYN human *herpesvirus* 5.

salivary gland v., SYN human *herpesvirus* 5.

sandfly fever viruses, SYN phlebotomus fever viruses.

San Miguel sea lion v., a calicivirus, family Caliciviridae, first isolated from sea lions on San Miguel island off the California coast, which is indistinguishable from the vesicular exanthema of swine v. both biophysically and clinically in terms of the vesicular disease syndrome that it produces in swine.

Semliki Forest v., an alphavirus in the family Togaviridae rarely associated with human disease.

Sendai v., a parainfluenza v. type 1 reported to cause inapparent infection in many animals; also used extensively to effect fusion of tissue culture cells.

Seoul v., a species of Hantavirus in the Far East causing hemorrhagic fever with renal syndrome. [the virus was named after Seoul in South Korea, the city where it was first isolated.]

serum hepatitis v., SYN hepatitis B v.

sheep-pox v., a poxvirus of the genus Capripoxvirus causing sheep-pox.

shipping fever v., a bovine strain of parainfluenza v. type 3. SEE parainfluenza viruses.

Shope fibroma v., SYN rabbit fibroma v.

major groups of viruses

DNA viruses virus family	envelope present	capsid symmetry	particle size (nm)	DNA structure*	medically important viruses
Parvoviridae	no	icosahedral	22	ss linear	B19 virus
Papovaviridae	no	icosahedral	55	ds circular, supercoiled	papillomavirus, polyomavirus (JC, BK)
Adenoviridae	no	icosahedral	75	ds linear	adenovirus
Hepadnaviridae	yes	icosahedral	42	ds incomplete circular	hepatitis B virus
Herpesviridae	yes	icosahedral	100**	ds linear	herpes simplex virus, Varicella-Zoster virus, cytomegalovirus, Epstein-Barr virus
Poxviridae	yes	complex	250×400	ds linear	smallpox virus, vaccinia virus

RNA viruses virus family	envelope present	capsid symmetry	particle size (nm)	RNA structure†	medically important viruses
Picornaviridae	no	icosahedral	28	ss linear, nonsegmented, +ve sense	poliovirus, rhinovirus, hepatitis A virus, enteroviruses
Reoviridae	no	icosahedral	75	ds linear, 10 segments	reovirus, rotavirus, Colorado tick fever virus
Togaviridae	yes	icosahedral	40–70	ss linear, nonsegmented, +ve sense	rubella virus, yellow fever virus
Retroviridae	yes	icosahedral	100	ss linear, 2 segments, +ve sense	HIV, human T-cell lymphotrophic virus (HTLV)
Coronaviridae	yes	helical	100	ss linear, nonsegmented, +ve sense	coronavirus
Calciviridae	no	icosahedral	35–40	ss RNA +ve sense	Norwalk agent
Orthomyxoviridae	yes	helical	80–120	ss linear, 8 segments, – ve sense	influenza virus
Paramyxoviridae	yes	helical	150	ss linear, nonsegmented, +ve sense	measles, mumps, parainfluenza, respiratory syncytial viruses
Rhabdoviridae	yes	helical	75 × 180	ss linear, nonsegmented, -ve sense	rabies virus
Arenaviridae	yes	helical	80–130	ss circular, 2 segments with cohesive ends, –ve sense	lymphocytic choriomeningitis virus
Bunyaviridae	yes	helical	100	ss circular, 3 segments with cohesive ends, –ve sense	California encephalitis, sandfly fever viruses
Filoviridae	yes	complex	80 × (800–900)	ss RNA, –ve sense	Marburg, Ebola virus

* ss, single stranded; ds, double stranded

** the herpesvirus nucleocapsid is 100 nm, but the envelope varies in size; the entire virus can be as large as 200 nm in diameter

† retrovirus RNA contains 2 identical molecules of mol. wt. 3.5×10^6

Shope papilloma v., a papillomavirus infecting wild cottontail rabbits. SEE Shope *papilloma*.

Simbu v., a serologic group of the genus Bunyavirus, comprising a number of species including the type strain, Simbu v.

simian v. (SV), any of a number of viruses, belonging to various families, isolated from monkeys or from cultures of monkey cells. SYN vacuolating v.

simian v. 40, SYN simian vacuolating v. No. 40.

simian vacuolating v. No. 40 (SV40), a small (40–45 nm) DNA v. of the genus Polyomavirus, family Papovaviridae; the cause of seemingly inapparent infections in monkeys, especially rhesus, and a common contaminant of monkey cell cultures; the v. may cause inapparent infection in humans and may be excreted in stools of children for several weeks; it can produce fibrosarcoma in suckling hamsters, and transformation may occur in human diploid cells; it may also form "hybrid" v. in cells also infected with certain adenoviruses. SYN simian v. 40.

Sindbis v., the type species of the genus Alphavirus, in the family Togaviridae, usually transmitted by mosquitoes of the genus *Culex;* and causative agent of Sindbis fever. [village in Egypt where first isolated]

Sin Nombre v., a species of Hantavirus in North America causing hantavirus pulmonary syndrome. SYN Four Corners v. [Spanish, without a name]

slow v., a v., or a viruslike agent, etiologically associated with a disease having a long incubation period of months to years with a gradual onset frequently terminating in severe illness and/or death.

smallpox v., SYN variola v.

snowshoe hare v., a member of the California group of arboviruses, genus Bunyavirus, family Bunyaviridae, causing fever, severe headache, and nausea in humans in North America.

soremouth v., SYN contagious ecthyma (pustular dermatitis) v. of sheep.

Spondweni v., an arbovirus of the genus Flavivirus isolated from mosquitoes in Africa; may cause disease in humans.

St. Louis encephalitis v., a group B arbovirus, genus Flavivirus in the family Flaviviridae, occurring in the U.S., Trinidad, and Panama; normally present as inapparent infection in humans, but sometimes a cause of encephalitis; the v. has been isolated from birds in Panama and from several mosquito species, especially *Psorophora*.

street v., an isolate of rabies v. from a naturally infected domestic animal.

Sudan v., a variant of Ebola v. SYN Ebola v. Sudan.

swine encephalitis v., a coronavirus, in the family Coronaviridae, that causes swine encephalitis.

swine fever v., SYN hog cholera v.

swine influenza viruses, strains of influenza v. type A which cause influenza of swine and can infect humans.

swinepox v., a poxvirus genus Suipoxvirus distinct from vaccinia v. and the cause of swinepox; the pig louse plays an important role in transmission.

Swiss mouse leukemia v., SYN Friend v.

Tacaribe v., the type v. of the Tacaribe complex of viruses of genus Arenaviruses isolated from bats and mosquitoes in Trinidad.

Tahyna v., a California group arbovirus genus Bunyavirus, in the family Bunyaviridae, from central Europe, known to infect humans.

Taiwan Dobrava-Belgrade v., a species of Hantavirus in the Balkans causing hemorrhagic fever with renal syndrome. [after Dobrava, Slovenia (where first isolated from field mice) and Belgrade, Yugoslavia (where first isolated from humans)]

temperate v., referring to a phage that does not lyse its host immediately but may persist in latent form and eventually lyse its host. SEE lysogeny.

Teschen disease v., a picornavirus causing Teschen disease of pigs; the v. is normally a harmless inhabitant of the intestinal tract, but virulent strains cause epizootics of the disease. SYN infectious porcine encephalomyelitis v.

Tete viruses, a serologic group of the genus Bunyavirus, comprising a number of types.

TGE v., SYN transmissible gastroenteritis v. of swine.

Theiler v., SYN mouse encephalomyelitis v.

Theiler mouse encephalomyelitis v., a virus genus Cardiovirus in the family Picornaviridae. SYN Theiler original v.

Theiler original v., SYN Theiler mouse encephalomyelitis v.

tick-borne v., SYN tick-borne encephalitis v.

tick-borne encephalitis v., arboviruses of the genus Flavivirus that occur in Central Europe and Russia in multiple subtypes, causing two forms of encephalitis in humans: tick-borne encephalitis (Central European subtype) and tick-borne encephalitis (Eastern subtype); the vectors are ticks of the genus *Ixodes*. SYN Russian spring-summer encephalitis v., tick-borne v.

TO v., theiler Original v. SEE mouse encephalomyelitis v.

Topografov v., a Hantavirus species found in Siberia.

trachoma v., former name for *Chlamydia trachomatis*.

transmissible gastroenteritis v. of swine, a genus Coronavirus that causes transmissible gastroenteritis of swine. SYN TGE v.

tumor v., SYN oncogenic v.

Turlock v., an unclassified serologic group of arboviruses in the genus Bunyavirus but antigenically unrelated to it.

Umbre v., a Bunyavirus related serologically to the Turlock v.

vaccine v., SEE vaccine.

vaccinia v., the poxvirus (genus Orthopoxvirus) used in the immunization of people against variola (smallpox), usually causing a local reaction but sometimes generalized vaccinia, especially in children; the v. is closely related serologically to the viruses of variola and cowpox, but certain differences have been demonstrated which indicate that they are perhaps distinct but closely related strains of a variola-vaccinia-cowpox complex; the lineage of vaccinia v. is uncertain, and it is very unlikely that it descended from Jenner original v. SYN poxvirus officinalis.

vacuolating v., SYN simian v.

varicella-zoster v., a herpesvirus, morphologically identical to herpes simplex v., that causes varicella (chickenpox) and herpes zoster in man; varicella results from a primary infection with the v.; herpes zoster results from secondary invasion by the same v. or by reactivation of infection which in many instances has been latent for many years. SYN chickenpox v., herpes zoster v., human herpesvirus 3, Varicellovirus.

variola v., a poxvirus of the genus Orthopoxvirus, the pathogen of smallpox in humans. SYN smallpox v.

VEE v., SYN Venezuelan equine encephalomyelitis v.

Venezuelan equine encephalomyelitis v., a group A arbovirus of the genus Alphavirus, family Togaviridae, occurring in Venezuela and several other South American countries, in Panama and Trinidad, and occasionally the U.S. causing Venezuelan equine encephalomyelitis in horses and humans; it seems to be more viscerotropic than neurotropic; the v. is transmitted by *Culex* mosquitoes. SYN VEE v.

vesicular exanthema of swine v., a Calicivirus causing vesicular exanthema of swine. SEE ALSO San Miguel sea lion v.

vesicular stomatitis v., an RNA v. of the genus Vesiculovirus, in the family Rhabdoviridae, causing vesicular stomatitis in horses, cattle, sheep, and pigs. SYN VS v.

viral hemorrhagic fever v., any one of more than 15 different viruses that cause hemorrhagic fever.

visceral disease v., SYN Cytomegalovirus.

visna v., an RNA v. a Lentivirus (family Retroviridae) that causes visna; it is closely related antigenically to the similar maedi v.

VS v., SYN vesicular stomatitis v.

WEE v., SYN western equine encephalomyelitis v.

Wesselsbron disease v., a mosquito-borne group B arbovirus of the genus Flavivirus causing Wesselsbron fever.

western equine encephalomyelitis v., a group A arbovirus of the genus Alphavirus, family Togaviridae, occurring in the western U.S. and parts of South America; it occurs naturally, usually as a symptomless infection in birds, but causes western equine encephalomyelitis in horses and humans following transfer by the bites of mosquitoes, chiefly *Culex tarsalis*. SYN WEE v.

West Nile v., SYN West Nile encephalitis v.

West Nile encephalitis v., a Flavivirus in the family Flaviviridae. SYN West Nile v.

xenotropic v., a retrovirus that does not produce disease in its natural host and replicates only in tissue culture cells derived from a different species.

Yaba v., a poxvirus from the Yatapoxvirus, family Poxviridae, distinct from monkeypox v., that causes Yaba tumors in monkeys. SYN Yaba monkey v.

Yaba monkey v., SYN Yaba v.

yellow fever v., an arbovirus, the type species of the genus Flavivirus, in the family Flaviviridae, endemic in tropical Africa south of the Sahara and in tropical South America, occasionally spreading to countries outside these areas; it is the cause of yellow fever of humans and other primates; the v. exists in wild primates, and probably also in edentates, marsupials, and rodents, and is transmitted to humans by *Aedes aegypti* and the *Haemagogus* complex of tree-top mosquitoes that feed on arboreal mammals.

Zaire v., a variant of Ebola v. SYN Ebola v. Zaire.

Zika v., a mosquito-borne virus of the genus Flavivirus (family Flaviviridae), found in parts of Africa and in Malaysia, that causes Zika fever. [*Zika,* forest in Uganda, where first isolated]

⌂**-virus.** A genus of viruses.

vi·rus·oid (vī′rŭs-oyd). A plant pathogen resembling a viroid but having a much larger circular or linear RNA segment and a capsid; it is a satellite agent requiring an associated virus (helper virus) for replication. [virus + G. *eidos,* resembling]

vi·rus shed·ding. Excretion of virus by any route from the infected host; route and duration of excretion vary according to the pathogenesis of the infection or disease.

vis, pl. **vi·res** (vis, vī′rēs). Force, energy, or power. [L. force]

v. conserva′trix, the inherent power in the organism resisting the effects of injury.

v. a fron′te, a force acting from in front; an obstructive, restraining, or impeding force.

v. a ter′go, a force acting from behind; a pushing or accelerating force.

v. vi′tae, v. vita′lis, SYN vitalism.

vis·cance (vis′kans). A measure of the energy dissipation due to a flow in a viscous system. In medicine and physiology, usually a measure of the energy dissipation in the flow of liquids, sols, or gels within cells and tissues, or of fluids (e.g., blood, respiratory gases) in tubes. The v. is the pressure gradient from one end to the other of the flow path when unit flow occurs. The relationship between viscosity and v. is of the same nature as that between specific resistance, or resistivity, of a conductor material and the resistance of a particular conductor made from that material.

vis·cera (vis′er-ă). Plural of viscus. SYN vitals.

vis·cer·ad (vis′er-ad). In a direction toward the viscera. [viscera + L. *ad,* to]

vis·cer·al (vis′er-ăl). Relating to the viscera. SYN splanchnic.

vis·cer·al·gia (vis-er-al′jē-ă). Pain in any viscera. [viscera + G. *algos,* pain]

vis·cer·i·mo·tor (vis′er-i-mō′ter). SYN visceromotor.

⌂**viscero-.** The viscera. SEE ALSO splanchno-. [L. *viscus,* pl. *viscera,* the internal organs]

vis·cer·o·cra·ni·um (vis′er-ō-krā′nē-ŭm) [TA]. That part of the skull derived from the embryonic pharyngeal arches; it comprises the facial bones of the facial skeleton (under *bone*) and is distinct from that part of the skull which forms the neurocranium or braincase. SYN facial skeleton✩, cranium viscerale, visceral cranium, jaw skeleton, splanchnocranium. [viscero- + cranium]

cartilaginous v., those elements of the fetal skull derived from the pharyngeal arch cartilages.

membranous v., components of v. that do not arise from a cartilagenous precursor; most of the mandible is a membrane bone, developing around and not from the first pharyngeal arch cartilage.

vis·cer·o·gen·ic (vis′er-ō-jen′ik). Of visceral origin; denoting a

number of sensory and other reflexes. [viscero- + G. *-gen,* producing]

vis·cer·o·graph (vis′er-ō-graf). An instrument for recording the mechanical activity of the viscera. [viscero- + G. *graphō,* to write]

vis·cer·o·in·hib·i·to·ry (vis′er-ō-in-hib′i-tōr-ē). Restricting or arresting the functional activity of the viscera.

vis·cer·o·meg·a·ly (vis′er-ō-meg′ă-lē). Abnormal enlargement of the viscera, such as may be seen in acromegaly and other disorders. SYN organomegaly, splanchnomegaly. [viscero- + G. *megas,* large]

vis·cer·o·mo·tor (vis′er-ō-mō′ter). **1.** Relating to or controlling movement in the viscera; denoting the autonomic nerves innervating the viscera, especially the intestines. **2.** Denoting a movement having a relation to the viscera; referring to reflex muscular contractions of the abdominal wall in cases of visceral disease. SYN viscerimotor.

vis·cer·o·pa·ri·e·tal (vis′er-ō-pă-rī′ĕ-tăl). Relating to the viscera and the wall of the abdomen. [viscero- + L. *paries,* wall]

vis·cer·o·per·i·to·ne·al (vis′er-ō-per-i-tō-nē′ăl). Relating to the peritoneum and the abdominal viscera.

vis·cer·o·pleu·ral (vis′er-ō-ploo′răl). Relating to the pleural and the thoracic viscera. SYN pleurovisceral.

vis·cer·op·to·sis, vis·cer·op·to·sia (vis′er-op-tō′sis, -tō′sē-ă). Descent of the viscera from their normal positions. SYN splanchnoptosis, splanchnoptosia. [viscero- + G. *ptōsis,* a falling]

vis·cer·o·sen·so·ry (vis′er-ō-sen′sōr-ē). Relating to the sensory innervation of internal organs.

vis·cer·o·skel·e·tal (vis-er-ō-skel′ĕ-tăl). Relating to the visceroskeleton. SYN splanchnoskeletal.

vis·cer·o·skel·e·ton (vis-er-ō-skel′ĕ-tŏn). **1.** Any bony formation in an organ, as in the heart, tongue, or penis of certain animals; the term also includes, according to some anatomists, the cartilaginous rings of the trachea and bronchi. **2.** The bony framework protecting the viscera, such as the ribs and sternum, the pelvic bones, and the anterior portion of the skull. SYN splanchnoskeleton, visceral skeleton.

vis·cer·o·so·mat·ic (vis′er-ō-sō-mat′ik). Relating to the viscera and the body. SYN splanchnosomatic. [viscero- + G. *sōma,* body]

vis·cer·o·tome (vis′er-ō-tōm). An instrument by means of which a section of an organ, e.g., the liver, can be removed from a cadaver for examination without performing a general autopsy. [viscero- + G. *tomos,* cutting]

vis·cer·ot·o·my (vis-er-ot′ō-mē). Dissection of the viscera by incision, especially postmortem. [viscero- + G. *tomē,* incision]

vis·cer·o·to·nia (vis′er-ō-tō′nē-ă). Personality traits of love of food, sociability, general relaxation, friendliness, and affection. [viscero- + G. *tonos,* tone]

vis·cer·o·tro·phic (vis′er-ō-trof′ik). Relating to any trophic change determined by visceral conditions. [viscero- + G. *trophē,* nourishment]

vis·cer·o·tro·pic (vis′er-ō-trop′ik). Affecting the viscera. [L. *viscero,* internal organs, + G. *tropē,* a turning]

vis·cid (vis′id). Sticky; glutinous. [L. *viscidus,* stick, fr. *viscum,* birdlime]

vis·cid·i·ty (vi-sid′i-tē). Stickiness; adhesiveness.

vis·ci·do·sis (vis-i-dō′sis). SYN cystic *fibrosis.*

vis·co·e·las·tic·i·ty (vis′kō-ē-las-tis′i-tē). The property of a viscous material that also shows elasticity.

vis·com·e·ter (vis-kom′ě-ter). SYN viscosimeter.

vis·co·sim·e·ter (vis-kō-sim′ě-ter). An apparatus for determining the viscosity of a fluid; in medicine, usually of the blood. SYN viscometer.

vis·co·sim·e·try (vis-kō-sim′ě-trē). Determination of the viscosity of a fluid, such as the blood. [viscosity + G. *metron,* measure]

vis·cos·i·ty (vis-kos′i-tē). In general, the resistance to flow or alteration of shape by any substance as a result of molecular cohesion; most frequently applied to liquids as the resistance of a fluid to flow because of a shearing force. [L. *viscositas,* fr. *viscosus,* viscous]

absolute v., force per unit area applied tangentially to a fluid, causing unit rate of displacement of parallel planes separated by a unit distance; units in CGS system: poise.

anomalous v., the viscous behavior of nonhomogenous fluids or suspensions, e.g., blood, in which the apparent v. increases as flow or shear rate decreases toward zero.

apparent v., the v. calculated from Poiseuille law at any particular flow and tube diameter; it is used for suspensions, such as blood, that exhibit anomalous v. and the Fahraeus-Lindqvist effect.

dynamic v. (μ), the internal or molecular frictional resistance of a fluid by Newton law of v. as the ratio of the applied force per unit area to the relative velocity of adjacent fluid layers (produced by the force).

kinematic v. (ν, υ), a measure used in studies of fluid flow; it is the dynamic viscosity, μ, in poises, divided by the density of the material; unit; stoke.

newtonian v., the v. characteristics of a newtonian fluid.

relative v., the ratio of the v. of a solution or dispersion to the v. of the solvent or continuous phase.

vis·co·tox·ins (vis′kō-toks′ins). A class of phytotoxins that have a hypotensive activity and slow the heart beat.

vis·cous (vis′kŭs). Sticky; marked by high viscosity. [see viscid, viscosity]

vis·cum (vis′kŭm). **1.** The berries of *Viscum album* (family Loranthaceae), a parasitic plant growing on apple, pear, and other trees; has been used as an oxytocic. SYN mistletoe. **2.** Herbage of *Phoradendron flavescens*, American mistletoe; has been used as an oxytocic and emmenagoque.

vis·cus, pl. **vis·cera** (vis′kŭs, vis′er-ă). An organ of the digestive, respiratory, urogenital, and endocrine systems as well as the spleen, the heart, and great vessels; hollow and multilayered walled organs studied in splanchnology. [L. the soft parts, internal organs]

¶ vi·sion (vizh′ŭn). The act of seeing. SEE ALSO sight. [L. *visio,* fr. *video,* pp. *visus,* to see]

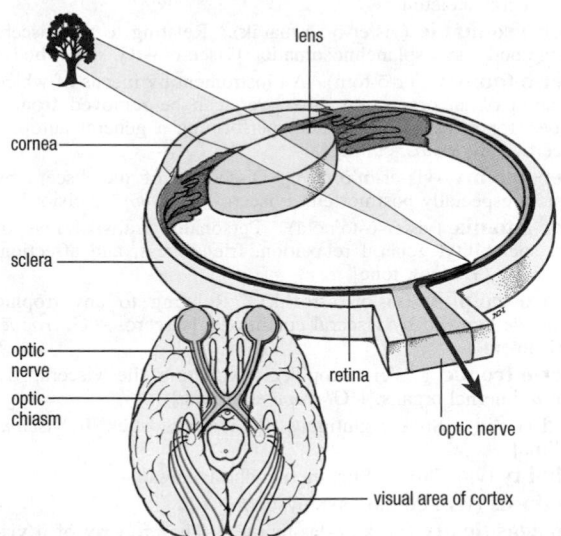

vision: light passes through the cornea and is focused onto the retina by the lens; cells in the retina then transmit this information through the optic nerve to the visual area of the cortex

achromatic v., SYN achromatopsia.

binocular v., v. with a single image, by both eyes simultaneously.

blue v., SYN cyanopsia.

central v., v. stimulated by an object imaged on the fovea centralis. SYN direct v.

chromatic v., SYN chromatopsia.

colored v. (VC), SYN chromatopsia.

cone v., SYN photopic v.

direct v., SYN central v.

double v., SYN diplopia.

facial v., sensing the proximity of objects by the nerves of the face, presumed in the case of the blind and also in sighted persons who are blindfolded or in darkness.

green v., SYN chloropsia.

halo v., a condition in which colored or luminous rings are seen around lights.

haploscopic v., stereoscopic v. produced by the haploscope, or mirror-type stereoscope.

indirect v., SYN peripheral v.

multiple v., SYN polyopia.

night v., SYN scotopic v.

oscillating v., SYN oscillopsia.

peripheral v., v. resulting from retinal stimulation beyond the macula. SYN indirect v.

photopic v., v. when the eye is light-adapted. SEE light *adaptation,* light-adapted *eye.* SYN cone v., photopia.

red v., SYN erythropsia.

rod v., SYN scotopic v.

scotopic v., v. when the eye is dark-adapted. SEE ALSO dark *adaptation,* dark-adapted *eye.* SYN night v., rod v., scotopia, twilight v.

stereoscopic v., the single perception of a slightly different image from each eye. SYN stereopsis.

subjective v., visual impressions that arise centrally and do not originate with ocular stimuli.

tinted v., SYN chromatopsia.

triple v., SYN triplopia.

tubular v., a constriction of the visual field, as though one were looking through a hollow cylinder or tube. SYN tunnel v.

tunnel v., SYN tubular v.

twilight v., SYN scotopic v.

yellow v., SYN xanthopsia.

vi·su·al (vizh′oo-ăl). **1.** Relating to vision. **2.** Denoting a person who learns and remembers more readily through sight than through hearing. SEE ALSO internal *representation.* [Late L. *visualis,* fr. *visus,* vision]

functional v. loss, an apparent loss of visual acuity or visual field with no substantiating physical signs; often due to a natural concern about visual loss combined with suggestibility and a fear of the worst; best treated with reassurance.

vi·su·al·ize (vizh′oo-ă-līz). To picture in the mind or to perceive; commonly misused by ascribing to the technique the act of making visible.

vi·su·o·au·di·tory (vizh′ū-ō-aw′di-tōr-ē). Relating to both vision and hearing; denoting nerves connecting the centers for these senses.

vi·su·og·no·sis (vizh′ū-og-nō′sis). Recognition and understanding of visual impressions. [L. *visus,* vision, + G. *gnōsis,* knowledge]

vis·u·o·mo·tor (viz′ū-ō-mō′ter). Denoting the ability to synchronize visual information with physical movement, e.g., driving a car or playing a video game of skill.

vi·su·o·psy·chic (vizh′ū-ō-sī′kik). Pertaining to the portion of the cerebral cortex concerned with the integration of visual impressions. [L. *visus,* vision, + G. *psychē,* mind]

vi·su·o·sen·so·ry (vizh′ū-ō-sen′sōr-ē). Pertaining to the perception of visual stimuli.

vis·u·o·spa·tial (viz′ū-ō-spā′shăl). Denoting the ability to comprehend and conceptualize visual representations and spatial relationships in learning and performing a task.

vi·su·scope (viz′ū-skōp). A modified ophthalmoscope that projects a black star on the patient's fundus.

vi·tal (vīt-ăl). Relating to life. [L. *vitalis,* fr. *vita,* life]

vi·tal·ism (vīt′ăl-izm). The theory that animal functions are dependent upon a special form of energy or force, the vital force, distinct from the physical forces. SYN vis vitae, vis vitalis. [L. *vitalis,* pertaining to life]

vi·tal·is·tic (vīt′ă-lis′tik). Pertaining to vitalism.

vi·tal·i·ty (vīt-al'i-tē). Vital force or energy.

vi·tal·ize (vīt'ăl-īz). To endow with vital force.

vi·ta·lom·e·ter (vī-tă-lom'ĕ-ter). An electrical device for determining the vitality of the tooth pulp.

vi·tal red [C.I. 23570]. Trisodium salt of a sulfonated diazo dye (a ditolyl group diazotized to sulfonated aminonaphthalene residues), used as a vital stain. SYN brilliant vital red.

vi·tals (vīt'ălz). SYN viscera.

vi·ta·mer (vī'tă-mer). One of two or more similar compounds capable of fulfilling a specific vitamin function in the body; e.g., niacin, niacinamide.

VITAMIN

---

vi·ta·min (vīt'ă-min). One of a group of organic substances, present in minute amounts in natural foodstuffs, that are essential to normal metabolism; insufficient amounts in the diet may cause deficiency diseases. [L. *vita*, life, + amine]

v. A, (1) any β-ionone derivative, except provitamin A carotenoids, possessing qualitatively the biological activity of retinol; deficiency interferes with the production and resynthesis of rhodopsin, thereby causing night blindness, and produces a keratinizing metaplasia of epithelial cells that may result in xerophthalmia, keratosis, susceptibility to infections, and retarded growth; **(2)** the original v. A, now known as retinol. SYN axerophthol.

v. A$_1$, SYN retinol.

v. A$_2$, SYN dehydroretinol.

v. A$_1$ acid, SYN retinoic acid.

v. A$_1$ alcohol, SYN retinol.

v. A aldehyde, SYN retinaldehyde.

v. A$_2$ aldehyde, SYN dehydroretinaldehyde.

antiberiberi v., SYN thiamin.

antihemorrhagic v., SYN v. K.

antineuritic v., SYN thiamin.

antirachitic v.'s, ergocalciferol (v. D$_2$) and cholecalciferol (v. D$_3$).

antiscorbutic v., SYN ascorbic acid.

antisterility v., SYN v. E (2).

v. B, a group of water-soluble substances originally considered as one v.

v. B$_1$, SYN thiamin.

v. B$_2$, (1) SYN riboflavin; **(2)** obsolete term for a complex of folic acid, nicotinic acid, nicotinamide, pantothenic acid, and riboflavin.

v. B$_3$, (1) obsolete term for nicotinamide and/or nicotinic acid; **(2)** obsolete term for pantothenic acid.

v. B$_4$, (1) once believed to be a factor necessary for nutrition of the chick, now identified simply as certain essential amino acids and/or adenine; **(2)** obsolete term for adenine.

vitamins and minerals: sources, etc.

vitamin/ mineral	sources	benefits	deficiency	recommended dietary allowance (RDA)
vitamin A*	sweet potatoes, carrots, milk	improved skin resistance to infection; good eyesight	night blindness, xerophthalmia	1000 µg retinol equivalents (5000 IU)
vitamin D*	sunlight, dairy products	strengthens bone development	rickets	5–10 µg (1000–1200 IU)
vitamin E*	green leafy vegetables, nuts, whole grains, wheat germ	oxidative protection of red blood cells	anemia	8–10 mg (30 IU)
vitamin K*	green leafy vegetables, tomatoes	blood clotting cascade	bleeding diathesis	70–140 µg
vitamin B$_1$† (thiamine)	whole grains, vegetables, nuts, wheat germ	carbohydrate metabolism	beriberi	1–1.5 mg
vitamin B$_2$† (riboflavin)	animal products, mushrooms, broccoli	protein metabolism, skin and eye protectant	angular stomatitis/ blepharitis	1.2–1.5 mg
vitamin B$_6$† (pyridoxine)	brewer's yeast, whole grains, nuts, meat	helps regulate central nervous system	peripheral neuropathy, seizures	1.7–2 mg
vitamin B$_{12}$†	animal products, fish, soybeans	red blood cell formation	mental status changes	3 µg
folic acid	green leafy vegetables, liver, yeast	protect against birth defects, red blood cell production	anemia	0.4 mg (or 400 µg)
vitamin C†	broccoli, tomatoes, Brussels sprouts, citrus fruits	resistance to stress; oral hygiene; wound healing	scurvy	60 mg
niacin†	nuts, poultry, fish	cholesterol-lowering agent, coenzyme in oxidations, reductions	pellagra	13–16 mg
calcium	dairy products	bone growth; nerve, muscle function	rickets, osteomalacia, osteoporosis	800 mg
potassium	tomatoes, citrus fruits	cellular function	Ileus, muscle weakness	1.8–6 g
sodium	most foods	cellular function	weakness, confusion	1–3.3 g
phosphorus	cereals, dairy products	cellular function	mental status changes, osteomalacia	800 mg
iron	green leafy vegetables, dried fruits, meat, wheat germ	red blood cell formation	anemia	10–18 mg
iodine	some dairy products, seafood, iodized salt	normal thyroid function, topical antiseptic	goiter	150 µg

* fat soluble
† water soluble

vi

v. B₅, term once used to describe biologic activities now ascribed to pantothenic acid or nicotinic acid.

v. B₆, pyridoxine and related compounds (pyridoxal; pyridoxamine).

v. B₁₂, generic descriptor for compounds exhibiting the biological activity of cyanocobalamin (cyanocob(III)alamin); the antianemia factor of liver extract that contains cobalt, a cyano group, and corrin in a cobamide structure. Several substances with similar formulas and with the characteristic hematinic action have been isolated and designated: B_{12a}, hydroxocobalamin; B_{12b}, aquacobalamin; B_{12c}, nitritocobalamin; B_{12r}, cob(II)alamin; B_{12s}, cob(I)alamin; B_{12III}, factors A and V_{1a} (cobyric acid) and pseudovitamin B_{12}. Vitamins B_{12a} and B_{12b} are known to be tautomeric compounds; B_{12b} has been obtained from cultures of *Streptomyces aureofaciens;* B_{12c} has been obtained from cultures of *Streptomyces griseus* and is distinguishable from B_{12} by differences in its absorption spectrum. The physiologically active v. B_{12} coenzymes are methylcobalamin and deoxyadenosinecobalamin. A deficiency of v. B_{12} is often associated with certain methylmalonic acidurias. SYN animal protein factor, antianemic factor, antipernicious anemia factor (1), erythrocyte maturation factor, maturation factor, methylcobalamin.

v. B_T, SYN carnitine.

v. B_x, SYN *p*-aminobenzoic acid.

v. B complex, a pharmaceutical term applied to drug products containing a mixture of the B v.'s, usually B_1, B_2, B_3, B_5, and B_6.

v. B_c conjugase, an enzyme catalyzing the hydrolysis of the pteroylpolyglutamic acids to pteroylmonoglutamic acid, with consequent increase in vitamin activity; v. B_c is an obsolete term for folic acid.

v. B₁₂ with intrinsic factor concentrate, a combination of v. B_{12} with suitable preparations of the mucosa of the stomach or intestine of domestic animals used for food by humans.

v. C, SYN ascorbic acid.

coagulation v., obsolete term for v. K.

v. D, generic descriptor for all steroids exhibiting the biologic activity of ergocalciferol or cholecalciferol, the antirachitic v.'s popularly called the "sun-ray v.'s." They promote the proper utilization of calcium and phosphorus, thereby producing growth, together with proper bone and tooth formation, in young children; the sulfate, a water-soluble conjugate, is found in the aqueous phase of human milk; v. D_1 is a 1:1 mixture of lumisterol and v. D_2.

v. D₂, SYN ergocalciferol.

v. D₃, SYN cholecalciferol.

v. E, (1) SYN α-tocopherol; (2) generic descriptor of tocol and tocotrienol derivatives possessing the biologic activity of α-tocopherol; contained in various oils (wheat germ, cotton seed, palm, rice) and whole grain cereals where it constitutes the nonsaponifiable fraction; also contained in animal tissue (liver, pancreas, heart) and lettuce; deficiency produces resorption or abortion in female rats and sterility in males. SYN antisterility factor, antisterility v., fertility v.

v. F, term sometimes applied to the essential unsaturated fatty acids, linoleic, linolenic, and arachidonic acids.

fat-soluble v.'s, those v.'s, soluble in fat solvents (nonpolar solvents) and relatively insoluble in water, marked in chemical structure by the presence of large hydrocarbon moieties in the molecule; e.g., v.'s A, D, E, K.

fertility v., SYN v. E (2).

v. G, obsolete term for riboflavin.

v. H, SYN biotin. [Ger, H for *Haut*, skin]

v. K, generic descriptor for compounds with the biologic activity of phylloquinone; fat-soluble, thermostable compounds found in alfalfa, hog liver, fish meal, and vegetable oils, essential for the formation of normal amounts of prothrombin. SYN antihemorrhagic factor, antihemorrhagic v.

v. K₁, v. K₁(20), SYN phylloquinone.

v. K₂, v. K₂(30), SYN menaquinone-6.

v. K₃, SYN menadione.

v. K₄, SYN menadiol diacetate.

v. K₅, an antihemorrhagic v.

v. K₂(35), SYN menaquinone-7.

microbial v., a substance necessary for the growth of certain microorganisms, e.g., biotin, *p*-aminobenzoic acid.

v. P, a mixture of bioflavonoids extracted from plants (especially citrus fruits). It reduces the permeability and fragility of capillaries and is useful in the treatment of certain cases of purpura that are resistant to v. C therapy. SEE ALSO hesperidin, quercetin, rutin. SYN capillary permeability factor, citrin, permeability v.

permeability v., SYN v. P.

v. PP, SYN nicotinic acid.

v. U, term given to a factor in fresh cabbage juice that encourages the healing of peptic ulcer, (3-amino-3-carboxypropyl)-dimethylsulfonium chloride, a methionine derivative.

---

vi·tel·lar·i·um (vit'ĕl-lar'ē-ŭm). In cestodes and trematodes, a common chamber receiving vitelline (yolk) material from the two vitelline ducts; the yolk material then passes into the ootype to surround the ovum with nutritive vitelline granules that are enclosed by a characteristically formed eggshell. SYN vitelline reservoir.

vi·tel·li·form (vī-tel'i-fōrm). Relating to or resembling the yolk of an egg.

vi·tel·lin (vī-tel'in). A lipophosphoprotein combined with lecithin in the yolk of egg. SYN lipovitellin, ovovitellin.

vi·tel·line (vī-tel'in, -ēn). Relating to the vitellus. SEE yolk *sac.*

vi·tel·lo·gen·e·sis (vī-tel'lō-jen'ĕ-sis, vī'tĕ-lō-). Formation of the yolk and its accumulation in the yolk sac. [L. *vitellus,* yolk, + G. *genesis,* production]

vi·tel·lo·gen·in (vī'tel-ō-jen'in). An egg yolk precursor protein; production is stimulated by estrogens. [L. *vitellus,* egg yolk, + -*gen* + -in]

vi·tel·lo·lu·te·in (vī-tel-ō-loo'tē-in). Lutein from the yolk of egg.

vitel·lo·ru·bin (vī-tel-ō-roo'bin). A reddish pigment from the yolk of egg.

vi·tel·lose (vī-tel'ōs). A protein fragment from vitellin.

vi·tel·lus (vī-tel'ŭs). SYN yolk (1). [L.]

v. o′vi, yolk of egg; used in pharmacy for emulsifying oils and camphors.

vi·ti·a·tion (vish-ē-ā'shŭn). A change that impairs utility or reduces efficiency. [L. *vitiatio* fr. *vitio,* pp. *vitiatus,* to corrupt, fr. *vitium,* vice]

vit·i·lig·i·nes (vit-i-lij'i-nēz). Plural of vitiligo.

vit·i·lig·i·nous (vit-i-lij'i-nŭs). Relating to or characterized by vitiligo.

vit·i·li·go, pl. **vit·i·lig·i·nes** (vit-i-lī'gō, vit-i-lij'i-nēz). The appearance on otherwise normal skin of nonpigmented white patches of varied sizes, often symmetrically distributed and usually bordered by hyperpigmented areas; hair in the affected areas is usually white. Epidermal melanocytes are completely lost in depigmented areas by an autoimmune process. SYN acquired leukoderma. [L. a skin eruption, fr. *vitium,* blemish, vice]

v. i′ridis, small white patches in brown irides.

vit·rec·to·my (vi-trek'tō-mē). Removal of the vitreous by means of an instrument that simultaneously removes vitreous by suction and cutting, and replaces it with saline or some other fluid. [vitreous + G. *ektomē,* excision]

anterior v., removal of the central vitreous gel.

posterior v., removal of the posterior cortical vitreous; sometimes the preretinal membranes are removed.

vit·re·in (vit'rē-in). A collagen-like protein that, with hyaluronic acid, accounts for the gel state of the vitreous humor. SYN vitrosin.

vit·re·i·tis (vit-rē-ī'tis). Inflammation of the corpus vitreum. SYN hyalitis. [L. *vitreus,* glassy, + G. -*itis,* inflammation]

vitreo-. Vitreous. [L. *vitreus,* glassy]

vit·re·o·den·tin (vit'rē-ō-den'tin). Dentin of a particularly brittle character.

vit·re·o·ret·i·nal (vit'rē-ō-ret'i-năl). Pertaining to the retina and the vitreous body.

vit·re·o·ret·i·nop·a·thy (vit′rē-ō-ret′i-nop′ă-thē). Retinopathy with vitreous complications.

exudative v. [MIM*193220], a familial, slowly progressive ocular disease; characterized by posterior vitreous detachment, vitreous membranes, heterotopia of macula, retinal detachment, neovascularization, and recurrent hemorrhage.

vit·re·ous (vit′rē-ŭs). **1.** Glassy; resembling glass. **2.** SYN vitreous body. [L. vitreus, glassy, fr. vitrum, glass]

persistent anterior hyperplastic primary v., a unilateral congenital abnormality occurring in full-term infants; characterized by a retrolental fibrovascular membrane formed by persistent primary v. with remnants of the hyaloid artery and tunica vasculosa lentis; associated with leukokoria, microphthalmos, shallow anterior chamber, and elongated ciliary processes.

persistent posterior hyperplastic primary v., a unilateral congenital anomaly in full-term infants; associated with a congenital retinal fold and a v. membranous stalk containing remnants of the hyaloid artery.

primary v., the v. first formed in the embryo between the optic cup and the lens vesicle, and later vascularized by the hyaloid artery and its branches.

secondary v., avascular v. formed around the primary v.

tertiary v., v. fibrils derived from the neuroepithelium of the ciliary body and forming the ciliary zonule.

vit·re·um (vit′rē-ŭm). SYN vitreous body. [L. ntr. of vitreus, glassy]

vit·ri·fi·ca·tion (vit′ri-fi-kā′shŭn). Conversion of dental porcelain (frit) to a glassy substance by heat and fusion. [L. vitrium, glassy, + facio, to make]

vit·ri·ol (vit′rē-ol). Any of the various salts of sulfuric acid, e.g., blue v. (cupric sulfate), green v. (ferrous sulfate), white v. (zinc sulfate). [L. vitreolus, glassy]

vitronectin (vit′rō-nek′tin). A plasma glycoprotein involved in inflammatory and repair reactions at sites of tissue damage.

vit·ro·sin (vit′rō-sin). SYN vitrein.

Vit·ta·for·ma (vē-ta-fōr′ma). A genus of microsporidia that can infect humans and can cause keratitis in the immunocompetent and disseminated infection in the immunocompromised; formerly Nosema.

vi·var·i·um, pl. **vi·var·ia** (vī-var′ē-ŭm, -ă). Quarters in which animals are housed, particularly animals used in medical research. [L. vivarius, pertaining to living creatures]

⚠**vivi-.** Living. [L. vivus, alive]

viv·i·di·al·y·sis (viv′i-dī-al′i-sis). Removal by dialysis, as by lavage of peritoneal cavity.

viv·i·dif·fu·sion (viv′i-di-fū′zhŭn). Archaic term for a method by which circulating blood may be submitted to dialysis outside the body and returned to the circulation without exposure to the air or to any noxious influences; the principle used in the performance of renal dialysis with the artificial kidney. [vivi- + diffusion]

viv·i·fi·ca·tion (viv′i-fi-kā′shŭn). SYN revivification (2). [L. vivifico, pp. -atus, fr. vivus, alive, + facio, to make]

viv·i·par·i·ty (viv′i-pār′i-tē). The quality or state of being viviparous, i.e., producing offspring that are living at the time of birth. SYN zoogony.

vi·vip·a·rous (vī-vip′ă-rŭs). Giving birth to living young, in distinction to oviparous, or egg-laying. SYN zoogonous. [vivi- + L. pario, to bear]

viv·i·per·cep·tion (viv′i-per-sep′shŭn). Observation of the vital processes in the organism without the aid of vivisection. [vivi- + perception]

viv·i·sect (viv-i-sekt′). To practice vivisection.

viv·i·sec·tion (viv-i-sek′shŭn). Any cutting operation on a living animal for purposes of experimentation; often extended to denote any form of animal experimentation. [vivi- + section]

viv·i·sec·tion·ist, viv·i·sec·tor (vi-vi-sek′shŭn-ist, -tŏr; vi-vi-sek′tŏr). One who practices vivisection.

Vladimiroff, Vladimir D., Russian surgeon, 1837–1903. SEE Mikulicz-V. amputation; V.-Mikulicz amputation.

VLDL Abbreviation for very low density lipoprotein. SEE lipoprotein.

VMA Abbreviation for vanillylmandelic acid.

V-max. SEE V_{max}.

VMC Abbreviation for void metal composite.

V-MI Abbreviation for Volpe-Manhold Index.

vo·cal (vō′kăl). Pertaining to the voice or the organs of speech. [L. vocalis]

vo·cal fry (vō′kal frī). Phonation at an unnaturally low frequency resulting in low-frequency popping and ticking sounds. SYN glottalization.

Vogel law. See under law.

Voges, Otto, German physician, *1867. SEE V.-Proskauer reaction.

Vogt, Alfred, Swiss ophthalmologist, 1879–1943. SEE V.-Koyanagi syndrome.

Vogt, Cécile, German neurologist, 1875–1962. SEE V. syndrome.

Vogt, Heinrich W., German neurologist, *1875. SEE Spielmeyer-V. disease.

Vogt, Karl C., German physiologist, 1817–1895. SEE V. angle.

Vogt, Oskar, German neurologist, 1870–1959. SEE V. syndrome.

Vogt ceph·a·lo·dac·ty·ly. SYN type II acrocephalosyndactyly.

Vohwinkel, H.H., 20th century German dermatologist. SEE Vohwinkel syndrome.

voice (voys). The sound made by vibration of the vocal folds caused by air passing out through the larynx and upper respiratory tract, the vocal folds being approximated. SYN vox. [L. vox]

amphoric v., a v. sound having a hollow, blowing character, heard over a pulmonary cavity when the patient speaks or whispers. SYN amphorophony.

bronchial v., SYN bronchophony.

cavernous v., the hollow or metallic v. sound heard over a pulmonary cavity.

epigastric v., the delusion of a v. proceeding from the epigastrium.

eunuchoid v., high-pitched v. in the adult male resembling the v. of a young boy; usually functional in origin.

myxedema v., the forced, rough, raucous v. of subjects of myxedema, probably due to myxedematous thickening of the vocal folds.

void (voyd). To evacuate urine or feces.

flow v., in magnetic resonance imaging, the absence of signal from blood whose activated protons leave a region before their magnetization is measured. SEE ALSO signal v.

signal v., in magnetic resonance imaging, a region emitting no radiofrequency signal, because there are no activated protons in the region (such as flowing blood), because a different element predominates, particularly calcium, or because of uncompensated dephasing, such as occurs at air-tissue interfaces in the lung.

void met·al com·pos·ite (VMC). A porous metal structure that enables tissue growth within the openings to establish long-term attachment between prosthesis and tissue.

vol. Abbreviation for [L.] volatilis, volatile.

vo·la (vō′lă). Palm of the hand or sole of the foot. [L.]

vo·lar (vō′lăr) [TA]. Referring to the vola; denoting either the palm of the hand or sole of the foot. SYN volaris [TA].

vo·la·ris (vō-lā′ris) [TA]. SYN volar.

vol·a·tile (vol.) (vol′ă-til). **1.** Tending to evaporate rapidly. **2.** Tending toward violence, explosiveness, or rapid change. [L. volatilis, fr. volo, to fly]

vol·a·til·i·za·tion (vol′ă-til-i-zā′shŭn). SYN evaporation. [fr. L. volatilis, volatile, fr. volo, pp. volatus, to fly]

vol·a·til·ize (vol′ă-til-īz). SYN evaporate.

Volhard, Franz, German physician, 1872–1950. SEE V. test.

vo·li·tion (vō-lish′ŭn). The conscious impulse to perform any act or to abstain from its performance; voluntary action. [L. volo,, to wish]

vo·li·tion·al (vo-lish′ŭn-ăl). Done by an act of will; relating to volition.

VO

Volkmann, Alfred W., German physiologist, 1800–1877. SEE V. *canals*, under *canal*.

Volkmann, Richard, German surgeon, 1830–1889. SEE V. *cheilitis, contracture, spoon*.

vol·ley (vol′ē). A synchronous group of impulses induced simultaneously by artificial stimulation of either nerve fibers or muscle fibers. [Fr. *volée,* fr. L. *volo,* to fly]

Vollmer, Herman, U.S. pediatrician, 1896–1959. SEE V. *test*.

Volpe, Anthony R., U.S. dentist, *1932. SEE V.-Manhold *Index*.

vol·sel·la (vol-sel′ă). SYN vulsella *forceps*. [see vulsella]

volt (v, V) (vōlt). The unit of electromotive force; the electromotive force that will produce a current of 1 A in a circuit that has a resistance of 1 ohm; i.e., joule per coulomb. [Alessandro *Volta,* It. physicist, 1745–1827]

volt·age (vōl′tej). Electromotive force, pressure, or potential expressed in volts.

vol·ta·ic (vōl-tā′ik). SYN galvanic.

vol·ta·ism (vōl′tă-izm). SYN galvanism.

vol·tam·e·ter (vōl-tam′ĕ-ter). An apparatus for measuring the strength of a galvanic current by its electrolytic action. [volt + G. *metron,* measure]

volt·am·pere (vōlt′am-pēr). A unit of electrical power; the product of 1 V by 1 A; equivalent to 1 W or $\frac{1}{1000}$ kW.

volt·me·ter (vōlt′mē-ter). An apparatus for measuring the electromotive force or difference of potential.

Voltolini, Friedrich E.R., German laryngologist, 1819–1889. SEE V. *disease*.

vol·ume (V, V) (vol′yŭm). Space occupied by matter, expressed usually in cubic millimeters, cubic centimeters, liters, etc. SEE water. SEE ALSO capacity. [L. *volumen,* something rolled up, scroll, fr. *volvo,* to roll]

atomic v., the atomic weight of an element divided by its density in the solid state; the v. of the gram-atomic weight of a solid element.

v. averaging, in computed tomography or magnetic resonance imaging, the effect of expressing the average density of a voxel as a pixel in the image; the greater the slice thickness, the more averaging is necessary, with loss in density resolution.

closing v. (CV), the lung v. at which the flow from the lower parts of the lungs becomes severely reduced or stops during expiration, presumably because of airway closure; measured by the sharp rise in expiratory concentration of a tracer gas that had been inspired at the beginning of a breath that started from residual volume.

distribution v., the v. throughout which an added tracer substance appears to have been evenly distributed, calculated by dividing the amount of tracer added by its concentration after equilibration.

end-diastolic v., the capacity or the amount of blood in the ventricle immediately before a cardiac contraction begins; a measurement of cardiac filling between beats, related to diastolic function.

end-systolic v., the capacity or the amount of blood in the ventricle at the end of the ventricular ejection period and immediately preceding the beginning of ventricular relaxation; a measurement of the adequacy of cardiac emptying, related to systolic function.

expiratory reserve v. (ERV), the maximal v. of air (about 1000 mL) that can be expelled from the lungs after a normal expiration. SYN reserve air, supplemental air.

extracellular fluid v. (ECFV), the fraction of body water not in cells, about 25% of body weight: it consists of plasma water (4.5% of body weight), water between cells (interstitial water-lymph, 11.5% of body weight), water in dense bone and connective tissue (7.5% of body weight), and water secretions. See entries under entries under water.; SEE ALSO intracellular *fluid*.

forced expiratory v. (FEV), the maximal v. that can be expired in a specific time interval when starting from maximal inspiration. A subscript annotation normally indicates the number of seconds the patient has been expiring e.g., FEV_{30-60}.

inspiratory reserve v. (IRV), the maximal v. of air that can be

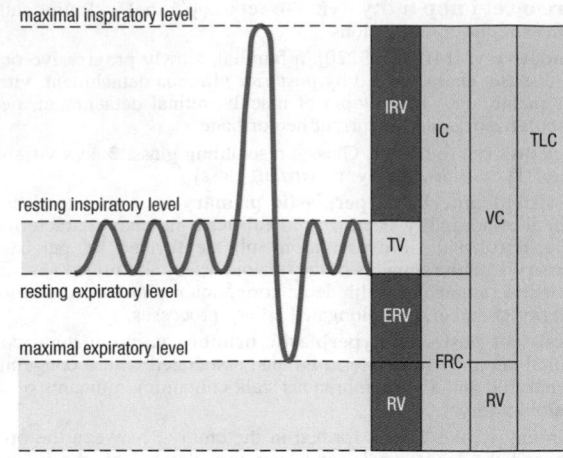

lung volume compartments and subdivisions: (based on a volume-time spirogram) **ERV:** expiratory reserve volume; the maximal amount of air that can be exhaled from the resting end-tidal (end-expiratory) position. **FRC:** functional residual capacity; the volume of air in the lungs at tidal volume end-expiratory position, or the sum of RV and ERV. **IC:** inspiratory capacity; the maximum volume of air that can be inhaled from the tidal volume end-expiratory position, or the sum of IRV and TV. This capacity usually makes up 60–70% of the vital capacity in healthy individuals. **IRV:** inspiratory reserve volume; the maximal amount of air inhaled from the end-inspiratory position. **RV:** residual volume; that volume of air remaining in the lungs after maximal exhalation, or TLC – VC. **TLC:** total lung capacity; the sum of all volume compartments or the volume of air in the lungs after maximal inspiration. **TV:** tidal volume; that volume of air inhaled or exhaled with each breath during quiet breathing. **VC:** vital capacity; the maximum volume of air exhaled from the point of maximum inspiration. VC can also be described as the sum of the TV, IRV, and ERV. In healthy individuals, VC makes up about 70% of total lung volume.

inspired after a normal inspiration; the inspiratory capacity less the tidal v. SYN complemental air.

mean corpuscular v. (MCV), the average v. of red cells, calculated from the hematocrit and the red cell count, in erythrocyte indices.

minute v., the v. of any gas or fluid moved per minute; e.g., cardiac output or the respiratory minute v.

packed cell v., the v. of the blood cells in a sample of blood after it has been centrifuged in the hematocrit; normally, it amounts to 45% of the blood sample.

partial v., the actual v. occupied by one species of molecule or particle in a solution; the reciprocal of the density of the molecule.

residual v. (RV), the v. of air remaining in the lungs after a maximal expiratory effort. SYN residual air, residual capacity.

respiratory minute v. (RMV), the minute v. of breathing; the product of tidal v. times the respiratory frequency. SEE pulmonary *ventilation*.

resting tidal v., the tidal v. under normal conditions, i.e., in the absence of exercise or other conditions that stimulate breathing.

standard v., the v. of an ideal gas at standard temperature and pressure, approximately 22.414 L.

stroke v., the v. pumped out of one ventricle of the heart in a single beat. SYN stroke output.

tidal v. (V_T), the v. of air that is inspired or expired in a single breath during regular breathing. SYN tidal air.

vol·ume·nom·e·ter (vol′ū-mĕ-nom′ĕ-ter). A device for determining the volume of a solid by measuring the amount of liquid it displaces. SYN volumometer. [volume + G. *metron,* measure]

vol·u·met·ric (vol-ū-met′rik). Relating to measurement by volume.

vol·u·mom·e·ter (vol-ū-mom′ĕ-ter). SYN volumenometer.

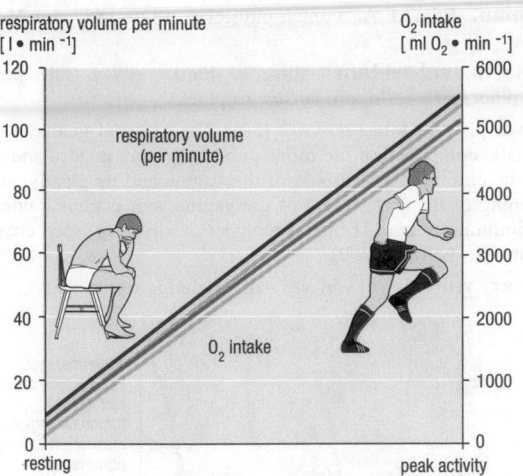

respiratory volume per minute
[l • min⁻¹]

O₂ intake
[ml O₂ • min⁻¹]

respiratory volume (per minute): oxygen intake and respiratory volume per minute of a 160 lb.(70 kg.) man, resting and at peak activity

---

vol·un·tary (vol′ŭn-tār-ē). Relating or acting in obedience to the will; not obligatory. [L. *voluntarius,* fr. *voluntas,* will, fr. *volo,* to wish]

vo·lup·tu·ous (vŏ-lŭp′tū-ŭs). Causing or caused by sensual pleasure; given to gratification of the senses. [L. *voluptuosus,* fr. *voluptas,* pleasure]

vo·lute (vŏ-loot). Rolled up; convoluted. [L. *voluta,* a scroll, fr. *volvo,* pp. *volutus,* to roll]

vol·u·tin (vol′oo-tin). A nucleoprotein complex found as cytoplasmic granules in certain bacteria, yeasts, and protozoa (such as trypanosome flagellates) which serves as food reserves. SYN volutin granules.

Vol·vox (vol′voks). A genus of highly organized colonial green flagellates of the class Phytomastigophorea. [L. *volvo,* to roll]

vol·vu·lo·sis (vol-voo-lō′sis). SYN onchocerciasis.

vol·vu·lus (vol′vū-lŭs). A twisting of the intestine causing obstruction; if left untreated may result in vascular compromise of the involved intestine. [L. *volvo,* to roll]

cecal v., rotation and twisting of the cecum toward the left upper quadrant, with ascending colon obstruction; associated with a cecum on a long mesentery.

gastric v., twisting of the stomach that may result in obstruction and impairment of the blood supply to the organ; it can occur in paraesophageal hernia and occasionally in eventration of the diaphragm. SEE organoaxial.

mesenteroaxial v., a type of gastric v. in which the axis of twist is parallel to the line of the gastric mesentery. SEE ALSO organoaxial.

sigmoid v., relatively common location of v., with obstruction either proximal or distal to the sigmoid segment.

vo·mer, gen. **vo·me·ris** (vō′mer, vō′mer-is) [TA]. A flat bone of trapezoidal shape forming the inferior and posterior portion of the nasal septum; it articulates with the sphenoid, ethmoid, two maxillae, and two palatine bones. [L. ploughshare]

v. cartilagin′eus, SYN vomeronasal *cartilage.*

vo·mer·ine (vō′mer-ēn). Relating to the vomer.

vom·er·o·bas·i·lar (vō′mer-ō-bas′i-lăr). Relating to the vomer and the base of the skull.

vom·er·o·na·sal (vō′mer-ō-nā′săl). Relating to the vomer and the nasal bone.

vom·it (vom′it). **1.** To eject matter from the stomach through the mouth. **2.** Vomitus; the matter so ejected. SYN vomitus (2). [L. *vomo,* pp. *vomitus,* to vomit]

Barcoo v., attacks of nausea and vomiting accompanied by bulimia affecting those living in the interior of the southern part of Australia.

bilious v., v. containing large amounts of bile suggestive of bowel obstruction distal to the papilla of Vater.

black v., the coffee-ground-colored material that is vomited, specifically, in severe yellow fever. SEE ALSO coffee-ground v. SYN vomitus niger.

coffee-ground v., v. consisting of fresh or old blood. SEE ALSO black v.

vom·it·ing (vom′i-ting). The ejection of matter from the stomach in retrograde fashion through the esophagus and mouth. SYN emesis (1), vomition, vomitus (1).

causes of vomiting

functional causes
psychogenic, pregnancy, functional esophageal disease

organic causes
esophagus: tumors, infections, stenoses, diverticula, mediastinal tumors, including bronchogenic carcinoma

stomach: acute gastritis, ulcer, stenosis by scars or tumors (postoperative gastric atony), pylorospasm (in children)

small and large intestines: acute gastroenteritis, mechanical ileus, obstruction

liver, gallbladder, pancreas: infections, gallstones, tumors; peritoneum: acute peritonitis (diffuse and local)

extraabdominal diseases
cerebral: meningitis, encephalitis, Ménière's disease, migraine headache, glaucoma, tumors, skull-brain injury, bleeding, hypertensive crises

disturbances of metabolism: diabetic precoma, lactic acidosis, uremia, thyrotoxicosis, Addison disease

exogenous causes
numerous drugs (digitalis, antibiotics, opiates, etc.)

intoxications (mushroom poisoning, alcohol, spoiled food, etc.)

---

cerebral v., v. due to intracranial disease, especially elevated intracranial pressure.

cyclic v., a syndrome of recurrent bouts of v. seen especially in preverbal children; many affected children later develop typical migraine headaches.

dry v., SYN retching.

epidemic v., v. caused by Norwalk virus, a 27-nm RNA virus in the family Caliciviridae frequently occurring in a group of people (e.g., in a school or small community) suddenly and without prodromal illness or malaise, is intense while it lasts, but ceases abruptly after 24–48 hours; symptoms are headache, abdominal pain, giddiness, and diarrhea in most of the cases, and extreme prostration in about 75%. SYN epidemic nausea.

fecal v., vomitus with appearance and/or odor of feces suggestive of long-standing distal small bowel or colonic obstruction. SYN copremesis, stercoraceous v.

morning v., v. occurring on rising or immediately after breakfast in some women during early pregnancy. SYN morning *sickness.*

pernicious v., uncontrollable v.

v. of pregnancy, v. occurring in the early months of pregnancy.

projectile v., expulsion of the contents of the stomach with great force.

psychogenic v., v. associated with emotional distress and anxiety.

retention v., v. due to mechanical obstruction, usually hours after ingestion of a meal.

stercoraceous v., SYN fecal v.

vo·mi·tion (vō-mish′ŭn). SYN vomiting. [L. *vomitio,* fr. *vomo,* to vomit]

vom·i·tu·ri·tion (vom′i-too-rish′ŭn). SYN retching.

vom·i·tus (vom′i-tŭs). **1.** SYN vomiting. **2.** SYN vomit (2). [L. a vomiting, vomit]

v. cruen′tes, SYN hematemesis.

VO

v. mari′nus, SYN seasickness.

v. ni′ger, SYN black *vomit.*

von. Often abbreviated to v. For names with this prefix not found here, see under the principal part of the name.

von Bruns, SEE Bruns.

von Ebner, Victor, Austrian histologist, 1842–1925. SEE Ebner *glands,* under *gland;* Ebner *reticulum;* imbrication *lines* of von E., under *line;* incremental *lines* of von E. under *line.*

von Economo, Constantin F., Austrian neurologist, 1876–1931. SEE von E. *disease.*

von Hansemann, D. P., German pathologist, 1858–1920. SEE Hansemann *macrophage.*

von Hippel, Eugen, German ophthalmologist, 1867–1939. SEE von H.-Lindau *syndrome.*

von Kossa, Julius, 19th century Austro-Hungarian pathologist. SEE von K. *stain.*

von Linné, SEE Linné.

von Meyenburg, SEE Meyenburg.

von Recklinghausen, SEE von Recklinghausen *disease.* SEE Recklinghausen.

von Schrötter, Leopold, Austrian laryngologist, 1837-1908. SEE Paget-von S. *syndrome.*

von Willebrand, E.A., Finnish physician, 1870–1949. SEE von W. *disease.*

Voorhoeve, N., Dutch radiologist, 1879–1927. SEE V. *disease.*

vor·tex, pl. **vor·ti·ces** (vōr′teks, vōr′ti-sēz). **1.** SYN verticil. **2.** SYN whorl (5). **3.** SYN v. lentis. [L. whirlpool, whorl, fr. *verto* or *vorto,* to turn around]

v. coccy′geus, a spiral arrangement of coarse hairs sometimes present over the region of the coccyx. SYN coccygeal whorl.

v. cor′dis [TA], SYN v. of heart.

Fleischer v., SYN *cornea* verticillata.

v. of heart [TA], a spiral arrangement of muscular fibers at the apex of the heart. SYN v. cordis [TA], whorl (2).

v. len′tis, one of the stellar figures on the surface of the lens of the eye. SYN vortex (3).

vor′tices pilo′rum [TA], SYN hair *whorls,* under *whorl.*

Vor·ti·cel·la (vōr-ti-sel′ă). A genus of Ciliata of the order Peritrichida, bell-shaped and with a spiral of cilia around the adoral zone; various free-living species have been found at times in the feces, urine, and mucous discharges. [Mod. L. dim. of L. *vortex,* a whorl]

vor·ti·ces (vōr′ti-sēz). Plural of vortex.

vor·ti·cose (vōr′ti-kōs). Arranged in a whorl. [L. *vorticosus,* fr. *vortex,* a whorl]

Vossius, Adolf, German pathologist, 1855–1925. SEE V. lenticular *ring.*

vox (voks). SYN voice. [L.]

v. cholera′ica, a peculiar, hoarse, almost inaudible voice of a sufferer in the last stage of Asiatic cholera.

vox·el (vok′sel). A contraction for volume element, which is the basic unit of CT or MR reconstruction; represented as a pixel in the display of the CT or MR image.

voy·eur (vwah-yer′). One who practices voyeurism.

voy·eur·ism (vwah-yer′izm). The practice of obtaining sexual pleasure by looking, especially at the naked body or genitals of another or at erotic acts between others. SYN scopophilia. [Fr. *voir,* to see]

VP Abbreviation for vasopressin; variegate *porphyria.*

VR Abbreviation for vocal *resonance.*

VS Abbreviation for volumetric *solution.*

VU Abbreviation for volume *unit.*

vul·ga·ris (vŭl-gā′ris). Ordinary; of the usual type. [L. fr. *vulgus,* a crowd]

Vulpian, Edme F.A., French physician, 1826–1887. SEE V. *atrophy.*

vul·sel·la, vul·sel·lum (vŭl-sel′ă, -lŭm). SYN vulsella *forceps.* [L. pincers, fr. *vello,* pp. *vulsus,* to pluck]

vul·va, pl. **vul·′vae** (vŭl′vă). [NA] The external genitalia of the female, comprised of the mons pubis, the labia majora and minora, the clitoris, the vestibule of the vagina and its glands, and the opening of the urethra and of the vagina. SYN cunnus, pudendum femininum, trema (2). [L. a wrapper or covering, seed covering, womb, fr. *volvo,* to roll]

vul·var, vul·val (vŭl′văr, vŭl′văl). Relating to the vulva.

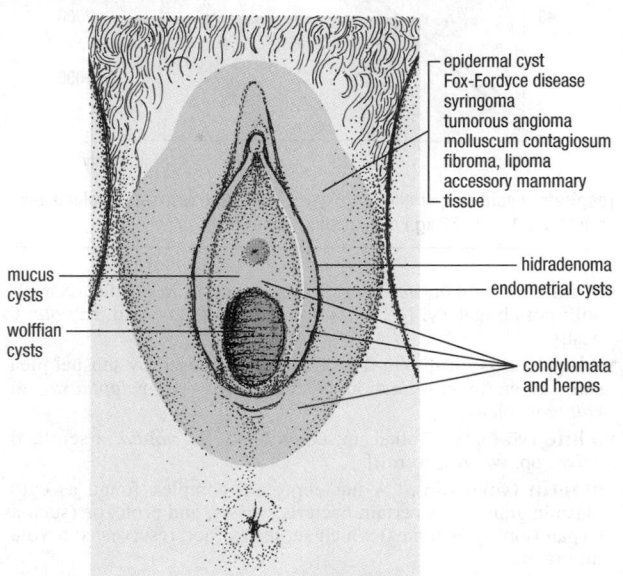

epidermal cyst
Fox-Fordyce disease
syringoma
tumorous angioma
molluscum contagiosum
fibroma, lipoma
accessory mammary
tissue

mucus cysts

wolffian cysts

hidradenoma
endometrial cysts

condylomata and herpes

differentiation of tumors and cysts of the **vulva:** according to location, (purple) vagina and urethra, (blue) vestibule, (yellow) labia minora, (pink) labia majora

vul·vec·to·my (vŭl-vek′tō-mē). Excision (either partial, complete, or radical) of the vulva. [vulva + G. *ektomē,* excision]

vul·vis·mus (vŭl-viz′mŭs). SYN vaginismus.

vul·vi·tis (vŭl-vī′tis). Inflammation of the vulva. [vulva + G. *-itis,* inflammation]

chronic atrophic v., an inflammation of atrophic vulvar skin, usually with severe pruritus.

chronic hypertrophic v., obsolete term for swelling of the vulval tissues due to lymphatic obstruction; in some cases it may be caused by filariasis, with induration or ulceration of the skin. SYN elephantiasis vulvae.

follicular v., inflammation of the vulvar hair follicles.

vulvo-. The vulva. [L. *vulva*]

vul·vo·cru·ral (vŭl′vō-kroo′răl). Relating to the vulva and the clitoris.

vul·vo·dyn·ia. Chronic vulvar discomfort with complaints of burning and superficial irritation.

vul·vo·u·ter·ine (vŭl-vō-ū′ter-in). Relating to the vulva and the uterus.

vul·vo·vag·i·nal (vŭl-vō-vaj′i-năl). Relating to the vulva and the vagina.

vul·vo·vag·i·ni·tis (vŭl′vō-vaj-i-nī′tis). Inflammation of both vulva and vagina.

Vve·den·skii. Alternative surname of Wedensky, Nikolai I.

V-Y plas·ty. SYN V-Y *flap.*

W Symbol for tungsten; watt; tryptophan; tryptophanyl.

Waage, P., Norwegian chemist, 1833–1900. SEE Guldberg-W. *law.*

Waaler, Erik, Norwegian biologist, *1903. SEE Rose-W. *test.*

Waardenburg, Petrus Johannes, Dutch ophthalmologist, 1886–1979. SEE W. *syndrome.*

Wachendorf, Eberhard J., German botanist and anatomist, 1702–1758. SEE W. *membrane.*

Wachstein, Max, U.S. histologist and pathologist, 1905–1965. SEE W.-Meissel *stain* for calcium-magnesium-ATPase.

Wächter, Herman J.G., German pathologist, *1878. SEE Bracht-W. *lesion.*

Wada, Juhn A., 20th century Japanese-Canadian neurologist. SEE W. *test.*

wad·ding (wahd′ing). **1.** Carded cotton or wool in sheets, used for surgical dressings. **2.** Fibrous material that is part of a shotgun shell, which is often found within the wound if the injury was inflicted at close range.

Waddington, Conrad H., British embryologist and geneticist, 1905–1975. SEE waddingtonian *homeostasis.*

wad·dle (wod′l). SYN waddling *gait.*

wa·fer (wā′fer). A thin sheet of dried flour paste, used to enclose a powder, the wafer being moistened and folded over the drug, so that it can be swallowed without taste. [M.E., fr. O.Fr. *waufre,* fr. Germanic]

Wagner, Hans, Swiss ophthalmologist, *1905. SEE W. *disease, syndrome.*

Wagstaffe, William, English surgeon, 1843–1910.

waist (wāst). The portion of the trunk between the ribs and the pelvis. [A.S. *waext*]

Walcher, Gustav A., German obstetrician, 1856–1935. SEE W. *position.*

Waldenström, Jan G., Swedish physician, *1906. SEE W. *macroglobulinemia, purpura, syndrome, test.*

Waldeyer (Waldeyer-Hartz), Heinrich W.G. von, German anatomist and pathologist, 1836–1921. SEE W. *fossae,* under *fossa, glands,* under *gland,* zonal *layer,* throat *ring, sheath, space, tract.*

walk. 1. To move on foot. **2.** The characteristic manner in which one moves on foot. SEE ALSO gait. [M.E. *walken,* fr. O.E. *wealcen,* to roll]

Walker, Arthur Earl, U.S. neurologist, *1907. SEE W. *tractotomy;* Dandy-W. *syndrome.*

Walker, J.T. Ainslie, English chemist, 1868–1930. SEE Rideal-W. *coefficient, method.*

Walker, James, British gynecologist, *1916. SEE W. *chart.*

wall (wawl) [TA]. An investing part enclosing a cavity such as the chest or abdomen, or covering a cell or any anatomic unit. A wall, as of the chest, abdomen, or any hollow organ. SYN paries [TA]. [L. *vallum*]

anterior w. of middle ear, SYN carotid w. of tympanic cavity.

anterior w. of stomach [TA], the part of the gastric w. that faces the peritoneal cavity. SYN paries anterior gastris [TA].

anterior w. of tympanic cavity, SYN carotid w. of tympanic cavity.

anterior w. of vagina [TA], somewhat shorter than the posterior w. and at its upper end penetrated by the cervix of the uterus. SYN paries anterior vaginae [TA].

axial w.'s of the pulp chambers, the w.'s parallel with the long axis of a tooth: the mesial, distal, buccal, and lingual w.'s.

carotid w. of middle ear, SYN carotid w. of tympanic cavity.

carotid w. of tympanic cavity [TA], it contains the carotid canal and the opening of the auditory tube. SYN paries caroticus cavi tympani [TA], anterior w. of middle ear, anterior w. of tympanic cavity, carotid w. of middle ear.

cavity w., one of the surfaces bounding a cavity.

cell w., (1) the outer layer or membrane of some animal and plant cells; in the latter, it is mainly cellulose. **(2)** in bacteria, the rigid structure, usually containing a peptidoglycan layer, that provides osmotic protection and defines bacterial shape and staining properties.

chest w., in respiratory physiology, the total system of structures outside the lungs that move as a part of breathing; it includes the rib cage, diaphragm, abdominal w., and abdominal contents. SYN thoracic w.

enamel w., in dentistry, the part of the w. of a cavity consisting of enamel.

external w. of cochlear duct, SYN external *surface* of cochlear duct.

inferior w. of orbit, SYN *floor* of orbit.

inferior w. of tympanic cavity, SYN jugular w. of middle ear.

jugular w. of middle ear [TA], the floor of the tympanic cavity; a thin plate of bone separating the tympanic cavity from the jugular fossa. SYN paries jugularis cavi tympani [TA], floor of tympanic cavity☆, fundus tympani, inferior w. of tympanic cavity.

labyrinthine w. of middle ear, SYN labyrinthine w. of tympanic cavity.

labyrinthine w. of tympanic cavity [TA], a bony layer separating the middle from the internal ear or labyrinth; it contains the fenestra vestibuli and the fenestra cochleae. SYN paries labyrinthicus cavi tympani [TA], medial w. of tympanic cavity☆, labyrinthine w. of middle ear, medial w. of middle ear.

lateral w. of middle ear, SYN membranous w. of tympanic cavity.

lateral w. of orbit [TA], a triangular w. of the orbit formed by the zygomatic bone, the greater wing of the sphenoid bone, and a small part of the frontal bone; posteriorly it is bounded by the superior and inferior orbital fissures. SYN paries lateralis orbitae [TA].

lateral w. of tympanic cavity, ☆official alternate term for membranous w. of tympanic cavity.

mastoid w. of middle ear, SYN mastoid w. of tympanic cavity.

mastoid w. of tympanic cavity [TA], it contains the opening into the mastoid antrum. SYN paries mastoideus cavi tympani [TA], posterior w. of tympanic cavity☆, mastoid w. of middle ear, posterior w. of middle ear.

medial w. of middle ear, SYN labyrinthine w. of tympanic cavity.

medial w. of orbit [TA], the thin, rectangular w. of the orbit formed by the orbital plate of the ethmoid, lacrimal, frontal and a small part of the sphenoid bones; the fossa for the lacrimal sac lies at its anterior limit. SYN paries medialis orbitae [TA].

medial w. of tympanic cavity, ☆official alternate term for labyrinthine w. of tympanic cavity.

membranous w. of middle ear, SYN membranous w. of tympanic cavity.

membranous w. of trachea [TA], the part of the tracheal w. posteriorly that is not reinforced by tracheal cartilages. SYN paries membranaceus tracheae [TA].

membranous w. of tympanic cavity [TA], the wall formed mainly by the tympanic membrane. SYN paries membranaceus cavi tympani [TA], lateral w. of tympanic cavity☆, lateral w. of middle ear, membranous w. of middle ear.

nail w. [TA], the fold of skin overlapping the lateral and proximal margins of the nail. SYN vallum unguis [TA], nail fold.

parietal w., the body w. or the somatopleure from which it is formed.

△ **Combining Forms**	☆ **Official alternate Terminologia Anatomica term**
▣ **Indicates term is illustrated, see Illustration Index**	
SYN Synonym	**[MIM] Mendelian Inheritance in Man**
Cf. Compare	**C.I. Colour Index**
[NA] Nomina Anatomica	
[TA] Terminologia Anatomica	**High Profile Term**

wa

posterior w. of middle ear, SYN mastoid w. of tympanic cavity.

posterior w. of stomach [TA], that part of the gastric w. that faces the omental bursa. SYN paries posterior gastris [TA].

posterior w. of tympanic cavity, �star official alternate term for mastoid w. of tympanic cavity.

posterior w. of vagina [TA], it is longer than the anterior w. and has a low ridge in the midline throughout most of its length. SYN paries posterior vaginae [TA].

pulpal w., (1) one of the w.'s of the pulp cavity; (2) the w. of a cavity preparation adjacent to the pulp space; e.g., mesial pulpal w.

splanchnic w., the w. of one of the viscera or the splanchnopleure from which it is formed.

superior w. of orbit, SYN *roof* of orbit.

tegmental w. of middle ear, SYN tegmental w. of tympanic cavity.

tegmental w. of tympanic cavity [TA], the superior wall, or roof, of the tympanic cavity, formed by the tegmen tympani of the temporal bone. SYN paries tegmentalis cavi tympani [TA], tegmental root of tympanic cavity✫, roof of tympanic cavity, tegmental w. of middle ear.

thoracic w., SYN chest w.

tympanic w. of cochlear duct, SYN tympanic *surface* of cochlear duct.

vestibular w. of cochlear duct, SYN vestibular *surface* of cochlear duct.

Wallenberg, Adolf, German physician, 1862–1949. SEE W. *syndrome.*

Waller, Augustus V., English physiologist, 1816–1870. SEE wallerian *degeneration,* wallerian *law.*

wal·le·ri·an (waw-ler′ē-an). Relating to or described by A.V. Waller.

wall-eye (wawl′ī). **1.** SYN exotropia. **2.** Absence of color in the iris, or leukoma of the cornea.

Walsh, Patrick Craig, U.S. urologist, *1938. SEE neurovascular *bundle* of Walsh, Walsh *procedure.*

Walthard, Max, Swiss gynecologist, 1867–1933. SEE W. cell *rest.*

Walther, August F., German anatomist, 1688–1746. SEE W. *dilator, canals,* under *canal, ducts,* under *duct, ganglion, plexus.*

wan·der·ing (wahn′der-ing). Moving about; not fixed; abnormally motile. [A.S. *wandrian,* to wander]

Wang, Chung Yik, Chinese pathologist, 1889–1931. SEE W. *test.*

Wangensteen, Owen H., U.S. surgeon, 1898–1981. SEE W. *drainage, suction, tube.*

Wang·i·el·la (wang-gē-el′ă). A dematiaceous genus of fungi characterized by phialides without collarettes, a black yeastlike colony with yeast forms, and later hyphae; the fungi grow well at 40°C. *W. (Exophiala) dermatitidis* is an etiologic agent of chromoblastomycosis.

Warburg, Otto H., German biochemist and Nobel laureate, 1883–1970. SEE W. *apparatus,* respiratory *enzyme,* old yellow *enzyme, theory;* W.-Lipmann-Dickens-Horecker *shunt;* Barcroft-W. *apparatus, technique.*

Ward, Frederick O., British osteologist, 1818–1877. SEE w.W. *triangle.*

Ward, Owen C., 20th century pediatrician. SEE Romano-W. *syndrome.*

ward (wōrd). A large room or hall in a hospital containing a number of beds. SEE ALSO unit. [A.S. *weard*]

Wardrop, James, British surgeon, 1782–1869. SEE W. *method.*

war·fa·rin so·di·um (war′fă-rin). An anticoagulant with the same actions as dicumarol; also used as a rodenticide; also available as the potassium salt, with the same actions and uses. [*Wis*consin *A*lumni *R*esearch *F*oundation + coum*arin*]

warm-blood·ed (wărm′blŭd-ed). SYN homeothermic.

Warren, Dean, U.S. surgeon, 1924–1989. SEE W. *shunt.*

wart (wōrt). SYN verruca.

anatomic w., SYN postmortem w.

asbestos w., SYN asbestos *corn.*

common w., SYN *verruca* vulgaris.

digitate w., SYN *verruca* digitata.

filiform w., SYN *verruca* filiformis.

flat w., SYN *verruca* plana.

fugitive w., a transitory w.; one that does not persist.

genital w., SYN *condyloma* acuminatum.

Henle w.'s, SYN Hassall-Henle *bodies,* under *body.*

infectious w., SYN *verruca* vulgaris.

mosaic w., plantar growth of numerous closely aggregated w.'s forming a mosaic appearance, frequently caused by human papillomavirus type 2.

Peruvian w., SYN *verruga* peruana.

pitch w., a precancerous keratotic epidermal tumor, common among workers in pitch and coal tar derivatives. SEE pitch-worker's *cancer.*

plane w., SYN *verruca* plana.

🅸**plantar w.,** an often painful w. on the sole, usually caused by human papillomavirus type 1. SYN verruca plantaris.

postmortem w., a tuberculous warty growth (tuberculosis cutis verrucosa) on the hand of one who performs postmortem examinations. SYN anatomic tubercle, anatomic w.

senile w., SYN actinic *keratosis.*

soot w., the precancerous lesion of chimney sweep's cancer.

telangiectatic w., SYN angiokeratoma.

tuberculous w., SYN *tuberculosis* cutis verrucosa.

venereal w., SYN *condyloma* acuminatum.

viral w., SYN *verruca* vulgaris.

Wartenberg, Robert, German neurologist, 1887–1956. SEE W. *symptom.*

Warthin, Aldred S., U.S. pathologist, 1866–1931. SEE W. *tumor;* W.-Finkeldey *cells,* under *cell;* W.-Starry silver *stain.*

wart·pox (wōrt′poks). SYN *variola* verrucosa.

warty (wōrt′ē). Relating to or covered with warts.

wash (wosh). A solution used to clean or bathe a part. For types of w.'s, see the specific term; e.g., eyewash, mouthwash.

Wasmann, Adolphus, 19th century German anatomist. SEE W. *glands,* under *gland.*

Wassermann, August P. von, German bacteriologist, 1866–1925. SEE W. *antibody, reaction, test;* provocative W. *test.*

Wassermann-fast. A term used to designate a case in which the Wassermann reaction remains positive despite all treatment.

wast·ing (wāst′ing). **1.** SYN emaciation. **2.** Denoting a disease characterized by emaciation.

salt w., inappropriately large renal excretion of salt despite the apparent need of the body to retain it.

wa·ter (wah′ter). **1.** H_2O; a clear, odorless, tasteless liquid, solidifying at 32°F (0°C, 0°R), and boiling at 212°F (100°C, 80°R), that is present in all animal and vegetable tissues and dissolves more substances than any other liquid. SEE volume. **2.** Euphemism for urine. **3.** A pharmacopeial preparation of a clear, saturated aqueous solution (unless otherwise specified) of volatile oils, or other aromatic or volatile substances, prepared by processes involving distillation or solution (agitation followed by filtration). SYN aromatic w. [A.S. *waeter*]

w. of adhesion, w. held by molecular attraction in contact with solid surfaces, but not forming an essential part of their constitution.

alkaline w., a w. that contains appreciable amounts of the bicarbonates of calcium, lithium, potassium, or sodium.

aromatic w., SYN water (3).

baryta w., a saturated aqueous solution of barium hydroxide; used as an alkaline reagent.

bitter w., a natural mineral w. containing Epsom salt.

bound w., w. held to colloids and other substances and not removed by simple filtration.

bromine w., a w. containing the bromides of magnesium, potassium, or sodium in therapeutic amounts.

calcic w., a w. containing appreciable quantities of calcium salts in solution.

carbonated w., carbonic w., w. that contains a considerable amount of carbonic acid in solution.

carbon dioxide-free w., purified w. that has been boiled vigorously for 5 min or more.

chalybeate w., a w. that contains salts of iron in appreciable quantities.

chlorine w., a w. that contains the chlorides of sodium, potassium, calcium, and magnesium in varying amounts.

w. of combustion, SYN w. of metabolism.

w. of constitution, w. held by a unit of structure as an essential part of its constitution, though not an ingredient of its molecules. SEE w. of crystallization.

w. of crystallization, w. of constitution that unites with certain salts and is essential to their arrangement in crystalline form; e.g., $CuSO_4 \cdot 5H_2O$.

deionized w., w. purified by passing through ion-exchange columns.

distilled w., w. purified by distillation.

earthy w., a w. containing a large amount of mineral matter, chiefly sulfate, in solution.

free w., w. in the body that can be removed by ultrafiltration and in which substances can be dissolved.

gentian aniline w., gentian violet with saturated aniline w., a more effective stain than simple gentian violet.

hard w., w. containing ions, such as Mg^{2+} and Ca^{2+}, that form insoluble salts with fatty acids so that ordinary soap will not lather in it.

heavy w., D_2O; w. in which the hydrogen atoms are deuterium, or heavy hydrogen (^2H), with physical properties that differ noticeably from those of ordinary w.; an elevated presence will cause a decrease in metabolic activity; used as a moderator in nuclear reactors because of its capacity to absorb neutrons. SYN deuterium oxide.

indifferent w., a mineral w. containing only a small quantity of saline matter.

w. for injection, w. purified by distillation for the preparation of products for parenteral use.

intracellular w., SYN intracellular *fluid*.

lime w., calcium hydroxide solution; a saturated solution prepared by mixing 3 g of calcium hydroxide in a liter of purified cool w. Undissolved calcium hydroxide is allowed to precipitate and the solution is dispensed without agitation; lime w. is a common ingredient in lotions and is used internally extensively in veterinary medicine.

w. of metabolism, the w. formed in the body by oxidation of the hydrogen of the food, the greatest amount being produced in the metabolism of fat (about 117 g per 100 g of fat). SYN w. of combustion.

mineral w., w. that contains appreciable amounts of certain salts, which give it therapeutic properties.

potable w., a w. fit for drinking, being free from contamination and not containing a sufficient quantity of saline material to be regarded as a mineral w.

purified w., w. obtained by distillation or deionization.

saline w., a w. that contains neutral salts (chlorides, bromides, iodides, sulfates) in appreciable amounts.

Selters w., Seltzer w., a mineral w. containing carbonates of sodium, calcium, and magnesium, and chloride of sodium. [Nieder *Selters,* a mineral spring in Prussia]

soft w., w. lacking those ions, such as Mg^{2+} and Ca^{2+}, that form insoluble salts with fatty acids, so that ordinary soap will lather easily in it.

sulfate w., a w. holding in solution appreciable quantities of the sulfates of calcium, magnesium, or sodium.

sulfur w., a w. containing hydrogen sulfide or the metallic sulfides.

total body w. (TBW), the sum of intracellular w. and extracellular w. (volume); about 60% of body weight.

transcellular w., that fraction of extracellular w. in cerebrospinal,

digestive, epithelial, introcular, pleural, sweat, and synovial secretions; about 1.5% of body weight.

wa·ter·fall (wah'ter-fawl). A term used to describe flow in vascular beds where lateral pressure tending to collapse vessels greatly exceeds venous pressure. Flow is independent of venous pressure and occurs only when arterial pressure exceeds lateral pressure; likened to flow making a waterfall from a sluice or spillway over a dam, with arterial pressure being height of water behind the dam, lateral pressure being spillway height, and venous pressure being height of outflow stream below the dam. SYN sluice.

Waterhouse, Rupert, British physician, 1873–1958. SEE W.-Friderichsen *syndrome.*

Waters, Charles Alexander, U.S. radiologist, 1885-1961. SEE W. view *radiograph.*

Waters, Edward G., U.S. obstetrician and gynecologist, *1898. SEE W. *operation.*

wa·ters (wah'terz). Colloquialism for amnionic *fluid.*

  bag of w., SEE *bag* of waters.

  false w., a leakage of fluid prior to or in beginning labor, before the rupture of the amnion.

wa·ter·shed. 1. The area of marginal blood flow at the extreme periphery of a vascular bed. 2. Slopes in the abdominal cavity, formed by projections of the lumbar vertebrae and the pelvic brim that determine the direction in which a free effusion will gravitate when the body is in a supine position.

Waterston, David J., British thoracic and pediatric surgeon, *1910. SEE W. *operation, shunt.*

Watson, Cecil J., U.S. physician, 1901–1983. SEE Watson-Schwartz *test.*

Watson, James Dewey, U.S. geneticist and Nobel laureate, *1928. SEE W.-Crick *helix.*

watt (W) (waht). The SI unit of electrical power; the power available when the current is 1 ampere and the electromotive force is 1 volt; equal to 1 joule (10^7 ergs) per second or 1 voltampere. [James *Watt,* Scot. engineer, 1736–1819]

wave (wāv). 1. A movement of particles in an elastic body, whether solid or fluid, whereby an advancing series of alternate elevations and depressions, or rarefactions and condensations, is produced. 2. The elevation of the pulse, felt by the finger, or represented in the curved line of the sphygmograph. 3. The complete cycle of changes in the level of a source of energy that is repetitively varying with respect to time; in the electrocardiogram and the electroencephalogram, the w. is essentially a voltage-time graph. SEE ALSO rhythm. [A.S. *wafian,* to fluctuate]

A w., (1) the initial negative deflection in the electroretinogram, presumably reflecting retinal photoreceptor activity; (2) an atrial deflection in an electrogram recorded from within the atrium of the heart; (3) the first positive deflection of the atrial and venous pulses due to atrial systole.

acid w., SYN acid *tide.*

alkaline w., SYN alkaline *tide.*

alpha w., SYN alpha *rhythm.*

arterial w., a w. in the jugular phlebogram due to transmission of carotid artery pulsation.

B w., the initial positive deflection in the electroretinogram, possibly arising from the inner nuclear layer of the retina.

beta w., SYN beta *rhythm.*

brain w., colloquialism for electroencephalogram.

C w., (1) a monophasic positive deflection in the electroretinogram arising in the pigment epithelium of the retina. (2) w. in the venous and atrial pulses occurring during isovolumic ventricular contraction in which the closed atrioventricular valves (mitral and tricuspid) are abruptly displaced into the atria with creation of a pressure transient.

cannon w., an exaggerated A w. in the jugular pulse caused by right atrial contraction occurring after ventricular contraction has closed the tricuspid valve, as in ventricular premature beats and in complete A-V block.

D w., a positive or negative deflection in the electroretinogram occurring when a light stimulus is removed (off-response).

wa

delta w., a premature upstroke of the QRS complex due to an atrial ventricular bypass tract as in WPW syndrome.

dicrotic w., the second rise in the tracing of a dicrotic pulse. SYN recoil w.

electrocardiographic w., a deflection of special shape and extent in the electrocardiogram representing the electric activity of a portion of the heart muscle.

epsilon w., late R w. (in lead V_1) of delayed right ventricular activation in arrhythmogenic RV dysplasia.

excitation w., a w. of altered electrical conditions that is propagated along a muscle fiber preparatory to its contraction.

F w.'s, the w.'s of atrial flutter usually best seen in ECG leads 2, 3, and AVF. (A small f indicates atrial fibrillation).

f w., ff w.'s, atrial fibrillation w. SYN fibrillary w.'s, fibrillatory w.'s, flutter-fibrillation w.'s.

fibrillary w.'s, SYN f w.

fibrillatory w.'s, SYN f w.

flat top w.'s, activity in the electroencephalogram having a pattern suggesting a flat top; these w.'s are often found in temporal lobe discharges.

fluid w., a sign of free fluid in the abdominal cavity; percussion on one side of the abdomen transmits a w. that is felt on the opposite side.

flutter-fibrillation w.'s, SYN f w.

microelectric w.'s, SYN microwaves.

mucosal w., the movement of the mucous membrane of the vocal cord during phonation.

overflow w., the descending w. of the sphygmogram from the apex to the first anacrotic break.

P w., the first complex of the electrocardiogram, during sinus and atrial rhythms, representing depolarization of the atria; if the P w. is retrograde or ectopic in axis or form, it is labeled P'.

percussion w., the main positive w. of an arterial pulse tracing.

postextrasystolic T w., the modified T w. of the beat immediately following an extrasystole.

pulse w., the progressive expansion of the arteries occurring with each contraction of the left ventricle of the heart.

Q w., the initial deflection of the QRS complex when such deflection is negative (downward).

R w., the first positive (upward) deflection of the QRS complex in the electrocardiogram; successive upward deflections within the same QRS complex are labeled R', R'', etc.

random w.'s, w.'s in the electroencephalogram which occur paroxysmally and asynchronously.

recoil w., SYN dicrotic w.

retrograde P w., the P w. pattern in the electrocardiogram representing retrograde depolarization of the atria, the impulse spreading from the AV junction or the lower atrium upward.

S w., a negative (downward) deflection of the QRS complex following an R w; successive downward deflections within the same QRS complex are labeled S', S'', etc.

sonic w.'s, audible sound w.'s, as distinguished from ultrasonic w.'s.

supersonic w.'s, sound w.'s of higher frequency than the level of audibility.

T w., the next deflection in the electrocardiogram following the QRS complex; represents ventricular repolarization.

theta w., SYN theta *rhythm.*

tidal w., the w. between the percussion w. and the dicrotic w. in the downward limb of the arterial pulse tracing.

Traube-Hering w.'s, SYN Traube-Hering *curves,* under *curve.*

U w., a positive w. following an upright T w. of the electrocardiogram. It is negative following an inverted T wave.

ultrasonic w.'s, the periodic configuration of energy produced by sound having a frequency greater than 30,000 Hz.

V w., a large pressure w. visible in recordings from either atrium or its incoming veins, normally produced by venous return but apparently becoming very large when blood regurgitates through the AV valve beyond the chamber from which the recording is made. This regurgitant wave is not a true V w., which is a passive (filling) wave.

x w., the negative w. in the atrial and venous pulse curves produced when ventricular ejection moves the floors of the atria toward the ventricular apices.

y w., the negative w. in the atrial and venous pulse curves reflecting rapid filling of the ventricles just after the atrioventricular valves open.

waveform. The form of a pulse; e.g., an arterial pressure or displacement wave; or of the pacemaker pulse as demonstrated on the oscilloscope under a specified load.

pressure w., a graphic representation of intravascular or intracardiac pressure related to phases of the cardiac cycle, displayed on an oscilloscope monitor or paper copy.

wave·length (Λ) (wāv'length). The distance from one point on a wave (frequently shaped like a sine curve) to the next point in the same phase; i.e., from peak to peak or from trough to trough.

wave·num·ber (σ) (wāv'nŭm-ber). The number of waves per centimeter (cm^{-1}), used to simplify the large and unwieldy numbers heretofore used to designate frequency.

wave·shape (wāv'shāp). SYN wave *form.*

wax (waks). **1.** A thick, tenacious substance, plastic at room temperature, secreted by bees for building the cells of their honeycomb. SYN beeswax, cera. **2.** Any substance with physical properties similar to those of beeswax, of animal, vegetable, or mineral origin (oils, lipids, or fats that are solids at room temperature). **3.** Esters of high molecular weight fatty acids with monohydric or dihydric alcohols (aliphatic or cyclic), that are solid at room temperature. Often accompanied by free fatty acids. [A.S. *weax*]

animal w., beeswax, spermaceti, and any w. derived from the animal kingdom.

baseplate w., a hard pink w. used in dentistry for making occlusion rims.

bleached w., SYN white w.

bone w., a mixture of antiseptic agents, oil, and w. used to stop bleeding by plugging bone cavities or haversian canals. SYN Horsley bone w.

boxing w., w. used for boxing impressions. SEE ALSO boxing.

Brazil w., SYN carnauba w.

carnauba w., a w. obtained from the Brazilian w. palm, *Copernica cerifera;* used in pharmaceuticals to coat medicaments in sustained release preparations and surfaces of tablets; used in waxes for wood and metal. SYN Brazil w., palm w.

casting w., any soft solid w. used in dentistry for patterns of all types and for many other purposes; most are basically paraffin but are modified by addition of gum dammar, carnauba w., or other ingredients, to meet various requirements. SYN inlay w.

Chinese w., (1) a vegetable w.; (2) a w. secreted by a scale insect, *Coccus ceriferus* or *C. pela,* and deposited in the twigs of a species of ash tree; used in China to make candles and also medicinally.

ear w., SYN cerumen.

earth w., SYN ceresin.

emulsifying w., a washable ointment base consisting of a mixture of cetostearyl alcohol, sodium lauryl sulfate, and water.

grave w., SYN adipocere.

Horsley bone w., SYN bone w.

inlay w., SYN casting w.

Japan w., a vegetable w. derived from *Rhus succedanea* and *Toxicodendron verniciferum.*

mineral w., (1) SYN paraffin w; (2) SYN ceresin; (3) a mineral substance whose physical properties are similar to wax.

montan w., a mineral w. extracted from lignite. [L. *montanus,* of a mountain, fr. *mons,* mountain]

palm w., SYN carnauba w.

paraffin w., a w. derived from petroleum. SYN mineral w. (1).

vegetable w., palm w. or any w. derived from plants such as the bayberry.

white w., yellow w. bleached by being rolled very thin and exposed to the light and air, or bleached by chemical oxidants; same uses as yellow w. SYN bleached w., white beeswax.

wool w., SYN *adeps* lanae.

yellow w., a yellowish, solid, brittle substance prepared from the honeycomb of the bee, *Apis mellifera;* the chief constituent is myricin (myricyl palmitate); others are cerotic acid (cerin), melissic acid, heptacosane, and hentriacontane; used in the preparation of ointments, cerates, plasters, and suppositories.

wax·ing, wax·ing-up (wak′sing). The contouring of a pattern in wax, generally applied to the shaping in wax of the contours of a trial denture or a crown prior to casting in metal.

Wb Symbol for weber.

WBC Abbreviation for white blood *cell.*

weak·ness (wēk′nes). **1.** Lack of strength or potency. **2.** Inability to perform normally.

  directional w., a right or left decrement of nystagmus, calculated from the responses to the binaural, bithermal caloric test.

wean (wēn). To implement weaning. [A.S. *wenian*]

wean·ing (wēn′ing). **1.** Permanent deprivation of breast milk and commencement of nourishment with other food. **2.** Gradual withdrawal of a patient from dependency on a life support system or other form of therapy.

wean·ling (wēn′ling). A young animal that has become adjusted to food other than its mother's milk.

wear (wār). Wasting or deterioration caused by friction.

  occlusal w., attritional loss of substance on opposing occlusal units or surfaces. SEE ALSO abrasion (3).

web (wĕb). A tissue or membrane bridging a space. SEE ALSO tela. [A.S.]

  esophageal w., a cribriform or w. formation in the esophagus caused by an irregular atrophy.

  w. of fingers/toes, one of the folds of skin, or rudimentary web, between the fingers and toes. SYN interdigital folds, plica interdigitalis.

  laryngeal w., congenital anomaly consisting of mucous membrane–covered connective tissue between the vocal cords located ventrally and extending dorsally for varying distances; it causes airway obstruction and hoarse cry in the newborn.

  terminal w., a network of actin filaments in the apical end of columnar epithelial cells that anchor in the zonula adherens.

web·bing (web′ing). Congenital condition apparent when adjacent structures are joined by a broad band of tissue not normally present to such a degree.

Weber, Rainer, 20th century U.S. pathologist. SEE W. *stain.*

Weber, Ernst Heinrich, German physiologist and anatomist, 1795–1878. SEE W. *glands,* under *gland, law, paradox, test* for hearing; Fechner-Weber *law;* W.-Fechner *law.*

Weber, Frederick Parkes, English physician, 1863–1962. SEE W.-Christian *disease;* W.-Cockayne *syndrome;* Rendu-Osler-W. *syndrome;* Sturge-Kalischer-W. *syndrome;* Sturge-W. *disease, syndrome;* Klippel-Trenaunay-W. *syndrome.*

Weber, Moritz Ignaz, German anatomist, 1795–1875. SEE W. *organ.*

Weber, Sir Hermann, English physician, 1823–1918. SEE Weber *sign;* Weber *syndrome.*

Weber, Wilhelm E., German physicist, 1804–1891. SEE W. *point, triangle.*

we·ber (Wb) (web′er). SI unit of magnetic flux, equal to volt-seconds (V·s). [Wilhelm E. Weber, 1804–1891]

WEBINO Acronym for wall-eyed bilateral internuclear *ophthalmoplegia.*

Webster, John C., U.S. gynecologist, 1863–1950.

Webster, John, English chemist, 1878–1927. SEE W. *test.*

Wechsler, David, U.S. psychologist, *1896. SEE W. intelligence *scales,* under *scale;* W.-Bellevue *scale.*

wed·del·lite (hwed′del-īte). A dihydrate of calcium oxalate; found in renal calculi. Cf. whewellite. [for *Weddell* Sea, after James Weddell, Eng. navigator (1787–1834), + -ite]

Wedensky (Vve·den·skii), Nikolai I., Russian neurophysiologist, 1852–1922. SEE W. *effect, facilitation, inhibition.*

wedge (wej). A solid body having the shape of an acute-angled triangular prism. [A.S. *weeg*]

  dental w., a double inclined plane used for separating the teeth,

maintaining the separation once obtained, or holding a matrix in place.

WEE Abbreviation for western equine *encephalomyelitis.*

Weeks, John E., U.S. ophthalmologist, 1853–1949. SEE W. *bacillus;* Koch-W. *bacillus.*

Weeksella (wēk-sel′a). A genus of nonoxidative, aerobic Gram-negative rods.

  w. zoohelcum, a bacterium producing infections in bites or scratches by dogs or cats.

Wegener, Friedrich, German pathologist, 1907–1990. SEE W. *granulomatosis.*

Wegner, Friedrich R.G., German pathologist, 1843–1917. SEE W. *disease, line.*

Weibel, Ewald R., Swiss physician, *1929. SEE W.-Palade *bodies,* under *body.*

Weichselbaum, Anton, Austrian pathologist, 1845–1920. SEE W. *coccus.*

Weidel, Hugo, Austrian chemist, 1849–1899. SEE W. *reaction.*

Weigert, Carl, German pathologist, 1845–1904. SEE W. *law,* iodine *solution.* See entries under stain.

weight (wāt). The product of the force of gravity, defined internationally as 9.80665 m/s^2, times the mass of the body. [A.S. *gewiht*]

  apothecaries w., an obsolescent system of w.'s based upon the w. of a grain of wheat. Has been used for centuries in weighing medicines and precious metals (Troy measure). Some drugs which have been available for long periods are still often designated as grains (e.g., 5 grains of aspirin, 1/2 grain of codeine, 1/100 grain nitroglycerin). This w. system has been largely superseded by the metric system (based on grams). One grain is the equivalent of 64.8 milligrams. One scruple contains 20 grains; one dram contains 60 grains; one apothecary ounce contains 8 drams (480 grains); one apothecary pound contains 12 ounces (5760 grains).

  atomic w. (at. wt., AW), the mass in grams of 1 mol (6.02×10^{23} atoms) of an atomic species; the mass of an atom of a chemical element in relation to the mass of an atom of carbon-12 (^{12}C), which is set equal to 12.000, thus a ratio and therefore dimensionless (although the actual mass, numerically the same, is sometimes expressed in daltons); not necessarily the w. of any individual atom of an element, since most elements are made up of several isotopes of different masses; e.g., the atomic w. of chlorine is 35.4527, because it is composed of ^{35}Cl and ^{37}Cl in proportions that give an average of 35.4527. SEE ALSO molecular w.

  birth w., in humans, the first w. of an infant obtained within less than the first 60 completed minutes after birth; a full-size infant is one weighing 2500 g or more; a low birth w. is less than 2500 g.; very low birth w. is less than 1500 g.; and extremely low is less than 1000 g.

  combining w., SYN gram *equivalent.*

  dry w., the w. of material remaining after removing the water (e.g., after heating above 100°C).

  equivalent w., SYN gram *equivalent.*

  gram-atomic w., atomic w. expressed in grams. Cf. mole.

  gram-molecular w., molecular w. expressed in grams. Cf. mole.

  molecular w. (mol wt, MW), the sum of the atomic w.'s of all the atoms constituting a molecule; the mass of a molecule relative to the mass of a standard atom, now ^{12}C (taken as 12.000). Relative molecular mass (M_r) is the mass relative to the dalton and has no units. SEE ALSO atomic w. SYN molecular mass, molecular weight ratio, relative molecular mass.

weight·less·ness (wāt′les-nes). The psychophysiologic effect of zero gravity, as experienced by someone falling freely in a vacuum (e.g., astronauts in a stable orbit). A temporary state of simulated w. can be achieved during powered flight within the earth's atmosphere by traversing an inverted parabolic curve where gravitational pull and centrifugal force cancel each other out.

Weil, Adolf, German physician, 1848–1916. SEE W. *disease.*

Weil, Edmund, Austrian physician, 1880–1922. SEE W.-Felix *reaction, test.*

We

Weil, Ludwig A., German dentist, 1849–1895. SEE W. basal *layer*, basal *zone.*

Weill, Georges J., French ophthalmologist, 1866–1952. SEE W.-Marchesani *syndrome.*

Weill, Jean A., French physician, *1903. SEE Leri-W. *disease*, *syndrome.*

Weinberg, Michel, French pathologist, 1868–1940. SEE W. *reaction.*

Weinberg, Wilhelm, German physician, 1862–1937. SEE Hardy-W. *equilibrium*, *law.*

Weingrow re·flex. See under reflex.

Weir Mitchell, Silas, U.S. neurologist, poet, and novelist, 1829–1914. SEE Mitchell *treatment;* Gerhardt-Mitchell *disease;* W. M. *treatment.*

Weisbach, Albin, Austrian anthropologist, 1837–1914. SEE W. *angle.*

Weismann, August Friedrich Leopold, German biologist, 1834–1914. SEE weismannism.

weis·mann·ism (vīs′man-izm). Theory of the noninheritance of acquired characteristics.

Weiss, Nathan, Austrian physician, 1851–1883. SEE W. *sign.*

Weiss, Soma, U.S. physician, 1898–1942. SEE Charcot-W.-Baker *syndrome;* Mallory-W. *lesion*, *syndrome*, *tear.*

Weitbrecht, Josias, German-Russian anatomist in St. Petersburg, 1702–1747. SEE W. *cartilage*, *cord*, *fibers*, under *fiber*, *foramen*, *ligament; apparatus* ligamentosus weitbrechti.

Welander, Lisa, Swedish neurologist, *1909. SEE Kugelberg-W. *disease;* Wohlfart-Kugelberg-W. *disease.*

Welch, William H., U.S. pathologist, 1850–1934. SEE W. *bacillus.*

Welcker, Hermann, German anthropologist and anatomist, 1822–1898. SEE W. *angle.*

well·ness (wel′nĕs). A philosophy of life and personal hygiene that views health as not merely the absence of illness but the fullest realization of one's physical and mental potential, as achieved through positive attitudes, fitness training, a diet low in fat and high in fiber, and the avoidance of unhealthful practices (smoking, drug and alcohol abuse, overeating).

> Wellness programs are widely offered by employers, health insurance programs, and social service agencies. Formal programs typically include preventive measures (e.g., immunizations against pneumococcal pneumonia and influenza in the elderly) and surveillance for common diseases (e.g., hypertension, diabetes mellitus, and breast and colon cancer). Such programs tend to attract persons already attuned to healthful attitudes and practices. Little clinical evidence exists to support their usefulness or justify their expense.

Wells, G.C., 20th century British dermatologist. SEE W. *syndrome.*

Wells, Michael Vernon, 20th century English physician. SEE Muckle-W. *syndrome.*

welt (wĕlt). SYN wheal. [O.E. *waelt*]

wen (wĕn). Old term for pilar *cyst.* [A.S.]

Wenckebach, Karel F., Dutch internist, 1864–1940. SEE W. *block*, *period*, *phenomenon.*

Wenzel, Joseph, German anatomist and physiologist, 1768–1808. SEE W. *ventricle.*

Wepfer, Johann J., 1620–1695. SEE W. *glands*, under *gland.*

Werdnig, Guido, Austrian neurologist, 1862–1919. SEE W.-Hoffmann *disease;* Werdnig-Hoffmann muscular *atrophy.*

Werlhof, Paul G., German physician, 1699–1767. SEE Werlhof *disease.*

Wermer, Paul L., U.S. internist, 1898–1975. SEE Wermer *syndrome.*

Wernekinck (Werneking), Friedrich C.G., German anatomist and physician, 1798–1835. SEE W. *commissure*, *decussation.*

Werner, F.F., early 20th century German chemist. SEE W. *test.*

Werner, Otto, German physician, *1879. SEE W. *syndrome.*

Wernicke, Karl, German neurologist, 1848–1905. SEE W. *aphasia*, *area*, *center*, *disease*, *encephalopathy*, *field*, *radiation*, *reaction*, *region*, *sign*, *syndrome*, *zone;* W.-Korsakoff *encephalopathy*, *syndrome.*

Wertheim, Ernst, Austrian gynecologist, 1864–1920. SEE W. *operation.*

Werther, J., 20th century German physician. SEE W. *disease.*

West, Charles, English physician, 1816–1898. SEE W. *syndrome.*

West, John B., Australian-U.S. pulmonary physiologist, *1928.

Westberg, Friedrich, 19th century German physician. SEE W. *space.*

Westergren, Alf, Swedish physician, *1891. SEE W. *method.*

West·ern blot, West·ern blot·ting. SYN Western blot *analysis.*

Westphal, Karl F.O., German neurologist, 1833–1890. SEE W. pupillary *reflex;* W.-Piltz *phenomenon;* Edinger-W. *nucleus.*

Wetzel, Norman C., U.S. pediatrician, *1897. SEE W. *grid.*

Wever, Ernest Glen, U.S. psychologist, *1902. SEE W.-Bray *phenomenon.*

Weyers, Helmut, 20th century German pediatrician. SEE W.-Thier *syndrome.*

WF Abbreviation for Working Formulation for Clinical Usage.

Wharton, Thomas, English anatomist and physician, 1614–1673. SEE W. *duct*, *jelly.*

wheal (hwēl). A circumscribed, evanescent papule or irregular plaque of edema of the skin, appearing as an urticarial lesion, slightly reddened, often changing in size and shape and extending to adjacent areas, and usually accompanied by intense itching; produced by intradermal injection or test, or by exposure to allergenic substances in susceptible persons; also encountered in dermatitis herpetiformis (Darier sign). SYN hives (2), welt. [A.S. *hwēle*]

wheat germ oil (hwēt jerm). An oil obtained by expression from the germ of the wheat seed, *Triticum aestivum* (family Gramineae); one of the richest sources of natural vitamin E; used as a nutritional supplement.

Wheatstone, Charles, English physicist, 1802–1875. SEE W. *bridge.*

wheel (hwēl). A circular frame or disk designed to revolve around an axis.

Burlew w., SYN Burlew *disk.*

Wheeler, Henry Lord, U.S. chemist, 1867–1914. SEE Wheeler-Johnson *test.*

Wheeler, John M., U.S. ophthalmologist, 1879–1938. SEE W. *method.*

wheeze (hwēz). **1.** To breathe with difficulty and noisily. **2.** A whistling, squeaking, musical, or puffing sound made on exhalation by air passing through the fauces, glottis, or narrowed tracheobronchial airways. [A.S. *hwēsan*]

asthmatoid w., a puffing or musical sound heard on exhalation in front of the patient's open mouth in a case of foreign body in the trachea or a bronchus.

whe·wel·lite (hwa′wel-īt). A monohydrate of calcium oxalate; found in renal calculi. Cf. weddellite. [William *Whewell*, Eng. philosopher (1794–1866), + -ite]

whey (hwā). The watery part of milk remaining after the separation of the casein. SYN serum lactis. [A.S. *hwaeg*]

alum w., w. produced by curdling milk by means of powdered alum.

w. protein, SEE whey *protein.*

whip·lash (hwip′lash). SEE whiplash *injury.*

Whipple, Allen O., U.S. surgeon, 1881–1963. SEE W. *operation.*

Whipple, George H., U.S. pathologist and Nobel laureate, 1878–1976. SEE W. *disease.*

whip·worm (hwip′werm). SEE *Trichuris trichiura.*

whis·ky, whis·key (hwis′kē). An alcoholic liquid obtained by the distillation of the fermented mash of wholly or partly malted cereal grains, containing 47 to 53% by volume of C_2H_5OH, at

15.56°C; it must have been stored in charred wood containers for not less than 2 years. The various grains used in the manufacture of w. are barley, maize, rye, and wheat. [Gael, *usquebaugh,* water of life]

whis·per (hwis′per). To speak without phonation, as with an open posterior part of the glottis. [A.S. *hwisprian*]

whis·tle (hwis′l). **1.** A sound made by forcing air through a narrow opening. **2.** An instrument for producing a w. [A.S. *hwistle*]

Galton w., a cylindrical w., attached to a compressible bulb, with a screw attachment that changes the frequency; used to test the hearing.

Whitaker, Robert, Br. surgeon, *1939. SEE W. *test.*

White, Paul Dudley, U.S. cardiologist, 1886–1973. SEE Lee-W. *method;* Wolff-Parkinson-W. *syndrome.*

white (hwīt). The color resulting from commingling of all the rays of the spectrum; the color of chalk or of snow. SYN albicans (1). [A.S. *hwīt*]

w. of eye, the visible portion of the sclera.

Whitehead, Walter, English surgeon, 1840–1913. SEE W. *deformity, operation.*

white·head (hwīt′hed). **1.** SYN milium. **2.** SYN closed *comedo.*

white·pox (hwīt′poks). SYN alastrim.

whites (hwīts). Colloquialism for leukorrhea or blennorrhea.

whit·ing (hwīt′ing). Chalk (CaCO₃) used for polishing metals or plastic appliances.

whit·loc·kite (hwit′lok-īt). SYN tribasic *calcium* phosphate. [Herbert P. *Whitlock,* Am. mineralogist (*1868), + -ite]

whit·low (hwit′lō). Purulent infection through a perionychial fold causing an abscess of the bulbous distal end of a finger. SYN felon. [M.E. *whitflawe*]

herpetic w., painful herpes simplex virus infection of a finger from direct inoculation of the unprotected perionychial fold, often accompanied by lymphangitis and regional adenopathy, lasting up to several weeks; most common in physicians, dentists, and nurses as a result of exposure to the virus in a patient's mouth.

thecal w., suppurative lesion of distal phalanx; may involve tendon sheath and bone.

Whitman, Royal, U.S. surgeon, 1857–1946. SEE W. *frame.*

Whitmore, Alfred, English surgeon, 1876–1946. SEE W. *disease.*

Whitnall, Samuel E., English anatomist, 1876–1952. SEE W. *tubercle.*

WHO Abbreviation for World Health Organization.

whoop (hoop). The loud sonorous inspiration in pertussis with which the paroxysm of coughing terminates, due to spasm of the larynx (glottis).

systolic w., SYN systolic *honk.*

whorl (hwerl). **1.** A turn of the spiral cochlea of the ear. **2.** SYN *vortex* of heart. **3.** A turn of a concha nasalis. **4.** SYN verticil. **5.** An area of hair growing in a radial manner suggesting whirling or twisting. SYN vortex (2). SEE hair w.'s. **6.** One of the distinguishing patterns comprising the Galton system of classification of fingerprints. SYN digital w.

coccygeal w., SYN *vortex* coccygeus.

digital w., SYN whorl (6).

hair w.'s [TA], a spiral arrangement of the hairs, as at the crown of the head. SYN vortices pilorum [TA].

whorled (hwerld). Marked by or arranged in whorls. SEE ALSO vorticose, turbinate, convoluted, verticillate.

Wickham, Louis-Frédéric, French dermatologist, 1860–1913. SEE W. *striae,* under *stria.*

Widal, Georges F.I., French physician, 1862–1929. SEE W. *reaction, syndrome;* Gruber-W. *reaction;* Hayem-W. *syndrome.*

wide·band (wīd-band). A broad array of sound frequencies as opposed to a narrow array of frequencies.

wid·ow's peak. A sharp point of hair growth in the midline of the anterior scalp margin, usually resulting from recession of hair of the temple areas, or occurring as a congenital configuration of scalp hair.

width (width, with). Wideness; the distance from one side of an object or area to the other.

orbital w., the distance between the dacryon and the farthest point on the anterior edge of the outer border of the orbit (Broca), or between the latter point and the junction of the frontolacrimal suture and the posterior edge of the lacrimal groove.

window w., the range of CT numbers (in Hounsfield units) included in the gray scale video display of the CT image, ranging from 1 to 2000 or 3000, depending on the type of machine. Also, the range of electromagnetic energies passed by an electronic screening module of an imaging device, as by a scintillation camera. SEE ALSO window *level.*

Wiedemann, Hans Rudolf, German pediatrician, *1915. SEE Beckwith-W. *syndrome.*

Wiener, H. SEE *tract* of Münzer and W.

Wigand, Justus Heinrich, German obstetrician and gynecologist, 1769–1817. SEE W. *maneuver.*

Wilde, Sir William R.W., Irish oculist and otologist, 1815–1876. SEE W. *cords,* under *cord, triangle.*

Wilder, Helenor C., 20th century U.S. scientist. SEE W. *stain* for reticulum.

Wilder, Joseph F., U.S. neuropsychiatrist, 1895–1976.

Wilder, William H., U.S. ophthalmologst, 1860–1935. SEE W. *sign.*

Wildermuth, Hermann A., German psychiatrist, 1852–1907. SEE W. *ear.*

Wildervanck, L.S., 20th century Dutch geneticist. SEE W. *syndrome.*

wild·fire (wīld′fīr). SYN fogo selvagem.

Wilhelmy, Ludwig F., German scientist, 1812–1864. SEE W. *balance.*

Wilkie, David P.D., Scottish surgeon, 1882–1938. SEE W. *artery, disease.*

Wilkinson, Daryl Sheldon, 20th century English dermatologist. SEE Sneddon-W. *disease.*

Willebrand, E.A. von. SEE von Willebrand.

Willett, J. Abernethy, English obstetrician, †1932. SEE W. *forceps.*

Willi, Heinrich, 20th century Swiss pediatrician. SEE Prader-W. *syndrome.*

Williams, Anna W., U.S. bacteriologist, 1863–1955. SEE W. *stain;* Park-W. *fixative.*

Williams, J.C.P., 20th century New Zealand cardiologist. SEE W. *syndrome.*

Williamson, Carl S., U.S. surgeon, 1896–1952. SEE Mann-W. *operation, ulcer.*

Willis, Thomas, English physician, 1621–1675. SEE W. *centrum* nervosum, *cords,* under *cord, pancreas, paracusis, pouch; circle* of W.; *accessorius* willisii; *chordae* willisii, under *chorda.*

Williston, Samuel Wendell, U.S. paleontologist, 1852–1918. SEE W. *law.*

wil·low (wil′ō). A tree of the genus *Salix;* the bark of several species, especially *S. fragilis,* is a source of salicin. [A.S. *welig*]

Wilms, Max, German surgeon, 1867–1918. SEE W. *tumor.*

Wilson, Clifford, English physician, *1906. SEE Kimmelstiel-W. *disease, syndrome.*

Wilson, James, English anatomist, physiologist, and surgeon, 1765–1821. SEE W. *muscle.*

Wilson, Miriam G., U.S. pediatrician, *1922. SEE W.-Mikity *syndrome.*

Wilson, Samuel A. Kinnier, English neurologist, 1878–1937. SEE W. *disease.*

Wilson, Sir William J.E., English dermatologist, 1809–1884. SEE W. *disease.*

Wilson meth·od. See under method.

wind·age (win′dej). Internal injury with no surface lesion, caused by collision with the pressure of compressed air or with an object propelled by compressed air.

wi

wind·burn (wind′bern). Erythema of the face due to exposure to wind.

win·dow (win′dō) [TA]. **1.** SYN fenestra. **2.** Any opening in space or time. **3.** *Radiology.* A view especially contrived to accentuate tissue contrast.

aortic w., obsolete term for a radiolucent region below the aortic arch on a left anterior oblique chest radiograph, formed by the bifurcation of the trachea and crossed by the left pulmonary artery.

aorticopulmonary w., SYN aortic septal *defect.*

aortic-pulmonic w., SYN aortopulmonary w.

aortopulmonary w., the indentation of the left side of the mediastinum by the lung partially interposed between the aortic arch and the left pulmonary artery, seen on frontal radiographs of the chest. SYN aortic-pulmonic w.

cochlear w., SYN round w.

lung w., CT settings of w. level and width appropriate to showing lung detail.

mediastinal w., CT settings of w. level and width appropriate to showing soft tissue structures. SYN soft tissue w.

oval w. [TA], an oval opening on the medial wall of the tympanic cavity leading into the vestibule, closed in life by the foot of the stapes. SYN fenestra vestibuli [TA], fenestra of the vestibule, fenestra ovalis, vestibular w.

round w. [TA], an opening on the medial wall of the middle ear leading into the cochlea, closed in life by the secondary tympanic membrane. SYN fenestra cochleae [TA], cochlear w., fenestra of the cochlea, fenestra rotunda.

soft tissue w., SYN mediastinal w.

tachycardia w., in paroxysmal tachycardia of the reentry type, the interval of time (the window) between the earliest and latest premature activation that can excite the paroxysm.

vestibular w., SYN oval w.

wind·pipe (wind′pīp). SYN trachea.

wine (wīn). **1.** The fermented juice of the grape. SYN vinous liquor. **2.** A group of preparations consisting of a solution of one or more medicinal substances in w., usually white w. because of its comparative freedom from tannin. There are no official w.'s. [Fr. *vin;* L. *vinum*]

high w., the strong spirit obtained by rectification or redistillation of low w. in making whisky.

low w., the first weak distillate obtained from the mash in the process of making whisky.

red w., claret, an alcoholic liquor made by fermenting grapes, the fruit of *Vitis vinifera,* with their skins (which imparts color); has been used as a tonic.

sherry w., a w. of amber color, obtained originally from Jerez, Spain, containing about 20% alcohol; used in preparation of medicinal w.'s.

wing. The anterior appendage of a bird. SYN ala (1).

angel w., a deformity in which both scapulae project conspicuously. SEE ALSO winged *scapula.*

ashen w., SYN vagal (nerve) *trigone.*

w. of central lobule [TA], the lateral winglike projection of the central lobule of the cerebellum; made up of an inferior part [TA], which is the lateral portion of lobule II (of Larsell), and a superior part [TA], which is the lateral portion of lobule III (of Larsell). SYN ala central lobule [TA], ala lobulis centralis [TA], ala cerebelli.

w. of crista galli, SYN *ala* of crista galli.

gray w., SYN vagal (nerve) *trigone.*

greater w. of sphenoid (bone) [TA], strong squamous processes extending in a broad superolateral curve from the body of the sphenoid bone. The greater w. presents these surfaces (facies): 1) cerebral surface: forms anterior third of the floor of the lateral portion of the middle cranial fossa; 2) temporal surface: forms the deepest portion of the temporal fossa; 3) infratemporal surface, forms the "roof" of the infratemporal fossa; 4) orbital surface: forms posterolateral wall of orbit. The greater w. forms the inferior or border of the supraorbital fissure, and is perforated at its root by foramina rotundum ovale and spinosum and the pterygoid canal. SYN ala major ossis sphenoidalis [TA], ala temporalis.

w. of ilium, ✩official alternate term for *ala* of ilium.

lesser w. of sphenoid (bone) [TA], one of a bilateral pair of triangular, pointed plates extending laterally from the anterolateral body of the sphenoid bone. Forming the posteriormost portion of the floor of the anterior cranial fossa, their sharp posterior edge forms the sphenoidal ridge separating anterior and middle cranial fossae. The medial end of the lesser w. attaches to the body by means of two pedicles, thus forming the optic canal. The w. itself forms the superior margin of the supraorbital fissure. SYN ala minor ossis sphenoidalis [TA], ala orbitalis, Ingrassia process.

w. of nose, SYN *ala* of nose.

w. of sacrum, ✩official alternate term for *ala* of sacrum.

w. of vomer, SYN *ala* of vomer.

Winiwarter, Felix von, German surgeon, 1852–1931. SEE W.-Buerger *disease.*

wink (wink). SYN blink. [A.S. *wincian*]

Winslow, Jacques B., Danish anatomist, physicist, and surgeon in Paris, 1669–1760. SEE *foramen* of W.; W. *ligament, pancreas, stars,* under *star; stellulae* winslowii, under *stellula.*

Winterbottom, Thomas Masterman, English physician, 1765–1859. SEE W. *sign.*

win·ter·green oil (win′ter-grēn). SYN methyl salicylate.

Winternitz, Wilhelm, Austrian physician, 1835–1917. SEE W. *sound.*

Wintersteiner, Hugo, Austrian ophthalmologist, 1865–1918. SEE W. *rosettes,* under *rosette.*

wire (wīr). Slender and pliable rod or thread of metal.

arch w., SYN archwire.

guide w., SEE guidewire.

Kirschner w., an apparatus for skeletal traction in long bone fracture or for fracture fixation. SYN Kirschner apparatus.

ligature w., a soft thin w. of stainless steel used in dentistry to tie an archwire to band attachments or brackets.

separating w., a w., usually of soft brass, used to gain separation between teeth. SEE ALSO separation (2).

wrought w., a w. formed by drawing a cast structure through a die into a desired shape and size; used in dentistry for partial denture clasps and orthodontic appliances.

wir·ing (wīr′ing). Fastening together the ends of a broken bone by wire sutures.

circumferential w., fixation of mandibular fractures by passing wires around a section of bone and intraoral splint; i.e., circummandibular w. SEE ALSO circumzygomatic w.

circumzygomatic w., a means of fixation for mandibular fractures in which the mandible is fastened to the zygomatic arches with wire.

continuous loop w., the formation of wire loops on both maxillary and mandibular teeth, for the placement of intermaxillary elastics; used in reduction and fixation of fractures. SYN Stout w.

craniofacial suspension w., a method of w. using areas of bones not contiguous with the oral cavity for the support of fractured jaw segments (e.g., pyriform aperture, zygomatic arch, zygomatic process of the frontal bone).

Gilmer w., a method of intermaxillary fixation in which single opposing teeth are wired circumferentially, and the wires are twisted together.

Ivy loop w., placement of a wire around two adjacent teeth to provide an attachment for intermaxillary elastics.

perialveolar w., fixing a splint to the maxillary arch by passing a wire through the alveolar process from the buccal surface to the lingual surface.

pyriform aperture w., a method of w. from the area of the pyriform aperture for the stabilization of fractures of the jaw.

Stout w., SYN continuous loop w.

Wirsung, Johann G., German anatomist in Padua, 1589–1643. SEE W. *canal, duct.*

wiry (wīr′ē). Resembling or having the feel of a wire; filiform and hard; denoting a variety of pulse.

Wiskott, Arthur, 20th century German pediatrician. SEE W.-Aldrich *syndrome.*

Wissler, Hans, Swiss pediatrician, *1906. SEE W. *syndrome.*

Wistar, Caspar, U.S. biologist, 1761–1818, after whom the Wistar Institute is named. SEE W. *rats,* under *rat.*

witch ha·zel (wich hāz'l). SYN hamamelis.

with·draw·al (with-draw'ăl). **1.** The act of removal or retreat. **2.** A psychologic and/or physical syndrome caused by the abrupt cessation of the use of a drug in an habituated individual. **3.** The therapeutic process of discontinuing a drug so as to avoid the symptoms of w. (2). **4.** A pattern of behavior observed in schizophrenia and depression, characterized by a pathological retreat from interpersonal contact and social involvement and leading to self-preoccupation.

wit·kop (vit'kop). A favoid condition of the scalp seen in South Africans.

wit·zel·sucht (vit'sel-zŭkht). A morbid tendency to pun, make poor jokes, and tell pointless stories, while being oneself inordinately entertained thereby. [Ger. *witzeln,* to affect wit, + *Sucht,* mania]

wob·ble (wah'bl). In molecular biology, unorthodox pairing between the base at the 5′ end of an anticodon and the base that pairs with it (in the 3′ position of the codon); thus, the anticodon 3′-UCU-5′ may pair with 5′-AGA-3′ (normal or Watson-Crick pairing) or with 5′-AGG-3′ (wobble). Wobble pairings can occur between the unusual base hypoxanthine and adenine, uracil, or cytosine, between uracil and guanine, and between guanine and uracil, when in the 5′ position of an anticodon. SEE ALSO wobble *base.*

Wohl·fahr·tia (vōl-far'tē-ă). A genus of larviparous dipterous fleshflies (family Sarcophagidae), of which some species' larvae breed in ulcerated surfaces and flesh wounds of humans and animals. Important species include *W. magnifica,* a widely distributed obligatory fleshfly whose tissue-destroying maggots invade wounds or head cavities of domestic animals and humans; *W. nuba,* a facultative fleshfly of Old World distribution, also found in head wounds or head cavities but not in dermal sores; and *W. vigil* (*W. opaca*), which produces cutaneous myiasis in human infants in the northern U.S. and southern Canada by larvae that penetrate the skin and cause infected, boil-like, or furuncular lesions; mink and fox pups in fur farms, and probably rabbits and rodents, are attacked by this species. [P. *Wohlfahrt,* Ger. medical writer, †1726]

wohl·fahr·ti·o·sis (vōl-far-tē-ō'sis). Infection of animals and humans with larvae of flies of the genus *Wohlfahrtia.*

Wohlfart, Gunnar, Swedish neurologist, 1910–1961. SEE W.-Kugelberg-Welander *disease.*

Wolf, A., 20th century U.S. pathologist. SEE W.-Orton *bodies,* under *body.*

Wolfe, John R., Scottish ophthalmologist, 1824–1904. SEE W. *graft;* W.-Krause *graft.*

Wolff, Julius, German anatomist, 1836–1902. SEE Wolff *law.*

Wolff, Kaspar F., German embryologist in Russia, 1733–1794. SEE wolffian *body;* wolffian *cyst;* wolffian *duct;* wolffian *rest;* wolffian *ridge;* wolffian *tubules,* under *tubule.*

Wolff, Louis, U.S. cardiologist, 1898–1972. SEE W.-Chaikoff *block, effect;* W.-Parkinson-White *syndrome.*

wolff·i·an (wulf'ē-an). Relating to or described by Kaspar Wolff.

Wölfler, Anton, Bohemian surgeon, 1850–1917. SEE W. *gland.*

wolf·ram, wolf·ram·i·um (wulf'ram, wulf-ram'ē-ŭm). SYN tungsten. SEE Wolfram *syndrome.* [from *wolframite*]

Wolfring, Emilj F. von, Polish ophthalmologist, 1832–1906. SEE W. *glands,* under *gland.*

wolfs·bane (wulfs'bān). SEE aconite.

Wolinel·la (wō-li-nel'ah). Genus of Gram-negative, microaerophilic bacteria with helical to curved cells; exhibits motility by a single polar flagellum. Isolated from the gingival sulcus and from root canal infections in humans, and from the bovine rumen. Type species is *Wolinella succinogenes.*

Wollaston, William H., English physician and physicist, 1766–1828. SEE W. *doublet, theory.*

Wolman, Moshe, 20th century Israeli neuropathologist, *1914. SEE W. *disease, xanthomatosis.*

womb (woom). SYN uterus. [A.S. the belly]

falling of the w., SYN *prolapse* of the uterus.

Wood, Paul. SEE Wood *units,* under *unit.*

Wood, Robert, U.S. physicist, 1868–1955. SEE W. *glass, lamp, light.*

wood al·co·hol (wud). SYN methyl *alcohol.*

wood wool. A specially prepared, not compressed, wood fiber used for surgical dressings.

wool (wul). The hair of the sheep; sometimes, when defatted, used as a surgical dressing. SYN lana.

w. alcohols, wool wax alcohols prepared by saponification of the grease of sheep wool and separation of the fraction that contains cholesterol (not less than 30%) and other alcohols; used to prepare w. ointment.

w. fat, the purified, anhydrous, fatlike substance obtained from the wool of sheep. SEE ALSO *adeps* lanae.

hydrous w. fat, SYN *adeps* lanae.

Woolf, B., 20th-century British biochemist. SEE W.-Lineweaver-Burk *plot.*

Woolner, Thomas, English sculptor, 1826–1892. SEE W. *tip.*

word sal·ad (werd sal'ăd). A jumble of meaningless and unrelated words emitted by persons with certain kinds of schizophrenia.

Woringer, M.M.F., 20th century French dermatologist. SEE Woringer-Kolopp *disease.*

work (work). **1.** Physical and/or mental effort to achieve a result. **2.** That which is accomplished when a force acts against resistance to produce motion.

---

workaholic (werk-a-hawl'ik). A person who manifests a compulsive need to work, even at the expense of family responsibilities, social life, and health. [by analogy with *alcoholic*]

> Although increasingly recognized as a source of emotional distress, social malfunctioning, and physical illness, the pathologic need of some people to invest all their energy in goal-directed and intensive labor has not been deeply studied, nor is it named or defined in the Diagnostic and Statistical Manual of Mental Disorders (DSM-IV). The workaholic may engage in physical or mental work or a combination of the two, and may work for an individual or a company, be self-employed, or even engage in volunteer activities without remuneration. The typical workaholic seems incapable of relaxing, and uses work not only as a source of livelihood but also as a form of recreation, substituting it for leisure pastimes such as socialization, hobbies, sports, and artistic and cultural pursuits. In this sense, work assumes the function of an addictive drug. Workaholics tend to postpone or omit meals, stay at work after others have gone home and even keep working until late at night, put in excessive amounts of overtime (sometimes failing to claim due compensation), and abuse nicotine, caffeine, alcohol, and other agents to assuage stress and withstand fatigue. The workaholic lifestyle is a common feature of various personality disorders, including a compulsion to achieve success, recognition, or advancement in one's chosen field of endeavor; a morbid absorption in the acquisition of wealth; and a need to immerse oneself in work as a distraction from the stresses or dissatisfactions of daily life. Some workaholic behavior is driven by family, social, or cultural expectations. Many workaholics manifest a compulsion to work even in childhood; some seem to be influenced by the example of a successful, driving parent, relative, family friend, or public figure. In Japan, death from overwork (*karoshi*) is formally recognized as a compensable form of occupational disorder. Japanese courts have ruled that deaths from heart failure, stroke, and even suicide are examples of karoshi.

Working Formulation for Clinical Usage (WF). Classifi-

Wo

cation of malignant lymphomas introduced by the National Cancer Institute in 1982, based on the correlation of clinical and histopathologic features of various lymphomas; widely used in clinical practice.

work·ing out (werk′ing). In psychoanalysis, the state in the treatment process in which the patient's personal history and psychodynamics are uncovered.

work·ing through. In psychoanalysis, the process of obtaining additional insight and personality changes in a patient through repeated and varied examination of a conflict or problem; the interactions between free association, resistance, interpretation, and working out constitute the fundamental facets of this process.

work·sta·tion (werk′stā′shŭn). A computer or television monitor with controls for studying and manipulating graphical or clinical images.

World Health Or·ga·ni·za·tion (WHO). A unit of the United Nations devoted to international health problems.

Worm, Ole, Danish anatomist, 1588–1654. SEE wormian *bones*, under *bone*.

worm (werm). **1.** In anatomy, any structure resembling a w., e.g., the midline part of the cerebellum in the forms of "vermis" and "lumbrical." **2.** Term once used to designate any member of the invertebrate group or former subkingdom Vermes, a collective term no longer used taxonomically; now commonly used to designate any member of the separate phyla Annelida (the segmented or true w.'s), Nematoda (roundworms), and Platyhelminthes (flatworms). Important species include *Dracunculus medinensis* (dragon, guinea, Medina, or serpent w.), *Enterobius vermicularis* (seat w. or pinworm), *Loa loa* (African eye w.), *Moniliformis* (phylum Acanthocephala, thorny-headed w.'s), *Oxyspirura mansoni* (Manson eye w.), *Pentastomida* (tongue w.), *Strongylus* (palisade w.), *Thelazia* (eye w.), and *Trichinella spiralis* (pork or trichina w.). For some types of w.'s not listed as subentries here (because they are usually written as one word), see the full name. [A.S. *wyrm*]

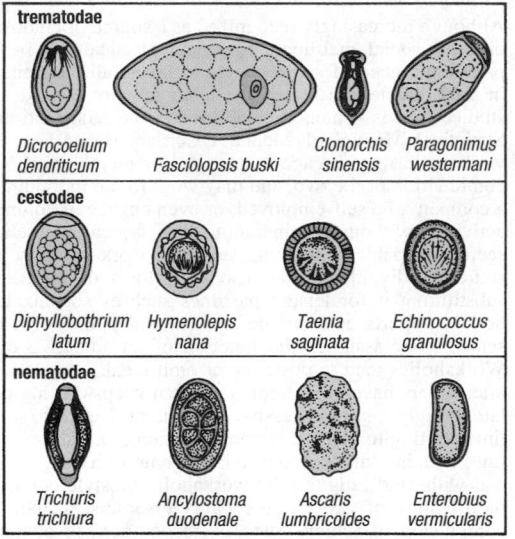

trematodae			
Dicrocoelium dendriticum	*Fasciolopsis buski*	*Clonorchis sinensis*	*Paragonimus westermani*

cestodae			
Diphyllobothrium latum	*Hymenolepis nana*	*Taenia saginata*	*Echinococcus granulosus*

nematodae			
Trichuris trichiura	*Ancylostoma duodenale*	*Ascaris lumbricoides*	*Enterobius vermicularis*

worms: eggs of various species

caddis w., aquatic larva in the insect order Trichoptera.

Manson eye w., SYN *Oxyspirura mansoni.*

meal w., the larva of beetles of the genus *Tenebrio;* both larvae and adults are important pests, destroying flour, meal, and other cereal products; they are also intermediate hosts of nematodes of the genus *Gongylonema,* and of various tapeworms of the genus *Hymenolepis.*

worm bark. SYN andira.

wor·mi·an (werm′ē-an). Relating to or described by Ole Worm.

Wormley, Theodore G., U.S. chemist, 1826–1897. SEE W. *test.*

worm·seed (werm′sēd). **1.** Santonica. **2.** SYN chenopodium.

worm·wood (werm′wud). SYN absinthium.

wort (wōrt). **1.** A suffix in the popular names of many plants, such as liverwort, lungwort, woundwort, etc. **2.** An infusion of malt. [A.S. *wyrt,* a plant]

St. John's w., a shrubby perennial (*Hypericum perforatum*) with numerous orange-yellow flowers whose petals may be speckled black along their margins; a herbal antidepressant that compares favorably with standard synthetic psychopharmaceutical agents in the treatment of mild to moderate depression.

In medieval folk-medicine this herb, traditionally gathered on the eve of the feast of St. John the Baptist (June 24), was used against various illnesses, including hysteria and epilepsy, as well as witches' spells and diabolical possession. In Europe, St. John's wort is widely prescribed for the treatment of depression. The herb has been shown in placebo-controlled trials to lessen depression, anxiety, apathy, sleep disturbances, insomnia, anorexia, and feelings of worthlessness. EEG studies have shown that it improves sleep intensity without increasing total sleep duration or interfering with REM sleep. In clinical comparisons it was only slightly inferior to the tricyclic agents imipramine, amitriptyline, and desipramine in abolishing depressive symptoms. In addition, memory and other mental functions may be improved instead of being blunted as with prescription antidepressants. No controlled studies comparing the efficacy of St. John's wort with that of selective serotonin reuptake inhibitors have been published. Fewer than 3% of subjects in clinical trials noted any side effects. Those most frequently experienced were gastrointestinal irritation, allergic reactions, fatigue, restlessness, and photodermatitis. The principal active ingredient of St. John's wort is believed to be hypericin, which has been shown in vitro to inhibit the uptake or biodegradation of several neurotransmitters, including serotonin, norepinephrine, and dopamine. It also binds to γ-aminobutyric acid receptors on CNS neurons and improves the signal produced by serotonin after it binds to its receptors. Ongoing studies seek to define the psychopharmaceutical potential of this agent more precisely and to confirm the safety of its use. Because it inhibits monoamine oxidase, at least in vitro, its use with other antidepressants is not recommended. It is not considered appropriate during pregnancy or in the treatment of severe depression with serious risk of suicide or of depression accompanied by psychosis.

Worth, Claud A., British ophthalmologist, 1869–1936. SEE W. *amblyoscope.*

Woulfe, Peter, English chemist, 1727–1803. SEE W. *bottle.*

wound (woond). **1.** Trauma to any of the tissues of the body, especially that caused by physical means and with interruption of continuity. **2.** A surgical incision. [O.E. *wund*]

abraded w., SYN abrasion (1).

avulsed w., a w. caused by or resulting from avulsion.

crease w., SYN gutter w.

glancing w., SYN gutter w.

gunshot w., a w. made with a bullet or other missile projected by a firearm.

gutter w., a tangential w. that makes a furrow without perforating the skin. SYN crease w., glancing w.

incised w., a clean cut, as by a sharp instrument.

nonpenetrating w., injury, especially within the thorax or abdomen, produced without disruption of the surface of the body.

open w., a w. in which the tissues are exposed to the air.

penetrating w., a w. with disruption of the body surface that extends into underlying tissue or into a body cavity.

perforating w., a w. with an entrance and exit opening.

puncture w., a w. in which the opening is relatively small as compared to the depth, as produced by a narrow pointed object.

septic w., a w. that has become infected.

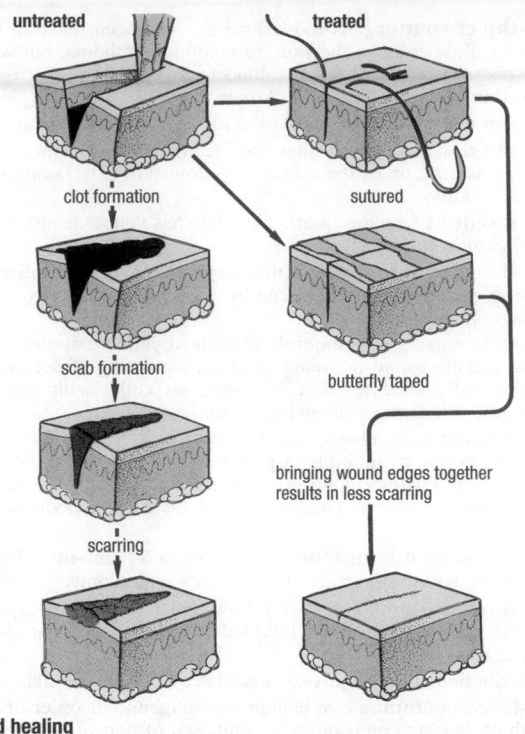

untreated   **treated**

clot formation   sutured

scab formation   butterfly taped

bringing wound edges together results in less scarring

scarring

wound healing

seton w., a tangential perforating w., the entrance and exit openings being on the same side of the body, head, or limb involved.

stab w., a puncture w. produced by the stabbing motion of a knife or similar object.

subcutaneous w., an injury or wound extending below the skin into the subcutaneous tissue, but not affecting underlying bones or organs.

sucking chest w., SYN open *pneumothorax*.

tangential w., a perforating w. or seton w. that involves only one side of the part.

W-plas·ty. Surgery to prevent the contracture of a straight-line scar; the edges of the wound are trimmed in the shape of a W, or a series of W's, and closed in a zig-zag manner.

W.r. Abbreviation for Wassermann *reaction*.

Wrᵃ Abbreviation for Wright *antigens*, under *antigen*. See low frequency blood groups, Blood Groups appendix.

wrap (rap). A cover, particularly one that enfolds or encloses.

cardiac muscle w., SYN cardiomyoplasty.

wreath (rēth). A structure resembling a twisted or entwined band or a garland. [A.S. *wraeth,* a bandage]

ciliary w., SYN *corona* ciliaris.

Wright, Basil Martin, 20th century British physician. SEE W. *respirometer*.

Wright, James Homer, U.S. pathologist, 1869–1928. SEE W. *stain*.

Wright, Marmaduke Burr, U.S. obstetrician, 1803–1879. SEE W. *version*.

wright·ine (rīt′ēn). SYN conessine.

wrin·kle (ring′kl). A furrow, fold, or crease in the skin, particularly with increasing occurrence as a result of sun exposure or, in perioral skin, cigarette smoking; associated with degeneration of dermal elastic tissue.

Wrisberg, Heinrich A., German anatomist and gynecologist, 1739–1808. SEE W. *cartilage, ganglia,* under *ganglion, ligament, nerve, tubercle*.

wrist (rist) [TA]. The proximal segment of the hand consisting of the carpal bones and the associated soft parts. SYN carpus (1) [TA]. [A.S. wrist joint, ankle joint]

w.-drop, paralysis of the extensors of the wrist and fingers; most often caused by lesion of the radial nerve. SYN carpoptosis, carpoptosia, drop hand.

wry·neck (rī′nek). SYN torticollis.

Wuch·er·e·ria (voo-ker-e′rē-ă). A genus of filarial nematodes (family Onchocercidae, superfamily Filarioidea) characterized by adult forms that live chiefly in lymphatic vessels and produce large numbers of embryos or microfilariae that circulate in the bloodstream (microfilaremia), often appearing in the peripheral blood at regular intervals. The extreme form of this infection (wuchereriasis or filariasis) is elephantiasis or pachydermia.

W. bancrof′ti, the bancroftian filaria, a species endemic in South Pacific islands, coastal China, India, and Burma, and throughout tropical Africa and northeastern South America (including certain Caribbean islands); transmitted to humans (apparently the only definitive host) by mosquitoes, especially *Culex quinquefasciatus* and *Aedes pseudoscutellaris,* but also by several other species of *Culex, Aedes, Anopheles,* and *Mansonia,* depending on the specific geographic area; adults are white, 40–100 mm cylindroid, threadlike worms, and the microfilariae are ensheathed, with rounded anterior end and tapered, nonnucleated tail; the adult worms inhabit the larger lymphatic vessels (e.g., in the extremities (especially lower), breasts, spermatic cord, and retroperitoneal tissues) and the sinuses of lymph nodes (e.g., the popliteal, femoral, and inguinal groups, and also the epitrochlear and axillary nodes), where they sometimes cause temporary obstruction to the flow of lymph and slight or moderate degrees of inflammation.

W. mala′yi, former name for *Brugia malayi*.

wu·cher·e·ri·a·sis (voo′ker-ē-rī′ă-sis). Infection with worms of the genus *Wuchereria*. SEE ALSO filariasis.

Wurster, Casimir, German chemist, 1856–1913. SEE W. *reagent, test*.

Wyburn-Mason, Roger, British physician. SEE Wyburn-Mason *syndrome*.

Wyman, Jeffries, U.S. biochemist, 1901–1995. SEE Monod-Wyman-Changeux *model*.

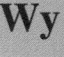

Wy

X Symbol for Kienböck *unit*; xanthosine; halogen atom; unspecified amino acid.

X Symbol for reactance.

Xaa Symbol for unspecified amino acid.

Xan Abbreviation for xanthine.

⌂**xanth-.** SEE xantho-.

xan·the·las·ma (zan-thĕ-laz'mă). SYN x. palpebrarum. [xanth- + G. *elasma*, a beaten metal plate]

generalized x., xanthoma planum of the neck, trunk, extremities, and eyelids in patients with normal plasma lipid levels.

x. palpebra'rum, soft, yellow-orange plaques on the eyelids or medial canthus, the most common form of xanthoma; may be associated with low-density lipoproteins, especially in younger adults. SYN xanthelasma, xanthoma palpebrarum.

xan·them·a·tin (zan-thĕm'ă-tin). A yellow substance derived from hematin by treating with nitric acid.

xan·the·mia (zan-thē'mē-ă). SYN carotenemia. [xanth- + G. *haima*, blood]

xan·thene (zan'thēn). **1.** The basic structure of many natural products, drugs, dyes (e.g., fluorescein, pyronin, eosins), indicators, pesticides, antibiotics, etc. **2.** A class of molecules based upon x. (1).

xan·thic (zan'thik). **1.** Yellow or yellowish in color. **2.** Relating to xanthine.

xan·thi·dy·lic ac·id (zan'thi-dil-ik). SYN *xanthosine 5'-monophosphate.*

xan·thine (Xan) (zan'thēn). 2,6-Dioxopurine; 2,6-(1*H*,3*H*)-purinedione; oxidation product of guanine and hypoxanthine, precursor of uric acid; occurs in many organs and in the urine, occasionally forming urinary calculi; elevated in molybdenum cofactor deficiency and in xanthinuria.

x. dehydrogenase, an oxidoreductase oxidizing x. to urate with NAD⁺ as the oxidant; lower activity in individuals with a deficiency of molybdenum cofactor.

x. nucleotide, SYN *xanthosine 5'-monophosphate.*

x. oxidase, a flavoprotein containing molybdenum; an oxidoreductase catalyzing the reaction of x., O_2, and H_2O to produce urate and superoxide; also oxidizes hypoxanthine, some other purines and pterins, and aldehydes. A lower activity is observed in molybdenum cofactor deficiency. SYN hypoxanthine oxidase, Schardinger enzyme.

x. ribonucleoside, SYN xanthosine.

xan·thi·nol ni·a·cin·ate, xan·thi·nol nic·o·tin·ate (zan'thi-nōl). A peripheral vasodilator.

xan·thi·nu·ria (zan-thi-noo'rē-ă). **1.** Excretion of abnormally large amounts of xanthine in the urine. **2.** A disorder [MIM*278300], characterized by urinary excretion of xanthine in place of uric acid, hypouricemia, and occasionally the formation of renal xanthine stones. There are two types: type I is due to xanthine dehydrogenase deficiency (XDH), and type II is due to deficiencies of both xanthine dehydrogenase and aldehyde oxidase. Autosomal recessive inheritance, caused by mutation in the XDH gene on chromosome 2p in some cases. SYN xanthiuria, xanthuria. [xanthine + G. *ouron*, urine]

xan·thism (zan'thizm) [MIM*278400]. A pigmentary anomaly of blacks, characterized by red or yellow-red hair color, copper-red skin, and often by dilution of iris pigment; autosomal recessive inheritance caused by mutation in the tyrosinase-related protein 1gene (TYRP1) on chromosome 9. SYN rufous albinism. [G. *xanthos,* yellowish]

xan·thi·u·ria (zan-thē-ū'rē-ă). SYN xanthinuria.

⌂**xantho-, xanth-.** Yellow, yellowish. [G. *xanthos*]

xan·tho·as·tro·cy·to·ma (zan'thrō-as'trō-sī-tō-mă). SYN pleomorphic x. [xantho + astrocytoma]

pleomorphic x., a rare variant of astrocytoma usually presenting early in life with seizures. The tumor is superficially located and composed of pleomorphic glial cells, lipidized astrocytes, and perivascular lymphocytes. SYN xanthoastrocytoma.

xan·tho·chro·mat·ic (zan'thō-krō-mat'ik). Yellow-colored. SYN xanthochromic.

xan·tho·chro·mia (zan-thō-krō'mē-ă). The occurrence of patches of yellow color in the skin, resembling xanthoma, but without the nodules or plates. SYN xanthoderma (1), yellow disease, yellow skin (1). [xantho- + G. *chrōma,* color]

xan·tho·chro·mic (zan-thō-krō'mik). SYN xanthochromatic.

xan·tho·der·ma (zan-thō-der'mă). **1.** SYN xanthochromia. **2.** Any yellow coloration of the skin. SYN yellow skin (2). [xantho- + G. *derma,* skin]

xan·tho·dont (zan'thō-dont). One who has yellow teeth. [xantho- + G. *odous,* tooth]

xan·tho·gran·u·lo·ma (zan'thō-gran'ū-lō'mă). A peculiar infiltration of retroperitoneal tissue by lipid macrophages, occurring most commonly in women.

juvenile x., single or multiple reddish to yellow papules or nodules, usually found in young children, consisting of dermal infiltration by histiocytes and Touton giant cells, with increasing fibrosis. SYN nevoxanthoendothelioma.

necrobiotic x., a cutaneous and subcutaneous x. with focal necrosis, presenting as multiple large, sometimes ulcerated, red to yellow granulomatous nodules with giant cells (often around the eyes) associated with paraproteinemia (usually monoclonal gammopathy).

xan·tho·gran·u·lo·ma·tous (zan'thō-gran'ū-lō'mă-tŭs). Relating to, of the nature of, or affected by xanthogranuloma.

xan·tho·ma (zan-thō'mă). A yellow nodule or plaque, especially of the skin, composed of lipid-laden histiocytes. [xantho- + G. *-oma,* tumor]

x. diabetico'rum, eruptive x. associated with severe diabetes.

x. dissemina'tum, a rare benign normolipemic disorder of adults with coalescent cutaneous x.'s composed of non-X histiocytes on flexural surfaces, often with mild diabetes insipidus.

eruptive x., the sudden appearance of groups of 1–4-mm waxy yellow or yellowish-brown papules with an erythematous halo, especially over extensors of the elbows and knees, and on the back and buttocks of patients with severe hyperlipemia, often familial or, more rarely, in severe diabetes.

fibrous x., SEE fibroxanthoma.

x. mul'tiplex, SYN xanthomatosis.

x. palpebra'rum, SYN *xanthelasma* palpebrarum.

x. pla'num, a form marked by the occurrence of yellow, flat bands or minimally palpable rectangular plates in the corium, either normolipemic or associated with type IIa or III hyperlipoproteinemia.

tendinous x., x. involving tendons, ligaments, and fascia, forming deep, smooth, sometimes painful nodules beneath normal-appearing freely movable skin of the extremities; associated with abnormal lipid metabolism, commonly familial increased β lipoproteins, or obstructive liver disease.

x. tubero'sum, xanthomatosis associated with familial type II, and occasionally type III, hyperlipoproteinemia. SYN x. tuberosum simplex.

x. tubero'sum sim'plex, SYN x. tuberosum.

verrucous x., histocytosis Y; a papilloma of the oral mucosa and skin in which squamous cell epithelium covers connective tissue papillae filled with large foamy histiocytes. SYN histiocytosis Y.

xan·tho·ma·to·sis (zan-thō-mă-tō'sis). Widespread xanthomas, especially on the elbows and knees, that sometimes affect mucous

---

⌂ **Combining Forms**	☆ **Official alternate Terminologia Anatomica term**
🔲 Indicates term is illustrated, see Illustration Index	
	[MIM] Mendelian Inheritance in Man
SYN Synonym	
Cf. Compare	**C.I. Colour Index**
[NA] Nomina Anatomica	
[TA] Terminologia Anatomica	**High Profile Term**

membranes and are sometimes associated with metabolic disturbances. SYN lipid granulomatosis, lipoid granulomatosis, xanthoma multiplex.

biliary x., x. with hypercholesterolemia, resulting from biliary cirrhosis. SYN Rayer disease.

x. bul′bi, ulcerative fatty degeneration of the cornea after injury.

cerebrotendinous x. [MIM*213700], a metabolic disorder associated with deposition of cholestanol and cholesterol in the brain and other tissues; plasma cholestanol level is high but plasma cholesterol level is normal; characterized by progressive cerebellar ataxia beginning after puberty, cataracts, spinal cord involvement, premature atherosclerosis, and tendinous or tuberous xanthomata; due to a defect in hepatic mitochondrial sterol 27-hydroxylase in bile acid biosynthesis; autosomal recessive inheritance, caused by mutation in the gene involved in cytochrome P-450 in the C27 position (CYP27) on chromosome 2q.

chronic idiopathic x., vague or indefinite term for inherited abnormalities of lipid metabolism leading to xanthoma formation (e.g., primary familial xanthomatosis).

familial hypercholesteremic x., SEE type II familial *hyperlipoproteinemia*.

generalized plane x., widespread x. associated with multiple *myeloma*, familial *hyperlipoproteinemia*, or less commonly with primary biliary *cirrhosis* or no underlying disease.

normal cholesteremic x., SYN Hand-Schüller-Christian *disease*.

Wolman x., SYN cholesterol ester storage *disease*.

Xan·tho·mo·nas (zan-thō-mō′as). Genus of the family Pseudomonadaceae; aerobic, Gram-negative, chemoorganotrophic, straight bacilli that exhibit motility by flagella. Type species is *Xanthomonas campestris*.

X. maltophil′ia, a species found primarily in clinical specimens but also in water, milk, and frozen food; frequent cause of infections in hospitalized and immunocompromised humans, it is resistant to many commonly used antibiotics; formerly called *Pseudomonas maltophilia*. SEE *Stenotrophomonas maltophilia*.

xan·tho·phyll (zan′thō-fil). Oxygenated derivative of carotene; a yellow plant pigment, occurring also in egg yolk and corpus luteum. SYN lutein (2), luteol, luteole.

xan·tho·pro·te·ic (zan-thō-prō′tē-ik). Relating to xanthoprotein.

xan·tho·pro·te·ic ac·id. A noncrystallizable yellow substance derived from proteins upon treatment with nitric acid.

xan·tho·pro·tein (zan-thō-prō′tēn). The yellow product formed upon treating protein with hot nitric acid, probably from nitration of phenyl groups.

xan·thop·sia (zan-thop′sē-ă). A condition in which objects appear yellow; may occur in picric acid and santonin poisoning, in jaundice, and in digitalis intoxication. SYN yellow vision. [xantho- + G. *opsis*, vision]

xan·tho·puc·cine (zan-thō-pŭk′sēn). SYN canadine.

xan·tho·sine (X, Xao) (zan′thō-sēn, -sin). 9-β-D-Ribosylxanthine; the deamination product of guanosine (O replacing –NH₂). SYN xanthine ribonucleoside.

x. 5′-monophosphate (XMP), the monophosphoric ester of x.; an intermediate in GMP biosynthesis. SYN xanthidylic acid, xanthine nucleotide, xanthylic acid.

x. 5′-triphosphate (XTP), x. with a triphosphoric acid esterified at its 5′ position.

xan·tho·sis (zan-thō′sis). A yellowish discoloration of degenerating tissues, especially seen in malignant neoplasms. [xantho- + G. *-osis*, condition]

xan·thous (zan′thŭs). Yellowish; yellow-colored. [G. *xanthos*, yellow]

xanth·u·ren·ic ac·id (zan-thoo-rēn′ik). The sulfur-yellow crystals form a red compound with Millon reagent, or an intensely green one with ferrous sulfate; excreted in the urine of pyridoxine-deficient animals after the ingestion of tryptophan, and of rats fed almost exclusively with fibrin.

xan·thu·ria (zan-thoo′rē-ă). SYN xanthinuria.

xan·thyl (zan′thil). A radical consisting of xanthine minus a hydrogen atom.

xan·thyl·ic (zan-thil′ik). Relating to xanthine.

xan·thyl·ic ac·id. SYN *xanthosine* 5′-monophosphate.

Xao Symbol for xanthosine.

Xe Symbol for xenon.

¹³³Xe Symbol for xenon-133.

xemilofiban (zem-il-of′ĭ-ban). A novel antiplatelet agent that blocks the binding of fibrinogen to specific membrane GPIIb/IIIa integrin receptors and thus prevents platelet aggregation induced by any known platelet agonist.

△**xeno-.** Strange; foreign material; parasite. SEE hetero-, allo-. [G. *xenos*, guest, host, stranger, foreign]

xen·o·bi·ot·ic (zen′ō-bī-ot′ik). **1.** A pharmacologically, endocrinologically, or toxicologically active substance not endogenously produced and therefore foreign to an organism. **2.** Pertaining to association of two animal species, usually insects, in the absence of a dependency relationship, as opposed to parasitism. [xeno- + G. *bios*, life + -ic]

xen·o·di·ag·no·sis (zen′ō-dī-ag-nō′sis). **1.** A method of diagnosing acute or early *Trypanosoma cruzi* infection (Chagas disease) in humans. Infection-free (laboratory-reared) triatomine bugs are fed on the tissue of the suspected person and the trypanosome is identified by microscopic examination of the intestinal contents of the bug after a suitable incubation period. **2.** A similar method of biologic diagnosis based upon experimental exposure of a parasite-free normal host capable of allowing the organism in question to multiply, enabling it to be more easily and reliably detected.

xen·o·gen·e·ic (zen′ō-jĕ-nē′ik). Heterologous, with respect to tissue grafts, especially when donor and recipient belong to widely separated species. SYN xenogenic (2), xenogenous (2). [xeno- + G. *-gen*, producing]

xen·o·gen·ic (zen-ō-jen′ik). **1.** Originating outside of the organism, or from a foreign substance that has been introduced into the organism. SYN xenogenous (1). **2.** SYN xenogeneic. [xeno- + G. *-gen*, producing]

xe·nog·e·nous (zĕ-noj′ĕ-nŭs). **1.** SYN xenogenic (1). **2.** SYN xenogeneic.

xen·o·graft (zen′ō-graft). A graft transferred from an animal of one species to one of another species. SYN heterograft, heterologous graft, heteroplastic graft, xenogeneic graft.

xe·non (Xe) (zē′non). A gaseous element, atomic no. 54, atomic wt. 131.29; present in minute proportion (0.087 ppm) in the dry atmosphere; produces general anesthesia in concentrations of 70 vol.%. [G. *xenos*, a stranger]

xe·non-133 (¹³³Xe). A radioisotope of xenon with a gamma emission at 81 keV and a physical half-life of 5.243 days; used in the study of pulmonary function and organ blood flow.

xen·o·par·a·site (zen-ō-par′ă-sīt). An ecoparasite that becomes pathogenic in consequence of weakened resistance on the part of its host.

xen·o·pho·bia (zen-ō-fō′bē-ă). Morbid fear of strangers. [xeno- + G. *phobos*, fear]

xen·o·pho·nia (zen-ō-fō′nē-ă). A speech defect marked by an alteration in accent and intonation. [xeno- + G. *phōnē*, voice]

Xen·o·psyl·la (zen-op-sil′ă). The rat flea; a genus of fleas parasitic on the rat and involved in the transmission of bubonic plague. The species *X. cheopis* serves as a potent vector of *Yersinia pestis*, largely because its gut becomes "blocked" by a mass of *Y. pestis* cells that prevents the flea from feeding normally, so that it is inclined to attack humans and other hosts; it is an important source of infection in traditional epidemic areas such as India. *X. astia* and *X. braziliensis* are also efficient vectors of plague. [xeno- + G. *psylla*, flea]

xen·yl (zen′il). A radical consisting of biphenyl minus a hydrogen atom.

xe·ran·sis (zē-ran′sis). A gradual loss of moisture in the tissues. [G. *xēransis*, fr. *xēros*, dry]

xe·ran·tic (zē-ran′tik). Denoting xeransis.

xe·ra·sia (zē-rā′zē-ă). A condition of the hair characterized by dryness and brittleness. [G. *xērasia*, fr. *xēros*, dry]

△**xero-.** Dry. [G. *xeros*]

xe

xer·o·chi·lia (zēr-ō-kī′lē-ă). Dryness of lips. [xero- + G. *cheilos,* lip]

xe·ro·der·ma (zēr′ō-der′mă). A mild form of ichthyosis characterized by excessive dryness of the skin due to slight increase of the horny layer and diminished water content of the stratum corneum from decreased perspiration, wind, or low humidity; seen with aging, atopic dermatitis, vitamin A deficiency, etc. [xero- + G. *derma,* skin]

x. pigmento′sum [MIM*278700], an eruption of exposed skin occurring in childhood and characterized by photosensitivity with severe sunburn in infancy and the development of numerous pigmented spots resembling freckles, larger atrophic lesions eventually resulting in glossy white thinning of the skin surrounded by telangiectases, and multiple solar keratoses that undergo malignant change at an early age; results from several rare autosomal recessive complementation groups in which DNA repair processes are defective, so that they are more liable to chromosome breaks and cancerous change when exposed to ultraviolet light. Severe ophthalmic and neurologic abnormalities are also found. SEE ALSO De Sanctis-Cacchione *syndrome.*

xe·ro·gram (zē′rō-gram). SYN xeroradiograph.

xe·rog·ra·phy (zēr-og′ră-fē). SYN xeroradiography.

xe·ro·ma (zē-rō′mă). SYN xerophthalmia.

xe·ro·mam·mog·ra·phy (zēr′ō-mam-og′ră-fē). Examination of the breast by xeroradiography.

xe·ro·me·nia (zēr-ō-mē′nē-ă). Obsolete term for occurrence of the usual constitutional symptoms at the menstrual period without any show of blood. [xero- + G. *mēniaia,* menses]

xe·ro·myc·te·ria (zēr′ō-mik-tēr′ē-ă). Extreme dryness of the nasal mucous membrane. [xero- + G. *myktēr,* the nose]

xe·ro·pha·gia, xe·roph·a·gy (zēr-ō-fā′jē-ă, zēr-of′ă-jē). The eating of dry foodstuffs; subsisting on a dry diet. [xero- + G. *phagō,* to eat]

xe·roph·thal·mia (zēr-of-thal′mē-ă). Excessive dryness of the conjunctiva and cornea, which lose their luster and become keratinized; may be due to local disease or to a systemic deficiency of vitamin A. SYN conjunctivitis arida, xeroma, xerophthalmus. [xero- + G. *ophthalmos,* eye]

xe·roph·thal·mus (zēr′of-thal′mŭs). SYN xerophthalmia.

xe·ro·ra·di·o·graph (zē-rō-rā′dē-ō-graf). The permanent record made by xeroradiography. SYN xerogram.

xe·ro·ra·di·og·ra·phy (zē′rō-rā′dē-og′ră-fē). Radiography using a specially coated charged plate instead of x-ray film, and developing with a dry powder rather than liquid chemicals, and transferring the powder image onto paper for a permanent record; edge enhancement is inherent. SYN xerography.

xe·ro·sis (zē-rō′sis). Pathologic dryness of the skin (xeroderma), the conjunctiva (xerophthalmia), or mucous membranes. [xero- + G. -*osis,* condition]

x. parenchymato′sus, superficial drying of the conjunctiva due to diffuse scarring, with closure of the lacrimal gland openings.

xe·ro·sto·mia (zēr′ō-stō′mē-ă). A dryness of the mouth, having a varied etiology, resulting from diminished or arrested salivary secretion, or asialism. [xero- + G. *stoma,* mouth]

xe·rot·ic (zē-rot′ik). Dry; affected with xerosis.

xe·ro·trip·sis (zēr-ō-trip′sis). Dry friction. [xero- + G. *tripsis,* a rubbing, fr. *tribō,* to rub]

Xg blood group. See Blood Groups appendix.

X-in·ac·ti·va·tion. SYN lyonization.

△**xiph-.** SEE xipho-.

xiph·i·ster·nal (zif-i-ster′năl). Relating to the xiphoid process.

xiph·i·ster·num (zif′i-ster′nŭm). SYN xiphoid *process.* [xiphoid + G. *sternon,* chest]

△**xipho-, xiph-, xiphi-.** Xiphoid, usually the processus xyphoideus. [G. *xiphos,* sword]

xiph·o·cos·tal (zif′ō-kos′tăl). Relating to the xiphoid process and the ribs. [xipho- + L. *costa,* rib]

xiph·o·dyn·ia (zif-ō-din′ē-ă). Pain of a neuralgic character, in the region of the xiphoid cartilage. SEE ALSO hypersensitive xiphoid *syndrome.* SYN xiphoidalgia. [xipho- + G. *odynē,* pain]

xi·phoid (zi′foyd) [TA]. Sword-shaped; applied especially to the xiphoid process. SYN ensiform, gladiate, mucronate. [xipho- + G. *eidos,* appearance]

xi·phoi·dal·gia (zif-oy-dal′jē-ă). SYN xiphodynia. [xiphoid + G. *algos,* pain]

xi·phoi·di·tis (zif′oy-dī′tis). Inflammation of the xiphoid process of the sternum. [xiphoid + G. -*itis,* inflammation]

xi·phop·a·gus (zi-fop′ă-gŭs). Conjoined twins united in the region of the xiphoid process of the sternum. SEE conjoined *twins,* under *twin.* [xipho- + G. *pagos,* something fixed]

X-linked. Pertaining to genes borne on the X chromosome. Commonly but erroneously used synonymously with sex-linked, which would also comprise Y-linked traits.

XMP Abbreviation for *xanthosine* 5′-monophosphate.

x-o·mat (eks′ō-mat). A trade name (of Kodak) that has become the generic designation of an automatic processor for x-ray films.

x-ra·di·a·tion. Radiant energy from an x-ray tube. SEE ALSO x-ray.

x-ray. **1.** The ionizing electromagnetic radiation emitted from a highly evacuated tube, resulting from the excitation of the inner orbital electrons by the bombardment of the target anode with a stream of electrons from a heated cathode. SYN roentgen ray. Cf. glass *rays,* under *ray,* indirect *rays,* under *ray.* **2.** Ionizing electromagnetic radiation produced by the excitation of the inner orbital electrons of an atom by other processes, such as nuclear delay and its sequelae. **3.** SYN radiograph.

XTP Abbreviation for *xanthosine* 5′-triphosphate.

Xy Abbreviation for xylose.

Xyl Abbreviation for xylose.

△**xyl-, xylo-.** Wood, woody; xylose, xylene. [G. *xylon*]

xy·la·zine (zī′la-zēn). A sedative/hypnotic/anesthetic widely used in veterinary medicine and in laboratory animals.

xy·lene (zī′lēn). SYN xylol.

x. cyanol FF [C.I. 43535], an acidic triphenylmethane dye used for histochemical staining of hemoglobin peroxidase and as a tracking dye for DNA sequencing in electrophoresis.

xy·le·nol (zī′lĕ-nol). Occurring in six isomeric forms; used in the manufacture of coal tar disinfectants and synthetic resins. SYN dimethylphenol.

xy·li·dine (zī′li-dēn). Aminodimethylbenzene; used as a reagent and in the manufacture of dyes.

xy·li·tol (zī′li-tol). An optically inactive sugar alcohol; often used as a sugar substitute in diabetic diets; the synthesis of x. from L-xylulose is blocked in individuals with idiopathic pentosuria.

xy·li·tol de·hy·dro·gen·ase. SYN *xylulose* reductase.

△**xylo-.** SEE xyl-.

xy·lo·bi·ose (zī′lō-bī′ōs). A disaccharide of two xylose residues linked β1→4, both in pyranose rings.

xy·loi·din (zī-loy′din). SYN pyroxylin.

xy·lo·ke·tose (zī-lō-kē′tōs). SYN xylulose.

xy·lol (zī′lol). A volatile liquid obtained from coal tar, having physical and chemical properties similar to those of benzene; it occurs as three isomers; *m-, o-,* and *p-*xylol; used as a solvent, in the manufacture of chemicals and synthetic fibers, and in histology as a clearing agent. SYN dimethylbenzene, xylene.

xy·lo·met·az·o·line hy·dro·chlo·ride (zī′lō-mĕ-taz′ō-lēn). A sympathomimetic drug used as a nasal decongestant.

xy·lon·ic ac·id (zi′lon-ik). A mild oxidation product of xylose.

xy·lo·py·ra·nose (zī-lō-pir′ă-nōs). Xylose in pyranose form.

xy·lose (Xy, Xyl) (zī′lōs). An aldopentose, isomeric with ribose, obtained by fermentation or hydrolysis of naturally occurring carbohydrate substances, e.g., in wood fiber. An important dietary component for herbivores. The D-isomer is also known as wood or beechwood sugar. SYN uridine diphosphoxylose.

xy·lu·lose (zī′loo-lōs). *threo-*Pentulose; a 2-ketopentose. L-Xylulose appears in the urine in cases of essential pentosuria; it is also an intermediate in the glucuronate pathway. SYN xyloketose.

x. 5-phosphate, the D-isomer is an intermediate in the pentose phosphate pathway and in transketolization.

x. reductase, an enzyme that reversibly converts x. to xylitol using either NADH (D-x. reductase) or NADPH (L-x. reductase); a deficiency of the L form is seen in individuals with essential pentosuria. SYN xylitol dehydrogenase.

L-xy·lu·lo·su·ria (zī′loo-lō-soo′rē-ă). SYN essential *pentosuria*.

xy·lyl (zī′lil). The radical consisting of xylene (xylol) minus a hydrogen atom.

    x. bromide, the *o*-, *m*-, and *p*-forms are powerful lacrimators.

xy·lyl·ene (zī′li-lēn). The radical consisting of xylene (xylol) minus two hydrogen atoms.

xys·ma (ziz′mă). Membranous shreds in the feces. [G. filings, shavings, fr. *xyō,* to scrape]

xy

Y Symbol for yttrium; tyrosine; pyrimidine nucleoside.

y⁺ SEE system (5).

YAC Abbreviation for yeast artificial *chromosomes*, under *chromosome*.

YAG Abbreviation for yttrium-aluminum-garnet.

yang (yang). SEE yin-yang.

yang·go·na (yang′gō-nǎ). SYN yaqona.

ya·qo·na (ya′kōnǎ). A Fijian drink made from the powdered root of *Piper methysticum* (family Piperaceae); excessive drinking of it causes a state of hyperexcitability and a loss of power in the legs; chronic intoxication induces roughening of the skin and a state of debility. SEE ALSO methysticum. SYN kava (2), yanggona. [Fijian name]

yaw (yau). An individual lesion of the eruption of yaws.

mother y., a large granulomatous lesion, considered to be the primary inoculation lesion in yaws, most commonly present on the hand, leg, or foot. SYN buba madre, frambesioma, protopianoma.

yawn (yaun). **1.** To gape. **2.** An involuntary opening of the mouth, usually accompanied by inspiration; it may be a sign of drowsiness or of vital depression, as after hemorrhage, but is often caused by suggestion. [A.S. *gānian*]

yawn·ing. The act of producing a yawn. SYN oscitation.

yaws (yawz). An infectious tropical disease caused by *Treponema pertenue* and characterized by the development of crusted granulomatous ulcers on the extremities; may involve bone, but, unlike syphilis, does not produce central nervous system or cardiovascular pathology. SEE ALSO nonvenereal *syphilis*. SYN boubas, frambesia tropica, granuloma tropicum, mycosis framboesioides, pian, zymotic papilloma. [of Caribbean origin; similar to Calinago yaya, the disease]

bosch y., SYN *pian* bois.

bush y., SYN *pian* bois.

foot y., y. of the feet with keratoderma of the palms and soles and ulcer formation.

Yb Symbol for ytterbium.

year.

disability-adjusted life y.'s (DALYs), a measure of the burden of disease on a defined population, based on adjustment of life expectancy to allow for long-term disability as estimated from official statistics. SEE ALSO global *burden* of disease. [Developed c.1990 by C.L. Murray and A. Lopez for the Harvard University/WHO Global Burden of Disease study.]

y.'s of potential life lost (YPLL), measure of the relative impact of various diseases and lethal forces on society, computed by estimating the years that people would have lived if they had not died prematurely from injury, cancer, heart disease, or other causes.

▣yeast (yēst). A general term denoting true fungi of the family Saccharomycetaceae that are widely distributed in substrates that contain sugars (such as fruits), and in soil, animal excreta, the vegetative parts of plants, etc. Because of their ability to ferment carbohydrates, some y.'s are important to the brewing and baking industries. [A.S. *gyst*]

brewers' y., y. produced by *Saccharomyces cerevisiae;* a by-product from the brewing of beer.

compressed y., the moist living cells of *Saccharomyces cerevisiae* combined with a starchy or absorbent base.

cultivated y., a form of y. propagated by culture and used in breadmaking, brewing, etc.

dried y., the dry cells of a suitable strain of *Saccharomyces cerevisiae;* brewers' dried y., debittered brewers' dried y., or primary dried y. are the sources of dried y.; it contains not less than 45% of protein, and in 1 g not less than 0.3 mg of nicotinic acid, 0.04 mg riboflavin, and 0.12 mg thiamin hydrochloride; used as a dietary supplement.

primary dried y., a source of dried y.; obtained from suitable strains of *Saccharomyces cerevisiae* grown in media other than those required for the production of beer.

wild y., any of the uncultivated forms of y.'s, useless as ferments and sometimes pathogenic.

yel·low (yel′ō). A color occupying a position in the spectrum between green and orange. For individual yellow dyes see specific name. [A.S. *geolu*]

corralin y., the sodium salt of rosolic acid.

indicator y., a compound formed in the bleaching of rhodopsin by light; it is chrome y. at pH 3.3–4.0 and pale y. at pH 9.0–10.0.

tumeric yellow, SYN curcumin.

visual y., SYN all-*trans*-retinal.

yel·low root. SYN hydrastis.

yer·ba san·ta (yer′bǎ san′tǎ). SYN eriodictyon. [Sp. sacred herb]

Yer·sin·ia (yer-sin′ē-ǎ). A genus of motile and nonmotile, non-spore-forming bacteria (family Enterobacteriaceae) containing Gram-negative, unencapsulated, ovoid to rod-shaped cells; Y. are nonmotile at 37°C, but some species are motile at temperatures below 30°C; motile cells are peritrichous; citrate is not used as a sole source of carbon; these organisms are parasitic on humans and other animals; the type species is *Y. pestis.* [A. J. E. *Yersin,* Swiss bacteriologist, 1862–1943]

Y. enterocolit′ica, a bacterial species that causes yersiniosis in humans; it is found in the feces and lymph nodes of sick and healthy animals, including humans, in material likely to be contaminated with feces, and in the cadavers of cattle, rabbits, hares, dogs, guinea pigs, horses, monkeys, pigs, and sheep; it replicates at refrigerator temperatures and has been associated with contamination of blood and blood products.

Y. frederikse′nii, reclassified from *Y. enterocolitica;* rare cause of enterocolitis in humans.

Y. interme′dia, reclassified from *Y. enterocolitica;* rare cause of enterocolitis in humans.

Y. kristense′nii, reclassified from *Y. enterocolitica;* pathogenicity uncertain.

Y. pes′tis, a bacterial species causing plague in humans, rodents, and many other mammalian species and transmitted from rat to rat and from rat to humans by the rat flea, *Xenopsylla;* it is the type species of the genus *Y.* SYN Kitasato bacillus, *Pasteurella pestis,* plague bacillus.

Y. pseudotuberculo′sis, a bacterial species causing pseudotuberculosis in birds, rodents, and, rarely, in humans. SYN *Pasteurella pseudotuberculosis.*

yer·sin·i·o·sis (yer-sin-ē-ō′sis). A common human infectious disease caused by *Yersinia enterocolitica* and marked by diarrhea, enteritis, pseudoappendicitis, ileitis, erythema nodosum, and sometimes septicemia or acute arthritis.

pseudotubercular y., SYN pseudotuberculosis.

yield (yēld). The amount or quantity produced or returned, often measured as a percentage of the starting material; e.g., a y. in an enzyme preparation is equal to the units of enzyme activity recovered at the end of the preparation divided by the total units observed in the starting material.

quantum y. (φ), the number of molecules transformed (e.g., via a reaction) per quantum of light absorbed; the inverse of the quantum requirement. SYN quantum efficiency.

yin-yang (yin′yang). In ancient Chinese thought, the concept of two complementary and opposing influences, Yin and Yang, underlying and controlling all nature, the aim of Chinese medicine

---

△ Combining Forms	☆ Official alternate Terminologia Anatomica term
▣ Indicates term is illustrated, see Illustration Index	
	[MIM] Mendelian Inheritance in Man
SYN Synonym	
Cf. Compare	C.I. Colour Index
[NA] Nomina Anatomica	
[TA] Terminologia Anatomica	**High Profile Term**

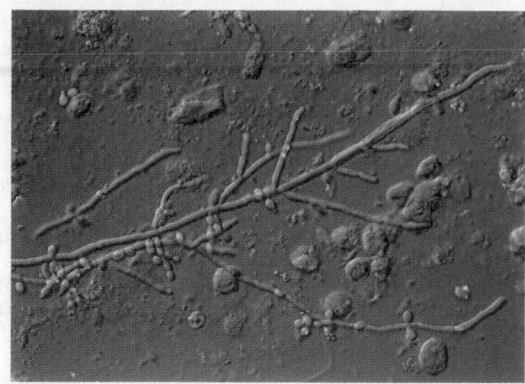

yeast

being to produce proper balance between them. Used in modern terms to characterize any dualistic, reciprocal control system in which one influence tends to promote things that the opposing influence tends to inhibit, and vice versa; e.g., the yin-yang hypothesis of biologic control in which cyclic GMP and cyclic AMP are supposed to act in this dualistic, reciprocal way in controlling cellular functions.

-yl. Chemical suffix signifying that the substance is a radical by loss of an H atom (e.g., alkyl, methyl, phenyl) or OH group (e.g., acyl, acetyl, carbamoyl).

-ylene. Chemical suffix denoting a bivalent hydrocarbon radical (e.g., methylene, $-CH_2-$) or possessing a double bond (e.g., ethylene, $CH_2=CH_2$).

yl·ides (il′idz). A class of compounds in which a positively charged negative element from group V or VI of the periodic table (e.g., N, O, S, P) is bonded to a carbon atom having an unshared pair of electrons; ylides have been observed in a number of enzyme-catalyzed reactions.

Y-link·age. The state of a genetic factor (gene) being borne on the Y chromosome. This idea is analogous with X-linkage, but since the Y chromosome does not fully take part in chiasma formation and recombination, it is not amenable to analysis by conventional linkage methods. Little is known about its content. There is a gene for the H-Y antigen, and indirect arguments suggest that there is a principle that determines the formation of the testis and masculinization of the fetus but its localization, though narrowing the limits, remains elusive.

yo·gurt, yo·ghurt (yō′gert). Fermented, partially evaporated, whole milk prepared by maintaining it at 50°C for 12 hours after the addition of a mixed culture of *Lactobacillus bulgaricus*, *L. acidophilus*, and *Streptococcus lactis;* used as a food. [Turkish]

yo·him·bine (yō-him′bēn). An alkaloid, the active principle of yohimbé, the bark of *Corynanthe yohimbi* (family Rubiaceae); it produces a competitive blockade, of limited duration, of adrenergic α-receptors; has also been used for its alleged aphrodisiac properties.

yoke (yōk) [TA]. SYN jugum (1). [A.S. *geoc*]

   alveolar y.'s [TA], one of the eminences on the outer surface of the alveolar process of the maxilla or mandible, formed by the roots of the incisor teeth. SYN juga alveolaria [TA].

   sphenoidal y., [☆]official alternate term for *jugum* sphenoidale.

yolk (yōk, yōlk). **1.** One of the types of nutritive material stored in the ovum for the nutrition of the embryo; y. is particularly abundant and conspicuous in the eggs of birds. SYN vitellus. **2.** Fatty material found in the wool of sheep; when extracted and purified, it becomes lanolin. [A.S. *geolca; geolu,* yellow]

   white y., y. consisting of much finer particles than those of yellow y.; thin layers of it lie between the zones of yellow y. and form the latebra.

   yellow y., the chief constituent of the y. in a bird's egg; it consists of relatively coarse particles of stored food materials and is laid down in concentric zones with interposed thin layers of white y.

Yorke au·to·lyt·ic re·ac·tion. See under reaction.

Young, Hugh H., U.S. urologist, 1870–1945. SEE Y. prostatic *tractor.*

Young, William John, 20th century Australian biochemist. SEE Harden-Y. *ester.*

Young, Thomas, English physician and physicist, 1773–1829. SEE Y. *modulus, rule;* Y.-Helmholtz *theory* of color vision.

YPLL Abbreviation for *years* of potential life lost, under *year.*

yp·sil·i·form (ip′si-li-fōrm). SYN hypsiloid. [G. *ypsilon, upsilon,* the letter u or y, + L. *forma,* form]

yt·ter·bi·um (Yb) (i-ter′bē-ŭm). A metallic element of the lanthanide group; atomic no. 70, atomic wt. 173.04. ¹⁶⁹Yb, with a half-life of 32.03 days, has been used in cisternography and in brain scans. [*Ytterby,* village in Sweden]

yt·tri·um (Y) (it′rē-ŭm). A metallic element, atomic no. 39, atomic wt. 88.90585. [*Ytterby,* village in Sweden]

yt·tri·um-90. An artificial radioactive isotope with a physical half-life of 2.67 days, which decays with the emission of a 2.282 MeV β particle; used as an implant in pituitary ablation.

Yvon, Paul, French physician and chemist, 1848–1913. SEE Y. *test.*

Yv

Z Abbreviation for benzyloxycarbonyl (carbobenzoxy-); symbol for an amino acid that is either glutamic acid, glutamine, or a substance that yields glutamic acid on acid hydrolysis of peptides (e.g., 4-carboxyglutamate or 5-oxoproline); carbobenzoxy; in italics, zusammen.

Z Abbreviation for atomic *number*.

z Abbreviation for zepto-.

Zaffaroni, Alejandro, Uruguayan-U.S. chemist and biochemist, *1923. SEE Zaffaroni *system*.

zafirlukast (za-fir-loo′kast). A blocker of leukotriene D$_4$ and E$_4$ (LTD$_4$ and LTE$_4$) components of a slow-reacting substance of anaphylaxis (SRSA); used for the prophylaxis of asthma attacks.

Zaglas, John, 19th century anatomist's assistant in Edinburgh. SEE Z. *ligament*.

Zahn, Friedrich W., German pathologist, 1845–1904. SEE Z. *infarct; lines* of Z., under *line; striae* of Z. under *stria*.

Zambusch, Leo von, 20th century German physician. SEE generalized pustular *psoriasis* of Z.

zanamivir (zan-am′ĭ-vir). An agent that inhibits neuraminidase of influenza virus.

Zappert, Julius, Austrian physician, 1867–1942. SEE Z. counting *chamber*.

Zavanelli, William, 20th century U.S. obstetrician. SEE Z. *maneuver*.

zea (zē′ă). The styles and stigmas of *Zea mays* (family Gramineae), Indian corn; formerly used as a diuretic and antispasmodic. SYN cornsilk. [Mod. L. maize]

ze·a·ral·e·none (zē′ă-ral-en-ōn). One of the resorcylic acid lactones; used in veterinary medicine as an anabolic.

ze·a·tin (zē′ă-tin). A cytokinin first isolated from kernels of sweet corn. SYN maize factor.

ze·a·xan·thin (zē′ă-zan′thin). A carotene found in corn, fruits, seeds, and egg yolk; isomeric with xanthophyll. SYN zeaxanthol. [Mod. L. *Zea*, Indian corn, fr. L. *zea*, grain + G. *xanthos*, yellow, + -in]

ze·ax·an·thol (zē-ă-za-thol). SYN zeaxanthin.

Zeeman, Pieter, Dutch physicist and Nobel laureate, 1865–1943. SEE Z. *effect*.

ZEEP Abbreviation for zero end-expiratory *pressure*.

ze·in (zē′in). A prolamine present in maize; it lacks chiefly the amino acids L-tryptophan and L-lysine and is also low in cysteine content. It is the main storage protein in maize.

Zeis, Eduard, Dresden ophthalmologist, 1807–1868. SEE Z. *glands*, under *gland; zeisian sty*.

zeis·i·an (zīs′ē-ăn). Relating to or described by Eduard Zeis.

Zeit·geist (zīt′gīst). In psychology, the climate of opinion, conventions of thought, covert influences, and unquestioned assumptions that are implicit in a given culture, the arts, or science at any point in time, and in which the individual operates and thus is influenced. [Ger. *zeit*, time, + *geist*, spirit]

Zellweger, Hans U., U.S. pediatrician, 1909–1990. SEE Z. *syndrome*.

ze·lo·pho·bia (zē-lō-fō′bē-ă). Morbid fear of jealousy. [G. *zēlos*, zeal, + *phobos*, fear]

ze·lo·typ·ia (zē-lō-tip′ē-ă). Excessive zeal, carried to the point of morbidity, in the advocacy of any cause. [G. *zēlotypia*; rivalry, envy, fr. *zēlos*, zeal, + *typtō*, to strike]

Zenker, Friedrich A., German pathologist, 1825–1898. SEE Z. *degeneration, diverticulum, fixative, paralysis*; formol-Z. *fixative*.

ze·o·lite (zē′ō-līt). A naturally occurring hydrated sodium aluminum silicate, Na$_2$O·Al$_2$O$_3$·(SiO$_2$)$_x$·(H$_2$O)$_x$, used for softening of hard water by exchanging its Na$^+$ for the Ca^{2+} of the water; thus z. is an ion exchanger. Some synthetic ion exchangers are termed synthetic z.'s, although there is no chemical relationship.

ze·o·scope (zē′ō-skōp). A device for determining the alcoholic content of a liquid by ascertaining its exact boiling point. [G. *zeō*, to boil, + *skopeō*, to examine]

zep·to- (z). Prefix used in the SI and metric systems to signify submultiples of 10^{-21}.

ze·ro (zē′rō). **1.** The figure 0, indicating the absence of magnitude, or nothing. **2.** In thermometry, the point from which the figures on the scale start in one or the other direction; in the Celsius and Réaumur scales, z. indicates the freezing point for distilled water; in the Fahrenheit scale, it is 32° below the freezing point of water. [Sp. fr. Ar. *sifr*, cipher]

absolute z., the lowest possible temperature, that at which the form of translational motion constituting heat is assumed no longer to exist, determined as −273.15°C or 0 kelvin.

ze·ro grav·i·ty (zē-rō-grav′i-tē). A physical state existing in space or at a time in flight when the centrifugal thrust of a parabolic glide or turn exactly counteracts the force of gravity.

ze·ta (zāt′a). **1.** The sixth letter of the Greek alphabet, ζ. **2.** In chemistry, denotes the sixth in a series, e.g., the sixth carbon from a functional group. **3.** Symbol for electrokinetic potential.

ze·ta·crit (zā′tă-krit). The packed cell volume produced by vertical centrifugation of blood in capillary tubes, allowing controlled compaction and dispersion of red blood cells; read with a hematocrit to produce the zeta sedimentation ratio.

ze·ta·pro·tein. SYN fibronectins.

zeug·ma·tog·ra·phy (zoog-mă-tog′ră-fē). Term coined by Lauterbur in 1972 for the joining of a magnetic field and spatially defined radiofrequency field gradients to generate a two-dimensional display of proton density and relaxation times in tissues, the first nuclear magnetic resonance image. [G. *zeugma*, that which joins together]

zi·do·vu·dine (zī-dō′voo-dēn). A thymidine analog that is an inhibitor of in vitro replication of HIV virus, the causative agent of AIDS and ARC, and is used in the management of these diseases. SYN azidothymidine.

Ziegler, Samuel L., U.S. ophthalmologist, 1861–1926.

Ziehen, Georg T., German psychiatrist, 1862–1950. SEE Z.-Oppenheim *disease*.

Ziehl, Franz, German bacteriologist, 1857–1926. SEE Z. *stain*; Z.-Neelsen *stain*.

Ziemann, Hans R.P., German pathologist, 1865–1939. SEE Z. *dots*, under *dot, stippling*.

Zieve, Leslie, U.S. physician, *1915. SEE Z. *syndrome*.

Zimmerlin, Franz, Swiss physician, 1858–1932. SEE Z. *atrophy*.

Zimmermann, Karl W., German histologist, 1861–1935. SEE Z. *corpuscle, granule*, elementary *particle*; polkissen of Z.

Zimmermann, Wilhelm, German physician, *1910. SEE Z. *reaction, test*.

zinc (Zn) (zingk). A metallic element, atomic no. 30, atomic wt. 65.39; an essential bioelement; a number of salts of z. are used in medicine; a cofactor in many proteins. [Ger. *Zink*]

z. acetate, an emetic, styptic, and astringent.

z. caprylate, a topical antifungal compound.

z. chloride, ZnCl$_2$; formerly used as a caustic for the removal of cutaneous cancers, nevi, etc., and in weak solution in the treatment of gonorrhea and conjunctivitis. SYN butter of zinc.

z. gelatin, z. oxide, gelatin, glycerin, and purified water; used topically as a protectant.

z. iodide, ZnI$_2$; has been used as an antiseptic and astringent.

medicinal z. peroxide, a mixture of z. peroxide, z. carbonate, and z. hydroxide; a topical disinfectant, astringent, and deodorant.

△ Combining Forms	☆ Official alternate Terminologia Anatomica term
▤ Indicates term is illustrated, see Illustration Index	
	[MIM] Mendelian Inheritance in Man
SYN Synonym	
Cf. Compare	C.I. Colour Index
[NA] Nomina Anatomica	
[TA] Terminologia Anatomica	**High Profile Term**

z. oxide, ZnO; used as a protective in ointment, as a dusting powder; also used in paint as a substitute for lead carbonate. SYN flowers of zinc, z. white.

z. oxide and eugenol, used as a base material beneath metallic dental restorations and as a temporary filling material or impression material; setting and hardening result from complex reactions between the powder and the eugenol.

z. permanganate, action is similar to that of potassium permanganate, but more astringent; used in urethritis, by injection or douche in a 1:4000 solution.

z. peroxide, ZnO_2; a yellowish white powder, insoluble in water and decomposed by acids; used in pharmaceutic preparations. SYN z. superoxide.

z. phenolsulfonate, used as an intestinal antiseptic and locally as an astringent in chronic inflammation of the mucous membranes. SYN z. sulfocarbolate.

z. phosphide, Zn_3P_2; used as a bait poison for the extermination of rats and mice.

z. stearate, a z. compound with variable proportions of stearic and palmitic acids; a water-repellent, protective agent used in powders and ointments in the treatment of eczema, acne, and other skin diseases.

z. sulfate, used as a local astringent in the treatment of gonorrhea, indolent ulcers, conjunctivitis, and various skin diseases, and internally as an emetic.

z. sulfocarbolate, SYN z. phenolsulfonate.

z. superoxide, SYN z. peroxide.

z. undecylenate, z. undecenoate, the z. salt of undecylenic acid; used in the treatment of fungal and other affections of the skin, including psoriasis.

z. white, SYN z. oxide.

zinc-65 (^{65}**Zn**). A radioactive zinc isotope that decays mainly by K-capture with a half-life of 243.8 days; used as a tracer in studies of zinc metabolism.

zinc·if·er·ous (zing-kif′er-ŭs). Containing zinc.

zinc·oid (zing′koyd). Relating to or resembling zinc. [G. *eidos,* resemblance]

zin·gi·ber (zin′ji-ber). SYN ginger.

Zinn, Johann G., German anatomist, 1727–1759. SEE Z. *artery,* vascular *circle, corona, ligament, membrane, ring, tendon, zonule.*

Zinsser, Hans, U.S. bacteriologist and immunologist, 1878–1940. SEE Brill-Z. *disease.*

zir·co·ni·um (Zr) (zir-kō′nē-ŭm). A metallic element, atomic no. 40, atomic wt. 91.224; widely distributed in nature, but never found in quantity in any one place. [*zircon,* a mineral, fr. Ar. *zarkūn,* cinnabar, Pers, *zargun,* goldlike]

zir·co·ni·um ox·ide. Used as a coating for the skin in dermatologic pharmaceuticals and as a pigment in paints.

zm Abbreviation for zeptometer.

Zn Symbol for zinc.

^{65}**Zn** Abbreviation for zinc-65.

Zo$_2$ Symbol for microliters of oxygen taken up per hour by 10^8 spermatozoa; can vary as a function of temperature.

zo-. SEE ZOO-.

zo·an·throp·ic (zō-an-throp′ik). Relating to or marked by zoanthropy.

zo·an·thro·py (zō-an′thrō-pē). A delusion that one is an animal, such as a dog. [G. *zōon,* animal, + *anthrōpos,* man]

zo·et·ic (zō-et′ik). Relating to life. [G. *zōē,* life]

zo·ic (zō′ik). Relating to living things; having life. [G. *zōikos,* relating to an animal]

zo·ite (zō′īt). SYN sporozoite. [G. *zōon,* animal]

Zollinger, Robert M., U.S. surgeon, *1903. SEE Z.-Ellison *syndrome, tumor.*

Zöllner, Johann F., German physicist, 1834–1882. SEE Z. *lines,* under *line.*

zol·pi·dem (zol′pē-děm). A sedative/hypnotic drug useful for treating anxiety and resembling benzodiazepines in its pharmacology but differing somewhat in chemical structure. Unlike benzodiazepines, z. lacks prominent anticonvulsant properties, and less tolerance may develop with its use.

zo·me·pir·ac so·di·um (zō-mě-pir′ak). An analgesic anti-inflammatory agent, no longer marketed.

zo·na, pl. **zo·nae** (zō′nă, zō′nē) [TA]. **1.** SYN zone. **2.** SYN *herpes* zoster. [L. fr. G. *zōnē,* a girdle, one of the zones of the sphere]

z. arcua′ta, SYN arcuate *zone.*

z. cilia′ris, SYN ciliary *zone.*

z. coro′na, SYN costal *fringe.*

z. dermat′ica, a ridge of thickened skin surrounding the protrusion in spina bifida.

z. epitheliosero′sa, the membranous ring, within the z. dermatica, surrounding the protrusion in spina bifida.

z. externa medullae renalis [TA], SYN outer *zone* of renal medulla.

z. fascicula′ta, the layer of radially arranged cell cords in the cortical portion of the suprarenal gland, between the z. glomerulosa and z. reticularis; secretes cortisol and dehydroepiandrosterone.

z. glomerulo′sa, the outer layer of the cortex of the suprarenal gland just beneath the capsule; secretes aldosterone.

z. hemorrhoida′lis, SYN hemorrhoidal *zone.*

zonae hypothalamicae [TA], SYN *zones* of hypothalamus, under *zone.*

z. incer′ta [TA], a flat, obliquely disposed plate of gray matter in the subthalamic region situated between the thalamic fasciculus (tegmental field H$_1$ of Forel) and the lenticular fasciculus (tegmental field H$_2$). Medially, cells of this nucleus are adjacent to the prerubral area (tegmental field H) and, laterally, they are continuous with the reticular nucleus of the thalamus. Z. i. is a derivative of the ventral thalamus; it receives afferents from the precentral motor cortex and the cerebellum.

z. interna medullae renalis [TA], SYN inner *zone* of renal medulla.

z. lateralis [TA], SYN lateral *zone*; SEE *zones* of hypothalamus, under *zone.*

z. medialis [TA], SYN medial *zone*; SEE *zones* of hypothalamus, under *zone.*

z. medullovasculo′sa, the fissured segment of the spinal cord that dorsally closes the sac in meningomyelocele.

z. ophthal′mica, herpes zoster in the distribution of the ophthalmic nerve.

z. orbicula′ris (articulationis coxae) [TA], fibers of the articular capsule of the hip joint encircling the neck of the femur. SYN orbicular zone of hip joint, ring ligament, zonular band.

z. pectina′ta, SYN pectinate *zone.*

z. pellu′cida, an extracellular coat, rich in glycoprotein, surrounding the oocyte; it contains microvilli of the oocyte and cellular processes of follicular cells and appears homogeneous and translucent under the light microscope. SYN pellucid zone.

z. perfora′ta, SYN *foramina* nervosa, under *foramen.*

z. periventricularis [TA], SYN periventricular *zone*; SEE *zones* of hypothalamus, under *zone.*

z. pupilla′ris, SYN pupillary *zone.*

z. radia′ta, SYN z. striata.

z. reticula′ris, the inner layer of the cortex of the adrenal gland, where the cell cords anastomose in a netlike fashion.

z. stria′ta, the thickened cell membrane of the ovum in forms, such as certain amphibia, in which it appears radially striated under the light microscope; with the electron microscope the striations can be seen to be microvilli. SYN membrana striata, striated membrane, z. radiata.

z. tec′ta, SYN arcuate *zone.*

z. transitionalis analis [TA], SYN anal transitional *zone.*

z. vasculo′sa, SYN vascular *zone.*

zon·al (zō′năl). Relating to a zone.

zo·na·ry (zō′nar-ē). Relating to or having the form of a zone or belt.

zon·ate (zō′năt). Zoned; ringed; having concentric layers of differing texture or pigmentation.

ZO

ZONE

zone (zōn) [TA]. A segment; any encircling or beltlike structure, either external or internal, longitudinal or transverse. SEE ALSO area, band, region, space, spot. SYN zona (1) [TA]. [L. *zona*]

abdominal z.'s, SYN abdominal *regions*, under *region*.

anal transitional z. [TA], region of anal canal in which the epithelium changes from the simple columnar epithelium of a mucosa to the stratified squamous epithelium of the anoderm (skin); this region is susceptible to a variety of carcinomas. SYN zona transitionalis analis [TA].

androgenic z., (1) SYN X z. (1); (2) SYN fetal reticularis (2). SYN fetal adrenal *cortex*. [Named in the belief (as yet unsubstantiated) that the cells within this zone secrete androgens.]

arcuate z., the inner third of the basilar membrane of the cochlear duct extending from the tympanic lip of the osseous spiral lamina to the outer pillar cell of the spiral organ (of Corti). SYN zona arcuata, zona tecta.

Barnes z., the lower fourth of the pregnant uterus, attachment of the placenta to any part of which may cause dangerous hemorrhage. SYN cervical z.

cervical z., SYN Barnes z.

cervical z. of tooth, SYN *neck* of tooth.

ciliary z., the outer, wider z. of the anterior surface of the iris, separated from the pupillary z. by the collarette. SYN zona ciliaris.

comfort z., the temperature range between 28°C and 30°C at which the naked body is able to maintain the heat balance without either shivering or sweating; in the clothed body the range is from 13°C to 21°C.

z.'s of discontinuity, concentric z.'s of varying optical density in the lens of the eye, as seen in slitlamp biomicroscopy.

dolorogenic z., SYN trigger *point*.

entry z., the area of the dorsal funiculus of the spinal cord, medial to the tip of the posterior horn, in which the entering fibers of the posterior nerve root divide into ascending and descending branches.

ependymal z., SYN ependymal *layer*.

epileptogenic z., a cortical region that on stimulation reproduces the patient's spontaneous seizure or aura.

equivalence z., in a precipitin reaction, the z. in which neither antibody nor antigen is in excess. SEE ALSO precipitation. SYN equivalence point.

erogenous z.'s, erotogenic z.'s, areas of the body, such as genitals and nipples, which elicit sexual arousal when stimulated.

fetal z., SYN fetal adrenal *cortex*.

gingival z., that portion of the oral mucosa which surrounds the teeth and is firmly attached to the underlying alveolar bone.

Golgi z., (1) part of the cytoplasm occupied by the Golgi apparatus; (2) in secretory cells of exocrine glands, a z. between the nucleus and the luminal surface.

grenz z. (grents), in histopathology, a narrow layer beneath the epidermis that is not infiltrated or involved in the same way as are the lower layers of the dermis. [Ger. *Grenze,* borderline, boundary]

Head z.'s, SYN Head *lines*, under *line*.

hemorrhoidal z., the part of the anal canal that contains the rectal venous plexus. SYN anulus hemorrhoidalis, zona hemorrhoidalis.

z.'s of hypothalamus [TA], rostrocaudally oriented regions of the hypothalamus characterized by their position and cell groups. The periventricular z. [TA] (zona periventricularis [TA]) is a thin sheet of small neurons located in the wall of the third ventricle. The medial z. [TA] (zona medialis [TA]) lies between the periventricular z. and a rostrocaudal line drawn between the mammillothalamic tract and the postcommissural fornix, and consists of supraoptic, tuberal, and mammillary regions. The lateral z. [TA] (zona lateralis [TA]) is lateral to the medial zones, and contains the tuberal nuclei and the fibers of the medial forebrain bundle. SYN zonae hypothalamicae [TA].

inner z. of renal medulla [TA], apical portion of renal pyramids, including renal papilla. SYN zona interna medullae renalis [TA].

intermediate z. [TA], SYN intermediate *column*.

intermediate z. of iliac crest [TA], the line on the crest of the ilium between the outer and inner lips, for origin of internal oblique muscle. SYN linea intermedia cristae iliacae [TA], intermediate line of iliac crest.

interpalpebral z., the exposed area of the cornea and sclera between the lids of the open eye.

intertubular z., the dentinal matrix that lies between z.'s of peritubular dentin; it is less calcified and contains larger collagen fibers than does peritubular dentin.

isoelectric z., the range of H+ ion concentration (pH) over which isoelectric precipitation occurs.

isopycnic z., the region in density gradient centrifugation having the same density as the buoyant density of the macromolecule.

language z., a large area of the cerebral cortex on the left side (in right-handed persons) considered by some to embrace all the centers of memories and associations connected with language.

latent z., that portion of the cerebral cortex, the stimulation of which produces no movement and a lesion of which produces no symptoms; mainly the more anterior areas of the frontal lobes.

lateral z. [TA], SEE z.'s of hypothalamus. SYN zona lateralis [TA].

Lissauer marginal z., SYN dorsolateral *fasciculus*.

Looser z.'s, SYN Looser *lines*, under *line*.

mantle z., (1) SYN mantle *layer*; (2) a layer of small B lymphocytes surrounding the paler-staining germinal centers of lymphoid follicles.

Marchant z., the area on the sphenoid and occipital bones at the base of the skull from which the dura mater is readily detached.

marginal z., (1) A z. between the red and white pulp of the spleen containing numerous macrophages and a rich plexus of sinusoids supplied by white pulp arterioles carrying blood-borne antigens. (2) SYN marginal *layer*.

medial z. [TA], SEE z.'s of hypothalamus. SYN zona medialis [TA].

motor z., that portion of the cerebral cortex, primarily the posterior region of the frontal lobe, near the central sulcus, which when stimulated produces a movement and when injured produces spasticity or paralysis.

neutral z., in dentistry, the potential space between the lips and cheeks on one side and the tongue on the other; natural or artificial teeth in this z. are subject to equal and opposite forces from the surrounding musculature.

nucleolar z., SYN nucleolar *organizer*.

Obersteiner-Redlich z., the narrow line along the course of a nerve (or nerve root) where the Schwann cells and connective tissue that support its axons are replaced by glia cells. The z. marks the true boundary between the central and the peripheral nervous system. Usually located at or near the surface of the spinal cord or brainstem, it can extend (e.g., in the eighth nerve) several millimeters out along the nerve. SYN Obersteiner-Redlich line.

orbicular z. of hip joint, SYN *zona* orbicularis (articulationis coxae).

outer z. of renal medulla [TA], basal portion of renal pyramid. SYN zona externa medullae renalis [TA].

pectinate z., the outer two-thirds of the basilar membrane of the cochlear duct. SYN zona pectinata.

pellucid z., SYN *zona* pellucida.

peritubular z., the dentinal matrix surrounding the odontoblastic process; it is more highly calcified and contains finer collagen fibers than does the rest of the dentinal matrix.

periventricular z. [TA], SEE z.'s of hypothalamus. SYN zona periventricularis [TA].

polar z., the region in the vicinity of an electrode applied to the body. SEE ALSO electrotonus.

protective z., the time in the cardiac cycle, immediately following the vulnerable period, during which a second stimulus will prevent the initiation of ventricular fibrillation by a previous stimulus applied during the vulnerable period, probably by blocking a reentrant pathway.

pupillary z., the central region of the anterior surface of the iris located between the collarette and the pupillary margin. SYN zona pupillaris.

reflexogenic z., the area or z. where stimulation will elicit a given reflex.

secondary X z., an adrenocortical z., situated in the inner zona fasciculata, that appears upon postpubertal gonadectomy in some male rodents, most notably the mouse; the development of this z. is believed to be stimulated by pituitary gonadotropins.

segmental z., in a young embryo, the thickened dorsal portion of the undifferentiated paraxial mesoderm that becomes metamerically divided to form the mesodermal somites. SYN segmental plate.

Spitzka marginal z., SYN dorsolateral *fasciculus.*

subplasmalemmal dense z., SYN corneocyte *envelope.*

sudanophobic z., a z. of cells, at the periphery of the zona fasciculata in the adrenal cortex of the rat, that is not stained by Sudan dyes.

tender z.'s, SYN Head *lines,* under *line.*

thymus-dependent z., SYN paracortex.

trabecular z., SYN trabecular *tissue* of sclera.

transformation z., z. on the cervix at which squamous epithelium and columnar epithelium meet; changes location in response to a woman's hormonal status.

transitional z., (1) the equatorial region of the lens of the eye where the anterior epithelial cells become transformed into lens fibers; (2) that portion of a scleral contact lens between the corneal and scleral sections.

transitional z. of lips [TA], hairless thin skin beginning at the vermillion border of the lips; appears red because of underlying capillary bed.

trigger z., SYN trigger *point.*

trophotropic z. of Hess, an area in the hypothalamus concerned with rewarding bodily sensations.

vascular z., an area in the external acoustic meatus where a number of minute blood vessels enter from the mastoid bone. SYN spongy spot, zona vasculosa.

vermilion z., vermilion transitional z., SYN vermilion *border.*

Weil basal z., SYN Weil basal *layer.*

Wernicke z., SYN Wernicke *center.*

z. 1, 2, 3, 4 of West, in pulmonary physiology, defines the levels in a vertical lung according to the relationships of alveolar gas pressure, capillary blood pressure, and pulmonary venous pressure.

X z., (1) a transient adrenocortical z. present in some rodents at birth, most notably in mice, situated between the zona reticularis and the adrenal medulla; it degenerates in males with the secretion at puberty and in females during their first pregnancy; it slowly enlarges in unmated females after puberty and does not degenerate until middle age; the X z. appears to secrete no hormone; SYN androgenic z. (1). **(2)** misnomer for the fetal adrenal *cortex* of primates. SYN fetal reticularis (3).

zo·nes·the·sia (zōn-es-thē'zē-ă). A sensation as if a cord were drawn around the body, constricting it. SYN girdle sensation, strangalesthesia. [G. *zōnē,* girdle, + *aisthēsis,* sensation]

zon·ing (zōn'ing). The occurrence of a stronger reaction in a lesser amount of suspected serum, observed sometimes in serologic tests used in the diagnosis of syphilis, and probably the result of high antibody titer.

zon·og·ra·phy (zō-nog'ră-fē). A form of tomography with a relatively thick plane of focus; especially used in renal radiography. [zone + G. *graphō,* to write]

zo·no·skel·e·ton (zō'nō-skel'ĕ-tŏn). The proximal skeletal segments of the limbs, i.e., scapula, clavicle, hip *bone.* [L. *zona,* zone, + skeleton]

zo·nu·la, pl. **zo·nu·lae** (zō'nū-lă, zon'ū-; -lē). SYN zonule. [L. dim. of *zona,* zone]

z. adhe′rens, a beltlike desmosomal attachment between colum-

nar epithelial cells, upon which filaments attach. SYN intermediate junction.

z. cilia′ris [TA], SYN ciliary *zonule.*

z. occlu′dens, tight junctions formed by the fusion of integral proteins of the lateral cell membranes of adjacent epithelial cells, limiting transepithelial permeability. SYN impermeable junction, tight junction.

zo·nu·lar (zō'nū-lăr, zon'ū-). Relating to a zonula.

zon·ule (zō'nūl, zon'ūl). A small zone. SYN zonula.

ciliary z. [TA], a series of delicate meridional fibers arising from the inner surface of the orbiculus ciliaris that run in bundles between, and in a very thin layer over, the ciliary processes; at the inner border of the corona, the fibers diverge into two groups that are attached to the capsule on the anterior and posterior surfaces of the lens close to the equator; the spaces between these two layers of fibers are filled with aqueous humor. SYN zonula ciliaris [TA], apparatus suspensorius lentis, suspensory ligament of lens, Zinn z.

Zinn z., SYN ciliary z.

zo·nu·li·tis (zō-nū-lī'tis). Assumed inflammation of the zonule of Zinn, or suspensory ligament of the lens of the eye. [zonule + G. *-itis,* inflammation]

zo·nu·lol·y·sis, zo·nu·ly·sis (zō'nū-lol'i-sis, -lī'sis). Dissolution of the zonula ciliaris by enzymes (α-chymotrypsin) to facilitate surgical removal of a cataract. SYN Barraquer method. [zonule + G. *lysis,* dissolution]

△**zoo-, zo-.** Animal, animal life. [G. *zōon*]

zo·o·an·thro·po·no·sis (zō'ō-an'thrō-pō-nō'sis). A zoonosis normally maintained by humans but that can be transmitted to other vertebrates (e.g., amebiasis to dogs, tuberculosis). Cf. anthropozoonosis, amphixenosis. [zoo- + G. *anthrōpos,* man, + *nosos,* disease]

zo·o·blast (zō'-ō-blast). An animal cell. [zoo- + G. *blastos,* germ]

zo·o·chrome (zō'ō-krōm). A naturally occurring animal pigment; includes human pigments.

zo·o·der·mic (zō-ō-der'mik). Relating to the skin of an animal. [zoo- + G. *derma,* skin]

zo·o·e·ras·tia (zō'ō-ĕ-ras'tē-ă). SYN zoophilia. [zoo- + G. *erastēs,* lover]

zo·o·ful·vin (zō'ō-fŭl'vin). A yellow pigment obtained from the feathers of certain birds.

zo·o·gen·e·sis (zō-ō-jen'ĕ-sis). The doctrine of animal production or generation. [zoo- + G. *genesis,* origin]

zo·o·ge·og·ra·phy (zō'ō-jē-og'ră-fē). The geography of animals; the study of the distribution of animals on the earth's surface.

zo·o·glea (zō-og'lē-ă, zō'ō-glē'ă). In bacteriology, an old term for a mass of bacteria held together by a clear gelatinous substance. [zoo- + G. *glia,* glue]

zo·og·o·nous (zō-oj'ŏ-nŭs). SYN viviparous.

zo·og·o·ny (zō-oj'ŏ-nē). SYN viviparity.

zo·o·graft (zō'ō-graft). A graft of tissue from an animal to a human. SYN animal graft, zooplastic graft.

zo·o·graft·ing (zō-ō-graft'ing). SYN zooplasty.

zo·oid (zō'oyd). 1. Resembling an animal; an organism or object with an animal-like appearance. 2. An animal cell capable of independent existence or movement, as the ovum or a spermatozoon, or the segment of a tapeworm. 3. An individual of a colonial invertebrate, such as a coral. [G. *zoōdēs,* fr. *zōon,* animal, + *eidos,* resemblance]

zo·o·lag·nia (zō-ō-lag'nē-ă). An older term for sexual attraction toward animals. [zoo- + G. *lagneia,* lust]

zo·o·lite, zo·o·lith (zō'ō-līt, zō-ō-lith). A petrified animal. [zoo- + G. *lithos,* stone]

zo·ol·o·gist (zō-ol'ō-jist). One who specializes in zoology.

zo·ol·o·gy (zō-ol'ō-jē). The branch of biology that deals with animals. [zoo- + G. *logos,* study]

zoom (zoom). The action of a varifocal lens system in a camera or microscope that maintains an object in focus while approaching it or receding from it; this effect may be obtained by moving two or

ZO

more of the lens components at rates bearing a linear relation to one another.

zo·o·ma·nia (zō-ō-mā'nē-ă). An excessive, abnormal love of animals. [zoo- + G. *mania,* frenzy]

zo·o·mar·ic ac·id (zō'ō-mer-ik). SYN palmitoleic acid.

Zo·o·mas·tig·i·na (zō'ō-mas-ti-jī'nă). SYN Zoomastigophorea. [zoo- + G. *mastix,* whip]

Zo·o·mas·ti·go·pho·ras·i·da (zō'ō-mas-ti-gō-fō-ras'i-dă). SYN Zoomastigophorea.

Zo·o·mas·ti·go·pho·rea (zō'ō-mas-ti-gō-fō'rē-ă). A class of flagellates (superclass Mastigophora) within the phylum Sarcomastigophora (flagellate and ameboid protozoans), of animal-like as opposed to plantlike characteristics. Chromatophores are absent; one to many flagella are found, although they may be absent in ameboid forms; sexuality is known in some groups. It includes many human parasites such as the trypanosomes and trichomonads, as well as a number of other parasitic and symbiotic forms. SYN Zoomastigina, Zoomastigophorasida. [zoo- + G. *mastix,* whip, + *phoros,* bearing]

zo·o·no·sis (zō-ō-nō'sis). An infection or infestation shared in nature by humans and other animals. SEE ALSO anthropozoonosis, cyclozoonosis, metazoonosis, saprozoonosis, zooanthroponosis. [zoo- + G. *nosos,* disease]

direct z., a z. transmitted between humans and other animals from an infected to a susceptible host by contact, by airborne droplets or droplet nuclei, or by some vehicle of transmission; the agent requires a single vertebrate host for completion of its life cycle and does not develop or show significant change during transmission; may include anthropozoonoses (rabies), zooanthroponoses (amebiasis), and amphixenoses (certain streptococcoses).

zo·o·not·ic (zō'ō-not'ik). Relating to a zoonosis.

zo·o·par·a·site (zō-ō-par'ă-sīt). An animal parasite; an animal existing as a parasite.

zo·o·pa·thol·o·gy (zō-ō-pă-thol'ō-jē). The study or science of diseases of the lower animals.

zo·oph·a·gous (zō-of'ă-gŭs). SYN carnivorous. [G. *zōophagos,* fr. *zōon,* animal, + *phagein,* to eat]

zo·o·phile (zō'ō-fīl). **1.** A lover of animals; especially one more fond of animals than of humans. **2.** One opposed to any animal experimentation; an antivivisectionist. [zoo- + G. *philos,* fond]

zo·o·phil·ia (zō-ō-fil'ē-ă). A paraphilia in which sexual arousal and orgasm are facilitated by engaging in sexual activities with animals. SYN bestiality, zooerastia.

zo·o·phil·ic (zō-ō-fil'ik). **1.** Relating to or displaying zoophilism. **2.** Animal-seeking or animal-preferring; denoting preference of a parasite for an animal host over a human. [zoo- + G. *philos,* fond, loving]

zo·oph·i·lism (zō-of'i-lizm). Fondness for animals, especially an extravagant fondness for them.

erotic z., the deriving of sexual pleasure by patting or stroking animals. SEE ALSO zoophilia, bestiality.

zo·o·pho·bia (zō-ō-fō'bē-ă). Morbid fear of animals. [zoo- + G. *phobos,* fear]

zo·o·phyte (zō'ō-fīt). An animal that resembles a plant, such as the sponges or sea anenomes. [zoo- + G. *phyton,* plant]

zo·o·plas·ty (zō'ō-plas-tē). Grafting of tissue from an animal to a human. SYN zoografting.

zo·o·sa·dism (zō-ō-sā'dizm). Sexual pleasure from cruelty to animals.

zo·os·mo·sis (zō-os-mō'sis). The process of osmosis in living tissues. [G. *zōos,* living, + osmosis]

zo·o·sperm·ia (zō-ō-sper'mē-ă). The presence of live spermatozoa in the ejaculated semen. [G. *zoon,* living, + *sperma,* seed, + -ia]

zo·o·ster·ol (zō'ō-stēr'ol). An animal sterol.

zo·o·tech·nics (zō-ō-tek'niks). The art of managing domestic or captive animals, including handling, breeding, and keeping. [zoo- + G. *technē,* art]

zo·ot·ic (zō-ot'ik). Pertaining to animals other than humans.

zo·o·tox·in (zō-ō-tok'sin). A substance, resembling the bacterial

toxins in its antigenic properties, found in the fluids of certain animals; e.g., in snake venom, the secretions of poisonous insects, eel blood. SYN animal toxin.

zo·o·tro·phic (zō-ō-trof'ik). Relating to or serving for the nutrition of the lower animals. [zoo- + Gr. *trophē,* nourishment]

zor·ub·i·cin (zō-roo-bǐ-sin). Semisynthetic derivative of daunorubicin; also similar to doxorubicin. Like those agents, zorubicin exerts significant myocardial toxicity. Used as an antineoplastic in breast cancer.

zos·ter (zos'ter). SYN *herpes* zoster. [G. *zōstēr,* a girdle]

geniculate z. (jen-i'kyu-lāt zos'ter), SYN *herpes* zoster oticus.

zos·ter·i·form (zos-ter'i-fōrm). SYN zosteroid.

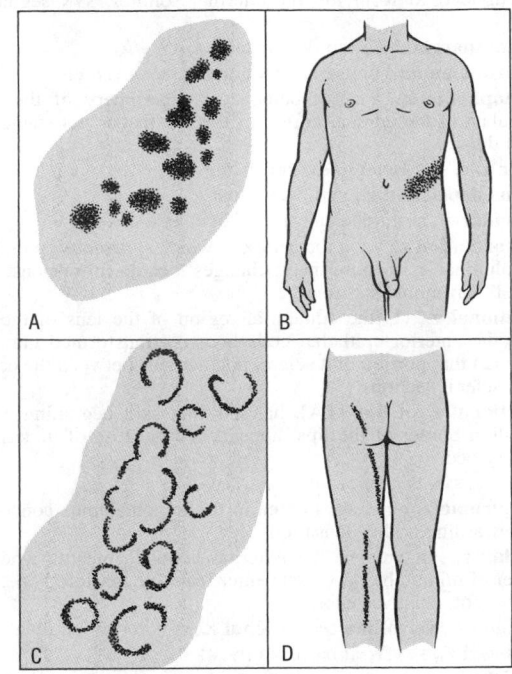

different configurations of skin lesions: (A) grouped; (B) zosteriform; (C) annular (circular) and arciform (arc); (D) linear

zos·ter·oid (zos'ter-oyd). Resembling herpes zoster. SYN zosteriform. [zoster + G. *eidos,* resemblance]

zox·a·zo·la·mine (zok-să-zō'lă-mēn). A centrally acting skeletal muscle relaxant that is no longer used because of its hepatic toxicity.

Z-plas·ty. Technique to elongate a contracted scar or to rotate tension 90°; the middle line of a Z-shaped incision is made along the line of greatest tension or contraction, and triangular flaps are raised on opposite sides of the two ends and transposed.

Zr Symbol for zirconium.

Zsigmondy, Richard A., Austro-German chemist and Nobel laureate, 1865–1929. SEE Z. *test;* brownian-Z. *movement.*

ZSR Abbreviation for zeta sedimentation *ratio.*

Zuckerkandl, Emil, Austrian anatomist, 1849–1910. SEE Z. *bodies,* under *body, convolution, fascia; organs* of Z., under *organ.*

zu·sam·men (Z) (zu-sam'men). **1.** SYN cis- (4). **2.** A form of geometric isomerism with regard to carbon-carbon double bonds in which all four moieties attached to the carbons are different. If the substituents with the higher ranking (based on established rules) are on the same side of the double bond, Z is used. SEE entgegen. [Ger. together]

zwie·back (zwī'bak). Sweetened bread that has been baked twice, preferred for infant feeding during teething. [Ger. twice-baked]

Zwis·chen·fer·ment (tsvish'en-fer-ment'). SYN glucose-6-phos-

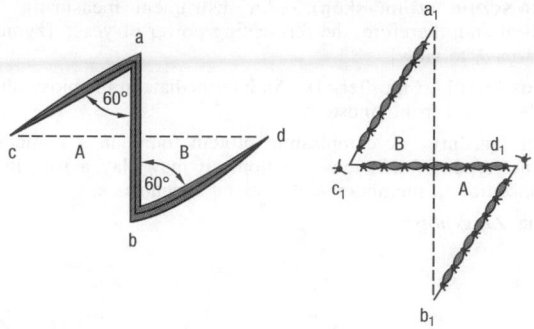

z-plasty: triangular flaps (A) and (B) are transposed to rotate line of tension 90 degrees (from c- -d to a¹- -b¹)

phate dehydrogenase. [Ger. *zwischen,* between, + *Ferment,* fermentation]

zwit·ter·gents (tsvit′er-jents). Detergents that are zwitterionic; often used as surfactants and in the release of proteins from biomembranes. SYN zwitterionic detergent. [*zwitter*ion + deter-*gent*]

zwit·ter·i·on·ic (tsvit′er-ī-on′ik). Denoting a substance with the properties of a zwitterion; e.g., at pH value of 6.11, alanine is z.

zwit·ter·i·ons (tsvit′er-ī-onz). SYN dipolar *ions,* under *ion.* SEE ALSO zwitter *hypothesis.* [Ger. *Zwitter,* hermaphrodite, mongrel + ion]

△**zyg-.** SEE zygo-.

zy·gal (zī′găl). Relating to or shaped like a zygon or yoke; H-shaped.

zyg·a·poph·y·si·al, zyg·a·poph·y·se·al (zī′gă-pō-fiz′ē-ăl, zī-gă-pof′i-se′ăl). Relating to a zygapophysis or articular process of a vertebra.

zyg·a·poph·y·sis, pl. **zyg·a·poph·y·ses** (zī′gă-pof′i-sis, -sēz). SYN articular *process,* articular *process.* [G. *zygon,* yoke, + *apophysis,* offshoot]

z. inferior [TA], SYN inferior articular *process.*

z. superior [TA], SYN superior articular *process.*

zyg·i·on (zig′ē-on). In cephalometrics and craniometrics, the most lateral point of the zygomatic arch. [G. a later form of *zygon,* yoke]

△**zygo-, zyg-.** A yoke, a joining. [G. *zygon,* yoke, *zygōsis,* a joining]

zy·go·ma (zī-gō′mă). **1.** SYN zygomatic *bone.* **2.** SYN zygomatic *arch.* [G. a bar, bolt, the os jugale, fr. *zygon,* yoke]

zy·go·mat·ic (zī′gō-mat′ik). Relating to the zygomatic bone.

△**zygomatico-.** Zygomatic; relating usually to the zygomatic bone. SEE zygo-. [G. *zygōma*]

zy·go·mat·i·co·au·ric·u·lar (zī′gō-mat′i-kō-aw-rik′ū-lăr). Relating to the zygomatic bone and the auricle.

zy·go·ma·ti·co·au·ri·cu·la·ris (zī′gō-mat′i-kō-aw-rik′ū-lār′is). SYN auricularis anterior *(muscle).*

zy·go·mat·i·co·fa·cial (zī′gō-mat′i-kō-fā′shăl). Relating to the zygomatic bone and the face.

zy·go·mat·i·co·fron·tal (zī′gō-mat′i-kō-fron′tăl). Relating to the zygomatic and frontal bones.

zy·go·mat·i·co·max·il·lary (zī′gō-mat′i-kō-mak′si-lār-ē). Relating to the zygomatic bone and the maxilla.

zy·go·mat·i·co·or·bi·tal (zī′gō-mat′i-kō-ōr′bi-tăl). Relating to the zygomatic bone and the orbit.

zy·go·mat·i·co·sphe·noid (zī′gō-mat′i-kō-sfē′noyd). Relating to the zygomatic and sphenoid bones.

zy·go·mat·i·co·tem·po·ral (zī′gō-mat′i-kō-tem′pŏ-răl). Relating to the zygomatic and temporal bones.

zy·go·max·il·la·re (zī′gō-mak-si-lā′rē). A craniometric point located externally at the lowest extent of the zygomaticomaxillary suture. SYN key ridge, zygomaxillary point.

zy·go·max·il·lary (zī-gō-mak′si-lār-ē). Relating to the zygomatic bone and the maxilla.

▣**Zy·go·my·ce·tes** (zī′gō-mī-sē′tēz). A class of fungi characterized by sexual reproduction resulting in the formation of a zygospore, and asexual reproduction by means of nonmotile spores called sporangiospores or conidia. SYN Phycomycetes. [zygo- + G. *mykēs* (*mykēt*-), fungus]

zy·go·my·co·sis (zī′gō-mī-kō′sis). A broad term that includes mucormycosis and entamophthoramycosis; usually applied when culture is not available and the clinical entity is unclear. SYN phycomycetosis, phycomycosis.

zy·gon (zī′gon). The short crossbar connecting the branches of a zygal fissure. [G. crossbar, yoke]

zy·go·ne·ma (zī-g-ō-nē′mă). SYN zygotene. [zygo- + G. *nēma,* thread]

zy·go·po·di·um (zī-gō-pō′dē-ŭm). The distal intermediate segment of the limb skeleton, i.e., radius and ulna, tibia and fibula. [zygo- + G. *podion,* small foot]

zy·go·sis (zī-gō′sis). True conjugation or sexual union of two unicellular organisms, consisting essentially in the fusion of the nuclei of the two cells. [G. a joining]

zy·gos·i·ty (zī-gos′i-tē). The nature of the zygotes from which individuals are derived; e.g., whether by separation of the division of one zygote (monozygotic), in which case they will be genetically identical, or from two separate fertilized ova (dizygotic).

zy·go·sperm (zī′gō-sperm). SYN zygospore. [zygo- + G. *sperma,* seed]

zy·go·spore (zī′gō-spōr). Among the Phycomycetes, a thick-walled sexual spore arising from fusion of two morphologically identical structures, generally hyphal tips, bearing nuclei of opposite mating types (gametangia). SYN zygosperm.

zygosyndactyly (zī-gō-sin-dak′til-ē). Complete or incomplete webbing of the fingers or toes. [zygo- + syndactyly]

zy·gote (zī′gōt). **1.** The diploid cell resulting from union of a sperm and an ovum. Cf. conceptus. **2.** The individual that develops from a fertilized ovum. [G. *zygōtos,* yoked]

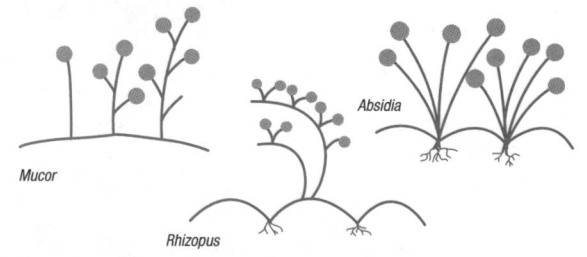

Zygomycetes: differentiating features of three genera

zy·go·tene (zī′gō-tēn). The stage of prophase in meiosis in which precise point for point pairing of homologous chromosomes begins. SYN zygonema. [zygo- + G. *tainia* (L. *taenia*), band]

zy·got·ic (zī-got′ik). Pertaining to a zygote, or to zygosis.

zy·go·to·blast (zī-gō′tō-blast). SYN sporozoite. [G. *zygōtos,* yoked, + *blastos,* germ]

zy·go·to·mere (zī-gō′tō-mēr). SYN sporoblast. [G. *zygōtos,* yoked, + *meros,* part]

△**zym-.** SEE zymo-.

zy·mase (zī′mās). **1.** Obsolete term for a mixture of enzymes. **2.** Specifically, the intracellular enzymes of yeast that promotes alcoholic fermentation.

△**zymo-, zym-.** Fermentation, enzymes. [G. *zymē,* leaven]

zy·mo·deme (zī′mō-dēm). An isoenzyme pattern, as identified by isoenzyme electrophoresis. [zymo- + G. *dēmos,* populace]

zy·mo·gen (zī′mō-jen). SYN proenzyme.

zy·mo·gen·e·sis (zī-mō-jen′ĕ-sis). Transformation of a proenzyme (zymogen) into an active enzyme. [zymo- + G. *genesis,* production]

zy

zy·mo·gen·ic (zī-mō-jen′ik). **1.** Relating to a zymogen or to zymogenesis. SYN zymogenous. **2.** Causing fermentation.

zy·mog·e·nous (zī-moj′ĕ-nŭs). SYN zymogenic (1).

zy·mo·gram (zī′mō-gram). Strips of paper, gels, etc., in which the locations of enzymes, separated electrophoretically or by other means, are demonstrated by histochemical methods. [zymo- + G. *gramma,* something written]

zy·mo·san (zī′mō-san). A carbohydrate (glucose polymer) obtained from the walls of yeast cells that interferes with complement.

zy·mo·scope (zī′mō-skōp). An instrument measuring CO_2 evolved and, therefore, the fermenting power of yeast. [zymo- + G. *skopeō,* to view]

zy·mos·ter·ol (zī-mos′ter-ol). An intermediate in the biosynthesis of cholesterol from lanosterol.

zy·xin (ziks′in). A cytoplasmic protein found in a number of distinct types of adherens junctions; it may play a role in the organization of membrane-cytoskeletal attachments.

ZZ SEE ZZ *genotype.*

CONTENTS TO THE APPENDICES

Medical Prefixes, Suffixes, and Combining Forms

a- not, without, less
ab- from, away from, off
abs- from, away from, off
acantho- thorn
acou- hearing
acro- extremity
acu- hearing
ad- increase, adherence, motion toward; very
-ad toward, in the direction of; -ward
adeno- gland
adip- fat
adipo- fat
-agog, **-agogue** promoter, stimulator
aidoio- genitals
-al pertaining to
alb- white
albo- white
alge- pain
algesi- pain
algio- pain
algo- pain
allo- other, different
ambi- around, on (both) sides, on all sides, both
ambly- dull
amblyo- dull
amyl- starch, polysaccharide
amylo- starch, polysaccharide
an- not, without, -less
ana- up, toward, apart
andro- male
angi- vessel
angio- vessel
ankylo- crooked
ante- before
anthraco- coal, carbon
anti- 1 against, opposing; 2 curative; 3 antibody
apo- separated from, derived from
aque- water
aqueo- water
-ar pertaining to
-arche beginning
arteri- artery
arterio- artery
arthr- joint, articulation
arthro- joint, articulation
-ary pertaining to
-ase an enzyme
-ate a salt or ester of an "-ic" acid
athero- pasty, fatty
atto- one-quintillionth (10^{-18})
audi- hearing
audio- hearing
aur- ear
auri- ear

auro- ear
aut- self, same
auto- self, same
bacteri- bacteria
bacterio- bacteria
balano- glans penis
bi- twice, double
bio- life
blasto- budding by cells or tissue
blephar- eyelid
blepharo- eyelid
brachi- arm
brachio- arm
brachy- short
bronch- bronchus
bronchi- bronchus
broncho- bronchus
carcin- cancer
carcino- cancer
cardi- 1 heart; 2 esophageal opening of stomach
cardio- 1 heart; 2 esophageal opening of stomach
carpo- wrist
cata- down
caud- tail, lower part of body
caudo- tail, lower part of body
-cele hernia, swelling
celio- abdomen
-centesis surgical puncture
centi- one-hundredth (10^{-2})
cephal- the head
cephalo- the head
cervic- 1 neck; 2 uterine cervix
cervico- 1 neck, 2 uterine cervix
cheil- lip
cheilo- lip
cheir- hand
cheiro- hand
chem- 1 chemistry; 2 drug
chemo- 1 chemistry; 2 drug
chir- hand
chiro- hand
chlor- 1 green; 2 chlorine
chloro- 1 green; 2 chlorine
chol- bile
chondrio- 1 cartilage; 2 granular; 3 gritty
chondro- 1 cartilage; 2 granular; 3 gritty
chrom- color
chromat- color
chromo- color
chron- time
chrono- time
-cidal killing, destroying
-cide killing, destroying
cis- on this side, on the near side

-clast breaker
-clysis washing
co- with, together, in association, very, complete
col- with, together, in association, very, complete
colp- vagina
colpo- vagina
com- with, together, in association, very, complete
con- with, together, in association, very, complete
conio- dust
cor- with, together, in association, very, complete
coreo- pupil
cost- rib
costo- rib
crani- cranium
cranio- cranium
-crine secretion
cry- cold
cryo- cold
crypt- hidden
crypto- hidden
culdo- cul-de-sac
cyan- 1 blue; 2 cyanide
cyano- 1 blue; 2 cyanide
cycl- 1 circle, cycle; 2 ciliary body
cyst- 1 bladder; 2 cyst; 3 cystic duct
cysti- 1 bladder; 2 cyst; 3 cystic duct
cysto- 1 bladder; 2 cyst; 3 cystic duct
cyt- cell
-cyte cell
cyto- cell
dacry- tears
dacryo- tears
dactyl- finger, toe
dactylo- finger, toe
de- away from, cessation
deca- ten
deci- one-tenth (10^{-1})
deka- ten
dent- tooth
denti- tooth
derm- skin
derma- skin
dermat- skin
dermato- skin
dermo- skin
-desis binding
dextr- right, toward or on the right side
dextro- right, toward or on the right side
di- separation, taking apart, reversal, not, un-

dif- separation, taking apart, reversal, not, un-
dipso- thirst
dir- separation, taking apart, reversal, not, un-
dis- separation, taking apart, reversal, not, un-
duo- two
duodeno- duodenum
-dynia pain
dynamo- force, energy
dys- bad, difficult
ect- outer, on the outside
-ectasia dilatation, stretching
-ectasis dilatation, stretching
ecto- outer, on the outside
-ectomy excision
-emphraxis obstruction
encephal- brain
encephalo- brain
end- within, inner
endo- within, inner
enter- intestine
entero- intestine
ent- inner, within
ento- inner, within
epi- upon, following, subsequent to
ergo- work
erythr- red, redness
erythro- red, redness
eso- inward
esthesio- sensation, perception
eu- good, well
ex- out of, from, away from
exo- exterior, external, outward
extra- without, outside of
ferri- ferric ion (Fe^{3+})
ferro- 1 metallic iron; 2 ferrous ion (Fe^{2+})
fibr- fiber
fibro- fiber
-form in the form or shape of
galact- milk
galacto- milk
gastr- 1 stomach; 2 belly
gastro- 1 stomach; 2 belly
-gen 1 producing, coming to be; 2 precursor
gen- 1 producing, coming to be; 2 precursor
giga- one billion (10^9)
gingiv- gums
gingivo- gums
gloss- tongue
glosso- tongue
gluco- glucose
glyco- sugars
gnath- jaw

gnatho- jaw
gon- seed, semen
gonio- angle
gono- seed, semen
-gram a recording
granul- granular, granule
granulo- granular, granule
-graph recording instrument
gyn- woman
gyne- woman
gyneco- woman
gyno- woman
hecto- one hundred (10^{10})
hem- blood
hema- blood
hemat- blood
hemato- blood
hemi- one-half
hemo- blood
hepat- liver
hepatico- liver
hepato- liver
hept- seven
hepta- seven
hidr- sweat
hidro- sweat
hist- tissue
histio- tissue
histo- tissue
homeo- same, constant
hydr- water; hydrogen
hydro- water; hydrogen
hyper- excessive, above normal
hypo- beneath; diminution, deficiency; the lowest
hyster- 1 uterus; hysteria; 2 late, following
hystero- 1 uterus; hysteria; 2 late, following
-ia a condition
-iasis condition, state
-ic pertaining to
-ics organized knowledge, practice, treatment
ileo- ileum
ilio- ilium
in- 1 in; 2 not
-in chemical suffix
-ine chemical suffix
infra- below
inguino- groin
inter- between, among
intra- within
intro- within
irid- iris
irido- iris
ischi- ischium
ischio- ischium
-ism 1 condition, disease; 2 practice, doctrine
-ismus spasm; contraction
iso- 1 equal, like; 2 isomer; 3 sameness

-ite the nature of, resembling
-ites -y, -like
-itides plural of -itis
-itis inflammation
kal- potassium
kali- potassium
karyo- nucleus
kerat- cornea
kerato- cornea
kilo- one thousand (10^3)
kin- movement
kine- movement
kinesi- motion
kinesio- motion
kineso- motion
kino- movement
labio- lip
lacrim- tears
lacrimo- tears
lact- milk
lacti- milk
lacto- milk
laparo- abdomen, abdominal wall
laryng- larynx
laryngo- larynx
lateri- lateral, to one side, side
latero- lateral, to one side, side
-lepsis seizure
-lepsy seizure
lepto- light, slender, thin, frail
leuk- white
leuko- white
linguo- tongue
lip- fat, lipid
lipo- fat, lipid
lith- stone, calculus, calcification
litho- stone, calculus, calcification
-log speech, words
log- speech, words
logo- speech, words
-logy 1 study of; 2 collecting
lymph- lymph
lympho- lymph
lys- lysis, dissolution
lyso- lysis, dissolution
macr- large; long
macro- large; long
mal- bad, deficient
-malacia softening
mamm- breast
mamma- breast
mammo- breast
mast- breast
masto- breast
meg- large, oversize
mega- 1 large, oversize; 2 one million (10^6)
megal- large
megalo- large
-megaly, enlargement

melan- black
melano- black
men- menstruation
mening- meninges
meningo- meninges
meno- menstruation
ment- chin
mento- chin
-mer member of a series
mes- 1 middle, mean, intermediate; 2 attaching membrane
meso- 1 middle, mean, intermediate; 2 attaching membrane
meta- 1 after, behind; 2 joint action, sharing
-meter measurement, measuring device
metr- uterus
metro- uterus
micr- 1 small, microscopic
micro- 1 small, microscopic; 2 one-millionth (10^{-6})
milli- one-thousandth (10^{-3})
mon- single
mono- single
morph- form, shape, structure
morpho- form, shape, structure
my- muscle
myo- muscle
myel- 1 bone marrow; 2 spinal cord
myelo- 1 bone marrow; 2 spinal cord
myring- tympanic membrane
myringo- tympanic membrane
myx- mucus
myxo- mucus
nano- 1 dwarf; 2 one-billionth (10^{-9})
nas- nose
naso- nose
natr- sodium
natri- sodium
necr- death, necrosis
necro- death, necrosis
neo- new
nephr- kidney
nephro- kidney
neur- nerve, nervous system
neuri- nerve, nervous system
neuro- nerve, nervous system
norm- normal
normo- normal
octo- eight
oculo- eye, ocular
odont- tooth
odonto- tooth
odyn- pain
odyno- pain
-oid resemblance to

olig- few, little
oligo- few, little
-oma tumor, neoplasm
-omata plural of -oma
oncho- onco-
onco- tumor, bulk, volume
-one ketone (–CO– group)
onych- fingernail, toenail
onycho- fingernail, toenail
oo- egg, ovary
oophor- ovary
oophoro- ovary
ophthalm- eye
ophthalmo- eye
-opia vision
-opsia vision
or- mouth
orchi- testis
orchido- testis
orchio- testis
ori- mouth
oro- mouth
-ose sugar
-oses plural of -osis
-osis process, condition, state
ossi- bone
osseo- bony
ost- bone
oste- bone
osteo- bone
ovari- ovary
ovario- ovary
ovi- egg
ovo- egg
oxa- oxygen
oxo- oxygen
oxy- 1 sharp, acid; 2 acute, shrill, quick; 3 oxygen
pachy- thick
pan- all, entire
pant- all, entire
panto- all, entire
para- 1 abnormal; 2 involvement of two like parts
pari- equal
path- disease
patho- disease
-pathy disease
ped- 1 child; 2 foot
pedi- 1 child; 2 foot
pedo- 1 child; 2 foot
-penia deficiency
penta- five
per- through, thoroughly, intensely
peri- around, about
-pexy fixation, usually surgical
phaco- lens
-phage eating, devouring
-phagia eating, devouring
phago- eating, devouring
-phagy eating, devouring

phako- lens
phanero- visible, evident
pharmaco- drugs, medicine
pharyng- pharynx
pharyngo- pharynx
phil- 1 attraction; **2** chemical affinity
-philia 1 attraction; **2** chemical affinity
philo- 1 attraction; **2** chemical affinity
phleb- vein
phlebo- vein
-phobia fear
phon- sound, speech
phono- sound, speech
phor- carrying, bearing
phoro- carrying, bearing
phos- light
phot- light
photo- light
phren- 1 diaphragm; **2** mind; **3** phrenic
phreni- 1 diaphragm; **2** mind; **3** phrenic
-phrenia of mind
phrenico- 1 diaphragm; **2** mind; **3** phrenic
phreno- 1 diaphragm; **2** mind; **3** phrenic
-phylaxis protection
phyll- leaf
phyllo- leaf
physi- 1 physical; **2** natural
physio- 1 physical; **2** natural
physo- 1 swelling, inflation; **2** air, gas
phyt- plants
phyto- plants
pico- one-trillionth (10^{-12})
plan- flat
plani- flat
plano- flat
-plasia formation
plasma- plasma
plasmat- plasma
plasmato- plasma
plasmo- plasma
platy- wide, flat
-plegia paralysis
pleo- more
plesio- near, similar
pleur- rib, side, pleura
pleura- rib, side, pleura
pleuro- rib, side, pleura
pluri- several, more
-pnea breath, respiration
pneo- breath, respiration
pneum- 1 air, gas; **2** lung; **3** breathing
pneuma- 1 air, gas; **2** lung; **3** breathing
pneumat- 1 air, gas; **2** lung; **3** breathing

pneumato- 1 air, gas; **2** lung; **3** breathing
pod- foot, foot-shaped
-pod foot, foot-shaped
podo- foot, foot-shaped
-poiesis production
poikilo- irregular, variable
polio- gray
poly- 1 multiplicity; **2** polymer
post- after, behind, posterior
pre- anterior, before
presby- old
pro- 1 before, forward; **2** precursor
proct- anus, rectum
procto- anus, rectum
prot- first
proto- first
pseud- false
pseudo- false
psych- mind
psyche- mind
psycho- mind
-ptosis sagging, falling
pyel- (renal) pelvis
pyelo- (renal) pelvis
pykn- dense, compact
pykno- dense, compact
pyo- suppuration, pus
pyreto- fever
pyro- fire, heat, fever
quadr- four
quadri- four
rachi- spinal column
rachio- spinal column
radio- 1 radiation, x-ray; **2** radius
re- again, backward
rect- rectum, straight
recto- rectum, straight
ren- kidney
reno- kidney
retro- backward, behind
rhin- nose
rhino- nose
-rrhagia discharge
-rrhaphy surgical suturing
-rrhea flow
-rrhexis rupture
salping- tube
salpingo- tube
sarco- flesh, muscle
schisto- split, cleft
schiz- split, cleft, division
schizo- split, cleft, division
scler- hardness (induration), sclerosis, ocular sclera
sclero- hardness (induration), sclerosis, ocular sclera
scolio- crooked
-scope instrument for viewing
-scopy viewing
scot- shadow, darkness
scoto- shadow, darkness

semi- one-half; partly
sept- 1 seven; **2** septum; **3** sepsis, infection
septi- seven
septo- 1 seven; **2** septum; **3** sepsis, infection
sial- saliva, salivary gland
sialo- saliva, salivary gland
sider- iron
sidero- iron
sigmoid- 1 S-shaped; **2** sigmoid colon
sigmoido- 1 S-shaped; **2** sigmoid colon
sin- sinus
sino- sinus
sinu- sinus
sito- food, grain
somat- body, bodily
somato- body, bodily
somatico- body, bodily
somno- sleep
son- 1 sound; **2** ultrasound
sono- 1 sound; **2** ultrasound
spasmo- spasm
spermato- semen, spermatozoa
spermo- semen, spermatozoa
sperma- semen, spermatozoa
sphygmo- pulse
spir- breathing
spiro- breathing
splanchn- viscera
splanchni- viscera
splanchno- viscera
splen- spleen
spleno- spleen
staphyl- grape, bunch of grapes; staphylococci
staphylo- grape, bunch of grapes; staphylococci
-stasis stopping
-stat arresting change or movement
steno- narrowness, constriction
stereo- solid
stheno- strength, force, power
stom- mouth
stoma- mouth
stomat- mouth
stomato- mouth
sub- beneath, less than normal, inferior
super- in excess, above, superior, in the upper part
supra- above
sy- together
syl- together
sym- together
syn- together
sys- together
tachy- rapid
tel- distant
tele- distant

ten- tendon
tendin- tendon
teno- tendon
tenont- tendon
tenonto- tendon
tera- one quadrillion (10^{15})
tetra- four
thel- nipple
thelo- nipple
therm- heat
thermo- heat
thorac- chest, thorax
thoracico- chest, thorax
thoraco- chest, thorax
thromb- blood clot
thrombo- blood clot
thyr- thyroid gland
thyro- the thyroid gland
toco- childbirth
-tome 1 cutting instrument; **2** segment, section
-tomy cutting operation
tono- tone, tension, pressure
top- place, topical
topo- place, topical
tox- toxin, poison
toxi- toxin, poison
toxico- toxin, poison
toxo- toxin, poison
trache- trachea
tracheo- trachea
trans- across, through, beyond
tri- three
trich- hair
trichi- hair
-trichia hair
tricho- hair
tris- three
-trophic food, nutrition
tropho- food, nutrition
-trophy food, nutrition
-tropia turning
-tropic turning toward, affinity
ultra- beyond
uni- one, single
uri- uric acid
-uria urine, urination
uric- uric acid
urico- uric acid
uro- 1 urine; **2** urinary tract
vas- duct, blood vessel
vasculo- blood vessel
vaso- duct, blood vessel
vesic- urinary bladder, vesicle
vesico- urinary bladder, vesicle
xanth- yellow, yellowish
xantho- yellow, yellowish
xero- dry
zo- 1 animal; **2** life
zoo- 1 animal; **2** life
zym- fermentation, enzymes
zymo- fermentation, enzymes

Appendices

α alpha: Bunsen's solubility coefficient; first in a series; specific rotation term; heavy chain class corresponding to IgA

a (specific) absorption (coefficient) (USUALLY ITALIC); (total) acidity; area; (systemic) arterial (blood) (SUBSCRIPT); asymmetric; atto-

A absorbance

A adenosine (or adenylic acid); alveolar gas (SUBSCRIPT); ampere

Å angstrom; Ångström unit

a̅a̅ [G.] *ana* of each (USED in prescriptions)

AA amino acid; aminoacyl

AB abortion

Ab antibody

ABG arterial blood gas

abl Abelson murine leukemia virus

ABLB alternate binaural loudness balance (test)

ABO blood group system

ABR abortus-Bang-ring (test); auditory brainstem response (audiometry)

abs. feb. [L.] *absente febre,* when fever is absent

γ-Abu γ-aminobutyric acid

ABVD Adriamycin (doxorubicin), bleomycin, vinblastine, and dacarbazine

ac acetyl; [L.] *ante cibum,* before a meal

aC arabinosylcytosine

Ac acetyl; actinium

AC acetate; acromioclavicular; atriocarotid

AC/A accommodation convergence-accommodation (ratio)

ACE angiotension-converting enzyme

ACEI angiotensin-converting enzyme inhibitor

ac-g accelerator globulin

AcG accelerator globulin

Ach acetylcholine

aCL anticardiolipin (antibody)

ACP acyl carrier protein

ACTH adrenocorticotropic hormone (corticotropin)

AD [L.] *auris dextra,* right ear; Alzheimer disease

add. [L.] *adde,* add

Ade adenine

ADH antidiuretic hormone

adhib. [L.] *adhibendus,* to be administered

ADL activities of daily living

ad lib [L.] *ad libitum,* freely, as desired

admov. [L.] *admove,* apply

Ado adenosine

ADP adenosine 5′-diphosphate

ad sat. [L.] *ad saturatum, ad saturandum,* to saturation

adst. feb. [L.] *adstante febre,* when fever is present

ad us. ext. [L.] *ad usum externum,* for external use

adv. [L.] *adversum,* against

A-E above-the-elbow (amputation)

AFB acid-fast bacillus

AFORMED alternating failure of response, mechanical, to electrical depolarization

AFP α-fetoprotein

Ag antigen; [L.] *argentum,* silver

A/G R albumin-globulin ratio

AHF antihemophilic factor

AHG antihemophilic globulin

AID artificial insemination donor

AIDS acquired immunodeficiency syndrome

AIH artificial insemination by husband; artificial insemination, homologous

A-K above-the-knee (amputation)

Al aluminum

Ala alanine (or its mono- or diradical)

ALA δ-aminolevulinic acid

ALD adrenoleukodystrophy

ALL acute lymphocytic leukemia

ALS antilymphocyte serum; advanced life support

ALT alanine aminotransferase

alt. hor. [L.] *alternis horis,* every other hour

Am americium

AML acute myelogenous leukemia

AMP adenosine monophosphate (adenylic acid)

amu atomic mass unit

ANA antinuclear antibody

ANF antinuclear factor

ANOVA analysis of variance

ANS autonomic nervous system

ANUG acute necrotizing ulcerative gingivitis

APA antipernicious anemia (factor)

APC antigen-presenting cell

A-P-C adenoidal-pharyngeal-conjunctival (virus)

aPS antiphospholipid antibody syndrome

APTT activated partial thromboplastin time

Ar argon

araC arabinosylcytosine (cytarabine)

ARDS adult respiratory distress syndrome

ARF acute renal failure; acute rheumatic fever

Arg arginine (or its mono- or diradical)

As arsenic

AS [L.] *auris sinistra,* left ear

ASA acetylsalicylic acid (aspirin)

ASCUS abnormal squamous cells of undetermined significance

ASHD arteriosclerotic heart disease

Asn asparagine (or its mono- or diradical)

ASO antistreptolysin O

Asp aspartic acid (or its radical forms)

AST aspartate aminotransferase

At astatine

ATFL anterior talofibular ligament

ATL adult T-cell leukemia; adult T-cell lymphoma

atm (standard) atmosphere

ATP adenosine 5′-triphosphate

ATPase adenosine triphosphatase

ATPD ambient temperature and pressure, dry

ATPS ambient temperature and pressure, saturated (with water vapor)

at. wt. atomic weight

Au [L.] *aurum,* gold

AU [L.] *auris utraque,* each ear, both ears

AV arteriovenous

A-V arteriovenous; atrioventricular

AVN atrioventricular node

AVP antiviral protein

AW atomic weight

ax. axis

AZT azidothymidine (zidovudine)

b second in a series

b blood (SUBSCRIPT)

B barometric (pressure) (SUBSCRIPT); boron

Ba barium

BADL basic activities of daily living

BAER brainstem auditory evoked response

BAL British anti-Lewisite (dimercaprol); bronchoalveolar lavage

BALB binaural alternate loudness balance (test)

BBB blood-brain barrier

BCG bacille bilié de Calmette-Guérin (vaccine)

BE barium enema

Be beryllium

B-E below-the-elbow (amputation)

Bi bismuth

bib. [L.] *bibe,* drink

b.i.d. [L.] *bis in die,* twice a day

BIDS brittle hair, impaired intelligence, decreased fertility, and short stature (syndrome)

BIPAP bilevel positive airway pressure

Bk berkelium

BM bowel movement

BMI body mass index

bp base pair

BP blood pressure; boiling point; *British Pharmacopoeia*

BPF bronchopleural fistula

BPH benign prostatic hyperplasia

Bq becquerel (SI unit of radionuclide activity)

Br bromine

BRAT (diet) banana, rice cereal, applesauce, toast

BSA body surface area

BSER brainstem evoked response (audiometry)

BT bleeding time

BTPS body temperature, ambient pressure, saturated (with water vapor)

BTU British thermal unit

BUN blood urea nitrogen

BUS Bartholin glands, urethra, Skene glands

C calorie (large); carbon; Celsius; centigrade; clearance (rate, renal) (followed by a SUBSCRIPT); compliance; concentration; cylindrical (lens); cytidine

c calorie (small); capillary (blood) (SUBSCRIPT); centi-

ca. [L.] *circa,* about, approximately

c-a cardioarterial

Ca calcium; cathodal; cathode

CA cancer; carcinoma; cardiac arrest; chronologic age; croup-associated (virus); cytosine arabinoside

CABG coronary artery bypass graft

cal calorie (small)

Cal calorie (large)

cAMP cyclic AMP (adenosine monophosphate)

CAP catabolite (gene) activator protein

CAPD continuous ambulatory peritoneal dialysis

CAT computerized axial tomography

CBC complete blood (cell) count

CBG corticosteroid-binding globulin

Cbz carbobenzoxy (chloride)

cc, c.c. cubic centimeter

C.C. chief complaint

CCK cholecystokinin

CCNU chloroethylcyclohexylnitrosourea (lomustine)

CCU coronary care unit; critical care unit

cd candela

Cd cadmium

CDC Centers for Disease Control and Prevention

cDNA complementary DNA

CDP cytidine 5′-diphosphate

Ce cerium

CEA carcinoembryonic antigen

CELO chicken embryo lethal orphan (virus)

CEP congenital erythropoietic porphyria

Cf californium

CF complement fixation; cystic fibrosis; coupling factor

CG chorionic gonadotropin

CGA catabolite gene activator

cGMP cyclic GMP

cgs, CGS centimeter-gram-second (system, unit)

Ch¹ Christchurch (chromosome)

CHF congestive heart failure

CHO carbohydrate

μCi microcurie

Ci curie

CI color index; *Colour Index*

CIB [L.] *cibus,* food

CIQ cognitive laterality quotient

CJD Creutzfeldt-Jakob disease

CK creatine kinase

Cl chlorine

CL cardiolipin

CLIA Clinical Laboratory Improvement Amendments

CLL chronic lymphocytic leukemia

cm centimeter

cM centimorgan

Cm curium

CMA Certified Medical Assistant

CMC carpometacarpal

CMI cell-mediated immunity

CML chronic myelogenous leukemia

CMP cytidine 5′-phosphate (or any cytidine monophosphate)

CMT Certified Medical Transcriptionist

CMV controlled mechanical ventilation; cytomegalovirus

CNM Certified Nurse Midwife

CNS central nervous system

Co cobalt

c/o complains of

CoA coenzyme A

COG center of gravity

conA concanavalin A

cont. rem. [L.] *continuetur remedium,* let the medicine be continued

COPD chronic obstructive pulmonary disease

CP cerebral palsy; costophrenic

CPAP continuous (or constant) positive airway pressure

CPD cephalopelvic disproportion

CPM continuous passive motility

CPPB continuous (or constant) positive-pressure breathing

CPPV continuous positive-pressure ventilation

CPR cardiopulmonary resuscitation

cps cycles per second

Cr chromium; creatinine

CR conditioned reflex; crown-rump (length)

CRD chronic respiratory disease

CRH corticotropin-releasing hormone

CRL crown-rump length

CRNA Certified Registered Nurse Anesthetist

CRP cross-reacting protein

CRST calcinosis cutis, Raynaud's phenomenon, sclerodactyly, and telangiectasia (syndrome)

Cs cesium

C&S culture and sensitivity

CSD catscratch disease

CSF cerebrospinal fluid

CT computed tomography

CTP cytidine 5′-triphosphate

CTR cardiothoracic ratio

Cu [L.] *cuprum,* copper

CV cardiovascular

CVA cerebral vascular accident

CVP central venous pressure

CXR chest x-ray

Cyd cytidine

cyl cylinder; cylindrical (lens)

CYP cytochrome P-450 (enzyme)

Cys cysteine

Cyt cytosine

δ delta; heavy chain class corresponding to IgD

Δ delta; change; heat

d deci-

d deuterium

d- dextrorotatory

D dead (space gas) (SUBSCRIPT); deciduous; deuterium; diffusing (capacity); dihydrouridine (in nucleic acids); diopter; [L.] *dexter,* right (opposite of left); vitamin D potency of cod liver oil

D- prefix indicating that a molecule is sterically analogous to D-glyceraldehyde

da deca-

dA deoxyadenosine

Da dalton

DA developmental age

dAdo deoxyadenosine

dAMP deoxyadenylic acid

DANS 1-dimethylaminonaphthalene-5-sulfonic acid

db decibel

dB decibel

DC Dental Corps; Doctor of Chiropractic

D & C dilation and curettage

DCG dacryocystography

DCI dichloroisoproterenol

dCMP deoxycytidylic acid

DDS Doctor of Dental Surgery

DDT dichlorodiphenyltrichloroethane (chlorophenothane)

D & E dilation and evacuation

def decayed, extracted, or filled (deciduous teeth)

DEF decayed, extracted, or filled (permanent teeth)

deglut. [L.] *degluttiatur,* let it be swallowed

DES diethylstilbestrol

det. [L.] *detur,* let it be given

DET diethyltryptamine

DEV duck embryo vaccine; duck embryo virus

DEXA dual-energy x-ray absorptiometry

df decayed and filled (deciduous teeth)

Df deficiency (absence or inactivation of a gene)

DF decayed and filled (permanent teeth)

dGMP deoxyguanosine monophosphate (deoxyguanylic acid)

DHEA dehydro-3-epiandrosterone

DIC disseminated intravascular coagulation

dieb. alt. [L.] *diebus alternis,* every other day

dil. [L.] *dilue,* dilute

dim. [L.] *dimidius,* one-half

DIP desquamative interstitial pneumonia; distal interphalangeal (joint)

dir. prop. [L.] *directione propria,* with proper direction

div. in par. aeq. [L.] *divide in partes aequales,* divide into equal parts

DJD degenerative joint disease

dk deca-, deka-

dM decimorgan

DMD Doctor of Dental Medicine; Duchenne muscular dystrophy

dmf decayed, missing, or filled (deciduous teeth)

DMF decayed, missing, or filled (permanent teeth)

DMSO dimethyl sulfoxide

DMT *N,N*-dimethyltryptamine

DN dibucaine number

DNA deoxyribonucleic acid

DNAase deoxyribonucleic acid nuclease

DNase deoxyribonuclease

DNAse deoxyribonuclease

DNP deoxyribonucleoprotein; 2,4-dinitrophenol

DNR do not resuscitate

DNS Director of Nursing Service(s)

DO Doctor of Osteopathy

DOA dead on arrival

DOC deoxycholic acid

DOC deoxycorticosterone

DOM 2,5-dimethoxy-4-methylamphetamine

Dp duplication of a gene or chromosomal segment

DP Doctor of Podiatry

2,3-DPG 2,3-diphosphoglycerate

DPH Doctor of Public Health; Doctor of Public Hygiene

DPI dry powder inhaler

DPM Doctor of Physical Medicine; Doctor of Podiatric Medicine

DPN diphosphopyridine nucleotide

DPT dipropyltryptamine; diphtheria, pertussis, and tetanus (vaccines)

dr dram

DR degeneration reaction, reaction of degeneration

DRG diagnosis-related group

DrPH Doctor of Public Health; Doctor of Public Hygiene

DRVVT dilute Russell's viper venom test

D-S Doerfler-Stewart (test)

DSA digital subtraction angiography

dsDNA double-stranded DNA

dT deoxythymidine

DT delirium tremens; duration of tetany

dTDP deoxythymidine 5-diphosphate

dThd thymidine

DTIC dimethyltrizenoimidazole carboxamide (dacarbazine)

dTMP deoxythymidylic acid

DTP diphtheria and tetanus toxoids and pertussis vaccine; distal tingling on percussion (Tinel sign)

DTPA diethylenetriamine pentaacetic acid

DTR deep tendon reflex

dTTP deoxythymidine 5′-triphosphate

dur. dol. [L.] *durante dolore,* while pain lasts

DVM Doctor of Veterinary Medicine

Dx diagnosis

Dy dysprosium

ε epsilon; molar absorption coefficient; heavy chain class corresponding to IgE

E exa-; extraction (ratio)

EB Epstein-Barr (virus)

EBV Epstein-Barr virus

ECF extracellular fluid

ECF-A eosinophilic chemotactic factor of anaphylaxis

ECG electrocardiogram

ECHO enterocytopathogenic human orphan (virus)

ECM erythema chronicum migrans

ECMO extracorporeal-membrane oxygenation

ECS electrocerebral silence

ECT electroconvulsive therapy

ED effective dose

EDTA ethylenediaminetetraacetic acid (edathamil, edetic acid)

EEG electroencephalogram

EENT eye, ear, nose, and throat

EIA enzyme immunoassay

EKG [German] *Elektrokardiogramme,* electrocardiogram

EKY electrokymogram

ELISA enzyme-linked immunosorbent assay

EMC encephalomyocarditis (virus)

EMF electromotive force

EMG electromyogram; exomphalos, macroglossia, and gigantism (syndrome)

emp. [L.] *emplastrum, plaster; ex modo praescripto,* in the manner prescribed

ENG electronystagmography

ENT ear, nose, and throat

EOG electrooculography

EPAP expiratory positive airway pressure

Er erbium

ER endoplasmic reticulum; emergency room

ERBF effective renal blood flow

ERCP endoscopic retrograde cholangiopancreatography

ERG electroretinogram

ERPF effective renal plasma flow

ERV expiratory reserve volume

Es einsteinium

ESEP extreme somatosensory evoked potential

ESP extrasensory perception

ESR electron spin resonance; erythrocyte sedimentation rate

ESRD end-stage renal disease

EtOH ethyl alcohol

Eu europium

ev electron-volt

eV electron-volt

f femto-; (respiratory) frequency

F Fahrenheit; faraday (constant); fertility (factor); field (of vision); fluorine; force; fractional (concentration); free (energy)

F1.2 (prothrombin) fragment 1.2

F₁ first filial generation

Fab fragment of antibody molecule involved in antigen binding

FAD flavin(e) adenine dinucleotide; familial Alzheimer disease

FANA fluorescent antinuclear antibody (test)

FB foreign body

FBS fasting blood sugar

Fc constant fragment of an antibody molecule

FDA Food and Drug Administration

Fe [L.] *ferrum,* iron

FEF forced expiratory flow

FET forced expiratory time

FEV forced expiratory volume

FF filtration fraction

FFD focus-film distance

FHR fetal heart rate

FHT fetal heart tones

FIA fluorescent immunoassay

FIGLU formiminoglutamic (acid)

FISH fluorescent in situ hybridization

Fm fermium

FMN flavin(e) mononucleotide

fps, FPS foot-pound-second (system, unit)

Fr francium; French (gauge, scale)

FRC functional residual capacity (of lungs)

FRF follicle-stimulating hormone-releasing factor

FRS first-rank symptom

Fru fructose

FSH follicle-stimulating hormone

FSH-RF follicle-stimulating hormone-releasing factor

FSH-RH follicle-stimulating hormone-releasing hormone

ft. [L.] *fiat,* let it be done, let there be made

FTA-ABS fluorescent treponemal antibody-absorption (test)

FU fluorouracil

FUO fever of unknown origin

FVC forced vital capacity

Fw F wave (fibrillary wave, flutter wave)

Fx fracture

γ gamma; Ostwald's solubility coefficient; the third in a series; heavy chain class corresponding to IgG

μg microgram

g gram

G giga-; glucose; gravitation (newtonian constant of); guanosine (or guanylic acid) residues in polynucleotides; gravida (obstetric history)

G 1 gap 1

G 2 gap 2

G6P glucose 6-phosphate

Ga gallium

GABA γ-aminobutyric acid

GABHS group-A β-hemolytic streptococcus

Gal galactose

GC gonococcus, gonorrhea

Gd gadolinium

GDP mannose-1-phosphate guanylyltransferase

Ge germanium

GERD gastroesophageal reflux disease

GFR glomerular filtration rate

GGT γ-glutamyl transferase

GH glenohumeral; growth hormone

GHB γ-hydroxybutyrate

GHRF growth hormone-releasing factor

GH-RF growth hormone-releasing factor

GHRH growth hormone-releasing hormone

GH-RH growth hormone-releasing hormone

GI gastrointestinal; Gingival Index

GIP gastric inhibitory polypeptide

GLC gas-liquid chromatography

Gln glutamine; glutaminyl

Glu glutamic acid; glutamyl

Gly glycine; glycyl

GMP guanosine monophosphate (guanylic acid)

GMS Gomori (or Grocott) methenamine silver (stain)

GnRH gonadotropin-releasing hormone

GOT glutamic-oxaloacetic transaminase (aspartate aminotransferase)

GPI Gingival-Periodontal Index

GPT glutamic-pyruvic transaminase (alanine aminotransferase)

gr grain

grad. [L.] *gradatim,* gradually

GSH reduced glutathione

GSR galvanic skin response

GSSG oxidized glutathione

gt. [L.] *gutta,* a drop

GTP guanosine 5'-triphosphate

gtt. [L.] *guttae,* drops

GTT glucose tolerance test

GU genitourinary

Guo guanosine

guttat. [L.] *guttatim,* drop by drop

GVHD graft-versus-host disease

Gy gray (unit of absorbed dose of ionizing radiation)

GYN gynecology

h hecto-

h Planck's constant

α-h the right-handed helical form assumed by many proteins

H henry; hydrogen; hyperopia; hyperopic

^{1}H hydrogen-1 (protium, light hydrogen)

^{2}H hydrogen-2 (deuterium, heavy hydrogen)

^{3}H hydrogen-3 (tritium, radioactive hydrogen)

H$^+$ hydrogen ion

Ha hahnium

HA hyaluronic acid; hemagglutinin

HAV hepatitis A virus

Hb hemoglobin

HbA adult hemoglobin

HbA$_1$ major component of adult hemoglobin

HbA$_2$ minor fraction of adult hemoglobin

HbAS heterozygosity for hemoglobin A and hemoglobin S (sickle cell trait)

HB$_c$Ag hepatitis B core antigen

HbCO carboxyhemoglobin

HB$_e$ hepatitis B early antigen

HB$_e$Ab hepatitis B early antibody

Hb$_e$Ag hepatitis B early antigen

HBIG hepatitis B immune globulin

HbF fetal hemoglobin

HbO$_2$ oxyhemoglobin, oxygenated hemoglobin

HbS sickle-cell hemoglobin

HB$_s$Ab hepatitis B surface antibody

HB$_s$Ag hepatitis B surface antigen

HBV hepatitis B virus

HCFA Health Care Financing Administration

HCG human chorionic gonadotropin

HCS human chorionic somatomammotropin (human placental lactogen)

Hct hematocrit

h. d. [L.] *hora decubitus,* at bedtime

HDL high-density lipoprotein

HDRV human diploid (cell strain) rabies vaccine

He helium

H&E hematoxylin and eosin

HEMPAS hereditary erythroblastic multinuclearity associated with positive acidified serum

Hf hafnium

HFJV high-frequency jet ventilation

HFOV high-frequency oscillatory ventilation

HFPPV high-frequency positive pressure ventilation

HFV high-frequency ventilation

Hg [L.] *hydrargyrum,* mercury

HGE human granulocytic ehrlichiosis

HGH human (pituitary) growth hormone

HGSIL high-grade squamous intraepithelial lesion

HI hemagglutination inhibition (test, titer)

His histidine

His- histidyl

-His histidino

HIV human immunodeficiency virus

Hl hyperopia, latent

HLA human lymphocyte antigen

Hm hyperopia, manifest (hypermetropia)

HME human monocytic ehrlichiosis

HMG human menopausal gonadotropin

HMG CoA 3-hydroxy-3-methylglutaryl coenzyme A

HMO Health Maintenance Organization

HMWK high molecular weight kininogen (Fletcher factor)

Ho holmium

hor. decub. [L.] *hora decubitus,* at bedtime

hor. som. [L.] *hora somni,* at bedtime

HPF high-power field

HPI history of present illness

HPL human placental lactogen

HPLC high-performance liquid chromatography

HPV human papilloma virus

h. s., HS [L.] *hora somni,* at bedtime

HSV herpes simplex virus

Ht hyperopia, total

5-HT 5-hydroxytryptamine (serotonin)

HTLV human T-cell lymphocytrophic virus; human T-cell lymphoma/leukemia virus

HVL half-value layer

Hx (medical) history

Hyp hydroxyproline

Hz hertz

I inspired (gas) (SUBSCRIPT); iodine

^{123}I iodine-123 (radioisotope)

^{125}I iodine-125

^{131}I iodine-131

IADL instrumental activities of daily living

IAP intermittent acute porphyria

ICD *International Classification of Diseases of the World Health Organization*

ICDA *International Classification of Diseases, Adapted for Use in the United States*

ICF intracellular fluid

ICP intracranial pressure

ICSH interstitial cell-stimulating hormone

ICU intensive care unit

ID infective dose

I&D incision and drainage

IDU idoxuridine

IF initiation factor; intrinsic factor

IFN interferon

Ig immunoglobulin

IGF insulin-like growth factor

IH infectious hepatitis

IL interleukin

ILA insulin-like activity

Ile isoleucine

IM internal medicine; intramuscular(ly); infectious mononucleosis

IMP inosine monophosphate (inosinic acid)

IMV intermittent mandatory ventilation

in d. [L.] *in dies,* daily

In indium

Ino inosine

INR international normalized ratio

int. cib. [L.] *inter cibos,* between meals

I&O (fluid) intake and output

IOML infraorbitomeatal line

IP interphalangeal; intraperitoneal(ly)

IPAP inspiratory positive airway pressure

IPPB intermittent positive-pressure breathing

IPPV intermittent positive-pressure ventilation

IPV inactivated poliovirus vaccine

IQ intelligence quotient

Ir iridium

IRV inspiratory reserve volume

ISI International Sensitivity Index

ITP idiopathic thrombocytopenic purpura; inosine 5'-triphosphate

IU International Unit

IUCD intrauterine contraceptive device

IUD intrauterine device

IV intravenous, intravenously; intraventricular

J joule

J flux (density)

k kilo-

K [Modern L.] *kalium,* potassium; kelvin

K$_M$ Michaelis constant

kat katal

kb kilobase

kc kilocycle

kcal kilocalorie

KCT kaolin clotting time
kDa kilodalton
kg kilogram
KJ knee jerk
Kr krypton
KS Kaposi sarcoma
17-KS 17-ketosteroid
kv kilovolt
kVp kilovolt peak
KW Kimmelstiel-Wilson (disease); Keith-Wagener (retinal changes)
μl, μL microliter
l liter
L inductance; left; [L.] *limes*, boundary, limit; liter
L- prefix indicating that a molecule is sterically analogous to L-glyceraldehyde
La lanthanum
LA lupus anticoagulant
LAP leucine aminopeptidase
LATS long-acting thyroid stimulator
LBT lupus band test
LC lethal concentration
LCAT lecithin-cholesterol acyltransferase
LCM lymphocytic choriomeningitis (virus)
LD lethal dose
LDH lactate dehydrogenase
LDL low-density lipoprotein
LE left eye; lupus erythematosus
LEEP loop electrosurgical excision procedure
LES lower esophageal sphincter
LETS large external transformation-sensitive (fibronectin)
Leu leucine
LFA left frontoanterior (fetal position)
LFP left frontoposterior (fetal position)
LFT left frontotransverse (fetal position)
LGSIL low-grade squamous intraepithelial lesion
LGV lymphogranuloma venereum
LH luteinizing hormone
LH/FSH-RF luteinizing hormone/follicle-stimulating hormone-releasing factor
LH-RF luteinizing hormone-releasing factor
LH-RH luteinizing hormone-releasing hormone
Li lithium
LLQ left lower quadrant
LM Licentiate in Midwifery

LMA left mentoanterior (fetal position)
LMP left mentoposterior (fetal position)
LMT left mentotransverse (fetal position)
LNPF lymph node permeability factor
LOA left occipitoanterior (fetal position)
LOP left occipitoposterior (fetal position)
LOT left occipitotransverse (fetal position)
LPF low-power field
LPH lipotropic pituitary hormone (lipotropin)
LPN Licensed Practical Nurse
Lr lawrencium
LRH luteinizing hormone-releasing hormone
LSA left sacroanterior (fetal position)
LSD lysergic acid diethylamide
LSP left sacroposterior (fetal position)
L/S R lecithin/sphingomyelin ratio
LST left sacrotransverse (fetal position)
LTH luteotropic hormone
LTM long-term memory
LTR long terminal repeat
Lu lutetium
LUQ left upper quadrant
LVET left ventricular ejection time
LVH left ventricular hypertrophy
LVN Licensed Visiting Nurse; Licensed Vocational Nurse
Lw (former symbol for) lawrencium (now Lr)
Lys lysine (or its radicals in peptides)
μ mu; micro-; heavy chain class corresponding to IgM
m mass; meter; milliminim; molar
m- *meta-*
M mega-, meg-; molar; moles (per liter); morgan; myopic; myopia
M molar; moles (per liter)
m moles (per liter)
μμ micromicro-
μm micrometer
mμ millimicron
mA milliampere
MA mental age
MAA macroaggregated albumin

M + Am compound myopic astigmatism
MAC *Mycobacterium avium* complex
MAI *Mycobacterium avium-intracellulare*
man. pr. [L.] *mane primo*, early morning, first thing in the morning
MAO monoamine oxidase
MAOI monoamine oxidase inhibitor
MAP morning-after pill
mA-S milliampere-second
Mb myoglobin
MBC maximum breathing capacity
MbCO carbon monoxided myoglobin
MbO₂ oxymyoglobin
MC Medical Corps
MCH mean corpuscular hemoglobin
MCHC mean corpuscular hemoglobin concentration
mCi millicurie
MCP metacarpophalangeal
MCV mean corpuscular volume
Md mendelevium
MD [L.] *Medicinae Doctor,* Doctor of Medicine
MDF myocardial depressant factor
MDI metered-dose inhaler
Me methyl
MEDLARS Medical Literature Analysis and Retrieval System
MEP maximal expiratory pressure
meq, mEq milliequivalent
Met methionine
MET metabolic equivalent of task
metHb methemoglobin
metMb metmyoglobin
MEV million electron-volts (10^6 ev)
mg milligram
Mg magnesium
MHC major histocompatibility complex
mho siemens unit
MHz megahertz
MI myocardial infarction
MID minimal infecting dose
MIP maximum inspiratory pressure
MK menaquinone (vitamin K_2)
mks, MKS meter-kilogram-second (system, unit)
ml, mL milliliter

MLC mixed lymphocyte culture (test)
MLD minimal lethal dose
mm millimeter
mmol millimole
MMPI Minnesota Multiphasic Personality Inventory
MMR measles-mumps-rubella (vaccine)
Mn manganese
Mo molybdenum
MO Medical Officer; mineral oil
mol mole
mol wt molecular weight
MOM Milk of Magnesia
MOPP Mustargen (mechlorethamine hydrocholoride), Oncovin (vincristine sulfate), procarbazine hydrochloride, and prednisone
mor. dict. [L.] *more dicto,* in the manner stated
mor. sol. [L.] *more solito,* as usual, as customary
MPD maximal permissible dose
MPS mononuclear phagocyte system
MR milk-ring (test)
*M*ᵣ molecular (weight) ratio
mrd, MRD minimal reacting dose
MRI magnetic resonance imaging
mRNA messenger RNA
ms millisecond
MS multiple sclerosis; morphine sulfate
msec millisecond
MSG monosodium glutamate
MSH melanocyte-stimulating hormone
mtDNA mitochondrial DNA
MTP metatarsophalangeal (joint)
Mu Mache unit
MUGA multiple-gated acquisition (imaging)
mV millivolt
Mv mendelevium
MVE Murray Valley encephalitis (virus)
MVV maximal voluntary ventilation
MW molecular weight
My myopia
ν nu; kinematic viscosity
n index of refraction; nano-
N newton; nitrogen; normal (concentration)
N normal (SMALL caps)
Na [Modern L.] *natrium,* sodium

NAD nicotinamide adenine dinucleotide; no acute distress

NAD⁺ nicotinamide adenine dinucleotide (oxidized form)

NADH nicotinamide adenine dinucleotide (reduced form)

NADP nicotinamide adenine dinucleotide phosphate

NADP⁺ nicotinamide adenine dinucleotide phosphate (oxidized form)

NADPH nicotinamide adenine dinucleotide phosphate (reduced form)

NAME nevi, atrial myxoma, myxoid neurofibromas, and ephelides (syndrome)

Nb niobium

NCV nerve conduction velocity

Nd neodymium

Ne neon

NE norepinephrine; not examined

NEEP negative end-expiratory pressure

NF National Formulary

ng nanogram

NGF nerve growth factor (antigen)

Ni nickel

NIH National Institutes of Health

NK natural killer (cell)

NKA no known allergies

NLM National Library of Medicine

nm nanometer

NMN nicotinamide mononucleotide

No nobelium

noc. maneq. [L.] *nocte maneque,* at night and in the morning

Np neptunium

NREM non-rapid eye movement (sleep)

nRNA nuclear RNA

NS normal saline

NSAID nonsteroidal anti-inflammatory drug

NSR normal sinus rhythm

NUG necrotizing ulcerative gingivitis

Ω omega; ohm

o- ortho-

O [L.] *oculus,* eye; opening (in formulas for electrical reactions); oxygen

OAV oculoauriculovertebral (dysplasia, syndrome)

OB obstetrics

OB/GYN obstetrics (and) gynecology

OBS organic brain syndrome

OC oral contraceptive

OCD obsessive-compulsive disorder

OD Doctor of Optometry; [L.] *oculus dexter,* right eye; overdose

ODD oculodentodigital (dysplasia, syndrome)

Oe oersted (centimeter-gram-second unit of magnetic field strength)

OFD orofaciodigital (dysostosis, syndrome)

OKT Ortho-Kung T (cell)

OML orbitomeatal line

OMM ophthalmomandibulomelic (dysplasia, syndrome)

omn. hor. [L.] *omni hora,* every hour

OMS organic mental syndrome

OP osmotic pressure; outpatient

O&P ova and parasites

OPV oral poliovirus vaccine

OR operating room

ORD optical rotatory dispersion

Orn ornithine (or its radical)

Oro orotate; orotic acid

Os osmium

OS [L.] *oculus sinister,* left eye

OSHA Occupational Safety and Health Administration

OT occupational therapy; Koch's old tuberculin

OTC over the counter (non-prescription drug)

OU [L.] *oculus uterque,* each eye (both eyes)

OXT oxytocin

oz ounce

p pico-; pupil

p- para-

P partial (pressure); peta-; phosphorus, phosphoric (residue); plasma (concentration); pressure; para (obstetric history)

³²P phosphorus-32

P₁ first parental generation

Pa pascal; protactinium

PA Physician's Assistant

PABA para-aminobenzoic acid

PAF platelet-aggregating (or -activating) factor

PAH para-aminohippuric (acid)

PAO₂ partial pressure of arterial oxygen

part. aeq. [L.] *partes aequales,* equal parts (amounts)

part. vic. [L.] *partitis vicibus,* in divided doses

PAS para-aminosalicylic (acid), periodic acid-Schiff (reagent)

PASA para-aminosalicylic acid

PAT paroxysmal atrial tachycardia

Pb [L.] *plumbum,* lead

PBG porphobilinogen

pc [L.] *post cibum,* after a meal

PCB polychlorinated biphenyl

Pco₂ partial pressure of carbon dioxide

PCP phencyclidine

Pd palladium

PD prism diopter

PDGF platelet-derived growth factor

PDLL poorly differentiated lymphocytic lymphoma

PEEP positive end-expiratory pressure

PEG polyethylene glycol

PET positron emission tomography

PF₄ platelet factor 4

PFT pulmonary function test

pg picogram

PG prostaglandin

PGA prostaglandin A

PGB prostaglandin B

PGE prostaglandin E

PGF prostaglandin F

pH hydrogen ion concentration; p (power) of $[H^+]_{10}$

Ph phenyl

Ph¹ Philadelphia (chromosome)

PHA phytohemagglutinin (antigen)

Pharm D [L.] *Pharmaciae Doctor,* Doctor of Pharmacy

PhD [L.] *Philosophiae Doctor,* Doctor of Philosophy

Phe phenylalanine (or its radical)

PhG Graduate in Pharmacy

PhG [L.] *Pharmacopoeia Germanica,* German Pharmacopeia

PICC peripherally inserted central catheter

PID pelvic inflammatory disease

PIF prolactin-inhibiting factor

PIP proximal interphalangeal (joint)

pK negative logarithm of the ionization constant (K_a) of an acid

PK pyruvate kinase

PKU phenylketonuria

pm picometer

Pm promethium

PM post mortem

PMN polymorphonuclear (leukocyte)

PMS premenstrual syndrome

PND paroxysmal nocturnal dyspnea; postnasal drip

PNP platelet neutralization procedure

PNPB positive-negative pressure breathing

Po polonium

PO [L.] *per os,* by mouth

PO₂, Po₂ partial pressure of oxygen

POEMS polyneuropathy, organomegaly, endocrinopathy, monoclonal protein, and skin changes (syndrome)

POMP prednisone, Oncovin (vincristine sulfate), methotrexate, and Purinethol (6-mercaptopurine)

POR problem-oriented (medical) record

PP pyrophosphate

PPCA proserum prothrombin conversion accelerator

PPD purified protein derivative (of tuberculin)

PPLO pleuropneumonia-like organism

ppm parts per million

PPO 2,5-diphenyloxazole

PPPPP pain, pallor, pulselessness, paresthesia, paralysis

PPPPPP pain, pallor, pulselessness, paresthesia, paralysis, prostration

PPV positive pressure ventilation

Pr praseodymium; presbyopia

PRA plasma renin activity

PRF prolactin-releasing factor

PRL prolactin

prn [L.] *pro re nata,* as needed

PRN [L.] *pro re nata,* as needed

pro rat. aet. [L.] *pro ratione aetatis,* according to (patient's) age

Pro proline (or its radicals)

psi pounds per square inch

PSV pressure-supported ventilation

Pt platinum

PT physical therapy; prothrombin time

PTA plasma thromboplastin antecedent; phosphotungstic acid; prior to admission

PTAH phosphotungstic acid hematoxylin

PTCA percutaneous transluminal coronary angioplasty

PTH parathyroid hormone

PTU prophylthiouracil

Pu plutonium

PUO pyrexia of unknown origin

PUPPP pruritic urticarial papules and plaques of pregnancy

PUVA (oral administration of) psoralen (and subsequent exposure to) ultraviolet light of A wavelength (UV-A)

PVC polyvinyl chloride; premature ventricular contraction

PVP polyvinylpyrrolidone (povidone)

Q volume of blood flow

Q coulomb

Qco$_2$ microliters CO_2 given off per milligram of dry weight of tissue per hour

qd [L.] *quaque die,* every day

qh [L.] *quaque hora,* every hour

qid [L.] *quater in die,* four times a day

q. l. [L.] *quantum libet,* as much as desired

QNS quantity not sufficient

Qo oxygen consumption

Qo$_2$ oxygen consumption

q. s. [L.] *quantum satis,* as much as is enough; [L.] *quantum sufficiat,* as much as may suffice; quantity sufficient

r racemic; roentgen

R gas constant (8.315 joules); (organic) radical; Réamur (scale) ; [L.] *recipe,* take; resistance determinant (plasmid); resistance (electrical); resistance (unit) (in the cardiovascular system); resolution; respiration; respiratory (exchange ratio); roentgen

Ra radium

RA rheumatoid arthritis

rad radian

RAS reticular activating system

RAST radioallergosorbent test

RAV Rous-associated virus

RAW resistance, airway

Rb rubidium

rbc red blood cell; red blood (cell) count

RBC red blood cell; red blood (cell) count

RBF renal blood flow

RD reaction of degeneration; reaction of denervation; Registered Dietician

RDA recommended daily allowance

rDNA ribosomal DNA

RDH Registered Dental Hygienist

RDS respiratory distress syndrome

RDW red (cell) diameter (or distribution) width

Re rhenium

RE right ear; right eye

rem roentgen equivalent, man

REM rapid eye movement (sleep); reticular erythematous mucinosis

rep roentgen equivalent, physical

RF release factor; rheumatoid factor

RFA right frontoanterior (fetal position)

RFLP restriction fragment length polymorphism

RFP right frontoposterior (fetal position)

RFT right frontotransverse (fetal position)

Rh Rhesus (Rh blood group); rhodium

RH releasing hormone

RIA radioimmunoassay

Rib ribose

RLL right lower lobe

RLQ right lower quadrant

RMA right mentoanterior (fetal position)

RML right middle lobe

RMP right mentoposterior (fetal position)

RMT right mentotransverse (fetal position)

Rn radon

RN Registered Nurse

RNA ribonucleic acid

RNase ribonuclease

RNP ribonucleoprotein

ROA right occipitoanterior (fetal position)

ROM range of motion

ROP right occipitoposterior (fetal position)

ROT right occipitotransverse (fetal position)

RP retinitis pigmentosa

RPF renal plasma flow

RPh Registered Pharmacist

rpm revolutions per minute

RPR rapid plasma reagent (test)

RQ respiratory quotient

rRNA ribosomal RNA

Rs resolution

RS respiratory syncytial (virus)

RSA right sacroanterior (fetal position)

RSP right sacroposterior (fetal position)

RST right sacrotransverse (fetal position)

RSV Rous-sarcoma virus; respiratory syncytial virus

rTMP ribothymidylic acid

Ru ruthenium

RUL right upper lobe

RUQ right upper quadrant

RV residual volume

RVH right ventricular hypertrophy

R$_x$ [L.] *recipe,* (the first word on a prescription), take; prescription; treatment

σ sigma; reflection coefficient; standard deviation; 1 millisecond (0.001 sec)

s [L.] *semis,* half; steady state (SUBSCRIPT); [L.] *sinister,* left

S [L.] *sinister,* left; saturation of hemoglobin (percentage of) (followed by subscript o_2 OR co_2); siemens; spherical; spherical (lens); sulfur; Svedberg (unit)

S$_1$ first selfing generation

S-A sinoatrial

SaO$_2$ oxygen saturation (of) arterial (oxyhemoglobin)

sat. saturated

sat. sol. saturated solution

Sb [L.] *stibium,* antimony

SBE subacute bacterial endocarditis

sc subcutaneous(ly)

Sc scandium

SC sternoclavicular; subcutaneous(ly)

SCID severe combined immunodeficiency

SD standard deviation; streptodornase

SDA specific dynamic action

Se selenium

Ser serine

Sf Svedberg flotation (constant, unit)

SGOT serum glutamic-oxaloacetic transaminase (aspartate aminotransferase)

SGPT serum glutamic-pyruvic transaminase (alanine aminotransferase)

SH serum hepatitis

Si silicon

SI [French] Système International d'Unités; International System of Units

SID source-to-image (-receptor) distance

SIDS sudden infant death syndrome

sig. [L.] *signa,* affix a label, inscribe

SIMV spontaneous intermittent mandatory ventilation; synchronized intermittent mandatory ventilation

SIRD source-to-image-receptor distance

SISI small-increment (or short-increment) sensitivity index (test)

SK streptokinase

SLE systemic lupus erythematosus

SLR straight leg raising

Sm samarium

Sn [L.] *stannum,* tin

SOAP subjective data, objective data, assessment, and plan (problem-oriented medical record)

SOB short(ness) of breath

sol. solution

soln. solution

s.o.s. [L.] *si opus sit,* if needed

sp. species

SPCA serum prothrombin conversion accelerator (factor VII)

SPECT single photon emission computed tomography

SPF sun protection (or protective) factor

sp. gr. specific gravity

sph spherical (lens)

spm suppression and mutation

spp. species (plural)

SQ subcutaneous

Sr strontium

SRF somatotropin-releasing factor

SRF-A slow-reacting factor of anaphylaxis

SRIF somatotropin-release-inhibiting factor

sRNA soluble RNA

SRS slow-reacting substance (of anaphylaxis)

SRS-A slow-reacting substance of anaphylaxis

ssDNA single-stranded DNA

ssp. subspecies

SSRI selective serotonin reuptake inhibitor

ST scapulothoracic

stat [L.] *statim,* immediately, at once

STD sexually transmitted disease

STEL short-term exposure limit

STH somatotropic hormone

STM short-term memory

STPD standard temperature (0° C) and pressure (760 mm Hg absolute), dry

Sv sievert (unit)

SV sievert (unit)

SVT supraventricular tachycardia

t metric ton

t temperature (Celsius); tritium

α-T α-tocopherol

T temperature, absolute (Kelvin); tension (intraocular); tera-; tesla; tetanus (toxoid); tidal (volume) (SUBSCRIPT); tocopherol; transverse (tubule); tritium; tumor (antigen)

T absolute temperature (Kelvin)

T_3 3,5,5′-triiodothyronine

T_4 tetraiodothyronine (thyroxine)

T ! decreased tension (pressure)

T+ increased tension (pressure)

Ta tantalum

TA *Terminologia Anatomica*

TAD transient acantholytic dermatosis

TAF tumor angiogenesis factor

TAR thrombocytopenia with absent radii (syndrome)

TAT thematic apperception test

Tb terbium

TB tuberculosis

TBP thyroxine-binding protein

TBV total blood volume

Tc technetium

^{99m}**Tc** technetium-99m

T&C type and crossmatch

TCA tricarboxylic acid; trichloracetic acid

TCN talocalcaneonavicular (joint)

Td tetanus-diphtheria (toxoids, adult type)

TDP ribothymidine 5′-diphosphate

Te tellurium

TEDD total end-diastolic diameter

TEN toxic epidermal necrolysis

TESD total end-systolic diameter

Th thorium

THC tetrahydrocannabinol

Thr threonine (or its radicals)

t_i/t_{tot} duty cycle

Ti titanium

TIA transient ischemic attack

t.i.d. [L.] *ter in die,* three times a day

tinct. tincture

TITh 3,5,3′-triiodothyronine

TKO to keep (venous infusion line) open

Tl thallium

TLC thin-layer chromatography; total lung capacity; tender, loving care

TLV threshold-limit value

t_m temperature midpoint (Celsius)

Tm thulium; tubular maximal (excretory capacity of kidneys)

T_m temperature midpoint (Kelvin)

TM transport maximum

TMJ temporomandibular joint

TMP ribothymidine 5′-monophosphate

TMT tarsometatarsal

TMV tobacco mosaic virus

Tn (ocular) tension; (intraocular) tension normal

TNF tumor necrosis factor

TNM tumor, node, metastasis (tumor staging)

TORCH toxoplasmosis, other, rubella, cytomegalovirus, and herpes simplex (maternal infections)

t-PA, TPA tissue plasminogen activator

TPHA *Treponema pallidum* hemagglutination (test)

TPI *Treponema pallidum* immobilization (test)

TPN total parenteral nutrition

TPR temperature, pulse, and respirations

tr. tincture

TRH thyrotropin-releasing hormone (stimulation test)

TRIC trachoma inclusion conjunctivitis (organism)

tRNA transfer RNA

Trp tryptophan (and its radicals)

TSH thyroid-stimulating hormone

TSS toxic shock syndrome

TSTA tumor-specific transplantation antigen

TTP thrombotic thrombocytopenic purpura

TU toxic unit, toxin unit

Tyr tyrosine (and its radicals)

U unit; uranium; uridine (in polymers); urinary (concentration)

UA urinalysis

UDP uridine diphosphate

UDPG UDP-glucose

UGIS upper gastrointestinal series

UMP uridine monophosphate (uridylic acid)

ung. [L.] *unguentum,* ointment

u-PA urokinase

Urd uridine

URI upper respiratory infection

USAN United States Adopted Names (Council)

USP *United States Pharmacopeia*

USPHS United States Public Health Service

UTI urinary tract infection

UTP uridine triphosphate

UV ultraviolet

v venous (blood); volt

V vanadium; vision; visual (acuity); volt; volume (frequently with subscripts denoting location, chemical species, and conditions)

$\dot{V}$ ventilation; gas flow (frequently with subscripts indicating location and chemical species); ventilation;

V_1CV_6 unipolar precordial electrocardiogram chest leads

VA viral antigen

$\dot{V}_A$ alveolar ventilation

V-A ventriculoatrial

Val valine (and its radicals)

$\dot{V}a/\dot{Q}$ ventilation/perfusion ratio

VATER vertebral defects, imperforate anus, tracheoesophageal fistula with esophageal atresia, and radial and renal dysplasia (complex)

VC vision, color; vital capacity

VCE vagina, (ecto)cervix, endocervical canal

V_D (physiologic) dead space

VDRL Venereal Disease Research Laboratory (test)

VHDL very-high-density lipoprotein

VIP vasoactive intestinal polypeptide

VLDL very-low-density lipoprotein

VMA vanillylmandelic acid (test)

V_{max} maximal velocity

VP vasopressin

VR vocal resonance

VS volumetric solution

V_T tidal volume

W watt; [German] *Wolfram,* tungsten

Wb weber

WBC white blood cell; white blood (cell) count

WD well-developed

WDLL well-differentiated lymphocytic (or lymphatic) lymphoma

WHO World Health Organization

WN well-nourished

X xanthosine

Xao xanthosine

Xe xenon

^{133}**Xe** xenon-133

XU excretory urogram

Y yttrium

YAG yttrium-aluminum-garnet (laser)

Yb ytterbium

Z carbobenzoxy (chloride)

ZEEP zero end-expiratory pressure

ZES Zollinger-Ellison syndrome

Zn zinc

^{65}**Zn** zinc-65

Zr zirconium

ZSR zeta sedimentation ratio

Appendices

SYMBOLS

Angles, Triangles, and Circles

∧   above • diastolic blood pressure (anesthesia records) • elevated • enlarged • improved • increased • superior (position) • upper

∨   below • decreased • deficiency • deficit • depressed • deteriorated • diminished • down • inferior (position) • lower • systolic blood pressure (anesthesia records)

>   causes • demonstrates • distal • followed by • derived from • greater than • indicates • leads to • more severe than • produces • radiates to • radiating to • results in • reveals • shows • to • toward • worse than • yields

<   caused by • derived from • less severe than • less than • produced by • proximal

∠   angle • flexion • flexor

∠E   angle of entry

∠x   angle of exit

∟   factorial product • right lower quadrant

⌐   right upper quadrant

¬   left upper quadrant

⌐   left lower quadrant

Δ   anion gap • centrad prism • change • delta gap • heat • increment • occipital triangle • prism diopter • temperature (anesthesia records)

Δ+   time interval

Δ A   change in absorbance

Δ dB   difference in decibels

Δ P   change in (intraocular) pressure

Δ pH   change in pH

Δ t   time interval

ΔH, HΔ   Hesselbach triangle

○   respiration (anesthesia records)

♀   female • female sex

♂   male • male sex

(A), (ax)   axilla (temperature)

(H), (h)   hypodermic • hypodermically

(IM)   intramuscular • intramuscularly

(IV)   intravenous • intravenously

(L)   left

(M)   murmur

(m)   by mouth • mouth (temperature) • murmur

√(m)   factitial murmur

(O)   by mouth • oral • orally

(R)   rectal • rectally • rectum (temperature) • right

(X)   end of anesthesia (anesthesia records • end of operation

Arrows

↑   above • elevated • elevation • enlarged • gas • greater than • improved • increase • increased • increases • more than • rising • superior (position) • up • upper

↑g   increasing • rising

↑V   increase due to in vivo effect (lab)

↓   below • decrease • decreased • deficiency • deficit • depressed • depression • deteriorating • diminished • diminution • down • falling • inferior (position) • less than • low • slower • normal plantar reflex • precipitate • precipitates

↓g   decreasing • diminishing • falling • lowering

↓V   decrease due to in vivo effect (lab)

↗   deviated • displaced • increasing

↘   decreasing

→   approaches limit of • causes demonstrates • direction of flow or reaction • distal • due to • followed by • indicates • leads to • produces • radiating to • results in • reveals • shows • to • to right • toward • yields

←   caused by • derived from • direction of flow or reaction • due to • produced by • proximal • resulting from • secondary to • to left

↑↑   extensor response (Babinski sign) • positive Babinski • testes undescended

↓↓   down bilaterally • plantar response (Babinski sign) • testes descended

↓↑   reversible reaction • up and down

⇆, ⇌   reversible (chemical) reaction

Genetic Symbols

Symbol	Meaning
□	male
○	female
◇	sex unspecified
□ ○	normal individuals
■ ● ◆	affected individual (with ≥ 2 conditions, the symbol is partioned and shaded with a different fill defined in a key or legend)
5 ⑤ ⟨5⟩	multiple individuals, number known (number of siblings written inside symbol)
n ⓝ ⟨n⟩	multiple individuals, number unknown ("n" used in place of specific number)
□—○	mating
□═○	consaguinity
(+)	uncommon or uncertain mode of inheritance
I □—○ II □ ○	parents and offspring, in generations
□ ○ (dizygotic)	dizygotic twins
□ ○ (monozygotic)	monozygotic twins
④ ③	number of children of sex indicated
□ ○ (adopted)	adopted individuals
⚲ ⚲	individual died without leaving offspring
□ ○ (no issue)	no issue
■ ●	affected individuals

Symbol	Meaning
↗■ ↗●	proband or propositus (first affected family member coming to medical attention)
⊞	examined professionally • normal for trait
⊡	not examined • dubiously reported to have trait
◫	not examined • reliably reported to have trait
◧ ◖	heterozygotes for autosomal recessive
⊙	carrier of sex-linked recessive
⊘ ⊘	death
⊘ SB 28 wk	⊘ SB 30 wk	⬦ SB 34 wk	stillbirth (SB)
▨ LMP 7/1/94	Ⓟ 20 wk	Ⓟ	pregnancy (P); gestational age and karotype (if known) below symbol
↗□ ↗○	consultand (individual seeking genetic counseling/testing)
△ male	△ female	△ ECT	spontaneous abortion (SAB); ECT below symbol indicates ectopic pregnancy
▲ male	▲ female	▲ 16 wk	affected SAB (gestational age, if known, below symbol, and key or legend used to define shading)
⧄ male	⧄ female	termination of pregnancy (TOP)
◣ male	◣ female	affected TOP (key or legend used to define shading)

Source: Genetic symbols are public domain: we credit and gratefully acknowledge the *American Journal of Human Genetics* (56:746–747, 1995) as our source for these symbols.

Numbers

0	completely absent (pulse) no response (reflexes)
+1, 1+	markedly impaired (pulse)
1+	low normal or somewhat diminished (reflexes) slight reaction or trace (lab tests)
+2, 2+	moderately impaired (pulse)
2+	average or normal (reflexes) noticeable reaction or trace (lab tests)
+3, 3+	slightly impaired (pulse)
3+	moderate reaction (lab tests) more brisk than average (reflexes)
+4, 4+	normal (pulse)
4+	hyperactive (reflexes) large amount (lab tests) pronounced reaction (lab tests)
•	very brisk (reflexes)
$\bar{1}$	bowel movement (numeral indicates number of stools in a given period)
1×	once one time
2×, ×2	twice two times
3×, ×3	three times, etc.

Appendices

Arabic	Roman		Arabic	Roman
0			17	XVII
1	I,		18	XVIII
2	II, ii		19	XIX
3	III, iii		20	XX
4	IV, iv		30	XXX
5	V, v		40	XL
6	VI, vi		50	L
7	VII, vii		60	LX
8	VIII, viii		70	LXX
9	IX, ix		80	LXXX
10	X, x		90	XC
11	XI, xi		100	C
12	XII, xii		1,000	M
13	XIII, xiii		5,000	$\overline{V}$
14	XIV, xiv		10,000	$\overline{X}$
15	XV		100,000	$\overline{C}$
16	XVI		1,000,000	$\overline{M}$

Pluses, Minuses, and Equivalencies

+	acid (reaction) • added to • convex lens • decreased or diminished (reflexes) • excess • less than 50% • inhibition of • hemolysis (Wassermann) • low normal (reflexes) • markedly impaired (pulse) • mild (severity) • plus • positive (lab tests) • present • slight reaction or trace (lab tests) • sluggish (reflexes) • somewhat diminished (reflexes)
(+)	significant
(+)ive	positive
+ to ++	slight pain
++	average (reflexes) • 50% inhibition of hemolysis (Wassermann) • moderate (pain, severity) • moderately impaired (pulse) • normally active (reflexes) • noticeable reaction or trace (lab tests)
+++	increased reflexes 75% inhibition of • hemolysis (Wassermann) • moderate amount • moderate reaction (lab tests) • moderately, hyperative (reflexes) • moderately severe (pain, severity) • more brisk than average (reflexes) • slightly impaired (pulse)
++++	complete inhibition of hemolysis (Wassermann) • large amount (lab tests) • markedly hyperactive (reflexes) • markedly severe (pain, severity) • normal (pulse) • pronounced reaction (lab tests) • very brisk (reflexes)
−	absent • alkaline (reaction) • concave lens • deficiency • deficient • minus • negative (lab test) • none • subtract • without

(−)	insignificant
±	doubtful • either positive or negative • equivocal (reflexes, qualitative tests) • flicker (reflexes) • indefinite • more or less • plus or minus • possibly significant • questionable • suggestive • variable • very slight (reaction, severity, trace) • with or without
(±)	possibly significant
± to +	minimal pain
∓	minus or plus
‡	moderate (severity) • normally active (reflexes)
#	fracture • gauge • number • pound(s) • weight
~	about • approximate • approximately • proportionate to
≈	approximately equal to
=	equal to
≠	not equal to
⌒	combined with
⇌	equivalent
⇎	not equivalent to
≡	identical • identical with
≢	not identical • not identical with
≒	nearly equal to
≑	approximately equal

(continued)

	Pluses, Minuses, and Equivalencies (*continued*)		
$\cong$	approximately • approximately equals • congruent to	$\not>$	not greater than
$\doteq$	approaches	$<$	less than
$\overset{=}{\_}$	equilateral	$\not<$	not less than
$\triangleq$	equiangular	$\geq, \geqslant$	greater than or equal to
$>$	greater than	$\leq, \leqslant$	less than or equal to

	Primes, Checks, Dots, Roots, and Other Symbols		
?	doubtful • equivocal (reflexes) • flicker (reflexes) • not tested (severity) • possible • questionable • question of • suggested • suggestive (severity) • unknown	$\sqrt{g}, \sqrt{\text{ing}}$	checking
!	factorial product	$\sqrt{\text{qs}}$	voided sufficient quantity
†	death • deceased	$\sqrt{}$	radical root
/	divided by • either meaning • extension • extensors fraction • of • per • to	$\sqrt[2]{}$	square root
'	foot • hour • univalent	$\sqrt[3]{}$	cube root
"	bivalent • ditto • inch • minute • second (1/60 degree)	*	birth • multiplication sign (genetics) • not verified • presumed • supposed
'''	line (1/12 inch) • trivalent	°	degree • measurement (1/360 of circle) • severity (burns, wounds) • temperature • time (hour)
$\sqrt{}$	check • observe for • urine • voided (urine)	:	is to • ratio
$\sqrt{\cdot}$	urine and defecation • voided and bowels moved	...	no data (in given category)
$\sqrt{\bar{c}}$	check with	∴	therefore
$\sqrt{d}$	checked • observed	∵	because • since
		::	as • equality between ratios • proportion • proportionate to

	Statistical Symbols		
α	probability of Type I error significance level	O	observed frequency in a contingency table
β	probability of Type II error	ϕ	ability continuum phi coefficient
$1-\beta$	power of statistical test	P	probability
$nCk; \binom{n}{k}$	binomial coefficient number of combination of n things taken k at a time	p	probability of success in independent trials
χ^2	chi-squared statistic	$P(A)$	probability that event A occurs
E	expected frequency in cell of contingency table	$P(A\backslash B)$	conditional probability that A occurs given that B has occurred
$E(X)$	expected value of random variable X	r	sample correlation coefficient, usually the Pearson product-moment correlation
F	F statistic (variance ratio)	r^2	coefficient of determination
f	frequency	r_s	Spearman rank correlation coefficient
H_0	null hypothesis		
H_1	alternative hypothesis	ρ	population correlation coefficient
μ	population mean	s	sample standard deviation
N	population size	s^2	sample variance
n	sample size	SE	standard error of estimate
$n!$	n factorial	σ	population standard deviation
		σ^2	population variance

$\sigma_{diff.}$	standard error of difference between scores		z	standard score
$\sigma_{est.}$	standard error of estimate		$=$	equal
$\sigma_{meas.}$	standard error of measurement		$\neq$	not equal
$\sum_{i=1}^{n} x_1, \sum_{i}^{n} x_i$	$x_1 + x_2 + \ldots + x_n$		$\approx$	approximately equal
t	Student t statistic Student test variable		$>$	greater than
			$\ngtr$	not greater than
θ	latent trait		$<$	less than
U	Mann-Whitney rank sum statistic		$\nless$	not less than
W	Wilcoxon rank sum statistic		$\geq, \geqslant$	greater than or equal to
$\overline{X}$	sample mean		$\leq, \leqslant$	less than or equal to
$|x|$	absolute value of x		∞	infinity
$\sqrt{x}$	square root of x			

ARTERIES OF THE HUMAN BODY

Artery/Arteries	Origin	Course	Branches/Distribution
Abdominal aorta	Continuation of thoracic aorta	Runs on anterior aspect of bodies of lumbar vertebrae	Visceral branches: celiac, superior and inferior mesenteric, renal, middle suprarenal, gonadal Parietal branches: lumbar, median sacral
Angular	Terminal branch of facial artery	Passes to medial angle (canthus) of eye	Superior part of cheek and lower eyelid
Anterior cerebral	Terminal branch (with middle cerebral) of internal carotid artery	Passes anteriorly, loops around genu of corpus callosum, then passes posteriorly in interhemispheric fissure	A1 segment: thalamus and corpus striatum A2 segment: cortex of medial aspects of frontal and parietal lobes
Anterior ciliary	Muscular (rectus) branches of ophthalmic artery	Pierces sclera at attachments of rectus muscles and forms network in iris and ciliary body	Iris and ciliary body
Anterior communicating	Anterior cerebral artery	Connects anterior cerebral arteries in prechiasmatic cistern, to complete cerebral arterial circle	Anteromedial central perforating arteries
Anterior division of internal iliac	Internal iliac	Passes anteriorly along lateral wall of lesser pelvis in hypogastric sheath and divides into visceral and parietal branches	Parietal branch: obturator artery Visceral branches: umbilical artery, inferior vesical, uterine, vaginal, middle rectal and pudendal
Anterior ethmoidal	Ophthalmic artery	Passes through anterior ethmoidal foramen to anterior cranial fossa and into nasal cavity, sending branches to skin of nose	Supplies anterior and middle ethmoidal cells, dura of anterior cranial fossa, anterosuperior nasal cavity, and skin on dorsum of nose
Anterior inferior cerebellar	Lower (initial) part of basilar artery	Runs posterolaterally, often looping in and out of internal acoustic meatus	Supplies inferior aspect of lateral lobes of cerebellum, inferolateral pons, and choroid plexus in cerebellopontine angle; usually gives rise to labyrinthine artery
Anterior intercostal (brs.)	Internal thoracic (intercostal spaces 1–6) and musculophrenic arteries (intercostal spaces 7–9)	Pass between internal and innermost intercostal muscles	Intercostal muscles, overlying skin, and underlying parietal pleura
Anterior interventricular (br.)	Left coronary artery	Passes along anterior IV groove to apex of heart	Walls of right and left ventricles including most of IV septum and contained atrioventricular bundle and branches (conducting tissue)
Anterior spinal	Superiorly, by a merger of intra-cranial branches, one from each vertebral artery; it is continued inferiorly by bifurcations of anterior segmental medullary arteries at various levels	Forms a continuous anastomotic chain that descends the length of the spinal cord in the entrance to the anterior median fissure	Supplies the anterior portion of the spinal cord by means of sulcal branches, which extend into the anterior median fissure, and the pial plexus, which ramifies over the surface of the cord
Anterior superior alveolar	Infraorbital artery	Arises within infraorbital canal and ascends through anterior alveolar canals	Supplies mucosa of maxillary sinus, and maxillary superior incisor and canine teeth
Anterior tibial	Terminal branch (with posterior tibial) of popliteal artery	Passes between tibia and fibula into anterior compartment through gap in superior part of interosseous membrane and descends this membrane between tibialis anterior and extensor digitorum longus	Anterior compartment of leg
Appendicular	Ileocolic artery	Passes between layers of mesoappendix	Vermiform appendix
Arch of aorta	Continuation of ascending aorta	Arches posteriorly on left side of trachea and esophagus and superior to root of left lung	Brachiocephalic, left common carotid, left subclavian
Arcuate (of foot)	Continuation of dorsalis pedis	Passes laterally, dorsal to the bases of the metatarsals	2nd, 3rd and 4th dorsal metatarsal arteries

Artery/Arteries	Origin	Course	Branches/Distribution
Artery of bulb of penis or vestibule of vagina	Internal pudendal artery	Pierces perineal membrane to reach bulb of penis or vestibule of vagina	Supplies bulb of penis or vestibule and bulbourethral gland (male) and greater vestibular gland (female)
Artery to ductus deferens	Inferior (or superior) vesical	Runs retroperitoneally to ductus deferens	Ductus deferens
Ascending aorta	Aortic orifice of left ventricle	Ascends approximately 5 cm to level of sternal angle where it becomes arch of aorta	Right and left coronary arteries
Ascending cervical	Terminal branch (with inferior thyroid artery) of thyrocervical trunk	Ascends on prevertebral fascia	Supplies anterior prevertebral muscles; anastomoses widely with other arteries of neck
Ascending palatine	Facial artery	Ascends alongside and crosses over superior border of superior constrictor of pharynx to reach soft palate and tonsillar fossa	Supplies lateral wall of pharynx, tonsils pharyngotympanic (auditory) tube, and soft palate
Ascending pharyngeal	Medial aspect of external carotid artery	Ascends between internal carotid artery and pharynx to cranial base, sending branches through jugular foramen and hypoglossal canal	Supplies pharyngeal wall, palatine tonsil, soft palate, and dura of posterior cranial fossa
Atrioventricular (AV) nodal (br.)	Right coronary artery near origin of posterior IV artery	Runs anteriorly in uppermost part of interventricular septum to AV node	AV node
Axillary	Continuation of subclavian artery after crossing 1st rib	Runs inferolaterally through axillary fossa, changing to brachial artery when it crosses the inferior border of teres major; parts are medial (1st), posterior (2nd), and lateral (3rd) to pectoralis minor	1st part: superior thoracic 2nd part: thoracoacromial and lateral thoracic arteries 3rd part: subclavian and anterior and posterior circumflex humeral arteries
Basilar	Formed by intracranial union of vertebral arteries	Ascends clivus in pontine cistern; terminates by bifurcating into posterior cerebral arteries	Branches: anterior inferior cerebellar, labyrinthine, pontine, mesencephalic, and superior cerebellar arteries
Brachial	Continuation of axillary artery past inferior border of teres major	Courses in medial intermuscular septum with median nerve; ends by bifurcating into radial and ulnar arteries in cubital fossa	Main artery of arm; branches: deep artery of arm, muscular and nutrient branches, superior and inferior ulnar collateral
Brachiocephalic (trunk)	1st and largest branch of arch of aorta	Ascends posterolaterally to the right, running anterior and then to the right of the trachea; deep to the sternoclavicular joint, it bifurcates into terminal branches	Right common carotid and right subclavian arteries
Bronchial (1–2 branches)	Anterior aspect of 1st part of thoracic aorta or 3rd rt. posterior intercostal artery	Run on the posterior aspects of the primary bronchi and follow the tracheobronchial tree	Bronchial and peribronchial tissue, visceral pleura
Buccal	Maxillary artery	Runs anterolaterally with buccal nerve, emerging from beneath anterior border of ramus of mandible	Supplies buccinator muscle, overlying skin, and underlying oral mucosa; anastomoses with branchs of facial and infraorbital arteries
Carpal branches, dorsal and palmar	Radial and ulnar arteries at level of wrist	Anastomose with corresponding branches of counterpart artery (ulnar or to form dorsal and palmar carpal arches	Provide collateral circulation at wrist
Celiac	Abdominal aorta just distal to aortic hiatus of diaphragm	Runs a short course (1.25 cm), giving rise to left gastric, and bifurcating into splenic and common hepatic arteries	Supplies inferiormost esophagus, stomach, duodenum (proximal to bile duct), liver and biliary apparatus, and pancreas
Central artery of retina	Ophthalmic artery	Runs in dural sheath of optic nerve and pierces nerve near eyeball; ramifying from center of optic disc into retinal arterioles	Supplies optic retina (except cones and rods); branches: macular, nasal and temporal retinal arterioles

Artery/Arteries	Origin	Course	Branches/Distribution
Circumflex (branch)	Left coronary artery	Passes to left in atrioventricular groove and runs to posterior surface of heart	Primarily left atrium and left ventricle; branches: left ventricular, atrial, and marginal
Circumflex humeral, anterior and posterior	Third part of axillary artery, typically opposite origin of subscapular artery	These arteries anastomose to form a circle around surgical neck of humerus; the larger posterior circumflex humeral artery passes through quadrangular space with axillary nerve	Supply shoulder joint, and muscles of proximal arm: deltoid, teres major and minor, and long and lateral heads of triceps
Circumflex scapular artery	Terminal branch (with thoracodorsal artery) of subscapular artery	Curves around axillary border of scapula and enters infraspinous fossa	Supplies subscapular and infraspinatus muscles; joins collateral anastomosis of shoulder around scapula
Common carotid, left and right	Left: 2nd branch of arch of aorta Right: terminal branch (with right subclavian) of brachiocephalic artery	Ascend from/pass deep to sterno-clavicular joint in carotid sheath under cover of sternocleidomastoid to level of C4 vertebra (or hyoid bone)	Terminal branches: internal and external carotid arteries
Common hepatic	Terminal branch (with splenic artery) of celiac artery (trunk)	Passes to right along superior border of pancreas, running anterior to portal vein	Terminal branches: hepatic artery proper and gastroduodenal artery
Common iliac, left and right	Terminal branches of abdominal aorta	Begin anterior to L4 vertebral body, diverging as they descend to terminate at L5/S1 level, anterior to sacroiliac joints	Terminal branches: external and internal iliac arteries
Common interosseous	Ulnar artery, just distal to bifurcation of brachial artery in cubital fossa	Passes deep to bifurcate into terminal branches after a very short course	Terminal branches: anterior and posterior interosseous arteries
Common palmar digital	Superficial palmar arch	Pass distally anterior to lumbricals to bifurcate proximal to webbings between digits	Receive palmar metacarpal arteries from deep palmar arch; terminal branches: proper palmar digital arteries
Common plantar digital arteries	Terminal portions of plantar metatarsal arteries	Short segments distal to transverse head of adductor hallucis proximal to webs between toes	Terminal branches: plantar digital arteries proper
Costocervical (trunk)	2nd part of subclavian artery	Very short artery passes posteriorly superior to cervical pleura to neck of 1st rib, and bifurcates into terminal branches	Terminal branches: supreme intercostal and deep cervical arteries
Cremasteric	Inferior epigastric	Accompanies spermatic cord through inguinal canal and into scrotal sac	Supplies cremaster muscle and other coverings of cord in males; round ligament in females
Cystic	Right hepatic artery	Arises within hepatoduodenal ligament	Gallbladder and cystic duct
Deep artery of arm	Brachial artery near its origin	Accompanies radial nerve through radial groove in humerus; terminal branches take part in anastomosis around elbow joint	Branches: deltoid, muscular (to head of triceps) and nutrient (to humerus) branches Terminal branches: middle and radial collateral arteries
Deep artery of penis or clitoris	Terminal branch of internal pudendal artery	Pierces perineal membrane to reach erectile bodies of clitoris or penis (corpora cavernosa)	Terminations (helicine arteries) uncoil to engorge erectile sinuses with arterial blood
Deep artery of thigh	Femoral artery in femoral triangle (about 4 cm distal to inguinal ligament)	Passes inferiorly on medial intermuscular septum, deep to adductor longus	Perforating branches pass through adductor magnus muscle to posterior and lateral part of anterior compartments of thigh
Deep auricular	1st part of maxillary artery	Ascends in parotid gland posterior to temporomandibular joint, piercing wall of external acoustic meatus	Supplies temporomandibular joint and skin of external acoustic meatus and tympanic membrane
Deep cervical	Costocervical trunk	Passes posteriorly between transverse process of C7 and neck of 1st rib and ascends between semispinalis cervicis and capitis to C2 level	Supplies deep posterior muscles of neck and anastomoses with descending branch of occipital artery and branches of vertebral artery

Appendices

Artery/Arteries	Origin	Course	Branches/Distribution
Deep circumflex iliac	External iliac artery	Runs on deep aspect of anterior abdominal wall, parallel to inguinal ligament	Supplies iliacus muscle and inferior part of anterolateral abdominal wall
Deep lingual	Continuation (third part of) lingual artery	Turns superiorly near anterior border of hyoglossus and then passes anteriorly flanking frenulum just deep to mucosa	Supplies genioglossus, inferior longitudinal muscle and mucosa of underside of tongue, tip of tongue
Deep palmar arch	Direct continuation of radial artery, completed on medial side by deep branch of ulnar artery	Curves medially, deep to long flexor tendons in contact with bases of metacarpals	Branches: palmar metacarpal arteries
Deep plantar arch	Continuation of lateral plantar artery	Courses anteromedially, between 3rd and 4th layers of muscles of sole of foot; anastomoses with dorsalis pedis via deep plantar artery between 1st and 2nd metatarsal bases	Branches: plantar metatarsal arteries
Deep temporal, anterior and posterior	2nd part of maxillary artery	Ascend between temporalis and bone of temporal fossa	Supplies temporalis muscle, periosteum and bone
Descending genicular	Femoral artery, in adductor canal	Descends in vastus medialis, just anterior to tendon of adductor magnus, to anastomose with superior medial genicular artery	Branches: saphenous branch, accompanying saphenous nerve to medial skin of leg; muscular branches to vastus medialis and adductor magnus
Descending palatine	3rd part of maxillary artery	Arises in pterygopalatine fossa; descends in palatine canal	Branches: greater and lesser palatine arteries
Dorsal artery of penis or clitoris	Terminal branch of internal pudendal artery	Pierces perineal membrane and passes through suspensory ligament of penis or clitoris to run on dorsum of penis or clitoris	Skin of penis and erectile tissue of penis or clitoris
Dorsal carpal arch	Radial and ulnar arteries	Arches within fascia on dorsum of hand	Branches: dorsal metacarpal arteries
Dorsal digital arteries (of fingers)	Dorsal metacarpal arteries	Run distally on the posterolateral aspects of the proximal one and a half phalanges	Supply dorsal aspects of proximal one and a half phalanges of fingers
Dorsal digital arteries (of toes)	Dorsal metatarsal arteries	Run distally on the posterolateral aspects of the proximal one and a half phalanges	Supply dorsal aspects of proximal one and a half phalanges of toes
Dorsal metacarpal	Dorsal carpal arch	Run on 2nd–4th dorsal interossei	Bifurcate into dorsal digital arteries; supply skin, muscle and bone of dorsum of hand and fingers to center of middle phalanx
Dorsal metatarsal	1st: termination of dorsalis pedis 2nd, 3rd and 4th: arcuate artery	Run distally on the superficial aspect of the corresponding dorsal interosseous muscles	Branches: dorsal digital arteries (of toes)
Dorsal nasal	Ophthalmic artery	Courses along dorsal aspect of nose and supplies its surface	Courses along dorsal aspect of nose and supplies its surface
Dorsal pancreatic	Splenic artery	Descends posterior to pancreas, dividing into right and left branches	Supplies middle portion of pancreas
Dorsal scapular (variation—1/3 of time it is replaced by a deep branch of the transverse cervical a.)	3rd (or 2nd) part of subclavian artery	Passes laterally through brachial plexus then deep to levator scapulae; joins dorsal scapular nerve running along vertebral border of scapula, deep to rhomboid muscles	Supplies branches to the trapezius, rhomboids, latissimus dorsi; participates in anastomoses around scapula (shoulder)
Dorsalis pedis	Continuation of anterior tibial artery distal to inferior extensor retinaculum	Descends anteromedially to first interosseous space and divides into plantar and arcuate arteries	Muscles on dorsum of foot; pierces first dorsal interosseous muscle as deep plantar artery to contribute to formation of plantar arch
Esophageal (4–5 branches)	Anterior aspect of thoracic aorta	Run anteriorly to esophagus	Esophagus

Artery/Arteries	Origin	Course	Branches/Distribution
External carotid	Common carotid artery at superior border of thyroid cartilage	Ascends slightly anteriorly and then inclines posteriorly and laterally, passing between mastoid process and mandible; enters substance of parotid gland, bifurcating into terminal branches deep to neck of mandible	Anterior branches: superior thyroid, facial and lingual aa. Posterior branches: occipital and posterior auricular arteries Medial branch: ascending pharyngeal Terminal branches: maxillary and superficial temporal arteries
External pudendal, superficial, and deep branches	Femoral artery	Pass medially across the thigh to reach the scrotum or labia majora	Skin of mons pubis and anterior labia (female); or root of penis and anterior scrotum (male)
Facial	External carotid artery	Ascends deep to submandibular gland, winds around inferior border of mandible and enters face, ascending obliquely across cheek, and side of nose to medial angle of eye	Branches: ascending palatine, tonsillar, glandular, submental, inferior and superior labial, and lateral nasal Terminal branch (continuation): angular artery
Femoral	Continuation of external iliac artery distal to inguinal ligament	Descends through femoral triangle, traverses adductor canal, and changes name to "popliteal" at adductor hiatus	Supplies anterior and anteromedial surfaces of thigh
Fibular (peroneal)	Posterior tibial	Descends in posterior compartment adjacent to posterior intermuscular septum	Posterior compartment of leg: perforating branches supply lateral compartment of leg
Gastroduodenal	Hepatic artery	Descends retroperitoneally, posterior to gastroduodenal junction	Stomach, pancreas, first part of duodenum, and distal part of bile duct
Genicular (superior lateral and medial, inferior lateral and medial, and middle)	Popliteal	Arise and run to "four corners" of knee joint (viewed anteriorly) around the patella and femoral and tibial condyles; middle genicular pierces oblique popliteal ligament in posterior center of joint capsule	Form, with participation also of descending genicular, descending branch of lateral circumflex femoral, circumflex fibular and recurrent tibial arteries, the genicular articular anastomosis
Greater pancreatic	Splenic artery	Penetrates left portion of pancreas, splitting into right and left branches which parallel pancreatic duct	Anastomoses with other pancreatic branches; supplies mostly the tail of the pancreas and contained duct
Hepatic artery proper	Celiac trunk	Passes retroperitoneally to reach hepatoduodenal ligament and passes between its layers to porta hepatis; bifurcates into right and left hepatic arteries	Branches: (right gastric, supraduodenal), right and left hepatic arteries; supplies liver and gallbladder, (stomach, pancreas, duodenum)
Ileocolic	Terminal branch of superior mesenteric artery	Runs along root of mesentery and divides into ileal and colic branches	Ileum, cecum, and ascending colon
Iliolumbar	Posterior division of internal iliac	Ascends anterior to sacroiliac joint and posterior to common iliac vessels and psoas major	Psoas major, iliacus and quadratus lumborum muscles, cauda equina in vertebral canal
Inferior alveolar	1st part of maxillary artery	Descends posterior to nerve of same name between medial pterygoid and ramus of mandible to enter mandibular canal via mandibular foramen	Branches: mylohyoid branch, dental branches, mental branch; Supplies muscles of floor of mouth, mandible and lower teeth, soft tissue of chin
Inferior epigastric	External iliac artery	Runs superiorly and enters rectus sheath; runs deep to rectus abdominis	Rectus abdominis and medial part of anterolateral abdominal wall
Inferior gluteal	Anterior division of internal iliac	Exits pelvis to enter gluteal region through greater sciatic foramen inferior to piriformis and descends on medial side of sciatic nerve; anastomoses with superior gluteal artery and participates in cruciate anastomosis of thigh, involving first perforating artery of deep femoral and medial and lateral circumflex femoral arteries	Pelvic diaphragm (coccygeus and levator ani), piriformis, quadratus femoris, uppermost hamstrings, gluteus maximus, sciatic nerve

Appendices

Artery/Arteries	Origin	Course	Branches/Distribution
Inferior labial	Facial artery near angle of mouth	Runs medially in lower lip	Lower lip and chin
Inferior mesenteric	Abdominal aorta	Descends retroperitoneally to left of abdominal aorta	Supplies part of gastrointestinal tract derived from hindgut
Inferior pancreaticoduodenal, anterior and posterior	Superior mesenteric artery	Ascends retroperitoneally on head of pancreas	Distal portion of duodenum and inferior head and uncinate process of pancreas
Inferior phrenic	As 1st branches of abdominal aorta (sometimes via a common stem, or from celiac trunk)	Ascend crus to underside of domes; medial branches anastomoses with each other and pericardiacophrenic arteries; lateral branches approach thoracic wall, anastomose with posterior intercostal and musculophrenic arteries	Branches: superior suprarenal arteries Supplies: diaphragm, inferior vena cava (right branch), esophagus (left branch), suprarenal glands
Inferior rectal	Internal pudendal artery	Leaves pudendal canal, and crosses ischioanal fossa to anal canal	Distal portion of anal canal (mainly inferior to pectinate line)
Inferior suprarenal	Renal	Ascends vertically to gland	Posterior and inferior aspects of suprarenal gland
Inferior thyroid	Terminal branch (with ascending cervical artery) of thyrocervical trunk	Ascends anterior to anterior scalene, turns medially passing between vertebral vessels and carotid sheath, then descends on longus colli to lower border of thyroid gland	Branches: inferior laryngeal artery; pharyngeal, tracheal, esophageal, and inferior and ascending glandular branches (latter to parathyroid glands); Main visceral artery of neck
Inferior vesical (male)	Anterior division of internal iliac	Passes retroperitoneally to inferior aspect of male urinary bladder	Inferior aspect of urinary bladder, ductus deferens, seminal vesicle, and prostate
Infraorbital	Third part of maxillary artery	Passes along infraorbital groove and foramen to face	Supplies inferior rectus and oblique muscles, inferior eyelid, lacrimal sac, maxillary sinus, maxillary incisor and canine teeth, and anterior cheek
Internal carotid	Common carotid artery at superior border of thyroid cartilage	Ascends vertically in neck to enter carotid canal, becomes horizontal and runs anteromedially through cavernous sinus, makes a 180 degree turn under anterior clinoid process, bifurcates into anterior and middle cerebral arteries	Gives branches to walls of cavernous sinus, pituitary gland, and trigeminal ganglion; provides primary blood supply to the orbit/eyeball, upper nasal cavity/nose and brain
Internal iliac	Common iliac	Passes over pelvic brim to reach pelvic cavity	Main blood supply to pelvic organs, gluteal muscles, and perineum
Internal pudendal	Anterior division of internal iliac	Leaves pelvis through greater sciatic foramen; hooks around ischial spine and enters perineum by way of lesser sciatic foramen and runs in pudendal canal to urogenital (UG) triangle	Main artery to perineum, including muscles and skin of anal and urogenital triangles; erectile bodies (does not supply branches to gluteal region)
Internal thoracic	Inferior surface of subclavian artery	Descends, inclining anteromedially, posterior to sternal end of clavicle and costal cartilages, lateral to sternum, and anterior to slips of transversus thoracis; divides at level of 6th costal cartilage into superior epigastric and musculophrenic arteries	Sternum and skin anterior to it; by way of anterior intercostal arteries to intercostal spaces 1–6; by way of perforating arteries, to medial aspect of breast
Interosseous, anterior and posterior	Common interosseous artery	Pass to anterior and posterior sides of interosseous membrane	Anterior and posterior compartments of forearm; anterior interosseous artery supplies both anterior and posterior compartments in distal forearm; the posterior interosseous artery gives off the recurrent interosseous artery, which participates in the arterial anastomoses around the elbow

Artery/Arteries	Origin	Course	Branches/Distribution
Intestinal (n = 15–18)	Superior mesenteric artery	Passes between the two layers of mesentery	Jejunum and ileum
Labyrinthine	Basilar or via a common trunk with anterior inferior cerebellar	Exits cranial cavity via internal acoustic meatus; enters bony labyrinth	Membranous labyrinth
Lacrimal	Ophthalmic artery	Passes along superior border of lateral rectus muscle to supply lacrimal gland, conjunctiva, and eyelids	Passes along superior border of lateral rectus muscle to supply lacrimal gland, conjunctiva, and eyelids
Lateral circumflex femoral	Deep artery of thigh; may arise from femoral artery	Passes laterally deep to sartorius and rectus femoris and divides into three branches	Ascending branch supplies anterior part of gluteal region; transverse branch winds around femur; descending branch descends to knee and joins genicular anastomoses
Lateral nasal	Facial artery as it ascends alongside nose	Passes to ala of nose	Skin on ala and dorsum of nose
Lateral plantar	Terminal branch (with medial plantar artery) of posterior tibial artery	Forms medial to calcaneus, courses anterolaterally between 1st and 2nd muscle layers of sole of foot to base of 5th metatarsal, then passes anteromedially between 3rd and 4th layers as deep plantar arch	Branches: muscular, to muscles of 1st and 2nd layers; superficial, to skin and subcutaneous tissue of lateral sole; anastomotic, with lateral tarsal and arcuate arteries; and calcaneal, to calcaneus
Lateral sacral (superior and inferior)	Posterior division of internal iliac	Runs on anteromedial aspect of piriformis to send branches into pelvic sacral foramina	Piriformis, structures in sacral canal, erector spinae and overlying skin
Lateral thoracic	Second part of axillary artery	Descends along axillary border of pectoralis minor and follows it onto thoracic wall	Lateral chest wall (pectoral muscles, serratus anterior, intercostals) and breast
Left colic	Inferior mesenteric artery	Passes retroperitoneally toward left to descending colon	Descending colon
Left coronary	Left aortic sinus	Runs in AV groove and gives off anterior interventricular and circumflex branches	Most of left atrium and ventricle, IV septum, and AV bundles; may supply AV node
Left gastric	Celiac trunk	Ascends retroperitoneally to esophageal hiatus, where it passes between layers of hepatogastric ligament	Distal portion of esophagus and lesser curvature of stomach
Left gastroomental (gastroepiploic)	Splenic artery in hilum of spleen	Passes between layers of gastrosplenic ligament to greater curvature of stomach	Left portion of greater curvature of stomach
Left marginal (br.)	Circumflex branch	Follows left border of heart	Left ventricle
Left pulmonary	Pulmonary trunk	Joins left bronchus and pulmonary veins to form root of left lung; descends in lung	Supplies the left lung; Branches: (ductus arteriosus in fetus), superior and inferior lobar arteries (in turn give rise to segmental arteries)
Lesser palatine	Descending palatine	Descend inferoposteriorly through lesser palatine foramen	Supply soft palate
Lingual	External carotid artery	Loops over greater horn of hyoid, passes medial to hyoglossus, and ascends to run along side of tongue	Branches: suprahyoid branch, dorsal lingual arteries, and sublingual artery; continues as deep lingual artery
Lingular, inferior and superior	Superior lobar artery (of left lung), in oblique fissure	Descends anteriorly to lingula	Lingular division (superior [S4] and inferior [S5] bronchopulmonary segments) of left lung
Long posterior ciliaries	Ophthalmic artery	Pierce sclera to supply ciliary body and iris	Pierce sclera to supply ciliary body and iris

Artery/Arteries	Origin	Course	Branches/Distribution
Lumbar	Abdominal aorta	Run horizontal courses posteriorly around sides of lumbar vertebrae and then laterally on posterior abdominal wall	Branches: dorsal, to deep muscles of back and overlying skin; spinal, to vertebrae, contents of vertebral canal, roots, and some (as segmental medullary arteries) to spinal cord
Marginal artery (of colon)	Formed by anastomoses (arcades) between right, middle, and left colic and sigmoid arteries	Rarely interrupted anastomotic channel parallels the colon at its mesenteric border	Branches passing to anterior and posterior aspect of colon
Masseteric	2nd part of maxillary artery	Passes posterior to temporalis tendon accompanying masseteric nerve through mandibular notch	Supplies masseter and temporo-mandibular joint; anastomoses with facial and transverse facial arteries
Maxillary	Terminal branch (with superficial temporal artery) of external carotid	Passes posterior and medial to neck of mandible (1st part), superficial or deep to inferior head of lateral pterygoid (2nd part), and into pterygopalatine fossa (3rd part)	1st part: deep auricular, anterior tympanic, middle meningeal, accessory meningeal, inferior alveolar 2nd part: deep temporal, pterygoid (branches), masseteric, buccal 3rd part: posterior superior alveolar, descending palatine, artery of pterygoid canal, pharyngeal, sphenopalatine, infraorbital
Medial circumflex femoral	Deep artery of thigh; may arise from femoral artery	Passes medially and posteriorly between pectineus and iliopsoas, enters gluteal region, and divides into two branches	Supplies most blood to head and neck of femur; transverse branch takes part in cruciate anastomosis of thigh; ascending branch joins inferior gluteal artery
Medial plantar	Terminal branch (with lateral plantar artery) of posterior tibial artery	Arises medial to calcaneus, passes distally along medial side of foot between 1st and 2nd layers of plantar muscles	Branches: muscular, to flexor hallucis brevis and abductor hallucis; superficial, to skin and subcutaneous tissue of medial sole; and superficial digital, that join 1st–3rd plantar metatarsals
Median sacral	Posterior aspect of abdominal aorta	Descends in median line over L4 and L5 vertebrae and the sacrum and coccyx	Lower lumbar vertebrae, sacrum, and coccyx
Mental (branch)	Terminal branch of inferior alveolar artery	Emerges from mental foramen and passes to chin	Facial muscles and skin of chin
Middle cerebral	Larger terminal branch (with anterior cerebral artery) of the internal carotid artery	Runs in lateral cerebral sulcus, then posterosuperiorly on the insula	Insula and most of lateral surface of cerebral hemispheres
Middle colic	Superior mesenteric artery	Ascends retroperitoneally and passes between layers of transverse mesocolon	Transverse colon
Middle collateral	Deep artery of arm	Descends to anastomose with recurrent interosseous artery	Part of collateral pathway around elbow; supplies lateral and medial heads of triceps
Middle meningeal	1st part of maxillary artery	Ascends vertically through foramen spinosum into middle cranial fossa; runs laterally dividing into frontal and parietal branches, which in turn ramify, ascending the lateral walls in the cranial dura mater	Branches: ganglionic branches, petrosal branches, superior tympanic artery, temporal branches, anastomotic branch to lacrimal artery; most blood is distributed to periosteum, bone and red bone marrow
Middle rectal	Anterior division of internal iliac	Descends in pelvis to lower part of rectum	Seminal vesicles and lower part of rectum
Middle suprarenal	Abdominal aorta	Arise at level of superior mesenteric artery; run very short course over crura of diaphragm	Supply suprarenal glands; anastomose with suprarenal branches of inferior phrenic and renal arteries
Musculophrenic	Terminal branch (with superior epigastric) of internal thoracic artery	Arising in 6th intercostal space, descends inferolaterally, paralleling costal margin	Branches: anterior intercostal arteries of 7th–9th intercostal spaces; also supplies upper abdominal muscles and the pericardium

Artery/Arteries	Origin	Course	Branches/Distribution
Mylohyoid (branch)	Inferior alveolar (before it enters mandibular foramen)	Pierces sphenomandibular ligament to run anteroinferiorly with nerve in groove on medial aspect of ramus of mandible	Muscles of floor of mouth; anastomoses with submental artery
Obturator	Anterior division of internal iliac	Runs anteroinferiorly on lateral pelvic wall to exit pelvis via obturator canal	Pelvic muscles, nutrient artery to ilium, head of femur, muscles of medial compartment of thigh
Occipital	External carotid artery	Passes medial to posterior belly of digastric and mastoid process; accompanies occipital nerve in occipital region	Scalp of back of head, as far as vertex
Ophthalmic	Internal carotid artery	Traverses optic foramen to reach orbital cavity	Traverses optic foramen to reach orbital cavity
Ovarian	Abdominal aorta, inferior to renal arteries	Run inferolaterally on psoas major, then pass medially to cross pelvic brim and descend in suspensory ligament of ovary	Branches: ureteric, tubal (to uterine tubes) and ovarian; the latter two anastomose branches of uterine artery of same name
Palmar metacarpal	Deep palmar arch (from radial artery)	Run distally on plane between adductor pollicis and interosseus muscle	Anastomose distally with common palmar digital arteries
Pericardiacophrenic	Internal thoracic artery	Descends parallel to phrenic nerve between mediastinal parietal pleura and pericardium	Supplies mediastinal parietal pleura and pericardium; anastomoses with phrenic and musculophrenic arteries
Perineal	Internal pudendal artery	Leaves pudendal canal and enters superficial perineal space	Supplies superficial perineal muscles and scrotum or labia
Plantar metatarsal	1st: junction between lateral plantar and dorsalis pedis arteries 2nd–4th: deep plantar arch	Extend distally between metatarsal bones on plantar aspect of interosseous muscles	Branches: perforating branches, common plantar digital arteries
Popliteal	Continuation of femoral artery at adductor hiatus in adductor magnus	Passes through popliteal fossa to leg; ends at lower border of popliteus muscle by dividing into anterior and posterior tibial arteries	Superior, middle, and inferior genicular arteries to both lateral and medial aspects of knee
Posterior auricular	External carotid artery	Passes posteriorly, deep to parotid, along styloid process between mastoid process and ear	Scalp posterior to auricle and auricle
Posterior cerebral	Terminal branch of basilar artery	Passes laterally, winding around cerebral peduncle to reach the tentorial cerebral surface	Inferior aspect of temporal lobe and occipital lobe of cerebrum
Posterior communicating	Anastomosis between internal carotid and posterior cerebral arteries	Passes superior to oculomotor nerve (CN III)	Optic tract, cerebral peduncle, internal capsule, and thalamus
Posterior division of internal iliac	Internal iliac	Passes posteriorly and gives rise to parietal branches	Pelvic wall and gluteal region
Posterior ethmoidal	Ophthalmic artery	Passes through posterior ethmoidal foramen to posterior ethmoidal cells	Passes through posterior ethmoidal foramen to posterior ethmoidal cells
Posterior gastric	Splenic artery	Ascends retroperitoneally (in posterior wall of omental bursa) to pass to gastric fundus via gastrophrenic fold (ligament)	Posterior wall of stomach
Posterior inferior cerebellar	Intracranial portion of vertebral artery	Passes posteriorly around side of medulla to reach inferior aspect of cerebellum	Supplies medial portion of inferior aspect of cerebellum (cerebellar tonsil and dentate nucleus), posterolateral medulla oblongata, and choroid plexus of fourth ventricle
Posterior intercostal	Posterior aspect of thoracic aorta	Pass laterally, and then anteriorly parallel to ribs	Lateral and anterior cutaneous branches

Artery/Arteries	Origin	Course	Branches/Distribution
Posterior intercostals	Superior intercostal artery (intercostal spaces 1 and 2) and thoracic aorta (remaining intercostal spaces)	Pass between internal and innermost intercostal muscles	Intercostal muscles and overlying skin, parietal pleura
Posterior interventricular (IV)	Right coronary artery	Runs from posterior IV groove to apex of heart	Right and left ventricles and IV septum
Posterior lateral nasal	Sphenopalatine artery	Ramify over conchae and meatuses; anastomoses with nasal branches of ethmoidal and greater palatine arteries	Supplies lateral walls of posterointerior nasal cavity, contributing also to supply of ethmoidal cells and maxillary and sphenoidal paranasal sinuses
Posterior scrotal or labial	Terminal branches of perineal artery	Runs in superficial fascia of posterior scrotum or labium majus	Skin of scrotum or labium majus
Posterior septal	Sphenopalatine artery	Crosses inferior surface of body of sphenoid to reach nasal septum, courses anteroinferiorly on vomer to incisive canals	Supplies nasal septum; anastomoses with greater palatine artery and septal branch of superior labial artery
Posterior spinal	Superiorly, from an intracranial branch of the vertebral artery; it is continued inferiorly by bifurcations of posterior segmental medullary arteries at various levels	Forms a continuous anastomotic chain that descends the length of the spinal cord in the posterolateral sulcus, adjacent to the emerging dorsal roots (rootlets) of the spinal nerves	Supplies posterolateral aspect of spinal cord, via the pial plexus and its peripheral branches
Posterior superior alveolar	3rd part of maxillary artery	Exits from pterygopalatine fossa via pterygomaxillary fissure; ramifies and penetrates infratemporal surface of maxilla, with some branches entering alveolar canals and others continuing over alveolar process	Supplies mucosa of maxillary sinus, maxillary molar and premolar teeth, and adjacent gingiva
Posterior tibial	Popliteal	Passes through posterior compartment of leg and terminates distal to flexor retinaculum by dividing into medial and lateral plantar arteries	Posterior and lateral compartments of leg; circumflex fibular branch joins anastomoses around knee; nutrient artery passes to tibia
Princeps pollicis	Radial artery as it turns into palm	Descends on palmar aspect of first metacarpal and divides at the base of proximal phalanx into two branches that run along sides of thumb	Thumb
Proper palmar digitals	Common palmar digital arteries	Run along sides of digits 2–5; at base of middle phalanx, gives rise to dorsal branch which replaces dorsal digital arteries	All of palmar and distal part (including nail beds) of dorsal aspect of fingers
Prostatic (branches)	Inferior vesical artery	Descends on posterolateral aspect of prostate	Prostate
Artery of pterygoid canal	3rd part of maxillary artery, or from greater palatine	Passes posteriorly through pterygoid canal	Mucosa of uppermost pharynx (pharyngeal recess), pharyngotympanic (auditory) tube and tympanic cavity
Radial	Smaller terminal division (with ulnar artery) of brachial artery in cubital fossa	Runs inferolaterally under cover of brachioradialis and distally lies lateral to flexor carpi radialis tendon; winds around lateral aspect of radius and crosses floor of anatomical snuff box to pierce fascia; ends by forming deep palmar arch	Supplies muscles of lateral portions of both anterior and posterior compartments of forearm, lateral aspect of wrist, skin of dorsum of hand and proximal portions of digits, deep muscles of palm
Radial collateral	Terminal branch (with middle collateral artery) of deep artery of arm	Perforates lateral intermuscular septum with radial nerve, runs between brachialis and brachioradialis to anastomose with radial recurrent, anterior to lateral epicondyle of humerus	Forms part of cubital anastomosis; supplies upper brachialis and brachioradialis, and anterolateral aspect of elbow joint

Artery/Arteries	Origin	Course	Branches/Distribution
Radial recurrent	Lateral side of radial artery, just distal to its origin	Ascends on supinator and then passes between brachioradialis and brachialis to anastomose with radial collateral, anterior to lateral epicondyle of humerus	Forms part of cubital anastomosis; supplies supinator, lower brachialis and brachioradialis, and anterolateral aspect of elbow joint
Radialis indicis	Radial artery, but may arise from princeps pollicis artery	Passes along lateral side of index finger to its distal end	All of lateral palmar and distal part (including nail bed) of dorsal aspect of index finger
Radicular, anterior and posterior	Spinal branches of segmental arteries (vertebral, posterior intercostal, lumbar and sacral arteries)	Course along anterior and posterior roots of spinal nerves, exhausting before reaching the longitudinal anterior and posterior spinal arteries	Supply anterior and posterior roots of spinal nerves and coverings (dural sheaths and arachnoid)
Renal, left and right	Posterolateral aspect of abdominal aorta, usually at the L2 vertebral level	Run horizontally and laterally across crura of diaphragm and psoas major, lying posterior to the renal vein, bifurcating into anterior and posterior divisions, or ramifying into segmental arteries near renal hilus	Source of blood to kidneys; Branches: inferior suprarenal, capsular branches, an anterior division giving rise to superior, anterior superior, anterior inferior and inferior segmental arteries; posterior division becomes posterior segmental artery
Retroduodenal	Gastroduodenal artery	Arise and run posterior to the first part of the duodenum	Supply the first part of the duodenum, the (common) bile duct, and head of the pancreas
Right colic	Superior mesenteric artery	Passes retroperitoneally to reach ascending colon	Ascending colon
Right coronary	Right aortic sinus	Follows coronary (AV) groove between the atria and ventricles	Right atrium, SA and AV nodes, and posterior part of IV septum
Right gastric	Hepatic artery	Runs between layers of hepatogastric ligament	Right portion of lesser curvature of stomach
Right gastroomental (gastroepiploic)	Gastroduodenal artery	Passes between layers of greater omentum to greater curvature of stomach	Right portion of greater curvature of stomach
Right marginal	Right coronary artery	Passes to inferior margin of heart and apex	Right ventricle and apex of heart
Right pulmonary	Pulmonary trunk	Passes beneath arch of aorta to join right bronchus and pulmonary veins to form root of right lung; descends in lung	Supplies the right lung; Branches: superior, middle and inferior lobar arteries (in turn give rise to segmental arteries)
Segmental arteries of kidney (superior, anterior superior, anterior inferior, inferior, and posterior)	Anterior and posterior divisions (or directly from) renal arteries	Arise at hilum, course through perirenal fat of renal sinus around renal pelvis to reach renal segment	Renal segment (segmental arteries are end arteries; no significant anastomoses occur between segments)
Segmental arteries of liver (right anterior, right posterior, left medial, and left lateral)	Left and right branches of hepatic artery proper	Arise within liver; right and left branches course horizontally, the right branch giving rise to anterior and posterior segmental arteries, the left to medial and lateral segmental arteries	Each segmental artery serves a division of the liver which, except for the medial division, is further subdivided into two hepatic segments; both right and left branches of hepatic artery send an artery to the caudate lobe
Segmental arteries of lung	Lobar arteries	Arise within the lung as tertiary branches of the right and left pulmonary arteries	Each segmental artery serves a broncho-pulmonary segment of the lung
Segmental medullary, anterior and posterior	Spinal branches of segmental arteries (vertebral, posterior intercostal, lumbar and sacral arteries)	Course along anterior and posterior roots of spinal nerves, and continue medially to anastomose with the longitudinal anterior and posterior spinal arteries	Dorsal and ventral roots of certain spinal nerves, and the spinal cord; the major anterior segmental medullary artery (Adamkiewicz) is largest, occurring at the lower thoracic, upper lumbar level, on the left side 65% of the time

Appendices

Artery/Arteries	Origin	Course	Branches/Distribution
Sinuatrial (SA) nodal	Right coronary artery near its origin (in 60%); circumflex branch of left coronary (in 40%)	Winds around right (60%) or left (40%) side of ascending aorta and ascends to SA node	Left atrium and SA node
Short gastric (n = 4–5)	Splenic artery in hilum of spleen	Passes between layers of gastrosplenic ligament to fundus of stomach	Fundus of stomach
Short posterior ciliaries	Ophthalmic artery	Pierce sclera at periphery of optic nerve to supply choroid, which in turn supplies cones and rods of optic retina	Pierce sclera at periphery of optic nerve to supply choroid, which in turn supplies cones and rods of optic retina
Sigmoid (n = 3–4)	Inferior mesenteric artery	Passes retroperitoneally toward left to descending colon	Descending and sigmoid colon
Sphenopalatine	3rd part of maxillary artery	Passes medially through sphenopalatine foramen, dividing immediately into septal and posterior lateral nasal arteries	Mucosa of posteroinferior half of nasal cavity, ethmoidal cells, and maxillary and sphenoidal paranasal sinuses
Splenic	Celiac trunk	Runs retroperitoneally along superior border of pancreas; it then passes between layers of splenorenal ligament to hilum of spleen	Body of pancreas, spleen, and greater curvature of stomach
Stylomastoid	Posterior auricular	Enters stylomastoid foramen and ascends facial canal, running with (and supplying) the facial nerve	Branches: posterior tympanic artery (to tympanic membrane); mastoid (to mastoid cells) and stapedial (to stapedius, stapes, and secondary tympanic membrane) branches
Subclavian	Left: aortic arch Right: brachiocephalic trunk	Arises—or passes—posterior to sternoclavicular joint, arches over cervical pleura anterior to apex of lung, and crosses first rib posterior to anterior scalene, becoming axillary artery at rib's outer edge	Branches: 1st part: vertebral, internal thoracic, thyrocervical (and costocervical on right side) 2nd part: dorsal scapular (and costocervical on left side) [Parts: medial (1st), posterior (2nd) and lateral (3rd) to scalenus anterior muscle]
Subcostal	Thoracic aorta	Courses along inferior border of 12th rib	Muscles of anterolateral abdominal wall
Sublingual	Terminal branch (with deep lingual artery) of lingual artery	Runs on genioglossus muscle superior to mylohyoid	Supplies muscles and mucous membrane of floor of mouth, and anterior lingual gingiva
Submental	Facial artery, distal to submandibular gland in submental triangle	Courses along inferior aspect of mylohyoid, adjacent to its attachment to the mandible, to the mandibular symphysis	Supplies mylohyoid, anterior belly of digastric, submental lymph nodes and, via its anastomoses with inferior labial and mental arteries, lower lip
Subscapular	Third part of axillary artery	Largest (but short—4 cm) branch of axillary artery, it descends along lateral border of subscapularis and axillary border of scapula to bifurcate at the level of the inferior angle	Via its terminal branches, the circumflex scapular and thoracodorsal arteries, it supplies muscles on both sides of the scapula, the latissimus dorsi, and posterior chest wall
Superficial cervical (variant, replacing superficial branch of transverse cervical artery)	Thyrocervical trunk	Passes laterally between sternocleidomastoid and anterior scalene, across brachial plexus and posterior triangle of neck, to bifurcate and run with accessory nerve on deep aspect of trapezius	Anterior scapene, sternocleidomastoid, brachial plexus, muscles of posterior triangle of neck, and—mainly—the trapezius
Superficial circumflex iliac	Femoral artery	Runs in superficial fascia along inguinal ligament	Subcutaneous tissue and skin over inferior part of anterolateral abdominal wall
Superficial epigastric	Femoral artery	Runs in superficial fascia toward umbilicus	Subcutaneous tissue and skin over suprapubic region

Artery/Arteries	Origin	Course	Branches/Distribution
Superficial palmar arch	Direct continuation of ulnar artery; arch is completed on lateral side by superficial branch of radial artery or another of its branches	Curves laterally deep to palmar aponeurosis and superficial to long flexor tendons; curve of arch lies across palm at level of distal border of extended thumb	Branches: three common palmar digital arteries
Superficial temporal	Smaller terminal branch of external carotid artery	Ascends anterior to ear to temporal region and ends in scalp	Facial muscles and skin of frontal and temporal regions
Superior cerebellar	Upper (terminal) part of basilar artery	Curves around cerebral peduncle	Supplies superior aspect of cerebellum, colliculi, and most cerebellar nuclei; pons; pineal body; superior medullary velum; and choroid plexus of third ventricle
Superior epigastric	Internal thoracic artery	Descends in rectus sheath deep to rectus abdominis	Rectus abdominis and superior part of anterolateral abdominal wall
Superior gluteal	Posterior division of internal iliac	Enters gluteal region through greater sciatic foramen superior to piriformis and divides into superficial and deep branches; anastomoses with inferior gluteal and medial circumflex femoral arteries (not shown above)	Piriformis muscle Superficial branch: supplies gluteus maximus Deep branch: runs between gluteus medius and minimus muscles, supplying both, as well as the tensor of the fascia lata
Superior labial	Facial artery near angle of mouth	Runs medially in upper lip	AUpper lip and ala (side) and septum of nose
Superior laryngeal	Superior thyroid	Runs deep to thyrohyoid to pierce thyrohyoid membrane with internal laryngeal nerve	Supplies larynx
Superior mesenteric	Abdominal aorta	Runs in root of mesentery to ileocecal junction	Part of gastrointestinal tract derived from midgut
Superior pancreaticoduodenal, anterior and posterior	Gastroduodenal artery	Descends on head of pancreas	Proximal portion of duodenum and head of pancreas
Superior phrenic (vary in number)	Anterior aspects of thoracic aorta	Arise at aortic hiatus and pass to superior aspect of diaphragm	Supply diaphragm and diaphragmatic parts of pericardium and parietal pleura
Superior rectal	Terminal branch (continuation of) inferior mesenteric artery	Crosses left common iliac vessels and descends into the pelvis between the layers of the sigmoid mesocolon	Upper part of rectum; anastomoses with middle and inferior rectal arteries
Superior suprarenal	Inferior phrenic	Short, multiple branches arising from the trunks of the inferior phrenic arteries as they ascend diaphragmatic crura, running along superomedial aspect of the gland	Superior part of suprarenal glands
Superior thoracic	Only branch of first part of axillary artery	Runs anteromedially along superior border of pectoralis minor and then passes between it and pectoralis major to thoracic wall	Helps to supply 1st and 2nd intercostal spaces and superior part of serratus anterior
Superior thyroid	1st branch from anterior aspect of external carotid artery	Passes inferomedially deep to infrahyoid muscles to the superior pole of the thyroid gland; its anastomosis with the inferior thyroid artery provide an important collateral pathway between external carotid and subclavian arteries	Branches: superior laryngeal artery, and infrahyoid, sternocleidomastoid, cricothyroid, and anterior, posterior and lateral glandular branches
Superior vesical	Patent (proximal) part of umbilical	Usually multiple, these arteries pass to the superior aspect of the urinary bladder	Superior aspect of urinary bladder, pelvic portion of ureter

Artery/Arteries	Origin	Course	Branches/Distribution
Supraduodenal	Gastroduodenal, hepatic, right gastric, or retroduodenal arteries	Often double, pass(es) superior to 1st part of duodenum	Supplies upper, proximal portion of superior part of duodenum
Supraorbital	Terminal branch of ophthalmic artery	Passes superiorly and posteriorly from supraorbital foramen to forehead and scalp	Supplies muscles and skin of most of forehead and anterior scalp (to vertex)
Suprascapular	Thyrocervical trunk	Passes inferolaterally over anterior scalene muscle and phrenic nerve, crosses subclavian artery and brachial plexus, and runs laterally posterior and parallel to clavicle; it then passes superior to transverse scapular ligament into supraspinous fossa, and then under acromion to infraspinous fossa	Supplies supraspinatus and infraspinatus muscles and participates in anastomosis around scapula
Supratrochlear	Terminal branch (with supraorbital artery) of ophthalmic artery	Passes from supratrochlear notch to medial forehead and anterior scalp	Skin and muscles of medial part of forehead and adjacent scalp
Supreme intercostal	Costocervical trunk	Descends between pleura and necks of 1st two ribs; anastomoses with 3rd posterior intercostal artery	Branches: 1st and 2nd posterior intercostal arteries, to muscles of and ribs bounding 1st and 2nd intercostal spaces
Sural, right and left	Popliteal	Large branches arise at level of femoral condyles and pass directly to heads of gastrocnemius, sending branches on to soleus	Supply medial and lateral heads of gastrocnemius, plantaris and soleus muscles
Testicular	Abdominal aorta, inferior to renal arteries	Descend inferolaterally across psoas muscles, pass through inguinal canal as part of spermatic cord, and reach testis in scrotum	Abdominal part provides branches/arterial blood to ureters, iliac lymph nodes; inguinal/scrotal part supplies cremaster and other coverings of cord, and testis
Thoracic aorta	Continuation of arch of aorta	Descends in posterior mediastinum to left of vertebral column; gradually shifts to right to lie in median plane at aortic hiatus	Posterior intercostal arteries, subcostal, some phrenic arteries and visceral branches (tracheal and esophageal)
Thoracoacromial	Second part of axillary artery deep to pectoralis minor	Curls around superomedial border of pectoralis minor, pierces clavipectoral fascia, and divides into four branches	Branches: acromial, clavicular, pectoral, and deltoid
Thoracodorsal	Subscapular artery	Continues course of subscapular artery and accompanies thoracodorsal nerve to latissimus dorsi	Latissimus dorsi
Thyrocervical trunk	Anterior aspect of first part of subclavian artery	Ascends as a short, wide trunk near the medial border of the anterior scalene and posterior to carotid sheath	Branches from trunk: transverse cervical (or superficial cervical) and suprascapular; terminal branches: ascending cervical and inferior thyroid arteries
Thyroid ima	Brachiocephalic trunk or arch of aorta	Ascends on anterior aspect of trachea to thyroid gland	Supplies medial aspect of both lobes of thyroid
Transverse cervical (variant: may be replaced by superficial cervical and dorsal scapular arteries	Thyrocervical trunk	Runs across anterior scalene, brachial plexus and posterior triangle of neck and passes deep to trapezius, dividing into deep and superficial branches	Superficial branch bifurcates into ascending and descending branches that run with accessory nerve on underside of trapezius; deep branch runs with dorsal scapular nerve, deep to rhomboids
Transverse facial	Superficial temporal artery within parotid gland	Crosses face superficial to masseter and inferior to zygomatic arch	Parotid gland and duct, muscles and skin of face

Artery/Arteries	Origin	Course	Branches/Distribution
Ulnar	Larger terminal branch of brachial artery in cubital fossa	Passes inferomedially and then directly inferiorly, deep to pronator teres, palmaris longus, and flexor digitorum superficialis to reach medial side of forearm; passes superficial to flexor retinaculum at wrist and gives a deep palmar branch to deep arch and continues as superficial palmar arch	Supplies medial (ulnar) part of anterior compartment of forearm, wrist and hand; supplies superficial structures of central palm, and most of palmar and distal dorsal aspects of fingers
Ulnar collateral (superior and inferior)	Superior ulnar collateral artery arises from brachial artery near middle of arm; inferior ulnar collateral artery arises from brachial artery just superior to elbow	Superior ulnar collateral artery accompanies ulnar nerve to posterior aspect of elbow; inferior ulnar collateral artery divides into anterior and posterior branches; both ulnar collateral arteries take part in anastomosis around elbow joint	Anastomose distally with anterior and posterior ulnar recurrent arteries
Ulnar recurrent, anterior and posterior	Ulnar artery, just distal to elbow joint	Anterior ulnar recurrent artery passes superiorly and posterior ulnar collateral artery passes posteriorly	Anastomose with anterior and posterior ulnar collateral arteries
Umbilical	Anterior division of internal iliac	Obliterates becoming medial umbilical ligament after running a short pelvic course during which it gives rise to superior vesical arteries	Superior aspect of urinary bladder (via superior vesical arteries); occasionally artery to ductus deferens (males)
Uterine	Anterior division of internal iliac	Runs medially in base of broad ligament superior to cardinal ligament, crossing superior to ureter, to sides of uterus	Uterus, ligaments of uterus, uterine tube, and vagina
Vaginal	Uterine artery	Arises lateral to ureter and descends inferior to it to lateral aspect of vagina	Vagina; branches to inferior part of urinary bladder and termination of ureter
Vertebral	1st part of subclavian artery	Ascends vertically through the transverse foramina of vertebrae C6–C2, passes laterally to traverse that of C1, then runs horizontal and medial to enter foramen magnum; intracranially, merges with contralateral artery to form basilar artery	Cervical branches: spinal (giving rise to radicular and segmental medullary arteries) and muscular (to suboccipital muscles) Intracranial branches: meningeal, anterior and posterior spinal, posterior inferior cerebellar, medial and lateral medullary

Appendices

MUSCLES OF THE HUMAN BODY

Muscle(s)	Origin	Insertion	Innervation	Main Action(s)
Abductor digiti minimi of foot	Medial and lateral tubercles of tuberosity of calcaneus, plantar aponeurosis, and intermuscular septa	Lateral side of base of proximal phalanx of 5th digit	Lateral plantar nerve (S2 and S3)	Abducts and flexes 5th digit
Abductor digiti minimi of hand	Pisiform, pisohamate ligament, flexor retinaculum	Medial side of base of proximal phalanx of little finger	Deep branch of ulnar nerve (C8 and T1)	Abducts digit 5
Abductor hallucis	Medial tubercle of tuberosity of calcaneus, flexor retinaculum, and plantar aponeurosis	Medial side of base of proximal phalanx of 1st digit	Medial plantar nerve (S2 and S3)	Abducts and flexes 1st digit (great toe, hallux)
Abductor pollicis brevis	Flexor retinaculum and tubercles of scaphoid and trapezium	Lateral side of base of proximal phalanx of thumb	Recurrent branch of median nerve (C8 and T1)	Abducts thumb and helps oppose it
Abductor pollicis longus	Posterior surfaces of ulna, radius, and interosseous membrane	Base of 1st metacarpal	Posterior interosseous nerve (C7 and C8), the continuation of deep branch of radial nerve	Abducts thumb and extends it at carpo-metacarpal joint
Adductor brevis	Body and inferior ramus of pubis	Pectineal line and proximal part of linea aspera of femur	Obturator nerve (L2, L3, and L4), branch of anterior division	Adducts thigh and to some extent flexes it
Adductor hallucis	Oblique head: bases of metatarsals 2–4 Transverse head: plantar ligaments of metatarso-phalangeal joints	Tendons of both heads attach to lateral side of base of proximal phalanx of 1st digit	Deep branch of lateral plantar nerve (S2 and S3)	Adducts 1st digit; assists in maintaining transverse arch of foot
Adductor longus	Body of pubis inferior to pubic crest	Middle third of linea aspera of femur	Obturator nerve, branch of anterior division (L2, L3, and L4)	Adducts thigh
Adductor magnus	Adductor part: inferior ramus of pubis, ramus of ischium; Hamstrings part: ischial tuberosity	Adductor part: gluteal tuberosity, linea aspera, medial supracondylar line; Hamstrings part: adductor tubercle of femur	Adductor part: obturator nerve (L2, L3, and L4), branches of posterior division; Hamstrings part: tibial part of sciatic nerve (L4)	Adducts thigh; Adductor part: flexes thigh; Hamstrings part: extends thigh
Adductor minimus	Inferior pubic ramus	Medial lip, uppermost linea aspera of femur	Obturator nerve (L2, 3 & 4)	Adducts and laterally rotates thigh
Adductor pollicis	Oblique head: bases of 2nd and 3rd metacarpals, capitate, and adjacent carpals; Transverse head: anterior surface of body of 3rd metacarpal	Medial side of base of proximal phalanx of thumb	Deep branch of ulnar nerve (C8 and T1)	Adducts thumb toward middle digit
Anconeus	Lateral epicondyle of humerus	Lateral surface of olecranon and superior part of posterior surface of ulna	Radial nerve (C7, C8, and T1)	Assists triceps in extending forearm; stabilizes elbow joint; abducts ulna during pronation
Articularis cubiti	Distal portion of posterior aspect of shaft of humerus	Posterior fibrous capsule of elbow joint	Radial nerve (C7 and C8)	Retracts posterior joint capsule during extension of elbow
Articularis genus	Distal portion of anterior aspect of shaft of femur	Synovial membrane of suprapatellar bursa of knee joint	Femoral nerve (L2–L4)	Retracts synovial membrane during extension of knee
Arytenoid, transverse and oblique	Posterolateral border of one arytenoid cartilage	Posterolateral border of opposite arytenoid cartilage	Recurrent laryngeal nerve (branch of vagus (CN X))	Closes intercartilaginous portion of rima glottidis
Auricularis anterior, posterior, and superior	Epicranial aponeurosis and mastoid part of temporal bone	Auricle (external ear)	Facial nerve (CN VII)	Protraction, retraction and elevation of auricle on side of head

2038

Muscle(s)	Origin	Insertion	Innervation	Main Action(s)
Biceps brachii	Short head: tip of coracoid process of scapula; Long head: supraglenoid tubercle of scapula	Tuberosity of radius and fascia of forearm via bicipital aponeurosis	Musculocutaneous nerve (C5 and C6)	Supinates forearm and, when it is supine, flexes forearm
Biceps femoris	Long head: ischial tuberosity Short head: linea aspera and lateral supracondylar line of femur	Lateral side of head of fibula; tendon is split at this site by fibular collateral ligament of knee	Long head: tibial division of sciatic nerve (L5, S1, and S2) Short head: common fibular (peroneal) division of sciatic nerve (L5, S1, and S2)	Flexes leg and rotates it laterally when knee is flexed; extends thigh (e.g., when starting to walk)
Brachialis	Distal half of anterior surface of humerus	Coronoid process and tuberosity of ulna	Musculocutaneous nerve (C5 and C6)	Flexes forearm in all positions
Brachioradialis	Proximal two-thirds of lateral supracondylar ridge of humerus	Lateral surface of distal end of radius	Radial nerve (C5, C6, and C7)	Flexes forearm
Buccinator	Mandible, pterygomandibular raphe, and alveolar processes of maxilla and mandible	Angle of mouth	Facial nerve (CN VII)	Presses cheek against molar teeth, thereby aiding chewing; expels air from oral cavity as occurs when playing a wind instrument; draws mouth to one side when acting unilaterally
Bulbospongiosus	Male: median raphe, ventral surface of bulb of penis, and perineal body Female: perineal body	Male: corpora spongiosum and cavernosa and fascia of bulb of penis Female: fascia of corpus cavernosa	Deep branch of perineal nerve, a branch of pudendal nerve (S2, 3 & 4)	Works with external anal sphincter to support/fix perineal body; Male: compresses bulb of penis to expel last drops of urine/semen; assists erection by pushing blood into body of penis and compressing outflow veins; Female: "sphincter" of vagina and assists in erection of clitoris
Ciliary	Scleral spur	Meridional, radial and ciircular fibers are instrinsic to ciliary body	Parasympathetic fibers of oculomotor nerve and ciliary ganglion	Relieve tension on lens of eye, allowing it to become more convex for near vision
Coccygeus (ischiococcygeus)	Ischial spine	Inferior end of sacrum	Branches of S4 and S5 nerves	Forms small part of pelvic diaphragm that supports pelvic viscera; flexes coccyx
Coracobrachialis	Tip of coracoid process of scapula	Middle third of medial surface of humerus	Musculocutaneous nerve (C5, C6, and C7)	Helps to flex and adduct arm
Corrugator supercilii	Medial end of superciliary arch of frontal bone	Skin above middle of eyebrow	Facial nerve (CN VII)	Draws eyebrow medially and inferiorly, producing vertical wrinkles above nose
Cremaster	Internal oblique muscle and inguinal ligament	Spermatic cord and tunica vaginalis	Genital branch of genitofemoral nerve (L1–L2)	Elevation of testis
Cricopharyngeus	Posterolateral cricoid cartilage on one side	Posterolateral cricoid cartilage of other side	Vagus (CN X)	Serves as upper esophageal sphincter
Cricothyroid	Anterolateral part of cricoid cartilage	Inferior margin and inferior horn of thyroid cartilage	External laryngeal nerve	Stretches and tenses vocal fold

Muscle(s)	Origin	Insertion	Innervation	Main Action(s)
Deep transverse perineal muscle	Internal surface of ischiopubic ramus and ischial tuberosity	Median raphe, perineal body, and external anal sphincter	Deep branch of perineal nerve, a branch of pudendal nerve (S2, 3 & 4)	Support and fix perineal body (pelvic floor) to support abdominopelvic viscera and resist increased intraabdominal pressure
Deltoid	Lateral third of clavicle, acromion, and spine of scapula	Deltoid tuberosity of humerus	Axillary nerve (C5 and C6)	Anterior part: flexes and medially rotates arm; Middle part: abducts arm; Posterior part: extends and laterally rotates arm
Depressor labii inferioris/anguli oris	Anterolateral aspect of body of mandible	Lower lip/angle of mouth	Marginal mandibular branch of facial nerve (CN VII)	Depresses and/or everts lower lip/pulls angle of mouth and modiolus inferiorly
Depressor septi nasi	Incisor fossa of maxilla	Mobile part of nasal septum	Facial nerve	Helps to dilate nostril during deep inspiration and depresses nasal septum
Diaphragm	Xiphoid process; inferior 6 costal cartilages and adjoining ribs; arcuate ligaments; anterior longitudinal ligaments and bodies and discs of lumbar vertebrae 1–3	Central tendon of diaphragm	Phrenic nerve (C3–C5)	Diaphragm descends, causing decreased intrathoracic pressure resulting in inhalation and assisting return of venous blood to heart
Digastric	Anterior belly: digastric fossa of mandible Posterior belly: mastoid notch of temporal bone	Intermediate tendon to body and greater horn of hyoid bone	Anterior belly: mylohyoid nerve, a branch of inferior alveolar nerve Posterior belly: facial nerve (CN VII)	Depresses mandible; raises hyoid bone and steadies it during swallowing and speaking
Dorsal interossei (four muscles) of foot	Adjacent sides of metatarsals 1–5	First: medial side of proximal phalanx of 2nd digit; Second to fourth: lateral sides of 2nd to 4th digits	Lateral plantar nerve (S2 and S3)	Abduct digits (2–4) and flex metatarso-phalangeal joints
Dorsal interossei 1–4 of hand	Adjacent sides of two metacarpals (bipennate muscles)	Extensor expansions and bases of proximal phalanges of digits 2–4	Deep branch of ulnar nerve (C8 and T1)	Abduct digits from axial line and act with lumbricals to flex meta-carpophalangeal joints and extend inter-phalangeal joints
Erector spinae	Arises by a broad tendon from posterior part of iliac crest, posterior surface of sacrum, sacral and inferior lumbar spinous processes, and supraspinous ligament	Iliocostalis—lumborum, thoracis, and cervicis: fibers run superiorly to angles of lower ribs and cervical transverse processes Longissimus—thoracis, cervicis, and capitis: fibers run superiorly to ribs between tubercles and angles, to transverse processes in thoracic and cervical regions, and to mastoid process of temporal bone Spinalis—thoracis, cervicis, and capitis: fibers run superiorly to spinous processes in the upper thoracic region and to skull	Posterior rami of spinal nerves	Acting bilaterally, they extend vertebral column and head; as back is flexed they control movement by gradually lengthening their fibers; acting unilaterally, they laterally bend vertebral column
Extensor carpi radialis brevis	Lateral epicondyle of humerus	Base of 3rd metacarpal bone	Deep branch of radial nerve (C7 and C8)	Extend and abduct hand at wrist joint

Muscle(s)	Origin	Insertion	Innervation	Main Action(s)
Extensor carpi radialis longus	Lateral supracondylar ridge of humerus	Base of 2nd metacarpal bone	Radial nerve (C6 and C7)	Extend and abduct hand at wrist joint
Extensor carpi ulnaris	Lateral epicondyle of humerus and posterior border of ulna	Base of 5th metacarpal bone	Posterior interosseous nerve (C7 and C8), the continuation of deep branch of radial nerve	Extends and adducts hand at wrist joint
Extensor digiti minimi	Lateral epicondyle of humerus	Extensor expansion of 5th digit	Posterior interosseous nerve (C7 and C8), the continuation of deep branch of radial nerve	Extends 5th digit at metacarpophalangeal and interphalangeal joints
Extensor digitorum	Lateral epicondyle of humerus	Extensor expansions of medial four digits	Posterior interosseous nerve (C7 and C8), the continuation of deep branch of radial nerve	Extends medial four digits at metacarpo-phalangeal joints; extends hand at wrist joint
Extensor digitorum brevis	Anteriormost portions of lateral and superior surfaces of calcaneus	Lateral side of long extensor tendons, with slips to proximal phalanges of 2nd–4th toes	Deep fibular (peroneal) nerve (L5 and S1)	Assists in extending middle three toes
Extensor digitorum longus	Lateral condyle of tibia and superior three-fourths of medial surface of the fibula and interosseous membrane	Middle and distal phalanges of lateral four digits	Deep fibular (peroneal) nerve (L5 and S1)	Extends lateral four digits and dorsiflexes ankle
Extensor hallucis brevis	Anteriormost portion of superior surface of calcaneus	Dorsal aspect of base of proximal phalanx of great toe (hallux)	Deep fibular (peroneal) nerve (L5 and S1)	Extends great toe
Extensor hallucis longus	Middle part of anterior surface of fibula and interosseous membrane	Dorsal aspect of base of distal phalanx of great toe (hallux)	Deep fibular (peroneal) nerve (L5 and S1)	Extends great toe and dorsiflexes ankle
Extensor indicis	Posterior surface of ulna and interosseous membrane	Extensor expansion of 2nd digit	Posterior interosseous nerve (C7 and C8), the continuation of deep branch of radial nerve	Extends 2nd digit and helps to extend hand
Extensor pollicis brevis	Posterior surface of radius and interosseous membrane	Base of proximal phalanx of thumb	Posterior interosseous nerve (C7 and C8), the continuation of deep branch of radial nerve	Extends proximal phalanx of thumb at carpometacarpal joint
Extensor pollicis longus	Posterior surface of middle third of ulna and interosseous membrane	Base of distal phalanx of thumb	Posterior interosseous nerve (C7 and C8), the continuation of deep branch of radial nerve	Extends distal phalanx of thumb at metacarpo-phalangeal and inter-phalangeal joints
External anal sphincter	Skin and fascia surrounding anus and coccyx via anococcygeal ligament	Perineal body	Inferior anal nerve	Closes anal canal; works with bulbospongiosus to support and fix perineal body
External intercostal	Inferior border of ribs, from tubercle to costochondral junction	Superior border of ribs below	Intercostal nerves	Elevate ribs (when upper ribs are fixed by scalene and sterocleidomastoid muscles)
External oblique	External surfaces of 5th–2th ribs	Linea alba, pubic tubercle, and anterior half of iliac crest	Thoracoabdominal nerves (inferior 6 thoracic nerves) and subcostal nerve	Compress and support abdominal viscera, a flex and rotate trunk
External urethral sphincter	Internal surface of ischiopubic ramus and ischial tuberosity	Surrounds urethra; in males, also ascends anterior aspect of prostate; in females, some fibers also enclose vagina (urethrovaginal sphincter)	Deep branch of perineal nerve, a branch of pudendal nerve (S2, 3 & 4)	Compresses urethra to maintain urinary continence; in females urethrovaginal sphincter portion also compresses vagina

Appendices

Muscle(s)	Origin	Insertion	Innervation	Main Action(s)
Fibularis (peroneus) brevis	Inferior two-thirds of lateral surface of fibula	Dorsal surface of tuberosity on lateral side of base of 5th metatarsal	Superficial fibular (peroneal) nerve (L5, S1, and S2)	Everts foot and weakly plantarflexes ankle
Fibularis (peroneus) longus	Head and superior two-thirds of lateral surface of fibula	Base of 1st metatarsal and medial cuneiform	Superficial fibular (peroneal) nerve (L5, S1, and S2)	Everts foot and weakly plantarflexes ankle
Fibularis (peroneus) tertius	Inferior third of anterior surface of fibula and interosseous membrane	Dorsum of base of 5th metatarsal	Deep fibular (peroneal) nerve (L5 and S1)	Dorsiflexes ankle and aids in eversion of foot
Flexor carpi radialis	Medial epicondyle of humerus	Base of 2nd metacarpal bone	Median nerve (C6 and C7)	Flexes and abducts hand (at wrist)
Flexor carpi ulnaris	Humeral head: medial epicondyle of humerus Ulnar head: olecranon and posterior border of ulna	Pisiform bone, hook of hamate bone, and 5th metacarpal bone	Ulnar nerve (C7 and C8)	Flexes and adducts hand (at wrist)
Flexor digiti minimi brevis of foot	Base of the 5th metatarsal	Base of proximal phalanx of 5th digit	Superficial branch of lateral plantar nerve (S2 and S3)	Flexes proximal phalanx of 5th digit, thereby assisting with its flexion
Flexor digiti minimi brevis of hand	Hook of hamate and flexor retinaculum	Medial side of base of proximal phalanx of little finger	Deep branch of ulnar nerve (C8 and T1)	Flexes proximal phalanx of digit 5
Flexor digitorum brevis	Medial tubercle of tuberosity of calcaneus, plantar aponeurosis, and intermuscular septa	Both sides of middle phalanges of lateral four digits	Medial plantar nerve (S2 and S3)	Flexes lateral four digits
Flexor digitorum longus	Medial part of posterior surface of tibia inferior to soleal line and by a broad tendon to fibula	Bases of distal phalanges of lateral four digits	Tibial nerve (S2 and S3)	Flexes lateral four digits and plantarflexes ankle; supports longitudinal arches of foot
Flexor digitorum profundus	Proximal three-fourths of medial and anterior surfaces of ulna and interosseous membrane	Bases of distal phalanges of medial four digits	Medial part: ulnar nerve (C8 and T1); Lateral part: median nerve (C8 and T1)	Flexes distal phalanges at distal interphalangeal joints of medial four digits; assists with flexion of hand
Flexor digitorum superficialis	Humeroulnar head: medial epicondyle of humerus, ulnar collateral ligament, and coronoid process of ulna Radial head: superior half of anterior border of radius	Bodies of middle phalanges of medial four digits	Median nerve (C7, C8, and T1)	Flexes middle phalanges at proximal inter-phalangeal joints of medial four digits; acting more strongly, it also flexes proximal phalanges at metacarpophalangeal joints and hand at wrist
Flexor hallucis brevis	Plantar surfaces of cuboid and lateral cuneiforms	Both sides of base of proximal phalanx of 1st digit	Medial plantar nerve (S2 and S3)	Flexes proximal phalanx of 1st digit
Flexor hallucis longus	Inferior two-thirds of posterior surface of fibula and inferior part of interosseous membrane	Base of distal phalanx of great toe (hallux)	Tibial nerve (S2 and S3)	Flexes great toe at all joints and weakly plantarflexes ankle; supports medial longitudinal arches of foot
Flexor pollicis brevis	Flexor retinaculum and tubercles of scaphoid and trapezium	Lateral side of base of proximal phalanx of thumb	Recurrent branch of median nerve (C8 and T1)	Flexes thumb
Flexor pollicis longus	Anterior surface of radius and adjacent interosseous membrane	Base of distal phalanx of thumb	Anterior interosseous nerve from median (C8 and T1)	Flexes phalanges of 1st digit (thumb)

Muscle(s)	Origin	Insertion	Innervation	Main Action(s)
Gastrocnemius	Lateral head: lateral aspect of lateral condyle of femur Medial head: popliteal surface of femur, superior to medial condyle	Posterior surface of calcaneus via calcaneal tendon	Tibial nerve (S1 and S2)	Plantarflexes ankle when knee is extended, raises heel during walking, and flexes leg at knee joint
Gemelli superior and inferior	Superior: ischial spine Inferior: ischial tuberosity	Medial surface of greater trochanter (trochanteric fossa) of femur	Superior gemellus: nerve to obturator internus (L5 and S1); Inferior gemellus: nerve to quadratus femoris (L5 and S1)	Laterally rotate extended thigh and abduct flexed thigh; steady femoral head in acetabulum
Genioglossus	Superior part of mental spine of mandible	Dorsum of tongue and body of hyoid bone	Hypoglossal nerve (CN XII)	Depresses tongue; its posterior part pulls tongue anteriorly for protrusion
Geniohyoid	Inferior mental spine of mandible	Body of hyoid bone	C1 via the hypoglossal nerve	Pulls hyoid bone anterosuperiorly, shortens floor of mouth, and widens pharynx
Gluteus maximus	Ilium posterior to posterior gluteal line, dorsal surface of sacrum and coccyx, and sacrotuberous ligament	Most fibers end in iliotibial tract that inserts into lateral condyle of tibia; some fibers insert on gluteal tuberosity of femur	Inferior gluteal nerve (L5, S1, and S2)	Extends thigh (especially from flexed position) and assists in its lateral rotation; steadies thigh and assists in rising from sitting position
Gluteus medius	External surface of ilium between anterior and posterior gluteal lines	Lateral surface of greater trochanter of femur	Superior gluteal nerve (L5 and S1)	Abducts and medially rotates thigh; keeps pelvis level when opposite leg is raised off ground
Gluteus minimus	External surface of ilium between anterior and inferior gluteal lines	Anterior surface of greater trochanter of femur	Superior gluteal nerve (L5 and S1)	Abducts and medially rotates thigh; keeps pelvis level when opposite leg is raised off ground
Gracilis	Body and inferior ramus of pubis	Superior part of medial surface of tibia	Obturator nerve (L2 and L3)	Adducts thigh, flexes leg, and helps rotate it medially
Hyoglossus	Body and greater horn of hyoid bone	Side and inferior aspect of tongue	Hypoglossal nerve (CN XII)	Depresses and retracts tongue
Iliacus	Iliac crest, superior two-thirds of iliac fossa, ala of sacrum, and anterior sacroiliac ligaments	Lesser trochanter of femur and shaft inferior to it, and to psoas major tendon	Femoral nerve (L2–L4)	Flexes thigh and stabilizes hip joint; acts with psoas major
Inferior constrictor of pharynx	Oblique line of thyroid cartilage and side of cricoid cartilage	Median raphe of pharynx	Cranial root of accessory nerve (CN XI) as above, plus branches of external and recurrent laryngeal nerves of vagus (CN X)	Constricts wall of pharynx during swallowing
Inferior longitudinal muscle of tongue	Root of tongue and body of hyoid bone	Apex of tongue	Hypoglossal nerve (CN XII)	Curls tip of tongue inferiorly and shortens tongue
Inferior oblique	Anterior part of floor of orbit	Sclera deep to lateral rectus muscle	Oculomotor nerve (CN III)	Abducts, elevates, and laterally rotates eyeball
Inferior rectus	Common tendinous ring	Sclera just posterior to cornea	Oculomotor nerve (CN III)	Depresses, adducts, and rotates eyeball medially

Muscle(s)	Origin	Insertion	Innervation	Main Action(s)
Infraspinatus	Infraspinous fossa of scapula	Middle facet on greater tubercle of humerus	Suprascapular nerve (C5 and C6)	Laterally rotate arm; help to hold humeral head in glenoid cavity of scapula
Innermost intercostal	Inferior border of ribs	Superior border of ribs below	Intercostal nerves	Probably elevate ribs
Innermost intercostal	Inner surface of ribs, from angles to costochondral junction	Superior border of ribs below	Intercostal nerves	Probably depress ribs
Internal intercostal	Inner surface of ribs, from angles to sternum	Superior border of ribs below	Intercostal nerves	Interchondral portion elevates ribs (when upper ribs are fixed), interosseous portion depresses ribs (when lower ribs are fixed)
Internal oblique	Thoracolumbar fascia, anterior two-thirds of iliac crest, and lateral half of inguinal ligament	Inferior borders of 10th–12th ribs, linea alba, and pecten pubis via conjoint tendon	Thoracoabdominal (anterior rami of inferior 6 thoracic) and first lumbar nerves	Compresses and supports abdominal viscera, and flexes and rotates trunk
Interspinales	Superior surfaces of spinous processes of cervical and lumbar vertebrae	Inferior surfaces of spinous processes of vertebrae superior to vertebrae of origin	Posterior rami of spinal nerves	Aid in extension and rotation of vertebral column
Intertransversarii	Transverse processes of cervical and lumbar vertebrae	Transverse processes of adjacent vertebrae	Posterior and anterior rami of spinal nerves	Aid in lateral bending of vertebral column; acting bilaterally, they stabilize vertebral column
Ischiocavernosus	Internal surface of ischiopubic ramus and ischial tuberosity	Crus of penis or clitoris	Deep branch of perineal nerve, a branch of pudendal nerve (S2, 3 & 4)	Maintains erection of penis or clitoris by compressing outflow veins and pushing blood into body of penis or clitoris
Lateral cricoarytenoid	Arch of cricoid cartilage	Muscular process of arytenoid cartilage	Recurrent laryngeal nerve (branch of vagus (CN X))	Adducts vocal fold (interligamentous portion)
Lateral pterygoid	Superior head: infratemporal surface and infratemporal crest of greater wing of sphenoid bone Inferior head: lateral surface of lateral pterygoid plate	Neck of mandible (pterygoid fovea); articular disc and capsule of temporomandibular joint	Mandibular nerve (CN V3) via lateral pterygoid nerve from anterior trunk, which enters its deep surface	Acting together, they protrude mandible and depress chin; acting alone and alternately, they produce side-to-side movements of mandible
Lateral rectus	Common tendinous ring	Sclera just posterior to cornea	Abducent nerve (CN VI)	Abducts eyeball
Latissimus dorsi	Spinous processes of inferior 6 thoracic vertebrae, thoraco-lumbar fascia, iliac crest, and inferior 3 or 4 ribs	Floor of intertubercular groove of humerus	Thoracodorsal nerve (C6, C7, and C8)	Extends, adducts, and medially rotates humerus; raises body toward arms during climbing
Levator anguli oris	Canine fossa of maxilla	Orbicularis oris and skin at angle of mouth	Facial nerve (CN VII)	Raises angle of mouth, as in smiling
Levator ani (pubococcygeus, puborectalis, and iliococcygeus)	Body of pubis, tendinous arch of obturator fascia, and ischial spine	Perineal body, coccyx, anococcygeal ligament, walls of prostate or vagina, rectum, and anal canal	Nerve to levator ani (branches of S4) and inferior anal (rectal) nerve and coccygeal plexus	Helps to support the pelvic viscera and resists increases in intraabdominal pressure

Muscle(s)	Origin	Insertion	Innervation	Main Action(s)
Levatores costarum	Tips of transverse processes of C7 and T1–T11 vertebrae	Pass inferolaterally and insert on subjacent rib between its tubercle and angle	Posterior rami of C8–T11 spinal nerves	Elevate ribs, assisting inspiration; assist with lateral bending of vertebral column
Levator labii superioris	Frontal process of maxilla and infraorbital region	Skin of upper lip and alar cartilage of nose	Facial nerve (CN VII)	Elevates lip, dilates nostril, and raises angle of mouth
Levator palpebrae superioris	Lesser wing of sphenoid bone, superior and anterior to optic canal	Tarsal plate and skin of superior (upper) eyelid	Oculomotor nerve (CN III); deep layer (superior tarsal muscle) is supplied by sympathetic fibers	Elevates superior (upper) eyelid
Levator scapulae	Posterior tubercles of transverse processes of C1–C4 vertebrae	Superior part of medial border or scapula	Dorsal scapular (C5) and cervical (C3 and C4) nerves	Elevates scapula and tilts its glenoid cavity inferiorly by rotating scapula
Levator veli palatini	Cartilage of pharyngotympanic (auditory) tube and petrous part of temporal bone	Palatine aponeurosis	Cranial part of CN XI through pharyngeal branch of vagus nerve (CN X) via pharyngeal plexus	Elevates soft palate during swallowing and yawning
Longus capitis	Basilar part of occipital bone	Anterior tubercles of C3–C6 transverse processes	Anterior rami of C1–C3 spinal nerves	Flexes head
Longus colli	Anterior tubercle of C1 vertebra (atlas); bodies of C1–C3 and transverse processes of C3–C6 vertebrae	Bodies of C5–T3 vertebrae, transverse process of C3–C5 vertebrae	Anterior rami of C2–C6 spinal nerves	Flexes neck with rotation (torsion) to opposite side if acting unilaterally
Lumbrical muscles of foot	Tendons of flexor digitorum longus	Medial aspect of expansion over lateral four digits	Medial one: medial plantar nerve (S2 and S3) Lateral three: lateral plantar nerve (S2 and S3)	Flex proximal phalanges and extend middle and distal phalanges of lateral four digits
Lumbricals 1 and 2 of hand	Lateral two tendons of flexor digitorum profundus (unipennate muscles)	Lateral sides of extensor expansions of digits 2 & 3	Median nerve (C8 and T1)	Flex digits at metacarpophalangeal joints and extend interphalangeal joints
Lumbricals 3 and 4 of hand	Medial three tendons of flexor digitorum profundus (bipennate muscles)	Lateral sides of extensor expansions of digits 4 & 5	Deep branch of ulnar nerve (C8 and T1)	Flex digits at metacarpophalangeal joints and extend interphalangeal joints
Masseter	Inferior border and medial surface of zygomatic arch	Lateral surface of ramus of mandible and its coronoid process	Mandibular nerve (CN V3) via masseteric nerve, which enters its deep surface	Elevates and protrudes mandible, thus closing jaws; deep fibers retrude it
Medial pterygoid	Deep head: medial surface of lateral pterygoid plate and pyramidal process of palatine bone Superficial head: tuberosity of maxilla	Medial surface of ramus of mandible, inferior to mandibular foramen	Mandibular nerve (CN V3) via medial pterygoid nerve	Acting bilaterally, elevates mandible, closing jaws; assists in protruding mandible; acting alone, assists in protruding same side of jaw; acting alternately, produce a grinding motion
Medial rectus	Common tendinous ring	Sclera just posterior to cornea	Oculomotor nerve (CN III)	Adducts eyeball
Mentalis	Incisive fossa of mandible	Skin of chin	Facial nerve (CN VII)	Elevates and protrudes lower lip

Muscle(s)	Origin	Insertion	Innervation	Main Action(s)
Middle constrictor of pharynx	Stylohyoid ligament and superior (greater) and inferior (lesser) horns of hyoid bone	Median raphe of pharynx	Cranial root of accessory nerve (CN XI) plus branches of external and recurrent laryngeal nerves of vagus (CN X)	Constricts wall of pharynx during swallowing
Mylohyoid	Mylohyoid line of mandible	Raphe and body of hyoid bone	Mylohyoid nerve, a branch of inferior alveolar nerve of CN V3	Elevates hyoid bone, floor of mouth, and tongue during swallowing and speaking
Nasalis	Superior part of canine ridge of maxilla	Nasal cartilages	Facial nerve (CN VII)	Draws ala (side) of nose toward nasal septum
Obliquus capitis inferior	Spinous process of axis (C2 vertebra)	Transverse process of atlas (C1 vertebrae)	Suboccipital nerve	Rotation of head at atlantoaxial joint
Obliquus capitis superior	Spinous process of atlas (C1 vertebra)	Lateral third of inferior nuchal line of occipital bone	Suboccipital nerve	Rotation of head at atlantoaxial joint
Obturator externus	Margins of obturator foramen and obturator membrane	Trochanteric fossa of femur	Obturator nerve (L3 and L4)	Laterally rotates thigh; steadies head of femur in acetabulum
Obturator internus	Pelvic surface of obturator membrane and surrounding bones	Medial surface of greater trochanter (trochanteric fossa) of femur	Nerve to obturator internus (L5 and S1)	Laterally rotates extended thigh and abducts flexed thigh; steadies femoral head in acetabulum
Occipitofrontalis (Occipital belly/frontal belly)	Lateral 2/3 of superior nuchal line & mastoid temporal bone/epicranial aponeurosis	Epicranial aponeurosis/skin of forehead and eyebrows	Posterior branch/temporal branch of facial nerve (CN VII)	Retracts scalp/elevates eyebrows and skin of forehead
Omohyoid	Superior border of scapula near suprascapular notch	Inferior border of hyoid bone	C1–C3 by a branch of ansa cervicalis	Depresses, retracts, and steadies hyoid bone
Opponens digiti minimi	Hook of hamate and flexor retinaculum	Medial border of 5th metacarpal	Deep branch of ulnar nerve (C8 and T1)	Draws 5th metacarpal anteriorly and rotates it, bringing digit 5 into opposition with thumb
Opponens pollicis	Flexor retinaculum and tubercles of scaphoid and trapezium	Lateral side of 1st metacarpal	Recurrent branch of median nerve (C8 and T1)	Draws 1st metacarpal bone laterally to oppose thumb toward center of palm and rotates it medially
Orbicularis oculi	Medial orbital margin, medial palpebral ligament, and lacrimal bone	Skin around margin of orbit; tarsal plate	Facial nerve (CN VII)	Closes eyelids; palpebral part gently closes lids; orbital part tightly closes them
Orbicularis oris	Some fibers arise near median plane of maxilla superiorly and mandible inferiorly; other fibers arise from deep surface of skin	Mucous membrane of lips	Facial nerve (CN VII)	As sphincter of oral opening, compresses and protrudes lips (e.g., purses them during whistling and sucking)
Palatoglossus	Palatine aponeurosis	Side of tongue	Cranial part of accessory nerve (CN XI) through pharyngeal branch of vagus nerve (CN X) via pharyngeal plexus	Elevates posterior part of tongue and draws soft palate onto tongue

Muscle(s)	Origin	Insertion	Innervation	Main Action(s)
Palatopharyngeus	Hard palate and palatine aponeurosis	Lateral wall of pharynx	Cranial part of accessory nerve (CN XI) through pharyngeal branch of vagus nerve (CN X) via pharyngeal plexus	Tenses soft palate and pulls walls of pharynx superiorly, anteriorly, and medially during swallowing
Palmar interossei 1–3	Palmar surfaces of 2nd, 4th, and 5th metacarpals (unipennate muscles)	Extensor expansions of digits and bases of proximal phalanges of digits 2, 4, and 5	Deep branch of ulnar nerve (C8 and T1)	Adduct digits toward axial line and assist lumbricals in flexing metacarpophalangeal joints and extending interphalangeal joint
Palmaris brevis	Ulnar side of central portion of palmar aponeurosis	Skin of ulnar side of hand	Superficial ulnar nerve (T1)	Wrinkles skin on palmar side of hand
Palmaris longus	Medial epicondyle of humerus	Distal half of flexor retinaculum and palmar aponeurosis	Median nerve (C7 and C8)	Flexes hand (at wrist) and tightens palmar aponeurosis
Pectineus	Superior ramus of pubis	Pectineal line of femur, just inferior to lesser trochanter	Femoral nerve (L2 and L3); may receive a branch from obturator nerve	Adducts and flexes thigh; assists with medial rotation of thigh
Pectoralis major	Clavicular head: anterior surface of medial half of clavicle; Sternocostal head: anterior surface of sternum, superior six costal cartilages, and aponeurosis of external oblique muscle	Lateral lip of intertubercular groove of humerus	Lateral and medial pectoral nerves; clavicular head (C5 and C6), sternocostal head (C7, C8, and T1)	Adducts and medially rotates humerus; draws scapula anteriorly and inferiorly; Acting alone: clavicular head flexes humerus and sternocostal head extends it
Pectoralis minor	3rd to 5th ribs near their costal cartilages	Medial border and superior surface of coracoid process of scapula	Medial pectoral nerve (C8 and T1)	Stabilizes scapula by drawing it inferiorly and anteriorly against thoracic wall
Piriformis	Anterior surface of sacrum and sacrotuberous ligament	Superior border of greater trochanter of femur	Branches of anterior rami of S1 and S2	Laterally rotate extended thigh and abduct flexed thigh; steady femoral head in acetabulum
Plantar interossei 1–3	Bases and medial sides of metatarsals 3–5	Medial sides of bases of proximal phalanges of 3rd to 5th digits	Lateral plantar nerve (S2 and S3)	Adduct digits (2–4) and flex metatarso-phalangeal joints
Plantaris	Inferior end of lateral supra-condylar line of femur and oblique popliteal ligament	Posterior surface of calcaneus via calcaneal tendon	Tibial nerve (S1 and S2)	Weakly assists gastrocnemius in plantarflexing ankle and flexing knee
Platysma	Superficial fascia of deltoid and pectoral regions	Mandible, skin of cheek, angle of mouth, and orbicularis oris	Facial nerve (CN VII)	Depresses mandible and tenses skin of lower face and neck
Popliteus	Lateral surface of lateral condyle of femur and lateral meniscus	Posterior surface of tibia, superior to soleal line	Tibial nerve (L4, L5, and S1)	Weakly flexes knee and unlocks it
Posterior cricoarytenoid	Posterior surface of laminae of cricoid cartilage	Muscular process of arytenoid cartilage	Recurrent laryngeal nerve (branch of Vagus (CN X))	Abducts vocal fold
Procerus	Aponeurosis covering bridge of nose	Skin of lower forehead between eyebrows	Facial nerve (CN VII)	Depresses medial end of eyebrow; produces transverse wrinkles over bridge of nose; produces look of concentration

Muscle(s)	Origin	Insertion	Innervation	Main Action(s)
Pronator quadratus	Distal fourth of anterior surface of ulna	Distal fourth of anterior surface of radius	Anterior interosseous nerve from median (C8 and T1)	Pronates forearm; deep fibers bind radius and ulna together
Pronator teres	Medial epicondyle of humerus and coronoid process of ulna	Middle of lateral surface of radius	Median nerve (C6 and C7)	Pronates and flexes forearm (at elbow)
Psoas major	Sides of T12–L5 vertebrae and discs between them; transverse processes of all lumbar vertebrae	Lesser trochanter of femur	Anterior rami of lumbar nerves (L1, L2, and L3)	Flexes and rotates thigh lateral at hip joint; when thigh is fixed, flexes lumbar vertebrae anteriorly and laterally
Psoas minor	Sides of T12–L1 vertebrae and intervertebral disc	Pectineal line, iliopectineal eminence via iliopectineal arch	Anterior rami of lumbar nerves (L1 and L2)	Acts conjointly with psoas major in flexing thigh at hip joint and in stabilizing this joint
Pyramidalis	Crest of pubis	Lower portion of linea alba	Subcostal nerve	Tenses linea alba
Quadratus femoris	Lateral border of ischia tuberosity	Quadrate tubercle on intertrochanteric crest of femur and area inferior to it	Nerve to quadratus femoris (L5 and S1)	Laterally rotates thigh; steadies femoral head in acetabulum
Quadratus lumborum	Medial half of inferior border of 12th rib and tips of lumbar transverse processes	Iliolumbar ligament and internal lip of iliac crest	Ventral branches of T12 and L1–L4 nerves	Extends and laterally flexes vertebral column; fixes 12th rib during inspiration
Quadratus plantae	Medial surface and lateral margin of plantar surface of calcaneus	Posterolateral margin of tendon of flexor digitorum longus	Lateral plantar nerve (S2 and S3)	Assists flexor digitorum longus in flexing lateral four digits
Rectus abdominis	Pubic symphysis and pubic crest	Xiphoid process and 5th–7th costal cartilages	Thoracoabdominal nerves (anterior rami of inferior six thoracic nerves)	Flexes trunk (lumbar vertebrae) and compresses abdominal viscera (indirectly opposing diaphragm)
Rectus capitis anterior	Anterior surface of lateral mass of C1 vertebra (atlas)	Base of skull, just anterior to occipital condyle	Branches from loop between C1 and C2 spinal nerves	Flexes head at atlanto-occipital joint
Rectus capitis lateralis	Transverse process of C1 vertebra (atlas)	Jugular process of occipital bone	Branches from loop between C1 and C2 spinal nerves	Flexes head and helps to stabilize it
Rectus capitis posterior major	Spinous process of axis (C2 vertebra)	Middle of inferior nuchal line of occipital bone	Suboccipital nerve	Extends head at atlanto-occipital joint
Rectus capitis posterior minor	Dorsal tubercle of atlas (C1 vertebra)	Medial third of inferior nuchal line of occipital bone	Suboccipital nerve	Extends head at atlanto-occipital joint
Rectus femoris	Anterior inferior iliac spine and ilium superior to acetabulum	Base of patella and by patellar ligament to tibial tuberosity	Femoral nerve (L2, L3, and L4)	Extend leg at knee joint; rectus femoris also steadies hip joint and helps iliopsoas to flex thigh
Rhomboid minor and major	Minor: nuchal ligament and spinous processes of C7 and T1 vertebrae. Major: spinous processes of T2–T5 vertebrae	Medial border of scapula from level of spine to inferior angle	Dorsal scapular nerve (C4 and C5) rotate	Retract scapula and rotate it to depress glenoid cavity; fix scapula to thoracic wall
Risorius	Platysma and fascia of masseter	Orbicularis oris, skin of corner of mouth, modiolus	Facial nerve (CN VII)	Retracts angle of mouth lengthening rima oris

Muscle(s)	Origin	Insertion	Innervation	Main Action(s)
Salpingopharyngeus	Cartilaginous part of auditory tube	Blends with palatopharyngeus	Cranial root of accessory nerve via pharyngeal branch of vagus and pharyngeal plexus	Elevate (shorten and widen) pharynx and larynx during swallowing and speaking
Sartorius	Anterior superior iliac spine and superior part of notch inferior to it	Superior part of medial surface of tibia	Femoral nerve (L2 and L3)	Flexes, abducts, and laterally rotates thigh at hip joint; flexes leg at knee joint
Scalenus anterior	Transverse processes of C4–C6 vertebrae	1st rib	Cervical spine nerves C4, C5, and C6	Elevates 1st rib; laterally flexes and rotates neck
Scalenus medius	Posterior tubercles of transverse processes of C4–C6 vertebrae	Superior surface of 1st rib, posterior groove for subclavian artery	Anterior rami of cervical spinal nerves	Flexes neck laterally; elevates 1st rib during forced inspiration
Scalenus posterior	Posterior tubercles of transverse processes of C4–C6 vertebrae	External border of 2nd rib	Anterior rami of cervical spinal nerves C7 and C8	Flexes neck laterally: elevates 2nd rib during forced inspiration
Semimembranosus	Ischial tuberosity	Posterior part of medial condyle of tibia; reflected attachment forms oblique popliteal ligament (to lateral femoral condyle)	Tibial division of sciatic nerve (L5, S1, and S2)	Extends thigh; flexes leg and, when knee is flexed, rotates it medially; when hip is flexed and knee is extended, can raise trunk against gravity
Semitendinosus	Ischial tuberosity	Medial surface of superior part of tibia	Tibial division of sciatic nerve (L5, S1, and S2)	Extends thigh; flexes leg and, when knee is flexed, rotates it medially; when hip is flexed and knee is extended, can raise trunk against gravity
Serratus anterior	External surfaces of lateral parts of 1st to 8th ribs	Anterior surface of medial border of scapula	Long thoracic nerve (C5, C6, and C7)	Protracts scapula and holds it against thoracic wall; rotates scapula
Serratus posterior inferior	Spinous processes of T11 to L2 vertebrae	Inferior borders of 8th to 12th ribs near their angles	Anterior rami of 9th to 12th thoracic spinal nerves	Depress ribs
Serratus posterior superior	Ligamentum nuchae, spinous processes of C7 to T3 vertebrae	Superior borders of 2nd to 4th ribs	2nd to 5th intercostal nerves	Elevate ribs
Soleus	Posterior aspect of head of fibula, superior fourth of posterior surface of fibula soleal line and medial border of tibia	Posterior surface of calcaneus via calcaneal tendon	Tibial nerve (S1 and S2)	Plantarflexes ankle independent of position of knee and steadies leg on foot
Splenius capitis et cervicis	Arises from inferior half of ligamentum nuchae and spinous processes of C7–T3 of T4 vertebrae	Splenius capitis: fibers run superolaterally to mastoid process of temporal bone and lateral third of superior nuchal line of occipital bone Splenius cervicis: posterior tubercles of transverse of C1–C3 or C4 vertebrae	Posterior rami of spinal nerves	Acting alone, they laterally bend and rotate head to side of active muscles; acting together, they extend head and neck
Stapedius	Internal walls of pyramidal eminence of posterior wall of tympanic cavity	Neck of the stapes	Facial nerve (CN VII)	Dampens vibrations of stapes reflexively in response to loud noise

Muscle(s)	Origin	Insertion	Innervation	Main Action(s)
Sternocleidomastoid	Lateral surface of mastoid process of temporal bone and lateral half of superior nuchal line	Sternal head: anterior surface of manubrium of sternum Clavicular head: superior surface of medial third of clavicle	Spinal root of accessory nerve (motor) and C2 and C3 nerves (pain and proprioception)	Tilts head to one side, i.e., laterally; flexes neck and rotates it so face is turned superiorly toward opposite side; acting together, the two muscles flex the neck so chin is thrust forward
Sternohyoid	Manubrium of sternum and medial end of clavicle	Body of hyoid bone	C1–C3 by a branch of ansa cervicalis	Depresses hyoid bone after it has been elevated during swallowing
Sternothyroid	Posterior surface of manubrium of sternum	Oblique line of thyroid cartilage	C2 and C3 by a branch of ansa cervicalis	Depresses hyoid bone and larynx
Styloglossus	Styloid process and stylohyoid ligament	Side and inferior aspect of tongue	Hypoglossal nerve (CN XII)	Retracts tongue and draws it up to create a trough for swallowing
Stylohyoid	Styloid process of temporal bone	Body of hyoid bone	Cervical branch of facial nerve (CN VII)	Elevates and retracts hyoid bone, thereby elongating floor of mouth
Stylopharyngeus	Styloid process of temporal bone	Posterior and superior borders of thyroid cartilage with palatopharyngeus	Glossopharyngeal nerve (CN IX)	Elevate (shorten and widen) pharynx and larynx during swallowing and speaking
Subclavius	Junction of 1st rib and its costal cartilage	Inferior surface of middle third of clavicle	Nerve to subclavius (C5 and C6)	Anchors and depresses clavicle
Subcostal	Internal surface of lower ribs near their angles	Superior borders of 2nd or 3rd ribs below	Intercostal nerves	Elevate ribs
Subscapularis	Subscapular fossa	Lesser tubercle of humerus	Upper and lower subscapular nerves (C5, C6, and C7)	Medially rotates arm and adducts it; helps to hold humeral head in glenoid cavity
Superficial transverse perineal muscle	(Compressor urethrae portion only)	Perineal body	Deep branch of perineal nerve, a branch of pudendal nerve (S2, 3 & 4)	Support and fix perineal body (pelvic floor) to support abdominopelvic viscera and resist increased intra-abdominal pressure
Superior longitudinal muscle of tongue	Submucous fibrous layer and median fibrous septum	Margins of tongue and mucous membrane	Hypoglossal nerve (CN XII)	Curls tip and sides of tongue superiorly and shortens tongue
Superior oblique	Body of sphenoid bone	Its tendon passes through a fibrous ring or trochlea, changes its direction, and inserts into sclera deep to superior rectus muscle	Trochlear nerve (CN IV)	Abducts, depresses, and medially rotates eyeball
Superior pharyngeal constrictor	Pterygoid hamulus, pterygomandibular raphe, posterior end of mylohyoid line of mandible, and side of tongue	Median raphe of pharynx and pharyngeal tubercle on basilar part of occipital bone	Cranial root of accessory nerve via pharyngeal branch of vagus and pharyngeal plexus	Constrict wall of pharynx during swallowing
Superior rectus	Common tendinous ring	Sclera just posterior to cornea	Oculomotor nerve (CN III)	Elevates, adducts, and rotates eyeball medially

Muscle(s)	Origin	Insertion	Innervation	Main Action(s)
Supinator	Lateral epicondyle of humerus, radial collateral and anular ligaments, supinator fossa, and crest of ulna	Lateral, posterior, and anterior surfaces of proximal third of radius	Deep branch of radial nerve (C5 and C6)	Supinates forearm (i.e., rotates radius to turn palm anteriorly)
Supraspinatus	Supraspinous fossa of scapula	Superior facet on greater tubercle of humerus	Suprascapular nerve (C4, C5, and C6)	Initiates and assists deltoid in abduction of arm and acts with rotator cuff muscles
Temporalis	Floor of temporal fossa and deep surface of temporal fascia	Tip and medial surface of coronoid process and anterior border of ramus of mandible	Deep temporal branches of mandibular nerve (CN V3)	Elevates mandible closing jaws; its posterior fibers retrude mandible after protrusion
Tensor of fascia lata	Anterior superior iliac spine and anterior part of iliac crest	Iliotibial tract that attaches to lateral condyle of tibia	Superior gluteal (L4 and L5)	Abducts, medially rotates, and flexes thigh; helps to keep knee extended; steadies trunk on thigh
Tensor tympani	Canal for tensor tympani of petrous part of temporal bone and cartilage of pharyngo-tympanic (auditory) tube	Handle of malleus	Branch of mandibular nerve (CN V3) via otic ganglion	Tenses tympanic membrane to dampen excessive vibration caused by loud noise
Tensor veli palatini	Scaphoid fossa of medial pterygoid plate, spine of sphenoid bone, and cartilage of pharyngotympanic (auditory) tube	Palatine aponeurosis	Medial pterygoid nerve (a branch of mandibular nerve—CN V3) via otic ganglion	Tenses soft palate and opens mouth of auditory tube during swallowing and yawning
Teres major	Dorsal surface of inferior angle of scapula	Medial lip of intertubercular groove of humerus	Lower subscapular nerve (C6 and C7)	Adducts and medially rotates arm
Teres minor	Superior part of lateral border of scapula	Inferior facet on greater tubercle of humerus	Axillary nerve (C5 and C6)	Laterally rotate arm; help to hold humeral head in glenoid cavity of scapula
Thyroarytenoid	Posterior surface of thyroid cartilage	Muscular process of arytenoid cartilage	Recurrent laryngeal nerve	Relaxes vocal fold
Thyrohyoid	Oblique line of thyroid cartilage	Inferior border of body and greater horn of hyoid bone	C1 via hypoglossal nerve	Depresses hyoid bone and elevates larynx
Tibialis anterior	Lateral condyle and superior half of lateral surface of tibia and interosseous membrane	Medial and inferior surfaces of medial cuneiform and base of 1st metatarsal	Deep fibular (peroneal) nerve (L4 and L5)	Dorsiflexes ankle and inverts foot
Tibialis posterior	Interosseous membrane, posterior surface of tibia inferior to soleal line, and posterior surface of fibula	Tuberosity of navicular, cuneiform, and cuboid and bases of 2nd, 3rd, and 4th metatarsals	Tibial nerve (L4 and L5)	Plantarflexes ankle and inverts foot
Transverse muscle of tongue	Median fibrous septum	Fibrous tissue at margins of tongue	Hypoglossal nerve (CN XII)	Narrows and elongates the tongue Act simultaneously to protrude tongue

Appendices

Muscle(s)	Origin	Insertion	Innervation	Main Action(s)
Transversospinal	Transverse processes: Semispinalis arises from transverse processes of C4–T12 vertebrae Multifidus arises from sacrum and ilium, transverse processes of T1–T3, and articular processes of C4–C7 Rotatores arise from transverse processes of vertebrae; are best developed in thoracic region	Spinous processes: Semispinalis—thoracis, cervicis, and capitis: fibers run superomedially to occipital bone and spinous processes in thoracic and cervical regions, spanning 4–6 segments; Multifidus: fibers pass superomedially to spinous processes of vertebrae above, spanning 2–4 segments; Rotatores: pass superomedially to attach to junction of lamina and transverse process, or spinous process, of vertebra above their origin, spanning 1–2 segments	Posterior rami of spinal nerves	Extend head and thoracic and cervical regions of vertebral column and rotate them contralaterally; Stabilizes vertebrae during local movements of vertebral column; Stabilize vertebrae and assist with local extension and rotary movements of vertebral column; may function as organs of proprioception
Transversus abdominis	Internal surfaces of 7th–12th costal cartilages, thoracolumbar fascia, iliac crest, and lateral third of inguinal ligament	Linea alba with aponeurosis of internal oblique, pubic crest, and pecten pubis via conjoint tendon	Thoracoabdominal (anterior rami of inferior 6 thoracic) and first lumbar nerves	Compresses and supports abdominal viscera
Transversus thoracis	Posterior surface of lower sternum	Internal surface of costal cartilages 2–6	Intercostal nerves	Depress ribs
Trapezius	Medial third of superior nuchal line; external occipital protuberance, nuchal ligament, and spinous processes of C7–T12 vertebrae	Lateral third of clavicle, acromion, and spine of scapula	Spinal root of accessory nerve (CN XI) (motor) and cervical nerves (C3 and C4) (pain and proprioception)	Elevates, retracts, and rotates scapula; superior fibers elevate, middle fibers retract, and inferior fibers depress scapula; superior and inferior fibers act together in superior rotation of scapula
Triceps brachii	Long head: infraglenoid tubercle of scapula Lateral head: posterior surface of humerus, superior to radial groove Medial head: posterior surface of humerus, inferior to radial groove	Proximal end of olecranon of ulna and fascia of forearm	Radial nerve (C6, C7, and C8)	Chief extensor of forearm at elbow; long head steadies head of abducted humerus
Uvula muscles	Posterior nasal spine and palatine aponeurosis	Mucosa of uvula	Cranial part of CN XI through pharyngeal branch of vagus nerve (CN X) via pharyngeal plexus	Shortens uvula and pulls it superiorly
Vastus intermedius	Anterior and lateral surfaces of body of femur	Base of patella and by patellar ligament to tibial tuberosity	Femoral nerve (L2, L3, and L4)	Extend leg at knee joint; rectus femoris also steadies hip joint and helps iliopsoas to flex thigh
Vastus lateralis	Greater trochanter and lateral lip of linea aspera of femur	Base of patella and by patellar ligament to tibial tuberosity	Femoral nerve (L2, L3, and L4)	Extend leg at knee joint; rectus femoris also steadies hip joint and helps iliopsoas to flex thigh
Vastus medialis	Intertrochanteric line and medial lip of linea aspera of femur	Base of patella and by patellar ligament to tibial tuberosity	Femoral nerve (L2, L3, and L4)	Extend leg at knee joint; rectus femoris also steadies hip joint and helps iliopsoas to flex thigh

Muscle(s)	Origin	Insertion	Innervation	Main Action(s)
Vertical muscle of tongue	Superior surface of borders of tongue	Inferior surface of borders of the tongue	Hypoglossal nerve (CN XII)	Flattens and broadens the tongue Act simultaneously to protrude tongue
Vocalis	Vocal process of arytenoid cartilage	Vocal ligaments	Recurrent laryngeal nerve (branch of Vagus (CN X))	Relaxes posterior vocal ligament while maintaining (or increasing) tension of anterior part
Zygomaticus major/minor	Zygomatic bone anterior/posterior to temporozygomatic suture	Muscles at angle of mouth/orbicularis oris of upper lip	Facial nerve (CN VII)	Elevate and evert upper lip

Nerve(s)/Nerve branch(es)	Origin	Course	Structures Innervated
Abdominopelvic splanchnic	Lower thoracic and lumbar segments of sympathetic trunk	Pass medially and inferiorly to prevertebral ganglion of para-aortic plexus	Motor: presynaptic sympathetics for innervation of abdominopelvic blood vessels and viscera
Abducent (CN VI)	Pons	Become intradural on clivus; traverse cavernous sinus and superior orbital fissure to enter orbit	Motor: lateral rectus
Accessory (CN XI)	Cranial root: medulla Spinal root: cervical spinal cord	Spinal root ascends into cranial cavity via foramen magnum; exits via jugular foramen; traverses posterior triangle of neck	Motor: sternocleidomastoid and trapezius
Ansa cervicalis	Superior root: hypoglossal nerve (C1 and C2 fibers) Inferior root: cervical plexus (C2 and C3 fibers)	Descends on external surface of carotid sheath	Motor: omohyoid, sternohyoid, and sternothyroid
Anterior ethmoidal	Nasociliary nerve (CN V1)	Arises in orbit, passes via anterior ethmoidal foramen to cranial cavity, then via cribriform plate of ethmoid to nasal cavity	Sensory: dural of anterior cranial fossa; mucous membranes of sphenoidal sinus, ethmoidal cells, and upper nasal cavity
Anterior femoral cutaneous	Femoral nerve (L2 and L3 fibers)	Arise in femoral triangle and pierce fascia lata of thigh along path of sartorius muscle	Sensory: skin on medial and anterior aspects of thigh
Anterior interosseous	Median nerve in distal part of cubital fossa	Passes inferiorly on interosseous membrane	Motor: flexor digitorum profundus, flexor pollicis longus, and pronator quadratus
Auriculotemporal	Mandibular nerve (CN V3)	From posterior division of CN V3, it passes between neck of mandible and external acoustic meatus to accompany superficial temporal artery	Sensory: skin anterior to auricle and posterior temporal region, tragus and part of helix of auricle, and roof of exterior acoustic meatus and upper tympanic membrane
Axillary	Terminal branch of posterior cord of brachial plexus (C5 and C6 fibers)	Passes to posterior aspect of arm through quadrangular space in company with posterior circumflex humeral artery and then winds around surgical neck of humerus; gives rise to lateral brachial cutaneous nerve	Motor: teres minor and deltoid Sensory: shoulder joint, and skin over inferior part of deltoid
Buccal	Mandibular nerve (CN V3)	From the anterior division of CN V3 in infratemporal fossa, it passes anteriorly to reach cheek	Sensory: skin and mucosa of cheek, buccal gingiva adjacent to 2nd and 3rd molar teeth
Calcaneal branches	Tibial and sural nerves	Pass from distal part of the posterior aspect of leg to skin on heel	Sensory: skin of heel
Cardiac plexus	Cervical and cardiac branches of vagus nerve and cardiopulmonary splanchnic nerves from sympathetic trunk	From arch of aorta and posterior surface of heart, fibers extend along coronary arteries and to SA node	SA nodal tissue and coronary arteries; parasympathetic fibers slow rate, reduce force of heartbeat, and constrict arteries; sympathetic fibers have opposite effect
Cardiopulmonary splanchnic	Cervical and upper thoracic ganglia of sympathetic trunk	Descend anteromedially to cardiac, pulmonary and esophageal plexuses	Motor: convey postsynaptic sympathetic fibers to nerve plexuses of thoracic viscera
Cavernous nerves	Parasympathetic fibers of prostatic nerve plexus	Perforates perineal membrane to reach erectile bodies of penis	Motor: helicine arteries of cavernous bodies; stimulation produces engorgement at arterial pressure (erection)
Cervical splanchnic	Cervical ganglia of sympathetic trunk	Pass medially and inferiorly to cardiac and pulmonary plexuses	Conducting tissue (SA and AV nodes) and coronary arteries

Nerve(s)/Nerve branch(es)	Origin	Course	Structures Innervated
Chorda tympani	Facial nerve (CN VII) within facial canal	Traverses tympanic cavity, passing between incus and malleus; exits temporal bone via petrotympanic fissure to enter infratemporal fossa where it merges with the lingual nerve	Motor: submandibular and sublingual (salivary) glands Sensory: taste sensation from anterior 2/3 of tongue
Ciliary (long, short)	Long ciliary: nasociliary nerve (CN V1) Short ciliary: ciliary ganglion	Pass to posterior aspect of eyeball	Sensory: cornea, conjunctiva Motor: ciliary body and iris
Clunial (superior, middle, and inferior)	Superior: posterior rami of L1, 2 and 3 Middle: posterior rami of S1, 2 and 3 Inferior: posterior cutaneous nerve of thigh	Superior nerves cross iliac crest; middle nerves exit through posterior sacral foramina and enter gluteal region; inferior nerves curve around inferior border of gluteus maximus	Sensory: skin of buttock or gluteal region as far as greater trochanter
Coccygeal (Co)	Conus medullaris of spinal cord	Anterior and posterior rami join adjacent rami of S4 and S5; anterior rami form coccygeal plexus, which gives rise to anococcygeal nerve	Sensory: skin over coccyx
Cochlear nerve	As a division of the vestibulo-cochlear nerve (CN VIII)	Traverses internal acoustic meatus, entering modiolus with spiral ganglia and peripheral processes in spiral lamina	Sensory: spiral organ (for hearing)
Common fibular (peroneal)	Terminal branch (with tibial nerve) of sciatic nerve (L4–S2 fibers)	Begins at apex of popliteal fossa; follows medial border of biceps femoris muscle to posterior aspect of head of fibula; bifurcates into superficial and deep fibular nerves as it winds around neck of fibula	Sensory: skin on lateral part of posterior aspect of leg via its branch, the lateral sural cutaneous nerve; knee joint via its articular branch Motor: short head of biceps femoris
Common palmar digital	Median and superficial branch of ulnar nerves	Run distally between long flexor tendons of palm, bifurcating in distal palm	branches: proper palmar digital nerves, supplying skin and joints of palmar and distal dorsal aspect of fingers
Common plantar digital	Medial and lateral plantar nerves	Run anteriorly in sole of foot between flexor tendons, bifurcating in distal sole	branches: proper plantar digital nerves, supplying skin and joints of plantar and distal dorsal aspect of toes
Deep branch of radial nerve	Radial nerve just distal to elbow	Winds around neck of radius in supinator; enters posterior compartment of forearm becoming posterior interosseous nerve	Motor: extensor carpi radialis brevis and supinator
Deep branch of ulnar nerve	Ulnar nerve at wrist as it passes between pisiform and hamate bones (T1 fibers)	Passes deep between muscles of hypothenar eminence then across palm with deep palmar (arterial) arch	Motor: hypothenar muscles (abductor, flexor, and opponens digiti minimi), lumbricals of digits 4 and 5, all interossei, adductor pollicis, and deep head of flexor pollicis brevis
Deep fibular (peroneal)	Common fibular (peroneal) nerve	Arises between fibularis longus and neck of fibula; passes through extensor digitorum longus and descends on interosseous membrane; passes deep to extensor retinaculum, crosses distal end of tibia and enters dorsum of foot	Motor: muscles of anterior compartment of leg and dorsum of foot Sensory: skin of first interdigital cleft (i.e., skin on adjacent sides of 1st and 2nd toes); and sends articular branches to the joints it crosses
Deep petrosal	Internal carotid plexus	Traverses cartilage of foramen lacerum to join greater petrosal nerve at entrance to pterygoid canal	Conveys the postsynaptic sympathetic fibers destined for the lacrimal gland and mucosa of the nasal cavity, palate, and upper pharynx
Deep temporal	Mandibular nerve (CN V3)	Ascend temporal fossa deep to temporalis muscle	Motor: temporalis Sensory: periosteum of temporal fossa

Nerve(s)/Nerve branch(es)	Origin	Course	Structures Innervated
Dorsal branch of ulnar nerve	Ulnar nerve about 5 cm proximal to flexor retinaculum	Passes distally deep to flexor carpi ulnaris, then dorsally to perforate deep fascia and course along medial side of dorsum of hand, dividing into 2 to 3 dorsal digital nerves	Sensory: skin of medial aspect of dorsum of hand and proximal portions of little and medial half of ring finger (occasionally also adjacent sides of proximal portions of ring and middle fingers)
Dorsal scapular	Anterior ramus of C5 with a frequent contribution from C4	Pierces scalenus medius, descends deep to levator scapulae, and enters deep surface of rhomboids	Motor: rhomboids and occasionally supplies levator scapulae
Esophageal plexus	Vagus nerve, sympathetic ganglia, greater splanchnic nerve	Distal to tracheal bifurcation, the vagus and sympathetic nerves form a plexus around the esophagus	Vagal (parasymp.) and sympathetic fibers to smooth muscle and glands of inferior two-thirds of esophagus
External nasal	Anterior ethmoidal nerve (CN V1)	Runs in nasal cavity and emerges on face between nasal bone and lateral nasal cartilage	Sensory: skin on dorsum of nose, including tip of nose
Facial (VII)	Posterior border of pons	Runs through internal acoustic meatus and facial canal of petrous part of temporal bone, exiting via stylomastoid foramen; main trunk forms intraparotid plexus	Motor: stapedius, posterior belly of digastric, stylohyoid, facial and scalp muscles Sensory: some skin of external acoustic meatus SEE ALSO: intermediate nerve
Femoral	Lumbar plexus (L2–L4 fibers)	Passes deep to midpoint of inguinal ligament, lateral to femoral vessels, and divides into muscular and cutaneous branches	Motor: anterior thigh muscles Sensory: hip and knee joints; skin on anteromedial side of thigh and leg
Frontal	Ophthalmic nerve (CN V1)	Crosses orbit on superior aspect of levator palpebrae superioris; divides into supraorbital and supratrochlear branches	Sensory: skin of forehead, scalp, upper eyelid, and nose; conjunctiva of upper lid and mucosa of frontal sinus
Genitofemoral	Lumbar plexus (L1 and L2 fibers)	Descends on anterior surface of psoas major and divides into genital and femoral branches	Sensory: Femoral branch supplies skin over femoral triangle; genital branch supplies scrotum or labia majora Motor: genital branch to cremaster muscle
Glossopharyngeal (CN IX)	Rostral end of medulla	Exits cranium via jugular foramen, passes between superior and middle constrictors of pharynx to tonsillar fossa, enters posterior third of tongue	Motor: somatic to stylopharyngeus; visceral (presynaptic parasympathetic) to parotid gland Sensory: posterior 2/3 of tongue (incl. taste), pharynx, tympanic cavity, auditory tube, carotid body and sinus
Great auricular	Cervical plexus (C2 & C3 fibers)	Ascends vertically over sterno-cleidomastoid, anterior and parallel to external jugular vein	Sensory: skin of auricle, adjacent scalp, and over angle of jaw; parotid sheath
Greater occipital	As medial branch of posterior ramus of spinal nerve C2	Pierces deep muscles of neck and trapezius to ascend posterior scalp to vertex	Motor: multifidus cervicis, semispinalis capitis Sensory: posterior scalp
Greater palatine	Branch of pterygopalatine ganglion (maxillary nerve)	Passes inferiorly through greater palatine canal and foramen	Motor: postsynaptic parasympathetics to palatine glands Sensory: mucosa of hard palate
Greater petrosal	Genu of facial nerve (CN VII)	Exits facial canal via hiatus for greater petrosal nerve; courses across tegmen tympani and passes through cartilage of foramen lacerum to join deep petrosal nerve at opening of pterygoid canal	Motor: presynaptic parasympathetics to pterygopalatine ganglion for innervation of lacrimal and nasal, palatine, and upper pharyngeal mucous glands
Greater splanchnic	5th–6th through 9th–10th thoracic sympathetic ganglia	Highest abdominopelvic splanchnic nerve; passes anteromedially on bodies of thoracic vertebrae, piercing diaphragm to converge on root of celiac trunk	Motor: conveys presynaptic sympathetics to celiac ganglia for innervation of celiac arteries and derivatives, and of the portion of the gut they supply

Nerve(s)/Nerve branch(es)	Origin	Course	Structures Innervated
Hypogastric	As continuation of superior hypogastric plexus into pelvis	Course anterior to sacrum within the hypogastric sheath to merge with pelvic splanchnic nerves in inferior hypogastric plexus	Motor: convey pre- and postsynaptic sympathetic fibers destined for pelvic viscera Sensory: conveys pain fibers from intraperiteoneal pelvic viscera (e.g., fundus/body of uterus)
Hypoglossal (CN XII)	Between pyramid and olive of myencephalon	Passes through hypoglossal canal then runs inferiorly and anteriorly, passing medial to the angle of the mandible and between mylohyoid and hyoglossus to reach muscles of tongue	Motor: intrinsic and extrinsic muscles of tongue (exception: palatoglossus)
Iliohypogastric	Lumbar plexus (L1 fibers)	Parallels iliac crest; pierces transverse abdominal muscle; branches pierce external oblique aponeurosis to reach inguinal and pubic regions	Motor: internal oblique and transverse abdominal muscles Sensory: lateral cutaneous branch supplies superolateral quadrant of buttock; skin over iliac crest and hypogastric region
Ilioinguinal	Lumbar plexus (L1 fibers)	Passes between 2nd and 3rd layers of abdominal muscles and passes through inguinal canal and divides into femoral and scrotal or labial branches	Motor: lowermost part of internal oblique and transverse abdominal muscles Sensory: femoral branch supplies skin over femoral triangle; genital branch supplies mons pubis and adjacent skin of labia majora or scrotum
Inferior alveolar	As terminal branch (with lingual nerve) of posterior trunk of mandibular nerve (CN V3)	Descends between lateral and medial pterygoid muscles of infratemporal fossa to enter mandibular canal of mandible	Sensory: lower teeth, periodontium, periosteum, and gingiva of lower jaw SEE ALSO: nerve to mylohyoid, mental nerve
Inferior anal (rectal)	Pudendal nerve (S2–S4 fibers)	Arises at entry to pudendal canal (ischial spine), courses medially through ischioanal fat pad to anal canal	Motor: external anal sphincter Sensory: anoderm, perianal skin
Inferior gluteal	Sacral plexus (L5–S2 fibers)	Leaves pelvis through greater sciatic foramen inferior to piriformis and divides into several branches	Motor: gluteus maximus
Infraorbital	Terminal branch of maxillary nerve (CN V2)	Runs in floor of orbit and emerges at infraorbital foramen	Sensory: skin of cheek, lower lid, lateral side of nose and inferior septum and upper lip, upper premolar incisors and canine teeth; mucosa of maxillary sinus and upper lip
Infratrochlear	Nasociliary nerve (CN V1)	Follows medial wall of orbit to upper eyelid	Sensory: skin/conjunctiva (lining) of upper eyelid
Intercostals	Anterior rami of T1 to T11 nerves	Run in intercostal spaces between internal and innermost layers of intercostal muscles	Motor: intercostal muscles; lower nerves supply muscles of anterolateral abdominal wall Sensory: skin overlying and pleura/peritoneum deep to muscles innervated
Intermediate	From the pons as a smaller root of the facial nerve (CN VII)	Traverses internal acoustic meatus merging at its distal end with the larger (root of the) facial nerve	Motor: presynaptic parasympathetics destined for pterygopalatine and submandibular ganglia via greater petrosal nerve and chorda tympani, respectively Sensory: taste from anterior 2/3 of tongue and soft palate
Lacrimal	Ophthalmic nerve (CN V1)	Passes through palpebral fascia of upper eyelid near lateral angle (canthus) of eye	Sensory: a small area of skin and conjunctiva of lateral part of upper eyelid

Appendices

Nerve(s)/Nerve branch(es)	Origin	Course	Structures Innervated
Lateral branch of median nerve	Median nerve as it enters palm of hand	Runs laterally to palmar thumb and radial side of index finger	Motor: 1st lumbrical Sensory: skin of palmar and distal dorsal aspects of thumb and radial half of index finger
Lateral cutaneous nerve of forearm	Continuation of musculocutaneous nerve (C6 and C7 fibers)	Descends along lateral border of forearm to wrist	Sensory: skin of lateral aspect of forearm
Lateral cutaneous nerve of thigh	Lumbar plexus (L2 and L3 fibers)	Passes deep to inguinal ligament, 2–3 cm medial to anterior superior iliac spine	Sensory: skin on anterior and lateral aspects of thigh
Lateral pectoral	Lateral cord of brachial plexus (C5–C7 fibers)	Pierces clavipectoral fascia to reach deep surface of pectoral muscles	Motor: primarily pectoralis major but sends a loop to medial pectoral nerve that innervates pectoralis minor
Lateral plantar	Smaller terminal branch of the tibial nerve (S1–S2 fibers)	Passes laterally in foot between quadratus plantae and flexor digitorum brevis muscles and divides into superficial and deep branches	Motor: quadratus plantae, abductor digiti minimi, and flexor digiti minimi brevis; deep branch supplies plantar and dorsal interossei, lateral three lumbricals, and adductor hallucis Sensory: skin on sole lateral to a line splitting 4th digit
Least splanchnic	12th (lowest) thoracic ganglion of sympathetic trunk	Passes through diaphragm with sympathetic trunk and ends in renal plexus	Motor: presynaptic sympathetic to renal arteries and deriviatives
Lesser occipital	Cervical plexus (C2 & C3 fibers)	Ascends posterosuperiorly, parallel to anterosuperior border of sternocleidomastoid	Sensory: skin of posterior surface of auricle and adjacent scalp
Lesser palatine	Pterygopalatine ganglion (maxillary nerve—CN V2)	Passes inferiorly through palatine canal and lesser palatine foramen	Motor: postsynaptic parasympathetics to glands of soft palate Sensory: mucosa of soft palate
Lesser petrosal	Tympanic plexus (glossopharyngeal nerve—CN IX)	Perforates tegmen tympanii to exit tympanic cavity into middle cranial fossa; runs anteriorly to descend through sphenopetrosal fissure or foramen ovale	Motor: conveys presynaptic parasympathetic fibers to otic ganglion for secretomotor innervation of parotid gland
Lesser splanchnic	10th and 11th thoracic gangia of sympathetic trunk	Descends anteromedially to perforate diaphragm to reach aorticorenal ganglion	Motor: presynaptic sympathetics to prevertebral ganglia Sensory: visceral afferents from upper GI tract
Lingual	Terminal branch (with inferior alveolar nerve) of posterior trunk of mandibular nerve (CN V3)	Joined by chorda tympani in infra-temporal fossa; passes anteroinferiorly between lateral and medial pterygoid muscles, and above mylohyoid to enter oral cavity	Motor: presynpatic parasympathetic fibers to submandibular ganglion for submandibular and sublingual salivary glands Sensory: anterior 2/3 of tongue, floor of mouth, and lingual mandibular gingiva
Long thoracic	Anterior rami of C5–C7	Descends posterior to C8 and T1 rami and passes distally on external surface of serratus anterior	Motor: serratus anterior
Lower subscapular	Posterior cord of brachial plexus (C5 and C6 fibers)	Passes inferolaterally, deep to subscapular artery and vein, to subscapularis and teres major	Motor: inferior portion of subscapularis and teres major
Lumbar splanchnic	Lumbar ganglia of sympathetic trunks	Pass anteromedially on bodies of lumbar vertebrae to prevertebral ganglia of paraaortic plexus	Motor: presynaptic sympathetics for lower abdominal and pelvic viscera Sensory: visceral afferents from same

Nerve(s)/Nerve branch(es)	Origin	Course	Structures Innervated
Mandibular (CN V3)	Trigeminal ganglion (motor root from pons)	Descends through foramen ovale into infratemporal fossa; divides into anterior and posterior trunks, the former ramifying immediately into a number of smaller branches, the latter bifurcating into the lingual and inferior alveolar nerves	Motor: muscles of mastication, mylohyoid, anterior belly of digastric, tensor tympani and tensor veli palatini Sensory: skin overlying mandible (except angle), lower half of mouth (including teeth, gingiva, mucosa of floor and vestibule, and anterior 2/3 of tongue) and temporomandibular joint
Masseteric	Anterior trunk of mandibular nerve (CN V3)	Passes laterally through mandibular notch	Motor: masseter Sensory: temporomandibular joint
Maxillary (CN V2)	Trigeminal ganglion	Runs anteriorly through foramen rotundum into pterygopalatine fossa, sending sensory roots to the pterygopalatine ganglion (branches of the ganglion are considered branches of the maxillary nerve); main trunk continues anteriorly through infraorbital fissure as infraorbital nerve	Motor: no motor fibers initially; branches of pterygopalatine ganglion distribute postsynaptic parasympathetic fibers to lacrimal gland and mucosal glands of nasal cavity, palate and upper pharynx Sensory: skin overlying maxilla, mucosa of posteroinferior nasal cavity and maxillary sinus; upper half of mouth (including teeth, gingiva, and mucosa of palate, vestibule, and cheek)
Medial branch of median nerve	Median nerve as it enters palm of hand	Runs medially to adjacent sides of index, middle, and ring fingers	Motor: 2nd lumbrical Sensory: skin of palmar and distal dorsal aspects of adjacent sides of index, middle, and ring fingers
Medial cutaneous nerve of arm	Medial cord of brachial plexus (C8 and T1 fibers)	Runs along the medial side of axillary vein and communicates with intercostobrachial nerve	Sensory: skin on medial side of arm
Medial cutaneous nerve of forearm	Medial cord of brachial plexus (C8 and T1 fibers)	Runs between axillary artery and vein	Sensory: skin over medial side of forearm
Medial cutaneous nerve of leg	Saphenous nerve	Descends medial side of leg with greater saphenous vein	Skin of anteromedial side of leg and medial side of foot
Medial dorsal cutaneous nerve	Superficial fibular (peroneal) nerve	Descends across ankle anteriorly running onto medial aspect of dorsum of foot	Supplies most of skin of dorsum of foot proximal portion of toes, except for web between great and 2nd toes
Medial pectoral	Medial cord of brachial plexus (C8 and T1 fibers)	Passes between axillary artery and vein and enters deep surface of pectoralis minor	Motor: pectoralis minor and part of pectoralis major
Medial plantar	Larger terminal branch of the tibial nerve (L4 and L5 fibers)	Passes distally in foot between abductor hallucis and flexor digitorum brevis and divides into muscular and cutaneous branches	Motor: abductor hallucis, flexor digitorum brevis, flexor hallucis brevis, and first lumbrical Sensory: skin of medial side of sole of foot and sides of first three digits
Median	Arises by two roots, one from the lateral cord of the brachial plexus (C6 and C7 fibers) and one from the medial cord (C8 and T1 fibers); roots join lateral to axillary artery	Over length of arm, crosses to medial side of brachial artery; exits cubital fossa between heads of pronator teres, running between intermediate and deep layers of anterior forearm compartment; becomes superficial proximal to the wrist and passes deep to the flexor retinaculum (transverse carpal ligament) as it passes through the carpal tunnel to the hand	Motor: flexor muscles in forearm (except flexor carpi ulnaris, ulnar half of flexor digitorum profundus); thenar muscles (except adductor pollicis and deep head of flexor pollicis brevis), lateral lumbricals (for digits 2 and 3) Sensory: skin of the palmar and distal dorsal aspects of the lateral (radial) 3 1/2 digits and adjacent palm
Mental	Terminal branch of inferior alveolar nerve (CN V3)	Emerges from mandibular canal at mental foramen	Sensory: skin of chin; skin and mucosa of lower lip
Musculocutaneous	Lateral cord of brachial plexus (C5–C7 fibers)	Enters deep surface of coracobrachialis and descends between biceps brachii and brachialis	Motor: flexor muscles of arm (coraco-brachialis, biceps brachii, and brachialis) Sensory: continues as lateral ante-brachial cutaneous nerve

Nerve(s)/Nerve branch(es)	Origin	Course	Structures Innervated
Nasociliary	Ophthalmic nerve (CN V1)	Arises in superior orbital fissure, passes anteromedially across retrobulbar orbit, providing sensory root to ciliary ganglion and terminating as infratrochlear nerve and nasal branches	Motor: no motor fibers initially; branches of ciliary ganglion (short ciliary nerves) convey postsynaptic sympathetics and parasympathetics to ciliary body and iris Sensory: tactile sensation from eyeball (conjunctiva and cornea); mucous membrane of ethmoidal cells and anterosuperior nasal cavity; skin of root, dorsum and apex of nose
Nasopalatine	Pterygopalatine ganglion (maxillary nerve—CN V2)	Exits pterygopalatine fossa via sphenopalatine foramen; crossing to and then running anteroinferiorly across nasal septum; passes through incisvie foramen to palate	Motor: postsynaptic parasympathetics to mucosal glands of nasal septum Sensory: mucosa of nasal septum, anteriormost hard palate
Nerve to obturator internus	Sacral plexus (L5, S1, and S2)	Enters gluteal region through greater sciatic foramen inferior to piriformis; descends posterior to ischial spine; enters lesser sciatic foramen and passes to obturator internus	Motor: superior gemellus and obturator internus
Nerves to lateral/medial pterygoid	Anterior trunk of mandibular nerve (CN V3)	Arise in infratemporal fossa immediately inferior to foramen ovale	Motor: lateral and medial pterygoid muscles
Nerve to mylohyoid	Inferior alveolar nerve	Arises from posterior aspect of inferior alveolar nerve immediately outside mandibular foramen; descends in bony groove on medial aspect of ramus of mandible	Motor: mylohyoid and anterior belly of digastric muscle
Nerve of pterygoid canal	Formed by merger of greater and deep petrosal nerves	Traverses pterygoid canal to reach pterygopalatine ganglion in pterygopalatine fossa	Motor: conveys postsynaptic sympathetic and presynaptic parasympathetic fibers to pterygopalatine ganglion
Nerve to quadratus femoris	Sacral plexus (L5, S1, and S2)	Leaves pelvis through greater sciatic foramen deep to sciatic nerve	Motor: inferior gemellus and quadratus femoris Sensory: hip joint
Nerve to stapedius	Facial nerve (CN VII)	Arises as facial inerve descends posterior to muscle in facial canal	Motor: stapedius
Nerve to tensor tympani	Otic ganglion (mandibular nerve–CN V3)	Courses along cartilagenous portion of pharyngotympanic (auditory) tube to hemicanal for tensor tympani	Motor: tensor tympani
Nerve to tensor veli palatini	Anterior trunk of mandibular nerve—CN V3	Arises as a branch of nerve to medial pterygoid	Motor: tensor veli palatini
Obturator	Lumbar plexus (L2—L4 fibers)	Enters thigh through obturator foramen and divides; its anterior branch descends between adductor longus and adductor brevis; its posterior branch descends between adductor brevis and adductor magnus	Motor: Anterior branch supplies adductor longus, adductor brevis, gracilis, and pectineus; posterior branch supplies obturator externus and adductor magnus Sensory: skin of medial thigh above knee
Oculomotor (CN III)	Interpeduncular fossa of mesencephalon	Pierces dura lateral to posterior clinoid process, runs in lateral wall of cavernous sinus, enters orbit through superior orbital fissure and divides into superior & inferior branches	Motor: somatic: all extraocular muscles except superior oblique and lateral rectus; presynaptic parasympathetic fibers to ciliary ganglion for ciliary body and sphincter pupillae
Olfactory (CN I)	Olfactory cells in olfactory epithelium (mucosa) of roof of nasal cavity	Approximately 20 bundles of nerve fibers ascend through foramina of cribriform plate of ethmoid to reach olfactory bulbs (anterior cranial fossa)	Sensory: olfactory mucosa (sense of smell)

Nerve(s)/Nerve branch(es)	Origin	Course	Structures Innervated
Ophthalmic (CN V1)	Trigeminal ganglion	Passes anteriorly in lateral wall of cavernous sinus to enter orbit through superior orbital fissue, branching into frontal, nasociliary and lacarimal nerves	Sensory: general sensation from eyeball (conjunctiva and cornea); mucous membrane of ethmoidal cells and frontal sinus, dura of anterior cranial fossa, falx cerebri and tentorium cerebelli, anterosuperior nasal cavity; skin of forehead, upper lid, root, dorsum and apex of nose
Optic (CN II)	Ganglion cells of retina	Exits orbit via optic canals; fibers from nasal half of retina cross to contralateral side at chiasm; fibers pass via optic tracts to geniculate bodies, superior colliculus and pretectum	Sensory: vision from retina
Palmar cutaneous branch of median nerve	Arises from median nerve just proximal to flexor retinaculum	Passes between tendons of palmaris longus and flexor carpi radialis and runs superficial to flexor retinaculum	Sensory: skin of central palm
Palmar cutaneous branch of ulnar nerve	Arises from ulnar nerve near middle of forearm	Descends on ulnar artery and perforates deep fascia in the distal third of forearm	Sensory: skin at base of medial palm, overlying the medial carpals
Pelvic splanchnic	Sacral plexus (S2–S4 fibers)	Run anteriorly and inferiorly to merge with inferior hypogastric plexus	Motor: Presynaptic parasympathetic fibers for pelvic viscera, descending and sigmoid colon Sensory: visceral afferent fibers from subperitoneal pelvic viscera (cervix of uterus and upper vagina, floor of bladder, rectum and upper anal canal; prostate)
Perineal	Terminal branch (with dorsal nerve of penis/clitoris) of pudendal nerve (S2–S4 fibers)	Separates from pudendal nerve on exit from pudendal canal; runs to superficial perineum dividing into a superficial cutaneous (posterior labial/ scrotal) and a deep motor branch	Motor: muscles of urogenital triangle (superficial and deep perineal muscles) Sensory: skin of posterior urogenital triangle (posterior portion of labia majora and minora, vestibule of vagina; posterior aspect of scrotum
Pharyngeal	Pterygopalatine ganglion	Passes posteriorly through palatovaginal canal	Supplies mucosa of nasopharynx posterior to the pharyngotympanic (auditory) tubes
Phrenic	Cervical plexus (C3–C5 fibers)	Passes through superior thoracic aperture and runs between mediastinal pleura and pericardium	Motor: diaphragm Sensory: pericardial sac, mediastinal and diaphragmatic pleura, and diaphragmatic peritoneum
Posterior auricular	As first extracranial branch of facial nerve (CN VII)	Passes posterior to ear, sending branch to occipital region	Motor: posterior auricular muscle and intrinsic auricular muscles, occipital belly of occipitofrontalis (epicranius)
Posterior cutaneous nerve of arm	Radial nerve (C5–C8 fibers)	Emerges from under posterior border of deltoid, between long and lateral heads of triceps brachii	Sensory: skin of posterior aspect of arm
Posterior cutaneous nerve of forearm	Arises in arm from radial nerve (C5–C8 fibers)	Perforates lateral head of triceps and descends along lateral side of arm and posterior aspect of forearm to wrist	Sensory: skin of distal posterior arm, posterior aspect of forearm
Posterior cutaneous nerve of thigh	Sacral plexus (S1–S3 fibers)	Leaves pelvis through greater sciatic foramen inferior to piriformis, runs deep to gluteus maximus, and emerges from its inferior border	Sensory: skin of buttock through inferior cluneal branches and skin over posterior aspect of thigh and calf; lateral perineum, upper medial thigh via perineal branch
Posterior ethmoidal	Nasociliary	Leaves orbit via posterior ethmoidal foramen	Supplies ethmoidal and sphenoidal paranasal sinuses
Posterior inferior nasal	Greater palatine	Arise in greater palatine canal, pierce through perpendicular plate of palatine bone	Mucosa of inferior nasal concha and walls of inferior and middle nasal meatuses

Nerve(s)/Nerve branch(es)	Origin	Course	Structures Innervated
Posterior interosseous	Terminal branch of deep branch of radial nerve (continuation of deep radial after emerging from supinator)	Runs between superficial and deep layers of posterior forearm, then passes between extensor pollicis longus and interosseous membrane	Motor: extensor carpi ulnaris, extensors of digits (including thumb), and abductor pollicis longus
Posterior labial	Perineal nerve	Emerge from pudendal canal and ramify in subcutaneous tissue	Skin of posterior portion of labium majus
Pudendal	Sacral plexus (S2–S4)	Enters gluteal region through greater sciatic foramen inferior to piriformis; descends posterior to sacrospinous ligament; enters perineum through lesser sciatic foramen	Supplies most motor and sensory innervation to the perineum; (supplies no structures in gluteal region)
Pulmonary plexus	Vagus nerve and cardiopulmonary splanchnic nerves from sympathetic trunk	Forms on primary bronchi and extends along root of lung and bronchial subdivisions	Motor: Parasympathetic fibers constrict bronchioles; sympathetic fibers dilate them
Radial	Terminal branch of posterior cord of brachial plexus (C5–C8 and T1 fibers)	Descends posterior to axillary artery; enters radial groove with deep brachial artery to pass between long and medial heads of triceps; bifurcates in cubital fossa into superficial and deep radial nerves	Motor: proximal to bifurcation, it innervates triceps brachii, anconeus, brachioradialis, and extensor carpi radialis longus muscles Sensory: skin on posterior aspect of arm and forearm via posterior cutaneous nerves of arm and forearm
Recurrent (thenar) branch of median nerve	Median nerve immediately distal to the flexor retinaculum	Loops around distal border of flexor retinaculum and enters thenar muscles	Motor: abductor pollicis brevis, opponens pollicis, and superficial head of flexor pollicis brevis
Recurrent laryngeal	Vagus nerve (CN X)	Loops around subclavian on right; on left runs around arch of aorta and ascends in tracheoesophageal groove	Motor: intrinsic muscles of larynx (except cricothyroid) Sensory: inferior to level of vocal folds
Saphenous	Femoral nerve	Descends with femoral vessels through femoral triangle and adductor canal and then descends with great saphenous vein	Sensory: skin on medial side of leg and foot
Sciatic	Sacral plexus (L4–S3 fibers)	Enters gluteal region through greater sciatic foramen inferior to piriformis, descends along posterior aspect of thigh, and divides proximal to knee into tibial and common fibular peroneal nerves	Motor: hamstrings by its tibial division (except for short head of biceps femoris, which is innervated by its common fibular division) Sensory: provides articular branches to hip and knee joints
Subclavian nerve	Superior trunk of brachial plexus (C5–C6; often C4 also)	Descends posterior to clavicle and anterior to brachial plexus and subclavian artery	Motor: subclavius Sensory: sternoclavicular joint
Subcostal	Anterior ramus of T12 spinal nerve	Courses along inferior border of 12th rib in same manner as intercostal nerves	Motor: muscles of anterolateral abdominal wall Sensory: Lateral cutaneous branch supplies skin inferior to anterior iliac rest
Suboccipital	Posterior ramus of C1 spinal nerve	Emerges between occipital bone and atlas, inferior to transverse part of vertebral artery, into suboccipital triangle; communicates with occipital nerve (C2)	Motor: suboccipital muscles (rectus capitis major and minor, obliquus capitis inferior and superior)
Superficial branch of radial nerve	Continuation of radial nerve after deep branch is given off in cubital fossa	Passes distally, anterior to pronator teres and deep to brachioradialis; emerging to pierce deep fascia at wrist and pass onto dorsum of hand	Sensory: skin of the lateral (radial) half of dorsum of hand and thumb, the proximal portions of the dorsal aspects of digits 2 and 3, and of the lateral (radial) half of digit 4

Nerve(s)/Nerve branch(es)	Origin	Course	Structures Innervated
Superficial branch of ulnar nerve	Arise from ulnar nerve at wrist as they pass between pisiform and hamate bones	Passes palmaris brevis and divides into two common palmar digital nerves	Motor: palmaris brevis Sensory: skin of the palmar and distal dorsal aspects of digit 5 and of the medial (ulnar) side of digit 4 and proximal portion of palm
Superficial fibular (peroneal)	Common fibular (peroneal) nerve	Arises between fibularis longus and neck of fibula and descends in lateral compartment of the leg; pierces deep fascia at distal third of leg to become cutaneous and send branches to foot and digits	Motor: fibularis (peroneus) longus and brevis Sensory: skin on distal third of anterior surface of leg and dorsum of foot and all digits, except lateral side of 5th and adjoining sides of the 1st and 2nd digits
Superior alveolar	Maxillary nerve (CN V2) or its continuation as the infraorbital nerve	Posterior: emerge from pterygomaxillary fissure into infratemporal fossa; pierce posterior aspect of maxilla Middle and anterior: arise from infra-orbital nerve in roof of maxillary sinus, descend walls of sinus	Sensory: mucosa of maxillary sinus, maxillary teeth and gingiva
Superior gluteal	Sacral plexus (L4–S1 fibers)	Leaves pelvis through greater sciatic foramen superior to piriformis and runs between gluteus medius and minimus	Motor: gluteus medius, gluteus minimus, and tensor fasciae latae
Superior laryngeal	Vagus (CN X)	Descends in parapharyngeal space; lateral to thyroid cartilage divides into internal and external laryngeal nerves; former pierces thyrohyoid membrane; latter runs inferomedially to gap between cricoid and thyroid cartilages	Motor: cricothyroid muscle (external laryngeal nerve) Sensory: supraglottic
Supraclavicular (lateral, intermediate, medial)	Cervical plexus (C3 & C4 fibers)	Arise via a common trunk that emerges at center of posterior border of sternocleido-mastoid; fan out as they descend onto lower neck, upper thorax and shoulder	Sensory: skin of lower anterolateral neck, uppermost thorax and shoulder
Supraorbital	Continuation of frontal nerve (CN V1)	Emerges through supraorbital notch, or foramen, and breaks up into small branches	Sensory: mucous membrane of frontal sinus and conjunctiva (lining) of upper eyelid; skin of forehead as far as vertex
Suprascapular	Superior trunk of brachial plexus (C5–C6; often C4 also)	Passes laterally across posterior triangle of neck, through scapular notch under superior transverse scapular ligament	Motor: supraspinatus, infraspinatus muscles Sensory: superior and posterior gleno-humeral (shoulder) joint
Supratrochlear	Frontal nerve (CN V1)	Passes superiorly on medial of supra-orbital nerve and divides into two or more branches	Sensory: skin in middle of forehead to hairline
Sural	Usually arises from merging of medial and lateral sural cutaneous nerves (from tibial and common fibular (peroneal) nerves, respectively)	Descends between heads of gastrocnemius and becomes superficial at the middle of the leg; descends with small saphenous vein and passes posterior to the lateral malleolus to the lateral side of foot	Sensory: skin on posterior and lateral aspects of leg and lateral side of foot
Tentorial	Intracranial portion of ophthalmic nerve (CN V1)	Arises as recurrent branch passing abruptly posteriorly around margins of tentorial notch onto superior aspect of tentorium cerebelli and ascending posterior limb of falx cerebri	Sensory: supratentorial dura mater (superior aspect of tentorium cerebri and falx cerebri)
Thoracic splanchnic	Thoracic ganglia of sympathetic trunk	Pass anteromedially on bodies of thoracic vertebrae as lower cardio-pulmonary splanchnic nerves to thoracic autonomic plexuses (cardiac, pulmonary, and esophageal) and as upper abdominopelvic splanchnic nerves to the prevertebral ganglia of paraaortic plexus	Motor: splanchnic nerves from 1st through 5th thoracic ganglia convey postsynaptic sympathetic fibers to heart, lungs and esophagus; those from 6th through 12th thoracic ganglia (i.e., the greater, lesser, and least splanchnic nerves) convey presynaptic sympathetic fibers to prevertebral ganglia

Appendices

Nerve(s)/Nerve branch(es)	Origin	Course	Structures Innervated
Thoracoabdominal	Continuation of lower intercostal nerves (T7–T11)	Cross costal margin to run between 2nd and 3rd layers of abdominal muscles	Motor: anterolateral abdominal muscles Sensory: overlying skin, underlying peritoneum, and periphery of diaphragm
Thoracodorsal	Posterior cord of brachial plexus (C6–C8 fibers)	Arises between upper and lower sub-scapular nerves and runs inferolaterally along posterior axillary wall to latissimus dorsi	Motor: latissimus dorsi
Tibial	Sciatic nerve (L4–S3 fibers)	Forms as sciatic bifurcates at apex of popliteal fossa; descends through popliteal fossa and lies on popliteus; runs inferiorly on the tibialis posterior with the posterior tibial vessels; terminates beneath the flexor retinaculum by dividing into the medial and lateral plantar nerves	Motor: muscles of posterior compartment of thigh (except short head of biceps), popliteal fossa, posterior compartment of leg, and sole of foot Sensory: knee joint; skin of leg (via medial sural) and sole of foot (via medial and lateral plantar nerves)
Transverse cervical	Cervical plexus (C2 & C3 fibers)	Emerges from middle of posterior border of sternocleidomastoid muscle; runs anterior across muscle	Sensory: skin overlying anterior triangle of neck
Trigeminal (CN V)	Lateral surface of pons by two roots: motor and sensory	Roots cross medial part of crest of petrous part of temporal bone, entering trigeminal cave of dura mater lateral to body of sphenoid and cavernous sinus; sensory root leads to trigeminal ganglion; motor root bipasses ganglion, becoming part of mandibular nerve (CN V3)	Motor: somatic: muscles of mastication, mylohyoid, anterior belly of digastric, tensor tympani and tensor veli palatini; visceral: distributes postsynaptic para-sympathetic fibers of head to their destinations Sensory: dura of anterior and middle cranial fossae, skin of face, teeth, gingiva, mucosa nasal cavity, paranasal sinuses, and mouth
Trochlear (CN IV)	Dorsolateral aspect of mesencephalon below inferior colliculus (only cranial nerve to emerge from dorsal aspect of brain stem)	Runs longest intracranial course, passing around brainstem to enter dura in free edge of tentorium close to posterior clinoid process; runs in lateral wall of cavernous sinus, entering orbit via superior orbital fissure	Motor: superior oblique muscle
Tympanic	As first extracranial branch of glossopharyngeal nerve (CN IX), from inferior (petrosal) glossopharyngeal ganglion	Passes in recurrent manner into tympanic canaliculus, entering tympanic cavity and ramifying on promontory of labyrinthine wall as tympanic plexus	Motor: conveys presynaptic para-sympathetic fibers that will reach otic ganglion for secretomotor innervation of parotid gland Sensory: mucosa of tympanic cavity, mastoid cells and pharyngotympanic (auditory) tube
Ulnar	Terminal branch of medial cord of brachial plexus (C8 and T1 fibers; often also receives C7 fibers)	Terminal branch of medial cord of brachial plexus (C8 and T1 fibers; often also receives C7 fibers)	Motor: majority of intrinsic muscles of hand (hypothenar, interosseous, adductor pollicis, and deep head of flexor pollicis brevis, plus the medial lumbricals [for digits 4 and 5]) Sensory: skin of the palmar and distal dorsal aspects of medial (ulnar) 1 1/2 digits and adjacent palm
Upper subscapular	Branch of posterior cord of brachial plexus (C5 and C6 fibers)	Passes posteriorly and enters subscapularis	Motor: superior portion of subscapularis
Vagus (CN X)	Via 8 to 10 rootlets from medulla of brainstem	Enters superior mediastinum posterior to sternoclavicular joint and brachiocephalic vein; gives rise to recurrent laryngeal nerve; continues into abdomen	Motor: voluntary muscle of larynx and upper esophagus; involuntary muscle and glands of tracheobronchial tree, gut (to left colic flexure) and heart via pulmonary plexus, esophageal plexus, and cardiac plexus; Sensory: pharynx, larynx, reflex afferents from same areas as above

Nerve(s)/Nerve branch(es)	Origin	Course	Structures Innervated
Vestibular	As a division of the vestibulocochlear nerve (CN VIII)	Traverses internal acoustic meatus to reach vestibular ganglion at fundus; branches pass to vestibule of bony labyrinth	Sensory: cristae of ampullae of semi-circular ducts, maculae of the saccule and utricle (for sense of equilibration)
Vestibulocochlear (CN VIII)	Groove between pons and myencephalon	Traverses internal acoustic meatus, dividing into cochlear and vestibular nerves	Sensory: spiral organ (for sense of hearing) and cristae of ampullae of semicircular ducts, maculae of the saccule and utricle (for sense of equilibration)
Zygomatic	Maxillary nerve (CN V2)	Arises in floor of orbit, divides into zygomaticofacial and zygomatico-temporal nerves, which traverse foramina of same name; communicating branch joins lacrimal nerve	Sensory: skin over zygomatic arch and anterior temporal region Motor: conveys secretory postsynaptic parasymp. fibers from pterygopalatine ganglion to lacrimal gland

TABLE OF ELEMENTS AND THEIR ATOMIC WEIGHTS

(Alphabetical Order)

Element	Symbol	Atomic Number	Atomic Weight	Element	Symbol	Atomic Number	Atomic Weight
Actinium	Ac	89	227.0278*	Neodymium	Nd	60	144.24
Aluminum	Al	13	26.981539	Neon	Ne	10	20.1797
Americium	Am	95	243.0614*	Neptunium	Np	93	237.0482*
Antimony	Sb	51	121.760	Nickel	Ni	28	58.6934
Argon	Ar	18	39.948	Niobium	Nb	41	92.90638
Arsenic	As	33	74.92159	Nitrogen	N	7	14.00674
Astatine	At	85	209.9871*	Nobelium	No	102	259.1009*
Barium	Ba	56	137.327	Osmium	Os	76	190.23
Berkelium	Bk	97	247.0703*	Oxygen	O	8	15.9994
Beryllium	Be	4	9.012182	Palladium	Pd	46	106.42
Bismuth	Bi	83	208.98037	Phosphorus	P	15	30.973762
Boron	B	5	10.811	Platinum	Pt	78	195.08
Bromine	Br	35	79.904	Plutonium	Pu	94	244.0642*
Cadmium	Cd	48	112.411	Polonium	Po	84	208.9824*
Calcium	Ca	20	40.078	Potassium	K	19	39.0983
Californium	Cf	98	251.0796*	Praseodymium	Pr	59	140.90765
Carbon	C	6	12.011	Promethium	Pm	61	144.9127*
Cerium	Ce	58	140.115	Protactinium	Pa	91	231.0388*
Cesium	Cs	55	132.90543	Radium	Ra	88	226.0254*
Chlorine	Cl	17	35.4527	Radon	Rn	86	222.0176*
Chromium	Cr	24	51.9961	Rhenium	Re	75	186.207
Cobalt	Co	27	58.93320	Rhodium	Rh	45	102.90550
Copper	Cu	29	63.546	Rubidium	Rb	37	85.4678
Curium	Cm	96	247.0703*	Ruthenium	Ru	44	101.07
Dysprosium	Dy	66	162.50	Samarium	Sm	62	150.36
Einsteinium	Es	99	252.083*	Scandium	Sc	21	44.955910
Erbium	Er	68	167.26	Selenium	Se	34	78.96
Europium	Eu	63	151.965	Silicon	Si	14	28.0855
Fermium	Fm	100	257.0951*	Silver	Ag	47	107.8682
Fluorine	F	9	18.9984032	Sodium	Na	11	22.989768
Francium	Fr	87	223.0197*	Strontium	Sr	38	87.62
Gadolinium	Gd	64	157.25	Sulfur	S	16	32.066
Gallium	Ga	31	69.723	Tantalum	Ta	73	180.9479
Germanium	Ge	32	72.61	Technetium	Tc	43	97.9072*
Gold	Au	79	196.96654	Tellurium	Te	52	127.60
Hafnium	Hf	72	178.49	Terbium	Tb	65	158.92534
Helium	He	2	4.002602	Thallium	Tl	81	204.3833
Holmium	Ho	67	164.93032	Thorium	Th	90	232.0381
Hydrogen	H	1	1.00794	Thulium	Tm	69	168.93421
Indium	In	49	114.818	Tin	Sn	50	118.710
Iodine	I	53	126.90447	Titanium	Ti	22	47.867
Iridium	Ir	77	192.217	Tungsten	W	74	183.84
Iron	Fe	26	55.845	Unnilquadium	Unq	104	261.11*
Krypton	Kr	36	83.80	Unnilpentium	Unp	105	262.114*
Lanthanum	La	57	138.9055	Unnilhexium	Unh	106	263.118*
Lawrencium	Lr	103	262.11*	Unnilseptium	Uns	107	262.12*
Lead	Pb	82	207.2	Uranium	U	92	238.0289
Lithium	Li	3	6.941	Vanadium	V	23	50.9415
Lutetium	Lu	71	174.967	Xenon	Xe	54	131.29
Magnesium	Mg	12	24.3050	Ytterbium	Yb	70	173.04
Manganese	Mn	25	54.93805	Yttrium	Y	39	88.90585
Mendelevium	Md	101	258.10*	Zinc	Zn	30	65.39
Mercury	Hg	80	200.59	Zirconium	Zr	40	91.224
Molybdenum	Mo	42	95.94				

Based on 1993 IUPAC Table of Standard Atomic Weights of the Elements.
* Relative atomic mass of the isotope of that element with the longest known half-life.

TABLE OF ELEMENTS AND THEIR ATOMIC WEIGHTS

(Order of Atomic Number)

Atomic Number	Element	Symbol	Atomic Weight	Atomic Number	Element	Symbol	Atomic Weight
1	Hydrogen	H	1.00794	55	Cesium	Cs	132.90543
2	Helium	He	4.002602	56	Barium	Ba	137.327
3	Lithium	Li	6.941	57	Lanthanum	La	138.9055
4	Beryllium	Be	9.012182	58	Cerium	Ce	140.115
5	Boron	B	10.811	59	Praseodymium	Pr	140.90765
6	Carbon	C	12.011	60	Neodymium	Nd	144.24
7	Nitrogen	N	14.00674	61	Promethium	Pm	144.9127*
8	Oxygen	O	15.9994	62	Samarium	Sm	150.36
9	Fluorine	F	18.9984032	63	Europium	Eu	151.965
10	Neon	Ne	20.1797	64	Gadolinium	Gd	157.25
11	Sodium	Na	22.989768	65	Terbium	Tb	158.92534
12	Magnesium	Mg	24.3050	66	Dysprosium	Dy	162.50
13	Aluminum	Al	26.981539	67	Holmium	Ho	164.93032
14	Silicon	Si	28.0855	68	Erbium	Er	167.26
15	Phosphorus	P	30.973762	69	Thulium	Tm	168.93421
16	Sulfur	S	32.066	70	Ytterbium	Yb	173.04
17	Chlorine	Cl	35.4527	71	Lutetium	Lu	174.967
18	Argon	Ar	39.948	72	Hafnium	Hf	178.49
19	Potassium	K	39.0983	73	Tantalum	Ta	180.9479
20	Calcium	Ca	40.078	74	Tungsten	W	183.84
21	Scandium	Sc	44.955910	75	Rhenium	Re	186.207
22	Titanium	Ti	47.867	76	Osmium	Os	190.23
23	Vanadium	V	50.9415	77	Iridium	Ir	192.217
24	Chromium	Cr	51.9961	78	Platinum	Pt	195.08
25	Manganese	Mn	54.93805	79	Gold	Au	196.96654
26	Iron	Fe	55.845	80	Mercury	Hg	200.59
27	Cobalt	Co	58.93320	81	Thallium	Tl	204.3833
28	Nickel	Ni	58.6934	82	Lead	Pb	207.2
29	Copper	Cu	63.546	83	Bismuth	Bi	208.98037
30	Zinc	Zn	65.39	84	Polonium	Po	208.9824*
31	Gallium	Ga	69.723	85	Astatine	At	209.9871*
32	Germanium	Ge	72.61	86	Radon	Rn	222.0176*
33	Arsenic	As	74.92159	87	Francium	Fr	223.0197*
34	Selenium	Se	78.96	88	Radium	Ra	226.0254*
35	Bromine	Br	79.904	89	Actinium	Ac	227.0278*
36	Krypton	Kr	83.80	90	Thorium	Th	232.0381*
37	Rubidium	Rb	85.4678	91	Protactinium	Pa	231.0388*
38	Strontium	Sr	87.62	92	Uranium	U	238.0289
39	Yttrium	Y	88.90585	93	Neptunium	Np	237.0482*
40	Zirconium	Zr	91.224	94	Plutonium	Pu	244.0642*
41	Niobium	Nb	92.90638	95	Americium	Am	243.0614*
42	Molybdenum	Mo	95.94	96	Curium	Cm	247.0703*
43	Technetium	Te	97.9072*	97	Berkelium	Bk	247.0703*
44	Ruthenium	Ru	101.07	98	Californium	Cf	251.0796*
45	Rhodium	Rh	102.90550	99	Einsteinium	Es	252.083*
46	Palladium	Pd	106.42	100	Fermium	Fm	257.0951*
47	Silver	Ag	107.8682	101	Mendelevium	Md	258.10*
48	Cadmium	Cd	112.411	102	Nobelium	No	259.1009*
49	Indium	In	114.818	103	Lawrencium	Lr	262.11*
50	Tin	Sn	118.710	104	Unnilquadium	Unq	261.11*
51	Antimony	Sb	121.760	105	Unnilpentium	Unp	262.114*
52	Tellurium	Te	127.60	106	Unnilhexium	Unh	263.118*
53	Iodine	I	126.90447	107	Unnilseptium	Uns	262.12*
54	Xenon	Xe	131.29				

The Merck Index: An Encyclopedia of Chemicals, Drugs, and Biologicals, Twelfth Edition, Susan Budavari, Maryadele J. O'Neil, Ann Smith, Patricia E. Heckelman, Joanne F. Kinneary, Eds. (Merck & Co., Inc., Whitehouse Station, NJ, USA, 1996).

Appendices

COMPARATIVE TEMPERATURE SCALES

Celsius °C	Fahrenheit °F	Kelvin °K
100	220	
	210	370
90	200	
	190	360
80	180	
	170	350
70	160	
	150	340
60	140	
	130	330
50	120	
	110	320
40	100	310
30	90	
	80	300
20	70	
	60	290
10	50	
	40	280
0	30	
	20	270
−10	10	260
	0	
−20	−10	250

To convert Celsius or Fahrenheit to Kelvin:

C to K: add 273.16
10°C to K: 10 + 273.16 = 283.16 K

F to K: convert to C, add 273.16
63°F = 17.2°C + 273.16 = 290.36 K

To convert Fahrenheit to Celsius, Celsius to Fahrenheit:

Above 0°C or 32°F

F to C: subtract 32, multiply by 5, divide by 9
63°F to C: 63 − 32 = 31 × 5 = 155 ÷ 9 = 17.2°C

C to F: multiply by 9, divide by 5, add 32
37°C to F: 37 × 9 = 333 ÷ 5 = 66.6 + 32 = 98.6°F

TEMPERATURE EQUIVALENTS

Celsius to Fahrenheit					Fahrenheit to Celsius					
°C	°F	°C	°F		°F	°C	°F	°C	°F	°C
−50	−58.0	49	120.0		−50	−46.7	99	37.2	157	69.4
−40	−40.0	50	122.0		−40	−40.0	100	37.7	158	70.0
−35	−31.0	51	123.8		−35	−37.2	101	38.3	159	70.5
−30	−22.0	52	125.6		−30	−34.4	102	38.8	160	71.1
−25	−13.0	53	127.4		−25	−31.7	103	39.4	161	71.6
−20	−4.0	54	129.2		−20	−28.9	104	40.0	162	72.2
−15	5.0	55	131.0		−15	−26.6	105	40.5	163	72.7
−10	14.0	56	132.8		−10	−23.3	106	41.1	164	73.3
−5	23.0	57	134.6		−5	−20.6	107	41.6	165	73.8
0	**32.0**	58	136.4		0	−17.7	108	42.2	166	74.4
1	33.8	59	138.2		1	−17.2	109	42.7	167	75.0
2	35.6	60	140.0		5	−15.0	110	43.3	168	75.5
3	37.4	61	141.8		10	−12.2	111	43.8	169	76.1
4	39.2	62	143.6		15	−9.4	112	44.4	170	76.6
5	41.0	63	145.4		20	−6.6	113	45.0	171	77.2
6	42.8	64	147.2		25	−3.8	114	45.5	172	77.7
7	44.6	65	149.0		30	−1.1	115	46.1	173	78.3
8	46.4	66	150.8		31	−0.5	116	46.6	174	78.8
9	48.2	67	152.6		**32**	**0**	117	47.2	175	79.4
10	50.0	68	154.4		33	0.5	118	47.7	176	80.0
11	51.8	69	156.2		34	1.1	119	48.3	177	80.5
12	53.6	70	158.0		35	1.6	120	48.8	178	81.1
13	55.4	71	159.8		36	2.2	121	49.4	179	81.6
14	57.2	72	161.6		37	2.7	122	50.0	180	82.2
15	59.0	73	163.4		38	3.3	123	50.5	181	82.7
16	60.8	74	165.2		39	3.8	124	51.1	182	83.3
17	62.6	75	167.0		40	4.4	125	51.6	183	83.8
18	64.4	76	168.8		41	5.0	126	52.2	184	84.4
19	66.2	77	170.6		42	5.5	127	52.7	185	85.0
20	68.0	78	172.4		43	6.1	128	53.3	186	85.5
21	69.8	79	174.2		44	6.6	129	53.8	187	86.1
22	71.6	80	176.0		45	7.2	130	54.4	188	86.6
23	73.4	81	177.8		46	7.7	131	55.0	189	87.2
24	75.2	82	179.6		47	8.3	132	55.5	190	87.7
25	77.0	83	181.4		48	8.8	133	56.1	191	88.3
26	78.8	84	183.2		49	9.4	134	56.6	192	88.8
27	80.6	85	185.0		50	10.0	135	57.2	193	89.4
28	82.4	86	186.8		55	12.7	136	57.7	194	90.0
29	84.2	87	188.6		60	15.5	137	58.3	195	90.5
30	86.0	88	190.4		65	18.3	138	58.8	196	91.1
31	87.8	89	192.2		70	21.1	139	59.4	197	91.6
32	89.6	90	194.0		75	23.8	140	60.0	198	92.2
33	91.4	91	195.8		80	26.6	141	60.5	199	92.7
34	93.2	92	197.6		85	29.4	142	61.1	200	93.3
35	95.0	93	199.4		86	30.0	143	61.6	201	93.8
36	96.8	94	201.2		87	30.5	144	62.2	202	94.4
37	**98.6**	95	203.0		88	31.0	145	62.7	203	95.0
38	100.4	96	204.8		89	31.6	146	63.3	204	95.5
39	102.2	97	206.6		90	32.2	147	63.8	205	96.1
40	104.0	98	208.4		91	32.7	148	64.4	206	96.6
41	105.8	99	210.2		92	33.3	149	65.0	207	97.2
42	107.6	**100**	**212.0**		93	33.8	150	65.5	208	97.7
43	109.4	101	213.8		94	34.4	151	66.1	209	98.3
44	111.2	102	215.6		95	35.0	152	66.6	210	98.8
45	113.0	103	217.4		96	35.5	153	67.2	211	99.4
46	114.8	104	219.2		97	36.1	154	67.7	**212**	**100.0**
47	116.6	105	221.0		98	36.6	155	68.3	213	100.5
48	118.4	106	222.8		**98.6**	**37.0**	156	68.8	214	101.1

Scale of the Metric System and SI

Prefix	Symbol	Power
yotta-	Y	10^{24}
zetta-	Z	10^{21}
exa-	E	10^{18}
peta-	P	10^{15}
tera-	T	10^{12}
giga-	G	10^{9}
mega-	M	10^{6}
kilo-	k	10^{3}
hecto-	h	10^{2}
deca-	da	10^{1}
UNIT		
deci-	d	10^{-1}
centi-	c	10^{-2}
milli-	m	10^{-3}
micro-	μ	10^{-6}
nano-	n	10^{-9}
pico-	p	10^{-12}
femro-	f	10^{-15}
atto-	a	10^{-18}
zepto-	z	10^{-21}
yocto-	y	10^{-24}

SI Base Units

Quantity	Name	Symbol
length	meter	m
mass*	kilogram†	kg
time	second	s
electric current	ampere	A
thermodynamic temperature	kelvin‡	K
luminous intensity	candela	cd
amount of substance	mole	mol

* In commercial and everyday use, "weight" usually means mass; *e.g.,* when speaking of a person's weight, the quantity referred to is mass.

† For historic reasons, kilogram is the only base unit with a prefix. Multiples and submultiples of the kilogram are formed by attaching the appropriate prefix to the stem word "gram" (*e.g.,* milligram) and the appropriate prefix symbol to the symbol "g" (*e.g.,* mg.).

‡ The degree Celsius (°C) is still widely accepted usage for expressing temperature and temperature intervals. Celsius (formerly centigrade) *temperature* is converted to kelvin (K) thermodynamic temperature by adding 273.16 to the Celsius scale. For *temperature interval,* 1°C equals K.

Some SI Derived Units
Expressed in Terms of Base Units

Quantity	Name	Symbol
area	square meter	m^2
volume*	cubic meter	m^3
specific volume	cubic meter per kilogram	m^3/kg
speed, velocity	meter per second	m/s
acceleration	meter per second squared	m/s^2
mass density	kilogram per cubic meter	kg/m^3
concentration	mole per cubic meter	mol/m^3
luminance	candela per square meter	cd/m^2

* Liter (L, l). 10^{-3} m^3, is regarded as a special name for the cubic decimeter.

Some SI Derived Units with Special Names

Quantity	Name	Symbol	Expression
Frequency	hertz	Hz	s^{-1}
force	newton	N	$m\ kg\ s^{-2}$
pressure, stress	pascal	Pa	$m^{-1}\ kg\ s^{-2}$
energy	joule	J	$m^2\ kg\ s^{-2}$
power	watt	W	$m^2\ kg\ s^{-3}$
quantity of electricity, electric charge	coulomb	C	$s\ A$
electric potential, electromotive force	volt	V	$m^2\ kg\ s^{-3}\ A^{-1}$
capacitance	farad	F	$m^{-2}\ kg^{-1}s^4\ A^2$
electrical resistance	ohm	Ω	$m^2\ kg^{-2}\ A^{-2}$
electrical conductance	siemens	S	$m^{-2}\ kg\ s^{-2}\ A^{-1}$
magnetic flux	weber	Wb	$m^2\ kg\ s^{-2}\ A^{-1}$
magnetic flux density	tesla	T	$kg\ s^{-2}\ A^{-1}$
activity of radionuclide	becquerel*	Bq	s^{-1}
absorbed dose of radiation	gray†	Gy	$m^2\ s^{-2}$
exposure (x and γ radiation)	coulomb per kilogram‡	C kg	$kg^{-1}\ s\ A$

* Replacing the curie (Ci), 3.7×10^{10} s^{-1}.

† Replacing the rad (rad), 10^{-2} J kg^{-1}.

‡ Replacing the roentgen (R), 2.58×10^{-4} C kg^{-1}.

Measures of Length

Micrometers	Millimeters	Centimeters	Meters	Kilometers	Miles	Yards	Feet	Inches
1	0.001	10^{-4}						0.000039
10^3	1	10^{-1}					0.00328	0.03937
10^4	10	1	0.01			0.0109	0.03281	0.3937
254,000	25.4	2.54	0.0254			0.0278	0.0833	1
	304.8	30.48	0.3048			0.333	1	12
10^6	10^3	10^2	1	0.001	0.0006213	1.0936	3.2808	39.37
914,400	914.40	91.44	0.9144	0.009	0.0005681	1	3	36
10^9	10^6	10^5	10^3	1	0.6215	1093.6121	3280.8	
			1609.0	1.609	1	1760.0	5280.0	

To convert:

Millimeters to inches: divide by 25.4
Inches to millimeters: multiply by 25.4

Centimeters to feet: divide by 30.7
Feet to centimeters: multiply by 30.7

Meters to yards: multiply by 1.09375
Yards to meters: multiply by 0.9143

Kilometers to miles: multiply by 0.625
Miles to kilometers: multiply by 1.6

Measures of Mass (Weight)

Avoirdupois Weights

				Metric Equivalents		
Grains	Drams	Ounces	Pounds	Milligrams	Grams	Kilograms
1	0.0366	0.0023	0.00014	64.8	0.0648	0.000065
27.34	1	0.0625	0.0039		1.772	0.001772
437.5	16	1	0.0625		28.350	0.028350
7,000	256	16	1		453.5924	0.453592
0.0154				1	0.001	
15.4324	0.5648	0.0353	0.002205	1000	1	0.001
15,432.358	564.32	35.27	2.2046		1000	1

To convert (approximately):

Kilograms to pounds: multiply by 2.2
Pounds to kilograms: multiply by 0.454

Grams to ounces: multiply by 0.03527
Ounces to grams: multiply by 28.35

Apothecaries' Weights

Grains	Scruples	Drams	Ounces	Pounds	Metric Equivalents		
					Milligrams	Grams	Kilograms
1	0.05	0.0167	0.0021	0.00017	64.8	0.0648	0.000065
20	1	0.333	0.042	0.0035		1.296	0.001296
60	3	1	0.125	0.0104		3.888	0.000389
480	24	8	1	0.0833		31.103	0.031103
5,760	288	96	12	1		373.2418	0.373242
0.0154					1	0.001	
15.4324		0.2572	0.0322	0.0027	1000	1	0.001
15,432.358		257.2	32.15	2.6792		1000	1

Measures of Capacity

Apothecaries' Measures

Minims	Fluid Drams	Fluid Ounces	Pints	Quarts	Gallons	Metric Equivalents	
						Liters	Milliliters
1	0.0166	0.002	0.00013			0.0006	0.06161
60	1	0.125	0.0078	0.0039		0.0037	3.6967
480	8	1	0.0625	0.0312	0.0078	0.0296	29.5737
7,680	128	16	1	0.5	0.125	0.4732	473.166
15,360	256	32	2	1	0.25	0.9464	946.358
61,440	1024	128	8	4	1	3.7854	3785.434
16,230	270.52	33.8418	2.1134	1.0567	0.2642	1	1000
16.23	0.2705	0.0338	0.00212	0.00106	0.000265	0.001	1

To convert (approximately):

1 British imperial gallon = 1.201 U.S. gallon
1 U.S. gallon = 0.8327 British imperial gallon

Liters to gallons: multiply by 0.264
Gallons to liters: multiply by 3.788

Liters to pints: multiply by 2.1
Pints to liters: multiply by 0.4762

Approximate Household Measures and Weights*

Teaspoons	Tablespoons	Cups or Glasses	Drams	Fluid Ounces	Milliliters	Grams
1			1	0.125	5	5
3	1		4	0.50	15	15
48	16***	1	64	8	237	240

* A drop is a measure of uncertain quantity, depending on the nature of the liquid as well as the shape of the container and of the opening from which the liquid falls. One drop of water is roughly equivalent to 1 minim.

** Tumbler or glass is generally intended to mean 8 fl. oz.

*** For dry measure, 12 tablespoons equals 1 cup.

Show-Hong Duh, PhD, DABCC, Department of Pathology,
University of Maryland School of Medicine
Janine Denis Cook, PhD, Department of Medical and Research Technology,
University of Maryland School of Medicine

Reference range values are for apparently healthy individuals and often overlap significantly with values for persons who are sick. Actual values may vary significantly due to differences in assay methodologies and standardization. Institutions may also set up their own reference ranges based on the particular populations that they serve, thus there can be regional differences. Consequently, values reported by individual laboratories may differ from those listed in this appendix.

All values are given in conventional and SI units. However, where the SI units have not been widely accepted, conventional units are used. In case of the heterogenous nature of the materials measured or uncertainty of the exact molecular weight of the compounds, the SI system cannot be followed, and mass per volume is used as the unit of concentration.

Abbreviations:

ACD, acid-citrate-dextrose; **CHF,** congestive heart failure; **Cit,** citrate; **CNS,** central nervous system; **CSF,** cerebrospinal fluid; **cyclic AMP,** adenosine 3′,5′-cyclic phosphate; **EDTA,** ethylenediaminetetraacetic acid; **HDL,** high-density lipoprotein; **Hep,** heparin; **LDL-C,** low-density lipoprotein-cholesterol; **Ox,** oxalate; **RBC,** red blood cell(s); **RIA,** radioimmunoassay; **SD,** standard deviation

References:

Reference Intervals. In Tietz Textbook of Clinical Chemistry. 3rd ed., C.A. Burtis and E.R. Ashwood, Ed. Philadelphia, W.B. Saunders Co., 1998.

Hematologic Values. In Clinical Hematology and Fundamentals of Hemostasis. 2nd ed., D.M. Harmening, Ed. Philadelphia, F.A. Davis Co., 1992.

National Cholesterol Education Program: Report of the expert panel on detection, evaluation, and treatment of high blood cholesterol in adults. Arch. Intern. Med. 1988; 148:36-69.

Clinical Chemistry Laboratory: Reference Range Values in Clinical Chemistry. Professional services manual. Baltimore, Department of Pathology, University of Maryland Medical System, 1999.

Triglyceride, High Density Lipoprotein, and Coronary Heart Disease. National Institute of Health Consensus Statement, NIH Consensus Development Conference, 1992, Volume 10, Number 2.

Tests	Conventional Units	SI Units
Acetaminophen, serum or plasma (Hep or EDTA)		
Therapeutic	10–30 µg/mL	66–199 µmol/L
Toxic	>200 µg/mL	>1324 µmol/L
Acetone		
Serum		
Qualitative	Negative	Negative
Quantitative	0.3–2.0 mg/dL	0.05–0.34 mmol/L
Urine		
Qualitative	Negative	Negative
Acid hemolysis test (Ham)	<5% lysis	<0.05 lysed fraction
Adrenocorticotropin (ACTH), plasma		
8 AM	<120 pg/mL	<26 pmol/L
Midnight (supine)	<10 pg/mL	<2.2 pmol/L
*Alanine Aminotransferase (ALT, SGPT), serum		
Male	13–40 U/L (37°C)	0.22–0.68 µkat/L (37°C)
Female	10–28 U/L (37°C)	0.17–0.48 µkat/L (37°C)
Albumin		
Serum		
Adult	3.5–5.2 g/dL	35–52 g/L
>60 y	3.2–4.6 g/dL	32–46 g/L
	Avg. of 0.3 g/dL higher in upright individuals	Avg. of 3 g/L higher in upright individuals
Urine		
Qualitative	Negative	Negative
Quantitative	50–80 mg/24 h	50–80 mg/24 h
CSF	10–30 mg/dL	100–300 mg/L
*Aldolase, serum	1.0–7.5 U/L (30°C)	0.02–0.13 µkat/L (30°C)
Aldosterone		
Serum		
Supine	3–16 ng/dL	0.08–0.44 nmol/L
Standing	7–30 ng/dL	0.19–0.83 nmol/L
Urine	3–19 µg/24 h	8–51 nmol/24 h
Amikacin, serum or plasma (EDTA)		
Therapeutic		
Peak	25–35 µg/mL	43–60 µmol/L
Trough		
Less severe infection	1–4 µg/mL	1.7–6.8 µmol/L
Life-threatening infection	4–8 µg/mL	6.8–13.7 µmol/L
Toxic		
Peak	>35–40 µg/mL	>60–68 µmol/L
Trough	>10–15 µg/mL	>17–26 µmol/L
∂-Aminolevulinic acid, urine	1.3–7.0 mg/24 h	10–53 µmol/24 h
Amitriptyline, serum or plasma (Hep or EDTA); trough (≥12 h after dose)		
Therapeutic	80–250 ng/mL	289–903 nmol/L
Toxic	>500 ng/mL	>1805 nmol/L
Ammonia		
Plasma (Hep)	9–33 µmol/L	9–33 µmol/L
*Amylase		
Serum	27–131 U/L	0.46–2.23 µkat/L
Urine	1–17 U/h	0.017–0.29 µkat/h
Amylase/creatinine clearance ratio	1–4%	0.01–0.04

*Test values are method dependent.

Tests	Conventional Units	SI Units
Androstenedione, serum		
Male	75–205 ng/dL	2.6–7.2 nmol/L
Female	85–275 ng/dL	3.0–9.6 nmol/L
Anion gap		
(Na – (Cl + HCO$_3$))	7–16 mEq/L	7–16 mmol/L
((Na + K) – (Cl + HCO$_3$))	10–20 mEq/L	10–20 mmol/L
α_1-Antitrypsin, serum	78–200 mg/dL	0.78–2.00 g/L
Apolipoprotein A-I		
Male	94–178 mg/dL	0.94–1.78 g/L
Female	101–199 mg/dL	1.01–1.99 g/L
Apolipoprotein B		
Male	63–133 mg/dL	0.63–1.33 g/L
Female	60–126 mg/dL	0.60–1.26 g/L
Arsenic		
Whole blood (Hep)	0.2–2.3 µg/dL	0.03–0.31 µmol/L
Chronic poisoning	10–50 µg/dL	1.33–6.65 µmol/L
Acute poisoning	60–930 µg/dL	7.98–124 µmol/L
Urine, 24 h	5–50 µg/d	0.07–0.67 µmol/d
Ascorbic acid, plasma (Ox, Hep, EDTA)	0.4–1.5 mg/dL	23–85 µmol/L
*Aspartate aminotransferase (AST, SGOT), serum	10–59 U/L (37°C)	0.17–1.00 -2 to +3 kat/L (37°C)
Base excess, blood (Hep)	−2 to +3 mEq/L	−2 to +3 mmol/L
Bicarbonate, serum (venous)	22–29 mEq/L	22–29 mmol/L
*Bilirubin		
Serum		
Adult		
Conjugated	0.0–0.3 mg/dL	0–5 µmol/L
Unconjugated	0.1–1.1 mg/dL	1.7–19 µmol/L
Delta	0–0.2 mg/dL	0–3 µmol/L
Total	0.2–1.3 mg/L	3–22 µmol/L
Neonates		
Conjugated	0–0.6 mg/dL	0–10 µmol/L
Unconjugated	0.6–10.5 mg/dL	10–180 µmol/L
Total	1.5–12 mg/dL	1.7–180 µmol/L
Urine, qualitative	Negative	Negative
Bone marrow, differential cell count		
Adult		
Undifferentiated cells	0–1%	0–0.01
Myeloblast	0–2%	0–0.02
Promyelocyte	0–4%	0–0.04
Myelocytes		
Neutrophilic	5–20%	0.05–0.20
Eosinophilic	0–3%	0–0.03
Basophilic	0–1%	0–0.01
Metamyeolocytes and bands		
Neutrophilic	5–35%	0.05–0.35
Eosinophilic	0–5%	0–0.05
Basophilic	0–1%	0–0.01
Segmented neutrophils	5–15%	0.05–0.15
Pronormoblast	0–1.5%	0–0.015
Basophilic normoblast	0–5%	0–0.05
Polychromatophilic normoblast	5–30%	0.05–0.30
Orthochromatic normoblast	5–10%	0.05–0.10
Lymphocytes	10–20%	0.10–0.20
Plasma cells	0–2%	0–0.02
Monocytes	0–5%	0–0.05

*Test values are method dependent.

Tests	Conventional Units	SI Units
CA 125, serum	<35 U/mL	<35 kU/L
CA 15-3, serum	<30 U/mL	<30 kU/L
CA 19-9, serum	<37 U/mL	<37 kU/L
Cadmium, whole blood (Hep)	0.1–0.5 µg/dL	8.9–44.5 nmol/L
Toxic	10–300 µg/dL	0.89–26.70 µmol/L
Cadmium, urine, 24 h	<15 µg/d	<0.13 µmol/d
Calcitonin, serum or plasma (Hep, EDTA)		
Male	≤100 pg/mL	≤100 ng/L
Female	≤30 pg/mL	≤30 ng/L
Calcium, serum	8.6–10.0 mg/dL (Slightly higher in children)	2.15–2.50 mmol/L (Slightly higher in children)
Calcium, ionized, serum	4.64–5.28 mg/dL	1.16–1.32 mmol/L
Calcium, urine		
Low calcium diet	50–150 mg/24 h	1.25–3.75 mmol/24 h
Usual diet; trough	100–300 mg/24 h	2.50–7.50 mmol/24 h
Carbamazepine, serum or plasma (Hep or EDTA), trough		
Therapeutic	4–12 µg/mL	17–51 µmol/L
Toxic	>15 µg/mL	>63 µmol/L
Carbon dioxide, total, serum/ plasma (Hep)	22–28 mmol/L	Same
Carbon dioxide (PCO_2), blood, arterial	Male 35–48 mm Hg Female 32–45 mm Hg	4.66–6.38 kPa 4.26–5.99 kPa
Carbon monoxide as carboxyhemoglobin (HbCO), whole blood (EDTA)		
Nonsmokers	0.5–1.5% total Hb	0.005–0.015 HbCO fraction
Smokers		
1–2 packs/d	4–5% total Hb	0.04–0.05 HbCO fraction
>2 packs/d	8–9% total Hb	0.08–0.09 HbCO fraction
Toxic	>20% total Hb	>0.20 HbCO fraction
Lethal	>50% total Hb	>0.5 HbCO fraction
Carotene, serum	10–85 µg/dL	0.19–1.58 µmol/L
Catecholamines, plasma (EDTA)		
Dopamine	< 30 pg/mL	<196 pmol/L
Epinephrine	<140 pg/mL	<764 pmol/L
Norepinephrine	<1700 pg/mL	<10,047 pmol/L
Catecholamines, urine		
Dopamine	65–400 µg/24 h	425–2610 nmol/24 h
Epinephrine	0–20 µg/24 h	0–109 nmol/24 h
Norepinephrine	15–80 µg/24 h	89–473 nmol/24 h
CEA, serum		
Nonsmokers	<5.0 ng/mL	<5.0 µg/L
*Cell counts, adult		
RBC Male	4.7–6.1 × 10⁶/µL	4.7–6.1 × 10¹²/L
Female	4.2–5.4 × 10⁶/µL	4.2–5.4 × 10¹²/L
Leukocytes		
Total	4.8–10.8 × 10³/µL	4.8–10.8 × 10⁶/L
Differential	Percentage Absolute	Absolute (SI)
Myelocytes	0 0/µL	0/L
Neutrophils		
Band	3–5 150–400/µL	150–400 × 10⁶/L
Segmented	54–62 3000–5800/µL	3000–5800 × 10⁶/L
Lymphocytes	20.5–51.1 1.2–3.4 × 10³/µL	1.2–3.4 × 10⁹/L
Monocytes	1.7–9.3 0.11–0.59 × 10³/µL	0.11–0.59 × 10⁹/L
Granulocytes	42.2–75.2 1.4–6.5 × 10³/µL	1.4–6.5 × 10⁹/L
Eosinophils	0–0.7 × 10³/µL	0–0.7 × 10⁹/L
Basophils	0–0.2 × 10³/µL	0–0.2 × 10⁹/L

*Test values are method dependent.

Appendices

Tests	Conventional Units	SI Units
Platelets	130–400 × 10³/μL	130–400 × 10⁹/L
Reticulocytes	0.5–1.5% red cells	0.005–0.015 of RBC
	24,000–84,000/μL	24–84 × 10⁹/L
Cells, CSF	0–10 lymphocytes/mm³	Same
	0 RBC/mm³	Same
Ceruloplasmin, serum	20–60 mg/dL	0.2–0.6 g/L
Chloramphenicol, serum or plasma (Hep or EDTA); trough		
Therapeutic	10–25 μg/mL	31–77 μmol/L
Toxic	>25 μg/mL	>77 μmol/L
Chloride		
Serum or plasma (Hep)	98–107 mmol/L	98–107 mmol/L
Sweat		
Normal	5–35 mmol/L	Same
Cystic fibrosis	60–200 mmol/L	Same
Urine, 24 h (vary greatly with Cl intake)		
Infant	2–10 mmol/24 h	Same
Child	15–40 mmol/24 h	Same
Adult	110–250 mmol/24 h	Same
CSF	118–132 mmol/L (20 mmol/L higher than serum)	Same
Cholesterol, serum		
Adult desirable	<200 mg/dL	<5.2 mmol/L
borderline	200–239 mg/dL	5.2–6.2 mmol/L
High risk	≥240 mg/dL	≥6.2 mmol/L
*Cholinesterase, serum	4.9–11.9 U/mL	4.9–11.9 kU/L
Dibucaine inhibition	79–84%	0.79–0.84
Fluoride inhibition	58–64%	0.58–0.64
*Chorionic gonadotropin, intact		
Serum or plasma (EDTA)		
Male and nonpregnant female	<5.0 mIU/mL	<5.0 IU/L
Pregnant female	Varies with gestational age	
Urine, qualitative		
Male and nonpregnant female	Negative	Negative
Pregnant female	Positive	Positive
Clonazepam, serum or plasma (Hep or EDTA); trough		
Therapeutic	15–60 ng/mL	48–190 nmol/L
Toxic	>80 ng/mL	>254 nmol/L
Coagulation tests		
Antithrombin III (synthetic substrate)	80–120% of normal	0.8–1.2 of normal
Bleeding time (Duke)	0–6 min	0–6 min
Bleeding time (Ivy)	1–6 min	1–6 min
Bleeding time (template)	2.3–9.5 min	2.3–9.5 min
Clot retraction, qualitative	50–100% in 2 h	0.5–1.0/2 h
Coagulation time (Lee-White)	5–15 min (glass tubes)	5–15 min (glass tubes)
	19–60 min (siliconized tubes)	19–60 min (siliconized tubes)
Cold hemolysin test (Donath-Landsteiner)	No hemolysis	No hemolysis

*Test values are method dependent.

Tests	Conventional Units	SI Units
Complement components		
Total hemolytic complement activity, plasma (EDTA)	75–160 U/mL	75–160 kU/L
Total complement decay rate (functional), plasma (EDTA)	10–20% Deficiency: >50%	Fraction decay rate: 0.10–0.20 >0.50
C1q, serum	14.9–22.1 mg/dL	149–221 mg/L
C1r, serum	2.5–10.0 mg/dL	25–100 mg/L
C1s(C1 esterase), serum	5.0–10.0 mg/dL	50–100 mg/L
C2, serum	1.6–3.6 mg/dL	16–36 mg/L
C3, serum	90–180 mg/dL	0.9–1.8 g/L
C4, serum	10–40 mg/dL	0.1–0.4 g/L
C5, serum	5.5–11.3 mg/dL	55–113 mg/L
C6, serum	17.9–23.9 mg/dL	179–239 mg/L
C7, serum	2.7–7.4 mg/dL	27–74 mg/L
C8, serum	4.9–10.6 mg/dL	49–106 mg/L
C9, serum	3.3–9.5 mg/dL	33–95 mg/L
Coombs' test		
Direct	Negative	Negative
Indirect	Negative	Negative
Copper		
Serum		
Male	70–140 μg/dL	11–22 μmol/L
Female	80–155 μg/dL	13–24 μmol/L
Urine	3–35 μg/24 h	0.05–0.55 μmol/24 h
Corpuscular values of erythrocytes (values are for adults; in children, values vary with age)		
Mean corpuscular hemoglobin (MCH)	27–31 pg	0.42–0.48 fmol
Mean corpuscular hemoglobin concentration (MCHC)	33–37 g/dL	330–370 g/L
Mean corpuscular volume (MCV)	Male 80–94 μ³ Female 81–99 μ³	80–94 fL 81–99 fL
Cortisol, serum		
Plasma (Hep, EDTA, Ox)		
8 AM	5–23 μg/dL	138–635 nmol/L
4 PM	3–16 μg/dL	83–441 nmol/L
10 PM	<50% of 8 AM value	<0.5 of 8 AM value
Free, urine	<50 μg/24 h	<138 mmol/24 h
*†**Creatine kinase (CK), serum**		
Male	15–105 U/L (30°C)	0.26–1.79 μkat/L (30°C)
Female	10–80 U/L (30°C)	0.17–1.36 μkat/L (30°C)
Note: Strenuous exercise or intramuscular injections may cause transient elevation of CK.		
*__Creatine kinase MB isoenzyme, serum__	0–7 ng/mL	0–7 μg/L
*__Creatinine__		
Serum or plasma, adult		
Male	0.7–1.3 mg/dL	62–115 μmol/L
Female	0.6–1.1 mg/dL	53–97 μmol/L
Urine		
Male	14–26 mg/kg body weight/24 h	124–230 μmol/kg body weight/24 h
Female	11–20 mg/kg body weight/24 h	97–177 μmol/kg body weight/24 h

*Test values are method dependent.
†Test values are race dependent.

Appendices

Tests	Conventional Units	SI Units
*Creatinine clearance, serum or plasma and urine		
Male	94–140 mL/min/1.73 m²	0.91–1.35 mL/s/m²
Female	72–110 mL/min/1.73 m²	0.69–1.06 mL/s/m²
Cryoglobulins, serum	0	0
Cyanide		
Serum		
Nonsmokers	0.004 mg/L	0.15 µmol/L
Smokers	0.006 mg/L	0.23 µmol/L
Nitroprusside therapy	0.01–0.06 mg/L	0.38–2.30 µmol/L
Toxic	>0.1 mg/L	>3.84 µmol/L
Whole blood (Ox)		
Nonsmokers	0.016 mg/L	0.61 µmol/L
Smokers	0.041 mg/L	1.57 µmol/L
Nitroprusside therapy	0.05–0.5 mg/L	1.92–19.20 µmol/L
Toxic	>1 mg/L	>38.40 µmol/L
Cyclic AMP		
Plasma (EDTA)		
Male	4.6–8.6 ng/mL	14–26 nmol/L
Female	4.3–7.6 ng/mL	13–23 nmol/L
Urine, 24 h	0.3–3.6 mg/d or 0.29–2.1 mg/g creatinine	1.0–10.9 µmol/d or 100–723 µmol/mol creatinine
Cystine or cysteine, urine, qualitative	Negative	Negative
*C-Peptide, serum	0.78–1.89 ng/mL	0.26–0.62 nmol/L
C-Reactive protein, serum	<0.5 mg/dL	<5 mg/L
*≠Cyclosporine, whole blood		
Therapeutic, trough	100–200 ng/mL	83–166 nmol/L
Dehydroepiandrostereone (DHEA), serum		
Male	180–1250 ng/dL	6.2–43.3 nmol/L
Female	130–980 ng/dL	4.5–34.0 nmol/L
Dehydroepiandrosterone sulfate (DHEAS), serum or plasma (Hep, EDTA)		
Male	59–452 µg/mL	1.6–12.2 µmol/L
Female		
Premenopausal	12–379 µg/mL	0.8–10.2 µmol/L
Postmenopausal	30–260 µg/mL	0.8–7.1 µmol/L
Desipramine, serum or plasma (Hep or EDTA); trough (12 h after dose)		
Therapeutic	75–300 ng/mL	281–1125 nmol/L
Toxic	>400 ng/mL	>1500 nmol/L
Diazepam, serum or plasma (Hep or EDTA); trough		
Therapeutic	100–1000 ng/mL	0.35–3.51 µmol/L
Toxic	>5000 ng/mL	>17.55 µmol/L
Digitoxin, serum or plasma (Hep or EDTA); 7.8 h after dose		
Therapeutic	20–35 ng/mL	26–46 nmol/L
Toxic	>45 ng/mL	>59 nmol/L
Digoxin, serum or plasma (Hep or EDTA); ≥12 h after dose		

*Test values are method dependent.
≠Actual therapeutic range should be adjusted for individual patient.

Tests	Conventional Units	SI Units
Therapeutic		
CHF	0.8–1.5 ng/mL	1.0–1.9 nmol/L
Arrhythmias	1.5–2.0 ng/mL	1.9–2.6 nmol/L
Toxic		
Adult	>2.5 ng/mL	>3.2 nmol/L
Child	>3.0 ng/mL	>3.8 nmol/L
Disopyramide, serum or plasma (Hep or EDTA); trough		
Therapeutic arrhythmias		
Atrial	2.8–3.2 μg/mL	8.3–9.4 μmol/L
Ventricular	3.3–7.5 μg/mL	9.7–22 μmol/L
Toxic	>7 μg/mL	>20.7 μmol/L
Doxepin, serum or plasma (Hep or EDTA); trough (≥12 h after dose)		
Therapeutic	150–250 ng/mL	537–895 nmol/L
Toxic	>500 ng/mL	>1790 nmol/L
*Estradiol, serum		
Adult		
Male	10–50 pg/mL	37-184 pmol/L
Female	Varies with menstrual cycle	
Ethanol, whole blood (Ox) or serum		
Depression of CNS	>100 mg/dL	>21.7 mmol/L
Fatalities reported	>400 mg/dL	>86.8 mmol/L
Ethosuximide, serum or plasma (Hep or EDTA); trough		
Therapeutic	40–100 μg/mL	283–708 μmol/L
Toxic	>150 μg/mL	>1062 μmol/L
Euglobin lysis	No lysis in 2 h	No lysis in 2 h
α-Fetoprotein (AFP), serum	<15 ng/mL	<15 μg/L
Fat, fecal, F, 72 h		
Infant, breast-fed	<1 g/d	Same
0–6 y	<2 g/d	Same
Adult	<7 g/d	Same
Adult (fat-free diet)	<4 g/d	Same
§Fatty acids, total, serum	190–420 mg/dL	7–15 mmol/L
Nonesterified, serum	8–25 mg/dL	0.28–0.89 mmol/L
Ferritin, serum		
Male	20–250 ng/mL	20–250 μg/L
Female	10–120 ng/mL	10–120 μg/L
Ferritin values of <20 ng/mL (20 μg/L) have been reported to be generally associated with depleted iron stores		
Fibrin degradation products	<10 μg/mL	<10 mg/L
*Fibrinogen, plasma (NaCit)	200–400 mg/dL	2–4 g/L
Fluoride		
Plasma (Hep)	0.01–0.2 μg/mL	0.5–10.5 μmol/L
Urine	0.2–3.2 μg/mL	10.5–168 μmol/L
Urine, occupational exposure	<8 μg/mL	<421 μmol/L
*Folate, Serum	3–20 ng/mL	7–45 nmol/L
Erythrocytes	140–628 ng/mL RBC	317–1422 nmol/L RBC

*Test values are method dependent.
§"Fatty acids" include a mixture of different aliphatic acids of varying molecular weight; a mean molecular weight of 284 daltons has been assumed.

Appendices

Tests	Conventional Units	SI Units
*Follicle-stimulating hormone (FSH), serum and plasma (Hep)		
Male	1.4–15.4 mIU/mL	1.4–15.4 IU/L
Female		
Follicular phase	1–10 mIU/mL	1–10 IU/L
Mid-cycle	6–17 mIU/mL	6–17 IU/L
Luteal phase	1–9 mIU/mL	1–9 IU/L
Postmenopausal	19–100 mIU/mL	19–100 IU/L
*Free Thyroxine Index (FTI), serum	4.2–13	same
Gastrin, serum	<100 pg/mL	<100 ng/L
Gentamicin, serum or plasma (EDTA)		
Therapeutic		
Peak		
Less severe infection	5–8 µg/mL	10.4–16.7 µmol
Severe infection	8–10 µg/mL	16.7–20.9 µmol/L
Trough		
Less severe infection	<1 µg/mL	<2.1 µmol/L
Moderate infection	<2 µg/mL	<4.2 µmol/L
Severe infection	<2–4 µg/mL	<4.2–8.4 µmol/L
Toxic		
Peak	>10–12 µg/mL	>21–25 µmol/L
Trough	>2–4 µg/mL	>4.2–8.4 µmol/L
Glucose (fasting)		
Blood	65–95 mg/dL	3.5–5.3 mmol/L
Plasma or serum	74–106 mg/dL	4.1–5.9 mmol/L
Glucose, 2 h postprandial, serum	<120 mg/dL	<6.7 mmol/L
Glucose, urine		
Quantitative	<500 mg/24 h	<2.8 mmol/24 h
Qualitative	Negative	Negative
Glucose, CSF	40–70 mg/dL	2.2–3.9 mmol/L
*Glucose-6-phosphate dehydrogenase (G-6-PD) in erythrocytes, whole blood (ACD, EDTA, or Hep)	12.1 ± 2.1 U/g Hb (SD) 351 ± 60.6 U/10^{12} RBC 4.11 ± 0.71 U/mL RBC	0.78 ± 0.13 mU/mol Hb 0.35 ± 0.06 nU/RBC 4.11 ± 0.71 kU/L RBC
γ-Glutamyltransfersae (GGT), serum		
Males	2–30 U/L (37°C)	0.03–0.51 µkat/L (37°C)
Females	1–24 U/L (37°C)	0.02–0.41 µkat/L (37°C)
Glutethimide, serum		
Therapeutic	2–6 µg/mL	9–28 µmol/L
Toxic	>5 µg/mL	>23 µmol/L
Glycated hemoglobin (Hemoglobin A1c), whole blood (EDTA)	4.2% - 5.9%	0.042–0.059
Growth hormone, serum		
Male	<5 ng/mL	<5 µg/L
Female	<10 ng/mL	<10 µg/L
Haptoglobin, serum	30–200 mg/dL	0.3–2.0 g/L
HDL-cholesterol (HDL-C), serum or plasma (EDTA)		
Adult desirable	>40 mg/dL	>1.04 mmol/L
borderline	35–40 mg/dL	0.78–1.04 mmol/L
high risk	<35 mg/dL	<0.78 mmol/L

*Test values are method dependent.

Tests	Conventional Units	SI Units
Hematocrit		
Males	42–52%	0.42–0.52
Females	37–47%	0.37–0.47
Newborn	53–65%	0.53–0.65
Children (varies with age)	30–43%	0.30–0.43
Hemoglobin (Hb)		
Males	14.0–18.0 g/dL	2.17–2.79 mmol/L
Females	12.0–16.0 g/dL	1.86–2.48 mmol/L
Newborn	17.0–23.0 g/dL	2.64–3.57 mmol/L
Children (varies with age)	11.2–16.5 g/dL	1.74–2.56 mmol/L
Hemoglobin, fetal	≥1 y old: <2% of total Hb	≥1 y old: <0.02% of total Hb
Hemoglobin, plasma	<3 mg/dL	<0.47 μmol/L
Hemoglobin and myoglobin, urine, qualitative	Negative	Negative
Hemoglobin electrophoresis, whole blood (EDTA, Cit or Hep)		
HbA	>95%	>0.95 Hb fraction
HbA$_2$	1.5–3.7%	0.015–0.037 Hb fraction
HbF	<2%	<0.02 Hb fraction
Homogentisic acid, urine, qualitative	Negative	Negative
β-Hydroxybutyric acid, serum, plasma	0.21–2.81 mg/dL	20–270 μmol/L
17-Hydroxycorticosteroids		
Urine		
Males	3–10 mg/24 h	8.3–27.6 μmol/24 h (as cortisol)
Females	2–8 mg/24 h	5.5–22 μmol/24 h (as cortisol)
5-Hydroxyindoleacetic acid, urine		
Qualitative	Negative	Negative
Quantitative	2–7 mg/24 h	10.4–36.6 μmol/24 h
Imipramine, serum or plasma (Hep or EDTA); trough (≥12 h after dose)		
Therapeutic	150–250 ng/mL	536–893 nmol/L
Toxic	>500 ng/mL	>1785 nmol/L
Immunoglobulins, serum		
IgG	700–1600 mg/dL	7–16 g/L
IgA	70–400 mg/dL	0.7–4.0 g/L
IgM	40–230 mg/dL	0.4–2.3 g/L
IgD	0–8 mg/dL	0–80 mg/L
IgE	3–423 IU/mL	3–423 kIU/L
Immunoglobulin G (IgG), CSF	0.5–6.1 mg/dL	0.5–6.1 g/L
Insulin, plasma (fasting)	2–25 μU/mL	13–174 pmol/L
*Iron, serum		
Males	65–175 μg/dL	11.6–31.3 μmol/L
Females	50–170 μg/dL	9.0–30.4 μmol/L
Iron binding capacity, serum, total (TIBC)	250–425 μg/dL	44.8–71.6 μmol/L
Iron saturation, serum		
Male	20–50%	0.2–0.5
Female	15–50%	0.15–0.5
17-Ketosteroids, urine		
Males	10–25 mg/24 h	38–87 μmol/24 h
Females	6–14 mg/24 h (decrease with age)	21–52 μmol/24 h (decrease with age)

*Test values are method dependent.

Tests	Conventional Units	SI Units
L-Lactate		
Plasma (NaF)		
Venous	4.5–19.8 mg/dL	0.5–2.2 mmol/L
Arterial	4.5–14.4 mg/dL	0.5–1.6 mmol/L
Whole blood (Hep), at bed rest		
Venous	8.1–15.3 mg/dL	0.9–1.7 mmol/L
Arterial	<11.3 mg/dL	<1.3 mmol/L
Urine, 24 h	496–1982 mg/d	5.5–22 mmol/d
CSF	10–22 mg/dL	1.1–2.4 mmol/L
*Lactate dehydrogenase (LDH)		
Total (L→P), 37°C, serum		
Newborn	290–775 U/L	4.9–13.2 μkat/L
Neonate	545–2000 U/L	9.3–34 μkat/L
Infant	180–430 U/L	3.1–7.3 μkat/L
Child	110–295 U/L	1.9–5 μkat/L
Adult	100–190 U/L	1.7–3.2 μkat/L
>60 y	110–210 U/L	1.9–3.6 μkat/L
*Isoenzymes, serum by agarose gel electrophoresis		
Fraction 1	14–26% of total	0.14–0.26 fraction of total
Fraction 2	29–39% of total	0.29–0.39 fraction of total
Fraction 3	20–26% of total	0.20–0.26 fraction of total
Fraction 4	8–16% of total	0.08–0.16 fraction of total
Fraction 5	6–16% of total	0.06–0.16 fraction of total
*Lactate dehydrogenase, CSF	10% of serum value	0.10 fraction of serum value
LDL-cholesterol (LDL-C), serum or plasma (EDTA)		
Adult desirable	<130 mg/dL	<3.37 mmol/L
borderline	130–159 mg/dL	3.37–4.12 mmol/L
high risk	≥160 mg/dL	≥4.13 mmol/L
Lead,		
Whole blood (Hep)	<10 μg/dL	<0.48 μmol/L
Urine, 24 h	<80 μg/d	<0.39 μmol/d
Lecithin-sphingomyelin (L/S) ratio, amniotic fluid	2.0–5.0 indicates probable fetal lung maturity; >3.5 in diabetics	Same
Lidocaine, serum or plasma (Hep or EDTA); 45 min after bolus dose		
Therapeutic	1.5–6.0 μg/mL	6.4–26 μmol/L
Toxic		
CNS, cardiovascular depression	6–8 μg/mL	26–34.2 μmol/L
Seizures, obtundation, decreased cardiac output	>8 μg/mL	>34.2 μmol/L
*Lipase, serum	23–300 U/L (37°C)	0.39–5.1 μkat/L (37°C)
Lithium, serum or plasma (Hep or EDTA); 12 h after last dose		
Therapeutic	0.6–1.2 mEq/L	0.6–1.2 mmol/L
Toxic	>2 mEq/L	>2 mmol/L
Lorazepam, serum or plasma (Hep or EDTA), therapeutic	50–240 ng/mL	156–746 nmol/L
*Luteinizing hormone (LH), serum or plasma (Hep)		

*Test values are method dependent.

Tests	Conventional Units	SI Units
Male	1.24–7.8 mIU/mL	1.24–7.8 IU/L
Female		
Follicular phase	1.68–15.0 mIU/mL	1.68–15.0 IU/L
Mid-cycle peak	21.9–56.6 mIU/mL	21.9–56.6 IU/L
Luteal phase	0.61–16.3 mIU/mL	0.61–16.3 IU/L
Postmenopausal	14.2–52.5 mIU/mL	14.2–52.3 IU/L
Magnesium		
Serum	1.3–2.1 mEq/L	0.65–1.07 mmol/L
	1.6–2.6 mg/dL	16–26 mg/L
Urine	6.0–10.0 mEq/24 h	3.0–5.0 mmol/24 h
Mercury		
Whole blood (EDTA)	0.6–59 μg/L	<0.29 μmol/L
Urine, 24 h	<20 μg/d	<0.1 μmol/d
Toxic	>150 μg/d	>0.75 μmol/d
Metanephrines, total, urine	0.1–1.6 mg/24 h	0.5–8.1 μmol/24 h
Methemoglobin (MetHb, hemoglobin), whole blood (EDTA, Hep or ACD)	0.06–0.24 g/dL or 0.78 ± 0.37% of total Hb (SD)	9.3–37.2 μmol/L or Mass fraction of total Hb: 0.008 ± 0.0037 (SD)
Methotrexate, serum or plasma (Hep or EDTA)		
Therapeutic	Variable	Variable
Toxic		
1–2 wk after low dose therapy	≥0.02 μmol/L	Same
post IV infusion 24 h	≥5 μmol/L	Same
48 h	≥0.5 μmol/L	Same
72 h	≥0.05 μmol/L	Same
Myelin basic protein, CSF	<2.5 ng/mL	<2.5 μg/L
Myoglobin, serum	<85 ng/mL	<85 μg/L
Nortriptyline, serum or plasma (Hep or EDTA); trough (≥12 h after dose)		
Therapeutic	50–150 ng/mL	190–570 nmol/L
Toxic	>500 ng/mL	>1900 nmol/L
*5′-Nucleotidase, serum	2–17 U/L	0.034–0.29 μkat/L
N-Acetylprocainamide, serum or plasma (Hep or EDTA); trough		
Therapeutic	5–30 μg/mL	18–108 μmol/L
Toxic	>40 μg/mL	>144 μmol/L
Occult blood, feces, random	Negative (<2 mL blood/150 g stool/d)	Negative (<13.3 mL blood/kg stool/d)
Qualitative, urine, random	Negative	Negative
Osmolality		
Serum	275–295 mOsm/kg serum water	275–295 mmol/kg serum water
Urine	50–1200 mOsm/kg water	50–1200 mmol/kg water
Ratio, urine/serum	1.0–3.0, 3.0–4.7 after 12 h fluid restriction	Same
Osmotic fragility of erythrocytes	Begins in 0.45–0.39% NaCl Complete in 0.33–0.30% NaCl	Begins in 77–67 mmol/L NaCl Complete in 56–51 mmol/L NaCl
Oxazepam, serum or plasma (Hep or EDTA), therapeutic	0.2–1.4 μg/mL	0.70–4.9 μmol/L

*Test values are method dependent.

Appendices

Tests	Conventional Units	SI Units
Oxygen, blood		
Capacity	16–24 vol% (varies with hemoglobin)	7.14–10.7 mmol/L (varies with hemoglobin)
Content		
Arterial	15–23 vol%	6.69–10.3 mmol/L
Venous	10–16 vol%	4.46–7.14 mmol/L
Saturation		
Arterial and capillary	95–98% of capacity	0.95–0.98 of capacity
Venous	60–85% of capacity	0.60–0.85 of capacity
Tension		
pO_2 arterial and capillary	83–108 mm Hg	11.1–14.4 kPa
Venous	35–45 mm Hg	4.6–6.0 kPa
P50, blood	25–29 mm Hg (adjusted to pH 7.4)	3.33–3.86 kPa
Partial thromboplastin time, activated (APTT)	<35 sec	<35 sec
Pentobarbital, serum or plasma (Hep or EDTA); trough		
Therapeutic		
Hypnotic	1–5 μg/mL	4–22 μmol/L
Therapeutic coma	20–50 μg/mL	88–221 μmol/L
Toxic	>10 μg/mL	>44 μmol/L
pH		
Blood, arterial	7.35–7.45	7.35–7.45
Urine	4.6–8.0 (depends on diet)	Same
Phenacetin, plasma (EDTA)		
Therapeutic	1–30 μg/mL	6–167 μmol/L
Toxic	50–250 μg/mL	279–1395 μmol/L
Phenobarbital, serum or plasma (Hep or EDTA); trough		
Therapeutic	15–40 μg/mL	65–172 μmol/L
Toxic		
Slowness, ataxia, nystagmus	35–80 μg/mL	151–345 μmol/L
Coma with reflexes	65–117 μg/mL	280–504 μmol/L
Coma without reflexes	>100 μg/mL	>430 μmol/L
Phenolsulfonphthalein excretion (PSP), urine	28–51% in 15 min	0.28–0.51 in 15 min
	13–24% in 30 min	0.13–0.24 in 30 min
	9–17% in 60 min	0.09–0.17 in 60 min
	3–10% in 2 h	0.03–0.10 in 2 h
	(After injection of 1 mL PSP intravenously)	(After injection of 1 mL PSP intravenously)
Phenylalanine, serum	0.8–1.8 mg/dL	48–109 μmol/L
Phenytoin, serum or plasma (Hep or EDTA); trough		
Therapeutic	10–20 μg/mL	40–79 μmol/L
Toxic	>20 μg/mL	>79 μmol/L
*Phosphatase, acid, prostatic, serum		
RIA	<3.0 ng/mL	<3.0 μg/L
*Phosphatase, alkaline, total, serum	38–126 U/L (37°C)	0.65–2.14 μkat/L
Phosphate, inorganic, serum		
Adults	2.7–4.5 mg/dL	0.87–1.45 mmol/L
Children	4.5–5.5 mg/dL	1.45–1.78 mmol/L
Phosphatidylglycerol (PG), amniotic fluid		
Fetal lung immaturity	Absent	Same
Fetal lung maturity	Present	Same
Phospholipids, serum	125–275 mg/dL	1.25–2.75 g/L
Phosphorus, urine	0.4–1.3 g/24 h	12.9–42 mmol/24 h

*Test values are method dependent.

Tests	Conventional Units	SI Units
Porphobilinogen, urine		
Qualitative	Negative	Negative
Quantitative	<2.0 mg/24 h	<9 μmol/24 h
Porphyrins, urine		
Coproporphyrin	34–230 μg/24 h	52–351 nmol/24 h
Uroporphyrin	27–52 μg/24 h	32–63 nmol/24 h
Potassium, plasma (Hep)		
Males	3.5–4.5 mEq/L	3.5–4.5 mmol/L
Females	3.4–4.4 mEq/L	3.4–4.4 mmol/L
Potassium		
Serum		
Premature		
Cord	5.0–10.2 mEq/L	5.0–10.2 mmol/L
48 h	3.0–6.0 mEq/L	3.0–6.0 mmol/L
Newborn, cord	5.6–12.0 mEq/L	5.6–12.0 mmol/L
Newborn	3.7–5.9 mEq/L	3.7–5.9 mmol/L
Infant	4.1–5.3 mEq/L	4.1–5.3 mmol/L
Child	3.4–4.7 mEq/L	3.4–4.7 mmol/L
Adult	3.5–5.1 mEq/L	3.5–5.1 mmol/L
Urine, 24 h	25–125 mEq/d, varies with diet	25–125 mmol/d; varies with diet
CSF	70% of plasma level or 2.5–3.2 mEq/L; rises with plasma hyperosmolality	0.70 of plasma level or 2.5–3.2 mmol/L; rises with plasma hyperosmolality
Prealbumin (Transthyretin), serum	10–40 mg/dL	100–400 mg/L
Primidone, serum or plasma (Hep or EDTA); trough		
Therapeutic	5–12 μg/mL	23–55 μmol/L
Toxic	>15 μg/mL	>69 μmol/L
Procainamide, serum or plasma (Hep or EDTA); trough		
Therapeutic	4–10 μg/mL	17–42 μmol/L
Toxic (also consider effect of metabolite (NAPA))	>10–12 μg/mL	>42–51 μmol/L
*Progesterone, serum		
Adult		
Male	13–97 ng/dL	0.4–3.1 nmol/L
Female		
Follicular phase	15–70 ng/dL	0.5–2.2 nmol/L
Luteal phase	200–2500 ng/dL	6.4–79.5 nmol/L
Pregnancy	Varies with gestational week	
*Prolactin, serum		
Males	2.5–15.0 ng/mL	2.5–15.0 μg/L
Females	2.5–19.0 ng/mL	2.5–19.0 μg/L
Propoxyphene, plasma (EDTA)		
Therapeutic	0.1–0.4 μg/mL	0.3–1.2 μmol/L
Toxic	>0.5 μg/mL	>1.5 μmol/L
Propranolol, serum or plasma (Hep or EDTA); trough		
Therapeutic	50–100 ng/mL	193–386 nmol/L
*Prostate-specific antigen (PSA), serum		
Male	<4.0 ng/mL	<4.0 μg/L
*Protein, serum		
Total	6.4–8.3 g/dL	64–83 g/L
Albumin	3.9–5.1 g/dL	39–51 g/L
Globulin		
α_1	0.2–0.4 g/dL	2–4 g/L
α_2	0.4–0.8 g/dL	4–8 g/L
β	0.5–1.0 g/dL	5–10 g/L
γ	0.6–1.3 g/dL	6–13 g/L

*Test values are method dependent.

Appendices

Tests	Conventional Units	SI Units
Urine		
Qualitative	Negative	Negative
Quantitative	50–80 mg/24 h (at rest)	Same
CSF, total	8–32 mg/dL	80–320 mg/dL
Prothrombin consumption	>20 sec	>20 sec
*Prothrombin time (PT)	12–14 sec	12–14 sec
Protoporphyrin, total, WB	<60 µg/dL	<600 µg/L
Pyruvate, blood	0.3–0.9 mg/dL	34–103 µmol/L
Quinidine, serum or plasma		
(Hep or EDTA); trough		
Therapeutic	2–5 µg/mL	6–15 µmol/L
Toxic	>6 µg/mL	>18 µmol/L
Salicylates, serum or plasma		
(Hep or EDTA); trough		
Therapeutic	150–300 µg/mL	1.09–2.17 mmol/L
Toxic	>500 µg/mL	>3.62 mmol/L
Sedimentation rate		
Wintrobe		
Males	0–10 mm in 1 h	0–10 mm/h
Females	0–20 mm in 1 h	0–20 mm/h
Westergren		
Males (<50 yr)	0–15 mm in 1 h	0–15 mm/h
Females (<50 yr)	0–20 mm in 1 h	0–20 mm/h
Sodium		
Serum or plasma (Hep)		
Premature		
Cord	116–140 mEq/L	116–140 mmol/L
48 h	128–148 mEq/L	128–148 mmol/L
Newborn, cord	126–166 mEq/L	126–166 mmol/L
Newborn	133–146 mEq/L	133–146 mmol/L
Infant	139–146 mEq/L	139–146 mmol/L
Child	138–145 mEq/L	138–145 mmol/L
Adult	136–145 mEq/L	136–145 mmol/L
Urine, 24 h	40–220 mEq/d (diet dependent)	40–220 mmol/d (diet dependent)
Sweat		
Normal	10–40 mEq/L	10–40 mmol/L
Cystic fibrosis	70–190 mEq/L	70–190 mmol/L
Specific gravity, urine	1.002–1.030	1.002–1.030
*Testosterone, serum		
Male	280–1100 ng/dL	0.52–38.17 nmol/L
Female	15–70 ng/dL	0.52–2.43 nmol/L
Pregnancy	3–4 × normal	3–4 × normal
Postmenopausal	8–35 ng/dL	0.28–1.22 nmol/L
Theophylline, serum or plasma		
(Hep or EDTA)		
Therapeutic		
Bronchodilator	8–20 µg/mL	44–111 µmol/L
Prem. apnea	6–13 µg/mL	33–72 µmol/L
Toxic	>20 µg/mL	>110 µmol/L
Thiocyanate		
Serum or plasma (EDTA)		
Nonsmoker	1–4 µg/mL	17–69 µmol/L
Smoker	3–12 µg/mL	52–206 µmol/L

*Test values are method dependent.

Tests	Conventional Units	SI Units
Therapeutic after nitroprusside infusion	6–29 µg/mL	103–499 µmol/L
Urine		
Nonsmoker	1–4 mg/d	17–69 µmol/d
Smoker	7–17 mg/d	120–292 µmol/d
Thiopental, serum or plasma (Hep or EDTA); trough		
Hypnotic	1.0–5.0 µg/mL	4.1–20.7 µmol/L
Coma	30–100 µg/mL	124–413 µmol/L
Anesthesia	7–130 µg/mL	29–536 µmol/L
Toxic concentration	>10 µg/mL	>41 µmol/L
*Thyroid-stimulating hormone (TSH), serum	0.4–4.2 µU/mL	0.4–4.2 mU/L
Thyroxine (T₄) serum	5–12 µg/dL (varies with age, higher in children and pregnant women)	65–155 nmol/L (vaires with age, higher in children and pregnant women)
*Thyroxine, free, serum	0.8–2.7 ng/dL	10.3–35 pmol/L
Thyroxine binding globulin (TBG), serum	1.2–3.0 mg/dL	12–30 mg/L
Tobramycin, serum or plasma (Hep or EDTA)		
Therapeutic		
Peak		
Less severe infection	5–8 µg/mL	11–17 µmol/L
Severe infection	8–10 µg/mL	17–21 µmol/L
Trough		
Less severe infection	<1 µg/mL	<2 µmol/L
Moderate infection	<2 µg/mL	<4 µmol/L
Severe infection	<2–4 µg/mL	<4–9 µmol/L
Toxic		
Peak	>10–12 µg/mL	>21–26 µmol/L
Trough	>2–4 µg/mL	>4–9 µmol/L
Transferrin, serum		
Newborn	130–275 mg/dL	1.30–2.75 g/L
Adult	212–360 mg/dL	2.12–3.60 g/L
>60 yr	190–375 mg/dL	1.9–3.75 g/L
Triglycerides, serum, fasting		
Desirable	<250 mg/dL	<2.83 mmol/L
Borderline high	250–500 mg/dL	2.83–5.67 mmol/L
Hypertriglyceridemic	>500 mg/dL	>5.65 mmol/L
*Triiodothyronine, total (T₃) serum	45–137 ng/dL	0.69–2.1 nmol/L
*Troponin-I, cardiac, serum	undetectable	undetectable
Troponin-T, cardiac, serum	undetectable	undetectable
*Uric acid		
Serum, enzymatic		
Male	4.5–8.0 mg/dL	0.27–0.47 mmol/L
Female	2.5–6.2 mg/dL	0.15–0.37 mmol/L
Child	2.0–5.5 mg/dL	0.12–0.32 mmol/L
Urine	250–750 mg/24 h (with normal diet)	1.48–4.43 mmol/24 h (with normal diet)
Urea nitrogen, serum	6–20 mg/dL	2.1–7.1 mmol Urea/L
Urea nitrogen/creatinine ratio, serum	12:1 to 20:1	48–80 urea/creatinine mole ratio
Urobilinogen, urine	0.1–0.8 Ehrlich unit/2 h	Same
	0.5–4.0 mg/24 h	Same

*Test values are method dependent.

Tests	Conventional Units	SI Units
Valproic acid, serum or plasma (Hep or EDTA); trough		
Therapeutic	50–100 µg/mL	347–693 µmol/L
Toxic	>100 µg/mL	>693 µmol/L
Vancomycin, serum or plasma (Hep or EDTA);		
Therapeutic		
Peak	20–40 µg/mL	14–28 µmol/L
Trough	5–10 µg/mL	3–7 µmol/L
Toxic	>80–100 µg/mL	>55–69 µmol/L
Vanillylmandelic acid (VMA), urine (4-hydroxy-3-methoxymandelic acid)	1.4–6.5 mg/24 h	7–33 µmol/d
Viscosity, serum	1.00–1.24 cP	1.00–1.24 cP
Vitamin A, serum	30–80 µg/dL	1.05–2.8 µmol/L
Vitamin B_{12}, serum	110–800 pg/mL	81–590 pmol/L
Vitamin E, serum		
Normal	5–18 µg/mL	12–42 µmol/L
Therapeutic	30–50 µg/mL	69.6–116 µmol/L
Zinc, serum	70–120 µg/dL	10.7–18.4 µmol/L

Linda A. Smith, PhD, CLS(NCA), Associate Professor and Graduate Program Director, Department of
Clinical Laboratory Sciences, University of Texas Health Science Center, San Antonio, TX.

In this appendix, and in the related terms defined in the dictionary proper, blood group is used to refer to an entire group system consisting of heritable antigens whose specificity is controlled by a series of allelic genes. Traditionally, blood group is used in reference to erythrocyte antigens; however, most blood components, including erythrocytes, leukocytes, and platelets, possess heritable antigens identified as belonging to systems. The term blood type or phenotype is used to refer to a specific reaction pattern to testing antisera within a system. The term blood group factor is used to refer to a specific antigen within a system; however, this usage is not universal. It should be noted that in current literature, a single system may be referred to in the plural (i.e., ABO blood groups) and the term blood group may be assigned to a single phenotype (i.e., blood group A).

Each blood group is defined in terms of reaction to the original antisera with which the system was discovered. Changes in, and additions to, a system occur by the discovery of additional antisera proven to be related to the same system. A new blood group antigen or factor can be defined by demonstrating that it is detected by an antiserum with reactions different from those of previously known antisera. If it is shown that the new antigen is genetically independent of known blood group systems, it may qualify as a prototype antigen for a new blood group. Alternatively, if it can be shown that the new antigen is controlled by a gene allelic to one of the known blood group genes, it is assigned to the blood group system of its alleles.

In the blood group definitions, emphasis has been placed on identification of symbols for genes, antigens, antisera, and phenotypes. The general convention that symbols for genes and genotypes are set in italics, whereas symbols for gene products or antigens, antisera, and phenotypes are set in Roman type is followed here. In the Rh-Hr terminology for the Rh blood group, Roman type is used to designate antigen substances, and boldface type is used to designate serological factors and their corresponding antibodies. These are in wide use but are not consistently followed by all authors.

Nomenclature

The designation of blood group systems and antigens has been based on alphabetical assignment of names or initials of first antibody producer, reactive or nonreactive red cell source, or derivation of name, location or discovering institution. The International Society of Blood Transfusion (ISBT) developed a Working Party on Terminology of Red Cell Surface Antigens to establish a uniform nomenclature, while not modifying historical designations and guidelines. Part of the Working Party's charge is to review periodically the available data and report additions, alterations, or deletions to those blood group antigens considered extinct. In addition, the Working Party developed a nomenclature coding system, based on order of discovery of the blood group systems, to aid in the computerization of data. Reports of the Working Party and updates are published in Vox Sanguinis (1990; 58:152-169, 1993; 65:77-80,1995; 69:265-279 1996; 71:246-248).

The ISBT classifies all antigens into one of four classifications: systems, collections, high-incidence antigens, and low-incidence antigens. Currently, there are 23 blood group systems. Each system is serologically, immunochemically, and genetically proven to be products of distinct independent genes. Although 52 Rh antigens have been identified, some have been removed from the system because initial identification and the system currently has 45 antigens. Other systems (i.e., P, Xg, Hh, and Kx systems) have only one antigen associated with the system. Table 1 lists the approved system names, abbreviated symbol, and numerical designation developed by the ISBT. For clinical considerations, the ABO and Rh are of most importance; others are useful for genetic linkage or red cell membrane protein studies.

In addition to the defined blood group system, there are other blood group antigens that fail, as of yet, to fit the system criteria. Some are related genetically or loosely associated by serological and immunochemical reactivity, but insufficient data exist to classify them as a system. Hence, they are referred to as collections. There are now five collections recognized by the ISBT (Table 2).

The remaining classifications of high-incidence and low-incidence antigens contain antigens that cannot be included in either a system or collection. Antigens occurring with a high incidence in the random population are collectively referred to as high-incidence or public antigens. These occur in almost all individuals, but are absent in a few. Antibodies to these antigens usually have been found in the serum of patients who lack the antigen and who have become immunized by transfusion or pregnancy. There are 12 distinct high-incidence antigens and some of the symbols applied to public antigens include Vel, Lan, Ata, Jra, and JMH.

Other erythrocyte antigens are uncommon and may be found only in members of a very few families. Because of their rarity, they are often referred to as low-incidence or private antigens. Antibodies to these antigens usually have been found in the serum of patients who have received transfusions or in mothers of infants with Hemolytic Disease of the Newborn. They are often named for the family in which they were first discovered. There are 34 distinct low-incidence antigens, and some symbols assigned to the private antigens are: By, Swa, Bi, NFLD, RASM, HJK, and ELO.

Appendices

Table 1. Designation of Blood Group Systems

No.	System Name	System Symbol	Gene name(s)
001	ABO	ABO	ABO
002	MNS	MNS	GYPA, GYPB, GYPE
003	P	PI	PI
004	Rh	RH	RHD, RHCE
005	Lutheran	LU	LU
006	Kell	KEL	KEL
007	Lewis	LE	FUT3
008	Duffy	FY	FY
009	Kidd	JK	JK
010	Diego	DI	AE1
011	Yt	YT	ACHE
012	Xg	XG	XG
013	Scianna	SC	SC
014	Dombrock	DO	DO
015	Colton	CO	AQPI
016	Landsteiner-Wiener	LW	LW
017	Chido/Rodgers	CH/RG	C4A, C4B
018	Hh	H	FUTI
019	Kx	XK	XK
020	Gerbich	GE	GYPC
021	Cromer	CROM	DAF
022	Knops	KN	CRI
023	Indian	IN	CD44

Table 2. Designation of Collections

Collection			Antigen		
No.	Name	Symbol	No.	Symbol	Incidence %
205	Cost	COST	205001	Cs^a	95
			205002	Cs^b	34
207	Ii	I	207001	I	>99
			207002	i	*
208	Er	ER	208001	Er^a	>99
			208002	Er^b	<1
209		GLOB	209001	P	>99
			209002	P^k	*
			209003	LKE	98
210			210001	Le^c	1
			210002	Le^d	6

Adapted from: Daniels, GL, Anstee, DJ, Cartron, JP et. al. Blood Group
Terminology 1995. *Vex Sang* 1995;69:265–279.

DRG	DRG Description
1.	Craniotomy, Age Greater than 17 Except for Trauma
2.	Craniotomy for Trauma, Age Greater than 17
3.	Craniotomy, Age 0–17
4.	Spinal Procedures
5.	Extracranial Vascular Procedures
6.	Carpal Tunnel Release
7.	Peripheral and Cranial Nerve and Other Nervous System Procedures with CC
8.	Peripheral and Cranial Nerve and Other Nervous System Procedures without CC
9.	Spinal Disorders and Injuries
10.	Nervous System Neoplasms with CC
11.	Nervous System Neoplasms without CC
12.	Degenerative Nervous System Disorders
13.	Multiple Sclerosis and Cerebellar Ataxia
14.	Specific Cerebrovascular Disorders Except Transient Ischemic Attack
15.	Transient Ischemic Attack and Precerebral Occlusions
16.	Nonspecific Cerebrovascular Disorders with CC
17.	Nonspecific Cerebrovascular Disorders without CC
18.	Cranial and Peripheral Nerve Disorders with CC
19.	Cranial and Peripheral Nerve Disorders without CC
20.	Nervous System Infection Except Viral Meningitis
21.	Viral Meningitis
22.	Hypertensive Encephalopathy
23.	Nontraumatic Stupor and Coma
24.	Seizure and Headache, Age Greater than 17 with CC
25.	Seizure and Headache, Age Greater than 17 without CC
26.	Seizure and Headache, Age 0–17
27.	Traumatic Stupor and Coma, Coma Greater than One Hour
28.	Traumatic Stupor and Coma, Coma Less than One Hour, Age Greater than 17 with CC
29.	Traumatic Stupor and Coma, Coma Less than One Hour, Age Greater than 17 without CC
30.	Traumatic Stupor and Coma, Coma Less than One Hour, Age 0–17
31.	Concussion, Age Greater than 17 with CC
32.	Concussion, Age Greater than 17 without CC
33.	Concussion, Age 0–17
34.	Other Disorders of Nervous System with CC
35.	Other Disorders of Nervous System without CC
36.	Retinal Procedures
37.	Orbital Procedures
38.	Primary Iris Procedures
39.	Lens Procedures with or without Vitrectomy
40.	Extraocular Procedures Except Orbit, Age Greater than 17
41.	Extraocular Procedures Except Orbit, Age 0–17
42.	Intraocular Procedures Except Retina, Iris, and Lens
43.	Hyphema
44.	Acute Major Eye Infections
45.	Neurological Eye Disorders
46.	Other Disorders of the Eye, Age Greater than 17 with CC
47.	Other Disorders of the Eye, Age Greater than 17 without CC
48.	Other Disorders of the Eye, Age 0–17
49.	Major Head and Neck Procedures
50.	Sialoadenectomy

DRG	DRG Description
51.	Salivary Gland Procedures Except Sialoadenectomy
52.	Cleft Lip and Palate Repair
53.	Sinus and Mastoid Procedures, Age Greater than 17
54.	Sinus and Mastoid Procedures, Age 0–17
55.	Miscellaneous Ear, Nose, Mouth, and Throat Procedures
56.	Rhinoplasty
57.	T and A Procedures Except Tonsillectomy and/or Adenoidectomy Only, Age Greater than 17
58.	T and A Procedures Except Tonsillectomy and/or Adenoidectomy Only, Age 0–17
59.	Tonsillectomy and/or Adenoidectomy Only, Age Greater than 17
60.	Tonsillectomy and/or Adenoidectomy Only, Age 0–17
61.	Myringotomy with Tube Insertion, Age Greater than 17
62.	Myringotomy with Tube Insertion, Age 0–17
63.	Other Ear, Nose, Mouth, and Throat OR Procedures
64.	Ear, Nose, Mouth, and Throat Malignancy
65.	Dysequilibrium
66.	Epistaxis
67.	Epiglottitis
68.	Otitis Media and URI, Age Greater than 17 with CC
69.	Otitis Media and URI, Age Greater than 17 without CC
70.	Otitis Media and URI, Age 0-17
71.	Laryngotracheitis
72.	Nasal Trauma and Deformity
73.	Other Ear, Nose, Mouth, and Throat Diagnoses, Age Greater than 17
74.	Other Ear, Nose, Mouth, and Throat Diagnoses, Age 0–17
75.	Major Chest Procedures
76.	Other Respiratory System OR Procedures with CC
77.	Other Respiratory System OR Procedures without CC
78.	Pulmonary Embolism
79.	Respiratory Infections and Inflammations, Age Greater than 17 with CC
80.	Respiratory Infections and Inflammations, Age Greater than 17 without CC
81.	Respiratory Infections and Inflammations, Age 0–17
82.	Respiratory Neoplasms
83.	Major Chest Trauma with CC
84.	Major Chest Trauma without CC
85.	Pleural Effusion with CC
86.	Pleural Effusion without CC
87.	Pulmonary Edema and Respiratory Failure
88.	Chronic Obstructive Pulmonary Disease
89.	Simple Pneumonia and Pleurisy, Age Greater than 17 with CC
90.	Simple Pneumonia and Pleurisy, Age Greater than 17 without CC
91.	Simple Pneumonia and Pleurisy, Age 0–17
92.	Interstitial Lung Disease with CC
93.	Interstitial Lung Disease without CC
94.	Pneumothorax with CC
95.	Pneumothorax without CC
96.	Bronchitis and Asthma, Age Greater than 17 with CC
97.	Bronchitis and Asthma, Age Greater than 17 without CC
98.	Bronchitis and Asthma, Age 0–17
99.	Respiratory Signs and Symptoms with CC
100.	Respiratory Signs and Symptoms without CC
101.	Other Respiratory System Diagnoses with CC

Appendices

DRG	DRG Description
102.	Other Respiratory System Diagnoses without CC
103.	Heart Transplant
104.	Cardiac Valve and Other Major Cardiothoracic Procedures with Cardiac Catheterization
105.	Cardiac Valve and Other Major Cardiothoracic Procedures without Cardiac Catheterization
106.	Coronary Bypass with PTCA
107.	Coronary Bypass with Cardiac Catheterization
108.	Other Cardiothoracic Procedures
109.	Coronary Bypass without Cardiac Catheterization
110.	Major Cardiovascular Procedures with CC
111.	Major Cardiovascular Procedures without CC
112.	Percutaneous Cardiovascular Procedures
113.	Amputation for Circulatory System Disorders Except Upper Limb and Toe
114.	Upper Limb and Toe Amputation for Circulatory System Disorders
115.	Permanent Cardiac Pacemaker Implant with Acute Myocardial Infarction, Heart Failure, or Shock or AICD Lead or General Procedure
116.	Other Permanent Cardiac Pacemaker Implant or PTCA with Coronary ART Stent
117.	Cardiac Pacemaker Revision Except Device Replacement
118.	Cardiac Pacemaker Device Replacement
119.	Vein Ligation and Stripping
120.	Other Circulatory System OR Procedures
121.	Circulatory Disorders with Acute Myocardial Infarction and Major Cardiovascular Complication, Discharged Alive
122.	Circulatory Disorders with Acute Myocardial Infarction without Major Cardiovascular Complication, Discharged Alive
123.	Circulatory Disorders with Acute Myocardial Infarction, Expired
124.	Circulatory Disorders Except Acute Myocardial Infarction with Cardiac Catheterization and Complex Diagnosis
125.	Circulatory Disorders Except Acute Myocardial Infarction with Cardiac Catheterization without Complex Diagnosis
126.	Acute and Subacute Endocarditis
127.	Heart Failure and Shock
128.	Deep Vein Thrombophlebitis
129.	Cardiac Arrest, Unexplained
130.	Peripheral Vascular Disorders with CC
131.	Peripheral Vascular Disorders without CC
132.	Atherosclerosis with CC
133.	Atherosclerosis without CC
134.	Hypertension
135.	Cardiac Congenital and Valvular Disorders, Age Greater than 17 with CC
136.	Cardiac Congenital and Valvular Disorders, Age Greater than 17 without CC
137.	Cardiac Congenital and Valvular Disorders, Age 0–17
138.	Cardiac Arrhythmia and Conduction Disorders with CC
139.	Cardiac Arrhythmia and Conduction Disorders without CC
140.	Angina Pectoris
141.	Syncope and Collapse with CC
142.	Syncope and Collapse without CC
143.	Chest Pain
144.	Other Circulatory System Diagnoses with CC
145.	Other Circulatory System Diagnoses without CC
146.	Rectal Resection with CC
147.	Rectal Resection without CC

DRG	DRG Description
148.	Major Small and Large Bowel Procedures with CC
149.	Major Small and Large Bowel Procedures without CC
150.	Peritoneal Adhesiolysis with CC
151.	Peritoneal Adhesiolysis without CC
152.	Minor Small and Large Bowel Procedures with CC
153.	Minor Small and Large Bowel Procedures without CC
154.	Stomach, Esophageal, and Duodenal Procedures, Age Greater than 17 with CC
155.	Stomach, Esophageal, and Duodenal Procedures, Age Greater than 17 without CC
156.	Stomach, Esophageal, and Duodenal Procedures, Age 0–17
157.	Anal and Stomal Procedures with CC
158.	Anal and Stomal Procedures without CC
159.	Hernia Procedures Except Inguinal and Femoral, Age Greater than 17 with CC
160.	Hernia Procedures Except Inguinal and Femoral, Age Greater than 17 without CC
161.	Inguinal and Femoral Hernia Procedures, Age Greater than 17 with CC
162.	Inguinal and Femoral Hernia Procedures, Age Greater than 17 without CC
163.	Hernia Procedures, Age 0–17
164.	Appendectomy with Complicated Principal Diagnosis with CC
165.	Appendectomy with Complicated Principal Diagnosis without CC
166.	Appendectomy without Complicated Principal Diagnosis with CC
167.	Appendectomy without Complicated Principal Diagnosis without CC
168.	Mouth Procedures with CC
169.	Mouth Procedures without CC
170.	Other Digestive System OR Procedures with CC
171.	Other Digestive System OR Procedures without CC
172.	Digestive Malignancy with CC
173.	Digestive Malignancy without CC
174.	GI Hemorrhage with CC
175.	GI Hemorrhage without CC
176.	Complicated Peptic Ulcer
177.	Uncomplicated Peptic Ulcer with CC
178.	Uncomplicated Peptic Ulcer without CC
179.	Inflammatory Bowel Disease
180.	GI Obstruction with CC
181.	GI Obstruction without CC
182.	Esophagitis, Gastroenteritis, and Miscellaneous Digestive Disorders, Age Greater than 17 with CC
183.	Esophagitis, Gastroenteritis, and Miscellaneous Digestive Disorders, Age Greater than 17 without CC
184.	Esophagitis, Gastroenteritis, and Miscellaneous Digestive Disorders, Age 0–17
185.	Dental and Oral Diseases Except Extractions and Restorations, Age Greater than 17
186.	Dental and Oral Diseases Except Extractions and Restorations, Age 0–17
187.	Dental Extractions and Restorations
188.	Other Digestive System Diagnoses, Age Greater than 17 with CC
189.	Other Digestive System Diagnoses, Age Greater than 17 without CC
190.	Other Digestive System Diagnoses, Age 0–17

DRG	DRG Description
191.	Pancreas, Liver, and Shunt Procedures with CC
192.	Pancreas, Liver, and Shunt Procedures without CC
193.	Biliary Tract Procedures Except Only Cholecystectomy with or without Common Duct Exploration with CC
194.	Biliary Tract Procedures Except Only Cholecystectomy with or without Common Duct Exploration without CC
195.	Cholecystectomy with Common Duct Exploration with CC
196.	Cholecystectomy with Common Duct Exploration without CC
197.	Cholecystectomy Except by Laparoscope without Common Duct Exploration with CC
198.	Cholecystectomy Except by Laparoscope without Common Duct Exploration without CC
199.	Hepatobiliary Diagnostic Procedure for Malignancy
200.	Hepatobiliary Diagnostic Procedure for Nonmalignancy
201.	Other Hepatobiliary or Pancreas OR Procedures
202.	Cirrhosis and Alcoholic Hepatitis
203.	Malignancy of Hepatobiliary System or Pancreas
204.	Disorders of Pancreas Except Malignancy
205.	Disorders of Liver Except Malignancy, Cirrhosis and Alcoholic Hepatitis with CC
206.	Disorders of Liver Except Malignancy, Cirrhosis, and Alcoholic Hepatitis without CC
207.	Disorders of the Biliary Tract with CC
208.	Disorders of the Biliary Tract without CC
209.	Major Joint and Limb Reattachment Procedures of Lower Extremity
210.	Hip and Femur Procedures Except Major Joint, Age Greater than 17 with CC
211.	Hip and Femur Procedures Except Major Joint, Age Greater than 17 without CC
212.	Hip and Femur Procedures Except Major Joint, Age 0–17
213.	Amputation for Musculoskeletal System and Connective Tissue Disorders
214.	No Longer Valid
215.	No Longer Valid
216.	Biopsies of Musculoskeletal System and Connective Tissue
217.	Wound Debridement and Skin Graft Except Hand for Musculoskeletal and Connective Tissue Disorders
218.	Lower Extremity and Humerus Procedures Except Hip, Foot, and Femur, Age Greater than 17 with CC
219.	Lower Extremity and Humerus Procedures Except Hip, Foot, and Femur, Age Greater than 17 without CC
220.	Lower Extremity and Humerus Procedures Except Hip, Foot, and Femur, Age 0–17
221.	No Longer Valid
222.	No Longer Valid
223.	Major Shoulder/Elbow Procedures or Other Upper Extremity Procedures with CC
224.	Shoulder, Elbow, or Forearm Procedures Except Major Joint Procedures without CC
225.	Foot Procedures
226.	Soft Tissue Procedures with CC
227.	Soft Tissue Procedures without CC
228.	Major Thumb or Joint Procedures or Other Hand or Wrist Procedures with CC
229.	Hand or Wrist Procedures, Except Major Joint Procedures without CC

DRG	DRG Description
230.	Local Excision and Removal of Internal Fixation Devices of Hip and Femur
231.	Local Excision and Removal of Internal Fixation Devices Except of Hip and Femur
232.	Arthroscopy
233.	Other Musculoskeletal System and Connective Tissue OR Procedures with CC
234.	Other Musculoskeletal System and Connective Tissue OR Procedures without CC
235.	Fractures of Femur
236.	Fractures of Hip and Pelvis
237.	Sprains, Strains, and Dislocations of Hip, Pelvis and Thigh
238.	Osteomyelitis
239.	Pathological Fractures and Musculoskeletal and Connective Tissue Malignancy
240.	Connective Tissue Disorders with CC
241.	Connective Tissue Disorders without CC
242.	Septic Arthritis
243.	Medical Back Problems
244.	Bone Diseases and Specific Arthropathies with CC
245.	Bone Diseases and Specific Arthropathies without CC
246.	Nonspecific Arthropathies
247.	Signs and Symptoms of Musculoskeletal System and Connective Tissue
248.	Tendonitis, Myositis, and Bursitis
249.	Aftercare, Musculoskeletal System and Connective Tissue
250.	Fractures, Sprains, Strains, and Dislocations of Forearm, Hand, and Foot, Age Greater than 17 with CC
251.	Fractures, Sprains, Strains, and Dislocations of Forearm, Hand, and Foot, Age Greater than 17 without CC
252.	Fractures, Sprains, Strains, and Dislocations of Forearm, Hand, and Foot, Age 0–17 with CC
253.	Fractures, Sprains, Strains, and Dislocations of Upper Arm and Lower Leg Except Foot, Age Greater than 17 with CC
254.	Fractures, Sprains, Strains, and Dislocations of Upper Arm and Lower Leg Except Foot, Age Greater than 17 without CC
255.	Fractures, Sprains, Strains, and Dislocations of Upper Arm and Lower Leg Except Foot, Age 0–17 with CC
256.	Other Musculoskeletal System and Connective Tissue Diagnoses
257.	Total Mastectomy for Malignancy with CC
258.	Total Mastectomy for Malignancy without CC
259.	Subtotal Mastectomy for Malignancy with CC
260.	Subtotal Mastectomy for Malignancy without CC
261.	Breast Procedure for Nonmalignancy Except Biopsy and Local Excision
262.	Breast Biopsy and Local Excision for Nonmalignancy
263.	Skin Graft and/or Debridement for Skin Ulcer or Cellulitis with CC
264.	Skin Graft and/or Debridement for Skin Ulcer or Cellulitis without CC
265.	Skin Graft and/or Debridement Except Skin Ulcer or Cellulitis with CC
266.	Skin Graft and/or Debridement Except Skin Ulcer or Cellulitis without CC
267.	Perianal and Pilonidal Procedures

Appendices

DRG	DRG Description
268.	Skin, Subcutaneous Tissue, and Breast Plastic Procedures
269.	Other Skin, Subcutaneous Tissue, and Breast Procedures with CC
270.	Other Skin, Subcutaneous Tissue, and Breast Procedures without CC
271.	Skin Ulcers
272.	Major Skin Disorders with CC
273.	Major Skin Disorders without CC
274.	Malignant Breast Disorders with CC
275.	Malignant Breast Disorders without CC
276.	Nonmalignant Breast Disorders
277.	Cellulitis, Age Greater than 17 with CC
278.	Cellulitis, Age Greater than 17 without CC
279.	Cellulitis, Age 0–17
280.	Trauma to Skin, Subcutaneous Tissue, and Breast, Age Greater than 17 with CC
281.	Trauma to Skin, Subcutaneous Tissue, and Breast, Age Greater than 17 without CC
282.	Trauma to Skin, Subcutaneous Tissue, and Breast, Age 0–17
283.	Minor Skin Disorders with CC
284.	Minor Skin Disorders without CC
285.	Amputation of Lower Limb for Endocrine, Nutritional, and Metabolic Disorders
286.	Adrenal and Pituitary Procedures
287.	Skin Grafts and Wound Debridement for Endocrine, Nutritional, and Metabolic Disorders
288.	OR Procedures for Obesity
289.	Parathyroid Procedures
290.	Thyroid Procedures
291.	Thyroglossal Procedures
292.	Other Endocrine, Nutritional, and Metabolic OR Procedures with CC
293.	Other Endocrine, Nutritional, and Metabolic OR Procedures without CC
294.	Diabetes, Age Greater than 35
295.	Diabetes, Age 0–35
296.	Nutritional and Miscellaneous Metabolic Disorders, Age Greater than 17 with CC
297.	Nutritional and Miscellaneous Metabolic Disorders, Age Greater than 17 without CC
298.	Nutritional and Miscellaneous Metabolic Disorders, Age 0–17
299.	Inborn Errors of Metabolism
300.	Endocrine Disorders with CC
301.	Endocrine Disorders without CC
302.	Kidney Transplant
303.	Kidney, Ureter, and Major Bladder Procedures for Neoplasm
304.	Kidney, Ureter, and Major Bladder Procedures for Non-neoplasms with CC
305.	Kidney, Ureter, and Major Bladder Procedures for Non-neoplasms without CC
306.	Prostatectomy with CC
307.	Prostatectomy without CC
308.	Minor Bladder Procedures with CC
309.	Minor Bladder Procedures without CC
310.	Transurethral Procedures with CC
311.	Transurethral Procedures without CC

DRG	DRG Description
312.	Urethral Procedures, Age Greater than 17 with CC
313.	Urethral Procedures, Age Greater than 17 without CC
314.	Urethral Procedures, Age 0–17
315.	Other Kidney and Urinary Tract OR Procedures
316.	Renal Failure
317.	Admission for Renal Dialysis
318.	Kidney and Urinary Tract Neoplasms with CC
319.	Kidney and Urinary Tract Neoplasms without CC
320.	Kidney and Urinary Tract Infections, Age Greater than 17 with CC
321.	Kidney and Urinary Tract Infections, Age Greater than 17 without CC
322.	Kidney and Urinary Tract Infections, Age 0–17
323.	Urinary Stones with CC and/or ESW Lithotripsy
324.	Urinary Stones without CC
325.	Kidney and Urinary Tract Signs and Symptoms, Age Greater than 17 with CC
326.	Kidney and Urinary Tract Signs and Symptoms, Age Greater than 17 without CC
327.	Kidney and Urinary Tract Signs and Symptoms, Age 0–17
328.	Urethral Stricture, Age Greater than 17 with CC
329.	Urethral Stricture, Age Greater than 17 without CC
330.	Urethral Stricture, Age 0–17
331.	Other Kidney and Urinary Diagnoses, Age Greater than 17 with CC
332.	Other Kidney and Urinary Diagnoses, Age Greater than 17 without CC
333.	Other Kidney and Urinary Diagnoses, Age 0–17
334.	Major Male Pelvic Procedures with CC
335.	Major Male Pelvic Procedures without CC
336.	Transurethral Prostatectomy with CC
337.	Transurethral Prostatectomy without CC
338.	Testes Procedures, For Malignancy
339.	Testes Procedures, For Nonmalignancy, Age Greater than 17
340.	Testes Procedures, For Nonmalignancy, Age 0–17
341.	Penis Procedures
342.	Circumcision, Age Greater than 17
343.	Circumcision, Age 0–17
344.	Other Male Reproductive System OR Procedures for Malignancy
345.	Other Male Reproductive System OR Procedures Except for Malignancy
346.	Malignancy of Male Reproductive System with CC
347.	Malignancy of Male Reproductive System without CC
348.	Benign Prostatic Hypertrophy with CC
349.	Benign Prostatic Hypertrophy without CC
350.	Inflammation of the Male Reproductive System
351.	Sterilization, Male
352.	Other Male Reproductive System Diagnoses
353.	Pelvic Evisceration, Radical Hysterectomy, and Radical Vulvectomy
354.	Uterine and Adnexal Procedures for Nonovarian/Adnexal Malignancy with CC
355.	Uterine and Adnexal Procedures for Nonovarian/Adnexal Malignancy without CC
356.	Female Reproductive System Reconstructive Procedures
357.	Uterine and Adnexal Procedures for Ovarian or Adnexal Malignancy

DRG	DRG Description
358.	Uterine and Adnexal Procedures for Nonmalignancy with CC
359.	Uterine and Adnexal Procedures for Nonmalignancy without CC
360.	Vagina, Cervix, and Vulva Procedures
361.	Laparoscopy and Incisional Tubal Interruption
362.	Endoscopic Tubal Interruption
363.	D and C, Conization, and Radioimplant for Malignancy
364.	D and C, Conization Except for Malignancy
365.	Other Female Reproductive System OR Procedures
366.	Malignancy of Female Reproductive System with CC
367.	Malignancy of Female Reproductive System without CC
368.	Infections of Female Reproductive System
369.	Menstrual and Other Female Reproductive System Disorders
370.	Cesarean Section with CC
371.	Cesarean Section without CC
372.	Vaginal Delivery with Complicating Diagnoses
373.	Vaginal Delivery without Complicating Diagnoses
374.	Vaginal Delivery with Sterilization and/or D and C
375.	Vaginal Delivery with OR Procedures Except Sterilization and/or D and C
376.	Postpartum and Postabortion Diagnoses without OR Procedures
377.	Postpartum and Postabortion Diagnoses with OR Procedures
378.	Ectopic Pregnancy
379.	Threatened Abortion
380.	Abortion without D and C
381.	Abortion with D and C, Aspiration Curettage or Hysterotomy
382.	False Labor
383.	Other Antepartum Diagnoses with Medical Complications
384.	Other Antepartum Diagnoses without Medical Complications
385.	Neonates, Died or Transferred to Another Acute Care Facility
386.	Extreme Immaturity or Respiratory Distress Syndrome of Neonate
387.	Prematurity with Major Problems
388.	Prematurity without Major Problems
389.	Full-Term Neonate with Major Problems
390.	Neonate with Other Significant Problems
391.	Normal Newborn
392.	Splenectomy, Age Greater than 17
393.	Splenectomy, Age 0–17
394.	Other OR Procedures of the Blood and Blood Forming Organs
395.	Red Blood Cell Disorders, Age Greater than 17
396.	Red Blood Cell Disorders, Age 0–17
397.	Coagulation Disorders
398.	Reticuloendothelial and Immunity Disorders with CC
399.	Reticuloendothelial and Immunity Disorders without CC
400.	Lymphoma and Leukemia with Major OR Procedure
401.	Lymphoma and Nonacute Leukemia with Other OR Procedure with CC
402.	Lymphoma and Nonacute Leukemia with Other OR Procedure without CC
403.	Lymphoma and Nonacute Leukemia with CC
404.	Lymphoma and Nonacute Leukemia without CC

DRG	DRG Description
405.	Acute Leukemia without Major OR Procedure, Age 0–17
406.	Myeloproliferative Disorders or Poorly Differentiated Neoplasms with Major OR Procedures with CC
407.	Myeloproliferative Disorders or Poorly Differentiated Neoplasms with Major OR Procedures without CC
408.	Myeloproliferative Disorders or Poorly Differentiated Neoplasms with Other OR Procedures
409.	Radiotherapy
410.	Chemotherapy without Acute Leukemia as Secondary Diagnosis
411.	History of Malignancy without Endoscopy
412.	History of Malignancy with Endoscopy
413.	Other Myeloprolifeative Disorders or Poorly Differentiated Neoplasm Diagnoses with CC
414.	Other Myeloprolifeative Disorders or Poorly Differentiated Neoplasm Diagnoses without CC
415.	OR Procedure for Infections and Parasitic Diseases
416.	Septicemia, Age Greater than 17
417.	Septicemia, Age 0–17
418.	Postoperative and Posttraumatic Infections
419.	Fever of Unknown Origin, Age Greater than 17 with CC
420.	Fever of Unknown Origin, Age Greater than 17 without CC
421.	Viral Illness, Age Greater than 17
422.	Viral Illness and Fever of Unknown Origin, Age 0–17
423.	Other Infections and Parasitic Diseases Diagnoses
424.	OR Procedure with Principal Diagnoses of Mental Illness
425.	Acute Adjustment Reactions and Disturbances of Psychosocial Dysfunction
426.	Depressive Neuroses
427.	Neuroses Except Depressive
428.	Disorders of Personality and Impulse Control
429.	Organic Disturbances and Mental Retardation
430.	Psychoses
431.	Childhood Mental Disorders
432.	Other Mental Disorder Diagnoses
433.	Alcohol/Drug Abuse or Dependence, Left Against Medical Advice
434.	Alcohol/Drug Abuse or Dependence, Detoxification, or Other Symptomatic Treatment with CC
435.	Alcohol/Drug Abuse or Dependence, Detoxification, or Other Symptomatic Treatment without CC
436.	Alcohol/Drug Abuse or Dependence with Rehabilitation Therapy
437.	Alcohol/Drug Abuse or Dependence with Combined Rehabilitation and Detoxification Therapy
438.	No Longer Valid
439.	Skin Grafts for Injuries
440.	Wound Debridements for Injuries
441.	Hand Procedures for Injuries
442.	Other OR Procedures for Injuries with CC
443.	Other OR Procedures for Injuries without CC
444.	Traumatic Injury, Age Greater than 17 with CC
445.	Traumatic Injury, Age Greater than 17 without CC
446.	Traumatic Injury, Age 0–17
447.	Allergic Reactions, Age Greater than 17
448.	Allergic Reactions, Age 0–17
449.	Poisoning and Toxic Effects of Drugs, Age Greater than 17 with CC
450.	Poisoning and Toxic Effects of Drugs, Age Greater than 17 without CC

Appendices

DRG	DRG Description
451.	Poisoning and Toxic Effects of Drugs, Age 0–17
452.	Complications of Treatment with CC
453.	Complications of Treatment without CC
454.	Other Injury, Poisoning, and Toxic Effect Diagnoses with CC
455.	Other Injury, Poisoning, and Toxic Effect Diagnoses without CC
456.	No Longer Valid
457.	No Longer Valid
458.	No Longer Valid
459.	No Longer Valid
460.	No Longer Valid
461.	OR Procedures with Diagnoses of Other Contact with Health Services
462.	Rehabilitation
463.	Signs and Symptoms with CC
464.	Signs and Symptoms without CC
465.	Aftercare with History of Malignancy as Secondary Diagnosis
466.	Aftercare without History of Malignancy as Secondary Diagnosis
467.	Other Factors Influencing Health Status
468.	Extensive OR Procedure Unrelated to Principal Diagnosis
469.	Principal Diagnosis Invalid as Discharge Diagnosis
470.	Ungroupable
471.	Bilateral or Multiple Major Joint Procedures of Lower Extremity
472.	No Longer Valid
473.	Acute Leukemia without Major OR Procedure, Age Greater than 17
474.	No Longer Valid
475.	Respiratory System Diagnosis with Ventilator Support
476.	Prostatic OR Procedure Unrelated to Principal Diagnosis
477.	Nonextensive OR Procedure Unrelated to Principal Diagnosis
478.	Other Vascular Procedures with CC
479.	Other Vascular Procedures without CC
480.	Liver Transplant
481.	Bone Marrow Transplant
482.	Tracheostomy for Face, Mouth, and Neck Diagnoses

DRG	DRG Description
483.	Tracheostomy Except for Face, Mouth, and Neck Diagnoses
484.	Craniotomy for Multiple Significant Trauma
485.	Limb Reattachment, Hip and Femur Procedures for Multiple Significant Trauma
486.	Other OR Procedures for Multiple Significant Trauma
487.	Other Multiple Significant Trauma
488.	HIV with Extensive OR Procedure
489.	HIV with Major Related Condition
490.	HIV with or without Other Related Condition
491.	Major Joint and Limb Reattachment Procedures of Upper Extremity
492.	Chemotherapy with Acute Leukemia as Secondary Diagnosis
493.	Laparoscopic Cholecystectomy without Common Duct Exploration with CC
494.	Laparoscopic Cholecystectomy without Common Duct Exploration without CC
495.	Lung Transplant
496.	Combined Anterior/Posterior Spinal Fusion
497.	Spinal Fusion with CC
498.	Spinal Fusion without CC
499.	Back and Neck Procedures Except Spinal Fusion with CC
500.	Back and Neck Procedures Except Spinal Fusion without CC
501.	Knee Procedures with PDX of Infection with CC
502.	Knee Procedures with PDX of Infection without CC
503.	Knee Procedures without PDX of Infection
504.	Extensive 3rd Degree Burn with Skin Graft
505.	Extensive 3rd Degree Burn without Skin Graft
506.	Full Thick Burn with Skin Graft or Internal Injuries with CC or Significant Trauma
507.	Full Thick Burn with Skin Graft or Internal Injuries without CC or Significant Trauma
508.	Full Thick Burn without Skin Graft or Internal Injuries with CC or Significant Trauma
509.	Full Thick Burn without Skin Graft or Internal Injuries without CC or Significant Trauma
510.	Nonextensive Burns with CC or Significant Trauma
511.	Nonextensive Burns without CC or Significant Trauma